KT-522-029

Contents

Volume One

Volume Two

Abbreviations

*	Indicates provisional registration
AB	Bachelor of Arts
ABPsS	Associate British Psychological Society
ADMS	Assistant Director Medical Services
AE	Air Efficiency Award
AFC	Air Force Cross
AFOM	Associate Faculty of Occupational Medicine
AFPM	Associate Faculty Pharmaceutical Medicine
AHA	Area Health Authority or Associate Institute of Hospital Administrators
AKC	Associate King's College (London)
AM	Albert Medal (Gold)
AMQ	American Medical Qualification
AMS	Army Medical Service
AO	Officer Order of Australia
ARIC	Associate Royal Institute of Chemistry
BA	Bachelor of Arts
BAc	Bachelor of Acupuncture
BAO	Bachelor of the Arts of Obstetrics
BASc	Bachelor of Applied Science
BC, BCh	Bachelor of Surgery
BChir	Bachelor of Surgery
BChD	Bachelor of Dental Surgery
BDA	British Dental Association
BDS	Bachelor of Dental Surgery
BDSc	Bachelor of Dental Science
BDentSc	Bachelor of Dental Science
BEM	British Empire Medal
BHy	Bachelor of Hygiene
BHyg	Bachelor of Hygiene
BM	Bachelor of Medicine
BMA	British Medical Association
BMedBiol	Bachelor of Medical Biology
BMedSc	Bachelor Medical Science
BMedSci	Bachelor of Medical Science
BPharm	Bachelor of Pharmacy
BS	Bachelor of Surgery
BSc	Bachelor of Science
BSc (MedSci)	Bachelor of Science (Medical Sciences)
BVMS	Bachelor of Veterinary Medicine & Surgery
CAA	Civil Aviation Authority
CAS Applied Immunol.	Certificate of Advance Study in Applied Immunology
CB	Companion Order of the Bath
CBE	Commander Order of British Empire
CC	County Council
CCFP	Certificate College of Family Physicians
CChem	Chartered Chemist
CCST	Certificate of Completion of Specialist Training
CD	Canadian Forces Decoration
Cert AvMed	Certificate in Aviation Medicine
CH	Companion of Honour
ChB	Bachelor of Surgery
CIH	Certificate in Industrial Health
CM, ChM	Master of Surgery
CMF	Christian Medical Fellowship
CMG	Companion Order of St Michael & St George
CMS	Church Missionary Society
CNAA	Council for National Academic Awards
CPH	Certificate in Public Health
CRAMC	Commander Royal Army Medical Corps
CRCP	Certificant Royal College of Physicians
CRCS	Certificant Royal College of Surgeons
CStJ	Commander Venerable Order of St John of Jerusalem
CTCM&H	Certificate in Tropical Community Medicine & Hygiene
CVO	Commander Royal Victorian Order
DA	Diploma in Anaesthetics
DADMS	Deputy Assistant Director Medical Services
DADH	Deputy Assistant Director of Health
DAP & E	Diploma in Applied Parasitology & Entomology
DAvMed	Diploma in Aviation Medicine
DBE	Dame Commander Order of British Empire
DipBMS	Diploma in Basic Medical Sciences
DC	District Council
DCC	Diploma of Chelsea College
DCCH	Diploma in Child & Community Health
DCD	Diploma in Chest Diseases
DCDH	Diploma in Community Dental Health
DCh	Doctor of Surgery
DCH	Diploma in Child Health
DChD	Doctor of Dental Surgery
DCHT	Diploma in Community Health in the Tropics
DCL	Doctor of Civil Law
DCM	Distinguished Conduct Medal
DCMT	Diploma in Clinical Medicine of Tropics
DCP	Diploma in Clinical Pathology
DCPath	Diploma College of Pathologists
DDerm	Diploma in Dermatology
DDM	Diploma in Dermatological Medicine
DDMS	Deputy Director Medical Services
DDO	Diploma in Dental Orthopaedics
DDR	Diploma in Diagnostic Radiology
DDS	Doctor of Dental Surgery
DDSc	Doctor of Dental Science
DFC	Distinguished Flying Cross
DFHom	Diploma Faculty of Homoeopathy
DFM	Distinguished Flying Medal
DFM	Diploma in Forensic Medicine
DGDP	Diploma in General Dental Practice
DGM	Diploma in Geriatric Medicine
DGMS	Director-General Medical Services
DGO	Diploma in Gynaecology & Obstetrics
Dip GU Med	Diploma in Genitourinary Medicine
DHA	District Health Authority
DHMSA	Diploma in History of Medicine, Society of Apothecaries
DHyg	Doctor of Hygiene
DIC	Diploma of Membership of Imperial College of Science & Technology (London)
DIH	Diploma in Industrial Health
Dip IMC RCS Ed	Diploma in Immediate Medical Care, Royal College of Surgeons, Edinburgh
DL	Deputy Lieutenant
DLO	Diploma in Laryngology & Otology
DM	Doctor of Medicine
DMC	District Medical Committee
DMD	Director of Dental Medicine
DMedRehab	Diploma Medical Rehabilitation
DMHS	Director Medical & Health Services

DMJ	Diploma in Medical Jurisprudence
DMO	District Medical Officer
DMR	Diploma in Medical Radiology
DMRD	Diploma in Medical Radio-Diagnosis
DMRE	Diploma in Medical Radiology & Electrolysis
DMRT	Diploma in Medical Radio-Therapy
DMS	Director Medical Services or Doctor of Medicine & Surgery
DMSA	Diploma in Medical Services Administration
DMSS	Director Medical & Sanitary Services
DMV	Doctor of Veterinary Medicine
DO	Diploma in Ophthalmology
DObst	Diploma Obstetrics
DObstRCOG	Diploma Royal College Obstetrics & Gynaecology
DOMS	Diploma in Ophthalmic Medicine & Surgery
DOrth	Diploma in Orthodontics
DPA	Diploma in Public Administration
DPath	Diploma in Pathology
DPD	Diploma in Public Dentistry
DPhil	Doctor of Philosophy
DPhilMed	Diploma in Philosophy of Medicine
DPhysMed	Diploma in Physical Medicine
Dip Pract Derm	Diploma of Practical Dermatology
DPH	Diploma in Public Health
DPM	Diploma in Psychological Medicine
DPMSA	Diploma in Philosophical Medicine Society of Apothecaries
DrAc	Doctor of Acupuncture
DR	Diploma in Radiology
DRACOG	Diploma Royal Australian College of Obstetrics & Gynaecology
DFACR	Diploma Royal Australasian College of Radiologists
DRCOG	Diploma Royal College of Obstetrics & Gynaecology
DRCPath	Diploma Royal College of Pathologists
DRM	Diploma in Radiation Medicine
DRS	Doctorandus
DS	Doctor of Surgery
DSC	Distinguished Service Cross
DSc	Doctor of Science
DSM	Diploma in Social Medicine
DSO	Companion Distinguished Service Order
DSSc	Diploma in Sanitary Science
DStJ	Dame Order of St John of Jerusalem
DTCD	Diploma in Tuberculosis & Chest Diseases
DTCH	Diploma in Tropical Child Health
DTD	Diploma in Tuberculous Diseases
DTM & H	Diploma in Tropical Medicine & Hygiene
DTPH	Diploma in Tropical Public Health
DV & D	Diploma in Venereology & Dermatology
ECFMG	Education Council for Foreign Medical Graduates
ED	Efficiency Decoration
EMAS	Employment Medical Advisory Service
EMS	Emergency Medical Service
ENT	Ear, Nose & Throat
ERD	Emergency Reserve Decoration
ESMI	Elderly Subnormal Mentally Infirm
FACA	Fellow American College of Anesthetists
FACC	Fellow American College of Cardiologists
FACDS	Fellow Australian College of Dental Surgeons
FACG	Fellow American College of Gastroenterology
FACMA	Fellow Australian College of Medical Administrators
FACO	Fellow American College of Otolaryngology
FACOG	Fellow American College of Obstetrics & Gynecology
FACP	Fellow American College of Physicians
FACR	Fellow American College of Radiologists
FACS	Fellow American College of Surgeons
FACTM	Fellow American College of Tropical Medicine
FAGO	Fellow in Australia in Obstetrics & Gynaecology
FANZCP	Fellow Australian & New Zealand College of Psychiatrists
FBIM	Fellow British Institute of Management
FBCO	Fellow British College of Ophthalmic Opticians
FBPsS	Fellow British Psychological Society
FCAP	Fellow College of American Pathologists
FCCP	Fellow American College of Chest Physicians
FCGP	Fellow College of General Practitioners
FCOphth	Fellow College of Ophthalmology
FCMS	Fellow College of Medicine & Surgery
FCPath	Fellow College of Pathologists
FCP	Fellow College of Clinical Pharmacology or Fellow College Physicians
FCPS	Fellow College of Physicians & Surgeons
FCS	Fellow Chemical Society
FCRA	Fellow College of Radiologists of Australia
FDS	Fellow in Dental Surgery
FETCS	Fellow European Board of Thoracic & Cardiovascular Surgeons
FFA	Fellow Faculty of Anaesthetists
FFCM	Fellow Faculty of Community Medicine
FFCMI	Fellow Faculty of Community Medicine in Ireland
FFD	Fellow Faculty of Dental Surgery
FFHom	Fellow Faculty of Homoeopathy
FFOM	Fellow Faculty of Occupational Medicine
FFPath	Fellow Faculty of Pathology
FFPHM	Fellow Faculty of Public Health Medicine
FFPM RCP (UK)	Fellow Faculty Pharmaceutical Medicine Royal College of Physicians UK
FFR	Fellow Faculty of Radiologists
FIHA	Fellow Institute of Hospital Administrators
FIBiol	Fellow Institute of Biology
FICS	Fellow International College of Surgeons
FKC	Fellow King's College London
FLCO	Fellow London College of Osteopathy
FLCOM	Fellow London College of Osteopathic Medicine
FLEXLic(USA)	Federal Licensing Examination (USA)
FLS	Fellow Linnean Society
FMC	Fellow Medical Council
FMCGP(Nigeria)	Fellow Medical Council of General Practitioners (Nigeria)
FOM	Faculty of Occupational Medicine
FPA	Family Planning Association
FPC	Family Practitioner Committee
FPHM	Faculty of Public Health Medicine
FPS	Fellow Pharmaceutical Society
FRACDS	Fellow Royal Australasian College of Dental Surgery
FRACGP	Fellow Royal Australian College of General Practitioners
FRACO	Fellow Royal Australasian College of Ophthalmologists
FRACOG	Fellow Royal Australian College of Obstetricians & Gynaecologists
FRACP	Fellow Royal Australasian College of Physicians
FRACR	Fellow Royal Australasian College of Radiologists
FRACS	Fellow Royal Australasian College of Surgeons
FRAI	Fellow Royal Anthropological Institute

FRANZCP Fellow Royal Australian & New Zealand College of Psychiatrists
FRC Anaesth Fellow Royal College of Anaesthetists
FRCD Fellow Royal College of Dentists
FRCGP Fellow Royal College of General Practitioners
FRCOG Fellow Royal College of Obstetricians & Gynaecologists
FRCP Fellow Royal College of Physicians
FRCPA Fellow Royal College of Pathologists Australasia
FRCPath Fellow Royal College of Pathologists
FRCPC Fellow Royal College of Physicians of Canada
FRCPI Fellow Royal College of Physicians of Ireland
FRCPS Fellow Royal College of Physicians & Surgeons
FRCPsych Fellow Royal College of Psychiatrists
FRCR Fellow Royal College of Radiologists
FRCRA Fellow Royal College of Radiologists of Australasia
FRCS Fellow Royal College of Surgeons
FRCSI Fellow Royal College of Surgeons of Ireland
FRES Fellow Royal Entomological Society
FRFPS Fellow Royal Faculty of Physicians & Surgeons
FRIC Fellow Royal Institute of Chemistry
FRIPHH Fellow Royal Institute of Public Health & Hygiene
FRMS Fellow Royal Microscopical Society
FRS Fellow Royal Society
FRSC Fellow Royal Society of Chemistry
FRSE Fellow Royal Society of Edinburgh
FRSH Fellow Royal Society of Health
FSS Fellow Royal Statistical Society
FZS Fellow Zoological Society
GBE Knight Grand Cross Order of the British Empire
GC George Cross
GCMG Knight Grand Cross Order of St Michael and St George
GCSI Knight Grand Commander Order of the Star of India
GCStJ Knight Grand Cross Venerable Order of St John of Jerusalem
GCVO Knight Grand Cross Royal Victorian Order
GLC Greater London Council
GM George Medal
GMC General Medical Council
GP General Practitioner
HA Health Authority
HDD Higher Dental Diploma
HSE Health & Safety Executive
IAMC Indian Army Medical Corps
i/c In Charge
IC Intensive Care
ICRF Imperial Cancer Research Fund
ICU Intensive Care Unit
ILEA Inner London Education Authority
IMA Irish Medical Association
IMS Indian Medical Service
ISO Imperial Service of Order
JCC Joint Committee on Contraception
JCHMT Joint Committee for Higher Medical Training
JCPTGP Joint Committee on Postgraduate Training in General Practice
JHMO Junior Hospital Medical Officer
JP Justice of the Peace
KBE Knight Commander British Empire
KCB Knight Commander Order of the Bath
KCMG Knight Commander Order of St Michael and St George
KCSI Knight Commander Order of the Star of India
KCVO Knight Commander Royal Victorian Order
KStG Knight Commander Order St Gregory the Great
KStJ Knight Commander Venerable Order of St John of Jerusalem
LAH Licentiate Apothecaries Hall, Dublin
LCPS Licentiate College of Physicians & Surgeons
LDSc Licentiate in Dental Science
LDS Licentiate in Dental Surgery
LicAc Licentiate in Acupuncture
LIHSM Licentiate of Institute of Health Services Management
LLB Bachelor of Laws
LLCO Licentiate London College of Osteopathy
LLCOM Licentiate London College of Osteopathic Medicine
LLD Doctor of Laws
LLM Master of Laws
LM Licentiate in Midwifery
LMC Local Medical Committee
LMCC Licentiate Medical Council of Canada
LMS Licentiate in Medicine & Surgery
LMSSA Licentiate in Medicine & Surgery Society of Apothecaries London
LRCP Licentiate Royal College of Physicians
LCRPI Licentiate Royal College of Physicians of Ireland
LRCPS Licentiate Royal College Physicians & Surgeons
LRCS Licentiate Royal College of Surgeons
LRCSI Licentiate Royal College of Surgeons of Ireland
LRFPS Licentiate Royal Faculty of Physicians & Surgeons
LSA Licentiate Society of Apothecaries London
LSM Licentiate School of Medicine
LVO Lieutenant Royal Victorian Order
M Member
MA Master of Arts
MACD Member Australasian College of Dermatology
MACGP Member Australasian College of General Practitioners
MACO Member Australian College of Ophthalmologists
MACR Member American College of Radiology
MANZCP Member Australian & New Zeland College of Psychiatrists
MAO Master of the Art of Obstetrics
MAustCOG Member Australian College Obstetrics & Gynaecology
MB Bachelor of Medicine
MBA Master in Business Administration
MBAcA Member British Acupuncture Association
MBE Member Order of British Empire
MC Military Cross
M-C Medico-Chirurgical
MC, MCh, MChir Master of Surgery
MCB Master of Clinical Biochemistry
MCCM Member College of Community Medicine (New Zealand)
MCCP Member Ceylon College of Physicians
MCDH Mastership in Community Dental Health
MCFP Member College of Family Practitioners
MCh Master of Surgery
MChir Master of Surgery
MChD Master of Dental Surgery
MChOrth Master of Orthopaedic Surgery
MChOtol Master of Otology
MClSc Master of Clinical Science
MClinPsychol Master of Clinical Psychology
MCommH Master of Community Health
MCPA Member College of Pathologists of Australia
MCPath Member College of Pathologists

MCPS Member College of Physicians & Surgeons
MCRA Member College of Radiologists of Australia
MD Doctor of Medicine
MDD Doctor of Dental Science
MDentSc Master of Dental Surgery
MDS Master of Dental Surgery
MDSc Master of Dental Science
MFCM Member Faculty of Community Medicine
MFCMI Member Faculty of Community Medicine, Ireland
MFHom Member Faculty of Homoeopathy
MFOM Member Faculty of Occupational Medicine
MFPaedRCPI Member Faculty of Paediatrics, Royal College of Physicians of Ireland
MFPM Member Faculty Pharmaceutical Medicine
MFPHM Member Faculty Public Health Medicine
MFPM RCP (UK) Member Faculty Pharmaceutical Medicine Royal College Physicians UK
MGDS Member in General Dental Surgery
MHyg Master of Hygiene
MIBiol Member Institute of Biology
MICGP Member of Irish College of General Practitioners
MIH Master of Industrial Health
MLCO Member London College of Osteopathy
MLCOM Member London College of Osteopathic Medicine
MM Military Medal
MMed Master of Medicine
MMedSc Master of Medical Science
MMF Member Medical Faculty
MMSA Master of Midwifery Society of Apothecaries
MMSc Master of Medical Science
MO Master of Obstetrics
MOD Ministry of Defence
MO & G. MObstG Master Obstetrics & Gynaecology
MOH Medical Officer of Health
MPhil Master of Philosophy
MPH Master of Public Health
MPS Member Pharmaceutical Society
MPSI Member Pharmaceutical Society of Ireland
MPsy Master of Psychiatry
MPsychMed Master of Psychological Medicine
MRACGP Member Royal Australasian College of General Practitioners
MRACO Member Royal Australasian College of Ophthalmologists
MRACP Member Royal Australasian College of Physicians
MRACR Member Royal Australasian College of Radiologists
MRad(D) Master of Radiodiagnosis
MRad(T) Master of Radiotherapy
MRANZCP Member Royal Australian & New Zealand College of Psychiatrists
MRC Medical Research Council
MRCGP Member Royal College of General Practitioners
MRCOG Member Royal College of Obstetricians & Gynaecologists
MRCP Member Royal College of Physicians
MRCPA Member Royal College of Pathologists Australasia
MRCPath Member Royal College of Pathologists
MRCPI Member of Royal College of Physicians of Ireland
MRCPsych Member Royal College of Psychiatrists
MRCS Member Royal College of Surgeons
MRCVS Member Royal College of Veterinary Surgeons
MRNZCGP Member Royal New Zealand College General Practitioners
MRO Member Register of Osteopaths
MRSH Member Royal Society of Health
MS Master of Surgery
MSc Master of Science
MScD Master of Dental Science
MSSc Master of Surgical Science
MSMF Member of State Medical Faculty
MVO Member Royal Victorian Order
NHI National Health Insurance
NHS National Health Service
NUI National University of Ireland
OBE Officer Order of British Empire
OSJ Knight Sovereign Order of St John
OStJ Officer Venerable Order of St John of Jerusalem
PAMC Pakistan Army Medical Corps
PC Privy Councillor, Pharmaceutical Chemist
PCT Primary Care Trust
PhD Doctor of Philosophy
PHLS Public Health Laboratory Service
PMO Principal Medical Officer
QC Queen's Counsel
QGM Queen's Gallantry Medal
QJM Queen's Jubilee Medal
QSM Queen's Service Medal
QSO Queen's Service Order
RADC Royal Army Dental Corps
RAMC Royal Army Medical Corps
RAuxAF Royal Auxiliary Air Force
RCAMC Royal Canadian Army Medical Corps
RCOG Royal College of Obstetricians & Gynaecologists
RCP Royal College of Physicians
RCS Royal College of Surgeons
RD Reserve Decoration
RHA Regional Health Authority
RNVR Royal Naval Volunteer Reserve
SA College of Medicine of South Africa
SBStJ Serving Brother Venerable Order of St John of Jerusalem
ScD Doctor of Science
SCMO Senior Clinical Medical Officer
SHO Senior House Officer
SHMO Senior Hospital Medical Officer
SpR Specialist Registrar
SSStJ Serving Sister Venerable Order of St John of Jerusalem
SMO Sovereign Military Order
TAVR Territorial & Army Volunteer Reserve
TC Dub Trinity College Dublin
TD Territorial Decoration
TDD Tuberculosis Diseases Diploma
T (M) Trained Medically (also T (GP) or T(specialty)) superseded by CCST
UGM Unit General Manager
VAD Voluntary Aid Detachment
VC Victoria Cross
VD Volunteer Decoration
VQE Visa Qualifying Examination USA
VRD Volunteer Reserve Decoration
VTS Vocational Training Scheme
VTSO Vocational Training Scheme Organiser
WHO World Health Organisation

The Medical Directory 2005

Part One

Medical Practitioners in the UK

N-Z

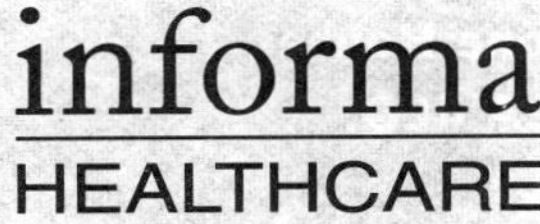

N'DOW, Kathleen Elizabeth 32 Westfield Park, Stonehaven AB39 2EF — MB ChB Aberd. 1991. Trainee GP/SHO Kincardinesh. VTS.

NAASAN, Mr Anas Department of Plastic Surgery, Ninewells Hospital and Medical Schools, Dundee DD1 9SY Tel: 01382 425644 Fax: 01382 223136 Email: a.naasan@dundee.ac.uk; Denehurst, Kincarrathie Crescent, Perth PH2 7HH Tel: 01738 621455 Fax: 01738 635255 Email: anaasan@doctors.org.uk — MB BCh Ain Shams 1979; FRCS Glas. 1987; T(S) 1994. Cons. Plastic Surg. Tayside Univ. Hosp. NHS Trust; Hon. Sen. Lect. Univ. Dundee. Specialty: Plastic Surg. Socs: Brit. Assn. Plastic Surg.; Brit. Soc. Surg. Hand. Prev: Sen. Regist. N. Gen. Hosp. Sheff.; Regist. Bangour Gen. Hosp. & Roy. Hosp. Sick Childr. Edin.; SHO St. And. Hosp. Billericay.

NABAR, Mr Bhalchandra Vasudeo (retired) 18 Elias Drive, Bryncoch, Neath SA10 7TG Tel: 01639 642068 — MB BS Bombay 1949; MS Bombay 1953; FRCS Ed. 1954; FRCS Eng. 1959; DLO Eng. 1965. Prev: Cons. Surg. (ENT) Singleton Hosp. Swansea, Neath Gen. Hosp. & Port Talbot Gen. Hosp.

NABARRO, Ruth Mary Grace Hadleigh Health Centre, Market Place, Hadleigh, Ipswich IP7 5DN Tel: 01473 822961 — MB BS Lond. 1988; BSc Lond. 1985; DRCOG 1991; MRCGP 1992. p/t Principal GP. Prev: Princip. EP Potteb. Boui.

NABI, Dewan Wahedun 17 Church Street, Wales, Sheffield S26 5LQ — MB BS Rajshahi 1967; MB BS Rajshahi Bangladesh 1967; MRCPsych 1983.

NABI, Ijaz Mahmood 403 Rochfords Gardens, Slough SL2 5XE — MB BS Lond. 1994 (Charing Cross & Westm. Med. Sch.) Specialty: Gen. Pract. Prev: Ho. Phys. Chelsea & Westm. Hosp. Lond.; Ho. Surg. Watford Gen. Hosp.

NABIJEE, Abdul Hussain Asgar Ali Alexandra Surgery, 39 Alexandra Road, London SW19 7JZ Tel: 020 8946 7578 Fax: 0845 330 8569; 235 West Barnes Lane, New Malden KT3 6JD Tel: 020 8395 9292 — MB BS Rajasthan 1974 (SMS Medical College Jarpur Royaslhan) GP Princip.; Clin. Asst. (A & E). Specialty: Accid. & Emerg. Socs: MDU.

NABILI, Aqdas 26 Penerley Road, London SE6 2LQ Tel: 020 8698 2398 Mob: 07909 990009 Fax: 020 8698 2398 Email: aqdas@doctors.net — Ptychio Iatrikes Ioannina 1989; Specialist Train. (SR) in Paediat.; MSc (Community Child Health); FRCPCH. Cons. Paediat. Barnet & Chase Farm Hosp. NHS Trust; PhD Research Project in Platelet Agrigation Univ. Ioannina Med. Sch., Greece; MSc in Community Paediat. on going; Cons. Paediat. in Acute & Community. Specialty: Paediat. Special Interest: Child Neurodisabilities; Behavioural Paediat.; Adoption & Fostering. Socs: BMA; Autistic Soc.; Brit. Assn. for Adoption & Fostering (BAAF). Prev: Cons. (Paediat.) Morecambe Bay PCT NHS Trust; Specialist Regist. (Paediat.) 1998 with Greek Min. of Health; Specialist Regist. (Paediat.) GMC as Specialist Register 1998.

NACHEV, Parashkev Choudomirov 321 Hills Road, Cambridge CB2 2QT — BM BCh Oxf. 1998.

NACKASHA, Evelyn Petrous 10 Erin Close, Bromley BR1 4NX — MB ChB Mosul, Iraq 1970; MRCOG 1978.

NACKASHA, Wajdi Louis Children's Unit, St. Peters Hospital, Guildford Road, Chertsey KT16 0PZ Tel: 01483 728201 Fax: 01483 776957; 23 Cross Acres, Pyrford Woods, Pyrford, Woking GU22 8QS Tel: 01932 341986 Fax: 01483 776957 — MB ChB Baghdad 1973; MRCP (UK) 1981; FRCP Lond. 1996. Cons. Paediat. (Community Child Health) Goldsworth Pk. Health Centre Woking & St. Peter's Hosp. Chertsey; Cons. Paediat. Ashford & St Peters NHS Trust. Specialty: Paediat. Prev: Sen. Regist. (Community Child Health) St. Leonard's Hosp. Lond.; Clin. Asst. Roy. Lond. Hosp.

NACZK, Antoni The Health Centre, 2 The Tanyard, Cumnock KA18 1BF Tel: 01290 422723 Fax: 01290 425444 — MB ChB Ed. 1985 (Edinburgh) DRCOG 1989; MRCGP 1991; DFFP 1993; Dip IMC RCS Ed 1998; Ass. FFAEM 1999. Gen. Prac.; Staff Grade Phys. (A & E) CrossHo. Hosp. Kilmarnock. Specialty: Gen. Pract.; Accid. & Emerg.; Care of the Elderly. Prev: Med. Adv. Bens. Agen. Med. Serv.; Med. Dir. Blairston Ho. Nursery Home, Bothwell S. Lancs.; Part. Gen. Prac. Isle of Bute.

NADA, Mr Esmael Mokhtar Esmael 239 Wrotham Road, Gravesend DA11 7LL — MB BCh Mansoura, Egypt 1975; FRCSI 1986.

NADAL, Miguel Jose 22 The Park, London NW11 7SU — MB BS Lond. 1982.

NADARAJAH, Kamalini 3 Martingale Road, Billericay CM11 1SG — MB ChB Aberd. 1997.

NADARAJAH, Mahendran 17 Longmeade Gardens, Wilmslow SK9 1DA — MB BS Lond. 1997.

NADARAJAH, Ramalingam Frimley Park Hospital, Portsmouth Road, Frimley, Camberley GU16 7UJ Tel: 01276 604544 Fax: 01276 604297; 46 Elvetham Road, Fleet, Aldershot GU12 8HL — MB BS Colombo 1978; MRCP (UK) 1985; MRCS Eng. LRCP Lond. 1987; FRCP (UK) 1997. Cons. Genitourin. Med. Frimley Pk. Hosp. NHS Trust Camberley. Specialty: Genitourinary Medicine. Socs: BMA; British Association for Sexual Health and HIV. Prev: Sen. Regist. (Genitourin. Med.) MRI Withington & Hope Hosp. Manch.; Regist. (Genitourin. Med.) St. Helier Hosp. Carshalton.

NADARAJAH, Srimalini Department of Public Health, Camden & Islington HA, 110 Hampstead Road, London NW1 2LJ Tel: 020 7853 5353 Fax: 020 7853 5355; 85 Weirdale Avenue, Whetstone, London N20 0AJ Tel: 020 8368 7500 — MB BS Sri Lanka 1974; LRCP LRCS Ed. LRCPS Glas. 1984. SCMO (Pub. Health) Camden & Islington HA. Specialty: Pub. Health Med. Prev: Clin. Med. Off. (Community Med.) Islington HA; SHO (Geriat. Med.) ChristCh. Hosp.; SHO (Geriat. Med.) New Cross Hosp. Wolverhampton.

NADARAJAH, Thambiayah (retired) Flat 23 Elderfield Place, Church Lane, London SW17 6EB Tel: 020 8672 0653 — MB BS Ceylon 1957 (Colombo) DA Eng. 1975. Prev: GP MexBoro.

NADARAJAN, Mr Periasamy 26 Prospect Road, Lowestoft NR32 3PT — MB BS Madurai 1976; MS (Orth.) Madras 1979; FRCS (Orth.) 1987. Cons. Orthop. Surg. Jas. Paget Hosp. Gt. Yarmouth. Specialty: Orthop.

NADEEM, Faris 222 Stanford Road, Norbury, London SW16 4QW Tel: 020 8764 7161 — MB BS Punjab 1976; BSc Punjab 1970, MB BS 1976; DA Eng. 1984; FFA RCSI 1985. Specialty: Anaesth.

NADEEM, Mr Rana Dilawaiz Postgraduate Centre, Falkirk & District Royal Infirmary, Falkirk FK1 5QE — MB BS Punjab 1985; FRCS Ed. 1992; FRCS Glas. 1993.

NADEL, Simon Department of Paediatrics, St Mary's Hospital, London W2 1NY Tel: 020 7886 6077; 18 Summerfield Road, London W5 1ND Tel: 020 8537 2715 Email: s.nadel@ic.ac.uk — MB BS Lond. 1985 (King's Coll.) MRCP (UK) Paediat. 1988. Cons. & Paediat. IC & Paediat. Infec. Disc. St. Mary Hosp. Lond. Specialty: Paediat. Socs: Fell. Clin. Research Paediat. St. Mary's Hosp. Lond.; MRCPCH; Intens. Care Soc. Prev: Fell. Paediat. Infec. Dis. Childr. Hosp. Philadelphia; SHO Hosp. for Sick Childr. Gt. Ormond St. Lond.; SHO (Paediat.) Whipps Cross Hosp. Lond.

NADERSEPAHI, Ali 6 Beverley Place, 38 Eton Rise, London W5 2ER — MB BS Lond. 1991.

NADIN, John Charles Kenneth Preston Grove Medical Centre, Preston Grove, Yeovil BA20 2BQ Tel: 01935 474353 Fax: 01935 425171 — MB BChir Camb. 1976; MA Camb. 1977, MB 1976, BChir 1975; DRCOG 1979; DCH Eng. 1980; MRCGP 1983.

NADKARNI, Sanjay c/o Department of Radiology, Royal Hallamshire Hospital, Glossop Road, Sheffield S10; 9 Fuler Road, Sheffield S11 8UF — MB BS West. Austral. 1992 (Univ. of Western Australia) MB BS Western Australia 1992; DA (UK) 1995; MRCP (UK) 1996; FRCR 1997. Specialist Regist. (Radiol.). Specialty: Radiol. Socs: Austral. Med. Assn.

NADLACAN, Liviu Mircea Flat 112, Room 1, Osler Road, Headington, Oxford OX3 9JW — State Exam Rome 1993.

NADRA, Aida Mary 6 Westminster Drive, Wrexham LL12 7AU — MB BCh Wales 1994.

NADRA, Asmat Nadra and Partners, The Surgery, Gardden Road, Wrexham LL14 2EN Tel: 01978 840034 Fax: 01978 845782 — MD Komensky 1973; MD Komensky 1973; LRCP LRCS Ed. LRCPS Glas. Edinburgh & Glasgow 1982.

NADRA, Azmi Baddow Road Surgery, 115 Baddow Road, Chelmsford CM2 7QD Tel: 01245 351351 Fax: 01245 494192 — MD Warsaw 1969 (Med. Acad. Warsaw) DCH Eng. 1973; LRCP LRCS Ed. LRCPS Glas. 1976. Prev: SHO (Paediat.) Stepping Hill & Cherry Tree Hosps. Stockport & Roy.; Alexandra Hosp. Rhyl; Regist. (Paediat.) Maelor Gen. Hosp. Wrexham.

NAEEM, Abdul The Surgery, 64 Dog Kennel Lane, Oldbury B68 9LZ Tel: 01922 552 1713 Fax: 01922 552 9980 — MRCS Eng. LRCP Lond. 1978 (Khyber Med. Coll.) SHO (Anaesth.) Roy. Gwent Hosp. Newport. Prev: SHO (Gen. Med.) St. Woolos Hosp.

Newport; SHO (Gyn. & Obst.) Aberdare Gen. Hosp.; Ho. Off. (Gen. Med.) Merthyr Gen. Hosp. Merthyr Tydfil.

NAEEM, Ajaz Ahmed The New Surgery, 8 Shenfield Road, Brentwood CM15 8AB Tel: 01277 218393 Fax: 01277 201017 — MB BCh Wales 1991; BSc Wales 1988; MRCP (UK) 1994. Specialty: Gen. Pract. Prev: Clin. Med. Off. Community Paediat. SE Lond.

NAEEM, Asim 7 Eton Avenue, Westlands, Newcastle ST5 3JL Tel: 01782 613667 — MB BS Lond. 1997 (St Georges University of London) MRCPsych 2001. SpR (Psychiat.) St. George's Train. Sch. Lond. Specialty: Gen. Psychiat. Socs: Roy. Coll. Psychiatr. Prev: SHO Rotat. (Psychiat.) Univ. of Lond., St Geo.'s Train. Scheme; Ho. Off. (Surg./Orthop.) St. Helier Hosp. Lond.; Ho. Off. (Gen. Med.) Manor Hosp. Walsall.

NAEEM, Muhammed The Surgery, High Street, Talke Pits, Stoke-on-Trent ST7 1QH Tel: 01782 782440 Fax: 01782 763884 — MB BS Karachi 1963 (Dow Med. Coll.) BSc, MB BS Karachi 1963.

NAEEM, Naushene Sara 241 Kingsway, Cheadle SK8 1LA Tel: 0161 428 9795 — MB ChB Dundee 1991; MRCGP 1997. Specialty: Gen. Pract.

NAERGER, Mr Harry Guy Anthony Motley Bank, Earls Grove, Camberley GU15 2EN Tel: 01276 509600 Fax: 01276 709555 — MB BS Lond. 1984 (Middlx.) FRCS Eng. 1988; FRCS Eng. 1988; FRCS (Urol.) 1997; FRCS Urol 1997. Cons. Urol. Frimley Pk. Hosp. Surrey & the Min. Defence. Specialty: Urol. Prev: Sen. Regist. (Urol.) St. Thos. Hosp. Lond.; Sen. Regist. (Urol.) Battle Hosp. Reading.

NAFIE, Sami Abdel El-Alim Abdo 57 Brunswick Road, Ealing, London W5 1AQ; 47 Ashdown Drive, Stourbridge DY8 5QY — MB BCh Ain Shams 1977; MChOrth Liverp. 1986; MRCS Eng. LRCP Lond. 1988. Regist. (Orthop. Surg.) Russells Hall/Corbett Hosps. Dudley HA. Specialty: Transpl. Surg.

NAFIS, Muhammad Amer Luton and Dunstable Hospital NHS Trust, Lewsey Road, Luton LU4 0DZ Tel: 01582 497973 Email: amer.nafis@idh-tr.anglox.nhs.uk — MB BS Pakistan; FFAEM; FRCS. Cons. in Accid. and Emerg. Med.; Northwest Thames SPR Rotat. Specialty: Accid. & Emerg. Special Interest: Soft Tissue Injury; Trauma Managem. Socs: BAEM; FAEM.

NAFTALIN, Adrian Paul Gray's Inn Medical, (surg.) 79 Gray's Inn Road, London WC1X 8TP Tel: 020 7405 9360 Fax: 020 7831 1964; 5 Ardwick Road, London NW2 2BX Tel: 020 7435 5781 Fax: 020 7435 9635 — MB BChir Camb. 1963 (Camb. & Middlx.) BA Camb. 1959, MA; FRCS Eng. 1968. Forens. Med. Examr. (Metrop. Police); Med. Off. Legal Educat. Lond.; Med. Off. Jewish Care; Vis. Med. Off. Camden Mens Hostels. Specialty: Gen. Pract.; Alcohol & Substance Misuse; Care of the Elderly. Socs: Fell. Hunt. Soc.; BMA; (Counc.) Hampstead Med. Soc. Prev: Cons. Health Screening Wellington Hosp. Lond.; Med. Off. Reader's Digest Assn.; Regist. (Plastic Surg.) Mt. Vernon & Middlx. Hosps.

NAFTALIN, Alan Avrom Newham University Hospital NHS Trust, Glen Road, London E13 8SL Tel: 020 7363 8036 Fax: 020 7363 8314 Email: alan.naftalin@newhamhealth.nhs.uk — MB ChB Glas. 1972; FRCOG 1991, M 1979. Director Med. Educat. Newham Healthcare Trust; Hon. Sen. Lect. (Obst. and Gyn.) at Roy. Lond. and St Bart. Sch. of Med. Specialty: Obst. & Gyn. Prev: Cons. O & G Newham Gen. Hosp. Lond.; Lect. & Sen. Regist. (O & G) Roy. Free Hosp. Lond.; Clin. Tutor Qu. Vict. Hosp. Melbourne, Austral.

NAFTALIN, Leslie (retired) Woodend, 3c 19 Milverton Road, Giffnock, Glasgow G46 7JN — LRCP LRCS Ed. LRFPS Glas. 1938; LDS RFPS Glas. 1936; MRCGP 1956. Prev: Med. Off. Attend. Allowance Bd. & Mem. Med. Bd. Panel Dept. Health & Social Security.

NAFTALIN, Lionel 4 Whitegables, 116 St. Andrews Drive, Glasgow G41 4RB Tel: 0141 427 1395 — LRCP LRCS Ed. LRFPS Glas. 1942; BSc Glas. 1942; FRCPath 1963. Chem. Path. Emerit. Lincoln Gp. Hosps.; Hon. Research Fell. Univ. Strathclyde. Specialty: Chem. Path. Socs: Biochem. Soc. Prev: Capt. RAMC.

NAFTALIN, Mr Nicholas Jonathan, OBE University Hospitals of Leiceister NHS Trust, Leicestershire Royal Infirmary, Infirmary Square, Leicester LE1 5WW Tel: 0116 258 6476 Fax: 0116 258 7560; 15 Knighton grange Road, Oadby, Leicester LE2 2LF Tel: 011602703358 Fax: 0116 270 6513 Email: naftalin@nascr.net — MB ChB Glas. 1965; FRCOG 1983, M 1970. Cons. Gyn. Leicester Roy. Infirm. Leicester. Specialty: Obst. & Gyn. Prev: Sen. Lect. Dept. O & G Univ. Leicester; Hall Fell. Dept. O & G Univ. Glas.; Research Fell. in Anesth. Harvard Med. Sch. Boston, U.S.A.

NAFTALIN, Professor Richard Julian Department of Physiology, University of London new Hunts House, King's College, Guy's Campus, London SE1 1OL Tel: 02078486216 Fax: 020 7848 6002 Email: richard.naftalin@kcl.ac.uk; 50 Wood Vale, London N10 3DN Tel: 020 8883 5602 — MB ChB Glas. 1962; PhD Lond. 1969, MSc 1965; DSc Glas. 1990. Prof. Physiol. Kings Coll. Lond. Specialty: Gastroenterol. Socs: Biochem. Soc.; Physiol. Soc. Prev: Reader (Physiol.) King's Coll. Lond.; Lect. (Physiol.) Univ. Leicester; Ho. Surg. Glas. Roy. Infirm.

NAG, Shipra 2 Sark Close, Heston, Hounslow TW5 0PZ Tel: 020 8572 3216 — MB BS Indore 1966; MS Indore 1969.

NAG-CHAUDHURY, Satya Ranjan 121 Harley Street, London W1N 1DH Tel: 020 7224 0130; 11 Bentley Way, Woodford Green IG8 0SE Tel: 020 8504 7920 Fax: 020 8504 3879 — MB BS Calcutta 1953; FFA RCS Eng. 1970; FRCOG 1993, M 1978. Assoc. Specialist (O & G) N. Middlx. Hosp. Lond. Specialty: Obst. & Gyn. Socs: BMA. Prev: Asst. (O & G) Barking Hosp. & N. Middlx. Hosp. Lond.; Regist. (O & G) Shrewsbury Gp. Hosps. & Groundslow Hosp. Tittensor.

NAGABHYRU, Anita 2 Pethill Close, Plymouth PL6 8NL Tel: 01752 784480 Fax: 01752 309716 — MB ChB Dundee 1994 (Dundee University) SHO (ENT) Derriford Hosp. Plymouth. Specialty: Gen. Pract. Prev: A & E Derriford Hosp. Plymouth; SHO (Gen. Med.) Derriford Hosp. Plymouth; SHO (Gen. Surg.) Derriford Hosp. Plymouth.

NAGABHYRU, Apparao Trelawny Surgery, 45 Ham Drive, Plymouth PL2 2NJ Tel: 01752 350700 Fax: 01752 784480; 2 Prethill Close, Earlswood, Plymouth PL6 8NL Tel: 01752 784480 Fax: 01752 309716 Email: anagabhyru@mcmail.com — MB BS Andhra 1968 (Rangaraya Med. Coll.) DLO Eng. 1976. GP. Specialty: Otolaryngol. Prev: Trainee GP Exeter VTS; Regist. (ENT) Warrington Gen. Hosp.; Clin. Asst. (ENT) Roy. Devon & Exeter Hosp.

NAGANATHAR, Indira 18 Glenham Drive, Ilford IG2 6SG — MB BS Ceylon 1971.

NAGAR, Mahesh Prabhashanker 74 Aberford Road, Wakefield WF1 4AL — MB BS Jabalpur, India 1983.

NAGARAJ, Channanagowd Basavaraj Om Shakthi, 7 Freemans Walk, Pembroke SA71 4AS — MB BS Mysore 1977; BSc Mysore 1968; DGM RCP Lond. 1987; DMedRehab RCP Lond 1988; T(GP) 1992. Med. Examr. (Assessor) Benefits Agency Med. Servs. DSS Swansea; Police Surg. HaverfordW.; Assoc. Psychiat. St. David's Hosp. Carmarthen; Deputising GP, Healthcall, Swansea Med. Serv.s; Medico-Legal Report Writer. Specialty: Rehabil. Med.; Rheumatol. Socs: BMA; Mem. Of Assoc of Police Surg., APS 5078. Prev: Staff. Phys. (Geriat. Med.) S. Pembrokesh. Hosp. Pembroke Dock.; Trainee GP Porthcawl; Regist. (Geriat. & Gen. Med.) Vict. Hosp. Blackpool.

NAGARAJ, Hutchappa Nandeesh 39 Drummond Way, Macclesfield SK10 4XJ — MB BS Bangalore 1984.

NAGARAJA, Etagi Gugupadappa Alim and Partners, 151 North Street, Keighley BD21 3AU Tel: 01535 607444 Fax: 01535 691201 — MB BS Mysore 1974. GP Keighley, W. Yorks.

NAGARAJAH, Kugan — MB ChB Aberd. 1998.

NAGARAJAN, Srikantiah Department of Histopathology, Middlesbrough General Hospital, Ayresome Green Lane, Middlesbrough TS5 5AZ Tel: 01642 850222 Fax: 01642 825071 — MB BS Bangalore 1974; MRCPath 1990.

NAGASUBRAMANIAN, Suryanarayanan London Eye Diagnostic Centre, 23 Harley St., London W1G 9QN Tel: 020 7323 5967 Fax: 020 7323 5972 Email: ledc@compuserve.com — (Madurai Med. Coll.) MB BS Madras 1962; DO Madras 1966; PhD Lond. 1974. Ophth. Lond. Eye Diagnostic Centre Lond.; Clin. Asst. Moorfields Eye Hosp. (City Rd. Br.); Sen. Lect. Inst. Ophth. Univ. Lond. Socs: Sec. Glaucoma Soc.; Comm. Mem. Internat. Glaucoma Soc. of Internat. Congr. of Ophth.; Fell. Amer. Acad. of Ophth. Prev: Sen. Lect. Inst. of Ophth.; Dept. of Clin. Ophth.; Lister Research Fell. Moorfields Eye Hosp. Lond.

NAGDEE, Khadija Amiena 6 Newstead Road, St. John's, Wakefield WF1 2DE — MB BCh Witwatersrand 1946; BSc, MB BCh Witwatersrand 1946; DPM Eng. 1975.

NAGEH, Thuraia 104 Gowan Avenue, Fulham, London SW6 6RG Tel: 020 7731 6132 — MB BS Lond. 1993 (St. Bart. Hosp. Med. Sch.) MRCP (UK) 1996. Spec. Registrar in Cardiology, Kings Coll. Hosp., Lond. Specialty: Cardiol.

NAGENDAR, Kopparam Flat 2, Married Accommodation, General Hospital, Ayresome Gree Lane, Middlesbrough TS5 5AZ — MB BS Bangalore 1983.

NAGENDRA, Kyle Hadley Victor Newtons, The Health Centre, Heath Road, Haywards Heath RH16 3BB Tel: 01444 412280 Fax: 01444 416943; The Magpies, The St, Bolney, Haywards Heath RH17 5PF — MB BS Lond. 1990 (St Georges Hosp. M S Univ. Liver'pl.) DFFP 1994; DRCOG 1994; MRCGP 1995. Specialty: Gen. Pract.

NAGENDRAN, Kulandavelu Department of Clinical Neurosciences, 38 Little Britain, St Bartholomews Hospital, London EC1A 7BE Tel: 020 7601 8859 Fax: 020 7601 7875 Email: nagendran01@hotmail.com — MB BS Sri Lanka 1978; MRCP (UK) 1983; FRCP Lond. 1996. Cons. Clin. Neurophysiol. St. Bart. Hosp. Lond. & Roy. Lond. Hosp.; Cons. Clin. Neurophysiologist Broomfield Hosp. Chelmsford Essex; Clin. Neurophysiologist Lond. Clinic 20 Devonshire Pl. W1G 6BW 020 7616 7653; Clin. Neurophysiologist Clementine Churchill Hosp. Harrow HA1 3RX. Specialty: Clin. Neurophysiol. Socs: Assn. Brit. Clin. Neurophysiol.; Brit. Soc. Clin. Neurophysiol.

NAGENDRAN, Ravindra Department of Radiology, Queen Elizabeth Hospital, Stadium Road, Woolwich, London SE18 4QH Tel: 0208 836 4766 — MB BS Ceylon 1971; FRCS Eng. 1979; FRCR 1984. Cons. Radiol.Qu. Eliz. Hosp. Lond. Specialty: Radiol.

NAGENDRAN, Mr Sivanandy c/o Drive K. Puvanachandra, Department of Ophthalmology, H. M. Stanley Hospital, St Asaph LL17 0RS Tel: 01745 583910 Fax: 01745 583143; Brindavan, 8 Clos Aberconway, Prestatyn LL19 9HU — MB BS Peradeniya 1985; FRCS Ed. 1993. Assoc. Specialist in Ophth., HM Stanley Hosp. St Asaph. Specialty: Ophth. Prev: Staff Grade HM Stanley Hosp. St Asaph.

NAGESH, Kalakonda 7 Hillside Road, Wallasey CH44 2DZ — MB BS Madras 1988; MRCP (UK) 1992.

NAGESH RAO, Mr Gadiyar William Harvey Hospital, Kennington Road, Willesborough, Ashford TN24 0LZ — MB BS Madras 1981; FRCS Ed. 1986; FRCS Glas. 1986; MD Hull 1997. Specialty: Gen. Surg. Socs: Med. Defence Union; BMA. Prev: Sen. Regist. (Colorectal Surg.) E. Glam. Hosp.; Regist. (Gen. Surg.) Sunderland Dist. Gen. Hosp., Aberd. Roy. Infirm., Bradford Roy. Infirm. & St. Lukes Hosp. Bradford.

NAGESWARAN, Ananda Sundram Department of Genitourinary Medicine, St. Anns General Hospital, St Anns Road, London N15 3TH Tel: 020 8442 6536 Fax: 020 8442 6811 Email: ana.nageswaran@haringey.nhs.uk; 47 Merryhills Drive, Enfield EN2 7NY — MB BS Sri Lanka 1975; MRCP (UK) 1983; FRCP 1999. Cons. Phys. (Genitourin. Med.) St. Anns Gen. Hosp. Lond.; Hon. Cons. Phys. (HIV) N. Middlx. Hosp. Lond; Cons. Phys. (Genitourn. Med.) Roy. Free Hosp. Lond. Specialty: Genitourinary Medicine; HIV Med. Socs: Med. Soc. Study VD; Brit. HIV Assn. Prev: Sen. Regist. & Regist. (Genitourin. Med.) Sheff.; Regist. (Infec. Dis.) Manch.

NAGI, Dinesh Kumar Pinderfields Hospital, Edna Coates Diabetes & Endocrine Unit, Wakefield WF1 4DG Tel: 01924 213901 Fax: 01924 814977 — MB BS Amritsar India 1980; FRCP; PhD Lond. Cons. (Diabetes/Endocrinol.); Hon. Sen. Lect. Univ. Leeds. Specialty: Diabetes; Endocrinol.

NAGI, Hussein Mostafa City Hospital, Dudley Road, Birmingham B60 1QH — MB BCh Cairo 1980; FRCA 1980; FFA RCSI 1988; MSc (Pain) 2001. Cons. Anaesth. Grimsby Dist. Hosp.; Cons. in Chromic Pain Managem. Specialty: Anaesth.; Chronic Pain. Socs: Pain Soc.; IARS.

NAGI, Sukhwinder Singh Browney House Surgery, Front Street, Langley Park, Durham DH7 9YT Tel: 0191 373 2860; Magadi, Cadger Bank, Lanchester, Durham DH7 0HE Tel: 0191 520774 — MB BS Calicut 1974 (Med. Sch. Calicut) DRCOG 1978; MRCGP 1980. GP Trainer Durh. Socs: Med. Protec. Soc. Prev: SHO (Obst. & Coronary Care) Dryburn Hosp. Durh.; SHO (Cardiol.) Shotley Bridge Gen. Hosp. Consett.

NAGINGTON, Jack (retired) 20 Gog Magog Way, Stapleford, Cambridge CB2 5BQ — MB ChB Manch. 1947; MRCS Eng. LRCP Lond. 1947; Dip. Bact. 1950; MD (Commend.) Manch. 1956. Prev: Cons. Virol. Pub. Health Laborat. Serv.

NAGLE, Christopher James 12 Rotton Park Road, Edgbaston, Birmingham B16 9JJ — MB ChB Bristol 1982.

NAGLE, Conor James Cliff Road Surgery, 10A Cliff Road, London NW1 9AN Tel: 020 7485 2276 Fax: 020 7428 9602; 13 Carlingford Road, London NW3 1RY — MB BS Lond. 1975; MRCS Eng. LRCP Lond. 1975; MRCPsych 1980; MRCGP 1988.

NAGLE, Lionel Richard Pall Mall Surgery, 178 Pall Mall, Leigh-on-Sea SS9 1RB Tel: 01702 478338 Fax: 01702 471294 — MB ChB Bristol 1987; DRCOG 1991.

NAGLE, Robert Emerson (retired) 12 Rotton Park Road, Birmingham B16 9JJ Tel: 0121 454 2136 — MB BChir Camb. 1955 (Univ. Coll. Hosp.) FRCP Lond. 1974, M 1963. Cons. Cardiol. Qu. Eliz. & Selly Oak Hosps. Birm. Prev: Research Asst. Univ. Coll. Hosp. Lond.

NAGLE, Robert Sharp 10 Kirk Park, Liberton, Edinburgh EH16 6HZ — MB ChB Ed. 1951; DTM & H 1957.

NAGPAL, Inderjeet Singh Flat 103, Doctors' Residences, Alder Hey Children's Hospital, Liverpool L12 2AP — MB BS Delhi 1988; MRCP (UK) 1994.

NAGPAL, Mr Iqbal Chand Adwick Road Surgery, 24 Adwick Road, Mexborough S64 0DB Tel: 01709 514443 — MB BS All India Inst. Med. Sci. 1964; M.Ch (Orth) L.Prof; FRCS Ed. 1968.

NAGPAL, Kanval Kant Stanhope Surgery, Stanhope Road, Waltham Cross EN8 7DJ Tel: 01992 635300 Fax: 01992 624292; 6 Homewood Avenue, Cuffley, Potters Bar EN6 4QG — MB BS Dibrugarh 1974 (Assam Med. Coll. Dibrugarh) DRCOG 1982. Prev: Trainee GP Enfield & Haringey VTS; SHO Dartford & Gravesham Health Dist.

NAGPAL, Nirmala William Hopwood Street Surgery, William Hopwood Street, Audley, Blackburn BB1 1LX; Arley Oaks, Wyfordby Avenue, Blackburn BB2 7AR Tel: 01254 582628 Fax: 01254 582646 — MB BS Rajasthan 1973 (R.N.T. Med. Coll. Udaipur) FRSH Rajasthan. GP. Specialty: Paediat. Socs: BMA; Overseas Doctors Assn.; Med. Protec. Soc. Prev: Trainee GP Preston; SHO (O & G) Qu. Pk. Hosp. Blackburn; SHO (A & E) Roy. Infirm. Blackburn.

NAGPAL, Satish William Hopwood Street Surgery, William Hopwood Street, Audley, Blackburn BB1 1LX; Arley Oaks, Wyfordby Avenue, Blackburn BB2 7AR Tel: 01254 582628 Fax: 01254 582646 — MB BS Rajasthan 1969 (R.N.T. Med. Coll. Udaipur) FRSH; MS (Ophth.) Rajasthan 1973; DO RCPSI 1979; DO Eng. 1979; MCOphth 1988. Sen. Clin. Med. Off. (Ophth.) Blackburn. Specialty: Ophth. Socs: BMA; Med. Protec. Soc.; Overseas Doctors Assn. Prev: Clin. Asst. (Ophth.) Roy. Infirm. Blackburn; Regist. (Ophth.) Roy. Infirm. Blackburn.

NAGPAL, Suman South Quay Surgery, 35-36 South Quay, Great Yarmouth NR30 2RG Tel: 01493 843196; 94 Victoria Road, Gorleston, Great Yarmouth NR31 6EA Tel: 01493 650772 — LMSSA Lond. 1985. Socs: MDU.

NAGPAL, Sunita South Quay Surgery, 35-36 South Quay, Great Yarmouth NR30 2RG Tel: 01493 843196 — MB BS Delhi 1977; MB BS Delhi 1977.

NAGPAL, Vidya Sagar (retired) 21 The Warren Drive, London E11 2LR Tel: 020 8989 0966 — MB BS Calcutta 1954 (Calcutta Med. Coll.) DGO 1956, DCH 1957; MRCOG 1961; MRCGP 1968. Prev: Ho. Off. & SHO Med. Coll. Calcutta.

NAGPAUL, Chaand The Surgery, 404 Honeypot Lane, Stanmore HA7 1JP Tel: 020 8204 1363 Fax: 020 8905 0286 — MB BS Lond. 1985 (St. Bart.) BSc (Hons.) Lond. 1982; DRCOG 1987; MRCGP 1990; FRCGP 2000. Chairm. Harrow E. & Kingsbury PCG. Specialty: Gen. Pract. Socs: Exec. Mem. NHS Primary Care Gp. Alliance; GMSC; RCGP Counc. Prev: Trainee GP Char. Cross Hosp. Lond. VTS.

NAGPAUL, Seema Watling Medical Centre, 108 Watling Avenue, Burnt Oak, Edgware HA8 0NR Tel: 020 8906 1711 Fax: 020 8201 1283 — MB BS Lond. 1986 (Guy's) DRCOG 1988; DCH RCP Lond. 1989; MRCGP 1990. Prev: Trainee GP Barnet; Trainee GP Ilford VTS; Ho. Surg. Guys Hosp. Lond.

NAGRA, Amarjit Singh Oakham Surgery, 213 Regent Road, Tividale, Oldbury B69 1RZ Tel: 01384 252274 Fax: 01384 240088 — BM Soton. 1986 (Southampton) MRCGP 1990; DRCOG 1990. Hon. Clin. Lect. Birm. Uni. Specialty: Gen. Pract.

NAGRA, Arvind 12 Berkeley Avenue, Cranford, Hounslow TW4 6LA — MB ChB Leeds 1988.

NAGRA, Indarjit Singh Solihull Hospital, Lode Lane, Solihull B91 2JL Tel: 0121 711 4455; 56 Wells Green Road, Olton, Solihull B92 7PG Tel: 0121 743 8812 — BM BS Nottm. 1988; BMedSci. Nottm. 1986; Cert. Family Plann. JCC 1991; DCCH RCP Ed. 1992;

DRCOG 1992; DFFP 1995; M.Sc. Sports Med 1997. SHO (Med.) Solihull Hosp. Specialty: Gen. Pract.

NAGRANI, P Ince Green Lane Surgery, 238 Ince Green Lane, Ince, Wigan WN3 4RP Tel: 01942 246263 Fax: 01942 824084 — MB BS Lucknow 1968; MB BS Lucknow 1968.

NAGRANI, Rani 8 Pavenham Drive, Birmingham B5 7TW — MB BS Delhi 1979; MRCOG 1993.

NAGRATH, Krishan Dass The Surgery, 21 Brownfield Street, London E14 6ND Tel: 020 7987 2774; The Manor House, Rectory Road, Orsett, Grays RM16 3EH Tel: 01375 891419 Fax: 01375 892825 — (Amritsar Med. Coll.) MB BS Panjab (India) 1954. Princip. Gen. Med. Practitioner Reader NHS. Specialty: Gen. Med.; Alcohol & Substance Misuse; Gen. Pract. Socs: ODA; BMA; Indian Med. Assn. Prev: Med. Off. Kenya.; Regist. (A & E) Kiddermister Gen. Hosp.

NAGREH, Baljit Kaur 237 London Road, Bedford MK42 0PX — MB ChB Sheff. 1993.

NAGUIB, Magdi Fouad Department of Medicine for Elderly, Norfolk & Norwich University Hospital, Colney Lane, Norwich NR4 7UY Tel: 01603 288011; 385 Unthank Road, Norwich NR4 7QG — MB BCh Cairo 1972; MRCP (UK) 1976; FRCP Lond. 1994. Cons. Phys. (elderly) Norf. & Nowich Univ. Hosp.; Clin. Teach. Univ. Camb. Specialty: Care of the Elderly. Prev: Sen. Regist. Roy. Vict. Hosp. Edin.; Regist. (Med.) Roy. Infirm. & Chalmers Hosp. Edin.; SHO (Med.) Hope Hosp. Salford.

NAGUIB, Meena Elshaher Nassef Charing Cross Hospital, Fulham Palace Road, London W6 8RF Tel: 020 8846 1234 — MB BCh Ain Shams 1976.

NAGUIB, Mr Mohamed Abd El-Aziem Ahmed 98 Preston New Road, Blackpool FY4 4HF Tel: 01253 698313 Fax: 01253 698313 Email: mnaguib@onetel.net.uk — MB BCh Ain Shams 1975; DLO (Dip. Laryngo. Otology) Roy. Coll. of Surgeons of Eng. 1989; FRCSI 1990. Specialty: Otolaryngol.

NAGVEKAR, Vidyalaxmi Fareham Health Centre, Fareham PO16 7ER; 2 Wightways Mews, Warsash, Southampton SO31 9AF — BM Soton. 1981. GP Retainer. Specialty: Gen. Med.

NAHA, Bishwajit 11 Sandbourne Avenue, London SW19 3EW — BM BS Nottm. 1985.

NAHA-BISWAS, Papiya 2 Pendlefields, Fence, Burnley BB12 9HN — MB ChB Ed. 1998.

NAHABEDIAN, Arakel M Orthopaedic Department, Mid Cheshire Hospitals Trust, Leighton Hospital, Crewe CW1 7QJ Tel: 01270 255141; High Doon, Moss Lane, Leighton, Crewe CW1 4RN Tel: 01270 522319 — MD Beirut 1981 (Amer. Univ. Beirut. Lebanon) BSc (Biol. & Chem.) Amer. Univ. Beirut 1974, MSc (Human Morphol.) 1976. Clin. Specialist (Orthop.) Mid Chesh. Hosp. Trust Crewe. Specialty: Orthop. Socs: BMA; AMA. Prev: Regist. (Orthop.) Crewe HA.

NAHAI, Simine Chantal Mount Tyndal, Spaniards Road, London NW3 7JH Tel: 020 8458 5543 — MB ChB Bristol 1972; BSc Bristol 1969, MB ChB 1972. Nutritional Medicine. Prev: Ho. Off. (Paediat.) Southmead Hosp. Bristol.

NAHAMI, G R Sheffield Medical Centre, 21 Spital Street, Sheffield S3 9LB Tel: 0114 272 6245.

NAHAR, Prem Nath Kildrum Health Centre, Afton Road, Cumbernauld, Glasgow G67 2EU Tel: 01236 721354 — MB ChB Glas. 1974.

NAHEED, Yasara 52 Lomeshaye Road, Nelson BB9 7AR — MB ChB Leeds 1998.

NAHHAS, Aktham Sobhi 110 Larkspur Drive, Langney, Eastbourne BN23 8EH — MD Aleppo, Syria 1983.

NAHL, Mr Sukhdev Singh Telfer Road, 190 Telfer Road, Coventry CV6 3DJ Tel: 024 7659 6060 Fax: 024 7660 1607 — MB ChB Birm. 1979; FRCS Glas. 1986; FRCS Ed. 1988. Prev: Regist. (ENT) W. Midl. Scheme.

NAHSER, Hans-Christean Walton Centre for Neurology & Neurosurgery, Lower Lane, Fazakerley, Liverpool L9 7LJ Tel: 0151 529 5538 Fax: 0151 529 5505 Email: hans.nahser@thewaltoncentre.nhs.uk — State Exam Med Dusseldorf 1977; D Med Essen 1982; ARZT (Neurochirureie) 1985; ARZT (Radiologische Diagnostik) 1988; Teilebiet Neuroradiologie 1989. Cons. Neuroradiol. & Hon. Sen. Lect. The Walton Centre for Neurol. & Neurosurg. Liverp.; Hon. Cons. Neuroradiologist Manch. Neurosci. Center Hope Hosp. Salford. Specialty: Neurosurg.; Radiol. Special Interest: Interventional Neuroradiology. Socs: British Society of Neuroradiology; UK Neurointerventional Group; Royal College of Radiologists.

NAIDOO, Arunavema Sathyadatta The Valley Surgery, 81 Bramcote Lane, Chilwell, Nottingham NG9 4ET Tel: 0115 943 0530 Fax: 0115 943 1958; 360 Musters Road, West Bridgford, Nottingham NG2 7DA — MB ChB Manch. 1978; BSc (Anat.) (Hons.) St. And. 1975; FRCGP 1982; DCH RCPS 1982; DRCOG 1983. Princip. GP Beeston & Chillwell Nottm.; Course Organiser Nottm. VTS. Socs: Panel Examr. Roy. Coll. Gen. Pract.

NAIDOO, Govindarajaloo Ramamurthie 1 Ludworth Road, Southport PR8 2AS Tel: 01704 77866; 2 Leamington Road, Ainsdale, Southport PR8 5LB — MB BCh Witwatersrand 1948. Mem. Sefton Med. Servs. Comm. Socs: BMA & S. Afr. Med. Assn. Prev: Clin. Asst. (Dermat.) Southport Infirm.

NAIDOO, Kebalanandha Ramamurthie Liverpool Road Practice, 107 Liverpool Road, Southport PR8 4DB Tel: 01704 566646 Fax: 01704 550858; Hilltop, 13 Selworthy Road, Birkdale, Southport PR8 2NS Tel: 01704 564666 Fax: 01704 550858 — MB BCh BAO NUI 1983 (RCS Irel.) Dip. Trop. Med. RCSI 1982; Dip. Radiol. RCSI 1983; LRCPI LM, LRCSI & LM 1983; Cert. Family Plann. JCC 1986; DRCOG 1988. GP Southport. Specialty: Obst. & Gyn. Socs: Vice-Chairm. Sefton LMC; (Comm.) S.port Med. Soc.

NAIDOO, Nirmala Kausilya Nuffield Health Centre, Welch Way, Witney OX28 6JQ Tel: 01993 703641; 5 Leys Villas, The Leys, Witney OX28 4DH Tel: 01993 702316 — MB ChB Manch. 1975; BSc St. And. 1972; MRCGP 1982; DRCOG 1983.

NAIDOO, Padhmanaba (retired) 49 Hillmorton Road, Rugby CV22 5AB Tel: 01788 330470 — MB BCh Witwatersrand 1950; DCH Eng. 1956. Prev: Regist. (Paediat.) Whittington Hosp. Lond.

NAIDOO, Rajan Olof Magnus 63 Leicester Road, London N2 9DY — MB BS Lond. 1990; BSc Psychol. Lond. 1987, MB BS 1990.

NAIDOO, Ramamurthie Surendra Kew Medical Centre, 66 Folkstone Road, Southport PR8 5PH Tel: 01704 546800 Fax: 01704 540486 — MB BCh BAO NUI 1978; LRCPI & LM, LRCSI & LM 1978. Specialty: Gen. Pract. Socs: DRCOG.

NAIDOO, Rani Kristina Anita Warrell Unit, St Mary's Hospital, Manchester M13 0JH Tel: 0161 276 6119 Fax: 0161 276 6140 Email: knaidoo@ugynae.cmht.nwest.nhs.uk; Foden Bank Farm, Byrons Lane, Macclesfield SK11 0HA Tel: 01625 614102 — MB ChB Sheff. 1985 (Sheffield) BMedSci Sheff. 1984; MRCOG 1992. Cons. Gynaecologist, St. Mary's Hosp., Manch.. Specialty: Obst. & Gyn. Prev: Sen. Regist. St. Mary's Hosp. Manch.

NAIDOO, Tharuna Maya St Anns Hospital, London N15 Tel: 020 8442 6467 — MB ChB Dundee 1972 (Lond.) DCH Eng. 1975; MRCPsych 1979. Cons. Child & Adolesc. Psychiat. Haringey Heathcare Trust; Cons.child & Adolesc.Psychiat. N. Middlx. Hosp. Trust, Lond. Specialty: Child & Adolesc. Psychiat. Socs: Assoc. Mem. Brit. Psychoanal. Soc. Prev: Sen. Regist. (Child Psychiat.) St. Mary's Hosp. Lond.; Regist. (Psychol. Med.) Univ. Coll. Hosp. Lond.

NAIDOO, Vishal — MB BCh Witwatersrand 1998; MRCGP Lond. Special Interest: Complementary Med.; Nutrit.; Cardiovasc. Risk Assessm. Prev: Chelsea & Westm. Hosp.

NAIDU, Govindarajalu Cupswami Perumal General Hospital, St Helier, Jersey JE2 3QS Tel: 01534 59000 Fax: 01534 622880; Fiorano House, Mont Gras D'Eau, St Brelade, Jersey JE3 8ED Tel: 01534 744175 Email: govnaidu@aol.com — MB BS Lond. 1981 (Univ. Coll. Hosp.) Assoc. Specialist (Orthop. & Trauma) Gen. Hosp. Jersey. Specialty: Trauma & Orthop. Surg. Socs: BOA; BASK; AAOS. Prev: Regist. (Orthop., A & E & Trauma) Gen. Hosp. Jersey; Regist. (Surg.) Roy. Masonic Hosp. Lond.; SHO (Orthop.) Hammersmith Hosp. Lond.

NAIDU, Vasanampalli 4 Beaulieu Close, London SE5 8BA — MB BS Lond. 1994.

NAIK, Caroline Susheila Barrington Medical Centre, 68 Barrington Road, Altrincham WA14 1JB Tel: 0161 928 9621 Fax: 0161 926 9317 — MB ChB Liverp. 1991.

NAIK, Darshana Rupal St Oswalds Surgery, The Parade, Pembroke SA71 4LD; 'Ty Arianna', 38 Parklands, St Florence, Tenby SA70 8NL — MB BCh Wales 1996. GP Principal. Specialty: Gen. Pract. Socs: MPS; BMA. Prev: SHO O & G Carmarithen; SHO Gen. Med. Princess of Wales. Bridgend; SHO Neoratol. Uni. Hosp. Wales.

NAIK, Dineshchandra Rameschandra White Lodge, 11 Denbank Avenue, Sheffield S10 5NZ Tel: 0114 230 1254 — MB ChB Sheff.

1962; DMRD Eng. 1967; FFR 1970; FRCR 1975. Cons. Radiol. & Hon. Clin. Lect. Univ. Sheff. N. Gen. Hosp. Sheff. Specialty: Radiol. Socs: BMA (Chairm. Sheff. Div.); Brit. Inst. Radiol. Prev: Edr. Brit. Med. Ultrasound Bull. BMU Soc.; Sen. Regist. (Radiol.) North. Gen. Hosp. Sheff. & United Sheff. Hosps.; Regist. Radiol. United Sheff. Hosps.

NAIK, Jay St James's Hospital, Beckett Street, Leeds LS9 7TF; 17 Carnoustie Close, New Moston, Manchester M40 3NF — MB ChB Leeds 1998; BSc Leeds 1996; MRCP UK 2001. Specialist Regist. (Med. Oncol.) North. Yorks. Rotat. Prev: PRHO, Vasc. Surg., Hull Roy. Infirm., Hull.

NAIK, Jayant Narayan Albion Street Surgery, 1 Albion Street, Liverpool L5 3QN Tel: 0151 263 1176 Fax: 0151 261 1295; 5 Cromptons Lane, Liverpool L18 3EU Tel: 0151 722 3101 — MB BS Karnatak 1961; DA Eng. 1963. Clin. Asst. (Dent. Anaesth.) Liverp.; Clin. Asst. (A & E) Walton Hosp. Liverp. Specialty: Anaesth. Socs: BMA; Liverp. Med. Inst.; Roy. Coll. Anaesth. Prev: Regist. (Anaesth.) Liverp. Roy. Infirm., Sefton Hosp. Liverp. & Cumbld. Infirm. Carlisle.

NAIK, Katherine Sunita Huddersfield Royal Infirmary, Acre Street, Lindley, Huddersfield HD3 3EA Tel: 01484 342762; 34 The Drive, Roundhay, Leeds LS8 1JH Tel: 0113 293 5042 — MB ChB (Hons.) Leeds 1989; BSc (Hons.) Leeds 1986; MRCP (UK) 1992; FRCR 1995. Cons. Radiol. Huddersfield Roy. Infirm. Specialty: Radiol.

NAIK, Purushottam Narayan c/o Drive S. Phadnis, 141 New Park Avenue, Palmers Green, London N13 5NA — MD Poona 1981; MB BS Ponna 1975; MRCPI 1984.

NAIK, Rajan Northern Gynaecological Oncology Centre, Queen Elizabeth Hospital, Sheriff Hill, Gateshead NE9 6SX Tel: 0191 445 2392; 50 St Georges Terrace NE2 2SY Tel: 0191 209 2960 — MB ChB Manch. 1986; MRCOG 1992; MD Newcastle 1997. Cons. Gyn. Oncologist, North. Gyn. Oncol. Centre. Specialty: Obst. & Gyn. Prev: Sen. Regist. Rotat. (O & G) Newc. & N. Region.

NAIK, Ramachandra Krishna Beechdrive Surgery, 17-19 Beechdrive, Fulwood, Preston PR2 3NB Tel: 01772 863033 — MB BS Mysore 1972 (Govt. Med. Coll. Mysore) Prev: GP Wrexham; SHO (Geriat.) Hallam & Heath La. Hosps. W. Bromwich; Clin. Asst. (Psych.) Winwick Hosp. Warrington.

NAIK, Ramesh Bhagwanji The Lawns, Old Bath Road, Sonning-on-Thames, Reading RG4 6TQ — MB ChB Birm. 1968 (Rhodesia) MRCP (UK) 1973. Cons. Phys. & Nephrol. Roy. Berks. Hosp. Reading. Specialty: Gen. Med. Socs: RCP Comm. Renal Dis. Assoc. Edr. Proc. Europ. Dialysis & Transpl Assn. Prev: Sen. Regist. Wessex Renal Unit Portsmouth & Roy. S. Hants. Hosp.; Soton.; Regist. Renal Unit E. Birm. Hosp.; Hon. Sen. Regist. E. Birm. Hosp. & Hon. Clin. Lect. Univ. Birm.

NAIK, Ravin Wadsley Bridge Medical Centre, 103 Halifax Road, Sheffield S6 1LA; Broom House, 12 Broomgrove Road, Sheffield S10 2LR — MB ChB Sheff. 1985; DCH RCP Lond. 1990; MRCGP 1994.

NAIK, Sandhia 58 Sancroft Road, Harrow HA3 7NT — MB ChB Manch. 1989.

NAIK, Sandra Valerie Isabella (retired) White Lodge, 11 Denbank Avenue, Sheffield S10 5NZ Tel: 0114 230 1254 — MB ChB Sheff. 1962; DA RCPSI 1968. Prev: Asst. Specialist (Endocrinol.) Sheff. HA (T).

NAIK, Sarita — BM BS Nottm. 1997. SHO Rotat. (Med.) Ashford Kent. Specialty: Gen. Med. Prev: SHO (Med.) Derby; SHO (Surg.) Reading.

NAIK, Sharatchandra Manohar (retired) The Garth, 93 Oldfield Road, Altrincham WA14 4BL Tel: 0161 928 9621 — (Grant Med. Coll.) MB BS Bombay 1950. Prev: Regist. Orthop. Surg. City Gen. Hosp. Sheff. & Regist. Plas. Surg. Wythenshawe Hosp, Manch.

NAIM, Tahir 17 Museum Mansion, 63a Great Russell St., London WC1B 3BJ — MB BS Punjab 1985.

NAIMA, Mr Sabah Jassim 66 Shelford Road, Fulbourn, Cambridge CB1 5HJ — MB ChB Baghdad 1976; FRCS Glas. 1990; FRCS (Orth.) 2001; MSc (Orth.) 2001.

NAINBY-LUXMOORE, Jonathan Chave The Surgery, Hill Terrace, Middleton-in-Teesdale, Barnard Castle DL12 0QE Tel: 01833 640217; Heatherbrae, Snaisgill Road, Middleton-in-Teesdale, Barnard Castle DL12 0RP Tel: 01833 640420 — MB BS Lond. 1983 (St. Bartholomew's Hosp.) MA Oxf. 1989, BA 1980; DRCOG 1988; MRCGP 1991. Specialty: Gen. Pract. Socs: BMA. Prev: Maj. RAMC GP Roy. Milit. Acad. Sandhurst; Ho. Off. (Surg.) St. Barts Hosp. Lond.

NAINBY-LUXMOORE, Richard Chave (retired) The Old Vicarage, Fareham Road, Southwick Village, Fareham PO17 6DY Tel: 023 9232 7792 — MRCS Eng. LRCP Lond. 1954 (Camb. & St. Bart.) MA Camb. 1956, BA 1950, MB 1955, BChir 1954; DA Eng. 1956; FFA RCS Eng. 1961. Prev: Cons. Anaesth. Portsmouth & S.E. Hants. Health Dist.

NAING, Sao Yan Dunsbury Way Clinic, Dunsbury Way, Leigh Park, Havant PO9 5BG Tel: 023 9248 2154 Fax: 023 9247 1892; 36 Breach Avenue, Emsworth PO10 8NB Tel: 01243 373608 — MB BS Rangoon 1960; DCH RCPS Glas. 1966. Clin. Med. Off. Dunsbury Way Clinic Hants.

NAIR, Amanda Lesley 17 Harness Close, Springfield, Chelmsford CM1 6UU — BM Soton. 1996.

NAIR, Balgopal 5-A Templebank Flats, Duckworth Lane, Bradford BD9 6RJ — MB BS Aligarh Muslim U India 1979.

NAIR, Divakaran Vakkappulathu Gopalain 16 Brunel Road, Chigwell IG8 8BE Tel: 0831 614508 — Vrach Moscow 1973; Vrach Peoples' Friendship U Moscow 1973. Prev: Regist. & SHO (Chest & Gen. Med.) Ipswich Hosp. Suff.

NAIR, Hemant Thankappan 11 Gambier Parry Gardens, Gloucester GL2 9RD — MB BS Bombay 1980.

NAIR, Indira Havering Hospitals NHS Trust, Waterloo Road, Romford RM7 0BE; 40 The Bowls, Vicarage Lane, Chigwell IG7 6NB — MB BS Lond. 1982; FFA RCSI 1992; FRCA 1992. Cons. (Anaesth.) Havering Hosp. NHS Trust Romford, Essex. Specialty: Anaesth. Socs: Assn. Anaesth.; BMA.

NAIR, Karal Venugopalan Chesterfield & North Derbyshire Royal Hospital, Calow, Chesterfield S44 5BL — MB BS Kerala 1969 (Med. Coll. Calicut) DMRD Eng. 1978; FRCR Eng. 1980. Cons. Radiol. Chesterfield & N. Derbysh. Roy. Hosp. Specialty: Radiol. Prev: Sen. Regist. (Diag. Radiol.) Newc. AHA (T).

NAIR, Prakash Peterborough District Hospital, Thorpe Road, Peterborough PE3 6DA Tel: 01733 875948 Fax: 01733 875967 — MB BCh Wales 1987 (University of Wales College of Medicine) MRCP (UK) 1991; FRCP (UK) 2002. Cons. Phys. (Gen. Med./Gastroenterol.). Specialty: Gen. Med.; Gastroenterol. Socs: Brit. Soc. Gastroenterol.; Roy. Coll. of Phys.s. Prev: SHO Leicester Med. Rotat.; Regist. E. of Eng. Gastroenterol. Rotat./Leicester/Peterboro; Sen. Reg. S.W. Rotat.

NAIR, Rajasekhararan Ramakrishnan Department of Anaesthetics, Airedale General Hospital, Skipton Road, Steeton, Keighley BD20 6TD Tel: 01535 652511; Rose Tor, 19 View Road, Keighley BD20 6JN Tel: 01535 602260 — MB BS Kerala 1974; BSc Kerala 1968; DLO RCS Eng. 1981; DA (UK) 1989. Assoc. Specialist Anaesthetics & Intens. Care Airedale Gen. Hosp. Keighley. Specialty: Anaesth. Prev: Staff Grade (Anaesth.) Airedale Gen. Hosp. Steeton; Clin. Asst. (ENT) Roy. Devon & Exeter Hosp.; Regist. (Anaesth.) King Geo. Hosp. Ilford.

NAIR, Mr Rajeev Gopal 8 Clare Drive, Macclesfield SK10 2TX — MB BS Bombay 1986; FRCS Glas. 1993.

NAIR, Raveendran Raghavan Pelton Fell Surgery, 21 Gardner Crescent, Pelton Fell, Chester-le-Street DH2 2NJ Tel: 0191 368 0614 Fax: 0191 387 4644 — MB BS Kerala 1974. GP CHester-le-St., Co. Durh.

NAIR, Mr Salil Baskaran Royal Hampshire Country Hospital, ENT Department, Romsey Road, Winchester SO22 5DG Tel: 01962 824302 Fax: 01962 825676 Email: salil.nair@weht.swest.nhs.uk; Southampton University Hospitals NHS Trust, Tremona Road, Southampton SO16 6YD — MB ChB Dundee 1991; FRCS Eng 1996; FRCS Ed 1996; FRCS (ORL-HNS) Lond 2000; MD Newc. 2002. SHO (ENT) Leeds Infirm. Specialty: Otorhinolaryngol. Prev: SHO (Neurosurg.) Addenbrooke's Hosp. Camb.; SHO (A & E) Bristol; SHO (Plastic Surg.) Bradford Roy. Infirm.

NAIR, Shanta 11 Gambier Parry Gardens, Gloucester GL2 9RD — MB BS Bombay 1985.

NAIR, Sindhu 96 Bay Horse Lane, Scarcroft, Leeds LS14 3JQ — MB ChB Leeds 1998.

NAIR, Mr Sunil 73 Evergreen Way, Hayes UB3 2BH — MB BS All India Inst. Med. Sci. 1990; FRCS Glas. 1994. Specialty: Orthop.

NAIR, Mr Unnikrishnan Ramanpillai The Yorkshire Heart Centre, Leeds General Infirmary, Great George St., Leeds LS1 3EX Tel: 0113 392 5792 Fax: 0113 392 5408 Email:

unnikrishnan.nair@leedsth.nhs.uk — (Trivandrum Med. Coll.) MB BS Kerala 1970; MS Kerala 1973; FRCS Ed. 1976; FRCS Eng. 1977; FETCS 1998. Cons. Cardiothoracic Surg. Yorks. Heart Centre, Leeds Gen. Infirm.; Hon. Sen. Lect. (Cardiothoracic Surg.) St. James'. Univ. Hosp.Leeds. Specialty: Cardiothoracic Surg. Socs: Soc. Thoracic & Cardiovasc. Surg. GB & Irel.; Eur. Assn. Cardiothoracic Surg.; Yorks. Thoracic Soc. Prev: Sen. Regist. (Cardiothoracic Surg.) Wythenshawe Hosp. Manch.; Sen. Regist. (Cardiothoracic Surg.) Killingbeck Hosp. Leeds; Cons. Surg. Palghat Polyclinic & Assisi Hosp. Kanjikode.

NAIR, Velayudhan Pillai Raghunadhan 5 Kensington Close, Mansfield Woodhouse, Mansfield NG19 9GZ — MB BS Andhra 1967. Specialty: Otolaryngol.

NAIRAC, Bertrand Laurence Orchard House, 17 Church St., St Peters, Broadstairs CT10 2TT Tel: 01843 604777 Fax: 01843 862211; Napier Lodge, Monkton Road, Minster, Ramsgate CT12 4EB — BM BCh Oxf. 1980; BA (Hons.) Oxf. 1977; MRCPsych 1985. Cons. Psychiat. (Child & Adolesc.) Canterbury & Thanet Community Healthcare NHS Trust. Specialty: Child & Adolesc. Psychiat. Prev: Sen. Regist. (Child & Adolesc. Psychiat.) Nottm.; Assoc. Research Fell. Univ. Coll. Lond.; Regist. (Psychiat.) Roy. Free, Friern & Whittington Hosps. Lond.

NAIRN, Mr David Sherwood Princess Alexandra Hospital, Hamstel Road, Harlow CM20 1QX Tel: 01279 827061 — MB BChir Camb. 1968; BA Camb. 1964; FRCS Eng. 1972. Cons. Orthop. & Hand Surg. Princess Alexandra Hosp. NHS Trust Harlow. Specialty: Orthop. Special Interest: Hand Surg.; Upper Limb & Foot Surg. Socs: BOA; Brit. Soc. Surg. of Hand; Brit. Foot Surg. Soc. Prev: Cons. Orthop. Surg. Herts. & Essex Hosp. Bishop's Stortford & St. Margt. Hosp. Epping; Cons. Hand Surg. Princess Alexandra Hosp. Harlow; Sen. Regist. (Orthop.) King's Coll. Hosp. Lond.

NAIRN, Edwin Robert Department of Histopathology, Crosshouse Hospital, Kilmarnock KA2 0BE Tel: 01563 577426 Fax: 01563 572407; 8 Lady Margaret Drive, Troon KA10 7AL Tel: 01292 311597 Email: rnairn@iname.com — MB ChB Manch. 1981; BSc St. And. 1978; MRCPath 1988; DFM Glas. 1990. Cons. Path. CrossHo. Hosp. Kilmarnock. Specialty: Histopath. Prev: Sen. Regist. (Histopath.) Dept. Histopath. Univ. Birm.; Sen. Regist. Dudley Rd. Hosp.; Sen. Regist. E. Birm. Hosp & Childr. Hosp. Birm.

NAIRN, Lesley May 119 Balshagray Avenue, Glasgow G11 7EG — MB ChB Glas. 1990; MRCP (UK) 1993. Specialty: Paediat.

NAIRN, Robert Martin Clarendon Medical, 35 Northland Avenue, Londonderry BT48 7JW Tel: 028 7126 5391 Fax: 028 7126 5932 — MB BCh BAO NUI 1979; BSc (Hons.) NUI 1976; DRCOG 1986; Dip. Family Plann. 1986; MRCGP 1987. Chairperson Foyle Young Pract. Gp.

NAIRN, Stuart Angus (retired) Filin, Lochinver, Lairg IV27 4LP Tel: 01571 844439 — MB ChB St. And. 1959. Prev: GP Lochinver.

NAIRNE, Angela Alice Clinical Neurology, Radcliffe Infirmary, Woodstock Road, Oxford — MB BS Lond. 1984 (Guy's) BSc Lond. 1978, MB BS 1984; DRCOG 1987; MRCP (UK) 1994. Assoc. Specialist. Neurol. Specialty: Neurol. Prev: Regist. (Neurol.) Oxf. Region Train Scheme.; SHO (Med.) Roy. Berks. Hosp. Reading; Clin. Asst. (Ophth.) Stoke Manderville Hosp. Aylesbury.

NAISBY, Geoffrey Philip South Cleveland Hospital, Marton Road, Middlesbrough TS4 3BW Tel: 01642 850850 Fax: 01642 700153 — MB BS Newc. 1981; FRCR 1988. Cons. Radiol. S. Cleveland Hosp. N. RHA. Specialty: Radiol. Prev: Sen. Regist. (Radiol.) Newc. u Tyne.

NAISBY, Mary Gwendoline Tennatn Street Medical Practice, Stockton-on-Tees TS18 2AT Tel: 01642 613331 — MB BS Newc. 1981; DRCOG 1983; DCCH RCGP 1984; MRCGP 1985; Dip. Ther. Newc. 1995.

NAISH, Clare Surgery, 65D Midland Road, Royston, Barnsley S71 4QW Tel: 01226 722418 Fax: 01226 700648; 30 Far Croft, Lepton, Huddersfield HD8 0LS Tel: 01484 5552 — MB BS Lond. 1972 (Roy. Free) MRCS Eng. LRCP Lond. 1972; MRCGP 1977; DRCOG 1977.

NAISH, Mrs Jeannette Chung-Meng Market Street Health Group, 52 Market Street, East Ham, London E6 2RA Tel: 020 8548 2200 Fax: 020 8548 2288 — MRCS Eng. LRCP Lond. 1965; MSc Lond. 1989, MB BS 1966; MRCGP 1981. Sen. Lect. Dept. Gen. Pract. & Primary Care St. Bart. & Lond. Hosp. Prev: Sen. Lect. Dept. Pub. Health & Primary Care Roy. Free Hosp. Lond.; Clin. Asst. Ment. Handicap Unit Enfield Dist. Hosp.; Chairm. N. E. Lond. Fac. Bd.

NAISH, John Michael Algars Manor, Iron Acton, Bristol BS37 9TB Tel: 01454 228372 — MD Camb. 1947 (King's Coll. Hosp.) MA Camb. 1940, MD 1947, MB BChir 1939; FRCP Lond. 1954, M 1945. Emerit. Cons. Gen. Med. Avon HA (T). Specialty: Gen. Med. Socs: Assn. Phys. Gt. Brit. & Irel. Prev: Cons. Phys. Frenchay Hosp. Bristol; Lect. in Med. Univ. Bristol; Prof. & Head Dept. Med. Univ. Lagos, Nigeria.

NAISH, Nora (retired) — (King's Coll. Hosp.) MB BS Lond. 1938; MRCS Eng. LRCP Lond. 1938; DCH Eng. 1948.

NAISH, Richard Hanwell Health Centre, 20 Church Road, Hanwell, London W7 1DR Tel: 020 8567 5738; Old Coach House, Bray, Maidenhead SL6 2AE — LMSSA Lond. 1975.

NAISH, Sonya — MB ChB Birm. 1998; DTM & H 2000; DGM 2001; DFSP 2002; DCH 2002; MRCGP 2003. GP Bristol.

NAISMITH, Alastair James William 27 Otterburn Drive, Glasgow G46 6PZ — MB ChB Glas. 1972; FFA RCSI 1978. Cons. Anaesth. Monklands Dist. Gen. Hosp. Airdrie. Specialty: Anaesth. Prev: Sen. Anaesth. Qu. Eliz. Centr. Hosp. Blantyre, Malawi; Sen. Regist. (Anaesth.) Stobhill Hosp. Glas.; Regist. (Anaesth.) Glas. Roy. Infirm.

NAISMITH, Alison Jane Dept. Psychiatry, Southern General Hospital, 1345 Govan Road, Glasgow G51 4TF Tel: 0141 201 1942 Fax: 0141 201 1920 Email: jane.naismith@glacomen.scot.nhs.uk; 12 Wykeham Road, Glasgow G13 3YT Tel: 0141 954 9885 Fax: 0141 954 9885 — MB ChB Dundee 1980; DObst 1982; MRCGP 1985; MRCPsych 1987. Cons. Psychotherapist Dept. Of Psychiat., Southern Gen. Hosp., Glas. Specialty: Psychother. Socs: Scott. Assn. Psychoan. Psychother.; Assoc. Mem. Brit. Psychoan. Soc.; Roy. Coll. of Psychiatrists. Prev: Sen. Regist. (Psychiat.) Gtr. Glas. HB.

NAISMITH, Douglas Stuart Low Waters Medical Centre, 11 Mill Road, Hamilton ML3 8AA Tel: 01698 283626 Fax: 01698 282839; 2 Gleneagles Park, Castle Park, Bothwell, Glasgow G71 8UT — MB ChB Glas. 1973; DObst RCOG 1975.

NAISMITH, James Henderson Wishaw Health Centre, Kennilworth Avenue, Wishaw ML2 7BQ Tel: 01698 372201; 119 Old Manse Road, Wishaw ML2 0EW Tel: 01698 372201 — MB ChB Glas. 1961.

NAISMITH, Karen Isobel Department Community Child Health, Strathmartine Hospital, Dundee — MB ChB Glas. 1984; FRCP FRCPCH; DCH RCPS Glas. 1986. Cons. Paediat. & Complex Disabil. Specialty: Disabil. Med.

NAISMITH, Laurence James Hutton Centre, St Luke's Hospital, Marton Road, Middlesbrough TS4 3AF Tel: 01642 854978 Fax: 01642 829542 — MRCS Eng. LRCP Lond. 1976; MRCPsych 1982; DPM Eng. 1982. Cons. Forens. Psychiat. St Luke's Hosp. Middlesbrough. Specialty: Forens. Psychiat. Prev: Cons. Forens. Psychiat. AMI Stockton Hall, Pk. La. Special Hosp. Merseyside; Sen. Regist. (Forens. Psychiat.) Yorks. RHA.

NAISMITH, Shelagh Margaret The Surgery, Denmark Street, Darlington DL3 0PD Tel: 01325 460731 Fax: 01325 362183; 119 Old Manse Road, Wishaw ML2 0EW Tel: 01698 375573 — MB ChB Glas. 1988. Resid. (Surg.) Monklands Dist. Gen. Hosp. Airdrie & Law Hosp. Carluke.

NAISMITH, Mr William Cairns McLean Kerr (retired) Innesfallen, 146 Mugdock Road, Milngavie, Glasgow G62 8NP Tel: 0141 571 7117 — MB ChB Glas. 1964; FRCOG 1981, M 1967; FRCS Glas. 1993. Cons. (O & G) South. Gen. Hosp. Glas.; Hon. Clin. Sen. Lect. Univ. Glas.

NAJADA, Salim Fadel (Surgery), 131 Addison Road, Kings Heath, Birmingham B14 7ER Tel: 0121 444 2729; 12 Manor Park Road, Castle Bromwich, Birmingham B36 0DL — LMS Madrid 1968. Prev: Regist. (O & G) Preston Hosp.; Regist. (O & G) Grimsby Gen. Hosp.

NAJAK, Bahadurali Gulam Hussein Blakesley Surgery, 39 Blakesley Road, Yardley, Birmingham B25 8XU Tel: 0121 783 4224 Fax: 0121 785 0423 — MB BS Madras 1973 (Madras Med. Coll.) Prev: Ho. Off./SHO (Med.) Newham Gp. Hosps. Lond.; Rotating Res. Ho. Off.; Govt. Gen. Hosp. & Govt. Hosp. Wom. & Childr. Madras India; Regist. (Med.) & SHO (Paediat.) St. Bart. Hosp. Lond.

NAJAM UD DIN, Dr 66 Henniker Point, Stratford, London E15 1LQ — MB BS Punjab 1985; FRCR 1994.

NAJIB, Riad Ahmad Mahamad Department of Haematology, Singleton Hospital, Swansea SA2 8QA Tel: 01792 205666; c/o Radam, First Floor, 75 Kimberley Gardens, London N4 1LD Email: drrnajib@hotmail.com — MB ChB Basrah 1985; MSc (Haemat.) Lond. 1995; MRCPI 1995. Staff Haemat. Singleton Hosp. Swansea.

Specialty: Haematology. Socs: Brit. Soc. Haematol. Prev: Regist. (Med.) Hull & York; SHO (Haemat.) Birm.

NAJIM, Hellme Abdullah Mental Health Unit, Basildon Hospital, Nethermayne, Basildon SS16 5NL — MB ChB Mosul 1977; MRCPsych 1984.

NAJIM, Zahair Nahi The Surgery, 59 Anson Road, London NW2 3UY Tel: 020 8208 4141 Fax: 020 8208 3536 — MB ChB Basrah 1974; MRCP (UK) 1987; (DPD) Cardiff 1997. GP Princip.; Trial in IDDM & Nephropathy. Specialty: Diabetes. Prev: Regist. (Acting Sen. Regist.) Edgware Gen. Hosp.

NAJM AL-DIN, Amir Salim Neurology Department, Pinderfields General Hospital, Aberford Road, Wakefield WF1 4DG Tel: 01924 212359 Fax: 01924 212359 — MB ChB Baghdad 1972; FRCP Lond.; FRCP Edin. Consultant Neurologist. Specialty: Neurol. Socs: ABN; IHS; Amer. Acad. of Neurol.

NAJMALDIN, Mr Azad The Leeds Teaching Hospitals, Department of Paediatric Surgery, Gledhow Wing, St. James's University Hospital, Leeds LS9 7TF Tel: 0113 206 4014 Fax: 0113 206 5496 Email: parmjit.jajuha@leedsth.nhs.uk — MB ChB Baghdad 1973; FRCS Ed. 1982; MS Soton. 1991; FRCS Eng 1998. Cons. Paediatric & Neonat. Surg. Leeds Teachg. Hosps.; Hon. Lect. Leeds Univ.; Chairm. Brit. Assn. Paediatric Endoscopic Surgeons. Specialty: Paediat. Surg. Special Interest: Minimally Invasive Surg. & Urol. Socs: Brit. Assn. Paediat. Surg.; Brit. Assn. of Paediat. Urologists; Chairm. Brit. Assn. of Paediatric Endoscopic Surg. Prev: Sen. Regist. Wessex Regional Centre for Paediat. Surg. Soton. & Roy. Childr. Hosp. Melbourne. Australia.

NAJMI, Syed Muhammad Azizullah Skegness and District Hospital, Dorothy Avenue, Skegness PE25 2BS Tel: 01754 762401 Fax: 01754 760132; 43 Amanda Drive, Louth LN11 0AZ Tel: 01507 604499 Fax: 01507 602005 — MB BS Sind 1962; MB BS Sind, Pakistan 1962. Assoc. Specialist (A & E & Orthop.) Pilgrim & Assoc. Hosps. NHS Trust. Prev: Regist. (Orthop.) Lonsdale Hosp. Barrow in Furness, Barnsley Dist. Gen. Hosp. & Lancaster Roy. Infirm.

NAKHLA, Labib Shehata (retired) 40 Mount Avenue, Ealing, London W5 2QJ — MB BCh Ein Shams Univ. Cairo 1957; DLO 1959; PhD Lond. 1966; LMSSA Lond. 1969; ECFMG Cert 1969; FRCPath 1986, M 1973. Prev: Cons. Microbiol. Mt. Vernon Hosp. Northwood & Harefield Hosp.

NAKHLA, Miss Venice 12 Cherrington Way, Solihull B91 3TH Tel: 0121 705 6890 Fax: 0121 705 6890; 40 Mount Avenue, Ealing, London W5 2QJ Tel: 020 8998 5434 Fax: 020 8991 1548 — MB ChB Liverp. 1990. SHO (ENT) Roy. Liverp. Univ. Hosp.; Specialist Regist. Warwick Hosp. Specialty: Otolaryngol. Socs: Brit. Assn. Otorhinolaryngol.; BMA; MDU.

NAKIELNY, Edward Antoni Blaennant, Talley, Llandeilo SA19 7YW Tel: 015583 354 — MB Camb. 1974 (Univ. Coll. Hosp.) BChir 1973. Prev: Ho. Phys. Kingston Gen. Hosp. Hull; Ho. Surg. Hull Roy. Infirm.

NAKIELNY, Edward Antoni (retired) 9 Braids Walk, Kirkella, Hull HU10 7PB Tel: 01482 657963 — MB ChB Polish Sch. of Med. 1945. Prev: Cons. Chest Phys. Chest Clinic Hull, Castle Hill Hosp.

NAKIELNY, Joanna Margaret — MB ChB Sheff. 1985 (Shef.) BMedSci Shef. Univ. 1983; DRCOG RCOG 1987; MRCPsych RCP 1992; MSc Univ. Lond. 1995. Director Europ. Regulatory Affairs Eli Lilley & Co Windlesham; Clin. Ass. Richmond Roy. Hosp. Kew Fort Rd. Richmond. Special Interest: Pharmaceutical Med.; Psychiat.

NAKIELNY, Richard Alexander 47 Brooklands Avenue, Sheffield S10 4GB — BM BCh Oxf. 1977; MA (Camb.) 1975; FRCR 1982. Cons. Radiol. (C.T. Scanning) Roy. Hallamsh. Hosp. Sheff. Specialty: Radiol.

NALINASEGAREN, Govindasamy Summerlee Medical Centre, Summerlee Road, Finedon, Wellingborough NN9 5LJ Tel: 01933 682203 Fax: 01933 682205; 136 Rothwell Road, Kettering NN16 8UP Tel: 01536 516828 — MB BS Madras 1976 (Christian Med. Coll. Vellore, Madras) MB BS Madras 1973; MRCS Eng. LRCP Lond. 1979; DTCH Liverp. 1982; DCH RCPS Glas. 1984; DGM RCP Lond. 1989. Hosp. Pract. (Paediat.) Ketting Gen. Hosp. N.ants. Socs: BMA; (Counc.) Small Pract.s Assn.; Christ. Med. Fellowsh. Prev: Regist. (Paediat.) Kettering Gen. Hosp.; Research Asst. (Paediat. Nephrol.) Alder Hey Hosp. Liverp.; SHO Rotat. (Paediat.) Alder Hey Hosp. Liverp.

NALINI, Velagapudi The Gables, Harold Road, Abergavenny NP7 7DG Tel: 018730 852374 — MB BS Andhra 1972 (Guntur Med. Coll.) DGO Andhra 1974. Clin. Asst. & Hosp. Specialist (Anaesth.) Gwent HA. Prev: SHO (Anaesth.) New Cross Hosp. Wolverhampton; SHO (Anaesth.) Ipswich Hosp. & Enfield Dist. Hosp.

NALIYAWALA, Abdul Hamid — MB BS Karachi 1985 (Dow Med. Coll., Karachi, Pakistan) MRCPsych Lond. 1993. Cons. Psychiat., E. Sussex Co. NHS Trust Hailsham; Med. Dir. Specialty: Gen. Psychiat. Socs: BMA; Roy. Coll. of Psychiatrists; GMC.

NALL, Peter Thomas Robin Hood Surgery, 1493 Stratford Road, Hall Green, Birmingham B28 9HT Tel: 0121 744 1731 — BM BCh Oxf. 1983. GP Birm.

NALLA, Jayasree 7 Hurley Crescent, Marlow Way, Rotherhithe, London SE16 6AL Tel: 020 7231 7387 — MB BS Andhra 1973; DA (UK) 1983.

NALLA, Mr Ramachandra Rao 5 Dorney Close, Appleton, Warrington WA4 5HY — MB BS Andhra 1971; FRCS Ed. 1980.

NALLETAMBY, Xavier Philippe 16 Raphael Road, Hove BN3 5QQ Tel: 01273 729607 — MB BS Lond. 1981; DCH RCP Lond. 1984; DRCOG 1986; MRCGP 1987. Med. Dir. Brightdocc. Specialty: Paediat. Prev: SHO (O & G) Brighton HA; SHO (Paediat.) Westm. Hosp. Lond. & Brighton HA.

NALLIAH, Stanley Jeyaratnam 94 Croydon Road, London SE20 7AB — MB BS Ceylon 1963.

NALLY, Rhiannon Elise Wansford Surgery and Kings Cliffe Practice, Yarwell Road, Wansford, Peterborough PE8 6PL Tel: 01780 782342 Fax: 01780 783434; 9 Wansford Road, Elton, Peterborough PE8 6RZ Tel: 01832 280361 — MB BCh Wales 1988 (Univ. Coll. Wales) DRCOG 1991; DCH RCP Lond. 1992; MRCGP 1993. Specialty: Gen. Pract. Prev: Trainee GP St. Mary's Med. Centre; SHO (Psychiat. & Paediat.) P'boro. Dist. Hosp.; SHO (ENT) UHW Heath Pk. Cardiff Hosp.

NAM, Sidney 68 Cathedral Road, Cardiff CF11 9LL Tel: 029 2038 8377 Fax: 029 2034 4033 — MB BCh Wales 1960; DPM Eng. 1965; MRCPsych 1972. Specialty: Forens. Psychiat. Socs: Welsh Psychiat. Soc.; Rhondda Med. Soc. Prev: Self Employed Medico-Legal Psychiat.; Cons. Psychiat. Mid Glam. HA; Resid. Clin. Path. St. Mary's Hosps. Manch.

NAMASIVAYAM, Kumutha Horsham Community Mental Health Farm, Horsham Hospital, Hurst Road, Horsham RH12 2DR; 3 Quantock Drive, Worcester Park KT4 8JN Tel: 0208 337 7555 — MB BS Sri Lanka 1977; LMSSA Lond. 1991. Specialty: Gen. Psychiat.; Alcohol & Substance Misuse.

NAMASIVAYAM, Sivakumar Macclesfield District General Hospital, Victoria Road, Macclesfield, Macclesfield SK10 3BL Tel: 01625 661244; 25 Manor Close, Buckden, St Neots, Huntingdon PE19 5XR — BChir Camb., MA 1989 1987 (Univ. of Camb.) FRCS Eng. 1992; ChM Leeds 1999; FRCS (Urol.) 1999. Cons. Urological Surg., Macclesfield Dist. Gen. Hosp.; Surgic. Coll. Tutor, Macclesfield Dist. Gen. Hosp. Specialty: Urol. Special Interest: Female Urol.; Incontinense. Socs: Brit. Assn. Urological Surg.; Roy. Coll. of Surg. of Eng.; Europ. Assn. of Urol. Prev: Specialist Regist. Urol., St James Univ. Hosp., Leeds.

NAMBIAR, Suresh Chandroth The Health Centre, Welbeck Street, Castleford WF10 1DP Tel: 01977 465777 Fax: 01977 519342; 51 Shelley Crescent, Oulton, Leeds LS26 8ER — MB BS Kerala 1977; BSc Kerala 1970; LRCP LRCS Ed. LRCPS Glas. 1987; MRCP (UK) 1990. GP Princip., W. Yorks. Specialty: Gen. Pract. Socs: Roy. Coll. Phys. Prev: Trainee GP Manch.; Clin. Asst. (Rheum.) W. Yorks.

NAMBISAN, Lakshmanan Sumathy Chapel Street Surgery, 1 Chapel Street, Pelsall, Walsall WS3 4LN Tel: 01922 685858 Fax: 01922 694763 — MB BS Madras 1969.

NAMDARAN, Mr Farshid (retired) 2/6 Craufurdland, Braepark Road, Edinburgh EH4 6DL Tel: 0131 317 8283 — MB ChB Glas. 1964 (Glasgow University) FRCS Ed. 1968; MSc Ed. 1983; MFCM RCP (UK) 1985. Prev: Asst. Prof. Shiraz Univ. Iran.

NAMJOSHI, Suhas Hillingdon Hospital, X-Ray Department, Field Heath Road, Uxbridge UB8 3NN Email: sunamjoshi@hotmail.com — MB BS Bombay 1974. Locum Cons. (Radiol.) Hillingdon Hosp. Uxbridge.

NAMMEN, Mr Kim Jacob — MB BS Kerala 1980. Cons. (Urol.) Sunderland Roy. Hosp. Sunderland. Specialty: Urol.

NAMNYAK, Simon Sandett Department of Medical Microbiology, Harold Wood Hospital, Gubbins Lane, Romford RM3 0BE Tel: 01708 345533 Fax: 01708 381486; 30 Sunbury Avenue, Mill Hill, London NW7 3SJ Tel: 020 8906 8493 Fax: 020 8906 8493 Email:

100142.744@compuserve.com — MD Dar-es-Salaam, Tanzania 1975 (Univ. Dar-es-Salaam, Tanzania) PhD Lond. 1981; FRCPath 1994, M 1983; T(Path) 1991. Cons.Infec. control doctor. Microbiol. Havering Hosps. NHS Trust Romford Essex. Specialty: Med. Microbiol. Socs: Assn. Clin. Path.; Assn. Med. Microbiol.; Hosp. Infec. Soc. Prev: Cons. Med. Microbiol. Altnagelvin Area Hosp. Londonderry; Cons. Med. Microbiol. Regional Laborat. & Blood Bank, Saudi Arabia; Regist. (Med. Microbiol.) St Stephen's Hosp. Lond.

NANA, Ahmed 32 New Way Road, Leicester LE5 5UA — MB ChB Birm. 1994; MRCP (UK); DCH.

NANABAWA, Hashim Ismail (branch Surgery) The Mount, 60 High Road, Earlsheaton, Dewsbury WF13 4HR Tel: 01924 465511; Hyrst House, 8 Track Road, Batley WF17 7AA — MB BS Baroda 1960 (Med. Coll. Baroda) DLO Baroda 1962.

NANAVATI, B T John Amery Drive Surgery, 14 John Amery Drive, Rising Brook, Stafford ST17 9LZ Tel: 01785 252244 — MB BS Gujarat 1971; MB BS Gujarat 1971.

NANAVATI, Bharatkumar Anant Ailsa Craig Medical Group, 270 Dickenson Road, Longsight, Manchester M13 0YL Tel: 0161 224 5555 Fax: 0161 248 9112; 60 Hilltop Ave, Cheadle Hulme, Cheadle SK8 7HY Tel: 0161 486 1804 Fax: 0161 486 1804 — MB ChB Manch. 1980; DRCOG 1983; MRCGP 1984; Dip. Occ. Med. 1998. Clin. Asst. Pheum. - Univ. Hosp. S. Manch.; Hosp. Practitioner Univ. Hosp. S. Manch.

NANAVATI, C B John Amery Drive Surgery, 14 John Amery Drive, Rising Brook, Stafford ST17 9LZ Tel: 01785 252244 — MB BS Indore 1973; MB BS Indore 1973.

NANAVATI, Mayur Kumar Glendale Medical Centre, 155 High Street, Harlington, Hayes UB3 5DA Tel: 020 8897 8288 Fax: 020 8754 1539 — MB ChB Manch. 1983 (Manchester) DA 1985; MRCGP 1989. GP Princip.; Clin. Asst. (Anaesth.) Hillingdon Hosp. Specialty: Anaesth.

NANAVATI, Nayan Arvindbhai Galleries Health Centre, Washington Centre, Washington NE38 7NQ Tel: 0191 419 0333 Fax: 0191 419 0444 — MB BS Gujarat 1971 (B.J. Med. Coll. Ahmedabad)

NANAYAKKARA, Charithananda Surasena Paediat. Directorate, Kettering General Hospital, Rothwell Road, Kettering NN16 8UZ Tel: 01536 492112 Email: charith.nanayakkara@kgh.nhs.uk — MB BS Ceylon 1965 (Fac. Med. Colombo (Univ. Ceylon)) DCH RCP Lond.; MRCP (UK) 1980; T(M) 1991; FRCP Lond. 1994; FRCPCH 1997. Cons. Paediat. Kettering Gen. Hosp. N.ants. Specialty: Paediat.; Neonat. Special Interest: Chronic Neonatology. Socs: MDU; Brit. Med. Assn. Prev: Cons. Paediat. Grantham & Kesteven Hosps.; Sen. Regist. (Paediat.) Radcliffe Infirm. Oxf.

NANAYAKKARA, Gamini (retired) 4 Elliswick Road, Harpenden AL5 4TP — MB BS Ceylon 1963 (Colombo) MB BS (2nd Cl. Hons.) Ceylon 1963; DPM Eng. 1975; MRCPsych 1977. Gen. Hosp. Hemel Hempstead. Prev: Cons. Psychiat. Ment. Illness Hill End Hosp. St. Albans & W. Herts Gen. Hosp. Hemel Hempstead.

NANCARROW, Mr Jeffrey Douglas Department of Plastic Surgery, Selly Oak Hospital, Raddlebarn Road, Selly Oak, Birmingham B29 6JD Tel: 0121 627 8197 — MRCS Eng. LRCP Lond. 1969 (St. Thos.) BSc (Anat.) Lond. 1966, MB BS 1969; FRCS Eng. 1975. Cons. Plastic Surg. Selly Oak Hosp., Birm.; Cons. Plastic & Reconstruc. Surg., Qu.s Hosp., Burton NHS Trust Burton-on-Trent, Staffs. Specialty: Plastic Surg. Special Interest: Dupoytren's Disease. Socs: Brit. Assn. Plastic Surg.; Brit. Soc. Surg. Hand.; Brit. Med. Assn. Prev: Cons. Plastic & Reconstruc. Surg. W. Midl. Regional Plastic Surg. Unit, Wordsley Hosp., Stourbridge.

NANCARROW, Jenny Georgina Ground Floor Flat, 33 Wrentham Avenue, London NW10 3HS — MB ChB Birm. 1992; DRCOG 1996; MRCGP 1997.

NANCARROW, Julie Accident and Emergency, Warwick HoSPITAL, Lakin Rd, Warwick CV34 5BW Tel: 01926 495321; Rowans, Longworth Road, Billington, Clitheroe BB7 9TS — MB ChB Manch. 1986; MRCGP 1990; DRCOG 1990; FRCS Ed. 1994; DA 1994; Dip. IMC RCS Ed. 1995. Cons. (A & E) Warwick Hosp. Specialty: Accid. & Emerg. Socs: FFAEM. Prev: Sen. Regist. (A & E) N. W. Region; Cons. (A & E) Blackburn Roy. Infirm.

NANCEKIEVILL, David Guy 50 Ormonde Terrace, Regents Park, London NW8 7LR Tel: 020 7586 5685 Fax: 020 7586 5685; Cintra, Marley Lane, Haslemere GU27 3RG — MB BS Lond. 1964 (Guy's) MRCS Eng. LRCP Lond. 1964; DA Eng. 1966; FFA RCS Eng. 1967. Cons. Anaesth. Harley St. Lond. Specialty: Anaesth. Socs: Assn. of Amaesthetists; Assn. of Dent. Anaesth.s; Dent. Soc. of Lond. Prev: Dir. (Anaesth. Servs.), Cons. Anaesth. & Sen. Cons. ITU St. Bart. Hosp. Lond.; Sen. Regist. & Resid. Anaesth. Guy's Hosp.; Regist. (Anaesth.) Guy's Hosp., St. Bart. Hosp. & Roy. North. Hosp. Lond.

NANCEKIEVILL, Leslie (retired) Gibbs Corner, Oak Hill, East Budleigh, Budleigh Salterton EX9 7DW Tel: 01395 442101 — MB BS Lond. 1939 (Guy's) MRCS Eng. LRCP Lond. 1938; FRCP Lond. 1969, M 1946; MD Lond. 1947. Prev: Sen. Regist. (Med.) United Sheff. Hosps.

NANCEKIEVILL, Martin Leslie Fairacre, Fairfield Road, Shawford, Winchester SO21 2DA Tel: 01962 714320 Fax: 01962 714264 — MB BS Lond. 1972 (Guy's) MRCS Eng. LRCP Lond. 1972; DA Eng. 1974; FFA RCS Eng. 1977. Cons. Anaesth. Winchester Health Dist. Specialty: Anaesth.; Intens. Care. Socs: Assn. Anaesths. Gt. Brit. & Irel.; BMA. Prev: Sen. Regist. (Anaesth.) Winchester & Soton. Health Dist. Regist.; (Anaesth.) Guy's Hosp. Lond. & Brighton Health Dist.; Resid. Anaesth. Guy's Hosp. Lond.

NANCHAHAL, Mr Jagdeep Department of Plastic Surgery, Charing Cross Hospital, Fulham Palace Road, London W6 8RF Tel: 020 8846 1790 Fax: 020 8846 1719 — MB BS Lond. 1985; PhD Lond. 1982, BSc 1980; FRCS Ed. 1989; FRCS Eng. 1989; FRCS (Plast) 1996. Sen. Lect. And Hon. Cons. (Plastic Surg.) Char. Cross Hosp. Lond. & Chelsea & W.minister Hosp. Specialty: Plastic Surg.

NANCOLLAS, Christopher Edward Yorkley Health Centre, Bailey Hill, Yorkley, Lydney GL15 4RS Tel: 01594 562437 — MB BS Lond. 1978; FFA RCSI 1984. Specialty: Anaesth.

NANDA, Deepak 51 Ash Grove, Heston, Hounslow TW5 9DU — MB BS Lond. 1987.

NANDA, Mr Kalyan Kumar (retired) Burton Hospital NHS Trust, Department of Radiology, Burton-on-Trent Tel: 01283 66333 — MB BS Calcutta 1968 (Med. Coll. Calcutta) MS Delhi 1972; FRCS Ed. 1976; FRCR 1986. Cons. Radiol. Burton Hosp. NHS Trust. Prev: Regist. (Diag. Radiol.) W. Midl. RHA.

NANDA, Nibedita Rickleton Medical Centre, Vigo Lane, Rickleton, Washington NE38 9EH Tel: 0191 415 0576 — LRCP LRCS Ed. LRCPS Glas. 1982; MB BS Utkal 1979.

NANDA, Umesh Chandra Rickleton Medical Centre, Vigo Lane, Rickleton, Washington NE38 9EJ Tel: 0191 415 0576 — MB BS Utkal 1973.

NANDADEVA, Mr Pinnawalalage Gedara 562 Green Lanes, London N13 5SA — MB BS Ceylon 1967; FRCS Eng. 1976.

NANDAKUMAR, Calathur Ganapathy Huddersfield Royal Infirmary , Department of Anaesthesia, Acre Street, Lindley, Huddersfield HD3 3EA Tel: 01484 342549 Fax: 01484 347107 Email: cnandu@doctors.org.uk — MB BS Madras 1979; DA; FRCA; FFA RCSI 1992. Consultan Anaesth., Hudderfield Roy. Infirm.; lead Clinician, ICU, Huddersfield Roy. Infirm. Specialty: Anaesth.; Intens. Care. Socs: SCATA; HCSA; SEAUK. Prev: Coll. Tutor, Huddersfield Roy. Infirm.

NANDAKUMAR, Elamana Department of Diagnostic Radiology, Blackburn Royal Infirmary, Bolton Road, Blackburn BB2 3LR Tel: 01254 63555; 95 Rogersfield, Langho, Blackburn BB6 8HD Tel: 01254 240767 — MD Madras 1982; MB BS Kerala 1978; FRCR 1986. Cons. Radiol. Blackburn Roy. Infirm.; Hon. Clin. Lect. in Radiol. Univ. of Manch. Specialty: Radiol. Prev: Sen. Regist. (Radiol.) Withington Hosp. Manch.; Regist. (Radiol.) Manch. Gp. Hosps.

NANDAKUMAR, Kalyana Naidu Department of Anaesthesia, Kingston Hospital, Galsworthy Road, Kingston upon Thames KT2 7QB — MB BS Madras 1980; FFA RCSI 1989.

NANDAKUMAR, Komath Marshall's Road Surgery, 7 Marshall's Road, Raunds, Wellingborough NN9 6ET Tel: 01933 622349 Fax: 01933 625421 — MB BS Mysore 1972 (Kasturba Med. Coll.) DA Eng. 1979. Regist. (Anaesth.) Kettering Dist. Gen. Hosp. Specialty: Anaesth. Prev: SHO (Anaesth.) St. Chas. Hosp. Lond.; SHO & Regist. (Anaesth.) Kettering & Dist. Gen. Hosp.

NANDANWAR, Chetana 34 Princes Way, London SW19 6QP — MB ChB Manch. 1976; DA 1980; FFA RCS 1982. Specialty: Anaesth.

NANDAPALAN, Mr Velanthapillai 6 Pinnington Road, Whiston, Prescot L35 3TY — MRCS Eng. LRCP Lond. 1986; FRCS Ed. 1992.

NANDASOMA, Udvitha Charatha 23 Worcester Road, Lodge Moor, Sheffield S10 4JH — BChir Camb. 1996.

NANDHA, Rakesh Kumar 84 Earles Meadow, Roffey, Horsham RH12 4HR Tel: 01403 241549 — MB ChB Leeds 1985; DRCOG 1990; DGM RCP Lond. 1990; Cert. Family Plann. JCC 1990; MRCGP 1991; DA 1991. Trainee GP Northallerton VTS. Prev: SHO (Anaesth.) Darlington Memor. Hosp.

NANDHABALAN, Kanagasingham Preston Road Surgery, 56 Preston Road, Wembley HA9 8LB — MB BS Sri Lanka 1972; DLO RCS Eng. 1981; LRCP LRCS Ed. LRCPS Glas. 1983.

NANDI, Ann Christine Surrey & Sussex Healthcare Trust, Crawley Hospital, Department of Haematology, West Green Drive, Crawley RH11 7DH Tel: 01293 600300 Fax: 01293 525716 Email: ac.nandi@doctors.org.uk — MB BS Lond. 1979 (University College London) MRCP (UK) 1982; MRCPath 1987; FRCPath 1997; FRCP 1998. Cons. Haemat. Crawley Hosp. Specialty: Haematology. Prev: Sen. Regist. (Haemat.) Roy. Marsden Hosp. Sutton & St. Geo. Hosp. Tooting.

NANDI, Bipul Chandra Dr B C Nandi Surgery, 93 The Ridgeway, Chingford, London E4 6QW Tel: 020 8529 6479 Fax: 020 8523 7341 — MB BS Calcutta 1972.

NANDI, Debal K Tower Hill Medical Centre, 25 Tower Hill, Great Barr, Birmingham B42 1LG Tel: 0121 357 1077 — MB BS Calcutta 1967; MB BS Calcutta 1967.

NANDI, Lisa Reema Sarah Neera Flat 4, 19 Shepherds Hill, London N6 5QJ — MB BS Lond. 1992.

NANDI, Paul Romen Department of Anaesthetics, National Hospital for Neurology & Neurosurgery, Queen Square, London WC1N 3BG Email: paul.nandi@uclh.org — MB BS Lond. 1977; MRCP (UK) 1982; FFA RCS Eng. 1986. Cons. Anaesth. Nat. Hosp. Neurol. & Neurosurg. Lond. Specialty: Anaesth. Prev: Sen. Regist. (Anaesth.) Bloomsbury HA.

NANDI, Runa 19 Bittacy Rise, London NW7 2HH — MB BS Lond. 1992.

NANDI, Santi Ranjan Wigan & Leigh Health Services NHS Trust, Wigan Infirmary, Wigan Lane, Wigan WN1 2NN Tel: 01942 822390 — MB BS Gauhati 1967; DCH Eng. 1970; MRCP (UK) 1977; FRCPS Glas. 1991; FRCP Lond. 1999. Cons. Phys. (Elderly Med.) Wigan Infirm. & Leigh Infirm. Lancs. Specialty: Care of the Elderly. Special Interest: heart Failure in the Elderly; Orthogeriatric; Stroke. Socs: Brit. Geriat. Soc.

NANDI, Mr Satyanarayan The Avenue Medical Centre, 149-153 Chanterlands Ave., Hull HU5 3JT Tel: 01482 3436 — MB BS Calcutta 1961 (N.R.S. Med. Coll. Calcutta) FRCS Ed. 1973. Socs: Hull Med. Soc.; BMA. Prev: Clin. Asst. (Gen. Surg.) Kingston Gen. Hosp. Hull; Clin. Asst. (Venereol.) Hull Roy. Infirm.; Regist. (Gen. Surg.) Hull Roy. Infirm.

NANDRA, Hardip Singh Saffron Manor, 35 Alderton Hill, Loughton, Ilford IG10 3JD — MB ChB Glas. 1985; MRCGP 1989; DRCOG 1989; DFFP 1996; MBA Univ. Keele 1996. Vice Chair N. E. Lond. Strategic Health Auth. Socs: Appeals Tribunal Service; Commission of Health Improvement. Prev: GP Auckland, NZ; GP Ilford; Trainee GP/SHO Newham Hosp. Lond. VTS.

NANDRA, Kanwalpal Singh Bulbanks Medical Centre, 62 Battle Road, Erith DA8 1BJ Tel: 01322 432997 Fax: 01322 442324 — MB BS Bihar 1981.

NANDWANI, Naresh 35 Ravenswood Road, Bristol BS6 6BW — BM BS Nottm. 1988.

NANDWANI, Rak Department of Genitourinary Medicine, The Sandyford Iniative, 6 Sandyford Place, Glasgow G3 7NB Tel: 0141 211 8608/0141 211 8610 Fax: 0141 211 8609 Email: Rak.Nandwani@glacomen.scot.nhs.uk — MB BS Lond. 1985 (Middlx. Hosp.) FRCP Glas.; MRCP (UK) 1991; DFFP 1993. Assoc. Director, The Sandyford Initiative, Greater Glas. Primary Care NHS Trust; Hon. Clin. Sen. Lect. Univ. Glas. Specialty: Genitourinary Medicine; HIV Med. Socs: Med. Soc. Study VD Fell.; Med Soc Stud VD Counc. Mem.; Med Soc Stud VD Scott. Br. Sec. Prev: Cons. HIV & Genitourin. Med. Glas. Roy. Infirm.; Regist. (HIV Med.) St. Stephens Clinic & Chelsea & Westm. Hosp. Lond.; Sen. Regist. (HIV & Genitourin Med.) King's Coll. Hosp. Lond. & Roy. Sussex Co. Hosp. Brighton.

NANDY, Anita Margaret 4 St Johns Close, Welwyn AL6 9RB — BM BS Nottm. 1993.

NANDY, Debanjan 10 Steping Stone, Highfield, Goytre, Usk NP5 0RP — MB BS Dacca 1970.

NANDY, Diptish C The Clinic, Muirkirk, Cumnock KA18 3RQ.

NANDY, Mihir Kanti Doctor's Residence, Hexham General Hospital, Hexham NE46 1QJ — MB BS Dacca 1963. Assoc. Specialist Spinal Injuries Unit Hexham Gen. Hosp. Prev: SHO (Orthop. Surg.) Sanderson (W.J.) Orthop. Hosp. Gosforth; SHO (Orthop. Surg.) St. Hilda's Hosp. Hartlepool; SHO (Orthop. Surg.) Peel Hosp. Galashiels.

NANDY, Sudip Kumar Island Health, 145 East Ferry Road, London E14 3BQ Tel: 020 7363 1111 Fax: 020 7363 1112 — MB BS Lond. 1991 (Lond. Hosp.) DCH RCP Lond. 1994; Dip. Obst. Auckland 1994; MRCGP 1996.

NANGALIA, Mr Ramlal 215 Hinckley Road, Nuneaton CV11 6LL — MB BS Utkal 1972; MS Utkal 1977; FRCS Ed. 1980.

NANJIANI, Mr Magsoodali (retired) Ross Hall Hospital, Crookston Road, Glasgow G52 3NQ Tel: 0141 810 3151; 24 Dunobin Avenue, Elderslie, Johnstone PA5 9NW Tel: 01505 346038 — MB BS Punjab 1958 (King Edwd. Med. Coll. Lahore) MB BS Punjab (Pakistan) 1958; DO Eng. 1963; DOMS RCPSI 1964; FRCS Ed. 1972; FCOphth 1988. JP.; Cons. Ophth. Surg. Eye Dept. Roy. Ross Hall Hosp. Crookston Rd. Glas. Prev: Ho. Surg. St. Helen's Hosp. Hastings.

NANKANI, Angana Jay 6 Ffordd Ystrad, Wrexham LL13 7QQ — MB ChB Liverp. 1998; DTM & H Liverp. 1999.

NANKANI, Mr Jayprakash Navalram Hill Crest Medical Centre, 86 Holt Road, Wrexham LL13 8RG Tel: 01978 262193 Fax: 01978 310193 (Call before faxing); 6 Ffordd Ystrad, Coed-y-Glyn, Wrexham LL13 7QQ Tel: 01978 262893 Fax: 01978 262893 — MB BS Gujarat 1972; MS Gujarat 1976, MB BS 1972. Clin. Asst. (Orthop.) Maelor Gen. Hosp. Wrexham.

NANKHONYA, Joseph McLagen Stepping Hill Hospital, Poplar Grove, Stockport SK2 7JE Tel: 0161 483 1010 Fax: 0161 419 4356 Email: jnankhonya@aol.com — MB ChB Manch. 1981 (Manchester) BSc Malawi 1976; MRCP Irel. 1988; FRCP Irel. 1998. Cons. Phys. Gen. & Geriat. Med. Stepping Hill Hosp. Stockport; Cons. Phys. Consg. Suite Alexandra Hosp. Cheadle. Specialty: Gen. Med.; Care of the Elderly; Rehabil. Med. Special Interest: Acute Stroke/TIA; Hypertens. Socs: Fell. Roy. Soc. Med.; BMA; Brit. Geriat. Soc. Prev: Cons. Phys. Gen. & Geriat. Med. St Thomas Hosp. Stockport; Sen. Regist. (Gen. & Geriat. Med.) N. West. RHA; Regist. Rotat. (Med.) Liverp. & Wirral.

NANKIVELL, Muriel (retired) 77 Pereira Road, Birmingham B17 9JA — MB ChB Birm. 1957; DObst RCOG 1975. Med. Assessor Benefits Agency. Prev: GP Kingstanding.

NANSON, Eileen Margaret (retired) 71 Kingswood Road, Wimbledon, London SW19 3ND Tel: 020 8542 4004 — MB BCh Camb. 1962 (St. Bart.) Prev: Med. Advis. DSS Lond.

NANSON, Justine Katherine La Playa, Coast Road, St Clement, Jersey JE2 6SB — MB ChB Bristol 1990 (Univ. Bristol) DCH RCP Lond. 1995; FRCA 1996. Specialist Regist. (Anaesth.) Soton. Gen. Hosp. Specialty: Anaesth.

NANSON, Patricia 20 Mitchell Avenue, Jesmond, Newcastle upon Tyne NE2 3LA — MB BS Newc. 1977; DRCOG 1980; MRCGP 1981. GP DSS.

NANU KANDIYIL, Vaniya 5-7 Norcot Road, Tilehurst, Reading RG30 6BP — MRCOG Lond.; FRCOG Lond.; MB BS Kerala 1971. Specialty: Gynaecology.

NAOROSE-ABIDI, Syed Majid Central Middlesex Hospital, Park Royal, London NW10 7NS Mob: 07905 714029 — MB BS Lahore 1970; BSc Punjab 1968; MRCPath Lond. 1984; FRCPath Lond. 1995. Cons. Haematologist, Centr. Middlx. Hosp., Lond. Specialty: Haematology. Prev: Cons. Haematologist, Whipps Cross Univ. Hosp., Lond.

NAOUMOV, Nikolai Vesselinov Institute of Hepatology, University College London Medical School, 69-75 Chenies Mews, London WC1E 6HX Tel: 020 7388 2013 Fax: 020 7380 0405 Email: n.naoumov@ucl.ac.uk; 78 Lavenham Road, Southfields, London SW18 5HE Tel: 020 8870 6086 Fax: 020 8870 6086 — State Exam Med Sofia 1978; MD Med. Acad. Sofia 1985; DSc Med. Acad. Sofia 1991; MRCPath Lond. 1998. Sen. Lect. (Hepat.) Univ. Coll. Lond. Med. Sch.; Hon. Cons. Phys. UCL. Hosps. NHS Trust. Specialty: Gastroenterol.; Virology. Socs: BASL; EASL; AASLD.

NAOUMOVA, Rossitza Petkova MRC Molecular Medicine, MRC Clinical Sciences Centre, Hammersmith Hospital, Du Cane Road, London W12 0NN Tel: 0208 383 1346 Fax: 0208 383 2028 — State Exam Med Acad. Med. Sofia, Bulgaria 1978 (Sofia, Bulgaria)

Dip Metabol Dis State Exam Med. Academy Sofia, Bulgaria 1981; Dip Internal Med State Exam Bd Sofia, Bulgaria 1985; U.K 1998. MRC Clin. Scientist Lipid Clinic,Hammersmith Hosp. and Hon. Cons. Phys. In Molecular Med. Hammersmith Hosp. Lond. Specialty: Gen. Med. Socs: Comm. Mem. Brit. Hyperlipidaemia Assn.; Amer. Heart Assn.; Brit. Med. Soc.

NAPIER, Alex James — MB ChB Liverp. 1998.

NAPIER, Anne Christine 8 Woodhead Drive, Orpington BR6 9RD — MB ChB Aberd. 1968.

NAPIER, David Charles The Surgery, Marlborough, Seaham SR7 7TS Tel: 0191 581 2866 Fax: 0191 513 0393 — MB ChB Sheffield 1979; MB ChB Sheff 1979. GP Seaham, Co. Durh.

NAPIER, Donna Elizabeth The Crescent Medical Practice, 12 Walmer Crescent, Glasgow G51 1AT Tel: 0141 427 0191 Fax: 0141 427 1581; 38 Addison Road, Glasgow G12 0TT — MB ChB Glas. 1979. Specialty: Paediat. Neurol.

NAPIER, Elizabeth Susan 11 Polnoon Street, Eaglesham, Glasgow G76 0BH — MB ChB Ed. 1965; MB ChB Ed. 1965.

NAPIER, Eoin Dominic 13 St Patricks Road, Saul, Downpatrick BT30 7JG — MB BCh BAO Belf. 1995.

NAPIER, Hilary Barbara Bridge Cottage Surgery, 41 High Street, Welwyn AL6 9EF Tel: 01438 715044 Fax: 01438 714013 — MB BS Lond. 1981 (Univ. Coll. Hosp.) BSc (Psychol.) Lond. 1978; DRCOG 1983; MRCGP (Distinc.) 1986. Trainee GP Lond. Prev: SHO (Paediat.) & (O & G) Edgware Gen. Hosp.; Ho. Phys. (Cardiol.) Whittington Hosp. Lond.

NAPIER, Ian Gordon Donnybrook House Group Practice, Clarendon Street, Hyde SK14 2AH Tel: 0161 368 3838 Fax: 0161 368 2210; Rye Flatt, Combs, Chapel-en-le-Frith, High Peak SK23 9UY Tel: 01298 812844 — MB ChB Manch. 1970. GP Hyde; Clin. Asst. (Anaesth.) Tameside Gen. Hosp. Prev: SHO (Anaesth.) Manch. Roy. Infirm.; SHO (O & G) Crumpall Hosp.; GP Stockport.

NAPIER, Isabella Ross (retired) Rothmar, 43 South Avenue, Thornly Park, Paisley PA2 7SG Tel: 0141 884 3201 — MB ChB Ed. 1948; MRCOG 1958; DPH 1960. Prev: Cons. (Genitourin. Med.) Roy. Infirm. Glas.

NAPIER, Jacqueline Claire Schering Health Care Ltd, The Brow, Burgess Hill RH15 9NE — MB ChB Birm. 1987; BSc (Hons.) Birm. 1984; MB ChB Hons.) Birm. 1987; MRCP (UK) 1990; Dip. Pharm. Med. RCP (UK) 1992; MFPM RCP Lond. 1997; FFPM RCP London 2003. Med.Dir.Sp.Care, Schering Healthcare Ltd. W. Sussex. Specialty: Pharmaceutical Medicine. Prev: SHO (Gen. Med.) Sandwell Dist. Gen. Hosp.; Ho. Off. (Gen. Surg.) E. Birm. Hosp.; Ho. Off. (Gen. Med. & Neurol.) Qu. Eliz. Hosp. Birm.

NAPIER, James Alexander 86 Ennerdale Road, Richmond TW9 2DL — MB ChB Ed. 1993.

NAPIER, Jane Margaret 11 Polnoon Street, Eaglesham, Glasgow G76 0BH — MB ChB Ed. 1992.

NAPIER, Janet Elizabeth Manchester Road Surgery, 280 Manchester Road, Warrington WA1 3RB Tel: 01925 230022 Fax: 01925 575069; 80 Whitbarrow Road, Lymm WA13 9BA Tel: 01925 754825 — (St. Bart.) MB BS Lond. 1968; MRCS Eng. LRCP Lond. 1968; DObst RCOG 1970; DCH Eng. 1971; DMJ(Clin) Soc. Apoth. Lond. 1993. Principle FME Merseyside Police Surgeon Cheshire; Deputy Coroner Cheshire. Socs: BMA; Assn. Police Surg.; Jun. Sec. Sect. Clin. Forens. & Legal Med. Roy. Soc. Med. Prev: SHO (Obst.) Luton & Dunstable Hosp.; Ho. Phys. (Child Health) St. Bart. Hosp. Lond.; Ho. Surg. (Orthop.) St. Bart. Hosp. Lond.

NAPIER, John Anthony Francis (retired) Rhyd-Y-Gwern Farm, Lower Machen, Newport NP10 8GJ Tel: 01633 441194 Email: napier@which.net — MB BS Lond. 1964 (Char. Cross) BSc Lond. 1961, MB BS 1964; PhD Camb. 1972; FRCPath M 1972. Cons. Haematolog. Prev: Wellcome Research Fell. Dept. Pathol. Univ. Camb.

NAPIER, John Francis (retired) Alderslade, 125 Derby Road, Aston-on-Trent, Derby DE72 2AE Tel: 01332 792657 — LRCPI & LM, LRCSI & LM 1949. Vis. Gen. Pract. Aston Hall Hosp. Aston-on-Trent. Prev: Dep. Civil. Med. Off. RAF.

NAPIER, Mr John Gordon (retired) 68 Wragby Road, Lincoln LN2 4PH Tel: 01522 526083 — (Ed.) MB ChB Ed. 1940; FRCS Ed. 1948; FRCOG 1964, M 1950. Prev: Cons. O & G Lincoln Co. Hosp.

NAPIER, Karen Claire The Redcliffe Surgery, 10 Redcliffe Street, London SW10 9DT Tel: 020 7460 2222 Fax: 020 7460 0116 — MB BChir Camb. 1988; MRCGP 1992.

NAPIER, Mark Peter Royal Devon & Exeter Hospital, Exeter Oncology Centre, Barrack Rd, Exeter EX2 5DW Tel: 01392 402825 Fax: 01392 402713 Email: mark.napier@rdehc-tr.swest.nhs.uk — MB BS Queensland 1985. Cons. (Med. Oncol.) Roy. Devon & Exeter Hosp. & N. Devon Dist. Hosp. Specialty: Oncol. Special Interest: Gastrointestinal Cancer; Sarcoma.

NAPIER, Noel Joseph 13 St Patricks Road, Downpatrick BT30 7JG — MB BCh BAO Belf. 1997.

NAPIER, Ramsay Brotchie (retired) 4 Sletts Park, Lerwick ZE1 0LN Tel: 01595 693716 — MB ChB Glas. 1960; DObst RCOG 1963.

NAPIER, Thomas George (retired) 11 Polnoon Street, Eaglesham, Glasgow G76 0BH — MB ChB St. And. 1960; MRCOG 1969; MRCGP 1978.

NAPIER-HEMY, Mr Richard Donald Department of Urology, Manchester Royal Infirmary, Oxford Road, Manchester M13 9WL Tel: 0161 276 4312 Fax: 0161 276 4221; 73 Higher Lane, Lymm WA13 0BZ Tel: 01925 753222 — MB ChB Manch. 1988 (Manchester) BSc (Med. Sci.) St. And. 1985; FRCS Ed. 1994; FRCS (Urol) 1998. Cons. (Urol.Surg.) Mans. Roy. Infrim. Specialty: Urol. Socs: Brit. Assn. Urol. Surg.; Brit. Soc. for Endocrinol. Prev: Specialist Regist. (Urol.) Manch. Roy. Infirm., Specialists Regist. (Urol.) Preston Roy. Hosp.; Regist. (Urol.) Hope Hosp. Salford Roy. Hosp., Specialists Regist. (Urol.) Withington. Hosp.; Regist. (Urol.) Stockport Acute Servs. NHS Trust.

NAPPER, Adrian John Drumhar Health Centre, North Methven Street, Perth PH1 5PD Tel: 01738 621726 — MB ChB Aberd. 1970; MRCGP 1976. GP Princip., Perth. Prev: SHO Tayside Health Bd.; SHO (Paediat.) Darlington Memor. Hosp.; Med. Off. Ch. of Scotl. Miss. Hosp. Qumbu, S. Africa.

NAPPER, Alexandra Mary Sophia Plenty House, Shipton Lane, Burton Bradstock, Bridport DT6 4NQ Tel: 01308 898259; Joseph Weld Hospice, Herringston Road, Dorchester DT1 2 — BM Soton. 1991; MRCGP 1995. Med. Off. Joseph Weld Hospice Dorchester. Specialty: Palliat. Med.

NAQESH-BANDI, Mr Hasan Abdulla University Hospital of Hartlepool, Holdforth Road, Hartlepool TS24 9AH; 26 Pinewood Close, Hartlepool TS27 3QU — MB ChB Baghdad 1969; FRCS Glas. 1980; FRCS Ed. 1981. Cons. Gen. Surg. (Surgic. Gastroenterol., Gastrointestinal Endoscopy & Lazerscopic Surg.), Univ. Hosp. of Hartlepool. Specialty: Gen. Surg.; Gastroenterol. Socs: Fell. Assn. Surgs.; Assn. Coloproctol.; N. Eng. Surgic. Soc.

NAQUI, Fatima Ahmed Parkside Surgery, 187 Northmoor Road, Longsight, Manchester M12 5RU Tel: 0161 257 3338 Fax: 0161 257 3338; 387 Wilbraham Road, Chorlton, Manchester M21 0UT Tel: 0161 881 3969 Fax: 0161 257 0205 — MB BS Punjab 1970 (Nishtar Med. Coll. Multan, Pakistan) MB BS (Hons.) Punjab 1970; MRCS Eng. LRCP Lond. 1979; DRCOG 1981; Cert. Prescribed Equiv. Exp. JCPTGP 1982. Socs: BMA; Fam. Plann. & Contracep. Assn.; Pakistan Med. Assn. Prev: Wom. Med. Off. Burewala, Multan; SHO (Geriat. & O & G) Tameside Gen. Hosp. Ashton-under-Lyne; SHO (O & G) Pk. Hosp. Davy Hulme.

NAQVI, Ahmad Tunveer Cromwell Medical Centre, 11-11A Cromwell Avenue, Cheshunt, Waltham Cross EN7 5DL Tel: 01992 624732 — MB BS Punjab 1970 (King Edwd. Med. Coll. Lahore) MB BS Punjab (Pakistan) 1970; DPH Eng. 1976. Socs: FRIPHH.

NAQVI, Nayyar Royal Albert Edward Infirmary, Wigan WN1 2NN Tel: 01942 44000 — MB BS Karachi 1968 (Dow Med. Coll. Karachi) MRCP (UK) 1975; FRCP Ed. 1986; FRCP Lond. 1995. Cons. Phys. & Cardiol. Roy. Albert Edwd. Infirm. Wigan. Specialty: Gen. Med. Socs: Fell. Europ. Soc. of Cardiol.; BMA & Mem. Brit. Cardiac Soc. Prev: Regist. Rotat. (Cardiothoracic Med.) Wythenshawe Hosp. Manch.; Kleinwort Research Fell. Dept. Cardiol. & Sen. Cardiac Research Fell.; (Hon. Sen. Regist.) St. Thos. Hosp. Lond.

NAQVI, Salma Batool 26 Chertsey Street, Tooting Broadway, London SW17 8LG — MB BS Karachi 1973.

NAQVI, Syed Mohammad Haider 54 Kilworth Drive, Lostock, Bolton BL6 4RL Tel: 01204 494931; 7 Manchester Road, Walkden, Worsley, Manchester M28 3NS Tel: 0161 790 3132 — MB BS Aligarh 1979; Dip. Orthop. Surg. Aligarh Muslim 1972; MB BS Aligarh Muslim 1979. Clin. Asst. (Orthop. Surg.) Bolton Roy. Infirm. Specialty: Accid. & Emerg. Prev: Regist. (Orthop. Surg.) Walton Hosp. Liverp.; Regist. (Accid. & Orthop.) Coventry & Warks. Hosp.; SHO (Geriat. Med.) Billinge Hosp.

NAQVI, Syed Mohammed Asim — MB BS Lond. 1996.
NAQVI, Syed Naseer Haider Chorley & South Ribble NHS Trust, Preston Road, Chorley PR7 1PP Tel: 01257 245286 Fax: 01257 245575 — MB BS Lucknow 1970; MD, India 1974; MRCP, UK 1977; FRCP, Glas. 1988; FRCP, Lond. 1990. Cons. Phys. in Med., Chorley Hosp., Lancs. Specialty: Gen. Med. Special Interest: Geriat. Socs: Med. Defence Union; BIDA; Pakistan Med. Soc.
NAQVI, Syed Nasim Hasan (retired) Heaton Grange Cottage, Heaton Grange Drive, Bolton BL1 5DA Tel: 01204 847111 — MB BS Punjab (Pakistan) 1962 (Nishtar Med. Coll. Multan) DA Eng. 1967; FRCA Eng. 1970. Prev: Cons. Anaesth. Bolton Roy. Infirm.
NARAD, Parveen Kumari 95 Himley Road, Dudley DY1 2QF — MB BS Lond. 1996.
NARAIN, Mr Bipin Garrick Hospital, Edinburgh Road, Stranraer DG9 7HQ Tel: 01776 702323 Fax: 01776 889102; 16 Abington Road, Dunfermline KY12 7XU Tel: 01383 621855 — State DMS Rome 1972; FRCS Ed. 1987; Dip. Urol. Lond 1992. Assoc. Specialist (Gen. Surg. & Urol.) Garrick Hosp. Stranraer. Specialty: Gen. Surg. Prev: Regist. (Gen. Surg.) W. Fife Hosp. Dunfermline.
NARAIN, Ishwar (retired) 1 Plas Elwy Orchard, The Roe, St Asaph LL17 0LT Tel: 01745 582048 — MB BS Calcutta 1956 (R.G. Kar Med. Coll.) DLO Eng. 1958. Prev: Regist (ENT) N. Staffs. Roy. Infirm. Stoke-on-Trent & Qu. Eliz. Hosp.Birm.
NARAIN, Mark Andrew Ceredigion & Mid Wales NHS Trust, Bronglais General Hospital, Aberystwyth SY23 1ER Tel: 01970 635981 Fax: 01970 635955 Email: mark.narain@ceredigion-tr.wales.nhs.uk — MB BS Lond. 1989 (St Mary's Lond.) MRCP (UK) 1994. Cons. Phys. & Gastroenterologist, Bronglais Gen. Hospita, Aberystwyth. Specialty: Gastroenterol.; Gen. Med. Prev: Specialist Regist. Gen. Med. & Gastroenterol., W. Midl.s Rotat.
NARAN, Kishore B Whitley Villa Surgery, 1 Christchurch Road, Reading RG2 7AB Tel: 0118 987 1645 Fax: 0118 931 4046 Email: kbnaran@doctors.org.uk; Cedar Lodge, Elm Lane, Reading RG6 5UH Tel: 0118 987 6084 — MB ChB Birmingham 1974; MRCP (UK) 1982; MRCGP (UK) 1985. Princip. in Gen. Pract., Reading; Hosp. Practitioner, Genitourin. Med., Roy. Berks. Hosp., Reading. Specialty: Gen. Pract. Socs: Reading Path. Soc. - Exec. Comm. Mem.
NARANG, Indra 15 Africa Gardens, Cardiff CF14 3BT Tel: 029 2061 3874 — MB BCh Wales 1993; BMedSci Cardiff 1993. SHO (Paediat.) Univ. Hosp. Wales, Cardiff. Specialty: Paediat. Prev: SHO (A & E) Cardiff; Ho. Off. (Gen. Med.) Cardiff; Ho. Off. (Paediat. Surg.) Edin.
NARANG, Mr Kush Kumar 16 Woodcote Lodge, 32 Woodcote Green Road, Epsom KT1S 7DW Tel: 01372 735735 Email: kushnarang@aol.com; 138 Edge Hill, Darras Hall Est., Ponteland, Newcastle upon Tyne NE20 9JL Tel: 01661 872603 — MB BS Delhi 1982 (Maulania Azad Med. Coll. N Delhi India) MS Delhi 1985; FRCS Eng. 1990; FRCS Glas. 1990; FRCS Ed. 1990; FRCS (Tr. & Orth.) 1999. Assoc. Specialist Worthing & Southlands Hosp. NHS Trust Worthing; Specialist Regist. SW Thames Region Rot. St Geo. Hosp. Specialty: Orthop. Socs: BMA. Prev: Staff Grade (Orthop.) Worthing & Southlands Hosp. Shoreham-by-Sea; Regist. (Orthop.) W. Hill Dartford; Regist. Rotat. (Orthop.) W. Midl.
NARANG, Radhe Sham 3 Lilian Board Way, Greenford UB6 0SA — MB BS Madras 1951 (Madras Med. Coll.) FFA RCS Eng. 1972. Cons. Anaesth. Roy. Albert Edwd. Infirm. Wigan. Specialty: Anaesth.
NARANG, Satish Kumar Aberbeeg Medical Centre, The Square, Aberbeeg, Abertillery NP13 2AB Tel: 01495 320520 Fax: 01495 320084 — MB BS Lucknow 1974.
NARANG, Satwant Kaur 30 Moorhead Lane, Shipley BD18 4JW — MB ChB Manch. 1995.
NARANG, Verinder Pal Singh 22 Northleigh, Bradford-on-Avon BA15 2RG — MB BS Lond. 1980 (Char. Cross) FFA RCS Eng. 1985. Regist. (Anaesth.) Soton Gen. Hosp. Specialty: Anaesth.
NARAVI, Maya Krishnanand 154 Lower Fairmead Road, Yeovil BA21 5SS Tel: 01935 427452 — BM Soton. 1993 (Southampton) MRCPI 1997. Specialist Regist. (A & E) N. Staffs. Roy. Infirm. Stoke on Trent; SHO (A & E) City Hosp. Dudley Rd. Birm.; SHO (Med.) Wolverhampton New Cross Hosp. Wolverhampton. Specialty: Accid. & Emerg. Socs: Assoc. Mem. BAEM; BMA; MPS. Prev: SHO (A & E) Birm. Heartlands Hosp. Birm.
NARAYAN, Mr Badri Singh The Old Mill Surgery, 22 Speedwell Road, Edgbaston, Birmingham B5 7QA Tel: 0121 440 4215 Fax: 0121 446 4302 — (Rajendra Med. Coll. Ranchi) MB BS Ranchi 1967; FRCS Glas. 1976. Specialty: Dermat.; Gen. Surg. Socs: BMA; ODA.
NARAYAN, Harini Department of Obstetrics & Gynaecology, Princess Margaret Hospital, Okus Road, Swindon SN1 4JU Tel: 01793 604937 Email: harini.narayan@virgin.net — MB BS Bangalore 1980; DGO Mangalore 1983; MRCOG 1989; FRCOG 2002. Cons. (O & G) The Grat West. Hosp. Marlborough Rd., Swindon SN3 6BB. Specialty: Obst. & Gyn. Socs: Roy. Coll. Obst. & Gyn. Prev: Sen. Lect. Univ. Leic.; Sen. Regist./Lect. Univ. Leic.
NARAYAN, Mrs Kamalini (retired) c/o Lloyds Bank Ltd., Bromley BR1 1LJ; 9 West Drive, Heathfield Park, Handsworth, Birmingham B20 3ST Tel: 0121 554 0018 — (Lucknow University India) BSc Lucknow 1947; MB BS Lucknow 1952; DObst RCOG 1956; DCH Eng. 1961. Prev: GP Birm.
NARAYAN, Prakash (retired) 9 West Drive, Heathfield Park, Handsworth, Birmingham B20 3ST Fax: 0121 554 0018 — MB BS Lucknow 1951; DTM & H Liverp. 1960. Prev: GP Birm.
NARAYAN, Prasanna Lakshmi 238 Birmingham Road, Wylde Green, Sutton Coldfield B72 1DH — MB ChB Birm. 1996; ChB Birm. 1996.
NARAYAN, Ramnath Eldon Square Surgery, 9 Eldon Square, Reading RG1 4DP Tel: 0118 957 4891 — MB BS Poona 1971; MB BS Poona 1971.
NARAYAN, Ravindra D Porth Farm Surgery, Porth Street, Porth CF39 9RR Tel: 01443 682579 Fax: 01443 683667 — (Darbhanga Medical College, Bihar, India) MB BS; BSc.
NARAYAN, Shalini 91 Lascelles Drive, Pontprennav, Cardiff CF23 8NZ Tel: 01222 541093 — MB BCh Wales 1993 (University of Wales College of Medicine) MRCP. SHO (Dermat.) Glas. Roy. Infirm. Specialty: Dermat. Socs: BMA; Med. Sickness Soc.; MDU. Prev: SHO (Med. Oncol.) Derby City Gen. Hosp.; SHO (Renal Med.) Derby City Gen. Hosp.; SHO (Respirat. Med.) Derby City Gen. Hosp.
NARAYAN, Vishwa Department of Paediatrics, Withybush Hospital, Haverfordwest SA61 2PZ Tel: 01437 764545 Fax: 01437 773579 Email: vnarayan25@hotmail.com — MB BS India 1986; DCH 1988; MD 1991; MRCP UK 1995. Cons. Paediat. Specialty: Respirat. Med.
NARAYANA, Venkataswamy Thursby Surgery, 2 Browhead Road, Burnley BB10 3BF Tel: 01282 422447 Fax: 01282 832575 — MB BS Bangalor 1971 (Bangalore Med. Coll.) MB BS Bangalore 1971. GP Burnley; Clin. Asst. (Rheum.) Burnley Gen. Hosp. Prev: Regist. (Med.) Burnley Gen. Hosp.; SHO (Gen. Med.) Vict. Hosp. Burnley.
NARAYANAN, Anushree Noorsaloman Department of Elderly Medicine, Northern General Hospital N H S Trust, Herries Rd, Sheffield S5 7AU; 32A Parkers Lane, Sheffield S10 1BR — MB ChB Sheff. 1997.
NARAYANAN, Gopalan Medicines & Healthcare Products, Regulatory Agency, London SW8 5NQ — MD Madras 1982; MB BS 1978; MRCP (UK) 1984. Med. Assessor Regulatory Agency Lond. Specialty: Gen. Med. Prev: Sen. Regist. Armed Forces Hosp. Riyadh, Saudi Arabia; Research Regist. Univ. Hosp. Wales Cardiff.
NARAYANAN, Mrs Janaki (retired) 1 St Margaret's Avenue, Leeds LS8 1RY Tel: 0113 686979 — MB BS Madras 1945; DPH Newc. 1966; MFCM 1974. Prev: SCM (Child Health) Sunderland AHA.
NARAYANAN, Mekkali Narayanan Department of Haematology, George Eliot Hospital, College Street, Nuneaton CV10 7DJ Tel: 024 7635 1351 Email: mekkali.narayanan@geh-tr.wmids.nhs.uk; 15 Poppyfield Court, Gibbet Hill, Coventry CV4 7HW Tel: 024 7669 7217 — MB BS Calicut 1978; MD Chandigarh 1982; MRCP (UK) 1985; FRCPath (Haemat.) 1997, M 1988; FRCP 1999. Cons. Haemat. Geo. Eliot Hosp. Nuneaton; Cons. Haematologist, Walsgrave Hosp., coventry. Specialty: Haematology. Socs: Brit. Soc. Haematol. Prev: Sen. Regist. (Haemat.) N. West. RHA; Tutor (Clin. Haemat.) Univ. Manch. & Manch. Roy. Infirm.
NARAYANAN, Seetha Flat B, 153 Southgate Road, London N1 3LE Tel: 020 7359 2744 Email: nseetha@aol.com — MB ChB Liverp. 1983; DCH RCP Lond. 1989; DTCH Liverp. 1990; MRCP (UK) 1990; FRCPCH 1997. Cons. - Community Paediat. Tower Hamlets Healthcare Trust Lond. Specialty: Community Child Health.
NARAYANAN, Shanmuganathan 67 Prince of Wales Drive, Ipswich IP2 9BP Tel: 01473 275306 — MB BS Malaya 1987; MRCP (UK) 1996. Specialist Regist. (Com. Paed) Loc. Heath Partn'shp, NHS Trust, Ipswich. Specialty: Paediat. Socs: BMA. Prev:

Locum Lect. Dept. of Paediat. Camb. Uni.; Sen. SHO, Princess Margeret Hosp. Swind.

NARAYNSINGH, Priya Aan 95 Fawnbrake Avenue, London SE24 0BG — MB BS West Indies 1987.

NARBOROUGH, Geoffrey Charles The Hawthorne, Cumberhills Road, Duffield, Belper DE56 4HA — MB ChB Manch. 1980; MRCP (UK) 1983; FRCR 1989. Cons. Radiol. Derbysh. Roy. Infirm. Specialty: Radiol. Prev: Sen. Regist. (Radiol.) Nottm.

NAREN, Mudigonda 28 Compton Hill Drive, Wolverhampton WV3 9DL — MB BS Osmania 1972; MRCPsych 1985.

NARENDRAN, Partheepan 110 Deans Lane, Edgware HA8 9NR — MB BS Lond. 1992; BSc (Basic Med. Sci. & Immunol.) Lond. 1989; MRCP (UK) 1995. Clin. Research Fell. Univ. of Bristol. Specialty: Endocrinol.; Diabetes; Immunol. Socs: Brit. Soc. Endocrinol.; Brit. Soc. Immunol.; Brit. Diabetic Assn. Prev: Med. Regist. Weston Gen. Hosp.; Med. SHO N. Manch. Gen. Hosp.

NARGOLWALA, Mr Viraf Sohrabji Newcastle Clinic, 4 Towers Avenue, Jesmond, Newcastle upon Tyne NE2 3QE Tel: 0191 281 2636 Fax: 0191 239 9922; Coppertop, 16 Holburn Gardens, Ryton NE40 3DZ Tel: 0191 413 2103 — (Osmania Med. Coll. Hyderabad) MB BS Osmania 1958; FRCS Eng. 1963; FRCS Ed. 1963. Hon. Cons. Orthop. Surg. NW Durh. Health Dist.; Spinal Surg. Washington Hosp. Tyne & Wear; Cons. Orthop. Surg. Newc. Nuffield Hosp. Specialty: Orthop.; Trauma & Orthop. Surg. Socs: Fell. BOA. Prev: Sen. Regist. Roy. Vict. Infirm. Newc.

NARGUND, Mrs Geeta Vinod — MB BS Karnatak 1983. Specialty: Obst. & Gyn.

NARGUND, Mr Vinod Hanamantrao Department of Urology, St Bartholomews Hospital, West Smithfield, London EC1A 7BE Tel: 020 7601 8394 Fax: 020 7601 7844 Email: vinod.nargund@bartsandthelondon.nhs.uk; 38 Ash Grove, Headington, Oxford OX3 9JL Tel: 01865 69758 Fax: 01865 69758 — MB BS Karnatak 1978 (Karnatak Med. Coll., Hubli) MS Karnatak 1981; FRCS Ed. 1985; PhD Bradford 1995; FRCS (Urol.) 1996. Cons. Urological Surg. (Urological Oncol.) Barts and Homerton Hosps.; Hon. Sen. Lect., Surg., Qu. Mary Sch. of Med. & Dent. Specialty: Urol. Special Interest: Andrology; Laparoscopic Uro-Oncology; Urological Oncology. Socs: Amer. Urological Assn.; Brit. Assn. of Urological Surg.; Brit. Med. Assn. Prev: Clin. Lect. (Urol.) Nuffield Dept. Surg. Univ. Oxf. & Oxf. Radcliffe Hosp.

NARHLYA, Nerinder Kumar 85 Fountain Road, Edgbaston, Birmingham B17 8NP — MB ChB Dundee 1996.

NARHLYA, Pawn Kumar 68 Fountain Road, Birmingham B17 8NR — MB ChB Aberd. 1991.

NARNOR, Francis William Dornu 4 Park Avenue, Woodthorpe, Nottingham NG5 4HS — MB BS Lond. 1967; DO Eng. 1972.

NARODDEN, Mohamad Noorsalomon 4 Parsonage Ct, Sheffield S6 5BU — MB ChB Sheff. 1997.

NAROUZ, Noshi Crewley Hospital, Sexual Health Clinic, West Green Drive, Crawley RH11 7DH Tel: 01293 600328 Fax: 01293 600405 — MB BCh Cairo 1979; MRCOG Lond. 1997; DFFP Lond. 1999; Dip GU Med Lond. 2000. Cons. (Genitourin., HIV Med.) Crawley Hosp. Crawley. Specialty: Family Plann. & Reproduc. Health. Special Interest: HIV.

NAROZ, Nabil Awadalla St George Medical Centre, New George Street, South Shields NE33 5DU Tel: 0191 455 5958 Fax: 0191 456 5828 — MB BCh Assiut 1971; DO RCPSI 1981; DRCOG 1983; DFFP 1993; MFFP 1993. Family Plann. Off. & Instruc. S. & NW Durh. HAs & S. Tyneside; Med. Off. (Maj.) Territorial Army; Police Surg. Durh. Constab. Specialty: Family Plann. & Reproduc. Health. Socs: Med. Protec. Soc.; BMA. Prev: Regist. (Oncol. & O & G) Shotley Bridge Gen. Hosp. Consett.

NARRAINEN, Marreemootoo (retired) 94 Andrew Lane, High Lane, Stockport SK6 8HY — MD Malta 1968 (Roy. Univ. Malta) DCH RCPS Glas. 1981. Assoc. Specialist (Paediat.) Stepping Hill Hosp. Stockport; Barrister-at-Law Lincoln's Inn. Prev: SHO (Obst.) Grimsby Matern. Hosp.

NARSAPUR, Surendra Laxmanrao Nethergate Medical Centre, 2 Tay Square, Dundee DD1 1PB Tel: 01382 21527 Fax: 01382 26772 — (Grant medical College) MBBS; Mumbai 1975; MRCGP UK 1987. GP Dundee; Med. Office, Pens. & DHSS. Specialty: Gen. Psychiat.; Gen. Surg.; Disabil. Med. Socs: Med. & Dent. Defence Union, Scotl.

NARULA, Mr Antony Ajay Pall St Mary's Hospital, Praed Street, London W2 1NY Tel: 020 7886 7566 Email: tony.narula@btinternet.com; Private Rooms, Princess Grace Hospital, 42-52 Nottingham Place, London W1U 5NY Tel: 020 7409 2377 — MB BChir Camb. 1980; MA Camb. 1980; FRCS Eng. 1984; FRCS Ed. 2001. Cons. ENT Surg. St Mary's Hosp. Lond.; 2004 on the Counc. of the Roy. Coll. of Surgeons; Hon. Prof. Otolaryngol. Middlx. Univ. Specialty: Otolaryngol. Socs: Fell. Brit. Soc. Audiol.; Fell. Roy. Soc. Med.; Fell. Amer. Acad. ORL-HNS. Prev: Cons. Otolaryngol. Leicester Roy. Infirm.

NARULA, Harmohan Singh Bryngwyn Surgery, 4 Bryngwyn Road, Newport NP20 4JS Tel: 01633 263463 Fax: 01633 252268 — MB BS Panjab 1971; Dip. Ther. Wales; MS (Ophth.) Rajasthan, India 1974; DO RCS Eng. 1977. Mem. LMC (Ophth. Comm.). Specialty: Ophth. Socs: SW Ophth. Soc.; Overseas Doctors Assn.; Treas. SDA UK.

NARULA, Surinder Kaur Bryngwyn Surgery, 4 Bryngwyn Road, Newport NP20 4JS Tel: 01633 263463 Fax: 01633 221421 — MB BS Guru Nanak Dev. 1975; Dip. Therap. 2000 Wales; Dip. Therap. Wales (2000); DObst RCPI 1978; DRCOG 1992; MRCOG 1992. Clin. Asst. (Gyn.) glan Hafru Trust; Mem. LMC. Specialty: Obst. & Gyn.

NARVANI, Amir Ali 8 Reynolds Close, London NW11 7EA — MB BS Lond. 1996.

NASAH, Tony Feuko — MB BS Ibadan 1986; MRCOG 1994. Specialty: Obst. & Gyn.

NASAR, Mohammad Abu Bridlington & Distrct Hospital, Bessingby Road, Bridlington YO16 4QP Tel: 01262 423166 Fax: 01262 400583; 4 Roundhay Road, Bridlington YO15 3JY Tel: 01262 672809 Fax: 01262 672809/400583 — MB BS Dacca Bangladesh 1965 (Chittagong Med. Coll.) MRCP (UK) 1977; FRCP Lond. 1993; FRCP Ed. 1993; FRCP Glas. 1994. Cons. Phys. Dept. Med. Elderly Bridlington & Dist. Hosp. Specialty: Care of the Elderly; Rehabil. Med.; Gen. Med. Socs: Fell. Roy. Soc. Health; Brit. Geriat. Soc.; Fell. Roy. Coll. of Phys.s (Lond. Ed.). Prev: Sen. Regist. (Geriat. Med. & Gen. Med.) St. John's Hosp. & Westm. Hosp. Lond.; Regist. Geriat. Research Unit St. John's Hosp. Lond.; Assoc. Prof. (Med.) Rangpur Med. Coll., Bangladesh.

NASAR, Muhammad Akram Paediatric Department, Conquest Hospital, St Leonards-on-Sea TN37 7RD Tel: 01424 755255 Fax: 01424 758014 Email: muhammad.nasar@esht.nhs.uk — MB BS Karachi 1974 (Dow Med. Coll., Karachi) DTM & H RCP Lond. 1978; MRCPI 1986; FRCPCH 1997; FRCPI 2001; FRCP (Hon.) 2002. Cons. Paediat. Conquest Hosp. St Leonards on Sea. Specialty: Paediat. Special Interest: Paediatric Allergy and Gastroenterol. Socs: Fell. Roy. Soc. Med. Prev: Regist. (Paediat.) Ipswich Hosp.; Community Hosp. Regist. Ipswich.

NASAR, Razia Begum 171 Ferrymead Avenue, Greenford UB6 9TP Tel: 020 8575 0163 — MB BS Punjab 1967; MRCOG 1977.

NASEEM, Mohammad (retired) 177 Church Hill Road, Birmingham B20 3PX Tel: 0121 515 2459; Greenways, 20 Highland Ridge, Halesowen B62 8PH Tel: 0121 423 1607 — (K.E. Med. Coll. Lahore) MB BS Punjab (Pakistan) 1953. Med. Pract.; Clin. Asst. Birm. & Midl. Eye Hosp. Prev: Clin. Asst. (Cas.) Gen. Hosp. Birm.

NASEEM, Mohammad Arfan — MB BCh Wales 1996; DRCOG; MRIS Glas. GP Registrar.

NASEEM, Muhammad Thorpe House Farm, Middleton Lane, Thorpe, Wakefield WF3 3BU — MB BS Punjab 1968.

NASEEM, Mr Muhammed Saleem Medway Hospital, Windmill Road, Gillingham ME7 5NY Tel: 01634 830000; 4 Smithys Close, St Leonards-on-Sea TN37 7SU Tel: 01424 753487 — MB BS Punjab 1985 (King Edward Med. Coll. Lahore, Pakistan) FRCSI 1991; FRCS Eng. 1991; Dip. Urol. Lond 1993. Staff Grade (Urol.) Medway Hosp. Gill'ham, Kent. Specialty: Urol. Prev: Regist. (Urol.) St Barts. Hosp. Lond.; Reg. (Urol.) Conquest Hosp. Hastings; Reg. (Urol.) Whipps Cross. Hosp. Lond.

NASH, Andrew Paul The Surgery, 18 Fouracre Road, Bristol BS16 6PG Tel: 0117 970 2033; (branch Surgery), 42 Abbortswood, Yate, Bristol Tel: 01454 313577 — MB ChB Bristol 1972.

NASH, Mr Anthony Gordon Hatherleigh, 13 Devonshire Road, Sutton SM2 5HQ — MB ChB Bristol 1959; FRCS Eng. 1966. Cons. Surg. Roy. Marsden Hosp.; Cons. Surg. St. Helier Hosp. Carshalton; Sen. Lect. (Surg.) St. Geo. Hosp. Lond. Specialty: Gen. Surg. Prev:

Sen. Regist. Roy. Marsden Hosp. Lond. & St. Geo. Hosp. Lond.; Fell. Surg. Memor. Hosp., New York.

***NASH, Audrey Ann** 9 Whirlow Court Road, Sheffield S11 9NS Tel: 0114 236 2296 — MB ChB Sheff. 1998; MB ChB Sheff 1998. Orthop. Ho. Off., Barnsley Gen. Dist., Barnsley Hosp. Specialty: Orthop.

NASH, Carey Helen Dr. Grays Hospital, Elgin IV30 1SN — BM BS Nottm. 1980. Staff Grade (Psychiat.) Grampian Primary Care NHS Trust. Specialty: Gen. Psychiat. Prev: Staff Grade (Psychiat.) Moray Health Servs.

NASH, Catherine Mary The Central Family Planning Clinic, Grove Road, Norwich NR1 3RH Tel: 01603 287345 Fax: 01603 287636 Email: kate.nash@nnuh.nhs.uk — MB BS Lond. 1972 (Roy. Free Hosp. Med. Sch. Lond.) MRCS Eng. LRCP Lond. 1972; DRCOG 1977; MFFP 1993. Cons. Family Plann. Norf. & Norwich Hosp. NHS Health Care Trust. Specialty: Family Plann. & Reproduc. Health. Prev: Clin. Asst. (Psychiat.) St. And. Hosp. Norwich & Hellesdon Hosp.; Trainee GP Norwich VTS.

NASH, Mr Charles John Amersham Health Centre, Chiltern Avenue, Amersham HP6 5AY Tel: 01494 434344; Oakfield, 2 Church Grove, Little Chalfont, Amersham HP6 6SH — MB BS Lond. 1982 (Middlx. Hosp.) FRCS Eng. 1986; DRCOG 1988; MRCGP 1989. Hosp. Practitioner, Urol., Wycombe Gen. Hosp. Specialty: Gen. Pract.

NASH, Mr Desmond Tyrie Llewellyn 34 Victoria Square, Rostrevor, Newry BT34 3EU — MB BCh BAO Dub. 1946 (T.C. Dub.) FRCSI 1951; LMCC 1956. Socs: BMA. Prev: Cons. Surg. Daisy Hill Hosp. Newry; Sen. Regist. (Surg.) Belf. Hosp. Gp.; Res. Surg. Off. Roy. Devon & Exeter Hosp.

NASH, Dylan Llywelyn The Cripps Health Centre, University Park, Nottingham NG7 2QW Tel: 0115 950 1654 — BM BS Nottm. 1985.

NASH, Edward Fairbairn — MB BS Lond. 1998.

NASH, Elizabeth Jane — BM BS Nottm. 1997.

NASH, Guy Fairbairn 40 More Close, London W14 9BN — MB BS Lond. 1992.

NASH, Ian Trevor The Old School Surgery, Bolts Hill, Chartham, Canterbury CT4 7JY Tel: 01227 738282 Fax: 01227 732122; White Ladies, White Hill, Bilting, Ashford TN25 4HB Tel: 01233 812360 Fax: 01233 813852 — MB BS Lond. 1969 (Guy's) MRCS Eng. LRCP Lond. 1969. Prev: Regist. (Anaesth.) Hastings Gp. Hosp.; Ho. Surg. Roy. E. Sussex Hosp. Hastings.

NASH, Joanna Clare Jeanne House, Dauntsey School, High St., West Lavington, Devizes SN10 4HE — MB ChB Birm. 1993.

NASH, John Martin Western Elms Surgery, 317 Oxford Road, Reading RG30 1AT Tel: 0118 959 0257 Fax: 0118 959 7950 — MB BS Newc. 1970; DObst RCOG 1974.

NASH, Mr John Roderick East Midlands Nuffield Hospital, Rykneld Road, Littleover, Derby DE23 7SN Tel: 07799 714 802 Fax: 01332 865 505 — MB BS Lond. 1972 (Middlx.) FRCS Ed 1977; MD Leics. 1979; FRCS Eng 1988. Cons. Gen. Vasc. & Endocr. Surg. Specialty: Gen. Surg. Socs: Assn. Surg. & Vasc. Soc.; 1921 Surg. Club GB (GB); Service Improve. Team, NHS Modern. Agency. Prev: Chief Exec. Derbysh. Roy. Infirm. NHS Trust; Med. Director Derbysh. Roy. Infirm. NHS Trust; Cons. Surg. South. Derbysh. HA.

NASH, John Rupert Gifford Liverpool University Department of Pathology, Duncan Building, Daulby St., Liverpool L69 3GA Tel: 0151 706 4483 Fax: 0151 706 5859 — BM BCh Oxf. 1975; MA, DPhil Oxf. 1973; FRCPath 1996, M 1983. Sen. Lect. (Path.) Univ. Liverp.; Hon. Cons. Path. Roy. Liverp. Univ. Hosps. Trust. Specialty: Histopath. Special Interest: Lymphoma Path. Socs: Fell. Roy. Coll. Pathol.; BMA; Internat. Acad. Path. Prev: Clin. Tutor & Clin. Lect. (Path.) Univ. Oxf.

NASH, Julian Trevor Royal NATIONAL Orthopaedic Hospital, Brockley Hill, Stanmore HA7 4LP — MB BCh Wales 1990; BSc (Hons.) Univ. Coll. Wales 1987; MRCP UK 1993; PhD Imperial Coll. Of Science & Technology 1999; CCST Rheumatology & Gen. Internal Med. 2002. Cons. Rheumatologist, Royal Nat. Orthopaedic Hosp. & Barnet Hosp. Specialty: Gen. Med.; Rheumatol. Socs: Med. Protec. Soc.; Brit. Soc. of Rheum.; Roy. Soc. of Med. Prev: Regist. (Med.) Stoke Mandeville Hosp. Aylesbury.; MRC Clin. Train. Fell. & Hon. Regist. (Rheum.) RPMS Hammersmith Hosp. Lond.; Specialist Regist. Rheum. and Gen. Med. Homerton Hosp. Lond.

NASH, Kathryn Louise 14 Fourth Avenue, Denvilles, Havant PO9 2QX — BChir Camb. 1995.

NASH, Pamela Elaine 47 Owls Lodge Lane, Mayals, Swansea SA3 5DP — MB BS Lond. 1980 (St. Mary's Hosp. Lond.) MRCP (UK) 1983; FFAEM 1992; FRCP Lond. 1995. Cons. A & E Neath Hosp. W. Glam. Specialty: Accid. & Emerg. Prev: Cons. A & E Hillingdon Hosp. Uxbridge; Sen. Regist. (A & E) Centr. Middlx. Hosp. Lond.

NASH, Peter James, CStJ 1 Rectory Close, Eastbourne BN20 8AQ Tel: 01323 411220 Fax: 01323 411575 — MB ChB Sheff. 1967; DA Eng. 1971; FFA RCS Eng. 1974. Cons. Anaesth. & Eastbourne Hosps. NHS Trust. Specialty: Anaesth. Socs: BMA; Assn. Anaesth. Prev: Sen. Regist. Roy. Sussex Co. Hosp. Brighton; Squadron Ldr. RAF Med. Br.; Direct Med. Servs. Eastbourne Hosp. NHS Trust.

NASH, Ruth Mary Dept Histopathology, King's College School of Medicine and Dentistry, Bessemer Road, London SE5 9PJ Tel: 020 7346 3005 Fax: 020 7346 3670; 157 Underhill Road, E. Dulwich, London SE22 0PG — (Sen. Lect. (Perinatal/Paediat. Path.)) BSc (Hons) Ed. 1975; MB BS Lond. 1978; MRCPath 1992; DRCPath (Cytol.) 1996. Specialty: Histopath. Socs: MRCPath.; Brit. Soc. Clin. Cytol.; Paediat. Path. Soc.

NASH, Sally Marion Katherine 44 Pinner Court, Pinner HA5 5RL — MB ChB Birm. 1994; ChB Birm. 1994.

NASH, Steven Roy Lanescot House, Lanescot, Par PL24 2RS — MB BS Lond. 1984; MRCGP 1989. Trainee GP Liskeard VTS.

NASH, Mr Thorolf Guy (retired) Westlands, 36 Collington Avenue, Bexhill-on-Sea TN39 3NE Tel: 01424 221886 Fax: 01424 213249 Email: tgnash@aol.com — MB BS Lond. 1960 (Guy's) MRCS Eng. LRCP Lond. 1959; FRCOG 1979, M 1966, DObst 1961; FRCS Ed. 1969; FRCS Eng. 1970. Gynaecologist in Private Pract.; Authorised Med. Examr. Civil Aviat. Auth. Prev: Regist. (Gen. Surg.) Roy. Vict. Hosp. Bournemouth.

NASH, Timothy Paul The Walton Centre, Lower Lane, Fazakerley, Liverpool L9 7LJ Tel: 0151 529 5749 Fax: 0151 529 5486 Email: tim.nash@thewaltoncentre.nhs.uk; Danesfield, 21 Stanley Road, Hoylake, Wirral CH47 1HN Tel: 0151 632 6985 Fax: 0151 632 0307 Email: nashtp@liv.ac.uk; tim.nash@which.net — (Univ. Coll. Hosp.) MB BS Lond. 1969; DObst RCOG 1971; FRCA Eng. 1974. Cons. in Pain Med., Walton Centre Liverp.; Hon. Sen. Lect., Univ. of Liverp.; Hon. Director of Pain Studie, Univ. of Liverp. Specialty: Anaesth. Socs: Assn. Anaesths.; IASP; Sect. Anaesth. RSM. Prev: Cons. Anaesth. & Pain Managem. Basingstoke Dist. Hosp.; Sen. Regist. (Anaesth.) Addenbrooke's Hosp. Camb.; Regist. (Anaesth.) Univ. Coll. Hosp. Lond.

NASH, William Norman Cecil Old Harlow Health Centre, Jenner House, Garden Terrace Road, Harlow CM17 0AX Tel: 01279 418136 Fax: 01279 429650 — MB BCh BAO Dub. 1965; MA.

NASHEF, Alexandra Jean Alconbury and Brampton Surgeries, The Surgery, School Lane, Alconbury, Huntingdon PE28 4EQ Tel: 01480 890281 Fax: 01480 891787 — MB ChB Glas. 1984; DRCOG 1986; MRCGP 1989. Clin. Med. Off. (Genitourin. Med.) Hinchingbrooke Hosp. Huntingdon. Specialty: Genitourinary Medicine.

NASHEF, Lina Neurology Department, King's College Hospital,, Denmark Hill, London SE5 9RS — MB ChB Bristol 1980; MRCP UK 1984; MD 1995; FRCP UK 2000. Cons. Neurol., King's Coll. Hosp. Lond.; Hon. Sen. Lect. GKT School of Med. Specialty: Neurol.

NASHEF, Mr Samer Abdel-Malik Papworth Hospital, Cambridge CB3 8RE Tel: 01480 364299 Fax: 01480 364744 Email: sam.nashef@papworth.nhs.uk; 16 Allen's Orchard, Brampton, Huntingdon PE28 4NW Tel: 01480 414966 — MB ChB Bristol 1980; BSc AUB 1976; FRCS Eng. 1984; FRCS Glas. 1984. Cons.(Cardiothoracic Surg.) Papworth Hosp. Camb.; Hon. Cons.(Cardiothoracic Surg.) Addenbrooke's Hosp. Camb.; Med. Exec. Director (Ectsia). Specialty: Cardiothoracic Surg. Socs: Eur. Club, Young Cardiac Surg. (Scientif. Sec.); EACTS Audit & Guidelines Comm. (Chairm.). Prev: Sen. Regist. (Cardiothoracic Surg.) Wythenshawe Hosp. Manch.; Attached Surg. Xavier Arnozan & Haut-Leveque Hosps. Bordeaux France.

NASIB, Asif 12 Glencairn Drive, Glasgow G41 4QN Tel: 0141 423 8179 — MB ChB Glas. 1995 (University of Glasgow) SHO (ENT Surg.). Specialty: Otolaryngol.

NASIM, Mr Akhtar South Manchester University Hospitals Trust, Wythenshawe Hospital, Southmoor Road, Wythenshawe, Manchester M23 9LT Tel: 0161 291 6642 — MB ChB Aberd.

1990; FRCS Ed. 1994; MD Leic. 1998. Cons. Vasc. Surg.; Hon. Lect. Univ. of Manch. Specialty: Gen. Surg. Socs: Europ. Soc. Vasc. & Endovasc. Surg.; Vasc. Surg. Soc. GB & Irel.; Assn. Surgs. GB & Irel. Prev: Specialist Regist. (Surg.) Leicester Roy. Infirm.; Clin. Research Fell. (Surg.) Univ. Leicester; SHO Rotat. (Surg.) Leicester.

NASIR, Taqleed Ullah Khan (retired) 8 Highfield Gardens, Heaton, Bradford BD9 6LY Tel: 01274 491573 — MB BS Sind 1963 (Liaquat Med. Coll. Hyderabad) DPM Eng. 1969; MRCPsych 1972. Cons. Psychiat. W.wood Hosp. Bradford. Prev: Regist. & Med. Asst. (Psychiat.) Whittingham Hosp. Preston.

NASIRI, Ahmed Zafar Sovereign Medical Centre, Sovereign Drive, Pennyland, Milton Keynes MK15 8AJ Tel: 01908 661166 Fax: 01908 233921; 26 Saddlers Place, Downs Barn, Milton Keynes MK14 7RS Tel: 01908 605265 — MB BChir Camb. 1988 (Cambridge) DCCH RCGP 1992; DRCOG 1992; MRCGP 1992. GP Partner; Prison Med. Off. HMP Woodhill, Milton Keynes. Specialty: Gen. Pract.; Forens. Psychiat. Prev: SHO Milton Keynes Gen. Hosp. GP VTS; Ho. Off. Ipswich Gen. Hosp.; Ho. Off. (Surg.) P'boro. Dist. Hosp.

NASIRUDDIN, Ismat Jehan 72 Gayville Road, London SW11 6JP Email: ismat@rocketmail.com — MB BS Lond. 1994; DFFP; DRCOG.

NASMYTH, Mr David George Department of Surgery, Furness General Hospital, Dalton Lane, Barrow-in-Furness LA14 4LF Tel: 01229 870870; Fellwood Head, Hooks Lane, Little Urswick, Ulverston LA12 0TH — MB BS Lond. 1976 (Oxf. & Middlx.) MA Oxf. 1973; FRCS Ed. 1982; FRCS Eng. 1982; MS Lond. 1988. Cons. Gen. Surg. Furness Gen. Hosp.; Clin. Tutor Furness Gen. Hosp.; Lead Clinician (Colorectal Cancer Unit) Morecambe Bay NHS Trust. Specialty: Gen. Surg. Socs: Fell. Roy. Soc. Med.; Assn. Coloproctol.; Assn. Surg.s GB & I. Prev: Sen. Regist. (Surg.) Roy. Liverp. Hosp.; Research Fell. Univ. Dept. Surg. Gen. Infirm. Leeds; Regist. (Surg.) Leicester Roy. Infirm.

NASR, Ehab Fayez 32 Whinney Heys Road, Blackpool FY3 8NP — MB BCh Ain Shams 1984.

NASR, Ibrahim Sobhy Ibrahim Mohamed Scunthorpe General Hospital, Dermatology Department, Cliff Gardens, Scunthorpe DN15 7BH Tel: 01724 282282 — (Alexandria University, Egypt) MBChB 1978; MA in Dermatology & Venereology 1985; MRCP (UK) 1995. DermpatologistScunthorpe Gen Hosp Scunthorpe; Cons Dermatol. The Roy. Hallamshire Hosp The Centr. Sheff. Univ, Hosps Sheff.; Hon Clin.Lec. Sheff. Univ Med Sch. Sheff.; Asst. Med. Director, Scunthorpe Gen. Hosp., Scunthorpe. Specialty: Dermat. Socs: Fell.of the Roy. Soc. of Med.; Brit. Assoc. of Dermatol.s; N. Eng. Dermatol. Soc. Prev: Cons. Dermatol., St Mary's Hosp., Newport, Isle of Wight; Cons. Dermatol., Alexandria, Egypt; Cons. Dermato. Wwales Gen Hosp Carmarthen.

NASR, Mr Mohamed Sayed Ahmed Department of Genito-Urinary Medicine, Royal South Hants Hospital, Southampton SO14 0YG; The Pines, Hadrian Way, Chilworth, Southampton SO16 7HZ — MRCOG 1977; MRCS Eng. LRCP Lond. 1978; FRCOG 1998. Cons. Genitourin. Med. Soton. Univ. Hosps. NHS Trust Salisbury NHS Trust. Specialty: Genitourinary Medicine.

NASRA, Mr Salim Elias St Mary's Hospital, Newport PO30 5TG Email: senasra@hotmail.com; La Paz, Kite Hill, Wootton, Ryde PO33 4LE Tel: 01983 882545 Fax: 01983 882545 — MD Damascus 1977; FRCS Glas. 1986; MRCS Eng. LRCP Lond. 1988; FRCS (Trauma & Orthop.) 1999. Cons. Orthop. Surg. St Mary's Hosp Isle of Wight. Specialty: Trauma & Orthop. Surg. Socs: Overseas Fell. BOA; Fell. BOA.

NASRALLA, A H K Wordsworth Health Centre, 19 Wordsworth Avenue, Manor Park, London E12 6SU Tel: 020 8548 5960 Fax: 020 8548 5983 — MB BS Lucknow 1969.

NASRALLAH, Di. Fayez K. 4 Underwood Road, Bassett, Southampton SO16 7BU Tel: 02380 790535 — MB BCh Alexandria 1958; DCH Eng. 1974; MRCS Eng. LRCP Lond. 1977; MRCPsych 1996. SCMO Child Health, Soton. Community Trust. Socs: BMA; Assoc. Mem. Brit. Paediat. Assn. Prev: Clin. Med. Off. (Child Health) Mid Surrey Health Dist.; SHO (Paediat.) N. Devon Dist. Hosp. Barnstaple.; SCMO (Child Health) Soton. & S.W. Hants. Health Dist. (T).

NASRUDDIN, Imelda Nasreen 31 Fore Street, Roche, St Austell PL26 8EP — MB ChB Manch. 1997.

NASSAR, Mr Ahmad Hafez Mohamed Vale of Leven District General Hospital, Alexandria G83 0UA Tel: 01389 754121 Fax: 01389 711150 Email: anassar@vol.scot.nhs.uk; 3 Courthill, Bearsden, Glasgow G61 3SN Tel: 0771 134 6603 Email: anassar@clinmed.gla.ac.uk — MB BCh Zagazig 1977; FRCS Ed. 1986. Cons. Surg. (Upper Gastrointestinal & Laparoscopic Surg.) Vale of Leven Dist. Gen. Hosp. Alexandria; Tutor (Minimal Access Ther. Train. Unit) RCS Eng.; Hon Clin Sen Lec Univ of Glas. Specialty: Gen. Surg. Socs: Soc. Minimally Invasive Ther.; Assn. Endoscopic Surgs.; Eur. Assn. Endoscopic Surgs. Prev: Lect. (Surg.) Univ. Coll. Cork; Cons. (Surg.) Nat. Guard Hosp. Jeddah, Saudi Arabia.

NASSAR, Mr Wadi Yusuf The Beeches Consulting Centre, Mill Lane, Cheadle SK8 2PY Tel: 0161 491 2470 Fax: 0161 428 1692; (rooms), 21 St. John St, Manchester M3 4DT Tel: 0161 834 4242 — MD Amer. Univ. Beirut 1956; DLO Eng. 1964; LAH Dub. 1967; MCh (Orl.) Liverp. 1967; FRCS Eng. 1969. Cons. ENT Surg. S. Manch. Health Dist. (T) S. Manch. Univ. Hosps. NHS Trust; Hon Lect. (Clin. Otolaryngol.) Manch. Univ. Specialty: Otolaryngol. Socs: Fell. Roy. Soc. Med.; Brit. Soc. Audiol.; Brit. Med. Assn. Prev: Regist. Warrington Gen. Hosp.; Lect. Univ. Manch.; Sen. Regist. Manch. Roy. Infirm.

NASSEF, Ahmed Hussein Kamel Northern General Hospital, Department of General Surgery, Herries Road, Sheffield S5 7AU — MB BCh Cairo 1986. Specialty: Gen. Surg.

NASSER, Abdul South Tyneside District Hospital, Harton Lane, South Shields NE34 0PL — MB BS Peshawar 1987; MRCP. Cons. Cardiol. Specialty: Cardiol. Socs: Brit. Cardiac. Soc.; Scott. Cardiac Soc.; BMA.

NASSER, Mr Nasser Ahmed Suite 15, 103-105 Harley Street, London W1G 6AJ Tel: 020 7224 1033; Flat 15, 103-105 Harley Street, London W1G 6AJ Tel: 020 7486 9402 — LMSSA Lond. 1977 (Char. Cross) BDS Glas. 1965; MRCS Eng. LRCP Lond. 1977; FDS RCPS Glas. 1980; FRCS Eng. 1980. p/t Cons. Oral & Maxillofacial Surg. Char. Cross Hosp. Lond.; Vis. Cons. Surg. to Govt. Cyprus. Specialty: Oral & Maxillofacial Surg.; Oncol.; Plastic Surg. Socs: Eur. Acad. Aesthetic Facial Surg.; Brit. Assn. Cosmetic Surg.; Amer. Acad. Facial Plastic & Reconstr. Surg. Prev: Cons. Oral & Maxillofacial Surg. Barnet & Edgware Hosps.; Sen. Regist. (Maxillofacial Surg.) King's Coll. Hosp. Lond. & ABU Hosp. Kaduna, Nigeria; SHO (Plastic, Head & Neck) St Geo. Hosp. Lond.

NASSER, Syed Muhammad Shuaib Addenbrookes Hospital, Allergy Clinic, Cambridge CB2 2QQ — MB BS Lond. 1985 (Guys Hosp.) MRCP (UK) 1989; MD London 1999. Cons.(Allergy & Astma) Addenbrooke's NHS Trust Camb. Specialty: Respirat. Med.; Immunol.; Allergy. Special Interest: All types of allergy; Asthma. Socs: Brit. Soc. Allergy & Clin. Immunol. Prev: Sen. Regist. Papworth Hosp.; Research Regist. & Regist. (Clin. Med.) Guy's Hosp. Lond.; Sen. Regist. & Clin. Lect. (Allergy Clin. Immunol. & Thoracic Med.) Addenbrooke's NHS Trust Univ. Camb.

NASSER, Zeinab Abdel-Aziz Ibrahim The Medical Centre, 2 Manor Court Avenue, Nuneaton CV11 5HX — MB BCh Cairo 1983; MSc Cairo 1989. SCMO Med. Centre Nuneaton. Specialty: Gen. Psychiat. Prev: Staff Grade (Psychiat.) Ashworth Hosp. Liverp.

NASSIF, Manhal Georges Georges Orthopaedic Department, Ninewells Hospital, Dundee DD1 9SY — MD (Damascus Univ.) FRCS; MChOrth. Cons. Ortopaedic Surg.; Sen. Clin. Teach. Specialty: Orthop. Special Interest: Lower Limb Arthroplasty; Revision Surg.

NASSIM, Michael Arnold The Croft, 10 Chapel Lane, Old Dalby, Melton Mowbray LE14 3LA — BM BCh Oxf. 1968 (St. Geo.) BSc, MA Oxf. 1968; MRCP (UK) 1971. Specialty: Pharmaceutical Medicine; Nephrol. Special Interest: 3D Lung Imaging and Models; Atherdmatous Dis.; Cardiovasc. Changes during Pregn. Socs: Collegiate Mem. RCP Lond. Prev: Sen. Clin. Pharmacol. Astra Charnwood Pharmaceuts. LoughBoro.; Lect. (Nephrol.) Inst. Urol. Lond.; Hon. Sen. Regist. St. Peter's Hosps. Lond.

NATALE, Salvatore Buckleigh House, 127 Devonport Road, Plymouth PL1 5RQ — State Exam Messina 1982.

NATALI, Colin Royal London Hospital, Whitechapel, London E1 1BB Tel: 020 7377 7197 Email: colin@backquack.demon.co.uk — MB BS Lond. 1986 (Lond. Hosp. Med. Coll.) BSc (Hons.) Lond. 1983, MB BS 1986; FRCS Eng. 1991; FRCS (Orth.) 1996. Cons. (Orthop. Surg.) Roy. Lond. Hosp. Specialty: Orthop. Special Interest: Disorders of the low back; Neck disorders.

NATALWALA, Siraj Block 47, Flat 3, Good Hope Hospital, Rectory Road, Sutton Coldfield B75 7RR; 50 West View Road, Sutton

Coldfield B75 6AY — MB BS Devi Ahilya India 1983; FRCS Glasgow. Staff Grade Urol., Good Hope Hosp.

NATARAJ, Vasudevan Bolton Road Surgery, 431-433 Bolton Road, Ewood, Blackburn BB2 4HY Tel: 01254 679781 Fax: 01254 693031; (Surgery) 2 Velvet Street, Ewood, Blackburn — MB BS Bihar 1972 (Darbhanga Med. Coll.)

NATARAJAN, Dhanapal c/o Dr S Anand, 2 Maindiff Court House, Ross Road, Abergavenny NP7 5LT — MB BS Madras 1984.

NATARAJAN, Ramanathan Northampton General Hospital, Cliftonville, Northampton NN1 5BD Fax: 01604 545588 — MB BS Madras Med. Coll. India 1984; FRCS (Trauma & Orthop.); FRCS Glas.; MS (Orthop.). Cons. Orthop. Surg. BMI Three Shire Hosp. Northampton. Specialty: Trauma & Orthop. Surg. Special Interest: Limb Reconstruction; Lower Limb Arthroplasty; Paediatric Orthop. Socs: Brit. Orthop. Assn.; Brit. Soc. Of Childrens Orthop.

NATARAJAN, Sivakumar Royal Hospital, Kayall Road, Sunderland SR4 7TP Tel: 0191 569 0004 Fax: 0191 569 9201; 9 West Farm Road, Cleadon, Sunderland SR6 7UG Tel: 0191 536 6111 Fax: 0191 536 6111 — MB BS Madras 1976; MD (Dermat.) Madras 1980; MRCP (UK) 1990; FRCP 1999. Cons. Dermat. Roy. Hosp. Sunderland. Specialty: Dermat. Socs: BMA; Brit. Assn. Dermat.; Scott. Dermat. Soc. Prev: Regist. (Dermat.) P'boro. Dist. Hosp.; Resid. (Dermat.) Jipmer, Pondicherry, India; Regist. (Dermat.) Stobhill Hosp. Glas.

NATARAJU, Manni Rathna (Surgery), 38 Wentworth Avenue, London N3 1YL Tel: 020 8346 1242 — MB BS Bangalore 1973.

NATAS, Sarah Anne 38 Kingfisher Drive, Ham, Richmond TW10 7UD — MB BS Lond. 1998.

NATERWALLA, Mr Russi Hormusji Frenesi, 68 Lyndhurst Road, River, Dover CT17 0NH Tel: 01304 825104 — MB BS Bombay 1965 (Topiwala Nat. Med. Coll.) FRCS Ed. 1975. Assoc. Specialist (A & E) Buckland Hosp. Dover. Prev: Clin. Asst. (Accid. Surg.) Buckland Hosp. Dover; Regist. (Gen. & Thoracic Surg.) B.Y.L. Nair Hosp. Bombay, India; SHO (Gen. Surg.) & SHO (Accid. & Orthop.) Buckland Hosp. Dover.

NATH, Abdulrehman Ramji 1 Hunters Park, Berkhamsted HP4 2PT; Royal Brompton and Harefield NHS Trust, Department Thoracic Medicine, Harefield Hospital, Hill End Road, Uxbridge UB9 6JH Tel: 01895 828692 Fax: 01895 822870 — (Guy's) MD Lond. 1973, MB BS 1962; MRCS Eng. LRCP Lond. 1962; MRCP Lond. 1968. Cons. Phys. (Thoracic Med.) Harefield Hosp. & Hemel Hempstead Gen. Hosp. Specialty: Gen. Med. Socs: Thoracic Soc.; FRCP (Lond.). Prev: Ho. Surg. Guy's Hosp. Lond.; Regist. (Med.) Qu. Mary's Hosp. Sidcup; Sen. Regist. Lond. Chest Hosp.

NATH, Basdeo Karamchand The Baird Health Centre, Gassiot House, St. Thomas' Hospital, London SE1 7EH Tel: 020 7202 8300; 27 Rosemont Avenue, London N12 0BY Tel: 020 8446 2156 — MB ChB Glas. 1967; T(GP) 1992. Sen. Med. Off. Baird Health Centre St Thomas' Hosp. Lond. Socs: BMA & Med. Defence Union. Prev: Lect. Univ. Guyana S. Amer. Fac. Health Sci.; Civil. GP MoD Middlx.

NATH, Mr Fredrik Prem Department of Neurosurgery, James Cook University Hospital, Manton Road TS4 3BW Tel: 01642 854317 Fax: 01642 854118 Email: fred.nath@onyx.octacon.co.uk — MB ChB Liverp. 1974; FRCS Ed. 1980. Cons. Neurosurg. Middlesbrough Gen. Hosp.; Cons. to the N. of Eng. Spinal Injuries Unit. Specialty: Neurosurg. Socs: Soc. of Brit. Neurol. Surgeons. Prev: Sen. Regist. (Neurosurg.) South. Gen. Hosp. Glas.

NATH, Jaharlal Doctor's Mess, Princess Royal Hospital, Lewes Road, Haywards Heath RH16 4EX; 14 Colwell Gardens, Haywards Heath, Haywards Heath RH16 4HG Tel: 01444 417040 — MB BS Calcutta 1974; DRCOG 1990; MRCOG 1990. Staff Obst. (O & G) Princess Roy. Hosp. Haywards Heath. Specialty: Obst. & Gyn.

NATH, Kantimon The Maerdy Ferndale Practice, Ferndale Medical Centre, 65-68 High Street, Ferndale CF43 4XX Tel: 01443 733202 Fax: 01443 733730.

NATH, Mahendra Aston Hall Hospital, Aston-on-Trent, Derby DE72 2AL; 77 Wollaton Vale, Nottingham NG8 2PD — MB BS Bangalore 1972 (Bangalore Medical College, India) MRCPsych 1989. Sen. Cons. Psychiat./Clin Dir. Specialty: Gen. Psychiat. Prev: Sen. Regist.N. E. Thames Rotat. Scheme; Cons. Psychiat. Ballamona Hosp. Douglas Isle of Man.

NATH, Mohan Lal Treharris Health Centre, Bargoed Terrace, Treharris CF46 5RB Tel: 01443 410242 Fax: 01443 413312; 9 Glybargfed Close, Treharris CF46 6AJ — MB BS Calcutta 1965 (R.G. Kar Med. Coll.)

NATH, Nirmal Kumar 51 Church Hill, Loughton IG10 1QP Tel: 020 8508 7477 — MB BS Calcutta 1960 (R.G. Kar Med. Coll.) DA Eng. 1965. Assoc. Specialist (Anaesth.) Moorfields Hosp. Lond. Prev: Regist. (Anaesth.) Moorfields Eye Hosp. (City Rd. Br.) Lond.; Jun. Ho. Off. (Med.) & SHO (Anaesth.) St. Jas. Hosp. Leeds; Regist. (Anaesth.) Hackney Hosp. Lond.

NATH, Pathikonda Uma 21 Beamish View, East Stanley, Stanley DH9 0XB — MB BS Newc. 1991; BMedSc Newc. 1989; MRCP (UK) 1994. Regist. (Neurol.) RVI Newc. Specialty: Neurol.

NATH, Pathikonda Viswambara, MBE Front Street Surgery, 1 Front Street, Craghead, Stanley DH9 6DS Tel: 01207 232698; Tapaswi, 21 Beamish View, Stanley DH9 0XB Tel: 01207 290606 Fax: 01207 230712 — MB BS Mysore 1965; DLO Eng. 1970. GP. Specialty: Aviat. Med.; Anaesth. Socs: Acupunc. Soc.

NATH, R Queens Park and Moredon Surgeries, 146 Drove Road, Swindon SN1 3AG Tel: 01793 487394 Fax: 01793 342011 — MB BS Agra 1962; MB BS Agra 1962.

NATH, Rahul Abbotswood, Bridle Way, Croydon CR0 5AH — MB BCh Wales 1992; BSc (Hons.) Pharmacol. Wales 1991, MB BCh 1992.

NATH, Samiran 10 Park Avenue, Grange Park, Gosforth, Newcastle upon Tyne NE3 2HL — MB ChB Ed. 1994; BSc (Med. Sci.) Ed. 1992. Ho. Off. (Med.) Roy. Infirm. Edin.; Ho. Off. (Surg.) Qu. Margt. Hosp. Trust Dunfermline.

NATHA, Liaqat Ali 67 Swan Lane, Bolton BL3 6TQ; 60 Swan Lane, Bolton BL3 6TQ — MB ChB Liverp. 1997 (Liverpool) SHO O & G, Bolton Roy. Hosp., Bolton. Specialty: Obst. & Gyn. Prev: SHO A & E Fazakerely Hosp., Liverp.; PRHO Med. & Surg., Roual Liverp. Univ. Hosp., Liverp.

NATHA, Maksood Ibrahim 2 Victoria Terrace, Hathersage Road, Longsight, Manchester M13 0HY — MB ChB Leeds 1995.

NATHA, Mr Salim Christopher Home Eye Unit, Wigan Infirmary, Wigan Lane, Wigan WN1 2NN Tel: 01942 822503 — MB ChB Liverp. 1992; FRCOphth 1996. Cons. Opthamologist Roy. Albert Edwd. Infirm. Wigan. Specialty: Ophth. Socs: Med. Retina Gp. Prev: Specialist Regist. Mersey Rotat.

NATHAN, Anita Rama 32 Claremont Av, Beeston, Nottingham NG9 3DG — MB ChB Birm. 1997.

NATHAN, Bernard Edward 31 Langland Gardens, London NW3 6QE Tel: 020 7794 7136 — MB BCh Witwatersrand 1962; DMRD Eng. 1968; FFR 1970; FRCR 1975. Cons. Radiol. Edgware Gen. Hosp. & Hammersmith Hosp. Lond. Specialty: Radiol. Socs: Brit. Inst. Radiol. Prev: Sen. Regist. Hammersmith Hosp. Lond.

NATHAN, James Alexander — MB ChB Bristol 1998.

NATHAN, Joanna Mary 160 Hatfield Road, St Albans AL1 4JD — BM Soton. 1996.

NATHAN, John Joseph Summerhill, 39 Detillens Lane, Limpsfield, Oxted RH8 0DH Mob: 08705 441131 — MB BS Lond. 1967 (King's Coll. Lond. & King's Coll. Hosp.) MRCS Eng. LRCP Lond. 1966; DObst RCOG 1973. Specialty: Orthop. Prev: Regist. Rotat. (Surg.) Wessex RHB; SHO (Orthop.) Norf. & Norwich Hosp.; Ho. Surg. King's Coll. Hosp. Lond.

NATHAN, Laurence Andrew Longcroft Clinic, 5 Woodmansterne Lane, Banstead SM7 3HH Tel: 01737 359332 Fax: 01737 370835 — MB BS Lond. 1973 (Westm.) MRCS Eng. LRCP Lond. 1973; MRCP (UK) 1976. Prev: Regist. (Radiother. & Oncol.) Roy. Marsden Hosp. Lond.; Regist. (Gen. Med.) Orpington Hosp.; Ho. Surg. Gordon Hosp. Lond.

NATHAN, Mark Peter Flat 1, 18 The Avenue, London NW6 7YD — MB ChB Manch. 1991.

NATHAN, Mr Nathan Walderslade Village Surgery, 62A Robin Hood Lane, Walderslade, Chatham ME5 9LD Tel: 01634 687250; 6 Meteor Road, Kate Reed Wood, West Malling, Maidstone ME18 6TH — MB BS Lond. 1981; FRCS 1984; DCH Lond. 1986; DRCOG 1987. Prev: Trainee Bournehall Health Centre Ewell Epsom.; SHO (Cas.) St. Geo.'s Hosp.; SHO (Neurol. & Neuro-surg.) Atkinson Morley's Hosp. Wimbledon.

NATHAN, Nicholas John — MB ChB Leeds 1971; MRCP (UK) 1976; Dip. Pract. Dermat. 1997; FRCP 2003. p/t GPwSI Dermat.; Medically Qualified Panel Mem. Appeals Serv. Specialty: Dermat. Socs: Primary Care Dermat. Soc. Prev: Hosp. Pract. (Genitourin.

Med.) Leeds Gen. Infirm.; GP Chevin Med. Pract., Otley; Regist. (Gen. Med.) Wharfedale Gen. Hosp. Otley.

NATHAN, Nicki Lisa 160A High Road, London N2 9AS — MB BS Lond. 1990.

NATHAN, Paul Andrew Hollybrook Medical Centre, Hollybrook Way, Littleover, Derby DE23 3TX; Meadow House, Church View, Derby Road, Duffield, Belper DE56 4FL Email: paul. Nathan@nhs.net — BM BS Nottm. 1986. Chair. Centr. Derby PCG.

NATHAN, Paul Daniel — MB BS Lond. 1996.

NATHAN, Rajan Neil Scott Clinic, Rainhill Road, St Helens CH3 8JR Tel: 0151 4306300 — MB BCh Wales 1991; MRCPsych; Dip Foren Sc; MMed Sc. Cons. Forens. Psychiat. Specialty: Gen. Psychiat.

NATHAN, Mr Senthil — BM BS Madras 1983 (Madras Medical College) MS 1987; FRCS Edin RCS Edin 1990; MPhil Lond. 1997; FRCS RCS Edin 1998; FEBU European Board of Urology 2000. Cons Urol., & Hon. Sen. Lect.; Hon. Cons., Roy. Free Hosp., Lond. Specialty: Urol. Special Interest: Uro Oncol. Socs: Roy. Soc. of Med.; Brit. Med. Assn.; Brit. Assn. of Urol. Surg.

NATHAN, Shirley Evelyn Brown Gables, Barnet Lane, Elstree, Borehamwood WD6 3RQ Tel: 020 8953 2350 Fax: 0208 953 7687 — MB BS Lond. 1951 (Univ. Coll. Hosp.) DObst RCOG 1953; FRCGP 1981, M 1965. Prev: Contract Med. Assessor for Hestor Disabil. Anal.

NATHAN, Thevakunchary 1 Aldridge Rise, New Malden KT3 5RJ — MB BS Ceylon 1971.

NATHAN, Yashica — MB BS Lond. 1998.

NATHANSON, Michael Harvey Department of Anaesthesia, University Hospital, Queen's Medical Centre, Nottingham NG7 2UH Tel: 0115 970 9195 Fax: 0115 978 3891 — MB BS Lond. 1984 (Middlesex Hospital Medical School) MRCP (UK) 1988; FRCA 1991. Cons. Anaesth. Univ. Hosp. Qu. Med. Centre Nottm. Specialty: Anaesth. Socs: Assn. Anaesth.; Amer. Soc. Anesthesiol.; Anaesth. Res. Soc. Prev: Sen. Regist. (Anaesth.) Univ. Hosp. Qu. Med. Centre Nottm.; Vis. Asst. Prof. Univ. Texas S.W.ern Med. Center, USA; Regist. (Anaesth.) St. Bart. Hosp. Lond.

NATHANSON, Vivienne Hilary BMA House, Tavistock Square, London WC1H 9JP Tel: 020 7387 4499 Fax: 020 7383 6710 Email: vivn@bma.org.uk — MB BS Lond. 1978. Director of Professional Resources. Prev: Regist. (Med.) Glan Clwyd Hosp. Bodelwyddan; Head of Prof. Resources & Research GP BMA.

NATHAVITHARANA, Chandrika Priyani Geethamala 293 Quinton Road, Harborne, Birmingham B17 0RB — MB BS Peradeniya 1979; MB BS Peradeniya, Sri Lanka 1979.

NATHAVITHARANA, Kamal Augustine Alexandra Hospital NHS Trust, Woodrow Drive, Redditch B98 7UB Tel: 01527 512163 Fax: 01527 503855; The Gables, 232 Bristol Road, Edgbaston, Birmingham B5 7TA Tel: 0121 472 1896 — MB BS Sri Lanka 1980 (Univ. Peradeniya) MRCP UK 1986; DCH RCP Lond. 1987; PhD Birm. 1989; FRCPCH Lond. 1996. Cons. (Paediat. & Gastroenterol.); Hon. Sen. Lect. Univ. Birm.; Sen. Lect. Univ. Warwick. Specialty: Gastroenterol.; Paediat. Special Interest: Gastroenterol. & Food Allergy. Prev: Lect. (Paediat. & Child Health) Univ. Birm.; Tutor (Child Health) Univ. Manch.; Lect. (Paediat.).

NATHDWARAWALA, Mr Yogesh Ramdas nevill Hall Hospital, Abergavenny NP7 7EG — MB BS Baroda 1986; MS (Orthop.) Baroda 1990, MB BS 1986. Regist. (Orthop.) Glan Clwyd Hosp. Rhyl. Specialty: Orthop. Prev: Regist. (Orthop.) Roy. Gwent Hosp. Newport.

NATHOO, Vijay 2 Glenholme Road, Bramhall, Stockport SK7 2BR — MB BCh Wales 1982; BSc Salford 1976; MSc Manch. 1977; DRCOG 1986; MRCGP 1989; LLM (LAMP) Wales 2001.

NATHOO, Yasmin 50 Grove Farm Park, Northwood HA6 2BQ — MB BS Newc. 1979.

NATHU, Azmeena Pennygate Surgery, 210 Pennygate, Spalding PE11 1LT Tel: 01775 710133.

NATHWANI, Ameet SmithKline Beecham R+D, New Frontiers Science Park (South), Harrow CM19 5AW Tel: 01279 646656 Fax: 01279 644976 Email: ameet_nathwani-1@sbphrd.com; 2 Axen Way, Osbourne Park, Welwyn Garden City AL7 1HR Tel: 01707 323638 Email: ameetnathwani@compuserve.com — MB BS Lond. 1987 (Middlx. Hosp.) MRCP (UK) 1991. Dir. & Vice-Pres. (Cardio. Therepu.Team). Specialty: Pharmaceutical Medicine. Prev: Sen. Clin. Research Phys. (Cardiopulm. & Anti-infec.) SmithKline Beecham Pharmaceut. Welwyn Garden City.; Cardiovasc. Research Phys. Glaxo Research & Developm.; SHO (Path. & Haemat.) Ashford Hosp. Middlx., Gp. Dir. Cardiovasc. Clin. Developm. SmithKline Beecham Pharmaceut. Harlow.

NATHWANI, Amit Chunilal The Coppice, Kingfisher Lyre, Loudwater, Rickmansworth WD3 4ET — MB ChB Aberd. 1984 (Univ. Aberd.) MRCP (UK) 1988; MRCPath 1995.

NATHWANI, Deepak Chandrakant 7A High Worple, Rayners Lane, Harrow HA2 9SJ — MB ChB Dundee 1987; FRCA 1994. Sen. Regist. (Anaesth. & IC) The Roy. Free Hosp. Rotat. Lond. Specialty: Anaesth. Prev: Sen. Regist. (Anaesth. & IC) The Nat. Hosp. for Nerv. Dis.s & Neurosurg. Lond.; Lect. Hon. Sen. Regist. (Anaesth.) Northwick Pk. & St. Marks Hosp. Harrow.

NATHWANI, Dilip Infection and Immunodeficiency Unit, Dundee Teaching Hospitals, Dundee DD3 8EA Tel: 01382 660111 Fax: 01382 816178; 3 William Street, Carnoustie DD7 6DG Email: nathwani@globalnet.co.uk — MB ChB Aberd. 1984; MRCP (UK) 1988; DTM & H RCP Lond. 1992; FRCP Ed. 1995. Cons. Phys. (Infec.) & Hon. Sen. Lect. (Med.) Univ. Dundee Med. Sch.; Edr. in Chief CME Bull.-Infec. Dis. & Trop. Med.; Sec. Specialist Advis. Comm. for Train. in Infect Dis. & Trop. Med. Specialty: Infec. Dis. Socs: Brit. Soc. Study of Infec.; Brit. Soc. Antimicrob. Chemother. Prev: Edr. Jl. Antimicrobial Chemother.

NATHWANI, Dinesh Kantilal 54 Kingsbridge Crescent, Southall UB1 2DL — MB ChB Sheff. 1991; FRCS Irel. 1996. Specialist Regist. (Orthop. & Trauma Surg.) Roy. Liverp. Univ. Hosp. Specialty: Orthop.

NATHWANI, Nahendra 2 Bayons Avenue, Scartho, Grimsby DN33 3LN Tel: 01472 750143 — MB BS Calcutta 1975.

NATIN, Daniel Joseph Mary Warwick Hospital, Department of Genitourinary Medicine, Lakin Road, Warwick CV34 5BW Tel: 01926 495321 Ext: 4405 Fax: 01926 482638 — MB BCh BAO NUI 1982; LRCPI, LRCSI 1982; MRCPI 1988. Cons. Phys. Genitourin. Med. & HIV Med. Specialty: Genitourinary Medicine; HIV Med. Socs: Brit. Assn. Of Sexual Health & HIV. Prev: Sen. Regist. (Genitourin. Med.) N. Staffs. Hosp. Centre Stoke-on-Trent.

NATION, Caroline Barbara May 63 Shortwood Main Road, Mangotsfield, Bristol BS16 9NQ — MB ChB Bristol 1996. VTS (Gen. Pract.) Univ. Bristol. Specialty: Gen. Pract.

NATKUNARAJAH, Sarathadevi 1 Old Orchard Close, Barnet EN4 0ND — MB BS Sri Lanka 1974; MRCS Eng. LRCP Lond. 1984; FFA RCSI 1984. Specialty: Anaesth.

NATKUNARAJAH, Sellathurai 1 Old Orchard Close, Barnet EN4 0ND — MB BS Sri Lanka 1973; MRCS Eng. LRCP Lond. 1983.

NATORFF, Benona Lillian Consultant in Pharmaceutical Medicine, 28 Coventh Close, Sunningdale, Ascot SL5 0NR Tel: 01344 624746 Mob: 07770942819 Fax: 01344 875060; 28 Coworth Close, Sunningdale, Ascot SL5 0NR Tel: 01344 624746 Fax: 01344 875060 — Lekarz Warsaw 1973 (Warsaw Med. Acad., Poland) Con. Pharm. Med.; Clin. Research Off. Centr. & E. Europ. Specialty: Pharmaceutical Medicine. Socs: Brit. Assn. Psychopharmacol.; Fac. Pharmaceut. Med. RCP (UK); Drug Informat. Assn. Prev: Med. Dir. Glaxo E. Europe Glaxo. Gp. Research Stockley Pk.; Clin. Research Phys. CNS Lilly Research Centre Windlesham; Clin. Research Fell. Human Psychopharm. Unit Med. Coll. St. Bart. & Roy. Lond. Med. Coll.

NATRAJAN, Krishnamoorthy 46 Abbotts Walk, Fleetwood FY7 6QG; 57 The Esplanade, Fleetwood FY7 6QE — MB BS Madras 1971; FFA RCS Eng. 1978. Cons. (Cardiothoracic Anaesth.) S. Cleveland Hosp. Middlesbrough; Clin. Dir. Cardiothoracic IC S. Cleveland Hosp. Middlesbrough. Specialty: Anaesth. Prev: Cons. Cardiothoracic Anaesth. Vict. Hosp. Blackpool; Sen. Regist. Qu. Eliz. Hosp. Birm. & Birm. Childr. Hosp.; Regist. (Anaesth.) N. Staffs Roy. Infirm. Stoke-on-Trent.

NATT, Antony Leo St Lawrence Road Doctors Surgery, 17-19 St. Lawrence Road, North Wingfield, Chesterfield S42 5LH Tel: 01246 851029 — MB BS Lond. 1978 (St Bartholomew's) MRCS Eng. LRCP Lond. 1978; MRCP (UK) 1982; DMedRehab RCP Lond. 1983; DRCOG 1984; DCH RCP Lond. 1985. Prev: Clin. Asst. (Rheum.) N. Derbysh. Dist. Gen. Hosp.

NATTRASS, John James (retired) 20 Landmere Grove, Lincoln LN6 0PD Tel: 01522 684545 — MB ChB Manch. 1959; DObst. RCOG 1961. Prev: GP Lincoln.

NATTRASS, Malcolm Selly Oak Hospital, Raddlebarn Road, Birmingham B29 6JD Tel: 0121 627 1627 Fax: 0121 627 8758 — BSc Leeds 1967; MB ChB Leeds 1970; MRCP (UK) 1974; PhD Soton 1982; FRCP Lond. 1987; FRCPath 1993. Cons. Phys. Univ. Hosp. Birm. NHS Trust. Specialty: Gen. Med.; Diabetes. Prev: Lect. (Chem. Path. & Human Metab.) Soton. Univ.

NATUCCI, Matteo Ovarian Scanning Clinic, 7th Floor, New World Block, Kings Cross Hospital, Denmark Hill, London SE5 9RS — State Exam Pavia 1991.

NATUSCH, Douglas Ian Torbay Hospital, Lawes Bridge, Torquay TQ2 7AA — MB ChB Manch. 1990; BSc (Med. Sci.) St Andrews 1987; MSc (Pain Management) University of Wales College of Medicine 2001. Cons. (Anaes & Pain Manag.) Torbay Hosp. Torquay. Specialty: Anaesth. Socs: Pain. Soc; Int. Assoc. Study of Pain; Assoc. Anaes.

NAUDEER, Sarah Fatimah Mariam 18 Carmalt Gardens, London SW15 6NE — MB BS Lond. 1993.

NAUGHTON, Anthony The Thornton Practice, Church Road, Thornton-Cleveleys FY5 2TZ Tel: 01253 827231 Fax: 01253 863478 — MB ChB Manch. 1989.

NAUGHTON, Carol Ann The Surgery, Heywood, Lodway Gdns, Pill, Bristol BS20 0DN Tel: 01275 372105 Fax: 01275 373879 — MB ChB Bristol 1978; MRCP (UK) 1981; DRCOG 1985; MRCGP 1986.

NAUGHTON, Mary Deidre Adcote House, Columbia Road, Oxton, Birkenhead CH43 6TU Tel: 0151 670 0031 Fax: 0151 670 6031 — MB BCh BAO NUI 1985; MRCPsych 1990. Cons. Child & Adolesc. Psychiat. Specialty: Child & Adolesc. Psychiat. Prev: Lect. (Child & Adolesc. Psychiat.) Univ. Liverp.; Regist. St. Finans Hosp. Killarney Eire; Regist. Roy. Hosp. Sick Childr. Yorkhill Glas.

NAUGHTON, Michael Anthony Department of Rheumatology, Ealing Hospital, Uxbridge Road, Southall UB1 3HW — MB BCh BAO NUI 1986 (Univ. Coll. Dub. Med. Sch.) MRCPI 1988; PhD Lond. 1997. Cons. Rheumat. Ealing Hosp.; Hon. Sen. Lect. Imperial Coll. Sc. Med. Hammersmith. Specialty: Rheumatol.; Gen. Med. Prev: Sen. Regist. (Rheum.) Char. Cross Hosp. Lond.; ARC Research Fell. Roy. Postgrad. Med. Sch. Lond.; Regist. (Rheum.) Univ. Hosp. Wales Cardiff.

NAUGHTON, Pauline Elizabeth Medical Services Examination Centre, Disability Benifit Centre, Fireways Complex, Islington Road, Middleway, Birmingham B15 1UT — MB BS Lond. 1981 (Char. Cross) DRCOG 1984; MRCGP 1986; MBA (Pub. Serv.) Birm. 1995. Disabil. Analyst. Med. Serv.s Exam. Centre, Fireways Complex. Specialty: Disabil. Med. Prev: Med. Off. DSS Edgbaston.; GP BRd.meadow; Police Surg. W. Midl.

NAUGHTON-DOE, Patrick Edward George Health Centre, Marmaduke Street, Hessle Road, Hull HU3 3BH Tel: 01482 327708 Fax: 01482 210250; 44 Wellesley Avenue, Beverley High Road, Hull HU6 7LW — MB ChB Leic. 1985. SHO (Gen. Med.) Leicester HA (T). Prev: Ho. Off. (Gen. Med./Cardiol.) & Ho. Off. (Gen. Surg./Neurosurg.) Hull HA.

NAUMANN, Ulrike The Surgery, Patwell Lane, Bruton BA10 0EG Tel: 01749 812310 Fax: 01749 812938 Email: ulrike.naumann@brutonsurgery.nhs.uk — State Exam Erlangen 1986; MD (Surg.) Erlangen; Approbation Erlangen 1986; Dobst RCOG 1989; MRCGP exam (not membership) 1990. GP.

NAUNTON, Andrew — MB ChB Manch. 1974; FFA RCS Eng. 1979. Specialty: Anaesth.

NAUNTON, William Johnson 182 Newmarket Road, Norwich NR4 6AR Tel: 01603 452035 — MRCS Eng. LRCP Lond. 1943 (Cambs. & Manch.) MA, MB BChir Camb. 1945; DOMS Eng. 1948. Specialty: Ophth. Prev: Emerit. Sen. Cons. Ophth. Surg. United Norwich Hosps.; Sen. Regist. Dept. Ophth. Univ. Manch.; Temp. Surg. Lt. RNVR.

NAUNTON MORGAN, Jonathan Clifford Bodnant Surgery, Menai Avenue, Bangor LL57 2HH Tel: 01248 364567 Fax: 01248 370654 — MB BS Lond. 1990.

NAUNTON MORGAN, Thomas Clifford Department of Diagnostic Radiology, West Middlesex University Hospital, Twickenham Road, Isleworth TW7 6AF Tel: 020 8565 5865 Fax: 020 8565 5251; 3 Campion Road, Putney, London SW15 6NN Tel: 020 8789 5211 — MB BS Lond. 1973 (St. Bart.) MRCS Eng. LRCP Lond. 1973; FRCS Eng. 1979; FRCR 1987. Cons. Radiol. W. Middlx. Univ. Hosp. Isleworth; Cons. Radiol. Stamford Hosp.; Hon. Cons. Radiol. Princess Margt. Hosp. Windsor. Specialty: Radiol. Socs: BMA; Worshipful Co. Barbers. Prev: Sen. Regist. (Radiol.) Char. Cross Hosp. Lond.; Regist. (Radiol.) Westm. Hosp. Lond.; Regist. (Surg.) Lond. Hosp. & Ipswich Hosp.

NAUTH-MISIR, Mr Rohan Ravindra University College London Hospitals NHS Trust, The Institute of Urology, 48 Riding House St., London W1P 7PN Tel: 020 7636 8333 Fax: 020 7637 7076 Email: rohan.nauth@ucl.ac.uk — MB BS Lond. 1983 (Lond. Hosp.) BSc (Hons.) (Pharmacol.) Lond. 1980, MB BS 1983; FRCS Eng. 1987; FRCS (Urol.) 1995. Cons. (Urol. & Transp. Surg.) Univ. Coll. Lond. Hosp. Trust Lond.; Hon. Sen. Lect. (Urol.) Inst. Urol. Lond. Specialty: Urol. Socs: Brit. Assn. Urol. Surg.; Brit Transpl. Soc.

NAUTH-MISIR, Tikai Narendra (retired) Owlets, The Glade, Hutton Mount, Brentwood CM13 2JL Tel: 01277 222443 — (Lond. Hosp) MRCS Eng. LRCP Lond. 1940; MB BS Lond. 1941; DCH Eng. 1947; FRCP Lond. 1973, M 1949. Prev: Cons. Paediatr. OldCh. Hosp. Romford & Harold Wood Hosp.

NAVA, Gillian Manor Farm House, Stratford Road, Honeybourne, Evesham WR11 5PP — MB ChB Birm. 1976; MRCOG 1983.

NAVA, Peter Linton The Health Centre, High Street, Bidford-on-Avon, Alcester B50 4BQ Tel: 01789 773372 Fax: 01789 490380 — MB ChB Birm. 1981; PhD Birm. 1981, BSc (Hons.) 1974, MB ChB 1981; MRCGP 1986.

NAVAMANI, Alexander Sharon Mayfield Surgery, 246 Roehampton Lane, Roehampton, London SW15 4AA Tel: 020 8780 5770; 14 Queen's Court, Queen's Road, Richmond TW10 6LA Tel: 020 8332 6489 — MB BS Lond. 1994 (St. Bartholomew's Hospital Medical College) MRCGP; DRCOG 1997. GP Regist. Specialty: Gen. Pract.

NAVAMANI, Sterlin Bretton Health Centre, Rightwell, Bretton, Peterborough PE3 8DT Tel: 01733 264506 Fax: 01733 266728 — MB BS Madras 1967 (Madurai Med. Coll.) DLO Madurai 1970.

NAVAN EETHA RAJAH, Prithiva 45 Granville Park W., Aughton, Ormskirk L39 5HS — MB ChB Liverp. 1992; MRCP UK 1997.

NAVANEETHAM, Neena George Eliot Hospital, Nuneaton Tel: 02476 865013 Email: neena.navaneetham@geh.nhs.uk — MB BS Bangalore 1984; MSc Birmingham; MRCOG India 1994. Cons., Obst. & Gyn., Geo. Eliot Hosp., Nuneaton; Clinical Director. Specialty: Obst. & Gyn. Socs: BMA; ICS.

NAVANEETHARAJA, Nadarajah Ethelbert Gardens Surgery, 63-65 Ethelbert Gardens, Ilford IG2 6UW Tel: 020 8550 3740 Fax: 020 8550 4300 — MB BS Colombo 1981; MB BS Colombo 1981.

NAVANEETHARAJAH, Beatrice Mary Jessie 45 Granville Park W., Aughton, Ormskirk L39 5HS — MB BS Ceylon 1962; DPH Liverp. 1972.

NAVANEETHARAJAH, Navaratnam Britonside Avenue Surgery, 41 Britonside Avenue, Southdene, Kirkby, Liverpool L32 6RZ Tel: 0151 546 2409 Fax: 0151 548 1941 — MB BS Ceylon 1963.

NAVANI, L High Street Surgery, 190 High Street, Feltham TW13 4HY Tel: 020 8751 3404 Fax: 020 8890 4858 — MB BS Rajasthan 1969; MB BS Rajasthan 1969.

NAVAPURKAR, Vilas Umesh 7 Russell Road, Moor Park, Northwood HA6 2LJ — MB ChB Dundee 1986; DA (UK) 1988; FRCA 1992. Sen. Regist. (Anaesth.) Addenbrooke's NHS Trust Camb. Specialty: Anaesth. Socs: Intens. Care Soc.; Assn. Anaesth. Prev: Research Fell. (Clin. Intens. Care) Camb.; Regist. (Anaesth.) Trent RHA; SHO (Neonat. & Adult Intens. Care) Camb.

NAVARATNAM, Anton Elmo Devanayagam (retired) 28 Chestnut Close, Duffield Hall, Duffield, Derby DE56 4HD — MB BS Ceylon 1956; MRCP Ed. 1969; MRCP (U.K.) 1969; FRCP Lond. 1980. Mem. Indep. Tribunal. Serv. Prev: Cons. Dermat. Derbysh. Gp. Hosps. Derby.

NAVARATNAM, Manchula 8 Valley Park, Hermitage Park, Wrexham LL13 7GW — MB ChB Ed. 1997.

NAVARATNAM, Romesh Marino 28 Chestnut Close, Duffield, Derby DE56 4HD; 66 Nursey Road, Pinner, Harrow HA5 2AR — BM BS Nottm. 1990; BmedSci (Hons) Nottm 1988; FRCS (Lond) 1994; MSC (Lond) 1998. Specialist Regist. Clin. Research Fell. Roy. Free Hosp. Lond. NW3. Specialty: Gen. Surg.

NAVARATNAM, Seeniar 5 Windy Hill, Hutton, Brentwood CM13 2HF Tel: 01277 223981 — MB BS Ceylon 1964 (Colombo) DCH Eng. 1969; FRCP Lond. 1971; DPhysMed Eng. 1971. Honary Cons. Rheumatologist, Roy. Free Hosp. Med. Sch., Hampstead, Lond.; Cons. Essex Nuffield Hosp Brentwood; BUPA Hartswood

Hosp. Brentwood; Chelsfield Pk. Hosp. Orpington Kent. Specialty: Rehabil. Med.; Rheumatol. Socs: Fell. Roy. Soc. Med.; Brit. Soc. Rheum. & BMA. Prev: Sen. Regist. Dept. Rheum. & Rehabil. Univ. Coll. Hosp. Lond.; Regist. Dept. Rheum. & Rehabil. Roy. Free Hosp. Lond.; SHO (Gen. Med.) Tottenham Gp. Hosps.

NAVARATNAM, Visvanathan (retired) University, School of Anatomy, Downing Street, Cambridge CB2 3DZ Tel: 01223 333750 Fax: 01223 333786; 93 Gilbert Road, Cambridge CB4 3NZ — (Colombo) MB BS Ceylon 1957; PhD Camb. 1964. Univ. Lect. (Anat.) & Dir. Med. Studies Christ's Coll. Camb. Prev: Ho. Off. Gen. Hosp. Kandy, Ceylon.

NAVARATNAM, Yogaranjitham 3 Kilmaine Drive, Ladybridge, Bolton BL3 4RU — MB BS Sri Lanka 1975; LRCP LRCS Ed. LRCPS Glas. 1988.

NAVARATNARAJAH, Grace Chandraranee Medical Centre, Woodfield Road, London W9; 69 Hayes Lane, Kenley CR8 5JR Tel: 020 8668 5461 — MB BS Ceylon 1967. Clin. Med. Off. (Community Paediat.) Pk. Side AHA. Prev: SHO Rotat. (Psychiat.) St. Bart. Hosp. Lond.

NAVARATNARAJAH, Murugesu Anaesthetic Department, May Day Hospital, Croydon — MB BS Ceylon 1973; MRCS Eng. LRCP Lond. 1979; FFA RCS Lond. 1980. Cons. (Anaesth.) Croydon Dist. HA; Sen. Regist. (Anaesth.) (Rotat.) Roy. Free Hosp. Lond., Northwick Pk. Hosp. & Clin. Research Centre Harrow. Specialty: Anaesth. Socs: Croydon Med Soc. Prev: Regist. (Anaesth.) Whittington Hosp. & Whipps Cross Hosp. Lond.

NAVARATNE, Lesley Amy 9 Birch Grove, Pyrford, Woking GU22 8NB — MB BS Lond. 1992 (The London Hospital Medical College) MRCP Lond. 1998. Specialty: Genitourinary Medicine; HIV Med.

NAVARATNE, Mohottalage Flat 7,Rowan House, Oakapple Lane, Maidstone ME16 9QQ — LRCP LRCS Ed. 1987; LRCP LRCS Ed. LRCPS Glas. 1987.

NAVARRO-WEITZEL, Ilona Claudia Royal London Hospital, Department of Anaesthetics, Whitechapel, London E1 1BB Tel: 020 7377 7700; 55 Highbury New Park, Basement Flat, London N5 2ET Tel: 020 7226 5415 — State Exam Med Freiburg 1992. SHO (Cardiothoracic Surg.) Roy. Brompton Hosp. Lond. Prev: SHO (A & E) St Bart. Hosp. Lond.

NAVAS, Frank (retired) Alviento, Gorsewood Drive, Hakin, Milford Haven SA73 3EP Tel: 01646 695804 — (Cardiff) MB BCh Wales 1958; DObst RCOG 1963. Prev: SHO (O & G) H.M. Stanley Hosp. St. Asaph.

NAVE, Elmar Ward Medical Centre, Medomsley Road, Consett DH8 5HR Tel: 01207 502266 Fax: 01207 506077; Haining Bank, Strathmore Road, Rowlands Gill NE39 1JA Tel: 01207 542678 — MB BS Durh. 1960. Specialty: Gen. Pract.

NAVEN, Tom Oaks Medical Centre, 1 Paisley Road, Barrhead G78 1HG Tel: 0141 580 1002; 8a Glen Avenue, Uplawmoor, Glasgow G78 4DF Tel: 01505 850605 — MB BCh BAO NUI 1976 (Galway, Ireland) MRCGP 1991. GP Glas.

NAVEY, Fleur Louise — MB BS Lond. 1982 (Lond. Hosp.) MRCGP 1988; Cert. Family Plann. JCC 1988. Locum GP (Freelance); Mem. A & E Primary Care Team St. Mary's Hosp. Lond.; Health Screening Doctor Clementine Churchill Hosp. (p/t). Socs: BMA; Roy. Coll. Gen. Pract. Prev: Princip. GP The Gr. Health Centre Lond.; SHO (Infec. Dis.) St. Ann's Hosp. Tottenham; Ho. Off. The Lond. Hosp. Mile End.

NAVIN, William Patrick 57 Walsgrave Road, Gosford Green, Coventry CV2 4HF Tel: 024 76 222271 — MB BCh BAO NUI 1940.

NAWAL, Hari Charan Singh Goldington Road Surgery, 12 Goldington Road, Bedford MK40 3NE Tel: 01234 352493 — MB BS Vikram 1962; DPM London 1974; DPM Dublin 1974.

NAWARSKI, Bernard John 14 Highfield Crescent, Northwood HA6 1EZ — MB BS Lond. 1996.

NAWAZ, Mohamed 34 Rennishaw Way, Links View, Northampton NN2 7NE — MB BS Ceylon 1964 (Colombo) Clin. Asst. (Psychogeriat.) Northampton HA. Prev: Med. Off. Gen. Hosp. Kurunagala, Sri Lanka; Ho. Off. Govt. Hosp. Matale, Sri Lanka & Govt. Hosp. Avissawella, Sri; Lanka.

NAWAZ, Mohammad 14 Park Lane, Aberdare CF44 8HN — MB BS Peshawar 1966.

NAWAZ, Rashad Mehmood 25 Wingfield Mount, Bradford BD3 0AG — MB ChB Manch. 1992.

NAWAZ, Mr Shah Clinical Sciences Centre, Hermes Road, Northern General Hospital, Sheffield S5 7AU Tel: 0114 271 4648 Email: s.nawaz@sheffield.ac.uk; 11 Ferrars Drive, Sheffield S9 1WU Tel: 0114 244 6069 — MB ChB Aberd. 1991; FRCS 1995. Lect. Univ. of Sheff. Specialty: Gen. Surg.; Vasc. Med. Socs: Rouceaux Club; SRS. Prev: SHO (Surg.) York. Dist. Hosp.

NAWAZ, Shahid 1 St Andrews Drive, Alwoodley, Leeds LS17 7TR — MB BS Punjab 1972 (King Edwd. Med. Coll. Lahore) MB BS Punjab (Pakistan) 1972; MRCPI 1977; MRCP (UK) 1977; LMSSA Lond. 1977.

NAWAZ, Shokat 87 St Lawrence Road, Sheffield S9 1SB — MB ChB Sheff. 1998.

NAWIMANA, Thamara — MB BS Colombo 1991. Clin. Fell. (Med. Microbiol.) Frenchay Hosp. Bristol. Specialty: Med. Microbiol.

NAWROCKI, Albert Sharmont, Deepdene Avenue, Croydon Tel: 020 8688 3634 — MB ChB St. And. 1963; MRCGP 1977. Prev: Clin. Adviser (Rhuematol.) S.W. Thames Region; Clin. Asst. Roy. Marsden Hosp. Lond.; Resid. in Med. Mayo Clinic U.S.A.

NAWROCKI, Mr Jan Dominik Princess Royal Hospital, Lewes Road, Haywards Heath RH16 4EX Tel: 01444 441881 Fax: 01444 455895; Royal Sussex County Hospital, Brighton BN2 5BE Tel: 01273 696955 — MB BS Lond. 1985 (King's College London) FRCS Eng. 1989; MS Lond. 1995; FRCS (Urol.) 1996. Cons. Urol. Princess Roy. Heath & Roy. Sussex Co. Hosp. Brighton. Specialty: Urol. Prev: Sen. Regist. Urol., Guy's Hosp. Lond.; Regist. Urol. Inst. Urol., Middlx. Hosp. Lond.; Regist. Gen. Surg., King's Coll. Hosp.

NAWROOZ, Neamat Mohamad Jawad 7 Brookview, Fulwood, Preston PR2 8FG — MB ChB Basrah, Iraq 1979; DCH Glas. 1985. Staff Grade (Community Child Health) Blackburn Communicare NHS Trust. Specialty: Community Child Health.

NAY WIN, Dr 7 Langley Grove, New Malden KT3 3AL — MB BS Rangoon 1979; MRCP (UK) 1985; MRCPath 1992; FRCP (UK) 1996. Cons. Haemat. NBS, S. Thames Centre Lond. Specialty: Blood Transfus.

NAYAGAM, Andrew Thanaraj 93 Woodland Drive, Hove BN3 6DF Tel: 01273 501894 — MB BS Ceylon 1972; MRCS Eng. LRCP Lond. 1981; MRCP (UK) 1983; FRCP (UK) 1996. Cons. Genitourin. Med. Southlands Hosp. Shoreham. Specialty: Genitourinary Medicine. Socs: Med. Soc. Study VD; Brit. Soc. Of Colposcopy & Cervial Path.; BMA. Prev: Sen. Regist. (Genitourin. Med.) Univ. Coll. Hosp. Lond.; Regist. (Genitourin. Med.) Roy. Lond. Hosp.; Regist. (Dermat.) Hull Roy. Infirm.

NAYAGAM, Mr Selvadurai 30 Eshe Road N., Crosby, Liverpool L23 8UF Tel: 0151 924 3019 Fax: 0151 931 5405 — MB ChB Manch. 1984; BSc St. And. 1981; FRCS Ed. 1989; MCh (Orth.) Liverp. 1995; FRCS (Orth.) 1996. Cons. (Orthop. & Trauma Surg.) Roy. Liverp. Univ. Hosp. Roy. Liverp. Childr. Hosp. Specialty: Orthop. Socs: Fell. Roy. Soc. Med.; Brit. Limb Reconstruc. Soc.; Fell. BOA. Prev: Career Regist. (Orthop. Surg.) Mersy RHA; SHO (Orthop. & Gen. Surg.) Roy. Liverp. Hosp.; Sen. Resid. (Orthop. Surg.) Mass. Gen. Hosp. Boston, USA.

NAYAK, Baidya Nath Wigan Infirmary, Wigan Lane, Wigan WN1 Tel: 01942 244000; 71 Ormskirk Road, Knowsley, Prescot L34 8HB Tel: 0151 546 1151 — MB BS Calcutta 1962; MRCP (UK) 1971; FRCP Lond. 1994. Specialty: Care of the Elderly. Socs: BMA & Brit. Geriat. Soc. Prev: Cons. Phys. Med. for Elderly Leigh & Wigan Trust; Cons. Phys. Med. for Elderly St. Helens & Knowsley HA.

NAYAK, Geeta Prashant Roby Medical Centre, 70-72 Pilch Lane East, Roby, Liverpool L36 4NP Tel: 0151 449 1972 Fax: 0151 489 4020; 1 Calderfield Road, Calderstones, Liverpool L18 3HB Tel: 0151 722 8800 — MB BS Baroda 1972 (M.S. Univ. Med. Coll.) Princip. GP Roby. Prev: Regist. (Chest Med.) Liverp. AHA (T).

NAYANI, Guruprasada Rao 2 Solar Court, Great Linford, Milton Keynes MK14 5HD — MB BS Bombay 1969.

NAYANI, Salim Wellingborough Community Mental Health Team, The Redcliffe, 51 Hatton Park Road, Wellingborough NN8 5AH — MB BS Karachi 1977; MRCPsych 1985; MMedSc Leeds 1987. Cons. Psychiat. Northants. Healthcare NHS Trust. Specialty: Gen. Psychiat. Prev: Cons. Psychiat. Leicestersh. Ment. Health NHS Trust; Sen. Regist. (Psychiat.) Leicester Gen. Hosp.

NAYANI, Tanveer Husein 6 Colville Terrace, London W11 2BE — MB BS Lond. 1986.

NAYAR, Asha Woodley Health Centre, Hyde Road, Woodley, Stockport SK6 1ND Tel: 0161 494 0213 Fax: 0161 406 9231; 43

Winnington Road, Marple, Stockport SK6 6PT Tel: 0161 427 7181 — MB BS Rajasthan 1967 (S.M.S. Med. Coll. Jaipur) MSc Audiol. Med. Manch. 1992. SCMO Stockport AHA. Specialty: Community Child Health. Socs: Fac. Community Health. Prev: Clin. Med. Off. Stockport & Tameside AHA.

NAYAR, Janaky Kutty Newland Health Centre, 187 Cottingham Road, Hull HU5 2EG Tel: 01482 492219 Fax: 01482 441418 — MB BS Kerala 1970. GP Sen. Partner.

NAYAR, Omesh Kumar Uttoxeter Road Surgery, 669 Uttoxeter Road, Meir, Stoke-on-Trent ST3 5PZ Tel: 01782 313884; Langdale, 963 Lightwood Road, Lightwood, Stoke-on-Trent ST3 7NE Tel: 01782 392702 — MB BS Bombay 1961 (Grant Med. Coll.) DCH Eng. 1962; MRCGP 1976. Clin. Asst., Geriat.s, Longton Cottage Hosp., Stoke on Trent. Specialty: Paediat.; Dermat.; Diabetes.

NAYAR, Pritibala — MB BS Lond. 1997.

NAYAR, Rahul 336 Wilbraham Road, Manchester M21 0UX — MB ChB Manch. 1993.

NAYAR, Rosebind Noreen 49 Highfields, Llandaff, Cardiff CF5 2QB — MB BS Punjab 1961; DA 1964.

NAYAR, Vijay Krishan Bedford Road Surgery, 273 Bedford Road, Kempston, Bedford MK42 8QD Tel: 01234 852222 Fax: 01234 843558; 126 Putnoe Lane, Bedford MK41 8LA Tel: 01234 402998 — MB BS Lond. 1986 (Middlx. & Univ. Coll. Hosp.) BSc (Hons.) Lond. 1983; FP Cert 1989; DCH 1989; Cert. Family Plann. JCC 1989; MRCGP 1990; DRCOG 1990; ILTM 2001. Course Organiser Bedford GP VTS.

NAYEEM, Mr Nadeem Accident & Emergency Department, Lewisham Hospital, Lewisham High St., London SE13 6LH Tel: 0208 333 3060 Fax: 0208 333 3109 Email: nadeem.nayeem@uhl.nhs.uk — MB BS Karachi 1980; FRCS Ed. 1986. Cons. A & E Lewisham Hosp. Lond. Specialty: Accid. & Emerg. Socs: Brit. Assn. Accid. & Emerg. Med.; Roy. Soc. Med. Lond. Prev: Sen. Regist. (A & E) Guy's Hosp. Lond.; Regist. (A & E) Milton Keynes Gen. Hosp.; Regist. (Gen. Surg.) OldCh. Hosp. Romford.

NAYEEMUDDIN, Farzana Anjum 11 Bromsberrow Way, Stoke-on-Trent ST3 7UE Tel: 01782 388600 — MB ChB Leeds 1995. SHO (Med.) Stoke-on-Trent. Specialty: Rheumatol.

NAYLER, Lisa — MB BS Lond. 1998.

NAYLOR, Andrew Ian The Surgery, Ferry Road, Leverburgh, Isle of Harris HS5 3UA Tel: 01859 520278 Fax: 01859 520202; 18 Ferry Road, Leverburgh, Isle of Harris HS5 3UA Tel: 01859 520200 — MB BS Newc. 1985; DGM RCP Lond. 1989; MRCGP 1989. Specialty: Gen. Pract. Socs: BASICS; Brit. Geriat. Soc. Prev: Trainee GP Cleveland VTS.

NAYLOR, Andrew Mark Antony, Surg. Lt.-Cdr. RN Grove House Surgery, 80 Pryors Lane, Rose Green, Bognor Regis PO21 4JB Tel: 01243 265222/266413 Fax: 01243 268693 — MB BS Lond. 1985 (Guy's)

NAYLOR, Professor Andrew Ross Department of Surgery, Clinical Sciences Building, Leicester Royal Infirmary, Leicester LE1 5WW Tel: 0116 252 3252 Fax: 0116 252 3179; 9 Dalby Avenue, Bushby, Leicester LE7 9RE Tel: 0116 241 7318 — MB ChB Aberd. 1981 (Aberdeen) FRCS Ed. 1986; MD Aberd. 1990; FRCS Eng. 1996. Prof. Vasc. Surg., Leicester Univ.; Hon. Sen. Lect. (Surg.) Leicester Univ. Specialty: Surgery, Vascular. Socs: Vasc. Surgic. Soc.; Eur. Vasc. Soc. Prev: Cons. Surg. Vasc. Leicester Roy. Infirm.; Cons. Surg. Vasc. Unit Aberd. Roy. Infirm.; Lect. (Surg.) Leicester Univ.

NAYLOR, Arthur (retired) Moat Cottage, Midgley Lane, Goldsborough, Knaresborough HG5 8NN Tel: 01423 865775 — MB ChB Sheff. 1937; FRCS Ed. 1939; MSc Sheff. 1935, BSc (Hons.) 1934. MD 1989, ChM 1940; FRCS Eng. 1944. Hon. Cons. Surg. Orthop. Roy. Infirm. Bradford, Bradford Hosp., Woodlands Orthop. Hosp. Rawdon & St. Luke's Hosp. Bradford. Prev: Temp. Maj. RAMC.

NAYLOR, Carolyn Ruth Yew Tree Medical Centre, 100 Yew Tree Lane, Solihull B91 2RA Tel: 0121 705 8787 Fax: 0121 709 0240 — MB ChB Birm. 1991; ChB Birm. 1991.

NAYLOR, Mr Christopher Hardy The Portland Hospital, 212-214 Great Portland Street, London W1W 5QN Tel: 020 8905 2412 Fax: 020 8905 2412 Email: dr@nayor.demon.co.uk; 35 Chiswick Quay, Hartington Road, London W4 3UR Tel: 020 8995 8701 Fax: 020 8995 1233 Email: dr@naylor0.demon.co.uk — MB BCh Wales 1958 (Cardiff) FRCOG 1981, M 1968, DObst. 1961. Cons. O & G Centr. Middlx. Hosp. Lond.; Hon. Sen. Lect. Univ. Coll. Hosp., Lond. Specialty: Obst. & Gyn. Socs: Indep. Doctors Forum. Prev: Sen. Regist. Qu. Charlotte's Hosp. & Chelsea Hosp. Wom. Lond.; Regist. King's Coll. Hosp. Lond.; Ho. Off. Matern. Hosp. Cardiff.

NAYLOR, Doris Helen Ruth 86 Blockley Road, Sudbury Court, Wembley HA0 3LW Tel: 020 8904 3073 — MB ChB Liverp. 1964; DA Eng. 1973. Clin. Asst. Anaesth. Centr. Middlx. Hosp. Lond. Prev: Ho. Surg. & Ho. Phys. Roy. S. Hosp. Liverp.; SHO (Anaesth.) Nottm. City Hosp.; Clin. Asst. Anaesth. Northwick Pk. Hosp.

NAYLOR, Edwin Gilderdale (retired) 18 Little Dene Copse, Pennington, Lymington SO41 8EW Tel: 01590 72021 — MB ChB St. And. 1945.

NAYLOR, Emma Louise 16 The Paddocks, Nuthall, Nottingham NG16 1DR — MB ChB Sheff. 1998.

NAYLOR, Frances Louise Pelaw Medical Practice, 7&8 Croxdale Terrace, Pelaw, Gateshead NE10 0RR; 83 St. Marys Field, Morpeth NE61 2QQ — MB BS Newc. 1991; MRCGP; DRCOG 1994; DFFP 1996. GP Princip. 6/9 Time. Socs: MRCGP; Dip. Roy. Coll. Obs & Gyn.; Dip. Fac. Fam. Plan. & Repro. Health c/o RCOG.

NAYLOR, Mr Gerald Victoria Hospital, Whinney Heys Road, Blackpool FY3 8NR Tel: 01253 303845 Fax: 02153 306743 Email: mr.naylor@exch.buh-tr.nwest.nhs.uk — MB ChB Leeds 1981; FRCS Ed. 1986; FRCOphth 1989. Cons. Ophth. Blackpool. Vict. Hosp. Specialty: Ophth. Socs: Europ. Soc. Of Cataract & Refractive Surd.; Mem. Oxf. Ophthalmological Congr. Prev: Sen. Regist. (Ophth.) Birm. & Midl. Eye Hosp.

NAYLOR, Graham John (retired) Little Acres, Baltic Road, Kirk Michael IM6 1EF Tel: 01624 878377 — MB ChB Sheff. 1962; DPM Ed. & Glas. 1967; FRCPsych 1976, M 1970; BSc Sheff. 1965, MD 1970. Prev: Cons. Psychiat. Tayside HB.

NAYLOR, Gregory Michael Plumtree House, Prescot Road, Aughton, Ormskirk L39 6TA — MB ChB Sheff. 1990.

NAYLOR, Heather Ann Doctors Surgery, Hinnings Road, Distington, Workington CA14 5UR Tel: 01946 830207 — MB BS Newc. 1989; DRCOG 1992; MRCGP 1993. Prev: SHO (Elderly Care) W. Cumbld. Hosp. Whitehaven; SHO (O & G) N. Tyneside Hosp. N. Shields.

NAYLOR, Mr Henry Gordon (retired) Timbers, 63 Ardleigh Green Road, Hornchurch RM11 2JZ Tel: 01708 449524 Fax: 01708 453488 — (Roy. Free) MB BS Lond. 1960; MRCS Eng. LRCP Lond. 1960; FRCS Eng. 1967. Prev: Cons. Surg. Basildon & Thurrock Gen. Hosps. NHS Trust.

NAYLOR, Howard Christopher — MB ChB Bristol 1979; FFA RCS Eng. 1984. Cons. Anaesth. Southend HA. Specialty: Anaesth. Prev: Sen. Regist. (Anaesth.) Mersey RHA.

NAYLOR, Jane Mary Pool Health Centre, Station Road, Pool, Redruth TR15 3DU Tel: 01209 717471; 33 Higher Penponds, Camborne TR14 0QG — BM BS Nottm. 1986; BMedSci (Hons.) Nottm. 1984. Prev: Trainee GP Pool Health Centre Cornw.; SHO (O & G) Redruth & Truro Hosp.; SHO (A & E) Derbysh. Roy. Infirm.

NAYLOR, Janet Sarah 2 Monarch Close, Locks Heath, Southampton SO31 6UG — BM Soton. 1992.

NAYLOR, John Richard Medicine For The Elderly, St Luke's Hospital, Blackmoorfoot Road, Huddersfield HD4 5RQ — MB ChB Leeds 1985; MRCP (UK) 1988.

NAYLOR, Karen Jacqueline 32 Mandeville Close, Weymouth DT4 9HP — BM Soton. 1989.

NAYLOR, Kathryn Phyllis Ashworth Hospital, Maghull, Liverpool L31 1HW Tel: 0151 473 0303 — MB ChB Liverp. 1991. Specialty: Forens. Psychiat.

NAYLOR, Kevin Michael Thomas 5 Carlton Road, Worsley, Manchester M28 7TT — MB ChB Sheff. 1985; MRCGP 1989.

NAYLOR, Professor Paul Francis Dorian Manor Park, Broadway, Sidmouth EX10 8HS Tel: 01395 516131 — MB BChir Camb. 1948 (Camb. & St. Thos) MD Camb. 1954, MA 1948. Emerit. Prof. Dermat. Univ. Lond.; Hon. Cons. Dermat. St. Thos. Hosp. Lond. Specialty: Dermat. Socs: Brit. Assn. Dermat. Prev: Prof. Dermat. St. Thos. Hosp. Med. Sch. Lond.; Hon. Cons. St. Thos. Hosp. Lond.; Adviser (Clin. Studies) St. Thos. Hosp. Med. Sch. Lond.

NAYLOR, Roger 18 Lakeside, Wickham Road, Beckenham BR3 6LX — MB BS Lond. 1956; MRCP Lond. 1968. Cons. Phys. (Geriat. Med.) Mayday Healthcare Croydon. Specialty: Care of the Elderly. Prev: Cons. Phys. Geriat. Med. Bromley HA.; Sen. Regist. (Geriat. Med.) Guy's Hosp. Lond.

NAYLOR, Sally Elizabeth Shay Lane Medical Centre, Shay Lane, Hale Barns WA15 8NZ Tel: 0161 980 3835 Fax: 0161 980 9215; 12 Kensington Gardens, Hale, Altrincham WA15 9DP Tel: 0161 904 8921 Fax: 0161 904 8921 — MB ChB Liverp. 1988; DRCOG 1991; MRCGP 1995. Specialty: Gen. Pract.

NAYLOR, Stanley (retired) 99 Windleshaw Road, St Helens WA10 6TR Tel: 01744 26997; 377 Gathurst Road, Orrell, Wigan WN5 0LL Tel: 01942 226938 — (Liverp.) BSc Lond. 1953; MB ChB Liverp. 1953; DPH 1958. Prev: Clin. Med. Off. Wigan AHA.

NAYLOR, Steven Roy Trengweath Hospital, Penryn St., Redruth TR15 2SP — BM BS Nottm. 1983; BMedSci (Hons.) Nottm. 1981; DGM RCP Lond. 1986; DRCOG 1987; MRCGP 1987; MRCPsych 1998. Cons. (Psychiat.) Cornw. Partnership Trust. Specialty: Gen. Psychiat. Prev: GP Camborne Cornw.

NAYLOR, Ursula Veronica Peggy Birchwood, 39 Tranby Lane, Swanland, North Ferriby HU14 3NE — MB ChB Liverp. 1962; DPM Eng. 1969. Cons. Psychiat. Broadgate Hosp. Specialty: Gen. Psychiat. Socs: Roy. Med.-Psych. Assn. Prev: Sen. Regist. (Psychiat.) & Med. Asst. Broadgate Hosp.; Regist. Psychiat. United Leeds Hosps.

NAYLOR, William Geoffrey Knowle Surgery, 1500 Warwick Road, Knowle, Solihull B93 9LE Tel: 01564 772010 — MB ChB Birm. 1990; BSc 1989; ChB Birm. 1990; MRCGP 1995. G P Princ. (F/T). Specialty: Gen. Pract. Prev: Med. Asst. Solihull Hosp.

NAYSMITH, Anne Pembridge Palliative Care Centre, St. Charles Hospital, Exmoor St., London W10 6DZ Tel: 020 8962 4405 Fax: 020 8962 4407 — MB ChB Ed. 1973; MRCP (UK) 1976; FRCP Ed. 1991. Cons. Palliat. Med. St Chas. Hosp. Specialty: Palliat. Med. Socs: Assn. Palliat. Med. Prev: Med. Dir. Parkside Health NHS Trust.

NAYSMITH, Cumming 77 Eastgate Street, Cowbridge CF71 7AA — MB ChB Glas. 1942; BSc Glas. 1939, MB ChB 1942.

NAYSMITH, James Hall (retired) 7 Berrymead Road, Cyncoed, Cardiff CF23 6QA Tel: 029 2075 1754; 22 Mead Lane, Thurlestone, Kingsbridge TQ7 3PB Tel: 01548 560575 — MB BCh Wales 1952 (Cardiff) BSc Wales 1948; DObst RCOG 1956; MRCGP 1964.

NAYSMITH, Margaret Caroline Southmead Health Centre, Ullswater Road, Bristol BS10 6DF Tel: 0117 950 7150 Fax: 0117 959 1110; 9 Belvoir Road, Bristol BS6 5DG Tel: 0117 942 2775 — MB ChB Bristol 1983; BSc Ed. 1965; MSc Leic. 1967; DRCOG 1987; MRCGP 1987.

NAYYAR, Nadim Ahmed 6 Helensburgh Close, Barnsley S75 2EU Tel: 01226 730000; 51 Green Hey, Much Hoole, Preston PR4 4QH — MB ChB Leic. 1991.

NAZ, Evelyn Mary Burley Street Surgery, Burley Street, Elland HX5 0AQ Tel: 01422 372057 Fax: 01422 311563 — MB ChB Ed. 1969; DObst RCOG 1973.

NAZ, Falak Burley Street Surgery, Burley Street, Elland HX5 0AQ Tel: 01422 372057 Fax: 01422 311563 — MB BS Peshawar 1965 (Khyber Med. Coll.)

NAZARE, Joao Caetano Felix 46 Arundel Drive, Worcester WR5 2HU — MB BS Bombay 1973.

NAZARETH, Hubert Anthony Agnelo Waterloo Surgery, 617 Wakefield Road, Waterloo, Huddersfield HD5 9XP Tel: 01484 531461; 6 School Hill, Kirkburton, Huddersfield HD8 0SG Tel: 01484 602814 — MB ChB Liverp. 1987; DCH RCP Lond. 1990; DRCOG 1990; MRCGP 1991. Specialty: Dermat. Socs: BMA; Hudds. Med. Soc. Prev: Trainee GP Kirby Liverp. VTS; SHO (Gen. Med.) Whiston Hosp. Prescot GP VTS.

NAZARETH, Irwin The Keats Group Practice, 1B Downshire Hill, London NW3 1NR Tel: 020 7435 1131 Email: i.nazareth@ucl.ac.uk — MB BS Bombay 1984; LRCP LRCS Ed. LRCPS Glas. 1986; PhD Lond. 1987; DRCOG 1988; MRCGP 1989. Sen. Lect. (Primary Health Care) Univ. Coll. Lond. Med. Sch.; GP Partner.

NAZEER, Anisa Fatima Salisbury District Hospital, c/o Eye Clinic, Salisbury District Hospital, Salisbury SP2 8BJ — MB BS Peshawar, Pakistan 1985; FRCSI 1992. Staff Ophth. Specialty: Ophth.

NAZEER, Shaukat Mayfair Medical Centre, 3-5 Weighhouse, London W1K 5LS Tel: 020 7493 1647 Fax: 020 7493 3169 — LMSSA Lond. 1989; MA Oxf. 1990. Socs: BMA. Prev: Ho. Phys. Univ. Coll. & Middlx. Sch. Med. Lond.

NAZERALI, Gulzar Abdullah 80 The Knoll, London W13 8HY — LRCPI & LM, LRSCI & LM 1958 (RCSI) LRCPI & LM, LRCSI & LM 1958; DObst RCPI 1962.

NAZIR, Masood 88 Nansen Road, Sparkhill, Birmingham B11 4DT Tel: 0121 778 5192; 88 Nansen Road, Sparkhill, Birmingham B11 4DT Tel: 0121 778 5192 — MB ChB Birm. 1997 (Birm. Med. Sch.) SHO Med. Birm. Healthcare Hosp. Specialty: Gen. Med. Socs: BMA. Prev: Boldesley Green E. - B'Ham.

NAZIR, Nargas Harrogate Road Surgery, 355 Harrogate Road, Leeds LS17 6PZ Tel: 0113 268 0066 Fax: 0113 288 8643 — MB ChB Leeds 1992.

NAZIR, Tallat Yausmine Department of Anaesthesia, Stepping Hill Hospital, Poplar Grove, Stockport SK2 7JE Tel: 0161 419 5869 — MB ChB Manch. 1989; BSc St. And. 1986. Cons. Anaesth., Stepping Hill Hosp., Stockport. Specialty: Anaesth. Socs: Fell. of the Roy. Coll. of Anaesth.s; OAA; DAS.

NAZKI, Mohamed Tariq Stockland Green Health Centre, 192 Reservoir Road, Erdington, Birmingham B23 6DJ Tel: 0121 373 5405 Fax: 0121 386 4909; 100 Wake Green Road, Moseley, Birmingham B13 9PX Tel: 0121 449 5211 — MB BS Patna 1967. Sen. GP, Stockland Green Health Centre, Erdington, Birm. Specialty: Diabetes; Family Planning. Socs: LMC; MDU.

NAZROO, Professor Jacques Yzet University College London, Department of Epidemiology and Public Health, 1-19 Torrington Place, London WC1E 6BT Tel: 020 7391 1705 Fax: 020 7813 0242 Email: j.nazroo@ucl.ac.uk — MB BS Lond. 1986 (St. George's Hospital Medical School) MSc Lond. 1989, BSc (Hons.) 1983; PhD 1999. Prof. Med. Sociology, Dept. Epidemiol. & Pub. Health, Univ. Coll. Lond. Specialty: Epidemiol. Socs: Mem. Fac. Of Public Health Med. through Distinction. Prev: Sen. Research Fell. Policy Studies Inst. Lond.; Reader (Sociology) Univ. Coll. Lond.; Hon. Lect. (Psychiat.) Univ. Coll.

NCUBE, William Alexandra Group Medical Practice, Glodwick Health Centre, 137 Glodwick Road, Oldham OL4 1YN Tel: 0161 909 8377 Fax: 0161 909 8414 — MUDr Charles Univ. Prague 1982; DRCOG 1992; DFFP 1993. Cosmetic Med. Practitioner, Pioneer Laser Clinic, 19 Buxton Rd, Stockport, Chesh. SK2 6LS. Socs: Assoc. Mem. RCGP; Fell. Roy. Soc. of Med.; Mem. of Brit. Assn. of Cosmetic Doctors.

NDEGWA, David Gituma South London and Maudsley NHS Trust, 108 Landor Road, London SW9 9NT — MB ChB Ghana 1979; MRCPsych 1985. Cons. Forens. Psychiat. S Lond. and Maudsley NHS Trust Care NHS Trust; Hon. Sen. Lect. King's Coll., Guy's, St Thos Med. Sch. Specialty: Forens. Psychiat. Prev: Cons. Forens. Psychiat. NE Thames RHA; Sen. Lect. (Forens. Psychiat.) St. Bart. Hosp. Med. Coll.

NDIRIKA, Amelia Chinwe Charlotte Keel Health Centre, Seymour Road, Easton, Bristol BS5 — MB BS Lond. 1989 (St. Geo. Hosp. Lond.) MA Physiol., BA Oxf. 1984; DRCOG 1991; MRCGP 1993. Socs: BMA.

NDUKA, Charles Chukwuemeka 30 Bellew Street, London SW17 0AD — MB BS Lond. 1994; MA Oxf. 1991; MRCS Lond. 1999; MD Lond. 2001.

NDUKA, Stella Aleruchi Maple Ward, Chase Farm Hospital, The Ridgeway, Enfield EN2 8JL Tel: 020 8366 6600; 20 The Larches, Long Lane, Hillingdon, Uxbridge UB10 0DJ Tel: 01895 251093 — MB BS Nigeria 1982; MB BS U. Nigeria 1982; DGM RCP Lond. 1995.

NE WIN, Dr 222 Preston Road, Chorley PR6 7BA — MB BS Med. Inst. (I) Rangoon 1976.

NÉVIN, Judith Alexandra 20 Ryeland Street, Crosshills, Keighley BD20 8SR — MB BS Lond. 1994 (RFHSM)

NEADES, Mr Glyn Thomas 2 Hillview Terrace, Edinburgh EH12 8RA — MB ChB Aberd. 1983; BMedBiol 1983; FRCS Glas. 1988; FRCS Ed. 1988; ChM Aberd. 1993. Cons. Surg. West. Gen. Hosp. Edin. Specialty: Gen. Surg.

NEAGLE, Elaine Heather 73 Kensington Road, Belfast BT5 6NL — MB BCh BAO Belf. 1990; MB BCh Belf. 1990.

NEAGLE, William Brian Birch Hill House, 26 Mullaghcarton Road, Ballinderry Upper, Lisburn BT28 2NP — MB BCh BAO Belf. 1991.

NEAL, Alistair John Duncan, Surg. Lt.-Cdr. RN 9 Devonshire Place, London W1G 6HR Tel: 020 7935 8425 — MB ChB Aberd. 1983; DAvMED RCol. 1993. Specialty: Gen. Pract.

NEAL, Anthony James St Luke's Cancer Centre, Royal Surrey County Hospital, Guildford GU2 7XX Tel: 01483 406767 Fax: 01483 406767 Email: anthony.neal@royalsurrey.nhs.uk — MB BS Lond. 1985 (St. Thom. Hosp. Med. Sch. Lond.) MRCP (UK) 1988;

FRCR 1992; MD Lond. 1995. Cons Clin Oncol. St Luke's Cancer Centre Guildford Surrey. Specialty: Oncol.; Radiother. Special Interest: Breast Cancer; Chemother.; Radiother. Prev: Cons. Clin. Oncol. Roy. Marsden NHS Trust Sutton; Sen. Regist. (Clin. Oncol.) Roy. Marsden Hosp. Lond. & Sutton; Lect. (Med. Oncol.) & Regist. (Radiother. & Oncol.) Roy. Lond. Hosp.

NEAL, Beryl Rose 25 Arlington Crescent, Wilmslow SK9 6BH — MB ChB St. And. 1961.

NEAL, Brynmor Lloyd Rectory Meadow Surgery, School Lane, Amersham HP7 0HG Tel: 01494 727711 Fax: 01494 431790; Hawthorn, Weedon Hill, Hyde Heath, Amersham HP6 5RN Tel: 01494 774421 — MB BS Lond. 1972 (Westm.) MRCS Eng. LRCP Lond. 1972; DObst RCOG 1975; FRCGP 1994, M 1977. GP Bucks.; Chairm. Educat. Div. Thames Valley Fac. RCGP; CPD Tutor Wycombe Dist.; Chairm. Thames Valley Fac. RCGP. Socs: Chiltern Med. Soc. Prev: GP Represen. on Community Unit Wycombe HA; Med. Adviser MPS Soc.; Clin. Asst. Psychiat.

NEAL, Christine Mary 65 Shoot-up-Hill, London NW2; 11 Silver Cres., London W4 5SF — MB BS Lond. 1984; MA Camb. 1986; DRCOG 1987.

NEAL, Christopher John Marlborough Park Avenue Surgery, 82 Marlborough Park Avenue, Sidcup DA15 9DX Tel: 020 8300 1197 Fax: 020 8309 7187 — MB ChB Manch. 1979.

NEAL, David Andrew James 35 Upper High Street, Thame OX9 2DN — BM Soton. 1990.

NEAL, Professor David Edgar Addenbrooke's Hospital, Box 193, Oncology Centre, Hills Road, Cambridge CB2 2QQ Tel: 01223 331940 — MB BS Lond. 1975; BSc (Anat.) Lond. 1972; FRCS Eng. 1980; MS Lond. 1983; FRCS Ed. 1994; Med Sci Acad. of Med. Sci. 1998. Prof. of Surgic. Oncol., Univ. of Camb. Specialty: Urol. Special Interest: Urological Oncol. Socs: Amer. Assn.. of Genito-Urin. Surg.s; Austral. Urological Assci.; Amerial Assoc. for Cancer Research. Prev: Sen. Lect. & Cons. Urol Surg. Univ. Newc. u Tyne; 1st Asst. Urol. Univ. Newc. upon Tyne & Lect. Surg. The Gen. Infirm. Leeds.

NEAL, David Mark Top Floor Flat, 4 Clifton Park Road, Clifton, Bristol BS8 3HL; Lauriston House, 43 Shepherds Way, Liphook GU30 7HH — MB ChB Manch. 1994. SHO (Cardiac Surg.) Bristol Roy. Infirm. Specialty: Otorhinolaryngol. Prev: SHO (Thoracic Surg.) Frenchay Hosp.; SHO (ENT Surg.) Southmead Hosp. Bristol; SHO (A & E) Frenchay Hosp.

NEAL, Frank Edward (retired) Sharon, Doncaster Road, Rotherham S65 1NN Tel: 01709 382300 — MB ChB Sheff. 1950; DMRT Eng. 1953; FFR 1959; FRCR 1976. Prev: Gen. Manager Weston Pk. Hosp. Sheff.

NEAL, Frank Richard Honor Oak Health Centre, 20 Turnham Road, London SE4 2LA Tel: 020 7639 9797 — MB Camb. 1983; MA Camb. 1984, MB 1983, BChir 1982. GP since 1987. Prev: SHO (O & G) Lewisham Hosp. Lond.; SHO (Psychiat.) S. West. Hosp. Lond.; SHO (ENT) Hither Green Hosp. Lond.

NEAL, Gillian 7 Dykes Terrace, Stanwix, Carlisle CA3 9AS — MB BS Newc. 1991; DRCOG 1994.

NEAL, James William Department of Histopathology, University Hospital of Wales, Cardiff CF4 4XN — MB ChB Bristol 1978; FRCS Eng. 1984; DPhil Oxf. 1988; FRC Path 2000. Sen. Lect. & Hon. Cons. Neuropath. Univ. Hosp. Wales Cardiff. Specialty: Neuropath.

NEAL, Janet Christine — MB BS Lond. 1988 (UMDS Guy's Hosp. Lond.) DRCOG 1992; MRCGP 1994; DA (UK) 1996; MRCP Lond. 2002. Specialty: Oncol.

NEAL, Keith Richard Dept. of Public Health & Epidemiology, University of Nottingham, Queens Medical Centre, Nottingham NG7 2UH; 8 Windley Crescent, Darley Abbey, Derby DE22 1BZ — BM Soton. 1981; MRCP (UK) 1985. Sen. Lect., Dept of Health & Epidemiol., Univ. Nott.

NEAL, Lesley Margaret Flash Cottage, Stannington, Sheffield S6 6GR — MB ChB Bristol 1976.

NEAL, Margaret Mary (retired) Sharon, Doncaster Road, Rotherham S65 1NN Tel: 01709 382300 — MRCS Eng. LRCP Lond. 1950 (Sheff.)

NEAL, Matthew Russell 128 High Storrs Road, Sheffield S11 7LF Tel: 01142 685746 Email: mattneal@compuserve.com — BM Soton. 1990; DA (UK) 1993; FRCA 1997. Specialist Regist. (Anaesth.) N. Trent Rotat. Centr. Sheff. Univ. Hosps. Specialty: Anaesth. Socs: Train. Mem. Assn. AnE.h.; Brit. Med. Acupunct. Soc.

NEAL, Richard David Meanwood Group Practice, 548 Meanwood Road, Leeds LS6 4JN Tel: 0113 295 1737 Fax: 0113 295 1736; Meanwood Group Practice, 548 Meanwood Road, Leeds LS6 4JN Tel: 0113 295 1730 Fax: 0113 295 1736 — MB ChB Birm. 1988; DFFP 1992; DRCOG 1992; MRCGP 1994. Lect. in Primary Care Research Centre for Research in Primary Care Leeds.; GP Princip. Meanwood Gp. Pract. Specialty: Gen. Pract. Prev: Research Train. Fell. Centre for Research in Primary Care; Trainee GP ScarBoro. VTS; SHO (Gen. Med.) Southport & Formby Dist. Gen. Hosp.

NEAL, Roger Charles Toddington Medical Centre, Luton Road, Toddington, Dunstable LU5 6DE Tel: 01525 872222 Fax: 01525 876711 — MB BCh Wales 1985; MRCGP 1989.

NEAL, Shona McDonald St John's Hospital, Howden, Livingston EH54 6PP — MB ChB Ed. 1991; BSc (Hons.) Ed. 1989. Specialist Regist. (Anaesth.) Dundee Teachg. Hosps. Specialty: Anaesth.

NEAL, Timothy James Department of Medical Microbiology, Royal Liverpool University Hospital, Prescot St., Liverpool L7 8XP Tel: 0151 706 5849 Email: tjneal@liv.ac.uk; 3 Holkham Gardens, St Helens WA9 5SS — MB ChB Liverp. 1987; MSc Manch. 1994; MRCPath 1997. Cons. Microbio. Liv'pl. Specialty: Med. Microbiol.

NEAL-DERKS, Jacinta Anna Maria Byways, Forestside, Rowlands Castle PO9 6EQ Tel: 023 9241 2355 — MB BS Adelaide 1980; DRCOG 1983.

NEAL-SMITH, Gillian Ann (retired) 5 Martineau Close, Esher KT10 9PW Tel: 01372 468523 — MB BS Lond. 1964 (Char. Cross) MRCS Eng. LRCP Lond. 1964; DObst RCOG 1966. Prev: Ho. Phys. (Gen. Med. & Paediat.) & Ho. Surg. Fulham Hosp.

NEALE, Aileen Winifred The Red House, Great Plumstead, Norwich NR13 5ED — MB ChB Birm. 1950; DPM Eng. 1973. Prev: Clin. Asst. St Nicholas Hosp. Gt. Yarmouth.

NEALE, Alastair James Brynallt, Polesgate, Pontesbury Hill, Pontesbury, Shrewsbury SY5 0YL — MB ChB Birm. 1987; MRCPsych 1992. Sen. Regist. (Child & Adolesc. Psychiat.) SW Peninsula. Specialty: Child & Adolesc. Psychiat.

NEALE, David Vivian Greenways, Main St., Northam, Rye TN31 6ND — BM Soton. 1984; DGM RCP Lond. 1988; DRCOG 1989; MRCGP 1989; Dip. Palliat. Med. Wales 1993. Socs: BMA; Assoc. Mem. Palliat. Med. Assn. Prev: Med. Dir. St. Michaels Hospice St. Leonards-on-Sea; GP Headcorn Kent; Trainee GP William Harvey Hosp. Ashford VTS.

NEALE, Mr Edmund John Bedford Hospital NHS Trust, Kempston Road, Bedford MK42 9DJ Tel: 01234 792065 Email: ed.neale@bedhos.anglox.nhs.uk — MB BS Lond. 1982 (St. Geo.) FRCOG; BSc Lond. 1979; MRCOG 1988. Cons. O & G Bedford Hosp.; Divisional Clin. Director for Womens and Childrens Servs., Bedford Hosp.; Dep. Med. Director, Bedford Hosp. Specialty: Obst. & Gyn. Socs: Nuffield Vis. Soc. Prev: Lect. & Hon. Sen. Regist. (O & G) Univ. Leicester; Vis. Lect. (O & G) Chinese Univ. Hong Kong.

NEALE, Graham (retired) St. Mary's Hospital, Clinical Safety Research Unit (Academic Dept of Surgery), 10th floor QEQM Building, Praed Street, London W2 1NY Tel: 020 7886 7814 Fax: 020 7413 0470 Email: g.neale@ic.ac.uk; 30 Bevin Sqaure, London SW17 7BB Tel: 020 8767 0159 — MB ChB Bristol 1960; BSc Lond. 1950; FRCP Lond. 1971, M 1963; FRCPI 1979; MA Camb. 1987. Vis. Prof. Acad. Dept. Surg. Imperial Coll. Lond. Prev: Lect. (Med.) Univ. Camb.

NEALE, Gregory 16 Cecilia Road, Clarendon Park, Leicester LE2 1TA — MB ChB Leic. 1996.

NEALE, Ian Andrew Brook Surgery, Chalgrove, Oxford OX44 7AF Tel: 01865 890760 Fax: 01865 893509 Email: ian@nealedesign.freeserve.co.uk — BM BCh Oxf. 1977 (Oxford) MA Camb. 1978; DRCOG 1980. Fitness to Practice Comm GMC; Performance Assessor NCAA; Clinical Governance Reviewer CHAI; PLAB Examr. GMC; Complaints Reviewer Health Commiss. Specialty: Gen. Pract. Socs: BMA; Chalgrove Charity Trustees. Prev: Performance Assessor GMC; Med. Dir. OXDOC S. GP Out of Hours Coop; Sec. Oxon. LMC 1987-94.

NEALE, Jacqueline Suzanne Gable House Surgery, High Street, Malmesbury SN16 9AT Tel: 01666 825825 — MB ChB Birm. 1983; DA (UK) 1988; DRCOG 1991. GP Princip. Specialty: Gen. Pract.

NEALE, Michael Lawrence (retired) 30 Roydscliffe Road, Heaton, Bradford BD9 5PS Tel: 01274 492115 Fax: 01274 492115 — MB ChB Manch. 1960; DObst RCOG 1962. Prev: Ho. Phys. City Hosp. York.

NEALE, Richard John Horace Herschel Medical Centre, 45 Osborne Street, Slough SL1 1TT Tel: 01753 520643 Fax: 01753 554964; Three Hollies, Cherry Tree Road, Farnham Royal, Slough SL2 3EF Tel: 01753 645757 — MB ChB St. And. 1966 (Queen's Coll. Dundee) Socs: BMA. Prev: SHO Upton Hosp. Slough & St. Mary Abbot's Hosp. Lond.; Resid. Med. Off. Fitzroy Nuffield Hosp. Lond.

NEALE, Robert Desmond (retired) 74 Parrys Lane, Stoke Bishop, Bristol BS9 1AQ Tel: 0117 968 2484 — MB ChB Bristol 1957; DPM Eng. 1962. Prev: Sen. Hosp. Med. Off. Barrow Hosp. Bristol.

NEALE, Ruth (retired) Bridlecroft, 314 Spring Lane, Mapperley Plains, Nottingham NG3 5RQ Tel: 0115 926 8956 — MB ChB Leeds 1954.

NEALE, Thomas William Kings Pond Cottage, Chesham Road, Hyde End, Great Missenden HP16 0RD — MB BS Lond. 1992.

NEALES, Kate Elisabeth Kent & Canterbury Hospital, Canterbury CT1 3NG Tel: 01227 766877; 4 The Grove, Barham, Canterbury CT4 6PP Tel: 01227 831363 — MB BS Melbourne 1980 (Univ. Melbourne Vict., Austral.) FRACOG 1992, M 1987; MRCOG 1989. Cons. O & G Kent & Canterbury Hosp. Specialty: Obst. & Gyn. Socs: Brit. Med. Soc.; Brit. Soc. Colpos. & Cerv. Path. Prev: Sen. Regist. (O & G) NW RHA; Research Regist. (Fetal Med.) Guy's Hosp. Lond.

NEAMAN, Gillian Mary The Surgery, 66 Long Lane, London EC1A 9EJ; 11 Chadwell Street, London EC1R 1XD Tel: 020 7837 4455 Fax: 020 7833 0268 — BM BCh Oxf. 1958 (Guy's) MA, BM BCh Oxf. 1958. Med. Off. to Reuters (p/t), Lond. Prev: Ho. Surg. New End Hosp. Hampstead; Ho. Phys. Whittington Hosp. Highgate; Resid. Med. Off. Hornsey Centr. Hosp.

NEAME, Mr John Humphrey (retired) Till's End, Stapleford, Salisbury SP3 4LT Tel: 01722 790484 — (Univ. Coll. Hosp.) BA Camb. 1946, MA 1958, MB BChir 1949; FRCS Eng. 1958. Prev: Cons. Otolaryngol. Salisbury Hosp Gp. & Swindon & MarlBoro. Hosps.

NEAME, Kenneth Dell (retired) Marlowe, Hessle Drive, Lower Heswall, Wirral CH60 8PS Tel: 0151 342 2132 — MB BS Lond. 1954 (St. Mary's) PhD Sheff. 1959. Prev: Sen. Lect. Univ. Liverp.

NEAME, Rebecca Louise 2 Mountbatten Way, Raunds, Wellingborough NN9 6PA — MB ChB Leic. 1995.

NEAME, Mr Robert Lawrence Hollands and Partners, Bridport Medical Centre, North Allington, Bridport DT6 5DU Tel: 01308 421896 Fax: 01308 421109 — MB BS Lond. 1986; FRCS Eng. 1991; DRCOG 1993; MRCGP 1994. Prev: Trainee GP Salisbury; Regist. (Surg.) Soton. Gen. Hosp.; SHO (Surg.) Bristol & Weston HA.

NEARY, Bruce Richard The Wicketts, 9 Dower Park, Escrick, York YO19 6JN — MB ChB Liverp. 1997.

NEARY, Professor David Hope Hospital, Greater Manchester Neurosciences, Stott Lane, Salford M6 8HD Tel: 0161 206 2561 Fax: 0161 206 2993; 8 Bollington Mill, Park Lane, Altrincham WA14 4TJ Tel: 0161 929 4694 Email: ann.hodson@srht.nhs.uk — MB ChB Manch. 1967; MD Manch. 1977; FRCP Manch. 1980. Cons. Neurol. Salford NHS Trust. Specialty: Neurol. Socs: Assn. Brit. Neurol.; Brit. Neurol. Path. Soc.; Assn. Phys.

NEARY, Dermot Mellotte Tramways Medical Centre, Newtownabbey BT36 7XX Tel: 02890 342131 Fax: 02890 839111; 27 Downview Avenue, Belfast BT15 4FB Tel: 02890 777311 — MB BCh BAO Belf. 1973.

NEARY, John Gerard Tramways Medical Centre, Farmley Road, Newtownabbey BT36 7XX Tel: 028 9034 2131 Fax: 028 9083 9111 — MB BCh BAO Belf. 1974. GP Princip. Belf./Newtonabbey; Chairm. of SEAL; S. E. Antrim Locality, Total purchasing project. Specialty: Sports Med.

NEARY, John Taaffe (retired) 28 Downview Avenue, Belfast BT15 4FB — MB BCh BAO NUI 1941.

NEARY, Joseph Mary Trinity Surgery, Norwich Road, Wisbech PE13 3UZ Tel: 01945 476999 Fax: 01945 476900; 66 North Brink, Wisbech PE13 1LN Tel: 01945 585884 Fax: 01945 474189 — MB BCh BAO NUI 1981; MRCGP 1983; DCH RCP Lond. 1986; MSc UEA 1998. Princip. Gen. Pract. Trinity Surg. Wisbech. Specialty: Gen. Pract. Socs: GP Asthma Gp.; Vice-Chairm. Camb. LMC; Nat. Counc. RCGP. Prev: Surg. Lt. RN; SMO HMS Glam..

NEARY, Peter Joseph Lytham Road Surgery, 352 Lytham Road, Blackpool FY4 1DW Tel: 01253 402800 Fax: 01253 402994; Flat 1, Cyprus Court, Cuprus Avenue, Lytham St Annes FY8 1DZ Tel: 01253 712968 — MB ChB Manch. 1964.

NEARY, Richard Henry 37 Chancery Lane, Alsager, Stoke-on-Trent ST7 2HE — MD Manch. 1991; MB ChB 1979; MRCPath 1986. Cons. Chem. Path. N. Staffs. Hosp. Centre Stoke-on-Trent. Specialty: Chem. Path.

NEARY, Wanda Janetta Child & Family Services Unit, Guardian House, Guardian St., Warrington WA5 1TP Tel: 01925 405717 Fax: 01925 405725; 36 Brooklands Road, Sale M33 3SJ Tel: 0161 973 5950 — MB ChB Manch. 1968; MSc (Audiol. Med.) Manch. 1990; MD Manch. 1995. Cons. Community Paediat. (Paediat. Audiol.) Warrington Community Health Care (NHS) Trust. Specialty: Paediat. Prev: SCMO Warrington HA; Clin. Med. Off. Manch. HA; Lect. (Path.) Univ. Manch.

NEARY, William David 36 Brooklands Road, Sale M33 3SJ — MB ChB Bristol 1995.

NEASHAM, John (retired) 26 Carr Bottom Road, Greengates, Bradford BD10 0BB — MB ChB Leeds 1968; DA Eng. 1971; FFA RCS Eng. 1973. Prev: Cons. Anaesth. Gen. Infirm. Leeds.

NEASHAM, John Percival Ilkley Health Centre, Springs Lane, Ilkley LS29 8TQ Tel: 01943 609255 Fax: 01943 430005; 4 Lakeside Close, Middleton, Ilkley LS29 0AG Tel: 01943 816271 Fax: 01943 816271 — MB ChB Birm. 1956; DObst RCOG 1961; MRCGP 1978. Clin. Asst. (Orthop.) Ilkley Coronation Hosp.; Med. Adviser Internat. Wool Secretariat, Ilkley; Clin. Asst. (Med.) Wharfedale Gen. Hosp. Specialty: Diabetes. Prev: Ho. Surg. Worcester Roy. Infirm.; Ho. Phys. St. Mary's Hosp. Portsmouth; Ho. Surg. (O & G) Dudley Rd. Hosp. Birm.

NEATBY, Guy Oliver Miller (retired) 7 Leighwood House, Church Road, Leighwoods, Bristol BS8 3PQ Tel: 0117 973 8398 — (St. Bart.) BA (1st cl. Classic Trip. Pt. I) Camb. 1932, MA; MRCS Eng. LRCP Lond. 1938; DOMS Eng. 1942. Prev: Ophth. Bath Clin. Area.

NEAVE, Farhad 81 Lynwood Road, Ealing, London W5 1JG Tel: 020 8998 3409 — MD Iran 1973; DMRT Ed. 1980; MPhil Lond. 1986; FRCR 1992. Cons. Radiother. & Oncol. N. Middlx. Hosp. Lond. Specialty: Oncol.; Radiother.

NEAVE, Sandra Margaret The Adam Practice, 306 Blandford Road, Hamworthy, Poole BH15 4JQ Tel: 01202 679234 — BM Soton. 1989; MRCGP 1995; DRCOG 1995. Specialty: Family Plann. & Reproduc. Health. Socs: Roy. Coll. Gen. Pract.; BMA.

NEAVES, Christopher Henry (retired) 18 Stepney Drive, Scarborough YO12 5DH Tel: 01723 376650 — MB BS Lond. 1949 (King's Coll. Hosp.) Prev: Ho. Surg. ENT Dept. King's Coll. Hosp.

NEAVES, Judith Mary Hemsby Medical Centre, Hemsby, Great Yarmouth NR2 Tel: 01493 730449 — MB BS Lond. 1983; DRCOG 1988; MRCGP 1990; DA (UK) 1996; MSc Lond. 2000. Med. Off. & Ltd. Specialist Anaesth. Daliburgh Hosp.; Trust Practitioner in Rheum., Norf. and Nomian Univ. Hosp.; Osteopath in private practice. Specialty: Gen. Med. Socs: Lond. Coll. of Osteopatric Med. 2000. Prev: GP Woking; SHO (Anaesth.) Chesterfield Hosp. Derbysh.

NECATI, Guner 17 Durham Avenue, Willenhall WV13 1JH — LMSSA Lond. 1975.

NEDEN, Catherine Anne Mildmay Court Surgery, Mildmay Court, Bellevue Road, Ramsgate CT11 8JX Tel: 01843 592576 Fax: 01843 852980 Email: catherie.neden@mildmaysurgery.co.uk — BM BCh Oxf. 1984; MA Camb. 1985; DRCOG 1987; DGM RCP Lond. 1988; DCH RCP Lond. 1988; FRCGP 1999; FRCP 2000. Prev: SHO (Rheum.) Middlx. Hosp.; SHO (Paediat.) Char. Cross Hosp. Lond.; Trainee GP Bath VTS.

NEDEN, David Arthur John Langham, 33 St. Mildreds Avenue, Ramsgate CT11 0HS Tel: 01843 593836 — (Univ. Coll. Hosp.) MB BS Lond. 1952; DObst RCOG 1956; FRCGP 1993. Local Med. Off. Civil Serv. Dept. Specialty: Palliat. Med. Prev: Ho. Surg., Ho. Phys. & Resid. Med. Off. Univ. Coll. Hosp. Lond.

NEDEN, John Wilfred David Mildmay Court Surgery, Mildmay Court, Bellevue Road, Ramsgate CT11 8JX Tel: 01843 592576 Fax: 01843 852980; The Surgery Flat, Grange Road, Ramsgate CT11 9NB Tel: 01843 852853 — MB BS Lond. 1984; MA Camb. 1985; DRCOG 1987; MRCGP 1988; DCH RCP Lond. 1989; FRCGP 1999; Dip. Pale (Med) 2001. Macriellan GP facilitator. Specialty: Infec. Dis.; Palliat. Med. Prev: Trainee GP Soton. & Bath VTS; SHO (Med. Microbiol.) Roy. Free Hosp. Lond.; Ho. Surg. King's Coll. Hosp. Lond.

NEE, Mr Patrick Anthony Michael Whiston Hospital, Prescot L35 5DR Tel: 0151 430 1853; 5 Peter's Close, Prestbury, Macclesfield SK10 4JQ Tel: 01625 828988 — MB ChB Liverp.

1982; MRCP (UK) 1987; FRCS Ed. (A&E) 1989; FFAEM 1994; FRCP 1998. Cons. Emerg. Med. & Critical Care Whiston Hosp. Prescot. Specialty: Accid. & Emerg. Socs: Intens. Care Soc.; Brit. Assn. Accid. & Emerg. Med.; UK Trauma (Audit & Research) Network. Prev: Sen. Regist. (A & E) NW RHA; Regist. (A & E) Univ. Hosp. S. Manch.; Regist. (Gen. Med.) Derbysh. Roy. Infim.

NEED, Rachel Elisabeth (retired) 2 Damer Gardens, Henley-on-Thames RG9 1HX Tel: 01491 572898 — MB BS Lond. 1954; DO RCS Eng. 1967; MCOphth 1989. Prev: Ho. Surg. (Ophth.) St. Bart. Hosp. Lond.

NEEDHAM-BENNETT, Humphrey Bethlem Royal Hospital, Denis Hill Unit, Monks Orchard Road, Beckenham BR3 3BX Tel: 020 8777 6611 Fax: 020 8776 4403 Email: humphrey.needham-bennett@slam.nhs.uk — MB BS Lond. 1987 (UMDS Guys and St Thomas') MRCPsych 1992. Cons. Forens. Psychiat. Bethlem Roy. Hosp. Specialty: Forens. Psychiat.; Gen. Psychiat.; Rehabil. Med. Special Interest: Forens. Addic.; Older Offenders.

NEEDHAM, Andrew Donald Department of Ophthalmology, Royal Liverpool Hospital, Prescot Road, Liverpool L7 8XP; The Laurels, Burton Road, Little Neston, South Wirral CH64 4AG — MB ChB Liverp. 1989; BSc Liverp. 1985; FRCOphth 1993. Glaucoma Fell. Liverp. Specialty: Ophth. Socs: BMA. Prev: Specialist Regist. (Ophth.) Dundee.

NEEDHAM, David Jonathan Tregenna Group Practice, 399 Portway, Woodhouse Park, Manchester M22 0EP Tel: 0161 499 3777 Fax: 0161 493 9119; 23 Grosvenor Square, Sale M33 6QU Tel: 0161 905 2229 — MB ChB Manch. 1988; BSc St. And. 1985; DRCOG 1991; DCH 1991; MRCGP 1992. Trainee GP Stepping Hosp. Stockport.

NEEDHAM, Elizabeth Albion Medical Practice, 1 Albion Street, Ashton-under-Lyne OL6 6HF Tel: 0161 339 9161 Fax: 0161 343 5131; Broomland, 5 Gallowsclough Road, Stalybridge SK15 3QS Tel: 01457 764505 — MB ChB Liverp. 1975 (Liverpool) MB ChB (Hons.) Liverp. 1975; DRCOG 1977; DCH RCPS Glas. 1978; MRCGP 1979. Clin. Asst. Diabetes Centre Tameside Gen. Hosp. Socs: Manch. Med. Soc. Prev: SHO (Obst.) Crumpsall Hosp. Manch.; SHO (Gyn.) St. Mary's Hosp. Manch.; SHO (Paediat.) Booth Hall Childr. Hosp. Manch.

NEEDHAM, Geoffrey Kenneth Holmside Medical Group, 142 Armstrong Road, Benwell, Newcastle upon Tyne NE4 8QB Tel: 0191 273 4009 Fax: 0191 273 2745 — MB ChB Liverp. 1977; FRCS Eng. 1982; MD Newc. 1988; MRCGP 1991. Specialty: Gen. Pract. Prev: Regist. (Surg.) S. Cleveland Hosp.; Sen. Research Assoc. (Surg.) Univ. Newc. u. Tyne.

NEEDHAM, Professor Gillian Westbank, 180 Nrthdeeside Road, Milltimber, Aberdeen AB13 0HL — MB ChB Manch. 1981; BSc (Hons.) Anat. Manch. 1978; FRCR 1986; FRCP (EDIN) 1999. PostGrad. Med. Dean Univ. of Aberd.; Hon. Cons. Radiologist Grampian Univeristy Hosp.s Trust Aberd. Specialty: Radiol.; Educat. Prev: Sen. Regist. (Radiol.) N. W. RHA; Regist. (Radiol.) N. West. RHA.; Cons. Radiologist Aberd. Roy. Hosp.s.

NEEDHAM, Hazel Joan Woodlands Park Health Centre, Canterbury Way, Wideopen, Newcastle upon Tyne NE13 6JL Tel: 0191 236 2366 Fax: 0191 236 7619; 34 Clayworth Road, Brunton Park, Newcastle upon Tyne NE3 5AB — MB ChB Dundee 1981; MRCGP 1985.

NEEDHAM, Hazel Maria 122 Alfreton Road, Newton, Alfreton DE55 5TR — MB ChB Dundee 1997.

NEEDHAM, Ian Charles 5 Greenways, Wolsingham, Bishop Auckland DL13 3HN Tel: 01388 527300 — MB ChB Sheff. 1973.

NEEDHAM, John Allan Peter House Surgery, Captain Lees Road, Westhoughton, Bolton BL5 3UB Tel: 01942 812525; 30 Lakelands Drive, Ladybridge, Bolton BL3 4NN Tel: 01204 653691 — MB ChB Manch. 1970; DObst RCOG 1973.

NEEDHAM, Karen Lesley College Lane Surgery, Barnsley Road, Ackworth, Pontefract WF7 7HZ Tel: 01977 611023 Fax: 01977 612146; Moat Cottage, 76 Sherburn St, Cawood, Selby YO8 3SS Tel: 01757 268893 — BM BS Nottm. 1982 (Nottingham) DCH RCP Lond. 1986; MRCGP 1989. GP. Specialty: Gen. Pract.

NEEDHAM, Morag Jane The Congregational Hall, Town Street, Marple Bridge, Stockport SK6 5AA Tel: 0161 427 2049/1074 Fax: 0161 427 8389 — MB ChB Sheff. 1990; MRCGP 1995; DFFP 1997. Specialty: Gen. Pract. Prev: Trainee GP Chesh.

NEEDHAM, Patricia Ruth Dorothy House Foundation, Winsley, Bradford-on-Avon BA15 Tel: 01225 311335 Email: trisha.needham@dorothyhouse-hospice.org.uk — MB BS Lond. 1986 (London) FRCP UK 2000. Cons. Palliat. Med. Bath. Specialty: Palliat. Med. Prev: Sen. Regist. (Palliat Med.) Avon; Regist. (Palliat. Med., Radiother. & Oncol.) Roy. Lond. Hosp.; Regist. (Palliat. Med.) St. Bart. Hosp. Lond.

NEEDHAM, Paul Jonathan 26 North Road, Williton, Taunton TA4 4SN — MB ChB Manch. 1996.

NEEDHAM, Mr Peter Grenville (retired) Solihull Hospital, Lode Lane, Solihull B91 2JL — MB Camb. 1965 (St. Bart.) BChir 1964; FRCS Eng. 1970; FRCOG 1986, M 1974. Prev: Cons. O & G Solihull Hosp. W. Midl.

NEEDHAM, Peter Ronald George (retired) Bryn y Gwynt Isaf, Prion, Denbigh LL16 4RW Tel: 01745 812805 — MB BS Lond. 1966 (Guy's) LMSSA Lond. 1964; MRCS Eng. LRCP Lond. 1966; FRCPath 1984, M 1972. Prev: Cons. Histopath. Ysbyty Glan Clwyd, Bodelwyddan Rhyl Denbighsh.

NEEDHAM, Philip Stapenhill Surgery, Fyfield Road, Stapenhill, Burton-on-Trent DE15 9QD — BM BS Nottm. 1985; MRCGP 1990. GP Princip. Stapenhill & Roshston Med. Centres; Appraiser E. Staffs. P.C.T. Prev: Trainee GP Nottm. VTS.; SHO (A & E) Burton Dist. Hosp.

NEEDHAM, Sravoni Bonny 23 Grosvenor Square, Sale M33 6QU Tel: 0161 905 2229 — MB ChB Manch. 1988; BSc St. And. 1985. SHO (Paediat.) Withington & Wythenshawe Hosp. S. Manch. Prev: Ho. Off. (Surg.) Withingtron Hosp. Manch.; Ho. Off. (Med.) Stepping Hill Hosp. Stockport HA.

NEEDHAM, Stephanie Jane 1 The Leas, Sedgefield, Stockton-on-Tees TS21 2DS — MB BS Lond. 1992.

NEEDHAM, Vernon Harold Charlton Hill Surgery, Charlton Road, Andover SP10 3JY Tel: 01264 337979 Fax: 01264 334251 — MB BS Lond. 1978; BSc Lond. 1975; MRCGP 1982; DRCOG 1984; FRCGP 1999. Med. Adviser Coke Hole Trust Andover; GP Trainer. Prev: Regtl. Med. Off. 15/19 Hussars; Regtl. Med. Off. 3rd Regt. Roy. Horse Artillery; Trainee Anaesth. Camb. Milit. Hosp. Aldershot.

NEEDOFF, Joseph (retired) 52 Middlefield Lane, Hagley, Stourbridge DY9 0PX Tel: 01562 883624 — MB ChB Manch. 1946. Prev: GP & Hosp. Pract. (Dermat.) Dudley & Stourbridge Hosps.

NEEDOFF, Mr Maurice King's Mill Hospital, Mansfield Road, Sutton-in-Ashfield NG17 4JL Tel: 01623 672378 — MB ChB Birm. 1981; FRCS Ed. 1986; FRCS (Orth.) 1994. Cons. Orthop. & Trauma Surg. King's Mill Hosp. Mansfield. Specialty: Orthop. Socs: Brit. Trauma Soc.; Brit. Assn. Surg. Knee. Prev: Sen. Regist. (Orthop.) Derby & Nottm.; Regist. (Orthop.) Nottm. & Mansfield.

NEEDS, John David (retired) The Old Rectory, Little Wenlock, Telford TF6 5BD — MB BS Lond. 1970 (St. Geo.) DA Eng. 1974. Prev: Surg. Lt.-Cdr. RN.

NEEHALL, Mr David John 3 Knoll Drive, Southgate, London N14 5LU Tel: 0208 368 7184; 6 Montserrat Avenue, Federation Park, Port-of-Spain, Trinidad, West Indies Tel: 0101 868 628 0635 — MB BS West Indies 1991; MRCOG 1998. Specialty: Obst. & Gyn.

NEELAMKAVIL, Devassy Paul Sunny 6 Plaxtol Close, Bromley BR1 3AU — State Exam Padua 1973; BSc (Chem.) Kerala 1964; DObst RCPSI 1982; Cert. Prescribed Equiv. Exp. JCPTGP 1985; Cert. Occupat. Med. 1992; DFFP 1993; Dip. Addic. Behaviour Lond. 1996; DPM 2000. Specialty: Gen. Pract.

NEELY, Mr Julian Alexander Cavendish (retired) 27 Springfield Park, North Parade, Horsham RH12 2BF Tel: 01403 248355 — MB BS Lond. 1958 (St. Bart.) FRCS Eng. 1963; MS Lond. 1968. Prev: Cons. Surg. Crawley Hosp., Qu. Vict. Hosp. E. Grinstead & Horsham Hosp.

NEELY, Robert Dermot Garmany 52 Albert Street, Durham DH1 4RJ — MB BCh Belf. 1983; BSc (1st cl. Hons.) (Biochem.) Belf. 1980, MB BCh BAO 1983; MRCP (UK) 1986; MRCPath 1991. Regist. (Chem. Path.) Roy. Vict. Hosp. Belf. Specialty: Chem. Path.

NEEP, Richard James Chatsworth Road Medical Centre, Chatsworth Road, Brampton, Chesterfield S40 3PY Tel: 01246 568065 Fax: 01246 567116 — MB ChB Manch. 1981; MRCGP 1986; DRCOG 1986.

NEERKIN, Jane Flat 4, 61 Fordwych Road, London NW2 3TL; St. Thomas's Hospital, Lambeth Palace Road, London SE1 7EH — MB BS Lond. 1997 (Guy's & St Thos.) BSc (Hons.) Leeds 1992.

NEESON, Conor Clifton Street Surgery, 15-17 Clifton Street, Belfast BT13 1AD Tel: 028 9032 2330 Fax: 028 9043 9812 — MB BCh BAO Belf. 1981; DRCOG 1983; MRCGP 1985.

NEESON, Lilwen Elonwy The Clears House, Colley Lane, Reigate RH2 9JJ Tel: 0173 72 47277 — (Ed.) MRCS Eng. LRCP Lond. 1945. Clin. Asst. (Cas. Dept.) St. Helier Hosp. Carshalton.

NEEVES, Zofia Wanda St Peter's Surgery, 58 Leckie Road, Walsall WS2 8DA Tel: 01922 623755 Fax: 01922 746477 — LRCP LRCS Ed. 1969; LRCPS Glas. 1969. Socs: BMA.

NEGANDHI, Damodar Bhagwandas Rugelian, 4 Toley Avenue, Wembley HA9 9TB Tel: 020 8908 6690 — MB BS Bombay 1952 (G.S. Med. Coll.) MRCGP 1962; Cert JCC (with IUD) Lond 1978. Socs: BMA.

NEGARGAR, Aryan 219 Burbury Street, Birmingham B19 1TW — MB ChB Birm. 1995; ChB Birm. 1995.

NEGRETTE, Jacinto Joseph Royal Alexandra Hospital, Corsebar Road, Paisley PA2 9PN Tel: 0141 887 9111 — MB ChB Manch. 1976; DMRD Lond. 1980; FRCR 1983. Cons. Radiol. Roy. Alexandra Hosp. Paisley. Specialty: Radiol.

NEGRYCZ, Roslyn Jane University Hospital of North Staffordshire NHS Trust, Community Paediatrics, 6th Floor, Maternity building, Stoke-on-Trent ST4 6QG Tel: 01782 553352 — MB BCh Wales 1983; DCH RCP Lond. 1987; MRCGP 1988; MA Keele University 1996. Locum Cons. Community Paediat., Univ. Hospt. N. Staffs. NHS Trust. Specialty: Community Child Health. Prev: Assoc. Specialist N. Staffs. Hosps. NHS Trust.

NEGUS, Andrew Graham Whitchurch Health Centre, Armada Road, Whitchurch, Bristol BS14 0SU Tel: 01275 832285 Fax: 01275 540035 — MB ChB Bristol 1969; DRCOG 1971. Socs: BMA; Sec. S. Bristol Med. Soc. Prev: Ho. Surg. Frenchay Hosp. Bristol; SHO (Paediat.) Bristol Childr. Hosp.; SHO (Obst.) Bristol Matern. Hosp.

NEGUS, Mr David Lister Hospital, Chelsea Bridge Road, London SW1W 8RH Tel: 020 7730 3417 Fax: 020 7824 8867; 10 Deamark Avenue, Wimbledon, London SW19 4HF Tel: 020 8946 9371 Fax: 020 8946 8034 — (St. Thos.) BM BCh Oxf. 1958; MRCS Eng. LRCP Lond. 1958; FRCS Eng. 1962; MA Oxf. 1958, DM, MCh 1967. Emerit. Cons. Surg. Lewisham Hosp. Lond. Specialty: Gen. Surg. Socs: Hon. Mem. Soc. Francaise De Phlébologie; Fell. Roy. Soc. Med. (Ex-Mem. Counc. Surg. & Clin. Sects. & Ex-Chairm.Venous Forum); Hon. Mem. Soc. Francaise De Phlébologie. Prev: Edr. Emerit. Phlebol.; Cons. Surg. Lewisham Hosp. Lond.; Sen. Regist. & Lect. (Surg.) St. Thos. Hosp.

NEGUS, Rupert Peter Michael 17 Keyes Road, London NW2 3XB Tel: 020 8450 8327 — MB BS Lond. 1986; BA Oxf. 1983; MRCP (UK) 1990; PhD (Lond.) 1998. Specialist Regist. (Gastroenterol. & Gen. Med.) N. W. thames Train. Progr. Specialty: Oncol.; Gastroenterol.; Gen. Med. Socs: Young Fell. Roy. Soc. Med.; Roy. Coll. Phys.; Brit. Cytokine Gp. Prev: Clin. Research Fell. Imperial Cancer Research Fund, Lond.; Regist. (Gen. Med. & Nephrol.) St Mary's & St Chas. Hosps. Lond.; SHO (Neurol.) Roy. Free Hosp. Lond.

NEHAUL, John Jaikaran Harrogate Clinic, 23 Ripon Road, Harrogate HG1 2JL Tel: 01423 500599 — LRCPI & LM, LRSCI & LM 1973 (RCSI) FRCPsych 1995, M 1979; DPM Leeds 1979. Cons. Psychiat. Leeds Community & Ment. Health Trust, St James Univ. Hosp. Leeds; Sen. Clin. Lect. (Psychiat.) Univ. Leeds. Specialty: Gen. Psychiat. Prev: Sen. Regist. Yorks. HA; Regist. (Psychiat.) Leeds AHA; Regist. Rotat. (Med.) St. Jas. Univ. Hosp. Leeds.

NEHAUL, Lika Kevin 5 Romsley Drive, The Farthings, Shrewsbury SY2 6TG — LRCPI & LM, LRSCI & LM 1975; LRCPI & LM, LRCSI & LM 1975; DCH Eng. 1979. Sen. Regist. (Community Med.) W. Midl. RHA. Specialty: Pub. Health Med. Prev: Regist. (Community Med.) S.E. Thames RHA.

NEHIKHARE, Friday Oghoghoaibi West Park Rehabilitation Hospital, Park Road West, Wolverhampton WV1 4PW Tel: 01902 444000 Fax: 01902 444318 — MB BS Nigeria 1982; MRCP UK 1994. Cons. Phys. in Geraitric Med. Specialty: Care of the Elderly. Socs: BGS; BASP.

NEHRA, Mr Dhiren Epson and St Helier NHS Trust, Wrythe Lane, Carshalton SM5 1AA Tel: 020 8296 3131 Fax: 020 8288 1838 Email: dhirennehra@epsom-sthelier.nhs.uk — MB BS Bombay 1983; FRCS Glas. 1990; MPhil Cardiff 1996. Cons. Gen. Surg. (Upper GI) Epsom and St Helier Hosps.; Private Consultations at St Anthonys Hospital Cheam; Private Consultations at Ashtead Hosp. Specialty: Gen. Surg. Special Interest: hernia repair; laparoscopic Gastrointestinal and Biliary Surg.; Upper GI. Socs: Surg. Soc. Alimentary Tract (USA); Assn. of Surgeons of Gt. Britain and Irel.; Assn. of Upper GI Surgeons of Gt. britain and Irel. Prev: Regist. (Gen. Surg.) Singleton Hosp.; Regist. (Gen. Surg.) Neath Gen. Hosp.; Regist. (Gen. Surg.) Wrexham Maelor Hosp.

NEHRING, Julia Valerie Prospect Park Hospital, Honey End Lane, Reading RG30 4EJ Tel: 0118 960 5000 — MB BS Lond. 1985; BA Oxf. 1980; MRCPsych 1989. Cons. Psychiat. Berks. Healthcare NHS Trust. Specialty: Gen. Psychiat. Prev: Clin. Research Fell. UMDS; Sen. Regist. (Psychiat.) St. Thos. Hosp. Lond.; Regist. (Psychiat.) Littlemore & Warneford Hosps. Oxf.

NEHRING, Sandra Jane Beighton Health Centre, Queens Road, Beighton, Sheffield S20 1BJ Tel: 0114 269 5061; Cloonmore, 29 Meadowhead, Sheffield S8 7UA — MB BS Lond. 1982; MRCGP 1986.

NEIGHBOUR, Roger Harvey (retired) Royal College of General Practitioners, 14 Princes Gate, London SW7 1PU; Argowan, Bell Lane, Bedmond, Abbots Langley WD5 0QS Tel: 01923 263961 Fax: 01923 264511 Email: roger.neighbour@dial.pipex.com — MB BChir Camb. 1971; MA Camb. 1972; DObst RCOG 1973; FRCGP 1986, M 1975. Pres., Roy. Coll. of Gen. Practitioners; Developm. Convenor Examrs.M RCGP 2002. Prev: Couvenor, Panel of MRCGP Examr.s, 1997-2002.

NEIL, Agnes Emily (retired) 1 Wolseley Gardens, Edinburgh EH8 7DG Tel: 0131 659 6545 — LRCP LRCS 1946 Ed (Roy. Colls. Ed.) LRFP LRFS Ed. LRFPS Glas. 1946. Prev: Cas. Off. Bootle Gen. Hosp.

NEIL, Andrew Fulton 55 Merton Hall Road, Wimbledon, London SW19 3PR — MB BS Lond. 1978 (Middlesex Hospital) MRCP (UK) 1981; FRCP 1995. Cons. Geriat. Qu. Mary's Hosp. Roehampton. Specialty: Care of the Elderly.

NEIL, Andrew Jardine (retired) 1 Wolseley Gardens, Edinburgh EH8 7DG Tel: 0131 659 6545 — LRCP LRCS Ed. LRFPS Glas. 1944 (Roy. Colls. Ed.) Prev: Surg. Lt. RNVR.

NEIL, Mrs Anne Baron (retired) 53 Talbot Road, Highgate, London N6 4QX Tel: 020 8340 0543 — MB ChB Leeds 1949. Prev: Sen. Community Med. Off. Lond. Boro. Ealing.

NEIL, Duncan 12 Colletts Green, Powick, Worcester WR2 4SB — MB ChB Glas. 1962 (Glas. & Brit. Columbia) DObst RCOG 1964. Socs: BMA. Prev: Surg. Resid. Joyce Green Hosp. Dartford; Med. Resid. Ballochmyle Hosp. Mauchline; Obst. Resid. Bellshill Matern. Hosp.

NEIL, Professor Hugh Andrew Wade, RD University of Oxford, Division of Public Health & Primary Health Care, Rosemary Rue Building, Old Road Campus, Headington, Oxford OX3 7LF Tel: 01865 226777 Fax: 01865 226777 Email: andrew.neil@wolfson.ox.ac.uk; 40 Beechcroft Road, Summertown, Oxford OX2 7AZ Tel: 01865 513348 — MB BS Lond. 1976 (St Thos. & Camb.) MA Camb. 1974, BA 1970; MRCS Eng. LRCP Lond. 1976; MRCP (UK) 1979; MSc Lond. 1981; MFCM 1987; FRCP Lond. 1995; FFPHM RCP (UK) 1995; DSc Lond. 2004. Prof. of Clin. Epidemiol.; Hon. Cons. Phys. Oxf. Centre for Diabetes, Endocrinol. & Metab, Churchill Hosp., Oxf. Specialty: Gen. Med.; Diabetes. Socs: Fell. Wolfson Coll. Univ. Oxf.; Trustee & Bd. Mem. HEART UK; Diabetes UK. Prev: Hon. Sen. Regist. & Lect. (Med.) Univ. Newc. Med. Sch.; Hon. Regist.(Med.) & Clin.Lect Univ.Oxf.

NEIL, Mr James Fulton (retired) Quaker Cottage, Quaker Lane, Farnsfield, Newark NG22 8EE Tel: 01623 882281 — (Camb. & Middlx.) MRCS Eng. LRCP Lond. 1942; MA, MB BChir Camb. 1943; FRCS Ed. 1947; DLO Eng. 1951. Prev: Cons. ENT Surg. Nottm. Univ. Hosp. & Kings Mill Hosp. Sutton-in-Ashfield.

NEIL, James Morton 4 Mid Brae, Mount Melville, Graigtoun, St Andrews KY16 8NT — MB ChB Manch. 1990.

NEIL, John Robert Knox GP - Plus, One Wemyss Place, Edinburgh EH3 6DH Tel: 0845 1196 049 Fax: 0845 1196 050 Email: johnneil@gpplus.com — MB ChB Glasgow 1971; MB ChB Glas 1971; MRCP (UK) 1977; MRCGP 1978; MFHom 1988. Private Gen. Practitioner and Specialist in Homeopathic Med. Socs: BMA.

NEIL, Lindsay Douglas (retired) Woodlands, Selkirk TD7 4ND Tel: 01750 20841 Email: neils@inigo.net — (Ed.) MB ChB Ed. 1965; DA Eng. 1972. Freelance GP Selkirk. Prev: Lt.-Col. RAMC, 205 Gen. Hosp. Gulf War.

NEIL, Shelagh Patricia Glenkens Medical Practice, The Surgery, High Street, New Galloway, Castle Douglas DG7 3RN Tel: 01644 420234 — MB ChB Aberd. 1972; MRCGP 1978. GP, New Galloway, Kirkcudbrightshire.

NEIL, Mr Thomas Kings Lane Surgery, 100 Kings Lane, Wirral CH63 5LY Tel: 0151 608 4347 Fax: 0151 608 9095 — MB ChB Leeds 1984; FRCS Ed. 1989; DRCOG 1991. Prev: Trainee GP Wirral VTS; SHO (Paediat.) Chester; SHO (Obst.) Warrington.

NEIL, Vanessa Shena (retired) Half Acre House, Lower Weald, Calverton, Milton Keynes MK19 6EQ Tel: 01908 560715 — MB BChir Camb. 1974; MA, MB Camb. 1974, BChir 1973; MRCP (UK) 1977; MRCPath 1982. Cons. Haemat. Bedford Gen. Hosp. Prev: Sen. Regist. (Haemat.) Oxon AHA (T).

NEIL, Wendy Jane Farthings, Pinfold Watering, Cookley, Halesworth IP19 0LT — MB ChB Ed. 1996. Specialty: Geriat. Psychiat.

NEIL, Mr William Fulton Head and Neck Centre, Royal Shrewsbury Hospital, Mytton Oak Road, Shrewsbury SY3 8XQ Tel: 01743 261499 Fax: 01742 261006 — (Middlx.) MB BS Lond. 1969; FRCS Eng. 1975. Cons. ENT Surg. Roy. Shrewsbury Hosp. NHS Trust. Specialty: Otolaryngol. Socs: Roy. Soc. Med. (Sects. Laryngol. & Otol.). Prev: Sen. Regist. (ENT) Roy. Berks. Hosp. Reading; Sen. Regist. Roy. Nat. Throat, Nose & Ear Hosp. Lond.

NEIL-DWYER, Mr Glenn Wessex Neurological Centre, Southampton General Hospital, Southampton SO16 6YD Tel: 023 8027 7222; Annesley Glade, Bank, Lyndhurst SO43 7FD Tel: 0142 128 3352 — MB BS Lond. 1963 (St. Mary's) FRCS Ed. 1967; FRCS Eng. 1969; MS Lond. 1974. Cons. Neurosurg. Wessex Neurol. Centre Soton. Gen. Hosp.; Hon. Cons. Neurosurg. Army. Specialty: Neurosurg. Socs: (Counc. Mem.) Brit. Soc. Neurol. Surgs. Prev: Cons. Neurosurg. SE Regional Neurosurg. Unit Brook Gen. Hosp. Lond.; Cons. Neurosurg. Cornw. Regional Hosp., Jamaica; Sen. Regist. (Neurosurg.) Wessex Neurosurg. Unit Soton. Gen. Hosp.

NEIL-DWYER, Jason Glen Annesley Glade, Bank, Lyndhurst, Southampton SO4 7FD — MB BS Lond. 1992; BSc (Hons. Surg.) Lond. 1989, MB BS 1992. SHO (Plastic Surg.) Qu. Vict. Hosp. E. Grinstead. Specialty: Accid. & Emerg. Socs: BMA. Prev: Ho. Off. (Gen. Med.) Roy. Sussex Co. Hosp.; Ho. Surg. Guy's Hosp. Lond.

NEIL-DWYER, Jennifer Susan Edith Annesley Glade, Bank, Lyndhurst SO43 7FD Tel: 023 8028 3352 — MB BS Lond. 1964 (St. Mary's) MRCS Eng. LRCP Lond. 1964; DO Eng. 1967. Clin. Asst. Soton. Eye Hosp. Prev: Clin. Asst. Guy's Hosp. Lond.; SHO Eye Unit Mayday Hosp. Croydon; SHO West. Ophth. Hosp. Lond.

NEILD, Professor Guy Hume Institute of Urology and Nephrology, University College and Middlesex School of Medicine, Middlesex Hospital, Mortimer Road, London W1T 3AA Tel: 020 7380 9366 Fax: 020 7380 9199 Email: g.neild@ucl.ac.uk — MB BS Lond. 1971 (St. Thos.) MD Lond. 1985; FRCP Lond. 1988; FRCPath Lond. 1999. Prof. Nephrol. UCMSM; Hon. Cons. St. Peter's Renal Unit UCL Hosps. (Middlx Hosp.) Lond. Specialty: Nephrol. Prev: Sen. Lect. (Nephrol.) Inst. of Urol.

NEILD, Penelope Jane — MB ChB Birm. 1987; BSc (Hons) 1984; MRCP 1991; MD Birm. 2000. Cons. & Hon. Sen. Lect. in Med. & Gastroenterol. Specialty: Gastroenterol. Special Interest: GI Physiol.; Nutrit. Socs: RSM; BMA; RCP.

NEILD, Valerie Susan Royal Victoria Hospital, Folkestone CT19 5HL; Swarling Manor, Petham, Canterbury CT4 5QP Tel: 01227 700377 — MB BS Lond. 1973 (St. Thos.) MRCP (UK) 1976; FRCP Lond. 1993. Cons. Dermat. SE Kent HA. Specialty: Dermat.

NEILL, Adrian K Site 3, Orchardvale, Upper Knockbreda Road, Belfast BT6 XXX — MB BCh BAO Belf. 1996.

NEILL, Alexander Edward (retired) Pound Cottage, South Stoke, Bath BA2 7DN — MB BChir Camb. 1949 (Lond. Hosp.) BA Camb. 1949. Prev: Med. Ref. BPA.

NEILL, Anne-Marie Grove House, Bury Road, Stapleford, Cambridge CB2 5BP Tel: 01223 846249 — MB ChB Sheff. 1988; MRCOG 1993. Locum Cons. W. Suff. Hosp. Specialty: Obst. & Gyn. Prev: Regist. (O & G) Rosie Matern. Hosp. Camb. & W. Suff. Hosp. Bury St. Edmunds; Regist. (O & G) N. Gen. Hosp. Sheff.; SHO (O & G) Jessop Hosp. Sheff.

NEILL, Fiona Elizabeth Silver Lodge, 44 Chatsworth Heights, Camberley GU15 1NH — MB BS Lond. 1990 (St. Bart. Hosp. Lond.) DCH RCP Lond. 1995. Specialist Regist. (Anaesth.) Kettering & Oxf. Specialty: Anaesth.

NEILL, Hugh Western Infirmary, Glasgow G11 6NT; 15 Raasay Gardens, Newton Mearns, Glasgow G77 6TH Tel: 0141 639 7535 — MB ChB Glas. 1992; BSc Glas. 1990; FRCA Lond. 1996. SPE(Anaesth.) N. Glas. Univ. Trust. Specialty: Anaesth. Socs: Glas. & W. Scot. Soc. Anaesth.; Scott. Soc. Anaesth.; Assoc. of Anaesth. Prev: SHO (Anaesth.) West. Infirm. Trust Hosps. Glas.

NEILL, James Hood (retired) 17 Hayne Park, Tipton St John, Sidmouth EX10 0TA Tel: 01404 811038 — MB ChB Ed. 1949. Prev: GP Eyam Derbysh.

NEILL, Leslie Gary Eskdaill Medical Centre, Eskdaill Street, Kettering NN16 8RA Tel: 01536 513053 Fax: 01536 417572; Beech House, Rectory Hill, Cranford, Kettering NN14 4AH Fax: 01536 330445 — MB ChB Sheff. 1981; DRCOG 1983. Specialty: Ment. Health.

NEILL, Margaret Philomena 4 Colbern Close, Brook Road, Maghull, Liverpool L31 3EP Tel: 0151 526 3726 — MB BCh BAO NUI 1952; DCH Dub. 1958; DPH NUI 1958; MRCPsych 1974. Prev: Cons. Psychiat. Moss Side Hosp. Liverp.

NEILL, Robert Alfred Bloomfield Surgery, 95 Bloomfield Road, Bangor BT20 4XA — MB BCh BAO Belf. 1980; DRCOG 1985; MRCGP 1986.

NEILL, Mr Robert Watson Kerr (retired) Grune House, Jarman Lane, Sutton, Macclesfield SK11 0HJ Tel: 01260 253172 — MB ChB Manch. 1957; FRCS Eng. 1968. Prev: Cons. Surg. Macclesfield Dist. Gen. Hosp.

NEILL, Sarah (Sallie) Mary Ashford & St Peters NHS Trust, Guildford Road, Chertsey KT16 0PZ; St Thomas's Hospital, St John's Dermatology Centre, Lambeth Palace Road, London SE1 7EH — MB ChB Manch. 1973; FRCP Lond.; MRCP (UK) 1981. Cons. Dermat. Ashford & St Peters NHS Trust, Guy's & St Thos. NHS Trust & Chelsea & Westm. NHS Trust. Specialty: Dermat. Special Interest: Anogenital Dermatoses. Socs: Brit. Assn. Dermat.; RSM; Internat. Soc. for the Study of Vulvovaginal Dis.

NEILL, Sarah Valerie 155A High Street, Brentwood CM14 4SD — MB ChB Glas. 1991.

NEILLIE, Jane Louise Worcester Royal Infirmary NHS Trust, Castle St., Worcester WR1 3AS; Apartment 6, Albemarle, Norton Barracks, Norton, Worcester WR5 2NZ — MB ChB Glas. 1993. Staff Grade (Psychiat.) Worcester Roy. Infirm. NHS Trust. Specialty: Gen. Psychiat. Prev: SHO (Dermat.) Monklands NHS Trust Airdrie; SHO (Dermat.) Stobhill NHS Trust Airdrie; SHO (Geriat.) Stobhill NHS Trust Glas.

NEILLY, Ian Joseph Wansbeck General Hospital, Woodhorn Lane, Ashington NE63 9JJ Tel: 01670 521212; 2 Swinton Close, Morpeth NE61 2XD Tel: 01670 518202 Email: ineilly@aol.com — MB ChB Aberd. 1982 (Aberdeen) MRCP (UK) 1985; MRCPath 1992; MD Aberdeen 1997; FRCP 1998; FRCPath 2000. Cons. Haemat. Wansbeck Gen. Hosp. Ashington. Specialty: Haematology. Prev: Sen. Regist. (Haemat.) Roy. Vict. Infirm. Belf.; Regist. (Haemat.) Aberd. Roy. Infirm.; Regist. (Med.) Roy. Alexandra Infirm. Paisley & West. & Gartnaval Infirms. Glas.

NEILSON, Angela Brasch — MB ChB Dundee 1981. GP Regist., Elmbank Gp., Foresterhill Health Centre, Aberd. Specialty: Gen. Pract. Prev: SHO Psychiat., Roy. Cornhill Hosp., Aberd.; Clin. Asst., Subst. Misuse, Roy. Cornhill Hosp., Aberd.; GP Assistance, Fyvie/Old Meldrum Med. Gp.

NEILSON, Anna Marguerite Craigwell Cottage, Barrhill Road, Dalbeattie DG5 4JB — MB ChB Glas. 1996; MRCPsych 2001.

NEILSON, David William 1/2 72 Novar Drive, Hyndland, Glasgow G12 9TZ Tel: 0141 357 2489 — MB ChB Glas. 1983.

NEILSON, Derek James Currer The Clinic, Mill Isle, Craignair Street, Dalbeattie DG5 4HE Tel: 01556 610331; Craggie, Dalbeattie DG5 4QT Tel: 01556 610455 — (St. And.) MB ChB St. And. 1967; DObst RCOG 1970. Specialty: Forens. Path. Prev: Ho. Off. (Med.) Falkirk & Dist. Roy. Infirm.; Ho. Off. (Obst.) Elsie Inglis Matern. Hosp. Edin.; Ho. Off. (Surg. & Paediat.) Roy. Hosp. Sick Childr. Edin.

NEILSON, Mr Donald Blackburn Royal Infirmary, Bolton Road, Blackburn BB2 3LR Tel: 01254 687262 — MB ChB Liverp. 1981; FRCS Ed. 1986; FRCS (Urol.) 1996; MD 1997. Cons. Urol. Blackburn Roy. Infirm. Blackburn. Specialty: Urol. Prev: Sen. Regist. (Urol.) Manch. Roy. Infirm.; Sen. Regist. (Urol.) Stepping Hill Hosp. Stockport; Sen. Regist. (Urol.) Withington Hosp. Manch.

NEILSON, Ewan Graham 55 Deanwood Avenue, Netherlee, Glasgow G44 3RQ — MB ChB Glas. 1996.

NEILSON, Frances Marguerite Currer The Sycamores, 5 Almoners Barn, Potters Bank, Durham DH1 3TZ — MB ChB Ed. 1967; DObst RCOG 1970; DPH Glas. 1971. Clin. Med. Off. (Community Child Health) Durh. Specialty: Community Child Health.

NEILSON, Frances Mary 63 Beatty Avenue, Coldean, Brighton BN1 9EP — MB ChB Aberd. 1976; MRCPsych 1982.

NEILSON, Graham Alexander 27 Turnberry Drive, Newton Mearns, Glasgow G77 5SE — MB ChB Glas. 1997. SHO (Anaesth.) Stobhill Hosp., Glas. Specialty: Anaesth. Socs: BMA. Prev: SHO A & E SHO Orthop.; Jun. Ho. Off. Med.; Jun. Ho. Off. Surg.

NEILSON, Professor James Purdie University of Liverpool, School of Reproductive & Developmental Medicine, Liverpool L69 3BX Tel: 0151 702 4100 Fax: 0151 702 4024 Email: jneilson@liv.ac.uk; 10 Oldfield Road, Heswall, Wirral CH60 6SE Tel: 0151 342 2796 — MB ChB Ed. 1975; MD Ed. 1985, BSc 1972; MRCOG 1981; FRCOG 1997. Prof. O & G Univ. Liverp.; Hon. Cons. Obst. & Gyn. Liverp. Wom. Hosp. Specialty: Obst. & Gyn. Prev: Sen. Lect. (O & G) Univ. Edin.; Lect. (Obst.) Univ. Glas.; Sen. Regist. Harare Centr. Hosp., Zimbabwe.

NEILSON, Jeffrey Roy Department of Heamatology, Leicester Royal Infirmary, Leicester LE1 5WW; 43 Main Street, Snarestone, Swadlincote DE12 7DB — MB ChB Manch. 1987; MRCP (UK) 1991; MRCPath 1998. Sen. Regist. (Haemat.) Leicester Roy. Infirm. Specialty: Haematology. Prev: Research Fell. (Haemat.) Birm. Heartlands Hosp.; Regist. Rot. (Haemat.) W. Midl.; SHO Rotat. (Gen. Med.) Blackburn Roy. Infirm.

NEILSON, Mr John Rosewood, Park St., Dumfries DG2 7PH Tel: 01387 255678 — (Univ. Glas.) MB ChB Glas. 1937, DPH 1939; FRFPS Glas. 1947; FRCS Ed. (ad eund.) 1961; FRCS Glas. 1962. Specialty: Gen. Surg. Socs: Fell. Assn. Surgs. Gt. Brit.; BMA. Prev: Sen. Cons. Surg. Dumfries & Galloway Roy. Infirm.; Sen. Clin. Lect. Aberd. Univ.; Med. Off. Hackney LCC Hosp.

NEILSON, Roderick Forsyth Falkirk & District Royal Infirmary, Department of Haematology, Majors Loan, Falkirk FK1 5QE Tel: 01360 624000 Ext: 5368 Email: roddy.neilson@fvah.scot.nhs.uk; 182 Southbrae Drive, Glasgow G13 1TX Tel: 0141 959 2449 Email: roddy@arneilson.demon.co.uk — MB ChB Glas. 1985; MRCP (UK) 1988; DFM Glas. 1994; MRCPath 1995; FRCP Glas. 1999; FRCP Ed. 1999; MPhil Glas. 2002; FRCPath 2003. Cons. (Haemat.) Falkirk & Dist. Roy. Infirm. Specialty: Haematology. Prev: Cons. Haematologist and Haemophilia Centre Director N. Hants. Hosp. Basingstoke; Med. Adviser Med. & Dent. Defence Union Scotl.; Sen. Regist. (Haemat.) Glas. Roy. Infirm.

NEILSON, William Robert 15 Mermaid Street, Rye TN31 7ET — MB BS Lond. 1975; MRCS Eng. LRCP Lond. 1975.

NEININGER, Patrick David Roger Woodbank Surgery, 2 Hunstanton Drive, Bury BL8 1EG Tel: 0161 705 1630 Fax: 0161 763 3221 Email: patrick.neininger@gp-p83017.nhs.uk; 11 Tonbridge Close, Bury BL8 1YH Email: patrick.neininger@virgin.net — MRCS Eng. LRCP Lond. 1972 (Birm.) DObst RCOG 1975; MRCGP 1978. Gen. Practitioner, Bury, Lancs. Specialty: Gen. Pract. Socs: BMA; Sands Cox Soc. Prev: Trainee GP Bury VTS; Ho. Surg. Dorset Co. Hosp. Dorchester; Ho. Phys. Whiston Hosp. Prescot.

NEITHERCUT, Margaret Stewart (retired) 4 Albany Drive, Burnside, Rutherglen, Glasgow G73 3QN Tel: 0141 647 6823 — MB ChB Glas. 1942; MD Glas. 1947. Prev: Cytol. Monklands Gen. Hosp. Airdrie.

NEITHERCUT, William Duncan Department of Chemical Pathology, Arrowe Park Hospital, Arrowe Park Road, Upton, Wirral CH49 5LN; Department of Chemical Pathology, Clatterbridge Hospital, Bebington, Wirral CH63 4JY — MB ChB Glas. 1980.

NEJIM, Mr Ali Airedale General Hospital, Steeton, Keighley BD20 6TD; Shay Croft, Shay Lane, Heaton, Bradford BD9 6SQ — MB ChB Baghdad 1979; FRCS Eng. 1991. Cons. Gen. Surg. Airedale Gen. Hosp. Keighley; Hon. Lect. Surg. Leeds Univ. Specialty: Gen. Surg. Socs: BMA; BASO; VSS. Prev: Sen. Regist. (Gen. Surg.) St. Jas. Univ. Hosp.; Regist. Rotat. W. Yorks.; SHO (Urol.) Wakefield.

NEJO, Tunde Akinwale Surrey Hampshire Borders NHS Trust, Briarwood Rehabilitation Unit, Broadhurst, Cove, Farnborough GU14 9XW — MB BCh BAO NUI 1985; MRCPsych 1993. Cons. Psychiat. Surrey Hants. Borders NHS Trust Briarwood Rehabil. Unit Broadhurst Cove Farnboro. Specialty: Gen. Psychiat.; Geriat. Psychiat. Socs: BMA; Roy. Coll. Psychiat.; Fell. Roy. Soc. Med. Prev: Cons./Sen. Regist. Gen. Psychiat. Norf. Ment. Health Care NHS Trust Norwich; Sen. Regist. (Geriat. Psychiat.) W. Suff. Hosp. Mid-Anglia NHS Trust.

NEL, George Department of Orthopaedic Surgery, Bedford Hospital, South Wing, Kempston Road, Bedford MK42 9DJ Tel: 01234 792201 Fax: 01234 340122; 62 Putnoe Heights, Bedford MK41 8EB Tel: 01234 352966 Fax: 01234 343202 — (Univ. of Cape town, S Africa) MB ChB Cape Town 1964; FCS(SA) (Orth) 1981. Clin Dir Orthop.Dept. Bedford Hosp. Specialty: Orthop. Socs: Brit. Orthop. Assn.; Roy. Soc. Med. Prev: Orthop. Cons. Mines Benefit Soc. S. Africa.

NEL, Mark Reginald Department of Anaesthesia, The Hillingdon Hospital, Pield Heath Road, Uxbridge UB8 3NN Tel: 01895 238282 Email: mark.nel@thh.nhs.uk — MB BCh Witwatersrand 1987; FRCA Roy. Coll. of Anaesthetists 1995 (Univ. of Witwatersrand) Cons. Anaesth., The Hillingdon Hosp., Uxbridge. Specialty: Anaesth. Special Interest: Obstetric Amaesthesia; Preoperative Assessment; Trauma & Orthopaedic Surgery. Socs: Soc. for Intravenous Anaesth.; Obstetric Anaesth. Assn.; Roy. Soc. of Med.

NELEMANS, Ian St Albans Medical Centre, 26-28 St. Albans Crescent, Bournemouth BH8 9EW Tel: 01202 517333; 34 Castlemain Avenue, Bournemouth BH6 5EJ — Artsexamen Nijmegen 1980; FRCGP 1996, M 1987. Clin. Asst. Pacing Dept., Dept. of Cardiol. Roy. Bournemouth Hosp. Specialty: Gen. Pract. Prev: Med. Off. i/c Consolata Hosp. Kyeni, Kenya.

NELIGAN, Patrick Hugh School House Farm, 2 Main Street, Copmanthorpe, York YO23 3SU Tel: 01904 703197 Email: paddy.neligan@btopenworld.com — MB ChB Birm. 1972; MRCP (UK) 1977; FRCP Lond. 1991. Assoc. Postgrad. Dean, Yorks. Specialty: Care of the Elderly. Socs: Brit. Geriat. Soc. Prev: Lect. (Med.) Univ. Dundee; SHO (Med.) Roy. Hosp. Wolverhampton; Ho. Phys. Childr. Hosp. Birm.

NELKI, Julia Sibyl Seymour House, 43 Seymour Terrace, Liverpool L3 5TE Tel: 0151 707 0101 Fax: 0151 708 9200 — MB ChB Bristol 1979; MA Oxf. 1975; DRCOG 1981; MRCPsych 1985; MSc 1990. p/t Cons. Child & Adolesc. Psychiat. Roy. Liverp. Child. NHS Trust; Project Director Family Refugee Support Project; Course Comm. Mem. for MA PsychoAnalyt. Observational Studies Merseyside Psychother. Inst. Specialty: Child & Adolesc. Psychiat. Socs: Assn. Family Ther.; Med. Foundat. for Care of Victims of Torture; NHS Consultants Assn. Prev: Sen. Regist. (Child & Adolesc. Psychiat.) Tavistock Clin.; SHO & Regist. (Adult Psychiat.) Lond. Hosp. Whitechapel.

NELKI, Michael Fenner Hermann Yatton Family Practice, 155 Mendip Road, Yatton, Bristol BS49 4ER Tel: 01934 832277; The Courtyard Flat, 41 Royal York Crescent, Bristol BG8 3JS — (St. Geo.) MB BS Lond. 1969; MRCS Eng. LRCP Lond. 1970; DObst RCOG 1971. Socs: MN.

NELLIST, Paul John Gibson Court Medical Centre, Gibson Court, Boldon Colliery NE35 9AN Tel: 0191 454 0421; 111 Victoria Road W., Hebburn NE31 1UX — MB BS Newc. 1989.

NELMS, Mark Thomas Carlisle House, 53 Lagland Street, Poole BH15 1QD Tel: 01202 678484 Fax: 01202 660507; 52 Twemlow Avenue, Parkstone, Poole BH14 8AN — BM Soton. 1985; DRCOG 1989.

NELSON, Alan Rache Harley House Surgery, 2 Irnham Road, Minehead TA24 5DL Tel: 01643 703441 Fax: 01643 704867 — MB BS Lond. 1977 (St. Thomas' Hospital London) MRCS Eng. LRCP Lond. 1977; DRCOG 1981; MRCGP 1981. Clin. Governance Lead Som. Coast PCT. Specialty: Gen. Pract.; Psychother.

NELSON, Alys Patricia (retired) Newby, 25 The Northern Road, Great Crosby, Liverpool L23 2RA — MB ChB Glas. 1943 (Univ. Glas.) BSc, MB ChB Glas. 1943. Prev: Ho. Phys. Roy. Infirm. Glas.

NELSON, Andrew Moore (retired) Sunny Meed Surgery, 15-17 Heathside Road, Woking GU22 7EY Tel: 01483 772760 — MB BS Lond. 1956. Police Surg. Woking.

NELSON, Brian Lynn Powell (retired) West Haven, Ton Kenfig Pyle, Bridgend CF33 4PT Tel: 01656 742159 — MB BCh Wales 1955 (Cardiff) Prev: GP Port Talbot.

NELSON, Christopher Sinclair 6 Park Lane, Allestree, Derby DE22 2DR Tel: 01332 557675 — MB ChB Glas. 1970; MRCP (UK) 1975; FRCP Glas. 1986. Cons. Paediat. & Paediat. Nephrol. Derby Childr. Hosp. & Nottm. City. Specialty: Nephrol. Prev: Lect. in Child Health Univ. Glas. Dept. Child Health Roy. Hosp. Sick; Childr. Glas.;

Regist. (Gen. Med.) Roy. Alexandra Infirm. Paisley; Regist. (Med. Paediat.) Roy. Hosp. Sick Childr. Glas.

NELSON, Cyril Anthony 3 Highbridge Road, Sutton Coldfield B73 5QA — MB ChB Birm. 1984; BSc Birm. 1981; FRCR 1993. Cons. Radiol. Good Hope NHS Trust. Specialty: Radiol. Socs: Fell. Roy. Coll. Radiol.

NELSON, Cyril Ellis 31 Avondale Road, Southport PR9 0NH — MRCS Eng. LRCP Lond. 1953 (Sheff.) Prev: Med. Regist. & Sen. Ho. Phys. Sharoe Green Hosp. Fulwood; SHO (Obst.) & Ho. Phys. Preston Roy. Infirm.

NELSON, David (retired) 101 Gledhow Lane, Roundhay, Leeds LS8 1NE Tel: 0113 294 8198 — MRCS Eng. LRCP Lond. 1961 (Liverp.) Prev: Regional Sec. Med. Protec. Soc.

NELSON, Deborah Elizabeth Palmerston House, 44Colinton Road, Edinburgh EH14 1AH Tel: 0131 337 5949 Email: dr_debbie_nelson@yahoo.com — MB ChB Ed. 1990; MRCPsych 1996; Dip. FMSA 1998. p/t Cons. Psychiat., Falkirk Roy. Infirm., Falkirk. Specialty: Forens. Psychiat.; Gen. Psychiat. Socs: BMA; Scottish Medicolegal Association. Prev: Specialist Regist. in Forens. Psychiat., Orchard Clinic, Roy. Edin. Hosp.

NELSON, Doreen Elizabeth Auskaird, 5 Greenwood, Culmore, Londonderry BT48 8NP — MB BCh BAO Belf. 1959.

NELSON, Elizabeth Christina 79 Cloch Road, Gourock PA19 1AU Tel: 01475 32332 — MB ChB Ed. 1948; DPH Ed. 1952; DCH Eng. 1957; DPM Leeds 1963. Prev: Cons. Child Psychiat. Argyll & Clyde HB; Sen. Regist. Wessex RHB & West. RHB (Scotl.); Regional Med. & Health Off. Sask., Canada.

NELSON, Fiona Gray The Surgery, Hounsfield Way, Sutton-on-Trent, Newark NG23 6PX Tel: 01636 821023 Fax: 01636 822308 — MB ChB Sheff. 1971. Asst. GP Sutton-on-Trent, Newark; Clin. Med. Off. Bassetlaw & Centr. Notts. HAs.

NELSON, Fiona Rosalind 22 Gilmour Road, Edinburgh EH16 5NT Tel: 0131 667 1173 Email: fiona.barry@tinyworld.co.uk — MB ChB Ed. 1992 (Edin.) M.Phil (Law & Med. Eth.) Glas. 1998; DFFP 1999; MRCOG 2002. Specialist Regist. (O & G) S.E. Scot. Rot. New Roy. Infrim. of Edin.; Sessional Doctor (Sexual Health) Midlothian Young Person Advis. Serv. Dalkeith and Penicuik, Midlothian; Dalkeith and Penicuilk, Midlothian. Specialty: Obst. & Gyn.; Family Plann. & Reproduc. Health; Medico Legal. Socs: Edin. Obst. Soc.; Scott. Medico-Legal Soc. Prev: Res. Fell. (O & G) Roy. Infirm. Edin.; Sen. SHO (O & G) Princess Anne Hosp. Soton.; SHO (A & E) Jersey Gen. Hosp.

NELSON, Professor George Stanley Snarlton House, Wingfield, Trowbridge BA14 9LH Tel: 01225 754763 — MB ChB St. And. 1948; DTM & H Liverp. 1953; DSc St. And. 1966, MD 1956; Dip. Applied Parasitol. & Entomol. Univ. Lond 1960; FRCP 1981, M 1971; FRCPath 1979. Emerit. Prof. Trop. Med. Infec. Dis. Liverp. Sch. Med. Specialty: Trop. Med. Socs: Fell. (Pres.) Roy. Soc. Trop. Med. & Hyg.; Hon. Fell. Amer. Soc. Trop. Med. & Hyg. Prev: Walter Myers Prof. Parasitol. Liverp. Sch. Trop. Med.; Prof. Helminthol. Lond. Sch. Hyg. & Trop. Med.; Sen. Parasitol. Nairobi.

NELSON, Gillian Louise Perrott End, New Yatt Road, North Leigh, Witney OX29 6TT — MB ChB Leic. 1991.

NELSON, Helen Margaret Queen's Hospital, Burton, Belvedere Road, Burton-on-Trent DE13 0RB Tel: 01283 566333 Fax: 01283 593014; 6 Park Lane, Allestree, Derby DE22 2DR — MB ChB Glas. 1974; FRCP Glas. 1989. Cons. Dermat. Burton Hosp. NHS Trust. Specialty: Dermat. Socs: Orindary Mem. Brit. Assn. Dermat.; Brit. Soc. Paediat. Dermatol.; Brit. Contact Dermatitis Gp. Prev: Sen. Regist. (Dermat.) Univ. Hosp. Nottm., Glas. Roy. Infirm. & West. Infirm. Glas.

NELSON, Hugh Francis John 99 Magheralane Road, Randalstowwn, Antrim BT41 2PA — MB BCh BAO Belf. 1991.

NELSON, Mr Ian Wilkie Frenchay Hospital, Department of Orthopaedic Surgery, Frenchay Park Road, Bristol BS16 1LE Tel: 0117 918 6514 Fax: 0117 918 6641 Email: ian.nelson@nbt.nhs.uk — MB BS Lond. 1979 (Westm.) MRCS Eng. LRCP Lond. 1979; FRCS Eng. 1984; MCh Orth. Liverp. 1990. Cons. Orthop. Surg. N. Bristol NHS Trust. Specialty: Trauma & Orthop. Surg. Special Interest: Spine. Socs: Brit. Scoliosis Soc.; Brit. Assn. Spine Surg.; Brit. Orthop. Assn. Prev: Lect. (Orthop.) Nuffield Orthop. Centre Oxf.; Regist. (Orthop.) Univ. Coll. Hosp. Lond.; Ho. Surg. & Cas. Off. Westm. Hosp. Lond.

NELSON, Ivan Douglas Magill (retired) 8 Leveson Close, Gosport PO12 2QJ Tel: 023 9235 8363 — (Qu. Univ. Belf.) MB BCh BAO Belf. 1941, DPH 1947; MFCM 1974. Hon. Clin. Teach. Soton. Univ. Med. Sch. Prev: SCM Hants. AHA (T).

NELSON, Jagbir Cheviot Way Health Centre, Cheviot Way, Bourtreehill South, Irvine KA11 1JU — MB ChB Glas. 1991. Clin. Asst. (Diabetes) CrossHo. Hosp. Kilmarnock. Specialty: Gen. Pract.

NELSON, James Prestwich The Nelson Practice, Amersall Road, Scawthorpe, Doncaster DN5 9PQ Tel: 01302 780704 Fax: 01302 390512; Grove Cottage, The Grove, Barnby Dun, Doncaster DN3 1EB — MB ChB Sheff. 1965.

NELSON, James Spiers 19 Trevose Gardens, Sherwood, Nottingham NG5 3FU Tel: 0115 960 9834 — MB BCh BAO Belf. 1949; LRCP LRCS Ed. LRFPS Glas. 1949; DMJ (Clin.) Soc. Apoth. Lond. 1971. Sen. Police Surg. Notts. Constab.; Phys. i/c BUPA Med. Centre Nottm.. Prev: Ho. Phys. City Hosp. Nottm.; Res. Ho. Off. Childr. Hosp. Nottm.

NELSON, James William 39 Parkside View, Leeds LS6 4NS — MB ChB Leeds 1998 (University of Leeds Medical School) BSc Leeds 1986; PhD Edinburgh 1990. Specialty: Gen. Pract.

NELSON, Jennifer Jane Ashworth Street Surgery, 85 Spotland Road, Rochdale OL12 6RT; 5 Beaumonds Way, Rochdale OL11 5NL Tel: 01706 646081 — MB ChB Manch. 1993 (Mans.) BSc St. And. 1990; MRCGP 1998. Specialty: Gen. Pract.

NELSON, Joanne Katherine Cupar Street Clinic, 91 Cupar Street, Belfast BT12 2LJ Tel: 028 9032 7613 — BM BCh Oxf. 1990; MRGPCH; FRCP Edin.; MA Camb. 1987; MD Queens Univ. Belfast 1999. Cons. (Paeds). Specialty: Paediat. Socs: Ulster Med. Soc.; RCPCH; Paediat. Res. Soc.

NELSON, John Kenneth The Ulster Hospital, Dundonald, Belfast BT16 1RH Tel: 028 9056 1384 Fax: 028 9055 0436 Email: susan.williams@nda.n-i.nhs.uk; 4 Rosepark East, Belfast BT5 7RL Tel: 028 9048 3221 Fax: 028 9048 7131 — (Qu. Univ. Belf.) MB BCh BAO (Hons.) Belf. 1960; MD Belf. 1963; FRCP Ed. 1971, M 1964; FRCP Lond. 1988. p/t Cons. Phys. Ulster Hosp. Dundonald, Belf.; Sen. Lect. (Med.) Qu. Univ. Belf.; Regional Adviser North. Irel. & Adviser RePub. Irel. for Roy. Coll. of Phys. Ed. Specialty: Gen. Med.; Diabetes; Endocrinol. Special Interest: Heart Failure; Hypertens.; Insulin Ther. in Type 2 Diabetes. Socs: Fell. Roy. Soc. Med.; Sen. Mem. Assn. Phys.; Diabetes UK (Med. & Scientif. Sect.). Prev: Sen. Regist. Sir Geo. E. Clark Metab. Unit Roy. Vict. Hosp. Belf.; Research Fell. Johns Hopkins Univ. Hosp. Baltimore, USA; Research Fell. (Med.) Qu. Univ. Belf.

NELSON, John Kenneth Mackenzie 3/2, 8 Cowan Street, Hillhead, Glasgow G12 8PF — MB ChB Glas. 1995.

NELSON, John Steven Department of Anaesthetics, Charing Cross Hospital, Gulham Palace Road, London SW1; 18 Manchuria Road, Battersea, London SW11 6AE — MB ChB Glas. 1988 (Glasgow University) FRCA (UK). Specialist Regist. (Anaesth.) St. Mary's Sch. Anaesth. Lond. Specialty: Anaesth.

NELSON, Joyce Marjorie (Surgery), 262 Stockport Road, Cheadle Heath, Stockport Tel: 0161 428 6729; 89 Gatley Road, Cheadle SK8 1LX — MB ChB Liverp. 1959; DObst RCOG 1962.

NELSON, Juliet Deborah 31 Tantallon Road, London SW12 8DF — MB ChB Bristol 1988; BSc (Hons.) Bristol 1986; MRCP (UK) 1992. GP Partner Wimbledon. Prev: GP Trainer Lond. Deanery; Ho. Surg. Bristol Roy. Infirm.; SHO (A & E) Bristol Roy. Infirm.

NELSON, Katherine Wendy 237 Spring Vale Road, Sheffield S10 1LG — MB ChB Sheff. 1991.

NELSON, Kenneth Alexander (retired) Clonvara, 17 Glenarm Road, Larne BT40 1BN — MB BCh BAO Belf. 1949. Prev: Res. Ho. Off. Roy. Vict. Hosp. Belf. & Roy. Hosp. Sick Childr. Belf.

NELSON, Kenneth Andrew Shankill Road Surgery, 136-138 Shankill Road, Belfast BT13 2BD Tel: 028 9032 4524; 5 Locksley Park, Belfast BT10 0AR — MB BCh BAO Belf. 1979; DCH Dub. 1983; MRCGP 1984.

NELSON, Mrs Margaret Elizabeth Kelsey (retired) Ivy House, Castlecaulfield, Dungannon BT70 3NP Tel: 0186 87 61240 — MB BCh BAO Dub. 1954 (T.C. Dub.) BA, MB BCh BAO Dub. 1954. SCMO South. Health & Social Servs. Bd. Prev: Princip. in Gen. Pract. Fivemiletown Co. Tyrone.

NELSON, Mark Richard Chelsea & Westminster Hospital, 369 Fulham Road, London SW10 — MB BS Lond. 1986; MA Camb. 1982. Cons. HIV Chelsea & Westm. Hosp. Lond. Specialty:

Genitourinary Medicine. Socs: Roy. Coll. Phys. Prev: Sen. Regist. (HIV & Genitourin. Med.) Chelsea & Westm. Hosp. Lond.; Regist. (HIV Med., Neurol. & Gastroenterol.) Westm. Hosp. Lond.

NELSON, Professor Maurice Gerald (retired) Rosefield, Ballylesson, Belfast BT8 8JX Tel: 0123 126433; Rosefield, Ballylesson, Belfast BT8 8JX Tel: 0123 126433 — MD Belf. 1940; MD (Gold Medal) Belf. 1940, MB BCh BAO (Hnrs.); FRCP Lond. 1961, M 1940; FRCPI 1955, M 1946; DTM & H Eng. 1947; FRCPath 1963. Prev: Cons. Clin. Pathol. Belf. Gp. Hosps.

NELSON, Michael Department of Neuroradiology, Clarendon Wing, Leeds General Infirmary, Leeds LS1 3EX Tel: 0113 392 3683 Fax: 0113 392 5196 Email: mike.nelson@leedsth.nhs.uk — MB BChir Camb. 1974; MRCP (UK) 1977; FRCR 1982. Cons. Neuroradiol. Yorks. RHA & ULTH NHS Trust; Clin. Sen. Lect. Univ. Leeds. Specialty: Radiol. Socs: Brit. Soc. Neuroradiol.; N. Eng. Neurol. Assn. Prev: Sen. Regist. (Radiodiagn.) Oxf. HA (T); Hon. Clin. Asst. Nat. Hosp. Nerv. Dis. Lond.

NELSON, Mr Michael Eric Dept. Ophthalmology, Royal Hallamshire Hospital, Glossop Rd, Sheffield S10 2JF Tel: 0114 271 2223 — MB ChB Liverp. 1980; FRCS Eng. 1985; FCOphth 1989; BSc (Hons.) Open 1995; Masters in Education 2000. Cons. Ophth. Roy. Hallamsh. Hosp. Sheff.; Hon. Sen. Lect. (Ophth.) Univ. Sheff. Specialty: Ophth.

NELSON, Philip David Flat 2, 27 Essendine Road, Maida Vale, London W9 2LT Tel: 020 7286 6282 — MB ChB Leeds 1988; FRCA 1995. Specialist Regist. (Anaesth.) St. Mary's Hosp. Lond. Specialty: Anaesth. Socs: BMA; Anaesth. Res. Soc.; Intens. Care Soc. Prev: Specialist Regist. (Anaesth.) Roy. Brompton Hosp. Lond.; Specialist Regist. (Anaesth.) Luton & Dunstable Hosp.; Specialist Regist. (Anaesth.) Qu. Charlotte's Hosp. Lond.

NELSON, Richard Andrew Countess of Chester Hospital, Liverpool Road, Chester CH2 1UL Tel: 01244 365000 Fax: 01244 365112 Email: richard.nelson@coch.nhs.uk — BM (Hons.) Soton. 1982; FRCA; MRCP (UK) 1985; FCAnaesth 1990. Cons. Anaesth. Countess of Chester Hosp. Specialty: Anaesth.; Intens. Care. Prev: Sen. Regist. Rotat. (Anaesth.) Mersey RHA.; Research Fell. (Clin. Pharmacol.) Vanderbilt Univ. Nashville, Tennessee, USA; Regist. Rotat. (Anaesth.) Mersey RHA.

NELSON, Robert (retired) 33 Beech Grove, Benton, Newcastle upon Tyne NE12 8LA Tel: 0791 266 6114; 33 Beech Grove, Benton, Newcastle upon Tyne NE12 8LA — MB ChB Manch. 1962; DCH Eng. 1964; FRCP Lond. 1979, M 1967. Cons. Paediatr. Roy. Vict. Infirm. Newc. u. Tyne. Prev: Lect. (Paediat.) Univ. Birm.

NELSON, Russell Ravenswood House, Knowle, Fareham PO17 5NA — BM Soton. 1985; MRCPsych 1997. Specialty: Forens. Psychiat. Socs: Roy. Coll. Psychiat.

NELSON, Samuel David (retired) Haematology Department, Craigavon Area Hospital, Craigavon BT63 5QQ Tel: 01762 334444 Fax: 01762 334582 — MB BCh BAO Belf. 1956; FRCPI 1970, M 1962; FRCPath 1979, M 1967. Cons. Haemat. Craigavon Area Hosp. Prev: Dep. Dir. Nat. Tissue Typing Ref. Laborat. Bristol.

NELSON, Sarah Ann The Strand Practice, 2 The Strand, Goring-by-Sea, Worthing BN12 6DN Tel: 01903 243351 Fax: 01903 705804 — BM Soton. 1987; BSc (Biochem.) Lond. 1976; DRCOG 1991; MRCGP 1991. Prev: Trainee GP Kent & Canterbury Hosp. VTS; Community Med. Off. (Community Child Health) Thameslink NHS Trust.

NELSON, Simon Charles Sid House, Sid Rd, Sidmouth, Sidmouth EX10 9AH — MB BS Lond. 1997.

NELSON, Stephen Ralph Department of Renal Medicine, St Georges Healthcare NHS Trust, Blackshaw Road, London SW17 0QT Tel: 020 8725 2705 Fax: 020 8725 2068 — MB ChB (Hons.) Leeds 1982; MD Leeds 1991; FRCP 1997. Cons. Nephrol. St. Geo. Healthcare NHS Trust Lond. Specialty: Nephrol. Prev: Cons. Nephrol. King's Coll. Hosp. Lond.

NELSON, Stuart Angus Barrons Overton Park Surgery, Overton Park Road, Cheltenham GL50 3BP Tel: 01242 580511; Bourneside, Bourne Lane, Brimscombe, Stroud GL5 2RQ — MB BS Lond. 1983 (St. Geo.) DRCOG 1986; MRCGP 1987; DCH 1988; DFFP 1994. Trainer (Gen. Pract.) Cheltenham. Specialty: Gen. Pract. Socs: (Treas.) Severn Fac. RCGP. Prev: Trainee GP Suff. VTS.

NELSON, Susan Priory View Medical Centre, 2A Green Lane, Leeds LS12 1HU; 40 Denton Ave, Leeds LS8 1LE — MB ChB Leeds 1991; DFFP 1994; MRCGP 1998. GP Princip. Specialty: Gen. Pract. Prev: Non-Princip. GP Leeds; SHO (A & E) Halifax Roy. Infirm.; SHO (O & G) Leeds Gen. Infirm.

NELSON, Susan Elizabeth Tippitiwitchet Cottage, Hall Road, Outwell, Wisbech PE14 8PE — MB BS Lond. 1974 (Univ. Coll. Hosp.) DCH Eng. 1976; MRCGP 1979.

NELSON, Tanya Rose Wonford House Hospital, Crisis Resolution Team, Dryden Road, Exeter EX2 5AF — MB BS Lond. 1992. Cons. Psychiat. Devon Partnership NHS Trust. Specialty: Gen. Psychiat.

NELSON, Terence Edward (retired) High Bank House, 46 Main St., Addingham, Ilkley LS29 0PL — MB BS Durh. 1959 (Newc.) DPM Eng. 1965; MRCP Lond. 1968; FRCPsych 1983, M 1971; FRCP London 1999. Prev: Med. Dir. Leeds CMH Teach. Hosp.

NELSON, Vivienne Margaret Anaesthetic Department, Whiston Hospital, Warrington Road, Prescot L35 5DS — MB ChB Leeds 1981; FFA RCS Eng. 1987. Specialty: Anaesth.

NELSON, William Edward Renal Unit, Belfast City Hospital, Belfast BT9; 2 Rosevale Gardens, Drumbeg, Dunmurry, Belfast BT17 9LH — MD Belf. 1983; MB BCh BAO 1974; DRCOG 1976; DCH RCPSI 1976; MRCP (UK) 1980. Cons. Nephrol. Belf. City Hosp. Specialty: Nephrol.

NELSON, William McClure 14 Rosepark, Belfast BT5 7RG Tel: 0123 183889 — MB BCh BAO Belf. 1958; MRCPI 1965; DPM Eng. 1965; MRCPsych 1971.

NELSON, William Myles Antrim Hospital, 45 Bush Road, Antrim BT41; 137 Whitesides Road, Ballymena BT42 2JG — MB BCh BAO Belf. 1992 (Qu. Univ. Belf.) BSc (Hons.) Belf. 1989; FRCR 2001. Cons. Radiologist. Specialty: Radiol. Socs: Fell. of Roy. Coll. of Radiologist. Prev: Specialist Regist. (Radiol.) Hull Roy. Infirm.; SHO (Gen. Surg.) Ards Hosp.; SHO (Orthop. Surg.) Musgrave Pk. Hosp.

NELSON-IYE, Ada Comfort 38 Moray Avenue, Hayes UB3 2AX — MB ChB Sheff. 1991.

NELSON-OWEN, Margot Esther Constance c/o Count & Countess De Lucovich, Llan Farm, Lisvane, Cardiff CF14 0RP — MB BCh Wales 1985.

NELSON-PIERCY, Catherine Department of Obstetrics, 10th Floor, N. Wing, St Thomas' Hospital, Lambeth Palace Road, London SE1 7CH Tel: 020 7928 9292 Ext: 6972 Fax: 020 7628 2322; 392 Shakespeare Tower, Barbican, London EC2Y 8NJ — MB BS Lond. 1986 (Camb. Univ. & St. Barts. Hosp.) MA Camb. 1987; MRCP (UK) 1989; FRCP (UK) 2000. Cons. Obst. Phys. Guy's & St. Hosp. Trust & Qu. Charlotte's Hosp.; Flexible Working Off. RCP. Specialty: Gen. Med. Socs: BMA. Prev: Sen. Regist. (Obst. Med.) NE Thames RHA; Regist. (Obst. Med.) NE Thames RHA; Regist. (Endocrinol.) Hammersmith Hosp. Lond.

NELSTROP, George Anthony West Herts Hospital NHS Trust, Watford General Hospital, Vicarage Road, Watford WD18 0HB — MB ChB Manch. 1962. Specialty: Nephrol.; Diabetes; Gen. Med. Prev: Cons. Phys. Watford Gen. Hosp.

NEMETH, Andrea Hilary The Wellcome Trust, Centre for Human Genetics, Windmill Road, Oxford OX3 7BN Tel: 01865 740021 Fax: 01865 742186; Department of Clinical Neurology, The Radcliffe Infirmary, Woodstock Road, Oxford OX2 6HE Tel: 01865 311188 — MB BS Lond. 1987; BSc Lond. 1984; MRCP (UK) 1991; DPhil Oxf. 1995. MRC Clinician & Scientist Fell. Wellcome Trust Centre for Human Genetics Oxf.; Hon. Sen. Regist. (Neurol.) Radcliffe Infirm. Oxf. Specialty: Neurol. Prev: MRC Train. Fell. (Molecular Genetics) John Radcliffe Hosp. Oxf.; Regist. (HIV & AIDS) Roy. Free Hosp. Lond.; SHO (Neurol.) Radcliffe Infirm. Oxf.

NEMETH, Cyril Hubert 10 Harley Street, London W1N 1AH Tel: 020 7636 6504 Fax: 020 7286 2633; 1 Langford Place, London NW8 0LJ Tel: 020 7286 2669 Fax: 020 7286 2633 — MRCS Eng. LRCP Lond. 1951 (Camb. & Westm.) MA Camb. 1951; MRCGP 1962. Phys. N.wood, Pinner & Dist. Hosp.; Lord Mayor City of Westminster; JP; Dep. High Steward Westm. Abbey. Socs: Fell. Roy. Soc. Arts; Med. Soc. Lond. & Hunt. Soc.; Fell. Roy. Geogr. Soc. Prev: Mem. (Chairm.) Hillingdon FPC; Mem. (Chairm.) Hillingdon Med. Advis. Comm.; Mem. (Chairm.) Lond. Boro. Hillingdon Soc. Servs. Comm.

NEMETH, Gabor 34 Derwent Court, District General Hospital, Moorgate Road, Rotherham S60 2UD — MD Budapest 1960; DA Eng. 1981.

NEMETH, William Department of Anaesthetics, St. George's Hospital, London SW17 0QT; 85 Montholme Road, London SW11 6HX — MB BS Sydney 1959; DA Eng. 1962; FFA RCS Eng.

1967. Cons. (Anaesth.) St. Geo. Hosp. Lond.; Hon. Sen. Lect. St. Geo. Med. Sch. Univ. Lond. Specialty: Anaesth.

NENSEY, Minaz Flat 4, Park Court, West Pk., 32 Ring Road, Leeds LS16 6EJ — MB BS Dacca 1969 (Dacca Med. Coll.)

NEOFYTOU, Stavros Kleopas Talliadoros High Street Surgery, 117 High Street, Clay Cross, Chesterfield S45 9DZ — MB BS Lond. 1972 (Univ. Coll. Lond. & St. Geo.) DObst RCOG 1974. Prev: Ho. Surg. Salisbury Gen. Infirm.; Ho. Phys. St. Geo. Hosp. Lond.; Res. Obstetr. Guy's Hosp. Lond.

NEOH, Kathleen Hong Peng Kosan, 1 Brooklyn Avenue, Bangor BT20 5RB — MB BCh BAO Belf. 1993; MRCGP. Specialty: Gen. Pract.

NEOH, Leng Chuan Brean Down, The Spital, Yarm TS15 9EX — MB BCh BAO Dub. 1975; DRCOG 1979; MRCGP 1980.

NEOMAN, Isis Fouad Zaki The Surgery, 9 Dollis Hill Lane, London NW2 6JH Tel: 020 8450 4040 Fax: 020 8450 7334; 8 Old Church Lane, London NW9 8TD Tel: 020 8205 2052 Fax: 020 8205 2205 — MB BCh Cairo 1972; MRCS Eng. LRCP Lond. 1979. Specialty: Gen. Pract.; Obst. & Gyn.; Family Plann. & Reproduc. Health. Prev: Trainee GP Wembley; Ho. Off., SHO & Regist. (O & G) St. Mary's Hosp. Lond.; Clin. Asst. (Gen. Med. & Geriat. Med.) Whipps Cross Hosp. Lond.

NEOPTOLEMOS, Professor John P University of Liverpool, Division of Surgery, 5th Floor UCD Block, Daulby Street, Liverpool L69 3GA Tel: 0151 706 4175 Fax: 0151 706 5798 Email: j.p.neoptolemos@liv.ac.uk — MB BChir Camb. 1977 (Camb. & Guy's) MA Camb. 1977; FRCS Eng. 1981; MD Leic. 1985; T(S) 1991. Prof. of Surg. & Head Div. of Surg. Roy. Liverp. Univ.; Hon. Cons. Surg.; General Surgeon (Pancreatic). Specialty: Gen. Surg. Special Interest: Acute Pancreatitis; Chronic Pancreatitis; Familial Pancreatic Dis. Socs: (Pres.) Pancreatic Soc. Of GB & I; (Sec.) Eur. Pancreatic Club; (Treas.) Europ. Digestive Surg. Soc. Prev: Prof. of Surg. City Hosp. Birm. 1994; Hon. Cons. Surg. Qu. Eliz. Hosp. Birm. 1996.

NEPALI, Panna Kaji 8 Meadow Lane, E. Herrington, Sunderland SR3 3RQ Tel: 0191 528 0060 — MB BS Kerala 1961 (Trivandrum Med. Coll.) DA Eng. 1963. Med. Asst. (Anaesth.) Sunderland AHA.

NERELI, Besim Evren Garden Flat, 8 Cowper Road, Bristol BS6 6NY — MB ChB Bristol 1983.

NERI, Mauro Suite 675, 2 Old Brompton Road, London SW7 3DQ — State DMS Turin 1987. Staff Grade Phys., A&E, Barnet Hosp. Specialty: Accid. & Emerg.

NERMINATHAN, Veerasingam Southend Hospital Trust, Southend on Sea, Southend-on-Sea SS0 0RY Tel: 01702 221253 Fax: 01702 221252 Email: nermi75@homtail.com — MB BS Sri Lanka 1972 (Fac. of Med., Colombo) FRCP, FRCPCH, DCH. Cons. Paediat., Southend Hosp. Trust, Southend; Cons. Paediat., BUPA Wellesley Hosp., Southend-on-sea. Specialty: Paediat. Socs: Roy. Coll. of Paediat. & Child Health; Roy. Coll. of Phys.

NERURKAR, Ian David Janardan Foxhill Medical Centre, 363 Halifax Road, Sheffield S6 1AF Tel: 0114 232 2055 Fax: 0114 285 5963 — MB ChB Bristol 1987; MRCGP; MRCP (UK); BSc (Hons.) Bristol 1984.

NERURKAR, Maya Jane 184 Doncaster Road, Newcastle upon Tyne NE2 1RB — MB ChB Bristol 1992.

NESA, Quamar Un 8 The Crescent, London NW2 6HA Tel: 020 8452 6892 — MB BS Bangladesh 1968; DFFP UK 1991.

NESARATNAM, Sakunthala Department of Anaesthetics, Luton & Dunstable Hospital NHS Trust, Lewsey Road, Luton LU4 0DZ Tel: 01582 491122 Fax: 01582 598990; 10 Simpson Road, Walton Park, Milton Keynes MK7 7HN Tel: 01908 691097 — MB BS Colombo 1978; FFA RCS Eng. 1986; MRCS Eng. LRCP Lond. 1987. Staff Grade (Anaesth.) Luton & Dunstable Hosp. NHS Trust. Specialty: Anaesth.

NESBITT, Anne 10 Talisman Square, London SE26 6XY Tel: 020 8778 4960 Fax: 020 8778 4960; Community Health South London, Elizabeth Blackwell House, Avonly Road, London SE14 5ER Tel: 020 7771 5212 Fax: 020 7771 5115 — BM BCh Oxf. 1971; DObst RCOG 1973; DCH Eng. 1975; MSc Lond. 1990; FRCP 1996; FRCPCH 1997. Cons. Community Paediat.Community health S. Lond.; Med. Dir. Specialty: Community Child Health. Prev: Clin. Med. Off. Camberwell HA; Lect. (Paediat.) Univ. Nairobi, Kenya; Lect. (Paediat.) Ahmadu Bello Univ. Hosp. Kaduna, Nigeria.

NESBITT, Deborah Joanne 72 Tranmere Road, Earlsfield, London SW18 3QW Tel: 020 8947 1389 — MB ChB Manch. 1992; MRCP 1996. Specialist Regist. (Paeds); Specialist Regist. (Paediat) Kingston Gen. Hosp. Kingston. Surrey. Specialty: Paediat. Socs: MRCPCH.

NESBITT, Kenneth (retired) Tarras, 21 Tobermore Road, Magherafelt BT45 5HB Tel: 028 7963 2713 Fax: 028 7963 2713 — MB ChB Ed. 1964; DO RCPSI 1976; FFAEM 1993. Prev: SHO Sunderland Eye Infirm.

NESBITT, Lindsey Elizabeth 5 Ava Lodge, Castle Terrace, Berwick-upon-Tweed TD15 1NP — MB BS Newc. 1991; DRCOG 1995; MRCGP 1996; DFFP 1997. GP Retainer (Glenpark Surg.) Dunston Gateshead. Socs: MRCGP 1996. Prev: Gen. Pract. Asst. (Centr. Surg.) S. Shields.

NESBITT, Mary Elizabeth Tarras, 21 Tobermore Road, Magherafelt BT45 5HB Tel: 028796 32713 Fax: 028796 32713 — MB ChB Ed. 1964; MFFP; Dip. Med. Acupunc. SCMO Reproduc. Healthcare; Indep. GP Acupunc. & Hypnother. Maagherafelt; EMO DHSS. Specialty: Family Plann. & Reproduc. Health. Socs: Brit. Med. Acupunct. Soc.; Brit. Soc. Med. & Dent. Hypn. Prev: Med. Off. DHSS; GP Magherafelt.

NESBITT, Sharon Fiona 110 Rosses Lane, Tullygarley, Ballymena BT42 2SB Tel: 01247 852387 — MB BCh BAO Belf. 1996 (QUB) DCH; DFFP 1999; DRCOG 1999; MRCGP 2001. G.P. Locum. Specialty: Gen. Pract. Prev: SHO (Gen. Pract.).

NESBITT, Sidney James 56 Hargrave Mansions, Hargrave Road, London N19 5SR — MB BCh BAO Dub. 1989; MRCP (UK) 1994.

NESDALE, Annette Deborah Flat 1, 39 Kyrle Road, London SW11 6BB — MB ChB Otago 1992.

NESHA, Marium Rotherham District General Hospital, 'B' Level Maternity Unit, Moorgate, Rotherham S60 2UD Tel: 01709 820000; 75 Spinneyfield, Rotherham S60 3HT Tel: 01709 531848 — MB BS Dacca 1973 (Dhaka, Bangladesh) MB BS Dacca, Bangladesh 1973. Clin. Asst. Rotherham Gen. Hosp.; Rotherham Priority Health Family Plann. Specialty: Obst. & Gyn. Prev: Specialist Gyn. Conisbrough Health Auth.

NESLING, Peter Mark Department of Anaesthetics, Singleton Hospital, Sketty Lane, Swansea SA2 8QA Tel: 01792 285427 Fax: 01792 285427; 356 Gower Road, Killay, Swansea SA2 7AE Fax: 01792 205691 — MB BCh Wales 1983; FRCA 1991. Cons. Anaesth. Singleton Hosp. Swansea. Specialty: Anaesth. Socs: Assn. Anaesth.; Obst. Anaesth. Assn. Prev: Sen. Regist. (Anaesth.) Cardiff & Merthyr Tydfil; Regist. (Anaesth.) Swansea; Regist. & SHO (Anaesth.) Birm.

NESS, Andrew Robert Department of Social Medicine, Canynge Hall, Whiteladies Road, Bristol BS8 2PR — BM BS Nottm. 1986 (Nottingham) DA 1990; MRCP (UK) 1991; DPH Camb. 1994; PhD Camb. 1997. Sen. Lect. Epidemiol. Specialty: Epidemiol.

NESS, Lawrence McKinnon Radiology Department, Royal Lancaster Infirmary, Ashton Road, Lancaster LA1 4RP Tel: 01524 65944; 15 Scotforth Road, Lancaster LA1 4TS — MB ChB Leeds 1982; FRCR 1989; T(R) (CR) 1991. Cons. Radiol. Roy. Lancaster Infirm. & Westmorland Gen. Hosp. Specialty: Radiol. Prev: Sen. Regist. (Diag. Radiol.) Yorks. RHA.

NESSIM, Amir Adly Portsmouth City Teaching Primary Care Trust, Finchdean House, Milton, Portsmouth PO3 6DP Tel: 023 9283 8340 — MB BCh Ain Shams 1972; DCH RCP Lond. 1980; MRCGP 1982; MRCOG 1987; DCCH RCP Ed. 1987; Spec. Accredit. Community Child Health JCHMT 1990; Docc Med. Lond. 2000. Salaried GP Portsmouth PCT; Medico-Legal Work. Specialty: Gen. Pract.; Occupat. Health. Socs: Fac. Comm. Health. Prev: SCMO & Assoc. Specialist (Community Paediat.) N. Downs Community Care Unit.; Wide range of Hosp. Med. and Surgic. posts; GP Vocational Train.

NESSIM MORCOS, Isis Bulwell Health Centre, Bulwell, Nottingham NG6 8QJ; 4 Rectory Gardens, Nottingham NG8 2AR — LMSSA Lond. 1964.

NETHERCLIFFE, Janine Mary-Sue 67 Goldney Road, Camberley GU15 1DW — MB BS Lond. 1990.

NETHERCOTT, Albert Stephen (retired) Caledon House, Marton, Welshpool SY21 8JX Tel: 01743 891340 — MB ChB Bristol 1944; DPH Bristol 1966; DIH Dund 1970. Prev: Sec. Health & Welf. Kwazulu Govt. Serv. S. Afr.

NETHERCOTT, Raymond Gerard 12 Ardmore Park S., Belfast BT10 0JF — MB BCh BAO Belf. 1992.

NETHERSELL, Anthony Barry Walter North Wales Cancer Treatment Centre, Glan Clwyd Hospital, Rhyl LL18 5UJ Tel: 01745 445156 Fax: 01745 445212; Dilysdale, Gannock Road, Deganwy, Conwy LL31 9HJ Tel: 01492 573447 Email: anthony.nethersell@medix-uk.com — MB BChir Camb. 1974 (Camb. & St. Bart.) MA Camb. 1972, BA (Nat. Sc.) 1968; MRCP (UK) 1978; FRCR 1982; FRCP 1998. Cons. Clin. Oncol. N. Wales Cancer Treatm. Centre. Specialty: Oncol.; Radiother. Socs: Fell. Roy. Soc. Med.; Eur. Sch. Therapeutic Radiol. & Oncol.; Mem. Amer. Soc Clin. Oncol. Prev: Head Sect. Oncol. Wellcome Research Laborat. & Hon. Cons. Radiother. & Oncol. King's Coll. & St. Thos. Hosps. Lond.; Sen. Regist. (Radiother. & Oncol.) Addenbrooke's Hosp. Camb.; Ho. Phys. (Med. Oncol.) St. Bart. Hosp. Lond.

NETHISINGHE, Shelton Wennel Ways, Southam Road, Dunchurch, Rugby CV22 6NW — LMSSA Lond. 1978; FFA RCSI 1977. Cons. Anaesth. Coventry & Warks. AHA's. Specialty: Anaesth. Prev: Sen. Regist. (Anaesth.) Newc. AHA (T); SHO (Anaesth.) Leighton Hosp. Crewe; Regist. (Anaesth.) Killingbeck Hosp. Leeds.

NETHISINGHE, Somanathage Kamala Nandani Wennel Ways, Southam Road, Dunchurch, Rugby CV22 6NW — LMSSA Lond. 1976 (Friendship Univ. Moscow) Dip. Community Paediat. Warwick 1988; MSc (Audiol. Med.) Manch. 1995. SCMO (Audiol. Med.) Northampton HA. Specialty: Audiol. Med. Prev: Ho. Off. (Gen. Med. & Gen. Surg.) Vict. Centr. Hosp. Wallasey; Clin. Med. Off. Barnsley HA.

NETSCHER, Margaret May 30 Braintree Road, Witham CM8 2DD — MB BS Lond. 1962 (Char. Cross) MRCS Eng. LRCP Lond. 1962; DObst RCOG 1964. Prev: Teachg. Fell. (Family Pract. & Paediat.) McGill Univ. Montreal; Canada; Sen. Ho. Phys. Musgrave Pk. Hosp. Belf.; Ho. Surg. City Hosp. & Jubilee Matern. Hosp. Belf.

NETTLE, Christopher John Harcourt Medical Centre, Crane Bridge Road, Salisbury SP2 7TD Tel: 01722 333214 Fax: 01722 421643 — MB BS Lond. 1971 (King's Coll. Hosp.) BSc Lond. 1968; DObst RCOG 1974; Cert. Family Plann. JCC 1974. Prev: SHO (Obst & Gyn. & Paediat.) Nottm. City Hosp.; Ho. Phys. King's Coll. Hosp.; Ho. Surg. Kent & Sussex Hosp. Tunbridge Wells.

NETTLETON, Mark Andrew Bridge Road Surgery, 1A Bridge Road, Oulton Broad, Lowestoft NR32 3LJ Tel: 01502 565936 Fax: 01502 567359 — MB BS Lond. 1988 (Charing Cross and Westminster London) DGM RCP Lond. 1992; Dip. IMC RCS Ed. 1993; MRCGP 1996. GP Norf. Specialty: Gen. Pract.; Aviat. Med.

NETTS, Paul Henry The Medical Centre, 37A Heaton Road, Heaton, Newcastle upon Tyne NE6 1TH Tel: 0191 265 8121 Fax: 0191 276 6085 — MB ChB Leeds 1988.

NEUBER, Miriam 25 Offerton Road, London SW4 0DJ — State Exam Med Lubeck 1993; Med State Exam Lubeck 1993. Specialty: Gen. Psychiat. Socs: Roy. Coll. Psychiats. (Inceptor). Prev: SHO Rotat. (Gen. Psychiat. & Psychiat. of Old Age) St. Geo.'s Tooting Lond.

NEUBERG, Kim Daniel 9 Barrington Road, Leicester LE2 2RA — MB ChB Leic. 1992. SHO (Geriat.) Leicester Gen. Hosp. Prev: Trainee GP Market HarBoro. Med. Centre Leics.; SHO (A & E Med.) Arrowe Pk. Hosp. Wirral.

NEUBERG, Roger Wolfe 9 Barrington Road, Stoneygate, Leicester LE2 2RA Tel: 0116 255 3933 — MB BS Lond. 1965 (Middlx.) MRCS Eng. LRCP Lond. 1965; FRCOG 1983, M 1970, DObst 1967. Cons. O & G Leicester Roy. Infirm. Specialty: Obst. & Gyn. Socs: Brit. Fertil. Soc.; BMA; Assn. BRd.casting Doctors. Prev: Sen. Regist. (O & G) John Radcliffe Hosp. Oxf. & Roy. Berks. Hosp. Reading; Regist. (O & G) Middlx. Hosp. & Hosp. for Wom. Lond.

NEUBERGER, Professor James Max Queen Elizabeth Hospital, Edgbaston, Birmingham B15 2TH Tel: 0121 472 1311 Fax: 0121 627 2449; The Moat House, Radford Road, Alvechurch, Birmingham B48 7ST Tel: 0121 445 1773 — BM BCh Oxf. 1974 (Oxford University and University College Hospital London) MRCP (UK) 1977; DM Oxf. 1982; FRCP Lond. 1991. Cons. Phys. Qu. Eliz. Hosp. Birm. Specialty: Gastroenterol.; Gen. Med. Prev: Sen. Wellcome Clin. Research Fell. Liver Unit King's Coll. Hosp. Lond.

NEUGEBAUER, Mr Mark Andrew Zygmunt Department of Ophthalmology, Leighton Hospital, Middlewich Road, Crewe CW1 4QJ Tel: 01270 255141; Church Farm, Willbank Lane, Faddiley, Nantwich CW5 8JG — MB ChB Manch. 1977; DO 1983; FRCS RCPS Glas. 1984; FCOphth 1988. Cons. Ophth. Crewe & Macclesfield HAs. Specialty: Ophth. Prev: Sen. Regist. Univ. Hosp., Nottm.; Regist. Roy. Vic. Infirm. Newc.

NEUKOM, Christopher Ralph City Walls Medical Centre, St. Martin's Way, Chester CH1 2NR Tel: 01244 357800 — MB ChB Liverp. 1980; MRCS Eng. LRCP Lond. 1980; MRCGP 1984; DRCOG 1985.

NEULING, Kim Fiona Susamme 25 Grand Avenue, Muswell Hill, London N10 3BD — MB ChB Leeds 1996.

NEUMANN, Kai Michael Solva Surgery, Cysgod-Yr-Eglwys, Solva, Haverfordwest SA62 6TW Tel: 01437 721306 Fax: 01437 720046; No Name Cottage, Llanddinog, Solva, Haverfordwest SA62 6NA — State Exam Med Hamburg 1984; MD Hamburg 1986; T(GP) 1994. GP Princip. Specialty: Gen. Med.

NEUMANN, Mr Lars The Nottingham Shoulder & Elbow Unit, Nottingham City Hospital NHS Trust, Hucknall Road, Nottingham NG5 1PB Tel: 0115 969 1169 Fax: 0115 962 8062 Email: larsneumann@rcsed.ac.uk; The BMI Park Hospital, Sherwood Lodge Drive, Burntstump Country Park, Nottingham NG5 8RX Tel: 0870 163 2851 Fax: 0870 190 9392 Email: lars.neumann@phf.uk.com — MD Odense 1980 (University of Odense, Denmark) FRCS Ed. 1997. Cons. Orthop. Surg. Nottm. Shoulder & Elbow Unit Nottm. City Hosp. Specialty: Orthop. Special Interest: Degenerative and Traum. Condits. of the shoulder and elbow, including sports injuries, Jt. replacement Surg. and arthroscopic Surg. Socs: Fell. BOA; Eur. Soc. Surg. Shoulder & Elbow (Educat. Comm.); Brit. Elbow & Shoulder Soc. (Hon. Treas.). Prev: Sen. Regist. (Orthop.) Univ. Hosp. Odense, Denmark; Cons. Orthop. Surg. & Hon. Sen. Lect. (Orthop. & Trauma Surg.) Qu. Med. Centre Nottm.; Shoulder Fell. to Prof. W. Angus Wallace Qu. Med. Centre Nottm.

NEUMANN, Vera Camilla Margit Chapel Allerton Hospital, Chapeltown Road, Leeds LS7 4SA Tel: 0113 392 4614 Fax: 0113 392 4653 Email: vera.neumann@leedsth.nhs.uk — MD Lond. 1990 (Westm.) FRCP; BA (Hons.) Oxf. 1973; MB BS 1976; MRCP (UK) 1979. Sen. Lect. & Cons. Rehabil. Med. Univ. Leeds & United Leeds Teach. Hosp. Trust. Specialty: Rheumatol.; Rehabil. Med. Socs: Soc. Research in Rehabil.; Internat. Soc. Prosth.s & Orthotics.; Exec. Bd. - Brit. Soc. Rehabil. Med. Prev: Sen. Regist. (Rheum. & Rehabil.) Leeds & Harrogate HAs; Research Fell. Rheum. Research Unit Leeds Univ.; SHO (Med.) Dudley Rd. Hosp. Birm.

NEUMEGEN, Joanna Louise 66 East Grove Road, St Leonards, Exeter EX2 4LX — BM BS Nottm. 1993; MRCGP 1990; DRCOG 1998. Specialty: Gen. Pract.

NEVARD, Richard Spencer Charles The Sollershott Surgery, 44 Sollershott East, Letchworth SG6 3JW Tel: 01462 683637 Fax: 01462 481348 — MB BS Lond. 1981 (Univ. Coll. Hosp.) GP Letchworth.

NEVE, Hilary Ann Waterloo Surgery, 191 Devonport Road, Stoke, Plymouth PL1 5RN Tel: 01752 563147 Fax: 01752 563304 — MB ChB Bristol 1983; DRCOG 1985; DA (UK) 1989; MRCGP 1991; M.Ed. Bristol 1993. Specialty: Gen. Pract.

NEVE, Janet Mair 5 Leonard Place, Westerham Road, Keston BR2 6HQ — MB BS Lond. 1982.

NEVILL, Christopher Gerald Newtown Surgery, Park Street, Newtown SY16 1EF Tel: 01686 611611/611622 Fax: 01686 611650; Newtown Medical Practice, Park St, Newtown SY16 1EF — (Univ. Camb. & St. Thos. Hosp.) MB BChir Camb. 1980; DRCOG 1983; MRCGP 1984. Specialty: Infec. Dis. Socs: Roy. Soc. Trop. Med. & Hyg. Prev: Research Dir. AMREF Nairobi, Kenya.

NEVILLE, Professor Alexander Munro (retired) Ludwig Institute for Cancer Research, Horatio House, 5th Floor South, London W6 8JC Tel: 020 8735 9240 Fax: 020 8741 4990 Email: munro.neville@lno.licr.org; 6 Woodlands Park, Tadworth KT20 7JL Tel: 01737 844113 Fax: 01737 844287 — MB ChB Glas. 1959; PhD Glas. 1965, MD 1969; FRCPath 1980, M 1969; DSc Lond. 1985. Prev: Assoc. Dir. Ludwig Inst. for Cancer Research Zürich, New York & Lond.

NEVILLE, Amanda Joyce St. Anns Health Centre, St. Anns, Well Road, Nottingham NG3 3PX Email: mandy.neville@gp-c4072.nhs.uk — MB BS Lond. 1985. Specialty: Gen. Pract.

NEVILLE, Anne Caroline Greatwood, Gainford, Darlington DL2 3EU — MB ChB Sheff. 1979; MRCGP 1987. Indep. GP Darlington.

NEVILLE, Anne Eleanor Pen y Gadlas, Ffordd Bryniau, Prestatyn LL19 8RD Tel: 01745 571626 — MB ChB Manch. 1980; DRCOG 1983; MRCGP 1984.

NEVILLE, Professor Brian George Richard Institute of Child Health, Wolfson centre, Mechlenburgh Square, London WC1N 2AP Tel: 020 7837 7618 Fax: 020 7833 9469; 10 the Chenies, Petts Wood, Orpington BR6 0ED Tel: 01689 825811 — MB BS Lond. 1964 (Guy's) FRCP Lond. 1979, M 1966. Prof. Paediat. Neurol. Inst. Child Health Lond.; Hon. Cons. Paediat. Neurol. Hosp. Sick Childr. Gt. Ormond St. Lond. Specialty: Paediat. Neurol. Prev: Cons. Paediat. Neurol. & Dir. Newcomen Centre Guy's Hosp. Lond.; Sen. Regist. (Paediat. Neurol.) Hosp. Sick Childr. Gt. Ormond St. & Nat. Hosp. Nerv. Dis. Qu. Sq. Lond.

NEVILLE, Catherine Ellen 44 Langstone Road, Langstone, Havant PO9 1RF — BChir Camb. 1996.

NEVILLE, Edmund Queen Alexandra Hospital, Respiratory Centre, Portsmouth Tel: 023 92 866782 Fax: 023 92 866735 Email: edmund.neville@porthosp.nhs.uk — (Guy's) MRCS Eng. LRCP Lond. 1970; MD Lond. 1979, MB BS 1970; MRCP (UK) 1973; FRCP Lond. 1989. p/t Cons. Phys. (Respirat. & GIM) Portsmouth Hosps. Portsmouth; Dir. of Train. at RCP; Chairm. of Exec. Comm. Brit. Toracic Soc. Specialty: Gen. Med.; Respirat. Med. Socs: Brit. Thoracic Soc.; Roy. Soc. of Med.

NEVILLE, Edmund Andrew (retired) 7 Heriot Road, Lenzie, Kirkintilloch, Glasgow G66 5AX Tel: 0141 776 2543 — MB ChB Glas. 1958 (Glasgow) DObst RCOG 1960; FRCP Glas. 1981, M 1962; FRCGP 1984, M 1978. GP. Prev: Assoc. Adviser (Gen. Pract.) W. Scotl. Comm. Postgrad. Med. Educat.

NEVILLE, Joseph Godfrey (retired) 2 Mile End Road, Newmarket Road, Norwich NR4 7QY Tel: 01603 452179 — MB BS Lond. 1948 (Char. Cross) MRCS Eng. LRCP Lond. 1948; MRCP Lond. 1951; DCH Eng. 1950, DPM 1954; MRCPsych 1971. Prev: Cons. Psychiat. (Child & Family Psychiat.) Bethel Hosp. Norwich.

NEVILLE, Kathleen Mary 73 Burdon Lane, Cheam, Sutton SM2 7BY Tel: 020 8642 9744 — MB ChB Birm. 1952; MRCS Eng. LRCP Lond. 1952.

NEVILLE, Kevin Francis Mill Cottage, Blaina, Abertillery NP13 3HL Tel: 01495 290226 — MB BCh BAO NUI 1950.

NEVILLE, Lisa Ann 10 The Chenies, Orpington BR6 0ED — MB ChB Bristol 1994; MRCP (UK) 1998.

NEVILLE, Louise Olwen Department of Medical Microbiology, Kingston NHS Trust, Galsworthy Rd, Kingston upon Thames KT2 7QB Tel: 020 8934 3070 Email: louise.neville@kingstonhospital.nhs.uk — MB BS Lond. 1979 (University College Hospital) MA Camb. 1980, BA 1976; MRCP (UK) 1983; MRCPath 1993; FRCPath 2002. Cons. (Med. MicroBiol.) Kingston NHST. Specialty: Med. Microbiol. Socs: Hosp. Infec. Soc.; Assn. Med. Microbiol.; Brit. Travel Health Assn. Prev: Temp. Sen. Lect. (Med. MicroBiol.) Roy. Hosps. Trust Lond.; Sen. Regist. & Regist. (Med. MicroBiol.) Roy. Free Hosp. Lond.; Research Fell. (Med. MicroBiol.) Roy. Free Hosp. Lond.

NEVILLE, Mary Louise (retired) Elm Court, Wychbold, Droitwich WR9 0DF Tel: 01527 861237 — MB BCh BAO NUI 1940 (Cork) FRCOG 1969, M 1947. Prev: Asst. Med. Off. St. Mary's Hospice Selly Oak.

NEVILLE, Michael James Gainford Surgery, Main Road, Gainford, Darlington DL2 3BE Tel: 01325 730204 — MB ChB Sheff. 1978; DRCOG 1982.

NEVILLE, Peter George 191 Main Street, Thornton, Coalville LE67 1AU Tel: 01530 230768; Bennion Centre, Glenfield Hospital, Groby Road, Leicester LE3 9DZ Tel: 0116 250 2761 — BM Soton. 1977; MRCPsych 1981. Cons. Psychiat. Leicester Ment. Health Servs. Trust. Specialty: Geriat. Psychiat. Prev: Sen. Regist. (Psychiat.) Leics. Rotat. Scheme.

NEVILLE, Peter Michael Nevill Hall Hospital, Breton Road, Abergavenny NP7 7EG Tel: 01873 732455 — MB ChB Leeds 1989; BSc Leeds 1986; FRCP (London) 2004. Cons. Gastroenterologist / Phys. Gwent Hosps. NHS Trust. Specialty: Gastroenterol.; Gen. Med. Socs: Brit. Soc. of Gastroneterology. Prev: SHO Rotat. (Med.) St. Jas. Univ. Hosp. Leeds.; Regist. Rotat. (Gastroenterol.) Hull Roy. Infirm., Bradford Roy. Infirm. & Leeds Gen. Infirm.

NEVILLE, Philippa Susan Harley House Surgery, 2 Irnham Road, Minehead TA24 5DL Tel: 01643 703441 Fax: 01643 704867; Higher Moor, Moor Road, Minehead TA24 5RY Tel: 01643 706875 — MB ChB Birm. 1980; DRCOG 1982; MRCGP 1985; DFFP 1996.

NEVILLE, Richard James (retired) Garden House, Rockmount, Pimlico, Clitheroe BB7 4PZ Tel: 01200 24129 — MB ChB St. And. 1963; DObst RCOG 1966; MRCGP 1972. Prev: GP Clitheroe Health Centre Lancs.

NEVILLE, Ronald Gilmour West Gate Health Centre, Charleston Drive, Dundee DD2 4AD Tel: 01382 668189 Fax: 01382 665943 — MB ChB Dundee 1980; MRCGP (Distinction) 1984; DRCOG 1985; MD 1990; FRCGP 1998. GP Dundee.

NEVILLE, Theresa Patricia 1 Blenheim Close, Bidford on Avon, Alcester B50 4HW — MB ChB Manch. 1946.

NEVILLE, Thomas Eugene Blackley Health Studio, 25 Old Market Street, Blackley, Manchester M9 3DT Tel: 0161 721 4865 Fax: 0161 740 6532 — MB BCh BAO NUI 1978 (Royal College of Surgeons Ireland) LRCPI & LM, LRCSI & LM 1978.

NEVILLE, William Peter 43 Ffordd Ffynnon, Prestatyn LL19 8BD — LMSSA Lond. 1954.

NEVILLE, William Thomas Abbey Road Surgery, 63 Abbey Road, Waltham Cross EN8 7LJ Tel: 01992 762082 Fax: 01992 717746 Email: bill.neville@gp-E82042.nhs.uk — MB BS Newc. 1978; MRCGP 1988; T(GP) 1991. Princip. GP Abbey Rd. Surg. Herts. Specialty: Gen. Pract. Prev: RAMC 1981-89.

NEVILLE-SMITH, Roger Fairfax — MB ChB Manch. 1975; DRCOG 1978; MFHom 1998; RCP Lond. 1998. Prev: SHO (Paediat.) Alder Hey Childr. Hosp. Liverp.; SHO (O & G & Psychiat.) Tameside Gen. Hosp.

NEVILLE-TOWLE, Andrew Ship House Surgery, The Square, Liphook GU30 7AQ Tel: 01428 723296 Fax: 01420 724022 — MB BS Lond. 1975 (Middlx.) MRCS Eng. LRCP Lond. 1975; FRACGP 1980; DRCOG 1986. Prev: SHO Portway Hosp. Weymouth; Resid. Med. Off. Ryde Hosp. Sydney, Australia; Ho. Phys. Mt. Vernon Hosp. N.wood.

NEVIN, Linda Joyce 9 Ballymadigan Road, Castlerock, Coleraine BT51 4RR — MB BCh BAO Belf. 1981. Specialty: Paediat.; Community Child Health; Family Plann. & Reproduc. Health.

NEVIN, Michael Gables, Oaklands Way, Bassett, Southampton SO16 7PA — MB BS Lond. 1978.

NEVIN, Professor Norman Cummings (retired) 17 Ogles Grove, Hillsborough BT26 6RS Tel: 01846 689126 — MB BCh BAO Belf. 1960; BSc Belf. 1957, MD 1965; FRCP Ed. 1976, M 1968; FRCPath 1981; FFCM 1981; FRCP Lond. 1990. Prof. Emerit. Med. Genetics Qu. Univ. Belf. Prev: John Dunville Fell. (Path.) Qu. Univ. Belf.

NEVISON, Jennifer 33 Wedon Way, Bygrave, Baldock SG7 5DX Tel: 01462 894743 Fax: 01462 894743 — MB BS Lond. 1968 (King's Coll. Hosp.) Indep. Specialist (Allergy & Environm. Med.) Herts. Prev: Unit Med. Off. RAF; Ho. Surg. (Ophth.) King's Coll. Hosp.; Ho. Phys. Greenbank Hosp. Plymouth.

NEVISON-ANDREWS, David Gordon St. Andrew's Hospital, Billing Road, Northampton NN1 5DG — MB ChB Ed. 1975; BSc Ed. 1972; MRCPsych. 1981. Cons. Psychiat. St. And. Hosp. N.ampton. Specialty: Gen. Psychiat. Prev: Sen. Regist. (Psychiat.) Guy's Hosp. Lond.

NEVITT, Gerald John Austin and Partners, 4 Market Place, Billesdon, Leicester LE7 9AJ Tel: 0116 259 6206 Fax: 0116 259 6388; Hill Rise, Gaulby Road, Gaulby, Leicester LE7 9BB — MB BS Lond. 1974 (Roy. Free) BSc (Anat.) Lond. 1971; MRCP (UK) 1978; FRCP 2001. Clin. Asst. (Dermat.) Leicester Gen. Hosp.

NEVRKLA, Elizabeth Julia (retired) — BSc Lond. 1964 (Univ. Coll. Hosp.) MB BS Lond. 1967; MRCP 1970; FRCPCH 1997. Cons. Developm. Paediat. (locum), The Wolfson Centre, GOSH. Prev: Sen. Regist. (Paediat.) Centr. Middlx. Hosp.

NEW, Alison Caroline 9 Battenhall Road, Worcester WR5 2BJ — BM BS Nottm. 1986. VTS Worcester.

NEW, Helen Vivien St Mary's Hospital, Department of Paediatrics, Praed Street, London W2 1NY Email: helen.new@st-marys.nhs.uk — MB BS Lond. 1989 (University College London) PhD Lond. 1986, BSc 1983; MRCP (UK) 1995; MRCPath 2000. p/t Cons. Paediatric Haematologist, St. Mary's Hosp., Lond. (9 sessions). Specialty: Haematology. Special Interest: Paediatric Transfus. Med. Socs: Brit. Soc. for Haemat.; UKCCSG Assoc. Mem. Prev: Specialist Regist. (Haemat.) Univ. Coll. Lond. Hosp. Lond.; Regist. (Haemat.) Hammersmith Hosp. Lond.; Post-doctoral Research Scientist Nat. Inst. Med. Research Mill Hill Lond.

NEW, John Wickham St James Surgery, Gains Lane, Devizes SN10 1QU Tel: 01380 722206 Fax: 01380 734541 — MB BChir Camb. 1972 (Lond. Hosp.) MA Camb. 1973; FRCS Eng. 1976; AFOM RCP Lond. 1993. GP, (Sen. Partner); Co. Med. Off. Wilts. Red Cross; Force Med. Off. Wilts. Constab. Specialty: Gen. Surg.; Orthop. Socs: ALAMA; BMA. Prev: Regist. (Surg.) Mt. Vernon Hosp. Northwood; SHO Roy. Nat. Orthop. Hosp. Stanmore; Ho. Phys. & Ho. Surg. Lond. Hosp.

NEW, Linda Carol 48 Durleston Park Drive, Bookham, Leatherhead KT23 4AJ — MB BS Lond. 1983; MSc Clin. Microbiol. Lond. 1990, BSc (1st cl. Hons.) 1980; MB BS (Distinc.) Lond. 1983; MRCP (UK) 1987. p/t Sen. Reg. Microbiology, Epsom & St Helier NHS Trust. Specialty: Med. Microbiol. Prev: Asst. Med. Microbiol. & Hon. Sen. Regist. Pub. Health Laborat. Serv. St. Geo. Hosp. Lond.

NEW, Norman Edwin Department of Cellular Pathology, Hull Royal Infimary, Anlaby Road, Hull HU3 2JZ — MB ChB Ed. 1983; BMedBiol. Aberd. 1980; FRCS Ed. 1988; MRCPath 1993; FRCPath 2001. Cons. Histopath, Hull and E. Yorks. NHS Trust. Specialty: Histopath. Prev: Sen. Regist. Rotat. (Histopath.) NW RHA; Cons. Histopath. King's Lynn & Wisbech NHS Trust.

NEWALL, Nicholas 5a Leigh Road, West Kirby, Wirral CH48 5DZ Email: newall@attglobal.net — MB BS Newc. 1992.

NEWBEGIN, Mr Christopher John Richard Lingards Wood House, Manchester Road, Marsden, Huddersfield HD7 6LR Tel: 01484 846506 Fax: 01484 482147 Email: newbegin@bigfoot.com — MB BS Lond. 1976 (St. Mary's) FRCS Eng. 1982. Cons. (ENT Surg.) Calderdale + Huddersfield NHS Trust; Regional Speciality Adviser in OtoLaryngol. Specialty: Otolaryngol. Prev: Sen. Regist. (ENT Surg.) Yorks. Region; Regist. (ENT Surg.) Char. Cross Hosp. Lond.

NEWBEGIN, Hilary Eileen Lingards Wood House, Manchester Road, Marsden, Huddersfield HD7 6LR — MB BS Lond. 1978 (St. Mary's) MSc; BA Oxf. 1975; FFA RCS Eng. 1982. Cons. Anaesth. Roy. Halifax Infirm. Specialty: Anaesth. Prev: Cons. Anaesth. Huddersfield Roy. Infirm.; Sen. Regist. (Anaesth.) Yorks. Region; Lect. (Anaesth.) Leeds Univ.

NEWBERRY, Douglas John Ashford and St Peter's Hospital, Ashford TW15 3AA Tel: 01784 884246 Fax: 01784 884437; 25 Fordbridge Road, Ashford TW15 2TD — MD McMaster Univ., Canada 1974; BSc 1971; CCFP 1980; MSc Epidemiol. Lond. 1988; MRCP (UK) 1991. Cons. Respiratory Phys. (Gen., Thoracic & Geriat. Med.) Ashfod & St Peter's Hosp. Middlx. Specialty: Respirat. Med.; Care of the Elderly. Socs: Brit. Geriat. Soc.; Brit. Thorac. Soc.

NEWBERRY, Juliam 33 West Dhuhill Drive, Helensburgh G84 9AW Tel: 01436 676572 Fax: 01434 676572 — MB ChB Glas. 1996. SHO (O & G) Ayrsh. Centr. Hosp. Irvine. Prev: SHO (Surg.) Gartnavel Gen. Hosp.; SHO (A & E) Hairmyres Hosp.; SHO (Med.) Ayr Hosp.

NEWBERRY, Roger Garstang (retired) 75 Sheepdown Drive, Petworth GU28 0BX Tel: 01798 343390 — MB BS Lond. 1952 (St. Bart.) DPH Eng. 1958; MFCM 1974. Prev: Dist. Community Phys. Gt. Yarmouth & Waveney Health Dist. MOH & Port. Med. Off. Gt. Yarmouth Co. Boro.

NEWBERY, Frederica Erna Failand House, Ox House Lane, Failand, Bristol BS8 3SL — MB ChB Bristol 1975; DRCOG 1978.

NEWBERY, John Michael (retired) 68 Victoria Place, Carlisle CA1 1LR Tel: 01228 532987; 68 Victoria Place, Carlisle CA1 1LR Tel: 01228 532987 — MB BChir Camb. 1964 (Westm.) MRCS Eng. LRCP Lond. 1963; DA Eng. 1968; FFA RCS Eng. 1971. Prev: Cons. Anaesth. Cumbld. Infirm. Carlisle & E. Cumbria Hosps.

NEWBERY, Sarah Ruth Medical Centre, 1 Oxford Drive, Eastcote, Ruislip HA4 9EY Tel: 020 8866 6589 Fax: 020 8868 3317 — MB BS Lond. 1989; DCH RCP Lond. 1992; DRCOG 1993; DFFP 1993; MRCGP 1993.

NEWBOLD, George Frank (retired) Golden Hill, Windmill Lane, Llantwit Major CF61 2SU Tel: 01446 792480 — (King's Coll. Lond. & St. Geo.) MRCS Eng. LRCP Lond. 1945; DObst RCOG 1947; MMSA Lond. 1948; MB BS Lond. 1949; DCH Eng. 1951. Prev: Obst. & Gyn Orsett Lodge Hosp. Essex.

NEWBOLD, Kenneth (retired) 6 Wrights Close, Quorn, Loughborough LE12 8TU Tel: 01509 412786 — MB ChB Birm. 1958; DObst RCOG 1963; MRCGP 1970. Prev: GP LoughBoro.

NEWBOLD, Kenneth Mark Walsgrave Hospital, Histology Department, Clifford Bridge Road, Coventry CV2 2DX Tel: 024 7653 8855 Fax: 024 7653 8715 Email: mark.newbold@uhcw.nhs.uk — MB ChB Birm. 1983; MRCPath 1989; MD Birm. 1991; Dip. BA Warwick 1998; FRCPath 1998. Cons. (Histopath. & Cytopath.); Managing Director, Hosp. of St Cross, Rugby; Hon. Sen. Clin. Lect. Warwick Univ. Specialty: Histopath. Special Interest: Colorectal cancer; Clin. Managem. & Leadership. Socs: Brit. Soc. of Gastroenterol. Prev: Clin. Director of Path., Univ. Hosps. Coventry and Warks. NHS Trust; Head Clin. Servs. / Ambulatory Care Div. & Assoc. Med. Director Univ. Hosps. Coventry & Warks. NHS Trust; Cons. (Histopath. and CytoPath.) Warwick Hosp. Warwick.

NEWBOLD, Sandra Margaret 22 Engliff Lane, Pyrford, Woking GU22 8SU — MB BS Lond. 1983 (St Bart.) MRCOG 1991; MD Lond. 1993. Cons. O & G St. Peter's Hosp. Chertsey, Surrey. Specialty: Obst. & Gyn. Prev: Sen. Regist. (O & G) John Radcliffe Hosp. Oxf.; Sen. Regist. Acad. Dept. Wellington Wom. Hosp., NZ; Regist. (O & G) Gloucester & Bristol Matern. Hosp.

NEWBON, Sarah 90 Ack La W., Cheadle Hulme, Cheadle SK8 7ES — MB BS Newc. 1997.

NEWBOULD, Melanie Joy Department of Pathology, Royal Manchester Children's Hospital, Hospital Road, Pendlebury, Manchester M27 4HA — MB BS Lond. 1979. Specialty: Histopath.

NEWBOULD, Ruth Anne (retired) 37 Daleside, Pudsey LS28 8HA Tel: 01274 667430 — MB ChB Leeds 1963.

NEWBOUND, Andrew David Meanwood Group Practice, 548 Meanwood Road, Leeds LS6 4JN Email: chriskinchin@talk21.com; The Beeches, Allerton Hill, Leeds LS7 3QB Tel: 01242 582372 — MB ChB Leeds 1979; DCH RCP Lond. 1982; DRCOG 1982; MRCGP 1983. GP Princip.; GP Trainee; Medico Legal Reporting.

NEWBURY, Anna Louise Beech Cottage, Raby Drive, Bebington, Wirral CH63 0NL — BM BS Nottm. 1992; DRCOG 1997.

NEWBURY, Louise The Cottage, Thorns Beach, Beaulieu, Brockenhurst SO42 7XN Email: newburyl@hotmail.com — MB BS Lond. 1994; MRCP (Lond.) 1997. E. Anglian Specialist Regist. Rotat. (Paediat.) Qu. Eliz. Hosp. Kings Lynn, Norf. Specialty: Paediat. Socs: MRCP; MRCPCH.

NEWBURY-ECOB, Ruth Angela Department of Clinical Genetics, St. Michaels Hospital, Southwell Street, Bristol BS2 8EG Tel: 0117 928 5107 Fax: 0117 928 5108 — MB ChB Sheff. 1983 (Sheffield) MRCP (UK) 1988; FRCPCH 1996; FRCP 2000; MD Sheffield 2002. Consultant in Clinical Genetics, Bristol. Specialty: Genitourinary Medicine. Socs: BMA; MDU; BSHG. Prev: Clin. Research Fell., Univ. of Nottm.; Sen. Regist. Clin. Genetics, Nottm.; Sen. Regist. (Clin. Genetics) Leicester.

NEWBY, David Ernest Royal Infirmary of Edinburgh, 1 Lauriston Road, Edinburgh EH3 9YW Tel: 0131 536 1000 Fax: 0131 536 2021; Upper Flat, 34 Mansion House Road, Edinburgh EH9 2JD — BM Soton. 1991; BSc (Hons.) Soton. 1990; MRCP (UK) 1994. Research Fell. Edin. Specialty: Cardiol. Socs: BMA. Prev: SHO (CCU & Med.) Roy. Infirm. Edin.; SHO (Med.) Borders Gen. Hosp.

NEWBY, David Malcolm Rotherham District General Hospital, Moorgate Road, Rotherham S60 2UD — MB ChB Leeds 1971; FFA RCS Eng. 1976. Cons. Anaesth. (IC) Rotherham AHA. Specialty: Anaesth. Prev: Staff Anaesth. Univ. Hosp. Groningen, Netherlands; Sen. Regist. (Anaesth.) Leeds AHA (T); Regist. Anaesth. Sheff. AHA (T).

NEWBY, Elizabeth Ann Brewers Home, 2 Burnside, Addingham, Ilkley LS29 0PJ — MB ChB Manch. 1995. SHO (Paediat.). Specialty: Paediat.

NEWBY, Jacqueline Clare Department of Oncology, Royal Free Hospital, Pond St, London NW3 2QG Email: jcnewby@mera-peak.freeserve.co.uk — MB ChB Manch. 1988 (Camb./Manch.) MA Camb. 1990; MRCP (UK) 1991; MD Manch 1997. Locum Cons., Med. Oncollogy, Roy. Free Hosp., Lond. Specialty: Oncol. Prev: Clin. Research Fell. Roy. Marsden Hosp. Lond.; Sen. Reg. N. Lond. Cancer network, Med. Oncol.

NEWBY, Martin Rodney Eaton Socon Health Centre, 274 North Road, Eaton Socon, Huntingdon PE19 8BB Tel: 01480 477111 Fax: 01480 403524; 3 Gordon Road, Little Paxton, Huntingdon PE19 6NU — MB ChB Sheff. 1970; DObst RCOG 1972. Prev: Ho. Phys. Roy. Hosp. Chesterfield; Ho. Surg. ENT & Cas. Roy. Infirm. Sheff.; SHO (Obst.) N. Gen. Hosp. Sheff.

NEWBY, Michael Paul — MB BS Newc. 1994 (Newcastle) FRCR. Consultant Radiologist Gateshaed Health. Specialty: Radiol. Prev: Specialist Regist. (Radiol.) S. Tyneside Health Care Trust.

NEWBY, Robert Thomas 32 Rose Glen, London NW9 0JS — MB BS Lond. 1991.

NEWBY, Vanessa Jane Newcastle General Hospital, Old Age Psychiatry, Akenside Unit, Newcastle upon Tyne NE4 6BE — MB BS Newc. 1994 (Newcastle) Specialist Reistrar, Newcastle General Hospital. Specialty: Gen. Psychiat. Prev: Sen. SHO (Psychiat.) S. Tyneside Health Care Trust.

NEWCOMBE, Charles Patrick (cons. rooms), 27 High Petergate, York YO1 7HP Tel: 01904 624007; 7 Thorn Nook, York YO31 9LH Tel: 01904 423163 — MRCS Eng. LRCP Lond. 1946 (St. Bart.) MD Lond. 1952, MB BS 1946; FRCP Lond. 1972, M 1954. Chief Med. Off. Gen. Accid. Life Assur. Co. Socs: Brit. Cardiac. Soc. & Thoracic Soc. Prev: Cons. Phys. York Health Dist.; Cons. Phys. Cardio-Thoracic Centre Killingbeck; Sen. Med. Regist. Leeds Gen. Infirm.

NEWCOMBE, Guy Lister Well Cottage, Bodenham, Hereford HR1 3JT Tel: 01568 797309 Fax: 01568 797309 — MB BS Lond. 1973 (Char. Cross) MRCGP 1980. Prev: Surg. Lt.-Cdr. RN.

NEWCOMBE, Mr John Fernley (retired) 36 Sandy Lodge Road, Rickmansworth WD3 1LJ Tel: 01923 822370 Email: newcombe@uppercourt.demon.co.uk — (Camb. & St. Bart.) MB BChir Camb. 1952; FRCS Eng. 1957; MA Camb. 1955, MChir 1963. Prev: Cons. Surg. Centr. Middlx. Hosp. Lond. & Wembley Hosp.

NEWELL, Antonia Gay Priory Road Surgery, Priory Road, Park South, Swindon SN3 2EZ Tel: 01793 521154 Fax: 01793 512562 — MB BS Lond. 1981 (Char. Cross) DRCOG 1984; MRCGP 1985. Specialty: Gen. Pract.

NEWELL, Antony Maxwell Barrett 66 Norfolk House Road, Streatham, London SW16 1JH; Mayday University Hospital, London Road, Thornton Heath CR7 7YE Tel: 020 8401 5033 Fax: 020 8402 3003 — MB BS Lond. 1987; MRCOG 1993. Cons. (HIV & Genitorinary Med.) Mayday Univ. Hosp. Specialty: Genitourinary Medicine; HIV Med. Prev: Sen. Regist. (HIV & Genitourin. Med.) St. Stephen's Clinic Lond.

NEWELL, Barry Anthony Thomas 50 Carlton Road, Grays RM16 2YA — MB BS Lond. 1996 (Roy. Free Hosp. Sch. of Med.) BSc (Hons) Lond. 1993; MRCP (UK) 1999.

NEWELL, David Nicholas The Surgery, 24 Albert Road, Bexhill-on-Sea TN40 1DG Tel: 01424 730456/734430 Fax: 01424 225615 — MB ChB Bristol 1982; MRCGP 1986.

NEWELL, Debra Moorcroft Surgery, 646 King Lane, Leeds LS17 7AN Tel: 0113 295 2750 Fax: 0113 295 2761; Milestones, 5 Creskeld Park, Bramhope, Leeds LS16 9EZ — MB ChB Leeds 1980; DRCOG 1982; MRCGP 1985. Prev: Princip. GP Birm.; Asst. GP Guiseley.

NEWELL, Emma Louise 145 North Road, St Andrews, Bristol BS6 5AH — MB ChB Manch. 1998; MRCP.

NEWELL, Janet 30 Sourhill, Dan's Road, Ballymena BT42 2LG — MB BCh BAO Belf. 1990; DGM RCP Ed. 1993; DRCOG 1994; MRCGP 1995. Specialty: Gen. Pract.

NEWELL, Jennifer Rachel Dolphins, Rue De St Jean, St Lawrence, Jersey JE3 1ND — MB BS Lond. 1962 (Univ. Coll. Hosp.) MRCS Eng. LRCP Lond. 1962. Community Health Jersey.

NEWELL, Jennifer Rachel Le Warne Clive House, The Street, Walsham Le Willows, Bury St Edmunds IP31 3AZ — MB BS Lond. 1993.

NEWELL, John Philip (retired) 34 Pierce Lane, Fulbourn, Cambridge CB1 5DL — MB ChB Leeds 1969; FFA RCS Eng. 1974; MA Camb. 1979; PhD Leeds 1983, BSc (Hons.) 1966. Cons. Anaesth. Camb. HA (T). Prev: Clin. Lect. (Anaesth.) Univ. Camb. Sch. Clin. Med.

NEWELL, Kathryn Anne 15 Gransha Close, Comber, Newtownards BT23 5RB Tel: 028 9044 8174 — MB ChB Ed. 1992 (Edinburgh) DRCOG 1994; MRCGP 1996. Primary Care Doctor (A & E) GP Geo.town Grand Cayman. Specialty: Gen. Pract. Socs: BMA; RCGP; MDU.

NEWELL, Richard Andrew 25 Belle Vue Gardens, Shrewsbury SY3 7JG — BChir Camb. 1996.

NEWELL, Richard Jonathan West Malling Group Practice, 116 High Street, Milverton, West Malling ME19 6LX Tel: 01732 870212 Fax: 01732 742437; Ladham Oast, Ladham Road, Goudhurst, Cranbrook TN17 1DE — MB ChB Liverp. 1985.

NEWELL, Mr Richard Leonard Martyn (retired) 11 Windsor Terrace, Penarth CF64 1AA — MB BS Lond. 1968 (Guy's) BSc Lond. 1965; MRCS Eng. LRCP Lond. 1968; FRCS Eng. 1973. Hon. Cons. Orth. Surg .Roy .Devon & Exeter. NHS.Trust. Prev: Cons. Orthop. Surg. N. Devon Dist. Hosp. Barnstaple & Princess Eliz. Orthop. Hosp. Exeter.

NEWELL, Simon James St. James's University Hospital, Leeds Teaching Hospitals, Leeds LS9 7TF Tel: 0113 206 6959 Fax: 0113 206 5405 Email: simon.newell@leedsth.nhs.uk; Milestones, 5 Creskeld Park, Bramhope, Leeds LS16 9EZ Tel: 0113 230 1170 — MB ChB Leeds 1980; MRCP (UK) 1983; DTM & H Liverp. 1989; MD Leeds 1996; FRCP Lond. 1996. Cons. And Sen. Clin. Lect., Neonat. Med. & Paediat. Gastroenterol. St. Jas. Univ. Hosp. Leeds; Sen. Clin. Lect. Univ. of Leeds; Acad. Sub-Dean Sch. of Med. Univ. of Leeds; Chair, MCPCH Clin. Exam. Bd., RCPCH. Specialty: Paediat.; Neonat. Socs: Paediat. Research Soc.; Fell. Roy. Coll. Paediat. & Child Health; Brit. Soc. Paediat. Gastroenterol. & Nutrit. Prev: Lect. (Paediat.) Univ. Birm.; Clin. Research Fell. Inst. Child Health Univ. Birm.; Regist. (Paediat.) Childr. Hosp. Birm. & York Dist. Hosp.

NEWELL, Stephen John North Street Medical Care, 274 North Street, Romford RM1 4QJ Tel: 01708 764477 Fax: 01708 757656 Email: stephen.newell@nhs.net; 3 Wayside Close, Romford RM1 4ES Tel: 01708 760736 Fax: 01708 788650 Email: doctorsjn@aol.com — MB BS Lond. 1980 (Roy. Lond. Hosp.) BSc Lond. 1977; Cert. Family Plann. JCC 1982; DRCOG 1982; DFFP 1995; MRCGP 1985, FRCGP 1999; Mem. Inst. Learn. & Teach. 2002. GP Princip.; Course Organiser for Havering VTS; Clin. Asst. Diabetic Clinic OldCh. Hosp. Romford; Univ. Tutor (Gen. Pract.) St. Bart. & The Lond. Med. Schs.; GP Appraiser. Specialty: Gen. Pract.; Diabetes. Prev: Trainer (Gen. Pract.) Romford; Mem. Barking & Havering LMC; Non-executive Director, Barking and Havering Health Auth.

NEWELL PRICE, John Charles (retired) Dragon Lodge, Millbridge, Frensham, Farnham GU10 3DQ — MB Camb. 1954 (King's Coll. Hosp.) MRCGP; BChir 1953. Clin. Asst. (Rheum.) Frimley Pk. Hosp. Prev: Med. Off. RAMC.

NEWELL-PRICE, John David Charles Department of Endocrinology, 5th Floor, King George V Block, St Bartholomew's Hospital, West Smithfield, London EC1A 7BE Tel: 020 7601 8343 Fax: 020 7601 8505; 77 Lyal Road, Bow, London E3 5QQ — MB BChir Camb. 1990 (Cambridge University) MA Camb. 1991, BA (Hons.) 1987; MRCP (UK) 1993. Lect. in Endocrinol. Specialty: Endocrinol.; Diabetes; Gen. Med. Socs: Soc. for Endocrinol.

NEWELL PRICE, Rebecca Jane Kibbear Barton, Trull, Taunton TA3 7LN — BM Soton. 1990; MRCGP 1995. GP Retainer.

NEWEY, Charlotte Anne — MB BS Lond. 1997.

NEWEY, James Arthur Drs. Beynon, Cottier, Fearon, Frood, Johnson & Newey Weaver Vale Practice, Hallwood Health Centre, Hospital Way, Runcorn WA7 2UT Tel: 01928 711911 Fax: 01928 717368 Email: james.newey@nhs.net; 61 Beech View Road, Kingsley, Frodsham WA6 8DG Tel: 01928 788132 — MB ChB Liverp. 1972; DCH Eng. 1974; DObst RCOG 1975; MRCGP 1977.

NEWEY, Mr Martyn Leslie 32 Twmpath Lane, Gobowen, Oswestry SY10 7AQ — MB BS Lond. 1986; BSc (Hons.) Sussex 1981; FRCS Ed. 1990; FRCS (Orth.) 1996. Sen. Regist. Robt. Jones & Agnes Hunt Orthop. Hosp. Oswestry. Specialty: Orthop. Socs: Sekforde Club; Roy. Soc. Med. Prev: Sen. Regist. (Orthop.) N. Staffs. Roy. Infirm.; Regist. (Orthop.) St. Geo. Hosp. Train. Scheme; SHO (Gen. Surg.) William Harvey Hosp. Ashford Kent.

NEWEY, Sarah Francesca 302 Ombersley Road, Worcester WR3 7HD — MB ChB Birm. 1989.

NEWGROSH, Bernard Stephen Great Lever Health Centre, Rupert St., Bolton — MB BS Lond. 1975.

NEWHAM, Mr John Reginald Turner Health Centre, Old Hall, Cowbridge CF71 7AD Tel: 01446 774008; Caecady House, 58 High St, Cowbridge CF71 7AH Tel: 01446 773878 — MB ChB Cape Town 1946; BSc Cape Town 1946; FRCS Eng. 1952.

NEWHOUSE, Robert Guy (retired) Ashlea, Rising Sun, Callington PL17 8JD Tel: 01579 350145 — MB ChB Bristol 1964; DObst RCOG 1966. Prev: Regist. (Med.) Plymouth Gen. Hosp.

NEWHOUSE, Ruth Elizabeth Handforth Health Centre, The Green, 166 Wilmslow Road, Handforth, Wilmslow SK9 3HL Tel: 01625 529421/01625 536560 — MB ChB Manch. 1980; MRCP (UK) 1983; MRCGP 1985; DRCOG 1986. Specialty: Gen. Pract.

NEWHOUSE, Shân Margaret ThE Elizabeth Courtauld Surgery, Factory Lane West, Halstead CO9 1EX Tel: 01787 475944 Fax: 01787 474506; Hare House, Wethersfield Road, Sible Hedingham,

Halstead CO9 3LA — BM (Hons.) Soton. 1984; BA (Social Philosophy) CNAA 1982; MRCGP 1989. GP Princip. Specialty: Gen. Pract. Socs: BMA. Prev: Trainee GP Soton. VTS; SHO (O & G) Princess Anne Hosp. Soton.

NEWINGTON, Mr David Peter 260 Gower Road, Sketty, Swansea SA2 9JL — MB BS Lond. 1985; FRCS Eng. 1989; FRCS (Orth.) 1993. Cons. Orthop. Surg. Morriston Hosp. Swansea. Specialty: Orthop. Socs: Brit. Orthop. Assn.; Brit. Soc. Surg. Hand. Prev: Sen. Regist. (Orthop.) Cardiff; Regist. (Orthop.) Glas. Roy. Infirm.

NEWISS, Louise Patricia Thornton Medical Centre, Church Road, Thornton-Cleveleys, Blackpool FY5 2TZ Tel: 01253 854321 Fax: 01253 862854; Overdale, The Spinney, Poulton-le-Fylde FY6 7EZ — MB ChB Manch. 1988.

NEWLAND, Professor Adrian Charles Department of Haematology, Royal London Hospital, Whitechapel, London E1 1BB Tel: 020 7377 7180 Fax: 020 7377 7016 Email: a.c.newland@qmul.ac.uk; 41 Elmwood Road, London SE24 9NS Tel: 020 7274 3295 — MB BChir Camb 1974 (Camb. and Lond. Hosp.) MA Camb. 1975; MRCP (UK) 1976; FRCPath 1992, M 1980; FRCP Lond. 1992. Prof. Haemat. St. Barts. & The Lond. Qu. Mary Sch. of Med. & Dent.; Assoc. Director for Path., BLT NHS Trust; Hon. Cons. BLT; Hon. Cons. RAMC. Specialty: Haematology. Socs: Vice-Pres. Roy. Coll. of Pathologists; BMA; Assn. Phys. Prev: Clin. Dir. N. E. Thames Cancer Network; Ex Dir. for Research & Developm. BLT; Clin. Dir. N. E. Thanet Cancer Network.

NEWLAND, Anthony David Lydiate Farm, Village Road, Lower Heswall, Wirral L60 8PR Tel: 0151 342 8733; 11 Silverdale Road, Oxton, Wirral CH43 2JS Tel: 0151 652 6566 — MB ChB Liverp. 1986; ECFMG Cert, FMGEMS 1988; FRCS Ed. 1991. SHO (A & E) Arrowe Pk. Hosp. Specialty: Gen. Surg. Prev: SHO (Surg./Urol.) Chester Roy. Infirm.; Demonst. (Anat.) Liverp. Med. Sch.

NEWLAND, Carol Jean X-Ray Department, Leicester General Hospital, Gwendolin Road, Leicester LE5 4PW Tel: 0116 249 0490; 3 Church Lane, Ashby Folville, Melton Mowbray LE14 2TA Tel: 01664 840519 — BM Soton. 1981; MRCP (UK) 1985; FRCR 1989. Cons. (Diag. Radiol.) Leicester Gen. Hosp. Specialty: Radiol. Prev: Sen. Regist. (Diag. Radiol.) Leicester Roy. Infirm.

NEWLAND, Lesley Ann Ash Grove Surgery, Cow Lane, Knottingley WF11 9BZ — MB BS Lond. 1978.

NEWLAND, Michael Arthur 14 Breakspeare, College Road, London SE21 Tel: 020 8693 7917 — MB BChir Camb. 1954 (St. Thos.) DTM & H Liverp. 1959; DA Eng. 1966; DObst RCOG 1967. Specialty: Gen. Med. Socs: Fac. Anaesth. RCS Eng. Prev: Cons. Primary Care Phys. Riyadh Al-Kharj Hosp. Progr., Saudi Arabia; Asst. Health Adviser Aden Protectorate Health Serv.; Med. Supt. Govt. Hosp. Dubai.

NEWLAND, Rita Anne London Road Surgery, 501 London Road, Thornton Heath CR7 6AR Tel: 020 8684 1172 Fax: 020 8665 5011; 37 Essendene Road, Caterham CR3 5PB — MB BS Lond. 1977; MRCGP 1981; DRCOG 1981.

NEWLAND, Tadeusz Michal The Hamlet, Tollerton, York YO61 1QR Tel: 01347 838462 — (Polish Sch. of Med. Ed.) MB ChB Polish Sch. of Med. 1948 Ed. Socs: Past Chairm. BMA - York Div.; Past Pres. York Med. Soc.; Anglo-Amer. Med. Soc. Prev: Regist. City Hosp. York; Hosp. Med. Off. St. Mary's Hosp. York; Cas. Off. & Anaesth. Harrogate Gen. Hosp.

NEWLANDS, Edward Stewart Charing Cross Hospital, Fulham Palace Road, London W6 8RF Tel: 020 8846 1419 Fax: 020 8846 1443 Email: e.newlands@ic.ac.uk; 3 Newington Green Road, London N1 4QP Tel: 020 7226 7211 Fax: 020 7226 7211 — (Middlx.) BA, BM BCh Oxf. 1966; MRCP (UK) 1970; PhD Lond. 1976; FRCP Lond. 1984. Prof. Cancer Med. Char. Imperial Coll. Sch. Med. Lond.; Dir. DoH Chorio Carcinoma Unit; Dir. Supra Regional Tumour Marker Assay Laborat. Specialty: Oncol. Socs: Fell. Roy. Soc. Med.; Assn. Cancer Phys.s; Amer. Assn. Cancer Research. Prev: Reader (Med. Oncol.) Char. Cross & Westm. Med. Sch.; Sen. Lect. & Hon. Cons. Med. Oncol. Char. Cross Hosp. Med. Sch. Lond.; Lect. (Med. Oncol.) Char. Cross Hosp. Med. Sch. Lond.

NEWLANDS, Linda Caroline 42 Cranmore Gardens, Belfast BT9 6JL — MB BCh BAO Belf. 1994.

NEWLANDS, Peter William 32 Foxley Lane, Purley CR8 3EE Tel: 020 8660 1304; 140 Chipstead Valley Road, Coulsdon CR5 3BB Tel: 020 8660 1305 — MRCS Eng. LRCP Lond. 1977 (Roy. Free) DRCOG 1980. GP Purley & Coulsdon. Prev: SHO (Gen. Med.) Croydon Gen. Hosp.; Ho. Surg. W. Norf. & Kings Lynn Gen. Hosp.; Ho. Phys. Shrewsbury Hosp.

NEWLANDS, Mr William Jeffrey Aberdeen Royal Infirmary, Foresterhill, Aberdeen AB25 2ZN Tel: 01224 681818; 43 Westholme Avenue, Aberdeen AB15 6AB Tel: 01224312987 — MB ChB Ed. 1952; FRCS Ed. 1961. Cons. Otolaryngol. Aberd. Roy. Hosp. (NHS Trust) & Orkney & Shetland HBs; Clin. Sen. Lect. (Otolaryngol.) Univ. Aberd. Specialty: Otorhinolaryngol. Prev: Prof. Otolaryngol. King Faisal Univ. Coll. Med. Dammam, Saudi Arabia; Cons. Otolaryngol. Co. Hosp. Uddevalla Sweden; Otolaryngol. Brown Clinic Calgary, Canada.

NEWLEY, Kevin Peter Evington Road Medical Centre, 71 Evington Road, Leicester LE2 1QH Tel: 0116 212 0212 — MB ChB Leic. 1982. GP Leicester.

NEWLOVE, Russell Martin 11 Carlton Street, Monton, Eccles, Manchester M30 9QE — MB ChB Manch. 1996.

NEWMAN, Anthony James 36 Parkstone Road, Poole BH15 2PG Tel: 01202 682174 Fax: 01202 660718; 4 Alton Road, Lower Parkstone, Poole BH14 8SJ Tel: 01202 723460 — MB BS Lond. 1982; DRCOG 1986; Cert. Family Plann. JCC 1986. Med. Off. Bombardier Support Servs.; Med. Off. Marconi plc Poole; Med. Off. Siemens plc Poole; Dorset Occupat. Care Servs. Specialty: Gen. Pract. Prev: SHO (A & E) St. Geo. Hosp. Lond.; SHO Poole Gen. Hosp.; Trainee GP E. Dorset HA.

NEWMAN, Barbara Joyce (retired) 62 Hazelwood Avenue, Newton Mearns, Glasgow G77 5QS Tel: 0141 639 2986 — MB ChB Glas. 1956; FFA RCS Eng. 1972. Prev: Cons. Anaesth. Inverclyde Roy. Hosp. Greenock.

NEWMAN, Barbara Mary (retired) Wyevale, 11 Primrose Way, Sandhurst GU47 8PL — (Roy. Free) MRCS Eng. LRCP Lond. 1947. Prev: Assoc. Specialist W. Middlx. Hosp. Isleworth.

NEWMAN, Mr Brian Maurice Newlands Medical Centre, Chorley New Road, Bolton BL1 5BP Tel: 01204 846909 Fax: 01204 847073 — MB ChB Manch. 1968; FRCS Ed. 1973; MD Manch. 1977. Indep. Cons. Surg. Bolton; Chairm. Med. Innovations; Dir. Newlands Med. Serv. Specialty: Gen. Surg. Prev: Cons. Surg. Bolton Dist. Hosp. HA; Sen. Regist. (Surg.) Manch. Roy. Infirm.; Lect. (Surg.) Dept. Gastroenterol. Manch. Roy. Infirm.

NEWMAN, Carole Ann Park Cottage, Farrington Road, Paulton, Bristol BS39 7LW Tel: 01761 412312 Email: carole.newman@mcmail.com — (Bristol) MB ChB Bristol 1966.

NEWMAN, Christopher John Forest Gate Surgery, Hazel Farm Road, Totton, Southampton SO40 8WU Tel: 023 8066 3839 Fax: 023 8066 7090 — MB BCh Wales 1974; DRCOG 1978.

NEWMAN, Christopher Leonard Royal Berkshire & Battle Hosps. NHS Trust, Royal Berkshire Hospital, Department of Paediatrics, Reading RG1 5AN Tel: 0118 987 5111 Fax: 0118 987 8383; Kiln House, The Street, Aldermaston Village, Reading RG7 4LN Tel: 0118 971 3525 — MB BS Lond. 1966 (Guy's) FRCPCH; MRCS Eng. LRCP Lond. 1966; DObst RCOG 1968; MRCP (UK) 1971; FRCP Lond. 1986. Cons. Paediat. Roy. Berks. Hosp. Reading. Specialty: Paediat. Socs: Fell of Roy. Coll of Paediat. & Child Health; Fell. & Collegiate Mem. Roy. Coll. Phys. Lond.; Fell. Roy. Soc. Med. Prev: Sen. Regist. (Paediat.) Hosp. Sick Childr. Gt. Ormond St.; Regist. (Paediat.) Roy. Hosp. Sick Childr. Glas.; SHO (Neonat. Paediat.) Hammersmith Hosp. Lond.

NEWMAN, Christopher Mark Howard Clinical Services Centre, Northern General Hospital, Sheffield S5 7AY Tel: 0114 271 4456 Fax: 0114 261 9587 Email: c.newman@sheffield.ac.uk; 58 Devonshire Road, Dore, Sheffield S17 3NW Tel: 0114 236 0219 — MB BS Lond. 1983; MA Camb. 1984, BA 1980; MRCP (UK) 1986; PhD CNAA 1992; FRCP 1999. Sen. Lect. (Cardiol.) Univ. Sheff. & Hon. Cons. Cardiol. N. Gen. Hosp. Sheff. Specialty: Cardiol. Prev: MRC Clinician Sci. Fell 1995; Reg. (Cardio) RPMS/Hamm'smth Hosp. 1989.

NEWMAN, Mr Christopher Patrick St John 1 Willow Garth, Ferrensby, Knaresborough HG5 0QD Tel: 01423 340534 — MB BS Lond. 1966; MRCS Eng. LRCP Lond. 1966; FRCS Eng. 1972.

NEWMAN, Cicely Emmeline 783 Faranseer Park, Macosquin, Coleraine BT51 4NB — MB BCh BAO Dub. 1958 (T.C. Dub.) Prev: Med. Asst. (Anaesth.) Altnagelvin Hosp. Londonderry; Med. Asst. (Gen. Med.) Roe Valley Hosp. Limavady.

NEWMAN, Claude Gerald Hugh Chelsea & Westminster Hospital, London SW10 9NH; 31 Southwood Lawn Road, Highgate, London

N6 5SD Tel: 020 8340 3516 Fax: 020 8340 1457 — MB BS Lond. 1953 (Middlx.) MRCS Eng. LRCP Lond. 1953; FRCP Lond. 1976, M 1955; DCH Eng. 1957; FRCPCH 1997. Emerit. Cardiol. Paediat. Chelsea & Westm. Hosp. Lond.; Hon. Cons. Paediat. Qu. Mary's Univ. Hosp. Roehampton; Med. Advis. Thalidomide Soc. Specialty: Paediat. Socs: Fell. Roy. Soc. Med.; Brit. Soc. Rehabil. Med. Prev: Dir. Leon Gillis Unit & Cons. Paediat. Qu. Mary's Hosp. Roehampton; Sen. Regist. (Paediat.) St. Thos. Hosp. Lond.; Cons. Paed. Cardiol. Chelsea & Westm. Hosp. Lond. SW10.

NEWMAN, Clive George Medical Centre, Cambridge Avenue, Bottesford, Scunthorpe DN16 3LG Tel: 01724 842415 Fax: 01724 271437; Briggate Farm House, Old Brigg Road, Messingham, Scunthorpe DN17 3RJ — MB ChB Sheff. 1979; MRCGP 1983; Dip. Palliat. Med. Wales. 1995.

NEWMAN, David Anthony King Street Surgery, 84 King Street, Maidstone ME14 1DZ Tel: 01622 756721/756722/3 — BM BCh Oxf. 1984 (Oxford) MA Oxf. 1987, BA 1981; DCH RCP Lond. 1986; MRCGP 1989. GP Maidstone. Prev: SHO (Paediat.) Maidstone Hosp.; Ho. Surg. Dorset Co. Hosp. Dorchester; Ho. Phys. Roy. Cornw. Hosp. Truro.

NEWMAN, David John Forest Road Health Centre, 8 Forest Road, Hugglescote, Coalville LE67 3SH Tel: 01530 832109 — MB ChB Sheff. 1976.

NEWMAN, Douglas Keith Addenbrooke's Hospital, Department of Ophthalmology (Box 41), Hills Road, Cambridge CB2 2QQ — BM BCh Oxf. 1990; MA Camb. 1987; FRCOphth 1994. Cons. Ophth. Surg. Addenbrooke's NHS Trust Camb. Specialty: Ophth. Socs: Fell. Roy. Coll. Ophth.; Fell. Roy. Soc. Med.; Amer. Acad. Ophth. Prev: Specialist Regist. (Ophth.) Addenbrooke's Hosp.; Fell. (Med. Retina) Moorfields Eye Hosp.; Fell. (Itreoretinal Surg.) Manch. Roy. Eye Hosp.

NEWMAN, Francesca St Thomas Surgery, Ysgol Street, St. Thomas, Swansea SA1 8LH Tel: 01792 653992 — MB BS Lond. 1987 (London St. Bartholomews) MRCGP 1991. GP Princip. St. Thos. Surg. Swansea. Socs: Roy. Coll. Gen. Pract.; BMA. Prev: Trainee GP Briton Ferry Health Centre Neath W. Glam.; SHO (Paediat. & O & G) Neath Gen. Hosp.

NEWMAN, Geoffrey Hannell Sussex Oncology Centre, Royal Sussex County Hospital, Eastern Road, Brighton BN2 5BE Tel: 01273 696955 — MB ChB Bristol 1976; MRCP (UK) 1979; FRCR 1989. Cons. Clin. Oncol. Roy. Sussex Co. Hosp. Brighton. Specialty: Oncol.; Radiother. Prev: Sen. Regist. Bristol.

NEWMAN, Gwyneth Margaret (retired) Crwys Road Surgery, 151 Crwys Road, Cathays, Cardiff CF24 4XT Tel: 029 2039 6987 Fax: 029 2064 0523 — MB BCh Wales 1962; DObst RCOG 1964; DPH Wales 1966.

NEWMAN, Helena Hillview Medical Centre, 3 Heathside Road, Woking GU22 7QP Tel: 01483 760707 — MB BS Lond. 1981; Cert. Family Plann. JCC 1987; DRCOG 1987; LFHom 1999.

NEWMAN, Hugh Francis Vernon Bristol Oncology Centre, Bristol BS2 8ED Tel: 0117 928 2412 Email: hugh.newman@ubht.swest.nhs.uk; Trunders, Upper Lansdown Mews, Bath BA1 5HF Tel: 01225 480491 — MB ChB Sheff. 1977; B. Jur. Sheff. 1972; FRCR 1983; MD Sheff. 1988. Cons. Clin. Oncol. Roy. Infirm. Bristol & Roy. United Hosp. Bath. Specialty: Oncol.; Radiother. Socs: Brit. Inst. Radiol. & Brit. Oncol. Assn. Prev: Clin. Sci MRC Clin. Oncol. Unit & Hon. Sen. Regist. (Oncol.) Addenbrooke's Hosp. Camb.; Regist. (Radiother. & Oncol.) Velindre Hosp. Cardiff; Hon. Fell. (Therap. Radiol.) Univ. Minnesota Hosp.

NEWMAN, Jennifer — MB ChB Dundee 1998.

NEWMAN, John Henry 10 Harley Street, London W1G 9PF Tel: 020 7636 6504; 6 Johnsons Drive, Hampton TW12 2EQ — MB ChB Ed. 1973; BSc (Med. Sci.) Ed. 1970, MB ChB 1973; AFOM RCP Lond. 1981. Sen. Phys. (Occupat. Med.) Char. Cross Hosp. Lond. Socs: Assoc. Mem. RCGP; Soc. Occupat. Med. Prev: Sen. Med. Advider BBC TV Lond.; Phys. (Occupat. Med.) St. Stephens Hosp. Lond.; Phys. (Occupat. Med.) Banstead Psychiat. Hosp.

NEWMAN, Mr John Howard 2 Clifton Park, Bristol BS8 3LH Tel: 0117 906 4213 Fax: 0117 973 0887 Email: newman2cp@aol.com; Cornerstones, 41 Canynge Road, Bristol BS8 3LH Tel: 0117 973 6030 Email: newmancorner@doctors.org.uk — MB BChir Camb. 1967 (Guy's) FRCS Eng. 1971; T(S) 1991. p/t Cons. Orthop. Surg. Bristol Roy. Infirm.; Cons. Orthopaedic Surg. N. Bristol NHS Trust Bristol. Specialty: Orthop. Special Interest: Knee Surg. Socs: Brit. Orthop. Assn.; Brit. Assn. Surg. of Knee. Prev: Sen. Regist. (Orthop.) Nottm. Gen. Hosp.; Regist. (Orthop.) Oxf.

NEWMAN, Joseph Department of Cellular Pathology, Birmingham Heartlands Hospital, Bordesley Green E., Birmingham B9 5SS Tel: 0121 685 5877 Fax: 0121 685 5898 Email: newmanj@heartsol.wmids.nhs.uk — (Cape Town) MB ChB Cape Town 1966; MMed (Path.) Cape Town 1971; FRCPath 1986, M 1974. Cons. Histopath.& Cytopath Birm. Heartlands Hosp. Specialty: Histopath. Socs: Brit. Soc. Gastroenterol.; Brit Soc. Clin. Cytol.

NEWMAN, Joshua Leslie (retired) Flat 5, Millo Lodge, 17 Derby Road, Bournemouth BH1 3PZ Tel: 01202 316198 — (Middlx.) MRCS Eng. LRCP Lond. 1942. Prev: Ho. Surg. Nelson Hosp. Merton.

NEWMAN, Joycelyn Helen Westwood (retired) 2 Makepeace Avenue, Highgate, London N6 6EJ — MB ChB Ed. 1948 (Univ. Ed.) DObst RCOG 1951; DPH Lond. 1954. Prev: Sen. Med. Off. (Child Health) Enfield & Haringey HA.

NEWMAN, Karen Louise 9 Woodlea Court, Woodlea Village, Meanwood Park, Leeds LS6 4SL — MB ChB Leeds 1997.

NEWMAN, Mr Kevin John Hanmer St. Peter's Hospital, Guildford Road, Chertsey KT16 0PZ Tel: 01932 872000 Fax: 01932 874757; 6 Greenside Close, Merrow Park, Guildford GU4 7EU Tel: 01483 574364 Email: kevinnewmanortho@hotmail.com — (Char. Cross Hosp. Lond.) MB BS Lond. 1984; FRCS Eng. 1988; FRCS (Orth.) 1995. Cons. Orthop. & Trauma St. Peter's Hosp. Chertsey. Specialty: Trauma & Orthop. Surg. Socs: Fell. BOA; Brit. Assn. Surg. of the Knee. Prev: Sen. Regist. (Orthop.) St. Geo. Hosp. Lond.; Regist. (Orthop.) St. Geo. Hosp. Lond.

NEWMAN, Mr Laurence Department Oral & Maxillofacial Surgery, Univeristy College London Hospitals Maxillofacial Unit, Mortimer Market, London WC1E 6AU Tel: 020 7380 9859 Fax: 020 7380 9855 Email: laurence.newman@uclh.org; 112 Harley Street, London W1G 7JQ — MB BS Lond. 1990 (Lond. Hosp. Med. Coll.) BDS Lond. 1981; FFD 1984; FDS RCS Eng. 1988; FRCS Eng. 1992. Cons. Maxillofacial Surg. UCL Hosps. Lond. Specialty: Oral & Maxillofacial Surg. Special Interest: Head & neck Oncol. Socs: Brit. Assn. Head & Neck Orcol.; Fell. Brit. Assn. Oral & Maxillofacial Surg.; Graisofacial Soc. Gt. Brit. Prev: Sen. Regist. Qu. Vict. Hosp. E. Grinstead.

NEWMAN, Lotte Therese, CBE The White House, 1 Ardwick Road, Hampstead, London NW2 2BX Tel: 020 7435 6630 Fax: 020 7435 6672 Email: jh44@dial.pipex.com; Wellington Hospital South, Wellington Place, London NW8 9LE Tel: 020 7586 3213 — MB BS Lond. 1957 (Westm.) BSc Birm. 1951; MRCS Eng. LRCP Lond. 1957; FRCGP 1977; FRNZCGP 1998. Specialty: Gen. Pract. Socs: Liveryman Worshipful Soc. Apoth. (Mem. Livery Comm.); Fell. Roy. Soc. Med.; Hon. Fell. BMA. Prev: Med. Advis. St John Amb.; Mem. GMC (Ex-Chair Registration Comm.); Pres. RCGP.

NEWMAN, Lynn Hazel Department of Anaesthesia, Southern General Hospital, 1345 Govan Road, Glasgow G51 4TF Tel: 0141 201 1658 — MB ChB Liverp. 1980; FCAnaesth 1984. Cons. Anaesth. South. Gen. Hosp. Glas. Specialty: Anaesth. Prev: Cons. Anaesth. & Dir. of Intens. Care Broadgreen Hosp. Liverp.; Sen. Regist. Rotat. (Anaesth.) Merseyside; Research Regist. (Clin. Shock Study Gp.) West. Infirm. Glas.

NEWMAN, Margaret Joy Queen Elizabeth II Hospital, Childrens Community Services, Mezzanine floor Q66, Howlands, Welwyn Garden City AL7 4HQ Tel: 01707 328111 Fax: 01707 365329 — MB BS Lond. 1976 (UCHMS) Clin. Med. Off. (Community Health) E. Herts. NHS Trust. Specialty: Community Child Health; Family Plann. & Reproduc. Health. Prev: GP St. Albans.

NEWMAN, Mrs Marianna (retired) 15 Wickham Way, Park Laugley, Beckenham BR3 3AA — MB BS Lond. 1951 (Roy. Free) MRCS Eng. LRCP Lond. 1951; DCH Eng. 1953. Prev: Clin. Med. Off. Bromley HA.

NEWMAN, Martin Charles — MB ChB Bristol 1979; MRC Psych. 1992. Cons. & Hon. Sen. Lect. (Child & Adol. Psychia) S.&W. Lond. & St Geo.s Ment. Health, NHS Trust, Lond. SW17. Specialty: Child & Adolesc. Psychiat.

NEWMAN, Michael Roland Blair Eyebrook House, Stoke Dry, Oakham LE15 9JG Tel: 01572 821796 Fax: 01572 821268 — MB BChir Camb. 1975; MA 1975; DA Eng. 1979; FRCOG 1994. Cons. (O & G) Kettering Gen. Hosp. NHS Trust. Specialty: Obst. & Gyn. Socs: BMA; BFS; BSCCP.

NEWMAN, Michelle Julia 6 Sunnyfield, Mill Hill, London NW7 4RG — MB BS Lond. 1988; DRCOG 1991. GP Winchmore Hill.

NEWMAN, Myra Claremont Surgery, 2 Cookham Road, Maidenhead SL6 8AN Tel: 01628 673033 Fax: 01628 673432; Willow Corner, Poyle Lane, Burnham, Slough SL1 8LA Tel: 01628 602589 Email: myra.newman@btinternet.com — MB BS Lond. 1967 (St. Geo.) DObst RCOG 1969. Clin. Asst.Obst. Wexham Pk. Hosp. Slough. Socs: Windsor Med. Soc. & BMA. Prev: SHO (Paediat.) Wexham Pk. Hosp. Slough; SHO (O & G) Upton Hosp. Slough; Ho. Phys. & Ho. Surg. (ENT & Eye) St. Geo. Hosp. Tooting.

NEWMAN, Nathan The Wick Clinic, 200 Wick Road, London E9 Tel: 020 8986 6341; 18 Palace Court, Finchley Road, London NW3 Tel: 020 7431 0892 — MB ChB Leeds 1926 (Univ. Leeds) Prev: Ho. Surg. Centr. Hosp. Plymouth; Sen. Res. Med. Off. Weir Hosp. Balham; Ho. Surg. St. Mark's Hosp. For Rectal Dis.

NEWMAN, Paul Leslie 141 Surrenden Road, Brighton BN1 6ZA — MB BS Lond. 1983.

NEWMAN, Paul Mark 19 Dinmont Road, Shawlands, Glasgow G41 3UJ Tel: 0141 632 1233 — MB ChB Liverp. 1991; PhD Glas. 1986; DA 1996; DRCOG 1998; MRCGP 1999; Diploma Diabetes 2002. GP Princip.; Vocational Studies Tutor, Univ. of Glas. Specialty: Gen. Pract. Special Interest: Diabetes; Med. Educat.; Minor Surg. Prev: SHO (Anaesth.) Glas. Roy. Infirm.

NEWMAN, Penelope Jane 68B Finsbury Park Road, London N4 2JX Tel: 020 7704 1531 — MB BS Lond. 1985; MSc Lond. 1991. Cons. Pub. Health Med. Havering Hosp. NHS Trust; Fell. Kings Fund. Specialty: Pub. Health Med. Prev: Trainee (Pub. Health) N. Thames (W.); Regist. (Paediat.) Wellington, NZ; SHO (O & G) Roehampton.

NEWMAN, Penelope Mary Old Farm, Newby, Middlesbrough TS8 0AD Tel: 01642 325999 — MB BS Lond. 1974.

NEWMAN, Percival Peter 16 North Park Grove, Leeds LS8 1JJ Tel: 0113 266 3654 — MD Liverp. 1952; MB ChB 1941. Sen. Lect. Neurophysiol. Univ. Leeds. Socs: Fell. Roy. Soc. Med.; Physiol. Soc. Prev: Fulbright Schol. 1959; Vis. Prof. Physiol. Einstein Coll. Med. New York U.S.A.; Asst. Neurosurg. Off. Walton Hosp. Liverp.

NEWMAN, Peter Kevin Department of Neurology, James Cook University Hospital, Marton Road, middlesbrough TS4 3BW Tel: 01642 854395 Fax: 01642 282770 Email: peter.newman@stees.nhs.uk; Old Farm, Newby, Middlesbrough TS8 0AD Email: dr.p.newman@doctors.org.uk — MB ChB Birm. 1973; MRCP (UK) 1977; FRCP Lond. 1989. Cons. Neurol. & Hon. Sen. Lect., James Cook Univ. Hosp., Middlesbrough; Assoc. Med. Director, James Cook Univ. Hosp., Middlesbrough. Specialty: Neurol. Socs: Assn. Brit. Neurol.

NEWMAN, Peter William Hawthornden Surgery, Wharf Lane, Bourne End SL8 5RX Tel: 01628 522864 Fax: 01753 646448 Email: newmedsurgery@hotmail.com — MB BS Lond. 1985 (Char. Cross) BSc (Hons.) Lond. 1979; DRCOG 1988; Cert Family Plann. JCC 1989; Cert Managem. Open Univ. 1998; Basic AvMed CAA 1999; Dip Managem. Open Univ. 2000. GP Princip. Bucks.; Co. Doctor M W Kellogg Ltd. Greenfd.; Medico-legal Expert Witness. Specialty: Occupat. Health; Medico Legal; Aviat. Med. Socs: Brit. Assn. Performing Arts Med.; Hon. Sec. E. Berks. Div. BMA; Windsor Med. Soc. Prev: GP Slough (Single-Handed); Chairm. (Hon. Sec.) Conf. 1999; Lead GP Slough Commiss. Pilot 1998-99.

NEWMAN, Philip Jonathon 104 Durlston Road, Kingston upon Thames KT2 5RU — MB BS Lond. 1987; FRCA. 1991. Cons. Anaesth. & Intens. Care Research Fell. (Anaesth.) St. Geo. Hosp. Lond. Specialty: Anaesth.

NEWMAN, Philippa Mary North Street House Surgery, 6 North Street, Emsworth PO10 7DD Tel: 01243 373538 Email: pip.newman@virgin.net; 110 Station Road, Liss GU33 7AQ Tel: 01730 895056 — MB BS Lond. 1984 (Lond. Hosp. Med. Coll.) DRCOG 1995. Specialty: Gen. Pract. Prev: Trainee GP Hastings VTS; SHO (A & E) Roy. E. Sussex Hosp.; SHO (O & G) St. Mary's Hosp. Portsmouth.

NEWMAN, Piers Fenton Princess Royal Hospital, Apley Castle, Telford TF1 6TF Tel: 01952 641222 — MB BS Lond. 1988; BSc 1985; MRCP (UK) 1992. Neurol. Specialty: Neurol.

NEWMAN, Rachel Maria Royal Cornwall Hospital, Treliske, Truro Tel: 01872 250000 — MB ChB Ed. 1985; MRCP (UK) 1994. Cons. In Palliative Med. Specialty: Palliat. Med. Socs: Assoc. Palliat. Med.; Palliat. Care Research Soc. Prev: Specialist Regist. (Palliat. Med.) Salisbury Dist. Hosp.; Macmillan Fell. (Oncol., Palliat. Care & Gen. Med.) Roy. Lancaster Infirm.; Regist. (Med.) Birch Hill Hosp. Rochdale.

NEWMAN, Mr Raymond Julian Harrogate District Hospital, Lancaster Park Road, Harrogate HG2 7SX Tel: 01423 885959 Fax: 01423 555443; Wingfield House, 22 Street Lane, Roundhay, Leeds LS8 2ET Tel: 0113 237 0327 Fax: 0113 237 0336 — MB ChB Leeds 1975; BSc Leeds 1972; FRCS Eng. 1980; FRCS Ed. 1980; DPhil Oxf. 1983; FRSH 1990. Cons. Orthop. Surg. Harrogate Dist. Hosp.; Hon. Lect. (Orthop. Surg.) Univ. Leeds; Mem. Ct. of Examiners Roy. Coll. Surg. Specialty: Trauma & Orthop. Surg. Socs: Fell. BOA; Brit. Orthop. Research Soc.; Brit. Elbow & Shoulder Soc. Prev: Sen. Lect. (Orthop. Surg.) Univ. Leeds. & Cons. St. Jas. Hosp. Leeds; Lect. (Orthop. Surg.) & Hon. Sen. Regist. Univ. Glas.; MRC Research Fell. & Hon. Sen. Regist. Nuffield Orthop. Centre Oxf.

NEWMAN, Richard Roderick Churchfield Surgery, 14 Iburndale Lane, Sleights, Whitby YO22 5DP Tel: 01947 810466 Fax: 01947 811375; 190 Coach Road, Sleights, Whitby YO22 5EN Tel: 01947 810866 — MB BChir Camb. 1979.

NEWMAN, Roy John Old Mill & Millgates Surgery, Stoke Road, Poringland, Norwich NR14 7JL; Church Farm, Wymondham Road, Wramplingham, Wymondham NR18 0RH — MB BS Lond 1978 (Roy. Free) BSc Biochem. (1st cl. Hons.) Lond. 1978; DRCOG 1985; DCH RCP Lond. 1986; MRCP (UK) 1987; MRCGP 1994. GP. Specialty: Gen. Pract.

NEWMAN, Ruth (retired) 19 Hayes End, South Petherton TA13 5AG Tel: 01460 41044 — MB ChB Liverp. 1932; MA, MB ChB Liverp. 1932.

NEWMAN, Terence Anthony Stanley Road Surgery, 204 Stanley Road, Bootle L20 3EW Tel: 0151 922 5719 — MB ChB Manch. 1978; DRCOG 1983; DCH RCP Lond. 1985.

NEWMAN, Valerie Jean Crawley Hospital, West Green Drive, Crawley RH11 7DH Tel: 01293 600300; 16 Smithbarn, Horsham RH13 6EB Tel: 01403 211154 — MB BS Lond. 1972 (St. Thos.) FFA RCS Eng. 1976. Cons. Anaesth. & Lead Clin. Anaesth. Theatres & ITU Surrey & Sussex Healthcare NHS Trusst. Specialty: Anaesth. Prev: Sen. Regist. (Anaesth.) Guildford Hosp. Surrey.

NEWMAN, Vanessa Ruth Wayside, Moushill Lane, Milford, Godalming GU8 5BQ — MB BS Lond. 1988; MRCP (Paediat.) (UK) 1992; FRCR I 1997. Assoc. Specialist Jacob Breast Screening Guildford. Specialty: Radiol. Prev: Regist. (Paediat.) Roy. Surrey Co. Hosp. Guildford.

NEWMAN, Mr William David Tennent Institute of Ophthalmology, Western Infirmary, Dumbarton Road, Glasgow G11 6NT; 22 Arthurlie Drive, Uplawmoor, Glasgow G78 4AH Tel: 01505 850584 — MB BS Lond. 1987 (Lond. Hosp. Med. Coll.) FRCOphth 1996, M 1993; FRCS Glas. 1995. Specialist Regist. (Ophth.) Tennent Inst. Ophth. Glas. Specialty: Ophth. Prev: SHO III (Ophth.) Glas. Roy. Infirm.; SHO (Ophth.) W.bourne Eye Hosp. Bournemouth; SHO Rotat. (Gen. Med.) Roy. Vic. Hosp. Bournemouth.

NEWMAN, William Gerard James St Mary's Hospital, Hathersage Road, Manchester M13 0JH — MB ChB Manch. 1992 (Specialist Regist. (Clin. Genetics) St. Mary's Hosp. Manch.) BSc (Hons.) Manch. 1989; MB ChB (Hons.) Manch. 1992; MRCP (UK) 1995; MA Healthcare Ethics & Law. Manch. 1999. Wellcome Trust Clin. Train. Fell. Univ. of Manch. Specialty: Genetics. Socs: BSHG.

NEWMAN, William James 110 Freehold Street, Lower Heyford, Kidlington OX5 3NT — BM Soton. 1990.

NEWMAN-SANDERS, Anthony Paul Gerard Mayday University Hospital NHS Trust, Department of Diagnostic Imaging, London Road, Thornton Heath CR7 7YE Tel: 020 8401 3000 Ext: 4749 Fax: 020 8401 3454 Email: tony.newman-sanders@mayday.nhs.uk — MB BS Lond. 1987; MA Cambs. 1987; MRCP (UK) 1991; FRCR 1997. Cons. Radiologist, Mayday Univ. Hosp., Croydon. Specialty: Radiol. Special Interest: Musculo-Skeletal Radiol. Socs: Brit. Soc. of Skeletal Radiol.; Croydon Med. Soc.; Magnetic Resonance Radiologists Assn. Prev: Regist. (Radiol. & Renal & Gen. Med.) St. Mary's Hosp. Lond.; Sen. Regist. (Radiol.) St. Mary's Hosp. Lond.

NEWMAN TAYLOR, Professor Anthony John, CBE Royal Brompton Harefield NHS Trust, Sydney St., London SW3 6NP Tel: 020 7351 8328 Fax: 020 7351 8336 Email: a.newmant@rbh.nthames.nhs.uk; 11 Waldegrave Road, Bickley,

Bickley BR1 2JP — (St. Bart.) MB BS Lond. 1970; MRCP (UK) 1973; MSc (Occupat. Med.) Lond. 1979; FFOM RCP Lond. 1987, MFOM 1983; FRCP Lond. 1986; F Med Sci 1999; FRCP (Edin.) 2000. Prof. Occupat. & Environm. Med. & Head Dept. Occupat. Environm. Med. Brompton Hosp & Imperial Coll. Sch. Med. Nat. Heart & Lung Inst. Lond.; Scientif. Adviser to Colt Foundat.; Mem. (Chairm.) Injuries Advis. Counc.; Civil. Cons. in Chest Med. RAF; Med. Dir. & Dir. of Research Roy Brompton & Harefield NHS Trust; Chairm. CORDA Charity. Specialty: Respirat. Med. Socs: Brit. Thorac. Soc.; Brit. Soc. Allergy & Clin. Immunol.; Amer. Thoracic Soc. Prev: Sen. Regist. (Med.) Brompton & Westm. Hosps. Lond.; Lect. (Clin. Immunol.) Cardiothoracic Inst. Brompton Hosp. Lond.; Regist. (Med.) St. Bart. Hosp. Lond.

NEWMARCH, Bernard Wellington Medical Centre, Bulford, Wellington TA21 8PW Tel: 01823 663551 Fax: 01823 660650 — MB BS Lond. 1979 (Guy's) MRCS Eng. LRCP Lond. 1978; DRCOG 1981; Cert. Family Plann. 1981. NHS Direct W. Country Med. Dir. Prev: GP Trainee Soton. Univ. Hosps. VTS.; Chairm. Som. Local Med. Comm.

NEWMARK, James Christopher Paul Farrow Medical Centre, 177 Otley Road, Bradford BD3 0HX Tel: 01274 637031 — MB ChB Leeds 1976; MRCGP 1988; MPH Leeds 1996. JP.

NEWMARK, Patricia Ann Farrow Medical Centre, 177 Otley Road, Bradford BD3 0HX Tel: 01274 637031 — MB ChB Leeds 1976; DRCOG 1978; MRCGP 1989.

NEWMARK, Robert Walter (retired) 85 Woodlands Road, Cleadon, Sunderland SR6 7UB Tel: 0191 536 2066 Email: rownew@compuserve.com — (Durh.) MB BS Durh. 1952.

NEWNAM, Peter Thomas Frank The Grange, Hutton Gate, Guisborough TS14 8EQ Tel: 01287 633928 — MB BS Durh. 1960 (Newc.) FFA RCS Eng. 1964. Cons. Anaesth. N & S Tees Hosp. Gps. Specialty: Anaesth. Prev: Asst. Clin. Tutor (Anaesth.) United Birm. Hosps.; Regist. (Anaesth.) Roy. Hosp. Wolverhampton; Regist. (Anaesth.) Newc. Gen. Hosp.

NEWNHAM, Claude Tristram Mead Cottage, Mackney Lane, Brightwell-cum-Sotwell, Wallingford OX10 0SQ — MRCS Eng. LRCP Lond. 1943 (St. Mary's) DOMS Eng. 1947. CStJ; Mem. Med. Counc. on Alcoholism. Prev: Regional Med. Off. West. Region Brit. Rly.; Ho. Surg. St. Mary's Hosp. Lond.; Squadron Ldr. RAF, Graded Ophth. & Venereol.

NEWNHAM, Donald Mackenzie Woodend Hospital, Eday Road, Aberdeen AB15 6XS Tel: 01224 663131 Ext: 56860 Fax: 01224 556339 — MB ChB Aberd. 1983 (Aberdeen University) MRCP (UK) 1988; MD Aberd. 1995. Cons. in Med. for the Elderly, Woodend Hosp., Aberd. Specialty: Care of the Elderly. Special Interest: Community Geriat.; Drug Prescribing. Socs: Brit. Geriat. Soc.

NEWNHAM, John Alan Victoria Road Surgery, 50 Victoria Road, Worthing BN11 1XB Tel: 01903 230656 Fax: 01903 520094; Walton House, 61 Grand Avenue, Worthing BN11 5BA Tel: 01903 247596 — MB ChB Ed. 1973; BSc (Med. Sci.) Ed. 1970. Specialty: Gen. Pract. Prev: Trainee GP Brighton VTS.

NEWNS, George Reginald (retired) Thatch Dyke, Whimpwell Green, Happisburgh, Norwich NR12 0QF — MB ChB Birm. 1938; FRCP Lond 1970, M 1945. Prev: Cons. Phys. Sheff. Centre for Investig. & Treatm. Of Rheum. Dis.

NEWPORT, Barry — MB ChB Birm. 1970; DObst RCOG 1973. GP Princip. Prev: SHO Dept. Communicable Dis. & SHO (Paediat.) E. Birm. Hosp.; Ho. Off. (Obst.) Cheltenham Matern. Hosp.

NEWPORT, Melanie Jane Cambridge Institute For Medical Research, Addenbrookes Hospital, Cambridge CB2 2XY Tel: 01223 331153 Email: melanie.newport@cimr.cam.ac.uk; 78 Stanley Road, Cambridge CB5 8LB — MB BS Lond. 1986 (St Marys Hopsital Med School) MRCP (UK) 1989; DCH RCP Lond. 1990; PhD Lond. Uni. 1996. Research Assoc.(Dept. of Med) Addenbrookes Hosp. Camb.; Hon. Cons. in Infec. Dis. Specialty: Infec. Dis. Special Interest: Genetic Immunodeficiency; Mycobacterial infections. Prev: Research Assoc. MRC Labs. The Gambia, W. Africa.

NEWPORT, Sheila Mary Ivy Grove Surgery, 1 Ivy Grove, Ripley DE5 3HN Tel: 01773 742286 Fax: 01773 749812; Redhill Cottage, Duffield Bank, Makeney, Derby DE56 0RT Tel: 01332 841304 — BM BS Nottm. 1980.

NEWRICK, Charles William, Group Capt. RAF Med. Br. (retired) 5 Brays Lane, Ely CB7 4QJ Tel: 01353 665202 — MB BChir Camb. 1962 (St. Geo.) DCP Lond 1972; MA Camb. 1974; FRCPath 1986, M 1975.

NEWRICK, Paul Gerrard Department of Medicine, Worcestershire Acute Hospitals NHS Trust, Kidderminster DY11 6RJ Tel: 01905 760243 Fax: 01905 760244 Email: drpgn@bigfoot.com — MB ChB Bristol 1979; MRCP (UK) 1982; MD Bristol 1988; T(M) 1992; FRCP Lond. 1998. Cons. Phys. (Diabetes & Endocrinol.) Worcs. Acute Hosp. Specialty: Diabetes; Endocrinol. Prev: Sen. Regist. (Diabetes & Endocrinol.) Bristol Roy. Infirm. & Roy. Devon & Exeter Hosp.; Research Fell. (Diabetes) Roy. Hallamsh. Hosp. Sheff.; Regist. (Med.) Frenchay Hosp. Bristol.

NEWRITH, Christopher Russell Francis Birmingham Therapeutic Community Service, Bridger House, 22 Summer Road, Acocks Green, Birmingham B27 7UT Tel: 0121 678 3244 Fax: 0121 678 3245 — MB ChB Manch. 1990; BSc St. And. 1987; MRCPsych 1996; MSc Oxford Brookes (Psychodynamic Psychotherapy in NHS settings) 2000. Cons. Psychiat. Birm.Therapeutic Community Serv. Birm. Specialty: Psychother. Prev: Regist. Oxf. Rotat. (Psychiat.); Specialist Regist. Oxf. Rotat. (Psychother.).

NEWRITH, Stella Fiona c/o Winterbourne House, 53-55 Argyle Road, Reading RG1 7YL — MB ChB Manch. 1990; BSc St. And 1987. Specialty: Gen. Psychiat.

NEWS, Marie Therese St. Johns Wood, 10 Woodville Avenue, Lurgan, Craigavon BT66 6JP — MB BCh BAO Belf. 1995.

NEWSAM, Avril Gladys, MBE (retired) 14 Comely Bank, Edinburgh EH4 1AN Tel: 0131 332 6307 — MB ChB Ed. 1954 (Edinburgh)

NEWSAM, Mr John Ernest (retired) 14 Comely Bank, Edinburgh EH4 1AN Tel: 0131 332 6307 — MB ChB Ed. 1949 (Edinburgh) FRCS Ed. 1955. Prev: Cons. Urol. Surg. West. Gen. Hosp. Edin.

NEWSHAM, Julie Ann 17 Grisedale Close, Formby, Liverpool L37 2YE — MB ChB Leeds 1984; DO RCS Eng. 1987.

NEWSHOLME, George Adam (retired) Yew Tree Cottage, Pentre Lane, Bredwardine, Hereford HR3 6BY Tel: 01981 500366 — MD Camb. 1951 (Camb. & Birm.) MA Camb. 1945, MD 1951, MB BChir 1945; FRCP Lond. 1970, M 1948; DMRT Eng. 1957; FRCR 1975. Prev: Radiotherap. United Birm. Hosps.

NEWSHOLME, Richard George Droitwich Medical Practice, Ombersley Street, Droitwich WR9 8RD — MB ChB Birm. 1979; BA Oxf. 1976.

NEWSHOLME, William Arthur 72 Holmefield Court, Belsize Grove, London NW3 4TU — MB BS Lond. 1992.

NEWSOM, Richard Samuel Babington Southampton Eye Unit, Tremona Road, Southampton SO16 6YD Tel: 02380 794758 — MB BS Lond. 1987; BSc Lond. 1984, MD 1994; FRCOphth 1994. p/t Cons. Ophth. Soton. Eye Unit. Specialty: Ophth. Special Interest: Diabetic Retinopathy; Retinal Dis. Socs: Apoth. Prev: Fell. New Eng. Eye Center Boston; Fell. Moorfields Eye Hosp.

NEWSOM, Rose Aylmer (retired) 11 The Footpath, Coton, Cambridge CB3 7PX Tel: 01954 210228 Fax: 01954 211871 Email: rose@newsom.demon.co.uk — MB BCh BAO Dub. 1957; MA Dub. 1957; DObst RCOG 1959; MFFP 1993. Prev: Sen. Clin. Med. Off. Cambs. HA.

NEWSOM, Samuel William Babington (retired) 11 The Footpath, Coton, Cambridge CB3 7PX Tel: 01954 210228 Fax: 01954 211871 — (Camb. & Westm.) MB BChir Camb. 1957; MD Camb. 1977, MA 1957; FRCPath 1976, M 1964; DTM & H Eng. 1964; T(Path.) 1991. Pres. Inst. Sterile Serv. Managers; Asst. Edr. Jl. Hosp. Infec. Prev: Cons. Microbiol. Camb. RHA.

NEWSOM-DAVIS, Professor John Michael, CBE Department of Clinical Neurology, University Oxford, Radcliffe Infirmary, Woodstock Road, Oxford OX2 6HE Tel: 01865 224940 Fax: 01865 224273 — MB BChir Camb. 1961 (Middlx.) FRCP Lond. 1973, M 1962; MA Camb. 1957, MD 1966; FRS 1991. Prof. Emerit. Clin. Neurol. Univ. Oxf. Specialty: Neurol. Special Interest: Disorders of the neuromuscular junction. Socs: Assn. Brit. Neurol.; Eur. Neurol. Soc.; Amer. Neurol. Assn. Prev: Edr. of Brain; MRC Clin. Research Prof. Neurol.; Hon. Cons. Roy. Free Hosp. & Nat. Hosp. Nerv. Dis. Lond.

NEWSON, Christopher Douglas Walsall Manor Hospital, Department of Anaesthetics, Moat Road, Walsall WS2 9PS Tel: 01922 721172 Ext: 7388 Email: newson.chris@walsallhospitals.nhs.uk; 10 Thornhill Road, Streetly, Sutton Coldfield B74 3EH Tel: 0121 353 5948 — MB BS Lond. 1984 (Guy's) MRCS Eng. LRCP Lond. 1984; FRCA 1991. Cons.

Anaesth. Walsall Manor Hosp.; Vis. Asst. Prof. Univ. Texas S. West. Med. Centre, Dallas. Specialty: Anaesth. Socs: Assn. Anaesth.; Christian Med. Fellowsh.; Obst. Anaesth. Assn. Prev: SHO (Anaesth.) MusGr. Pk. Hosp. Taunton & Frenchay Hosp. Bristol; SHO (Cardiol. & Chest Med.) Harefield Hosp. Middlx.

NEWSON, David Heath 39 Yeldham Road, London W6 8JF Tel: 020 8748 6840 — MB BS Lond. 1991 (Char. Cross & Westm.) BSc (Pharmacol.) Lond. 1988; MRCP (UK) 1995. Resid. (Paediat. ICU) Guy's Hosp. Lond. Specialty: Paediat. Socs: Christian Med. Fellowsh.; Brit. Paediat. Assn. Prev: Regist. (Paediat.) Mater Miser. Childr Hosp. Brisbane, Austral.; Regist. (Paediat.) Lewisham Gen. Hosp. Lond.; SHO (Paediat. Neonates) Univ. Coll. Hosp. Lond.

NEWSON, Diana Charmian Westgate Practice, Greenhill Health Centre, Church Street, Lichfield WS13 6JL Tel: 01543 414311 Fax: 01543 256364 — MB BS Lond. 1984 (Guy's) MRCGP 1988.

NEWSON, Edward James Cedar House Surgery, 14 Huntingdon Street, St Neots PE19 1BQ Tel: 01480 406677 Fax: 01480 475167 — BM Soton. 1998.

NEWSON, Mrs Elizabeth Rachel Alberta Hebblethwaite Hall, Cautley, Sedbergh LA10 5LX Tel: 01539 621307 — BM BCh Oxf. 1967 (Oxf. & Lond. Hosp.) Prev: Ho. Phys. Childr. Dept. & Receiv. Room Off. Lond. Hosp.; GP & Postgrad. Trainer (Gen. Pract.) Lond.

NEWSON, Louise Rachel 22 Finchley Road, Hale, Altrincham WA15 9RD Tel: 0161 928 0483 — MB ChB Manch. 1994; BSc (Hons.) Manch. 1992; MB ChB (Hons.) Manch. 1994; MRCP 1996. GP Regist. Specialty: Gen. Pract. Socs: Med. Wom. Federat. Prev: SHO (O & G) Chester; SHO (Med.) Mans.

NEWSON, Mary Penelope Valley Medical Centre, 14 Waller Close, Liverpool L4 4QJ Tel: 0151 207 3447 — MB ChB Liverp. 1986 (Liverpool) MRCGP 1990; DRCOG 1990. GP Liverp.; Clin. Asst. (Dermat.) Roy. Liverp. Univ. Hosp. Specialty: Gen. Pract. Prev: SHO (O & G) Wom. Hosp. Liverp.

NEWSON, Timothy Peter Kent & Canterbury Hospitals, NHS Trust, Canterbury CT1 3NG Tel: 01227 766877; 2 The Granary, Limetree Farm, Stone St, Petham, Canterbury CT4 5PW — BM BS Nottm. 1986; MRCP (UK) 1991. Cons. (Paed) Kent & Cantb. Hosp. Cantab. Kent. Specialty: Paediat. Prev: Regist. (Paediat.) Qu. Eliz. Hosp. for Childr. Hackney; Sen. Med. Off. (Paediat.) Jane Furse Memor. Hosp. Transvaal, S. Afr.; Sen. Regist. (Paediat.) Newc. Gen. Hosp.

NEWSON-SMITH, Grevile Robin Farnham Road Surgery, 301 Farnham Road, Slough SL2 1HD Tel: 01753 520917 Fax: 01753 550680; 3 Braybank, Old Mill Lane, Bray, Maidenhead SL6 2BQ Tel: 01628 624085 Fax: 01628 624085 — MB BS Lond. 1967 (St. Geo.) DObst RCOG 1973. Socs: Brit. Soc. Med. & Dent. Hypn. Prev: Ho. Phys. & Ho. Surg. Wycombe Gen. Hosp. High Wycombe; Resid. Obst. Asst. St. Geo. Hosp. Lond.; Squadron Ldr. RAF Med. Br.

NEWSON-SMITH, Jane Grace Beatrice Sevenacres, St. Mary's Hospital, Newport PO30 5TG Tel: 01983 524081 — MB BS Lond. 1970 (Char. Cross) MRCS Eng. LRCP Lond. 1970; MRCPsych 1976; FRCPsych 1999. Cons. Psychiat. St Mary's Hosp. Newport, I. of Wight. Specialty: Gen. Psychiat. Socs: BMA. Prev: Cons. Psychiat. Knowle Hosp. Fareham; Sen. Regist. (Psychiat.) St. Geo. Hosp. Lond.; Regist. (Psychiat.) & Clin. Research Fell. Char. Cross Hosp. Lond.

NEWSTEAD, Charles George Renal Unit, St James' University Hospital, Beckett St., Leeds LS9 7TF Tel: 0113 243 3144 Fax: 0113 244 0499 — MB BS Lond. 1981 (Guy's) MRCP (UK) 1986; BSc Lond. 1978, MD 1991; FRCP 1997. Cons. Renal Phys. St. Jas. Univ. Hosp. Leeds. Specialty: Nephrol. Socs: Physiol. Soc. & Internat. Soc. Nephrol.; Renal Assn.; Brit. Transpl. Soc.

NEWSTEAD, Mr Mark Roberts Coastal Villages Practice, Pippin Close, Ormesby St. Margaret, Great Yarmouth NR29 3RW Tel: 01493 730205 Fax: 01493 733120; North End Farm, Long Lane, Ingham, Stalham, Norwich NR12 0TJ — MB ChB Liverp. 1983; FRCS Eng. 1988; FRCS Ed. 1988; MRCGP 1993; T(GP) 1993. Specialty: Gen. Pract.

NEWSTEAD, Peter Oakmeadow Surgery, 87 Tatlow Road, Glenfield, Leicester LE3 8NF Tel: 0116 287 7911 — MB BS Lond. 1983; DRCOG 1988. GP Leicester FPC.

NEWSTEAD, Sheila Mary Setters, Hyde, Fordingbridge SP6 2QB Tel: 01425 52993 — MB BS Lond. 1940 (King's Coll. Hosp.) MRCS Eng. LRCP Lond. 1940; FRCP Lond. 1973, M 1943; FRCPath 1971. Socs: Assn. Clin. Pathols. & Brit. Soc. Haemat. Prev: Cons. Pathol. Bromley Gp. Hosps.; Asst. Clin. Pathol. King's Coll. Hosp.

NEWSTONE, Justin 67 Lance Lane, Liverpool L15 6TU — MB ChB Leic. 1995 (Glasgow) MRCP (UK) 1998.

NEWTH, Jeffrey Bernard 16 Springfield Crescent, Parkstone, Poole BH14 0LL — MB BChir Camb. 1961 (Camb. & Lond. Hosp.) BA Camb. 1958, MB BChir 1961; MRCP Lond. 1965; DTM & H Liverp. 1967. Med. Adviser Dorset Health Commiss. Socs: BMA. Prev: GP S. Molton; Regist. (Paediat.) Bath Gp. Hosps.; Directeur Centre Nutrit. EAR Kigeme, Rwanda.

NEWTH, Sarah Jane — MB ChB Birm. 1979; BSc (Anat.) Birm. 1975; MRCPsych 1984. Cons. Child Psychiat. Privat. Pract. Specialty: Child & Adolesc. Psychiat.; Medico Legal. Socs: Roy. Coll. Psychiat. Prev: Cons. Developm. Psychiat. S. Birm. Health Dist.; Cons. Child Psychiat. Solihull Healthcare NHS Trust.

NEWTON, Adrienne Ashley Tina The Surgery, 4 Hardell Rise, Tulse Hill, London SW2 3DX Tel: 020 8674 6586 — MB BS Lond. 1986 (Uni. Coll. Hosp. (Lond)) BSc Manch. 1980; MRCGP 1992. Specialty: Gen. Pract.

NEWTON, Alastair Inglis 29 Munro Road, Glasgow G13 1SQ — MB ChB Glas. 1990.

NEWTON, Andrew Paul Accident and Emergency Department, Weston General Hospital, Grange Road, Uphill, Weston Super Mare BS23 4TQ Tel: 01934 647103; Fair View, Top Road, Shipham, Winscombe BS25 1TB Tel: 0934 843246 — BM BS Nottm. 1985; BMedSci Nottm. 1983; MRCGP 1993; DCCH Ed. 1998; MSc (Child Health) Cardiff 2001. Assoc. Specialist A&E (Paediat.) Weston Gen. Hosp.; On-call Doctor Mendip Rescue Organisation (Cave Rescue); Med. Adviser Dyslexia Assn. N. Som.; Hon. Med. Adviser RNLI W.on; Nat. Chair of BAEM Forum for Assoc. Specs and Staff Grades in A&E. Specialty: Accid. & Emerg.; Paediat.; Community Child Health. Socs: Brit. Dyslexia Assn.; Roy. Coll. Surg. Ed. (Fac. Immediate Med. Care); Brit. Assn. Community Child Health. Prev: Squadron Med. Off. to Sixth Frigate Squadron RN; Gen. Pract. Avon FHSA.

NEWTON, Angela Francesca Woodbrook Medical Centre, 28 Bridge Street, Loughborough LE11 1NH Tel: 01509 239166 Fax: 01509 238747; Vine Cottage, 69 Brook St, Wymeswold, Loughborough LE12 6TT — MB BS Lond. 1973 (Char. Cross)

NEWTON, Anthony Simon Merchiston Surgery, Highworth Road, Swindon SN3 4BF Tel: 01793 823307 Fax: 01793 820923 — MB BS Lond. 1985; MA Camb. 1982; DA (UK) 1988; MRCGP 1990. Prev: Trainee GP Winchester VTS; SHO (Anaesth.) Whipps Cross Hosp. Lond.

NEWTON, Anthony Winston Lichfield Street Surgery, 19 Lichfield Street, Walsall WS1 1UG Tel: 01922 20532 Fax: 01922 616605 — MB ChB Birm. 1974; BSc (Hons.) (Physiol.) Birm. 1971, MB ChB 1974; DRCOG 1978; DCH Eng. 1978; MRCGP 1979.

NEWTON, Catherine Elizabeth Carn Cottage, Town Hill, St Agnes TR5 0QT — MB ChB Bristol 1997.

NEWTON, Charmian Rosemary St. George's Hospital, Blackshaw Road, London SW17 0QT Tel: 020 8725 3032 Fax: 020 8725 0830 Email: charmain.newton@stgeorges.nhs.uk — (Westm.) MB BS Lond. 1965; MRCS Eng. LRCP Lond. 1965; MRCP Lond. 1967; DObst RCOG 1967; FRCP Lond. 1993. Cons. Phys. St. Geo. Hosp. & Bolingbroke Hosp. Lond. Specialty: Gastroenterol.; Gen. Med.; Diabetes. Socs: Brit. Soc. Gastroenterol.; Brit. Diabetic Assn. Prev: Sen. Regist. (Med.) Middlx. Hosp. Lond. 1975-77; Sen. Regist. (Gastroenterol.) Centr. Middlx. Hosp. Lond. 1973-75; Research Asst. St. Mark's Hosp. Dis. of Rectum Lond. 1969-72.

NEWTON, David John — MD Birm. 1984; MB ChB 1972; MRCP (UK) 1976. Specialty: Diabetes. Socs: BMA; Diabetes U.K. Prev: Regist. (Endocrinol.) Radcliffe Infirm. Oxf.; Regist. (Gen. Med. & Diabetes) John Radcliffe Hosp. Oxf.; Clin. Research Fell. (Therapeut.) Roy. Hallamsh. Hosp. Sheff.

NEWTON, David John Highfield Surgery, Highfield Way, Hazlemere, High Wycombe HP15 7UW Tel: 01949 813396 Fax: 01949 814107; 74 Baring Road, Beaconsfield HP9 2NF Tel: 01494 675359 — (Univ. Coll. Hosp.) BM BCh Oxf. 1965; MRCP (U.K.) 1970. Prev: Research Fell. & Hon. Sen. Regist. MRC Rheum. Research Unit Canad.; Red Cross Memor. Hosp. Taplow; Med. Regist. Hammersmith Hosp. Lond. Ho. Phys. & Ho. Surg. Univ.

NEWTON, Duncan Angus Gray (private rooms), The Yorkshire Clinic, Bradford Road, Bingley BD16 1TW Tel: 01274 560311;

Tiverton, Southfield Road, Burley-in-Wharfedale, Ilkley LS29 7PA Tel: 01943 862258 — MB BS Newc. 1968; MRCP (UK) 1971; FRCP Lond. 1990. Cons. Phys. St. Luke's Hosp. Bradford. & Bradford Roy. Infirm. Specialty: Gen. Med. Prev: Sen. Med. Regist. St. Jas. Hosp. Leeds; Med. Regist. Hammersmith Hosp. Lond.; Res. Med. Off. Nat. Heart Hosp. Lond.

NEWTON, Elizabeth Mary Gray Tiverton, Southfield Road, Burley-in-Wharfedale, Ilkley LS29 7PA Tel: 01943 862258 — MB BS Newc. 1967. Prev: Regist. Roy. Hosp. Sick Childr. Glas.

NEWTON, Ellen Rosemary The David Lewis Centre, Mill Lane, Gt Warford, Alderley Edge SK9 7UD Tel: 01983 295251; The White Cottage, Parkfield Road, Knutsford WA16 8 Email: simon-mganga@doctors.org.uk — MB BS Lond. 1976. Assoc. Specialist in Childh. Epilepsy/ Manager Childr.'s Assesment Serv. Specialty: Paediat. Prev: Clin. Med. Off. Child Health Stockport HA; Trainee GP Macclesfield VTS; Princip. GP Knutsford, Chesh.

NEWTON, Mr Eric Joseph (retired) 237 Eccleshall Road, Stafford ST16 1PE Tel: 01785 251841 — MB BS Madras 1942; MRCS Eng. LRCP Lond. 1949; FRCS Eng. 1950. Prev: Cons. Neurosurg. Stoke-on-Trent Hosp. Gp.

NEWTON, Eric Michael (retired) Netherfield, Round St., Cobham, Gravesend DA13 9BA Tel: 01474 814247 — MRCS Eng. LRCP Lond. 1951 (Guy's) DObst RCOG 1958. Prev: Regtl. Med. Off. 2nd Btn. Black Watch.

NEWTON, Eva Katharina Stoke Mandeville Hospital NHS Trust, Mandeville Road, Aylesbury HP21 8AL; Ribbleton, Foxcombe Lane, Boars Hill, Oxford OX1 5DH Tel: 01865 735307 — MB BS Lond. 1982 (Kings Coll.) BSc (Physiol.) Lond. 1979; MRCOphth 1995. Staff Grade (Ophth.) Stoke Mandeville Hosp. Aylesbury. Specialty: Ophth.

NEWTON, Frank Antony (retired) Grafton Leys, 39 Cattle End, Silverstone, Towcester NN12 8UX Tel: 01327 857415 Fax: 01327 857415 Email: frank@sorebones.freeserve.co.uk — MRCS Eng. LRCP Lond. 1956 (Manch.) DA Eng. 1958; MSc (Sports Med.) Nottm. 1994. Hon. Med. Off. UK: Athletics; Resid. Hon. Med. Off. Silverstone Circuit; Med. Comm. Internat. Sailing Federat. Prev: Regist. (Anaesth.) Dudley Rd. Hosp. Birm.

NEWTON, Fraser Leigh — MB ChB Liverp. 1997; MRCGP 2003.

NEWTON, Mr Geoffrey (retired) The School House, The Green, Bretby, Burton-on-Trent DE15 0RE Tel: 01283 703721 — MB ChB Manch. 1954; FRCS Eng. 1965. Prev: Cons. Orthop. Surg. Derbysh. Roy. Infirm.

NEWTON, Helen Great Western Hospital, Swindon SN3 6BB Tel: 01793 605 106 Email: helen.newton@smnhst.swest.nhs.uk; Grove Farm House, Bourton, Swindon SN6 8JA Tel: 01793 784413 Email: helen.newton@lineone.net — BM Soton. 1982; MRCP (UK) 1985; FRCP 1997. p/t Cons. Stroke Phys., Dept. of Med. for the Elderly, Gt. West. Hosp., Swindon. Specialty: Care of the Elderly; Gen. Med. Socs: Brit. Geriat. Soc.; Brit. Assn. of Stroke Phys.s. Prev: Hon. Lect. & Sen. Regist. (Geriat. Med.) Portsmouth & Soton.

NEWTON, Helen Agnes (retired) 35 Bay Street, Fairlie, Largs KA29 0AL Tel: 01475 568355 — MB ChB Glas. 1954.

NEWTON, Hilary Skardon (retired) 20 Castle Street, Thornbury, Bristol BS35 1HB Tel: 01454 418698 — MB ChB Bristol 1957. Prev: Ho. Surg. Bristol Roy. Infirm.

NEWTON, James Douglas 142 Howard Road, Leicester LE2 1XJ — MB ChB Leic. 1998.

NEWTON, James Evelyn Watton Place Clinic, 60 High Street, Watton-at-Stone, Hertford SG14 3TA Tel: 01920 830232; Garden Cottage, Rectory Lane, Datchworth, Knebworth SG3 6RD — MB BS Lond. 1980; DRCOG 1984; MRCGP 1986. Socs: BMA. Prev: Ho. Surg. St. Bart. Hosp. Lond.; Ho. Phys. Hackney Hosp. Lond.

NEWTON, Janet Suzanne Red Bank Group Practice, Red Bank Health Centre, Unsworth Street, Manchester M26 3GH Tel: 0161 724 0777 Fax: 0161 724 8288; 1 Delbooth Avenue, Flixton, Urmston, Manchester M41 8SD — MB ChB Birm. 1986; DFFP 1990; DRCOG 1991; MRCGP 1992.

NEWTON, Joan Marie (retired) 231 Lauderdale Tower, Barbican, London EC2Y 8BY Tel: 020 7628 6781 — MB BS Lond. 1952 (Guy's) MRCS Eng. LRCP Lond. 1952; DA Eng. 1955.

NEWTON, Joan Victoria (retired) 6 Briar Rigg, Keswick CA12 4NW Tel: 017687 73242 — MB BS Lond. 1939 (Univ. Coll. Hosp.) MRCS Eng. LRCP Lond. 1939. Prev: Hon. Clin. Asst. Psychiat. Dept. Bromley Hosp.

NEWTON, John 72 Clober Road, Milngavie, Glasgow G62 7SR — MB ChB Glas. 1941 (Univ. Glas.) Prev: Ho. Surg. Vict. Infirm. Glas.; Squadron Ldr. RAFVR (Ret.).

NEWTON, John Henry (retired) — MB BS Lond. 1964 (Char. Cross) MRCS Eng. LRCP Lond. 1964; LRCP Lond. 1964; MRCS Eng. 1964; DMRD Eng. 1969; DMRD Eng. 1969; FFR 1971; FFR 1971; FRCR 1975; FRCP 1975. Cons. Radiol. Bedford Hosp. Prev: Chairm. NW Thames RHA Radiol. Sub-Comm.

NEWTON, John Hotham (retired) The Coach House, Landridge Road, London SW6 4LF Tel: 020 7736 8017 Fax: 020 7731 1801 — MB BChir Camb. 1952 (Lond. Hosp.) MRCS Eng. LRCP Lond. 1951; DPM Eng. 1973; MRCPsych 1974. Hon. Vis. Lect. Dept. Psychiat. Nat. Univ. Malaysia, Kuala Lumpur. Prev: Cons. Adolesc. Psychiat. E. Berks.

NEWTON, John Murray Endekiln, Strathblane, Glasgow Tel: 0141 70340 — MB ChB Glas. 1954.

NEWTON, John Norman Unit of Health-Care Epidemiology, University of Oxford, Old Road, Oxford OX3 7LF Tel: 01865 226991 Fax: 01865 226993; Ribbleton, Foxcombe Lane, Boars Hill, Oxford OX1 5DH — MB BS Lond. 1982; MA Oxf. 1979; MRCP (UK) 1985; MSc Lond. 1989; MFPHM RCP (UK) 1991; FRCP (UK) 1999; FFPHM RCP (UK) 2000. Cons. Epidemiol. Univ. Oxf. Unit of Healthcare Epidemiol.; Hon. Cons. Pub. Health Med. Oxf. HA; Univ. Research Lect. Univ. Oxf.; Hon. Sen. Lect. Univ. S.on; Director of Research & Developm., Oxf. Radcliffe Hosp. NHS Trust. Specialty: Epidemiol.; Pub. Health Med.; Research. Prev: Sen. Regist. (Pub. Health Med.) Oxf. RHA; Regist. (Dermat.) Wycombe Gen. Hosp.

NEWTON, Professor John Richard 25 Westfield Road, Edgbaston, Birmingham B15 3QF Tel: 0121 455 0263 Fax: 0121 684 2141 Email: johnnewton@hilltrees.freeserve.co.uk — (St. Bart.) MB BS Lond. 1962; MRCS Eng. LRCP Lond. 1962; FRCOG 1980, M 1967, DObst 1964; MD Lond. 1972; LLM 1994. Hon. Cons. Birmongham Womens Healthcare NHS Trust; Examr. Univs. Birm. Specialty: Obst. & Gyn.; Family Plann. & Reproduc. Health. Socs: (Comm.) ESGE & ISGE; Chairm. Scienti. Comm. ISGE; Past Pres. Fac. Family Plann. & Reproduc. Health Care. Prev: Sen. Lect. (O & G) King's Coll. Hosp. Lond.; Prof. & Cons. O& G Univ. Birm. Dir. Laser & Endoscopy Train. Centre W. Midl. 1979 - 2000.

NEWTON, John Roland 126 Harley Street, London W1N 1AH Tel: 020 7580 3383; 158 Sheen Lane, East Sheen, London SW14 8LZ Tel: 020 8876 7590 — MRCS Eng. LRCP Lond. 1962; MB ChB Manch. 1962; DMRD Eng. 1969; FFR 1972; FRCR 1975. Cons. Radiol. Char. Cross Hosp. & Westm. Hosp. Lond. Specialty: Radiol. Socs: BMA; Fell. Roy. Coll. Radiologists; Brit. Inst. Radiol.

NEWTON, Jonathan Ray 70 Seafield Road, Broughty Ferry, Dundee DD5 3AQ Tel: 01382 776239; 6 Bellefield Avenue, Dundee DD1 4NQ Tel: 01382 642535 — MB ChB Ed. 1994. SHO (Paediat.) Ninewells Hosp. Dundee Teach. Hosps. Specialty: Paediat. Prev: Resid. Med. Off. Mater Miser. Hosp. Brisbane, Austral.

NEWTON, Josephine Clare Fairview, Top Road, Shipham, Winscombe BS25 1TB — BM Soton. 1989; BA (1st cl. Hons. Human Scis.) Oxf. 1983; DCH RCP Lond. 1992; DRCOG 1993; MRCGP 1994.

NEWTON, Joyce (retired) Hegglehead, Hutton Roof, Penrith CA11 0XS Tel: 01768 484566 — MB ChB Manch. 1958.

NEWTON, Julia Lindsey 51 Castledene Court, Newcastle upon Tyne NE3 1NZ Tel: 0191 284 1762 — MB BS Newc. 1990; MRCP (UK) 1993. Clin. Research Assoc. (Physiol. & Med.) Med. Sch. Newc. u. Tyne. Specialty: Care of the Elderly. Socs: Brit. Geriat. Soc. Prev: Clin. Regist. (Med. & Geriat.) Qu. Eliz Hosp. Gateshead.

NEWTON, Julian Charles Barker Ashenfell Surgery, Church Lane, Baslow, Bakewell DE45 1SP Tel: 01246 582216 Fax: 01246 583867 — MB ChB Manch. 1972; DCH Eng. 1975; DRCOG 1976; MRCGP 1977; Dip. Palliat. Med. Wales 1991; BSc (Medical Sciences) St. Andrews 2003. Specialty: Palliat. Med. Prev: Assoc. Med. Dir. Ashgate Hospice Chesterfield.

NEWTON, Kay Jocelyn Welsby The Waterfield Practice, Ralphs Ride, Harmanswater, Bracknell RG12 9LH Tel: 01344 454626 Fax: 01344 303929; 4 Walnut Close, Wokingham RG41 4BG Tel: 0118 978 7962 Fax: 01344 303929 — MB BS Lond. 1968 (Char. Cross) MB BS London 1968 (Honours); MRCS England LRCP London 1968; DCH England 1972.

NEWTON, Kenneth Arthur (retired) Tumbling Bay, Underriver, Sevenoaks TN15 0SD Tel: 01732 832016 — MB BS Lond. 1945

(Guy's) FRCP Lond. 1967, M 1949; DMR 1952; DMRT Eng. 1952; FFR 1955; FRCR 1975. Prev: Hon Civil Cons. Radiother. RAF.

NEWTON, Lisa Jane Ward 7, Bradford Royal Infirmary, Duckworth Road, Bradford BD9 6RJ Tel: 01274 364367 Email: ljnewts@hotmail.com — MB ChB Sheff. 1991 (Sheffield) MRCP (UK) 1994; Dip RCPath 1996; MRCPATH 1999. Cons. Haematologist, Bradford Roy. Infirm., Bradford. Specialty: Haematology. Prev: Specialist Regist. in Haemat. Leeds Region; SHO (Gen. Med.) Roy. Hallamsh. Hosp. Sheff.

NEWTON, Magda Oldchurch Hospital, BHR Trust, Waterloo Road, Romford RM7 0BE Tel: 01708 708224 Fax: 01708 651506 Email: magda.smith@bhrhospitals.nhs.uk — MB BS Lond. 1987 (St Bartholomew's Hosp. Med. Sch.) FRCP London 2003. Cons. Phys. & Gastroenterol., Old Ch. Hosp., Ramford. Specialty: Gastroenterol. Socs: Brit. Soc. of Gastroenterol.

NEWTON, Margaret (retired) Tigh-na-Gaoith, Achterneed, Strathpeffer IV14 9AE Tel: 01997 421241 — (Univ. Ed.) MB ChB Ed. 1943. Prev: Ho. Phys. Roy. Edin. Hosp. Sick Childr.

NEWTON, Margaret Patricia The Schoolhouse, The Green, Bretby, Burton-on-Trent DE15 0RE Tel: 01283 703721 — MB ChB Manch. 1954; DObst RCOG 1960.

NEWTON, Marjorie Stella (retired) 30 Silverknowes Hill, Edinburgh EH4 5HD Tel: 0131 336 3785 — MB ChB Ed. 1956; DObst RCOG 1960. Prev: GP Edin.

NEWTON, Mary Constance National Hospital for Neurology and Neurosurgery, Department of Anaesthesia, Queen Square, London WC1N 3BG Tel: 020 7837 3611 — MB BS Lond. 1979 (St. Geos. Hosp. Med. Sch. Lond.) FFA RCS Eng. 1985. Cons. Neuroanaesth. Nat. Hosp. Neurol. & Neurosurg. Lond. Specialty: Anaesth. Prev: Cons. Anaesth. St. Bart. Hosp. Lond.; Regist. (Anaesth.) Univ. Coll. Hosp., Hosp. for Sick Childr. Gt. Ormond St. & St. Geo. Hosp. Med. Sch. Lond.

NEWTON, Mathew Laurence 80 Knutsford Road, Wilmslow SK9 6JD Tel: 01625 548534 Fax: 01625 529152 — MB ChB Manch. 1981; MBA Keele 1995. Dir., Pterion Ltd.; Clin. Asst. Cardiol. Stepping Hill Hosp. Prev: Sen. Assoc. Coopers & Lybrand Manch.

NEWTON, Nicholas Ian Department of Anaesthetics, Guy's Hospital, London SE1 9RT Tel: 020 7955 4051 Fax: 020 7955 8844; 41 Grange Grove, London N1 2NP — BM BCh Oxf. 1969; DA Eng. 1972; FRCA 1976; BA (Hons.) Camb. 1966, MA 1980. Cons. Anaesth. Guy's & St. Thos. NHS Hosp. Trust. Specialty: Anaesth. Socs: Assn. Anaesths.; Roy. Soc. Med.; BMA. Prev: Sen. Regist. (Anaesth.) St. Bart. Hosp. Lond.; Regist. (Anaesth.) Nuffield Dept. Anaesth. Radcliffe Infirm. Oxf.; Regist. (Anaesth.) Groote Schuur Hosp. Cape Town, S. Afr.

NEWTON, Paul (retired) 3 Constable Close, London NW11 6UA — MB ChB Ed. 1974; MRCP (UK) 1977; FRCP 1996. Prev: Cons. Rheum. Roy. Wolverhampton Hosps. NHS Trust.

NEWTON, Paul Gregory 19 Peel Road, Douglas IM1 4LS — MB ChB Birm. 1967; MCPS Sask. 1975; MSc Columbia Pacific Univ. 1989. Specialty: Gen. Pract. Socs: Fell. Inst. for Supervis. & Managem.; World Assn. for Disaster & Emerg. Med. Prev: Employee Health Phys. King Fahd Milit. Hosp. Dhahran, Saudi Arabia; Ships Surg. Roy. Fleet Auxil.; Med. Off. Canad. Forces Base Trenton, Ontario.

NEWTON, Paul Nicholas 90 Crescent Road, Oxford OX4 2PD — BM BCh Oxf. 1989 (University of Oxford) MRCP (UK) 1992; DTM & H (Lond.) 1996. Specialty: Gen. Med.; Infec. Dis.; Trop. Med.

NEWTON, Paula Jane Bartlett, Cronk and Newton, Chequers Lane, Papworth Everard, Cambridge CB3 8QQ Tel: 01480 830888 Fax: 01480 830001; 31 Victory Way, Cottenham, Cambridge CB4 8TG Tel: 01954 200667 — MB BChir Camb. 1990; DCH RCP Lond. 1992; MRCGP 1994. Prev: Trainee GP/SHO Hinchingbrooke Trust Hosp. Camb. VTS.

NEWTON, Peter Michael Carlton House Surgery, 28 Tenniswood Road, Enfield EN1 3LL Tel: 020 8363 7575 Fax: 020 8366 8228 — MB BS Lond. 1976; MRCGP 1982; DRCOG 1982. GP Enfield.; Trainer Cons. Deaney.

NEWTON, Philippa Jane Clock House, Lea Road, Lea Town, Preston PR4 0RA — MB BS Lond. 1992.

NEWTON, Professor Ray William 70 Seafield Road, Broughty Ferry, Dundee DD5 3AQ Tel: 01385 76239 — MB ChB Ed. 1969; MRCP (UK) 1972; FRCP Ed. 1981; FRCP Glasgow 1995. Cons. Phys. Ninewells Hosp.; PostGrad. Dean E. of Scotl. Specialty: Gen. Med. Socs: Brit. Diabetic Assn.; Scott. Soc. Phys.; Brit. Diabetic Assn. Prev: Regist. Roy. Infirm. Edin.

NEWTON, Richard Charles Feakes RCF Newton, St. Peter's Hospital, Guildford Road, Chertsey KT16 0PZ Tel: 01932 87200; Woodhambury, Woodham Lane, Woking GU21 5SR — MB Camb. 1963, BChir 1962 (Univ. Coll. Hosp.) DObst RCOG 1964; DCH Eng. 1969; MRCP (UK) 1969; FRCP 1994; FRCPCH 1997. Cons. Paediat. St. Peters Hosp. Chertsey & Ashford Hosp. Middlx. Specialty: Paediat. Prev: Ho. Off. Qu. Eliz. Hosp. Childr. Lond.; Resid. Med. Off. Westm. Childr. Hosp. Lond.; Sen. Regist. (Paediat.) Char. Cross Hosp. Lond.

NEWTON, Richard Ward Royal Manchester Childrens Hospital, Pendlebury, Manchester M27 4HA Tel: 0161 794 4696 Fax: 0161 727 2555; 7 Oakwood Drive, Heaton, Bolton BL1 5EE Tel: 01204 843303 — MB BS Lond. 1973 (King's Coll. Hosp.) MRCS Eng. LRCP Lond. 1973; DCH Eng. 1976; MRCP (UK) 1977; MRCGP 1977; DRCOG 1977; MD Lond. 1982; FRCP Lond. 1990; FRCPCH 1997. Cons. Paediat. Neurol. Roy. Manch. Childr. Hosp. & Booth Hall Childr. Hosp. Specialty: Paediat. Neurol. Socs: MAMH Euro Assoc of Intellectual Disabil. med. (Past Pres.); Brit. Paediat. Neurol. Assn. (Past Pres.). Prev: Trainee GP Hull VTS; Tutor (Child Health) St. Mary's Hosp. Manch.; Regist. (Paediat.) Hull Roy. Infirm.

NEWTON, Robert Edward ICRF Cancer Epidemiology Unit, Gibson Building, Radcliffe Infirmary, Oxford OX2 6HE — MB BS Lond. 1991. MRC Clin. Research Fell. ICRF Cancer Epidemiol. Unit Oxf. Specialty: Epidemiol. Prev: Ho. Off. (Surg.) Medway Hosp. Kent; Ho. Off. (Med.) Qu. Eliz. Hosp. King's Lynn.

NEWTON, Robert George (retired) 58 Moor Lane, Bramcote, Beeston, Nottingham NG9 3FH Tel: 0115 925 6987 Fax: 0115 925 6987 — (Westm.) AKC; MB BS Lond. 1952. Prev: GP Nottm.

NEWTON, Robin Archibald Houston (retired) 35 Bay Street, Fairlie, Largs KA29 0AL Tel: 01475 568355 — MB ChB Glas. 1954.

NEWTON, Roger John Dr N R Williams and Partners, Egginton Road, Etwall, Derby DE65 6NB Tel: 01283 732257 Fax: 01283 734876; 131 Station Road, Mickleover, Derby DE3 5FN Tel: 01332 514176 — MB BS Newc. 1974 (Newc. u. Tyne) DCH RCPS Glas. 1976; DRCOG 1979. Specialty: Gen. Pract. Socs: Derby Med. Soc. Prev: Trainee GP Derby VTS; Ho. Phys. Nottm. City Hosp.; Ho. Surg. Burton-on-Trent Gen. Hosp.

NEWTON, Sally Eelin (retired) 107 Randolph Avenue, London W9 1DL — MB BS Lond. 1957. Prev: Ho. Surg. & Ho. Phys. St. Bart. Hosp. Lond.

NEWTON, Sheelin Jane The Surgery, Trimperley, Ellesmere SY12 0DB Tel: 01691 622798 Fax: 01691 623294 — MB ChB Bristol 1983; MRCGP 1990. Specialty: Otorhinolaryngol.

NEWTON, Tina Birmingham Childrens' Hospital, Steelhouse Lane, Birmingham B4 6NH; Sunrise Cottage, 2 The Rocks, Holy Cross Clent, Stourbridge DY9 9QE Email: tinanewton.home@virgin.net — MB ChB Birm. 1991; ChB Birm. 1991; MRCP CH 1999. SpR (Paed.) Birm.

NEWTON, Professor Emerita Valerie Elizabeth (retired) Human Communication and Deafness, Manchester University, Manchester M13 9PL Tel: 0161 275 3370 Fax: 0161 275 3373 Email: valerie.newton@man.ac.uk — MB ChB Sheff. 1960; MSc Manch. 1979; MD Sheff. 1987. Prev: Hon. Cons. Paediat. Audiol. Univ. Manch.

NEWTON, Mr Walter Dick 14 Bonnyton Drive, Eaglesham, Glasgow G76 0LU — MB ChB Glas. 1970; FRCS Glas. 1975. Cons. Orthop. Surg. StoneHo. Hosp. & Hairmyres Hosp. Lanarksh. Specialty: Orthop.

NEWTON, William Boyd (retired) Kilbrennan, Brockham Green, Betchworth RH3 7HJ Tel: 0173 784 3609 — MB ChB Glas. 1941; MB ChB (Commend.) Glas. 1941.

NEWTON, William Kenneth 79 Harley Street, London W1G 8PZ Tel: 020 7935 0871 Fax: 020 7935 3417 — MB BS Lond. 1979 (Westm.) MB BS Lond. 1949; MRCP Lond. 1954. Socs: Fell. Harv. Soc. & Roy. Soc. Med. Prev: Regist. (Med.) Nat. Hosp. Nerv. Dis. Lond.; Resid. Med. Off. Nat. Heart Hosp. Lond.; Ho. Phys. Westm. Hosp.

NEWTON BISHOP, Julia Ann Department of Dermatology, St. James' University Hospital, Beckett St., Leeds LS9 7TF Tel: 0113 206 5816 Fax: 0113 242 9886 — MB ChB Sheff. 1978 (Sheffield)

MB ChB (Hons.) Sheff. 1978; MRCP (UK) 1980; MD (Commend.) Sheff. 1987; FRCP Lond. 1994. Cons. Dermat. & CR-Uk Sen. Clin. Scientist St. Jas. Univ. Hosps.; Honorary Reader in Oncological Demeology, University of Leeds. Specialty: Dermat.; Oncol. Socs: Brit. Assn. Dermat.; Brit. Assn. Cancer Research. Prev: Sen. Lect &. Hons. Cons. (Dermat.) Roy. Lond. Hosp. Med. Coll.; Regist (Dermat.) St. Thos. Hosp.; Regist. Rotat. (Med.) & SHO The Lond. Hosp.

NEWTON DUNN, Alan Richard Dr R G Mann and Partners, 61 New Street, Salisbury SP1 2PH — MB BS Lond. 1972 (St. Bart.) MRCS Eng. LRCP Lond. 1972; DObst RCOG 1975. Socs: BMA. Prev: Ho. Surg. N. Middlx. Hosp. Edmonton; Ho. Phys. Salisbury Gen. Infirm.; SHO (O & G) Soton. Gen. Hosp.

NEYLAN, Catherine Margaret Mary Angela Brennan and Neylan, The GP Centre, 322 Malden Road, North Cheam, Sutton SM3 8EP Tel: 020 8644 0224 — MB BS Lond. 1966 (St. Mary's) MRCS Eng. LRCP Lond. 1966; DCH RCP Lond. 1992; DFFP Lond. 1993. Specialty: Gen. Pract. Socs: Assoc. Mem. Brit. Roy. Coll. Paediat. & Child Health. Prev: Clin. Med. Off. Merton & Sutton HA.

NEYLON, Jonathan James St James Surgery, Harold Street, Dover CT16 1SF Tel: 01304 225559 Fax: 01304 213070; 3 Guthrie Gardens, Common Lane, River, Dover CT17 0PW — MB ChB Birm. 1979 (Birmingham) GP Dover. Specialty: Accid. & Emerg. Prev: Cas. Off. Roy. Vict. Hosp. Folkestone.

NEYLON, Kerri Louise — MB ChB Glas. 1998.

NG, Biing Yann Musgrave and Clark House, Royal Victoria Hospital, Grosvenor Road, Belfast BT12 6BA — MB BCh BAO Belf. 1995.

NG, Mr Bobby Kin Wah 16 Park Court, Cardrew Avenue, Friern Park, London N12 9UH — MB ChB Bristol 1984; FRCS Ed. 1992. Ho. Off. (Gen. Surg.) Dewsbury Gen. Hosp; Ho. Off. (Gen Med.) Frenchay Hosp. Brist.; SHO (Orthop.) St. Ann's Hosp. Lond.; SHO (A & E) N. Middlx. Hosp. Lond.

NG, Calvin Shin Haw 315 Sir John Henry Biggart House, Broadway, Belfast BT12 6HQ; 31 Cloona Park, Upper Dunmurry Lane, Lisburn BT17 0HQ Tel: 07801 351907 Email: u9310665@hotmail.com — MB BCh Belf. 1998. SHO Roy.Vic. Hosp. (Med) Belf. Prev: BMA; MPS.

NG, Chi Hwa — MB ChB Glas. 1998.

NG, Cho Yiu 67 Gordon Mansions, Torrington Place, London WC1E 7HH — BChir Camb. 1990.

NG, Chong Sum HM Stanley Hospital, St Asaph LL17 0RS Tel: 01745 589725 — MB ChB Leic. 1987; FRCOphth 1993. Cons Ophthamology Conwy & Denbighsh. NHS Trust Bodelwyddan. Specialty: Ophth.

NG, Chung Hong Selwyn Stoke Mandeville Hospital, Department of Cellular Pathology, Mandeville Road, Aylesbury HP21 8AL — MB ChB Sheff. 1998.

NG, Mr Colin Leong Liong 119 Turnpike Link, Croydon CR0 5NU — MB ChB Liverp. 1988; FRCS Glas. 1994. Regist. (Surg.) John Radcliffe Hosp. Oxf. Socs: Fell. Roy. Soc. Med.

NG, David Pak-Ken 1 Mooreway, Rainhill, Prescot L35 6PD — MB ChB Liverp. 1985.

***NG, David Palkin** 12 Richmond Way, Ponteland, Newcastle upon Tyne NE20 9HU — MB ChB Dund. 1998 (Dundee University) MB ChB Dund 1998. PRHD Medicene, Wansbeck Gen. Hosp. Specialty: Gen. Med. Prev: PRHO Surg., S. Cleveland Hosp.

NG, Ernest Wee Oon 183 Knighton Church Road, Leicester LE2 3JP — MB ChB Leic. 1996.

NG, Geraldine Yin Taeng Neonatal Intensive Care Unit, St. Thomas' Hospital, London SE1 7EH Tel: 020 7928 9292 — MB BS Lond. 1994; BSc (Hons.) Neurosci. Lond. 1991; MRCP (Lond) 1997; MRCPCH 1997. Specialist Regist. (Neonatology) St. George's Hosp. Lond. Specialty: Paediat. Prev: Fell. Neonat. - Perinatal Med., Hosp. Sick Childr., Toronto, Canada.

NG, Ghulam Andre Glenfield Hospital, Department of Cardiovascular Sciences, Clinical Sciences Wing, Leicester LE3 9QP Tel: 0116 2502438 Fax: 0116 2875792 Email: gan1@le.ac.uk — MB ChB Glas. 1989; MRCP (UK) 1992; PhD Glas. 1998. Sen. Lect./Cons. Cardiol., Cardiol., univ hosp leic. Specialty: Cardiol. Special Interest: Cardiac Electrophysiol.; Catheter Ablation; Implantable Devices. Socs: Brit. Cardiac Soc.; BMA; BPEG. Prev: Clin. Lect./Sen. Regist.. Qu. Eliz hosp. Birming; Research Fell. (Med. Cardiol.) Glas. Roy. Infirm.; SHO Rotat. (Med.) Stobhill Gen. Hosp. Glas.

NG, Hon Wah Kelvin Kent Elms Health Centre, Rayleigh Road, Leigh-on-Sea SS9 5UU Tel: 01702 522012 Fax: 01702 512375 — MB ChB Sheff. 1984; MRCP (UK) 1987; T(M) 1993; Spec. Accredit. Gen. Med. & Clin. Pharmacol. JCHMT 1993; MD Liverp. 1994; T(GP) 1995. Specialty: Gen. Med. Socs: Med. Defence Union; BMA. Prev: Lect. & Hon. Sen. Regist. (Gen. Med., Clin. Pharmacol. & Therap.) Univ. Liverp. & Roy. Liverp. Univ. Hosp.; Research Fell. & Hon. Sen. Regist. (Clin. Pharmacol. & Therap.) Univ. Liverp. & Roy. Liverp. Univ. Hosp.; Regist. (Gen. Med., Haemat. & Coronary Care) Southport Dist. Gen. Hosp.

NG, Jonathan Chun Man 81 Hornsey Lane Gardens, Highgate, London N6 5PA — MB ChB Liverp. 1994.

NG, Joo Li 3 Hunters Lodge, The Green, Wallsend NE28 7ES — MB BS Newc. 1992.

NG, Julia Mae-Zsianne Calremont House, 51 London Road, Liphook GU30 7SG — MB BS Lond. 1996.

NG, Karl Keow Giong — MB BS (Hons.) New South Wales 1992; MRCP (UK) 1997; FRACP 2002. Specialist Regist. (Neurophysiol.) Nat. Hosp. Neurol. & Neurosurg. Lond. Specialty: Neurol.; Clin. Neurophysiol.

NG, Mr Keng Jin Apartment 45, Bishop Court, 76 Bishops Bridge Road, London W2 6BE — MB BCh Wales 1986; FRCS Ed. 1990. Specialty: Urol.

NG, Kerry Shin Lih 86 Upper Malone Park, Belfast BT9 6PP — MB BCh BAO Belf. 1994.

NG, Lenny Vi-Lynn 63 Cloisters Avenue, Bromley BR2 8AN — MB BCh Wales 1996.

NG, Professor Leong Loke Department of Pharmacology, Clinical Sciences Building, Leicester Royal Infirmary, Leicester LE2 7LX Tel: 01162 523108 Fax: 01162 523108 — MB BChir Camb. 1979 (University of Cambridge) MRCP (UK) 1982; MA Camb. 1982, MD 1988; FRCP Lond 1996. Prof. of Med. and Therap. Specialty: Pharmacology; Cardiol. Socs: Brit. Pharmacological Soc. Prev: Lect. Radcliffe Infirm. Oxf.; MRC Train. Fell., Radcliffe Infirm. Oxf.; Regist. (Med.) Addenbrooke's Hosp. Camb.

NG, Nicola Su-Han 30 Montagu Mansions, London W1U 6LB — MB BS Lond. 1998.

NG, Pang Han 18 Chandos Avenue, Southgate, London N14 7ET — MB ChB Sheff. 1996.

NG, Raymond Sai Ho — MB BS Lond. 1997; MRCP.

NG, Mr Roy Lip Hin Dept of Plastic Surgery, UCL Hospitals, Pond St., London NW3 2QG Tel: 020 7794 0500; 18 Parkgate Mews, 14-16 Stanhope Road, Highgate, London N6 5NB Tel: 020 8347 7853 — BM BCh Oxf. 1989; MA Camb. 1990; FRCS Eng. 1993. Specialist Regist. (Plastic Surg.)Roy. Free Hosps. Lond. Specialty: Plastic Surg. Prev: Research Regist. (Plastic Surg.) Blond McIndoe Centre Qu. Vict. Hosp. E. Grinstead; Specialist Regist. Pastic surg.UCH; Specialist Regist. Plastic Surg.Mt. Vernon Hosp.

NG, Sui Yin 2 Kensington Place, Bristol BS8 3AH Email: syng@lineone.net; 9 Gerbang Ampang Hilir 55000, Malaysia — MB ChB Bristol 1994; MRCP (Lond.) 1998. SHO (Lect.) Univ. Putra Malaysia. Specialty: Paediat. Socs: MRCPCH. Prev: SHO (Paediat.) St. Geo.s Hosp. Lond.; SHO (Paediat.) Roy. Lond. Hosp.; SHO (Paediat.) Mayday Univ. Hosp.

NG, Sze Hing (retired) 115 Turnpike Link, Croydon CR0 5NU Tel: 020 8686 5020 — (Singapore) MB BS Malaya 1961; DCH Eng. 1963; FRCP Lond. 1987, M 1967. Prev: Sen. Regist. (Paediat.) King's Coll. Hosp. Lond.

NG, Thomas Siu Fai — MB ChB Dundee 1990 (Univ. of Dundee, Scotl.) BMSc Dund 1987; MRCPI 1996; MRCP 1996. Med. Advis. Manager, Roche Product Ltd. (UK), Welwyn Garden City, Herts AL7 3AY. Specialty: Pharmaceutical Medicine. Socs: Fell. of Roy. Soc. of Med.; Soc. of Pharmaceutical Med.; Europ. Soc. of Pharmacol. Prev: Regist. (Gen. Med.) Warrington Hosp.; Regist. Rotat. (Haemat.) Pembury Hosp., Kent & Sussex Hosp. & King's Coll. Hosp. Lond.

NG, Tony Tsz Cheong Cell Biophysics Laboratory, Imperial Cancer Research Fund, 44 Lincoln's Inn Fields, London WC2A 3PX Tel: 020 7269 3082 — MB ChB Aberd. 1989; MRCP (UK) 1992; PhD Lond. 1997. Gp. Ldr./ MRC Clin. Scient./ Hon. Sen. Clin. Lect. Kings Coll. Lond. Specialty: Immunol. Prev: MRC AIDS Progr. Clin. Fell. Dept. Immunol. St. Bart. Hosp. Lond.; Translational Clin. Research Fell. Imperial Cancer Research Fund Lond.

NG, Virginia Wun Kum Maudsley Hospital, Center for Neuroimaging Sciences, Denmark Hill, London SE5 8AZ Tel: 020

7919 3084 Fax: 020 7919 2477 Email: v.ng@iop.kcl.ac.uk — MB BS Lond. 1987 (St. Bart. Med. Sch.) MRCP (UK) 1991; FRCR 1995; MD Lond. 2000. Cons. Neuro. Maudsley Hosp. Lond. 1/2000; Hon. Sen. Lect. Inst. of Psychiat. Lond. Specialty: Radiol. Special Interest: Contemporary neuroimaging techniques as applied to Psychiat. and Neurol. Prev: Wellcome Clin. Train. Fell. (Neuroimaging) Inst. of Psychiat. Lond.; Specialist Regist. Nat. Hosp. Neurol. (Neuroradiolo.) Lond.; Sen. Regist. (Radiol.) St. Geo. Hosp. Lond.

NG, Wang Tat 9 Woodvale Avenue, Cardiff CF23 6SP — MB BCh Wales 1984.

NG, Wei Seng 1B The Green, Twickenham TW2 5TU Tel: 020 8894 6870 Fax: 020 8893 8579; 8 Fairwater House, Twickenham Road, Teddington TW11 8AY Tel: 020 8977 1704 — MB BS Lond. 1989.

NG, Wing Shang (retired) 6 Park Road, Radyr, Cardiff CF15 8DG Tel: 029 2084 2318 — MB BCh Wales 1961 (Cardiff) FFA RCS Eng. 1966. Cons. Anaesth. Univ. Hosp. Wales Cardiff. Prev: Assoc. Prof. Anaesth. Thos. Jefferson Univ. Philadelphia, USA.

***NG, Yeung Hwa** — MB ChB Glas. 1998; BSc (Hons) Glas. 1998; MRCS (Ed.) 2001.

NG, Yin Khow Dovecote House, 38 Wollaton Road, Beeston, Nottingham NG9 5NR Tel: 0115 8752104 Fax: 0115 925 3361 — MB BS Lond. 1977 (King's Coll. Hosp.) BSc (Physiol.) Lond. 1974; DRCOG 1979; DCH Eng. 1980; MRCP (UK) 1981; MD Leic. 1996; FRCPCH 1997. Cons. Paediat. (Community Child Health) Qu.s Med. Centre Nottm. Univ. Hosp. NHS Trust. Specialty: Community Child Health. Socs: Med. Wom.'s Federat.; Nottm. Med. Chirurgical Soc.; Brit. Assn. Community Child Health. Prev: Lect. (Community Paediat.) Univ. Nottm.; Clin. Research Fell. Univ. Leic.; Ho. Phys. Hosp. for Sick Childr. Gt. Ormond St. Lond.

NG CHENG HIN, Alan Kenneth Woodside, Kincraig, Invergordon IV18 0PW — MB ChB Dundee 1986; Dip. Obst. Otago 1989; DCH RCP Lond. 1991; MRCGP 1992; DFFP 1993; DTM & H Liverp. 1996; CCFP Canada 2001.

NG CHENG HIN, Harold Sinkwee Lehman and Partners, Hightown Surgery, Hightown Gardens, Banbury OX16 9DB Tel: 01295 270722 Fax: 01295 263000; Durrel Cottage, Chapel Lane, Bodicote, Banbury OX15 4DB — MB ChB Birm. 1980; MRCP (UK) 1983. Specialty: Paediat.

NG CHENG HIN, Mr Philip c/o Drive Ah Kye, 8 Rockwells Gardens, London SE19 1HW — MD Lyon 1977; ECFMG Cert. 1975; MD (Hons.) Lyon 1977; FRCS Ed. 1983. Cons. Surg. Dallah Hosp. Riyadh. Specialty: Gen. Surg. Socs: Fell. Roy. Soc. Med. Prev: Cons. Surg. Tawam Hosp. Al Ain, UAE; Vis. Lect. Chinese Univ. Hong Kong; Regist. Rotat. (Surg.) Guy's Hosp. Lond.

NG CHIENG HIN, Mr Steve Miow Cheong 25 Leybourne Road, Kingsbury, London NW9 9QG — MB ChB Leeds 1985; FRCS Ed. 1989.

NG HOCK OON, Paul Flat D, 125 Grove Park, London SE5 8LD — MB ChB Leic. 1992.

NG HUANG, Stephen Chee Peng — MB BS Singapore 1986; MRCGP 1992; MFPM 2003.

NG MAN KWONG, Georges Stepping Hill Hospital, Poplar Grove, Stockport SK2 7JE — MB ChB Manch. 1990; MRCP (UK) 1993; Dip Mgt(open) 2002. Cons. Fairfield Gen. Hosp. Bury Pennnine Acute Hosps. NHS Trust. Specialty: Respirat. Med.; Genitourinary Medicine. Prev: Cons. Phys. Stepping Hill Hosp.; Clin. Research Fell. (Respirat. Med.) Univ. Sheff. 1999-2001; Specialist Regist. (Respirat. & Gen. Internal Med.) Roy. Bolton Hosps. NHS Trust.

NG PING CHEUNG, Jean-Pierre Department of Haematology, Barnsley District General Hospital, Gawber Road, Barnsley S75 2EH; 39 Moorbank Road, Sandygate, Sheffield S10 5TQ Email: jean-pierre@lineone.net — MB ChB Glas. 1981; MRCPath 1989 FRC Path; FRCP Lond.; FRCP Glas.; MRCP (UK) 1984. Cons. Haemat. Barnsley Dist. Gen. Hosp. Specialty: Haematology. Prev: Sen. Regist. (Haemat.) W. Midl. RHA.

NG SUI HING, Ng You Kwong 51 Cathles Road, London SW12 9LE — MB ChB Glas. 1977.

NGAN, Cheung Yuen 41 The Avenue, Sale M33 4PJ — MB ChB Manch. 1982.

NGAN, Henry 22 Lavington Court, 77 Putney Hill, London SW15 3NU Tel: 020 8789 8417 — MB BS Lond. 1962 (Westm.) MRCS Eng. LRCP Lond. 1962; MRCP Ed. 1965; MRCP Lond. 1967; DMRD Eng. 1969; FFR 1971. Cons. Radiol. Qu. Mary's Hosp. Roehampton. Specialty: Radiol. Socs: Fell. Roy. Soc. Med. Prev: Sen. Regist. Radiol. Westm. Hosp.; Regist. Med. Roy. Marsden Hosp.; Regist. Radiol. Hammersmith Hosp.

NGAN, Sarah — MB BS Lond. 1998.

NGAN-SOO, Eleanor Mei-San 94 Higher Drive, Banstead SM7 1PQ — MB BS Lond. 1998.

NGEH, Joseph Kho Tong Department of Medicine, Warwick Hospital, Lakin Road, Warwick CV34 5BW Tel: 01926 495321 Fax: 01926 482609 Email: joseph.ngeh@swh.nhs.uk — MB BCh BAO (Hons.) 1993; MRCP UK 1998; MSc (Geriatric med.) Keele 2000. Cons. Phys., Geriat. and Gen. Med. Specialty: Gen. Med.; Care of the Elderly. Socs: Brit. Geriat. Soc.; Brit. Assn. of Stroke Physicians; Roy. Coll. of Physicians. Prev: Specialist Regist., Geriat. and Gen. Med., Lond. and Oxf. Deaneries.

NGUYEN, Anthony Long 10A Fairview Road, Wednesfield, Wolverhampton WV11 1BY — MB ChB Leeds 1993.

NGUYEN, Chinh Truong 20B Anson Road, London N7 0RD — MB BS Lond. 1993.

NGUYEN, Cuong Tuan 40 Downsview Road, London SE19 3XB — MB BS Lond. 1995.

NGUYEN, Dai Quoc Anh 22 Sidcup Road, London SE12 8BW — MB ChB Bristol 1998.

NGUYEN, Duke Duc Hoang 210 Gurney Close, Barking IG11 8JZ — MB BS Lond. 1996; BSc 1994.

NGUYEN, Dzung Manh 7 St Andrews Gardens, Cobham KT11 1HG — MRCS Eng. LRCP Lond. 1985; DRCOG 1990. Specialty: Gen. Pract.

NGUYEN, Hiep 32 Maran Way, Erith DA18 4BP — MB BS Lond. 1993.

NGUYEN, Hoa Binh 7 St Andrews Gardens, Cobham KT11 1HG — MRCS Eng. LRCP Lond. 1985.

NGUYEN, Michael Loc 10A Fairview Road, Wednesfield, Wolverhampton WV11 1BY — MB ChB Birm. 1997.

NGUYEN, Tan Dung The Surgery, 80 Torridon Road, London SE6 1RA Tel: 020 8698 5281 Fax: 020 8695 1841 — MB BS Lond. 1991.

NGUYEN-VAN-TAM, Jonathan Stafford Department of Public Health Medicine & Epidemiology, University of Nottingham Medical School, Queen's Medical Centre, Nottingham NG7 2UH Tel: 0115 970 9320 Fax: 0115 970 9316; 14 Greengate Lane, Birstall, Leicester LE4 3DJ Tel: 0116 267 1004 — BM BS Nottm. 1987; BMedSci (Hons) 1985. Sen. Lect. (Pub. Health Med.) Univ. Nottm.; Hon. Sen. Regist. N. Lincs. HA; Clin. Med. Off. Lincs. Army Cadet Force (TA). Specialty: Pub. Health Med. Prev: Hon. Regist. (Pub. Health Med.) Nottm. HA; SHO (Pub. Health Med.) Leicester HA; SHO (Anaesth.) Univ. Hosp. Nottm. & Co. Hosp. Lincoln.

NGWU, Mr Uchechukwu Okoronkwo Newbold Verdon Medical Practice, St George's Close, Newbold Verdon, Leicester LE9 9PZ Tel: 01445 822171 Fax: 01445 824968 — BM BCh Nigeria 1977 (University of Nigeria, Enugu) FRCS Ed. 1986. Specialty: Gen. Pract.; Gen. Surg.; Urol.

NHEMACHENA, Charles Musena 174 Aberford Road, Stanley, Wakefield WF3 4NP Tel: 01924 828924 — MB ChB Birm. 1979. Assoc. Specialist Anaesth. Fairfield Gen. Hosp. Bury. Specialty: Anaesth. Socs: Med. Protec. Soc.; BMA.

NI BHROLCHAIN, Cliona Maire Huntingtonshire PCT, Primrose Lane, Huntingdon PE29 1WG Tel: 01480 415207 Fax: 01480 415212; 104 Bridgwater Drive, Northampton NN3 3BB — MB BCh BAO NUI 1981; DCH RCSI 1983; MRCPI 1985; DObst RCPI 1985; MRCGP 1986; FRCPCH 1996. Cons. Community Paediat. Huntingtonshire PCT. Specialty: Community Child Health. Socs: Brit. Assn. Community Child Health (Treas.); Fell. Roy. Coll. Paediat.s & Child Health. Prev: Cons. Community Paediat. Northampton Gen. Hosp.; Sen. Regist. (Community Paediat.) Northampton; Clin. Med. Off. S. Sefton HA.

NI CHUILEANNAIN, Fiona Maire 2B Tarn House, Abbey Way, Barrow-in-Furness LA14 1BP; 14 Avondale Lawn, Blackrock, County Dublin, Republic of Ireland — MB BCh BAO NUI 1989; MRCOG 1994. Regist. (O & G) Furness Gen. Hosp. Cumbria. Specialty: Obst. & Gyn.

NI'MAN, Mufeed Na'eem 15 Kings Avenue, Christchurch BH23 IL2 Tel: 01202 773267 — MD Aleppo 1985; LMSSA LRCS LRCP Lond. 1998. ENT SHO, Poole Gen. Hosp.

NIAYESH, Mr Mohammad Hossein Yeovil District Hospital, Higher Kingston, Yeovil BA21 4AT Tel: 01935 475122; 34 Mitchelmore Road, Yeovil BA31 4BA Tel: 01935 420808 Fax: 01935 420808 Email: mhniayesh@hotmail.com — MD Pahlavi 1984; MRCS Eng. LRCP Lond. 1988; FRCS Ed. 1988; FRCS (Gen. Surg.) 2001. Cons. Surg. Yeovil Dist. Hosp. Specialty: Gen. Surg. Special Interest: Breast. Prev: Sen. Regist. (Gen.Surg.) Horneton Hosp.; Regist. (Gen. Surg.) Greater Manch. Hosp.

NIBLETT, David John Department of Anaesthesia, Bedford Hospital, Kempston Road, Bedford MK42 9DJ Tel: 01234 355122 Fax: 01234 795910 Email: david.niblett@bedhos.anglox.nhs.uk; Alberta, Station Road, Turvey, Bedford MK43 8BH Tel: 01234 881468 — MB BS Lond. 1977 (Univ. Coll. Hosp.) FFA RCS Eng. 1982. Cons. Anaesth. & Intens. Care Bedford Hosp. Specialty: Anaesth.; Intens. Care. Prev: Sen. Regist. Nuffield Dept. Anaesth. Oxf.; Lect. (Anat.) Stanford Univ. Med. Sch. Calif., USA.

NIBLOCK, James Logan Barns Street Surgery, 3 Barns Street, Ayr KA7 1XB Tel: 01292 281439 Fax: 01292 288268; 13 Doonholm Road, Alloway, Ayr KA7 4QQ Tel: 01292 443112 — MB ChB Glas. 1969; DObst RCOG 1973. Med. Off. Marks & Spencer plc & Dana Glacier Vandervell, Kilmarnock. Socs: Soc. Occupat. Med. Prev: Regist. (O & G) Robroyston Hosp. Glas.; Ho. Phys. Falkirk & Dist. Roy. Infirm.; Ho. Surg. West. Infirm. Glas.

NICE, Alison Mary The Priory Surgery, 24-26 Priory Avenue, High Wycombe HP13 6SH Tel: 01494 448132 — MB ChB Leeds 1988; DCH RCPS Glas. 1992; DFFP 2003. Prev: Trainee GP Wakefield VTS; Ho. Off. (Gen. Med.) Bradford Roy. Infirm.; Ho. Off. (Gen. Surg.) St. Jas. Univ. Hosp.

NICE, Colin Andrew 29 Roundstone Close, Haydon Grange, Newcastle upon Tyne NE7 7GH Tel: 0191 270 2721 — MB ChB Dundee 1991; FRCS Ed 1996; FRCR 2001. Cons. Radiologist Qu. Eliz. Hosp. Gateshead.

NICELL, Donald Thomas 5 Penbrey Path, St. Dial's, Cwmbran NP44 4RR — MB ChB Cape Town 1982.

NICHANI, Sanjiv Hari Leicester Royal Infirmary, Infirmary Square, Leicester LE1 5WW — MB BS Univ. Poona 1986; MRCP (UK) 1991.

NICHOL, Frank Edward Department of Rheumatology, Leicester Royal Infirmary, Infirmary Square, Leicester LE1 5WW Tel: 0116 258 6473 — MB ChB Liverp. 1973; MD Liverp. 1981; FRCP Ed. 1988; FRCP Lond. 1993. Cons. Rheum. Leicester Roy. Infirm. Specialty: Rheumatol. Socs: Brit. Soc. Rheum. Prev: Sen. Regist. Leicester Roy. Infirm.; Research Fell. & Hon. Sen. Regist. (Med.) Univ. Liverp. & Roy. Liverp. Hosp.

NICHOL, Ian Edward 104 Rayleigh Drive, Wideopen, Newcastle upon Tyne NE13 6AJ — MB BS Newc. 1992.

NICHOL, Mr Neil Macpherson A&E Department, Ninewells Hospital, Dundee DD1 9SY — MB ChB Ed. 1983 (Edin.) BSc (Med. Sci.) Ed. 1980; DRCOG 1986; Cert. Family Plann. JCC 1986; MRCGP 1987; FRCS Ed. 1994; FFAEM 1999. Cons.(A & E Dept) Ninewells Hosp. Dund.; Hon. Sen. Lect., Dundee Univ. Med. Sch. Specialty: Accid. & Emerg. Prev: SHO III (A & E) Roy. Infirm. Edin.; Sen. Reg. (A&E) Roy. Infirm. Edin.; Chief Med. Off. St. Helena.

NICHOLAOU, Theodorakis Andrew 2 Ulster Gardens, Palmers Green, London N13 5DW — MB BS Lond. 1993 (Lond. Hosp. Med. Coll.) BSc (Hons. Psych.); BSc (Hons.) 1992. Research Fell. The Ludwig Inst. Melbourne Austral. Specialty: Oncol.; Radiother. Socs: BMA; Hellenic Med. Soc.; RCP. Prev: Dep. Clin. Off. Antisoma; Dep. Clin. Off. Astrozeneca; Radiother. Oncol. Train. Mt. Vernon, Char. Cross & Hammersmith Hosps. Lond.

NICHOLAS, Angela Patricia 95 Lander Close, Poole BH15 1UL — MB ChB Manch. 1992 (Manchester) BSc (Hons.) Manch. 1988.

NICHOLAS, Anne Mary 1 Seymour Road, London SW18 5JB — MB BS Lond. 1979.

NICHOLAS, Annette Christaline Shandhini Woodsley Road Surgery, 144 Woodsley Road, Leeds LS2 9LZ Tel: 0113 245 4038 Fax: 0113 244 2084 — MB BS Ceylon 1964; DCH Ceylon 1972; MRCP (UK) 1979. Specialty: Pharmacology; Gen. Med. Socs: BMA.

NICHOLAS, Arthur Stuart 1 Tower Lane, Colehill, Wimborne BH21 2QP Tel: 01202 841505 — MB ChB Manch. 1952; MRCS Eng. LRCP Lond. 1952.

NICHOLAS, Audrey (retired) 1 Devereux Way, Billericay CM12 0YS Tel: 01277 626295 — MB BS Durh. 1960 (Newc.)

NICHOLAS, Bridget Mary Child & Family Unit, St James University Hospital, Beckett St., Leeds LS9 7TF — MB ChB Sheff. 1985; DCH RCP Lond. 1988; DRCOG 1989; MRCGP 1989; MRCPsych 1994. Sp. Regist. Rotat. (Child & Adolesc. Psychiat.) Leeds. Specialty: Child & Adolesc. Psychiat. Prev: Sen. Regist. Rotat. (Child & Adolesc. Psychiat.) Oxf.; Regist. Rotat. (Psychiat.) Oxf.; Sp. Regist. Rotat C & A Psych Bristol.

NICHOLAS, David Stuart Pathology Department, Poole Hospital NHS Trust, Longfleet Road, Poole BH15 2JB Tel: 01202 442211 Fax: 01202 448452 Email: david.nicholas@poole.nhs.uk — MB BS Lond. 1979; BA Oxf. 1976. Cons. Histopath. Poole Hosp. NHS Trust. Specialty: Histopath.

NICHOLAS, Dorothy Joy (retired) 9 Orchard Drive, Durham DH1 1LA Tel: 0191 384 3598 Email: ken@kendor32.freeserve.co.uk — MB ChB Birm. 1961. Prev: Dent. Anaesth. Sunderland HA.

NICHOLAS, Florence Eileen Woodmount, Linden Road, Clevedon BS21 — MB ChB Bristol 1946. Med. Off. Family Plann. Assn. Socs: BMA. Prev: Ho. Surg. Bristol Roy. Hosp.

NICHOLAS, Ivor Hugh 42 Doddington Road, Wellingborough NN8 2JH — MB BS Lond. 1973; MRCS Eng. LRCP Lond. 1973; MRCP (UK) 1977.

NICHOLAS, Jacob 6 Castlehill Manor, Belfast BT4 3QH — MB BS Kerala 1974.

NICHOLAS, Jeffery John, Surg. Cdr. RN (retired) Hope Cottage, Exton, Southampton SO32 3LT Tel: 01489 877347 — MB ChB Bristol 1961; DIH Eng. 1976; MFOM RCP Lond. 1980. Prev: Late Roy. Naval Med. Serv.

NICHOLAS, Mr John Leyton (retired) Hull Royal Infirmary, Anlaby Road, Hull HU3 2JZ — BM BCh Oxf. 1960 (Oxf. & Lond. Hosp.) MA. 1960; FRCS Eng. 1967. Cons. Paediat. Surg. Hull Roy. Infirm. Prev: Sen. Surg. Regist. Hosp. Sick Childr. Gt. Ormond St. & Westm. Hosp.

NICHOLAS, John Richard Queens Park Medical Centre, Farrer Street, Stockton-on-Tees TS18 2AW Tel: 01642 679681 Fax: 01642 677124 — MB Camb. 1979, BChir 1978; MRCGP 1982; DCH RCP Lond. 1982. GP Qu. Pk. Med. Centre Stockton-on-Tees.

NICHOLAS, Keith Stuart Heswall Medical Centre, Telegraph Road, Heswall, Wirral CH60 7SG Tel: 0151 342 2230 — MB ChB Liverp. 1970; DObst RCOG 1974.

NICHOLAS, Martin Edward Leckhampton Surgery, Lloyd Davies House, 17 Moorend Park Road, Cheltenham GL53 0LA Tel: 01242 515363 Fax: 01242 253512; Home Farm, Foxcote, Cheltenham GL54 4LP Tel: 01242 820252 Fax: 01242 820173 — MB BS Lond. 1983 (St. George's Hospital) MRCGP 1987; DRCOG 1987; Dip. Sports Med. Scotl. 1995. Specialty: Sports Med.

NICHOLAS, Martin Paul Queen Margaret Hospital, Whitefield Road, Dunfermline KY12 0SU Tel: 01383 623623 — MB BS Lond. 1979; FFA RCS Eng. 1984. Cons. Anaesth. Qu. Margt. Hosp. Dunfermline. Specialty: Anaesth.

NICHOLAS, Michael 14 Hill View, Henleaze, Bristol BS9 4PZ Tel: 0117 962 3180 — (Bristol) MB ChB Brist. 1958 SR; DPM Eng. 1964; MRCP Lond. 1969; FRCPsych 1986, M 1971. Specialty: Gen. Psychiat. Prev: Cons. Psychiat. Glenside Hosp. Bristol.

NICHOLAS, Michelle 13 Castle View, Bridgend CF31 1HL Email: michellenicholas@doctors.org.uk — BM Soton. 1992; FRCA 1998. Cons. Anaesth. Specialty: Anaesth. Socs: Obstetric Anaesthetists Assn.; Brit. Med. Assn.; Vasc. Anaesth. Soc. Prev: Specialist Regist. (Anaesth.) All Wales Rotat. 1997; SHO (Anaesth.) Swansea Hosp. 1997; SHO (Accid. & Emerg.) Poole Hosp. 1994.

NICHOLAS, Nicos Sotiriou 41 Main Avenue, Moor Park, Northwood HA6 2LH Tel: 01923 820001 — MB BS Lond. 1977 (Guy's) MRCS Eng. LRCP Lond. 1977; Cert. Family Plann JCC 1979; FRCOG 1994, M 1981; BSc (Hons.) Lond. 1974, MD 1987. Cons. O & G Hillingdon Hosp.; Sen. Regist. (Obst. & Gyn.) Qu. Charlottes Hosp. & Chelsea Wom. Hosp. Lond. Specialty: Obst. & Gyn. Socs: Blair Bell Res. Soc.; Victor Bonney Soc. (Scientif. Sect.) Roy. Soc. Med.; (Pres.) Hellenic Med. Soc. Prev: Wellcome Surg. Research Fell. Guy's Hosp. Lond.; Regist. (O & G) Guy's Hosp. Lond.; Lect. (O & G) Guy's Hosp. Lond.

NICHOLAS, Paul Lindsay The Surgery, 298 Cavendish Road, Balham, London SW12 0PL Tel: 020 8672 3331; 43 Winterbrook Road, London SE24 9HZ Tel: 020 7274 3491 — MB BS Lond. 1976. Specialty: Gen. Pract.

NICHOLAS, Peter Thomas (retired) Cedarwood, 105 Highgate Lane, Lepton, Huddersfield HD8 0HQ Tel: 01484 605179 — MRCS

Eng. LRCP Lond. 1953 (Middlx.) FRCGP 1977, M 1963. Prev: Med. Off. DSS.

NICHOLAS, Philip Owen (retired) 22 Falmouth Avenue, Weeping Cross, Stafford ST17 0JH Tel: 01785 665896 — MB ChB (Distinc. Pub. Health) Bristol 1953; DCH Eng. 1958; DPH Leeds 1961; FFPHM 1980, M 1972. Prev: Community Phys. Wirral & Chester HAs.

NICHOLAS, Mr Reginald John 28 Broom Park, Teddington TW11 9RS Tel: 020 8977 9449 Fax: 020 8977 9449; 28 Broom Park, Teddington TW11 9RS Tel: 020 8977 9449 Fax: 020 8977 9449 — MB BS Durh. 1964 (King's College, Durham, UK) MD Newc. 1969; FRCS Ed. 1976. Locum Cons. Paediat. Surg. John Radcliffe Hosp. Specialty: Paediat. Surg. Prev: Cons. Paediat. Surg. Roy. Commiss. Med. Centre Yanbu al Sinaiyah, Saudi Arabia.

NICHOLAS, Richard Charles Melbourne Street Medical Centre, 56 Melbourne Street, Leicester LE2 0AS Tel: 0116 262 2721; 304 Victoria Park Road, Leicester LE2 1XE — MRCS Eng. LRCP Lond. 1978. Specialty: Gen. Psychiat.

NICHOLAS, Mr Richard Martin Royal Victoria Hospital, Belfast BT12 6BA Tel: 02890 634810 — MB BCh BAO Belf. 1985 (Qu. Univ. Belf.) BDS Lond. 1980; FRCS Ed. 1989; FRCSI 1989; MD Belf. 1992; FRCSI (Sports&Exercise Med.) 2003. Cons. Orthop. and Sports (Knee Injury) Surg. Roy. Vict.Hosp. Belf. & Musgrave Pk. Hosp. Belf. Specialty: Trauma & Orthop. Surg.; Sports Med. Socs: Brit. Orthop. Assn.; BMA; Ulster Med. Soc. Prev: Sen. Regist. Rotat. (Orthop. & Trauma Surg.) N. Irel.; Fell. Brisbane Orthop. & Sports Med. Centre; DHSS Research Fell. (Orthop. Surg.) Qu. Univ. Belf.

NICHOLAS, Richard St John 6 Kilmorey Road, St. Margarets, Twickenham TW1 1PX — MB BS Lond. 1991.

NICHOLAS, Saran Gwenllian Plas Maes y Groes, Talybont, Bangor LL57 3YD Email: NchS5@aol.com — MB BCh Wales 1997; MRCP 2002.

NICHOLAS, Shirley Pamela Kay (retired) 22 Falmouth Avenue, Weeping Cross, Stafford ST17 0JH Tel: 01785 665896 — MB ChB Liverp. 1955 (Liverpool) DObst RCOG 1957.

NICHOLAS, Simon Courtenay 2 Newport Road, Barnes, London SW13 9PE Tel: 020 8748 4845; Greek Court, 14A Old Compton St, London W1D 4TJ Tel: 020 7437 1772 Fax: 020 7437 1782 — (Camb. & Lond. Hosp.) MRCS Eng. LRCP Lond. 1965; MB BChir Camb. 1966; MA Camb. 1966. Clin. Asst. (Anaesth.) Centr. Middlx. Hosp. Lond. Specialty: Anaesth.

***NICHOLAS, Victor Selvaranjan Babapulle** 30 Whinmoor Gardens, Leeds LS14 1AF Tel: 0113 293 3558 — MB BS Lond. 1997 (Kings College School of Medicine London) Specialty: Accid. & Emerg. Prev: Ho. Surg. Greenwich Dist.; Ho. Phys. Brighton.

NICHOLAS-PILLAI, Anthonipillai Bush Hill Park Surgery, 24 Amberley Road, Enfield EN1 2QY Tel: 020 8360 2477; 24 Amberley Road, Enfield EN1 2QY Tel: 020 8360 2477 — (St. Johns Medical College India) MB BS Bangalore 1970; DRCOG 1980; LMSSA Lond. 1980; DTM & H Lond 1981; Dip.in Primary Care 1997. GP Enfield PCT. Socs: Hon. Sec. & Treas. Enfield & Haringey BMA div; Fellow of Royal Society of Medicine. Mem. LMC Enfield, Barts. Prev: Regist. (A & E) N. Middlx. Hosp. Lond.; SHO (Cardiothoracic Dept. N. Middlx. Hosp. Lond.; SHO (Orthop.) Princess Alexandra Hosp. Harlow.

NICHOLL, Anthony David Joseph 41 Graham Road, Ipswich IP1 3QE Tel: 01473 430563 — MRCS Eng. LRCP Lond. 1977 (St. Mary's) FFA RCSI 1983; FFA RCS Eng. 1984. Cons. Anaesth. Ipswich Hosps. Specialty: Anaesth. Socs: Assn. Anaesth. Prev: Sen. Regist. (Anaesth.) E. Anglian RHA.; Regist. Rotat. (Anaesth.) Sheff. HA; Post-Fellowsh. (Anaesth.) Killingbeck Cardiothoracic Unit Leeds.

NICHOLL, Betty, OBE (retired) 19 Runkerry Road, Bushmills BT57 8SZ Tel: 028207 32314 Email: betty.bailie@btinternet.com — MB BCh BAO Belf. 1952; MD Belf. 1960; FRCPath 1978, M 1967. Prev: Cons. Clin. Pathologist, Belvoir Pk. Hosp. Belf.

NICHOLL, Claire Gilmour Department of Medicine for the Elderly, Box 135 Addenbrooke's Hospital, Hills Road, Cambridge CB2 2QQ Tel: 01223 217784 Fax: 01223 217783 Email: claire.nicholl@addenbrookes.nhs.uk; Quanea Farm, Quanea Drove, Ely CB7 5TJ Email: nicholl.wood@btinternet.com — MB BS Lond. 1979 (St. Mary's) BSc Lond. 1976; MRCP (UK) 1982; DGM RCP Lond. 1986; FRCP Lond. 1994. Cons. Phys., Addenbrooke's Hosp. Camb.; Cons. Phys. Princess of Wales Hosp. Ely; Clin. Director (Med. for Elderly). Specialty: Care of the Elderly; Gen. Med. Socs: Brit. Geriat. Soc.; Nat. Train. Comm. Prev: Sen. Lect. in Med. ICSM & Chief of Serv. for Med. for the Elderly, Hon. Cons. Phys., Hammersmith Hosps. Trust.

NICHOLL, Geoffrey McKillop Joseph (retired) Pear Tree Cottage, South Carlton, Lincoln LN1 2RH Tel: 01522 730151 — MRCS Eng. LRCP Lond. 1942 (Middlx. & Camb.) MA Camb. 1944; MRCGP 1956; DPM Eng. 1960; MRCPsych 1971. Prev: Cons. Child Psychiat. Gwynedd AHA & Lincoln.

NICHOLL, Hilda Jane McKay Accid. & Emerg. Dept., Craigavon Area Hospital, Lurgan Road, Portadown Tel: 028 3861 2514 Email: hildanicholl@hotmail.com — MB ChB Ed. 1994 (Edin.) MRCP 1997; FFAEM 2003. Cons. Accid. & Emerg., Craigavon Area Hosp. Specialty: Accid. & Emerg. Prev: Specialist Regist. (Emerg. Med.) N Irel.

NICHOLL, Mr James Edward Kent & Sussex Hospital, Mount Ephraim, Tunbridge Wells TN4 8AT Tel: 01892 526111 — MB BChir Camb. 1989; MA Camb. 1989; FRCS Eng. 1992; FRCS (Orth.) 1996. Cons. (Orthop.) Kent & Sussex hosp. Specialty: Orthop.

NICHOLL, Joanne Louise Little Orchard, Franfield Road, Buxted, Uckfield TN22 4LE — MB BS Lond. 1996.

NICHOLL, Keith The General Medical Centre, PO Box 11962, Dubai, United Arab Emirates Tel: 00 971 43495959 Fax: 00 971 43495634; The Old Studio, West Green, Crail, Anstruther KY10 3RD Tel: 01333 450574 — MB ChB Dundee 1980 (Univ. Dundee) DCH RCPS Glas. 1986. Paediat. Specialist Gen. Med. Centre Dubai, UAE/ Med. Director. Specialty: Paediat. Socs: Roy. Coll. Paediat. & Child Health; Fell. of Roy. Soc. of Trop. Med. and Hygene.; Emirate Med. Assn. Prev: Regist. (Paediat.) Ninewells Hosp. Med. Sch. Dundee.

NICHOLL, Michael Eakin Lodge Health, 20 Lodge Manor, Coleraine BT52 1JX Tel: 028 7034 4494 Fax: 028 7032 1759; Iniskeel, 7 O'Hara Drive, Portstewart BT55 7PD — MB BCh BAO Belf. 1982; MB BCh Belf. 1982; DRCOG 1984; DCH Dub. 1985; MRCGP 1986. Socs: BMA.

NICHOLL, Mr Philip Thomas Flat 2, 18 Vernon Road, Birmingham B16 9SH — MB BCh BAO Belf. 1987; FRCS Ed. 1991. Research Regist. (Vasc. Surg.) Roy. Free Hosp. Lond. Specialty: Gen. Surg.

NICHOLL, Raymond Stuart (retired) 27 Throxenby Lane, Newby, Scarborough YO12 5HN Tel: 01723 503449 — MRCS Eng. LRCP Lond. 1957. Prev: Clin. Asst. (Geriat.) St. Mary's Hosp. ScarBoro.

NICHOLL, Richard Martin Northwick Park Hospital, Northwest London Hospitals NHS Trusts, Harrow HA1 3VJ Tel: 020 869 2642 Fax: 020 8889 2927 Email: drnicholl@aol.com — MB ChB Birm. 1983; DCH RCP Lond. 1989; MRCP (UK) 1990; FRCPCH 1993; MRCPCH 1996. Cons. Neonatologist Northwick Pk. Hosp. Harrow. Specialty: Neonat. Socs: Neonat. Soc.; Paediat. Research Soc.; Brit. Assn. of Perinatal Med. Prev: Lect. (Neonat.) & Sen. Regist. King's Coll. Hosp. Lond.

NICHOLL, Robert Martin (retired) 32 Deramore Drive, Malone Road, Belfast BT9 5JR Tel: 028 9066 9684 — MD Belf. 1965; MB BCh BAO 1952; FFA RCS Eng. 1958; FFA RCSI 1971. Prev: Cons. Anaesth. Roy. Vict. Hosp. Belf.

NICHOLL, Stuart 56 Houlgate Way, Axbridge BS26 2BY — MB BS Lond. 1995.

NICHOLLES, Maia — MB BS Lond. 1992 (Royal Free) BSc London 1989; DRCOG 1995; MRCGP 1996. GP Princip. Specialty: Gen. Pract.

NICHOLLS, Agnes Mary Hinshelwood 45 Middle Park Road, Selly Oak, Birmingham B29 4BH — MB ChB Birm. 1965; DA Eng. 1967. Staff Grade (Anaesth.) Roy. Orthop. Hosp. Birm.

NICHOLLS, Anne (retired) West Suffolk Hospital, Hardwick Lane, Bury St Edmunds IP33 2QZ Tel: 01284 713440 Fax: 01284 712519; The Old Rectory, Bradfield St George, Bury St Edmunds IP30 0DH Tel: 01284 386551 — (St. Mary's) MB BS Lond. 1962; MRCS Eng. LRCP Lond. 1962; FRCP Lond. 1983, M 1969. Prev: Cons. Rheum. & Rehabil. W. Suff. Hosp.

NICHOLLS, Anne Patricia (retired) 41 Dry Hill Park Road, Tonbridge TN10 3BU Tel: 01732 354009 — MB BS Lond. 1959 (Roy. Free) MRCS Eng. LRCP Lond. 1958. Prev: GP Tonbridge.

NICHOLLS, Anthony Jeffery Stephen Pinn Medical Centre, 8 Eastcote Road, Pinner HA5 1HF Tel: 020 8866 5766 Fax: 020 8429 0251 — MB BS Lond. 1968 (Westm.) MRCS Eng. LRCP Lond. 1968; DObst RCOG 1970; DCH Eng. 1971; MRCP (UK) 1972;

MRCGP 1983. Prev: SHO (Med.) Nottm. City Hosp.; SHO Cardio-Thoracic Unit Hosp. Sick Childr. Gt. Ormond St. Lond.; Paediat. Regist. Roy. Free Hosp. & Edgware Gen. Hosp. Lond.

NICHOLLS, Anthony Julian Royal Devon & Exeter Hospital, Barrack Road, Exeter EX2 5DW Tel: 01392 402535 Fax: 01392 402527 Email: anthony.nicholls@rdehc-tr.swest.nhs.uk — MB BS Lond. 1975 (Guy's) MRCP (UK) 1977; FRCP Lond. 1992; FRCP Ed. 1999. Cons. Phys. & Nephrol. Roy. Devon & Exeter Healthcare NHS Trust. Specialty: Nephrol.; Gen. Med. Socs: Renal Assn.; Europ. Renal Assn. Prev: Sen. Regist. (Nephrol.) Sheff. AHA; Lect. (Med.) Univ. Aberd.; Ho. Phys. Guy's Hosp. Lond.

NICHOLLS, Barry John Langholm, 10 Church St., Bishops Lydeard, Taunton TA4 3AT — MB ChB Liverp. 1977; FFA RCS Eng. 1983. Specialty: Anaesth.

NICHOLLS, Charles Sebastian Rose Cottage, 217 Whitchurch Road, Tavistock PL19 9DQ Tel: 01822 617684 — MB BCh Wales 1989; MRCGP 1997; DFFP 1997. Specialty: Gen. Pract.

NICHOLLS, Christopher William 8 Tromode Close, Douglas IM2 5PE Tel: 01623 452900/01624 662644 — MB ChB Liverpool 1974. G.P. Locum; M.O. To D.H.S.S. Socs: Isle Of Man Med. Soc. Prev: GP Douglas, Isle of Man.

NICHOLLS, Cicely Ruth Camelot, Tromode Close, Douglas IM2 5PE Tel: 01624 662644 Email: chrisnicholls@im25pe.freeserve.co.uk — MB ChB Liverp. 1967; BSc Liverp. 1964. Med. Adviser I. of Man Civil Serv. Commiss.; Adjudicating Off. Manx DHSS. Specialty: Occupat. Health. Socs: I. of Man Med. Soc.

NICHOLLS, Dasha Elizabeth Department of Psychological Medicine, Great Ormond Street Hospital, Great Ormond St., London WC1N 3JH Tel: 020 7829 8679 — MB BS Lond. 1988; MRCPsych 1993; MD Lond. 2002. Cons. (Child and Adolesc. Psychiat.) & Head of Feeding & Eating Disorders. Specialty: Child & Adolesc. Psychiat. Special Interest: Early onset eating disorders.

NICHOLLS, Professor David Paul Royal Victoria Hospital, Belfast BT12 6BA Tel: 028 90633323 Fax: 028 90633917 Email: paul.nicholls@royalhospitals.n-i.nhs.uk; 2 Printshop Road, Templepatrick, Ballyclare BT39 0HZ Tel: 028 9443 3351 Email: dpnicholls@compuserve.com — MB ChB Manch 1969 (manchester) MRCP (UK) 1974; MD Manch. 1984; FRCP Lond. 1991; DSc (QUB) 1999. Cons. (Phys.) Roy. Vict. Hosp. Belf.; Hon. Prof. Med. Qu.s Univ.Belf. Specialty: Gen. Med. Prev: Sen. Regist. (Cardiol.) Belf. City Hosp.; Regist. (Med.) Tameside Gen. Hosp. Ashton-under-Lyne; Tutor (Med.) Hope Hosp. Salford.

NICHOLLS, David Ronald The Witterings Health Centre, Cakeham Road, East Wittering, Chichester PO20 8BH Tel: 01243 673434 Fax: 01243 672563; The Gables, Tangmere Road, Shopwhyke, Chichester PO20 6BL — BM BCh Oxf. 1971; MA; DCH Eng. 1974; DObst RCOG 1975. Prev: Trainee GP Chichester VTS; Ho. Off. (Med.) Roy. United Hosp. Bath; Ho. Surg. Radcliffe Infirm. Oxf.

NICHOLLS, Elizabeth Anne St Clement's Surgery, 24 Marshland Street, Terrington St. Clement, King's Lynn PE34 4NE Tel: 01553 828475/827051 Fax: 01553 827594 — MB BCh Wales 1985; DRCOG 1990.

NICHOLLS, Fiona Michelle Department of Anesthesiology, St Mary's Hospital, Praed Street W2 1NY Tel: 020 7886 1556; 84 Waverley Road, Enfield EN2 7AQ Tel: 020 8367 5581 — MB BS Lond. 1989 (Lond. Hosp.) FRCA Lond. 1996; CCST Anaesthetics 2000. Cons. Anaesth., St Mary's Hosp., Lond. Specialty: Anaesth. Special Interest: Cardiothoracic; Ophth.; Vasc.

NICHOLLS, Francis Ambrose John Highdown Surgery, 1 Highdown Avenue, Worthing BN13 1PU Tel: 01903 265656 Fax: 01903 830450; 7 Modena Road, Hove BN3 5QF — MB BS Lond. 1988. GP Highdown Surg. Worthing; Clin. Asst. St. Barnabas Hospice Worthing. Specialty: Gen. Pract. Socs: BMA & Med. Defence Union. Prev: Trainee GP St. Lawrence Surg.; SHO (c/o the Elderly, O & G, Palliat. Med. & Padiat.) Worthing VTS; SHO (Orthop., A & E) Roy. Sussex Co. Hosp. Brighton.

NICHOLLS, Gail Catherine Rosebank Surgery, Pointer Court, Ashton Rd, Lancaster LA1 4JS Tel: 01524 842284 — MB ChB Manch. 1997 (St. And. and Manch.) BSc St. And. 1994. GP Regist, Lancaster. Specialty: Gen. Pract. Socs: Assoc. of CCGP. Prev: SHO. (Paediat.) New Zealand.; SHO. (A&E.) Lancaster.; SHO in Obst. & Gyn., Lancaster.

NICHOLLS, Mr Guy Department Paediatric Surgery, Bristol Royal Hospital for Sick Children, St. Micheal's Hill, Bristol BS2 8BJ Tel: 0117 921 5411; Flat 2, 13 Dowry Square, Clifton, Bristol B58 4SL — MB ChB Birm. 1986; BSc Birm. 1983, MB ChB 1986; FRCS Ed. 1990; MD Birm. 1997; FRCS (Paed. Surg.) 1998. Cons. in Paediat. Surg. & Urol., Bristol Childr.'s Hosp.; Hon. Clin. Lect., Univ. of Bristol. Specialty: Paediat. Surg.

NICHOLLS, Harriet Anne 3 Mount Drive, Park St., St Albans AL2 2NP — MB BChir Camb. 1993; FRCA 1996. Regist. (Anaesth.) The Middlx. Hosp. Specialty: Anaesth. Prev: SHO (ITU) Nat. Hosp. Neurol. & Neurosurg.; SHO (Anaesth.) Watford Gen. Hosp.

NICHOLLS, Heather Meddygfa'r Llan, Church Surgery, Portland Street, Aberystwyth SY23 2DX Tel: 01970 624855 Fax: 01970 625824; Llys Terfyn, Taliesin, Machynlleth SY20 8JR Tel: 01970 832251 — MB BCh Wales 1983; DRCOG 1987. GP Princip. Specialty: Community Child Health. Prev: SCMO E. Dyfed HA Aberystwyth Dyfed.

NICHOLLS, Hedley John Leslie (retired) Blackbarrow, Norton-sub-Hamdon, Taunton Tel: 0193 588236 — MB ChB Bristol 1955; MRCS Eng. LRCP Lond. 1955; DObst RCOG 1957. Prev: Ho. Phys. Frenchay Hosp. Bristol.

NICHOLLS, James Eric Church View Surgery, Burley House, 15 High Street, Rayleigh SS6 7DY Tel: 01702 202514 Fax: 01702 204110; The Myrtles, 215 Hockley Road, Rayleigh SS6 8BH Tel: 01268 777872 Fax: 01268 779333 Email: jamienicholls@compuserve.com — MB BS Lond. 1974 (Lond. Hosp.) DRCOG 1976. GP Princip.; GP Tutor Southend-on-Sea.

NICHOLLS, Janet Mary Epsom General Hospital, Dorking Road, Epsom KT18 7EG Tel: 01372 735261 — MB BS Lond. 1978; MRCP (UK) 1982; T(M) (Paed) 1991; FRCP Lond. 1996. Cons. Paediat. Epsom Gen. Hosp. Epsom. Specialty: Paediat.

NICHOLLS, Jeanette — MB ChB Birm. 1985; MB ChB Birmingham 1985. Term Time Staff Grade (Child Health) NBC Trust.; Staff Grade Community Paediatrician Clinical Assistant ENT. Specialty: Community Child Health. Prev: Clin. Med. Off. (Child Health) Birm. HA.

NICHOLLS, Jennifer Burnfield Medical Practice, Harris Road, Inverness IV2 3PF Tel: 01463 220077 Fax: 01463 714588 — MB ChB Dundee 1974; MRCGP UK 1991; Dip Palliat Med Cardiff 1994. Assoc. Adviser in Gen. Pract., N. of Scotl. Inst. for Postgrad. Med. & Dent. Educat., Railmore Hosp., Inverness. Specialty: Gen. Pract.; Hypnother. Socs: BMA; Assn. for Palliat. Med.

NICHOLLS, Mr John Charles Hemel Hempstead Hospital, Hemel Hempstead HP2 4AD Tel: 01442 213141 Fax: 01442 287405 — MB BS Lond 1963 (Char. Cross) MRCS Eng. LRCP Lond. 1963; FRCS Eng. 1969. Secondary Care Adviser HCAA. Specialty: Gen. Surg.; Paediat. Surg. Special Interest: Gen. Paediatric Surg.; Oncol. Socs: Fell. Assn. Surg.; BMA. Prev: Cons. Surg. Govt. of Seychelles; Med. Dir. St. Albans & Hemel Hempstead NHS Trust; Cons. Surg. Hemel Hempstead Hosp.

NICHOLLS, Jonathan Simon David Oxford Radcliffe Hospitals NHS Trust, Horton Hospital, Dept of Obst. & Gyn., Banbury OX16 9AL Email: jonathan.nicholls@orh.nhs.uk; Scotland Mount, Round Close Road, Banbury OX15 5NT Tel: 01608 737348 — (Westm.) MB BS Lond. 1985; MRCOG 1994; MD 2000. Cons. (Obst. & Gyn.) Horton Hosp., Banbury; Cons. (Obs & Gyn) John Racliffe Hosp., Oxf. Specialty: Obst. & Gyn. Socs: Brit. Soc. of Gyn. Endoscopy; Oxf. Medico-Legal Soc.; Bristol Obst. & Gyn. Soc. Prev: Sen. Regist. (Obst. & Gyn.) St Michaels Hosp. Bristol; Sen. Regist. (Obst. & Gyn.) Southmead Hosp. Bristol; Clin. Research Fell. Dept. Clin. Endocrinol. St. Mary's Hosp. Med. Sch. Lond.

NICHOLLS, Judith Elizabeth Ablewell House, 30 Birmingham Road, Walsall WS1 2LT Tel: 01922 775000 Fax: 01922 775002 — MB ChB Birm. 1986; MRCPsych 1990. Cons. (Child & Adolesc. Psychiat.) Walsall Community Health Trust. Specialty: Child & Adolesc. Psychiat. Prev: Sen. Regist. (Child Adolesc. Psychiat.) W. Midl. Rotat.

NICHOLLS, Kate Charlotte Keel Health Centre, Seymour Road, Easton, Bristol BS5 0UA Tel: 0117 9027155 Fax: 0117 951 2373 — MB ChB Bristol 1978; DRCOG 1981; MRCGP 1983. Specialty: Gen. Pract. Socs: Roy. Coll. Gen. Pract.

NICHOLLS, Kevin Roy — MB ChB Birm. 1988; BSc (Hons.) Birm. 1985; MRCPsych 1995; MPhil Keele 2000. Cons. Gen. Psych.

Specialty: Paediat. Neurol. Prev: Sen. Regist. Profess. Unit Stoke-on-Trent.

NICHOLLS, Kit-Mei Hebburn Health Centre, Campbell Park Road, Hebburn NE31 2SP Tel: 0191 483 5533 Fax: 0191 428 1826; 7 Townhead, Slaley, Hexham NE47 0AT — MB ChB Dundee 1989. GP Hebburn, Tyne & Wear.

NICHOLLS, Marcus John Heath End Cottage, Heath End, Berkhamsted HP4 3UE — MB ChB Manch. 1997.

NICHOLLS, Margot Jane — MB BS Lond. 1990 (UCMHMS) DRCOG 1992; MRCGP 1994. Specialist Regist. (Pub. Health.), Croydon Health Auth. Specialty: Pub. Health Med. Prev: Toxic. Reg. NPIS, Lond.; GP Reg. S. Harrow, Northwick Pk. Hosp. VTS.

NICHOLLS, Martyn John The Surgery, 59 Sevenoaks Road, Orpington BR6 9JN Tel: 01689 820159; 29 Goldfinch Close, Chelsfield, Orpington BR6 6NF Tel: 01689 860639 — MB ChB Manch. 1984.

NICHOLLS, Maxim Daniel William 23 Alan Drive, Barnet EN5 2PP — MB BS Lond. 1993.

NICHOLLS, Michael John (retired) 28 The Hamlet, Leek Wootton, Warwick CV35 7QW — MB BS Lond. 1959 (Univ. Coll. Hosp.) MRCS Eng. LRCP Lond. 1959; DObst RCOG 1962. Prev: Sen. Part. Or Nicholls and Partners Southampton.

NICHOLLS, Michael William Newbery (retired) Creekside, 28 Greenacres, Birdham, Chichester PO20 7HL Tel: 01243 512937 Fax: 01243 511087 Email: michael.nicholls@which.net — MB BS Lond. 1957 (Univ. Coll.) MRCS Eng. LRCP Lond. 1955; FRCPath 1980, M 1968. Trustee Tushinskaya Hosp. Trust Lond.; Dir. of Finance Fellowsh. PostGrad. Med. Lond. Prev: Dean Postgrad. Med. Educat. (SE Thames) Univ. Lond. & Asst. Dir. Brit. Postgrad. Med. Federat. Univ. Lond.

NICHOLLS, Peter Eric Department of Histopathology, Royal Shrewsbury Hospital, Shrewsbury SY3 8XQ Tel: 01743 261168 Fax: 01743 355963 Email: pen@rshhis.demon.co.uk; 36 Roman Road, Shrewsbury SY3 9AT Email: pe.nicholls@virgin.net — MB BS Lond. 1969 (Guy's) MRCS Eng. LRCP Lond. 1969; FRCPath 1989, M 1977. Cons. (Histopath.) Roy. Shrewsbury Hosp. Specialty: Histopath. Socs: Acad. Path. & Assn. Clin. Path.; Internat. Acad. Path.; Assn. Clin. Pathol. Prev: Lect. (Histopath.) Westm. Med. Sch. Lond.; SHO (Path.) Miller Gen. Hosp. Greenwich; Regist. (Clin. Path.) Guy's Hosp. Lond.

NICHOLLS, Professor Ralph John 149 Harley Street, London W1G 6DE Tel: 020 7935 4444 Fax: 020 7486 0665; 24 St Marks Crescent, London NW1 7TU — MB BChir Camb. 1968; FRCS Eng. 1972; BA Camb. 1964, MChir 1978; FRCS Glas. 1993. Cons. Surg. St Marks Hosp. Harrow; Edr. Colorectal Dis.; Sec. Div. of Coloproctol. UEMS. Specialty: Gen. Surg. Socs: Brit. Soc. Gastroenterol.; (Exec.) Assn. Coloproctol.; Mem. d'Honneur Assn. Fr. de Chirurgie. Prev: Cons. Surg. St. Thos. Hosp. Lond.; Sen. Lect. (Surg. Oncol.) St. Bart. Hosp. Med. Coll. Lond.; Clin. Asst. Univ. Heidelberg.

NICHOLLS, Robert David 31 Weald Way, Reigate RH2 7RG — MB ChB Manch. 1998.

NICHOLLS, Sarah Department of Sexual Health, Princess Alice Day Hospital, Carew Road, Eastbourne BN21 2AX; Ave. House, The Avenue, Eastbourne BN21 3XY — MB BS Lond. 1991.

NICHOLLS, Stuart Warren Department of Paediatrics, Worthing Hospital, Lyndhurst Road, Worthing BN11 2DH Tel: 01903 285176 — MB BCh Wales 1984 (Cardiff) FRCP Edin.; FRCPCH. Cons. (Paediat.) Worthing Hosp. Specialty: Paediat.

NICHOLLS-VAN VLIET, Maria Anna Theresia Winstanley Drive Surgery, 138 Winstanley Drive, Leicester LE3 1PB Tel: 0116 285 8435 Fax: 0116 275 5416 — Artsexamen Rotterdam 1978; PhD Nijmegen 1985; ONNACOJ 1987. Gen. Pract.

NICHOLS, David Borve Medical Practice, Borve, Isle of Lewis HS2 0RS Tel: 01851 850282 Fax: 01851 860333; 14 Port of Ness, Isle of Lewis HS2 0XA Tel: 01851 810794 — MB ChB Glas. 1974. Specialty: Acupunc. Prev: GP E. Kilbride; Regist. (Anaesth.) Glas. Roy. Infirm. & Roy. Alexandra Infirm.; SHO Paisley Matern. Hosp.

NICHOLS, David Martin Department Radiodiagnosis, Raigmore Hospital, Inverness IV2 3UJ Tel: 01463 704000 — MB ChB Aberd. 1974 (Aberdeen) MRCP (UK) 1978; DMRD Aberd. 1979; FFR RCSI 1981; FRCP (C) 1982; FRCR 1983; FRCP Ed. 1990; FRCS Ed. 1997. Cons. Radiol. Raigmore Hosp. Inverness.; Sen. Lect. Radiol. Univ. Aberd. Specialty: Radiol. Prev: Radiol. Vancouver Gen. Hosp. & Asst. Prof., Univ. Brit. Columbia; Sen. Regist. (Diag. Radiol.) Aberd. Hosps.

NICHOLS, Elizabeth Anne, Surg. Cdr. RN 25 Valletort Road, Millbridge, Plymouth PL1 5PH — MB BS Lond. 1990 (Guy's) DRCOG; MRCGP. Roy. Navy.

NICHOLS, Mr Geoffrey James Park Lane Surgery, 2 Park Lane, Allestree, Derby DE22 2DS Tel: 01332 552461 Fax: 01332 541500 — BM Soton. 1985; FRCS Ed. 1990; T(GP) 1994. Prev: SHO (O & G) Trafford Gen. Hosp.; SHO & Regist. (Gen. Surg.) Trafford & N. Manch. Gen. Hosp.; SHO (A & E & Orthop. Surg.) Hope Hosp. Salford.

NICHOLS, John Anthony Alvan Fairlands Medical Centre, Fairlands Avenue, Worplesdon, Guildford GU3 3NA Tel: 01483 594250 Fax: 01483 598767; 60 Manor Way, Onslow Village, Guildford GU2 7RR Tel: 01483 564967 — MB ChB Liverp. 1967; DObst RCOG 1970; DCH Eng. 1972; MRCGP 1973. Socs: Brit. Soc. Allergy & Environm. Med. Prev: Regist. (Gen. Med.) St. Luke's Hosp. Guildford; SHO (O & G & Paediat.) St. Luke's Hosp. Guildford; Ho. Phys. Sefton Gen. Hosp. Liverp.

NICHOLS, John Bowes (retired) Greenways, Moor End, Stibbard, Fakenham NR21 0EJ Tel: 01328 829225 Email: jbnichols@ukonline.co.uk — (Camb. & St. Bart.) MB Camb. 1958, BChir 1957; DObst RCOG 1960. Prev: Regist. (Med.), Ho. Surg. & Ho. Phys. St. Bart. Hosp.

NICHOLS, Kathleen Clare The Surgery, 18 Fouracre Road, Bristol BS16 6PG Tel: 0117 970 2033 — MB ChB Bristol 1975; DRCOG 1979; MRCGP 1995.

NICHOLS, Marion Jane The Parks Surgery, 116 Kings Rd, Herne Bay, Canterbury CT6 5RE Tel: 01227 771474/01926 513060 Email: cm.dallaway@talk21.com; 11 Juniper Close, Canterbury CT1 3LL Tel: 01227 455558 Email: marionnichols@btinternet.com — MB ChB Bristol 1995; BSc (Hons.) Bradford 1985. GP Princip., The Pk. Surg., Herne Bay. Specialty: Gen. Pract. Prev: GP Locum Whitstable Med. Pract.

NICHOLS, Mary Elizabeth Yelverton Surgery, Westella Road, Yelverton PL20 6AS — MB ChB Manch. 1989. GP Yelverton. Specialty: Gen. Pract. Prev: SHO (A & E) Derriford Hosp. Plymouth.

NICHOLS, Mary Patricia 76a Norwich Road, Wymondham NR18 0SZ Email: mary.nichols@bigfoot.com — MB BS Lond. 1982 (Roy. Free) DGM RCP Lond. 1985; MRCGP 1986; Cert. Family Plann. JCC 1987; DRCOG 1987; DFFP 1993; MSc (Dist) Oxf. Brookes Univ. 1999; ILTM 2002; Dip Med Educat Dundee 2003. p/t GP Non-Princip.; MRCGP Examr.; Appraiser, S. Norf., W. Norf. and Norwich PCTs; Progr. Director, HPE Scheme (Norfolk & Suffolk). Specialty: Gen. Pract.; Educat. Socs: BMA; AMEE. Prev: Trainee GP Oxf. VTS.

NICHOLS, Mr Paul Henry Department of Surgery, Southampton General Hospital, Tremont Road, Southampton SO16 6YD Tel: 023 8079 6606 Email: paul.nichols@suht.swest.nhs.uk — MB ChB Leeds 1989; MD Leeds 1999; FRCS (Eng.) 2001. Cons. Gen. and Colorectal Surg., Soton. Gen. Hosp. Specialty: Gen. Surg. Special Interest: laparoscopic and Rectal Surg. Socs: Assn. Coloproct.; Roy. Coll. of Surgeons (England); BMA.

NICHOLS, Paul Kenneth Trevor Royal Gwent Hospital, Newport NP20 2UB — MB BCh Wales 1982; FFA RCS Eng. 1987. Cons. Anaesth. Intens. Ther. Unit. Roy. Gwent Hosp. Specialty: Anaesth. Prev: Sen. Regist. (Anaesth.) W. Glam. HA.

NICHOLS, Roger William Townsend Station Road Surgery, 69 Station Road, Sidcup DA15 7DS Tel: 020 8309 0201 Fax: 020 8309 9040; 11 Buckingham Drive, Chislehurst BR7 6TB — MB BS Lond. 1975 (Guy's) MRCS Eng. LRCP Lond. 1975; FRCS Eng. 1980.

***NICHOLS, Thomas Arthur Edward** Royal United Hospital, Coombe Park, Bath BA1 3NG — MB BS Newc. 2003. PRHO (Gen. Med./Respirat. Med.).

NICHOLSON, Agnes Frances Barrhead Health Centre, 203 Main Street, Barrhead G78 1HG Tel: 0141 880 6161 Fax: 0141 881 7036; 11 Letham Drive, Glasgow G43 2SL Tel: 0141 637 2410 — MB ChB Glas. 1968.

NICHOLSON, Alexander Barnes Shropshire & Mid Wales Hospice, Bicton Heath, Shrewsbury SY3 8HS Tel: 01743 236565 Fax: 01743 261512 — MB BS Newc. 1993 (Newc. upon Tyne) DRCOG 1995; DCH 1997; JCPTGP Cert. Of Equiv. Exp. 1998; MRCGP 1998; Dip Palliat Med 2000. Specialist Regist. in Palliat. Med., W. Midl.s Rotat. Specialty: Palliat. Med. Socs: Assn. for

Palliat. Med.; Fell. of Roy. Soc. of Med. Prev: GP Princ. Wylam, N.umber. 1999; Locum cons. In Pall. Med, St. Benedicts Hospice, Sunderland 2000.

NICHOLSON, Andrew Gordon Department of Histopathology, Royal Brompton Hospital, Sydney Street, London SW3 6NP — MB BS Lond. 1987; FRCPath Oxon.

NICHOLSON, Anthony Andrew 75 Southfield, Hessle HU13 0EX Tel: 01482 645840 Fax: 01482 649938 Email: tonynick@tonynick.demon.co.uk — MB ChB Sheff. 1983 (Sheffield) FRCR 1988. Cons. Radiol. Hull Roy. Infirm. Specialty: Radiol. Socs: Brit. Soc. Interven.al Radiol. (Vice Pres. 1997-1999, Pres. 1999-2001); Soc. Cardiovasc. & Interven.al Radiolog. Soc. of N. Amer.; Fell.Cardiovasc. & Interven.al Soc. Europe. Prev: Sen. Regist. Univ. Hosp. Wales Cardiff; SHO (Gen. Med.) Roy. Hallamsh. Hosp. Sheff.

NICHOLSON, Professor Anthony Norman, OBE Applewood Island, Steep, Petersfield GU32 1AE Tel: 01730 233863 Fax: 01730 260610 Email: nicholson@btopenworld.com — MB ChB Birm. 1957; FRCPath 1978; PhD Birm. 1964, DSc 1980; FRCP Ed. 1986; FRAeS 1992; MD (hc) Russian Academey of Sci. 1996; FFOM 1997; FRCP Lond. 1998. Med. Dir. (Academic Clin. for Disorders of Sleep & Wakefulness) Univ. Surrey; Vis. Prof. Aviat Med. King's Coll. Lond.; Chairm. of Trustees, UK Confidential Air Human Factors Reporting Progr. Farnborough. Specialty: Occupat. Health. Special Interest: Aviation Medicine; Sleep Medicine. Socs: Brit. Pharmacol. Soc.; Liveryman Soc. of Apoth.; Physiol. Soc. Prev: Progr. Manager 'Med. Aspects of Fitness to Drive' UK Dept. Transport; Vis. Prof. Med. Imperial. Coll. Lond; Commandant & Dir. Research RAF Inst. Aviat. Med.

NICHOLSON, Anthony Paul Rosewood House, 200 Abbotswell Crescent, Aberdeen AB12 3DD — MB ChB Aberd. 1958. Med. Off. Stud. Health Aberd. Univ. Prev: Asst. MOH Aberd.sh. CC.

NICHOLSON, Arthur Robert (retired) Clifton Cross, Ashbourne DE6 2DH Tel: 0161 432 7382 — MB ChB Sheff. 1965; DObst RCOG 1967; MRCGP 1972. Prev: Ho. Phys. Profess. Cardiovasc. Unit & Ho. Surg. Urol. Unit City Gen.

NICHOLSON, Basil Sonoma, Valley, Holyhead LL65 3EY — MB ChB Manch. 1944; DTM & H Eng. 1948; DPH Lond. 1953; MFCM 1973. Asst. Dir. Med. Dept. Brit. Counc. Prev: Princip. Asst. Sen. Med. Off. (Computer Servs.) Birm. RHB; Sen. Med. Off. Glos. CC; Sen. Leprosy Off. Nigeria (W. Region).

NICHOLSON, Catherine Agnes Grove Road Surgery, 25 Grove Road, Borehamwood WD6 5DX Tel: 020 8953 2444 Fax: 020 8207 4060; 104 Aldenham Road, Bushey, Watford WD23 2EX Tel: 01923 229905 — MB BS Lond. 1978; DRCOG 1981; MRCGP 1983.

NICHOLSON, Claire Louise — MB ChB Glas. 1998.

NICHOLSON, David Andrew Ingledene, Richmond Green, Bowdon, Altrincham WA14 2UB — BM BS Nottm. 1983; BMedSci 1981; BMedSci 1981; FRCR 1990. Cons. Radiol. Hope Hosp. Manch.; Sen. Research Fell. Hammersmith Hosp. Lond. Specialty: Radiol. Prev: Sen. Regist. (Diagn. Radiol.) Manch.; Lect. (Anat.) Univ. Hosp. Nottm.; SHO (Surg.) Addenbrooke's Hosp. Camb.

NICHOLSON, David George Garden Lane Medical Centre, 19 Garden Lane, Chester CH1 4EN Tel: 01244 346677 Fax: 01244 310094 — MB ChB Sheff. 1989.

NICHOLSON, Elizabeth (retired) 48 Cornmoor Road, Whickham, Newcastle upon Tyne NE16 4PU Tel: 0191 488 7165 — MB BS Durh. 1950. Prev: Ho. Phys. & Ho. Surg. (Accid. Room) Roy. Vict. Infirm. Newc.

NICHOLSON, Elizabeth Mary (retired) abbots Leigh Manor, Manor Rd, Abbots Leigh, Bristol BS8 3RP Tel: 0117 374669 — MB BS Lond. 1952 (Roy. Free) DA Eng. 1959; MD Bristol 1982. Prev: Assoc. Specialist (Thoracic Med.) Bristol.

NICHOLSON, Felicity 13 Tidenham Gardens, Park Hill, Croydon CR0 5UT — MB BS Lond. 1984; BSc (1st cl. Hons.) Lond. 1981, MB BS 1984; MRCPath 1991; FRCPath 1999. Forens. Med. Examr. for Metrop. Police; Cons. in Travel Med. Trailfinders Immunisation Centre Lond. Specialty: Forens. Path.; Trop. Med. Socs: BMA; Medico-legal Soc.; Assn. of Police Surg.s. Prev: Sen. Regist. (Virol.) St. Thos. Hosp. Lond.; Regist. (Microbiol.) St. Thos. Hosp. Lond.; SHO Rotat. (Path.) & Ho. Phys. St. Thos. Hosp. Lond.

NICHOLSON, Geoffrey (retired) Ravenscar, 99 Broadbottom Road, Mottram-in-Longdendale, Hyde SK14 6JA Tel: 01457 763653 — MB ChB Birm. 1971; BSc (Hons.) (Physiol.) Birm. 1968, MD 1978, MB ChB; MRCP (UK) 1974. Prev: Cons. Phys. Roy. Oldham Hosp.

NICHOLSON, George 25 Witbank Road, Darlington DL3 6SB — MB BS Lond. 1983.

NICHOLSON, Gillian Marilyn 55 Sleepy Valley, Richhill, Armagh BT61 9LH Tel: 01762 871520 — MB BCh BAO Belf. 1988; MB BCh Belf. 1988; DRCOG 1992; Cert. Family Plann. JCC 1992; Cert. Adv. Family Plann. JCC 1993; MRCGP 1993; Cert. Prescribed Equiv. Exp. 1993; DCCH RCGP 1994. Prev: SHO (Psychiat.) Holyell Antrim; SHO (O & G) S. Tyrone Hosp. Dungannon; SHO (Paediat.) Craigavon Area Hosp. Portadown.

NICHOLSON, Mr Hamish Oliphant (retired) The Granary, Foss Home Farm, Foss, Pitlochry PH16 5NQ Tel: 01882 634307 Email: hamish@nicholson34.fsnet.co.uk — MB ChB Ed. 1957; FRCS Ed. 1965; FRCOG 1978, M 1966. Prev: Cons. O & G Centr. Birm. Health Dist.

NICHOLSON, Helen Diana Department of Anatomy, School of Medical Sciences, University of Bristol, Bristol BS8 1TD Tel: 0117 928 8692 Fax: 0117 929 1687 — MB ChB Bristol 1979; MD Bristol 1986. Sen. Lect. (Anat.) Univ. Bristol. Specialty: Anat.

NICHOLSON, Howard (retired) Chelwood, Laughton, Lewes BN8 6BE — (Univ. Coll. Hosp.) MB BS Lond. 1935; MD Lond. 1938; MRCS Eng. LRCP Lond. 1935; FRCP Lond. 1949, M 1938. Fell. Univ. Coll. Lond.; Consg. Phys. Univ. Coll. Hosp. & Brompton Hosp. Prev: Phys. Univ. Coll. Hosp. & Brompton Hosp.

NICHOLSON, Hugh Philip The Surgery, 4 Stone Street, Hastings TN34 1QD Tel: 01424 427015 Fax: 01424 427633 — BM Soton. 1983. Socs: Assoc. Inst. Med. Laborat. Scs.

NICHOLSON, Iain Gordon 8 Strouden Avenue, Bournemouth BH8 9HT Tel: 01202 517250 — MB BS Lond. 1976 (Guy's) DObst 1982. Prev: SHO (O & G) Middlx. Hosp. Lond.; Cas. Off. Guy's Hosp. Lond.; Resid. Med. Off. (Chest Med. & Tuberc.) Ruttonjee Sanat. Hong Kong.

NICHOLSON, Jacob Alexander 106 East Sheen Avenue, London SW14 8AU — MB BS Lond. 1966; MRCS Eng. LRCP Lond. 1966; MRCP Lond. 1969.

NICHOLSON, Jacqueline — (Sheff.) MB ChB (Hons.) Sheff. 1966; DCH Eng. 1969; Cert JCC Lond. 1976; FRCPCH 1997. Designated doctor special needs SDHA. Specialty: Community Child Health. Socs: Eur. Acad. Childh. Disabil.; Fell. Roy. coll. Paediat. and Child Health. Prev: SHO Profess. Unit Sheff. Childr. Hosp.; Ho. Off. Profess. Therap. Unit & Ho. Off. Surg. Unit Sheff. Roy. Infirm.; Cons. Community Paediat. Community Child & Family Health S. Derbysh.

NICHOLSON, James Christopher Addenbrookes Hospital (Box 181), Hills Road, Cambridge CB2 2QQ Tel: 01223 256298 Fax: 01223 586794 Email: james.nicholson@addenbrookes.nhs.uk — MB BChir Camb. 1989; MA Camb. 1990; MRCP (UK) 1992; DM (Southampton) 1999. Cons. (Paediat. Oncol.) Addenbrookes NHS Trust Camb. Specialty: Paediat. Socs: MRCPCH; UKCCSG; SIOP. Prev: Clin. Research Fell. (Paediat.) Soton.; Regist. Roy. Childr.'s Hosp. Melbourne, Australia.; Specialist Regist. (Paediat. Oncol.) Soton. & Roy. Marsden Hosp.

NICHOLSON, James Gordon (retired) 8 Strouden Avenue, Bournemouth BH8 9HT Tel: 01202 517250 Fax: 01202 517250 Email: jimmienich@amserve.net — MB BS Lond. 1951 (Univ. Coll. Hosp.) DObst RCOG 1956. Prev: Ho. Surg. Roy. Ear Hosp. (Univ. Coll. Hosp.).

NICHOLSON, John Antrim Hospital, Bush Road, Antrim BT41 2QB Tel: 018494 64921 — MB BCh BAO Belf. 1978; FRCP; FRCPaeds; MRCP (UK) 1982. Cons. Paediat. N. HSSB. Specialty: Paediat. Prev: Cons. Paediat. Worcester HA; Lect. (Paediat.) Univ. Sheff.

NICHOLSON, John Charles Woodland View Surgery, Woodland View, West Rainton, Houghton-le-Spring DH4 6RQ Tel: 0191 584 3809 Fax: 0191 584 9177 — MB ChB Glas. 1974; DRCOG 1976.

NICHOLSON, Jolyon Anthony Howard The Halliwell Surgery, Lindfield Drive, Bolton BL1 3RG Tel: 01204 523813 Fax: 01204 384204 Email: jolyon.nicholson@gp-p82029.nhs.uk — MB ChB St. And. 1963 (St andrews)

NICHOLSON, Julian 85 Holly Avenue, Breaston, Derby DE72 3BR Tel: 0133 172971; Health Centre, Midland St, Long Eaton, Nottingham NG10 1NY — MB ChB St. And. 1970; DObst RCOG 1974; MRCGP 1977.

NICHOLSON, Karl Graham 2 Huntsmans Close, Quorn, Loughborough LE12 8AR — MB BS Lond. 1973; MRCS Eng. LRCP Lond. 1973; MRCP (UK) 1975; FRCP Lond. 1988; FRCP 1988; FRCPath 1994, M 1989; MD Leics. 1990. Sen. Lect. & Hon. Cons.

Infec. Dis. Leicester Univ. & Leicester Roy. Infirm. Specialty: Infec. Dis. Socs: Assn. Phys.; (Sec.) Europ. Scientif. Working Gp. on Influenza. Prev: Lilly Research Fell. Nat. Centre for Dis. Control Atlanta, USA; Mem. Staff of MRC Div. Communicable Dis. Northwick Pk. Hosp.

NICHOLSON, Katrina Mary St Johns Medical Centre, 62 London Road, Grantham NG31 6HR Tel: 01476 590055 Fax: 01476 400042 — MB ChB Liverp. 1988; DRCOG 1991; DCH RCP Lond. 1992; MRCGP 1993.

NICHOLSON, Margaret Jean 6 Canton Court, Belfast BT6 9EL — MB BCh BAO Belf. 1984; MB BCh Belf. 1984.

NICHOLSON, Mark Edward James Imperical Medical Practice, 47-49 Imperial Road, Exmouth EX8 1DQ Tel: 01395 224555 Fax: 01395 279282 — MB ChB Bristol 1990; DGM RCP Lond. 1993; MRCGP 1994. Princip. Gen. Pract., Exmouth. Prev: Locum Clin. Asst. Exeter Hospice; SHO (Palliat. Care) Rowcroft Hospice Torquay; GP VTS Exeter.

NICHOLSON, Meriel Susan (retired) Ladymead, Huggett's Lane, Willingdon, Eastbourne BN22 0LH Tel: 01323 502793 Fax: 01323 521390 Email: merielnicholson@compuserve.com — (Middlx.) FRCPH; FRCP; FIPH; MB BS Lond. 1965; DCH Eng. 1979; MRCP (UK) 1982. p/t Project Director Child Friendly Healthcare Initiative Child Advocacy Internat. Prev: Cons. Child Health Dist. Gen. Hosp. E.bourne.

NICHOLSON, Professor Michael Lennard Department of Cardiovascular Sciences - Transplant, Leicester General Hospital, Glendolen Road, Leicester LE5 4PW Tel: 0116 258 4604 Fax: 0116 249 0064 Email: mln2@le.ac.uk — BM BS Nottm. 1982; BMedSci (Ist cl. Hons.) Nottm. 1980; FRCS Eng. 1986; MD Leic. 1990. Prof. (Transpl. Surg.) Leic. Gen. Hps. Specialty: Gen. Surg.; Transpl. Surg. Special Interest: Endocrine Surgery; Renal Transplantation. Socs: Assn. of Surgeons; BTS; BAES. Prev: Cons. Surg. & Sen. Lect. Leic. Gen. Hosp.; Sen. Regist. (Surg.) Univ. Hosp. Nottm.; Regist. (Surg.) Leicester Hosps.

NICHOLSON, Michael Robert Craigavon Psychiatric Unit, 68 Lurgan Road, Portadown, Craigavon BT63 5QQ — MB BCh BAO Belf. 1986; DCH RCPSI 1989; MRCPsych 1993. Cons. (Gen. Adult. Psychiat.) Craigdown Psychiatric Unit, Portadown. Specialty: Gen. Psychiat. Prev: Trainee GP Stranraer.

NICHOLSON, Olwen Patricia 8 Hardwick Court, Hartlepool TS26 0AZ Tel: 01429 263667 — MB BS Newc. 1994 (Univ. Newc. u. Tyne) BMedSc (Hons.) Newc. 1991. SHO (Psychiat.) Watford Gen. Hosp. Specialty: Gen. Psychiat. Socs: BMA; MPS; MSS. Prev: SHO (Psychiat.) Napsbury Hosp. St. Albans; SHO (Med.) Middlx. Hosp. Lond.; Ho. Off. (Med.) Roy. Vict. Infirm. Newc. u. Tyne.

NICHOLSON, Paul James Procter & Gamble, Whitehall Lane, Egham TW20 9NW Tel: 01784 474612 Fax: 01784 474547 — MB BS Newc. 1981; MFOM RCP Lond. 1992, AFOM 1986; MRCGP 1986; DAvMed FOM RCP Lond. 1990; FFOM RCP Lond. 1998; FRCP RCP London 2001. Assoc. Med. Director, Procter & Gamble. Specialty: Occupat. Health; Occupational Medicine. Special Interest: Occupational Asthma, Ergonomics. Socs: Soc. Occup. Med. (Past Pres. & Past Asst. Edr.). Prev: Occupat. Phys. ICI Chem. & Polymers Ltd. Teeside; Sqd. Ldr. RAF Med. Br.

NICHOLSON, Mr Richard Arthur Roselind, 3 Back Lane, Whizley YO26 8BG Tel: 01423 339902 Fax: 01423 339903 — MRCS Eng. LRCP Lond. 1963 (Guy's) FRCS Glas. 1972. Cons. Orthop. in Medico-Legal Pract. Specialty: Orthop. Prev: Cons. Orthop. Pontefract Gen. Infirm.; Sen. Regist. Orthop. Middlesbrough Gen. Hosp.; Orthop. Regist. Bradford Roy. Infirm.

NICHOLSON, Richard Hugh 6 Gallia Road, London N5 1LA Tel: 020 7359 8803 — (Oxf. & Lond. Hosp.) MA, BM BCh Oxf. 1974; DCH RCPS Glas. 1977. Edr. Bull. Med. Ethics. Socs: Fell. Roy. Soc. Med. (Pres. Open Sect.); Brit. Paediat. Assn. Prev: Clin. Med. Off. (Child Health) Tower Hamlets Health Dist.; Leverhulme Research Fell. in Med. Ethics; Regist. (Paediat. Audiol.) Roy. Nat. Throat, Nose & Ear Hosp. Lond.

NICHOLSON, Mr Robert Dunning (retired) Heale Cottage, Dunster, Minehead TA24 6RT Tel: 01643 821330 — MB BS Lond. 1947 (St. Bart.) MRCS Eng. LRCP Lond. 1943; FRCS Eng. 1956. Assoc. Specialist (Gen. Surg.) W. Som. Hosp. Gp. Prev: Surg. Regist. Vict. Hosp. Swindon.

NICHOLSON, Robert Gordon (retired) Meadow View, Holt Lane, Holt, Wimborne BH21 7DQ Tel: 01202 884292 — MB BS Lond. 1949 (Guy's) DObst RCOG 1953; FRCGP 1979, M 1965. Prev: Outpat. Off., Childr. Ho. Phys. & Res. Obstetr. Guy's Hosp.

NICHOLSON, Robert Stephen Barn Surgery, Hill Road, Watlington, Oxford OX49 5AF Tel: 01491 612444 Fax: 01491 613988; Forelands, 26 Hill Road, Watlington, Oxford OX44 5AD — BM BCh Oxf. 1976; BA Camb. 1974; MA, BM BCh Oxf. 1976; MRCGP 1981. GP Princip.; Bd. Mem. S.E. Oxf. PCG.

NICHOLSON, Mr Robert William Blackburn Royal Infirmary, Department of General Surgery, Bolton Road, Blackburn BB2 3LR; Ellisland, Station Road, Hoghton, Preston PR5 0DD — MB ChB Manch. 1971; FRCS Eng. 1976; MD Manch. 1980. Cons. Surg. Blackburn Roy. Infirm. Specialty: Gen. Surg. Prev: Sen. Regist. (Surg.) N. West. RHA; Regist. (Surg.) Bury Gen. Hosp.; C.P. Zochonis Research Schol. Manch. Roy. Infirm.

NICHOLSON, Roger David 72 Longwestgate, Scarborough YO11 1RG — MB ChB Leeds 1973; MRCPsych 1979.

NICHOLSON, Sandra 24 Townfoot Court, Carlisle Road, Brampton CA8 1SP Tel: 016977 3363 — MB ChB Leic. 1988; MRCGP 1993.

NICHOLSON, Sarah Mary 1 Wharf Hill, Winchester SO23 9NQ — MB BS Lond. 1986; Dip. Obst. Auckland 1989; DGM RCP Lond. 1990; MRCPsych 1993; DCH RCP Lond. 1994. Staff Grade Child Psychiat. Soton. Specialty: Child & Adolesc. Psychiat. Prev: Clin. Med. Off. (Child Psychiat.) Centr. Health Clinic Soton.; Regist. Rotat. (Psychiat.) Soton. HA.

NICHOLSON, Simon St. John's Hospital, Livingston, Edinburgh; Richmond, 13 Dreghorn Loan, Edinburgh EH13 0DF — MB BChir Camb. 1989; MD Camb. 1995; MRCOG 1995. Cons., St. John's Hosp., Livingston. Specialty: Obst. & Gyn. Prev: Regist. (O & G) Simpson Memor. Matern. Pavil. Edin.; Research Fell. Nuffield Dept. O & G John Radcliffe Matern. Hosp. Oxf.; SHO (O & G) John Radcliffe Matern. Hosp. Oxf.

NICHOLSON, Simon Dennis Fairfield Cottage, 8 Barbican Road, Barnstaple EX32 9HW — MB BS Lond. 1982; BSc (Hons.) Lond. 1978, MB BS 1982; DGM RCP Lond. 1986. Liaison (Psychiat.) Lewisham Hosp. Lond.

NICHOLSON, Spencer Pendlebury Health Centre, Nelson Fold Medical Centre, 659 Bolton Road, Manchester M27 8HP — MB ChB Leeds 1988. GP Princip. Swinton; Staff Grade (A & E) Chorley Dist. Gen. Hosp. Specialty: Gen. Pract. Prev: SHO (Elderly Med. & O & G) Bolton Dist. Gen. Hosp.

NICHOLSON, Mr Stewart Department of Surgery, York District Hospital, Wigginton Road, York YO31 8HE Tel: 01904 631313 Email: snicholson@doctors.org.uk — MB BS (Hons.) Newc. 1980; FRCS Eng. 1985; MD Newc. 1989. Cons. in Breast, Endocrine and Gen. Surg., York Hosp. Specialty: Gen. Surg. Special Interest: Endocrine Surg.; Oncoplastic Breast Surg. Socs: Assn. of Breast Surg.; Brit. Assn. of Surgic. Oncol.; Brit. Assn. of Endocrine Surgeons. Prev: Cons. Surg., Weston Gen. Hosp., Weston Super Mare; Lect. in Surg., Univ. of Bristol.

NICHOLSON, Teresa Felicity Claremont Medical Practice, Exmouth Health Centre, Claremont Grove, Exmouth EX8 2JF Tel: 01395 273001 Fax: 01395 273771; 13 Green Close, Exmouth EX8 3QH — MB ChB Bristol 1983; MRCGP 1987; DRCOG 1987. Clin. Asst. (Learning Disabil.) Exmouth. Socs: BMA. Prev: Trainee GP Exeter VTS; Ho. Phys. N. Devon Dist. Hosp. Barnstaple; Ho. Surg. MusGr. Pk. Hosp. Taunton.

NICHOLSON, Tonia Chrisula 35 Maidwell Way, Laceby Acres, Grimsby DN34 5UP Tel: 01475 752655 — MB BS Lond. 1992; BSc (Psych.) Lond. 1989; MRCP Ed. 1995. Regist. (ED) Sir Chas. Gairdrer Hosp., Perth, WA. Specialty: Accid. & Emerg. Prev: Regist. (Gen. Med.) Waikato Hosp. Hamilton, NZ; Regist. (Paediat.) ChristCh. Pub. Hosp. ChristCh., NZ; SHO (Med.) Bradford.

NICHOLSON, William Dallas (retired) Brookwood, 3 Brookwood Avenue, Sale M33 5BZ Tel: 0161 962 2172 — (Aberd.) MB ChB Aberd. 1949. Prev: Ho. Phys. Aberd. Roy. Infirm.

NICHOLSON-LAILEY, Thomas John Francis Dr Robson and Partners, Manzil Way, Cowley Road, Oxford OX4 1XD Tel: 01865 242109; 52 Aston Street, Oxford OX4 1EP — MB BS Lond. 1982; MA Camb. 1983; DRCOG 1986; MRCGP 1987.

NICHOLSON ROBERTS, Timothy Charles, Capt. RAMC Church House, Withington, Hereford HR1 3QE Tel: 01432 850260 — MB BS Lond. 1996 (Charing Cross and Westminster) BSc Lond. 1994. RMO 4 Regt. RA. Prev: SHO, A & E, RH Haslar; Ho. Off. Med, Char. Cross Hosp.; Ho. Off. Surg MDHU Derriford.

NICKALLS, Richard William Dye Department of Anaesthesia, City Hospital, Nottingham NG5 1PB — MB BS Lond. 1974 (Guy's) BSc (1st cl. Hons. Physics in Med.) Lond. 1971; FFA RCS Eng. 1979; PhD Leeds 1989. Cons. Anaesth. City Hosp. Nottm. Specialty: Anaesth. Socs: Mathematical Assn.; Soc. Computing & Technol. in Anaesth.; Hist. Anaesth. Soc. Prev: Sen. Lect. (Anaesth.) Univ. Nottm.; Sen. Regist. (Anaesth.) Newc. u. Tyne; MRC Research Fell. (Cardiovasc. Stud.) Leeds Univ.

NICKELLS, James Shaughn Sonamar, East Shalford Lane, Guildford GU4 8AF — MB BS Lond. 1990.

NICKERSON, Mr Christopher Bruce Sighthill Health Centre, 380 Calder Road, Edinburgh EH11 4AU Tel: 0161 998 3206 Fax: 0161 945 9173; 16 Palatine Crescent, Didsbury, Manchester M20 3LL — MB ChB Ed. 1982; FRCS Glas. 1987; FRCS Ed. 1987; DRCOG 1990; DCH RCP Lond. 1991; MRCGP 1992. GP Manch.

NICKERSON, Susan Mary 96 Craiglea Drive, Edinburgh EH10 5PH Tel: 0131 446 0628 — MB ChB Manch. 1989 (St. And. Manch.) MRCOG 1994. GP Regist. (Locum). Specialty: Obst. & Gyn. Prev: Regist. (O & G) Stepping Hill Hosp.

NICKFORD, Claire Louise — MB ChB Aberd. 1998.

NICKLESS, Stephen James — MB BS Lond. 1976 (St Marys Hospital London) DA Eng. 1978; MRCGP 1983; DTM & H RCP Lond. 1983; DRCOG 1984; T(GP) 1991. GP Asst., Brondesbury Med. Centre, Lond. NW6. Prev: SHO (Anaesth. & A & E) St. Richards Hosp. Chichester; SHO (Paediat.) City Gen. Hosp. Stoke-on-Trent.

NICKLIN, Michael John (retired) Caskgate Street Surgery, 3 Caskgate Street, Gainsborough DN21 2DJ Tel: 01427 612501 Fax: 01427 615459 — (Lond. Hosp.) MRCS Eng. LRCP Lond. 1964; MB BChir Camb. 1966; DIH Eng. 1969.

NICKLIN, Sean 85 Gorsey Lane, Cannock WS11 1EX — MB ChB Liverp. 1991.

NICKOL, Kenneth Hugh 415 Baddow Road, Great Baddow, Chelmsford CM2 7QL Tel: 01245 471349 Fax: 01245 477759 — MB BS Lond. 1946 (Lond. Hosp.) DIH Eng. 1963; FRCP Lond. 1974; FFOM RCP Lond. 1979; FRIPHH 1999. Specialty: Occupat. Health. Socs: Fell. Roy. Soc. Med.; Soc. Occupat. Med.; fFell.Roy.Inst..Pub.Health & Hyg. Prev: Sen. Med. Off. Ford Motor Company; Sen. Regist. Camb. Chest Clinic; Regist. (Med.) Brompton Hosp.

NICKSON, Harold (retired) 20 Hazlewood Road, Duffield, Derby DE56 4DQ Tel: 01332 841070 — MB ChB Manch. 1956; DObst RCOG 1959; MRCGP 1969.

NICKSON, Jack Warren Down, Peasemore, Newbury RG20 7JL Tel: 01635 248331 Fax: 01635 248331 — (King's Coll. Hosp.) MB BS Lond. 1953; MRCS Eng. LRCP Lond. 1953; DObst RCOG 1955. Phys. (Orthop.) Newbury. Specialty: Orthop.; Sports Med. Socs: Brit. Inst. Musculoskel. Med. Prev: Ho. Surg. (Cas.) King's Coll. Hosp. Lond.; Ho. Phys. Sutton & Cheam Gen. Hosp.; Ho. Off. (Obst.) Luton Matern. Hosp.

NICKSON, Paul Jeffrey Victoria Place Surgery, 11 Victoria Place, Bethesda, Bangor LL57 3AG Tel: 01248 600212 Fax: 01248 602790; 3 Cwlyn, Braichmelyn, Bethseda, Bangor LC57 3RG Tel: 01248 601627 — MB BS Lond. 1976 (Westminster) MRCS Eng. LRCP Lond. 1976; MFHom 1976; MSc (Nutrit.) Lond. 1978; DCH Eng. 1980; DRCOG 1981; MRCGP 1983. Clin. Asst. (Chronic Fatigue Syndrome Serv.) Eryn Hosp. Caernarfon; Clin. Asst. (Homoeop.) Colwyn Bay; Clin. Asst. (Subst. Misuse) Ysbyty Gwynedd Bangor. Specialty: Gen. Pract. Prev: GP Trainee Hayes; SHO (Obst.) Southmead Hosp. Bristol; SHO (Paediat.) Bronglais Gen. Hosp. Aberystwyth.

NICOL, Alan Peter Mayberry, CBE, LVO (retired) 11 Churchill Road, Whitchurch, Tavistock PL19 9BU Tel: 01822 614698 — (Camb. & King's Coll. Hosp.) BA Camb. 1940; MRCS Eng. LRCP Lond. 1943; DA Eng. 1956; FFA RCSI 1965; FFA RCS Eng. 1966. Prev: Cons. Anaesth. PeterBoro. Dist. Hosp.

NICOL, Alastair McPherson, Maj. RAMC Penanjong Garrison, RBAF (LS) BFPO 605 Tel: 00 673 4 233094 Fax: 00 673 4 233094; c/o Nicol, 10 Bridge Lane, Barnhill, Dundee DD5 2SZ Tel: 01382 779476 — MB ChB Dundee 1988; DRCOG 1992; DFFP 1993; MRCGP 1993; Dip. IMC RCS Ed. 1995. HM Forces Med. Off. Specialty: Gen. Pract.

NICOL, Alexander (retired) The Glebe House, Badgeworth, Cheltenham GL51 4UL Tel: 01452 712159 — MD Aberd. 1962; MD (Commend.) Aberd. 1962, MB ChB 1949; FRCPath 1976, M 1964. Prev: Hon. Cons. Path. Glos. Roy. Hosp. & Cheltenham Gen. Hosp.

NICOL, Alexandra Elizabeth Shona — MB BS Lond. 1998.

NICOL, Andrew The Surgery, 61 Wheatway, Abbeydale, Gloucester GL4 5ET Tel: 01452 383323 — MB ChB Sheff. 1977; DRCOG 1980; MFHom 1989. Clin. Asst. (Geriat. Med.) Glos. HA.

NICOL, Andrew Kingfisher House, Hellesdon Hospital, Norwich NR12 0BL Tel: 01603 421608 — MB ChB Sheff. 1986; MRCPsych 1990. Cons. Psychiat., Gen. & Community, Norf. Ment. Healthcare Trust, Norwich; Cons. Psychiat. To Home Treatm. of Crisis Resolution Serv., Norf. Specialty: Gen. Psychiat. Socs: Brit. Assoc. of PsychoPharmacol. Prev: Sen. Regist. (Psychiat.) Roy. Hallamsh. Sheff.; Research Fell., Bristol; Psychiat. Trainee (Sen/Reg.), Glenside Hosp. Bristol.

NICOL, Andrew Edward Leslie 42 Sutherland Avenue, Cuffley, Potters Bar EN6 4EQ — MB BS Lond. 1975; FFA RCS Eng. 1980. Specialty: Anaesth.

NICOL, Anne Department of Pathology, Leighton Hospital, Crewe CW1 4QS Tel: 01270 255141 — MB ChB Dundee 1977; MRCPath. 1984; Dip. Health Mgt. Keele 1994; FRCPath 1995. Cons. Path. Leighton Hosp. Crewe. Specialty: Pathology, General.

NICOL, Professor Arthur Rory WHO Collaborating Centre, Institute of Psychiatry, De Crespigny Park, London SE5 Tel: 020 7919 2546; 27 Springcroft Avenue, London N2 9JH Tel: 020 8883 8691 Fax: 020 8020 8883 8691 Email: rorynicol@lineone.net — (Univ. Coll. Hosp.) M Phil Lond. 1970, BSc 1960, MB BS 1963; FRCP 1985, M 1967; FRCPsych. 1981 M 1972; FRCPCH 1996. Vis. Prof. Inst. Psych. Lond. Specialty: Child & Adolesc. Psychiat. Prev: Prof. Cild Psychiat. Univ. Leicester.

NICOL, Barbara Jane Lapworth Surgery, Old Warwick Road, Lapworth, Solihull B94 6LH Tel: 01564 783983 Email: bjnicol@doctors.org.uk — MB ChB Birm. 1978; DRCOG 1980; MRCGP 1982. Specialty: Gen. Pract. Prev: Trainee GP E. Birm. VTS; Ho. Surg. Dudley Rd. Hosp. Birm.; Ho. Phys. E. Birm. Hosp.

NICOL, Barbara Josephine (retired) 194 Kimbolton Road, Bedford MK41 8DP Tel: 01234 353579 — (Manch.) MB ChB Manch. 1949; DCH Eng. 1953.

NICOL, Denys Bewdley The Swan Medical Centre, 4 Willard Road, Yardley, Birmingham B25 8AA Tel: 0121 706 0216 Fax: 0121 707 3105; Field House, 261 Blossomfield Road, Solihull B91 1TA Tel: 0121 705 3337 — MB BChir Camb. 1966 (Camb. & Char. Cross) MA, MB Camb. 1966, BChir 1965; DCH Eng. 1968; DObst RCOG 1968. Prev: SHO (Paediat.) Jenny Lind Hosp. Norwich; SHO (O & G) Ipswich & E. Suff. Hosp.; Family Pract. Sen. Resid. Fairview Hosp. Minneapolis, USA.

NICOL, Douglas Robert Hamilton Mintlaw Group Practice, Newlands Road, Mintlaw, Peterhead AB42 5GP Tel: 01771 623522 Fax: 01771 624349; 2 Anderson Drive, Longside, Peterhead AB42 4XG Tel: 01779 821560 — MB ChB Aberd. 1977; BMedBiol 1974; DRCOG 1980; MRCGP 1982. GP Mintlaw, Peterhead.; Hon. Tutor Univ. Aberd. Socs: Peterhead & Dist. Med. Soc. Prev: Trainee Asst. Peterhead Health Centre; Research Fell. (O & G) Univ. Aberd. SHO Aberd. Matern.; Hosp., Kingseat Hosp. & Roy. Aberd. Childr. Hosp.

NICOL, Eben Russell Macmillan (retired) 26 Mytchett Heath, Mytchett, Camberley GU16 6DP Tel: 01252 376571 — (St. Mungo's Coll. Glas.) LRCP LRCS Ed. LRFPS Glas. 1945. Prev: Ho. Surg. Glas. Roy. Infirm.

NICOL, Edith Fiona 11 West Carnethy Avenue, Edinburgh EH13 0ED Tel: 0131 225 9191 Fax: 0131 226 6549 — MB BS Lond. 1976; MRCS (Eng.); BSc (Hons.) Lond. 1973; LRCP Lond. 1976; MRCP (UK) 1979; MRCGP 1982; FRCP Ed. 1999. Director of Studies. Specialty: Gen. Med. Prev: Sen. Lect. Med. Educat. Univ. Edin.; Assoc. Adviser SE Scotl. Comm. for Postgrad. Med. & Dent. Educat.

NICOL, Gavin Lindsay James 34 Copstone Drive, Dorridge, Solihull B93 8DJ — MB ChB Birm. 1994; ChB Birm. 1994.

NICOL, Gillian Jane Catherine 30 Victoria Road, Grangemouth FK3 9JN Tel: 01324 486696 — MB ChB Ed. 1998; MRCGP; DFFP; DRCOG. Specialty: Gen. Pract.

NICOL, John (retired) 12 London Road, Kilmarnock KA3 7AE; 49 London Road, Kilmarnock KA3 7AG Tel: 23593 — MB ChB Glas. 1961.

NICOL, John William Maryhill Practice, Elgin Health Centre, Maryhill, Elgin IV30 1AT Tel: 01343 543788 Fax: 01343 551604 — MB ChB Ed. 1988; MRCGP 1995.

NICOL, Keith Mill Farm, Brigg Road, South Kelsey, Market Rasen LN7 6PH — MB BS Lond. 1969; St. Geo.).

NICOL, Kirstie M Barcaldine, Strathearn Terrace, Crieff PH7 3BZ.

NICOL, Leslie George (retired) 194 Kimbolton Road, Bedford MK41 8DP Tel: 01234 353579 — MRCS Eng. LRCP Lond. 1947 (Manch.) DPM Manch. 1950, DPH 1956. Prev: Community Phys. (Liaison Social Servs.) Beds. AHA.

NICOL, Malcolm John Manning Field House, 261 Blossom Field Road, Solihull B91 1TA — MB BS Lond. 1998.

NICOL, Margaret Elizabeth 6 Weybridge Walk, Shoeburyness, Southend-on-Sea SS3 8YJ — MB ChB Aberd. 1982; DA (UK) 1985; FFA RCS Eng. 1988. Specialty: Anaesth.

NICOL, Mark Fergus 30 Hertford Close, Congleton CW12 1TB — MB ChB Manch. 1987; BSc (Med. Sci.) St. And. 1984. Regist. Rotat. (Anaesth.) Stoke-on-Trent. Prev: SHO (Anaesth.) Wythenshawe Hosp. & Oldham Hosps.; SHO (A & E) Hope Hosp. Manch.

NICOL, Mrs Mary (retired) 8 Rowley Crescent, Stratford-upon-Avon CV37 6UT Tel: 01789 205084 — (Middlx.) MB BChir Camb. 1959; MA Camb. 1959. Prev: Cas. Off. Stratford-upon-Avon Gen. Hosp.

NICOL, Norman Thomas, OBE, TD Bracken Rigg, 5 Egton Road, Aislaby, Whitby YO21 1SU — MB ChB Aberd. 1950; DMRT Eng. 1954; FFR 1959; FRCR 1975. Emerit. Radiother. Leicester HA. Socs: Fell. Roy. Soc. Med.; BMA. Prev: Radiother. i/c Dept. Radiother. Roy. Infirm. Leic.; Assoc. Cons. Nat. Centre for Radiother.; Clin. Tutor. Fac. of Med. Univ. Leic.

NICOL, Peter Alan Bangor Health Centre, Newtownards Road, Bangor BT20 4LD Tel: 02891 515222 Fax: 02891 515397; 40 Sheridan Drive, Helens Bay, Bangor BT19 1LB Tel: 01247 853528 — MB BCh BAO Belf. 1982; DRCOG 1984; MRCGP 1986; DCH Dub. 1987. Socs: BMA.

NICOL, Rhoderic Eion Lapworth Surgery, Old Warwick Road, Lapworth, Solihull B94 6LH Tel: 01564 783983 — MB ChB Birm. 1978; DRCOG 1980; MRCGP 1982. Specialty: Gen. Pract. Prev: Trainee GP E. Birm. VTS; Ho. Surg. E. Birm. Hosp.; Ho. Phys. Dudley Rd. Hosp. Birm.

NICOL, Robert John Auld (retired) Mountain Ash, Viewlands Avenue, Off Grays Road, Westerham TN16 2JE Tel: 01959 532893 — (St. And.) MB ChB (Commend.) St. And. 1947. Prev: Regist. (Med.) Roy. Infirm. Perth.

NICOL, Stephen Graham 27 The Gallolee, Edinburgh EH13 9QL — MB ChB Ed. 1997.

NICOL, William Alan (retired) 24 Abbots Way, Doonfoot, Ayr KA7 4EY — MB ChB Glas. 1954; MRCGP 1966; MFCM RCP (UK) 1982; MFPHM RCP (UK) 1989. Prev: Cons. Pub. Health Med. Ayrsh. & Arran HB.

NICOL, Mr William James (retired) Abbey Royd, Bridge St., Kelso TD5 7JE Tel: 01573 25052 — (St. And.) MB ChB St. And. 1958; FRCS Ed. 1968; BA Open 1987; MSc (Afr. Studies) Ed. 1996. Prev: Sen. Regist. (Orthop.) Dundee Roy. Infirm.

NICOLA, Kyriacos Panayioutou 20 Woodland Way, London N21 3QA — MB BS Lond. 1998.

NICOLAIDES, Professor Kyprianos Herodotou 107 Alleyn Park, London SE21 8AA — MB BS Lond. 1978; BSc Lond. 1974; MRCOG 1984. Prof. Fetal Med. Univ. Lond. Specialty: Obst. & Gyn. Prev: Lect. Harris Birthright Research Centre for Fetal Med. King's Coll. Hosp. Med. Sch. Lond.

NICOLAIDES, Paulina Child Development Centre, Royal Liverpool Children's NHS Trust, Alder Road, Liverpool L12 2AP; Raby Glen, Blakeley Dell, Raby Mere, Wirral CH63 0NJ Tel: 0151 343 0573 Email: pnicolaides@btinternet.com — MB ChB Manch. 1985; MRCP (UK) 1991. Cons.. (Paediat. Neurol.) The Roy. Liverp. Childr.'s NHS Trust. Specialty: Paediat. Neurol. Socs: Brit. Paediat. Assn.; Paediat. Neurol. Assn. (BPNA); Europ. Paed. Neurol. Soc. (EPNS). Prev: Sen. Regist. (Paediat. Neurol.) The Roy. Liverp. Childr.'s NHS Trust; Regist. (Paediat. Neurol.) Roy. Manch. Childr. Hosp.; Regist. (Intens. Care) Hosp. for Sick Childr. Gt. Ormond St. Lond.

NICOLAOU, Andrew John St Georges Hospital, Blackshaw Road, London SW17 0QT — MB BS Lond. 1990 (Kings Coll. Hosp.) FRCA; BSc (Hons) Lond. 1997. Cons. (Anaes) St Geo.'s Hosp, Atkinson Morley's Hosp.& Trinity Hospice, Clapham Lond.; Cons. (Pain Specialist) St. Geo. Hosp., Atkinson Morley's Hosp.& Trinity Hospice, Clapham Lond. Specialty: Anaesth. Socs: Pain. Soc. Prev: Clin. Pain Fell. Guy's & St Thomas' Hosp.; Specialist Regist. (Anaesth.) Guy's Hosp.

NICOLAOU, Anthony Christopher Whaddon Way Surgery, 293 Whaddon Way, Bletchley, Milton Keynes MK3 7LW Tel: 01908 375341 Fax: 01908 374975 — MB BS Lond. 1981; DRCOG 1988.

NICOLAU, Marios — BM BS Nottm. 1998.

NICOLE, Thomasina Mary Street Farm, South Brewham, Bruton BA10 0JZ Tel: 01749 850524 Fax: 01749 850876 — MB BS Lond. 1975 (St. Thos.) MA Oxf. 1977; MRCPCH 1996. Assoc. Specialist (Paediat.) Yeovil Dist. Hosp. Specialty: Paediat. Socs: Brit. Assn. Preven. Child Abuse & Neglect. Prev: Clin. Asst. (Paediat. Med.) Yeovil Dist. Hosp.; SHO (Neonat. Paediat.) St. Thos. Hosp. Lond.; SHO (Paediat.) MusGr. Pk. Hosp. Taunton.

NICOLL, Angus Gordon Health Protection Agency, Communicable Disease Surveillance Centre, 61 Colindale Avenue, London NW9 5EQ Tel: 020 8200 6868 Fax: 020 8200 7868 Email: angus.nicoll@hpa.org.uk; 2 New House Park, St Albans AL1 1UB — MB Camb. 1977; BChir 1976; MRCP (Paediat.) (UK) 1980; MSc Epidemiol. Lond. 1986; MFPHM RCP (UK) 1996. Director Health Protec. Communicable Dis. Surveillance Centre Lond.; Prof. Univ. Lond. Specialty: Pub. Health Med. Socs: Med. Soc. Study VD; Fell. RCP. Prev: Sen. Lect. Lond. Sch. Hyg. & Trop. Med. Univ. Lond.

NICOLL, Ann Middleton (retired) Westlands, Eyemouth TD14 5BZ Tel: 018907 51040 — MB ChB Ed. 1955 (Edinburgh) Prev: Gen. Practioner Eyemouth Berwicksh.

NICOLL, David 2 Nevis Place, Broughty Ferry, Dundee DD5 3EL — MB ChB Dundee 1998.

NICOLL, David Melville Lister House, 473 Dunstable Road, Luton LU4 8DG Tel: 01582 571565 Fax: 01582 582074 — MB ChB Birm. 1958; BSc Queensld. 1972. Socs: BMA.

NICOLL, Derek Alan Proctor, Wing Cdr. RAF Med. Br. Retd. Menwith Hill Station, Menwith Hill, Harrogate HG3 2RF Tel: 01423 777885; Greenbanks, 5 Westgate, Rillington, Malton YO17 8LN Tel: 01944 758740 — MB ChB Dundee 1979; BSc (Hons.) Biochem. Dundee 1974; Cert. Occupat. Health Aberd. 1992. Med. Off. Prev: Sen. Med. Off. RAF Linton-on-Ouse, York.

NICOLL, Frederick James (retired) Westlands, Coldingham Road, Eyemouth TD14 5BZ Tel: 018907 51040 Email: fred.nicoll@exmouth.demon.co.uk — MB ChB Ed. 1956. Prev: GP Eyemouth Berwicksh.

NICOLL, James Alan Ramsay Department of Neuropathology, Institute of Neurological Sciences, Southern General Hospital, Glasgow G51 4TF Tel: 0141 201 2046 Fax: 0141 201 2998 Email: j.nicoll@clinmed.gla.ac.uk — MB ChB Bristol 1984; BSc (Physiol.) Bristol 1981, MD 1993, MB ChB 1984; MRCPath 1990. Cons. Sen. Lect. Neuropath. Glas. Univ. Specialty: Neuropath.

NICOLL, Janet Alison 8 Claremont Crescent, Edinburgh EH7 4HX — MB ChB Ed. 1988.

NICOLL, John Martin Vere 2 Manor Park, Hougham, Grantham NG32 2JJ Tel: 0140 025 0508 Fax: 01400 250508 Email: martinnic@btinternet.com; 2 Manor Park, Hougham, Grantham NG32 2JJ Tel: 0140 025 0508 Fax: 01400 250508 — MB BS Lond. 1965; MCRS Eng. LRCP Lond. 1965; DRCOG 1970. Cons. Anaesth. Univ. Hosp. Nottm. Specialty: Anaesth. Prev: Cons. Anaesth. King Fahad Nat. Guard Hosp., K. Khaled Eye Specialist Hosp. Riyadh & St. Jas. Univ. Hosp. Leeds; Princip. Anaesth. Johannesburg Hosp., S. Africa.

NICOLL, Jonathan James Bankdale Park, Wreay, Carlisle CA4 0RR — MB BS Lond. 1977 (Westm.) BA Camb. 1974, MA 1980; MRCP (UK) 1981; FRCR 1987; FRCP 1999. Cons. Radiother. & Oncol. Cumbld. Infirm. Carlisle. Specialty: Oncol.; Radiother.

NICOLL, Kirsteen Sheonagh Royal Camhill Hospital, Camhill Hospital, Aberdeen AB25 2RQ Tel: 01224 663131; The Bungalow, Hardhillock, Marycutler, Aberdeen AB12 5GQ Tel: 01224 733545 Email: kirsteen@tmcnamee.freeserve.co.uk — MB ChB Aberd. 1993; MRC Psych 1999. Specialist Regist. Roy. Cornhill Hosp. Aberd. Specialty: Gen. Psychiat. Prev: Locum GP Brisbane, Austral., SHO (Psychiat.) Roy. Cornhill Hosp. Aberd.; SHO (Surg.) Stirling; SHO (Med.) Inverness.

NICOLL, Lorna May West Gate Health Centre, Charleston Drive, Dundee DD2 4AD Tel: 01382 668189 Fax: 01382 665943 — MB ChB Dundee 1981; MRCGP 1985.

NICOLL, Sheila Margaret Ninewells Hospital & Medical School, Cytopathology, Directorate of Pathology, Dundee DD1 9SY Tel: 01382 633943 Fax: 01382 496215 Email: sheila.nicoll@tuht.scot.nhs.uk — MB ChB Dundee 1978; MRCPath 1989; FRCPath 1996. Cons. Cytol. Ninewells Hosp. & Med. Sch. Cons Cytopathologist Ninewells Hosp Dundee. Specialty: Pathology, General. Socs: Scott. Assn. Clin. Cytol.; Brit. Soc. Clin. Cytol.; Internat. Acad. Path. Prev: Sen. Regist. (Histopath.) John Radcliffe Hosp. Oxf.; Lect. (Path.) Ninewells Hosp. Dundee.

NICOLL, Stephanie Jane Barnes Eastbourne District General Hospital, Kings Drive, Eastbourne BN21 2UD Tel: 01323 413745 — MB ChB Glas. 1984 (Univ. Glas.) DA (UK) 1986; FFA RCS Eng. 1989. Cons. (anaesth.), Eastbourne Dist. Gen. Hosp. Specialty: Anaesth. Prev: Sen. Regist. (Anaesth.) Qu. Vict. Hosp. E. Grinstead.; Sen. Regist. (Anaesth.) Gt. Ormond St. Hosp. Sick Childr. Lond.; Sen. Regist. (Anaesth.) Guy's Hosp. Lond.

NICOLL, William Douglas (retired) 8Lochpark, Ayr KA7 4EU Tel: 01292 441657 — MB ChB Glas. 1945 (Univ. Glas.) FRCPath 1966, M 1963; FRCP Glas. 1975, M 1972. Prev: Cons. Haematol. Ayrsh. Area.

NICOLL, William Sim Galston Surgery, 5A Henrietta Street, Galston KA4 8JW Tel: 01563 820424 Fax: 01563 822380 — MB ChB Ed. 1982; BSc Ed. 1979, MB ChB 1982; MRCGP 1986.

NICOLLE, Annette Louise Royal Victoria Infirmary, Queen Victoria Road, Newcastle upon Tyne NE1 4LP — MB BS Newc. 1996; MRCP Ed. 1999. SpR (Haematol.) Roy. Vict. Hosp. Newc. Upon Tyne. Specialty: Gen. Med. Socs: BMA; RCP (Ed.). Prev: SHO (Gen. Med.) N. Tees Gen. Hosp. Hardwick Stockton.

NICOLLE, Mr Frederick Villeneuve Knighton Farmhouse, Knighton Farmhouse, Ramsbury, Marlborough SN8 2QB Tel: 01672 520471 Fax: 01672 520471 Email: frederick.nicolle@btopenworld.com — MB Camb. 1957 (Camb. & Middlx.) BA Camb. 1953, MChir 1972, MB 1957, BChir 1956; LMCC 1958; FRCS Canada 1962. Cons. Plastic Surg. Hosp. St. John & Eliz. Lond. Specialty: Plastic Surg. Socs: (Pres.) Brit. Assn. Aesthetic Plastic Surgs.; (Treas.) Internat. Soc. Aesthetic Plastic Surgs.; Brit. Assn. Plastic Surg. Prev: Cons. Plastic Surg. Hammersmith Hosp. & Lect. (Surg.) Roy. Postgrad. Med. Sch. Lond.; Sen. Regist. (Plastic Surg.) Hammersmith Hosp. Lond.; Chief Resid. Plastic Surg. & Trauma Unit Montreal Gen. Hosp.

NICOLLE, Penelope Upper Folds, Little Bognor, Fittleworth, Pulborough RH20 1JT — MB BS Lond. 1989 (St. Geo. Hosp.) MRCGP Lond. 1993; DRCOG Lond. 1993. Socs: BMA (Ex.-Hon. Sec. Hong Kong Br.).

NICOLLS, David Bruce Hilltops Medical Centre, Kensington Drive, Great Holm, Milton Keynes MK8 9HN Tel: 01908 568446 — MB BS Lond. 1987; MRCGP 1991; T(GP) 1991.

NICOLSON, Andrew 1 Morton Carr Lane, Nunthorpe, Middlesbrough TS7 0JU — MB ChB Manch. 1995; MRCPI 1997. SHO (Gen. Med.). Specialty: Gen. Med. Prev: Med. Rotat. Countess of Chester Hosp.

NICOLSON, Anne West Suffolk Hospital, Hardwick Lane, Bury St Edmunds IP33 2QZ — MB BS Adelaide 1976; MRCP (UK) 1983.

NICOLSON, Anne Law Skerryvore Practice, Health Centre, New Scapa Road, Kirkwall KW15 1BQ Tel: 01856 885440 Fax: 01856 870043 — MB ChB Aberd. 1990. Trainee GP Kirkwall. Prev: SHO (O & G & A & E) St. Johns Hosp. Livingston; SHO (Psychiat.) Argyll & Bute Hosp. Lochgilphead.

NICOLSON, Bridget Ruth Leckhampton Surgery, Lloyd Davies House, 17 Moorend Park Road, Cheltenham GL53 0LA Tel: 01242 515363 Fax: 01242 253512 — MB ChB Bristol 1987; DRCOG 1991. GP Glos. VTS.

NICOLSON, Helen Stewart (retired) — MB ChB St. And. 1947 (Dundee) DPM Manch. 1960; Dip. Psychother. Aberd. 1966; MRCPsych 1971. Prev: Cons. (Child & Adolesc. Psychiat.) Tayside Health Bd.

NICOLSON, Joan MacPherson 32 Netherview Road, Glasgow G44 3XH — MB ChB Glas. 1962; DObst RCOG 1965; Cert FPA 1971, IUD 1972. Community Paediat. (Community Health) Yorkhill Trust Glas.; Clin. Med. Off. (Family Plann.) Well Wom. Serv. Greater Glas. HB. Socs: Assoc. Mem. Fac. Homoeop; BMA. Prev: GP Glas.; Regist. (Dermat.) Vict. Infirm. Glas.; SHO Redlands Hosp. Glas.

NICOLSON, John Andrew Devon Road Surgery, 32 Devon Road, South Darenth, Dartford DA4 9AB Tel: 01322 862121 Fax: 01322 868794; Griffins, Sparepenny Lane, Eynsford, Dartford DA4 0JJ Tel: 01322 862977 Fax: 01322 868794 Email: johnandrewnicolson@lineone.net — MB BS Lond. 1972 (King's Coll. Hosp.) MRCS Eng. LRCP Lond. 1972; MRCGP 1980; FRCGP 1998. Clin. Governance Lead, Dartford, Gravesend and Swanley PCT.; Exec. Bd. Mem., Dartford, Gravesend and Swanley P.C.T.; Vice Chairm., W. Kent L.M.C. Prev: Course Organiser NW Kent Postgrad. Centre, Dartford & Gravesham VTS; Trainee GP Dartford VTS; Assoc. Adviser (Gen. Pract.) W. Kent.

NICOLSON, Kenneth Thomas (retired) The Old Rectory, West Camel, Yeovil BA22 7QB Tel: 01935 850214 — MB BS Lond. 1957 (Guy's) Prev: GP Qu. Camel.

NICOLSON, Marianne Coutts Anchor Unit, Aberdeen Royal Infirmary, Foresterhill, Aberdeen AB25 2ZN Tel: 01224 681818 Fax: 01224 554183 Email: m.nicolson@arh.grampian.scot.nhs.uk — MB ChB Ed. 1982; BSc (Med. Biol.) Ed. 1979; MRCP (UK) 1985; FRCP (Ed.) 1996; MD Edin. 1996. Cons. Med. Oncol. Aberd. Roy. Infirm. Specialty: Oncol. Socs: Assn. Cancer Phys.s(Treas.); Scott. Melanoma Gp. Prev: Sen. Regist. (Med. Oncol.) Roy. Marsden Hosp. Sutton.

NICPON, Mr Krzysztof Jozef 14 Meadowcroft Close, Otterbourne, Winchester SO21 2HD — BM (Hons.) Soton. 1984; FRCS Eng. 1988.

NICUM, Rupal 22 Alveston Gr, Knowle, Solihull B93 9NX — MB ChB Leic. 1997.

NICUM, Shibani 17 Kelton Court, Carpenter Road, Birmingham B15 2JX — MB ChB Birm. 1996; ChB Birm. 1996.

NIDA, Anne Mary Dunorlan Medical Group, 64 Pembury Road, Tonbridge TN9 2JG Tel: 01732 352907 Fax: 01732 367408; 24 Ridgeway Crescent, Tonbridge TN10 4NP Tel: 01732 362248 — MB BS Lond. 1977. GP Princip. Prev: GP Stansted.

NIEDER, Mary 636 Gleadless Rd, Sheffield S14 1PQ — MB ChB Sheff. 1995. GP Retainee Gleadless Med. Centre. Specialty: Gen. Pract. Prev: GP Regist. Chesterfield & N. Derbysh. Roy. Hosp.

NIELD, Mrs Dalia Virginia 149 Harley Street, London W1N 2DE Tel: 020 7935 4444 Fax: 020 7935 5091; 16 Wellfield Avenue, Muswell Hill, London N10 2EA Tel: 020 8883 1976 — Medico-Cirujano Andes Venezuela 1970; FRCS Ed. 1982; CSST(Plastic Surg.) 1991. Cons. Plastic & Reconstruc. Surg. The Lond. Clinic; Cons. Plastic Surg. Lond. Clinic; Recognised Teach. Univ. Lond. Specialty: Plastic Surg. Socs: Fell. Roy. Soc. Med. (Plastic Surg. Chapter); Brit. Assn. Plastic Surg.; Internat. Microsurg. Soc. Prev: Cons. Plastic Surg. St. Bart. & Homerton Hosps. Lond.; Sen. Regist. (Head, Neck and Breast Reconstruc. Surg.) Roy. Marsden Hosp.; Sen. Regist. & Regist. (Plastic Surg.) Wexham Pk. Hosp.

NIELSEN, Ebba 108 Station Road, Hampton TW12 2AS Tel: 020 8898 1696 Fax: 020 8898 1696 Email: nielsen@medical_vision@co.uk; Hans Place Practice, 43 Hans Place, Knightsbridge, London SW1X 0JZ Tel: 020 7584 1642 Fax: 020 7589 5862 — MD Copenhagen 1991; DFFP 1995; DRCOG 1997. GP Princip. Centr. Lond. Specialty: Gen. Pract.; Family Plann. & Reproduc. Health. Socs: BMA. Prev: Lizei GP Centr. Lond.; GP/Regist. Capelfield Surg. Esher; SHO (O & G) Qu. Mary's Hosp. Sidcup.

NIELSEN, Fiona 247 ThurnCt. Road, Leicester LE5 2NL Tel: 0116 243 2093; 247 Thurncourt Road, Leicester LE5 2NL Tel: 0116 243 2093 — MB ChB Ed. 1992 (Univ. Ed.) MRCPsych 2001. Staff Grade in Rehabil. Psychiat. Specialty: Gen. Psychiat. Socs: BMA; Mem. Roy. Coll. Psychiat. Prev: SHO (Liaison Psychiat.) Leicester Gen. Hosp.; SHO (Gen. Psychiat.) Leicester Gen. Hosp.; SHO (Therapeutic comm.) Francis Dixon Lodge, Leicester.

NIELSEN, Hugh John Village Medical Centre, 20 Quarry Street, Liverpool L25 6HE Tel: 0151 428 4282 Fax: 0151 421 0884; 25 Montclair Drive, Mossley Hill, Liverpool L18 0HA — BM BCh Oxf. 1979; MA Oxf. 1980, BM BCh 1979; MRCP (UK) 1986; MFHom 1990. Prev: Regist. (Med.) Roy. Liverp. Hosp.; Med. Dir. Outpats. Dept. Curtis Memor. Hosp. Newfld., Canada; SHO Roy. Brisbane Hosp. Austral.

NIELSEN, Karen Chinedu Grove Medical Group, 1 The Grove, Gosforth, Newcastle upon Tyne NE3 1NU Tel: 0191 210 6680 Fax: 0191 210 6682 — MB BS Newc. 1987; BMedSc Newc. 1984; MRCGP 1992; DRCOG 1992. Prev: Trainee GP Newc VTS.

NIELSEN, Karin Schoubo The Waterfield Practice, Ralphs Ride, Harmanswater, Bracknell RG12 9LH Tel: 01344 454626 Fax: 01344 303929 — MD Aarhus 1994.

NIELSEN, Michael Stewart Intensive Care Unit, Southampton General Hospital, Southampton SO16 6YD Tel: 023 8079 6117 Fax: 023 8079 4753; 7 Grosvenor Road, Chandlers Ford, Eastleigh SO53 5BU — MB BS Lond. 1971 (Guy's) MB BS (Hons., Distinc. Obst. & Gyn.) Lond. 1971; FFA RCS Eng. 1975. Cons. Anaesth. & Intens. Care Soton. Gen. Hosp. Specialty: Anaesth.

NIELSON, Paul Christian Okethampton Medical Centre, East Street, Okehampton EX20 1AY Tel: 01837 52233; The Glebe House, Exbourne, Okehampton EX20 3RD — MB BS Lond. 1985 (Charing Cross) BSc Lond. 1979, MB BS 1985; DRCOG 1988. GP Princip.; Hosp. Specialist (Gen. Med.). Specialty: Gen. Med.

NIEMAN, Eric Arnold (retired) 24 Woodside Avenue, London N6 4SS — (Liverp.) MB ChB Liverp. 1950; DCH Eng. 1952; FRCP Lond. 1974, M 1955; MD Liverp. 1958. Emeritus Cons. Neurol. St. Mary's Hosp. Lond. Prev: Cons. Neurol. St. Mary's, St. Chas. & Roy. Masonic Hosps. Lond.

NIEMCZUK, Peter Smith, Niemczuk, Puuirajasingham, 279-281 Mill Road, Cambridge CB1 3DG Tel: 01223 247812 Fax: 01223 214191 — MB ChB Leic. 1983.

NIEMIRO, Lorynda Aleksandra Krystyna Department of Anaesthetics, Frimley Park Hospital, Portsmouth Road, Frimley, Camberley GU16 7UJ Tel: 01276 604161; Oaklawn House, Star Hill Drive, Churt, Farnham GU10 2HP Tel: 01276 712207 — MB BS Lond. 1981 (St. Bartholomew's) DA (UK) 1986; FRCA 1989. Cons. Anaesth. Frimley Pk. Hosp. Surrey. Specialty: Anaesth. Prev: Cons. & Sen. Regist. (Anaesth.) Camb. Milit. Hosp.; Sen. Regist. (Anaesth.) Bristol & Frenchay Hosps.

NIEPEL, Graham Gerd — MB ChB Liverp. 1997.

NIESSER, Alison Janet Feddygfa Wen Surgery, Feddygfa Wen, Porthmadog LL49 4NU Tel: 01766 514207 Fax: 01766 514828 — MB BS Lond. 1979; MRCGP 1984.

NIESSER, Anton Arthur Fron Olau, Mersey St., Borth y Gest, Porthmadog LL49 9UB Tel: 01766 513041 Fax: 01766 514828; Y Feddygfa Wen, Hafod Y Gest, Porthmadog LL49 9NU Tel: 01766 514610 — State Exam Med Ulm 1978 (Ulm, Germany) MD Ulm 1980; T(GP) 1991. Specialty: Gen. Pract. Socs: Balint Soc.

NIETO VELILLAS, Jose Joaquin Norfolk & Norwich University Hospital, Colney Lane, Norwich NR4 7UZ Tel: 01603 288692 — LMS Saragossa 1986; BSc Saragossa 1987; MRCOG 1995. Specialty: Obst. & Gyn.

NIEVEL, John George Mayridge, 8 Brownlow Road, Croydon CR0 5JT Tel: 020 8681 0331 Fax: 020 8681 0331 — MD Budapest 1958; PhD Lond. 1967; FRIC 1976; FIBiol. 1976; FRSC 1980; FRCPI 1984, M 1981. Co-Dir. Dept. Clin. Pharmacol. & Therap. & The Hypertens. Unit & Sen. Regist. Roy. N. Hosp. Lond; Hon. Lect. (Med.) Acad. Dept. Med. Roy. Free Hosp. Sch. Med. Univ. Lond; Hon. Sen. Regist. Roy. Free Hosp. Lond. Specialty: Gen. Med.; Pharmacology. Prev: Dir. Med. Research Brit. Indust. Biol. Research Assn.; Sen. Clin. Research Fell. Dept. Med. King's Coll. Hosp. Med. Sch. Univ. Lond.; Prof. Clin. Pharmacol. & Therap. Jeddah Saudi Arabia.

NIEZYWINSKI, Wojciech Aleksander 36 Florence Road, West Bridgford, Nottingham NG2 5HR — Lekarz Gdansk 1984.

NIGAM, Mr Ajay Depart. Of Otolaryngology, Blackpool Victoria Hospital, Whinney Heys Road, Blackpool FY3 8NR Tel: 01253 306838 Email: nigam100@yahoo.com — MB BS Kanpur 1979; FRCS (Surg.) Ed. 1985; FRCS (Otol.) Ed. 1990; FRCS (Otol.) Lond 1990; FRCS (ORL) 1995. Sen. Regist. (Otolaryngol.) Freeman Hosp. Newc. upon Tyne; Cons. (OtoLaryngol.), Blackpool Vict. Hosp., Blackpool. Specialty: Otolaryngol. Socs: BMA & Otolaryngol. Research Soc. Prev: Regist. Rotat. (ENT) W. Midl.; SHO (ENT) Leicester Roy. Infirm.; Sen. Regist. (ENT), Freeman Hosp., Newc. Upon Tyne.

NIGAM, Mr Anurag Kishore Royal Surrey County Hospital, Dept. of Urol., Egerton Rd, Guildford GU2 7XX Tel: 01483 464045 Fax: 01483 402718 Email: raj.nigam@royalsurrey.nhs.uk — MB BS Lond. 1987 (Univ. Coll. Lond.) FRCS Eng. 1991; FRCS (Urol.) 1997; FEBU. 1998; MD Lond. 1999. Cons. Urological Surg., Roy. Surrey Co. Hosp., Guildford; Cons. Urological Surg. Specialty: Urol. Special Interest: Andrology; Male Infertility; Prostate Dis. Socs: Brit. Assn. of Urological Surg; Brit. Med. Assn.; Roy. Soc. of Med. Prev: Sen. Regist. (Urol.) St. Bart. Hosp. & Roy. Lond. Hosp.

NIGAM, Ashok Kumar Prince Philip Hospital, Bryngwynmawr, Dafen, Llanelli SA14 8QF Tel: 01554 756567; 83 Rhyd-y-Defaid Drive, Derwen Fawr, Swansea SA2 8AN Tel: 01792 296326 — MB BS Jabalpur 1969; DA Delhi 1973; FFA RCS 1978. Cons. Anaesth. P. Philip Hosp. Llanelli, Dyfed. Specialty: Anaesth. Prev: Cons. Anaesth. Llanelli Gen. Hosp. Dyfed; Regist. (Anaesth.) Singleton Hosp. Swansea & Univ. Hosp. Wales Cardiff.

NIGAM, Mr Keshav Mansfield Road, Sutton-in-Ashfield NG17 4JL Tel: 01623 622 515; Pytchley, Foxhole Road, Chelston, Torquay TQ2 6RY — MB BS Delhi 1983 (Maulana Azad Med. Coll. Delhi, India) MS (Gen. Surg.) Delhi 1986; FRCS Ed. 1991; FRCS Ed (Gen. Surg.) 2001. Cons. Surgeon,Kings Hill Hosp., Sutton-in-Ashfield. Specialty: Gen. Surg. Socs: Brit. Soc. Gastroenterol.; BMA. Prev: Regist. & SHO (Gen. Surg.) Torbay Hosp.; Regist. (Gen. Surg.) LNJPN Hosp. New Delhi; Staff Grade (Gen. Surg.) Torbay Hosp.

NIGAM, Ragni Wibsey and Queensbury Medical Practice, Fair Road, Wibsey, Bradford BD6 1TB Tel: 01274 677198 Fax: 01274 693389; 61 Hodgson Lane, Drighlington, Bradford BD11 1BW — MB BS Newc. 1988 (Univ. Newc. u. Tyne) DRCOG 1993. Partner Wibsey Med. Centre, Bradford; Clin. Asst. (Genito - Urin. Med.) St Lukes Hosp. Bradford. Specialty: Gen. Pract. Prev: Trainee GP Bradford Roy. Infirm. VTS.; SHO (Gen. Med., Microbiol. & Infec. Dis.) Hope Hosp. Salford.

NIGAM, Subhash Chandra 129 Straight Road, Harold Hill, Romford RM3 7JD Tel: 01708 342517; 94 Parkstone Avenue, Emerson Park, Hornchurch RM11 3LR Tel: 01708 455574 — MB BS Lucknow 1967 (G.S.V.M. Med. Coll. Kanpur) BSc Agra 1958.

NIGHTINGALE, Andrea Jane — MB ChB Ed. 1990; BSc (Med. Sci.) (Hons.) Ed. 1988; DRCOG 1994; MRCGP 1994. Prev: Trainee GP/SHO Carlisle VTS.

NIGHTINGALE, Angus Kullervo 12 Springfield Road, Portishead, Bristol BS20 6LH Tel: 01275 814016 — MB BChir Camb. 1993; MRCP (Lond) 1995. Specialty: Cardiol.

NIGHTINGALE, Anne Margaret Lansdowne Clinic, 3 Whittingehame Gardens, Great Western Road, Glasgow G12 0AA Tel: 0141 211 3558 Fax: 0141 232 0022 Email: anne.nightingale@glacomen.scot.nhs.uk — MB BChir Camb. 1980 (Cambridge University Addenbrooks Hosp) MA Camb. 1979; MRCPsych 1986. Cons. Psychotherapist Lansdowne Clinic Glas. Specialty: Psychother.

NIGHTINGALE, David Anthony — (Lond. Hosp.) BA Camb. 1954; MB BChir Camb. 1957; DA Eng. 1960; FRCA 1961. Emerit. Cons. Anaesth. Roy. Liverp. Childr. Hosp. Alder Hey. Specialty: Anaesth. Socs: Assn. Anaesth.; Assn. Paediat. Anaesth. Prev: Regional Educat. Adviser Coll. of Anaesth.; Dir. of Studies in Paediat. Anaesth. Univ. Liverp.; Sen. Fell. (Anaesth.) Childr. Hosp. Philadelphia, USA.

NIGHTINGALE, Doreen (retired) Flat 158, The White House, Albany St., London NW1 3UP — MRCS Eng. LRCP Lond. 1939 (Univ. Coll. Hosp.) MS Lond. 1945, MB BS 1940; FRCS Eng. 1945. Fell. UCL. Prev: Thoracic Surg. Univ. Coll. Hosp. & Examr. in Surg. Univ. Lond.

NIGHTINGALE, Elizabeth Anne Esslemont Richards and Partners, The Surgery, North Street, Langport TA10 9RH Tel: 01458 250464 Fax: 01458 253246; South Ham Farm, Muchelney Ham, Langport TA10 0DJ Tel: 01458 250816 — MB ChB Aberd. 1974; DObst RCOG 1976. Prev: SHO (Geriat.) High Carley Hosp. Ulverston; SHO (O & G) Risedale Matern. Hosp. Barrow-in-Furness; Ho. Phys. (Gen. Med.) & Ho. Surg. (Gen. Surg.) Roy. Hosp. Chesterfield.

NIGHTINGALE, Evelyn Agnes (retired) Ash House, 118 London Road, Bromley BR1 3RL Tel: 0181 313 1157 — (Lond. Sch. Med. Wom.) MB BS Lond. 1941; MRCS Eng. LRCP Lond. 1941.

NIGHTINGALE, Jeremy John — MB ChB Bristol 1978; FFA RCS Eng. 1983. Cons. Anaesth. Portsmouth Hosps. Specialty: Anaesth. Socs: Assn. Anaesth.; Anaesth. Res. Soc.; Obst. Anaesth. Assn. Prev: Cons. Stoke Mandeville Hosp. Aylesbury; Sen. Regist. (Anaesth.) Soton. Gen. Hosp.; Lect. (Anaesth.) Univ. Soton.

NIGHTINGALE, Jeremy Mark Darby Digestive Disease Centre, Leicester Royal Infirmary, Leicester LE1 5WW Tel: 0116 258 6324 Fax: 0116 258 6985 Email: jeremy.nightingale@uhl-tr.nhs.uk; Bosworth Mill, Barton Road, Carlton, Nuneaton CV13 0RL Tel: 01455 290438 — MB BS Lond. 1981 (Lond. Hosp. Med. Coll.) MRCP (UK) 1984; cert. MHS 1993; MD Lond. 1993; FRCP 2002. Cons. Gastroenterol. (Gen. Phys.) Leicester Roy. Infirm.; Hon. Sen. Lecturer; Cons. Gastroenterologist, Hinerk Hosp. Specialty: Gastroenterol. Socs: Brit. Soc. Gastroenterol.; Inst. Health Servs.

Managem.; BSG. Prev: Sen. Regist. (Gen. Med. & Gastroenterol.) Leicester Roy. Infirm. & Leicester Gen. Hosp.; Regist. (Gastroenterol.) St. Mark's Hosp. Lond.; Research Regist. (Gastroenterol.) St. Marks Hosp. Lond. & OldCh. Hosp. Romford.

NIGHTINGALE, John Alexander (retired) 1 Charney Fold, Charney Well Lane, Grange-over-Sands LA11 6DB — MB ChB Manch. 1947; MRCP Lond. 1949. Prev: Regist. (Cardiol.) & Resid. Clin. Path. Manch. Roy. Infirm.

NIGHTINGALE, John Halkon Grove Medical Practice, Shirley Health Centre, Grove Road, Shirley, Southampton SO15 3UA Tel: 023 8078 3611 Fax: 023 8078 3156 Email: john.nightingale@gp-j82088.nhs.uk; 1 Crofton Close, Oakmount, Highfield, Southampton SO17 1XB Tel: 02380 559274 — (Newcastle-upon-Tyne) MB BS Newc. 1970; DObst RCOG 1973; MRCGP 1976. Indep. Med. Assessor; Clin. Asst. Dermat. Specialty: Alcohol & Substance Misuse. Prev: Resid. Hosp. Sick Childr. Toronto, Canada; SHO (O & G) Soton. Univ. Gp. Hosps.; SHO (Psychiat.) Knowle Hosp. Fareham.

NIGHTINGALE, Julia Anne 146 Woodside Road, Huddersfield HD4 5JJ — BM BCh Oxf. 1991 (Oxford University) BA (Hons.) Oxf. 1988; MRCP (UK) 1994. Specialist Regist., Thoracic Medicene, NW Thames Region. Specialty: Respirat. Med. Prev: Research Fell. (Thoracic Med.) Nat. Heart & Lung Inst. Imperial Coll.

NIGHTINGALE, Michael Douglas Bourne Hall Health Centre, Chessington Road, Ewell, Epsom KT17 1TG Tel: 020 8394 1500 — MB BS Lond. 1966 (St. Bart.) MRCS Eng. LRCP Lond. 1966; FFA RCS Eng. 1970; MRCGP 1979. Specialty: Anaesth. Socs: Brit. Soc. Allergy, Environm. & Nutrit. Med. Prev: SHO (Anaesth.) Nuffield Dept. Anaesth. Oxf. & Poole Gen. Hosp.; SHO (Cas.) Redhill Gen. Hosp.

NIGHTINGALE, Paul Douglas Lakeside Medical Centre, Church Road, Perton, Wolverhampton WV6 7QL Tel: 01903 755329 Fax: 01902 755224 — MB ChB Birm. 1979.

NIGHTINGALE, Peter Intensive Care Unit, Wythenshawe Hospital, Southmoor Road, Manchester M23 9LT Tel: 0161 291 6420 Fax: 0161 291 6421 Email: peter.nightingale@smtr.nhs.uk — MB BS Lond. 1975 (Guy's Hosp. Lond.) MRCS Eng. LRCP Lond. 1975; FRCA 1980; FRCP Lond. 2000. Cons. Anaesth. and Intens. Care Wythenshawe Hosp. Manch. Specialty: Anaesth.; Intens. Care.

NIGHTINGALE, Peter Bryan Bentham Medical Practice, Grasmere Drive, High Bentham, Lancaster LA2 7JP Tel: 01524 261202 Fax: 01524 262222905; Fieldway, Mount Pleasant, High Bentham, Lancaster LA2 7LA Tel: 01524 262652 — MB BS Lond. 1982; DCH RCP Lond. 1985; DTM & H Liverp. 1986; MRCGP 1986; DRCOG 1986. Prev: Med. Off. St Francis Hosp. Katete, Zambia.

NIGHTINGALE, Peter John Health Clinic, 407 Main Road, Dovercourt, Harwich CO12 4ET Tel: 01255 201299 Fax: 01255 201270; Terling, Oakley Road, Little Oakley, Harwich CO12 5DR Tel: 01255 508397 — MB BChir Camb. 1976; BA Camb. 1973, MA, MB BChir 1976; Danish Med. Lic. 1978; DRCOG 1983. Gen. Med. Pract. DoverCt. Essex; Med. Off. Trinity Ho. Lond.; Police Surg. Essex Constab.; Med. Off. Harwich & DoverCt. Hosp.; Aviat. Med. Examr. Prev: Trainee GP Colchester Gp. VTS; Regist. (Anaesth. & IC) Bispebjerg Hosp. & Sundby Hosp. Copenhagen.

NIGHTINGALE, Peter John Richards and Partners, The Surgery, North Street, Langport TA10 9RH Tel: 01458 250464 Fax: 01458 253246; South Ham Farm, Muchelney Ham, Langport TA10 0DJ — MB ChB Sheff. 1974. Prev: SHO (O & G) Risedale Hosp. Barrow-in-Furness. Regist. Gen.; Med. N. Lonsdale Hosp. Barrow-in-Furness; Ho. Off. (Gen. Surg.) & Ho. Off. (Gen. Med.) Roy. Hosp. Chesterfield.

NIGHTINGALE, Robert Charles — MRCS Eng. LRCP Lond. 1973 (St. Mary's) MB Camb. 1974, BChir 1973; MRCP (UK) 1977; FRCR 1982. Cons. Radiol. Ipswich Hosp. Specialty: Nuclear Med. Socs: Brit. Med. Ultrasound Soc. Prev: Sen. Regist. (Radiol.) Addenbrookes Hosp. Camb.; SHO (Anaesth.) & (Renal Unit) Addenbrookes Hosp. Camb.; SHO (Chest Unit) Papworth Hosp. Camb.

NIGHTINGALE, Sharon Louise 14 Station Road, Denby, Ripley DE5 8ND — MB ChB Leeds 1993.

NIGHTINGALE, Simon Robert Severn Lodge, 58 New St., Shrewsbury SY3 8JQ — MD Lond. 1987 (UCHMS London) BSc Lond. 1970, MD 1987, MB BS 1973; MRCP (U.K.) 1976; FRCP 1996. Cons. Neurol. Roy. Shrewsbury Hosp. Specialty: Neurol. Prev: Hon. Sen. Clin. Lect. Univ. of Birm.

NIHAL, Mr Aneel Flat 4, 62 Sinclair Road, London W14 0NH Tel: 020 7603 8194 — MB BS Karachi, Pakistan 1986; FRCS Ed. 1992; FRCS Glas. 1992. Regist. (Orthop.) Roy. Surrey Co. Hosp. Guildford. Specialty: Orthop. Prev: Regist. (Orthop.) Kingston Hosp. Surrey.

NIHOYANNOPOULOS, Petros Cardiology Department, Hammersmith Hospital, Du Cane Road, London W12 0NN Tel: 020 8383 3948 Fax: 020 8740 8373 Email: petros@ic.ac.uk; 18 Endlesham Road, London SW12 8JU Tel: 020 8673 2095 — MD Strasbourg 1979 (Louis Pasteur Strasbourg, France) Cons. Cardiol. Hammersmith Hosp. Lond.; Reader, Imp. Coll. Sch. Med. Lond. Specialty: Cardiol. Special Interest: Cardiomyopathies; Coronary artery Dis.; Echocardiography. Socs: Fell. Roy. Coll. of Physicians; Fell. Amer. Heart Assn.; Fell. Amer. Coll. Cardiol. Prev: Sen. Lect., Sen. Regist. & Regist. Hammersmith Hosp. & Roy. Postgrad. Med. Sch. Lond.

NIJHAR, Amarjeet The Surgery, 1 Waynflete Square, London W10 6UX — MB ChB Liverp. 1980.

NIJJAR, Amarjit Singh 255 Nithsdale Road, Glasgow G41 5AQ — MB ChB Glas. 1976.

NIJJAR, Avtar Singh Family Doctor Unit Surgery, 92 Bath Road, Hounslow TW3 3LN Tel: 020 8570 6271 Fax: 020 8570 3243; 378 Jersey Road, Osterley, Isleworth TW7 5PL Tel: 020 8758 2288 — MB BChir Camb. 1987 (Addenbrooke's Hosp. Camb.) MA Camb. 1987; MRCGP 1991; Cert. Family Plann. JCC 1991; DCH RCP Lond. 1991. Asst. (Cardiol.) Ashford Hosp. Middlx. Specialty: Gen. Pract.

NIKAPOTA, Herath Mudiyanselage Vijita L B Barnet General Hospital, Barnet EN5 3DJ Tel: 020 8732 4496 Fax: 020 8732 4499; 90 Abbots Road, Abbots Langley WD5 0BH Tel: 01923 62228 Fax: 020 8732 4499 — MB BS Ceylon 1965; DMRD Eng. 1972; FFR 1974; FRCR 1975; MD Colombo 1982. Cons. Radiol. Barnet Gen. Hosp. Specialty: Radiol. Socs: FRCR; Sri Lanka Med. Assn.; Med. Defence Union. Prev: Sen. Regist. Roy. Free Hosp. Lond.; Sen. Regist. Childr. Hosp. Lond.; Regist. Northwick Pk. Hosp.

NIKLAUS, Lisa Justine Windsor House, Coleford, Crediton EX17 5DE — MB ChB Manch. 1993.

NIKOLAOU, Constantine Marios c/o V. Philips, 243 Hurst Road, Sidcup DA15 9AL — Ptychio Iatrikes Athens 1964.

NIKOLAOU, Dimitrios IVF Unit, Hammersmith Hospital, Du Cane Road, London W12 0NN Tel: 020 8383 8160 Email: dnikolaou@talk21.com; 54 Cavendish Road, Ealing, London W13 03Q Tel: 020 8997 2891 — Ptychio Iatrikes Athens 1993; MD Ptychio Iatrikes Athens 1993; DFFP 1996; MRCOG 1997. Clin. Rec. Fell. (Repro. Med.) IVF Unit Ham'smth Hosp. Lond. W12 0NN. Specialty: Obst. & Gyn. Socs: MBA. Prev: Specialist Regist. (O & G) Aber. Mater. Hosp.; Sen. SHO (O & G) Nevill Hall Hosp. Abergoreuus Wales.; SHO (O & G) St Jowes Hosp. Leeds.

NIKOLOPOULOS, John 41 Glasslyn Road, London N8 8RJ — Ptychio Iatrikes Athens 1981.

NILSSEN, Mr Erik Lars Kristian Department of Otolaryngology, Queen Alexandra Hospital, Cosham, Portsmouth Tel: 02392 286377 Fax: 02392 286708 Email: erik.nilssen@porthosp.nhs.uk — MB ChB UCT 1987; DLO 1992; FSC (SA), ORL 1996; FRCS Ed. 1997; FRCS ORL HMS 1998. Cons. Otolaryngologist, Portsmouth Hosp. NHS Trust, Portsmouth. Specialty: Gen. Surg. Socs: BAOHNS; Brit. Rhinological Soc.; Europ. Rhinological Soc.

NIMAN, Wilfred 6 Hilton Court, South Promenade, Lytham St Annes FY8 1LZ Tel: 01253 728408 — MRCS Eng. LRCP Lond. 1945 (Leeds) Prev: Ho. Surg. & Ho. Phys. Pinderfields Emerg. Hosp. Wakefield.

NIMMAGADDA, Seshagiri Rao Thornford Park Hospital, Crookham Hill, Thatcham RG19 8ET Tel: 01635 273868/01635 860072 Fax: 01635 874580 — MB BS India 1993; DPM Irel.; MRCPsych; MMed Sc Leeds. Cons. Forens. Psychiat., Thornford Pk. Hosp., Thatcham. Specialty: Forens. Psychiat. Special Interest: Ment. Health Law; Psychiatric aspects of crime; Prison Psychiat. Prev: Specialist Regist. (Foresnic Psychiat.) Reaside Clinic Birm.

NIMMO, Alastair Forbes Department of Anaesthesia, Royal Infirmary of Edinburgh, Lauriston Place, Edinburgh EH3 9YW Tel: 0131 536 3651 Fax: 0131 536 3672 Email: a.nimmo@ed.ac.uk; 3 Queens Avenue, Blackhall, Edinburgh EH4 2DG Tel: 0131 539 2130 Fax: 08700 347157 — MB ChB Aberd. 1983 (Aberdeen) FFA RCS Eng. 1988. Cons. Anaesth. Roy. Infirm. Edin. NHS Trust; Hon. Clin. Sen. Lect. Univ. of Edin. Specialty: Anaesth. Socs: Assn. Anaesth.; Vasc. Anaesth. Soc.; Soc. Intravenous Anaesth. Prev: Specialist

Anaesth. Charité Univ., Berlin; Sen. Regist. (Anaesth.) Lothian HB; Research Fell. (Anaesth.) Roy. Infirm. Edin.

NIMMO, David Henderson (retired) 46 Kelvin Walk, Netherhall, Largs KA30 8SJ Tel: 01475 675415 — MB ChB Glas. 1952; DPM Eng. 1957; MRCPsych 1971. Prev: Cons. Psychiat. Leverndale Hosp. Glas.

NIMMO, Graham Robert Acute Receiving Unit, Western General Hosp, Lothian University Hospitals NHS Trust, Edinburgh EH4 2XU Tel: 0131 534 1876 Fax: 0131 539 1021 Email: g.nimmo@ed.ac.uk; Kolvir, 79 Belgrave Road, Corstorphine, Edinburgh EH12 6NH Tel: 0131 334 1876 Email: g.nimmo@ed.ac.uk — MB ChB Ed. 1982 (Univ. Ed.) BSc (Med. Sci.) Ed. 1979; MRCP (UK) 1985; DA (UK) 1993; FFA RCSI 1996; MD Ed. 1996; FRCP Edin 1998. Cons.INT Med. & Intens. Care West. Gen. Hosp. Edin.; Hon. Sen. Lec. Univ of Edin. Specialty: Gen. Med.; Intens. Care. Prev: Career Regist. (Anaesth.) Vict. Infirm.Glas.; Career Regist. (Renal Med.) Glas. Roy. Infirm.; Regist. (Renal Med.) Roy. Infirm. Edin.

NIMMO, Isabelle Gardner Reid (retired) Flat 6, Dunard, 123 Grange Loan, Edinburgh EH9 2EA Tel: 0131 667 0094 — (St And) BSc 1945; MB ChB St. And. 1949 1949.

NIMMO, John Medical Unit, Western General Hospital, Crewe Rd, Edinburgh EH4 2XU Tel: 0131 537 1037 Fax: 0131 537 1728; 5A Wedderburn Terr, Inveresk, Musselburgh EH21 7TJ Tel: 0131 665 5432 — MB ChB Ed. 1965; FRCP Ed. 1976, M 1969; FFPM RCP (UK) 1995. Cons. Phys. Western Gen. Hosp., Edin.; Hon. Sen. Lect. (Med.) West. Gen. Hosp. Edin. Specialty: Gen. Med.; Gastroenterol. Prev: Cons Phys.E.ern. Gen. Hosp.Edin. 1974-1998.

NIMMO, Malcolm James Ninewells Hospital, Ninewells Avenue, Dundee DD1 9SY Tel: 01382 632651; The Court, 6 Farington St, Dundee DD2 1PJ Tel: 01382 668061 Email: mnimmo7128@aol.com — MB ChB Ed. 1981 (Ediburgh) FRCR 1989. Cons. Radiol. Ninewells Hosp. Dundee. Specialty: Radiol.; Nuclear Med.

NIMMO, Shirin Kingswood Medical Centre, Clayhill Road, Kingswood, Basildon SS16 5AD; 24 Wick Lane, Wickford SS11 8AR Tel: 01268 561047 — MB BCh Wales 1985. Prev: Trainee GP Cardiff; SHO (Obst.) Merthyr Gen. Hosp.; SHO (Gen. Med.) Carmarthen Hosps.

NIMMO, Steven Brian Barton Surgery, Barton, Horn Lane, Plymouth PL9 9BR Tel: 01752 407129 Fax: 01752 482620 — MB ChB Leic. 1988; BSc Leic. 1986; DRCOG 1995; DFFP 1995; MRCGP 1996. Specialty: Gen. Pract.

NIMMO, Susan Mary Kolvir, 79 Belgrave Road, Corstorphine, Edinburgh EH12 6NH — MB ChB Ed. 1985; BSc (Hons.) Ed. 1983; MRCP (UK) 1988; FRCA 1992. Cons. Anaesth. Roy. Infirm. Edin. Specialty: Anaesth. Prev: Sen. Regist. (Anaesth.) Roy. Infirm. Glas.; Regist. (Renal Med.) West. Infirm. Glas.; SHO (Anaesth.) Roy. Infirm. Edin.

NIMMO, Thomas William Camelon Medical Practice, 3 Baird Street, Camelon, Falkirk FK1 4PP Tel: 01324 622854 Fax: 01324 633858; 40 Majors Loan, Falkirk FK1 5QB Tel: 01324 26955 — BSc (Med. Sci.) Ed. 1975, MB ChB 1978; DRCOG 1980; DCH Glas. 1980; MRCGP 1982.

NIMMO, Walter Sneddon 1wn, 18 Alva Street, Edinburgh EH2 4QG Mob: 07710 762416 Email: walter@1wn.co.uk — MB ChB 1971; BSc (Med. Sci.) 1968; MRCP (UK) 1975; FFA RCS Eng. 1977; MD Ed. 1982; FRCP Glas. 1984; FRCP Ed. 1984; FANZCA 1993; FRCA 1993; FFPM RCP (UK) 1993; FRSE 2000. Specialty: Pharmaceutical Medicine; Pharmacology; Anaesth. Prev: Chief Exec. Inveresk Research; Prof. (Anaesth.) Univ. Sheff.; Sen. Lect. (Anaesth.) West. Infirm. Glas.

NINAN, Golda Mary 123C Newtown Road, Warsash, Southampton SO31 9GY — MB BCh Wales 1995 (Cardiff) GP Princip. Gosport, Hants. Specialty: Gen. Pract. Special Interest: Gen. Med., Med. Ethics/Law, Humanities. Socs: MRCGP. Prev: GP Locum; GP Regist. extension (Musculoskeletal Med., Management); GP Regist.

NINAN, Mammen c/o Mr V. Harihar, 49 Chapman Road, Coreys Mill Lane, Stevenage SG1 4RJ — MB BS Kerala, India 1992; MRCP (UK) 1992.

NINAN, Titus Kallupurackal Heartlands and Solihull NHS Trust, Borderley Green, Birmingham B9 5SS — MD Bombay 1982; MB BS Bombay 1979; DCH Bombay 1982; MRCP (UK) 1987.

NIND, Nicholas Robert 120 Shelford Road, Cambridge CB2 2NF — MB ChB Sheff. 1995. Specialty: Histopath.

NINES, Ronald John Nines and Partners, Shoreham Health Centre, Pond Road, Shoreham-by-Sea BN43 5US Tel: 01273 440550 — MB Camb. 1976; BChir 1975; DRCOG 1977; DCH Eng. 1977; MRCGP 1979.

NINHAM, Mark Charles Royal Manor Health Care, Park Estate Road, Easton, Portland DT5 2BJ Tel: 01305 820422 Fax: 01305 824143 — BM BS Nottm. 1992; MRCGP 1998. Specialty: Gen. Pract.

NINIS, Nelly 3 Monkfrith Way, London N14 5LG — MB BS Lond. 1989.

NINKOVIC, Mary — MB BChir Camb. 1987; BPharm Lond. 1978; Mps 1979; PhD Camb. 1982. Cons. Gastroenterol. P'boro. Dist. Hosp. Specialty: Gastroenterol. Prev: Sen. Regist. (Gastroenterol.) Addenbrooke's Hosp. Camb.; Foulkes Foundat. Fellowship 1984-86.; Sen. Regist. (Gastroenterol.) Roy. Free Hosp. Lond.

NIPPANI, Mrs Krishna Jyothi Warwickshire Nuffield Hospital, The Chase, Old Milverton Lane, Leamington Spa CV32 6RW Tel: 01926 427971 Fax: 01926 422659 Email: jyothi@doctors.org.uk — MB BS Andhra Med. Coll. 1986; MRCOG Lond. 1994. Cons. Obst. & Gyn. Warwick Hosp. Specialty: Obst. & Gyn.

NIRANJAN, Kantha King Georges Hospital, Barley Lane, Ilford IG3 8YB — MB BS Sri Lanka 1981 (Univ. Perdeniya, Sri-Lanka) MB BS Sri Lanka 1980; MRCS Eng LRCP Lond. 1988; MRCP (UK) 1990; MSc Gerontol. Lond. 1995. Cons. Physic. Redbridge NHS Healthcare, Essex Trust. Specialty: Gen. Med. Special Interest: Stroke & Parkinsons Dis. Socs: Brit Geriat. Soc.; Mem. of Brit. Assn. of Stroke Physicians; Roy. Coll. Physicians. Prev: Sen. Regist. Integrated Med. W. Mid. Rot. Birm.; Research Fell. (Neuro.) Old Ch. Hosp. Romford.

NIRANJAN, Nadarajah 12 Grosvenor Gardens, London N14 4TX — MB BS Colombo 1980.

NIRANJAN, Mr Nandagudi Shivaiah Broomfield Hospital, St. Andrews Centre for Plastic Surgery; Chelmsford CM1 7ET Tel: 01245 266985 Fax: 01245 266620 Email: niriniranjan@aol.com/niriniranjan@hotmail.com; Weatherby, Goat Hall Lane, Chelmsford CM2 8PG Tel: 01245 266985 Fax: 01245 263668 — MB BS Karnatak Univ. 1972 (JN Medical College Belgaum, India) MS Mysore 1975; MRCS Eng. LRCP Lond. 1979; FRCS Ed. 1979; FRCS Eng. 1980; FRCS (Plast) 1992. Cons. Plastic Surg. Broomfield Hosp.; Hon. Cons. Plastic Surg. Roy. Lond. Hosp. Specialty: Plastic Surg. Socs: Brit. Assn. Plastic Surg.; Brit. Assn. Aesthetic Plastic Surgs.; Brit. Soc. Surg. Hand. Prev: Cons. Plastic Surg. Roy. Lond. Hosp.; Sen. Regist. (Plastic Surg.) St. Lawrence Hosp. Chepstow; Regist. (Plastic & Reconstruc. Surg.) St. Lawrence Hosp., Chepstow.

NIRDOSH, Neetu 62 Elizabeth Road, Moseley, Birmingham B13 8QJ — MB ChB Birm. 1998.

NIRMAL, Divyabala Lalitkumar Fairwater Surgery, Fairwater, Cwmbran NP44 Tel: 0163 33 69544; (resid), 86 Glan Ryde, Coed Eva, Cwmbran NP44 6TZ Tel: 0163 33 66233 — MB BS Saurashtra 1970 (M.P. Shah Med. Coll. Jamnagar) DObst RCOG 1972. Prev: Regist. (O & G) & SHO (O & G) Wordsley Hosp.; Stourbridge.

NIRMALAN, Rajanayagam The Roehampton Surgery, 191 Roehampton Lane, London SW15 4HN Tel: 020 8788 1188 Fax: 020 8789 9914 — MB BS Lond. 1980 (Char. Cross) MRCS Eng. LRCP Lond. 1979. Specialty: Gen. Med.

NIRMALANANTHAN, Mr Sivaguru 50 Marlands Road, Clayhall, Ilford IG5 0JJ Tel: 020 8551 6906 — MB BS Ceylon 1963; DO RCS Eng. 1979; FRCS Ed. 1980; FRCOphth 1989. Hon. Cons. Ophth. Roy. Free Hosp. Lond.; Assoc. Specialist Moorfields Eye Hosp. Lond. Specialty: Ophth. Prev: Cons. Ophth. Govt. Gen. Hosp. Jaffna, Sri Lanka; Clin. Asst. Moorfields Eye Hosp. Lond.; Regist. Chelmsford & Essex Hosp. Chelmsford.

NIRODI, Gajanan Niranjan 31 Derby Street, Beverley Road, Hull HU3 1ST — MB ChB Manch. 1994.

NIRODI, Pratibha 5 Linden Close, Saintfield, Ballynahinch BT24 7BH — MB BCh BAO Belf. 1991.

NIRODI, Sandya 5 Linden Close, Saintfield, Ballynahinch BT24 7BH — MB ChB Ed. 1996.

NIRODI, Vinatha Niranjan 5 Linden Close, Saintfield, Ballynahinch BT24 7BH Tel: 01238 510839 — MB BS Bombay 1962 (Topiwalla Nat. Med. Coll. Bombay) DGO CPS Bombay 1964; Cert. Family Plann. JCC 1983.

NIRULA, Mr Harish Chandra Artificial Limb and Appliance Centre, Wrexham Maelor Hospital, Croesnewydd Rd, Wrexham LL13 7NT Tel: 01978 727288 Fax: 01978 727307; 9 Badgers Rake, Victoria Road, Formby, Liverpool L37 1XU Tel: 01704 870003 — (Govt. Med. Coll. Nagpur) MB BS Nagpur 1960; FRCS Eng. 1964. Cons. Rehabil. Med. Wrexham Maelor Hosp. Specialty: Rehabil. Med.

NIRULA, Neera H. M. Prison, 2 Ribbleton Lane, Preston PR1 5AB; 9 Badgers Rake, Victoria Road, Formby, Liverpool L37 1XU — MD Nagpur 1971 (Lady Hardinge Med. Coll.) MB BS Delhi 1966; DGO Nagpur 1969; MD (Obst. & Gyn.) Nagpur 1971; DA Eng. 1974. Sen. Med. Off. H.M Prison Preston. Specialty: Gen. Pract. Prev: Med. Off. H.M. Prison Wakefield; SHO (Obst.) & SHO (Anaesth.) Pontefract Gen. Infirm.; SHO (Anaesth.) Nevill Hall Hosp. Abergavenny.

NIRULA, Radhika Payal 9 Badgers Rake, Formby, Liverpool L37 1XU — BM BS Nottm. 1998.

NISBET, Alister Macgregor 32 Rosebery Avenue, Bridlington YO15 3PR Tel: 01262 675003 — MB ChB Aberd. 1954; DObst RCOG 1959; Cert Developm. Paediat. Univ. Leeds 1980; MFCH 1989. Sen. Clin. Off. (Child Health) Hull HA. Socs: Fac. Community Health.

NISBET, Angus Paul Department of Neurology, Brighton & Sussex University Hospitals NHS Trust, Eastern Road, Brighton BN2 5BE Tel: 01273 696955 Ext: 7985 Email: sarah.mansell@bsuh.nhs.uk — BM BS Nottm. 1986; BMedSci Nottm. 1984; MRCP (UK) 1990; CCST Neurol. 1997; FRCP 2003. Cons. Neurol., Brighton & Sussex Univ. Hosps. NHS Trust. Specialty: Neurol. Special Interest: Epilepsy; Multiple Sclerosis; Parkinson's Dis. Socs: Assn. of Brit. Neurol.; Hosp. Cons. & Specialist Assn. Prev: Sen. Regist. (Neurol.) Qu.'s Med. Centre, Nottm.; Research Regist., Nat. Hosp. for Neurol., & Neurosurg.

NISBET, Charlotte (retired) 2 Grey Gables, Southwood, Monkton, Prestwick KA9 1UR — MB ChB Glas. 1963; FRCPath 1987, M 1973. Prev: Cons. Haemat. Ayrsh. & Arran HB.

NISBET, Ian Gardner Old Brandon Road Surgery, Old Brandon Road, Feltwell, Thetford IP26 4AY Tel: 01842 828481 Fax: 01842 828172; The Old House, Feltwell, Thetford IP26 4DL Tel: 01842 828956 — MB BS Lond. 1968 (Lond. Hosp.) MRCS Eng. LRCP Lond. 1968; DObst RCOG 1970. Prev: SHO (Obst.) & Ho. Phys. Redhill Gen. Hosp.; Ho. Surg. (Accid. & Orthop.) Lond. Hosp.

NISBET, Nanette Hendry (retired) 6 High Street, Pittenweem, Anstruther KY10 2LA — (Univ. Glas.) MD (High Commend.) Glas. 1952, MB ChB 1948; FRCP Glas. 1977, M 1964. Prev: Cons. Geriat. Highland Health Bd.

NISBET, Mr Norman Walter (retired) 3 Canberra Court, Richmond Avenue, Bognor Regis PO21 2YH Tel: 01243 863555 — (Med School of the Royal Colleges of Edinburgh & Glasgow) LDS RCS Ed. 1932; LRCP LRCS Ed. LRFPS Glas. 1934; FRCS Ed. 1936; FRCS Eng. 1966. Prev: Dir. Research Robt. Jones & Agnes Hunt Orthop. Hosp. Oswestry Shrops.

NISBET, Ruth Kelso Medical Group Practice, Health Centre, Inch Road, Kelso TD5 7LS Tel: 01573 224424 Fax: 01573 226388; Eden House, Eden Road, Ednam, Kelso TD5 7QG — MB ChB Ed. 1981; DRCOG 1984; MRCGP 1985.

NISBET, Ruth Margaret OHSAS, Navy House, Stuart Road, Rosyth, Dunfermline KY12 2BJ — MB ChB Ed. 1988; MRCGP 1993; DLO 1998; FRCS Ed. 1999; AFOM 2004. SpR Occupat. Med. Socs: BMA; SOM; FOM. Prev: SHO ENT.

NISBET, William Henry (retired) 294 Ferry Road, Edinburgh EH5 3NP Tel: 0131 552 5390 — MB ChB Ed. 1947 (Univ. Ed.) Dip. Ven. Soc. Apoth. Lond. 1976. Prev: Clin. Asst. Sexually Transm. Dis. Roy. Infirm. Edin.

NISBET-SMITH, Ann Patricia (retired) 2 Middleton Buildings, Langham St., London W1W 7SZ Tel: 020 7636 6403 — (St. Mary's) MB BS Lond. 1959; MRCS Eng. LRCP Lond. 1959. Prev: Assoc. Specialist (Histopath.) Northwick Pk. Hosp. Harrow.

NISBET-SMITH, Catherine Heathgate Surgery, Poringland, Norwich NR14 7JT Tel: 01508 494343; Whitehouse Farm, 4 Edward Seago Place, Brooke, Norwich NR15 1HL Tel: 01508 558387 — MB BS Lond. 1987; BSc (Hons.) St. And. 1982; MA Camb. 1984.

NISCHAL, Mr Kanwal Ken Dept. of Ophthalmology, Great Ormond Street Hospital for Children, Great Ormond Street, London WC1N 3JH Tel: 020 7813 8524 Fax: 020 7829 8647 — MB BS Lond. 1988 (King's College Hospital, London University) FRCOphth 1993. p/t Cons., Gt. Ormond St. Hosp.; Mem. of the Standard Med. Advisery Comm. to The Dept. of Health; Mem. of the Scientif. Advisery Bd. of the Cornecia de Lange Soc.; Mem. of the Editorial Bd. of the Amer. Orthoptic Jl.; Hon. Sen. Lect., Inst. of Child Health, Lond. Specialty: Ophth.; Medico Legal. Special Interest: Anterior segment surger including cornea grafts in Childr.; Strabismus Surg. Socs: Foundat. of Sci. & Technol.; Brit. Med. Assn.; Roy. Soc. Med. Prev: Clin. Fell., Hosp. for Sick Childr., Toronto; Sen. Regist. Oxf. Eye Hosp. & P. Chas. Eye Unit Windsor; Regist. Birm. & Morland Eye Hosp.

NISCHAL, Vijaya Kumar 20 Blenheim Avenue, Gants Hill, Ilford IG2 6JQ — MB BCh BAO Belf. 1980; DRCOG 1983.

NISHITH, Shirish 4 College Close, Birkdale, Southport PR8 4DG — MB BS Madras 1983; FCOphth 1990.

NISSEN, Mr Justin James Department of Neurosciences, Newcastle General Hospital, Westgate Road, Newcastle upon Tyne NE4 6BE — BM BS Nottm. 1989; FRCS Eng. 1993. Cons. (Neurosurg.) Newc. Gen. Hosp. Newc.

NISSENBAUM, Hilary 10 Cheviot Gardens, London NW2 1QN — MB ChB Liverp. 1978; MA (Med. Law & Ethics, Keys Col. 1997); BSc (Hons.) (Physiol.) Liverp. 1975; MRCPsych 1982. Cons. (Old Age Psychiat.) Harrow and Hillingdon NHS Trust, Northwick Pk. Hosp.; Second Opinion Doctor Ment. Health Act Commiss.; Ment. Health Review Tribunal. Specialty: Geriat. Psychiat. Prev: Cons. Psychogeriat., S. Lond. and Maudsley Trust; Cons. Psychogeriat. Qu. Eliz. Psychiat. Hosp.; Regist. (Psychiat.) Withington Hosp. Manch.

NISSENBAUM, Simon Henry Welbeck Road Surgery, 1A Welbeck Road, Bolsover, Chesterfield S44 6DF Tel: 01246 823742 — MB ChB Manch. 1980; MRCGP 1984.

NITHIANANDAN, Mr Ponniah Kings Hill Hospital, Sutton-in-Ashfield NG17 4JL — MB BS Ceylon 1972; MRCS Eng. LRCP Lond. 1979; DO Eng. 1981; FRCS (Ophth.) Ed. 1982. Regist. (Ophth.) Kings Mill Hosp. Notts. Specialty: Ophth.

NITHIANANDAN, Sulochana Kings Mill Hospital, Sutton-in-Ashfield NG17 4JL — MB BS Sri Lanka 1976; MB BS Sri Lanka 1976 MRCS Eng. LRCP Lond. 1979; FFA RCS Eng. 1981 DA Eng. 1980. Regist. (Anaesth.) Qu. Univ. Med. Centre, Notts. Specialty: Anaesth.

NITHIANANTHAM, Vellore Thiruvengadam 70 Hither Green Lane, Redditch B98 9BW — MB BS Madras 1969.

NITHIYANANTHAN, Ratnasingam Birmingham Heartlands Hospital, Boardesly Green E., Birmingham B9 5SS Tel: 0121 766 6611; 20 King Henrys Road, Kingston upon Thames KT1 3QA Tel: 020 8241 3469 — MB ChB Leeds 1993; MRCP (UK) 1997. Specialist Regist. (Diabetes & Endocrinol. with Gen. Med.) Heartland & Solihull NHS Trust Birm. Specialty: Gen. Med. Socs: BMA; Med. Protec. Soc.

NITHYANANDARAJAH, Mr Gnanapragasam Antony Loyala 123 Waverly Roayd, Harrow HA2 9RQ Email: nithy.g@btinternet.com — MB BS Peradeniya 1982; FRCS Ed. 1989; FCOphth 1990. Specialty: Ophth.

NITZKE, Franciszek Jerzy (retired) 96 Timberley Lane, Birmingham B34 7EN Tel: 0121 747 2100 — MD Warsaw 1930.

NIVEN, Anne Pullar — MB ChB Cape Town 1975; MRCGP 1980; DRCOG 1980.

NIVEN, Christine Frances NHS Fife - Primary Care Division, Rosyth, Dunfermline KY11 2SE Tel: 01383 416181 — MB ChB Glas. 1980; BSc (Hons. Molecular Biol.) Glas. 1977; DCCH RCGP & FCM 1986; DRCOG 1986; MRCGP 1986. Staff Grade (Community Paediat.) NHS Fife - Prim. Care Div. Specialty: Community Child Health. Socs: BMA; Brit. Assn. of Community Doctors in Audiol. (BADA); Brit. Assn. for Community Child Health (BACCH). Prev: Trainee GP & Community Paediat. Edin. VTS.; SHO (Otorhinolaryngol.) Vict. Infirm. Glas.; GP Dumbarton Health Centre VTS.

NIVEN, Mr Peter Ashley Robertson 2 Clifton Park, Clifton, Bristol BS8 3BS Tel: 0117 9738446 & profess. 238206 — (Camb. & St. Bart.) MA, MB Camb. 1963, BChir 1962; FRCS Eng. 1966; FRCOG 1982, M 1969. Cons. O & G St. Michael's Hosp. Bristol United Bristol Healthcare Trust. Specialty: Obst. & Gyn. Prev: Eden Trav. Fellowship RCOG; Sen. Regist. (O & G) St. Bart. Hosp. Lond.; Cons. O & G Newc. Gen. & Hexham Gen. Hosps.

NIVEN, Robert McLay North West Lung Centre, Wythenshawe Hospital, Southmoor Road, Manchester M23 9LT Tel: 0161 998 7070 Fax: 0161 291 2832; 1 Stour Close, Altrincham WA14 4UE Tel: 0161 929 9448 — MD Manch. 1994; BSc St. And. 1981; MB ChB 1984; MRCP (UK) 1988; MFOM RCP Lond. 1995; FRCP (UK) 2001. Hon. Cons. (Phys. Respirat. Med.) Wythenshawe Hosp. Specialty: Respirat. Med. Prev: Sen. Regist. (Respirat. Med.) Wythenshawe Hosp.; Sen. Regist. Train. Post (Occupat. Med.) Manch. Univ. Wythenshaw Hosp. & Agrevo Ltd; Research Regist. Wythenshawe Hosp.

NIVEN, Sacha David The Walton Centre for Neurology & Neurosurgery, Lower Lane, Fazakerley, Liverpool L9 7LJ Tel: 0151 525 3611 Fax: 0151 529 5500 — MB ChB Liverp. 1993; FRCR; BSc (Hons.); MRCP 1997. Cons. Neuroradiol. Walton Centre Liverp. Specialty: Radiol. Special Interest: Neuroradiology. Prev: Specialist Regist. (Radiol.) Roy. Liverp. Univ. Hosp.

NIVEN-JENKINS, Nicholas Craig 26 High Street, Erdington, Birmingham B23 6RN Tel: 0121 373 0086; 86 Antrobus Road, Boldmere, Sutton Coldfield B73 5EL Tel: 0121 355 6511 — MB ChB Birm. 1978; BSc (Hons.) Birm. 1975, MB ChB 1978; MRCGP 1984. Specialty: Occupat. Health. Socs: Roy. Coll. Gen. Pract.; Soc. Occupat. Med. Prev: SHO VTS Birm. Dist.; Ho. Off. (Surg.) Qu. Eliz. Hosp. Birm.; Ho. Off. (Med.) Dudley Rd. Hosp. Birm.

NIWA, Khatim 85 Dolobran Road, Birmingham B11 1HL — MB BS Lond. 1998.

NIX, Amanda Louise 13 Stanmore Street, Burley, Leeds LS4 2RS — MB ChB Leeds 1993.

NIX, Anthony John Haunton (retired) 11 Willingale Way, Thorpe Bay, Southend-on-Sea SS1 3SL Tel: 01702 586440 — (Camb. & Lond. Hosp.) BA Camb. 1956; MB BChir Camb. 1960; MRCS Eng. LRCP Lond. 1960. Prev: GP Southend-on-Sea.

NIX, Paul Alan 14 Chestnut Green, Monk Fryston, Leeds LS25 5PN Tel: 01977 681162 — BM BCh Oxf. 1994; BA (Physiol. Sci.) Oxf. 1999; FRCS Eng. 2000. SHO Rotat. (Surg.) Leeds Gen. Infirm. Specialty: Gen. Surg. Prev: SHO (Orthop.) Leeds 1998; SHO (Vasc. Surg.) Leeds 1997; SHO (Neurosurg.) Leeds 1997.

NIXON, Alexander Allan Dr McElhone and Partners, Townhead Surgery, 6-8 High St., Irvine KA12 0AY Tel: 01294 273131 Fax: 01294 312832 — MB ChB Dundee 1981; BMSc 1978.

NIXON, Caroline Meryl The Medical Centre, Badgers Crescent, Shipston-on-Stour CV36 4BD Tel: 01608 661845 Fax: 01608 663614 — MB ChB Birm. 1983; MRCP (UK) 1986; MRCGP 1989.

NIXON, Caroline Violet Charlotte 15 Kingfisher Close, Hamble, Southampton SO31 4PE — BM Soton. 1990.

NIXON, Christopher John The Health Centre, Oliver St., Ampthill, Bedford MK45 2SB Tel: 01525 402302 Fax: 01525 840764 — MB BS Lond. 1970; MRCS Eng. LRCP Lond. 1971; MRCP (UK) 1973; DRCOG 1979; MRCGP 1983. Course Organiser Bedford VTS.

NIXON, Mr David Peter Wychwood Surgery, 62 High Street, Milton-under-Wychwood, Chipping Norton OX7 6LE Tel: 01993 830260 Fax: 01993 831867; Snowdon House, Fiddlers Hill, Shipton under Wychwood, Chipping Norton OX7 6DR — MB ChB Ed. 1979; FRCS Ed. 1985; FRCS Eng. 1985; DRCOG 1988; MRCGP 1990. Prev: Regist. (Surg.) Roy. Liverp. Hosp.; Trainee GP/SHO Roy. Utd. Hosp. Bath VTS; Princip. Med. Off. Gizo, Solomon Is.

NIXON, Dennis The Medical Centre, Pinkham, Cleobury Mortimer, Kidderminster DY14 8QE Tel: 01299 270209 Fax: 01299 270482; The Old Barns, Tenbury Road, Cleobury Mortimer, Kidderminster DY14 8RB Tel: 01299 270209 Email: dennis@oldbouns.freeserve.co.uk — MB ChB Birm. 1973; DObst RCOG 1976; MRCGP 1978. Med. Assessor Indep. Tribunal Serv.

NIXON, Desni Lee 10B Wester Coates Gardens, Edinburgh EH12 5LT Tel: 0131 337 0331 — MB ChB Aberd. 1995 (Aberdeen) Psychiat. Roy. Edin. Hosp. Edin. Specialty: Gen. Psychiat.; Geriat. Psychiat.; Psychother.

NIXON, Helena Katherine BUPA Occupational Health, 7th Floor, 102 New Street, Birmingham B2 4HQ Tel: 0121 695 5472 Fax: 0121 695 5471 Email: nixon@bupa.com — MB ChB Leic. 1985; Cert. Family Plann. JCC 1991; DRCOG 1991; AFOM RCP Lond. 1996; MFOM RCP Lond. 1998. Cons Ocupational Phys. BUPA Occupational Health; Assoc. Specialist Ocupational Health, Selly Oak Hosp., Birm. Specialty: Occupat. Health. Socs: Soc. Occupat. Med.; Roy. Soc. Med.; Diplomates Assn. RCOG. Prev: Med. Off. Lucas Indust. Birm., Post Office & Benefits Agency Birm.

NIXON, Professor James Robert 1 Hamilton Villa, Ballyholme, Bangor BT20 5PG Tel: 028 9147 4015 Fax: 028 9147 4043 Email: james.nixon@dnet.co.uk — MB BCh BAO Dub. 1967; FRCSI 1971; FRCS Eng. 1972; MChOrth Liverp. 1975; T(S) 1991. Cons. Orthop. Surg. Musgrave Pk. Hosp.; Hon. Prof. Qu. Univ. Belf. Specialty: Orthop. Socs: Fell. BOA; Irish Orthop. Assn.; Brit. Hip Soc. (Pres.). Prev: Med. Dir. GreenPk. Health Care Trust.

NIXON, Janet Ruth Schoolane Surgery, 2 Schoolane Road, Shard End, Birmingham B34 6RB — MB BS Lond. 1983; DRCOG 1988. GP Princip. Schoolane Surg., Birm.

NIXON, Jennifer Margaret (retired) 8 Cryon View, Gloweth, Truro TR1 3JT — MB BCh BAO NUI 1959; MRCOG 1967. Prev: Clin. Asst. (O & G) Roy. Cornw. Hosp. (Treliske) Truro.

NIXON, John (retired) 51 Riverpark Drive, Marlow SL7 1QT — MB ChB Bristol 1962. Clin. Asst. (Psychiat.) N. Middlx. Hosp. Lond.; Hosp. Pract. (Gen. Med.) N. Middlx. Hosp. Lond.

NIXON, John Department of Neurology, Royal United Hospital, Bath BA1 3NG — MB ChB Bristol 1989; BSc (Hons.) Bristol 1983, MB ChB 1989; MRCP (UK) 1992.

NIXON, Mr John Edwin 148 Harley Street, London W1G 7LG Tel: 020 7935 1207 Fax: 020 7224 1528; Department of Orthopaedic Surgery, Charing Cross Hospital, Fulham Palace Road, London W6 8RF Tel: 020 8846 1475 — MB ChB Ed. 1972; FRCS Eng. 1978; MA Oxf. 1980; ChM Ed. 1987. Sen. Examr. (Surg.) Univ. Lond.; Hon. Sen. Lect. Imperial Coll. Specialty: Orthop.; Trauma & Orthop. Surg. Socs: Fell. Roy. Soc. Med.; Fell. BOA; Brit. Assoication of Spinal Surg.s. Prev: Cons. Orthop. Surg. King's Coll. Hosp. Lond.; Clin. Reader & Hon. Cons. Orthop. Surg. Univ. Oxf. & Nuffield Orthop. Centre Oxf.

NIXON, Mr John Moylett Gerrard (retired) 13 Park Drive, Chilmark, Salisbury SP3 5AW — (T.C. Dub.) MB BCh BAO Dub. 1937; DOMS Eng. 1946; FRCS Eng. 1948. Hon. Cons. Ophth. Surg. W. Dorset Gp. Hosps. Prev: Sen. Ho. Surg. Moorfields, Westm. & Centr. Eye Hosp. (Centr. Br.).

NIXON, Jonathan Mark 18 Tay Ter., Newport-on-Tay DD6 8AZ Tel: 01382 542241 — MB ChB Ed. 1993. Specialty: Obst. & Gyn.

NIXON, Julian Robert 11 Admirals Court, Hamble, Southampton SO31 4LT — MB BS Lond. 1994.

NIXON, Keith Pinfold Health Centre, Field Road, Bloxwich, Walsall WS3 3JP Fax: 01922 775132; Brook House Farm, Audmore Road, Gnosall, Stafford ST20 0HA — MB ChB Manch. 1975. Prev: Trainee GP N. Staffs. VTS; Ho. Surg. Staffs. Roy. Infirm. Stoke-on-Trent; Ho. Phys. Gen. Hosp. Stoke-on-Trent.

NIXON, Kenneth Harry (retired) Rose Cottage, East St., Westbourne, Emsworth PO10 8SH Tel: 01243 373163 — MB BS Lond. 1955; DPhysMed Eng. 1958. Prev: Cons. Phys. (Rheum. & Rehabil.) Portsmouth Hosp. Gp.

NIXON, Marie Clare Department of Anaesthetics, Leicester General Hospital, Gwendolen Road, Leicester LE5 4PW — MB BS Lond. 1992.

NIXON, Neil Leslie Peter 14 Rusland Park Road, Harrow HA1 1UT — MB BS Lond. 1996.

NIXON, Paul 6 Barnacre Close, Fulwood, Preston PR2 9WN — MB BS Newc. 1994.

NIXON, Peter George Frederick (retired) Evenlode Cottage, Evenlode, Moreton-in-Marsh GL56 0NT Tel: 01608 651337 Fax: 01608 651337 Email: peter@evenlode-nixon.fsnet.co.uk — MB BS Durh. 1949; FRCP Lond. 1970, M 1955. Prev: Hon. Cons. Cardiol. Riverside HA.

NIXON, Robert Giles Ashington House, Ashington Way, Westlea, Swindon SN5 7XY Tel: 01793 614840; 24 Wrde Hill, Highworth, Swindon SN6 7BX Tel: 01793 764233 — MB BS Lond. 1978.

NIXON, Ronald John Church Lane Surgery, Church Lane, Boroughbridge, York YO51 9BD Tel: 01423 322309 Fax: 01423 324458 Email: ron.nixon@gp-b82032.nhs.uk; The Red House, Kirby Hill, Boroughbridge, York YO51 9DR Tel: 01423 322500 Fax: 01423 325388 Email: ronald_nixon@btopenworld.com — MB ChB Ed. 1967; DObst RCOG 1969. Socs: Life Mem. Roy. Med. Soc.

NIXON, Sarah Jane 9 Oakways, Appleton, Warrington WA4 5HD — MB BChir Camb. 1992. Trainee GP/SHO Yeovil Dist. Hosp.

NIXON, Mr Stephen James Western General Hospital, Crewe Road, Edinburgh EH4 2XU; 78 Greenbank Crescent, Edinburgh EH10 5SW — MB ChB Ed. 1973; FRCS Ed. 1978. Specialty: Gen. Surg.

NIXON, Susan Joanna The Surgery, 1 Manor Place, London SE17 3BD Tel: 020 7703 3988 Fax: 020 7252 4002 — MB ChB Bristol 1988; DRCOG 1991; MRCGP 1994; MA (Med. Law & Ethics) Lond. 1996. GP Partner; Advisory work for MDU; Researcher& Lecturer Med. Law & Ehtics. Specialty: Gen. Pract.; HIV Med.

NIXON, Susan Margaret 108 Roman Road, Broadstone BH18 9JU — MB ChB Sheff. 1990.

NIXSEAMAN, Mr David Hugh (retired) River Cottage, Denmark St., Diss IP22 4BE Tel: 01379 643659 — MB BChir Camb. 1950 (St. Geo.) MRCS Eng. LRCP Lond. 1949; FRCS Eng. 1957; DO Eng. 1959. Prev: Cons. Ophth. Ayrsh. & Galloway Area.

NIYADURUPOLA, Mr Thisara West Sussex Eye Unit, Worthing Hospital, Lyndhurst Road, Worthing BN11 2DH Tel: 01903 205111 Fax: 01903 285062 — MB BS Sri Lanka 1974 (Peradeniya, Sri Lanka) DO RCS Eng. 1983; FRCS (Ophth.) Ed. 1985; FRCOphth 1989. Cons. Ophth. Worthing Hosp. & St Richards Hosp. Chichester; Cons Ophthamologist Goring Hall Hosp. Goring by Sea W. Sussex; Cons Ophthamologist The Sherburne Hosp Chichester W. Sussex. Specialty: Ophth. Socs: S.ern Ophthamol. Soc.; Brighton & Sussex Medico-chirurgical Soc.; Comm. Mem. Sri Lankan Med & Dent. Assoc.

NIZAM, Mr Mazhar 246 Whitton Avenue E., Greenford UB6 0QA — FRCS Ed. 1989. Specialty: Plastic Surg.

NJOKU, Lucia Ihuoma 127 Long Elms, Harrow Weald, Harrow HA3 5LB — MB BS Benin 1983; MB BS Benin, Nigeria 1983; MRCOG 1990; MRCGP 1994. Specialty: Obst. & Gyn.

NJUKI, Frederick Ivan 16 Strandgeld Close, Plumstead, London SE18 1LA Email: fred.njuki@zetnet.co.uk — LMSSA Lond. 1994 (Univ. Coll. Lond.) LRCS Eng. LRCP Lond. 1994. SHO (Med.) Mayday Univ. Hosp. Croydon. Socs: Med. Defence Union. Prev: SHO (Geriat.) S. Manch. Univ. Hosp.

NKANZA, Kamona Margaret East Surrey Hospital, Three Arch Road, Redhill RH1 5RH — MB BS Delhi 1979; DO RCPSI 1982; FRCS Ed. (Ophth.) 1986. Assoc. Specialist (Ophth.) Surrey. Specialty: Ophth.

NKERE, Udim Uto 64 Halstead Road, London N21 3DS — MB BS Lond. 1981. Cardiac Unit Roy. Infirm. Glas. Specialty: Cardiothoracic Surg. Prev: SHO (Gen. Surg.) Leicester Gen. Hosp.; SHO (A & E) Crawley Hosp.

NKONDE, Petronella Mwamba 24 Plantation Avenue, Alwoodley, Leeds LS17 8TB Tel: 0113 225 1986 Fax: 0113 225 1986 — MB ChB Zambia 1978; MRCS Eng. LRCP Lond. 1988. Clin. Med. Off. (Psychiat.) Leeds. Specialty: Gen. Psychiat. Prev: Regist. Rotat. (Psychiat.) Leeds, Wakefield & Pontefract.

NKONGE, Frederick Michael Kiwanuka S Diabetey Unit, 5th Floor, Alexandra Wing, Royal London Hospital, London E1 1BB Tel: 0207 377 7000 — MB BChir Camb. 1977; MA Camb. 1977, MB BChir 1977; MRCP (UK) 1984. Diabetologist, Royal London Hospital, White Chapel, London. Prev: Regist. (Chest & Gen. Med.) St. Margt. Hosp. Epping; SHO OldCh. Hosp. Romford; SHO Roy. North. Hosp. Lond.

NNOCHIRI, Mr Cosmas Chiedozi Paschal Old Fletton Surgery, Rectory Gardens, Peterborough PE2 8AY Tel: 01733 343137; Marriotts Way, Ramsey Mereside, Huntingdon PE26 2TY — MB BChir Camb. 1980; MA Camb. 1982, MB BChir 1980; FRCS Ed. 1985; FRCS Eng. 1987. Bank Surg. PeterBoro. Hosp. NHS Trust, Cambs. Prev: Regist. (Surg.) The Middlx. Hosp. Lond., Regist. Rotat. (Surg.) Bloomsbury HA; Regist. (Surg.) Roy. Liverp. Hosp. & Alder Heys Hosp. Liverp.; Demonst. & Tutor Anat. Dept. Univ. Camb.

NOAH, Professor Norman David London School of Hygiene & Tropical Medicine, Keppel Street, London WC1E 7HT Tel: 020 7927 2812 Fax: 020 7436 4230 Email: norman.noah@lshtm.ac.uk; Orley Rise, Orley Farm Road, Harrow-on-The-Hill, Harrow HA1 3PE Tel: 020 8422 2649 Fax: 020 8423 8845 — MB BS Lond. 1963 (St Thos.) MRCP Lond. 1968; MFPHM RCP UK 1981; FFPHM RCP UK 1987; FRCP Lond. 1988. Prof. Epidemiol. & Pub. Health Lond. Sch. Hyg. & Trop. Med.; Sen. Edr. Epidemiol. & Infec. Specialty: Epidemiol. Special Interest: food poisoning; meningitis; Hyg. of skin piercing; vaccines; surveillance. Socs: Fell. Roy. Soc. Med.; Former Sec Internat.Epidemiol.Assn; BMA. Prev: Cons. (Epidemiol.) PHLS Communicable Dis. Surveillance Centre Colindale; Prof. Epidemiol. & Pub. Health Kings Healthcare; Research Asst. Inst. Dis. Chest. Brompton Hosp. Lond.

NOAKES, John Edward, OBE (retired) Old Church Cottage, Old Church Cottage, Chapel Lane, Long Marston, Tring HP23 4QT Tel: 01896 660072 — MB BS Lond. 1959 (Char. Cross) DObst RCOG 1962; FRCGP 1988, M 1977. Non-Exec. Dir. Health Educat. Auth.

NOAKES, John Peter Llewelyn Dolwar, High St., Cilgerran, Cardigan SA43 2SL — MB BS Lond. 1982.

NOAKES, Michael John Hollin House, 10 Combe Park, Weston, Bath BA1 3NP — MB BS Lond. 1970 (Char. Cross) MRCS Eng. LRCP Lond. 1970; DMRD Eng. 1977; FRCR 1978. Cons. (Radiol.) Roy. United Hosp. Bath. Specialty: Radiol. Prev: Sen. Regist. (Radiol.) Leeds Gen. Infirm.; SHO (Med. & Paediat.) Plymouth Gen. Hosp.; Ho. Off. Char. Cross Hosp. Lond.

NOAKES, Paul Christopher The Park Surgery, 4 Alexandra Road, Great Yarmouth NR30 2HW Tel: 01493 855672 — MB ChB Bristol 1986.

NOAMAN, Linda Ann 16 Lammerton Terrace, Dundee DD4 7BW — MB ChB Aberd. 1972.

NOBBS, William Michael Anthony Apartment 3, The Haie, Newnham GL14 1HW — MB BS Lond. 1965; MRCS Eng. LRCP Lond. 1965. Specialty: Accid. & Emerg.

NOBLE, Alastair Lockington Lodgehill Road Clinic, Lodgehill Road, Nairn IV12 4RF Tel: 01667 452096 Fax: 01667 456785 — MB ChB Glas. 1969; DObst RCOG 1972.

NOBLE, Alison Margaret Bankfield, 465 Garstang Road, Broughton, Preston PR3 5JA — MB ChB Bristol 1998.

NOBLE, Mr Anthony Douglas Upper Barford Farm, Bramshaw, Lyndhurst SO43 7JN Tel: 01794 390564 Fax: 01794 390592 — MB BS Lond. 1958 (Lond. Hosp.) MRCS Eng. LRCP Lond. 1958; DCH Eng. 1960; FRCOG 1981, M 1968, DObst. 1964; FRCS Ed. 1966. Medico-legal Expert witness Obst. & Gyn. Specialty: Obst. & Gyn. Socs: BMA. Prev: Cons. (O & G) Winchester & E. Leigh Health Care Trust; Hon. Clin. Teach. Med. Univ. Soton.

NOBLE, Barbara Sylvia Duncan Street Surgery, Duncan Street, Wolverhampton WV2 3AN Tel: 01902 458193 Fax: 01902 455309; 1 Rowley Park Farm House, Worfield, Bridgnorth WV15 5NT Tel: 01746 716584 Fax: 01746 716584 — MB ChB Liverp. 1977; DRCOG 1979; MRCGP 1983; MMedsci. Birm. 1995; FRCGP 2001. Clin. Asst. (Obst. & Gyn.) New Cross Hosp. Wolverhampton; Clin. Lect., Dept. of Primary Care and Gen. Pract., Univ. of Birm. Prev: GP Tutor Wolverhampton.

NOBLE, Mr Bruce Alexander Eye Department, General Infirmary at Leeds, Belmont Grove, Leeds LS2 9NS Tel: 0113 392 2750 — MB BS Lond. 1972 (St. Bart.) BSc Cape Town 1966; FRCS Eng. 1977; FRCOphth 1988. Cons. Ophth. Gen. Infirm. United Leeds Teachg. Hosps. Trust; Cons. Ophth., Yorks. Eye Hosp. Specialty: Ophth. Socs: Internat. Ophth. Microsurg. Study Gp. (Sec.). Prev: Chief Asst. (Eye) St. Bart. Hosp. Lond.; Regist. & SHO Bristol Eye Hosp.; Resid. Surg. Off. Moorfields Eye Hosp. Lond.

NOBLE, Colin 87 Colthill Circle, Milltimber AB13 0EH — MB ChB Aberd. 1996.

NOBLE, Dawn Louise Dryburn Hospital, North Road, Durham DH1 5TW Tel: 0191 333 2333; 16 The Oval, Hartlepool TS26 9QH Tel: 01429 861250 — MB BS Newc. 1997 (Newcastle) SHO (Med.) Dryburn Hosp. Durh. Specialty: Gen. Med. Prev: PRHO (Surg) RUI, Newc.1998.

NOBLE, Deborah Clare 6 Sergison Road, Haywards Heath RH16 1HS — BM BS Nottm. 1995.

NOBLE, Dilys Ann Birley Health Centre, 120 Birley Lane, Sheffield S12 3BP Tel: 0114 239 2541 Fax: 0114 264 5814; 92 Ashdell Road, Sheffield S10 3DB Tel: 0114 661372 — MB ChB Sheff. 1971; DRCOG 1973; DCH Eng. 1976. Prev: Regist. (Cas.) Sheff. Childr. Hosp.; SHO (O & G) Scarsdale Hosp. Chesterfield; Med. Off. St. Joseph's Hosp. Jirapa, Ghana.

NOBLE, Elizabeth Patricia Eastfield Group Practice, 1 Eastway, Eastfield, Scarborough YO11 3LS Tel: 01723 582297 Fax: 01723 582528; 16 Holbeck Avenue, Scarborough YO11 2XQ — MB ChB Aberd. 1983; DRCOG 1986. GP E.field Surg. ScarBoro. VTS. Prev: Clin. Med. Off. ScarBoro. HA; Trainee GP ScarBoro. Hosp. VTS; Ho. Off. (Surg.) Harrogate Dist. Hosp.

NOBLE, George Edward 6 Schofield Way, Eastbourne BN23 6HQ — MB BS Lond. 1983; MRCP (UK) 1986; LLB Lond. 1991; LLM Wales 1995; FRACP 1999.

NOBLE, Gillian Margaret White Medical Group, Thornhill Road, Ponteland, Newcastle upon Tyne NE20 9 Tel: 01661 822222 Fax: 01661 821994 — MB BS Newc. 1982; MRCGP 1988. GP Newc.

NOBLE, Hartley Marshall Sutherland (retired) 46 Broadway, Sheerness ME12 Tel: 01795 663481 — MB ChB Ed. 1949; MRCGP 1963. Div. Surg. St. John Ambul. Brig.; Med. Off. Red Cross I. of Sheppey Br. Prev: GP Sheerness.

NOBLE, Hilary Alison Appt. 1, The Gloster, The Parade, Cowes PO31 7QD Tel: 01983 280865 — BM Soton. 1977; FFA RCS Eng. 1984; FRCA (Eng.) 1984. Cons. Anaesth. St. Mary's Hosp. Newport I. of Wight. Specialty: Anaesth.

NOBLE, Iain Samuel The Diamond Medical Centre, The Diamond, Magherafelt BT45 6ED — MB ChB Bristol 1984; DRCOG 1986; MRCGP 1988.

NOBLE, Isabel Mary (retired) 17 Glenorchy Terrace, Edinburgh EH9 2DQ — MB ChB Aberd. 1954; MRCP Lond. 1963; FRCP Ed. 1973, M 1971. Cons. Phys. Roy. Infirm. & Chalmers Hosp. Edin. Prev: Cons. Phys. Bruntsfield, Longmore & Deaconess Hosps. Edin.

NOBLE, James Kelvingrove Medical Centre, 28 Hands Road, Heanor DE75 7HA Tel: 01773 713201 Fax: 01773 534380 — MB ChB Glas. 1974; BSc Glas. 1974; MRCGP 1985. Specialty: Plastic Surg.

NOBLE, James Gordon 201 Hesketh Lane, Tarleton, Preston PR4 6AT — LRCP LRCS Ed. 1953; LRCP LRCS Ed. LRFPS Glas. 1953; DPM Eng. 1962; MRCPsych 1971. Specialty: Gen. Psychiat. Prev: Cons. Psychiat. Greaves Hall Hosp.; Dep. Med. Supt. & Cons. Psychiat. Rampton Hosp. Retford & Moss Side Hosp.; Asst. Psychiat. Stoke Pk. Hosp. Bristol.

NOBLE, Jane Elizabeth 30 India Street, Montrose DD10 8PG — MB ChB Ed. 1991.

NOBLE, Jane Mary 6 Hambledon Gardens, High Heaton, Newcastle upon Tyne NE7 7AL — BM BCh Oxf. 1991.

NOBLE, Mr Jeremy Guy Churchill Hospital, Department of Urology, Oxford OX3 7LJ Tel: 01865 225942 Fax: 01865 226086 Email: jeremy.noble@orh.nhs.uk — MB BS Lond. 1984 (St. Bart. Hosp. Lond.) FRCS Ed. 1989; FRCS Eng. 1989; FRCS (Urol.) 1994; MD Lond. 1994. Cons. Urol. Surg. Oxf. Radcliffe Hosp. Trust; Hon. Clin. Sen. Lect. Fac. of Med. Univ. of Oxf. Specialty: Urol. Special Interest: Lower Urin. Tract Dysfunction; Pelvic Cancer; Reconstruction. Socs: Brit. Assn. Urol. Surgs.; Roy. Soc. Med.; RCS. Prev: Sen. Regist. (Urol.) Guy's Hosp. Lond., St. Peter's Hosp. & Inst. Urol. Lond.; Research Fell. (Urol.) Middlx Hosp. Lond.; Regist. (Surg.) Lond.

NOBLE, Joan Lamont Lodgehill Road Clinic, Lodgehill Road, Nairn IV12 4RF Tel: 01667 452096 Fax: 01667 456785 — MB ChB Aberd. 1971; MRCP (UK) 1973; BA (Hons.) Open Univ. 1994; FRCP Glas. 1994; FRCP Glas. 1994.

NOBLE, Joan Laura Manchester Royal Eye Hospital, Oxford Road, Manchester M13 9WH Tel: 0161 276 5567 Fax: 0161 272 6618; New Hall, Stocks Lane, Over Peover, Knutsford WA16 9HE Tel: 01565 722871 Fax: 01565 722871 — MB ChB Ed. 1971; DO Eng. 1976; FRCS Ed. 1976; FRCOphth 1989. p/t Cons. Ophth. Surg. Roy. Manch. Eye Hosp.; Cons. Ophth., Booth Hall Childrens Hosp. Specialty: Ophth. Socs: Eur. Occuloplastic & Reconstruc. Surgs.; Brit. Occuloplastic Soc.; Roy. Coll. of Ophthalmologists.

NOBLE, John Robinson Solstrand, Whiterock Bay, Killinchy, Newtownards BT23 6QA — MB BCh BAO Dub. 1953 (T.C. Dub.) MA Dub. 1971, BA 1951; DPM Eng. 1970; FRCPsych 1985, M 1972. Specialty: Gen. Psychiat. Prev: Cons. Psychiat. Holywell Hosp. Antrim & Whiteabbey Hosp., Belf.

NOBLE, John Stephen Cumine Flat 5, 60 Lumsden St., Over Newton Square, Glasgow G3 8RH Tel: 0141 357 3234; 19 Grattan Place, Fraserburgh AB43 9SD Tel: 01346 518115 — MB ChB Aberd. 1986; DRCOG 1990; MRCP (UK) 1990; MRCGP 1993; FRCA 1997; FFARCS 1997. Specialist Regist. (Anaesth.) Vict. Infirm. Glas. Specialty: Anaesth.

NOBLE, Mr Jonathan BUPA Hospital, Russell Road, Whalley Range, Manchester M16 8AJ Tel: 0161 232 2592; New Hall, Stocks Lane, Over Peover, Knutsford WA16 9HE Tel: 01565 722871 — (Ed.) MB ChB Ed. 1966; FRCS Ed 1972; ChM Ed. 1980; FRCS Eng. 1990. Cons. Orthop. Surg. Salford HA; Hon. Sen. Lect. (Orthop. Surg.) Univ. Manch. Specialty: Orthop. Socs: Fell. BOA; Brit. Soc. Surg. Hand; Past Pres. Brit. Assn. Surg. Knee. Prev: Reader (Orthop. Surg.) Univ. Manch; Sen. Lect. (Orthop. Surg.) Univ. Manch.; Lect. (Orthop. Surg.) Univ. Edin.

NOBLE, Katharine Louise New Sheepmarket Surgery, Ryhall Road, Stamford PE9 1YA Tel: 01780 758123 Fax: 01780 758102 — MB ChB Leic. 1988.

NOBLE, Kerr William Braids Medical Practice, 6 Camus Avenue, Edinburgh EH10 6QT Tel: 0131 445 5999 Fax: 0131 445 3553; 17 Foulis Crescent, Juniper Green EH14 5BN Tel: 0131 453 4041 — MB ChB Dundee 1982 (University of Dundee) DRCOG 1985; MRCGP 1986.

NOBLE, Margaret Bonney (retired) 3 Swinbrook Court, Langdale Gate, Witney OX28 6FN Tel: 01993 774836 — MB ChB (Commend.) St. And. 1944 (Univ. St. And.) BSc St. And. 1941; MRCOG 1952; MRCGP 1963.

NOBLE, Mr Mark Christopher Brian Scarborough Hospital, Scarborough YO12 6QL Tel: 01723 368111; Finistere, Hutton Buscel, Scarborough YO13 9LL — MB ChB Aberd. 1973; FRCOG 1996, M 1979. Cons. O & G ScarBoro. & N. E. Yorks. Healthcare Trust. Specialty: Obst. & Gyn. Socs: Blair Bell Res. Soc.; Spencer Wells Soc.; Brit. Soc. Colpos. & Cerv. Path. Prev: Sen. Regist. (O & G) Princess Mary Matern. Hosp. & Roy. Vict. Infirm. Newc.; Regist. (O & G) King's Coll. Hosp. Lond.; SHO (Obst.) St. Mary's Hosp. Lond.

NOBLE, Matthew Dominic 7 Charnwood Drive, Thurnby, Leicester LE7 9PD — MB BS Lond. 1988; DRCOG 1993. SHO (Adult Psychiat.) Peter Hodgkinson Centre Lincoln. Specialty: Alcohol & Substance Misuse.

NOBLE, Michael John Acle Medical Centre, Bridewell Lane, Acle, Norwich NR13 3RA Tel: 01493 750888 Fax: 01493 751652 — MB BChir Camb. 1988.

NOBLE, Paul David — MB BCh Wales 1987; DA (UK) 1991; FRCA 1993. Specialty: Anaesth. Socs: Assoc. Mem. Assn of Cardio-Thoracic Anaesth. Prev: Sen. Regist. (Anaesth.) King's Coll. Hosp. Lond.; Sen. Regist. (Anaesth.) Roy. Sussex Co. Hosp. Brighton.

NOBLE, Penelope Louise 46 Sunray Avenue, London SE24 9PX — MB BS Lond. 1991 (King's College Hospital London) BSc (Psychol.) Lond. 1988; MRCOG 1997. Research Fell. (Fetal Med.) King's Coll. Hosp. Lond. Specialty: Obst. & Gyn. Prev: SHO (O & G) Roy. Sussex Co. Hosp. Brighton.

NOBLE, Peter John The Maudsley Hospital, Denmark Hill, London SE5 8AZ Tel: 0207 733 6333 — MB BChir Camb. 1962; FRCP Lond. 1981, M 1964; DPM Lond. 1969; MA Camb. 1971, MD 1971; FRCPsych 1979, M 1971. Emerit. Cons. Psychiat. Bethlem Roy. & Maudsley Hosps. Lond. Specialty: Gen. Psychiat. Socs: Fell. Roy. Soc. Med.; Fell. Roy. Coll. Phys.; Fell. Roy. Coll. Psychiat. Prev: Cons. Psychiat. Bethlem Roy. & Mandsley Hosps. Lond.; Sen. Lect. Univ. Lond.; Lect. Inst. Psychiat. Lond.

NOBLE, Peter Richard 51 Grosvenor Park, London SE5 0NH — BM BCh Oxf. 1985.

NOBLE, Richard Simon c/o Haematology Department, Treliske Hospital, Truro TR1 3LJ Tel: 01872 74242 Email: richard.noble@cornwall.nhs.uk — MB ChB Bristol 1983; MRCP (UK) 1988; MRCPath 1996. Cons. Haemat. Treliske Hosp. Truro. Specialty: Haematology. Prev: Sen. Regist. (Haemat.) W. Yorks.; Regist. (Haemat.) Roy. Vict. Infirm. Newc.; Research Regist. (Haemat.) Sunderland Roy. Infirm.

NOBLE, Sandra Elizabeth — MB ChB St Au 1968; DCCH. Sen. Clin. Med. Off. Community Child Health.

NOBLE, Simon Ian Robert 2 Ladbroke Hurst, Dormansland, Lingfield RH7 6QB — MB BS Lond. 1993.

NOBLE, Stanley Charles The Health Centre, Marmaduke St., Hull HU3 3BH — MB ChB Leeds 1954.

NOBLE, Susan Grace Newlands Medical Centre, Borough Road, Middlesbrough TS1 3RX — MB ChB Glas. 1985; DRCOG 1988; DCH RCPS Glas. 1989; MRCGP 1990.

NOBLE, Thomas Cyril (retired) 2 Sycamore Close, Sedbergh LA10 5EB Tel: 01539 620100 Email: t.c.noble@talk21.com — MB ChB Ed. 1944 (Univ. Ed.) FRCP Ed. 1970, M 1949; DCH Eng. 1951; FRCPCH 1998. Prev: Cons. Paediat. Newc. AHA (T).

NOBLE, Thomas William Norwood Medical Centre, 360 Herries Road, Sheffield S5 7HD Tel: 0114 426208; 29 Fir Street, Sheffield S6 3TG — MB ChB Sheff. 1979; MRCGP 1985. Assoc. Specialist in Palliat. Care St. Luke's Nursing Home Sheff. Prev: Trainee GP Sheff. VTS; Ho. Surg. Sheff. Childr. Hosp.; Ho. Phys. Roy. Hallamsh. Hosp.

NOBLE, Timothy Charles University Medical Centre, Giles Lane, Canterbury CT2 7PB Tel: 01227 765682 Fax: 01227 780954 — MB BS Lond. 1986; DRCOG 1994; MRCGP 1995. Clin. Asst. Psychosexual Thearpy Canterbury. Specialty: Gen. Pract. Socs: Mem. Inst. Psychosexual Med. Prev: Regist. Gen. Hosp. St. Helier Jersey; Clin. Asst. (Med. Oncol.) Kent & Cantrerbury Hosp.

NOBLE, Timothy John 42 Walney Road, Heworth, York YO31 1AJ — MB BS Lond. 1989; MRCP (UK) 1995. Specialist Regist. (Resp.) Northern Gen. Hosp. Sheff. Specialty: Respirat. Med.; Gen. Med.

NOBLE, Vibert 19 Misterton Crescent, Ravenshead, Nottingham NG15 9AX Tel: 01623 797092 — MB BS Lond. 1980 (King's Coll. Hosp.) MRCP (UK) 1986. Cons. Paediat. King's Mill Centre for Healthcare Serv. Specialty: Paediat.; Neonat.

NOBLE, Warwick Stanley (retired) 516 Clive Court, Maida Vale, London W9 1SG — MRCS Eng. LRCP Lond. 1934 (Guy's) Prev: Ho. Surg. Gravesend & N. Kent Hosp.

NOBLE, Wendy Lou Oakhouse, 43 North Barr Without, Beverley HU17 7AG Tel: 01482 888099 — MB ChB Leic. 1985; BSc Biol. Chem. Essex 1980; MRCOG 1994; CCST 2000. Cons. Obsehician & Gynaecologist; Hull & E. Yorks. Hosp. Trust. Specialty: Obst. & Gyn.; Educat. Socs: RCOG; BSGE. Prev: Regist. (Genitourin. Med.) & SHO (O & G) St. Richards Hosp. Chichester; Regist. (O & G) St. Mary's Hosp. Portsmouth.; SR (OTG) Princess Anne Hosp. Southampton.

NOBLE, William Arthur (retired) Bankfield, Broughton, Preston PR3 5JA — MB BCh BAO NUI 1960; FFA RCS Eng. 1969.

NOBLE-MATHEWS, Priscilla Mary, OStJ (retired) Lovehill Cottage, Trotton, Petersfield GU31 5ER Tel: 01730 816583 Fax: 01730 816583 Email: priscillamary.nm@virgin.net — BM Soton. 1976; Barrister at Law Middle Temple 1953; Dip. Palliat. Med. Wales 1992; Dip. IMC (RCS Ed.) 1996; FIMC (RCS ed.) 2000. Prev: Clin. Asst. Diabetes Worthing Hosp.

NOBLETT, Angela Katherine Over Wyre Medical Centre, Wilkinson Way, Off Pilling Lane, Poulton-le-Fylde FY6 0EX Tel: 01253 810722 Fax: 01253 812039 Email: overwyremed.centre@btinternet.com; Brooklyn, Carr Lane, Hambleton, Poulton-le-Fylde FY6 9AZ Tel: 01253 700381 — MB BS Newc. 1985; Cert. Family Plann. JCC 1987; DRCOG 1988; MRCGP 1989. Specialty: Gen. Pract. Socs: Brit. Med. Soc. Prev: Trainee GP Preston VTS; SHO (Paediat.& Gen. Med.) Roy. Preston. Hosp.; SHO (A & E & O & G) Preston HA.

NOBLETT, John Joseph The Croft Surgery, The Croft, Kirkbridge, Carlisle CA7 5JH — MB ChB Liverp. 1986.

NOCK, Ian David 6 Widecombe Avenue, Stafford ST17 0HX — BM Soton. 1991.

NOCKLER, Ingeborg Barbara X-Ray Department, St Bartholomew's Hospital, West Smithfield, London EC1A 7BE Fax: 0207 601 8301; 48 Stanhope Road, Highgate, London N6 5AJ Tel: 020 8348 0026 Fax: 020 8348 0026 Email: ingenockler@hotmail.com — MB ChB Pretoria 1971; FRCR Lond. 1981. Cons. Radiol. (Breast Imaging) St Bart's Hosp W. Smithfield Lond.; Cons Radiologist (Breast Screening) Char. Cross Hosp Lond., The Lond. Clinic, Devonshire Pl., Lond., The Princess Grale Hosp., Nottm. Pl., The King Edwd. VII Hosp., Beaumont St., Lond. Specialty: Radiol. Socs: Roy. Coll. Radiol.; Roy. Soc. Med.; BMS.

NOCKOLDS, Claire Louise 55 Milton Av, King's Lynn PE30 2QQ — MB ChB Sheff. 1997.

NOCTON, John Marcus (retired) Cobdown, Five Ash Down, Uckfield TN22 3AR Tel: 01825 732175 — (St. Thos.) MB BS Lond. 1961; DObst RCOG 1963. Prev: Cas. Off., Ho. Surg. (Orthop.) & Ho. Phys. (O & G) St. Thos. Hosp. Lond.

NODDER, Elizabeth Mary Louise Dean Lane Surgery, Dean Lane, Sixpenny Handley, Salisbury SP5 5PA Tel: 01725 552500 Fax: 01725 552029; The White House, High St, Sixpenny Handley, Salisbury SP5 5ND — BM BCh Oxf. 1983 (Univ. Camb., John Radcliffe Hosp. Oxf.) DGM RCP Lond. 1985; DCH RCP Lond. 1986; MRCGP 1988. Socs: Assn. Med. Advisers Brit. Orchestras.

NODDER, James Henry Bennetts End Surgery, Gatecroft, Hemel Hempstead HP3 9LY Tel: 01442 263511 Fax: 01442 235419 — MB BS Lond. 1973; DRCOG 1976. Prev: Ho. Surg. (Neurosurg.) & SHO (O & G) Lond. Hosp.; Trainee Gen. Pract. Watford Vocational Train. Scheme.

NODEN, Jayne Belinda 10 Grange Holt, Alwoodley, Leeds LS17 7TY — MB ChB Leeds 1987.

NOEL, Isabel Department Pathology, Dryburn Hospital, North Road, Durham DH1 5TW — MB ChB Dundee 1978; MD Dundee 1996, BMedSci (Anat.) (Hons.) 1975; MSc (Med. Microbiol.) Lond. 1983. Assoc. Specialist (Med. Microbiol) Dryburn Hosp. Durh. Specialty: Med. Microbiol.

NOEL, Montague Geoffrey Bickersteth High Street Surgery, 137 High Street, Cranfield, Bedford MK43 0HZ Tel: 01234 750234; Monastery House, Little Crawley, Newport Pagnell MK16 9LT Tel: 01234 391228 — MRCS Eng. LRCP Lond. 1956 (Westm.) DA Eng. 1967; FFA RCS Eng. 1968. Specialty: Anaesth.

NOEL, Peter Roy Butlin (retired) 8 Church Street, Hemingford Grey, Huntingdon PE28 9DF — MB BS Lond. 1948 (Univ. Coll. Hosp.) Prev: Med. & Sci. Dir. Huntingdon Res. Centre.

NOEL-PATON, Mary Kezia Hewlett The South Wing, Holmbush House, Horsham RH12 4SE Tel: 01293 851578 Fax: 01293 852578 Email: noel.paton@solutions.inc.co.uk; The South Wing, Holmbrush House, Faygate, Horsham RH12 4SE Tel: 01293 851578 — MB BS Lond. 1964 (St. Thos.) Dobst RCOG 1967. Gen. practitioner Locum, Pk. Surg., Horsham. Socs: Brit. Soc. Allergy & Environm. Med.; Med. Off. Sch. Assn. Prev: Regist. (Psychiat.) Brookwood Hosp. Knaphill; Ho. Surg. (Obst.) Weir Hosp. Balham; Sch. Med. Off. Christ's Hosp. Horsham.

NOFAL, Mr Farhat Metwally Chesterfield & North Derbyshire Royal NHS Hospital, ENT Department, Calow, Chesterfield S44 5BL; Rosehill, 57 Chesterfield Road, Deconsfield, Dronfield S18 2XA Tel: 01246 413706 Fax: 01246 413706 — MB BCh Cairo 1972 (Cairo Uni.) DLO RCS Eng. 1979; FRCS Ed. 1980. Cons. ENT Chesterfield & N. Derbysh. Roy. Hosp. Specialty: Otorhinolaryngol.

NOFAL, Mr Magdy Abd-El Monem Saleh Torbay General Hospital, Lawe's Bridge, Torquay TQ2 7AA; 5 Stadium Drive, Kingskerswell, Newton Abbot TQ12 5HP — MB ChB Cairo 1975; FRCS (Ophth.) Ed. 1983.

NOGLIK, Anne Marga 26 Ford Road, Upton, Wirral CH49 0TF — MB ChB Liverp. 1992; MRCP (UK) 1997. Specialist Regist. (Paediat.) Alder Hey Child. Hosp. Liv'pl. Specialty: Paediat.; Neonat.

NOH, Mohamed Bin Md 22 Adelaide Park, Belfast BT9 6FX — MB BCh BAO Belf. 1992.

NOHL-OSER, Mr H Christian (retired) 23 Bracknell Gate, Frognal Lane, London NW3 7EA Tel: 020 7435 3376 — BM BCh Oxf. 1944; DM Oxf. 1960, MA, BM BCh 1944; FRCS Eng. 1951. Hon. Cons. Thoracic Surg. Harefield Hosp. Prev: Cons. Thoracic Surg. Harefield, Hillingdon & W. Middlx. (Univ.) Hosp.

NOHR, Karine Foxhill Medical Centre, 363 Halifax Road, Sheffield S6 1AF Tel: 0114 232 2055 Fax: 0114 285 5963; Foxhill MC, 363 Halifax Road, Sheffield S6 1AF Tel: 0114 232 2055 — MB ChB Sheff. 1982; MRCOG 1987; MRCGP 1993. GP Sheff.; Clin. Asst. (Psychosexual Med.); Hon. Lect. Clin. Tutor Dept. Gen. Pract. Univ. of Sheff. Specialty: Psychosexual Med.

NOKES, Leonard Derek Martin Cardiff School of Engineering, PO Box 917, Newport Road, Cardiff CF24 0XH; 35 Lon Isa, Rhiwbina, Cardiff CF14 6EE — MB BCh Wales 1990; BEng Wales 1980; MSc Wales 1982; PhD Wales 1983; MD Wales 1993. Dir. Med. Eng. Research Centre. Univ. Wales Coll. Cardiff; Hon. Lect. (Forens. Med.) Univ. Wales Coll. Med. Specialty: Orthop.; Sports Med.

NOKES, Timothy John Charles 32 Wynndale Road, London E18 1DX Tel: 020 8505 9684; Department of Haematology, UCLH, Grafton Way, London WC1 Tel: 020 7387 9300 — MB BS Lond. 1990 (Roy. Free Hosp.) MRCP (UK) 1993; DRCPath 1995; MRCPath 1997. Sen. Regist. (Haemat.) UCLH. Specialty: Haematology. Socs: Roy. Coll. Path.; Brit. Soc. Haematol. Prev: Sen. Regist. (Haemat.) Centr. Middlx. Hosp. Lond.; Sen. Regist. (Haemat.) Edgware & Barnet Gen. Hosp. Middlx.; Regist. (Haemat.) UCLH & Whipps Cross Hosp. Lond.

NOKTEHDAN, Niloufar Halliwick Psychotherapy Department, St Anne's Hospital, St Ann's Road, London N15 3TH — BM Soton. 1995.

NOLAN, Mr Bernard (retired) Wester Rubislaw, 79/1 Braid Avenue, Edinburgh EH10 6ED Tel: 0131 447 3383 — MB ChB Ed. 1949; FRCS Ed. 1955; FRCS Eng. 1957; ChM Ed. 1968. Prev: Cons. Surg. Roy. Infirm. Edin.

NOLAN, Catherine Mary Intensive Care Unit, Southampton General Hospital, Southampton SO16 6YD Tel: 023 8079 6117 Email: kathleen.nolan@suht.swest.nhs.uk — MB BCh BAO NUI

1982; FFA RCSI 1987. Cons. Intens. Care Soton. Gen. Hosp. Specialty: Intens. Care.

NOLAN, Christopher Paul 47 Sandhurst Gardens, Belfast BT9 5AX — MB BCh BAO Belf. 1987. Cons., Orthop.

NOLAN, Daniel Joseph (retired) — MB BCh BAO NUI 1965 (Univ. Coll. Dub.) LM Rotunda. 1966; DMRD Eng. 1970; MRCP (UK) 1971; FRCR 1972; MB BCh BAO NUI 1980; MD NUI 1980; FRCP 1998. Prev: Cons. Radiol. John Radcliffe Hosp. Oxf.

NOLAN, David Francis Luke Horstead House, Mill Road, Horstead, Norwich NR12 7AU — MB BS Lond. 1998.

NOLAN, Deborah Mary 34 Sandhurst Road, Didsbury, Manchester M20 5LR — MB ChB Manch. 1978; FFA RCS Eng. 1984. Cons. Anaesth. Univ. Hosp. S. Manch. Specialty: Anaesth. Prev: Sen. Regist. (Anaesth.) Roy. Perth Hosp., Australia.

NOLAN, Eileen Mary Aylestone Road Medical Centre, 705 Aylestone Road, Leicester LE2 8TG Tel: 0116 283 2325; Glennamaddy, 8 Link Road, Leicester LE2 3RA — MB ChB Glas. 1972.

NOLAN, Ellen Mary Oakengates Medical Practice, Limes Walk, Oakengates, Telford TF2 6JJ — MB BCh BAO NUI 1983; DCH RCP Lond. 1986; DRCOG 1987; MRCGP 1988.

NOLAN, Frances Carmel The Surgery, 939 Green Lanes, Winchmore Hill, London N21 2PB Tel: 020 8360 2228 Fax: 020 9360 5702 — MB BCh BAO NUI 1976; DRCOG 1980. Princip. in Gen. Pract. Lond. Prev: Trainee GP Brighton; Ho. Surg. St. Geo. Hosp. Lond.; Ho. Phys. Southlands Hosp. Shoreham-by-Sea.

NOLAN, James 31 Enfield Road, Old Swan, Liverpool L13 5TB — MB ChB Leeds 1983.

NOLAN, Jane Ann Brunswick House Medical Group, 1 Brunswick Street, Carlisle CA1 1ED Tel: 01228 515808 Fax: 01228 593048; 4 The Forge, Dalston, Carlisle CA5 7QL Tel: 01228 711183 — MB ChB Birm. 1979; DRCOG 1981; DCH RCP Lond. 1983; MRCGP 1984. Specialty: Obst. & Gyn. Prev: GP Birm.

NOLAN, Janet Anne Devonshire Road Surgery, 467 Devonshire Road, Blackpool FY2 0JP Tel: 01253 352233; 467 Devonshire Road, Blackpool FY2 0JP Tel: 01253 52233 — MB ChB Manch. 1985. Socs: Primary Care Rheum. Soc.; Brit. Menopause Soc. Prev: Trainee GP Preston; Trainee GP/SHO Truro VTS; Ho. Off. Blackburn.

NOLAN, Jeremy Paul Department of Anaesthetics, Royal United Hospital, Combe Park, Bath BA1 3NG Tel: 01225 825056 Fax: 01225 825061 — MB ChB Bristol 1983; FRCA 1989. Cons. Anaesth. Roy. United Hosp. Bath. Specialty: Anaesth.; Intens. Care. Socs: Assn. Anaesth.; Intens. Care Soc.; Resusc. Counc. Mem. of Exec. Comm. Prev: Sen. Regist. (Anaesth.) Roy. United Hosp. Bath.; Regist. Rotat. (Anaesth.) Bristol.

NOLAN, Joanne Elizabeth The Old Vicarage, The Street, Hempnall, Norwich NR15 2AD Tel: 01508 499641 Email: jfnolan@enterprise.net — MB BS Lond. 1989; MRCGP 1994.

NOLAN, Johanna Assumpta Cecilia Lochhead Cottage, Forfar DD8 2RL — MB BCh BAO Dub. 1975.

NOLAN, Mr John Francis Orthopaedic Department, Norfolk & Norwich Hospital, Brunswick Road, Norwich NR1 3SR Tel: 01603 287853 Fax: 01603 287498 Email: john.nolan@nnuh.nhs.uk — MB BS Lond. 1984; FRCS Eng. 1988; FRCS (Orth.) 1993. Cons. Orthop. & Trauma Norf. & Norwich Hosp.; Examr. (Speciality Bd. in Trauma & Orthop.). Specialty: Orthop. Socs: Brit. Hip Soc. - Mem.; Brit. Orthopaedic Assn. - Fell.; E. Anglian Orthopaedic Club - Sec.

NOLAN, Philip John (retired) Meltham Road Surgery, 9 Meltham Road, Lockwood, Huddersfield HD1 3UP Tel: 01484 432940 Fax: 01484 451423; 67 Kaye Lane, Almondbury, Huddersfield HD5 8XT Tel: 01484 432847 — MB ChB Manch. 1962; FRCGP 1980, M 1974.

NOLAN, William Patrick New Caple Street Surgery, Pontnewydd, Cwmbran NP44 1DU — MB BCh BAO NUI 1985.

NOLAN, Miss Winifred Patricia The Institute of Opthalmology, University of London, Bath St., London EC1V 9EL; 10 Apsley Road, Summertown, Oxford OX2 7QY — MB ChB Birm. 1991 (Uni. Birm.) FRCOphth 1997. Research Fell. (Ophth.) Inst. Ophth. Specialty: Ophth.

NOLAND, Deborah Jane Student Services Centre, 150 Mount Pleasant, Liverpool L69 3BX Tel: 0151 794 4720 — MB ChB Liverp. 1989; DRCOG 1991; MRCGP 1994.

NOLTIE, Anne Christina Kirsty Abbey Health Centre, Arbroath DD11 1EN Tel: 01241 872692 Fax: 01241 872976 — MB ChB Manch. 1981 (Manchester) BSc MedSci St. And. 1978; MRCGP 1986.

NONDY, Bissesswor c/o Lloyds Bank, Southampton Row, London WC1; 15 Saxon Road, South Norwood, Selhurst, London SE25 5EQ — MB BS Calcutta 1955; DLO Eng. 1966. Socs: BMA; Med. Protec. Soc. Prev: GP Lond.

NONHEBEL, Alice Charlotte Rowleys, Southwood Rd, Shalden, Alton GU34 4EB — MB ChB Leeds 1996.

NONIS, Chrisantha Nicholas Anthony 51 Gilling Court, Belsize Grove, London NW3 4XA — MB BS Lond. 1990; BSc Lond. 1989.

NONOO-COHEN, Cinderella Ground Floor Flat, 101 Talbot Road, Highgate, London N6 4QX Tel: 020 8347 7486 Fax: 020 8347 7486 — MB BS Lond. 1993; DRCOG 1998. GP Regist. Specialty: Gen. Med. Socs: LJMS. Prev: SHO (c/o Elderly) Univ. Coll. Hosp. Lond.; SHO (A & E) Whittington Hosp. Lond.; SHO Rotat. (Med.) St. Bart. Hosp. Lond.

NOOH, Ahmed Mohamed Mahdy Khaleel 11 Gayton Road, King's Lynn PE30 4EA — MB BCh Zagazig, Egypt 1981.

NOOHU KANNU, Abdulkhadir The Surgery, 33 Penrose Street, London SE17 3DW Tel: 020 7703 3677; 29 Fermoy Road, Greenford UB6 9HX Tel: 020 8578 3751 — MB BS Kerala 1971 (Med. Coll. Trivandrum) Cert. Prescribed Exp. JCC 1980; MICGP 1987. Prev: Tutor (Gen. Med.) Coll. Kottayam, India; Med. Off. Mwanza Consulat Hosp. Tanzania; SHO (Geriat. Med.) Linton Hosp. Maidstone.

NOOKARAJU, Kondru Nantyglo Medical Centre, Queen Street, Nantyglo, Brynmawr, Ebbw Vale NP23 4LW Tel: 01495 310381 Fax: 01495 310807; 2 Coed-Cae, Rassau, Ebbw Vale NP23 5TP Tel: 01495 303798 — MB BS Andhra 1963 (Guntur Med. Coll.) Cert FPA 1974. Specialty: Family Plann. & Reproduc. Health.

NOON, Adrian James 10 Church Close, Wythall, Birmingham B47 6JQ — MB ChB Birm. 1986.

NOON, Mr Charles Frederick (retired) 21 Lawrie Park Crescent, London SE26 6HH Tel: 020 8778 5174 Fax: 020 8249 5193 — (St. Bart.) BA (2nd cl. Nat. Sci. Trip. Pts. 1 & 2) Camb.; MRCS Eng. LRCP Lond. 1947; FRCS Eng. 1953. Prev: Cons. Surg. Redbridge HA.

NOON, Christopher Charles The Surgery, Pleasant Place, Hersham, Walton-on-Thames KT12 4HT Tel: 01932 229033 Fax: 01932 254706; 28 St. Martins Drive, Walton-on-Thames KT12 3BW — MB BS Lond. 1976 (St. Bart.) MRCS Eng. LRCP Lond. 1976. Clin. Asst. (Cardiol.) St. Peters Hosp. Chertsey. Prev: Trainee GP King's Lynn VTS; SHO (Cas.) Wexham Pk. Slough; Ho. Off. (Gen. Surg.) Norf. & Norwich Hosp.

NOONAN, Alex (retired) 20 St Nicholas Way, Abbots, Bromley WS15 3EB Tel: 01283 841090 Email: naranjaalex@aol.com — MB BS Lond. 1966 (St. Bart.) MRCS Eng. LRCP Lond. 1966. Prev: Ho. Phys. St. Bart. Hosp.

NOONAN, Walter John The Health Centre, Rikenel, The Park, Gloucester GL1 1XR Tel: 01452 891110 Fax: 01452 891111 — MB BS Sydney 1977; MRCGP 1986.

NOONE, Bridget Eleanor Mary 5 Nicholl Court, Mumbles, Swansea SA3 4LZ — MB BCh BAO NUI 1977.

NOONE, Catherine Stoke Mandeville Hospital, Mandeville Road, Aylesbury HP21 8AL Tel: 01296 315159 Fax: 01296 345163; 17 Haglis Drive, Wendover, Aylesbury HP22 6LY — MB BS Lond. 1976 (King's Coll. Hosp.) MRCP (UK) 1979; FRCP Lond. 1995. Cons. Paediat. Stoke Mandeville Hosp. Aylesbury. Specialty: Paediat.

NOONE, John Francis Elms Medical Centre, Green Lane, Whitefield, Manchester M45 7FD Tel: 0161 766 2311 Fax: 0161 767 9544; 15 Longley Drive, Worsley, Manchester M28 2TP — MB ChB Manch. 1971 (Manchester) MRCGP 1977. Lect. Dept. Gen. Pract. Univ. Manch.; Clin. Governance Lead Bury S. PCG.

NOONE, Martina Ann 12 Chappell Road, Droylsden, Manchester M43 7NA; University College London, 26 Rustat Road, Cambridge CB1 3QT — MB ChB Manch. 1992. Clin. Research. Fell. Uni. Coll. Lond. Specialty: Paediat.

NOONE, Oliver Pratap 25 Loddon Bridge Road, Woodley, Reading RG5 4AU — MB BS Kerala 1972; Dip. Thoracic Med. Lond 1983.

NOOR, Farah — MB BS Lond. 1996. Socs: MDU.

NOOR, Rizwana 20 The Orchard, Winchmore Hill, London N21 2DH — MB ChB Leeds 1986.

NOORANI, Farah 177 Rectory Road, Farnborough GU14 8AJ — MB BS Lond. 1998.

NOORANI, Mr Mohammed Ali (retired) 20 Littlebourne Road, Maidstone ME14 5QP Tel: 01622 209535 Fax: 01622 209535 — MB BS Karachi 1960; DLO RCS Eng. 1967; FRCS Ed. 1969. Prev: Locum Cons. ENT Surg., MiddlesBoro., Basingstoke, Whipps Cross Hosp., Crawley.

NOORDEEN, Mr Mohammed Hamza Hilali 107 Harley Street, London W1G 6AL Tel: 020 7487 2819 Fax: 020 7935 3036 Email: hilali.noordeen@virgin.net — BM BCh Oxf. 1985; MA Oxf. 1983; FRCS Eng. 1989; MCh (Orth.) 1993; FRCS (Orth.) 1993. Cons. Orthop. Surg. Roy. Nat. Orthop. Hosp. & Hosp. Childr. Gt. Ormond St. Lond.; Hon. Sen. Lect. Inst. of Orthop. Univ. of Lond.; Hon. Sen. Lect. Insititute of Child Health Univ. of Lond. Specialty: Orthop. Socs: Brit. Orthop. Assn.; Brit. Scoliosis Soc.; BMA. Prev: Cons. Orthop. Surg. Middlx. & Unit. Coll. Hosp. Lond.; Sen. Regist. Middlx. Hosp.; Regist. Univ. Coll. Hosp. Lond. and RNOH Stanmore.

NOORI, Muna 39 Scotts Lane, Shortlands, Bromley BR2 0LT Tel: 020 8658 2860 — MB BS Lond. 1998 (Char. Cross) BSc (Hons.) Lond. 1995. PRHO in Urol., Mayday Uni. Hosp. Thornton Heath, Lond. Specialty: Urol. Prev: PRHO in Gen. Surg. Mayday Uni. Hosp. Thornton Heath, Lond.; PRHO in Med. Kent & Canterbury Hosp. Canterbury.

NOORI, Sharifah Nuriyah c/o 166 Devonshire Road, London NW7 1DJ Email: snn71@yahoo.co.uk — MB BS Lond. 1997.

NOORI, Mr Zuhair Fadhel Abdul Salam RNOH Stanmore, Brockley Hill, Stanmore HA7 4LP — MB ChB Mosul 1973; LMSSA Lond. 1981; FRCS Glas. 1983. Sen. Regist. (Spinal Injuries & Neuro Rehabilitation) RNOH Stanmore. Specialty: Neurosurg. Special Interest: Neuro Rehabilitiation. Socs: Congr. of Neurol. Surgs. USA; Brit. Neurol. Soc.; Emirate Med. Assn. Prev: Cons. & Head Neurosurg. & Pain Clinic Al Jazerha & Centr. Hosp. Abu Dhabi UAE; Regist. (Neurosurg.) Nat. Hosp. Neurol. & Neurosurg. Dis. Lond.; Regist. (Neurosurg.) Old Ch. Hosp. Romford & Walton Hosp. Liverp.

NOORPURI, Ranbir Singh PO Box 53, Birkenhead L42 5ET — MB ChB Liverp. 1993. SHO (O & G) Wirral Hosp. NHS Trust. Specialty: Obst. & Gyn.

NOOTT, Gerald Guy Glenside, Scarrowscant Lane, Haverfordwest SA61 — LRCPI & LM, LRSCI & LM 1955; LRCPI & LM, LRCSI & LM 1955.

NORBROOK, Penelope Jane 12 Amenbury Lane, Harpenden AL5 2DF — MB BS Lond. 1974 (Roy. Free) MRCS Eng. LRCP Lond. 1974. Hosp. Practitioner Hemel Hempstead. Specialty: Dermat. Prev: GP Princip. Lond.; SHO (Med.) Whittington Hosp. Lond.; Ho. Phys. Roy. Free Hosp. Lond.

NORBURN, Peter Stuart Department of Radiology, Trafford District General Hospital, Moorside Road, Davyhulme, Manchester M41 5SL — MB ChB Manch. 1979; MRCP (UK) 1982; FRCR 1987. Cons. Radiol. Trafford Dist. Gen. Hosp. Manch. Specialty: Radiol.

NORBURY, Lynn Patricia Borcharot Medical Centre, 62 Whitchurch Road, Withington, Manchester M20 1EB Tel: 0161 445 5907 Fax: 0161 448 0466 — BM Soton. 1977; MRCGP 1984; DRCOG 1985; M Med. Sci. 1999.

NORCLIFFE, Pamela Jayne 17 Beech Road, Glinton, Peterborough PE6 7LA — MB ChB Bristol 1997; MRCP.

NORCOTT, Mr Harry Christopher Russells Hall Hospital, Dudley DY1 2HQ; 16 Dingle Road, Stourbridge DY9 0RS Tel: 01562 883239 — MB BS Lond. 1969 (Char. Cross) MRCS Eng. LRCP Lond. 1969; FRCS Eng. 1974. Cons. (Gen. Surg.) Russells Hall Hosp. Dudley. Specialty: Gen. Surg. Prev: Sen. Regist. (Gen. Surg.) Qu. Eliz. Hosp. Birm.; Regist. (Gen. Surg.) N. Staffs. Roy. Infirm. Stoke-on-Trent; Regist. (Gen. Surg.) Roy. Hosp. Wolverhampton.

NORCOTT, Margaret Beatrice Boyle (retired) 2 Chancellors Close, Edgbaston, Birmingham B15 3UJ Tel: 0121 454 1648 — MB ChB Manch. 1954; DObst RCOG 1965. Prev: GP Health Centre Birm.

NORDEN, Anthony George William Department of Clinical Pathology, Hinchingbrooke Hospital, Hinchingbrooke Park, Huntingdon PE29 6NT Tel: 01480 416266 Fax: 01480 416527; School Cottage, 10 School Lane, Watton-at-Stone, Hertford SG14 3SF Tel: 01920 830838 Fax: 01920 830838 — MB BS Lond. 1979 (Univ. Coll. Hosp.) BSc Lond. 1971; PhD Calif. 1974; T(Path) 1991; FRCPath 1996. Cons. Chem. Path. Hinchingbrooke, Addenbrooke's and Papworth Hosp.s. Specialty: Chem. Path. Prev: Sen. Regist. (Chem. Path.) Univ. Coll. Hosp. & Whittington Hosp. Lond.

NORDIN, Andrew John Chelsea & Westminster Hospital, 369 Fulham Road, Chelsea, London SW10 9NH; 38 Cross Gates Close, Marlins Heron, Bracknell RG12 9TY — MB BS Adelaide 1987; MRCOG 1994. Regist. (O & G) Chelsea & Westm. Hosp. Lond. Specialty: Obst. & Gyn. Prev: Regist. (O & G) N. Hants. Hosp. Basingstoke & MusGr.r Pk. Hosp. Taunton.

NORDSTROM, Monica Evelyn St. Peter's Hospital, Chest Department, Guildford Road, Chertsey KT16 0PZ Tel: 01932 722310 Fax: 01932 873983; Vellow Wood, Winterbourne Grove, Weybridge KT13 0PP Tel: 01932 854917 Fax: 01932 858291 Email: monicanordstrom@hotmail.com — MD Odense 1980 (Odense, Denmark) MD (Gen. Med. & Gerontol.) Odense 1980. Clin. Asst. (Chest) St. Peter's Hosp. Chertsey. Specialty: Gen. Med. Special Interest: Asthma, COPD, TB, PE, DVT, homocystein. Prev: Gen. Med. Univ. Hosp. Malmö, Sweden.

NORELL, Michael Simon The Mill House, The Holloway, Trysull, Wolverhampton WV5 7JA Tel: 01902 898188 Email: norellmike@aol.com — MB BS Lond. 1978 (University College London) FRCP; MD Lond. 1990. Cons. Interventional Cardiol. P.C.I. Progr. Director, The Heart Centre, New Cross Hosp., Wolverhampton. Specialty: Cardiol. Socs: Hon. Sec. Brit. Cardiovasc. Interven. Soc. (past); Brit. Cardiac Soc. 1996-2000; BCIS (Council 1994-2002). Prev: Cons. Cardiol., Hull Roy. Infirm., Hull; Sen. Regist. Harefield and Roy. Free Hosps.

NOREN, Claes Eric Steyning Health Centre, Tanyard Lane, Steyning BN44 3RJ Tel: 01903 843400 Fax: 01903 843440 — MB BS Lond. 1975 (St. Bart.) MRCP (UK) 1978; MRCGP 1984. Sch. Doctor Windlesham Hse. Findon, W. Sussex; Trainer (Gen. Pract.) W. Sussex; Hosp. Pract. (Diabetes) Roy. Sussex Co. Hosp. Brighton. Prev: SHO Rotat. (Gen. Med.) & Ho. Phys. (Gen. Med. & Cardiol.) St. Bart. Hosp. Lond.; Ho. Surg. (Gen. Surg.) Roy. Berks. Hosp. Reading.

NORFOLK, Derek Raymond Department of Haematology, The General Infirmary at Leeds, Leeds LS1 3EX Tel: 0113 292 3935 Fax: 0113 242 0881 Email: derek.norfolk@leedsth.nhs.uk — MB BS Lond. 1975 (Guy's) MRCS Eng. LRCP Lond. 1975; MRCP (UK) 1978; FRCPath 1994, M 1983; FRCP Lond. 1993. Cons. Haemat. Gen. Infirm. Leeds; Hon. Sen. Clin. Lect. (Med. & Path.) Univ. Leeds; Assoc. Director of Research and Developm. Leeds Teachg. Hosp.s NHS Trust. Specialty: Haematology. Socs: BMA; Brit. Soc. Haematol. Prev: Sen. Regist. (Haemat.) Gen. Infirm. Leeds; Regist. & SHO (Gen. Med.) Vict. Hosp. Blackpool.

NORFOLK, Guy Adrian Stockwood Health Clinic, Hollway Road, Bristol BS14 8PT Tel: 01275 833103 Fax: 01275 891637; Whitewood Lodge, Norton Lane, Whitchurch, Bristol BS14 0BU Tel: 01275 834888 — MB ChB Leeds 1980; MRCGP 1985; DMJ Soc. Apoth. Lond. 1991; LLM Cardiff 1995.

NORGAIN, Helen Ruth Rockwood, Sandy Lane, Helsby, Warrington WA6 9BD — BM BS Nottm. 1994.

NORGATE, Ian Francis Tristram (retired) 60 Chester Road, Salterswall, Winsford CW7 2NQ Tel: 01606 593387 — LRCP LRCS Ed. 1951 (Glas.) LRCP LRCS Ed. LRFPS Glas. 1951. Prev: Ho. Surg. Wrexham Memor. Hosp.

NORGREN, Priscilla Marie 47 Westbridge Cottages, Tavistock PL19 8DQ — MB BS Lond. 1992.

NORLEY, Ian White Gables, 4 Clennon Park, Paignton TQ4 5HL — MB BS Lond. 1977 (St ary's Hospital, London) FFA RCS Eng. 1982. Cons. Anaesth. Torbay Hosp. Torquay. Specialty: Anaesth.

NORMAN, Abraham Eric (retired) 2 Rockbourne Avenue, Liverpool L25 4TW Tel: 0151 428 1340 — (Liverp.) MB ChB Liverp. 1938; FRCGP 1979, M 1954. Hon. Capt. RAMC. Prev: Exam. Med. Off. Dept. Health & Social Security.

NORMAN, Aidan Thomas 9 Glebe Field Croft, Wetherby LS22 6WQ — MB ChB Manch. 1992; FRCA 1999.

NORMAN, Mr Alan Greaves (retired) Thatched Cottage, Clarks Yard, Cavendish, Sudbury CO10 8AZ Tel: 01787 281437 — MRCS Eng. LRCP Lond. 1947 (Camb. & St. Thos.) MA Camb. 1949, MChir 1961, MB BChir 1947; FRCS Eng. 1952. Prev: Cons. Thoracic Surg. Sheff. HA.

NORMAN, Alan Sellers Castle Surgery, 5 Darwin Street, Castle, Northwich CW8 1BU Tel: 01606 74863 Fax: 01606 784847; Findhorn, 10 Sandfield Lane, Hartford, Northwich CW8 1PU Tel:

01606 75208 Email: alan.norman@bigfoot.com — MB ChB Manch. 1988 (Manch. & St. And.) BSc St. And. 1985; MRCGP 1992.

NORMAN, Aleida Elisabeth Mabel May (retired) White Lodge, Heather Close, Kingswood, Tadworth KT20 6NY Tel: 01737 832626 — BM BCh Oxf. 1946; MA Oxf. 1946; DCH Eng. 1949. Prev: Ho. Phys. Radcliffe Infirm. Oxf.

NORMAN, Andrew Michael Clinical Genetics Unit, Birmingham Women's Hospital, Edgbaston, Birmingham B15 2TG Tel: 0121 607 4727 Fax: 0121 627 2618 Email: andrew.norman@bwhct.nhs.uk — MB BCh Wales 1981; MA Camb. 1982; MRCP (UK) 1984; MD Wales 1992; FRCP 2000. Cons. Clin. Genetics Birm. Wom.'s Hosp. Specialty: Genetics. Prev: Sen. Regist. (Clin. Genetics) Manch.; Clin. Research Off. Inst. Med. Genetics Cardiff; Regist. (Med.) Plymouth Gen. Hosp.

NORMAN, Andrew Richard Francis 121 Ladbroke Grove, London W11 1PN Tel: 020 7792 8060 Fax: 020 7792 3236; 4 Dewhurst Road, London W14 0ET — MB ChB Bristol 1972. Prev: GP Alderton; GP Trainee Cirencester VTS; Dep. to Chief Med. Adviser Commercial Union Assur. plc.

NORMAN, Andrew Spencer Wells Health Centre, Glastonbury Road, Wells BA5 1XJ Tel: 01749 672137 Fax: 01749 679833 — MB BS Lond. 1990; MRCGP 1996. Specialty: Gen. Pract.

NORMAN, Andrew William Market Deeping Health Centre, 2 Douglas Road, Market Deeping, Peterborough PE6 8PA — MB BS Lond. 1975; MRCS Eng. LRCP Lond. 1975; MRCGP 1979.

NORMAN, Annabel Le Sauteur Fairfield, Faldouet, Gorey, St Martin, Jersey JE3 6DP — MB BS Lond. 1993 (Lond. Hosp. Med. Coll.) BSc (Hons.) 1990; DFFP 1997; DRCOG 1997; DCH 1998. GP Regist. Bath. Specialty: Gen. Pract. Prev: SHO (Paediat.) Roy. Alexandra Hosp. Brighton; SHO (O & G) Jersey Gen.

NORMAN, Anthea Mary 4 Malvern Road, Southsea PO5 2NA Tel: 023 9283 3905 — BM BS Nottm. 1991; DRCOG 1995; T(GP) 1995; MRCGP 1997. Trainee GP Portsmouth VTS; Salaried GP John Pounds Med. Centre Portsmouth.

NORMAN, Archibald Percy, MBE (retired) White Lodge, Heather Close, Kingswood, Tadworth KT20 6NY Tel: 01737 832626 — (Camb. & Middlx.) MRCS Eng. LRCP Lond. 1937; MB BChir Camb. 1938; FRCP Lond. 1954, M 1947; DCH Eng. 1947; MA Camb. 1938, MD 1949; FRCPI 1995; FRCPCH 1996. Hon. Phys. Hosp. Sick Childr. Gt. Ormond St.; Hon. Paediat. Qu. Charlotte's Matern. Hosp. Lond. Prev: Resid. Asst. Phys. Westm. Childr. Hosp. Vincent Sq.

NORMAN, Benjamin Peter — MB ChB Ed. 1998.

NORMAN, Bernard John Charing Cross Hospital, Fulham Palace Road, London W6 8RF Tel: 020 8846 1234; 125 St. Albans Avenue, Chiswick, London W4 5JS — MB BS Lond. 1990; BSc (Hons.) Lond. 1987; FRCA 1994. Specialist Regist. (Anaesth.) Char. Cross Hosp. Lond. Specialty: Anaesth. Socs: Fell. Roy. Soc. Med.; Assn. Anaesth.; Obst. Anaesth. Assn. Prev: SHO (Anaesth.) St. Geo. Hosp. Lond.

NORMAN, Charles William 27 St Anns Lane, Godmanchester, Huntingdon PE29 2JE — MB BS Lond. 1996; DCH Lond. 2000; MRCGP Lond. 2001; DFFP Lond. 2002.

NORMAN, David Paul Ringmead Medical Practice, Great Hollands Health Centre, Great Hollands Square, Bracknell RG12 8WY Tel: 01344 454338 Fax: 01344 861050; 28 Avebury, Little Foxes, Bracknell RG12 8SQ — MA Camb. 1972; MRCS Eng. LRCP Lond. 1975; DCH Eng. 1978; DRCOG 1978.

NORMAN, Dorothy (retired) 1 Churchgate Mews, Bibby Road, Southport PR9 7PS — (Leeds) MB ChB Leeds 1953. Prev: SHO (O & G) Crewe Memor. Hosp. & Barony Hosp. Nantwich.

NORMAN, Hugh Michael McCormick (retired) Hillside, Vicarage Lane, Barrow Gurney, Bristol BS48 3RT Tel: 01275 462730 — MB BCh BAO Dub. 1954 (T.C. Dub.) DObst RCOG 1963. Prev: SHO (Obst.) Stafford Gen. Infirm.

NORMAN, James Marcus Charlotte Keel Health Centre, Seymour Road, Easton, Bristol BS5 0UA Tel: 0117 951 2244 Fax: 0117 951 2373; 1 Leigh Road, Clifton, Bristol BS8 2DA — MB ChB Bristol 1972; MRCGP 1978.

NORMAN, Jane Elizabeth Department Obstetrics & Gynaecology, University of Glasgow, Queen Elizabeth Building, Glasgow Royal Infirmary, 10 Alexandra Place, Glasgow G31 2ER Tel: 0141 211 4702 Fax: 0141 553 1367; 33 Southbrae Drive, Glasgow G13 1PU — MB ChB Ed. 1986; MD Ed. 1992; MRCOG 1992. Reader (O & G) Glas. Univ. Specialty: Obst. & Gyn. Prev: Lect. (O & G) Univs. Edin. & Glas.; Research Regist. (O & G) Edin.; Regist. (O & G) Borders Gen. Hosp. Melrose.

NORMAN, Joanne Louise 245 Upper Halliford Road, Shepperton TW17 8ST — MB BS Lond. 1994; BSc (Hons.) Lond. 1991, MB BS 1994.

NORMAN, John (retired) 2 Russell Place, Portswood, Southampton SO17 1NU Tel: 023 8055 5177 Email: johnnorman1@aol.com — MB ChB Leeds 1957; FRCA 1963; PhD Leeds 1969; FANZCA 1983. Prev: Prof. Anaesth. Univ. Soton.

NORMAN, Professor John Nelson 39 Morningfield Road, Aberdeen AB15 4AP Tel: 01224 316765 Fax: 01224 316765 Email: j.n.norman@abdn.ac.uk — MB ChB Glas. 1957; PhD Glas. 1964, MD 1961; FRCS Glas. 1967; FRCS Ed. 1967; DSc Aberd. 1976; FFOM RCP Lond. 1993, MFOM 1986. Emerit. Prof. Environ. Studies. Univ. Aberd.; Vis. Prof. Communit. Med. UAE. Specialty: Occupat. Health. Socs: Underwater Med. Soc. Prev: Med. Dir. Robt. Gordon's Inst. Technol. Survival Centre Ltd., Aberd.; Dir. Inst. Environm. & Offshore Med. Univ. Aberd.; Reader (Surg.) Univ. Aberd.

NORMAN, John Richard Nutwood Surgery, Windermere Road, Grange-over-Sands LA11 6EG Tel: 015395 32108 Fax: 015395 35986; The Old Parsonage, Grange Fell Road, Grange-over-Sands LA11 6BJ Tel: 01539 534428 Fax: 01539 536288 — MB ChB Leeds 1975; MB ChB (Hons.) Leeds 1975. Med. Off. Cartmel Racecourse.

NORMAN, John Robin Henfield Medical Centre, Deer Park, Henfield BN5 9JQ Tel: 01273 492255 Fax: 01273 495050; Clovelly, Cagefoot Lane, Henfield BN5 9HD Tel: 01273 492612 — MB BChir Camb. 1968 (Camb. & St. Thos.) MA Camb. 1968; DCH Eng. 1970; MRCP (UK) 1972; DObst RCOG 1974. Gen. Med. Pract. Henfield. Prev: Clin. Asst. (Child Psychiat.) Roy. Alexandra Hosp. Brighton; Regist. (Paediat.) St. Thos. Hosp. Lond.; Ho. Off. (O & G) King's Coll. Hosp. Lond.

NORMAN, Joseph Edward (retired) 55 Spylaw Bank Road, Colinton, Edinburgh EH13 0JB Tel: 0131 441 6643 — MB ChB Ed. 1945; DA Eng. 1951; FFA RCS Eng. 1954. Prev: Cons. Anaesth. Edin. North. Gp. Hosps.

NORMAN, Joseph Roger, RD (retired) Glenwood House, 33 Queens Road, Waterlooville PO7 7SB Tel: 023 9225 1624 — MB BS Lond. 1960 (Guy's) MRCS Eng. LRCP Lond. 1960; DCH Eng. 1963. Prev: Ho. Phys. & Ho. Surg. Pembury Hosp.

NORMAN, Justine Clare Casapeka, Low Road, Harwich CO12 3TS — MB ChB Leic. 1994.

NORMAN, Lucinda Kathryn Victoria — MB BS Lond. 1990; FRCS Lond. 1998; MRCGP (Distinc.) 2000.

NORMAN, Madeline Georgina Northcroft Surgery, Northcroft Lane, Newbury RG14 1BU Tel: 01635 31575 Fax: 01635 551857 — MB BS Lond. 1988; DRCOG 1992; MRCGP 1994. Princip. GP, Berks. Specialty: Gen. Pract.

NORMAN, Maria Louise The Briars, Farm Road, Bristol BS16 6DD — MB ChB Bristol 1991. SHO (O & G) Southmead Hosp. Bristol.

NORMAN, Mark 10 Hivings Park, Chesham HP5 2LG — MB BS Lond. 1993.

NORMAN, Mark Adrian Orchard Medical Centre, Macdonald Walk, Kingswood, Bristol BS15 8NJ Tel: 0117 980 5100 Fax: 0117 980 5104; Greystone Cottage, Bury Lane, Doynton, Bristol BS30 5SW — MB ChB Birm. 1983; DCH RCP Lond. 1988.

NORMAN, Michael Hayes (retired) 88 Humberstone Road, Luton LU4 9SS Tel: 01582 571131 — LMSSA Lond. 1951 (St. Bart.) DA Eng. 1956.

NORMAN, Michael Hugh University Medical Centre, Giles Lane, Canterbury CT2 7LR Tel: 01227 65682; Monks Hall, School Lane, Fordwich, Canterbury CT2 0DF — MB BChir Camb. 1981; MA Camb. 1983, MB BChir 1981; DRCOG 1987.

NORMAN, Patricia Mary National Hospital for Neurology & Neurosurgery, Queen Square, London WC1N 3BG Tel: 020 7837 3611; Queen's Lodge, Queen's Club Gardens, West Kensington, London W14 9TA Tel: 020 7385 3122 — MB BCh BAO Dub. 1958; FRCPath 1980, M 1968. Cons. Path. (Haemat., Microbiol. & Cytol.) Nat. Hosps. Nerv. Dis. Qu. Sq. & Maida Vale. Specialty: Haematology.

NORMAN, Paul Public Health Laboratory, Northern General Hospital, Herries Road, Sheffield S5 7AU Tel: 0114 271 4925 Fax: 0114 242 1385 — MB Camb. 1975; BChir 1974.

NORMAN, Paul Richard Minden Medical Centre, 2 Barlow Street, Bury BL9 0QP Tel: 0161 764 2652 Fax: 0161 761 5967 — MB ChB Liverp. 1991; DCH RCP Lond. 1993; MRCGP 1995; DRCOG 1995. Specialty: Family Plann. & Reproduc. Health. Prev: Trainee GP/SHO Bury VTS; Ho. Off. (Surg. & Med.) Wirral Hosps.

NORMAN, Peter Frank (retired) Barafundle, Down Park Drive, Tavistock PL19 9AH Tel: 01822 613834 — MB ChB Manch. 1960; DMRD Eng. 1965; FFR 1967; FRCR 1975. Prev: Cons. Neuroradiol. Plymouth Gen. Hosp.

NORMAN, Sarah Ann Medico -Legal Practice, Atlantic Business Centre, Atlantic St, Altrincham WA14 5NQ Tel: 0161 926 3660/ 0161 926 3661; 2 The Haven, Hale, Altrincham WA15 8SA — BM BS Nottm. 1988; DRCOG 1991; Cert. Family Plann. JCC 1991; MRCGP 1992; MEWI 1998. Medio-legal Cons. Specialty: Medico Legal. Socs: Expert Witnen Inst. Mem.; BMA Mem. Prev: Trainee GP Chester VTS; Gen. Practitioner Chester.

NORMAN, Simon Philip The Briars, Farm Road, Bristol BS16 6DD — MB ChB Bristol 1995.

NORMAN, Stephen George Medway Maritime Hospital, Windmill Road, Gillingham ME7 5NY Tel: 01634 830000 Fax: 01634 811250 — BM BS Nottm. 1984 (Nottingham) BSc Leeds 1974; PhD Camb. 1978; BMedSci Nottm. 1982; MRCOG 1989; FRCOG 2001. Cons. O & G Medway Maritime Hosp. Gillingham. Specialty: Obst. & Gyn. Prev: Cons. O & G All St.s Hosp. Chatham; Sen. Regist. (O & G) King's Coll. Hosp. Lond.

NORMAN, Stephen Grahame 12 Cardiff Road, Luton LU1 1QG Tel: 01582 22143 Fax: 01582 485721; 65 Stopsley Way, Stopsley, Luton LU2 7UU Tel: 01582 411726 — MB ChB Sheff. 1980; MRCGP 1988. Specialty: Gen. Pract. Socs: Christian Med. Fellowsh. & Caring Professions Concern. Prev: Trainee GP Luton & Dunstable Hosp. VTS; Paediat. North. Gen. Hosp. Sheff.; Ho. Phys. (Surg.) Rotherham Dist. Gen. Hosp.

NORMAN, Susan 1 Leigh Road, Clifton, Bristol BS8 2DA — MB ChB Bristol 1972; DObst RCOG 1975. Clin. Asst. (Venereol. & Colposcopy) Bristol Roy. Infirm.

NORMAN, Thomas (retired) The Old Rectory, Winterborne Houghton, Blandford Forum DT11 0PD Tel: 01258 880272 — (Middlesex Hospital) MA Camb.; MB BChir Camb. 1943; DTM & H Eng. 1951. Prev: PMO Jhanzie Tea Assn. & Amguri Tea Est.s.

NORMAN, Valerie Elizabeth (retired) 3 Princes Road, Clevedon BS21 7SY Tel: 01275 874124 — MB ChB Birm. 1963. Prev: Sen. Med. Off. (Family Plann.) United Bristol Healthcare & Weston Area Health Trusts.

NORMAN, William Anthony Cromer Group Practice, 48 Overstrand Road, Cromer NR27 0AJ Tel: 01263 513148 — MB Camb. 1964; BChir 1963; DRCOG 1965; DA Eng. 1966; CCFP Canada 1973.

NORMAN, William John The Rope Walk, Lyth Hill, Bayston Hill, Shrewsbury SY3 0BS Tel: 01743 872554; Fullers Cottage, Condover, Shrewsbury SY5 7BT Tel: 01743 872554 — MB BChir Camb. 1961 (Camb. & Guy's) MA, MB BChir Camb. 1961; DMRD Eng. 1969; FFR 1972. Cons. Radiol. Roy. Shrewsbury Hosp. Specialty: Radiol. Prev: Sen. Regist. (Radiol.) United Bristol Hosps.

NORMAN-NOTT, Arabella Gabriella The Limberlost, St Giles Hill, Winchester SO23 0HH — MB BS Lond. 1996.

NORMAN-TAYLOR, Mr Fabian Hugh 12 Maida Vale, Norwich NR2 3EP — MB BS Lond. 1988; FRCS Eng. 1992. Specialty: Orthop.

NORMAN-TAYLOR, Mr Julian Quentin Chelsea & Westminster Hospital, Fulham Rd, London SW10 9NH — MB ChB Leic. 1982; MRCOG. Cons. (Gynae.). Specialty: Obst. & Gyn. Socs: Roy. Coll. Obst. & Gyn.; Brit. Fertil. Soc.

NORMAND, Professor Ian Colin Stuart 23 St Thomas' Street, Winchester SO23 9HJ Tel: 01962 852550 — BM BCh Oxf. 1952 (Oxf. & St. Mary's) FRCP Lond. 1971, M 1956; MA Oxf. 1963, DM 1976; Hon. FRCPCH 1996. Emerit. Prof. Child Health Univ. Soton. Specialty: Paediat. Prev: Dean Fac. Med. Univ. Soton.; Cons. Paediat. & Hon. Sen. Lect. (Paediat.) Univ. Coll. Hosp. Lond.; Fell. (Pediat.) Johns Hopkins Hosp., USA.

NORMANDALE, Jeremy Philip Pear Tree Cottage, West Lane, Snainton, Scarborough YO13 9AR — MB BS Lond. 1978; FFARCS 1983. Cons. (Anaesth.) ScarBoro. & Bridlington Hosps. Specialty: Anaesth. Socs: Obst. Anaesth. Assn. Prev: Attend. Anaesth. Univ. Washington Seattle, USA; Sen. Regist. Dept. Anaesth. Middlx. Hosp. Lond.; Regist. Hammersmith Hosp. Lond.

NORMINTON, David Roger Harold Kings Corner Surgery, Kings Road, Ascot SL5 0AE Tel: 01344 623181 Fax: 01344 875129 — MB BS Lond. 1969; DObst RCOG 1971; Cert. FPA 1973; MRCGP 1986.

NORONHA, Mr Derek Thomas 28 Wallace Street, Spital Tongues, Newcastle upon Tyne NE2 4AU — MD Dar-es-Salaam 1986; FRCS Ed. 1992.

NORONHA, Enid Antoinette Manchester Road Surgery, 39 Manchester Road, Walkden Worsley, Manchester M28 3NS Tel: 0161 702 8595 Fax: 0161 702 8592; 39 Manchester Road, Walkden, Worsley, Manchester M28 3NS Tel: 0161 702 8595 Fax: 0161 702 8592 — MB BS Poona 1964 (B.J. Med. Coll.) GP Salford & Scafford SHSA. Specialty: Cardiol. Prev: SHO (Paediat.) Bradford Roy. Infirm.; Ho. Phys. St. Luke's Hosp. Bradford; Ho. Surg. Bury Gen. Hosp.

NORONHA, Hermes Dulci Santana 10 Woodbury Close, Croydon CR0 5PR — MB ChB Leeds 1973.

NORONHA, Michael Diago 2 Park Close, Shirland, Alfreton DE55 6AZ — MB BS Bangalore 1988.

NORONHA, Michael Joseph 35 Ellesmere Road, Eccles, Manchester M30 9FE Tel: 0161 789 3761 Fax: 0161 789 3761 — MRCS Eng. LRCP Lond. 1959 (RCSI) LRCPI & LM, LRCSI & LM 1958; MRCPI 1961; FRCP Ed. 1976, M 1963; FRCP Lond. 1981, M 1967. Hon. Cons. Paediat. Neurol. Roy. Manch. Childr. Hosp. & Booth Hall Childr. Hosp.Manch. Specialty: Paediat. Neurol. Socs: Assn. Brit. Neurol. & Assn. Brit. Paediat. Neurol. Prev: Research Regist. (Neurol.) Leeds Gen. Infirm.; Regist. (Med.) Bradford Roy. Infirm.; SHO Edin. Roy. Infirm.

NORRIE, Bruce Garland (retired) Eildonhurst, 500 Perth Road, Dundee DD2 1LS — MB ChB St. And. 1962. Prev: SHO (Paediat.) Inverness Hosp. Gp.

NORRIE, Douglas McKane Moorcroft, 16 Southway Lane, Roborough, Plymouth PL6 7DH Tel: 01752 774464 — MB ChB St. And. 1955; DA Eng. 1959. Adjudicating Med. Pract.; Examg. Med. Pract. War Pension Med. Bds.; Med. Adviser Incapacity Benefit Bds. Prev: GP Plymouth; Regist. (Anaesth.) S. Devon & E. Cornw. Hosps.

NORRIE, Iain Alexander The Health Centre, Campbeltown PA28 6AT Tel: 01586 552105 — MB ChB Leeds 1993. Specialty: Gen. Pract.

NORRIE, Mary Stella 8 Abbey Close, Fairfield, Stockton-on-Tees TS19 7SP Tel: 01642 654243 — MB BCh BAO Belf. 1972 (Queens University Belfast) MRCGP Ed. 1977. GP Princip. in Eston Teeside. Specialty: Occupat. Health; Psychother. Socs: Soc. Occupat. Med.; Brit. Soc. Med. and Dent. Hypn.

NORRIE, Muriel Kinnison (retired) Moorcroft, 16 Southway Lane, Roborough, Plymouth PL6 7DH Tel: 01752 774464 — MB ChB St. And. 1955. Med. Ref. DHSS.; Mem. Examr. Incapacity Benefit Bd. Prev: Adjudicating Med. Pract. Indust. Benefit Bds.

NORRIE, Stuart David Leek Health Centre, Fountain St., Leek ST13 6JB Tel: 01538 381022; Pinehurst, Sutherland Road, Longsdon, Stoke-on-Trent ST9 9QD Tel: 01538 399680 — MB ChB Birm. 1979; DRCOG 1983.

NORRIS, Alan Central Health Centre, North Carbrain Road, Cumbernauld, Glasgow G67 1BJ Tel: 01236 737214 Fax: 01236 781699; Craigmarloch Medical Centre, 17 Auchinsee Way, Craigmarloch, Cumbernauld G68 0EZ Tel: 01236 780700 Fax: 01236 780344 — MB ChB Glas. 1977.

NORRIS, Alan 13 Pickletullum Road, Craigie, Perth PH2 0LL — MB ChB Ed. 1987; BSc (Hons.) Ed. 1985; MRCP (UK) 1992. Assoc. Specialist (Blood Transfus.) Ninewells Hosp. Dundee. Specialty: Blood Transfus. Prev: Regist. (Haemat.) Glas. Roy. Infirm. & Stobhill Hosp. Glas.; Regist. (Med.) Raigmore Hosp. Inverness; SHO (Med.) Law Hosp. Carluke.

NORRIS, Alan Michael Lagan Valley Hospital, Hillsborough Road, Lisburn BT28 1JP Tel: 028 9266 5141 Fax: 028 9074 1342; 36 Royal Lodge Avenue, Purdysburn Road, Belfast BT8 7YR — MB BCh BAO Dub. 1985 (Trinity) MRCPI 1988; MRCP (UK) 1990; FRCR 1993. Cons. Radiol. Lagan Valley Hospital, Lisburn Belf. Specialty: Radiol.

NORRIS, Alexander Donald Craig Kings House, High Street, Charing, Ashford TN27 0LS Tel: 01233 714962 Fax: 01233 713340 Email: alex@charing.fsnet.co.uk — (Camb. & Lond. Hosp.) MB

BChir Camb. 1961; MA Camb. 1961; FRCP Lond. 1978, M 1963. Cons. Cardiol., Benenden Hosp., Cranbrook, Kent. Specialty: Gen. Med.; Cardiol. Socs: BMA & Brit. Cardiac Soc. Prev: Sen. Regist. (Gen. Med.), Regist. (Gen. Med. & Cardiol.) Lond. Hosp.; Cons. Phys. William Harvey Hosp. Ashford, Kent; Cons. Cardiac Guys Hosp. Lond.

NORRIS, Andrew Michael Top Hovel, Hockerton Road, Hockerton, Southwell NG25 0PP — MB ChB Sheff. 1986; FRCA 1993. Cons. (Anaesth.) Qu. Med. Centre Nottm. Specialty: Anaesth.

NORRIS, Carol Ann, MBE Borders General Hospital, Huntlyburn, Melrose TD6 9BS Tel: 01896 826000 — MB ChB Birm. 1969; MRCP (UK) 1974; FRCP Ed. 1993. Cons. Phys. (Med. for Elderly & Gen. Med.) NHS Borders. Specialty: Gen. Med.; Care of the Elderly; Cardiol. Socs: Scott. Cardiac Soc.; NHS Cons. Assn.

NORRIS, Christopher Stewart The Park Medical Practice, Cannands Grave Road, Shepton Mallet BA4 5RT Tel: 01749 342350 Fax: 01749 346845 — MB ChB Bristol 1972; DObst RCOG 1974; MRCGP 1976.

NORRIS, Clive Denis 1206 Christchurch Road, Boscombe East, Bournemouth BH7 6DZ — MB BS Lond. 1970 (Lond. Hosp.) MRCS Eng. LRCP Lond. 1970; DObst RCOG 1973; Cert FPA 1973; MRCGP 1981.

NORRIS, Elizabeth Angela (retired) 9 Melton Green, Wath Upon Dearne, Rotherham S63 6AA Tel: 01709 872051 — MB ChB Sheff. 1978; DA (UK) 1981; DRCOG 1985. Prev: GP Wombwell Barnsley S. Yorks.

NORRIS, Elizabeth Margaret St Sampson's Medical Centre, Grandes Maisons Road, St. Sampson, Guernsey GY2 4JS — MB ChB Bristol 1977; DRCOG 1980; MRCGP 1981. Prev: GP Westbury on Trym, Bristol; GP Whitecliff Mill St. Dorset.

NORRIS, Elizabeth Mary The Health Centre, Marbles Road, Newick, Lewes BN8 4LR Tel: 01825 722272 — MB ChB Bristol 1996 (Bristol Uni.) BSc Bristol 1992; MRCGP 2001. GP Principal. Specialty: Obst. & Gyn.

NORRIS, Geoffrey Francis, MBE GP Office, Medical Education Centre, Whipps Cross Hospital, Whipps Cross Road, London E11 1NR Tel: 020 8535 6417 Fax: 020 8535 6417 Email: sheilagped@aol.com; 21 Falmouth Avenue, Highams Park, London E4 9QL Tel: 020 8527 3544 — MB BChir Camb. 1960 (Westm.) MA Camb. 1960; DObst RCOG 1963; FRCGP 1988, M 1968. p/t GP; Tutor (Priamry Care) & Course Organiser Whipps Cross Hosp. VTS. Specialty: Gen. Pract. Socs: RCGP; Hosp. Convenor N. E. Lond. Fac. Prev: SHO (O & G), Ho. Phys. (Gen. Med. & Paediat.) & Ho. Surg. St. Margt. Hosp. Epping; Assoc. Dean Pan Thames; TPMDE Facilitator Extended VTS.

NORRIS, John Phillips, QGM (retired) 51 Moberly Road, Salisbury SP1 3BX Tel: 01722 322440; 51 moberly Road, Salisbury SP1 3BX Tel: 01722 322440 — MB ChB Bristol 1948; DObst RCOG 1952; FRCGP 1978, M 1960.

NORRIS, Mr John Samuel Princess Royal Hospital, Hurstwood Park Neurological Centre, Haywards Heath RH16 4EX Tel: 01444 441881 Ext: 4748 Fax: 01444 417995 — MB ChB Bristol 1986; FRCS Ed. 1990; FRCS (SN) 1995. Cons. Neuro. Surg.Hurstwood Pk. Neurosci.s Centre Princess Roy. Hosp. Haywards Heath; Fell. (Neurovasc.) Toronto Hosp. Canad. Specialty: Neurosurg. Socs: BMA; Roy. Soc. Med.; Soc. Brit. Neurol. Surgs. Prev: Regist. (Neurosurg.) Qu. Med. Centre Nottm.; Sen. Regist. (Neurosurg.) Roy. Lond. & OldCh. Hosps. Lond.; Fell. (Neurovasc.) Toronto Hosp., Canada.

NORRIS, Professor John William Department of Neurosciences, St Georges Hospital Medical School, London SW17 0RE, Canada Tel: 0208 725 2735 Email: carotid@btopenworld.com; 20 Onslow Square, London SW7 3NP Tel: 0207 225 1329 Fax: 0207 225 1329 — MB ChB Aberd. 1957; FRCP Ed. 1978, M 1962; FRCP Lond. 1982, M 1964. Specialty: Neurol. Socs: Assn. Brit. Neurols.; Amer. Neurol. Assn.; Amer. Acad. Neurol.

NORRIS, Jonathan Frazer Bate Denbie, Lockerbie DG11 1DU Tel: 01387 840333 — MB ChB Manch. 1974; DCH Eng. 1977; DRCOG 1977; MRCP (UK) 1979; FRCP Ed. 1996. Cons. Dermat. Dumfries & Galloway Roy. Infirm. Dumfries. Specialty: Dermat. Prev: Tutor (Dermat.) Leeds Univ.; Hon. Sen. Regist. (Dermat.) Leeds Gen. Infirm.

NORRIS, Jonathan Scott Fairlands Medical Centre, Fairlands Avenue, Worplesdon, Guildford GU3 3NA Tel: 01483 594250 Fax: 01483 598767; 32 Selbourne Road, Burpham, Guildford GU4 7JP — BM BS Nottm. 1978; MRCGP 1982. Trainer (Gen. Pract.) Guildford. Specialty: Gen. Pract. Prev: Trainee GP Derbysh. Family Pract. Comm. VTS.

NORRIS, Julia Constance Fircroft, Gladsmuir Road, Barnet EN5 4PJ — MB BCh Wales 1967; DA Eng. 1969.

NORRIS, Kate Louise St. Marys Street Surgery, 47 St Marys St., Ely CB7 4HF Tel: 01353 663434 Fax: 01353 669532; 66 Aldreth Road, Haddenham, Ely CB6 3PW — MB BS Lond. 1982 (CXHMS) DRCOG 1986. Partner in Gen. Pract.; Clin. Asst. in Gyn., Princess of Wales Hosp., Ely, Cambs. Prev: Asst. GP Cheltenham; Trainee GP Cheltenham VTS.

NORRIS, Katharine Joanne West Timperley Medical Centre, 21 Dawson Road, Altrincham WA14 5PF Tel: 0161 929 1515 Fax: 0161 941 6500; 3 Bankhall Lane, Hale, Altrincham WA15 0LA Tel: 0161 928 8979 — MB ChB Bristol 1986; DRCOG 1990; MRCGP 1991; T(GP) 1991. Prev: SHO (Paediat. & A & E) S. Manch. Hosp.; SHO (Geriat.) Chester City Hosp.

NORRIS, Margaret Jennifer 7 Endcliffe Grove Avenue, Sheffield S10 3EJ Tel: 0114 666568 — MB ChB Ed. 1969; BSc (Med. Sci.) Ed. 1966, MB ChB 1969. Prev: Ho. Phys. Leith Hosp. Edin.; Ho. Surg. Roodlands Hosp. Haddington; SHO (O & G) St. Mary's Hosp. Kettering.

NORRIS, Mark Christopher 46 The Willows, Newington, Sittingbourne ME9 7LS — MB ChB Leic. 1996.

NORRIS, Mr Michael Graham Hall Farm, Somerford Booths, Congleton CW12 2JR Tel: 01260 224261 — MB ChB St. And. 1965 (St. Andrews) DObst RCOG 1967; FRCS Ed. 1972. Cons. Orthop. Surg. E. Chesh. NHS Trust. Specialty: Orthop.; Medico Legal. Socs: Fell. BOA; BMA; HCSA. Prev: Regist. (Orthop.) Nuffield Orthop. Centre Oxf.; Sen. Regist. (Orthop.) Harlow Wood Orthop. Hosp. Mansfield.

NORRIS, Patricia Mary The Surgery, 212 Richmond Road, Kingston upon Thames KT2 5HF Tel: 020 8546 0400 Fax: 020 8974 5771; 4 Rosewood, 105 Manor Road North, Thames Ditton KT7 0BH Tel: 020 8398 8226 — MB ChB Liverp. 1970; MRCS Eng. LRCP Lond. 1970; DObst RCOG 1972; Cert. Family Plann. JCC 1986; Cert. Occupat. Med. 1988; MRCGP 1991; Cert. Av. Med. 1993; D.Occ. Med. 1997; Adv. Aviat. Med. Cert. 1999. Sen. Partner Gen. Pract.; Gp. Med. Adviser BAE Systems; Med. Adviser Lond. Gen. Holdings Kingston, Europe Worthing & AIM Avionics Byfleet; Local Med. Adviser Thames Water. Specialty: Occupat. Health; Aviat. Med. Special Interest: Occupational Med. Socs: Soc. Occupat. Med.

NORRIS, Paul Graham Department of Dermatology, Addenbrooke's Hospital, Cambridge CB2 2QQ — MB BChir Camb. 1981 (St George's) MRCP (UK) 1984. Cons. Dermat. Addenbrooke's Hosp. Camb. Specialty: Dermat. Socs: FRCP.

NORRIS, Paul Martin — MB BS Lond. 1998.

NORRIS, Peter Edward Riverside Surgery, Barnard Avenue, Brigg DN20 8AS Tel: 01652 650131 Fax: 01652 651551; 6 Barff Meadow, Glentham LN8 2FD Tel: 01673 875757 — BM BCh Oxf. 1977; MA Oxf. 1978.

NORRIS, Philip, Wing Cdr. RAF Med. Br. Retd. Church Park, Rhossili, Gower, Swansea SA3 1PL Tel: 01792 390540 — MB ChB Bristol 1952. Prev: Flying Personel Med. Off. RAF Inst. Aviat. Med. FarnBoro.; GP Camberley; Med. Adviser Dept. Transport DVLC Swansea.

NORRIS, Richard Lansdowne Road Surgery, 6 Lansdowne Road, Bedford MK40 2BU Tel: 01234 270170 Fax: 01234 214033; 47 The Glebe, Clapham MK41 6GB Tel: 01234 347423 Fax: 01234 347423 — BM BS Nottm. 1978; BMedSci Nottm. 1978; Cert. Family Plann. JCC 1981. GP Bedford. Prev: Dep. Police Surg. & Prison Med. Off.

NORRIS, Richard Martin Parkfield Medical Centre, The Walk, Potters Bar EN6 1QH Tel: 01707 651234 Fax: 01707 660452; 21 Mount Grace Road, Potters Bar EN6 1RD — MB BChir Camb. 1972 (Univ. Coll. Hosp.) BA Camb. 1968; MRCGP 1983. Bd. Mem. Hertsmere PCG. Prev: SHO St. Martin's Hosp. Bath; Cas. Surg. Off. Middlx. Hosp. Lond.; Ho. Surg. Whittington Hosp. Lond.

NORRIS, Mr Richard William BUPA Alexandra Hospital, Impton Lane, Walderslade, Chatham ME5 9PG Tel: 01634 687166; Torridon House, Church Cliff, Kingsdown, Deal CT14 8AT Tel: 01304 380684 — MB BS Lond. 1976 (Lond. Hosp.) MRCS Eng.

LRCP Lond. 1976; FRCS Eng. 1980; T(S) Lond. 1987. Cons. Plastic Surg. Chaucer Hosp Canterbury., BUPA Alexandra Hosp. Walderslade & Chaucer Hosp. Canterbury; Dir. of Surg. The Kent Hand & Plastic Surg. Unit Alexandra Hosp. Walderslade. Specialty: Plastic Surg. Socs: Brit. Assn. Plastic Surg.; Brit. Assn. Aesthetic Plastic Surgs.; Brit. Soc. For Surg. of the hand. Prev: Cons. Plastic Surg. Qu. Vict. Hosp. E. Grinstead; Regist. (Surg.) Lond. Hosp.; Demonst. (Anat.) Lond. Hosp. Med. Coll.

NORRIS, Robin MacKenzie (retired) Cardiac Department, The Royal Sussex County Hospital, Brighton BN2 5BE Tel: 01273 696955 Fax: 01273 673106; Chatfield, Lewes Road, Ringmer, Lewes BN8 5ER Tel: 01273 814403 — MB ChB New Zealand 1955; MRCP (UK) 1960; MD Birm. 1965; FRACP 1972; FRCP Lond. 1977. Hon. Cons. Cardiol. & Sen. Vis. Fell. (Cardiac) Roy. Sussex Co. Hosp. Prev: Cardiol. Coronary Care Unit Green La. Hosp. Auckland, NZ.

NORRIS, Stephanie Claire Denbie, Lockerbie DG11 1DU — MB ChB Manch. 1979; BSc (1st cl. Hons. Pharm.) Manch. 1973; MB ChB (Hons.) Manch. 1979; MRCP (UK) 1982. Med. Director N. Cumbria Acute Hosp. NHS Trust. Prev: Med. Adviser Primary Care Dumfries & Galloway HB.; Med. Adviser ICI Pharmaceut. Div. Alderley Pk.; Clin. Research Fell. ICI Pharmaceut. Div. Alderely Pk.

NORRIS, Mr Stephen Henley 7 Endcliffe Grove Avenue, Sheffield S10 3EJ Tel: 0114 266 0707 Fax: 0114 267 8600 Email: stephennorris@medix-uk.com — MD Bristol 1985 (Middlx.) MB BS Lond. 1970; FRCS Eng. 1974. p/t Cons. Orthop. Surg. N. Gen. Hosp. Sheff.; Mem. Ct. of Examr.s Roy. Coll. of Surg.s. Specialty: Orthop. Special Interest: Hand and Wrist Surg. Socs: Fell. BOA; Hand Soc.; Ct. Exam. RCS Eng. Prev: Sen. Lect. (Orthop. Surg.) Univ. Sheff.; Lect. (Orthop. & Traum. Surg.) Univ. Bristol; Resid. (Orthop.) Mass. Gen. Hosp., Boston.

NORRIS, Tessa Carolyn Margaret The Long Melford Practice, Cordell Road, Long Melford, Sudbury CO10 9EP — MB BS Lond. 1983; MA (Hons.) Camb. 1984; MRCGP 1987. Med. Adviser Schering-Plough Ltd. Mildenhall.; GP, The Surg., Sudbury. Prev: GP Richmond; SHO (Paediat., Med. & A & E) Qu. Mary's Hosp. Lond.

NORRIS, Willam Desmond — MB ChB Dundee 1997.

NORRIS, William Anderson, OBE (retired) 42 Bawn Hill Road, Ballynahinch BT24 8LD Tel: 01238 561266 Fax: 01238 561266 — MD Belf. 1952; MB BCh BAO 1948, DPM 1952; FRCPI 1981, M 1954; FRCPsych 1982, M 1971. Prev: Cons. Psychiat. Purdysburn Hosp., Roy. Vict. Hosp. & Day Hosp. Belf.

NORTH, Adrian C 19 Laithes Drive, Alverthorpe, Wakefield WF2 9TE Email: anorth@compuserve.com — MB ChB Manch. 1997 (Manchester University) VTS Pinderfield Gen. Hosp. Wakefield. Prev: Ho. Off. (Gen. Surg. & Orthop.); Ho. Off. (Elderly Med. & Respirat. Med.).

NORTH, Mr Andrew David Scarborough Hospital, Woodlands Drive, Scarborough YO12 6QL Tel: 01723 368111; The Old Station, Staintondale, Scarborough YO13 0EZ — BM BS Nottm. 1980; FRCS Glas. 1984; FRCS Orth. Glas. 1992. Cons. Orthop. Surg. ScarBoro. Hosp. N. Yorks. Specialty: Orthop. Prev: Sen. Regist. Guy's Hosp. Lond.; Regist. Qu. Med. Centre Nottm.

NORTH, Carolyn Elizabeth Nidderdale View, Burnt Yates, Harrogate HG3 3EG — MB BS Lond. 1998.

NORTH, Christopher Hill Brow Surgery, Long Croft, Mapplewell, Barnsley S75 6FH Tel: 01226 383131 Fax: 01226 380100; 136 Park Grove, Barnsley S70 1QG — MB ChB Sheff. 1977.

NORTH, Christopher Ivan The Doctors House, Victoria Road, Marlow SL7 1DN Tel: 01628 484666 Fax: 01628 891206 — MB BS Lond. 1979; DRCOG 1981; DCH RCP Lond. 1983.

NORTH, Claire Elizabeth Orchard Surgery, Cope Road, Banbury OX16 2EJ Tel: 01295 277220 Fax: 01295 273400; Aldsworth, Hook Norton Road, Sibford Ferris, Banbury OX15 5QR — MB ChB Leic. 1985; DRCOG 1987; MRCGP 1989. Prev: Trainee GP Qu. Eliz. II Hosp. Welwyn Gdn. City VTS.

NORTH, Clive Doyne Child and Family Consultation Service, 25 West Avenue, Clacton-on-Sea CO15 1EU Tel: 01255 207070 Fax: 01255 207088 — MB BS Lond. 1987; MA Oxf. 1992, BA 1983; MSc Manch. 1992; MRCPsych 1992; MD Lond. 1997. Cons. Child & Adolesc. Psychiat. N. Essex Ment. Health Partnership Trust. Specialty: Child & Adolesc. Psychiat.

NORTH, Derek The Surgery, 66-68 Stoke Road, Gosport PO12 1PA Tel: 023 9258 1529 Fax: 023 9250 1417; 3 Ellachie Road, Gosport PO12 2DP Tel: 02392 581529 — MB ChB Sheff. 1975; DCH Eng. 1977; DRCOG 1979; MRCGP 1980. GP Princip.; GP Trainer. Specialty: Gen. Pract. Socs: BMA.

NORTH, Elizabeth Ann Epsom & St Helier NHS Trust, Wrythe Lane, Carshalton SM5 1AA Email: elizabeth.north@epson_sthelier.nhs.uk; Cavendish Lodge, 1 Cavendish Road, Sutton SM2 5ET Tel: 020 8642 8027 Fax: 020 8770 0945 — MB ChB Liverp. 1970; DObst RCOG 1972; DMRD Liverp. 1974; FRCR 1975; BA (Hons.) Open 1988. Cons. Radiol. St. Heliers Hosp. Carshalton; Hon. Lect. St. Geo. Hosp. Tooting. Specialty: Radiol. Socs: (Ex-Pres.) Sutton & Merton Dist. Med. Soc.; Brit. Soc. Interven. Radiol.; Cardiovasc. & Interven. Soc. Europe. Prev: Sen. Regist. (Radiol.) St. Mary's Hosp. Paddington; Ho. Off. David Lewis North. Hosp. Liverp.

NORTH, Gillian Norma Shiregreen Medical Centre, 492 Bellhouse Road, Sheffield S5 0RG Tel: 0114 245 6123 Fax: 0114 257 0964; 38 Eagleton Drive, High Green, Sheffield S35 4DS Tel: 0114 284 5830 Email: gill@eagleton.demon.co.uk — MB ChB Leeds 1978; MRCGP 1982; DCH RCP Lond. 1982; Dip. Palliat. Med. Wales 1991. GP Trainer Sheff.; Hosp. Pract. Wheata Day Hospice Sheff. Specialty: Palliat. Med. Prev: Trainee GP/SHO Huddersfield Roy. Infirm. VTS; Ho. Phys. & Ho. Surg. St. Jas. Hosp. Leeds.

NORTH, Jennifer Rachel 61 Compton Road, London N21 3NU — MB ChB Sheff. 1993.

NORTH, Joan Lane End Farm, Hightown, Ringwood BH24 3DY Tel: 0142 542036 — MB ChB St. And. 1949; MRCOG 1958.

NORTH, Mr John Frederick (retired) Boundary Cottage, Kemerton, Tewkesbury GL20 7JD Tel: 01386 725376 — MRCS Eng. LRCP Lond. 1941 (Camb. & St. Thos.) BA Camb 1938, MA 1942, MB BChir 1941; FRCS Eng. 1947. Prev: Surg. i/c W. Midl. Regional Plastic Surg. Centre Wordsley Hosp.

NORTH, John Kingsley Rosebank Surgery, Ashton Road, Road, Lancaster LA1 4JS Tel: 01524 842284 Fax: 01524 844839; 5 Pinewood Close, Lancaster LA2 0AD Tel: 01524 68338 — MB BS Lond. 1982 (Guy's Hospital, London) DCH RCP Lond. 1986; DRCOG 1987; MRCGP 1988. GP Lancaster. Specialty: Gen. Pract.

NORTH, Jonathan Paul Immunology Department, City Hospital, Dudley Road, Birmingham B18 7QH Tel: 0121 507 4250 Fax: 0121 507 4567 Email: jpn@immunology.demon.co.uk — MB BCh Wales 1982; MRCPath 1992; DM Soton. 1993; FRCP (Path) 2000. Cons. Immunol. City Hosp. & NBS Birm.; Hon. Sen. Lect. Immunol. Birm. Med. Sch. Specialty: Immunol. Socs: Brit. Soc. Immunol.; Assn. Clin. Path.; Brit. Soc. Allergy and Clin. Immunol. Prev: Sen. Regist. (Immunol.) Leics. Roy. Infirm.; Regist. (Immunol.) Dudley Rd. Hosp. Birm.; Research Regist. Roy. Vict. Hosp. Bournemouth & Tenovus Research Inst. Soton.

NORTH, Michael Alan Maylandsea Medical Centre, Imperial Avenue, Maylandsea, Chelmsford CM3 6AH Tel: 01621 742233 Fax: 01621 742917; Downside Cottage, Summerhill, Althorne, Chelmsford CM3 6BY Email: mikenorth@equip.ac.uk — MB BS Lond. 1978 (Royal Free Hospital) DRCOG 1981; FRCGP 1996, M 1986.

NORTH, Penelope Claire Moregrove, Perrymead, Bath BA2 5AZ — BM Soton. 1991; BSc Sheff. 1986.

NORTH, Peter Edwin (retired) Long Meadow, 58 Burnham Road, Epworth, Doncaster DN9 1BY Tel: 01427 872422 — MB ChB St. And. 1957; FFA RCS Eng. 1964. Prev: Cons. Anaesth. Scunthorpe Health Dist.

NORTH, Peter John 9 Chadderton Drive, Unsworth, Bury BL9 8NL — MRCS Eng. LRCP Lond. 1964; DO Eng. 1970.

NORTH, Philipa Therese — MB ChB Ed. 1997.

NORTH, Professor Richard Alan Institute of Molecular Physiology, University of Sheffield, Alfred Denny Building, Western Bank, Sheffield S10 2TN Tel: 0114 222 4668 Fax: 0114 222 2360 Email: r.a.north@sheffield.ac.uk; 64 A Dore Road, Sheffield S17 3NE — MB ChB Aberd. 1969; BSc Aberd. 1969; PhD Aberd. 1973. Prof. Inst. Molecular Physiol. Univ. Sheff. Specialty: Pharmacology. Socs: Fell. Roy. Soc. Lond.; Fell. Roy. Coll. Phys. Prev: Prof. Vollum Inst.; Prof. Mass. Inst. Technol.; Princip. Scientist, Glaxo Wellcome Research and Developm., Geneva.

NORTH, Sarah Melody Putneymead Medical Centre, 350 Upper Richmond Road, London SW15 6TL Tel: 020 8788 0686; 9 Ellison Road, Barnes, London SW13 0AD — MB BS Lond. 1974.

NORTH, Serena Laura Peabody The Surgery, 3 Austin Road, Battersea, London SW11 5JP Tel: 020 7498 0232 Fax: 020 7498 0271 — BM BCh Oxf. 1975 (Oxford) MRCGP 1979. GP Battersea Fields Lond.; Med. Cons. to Christian Action Research & Educat. (CARE).

NORTH-COOMBES, David Paul The Bridge Practice, The Health Centre, Stepgates, Chertsey KT16 8HZ Tel: 01932 561199; Farthings, Brox Lane, Ottershaw, Chertsey KT16 0LL Tel: 01932 872220 — MB BS Lond. 1978 (Middlx.) DCH RCP Lond. 1980; DRCOG 1982; MRCGP 1984.

NORTH-SMITH, Margaret Holden (retired) 29 Esher Park Avenue, Esher KT10 9NX Tel: 01372 486784 — LRCP LRCS Ed. LRFPS Glas. 1949 (Roy. Colls. Ed.) DA Eng. 1954. Prev: Anaesth. NW Surrey Hosp. Gp.

NORTHCOTE, Robin John Department of Medicine, The Victoria Infirmary, Langside, Glasgow G42 9TY Tel: 0141 201 5396; Whinmuir, 11 Ewenfield Road, Ayr KA7 2QF — MD Glas. 1986; MB ChB 1978; MRCP (UK) 1982; FRCPS Glas. 1992; Dip. Sp. Med. 1997. Cons. Phys. & Cardiol. Vict. Infirm. Glas. Specialty: Cardiol. Socs: Brit. Cardiac Soc. & Med. Research Soc. Prev: Sen. Regist. (Cardiol. & Gen. Med.) & Research Fell. (Cardiol.) Vict. Infirm. Glas.

NORTHEAST, Mr Andrew David Roland Wycombe General Hospital, Queen Alexandra Road, High Wycombe HP11 2TT Tel: 01494 526161 Email: anortheast@compuserve.com — BM BCh Oxf. 1980; MA Oxf. 1981; FRCS Ed. 1986; FRCS Eng. 1987. Cons. Gen. Surg. S. Bucks. NHS Trust. Specialty: Gen. Surg. Socs: Fell. Roy. Soc. Of Med.; Vasc. Scrn. Soc.(GB); Assn. Surg. Prev: Sen. Regist. & Regist. St. Thos. Hosp. Lond.; Regist. (Gen. Surg.) St. Thos. Hosp. Lond.; SHO (Surg.) MusGr. Pk. Hosp. Taunton.

NORTHEN, Mary Ellen Lingfield Surgery, East Grinstead Road, Lingfield RH7 6ER Tel: 01342 833456 Fax: 01342 836347; Hadlow, Pk Road, Dormans Park, East Grinstead RH19 2NQ Tel: 01342 670646 — MB ChB Glas. 1971; MRCP (UK) 1974. GP Lingfield. Prev: GP Hitchin; Regist. (Gen. Med.) West. Infirm. Glas.

NORTHERN, David Graham Frank Oakengates Medical Practice, Limes Walk, Oakengates, Telford TF2 6JJ Tel: 01952 620077 Fax: 01952 620209; 8 Woodhouse Lane, Priorslee, Telford TF2 9SX Tel: 01952 293775 — MB ChB Manch. 1981; DRCOG 1983; DCH RCP Lond. 1984; MRCGP 1985.

NORTHFIELD, John William Hazelwood Farm, Doghurst La, Coulsdon CR5 3PL — MB BS Lond. 1997.

NORTHFIELD, Mark 574 Broadway, Chadderton, Oldham OL9 9NF — MB ChB Manch. 1982; BSc St. And. 1979.

NORTHFIELD, Rosemary Raymonde (retired) Hazelwood Farm, Doghurst Lane, Chipstead, Coulsdon CR5 3PL Tel: 01737 553209 Fax: 01737 551560 — (Guy's) MB BS Lond. 1961; MRCS Eng. LRCP Lond. 1961; DA Eng. 1964; DIH Eng. 1970; FFOM RCP Lond. 1997, MFOM 1978; T(OM) 1991. Prev: Med. Adviser Brit. Gas Croydon.

NORTHFIELD, Professor Timothy Clive (retired) Hazelwood Farm, Doghurst Lane, Chipstead, Coulsdon CR5 3PL Tel: 01737 553209 Fax: 01737 551560 — MB BChir Camb. 1963 (Guy's) MRCS Eng. LRCP Lond. 1962; FRCP Lond. 1977, M 1965; MA Camb. 1959, MD 1970. Cons. Phys. & Prof. Gastroenterol. St. Geo. Hosp. & Med. Sch. Lond. Prev: Regist. (Gastroenterol.) Centr. Middlx. Hosp. Lond.

NORTHMORE-BALL, Mr Martin Dacre The Robert Jones and Agnes Hunt, Othopaedic Hospital, Oswestry SY10 7AG; Higher Grange, Ellesmere SY12 9DH — MB BChir Camb. 1968 (Camb. & St. Thos.) MA Camb. 1968; FRCS Eng. 1973. Hon. Cons. Orthop. Surg. Robt. Jones & Agnes Hunt Orthop. Hosp. Oswestry. Specialty: Orthop. Prev: Sen. Regist. (Orthop.) Addenbrooke's Hosp. Camb.; Clin. Fell. (Orthop.) Univ. Toronto, Canada; Regist. (Orthop.) King's Coll. Hosp. Lond.

NORTHOVER, Catherine Sophia Cutlers Hill Surgery, Burgay Road, Halesworth IP19 8HP Tel: 01986 874618/01986 874908 — MB ChB Liverp. 1972; DCH Eng. 1976.

NORTHOVER, Professor John Martin Alban St. Mark's Hospital, Northwick Park, Watford Road, Harrow HA1 3UJ Tel: 020 8235 4250 Fax: 020 8235 4277 Email: john.northover@cancer.org.uk; 2 Park Avenue N., Priory Park, London N8 7RT Tel: 020 8342 9837 Fax: 020 8348 7605 — MB BS Lond. 1970 (King's Coll. Hosp.) MRCS Eng. LRCP Lond. 1970; FRCS Eng. 1975; MS Lond. 1980. Cons. Surg. St. Marks Hosp. Lond.; Director Cancer Research UK Cloorectal Cancer Unit; Prof. Imperial Coll. Lond. Specialty: Gastroenterol. Prev: Hon. Dir. ICRF Colorectal Cancer Unit.; Sen. Lect. Imp. Coll. Lond.

NORTHOVER, Julian Roy Little Thatches, Hill St., Calmore, Southampton SO40 2RX — BM Soton 1997.

NORTHOVER, Ruth Patricia St Thomas Health Centre, Cowick Street, St. Thomas, Exeter EX4 1HJ Tel: 01392 676677 Fax: 01392 676677; Home Farm, Oxton, Exeter EX6 8EX Tel: 01626 891162 — MB BS Lond. 1985 (St Bart.) MRCGP 1989; DRCOG 1989. GP Exeter. Specialty: Diabetes. Prev: Clin. Asst. (Diabetes) Exeter; Trainee GP Dartmouth; SHO (O & G & Med.) Harold Wood Hosp. Romford.

NORTHOVER, Susan Carolyn 17 Kyle Close, Bracknell RG12 7DF — BM Soton. 1998.

NORTHOVER, Tracy Heidi Royal Bolton Hospital, Minerva Road, Farnworth, Bolton BL4 0JR Tel: 01204 390390 Email: heidi.northover@boltonh-tr.nwest.nhs.uk — MB ChB Manch. 1986; DRCOG 1988; DCH RCP Lond. 1989; MRCP (UK) 1992; FRCPCH 1996. Cons. Paediat. Roy. Bolton Hosp. Specialty: Paediat. Prev: Sen. Regist. (Paediat.) Roy. Manch. Childr. Hosp.; Regist. (Paediat.) Roy. Manch. Childr. Hosp.; Regist. (Paediat.) Roy. Childr. Hosp. Melbourne, Austral.

NORTHRIDGE, Cecil Samuel Colne Health Centre, Market Street, Colne BB8 0LJ Tel: 01282 862451 — MB BCh BAO Dub. 1976 (TC Dub.) GP Princip.; E. Lancs. L.M.C. Mem. 1995.

NORTHRIDGE, David Bourke Department Cardiology, Western General Hospital, Edinburgh EH4 2XU Tel: 0131 537 1849 Fax: 0131 537 1849 — MB ChB Ed. 1983; MRCP (UK) 1986. Cons. Cardiol. Western Gen. Hosp. Edin.; Hon. Sen. Lect. Univ. of Edin. Specialty: Cardiol. Socs: Coun. Mem. Brit. Soc. Echocardigraphy. Prev: Sen. Regist. (Cardiol.) Univ. Hosp. Wales Cardiff.; Regist. (Cardiol.) West. Infirm. Glas.

NORTHRIDGE, Guy Hamilton 3 Basil Street, London SW3 1AU Tel: 020 7235 6642 Fax: 020 7235 6052 — BM BCh Oxf. 1978; MRCS Eng. LRCP Lond. 1977; MA Oxf. 1978; MRCP (UK) 1981; DCH Eng. 1981; MRCGP 1982. Specialty: Gen. Pract. Prev: Regist. (Med.) St. Bart. Hosp. Lond.; SHO (Paediat.) & Ho. Phys. St. Thos. Hosp. Lond.

NORTHROP, Michelle Marie 300A Victoria Drive, Eastbourne BN20 8XS — BM Soton. 1998.

NORTHWAY, Mr Jonathan Ross Berega Hospital, Morogoro PO BOX 320, Tanzania Email: northway@maf.or.tz; c/o 97 Shelvers Way, Tadworth KT20 5QQ Tel: 01737 354674 — BM Soton. 1988 (Liverpool Uni.) FRCS Eng. 1993; DTM + H Liv'pl Sch. Trop. Med. 1996. Med. Miss. Specialty: Paediat.; Trop. Med.; Obst. & Gyn. Prev: SHO (Gen. Surg.) Horton Gen. Hosp. Banbury; SHO (Accid. & Emerg., Gen. Surg. & Orthop.) Wycombe Gen. Hosp.; SHO (Paediat. Surg.) John Radcliffe Hosp. Oxf.

NORTHWOOD, David — LMSSA Lond. 1980; BSc Lond. 1977, MB BS 1981; FFA RCS Eng. 1985. Cons. (Anaesth.) Doncaster & Bassetlaw Hosps. NHS Trust. Specialty: Anaesth.

NORTLEY, Ernest Richmond Wulck Merton Medical Practice, 12-17 Abbey Parade, Merton High Street, London SW19 1DG Tel: 020 8540 1109 Fax: 020 8543 3353 — MB ChB Ghana 1978; LRCP LRCS Ed. LRCPS Glas. 1985; DObst RCPI 1985. Socs: MDU. Prev: Vis. Med. Off. Sticklan Lodge Lond.; Clin. Med. Off. (Family Plann.) St. Geo. Hosp. Lond.

NORTON, Alice Elizabeth 26 St Leodegars Way, Hunston, Chichester PO20 1PF — MB ChB Bristol 1997.

NORTON, Andrew Carey Department of Anaesthesia, Pilgrim Hospital, Sibsey Road, Boston PE21 9QS Email: andrew.norton@ulh.nhs.uk — MB BS Lond. 1981; BSc Lond. 1977; FFA RCS Eng. 1985. Cons. Anaesth. Pilgrim Hosp. Boston. Specialty: Anaesth. Socs: Soc. Computing & Technol. in Anaesth.; Obst. Anaesth. Assn. Prev: Lect. & Hon. Sen. Regist. (Anaesth.) Aberd. Univ. & Aberd. Roy. Infirm.; Regist. (Anaesth.) South. Gen. Hosp. Glas.

NORTON, Andrew John Department of Histopathology, St Bartholomew's Medical School, London EC1A 7BE Tel: 020 7601 8539 — MB BS Lond. 1981 (Char Cross) MRCPath 1987. Sen. Lect. & Hon. Cons. (Histopath.) St. Bart. Med. Sch. Specialty: Histopath. Prev: Lect. Univ. Coll. & Inst. Laryng. & Otol.; Graham Schol. Univ. Coll. Lond.

NORTON, Andrew McNeill Bonnyrigg Health Centre, High Street, Bonnyrigg EH19 2DA Tel: 0131 663 7272 Fax: 0131 660 5636; 81 Woodfield Avenue, Colinton, Edinburgh EH13 0QR — MB ChB Ed. 1974; BSc Ed. 1971, MB ChB 1974. Socs: Life Mem. Roy. Med. Soc. Prev: SHO (Gen. Surg.) Roodlands Gen. Hosp. Haddington; SHO Peripheral Vasc. Clinic Roy. Infirm. Edin.; SHO A & E Dept. Roy. Infirm. Edin.

NORTON, Anne Grove Medical Centre, 6 Uplands Terrace, Uplands, Swansea SA2 0GU Tel: 01792 643000 Fax: 01792 472800; 105 Bishopston Road, Bishopston, Swansea SA3 3EU Tel: 0144 128 2929 — MB ChB Dundee 1976; DCH Eng. 1978. The Gr. Med. Centre.

NORTON, Aurelia Mary 2 Topiary Square, Stanmore Road, Richmond TW9 2DB — MB BS Lond. 1991.

NORTON, Bernard Derbyshire Royal Infirmary NHS Trust, London Road, Derby DE1 2QY Tel: 01332 347141 Fax: 01332 254764; 67 Green Lane, Liverpool L13 7BA — MB ChB Liverp. 1986; MRCP (UK) 1989; MD Liverp. 1993; FRCP 2000. Cons. Phys. & Gastroenterol. Derbysh. Roy. Infirm. Specialty: Gastroenterol.; Gen. Med. Socs: BMA; Brit. Soc. Gastroenterol.; Brit. Assn. Paren. & Ente. Nutrit. Prev: Sen. Regist. (Gen. Med. & Gastroenterol.) Derbysh. Roy. Infirm. & Nottm. City Hosp.; Regist. (Gen. Med., Gastroenterol. & Clin. Nutrit.) Roy. Lond. Hosp.; Regist. (Gen. Med. & Gastroenterol.) Countess of Chester Hosp.

NORTON, Beverley Child and Family Psychiatry, St. John's Hospital, Livingston, Edinburgh EH54 6PP Tel: 01506 419666 — MB ChB Ed. 1974; MPhil Ed. 1982, BSc 1971; MRCPsych 1978. Cons. Child & Adolesc. Psychiat. Roy. Hosp. for Sick Childr., Lothian Primary Care Trust. Specialty: Child & Adolesc. Psychiat. Socs: Fell. Roy. Med. Soc. Edin. Prev: Cons. Child & Adolesc. Psychiat. Falkirk Roy. Infirm. Centr. Scotl. Healthcare; Sen. Regist. (Child & Adolesc. Psychiat.) Young People's Unit Roy. Edin. Hosp. & Roy. Hosp. Sick Childr. Edin.; Regist. (Psychiat.) Roy. Edin Hosp.

NORTON, Catherine Anne University Hospital of Wales, Heath Park, Cardiff CF14 4XW; 32 Heol y Delyn, Lisvane, Cardiff CF14 0SQ Tel: 01222 520640 — MB BCh Wales 1991 (University of Wales College of Medicine) DCH; BSc; MRCP. Specialist Regist. Specialty: Paediat.

NORTON, Jane Department of Histopathology, University Hospital Lewisham, Lewisham High St., London SE13 6LH Tel: 020 8333 3046 Fax: 020 8333 3254 Email: jane.norton@uhl.nhs.uk — MB BS Lond. 1984; MRCPath 1993; MD Lond. 1994. Cons. Histopath. Univ. Hosp. Lewisham Lond. Specialty: Histopath. Prev: Cons. Histopath. William Harvey Hosp. Ashford; Lect. (Histopath.) St. Marys' Hosp. Lond.; Regist. (Histopath.) Roy. Marsden Hosp. Sutton.

NORTON, John Christopher Gerard 27 Caledonia Road, Saltcoats KA21 5AJ Tel: 01294 63011; 17 South Crescent, Ardrossan Tel: 01294 63011 — MB BCh BAO NUI 1981; MRCGP 1985. GP Ardrossan.

NORTON, Keith John Kingsthorpe Medical Centre, Eastern Avenue South, Northampton NN2 7JN Tel: 01604 713823 Fax: 01604 721996 — MB ChB St. And. 1965; DRCOG 1967; Cert JCC Lond. 1976. Hosp. Pract. (Psycho.-Geriat.) St. Crispin Hosp. N.ampton. Prev: Clin. Asst. (Psycho Geriat.) St. Crispin Hosp. N.ampton.

NORTON, Kenneth Ross (retired) 25 Granville Road, Barnet EN5 4DS Tel: 020 8440 2581 — MB BS Lond. 1951 (St. Thos.) DObst RCOG 1952; DCH Eng. 1956; FRCP Lond. 1975, M 1958. Cons. Paediat. Barnet & Edgware Gen. Hosps. Prev: Regist. (Med.) Barnet Gen. Hosp.

NORTON, Kingsley Raymond William Henderson Hospital, 2 Homeland Drive, Brighton Road, Sutton SM2 5LT Tel: 020 8661 1611 Email: knorton@sghms.ac.uk — MB BChir 1976; BA Cantab. 1973; MA Cantab. 1976; MRCPsych 1980; MD Camb. 1988; FRCPsych 1995. Cons. Psychother. Henderson Hosp.; Reader Psychother., St. George's Hosp. Med. Sch., Lond. Specialty: Psychother. Prev: Cons. Psychiat. Sutton Hosp.; Lect. (Psychiat.) St. Geo. Hosp. Med. Sch. Lond.

NORTON, Margaret Alice (retired) 163 Malvern Road, St. John's, Worcester WR2 4NN Tel: 01905 423183 — MB ChB Birm. 1939; MRCGP 1953. Prev: Med. Off. Alice Ottley Sch. Worcester.

NORTON, Margot Lotte Sophie Park Gates, The Green, Richmond TW9 1QG Tel: 020 8940 4742 Fax: 020 8948 7211 — (Roy. Free) MRCS Eng. LRCP Lond. 1950; MB BS (Hons.) Lond. 1950.

NORTON, Mark Richard Cornerways Surgery, 50 Manor Road, Beckenham BR3 5LG Tel: 020 8650 2444; 61 Barnfield Wood Road, Beckenham BR3 6ST — MB BS Lond. 1984.

NORTON, Mark Ross Princess Elizabeth Orthopaedic Centre, Royal Devon & Exeter Hospital, Barrack Road, Exeter EX2 4UE Tel: 01392 411611; The Chapter House, 3 St Scholastica's Abbey, Teignmouth TQ14 8FF Tel: 01626 774734 Fax: 01626 774734 — MB ChB Cape Town 1988; FRCS Eng. 1995. Specialist Regist. (Trauma & Orthop. Surg.) Roy. Devon & Exeter Hosp. Exeter. Specialty: Trauma & Orthop. Surg. Socs: Assoc. Mem. BOA; Brit. Orthop. Train. Assn.

NORTON, Martyn Howard Shelfield Surgery, 144 Lichfield Road, Shelfield, Walsall WS4 1PW Fax: 01922 694069; 144 Lichfield Road, Shelfield, Walsall WS4 1PW Tel: 0121 353 6847 — MB ChB Liverp. 1971.

NORTON, Paul Gorvin Valley Medical Centre, Johnson Street, Stocksbridge, Sheffield S36 1BX Tel: 0114 288 3841 Fax: 0114 288 7897; 3 Royd Lane, Deepcar, Sheffield S36 2RZ — MB BS Lond. 1969; DObst RCOG 1972.

NORTON, Peter Malcolm Banksfield, Lands Lane, Knaresborough HG5 9DE Tel: 01423 863156 — MB ChB Leeds 1967; DA Eng. 1969; DObst RCOG 1969; FFA RCS Eng. 1972. Cons. (Anaesth.) Harrogate Health Care Trust. Specialty: Anaesth. Prev: Ho. Phys. & Ho. Surg. (Obst.) York 'A' Gp. Hosps.; Regist. (Anaesth.) United Sheff. Hosps.; Sen. Regist. (Anaesth.) Leeds Gps. Hosps.

NORTON, Richard Christopher 19 Dobbins Lane, Wendover, Aylesbury HP22 6BZ — MB BChir Camb. 1952 (Middlx.) DObst RCOG 1953. Prev: Sen. Princip. Med. Off. Med. Research Counc.; Ho. Phys. Middlx. Hosp.; Ho. Surg. O & G St. Mary Abbots Hosp. Kensington.

NORTON, Mr Robert Walsgrave Hospital, Coventry CV2 2DX Tel: 02476 538933 Fax: 02476 535105 Email: robert.noton@uhcw.nhs.uk; 6 Amherst Road, Kenilworth CV8 1AH Tel: 01926 857870 — MB BChir Camb. 1966 (St. Thos.) FRCS Eng. 1972. Cons. Cardiothoracic Surg. Walsgrave Hosp. Coventry. Specialty: Cardiothoracic Surg. Socs: Soc. Thoracic & Cardiovasc. Surgs. Of Gt. Britain and Irel. Prev: Cons. Thoracic Surg. Wentworth & King Geo. V Hosps. Durban, S. Afr.; Sen. Regist. (Cardiothoracic Surg.) Roy. Infirm. & City Hosps. Edin.

NORTON, Rosalind Jane — BM BS Nottm. 1997.

NORTON, Ruth Helen Redham House, Redham Lane, Pilning, Bristol BS35 4HQ — MB BS Newc. 1996.

NORTON, Miss Sally Alexis The Old Barn, Elberton, Nr. Olveston, Bristol BS35 4AQ — MB ChB Bristol 1989; FRCS Ed. 1993; MD Bristol 1999. Specialty: Gen. Surg.

NORTON, Samuel Edward — MB BS Lond. 1998; MRCS Ed. 2002.

NORTON, Stephen Charles Doctors Surgery, Pembroke Road, Framlingham, Woodbridge IP13 9HA Tel: 01728 723627 Fax: 01728 621064 — MB BS Lond. 1971 (Char. Cross) MRCS Eng. LRCP Lond. 1971; DObst RCOG 1973. Prev: SHO Profess. Obst. Unit Char. Cross Hosp. Lond.; Ho. Surg. Profess. Dept. Surg. Fulham Hosp.; Ho. Phys. Paediat. Dept. New Char. Cross Hosp. Fulham.

NORTON, William David Albany House Surgery, Albany Terrace, Barbourne, Worcester WR1 3DU Tel: 01905 26086 Fax: 01905 26888 — MB ChB Birm. 1980; DCH RCP Lond. 1983; DRCOG 1983; MRCGP 1984.

NORWELL, Nicholas Peter 4 Ladwell Close, Newbury RG14 6PJ — MB BS Lond. 1972 (Guy's & King's Coll. Hosp.) DA Eng. 1974; MRCGP 1977; DCH Eng. 1977. Socs: MDU Secretariat.

NORWICH, Roger Peter, RD (cons. rooms), Medico-Legal Consultancy plc, The Old Docks Office, Commercial Road, Gloucester GL1 2EB Tel: 01452 386242 Fax: 01452 304436; 17 Shrewsbury Road, Church Stretton SY6 6JB Tel: 01694 722951 — MB ChB Manch. 1982; MRCGP 1986. Med. Dir. (Medico-Legal Consult.) Glos. Socs: Roy. Soc. Med.

NORWOOD, Christine Child Health Department, Willow House, St Mary's Hospital, Greenhill Road, Leeds LS12 3QE Tel: 0113 279 0121; 31 Saxon Grove, Leeds LS17 5DY Tel: 0113 268 1365 — MB ChB Leeds 1982; BSc (Biochem.) Leeds 1979. Staff Grade (Community Child Health) Leeds. Specialty: Community Child Health. Socs: Guild of Catholic Doctors (Sec. Leeds Br.).

NORWOOD, Fiona Lucinda Margaret Wessex Neurological Centre, Southampton General Hospital, Tremona Road,

Southampton SO16 6YG — MB BS Lond. 1991 (Guy's) MRCP; PhD. Specialty: Gen. Med.

NORWOOD, Jeffrey Michael Walsall Health Authority, 27-31 Lichfield St., Walsall WS1 1TE Tel: 01922 720255 Fax: 01922 722051 — MB BChir Camb. 1974 (Cambridge University/St. Thomas's Hospital) DCH RCP Lond. 1975; MFPHM RCP (UK) 1994. Cons. Pub. Health Med. Walsall HA; Lect. (Med. Managem.) Keele Univ. Specialty: Pub. Health Med. Socs: (Exec. Comm.) Pub. Health & Primary Care Gp. Prev: Sen. Regist. & Regist. (Pub. Health Med.) SW RHA; GP; Sen. Med. Off. Solomon Is.s.

NORWOOD, Michael Geoffrey Austin The Rectory, Wiveton Road, Blakeney, Holt NR25 7NJ — MB ChB Leic. 1998.

NOSENZO, Ivana c/o Drive H. Paul, 45 Barton Road, Canterbury CT1 1YQ — MB BCh Witwatersrand 1985; MB BCh Wirwatersrand 1985.

NOSHIRVANI, Homa Fallah Flat 25, Sandringham Court, Maida Vale, London W9 1UA Tel: 020 7289 7680 — (Hamburg Uni.) State Exam Med. Hamburg 1969; DPM Eng. 1978; MRCPsych 1982. Assoc. Specialist. Specialty: Gen. Psychiat.; Psychother. Socs: MRCPsych.

NOSSEIR, Mohamed Nabil Abdel Hamid Queen Mary's Hospital, Sidcup DA14 6LT Tel: 020 8302 2678; 18 Langdon Shaw, Sidcup DA14 6AU — MB ChB Alexandria 1965; FFA RCSI 1987. Specialty: Anaesth.

NOTCUTT, William George James Paget Hospital, Gorleston, Great Yarmouth NR31 6LA Tel: 01493 452452 Fax: 01493 452753 Email: willy@tucton.demon.co.uk; 240 Brasenose Avenue, Gorleston, Great Yarmouth NR31 7EB Tel: 01493 665816 Fax: 0870 055 3847 — MB ChB Birm. 1970; DA Eng. 1973; FRCA. 1976. Cons. Anaesth. Jas. Paget Hosp. Gt. Yarmouth; Hon. Sen. Lect. Univ. E. Anglia. Specialty: Anaesth. Socs: BMA; Pain Soc.; Assn. Anaesth. Prev: Sen. Regist. (Anaesth.) Notts. AHA (T); Lect. (Anaesth. & Intens. Care) Univ. W. Indies Kingston, Jamaica; Med. Off. Lesotho Flying Doctor Serv.

NOTGHI, Alp City Hospital NHS Trust, Department of Nuclear Medicine, Dudley Road, Birmingham B18 7QH Tel: 0121 507 5228 Fax: 0121 507 5223 Email: alp.notghi@swbh.nhs.uk — MD Shiraz 1976; LRCP LRCS Ed. LRCPS Glas. 1984; MRCP (UK) 1985; MSc Nuclear Med. Lond. 1993; FRCP Ed. 1998; FRCP Lond. 1999. Cons. Nuclear Med. City Hosp. NHS Trust Birm. Specialty: Nuclear Med. Special Interest: Cardiol.; GI Tract. Socs: Brit. Nuclear Med. Soc. (Counc. Mem.); Europ. Assn. of Nuclear Med.; Brit. Inst. of Radiol. Prev: Sen. Regist. (Nuclear Med.) Dudley Rd. Hosp. Birm.

NOTGHI, Lesley Murray Birmingham Children's Hospital, Department of Clinical Neurophysiology, Steelhouse Lane, Birmingham B4 6NH Tel: 0121 333 9258 Fax: 0121 333 9261 Email: lesley.henderson@bch.nhs.uk — MB ChB Dundee 1981; MRCP (UK) 1985; FRCP 1999; FRCP Edin. 2002. Cons. Clin. Neurophysiologist, Birm. Childrens Hosp. NHS Trust. Specialty: Clin. Neurophysiol. Special Interest: paediatric neurophysiology. Socs: Roy. Coll. Phys. Edin.; Christian Med. Federat.; Brit. Soc. Clin. Neurophysiol. Prev: Cons. Clin. Neurophysiol. Univ. Hosp. Nottm.; Cons. Clin. Neurophysiologist, Coventry and Warks. NHS Trust.

NOTLEY, Mr Richard Guy (retired) Spindlewood, 59 Pewley Hill, Guildford GU1 3SW Tel: 01483 566295 Fax: 01483 579354 — (Guy's) MB BS Lond. 1959; MRCS Eng. LRCP Lond. 1959; FRCS Eng. 1963; MS Lond. 1968. Cons. Urol. Surg. Emerit. Roy. Surrey Co. & St. Luke's Hosp. Trust; Educational Adviser in Urol. to the Raven Dept. of Educat. Roy. Coll. of Surg.s of Eng. Prev: Cons. Urol. Surg. & Med. Dir. Roy. Surrey Co. & St. Luke's Hosp. Trust.

NOTMAN, Ian Andrew North Avenue Surgery, 18 North Avenue, Cambuslang, Glasgow G72 8AT Tel: 0141 641 3037 Fax: 0141 646 1905; 70 Stewarton Drive, Cambuslang, Glasgow G72 8DG — MB ChB Glas. 1977; Dip. Roy. Coll. Obst. & Gyn. Lond. 1980; MRCGP 1982.

NOTT, Mr David Malcolm c/o Department of Surgery, Chelsea & Westminster Hospital, 369 Fulham Road, London SW10 9NH Tel: 020 8746 8464 Fax: 020 8746 8294; 41 Ferryman's Quay, William Harris Way, London SW6 2UT — MD Manch. 1989 (St Andrews and Manchester) BSc St. And. 1979; MB ChB Manch. 1981; FRCS Eng. 1985. Cons. Surg. Chelsea & Westminster Hosp.; Cons. Vasc. Surg. Roy. Brompton & Harefield NHS Trust & Char. Cross Hosp. Lond.; Examr. (Surg.) Univ. Lond.; Extern. Examr. (Surg.) Univ. Glas.; Hon. Sen. Lect. (Surg.) Univ. Lond. Specialty: Gen. Surg. Socs: Vasc. Surg. Soc.; Surg. Research Soc.; BMA. Prev: Sen. Regist. (Gen. Surg.) Mersey RHA; Cancer Research Fell. Univ. Liverp.; Ho. Surg. Manch. Roy. Infirm. & Ho. Phys. Chapel Allerton Hosp. Leeds.

NOTT, James Gildon Harley Asplands Medical Centre, Apslands Close, Woburn Sands, Milton Keynes MK17 8QP Tel: 01908 582069 Fax: 01908 281597; Rush Hill, Tyrells End, Eversholt, Milton Keynes MK17 9DS — MB BS Lond. 1976; MA Camb. 1971; DRCOG 1980; DCH RCP Lond. 1982; MRCP (UK) 1983; MRCGP 1988. Mem. Heartlands PCT Exec. Comm.; Locality Clin. governance lead, Heartlands PCT. Prev: Trainee GP E. Lond. VTS; SHO (Neurol.) Harlow Dist.

NOTT, Michael Richardson Royal West Sussex Hospital, St. Richard's, Chichester PO19 6SE Tel: 01243 788122 Fax: 01243 531269; Chatsworth, 22 Church St, Littlehampton BN17 5PX Tel: 01903 713050 — (St. Geo.) MB BS Lond. 1966; DA Eng. 1970; FFA RCS Eng. 1972. Cons. Anaesth. Roy. W. Sussex Trust. Specialty: Anaesth. Socs: Anaesth. Res. Soc.; Roy. Soc. Med. (Anaesth. Sect.). Prev: Lect. (Anaesth.) Univ. Soton. Fac. Med.; SHO (Clin. Meas.) Westminster Hosp. Lond.; Regist. (Anaesth) Chelmsford Essex.

NOTT, Peter Norman (retired) The Limberlost, St. Giles Hill, Winchester SO23 0HH Tel: 01962 869674 — MRCS Eng. LRCP Lond. 1962; MD Camb. 1984, MB 1963, BChir 1962; DPM Eng. 1967; FRCP Ed. 1983, M 1969; FRCPsych 1984, M 1972. Cons. Psychiat. Dept. Psychiat. Soton. Prev: Sen. Lect. (Psychiat.) Univ. Soton.

NOTT-BOWER, William George Penn Hill Surgery, St Nicholas Close, Yeovil BA20 1SB Tel: 01935 74005 Fax: 01935 421841 — MB BS Lond. 1984; BA Oxf. 1981; DCH RCP Lond. 1987; DRCOG 1988; MRCGP 1989. Prev: Trainee GP Taunton VTS; Cas. Off. Qu. Mary's Hosp. Roehampton.

NOTTINGHAM, John Frank Department of Cellular Pathology, Northampton General Hospitals, Cliftonville, Northampton NN1 5BD — MB ChB Sheff. 1980; FRCPath 1997, M 1987. Cons. Histopath. Northampton Gen. Hosp. Trust, Northampton. Specialty: Histopath. Socs: Brit. Soc. Clin. Cytol.; Assn. Clin. Path. Prev: Sen. Regist. North. Gen. & Roy. Hallamsh. Hosps. Sheff.; Regist. BRd. Green & Alder Hey Hosps. Liverp.; Cons. Geo. Eliot Hosp., Nuneaton, Warks.

NOUR, Hilal The Surgery, 77 Pickford Lane, Bexleyheath DA7 4RN Tel: 020 8304 3660 Fax: 020 8298 7736 — MB ChB Baghdad 1961; MRCS Eng. LRCP Lond. 1971. Socs: Assur. Med. Soc.

NOUR, Mr Shawqui Abd El-Raheem Mohamed Leicester Royal Infirmary, Infirmary Square, Leicester LE1 5WW — MB BCh Cairo 1973; FRCS Glas. 1981; FRCS Ed. 1981; MD 1992; FRCS (Paediat.) 1993. Cons. Paediat. Surg. Leicester Roy. Infirm. Specialty: Paediat. Surg. Prev: Sen. Regist. Childr. Hosp. Sheff.; Career Regist. (Paediat. Surg.) Sheff. Childr. Hosp.

NOUR-ELDIN, Fawzy 4 Rutland House, Marloes Road, Kensington, London W8 5LE Tel: 020 7937 0685 — MB BCh Cairo 1946; PhD Manch. 1952; LMSSA Lond. 1958; FRCPath 1976, M 1963. Cons. Haemat. & Med. Writer; Vis. Cons. Blood Dis. Bakhsh Clinics & Hosps. Saudi Arabia; Edr. Excerpta Medica (Represen. UK Haemat. Sect.); Edr. Research Defence Soc. Lond.; Hon. Examr. (Path.) Brit. Sch. Osteop. Lond. Specialty: Haematology; Med. Publishing; Research. Socs: Fell. Roy. Soc. Med.; BMA; Brit. Soc. Haematol. Prev: Cons. Clin. Path. NW Thames RHA; Clin. Research Fell. (Haemat.) Roy. Infirm. Manch. & Unit. Manch. Hosps.; Med. Off. Blood Transfus. Centre Brentwood.

NOURI-DARIANI, Esmael County Hospital, Greetwell Road, Lincoln LN2 5QY Tel: 01522 512512; 16 Geralds Close, Lincoln LN2 4AL Tel: 01522 512838 — MD Iran 1971 (Nat. Univ. Iran) DLO Eng. 1976. Assoc. Specialist (ENT. Surg.) Co. Hosp. Lincoln; Cons. ENT Surg. John Coupland Hosp. GainsBoro. Specialty: Otolaryngol. Socs: BMA. Prev: Cons. ENT Surg. Bougshan Hosp., Jeddah; Regist. (ENT) William Harvey & Roy. Vict. Hosps. Ashford; SHO (ENT) Poole Gen. Hosp. Dorset.

NOURIEL, Henry — MD Tel-Aviv 1983; MRCP (UK) 1996. Specialty: Cardiol. Socs: Brit. Cardiac Soc.

NOURISH, Laura Mary — MB ChB Birm. 1998.

NOURSE, Christopher Henry (retired) 12 Fonnereau Road, Ipswich IP1 3JP Tel: 01473 250969 Fax: 01473 217159 Email: candjnourse@onetel.com; 110 Christchurch Street, Ipswich IP4 2DE Tel: 01473 250969 Fax: 01473 445096 — (Camb. & Middlx.) MB BChir Camb. 1958; MA Camb. 1958; DObst RCOG 1959; DCH Eng.

1960; FRCP Ed. 1977, M 1965; FRCP Lond. 1994. Prev: Cons. Paedia. & Med. Dir.

NOURY, Susana Ana Maria 28 Weller Grove, Chelmsford CM1 4YJ; 1 Digby Mansions, Hammersmith Bridge Road, London W6 9DE Tel: 020 8746 9883 — BM BCh Oxf. 1996; MA (Camb.) 1993; MRC Ophth 1997. SHO (Neurosurg.) W. Lond. Neurosci.s Centre Char. Cross Hosp. Specialty: Ophth. Prev: Ho. Phys. Glos. Roy. Hosp.; Ho. Surg. John Radcliffe Hosp. Oxf.

NOVAK, Alan Zdenek Scott Coastal Villages Practice, Pippin Close, Ormesby St. Margaret, Great Yarmouth NR29 3RW Tel: 01493 730205 Fax: 01493 733120; Willow House, 54 North Road, Ormesby-St-Margaret, Great Yarmouth NR29 3LE Tel: 01493 731943 — MB BS Lond. 1971; Cert Contracep. & Family Plann. RCOG, RCGP &; Cert FPA 1975. Prev: Trainee Gen. Pract. Mid-Sussex Vocational Train. Scheme.

NOVAK, Stephen Andrew 118B Wellsway, Bath BA2 4SD — MB BS Lond. 1985; MRCP (UK) 1990.

NOVAK, Thomas Vladimir Leavesden Road Surgery, 141A Leavesden Road, Watford WD2 5EP Tel: 01923 225128; 27 Cassiobury Park Avenue, Watford WD18 7LA — MRCS Eng. LRCP Lond. 1976.

NOVELL, Mr John Richard Luton & Dunstable NHS Trust, Lewsey Road, Luton LU4 0DZ Tel: 01582 497234 Fax: 01582 497234 — MB BChir Camb. 1981; MA Camb. 1982; FRCS 1986; MChir Camb. 1993. Cons. Coloproctol. Luton & Dunstable NHS Trust; Cons. Surg., BUPA Hosp., Harpenden. Specialty: Gen. Surg. Socs: Assn. Colproctol. Gt. Britain & Irel.; Assn. Surg. Gt. Britain & Irel.; Roy. Soc. Med. (Sec. Colproctol. Sect.; Mem. Acad. Bd.). Prev: Sen. Regist., The Roy. Free Hampstead NHS; Research Fell., Acad. Dept. of Surg., The Roy. Free Hampstead NHS Trust.

NOVELLI, Marco Riccardo Department of Histopathology, University College Hospitals, Rockefeller Building, University St., London WC1E 6JJ Tel: 020 7209 6033 Email: rmkdhmn.ucl.ac.uk; 29 Bardwell Road, St Albans AL1 1RQ — MB ChB Bristol 1987; MSc Experim. Path. (Toxicol.) 1989; PhD Lond. 1997; MRC Path, Royal Coll. Pattrologists, 1999. Lect. (Histopath.) Univ. Coll. Lond. Specialty: Histopath. Prev: Clin. Fell. Imperial Cancer Research Fund Lincoln's Inn Fields Lond.

NOVELLI, Vas Great Ormond Street Hospital for Children, Great Ormond Street, London WC1N 3JH Tel: 020 7813 8504 Fax: 020 7813 8552 Email: novelv@gosh.nhs.uk — MB BS Melbourne, Australia 1974; MRCP UK 1979; FRACP 1983; FRCP 1994; FRCPCH 1998. Cons. in Paediatric Infec. Dis.s, Gt. Ormord St. Childr.s Hosp. Lond.; Hon. Sen. Lect., ImumunoBiol. Unit, Inst. of Child Health, Lond. Specialty: Paediat. Socs: Brit. Paediatric Allergy, Immunol., Infec. Dis.s Gp.; Immunocompromised Host Soc.; Brit. HIV Assn. Prev: Cons. in Paediatric Infec. Dis.s, Roy. Hosp., Muscat, Oman, (1989-1991); Cons. in Paediatric Infec. Dis.s, Hamad Hosp., Doha, Qatar (1986-1989); Fell. In Pediatric Infec. Dis.s, Univ. Of Texas Health Sci. Centre, San Antonio, Texas 1984-1986.

NOVICK, Stephen Maxwell 14 Parc Caradog, Trewern, Welshpool SY21 8DS — MB ChB Manch. 1985. (Psychiat.) Shrops. PCT. Specialty: Psychother.

NOVOSEL, Steven Hartwood Hill Hospital, Hartwood, Shotts ML7 4LA Tel: 01501 823366 — MB ChB Aberd. 1978; MRCPysch. 1983; T(Psychiat.) 1991; MPhil Glasg. 1992. Cons. Community Psychiat. Specialty: Gen. Psychiat.; Forens. Psychiat. Socs: Roy. Coll. Psychiats.

NOWAK, Janik Josef Richard St Helen's Medical Centre, 151 St. Helens Road, Swansea SA1 4DF Tel: 01792 476576 Fax: 01792 301136 — MB BCh Wales 1982.

NOWAYHIO, Fadi Amin Department of Urology, University Hospital of Wales, Heath Park, Cardiff CF14 4XW — MD Lebabon 1985.

NOWELL, Hilary Jane Dormer Cottage, York Road, West Habbourne, Didcot OX11 0NG Tel: 01235 851236 — MB BS Lond. 1984; MRCGP 1989. GP Locum. Prev: GP Princip. Hanworth; Trainee GP W. Middlx. Hosp. Isleworth VTS.

NOWELL, Theresa Eve Long Furlong Medical Centre, 45 Loyd Close, Abingdon OX14 1XR Tel: 01865 61651 — BM BCh Oxf. 1988; DGM RCP Lond. 1991; DRCOG 1991; Cert. Family Plann. JCC 1991; MRCGP 1992. Prev: Trainee GP Oxf. VTS.

NOWERS, Christopher David Iver Medical Centre, High St., Iver SL0 9NU Tel: 01753 653008 Fax: 01753 650890; Elbury, Bassetbury Lane, High Wycombe Tel: 01494 523060/01494 523113 Email: christopher@nowers.com — MB BS Lond. 1975 (Westm.) BSc Lond. 1972; MRCS Eng. LRCP Lond. 1975. Specialty: Gen. Pract. Prev: Regist. (Psychiat.) Atkinson Morley Hosp. Lond.

NOWERS, Michael Peter Avon & Wiltshire Mental Health Trust, Directorate of Mental Health Services, Cossham Hospital, Lodge Road, Kingswood, Bristol BS15 1LF Tel: 0117 975 8053 Fax: 0117 975 8034 — MB BS Lond. 1977; MRCS Eng. LRCP Lond. 1977; FRCPsych 1997, M 1985; MPhil. Lond. 1990. Cons. Psychiat. (Old Age) Avon and Wilts. Ment. health trust; Hon. Sen. Lect. (Ment. Health) Univ. Bristol. Specialty: Geriat. Psychiat.

NOWIAK, Zofia (retired) 2 Dovedale Road, E. Dulwich, London SE22 0NF; 2 Dovedale Road, E. Dulwich, London SE22 0NF — MRCS Eng. LRCP Lond. 1951. Prev: Princip. GP Lond.

NOWICKI, Margaret Tennant 37 Nimrod Road, London SW16 6SZ — MB BS Lond. 1976; MRCS Eng. LRCP Lond. 1976; MFFP 1993. Specialty: Family Plann. & Reproduc. Health.

NOWICKI, Robert Waclaw Antoni 22 Baker Avenue, Nottingham NG5 8FU — MB BS Lond. 1991.

NOWLAN, William Anthony 24 High Street, Marshfield, Chippenham SN14 8LP — MB BS Lond. 1983; BA Oxf. 1978; MRCP (UK) 1986. Research & Developm. Cons. Hewlett Packard Mass, USA. Specialty: Pub. Health Med. Prev: Sen. Lect. (Epidemiol. & Pub. Health) & Clin. Research Fell. (Med. Informat.) Univ. Manch.

NOYELLE, Richard Mark Sandoz Pharmaceutics (UK) Ltd., Frimley Business Park, Frimley, Camberley GU16 5SG — MB BS Lond. 1977 (Univ. Coll. Hosp.) BSc (Pharmacol.) Lond. 1974, MB BS 1977; DRCOG 1980; DCH Eng. 1981; Dip. Pharm. Med. RCP (UK) 1985; MFPM 1989. Med. Dir. Sandoz Pharmaceut. UK Ltd. Specialty: Pharmaceutical Medicine.

NOYES, Kathryn Joan 19 Edderston Road, Peebles EH45 9DT — MB ChB Ed. 1987. Assoc. Specialist (Paediatric Diabetes) Roy. Hosp. Sick Childr. Edin. Specialty: Paediat. Prev: Research Fell. (Paediat.) Dept. Child Life & Health Edin.; Staff Grade (Paediat. Diabetes) Roy. Hosp. Sick Childr. Edin.

NQUMAYO, Christopher Carl Flat E2, 101 Manthorpe Road, Grantham NG31 8DG Tel: 01476 65232 Fax: 01476 590441 — MB ChB Zambia 1984; MRCOG 1993.

NRIALIKE, Patrick Olisa 21 Cumberland Road, Kirkholt, Rochdale OL11 2RP — MB BS Ibadan 1979; MRCOG 1993.

NSAMBA, Mr Christian Royal Albert Edward Infirmary, Wigan Lane, Wigan WN1 2NN Tel: 01942 244000 — MB ChB Ed. 1964; DLO Eng. 1966; FRCS Ed. 1969. Cons. Surg. (ENT) Wigan HA. Specialty: Otorhinolaryngol. Socs: Brit. Assn. Otol.; Otolaryngol. Research Soc. Prev: Research Fell. Inst. Laryng. & Otol. Lond.; Research Fell. Audio-Vestibular Unit Univ. Brit. Columbia Vancouver; Vis. Scientist Karoliska Inst. Sweden.

NTOUNTAS, Ioannis (John) c/o Paul Welsford Esq., 42 42 Willmore End, London SW19 3DF — State Exam Milan 1985.

NUBI, William Ajibola Olusegun The 157 Medical Practice, 157 Stroud Green Rd, Finsbury Park, London N4 3PZ Tel: 0207 2638950 — MB BS Newc. 1969; DCH RCPSI 1972; DPH Glas. 1978; Cert. Family Plann. JCC 1990. Specialty: Community Child Health. Socs: BMA & Med. Defence Union.

NUGENT, Ailish Gabrielle Craiganon Area Hospital, 68 Lurgan Rd, Portadown, Craigavon BT63 5QQ; 6 Cleaner Gardens, Belfast BT9 5HZ Email: agnugent@aol.com — MB BCh BAO Belf. 1989 (Queen's Univ. Belf.) MRCP (UK) 1992; MD 1996. Specialty: Diabetes; Gen. Med.

NUGENT, Anne Marie Royal Victoria Hosp, Grosvenor Road, Belfast BT12 6BA — MB BCh BAO Belf. 1987; MRCP (UK) 1990; MD Belf. 1994. Specialty: Respirat. Med.; Gen. Med.

NUGENT, Anthony Lowfield, Upton, Pontefract WF8 2RP — MB ChB Leeds 1950. Socs: BMA. Doncaster Med. Soc. Prev: Ho. Phys. Pontefract Gen. Infirm.; Res. Obst. Off. Gen. Hosp. Wakefield; Capt. RAMC.

NUGENT, Colette Marie Ainsdale Medical Centre, 66-68 Station Road, Ainsdale, Southport PR8 3HW Tel: 01704 574137 Fax: 01704 573875; 66 Burnley Road, Ainsdale, Southport PR8 3LR Tel: 01704 75466 — MB ChB Liverp. 1985. Prev: Trainee GP Southport VTS.

NUGENT, David 8 Cambridge Avenue, Middlesbrough TS5 5HQ — MB ChB Ed. 1990.

NUGENT, Desmond Andrew William (retired) Craigievar, 27 Golf Side, Cheam, Sutton SM2 7HA Tel: 020 8643 2052 — MB BS Madras 1944; DPH Liverp. 1949; DTM & H Liverp. 1952. Prev: WHO Country Represen..

NUGENT, Elizabeth Mary Dr Nugent and Partners, 243 Abbey Road, Barrow-in-Furness LA14 5JY Tel: 01229 821599; 25 Croslands Park, Barrow-in-Furness LA13 9NH — MB ChB Manch. 1975; DRCOG 1978. GP Barrow-in-Furness; Work for DHSS Bootle Merseyside. Socs: Disabil. Appeal Tribunals. Prev: SHO (Paediat.) Booth Hall Childr. Hosp. Manch.; SHO (O & G) N. Manch. Gen. Hosp.; SHO (Dermat.) Manch. Skin Hosp.

NUGENT, Mr Ian Michael The Royal Berkshire Hospital, London Road, Reading RG1 5AN Tel: 0118 987 5111 Email: ian.nugent@rbbh-tr.nhs.uk — MB BS Lond. 1983 (St. Thomass Hosp.) BSc (Hons.) Lond. 1980; FRCS Eng. 1987; FRCS (Orth.) 1994. Cons. Orthop. Surg. Roy. Berks. Hosp. Reading. Specialty: Orthop. Socs: Brit. Orthopaedic Foot Surg. Soc.; Brit. Orthopaedic Assn. Prev: Sen. Regist. Bath & Swindon; Regist. Oxf. & Swindon.

NUGENT, John Joseph Dr Nugent and Partners, 243 Abbey Road, Barrow-in-Furness LA14 5JY Tel: 01229 821599; 243 Abbey Road, Barrow-in-Furness LA14 5JY Tel: 01229 21599 — MB ChB Manch. 1975; DRCOG 1979; MRCGP 1980. Prev: SHO (Med./Neurol.) N. Manch. Gen. Hosp.; SHO (Paediat.) Booth Hall Childr. Hosp. Manch.; SHO (O & G) N. Manch. Gen. Hosp.

NUGENT, John Patrick Devonshire Road Surgery, 467 Devonshire Road, Blackpool FY2 0JP — MB ChB Manch. 1982; DRCOG 1985; MRCGP 1986.

NUGENT, Karen Patricia Professional Surgical Unit, Southampton General Hospital, Tremona Road, Southampton SO16 6YD Tel: 023 8079 6145 Fax: 023 8079 4020; 40 Porchester Road, Fareham PO16 8PT Tel: 01329 233849 — MB BS Lond. 1987; MA Camb. 1988; FRCS Eng. 1991; MS Lond. 1994. Lect. & Hon. Sen. Regist. (Gen. Surg.) Univ. Soton.; Sen. Lect. & Hon. Cons. Uni. Soton. Specialty: Gen. Surg. Prev: Research Regist. St. Mark's Hosp. Lond.

NUGENT, Theodore Patrick Joseph Errigal Medical Centre, Old Dungannon Road, Ballygawley, Dungannon BT70 2EY; 21 Killymorgan Road, Tirnaskea, Ballygawley, Dungannon BT70 2JJ — MB BCh BAO Belf. 1983; MB BCh Belf. 1983; DCH RCP Lond. 1985; DRCOG 1986; MRCGP 1988.

NUKI, George Western General Hospital, Edinburgh EH4 2XU Tel: 0131 537 1000 — MB BS Lond. 1960 (King's Coll. Lond. & King's Coll. Hosp.) MRCS Eng. LRCP Lond. 1960; FRCP Lond. 1978, M 1964; FRCP Ed. 1980. Prof. (Rheum.) Univ. Edin. & Hon. Cons. Phys. Rheum. Dis. Unit.; N.. Gen. Hosp. & Roy. Infirm. Edin. Specialty: Gen. Med. Socs: Brit. Soc. Rheumat. & Med. Research Soc. Prev: Reader Welsh Nat. Sch. Med. Cardiff & Hon. Cons. Phys. Univ. Hosp.; Wales Cardiff.

NULLIAH, Krishnamurthi The Brock Street Clinic, 29 Brock St., Bath BA1 2LN; 8 Upper Church Street, Bath BA1 2PT — MB BS Lond. 1977.

NUNAN, Thomas Oliver St Thomas' Hospital, Department of Nuclear Medicine, London SE1 7EH Tel: 020 7928 9292 Fax: 020 7928 5634 — MD NUI 1984; MB BCh BAO 1973; MRCP (UK) 1975; MSc Lond. 1979; BSc NUI 1970, MD 1984; FRCP Lond. 1991; FRCR 2000. Cons. Phys. St. Thos. Hosp. Lond.; Edr. Nuclear Med. Communications. Specialty: Nuclear Med.; Gen. Med. Socs: Brit. Nuclear Med. Soc.; Pres. Brit. Nuclear Med. Soc. Prev: Sen. Regist. (Renal Med.) St. Thos. Hosp. Lond.; Research Fell. St. Thos. Hosp. Lond.; SHO (Med.) Hillingdon Hosp. Uxbridge.

NUNES, Michelle Doreen Anne 4 Catherine's Drive, Richmond TW9 2BX Tel: 020 8332 9868 — (St. Mary's) BSc (Clin. Scis.) Lond. 1990, MS BS 1991.

NUNEZ, Mr Desmond Antonio Southmead Hospital, Department of Otolaryngology, Bristol BS10 5NB Tel: 0117 959 6222 Fax: 0117 959 5850 Email: d.a.nunez@bristol.ac.uk — MB BS West Indies 1982; FRCS Ed. 1986; DLO RCS Eng. 1986; FRCS (Orl.) 1994; MD 1998. Cons. Otolaryngol. N. Bristol NHS Trust; Sen. Lect. (Otolaryngol.) Univ. Bristol. Specialty: Otorhinolaryngol. Socs: Coun. Otolaryngol. Research Soc.; Brit. Assn. Paediat. Otol. Prev: Cons. & Sen. Lect. (Otolaryngol.) Aberd. Roy. Infirm. & Roy. Aberd. Childr. Hosp.; Sen. Regist. Univ. Hosp. Nottm.; Sen. Regist. Leicester Roy. Infirm.

NUNEZ MIRET, Olga 11 Gadwall Close, Worsley, Manchester M28 7AF; The Spinhey, Everest Road, Atherton, Manchester M96 9NT — LMS Barcelona 1992. Assoc. Spec. (Psychiat.) Manch. Specialty: Gen. Psychiat.; Forens. Psychiat. Socs: Colegio De Medicos, Barcelona; BMA. Prev: Regist. (Psychiat.) Halifax Gen. Hosp.; SHO (Acute Adult Psychiat.) Qu. Charlotte's Hastings & Eastbourne Dist. Gen. Hosp.

NUNN, Andrew Nigel 33 Heol Briwnant, Rhiwbina, Cardiff CF14 6QF — MB BCh Wales 1997.

NUNN, Bryan Roger Filey Surgery, Station Avenue, Filey YO14 9AE Tel: 01723 515881 Fax: 01723 515197 Email: roger.nunn@gp-b82037.nhs.uk; 9-11 Church Hill, Hunmanby, Filey YO14 0JU Email: roger_nunn@yahoo.co.uk — MB ChB Sheff. 1977; DRCOG 1981; Cert. Family Plann. JCC 1982; MRCGP 1982; DCH RCP Lond. 1982. GP Filey, N. Yorks.; Lifeboat Med. Off. Filey RNLI; GP Trainer. Socs: MRC GP Research Framework. Prev: GP Regist. ChristCh., New Zealand; Med. Off. Scotts Base Antartica; Emerg. Room Resid. Amer. Hosp. of Paris.

NUNN, Christopher Miles Hasler (retired) Barfad Beag, Ardfern, Lochgilphead PA31 8QN Tel: 01852 500321 Email: chrisnunn@compuserve.com — MB BS Lond. 1963 (St. Thos.) DPM Eng. 1966; FRCPsych 1985, M 1972; MD Lond. 1974. Prev: Cons. Psychiat. Roy. S. Hants. Hosp. Soton.

NUNN, David Spring Hall Group Practice, Spring Hall Medical Centre, Spring Hall Lane, Halifax HX1 4JG Tel: 01422 349501 Fax: 01422 323091 — MB ChB St. And. 1968; DA Eng. 1970.

NUNN, Mr David Department of Orthopaedics, Guy's Hospital, St Thomas St., London SE1 9RT Tel: 020 7955 5000 Fax: 020 7955 2759 — MB BS Lond. 1978 (St. Mary's) MRCS Eng. LRCP Lond. 1978; FRCS Ed. 1983; FRCS Ed. Orthop. 1990; FRCS Eng. 1997. Cons. Orthop. Surg. Guy's & St. Thos. Hosps. Lond. Specialty: Orthop. Prev: Lect. (Orthop.) Lond. Hosp. Med. Coll.; Regist. (Orthop.) St. Geo. Hosp. Lond.; Sen. Regist. (Orthop.) Guy's & St. Thos. Hosp. Lond.

NUNN, Geoffrey Francis Old Vicarage, The Ginnel, Bardsey, Leeds LS17 9DU — MB BS Lond. 1975; FRCA 1980. Cons. Anaesth. The Gen. Infirm. Leeds. Specialty: Anaesth. Prev: Cons. Anaesth. Wakefield Hosps.

NUNN, John Francis (retired) 3A Dene Road, Northwood, Northwood HA6 2AE Tel: 01923 826363 — MB ChB Birm. 1948; FRCA 1955; PhD Birm. 1958; MD 1970; FRCS (Eng.) 1983; FANZCA (Hon.) 1984; FGS; FCA RCSI (Hon.) 1985; DSc DSc 1992 1992; Laurea (Honoris Causa) Turin 1993; MD (Hon.) Uppsala 1996. Emerit. Cons. Northwick Pk. Hosp. Harrow. Prev: Head of Div. Anaesth. Clin. Research Centre (MRC) 1968-91.

NUNN, Nicola Kay Hawthorne House, Kilburn Road, Oakham LE15 6QL — MB ChB Liverp. 1993.

NUNN, Mr Paul Andrew 49 Highfield Hill, Upper Norwood, London SE19 3PT — MB BS Lond. 1983; BSc (Hons.) Lond. 1980, MB BS 1983; FRCS Ed. 1988.

NUNN, Richard Andrew The Surgery, Angel Lane, Dunmow CM6 1AQ Tel: 01371 872105 Fax: 01371 873679; Haydens, Onslow Green, Barnston, Dunmow CM6 3PP Tel: 01371 820429 — MB BS Lond. 1969 (Roy. Free) MRCS Eng. LRCP Lond. 1969; MRCGP 1978. Specialty: Gen. Med. Socs: Assoc. Mem. Roy. Coll. Homeop.

NUNN, Terence John 20 Cleghorn Road, Lanark ML11 7QR Tel: 01555 663139 — MB ChB Glas. 1971; DObst RCOG 1973; FFA RCS Eng. 1975. Assoc. Med. Dir. Wishaw Gen. Hosp. Specialty: Anaesth. Prev: Cons. (Anaesth.) Law Hosp. Carluke.; Sen. Regist. (Anaesth.) Regionsykehuset I Trondheim, Norway; Sen. Regist. (Anaesth.) Bristol Roy. Infirm.

NUNN, Thomas 90 Norsey Road, Billericay CM11 1BG — MB ChB Glas. 1998.

NUNN, Timothy Richard Haydens, Hounslow Green, Barnston, Dunmow CM6 3PP — MB BS Lond. 1996.

NUNNELEY, Joyce Beryl 1 Palace Gardens, Buckhurst Hill IG9 5PQ — MB BS Lond. 1952 (Roy. Free) MRCS Eng. LRCP Lond. 1952. Vis. Venereol. H.M. Prison Holloway. Specialty: Genitourinary Medicine. Socs: Fell. Roy. Soc. Med.; Med. Soc. Study VD. Prev: Cons. Venereol. S. Lond. Hosp.; Clin Asst. (Venereol.) Roy. North. Hosp. Lond.; Asst. Med. Off. Lond. Boros. Haringey & Barnet.

NUNNERLEY, Heather Bell (retired) 6 The Tudors, 10 Court Downs Road, Beckenham BR3 6LR Tel: 020 8658 8134 — (Liverpool) MB ChB Liverp. 1956; DCH Eng. 1958; DObst RCOG 1959; DMRD Eng. 1967; FRCR 1975; FRCP 1997. Chairm.

Ravensbourne NHS Trust. Prev: Cons. Radiol. King's Coll. Hosp. Lond.

NUNNS, David Nottingham City Hospital, Nottingham NG3 5EA Tel: 0115 845 7361 Email: d.nunns@virgin.net — MB ChB Manc. 1991 (Univ. Manch.) MD Manc 1995; MRCOG 1997. Cons. Gynaecologist Nottm. City Hosp. Specialty: Obst. & Gyn.; Gynaecology; Oncol. Socs: MRCOS. Prev: Subspenality Trainee Gyn. Lenetes Roy. Inirmary; Clin. Lect. (Pathol. Scis.) Manch. Med. Sch. Univ. Manch.; Regist. (O & G) St. Mary's Hosp. Manch.

NUNNS, Mary Eleanor Beatrice The Mission Practice, 208 Cambridge Heath Road, London E2 9LS Tel: 020 8983 7300 Fax: 020 8983 6800; 22 Hadley Court, Cazenove Road, Stoke Newington, London N16 6JU — MB BS Lond. 1978. Specialty: Gen. Pract. Prev: Trainee GP Hackney Hosp. VTS Lond.

NUNOO-MENSAH, Mr Joseph William 334 Manchester Road, Worsley, Manchester M28 3WE Tel: 0161 790 4069 Email: jwnm@thedoghousemail.com — BM BS Nottm. 1993 (Nottm. Med. Sch.) BMedSci Nottm. 1991; FRCS Eng. 1997. Specialist Regist. (Gen. Surg.) Manch.; USLME 1995. Specialty: Gen. Surg. Socs: Med. Protec. Soc. Prev: SHO (Gen. Surg.) Frimley Pk. Hosp. Frimley Surrey; SHO Rotat. (Surg.) John Radcliffe Hosp. Oxf.; Anat. Prosector Camb. Univ.

NUR, Mousa Ahmed Mohamed 13 Blantfell Drive, Burnley BD12 8AW Tel: 01282 715035 Email: musanur@hotmail.com — MB BS Khartoum 1976; MRCPI 1984. Locum Cons. Phys. Specialty: Rheumatol.

NUR, Mr Oomar Ali Withybush Hospital, Fishguard Road, Haverfordwest SA61 2PZ Tel: 01437 764545; Eastleigh, Treffgarne, Haverfordwest SA62 5PH Tel: 01437741429 — MB BS Karachi 1982 (Dow Med. Coll. Karachi) FRCS Glas. 1991; FRCSI 1991; Dip Urol UCL 1993. Assoc. Specialist Surg., Withaybush Hosp., Haverford W. Specialty: Gen. Surg. Prev: Regist.- Withaybush Hosp.; Regist., Urol., P. Phillip Hosp., Unaeup; SHO (Surg.) Princess of Wales Hosp. Bridgend.

NURBHAI, Suhail Pfizer Central Research, Sandwich CT13 9NJ — MB ChB Dundee 1988; MRCP (UK) 1992. Clin. Project Manager Pfizer Centr. Research Kent. Specialty: Pharmaceutical Medicine. Prev: Regist. (Med.) BRd. Green Hosp. Liverp.

NURENNABI, Abul Khair Mohamed 72 Half Edge Lane, Eccles, Manchester M30 9BA — MRCS Eng. LRCP Lond. 1968; MRCP (U.K.) 1971.

NURICK, Simon 40 Wilbury Road, Hove BN3 3JP Tel: 01273 206206 Fax: 01273 721411; 47 Park Crescent, Brighton BN2 3HB Tel: 01273 605795 — (Oxf. & Guy's) BM BCh Oxf. 1958; FRCP Lond. 1978, M 1964; MA Oxf. 1959, DM 1971. Hons. Cons. Neurol. Brighton Health Care NHS Trust & Hurstwood Pk. Neurol. Centre. Specialty: Neurol. Prev: Cons. Neurol. SE Thames RHA & Hurstwood Pk. Hosp. Haywards Heath; Sen. Regist. Nat. Hosp. Nerv. Dis. Maida Vale; Resid. Med. Off. Nat. Hosp. Qu. Sq. Lond.

NURMIKKO, Turo Juhani The Walton Centre for Neurology & Neurosurgery, Rice Lane, Liverpool L9 1AE — Lic Med Turku 1974.

NURMOHAMED, Akil GP Direct, 5/7 Welback Road, West Harrow, Harrow HA2 0RH Tel: 020 8515 9300 Fax: 020 8515 9300 — MB BS Lond. 1994; BSc; DRCOG.

NURSE, Diane Elizabeth Bromley Hospital, Cromwell Avenue, Bromley BR2 9AJ Tel: 020 8289 7010 — MB ChB Bristol 1979 (Univ. Bristol. Med. Sch.) FRCS Eng. 1985; FRCS (Urol.) 1990; ChM Bristol 1995. Cons. Urol. Bromley Hosps. NHS Trust. Specialty: Urol. Socs: Brit. Assn. Urol. Surgs.; Roy. Soc. Med. Prev: Sen. Regist. Rotat. (Urol.) Guy's Hosp. & Brighton HA; Regist. (Urol.) Adelaide Childr. Hosp., S. Austral.

NURSE, Joanna Mary 108 Alma Road, Southampton SO14 6UW — BM Soton. 1991. Specialty: Pub. Health Med.

NURUZZAMAN, Muhammad 61 Norman Road, Walsall WS5 3QS Tel: 01922 31782; 61 Norman Road, Walsall WS5 3QS Tel: 01922 31782 — MB BS Dacca 1959 (Dacca Med. Coll.) DTM & H Liverp. 1966; FRCP Ed. 1985, M 1967; FRCP Glas. 1984, M 1967; FCPS Bangladesh 1974. Cons. Phys. (Geriat. Med.) Walsall AHA. Specialty: Gen. Med. Prev: Research Fell. (Gastroenterol.) Nuffield Dept. Clin. Med. Radcliffe; Infirm. Oxf.; Sen. Regist. (Geriat. Med.) Soton. & Poole Gen. Hosps.

NUSAIR, Aber-Rahman Qassem — Medic Romania 1981; MD Romania 1981; DPM 1989; Board Psych. 1992; MPsych. Liverpool 1995. Cons. Psychiat. Burnley Gen. Hosp. Specialty: Geriat. Psychiat. Socs: Brit. Assn. Psychopharmacol.; CINP. Prev: SCMO (Psychiat.) Barnsley; Assoc. Specialist (Child Psychiat.) Nuneaton.

NUSEIBEH, Mr Isaac Mohamed National Spinal Injuries Centre, Stoke Mandeville Hospital, Mandeville Road, Aylesbury HP21 8AL Tel: 01296 315000 Fax: 01296 315868 — MB ChB Lond. 1960; LMSSA Lond. 1968; FRCS Ed. 1972. Cons. Surg. Spinal Injuries & Hon. Lect. BPMF Univ. Lond. Specialty: Orthop. Socs: Hon. Sec. Internat. Med. Soc. Paraplegia.

NUSSBAUM, Toni 31 Barlow Moor Court, West Didsbury, Manchester M20 2UU Tel: 0161 448 1327 — MB ChB Manch. 1992 (Manchester) MRCGP 1998.

NUSSEY, Andrew Paul Department of Anaesthetics, Addenbrooke's Hospital, Hills Road, Cambridge CB2 2QQ — MB BS Queensland 1986.

NUSSEY, Fiona Elizabeth Department of Clinical Oncology, Western General Hospital, Crewe Road, Edinburgh EH4 2XU Tel: 0131 537 1000; 7 Murrayfield Drive, Edinburgh EH12 6EB — MB ChB Aberd. 1995; MRCP UK (Edin) 1998. Clin. Lect. Med. Oncol., Edin. Cancer Centre, W.ern. Gen. Hosp. Edin. Specialty: Oncol. Prev: SHO (Med.Oncol.); SHO (Clin. Oncol.); SHO (Gen. Med.).

NUSSEY, Professor Stephen Spencer St. George's Hospital Medical School, London SW17 0RE Tel: 020 8725 5803 Fax: 020 8725 0240 Email: s.nussey@sghms.ac.uk; 51 Galveston Road, London SW15 2RZ — BM BCh Oxf. 1977; MA, DPhil Oxf. 1974; MRCP (UK) 1979; FRCP Lond. 1992. Professor (Endocrinol.) St. Geo.'s Hosp. Med. Sch. Lond.; Cons. Endocrinologist St. Geo. Hosp. Lond. Specialty: Endocrinol. Prev: Reader (Endocrinol.) St. Geo.'s Hosp. Med. Sch. Lond.; Sen. Lect. & Lect. St. Geo.'s Hosp. Med. Sch. Lond.; Sen. Regist. St. Jas. Hosp. Lond.

NUTBEAM, Helen Mary The Surgery, Pound Close, Oldbury, Warley B68 8LZ Tel: 0121 552 1632 Fax: 0121 552 0848; 287 Lordswood Road, Harborne, Birmingham B17 8PR Tel: 0121 429 9096 — MB ChB Ed. 1974; DCH RCPS Glas. 1976; MRCP (UK) 1976; MRCGP 1980. Specialty: Gen. Med. Prev: Lect. (Paediat.) Char. Cross Hosp. Lond.; Regist. (Paediat.) St. Stephen's Hosp. Lond.

NUTBOURNE, Patricia Anne (retired) Oulton House, Church St., Great Wilbraham, Cambridge CB1 5JQ — MB BS Lond. 1960 (St. Mary's) DA Eng. 1976; FFA RCS Eng. 1981.

NUTHALL, Timothy Richard Alexander 117 Shepards Bush Road, London W6 7LP — MB BS Lond. 1992.

NUTLEY, Peter Graham Bishops Park Health Centre, Lancaster Way, Bishop's Stortford CM23 4DA Tel: 01279 755057 — MB BS Lond. 1978 (Middlx.) MRCS Eng. LRCP Lond. 1978; DCH RCP Lond. 1982; DRCOG 1982; BA Open 1984; MFPHM 1990. GP Bishop's Stortford. Specialty: Gen. Med. Socs: Brit. Acupunc. Soc. Prev: Med. Dir. Til (Med.) Ltd.; Head of Quality Audit Med. & Clin. Managem. Ltd.

NUTT, Adrian Ernest Craig Thornhedge, 2 Kilcorig Road, Magheragall, Lisburn BT28 2QY Tel: 01846 621807 — MB BCh BAO Dub. 1977; DCH RCPSI 1979; DO RCPSI 1986.

NUTT, Christopher John 7 Fieldfare Road, Hartlepool TS26 0SA — MB ChB Dundee 1997.

NUTT, Professor David John Psychopharmacology Unit, University of Bristol, Dorothy Hodgkin Building, Whitson Street, Bristol BS1 3NY Tel: 0117 3313143 Fax: 0117 3313180 Email: david.j.nutt@bristol.ac.uk — MB BChir Camb. 1975 (Guy's) BA 1972; MRCP UK 1977; MA Camb. 1982; DM Oxf 1983; MB 1983; FRCPsych 1993; FRCP UK 2002; FMedSci UK 2002. Head of Dept. of Community Based Med., Bristol; Hon. Cons. Psychiat. United Bristol Health Trust; Prof. Psychopharmacol. Univ. Bristol; Edr. Jl. Psychopharmacol. Specialty: Gen. Psychiat. Special Interest: Psychopharmacology. Socs: (Pres.) Brit. Assn. Psychopharmacol.; Fell. CINP; Fell. ECNP. Prev: Head Div. Psychiat. Univ. Bristol; Dir. (Clin. Research) NIAAA, USA; Wellcome Sen. Fell. (Clin. Sc.) Warneford Hosp. Oxf.

NUTT, Desmond John Pattison Liffock Surgery, 69 Sea Road, Castlerock, Coleraine BT51 4TW Tel: 028 7084 8206 Fax: 028 7084 9146; 71 Killane Road, Limavady BT49 0DL — MB BCh BAO Belf. 1976; DRCOG 1979.

NUTT, Michael Neil The Dovercourt Surgery, 309 City Road, Sheffield S2 5HJ Tel: 0114 270 0997 Fax: 0114 276 6786 — MB ChB Sheff. 1984. Trainee GP Sheff. Prev: SHO (Paediat.) Sheff.; SHO (Psychiat.) Exeter.

NUTT, Michael Richard 61 Greenhill Road, Griffithstown, Pontypool NP4 5BG — BM BS Nottm. 1990.

NUTT, Nicholas Richard 47 Charlton Road, Keynsham, Bristol BS31 2JG Tel: 0117 986 4439 Email: nnutt@fsmail.net; 47 Charlton Road, Keynsham, Bristol BS31 2JG Tel: 0117 986 4439 Email: nnutt@fsmail.net — MB BS Lond. 1972 (King's Coll. Hosp.) MRCS Eng. LRCP Lond. 1972; DObst RCOG 1974; MRCGP 1977. Locums; Cons. Nat. Slimming Centres 2/3 Denmark St. Bristol BS1 5DG. Special Interest: Care of the elderly; Chronic Dis. Managem.; Computers. Socs: Counc. Mem. of Bath Inst. Med. Engin. Prev: Med. Off. (Geriat.) Keynsham Hosp.; Princip. Gen. Pract. Keynsham; SHO Princess Margt. Hosp. Swindon.

NUTTALL, Andrew Makepeace High Street Surgery, 2 High Street, Macclesfield SK11 8BX Tel: 01625 423692 — MB ChB Manch. 1980.

NUTTALL, Ian Douglas Lynwood, 63 Bramhall Park Road, Bramhall, Stockport SK3 3NA Tel: 0161 486 9600 — MD Manch. 1985; MB ChB 1972; FRCOG 1990, M 1977. Cons. O & G Stockport HA. Specialty: Obst. & Gyn. Prev: Sen. Regist. (O & G) N. Western RHA; Clin. Research Fell. (O & G) Withington Hosp. Manch.; Regist. (O & G) Univ. Cape Town, S. Africa.

NUTTALL, Jayne Sonia The Surgery, Ruckinge Road, HamSt., Ashford TN26 2NJ Tel: 0123 373 2262 — MB BS Lond. 1987; DRCOG 1991. Prev: Trainee GP Nottm. VTS.

NUTTALL, Joan Harston (retired) 4 Smithie Close, New Earswick, York YO32 4DG — MB BS Lond. 1954.

NUTTALL, John Barry Clarence Avenue Surgery, 14 Clarence Avenue, Northampton NN2 6NZ Tel: 01604 718464 Fax: 01604 721589; Church Cottage, 15 Church Street, Boughton, Northampton NN2 8SF — MRCS Eng. LRCP Lond. 1958 (Camb. & Leeds) MA Camb. 1959; DObst RCOG 1960; MRCGP 1968. Prev: Ho. Surg. St. Jas. Hosp. Leeds.

NUTTALL, Martin Chandler — MB BS Lond. 1998 (St Mary's) MA Cantab. Ho.. Off. Dept. Med. St Mary;s Med. Sch.

NUTTALL, Peter Julian Devaney Medical Centre, 40 Balls Road, Oxton, Birkenhead CH43 5RE Tel: 0151 652 4281 Fax: 0151 670 0445 — MB ChB Liverp. 1987; DRCOG 1990. Specialty: Gen. Pract. Socs: Birkenhead Med. Soc. Prev: Trainee GP Wirral VTS; Regist. (Psychiat.) Melbourne Australia.

NUTTEN, Horace Edward (retired) Pantiles, Felsham Road, Cockfield, Bury St Edmunds IP30 0HW Tel: 01284 828414 — (Aberd.) MB ChB Aberd. 1951; DPH Aberd. 1955; MFCM RCP Lond. 1974; AFOM RCP Lond. 1978. Prev: Regional Med. Off. Gen. Counc. Brit. Shipping Lond.

NUTTING, Christopher Martin Department of Radiotherapy, St Bartholomew's Hospital, West Smithfield, London EC1A 7BE Tel: 020 7377 7000 Fax: 020 7601 8364 — MB BS Lond. 1992 (Middlesex) BSc (Cell Path.) Lond. 1989; MRCP (UK) 1995; FRCR 1998. Sen. Regist. (Clin. Oncol.) St. Bart. Hosp., Lond.,. Specialty: Oncol.; Radiother. Prev: Regist. (Clin. Oncol.) Roy. Marsden Hosp. Lond.; SHO (Med.) Univ. Hosp. Nottm.; Ho. Phys. Middlx. Hosp. Lond.

NUTTING, Linda Mary 27 Park Terrace, Dunston, Gateshead NE11 9PA Tel: 0191 460 1284; The Health Centre, Prince Consort Road, Gateshead NE8 1NR Tel: 0191 477 2243 Fax: 0191 478 6728 — MB BS Newc. 1988; DRCOG 1991. GP Princip. Health Centre N. Tyneside. Specialty: Gen. Med. Prev: SHO (Community Paediat.) N. Tyneside.; SHO (Med.) N. Tyneside HA; Trainee GP N.d. VTS.

NUTTON, Miranda 49 Andes Close, Alexandra Quay, Ocean Village, Southampton SO14 3HS — BM BS Nottm. 1975.

NUTTON, Mr Richard William Royal Infirmary of Edinburgh, Littl France, Old Dalkeith Road, Edinburgh EH16 4SO Tel: 0131 242 3493 Fax: 0131 242 3466 Email: richard.nutton@luht.scot.nhs.uk; 5 Corrennie Gardens, Morningside, Edinburgh EH10 6DG Tel: 0131 447 3475 — MD Newc. 1984 (Newcastle upon Tyne) FRCS Eng. 1979; FRCS Ed. 1994. Hon. Sen. Lect. Orthop. and Trauma Univ. of Edin.; Cons. Orthop. Surg. Roy. Infirm. Edin. NHS Trust. Specialty: Orthop. Socs: Brit. Elbow & Shoulder Soc.; Brit. Assn. Surg. Knee; Brit. Orthop. Research Soc.

NUVOLONI, Maureen Colette Christine Ross Road Medical Centre, 85 Ross Road, Maidenhead SL6 2SR — MB ChB Manch. 1965; DObst RCOG 1967. GP.

NWABINELI, Mr Nwachukwu James South Tyneside District Hospital, Harton Lane, South Shields NE34 0PL Tel: 0191 454 8888 Fax: 0191 202 4067; Bethel, 4 Elsdon Road, Whickham, Newcastle upon Tyne NE16 5HZ Tel: 0191 488 7178 — MB BS Ibadan 1974 (Ibadan, Nigeria) MRCOG 1980; FWACS Accra 1986; FRCOG 1995. Cons. in O & G S. Tyneside Dist. Hosp.; Clin. Lead in Obst. and Gyn. Specialty: Obst. & Gyn. Socs: BMA; Internat. Continence Soc.; Eur. Menopause Soc. Prev: Train. Fell. (Gyn. & Oncol.) Stobhill Hosp. Glas.; Cons. Gyn. Univ. Benin Teach. Hosp. Nigeria; Research Fell. Freeman Hosp. Newc. u. Tyne.

NWABOKU, Mr Harold Chukwuemeka Ifeanyi 10 Tregothnan Road, London SW9 9JX — MB BS Lond. 1988 (Middlesex) FRCS Ed. 1992; FRCS Eng. 1992; FRCS (Orth.) 1997. Orthop. Specialty: Orthop. Socs: BOTA; BMA.

NWABUEZE, Emmanuel Dibua 1A Ffordd Ffrith, Prestatyn LL19 7UD — BM BCh Nigeria 1976. GP. Specialty: Gen. Pract.

NWACHUKU, Oludotun Mofolusho 143 Rectory Path Avenue, Northolt UB5 6SB — MB ChB Aberd. 1966.

NWACHUKWU, Mr Ikechukwu Augustine Warwick Hospital, Lakin Road, Warwick CV34 5BW Tel: 01926 495321 Ext: 4067 Fax: 02476 511168 Email: ike3@btinternet.com — MB BS Nigeria 1985; MB BS U. of Nigeria 1985; FRCS Eng 1991; FRCS (Tr & Orth) Eng. 1998. Cons. Shoulder and Upper Limb Surg., Warwick. Specialty: Orthop. Special Interest: Shoulder and Upper Limb Surg. Socs: BOA; BESS.

NWAKAKWA, Victor Chinedu 26A Rowley Way, St Johns Wood, London NW8 0SQ — MB BS Ibadan, Nigeria 1993; MRCP (UK) 1993.

NWAMARAH, Mr David Ezeakolam 91 Central Avenue, Welling DA16 3BG Tel: 020 8855 7238 — MB BS Lagos 1978; FRCS Ed. 1988; FRCS Glas. 1989.

NWEKE, Anny Joseph 28 Patch Close, Horninglow, Burton-on-Trent DE13 0GE — MB BS Lagos 1974.

NWOKOLO, Chukwuemeka Felix 25 Ashfield Crescent, Springhead, Oldham OL4 4NX Tel: 0161 652 8755 — MB BS Nigeria 1980; MB BS Nigeria Univ. 1980; MRCOG 1992.

NWOKOLO, Chukwuka Uchemefuna University Hospitals Coventry & Warwickshire, Clifford Bridge Road, Coventry CV2 2DX Tel: 024 76 538759; 57 St Bernards, Solihull B91 3PH Tel: 0121 706 9567 Fax: 0121 711 4967 — BM BCh Nigeria 1978; MD Birm. 1993; FRCP 1998; FRCP Ed 1998. Hon Sen Lec Dep of Biological Sci.s Univ. of Warwick; Vis. Clin. Sen. Lect. Sch. Postgrad. Med. Educat. Univ. Warwick. Specialty: Gastroenterol. Socs: Brit. Soc. Gastroenterol. & Midl. Gastrointestinal Soc.; Amer. Gastoenterol. Assn. Prev: Sen. Regist. (Med. & Gastroenterol.) Dudley Rd. Hosp. Birm.; Sen. Regist. (Med. & Gastroenterol.) Walsgrave Hosp. Coventry.; Clin. Research Fell. (Gastroenterol.) Roy. Free Hosp. Lond.

NWOKORA, Mr Gregory Ezennia Eye Department, The Royal Hospital, Haslar, Gosport PO12 2AA Tel: 023 9258 4255 Ext: 2411; 5 Orwell Close, Priddyi Hard, Gosport PO12 4GR Tel: 02392 525090 — MB BS Lagos 1977 (College of Medicine University of Lagos, Nigeria) DO RCPSI 1984; FRCSI 1986; FCOphth 1988; FRCOphth 1993. Assoc. Specialist (Ophth.) (Min. of Defence) Roy. Hosp. Haslar Gosport. Specialty: Ophth. Socs: BMA. Prev: Cons. (Ophth. Surg.) N W Armed Forces Hosp. Tabuk, KSA, and Altnagelvia Hosp. Londonderry.

NWOSU, Mr Ezechi Callistus Whiston Hospital, Warrington Road, Prescot L35 5DN Tel: 0151 427 1600 Fax: 0151 430 1335 Email: cally.nwosu@sthkhealth.nhs.uk — BM BCh Nigeria 1978 (Univ. Nigeria Med. Sch. Enugu Campus) FRCOG; MRCOG 1989; MObstG Liverp. 1992. Cons. O & G Whiston Hosp. Prescot; Hon. Lect. (Obst. & Gyn.) Univ. Liverp. Specialty: Obst. & Gyn. Special Interest: High Risk Obstetrics. Socs: BMA; Med. Assn. Nigerian Specialists & GPs; Med. Defense Union. Prev: Sen. Regist. (O & G) Liverp. Matern. Hosp.; Regist. Masters in Feto-Matern. Med. Mill Rd. Liverp. Matern. Hosp.; Regist. N. Tyneside Gen. Hosp. N. Shields & Princess Mary Matern. Hosp. Newc.

NWOZO, Mr James Chinyelu 180 Glastone Park Gardens, London NW2 6RL — MB BS Lond. 1962; MRCS Eng. LRCP Lond. 1962; FRCS Eng. 1966.

NWULU, Bernard Nchewa Rampton Hospital, Retford DN22 0PD Tel: 01777 247706 Email: nchewanwulu@aol.com; 146 Grange Road, Broom, Rotherham S60 3LL Tel: 0797 407 1721 Fax: 01709

519514 — MD National U, Zaire 1972 (University of Zaire) MRCPsych 1982; MPhil Ed. 1984; FRCPsych 1996; MA (Theology) 2003. Cons. Psychiat. Rampton Hosp. Retford; Hon. Lect. Univ. Sheff.; Med Mem. Ment. Health Review Tribunal Eng. Specialty: Ment. Health; Gen. Psychiat.; Forens. Psychiat. Socs: BMA & Soc. Clin. Psychiat.; Roy. Coll Psychiat. Prev: Sen. Regist. Balderton & E. Dale Unit Newark; Regist. (Psychiat.) Stratheden Hosp. Fife; Clin. Asst. Roy. Edin. Hosp.

NYAMUGUNDURU, Godfrey Bishop Auckland Hospital, Cockton Hill Road, Bishop Auckland DL14 6AD Tel: 01388 455000 — MB BS Lond. 1986 (St Geo.) MRCP UK 1991; FRCPCH 1999; MSc (Paediat.) Birm. 2001. Cons. Paediat. Specialty: Paediat. Special Interest: Respirat. Paediat. Socs: Roy. Coll. of Paediat.; Brit. Paediatric Respirat. Soc. Prev: Clin. Research Fell. Birm. Childr. Hosp.; Regist. (Paediat.) Birm. Heartlands Hosp.; Regist. (Med.) Jas. Paget Hosp. Gt. Yarmouth.

NYE, Alan David Hopwood House, The Vineyard, Lees Road, Oldham OL4 1JN Tel: 0161 628 3628 Fax: 0161 628 4970 — MB ChB Sheff. 1983; BMedSci (Hons.) Sheff. 1982. Trainee GP Oldham HA VTS.

NYE, Brenda Margaret Bradford Road Medical Centre, 60 Bradford Road, Trowbridge BA14 9AR Tel: 01225 754255 Fax: 01225 777342 — MB ChB Birm. 1980 (Birmingham Medical School) DCH 1984; DRCOG 1985; MRCGP 1985; DFFP 1996. Partnership in Gen. Pract. Bradford Rd. Med. Centre Trowbridge. Specialty: Gen. Pract. Prev: Retainer GP Bath; GP Fernville Surg. Hemel Hempstead.

NYE, Frederick John Tropical and Infectious Diseases Unit, Royal Liverpool University Hospital, Prescot Street, Liverpool L7 8XP; 23 Bonnington Ave, Great Crosby, Liverpool L23 7YJ — MRCS Eng. LRCP Lond. 1966 (St. Geo.) MD Lond. 1976, MB BS 1966; FRCP Lond. 1981, M 1969. Cons. Phys. & Clin. Lead, Chronic Fatigue Syndrome Serv., Roy. Liverp. Univ. Hosp. Specialty: Gen. Med.; Infec. Dis. Socs: Brit. Soc. Antimicrobial Chemother. & Brit. Infec. Soc. Prev: Cons. Phys. Infec. Dis. Unit, Univ. Hosp.. Liverp.; Clin. Lect. Dept. Trop. Med. & Infec. Dis. Univ. Liverp.; Sen. Med. Regist. St. Geo. Hosp. Lond. & Dept. Communicable Dis. E.

NYE, Matthew Yau Leung The Surgery, Aston University, The Aston Traingle, Birmingham B4 7ET Tel: 0121 359 3611 Fax: 0121 333 6023; Priory Hospital, Priory Road, Edgbaston, Birmingham B5 7UG Tel: 0121 440 6611 — MB ChB Sheff. 1981 (Sheff. Med. Sch.) Dip. Acupunc. 1984; MRCGP 1985; DRCOG 1986; DCH RCP Lond. 1988; Dip. Pract. Dermat. Wales 1990; AFOM 1994. Chief Univ. Phys. Univ. Aston.; VTS Course Organiser W. Birm.; Cons. Acupunc. Specialty: Dermat. Socs: Brit. Med. Acupunc. Soc. Prev: GP Birm.; GP Tutor.

NYEKO, Christopher UMDS, Boland House, Guy's Hospital, London SE1 9RT — LMSSA Lond. 1995.

NYHOLM, Elizabeth Shannon Yardley Green Medical Centre, 73 Yardley Green Road, Bordesley Green, Birmingham B9 5PU Tel: 0121 773 3838 Fax: 0121 506 2005; 35 Broad Oaks Road, Solihull B91 1JA Tel: 0121 705 5407 Fax: 0121 705 5407 — MB BS Lond. 1978; MFFP; DRCOG 1983; MRCGP 1983; DCH RCPS Glas. 1984. Princip. (Gen. Pract.) Hosp. Pract. (Gastroenterol.) Heartlands Hosp. Specialty: Gen. Pract.

NYHOLM, Rosemary Erica Denton Turret Medical Centre, 10 Kenley Road, Slatyford, Newcastle upon Tyne NE5 2UY Tel: 0191 274 1840; 24 Queensway, Ponteland, Newcastle upon Tyne NE20 9RZ Tel: 01661 871663 — MB BS Lond. 1985 (Univ. Coll. Sch. of Med.) BSc Reading 1975; MPhil Lond. 1980; DRCOG 1987; MRCGP 1990.

NYIRI, Polly Jennifer Flat 3, 26 Morwell St., London WC1B 3AZ — MB BChir Camb. 1990.

NYLANDER, Mr Arthur Gustavus Ekundayo Blackburn Royal Infirmary, Department of Ophthalmology, Bolton Road, Blackburn BB2 3LR Tel: 01254 687252 Email: anylander@doctors.org.uk — MB BS Nigeria 1980 (Ibadan, Nigeria) DO RCPSI 1984; FRCS Glas. 1987; FCOphth 1988. p/t Cons. Ophth. Blackburn Roy. Infirm.; Cons. Ophth. Burnley Gen. Hosp.; Coll. Tutor Ophth. E. Lancs NHS Trust, Burnley; FRCS Examr. Roy. Coll. of Physicians and Surgeons, Glas.; FRCC Examr., Roy. Coll. of Ophthalmologists. Specialty: Ophth. Special Interest: Anterior Segment; Glaucoma and Cataract; Oculoplastics. Socs: Amer. Acad. of Ophth.; UK & Irel. Soc. Cataract & Refractive Surg.; Oxf. Ophthalmological Soc. Prev: Anterior Segment Fellowsh., Roy. Hallamshire Hosp., Sheff.; Sen. Regist., Roy. Hallamshire Hosp., Sheff.

NYLANDER, David Leslie 176 Brantingham Road, Manchester M21 0TS — MB BS Newc. 1988; MRCP (UK) 1992.

NYLANDER, Harold Hercules 92 Kirkland Avenue, Ilford IG5 0TN — MB BS Newc. 1974; MRCPI 1982.

NYMAN, Cyril Richard Pilgrim Hospital NHS Trust, Sibsey Road, Boston PE21 9QS Tel: 01205 364801 Fax: 01205 359257; Stoke Lodge, 116 Tower Road, Boston PE21 9AU Tel: 01205 351748 Email: cnyman2@compuserve.com — MB BS Lond. 1968 (St. Mary's) MRCS Eng. LRCP Lond. 1968; DObst RCOG 1970; MRCP (UK) 1971; FRCP Lond. 1987; T (M) Roy. Coll. Physicians 1990; FESC European Soc. Of Cardiology 2000; FACC American Coll. Of Cardiology 2001. Cons. Phys. (Cardiorespirat. Med.) Pilgrim Hosp. Boston; Local Collaborator for "Search" and "Procardis" Studies Boston (Main Centre Oxf.). Specialty: Gen. Med.; Cardiol.; Respirat. Med. Socs: Brit. Cardiac Soc.; Brit. Thorac. Soc.; Brit. Soc. Echocardiogr. Prev: Sen. Regist. CardioRespirat. Med. Waller CardioPulm. Unit St Mary's Hosp. Lond.; Regist. (Gen. & Thoracic Med.) St. Thos. Hosp. Lond.

NYMAN, Lorraine Esther 22 Bridgewater Way, Bushey, Watford WD23 4UA — MB BS Lond. 1991.

NYMAN, Valerie Anne Royal Comwall Hospital, Truro TR1 3LJ Tel: 01872 274242; Harbourside, 29 Esplanade, Fowey PL23 1HY Tel: 01726 832556 Email: howardval.fowey@virgin.net — MB ChB Liverp. 1966. p/t Hosp. Practitioner, O & G Treliske Hosp. Truro; Clin. MO & Instruc. Dr. Fam. Plann. Cornw. Healthcare Trust. Specialty: Family Plann. & Reproduc. Health; Obst. & Gyn. Socs: Fac. Comm. Health; Fac. Fam. Plann. & Reproduc. Health Care. Prev: Lead Clin. Community Serv. for Wom. & Young People N. Devon.

NYSENBAUM, Anthony Michael 87 Palatine Road, West Didsbury, Manchester M20 3JQ Tel: 0161 434 9126; Fir Trees, 88 Moss Lane, Sale M33 5BT Tel: 0161 973 5995 — MD Manch. 1980; MB ChB 1977; MRCOG 1982. Cons. O & G Trafford HA. Specialty: Obst. & Gyn. Socs: Fell. N. Eng. Obst. & Gyn. Soc.; Blair Bell Soc. Prev: Lect. (O & G) The Lond. Hosp.; Regist. (O & G) St. Bart. Hosp. Lond.; Research Fell. Dept. Child Health Univ. Manch.

NYUNT, Aung Children Centre, 70 Walker Street, Hull HU3 2HE Tel: 01482 617639 Email: aung.nyunt@humber.nhs.uk — MB BS Rangoon; DLO 1984; DCH 1985; MSc 1991; MRCPCH 1996. Cons. Paediat. Audiologist (Audiological Med.) Hull & E. Riding Community Health NHS Trust. Specialty: Audiol. Med.

NZEGWU, Grace Olufunmilayo 27 Woodnook Road, Streatham, London SW16 6TZ — MB BS Lond. 1956.

NZELU, Ernest Nnoruka 25 Delacourt Road, Manchester M14 6BU — MB BS Ibadan 1980; MB BS Ibadan Nigeria 1980; MRCOG 1989.

NZEWI, Mr Onyekwelu Chibuike 4 Forest Drive, Bearsden, Glasgow G61 4SJ — BM BCh Nigeria 1980; FRCSI 1991.

O'BEIRN, Diarmuid Peadar Department of Medicine for Elderly, General Hospital, Llandudno LL30 1LB Tel: 01492 860066 Fax: 01492 871668 — MB BCh BAO NUI 1973; DCH Dub. 1976; MRCPI 1980; FRCPI 1989. Cons. Phys. (Med. for Elderly) Gen. Hosp. Llandudno. Specialty: Care of the Elderly. Socs: Brit. Geriat. Soc. Prev: Clin. Lect. & Sen. Regist. (c/o Elderly) Univ. Birm.; Regist. (Gen. Med.) Castlebar Gen. Hosp.; Regist. (Respirat. Med.) Merlin Pk. Hosp.

O'BOYLE, Ciaran Patrick 26 Townview Avenue S., Omagh BT78 1HX — MB BCh BAO Belf. 1996.

O'BOYLE, Mr Patrick John (retired) Wild Oak Cottage, Wild Oak Lane, Trull, Taunton TA3 7JS Tel: 01823 278057 Fax: 01823 343571 — MB ChB Glas. 1965; FRCS Ed. 1970; ChM Liverp. 1978. Prev: Cons. Urol. Taunton & Som. NHS Trust.

O'BRADY, Deirdre Siobhain 11 Rugby Mansions, Bishop Kings Road, London W14 8XD — MB BCh BAO NUI 1979; LRCPI & LM, LRCSI & LM 1979.

O'BRART, Mr David Phillip Saul Department of Ophthalmology, St Thomas' Hospital, Lambeth Palace Road, London SE1 7EH Tel: 020 7928 9292 Fax: 020 7922 0586 — MB BS Lond. 1985 (Guy's) FRCS Eng. 1990; FCOphth. 1990; DO RCS Eng. 1990; MD Lond. 1995. Cons. Ophth. Guy's & St. Thos. NHS Trust; Hon. Sen. Lect. Univ. of Lond. Specialty: Ophth. Socs: ARVO; UKIRCSS. Prev: Sen. Regist. (Ophth.) Addenbrooke's Hosp. Camb.; Regist. Rotat. & SHO (Ophth.) St. Thos. Hosp. Lond.

O'BRIEN, Mr Aidan Craigavon Area Hospital, Craigavon BT63 5QQ Tel: 028 3861 2634 Fax: 028 3833 3839 Email: aobrien@cah9t.n-i.nhs.uk; 12 Clover Hill, Moy, Dungannon BT71 7TP Tel: 028 8778 9494 Email: aidanpobrien@aol.com — MB BCh BAO Belf. 1978 (Queen's University, Belfast) FRCSI 1983. Cons. Urol. Craigavon Area Hosp. Gp. Trust Craigavon. Specialty: Urol. Socs: Irish Soc. Urol.; Fell. Roy. Acad. Med. Irel.; Fell. Ulster Med. Soc. Prev: Sen. Regist. (Paediat. Urol.) Bristol; Sen. Regist. (Urol.) Matern. Hosp. Dub.; Sen. Regist. (Urol.) Beaumont Hosp. Dub.

O'BRIEN, Aileen Ann Corwen Lodge, Castle Rising Road, South Wootton, King's Lynn PE30 — MB BS Lond. 1994.

O'BRIEN, Alastair John 6 The Hamlet, Champion Hill, London SE5 8AW.

O'BRIEN, Ambrose Patrick Harley Street Medical Centre, Hanley, Stoke-on-Trent ST1 3RX Tel: 01782 281806 — MB BCh BAO NUI 1952 (Univ. Coll. Dub.) Prev: Med. Off. Defence Forces of Irel. Att. Gen. Milit. Hosp. Curragh Camp; Sen. Res. Ho. Phys. St. Vincent's Hosp. Dub.; Res. Anaesth. City Gen. Hosp. Stoke-on-Trent.

O'BRIEN, Ann Elizabeth Oak Tree Medical Centre, 273-275 Green Lane, Seven Kings, Ilford IG3 9TJ Tel: 020 8599 3474 Fax: 020 8590 8277 Email: a.o'brien@virgin.net; 18 Hill Hall, Theydon Mount, Epping CM16 7QQ Tel: 01992 560 526 Email: a.o'brien@virgin.net — MB BS Lond. 1975 (Kings Coll.) DRCOG 1979; MRCGP 1980; DFFP 1993; FRCGP 2002. Director, Redbridge GP OnCall. Socs: Royal Society of Medicine, Fellow. Prev: Non-Exec. Dir. Redbridge & Waltham Forest HA; Chairm. Local Med. Comm.; Clin. Asst. (Paediat.) King Geo. Hosp. Ilford.

O'BRIEN, Anthony Aloysius John Department of Medicine for Elderly, Southend General Hospital, Prittlewell Chase, Westcliff on Sea SS0 0RY Tel: 01702 435555 Fax: 01702 221377 — MB BCh BAO Dub. 1980; MB BCh Dub. 1980; MRCPI 1983; MD 1992; FRCPI 1998. Cons. Phys. (Med.) Southend Gen. Hosp. Specialty: Care of the Elderly; Gen. Med. Socs: Brit. Geriat.s Soc.; Amer. Geriat. Soc. Prev: Hon. Sen. Regist. (Geriat. Med.) Hammersmith Hosp. Lond.

O'BRIEN, Anthony Timothy James Brae Cottage, Rosemary Lane, Freshford, Bath BA2 7UF — MB BChir Camb. 1993.

O'BRIEN, Mr Barry Shaun 33A Oaklands, Gosforth, Newcastle upon Tyne NE3 4YQ — MB BS (Hons.) Newc. 1990; FRCS Eng. 1994; FRCS (Tr & Orth) 1999. Cons., Sunderland Roy. Hosp. Specialty: Orthop. Prev: Regist. (Orthop.) N. Regional Train. Scheme.

O'BRIEN, Bernard William Beechcroft, Ruff Lane, Ormskirk L39 4 — MB ChB Liverp. 1972; DIH Lond. 1982.

O'BRIEN, Brendan Cornwall & Isles of Scilly Health Authority, John Kay House, St Austell PL25 4NQ Tel: 01726 627918 Fax: 01726 71777; 36 Lanyon Road, Playing Place, Truro TR3 6HF Tel: 01872 865801 — MB BCh BAO Belf. 1994; Dip. Ment. Health Belf. 1997. Specialist Regist. (Pub. Health Med.) Cornw. & Isles of Scilly Health Auth. St Austell. Specialty: Pub. Health Med.

O'BRIEN, Catherine Geraldine Mersey Care NHS Trust, Arundel House, Sefton General Hospital, Smithdown Road, Liverpool L9 7JP Tel: 0151 330 8015 Fax: 0151 280 0929 — MB BCh BAO NUI 1980; MRCPsych 1986. Adult Directorate Mersey Care NHS Trust. Specialty: Gen. Psychiat. Prev: Sen. Regist. (Psychiat.) Mersey RHA; Sen. Regist. Bloomsbury HA & UCH.; Cons. Psychiat. Sefton Gen. Hosp. Liverp.

O'BRIEN, Catherine Mary Bristol Childrens Hospital, Uppu Mandlin Street, Bristol — MB ChB Birm. 1991. Specialist Regist. (Paediat.) Bristol. Specialty: Paediat.

O'BRIEN, Miss Catherine Mary Brock Hall, Shawbury Lane, Shustoke, Birmingham B46 2SA Tel: 01676 540363 Fax: 01676 541175 — MB BS Lond. 1994 (Guy's & St. Thos. Hosp. Lond.) FRCS (Eng) 1998. SpR (Plast. Surg.) W. Midlands Rotat. Specialty: Plastic Surg. Prev: SHO Plastic Surg.; SHO Rotat. (Surg.) Frenchay Hosp. Bristol; Cas. Off. Kent & Canterbury Hosp.

O'BRIEN, Charles Joseph Daisy Hill Hospital, Newry BT35 8DR Tel: 028 3083 5167 Fax: 028 3025 7965 Email: c.j.o'brien@dhn.n-i.nhs.uk; 40 Drumreagh Road, Rostrevor, Newry BT34 3DS — MB BCh BAO Belf. 1979; MRCP (UK) 1982; MD Belf. 1988; FRCP Lond. 1997; FRCPI 1997. Cons. Phys. & Postgrad. Clin. Tutor Daisy Hill Hosp. Newry. Specialty: Gastroenterol. Socs: Brit. & Irish Soc. Gastroenterol.; Brit. Assn. Study Liver; BMA. Prev: Sen. Regist. (Med. & Gastroenterol.) Roy. Hallamsh. Hosp. Sheff.; Research Fell. Liver Unit King's Coll. Hosp. Lond.; Ho. Off. Mater Infirmorum Hosp. Belf.

O'BRIEN, Christine Department of Respiratory Medicine, George Eliot Hospital, College Street, Nuneaton CV10 7DJ — State Exam Med Hamburg 1988; MD Hamburg 1989; MRCP (UK) 1992; MD Birm. 2003. Cons. Phys. Respirat. and Gen. Med.; Royal College Tutor. Specialty: Gen. Med. Prev: Specialist Regist. (Respirat. Med.) W. Midl.

O'BRIEN, Christopher John Department of Paediatrics, Royal Victoria Infirmary, Queen Victoria Road, Newcastle upon Tyne NE1 4LP Tel: 0191 233 6161 Email: Christopher.o'brien@nuth.northy.nhs.uk — MB BS Lond. 1986 (Univ. of Lond.) Dip. Obst. Auckland 1989; MRCP (UK) 1991. Cons. Paediat. Roy. Vict. Infirm., Newc. Specialty: Respirat. Med.; Paediat. Prev: Research Fell. Roy. Vict. Infirm. Newc.; Clin. Fell., Mater Misericordial Hosp., Brisbane, Australia.

O'BRIEN, Ciaran Joseph Department of Pathology, Swansea NHS Trust Morriston Hospital, Swansea SA6 6NL Tel: 01792 702222 Fax: 01792 703051 Email: ciaran.obrien@swansea-tr.wales.nhs.uk — MB BCh BAO Dub. 1977 (Trinity Coll. Dub.) MRCPI 1980; FRCPath 1995, M 1985; FRCPI 2001. Cons. Histopath. Swansea NHS Trust, Morriston Hosp. Swansea. Specialty: Histopath. Prev: Lect. & Hon. Cons. Univ. Leeds.

O'BRIEN, David Charles 177 Russell Road, Moseley, Birmingham B13 8RR — MB BS Lond. 1977.

O'BRIEN, David John 53 Hickmans Avenue, Cradley Heath, Sandwell, Cradley Heath B64 5NH — MB ChB Liverp. 1981.

O'BRIEN, David Pascal Department of Neurosurgery, Hope Hospital, Stott Lane, Salford M6 8HD — MB BCh BAO NUI 1986.

O'BRIEN, David Vincent Haematology Department, Ormskirk and District General Hospital, Wigan Road, Ormskirk L39 2AZ Tel: 01695 656637 Fax: 01695656651 Email: davidobrien@soh-tr.nwest.nhs.uk — MB ChB Liverp. 1983; MRCP (UK) 1986; MRCPath 1994. Cons. Haemat. Southport & Ormskirk Hosp. NHS Trust. Specialty: Haematology. Prev: Sen. Regist. (Haemat.) Birm. Childr. Hosp.; LRF Fell. Qu. Eliz. Med. Centre Birm.; Regist. (Haemat.) Roy. Liverp. Hosp.

O'BRIEN, Deirdre Anne 55 High Street, Minster in Thanet, Ramsgate CT12 4BT — MB BCh BAO NUI 1977 (Univ. Coll. Dub.) DRCOG 1981. Clinical Lead for Contraception and Psychosexual therapy services in East Kent; Med. Off. (Psychosexual Med.) Margate & Broadstairs; Mem. Inst. Psychosexual Med.; Clin. Asst. (GUM)Ramsgate; MO (FPC) Ramsgate; Clin. Asst. (Dermat.) QEQMH Hosp. Margate Kent. Specialty: Dermat.; Genitourinary Medicine; Psychosexual Med. Prev: Trainee GP Thanet VTS; H.O. Surg. Laois Co. Hosp. Portlaoise; H.O. Med. St. Vincents Dub.

O'BRIEN, Denis Joseph Park Road Group Practice, The Elms Medical Centre, 3 The Elms, Liverpool L8 3SS Tel: 0151 727 5555 Fax: 0151 288 5016; Talka House, 42 Ullet Road, Liverpool L17 3BP Tel: 0151 733 4785 Fax: 0151 733 0765 — MB BCh BAO NUI 1982; DCH NUI 1985; DObst. RCPI 1985; MRCGP 1986.

O'BRIEN, Donogh Declan, OStJ, Brigadier late RAMC Retd. (retired) Park View, 38 Park Avenue, Bromley BR1 4EE Tel: 020 8464 0578 — (Univ. Coll. Dub.) MB BCh BAO NUI 1946; LM Coombe Hosp. Dub. 1948. Prev: Chief Med. Off. Brit. Red Cross Soc.

O'BRIEN, Edmund Noel (retired) 19 Beverley Gardens, Wargrave, Reading RG10 8ED Tel: 0118 940 2562 — MB BS Melbourne 1952 (Melb.) FRACP 1970, M 1959; FRCPath 1978, M 1966. Prev: Hon. Med. Adviser Brit. Olympic Assn.

O'BRIEN, Elizabeth McQuilkan Davidson (retired) 54 Abbotsbury Close, London W14 8EQ Tel: 020 7371 1327 — MB BChir Camb. 1950 (Camb. & Leeds) MRCS Eng. LRCP Lond. 1950; DPM Eng. 1967; FRCPsych 1987, M 1971. Prev: Cons. Child Psychiat. Newham HA Lond.

O'BRIEN, Fiona Geraldine Mary Light House, Newtonairds, Dumfries DG2 0JL — MB BCh BAO NUI 1987; DCH NUI 1989; DObst. RCPI 1990; MRCGP 1991. SHO (Geriat.) Edin. Specialty: Care of the Elderly. Prev: A & E Roy. Infirm. Edin.; Trainee GP Edin.; SHO (Geriat.) Roy. Vict. Hosp. Edin.

O'BRIEN, Frances Clare Town End Medical Practice, 41 Town End, Caterham CR3 5UJ Tel: 01883 345613 Fax: 01883 330142; 47 Hartscroft, Croydon CR0 9LB — MB ChB Birm. 1978; BA Camb. Specialty: Family Plann. & Reproduc. Health.

O'BRIEN, Hugh Anthony William 3 The Courtyard, Castle Carrock, Carlisle CA8 9LS — MB BS Lond. 1974; MRCP (UK) 1977; MRCPath 1982; FRCP 1996. Cons. (Haemat.) Cumbld. Infirm. Carlisle. Specialty: Haematology. Prev: Sen. Regist. St. Bart. Hosp. Lond.

O'BRIEN, Iain Anthony Daniel Law Hospital, Carluke ML8 5ER Tel: 01698 361100; Murrayfield, Broughton Road, Biggar ML12 6HA Tel: 01899 220036 — MB BS Lond. 1973; MRCP (UK) 1977; MD Bristol 1988; FRCP Glas. 1992; FRCP Ed. 1993. Cons. Gen. Med. Wishaw Gen. Hosp., Wishaw ML2 0DP. Specialty: Gen. Med.; Diabetes; Endocrinol. Prev: Sen. Regist. (Diabetes & Endocrinol.) Roy. Devon & Exeter Hosp. & Bristol Roy. Infirm.

O'BRIEN, Ian Michael 6 The Hamlet, Champion Hill, London SE5 8AW Tel: 020 7733 1792 — MB BS Lond. 1970 (Char. Cross) MRCS Eng. LRCP Lond. 1970; MRCP (UK) 1972; FRCP Lond. 1987. Cons. Phys. Medway Health Dist.; Sen. Lect. (Med.) St. Thos. Hosp. Med. Sch. Lond. Specialty: Gen. Med. Prev: Regist. (Med.) & Lect. (Med.) St. Thos. Hosp. Lond.; Lect. (Clin. Immunol.) Brompton Hosp. Lond.

O'BRIEN, James Anthony South and West Devon Health Authority, The Lescaze Offices, Shinners Bridge, Dartington, Totnes TQ9 6JE Tel: 01803 866665 Fax: 01803 861853; 3 Elm Grove, Taunton TA1 1EG Tel: 01823 259819 — MB BCh BAO NUI 1982; DObst. RCPI 1984; MFPHM RCP (UK) 1990. Cons. Pub. Health Med. Som. HA. Specialty: Pub. Health Med. Prev: Dir. Med. Servs. Guadalcanal, Solomon Is.s.

O'BRIEN, James Robert c/o The Fermoy Unit, Queen Elizabeth District General Hospital, King's Lynn Tel: 01533 766266 — MB BCh BAO NUI 1960 (Cork) DPM Eng. 1964; MRCPsych 1971. Cons. Psychiat. W. Norf. & Wisbech HA. Specialty: Gen. Psychiat. Prev: Sen. Regist. Long Gr. Hosp. Epsom; Regist. Whipps Cross Hosp. Leytonstone & Warley Hosp. Brentwood.

***O'BRIEN, Jennifer Mary** Royal Bolton Hospital, Minerva Road, Farnworth, Bolton BL4 0JR Tel: 01204 390390 — MB BS Lond. 1998 (University College London Medical School) DFFP; BSc; DRCOG. SHO(GP VTS), Roy. Bolton Hosp., Bolton. Specialty: Paediat. Dent. Socs: BMA. Prev: Ho. Off. (Med.), Darlington Memor. Hosp., Darlington.; Ho. Off.(Gen. Surg.), Roy. Bolton Hosp., Bolton.

O'BRIEN, Mrs Joan Elizabeth Mary (retired) Amerique, Castle St., Winchelsea TN36 4HU — MRCS Eng. LRCP Lond. 1950.

O'BRIEN, John Anthony Broad Lane Surgery, 684 Broad Lane, Coventry CV5 7BB Tel: 024 7646 6583 Fax: 024 7669 5972; Rose Cottage, Berryfields, Fillongley, Coventry CV7 8EX Tel: 01676 540312 — MB ChB Manch. 1968; MRCGP 1977. Clin. Asst. (Obst. & Gyn.) Coventry Hosps.; Clin. Asst. (Genitourin. Med.) Coventry, Nuneaton & Rugby Hosps.

O'BRIEN, John Ignatius Westgate Surgery, 15 Westgate, Chichester PO19 3ET Tel: 01243 782866 — MB ChB Aberd. 1990 (Kings Coll.) DRCOG; MRCGP; BSc (Hons.) Lond. 1984; MSc Aberd. 1985, MB ChB 1990. Clin. Asst. Ophthamology, Qu. Alexandra Hosp., Portsmouth.

O'BRIEN, Mr John Michael Brock Hall, Shawbury Lane, Shustoke, Coleshill, Birmingham B46 2SA Tel: 01676 540363 — MB BCh BAO Dub. 1958 (TC Dub.) MA, MB BCh BAO Dub. 1958; FRCS Ed. 1969; FRCS Eng. 1970. Cons. Surg. (Urol.) E. Birm. Gen. Hosp. & Solihull Hosp.; Mem. Panel Examr. RCS Ed. Specialty: Urol. Socs: Brit. Assn. Urol. Surgs. Prev: Sen. Clin. Lect. (Surg.) Univ. Birm.; Clin. Research Fell. Hosp. Sick Childr. Toronto, Canada; Sen. Regist. (Urol. Surg.) West. Gen. Hosp. Edin.

O'BRIEN, John Michael, QHP (retired) Catbells, 2 Ullswater Drive, Great Warford, Alderley Edge SK9 7WB Tel: 01565 872948 Fax: 01565 872948 Email: tja146@aol.com — DPH (Distinc. & Trevor Lloyd Hughes Gold Medal); MB ChB Manch. 1961; FFCM 1980, M 1973; FFPHM 1989; FRCP Ed. 1996; Lond. 1990; FRCPath 1992; FFOM (Hon.) 1993; FFPHMI (Hon.) 1998. Prev: Chairm. N.d. HA.

O'BRIEN, Mr John Patrick 149 Harley Street, London W1G 6DE Tel: 020 7935 4444 Fax: 020 7486 5222 Email: obrien.spine@btinternet.com; 12 Wyndham Place, London W1H 2PY — MB BS Sydney 1960; FRCS Ed. 1966; PhD Gothenburg 1975; FACS 1977; FRACS 1988. Socs: Internat. Soc. Study Lumbar Spine; Scoliosis Research Soc.; Cervical Spine Research Soc. Prev: Vis. Prof. Bioeng. Unit Strathclyde Univ. Glas. 1977-85; Dir. (Spinal Disorders) Robt. Jones & Agnes Hunt Orthop. Hosp. Oswestry; Lect. (Orthop. Surg.) Univ. Hong Kong.

O'BRIEN, John Temple 42 Angel Hill Drive, Sutton SM1 3BX Tel: 020 8641 2917 — MB BChir Camb. 1988; FRCS Eng. 1994. Specialist Regist. (Radiol.) Mersey. Specialty: Radiol. Prev: SHO (Surg.) William Harvey Hosp. Ashford; SHO (Surg.) Manch. Roy. Infirm.

O'BRIEN, Professor John Tiernan Wolfson Research Centre, Institute for Ageing & Health, Newcastle General Hospital, Newcastle upon Tyne NE4 6BE Tel: 0191 256 3323 Fax: 0191 219 5051 Email: j.t.o'brien@ncl.ac.uk — BM BCh Oxf. 1986 (Oxford) MA Camb. 1987; MRCPsych 1990; DM Oxf. 1996. Prof. & Cons. Old Age Psychiat. Newc. Gen. Hosp. & Univ. Newc. u. Tyne. Specialty: Geriat. Psychiat. Socs: Bd. Mem. Internat. Psychogeriatric Assn.

O'BRIEN, Joseph Dominic Department of Gastroenterology, Southend Hospital, Prittlewell Chase, Westcliff on Sea SS0 0RY Tel: 01702 221156 Fax: 01702 221379 — MB BS Lond. 1979 (Lond. Hosp.) BSc (1st cl. Hons. Physiol.) Lond. 1974, MD 1987; FRCP Lond. 1996. Cons. Phys. (Gastroenterol.) Southend Hosp. Trust. Specialty: Gastroenterol. Socs: Brit. Soc. Gastroenterol.; BMA. Prev: Sen. Regist. Rotat. W. Midl.; Clin. Research Fell. (Gastroenterol.) Lond. Hosp.; Regist. (Med.) St. Mark's Hosp. Lond.

O'BRIEN, Joyce Margaret (retired) 34 Torcross Road, South Ruislip, Ruislip HA4 0TB — MB BS Melbourne 1949 (Melb.) Prev: Resid. Med. Off. Qu. Vict. Memor. Hosp. Melb., Austral.

O'BRIEN, Katherine 6 Churchwood Road, Didsbury, Manchester M20 6TY — MB ChB Manch. 1986; MRCP (UK) 1989. Prev: SHO (Gen. Med.) Staffs. Gen. Infirm.

O'BRIEN, Katherine Mary 1 Saltcoats Road, London W4 1AR — BM Soton. 1995. GP Locum. Specialty: Gen. Med. Prev: Med. SHO diabetes.Roy.Hants Co. Hosp.Winchester.

O'BRIEN, Kathrine Mary Courtfield Medical Centre, 73 Courtfield Gardens, London SW5 0NL Tel: 020 7370 2453 Fax: 020 7244 0018 — MB BS Lond. 1985; BA Oxf. 1982; MB BS (Hons.) Lond. 1985; MRCP (UK) 1988; DRCOG 1989. Specialty: Gen. Pract.

O'BRIEN, Kevin (retired) 23 The Spinney, Handsworth Wood, Birmingham B20 1NR — MB ChB Aberd. 1941; DLO Eng. 1947. Prev: Regist. ENT Dept. United Birm. Hosps.

O'BRIEN, Laurence Stephen Ferndale Unit, University Hospital Aintree, Longmoor Lane, Liverpool L9 7AL — MB ChB Liverp. 1979; MRCS Eng. LRCP Lond. 1979; MRCPsych 1985. Clin. Dir. Ment. Health Servs., Mersey Care NHS Trust, Liverp. Specialty: Gen. Psychiat.; Alcohol & Substance Misuse.

O'BRIEN, Marion Kathryn New Court Surgery, Borough Fields, Wootton Bassett, Swindon SN4 7AX Tel: 01793 852302 — MB BCh BAO NUI 1991 (Univ. Coll. Cork) DCH RCP Lond. 1996; DGM RCP Lond. 1997; MRCGP Lond. 1998. GP NewCt. Surg. Wootton Bassett. Specialty: Gen. Pract.

O'BRIEN, Martin Joseph Brock End Surgery, Potton, Sandy SG19 2QS Tel: 01767 261777; 21 The Square, Potton, Sandy SG19 2NP Tel: 01767 261656 — MB BCh BAO NUI 1992 (Univ. Coll. Dub.) DObst RCPI 1995; MRCAP 1996. Specialty: Gen. Pract.

O'BRIEN, Mary 5 Kingsley Road, Dentons Green, St Helens WA10 6JN — MB BCh BAO NUI 1938.

O'BRIEN, Mary Bridget 55 Marian Terrace, Killarney, Newtown — MB BCh BAO NUI 1985.

O'BRIEN, Mary Elizabeth Rose Royal Marsden Hospital, Downs Rd, Sutton SM2 5PT Tel: 020 8661 3278 — MB BCh BAO Dub. 1980; MRCP (UK) 1983; MD Dub. 1990; FRCP 2000. Sen. Regist. (Med. Oncol.) Roy. Marsden Hosp.; Cons. (Med. Oncol.) Roy. Marsden Hosp.; Cons. (Med. Oncol.) Kent Cancer Centre. Specialty: Oncol. Socs: ACP; ASCO; IASLC. Prev: Research Regist. Birm.; Regist. (Med. Oncol.) Edin.; Foreign Med. Resid. Creteil, France.

O'BRIEN, Mary Sharon Geraldine Department of Gastroenterology, The Central Middlesex Hospital, Acton Lane, London NW10 7NS — MB ChB BAO 1984; MRCPI 1986; MD NUI 1992; FRCP 2003. Cons. Physican (Gastroenterol. & Gen. Med.) Centr. Middlx. Hosp. Lond. Specialty: Gastroenterol.; Gen. Med. Prev: Sen. Regist., (Gastroenterol. & Gen. Med.) Centr. Middlx. Hosp. Lond.; Lect. (Gastroenterol.) Middlx. Hosp. Lond.

O'BRIEN, Michael (retired) Eastville Health Centre, East Park, Eastville, Bristol BS5 6YA Tel: 0117 951 0046; 27 Druid Stoke Avenue, Stoke Bishop, Bristol BS9 1DB Tel: 0117 968 4849 — LRCPI & LM, LRSCI & LM 1957 (RCSI) LRCPI & LM, LRCSI & LM 1957.

O'BRIEN, Michael Dermod Department of Neurology, Guy's Hospital, London SE1 9RT Tel: 020 7955 4499 Fax: 020 7955 4864 Email: michael.obrien@gstt.sthames.nhs.uk — (Guy's) MB BS Lond. 1962; MRCS Eng. LRCP Lond. 1962; FRCP Lond. 1981, M 1967; MD Lond. 1973. Cons. Neurol. Guy's & St. Thos. Hosp. NHS Trust; Hon. Cons. Neurol. Nat. Hosp. for Neurol. & Neurosurg.; Hon. Cons. Neurol. Neurosci.s Centre Kings Healthcare Trust. Specialty: Neurol. Socs: Fell. Med. Soc. Lond.; Fell. Roy. Soc. Med.; Assn. Brit. Neurols. Prev: Acad. Regist. Nat. Hosp. Nerv. Dis. Qu. Sq. Lond.; Sen. Regist. Regional Neurol. Centre Newc.; MRC Trav. Fell. (Neurol.) Univ. Minnesota, USA.

O'BRIEN, Michael James 27 South Station Road, Gateacre, Liverpool L25 3QE — MB ChB Manch. 1997.

O'BRIEN, Neil John Daisy Cottage, Front St, Seghill, Cramlington NE23 7TG — MB ChB Dund. 1998.

O'BRIEN, Patricia Mary Brock Hall, Shawbury Lane, Shustoke, Birmingham B46 2SA Tel: 01676 540363 Fax: 01676 541175; Brock Hall, Shawbury Lane, Shustoke, Birmingham B46 2SA Tel: 01676 540363 Fax: 01676 541175 — MB ChB Liverp. 1966; DObst RCOG 1968; DA Eng. 1972. Clin. Asst. Anaesth. Dept. Birm. Heartlands Hosp. Specialty: Anaesth. Socs: Assn. Anaesth. Prev: Clin. Asst. (Anaesth.) Heartlands Hosp. Birm.; Regist. (Med.) St. Catherine's Hosp. Birkenhead; SHO (Anaesth.) West. Gen. Hosp. Edin.

O'BRIEN, Patrick David 30 Jermyn Road, King's Lynn PE30 4AE — MB BCh BAO NUI 1978 (Univ. Coll. Dub.) MRCPsych 1988; MRCGP 1989; MRCPI 1992; T(Psychiat.) 1994. Cons. Psychiat. Qu. Eliz. Psychiat. Hosp. Birm. Specialty: Gen. Psychiat. Prev: Sen. Regist. (Psychiat.) E. Anglia Higher Psychiat. Train. Scheme; Regist. (Psychiat.) Qu. Eliz. Hosp. Kings Lynn; Ho. Surg. & Ho. Phys. St. Michael's Hosp. Dun Laoghaire.

O'BRIEN, Patrick James AXA-PPP Healthcare, Occupational Health Services, MIS House, 23 St Leonards Road, Eastbourne BN21 3PX Tel: 01323 724889 Email: patrick.obrien@axa-pppohs.co.uk — MB ChB Glas. 1979; MRCGP 1985; T(GP) 1991; AFOM RCP Lond. 1994. Occupational Phys., AXA-PPP Healthcare. Specialty: Occupat. Health. Prev: Occupat. Phys. MTL Med. Servs.; Med. Adviser Shell UK Ltd.; GP Bootle.

O'BRIEN, Patrick Michael John (retired) Carlrayne, Burley Road, Menston, Ilkley LS29 6NX Tel: 01943 874093 — MB BS Lond. 1951 (Guy's) MRCS Eng. LRCP Lond. 1951; DPM Eng. 1957; MRCP Lond. 1960; MRCPsych 1971. Prev: Cons. Psychiat. Scalebor Pk. Burley-in-Wharefdale.

O'BRIEN, Professor Patrick Michael Shaughn Academic Obstetrics and Gynaecology Keele University School of Medicine, University Hospital North Staffordshire, Newcastle Road, Stoke-on-Trent ST4 0XG Tel: 01782 552472 Fax: 01782 552472 — MD Wales 1979; MB BCh 1972; FRCOG 1991, M 1979. Prof. Obst. and Gyn. Univ. Keele Sch. of Med.; Cons. N. Staffs. Hosp.; Vice Pres. Roy. Coll. of Obstetricians and Gynaecologists; Chairm. N. Staffs Med. Inst. Specialty: Obst. & Gyn. Special Interest: Gyn. Endocrinol. Socs: RSM; NSMI; BMS. Prev: Cons./Sen. Lect. Roy. Free Med. Sch.

O'BRIEN, Patrick William, VRD (retired) Heath Cottage, Herringswell, Bury St Edmunds IP28 6SS Tel: 01638 750252 — MB ChB St. And. 1950. Med. Adviser Albright & Wilson Ltd.; Surg. Lt.-Cdr. RNR. Prev: Regist. City Gen. Hosp. Sheff.

O'BRIEN, Paul Aloysius 19 Calthorpe Street, London WC1X 0JP — MB BCh BAO NUI 1978; LRCPI & LM, LRCSI & LM 1978; MSc (Econ.) Lond. 1983; DRCOG 1994.

O'BRIEN, Paul William Martin 151 Cedars Avenue, Coventry CV6 1DP — MB BS Lond. 1994.

O'BRIEN, Richard Andrew Dermod Babbs Farm, Westhill Lane, Watchfield, Highbridge TA9 4RF — MB BS Lond. 1987; BSc (Hons.) Soton. 1973; PhD Lond. 1977; MRCGP 1991; DRCOG 1991. Socs: BMA.

O'BRIEN, Russell James 98 Adderley Road, Leicester LE2 1WB Tel: 0116 2213 152; 36 Bowness Avenue, Bromborough, Wirral CH63 0EZ — MB ChB Leic. 1994; MRCP, UK 1998. Med. Specialist Regist. Leicester. Specialty: Gen. Med. Prev: SHO (A & E) P'boro.

O'BRIEN, Sarah Jane PHLS Communicable Disease Surveillance Centre, 61 Colindale Ave, London NW9 5EQ Tel: 0208 200 6868 Ext: 4422 Fax: 0208 200 7868 — MB BS Newc. 1986; DTM & H RCP Lond. 1989; MFPHM RCP (UK) 1992; FFPHM RCP (UK) 1999. Cons. Epidemiologist. Specialty: Pub. Health Med. Socs: Roy. Soc. of Med.; Internat. Epidemiol. Assn.; Brit. Infec. Soc. Prev: Cons. in Pub. Health Med., Scott. Centre for Infec. and Environm. Health and Hon. Sec. Clin, Lect. Univ. of Glas..; Sen. Lect. (Epidemiol. of Infec.) Univ. Birm.; Lect. (Pub. Health Med.) Univ. Newc. u. Tyne.

O'BRIEN, Stephen Gerard Department of Haematology, The Medical School, University of Newcastle, Newcastle upon Tyne NE1 4LP Tel: 0191 2824743/4262 Fax: 0191 201 0154 Email: s.g.o'brien@ncl.ac.uk — MB ChB Manch. 1987; BSc (Hons.) Manch. 1985; MRCP (UK) 1990; MRCPath 1997; PhD 1998. Sen.Lect./Hon.Cons.Haem.Univ.Newc. Specialty: Haematology. Prev: Lect. (Haemat.) Univ. Wales Coll. Med. Cardiff; Research Fell. LRF Leukaemia Unit Roy. Postgrad. Med. Sch. Hammersmith Hosp. Lond.; Regist. (Haemat.) Hammersmith Hosp. Lond.

O'BRIEN, Mr Terence Edward Brendan (retired) Oakbank, 90 Manchester Road, Accrington BB5 2BN Tel: 01254 233944 — MB ChB Liverp. 1965; DA Eng. 1972; DObst RCOG 1972; FRCS Ed. 1974; ChM Liverp. 1982. Cons. Surg. Blackburn, Hyndburn & Ribble Valley HA; Arris & Gale Lect. RCS Eng. Prev: Sen. Regist. (Surg.) Manch. AHA (T).

O'BRIEN, Terence Michael (retired) 84 Riseholme Road, Lincoln LN1 3SP Tel: 01522 524953 — MB BS Lond. 1951; DObst RCOG 1953; DA Eng. 1958.

O'BRIEN, Thomas Gerard 52 Croxteth Hall Lane, Croxteth, Liverpool L11 4UG — MB BCh BAO NUI 1982; DCH NUI 1986; DObst. RCPI 1988; MRCGP 1989. Trainee GP Crewe.

O'BRIEN, Thomas Patrick 38 Carisbrook Terrace, Chiseldon, Swindon SN4 — MB BCh BAO Dub. 1935 (Univ. Coll. Dub.) LM 1937; BSc NUI 1939; DPH 1939. Socs: B.M.A. Prev: Ho. Surg. Gt. Yarmouth Gen. Hosp.; Extern Matern. Asst. Coombe Hosp.; Med. Off. Oakwood Hall Sanat. Rotherham.

O'BRIEN, Timothy Desmond 6 The Nook, off Manchester Road, Greenfield, Oldham OL3 Tel: 0145 773859 — MD NUI 1971 (Cork) MB BCh BAO 1955. Cons. Phys. (Geriat.) Oldham & Dist. Gen. Hosp. Specialty: Gen. Med.

O'BRIEN, Timothy Philip 27 The Fairway, Leeds LS17 7QP — MB ChB Leeds 1993; BEng. (Hons) Liverp. 1985. SHO (Psychiat.) St. Jas. Univ. Hosp. Leeds.; Airedale VTS (GP). Specialty: Gen. Pract. Prev: SHO (Anaesth.); SHO (Paediat.); GP Regist.

O'BRIEN, Mr Timothy Stephen Department of Urology, Churchill Hospital, Oxford OX3 7DL Tel: 01865 225941; 16 Windsor Street, Oxford OX3 7AP Tel: 01865 741086 — BM BCh Oxf. 1986; MA Camb. 1988; FRCS Lond. 1990. Research Fell. (Urol.) Churchill Hosp. Oxf. Specialty: Urol. Socs: Brit. Assn. Urol. Surgs.

O'BRIEN, William, OBE, Maj.-Gen. late RAMC Retd. Kitfield Cottage, Ardingly, Haywards Heath RH17 6UP — MRCS Eng. LRCP Lond. 1941 (Char. Cross) MD (Distinc.) Lond. 1950, MB BS 1941; FRCP Lond. 1967, M 1948. Prev: Cons. Phys. to Army; Sen. Lect. Med. Univ. Coll. Khartoum; Med. Regist. Char. Cross Hosp.

O'BRYAN-TEAR, Charles Gillies 141-9 Staines Road, Hounslow TW3 3JA Tel: 020 8572 7422 Fax: 020 8754 3789; 2 Hereford Mansions, Hereford Road, London W2 5BA Tel: 020 7229 0789 — MB BS Lond. 1980; BA Camb. 1977; MRCP (UK) 1983; MFPM RCP (UK) 1990. Med. Dir. Bristol-Myers Squibb, Hounslow. Specialty: Pharmaceutical Medicine. Socs: RCP; Brit. Assn. Pharmaceut. Phys.; Fac. Pharmaecut. Med. Prev: Dir. Med. Affairs Sanofi Winthrop Guildford; Dir. Clin. Research Searle Skokie Illinois, USA; Regist. (Med.) St. Mary's Hosp. Lond.

O'BYRNE, Ella Karen 8 Goosebrook Close, Comberbach, Northwich CW9 6BX — MB ChB Leeds 1997.

O'BYRNE, John Joseph Westlands Medical Centre, 20B Westlands Grove, Portchester, Fareham PO16 9AD; 4 Woodstock Close, Fareham PO14 1NW — MB BS Lond. 1978 (Char. Cross) DCH RCP Lond. 1982; DRCOG 1983; MRCGP 1984; MLCOM 1991.

O'BYRNE, Kenneth John ICRF Clinical Oncology Unit, Churchill Hospital, Headington, Oxford OX3 7LJ — MB BCh BAO NUI 1984.

O'BYRNE, Kevin Patrick The Health Centre, Lawson Street, Stockton-on-Tees TS18 1HX Tel: 01642 676520 Fax: 01642 614720; 9 Orchard Road, Linthorpe, Middlesbrough TS5 5PN Tel: 01642 819837 — MB BS Newc. 1975; MRCGP 1979. Specialty: Paediat. Neurol. Prev: Trainee GP Cleveland VTS.

O'BYRNE, Sharon Rose Therese Department of Clinical Pharmacology, St Bartholemew's & The Royal London School of Medicine &, Dentistry, Chapterhouse Square, London EC1M 6BQ Tel: 020 7415 3416 Fax: 020 7415 3408 Email:

s.r.o'byrne@mds.qmw.ac.uk — MB BCh BAO NUI 1983 (Univ. Coll. Gallway Irel.) MRCPI 1986; MSc (Clin. Pharm.) Aberd. 1992; MD Dub. 1997. Lect./Gen. Regist. Clin. Pharmacol. St. Barts. Roy. Lond. Sch. Med. & Dent. Specialty: Pharmacology. Prev: Sen. Diabetes/Endocrinol. King's Coll. Hosp.; Postdoctoral Research Fell. Vanderbilt Univ. USA; Med. Regist. Aberd. Roy. Infirm.

O'CALLAGHAN, Abina Catherina P.O. Box 24488, London W5 2XT Tel: 020 8991 8198/07831 537835 Fax: 020 8991 8198 — MB BS Lond. 1977 (Roy. Free) MRCS Eng. LRCP Lond. 1977; FRCA Eng. 1981. Indep. Cons. Pain Managem. & Anaesth. Lond. Specialty: Anaesth. Prev: Cons. Anaesth. Centr. Middlx. Hosp.; Clin. & Research Fell. (Paediat. Anaesth.) Toronto Sick Childr. Hosp., Canada; Sen. Regist. (Anaesth.) Middlx., Centr. Middlx. & Northwick Pk. Hosps.

O'CALLAGHAN, Ann Mary Portsmouth Oncology Centre, St Mary's Hospital, Milton Road, Portsmouth PO3 6AD Tel: 023 92 286000 Ext: 3880 Fax: 023 92 866313 Email: ann.o'callaghan@porthosp.nhs.uk — MB BCh BAO NUI 1988 (UCD) MRCPI 1990. Cons. in Med. Oncol. Specialty: Oncol. Prev: CRC Clin. Research Fell. & Hon. Sen. Regist. (Med. Oncol.) Wessex Med. Oncol. Unit Soton.

O'CALLAGHAN, Christopher Liam — BM BS Nottm. 1982; BMedSci 1980; MRCP (UK) 1985; DM Nottm. 1992; FRCP 1996; PhD Leic. 1997; FRCPCH 1997. Prof. Of Paediat. Univ. Of Leicester. Prev: Sen. Lect. (Child Health) & Hon. Cons. Paediat. Univ. Leicester.; Cons. Thoracic Royd Childr. Hosp. Melbourne, Austral.; Lect. (Child Health) Univ. Nottm.

O'CALLAGHAN, Desmin Pierce Park Avenue Medical Centre, 166-168 Park Avenue North, Northampton NN3 2HZ Tel: 01604 716500 Fax: 01604 721685 — MB BCh BAO NUI 1982; DRCOG 1986; MRCGP (Distinc.) 1987. Clin. Asst. (Dermat.) Isebrook Hosp. WellingBoro.

O'CALLAGHAN, Eamonn Gabriel Winstree Road Surgery, 84 Winstree Road, Colchester CO3 5QF Tel: 01206 572372 Fax: 01206 764412; Greensleeves, Layer Breton Heath, Colchester CO2 0PP Tel: 01206 330668 — MB BCh BAO NUI 1965 (Univ. Coll. Dub.) DObst RCOG 1974. Princip.Gen.pract., Visit.clin.asst. Specialty: Gen. Med. Socs: Colchester Med. Soc. Prev: Regist. (O & G) Milit. Hosp. Colchester; Paediat. Ho. Phys. St. Kevin's Hosp. Dub.

O'CALLAGHAN, Ellen Maria Whipps Cross Hospital, Leytonstone, London E11 1NR Tel: 020 8535 6744 Email: maria.o'callaghan@whippsx.nhs.uk — MB BS Newc. 1983 (Univ. Newc. upon Tyne) MRCP (UK) 1986; FRCP 1997; FRCPCH 1997. Cons. Paediat. Whipps Cross Hosp. Lond. Specialty: Paediat. Prev: Lect. (Child Health) St. Geo. Hosp. Med. Sch. Lond.; Regist. (Paediat.) Leic. Roy. Infirm. & P'boro. Dist. Hosp.

O'CALLAGHAN, Finbar Joseph Kevin Southampton General Hospital, Southampton SO9 4X7 Tel: 0117 942 7373; 5 Alexandra Park, Redland, Bristol BS6 6QB — MB ChB Bristol 1990; MA Oxf. 1988; MRCP (UK) 1993. Research Fell. & Hon. Sen. Regist. (Paediat.) Univ. Bath. Specialty: Paediat. Socs: Brit. Paediat. Assn.; BMA. Prev: Clin. Fell. (Neonat.) Hosp. Sick Childr. Toronto, Canada; Regist. (Paediat.) Birm. Childr. Hosp.; SHO (Paediat.) Roy. Hosp. Sick Childr. Bristol.

O'CALLAGHAN, Kathleen Mary Unsworth Medical Centre, Parr Lane, Unsworth, Bury BL9 8JR Tel: 0161 766 4448 Fax: 0161 767 9811; 126 Manchester Road, Accrington BB5 2PD Tel: 01254 235348 — MB ChB Leeds 1980; MRCGP 1984.

O'CALLAGHAN, Mary Claremont, 2 Church Road, Evington, Leicester LE5 6FA — MB BCh BAO NUI 1973; DCH RCPSI 1975; DObst RCPI 1979. Staff Grade Paediat., Childrens Servs., Leicester, City W. PCT. Specialty: Community Child Health. Prev: SHO (Paediat.) St Finbarr's Hosp. Cork & Mercy Hosp. Cork; SHO (Obst.) Erinville Hosp. Cork.

O'CALLAGHAN, Nigel Graham Sowerby and Partners, The Health Centre, Park Road, Tarporley CW6 0BE Tel: 01829 733456 Fax: 01829 730124; Ivy Farm, Tattenhall, Chester CH3 9NH Tel: 01829 770491 Email: nigel.ocallaghan@btinternet.com — MB BS Lond. 1973 (Roy. Free) Dip. Med. Acupunc. 1995 BMAS. Socs: Brit. Acupunc. Soc. Prev: SHO (A & E) Roy. Free Hosp. Lond.; SHO (Paediat.) St. Albans City Hosp.; SHO (O & G) Barnet Gen. Hosp.

O'CALLAGHAN, Patrick Anthony Melbourne Street Medical Centre, 56 Melbourne Street, Leicester LE2 0AS Tel: 0116 262 2721; Claremont, 2 Church Road, Evington, Leicester LE5 6FA Tel: 0116 2215513 — MB BCh BAO NUI 1974 (Cork) DObst RCPI 1979. Prev: Trainee Gen. Pract. Leicester Vocational Train. Scheme; Intern S. Infirm. Cork.

O'CALLAGHAN, Peter Augustine Department of Cardiological Science, St. Georges Hospital Medical School, Cranmer Terrace, London SW17 0RE — MB BCh N U Ireland 1988. Specialty: Cardiol.

O'CALLAGHAN, Sarah Elizabeth Southlea Surgery, 276 Lower Farnham, Aldershot GU11 3RB — MB ChB Bristol 1975; MRCP (UK) 1978; MRCGP 1980.

O'CALLAGHAN, Timothy James Patrick (retired) The Arches, 515 Yarm Road, Eaglescliffe, Stockton-on-Tees TS16 9BG Tel: 01642 648348 Fax: 01642 866419 — (Newcastle-upon-Tyne) MB BS Durh. 1961; DObst RCOG 1964. Prev: Sen. Med. Practitioner Eaglescliffe.

O'CALLAGHAN, Una Catherine Parsons Heath Medical Practice, 35A Parsons Heath, Colchester CO4 3HS Tel: 01206 864395 Fax: 01206 869047; 90 Egret Crescent, Colchester CO4 3FP — MB BCh BAO NUI 1983; DCH NUI 1985; DObst RCPI 1987; MRCGP 1988.

O'CARROLL, Aisling Anne Woodlands Health Centre, Paddock Wood, Tonbridge TN12 6AR — MB BCh BAO NUI 1991.

O'CARROLL, Anne-Marie 9 St Mary's Avenue, London E11 2NR — MB BChir Camb. 1993.

O'CARROLL, Aodhan (retired) 22 St Mary's Garden, Worsbrough Village, Barnsley S70 5LU Tel: 01226 287930 — MB BCh BAO NUI 1972 (Galway)

O'CARROLL, Aongus Finian Ely 97 Browning Road, Manor Park, London E12 — MB BCh BAO NUI 1947 (Univ. Coll. Dub.) LM Coombe 1958. Med. Off. Refuge Insur. Co. & Britannia Insur. Co. Prev: Sen. Ho. Surg. Peace Memor. Hosp.; Sen. Ho. Phys. Salisbury Gen. Hosp.; Surg. Shaw Savill Shipp. Line.

O'CARROLL, Mr Charles Brian (retired) Fieldway, Woodbine Lane, Illogan, Redruth TR16 4ED — MB BS Lond. 1941 (St. Bart.) MB BS Lond. (Hnrs. in Surg.) 1941; MRCS Eng. LRCP Lond. 1941; FRCS Ed. 1943. Prev: Maj. RAMC, Surg. Specialist.

O'CARROLL, Daniel Joseph 14 Patterdale Road, Davyhulme, Manchester M41 7DW — MB ChB Sheff. 1996.

O'CARROLL, Geraldine Teresa 97 Browning Road, Manor Park, London E12 — MB BCh BAO NUI 1948 (Galw.) DPH Eng. 1956; DPH Manch. 1956. Prev: Ho. Surg. Peace Memor. Hosp. Watford; Med. Off. Pub. Health, Matern. & Child Welf. Servs. Birm.

O'CARROLL, Mary Geraldine Ridingleaze Medical Centre, Ridingleaze, Bristol BS11 0QE Tel: 0117 982 2693 Fax: 0117 938 1707 — MB BCh BAO NUI 1977.

O'CARROLL, Patrick Joseph Anthony Church Lane Surgery, 24 Church Lane, Brighouse HD6 1AS Tel: 01484 714349 Fax: 01484 720479 — MB BCh BAO NUI 1965 (Cork) Clin. Asst. (Diabetes) Roy. Infirm. Huddersfield. Specialty: Diabetes. Prev: Regist. (Gen. Med.) & SHO (O & G) Huddersfield Roy. Infirm.; Regist. (Med.) Huddersfield Roy. Infirm.; SHO (Med. & Geriat.) St. Luke's Hosp. Huddersfield.

O'CARROLL, Timothy Michael 21 Southernhay Road, Leicester LE2 3TN Tel: 0116 270 6221 — (St. Bart.) MB BS Lond. 1970; MRCS Eng. LRCP Lond. 1970; DObst RCOG 1974; FRCA 1975. Cons. Anaesth. Leicester Roy. Infirm. Specialty: Anaesth.

O'COLMAIN, Brendan Paul O'Colmain and Partners, Fearnhead Cross Medical Centre, 25 Fearnhead Cross, Warrington WA2 0HD Tel: 01925 847000 Fax: 01925 818650 — MB BCh BAO NUI 1974.

O'CONNELL, Brian Augustine 146 Kensington Park Road, London W11 2EP Tel: 020 7221 2725 — MB BCh BAO NUI 1950 (Univ. Coll. Dub.) DPM RCPSI 1953; FRCPsych 1971. Specialty: Gen. Psychiat. Socs: Founder Mem. Brit. Acad. Foren. Scs.; Trav. Fell. WHO. Prev: Med. Dir. & Cons. Psychiat. N.gate Clinic Lond.; Cons. Psychiat. Hammersmith & Fulham Health Auth. (T); Hon. Cons. Psychiat. St. Geo. Hosp. Lond.

O'CONNELL, Bridget 4 The Priory, Priory Park, London SE3 9XA Tel: 020 8852 3157 — (Cork) MD NUI 1964, MB BCh BAO 1956; DCH Eng. 1960; MRCP Ed. 1964; MRCP Lond. 1964; FRCP (Ed.) 1997; FRCPCH 1997. Hon. Cons. Paediat. Redbridge & N. Thames Health Auth. Specialty: Paediat. Socs: BMA; Fell. Roy. Soc. Med.; Fac. Paediat. Prev: Sen. Regist. (Paediat.) Hosp. Sick Childr. Gt. Ormond St. Lond.; Sen. Regist. (Paediat.) Lond. Hosp.; Lect. in Paediat. Dept. Physiol. Lond. Hosp. Med. Coll.

O'CONNELL, Cormac Roderic William 42 High Street, Sutton, Ely CB6 2RB — MB BCh BAO NUI 1978 (RCSI) LRCPI & LM, LRCSI & LM 1977.

O'CONNELL, Daniel, KM, KCSG (retired) 17 Rosscourt Mansions, 13 Buckingham Palace Road, London SW1W 0PR Tel: 020 7834 5121 — MB BCh BAO Dub. 1945; DMR Lond 1948; MD Dub. 1957; FFR 1958; FFR RCSI 1962; FRCR 1975. Prev: i/c Radiother. Dept. Char. Cross Hosp. Lond.

O'CONNELL, David Michael 321 Tettenhall Road, Wolverhampton WV6 0JZ; 1 Chilgrove Gardens, Tettenahll, Wolverhampton WV6 8XP — MB ChB Bristol 1966.

O'CONNELL, Edmund Joseph (retired) Inniscarra, Old Bath Road, Sonning-on-Thames, Reading RG4 6TE — MB BCh BAO NUI 1943 (Cork) Prev: Med. Adviser AdW. Engin., Western Thompson Controls & Harris Lebus.

O'CONNELL, Elizabeth Philomena Genitourin Clinic, District General Hospital, Stafford; The Hall, Bednall, Stafford ST17 0SA Tel: 01785 712621 Fax: 01785 661064 — MB BCh BAO NUI 1977 (Univ. Coll .Cork) DCH NUI 1980; DPH NUI 1981. Staff Grade, GuGenitourin. Med., Dist. Gen. hosp. Stafford; Clin. Asst. N. Stafford Hosp. Stoke-on-Trent. Specialty: Genitourinary Medicine.

O'CONNELL, Francis Joseph (retired) 8 Down End Road, Drayton, Portsmouth PO6 1HT — (St. Thos.) MB BS Lond. 1955; DObst RCOG 1957.

O'CONNELL, Gillian Sawrey Ground, Hawshead Hill, Ambleside LA22 0PP — MB ChB Dundee 1977; DA Eng. 1979; FFA RCS Eng. 1983. Staff Grade Clin. Asst. (Anaesth.) Northwick Pk. Hosp. Middlx. Specialty: Anaesth. Prev: Clin. Asst. & Regist. (Anaesth.) Lancaster Roy. Infirm.

O'CONNELL, Ian Patrick Michael Dept of Medicine, Royal Albert Edward Infirmary, Wigan Lane, Wigan WN1 2NN Tel: 01942 822292 — MB ChB Manch. 1987; BSc (Hons.) St. And. 1984; MRCP (UK) 1991. Cons. Phys. (Diabetes & Endocrinol., Gen. Med.) Roy. Albert Edwd. Infirm. Wigan. Specialty: Gen. Med.; Diabetes; Endocrinol. Socs: RCP Edin.; Soc. Endocrinol.; Brit. Diabetic Assn. (Med. & Scientif. Sect.). Prev: Specialist Regist. (Endocrinol. & Gen. Med.) Hope Hosp. Salford; Research Fell. NW Injury Research Centre Salford; Regist. (Endocrinol. & Gen. Med.) Hope Hosp. Salford.

O'CONNELL, Janet Elisabeth Consultant Otolaryngologist, Sandwell & West Birmingham Hospitals NHS Trust, Dudley Road, Birmingham B18 7QH — MB ChB Dundee 1976 (Dundee University) O.R.L. 1996 Intercollegiate Examination; FRCS (Gen.) Ed. 1984; FRCS (Oto.) Ed. 1986. Cons. Otolaryngologist City Hosp. NHS Trust Birm. Specialty: Otolaryngol. Socs: BMA; Brit. Assn. Paediat. Otol.; Brit. Assn. of Head and Neck Surg.s.

O'CONNELL, Janice Elizabeth Sunderland Royal Hospital, Sunderland SR4 7TP Tel: 0191 565 6256 Fax: 0191 569 9238 — MB ChB Glas. 1985; MRCP (UK) 1988; FRCP 1998; FRCP 1999. Sen. Lect. (Geriat. Med.) Univ. Newc. Specialty: Care of the Elderly. Prev: Cons. Phys. (c/o Elderly) S. Tyneside Dist. Hosp.

O'CONNELL, Mr John Michael 46 Vanderbilt Road, London SW18 3BQ — MB BS Lond. 1984 (Westm.) BSc Lond. 1981; FRCS (Otol.) 1990; MPhil Sussex 1993; FRCS (Orl.) 1996. Cons. ENT & Facial Plastic Surg., Brighton Healthcare NHS Trust, Brighton.; Edit. Bd. ENT News. Specialty: Otorhinolaryngol. Socs: Fell. Roy. Soc. Med.; Brit. Assn. Otol. Head & Neck Surg.; Coun. Mem. Europ. Acad. of Facial Plast. Surgs. Prev: Sen. Regist. Roy. Nat. Throat, Nose & Ear Hosp. Lond.; Sen. Regist. (Paediat. Otolaryngol.) Gt. Ormond St. Hosp.; SHO (Surg.) Profess. Unit Roy. Marsden Hosp. Lond.

O'CONNELL, John Paul Tramways Medical Centre, 54 Holme Lane, Sheffield S6 4JQ Tel: 0114 234 3418 Fax: 0114 285 5958 — MB ChB Sheff. 1985.

O'CONNELL, John Philip James 73 Harley Street, London W1N 1DE Tel: 07850 312252 Fax: 0208 788 8026 Email: johnpcon@aol.com; 69 Medfield St, Roehampton, London SW15 4JY — MB BS Lond. 1970 (Middx. Hosp.) MRCS Eng. LRCP Lond. 1970; DA Glasgow 1974; MRCP (UK) 1976; FRCP Lond. 1991; FRCPCH 1999. Cons. Paediat.Childr.'s Trust; Cons. Paediat. Epsom & St. Helier NHS Trust. Specialty: Paediat. Prev: Cons. Paediat. Epsom Health Care NHS Trust Lond.; Nat.Peadiat.Governm.Vanatu; Cons.peadiat/Sen. Lect. Child Health Fiji Sch. of Med.

O'CONNELL, Mary Elizabeth Ann Department of Radiotherapy, New Guy's House, Guy's Hospital, St Thomas' St., London SE1 9RT Tel: 020 7955 4400 Fax: 020 7955 4828; Flat 1 Ashleigh Court, 81 Lawrie Pk Road, Sydenham, London SE26 6EX Tel: 020 8659 9598 Fax: 020 8659 9598 — MB BS Lond. 1981 (Roy. Free) MRCP (UK) 1984; FRCR 1989; MD Lond. 1993. Cons. Radiother. & Oncol. Guy's and St Thomas's Cancer Centre Lond. Specialty: Oncol.; Radiother. Socs: Fell. Roy. Coll. Radiol.; Brit. Inst. Radiol.; Eur. Soc. Therap. Radiol. & Oncol. Prev: Sen. Regist. (Clin. Oncol.) Addenbrooke's Hosp. Camb.; Hon. Sen. Regist. & Research Fell. (Radiother.) Roy. Marsden Hosp. Sutton; Regist. (Radiother.) Roy. Marsden Hosp.

O'CONNELL, Mary Susanna Paynes Farm House, Salcott-cum-Virley, Maldon CM9 8HG — MB BS Lond. 1981 (Char. Cross Hosp.) MRCS Eng. LRCP Lond. 1980; DRCOG 1983.

O'CONNELL, Maureen Patricia c/o 1 Avington Close, London Road, Guildford GU1 1SL — MB BS Lond. 1964 (Roy. Free) MRCS Eng. LRCP Lond. 1964; DObst RCOG 1966.

O'CONNELL, Maurice Charles Beacon Surgery, Beacon Road, Crowborough TN6 1AF Tel: 01892 652233 Fax: 01892 668840; 6 Beacon Gardens, Crowborough TN6 1BD Tel: 01892 663418 — MB BS Lond. 1978; DA Eng. 1980; DRCOG 1982.

O'CONNELL, Morgan Ross, Surg. Capt. RN Combat Stress/Ex-Servicement's Mental Welfare Society, Tyrwhitt House, Oaklawn Road, Leatherhead KT22 0BX; Wickham House, Wickham, Fareham PO17 5JG Tel: 01329 834512 Fax: 01329 835150 Email: sprint@athene.co.uk — MB BCh BAO NUI 1968 (Galw.) DPM Eng. 1974; FRCPsych 1990, M 1976. Chief Cons. Psychiat. Combat Stress/Ex- Serv.men's Ment. Welf. Soc.; Hon. Cons. Psychiat. RNLI. Specialty: Gen. Psychiat. Socs: BMA; Fell., Roy. Soc., of Med.; Intern. Soc. Traum. Stress Studies. Prev: Cons. Adviser, Psychiat. to the Med. Dir. Gen. (Roy. Navy); Cons. Psych. Roy. Naval Hosp. Haslar, Gosport, Hants.; PMO HMS Fearless.

O'CONNELL, Niall John Woodley Centre Surgery, 106 Crockhamwell Road, Woodley, Reading RG5 3JY Tel: 0118 969 5011 Fax: 0118 944 0382 — MB BS Lond. 1980 (St. Mary's) DRCOG 1984; FRCGP 1995, M 1989; LLM 1991. Socs: Fell. Roy. Soc. Med.; BMA. Prev: SHO (Accid. & Traum. Surg.) Roy. Berks. Hosp. Reading; SHO (Obst.) Heatherwood Hosp.

O'CONNELL, Nicola Margaret 82 Moor Drive, Liverpool L23 2US — MB ChB Liverp. 1998.

O'CONNELL, Nuala Maria Department Laboratory Medicine, Salisbury District Hospital, Salisbury SP2 8BJ Tel: 01722 336262 — MB ChB Manch. 1980. Assoc. Specialist (Laborat. Med.). Specialty: Chem. Path.

O'CONNELL, Olivia 3 Woodvale, Ponteland, Newcastle upon Tyne NE20 9JR — MB ChB Sheff. 1998. SHO, A & E, Roy. Vic. Infirm., Newc. Gen. Hosp.,Newc. Specialty: Accid. & Emerg. Prev: Ho. Off.; Roy. Hallanshire Hosp. Weston Pk. Hosp. Sheff.

O'CONNELL, Paul Timothy Joseph St Martins, Griffinstown, Kinnegad, Mullingar, County Westmeath, Republic of Ireland; 22 Egmont Road, Sutton SM2 5JN Tel: 020 8642 4007 — MB BCh BAO NUI 1989; MRCPsych 1994. Sen. Regist. (Psychiat.) Maudsley Hosp. Lond. Specialty: Gen. Psychiat.

O'CONNELL, Peter James 27 Cricklade Road, Highworth, Swindon SN6 7BW — MB BS Lond. 1990.

O'CONNELL, Rebecca — MB BS Lond. 1993.

O'CONNELL, Shaun Michael 15 Queen's Down, Creech St Michael, Taunton TA3 5QY — BM Soton. 1990; DCH RCP Lond. 1994; MRCGP 1995. Specialty: Gen. Pract.

O'CONNELL, Thomas Joseph (retired) Kilcrea, 34 Laurel Road, St Helens WA10 4AZ Tel: 01744 609211 — MB BCh BAO NUI 1949 (Cork) LM Dub. 1953. Prev: Ho. Phys. S. Devon & E. Cornw. Hosp. Plymouth.

O'CONNELL, Una (retired) 17 Rosscourt Mansions, Buckingham Palace Road, London SW1W 0PR Tel: 020 7834 5121 — (King's Coll. Hosp.) MB BS Lond. 1948; DMRD Lond 1951. Prev: Cons. Radiol. Sutton & W. Merton (St. Helier) Health Dist.

O'CONNOR, Aidan Patrick The Family Medical Practice, 98 High St., Golborne, Warrington WA3 3DA — MB BCh BAO NUI 1983. Prev: SHO (Paediat.) Hartlepool Gen. Hosp.; SHO (O & G) Doncaster Roy. Infirm.; Ho. Off. Belf. City Hosp.

O'CONNOR, Alison Mary 64 Park Road, Prestwich, Manchester M25 0FA — MB ChB Liverp. 1990.

O'CONNOR, Anthony Paul (retired) Deddington Health Centre, Earls Lane, Deddington, Banbury OX15 0TQ Tel: 01869 338611 Fax: 01869 37009 — LMSSA Lond. 1965 (St. Mary's) DObst RCOG 1970; MRCGP 1974; DFFP 1995. Prev: Lt.-Col. RAMC.

O'CONNOR, Bernadette Sheila 14 Glencree Park, Newtownabbey BT37 0QS — MB BCh BAO Belf. 1997.

O'CONNOR, Brendan Bernard Department of Anaesthesia, Birmingham Heartlands Hospital, Bordesley Green, Birmingham B9 5SS Tel: 0121 424 3438 Email: oconnob@heartsol.wmids.nhs.uk — MB ChB Birm. 1987; BSc Physiol. (Hons.) Birm. 1984; ChB Birm. 1987; FRCA 1993. Cons. Anaesth. Birm. Heartlands & Solihull NHS Trust. Specialty: Anaesth. Prev: Sen. Regist. (Anaesth.) Coventry Sch. Anaesth.; Lect. (Anaesth.) Univ. Sheff.; Regist. (Anaesth.) N. Staffs. Hosp. Stoke-on-Trent & Wolverhamton Hosps.

O'CONNOR, Brendan Gerard 6 Butler Place, Belfast BT14 7NY — MB BCh BAO Belf. 1990; BDS Belf. 1983; MB BCh Belf. 1990.

O'CONNOR, Brendan Hayes — MB BS Lond. 1973 (St. Bart.) FFPHM RCP (UK) 1987, M 1980; T(PHM) 1991. Director of Pub. Health SW Kent PCT; Princip. Lect. in Pub. Health, PostGrad. Med. Sch. Univ. of Brighton. Specialty: Pub. Health Med. Socs: Fell. (Ex-Hon. Sec.) Roy. Soc. Med. (Sect. Epidemiol.). Prev: Dep. Director of Pub. Health, E. Sussex, Brighton & Hove HA; Dir. Pub. Health E. Sussex HA & E. Sussex FHSA; Dir. Pub. Health Tunbridge Wells HA.

O'CONNOR, Brian Dominic Greenbank Drive Surgery, 8 Greenbank Drive, Sefton Park, Liverpool L17 1AW Tel: 0151 733 5703; 69 Dovedale Road, Mossley Hill, Liverpool L18 5EP — MB ChB Liverp. 1985.

O'CONNOR, Brian Joseph Department of Respiratory Medicine, King's College School of Medicine & Dentistry, Bessemer Road, Denmark Hill, London SE5 9RS Tel: 020 7346 3583 Fax: 020 7346 3589; 14 Binns Road, Chiswick, London W4 2BS Tel: 020 7640 0945 Fax: 020 7498 4714 — MB BCh BAO NUI 1980 (Univ. Coll. Dub.) MRCPI 1984; DCH NUI 1987. Cons. Phys. (Respirat. Med.) King's Healthcare Lond.; Sen. Lect. King's Coll. Sch. Med. & Dent. Lond. Specialty: Respirat. Med. Socs: Fell. Roy. Soc. Med. (Pres. Counc. Respirat. Sect.); Brit. Thorac. Soc.; Amer. Thoracic Soc. Prev: Cons. Phys. & Sen. Lect. (Thoracic Med.) Roy. Brompton Hosp., Imperial Sch. Med. & Nat. Heart & Lung Inst. Lond.; Lect. (Med.) Univ. Coll. Dub.

O'CONNOR, Catherine Mary Ita The Surgery, 241 Westbourne Grove, London W11 2SE Tel: 020 7229 5800 Fax: 020 7243 2058 — MB BCh BAO NUI 1970.

O'CONNOR, David Orthopaedic Department, Royal Bournemouth Hospital, Castle Lane East, Bournemouth BH7 7DW Tel: 01202 4070 4927 — MB BCh Wales 1987.

O'CONNOR, Deirdre Mary Elizabeth Limes Medical Centre, The Plain, Epping CM16 6TL Tel: 01992 572727 Fax: 01992 574889 — MB BCh BAO NUI 1975; Cert. Family Plann. JCC 1979; DCH RCPSI 1979; DObst RCPI 1979; MRCGP 1981.

O'CONNOR, Dermot Charles The Surgery, 30 Old Road West, Gravesend DA11 0LL Tel: 01474 351557 Fax: 01474 333952 Email: dermotoconnor28@hotmail.com — MB BCh BAO Dub. 1973 (TC Dub.) BA; MRCGP 1979. GP Gravesend.; Covenor Dartford & Gravesham Trainers Gp. Prev: Ho. Off. (Surg.) & Ho. Off. (Med.) & Research Fell. in Vasc. Dis. Sir; P. Dun's Hosp. Dub.

O'CONNOR, Dominic James 1 Preston Close, Stanton under Bardon, Markfield LE67 9TX — MB ChB Manch. 1995. SHO Rotat. (Anaesth), Trafford Gen. Hosp., S. Manch. Specialty: Anaesth. Socs: Assoc. of Anaesth.s; Manch. Med. Soc.; RCA.

O'CONNOR, Eric Joseph Michael (retired) 25 Minterne Avenue, Norwood Green, Southall UB2 4HW Tel: 020 8574 1727 — LRCPI & LM, LRSCI & LM 1949; LRCPI & LM, LRCSI & LM 1949; DCH RCPSI 1951.

O'CONNOR, Mr Fergus ENT Out Patient Department, Fairfield General Hospital, Rochdale Old Road, Bury BL9 7TD Tel: 0161 705 3671 Fax: 0161 705 3671; 12 Nabbs Fold, Greenmount, Bury BL8 4EH Tel: 0120 488 6418 Fax: 0161 705 3671 — (Manch.) MRCS Eng. LRCP Lond. 1964; FRCS Ed. 1970; FRCS Eng. ad eundem 1998. Cons. Surg. (ENT) Bury Gen. Hosp. & Birch Hill Hosp. Rochdale. Specialty: Otolaryngol. Socs: Fell. Manch. Med. Soc.; Fell. Roy. Soc. Med. Prev: Sen. Regist. (ENT) Univ. Hosp. Wales Cardiff; Regist. (ENT) Liverp. ENT Infirm.; SHO (Surg.) Manch. Roy. Infirm.

O'CONNOR, Frances Patricia Carteknowle and Dore Medical Practice, 1 Carterknowle Road, Sheffield S7 2DW Tel: 0114 255 1218 Fax: 0114 258 4418 — MB BS Lond. 1986.

O'CONNOR, Francis Alexander Altnagelvin Area Hospital, Londonderry BT47 1JD Tel: 02871 345171 — MB BCh BAO Belf. 1969; MRCP (UK) 1972; MD Belf. 1976; FRCP Lond. 1987; FRCP(I) 1997; FACG (US) 1999. Cons. Phys. & Gastroenterol. Altnagelvin Hosp. Londonderry; Hon. Sen. Lect. Qu.'s Univ. Belf. Specialty: Gen. Med.; Gastroenterol. Socs: Brit. & Irish Soc. Gastroenterol.; Amer. Coll. Gastroenterol.; Amer. Soc. Dig. Endoscop. Prev: Sen. Tutor (Med.) Qu. Univ. Belf.; Sen. Fell. (Gastroenterol.) Univ. Washington Seattle, USA; Research Fell. Roy. Vict. Hosp. Belf.

O'CONNOR, Francis Anthony The Surgery, 9 Albion Street, Brighton BN2 2PS Tel: 01273 601122/601344 Fax: 01273 623450; 87 Stanford Avenue, Brighton BN1 6FA Tel: 01273 509535 — MB ChB Sheff. 1980; RMN 1968; RGN 1970. Specialty: Gen. Pract.

O'CONNOR, Ian Oak Tree Surgery, Whitethorn Drive, Brackla, Bridgend CF31 2PQ Tel: 01656 657134 — MB BS Lond. 1990 (St. Mary's) BSc (Hons.) Lond. 1986; DCH RCP Lond. 1994; MRCGP 1996. Socs: BMA; Brain Res. Assn.

O'CONNOR, Mr Ivan Mathew Thomas James, Group Capt. RAF Med. Br. Retd. (retired) 2 Vicarage Close, Wendover, Aylesbury HP22 6DS — MB BCh BAO NUI 1942 (Univ. Coll. Dub.) FRCOphth; BSc NUI 1944; MCh 1949, DPH 1944; DOMS Eng. 1948; FCOphth 1990. Prev: Cons. Adviser Ophth. RAF.

O'CONNOR, James Civic Medical Centre, Civic Way, Bebington, Wirral CH63 7RX Tel: 0151 645 6936 Fax: 0151 643 1698; Merlewood, 73 Church Road, Bebington, Wirral CH63 3EA Tel: 0151 334 2585 — MB ChB Liverp. 1974; DRCOG 1977. GP Princip.; Sec. Wirral Local Med. Comm. Specialty: Care of the Elderly. Socs: BMA; Birkenhead Med. Soc. Prev: Trainee GP Wirral VTS; Ho. Phys. & Ho. Surg. Wirral AHA.

O'CONNOR, James Patrick Bernard 10 Moss Lane, Timperley, Altrincham WA15 6SZ — MB BS Lond. 1998. SHO (Urol.) Pinderfields Gen. Hosp. Wakefield.

O'CONNOR, Janet Elizabeth Rosemary Medical Centre, 2 Rosemary Gardens, Parkstone, Poole BH12 3HF Tel: 01202 741300 Fax: 012020 721868 — MB BS Lond. 1970 (Univ. Coll. Hosp.) MRCS Eng. LRCP Lond. 1970; DA Eng. 1972; DObst RCOG 1974. Specialty: Dermat. Prev: Clin. Med. Off. (Paediat.) E. Dorset HA; SHO (Anaesth. & Paediat.) P'boro. Dist. Hosp.; SHO (O & G) Poole Gen. Hosp.

O'CONNOR, Joan Mary Ladybarn Group Practice, 177 Mauldeth Road, Fallowfield, Manchester M14 6SG Tel: 0161 224 2873 Fax: 0161 225 3276; 47 Moorland Road, Didsbury, Manchester M20 6BB Tel: 0161 434 5148 — MB ChB Manch. 1990 (Manc.) Dip Family Plann Lond. 1993; DCH RCP Lond. 1993; DRCO Lond. 1993; MRCGP 1995; Dip Pract Dermatol 1997. Princip. in Gen. Pract. Specialty: Gen. Pract. Socs: MRCGP. Prev: Regist. GP Withenshawe; SHO Withenshawe VTS.

O'CONNOR, John Brendan Grove Village Medical Centre, 4 Cleeve Court, Grove Village, Bedfont, Feltham TW14 8SN Tel: 020 8751 6282; 3 Churchill Avenue, Harrow HA3 0AX — LRCPI & LM, LRSCI & LM 1961; LRCPI & LM, LRCSI & LM 1961.

O'CONNOR, John Charles Rosemary Medical Centre, 2 Rosemary Gardens, Parkstone, Poole BH12 3HF Tel: 01202 741300 — MB BS Lond. 1971 (Univ. Coll. Hosp.) DObst RCOG 1975; MRCGP 1976. Clin. Asst. (Dermat.) Poole Gen. Hosp. Prev: GP Tutor & Trainee Course Organiser Poole.

O'CONNOR, Karen Ruth 1 High Leigh, Sheffield Road, Hathersage, Hope Valley S32 1DA Tel: 01433 659 979 — MB ChB Sheff. 1984; DFFP 1993; MRCGP 1994. Specialty: Gen. Pract.

O'CONNOR, Kathleen Ann 41 Slaidburn Street, Chelsea, London SW10 0JW— MB BCh BAO NUI 1979.

O'CONNOR, Kerry Michael Endless Street Surgery, 72 Endless Street, Salisbury SP1 3UH Tel: 01722 336441 Fax: 01722 410319 — MB ChB Bristol 1979; BSc Bristol 1976, MB ChB 1979; MRCOG 1984; MRCGP 1985. Prev: Trainee GP Portishead Health Centre; SHO (Geriat.) Ham Green Hosp.; SHO (O & G) Bristol Matern. Hosp.

O'CONNOR, Kerstin Birgit 154 Silverhere Road, Catford, London SE6 4QT — MB ChB Leic. 1996.

O'CONNOR, Leo Declan Williams, O'Connor and Morgan, New Quay Surgery, Church Road, New Quay SA45 9PB Tel: 01545 560203 Fax: 01545 560916; Vaynor, High Street, New Quay

SA45 9NY Tel: 01545 560203 — MB BCh BAO NUI 1984; DCH NUI 1986.

O'CONNOR, Louise Margaret 65 Gleneagles Road, Urmston, Manchester M41 8SB — MB ChB Leeds 1994.

O'CONNOR, Margaret Thanet, 257 Abington Avenue, Northampton NN3 2BU Tel: 01604 713542 — LRCPI & LM, LRSCI & LM 1934; LRCPI & LM, LRCSI & LM 1934. Sch. Med. Off. N.ants.

O'CONNOR, Margaret Mary 8 Homelands Road, Sale M33 4BE — MB ChB Liverp. 1998.

O'CONNOR, Mark Dennis 85 Aylward Road, Merton Park, London SW20 9AJ — MB BS Lond. 1989.

O'CONNOR, Mary Brigid 46 Poppythorn Lane, Prestwich, Manchester M25 3BY — BM BS Nottm. 1992; FRCA 2000. Anesthetic Research Fell. Queen's Med. Centre Nottm.

O'CONNOR, Mary Gerardine Royal Belfast Hospital for Sick Children, 180 Falls Road, Belfast BT12 6BE Tel: 028 90240503 Ext: 3976; 2 Sharman Road, Stranmills, Belfast BT9 5FW — MB BCh BAO Belf. 1984; MRCP (UK) 1988. Cons. Paediat. (Nephrol.) Roy. Belf. Hosp. Sick Childr. Specialty: Paediat.; Nephrol. Prev: Sen. Regist. (Paediat. Nephrol.) Southmead Hosp. Bristol.

O'CONNOR, Mary Regina Anaesthetic Department, Southern General Hospital, Glasgow G51 4TF Tel: 0141 201 1100 — MB BCh BAO NUI 1986; FFA RCSI 1990. Cons. Anaesth. Gtr. Glas. HB. Specialty: Anaesth. Prev: Sen. Regist. & Career Regist. (Anaesth.) Gtr. Glas. HB.

O'CONNOR, Michael Department of Anaesthetics, Princess Margaret Hospital, Okus Road, Swindon SN1 4JU Tel: 01793 536231 Fax: 01793 431023 — MB ChB Bristol 1978; FRCA 1982; T(Anaes.) 1991. Cons. Anaesth. Swindon & MarlBoro. NHS Trust. Specialty: Anaesth. Socs: Pain Soc.; BMA & Assn. Anaesth. Prev: Sen. Regist. (Anaesth.) Nuffield Dept. Anaesth. Oxf.; Sen. Regist. (Anaesth. & Intens. Care) Adelaide, S. Austral.; Regist. (Anaesth.) Sir Humphry Davy Dept. Anaesth. Bristol.

O'CONNOR, Mr Michael Andrew 12 Ferndene Road, Withington, Manchester M20 4TT Tel: 0161 434 5148 Email: mike@oconn49.freeserve.co.uk — MB ChB Manch. 1989; FRCS Ed. 1994. Orthop. Specialist Regist., Mersely Region, Liverp. Specialty: Orthop.

O'CONNOR, Michael John Christopher 5 Viewpoint, Sandbourne Road, Alum Chine, Bournemouth BH4 8JP — MB BS Lond. 1981 (Guy's) MRCS Eng. LRCP Lond. 1981.

O'CONNOR, Michael Pearse 47 Albany Road, New Malden KT3 3NY — MB BCh BAO NUI 1991.

O'CONNOR, Niall Finbarr Dublin Road Surgery, 4 Dublin Road, Castlewellan, Newcastle BT31 9AG Tel: 028 4372 3221 Fax: 028 4372 3162 — MB BCh BAO NUI 1979; DRCOG 1983; MRCGP 1983.

O'CONNOR, Nigel Timothy James 82 The Mount, Shrewsbury SY3 8PN Tel: 01743 343068 Fax: 01743 343068 — MB BS Lond. 1977 (St. Thos.) MRCP (UK) 1981; MD Lond. 1986; MRCPath 1988; FRCP Lond. 1996. Cons. Haemat. Roy. Shrewsbury Hosp. Specialty: Haematology. Prev: Sen. Regist. Roy. Free Hosp. Lond.; MRC Train. Fell. Nuffield Dept. Med. John Radcliffe Hosp. Oxf.; Regist. (Gen. Med.) Norf. & Norwich Hosp.

O'CONNOR, Patricia Accident & Emergency Unit, Hairmyres Hospital, East Kilbride, Glasgow G75 8RG Tel: 014120292; Nethershields Farm, Quarter, Hamilton ML3 7XP — MB ChB Dundee 1987; MRCP (UK) 1990; FRCS A&E 1995. Cons. (A & E) Hairmyres Hosp. Hairmyres E. Kilbride. Specialty: Accid. & Emerg.; Paediat. Socs: BAEM; BMA.

O'CONNOR, Patrick Denis Hugh 41 Wallace Road, London N1 2PQ; Friary View, Kildare, Republic of Ireland Tel: 0145 21218 — MB BCh BAO Dub. 1986; DCH NUI 1987; MRCPI 1989; MRCOG 1992. Research Regist. (Gyn. Endoscopic Surg.) Roy. Free Hosp. Lond. Specialty: Obst. & Gyn. Prev: Regist. Rotat. Univ. Coll. Hosp. Lond.; SHO (Obst.) Qu. Charlottes Hosp.; SHO Rotat. (O & G) Rotunda & Hammersmith Hosp.

O'CONNOR, Patrick Joseph Gilbert Bain Hospital, Lerwick ZE1 0TB Tel: 01595 743000 — MB ChB Leeds 1989; FRCA 1995. Cons. Anaesth. Specialty: Anaesth.

O'CONNOR, Peter Francis Michael 75 The Ridgeway, Watford WD17 4TJ — MB BS Lond. 1964 (Lond. Hosp.) MRCS Eng. LRCP Lond. 1963; FRCOG 1989, M 1970. p/t GP Locum. Prev: GP Watford.

O'CONNOR, Philip James Missy Cottage, Crag Lane, Huby, Leeds LS17 0BW — MB ChB Manch. 1987.

O'CONNOR, Phillip Joseph 33 Killeaton Park, Dunmurry, Belfast BT17 9HE — MB BCh Belf. 1998.

O'CONNOR, Rory Daniel 21 South Drive, Harrogate HG2 8AT Tel: 01423 527584 — MB ChB Manch. 1990; DTM & H Liverp.; MSc Robert Gordon Aberd. 1998. Med. Servs. Manager Agipkco Kazathstan. Prev: Med. Off. Brit. Antarctic Survey; SHO (A & E) Stoke Mandeville Hosp.

O'CONNOR, Ruth Christine 1 Hermitage Close, Appley Bridge, Wigan WN6 9JQ — MB ChB Ed. 1988; MRCP (UK) 1991. Specialty: Paediat.

O'CONNOR, Simon Philip John The Hollies Medical Centre, 20 St. Andrews Road, Sheffield S11 9AL Tel: 0114 255 0094 Fax: 0114 258 2863 — BM Soton. 1986.

O'CONNOR, Simon Roderick Department of Histopathology, Leicester Royal Infirmary, Leicester LE1 5WW Tel: 0116 254 1414; Chehalis, Ballyglan, Woodstown, Waterford, Republic of Ireland — MB BCh BAO NUI 1993 (University College Dublin) Dip RCPath 1998. Specialty: Histopath.

O'CONNOR, Siobhan Anne Downshire Hospital, Ardglass Road, Downpatrick BT30 6RA Tel: 01396 613311 — MB BCh BAO Belf. 1977; DRCOG 1980; MRCPsych 1984; MMedSci (Psychother.) 1989. Cons. Psychiat. Psychotherap. Downshire Hosp. Downpatrick. Specialty: Gen. Psychiat.; Psychother. Prev: Sen. Regist. (Psychother.) Day Hosp. Belf.

O'CONNOR, Susan Barrow Hospital, Long Ashton, Bristol BS48 3SG Tel: 0117 939 2811; Yew Tree House, Brinsea Road, Congresbury, Bristol BS49 5JQ — MB BChir Camb. 1975; BA Camb. 1972, MB BChir 1975; MRCPsych 1981. Clin. Dir. Ment. Health Servs. United Bristol Healthcare Trust. Specialty: Gen. Psychiat.

O'CONNOR, Terence Patrick 377 Garstang Road, Fulwood, Preston PR2 3LN Tel: 01772 863366 — MB ChB Manch. 1976; BSc St. And. 1973; DRCOG 1978; MRCGP 1986; FRCGP 1997.

O'CONNOR, Timothy John (retired) 4 Beauford House, The Hollow, Bamford, Hope Valley S33 0AU — MB BCh BAO NUI 1955 (Cork) Prev: Ho. Off. St. Luke's Matern. Hosp. Bradford.

O'CONOR, Helen Mary Nell Saltway Farm, Northleach, Cheltenham GL54 3QB Tel: 01285 720110 — MB BS Lond. 1975 (St. Mary's) MRCS Eng. LRCP Lond. 1975. Prev: Med. Dir. Hospice of St. Francis Berkhamsted.

O'DAIR, Graham Nelson 4 Avondale Gardens, West Bolden, East Boldon NE36 0PR — MB ChB Manch. 1994.

O'DAIR, Jonathan David 4 Avondale Gardens, West Boldon, East Boldon NE36 0PR — MB ChB Liverp. 1997.

O'DALY, Eamon Francis Savile Road Surgery, 90 Savile Road, Savile Town, Dewsbury WF12 9LP Tel: 01924 465725 — LRCPI & LM, LRSCI & LM 1958 (RCSI) LRCPI & LM, LRCSI & LM 1958. GP Dewsbury. Prev: Maj. RAMC, Regtl. Med. Off. Yorks. Brig. Depot Strensall; Ho. Surg. & Ho. Phys. Chesterfield Roy. Hosp.

O'DEA, Geraldine Anne Flat C, 1 Upper Hamilton Road, Brighton BN1 5DF — MB BCh BAO NUI 1984 (Univ. Coll. Galway) MRCGP 1990; MPH NUI 1993. Sen. Regist. Rotat. (Pub. Health Med.) Merton, Sutton & Wandsworth HA. Specialty: Pub. Health Med. Socs: BMA. Prev: Sen. Regist. (Pub. Health Med.) W. Sussex HA.

O'DEA, John Francis c/o Department of Anaesthetics, Dudley Road Hospital, Birmingham B18 7QH Fax: 0121 554 3801 Email: jfod@compuserve.com — MB BCh BAO NUI 1982 (Galway) FFA RCSI 1986. Cons. Anaesth. & Intens. Care Dudley Rd. Hosp. Birm.; Hon. Clin. Lect., Univ. of Birm. Specialty: Anaesth.; Intens. Care. Socs: Intens. Care Soc.; BMA. Prev: Sen. Regist. (Intens. Care Unit) Qu. Eliz. Hosp. Adelaide.

O'DELL, Ellen Guy's Hospital, PICU Guy's Hospital, St Thomas Street, London SE1 9RT Tel: 020 7955 5000 — MB BCh BAO NU Irel. 1996; BMedSci; MRCPCH. Fell. (Paediat. Intens. Care) Guy's Hosp. Lond. Specialty: Paediat. Special Interest: Paediatric Intens. Care.

O'DOHERTY, Andrew Hassengate Medical Centre, Southend Road, Stanford-le-Hope SS17 0PH Tel: 01375 673064 Fax: 01375 675196 — MB BS Lond. 1989; BSc Lond. 1986, MB BS 1989.

O'DOHERTY, Ann Jacinta 17 Oakwood Park, Malone Court, Belfast BT9 6SE — MB BCh BAO NUI 1981; LRCPI & LM, LRCSI & LM 1981; MRCPI 1983; FRCR 1987; FFR RCSI 1993. Cons. Radiol.

Roy. Vict. Hosp. Belf. Specialty: Radiol. Prev: Regist. (Radiol.) Roy. Vict. Hosp. Hosp. Belf.

O'DOHERTY, Catherine Anne St. Francis' Hospice, The Hall, Havering-atte-Bower, Romford RM4 1QH — MB BS Lond. 1992; BSc (Hons.) Lond. 1986; PhD Camb. 1990; MRCP (UK) 1995. Specialty: Palliat. Med.

O'DOHERTY, Catherine Mary 8 Kendal Road, Hove BN3 5HZ — MB BCh BAO Dub. 1982; MB BCh Dubl. 1982; MRCPI 1985.

O'DOHERTY, Conor St John 100 Harley Street, London W1G 7JA Tel: 0207 935 3468 — MB BCh BAO NUI 1970 (Univ. Coll., Dub.) MRCP (UK) 1979; MSc (Lond.) 1980; FRCP 1998. p/t Cons. Dermatol., E. & N. Herts Trust, QE II Hosp., Welywn Garden City. Specialty: Dermat. Special Interest: Eczema in Childr.; Functional Med.; Skin Surgery. Socs: Amer. Acad. Dermat.; Brit. Assn. Dermat.; Roy. Soc. Med. Prev: Lect. Dermat., Univ. of Edin.; Sen. Ho. Off., Roy. Marsdon Hosp., Lond.

O'DOHERTY, Mr Declan Patrick William Department of Orthopaedic Surgery, A4, University of Wales Hospital, Heath Park, Cardiff CF14 4XW Tel: 029 2074 3866 Fax: 029 2074 5399 — MD Sheff. 1994; MB BS Lond. 1981; MRCS Eng. LRCP Lond. 1981; FRCS Ed. 1985; MD Univ. Sheff. 1994. Cons. Orthop. Surg. Univ. of Wales Hosp. Specialty: Orthop. Socs: Fell.Brit. Orthopaedic Assoc.; Brit. Orth. Foot Surg.s Soc.; Brit. Soc. Child Orthopaedic Surg.s. Prev: Lect. (Orthop.) Surg. Sheff.; Clin. Research Fell. (Human Metab. & Clin. Biochem.ry) Sheff.

O'DOHERTY, Kim Saundersfoot Medical Centre, Westfield Road, Saundersfoot SA69 9JW Tel: 01834 812407 Fax: 01834 811131; Tanglewood, Narberth Road, Tenby SA70 8HX — MB BCh Wales 1979; MA Camb. 1979; DRCOG 1981; MRCGP 1990; Dip. Palliat. Med. Wales 1994; Dip. Therapeutics Wales 2001.

O'DOHERTY, Moya-Anne Mount Cottage, Shawclough Rd, Rochdale OL12 7HR — MB ChB Bristol 1997.

O'DOLAN, Carroll Anthony Temple Rusheen, Belcoo, Enniskillen BT93 5DU — MB BCh BAO Belf. 1990 (Queen's Belfast) LMCC (Ottowa, 1994); DFFP (UK) 1996; MRCGP (UK) 1997; DCH (UK) 1998.

O'DONNCHADHA, Benin Padhraic Cliff House, Ferryside SA17 5SP — MB BCh BAO Dub. 1979; MB BCh Dub. 1979; FFA RCS Eng. 1985; FFA RCSI 1986. Cons. Anaesth. P. Philip Hosp. LLa.lli. Specialty: Intens. Care; Anaesth.

O'DONNCHADHA, Mr Eamon Proinseas Royal Eye Hospital, Oxford Road, Manchester M13 9WL Tel: 0161 276 5226 Fax: 0161 272 6618 — MB BCh BAO NUI 1980; FRCS Ed. 1987; FRCOphth 1989. Cons. Ophth. Surg. Roy. Eye Hosp. Manch.; Lect. (Ophth.) Univ. Manch. Specialty: Ophth. Socs: Assn. for Research in Vision & Ophth., USA. Prev: Fell. Paediat. Ophth. Hosp. Sick Childr. Toronto, Canada; Fell. Glaucoma Moorfield Eye Hosp. Lond.; Resid. Moorfields Eye Hosp. Lond.

O'DONNELL, Aidan Mark St. John's Hospital at Howden, Howden Road W., Livingston EH54 6PP Tel: 01506 419666 — MB ChB Ed. 1996; BSc (Hons.) Ed. 1994. SHO (Anaesth.) St. John's Hosp. Livingston. Specialty: Anaesth. Socs: Ord. Mem. Assn. du Corps de Santé Internat. de Notre Dame de Lourdes.

O'DONNELL, Anne 63 Sandacre Road, Baguley, Wythenshawe, Manchester M23 1AP — MB ChB Dundee 1996.

O'DONNELL, Anthony John St. Martin's Health Centre, Les Camps du Moulin, St Martin's, Guernsey GY4 6DA Tel: 01481 237757 Fax: 01481 239591; Le Vieux Rouvet, St. Saviours, Guernsey GY7 9NB Tel: 01481 64414 — MB BS Lond. 1966 (Guy's) MRCS Eng. LRCP Lond. 1966; DObst RCOG 1968; DCH Eng. 1969; MRCGP 1976. Mem. Med. Staff Princess Eliz. Hosp. Guernsey. Socs: BMA (Ex-Chairm. Guernsey & Alderney Div.). Prev: Dep. Res. Med. Off. Middlx. Hosp. Lond.; SHO (Paediat.) King's Coll. Hosp.; Ho. Phys. Guy's-Evelina Hosp. Childr. Lond.

O'DONNELL, Catherine Anne-Marie The Chase, Heathlands Road, Wokingham RG40 3AS — MB BS Lond. 1991; MRCP; MRCGP; AFOM.

O'DONNELL, Charles James 75 Osprey Close, Snaresbrook, London E11 1SZ Tel: 020 8491 6510 — MB BS Lond. 1989; FFAEM; EOICM; DA (Lond.); MRCP (UK) 1993; FRCP 2003. Cons. (A & E) Whipps Cross Hosp. Lond. Specialty: Accid. & Emerg.; Intensive Care Medicine.

O'DONNELL, David Austen (retired) 21 Little Poulton Lane, Poulton-le-Fylde FY6 7ET — MB ChB Ed. 1968. Prev: GP Blackpool.

O'DONNELL, Declan Wake Green Surgery, 7 Wake Green Road, Moseley, Birmingham B13 9HD Tel: 0121 449 0300; 116 Oxford Road, Masbury, Birmingham B13 9SQ Tel: 0121 449 8778 — MB BCh BAO NUI 1987; LRCPI Leic. 1987. Police Surg. Prev: SHO (O & G) Good Hope Hosp. Birm.; SHO (Paediat.) Princess Roy. Hosp. Telford; SHO (A & E) Selly Oak Hosp. Birm.

O'DONNELL, Denis Rodney The Chase, Heathlands Road, Wokingham RG40 3AS — MB BCh BAO NUI 1965.

O'DONNELL, Elizabeth Ann 1 Maners Way, Cambridge CB1 8SL — MB BCh Wales 1980; DRCOG 1983; MRCGP 1985; DCH RCP Lond. 1986. Specialist Regist. Pub. Health Med. Anglia Regional Train. Scheme Ipswich. Specialty: Pub. Health Med.; Gen. Pract.; Gen. Psychiat. Socs: Med. Wom. Federat. Prev: GP Ruislip; Clin. Asst. (Community Adult Psychiat.) Mid-Anglia Community Health Trust Newmarket, Suff.

O'DONNELL, Emma Louise 16 Ashfield Road, Anderton, Chorley PR6 9PN — MB ChB Liverp. 1994.

O'DONNELL, Ennis Ignatius Ashton Health Centre, 67-69 Pedders Lane, Ashton-on-Ribble, Preston PR2 1HR Tel: 01772 726500 — MB ChB Glas. 1971; DObst RCOG 1973.

O'DONNELL, Helen Elizabeth 60 Upper Captain Street, Coleraine BT51 3LZ — MB BS Lond. 1998; MB BS Lond 1998.

O'DONNELL, Hugh, Surg. Lt.-Cdr. RN Retd. Farnham Health Centre, Brightwells, Farnham GU9 7SA Tel: 01252 723122; Silver Hill, 53 Dene Lane, Farnham GU10 3RJ Tel: 01252 737480 — MB ChB Ed. 1973; BSc (Med. Sci.) Ed. 1970, MB ChB 1973; MRCGP 1978; DRCOG 1981. Princip. Gen. Pract. Farnham. Prev: Gen. Pract. Vocational Trainee Helensburgh; Ho. Surg. Dunfermline & W. Fife Hosp.; Ho. Phys. (Cardiol.) West. Gen. Hosp. Edin.

O'DONNELL, Hugh Francis Deddington Health Centre, Earls Lane, Deddington, Banbury OX15 0TQ Tel: 01869 338611 Fax: 01869 37009; Grove Cottages, High St, Deddington, Banbury OX15 0SL Tel: 01869 — MB BS Lond. 1968.

O'DONNELL, James Gerard Mary Unilabs Clinical Trials Ltd., Bewlay House, 32 Jamestown Road, London NW1 7BY Tel: 020 7333 8436 Fax: 020 7424 0607; Ambleside, 90 London Road, Datchet, Slough SL3 9LQ Tel: 01753 548065 Fax: 01753 541325 — MB BCh BAO NUI 1978; DCH RCPSI 1981; DObst RCPI 1982; MRCGP 1985; Dip. Pharm. Med. RCP (UK) 1992; MFPM RCP (UK) 1993. Med. Dir. Chiltern Internat. Ltd.; Vis. Lect. Univ. Wales. Specialty: Pharmaceutical Medicine. Socs: Fell. Roy. Soc. Med.; Eur. Med. Research Gp. (Lond.). Prev: Sen. Clin. Research Regist. (Cardiol.) Wexham Pk. Hosp. Slough; Regist. (Med.) Ibn Al Bitar Parc, Baghdad; Regist. (Paediat.) Lourdes Hosp. Drogheda.

O'DONNELL, James Joseph, Col. late RAMC Retd. (retired) Primrose Cottage, Sandy Lane, Rushmoor, Farnham GU10 2ET Tel: 01252 790330 — LMSSA Lond. 1959 (St. Mary's) DA Eng. 1962; FFA RCS Eng. 1971. Prev: Cons. Anaesth. Army Med. Servs.

O'DONNELL, James Joseph Park House Surgery, 55 Higher Parr Street, St Helens WA9 1BP Tel: 01744 23705 Fax: 01744 454601; 9 Hard Lane, St Helens WA10 6JP Tel: 01744 611075 Fax: 01744 454601 Email: odonnell@gpiag-asthma.org — MB ChB Liverp. 1976; DRCOG 1978; T(GP) 1990. Chairm. St. Helens S. PCG; Med. Sec. St. Helens & Knowsley LMC. Specialty: Gen. Pract. Prev: SHO (Paediat.) Roy. Liverp. Child. Hosp. City Br.; Ho. Phys. & Ho. Surg. Birkenhead Gen. Hosp.; Ho. Off. Obst. Profess. Unit Mill Rd. Matern. Hosp. Liverp.

O'DONNELL, James Stewart 29 Five Acres, Dublin Road, Strabane BT82 9JD — MB BCh BAO Dub. 1990; MB BCh Dub. 1990.

O'DONNELL, Jill Frances The Valley Medical Centre, 14 Waller Close, Liverpool L4 4QJ Tel: 0151 207 3447; 280 Greenhill Road, Allerton, Liverpool L18 9SY — MB ChB Liverp. 1985; DRCOG 1992. GP Liverp. Prev: Clin. Med. Off./SHO (Community Paediat.) Sefton Gen. Hosp. Liverp.; SHO (Chest Med.) Regional Chest Unit Fazakerley Hosp. Liverp.; SHO (Med.) Arrowe Pk. Hosp. Wirral.

O'DONNELL, John White Lodge, Well Lane, Mollington, Chester CH1 6LD — MB ChB Manch. 1967; MRCGP 1978.

O'DONNELL, John Desmond Wingate Medical Centre, 79 Bigdale Drive, Liverpool L33 6YJ Tel: 0151 546 2958 Fax: 0151 546 2914 Email: johnodonnell@doctors.org.uk — MB ChB Liverp. 1981 (Liverpool) Socs: Assoc. Mem. RCGP. Prev: SHO (A & E & O & G) Whiston Hosp. Prescot; SHO (Gen. Med.) Morriston Hosp. Swansea.

O'DONNELL, John Gerald 11 Watersmeet, Northampton NN1 5SQ — MB ChB Glas. 1983; BSc (Hons.) Glas. 1980, MB ChB 1983.

O'DONNELL, John James Joseph Health Centre, Great James Street, Londonderry BT48 7DH Tel: 028 7137 8500; 5 Locarden, Culmore, Londonderry BT48 8RP Tel: 028 7135 1408 — MB BCh BAO NUI 1989; DRCOG 1993; MRCGP 1994.

O'DONNELL, Katrina Maria 179 St. Helens Road, Eccleston Park, Prescot L34 2QB — MB BCh BAO NUI 1987; LRCPI 1987.

O'DONNELL, Louise Virginia 52 Waterloo Road, Southport PR8 2NB — MB ChB Liverp. 1997.

O'DONNELL, Maire Teresa Kennedy Centre Surgery, 568 Falls Road, Belfast BT11 9AE Tel: 028 9061 1411 — MB BCh BAO NUI 1986.

O'DONNELL, Marie 28 Marine Drive, Hest Bank, Lancaster LA2 6EB — MB BCh Wales 1980.

O'DONNELL, Marie Department of Pathology, University of Edinburgh Medical School, Teviot Place, Edinburgh EH8 9AG Tel: 0131 650 2945 — MB BCh BAO NUI 1991. Regist. (Histopath.) Univ. Edin. Med. Sch. Specialty: Histopath.

O'DONNELL, Martin Antony Clarence House, 14 Russell Road, Rhyl LL18 3BY Tel: 01745 350680 Fax: 01745 353293; 1 Cwrt-y-Dderwen, Colwyn Bay LL29 7BF Tel: 01492 535431 — MB BCh BAO NUI 1985; MRCGP 1993. Mem. Denbighsh. A.C.P.C.; Vice-Chairm. N. Clwyd GP Co-op. Specialty: Diabetes. Socs: Roy. Coll. Gen. Pract.; Brit. Diabetic Assn.

O'DONNELL, Michael Handon Cottage, Markwick Lane, Loxhill, Godalming GU8 4BD Tel: 01483 208295 Fax: 01483 208270 — MB BChir Camb. 1952 (Camb. & St. Thos.) FRCGP 1990. Author & Broadcaster. Socs: GMC (Chairm. Professional Standards Comm.); BMA & Slagthorpe Med. Soc.; Hon. Mem. Alpha Omega Alpha Honor Med. Soc. Prev: GP; Edr. World Med.; Ho. Surg. St. Thos. Hosp. Lond.

O'DONNELL, Michael Joseph St. James Health Centre, 29 Great George Square, Liverpool L1 5DZ Tel: 0151 709 1120 — MB BCh BAO NUI 1943.

O'DONNELL, Michael Joseph Unum Provident, Milton Court, Dorking RH4 3LZ Tel: 01306 646032/07796 442366 Fax: 01306 873351 Email: michael.o'donnell@unumprovident.co.uk — MB ChB Manch. 1975; MFOM RCP Lond. 2001; DDAM 2004. CMO & Head of Med. Servs., Unum Provident; Hon. Vis. Prof., Univ. of Salford. Specialty: Occupat. Health. Socs: Occupat. Med. Soc.; Inst. Occupat. Health & Safety; Brit. Soc. Rehabil. Med. Prev: Force Med. Adviser (Occupat. Med.) Sussex Police; Med. Off. Brit. Nuclear Fuels Sellafield; Manager Med. Servs. Saudi Petrochem. Co. Saudi Arabia.

O'DONNELL, Neil Gerard Department of Anaesthesia, Western Infirmary, Dumbarton Drive, Glasgow G11 6NT Tel: 0141 211 2069 — MB ChB Glas. 1983; FFARCS 1988. Cons. Anaesth. West. Infirm. Glas. Specialty: Anaesth.

O'DONNELL, Patrick James Dept. of Histopathology, 2nd Floor, North Wing, St. Thomas's Hospital, Lambeth Palace Road, London SE1 7EH Fax: 020 7401 3661 — MB BCh BAO NUI 1975 (Univ. Coll. Galway Eire) MRCPath 1982; FRCPath 1994. Cons. Histopath. (Renal Path.) Guy's & St. Thos. Hosp. Trust Lond. Specialty: Histopath. Socs: Assn. of Clin. Pathologists; Renal Assn.; Europ. Renal Assn. Prev: Cons. (Histopath.) King's Coll. Hosp. Lond.; Lect. (Morbid. Anat.) St. Thos. Hosp. Lond.; Regist. (Path.) Sch. Med. Univ. Leeds.

O'DONNELL, Patrick Michael Joseph (retired) 6 Churchill Close, Streatley, Luton LU3 3PJ Tel: 01582 882502 Email: odon@ukonline.co.uk — MB BS Lond. 1961 (St. Mary's) DObst RCOG 1963; FRCGP 1981, M 1971. p/t Medical Officer, Benefit Agency; Locum GP.

O'DONNELL, Paul Noel Simon 67 Ashdon Road, Saffron Walden CB10 2AQ — BM BS Nottm. 1993; MRCP UK 1997.

O'DONNELL, Paula Anne Queen Street Surgery, 9-11 Queen Street, Whittlesey, Peterborough PE7 1AY Tel: 01733 204611 Fax: 01733 208926 — MB ChB Glas. 1989; MRCGP 1993. GP Whitlesey PeterBoro. Specialty: Gen. Pract.; Family Plann. & Reproduc. Health. Prev: SHO Psychiat. Boston; SHO Gynercology, PeterBoro.

O'DONNELL, Paula Sheila — MB BS Lond. 1984; BSc Lond. 1981; DCH RCP Lond. 1989. GP Princip., Brockley, Lond. Specialty: Gen. Pract. Prev: Clin. Asst. (Blood Transfus. & Apheresis) S. Thames Blood Transfus. Serv. Lond.

O'DONNELL, Peter John The Old Court House Surgery, Throwley Way, Sutton SM1 4AF Tel: 020 8643 8866 Fax: 020 8770 2629 — MB BS Lond. 1978 (St. Mary's) MRCS Eng. LRCP Lond. 1978; DRCOG 1984. Prev: GP Principle, GP Med. Unit, The Manor Dr.Worchester Par, Surrey.

O'DONNELL, Peter Sean Richard Binscombe Medical Centre, 106 Binscombe Lane, Godalming GU7 3PR Tel: 01483 415115 Fax: 01483 414925 — MB BS Lond. 1989.

O'DONNELL, Roddy Department of Paediatrics, Addenbrooke's Hospital, Hills Road, Cambridge CB2 2QQ Tel: 01223 245151 Email: drod@addenbrookes.nhs.uk — MB BS Lond. 1989 (UMDS (Guy's and St. Thomas' Hospital) London) MRCP; MRCP (UK) 1992; PhD Lond. 1997. Cons. in Paediatric Care, Addenbrooke's Hosp., Cambs. Specialty: Paediat.; Respirat. Med. Socs: MRCPCH. Prev: Lect. (Paediat. Infec. Dis.s) Imperial Coll. of Sci. Technol. & Med. St. Mary's Hosp. Lond.; Clin. Fell. (Pulm. Med.) Childr.'s Hosp. Med. Centre Cincinnati USA; Wellcome Train. Fell. (Respirat. Med.) St. Mary's Hosp. Med. Sch. Lond.

O'DONNELL, Ruaidhri (retired) Sunningdale, 7 Albany Avenue, Eccleston Park, Prescot L34 2QN Tel: 0151 426 5083 — MB BCh BAO NUI 1951.

O'DONNELL, Stanley John (retired) 39 Dean Road, South Shields NE33 4AS Tel: 0191 456 0232; 1 Primrose Drive, Oakdene Park Farm, Ashford TN23 3NP Tel: 01233 502758 — MB BS Durh. 1952 (Newc.) Prev: GP South Shields.

O'DONNELL, Valerie Anne Lancashire Teaching Hospitals & NHS Trust, Preston Acute Hospital, Shacoe Green Lane North, Fulwood, Preston PR2 9HT Tel: 01772 522055 Fax: 01772 522035 — MB ChB Leic. 1987 (Leic. Univ. Med. Sch.) MRCP (UK). Cons. (Palliative Med.) Lancs. Teachg. Hosps. NHS Trust.

O'DONOGHUE, Alison 9 Castlemead Walk, Kingsmead, Northwich CW9 8GP — MB ChB Ed. 1991 (Edinburgh) BSc Ed. 1991; DFFP 1994; DRCOG 1994; MRCGP 1995. Clin. Research Phys. Medeval Ltd. Manch. Specialty: Pharmacology.

O'DONOGHUE, Angela Elizabeth Marie Anna Derby City Hospital, Derby Tel: 01132 340141; The Coach House, Milicent Road, Nottingham NG2 7LD — BM BS Nottm. 1994; BMedSci (Hons) 1992; MRCP UK 1997. Specialist Regist. (Renal) Derby City Hosp. Specialty: Nephrol.

O'DONOGHUE, Beata Maria The Royal National Throat, Nose & Ear Hospital, Gray's Inn Road, London WC1X 8DA Tel: 020 7915 1300 Fax: 020 7833 5518; 150 Harley Street, London W1G 7LQ Tel: 020 7935 6000 Fax: 020 7584 4046 — MD Lodz, Poland 1969; FFA RCS Eng. 1980. Cons. Anaesth. Roy. Nat. Throat Nose & Ear Hosp. Lond. Specialty: Anaesth. Socs: Brit. Sleep Soc.; Roy. Soc. Med.

O'DONOGHUE, Charles Reid 34 Camperdown Street, Broughty Ferry, Dundee DD5 3AB — MB ChB Dundee 1991.

O'DONOGHUE, Dara Bartholomew 42 Hilltown Road, Mayobridge, Newry BT34 2HJ — MB BCh BAO Belf. 1993.

O'DONOGHUE, Dennis Michael 113 Cranley Gardens, London N10 3AE Tel: 020 8883 7090 Fax: 020 8883 7090 — MB ChB Otago 1946; DA Eng. 1950; FFA RCS Eng. 1953; FRCA 1992. Emerit. Cons. Anaesth. Univ. Coll. & Middlx. Hosp. Lond.; Hon. Cons. Anaesth. Roy. Nat. Orthop. Hosp. Lond. Specialty: Anaesth. Socs: Fell. Roy. Soc. Med.; BMA. Prev: Cons. Anaesth. Univ. Coll. Hosp., Roy. Nat. Orthop. Hosp. Lond. & Hosp. Trop. Dis.; Cons. Anaesth. Nat. Dent. Hosp.; Sen. Regist. (Anaesth.) Univ. Coll. Hosp.

O'DONOGHUE, Donal Joseph Department of Renal Medicine, Hope Hospital, Salford Royal Hospitals NHS Trust, Eccles New Road, Salford M6 8HD Tel: 0161 787 4389 Fax: 0161 787 5775; 6 Millstone Close, Poynton, Stockport SK12 1XS Tel: 01625 871381 — MB ChB Manch. 1980; BSc (1st cl. Hons. Physiol.) Manch. 1977; MRCP (UK) 1983; FRCP Lond. 1996. Cons. Renal & Gen. Phys. Hope Hosp. Salford; Hon. Lect. (Med.) Univ. Manch. Specialty: Nephrol. Socs: Amer. Soc. Nephrol.; RCP Edin.; Renal Assn. Exec. 2000-2004. Prev: Sen. Regist. (Nephrol. & Gen. Med.) Roy. Infirm. Edin.; MRC Trav. Fell. Hopital Necker Paris; Regist. (Nephrol.) Manch. Roy. Infirm.

O'DONOGHUE, Eamon 16 Daryngton Avenue, Birchington CT7 9PS Tel: 01843 42449 — MB BCh BAO NUI 1949 (Cork) LM Nat. Matern. Hosp. 1949; AFOM RCPI 1978. Dep. Chief Staff Med.

Serv. ILEA. Prev: Cas. Off. Radcliffe Infirm. Oxf.; Res. Med. Off. Osler Sanat. Oxf.; Ho. Surg. (Gyn.) Churchill Hosp. Oxf.

O'DONOGHUE, Mr Gerard Mary Department of ENT, Queen's Medical Centre, Derby Road, Nottingham N67 2UH Tel: 0115 970 9224 Fax: 0115 970 9748 Email: sarah.gregory@mail.qmcuh-tr.trent.nhs.uk — MB BCh BAO NUI 1975 (Univ. Coll. Dub.) FRCSI 1979. Cons. ENT Surg., Queens Med. Centre, Nottm. Specialty: Otolaryngol. Socs: Roy. Soc. of Med. Prev: Regist. (Gen. Surg.) Regional Hosp. & Mercy Hosp. Cork.; SHO (Neurosurg.) St. Finbarr's Hosp. Cork.; Regist. Roy. Nat. Throat, Nose & Ear Hosp. Lond.

O'DONOGHUE, James 1 Reddish Avenue, Whaley Bridge, High Peak SK23 7DP — MB ChB Liverp. 1948.

O'DONOGHUE, John Patrick Marsh House Medical Centre, 254 Marsh House Avenue, Billingham TS23 3EN Tel: 01642 561282/565068 Fax: 01642 565982; Redwalls, 15 Thornton Road, Thornton, Middlesbrough TS8 9BS Tel: 01642 597443 — MB BCh BAO NUI 1978; DRCOG 1980; DCH Dub. 1982; MRCGP 1982.

O'DONOGHUE, Maire Anne Therese Leighton Hospital, Middlewich Road, Crewe CW1 4QJ Tel: 01270 255141 — MB BCh BAO Dub. 1982; MA Dub. 1992, MB BCh 1982; MRCPath 1990; FRCPath 1998. Cons. Microbiol. Leighton Hosp. Crewe. Specialty: Med. Microbiol.

O'DONOGHUE, Margaret Mary (retired) Greetwell Cottage, 1 Greetwell Gate, Lincoln LN2 4AW Tel: 01522 532728 — MB BCh BAO NUI 1948; Cons. Anaesth. Co. Hosp. Lincoln; DA Eng. 1955. Prev: Cons. Anaesth. Lincoln Co. Hosp.

O'DONOGHUE, Michael Francis 1 Eaton Court, Water Eaton Road, Oxford OX2 7QT; Brentwood, Willoughby-on-the-Wold, Leicester LE12 6SZ Tel: 01509 880494 Fax: 01509 156467 — MB BS Lond. 1985 (Univ. Coll. Hosp.) BSc Lond. 1982; MRCP (UK) 1988. Cons. NeUrol., Nottm. Prev: SHO (Gen. Med.) Hammersmith Postgrad. Hosp. Lond. & Lond Chest Hosp.; Ho. Off. (Gen. Med.) Univ. Coll. Hosp. Lond.; SHO (Gen. Med.) John Radcliffe Hosp. Oxf.

O'DONOGHUE, Michael Geoffrey The Surgery, H. M. Tower of London, 2 Tower Green, London EC3N 4AB — LRCPI & LM, LRSCI & LM 1957; LRCPI & LM, LRCSI & LM 1957. Phys. BUPA Med. Centre Lond. Prev: Ho. Phys. & Ho. Surg. W. Cornw. Hosp. Penzance; Clin. Asst. Roy. Nat. Throat, Nose & Ear Hosp. Lond.

O'DONOGHUE, Mr Neil 99 Harley Street, London W1G 6AQ Tel: 020 7935 6200 Fax: 020 7224 6177 — MB BCh BAO NUI 1963; FRCS Eng. 1967. Cons. Urol. St. Peter's Hosp. Lond.; Sen. Lect. Inst. Urol. Lond. Specialty: Urol. Socs: Internat. Soc. Urol. & Brit. Assn. Urol. Surgs. Prev: Vis. Assoc. Univ. Iowa Hosps., USA; Sen. Regist. St. Bart. Hosp. Lond.; Resid. Hammersmith Hosp.

O'DONOGHUE, Nora Brigid 12 Sandileigh Avenue, Manchester M20 3LW — MB ChB Glas. 1994.

O'DONOGHUE, Patrick 5 Stanmore Road, Stevenage SG2 2QA Tel: 01438 749734 Fax: 01438 749734 — MB BCh BAO NUI 1982 (Cork) DCH RCPSI 1984; DObst RCPI 1985; MRCGP 1987.

O'DONOGHUE, Paula 42 Hilltown Road, Mayobridge, Newry BT34 2HJ — MB BCh BAO Belf. 1994. SHO (Med.) Antrim Area Hosp. Prev: Ho. Off. Belf. City Hosp.

O'DONOHOE, Jarlath Michael 21 Scaffog Avenue, Enniskillen BT74 7JJ — MB BCh BAO NUI 1978; MSc Lond. 1986; MRCP (UK) 1986. Cons. Paediat. & Community Paediat. Qu. Mary's Univ. Hosp. Roehampton & Roehampton, Twickenham & Richmond HA. Specialty: Paediat. Prev: Lect. (Paediat.) Char. Cross & Westm. Med. Sch.; Cons. Paediat. Taif Saudi Arabia; Regist. Roy. Hosp. for Sick Childr. Glas.

O'DONOHUE, John William University Hospital Lewisham, London SE13 6LH Tel: 020 8333 3000 Ext: 6182 Fax: 020 83333 3093 Email: johnod13@yahoo.com; 53 Lee Terrace, London SE3 9TA Tel: 020 8852 8717 Fax: 020 8333 1777 — MB BCh BAO Dub. 1987 (Univ Dub.) MRCPI 1989; MD 1998; MA 2000; FRCPI 2001; FRCP 2003. Cons. Gastroenterol. Univ. Hosp. Lewisham & King's Coll. Hosp. Specialty: Gastroenterol. Socs: Brit. Med. Assn. (BMA); (BSG) Brit. Soc. of Gastronetrology; (BASL) Brit. Assn. for the study of Liver Dis. W. Kent Chirurgic – Med. Soc. Prev: Sen. Regist. (Med & Gastroenterol.) W. Glas. Hosps. Trust; Research Fell. Inst. Liver Studies King's Coll. Hosp. Lond.; Regist. (Gastroenterol.) St. Bart. Hosp. Lond.

O'DONOHUE, Mary Bridget 2 Denbigh Road, Ealing, London W13 8PX — MB BCh BAO NUI 1957.

O'DONOVAN, Anne Louise (retired) Mill Farmhouse, Martlesham, Woodbridge IP12 4PB — MRCS Eng. LRCP Lond. 1962 (Roy. Free) Prev: GP Leighton Buzzard.

O'DONOVAN, Carmel Philomena 43 Taylor Avenue, Richmond TW9 4EB Tel: 020 8876 6661 Fax: 020 8876 6661 — MB BS Lond. 1981 (St. Mary's) MRCP (UK) 1984. Indep. Medico-Legal Cons. Richmond. Prev: Med. Secretariat Med. Defence Union.

O'DONOVAN, Dominic Gerard Oldchurch Hospital, Neuropathology Department, Waterloo Road, Romford RM7 0BE Tel: 01708 708121 Fax: 01708 708121 — MB ChB Liverp. 1983; MRCPath 1992; FRCPath 2000. Cons. Neuropath. Addenbrooke's Hosp. Camb. & Oldch. Hosp. Romford. Specialty: Neuropath.; Histopath. Special Interest: Muscle & Nerve Path.; Ocular Path. Socs: World Muscle Soc.; Brit. Neuropath. Soc.; Internat. Soc. Neuropath. Prev: Sen. Regist. (Neuropath.) Manch. Roy. Infirm. & Roy. Preston Hosp.; Regist. (Path.) South. Gen. Hosp. Glas.; SHO (Path.) Roy. Gwent Hosp. Newport.

O'DONOVAN, Ellen Christina The Corner House, Coates, Cirencester GL7 6NH Tel: 01285 770456 — MB BCh BAO NUI 1941.

O'DONOVAN, Gerard Barry (retired) The Cottage, Rainford, St Helens WA11 8NG Tel: 01744 882534 — (RCSI) LRCPI & LM, LRCSI & LM 1962. Prev: Clin. Med. Off. St. Helens & Knowsley HA.

O'DONOVAN, Isabel Andrea Mary Risedale Surgery, 2-4 Gloucester Street, Barrow-in-Furness LA13 9RX Tel: 01229 822332 Fax: 01229 433636; Well House, Bardsea, Ulverston LA12 9QY — MB BS Lond. 1989 (St Gearge's Hosp.Med.Sch.) DRCOG 1995; MRCGP 1995; DFFP 1995. GP Princ.

O'DONOVAN, Mr James John Market Street Surgery, 92 Market Street, Dalton-in-Furness LA15 8AB Tel: 01229 462591 Fax: 01229 468217; Well House, Bardsea, Ulverston LA12 9QY Tel: 01229 869573 — MB BS Lond. 1987 (Charing Cross & Westminster) FRCS Ed. 1992; MRCGP 1996. GP Full Partner. Prev: Trainee GP Cumbria Infirm., Carlisle.

O'DONOVAN, Mr John Peter Joseph, OBE(Mil), Lt.-Col. RAMC Retd. Ellengower, Garelochhead, Helensburgh G84 0EJ Tel: 01436 811085 Email: odonovan@btinternet.com — MB BS Lond. 1967 (Westm.) MRCS Eng. LRCP Lond. 1967; FRCS Ed. 1978. Specialty: Gen. Surg. Special Interest: G.I.Endoscopy, Trauma (Military and Civil). Socs: Founding Fell. Acad. Med. (Surg.) Hong Kong; Fell. Hong Kong Coll. Surgs.; Founder Vice-Pres. New Medico-Legal Soc. of Hong Kong. Prev: Priv. Cons. Gen. & Traum. Surg. Hong Kong; Sen. Cons. Surg. Brit. Milit. Hosp. Hong Kong; Sen. Regist. & Lect. (Surg.) St. Bart. Hosp. Lond.

O'DONOVAN, Maire Hammersmith Hospital, Du Cane Road, London W12 0HS — MB BCh BAO NUI 1992; LRCPSI 1992.

O'DONOVAN, Marie Rosarie 22 Olive Road, London NW2 6TX — MB BS Lond. 1997.

O'DONOVAN, Mary Josephine (retired) 22 Hogarth Way, Hampton TW12 2EL — MB BCh BAO NUI 1949; DCH NUI 1954; DPH NUI 1956; MFCM 1982.

O'DONOVAN, Michael Conlon Department of Psychological Medicine, University of Wales College of Medicine, Heath Park, Cardiff CF14 4XN Tel: 029 2074 3242 Fax: 029 2074 7839 Email: odonovanmc@cardiff.ac.uk — MB ChB Glas. 1983; BSc (Hons.) Glas. 1980, MB ChB 1983; MRCPsych 1987; PhD Wales 1994; FRCPsych 1999. Prof. (Psychiat. Genetics) Univ. Wales Coll. Med. Specialty: Gen. Psychiat.

O'DONOVAN, Nicholas Patrick Southlands, Park Lane, Barnstaple EX32 9AL — MB BCh BAO NUI 1973; FFA RCS Eng. 1981. Cons. Anaesth. N. Devon Dist. Hosp. Barnstaple. Specialty: Anaesth.

O'DONOVAN, Nicolas David 21 Orchard Road, Havant PO9 1AT Email: nick@thedonovans.freeserve.co.uk — MB ChB Birm. 1980; DRCOG 1983. GP; Med. Mem. Disabil. Appeal Tribunals for Indep. Tribunal Serv.; EMP for Benefits Agency. Socs: Assur. Med. Soc.

O'DONOVAN, Norah Mary (retired) Loreto, 57 York Avenue, Finchfield, Wolverhampton WV3 9BX Tel: 01902 656269 — MB BCh BAO NUI 1946.

O'DONOVAN, Patricia Anne Department of Obstetrics & Gynaecology, Queen's Park Hospital, Haslingden Road, Blackburn BB2 3HH — MB BCh BAO NUI 1980; BSc NUI 1975; MRCOG 1987; FRCS Ed. 1988; FRCOG 1999. Cons. O & G Qu. Pk. Hosp. Blackburn. Specialty: Obst. & Gyn. Prev: Lect. & Sen. Regist. (O &

G) St. Jas. Univ. Hosp. Leeds; Asst. Master Combe Lying-in Hosp. Dub.; Regist. (O & G) Mater Infirmorum Hosp. Belf.

O'DONOVAN, Patrick (retired) Loreto, 57 York Avenue, Finchfield, Wolverhampton WV3 9BX Tel: 01902 656269 — (Cork) MB BCh BAO NUI 1945.

O'DONOVAN, Mr Peter Joseph Cotswold, 3 Creskeld Crescent, Bramhope, Leeds LS16 9EH Tel: 01274 364888 Fax: 01274 366945 Email: podonovan@hotmail.com — MB BCh BAO NUI 1978 (National University of Ireland) FRCS Eng. 1982; MRCOG 1986. Cons. O & G Bradford Roy. Infirm. Specialty: Obst. & Gyn. Socs: Mem. Brit. Soc. Gyna. Endoscopy; Mem. Brit. Soc. Colposcopy and Cervical Pathol. Prev: Sen. Regist. (O & G) Leeds Gen. Infirm.; SHO (Perinatal Med.) Nat. Matern. Hosp. Dub.

O'DONOVAN, Timothy Joseph 160 Ribblesdale Road, Nottingham NG5 3HW Tel: 0115 263644 — MB BCh BAO NUI 1951 (Cork) Prev: Ho. Surg. Pk. Hosp. Davyhulme; SHO Paediat. Gen. Hosp. Burnley; Ho. Surg. Newc. Sanat. Co. Wicklow.

O'DOWD, Ruth Lena Royal Shrewsbury Hospital, Mytton Oak Road, Shrewsbury SY3 8XQ — MB ChB Dundee 1990; MB ChB Dundee 1990; FRCA 1996; FRCA 1996. Cons. Anaesth., Roy. Shrews. Hospt. Specialty: Anaesth. Prev: Regist. Rotat. (Anaesth.) Stoke-on-Trent.

O'DOWD, Clare Elizabeth Dr Ibrahim & Partners, Farnham Health Centre, Brightwells, Farnham GU9 7SA Tel: 01252 850018 Email: clare.odowd@virgin.net; Whitebridge, Redlands Lane, Crondall, Farnham GU10 5RF — MB BS Lond. 1991 (St Thomas' Hospital London) DRCOG 1995; DFFP 1995; MRCGP 1996. Specialty: Gen. Pract.

O'DOWD, Gerard Michael 444 Aigburth Road, Liverpool L19 3QE — MB BCh BAO Dub. 1987; MRCPath 1995, D 1994. Lect. (Path.) Univ. Liverp. Specialty: Histopath.

O'DOWD, John Gerard Mary Avenue Medical Centre, Wentworth Avenue, Slough SL2 2DG Tel: 01753 524549 Fax: 01753 552537 — MB BCh BAO Dub. 1981; MRCPI 1983; DCH RCP Lond. 1984; MRCGP 1985.

O'DOWD, John James Mallon 29 Ballater Crescent, Woodlands Gate, Wishaw ML2 7YJ — MB ChB Glas. 1996.

O'DOWD, John Joseph Department of Histopathology, Airedale General Hospital, Skipton Road, Steeton, Keighley BD20 6TD Tel: 01535 652511 — MB ChB Leeds 1982; MRCPath 1990; FRCPath 1999. Cons. Histopath. Airedale Gen. Hosp. Keighley. Specialty: Histopath.

O'DOWD, Mr John Kevin Centre for Spinal Studies & Surgery, Queens Medical Centre, Nottingham NG7 2UH Tel: 0115 924 9924 Fax: 0115 970 9991; 5 Tennis Drive, The Park, Nottingham NG7 1AE Tel: 0115 948 0760 — MB BS Lond. 1982; FRCS Ed. 1988; FRCS Eng. 1988; FRCS Orth. 1994. BOA Spinal Fell. Qu. Med. Centre Nottm. Specialty: Orthop. Socs: Fell. Roy. Soc. Med.; Brit. Trauma Soc. Prev: Sen. Regist. (Orthop.) St. Geo. Hosp. Lond.; Sen. Regist. Qu. Mary's Hosp. for Childr. Carshalton; Research Fell. Acad. Dept. (Orthop.) St. Thos. Hosp. Lond.

O'DOWD, Lorien Rachel Maudsley Hospital, Denmark Hill, London SE5 8AZ Tel: 020 7703 6333 Fax: 020 7919 2171 — BM BS Nottm. 1990; BMedSci Nottm. 1988. Regist. (Child Psychiat.) Maudsley Hosp. Lond. Specialty: Child & Adolesc. Psychiat.

O'DOWD, Sylvia 4 The Orchard, Malt House Lane, Wolverhampton WV6 9PF Tel: 01902 752311 — MRCS Eng. LRCP Lond. 1939 (Birm.) Prev: Sen. Med. Off. Wolverhampton Health Auth. Clin. Med. Off.; Wolverhampton Health Auth.; GP Wolverhampton.

O'DRISCOLL, Aisling Mary Department of Haematology, Worthing Hospital, Lyndhurst Road, Worthing BN11 2DH Tel: 01903 205111 Fax: 01903 285072 Email: aisling.o'driscoll@wash-tr.sthames.nhs.uk — MB BS Lond. 1986; MRCP (UK) 1989; DRCPath 1992; MRCPath 1997, D 1992. Cons. Haematologist. Worthing & Southlands Hosp. Trust, Worthing. Specialty: Haematology. Prev: Sen. Regist. St. Geo.'s Hosp., Lond..; Regist. & Jun. Lect. (Haemat.) Univ. Coll. Hosp. Lond..

O'DRISCOLL, Anthony Micael Birmingham & Midland Eye Centre, Western Road, Birmingham B18 7QU Tel: 0121 236 4911; 12 Fetherston Grange, Glasshouse Lane, Packwood, Lapworth, Solihull B94 6PX Tel: 0121 704 9187 — MB ChB Cape Town 1986; FRCOphth 1994. Regist. (Ophth.) Birm. & Midl. Eye Hosp. Specialty: Ophth. Socs: Midl. Ophth. Soc.; UK & Irel. Soc. of Cataract & Refractive Surgs.; Eur. Soc. Cataract & Refractive Surgs. Prev: SHO (Ophth.) Birm. & Midl. Eye Hosp. & Kent & Canterbury Hosp.; GP Canada; Regist. (Surg.) Vict. Hosp. Cape Town, S. Afr.

O'DRISCOLL, Anthony Micael Warwick Hospital, Lakin Road, Warwick CV34 5BW Tel: 01926 495321 Email: eyesurgeon@mac.com — MB ChB Cape Town 1986. Cons. Ophth. Surg., Warwick Hosp., Warwick; Hon. Cons. Vitreoretinal Surg., Coventry and Warks. Hosp., Coventry. Specialty: Ophth. Special Interest: Cataract Surg.; Vitreoretinal Surg. Socs: United Kingdom and Irel. Soc. of Cataract and Refractive Surgeons; Brit. and Eire Assn. of Vitreoretinal Surgeons; Europ. Soc. of Cataract and Refractive Surgeons. Prev: Vitreoretinal Fell., Birm. and Midl. Eye Centre 1999; Ophth. Regist., W. Midlands Rotat., 1994-1998.

O'DRISCOLL, Barry Joseph 1 Elm Grange, Cow Lane, Wilmslow Park, Wilmslow SK9 2AZ Tel: 01625 532828 Fax: 01625 537317 Email: barryjod@hotmail.com — MB ChB Manch. 1965. Clin. Asst. (Orthop.) Tameside Gen. Hosp. Prev: Ho. Off. (Med.) & Cas. Off. Salford Roy. Hosp.; Ho. Off. (Obst.) St. Mary's Hosp. Manch.

O'DRISCOLL, Bartholomew Ronan Campion Salford Royal Hospitals NHS Trust, Hope Hospital, Cardiorespiratory Medicine, Salford M6 8HD Tel: 0161 206 5154 Fax: 0161 206 4328 Email: ronan.odriscoll@srht.nhs.uk — MB BCh BAO (Hons.) NUI 1977; MD NUI 1983, BSc (1st cl. Hons.) 1974; MRCPI 1979; MRCP (UK) 1980; FRCP (UK) 1997. Cons. Phys. (Gen. & Respirat. Med.) Salford Roy. Hosps. NHS Trust. Specialty: Respirat. Med. Socs: Brit. Soc. Allergy & Clin. Immunol.; Brit. Thorac. Soc.; Eur. Respirat. Soc. Prev: Sen. Regist. (Thoracic Med.) Hope & Wythenshawe Hosps.; Clin. Lect. & Hon. Regist. Cardiothoracic Inst. & Brompton Hosp. Lond.; Regist. (Med.) Guy's Hosp. Lond. & Merlin Pk. Hosp. Galway.

O'DRISCOLL, Catherine Mary 114 Upper Street, Islington, London N1 1QN — MB BS Lond. 1978.

O'DRISCOLL, David Lawrence 52 Moorfield Road, Salford M6 7QD — MRCS Eng. LRCP Lond. 1986 (Univ. Columbia) Regist. (Psychiat.) Salford; NY State Licensing Auth. (Flex) 1992. Specialty: Gen. Psychiat. Prev: Intern & Resid. (Med.) Roosevelt Hosp., NY & Norwalk Hosp. Yale Univ.

O'DRISCOLL, Deirdre Patricia Springburn Health Centre, 200 Springburn Way, Glasgow G21 1TR Tel: 0141 531 9661 Fax: 0141 531 9666; 42 Upper Glenburn Road, Bearsden, Glasgow G61 4BN Tel: 0141 942 6976 — MB BCh BAO NUI 1986; MRCGP 1992; DRCOG 1992. Prev: SHO (O & G) City Hosp. Nottm.; SHO (Psychiat.) Pastures Hosp. Derby; Trainee GP Devon.

O'DRISCOLL, Denis Peter 13 Crescent Road, Hale, Altrincham WA15 9NB — MB BCh BAO NUI 1980.

O'DRISCOLL, Dilys Jane Fox Hollies Surgery, 511 Fox Hollies Road, Hall Green, Birmingham B28 8RJ Tel: 0121 777 1180; 6 Barbourne Close, Solihull B91 3TL — MB ChB Cape Town 1988; DRCOG 1992; DCH RCP Lond. 1993. Trainee GP Hall Green, Birm. Prev: SHO (Paediat.) Kent & Canterbury Hosp.; SHO (Geriat., A & E & O & G) Kent & Canterbury Hosp.

O'DRISCOLL, Fergal Alexander Westwood Surgery, 45-47 Westwood Avenue, Lowestoft NR33 9RW Tel: 01502 588854; 403 London Road S., Lowestoft NR33 0BJ Tel: 01502 584485 — MB BCh BAO NUI 1982. Clin. Asst. Lothingland Hosp.; Clin. Asst. LoW.oft & N. Suff. Hosp. Socs: BMA (Sec. Gt. Yarmouth & Waveney Div.). Prev: Trainee GP Merthyr & Cynon Valley HA VTS; SHO (Psychiat.) Bangour Village Hosp. W. Lothian Scotl.

O'DRISCOLL, Finnbarr Hugh Grange Road Welfare Centre, Grange Road, Widdrington, Morpeth NE61 5LX Tel: 01670 790229 Fax: 01670 791312 — MB BS Lond. 1968; MRCS Eng. LRCP Lond. 1968; DObst RCOG 1970. Prev: Hosp. Pract. (Psychiat.) St. Geo. Hosp. Morpeth.

O'DRISCOLL, Gary Captial Road Surgery, Higher Openshaw, Manchester M11 1LA Tel: 0161 370 2133 — MB BS Lond. 1997; BSc. GP; Med. Advisor/Team Phys. Ireland U21 Rugby Team. Specialty: Sports Med.

O'DRISCOLL, Jean Catherine Microbiology Department, Stoke Mandeville Hospital NHS Trust, Mandeville Road, Aylesbury HP21 8AL Tel: 01296 315330; 66 Woodstock Road S., St Albans AL1 4QH Fax: 01296 315389 Email: jean.o'driscoll@smh.nhs.uk — MB BCh BAO NUI 1984; MSc Lond. 1989; MRCPath 1991; FRCPath 2000. Cons. Microbiol. Stoke Mandeville Hosp. NHS Trust Aylesbury. Specialty: Med. Microbiol. Socs: Hosp. Infec. Soc.; Assn. Med. Microbiol.; Brit. Soc. Antimicrob. Chemother. Prev: Sen. Regist.

(Microbiol.) St. Geo. Hosp. Lond.; Regist. (Med. Microbiol.) Qu. Mary's Hosp. Lond.

O'DRISCOLL, John Brian The Beeches Consulting Centre, Alexandra Hospital Grounds, Mill Lane, Cheadle SK8 2PY Tel: 0161 428 4185 Fax: 0161 428 1692 — MB BS Lond. 1976 (Westm.) MRCS Eng. LRCP Lond. 1976; MRCP (UK) 1984; FRCP 1998. Cons. Dermatol. Stepping Hill Hosp., Stockport; Cons. Dermatol., Hope Hosp., Salford & Buxton Hosp., Buxton. Specialty: Dermat. Special Interest: Dermat. Prev: Regist. (Dermat.) Manch. Skin Hosp.

O'DRISCOLL, John Patrick Spring Gardens Health Centre, Providence Street, Worcester WR1 2BS Tel: 01905 681681 Fax: 01905 681699 — MB BS Lond. 1982; MRCGP 1987; DRCOG 1988. GP Worcester.

O'DRISCOLL, Maeve The Verwood Surgery, 54 Manor Road, Verwood BH31 7PY Tel: 01202 825353 Fax: 01202 829697; Ormiston, Moorside Road, West Moors, Ferndown BH22 0EJ — MB BS Lond. 1981. Specialty: Gen. Pract.

O'DRISCOLL, Margaret Christina 24 Gunterstone Road, London W14 9BU — MB BCh BAO Dub. 1979.

O'DRISCOLL, Melinda Jane The Brunswick Surgery, Oakhill Health Centre, Oakhill Road, Surbiton KT6 6EN Tel: 020 8390 5321 Fax: 020 8390 3223 — MB BS Lond. 1987 (St Georges Hospital Medical School) BSc (Hons.) Lond. 1984, MB BS 1987; DRCOG 1991; MRCGP 1992.

O'DRISCOLL, Mr Michael The South Cheshire Private Hospital, Leighton, Crewe CW1 4QP; The Old Croft, Legh Road, Knutsford WA16 8NR — MB ChB Leeds 1962; FRCS Eng. 1967; FRCS Eng. 1967; ChM Bristol 1973; ChM Bristol 1973. Cons. Orthop Surg. S. Chesh. - Indep. Pract. Specialty: Orthop. Socs: S.I.C.O.T. Prev: Indep. Pract. S. Chesh. Private Hosp. Crewe; Cons. Orthop. Leighton Hosp. Crewe & The Robt. Jones & Agnes Hunt Orthop. Hosp. Oswestry.

O'DRISCOLL, Patrick Michael 1 Harley Street, London W1N 1DA Tel: 020 7580 6191; Department of Oral & Maxillofacial Surgery, Guy's Hospital, London SE1 9RT Tel: 020 7955 4419 — MB BS Lond. 1961 (Guy's) FDS RCS Eng. 1963, L 1957; BDS (Hons.) Lond. 1958; MRCS Eng. LRCP Lond. 1961. Cons. Oral & Maxillofacial Surg. Guy's Hosp.; Head Dept. Oral & Maxillofacial Surg. Guy's Dent. Hosp. Specialty: Oral & Maxillofacial Surg. Socs: Fell. Brit. Assn. Oral & Maxillofacial Surg.; Chairm. Dent. Provident Soc.; BMA. Prev: Sen. Regist. (Dent. Surg.) & Ho. Surg. Dent. Dept. Qu. Vict. Hosp. E. Grinstead; Sen. Regist. (Oral Surg.) Inst. Dent. Surg. & Eastman Dent. Hosp.

O'DRISCOLL, Susan Catherine 2-6 Capital Road, Higher Openshaw, Manchester M11 1LA — MB BS Lond. 1976 (Westm.) BSc (Pharmacol.) Lond. 1973, MB BS 1976; DRCOG 1979. SHO (O & G) Heatherwood Hosp. Ascot. Prev: Ho. Surg. Westm. Hosp. Lond.; Ho. Phys. & Cas. Off. St. Stephen's Hosp. Lond.

O'DRISCOLL, Susan Leah (retired) The Old Croft, Legh Road, Knutsford WA16 8NR — MB ChB (Hons.) Leeds 1964; MRCP UK 1972; FRCP 1998.

O'DRISCOLL, Mr Thomas Gerard (retired) Calvert House, Greenway, Hutton Mount, Brentwood CM13 2NR Tel: 01277 223617 — MB BCh BAO NUI 1948; DO RCS Eng. 1951; FRCS Eng. (Ophth.) 1956; FCOphth. 1989. Prev: Cons. Ophth. Surg. Regional Eye Unit OldCh. Hosp. Romford.

O'DUCHON, Oscar 5 Linden Close, Saintfield, Ballynahinch BT24 7BH — MB BCh BAO NUI 1991.

O'DUFFY, Desmond Royal Gwent Hospital, Department of Ophthalmology, Block E, Cardiff Road, Newport NP20 2UB Tel: 01633 234234 Ext: 8443 — MB BCh BAO NUI 1985 (Dublin) FRCOphth. Cons. Ophth. Surg. at Roy. Gwent Hosp. with special interest in Glaucoma. Specialty: Ophth. Socs: SWOS.

O'DWYER, Anne-Marie 63 Grandison Road, London SW11 6LT — MB BCh BAO Dub. 1986 (Trinity Coll. Dublin.) MRCPsych 1991; MRCPL (Irl) 1998; MD (Trinity Coll. Dublin) 1999. Cons. Psychiat. Maudsley Hosp. Lond. Specialty: Gen. Psychiat.

O'DWYER, Mr Francis Gabriel Joseph Accident & Emergency Department, Burton Queens Hospital, Belverdere Road, Burton-on-Trent DE13 0RB Tel: 01283 511511 Ext: 5023 Email: frank.odwyer@burtonh-tr.wmids.nhs.uk — MB BCh BAO NUI 1981; FFAEM; BSc (Hons.) Dub. 1983; FRCSI 1987. Cons. A & E Burton Dist. Hosp. Specialty: Accid. & Emerg. Special Interest: Hand Injuries; Soft Tissue Injuries. Prev: Regist. (A & E) Leicester Roy. Infirm.

O'DWYER, Gearoid A Pontcae Surgery, Dynevor Street, Georgetown, Merthyr Tydfil CF48 1YE Tel: 01685 723931 Fax: 01685 377048.

O'DWYER, Hugh Studdert 1 Craig-yr-Haul Drive, Castleton, Cardiff CF3 2SA — MB BCh Wales 1970; FFA RCS Eng. 1975. Cons. (Anaesth.) Roy. Gwent Hosp. Newport. Specialty: Anaesth. Prev: Sen. Regist. (Anaesth.) Univ. Hosp. Wales Cardiff; SHO (Cas.) Cardiff Roy. Infirm.; SHO (O & G) Neath Gen. Hosp.

O'DWYER, Jane Mary Eileen Department of Psychiatry, University of Sheffield, Northern General Hospital, Sheffield S5 7AU Tel: 01142 715216; 46 Carter Knowle Road, Sheffield S7 2DX — MB BCh BAO NUI 1983 (Univ. Coll. Galway) MRCPsych 1991; MD 1997. Sen. Lect. (Psychiat. of Learining Disabil.) Univ. Sheff.; Hon. Cons. Psychiat. of Learning Disabil. Community Health Sheff. NHS Trust. Specialty: Gen. Psychiat.; Ment. Health. Prev: Sen. Regist. (Psychiat.) Leeds; Regist. (Psychiat.) Leicester.

O'DWYER, John Studdert (retired) Troed-y-Bryn, Abertridwr, Caerphilly CF83 4BH — MB BCh BAO NUI 1940 (Univ. Coll. Cork) Prev: Capt. RAMC.

O'DWYER, Joseph Patrick Department of Anaesthesia, Southlands Hospital, Upper Shoreham Road, Shoreham-by-Sea BN43 6TQ Tel: 01273 455622; Hillbrook, London Road, Albourne, Hassocks BN6 9BJ — MB BCh BAO NUI 1982; MRCP (UK) 1986; FCAnaesth 1989. Cons. Anaesth. Worthing & Southlands Hosps. NHS Trust. Specialty: Anaesth. Prev: Sen. Regist. (Anaesth.) Soton. Gen. Hosp.; Vis. Asst. Prof. Anesthesiol. Univ. Maryland, Baltimore, USA.

O'DWYER, Mr Kevin John Department of Orthopaedic Surgery, Worcester Royal Infirmary, Castle St., Worcester WR1 3AS Tel: 01905 760163 Fax: 01905 760163; Thurlesbeg, 224 Malvern Road, Worcester WR2 4PA Tel: 01905 425230 Fax: 01905 425230 — MB BCh BAO Dub. 1978 (Trinity Coll. Dublin) FRCS Eng. 1983; FRCS (Orth.) 1994. Cons. Orthop. Surg. Worcester Roy. Infirm. NHS Trust. Specialty: Orthop. Socs: Fell. BOA; Brit. Trauma Soc. Prev: Sen. Regist. Rotat. (Orthop.) Exeter & Truro; Regist. (Orthop.) Princess Eliz. Orthop. Hosp. Exeter & Roy. Cornw. Hosp. Truro.

O'DWYER, Patrick Dermot (retired) Eithinog Hall, Cyfronydd, Welshpool SY21 9ED — MB BS Lond. 1964 (Univ. Coll. Hosp.) MRCS Eng. LRCP Lond. 1964; MRCOG 1971.

O'DWYER, Professor Patrick Joseph University Department of Surgery, Western Infirmary, Glasgow G11 6NT Tel: 0141 339 8822 Fax: 0141 211 1972 Email: pjod25@clinmed.gla.ac.uk; 5 Fulton Gardens, Houston, Johnstone PA6 7NU Tel: 01505 324617 — MB BCh BAO NUI 1979; FRCSI 1983; MCh NUI 1986. Prof. (Gastrointestinal Surg.) Univ. Glas.; Hon. Cons. Surg. West. Infirm. Glas. Specialty: Gen. Surg. Socs: Surg. Research Soc.; Eur. Assn. Endoscopic Surg.; Assn. Surg. GB & Irel. Prev: Lect. (Surg.) Univ. Coll. Dub.

O'DWYER, Peter Francis The Surgery, 91 Dodworth Road, Barnsley S70 6ED Tel: 01226 282535 — MB BCh BAO NUI 1973 (Cork) DCH NUI 1975; DCH RCPSI 1975; DObst RCPI 1976; MRCGP 1977; DRCOG 1978; DGM RCP Lond. 1987; BA Open 1992. GP. Specialty: Gen. Pract. Socs: BMA. Prev: Intern St. Finbarr's Hosp. Cork; SHO (Gen. Pract.) Barnsley AHA.

O'DWYER, Sarah Theresa Patrice Christie Hospital, Wilmslow Road, Withington, Manchester M20 4BX Tel: 0161 446 3366 Fax: 0161 446 3365 Email: gill.harnson@christie-tr.nwest.nhs.uk — MB ChB Manch. 1979; BSc St. And. 1976; FRCS 1984; FRCS Edin. 1984; MD Manch. 1988. Cons. Surg. and Director of Surg. and Anaesthetics, Christie Hosp., Manch.; Cons. Surg. and Lead Colorectal Clinician, S. Manch. Univ. Hosp. Specialty: Gen. Surg. Special Interest: Colorectal Surgery. Socs: RSM; Manch. Med. Soc.; Assn. of Coloproctology. Prev: Cons. Surg. and Hon. Sen. Lect. Univ. Hosp. S. Birm.

O'DWYER, Teresa Mary Anderson Court, Berwick-upon-Tweed Tel: 01289 356910 — MB ChB Leeds 1986; MRCPsych 1991; MMedSci (Clin. Psychiat.) Leeds 1993. Community Psychiat. Anderson Ct., Berwick-upon-Tweed. Specialty: Gen. Psychiat. Socs: BMA; Roy. Coll. Psychiats. Prev: Cons. Psychiat. St. Geo. Hosp. N.d. Ment. Health Trust; Sen. Regist. Flexible Train. Scheme N. Deanary; Regist. Rotat. (Psychiat.) Leeds Train. Scheme.

O'FARRELL, Anne Marie — MB ChB Bristol 1997.

O'FARRELL, Brendan David West Bar Surgery, 1 West Bar Street, Banbury OX16 9SF Tel: 01295 256261 Fax: 01295 756848; 41

Church View, Banbury OX16 9NB Tel: 01295 264017 — MB BS Lond. 1971 (St. Bart.) MRCS Eng. LRCP Lond. 1971; DObst RCOG 1973; MRCGP 1976. Prev: Trainee GP Kettering & Dist. VTS; Ho. Phys. & Ho. Surg. Redhill Gen. Hosp.

O'FARRELL, Jeanne Mary Department Medicine for Elderly People, Whipps Cross Hospital, Whipps Cross Rd, Leytonstone, London E11 1NR Tel: 020 8539 5522 Fax: 020 8535 6970; Flat 2, 546 Caledonian Road, London N7 9SJ Tel: 020 7609 6712 — MB BCh BAO NUI 1977 (Univ. Coll. Dub.) MRCGP 1982; MRCP (UK) 1985; FRCP 2001. Cons. Med. for Elderly Whipps Cross Hosp. Lond. Specialty: Care of the Elderly. Socs: Brit. Geriat. Soc. Prev: Clin. Lect. (Geriat. Med.) Univ. Coll. & Middlx. Sch. Med. Univ. Coll. Hosp. Lond.; Regist. (Med.) Qu. Eliz. II Hosp. Welwyn Gdn. City Herts.; Ho. Surg. & Ho. Phys. Mater Miser. Hosp. Dub.

O'FARRELL, Nigel 44 Crookham Road, London SW6 4EQ — MB ChB Birm. 1976; MRCPI 1984; MRCGP 1986.

O'FARRELL, Thomas Denis Paul Flat 4 Chartwell, 4B Church Hill, Edinburgh EH10 6BQ Tel: 0131 452 8335 — (Univ. Coll. Dub.) MB BCh BAO NUI 1967; DPM Ed. & Glas. 1971; FRCPsych 1988, M 1972. Cons. Psychiat. (Psychother.) Roy. Edin. Hosp.; Traing. Psychoanal. Scott. Inst. of Human Relations Edin.; Hon. Sen. Lect. Univ. Edin. Specialty: Gen. Psychiat. Socs: Brit. Psychoanal. Soc. Prev: Sen. Lect. & Cons. (Psychother.) St. Geo. Hosp. Med. Sch. Lond.; Sen. Regist. (Adult) Tavistock Clinic Lond.; Sen. Regist. & Clin. Tutor (Psychiat.) Univ. Edin.

O'FLAHERTY, Gerard Martin Riverside Practice, Upper Main Street, Strabane BT82 8AS Tel: 00 353 73 7781268 — MB BCh BAO Dub. 1990; BSc Ulster 1978; DCH RCPS Glas. 1993; DRCOG 1993; MRCGP 1994; T(GP) 1994; MICGP 1996. Asst. GP NW HB. Socs: Donegal Clin. Soc. Prev: SHO (Psychiat.) Gartnavel Roy. Hosp. Glas.; SHO (Accid. & Emerg.) Ayr Hosp.; Trainee GP W. Kilbride.

O'FLAHERTY, Kenneth Anthony Waterside Health Centre, Glendermott Road, Londonderry BT47 6AU Tel: 028 7132 0100 Fax: 028 7132 0117 — (NUI Univ. Coll. Galway) MB BCh BAO 1983; DRCOG 1987; MRCGP 1989; DCH Glas. 1990. SHO (Med.) Altnagelvin Hosp. Lond.derry. Prev: SHO (O & G & Paediat.) Altnagelvin Hosp. Londonderry; Cas. Off. Roy. Preston Hosp.

O'FLANAGAN, Joyce Olwen 8 Marlfield Road, Grappenhall, Warrington WA4 2JT — MB ChB Birm. 1954; DPM Eng. 1962, DCH 1957; DObst RCOG 1958.

O'FLANAGAN, Paul Henry Appletree Medical Practice, 47a Town Street, Duffield, Belper DE56 4GG Tel: 01332 841219 — MB BCh BAO Dub. 1972; BA Dub. 1971; FRCGP 1988, M 1976; DObst RCOG 1976. Socs: BMA & Chairm. Primary Care Quality Gp. Derbysh. Prev: Chairm. Vale of Trent Fac. Bd.; Course Organiser Derby VTS; Trainee GP Derby VTS.

O'FLANAGAN, Peter Malpas 8 Marlfield Road, Grappenhall, Warrington WA4 2JT Tel: 01925 63247 — LRCPI & LM, LRSCI & LM 1945 (RCSI) LRCPI & LM, LRCSI & LM 1945; DPM RCPSI 1947; FRCPsych 1972. Prev: Cons. Psychiat. Winwick Hosp.; Psychiat. Regist. Pastures Hosp. Derby; Ho. Phys. Richmond Hosp. Dub.

O'FLANAGAN, William Joseph Dominic The Saltscar Centre, 22 Kirkleatham Street, Redcar TS10 1UA; 20 Hawthorn Road, Redcar TS10 3PA Tel: 01642 471436 — MB BS Newc. 1975; MRCGP 1979.

O'FLYNN, David William South London and Maudsley NHS Trust, Rehabilitation Services, Rehab Building, Lambeth Hospital, 108 Landor Rd, London SW9 9NT Tel: 020 7411 6306 Fax: 020 7411 6527 Email: david.o'flynn@slam-tr.nhs.uk — MB BS Lond. 1983; MRCPsych 1989. Cons. Psychiat., S. Lond. & Maudsley NHS Trust, Rehabil. Servs., Rehab Building. Lambeth Hosp., 108 Landor Rd, Lond. Specialty: Gen. Psychiat. Prev: Research Fell. UMDS; SHO & Regist. (Psych. Med.) Guy's Hosp. Lond.; Specialist Regist.

O'FLYNN, Kieran Gerard 47 Third Cross Road, Twickenham TW2 5DY — MB BS Lond. 1990.

O'FLYNN, Mr Kieran Jeremiah 14 Broomfield Road, Stockport SK4 4ND — MB BCh BAO NUI 1982; FRCSI 1986.

O'FLYNN, Mark William 6 Arum Close, Malvern WR14 2UT — MB BS Lond. 1992.

O'FLYNN, Nora Mary Flat 2, 27 Manville Road, London SW17 8JW — MB BCh BAO NUI 1985; DGM RCP Lond. 1991; DRCOG 1992; MRCGP 1993.

O'FLYNN, Mr Paul Edward The Royal National Throat, Nose & Ear Hospital, Grays Inn Road, London WC1X 8DA Tel: 020 7915 1300; 55 Harley Street, London W1G 8QR Tel: 020 7580 4111 Fax: 020 7436 4901 — MB BS Lond. 1982 (Univ. Coll. Lond.) FRCS Eng. 1988. Cons. Surg. Roy. Nat. Throat, Nose & Ear Hosp. Lond.; Hon. Sen. Lect., UCL. Specialty: Otorhinolaryngol. Prev: Sen. Regist. (ENT Surg.) Nottm. & Derby Hosps.; Regist. (ENT Surg.) Char. Cross Hosp. Lond.; SHO (ENT Surg.) Roy. Nat. Throat, Nose & Ear Hosp. Lond.

O'FLYNN, Richard Redmond Department of Psychiatry, West Suffolk Hospital, Hardwick Lane, Bury St Edmunds IP33 2QZ Tel: 01284 713390 Fax: 01284 713694 — MB BS Lond. 1981 (Char. Cross) MRCPsych 1985. Cons. Psychiat. W. Suff. Hosp. & Staff Cons. Psychiat. Priory Hosp. Chelmsford; Psychiat. Mem., the Parole Bd. for Eng. and Wales. Specialty: Gen. Psychiat. Prev: Sen. Regist. (Psychiat.) SE Thames HA; Sen. Regist. (Psychiat.) SE Thames HA.

O'GALLAGHER, Deirdre Mary Bernadette Rylett Road Surgery, 45 Rylett Road, Shepherds Bush, London W12 9ST Tel: 020 8749 7863 Fax: 020 8743 5161 — MB BS Lond. 1985; MRCGP 1993.

O'GARA, Mary Geraldine Small Heath Medical Practice, 2 Gt. Wood Road, Small Heath, Birmingham B10 9QE Tel: 0121 766 8828 Fax: 0121 772 0097 — MB BCh BAO NUI 1977; DRCOG 1981; MRCGP 1982. GP Partner, Small Heath Med. Pract., Small Heath, Birm.; Hosp. Practitioner, Diabetes, Heartlands Hosp., Birm.

O'GORMAN, Angela Jayne 21 Birchwood Avenue, Sidcup DA14 4JY — BM BS Nottm. 1998.

O'GORMAN, Ciaran 33 Hampton Parade, Sunnyside, Belfast BT7 3EQ — MB ChB Dundee 1995.

O'GORMAN, Clare Josephine Antrim Health Centre, Station Road, Antrim BT41 4BS Tel: 028 90413930 — MB BCh BAO Belf. 1986; MRCGP 1990; DRCOG 1991; DMH Queen's Univ. 1991. Princip. in Gen. Pract., Antrim. Socs: BMA.

O'GORMAN, Daniel Princess Royal Hospital, Telford TF1 6TF Tel: 01952 641222 Ext: 4520 — MB BCh N U Irel 1980. Cons. (Cardiol.) Princess Roy. Hosp. Telford and City Gen. Hosp. Stoke. Specialty: Cardiol.

O'GORMAN, Ethna Catherine 134 Monlough Road, Saintfield, Ballynahinch BT24 7EU; Department of Mental Health, Whitla Medical Builidng, Queens University, Belfast BT9 7BL Tel: 01232 272169 Fax: 01232 324543 — (Univ. Coll. Galway, Irel.) MB BCh BAO NUI 1966; MD NUI 1974; DPM RCPSI 1975; FRCPsych 1985, M 1978. Cons. Psychiat. Belf. City Hosp. Trust; Dir. Clinic Skills Educat. Centre Qu.'s Univ. Belf. Specialty: Gen. Psychiat.; Psychosexual Med. Socs: Fell. Rot. Soc. Med.; BMA; Ulster Med. Soc. Prev: Sen. Lect. Ment. Health Qu. Univ. Belf.; HA RVA RD Macy Schol. 1995; Clin. Research Fell. & Tutor/Regist. (Ment. Health) Belf.

O'GORMAN, Margaret (retired) 37 Hale Road, Hale, Liverpool L24 5RB Tel: 0151 425 2087 — MB BCh BAO NUI 1948.

O'GORMAN, Margaret Elizabeth Nelson (retired) Westholm, Low Town, Thornhill, Stirling FK8 3PX Tel: 01786 85295 — (Glas.) MB ChB Glas. 1963; DPM Ed. & Glas. 1967; MRCPsych 1971. Prev: Cons. Child & Adolesc. Psychiat. Forth Valley HB.

O'GORMAN, Mary Elizabeth Victoria Road Surgery, 21 Victoria Road, Acocks Green, Birmingham B27 7XZ Tel: 0121 706 1129 Fax: 0121 765 4927 — MB ChB Liverp. 1978; DRCOG 1980; DTM & H Liverp. 1982. Prev: Med. Off. Likuni Hosp. Malawi; Med. Off. Shisong Hosp. Cameroon.

O'GORMAN, William Joseph The Square House, Peppard, Henley-on-Thames RG9 5EJ — MB ChB Manch. 1996; MRCGP (Merit) 2003. Specialty: Gen. Pract.

O'GORMAN-LALOR, Olivia Anna Stephanie Nora Chelsea and Westminster Hospital, 369 Fulham Road, London W6 — MB BS Lond. 1994 (Char. Cross & Westm. Med. Sch.) BSc 1991; MRCP (UK) 1997. Specialty: Dermat.

O'GRADY, Catherine Josephine (retired) Flat 6, Princess Court, 10-12 Canning Road, Croydon CR0 6QB Tel: 020 8654 1547 — (NUI) MB BCh BAO NUI 1950. Prev: Ho. Phys. St. Luke's Hosp. Guildford.

O'GRADY, Elizabeth Anne 38 Harington Road, Formby, Liverpool L37 1NU — MB ChB Liverp. 1985.

O'GRADY, Professor Francis William, CBE, TD (retired) 32 Wollaton Hall Drive, Nottingham NG8 1AF Tel: 0115 978 3944 — (Middlx.) MB BS (Hons.) Lond. 1950; MSc Lond. 1956, BSc (1st cl. Hons.) 1947, MD 1957; FRCPath 1972, M 1963; FRCP Lond. 1976,

M 1971; Hon. FFPM RCP Lond. 1988. Chief Scientist Dept Health. Prev: Prof. Microbiol. Univ. Nottm.

O'GRADY, Professor John 47 Granville Road, Sevenoaks TN13 1HB Tel: 01732 453229 Fax: 01732 743122 — MB ChB Manch. 1967; MRCP (UK) 1976; MD Manch. 1983; FRCP Lond. 1988; FFPM 1989; T(M) 1991. Extern. Examr. Univ. Guildford; Vis. Prof. Univ. Lond.; Vis. Prof. Clin. Pharmacol. Univ. Vienna, Austria; Examr. Dip. Pharmaceut. Med. RCP; Cons. Health Protec. Br. Canada. Specialty: Pharmacology. Socs: Fell. Roy. Soc. Med.; Fell. Roy. Statistical Soc.; Brit. Pharm. Soc. Prev: Med. Dir. May & Baker Ltd.; Head (Clin. Human Pharmacol.) Wellcome Foundat. Ltd.; Sen. Regist. St. Bart. Hosp. Lond.

O'GRADY, John Charles Ravenswood Home, Medium Secure Unit, Knowle, Fareham PO17 5NA Tel: 01329 836009 Fax: 01329 834780 — MB BCh BAO NUI 1975; FRCPsych 1995, M 1979; MBA Durham 1995. Cons. Psychiat. (Forens. Psychiat.) Ravenswood Ho. Fareham. Specialty: Forens. Psychiat.

O'GRADY, John Gerard Mary King's College Hospital, Denmark Hill, London SE5 9PJ Tel: 020 7346 3367 Fax: 020 7346 3167 Email: john.g.o'grady@kcl.ac.uk — MB BCh BAO NUI 1978; MD NUI 1983; FRCPI 1996. Cons. (Hepat.) King's Coll. Hosp. Lond.; Hon. Sen. Lect. KCH Med. & Dent. Lond. Specialty: Gastroenterol. Socs: Brit. Soc. Gastroenterol.; Eur. Assn. Study Liver; Amer. Assn. Study Liver Dis. Prev: Cons. (Hepat.) & Sen. Clin. Lect. St. James' Hosp. Leeds; Sen. Lect. Inst. Liver Studies King's Coll. Hosp. Lond.

O'GRADY, Margaret Mary Martina 9 The Mews, Sundrum Castle, By Coylton, Ayr KA6 5JY — MB BCh BAO NUI 1990 (Galway) MRCPsych 1997. Cons. Psychiat. with s/i in Liason Psychiat. Specialty: Gen. Psychiat.; Forens. Psychiat. Socs: Roy. Coll. Psychiat. Prev: Specialist Regist. (Psychiat.) W. of Scot. Higher Train. Scheme.

O'GRADY, Michael Standish (retired) Spreets Rew, Arreton, Newport PO30 3AL Tel: 01983 865370 — MB BCh BAO Dub. 1948 (T.C. Dub.) DObst RCOG 1953. JP.

O'GRADY, Timothy John Peter Hodgkinson Centre, Lincoln County Hospital, Lincoln LN2 5UA — MB ChB Leic. 1980; MRCPsych 1984. Cons. Psychiat. Lincoln Co. Hosp. Specialty: Gen. Psychiat.

O'HAGAN, Art Henry Knockaconey Road, Armagh BT61 8DU — MB BCh BAO Belf. 1994.

O'HAGAN, David Patrick 28 Cumbrian Way, Burnley BB12 8UF — MB BS Lond. 1993.

O'HAGAN, Dorothy Winifred (retired) Sounion, Mill Lane, Thimbleby, Horncastle LN9 5JS Tel: 01507 522382 — MB BS Durh. 1941 (Newc.) Prev: Asst. Co. Med. Off., Sch. Med. Off. & Family Plann. Med. Off. Lindsey CC.

O'HAGAN, Frances Theresa Friary Surgery, Dobbin Lane, Armagh BT61 7OG Tel: 375 21500 — MB BCh BAO Belf. 1989 (Queens Belfast) MRCGP; DRCOG; DCH; DGM; DRCOG; DGM; DCH; MRCGP. GP. Specialty: Gen. Pract.

O'HAGAN, Julie Elizabeth Clatterbridge Centre of oncology, Clatterbridge Road, Bebington, Wirral CH63 4JY; 13 Norfolk Avenue, Burton-upon-Stather, Scunthorpe DN15 9EW — MB BS Lond. 1993; MRCP (UK) 1997. Specialty: Oncol.

O'HAGAN, Simon James 21 William Alexander Park, Belfast BT10 0LX — MB BCh Belf. 1998.

O'HALLORAN, Paul David The Health Centre, Charlton Road, Andover SP10 3LD Tel: 01264 365031 Fax: 01264 336701; South View House, Ragged Appleshaw, Andover SP11 9HX Fax: 01264 772071 — MRCS Eng. LRCP Lond. 1985 (Char. Cross. Hosp. Lond.) DObst Auckland 1989; MRCGP 1991; DFFP 1996. GP Partner & Princip. Specialty: Gen. Pract. Socs: (Sec.) Winchester & Andover Med. Golf Soc. Prev: Regist. (Psychiat.) Pk. Prewitt Hosp.; SHO (Psychiat.) Old Manor Hosp. Salisbury; SHO (O & G) & Regist. (Paediat.) Nat. Wom. Hosp. Auckland, NZ.

O'HANLON, Christopher Houghton Tower Farm, Ramsbrook Lane, Hale, Liverpool L24 5RP — MB ChB Liverp. 1970.

O'HANLON, Denise Patricia Arrowe Sports Injuries Clinic, Archers Health Club, 132 Ford Road,Upton, Wirral CH49 0TQ Tel: 0151 604 0604; 22 Heron Road, Meols, Wirral CH47 9RU Tel: 0151 632 3946 — BM BS Nottm. 1991; BMedSci 1989; Dip. Sports Med. (Scott. Roy. Colls.) 1997. Specialty: Sports Med. Socs: BMA; Brit. Assn. Sport & Med.

O'HANLON, Donal Thomas John 56 Dundalk Street, Newtownhamilton, Newry BT35 0PB — MB BCh BAO NUI 1990; LRCPSI 1990.

O'HANLON, John James 19 Richmond Court, Lisburn BT27 4QU — MB BCh BAO Belf. 1988; BSc Belf. 1985; FFARCSI 1992; Dip Pain Med 2001.

O'HANLON, Karen Christina Burnside, Closeburn Avenue, Heswall, Wirral CH60 4SP — BM BS Nottm. 1986.

O'HANLON, Sean 22 Sourhille, Ballymena BT42 2LG — MB BCh BAO Belf. 1989.

O'HANLON, Stephen Gray The White Cottage, Western Avenue, Reading RG5 3BN — BChir Camb. 1997; BChir Camb 1997.

O'HANLON, Sylvia North Tyneside General Hospital, Roke Lane, North Shields NE29 8NH Tel: 0191 253 6660 Fax: 0191 293 2563 — Approbation Halle 1980 (Univ. Halle Germany) MRCP equivalent (Germany) 1985; MSc (Pub. Health) Newc. 1993. Staff Grade (c/o Elderly) Newc. u. Tyne. Specialty: Care of the Elderly.

O'HANLON, Teresa Mary Old Hall Grounds Health Centre, Old Hall Grounds, Cowbridge CF71 7AH Tel: 01446 772237 Fax: 01446 775883; Stallcourt House, Stallcourt Close, Llanblethian, Cowbridge CF71 7JU — MB BS Lond. 1977; MRCGP 1982.

O'HARA, Ann Wilson 5 Marine Terrace, Muchalls, Stonehaven AB39 3RD — MB ChB Glas. 1975; DRCOG 1977; DCH RCPS Glas. 1978. Assocaite Specialist (Community Child Health) Aberd.

O'HARA, Arthur Gerard Gransha Hospital, Clooney Road, Londonderry BT47 6WJ Tel: 01504 860261 — MB BCh BAO Belf. 1974. Cons. Psychiat. Gransha Hosp. Lond.derry. Specialty: Gen. Psychiat.

O'HARA, Dermot Patrick Dr D P O'Hara & Partners, 46-48 Grey Road, Liverpool L9 1AY Tel: 0151 525 1644; 5 Granville Park, Aughton, Ormskirk L39 5DS Tel: 01695 422247 — MB BCh BAO NUI 1981; LRCPI & LM, LRCSI & LM 1981; DCH RCSI 1983; DRCOG 1988. GP Princip., Sen. Partner. Prev: Princip. GP Manch. & Warrington, Med. Off. DSS.

O'HARA, Fenella Rachel The Surgery, 119 Wrenway, Farnborough GU14 8TA Tel: 01252 541884; 22 Leawood Rd, Fleet GU51 5AL — MB BS Newc. 1990 (Newcastle) DRCOG 1994; MRCGP 1995. GP Retainee Wrenway Farnborough. Specialty: Gen. Pract. Prev: GP Retainee Judges Close Surgery E. Grinstead; GP Princip.Chester.

O'HARA, Gerard Vincent 71 Naishcombe Hill, Wick, Bristol BS30 5QS — MB ChB Sheff. 1991.

O'HARA, Helena 128 Wolseley Road, Rugeley WS15 2ET — MB BCh BAO NUI 1940 (Univ. Coll. Dub.)

O'HARA, Jean The Royal London Hospital, 130A Sewardstone Road, East London & the City Mental Health Trust, London E2 9HN Tel: 020 8981 7425 Fax: 020 8983 1026 — MB BS Lond. 1983; MRCPsych 1988. Cons. Psychiat. Roy. Lond. Hosp.; Hon. Cons. - Barts & the Lond. NHS Trust; Hon. Sen. Clin. Lect. - Qu. Mary & Westfield Coll. Univ. Of Lond. Socs: Fell. Roy. Soc. Med.; BMA; Roy. Coll. Psychiat. Prev: Sen. Regist. (Psychiat. of Ment. Handicap) Dept. Psychol. Med. St. Bart. Hosp. Lond. & Leytonstone Hse. S. Ockenden; SHO & Regist. Rotat. (Psychiat.) Waltham Forest & Enfield HA.

O'HARA, Mr John Neary Royal Orthopaedic Hospital, Northfield, Birmingham B31 2AP Tel: 0121 449 5177/0121 685 4210 Fax: 0121 442 4410 Email: jneary04@aol.com; Wind Flowers, The Drive, Burcot, Bromsgrove B60 1PP Tel: 0121 445 1386 — LRCPI & LM, LRSCI & LM 1976 (RCSI) MB BCh BAO Dublin; FRCS Eng. 1981; FRCSI Dub. 1981; MCh NUI 1991. Cons. Orthopaedic Surg., ROH, Birm.; Cons. Orthopaedic Surg., Birm. Childrens Hosp. Specialty: Orthop. Socs: BOA; FAAOS; BSCOS. Prev: Staff Sick Childr. Hosp. Toronto; Regist. Rotat. (Orthop.) Birm.; Regist. (Surg.) Bradford AHA.

O'HARA, Lawrence Joseph 18 Stonor Road, London W14 8RZ — MB BS Lond. 1991.

O'HARA, Liam Andrew 18 Melmerby Cl, Newcastle upon Tyne NE3 5JA — MB ChB Manch. 1997.

O'HARA, Mary Geraldine Ballymena Health Centre, Cushendall Road, Ballymena BT43 6HQ Tel: 028 2564 2181 Fax: 028 2565 8919; Leighinmohr Avenue, Ballymena BT42 2AT Tel: 01266 45974 — MB BCh BAO Belf. 1982; MRCGP 1987; DCH Dub. 1987; DRCOG 1987.

O'HARA, Michael Denis Department of Pathology, Queen's University Belfast, Grosvenor Road, Belfast BT12 6BN Tel: 028 9089

4744 Fax: 028 9023 3643 Email: d.ohara@qub.ac.uk — MB BCh BAO Belf. 1966 (Qu. Univ. Belf.) BSc (Hons. Anat.) Belf. 1963; FRCPath 1985, M 1973. Sen. Lect. Qu. Univ. Belf.; Cons. Roy. Vict. Hosp. Belf. Specialty: Histopath. Socs: Path. Soc.; Assn. Clin. Path.; (Treas.) Brit. Paediat. Path. Assn. Prev: Dunville Fellowship (Path.) Qu. Univ. Belf.; Sen. Regist. & Tutor Inst. Path. Qu. Univ. Belf.

O'HARA, Nora Patrica (retired) 118 St Marys Street, Latchford, Warrington WA4 1BH — MB, BCh BAO NUI 1946.

O'HARA, Richard James 31 Branksome Road, Coundon, Coventry CV6 1FW — BM BS Nottm. 1991; FRCS 1996. Specialist Regist. (Gen. Surg.) Oxf. Deanery. Specialty: Gen. Surg.

O'HARA, Sheila Valerie Portland Medical Centre, 184 Portland Road, London SE25 4JQ Tel: 020 662 1233 Fax: 020 8656 7984/ 020 8662 1223; Oakcroft, 12 Grimwade Avenue, Croydon CR0 5DG Tel: 020 8656 0213 — MB ChB Manch. 1969; Cert. Family Plann. JCC 1975. GP Trainer Lond.; GP Tutor KCH Med. Sch. Lond. Prev: Ho. Surg. Univ. Hosp. S. Manch. Withington Hosp.; Ho. Phys. St. Mary Abbots Hosp. Lond.

O'HARA, Simon David North Chevin Medical Practice, 3 Bridge Street, Otley LS21 1BQ — MB ChB Liverp. 1988; MRCGP; BA. GP Princip. Prev: SHO Rotat. (Med.) Leeds Gen. Infirm.

O'HARE, Adrian Gerard Mary 2 Rostrevor Road, Warrenpoint, Newry BT34 3RT — MB BCh BAO NUI 1981.

O'HARE, Anne Elizabeth 39 Grange Road, Edinburgh EH9 1UG — MB BS Newc. 1978; MRCP (UK) 1980; MD 1987; FRCP 1995; FRCPCH 1997.

O'HARE, Brendan Joseph Castlederg Surgery, 13A Lower Strabane Road, Castlederg BT81 7AZ Tel: 028 8167 1211 Fax: 028 8167 9700 — MB BCh BAO Belf. 1985; DGM RCP Lond. 1987; DCH RCPS Glas. 1988; DRCOG 1988; MRCGP 1989.

O'HARE, Conor Vincent 21 Barranderry Heights, Enniskillen BT74 6JW — MB BCh BAO Belf. 1990; MB BCh Belf. 1990.

O'HARE, Deborah Jayne 2 Stamford Road, Exton, Oakham LE15 8AZ — MB ChB Manch. 1990. Demonst. (Anat.) St. And. Univ.

O'HARE, Deirdre Mary McDonnell and Partners, 139-141 Ormeau Road, Belfast BT7 1DA Tel: 028 9032 6030; 125 Shandon Park, Belfast BT5 6NZ Tel: 01232 795295 — MB BCh BAO Belf. 1984; DRCOG 1988; MRCGP 1989.

O'HARE, Irene Paula 18 Drumnabey Road, Castlederg BT81 7NF — MB BCh BAO Belf. 1983; MB BCh Belf. 1983; DRCOG 1987; MRCGP 1989. Specialty: Dermat.

O'HARE, John 21 Floral Park, Newtownabbey BT36 7RU — MB BCh BAO Belf. 1996.

O'HARE, Joseph Paul Hospital of St Cross, Barby Road, Rugby CV22 5PX Tel: 01788 545180 Fax: 01788 545251; 32 Waverley Road, Kenilworth CV8 1JN Tel: 01926 853783 — MB BS Lond. 1979; MRCP (UK) 1982; MD Lond. 1986; FRCP Lond. 1994. Cons. Phys. (Diabetes & Endocrinol.) Hosp. St. Cross Rugby; Reader (Med. & Biol. Sci.) Univ. Warwick. Specialty: Diabetes.

O'HARE, Kevin John 3F1, 121 Novar Drive, Hyndland, Glasgow G12 9TA Tel: 0141 339 1055 Email: kevin.o'hare@virgin.net — MB ChB Ed. 1991; FRCA 1997; FFARCSI 1997. Specialist Regist. (Anaesth.) Glas. Roy. Infirm. NHS Trust. Specialty: Anaesth. Prev: Specialist Regist. (Anaesth.) Glas. Roy. Infirm. NhS Trust.

O'HARE, Martin 23 Spelga Park, Hilltown, Newry BT34 5UU — MB ChB Birm. 1993.

O'HARE, Mary Patricia Dufferin Wards (ENT), Belfast City Hospital, Lisburn Road, Belfast BT9 7A; 6 Deramore Park S., Belfast BT9 5JY — MB BCh BAO Belf. 1983; DGM RCP Lond. 1986; DRCOG 1986; Cert. Family Plann. JCC 1986; MRCGP 1988. GP Belf.

O'HARE, Michael Francis Daisy Hill Hospital, Newry BT35 8DR Tel: 028 3083 5000 Fax: 028 3026 8285 Email: m.f.ohare@btinternet.com; 39 Camlough Road, Newry BT35 7LS Tel: 028 3026 2445 Fax: 028 3026 8285 — MD Belf. 1983, MB BCh BAO 1970; DRCOG 1972; FRCOG 1989, M 1975; FRCPI 2001. Cons. O & G Daisy Hill Hosp. Newry. Specialty: Obst. & Gyn. Socs: Fell. Ulster Med. Soc. Prev: Sen. Tutor & Sen. Regist. Roy. Matern. Hosp. & Dept. Midw. & Gyn.; Qu.'s Univ. Belf.; Clin. Research Fell. Dept. Midw. & Gyn. Qu. Univ.; Belf.; Regist. (O & G) Harari Centr. Hosp. Salisbury, Rhodesia.

O'HARE, Patrick Austen — MB ChB Leeds 1977; DRCOG 1979. Socs: Leeds Med. Soc. Prev: Ho. Phys. St. Jas. Univ. Hosp. Leeds; Ho. Surg. Chapel Allerton Hosp. Leeds.

O'HARE, Mr Peter Melville Department of Plastic Surgery, Castle Hill Hospital, Castle Road, Cottingham HU16 Tel: 01482 875875 Fax: 01482 622353 — MB ChB Bristol 1973; BSc (Biochem., Hons.) Bristol 1970; FRCS Eng. 1977. Cons. (Plastic Surg.) Hull E. Yorks. NHS Trust. Specialty: Plastic Surg. Socs: Brit. Assn. Plastic Surg.; Mem. Spec. Advisery Comm. For Plastic Surg. To Jt. Comm. For Higher Surg. Train. (Roy. Coll. Surg.s). Prev: Sen. Regist. (Plastic Surg.) Roy. Vict. Hosp. Belf. & The Ulster; Hosp. Dundonald.; Regist. E. Anglian Regional Plastic Surg. Serv. W. Norwich Hosp.

O'HARE, Ronan Andrew 21 Barranderry Heights, Enniskillen BT74 6JW — MB BCh BAO Belf. 1992; MB BCh Belf. 1992.

O'HARE, Rosemary (retired) 6 Park Court, Giffnock, Glasgow G46 7PB Tel: 0141 638 5177 — BSc Glas. 1940; MB ChB Glas. 1943; MRCGP 1965. Prev: GP Glas.

O'HARE, Ruth The Surgery, 41 Connaught Square, London W2 2HL Tel: 020 7723 3338 Fax: 020 7402 3342 — MB BChir Camb. 1978; MA Camb. 1979; MRCP (UK) 1981. Lect. (Gen. Pract.) St. Mary's Med. Sch. Lond.

O'HEA, Anna-Marie Dormer Cotrtage, Green End St., Aston Clinton, Aylesbury HP22 5EX — MB BCh BAO Dub. 1977; MRCP (UK) 1980; MRCPath 1984. Cons. Haemat. Stoke Mandeville Hosp. Aylesbury. Specialty: Haematology.

O'HICKEY, Stephen Patrick Department of Respiratory Medicine, Worcester Royal Infirmary, Worcester WR1 3AS Tel: 01905 760240 Fax: 01905 760237 — MB ChB Manch. 1981; MRCP (UK) 1984; MD Manch. 1990; FRCP 1999. Cons. Phys. (Respirat. Med.) Worcester Roy. Infirm. Specialty: Respirat. Med.; Intens. Care. Prev: Cons. Phys. (Respirat. Med.) Solihull Hosp. W. Midl.; Sen. Regist. (Thoracic Med.) E. Birm. Hosp.; Research Asst. (Respirat. Med.) Guy's Hosp. Lond.

O'HIGGINS, Frances Margaret 27C Beaufort Road, Clifton, Bristol BS8 2JX — MB BS Lond. 1991; BSc Lond. 1989; MRCP (UK) 1994; FRCA 1997.

O'HIGGINS, Paul Department of Anatomy & Developmental Biology, University College London, Gower St., London WC1E 6BT — MB ChB Leeds 1982; PhD Leeds 1989. Reader (Anat.) Univ. Coll. Lond. Specialty: Anat. Prev: Sen. Lect. (Anat.) Univ. West. Austral.; Lect. (Anat.) Univ. Leeds.

O'HORAN, Patrick The Burns Medical Practice, 4 Albion Place, Bennetthorpe, Doncaster DN1 2EQ Tel: 01302 810888 Fax: 01302 812150 — MB BS Lond. 1982 (St. Mary's) Cert. Family Plann. JCC 1986. Princip. GP Doncaster.; Med. Adviser Doncaster MBC. Specialty: Gen. Pract.; Occupat. Health. Socs: BMA; Soc. of Occup. Med. Prev: Trainee GP Doncaster VTS.

O'KANE, Agnes Elizabeth The Bungalow, 118 Malone Road, Belfast BT9 5HR — MB BCh BAO Belf. 1985.

O'KANE, Anne Genevieve Diamond Medical Centre, Meeting Street, Magherafelt BT45 6ED Email: aokane@doctors.org.uk — MB BCh BAO Belf. 1983; DRCOG 1986; DCH Dub. 1987; DCCH RCP Ed. 1987; MRCGP 1988.

O'KANE, Bronagh Mary Wynne Hill Surgery, 51 Hill St., Lurgan, Craigavon BT66 6BW Tel: 01762 326333; 75 Steps Road, Donaghcloney, Craigavon BT66 7NZ — MB BCh BAO Belf. 1985; DRCOG 1988; DCH RCPSI 1989; MRCGP 1991.

O'KANE, Cecilia Majella 18 Foyle Av, Greysteel, Londonderry BT47 3EB — MB BCh BAO Belf. 1997.

O'KANE, Damian Joseph Crumlin Road Health Centre, 130-132 Crumlin Road, Belfast BT14 6AR — MB BCh BAO Belf. 1987; MRCGP 1992; DRCOG 1994.

O'KANE, Declan 13 The Cedars, Jordanstown, Belfast BT5 6LU — MB BCh BAO Belf. 1991. Specialty: Gen. Med.

O'KANE, Dermot Patrick 148 Priory Road, Dungiven, Londonderry BT47 4LR — MB BCh BAO Belf. 1995.

O'KANE, Ellen Maria 185 Ballymena Road, Doagh, Ballyclare BT39 0TW — MB BCh BAO Belf. 1990; MB BCh Belf. 1990.

O'KANE, Gerald St. Machar's House, Kilbarchan Road, Bridge of Weir PA11 3ET — MB ChB Glas. 1973.

O'KANE, Hugh Felix Gerald 9 Malone Park, Belfast BT9 6NH — MB BCh Belf. 1998.

O'KANE, Mr Hugh Oliver 9 Malone Park, Belfast BT9 6NH Tel: 028 9066 5778 — MB BCh BAO Belf. 1960; BSc Belf. 1957, MCh

1970, MB BCh BAO 1960; FRCS Ed. 1963. Cons. Cardiac Surg. Roy. Vict. Hosp. Belf. Specialty: Cardiothoracic Surg. Socs: Brit. Soc. Thoracic & Cardiovasc. Surg. & Brit. Cardiac Soc.; Pres. Irish Cardiac Soc. Prev: Asst. Prof. Surg. Washington Univ. St. Louis, USA; on Attend. Staff Jewish Hosp. St. Louis, USA; Resid. (Cardiothoracic Surg.) Mayo Clinic Rochester, USA.

O'KANE, Jacintha Grace — MB BCh Belf. 1998.

O'KANE, John Bernard The Oaks Family Medical Centre, 48 Orritor Road, Cookstown BT80 8BG Tel: 028 7976 2249 Fax: 028 7976 6793; 1 Tullagh Drive, Cookstown BT80 8ED — MB BCh BAO Belf. 1974; DObst RCOG 1976. Socs: GMSC (N. I.); GMC(N.I.); Northern LMC. Prev: Mem. United Hosps. Trust (GP Forum).

O'KANE, Judith Jane Bridge Street Medical Centre, 30 Bridge Street, Londonderry BT48 6LA Tel: 028 7126 1137 Fax: 028 7137 0723 — MB BCh BAO Dub. 1977; DRCOG 1980; DCH Dub. 1981. Socs: BMA.

O'KANE, Kevin Malachy — MB BCh BAO Belf. 1987; MRCGP.

O'KANE, Martin Patrick 180 Vow Road, Ballymoney BT53 7NS — MB BCh BAO Belf. 1997.

O'KANE, Maurice John Clinical Chemistry Laboratory, Altnagelvin Hospital, Glenshane Road, Londonderry BT47 6SB Tel: 01504 45171 — MB ChB Ed. 1985; BSc (Hons.) Ed. 1983; MRCP (UK) 1988; MRCPath 1993; MD Belf. 1995. Cons. Chem. Path. Altnagelvin Hosp. Londonderry. Specialty: Chem. Path. Socs: Assn. Clin. Biochem.

O'KANE, Michael John Cwmfelin Medical Centre, 298 Carmarthen Road, Swansea SA1 1HW Tel: 01792 653941 — MB BS Lond. 1966 (Middlx.) MRCS Eng. LRCP Lond. 1966; DCH Eng. 1968. Prev: Ho. Surg. O & G Middlx. Hosp.; Ho. Phys. Paediat. St. Albans City Hosp.

***O'KANE, Roisin Maira Teresa** 19 Innisfayle Road, Belfast BT15 4ES; 19 Innisfayle Road, Belfast BT15 4ES — MB BCh BAO Belf. 1997; DME 1999. SHO GP Rotat. Specialty: Gen. Pract.

O'KANE, William Patrick (retired) 6 Leighimohr Avenue, Ballymena — MB BCh BAO Belf. 1957. Prev: Clin. Med. Off. North. Health & Social Servs. Bd. (N. Irel.).

O'KEEFFE, Anthony Guy 26 Eaton Terrace, London SW1W 8TS Tel: 020 7730 5070 Fax: 020 7730 2780 Email: dr.gokeeffe@btconnect.com — MB BS Lond. 1986 (Guy's Hosp.) MA Camb. 1982; MRCP (UK) 1986; Cert. Family Plann. JCC 1988. Indep. GP Lond. Specialty: Gen. Pract. Socs: BMA; Lister Hosp. Private Pract. Gp. Prev: Trainee GP St. Thos. Hosp. VTS; Regist. (Med.) Roy. Masonic Hosp.; SHO (A & E) Guy's Hosp. Lond.

O'KEEFFE, Caroline Jane 244 Hammersmith Grove, London W6 7EP — MB ChB Bristol 1998.

O'KEEFFE, Charles James Maunsell (retired) 1 Brookedor, Kingskerswel, Newton Abbot TQ12 5BJ Tel: 01803 873861 — MB BS Lond. 1958 (St. Bart.) DObst RCOG 1961. Prev: Ho. Surg., Ho. Phys. & SHO O & G Norf. & Norwich Hosp.

O'KEEFFE, Daniel Finnbarr Churchward and Partners, Croft Medical Centre, 2 Glen Road, Oadby, Leicester LE2 4PE Tel: 0116 271 2564 Fax: 0116 272 9000; 63 Linden Drive, Evington, Leicester LE5 6AJ — MB BCh BAO NUI 1976; DCH RCPSI 1978; DObst RCPI 1979.

O'KEEFFE, Mr Declan (retired) 2 Roseville Apartments, Wandsworth Road, Bangor BT19 1DZ Tel: 01247 272143 — MB BS Lond. 1945 (Guy's) MRCS Eng. LRCP Lond. 1945; FRCS Eng. 1950; DTM & H Eng. 1952. Prev: Vis. Lect. Prof. Calif. Med. Centre, Los Angeles.

O'KEEFFE, Declan Barry Cardiac Unit, Belfast City Hospital, Lisburn Road, Belfast BT9 7AB Tel: 028 329241 — MD Lond. 1970 (Guys) BSc (1st cl. Hons. Anat.) Lond. 1970, MD, MB BS 1973; MRCP (UK) 1975; FRCP Lond. 1989. Cons. Cardiol. Belf. City Hosp. Specialty: Cardiol.

O'KEEFFE, Mr Leonard Joseph ENT Department, Royal Bolton Hospital, Minerva Road, Farnworth, Bolton BL4 0JR Tel: 01204 390018; 17 Greenmount Lane, Bolton BL1 5JE — MB BCh BAO NUI 1984; FRCSI 1988; FRCS Ed. 1994; FRCS (Orl.) 1996. Cons. Otorhinolaryngologists, Bolton. Specialty: Otolaryngol. Socs: Brit. Assoc. of OtorhinoLaryngol. and Head & Neck Surg.s; Roy. Soc. Med.; OtoLaryngol. Research Soc. Prev: Regist. (Gen. Surg.) Mercy Hosp. Cork; SHO (ENT) Bristol Roy. Infirm.; Sen. Regist. Rotat. NW Region.

O'KEEFFE, Nial John Manchester Royal Infirmary, Department of Anaesthesia, Oxford Road, Manchester M13 9WL Tel: 0161 276 4552 Fax: 0161 276 8027 Email: niall.okeeffe@man.ac.uk; 27 Elm Road, Didsbury, Manchester M20 6XD — MB BCh BAO NUI 1984; FFA RCSI 1988; FCAnaesth 1989. Cons. Anaesth. Manch. Roy. Infirm. Specialty: Anaesth. Prev: Sen. Regist. NW RHA; Regist. (Anaesth.) Withington Hosp. S. Manch. HA.

O'KEEFFE, Paul Timothy Andrew Great Western Hospital, Marlborough Road, Swindon SN3 6BB Tel: 01793 604020; High Street, Bampton — MB BS Lond. 1983; BSc Lond. 1980; MRCP (UK) 1987. Cons. Paediat. Specialty: Paediat. Prev: Paediat. Sen. Regist. John Radcliffe, Oxf.; Research Fell. (Paediat.) Princess Margt. Hosp. Perth, Austral.; Cons. Paediat. Princess Margt. Hosp., Swindon.

O'KEEFFE, Mr Terence Sidney University of Miami, Miami, USA; Fonbadet, Odstock, Salisbury SP5 4JB Tel: 01722 332083 Fax: 01722 332083 Email: tokeeffe@mac.com — MB ChB Ed. 1994; BSc (1st cl. Hons.) Ed. 1992; FRCS (Ed.) 1999. Tr. Fell. (Gen. Surg.). Specialty: Gen. Surg. Socs: SAGES; AMA; ACS. Prev: SHO (Orthop.) Salisbury Dist. Hosp.; SHO (Gen. Surg.) Salisbury Dist. Hosp.; SHO (A & E Med.) Roy. Infirm. Edin.

O'KEEFFE, Una Bridget — MB BCh BAO NUI 1960.

O'KEEFFE, Vincent Martin St. Winifrides School House, Llanasa Road, Glwespyr, Holywell CH8 9LU — MB BCh BAO NUI 1986.

O'KELLY, Mr D. Aeneas Ysbyty Glan Clwyd, Bodelwyddan LL18 5UJ Tel: 01745 583910 Ext: 3512 Email: aeneas.okelly@cd-tr.nhs.wales.uk — LRCPI & LM, LRCSI & LM 1982 (RCSI) FRCSI 1989; FRCS Ed. 1990; MSc (Orth.) Lond. 1994; FRCS (Orth.) 1997. Cons. Surg. in Trauma and Orthopaedic Surg. Special Interest: Trauma Care.

O'KELLY, Francis Joseph, OBE (retired) Large Barn, North Bersted St, Bognor Regis PO22 9AH Tel: 01243 826189 — MB BCh BAO NUI 1946; DPH 1961; FFCM 1977; MFOM RCP Lond. 1980; FACOM 1985. Prev: Cons. (Occupat. Health) Governm. of Hong Kong.

O'KELLY, Francis Patrick, MBE Clare House, Newport St., Tiverton EX16 6NJ Tel: 01884 252337; Villa Franca, 9 Park Road, Tiverton EX16 6AU Tel: 01884 256570 — MB BS Lond. 1987 (St. Bart. Hosp. Lond.) DA (UK) 1993; DCH RCP Lond. 1994; MRCGP 1995; DRCOG 1995. GP Princip.; Hosp. Pract. Anaesth. Specialty: Gen. Pract.; Anaesth. Prev: SHO (Anaesth.) Roy. United Hosp. Bath; Trainee GP Midsomer Norton; SHO (Med. & Geriat.) Jersey Gen. Hosp.

O'KELLY, John Kevin Aberfoyle Terrace Surgery, 3-5 Aberfoyle Terrace, Strand Road, Londonderry BT48 7NP Tel: 028 7126 4868; 3 Waterstone Park, Trench Road, Londonderry BT47 2AG — MB BCh BAO Belf. 1984; DCH RCP Lond. 1987; MRCGP 1989.

O'KELLY, Kate Francesca Bacon One Tree House, South Harting, Petersfield GU31 5NW — MB BS Lond. 1989; BA Oxf. 1986; Dip. Paediat. Auckland 1992; MRCGP 2001. GP Chichester.

O'KELLY, Lindsay Margaret 2 Moorgate, Lechlade GL7 3EH — BM Soton. 1982; DCH RCP Lond. 1986; DRCOG 1987; MRCGP 1994. GP Faringdon, Oxon; Fellow, Dept. of Primary Care, Oxford University. Prev: GP Soton.; Fell. (Family Pract.) Univ. Michigan, USA.

O'KELLY, Noel Ignatius The Surgery, Bull Yard, Simpson Street, Spilsby PE23 5LG Tel: 01790 752555 Fax: 01790 754457 — MB BCh BAO Belf. 1986; MRCGP 1990; DRCOG 1990.

O'KELLY, Rosaleen Mary 2 Burghley Road, Stone Manor Park, Lincoln LN6 7YE — MB BCh BAO NUI 1976 (Univ. Coll. Dub.) MRCGP 1981. Specialty: Gen. Psychiat.

O'KELLY, Sean William Princess Margaret Hospital, Okus Road, Swindon SN1 4JU Tel: 01793 426389 — BSc (Hons.) Bristol 1981, MB ChB 1984; DA (UK) 1988; DCH RCP Lond. 1989; FCAnaesth. 1991. Cons. Anaesth. Princess Margt. Hosp. Swindon. Specialty: Anaesth. Socs: Anaesth. Res. Soc.; Soc. Cardiovasc. Anaesth. Prev: Clin. Asst. Prof. Dept. Anaesth. Univ. Michigan, USA; Sen. Regist. (Anaesth.) Soton. & Portsmouth.

O'KELLY, Mr Terence James Whin Cottage, Ardoe, Aberdeen AB12 5XT — MB BS Lond. 1983; BSc Lond. 1980, MB BS 1983; FRCS Eng. 1987. Research Fell. (Pharmacol.) & Nuffield Dept. Surg. Univ. Oxf.; Hon. Clin. Lect. Nuffield Dept. Surg. Univ. Oxf.; Hon. Regist. John Radcliffe Hosp. Oxf. Specialty: Gen. Surg. Prev: Regist. (Surg.) John Radcliffe Hosp. Oxf.; SHO (Surg.) Glos. Roy. Hosp.

O'LEARY, Amanda Jane Obsacitynae Department, South Mead Hospital, Westbury-onTrym, Bristol BS10 5NB Mob: 01179 505050 Email: amandajoleary@hotmail.com — MB ChB Aberd. 1992 (Aberdeen) MRCOG 1998. Research Fell. S. Mead Hosp. Bristol. Specialty: Obst. & Gyn. Prev: Specialist Regist. (O & G) - Welsh Sotation.

O'LEARY, Catherine Anne 9 Buckingham Road, Bicester OX26 2NU — MB ChB Birm. 1996; ChB Birm. 1996.

O'LEARY, Clare Louise 25 Quarry Hills Lane, Lichfield WS14 9HL — BM BS Nottm. 1997.

O'LEARY, Clare Marie 24 Springbank Road, Cheltenham GL51 0LU — MB ChB Liverp. 1998.

O'LEARY, Colin Peter Department of Neurology, Inst. of Neurological Sciences, Southern General Hospital, 1345 Govan Road, Glasgow G51 4TF Tel: 0141 201 1100 Fax: 0141 201 2993 Email: cpol1j@clinmed.gla.ac.uk — MB BCh BAO NUI 1986 (Univ. Coll., Cork) MRCP (UK) 1990. Cons. (Neurol.) INS, SGH; Hon. Sen. Lect. (Neurol.), Univ. of Glas. Specialty: Neurol. Socs: Assn. Brit. Neurol.; Scott. Assn. Neurol. Scis.; RCP (Lond.). Prev: Clin. Lect. & Hon. Sen. Regist. (Neurol.) Inst. Neurol. Sci. South. Gen. Hosp. Glas.; Career Regist. (Neurol.) Inst. Neurol. Sci. South. Gen. Hosp. Glas.; Regist. (Gen. Med.) Nottm. City Hosp.

O'LEARY, Cornelia Frances Birchlands, 146 Forest Road, Liss GU33 7BU Tel: 01730 893741 Email: corneliaeiss@onetel.net.uk — MB BCh BAO NUI 1974 (Univ. Coll. Cork, Irel.) DCH Eng. 1977; FRCA RCS Eng. 1981; FFPM 1996. Sen. Med. Off. Med. Control Agency Lond. Specialty: Pharmaceutical Medicine; Paediat. Socs: FFPM.

O'LEARY, David Reginald Dean Street Surgery, 8 Dean Street, Liskeard PL14 4AQ Tel: 01579 343133 Fax: 01579 344933 — MB Camb. 1976; BA Camb. 1972, MB 1976, BChir 1975; DRCOG 1979; MRCGP 1984.

O'LEARY, Denis Andrew 3 Maybury Close, Frimley, Camberley GU16 7HH — MB ChB Liverp. 1994.

O'LEARY, Denis Anthony No. 34A Coton House, Addenbrooke's Hospital, Hills Road, Cambridge CB2 2QQ — MB BCh BAO NUI 1987.

O'LEARY, Gerard (retired) 22 Welford Road, Filey YO14 0AE Tel: 01723 514374 — MB BCh BAO NUI 1940 (Univ. Coll. Dub.)

O'LEARY, Martin Anthony 133 Richmond Park, Tuebrook, Liverpool L6 5AB Tel: 0151 263 9316 — MB ChB Leeds 1986.

O'LEARY, Maureen Loversall Hospital, Weston Road, Balby, Doncaster DN4 8NX Tel: 01302 796296 Fax: 01302 796134; 185 Chippinghouse Road, Nether Edge, Sheffield S7 1DQ Tel: 0114 258 2611 — MB ChB Bristol 1976; MRCPsych 1981. Cons. Psychiat. Rehabil. Doncaster. Specialty: Gen. Psychiat.; Rehabil. Med. Socs: BMA; Roy. Coll. Psychiat. Prev: Sen. Regist. Rotat. (Adult Psychiat.) Sheff. VTS.

O'LEARY, Mr Sean Thomas — MB BChir Camb. 1989 (St. Mary's Hosp.) FRCS Ed. 1994; FRCS Eng. 1994; FRCS (Tr & Orth) 1998. Cons. (Orthop.), Roy. Berks. Hosp. Reading. Specialty: Orthop. Socs: BMA; Assoc. Mem. BOA; Brit. Orthop. Train. Assn. Prev: Specialist Regist. St Mary's Hosp., Lond. W2; Specialist Reg. Centr. Middlx. Hosp., Lond.

O'LEARY, Thomas Dundalk Street Surgery, 53 Dundalk Street, Newtownhamilton, Newry BT35 0PB Tel: 028 3087 8204 Fax: 028 3087 8196; Bog Road, Mullaghbawn, Newry BT35 9TT — MB BCh BAO NUI 1981; DRCOG 1983; MRCGP 1985. GP Newtownhamilton. Specialty: Gen. Pract. Socs: BMA & Brit. Med. Acupunc. Soc. Prev: Trainee GP Warrenpoint Health Centre Newry; Trainee GP Daisy Hill Hosp. VTS Newry.

O'LEARY, Thomas Philip The Park Canol Group Practice, Park Canol Surgery, Central Park, Pontypridd CF38 1RJ Tel: 01443 203414 Fax: 01443 218218 — MB BCh Wales 1985.

O'LEARY, Tracey Diane Greenland Surgery, Greenland, Millbrook, Torpoint PL10 1BA Tel: 01752 822576 Fax: 01752 823155; 1 Whiteford Road, Mannamead, Plymouth PL3 5LU — MB ChB Aberd. 1992; DRCOG 1995; MRCGP 1996. GP Millbrook Surg. Millbrook Torpoint Cornw. Specialty: Gen. Pract. Prev: GP/Regist. (Gen. Pract.) Stonehaven Med. Centre.

O'LOAN, Aidan Aloysius 19 Salisbury Gardens, Antrim Road, Belfast BT15 5EL — MB BCh BAO NUI 1983.

O'LOAN, John Jackson Avenue Health Centre, Jackson Avenue, Culcheth, Warrington WA3 4DZ Tel: 01925 763077 — MB ChB Aberd. 1987.

O'LOAN, Maria Dolores Antrim Hospital, 45 Bush Road, Antrim BT41 2RL Tel: 02894 424 000 Fax: 02894 424 294; 48 Glen's Brae Road, Martinstown, Ballymena BT43 7LX Tel: 02821 758 361 — MB BCh BAO Belf. 1983 (Belfast) DCH RCPS Glas. 1986; DRCOG 1986; MRCGP 1988; DTM & H Liverp. 1990; MRCP & Glas. 1997. Staff Grade (Paediat.) Antrim Hosp. Specialty: Paediat. Socs: Ulster Paediat. Soc. Prev: Med. Off. Ortum Mission Hosp. Kitale, Kenya; Trainee GP/SHO Waveney Hosp. Ballymena Vocations Train. Scheme; Trainee GP New Galloway.

O'LOAN, Philip Raymond Portstewart Medical Centre, Mill Road, Portstewart BT55 7SW Tel: 028 7083 2600 Fax: 028 7083 6871 — MB BCh BAO Belf. 1982; MRCGP 1987. Specialty: Gen. Pract.

O'LOGHLEN, Niall Anthony Abbotswood Medical Centre, Defford Road, Pershore WR10 1HZ Tel: 01386 552424; The Pound House, Great Comberton, Pershore WR10 3DU — MB BS Lond. 1979; MA Camb. 1975; DRCOG 1982; DCH RCP Lond. 1983; MRCGP 1983.

O'LOUGHLIN, Anne Marie Mourne Family Surgery, Newry Street, Kilkeel, Newry BT34 4DN Tel: 028417 65422; 3 Ardaveen Drive, Newry BT35 8UH — MB BCh BAO Belf. 1995 (Qu. Univ. Belf.) DRCOG London 1977; MRCGP 1999. GP Locum. Specialty: Gen. Pract.

O'LOUGHLIN, Bernadette Ann Silver Lane Surgery, 1 Suffolk Court, Yeadon, Leeds LS19 7JN Tel: 0113 250 4953 Fax: 0113 250 9804; Beck House, Hebers Ghyll Drive, Ilkley LS29 9QH — MB ChB Leeds 1981; MRCP (UK) 1984; DRCOG 1986; MRCGP 1986.

O'LOUGHLIN, James Peter (retired) 2 Fern Clough, Hillside, Chorley New Road, Bolton BL1 5DX Tel: 01204 847087 Email: p.andm.oloughlin@ntlworld.com — MB ChB Manch. 1956; FRCP Lond. 1977, M 1963. Prev: Phys. Bolton Dist. Gen. Hosp. & Bolton Roy. Infirm.

O'LOUGHLIN, Michael Alfred Parkview Surgery, 14 Ballygawley Road, Dungannon BT70 1EL — MB BCh BAO NUI 1980; DCH 1983; MRCGP 1984. GP Dungannon.

O'MAHONY, Barbara Ann (retired) 2 Tranmere Drive, Guiseley, Leeds LS20 8NQ Tel: 01943 874888 — (Newc.) MB BS Durh. 1961; MRCP Lond. 1967.

O'MAHONY, Colm Pierce Department of Sexual Health, Countess of Chester Hospital NHS Trust, Liverpool Road, Chester CH2 1UL Tel: 01244 363097 Fax: 01244 363095 Email: colm.omahony@coch.nhs.uk — MB BCh BAO NUI 1981 (Univ. Coll. Dub.) BSc (Microbiol.) Dub. 1975; MD NUI 1986; Dip. Ven. Liverp. 1986; FRCPI 1995, M 1988; FRCP (Lond.) 2001. Cons. Sexual Health, Countess of Chester Hosp. NHS Trust, Chester. Specialty: Genitourinary Medicine.

O'MAHONY, Grania Anne Mary St Wulfstan Surgery, Southam Clinic, Pendicke Street, Southam CV47 1PF Tel: 01926 810939; Fieldgate View, Pillory Green, Napton, Southam CV47 8LN Tel: 01926 815739 — MB BS Lond. 1983 (St. Bart.) DRCOG 1987; DCH RCP Lond. 1988; MRCGP 1989. GP.

O'MAHONY, James Finbar 77 Old Park Road, London N13 4RG — MB BS Lond. 1973.

O'MAHONY, James Gerard Gastroenterology Unit, Leeds General Infirmary, Great George St., Leeds LS1 3EX Tel: 0113 392 6733 Fax: 0113 392 6968 — MD NUI 1991; MB BCh BAO 1983; MRCPI 1986; MRCP (UK) 1988; FRCP Ed 1998. Cons. Phys. Leeds Gen. Infirm. Specialty: Gastroenterol. Prev: Sen. Regist. (Gen. Med. & Gastroenterol.) Yorks. RHA.; Regist. (Gen. Med. & Gastroenterol.) Cork Regional Hosp.; Research Fell. & Hon. Regist. Gastrointestinal Unit West. Gen. Hosp. Edin.

O'MAHONY, Jeremiah B St. Annes Health Centre, Nottingham NG3 3PX; 49 Bridge Road, Welwyn Garden City AL8 6UH — MB BCh BAO NUI 1947 (Cork) Prev: Ho. Surg. N. Infirm. Cork.

O'MAHONY, Marcella Sinead Llandough Hospital, Penlan Road, Penarth CF64 2XX Tel: 029 2071 6984 Fax: 029 2071 1267 Email: omahonyms@cf.ac.uk — MB BCh BAO NUI 1986 (University College, Cork, National University of Ireland) BSc (Hon. Physiology) Ireland 1983; MRCPI Ireland 1989; FRCPI Ireland 2000; FRCP Lond. 2002. Sen. Lect. (Geriat. Med.) Univ. Wales Coll. Med. Cardiff.; Hon. Cons. Phys., Cardiff and Vale NHS Trust, Cardiff. Specialty: Care of the Elderly. Socs: Brit. Geriat. Soc.; Irish Gerontological Soc.; Brit. Geriat. Soc., Drugs and prescribing Sect. Prev: Lect. in Geriat.

Med., Univ. of Wales Coll. of Med., 1991-1995; Brit. Geriat. Soc./Nuffield Trav. Fell., Cell Biol. and Aeging, Univ. of Calif., San Francisco, 1993-1994; Regist. Respirat. Med., Med. Professional Unit, St. Vincent's Hosp., Dub., 1990-1991.

O'MAHONY, Mark Yves Cadbury Heath Health Centre, Parkwall Road, Cadbury Heath, Bristol BS30 8HS Tel: 0117 980 5700 Fax: 0117 980 5701; 8 Carnarvon Road, Redland, Bristol BS6 7DP Tel: 0117 924 3361 — BM Soton. 1979 (Southampton) Cert. Evidence Based Healthcare 1997 (Oxon.); MRCP (UK) 1982; DRCOG 1984; MRCGP 1986. Prev: Trainee GP Avon VTS; SHO Rotat. (Med.) Princess Margt. Hosp. Swindon; SHO Rotat. (Path.) John Radcliffe Hosp. Oxf.

O'MAHONY, Mary Catherine Health Protection Agency, Local and Regional Services Division, Level 11 The Adelphi, 1-11 John Adam Street, London WC2N 6HT Tel: 020 7339 1338 Fax: 020 7339 1309 Email: mary.o'mahoney@hpa.org.uk — MB BCh BAO Dub. 1975; MSc Lond. 1980; MRCPI 1981; FFPHM 1992, M 1984. Specialty: Pub. Health Med.

O'MAHONY, Patrick Henry Michael Abernethy House, 70 Silver Street, Enfield EN1 3EP Tel: 020 8366 1314 Fax: 020 8364 4176 — MB BS Lond. 1976 (St. Geo.) DPMSA 1998. Prev: GP Tutor Enfield Dist. Hosp. Postgrad. Centre.; Ho. Off. (Vasc. Surg.) St. Geo. Hosp. Lond.; SHO (O & G/Paediat.) Chase Farm Hosp. Enfield.

O'MALLEY, Brendan Peter Kettering General Hospital, Rothwell Road, Kettering NN16 8UZ Tel: 01858 462840; Pine Lodge, 91 Fairfield Road, Market Harborough LE16 9QH Tel: 01858 462840 — MB BChir Camb. 1973; BA (Hons.) Camb. 1969; MRCP (UK) 1976; MD Leic. 1987; FRCP (Lond.) 1995. Cons. Phys. Kettering Gen. Hosp. N.ants. Specialty: Endocrinol. Socs: Thyroid Club; Soc. Endocrinol.; Brit. Diabetic Assn. Prev: Lect. & Hon. Sen. Regist. (Therap.) Univ. Leicester; SHO Rotat. (Med.) Bath Health Dist.; Regist. (Med.) Leicester Roy. Infirm.

O'MALLEY, Daniel Noel Ballamona Hospital, Braddan IM4 4RF — MB BCh BAO Belf. 1975 (Queen's Univ. Belf.) MRCPsych 1982. Specialty: Gen. Psychiat. Socs: Roy. Coll. Psychiat.

O'MALLEY, Geraldine Washway Road Medical Centre, 67 Washway Road, Sale M33 7SS Tel: 0161 962 4354 Fax: 0161 905 4706 — MB ChB Sheff. 1986; DCH RCP Lond. 1989; MRCGP 1990. GP Princip. Specialty: Gen. Pract. Prev: Trainee GP Doncaster VTS.

O'MALLEY, Helen Anne 66 Tandle Hill Road, Royton, Oldham OL2 5UX — MB ChB Leic. 1995.

O'MALLEY, Helen Frances Medical Services, Grove House, 3 Grove Place, Swansea SA1 Tel: 01792 659840 — MB BCh Wales 1974. Med. Adviser Med. Serv.s, Swansea. Specialty: Disabil. Med. Socs: Brit. Med. Acupunct. Soc. Prev: Princip. GP Swansea; Dep. Disignated Doctor Cervical Cytol. West. Glam. HA; Regist. (Respirat. Med.) Morriston Hosp.

O'MALLEY, John Francis 17 Easingwold Gardens, Luton LU1 1UD — MB ChB Manch. 1991.

O'MALLEY, Michael Crofton Street Surgery, 1 Crofton Street, Oldham OL8 3DA Tel: 0161 624 4716 Fax: 0161 628 9513; Crofton House, 1 Crofton St, Oldham OL8 3BZ — MB ChB Birm. 1968; BSc (Hons.) Birm. 1964, MB ChB 1968. Sec. Oldham Med. Soc.

O'MALLEY, Patricia Anne Moorside, Trafford General Hospital, Moorside Road, Davyhulme, Urmaston, Manchester M41 5SL — MB ChB Manch. 1984; MRCPsych 1989; MSc Manch. 1992. Cons. Psychiat. In Old Age Psychiatry, Bolton, Salford & Trafford Mental Health NHS Trust. Specialty: Geriat. Psychiat.

O'MALLEY, Mr Steven Patrick Milton Keynes NHS Trust, Standing Way, Milton Keynes MK6 5LD Tel: 01908 243141 Fax: 01908 243141 Email: steven.o'malley@mkgeneral.nhs.uk; Deiter House, Chase Park Road, Yardley Hastings, Northampton NN7 1HF Tel: 01604 696045 Fax: 01908 243141 Email: steven.omalley@care.4free.net — MB BS Lond. 1977 (St. Thos.) FRCS Eng. 1983. Cons. Otol. Milton Keynes Gen. Hosp.; Cons. Otol. Northampton Gen. Hosp. Specialty: Otolaryngol. Prev: Lect. & Sen. Regist. Manch.

O'MARA, Lee 72 Suffield Way, King's Lynn PE30 3DL — MB BS Lond. 1986.

O'MARA, Lucy 29-53 Himley Road, Dudley DY1 2QD Tel: 01384 254423 — MB ChB Manch. 1996; DRCOG, RCOG 1998; MRCGP 2001. GP. Dudley; Clin. Asst. Palliat. Care, Mary Stevens Hospice Stourbridge.

O'MEARA, Margaret Mary (retired) P.O. Box No 17317, London SW3 4WJ Tel: 020 7730 2800 Fax: 020 7730 0818 — MB BCh BAO NUI 1943; CPH Liverp. 1948. Prev: Ho. Surg. Jervis St. Hosp. Dub. & Temple St. Childr. Hosp. Dub.

O'MEARA, Moira Elizabeth Primrose Cottage, Primrose Lane, Boston Spa, Wetherby LS23 6DL — MB ChB Leeds 1984.

O'MOORE, Gerald Roderick (Surgery), 279 Katherine Road, Forest Gate, London E7 8PP Tel: 020 8472 0803 Fax: 020 8503 4490; 21 Stradbroke Drive, Chigwell IG7 5QU Tel: 020 8500 6502 — MB BCh BAO NUI 1952 (Univ. Coll. Dub.) MICGP 1987. Socs: BMA; BMA. Prev: Ho. Phys. PeaMt. Sanat. Newc., Dub., Bon Secours Hosp. Glasnevin & Mater Hosp. Dub.

O'MOORE, John Charles Francis Devereux Upminster Bridge Surgery, 126 Upminster Road, Hornchurch RM12 6PL Tel: 01708 440642 Fax: 01708 477329 Email: johnomoore@doctors.org.uk; 2 Oaklands Avenue, Romford RM1 4DB Tel: 01708 765996 Fax: 01708 765996 Email: johnomoore@doctors.org.uk — MB BCh BAO NUI 1989 (Univ. Coll. Dub.) T.(GP) 1993; DFFP 1993; DRCOG 2002; MRCGP 2002. Princip. in Gen. Pract.; Med. Ref. - City of Lond. Crematorium. Specialty: Gen. Pract. Socs: Fell. Roy. Soc. Med.; BMA. Prev: Trainee GP Glos.; SHO Barking Hosp. & King Geo. Hosp. Essex; Ho. Off. (Med. & Surg.) Walton Hosp. Liverp.

O'MULLANE, Nicholas Matthew — MB ChB Birm. 1969; DObst RCOG 1972; DCH Eng. 1972; MRCP (UK) 1974; Cert. Higher Med. Train. in Diabetes, Endocrinol. & Gen. (Int.) Med. 1981; FRCP Lond. 1990. Cons. Phys. Tameside Gen. Hosp. Ashton-under-Lyne.; Cons. Phys. (Diabetes, Endocrinol. & Several Internal Med.). Specialty: Gen. Med.; Diabetes; Endocrinol. Prev: Clin. Tutor Tameside Gen. Hosp. Ashton-under-Lyne.

O'NEAL, Hugh Brighton General Hospital, Brighton BN2 3EW Tel: 01273 696955; 41 Wilbury Crescent, Hove BN3 6FJ Tel: 01273 724198 Email: hugh.oneal@cwcom.net — BM Soton. 1976; BSc (Hons.) (Physiol. & Biochem.) Soton. 1971; MRCP (UK) 1980; FRCP Lond. 1994. Cons. Geriat. Brighton Health Care NHS Trust. Specialty: Care of the Elderly. Prev: Cons. Geriat. SE Thames RHA.

O'NEIL, Helen Alison Earwicker and Partners, The Health Centre, 97 Derby Road, Nottingham NG9 7AT Tel: 0115 939 2444 Fax: 0115 939 5625 — MB BS Lond. 1979 (Univ. Coll.) DRCOG 1981; DCH RCP Lond. 1982; MRCGP 1983.

O'NEIL, James Edward Gerard 14 Alexandra Park, Lenzie, Glasgow G66 5BH — MB ChB Glas. 1983; MRCGP 1987; MPH Glas. 1995. Prev: Med. Dir. Glas. Emerg. Med. Serv.; Trainee (Pub. Health Med.) Gtr. Glas. HB.

O'NEIL, Michael Jeffrey (retired) Holly Bank, Haughs Road, Huddersfield HD3 4YS — MB ChB Leeds 1975; FFA RCS Eng. 1983. Prev: Sen. Regist. (Anaesth.) Nottm. & E. Midl. Train. Scheme.

O'NEIL, Michael John Earwicker and Partners, The Health Centre, 97 Derby Road, Nottingham NG9 7AT Tel: 0115 939 2444 Fax: 0115 939 5625 — MB BS Lond. 1980 (Univ. Coll. Hosp.) BSc (Anat II 1) Lond. 1977, MB BS 1980; MRCP (UK) 1983.

O'NEIL, Professor Raymund 49 Combemartin Road, Southfields, London SW18 5PP Tel: 020 8788 6609 — (Westm.) BDS Manch. 1948; FDS RCS Eng. 1952; MRCS Eng. LRCP Lond. 1957. Specialty: Oral & Maxillofacial Surg. Socs: Fell. Roy. Soc. Med.; BDA; BMA. Prev: Emerit. Prof. Oral Surg. Univ. Coll. Lond.

O'NEILL, Alice Elizabeth West Norfolk Primary Care Trust, St James, Exton's Road, King's Lynn PE30 5NU Tel: 01553 816293 Email: alice.oneill@westnorfolk-pct.nhs.uk; Smith's Farmhouse, Herne Lane, Toftwood, Dereham NR19 1QE — MB BS Lond. 1985 (Roy. Free) DCH RCP Lond. 1988; DRCOG 1989; Cert. Family Plann. JCC 1989; MRCP (UK) 1996; MSc (Health Sci.) UEA 2002. Cons. Community Paediat., Norwich. Specialty: Paediat. Socs: MRCPCH. Prev: Regist. (Paediat.) Addenbrooke's Hosp. Camb.; Specialist Regist. (Community Paediat.) Norwich; Regist. (Paediat.) Qu. Eliz. Hosp. King's Lynn.

O'NEILL, Ann-Marie St Catherine's, West Hill Road, Woking GU22 7UL — MB BCh BAO Dub. 1987; DRCPath 1995. Sen. Regist. (Med. Microbiol.) Roy. Hants. Co. Hosp Winchester. Specialty: Med. Microbiol.

O'NEILL, Anne 50 Stuart Road, Corby NN17 1RL — MB BS Lond. 1993.

O'NEILL, Anthony Peter Forest Surgery, 11 Station Road, Loughton IG10 4NZ Tel: 020 8508 3818 Fax: 020 8508 2539; 6 Theydon Park Road, Theydon Bois, Epping CM16 7LW Tel: 01992 813643 — MB BS Lond. 1980 (Roy. Free Hosp. Sch. Med.) MRCGP 1991. Clin. Asst. (Dermat.) St. Margt. Hosp. Epping. Specialty: Dermat.

O'NEILL, Anthony St John 12 Turnberry Road, Glasgow G11 5AE — MB BCh BAO NUI 1988.

O'NEILL, Ciara Anne Omagh Health Centre, Mountjoy Road, Omagh BT79 7BA Tel: 028 8224 3521; 12 Gleannan Park, Killyclogher, Omagh BT79 7XZ Tel: 01662 249026 — MB BCh BAO Belf. 1989; DGM RCPS Glas. 1991; DRCOG 1992; MRCGP 1993.

O'NEILL, Conor Patrick 26 Laurelvale, Crumlin BT29 4WW — MB BCh BAO Belf. 1994.

O'NEILL, Corneilus Omalley 27 Meeting Street, Magherafelt BT45 6BW — MB BCh BAO Belf. 1988; MB BCh Belf. 1988.

O'NEILL, Cyril Patrick Norton Medical Centre, Billingham Road, Norton, Stockton-on-Tees TS20 2UZ Tel: 01642 360111 Fax: 01642 558672 — MB BS Newc. 1982; DRCOG 1986; DCCH RCP Ed. 1986; MRCGP 1987. GP Norton Med. Centre. Prev: Trainee GP Cleveland VTS.; Med. Off. Makiungu Hosp. Singida, Tanzania.

O'NEILL, Mr Damian Patrick c/o Eye Department, Leeds General Infirmary, Leeds LS1 3EX — MB BCh BAO NUI 1986; LRCPI & LM LRCSI & LM 1986; MRCPI 1988; DO RCS Eng. 1989; FRCS Eng. 1990; FCOphth 1990; FRCOpth 1993. Sen. Regist. (Ophth.) Roy. Hallamsh. Hosp.; Cons. (Ophth.) Leeds Gen. Infirm.; Hon. Sen. Clin. Lect. Leeds Univ. Specialty: Ophth. Prev: Regist. Moorfields Eye Hosp. Lond.

O'NEILL, Daphne (retired) Merrion House, 5 Barley Hill Lane, Poulshot, Devizes SN10 1RS Tel: 01380 827095 Fax: 01380 827236 — MB BS Durh. 1953.

O'NEILL, David 10 Providence Road, Bromsgrove B61 8EL — MB BChir Camb. 1980; BA Camb. 1977, MA, MB BChir 1980; MRCP (UK) 1987.

O'NEILL, David Marnoch 10 Harling Drive, Troon KA10 6NF — MB ChB Glas. 1970; MRCP (U.K.) 1974.

O'NEILL, Declan Finbarr Bell Bungalow, High Street, Burwash, Etchingham TN19 7EH — MB BCh BAO NUI 1976; MPH Sydney 1988; MFPHM RCP (UK) 1993; FFPHM RCP (UK) 1998. Cons. Pub. Health Med. S. Thames RHA; 2000, Assoc. Director, Centre for Health Servs. Studies, Univ. of Kent. Specialty: Pub. Health Med. Socs: Fell. Roy. Austral. Coll. Med. Admin.; Fell. Austral. Fac. Pub. Health Med. Prev: Dep. Dir. Fremantle Hosp.; Med. Off. Health Dept. West. Austral.; Regist. Roy. Perth Hosp.

O'NEILL, Denis William James, TD, SBStJ (retired) 8 Oaklands Park, Warmwell, Dorchester DT2 8JQ Tel: 01305 852722 — (Sheff.) MRCS Eng. LRCP Lond. 1946; MRCGP 1953. Prev: Ho. Surg. & Ho. Phys. Roy. Infirm. Sheff.

O'NEILL, Mr Eamon Canice BMEC, City Hospital, Dudley Road, Birmingham Tel: 0121 554 3801 Email: eamon_oneill@hotmail.com — MB BCh BAO NUI 1970; FRCS Ed. 1976; FRCOphth Lond. 1979. Cons. Ophth. Surg., Birm. and Midl. Eye Centre; Director of Glaucoma Serv.; Hon. Sen. Clin. Lect., Univ. of Birm. Specialty: Ophth. Socs: RSM; BMA; Midlands Ophth. Soc.

O'NEILL, Eileen Moira 5 Amberley Gardens, Bedford MK40 3BT Tel: 01234 325800 — MD Sheff. 1961; MB ChB 1953; DCH Eng. 1957; FRCP Lond. 1976, M 1964. Cons. Paediat. Emerit. Specialty: Paediat. Socs: Fell. Roy. Coll. Phys. Lond.; Brit. Paediat. Assn. Prev: Sen. Regist. (Paediat.) Whittington Hosp. Lond.; Regist. (Med.) Fulham Hosp. Lond.; Regist. (Paediat. Clin. & Research) North. Gen. Hosp. Sheff.

O'NEILL, Elizabeth Mary 1 Marquis Close, Wembley HA0 4HF — MB ChB Liverp. 1985.

O'NEILL, Elizabeth Valerie Donmall and Partners, 87 Albion Street, London SE16 7JX Tel: 020 7237 2092 Fax: 020 7231 1435 — MB BCh BAO NUI 1994.

O'NEILL, Emma Jane — MB ChB Glas. 1989; MRCP (UK) 1994; FFARCSI 1998. GP LOCUM. Specialty: Gen. Pract. Socs: BMA; Med. & Dent. Defence Union Scotl.

O'NEILL, Francis Charles Friends House, Abbeystead, Lancaster LA2 9DT Tel: 01524 791770 Email: francis.oneill@ukonline.co.uk — MB ChB Manch. 1963; MRCP Lond. 1968. Disability Analyst; Medically Qualified Panel Mem., The Appeals Serv. Specialty: Respirat. Med.

O'NEILL, George Dermot Springfield Road Surgery, 66-70 Springfield Road, Belfast BT12 7AH Tel: 028 9032 3571 Fax: 028 9020 7707 — MB BCh BAO Belf. 1971.

O'NEILL, Gordon Francis Allen Flat 1 Emerson Bainbridge House, 47 Cleveland St., London W1T 4JQ — MB BS New South Wales 1987.

O'NEILL, Gregory Thomas John Dept of Radiology, Glasgow Royal Infirmary, Glasgow G4 0SF; 10 Main Street, Overtown, Wishaw ML2 0QA — MB ChB Ed. 1992. Specialist Regist. Radiol.

O'NEILL, Hilary Mary-Josephine Department of Radiology, North Hampshire Hospital, Aldermaston Road, Basingstoke RG24 9NA — MB BCh BAO NUI 1979; DCH NUI 1982; MRCPI 1983; FFR RCSI 1986. Cons. Radiol. N. Hants. Hosp. Specialty: Radiol. Prev: Sen. Regist. (Radiol.) Soton. Gen. Hosp.; Regist. (Radiol.) Mater Hosp. Dub.

O'NEILL, Hugh Blaise Horsford Medical Centre, 205 Holt Road, Horsford, Norwich NR10 3DX Tel: 01603 898300 Fax: 01603 891818; 130 Lower Street, Salhouse, Norwich NR13 6RX Tel: 01603 722035 — MB BCh BAO NUI 1980; MRCS Eng. LRCP Lond. 1980; Cert. Av. Med. 1987; AFOM 2002. C. Med. Off. Norf. Army Cadet Force; Med. Examr. of Divers HSE; Sen. Cons. Unity Med. Servs. Specialty: Occupat. Health. Socs: Assn. Police Surg.; Soc. Occupat. Med.; Soc. Orthop. Med. Prev: SHO (O & G, Orthop. & A & E) Norf. & Norwich Hosp.; Force Surg. Norf. Constab.; Sen. Cons. Clin. Forens. Med. B & C Div. Norf. Constab.

O'NEILL, Hugh Finbarr 11 Rosetta Drive, Belfast BT7 3HL — MB BCh BAO Belf. 1992; FFARCSI 1988. Specialty: Anaesth.

O'NEILL, James Dermot Willowbrook Health Centre, Cottingham Road, Corby NN17 2UR Fax: 01536 402153; 28 Skeffington Close, Geddington, Kettering NN14 1BA Tel: 01536 742305 — MB BCh BAO NUI 1974 (Galway) DRCOG 1977. Specialty: Gen. Pract.

O'NEILL, Jane Maria Bernadette Priory Court, Priory Hospital, Priory Lane, London SW15 5JJ — MB BCh BAO Dub. 1983; MB BCh Dub. 1983.

O'NEILL, Janet (retired) Rose Cottage, Gosforth, Seascale CA20 1JB Tel: 0194 67 25216 — BM BCh Oxf. 1963 (Oxf. & Middlx.) MA Oxf. 1963; DObst RCOG 1966; MRCP Lond. 1967; DPM Eng. 1972; MRCPsych 1973; FRCP 1999. Prev: Princip. GP.

O'NEILL, Mr John Joseph (retired) Arus Na Greine, Killuney, Portadown Road, Armagh BT61 9HE — MB BCh BAO Belf. 1958; FRCS Ed. 1965; FRCSI 1987. Prev: Cons. Surg. Craigavon Area Hosp. & Armagh City Hosp.

O'NEILL, John Marmion Radiology Department, Royal Infirmary, Lauriston Place, Edinburgh EH3 9HB Tel: 0131 536 2900; 17 Marchmount Road, Edinburgh EH9 1HY Tel: 0131 466 0639 — MB BCh BAO NUI 1992; MRCPI 1996; MSc 1999; FRCR 2001. Specialist Regist. (Radiol.) Roy. Infirm. Edin. Specialty: Radiol. Prev: Regist. (Gen. Med. & Nephrol.) & SHO (Med.) Univ. Coll. Cork.

O'NEILL, Mr John Stephen Borders General Hospital, Melrose TD6 9BS Tel: 01896 826000 Fax: 01896 826924 Email: john.oneill@borders.scot.nhs.uk; Grianan, Gattonside, Melrose TD6 9NB — MB ChB Glas. 1978; FRCS Ed. 1983; FRCS Glas. 1983; BSc (1st cl. Hons. Path.) Glas. 1976, MD 1989. Cons. Gen. Surg. Borders Gen. Hosp. Melrose. Specialty: Gen. Surg. Prev: Lect. (Surg). Univ. Edin. & Roy. Infirm. Edin.

O'NEILL, Joseph Marcus Margaret Thompson Medical Centre, 105 East Millwood Road, Speke, Liverpool L24 6TH Tel: 0151 425 2889 Fax: 0151 425 2772 Email: jmoneill@btinternet.com; 4 Hamilton Street, Chester CH2 3JG Tel: 01244 322440 — MB BCh BAO NUI 1984 (RCSI) CTCM & H RCSI 1983; LRCPI & LM, LRCSI & LM 1984; DCH NUI 1986; MRCGP 1991; Dip. Palliat. Med. Wales 1995; CCST (Palliative Medicine) 1996. Gen. Practitioner; Clin. Cancer Lead. Liverp. S PCG. 1 Childwall Pk Ave. Liverp. L16 0JE. Specialty: Palliat. Med.; Gen. Pract. Prev: Sen. Regist. (Palliat. Med.) Trent RHA; Assoc. Specialist (Palliat. Med.) S. Downs Health NHS Trust; SHO (Palliat. Med.) St. Joseph's Hospice Lond.

O'NEILL, Kareen Ann 7 Douglas Park Crescent, Bearsden, Glasgow G61 3DS; Beechwood, 19 The Balk, York YO42 2QQ — MB ChB Manch. 1987. Princip. GP Goole. Specialty: Gen. Pract.

O'NEILL, Kenneth Francis Midlock Medical Centre, 7 Midlock Street, Glasgow G51 1SL Tel: 0141 427 4271 Fax: 0141 427 1405 — MB ChB Glas. 1983; BSc (Holu Intercalate) 1980; MRCGP 1988.

O'NEILL, Kenneth Maurice Durham Road Surgery, 25 Durham Road, Edinburgh EH16 4DT Tel: 0131 669 1153 Fax: 0131 669

3633; 8 Hamilton Terrace, Edinburgh EH15 1NB Tel: 0131 669 1150 — MB ChB St. And. 1967. Socs: Clin. Club Edin. & Brit. Soc. Sport & Med. Prev: SHO (Gen. Med.) Edin. Roy. Infirm.; Ho. Phys. Maryfield Hosp. Dundee; Ho. Surg. Dundee Roy. Infirm.

O'NEILL, Kevin Peter Ipswich Hospital, Heath Road, Ipswich IP4 5PD Tel: 01473 712233; 12 Ipswich Road, Woodbridge IP12 4BU Tel: 01394 388308 — MB BS Lond. 1979; MRCP (UK) 1984. Cons. Paediat. Ipswich Hosp. Specialty: Paediat. Socs: Brit. Paediat. Assn. Prev: Sen. Regist. (Paediat.) Dept. Child Health Ninewells Hosp. Dundee; Regist. (Paediat.) Dept. Child Health Newc. u Tyne; Research Clin. MRC, The Gambia.

O'NEILL, Kevin Richard 1 Crossley Terrace, Arthurs Hill, Newcastle upon Tyne NE4 5NY — MB BS Lond. 1992.

O'NEILL, Kevin Sean 63 Woodfarm Close, Leigh-on-Sea SS9 4PF — MB BS Lond. 1989; BSc (Hons.) Lond. 1986, MB BS 1989. SHO (Orthop.) St. Geo. Hosp. Lond. Prev: SHO (Neurosurg.) Atkinson Morley's Hosp.; SHO (A & E) Ealing Gen. Hosp.; Ho. Surg. St. Mary's Hosp. Lond.

O'NEILL, Margaret Betty Edith 44 Salisbury Road, Cressington Park, Liverpool L19 0PJ Tel: 0151 427 2329 — MB BCh BAO Dub. 1949 (T.C. Dub.) BA, MB BCh BAO Dub. 1949. Clin. Med. Off. (Community Health) Liverp. HA. Prev: Ho. Surg. Pk. Hosp. Davyhulme; Ho. Phys. Vict. Hosp. Blackpool & Dorking Gen. Hosp.

O'NEILL, Mark Francis Joseph (retired) Merrion House, 5 Barley Hill Lane, Poulshot, Devizes SN10 1RS Tel: 01380 827095 Fax: 01380 827236 Email: mfoneill@ukonline.co.uk — MB BS Durh. 1954.

O'NEILL, Martin Patrick O'Malley Mourneside Medical Centre, 1A Ballycolman Avenue, Strabane BT82 9AF Tel: 028 7138 3737 Fax: 028 7138 3979; 6 Cedar Park, Urney Road, Strabane BT82 9ER — MB BCh BAO Belf. 1975.

O'NEILL, Mary Judith 16 Holborn Hall, Lisburn BT27 5AU — MB BCh BAO Belf. 1992; MRCPsych 1997. Specialty: Gen. Psychiat.

O'NEILL, Mary Margaret Meadowlands Surgery, Newry Health Village, Monaghan Street, Newry BT35 6BW Tel: 028 3026 7534; The Pines, 35 Windsor Hill, Newry BT34 1HS — MB BCh BAO Belf. 1983; DRCOG 1985; DCH NUI 1986; MRCGP 1987.

O'NEILL, Mary Siobhan Gerandine Alexandra Road Practice, 11 Alexandra Road, Harrogate HG1 5JS; 41 Duchy Road, Harrogate HG1 2HA — MB BChir Camb. 1980; MRCGP 1983; DRCOG 1983. Prev: GP Leeds.

O'NEILL, Maureen Patricia Mid-Ulster Hospital, 59 Hospital Road, Magherafelt BT45 5EX Tel: 028 796 31031 Fax: 028 793 66992 Email: maureenoneill@doctors.org.uk; The St, 65 Tobermore Road, Magherafelt BT45 5EJ — MB BCh BAO Belf. 1975; DCH RCPSI 1977; FFA RCS Irel. 1980. Cons. Anaesth. Mid Ulster Hosp. Magherafelt. Specialty: Anaesth. Socs: Assn. Anaesth.; Brit. Assn. Day Surg.; Med. Wom. Federat. Prev: Cons. Anaesth. Belf. City Hosp.; Sen. Regist. (Anaesth.) Roy. Vict. Hosp.; Hon. Lect. & Sen. Regist. Univ. Zambia.

O'NEILL, Michael Robert (retired) 11 Blakeley Brow, Raby Mere, Wirral CH63 0PS Tel: 0151 334 1905 Email: michaelgill2@onetel.com — MB BCh BAO Belf. 1960. Prev: Sen. Resid. Med. Off. Belf. City Hosp.

O'NEILL, Niamh Mary Deidre Rose Flat 1, 89 Elgin Avenue, London W9 2DA — MB BS Lond. 1998.

O'NEILL, Owen Brian 21 Claremont Crescent, Edinburgh EH7 4HX Tel: 0131 557 3444 — MB BCh BAO NUI 1971 (Univ. Coll. Cork) BSc NUI 1968; MRCPsych 1976; T(Psych) 1991. Hon. Cons. Psychother. Roy. Edin. Hosp. Specialty: Psychother. Socs: Brit. PsychoAnalyt. Soc.; Tavistock Soc. of Psychotherapists; N. Eng. Assn. for Train. in Psychother. Prev: Cons. Psychother. Portman Clinic Lond.; Dep. Dir. Lond. Clinic Psycho-Anal.; Cons. Psychother. Watford Gen. Hosp.

O'NEILL, Patricia Alice (retired) 145 Perry Hill, London SE6 4LR Tel: 020 8699 1062 — BM BCh Oxf. 1976; MRCS Eng. LRCP Lond. 1976.

O'NEILL, Patricia Josephine Grange Road Surgery, Grange Road, Bishopsworth, Bristol BS13 8LD Tel: 0117 964 4343 Fax: 0117 935 8422 — MB BChir Camb. 1989.

O'NEILL, Patricia Mary Royal Shrewsbury Hospital, Department of Microbiology, Mytton Oak Road, Shrewsbury SY3 8XQ Tel: 01743 261161 Fax: 01743 261165 Email: patricia.oneill@rsh.nhs.uk — MB BS Lond. 1983 (Westm. Med. Sch. Lond.) BA Oxf. 1980; MRCPath 1992. Cons. (Microbiology) Roy. Shrewsbury Hosp.; Cons. in Communicable Dis. Control, Shrops. and Staffs., Health Protec. Unit. Specialty: Med. Microbiol.; Pub. Health Med. Socs: Assn. Med. Microbiol.; Hosp. Infec. Soc.; FRCPath. Prev: Sen. Regist. Rotat. (Microbiol.) W. Midl.; Regist. (Microbiol.) Char. Cross Hosp. Lond.

O'NEILL, Patrick 22 Somersall Park Road, Chesterfield S40 3LD Tel: 01246 566395 — MB BCh BAO NUI 1965.

O'NEILL, Pauline (retired) Stone House, Blocklands, Langton Matravers, Swanage BH19 3LD — (Oxf. & St. Thos.) BM BCh Oxf. 1952; DM Oxf. 1977. Prev: Cons. Microbiol. Lewisham Hosp. Lond.

O'NEILL, Pauline Mary 6 Ardaluin Court, Newcastle BT33 0RT — MB BCh BAO NUI 1986 (Univ. Coll. Dub.) DCH RCPSI 1990; DRCOG 1991; DMH Belf. 1992; MRCGP 1994. Staff Grade Community Piediatrician & GP Locum. Specialty: Community Child Health. Socs: BMA. Prev: Clin. Med. Off. (Child Health) Kilkeel.

O'NEILL, Penelope Anne 12 Hall Walk, Cottingham HU16 4RL — MB ChB Liverp. 1994 (Liverpool) MB ChB (Hons.) Liverp. 1994; MRCP (UK) 1997. Specialist Regist. Clatterbridge Centre for Oncol. Wirral, Merseyside. Specialty: Oncol.

O'NEILL, Mr Peter Balfe (retired) 44 Salisbury Road, Cressington Park, Liverpool L19 0PJ — MB BS Lond. 1948 (Westm.) DLO Eng. 1950; FRCS Eng. 1954. Prev: Cons. ENT Surg. Warrington Dist. Gen. Hosp. & Whiston Hosp.

O'NEILL, Rory Conor O'Hagan Chard Road Surgery, Chard Road, St Budeaux, Plymouth PL5 2UE Tel: 01752 363111 Fax: 01752 363611 — MB BS Lond. 1972 (St. Bart.) MRCGP 1978. Prev: Surg. Lt.-Cdr. RN; Ho. Surg. Crawley Hosp.

O'NEILL, Ryan Joseph 4 Rannyglass, Dungiven, Londonderry BT47 4NE — MB BCh BAO Belf. 1997.

O'NEILL, Sarah Siobhan 14 Stanley Road, Stockport SK4 4HL — BM BCh Oxf. 1998; BM BCh Oxf 1998.

O'NEILL, Sheena Berenice 13 Ashbourne Park, Lanberg, Lisburn BT27 4NS — MB BCh BAO Belf. 1996.

O'NEILL, Sheila Maria Keswick, 13 Woodburn Road, Newlands, Glasgow G43 2TN — MB ChB Glas. 1962. Assoc. Specialist Dermat. Glas. Roy. Infirm. Univ. NHS Trust. Specialty: Dermat.

O'NEILL, Suzanne Louise Top Floor Flat, 1 Walker St., Edinburgh EH3 7JY — MB ChB Ed. 1998.

O'NEILL, Terence William 42 Downview Park W., Antrim Road, Belfast BT15 5HP — MB BCh BAO Dub. 1984; MRCPI 1986.

O'NEILL, Tracey Ann 9 Meadowside, Glenayy, Crumlin BT29 4FE Tel: 01849 459331 — MB BCh BAO Belf. 1996. Specialty: Gen. Med.

O'NEILL, Mr Trevor John Plastic Surgery Associates, Hill House, BUPA Hospital, Colney, Norwich NR4 7TD Tel: 01603 250368 Fax: 01603 250404 — MB BS Lond. 1972; MRCS Eng. LRCP Lond. 1972; FRCS Eng. 1976. Cons. Plastic Surg. Norwich. Specialty: Plastic Surg. Socs: BAPS; BAAPS; Craniofacial Soc. Prev: Sen. Regist. (Plastic Surg.) Qu. Vict. Hosp. E. Grinstead; Regist. (Plastic Surg.) Mt. Vernon Hosp. Northwood & Univ. Coll. Hosp. Lond.

O'NEILL, Vincent Mel 17 Norfolk Farm Road, Pyrford, Woking GU22 8LH — MB BCh BAO NUI 1980.

O'NEILL, William Mary British Medical Association, 14 Queen St., Edinburgh EH2 1LL Tel: 0131 247 3000 Fax: 0131 247 3011 Email: boneill@bma.org.uk; 4 North East, Circus Place, Edinburgh EH3 6SP — MB BCh BAO NUI 1979 (Univ. Coll. Dub.) BSc NUI 1974; DCH NUI 1980; MRCGP 1985, FRCGP 2001. Scott. Sec., BMA. Specialty: Gen. Med.; Medical Management. Prev: Developm. Cons. Primary Care Support Force; Cons. & Sen. Lect. (Palliat. Med.) St. Thos. Hosp. Lond. & Bristol Oncol. Centre; GP W. Lond.

O'NEILL-BYRNE, Katrina Erth Centre, Park Crescent, Erith DA8 3EE Tel: 01322 356110 — MB BCh BAO Dub. 1984; MRCPsych. 1988. Cons. Psychiat. Oxleas NHS Trust Bexley; Hon. Sen. Lect. Psychiat. KGT Med. Sch., Lond.. Specialty: Gen. Psychiat. Prev: Sen. Regist., Psychiat., Lewisham and Guy's NHS Trust.

O'NUNAIN, Sean Seosamh Cranfield Cottage, 27 Church St., Southwell NG25 0HQ — MB BCh BAO NUI 1979.

O'RAHILLY, Professor Stephen Patrick Addenbrooke's Hospital, Department of Clinical Biochemistry, Cambridge CB2 2QR Tel: 01223 336855 Fax: 01223 330598/so104@medschl.cam.ac.uk — MB BCh BAO NUI 1981; MRCPI 1983; MRCP (UK) 1984; MD NUI 1988; FRCPI 1996; FRCP Lond. 1996; FMedSci 1999; FRS 2003. Prof. Clin. Bioch. & Med. Univ. Camb.; Hon. Cons. Phys. Addenbrooke's Hosp. Camb.; Hon. Sen. Scient. MRC Human Nutrit.

Research Cam.; Dep. Dir. Wellcome Trust Clin. Addenbrooke's Hosp. Camb. Specialty: Endocrinol.; Diabetes; Gen. Med. Socs: Hon. Mem. Assn. Phys.; Diabetes UK; Soc. Endocrinol. Prev: Prof. Metab. Med. 96-2002 Univ. Camb.; Research Fell. Nuffield Dept. Med. Diabetes Research Laborats. Oxf.; Wellcome Sen. Clin. Research Fell. Addenbrooke's Hosp. Camb.

O'RAWE, Angela Marie 53 Castle Gardens, Belfast BT15 4GB Tel: 028 779893 — MB BCh BAO Belf. 1983; MRCP (UK) 1987; DCH RCPS Glas. 1987. Research Regist. (Paediat.) Dept. Child Health Qu. Univ. Belf. Specialty: Paediat. Socs: BMA & Nutrit. Soc.

O'RAWE, Martin Gerard Daniel Health Centre, 80 Cambridge Gardens, London W10 6HS Tel: 020 8969 5517 Fax: 020 8964 4766 Email: martinorawe@nhs.net — MB BCh BAO Belf. 1984; MB BCh Belf. 1984; DCH Dub. 1987; JCPTGP 1988. Dep. for Heathcall Med. Servs. Prev: GP Bletchley.

O'REGAN, Josephine Mary Martha (retired) 30 Moor Way, Hawkshaw, Bury BL8 4LF Tel: 01204 885536 — LRCPI & LM, LRSCI & LM 1946; LRCPI & LM, LRCSI & LM 1946. Prev: Clin. Med. Off. Blackburn Hyndburn & Ribble Valley HA.

O'REGAN, Mary Elizabeth 4 Millig Street, Helensburgh G84 9LA — MB BCh BAO Dub. 1983.

O'REGAN, Mary Helen 22 Cliftonville Road, Lowestoft NR33 7AY — MB BS Lond. 1993.

O'REGAN, Mr Michael Barry Queen Margaret Hospital, Whitefield Road, Dunfermline KY12 0SU; Glenlomond House, Glenlomond, Kinross KY13 9HF — MB BCh BAO NUI 1977; BDS NUI 1983; FFD RCSI 1986; FDS (Hon.) Ed. 1997. Cons. Oral & Maxillofacial Surg. Qu. Margt. Hosp. NHS Trust Dunfermline; Postgrad. Tutor Qu. Margt. Hosp. Dunfermline; Hon Sen. Lect. Univ. of Edin.; Fellowship Examr. (FDS) Univ. of Edin. Specialty: Oral & Maxillofacial Surg. Socs: Scott. Oral and Maxillofacial Soc.; Fell. and Inaurgural Sec.; Brit. Assn. Oral & Maxfacial Surgs. Prev: Regist. Univ. Coll. Hosp. Lond.; Sen. Regist. The Roy. Lond. Hosp. Lond.

O'REGAN, Rita 9 Oxford Mews, Cromwell Raod, Hove BN3 3NF — MB BS Lond. 1991 (UCMSM)

O'REILLY, Adrian James Newnham Walk Surgery, Wordsworth Grove, Cambridge CB3 9HS Tel: 01223 366811 Fax: 01223 302706 — MB BCh Wales 1984; DObst RCOG 1988; MRCGP 1988; DCH RCP Lond. 1989; MBA Cambs. 1992; DPH Camb. 1995; MFPHM Part I (I) 1996. Princip. GP Camb.; PCG Bd. Mem., Camb. City PCG; 1-deg. Care Cancer Lead, Camb. City PCG (Prelim. care). Specialty: Pub. Health Med. Socs: Local Med. Comm. (Camb.shire). Prev: Regist. (Pub. Health) Camb. & Huntingdon Health Commiss.; Trainee GP S. Gwent VTS.

O'REILLY, Aidan Patrick Hemel Hempstead General Hospital, Department of Histopathology, Hillfield Road, Hemel Hempstead HP2 4AD Tel: 01442 287841 Fax: 01442 287845 Email: mary.langford@whht.nhs.uk — MB BCh BAO Cork 1975; MRCPath 1984. Cons. Histopath. Specialty: Histopath. Socs: BMA; Internat. Acad. of Path.; Europ. Soc. of Path. Prev: Vis. Teach. Fac. of Med. Univ. of Singapore; Lect. in Path. Univ. of Lond., Roy. Free Hosp. Med. Sch.

O'REILLY, Mr Brian Francis 21 Newlands Road, Glasgow G43 2JD Tel: 0141 649 1961 Fax: 0141 201 3162 Email: brian.o'reilly@northglasgow.scot.nhs.uk — MB ChB Glas. 1972; FRCS Glas. 1977. Cons. ENT Surg. Stobhill Hosp. Glas.; Cons. Neuro-Otol. Inst. Neurol. Sci. S. Gen. Hosp. Glas. Specialty: Otorhinolaryngol. Socs: Scott. Otorhinolaryngological Soc.: Pat Sec.; Brit. Assn. of otorhinolaryngologists: Counc. Mem.; Roy. Soc. of Med.: Past Counc. Mem.

O'REILLY, Mr Brian Joseph, Wing Cdr. RAF Med. Br. Retd. Basildon Hospital, Basildon SS16 5NL Tel: 01268 598500 Fax: 01268 598501 Email: brain_oreilly@_; Glasshouse Cottages, Mapletree Lane, Ingatestone CM4 0PP Tel: 01277 355794 Fax: 01277 355794 — MB ChB Bristol 1978; DLO RCS Eng. 1982; FRCS Ed. 1984. Cons. Otorhinolaryngol. Orsett & Basildon Hosps. Essex. Specialty: Otorhinolaryngol. Special Interest: Sleep Disorders; Vertigo; Voice Disorders. Socs: Brit. Assn. Otol. Head & Neck Surg.; Roy. Soc. of Med.; Brit. Soc. Neurotology. Prev: Cons. Adviser (Otorhinolaryngol.) Princess Mary's Hosp. RAF Halton; Hon. Cons., The Lond. Hosp.

O'REILLY, Brian Nestor Wombwell Medical Centre, George St., Wombwell, Barnsley S73 0DD — MRCS Eng. LRCP Lond. 1976 (Univ. Coll. Dub.) BDS Dub. 1963; MB BCh BAO Dub. 1976; DObst RCPI 1979; DRCOG 1979; DCH NUI 1981.

O'REILLY, Colum Vincent c/o McGee, 5 Beverley Road, Newlands, Glasgow G43 2RT — MB ChB Glas. 1976.

O'REILLY, David Terence West Suffolk Hospital, Hardwick Lane, Bury St Edmunds IP33 2QZ — MB BChir Camb. 1981 (Cambridge) MA Camb. 1982, MB BChir 1981; MRCP (UK) 1984. Cons. Phys. & Rheum. W. Suff. Hosp. Specialty: Gen. Med.; Rheumatol. Prev: Sen. Regist. (Rheum.) Manch. Roy. Infirm.

O'REILLY, Denis St John Institute of Biochemistry, Royal Infirmary, Alexandra Parade, Glasgow G4 0SF Tel: 0141 211 4631 — MB BCh BAO NUI 1975 (Cork) MSc Birm. 1978; MD 1991; FRCPath 1995; MRCP 1997; FRCP (Glas) 1999. Cons. Clin. Biochem. Glas. Roy. Infirm. Specialty: Biochem. Socs: Assn. Clin. Biochem. & Soc. Endrocrinol.; Brit. Thyroid Assn.. Prev: Sen. Regist. (Chem. Path.) Bristol Roy. Infirm.; Regist. (Clin. Chem.) Qu. Eliz. Med. Centre Birm.

O'REILLY, Derval Maeve Martine Cornmarket Surgery, Newry Health Village, Monaghan Street, Newry BT35 6BW — MB BCh BAO Belf. 1985.

O'REILLY, Eugene (retired) 37 Crossfield Drive, Worsley, Manchester M28 2QQ — MB BCh BAO NUI 1949. Prev: Ho. Phys. & Ho. Surg. Hope Hosp. Salford.

O'REILLY, Fingal Erik 71 New Road, Bengeo, Hertford SG14 3JH — MB BS Lond. 1996.

O'REILLY, Garrett Vincent Friary Surgery, Dobbin Lane, Armagh BT61 7QG Tel: 028 3752 3165 Fax: 028 3752 1514; 8 Mullinure Park, Armagh BT61 9EJ — MB BCh BAO Belf. 1971; MRCGP 1975.

O'REILLY, Gerard Michael 21 Knockchree Road, Downpatrick BT30 6RP — MB BCh BAO NUI 1984.

O'REILLY, Mr James Alphonsus (retired) 27 Westland Road, Cookstown BT80 8BZ Tel: 0164 87 62351 — MB BCh BAO NUI 1948; FRCS Eng. 1960; FRCS Ed. 1960. Prev: Cons. ENT Surg. S. Tyrone Hosp. Dungannon.

O'REILLY, John Francis Blackpool Victoria Hospital, Whinney Heys Road, Blackpool FY3 8NR Tel: 01253 303477 Fax: 01253 303475 — MB Camb. 1977; MB Camb. 1976, BChir 1976; MA Camb. 1977; MRCP (UK) 1978. Cons. Gen. & Respirat. Med. Blackpool, Wyre & Fylde HA. Specialty: Gen. Med.; Respirat. Med. Socs: BMA; Brit. Thorac. Soc.

O'REILLY, Josephine Kate Maudsley Hospital, London SE15; 3 Fontarabia Road, London SW11 5PE — BSc (Hons.) Lond. 1985, MB BS 1988; DCH RCP Lond. 1991. Regist. (Psychiat.) Maudsley Hosp. Lond. Specialty: Gen. Psychiat. Prev: SHO (Paediat.) St. Mary's Hosp. Lond.; SHO (Psych.) Univ. Coll. Hosp.

O'REILLY, Karen Anastasia 21 Winston Rise, Four Marks, Alton GU34 5HP — MB BS Lond. 1984; MRCGP 1991.

O'REILLY, Kieran Miceal Leicester General Hospital, Gwendolen Road, Leicester LE5 4PW; Glennamaddy, 8 Link Road, Leicester LE2 3RA Tel: 0116 270 6334 — MB ChB Glas. 1972; MB ChB (Commend.) Glas. 1972; FRCPath 1992, M 1980. Cons. Histopath. Leicester Gen. Hosp. Specialty: Histopath.

O'REILLY, Maria Antoinette Wellfield Surgery, 291 Oldham Road, Rochdale OL16 5HX Tel: 01706 355111 — MB ChB Manch. 1990.

O'REILLY, Marian Dorothy House, Winsley House, Winsley, Bradford-on-Avon BA15 2LE Tel: 01225 722988 Fax: 01225 722907; 4 St Catherine's Close, Bath BA2 6BS Tel: 01225 428657 Email: david.hill@amserve.net — MB BS Lond. 1976; MRCS Eng. LRCP Lond. 1976; DCH Eng. 1979; DRCOG 1981; MRCGP 1984; Dip. Palliat. Med. 1996. Cons. (Palliat. Med.) Bath. Specialty: Palliat. Med.

O'REILLY, Mary Anastasia Regan Dept. of Radiology, Queen Mary's University Hospital, Roehampton, London SW15 5PN — MB BCh BAO NUI 1985; MSc NUI 1987, B Ed. 1978; DCH NUI 1988; MRCPI 1988; FRCR 1993; FFR RCSI 1993; FRCPI 1999. Cons. Radiol., Qu. Mary's Univ. Hosp., Lond.; Cons. Radiologist, Kingston Hosp., Surrey. Specialty: Radiol.

O'REILLY, Michael Fraser Lifeline Occupational Health, 172 Newbridge Street, Newcastle upon Tyne NE1 2TE Tel: 0191 230 4544 Fax: 0191 230 4744; Trinity House, Bridgend, Duns TD11 3ER — MB ChB Ed. 1989; Adv Dip Occ Med; MRCGP 1995. Clin. Dir. Lifeline Occupational Health Newc. u. Tyne. Specialty: Occupat. Health.

O'REILLY, Michael Kenneth 55 Burley Lane, Quarndon, Derby DE22 5JR — MB BCh BAO NUI 1980.

O'REILLY, Nial The Health Centre, Newry BT35 8DE Tel: 01693 61236; 28 Hawthorn Hill, Dublin Road, Newry BT35 8DE Tel: 01693 63320 — MB BCh BAO NUI 1949; LM Coombe 1951; DCH 1965.

O'REILLY, Mr Patrick Henry Stepping Hill Hospital, Hazel Grove, Stockport SK2 7JE Tel: 0161 419 5484 Fax: 0161 419 5699 — MRCS Eng. LRCP Lond. 1970 (Manch.) MD Manch. 1977, MB ChB 1970; FRCS Eng. 1974. Cons. Urol. Surg. Stepping Hill Hosp. Stockport; Vis. Prof. Austral. Kidney Foundat. 1993; Edit. Bd. Brit. Jl. Urol. Specialty: Urol. Socs: Fell. Europ. Bd. Urol.; Amer. Urol. Assn. Prev: Sen. Regist. (Urol.) United Manch. Hosps.; Regist. (Surg.) Wythenshawe Hosp. Manch.; Lect. (Anat.) Univ. Manch.

O'REILLY, Patrick Joseph Dermot 26 Brook Street, Enniskillen BT74 7EU — MB BCh BAO Belf. 1980.

O'REILLY, Paul Joseph 10 Albert Road, Harbourne, Birmingham B17 0AN — BM BCh Oxf. 1986.

O'REILLY, Pauline Veronica 21 Newlands Road, Glasgow G43 2JD Tel: 0141 649 1961 — MB ChB Glas. 1973.

O'REILLY, Ragnar Sean 2 Coeur de Lion, Colchester CO4 5WN — MB BS Lond. 1994.

O'REILLY, Rebecca Jane Glass House Cottages, Maple Tree Lane, Mill Green, Ingatestone CM4 0PP — MB ChB Bristol 1978. Specialty: Occupat. Health.

O'REILLY, Roisin 8 Mullinure Park, Armagh BT61 9EJ — MB BCh BAO Belf. 1996.

O'REILLY, Sean Talgarth Medical Centre, Talgarth, Brecon LD3 0AE Tel: 01874 711309 Fax: 01874 712033 — MB BCh BAO NUI 1983 (Dubl.) Dip. Geriat. Med. 1988; MRCGP 1990; DCH RCP Lond. 1990. Specialty: Ment. Health. Prev: Trainee GP Camberley & Talgarth.

O'REILLY, Sheila Catherine Derbyshire Royal Infirmary, Department of Rhematology, London Road, Derby DE1 2QY Tel: 01332 347141 Fax: 01332 254989 Email: sheila.o'reilly@sdah-tr.trent.nhs.uk — BM BS Nottm. 1988; MRCP (UK) 1991; DM Nottm. 1997. Cons. (Rheum.), Derbysh. Roy. Infirm. Specialty: Rheumatol. Prev: Sen. Regist. (Rheum.) Derbysh. Roy. Infirm.

O'REILLY, Susan Margaret Mary Clatterbridge Centre for Oncology, Bebington, Wirral CH63 4JY Tel: 0151 334 1155 Fax: 0151 482 7675; 4 Hawthorn Cottages, Dee View Road, Heswall, Wirral CH60 0DN — MB BCh BAO NUI 1981 (Dublin) MRCPI 1984; MD NUI 1992. Cons. Med. Oncol. Clatterbridge Centre for Oncol. Wirral. Specialty: Oncol. Prev: Sen. Regist. (Med. Oncol.) Char. Cross Hosp. Lond.; ICRF Research Fell. Clin. Oncol. Unit Guy's Hosp. Lond.

O'REILLY, Vivienne Halina 35 Svenskaby, Orton, Wistow, Peterborough PE2 6YZ — MB ChB Manch. 1977; DRCOG 1980.

O'RIORDAN, Mr Brendan Gerard Mary Department of Surgery, West Wales General Hospital, Carmarthen SA31 2AF Tel: 01267 227545 — MB BCh BAO NUI 1981 (Dublin) FRCSI 1985; FRACS 1992. Cons. Gen. & Specialist UGI Surg. W. Wales Gen. Hosp. Camarthen; Cons Gen Surg., Werndale Private Hosp., Camarthen. Specialty: Gen. Surg. Socs: ASGBI; AUGIS; HCSA. Prev: Clin. Research Fell. (Surg. Oncol.) Jefferson Hosp. Philadelphia, USA.

O'RIORDAN, Mr Dermot Charles West Suffolk Hospital, Hardwick Lane, Bury St Edmunds IP33 2QZ Email: dermot.o'riordan@wsh.nhs.uk — MB BS Lond. 1988 (St Bart.) FRCS Eng. 1993; FRCS Ed. 1993. Specialty: Gen. Surg. Prev: Specialist Regist. Rotat. Gen. Surg. NE Thames; Research Fell. Nat. Groin Hernia Outcomes Project RCS Eng. Lond.; Regist. Rotat. (Gen. Surg.) NE Thames.

O'RIORDAN, Donagh Kevin Flat 5, 22 Crawford Avenue, Wembley HA0 2JS — MB BCh BAO NUI 1984; MRCPI 1988.

O'RIORDAN, Jane Ann 28 Brodrick Road, London SW17 7DY — MB BS Lond. 1986; FRCA 1992. Cons. (Anaesth.) St. Geo. Hosp. Lond. Specialty: Anaesth.

O'RIORDAN, Professor Jeffrey Lima Hayes 14 Northampton Park, London N1 2PJ Tel: 020 7226 9676 Email: jeffrey@oriordan.demon.co.uk — (Middlx.) DM Oxf. 1970, MA, BSc, BM BCh 1957; FRCP Lond. 1971, M 1959. Emerit. Prof. Metab. Med. Univ. Coll. Lond.; Emerit. Hon. Cons. Phys. Middlx. Hosp. Lond. Specialty: Endocrinol. Socs: Assn. Phys.; Amer. Endocrine Soc. Prev: Regist. Middlx. Hosp. Lond.; Vis. Assoc. Nat. Inst. Arthritis & Metab. Dis. Bethesda, MD.

O'RIORDAN, Mr John Bosco Andrews 42 Brooklands Park, London SE3 9BL Tel: 020 8852 7237 — MB BCh BAO NUI 1965; FRCSI 1970. Cons. Cardiac Surg. St. Thos. Hosp. Lond. Specialty: Cardiothoracic Surg. Socs: BMA; Soc. Thoracic & Cardiovasc. Surg.; Brit. Cardiac Soc. Prev: Cons. Cardiac Surg. Brook Gen. Hosp.

O'RIORDAN, Jonathan Ignatius Department of Neurology, Nine Wells Hosp & Medical School, Dundee DD1 9SY Tel: 01382 660111 Email: j.oriordan@tuht.scot.nhs.uk — MB BCh BAO NUI 1989; MD Dub. 1998; FRCP Edin. 2001; FRCPI 2002. Cons. Neurologist, Director Tayside MS Research Unit. Special Interest: Multiple Sclerosis.

O'RIORDAN, Joseph Edward Gerard Picton Road Surgery, 194 Picton Road, Liverpool L15 4LL Tel: 0151 733 1347 — MB BCh BAO NUI 1978.

O'RIORDAN, Mary 2 First Avenue, Netherlee, Glasgow G44 3UB Tel: 0141 637 1819 — MB BCh BAO NUI 1987 (Univ. Coll. Galway, Irel.) Diploma in Palliative Medicine; BSc (Biochem.) NUI 1984; DCH RCPSI 1991; DRCOG 1993; MRCGP 1993. Specialist Regist. in Palliat. Med., W. of Scotl. Train. Scheme. Specialty: Palliat. Med.

O'RIORDAN, Mr Michael David 15 Cedar Court, Somerset Road, London SW19 5HU Tel: 020 8946 6837 — MB BS Lond. 1952 (Westm.) DO Eng. 1959; FRCP Ed. 1982, M 1963; FRCS Eng. 1964; LMCC 1967; FRCSC 1972; BA Open University 1989; FRCOphth. 1989. Emerit. Cons. Ophth. Croydon Eye Unit Mayday Univ. Hosp. Thornton Heath. Specialty: Ophth. Prev: Sen. Regist. Roy. Free Hosp. Lond.; Emerg. Off. Radcliffe Infirm. Oxf.; Ho. Phys. Westm. Hosp. Lond.

O'RIORDAN, Mr Sean Michael Consulting Rooms, 6 Avenue Road, Grantham NG31 6TA Tel: 01476 593919 Fax: 01476 593919; Consulting Rooms, Nuffield Hospital, Nettleham Road, Lincoln LN2 2QU; The Old Stone School, Carlton Scroop, Grantham NG32 3AU Tel: 01400 250730 — MB BS Lond. 1968 (Lond. Hosp.) BSc Lond. 1965; MRCS Eng. LRCP Lond. 1968; DObst RCOG 1970; FRCS Eng. 1975. Cons. Orthop. Surg. Co. Hosp. Lincoln. Specialty: Orthop. Prev: Sen. Regist. (Orthop.) Lond. Hosp.; Regist. (Orthop.) Broomfield Hosp. Chelmsford; Resid. Med. Off. Gambo Leprosy Control & Rural Health Centre.

O'RIORDAN, Sean Peter Great Ormond Street Hospital, Department Immunology & Infectious Diseases, Great Ormond Street, London WC1N 3JH Tel: 0207 405 9200 Email: oriors@gosh.nhs.uk — MB BChir Camb. 1993 (Char. Cross & Westm. Med. Sch.) MRCP Lond. 1995. SpR Paediatric Infec. Diseases. Specialty: Paediat.

O'RIORDAN, Shelagh Elizabeth 19 Azof Street, London SE10 0EG — MB BS Lond. 1990.

O'ROURKE, Alan John 72 Sandford Grove Road, Nether Edge, Sheffield S7 1RR Email: a.j.orourke@sheffield.ac.uk — MB ChB Sheff. 1986 (Sheffield) MSc Sheff. 1996. Non-Clin. Lect. Sheff. Univ. Specialty: Gen. Pract.; Med. Publishing; Research. Socs: BMA.

O'ROURKE, Brian 49 Lilybank Road, Port Glasgow PA14 5AW — MB ChB Aberd. 1992 (Aberdeen) MRCP (UK) Glas. 1995. Specialty: Cardiol.

O'ROURKE, Declan Martin Department of Pathology, Belfast City Hospital Trust, Lisbun Road, Belfast Tel: 028 9032 9241 Ext: 2332 — MB BCh BAO Belf. 1988 (Queen's University of Belfast) MRCP (UK) 1991; MRCPath 1998; Dip RCPath. (Cytopathology) 1998. Cons. Histo/Cytopatnologist, Belf. City Hosp. Trust. Specialty: Histopath.; Pathology, General. Socs: Mem. Of the Roy. Coll. Of Patrologists. Prev: Regist. (Histopath.) Roy. Vict. Hosp. Belf.; SHO (Histopath.) Roy. Vict. Hosp. Belf.

O'ROURKE, Edward Joseph 41 Grange Avenue, Derby DE23 8DH — MB ChB Leeds 1994.

O'ROURKE, Fintan Martin 2 Smalls Road, Warrenpoint, Newry BT34 3PL — MB BCh BAO Belf. 1995.

O'ROURKE, Jeremiah Gerard Ardlarich, 15 Culduthel Road, Inverness IV2 4AG — MB ChB Aberd. 1981; DRCOG 1983; DCH RCPS Glas. 1984; MRCGP 1985. GP Inverness.

O'ROURKE, Mr John Seanan Department of Urology, Treliske Hospital, Truro TR1 3LJ — MB BCh BAO NUI 1979; FRCSI 1983; BSc NUI 1981, MCh 1990.

O'ROURKE, Lucy Elizabeth Shoreditch Park Surgery, 10 Ruston Street, London N1 5DR Tel: 020 7739 8525 Fax: 020 7739 5352 — MB BS Lond. 1993 (UCMSM) BSc (Hons.) Lond. 1990; MRCGP 1997. GP Princip., ShoreditchPk. Surg., Hackney.; Mem. LMC, E. Lond. Specialty: Gen. Pract.

O'ROURKE, Michael Hugh Beds & Luton Comm. NHS Trust Learning Disability Sevice, Specialist Medical Department, Twinwoods Health Resource, Milton Rd, Clapham, Bedford MK41 6AT Tel: 01234 310582; 14 Princes Road, Bromham, Bedford MK43 8QD — MRCPsych 1982 Dublin; LRCPI & LM, LRCSI & LM 1976; DO Dublin 1978; DCH 1979. Clin. Dir. (Learning Disabil. Serv.) Beds & Luton Community NHS Trust. Specialty: Ment. Health.

O'ROURKE, Nicholas Peter The Surgery, 280 Havant Road, Drayton, Portsmouth PO6 1PA Tel: 02392 370422 Fax: 02392 618383 Email: nporourke@hotmail.com — BM Soton. 1989; DRCOG 1993; MRCGP 1994.

O'ROURKE, Noelle Patricia Beatson Oncology Centre, Western Infirmary, Glasgow G11 6NT — BM BCh Oxf. 1986; MA Camb. 1987; MRCP (UK) 1989; MD Sheff. 1994; FRCR (Oncol.) 1995. Sen. Lect. & Hon. Cons. Clin. Oncol. Glas.; Lead Clinician W. Scotl. Lung Cancer Network. Specialty: Oncol.; Radiother. Prev: Sen. Regist. (Radiother. & Clin. Oncol.) Oxf.; Regist. (Clin. Oncol.) Hammersmith Hosp. Lond.; Clin. Research Fell. (Human Metab.) Univ. Sheff.

O'RYAN, Michael Francis Nicholas 27 Central Avenue, Eccleston Park, Prescot L34 2QL Tel: 0151 426 5418 Fax: 0151 426 5418 Email: mfnoryan@hotmail.com — (Dub.) MB BCh BAO Dub. 1959; FRCGP 1990, M 1974; MA Dub. 1982; MICGP 1985. Indep. GP Merseyside; Med. Mem. & Assessor Indep. Trib. Serv.; Appraiser St Helens PCT; Clin. & Communications Skills Assessor. Specialty: Gen. Pract. Socs: Nat. Assn. Non-Princip. Prev: Hon. Clin. Tutor Univ. Liverp.; Course Organiser Mersey Regional Train. Scheme.

O'SHAUGHNESSY, Catherine Victoria 40 Gledholt Road, Huddersfield HD1 4HR — MB BS Newc. 1997.

O'SHAUGHNESSY, Donal Michael Kevin O'Shaughnessy, Rathfriland Health Centre, John Street, Rathfriland, Newry BT34 5QH Tel: 02840 630666 Fax: 02840 631198; 2 Barnmeen Road, Rathfriland, Newry BT34 5AW Tel: 02840 630666 Fax: 02840 631198 — MB BCh BAO NUI 1976 (University College Galway) MICGP 1987. GP; Mem. Fac. Sports & Exercise Med.; Hon. Med. Off. Rugby Union.; Hon. Med. Off. Barbarians RFC. Specialty: Gen. Pract.; Sports Med. Socs: Irish Coll. Gen. Pract.; Brit. Assn. of Sport Med.

O'SHAUGHNESSY, Kevin Michael Addenbrooke's Hospital, Clinical Pharmacology Unit, Level 6, ACCI, Box 110, Hills Road, Cambridge CB2 2QQ Tel: 01223 762578 Fax: 01223 762376 Email: kmo22@medschl.cam.ac.uk; Tanglewood House, Cherry House, Duton Hill, Dunmow CM6 2EE Tel: 01371 870239 — BM BCh Oxf. 1986; MA Camb. 1984, BA 1980; DPhil Oxf. 1983, BM BCh 1986; MRCP (UK) 1989. Univ. Lect. Clin. Pharmacol. Univ. Camb. & Hon. Cons. Phys. Addenbrookes Hosp., Camb. Specialty: Pharmacology. Socs: Brit. Hypertens. Soc. Prev: Sen. Regist. (Clin. Pharmacol.) Hammersmith Hosp. Lond.; Research Fell. & Hon. Sen. Regist. Hammersmith Hosp. Lond.; SHO (Med.) Centr. Middlx. Hosp. Lond.

O'SHAUGHNESSY, Terence Conleth Newham General Hospital, Glen Road, Plaistow, London E13 8SL Tel: 020 7476 4000 Fax: 020 7363 8081 — MB BChir Camb. 1983; MRCPI; BSc (Hons.) St. And. 1981. Cons. Respirat. & Gen. Med. Newham Gen. Hosp. Plaistow. Specialty: Respirat. Med.; Gen. Med.

O'SHEA, Diarmuid Donal Paschal 10 Hardwick Place, Gosforth, Newcastle upon Tyne NE3 4SH — MB BCh BAO NUI 1986; MRCPI 1988.

O'SHEA, Donal Brendan 145A Harbord Street, Fulham, London SW6 6PN — MB BCh BAO NUI 1989.

O'SHEA, Elaine Maria Anne 79 Broomgrove Gardens, Edgware HA8 5RJ — MB ChB Bristol 1996 (University of Bristol) SpR Anaesth. Soton Gen. NHS Trust. Specialty: Gen. Med. Prev: SHO (Gen. Med.) The Ipswich Hosp. NHS Trust.

O'SHEA, Mr John Gerard Birmingham and Midand Eye Centre, Dudley Road, Birmingham B18 4EJ — MB BS Monash 1983; DHMSA 1989; MRCOphth 1991; MD Monash 1991; FRCS Ed. 1991. Sen. Regist. Birm. & Midl. Eye Centre Dudley. Specialty: Ophth. Prev: Sen. Regist. (Ophth.) St. John Ophth. Hosp., Jerusalem.

O'SHEA, John Kevin West Sussex Health and Social Care NHS Trust, 72 Stockbridge Road, Chichester PO19 8QJ Tel: 01243 782919 Fax: 01243 783919; Flat 18 Lombard Court, Lombard St, Old Portsmouth, Portsmouth PO1 2HU — MB BCh BAO NUI 1986; DCH NUI 1988; MRCPsych 1994. Cons. Psychiat. Learning Disabil. Serv. W. Sussex Health & Social Care NHS Trust. Specialty: Ment. Health. Socs: Fell. Soc. Med.

O'SHEA, Judith Rowan 74 Mill Hill Road, Norwich NR2 3DS — MB BS Lond. 1990.

O'SHEA, Matthew James Birchwood Medical Centre, 15 Benson Road, Birchwood, Warrington WA3 7PJ — MB ChB Liverp. 1993; DRCOG; BSc (Hons). 1990. Specialty: Gen. Pract.

O'SHEA, Maureen Staplands, Hinderton Road, Neston, South Wirral CH64 9PW Tel: 0151 336 1422 — MB ChB Liverp. 1960; DObst RCOG 1964.

O'SHEA, Michael James 17 Kennedy Road, Shrewsbury SY3 7AB Tel: 01743 61148 — MD Camb. 1974; MB 1959, BChir 1958; FRCPath. 1980, M 1968. Cons. Haemat. Salop AHA. Specialty: Haematology. Socs: Brit. Soc. Haemat. & Assn. Clin. Path. Prev: Lect. Haemat. King's Coll. Hosp. Inst. Child Health; Sen. Lect. & Cons. Haemat. Roy. Free Hosp. Lond.

O'SHEA, Patrick John 48 Southmeade, Maghull, Liverpool L31 8EF — MB ChB Glas. 1996.

O'SHEA, Peter John Anaesthetic Department, The London Hospital, Whitechapel, London E1 1BB — MB BS Lond. 1968 (Lond. Hosp.) FFA RCS Eng. 1973. Cons. Anaesth. Lond. Hosp. Specialty: Anaesth.; Intens. Care.

O'SHEA, Roger Aloysius 194 Burton Street, Melton Mowbray LE13 1DN — MB BCh BAO NUI 1942 (Univ. Coll. Dub.) CPH 1948; LM Nat. Matern. Hosp. Dub. 1948; DObst RCOG 1949. Div. Surg. St. John Ambul. Brig. Socs: Foundat. Mem. Coll. of Gen. Pract.; Nottm. M-C Soc. & Derby Med. Soc. Prev: Res. Surg. Off. Leigh Infirm. Lancs.; Ho. Phys. Huddersfield Roy. Infirm.; O & G Regist. Stepping Hill Hosp. Stockport.

O'SHEA, Roger Michael John Ryle Health Centre, Southchurch Drive, Clifton, Nottingham NG11 8EW Tel: 0115 921 2970; 5 Manor Park, Ruddington, Nottingham NG11 6DS Tel: 0115 921 2177 — LRCPI & LM, LRCSI & LM 1972; DCH NUI 1976; DObst. RCPI 1977. Occupat. Health Phys. Jessop & Son. Ltd. Nottm. John Lewis Partnership.

O'SHEA, Sarah Jane 58 Manor Park South, Knutsford WA16 8AN — MB BS Lond. 1991; BSc Lond. 1989; MRCP (UK) 1994; FRCR (UK) 2000. Specialty: Radiol.

O'SHEA, Sean Brian 13 Pauls Row, Truro TR1 1HH — MB BS Lond. 1987; MRCGP 1994.

O'SHEA, Thomas Stephen Hyde Park Surgery, 3 Woodsley Road, Leeds LS6 1SG Tel: 0113 295 1235 Fax: 0113 295 1220 — MB BCh BAO NUI 1977; DRCOG 1980; MRCGP 1981.

O'SULLIVAN, Aideen Kathryn 25 Waterloo Park, Belfast BT15 5HU — MB BCh BAO Belf. 1996.

O'SULLIVAN, Anthony Gerard Priory Manor Child Development Centre, 1 Blagdon Road, Lewisham, London SE13 7HL Tel: 020 7771 4510 Fax: 020 7771 4540 Email: tony.o'sullivan@lewishampct.nhs.uk; 88 Erlanger Road, New Cross, London SE14 5TH Tel: 020 7732 0304 Email: tony@osullivan17.freeserve.co.uk — MB ChB Liverp. 1974; DCH RCP Lond. 1987; MRCP (UK) 1989. Cons. Community Paediat. Lewisham Primary Care Trust, Priory Manor Child Developm. Centre Lewisham. Specialty: Community Child Health. Socs: Fell.Roy. Coll. of Paediat. and Child Health; Brit. Paediat. Neurol. Assn.; BACCH.

O'SULLIVAN, Barbara Mary Philomena 57 Drones Road, Armoy, Ballymoney BT53 8YP — MB BCh BAO NUI 1981; LRCPSI 1981; MRCGP 1990.

O'SULLIVAN, Bernadette Mary The Surgery, 2 Oxford Street, Southampton SO14 3DJ Tel: 023 8033 5157 — MB BS Lond. 1977 (Roy. Free) DA Eng. 1981; MRCGP 2001.

O'SULLIVAN, Brian Columbanus Dalvennan Avenue Practice, 27 Dalvennan Avenue, Patna, Ayr KA6 7NA Tel: 01292 531367 Fax: 01292 531033; 14 Chalmer's Road, Ayr KA7 2RQ — MB BCh BAO NUI 1987 (Dublin) DRCOG 1990; MRCGP 1992. GP Princip.; Forens. Med. Examr. Strathclyde Police. Specialty: Gen. Pract. Socs: BMA. Prev: Trainee GP Peebles; Regist. (Psychiat.) Roy. Edin. Hosps.; SHO Ards Hosp. Newtownards.

O'SULLIVAN, Catherine Cecelia Pilgrim's Hospice, 56 London Road, Canterbury CT2 8JA Tel: 01227 459700; 3 Town Road, Petham, Canterbury CT4 5QT Tel: 01227 700898 — MB BCh BAO NUI 1973; DTM & H Liverp. 1977; MA (Psychother. & Counselling) Regent's Coll. 1994. Hospice Phys. (Palliat. Med.) Pilgrim's Hosp. Canterbury. Specialty: Palliat. Med. Socs: BMA. Prev: Clin. Med. Adviser Ellenor Foundat. Livingstone Community Hosp. Dartford.
O'SULLIVAN, Clare Jennifer The Surgery, 48 Mulgrave Road, Belmont, Sutton SM2 6LX Tel: 020 8642 2050 — MB BS Lond. 1987; DRCOG 1989; Cert. Family Plann. JCC 1989; MRCGP 1991. Prev: Trainee GP Wessex VTS.
O'SULLIVAN, Daniel John Wombwell Medical Centre, George Street, Wombwell, Barnsley S73 0DD Tel: 01226 752363; 29 South View Crescent, Nether Edge, Sheffield S7 1DG Tel: 0114 250 8035 Fax: 0114 250 8035 — MB BCh BAO Dub. 1987 (Trinity College Dublin) DGM RCP Lond. 1990; DCH NUI 1992; DFFP 1994; MRACGP 1994; MRCGP 1994; DFFP 1994. GP.
O'SULLIVAN, Dawn Alice Maple House, Rue de la Vista, St Lawrence, Jersey JE3 1ED — MB BS Lond. 1996.
O'SULLIVAN, Denis Michael 92 Cavendish Road, Cambridge CB1 3AF — MB BChir Camb. 1992 (Cambridge) MA Camb. 1992; MRCP (UK) 1995. Specialist Regist. (Cardiol.) Papworth Hosp. Camb. Specialty: Cardiol.
O'SULLIVAN, Desmond Patrick Llety Dawell, Greenhill Road, Griffithstown, Pontypool NP4 5BE — LRCPI & LM, LRSCI & LM 1937; LRCPI & LM, LRCSI & LM 1937.
O'SULLIVAN, Desmond Patrick Dominic Novartis Pharmaceuticals UK Ltd., Frimley Business Park, Frimley, Camberley GU16 7SR Tel: 01276 698276 Fax: 01276 698454 — MB BChir Camb. 1982; Dip. Pharm. Med. RCP (UK) 1985. Dir. Clin. Safety & Epidemiol. Novartis Pharmaceuts.UK LTD Surrey. Specialty: Pharmaceutical Medicine; Epidemiol.
O'SULLIVAN, Donal Gerard Mary Lambeth, Southwark and Lewisham Health Authority, 1 Lower Marsh, London SE1 7NT Tel: 020 7716 7030 Fax: 020 7716 7018 Email: donal.osullivan@ob.lslha.sthames.nhs.uk; Fairoaks, 221 Crofton Lane, Orpington BR6 0BL Tel: 01689 838125 — MB BCh BAO NUI 1982 (University College, Cork) MB BCh BAO (NUI) 1982; MSc Lond. 1987; MFPHM RCP (UK) 1990; FFPHM RCP (UK) 1997. Cons. Communicable Dis. Control Lambeth, Southwark & Lewisham HA. Specialty: Pub. Health Med. Socs: BMA; Internat. Epidemiol. Assn.; Pub. Health Med. Environm. Gp. Prev: Sen. Regist. (Pub. Health Med.) S. E. Thames RHA.
O'SULLIVAN, Eleanor Meriel 151 Finborough Road, London SW10 9AP Tel: 01926 492522/020 7373 6654 — MB BS Lond. 1966; MRCS Eng. LRCP Lond. 1966; FFR 1974; FRCR 1975. Cons. (Radiol.) Qu. Mary's Hosp. Roehampton; Cons. (Radiol.) St. Helier's Hosp. Carshalton Surrey. Specialty: Radiol.
O'SULLIVAN, Eoin Patrick 77 Yale Court, Honeybourne Road, London NW6 1JH — MB BChir Camb. 1990.
O'SULLIVAN, Fergus Timothy HMP Littlehey, Perry, Huntingdon PE18 0SR Tel: 01480 812202; 63 Elton Road, Wansford, Peterborough PE8 6JS — MB BCh BAO NUI 1977; DObst RCPI 1980; DPM RCPSI 1989. Sen. Med. Off. (Psychiat.) HMP Littlehey Cambs. Specialty: Gen. Psychiat. Prev: Managing Med. Off. HMP Albany; Med. Off. HMP Pk.hurst I. of Wight.
O'SULLIVAN, Finbar Eugene Flat 8, 183 Sussex Gardens, London W2 2RH — MB BS Lond. 1998.
O'SULLIVAN, Geraldine Frances Mary Northamphshire Hospital Trust, Aldermaston Road, Basingstoke RG24 9NA Tel: 01256 313492; Mallard's Close, Bourne Lane, Twyford, Winchester SO21 1NX Tel: 01962 713967 — MB BCh BAO Dub. 1973; DMRD Eng. 1977; FRCR 1982. Cons. Radiol. Basingstoke N. Hants. Hosps. Trust; Q.A. Radiologist, S. E. (W.) Region, Dir. Of Breast Screening. Specialty: Radiol. Socs: BMUS; Roy. Coll. of Raiologists Breast Grp. Prev: Sen. Regist. (Diag. Radiol.) Soton. Gen. Hosp.; Sen. Regist. (Diag. Radiol.) Lond. Hosp. Whitechapel; Regist. (Diag. Radiol.) Roy. Free Hosp. Lond.
O'SULLIVAN, Geraldine Helen Trust Head Office, 99 Waverley Rise, St Albans AL3 5TL Tel: 01727 897708 Email: geraldine.osullivan@hpt.nhs.uk — MB BCh BAO NUI 1981 (Univ. Coll. Cork Irel.) MRCPsych. 1986; MD 1993. Med. Dir. Cons. Community Psychiat. Herts. NHS Trust. Prev: Sen. Regist. Bethlem Roy. Maudsley Hosps.; Lect. & Research Work Inst. Psychiat. Lond.
O'SULLIVAN, Geraldine Mary Department of Anaesthetics, St Thomas Hospital, London SE1 7EH Tel: 020 7188 0652 Fax: 020 7188 0628 Email: geraldine.o'sullivan@gstt.sthames.nhs.uk — MB BCh BAO NUI 1975 (Univ. Coll. Cork) FRCA; MD NUI 1985. Cons. Anaesth., Guy's & St. Thomas NHS Turst Hosps., Lond. Specialty: Anaesth. Special Interest: Obst.
O'SULLIVAN, Gerard Patrick Delamere Street Health Centre, 45 Delamere Street, Crewe CW1 2ER Tel: 01270 214046 — MB ChB Birm. 1984; MRCGP 1988.
O'SULLIVAN, Jerry Patrick, TD (retired) 3 Wiston Avenue, Donnington, Chichester PO19 8RJ Tel: 01243 527797 — MB ChB Glas. 1966; BSc (Hons) Glas. 1961; FRCPath 1986, M 1973; BA (Hons) Open 1987. Cons. Histopath. St. Richard's Hosp. Chichester. Prev: Cons. Histopath. St. Jas. Hosp. Lond.
O'SULLIVAN, Mr John Conor 8 Pennant Mews, London W8 5JN Tel: 020 7580 6966 Fax: 020 7580 6966; 96 Arthur Road, Wimbledon, London SW19 7DT Tel: 020 8946 6242 — BM BCh Oxf. 1959 (Westm.) BA (Hons.) Oxf. 1955, MA 1959; FRCS Eng. 1967; FRCOG 1983, M 1970; T(GP) 1996. Cons. Gyn. Oncol. Hammersmith Hosp. Lond.; Sen. Lect. Roy. Postgrad. Med. Sch. Hammersmith Hosp. Lond. & Inst. Obst. & Gyn.; Examr. Bd. Eng. & Univs. Lond. & Camb.; Examr. RCOG & Prof. & Linguistics Assessm. Bd. Specialty: Obst. & Gyn. Socs: Founder Mem. Brit. Assn. Surg. Oncols.; Brit. Gyn. Cancer Soc. Prev: Sen. Regist. (O & G) Hammersmith Hosp. Lond.; Ho. Off. (Surg.) Qu. Charlotte's & Chelsea Hosps. Lond.; Cas. Off. & Ho. Off. (Surg.) Westm. Hosp. Lond.
O'SULLIVAN, John Francis Xavier The Surgery, 1 Balliol Road, Coventry CV2 3DR Tel: 024 7644 9111 — LRCPI & LM, LRSCI & LM 1951; LRCPI & LM, LRCSI & LM 1951. Clin. Asst. (Rheum.) Coventry & Warks. Hosp.; Co. Med. Off. Various Midl. Firms. Prev: SHO Friern Hosp. Lond.; Ho. Surg. & Cas. Off. Metrop Hosp. Lond.
O'SULLIVAN, John James M, RD Ashling Occupational Health Ltd., Ashling House, Works Lane, Lostock Gralam, Northwich CW9 7FA Tel: 01606 330660 Fax: 01606 330644 Email: drosullivan@ashling.co.uk; Ashling, 59 Mill Lane, Upton-by-Chester, Chester CH2 1BS Tel: 01244 372646 — MB BCh BAO NUI 1974; MSc (Occupat. Med.) Lond. 1977; DIH Eng. 1977; FFOM RCP Lond. 1993, MFOM 1983; LLM Cardiff 1996. Cons. Occupat. Health Ashling Occupat. Health Ltd N.wich; Tutor Distance Learning Course Manch. Univ.; Vis. Lect. Univ. Coll. Dub. Specialty: Occupat. Health. Prev: Cons. Occupat. Health Brunner Mond & Co. N.wich; Sen. Med. Off. Imperial Chem. Indust. Chem. Gp. N.wich; Works Med. Off. Castner-Kellner Works, Imp. Chem. Indust. PLC, Mond Div. Runcorn.
O'SULLIVAN, John Laurence Twyford Surgery, Hazeley Road, Twyford, Winchester SO21 1QY Tel: 01962 712202 Fax: 01962 715158; Mallard's Close, Bourne Lane, Twyford, Winchester SO21 1NX Tel: 01962 713967 — MB BCh BAO Dub. 1973; DCH Eng. 1977; DRCOG 1978; MRCGP 1981; DFP & RHC 1996. GP Winchester, Hants. Socs: BMA. Prev: Regist. St. Joseph's Hospice Lond.; MOH Ubon Refugee Camp Thailand (Save the Childr. Fund); SHO (Paediat.) Qu. Eliz. Hosp. Lond.
O'SULLIVAN, Joseph Philip (retired) 12 Upper Northgate Street, Chester CH1 4E — LRCPI & LM, LRSCI & LM 1948; LRCPI & LM, LRCSI & LM 1948. Prev: Ho. Surg. & Ho. Phys. Jervis St. Hosp. Dub.
O'SULLIVAN, Katherine Elizabeth — MB BS Lond. 1988; DRCOG 1992. GP, Non-Princip., Basingstoke; Health Screening BUPA. Specialty: Gen. Pract.
O'SULLIVAN, Kevin Aelred 32 Hawthorn Lane, Wilmslow SK9 5DG — MB BCh BAO NUI 1983; FFARCS 1988. Sen. Regist. (Anaesth.) NW RHA. Specialty: Anaesth. Prev: Regist. (Anaesth.) Roy. Lancaster Infirm.; Regist. (Anaesth.) Univ. Hosp. S. Manch.
O'SULLIVAN, Kevin Miceal c/o AIKMO Medical Ltd., 62-63 Westborough, Scarborough YO11 1TS — MB ChB Manch. 1982; DRCOG 1985. Managing Dir. AIKMO Med. Ltd. Specialty: Pharmaceutical Medicine. Prev: Med. Dir. BUPA Insur.; Regional Med. Dir. SmithKline Beecham Internat.; Med. Dir. The Harley Gp.
O'SULLIVAN, Maeve Coralie Banna House, 27 Heath End Road, Flackwell Heath, High Wycombe HP10 9DT — MB BS Newc. 1998; BSc (Hons), Physiology, Sheff 1987; PhD, Neurophysiology, Newc. 1991. SHO (Paediat.) Guy's & St Thomas' Hosp. Lond. Prev: JHO, Roy. Vichne Hosp. Belf.; SHO (Paediat.) St James Univ. Hosp., Leeds; LAT (Paediat.), Bury, Manch.

O'SULLIVAN, Margaret Marian Wrexham Maelor Hospital, Croesnewydd Road, Wrexham LL13 7TD Tel: 01978 725094 — MB BCh BAO NUI 1977; MRCPI 1979; DCH NUI 1980; MD NUI 1989. Cons. Rheum. Wrexham Maelor Hosp. Clwyd. Specialty: Rehabil. Med.; Rheumatol. Prev: Sen. Regist. (Rheum.) Univ. Hosp. Wales Cardiff; SHO Hosp. Sick Childr. Crumlin; SHO (Med.) Regional Hosp. Cork.

O'SULLIVAN, Mr Mark Jonathan Benjamin North Hampshire Hospital, Aldermaston Road, Basingstoke RG24 9NA Tel: 01256 313369; The Hampshire Clinic, Basing Road, Basingstoke RG24 7AL Tel: 01256 377694 — MB BS Lond. 1988 (Roy. Lond. Hosp.) MRCOG 1994; DM Soton. 1998. Cons. O & G Basingstoke. Specialty: Obst. & Gyn. Special Interest: Colposcopy; Infertil.; Polycystic Ovarian Syndrome. Socs: Brit. Fertil. Soc.; Brit. Soc. for Colposcopy & Cervical Path. (BSCCP). Prev: Sen. Regist. N. Hants. Hosp.; Regist. (O & G) Princess Anne Hosp. Soton. & Roy. Hants. Co. Hosp. Winchester.; Specialist Regist. (O & G) Salisbury Dist. Hosp. Salisbury.

O'SULLIVAN, Mary Countisbury Avenue Surgery, 152 Countisbury Avenue, Llanrumney, Cardiff CF3 5YS Tel: 029 2079 2661 Fax: 029 2079 4537 — MB BCh BAO NUI 1980. GP Cardiff Wales.

O'SULLIVAN, Mary Fiona East Surrey Hospital, Three Arch Road, Redhill RH1 5RH — MB BCh BAO NUI 1982 (Univ. Coll. Cork, NUI) FRCS (Ophth.) Glas. 1987; MD NUI 1994. Cons. Ophth. E. Surrey Hosp. Redhill. Specialty: Ophth. Prev: Research Fell. (Glaucoma) Moorfields Eye Hosp. Lond.; Sen. Regist. St. Geo. Hosp. Lond.; Regist. West. Ophth. Hosp. Lond.

O'SULLIVAN, Mary Josephine (retired) 11 Rowland Close, Wolvercote, Oxford OX2 8PW Tel: 01865 559269 — (Roy. Free) MRCS Eng. LRCP Lond. 1955; DPH Lond. 1962; BA Open Univ. 1974. Prev: Assoc. Specialist Blood Transfus. Serv. Oxf.

O'SULLIVAN, Mary Teresa Martin Ballamona Hospital, Braddan IM4 4RF Tel: 01624 642829 Fax: 01624 642833 — MB BCh BAO NUI 1959; MRCPsych 1974. Cons. Psychiat., Isle of Man. Specialty: Geriat. Psychiat. Socs: Isle of Man Med. Soc. Prev: Lead Cons., Dept. of Health and Social Security, Isle of Man; Clin. Director, South. Health Bd., Cork, South. Irel.

O'SULLIVAN, Michael Edward Howard Barton, Hittisleigh, Exeter EX6 6LP — MB ChB BAO NUI 1949.

O'SULLIVAN, Michael Gerard 140 Churchfields, Shoeburyness, Southend-on-Sea SS3 8TW — MB BCh BAO NUI 1983.

O'SULLIVAN, Michael John Bernard Shantallow Health Centre, Racecourse Road, Londonderry BT48 8NL Tel: 028 7135 3054; Aarhus, 27 Rock Road, Londonderry BT48 7NE Tel: 01504 265963 — MB BCh BAO NUI 1959. Prev: Ho. Surg. & Ho. Phys. Waterside Gen. Hosp. Londonderry; SHO Altnagelvin Hosp. Londonderry; Cas. & Admission Off. Limerick Regional Hosp.

O'SULLIVAN, Nicole Therese 21 Brockley View, Forest Hill, London SE23 1SN — MB BS Queensland 1991.

O'SULLIVAN, Nigel Noel Vincent Elm Park Clinic, 69 Elm Park, Stanmore HA7 4AU Tel: 020 8954 1333 Fax: 020 8420 7027; 61 Parson Street, Hendon, London NW4 1QT Tel: 020 8203 1258 — MRCS Eng. LRCP Lond. 1960 (Guy's) Specialty: Acupunc.

O'SULLIVAN, Patrick Finbarr (retired) High End, 33 Old Camp Road, Eastbourne BN20 8DL — (Cork) MB BCh BAO NUI 1960; DObst RCOG 1962; DCH NUI 1962; DMRD Eng. 1966; FRCR 1968. Prev: Cons. Radiol. Eastbourne HOsp. NHS Trust.

O'SULLIVAN, Patrick Joseph Gerard 44 Eight Avenue, Lancing BN15 9XD Tel: 01903 764769 — MB BCh BAO NUI 1950.

O'SULLIVAN, Mr William Joseph Orchard House, Three Gates Lane, Haslemere GU27 2LD Tel: 01428 654620 — (Galw.) MB BCh BAO NUI 1950; FRCOG 1971, M 1956, DObst 1953; MD NUI 1961, MAO 1955; FRCS Ed. 1963. Cons. (O & G) Sutton & W. Merton Health Dist.; Sen. Lect. St. Geo. Hosp. Med. Sch. Lond. Specialty: Obst. & Gyn. Prev: Sen. Regist. Postgrad. Med. Sch. Lond.

O'TIERNEY, Donal Padraig (retired) O'Tierney, Murphy and Ryan, Health Centre, Summerhill, Warrenpoint, Newry BT34 3JD; Belmont, 41 Seaview, Warrenpoint, Newry BT34 3NJ Tel: 028 4177 3630 — MB BCh BAO NUI 1958 (Univ. Coll. Dub.) LAH Dub. 1957; FRCGP 1987, M 1968. Prev: Med. Adviser SCA Packaging Ltd. Warrenpoint.

O'TOOLE, Conor Emmett Kevin 22 Blackstaff Road, Clough, Downpatrick BT30 8SW — MB BCh BAO Belf. 1994.

O'TOOLE, Mr Gregory Anthony 1 Eastcote View, Pinner HA5 1AT — MB ChB Sheff. 1992; FRCS Lond. 1996. Regist / Research Fell. (Plas Surg.) St Geo.s Hosp. Austral. Specialty: Plastic Surg. Prev: SHO (Plastic Surg.) Qu. Mary's Hosp. Roehampton Lond.; SHO (Plastic Surg.) Leicester Roy. Infirm.

O'TOOLE, James Gerard Cambria Surgery, Ucheldre Avenue, Holyhead LL65 1RA Tel: 01407 762735 Fax: 01407 766900 — MB ChB Ed. 1982; BSc Ed. 1989, MB ChB 1982; MRCGP 1989.

O'TOOLE, Mark Anthony 2 Tawell Mews, Tiptree, Colchester CO5 0QU — MB BS Lond. 1994.

O'TOOLE, Oliver Bartholomew Kirby Road Surgery, 58 Kirby Road, Dunstable LU6 3JH Tel: 01582 609121 Fax: 01582 472002; 11 Friars Walk, Dunstable LU6 3JA Tel: 01582 606956 — MB ChB Birm. 1974; DRCOG 1978; MRCGP 1979. GP Trainer NW Thames & Lond. Hosp. Train. Scheme. Prev: Clin. Asst. (Obst.) Luton & Dunstable Hosp. S. Beds. DHA; Trainee GP Luton & Dunstable VTS; SHO Luton & Dunstable Hosp. Beds.

O'TOOLE, Paul Anthony University Hospital Aintree, Longmoor Lane, Fazakerley, Liverpool L9 7AL Email: paul.otoole@aht.nwest.nhs.uk — (Oxford) BA (Hons) Oxf 1982; BM BCh Oxf. 1985; MRCP (UK) 1989; FRCP Lond. 2001. Cons. (Gastroenterol.) Univ. Hosp. Aintree Liverp.; Dep. Director Mersey Sch. Endoscopy Roy. Liverp. Univ. Hosp. Specialty: Gastroenterol. Special Interest: Endoscopy Train.; Nutrit.

O'TOOLE, Mr Stuart John 12 Cromwell Drive, East Leake, Loughborough LE12 6LZ — MB BS Newc. 1988; FRCS Glas. 1993.

OADE, Yvette Alison Halifax General Hospital, Salterhebble, Halifax HX3 0PW; 25 Fall Lane, Hartshead, Liversedge WF15 8AP — MB ChB Leeds 1984; BSc (Hons.) Leeds 1980; MRCP (UK) 1989. Cons. Paediat. Calderdale Healthcare NHS Trust. Specialty: Paediat. Prev: Sen. Regist. (Paediat.) Roy. Manch. Childr. Hosp.

OADES, Patrick John Royal Devon & Exeter Healthcare Trust (Wonford), Barrack Road, Exeter EX2 5DW Tel: 01392 411611 Fax: 01392 402715 — MB BCh Wales 1985; MA Camb. 1996, BA (Hons.) 1982; MRCP (UK) 1988; FRCPCH 1997. Cons. Paediat. Roy. Devon & Exeter Healthcare Trust. Specialty: Paediat.

OAKELEY, Penelope Susan Family Planning Services, Tooting Health Clinic, 63 Bevill Allen Close, Amen Corner, Tooting, London SW17 8PX Tel: 020 8700 0424 Fax: 020 8700 0426 — MRCS Eng. LRCP Lond. 1966 (RCSI & St. Thos.) MFFP 1993. Cons. Family Plann. & Reprod. Health S. W. Lond. Community NHS Trust; Hon. Sen. Lect. (Family Plann.) Dept. Obst. & Gyn. St. Geo. Hosp. Lond.; Sessional Med. Off. Amarant Menopause Clinic GainsBoro. Clinic Lond.; Clin. Asst. Genitourin. Med. St. Geogrs. Hosp. Lond. Specialty: Family Plann. & Reproduc. Health; Genitourinary Medicine. Socs: Bd. Mem. Fac. Community Health RIPHH; BASSH; Assoc. Mem. Inst. Psycho-Sexual Med. Prev: Clin. Asst. (Genitourin. Med. & Sexual Problems) St. Thos. Hosp. Lond.; Med. Off. (Family Plann.) W. Lambeth, Camberwell, Lewisham, N. Southwark & Wandsworth HA's; Ho. Phys. (Psychiat.) St. Thos. Hosp. Lond.

OAKENFULL, Andrew Gordon Perrin Ferryhill Medical Practice, Durham Road, Ferryhill DL17 8JJ Tel: 01740 651238 Fax: 01740 656291; 2 Acle Meadows, Newton Aycliffe DL5 4XD Tel: 01325 301820 — MB BS Newc. 1982; DRCOG 1986; MRCGP 1987. GP Ferryhill. Prev: Trainee GP W. Cumbld. VTS; SHO (Gen. Surg.) Qu. Eliz. Hosp. Gateshead; SHO (Neonat. Paediat.) Simpson Memor. Matern. Pavilion Edin.

OAKENFULL, Isabella Bethune (retired) Central House, 25 King St., Winterton, Scunthorpe DN15 9TP Tel: 01724 732278 — MB ChB Ed. 1951. Prev: Clin. Asst. (Dermat.) Gen. Hosp. Scunthorpe.

OAKERVEE, Heather Evelyn — MB BS Lond. 1993 (United Medical and Dental Schools) MRCP (UK) 1996; MRCPath 2002. Specialist Regist. /Research Fell. (Haemat.) Barts & The Lond. NHS Trust Lond. Specialty: Haematology. Prev: Specialist Regist. (Haemat.) Homerton Hosp. Lond.

OAKES, John Laurence 28 Castle Road, Hythe CT21 5HW — MB BS Lond. 1996.

OAKES, Mary (retired) Meadowsweet, Whitchurch Road, Horrabridge, Yelverton PL20 7TZ Tel: 01822 852585 — MB ChB Sheff. 1954. Private Med. Homeopath. Prev: Gen. Pract., Plymouth.

OAKES, Sarah Marie 23 Wollaton Avenue, Sheffield S17 4LA — MB ChB Liverp. 1998.

OAKES, Stuart Victor (retired) 16 Far View Bank, Almondbury, Huddersfield HD5 8EP Tel: 01484 424183 — MB ChB Leeds 1970; MRCPsych 1977. Prev: Cons. Psychiat. St. Lukes Hosp. Huddersfield.

OAKESHOTT, Philippa Community Health Sciences, General Practice & Primary Care, St. George's Hospital Medical School, London SW17 0RE Tel: 020 8672 9944 Fax: 020 8767 7697 Email: oakeshot@sghms.ac.uk; Manor Health Centre, 86 Clapham Manor St, London SW4 6EB Tel: 020 7411 6951 — MB BChir Camb. 1975 (Camb. & Barts.) MA Camb. 1975; MRCP (UK) 1979; MRCGP 1981; MD Camb. 1999; FRCP 2002. p/t Sen. Lect. (Gen. Pract. & Primary Care) St. Geo. Hosp. Med. Sch. Lond. Specialty: Gen. Pract. Special Interest: Hypertens.; STD's. Socs: RCP; RCGP; BMA. Prev: Trainee GP Lond. (St. Thos.) VTS; Ho. Surg. St. Bart. Hosp. Lond.; Ho. Phys. Northwick Pk. Hosp. & Clin. Research Centre Harrow.

OAKESHOTT, Simon 17 Hinton Way, Great Shelford, Cambridge CB2 5AX Tel: 01223 844961 — (St. Mary's) MA Oxf. 1959; MB BS Lond. 1966; MRCPsych 1978. Indep. Psychother. Camb. Specialty: Psychother. Prev: Sen. Regist. (Child & Family Psychiat.) Camb. AHA; Regist. Fulbourn Hosp. Camb.; Demonst. (Anat.) Univ. Camb.

OAKEY, Helen Mary 64 Circular Road, Jordanstown, Whiteabbey, Newtownabbey BT37 0RQ; 64 Circular Road, Jordanstown, Whiteabbey, Newtownabbey BT37 0RQ — MB BS Lond. 1988 (St. George's Hospital Medical School London) DRCOG 1992; MRCGP 1994. Med. Off. Roy. Flying Doctor Serv. Derby WA Australia. Specialty: Gen. Pract. Socs: MRCGP; DRCOG; FRACGP. Prev: Med. Off. Roy. Flying Doctor Serv. Broken Hill NSW, Australia; Emerg. Regist. Roy. N. Shore Hosp. Sydney; GP Regist. Camb.

OAKEY, John Stuckey (retired) 37 Burses Way, Hutton, Brentwood CM13 2PL — MB BS Sydney 1946; FRCPath. 1982, M 1970; FRCPA 1978. Prev: Cons. Haematol. Basildon & Thurrock Dist. Hosps.

OAKFORD, Andrew Charles 160 Newark Road, North Hykeham, Lincoln LN6 8LZ — MB ChB Sheff. 1990.

OAKHILL, Anthony Langford Cottage, Woollard, Pensford, Bristol BS39 4HT — MB ChB Birm. 1973; DCH Eng. 1975; MRCP (UK) 1976. Cons. Paediat. Oncol. Bristol Roy. Sick Childr. Hosp. Specialty: Paediat.

OAKLAND, Mr Christian David Hirst Accident & Emergency Department, Frenchay Hospital, Frenchay, Bristol BS16 1LE Tel: 0117 975 3840 Fax: 0117 918 6595; The Old Stables, The Street, Alveston, Bristol BS35 3SX Tel: 01454 416885 Fax: 01454 416881 Email: chris.oakland@btinternet.com — MB ChB Birm. 1978; FRCS Ed. 1982; FRCS Eng. 1983. Cons. A & E N. Bristol NHS Trust; Cahir 'Avonsafe' Accid. Precaution. Specialty: Accid. & Emerg. Socs: Fell. Fac. A & E Med. Prev: Sen. Regist. Basingstoke Dist. Hosp.

OAKLAND, Mr Desmond John (retired) 5 Breinton Lee, Hereford HR4 0SZ Tel: 01432 272262 Fax: 01432 272262 — MB ChB Birm. 1947; MRCS Eng. LRCP Lond. 1947; FRCS Eng. 1952; ChM Birm. 1959. Prev: Cons. Surg. Gen. & Co. Hosps. Hereford & Ledbury Cott. Hosp.

OAKLAND, Michael Hurst (retired) Coromandel, Auberrow, Wellington, Hereford HR4 8AL Tel: 01432 830799 Email: michael.oakland@btinternet.com — MB ChB Birm. 1954; BSc (Hons.) Birm. 1951; MRCGP 1963. Prev: Clin. Asst. United Birm. Hosps.

OAKLEY, Carol Jane The Surgery, 18 New Wokingham Road, Crowthorne RG45 6JL Tel: 01344 773418; Pinegrove, 100 Ellis Road, Crowthorne RG45 6PH Tel: 01344 762714 — BM Soton. 1984; DRCOG 1987; DCH RCP Lond. 1987; MRCGP (Distinc.) 1988. GP Crowthorne, Berks. Specialty: Gen. Pract. Prev: Clin. Med. Off. N. Herts. HA; SHO (O & G & Paediat.) Heatherwood Hosp. Ascot; Trainee GP Sunningdale Berks.

OAKLEY, Professor Celia Mary (retired) Hammersmith Hospital, Du Cane Road, London W12 0NN Tel: 020 8383 3141 Fax: 020 8740 8373; Long Crendon Manor, Long Crendon, Aylesbury HP18 9DZ Tel: 01844 208246 Fax: 01844 208246 — MB BS Lond. 1954 (Roy. Free) MB BS (Hons.) Lond. 1954; MRCS Eng. LRCP Lond. 1954; FRCP Lond. 1970, M 1956; MD Lond. 1965; FACC 1972; FESC 1988. Prof. Emerit. Clin. Cardiol. Roy. Postgrad. Med. Sch. Lond. & Hon. Cons. Cardiol. Hammersmith Hosp. & St. Mary's Hosp. Prev: MRC Fell. Mem. Hosp. Rochester USA.

OAKLEY, Clifton Douglas (retired) Apt. 7 St Anne's court, llanrhos, Llandudno LL30 15D — MB ChB Birm. 1952 (Birmingham) Local Treasury Med. Off.

OAKLEY, Dennis Elliott (retired) The Yetchleys, Lyneal, Ellesmere SY12 0QF Tel: 0194 875324 — MB ChB Birm. 1945; MRCS Eng. LRCP Lond. 1945; DIH Soc. Apoth. Lond. 1968.

OAKLEY, Donald Percy (retired) 5 Woodlands Way, Barton, Preston PR3 5DU — MB ChB Manch. 1952; DPM Eng. 1958; MD Manch. 1962; FRCPsych 1975, M 1971. Prev: Cons. Psychiat. Preston Health Dist.

OAKLEY, Edward Howard Nigel, Surg. Cdr. RN Brooklands Lodge, Park View Close, Wroxall, Ventnor PO38 3EQ Tel: 01983 853605 — MB BCh Wales 1979; BA Oxf. 1976; MSc Lond. 1987. Head of Survival & Thermal Med. Inst. Naval Med. Specialty: Clin. Physiol. Socs: Eur. Undersea Biomed. Soc.; Brit. Med. Informat. Soc. Prev: Med. Off. Jt. Serv. Expedition to Brabant Is., Antarctica.

OAKLEY, Gary Mark Flat C, 8 Hartham Road, London N7 9JG — MB BS Lond. 1992.

OAKLEY, George David Gastineau Cardiothoracic Unit, Northern General Hospital, Herries Road, Sheffield S5 7AU — MD Camb. 1984 (Westm.) MA 1972, MB BChir 1973; FRCP 1988, M 1975. Cons. (Cardiol.) N. Gen. Hosp. Sheff.; Hon. Clin. Lect. Univ. Sheff. Specialty: Cardiol. Socs: Brit. Cedrac Soc.; Brit. Cardiac Soc. Prev: Sen. Regist. (Cardiol.) North. Gen. Hosp. Sheff.; Regist. (Cardiol.); Roy. Postgrad. Med. Sch. Hammersmith Hosp. Lond.; Regist. (Gen. Med.); City Gen. Hosp. & N. Staffs Roy. Infirm. Stoke-on-Trent.

OAKLEY, Giles Anthony Montpelier Health Centre, Bath Buildings, Bristol BS6 5PT Tel: 0117 942 6811 Fax: 0117 944 4182 — MB ChB Leic. 1991; MRCP (UK) 1994. Specialty: Paediat.

OAKLEY, Hazel Monkwearmouth Health Centre, Dundas St., Sunderland SR6 0AB Tel: 0191 567 4459 Fax: 0191 565 3336; 17 Rectory Green, West Boldon, East Boldon NE36 0QD Tel: 0191 536 3276 — MB BS Durh. 1964; MFFP 1994.

OAKLEY, Helen Julia — MB BS Newc. 1990; MRCGP 1994; DFFP 1994. Prev: Trainee GP Doncaster VTS.

OAKLEY, John Richard 52 Bishops Way, Four Oaks, Sutton Coldfield B74 4XS Tel: 0121 308 8876; 161 Tamworth Road, Sutton Coldfield B75 6DY Tel: 0121 378 1251 — MB ChB Sheff. 1972; DCH RCPS Glas. 1974; MRCP (UK) 1974. Specialty: Gen. Med. Socs: Fell.Roy. Soc. of Med. Prev: Clin. Co-ordinator Multicentre PostNeonat. Study Project; Regist. (Med.) Childr. Hosp. Sheff.

OAKLEY, Judith Ellen (retired) Gibbs and Oakley, Doctors Surgery, Millend, Blakeney, Lydney GL15 4ED Tel: 01594 510225 Fax: 01594 516074 — MB BChir Camb. 1975; MRCP (UK) 1978. Prev: Sen. Regist. (Haemat.) W. Midl. Region.

OAKLEY, Louise Henderson 7 Lismore Close, Maidstone ME15 9SN; 7 Lismore Close, Maidstone ME15 9SN Tel: 01622 746217 — MB ChB Ed. 1970; DObst RCOG 1972; DCH RCP Lond. 1973; DTM & H Liverp. 1974; MRCGP 1983. GP working in Health Assessm. Prev: Princip. GP Brook La. Med. Mission Pract.; Med. Off. HEED Bangladesh.; GP Kent FHSA Retainer Scheme.

OAKLEY, Mr Matthew John 2 Pickwick Close, Merryoaks, Eluet Moor, Durham DH1 3QU Tel: 0191 384 7204 — MB ChB Glas. 1991; FRCS Ed 1996; FRCS Glas 1996; FRCS (Trauma & Orth) 2001. Specialist Regist. Trauma & Orthop. Surg. Northern Rotat. Specialty: Trauma & Orthop. Surg. Socs: BOA.

OAKLEY, Mr Neil Royal Hallamshire Hospital, Glossop Road, Sheffield S10 2JF Tel: 0114 271 2097 Email: neiloakleyqbtinternet.com; 56 High Storrs Crescent, Sheffield S11 7JZ Tel: 01742 687224 Email: neil.oakley@bigfoot.com — MB ChB Sheff. 1990 (Sheffield) FRCS Eng. 1994; FRCS (Urol) 1998. Consultant Urologist Surgeon. Specialty: Urol.

OAKLEY, Nigel Wingate London Medical London Diabetes, 49 Marylebone High Street, London W1U 5HJ Tel: 020 7467 5470 Fax: 020 7467 5471 Email: drnigeloakley@aol.com; The Homestead House, 113 Church Road, London SW13 9HL Tel: 020 8741 3311 Fax: 020 8563 0580 — MB BChir Camb. 1958 (Univ. Coll. Hosp.) MRCS Eng. LRCP Lond. 1958; FRCP Lond. 1978, M 1960; MA Camb. 1959, MD 1974. Hon. Cons. Phys. & Hon. Sen. Lect. St. Geo. Hosp. Lond.; Hon. Cons. Phys. St. Luke's Hosp. for the Clergy. Specialty: Diabetes; Endocrinol. Special Interest: Clin. Managem. of diabetes with special interest in diabetes and Pregn. Socs: Diabetes UK; Med. Soc. Lond.; Assn. of Brit. Clin. Diabetologists. Prev: Sen. Lect. & Hon. Cons. Phys. St. Mary's Hosp. & Med. Sch. Lond.; Sen. Regist. Middlx. Hosp. Lond.

OAKLEY, Peter Anthony North Staffordshire Hospital, Princes Road, Hartshill, Stoke-on-Trent ST4 7LN Tel: 01782 715444 Fax: 01782 554627 — BChir Camb. 1979 (Cambridge) MA (Physics) Oxf. 1979, BA 1975; MB 1980; MRCGP 1983; FFA RCS Eng. 1987. Cons. Anaesth. with s/i in Trauma & Intens. Care Stoke-on-Trent. Specialty: Anaesth.; Intens. Care. Socs: Internat. Trauma Anaesth. & Critical Care Soc.; Brit. Trauma Soc. (Pres. 1998-1999). Prev: Wellcome Inst. Sen. Research Fell. & Hon. Sen. Regist. (Anaesth.) Nuffield Dept. Anaesth. Oxf.; Regist. (Anaesth.) Sir Humphry Davy Dept. Anaesth. Bristol; Clin. Fell. (Emerg. Med. & Trauma) Sunnybrook Med. Centre Toronto, Canada.

OAKLEY, Richard John 18 Horn Park Lane, London SE12 8UU — MB BS Lond. 1997; BDS London 1988; FDSRCS (Eng) 1996; MRCS ED 2001; DLO 2001. ENT Specialist Regist., Lond., Kent, Surrey & Sussex Deanery.

OAKLEY, Robert Harvey 1 Oaklands Road, Bedford MK40 3AG — MB ChB Liverp. 1976; DMRD Liverp. 1980; FRCR Lond. 1982. Cons. Radiol. Bedford Gen. Hosp. Specialty: Radiol.

OAKLEY, Suzan Elizabeth — MB BCh Wales 1997.

OAKLEY, Timothy Neil Wallsend CMHC, The Green, Wallsend NE28 7PD Tel: 0191 262 4314 Fax: 0191 262 5228 — MB ChB Sheff. 1987; BMedSci 1986; MMedSci (Clin. Psychiat.) Leeds 1994. Cons. (Psychiat.) Wallsend Community Ment. Health Centre. Specialty: Gen. Psychiat. Prev: Sen. Regist. (Psychiat.) Newc. Gen. Hosp.

OAKLEY, Wendy Elizabeth Queens Hospital, Burton Hospitals NHS Trust, Belvedere Road, Burton-on-Trent DE13 0RB Tel: 01283 566333 — MB ChB Leic. 1987; MRCOG 1992; MD Warwick 1998. Cons. (Obst. & Gyn), Qu.s Hosp. Burton. Specialty: Obst. & Gyn. Socs: BMUS. Prev: Sen. Regist., W. Midl. Region; Research Fell. Assisted Conception Unit, Walsgrave Hosp. Coventry; Regist. Rotat. (O & G) Oxf. Region.

OAKSHOTT, Gordon Henry Leonard The Medical Physics & Bio Engineering Research Unit, Doncaster Royal Infirmary, Armthorpe Road, Doncaster DN2 5LT Tel: 01302 366666; 12 Bellwood Crescent, Thorne, Doncaster DN8 4BA Tel: 01405 812433 — MB ChB Leeds 1952; MRCGP 1960; BA Open 1974; MSc (Human Genetics) Ed. 1977; AFOM RCP Lond. 1981. Hon. Med. Adviser (Med. Phys.) & Bioeng. Research Unit Doncaster Roy. Infirm. Specialty: Genetics. Socs: Leeds & W. Riding Medico-Legal Soc. Prev: GP Thorne; Teach. (Gen. Pract.) Univ. Leeds; Indust. Med. Off. GEC Thorne.

OATES, Anita Paulette Hanscombe House Surgery, 52A St Andrew Street, Hertford SG14 1JA Tel: 01992 582025 Fax: 01992 305511; 117 Ware Road, Hertford SG13 7EE — MB BS Lond. 1983 (St. Geo.) DCH RCP Lond. 1986; MRCP (UK) 1987. Specialty: Gen. Med. Prev: Trainee GP Epsom VTS; Family Med. Duke Univ., USA.

OATES, Beverley Claire Dearden Brook, Edenwood Lane, Ramsbottom, Bury BL0 0EX — MB ChB Birm. 1993; ChB Birm. 1993.

OATES, Bridget Daphne Royal Hospital For Sick Children, Yourk Hill, Glasgow G15 6PX — MB ChB Ed. 1992; BSc (Hons.) Med. Sci. Ed. 1990; MRCP (UK) 1996. Regist., (Paediat.), RHSC, Yorkhill, Glas. Specialty: Paediat. Prev: SHO (Paediat.) Simpson Memor. Matern. Pavil. Edin.; SHO (Paediat.) Childr. Hosp. Birm.

OATES, Caroline Sinclair 71 Hunter House Road, Sheffield S11 8TU — MB ChB Sheff. 1997.

OATES, Christopher Glyn Mayford House Surgery, Boroughbridge Road, Northallerton DL7 8AW Tel: 01609 772105 Fax: 01609 778553; The Old Chapel, Newby Wise, Northallerton DL7 9EX — MB BS Newc. 1980; DRCOG 1983; DCCH RCGP & FCM 1984; MRCGP 1984. Prev: Trainee GP Northumbria VTS; Ho. Off. Newc. Teach. Hosps.

OATES, David Eden Rayner Oughtibridge Surgery, Church Street, Oughtibridge, Sheffield S35 0FW Tel: 0114 286 2145 Fax: 0114 286 4031 — MB ChB Sheff. 1971.

OATES, Mr Geoffrey Donald (cons. rooms), 81 Harborne Road, Edgbaston, Birmingham B15 3HG Tel: 0121 455 9496 Fax: 0121 455 0288; 14 Hintlesham Avenue, Edgbaston, Birmingham B15 2PH Tel: 0121 454 3257 Email: gdoates@doctors.org.uk — MB ChB Birm. 1953; BSc (Anat. & Physiol. 1st cl. Hons.) Birm. 1950; FRCS Eng. 1959; MS (Surg.) Univ. Illinois 1964. Emerit. Cons. Surgic. Oncol. & Gen. Surg. Univ. Birm. NHS Trust; NCRI - Colorectal Study Gp. Specialty: Gen. Surg. Socs: Fell. Roy. Soc. Med. (Mem. (Ex-Pres.) Sects. Oncol. & Colo-proctol., Mem. Sect. Surg.); Assn. Coloproctol. (Ex-Pres.); Europ. Assn. Coloproctol. Prev: Sen. Clin. Lect. (Surg.) Univ. Birm.; Capt. RAMC; Sen. Research Fell. & Instruc. (Surg.) Univ. Illinois, Chicago.

OATES, Mr John The ENT Department, Queen's Medical Burton, Belvedere Rd, Burton-on-Trent DE13 0RB Tel: 01889 504393 Fax: 01283 541683 — MB ChB Birm. 1979 (Birmingham) FRCS Ed. 1984. Cons. Otolaryngol. Burton, Lichfield & Tamworth Hosps.; Educational Monitoring Team, W. Midl.s PostGrad. Deanery; Hon. Clin. Tutor, Univ. of Leics. Med Sch.; Cons. Otolaryngol Heartlands Hosp. Specialty: Otorhinolaryngol. Socs: Brit. Assn. of Otolaryngologists, head & neck Surg.s; Roy. Soc. Med. (RSM); Young Cons. Otolaryngol. Head & Neck Surg. (Pres.). Prev: Cons. Otolaryngol. Burton Hosps. Burton-on-Trent; Sen. Regist. (Otolaryngol.) Univ. Hosp. Nottm. & Derby Roy. Infirm.; Regist. (Otolaryngol.) Qu. Eliz. Hosp. Birm. & E. Birm. Hosp.

OATES, John Gordon Parkfield Medical Centre, Sefton Road, New Ferry, Wirral CH62 5HS Tel: 0151 644 6665; 9 Buerton Close, Noctorum, Birkenhead CH43 9EA Tel: 0151 653 5014 — MB ChB Dundee 1980; MRCGP 1986. Prev: GP Bootle, Merseyside.

OATES, John Kenyon (retired) 76 Glengall Road, Woodford Green IG8 0DL Tel: 020 8504 7379 Email: jkoates@waitrose.com — (Lond. Hosp.) MB BS Lond. 1946; FRCP Ed. 1970, M 1956; MA Camb. 1973. Prev: Cons. Phys. (Genitourin. Med.) Addenbrooke's Hosp. Camb. & Westm. Hosp. Lond.

OATES, Jonathan David Lawson South Glasgow University Hospitals Division, NHS Greater Glasgow, Victoria Infirmary, Langside Road, Glasgow G42 9TY Tel: 0141 201 5320 — BM Soton. 1983; DA (UK) 1985; FFA RCSI 1988. Cons. Anaesth. S. Glas. Univ. Hosps. Div. Specialty: Anaesth.

OATES, Kenneth Raymond Highland Health Board, Public Health Medicine Department, Beechwood Park, Inverness IV2 3HG Tel: 01463 704886 Fax: 01463 717666 Email: ken.oates@hhb.scot.nhs.uk; 8 Mayfield Road, Inverness IV2 4AE Tel: 01463 226236 — MB ChB Aberd. 1985; DRCOG 1987; Cert. Family Plann. JCC 1989; MRCGP 1989; MFPHM RCP (UK) 1995; FFPH 2002. Cons. (Pub. Health Med.) Highland Health Bd. Inverness; Hon. Sen. Lect. (Pub. Health) Aberd. Univ. Specialty: Pub. Health Med. Prev: Sen. Regist. (Pub. Health Med.) Highland HB Inverness; Med. Audit Facilitator Highland HB Inverness; Trainee GP Inverness VTS.

OATES, Margaret Rose Department of Psychiatry, University Hospital, Queens Medical Centre, Nottingham NG7 2UH Tel: 0115 970 9339 — MB ChB Liverp. 1966; DPM Eng. 1970; FRCPsych 1990, M 1972. Hon. Cons. Psychiat. Univ. Hosp. Nottm.; Sen. Lect. (Psychiat.) Univ. Nottm. Med. Sch. Specialty: Gen. Psychiat. Prev: Lect. (Psychiat.) Univ. Nottm. Med. Sch.; Sen. Regist. (Psychiat.) Manch. Roy. Infirm.; Regist. Roy. Edin. Hosp.

OATES, Nathalie Roberta The Old Kiln House, 79 Haymeads Lane, Bishop's Stortford CM23 5JJ Tel: 01279 659287 — MB BS Lond. 1985.

OATES, Peter Edward Lister House Surgery, The Common, Hatfield AL10 0NL Tel: 01707 268822 Fax: 01707 263990 — MB ChB Sheff. 1973; DObst RCOG 1976.

OATES, Philip Damian Department of Anaesthesia, Southern General Hospital, Glasgow, 1345 Gosan Road, Glasgow G51 4CF Tel: 0141 201 1658 Fax: 0141 201 1320 Email: philip.oates@sgh.scot.nhs.uk — MB ChB Dundee 1983; DA (UK) 1985; FFA RCSI 1988. Cons. Anaesth. South. Gen. Hosp. NHS Trust. Glas.; Hon. Sen. Lect., Univ. of Glas. Med. Soc.. Specialty: Anaesth.

OATES, Sharon Elizabeth Royal Shrewsbury Hospital, Mytton Oak Road, Copthorne, Shrewsbury SY3 8XQ Tel: 01743 261669 Fax: 01743 261659; 181 Holyhead Road, Wellington, Telford TF1 2DP Tel: 01952 252498 — MB ChB Liverp. 1982; MRCOG 1987; Dip. Human Sex Manch. 1990; Dip Psychosexual Med 1991; FRCOG 2003. Cons. O & G Shrops. & Powys HA; Psychosexual Counsellor. Specialty: Obst. & Gyn. Socs: Shrewsbury Med. Institue; Brit. Assn. Sexual & Marital Ther. Prev: Lect. (O & G) St. Mary's Hosp. Manch.

OATES, Valerie Elizabeth Marshall 14 Craighlaw Avenue, Eaglesham, Glasgow G76 0EU — MB BS Lond. 1983; BSc (Hons.) Aberd. 1977; DRCOG 1986; MRCGP 1987; Dip. Palliat. Med. Wales 1995. Hospice Phys. P. & Princess of Wales Hospice, Glas. Specialty: Palliat. Med.

OATES, William Keith Health Centre, Whyteman's Brae, Kirkcaldy KY1 2NA Tel: 01592 642902 Fax: 01592 644814 — MB ChB Ed. 1972; MRCGP 1977.

OATWAY, Helen Beverley 58 Cambidge Road, Middlesbrough TS5 5HG — MB BS Newc. 1989. SHO (Anaesth.) S. Cleveland Hosp. Middlesbrough.

OBADIAH, Mercia (retired) 10 Windsor House, 2 Regency Crescent, London NW4 1NW Tel: 01702 430685 — MB BS Calcutta 1951; DObst RCOG 1959; MFCM 1974.

OBADIAH, Rachel 52 Eastbury Road, Northwood HA6 3AW — MB Calcutta 1937; DRCOG 1947.

OBAID, Matthew Paul 25 Celtic View, Bridgend CF31 1YG — MB BCh Wales 1994.

OBAID, Sarah Louise 25 Celtic View, Litchard, Bridgend CF31 1YG — MB BS Lond. 1996.

OBAID, Shaza 132 Woodway Lane, Coventry CV2 2EJ — MD Damascus 1986; MRCP (UK) 1994.

OBAIDULLAH, Mohammad The Surgery, Woodlands Terrace, Caerau, Bridgend CF32 7LB; 25 Celtic View, Litchard, Bridgend CF31 1YG — MB BS Peshawar 1968 (Khyber Med. Coll.) MRCOG 1976, DObst 1973; MRCGP 1978; Dip. Pract. Dermat. Wales 1990; FRCOG 1991; Dip. Palliat. Med. Wales 1991; LLM (Legal Aspects of Med. Practice) Wales 1997. Mem. of the Local Research Ethics Comm. of Iechyd Morgannwy Health; Mem. of the Appeals Tribunal; Mem. of the Multi Research Ethics Comm. of Wales; Mem. of the Buidford Local Health Gp. Prev: Hosp. Pract. (O & G) Bridgend Gen. Hosp. GP Trainer & Family.

OBAJI, Abdel Kader Kassem Horeb Street Surgery, Horeb Street, Treorchy CF42 6RU Tel: 01443 772185 Fax: 01443 773083 — MB BCh Al-Azhar Cairo 1971; MB BCh Al-Azhar Egypt 1971.

OBALE, Begho Agboraw Westmoreland General Hospital, Burton Road, Kendal LA9 7RG; 28 Scar View Road, Oxenholme, Kendal LA9 7EU — MB BS Ibadon 1989. Staff Grade Phys. Westmorland Gen. Hosp. Kendal. Specialty: Gen. Med. Special Interest: Diabetes.

OBARA, Lawrence Gordon 17 Maple Way, Cranfield, Bedford MK43 0DW — MB ChB East Africa 1970 (Makerere Univ. Coll.) DLO Eng. 1978. Regist. (ENT Surg.) Gen. Hosp. & Univ. Hosp. Nottm. Prev: SHO (ENT Surg.) Gen. Hosp. Nottm.

OBASI, Angela Ijeoma Nwabuche Chukwu The London School of Hygiene & Tropical Medicine, Keppel St., London WC1E 7HT Email: angela.obasi@ishtm.ac.uk — MB BS Lond. 1988; MSc (Distinc.) Lond. 1992; MRCP (UK) 1994; MSc Lond. 1996. Research Fell. Clin. Epidemiol. Lond. Sch. Hyg. & Trop. Med. Specialty: Epidemiol.

OBEID, Daisy Alexandra Hospital, Woodrow Drive, Redditch B98 7UB Tel: 01527 503030 Fax: 01527 512007; 111 Fitzroy Avenue, Harborne, Birmingham B17 8RG Tel: 0121 427 1955 — (Ain Shams) MB BCh Ain Shams 1965; DCH Eng. 1970; FRCPath 1990, M 1978. Cons. Haemat. W. Midl. RHA. Alexandra Healthcare NHS Trust Redditch. Specialty: Haematology. Prev: Sen. Regist. & Regist. (Haemat.) W. Midl. RHA; Gen. Duty Med. Off., Sudan.

OBEID, Mr El Moez Hayder Tameside General Hospital, Fountain Street, Ashton-under-Lyne OL6 9RW Tel: 0161 231 6823 Email: obeiduk@ntlworld.com — MB BCh Alexandria 1978 (Egypt) FRCSI 1990; MChOrth Liverp. 1993; FRCS (Tr & Orth). 1998. Cons. Orthopaedic Surg., Manch. Specialty: Orthop. Socs: BOA; BMA; AAOS.

OBEID, Mr Magdi Latif 111 Fitzroy Avenue, Harborne, Birmingham B17 8RG Tel: 0121 427 1955 — MRCS Eng. LRCP Lond. 1973 (E' In Shams Univ. Cairo) MB BCh E' In Shams Univ. 1965; FRCS Ed. 1969; FRCS Eng. 1971. Cons. Surg. Dudley Rd. Hosp. & St. Chads Hosp. Birm. Specialty: Gen. Surg. Socs: BMA & Brit. Transpl. Soc. Prev: Sen. Regist. (Surg.) Qu. Eliz. Hosp. Birm.; Regist. (Paediat. Surg.) Childr. Hosp. Birm.; Regist. (Surg.) Artific. Kidney & Renal Transpl. Unit Qu. Eliz. Hosp.

OBEL, Owen Abraham Flat 4, 68 Elmbourne Road, London SW17 8JJ — MB BCh Witwatersrand 1986; MRCP (UK) 1993.

OBENG, Francis 230 Chalklands, Wembley HA9 9DY — State Exam Med Erlangen 1977.

OBERAI, Bhavneet 55 Chesterfield Road, Ashford TW15 2NE — BM BCh Oxf. 1986; BSc Lond. 1983; DRCOG 1989. Trainee GP Ashford Middlx. VTS.

OBERAI, Surendra K Pant Surgery, 57 Aberdare Road, Cwmbach, Aberdare CF44 0HL Tel: 01685 872434 Fax: 01685 878158. GP Aberdare, M. Glam.

OBERMAN, Anthony Stephen 39 The Ridgeway, Golders Green, London NW11 8QP — MB BS Lond. 1981.

OBEROI, Arjun 11 Hogan Mews, London W2 1UP — MB ChB Ed. 1997.

OBERTHUR, Eric Pierre Andre Westlake Surgery, West Coker, Yeovil BA22 9AH Tel: 01935 862212 Fax: 01935 864196 — MB Camb. 1964 (Westm.) BChir 1963. Socs: BMA. Prev: Ho. Off. (Med.) St. Stephen's Hosp. Chelsea; SHO (Paediat.) Qu. Eliz. II Hosp. Welwyn Gdn. City; SHO (O & G) Centr. Middlx. Hosp. Lond.

OBEYESEKERA, Sharmin Lesrene 25 Barn Way, Wembley HA9 9NT — MB BS Lond. 1994.

OBHOLZER, Anton Meinhard Tavistock Clinic, 120 Belsize Lane, London NW3 5BA Tel: 020 7435 7111 Fax: 020 7447 3709 — MB ChB Cape Town 1963; DPM Cape Town 1969; FRCPsych 1987, M 1973; T(Psych) 1991. Chief Exec. Tavistock & Portman NHS Trust; Cons. Psychiat. Tavistock Clinic; Prof. Assoc. Brunel Univ.; Hon. Sen. Lect. Roy. Free Hosp. Med. Sch. Specialty: Child & Adolesc. Psychiat. Socs: Assoc. Mem. Brit. Psychoanalyt. Soc. Prev: Cons. Psychiat. Child Guid. Train. Centre Lond.; Sen. Regist. Adolesc. Dept. Tavistock Clinic Lond.; Regist. Groote Schuur Hosp. Cape Town, S. Afr.

OBHRAI, Mr Manjit Singh North Staffordshire Maternity Hospital, Hilton Road, Harpfields, Newcastle ST5 Tel: 01782 552402 Fax: 01782 552695; Little Croft, Tower Road, Ashley Health, Market Drayton TF9 4PU Tel: 01630 673723 — BM BS Nottm. 1975 (Nottingham University) MRCOG 1982. Cons. Obst. & Obst. & Med. Dir. Fertil. Centre N. Staffs. Hosps. NHS Trust; Sen. Clin. Lect. Univ. Keele. Specialty: Obst. & Gyn. Socs: Brit. Fertil. Soc.; Eur. Soc. Human Reproduc. & Embryol. Prev: Cons. & Sen. Lect. & Sen. Regist. & Lect. (O & G) Univ. Birm.

OBI, Benedict Chibuzor The Royal Surrey County Hospital, Egerton Road, Guildford GU2 7XX — MB BS Lond. 1991.

OBI, Bernard Chukwura Dr J E Barker and Partners, 85 Ross Road, Maidenhead SL6 2SR Tel: 01628 623767 Fax: 01628 789623 Email: bernardobi@doctors.org.uk — (St. Mary's) MRCS Eng. LRCP Lond. 1970; DObst RCOG 1975; DTM & H Eng. 1975; MRCOG 1982; MFFP 1993. Hosp. Pract. (O & G) Wexham Pk. Hosp. Slough. Socs: Christ. Med. Fellowsh.; BMA; Assn. Forensic Physicians. Prev: Regist. (O & G) Wexham Pk. Hosp. Slough; Sen. Med. Off. Iyi-Enu Miss. Hosp. Onitsha, Nigeria; Regist. (Gen. Med.) Croydon Gen. Hosp.

OBICHERE, Austin 28B Fairhazel Gardens, London NW6 3SJ — MB BS Lagos 1987.

OBIECHINA, Nonyelum Evangeline 56 Kingfisher Grove, Bradford BD8 0NP Tel: 01274 880181 — LRCP LRCS Ed. 1993; MB BS U. of Nigeria 1987; LRCP LRCS Ed. LRCPS Glas. 1993.

OBIEKWE, Margaret Ngozi Park Lodge Medical Centre, 3 Old Park Road, Palmers Green, London N13 4RG Tel: 020 8886 6866 Fax: 020 8882 8884 — MRCS Eng. LRCP Lond. 1989; BM BCh Nigeria 1984; MRCS Eng LRCP Lond. 1989. Regist. (O & G) Roy. Lond. Hosp. Specialty: Obst. & Gyn. Prev: SHO (O & G) Univ. Coll. Hosp. & Whipps Cross Hosp. Lond.

OBIN, Olive Mary (Surgery), 66A Portsmouth Road, Woolston, Southampton SO19 9AL Tel: 023 8043 6277 Fax: 023 8039 9751; Newstead, 32 Havelock Road, Warsash, Southampton SO31 9FX Tel: 01489 575970 — MB BS Lond. 1957 (Roy. Free) MRCS Eng. LRCP Lond. 1957. Specialty: Family Plann. & Reproduc. Health. Prev: Sen. Med. Off. (Family Plann.) Cosham & Fareham Health Centres; Ho. Surg. Mayday Hosp. Croydon; Ho. Phys. Croydon Gen Hosp.

OBINECHE, Professor Enyioma Nwaogu Acting \Chairman, Department of Internal Medicine, Faculty of Medicine & Health Sciences, United Arab Emirates University, PO Box 17666 Al-Ain, United Arab Emirates Tel: 971 3703 9420 Fax: 971 372995 Email: obineche@emirates.net.ae; 10 St Margarets Avenue, London N15 3DH Tel: 0208 881 0795 Fax: 0208 245 3498 — MB ChB Glas. 1963 (Glasgow University School of Medicine) DCH RCP Lond. 1965; FRCPS Glas. 1978, M 1968. Director Kidney Dialysis Centre King Fahad Hosp. Al Baha, Saudi Arabia; Prof. Fac. Med. & Health Sci. UAE Univ., Al-Ain.; Acting Chairm. Dept of Internal Med. Specialty: Nephrol. Socs: Int. Soc. Nephrol.; Eur. Dialysis & Transpl.

Assn.; BMA. Prev: Director Renal Unit K. Fahd Hosp., Al-Baha, Saudi Arabia; Cons. Nephrol. Milit. Hosp. Tabuk, Saudi Arabia; Asst. Dean & Prof. Med. Ahmadu Bello Univ. Med. Sch., Kaduna & Zaria, Nigeria.

OBONNA, Rex 53 Langdale Way, East Boldon NE36 0UF — MB ChB Dundee 1983. SHO (O & G) Edith Watson Matern. Unit Burnley Gen. Hosp. Prev: Ho. Off. (Surg.) Qu. Eliz. Hosp. Edgbaston; Ho. Off. S. Shields Gen. Hosp. Tyne & Wear.

OBONYO, Mr Henry Benjamin 36 Barringer Square, London SW17 8EE — MB ChB East Africa 1965; FRCS Ed. 1969; MD Nairobi 1985. Cons. Urol. Princess Roy. Hosp. Telford. Specialty: Urol. Socs: Fell. Assn. Surgs. of E. Afr.; BMA; Brit. Assn. Urol. Surgs. Prev: Cons. Urol. Mulago Hosp., Uganda; Lect. (Urol.) Nairobi Univ., Kenya.

OBOTH OWINO, Nimrod — MB ChB Glas. 1972; DObst RCOG Lond. 1974; MSc (Clin Trop. Med.) Lond. 1980; MSc (Clin. Microbiol.) Lond. 1987. GP Regist. Enfield & Haringey GPVTS. Specialty: Gen. Pract. Prev: Sen. Regist. (Microbiol.) Guy's & St. Thos. NHS Trust Lond.; Sen. Regist. (Microbiol.) Ashford PHL William Harvey Hosp. Kent; Regist. (Microbiol.) Lewisham Hosp. Lond., St. And. Hosp. & Lond. Hosp. Med. Coll.

OCANSEY, John Alfred Greencroft Medical Centre (South), Greencroft Wynd, Annan DG12 6GS Tel: 01461 202244; 7 Kirkland Road, Calside, Dumfries DG1 4EZ Tel: 01387 257015 Email: johnocansey@hotmail.com — MB ChB Ghana 1991; DFFP 2001; DRCOG 2003. GP Regist. Annan. Prev: SHO (Med.) Lorn & Is. Dist. Gen. Hosp. Oban; GP train. Dumfries & Galloway Roy. Infirm.; Regist. (O & G) Doncaster Roy. Infirm.

OCANSEY, Peter Trafford General Hospital, Department of Old Age Psychiatry, Moorside Unit, Moorside Road, Manchester M41 5SL Tel: 0161 746 2651; 44 Chelsfield Grove, Chorlton, Manchester M21 7SG — MB ChB Ghana 1993; MSc; MRCPsych; BSc Hons. Cons. Old Age Psychiat. Trafford Gen Hosp Manch. Specialty: Geriat. Psychiat. Prev: Specialist Regist. (Psychiat.) Manch. Roy. Infirm. Lancs.

OCHEFU, Oche Aaron University Hospital Aintree, Fazailerley, Liverpool L9 4AE Email: cooloche@yahoo.com; 32 Preston Road, Southport PR9 9EE — MB BS Benin 1982 (Univ. of Benin Nigeria) Staff Grade (Otorhinolaryng. & Head & Neck Surg.) Aintree Hosps. Liverp. Specialty: Otorhinolaryngol. Socs: S.port Med. Soc. Prev: Regist. (ENT) Roy. Preston Hosp.

OCHOA GRANDE, Juan 9B Barnsbury Avenue, Aylesbury HP20 1NL — LMS Extramadura 1982.

OCKELFORD, Olwyn Kathleen (retired) Flat 3, Burnage Court, 6 Martello Park, Canford Cliffs, Poole BH13 7BA Tel: 01202 701189 — (Camb. & Roy. Free) MRCS Eng. LRCP Lond. 1949; MB BChir Camb. 1950; MA Camb. 1950; DCH Eng. 1952; MRCPsych 1977. Prev: Cons. Psychiat. Avon AHA (T).

OCKELFORD, Stuart John 22 Robin Down Lane, Mansfield NG18 4SW — MB ChB Bristol 1995.

OCKENDEN, Barbara Georgina (retired) 4 Weavers Walk, Swynnerton, Stone ST15 0QZ — MB BS Lond. 1945 (King's Coll. Hosp.) FRCPath 1976, M 1964. Prev: Cons. Morbid Anat., Histopath. Centr. Path. Laborat. Stoke-on-Trent.

OCKRIM, Jeremy Louis 22 Braidholm Road, Giffnock, Glasgow G46 6HJ — MB ChB Glas. 1994.

OCKRIM, Jonathan Barry — MB ChB Glas. 1989; FRCS Glas. 1994; FRCS (Gen.) 2002.

OCKRIM, Zoe Kate — MB ChB Glas. 1996 (University of Glasgow) MRCOpth 2000. Research Regist. Moorfields Eye Hosp. Specialty: Ophth. Socs: RCOphth; BMA; MDDUS. Prev: SHO (Ophth.) S. Thames Rotat.; SHO (Ophth) Qu. Marys Hosp, Sidcup, Kent; SHO (Ophth.) Vict. Eye Hosp. Hereford.

ODAM, Richard (retired) Southfield Gate, 78 Sandy Lane, Charlton Kings, Cheltenham GL53 9DH Tel: 01242 582778 — (St. Mary's) MRCS Eng. LRCP Lond. 1965; MB BS Lond. 1966.

ODBER, Elizabeth Anne The Aldergate Medical Practice, The Mount, Salters Lane, Tamworth B79 8BH Tel: 01827 54775 Fax: 01827 62835 — BM Soton. 1983; DA (UK) 1987; MRCGP 1990. Specialty: Gen. Pract.

ODBERT, Reginald Massey Highcliffe Medical Centre, 248 Lymington Road, Highcliffe, Christchurch BH23 5ET Tel: 01425 271086 — MB ChB Sheff. 1976; FIMC RCS Ed.; BSc Wales 1971; MRCGP 1981; DRCOG 1982; DAvMed FOM RCP Lond. 1985. Clin. Asst. (Ophth.) Soton. Univ. Hosp. Trust. Specialty: Aviat. Med. Socs: Roy. Aeronaut. Soc.; RCS Edin.; Fac. Pre-Hosp. Care. Prev: Clin. Asst. (Ophth.) Roy. Bournemouth Hosp. Trust; Sen. Med. Off. RAF Akrotiri BFPO 57 & Aeromed Co-ordinating Off.; Sen. Med. Off. RAF Chivenor.

ODD, David Edward 160 Conway Avenue, Great Wakering, Southend-on-Sea SS3 0BJ — MB ChB Leic. 1996.

ODDIE, Samuel Joseph Ripley Newcastle Neonatal Service, Department of Child Health, Royal Victoria Infirmary, Newcastle upon Tyne NE1 4LP — MB BS Newc. 1991. Specialist Regist. Roy. Vict. Infirm.

ODDY, Alice Virtue Llanberis Surgery, High Street, Llanberis, Caernarfon LL55 4SU — MB ChB Dundee 1992; DRCOG 1995; MRCGP 1996; DCH RCP Lond. 1996.

ODDY, Clifford Gaunt (retired) 107 Pogmoor Road, Pogmoor, Barnsley S75 2LN Tel: 01226 206186 — MB ChB Sheff. 1956; DPH Leeds 1961; MFCM 1972. Prev: Cons. Pub. Health Med. & Communicable Dis. Control Barnsley HA.

ODDY, Michael Jonathan Flat 7, 1 Prince of Wales Road, London NW5 3LW — BChir Camb. 1996 (Univ. of Camb.) MB Camb. 1997; MA Camb. 1998; MRCS Eng. 2000; MSc UCL 2002.

ODEDRA, Nathalal Wolverton Health Centre, Gloucester Road, Wolverton, Milton Keynes MK12 5DF Tel: 01908 316633 Fax: 01908 225397 — MB BS Baroda 1972; MB BS Baroda 1972.

ODEDUN, Mr Titus Oyewole Brittania Medical Bureau, 12 Harley St., London W1G 9PG Tel: 020 7580 4903 Fax: 020 7580 4906; 6 Heather Drive, Rise Park, Romford RM1 4SP — MRCS Eng. LRCP Lond. 1978; FRCS Ed. 1981; FRCS Eng 1982; MD Malta 1989. Cons. Surg. Old Ct. Hosp. Lond.; Cons. Ormskirk & Dist. Hosp. Specialty: Accid. & Emerg. Prev: Regist. (Surg.) Pinderfield Hosp. Wakefield; Lect. (Surg.) Univ. Calabar, Nigeria.

ODEGAARD, Esten Reidar ASnaesthetic Department, West Suffolk Hospital, Hardwick Lane, Bury St Edmunds IP33 2QZ — Cand Med Bergen 1961.

ODEKA, Benjamin Olugbola Pennine Acute Hospitals NHS Trust, Child Health Department, Royal Oldham Hospital, Oldham OL1 2JH Fax: 0161 627 8309 Email: egware@aol.com — MB BS Ibadan 1980; DCH RCPS Glas. 1985; MRCP (UK) 1987; FRCPCH Eng. 1995; FRCP 2000. Cons. Paediat. Roy. Oldham Hosp.; Hon. Lect. Univ. of Manch.; Clin. Dir. (Child Health); UnderGrad. Tutor. Specialty: Paediat. Special Interest: Gastroenterol. Socs: Paediat. Research Soc.; Brit. Paediat. Assn.; Brit. Soc. Paediat. Gastroenterol. & Nutrit. Prev: Sen. Regist. Rotat. Special Care Baby Unit Roy. Gwent Hosp.; Research Fell. Child Health (Paediat. Gastroenterol.) Univ. Manch. Booth Hall Childr. Hosp. Manch.; Regist. Rotat. (Paediat.) Roy. Manch Childr. Hosp. (Metab. Unit.), Pendlebury & Burnley Gen. Hosp.

ODEKU, Katherine Jill (retired) 81 Linford Avenue, Newport Pagnell MK16 8BX Tel: 01908 616850 — (Roy. Free) MB BS Lond. 1961; MRCS Eng. LRCP Lond. 1961; DObst RCOG 1963. SCMO Milton Keynes Community NHS Trust. Prev: Clin. Med. Off. Bucks. AHA.

ODELL, Ruth Mary (retired) Elmbank, Church Lane, Ropley, Alresford SO24 0EA Tel: 01962 772499 — (Camb. & Roy. Free) MA Camb. 1955, BA (Nat. Sc. Trip.) 1944; MB BChir Camb. 1947; MRCS Eng. LRCP Lond. 1947. Prev: Clin. Asst. (ENT) Roy. Free Hosp. & Connaught Hosp.

ODEMUYIWA, Olusola Department of Cardiology, Epsom General Hospital, Dorking Road, Epsom KT18 7EG Tel: 01372 735735 Fax: 01372 743421 — MB BS Lagos 1979; MRCP (UK) 1983; MD Newc. 1991; FRCP 1999. Cons. Cardiol. Epsom Gen. Hosp. Specialty: Cardiol. Socs: Brit. Cardiac Soc.; Brit. Cardiovasc. Interven. Soc. Prev: Sen. Regist. Wessex Cardiothoracic Centre Soton. Gen. Hosp.; Research Fell. (Cardiol. Sci.) St. Geo. Hosp. Med. Sch. Lond.

ODETOYINBO, Olusegun Abayomi Spitalfields Practice, 20 Old Montague St, London E1 5PB Tel: 020 7247 7070 — MB BS Ibadan 1975; MRCP (UK) 1985; LMSSA Lond. 1986. GP City & E. Lond. FHSA. Specialty: Cardiol.; Diabetes. Prev: Med. Transpl. Off. Harefield Hosp.; Regist. (Med. of Elderly) Ealing Hosp.; SHO (Med.) Stepping Hill Hosp. Stockport.

ODGAARD, Mr Anders St Mary's Hospital, Praed Street, London W2 1NY Tel: 020 7886 1918 Fax: 020 7886 1766 — MD Aarhus 1987; DMSc. Cons. Orth. Surg. Specialty: Trauma & Orthop. Surg.

Special Interest: Foot & Ankle; Knee. Socs: Brit. Orth. Assn.; Orth. Research Soc.; Brit. Orth. Foot Surg. Soc.

ODGERS, Peter Brian The Cromwell Hospital, Cromwell Road, London SW5 0TU; 6 Devonshire Place, London W1G 6HN — MB ChB Leeds 1956. Med. Adviser King Edwd. VII Hosp. Fund, Globtik Tankers Ltd. & other Cos. Socs: Fell. Roy. Soc. Med.; (Ex-Sec.) Chelsea Clin. Soc. Prev: Surg. Lt.-Cdr. RN, Staff Med. Off. W. Indies Squadron; SHO (Med.) Roy. Postgrad. Med. Sch. Lond.; SHO (Surg.) Leeds Gen. Infirm.

ODGERS, Mr Robin Charles Blake Corton Denham House, Corton Denham, Sherborne DT9 4LR Tel: 01963 220205 — BM BCh Oxf. 1974 (Guy's) MA; FRCS Eng. 1979; DRCOG 1983. Specialty: Gen. Pract. Prev: Regist. Surg. Qu. Mary's Hosp. Roehampton; Regist. (Surg.) St. Helier Hosp. Carshalton; SHO (Cas.) Guy's Hosp. Lond.

ODLING-SMEE, Mr George William Department of Surgery, Queen's University, Belfast City Hospital Trust, Lisburn Road, Belfast BT9 7AB Tel: 028 263909 Fax: 028 263875 — (Newc.) MB BS Durh. 1959; FRCS Eng. 1968; FRCSI 1987. Sen. Lect. (Surg.) Qu. Univ. Belf.; Cons. Surg. Belf. City Hosp. Specialty: Gen. Surg. Prev: Sen. Tutor (Surg.) Qu. Univ. Belf.; Surg. & Act. Dir. Brit. Child Med. Care Unit Enugu; Surg. Unit Newc. Gen. Hosp.

ODLUM, Hugh Rupert Burgh Cottage, Burgh, Woodbridge IP13 6PT Tel: 01473 735226 — (Camb. & St. Bart.) BA Camb. 1945, MA; MRCS Eng. LRCP Lond. 1947; MB BChir. Camb. 1949. Socs: Fell. Roy. Soc. Med.; BMA. Prev: Ho. Surg. (Orthop.) Dept. St. Bart. Hosp.; Jun. Regist. (Anaesth.) Edgware Gen. Hosp.; Ho. Surg. Obst. St. Paul's Hosp. Hemel Hempstead.

ODOM, Mr Nicholas John Cardiothoracic Department, Manchester Royal Infirmary, Oxford Road, Manchester M13 9WL Tel: 0161 276 4519; 16 Grosvenor Gardens, Sharston, Manchester M22 4XA — MD Newc. 1988; BA Camb. 1971; MB BChir 1974; DA Eng. 1977; FRCS Eng. 1979. Cons. Cardiothoracic Surg. Manch. Roy. Infirm.; Vis. Surg., Roy. Bolton Hosp. Specialty: Cardiothoracic Surg. Socs: Soc. Carthoracic Surg. Gt. Brit. & Irel. Prev: Clin. Fell. CardioPulm. Transpl. Mayo Clinic USA; Sen. Regist. Freeman Hosp. Newc.

ODONGA, Florence 5 Smithills Drive, Bolton BL1 5RB — LRCP LRCS Ed. 1978; LRCP LRCS Ed. LRCPS Glas. 1978.

O'DONNELL, Mark John Victoria Hospital, Whinney Heys Road, Blackpool FY3 1NR Tel: 01253 303861 Fax: 01253 306810 — MB ChB Liverp. 1980; MD Birm. 1993; Dip. Rehabit. Med. 1993; FRCP 1998. Cons. Phys. Vict., Clifton & Wesham Pk. Hosps. Specialty: Care of the Elderly; Gen. Med.; Rehabil. Med. Socs: Hon. Life Mem. Liverp. Med. Stud.s Soc.; Liverp. Med. Inst.

ODUFUWA-BOLGER, Titilayo Olubola Professional Residents Room, Moorfields Eye Hospital, City Road, London EC1V 2PD — MB BS Lagos 1986; MB BS Lagos, Nigeria 1986; FRCS Ed. 1993; FRCOphth 1993.

ODUKOYA, Mr Abiodun Olusegun Department Obstetrics and Gynaecology, Scunthorpe District Hospital NHS Trust, Scunthorpe DN15 7BH Tel: 01724 282282 Fax: 01724 290435 Email: odukoya@doctors.org.uk — MB BS Ibadan 1980 (Ibadan, Nigeria) MBA; FMCOG (Nigeria) 1987; MRCOG 1990; FWACS 1991; MD Sheff. 1995; FRCOG 2003. Hon. Den. Clin. Lect. Sheff. Uni.; PostGrad. Clin. Tutor; Cons. (O & G) Minimal Access Surg. Specialty: Obst. & Gyn. Socs: BMA; Eur. Soc. Human Reproduc. & Embryol.; Brit. Fertil. Soc. Prev: Lect./Hon. Sen. Regist. (O & G) Jessop Hosp.; Centr. Univ. Teachg. Hosp. Sheff.

ODUM, Jonathan Renal Unit, New Cross Hospital, Wolverhampton WV10 0QP Tel: 01902 643086 Fax: 01902 643192 — MD Birm. 1993; MB ChB 1984; MRCP (UK) 1987; FRCP 1999. Clin. Director Med. Specialty: Nephrol. Socs: Brit. Renal Assn. & EDTA-ERA. Prev: Sen. Regist. Roy. Adelaide Hosp.; Regist. N. Staffs. Roy. Infirm.; Cons. Phys. & Nephrol. Roy. Wolverhampton Hosp. Trust.

ODUM, Simon Brooklea Clinic, Wick Road, Bristol BS4 4HU Tel: 0117 971 1211 Fax: 0117 972 3370; 14 Claverton Road, Saltford, Bristol BS31 3DP — MB ChB Birm. 1989. Specialty: Accid. & Emerg.

ODUNSI, L O (retired) Cater Street Surgery, 1 Cater Street, Kempston, Bedford MK42 8DR Tel: 01234 853461 Fax: 01234 840536 — MB BS Lagos 1978; MB BS Lagos 1978.

ODUNUGA, Bankole Abidemi 133 Inverness Terrace, London W2 6JF — MB BS Lond. 1997.

ODURNY, Allan Department of Radiology, Southampton General Hospital, Tremona Road, Southampton SO16 6YD Tel: 023 8079 6862 Fax: 023 8079 4038 — MB ChB Birm. 1974; FRCS Eng. 1978; FRCR 1986. Cons. Radiol. Soton. Gen. Hosp. Specialty: Radiol. Socs: Brit. Soc. Interven. Radiol.; Cardiovasc. & Interven. Soc. Europe. Prev: Cons. Radiol. E. Birm. Hosp.; Sen. Regist. (Radiol.) Soton. Gen. Hosp.; Fell. Angiogr. Toronto Gen. Hosp. & Univ. Toronto, Canada.

ODURO-DOMINAH, Asamoah Papworth Hospital NHS Trust, Papworth Hospital, Papworth Everard, Cambridge CB3 8RE Tel: 01480 830541 Fax: 01480 831143 — MB BS Newc. 1973 (Newcastle Upon Tyne) MRCP (UK) 1978; FRCA Eng. 1982; FFA RCS Eng. 1982; FRCP 1999. Cons. Anaesth. Papworth Hosp. Specialty: Anaesth. Socs: Assn. Cardiothoracic Anaesth.; Eur. Assn. Cardiothoracic Anaesth.; Eur. Soc. Intens. Care Med.

ODURO-YEBOAH, Adwoa Millway Medical Practice, Hartley Avenue, Mill Hill, London NW7 2HX Tel: 020 8959 0888 Fax: 020 8959 7050 — MB BS Lond. 1992 (Univ. Coll. & Middlx. Sch. of Med.) DGM RCP Lond. 1994; DCH RCP Lond. 1994; DRCOG 1995; MRCGP 1996. GP Lond. Specialty: Gen. Pract. Socs: (Chairm. & Asst. Sec.) Afr. Caribbean Soc. Prev: GP/Regist. Lond.

ODUTOLA, Taofeequat Abibayo Adedoyin c/o Mrs R F Bamgbala, 14 Sunnydene Lodge, Sunnydene Gardens, Wembley HA0 1AT — MB ChB Glas. 1965.

ODY, Catriona Luise McCormick 58 Shortheath Road, Farnham GU9 8SQ — MB BS Lond. 1994.

OELBAUM, Moses Hirsh (retired) 14 The Residences, Scholes Lane, Prestwich, Manchester M25 0NT Tel: 0161 773 6679 — (Manch.) BSc Manch. 1942, MD 1951, MB ChB (Hons., Distinc; Anat., Pharmacol. & Surg.) 1945; FRCP Lond. 1971, M 1947. Hon. Clin. Lect. Med. Univ. Manch. Prev: Cons. Phys. Crumpsall Hosp., N. Hosp. & Vict. Memor. Jewish Hosp.

OELBAUM, Raymond Stuart Ormskirk District General Hospital, Wigan Road, Ormskirk L39 2AZ Tel: 01695 656066 Fax: 01695 656484 — MB ChB Manc 1982 (Mancester) BSc (1st cl. Hons.) Med. Biochem. Manch. 1979; MRCP (UK) 1986; MD 1994. Cons. Phys. Diabetes & Endocrinol. Ormskirk Dist. Gen. Hosp. Specialty: Gen. Med.; Diabetes; Endocrinol. Prev: Sen. Regist. (Med.) St. Mary's Hosp. & Northwick Pk. Hosp.; Research Regist. (Diabetes & Lipid Research) St. Bart. Hosp. Lond.

OELBAUM, Sandra 14 Snaefell Avenue, Tuebrook, Liverpool L13 2EY Tel: 0151 228 2377 Email: sandra.oelbaum@free-internet.co.uk; 65 Dudlow Lane, Calderstones, Liverpool L18 2EY — MB ChB (Hons.) Manch. 1982; BSc (1st cl. Hons.) Physiol. Manch. 1979; MRCP (UK) 1988. Tutor, Univ. of Liverp. Socs: Brit. Med. Soc. Prev: Princip. GP N.olt Middlx.; Lect. (Med.) Univ. Coll. Hosp. Lond.; GP Princip., Harrow, Middx.

OELMANN, Gareth John 66 Llanfair Road, Cardiff CF11 9QB — MB BCh Wales 1994.

OEPPEN, Marion Heulwen (retired) Shelton House, Newton, Martley, Worcester WR6 6PR Tel: 01886 821497 — MB BCh Wales 1959 (Welsh Nat. Sch. Med.) DCH RCPS Glas. 1981. Prev: Sen. Clin. Med. Off (Community Child Health & Paediat. Audiol.) Hearing & Speech Centre Hereford.

OEPPEN, Rachel Suzanne Department of Radiology, Southampton General Hospital, Tremona Rd, Southampton SO16 6YD — MB ChB Bristol 1992; MRCP (UK) 1996; FRCR 2000. Specialist Regist. Wessex Radiol. Train. Scheme. Specialty: Radiol.

OETIKER, Ursula Kingsfield Medical Centre, 146 Alcester Road South, Kings Heath, Birmingham B14 6AA Tel: 0121 444 2054 Fax: 0121 443 5856; 22 Amesbury Road, Moseley, Birmingham B13 8LD — MB BS Lond. 1985 (St. Thos. Hosp. Lond.) DRCOG Lond. 1989; DCH RCP Lond. 1990; MRCGP 1994. GP Princip. Prev: GP Newc.; Trainee GP Lond.; SHO (Obst & Gyn., Paediat. & Geriat.) St. Geo. Hosp. Lond.

OFFEN, Mr David Nigel NHS Exec. Easter Region Office, Capital Park, Fulbourn, Cambridge CB1 5XB Tel: 01223 597500 Fax: 01223 597555; 83 Drury Road, Colchester CO2 7UU Tel: 01206 570058 Fax: 01206 523636 Email: david.offen@dtn.nh.com — MB BS Lond. 1966 (St. Bart.) LIHSM; FRCS Eng. 1971. Head of Clin. Qualiy E.R.O. NHS Exec. Socs: Chairm. Brit. Assn. Med. Managers; Fell. Roy. Soc. Med. & Hunt. Soc. Prev: Chier Exec., Essex Rivers NHS Trust; Cons. Clin. Audit & Quality Improvem. NE Thames RHA; Cons. Surg. Whipps Cross & Wanstead Hosps.

OFFER, Catherine Mary (retired) 26 The Close, Norwich NR1 4DZ — MB BS Lond. 1963 (St. Bart) MRCS Eng. LRCP Lond. 1963; DCH Eng. 1966; MRCP Lond. 1969. Prev: Cons. Phys. (Geriat. Med.) Soton. & SW Hants. Health Dist. (T).

OFFER, Mr Graham John 16 Lytham Road, Clarendon Park, Leicester LE2 1YD — MB ChB Leic. 1993; BSc (1st cl. Hons.) Leic. (Pharmacol.) 1990; FRCS (Eng.) 1997. Specialist Regist., (Lat), Plastic Surg. Specialty: Plastic Surg. Socs: Trent S. Jun. Doctor's Comm. BMA; Nat. Jun. Doctor's Comm. 1997; Full Mem., Brit. Burns Assoc. Prev: SHO (Neurosurg.) Qu.'s Med. Centre Nottm.; Demonst. (Anat.) Univ. Leic.; SHO (Plastic Surg.) Leic. Roy. Infirm.

OFFER, Mark 22 Malvern Road, London NW6 5PP — MB BS Lond. 1996.

OFFERMAN, Edward Leslie (retired) 11 Camden Row, Blackheath, London SE3 0QA Tel: 020 8852 7063 — MB BS Lond. 1959 (Univ. Coll. Hosp.) DObst RCOG 1961; FRCPath 1986, M 1973. Cons. Haemat. Qu. Mary's Hosp. Sidcup. Prev: Sen. Regist. (Haemat.) Univ. Coll. Hosp. & Whittington Hosp. Lond.

OFFORD, Catherine Mary Belmont Surgery, St James Square, Wadhurst TN5 6BJ Tel: 01892 782121 Fax: 01892 783989 — MB BS Lond. 1985; BSc Lond. 1982, MB BS 1985; DRCOG 1987; MRCGP 1989.

OFFORD, George Brian (retired) 41 Woodland Grove, Weybridge KT13 9EQ Tel: 01932 843180; (surgery) 290 Albert Drive, Sheerwater, Woking GU21 5TX Tel: 01932 343524 — MB BS Lond. 1963 (Westm.) MRCS Eng. LRCP Lond. 1963; DObst RCOG 1966; DA Eng. 1971. Prev: Clin. Asst. (A & E) Roy. Hosp. Portsmouth.

OFILI, Esther Adesomo The Surgery, 75 Union Street, Larkhall ML9 1DZ Tel: 01698 882105 — MB BS Ibadan 1979 (Univ. Coll. Hosp. Ibadan Nigeria) DCCH RCP Lond. 1988; MRCGP 1990; T(GP) 1992. GP Princip. Special Interest: Paediat.; Psychiat. in the Community. Socs: RCGP; MDDUS; BMA.

OFILI, Gregory Ubaka Wishaw General Hospital, 50 Netherton Street, Wishaw ML2 0DP Tel: 01698 361100 — MB BS Benin 1978; BSc (Hons.) (Biochem.) Ahmadu Bello 1975; MRCOG 1988; T(OG) 1995. Research Fell. (Colposcopy Clinic) Dept. O & G Roy. Infirm. Edin.; Temp. Lect. & Sen. Regist. (Obst. & Gyn.) Univ. Edin. Specialty: Obst. & Gyn. Socs: BMA & Glas. Obst. Soc. Prev: Regist. (O & G) E. Gen. Hosp. Edin.

OFOE, Victor Dotse 1 Valkyrie, Longfield, Grahame Park, Colindale, London NW9 5SN Tel: 020 8205 5908 — MB ChB Ghana 1983; MRCP (UK) 1991.

OFORI, Joakin Apeadu Bosompra (retired) 79 Friern Barnet Road, London N11 3EH — MB BS Lond. 1971 (Univ. Coll. Hosp.) Prev: Ho. Surg. Edgware Gen. Hosp.

OGAKWU, Michael Obioha c/o Mr. Emeka Agu, 152 Purves Road, Kensal Rise, London NW10 5TG — MB BS Nigeria 1980; MB BS U of Nigeria 1980; MRCOG 1992.

OGANWU, Sylvanus Oyeshine 4 Riverseide Close, London E5 9SP Tel: 020 8806 7707 — MB BS Ibadan 1978; MB BS Ibadan, Nigeria 1978; MRCOG 1991. Career Regist. (O & G) Edgware Gen. Hosp. Specialty: Obst. & Gyn.

OGBOBI, Sale Emeje Flat 33, 38 Windsor Park, Belfast BT9 6FS — MB BS Lagos, Nigeria 1983.

OGBORN, Anthony Douglas Ronald Riseley House, 10A Rotten Row, Bedford MK44 1EJ Tel: 01234 708010 — BM BCh Oxf. 1963 (Univ. Coll. Hosp.) MA Oxf. 1963; FRCOG 1982, M 1969, DObst 1966. Cons. O & G Bedford Gen. Hosp. Specialty: Obst. & Gyn. Prev: Sen. Regist. (O & G) Northampton Gen. & Hammersmith Hosps.; Regist. Radcliffe Infirm. Oxf.; Ho. Phys. Univ. Coll. Hosp. Lond.

OGBUEHI, Nwabueze John 2D Grove Park Road, Rainham RM13 7BX — MB BS Lond. 1962.

OGDEN, Adrian David Clifton Lane Health Centre, Clifton Lane, Doncaster Road, Rotherham S65 1DU Tel: 01709 382315 Fax: 01709 512646 — MRCS Eng. LRCP Lond. 1975.

OGDEN, Alan Stanley 10 Farrington, 54 Westcliff Road, Bournemouth BH4 8BE Tel: 01202 767115 — MB ChB Manch. 1939. Socs: Fell. BMA.

OGDEN, Mr Andrew Chester Broadlands, Lochmaben, Lockerbie DG11 1RL — MB ChB Glas. 1969; FRCS Glas. 1976.

OGDEN, Anne Barbara 21 Amberley Close, Send, Woking GU23 7BX Tel: 01483 223697 — MB ChB Bristol 1949.

OGDEN, Barbara Eileen Patricia 14 Burlington Road, Ipswich IP1 2EU Tel: 01473 211661; Windmill Lodge, Mill Lane, Witnesham, Ipswich IP6 9HR Tel: 01473 785309 — MB BS Lond. 1959 (Lond. Hosp.) DObst RCOG 1960; DCH Eng. 1962.

OGDEN, Mr Christopher William Department of Urology, Chelsea & Westminster Hospital, Fulham Road, London SW10 9NH Tel: 0208 746 8559 Fax: 0208 746 8846 Email: chrisogden@compuserve.com; 19 Queensdale Road, Holland Park, London W11 4SB Tel: 020 7603 7584 Fax: 020 8869 2446 Email: chrisogden@compuserve.com — MB BS Lond. 1984 (Char. Cross Hosp.) FRCS Ed. 1989; FRCS Eng. 1990; MS Lond. 1993; FRCS (Urol.) 1995; FEBU 1996. Cons. Urol., Chelsea & Westm. Hosp.; Senior Lecturer, Imperial College Medical School, London. Specialty: Urol. Socs: Brit. Assn. Urol.; RSM; RCSE. Prev: Sen. Regist. Roy. Marsden, St. Mary's, Char. Cross & Westm. Hosps.; Cons. Urol. and Clin. Lead in Urol. at Northwick Pk. and St. Marys Hosp. from 1995 to 2001.

OGDEN, David James Stoneycroft House, Broadgreen Hospital NHS Trust, Thomas Drive, Liverpool L14 3LB — MB ChB Liverp. 1994.

OGDEN, David John Rothschild House Surgery, Chapel Street, Tring HP23 6PU Tel: 01442 822468 Fax: 01442 825889 — MB BS Lond. 1969.

OGDEN, Elizabeth Claire Broadlands, Lochmaben, Lockerbie DG11 1RL — MB ChB Glas. 1976; DMRD Ed. 1980.

OGDEN, George Herbert, Surg. Lt.-Cdr. RN Retd. Kearsley Medical Centre, Jackson St., Kearsley, Bolton BL4 8EP Tel: 01204 573164; 2A Boothstown Drive, Worsley, Manchester M28 1UF — MB ChB Birm. 1989 (Birmingham) DRCOG 1994; MRCGP 1998. GP Princip. Kearsley Med. Centre. Specialty: Gen. Pract. Prev: Trainee GP Vanburgh Hill Health Centre Lond.

OGDEN, Jacqueline Noelle North Cardiff Medical Centre, Excalibur Drive, Thornhill, Cardiff CF14 9BB Tel: 029 2075 0322 Fax: 029 2075 7705; Pant y Gollen, Caerphilly Mountain, Caerphilly CF83 1LY — MB BCh Wales 1988; BSc (Hons.) Wales 1985, MB BCh 1988; DRCOG 1993; MRCGP 1994; T(GP) 1994. Socs: Roy. Coll. Obst. & Gyn. Prev: SHO (Gen. Med.) Univ. Hosp. Wales Cardiff.

OGDEN, James Rennie 14 Reedley Grove, Burnley BB10 2LA — MB ChB Manch. 1963; FRCOG 1982, M 1969, DObst 1965. Cons. (O & G) Burnley Gen. Hosp. Specialty: Obst. & Gyn.

OGDEN, Jane 50 Leamington Street, Sheffield S10 1LW — MB ChB Sheff. 1998.

OGDEN, Jean Sheila Margaret 45 Grove Road, Norwich NR1 3RQ — MB BS Lond. 1955 (St. Mary's) DObst RCOG 1957; DA Eng. 1962; FFA RCS Eng. 1966. Cons. Anaesth. United Norwich Hosps. Specialty: Anaesth.

OGDEN, Mrs Lynne Mary Commercial Road Surgery, 75 Commercial Road, Leeds LS5 3AT Tel: 0113 295 1380; 19 Batcliffe Drive, Leeds LS6 3QB Tel: 0113 278 4576 — MB ChB Leeds 1980.

OGDEN, Terence Lister c/o The Surgery, Caerffynnon, Dolgellau LL40 1LY — MB ChB Birm. 1972; Cert. Family Plann. JCC 1975. Mem. Wales LMC; Hon. Teach. Welsh Nat. Sch. Med. Prev: Trainer (Gen. Pract.) Gwynedd; Sec. Meirionydd Med. Soc.; SHO (Obst., Anaesth. & Paediat.) Good Hope Hosp. Sutton Coldfield.

OGDEN, Thomas Bull Hill, Cobden Edge, Mellor, Stockport SK6 5NL — MRCS Eng. LRCP Lond. 1962 (Manch.) Socs: BMA.

OGDEN, William Stewart Winoma, Orchehill Avenue, Gerrards Cross SL9 8QJ Tel: 01753 884273 — (Camb. & St. Bart.) MRCS Eng. LRCP Lond. 1954; MB BChir Camb. 1955; MA Camb. 1955. Specialty: Pharmaceutical Medicine; Gen. Pract. Socs: BMA; (Ex-Pres.) Chiltern Med. Soc.; Brit. Assn. Pharmaceut. Phys. Prev: Flight Lt. RAF Med. Br.; Ho. Surg. (ENT) St. Bart. Hosp.; Ho. Phys. OldCh. Hosp. Romford.

OGDEN-FORDE, Fiona Elizabeth 4 Savoylands Close, Liverpool L17 5BR — MB ChB Liverp. 1989.

OGEAH, John Chukwukadibia Fordwater, Cuddington Way, Sutton SM2 7JA — MB BS Ibadan 1984; MB BS Ibadan 1984.

OGEDEGBE, Mr Arikoge Joseph 17 Wynton Gardens, South Norwood, London SE25 5RS Tel: 020 8771 6955; 14 Crossways Road, Mitcham CR4 1DQ Tel: 0781 687 2859 Email: arikcoged@aol.com — MB BS Benin 1987; FRCS Ed. 1993. Surg. Research Regist. & Lect. (Surg.) Surg. Roy. Lond. & St. Barth. NHS Trust; Specialist Regist., UCL Hosp. NHS Trust, Lond. Specialty: Gen.

Surg. Socs: Assoc. Mem. Assn. Surg. GB & Irel.; Assn. Surg. Train.; Brit. Assn. Surg. Oncol. Prev: Specialist Regist. (Surg.) Newham Gen. Hosp. Lond.; Career Regist. (Surg.) Havering Hosps. Trust.

OGG, Mr Archibald John (retired) Clearbury Cottage, Woodgreen, Fordingbridge SP6 2QU — BM BCh Oxf. 1946 (Lond. Hosp.) BM BCh Oxon. 1946; DO Eng. 1951; FRCS Eng. 1954. Surg. Lt. RNR. Prev: Opthalmic Cons., Salisbury Infirm.

OGG, Chisholm Stuart Evelegh's, High St., Long Wittenham, Abingdon OX14 4QH Tel: 01865 407774 — (Guy's) BSc (Physiol.) Lond. 1958, MD 1967, MB BS; MRCS Eng. LRCP Lond. 1960; (Distinc. Med.) 1961; DObst RCOG 1963; FRCP Lond. 1975, M 1964. Emerit. Cons. Nephrol. Guys & St. Thomas Hosp. Trust. Specialty: Nephrol. Socs: Renal Assn. & Europ. Dialysis & Transp. Assn. Prev: Cons. Renal Phys. Guy's Hosp. Lond.; Dir. of Clin. Renal Servs. 1972-98; Civil Cons. Renal Dis. RN.

OGG, Elaine Catherine Serena, High Barrwood Road, Kilsyth, Glasgow G65 0EE — MB ChB Glas. 1983; DRCOG 1985; MRCGP 1987; MRCPsych 1990. Cons. Psychiat. (Psychother.) Larkfield Centre, Glas. Specialty: Gen. Psychiat.; Psychother. Socs: Roy. Coll. Psychiat.; Scott. Assn. of Analyt. Psychother.

OGG, Fiona Lindsay Mary Portlethen Medical Centre, Portlethen, Aberdeen AB12 4QP — MB ChB Aberd. 1991; MRCGP 1995; Diploma Family Plann. 1996. GP Princip. Portlethen Aberd. Specialty: Gen. Pract. Prev: Aberd. P VTS; Ho. Off. Rotat. Aberd. Roy. Hosp.

OGG, Graham Stuart Weatherall Institute of Molecular Medicine, Oxford OX3 9DS Tel: 01865 222443 — BM BCh Oxf. 1992; BA (Hons.) Oxf. 1989; MRCP (UK) 1995; DPhil 1998. MRC Sen. Clin. Fell. Nuffield Dept Clin Med. Oxf.; Hon. Cons. Dermatol. Specialty: Dermat.

OGG, Thomas Winchester (retired) 11 Worts Causeway, Cambridge CB1 8RJ Tel: 01223 248703 Fax: 01223 413005 — MB ChB Aberd. 1964; DA Eng. 1968; FFA RCS Eng. 1971; MA Camb. 1977. Assoc. Lect. Camb. Univ; Dir. Day Surg. Addenbrooke's Hosp. Camb. Prev: Cons. Anaesth. Addenbrooke's Hosp. Camb.

OGHOETUOMA, Jerry Oghenekevbe Bishop Auckland General Hospital, Cockton Hill Road, Bishop Auckland Tel: 01388 455186 Fax: 01388 455055 — MB BS Lagos 1985; MRCOG 1993. Consultant, Bishop Auckland. Socs: Brit. Fertil. Soc.

OGILVIE, Alan James East Hill Surgery, 78 East Hill, Colchester CO1 2RW Tel: 01206 866133 Fax: 01206 869054; 10 Fitzwalter Road, Colchester CO3 3SS Tel: 01206 768393 — MB ChB St. And. 1967; DObst RCOG 1969. Socs: (Hon. Treas.) Colchester Med. Soc. Prev: SHO (Paediat.) St. John's Hosp. Chelmsford; Ho. Off. (O & G) Essex Co. Hosp. Colchester.

OGILVIE, Alan Leonard Northampton General Hospital, Cliftonville, Northampton NN1 5BD Tel: 01604 545567; 26 Kingsley Road, Northampton NN2 7BL — MB BChir Camb. 1974 (Univ. Camb.) MRCP (UK) 1976; MA Camb. 1974, MD 1986; FRCP Ed. 1989; FRCP Lond. 1991. Cons. Phys. Northampton Gen. Hosp. Specialty: Gastroenterol. Socs: Fell. Roy. Coll. Of Phys.s, Lond; Fell. Roy. Coll. Of Phys.s, Edin.; Mem, Brit. Soc. Of Gastroenterol. Prev: Sen. Regist. Edin. Teach. Hosps.; Research Fell. Univ. Hosp. Nottm.; Regist. (Med.) Luton & Dunstable Hosp.

OGILVIE, Alexander Collingwood Fitzwilliams (retired) 37 Nackington Road, Canterbury CT1 3NP Tel: 01227 452232 — MB BS Lond. 1944 (Middlx.) MRCS Eng. LRCP Lond. 1944; MD Lond. 1952; FRCPath 1966. Hon. Cons. Path. Kent & Canterbury Hosp. Prev: Cons. Path. W. Cumbld. Hosps.

OGILVIE, Bruce Campbell Wessex Cardiothoracic Centre, Southampton General Hospital, Southampton SO16 6YD Tel: 023 8079 4833 Fax: 023 8079 6341; 14 Russell Place, Southampton SO17 1NU Tel: 02380 556762 — MB ChB Ed. 1965; DObst RCOG 1968; MRCP (UK) 1970; DMRD Ed. 1972; FRCR 1975; FRCP Ed. 1987. Cons. Radiol. Soton. Univ. Hosps. NHS Trust. Specialty: Radiol. Socs: Fell. Roy. Soc. Med.; Brit. Inst. Radiol.; Brit. Cardiac Soc. Prev: Sen. Regist. & Research Fell. (Radiodiag.) Roy. Infirm. Edin.; Regist. (Med.) Vict. Hosp. Kirkcaldy.

OGILVIE, Charles Keith Meadowbank Health Centre, 3 Salmon Inn Road, Falkirk FK2 0XF Tel: 01324 715753 Fax: 01324 717565 — MB ChB Glas. 1968.

OGILVIE, Mr Colin Taunton & Somerset NHS Trust, Musgrove Park Hospital, Taunton TA1 5DA Tel: 01823 342965 — MB ChB Leeds 1979; FRCS Eng. 1984; MD Leeds 1992. Cons. Orthop. Surg. Taunton & Som. NHS Trust Taunton. Specialty: Orthop. Socs: Fell. BOA. Prev: Sen. Regist. Bristol Hosps.; Action Research Fell. (BioMech.) Salford.

OGILVIE, Colin Macleod The Riffel, Woolton Park, Woolton, Liverpool L25 6DR Tel: 0151 428 3472 — MB ChB Liverp. 1944; FRCP Lond. 1968, M 1950; MD Liverp. 1954. Emerit. Cons. Phys. Roy. Liverp. Hosp. & King Edwd. VII Hosp. Midhurst. Specialty: Gen. Med. Socs: (Ex-Pres.) Brit. Thoracic Soc.; Assn. Phys.; (Ex-Pres.) Liverp. Med. Inst. Prev: Cons. Phys. Roy. Liverp. Hosp. & Regional Cardiothoracic Centre; Postgrad. Trav. Fell. Univ. Lond.; Sen. Regist. & Lect. (Med.) Lond. Hosp.

OGILVIE, Danuta Maria Helena Bedwell Medical Centre, Sinfield Close, Stevenage SG1 1YU; All Saints Lodge, 6 Myddelton Park, Whetstone, London N20 0HX Tel: 020 8446 4671 — MB BS Lond. 1963 (Guy's) MRCS Eng. LRCP Lond. 1963. GP Princip. 37/39 The Hyde Stevenage SG2 9SB. Socs: Med. Disab. Appeal Tribunals. Prev: Clin. Asst. (Rheum.) Lister Hosp. Stevenage.; Med. Disabil. Appeals Tribunal.

OGILVIE, David Queen Marys Hospital for Children, Wrythe Lane, Carshalton SM5 1AA Tel: 020 8296 3060 Fax: 020 8644 6878 — MB BS Lond. 1969 (Guy's) MRCS Eng. LRCP Lond. 1969; MRCP (UK) 1972; DCH Eng. 1977; FRCP Lond. 1990. Cons. Paediat. Qu. Mary's Hosp. for Childr. & St. Helier Hosp. Carshalton. Specialty: Paediat. Prev: Sen. Regist. Hosp. Sick Childr. Lond. & Qu. Eliz. Hosp. for Childr. Lond.; Regist. Hammersmith Hosp. Lond.

OGILVIE, David Bruce MRC Social and Public Health Sciences Unit, University of Glasgow, 4 Lilybank Gardens, Glasgow G12 8RZ Tel: 0141 357 3949 Fax: 0141 337 2389 Email: d.ogilvie@msoc.mrc.gla.ac.uk — MB BChir Camb. 1993; MA Camb. 1995; DRCOG 1996; MRCGP (Distinc.) 1998; DFFP 1998; MPH Glas. 2000; MFPHM 2003. MRC Fell. Specialty: Pub. Health Med. Socs: Soc. for Social Med.; Higher Educat. Acad. Prev: Specialist Regist. (Pub. Health Med.) W. of Scotl.; SHO and GP Regist., W. Suff.; Ho. Phys. Addenbrooke's Hosp. Camb.

OGILVIE, George Fleming Rhind (retired) Brooklands, Burnley Road, Crawshawbooth, Rossendale BB4 8BW Tel: 01706 215965 — MB ChB Manch. 1959; DObst RCOG 1961.

OGILVIE, Ian Maurice (retired) 11 Cherry Tree Gardens, Balerno EH14 5SP Tel: 0131 449 3960 — MB ChB Ed. 1948 (Univ. Ed.) DPH Lond. 1961; MFCM 1974; AFOM RCP Lond. 1980. Prev: Air Commodore RAF Med. Br.

OGILVIE, James Robertson The Medical Centre, 7 Hill Place, Arbroath DD11 1AE Tel: 01241 431144 Fax: 01241 430764 — MB ChB Ed. 1968.

OGILVIE, Katherine Elizabeth Ryehill Health Centre, St Peter Street, Dundee DD1 4JH Tel: 01382 644466 Fax: 01832 646302 Email: kogilvie@tyehill.tayside.scot.nhs.uk; Kirkton House, Balmerino, Newport-on-Tay DD6 8SA Tel: 01382 330205 Email: keogilvie@keogilvie.freeserve.co.uk — MB ChB Dundee 1983; DRCOG 1986; MRCGP 1987; DFFP 1997. Principal in General Practice; Designated Med. Practitioner to Austral., Canad. & New Zealand High Commissions. Specialty: Gen. Pract.; Family Plann. & Reproduc. Health; Obst. & Gyn. Special Interest: Family Plann. & Reproductive Health; Obst. & Gyn.

OGILVIE, Marie Matheson Department of Medical Microbiology, Medical School, Teviot Place, Edinburgh EH8 9AG Tel: 0131 650 3153 Fax: 0131 650 6531 Email: marie.ogilvie@ed.ac.uk; 62/3 Blacket Place, Edinburgh EH9 1RJ Tel: 0131 668 1759 — (Ed.) MB ChB Ed. 1965; BSc (Hons.) Ed. 1963, MD 1970; MRCPath 1991. Sen. Lect. (Virol.) Univ. Edin. & Hon. Cons. Virol. Roy. Infirm. Edin. NHS Trust. Specialty: Virology. Prev: Sen. Lect. & Hon. Cons. (Virol.) Univ. Soton.

OGILVIE, Patricia Joy Felin Bencoed, Llangybi, Pwllheli LL53 6SR — MB ChB Liverp. 1997.

OGILVIE, Paul Nicholas Felin Bencoed, Llangybi, Pwllheli LL53 6SR — MB ChB Liverp. 1994.

OGILVIE, William Alasdair (retired) 107 Balshagray Avenue, Glasgow G11 7EG Tel: 0141 959 1536 — LRCP LRCS Ed. 1942 (Anderson Coll. Glas.) LRCP LRCS Ed. LRFPS Glas. 1942. Prev: Resid. Surg. (ENT) & Resid. Asst. (Out.-Pats.) West. Infirm. Glas.

OGILVY, Andrew James 5 Huntsmans Close, Quorn, Loughborough LE12 8AR — MB ChB Leeds 1986; FRCA. 1992. Lect. (Anaesth.) Univ. Leicester. Specialty: Anaesth. Prev: Regist. (Anaesth.) Leeds Gen. Infirm.

OGILVY, Jennifer Elizabeth 14 Marlborough Square, Clifton Road, Ilkley LS29 8PU Tel: 01943 609424 — MB ChB Leeds 1985.

OGILVY, Kathleen Mary (retired) 46 Dorward Road, Montrose DD10 8SB Tel: 01674 677633 — MB ChB Ed. 1948. Prev: Assoc. Specialist (Psychiat.) Sunnyside Roy. Hosp. Montrose.

OGILVY-STUART, Amanda Lesley Neonatal Unit, Rosie Hospital, Addenbrooke's NHS Trust, Cambridge CB2 2SW Tel: 01223 245151 Fax: 01223 217064 Email: amanda.ogilvy-stuart@addenbrookes.nhs.uk — BM Soton. 1983; MRCP (UK) 1987; DM Soton. 1994; MRCPCH 1996; FRCP 2001. Cons. Neonatologist Addenbrooke's NHS Trust Camb. Specialty: Neonat. Socs: MRCPCH; Eur. Soc. Paediat. Endocrinol.; Brit. Soc. Paediat. Endocrinol. & Diabetes. Prev: Clin. Lect. (Paediat.) Univ. of Oxf.; Clin. Research Fell. (Paediat. Endocrinol.) Christie Hosp. & Holt Radium Inst. Manch.; Regist. (Paediat.) Taranaki Base Hosp. New Plymouth, NZ.

OGLE, John Lambert Cannington Health Centre, Mill Lane, Cannington, Bridgwater TA5 2HB Tel: 01278 652335; Old Vicarge, Bromfield, Bridgwater TA5 2EQ Tel: 01823 451296 — MB BS Lond. 1973 (Guy's) LRCP Lond. 1973; MRCS Eng. 1973; MRCS Eng. LRCP Lond. 1973; DRCOG 1979; DRCOG 1979; DA Eng. 1981; DA Eng. 1981. Mem. S. W. MREC; Mem. Plymouth LREC. Socs: BMA; Plymouth Med. Soc. (Ex. Hon. Sec.). Prev: Med. Off. Roy. Geogr. Expedition to Borneo 1978.

OGLESBY, Alfred Ian 20 School Lane, Copmanthorpe, York YO23 3SG — MB ChB Leeds 1959.

OGLESBY, Stuart David 39 Kildonan Road, Warrington WA4 2LJ — MB ChB Dundee 1995.

OGLETHORPE, Rachel Jane Lindsay Department of Child and Family Psychiatry, 187 Old Rutherglen Road, Gorbals, Glasgow G5 0RE Tel: 0141 300 6360 Fax: 0141 300 6399 — MB ChB Birm. 1977 (University of Birmingham) MRCPsych 1986; MSc University of Prtsmouth 2001. Cons. (Child Psychiat.) Dept. Child & Family Psychiat. Yorkhill NHS Trust Glas. Specialty: Child & Adolesc. Psychiat. Prev: Sen. Regist. (Child. & Adolesc. Psychiat.) WhitCh. Hosp. Cardiff & Roy. Hosp. Sick Childr. Edin.; Regist. (Psychiat.) Roy. Edin. Hosp. & WhitCh. Hosp. Cardiff; SHO (Paediat.) E. Birm. Hosp. & Bristol Roy. Hosp. Sick Childr.

OGLEY, Reginald 3 North Avenue, Ashbourne DE6 1EZ — MRCS Eng. LRCP Lond. 1942 (Univ. Coll. Hosp.) Prev: Ho. Surg. Leic. Roy. Infirm.; Obst. Ho. Surg. Matern. Hosp. Darlington; Capt. R.A.M.C. 1942-6.

OGSTON, Professor Derek, CBE (retired) 64 Rubislaw Den S., Aberdeen AB15 4AY Tel: 01224 316587 — MB ChB Aberd. 1957; DTM & H Ed. 1959; FRCP Ed. 1973, M 1963; FRCP Lond. 1977, M 1967; DSc Aberd. 1975, PhD 1962, MD 1969. Prev: Prof. Med. Univ. Aberd.

OGSTON, Keith Nicholas 64 Rubislaw Den S., Aberdeen AB15 4AY — MB ChB Aberd. 1992. Specialty: Gen. Surg.

OGUFERE, Mr Wallace Edafe Department of Ortropoedic Surgery, University Hospital, Lewishom High St., London SE13 6LH; 51 Uphill Grove, Mill Hill, London NW7 4NH — MB BS Benin 1985 (University of Berlin Teaching Hospital, Bernin, Higeria) MB BS Benin, Nigeria 1985; FRCS Ed. 1992; FRCS (Trauma & Orth.) 1998. Cons. Orthop. Surg., Univ. Hosp. Lewisham. Specialty: Orthop.; Trauma & Orthop. Surg. Prev: Specialist Regist. N. W. Thames Rotat.

OGUGUA, Viviene Obeagali 90 Wakeman Road, London NW10 5DH — MB ChB Bristol 1994; MRCP Paeds. 1998. Specialty: Paediat.

OGUNBIYI, Mr Olagunju Adeolo Royal Free & University College Medical School, University Department of Surgery, Royal Free Hospital, Pond St., London NW3 2QG Tel: 020 7794 0500 Ext: 8666 Fax: 0870 162 3930 Email: ogunbiyi@dircon.co.uk — MB BS Lond. 1986 (Charing Cross Hosp. Univ. of Lond) FRCS Eng. 1990; MD (Sheffield) 1994; CCST 1998. Sen. Lect./Cons. Surg. - colorectal Surg. Roy. Free & Univ. Coll. Sch. of Med. Specialty: Gen. Surg. Socs: Brit. Assn. of Surg. Oncol.; Roy. Soc. of Med.; Am. Soc. of Colon & Rectal Surg. Prev: Cold Rectal Fell. - The Roy. Lond. Hosp. 1997 - 1999; Lect./Sen. Regist. - The Univ. of Birm. In Surg. at Qu. Eliz. Hosp. Birm.; Colorectal Fell. - Washington Univ. Sch. of Med. St. Louis, Missouri, USA, 1995-97.

OGUNBIYI, Mr Theophilus Ayo James 28 Regent House, 43 Windsor Way, London W14 0UB — BM BCh Oxf. 1961; FRCS Eng. 1966.

OGUNDIPE, Enitan Modupe Flat G01, Beaux Arts Building, Manor Gardens, London N7 6JY — MB BS Lagos 1985; MRCP (UK) 1993. Clin. Research Fell. & Lect. (Child Health) King's Coll. Sch. Med. & Dent. UMDS Lond. Specialty: Neonat. Prev: Regist. (Paediat. & Neonat.) Lewisham Hosp.; SHO (Paediat.) Northwick Pk. Hosp. & King's Coll. Hosp. Lond.

OGUNLESI, Tolulola Olusesan Olusola Newland Avenue Surgery, 239-243 Newland Avenue, Hull HU5 2EJ Tel: 01482 448456 Fax: 01482 449536; 239-243 Newland Avenue, Hull HU5 2EJ Tel: 01482 448456 — MB BS Lond. 1967.

OGUNMUYIWA, Taiwo Adeyemi (retired) 125 Godric Crescent, New Addington, Croydon CR0 0HS Tel: 0802 482816; 16 Kano Street, Ebute-MettaNigeria, Lagos, Nigeria — (University of Glasgow) MB ChB Glas. 1967; DPH Glas. 1976. Prev: Dir. Health Servs. Univ. Lagos Nigeria.

OGUNREMI, Adeyemi Oluwakemi Department of Obstetrics & Gynaecology, Farnborough Hospital, Orpington BR6 8ND — MB BS Ibadan 1986; MRCOG 1994; MFFP 1994. Locum Cons. Gynaecologist & Obstetri.

OGUNSANWO, Olugbenga Adeleke Olarewaju HM Prison Service HQ, Cleland House, Page St., London SW1P 4LN Tel: 020 7217 3000 — MB BS Ibadan 1979; MRCOG 1985. Health Care Adviser (Princip. Med. Off.) Directorate of Health Care (S.) HM Prison HQ. Specialty: Civil Serv.; Obst. & Gyn. Socs: Med. Protec. Soc.; BMA; Eur. Assn. Obst. and Gyn. Prev: Sen. Med. Off. HM Prison Swaleside, E.Ch., Kent; Locum Cons. O & G Princess Roy. Hosp. Haywards Heath; Regist. (O & G) Cuckfield Hosp. Haywards Heath & MusGr. Pk. Hosp. Taunton.

OGUZ, Cenk Flat 1, 58 Fitzjohns Ave, Hampstead, London NW3 5LT — MB BS Lond. 1997.

OH, Colin Joo Eong The Oaks Surgery, Applegarth Avenue, Park Barn, Guildford GU2 8LZ Tel: 01483 563424 Fax: 01483 563789; Langley House, Gasden Copse, Witley, Godalming GU8 5QE — MB BS Lond. 1988; DRCOG 1991. Specialty: Gen. Pract.

OH, Sarah Yung An 9 Albany Court, 48 Oatlands Dr, Weybridge KT13 9JF — BM Soton. 1997.

OHIORENOYA, Mr Bamidele Accident & Emergency Department, Arrowe Park Hospital, Arrowe Park Road, Upton, Wirral CH49 5PE Tel: 0151 678 5111 Fax: 0151 604 7114 — MB BCh Wales 1980 (Cardiff) BSc (Hons.) Salford 1975; FRCS Ed. 1988; FFAEM 1995. Cons. A & E Arrowe Pk. Hosp. Wirral Merseyside. Specialty: Accid. & Emerg. Socs: Brit. Assn. Accid. & Emerg. Med.; Hosp. Cons. & Spec. Assn.; Fell. Fac. Acc. & Emmerg. Med. Prev: Sen. Regist. (A & E) Bristol Roy. Infirm. & Frenchay Hosp. Bristol; Regist. (A & E) Wythenshawe Hosp. Manch.; Regist. (Gen. Surg.) Bolton Gen. Hosp. & Bolton Roy. Infirm.

OHLSSON, Victoria Paediatric Department, Derriford Hospital, Plymouth PL6 8DA Tel: 01752 777111 Email: v.ohlsson@doctors.org.uk; 3 Willowby Park, Meavy Lane, Yelverton PL20 6AN — BM BS Nottm. 1995 (Nottingham) BMed. Sci. Nottm. 1993; MRCPCH Lond. 1999. Paediatric Specialist Regist. Derriford Hosp. Plymouth. Specialty: Paediat.

OHRI, Anil Kumar Elephanta, 18 Courtney Road, London SW19 2ED Tel: 020 8543 4804 — BM Soton. 1989. SHO Rotat. (Surg.) St. Geo. Hosp. Lond. Prev: SHO (Surg.) Roy. Marsden Hosp.; Anat. Prosector Oxf. Univ.; SHO (Orthop.) Qu. Eliz. Milit. Hosp. Lond.

OHRI, Chandrika K Ardoch Medical Centre, 6 Ardoch Grove, Cambuslang, Glasgow G72 8HA Tel: 0141 641 3729 Fax: 0141 641 4339 — MB BS Bombay 1969; MB BS Bombay 1969.

OHRI, Kamal Mohan Ardoch Medical Centre, 6 Ardoch Grove, Cambuslang, Glasgow G72 8HA Tel: 0141 641 3729 Fax: 0141 641 4339; 52 Hamilton Avenue, Pollokshields, Glasgow G41 4HD Tel: 0141 427 6503 — MB BS All India Med. Scis. 1972; MF HOM Faculty of Homoeopathy 1986. Specialty: Gen. Pract.; Homeop. Med. Socs: BMA; Fac. of Homoeopathy (Mem.).

OHRI, Prem Nath Eryri Hospital, Caernarfon LL55 2YE Tel: 01286 662734 Email: pnohri@hotmail.com; Bryn Awel, 3 Rhoslan, Penrhosgarnedd, Bangor LL57 2NH Tel: 01248 353984 — MB BS Rajasthan 1975. Assoc. Specialist (Med. & c/o Elderly) Gwynedd Hosp. Trust. Specialty: Care of the Elderly; Gen. Med. Prev: Regist.

(Geriat.) St. David's Hosp. Bangor; Clin. Asst. (Geriat.) Dist. Gen. Hosp. Bangor.

OHRI, Rita 107 Harley Street, London W1N 1DG Tel: 020 7580 3614 Fax: 020 7935 5187 — MB BCh Wales 1972; FRCOphth.; DO Lond. 1979; FRCS Ed. 1981. Cons. Ophth. Surg. Whipps Cross Hosp. Lond. Specialty: Ophth. Socs: Roy. Soc. Med. Prev: Sen. Regist. West. Ophth. Hosp. & Moorfields Eye Hosp.

OHRI, Mr Sunil Kumar Wessex Cardiac Centre, Southampton General Hospital, Tremona Road, Southampton SO16 6YD Tel: 023 8079 6233 Fax: 023 8079 6614; Hamtun House, 9A Westrow Road, Banister Park, Southampton SO15 2NA Tel: 023 8063 0885 Email: sunil@ohri.co.uk — MB BS Lond. 1985 (The Middlx. Hosp. Med. Sch.) FRCS Eng. 1989; FRCS Ed. 1989; MD Lond. 1994; FRCS (Cth.) 1996. Cons. Cardiac Surg. Dept. fo Cardiothoracic Surg., Soton. Gen. Hosp., Soton., Hants.; Hon. Clin. Sen. Lect., Univ. of Southampton. Specialty: Cardiothoracic Surg. Special Interest: Aortic Surg.; Off- Pump Cardiac Surg. Socs: Soc. Cardiothoracic Surgs. GB & Irel.; Internat. Mem. Soc. Thoracic Surgs. (USA). Prev: Sen. Regist. (Cardiac Surg.) Middlx. Hosp. Lond.; Sen. Regist. (Cardiac Surg.) Hammersmith Hosp. Lond.; Locum Cons. Harefield Hosp. Middlx.

OHUIGINN, Peadar South Croydon Medical Practice, 96 Brighton Road, South Croydon CR2 6AD Tel: 020 8688 0875; 50 Coombe Road, Croydon CR0 5SG — MB BCh BAO NUI 1978. Socs: BMA.; Roy. Soc. of Med. Prev: Trainee GP Redhill VTS; SHO (O & G) Wexford Gen. Hosp.; Ho. Surg. St. Vincents Hosp. Dub.

OIEN, Karin Anne Glasgow Royal Infirmary, University Department of Pathology, Castle Street, Glasgow G4 0SF Tel: 0141 211 4046 Email: k.oien@clinmed.gla.ac.uk; CR-UK Dept of Medical Oncology, CR-UK Beatson Labs, University of Glasgow, Garscube Estate, Switchback Road, Bearsden, Glasgow G61 1BD Tel: 0141 330 3506 Email: k.oien@beatson.gla.ac.uk — MB ChB Glas. 1992; BSc (Hons.) Glas. 1989; MRCPath 2001; PhD (Molecular Path.) Glas. 2002. Cancer Research UK Clinician Scientist; Sen. Lect. (Molecular Pathology) Univ. of Glas.; Hon. Cons. (Pathology) N. Glas. Hosps. Univ. NHS Trust. Specialty: Histopath.

OJAGBEMI, Festus Oluwole 101 Hathaway Crescent, Manor Park, London E12 6LS — MB BS Benin 1987.

OJAR, Davendra Hari 45/10 Caledonian Crescent, Edinburgh EH11 2AQ — MB BS W. Indies 1988.

OJHA, Abha All Saints Medical Centre, 1 Vicarage Road, Kings Heath, Birmingham B14 7QA Tel: 0121 784 5465; The Surgery, 196 Green Lane, Castle Bromwich, Birmingham B36 0BU Tel: 0121 749 5115 Fax: 0121 749 5198 — MB BS Rajasthan 1982; MRCOG 1992. Specialty: Obst. & Gyn. Socs: Fac. Family Plann. Prev: Trainee GP Altrincham VTS; SHO (O & G) Roy. Oldham Hosp. & Hull Matern. Hosp.; SHO (Radiother. & Oncol.) Princess Roy. Hosp. Hull.

OJHA, Rekha Rani Kusum Medical Centre, 274 Union Road, Oswaldtwistle, Accrington BB5 3JB Tel: 01254 232351; 3 The Pastures, Beardwood, Blackburn BB2 7QR Tel: 01254 682575 — MB BS 1970 (Darbharga Medical College, Caheriasarai) MBBS DRCOG FPCert. DFFP Roy. Coll. Obst. & Gyn. London. GP Princip.; Clin. Med. Off., Family Plann. and Sexual Health of Hythe & Bury Community Clinic. Specialty: Obst. & Gyn.; Family Plann. & Reproduc. Health. Prev: CMO in Basic Advanced Centre, Blackburn; CMO at Accrington Surg. Dept., Vict. Hosp., Accrington.

OJI, Mr Erasmus Oluchukwu — MRCS Eng. LRCP Lond. 1970 (St Mary's) FRCOphth; BSc Ibadan 1966; DO Eng. 1974; FRCS Eng. 1976; PhD Lond. 1980. Specialty: Ophth. Socs: FRCOphth. Prev: Cons. Ophth. Surg. Rotherham Dist. Gen. Hosp.; Sen. Regist. Moorfields Eye Hosp. Lond.; Prof. Ophth. Univ. of Jos, Nigeria.

OJI, Mr Kalu Nwokeka 42 Fairview Road, London N15 6LJ Tel: 020 8802 6015 — LRCPI & LM, LRSCI & LM 1953 (RCSI) LRCPI & LM, LRCSI & LM 1953; FRCS Ed. 1967.

OJO, Mr Akinyede Abraham King George's Hospital, Barley Lane, Goodmayes, Ilford IG3 8YB — MB BS Lagos 1975; FRCS Eng. 1983. Cons. Surg. King Geo. Hosp. Ilford. Specialty: Gen. Surg.

OJO, Oluropo Ebenezer 23 Bunkers Hill, Lincoln LN2 4QS — MB BS Nigeria 1978.

OJO, Olurotimi Ademuyiwa Mill View Hospital, South Down Health NHS Trust, Nevill Avenue, Hove BN3 7HZ Tel: 01273 242219 Email: ojo317@aol.com — MB BS Lagos 1990; MRCPsych 1996; MSc Lond. 1999. Cons. in Adult Gen. / Community Psychiat.; Hon. Therapist - Sex and Relationship Problems Clinic, Weston Rd. Lond.

OJO-AROMOKUDU, Mr Olumuyiwa Olugbenga — MB BS Ibadan 1987; MB BS Ibadan, Nigeria 1987; FRCS Ed. 1995; MSc (Surgic. Sci.) Lond. 1997. Prev: Specialist Regist. Rotat. (Surg.) N. Thames; Research Regist. Middlx. Hosp. Univ. Coll. Lond.

OJUKWU, Clifford Ikechukwu Gynaecology Department, Alexandra Hospital, Woodrow Drive, Redditch B98 7UB Tel: 01527 503030 Fax: 01527 512004 Email: cojukwu@aol.com; 114 Mercot Close, Redditch B98 7YY — MB BS Ibadan 1984; MB BS Ibadan, Nigeria 1984; MRCOG 1992; MFFP 1995. Staff Grade, Obst. of Gyn., Alexandra Hosp., Redditch. Worcs.. Specialty: Obst. & Gyn. Socs: Brit. Med. Assoc; Brit. Menopause Soc.; Bist. Soc. of Colposcopy & Cervical Path.

OJUKWU, Nnaemeka Jonathan St. Bartholmew's Surgery, 292A Barking Road, London E6 3BA Tel: 020 8472 0669 — MB BS Nigeria 1975; DRCOG 1987; FMCOG 1989; DFFP 1996. Specialty: Gen. Pract.; Obst. & Gyn.; Family Plann. & Reproduc. Health. Socs: Fell. Med. Coll. Obst. & Gyn. Nigeria. Prev: SHO (O & G) Char. Cross Hosp. Lond., Barking Hosp. & N. Middlx. Hosp. Lond.

OJURO, Mr Ifeanyi Valentine c/o Mr J. Ukemenam, 7 Oxford Road, London E15 1DD — MB BS Nigeria 1987; FRCS Glas. 1995.

OJUTIKU, Moboladale Aderogba Basildon & Thurrock University Hospitals NHS Trust, Directorate of Obstetrics, Gynaecology & Paediatrics, Basildon SS16 5NL Tel: 01268 598246 Fax: 01268 598640 Email: mr.oijutiku@btuh.nhs.uk — MB BS Ibadan 1985 (Univ. Coll. Hosp., Univ. of Ibadan, Nigeria) MFFP 1994; MRCOG 1994; MSc Lond. 1999. Cons. Obst. & Gyn., Basildon & Thurrock Univ. Hosps. NHS Trust, Essex. Special Interest: Menopause; Pelvic Floor Surgery; Perineal Injuries. Prev: Sen. Regist., Pembury Hosp., Tunbridge Wells, Kent; Sen. Regist. Medway Hosp., Kent.

OKAFOR, Mr Benignus Emeka 3 Sellincourt Road, Tooting, London SW17 9RX — MB BS Lond. 1987 (St. Bart.) FRCS Eng. 1991. Regist. Rotat. (Orthop.) Roy. Nat. Orthop. Hosp. & Basildon & OldCh. Hosps. Specialty: Orthop. Socs: BMA.

OKAGBUE, Mr Chuma Ernest 10 Lake Way, Huntingdon PE29 6SU — MB BS Ibadan 1977; FRCS Ed. 1992.

OKARO, Chukwuemeka Obianagha 2 Crescent Lodge, 15 Sunningfields Crescent, Hendon, London NW4 4RD — MB BS Nigeria 1991.

OKE, Anthony Olawale 56 Kingfisher Grove, Lower Grange, Bradford BD8 0NP — MB ChB Ife, Nigeria 1985; MRCPI 1994.

OKE, Olatokunbo Olutayo Queen Elizabeth Hospital, Stadium Road, Woolwich, London SE18 4QH Tel: 0208 836 5480 Fax: 0208 836 5436 — MB BS Ibadan 1987 (Univ. Coll. Hosp. Ibadan) FRCS Ed. 1993; FRCS (Gen.Surg.) 2000; MMed Sc Keele 2000. Gen. Surg. and ColoprOtol., Qu. Eliz. Hosp. Woolwich Lond. Specialty: Gen. Surg. Special Interest: Arorectal Sepsis; Colorectal Cancer; Endoscopy. Socs: BMA; Assoc. of Surg.s in Train.; W Midl.s Surg. Soc. Prev: Specialist Regist. Inaisall Manor Hosp., Walsall; Specialist Regist. Gen. Surg.; Colorectal Fell., the Roy. Lond. Hosp., Lond.

OKE, Peter Thompson (retired) 15 Gospelgate, Louth LN11 9JX Tel: 01507 602303 — MB BS Lond. 1957 (Char. Cross) MRCS Eng. LRCP Lond. 1957. Prev: Ho. Surg. (Gyn.) & Resid. Obst. Off. Char. Cross Hosp. Lond.

OKE, Sarah Cecile Barrow Hospital, Barrow Gurney, Bristol BS48 3SG Tel: 01275 392811 — MB BS Lond. 1984; BSc Lond. 1981; MRCPsych 1988. Cons. Psychiat. Barrow Hosp. Bristol (Mother & Baby Unit). Specialty: Gen. Psychiat. Prev: Sen. Regist. Rotat. (Psychiat.) Exeter; SHO Rotat. (Psychiat.) St. Mary's Hosp. Lond. W2.

OKEAHIALAM, Majella Gerard Department of Obstetrics & Gynaecology, Bradford Royal Infirmary, Duckworth Lane, Bradford BD9 6RJ Tel: 01274 542200; 33 Aireville Avenue, Bradford BD9 4ER — MB BS Nigeria 1982 (Univ. Nigeria) MRCOG 1992. Staff Grade Pract. (O & G) Bradford Roy. Infirm. Specialty: Obst. & Gyn. Socs: Fell. W. Afr. Coll. Surgs. (Obst. & Gyn. Sect.); BMA; Eur. Assn. Gyn. & Obst. Prev: Regist. (O & G) E. Glam. Gen. Hosp. Pontypridd.

OKECH, Mark Nuffield College of Surgical Sciences, Royal College of Surgeons of England, Lincoln's Inn Field, London WC2A 3PE — MB ChB East Africa 1968.

OKELL, Roger William Grove Cottage, Chester Road, Acton, Nantwich CW5 8LD — MB ChB Manch. 1980; FFA RCS Eng. 1985; MRCP (UK) 1988. Cons. Anaesth. Leighton Hosp. Crewe. Specialty: Anaesth. Prev: Sen. Regist. (Anaesth.) Univ. Hosp. Wales; Sen.

Regist. (Anaesth.) Gwynedd Hosp. Bangor; Regist. (Anaesth.) Arrowe Pk. Hosp. Wirral, Broadgreen Hosp. Liverp. & Walton Hosp. Liverp.

OKEREKE, Chikezie Dean Dewsbury & District Hospital, Accident & Emergency Department, Halifax Road, Dewsbury WF13 4HS Tel: 01924 816110 Fax: 01924 816079 Email: chikezie.okereke@midyorks.nhs.uk — MB BS Nigeria 1987; FRCSEd Edin. 1995; FFAEM Glas. 2000. Cons. (Emerg. Med.) Dewsbury & Dist. Hosp. Dewsbury; Hon. Sen. Lect. Sch. of Med. Leeds. Special Interest: Acute Emergencies. Socs: MPS; BAEM.

OKEREKE, Robert Amobi 8 Holt Way, Holt Park, Leeds LS16 7QP Tel: 0113 267 6400 — MB BS Ibadan 1978; MRCOG 1989. Specialty: Obst. & Gyn.

OKHAH, Mr Michael University Hospital Aintree, Accident & Emergency Department, Lower Lane, Liverpool L9 7AL; 11 Pondwater Close, Liverpool L32 9BD — MB BS Ibadan 1985; FRCS Ed. 1993.

OKHAI, Abdul Aziz Hassam 43 Dundee Road, Broughty Ferry, Dundee DD5 1NA Tel: 01382 739673 — MB ChB St. And. 1966.

OKHANDIAR, Ashok Department of Haematology, The Royal Hospital, Haslar, Gosport PO12 2AA Tel: 023 9258 4255 Fax: 023 9276 2549 Email: okhandiar@haslar.demon.co.uk; Aashray, 1 Shorwell Place, Lakeside, Brierley Hill DY5 3TZ Tel: 01384 486099 — MB BS Poona 1979 (Poona, India) LMSSA Lond. 1985; MRCPath 1993. Cons. Haemat. Roy. Hosp. Haslar, Gosport. Specialty: Haematology. Socs: Brit. Soc. Haematol.; Eur. Haemat. Assn. Prev: Staff Haemat. Russells Hall Hosp. Dudley.

OKHRAVI, Narciss Department of Clinical Ophthalmology, The Institute of Ophthalmology, 11-43 Bath St., London EC1V 9EL Tel: 020 7608 6872 Fax: 020 7608 6931; Flat 72, Elm Quay Court, Nine Elms Lane, London SW8 5DF — MB BS Lond. 1989; BSc Lond. 1986, MB BS (Hons.) 1989; FRCOphth 1994. Wellcome Vision Research Fell. Inst. Ophth. Lond. Specialty: Ophth. Socs: Roy. Soc. Med.; Med. Res. Soc. Prev: SHO (Ophth.) West. Eye Hosp. Lond. & Roy. Lond. Hosp.; SHO (Neurosurg.) Brook Gen. Hosp. Woolwich.

OKINE, Emmanuel Ashaley Health Centre, Little Lane, South Elmsall, Pontefract WF9 2NJ Tel: 01977 465331 — Artsexamen Amsterdam 1992. GP Pontefract, W. Yorks.

OKOCHA, Chike Oxleas House, Queen Elixabeth Hospital, London SE18 4QH Tel: 020 88366657 Fax: 020 88366659 — MB BS Ibadan 1985 (Univ. Coll Hosp. University of Ibadan, Nigeria) MB BS Ibadan, Nigeria 1985; MRCPsych 1992; PhD Lond. 1996. Cons. Qu. Eliz. Hosp. Lond. Specialty: Gen. Psychiat. Prev: Hon. Sen. Regist. MRC Unit Psychopharmacol. Inst. Psychiat. Lond.; Research Fell. King's Coll. Hosp. & Inst. of Psychiat.; Child & Adolesc. Psychiat. Elmsleigh Medway Hosp. Kent.

OKOH, Dennis Knightsbridge Medical Centre, 71-75 Pavilion Road, London SW1X OEP Tel: 020 8237 2600 Fax: 020 8237 2626 Email: dennisOkoh@hotmail.com — MB ChB Obafemi Awolowo 1990. GP. Specialty: Gen. Pract. Special Interest: Obst. & Gyn.

OKOKO, Acha Edegbanya Jeremiah Barnsley Primary Care Trust, Barnsley District General Hospital, Gawber Rd, Barnsley S75 2EP Tel: 01226 202859/01226 730000 — MB BS Ahmadu Bello Univ. Nigeria 1972; MSc Sheff.; MSc OU. Milton Keynes; MIBiol Lond.; MRCPsych 1976; DPM Eng. 1977. Cons. Psychiat. N. Gen. Hosp. Sheff. Specialty: Gen. Psychiat. Socs: Fell. Postgrad. Med. Coll. (Psychiat.) Nigeria; BMA; Nigerian Psychiat. Assn. Prev: Sen. Lect. (Psychiat.) Univ. Jos, Nigeria; Chief. Cons. Psychiat. MoH Jos, Nigeria.

OKOLO, Mr Stanley Obiora Department of Obstetrics and Gynaecology, Royal Free Hospital School of Medicine, Pond St., London NW3 2QG Tel: 020 7794 0500 Ext: 6274 Fax: 020 7830 2261 Email: okolo@rfhsm.ac.uk; 68 Northumberland Road, New Barnet, London EN5 1EE Tel: 0378 000097 — BM BCh Nigeria 1979; FWACS 1985; MRCOG 1987; PhD Lond 1995. Cons Gyn. N. Middlx. Hosp. Lond.; Sen. Lect, Gyn. Roy. Free Hosp. Lond. Specialty: Obst. & Gyn. Socs: ESHRE; RSM; BMS. Prev: Lect./Sen. Regist. Univ. of Bristol; Clin. Research Fell. (Reproduc. Endocrinol.) Roy. Free Hosp. Sch. Med. Lond.; Regist. (O & G) Roy. Sussex Co. Hosp. Brighton.

OKONKWO, Mr Alfred Chigbo Ogochukwu 14 Southbourne Avenue, Drayton, Portsmouth PO6 2HN — MB BS Ibadan 1974; FRCS Glas. 1980.

OKONKWO, Ndubisi Azubike 2 Victoria Avenue, London N3 1BD — MB BS Newc. 1982.

OKONKWO, Okechukwu Jonathan Dr. Outar and Partner, Orton Medical Practice, Orton Goldhay, Peterborough PE2 5RQ Tel: 01733 291022 Fax: 01733 391034 — BM BCh Nigeria 1978; MRCOG 1987; MFFP 1993. GP; GP Princip., Partner & Specialist GP (O&G). Specialty: Gen. Pract.; Obst. & Gyn.; Family Plann. & Reproduc. Health. Prev: GP Regist., Dr Moyce & Partners, Oakham Med. Pract.; Staff Grade (O & G) P'boro. Dist. Hosp.; Tutor (O & G) Aberd. Univ.

OKONKWO, Ozioma Obiageli Flat 23, 48-52 Coram St., Russel Square, London WC1N 1HE — MB BS Lond. 1996.

OKONKWO, Stella Ifeoma Health Centre, Brunswick Park Road, London N11 1EY Tel: 020 8368 1568; 2 Victoria Avenue, Fincheley Central, London N3 1BD — MB BS Newc. 1973; MRCP (UK) 1977; DCH Eng. 1977. Specialty: Gen. Med. Socs: Fell. Roy. Soc. Med.; BMA. Prev: Lect. & Hon. Cons. Paediat. Univ. Nigeria Teach. Hosp.

OKOREAFFIA, Affia Chidi Athena Medical Centre, 21 Atherden Road, London E5 0QP Tel: 020 8985 6675 Fax: 020 8533 7775 Email: aokoreaffia@nhs.net — MRCS Eng. LRCP Lond. 1980 (Sheff.) Specialty: Gen. Med. Prev: SHO (Gen. Surg.) Scunthorpe Gen. Hosp.; SHO (A & E) Chesterfield Roy. Hosp.

OKORIE, N M Okorie, The Medical Centre, 1a Ingfield Avenue, Sheffield S9 1WZ Tel: 0114 261 0623 Fax: 0114 261 0949.

OKORO, Mr Joseph Onyekachi Yare Valley Medical Practice, 202 Thorpe Road, Norwich NR1 1TJ Tel: 01603 437559 Fax: 01603 701773 — MB BCh Nigeria 1977; FRCS Glas. 1990. GP Norwich. Specialty: Gen. Pract. Prev: Regist. (Gen. Surg.) Watford Gen. Hosp.

OKOSUN, Onoage Henry 81B Lechmere Avenue, Woodford Green IG8 8QG — MB BS Benin 1992; MRCOG 1992.

OKUBADEJO, Adedeji Abiodun 183 Woodruff Way, Tame Bridge, Walsall WS5 4SB — MB BS Lagos, Nigeria 1987.

OKUBADEJO, Adeyoola Adrian Tejumade Peterborough District Hospital, Thorpe Road, Peterborough PE3 6DA Tel: 01733 874000; 50 West End, Langtoft, Peterborough PE6 9LU — MB BS Lond. 1986; MRCP (UK) 1991. Sen. Regist. (Med. for Elderly) Homerton Hosp. Lond.; Cons. (Med. for Elderly) PeterBoro. Dist. Hosp. Specialty: Care of the Elderly. Socs: Brit. Geriat. Soc. Prev: Research Regist. (Respirat. Med.) Lond. Chest Hosp.; Regist. (Med.) Basildon Hosp.

OKUBADEJO, Olumade Adetola (retired) 39 Solent Road, Portsmouth PO6 1HH — MD Lond. 1966 (King's Coll. Lond. & King's Coll. Hosp.) MB BS 1958; DCP Lond 1963; FRCPath. 1982, M 1972. Prev: Dir. Pub. Health Laborat. Portsmouth.

OKUGBENI, Gabriel Itobore South Tyneside District Hospital, Harton lane, South Shields NE34 0PL — MB BS Univ. Nigeria 1982; MRCP (UK) 1994. Cons. (Paediat.) S. Tyneside Dist. Hosp. Specialty: Paediat. Socs: FRCPCH; Coll. Mem. RCPCH. Prev: Staff Grade (Paediat.) Qu. Mary's Univ. Hosp. Lond.; Regist. (Paediat. & Gastroenterol.) Chelsea & Westm. Hosp.; Regist. (Paediat.) Ealing Hosp. Middlx.

OKUN, Taiwo Odion Stepney Health Centre, 79 Ben Jonson Road, London E1 4SA Tel: 020 7790 1059 Email: taiokun@hotmail.com — MB BS Univ. Lagos Nigeria 1977; DFFP Lond. GP Princip. Lond. Socs: BMA.

OKUNDI, Anne Josephine Adhiambo Flat C, 16 Stoneygate Road, Leicester LE2 2AB — MB ChB Leic. 1992.

OKUNOLA, Olufunmilayo Olayemi 218 Broxburn Drive, South Ockendon RM15 5QY — BM Soton. 1995.

OKUONGHAE, Humphrey Osarenren Obasuyi — MB BS Benin 1980 (RCPCH) FMCPaed 1988; FWACP 1989; MRCPCH 1996; DCH RCP Lond. 1996; MSc 1999; FRCPCH 2004. Cons. Paediat. P. Chas. Hosp. Merthyr Tydfil. Specialty: Paediat. Special Interest: Respirat.; diabetes. Socs: BMA; FWACP W. African Coll. Phys. 1989; Paediatric Asso of Nigeria 1989. Prev: Hon. Sen. Regist. Liverp. Matern. Hosp.; Cons. & Lect. Jos Univ. Teachg. Hosp., Nigeria.

OKUSI, Dolomena 75 Sarsfield Road, London SW12 8HS — MB BS Lond. 1993.

OKWERA, James Mathias Rotherham General Hospital, Moorgate, Rotherham S60 2UD Tel: 01709 304164 Fax: 01709 304419 Email: james.okwera@rothgen.nhs.uk — MB ChB Makerere 1974; Mmed (Internal Med.) Nairobi 1981; MRCPI 1992; FRCPI 2003. Cons. Phys. (Stroke & Elderly Med.) Rotherham Gen. Hosp. Specialty: Gen. Med. Special Interest: Stroke Med. & Cardiovasc.

Dis. in the Elderly. Socs: Brist. Assn. Stroke Phys.; Brit. Geriat. Soc. Prev: Cons. Phys. (Gen. Internal Med.) Bassetlaw Dist. Gen. Hosp. Worksop; Sen. Regist. (Geriat.) Qu. Med. Centre Nottingham.

OKYERE, Kwame Marfo 2 Grace Avenue, OldBrook, Milton Keynes MK6 2XN — MB ChB Ghana 1975; MB ChB U Ghana 1975. Staff Psychiat. Hellesdon Hosp. Norwich. Specialty: Gen. Psychiat. Socs: Fell. Roy. Soc. Med. Prev: Staff Psychiat. ScarBoro. & NE Yorks. Healthcare NHS Trust.

OLA, Ayodele Olusegun New Medical Centre, 264 Brentwood Road, Romford RM2 5SU Tel: 01708 478800 Fax: 01708 471422 — LRCP London; LMSSA London; MB BS Ibadan 1985; MB BS Ibadan 1985; LRCS England 1994.

OLADIPO, Mr Abiodun 25 Maple Leaf Close, Abbots Langley WD5 0SP — MB BS Lagos 1981; MRCOG 1993; MFFP 1994; FRCS Ed. 1995. Specialist Regist. (O & G) Roy. United Hosp. Bath; Cons. Gyn. (with s/i in Oncol.) Lead Colposcopist, Roy. coirnwall hosp. Truro, TRI 3LJ. Specialty: Obst. & Gyn. Socs: Brit. Med. Ultrasound Soc.; BMA; Brit. Menopause Soc. Prev: Regist. (O & G) Salisbury Dist. Hosp. & Roy. Gwent Hosp.; SHO Scunthorpe Gen. Hosp.; SpR (Gyn. Unit) Univ. of Southampton Teachg. Hosp. (P.ss Anne Hosp.) Southampton.

OLADIPO, Mr James Olarewaju Olagboyega 78 York Road, Linthorpe, Middlesbrough TS5 6LL Tel: 01642 812945 Fax: 01642 812945 — MB BS Ibadan 1987; FRCS Glas. 1992; FRCS Ed. 1992.

OLAITAN, Adeola Flat 13 Northgates, 445 High Road, London N12 0AR — MB BS Lond. 1987.

OLAJIDE, Oladele Olugbenga Maudsley Hospital, Denmark Hill, London SE5 8AZ Tel: 020 7919 2951 Fax: 020 7919 2643 Email: dele.olajide@slam-tr.nhs.uk — MB BS Ibadan 1977 (Ibadan, Nigeria) PhD Lond. 1985; T(Psych) 1991; MRCPsych 1987, FRCPsych 1997. Cons. Psychiat. Maudsley Hosp. Lond.; Clin. Sen. Lect. Dept. of Psychol. Med. Inst. of Psychiat. Lond.; Hon. Sen. Lect., Inst. of Psychiat., Lond. Specialty: Gen. Psychiat. Socs: Fell. Collegium Internat.e Neuro-Psychopharmacol.; Eur. Coll. Neuropsychopharm.; Brit. Assn. Psychopharmacol. Prev: Cons. Psychiat. & Sen. Lect. Maidstone Priority Care NHS Trust & King's Coll. Hosptial Inst. Psychiat. Lond.

OLAJIDE, Victoria Feyishola South Tyneside District Hospital, Harton Road, South Shields NE34 0PL Tel: 0191 454 8888 Fax: 0191 202 4180; 16 Rothwell Road, Gosforth, Newcastle upon Tyne NE3 1TY Tel: 0191 284 4666 Fax: 0191 285 4820 — MB BS Ibadan 1978; MB BS (Distinc. Obst. & Gyn.) Ibadan 1978; MRCOG 1986. Cons. O & G S. Tyneside Dist. Hosp. S. Shields. Specialty: Obst. & Gyn. Socs: BMA; Brit. Fertil. Soc. Prev: Cons. O & G Ealing Hosp. Lond.; Lect. Princess Mary & Roy. Vict. Infirm. Newc.; IVF Research Regist. St. Bart. Hosp. Lond.

OLAKANPU, Obasanmi Andrew 17 Ruskin Court, Winchmore Hill Road, London N21 1QJ — MB BS Lond. 1996.

OLAMIJULO, Joseph Ayodeji Department of Obstetrics & Gynaecology, Pilgrim Hospital, Sibsey Road, Boston PE21 9QS Tel: 01205 442112 Fax: 01205 442319 Email: ayolamijulo@hotmail.com — MB BS Univ. of Lagos Nigeria 1984 (Lagos) FMCOG; FWACS; MRCOG. Cons. Obst. & gynaecologist Pilgrim Hosp. Boston. Specialty: Obst. & Gyn. Special Interest: Gyn. Endoscopic Surg. Socs: British Society of Gynae. Endoscopy. Prev: Specialist Regist. Obst. & Gyn., Qu.'s Pk. Hosp..

OLATEJU, Mahmoud Abimbola Olatunji 3 Beachcroft Way, London N19 3HR — MB BS Lond. 1963.

OLAWO, Ayoola Oladoye 78 Bron-y-Nant, Croesnewydd Road, Wrexham LL13 7TZ Tel: 01978 291100 — MB BS Lagos, Nigeria 1987 (Coll. Med. Univ. Lagos) MRCOG 1995. Specialist Regist. (O & G) Wrexham Maelor Hosp. Specialty: Obst. & Gyn. Prev: Specialist Regist. (O & G) Ysbyty Gwynedd Bangor.

OLAYEMI, Agnes Oaikhohen 80 Hornby House, Clayton St., London SE11 5DB — MB BS Lond. 1986.

OLCZAK, Stephen Andrzej Pilgrim Hospital, Boston PE21 9QS Tel: 01205 442099 Email: stephen.olczak@nlh.nhs.uk — MB BS Lond. 1975 (Guy's) MD Lond. 1984, BSc (1st cl. Hons. Physiol.) 1972; MRCP (UK) 1978; FRCP Lond. 1994. Cons. Phys. Endocrinol. & Diabetes Pilgrim Hosp. Boston. Specialty: Endocrinol.

OLD, Eric Gordon (retired) 1 Glendower Street, Monmouth NP25 3DG Tel: 01600 712582 Email: eric.old@lineone.net — MB BS Lond. 1947 (Cardiff & Westm.) MRCS Eng. LRCP Lond. 1947; DObst RCOG 1954; DA Eng. 1966. Prev: GP Monmouth.

OLD, Francis Tristram Herland Farmhouse, Godolphin, Helston TR13 9RJ — MB ChB Leeds 1998.

OLD, Peter John Isle of Wight, Portsmouth & S.E. Hampshire Health Authority, Finchdean House, Milton Road, Portsmouth PO3 3DP Tel: 023 9283 5104 — MB BS Lond. 1978; DRCOG 1984; MRCGP 1984; DCH RCP Lond. 1985; LLM Wales 1992; MFPHM RCP (UK) 1993. Dir. Pub. Health Isle of Wight Portsmouth & S.E. Hants. Health Auth. Specialty: Pub. Health Med. Socs: Inst. Health Servs. Managem.; Medico-Legal Soc. Prev: Cons. Pub. Health Med. Soton. & SW Hants. Health Commiss.; GP Gosport; Med. Off. Save Childr. Fund Torit, S. Sudan.

OLD, Sally Emma 1 Merchants Walk, Baldock SG7 6TJ — MB BS Lond. 1991; MRCP (UK) 1994; FRCR (Clin. Oncol.) 1998. SHO (Clin. Oncol.) Mt. Vernon Hosp. Rickmansworth; Cons. Clin. Oncol. Addenbrookes Hosp. Camb. Specialty: Gen. Med. Socs: Roy. Coll. Phys. Lond.; BMA. Prev: SPR Clin. Oncol. Addenbrookes Hosp.; SHO (Med.) Lister Hosp.; SHO (A & E) Luton & Dunstable Hosp.

OLD, Simon York Hospital, Dept. of Anaesthesia, Wigginton Road, York YO31 8HE Tel: 01904 631313; Bilbrough House, Bilbrough House, Main Street, Bilbrough, York YO23 3PH Tel: 01937 832605 Email: alexis_simon.old@virgin.net — MB ChB Bristol 1988 (Brist.) MA Oxf. 1981; DA (UK) 1991; FRCA 1993. Cons., Anaesth., York Dist. Hosp. Specialty: Anaesth. Special Interest: Maxillo-Facial Anaesth.; Obst. Socs: World Anaesth.; Obst. Anaesth. Assn.

OLDALE, Mark Jonathan 69 Adswood Road, Cheadle Hulme, Cheadle SK8 5QY — MB ChB Manch. 1998.

OLDER, Mr Michael William John King Edward VII Hospital, Midhurst GU29 0BL Tel: 01730 811166 Fax: 01730 811168; Verdley Hill House, Henley, Haslemere GU27 3HG Tel: 01428 656652 — MB BS Lond. 1966 (Guy's) BDS Lond. 1960; LDS RCS Eng. 1960; MRCS Eng. LRCP Lond. 1965; FRCS Ed. 1971; FRCS Eng. 2002. Cons. Orthop. Surg. King Edwd. VII Hosp. Midhurst & Mt. Alvernia Hosp. Guildford; Hon. Cons. Orthop. Surg. Roy. Surrey Co. Hosp. Guildford; Clin. Anatomist (Acad. Dept. Anat.) Guy's King's & St Thos. Sch. Med., Dent. & Biomed. Sci., Guy's Campus Lond. Specialty: Orthop. Socs: Fell. Internat. Hip Soc.; Brit. Hip Soc.; Brit. Orthop. Assn. Prev: Sen. Regist. (Orthop. & Traum. Surg.) Bristol. Roy. Infirm.; Clin. Research Fell. (Orthop. Surg.) Univ. Toronto, Canada; Ho. Phys. & Ho. Surg. Guy's Hosp. Lond.

OLDERSHAW, Kenneth Leslie 6 Honor Oak, London SE23 3SF — MB BS Lond. 1949 (Lond. Hosp.) DObst RCOG 1954; MRCGP 1968. Socs: BMA. Prev: Receiv. Room Off. Lond. Hosp.; Obst. Ho. Off. Roy. Berks. Hosp.

OLDERSHAW, Paul John 76 Carlton Hill, London NW8 0ET — MD Camb. 1991 (St. Thos. & Camb.) MB 1974, BChir 1973; MRCP (UK) 1975; FRCP Lond. 1990. Cons. (Cardiol.) Brompton Hosp. Lond.; SHO & Regist. (Cardiol.) Brompton Hosp. Lond. Specialty: Cardiol. Socs: Fell.Amer. Coll. of Cardiol. (FACC); Fell.Europ. Soc. of Cardiol. (FESC). Prev: Sen. Regist. (Cardiol.) St. Geo. Hosp. Lond.

OLDERSHAW, William Henry (retired) 23 Conalan Avenue, Sheffield S17 4PG Tel: 0114 235 2272 — MB ChB Sheff. 1940; Specialist Accredit (Occupat. Med.) RCP Lond; MFOM RCP Lond. 1978.

OLDFIELD, Jessica Ann 72 Doeford Close, Culcheth, Warrington WA3 4DL — MB ChB Liverp. 1998.

OLDFIELD, Paul Douglas Weaverham Surgery, Northwich Road, Weaverham, Northwich CW8 3EU Tel: 01606 852168 Fax: 01606 854980 Email: oldfieldmanor@aol.com — MB ChB Liverp. 1969; FRCGP; DObst RCOG 1972; MRCGP 1977. GP. Socs: S. Chesh. LMC; Northwich Med. Soc. (Sec.). Prev: Clin. Asst. (Med.) Vict. Infirm. Northwich.

OLDFIELD, Raymond Henry 18 Roles Grove, Chadwell Heath, Romford RM6 5LT — MB BS Lond. 1950 (St. Thos.) MRCS Eng. LRCP Lond. 1946.

OLDFIELD, William Laurence George St. Mary's Hospital, Chest & Allergy Unit, Praed Street, London W2 INY — MB BS Lond. 1992 (St. Georges) BSc Lond. 1985; MSc Lond. 1987; MRCP (UK) 1995; PhD Imperial Coll., Lond. 2003. Cons. in Respirat. Med., St. Mary's Hosp. Lond.; Cons. in Respirat. Med., Roy. Brompton Hosp., Lond.; Hon. Sen. Lect. in Med., Imperial Coll. Sch. of Med., Lond. Specialty: Respirat. Med. Socs: Brit. Thoracic Soc.; Europ. Respirat. Soc.; Amer. Thoracic Soc. Prev: SpR in Intens. Care, St. Marys Hosp., Lond.; Senior SpR (Respirat. Med.) St Marys Hosp. Lond.; SpR in Respirat. Med., Roy. Brompton Hosp., Lond.

OLDHAM, Barbara Firwood, Leycester Road, Knutsford WA16 8QR — MRCS Eng. LRCP Lond. 1947; MB ChB Manch. 1949.

OLDHAM, Eileen Patricia (retired) Gorsebank, 152 Upton Road, Bidston, Prenton CH43 7QG Tel: 0151 652 4579 — MB ChB Liverp. 1950.

OLDHAM, Sir John, OBE Oldham and Partners, Manor House Surgery, Manor Street, Glossop SK13 8PS — MB ChB Manch. 1977; DCH Eng. 1980; MRCGP 1981; MBA (Distinc.) Manch. 1992. GP Glossop; Nat. Primary Care Developm. Team, NHS. Prev: Med. Adviser Mersey RHA; Med. Adviser Primary Care Div. NHS Exec. HQ; Fac. Mem. Inst. of Health Care.

OLDHAM, Jonathan Richard Dial House Medical Centre, 131 Mile End Lane, Offerton, Stockport SK2 6BZ Tel: 0161 456 9905 Fax: 0161 456 7127 — MB ChB Manch. 1975; MRCGP 1986.

OLDHAM, Judith Caroline Mount Pleasant Practice, Tempest Way, Chepstow NP16 5XR Tel: 01291 636500 Fax: 01291 636518 — MB ChB Manch. 1977. Specialty: Dermat.

OLDHAM, Kenneth William (retired) Three Gables, 53 Wrenbeck Drive, Otley LS21 2BP Tel: 01943 464914 — MRCS Eng. LRCP Lond. 1944 (St. Thos.) DA Eng. 1954. Asst. Anaesth. Northampton & Dist. Gp. Hosps. Prev: Regist. (Anaesth.) St. Peter's Hosp. Chertsey.

OLDHAM, Mary Marian New Cross Surgery, 48 Sway Road, Morriston, Swansea SA6 6HR Tel: 01792 771419 — MB BCh Wales 1972 (Welsh National School of Medicine) DObst RCOG 1974; MRCGP 1976. Socs: BMA. Prev: Clin. Med. Off. W. Glam. AHA; SHO (Cas.) Singleton Hosp. Swansea; SHO (Paediat.) Morriston Hosp. Swansea.

OLDHAM, Roger Department of Rheumatology, University Hospitals of Leicester NHS Trust, Leicester Royal Infirmary, Infirmary Square, Leicester LE1 5WW Tel: 0116 254 1414 Fax: 0116 258 6992 Email: roldham@talk21.com — MB BS Lond. 1969 (Char. Cross) BSc (Hons.) Lond. 1966; MRCS Eng. LRCP Lond. 1969; MRCP (UK) 1974; FRCP Lond. 1992; FRCP Ed. 1995. Cons. Rheum. Univ. Hosp.s of Leicester NHS Trust. Specialty: Rheumatol. Socs: Brit. Soc. Rheum.; Leic. Med. Soc. Prev: Sen. Regist. (Med.) Leicester Roy. Infirm.; Regist. (Med.) Groby Rd. Hosp. Leicester; Ho. Surg. & Ho. Phys. Char. Cross Hosp. Gp.

OLDHAM, Rosemary Ann Stepping Hill Hospital, Poplar Grove, Stockport SK2 7SE Tel: 0161 483 1010; 16 Gladstone Road, Sheffield S10 3GT Tel: 0114 230 2884 — MB ChB Manch. 1997. SHO Adult Med., Stepping Hill Hosp. Stockport. Specialty: Gen. Med.

OLDHAM, Thomas Anthony 12 The Avenue, Whitchurch, Cardiff CF14 2EG — MB BS Lond. 1989.

OLDHAM, Trevor Peter Bridgegate Medical Centre, Winchester Street, Barrow-in-Furness LA13 9SH Tel: 01229 820304 Fax: 01229 836984; Dove Cottage, Aldingham, Ulverston LA12 9RT — MB ChB Birm. 1976; DCH Eng. 1981; MRCP (UK) 1982.

OLDMAN, Lynne Elizabeth — MB ChB Birm. 1985; DRCOG 1988; MRCGP 1990; MA 1999; MRCPsych 2002.

OLDMAN, Matthew John Derriford Hospital, Plymouth PL6 8DH; Delamere, The Common, Shotesham All Saints, Norwich NR15 1YD Email: oldman@globalnet.co.uk — MB BS Lond. 1994 (St Georges Hosp.) Specialist Regist. Anaesth. Derriford Hosp., Plymouth. Specialty: Anaesth. Prev: SHO Neonat. Med., Roy. Devon & Exeter Hosp.; SHO Anaesth. Roy. Devon & Exeter Hosp.; Sen. Ho. Off., Elderly Med. Roy. Devon & Exeter Hosp.

OLDREIVE, Peter David (retired) Wildwood, 85 Island Road, Sturry, Canterbury CT2 0EF Tel: 01227 710232 — BM BCh Oxf. 1958.

OLDREY, Timothy Branston Nugent, Brigadier late RAMC (retired) The Cottage, Figheldean, Salisbury SP4 8JJ — (Middlx.) MB BS Lond. 1966; MRCS Eng. LRCP Lond. 1966; MRCP (UK) 1973; FRCP Lond. 1985. Prev: Dir. of Army Med. & Cons. Phys. to Army.

OLDRING, John Kennett Orchard Medical Practice, Orchard Road, Broughton Astley, Leicester LE9 6RG Tel: 01445 282599 Fax: 01445 286772; The White House, Main St, Ullesthorpe, Lutterworth LE17 5BT Tel: 01455 209337 — MRCS Eng. LRCP Lond. 1976; MA, BM BCh Oxf. 1976; MRCGP 1982; DRCOG 1982. GP Ullesthorpe.

OLDROYD, David The General Medical Centre, Surgery Lane, Hartlepool TS24 9DN Tel: 01429 266148 Fax: 01429 222416; Avis House, High Throston, Hartlepool TS26 0UG — MB ChB Birm. 1960.

OLDROYD, David Anthony Falsgrave Surgery, 33 Falsgrave Road, Scarborough YO12 5EB Tel: 01723 360835 Fax: 01723 503220; Overgreen Farm, Overgreen Lane, Burniston, Scarborough YO13 0HY Tel: 01723 870039 — (St. Thos.) MB BS Lond. 1971.

OLDROYD, Glenda Jacqueline 2 Highfold, Yeadon, Leeds LS19 7DN — MB ChB Leeds 1983; FRCA 1991. Cons. Anaesth. Bradford Hosps NHS Trust. Specialty: Anaesth.

OLDROYD, Jessica Claire Chainbridge Medical Partnership, Chainbridge House, The Precinct, Blaydon-on-Tyne NE21 5BT Tel: 0191 414 2856 — MB BS Newc. 1987. Specialty: Gen. Pract. Prev: GP Partner, Falcon Ho., Heaton Rd., Newc. upon Tyne; GP Partner, Saville Med. Gp., Saville Pl., Newc. upon Tyne.

OLDROYD, Keith George Department of Medical Cardiology, Hairmyres Hospital, East Kilbride, Glasgow G75 8RG Tel: 01355 72636; 5 Hamilton Drive, Cambuslang, Glasgow G72 8JG Tel: 0141 641 3759 — MB BS Aberd. 1982; MB ChB Aberd. 1982; MRCP (UK) 1985; MD (Hons.) Aberd. 1993; FRCP (Glas.) 1998. Cons. Phys. & Cardiol. Hairmyres Hosp. E. Kilbride. Specialty: Cardiol. Socs: Briitsh Cardiac Soc.; Scott. Cardiac Soc. Prev: Clin. Lect. (Med. Cardiol.) Glas. Roy. Infirm. & Univ. Glas.; Fell. Dept. of Cardiol., Toronto Gen. Hosp..

OLDROYD, Ruth Elizabeth New Street, Wem, Shrewsbury SY4 5AF — MB BS Newc. 1994; DCH RCPS Glas. 1996; DRCOG 1997; MRCGP 1999. GP Princip. Specialty: Gen. Pract. Prev: SHO Med. Shrewsbury; SHO (O & G) Shrewsbury.

OLDS, Elizabeth Mary Ninnis Farm, Lelant Downs, Hayle TR27 6NL — MB ChB Wales 1993; BSc (1st cl. Hons.) Pharmacol. Wales, 1992, MB BCh 1993. SHO (Paediat.) Univ. Hosp. Wales. Specialty: Paediat.

OLEESKY, David Alan 8 Carew Court, Curlew Close, Cardiff CF14 1BQ Tel: 029 2061 7760 Email: david.oleesky@gwent.wales.nhs.uk — MB BS Lond. 1979 (Westm.) BA (Hons.) Camb. 1976, MA 1980; MRCPath 1986. Specialty: Chem. Path.

OLEESKY, Samuel (retired) 1 Dunham Lawn, Bradgate Road, Altrincham WA14 4QJ Tel: 0161 928 8066 — MB ChB Manch. 1944 (Manch. & Washington Univ. St. Louis) MSc Manch. 1951, BSc 1941; MB ChB (Hons.) 1944; FRCP Lond. 1963, M 1946; MD (Hons.) Washington Univ. St. Louis 1949. Prev: Cons. Phys. Manch. Roy. Infirm.

OLEOLO, Misbahudeen — MB BS Ilorin 1992. Sen. Ho. Off. (Gen. Med.) Queens Hosp. Trent.

OLESHKO, Christopher George Moss Lane Surgery, Moss Lane, Madeley, Crewe CW3 9NQ Tel: 01782 750274 Fax: 01782 751835 — MB BS Lond. 1985.

OLFORD, Colin Arthur Chichester Road Surgery, 34 Chichester Road, Portsmouth PO2 0AD — MB BS Lond. 1964 (Middlx.) DObst RCOG 1971. Prev: Surg. Lt. RN; Ho. Phys. RN Hosp. Haslar; Ho. Surg. Roy. Portsmouth Hosp.

OLI, Professor Johnie Mbanefo c/o Dr B C Onyeabo, 25 Kelland Close, Park Road, London N8 8JS Tel: 020 8341 4874; Department of Medicine, University of Nigera Teaching Hospital, Enugy, Nigeria Tel: (00 23) (442) 451281 Fax: (00 23) (442) 451281 — (University of Manchester Medical School) MB ChB Manch. 1966; MRCP (U.K.) 1971; FRCP Ed 1984; FRCP (Lond.) 1986. Prof. Med. Univ. Nigeria Enugy, Nigeria; Hon. Cons. Phys. Univ. Nigeria Enugu, Nigeria. Specialty: Gen. Med.; Diabetes; Endocrinol. Socs: Diabetic Assn. Nigeria Trustee; Nigerian Soc. Endocrinol. & Metab.; Nutrit. Soc. Nigeria.

OLIN, Robert Henry 25 The Beeches, Park St., St Albans AL2 2PL Tel: 01727 74034; 1353 Hedman Way, White Bear Lake, Minnesota 55110, USA Tel: 612 653 1970 — MD Minnesota 1958. Specialty: Accid. & Emerg. Socs: Amer. Acad. Family Pjys.; Minnesota Med. Soc.

OLIPHANT, Christopher John Hebburn Health Centre, Campbell Park Road, Hebburn NE31 2SP — MB BS Newc. 1975; DRCOG 1977; MRCGP 1979.

OLIVE, John Edward Victoria House, 28 Alexandra Road, Lowestoft, Norwich NR32 1PL Tel: 01603 288104 Fax: 01502 532147 — MB ChB Birm. 1969; MRCPsych 1976; PG Dip. MH Law Northumb. 2003. Cons. Psychiat. Norf. Trust, Med. Health Care; Assoc. Clin. Prof. of Psychiat. St. Geo.s Med. Sch., Grenada.

Specialty: Gen. Psychiat. Prev: Sen. Regist. (Psychiat.) All St.s' Hosp. Birm.; Hon. Clin. Lect. Univ. Birm.; Resid. (Paediat.) Ottawa Gen. Hosp.

OLIVEIRA, Professor David Benjamin Graeme Division of Renal Medicine, St. George's Hospital Medical School, Cranmer Terrace, Tooting, London SW17 0RE Tel: 020 8725 5038 Fax: 020 8725 5036 Email: doliveir@sghms.ac.uk; 62 Coombe Lane W., Kingston upon Thames KT2 7BY Tel: 020 8336 2446 — MB BChir Camb. 1979; MA Camb. 1981; MRCP (UK) 1981; PhD 1987; FRCP Lond. 1996. Prof. Renal Med. & Hon. Cons. Nephrol. St. Geo. Hosp. Med. Sch. Lond. Specialty: Nephrol.

OLIVER, Alexander Neville 16 Court Drive, Uxbridge UB10 0BJ — MB BS Lond. 1992.

OLIVER, Ann Patricia (retired) 8 Lyme Park, Chinley, High Peak SK23 6AG — MB ChB Manch. 1965. Prev: GP Chapel-en-le-Frith.

OLIVER, Anne Stragrane House, Dyan, Caledon BT68 4YA — MB ChB Aberd. 1996.

OLIVER, Barbara Kathleen (retired) 96 Dorset House, Gloucester Place, London NW1 5AF Tel: 020 7935 4519 — (Guy's) MRCS Eng. LRCP Lond. 1954; DA Eng. 1962; FFA RCS Eng. 1969. Prev: Cons. Anaesth. The Roy. Lond. Hosp.

OLIVER, Barry John Barnard Medical Practice, 43 Granville Road, Sidcup DA14 4TA Tel: 020 8302 7721 Fax: 020 8309 6579 — MB BS Lond. 1974 (Middlx.) Cert JCC Lond. 1976. Sen. Partner NHS Gen. Pract.

OLIVER, Carol Anne Victoria Strathmore Medical Practice, 26-28 Chester Road, Wrexham LL11 2SA Tel: 01978 352055 Fax: 01978 310689; 4 Derwen Court, Wrexham LL13 7JA — MB ChB Manch. 1981; BSc (Med. Sci.) St. And. 1978; Cert. Family Plann. JCC 1984; DRCOG 1984. Prev: Trainee GP S. Clwyd VTS; Ho. Surg. Maelor Gen. Hosp. Clwyd; Ho. Phys. Univ. Hosp. S. Manch.

OLIVER, Caroline Diane The Surgery, 1 Glebe Road, Barnes, London SW13 0DR Tel: 020 8748 1065 — MB BS Lond. 1993.

OLIVER, Charles Henry Teviot Medical Practice, Teviot Road, Hawick TD9 9DT Tel: 01450 370999 Fax: 01450 371025; Broomieknowe, Stirches Road, Hawick TD9 7HF Tel: 01450 73240 — MB ChB Ed. 1972; DCH Eng. 1976; MRCP (UK) 1978. Clin. Tutor Gen. Pract. Univ. of Edin.; Police Surg. Lothian & Borders Police. Prev: Maj. RAMC.

OLIVER, Christopher John Russell Oliver and Partners, Millhill Surgery, 87 Woodmill Street, Dunfermline KY11 4JW Tel: 01383 621222 Fax: 01383 622862 — BM BCh Oxf. 1972; DObst RCOG 1974. Prev: SHO Raigmore Hosp. Inverness.; Ho. Off. Princess Margt. Hosp. Swindon.

OLIVER, Mr Christopher William Royal Infirmary of Edinburgh , Edinburgh Orthopaedic Trauma Unit, Old Dalkeith Road, Edinburgh EH16 4SU Tel: 0131 2423402 Fax: 0131 2423467 Email: c.w.oliver@ed.ac.uk; BUPA Murrayfield Hospital, 112 Corstorphine Road, Edinburgh EH12 6UD Tel: 0131 3340363 — MB BS Lond. 1985 (Univ. Coll. Hosp.) BSc (Physiol.) Lond. 1981; FRCS Eng. 1989; FRCS (Orth.) 1995; MD 1995; FRCS (Ed) 1998; FRCP (Ed) 2000; DMI (RCSEd) 2002. Cons. (Trauma & Orthop.Surg.) Roy. Infirm. Edin.; p/t Sen. Lect. (Orthop.) Univ. Edin. Specialty: Orthop. Special Interest: Hand Surg. Socs: Fell. Brit. Orthop. Assn.; AO Alumni; Orthopaedic Trauma Assoc. Prev: Fell. Musculoskeletal Trauma John Radcliffe Hosp. Oxf.; AO Fell. Harborview Med. Centre, Seattle, USA; Spinal Research Fell. (Orthop.) Middlesbrough Gen. Hosp.

OLIVER, Colin Barry Duncan Department of Clinical Radiology, Walsgrave Hospital, Coventry CV2 2DX Tel: 024 76 602020 Fax: 024 7684 4150 — BSc (Pharmacol.) Lond. 1983; MB BS Lond. 1986; MRCP (UK) 1990; FRCR 1994. Cons. (Diagn. Radiol.) Walsgrave Hosp. Coventry. Specialty: Radiol. Prev: Sen. Regist. (Diagn. Radiol.) Bristol Roy. Infirm.

OLIVER, David 46 Hitchen Hatch Lane, Sevenoaks TN13 3AU Tel: 01732 741233 — MB BChir Camb. 1990 (Univ. Camb. Trinty Hall. & Univ. Oxf. Qu. Coll.) BA Physiol. Oxf. 1987; MB BChir Camb. 1989; DGM RCP Lond. 1992; MRCP (UK) 1993. Sen. Regist. Rotat. (Geriat. & Gen. Med.) St. Thos. Hosp. Lond. Specialty: Care of the Elderly; Gen. Med. Socs: BMA; Med. Protec. Soc.; Brit. Geriat. Soc. Prev: Sen. Regist. (Geriat.) Kent & Canterbury Hosp.; Research Fell. & Regist. St. Thos. Hosp. Lond.

OLIVER, David John Wisdom Hospice, High Bank, Rochester ME1 2NU Tel: 01634 830456 Fax: 01634 845890 Email: david.oliver@medwaypct.nhs.uk — MB BS Lond. 1978 (Univ. Coll. Hosp.) BSc Lond. 1975; DRCOG 1981; FRCGP 1993, M 1982. Cons. Phys. (Palliat. Med.) Wisdom Hospice (Medway Primary Care Trust); Hon. Sen. Lect. in Palliat. Care at Kent Inst. of Med. & Health Sci. Univ. Kent Canterbury. Specialty: Palliat. Med. Socs: Fell. Roy. Soc. Med.; BMA; Assn. Palliat. Med. Prev: Trainee GP Swindon VTS; Sen. Regist. St. Christopher's Hospice Sydenham.

***OLIVER, David Jonathan** 60 York Close, Bournville, Birmingham B30 2HN Tel: 0121 486 2576 — MB ChB Birm. 1998 (Univ. of Birm.) DFFP; DRCOG; MRCGP. Ho. Off. in Surg.Birm. Heartlands Hosp., Over 6 months, Vasc., gerneral & Urol.; SHO in A & E, Selly Oak Hosp. Birm.; SHO in Elderly Care Med. W. Heath. Birm. Specialty: Accid. & Emerg. Socs: MDU; BMA. Prev: Ho. Off. in Med. Qu. Eliz. Hosp., Univ of Birm. NHS Trust, Birm UK.

OLIVER, David William Radcliffe Infirmary, Woodstock Road, Oxford OX2 6HE — MB ChB Birm. 1991; ChB Birm. 1991.

OLIVER, Edward James Hoblyn 36 Woodstock Road, Redland, Bristol BS6 7EP Tel: 0117 924 6296 Fax: 0117 940 6555 — MB ChB Bristol 1984 (Bristol Univ.) BSc Bristol 1981; DCH RCP Lond. 1987; MSc (IT) Bristol 1990. Managing Dir. Edit Ltd. Bristol. Specialty: Gen. Pract. Socs: BMA. Prev: Informat. Manager S & W RHA; Managem. Cons. Price WaterHo.

OLIVER, Elizabeth Hawthorn Medical Centre, May Close, Swindon SN2 1UU Tel: 01793 536541 Fax: 01793 421049 — MB ChB Aberd. 1977; MRCGP 1981. GP Swindon.

OLIVER, Elizabeth Mary Coleby Hall, Coleby, Scunthorpe DN15 9AL Tel: 01724 734531 — MB ChB Bristol 1972; MRCS Eng. LRCP Lond. 1971; DA Eng. 1974.

OLIVER, Fred Tameside & Glossop Community & Priority Services NHS Trust, Tameside General Hospital, Fountain St., Ashton-under-Lyne OL6 9RW Tel: 0161 331 5063; Northenden, 25 Netherwood Road, Manchester M22 4BW — MB ChB Manch. 1966; DObst RCOG 1968; DPM Eng. 1973; FRCPsych 1997, M 1974. Cons. Psychiat. Tameside Gen. Hosp. Specialty: Geriat. Psychiat. Socs: Manch. Med. Soc. (Mem. Counc. Psychiat. Sect.). Prev: Sen. Regist. (Psychiat.) United Manch. Hosps.; Regist. (Psychiat.) Univ. Hosp. Withington; Dist. Med. Off. St. Lucia, W. Indies.

OLIVER, Gillian The Health Centre, Lawson Street, Stockton-on-Tees TS18 1HX Tel: 01642 672351 Fax: 01642 618112 — MB ChB Leeds 1992.

OLIVER, Graeme Whickham Health Centre, Rectory Lane, Whickham, Newcastle upon Tyne NE16 4PD Tel: 0191 414 3384 — MB BS Newc. 1968; DObst RCOG 1971; MRCGP 1972.

OLIVER, Hugh Walter Latham, MBE (retired) 45 Tunwells Lane, Great Shelford, Cambridge CB2 5LJ Tel: 01223 842919 — MB BS Lond. 1954 (Lond. Hosp.) DObst RCOG 1959. Prev: GP Camb.

OLIVER, James 3 Kirkhill Drive, Oldmeldrum, Inverurie AB51 0FP — MB ChB Aberd. 1979.

OLIVER, James The Meads Surgery, Grange Road, Uckfield TN22 1QU Tel: 01825 765777 Fax: 01825 766220 — MB ChB Leic. 1986.

OLIVER, James John 83 East Claremont Street, Edinburgh EH7 4HU — MB ChB Birm. 1996; BSc Birm. 1994; MRCP 1999.

OLIVER, James Philip Nansmellion Road Health Centre, Nansmellion Road, Mullion, Helston TR12 7DQ Tel: 01326 240212 Fax: 01326 240420 — MB BChir Camb. 1987; MA Camb. 1989, BA 1984. Prev: Trainee GP Truro VTS; Ho. Surg. MusGr. Pk. Hosp. Taunton; Ho. Phys. Tehidy & Treliske Hosp.

OLIVER, Miss Jane Margaret Newham Healthcare NHS Trust, Glen Road, London E13 8SL Tel: 020 7476 4000 Email: jane.oliver@newhamhealth.nhs.uk — MB ChB Bristol 1985; BSc (Hons.) Bristol 1974; FRCS Ed. 1990; FFAEM 1997. Cons. & Clin. Director in Emerg. Med., Newham Univ. Hosp. Specialty: Accid. & Emerg.; Emergency Medicine. Socs: BAEM.

OLIVER, Jean Mary (retired) 15 Falcon Drive, Mudeford, Christchurch BH23 4BA — (Ed.) MB ChB Ed. 1938; DPM RCPSI 1949. Prev: Cons. Psychiat. Epsom Dist. Hosp. & W. Pk. Hosp. Epsom.

OLIVER, Jeffrey Enrique The Surgery, 218 Ifield Drive, Ifield, Crawley RH11 0EP Tel: 01293 547846 — BM BCh Oxf. 1978; MA Oxf. 1978; MRCP (UK) 1980; DRCOG 1982. Tutor (Gen. Pract. & Primary Care) St. Geo.'s Hosp. Med. Sch. Lond.; Trainer (Gen. Pract.) Crawley; Tutor GP Crawley & Horsham Dist. Prev: SHO

(Med.) Roy. Vict. Infirm. Newc.; Ho. Phys. John Radcliffe Infirm. Oxf..

OLIVER, Jill Rosemary 31 College Road, Isleworth TW7 5DJ — MB ChB Ed. 1965; DA Eng. 1968. Clin. Asst. (Anaesth.) W. Middlx. Hosp. Isleworth.

OLIVER, Juliet Flat 7, Parade Mansions, E. Preston, Littlehampton BN16 1NT — MB BS Lond. 1991; MRCP, Univ. Lond. Specialty: Paediat. Socs: RSM.

OLIVER, Karen Janet Captain French Surgery, Captain French Lane, Kendal LA9 4HR — MB BS Lond. 1989; DRCOG 1994; DFFP 1995; MRCGP 1995. GP Partner.

OLIVER, Kathryn Jane Quorn Medical Centre, 1 Station Road, Quorn, Loughborough LE12 8BP Tel: 01509 412232 Fax: 01509 620652 — MB ChB Manch. 1990; DFFP 1993; MRCGP 1995. GP Princip.; Macmillan GP Facilitater, Leisc. Specialty: Gen. Pract. Socs: (Treas.) Leic. Fac. RCGP. Prev: Course Organiser Leicesrer VTS; SHO (Palliat. Care) Loros Hospice Leics.; Trainee GP Leics. VTS.

OLIVER, Keith Robert (retired) Ailsa Hame, Cwrt Bryn-Y-Bia, Craigside, Llandudno LL30 3AU Tel: 01492 540263 — (St. Bart.) MA, MB BChir Camb. 1954. Prev: Ho. Surg. & Ho. Phys. Ashford Hosp. Middlx.

OLIVER, Krista 39 Oaklands Drive, Bebington, Wirral CH63 7NB — MB ChB Leic. 1993.

OLIVER, Lorna Sherbourne Medical Centre, 40 Oxford Street, Leamington Spa CV32 4RA Tel: 01926 424736 Fax: 01926 470884; 1, The Cedars, Warwick Place, Leamington Spa CV32 5YE — MB ChB Birm. 1992; DRCOG 1995; MRCGP 1996. Princip. GP Leamington Spa. Specialty: Gen. Pract.

OLIVER, Louise 60 York Close, Bournville, Birmingham B30 2HN — MB ChB Birm. 1998. MHO (Gen. Med. & Cardiol.) Walsall Manor Hosp. Specialty: Paediat. Prev: SHO, Gen. Surg. & Colorectal, Good Hope Hosp.

OLIVER, Louise Elizabeth Low Farm, Saxlingham Nethergate, Norwich NR15 1TE — MB BS Lond. 1985.

OLIVER, Lucinda Jane Swyllmers Barn, The Lee, Great Missenden HP16 9NA Tel: 01494 837317 — MB ChB Leic. 1991; MRCP (UK) 1996. Specialist Regist. (Palliat. Med.) Michael Sobell Ho. Oxf. Specialty: Palliat. Med. Prev: SHO (Palliat. Care) Priscilla Bacon Lodge Norwich; Regist. Waikato Hosp. New Zealand.

OLIVER, Margaret Yool Abbey (retired) East Morningside House, 5 Clinton Road, Edinburgh EH9 2AW Tel: 0131 447 1417; Easter Seven Gables, South St, Elie, Leven KY9 1DN Tel: 01333 330451 — MB ChB Ed. 1947. Prev: SCMO (Family Plann.) Lothian HB & Edin.

OLIVER, Mark David 10 Browning Street, Stafford ST16 3AT Tel: 01785 258240 Fax: 01785 253119 — MB ChB (Hons.) Sheff. 1984; MRCP (UK) 1987. Prev: Regist. (Renal Med.) Leeds Gen. Infirm.; Regist. (Med.) Edin. Roy. Infirm.

OLIVER, Matthew Charles 4 Pickhill Oast, Smallhythe Road, Tenterden TN30 7LZ — MB BS Lond. 1998; MRCS (Eng.).

OLIVER, Maurice Herbert (retired) 4 Rawcliffe Grove, York YO30 6NR Tel: 01904 654122 — (Sheff.) MB ChB (Hons.) Sheff. 1944; MRCGP 1956. SBStJ. Prev: Supernum Med. Regist. Leeds Gen. Infirm.

OLIVER, Max Trahearn Windmill Medical Practice, 65 Shoot Up Hill, London NW2 3PS Tel: 020 8452 7646 Fax: 020 8450 2319; 14 Parkhill Road, London NW3 2YN — MB BS Lond. 1969.

OLIVER, Professor Michael Francis, CBE — MB ChB Ed. 1947; FRCP Ed. 1957, M 1951; MD (Gold Medal) Ed. 1957; FRCP Lond. 1969, M 1963; Hon. FACC 1973; FFPHM 1974; MD (Hon. Causa) Karolinska 1980; MD (Hon. Causa) Bologna 1985; FRACP 1987; FRSE 1987; FRCPI 1987; FESC 1988. Emerit. Prof. Univ. Edin.; Hon. Prof. Nat. Heart & Lung Inst. Lond.; Cons. Cardiovasc. Div. WHO. Specialty: Cardiol. Socs: Assn. Phys.; Med. Res. Soc.; Brit. Cardiac Soc. (Pres. 1980-84). Prev: Dir. Wynn Inst. for Metabol. Research Inst. Lond.; Duke of Edin. Prof. Cardiol. Univ. Edin.; Pres. Brit. Cardiac Soc. & Roy. Coll. Phys. Edin.

OLIVER, Michael Henry North Devon District Hospital, Barnstaple EX31 4JB Tel: 01271 322577 Fax: 01271 322709; 7 Trafalgar Lawn, Barnstaple EX32 9BD Tel: 01271 374294 — MB BS (Hons.) Lond. 1976 (Univ. Coll. Hosp.) BA (Chem.) Oxf. 1971; MRCP (UK) 1978; MD Lond. 1993; FRCP Lond. 1996. Cons. Gen. & Chest Med. N Devon Dist. Hosp. Barnstaple. Specialty: Respirat. Med.; Gen. Med. Socs: (Ex-Treas.) Brit. Thoracic Soc.; (Ex-Sec.) W. Country Chest Soc.; (Ex-Chairm. N. Devon Div.) Brit. Med. Assoc. Prev: Sen. Regist. (Gen. & Chest Med.) Bristol Roy. Infirm.; Clin. Lect. Cardiothoracic Inst. Brompton Hosp. Lond.; Regist. & SHO (Gen. Med.) Stoke City Gen. Hosp.

OLIVER, Neil McCrae Dr Carson, Oliver and Greely, The Health Centre, Academy St, Castle Douglas DG7 1EE Tel: 0155650250; 1 Whitecraigs, Whitepard Rd, Castle Douglas DG7 1EX — MB ChB Ed. 1992. GP Princip. Specialty: Gen. Pract.

OLIVER, Paul Anthony David The Surgery, 577 Carlton Road, Nottingham NG3 7AF Tel: 0115 958 0415 Fax: 0115 950 9245 — BM BS Nottm. 1980; BMedSci Nottm. 1978; DRCOG 1983; MRCGP 1984. Lect. (Gen. Pract.) Univ. Nottm. Prev: GP Nottm.

OLIVER, Peter James Robert 22 Woodlands Close, Hawsley, Camberley GU17 9HZ — MB BS Lond. 1998.

OLIVER, Peter Owen, RD Mill House, Milton Mills, Milton Abbas, Blandford Forum DT11 0BQ Tel: 01258 880675 Fax: 01258 880178 — (King's Coll. & St. Geo.) MRCS Eng. LRCP Lond. 1948; MB BS Lond. 1949; DIH Soc. Apoth. Lond. 1958; DPH Eng. 1960; MD Lond. 1964; FFOM RCP Lond. 1982, M 1978. Cons. Occupat. Health & Nautical Med. Soton.; Surg. Lt.-Cdr. RNR. Specialty: Occupat. Health. Socs: Fell. Roy. Soc. Med.; Soc. Occupat. Med. Prev: Med. Dir. Cunard Line Ltd.; Chief Med. Off. Gillette Industs. Ltd.; Sen. Indust. Med. Off. Air Corps. Jt. Med. Serv. (BOAC).

OLIVER, Peter Stephen Russell's Hall Hospital, Dudley DY1 2HQ Tel: 01384 456111 Fax: 01384 244051; 9 The Heathlands, Old Swinford, Stourbridge DY8 1NR Tel: 01384 396062 — MB Camb. 1984; MB BChir Camb. 1984; MA Camb. 1986; MRCP (UK) 1987; FRCR 1992. Cons. Radiol. Dudley Gp. Hosps. NHS Trust. Specialty: Radiol.; Nuclear Med. Prev: Sen. Regist. (Diagn. Radiol.) W. Midl. RHA.; Regist. (Gen. Med.) Glos. Roy. Hosp. Gloucester; SHO (Gen. Med.) Norf. & Norwich Hosp.

OLIVER, Philip David Chard Road Surgery, Chard Road, St Budeaux, Plymouth PL5 2UE — MRCS Eng. LRCP Lond. 1984 (Guy's Hospital) MRCGP 1990.

OLIVER, Philip Peter Market Surgery, Warehouse Lane, Wath-On-Dearne, Rotherham S63 7RA Tel: 01709 877524 — MB ChB Bristol 1984; MRCGP 1988.

OLIVER, Raife Morgan Cromer Group Brachee, Ovestrand Road, Cromer Tel: 01263 513148 — MB ChB Leic. 1991 (Leicester) DCH RCP Lond. 1993; DRCOG 1995; MRCGP 1996. Gen. Practitioner. Specialty: Gen. Pract.

OLIVER, Raymond Ernest Willis (retired) 4 Crosslands Avenue, Ealing Common, London W5 3QH Tel: 020 8993 3345 — MRCS Eng. LRCP Lond. 1940 (Middlx.) FRCGP 1994, M 1953; DIH Soc. Apoth. Lond. 1962; DIH Eng. 1963; MFOM RCP Lond. 1978. Prev: Squadron Ldr. RAFVR.

OLIVER, Richard Ecclesfield Group Practice, 96A Mill Road, Ecclesfield, Sheffield S35 9XQ Tel: 0114 246 9151/0114 257 0935 Email: richard.oliver@gp-c88039.nhs.uk — MB ChB Sheff. 1983; MRCGP 1988; Dip. Occ. Med. RCP Lond. 1996. GP Partner; GP Mem. N. Sheff. PCT Exec. Comm. Lead Responsibil. for Prescribing/Commiss.ing. Specialty: Gen. Pract. Prev: Trainee GP Sheff.; SHO (Psychiat.) Middlewood Hosp. Sheff.; SHO (Geriat.) North. Gen. Hosp. Sheff.

OLIVER, Mr Richard Hywel Picton (retired) Cefn Llwyn, 26 Ffriddoedd Road, Bangor LL57 2TW — (Univ. Coll. Hosp.) MS Lond. 1966, MB BS 1948; FRCS Eng. 1954 MRCS Eng. LRCP Lond. 1948. Prev: Cons. Surg. Caernarvon & Anglesey Gen. Hosp. Bangor.

OLIVER, Richard Martin Cardiology Department, Castle Hill Hospital, Castle Road, Cottingham, Hull HU 16 5JQ Tel: 01482 622044 Fax: 01482 622045 — MB BS Lond. 1980 (St. George's Hospital Medical School London) MRCP (UK) 1985; DM Soton 1992; FRCP Lond. 1998; FESC 1999. Cons. Cardiol., Hull & E. Yorks. Hosps. NHS Trust, Hull, E. Yorks. Specialty: Cardiol. Socs: Brit. Cardiac Soc.; BMA; FESC. Prev: Sen. Regist. & Regist. (Cardiol.) Middlx. & Univ. Coll. Hosp. Lond.; Clin. Research Fell. (Cardiovasc. Med.) Soton. Gen. Hosp.; Regist. (Med.) Portsmouth Hosps.

OLIVER, Professor Roderick Timothy Desmond Department Medical Oncology, St. Bartholomew's Hospital & Royal Lond. School Med. & Dent., 1st Floor KGV, West Smithfield, London EC1A 7BE Tel: 020 7601 8522 Fax: 020 7796 0432 Email: r.t.oliver@qmul.ac.uk — MB BChir Camb. 1966 (Lond. Hosp.) MRCS Eng. LRCP Lond. 1966; FRCP Lond. 1986, M 1968; MD Camb. 1975. Prof. Med. Oncol. Med. Coll. Roy. Lond. Hosp.; Chair

N. E. Lond. Urological Oncol. Tumor Bd. Specialty: Oncol. Special Interest: Urological Cancers. Socs: Roy. Soc. of Med.; Brit. Assn. of Urological Surgeons; Brit. Oncol. Assn. Prev: Sen. Lect. (Med. Oncol.) Inst. Urol. Lond.; Sen. Scientif. Off. Dept. Med. Oncol. St. Bart. Hosp. Lond.; Lect. (Immunol.) Dept. Tissue Immunol. Lond. Hosp. Med. Coll.

OLIVER, Ronald Martin, CB, RD (retired) Greenhill House, Beech Avenue, Effingham, Leatherhead KT24 5PH Tel: 01372 452887 — (King's Coll. Lond. & St. Geo.) MD Lond. 1965, MB BS 1952; MRCS Eng. LRCP Lond. 1952; DCH Eng. 1954, DPH 1960, DIH 1961; MFOM RCP Lond. 1978; MFCM 1987; MRCP (UK) 1987; FRCP (UK) 1998. Prev: Dep. Chief Med. Off. Dept. of Health.

OLIVER, Rosalind Mary A Block, Medway Maritime Hospital, Windmill Rd, Gillingham ME7 5NY Tel: 01634 833828 Fax: 01634 830082; 18 King's Avenue, Rochester ME1 3DS — MB BS Lond. 1972; MRCS Eng. LRCP Lond. 1972; DPM Leeds 1975; MRCPsych 1977. Cons. Psychiat. Thames Gateway NHS Trust. Specialty: Gen. Psychiat. Socs: BMA; NHS Cons. Assn. Prev: Cons. Psychiat. Thameslink Healthcare NHS Trust; Cons. Psychiat. Centr. Notts. NHS Trust; Cons. Psychiat. Invicta Community NHS Trust.

OLIVER, Rosemary 28 Dawlish Road, Dudley DY1 4LU Tel: 01902 885926 — MB ChB Liverp. 1989; BSc (Hons.) Liverp. 1986, MB ChB 1989.

OLIVER, Sarah Elizabeth — MB BS Newc. 1993.

OLIVER, Shirley Mary Morven, Blackhall Colliery, Hartlepool TS27 4EE Tel: 01429 586 4331 — MB BS Durh. 1959.

OLIVER, Stephen Francis Oliver and Partners, The Guildhall Surgery, Lower Baxter Street, Bury St Edmunds IP33 1ET Tel: 01284 701601 Fax: 01284 702943 — MB BS Lond. 1964 (Middlx.) DObst RCOG 1968; FRCGP 1979, M 1972. Prev: Ho. Phys. Middlx. Hosp. Lond.; Ho. Surg. Centr. Middlx. Hosp.; Course Organiser W. Suff. VTS.

OLIVER, Steven Edward Bracken Hill Lodge, North Road, Leigh Woods, Bristol BS8 3PL — BM BS Nottm. 1989; MRCP (UK) 1992.

OLIVER, Stuart Dean Covance Clinical Research Unit, Springfield House, Hyde St., Leeds LS2 9NG Tel: 0113 244 8071 Fax: 0113 237 3546; 5 Forest Hill Gardens, Outlane, Huddersfield HD3 3GA — MB BChir Camb. 1982; MB Camb. 1982, BChir 1981; MA Camb. 1986; MRCGP 1986; Dip. Pharm. Med. RCP (UK) 1991; MFPM RCP (UK) 1996. Med. Dir. (Pharmaceut. Med.) Covance Clin. Research Unit. Specialty: Pharmaceutical Medicine.

OLIVER, Sybil Enid Kathleen (retired) 2 Courtenay House, Kingsway, Hove BN3 2WF Tel: 01273 732051 — (TC Dub.) BA, MB BCh BAO Dub. 1949. Prev: Sessional Med. Off. Brighton & Hove Family Plann. Assn.

OLIVER, Thomas Barry Clinincal Radiology Department, Ninewells Hospital and Medical School, Dundee Tel: 01382 660111 — MB ChB Ed. 1988; MRCP (UK) 1991; FRCR 1996. Cons. Radiologist, Clin. Radiol. Dept., Ninewellas Hosp. and Med. Sch., Dundee. Specialty: Radiol.

OLIWIECKI, Simone Department of Dermatology, New Cross Hospital, Wolverhampton WV10 0QP Tel: 01902 642830; Desmonde, Edgerton Road, Egerton, Huddersfield HD3 3AA — MB ChB Manch. 1982; MRCP (UK) 1985. Cons. Dermatol., Roy. Wolverhampton Hosps. NHS Trust. Specialty: Dermat. Prev: Research Regist. Bristol Roy. Infirm.

OLLERENSHAW, Katherine Judith 25 Meadowlands, Portstewart BT55 7FG — BM BS Nottm. 1988; BMedSci Nottm. 1986; DRCOG 1991; MRCGP 1992. Socs: BMA.

OLLERHEAD, Elizabeth — MB BS Lond. 1986; DCH RCP Lond. 1989; DRCOG 1991; MSc (Pub. Health Med.) Lond. 1994; MRCGP 1995; MFPHM 1998. Cons. in Pub. Health, Eastleigh and test Valley S. PCT. Specialty: Pub. Health Med.

OLLERHEAD, Mr Keith John New Chineham Surgery, Reading Road, Chineham, Basingstoke RG24 8ND Tel: 01256 479244 Fax: 01256 814190; The Barn House, Orchard Farm, Cowfold Lane, Rotherwick, Hook RG27 9BP Tel: 01831 818063 — MB ChB Manch. 1982; BSc Manch. 1977; MB ChB (Hons.) Manch. 1982; FRCS Ed. 1987; MRCGP 1989. Chair N. Hants. PCG. Specialty: Gastroenterol. Socs: Manch. Med. Soc. Prev: Trainee GP Manch. VTS; Research Fell. (Surgic. Gastroenterol.) Manch. Roy. Infirm.; Regist. Rotat. (Surg.) Roy. Hallamsh. Hosp. Sheff.

OLLERTON, Andrew Hawkley Brook Surgery, Highfield Grange Avenue, Wigan WN3 6SU Tel: 01942 234740 Fax: 01942 820037 — MB ChB Birm. 1982.

OLLERTON, Joanne Emma 1 Jacquemart Close, Coalville LE67 4QP Email: j.ollerton@doctors.org.uk — MB ChB Bristol 1993; RCS Ed.; RAMC; MRCP; Dip IMC.

OLLERTON, Stephen James Abraham 25 Chantrell Court, The Calls, Leeds LS2 7HA — MB ChB Leeds 1998. SHO in A & E, at St James, Leeds. Specialty: Accid. & Emerg. Socs: Affil. of Roy. Coll. of Surg.s. Prev: PRHO Surg., Roy. Halifax; PRHO Med. Halifax Gen.

OLLEY, Lorraine Michelle 166 Leesons Hill, Chislehurst BR7 6QL — MB BS Lond. 1998.

OLLEY, Peter William 29 Bridge Park, Gosforth, Newcastle upon Tyne NE3 2DX Tel: 0191 284 5560; The Village Green Surgery, The Green, Wallsend NE28 6BB Tel: 0191 295 8500 Fax: 0191 295 8519 — MB BS Newc. 1982 (Newc. u. Tyne) DRCOG 1992; MRCGP 1995. Specialty: Gen. Pract. Socs: Roy. Coll. Gen. Pract.; BMA. Prev: Trainee GP Northumbria VTS; Regist. (O & G) Bellshill Matern. Hosp. Lanarksh.; Regist. (O & G) South. Gen. & Qu. Mothers Hosps. Glas.

OLLEY, Mr Stephen Francis c/o The Oral Surgery Department, Shrewsbury Hospital (Copthorne North), Mytton Oak Road, Shrewsbury SY3 8BR Tel: 01743 231122; (resid.) Carmel House, 47 The Mount, Shrewsbury SY3 8PP Tel: 01743 361714 — MB BS Lond. 1972; BDS (Hons.) 1968; FDS RCS Eng. 1974; FRCS Ed. 1985. Cons. Oral & Maxillofacial Surg. W. Midl. RHA. Specialty: Oral & Maxillofacial Surg. Socs: Fell. BAOMS; EAOMFS.

OLLIFF, Jennifer Mary (retired) Grevels House, Chipping Campden GL55 6AG Tel: 01386 840395 — MB ChB Bristol 1949. Prev: Sen. Resid. Off. Bristol Eye Hosp.

OLLIFF, Julie Frances Caroline Clinical Radiology Department, Queen Elizabeth Hospital, Queen Elizabeth Medical Centre, Birmingham B15 2TH Tel: 0121 627 2458 Fax: 0121 697 8290 — BM BS Nottm. 1979; BMedSci Nottm. 1977; MRCP (UK) 1983; FRCR 1987. Cons. Radiol. Qu. Eliz. Hosp. & Univ. Hosp. Birm. NHS Trust. Specialty: Radiol. Prev: Sen. Lect. (Diagn. Radiol.) Roy. Marsden Hosp. Sutton; Sen. Regist. (Diagn. Radiol.) St. Geo. Hosp. Lond.

OLLIFF, Simon Piers Clinical Radiology Department, Queen Elizabeth Hospital, Queen Elizabeth Medical Centre, Birmingham B15 2TH Tel: 0121 697 8488 Fax: 0121 697 8290 Email: simon.olliff@uhb.nhs.uk; 57 Moor Green Lane, Moseley, Birmingham B13 8NE — MB BS Lond. 1979 (Camb. & Univ. Coll. Hosp.) MA Camb. 1980, BA 1976; MRCP (UK) 1983; FRCR 1988. Cons. Radiol. Qu. Eliz. Hosp. Birm. & Univ. Hosp. Birm. NHS Trust; Hon. Cons. Radiol., Birm. Childr.s Hosp. Specialty: Radiol. Socs: Liveryman Soc. Apoth. City Lond.; Brit. Soc. Interven. Radiol.; Special Interest Gp. For Gastrointestinal and Abdom. Radiol. Prev: Sen. Regist. (Radiol.) King's Coll. Hosp. Lond.

OLLIFF-COOPER, Anna Katharine Chalford Manor, Stoney Cross, Lyndhurst SO43 7GP Tel: 023 8081 2202 — MB BS Lond. 1973 (St. Bart.) MRCS Eng. LRCP Lond. 1973; MRCP (UK) 1979; MRCGP 1985. Clin. Asst. (A & E) Soton. Gen. Hosp. Specialty: Accid. & Emerg.

OLLIFFE, David James 5 Bryn y Gors, Morriston, Swansea SA6 6DQ — MB BCh Wales 1988; MRCGP 1992.

OLLIVER, Mary Elizabeth 11 Pitter Close, Littleton, Winchester SO22 6PD — MB BS Lond. 1987; T(GP) 1992; MFFP 1994. SCMO Margt. Pyke Centre Lond.; Clin. Asst Med./GUM Elderly Hosp.; Clin. Asst. Breast Unit Roy. Harb Co. Hosp. Winchester. Specialty: Family Plann. & Reproduc. Health; Genitourinary Medicine. Socs: Chairm. Lond. Soc. of Family Plann. Doctors.

OLLIVER, Richard John The Health Centre, Kings Road, Horley RH6 7DG Tel: 01293 772686 Fax: 01293 823950; 2 Limes Avenue, Horley RH6 9DH Tel: 01293 786710 — MB BS Lond. 1969 (St. Geo.) DCH Eng. 1971; DObst RCOG 1972; Cert. Family Plann. JCC 1974; MRCGP 1974; PHEC certificate RCS (Ed) 1998. Specialty: Gen. Pract. Socs: Co. Med.off.St John's Ambul. surrey. Prev: Trainee GP Wessex VTS; SHO (Paediat.) Qu. Mary's Hosp. Childr. Carshalton; SHO (O & G) Roy. Hants. Co. Hosp. Winchester.

OLNEY, Jonathan Simon Hurstwood Park Neuro Centre, Brighton and Sussex University Hospitals NHS Trust, Lewes Road, Haywards Heath RH16 4EX Tel: 01444 441881 — MB BS Lond. 1974; FRCR

1985. Cons. Radiol. Hurstwood Pk. Neurol. Centre. Specialty: Radiol. Prev: Sen. Regist. Nat. Hosp. Nerv. Dis. Lond.

OLNEY, Peter John (retired) 216 St Faith's Road, Old Catton, Norwich NR6 7AG Tel: 01603 426652 — MB BS Lond. 1953 (Lond. Hosp.) DObst RCOG 1956. Prev: SHO (Obst.) St. Mary's Hosp. Wom. & Childr. Manch.

OLNEY, Shelagh Mary The Surgery, 1 Glebe Road, Barnes, London SW13 0DR Tel: 020 8748 1065 Fax: 020 8741 8665 — MB BS Lond. 1986 (King's Coll. Sch. Med. & Dent.) BSc Warwick 1981; DRCOG 1989; DCH RCP Lond. 1990; MRCGP 1996. Gen. Practitioner, Barnes; Clin. Asst. (Dermat.) Qu. Mary's Hosp. Lond.; Hon.Sen. Lect. Primary Care Imperial Coll. of Sci., Technol. & Med. Prev: Occupat. Health Phys. BBC.

OLOBIA, Edirhiohwo Victoria Atamu 30 Mandarin Court, Edward St., London SE8 5HL — MB BS Lond. 1994.

OLOBO-LALOBO, James Henry 93 Harley Street, London W1N 1DF Tel: 020 7935 2627 Fax: 020 7935 4435; Obul, 49 Finchley Lane, London NW4 1BY — MB ChB Makerere 1973 (Makerere Univ. Med. Sch. Kampala) MSc Lond. 1978; MRCOG 1980. Cons. O & G Harley St. Lond.; Cons. Gyn. Populat. Servs. Europe. Specialty: Obst. & Gyn. Socs: BMA & Roy. Soc. Med. Prev: Regist. (O & G) Ealing Hosp.

OLOJUGBA, Mr Oladeji Henry 16 Shenton Park Avenue, Sale M33 4NZ — MB BS Benin 1988; MB BS Benin, Nigeria 1988; FRCS Ed. 1993.

OLORUNDA, Mr Harry Ladipo Olufemi Caithness General Hospital, Bankhead Road, Caithness, Wick KN1 5HS — MB BS Lagos 1971; FWACS; FRCOG 1995, M 1981. Cons.(Obst. & Gyno.) Caithness Gen. Hosp. Specialty: Obst. & Gyn. Special Interest: Womens Sexual Health.

OLOTO, Mr Emeka Josiah 74 Sunnigdale Ave, Alwoodley, Leeds W17 7SN Tel: 0113 269 1130 Fax: 0113 269 1130 Email: ejoloto@bigfoot.com — MB BS Nigeria 1982; MRCOG 1993; MFFP 1994. Specialist Regist. in D&G, Princess Roy. Hosp., Hull. Specialty: Obst. & Gyn. Socs: Fell. W. Afr. Postgrad. Med. Coll.; Eur. Soc. Contracep. Prev: Research Fell. & Hon. Sen. Regist. St. James Univ. Hosp. Leeds; Regist. (O & G) S. Tyneside Dist. Hosp., Furness Gen. Hosp., Roy. Vict. Infirm. & Princess Mary Matern. Hosp. Newc.

OLSBURGH, Bernard Whitley Road Health Centre, Whitley Road, Whitley Bay NE26 2ND; 12 Westfield Grove, Newcastle upon Tyne NE3 4YA Tel: 0191 213 0668 — MB BS Newc. 1966; DObst RCOG 1968; FRCGP 1993, M 1971. Local Med. Off. Whitley Bay; Train. Northumbria VTS.

OLSBURGH, Mr Jonathon David 28 Oakdene Drive, Leeds LS17 8XW — MB ChB Leeds 1993; FRCS Eng. 1997. Specialty: Urol.

OLSEN, Noel David Lyche Oakdale, Court Wood, Newton Ferrers, Plymouth PL8 1BW Tel: 01752 873054 Fax: 01752 872653 Email: noelolsen@clara.co.uk — (St. Geo.) FFPHM; MB BS Lond. 1969; MRCP (UK) 1973; MSc (Social Med.) Lond. 1978; FFCM 1986, M 1979; FRCP Lond. 1993. Indep. Pub. Health Phys.; Chairm. Alcohol Educat. & Research Counc. UK; Hon. Sec. Internat. Agency on Tobacco & Health; Hon. Treas. Nat. Heart Forum; Chairm. Watervoice SW; Cons. Adviser, Fuel Poverty DEFRA. Specialty: Pub. Health Med. Socs: (Ex.) BMA (Counc. 1993-98); (Ex. Hon. Sec.) Nat. Heart Forum; (Ex. Hon. Sec.) ASH (1975 - 1994). Prev: DPH Plymouth & Hampstead; DCP & Assoc. Lect. Camb.; Hon. Sen. Lect. Roy. Free Hosp. Sch. Med. Lond.

OLSON, Ian Alistair (retired) 20 Burns Road, Aberdeen AB15 4NS Tel: 01224 316497 — MD Aberd. 1969; MB ChB 1962. Prev: Vice-Dean & Prof. (Human Morphol. & Experim. Path.) Kuwait Med. Sch.

OLSON, James John 28 Leven Close, Chandlers Ford, Eastleigh SO53 4SH — MB BS Lond. 1997 (St Georges) SHO in Anaesth., Carshalton. Specialty: Anaesth.

OLSON, John Alexander The Eye Clinic, Aberdeen Royal Infirmary, Foresterhill, Aberdeen AB25 2ZN Tel: 0122468 1818 — MB ChB Aberd. 1987; MRCP UK 1990; MD Aberd. 2000; FRCP Edin. 2001. Cons. Med. Opthalmology Aberd. Roy. Hosp. Trust. Specialty: Ophth. Prev: Sen. Regist. Med. Opthalmology Aberd. Roy. Hosp. Trust; Research Fell. Diabetic Retinopathy Aberd. Roy. Hosp. Trust; Regist. Gen. Med. Aberd. Roy. Hosp. Trust.

OLSON, Shona Department of Radiology, Aberdeen Royal Infirmary, Foresterhill, Aberdeen AB25 2ZN Tel: 01224 681818 — MB ChB Aberd. 1991. Specialist Regist. inDiagnostic Radiol. Specialty: Radiol.

OLUFUNWA, Philip Bandele Harrow Road Health Centre, 263-265 Harrow Road, London W2 5EZ Tel: 020 7286 1231 Fax: 020 7266 1253 — MB BS Ibadan 1975; MB BS Ibadan 1975.

OLUGBILE, Adedapo Olumuyiwa Babatunde 27 Lucien Road, London SW17 8HS — MB ChB Leeds 1966; MRCPI 1972; FRCPI 1992.

OLUJOHUNGBE, Adebayo Babayide Kolade 16 Howard Avenue, Cheadle Hulme, Cheadle SU8 6HH Tel: 0151 529 2837 Fax: 0151 529 3310 Email: aoluohungbe@btclick.com — MB BS Ibadan 1985; MRCPath; MD; Dip. Haemat. Lond. 1989; MRCP (UK) 1992. Cons. Haematologist. Specialty: Haematology. Special Interest: Haemoglobinopathy; Myeloma. Socs: Royal College of Physicians; Royal College of Pathologists. Prev: Regist. (Haemat.) Edgware Gen. Hosp.; Regist. (Haemat.) Roy. Free Hosp. Lond.; Sen. Regist. Manch. Roy. Infirm.

OLUONYE, Ngozi Margaret Dept. of Clinical Health, Royal Free Hospital, NHS Trust, Pond St., London NW3 Tel: 020 7830 2440 Fax: 020 7830 200 3 Email: noluonye@rfhsm.ac.uk; 1 Holly Farm Close, Caddington, Luton LU1 4ET Tel: 01582 452998 — MB BS Ibadan 1986 (College of Medicine, Univ of Ibadau, Nigeria) MRCP (UK) 1993. Specialist Regist. Community Paediat., (p/t) - Roy. Free Hosp., NHS Trust, Pond St., Lond. Specialty: Community Child Health. Prev: Specialist Regist. Communitgy Paediat. (p/t), Roy. Free Hosp. Lond.; Specialist Regist. Community Paediat. (p/t), S. Beds. Community Health Care Trust., Lutton; Paediat. Regis., Lutton & Dunstable Hosp., Dutton.

OLUSANYA, Adolphus Akinola Adesanya 18 Waterloo Close, Jack Dunning Estate, London E9 6EF — LRCPI & LM, LRSCI & LM 1965; LRCPI & LM, LRCSI & LM 1965.

OLUWAJANA, Mr Folajogun Michael Department of Surgery, Chesterfield & North Derbyshire Royal Hospital, Chesterfield S44 5BL Email: jogunoluwajana@msn.com; 6 Fairfield Drive, Ashgate, Chesterfield S42 7PU — MB BS Ibadan 1979; MB BS Ibadan, Nigeria 1979; FRCS Ed. 1988. Staff Surg. (Gen. Surg.) Chesterfield & N. Derbysh. Roy. Hosp. NHS Trust. Specialty: Gen. Surg. Prev: Regist. (Surg.) Scunthorpe HA.

OLUWOLE, Mr Matthew Olufunso Kolawole City Hospital, Department of Otorlaryngology, Birmingham B60 2TQ Tel: 0121 5074559 Email: matthew.oluwole@swbh.net.uk — MB BS Ibadan 1983; FRCS (Otol.) Ed. 1991. Cons. E.N.T. Surg., City Hosp., Birm.. B18 &QH. Specialty: Otolaryngol. Special Interest: Rhinology. Socs: BAOL; HNS; Head & Neck Surg.s. Prev: Cons. Otolaryngol. Memor. Hosp. Darlington.

OLVER, Miss Jane Madeleine Charing Cross Hospital, Fulham Palace Road, London W6 8RF Tel: 0208 846 1497 Fax: 0208 846 1959; Western Eye Hospital, Marylebone Road, London NW1 5YE Tel: 0207 886 3264 Fax: 0207 886 3259 — MB BS Lond. 1979 (St. Thos.) BSc (Hons.) Lond. 1976; DO RCS Eng. 1983; FRCS Eng. 1984; FRCOphth St Thomas 1984. Cons. Ophth. & Oculoplastic Surg. Char. Cross Hosp. & West. Eye Hosp. Lond. Specialty: Ophth. Socs: Roy. Soc. Med.; Founder Sec. Brit. Oculoplastic Surg. Soc. Prev: Sen. Regist. Moorfields Eye Hosp. Lond.; Francis & Rene Hock Jun. Research Fell. Moorfields Eye Hosp.; Regist. (Ophth.) Univ. Hosp. Wales Cardiff & SHO (Neurosurg.) Brook Hosp. Lond.

OLVER, Julian John, TD 28 Oakleigh Park South, Whetstone, London N20 9JP Tel: 020 8446 4315 Email: medical@olver.org.uk — MB BS Lond. 1974 (St. Thos.) FFA RCS Eng. 1981. Cons. Anaesth. Chase Farm Hosp. Enfield. Specialty: Anaesth. Socs: Assn. Anaesth.; Intens. Care Soc.; BMA Armed Forces Comm. 2002-. Prev: Sen. Regist. (Anaesth.) Roy. Free Hosp. Lond.; Regist. (Anaesth.) Univ. Coll. Hosp. Lond.; SHO St. Thos. Hosp. Lond.

OLVER, Julie Diane 36 The Grove, Hales Road, Cheltenham GL52 6SX — MB ChB Birm. 1984; DRCOG 1989. GP Cheltenham & Staunton Retainer Scheme. Prev: Trainee GP Worcester.

OLVER, Michael John Middlewich Road Surgery, 6 Middlewich Road, Sandbach CW11 1DL Tel: 01270 767411 Fax: 01270 759305 — MB BS Lond. 1960 (Univ. Coll. Hosp.) MRCS Eng. LRCP Lond. 1960; DObst RCOG 1961. Socs: BMA. Prev: Ho. Off. Obst. St. Mary's Hosps. Manch.; Ho. Phys. Paediat. Duchess of York Hosp. Babies Manch.

OLVER, Richard Edmund 45 West Side, Wandsworth Common, London SW18 2EE — MB BS Lond. 1966; BSc (Physiol.) Lond.

1963, MB BS 1966; FRCP Lond. 1982, M 1970. Reader (Paediat.) Univ. Coll. Lond.; Cons. Paediat. Univ. Coll. Hosp. Lond. Specialty: Paediat. Prev: Ho. Phys. Med. Unit & Dept. Paediat. St. Thos. Hosp. Lond.; MRC Trav. Fell. Cardiovasc. Research Inst. Univ. Calif. San; Francisco USA; Vis. Prof. Physiol. Univ. New York USA.

OLVER, William John Department of Microbiology, Ninewells Hospital, Dundee Tel: 01382 632559 — MB ChB Aberd. 1993; BMedBiol. Aberd. 1992. Consultant (microbiology) Ninewells Hosp., Dundee. Specialty: Med. Microbiol. Socs: BMA; MDDUS. Prev: Specialist Regist. (Microbiol.) Qu. Med. Centre, Nottm.; SHO (Cas.) West. Infirm. Glas.; SHO (Infect. Dis.) Roy. Free Hosp.

OLVERMAN, George Nicholson Department of Accident and Emergency, Macclesfield District General Hospital, 3 Victoria Road, Macclesfield SK10 3BL — MB ChB Glas. 1984; BSc Hons. Glas. 1978; FFARCS Dub 1992. Cons. A & E Maeclesfield Dutet Gen. Hosp. Specialty: Accid. & Emerg. Socs: BMA.

OM PRAKASH, Manni 19 The Loning, Colindale, London NW9 6DR — MB BS Madras 1977.

OMARA-BOTO, Tom Cabin Adie University College Hospital, Huntley St., London WC1E 6DH; 221 Rosendale Road, West Dulwich, London SE21 8LW — MRCS Eng. LRCP Lond. 1980; Cert. Family Plann. RCOG 1982; MRCOG 1986. Sen. Regist. (O & G) Univ. Coll. Hosp. Lond.; Mem. Europ. Soc. Hysteroscopy (Lond. Represen.). Specialty: Obst. & Gyn. Socs: BMA. Prev: Research Fell. Lond. Hosp. Med. Coll. Newham Gen. Hosp.; Regist. (O & G) Whittington Hosp. Lond.; SHO (O & G) King's Coll. Hosp. Lond.

OMARI, Amy Anita Aika c/o Drive R. Morgan, 54 Rosemead Avenue, Pensby, Wirral CH61 9NW — MB BCh Wales 1989; DTM & H Liverp. 1990; MRCP (Paediat.) 1997. SHO (Paediat.) Wirral. Specialty: Paediat. Prev: Trainee GP Wirral.

OMAYER, Mr Abdalla Salim 12 The Greenway, Hounslow TW4 7AJ — MB BCh Cairo 1973; FRCS Glas. 1983.

OMER, Fazal The Headland Surgery, 113 Durham Street, Hartlepool TS24 0HU Tel: 01429 288100 Fax: 01429 282500; 21 Bankston Close, Hartlepool TS26 0PP — MB ChB Dundee 1984. Prev: Trainee GP Scunthorpe VTS; SHO (Anaesth.) Gen. Hosp. Hartlepool.

OMER, Salah El Din Mohamed Department of Neurology, Kingston Hospital, Galsworth Road, Kingston upon Thames KT2 7QB Tel: 020 8546 7711 Ext: 3348 Fax: 020 8934 3391 Email: sarah.omer@kingstonhospital.nhs.uk — MB BS 1980; MRCP UK 1985; FRCP Edin. 1996; FRCP Lond 2001. Cons. Neurologist, Kingston Hosp.; Cons. Neurologist, St Georges Hosp. Tooting. Specialty: Neurol. Special Interest: Epilepsy; headaches; neuro-Genetics. Socs: Assn. of Brit. Neurologists; Amer. Acad. of Neurol.; pan Arab Neurol. Soc. Prev: Cons. Neurologist, Halifax Gen. Hosp. and Leeds Gen. Infirm.; Cons. Neurologist, King Kahlid Nat. Guard Hosp., Saudi Arabia.

OMOKANYE, Adenike Musili Bassetlaw NHS Trust, Worksop S81 0BD Tel: 01909 481156 Email: omokanye@aol.com; Wentworth House, 57 Water Meadows, Worksop S80 3DB Tel: 01909 481156 Email: omokanye@aol.com — (Ahmadu Bello Univ. Zaria Nigeria) MBBS 1985; DCH 1993; MRCPI 1997; MRCPCH 1997. GP Regist., Bawtry health centre. Specialty: Gen. Pract.; Paediat. Prev: SHO Obst. & Gynae. Wom.s hosp, Dorchester Roy.; SHO Psychiat., Doncaster Roy. Infirminary; Staff grade Paediat., Bassetlaw Hosp.

OMOKANYE, Salmon Ajikanle South East Sheffield Primary Care Trust, Central Health Clinic, 1 Mulberry Street, Sheffield S1 2PJ Tel: 0114 271 6800 Email: salmon.omokanye@sheffieldse-pct.nhs.uk; Wentworth House, 57 Water Meadows, Worksop S80 3DB Tel: 01909 481156 Email: omokanye@aol.com — MB BS Ibadan 1980; FMCOG (Nigeria) 1989; MRCOG 1992; MFFP 1993. Cons. in Contracep. and Reproductive Health Care. Specialty: Gen. Pract.; Obst. & Gyn. Socs: Brit. Menopause Soc.; Europ. Soc. for Contracep.; Brit. Soc. for Colposcopy and Cervical Path. Prev: Vocational Train. scheme, Rotheram; Sen. Clin. Med. Off., family Plann. and reproductive health care, Nottg; Staff Grade in OBS and Gynal.Bassetlaw Hosp.

OMOLOLU, Mr Ajibade Gabriel 46 Pasquier Road, Walthamstow, London E17 6HB — MB BS Lagos 1983; FRCS Ed. 1992.

OMOREGBEE, Mr Anthony Igbinoghodua Kayode 71 Albany Road, Hornchurch RM12 4AE — MB BS Lagos 1975; FRCS Glas. 1990.

OMRAN, Hany Talaat Ibrahim Yeovil District Hospital, Higher Kingston, Yeovil BA21 4AT Tel: 01935 475122; 11 Oakleigh, Sampson Wood, Yeovil BA20 2SR Tel: 01935 422880 — MB BCh Cairo 1982; MRCOG 1994. Staff Grade Practitioner, O & G, Yeovil Dist. Hosp. Yeovil. Specialty: Obst. & Gyn. Socs: BMA.

ON, Fei Wen Flat 1/L, 314 St George's Road, Glasgow G3 6JR — MB ChB Glas. 1995.

ONAFOWOKAN, Jamilat Aduke Airedale General Hospital, Skipton Road, Steeton, Keighley BD20 6td — MB ChB Leeds 1980; MRCP (UK) 1983; MD Leeds 1988. Cons. (Elderly Med.) Airedale Gen. Hosp. Keighley.

ONEILL, Mary Frances 19 South Parade, Belfast BT7 2GL — MB BCh BAO Belf. 1983; DO RCPSI 1988.

ONEN, Tom Sunny 186 Orchards Way, Beckenham BR3 3EU Tel: 020 8650 7809 — MB ChB Makerere 1976; MRCPsych 1986. Cons. Psychiat. St. Thos. Hosp. Lond.; Hon. Sen. Lect. UMDS Guy's & St. Thos. Hosps. Lond. Specialty: Gen. Psychiat. Prev: Regist. (Psychiat.) Crawley Hosp; Sen. Regist. Rotat. (Psychiat.) St. Thos. & Guy's Hosps. Lond.

ONG, Albert Chee Meng Clinical Sciences Centre, Division of Clinical Sciences (North), University of Sheffield, Northern General Hospital, Herries Road, Sheffield S5 7AU — BM BCh Oxf. 1984 (Oxford) MA Oxf. 1986, BA (Hons.) 1981; MRCP (UK) 1987; DM Oxf. 1997; FRCP Lond. 2003. Sen. Lect. & Cons. Nephrol., Univ. of Sheff. Specialty: Nephrol. Prev: Sen. Regist., (Nephrol.), Oxf. Renal Unit; NKRF Sen. Research Fell., Oxf. Univ.; Clin. Lect. (Med.) Univ. Coll. Lond. Med. Sch.

ONG, Christina 9 West Heath Avenue, London NW11 7QS — MB BS Lond. 1997.

ONG, Mr Eng Kwee Western General Hospital, Department of Urology, Crewe Road South, Edinburgh EH4 2XU Tel: 0131 537 1000 Email: engong@doctors.org.uk — MB BCh BAO NUI 1995 (Cork) FRCSI 1999; MRCS Glas. 1999; MSc Liverp. 2003. Specialist Regist. (Urol.) West. Gen. Hosp. Edin. Specialty: Urol. Special Interest: Peri-operative nutritional supplementation. Prev: Specialist Regist. (Urol.) Aberd. Roy. Infirm.; Specialist Regist. (Urol.) Raigmore Hosp. Inverness; Surgic. Train. Mersey Deanery.

ONG, Miss Evelyn Geok Peng 9 Ridgeway Gardens, Highgate, London N6 5XR Tel: 020 7272 2841 — MB BS Lond. 1994 (Royal Free Hospital) BSc Lond. 1991; FRCS Eng. 1998. SHO Neonat. Unit, Chelsea & Westminster. Specialty: Paediat. Surg. Prev: SHO Surg., Derriford Hosp. Plymouth; SHO Paediat. Surg., Brist. Childr.s Hosp.

ONG, Florina Geok-Cheong 10 Holme Lacey Road, London SE12 0HR — MB BS Lond. 1992.

ONG, Grace May Leng 23 Martinville Park, Belfast BT8 7JH — MB BCh BAO Belf. 1993 (Qu. Univ. Belf.) SHO Microbiol. Roy. Vict. Dept. Belf. Specialty: Med. Microbiol. Socs: BMA; Med. Sickness Soc.

ONG, Hean Yee 18 Rossdale Road, Belfast BT8 6TG Tel: 028 9079 3198 Email: heanong@doctors.org.uk; Lot 71A Jalan Tasek, Kuala Lumpur 58100, Malaysia Tel: 00 603 7811740 — MB BCh BAO Belf. 1994; MRCP Edin. 1998. Specialty: Gen. Med.

ONG, Jeannie Peng Lan 5 Barnfield Close, Cardiff CF23 8LN — MB BCh Wales 1995.

ONG, Juling 136 The Colonnades, 34 Porchester Square, London W2 6AP — MB BS 1996; MRCS 2001.

ONG, Kar-Binh FLat 12 Cathedral Lodge, 110-115 Aldersgate St., London EC1A 4JE — MB BS Lond. 1995.

ONG, Kenneth Kian Leong 69 Glebe Road, Cambridge CB1 7TF Email: ko224@cam.ac.uk — MB BChir Camb. 1991 (Camb. & Guy's Hosp. Lond.) MA Camb. 1992; MRCP (UK) 1994. Clin. Lect. (Paed. Endocrinol.) Addenbrookes Hosp., Camb. Specialty: Paediat.

ONG, Liang Chai Edmund Department of Infection & Tropical Medicine, Newcastle General Hospital, Newcastle upon Tyne NE4 6BE Tel: 0191 273 8811 Fax: 0191 273 0900 Email: e.l.c.ong@ncl.ac.uk — MB BS Newc. 1983 (Univ. Newc. Med. Sch.) FRCPI 1993, M 1986; MSc Lond. 1987; DTM & H RCP Lond. 1987; FRCP 1997. Cons. Phys. & Sen. Lect. (Med.) with interest Infec. Dis. Newc. Gen. Hosp. Specialty: Infec. Dis.; Trop. Med.; HIV Med. Socs: Fell. Roy. Soc. Trop. Med. & Hyg.; Internat. AIDS Soc.; Brit. Infec. Soc. Prev: Sen. Regist. & Regist. (Infec. Dis. & Gen. Med.) Monsall

Hosp. Manch.; SHO Rotat. (Med.) S. Cleveland Hosp. Middlesbrough.

ONG, Poh Suan Queen's Hospital, Belvedere Road, Burton-on-Trent DE13 0RB Tel: 01283 566333 Fax: 01283 593010 — MB BS Lond. 1983 (Roy. Free) MRCPath 1990; FRCPath 1998. Cons. Histopath. Specialty: Histopath. Special Interest: Non-gynaecological Cytol.; botulinum toxin in aesthetic use. Socs: BMA; RSM; Med. Wom. Federat. Prev: Cons. Cellular Path. Joyce Green Hosp. Dartford; Sen. Regist. (Histopath.) Westm. & Char. Cross Med. Sch. Lond.; Regist. (Histopath.) Northwick Pk. Hosp. Middlx.

ONG, Thian Keh 17 Hazelmere Avenue, Melton Park, Gosforth, Newcastle upon Tyne NE3 5QL — MB ChB Sheff. 1993; BDS Sheff. 1984; FDS RCS Eng. 1988.

ONG, Tuyen Binh — MB BS Lond. 1998.

ONG, Voon Hong Room 700, Staff Residence, Hull Royal Infirmary, Anlaby Road, Hull HU3 2JZ Tel: 01482 328541 Ext: 4676; 17 Rmk Dusun Nylor, Seremban, Negeri Sembilan 70100, Malaysia — MS BS Melbourne 1996. SHO (Med.) Hull Roy. Infirm. Specialty: Gastroenterol. Socs: BMA; MDU. Prev: Med. SHO (Geriat.s) Hull Roy. Infirm.

ONG, Wei Wei Walsgrave Hospital, Clifford Bridge Road, Coventry CV2 2DX Tel: 024 76 602020; 5 Melina Court, Grove End Road, London NW8 9SB Tel: 0973 369250 — MB BS Lond. 1996. SHO (O & G). Specialty: Obst. & Gyn.

ONG, Yee Ean 19 Walsham Drive, Huddersfield HD3 3GS — MB BS Lond. 1993.

ONG, Yee Gan 19 Walsham Drive, Salendine Nook, Huddersfield HD3 3GS — MB BS Lond. 1991.

ONG, Yong Lee 101 Greer Park Avenue, Belfast BT8 7YF Email: ongyl@doctors.org.uk — (Queen's University of Belfast) MB BCh BAO Belf. 1991; MD 2001; MRCPath 2002. Cons. Haematologist. Specialty: Haematology. Prev: Specialist Regist. Haemat.

ONG, Yuen Li 6 Hugh Street, Belfast BT9 7HH — MB BCh BAO Belf. 1990; MB BCh Belf. 1990.

ONI, Mr John Queen's Medical Centre, Nottingham NG7 2UH — MB BCh BAO Dub. 1982; FRCS Glas. 1987; MA Dub. 1987; FRCS (Orthop.) 1996. Cons. (QMC Nottm.). Specialty: Trauma & Orthop. Surg.; Orthop. Socs: Roy. Soc. Med.; Assoc. Mem. BOA. Prev: Sen. Regist. (Orthop.) St. Jas. Hosp. Leeds; Regist. (Orthop.) Qu. Mary's Hosp. Sidcup, Huddersfield Roy. Infirm. & Roy. Halifax Infirm.

ONI, Mr Olusola Olumide Akindele Koro Lodge, 16 Sutherington Way, Meadowfields, Anstey, Leicester LE7 7TH Tel: 0116 236 7858 — MB BS Ibadan 1973; FRCS Ed. 1977; MSc Leic. 1994, MD 1987. Cons. Orthop. Surg. Glenfield Gen. Hosp. Leicester; Lect. (Orthop. Surg.) Univ. Leicester. Specialty: Orthop. Socs: Brit. Assn. Surg. Knee; Fell. Nigerian Postgrad. Med. Coll. 1984; Fell. W. African Coll. Surgs. 1983. Prev: Sen. Lect. Univ. Leicester; Sen. Regist. (Orthop.) Watford Gen. Hosp.; Lect. (Orthop. Surg.) Univ. Benin, Nigeria.

ONI-ORISAN, John Edward Adetokubo (retired) Airdrie Health Centre, Monkscourt Avenue, Airdrie ML6 0JU Tel: 01236 769333; 14 Woodview Drive, Cairnhill, Airdrie ML6 9HJ Tel: 01236 769333 — MB BS Lond. 1964 (Guy's) MRCS Eng. LRCP Lond. 1964; FRCOG 1989, M 1968. Prev: Med. Off. St. And.Hospice Airdrie.

ONION, Carl William Reginald Wirral Health Authority, St. Catherines Hospital, 1st Floor Admin. Block, Church Road, Tranmere, Birkenhead CH42 0LQ Tel: 0151 651 0011 Fax: 0151 652 2668; 10 Ploughmans Way, Great Sutton, South Wirral CH66 2YJ Tel: 0151 339 2154 — MB ChB Liverp. 1980; MRCGP 1989; MSc Liverp. 1991; MD Liverp. 1997. Med. Dir. & Med. Adviser Wirral HA; Hon. Lect. (Med. Educat.) Univ. Liverp.; Examr. Fac. Pub. Health RCP Lond., Ed., Glas. Socs: Assn. Primary Care Med. Advisers; Hon. Sec. Mersey Fac. RCGP. Prev: GP Birkenhead.

ONOCHE, Anne Ogugua 10 Arnal Crescent, Linstead Way, London SW18 5PX — MB BS Nigeria 1988; MRCP (UK) 1993.

ONON, Temujin Argyle Street Surgery, 141 Argyle Street, Heywood OL10 3SD Tel: 01706 366135 Fax: 01706 627706 — MB ChB Aberd. 1983. Specialty: Obst. & Gyn. Prev: Trainee GP Coleshill Birm.; SHO (A & E) Hull Roy. Infirm.; Ho. Off. (Surg.) & Ho. Off. (Med.) Hull Roy. Infirm.

ONORI, Kathleen Margaret The Richmond Practice, Health Centre, Dean Road, Bo'ness EH51 0DH Tel: 01506 822665 Fax: 01506 825939; 2 Kinglass Drive, Bo'ness EH51 9RB — MB ChB Ed. 1974; DRCOG 1976; MRCGP 1978.

ONSLOW, Julie Marie Anaesthetic Department, Southampton General Hospital, Tremona Road, Southampton SO16 6YD Tel: 023 8077 7222; 7 Hawthorn Close, Colden Common, Winchester SO21 1UX Tel: 01962 715383 — BM Soton. 1992; DCH 1995; FRCA 1999. Specialist Regist. (Anaesth.) Soton Gen. Hosp. Specialty: Anaesth. Prev: Specialist Regist., Perth, West. Australia.

ONUGHA, Chinye Okwudili Grantham & District Hospital, United Lincolnshire Trust, 101 Manthorpe Road, Grantham NG31 8DG Email: chibin@supanet.com — (Prince of Wales Med. Coll. Patna) MB BS Patna 1965; DA Ibadan 1971; FFA RCSI 1975. Cons. Anaesth. Trent RHA. Specialty: Anaesth. Socs: BMA & Soc. Anaesth. of Gt. Brit. & Irel.; Assn. Anaesth.; Soc. Low Flow Anaesth. Prev: Sen. Regist. (Anaesth.) N. Staffs. Hosps. Centre Stoke-on-Trent; Lect. (Anaesth.) Univ. Benin Teach. Hosp., Nigeria.

ONUGHA, Edwin Nwokedi 3 Wood Close, Salfords, Redhill RH1 5EE; East Surrey Hospital, Three Arch Road, Redhill RH1 5RH Tel: 01737 768511 — BM BCh Univ. Nigeria 1976 (University of Nigeria Medical School) DRCOG 1984. Assoc. Specialist (O & G). Specialty: Obst. & Gyn.

ONUOHA, Oyoyo Ogoegbunam 12 St Georges Avenue, London NW9 0JU — MB ChB Bristol 1996.

ONUZO, Obed Chukwunedum — MB BS Ibadan 1974; DCH Lond. 1980; DTCH Liverp. 1981; MRCP Lond. 1981; FWACP 1985. Cons. Paediatric Cardiol., Univ. Hosp. of Wales, Cardiff. Specialty: Cardiol. Prev: Locum Paediatric Cardiol., Birm. Childrens Hosp.; Assoc. Specialist in Paediatric Cardiol., Roy. Brompton, Harefield and Lond. Hosps.

ONWUBALILI, James Kenechukwu North Middlesex University Hospital, Sterling Way, London N18 1QX Tel: 020 8887 4648 Fax: 020 8887 4491; The Royal Free Hospital, Pond Street, Hampstead, London NW3 2QG; 44 Little Bornes, London SE21 8SE Tel: 020 8670 9206 Fax: 020 8670 9206 Email: james.onwubalili@nmh.nhs.uk — MB BS Ibadan 1975 (Ibadan Nigeria) MRCP (UK) 1979; MD Ibadan 1985; FRCP Lond. 1992; T(M) 1995. Specialty: Nephrol.; Gen. Med. Socs: Brit. Renal Assn.; Europ. Dialysis & Transpl. Assoc. Prev: Sen. Cons. Neprol. King Abdulaziz Hosp. Jeddah, Saudi Arabia; Cons. Nephrol. & Sen. Lect. (Med.) Univ. Nigeria Teach. Hosp. Enugu; MRC Research Fell Clin. Research Centre Harrow.

ONWUCHEKWA, Wilvar Ohiaeri 38 Bonsor House, Patmore Est., London SW8 4UR — MB BS Lond. 1963; DCH RCP Lond. 1966; DObst RCOG 1967; FMCGP (Nigeria) 1982; T(GP) 1993. Socs: Assoc. Mem. Roy. Coll. Gen. Pract. Prev: Chief Med. Off. i/c Staff Health at Nat. Orthop. Hosp. Enugu, Nigeria.

ONWUDE, Mr Joseph Loze Springfield Hospital, Lawn Lane, Springfield, Chelmsford CM1 7GU Tel: 01245 234004 Email: jlonwude@btconnect.com; St John's Hospital, Wood St., Chelmsford CM2 9BG Tel: 01245 513456 — MB BS Ibadan 1981 (Univ. of Ibadan, Nigena) DLSH TM (Lond.); MSc; T(OG) 1993; FRCOG 2000. Cons. Gyn. (Prviate Pract.). Specialty: Obst. & Gyn. Special Interest: Menopause; Pelvic Pain; Recurrent Prolapse. Prev: Cons. Obst. & Gyn., St Johns Hosp., Chelmsford.

ONWUDIKE, Mr Madu Dept of General Surgery, Bolton Hospitals NHS Trust, Royal Bolton Hospital, Bolton BL4 0JR Tel: 01204 390390 Fax: 01204 390109 — MB BS Ibadan 1984; FRCS Ed. 1992; MSc (Surg. Sci.) Lond. 1996; FRCS (Gen) 1999. Cons. Gen. and Vasc. Surg., Bolton Hosp. NHS Trust. Specialty: Gen. Surg. Socs: Assn. Surg. Of GB & Irel.; Fell. W. African Coll. & Surg. 1996; Vasc. Surg. Soc. GB & Irel. Prev: Sp. Reg. Whipps Cross Hosp.; Sp. Reg. Vasc. Surg., Barts and the Lond. NHS Trust.; Sp. Reg. Vasc. Surg., Univ. Coll. Lond. Hosp. NHS Trust.

ONWUZURIKE, Kaokwem Bennet 56 Bawdsey Avenue, Newbury Park, Ilford IG2 7TJ Mob: 07985 702057 Fax: 020 8598 8172 — MB BS Jos 1983; FWACS 1998. Specialist Regist. Darent Valley Hosp. Dartford Kent. Specialty: Obst. & Gyn. Socs: RCOG; MDU. Prev: SHO (O & G) N. Middlx. Hosp. Lond.

ONYALI, Mr Kenneth Obidigbo 30 Burwash Road, London SE18 7QZ Tel: 020 8855 9397 — MB BS Nigeria 1985; FRCS Ed. 1990.

ONYEABO, Benjamin Chukwunwuba 25 Kelland Close, Park Road, Hornsey, London N8 8JS Tel: 020 8341 4874 — MB BCh BAO Belf. 1953; DTM & H Liverp. 1955. Med. Specialist (Genitourin. Med.) Char. Cross Hosp. Gp. Lond. Socs: Fell. Roy. Soc. Trop. Med. & Hyg.

ONYEADOR, Miriam Ijeoma Walm Lane Surgery, 114 Walm Lane, London NW2 4RT Tel: 0208 451 4100 — MB BS Nigeria 1979; MRCOG 1988; MFFP 1995. GP Princip.; Forens. Med. Examr. for Victims of Sexual Assault for the Metrop. Police. Specialty: Gen. Pract.; Family Planning; Medico Legal. Socs: Fac. of Family Plann.; BMA.

ONYEAMA, Warwick Paul Joseph Chukwuma Cygnet Wing Blackheath, 80-82 Blackheath Hill, London SE3 9RQ Tel: 0208 694 2111 Fax: 0208 692 0570 — MB BS Lond. 1967; MRCS Eng. LRCP Lond. 1967; DPM Eng. 1972; T(Psych) 1991; FRCPsych 1991, M 1991; MAE (Eng) 1997. Independant Cons. Psychiat.,Hon.Cons., Slam (NHS) Trust. Specialty: Gen. Psychiat. Socs: Brit. Med. Assn. (Mem.); Acad. of Experts (Mem.); Roy. Coll. of Psychiat.s (Fell.). Prev: Sen. Lect. (Psychiat.) Univ. Nigeria Teachg. Hosp. Enugu, Nigeria; Med. Dir. Staff Psychiat. Hosp. Enugu, Nigeria; Cons. Psychiat..Lect.S. Lond. Maldsley NHS Trust & Glct Med. Sch.

ONYEKWULUJE, Chike Egbuonu Bedford Hospital NHS Trust, Department of Clinical Radiology, Kempston Road, Bedford MK42 9DJ Tel: 01234 355122 Fax: 01234 792106 Email: chaikoko@yahoo.co.uk — MB BS Ibadan, Nigeria 1976; DMRD 1984; FRCR 1985. Cons. Radiologist Bedford Hosp. NHS Trust; Cons. Radiologist Luton & Dunstable Hosp. Breast Centre. Specialty: Radiol. Special Interest: Breast Radiol.; Cross sectional imaging. Socs: Roy. Coll. of Radiol.; Brit. Inst. of Radiol. (Member); Radiological Soc. of N. America (Member). Prev: Cons. & Head of Radiol. Bakhsh Hosp. Jeddah Saudi Arabia.

ONYETT, Roger Martin Mount Pleasant Health Centre, Mount Pleasant Road, Exeter EX4 7BW Tel: 01392 55262 Fax: 01392 270497; 36 Monmouth Street, Topsham, Exeter EX3 0AJ Tel: 01392 873853 — MB BS Lond. 1973 (Roy. Free) BSc Nott. 1961; BSc Nottm. 1961; MRCS Eng. 1973; LRCP Lond. 1973; MRCS Eng. LRCP Lond. 1973; DCH Eng. 1975; DCH Eng. 1975; MRCGP 1979; MRCGP 1979. Trainer (Gen. Pract.) Exeter.

OO, Mg Mg Bedwell Medical Centre, Sinfield Close, Bedwell Crescent, Stevenage SG1 1LYU Tel: 01438 355551 Fax: 01438 749704.

OO, Myint South Cleveland Hospital, Marton Road, Middlesbrough TS4 3BW Tel: 01642 854869 Fax: 01642 854870; 46 The Green, Norton, Stockton-on-Tees TS20 1DU Tel: 01642 556291 Fax: 01642 556291 — MB BS Rangoon 1960 (Rangoon Med. Coll.) DCH Eng. 1962; FRCP Lond. 1982, M, 1966. Cons. Paediat. N. Tees Gen. Hosp. Stockton-on-Tees; Locum Cons. Comm. Paediat., Tees & N.E. Yorks. NHS Trust. Middlesbrough. Specialty: Paediat. Socs: BMA; Paediat. Assn.; N. Eng. Paediat. Soc.

OO, Myint Kyam Warrengate Medical Centre, Upper Warrengate, Wakefield WF1 4PR Tel: 01924 371011; 3 The Holloway, Amblecote, Stourbridge DY8 4DL — MB BS Med. Inst. (I) Rangoon 1987.

OOI, Mrs Jane Louise Royal Liverpool University Hospital, Prescot Street, Liverpool L7 8XP — MB ChB Liverp. 1990; FRCS Ed. 1995. Specialist Regist. (Gen. Surg.) Mersey Deanery. Specialty: Gen. Surg. Special Interest: Breast. Socs: Assn. Breast Surg. at BASU. Prev: Specialist Regist. (Gen. Surg.) NW Deanery; SHO Rotat. (Surg.) Merseyside.

OOI, Kao Hua Centenary Surgery, 9 Centenary Gardens, Coatbridge ML5 4BY Tel: 01236 423355 Fax: 01236 606345 — MB ChB Glas. 1981; DRCOG 1983; DCH RCPS Glas. 1984. GP Lanarksh.

OOI, Kheng Hong 40 North Linkside Road, Liverpool L25 9NT — MB ChB Liverp. 1977; DTM & H Liverp. 1979; MRCS Eng. LRCP Lond. 1979; Dip. Ven. Liverp. 1981; DRCOG 1984; MRCGP 1986.

OOI, Laureen Gek Sim — MB ChB Ed. 1982; FFA RCS Eng. 1988. Cons. Anaesth. Mid Essex Hosps. Trust. Specialty: Anaesth. Prev: Cons. Anaesth. Kingston Hosp.; Sen. Regist. (Anaesth.) Roy. Lond. Hosp.; Lect. (Anaesth.) Lond. Hosp. Med. Coll.

OOI, May May Flat 50, Richmond Hill Court, Richmond Hill, Richmond TW10 6BE — MB BS Lond. 1991.

OOI, Richard Gek Beng Stonecroft, Northgate Drive, Camberley GU15 2AP — MB ChB Bristol 1984; FRCA 1989. Cons. Anaesth. Chelsea & Westm. Healthcare Trust. Specialty: Anaesth. Prev: Asst. Prof. Anaesth. Duke Univ. & Med. Center, USA; Lect. (Anaesth.) Char. Cross & Westm. Med. Sch. Lond.

OOI, Yang Wern The Charlton Stores, Charlton, Pershore WR10 3LG — BM BCh Oxf. 1991.

OOLBEKKINK, Marjon St Catharine's Hospital, Church Road, Birkenhead CH42 0LQ; 25 Heronpark Way, Spital, Wirral CH63 9FN Tel: 0151 340680 — Artsexamen Utrecht 1985; PhD Amsterdam 1989. Clin. Asst. (Geriat. Med.) St Catharine's Hosp. Prev: SHO (Gen. Med.) Bussum, Netherlands; Research Fell. Diabetic Research Amsterdam, Netherlands.

OOMMEN, Mr Puthenparambil Korah 14 Merwood Avenue, Heald Green, Cheadle SK8 3DN; Department of Cardiothoracic Surgery, Wythenshawe Hospital, Southmoor Road, Manchester M22 9RL — MB BS Musore 1979; MB BS Mysore 1979; FRCS Ed. 1988; FRCS Eng. 1989. Staff Grade, Cardiothoracic Surg. & ICU Wythenshawe Hosp. Manch. Specialty: Cardiothoracic Surg.

OON, Lynette Lin Ean 25 Lisburne Road, London NW3 2NS; 3 Peach Garden, Singapore 437604, Singapore — MB BS Lond. 1992; BSc Lond. 1989; MRCP (UK) 1995. SHO (Neurol.) Lond. Specialty: Gen. Med. Socs: BMA; MDU.

OON, Vincent Jin Huat 6 Woodsford Square, London W14 8DP; Academic Department of Obstetrics and Gynaecology, Imperial College School of Medicine, Chelsea and Westminster Hospital, London SW10 9NH — MB BChir Camb. 1991; MA Camb. 1992, BA 1988. Research Lect. Acad. Dept. O & G Imperial Coll. Sch. Med. Chelsea & Westm. Hosp. Lond. Specialty: Obst. & Gyn. Prev: SHO (Obst.) UCL Hosps. Lond.

OOSTHUYSEN, Stefanus Adrian Van Rooyen Broadlands, Priory Road, St Olaves, Great Yarmouth NR31 9HQ — MB ChB Cape Town 1980.

OPANEYE, Abayomi Adegboyega Department of Genitourinary Medicine, Middlesbrough General Hospital, Middlesbrough TS5 5AZ Tel: 01642 854548 Fax: 01642 854328; 6 Mallowdale, Nunthorpe, Middlesbrough TS7 0QA Tel: 01642 318236 Fax: 01642 854328 — MB BS Ibadan 1974; MRCOG 1982; MPH Univ. Cali. Berkeley 1989; MFFP 1993; FRCOG 1997. Cons. Phys. (Genitourin. Med.) Middlesbrough Gen. Hosp. Cleveland; Cons. Phys. (Genitourin. Med.) Friarage Hosp. N.allerton. Specialty: Genitourinary Medicine. Socs: Fell. Roy. Soc. Health; Fell. W. African Coll. Surg.; Med. Soc. Study VD. Prev: Sen. Lect. & Cons. O & G Coll. Health Scs. Ogun State Univ, Nigeria; Cons. O & G King Khalid Hosp. Al-Kharj, Saudi Arabia; Regist. (Obst. Gyn.) Gen. Hosp. S. Shields.

OPDAM, Helen Ingrid Kent & Canterbury Hospital, Department of Anaesthetics, Ethelbert Road, Canterbury CT1 3NG — MB BS Monash 1990.

OPDEBEECK, Goedele Patricia Edwarda Maria T 15 Eden Park, Scotforth, Lancaster LA1 4SJ Tel: 01524 63459 — MB BCh BAO NUI 1975; MRCPsych 1989. Sen. Regist. (Psychogeriat.) NW RHA. Specialty: Geriat. Psychiat. Prev: Regist. (Psychiat.) Sheff.; Regist. (Psychiat.) Lancaster HA.

OPEMUYI, Isaac Olusoji Olumbamishe — MB BS Ibadan 1977; MRCOG 1988; FRCOG 2001. Cons. (O & G) Barking, Havering & Redbridge HA. Specialty: Obst. & Gyn.

OPENSHAW, Professor Peter John Morland Imperial College at St Mary's, Department of Respiratory Medicine, Paddington, London W2 1PG Tel: 020 7594 3854 Fax: 020 7262 8913 Email: p.openshaw@imperial.ac.uk — MB BS Lond. 1979 (Guy's) BSc (Physiol.) Lond. 1976; MRCP (UK) 1982; PhD Brunel Univ. 1989; FRCP 1994; FMedSci 1999. Prof. (Exp. Med.) Imperial Coll. of Sci. Technol. & Med. Nat. Heart & Lung Inst.; Hon. Cons. Phys. St. Mary's Hosp. Med. Sch. Lond.; Head Dept. of Respirat. Med. Specialty: Respirat. Med.; Immunol. Special Interest: Common colds. Socs: Assn. Phys.; FASEB/Amer. Soc. of Immunol.; Amer. Thoracic Soc. Prev: MRC Train. Fell.; Regist. Roy. Postgrad. Med. Sch. Lond.

OPENSHAW, Mrs Susan Elizabeth (retired) 104 Bove Town, Glastonbury BA6 8JG Tel: 01458 32181; 104 Bove Town, Glastonbury BA6 8JG — BM BCh Oxf. 1949 (Oxf. & King's Coll. Hosp.) BM BCh Oxon. 1949. Prev: GP.

OPENSHAW, William Arthur (retired) 104 Bove Town, Glastonbury BA6 8JG Tel: 01458 832181 — BM BCh Oxf. 1950 (Oxf. & Guy's) MA, BM BCh Oxon. 1950; MRCGP 1974.

OPHER, Simon Joseph The Westgate Surgery, 40 Parsonage Street, Dursley GL11 4AA Tel: 01453 545981 — MB BS Lond. 1988; MRCGP 1993.

OPIE, Neil John 45 Larch Way, Farnborough GU14 0QW — MB ChB Leeds 1998.

OPIE, Peter Michael The Surgery, Worsley Road, Immingham, Grimsby DN40 1BE Tel: 01469 572058 Fax: 01469 573043 Email:

peter.opie@virgin.net; Health Centre, Pelham Crescent, Keelby, Grimsby Tel: 01469 560202 Fax: 01469 573043 — MB BS Lond. 1981 (Westminster) BSc Lond. 1978; DRCOG 1985; MRCGP 1985.

OPIRA-ODIDA, Mr Francis Xavier Airedale General Hospital, Skipton Road, Steeton, Keighley BD20 6TD; 44 Currer Walk, Thornhill Road, Steeton, Keighley BD20 6TL — MD Dar-es-Salaam, Tanzania 1980; MMed Uganda 1989; MRCOG 1996. Staff Grade (O & G) Airedale NHS Trust Keighley W. Yorks. Specialty: Obst. & Gyn.

OPPE, Thomas Ernest, CBE 2 parkholme Cottages, Fife Road, Sheen common, London SW14 7ER Tel: 0208 392 1626 — (Guy's) MB BS (Hons., Distinc. Med.) Lond. 1947; FRCP Lond. 1966, M 1948; DCH Eng. 1950. Emerit. Prof. Paediat. Univ. Lond. Specialty: Paediat. Prev: Cons. Paediat. St. Mary's Hosp. Lond.; Sen. Censor (1st Vice-Pres.) RCP Lond.; Lect. (Child Health) Univ. Bristol.

OPPENHEIM, Audrey Isabelle Cons. Child Psychiat., North Team CAMHS, Spencer Street, Liverpool L6 Tel: 0151 222 5866 Fax: 0161 980 1773 Email: info@medicarta.com — MB ChB Manch. 1983; BSc Manch. 1983; MRCPsych 1988; FRCPsych 2002. Cons., Child & Adolesc. Psychiat., Roy. Liverp. Childr. Hosp.; Special Adviser to Nat. Youth Advocacy Serv. Specialty: Child & Adolesc. Psychiat. Socs: Mem. of the Disabil. Living Allowance Advis. Bd.

OPPENHEIM, Esther Margaret Jiggins Lane Surgery, 17 Jiggins Lane, Bartley Green, Birmingham B32 3LE Tel: 0121 477 7272 Fax: 0121 478 4319; 59 Weoley Park Road, Birmingham B29 6QZ Tel: 0121 472 1356 Fax: 0121 472 1356 — MB BCh Witwatersrand 1975; BSc Witwatersrand 1972; MPH Hebrew Univ. Jerusalem 1980; Cert. Prescribed Equiv. Exp. JCPTGP 1982. Socs: Assoc. Mem. RCGP. Prev: GP Ladywood Birm.; Trainee GP Glyncorrwg VTS; Med. Off. Moroka Hosp. Thaba Nchu, S. Afr.

OPPENHEIMER, Catherine Violet Rosalie P The Warneford Hospital, Oxford OX3 7JX Tel: 01865 226263 — (Oxf.) BM BCh Oxf. 1968; MRCP (UK) 1972; FRCPsych 1989, M 1978; FRCP Lond. 1992. Cons. Psychiat., Dept. of Psychiat. of Old Age, Warneford Hosp., Oxf.; Med. Dir. Oxon. Ment. Healthcare NHS Trust Oxf. Specialty: Geriat. Psychiat.

OPPENHEIMER, Christina Adrienne Women's Hospital, Leicester Royal Infirmary, Leicester LE1 5WW Tel: 0116 258 5923 Fax: 0116 258 7771 — MB BS Lond. 1980 (Cambridge, Westminster Medical School) MA Camb. 1981; FRCS Eng. 1984; MRCOG 1989; FRCOG 2003. Cons. O & G Leicester Roy. Infirm.; Hon. Sen. Lect. in Med. Educat., Univ. of Leicester. Specialty: Obst. & Gyn. Socs: Brit. Med. Ultrasound Soc.; Brit. Matern. and Fetal Med. Soc.; Brit. Soc. for Paediatirc and Adolesc. Gynae.

OPPENHEIMER, Matilda Magdalen Grenville Pangbourne Medical Practice, The Boat House Surgery, Whitchurch Road, Pangbourne, Reading RG8 7DP Tel: 0118 984 2234 Fax: 0118 984 3022 Email: mmgoppenheimer@aol.com; The White House, High St, Whitchurch-on-Thames, Reading RG8 7HA Tel: 01734 842915 Fax: 01734 841264 — MB BS Lond. 1981; MA Oxf. 1978; DRCOG 1984; MRCGP 1985. Gen. Practitioner. Specialty: Gen. Pract. Socs: Wom. Med. Federat.; Reading Path. Soc.; RCGP.

OPPONG, Amma Caroline Kyerewaa 1 Hoveton Close, Shelton Lock, Derby DE24 9QH Tel: 01332 732371 Fax: 01332 732371 — BM BS Nottm. 1988 (Nottingham University) DCH RCP Lond. 1990; MRCP (UK) 1992; MD Keele 1997. Sen. Regist. (Community Paediat.) South. Derbysh. NHS Trust. Specialty: Community Child Health. Socs: BACCH; RCPCH; BMA. Prev: Regist. (Paediat.) City Gen. Hosp. Stoke-on-Trent; SHO (Neonat. & Gen. Paediat.) Leicester Roy. Infirm.; SHO (Paediat.) Alder Hey & Roy. Liverp. Childr. Hosp.

OPPONG, Mr Fielding Christian Derriford Hospital, Derriford Road, Plymouth PL6 8DH Tel: 01752 763289 Email: chris.oppong@phnt.swest.nhs.uk; Nuffield Hospital, Plymouth Tel: 01752 761834 — MB ChB Ghana 1979 (Univ. of Ghana Med. Sch.) FRCS Eng. 1989; FRCS (Gen. Surg.) 2000. Cons. Colorectal Surg. Derriford Hosp. Plymouth; Cons. Gen. Surg., Plymouth Nuffield Hosp. Specialty: Gen. Surg. Special Interest: Pelvic Floor Surg.; Faecal Incontinence; Rectal Prolapse Surg. Socs: Fell. Roy. Coll. Surg. Eng.; Assn. Surg. GB & Irel.; Assn. Coloproctol. of Gr. Britain & N. Irel. Prev: Specialist Regist., Southmead Hosp., Bristol; Assoc. Specialist (Gen. Surg.) Derriford Hosp. Plymouth; Staff Grade Surg. (Gen. Surg.) Derriford Hosp. Plymouth.

OR, Christine — MB BS Lond. 1994 (UMDS) DRCOG 1996; DFFP 1997; Dip Ther 1999. GP Locum. Specialty: Gen. Pract. Socs: BMA. Prev: Vocationally Trained Acad. Assoc. VTAA Market Pl. Surg. Kent.

ORAELOSI, Florence Nwakaego Obiamaka Ecclesbourne, Warwick Terrace, Lea Bridge Road, London E17 9DP Tel: 020 8539 2077; 504 Chigwell Road, Woodford Green IG8 8PA Tel: 020 8504 2126 — MB BCh BAO NUI 1982. Prev: SHO (O & G) Birm. & Midl. Hosp. for Wom. & Birm. Matern. Hosp.; SHO (Paediat.) Roy. Gwent Hosp. Newport Wales; Regist. (O & G) Burton Dist. Hosp. Centre.

ORAKWE, Mr Samuel Ikemefuna 95 Berkeley Road, Shirley, Solihull B90 2HT — MB BS Univ. Nigeria 1986; FRCS Ed. 1992.

ORAM, David Andrew Tandon Medical Centre, Kent St., Upper Gornal, Dudley DY3 1UX Tel: 01902 882243; 5 Turf Cottages, Penn Common, Wolverhampton WV4 5LA — MB ChB Manch. 1980; DRCOG 1986.

ORAM, David Charles Sunnyside Doctors Surgery, 150 Fratton Road, Portsmouth PO1 5DH Tel: 023 9282 4725 Fax: 023 9286 1014 — MB BS Lond. 1979 (St Bart.) BSc (Hons.) (Pharmacol.) Lond. 1976; MRCS Eng. LRCP Lond. 1979; DRCOG 1984; DCH RCP Lond. 1985; MRCGP 1985. Specialty: Occupat. Health. Special Interest: occupational health and diabetes. Socs: BMA.

ORAM, Mr David Howard 121 Harley Street, London W1G 6AX Tel: 020 7935 7111 Fax: 020 7935 9001 Email: oram@gynaecology.freeserve.co.uk; Papplewick, 33 College Road, London SE21 7BG — MB BS Lond. 1971 (King's Coll. Hosp.) MRCS Eng. LRCP Lond. 1971; DObst RCOG 1974; FRCOG 1990, M 1977. Cons. Gyn. Oncol. Dept. Gyn. Oncol. St. Bart. Hosp. Lond. Specialty: Obst. & Gyn. Socs: Blair Bell Res. Soc.; Brit. Gyn. Cancer Soc.; Internat. Gyn. Cancer Soc. Prev: Sen. Regist. King's Coll. Hosp. Lond.; Sen. Regist. King Edwd. VIII Hosp. Durban, S. Afr.; Research Fell. Geo.town Univ. Washington DC, USA.

ORAM, Edmund George (retired) 47 Rodney Road, West Bridgford, Nottingham NG2 6JH Tel: 0115 923 2746 — MB ChB Glas. 1953; DPM Eng. 1959; FRCPsych 1980, M 1971. Emerit. Cons. Psychiat. Univ. Hosp. Qu. Med. Centre Nottm. Prev: Sen. Regist. Nuffield Research Unit Fulbourn Hosp. Camb.

ORAM, John Christopher 2 Devon Road, Failsworth, Manchester M35 0NR — MB ChB Leeds 1996.

ORAM, Julian John 40 Vincent Square, London SW1P 2NP Tel: 020 7630 5154 Fax: 020 7630 5164 — MB BS Lond. 1974 (Guy's) MRCS Eng. LRCP Lond. 1974; DObst RCOG 1976; MRCP (UK) 1977; FRCP Lond. 1991. Cons. Phys. (Geriat.) St. Geo. Hosp. Lond. Specialty: Gen. Med. Socs: Brit. Geriat. Soc.; Trustee Brit. Vasc. Foundat. Prev: Sen. Med. Regist. (Geriat.) St. Geo. Hosp. Lond.

ORAM, Muriel Churchill Holmes Caer Eden, 47 Slamannan Road, Falkirk FK1 5NF Tel: 01324 21170 — MB ChB Glas. 1939. Socs: BMA. Prev: Clin. Med. Off. Dept. Community Med. W. Lothian Health Dist. Res.; Med. Off. Stobhill Hosp. Glas. & Barnhill Inst. Glas.; Res. Obst. Surg. East. Dist. Hosp. Glas.

ORAM, Suzanne Burton (retired) 43 London Road, Harston, Cambridge CB2 5QQ Tel: 01209 870320 — MB BS Adelaide 1948; DObst RCOG 1956. Prev: Clin. Med. Off. Cambs. HA (T).

ORANGE, Gillian Valerie Department of Medical Microbiology, Ninewells Hospital, Dundee DD1 9SY — MB ChB Glas. 1979.

ORANGE, M Park Attwood Clinic, Trimpley, Bewdley DY12 1RE Tel: 01299 861444 Fax: 01299 861375 — Artsexamen Utrecht 1983.

ORANGE, Robert William — MB ChB Sheff. 1990; MMedSc (Clin. Psychiat.) Leeds; MRCPsych 1995. Cons. Psychi. Older People, Calderdale Roy. Hosp. Halifax.

ORANGE-LOHN, Bettina 41 Heath Street, Stourbridge DY8 1SE — State Exam Med Dusseldorf 1987.

ORBINSON, Helen Maureen 21 Calvertstown Road, Portadown, Craigavon BT63 5NY — MB BCh Belf. 1998.

ORCHARD, Ann Seymour (retired) 67 Croham Road, South Croydon CR2 7HF Tel: 020 8651 1222 — MB BS Lond. 1965 (Char. Cross) MRCS Eng. LRCP Lond. 1965; DObst RCOG 1970. Prev: SHO (Obst.) Char. Cross Hosp. Lond.

ORCHARD, Jennifer Ann Milford Hill Cottage, Milford Hill, Salisbury SP1 2QZ — MB BS Lond. 1975; MRCPath 1983. Specialty: Haematology.

ORCHARD, John Michael Limes Medical Centre, Limes Avenue, Alfreton, Derby DE55 7DW Tel: 01773 833133; Bramble Cottage, Main Road, Higham, Alfreton DE55 6EF Tel: 01773 831064 — MB ChB Liverp. 1980; DRCOG 1983; FRCGP 1995, M 1984. Adviser Dept. of Postgrad. Gen. Pract. Univ. of Sheff. Socs: Chairm.

Chesterfield Med. Soc. Prev: Course Organiser (Gen. Pract.) Chesterfield VTS.

ORCHARD, Kim Harold Cancer Research UK, Oncology Unit, Southampton University School of Medicine, Southampton SO16 6YD; 130 Great Preston Road, Ryde PO33 1AZ — MB BS Lond. 1985 (Royal Free) MRCP (UK); BSc (Hons.) Warwick 1977; MRCPath 1997. Dir. Transpl. Cancer Research Oncol. Unit Soton. Specialty: Haematology. Socs: Brit. Soc. Haematol. Prev: Research Fell. (Haemat.) Hammersmith & Roy. Free Hosp.; Sen. Regist. (Haemat.) Hammersmith Hosp. Trust; SHO (Med.) Rotat. Northwick Pk. Hosp. Middlx.

ORCHARD, Robin Theodore St Anthony's Hospital, London Road, North Cheam, Sutton SM3 9DW Tel: 020 8337 6691; 67 Croham Road, South Croydon CR2 7HF — (Char. Cross) MB BS Lond. 1965; MRCS Eng. LRCP Lond. 1965; FRCP Lond. 1982, M 1969. Cons. Phys. St. Helier, Sutton & Nelson Hosp.; Hon. Sen. Lect. St. Geo. Hosp. Med. Sch. Specialty: Gastroenterol.; Gen. Med. Socs: BMA; Brit. Soc. Gastroenterol. Prev: Sen. Regist. (Med.) Char. Cross Hosp. Lond.; Regist. (Med.) St. Stephen's Hosp. Chelsea; Ho. Phys. Lond. Chest Hosp.

ORCHARD, Timothy Robin 3 Wolsey Court, Woodstock Road, Woodstock OX20 1QP — MB BChir Camb. 1991 (Char. Cross & Westm.) MA Camb. 1992; MRCP (UK) 1994; MD Camb 1999; MA DM Oxford 1999. Clin. Research Fell. Gastroenterol. Unit Nuffield Dept. Med. Univ. Oxf.; Emmanoel Lee Research Fell. St. Cross Coll. Oxf. Specialty: Gastroenterol.; Gen. Med. Socs: Brit. Soc. of Gastroenterol. Prev: Regist. Rotat. (Med.) St. Geo. Hosp. Lond.; SHO Frimley Pk. Hosp.; Ho. Off. Westm. Hosp. Lond.

ORCHARTON, Alan MacKintosh (retired) 2 Glebe Avenue, Kilmarnock KA1 3DX Tel: 01563 524329 — (Glas.) MB ChB Glas. 1952; DObst RCOG 1956. Prev: Ho. Surg. W. Infirm. Glas.

ORCUTT, Roger Lee (retired) Tremorham House, Downderry, Torpoint PL11 3JX — BM BCh Oxf. 1952; MA, BM BCh Oxon. 1952. Prev: ENT Ho. Surg. St. Thos. Hosp. Lond.

ORD-HUME, Gail Celia Alma Road Surgery, 68 Alma Road, Portswood, Southampton SO14 6UX Tel: 023 8067 2666 Fax: 023 8055 0972; Cherry Tree Cottage, Coputhorne Crescent, Coputhorne, Southampton SO40 2PE — BM Soton. 1980; DA Eng. 1983; DRCOG 1984; MRCGP 1986.

ORDMAN, Anthony James Department of Anaesthetics, The Royal Free Hospital, Hampstead, London NW3 2QG Tel: 0207 830 2623 Fax: 0207 830 2245 Email: anthony.ordman@royalfree.nhs.uk — MB BS Lond. 1978 (Roy. Free) MRCS Eng. LRCP Lond. 1978; FFA RCS Eng. 1984. Cons. Anaesth. & Head Pain Managem. Serv. Roy. Free Hosp. Specialty: Anaesth. Prev: Cons. Anaesth. Roy. Lond. Hosp.; Sen. Regist. (Anaesth.) Univ. Coll. Hosp. Lond.; Clin. Fell. (Anaesth.) Univ. Toronto Mt. Sinai Hosp., Canada.

ORDUNA MONCUSI, Modesto Royal Preston Hospital, Doctors Mess, Sharoe Green Lane, Fulwood, Preston PR2 9HT; 13 Whitehouse Close, Heywood OL10 2QU — LMS Barcelona 1994.

OREN, Caroline Lucy Four Pads, California Lane, Bushey Heath, Watford WD23 1EP Tel: 020 8950 0643 — MB BS Lond. 1989; MRCP (UK) Paediat. 1993. Specialty: Paediat.

ORFORD, Christine Elizabeth 18 Myrtle Grove, Southport PR8 6BQ Tel: 01704 539930 — MB ChB Liverp. 1971 (Liverpool) DObst RCOG 1973. Clin. Med. Off. (Contracep. & Sexual Health) N. Mersey NHS Trust; Clin. Med. Off. (Contracep. & Sexual Health) Southport Community Health Serv. NHS Trust. Specialty: Family Plann. & Reproduc. Health. Socs: Foundat. Mem. Fac. Family Plann. & Reproduc. Health c/o RCOG. Prev: SCMO (Family Plann.) Wolverhampton HA.

ORFORD, Elaine Dawn 12 Mill Lane, Stock, Ingatestone CM4 9RY — MB ChB Leeds 1997.

ORGAN, Joan Mary (retired) 6 Bawnmore Court, Bilton, Rugby CV22 7QQ Tel: 01788 812811 — (Glas.) MB ChB Glas. 1965; DCH RCPS Glas. 1970. Prev: SCMO Warks. AHA.

ORGEE, Jane Margaret Ashleigh, Walwyn Road, Colwall, Malvern WR13 6QT — MB ChB Sheff. 1987.

ORGLES, Clive Somerset Airedale General Hospital, Steeton, Keighley BD20 6TD Tel: 01535 652511 Fax: 01535 292237 Email: clive.orgles@anhst.nhs.uk — MB ChB Leeds 1983 (Univ. Leeds Med. Sch.) DRCOG 1987; MRCGP 1991; FRCR 1996. Cons. Diagnostic Radiol. Airedale Gen. Hosp. Specialty: Radiol. Special Interest: Cross Sectional and Musculoskeletal Imaging. Prev: Leeds/Bradford Radiol. Train. Scheme; GP Shipley Health Centre Bradford; Trainee GP Bradford VTS.

ORIMOLOYE, Adekola Oluwole Market Street Health Group, 52 Market Street, East Ham, London E6 2RA Tel: 020 8548 2200 Fax: 020 8548 2288 — MB BS Lagos 1985; MRCOG 1993.

ORLANDI, Janet Robertson Aon Health Solutions, F1 Block, Wilton Centre, Redcar TS10 4RF Tel: 01642 430169 Fax: 01642 454599 — MB ChB Dundee 1985; MRCGP 1989; AFOM RCP Lond. 1992; MFOM Lond. 1998. Occupat. Phys. ICI Wilton Middlesbrough. Specialty: Occupat. Health.

ORLANDI, Martin Ferryhill Medical Practice, Durham Road, Ferryhill DL17 8JJ Tel: 01740 651238 Fax: 01740 656291 — MB ChB Dundee 1984.

ORLANDO, Antonio Plastic Surgery Department, Frenchay Hospital, Frenchay Park Road, Bristol BS16 1LE Tel: 0117 975 3873; Consulting Rooms, The Bristol Nuffield Hospital, At The Chesterfield, 3 Clifton Hill, Bristol BS8 1BP Tel: 0117 970 1212 Ext: 2762 Fax: 0117 975 3846 — State Exam Florence 1988 (Univ. Florence) Spec. Otolaryngology - Univ.of Florence, Italy, 1991; T(S) 1994; Spec. in Plastic Surgery, Univ of Parma, Italy 1996. Specialist Regist. Plastic Surg. Frenchay Hosp. Bristol; Hon. Sen. Lect. Sch. of Specialisation of Plastic Surg., Univ. Parma, Italy. Specialty: Plastic Surg.; Otorhinolaryngol. Socs: Brit. Assn. of Head & Neck Oncol.; Italian Soc. Plastic Reconstruct. & Aesthetic Surg.; Italian Soc. Otolarkingol. & Head & Neck Surg. Prev: Resid. Plastic Surg. Parma Gen. Hosp. Parma Italy.

ORLANS, David Anthony Childwall Valley Road Surgery, 70 Childwall Valley Road, Liverpool L16 4PE Tel: 0151 722 7321 — MB ChB Liverp. 1974.

ORLANS, Marian Childwall Valley Road Surgery, 70 Childwall Valley Road, Liverpool L16 4PE Tel: 0151 722 7321 — MB ChB Liverp. 1978; DRCOG 1980; MRCGP 1982.

ORME, Christopher Giles (retired) 16 Imperial Road, Matlock DE4 3NL Tel: 01629 582981 — MB ChB Sheff. 1955.

ORME, Gail Elizabeth 77 Gateland Lane, Shadwell, Leeds LS17 8LN — MB ChB Manch. 1984.

ORME, Leslie John The Health Centre, Fieldhead, Shepley, Huddersfield HD8 8DR Tel: 01484 602001 Fax: 01484 608125 — MB ChB Ed. 1974; BA Camb. 1971.

ORME, Nicholas John 42 Mariners Road, Blundellsands, Liverpool L23 6SX — MB ChB Liverp. 1988.

ORME, Richard Colin L'Estrange (retired) Department of Child Heath, Postgraduate Medical School, University of Exeter, Church La, Heavitree, Exeter EX2 5SQ Tel: 01392 403145 Fax: 01392 403158; 6 Glenthorne Road, Duryard, Exeter EX4 4QU — MB BChir Camb. 1961 (Camb. & King's Coll. Hosp.) MA, MB Camb. 1961; DCH Eng. 1966; FRCP Lond. 1981, M 1967; MRCP Ed. 1967; FRCPCH 1997. Hon. Sen. Lect. Dept. Child Health Postgrad. Med. Sch. Univ. Exeter. Prev: Sen. Regist. United Bristol Hosps. & S.W. RHB.

ORME, Richard Ian Royal Shrewsbury Hospital, Mytton Oak Road, Shrewsbury SY3 8XQ Tel: 01743 261000 — MB ChB Bristol 1986; MRCP (UK) 1989; FRCR 1993. Cons. Diagn. Radiol. Roy. Shrewsbury Hosps. NHS Trust. Specialty: Radiol. Socs: Brit. Soc. Interven. Radiol. Prev: Sen. Regist. (Diagn. Radiol.) W. Birm. HA.

ORME, Robert Martin L'Estrange John Radcliffe Hospital, Nuffield Department of Anaesthetics, Headley Way, Headington, Oxford OX3 9DU Tel: 01865 221590; 6 Wrightons Hill, Helmdon, Brackley NN13 5UF — MB ChB Dundee 1993; BMSc (Hons.) Dund 1989; FRCA 2000. Specialty: Anaesth. Socs: Assoc. of Anaesth. Of Britian & Ire.; Obst. Anaesth. Assn.; Intensive Care Society. Prev: SpR in Anaesthetics, Oxf. Region; Regist. in Med., Whangarei, New Zealand; Registar in Anaesthetics, Dunedin, New Zealand.

ORME, Susan Northern General Trust, Sheffield Tel: 0114 271 1900; 68 Charnock Hall Road, Sheffield S12 3HG — BM BS Nottm. 1991; BM BS Hons. Nottm. 1991; MRCP (UK) 1994. Sen. Regist. (Cent. & Geriat. Med.) Centre Sheff. Univ. Trust. Specialty: Care of the Elderly. Prev: Regist. (Gen. Med.) North. Gen. Trust.; SHO (Accid. & Med. & Dermat.) Roy. Hallamsh. Hosp. Sheff.; SHO (Med.) North. Gen. Hosp.

ORME-SMITH, Elizabeth Ann Heathcote Medical Centre, Heathcote, Tadworth KT20 5TH Tel: 01737 360202; Lion Hill, 3 Tadworth St, Tadworth KT20 5RP Tel: 01737 358983 Email:

100604.724@compuserve.com — MB BS Lond. 1957 (Guy's) FRCGP 1989, M 1981. Prev: Course Organiser Epsom GP VTS.

ORMEROD, Alex Edward 17 Harley Street, London W10 9QH Tel: 020 7580 9854 Fax: 020 7636 2836; 8 Claygate Avenue, Harpenden AL5 2HF Tel: 01582 764045 — BM BCh Oxford 1967 (Oxf.) MA Oxf. 1967; DObst RCOG 1970; AFOM RCP Lond. 1981. Occupat. Phys. Herts. Specialty: Occupat. Health. Socs: Fell. Roy. Soc. Med.; Soc. Occupat. Med. Prev: Sen. Med. Off. BRB Lond.; SHO & Ho. Off. Radcliffe Infirm. Oxf.

ORMEROD, Anthony David Ward 29, Aberdeen Royal Infirmary, Foresterhill, Aberdeen AB25 2ZN Tel: 01224 681818 Fax: 01224 840555 — MB ChB Manch. 1978; MRCP (UK) 1981; FRCP Ed. 1996; MD 2000. Cons. Dermat. Aberd. Roy. Infirm.; Reader Med. & Therap. (Dermat.) Univ. Aberd. Specialty: Dermat. Socs: Brit. Assn. Dermat.; Brit. Soc. Investig. Dermat.; Eur. Soc. Dermat. Res. Prev: Sen. Regist. (Dermat.) Aberd. Roy. Infirm.

ORMEROD, Fiona The Surgery, Northwick Road, Pilning, Bristol BS35 4JF Tel: 01454 632393 — MB BS Lond. 1979 (Middlx. Hosp.) DRCOG 1980; DA (UK) 1982; MRCGP 1988.

ORMEROD, I R Plane Trees Group Practice, 51 Sandbeds Road, Pellon, Halifax HX2 0QL Tel: 01422 330860 Fax: 01422 364830 — MB ChB Sheffield 1981; MB ChB Sheffield 1981.

ORMEROD, Ian Edward Charlton Frenchay Hospital, Frenchay, Bristol BS16 1LE Tel: 0117 970 1212 — MB BS Lond. 1978 (Middlx. Hosp.) FRCP; MD Lond. 1987; FRCP Lond. 1995. Cons. Neurol. Bristol Roy. Infirm (UBHT) N. Bristol NHS Trust. Specialty: Neurol. Socs: Assn. Brit. Neurol. Prev: Cons. Neurol. Nat. Hosp. Neurol. & Neurosurg. Qu. Sq. Lond. & St. Thos. Hosp. Lond.; Clin. Asst. Moorfields Eye Hosp. Lond.

ORMEROD, Jean Elizabeth Helen (retired) Silwood, Prescot Road, Hale, Altrincham WA15 9PZ Tel: 0161 928 0733 — MB ChB St. And. 1949; DCH Eng. 1952. Prev: Trainer in Gen. Pract. & Family Plann. Manch.

ORMEROD, Professor Lawrence Peter Chest Clinic, Blackburn Royal Infirmary, Blackburn BB2 3LR Tel: 01254 294338 Fax: 01254 294459 Email: peter.ormerod@mail.bhrv.nwest.nhs.uk — MB ChB Manch. 1974; BSc (Hons.) (Pharmacol.) Manch. 1971; MRCP (UK) 1977; MD Manch. 1986; FRCP Lond. 1990; DSc 2000. Cons. Resiratory Phys., E. Lancs NHS Trust, Blackburn; Prof. Lancs. PostGrad. Sch. of Med. & Health Univ. of Centr. Lancs. Specialty: Respirat. Med. Special Interest: Tuberc. and Myobacterial Diseases. Socs: Fell. Manch. Med. Soc.; Brit. Thorac. Soc. (Chairm. Jt. Tuberc. Comm.).; Internat. Union Against Tuberc. and Lung Diseases. Prev: Sen. Regist. N. Manch. Gen. Hosp.; Regist. (Gen. & Chest Med.) E. Birm. Hosp.; SHO (Gen. Med.) Univ. Hosp. S. Manch.

ORMEROD, Oliver John More Cardiac Department, John Radcliffe Hospital, Headington, Oxford OX3 9DU Tel: 01865 741166 Fax: 01865 221194; 4 Walton Crescent, Oxford OX1 2JG Tel: 01865 511957 — BM BCh Oxf. 1978; MRCP (UK) 1980; BA Oxf. 1975, MA 1986, DM 1986; FRCP 1996. Cons. Cardiol. John Radcliffe Hosp. Oxf. Specialty: Cardiol. Socs: BMA & Brit. Cardiac Soc. Prev: Clin. Lect. (Cardiovasc. Med.) Univ. Oxf.; Grimshaw Pk.inson Stud. (Cardiovasc. Dis.) Univ. Camb.; Regist. (Cardiol.) Papworth Hosp. Camb.

ORMEROD, Peter Stuart Medical Informatics Ltd., Ribble Bank Manor, Preston New Road Samlesbury, Preston PR5 0UL Tel: 01772 877111 Fax: 01772 877112 — MB ChB Glas. 1968; DAvMed. FOM RCP Lond. 1973; MSc Occupat. Med. Lond. 1981; FFOM RCP Lond. 1982; T(OM) 1991. Med. Dir. Med. Informatics Ltd. Specialty: Occupat. Health. Prev: Gp. Med. Off. WH Smith plc; Area Med. Off. CEGB; Sen. Med. Off. HM Naval Base Portsmouth.

ORMEROD, Raymond (retired) Silwood, Prescot Road, Hale, Altrincham WA15 9PZ Tel: 0161 928 0733 — MB ChB Manch. 1947; MRCGP 1968.

ORMEROD, Simon James Health Centre, Handsworth Avenue, Highams Park, London E4 9PD Tel: 020 8527 0913 Fax: 020 8527 6597 — MB BS Lond. 1985.

ORMEROD, Thomas Edward (retired) 40 Rectory Lane, Orlingbury, Kettering NN14 1JH Tel: 01933 678373; 40 Rectory Lane, Orlingbury, Kettering NN14 1JH Tel: 01933 678373 Fax: 01933 678373 — MB ChB Manch. 1952.

ORMEROD, Thomas Peter The Garden House, West Drive, Cheltenham GL50 4LB Tel: 01242 513896 Fax: 01242 512896 — (St. Bart.) MB BS Lond. 1956; DCH Eng. 1959; FRCP Lond. 1977, M 1962; MD Lond. 1966. Specialty: Gen. Med. Socs: Fell. Roy. Soc. Med.; BMA; Brit. Soc. of Gastroenerology. Prev: Cons. Phys. Cheltenham Gen. Hosp.; Chief Med. Off. Eagle Star Insur. Gp.; Chairm. Med. Panel Cheltenham Coll.

ORMEROD, William Paterson (retired) The Grey House, 102 West St., Corfe Castle, Wareham BH20 5HE — MB BChir Camb. 1961 (Camb. & Bristol) MA, MB Camb. 1961, BChir 1961. Medically Qualified Panel Mem. (MQPM) for the Appeals Serv., Wales and S. Western Region. Prev: GP Poole,Dorset 1965-1995.

ORMISTON, Ian Nigel Robert Milton House Surgery, Doctors Commons Road, Berkhamsted HP4 3BY Tel: 01442 874784 Fax: 01442 877694 — MB BS Lond. 1974; MRCP (UK) 1977; DRCOG 1982.

ORMISTON, Mr Ian William Department of Oral & Maxillofacial Surgery, Leicester Royal Infirmary, Infirmary Square, Leicester LE1 5WW Tel: 0116 258 5254 Fax: 0116 258 5205 — MRCS Eng. LRCP Lond. 1987; BDS Ed. 1981; FDS RCS Eng. 1992; FRCS Ed. 1994. Cons. Oral & Maxillofacial Surg., Maxillofacial unit, Leicester Roy. Infimary. Specialty: Oral & Maxillofacial Surg. Socs: Fell. Coll. Surgs. Hong Kong; Fell.Brit. Assoc. Oral & Maxillofacial Surgs.; Fell.Hong Kong Acad. of Med. Prev: SHO (Head & Neck, ENT & Oral & Maxillofacial Surg.) Leics. HA; Lect. (Oral & Maxillofacial Surg.) Univ. Hong Kong.

ORMISTON, Mr Michael Charles Elliott Hemel Hempstead General Hospital, Hillfield Road, Hemel Hempstead HP2 4AD Tel: 01442 213141 — MB BChir Camb. 1974; FRCS Eng. 1978; MChir Camb. 1984. Cons. Surg. St Albans & Hemel Hempstead NHS Trust. Specialty: Gen. Surg.; Vasc. Med. Socs: Vasc. Surgic. Soc. GB & Irel.; Assn. of Surg.s of Gt. Britain & Irel.; BMA. Prev: Sen. Regist. King's Coll. Hosp. Lond.

ORMISTON, Philip John Burnside Surgery, 365 Blackburn Road, Bolton BL1 8DZ Tel: 01204 528205 Fax: 01204 386409 — MB ChB Sheff. 1978; DRCOG 1981; MSc Manch. 1997.

ORMONDE, Susan Elizabeth Ophthalmology Department, Royal Berkshire Hospital, Reading RG1 5AN Tel: 01734 875111 — MB ChB Bristol 1992. SHO (Ophth.) Roy. Berks. Hosp. Specialty: Ophth. Prev: SHO (Ophth.) Roy. Berks. Hosp.; Ho. Phys. & Ho. Surg. Bristol Roy. Infirm.; Resid. Med. Off. BUPA Hosp. Sutton Coldfield.

ORMROD, Mr John Neville (retired) Malt House, Chart Road, Chart Sutton, Maidstone ME17 3RA — MB ChB Birm. 1944; MB ChB (Hon.) Birm. 1944; DO Eng. 1952; FRCS Eng. 1956; FRCOphth. 1988. Prev: Cons. Ophth. Surg. Kent Co. Ophth. Hosp. Maidstone & Gravesend & N. Kent Hosp.

ORMSBY, James Matthew Ravenswood House, Knowle, Fareham PO17 5NA — BM Soton. 1991; MRCPsyc 1996. Specialist Regist., Wessex. Specialty: Gen. Psychiat.; Forens. Psychiat.

ORMSTON, Brian John 6 Peckitt Street, York YO1 1SF Tel: 01904 639171; 322 Tadcaster Road, York YO24 1HF — MB BS Newc. 1968; MRCP (UK) 1974; FRCGP 1997. GP York; Dep. Dir. Postgrad. Med. Educat. Yorks.

ORMSTON, Ronald Mark Ayton 6 Dorset House, Gloucester Place, London NW1 5AB Tel: 020 7935 7299 — (Univ. & Roy. Colls. Ed. & Dub.) LRCP LRCS Ed. LRFPS Glas. 1933; DPM RCPSI 1936.

ORNADEL, Dan Department of Chest Medicine, Northwick Park Hospital, Watford Road, London E16 3QU Tel: 020 8869 2613 Email: dan.ornadel@lineone.net — MB BS Lond. 1987 (St Thomas' Hosp.) BA Oxf. 1985; MRCP (UK) 1990; MD (London) 1999. Cons. Respirat. Med. Northwick Pk. Hosp. Lond. Specialty: Gen. Med.; Respirat. Med.; Intens. Care. Socs: Brit. Thoracic Sosciety; Roy. Soc. Med.; Amer. Thoracic Soc.

ORNSTEIN, Mr Marcus Henry Consulting Rooms, 118 Harley Street, London W1G 7JN; The Hill Studio, 23 Crown Street, Harrow on the Hill, Harrow HA2 0HX Tel: 020 8423 8236 Fax: 020 8423 3339 Email: mark.ornstein@virgin.net — MB ChB Bristol 1968; FRCS Eng. 1973; Accredit. Surg. 1983. Indep. Cons. Lond.; Locum Cons. Surg. (Gen. & Breast Surg.) St Mary's Hosp. NHS Trust Lond. Specialty: Gen. Surg. Socs: Assn. Surg. GB. & Irel.; Roy. Soc. Med.; BMA. Prev: Hon. Clin. Teach. St. Mary's Hosp. Med. Sch. Lond.; Sen. Regist. (Surg.) St. Mary's Hosp. Lond.; Regist. (Surg.) Northwick Pk. Hosp. Middlx.

ORPEN, Ian Michael St James Surgery, 8-9 Northampton Buildings, Bath BA1 2SR Tel: 01225 422911 Fax: 01225 428398; 22 Hantone Hill, Bathampton, Bath BA2 6XD — MB ChB Cape

Town 1982; DGM RCP Lond. 1989; DCH RCP Lond. 1989; MRCGP 1990. Prev: Asst. GP Bath; Trainee GP Bath VTS.

ORPHANIDES, D The Surgery, 74 Perry Hall Road, Orpington BR6 0HS Tel: 01689 837366 Fax: 01689 872990.

ORPIN, Madeleine Mary Tower House Practice, St. Pauls Health Centre, High Street, Runcorn WA7 1AB Tel: 01928 567404; 8 Borrowdale Close, Frodsham, Warrington WA6 7LN Tel: 01928 733611 — MB BS Lond. 1978; DCH RCP Lond. 1981; MRCGP Lond. 1982; DRCOG 1983.

ORPIN, Richard Peter Ian Shelley Surgery, 23 Shelley Road, Worthing BN11 4BS; Green Banks, Mill Lane, Worthing BN13 3DE Tel: 01903 263813 — MB BS Lond. 1976 (Char. Cross) MRCS Eng. LRCP Lond. 1976; DCH Eng. 1978; MRCGP 1981; DRCOG 1981. Specialty: Paediat. Prev: Trainee GP Portsmouth; SHO (O & G) St. Mary's Hosp. Portsmouth; SHO (Med.) Brook Hosp. Lond.

ORR, Andrew William Townhead Surgery, Townhead, Murray Lane, Montrose DD10 8LE Tel: 01674 676161 Fax: 01674 673151 — MB BS Lond. 1971 (St. Bart.) MRCS Eng. LRCP Lond. 1971; DObst RCOG 1974; MRCGP 1977; DCH Eng. 1977; FRCGP 1999. Prev: SHO (Obst.) Rochford Gen. Hosp.; SHO (Paediat.) B.M.H. Munster; Maj. RAMC.

ORR, Anthony McNeill Moorfield House Surgery, 35 Edgar Street, Hereford HR4 9JP Tel: 01432 272175 Fax: 01432 341942; Highcroft, Longmeadow, Breinton, Hereford HR4 7PA Tel: 01432 354948 Email: amorr@doctors.org.uk — MB BS Lond. 1984 (The London Hospital Medical College) DRCOG; LHMC. Gen. Pract.-Princip.

ORR, Brian William Gordon (retired) 64 St Marys Road, Cowes PO31 7ST Tel: 01983 295527 Fax: 01983 295527 — MB BChir Camb. 1956 (Cambridge University, Middlesex Hospital) DRCOG 1961. Prev: Gen. Practioner, Portsmouth.

ORR, Charles James Kirkpatrick (retired) 13 Hillside Park, Ballymena BT43 5ND Tel: 0285 656068 — MB BCh BAO Belf. 1939 (Qu. Univ. Belf.) DA Eng. 1948; FFA RCS Eng. 1953; FRCA 1993. Hon. Cons. Anaesth. Mid Antrim Area Gp. Hosps. Prev: Sen. Cons. Anaesth. Mid-Antrim Area Gp. Hosps.

ORR, David Hugh Musgrave & Clark House, Royal Victoria Hospital, Grosvenor Road, Belfast BT12 6BA — MB BCh Belf. 1997.

ORR, David Samuel Alexander Garvagh Health Centre, 110 Main Street, Garvagh, Coleraine BT51 5AE Tel: 028 2955 8210 Fax: 028 2955 7089; 78 Drumsaragh Road, Kilrea, Coleraine BT51 5XR — MB BCh BAO Belf. 1985; DRCOG 1988; MRCGP 1990.

ORR, Desmond Alan Dept. Anaesthesia, Craigavon Area Hospital Group Trust, Craigavon BT63 5QQ Tel: 028 38 334444; 19 Corcreeny Road, Hillsborough BT26 6EH — MB BS Newc. 1979; FFA RCSI 1983; FFA RCS Eng. 1984. Cons. Anaesth. Craigavon Area Hosp. Specialty: Anaesth.

ORR, Donald Stuart (retired) Thatchers, Combe Raleigh, Honiton EX14 4TQ Tel: 01404 43198 — MRCS Eng. LRCP Lond. 1942 (Guy's) Prev: Ho. Phys. & Ho. Surg. EMS.

ORR, Mr Douglas James Glasgow Royal Infirmary, 84 Castle Street, Glasgow G4 0SF — MB ChB Glas. 1990; BSc (Hons.) Glas. 1987; FRCS Glas. 1994; FRCS Ed. 1994. Specialty: Gen. Surg.

ORR, Mr Frederick George Geoffrey 48 Esplanade, Greenock PA16 7SD Tel: 01475 787038 — MB ChB Birm. 1971; BSc (Hons.) Anat. Birm. 1968; FRCS Ed. 1976. Cons. Urol. Inverclyde Roy. Hosp. Greenock. Specialty: Urol. Socs: Brit. Assn. Urol. Surg.; Assn. Surg. Prev: Sen. Regist. (Gen. Surg.) Aberd. Hosp.

ORR, George Alfred Birleywood Health Centre, Birleywood, Skelmersdale WN8 9BW Tel: 01695 723333 Fax: 01695 556193; 236 Elmers Green Lane, Skelmersdale WN8 6SN — MB ChB Liverp. 1980. Socs: W Lancs. Med. Soc.

ORR, Gordon David Front Street Surgery, 14 Front Street, Acomb, York YO24 3BZ Tel: 01904 794141 Fax: 01904 788304 — MB ChB Ed. 1990; DRCOG 1994. Trainee GP/SHO Carlisle VTS.

ORR, Ian Alexander Craigavon Area Hospital, Craigavon BT63 5QQ Tel: 04428 3833 4444 Email: ianorr@cahgt.n-i.nhs.uk — MB BCh BAO Belf. 1975 (Queens University, Belfast) FFA RCSI 1978; DRCOG 1979; MD (Hons.) Belf. 1981. Cons. Anaesth. Craigavon Area Hosp. Specialty: Anaesth. Socs: Chairm., Educat. Comm., Coll. of Anaesthetists, RCSI Dub. Prev: Cons. Roy. Vict. Hosp. Belf.

ORR, Jacqueline Elizabeth Royal Alexandra Hospital Trust, Corsebar Road, Paisley PA2 9PN Tel: 0141 887 9111; 48 Esplanade, Greenock PA16 7SD Tel: 01475 787038 — MB ChB Aberd. 1976; FFA RCS Eng. 1980. Cons. Anaesth. Roy. Alexandra Hosp. Paisley. Specialty: Anaesth. Socs: Assn. Anaesth.; Obst. Anaesth. Assn.; Difficult Airway Soc.

ORR, James Henry (retired) c/o National Westminster Bank plc., 7 Manor Square, Otley LS21 3AP Email: jorr204459@aol.com — MB ChB Bristol 1955; DPM Eng. 1966; FRCPsych 1978, M 1972. Prev: Cons. Forens. Psychiat. W. Yorks.

ORR, James Thomas King Street Surgery, 38 King Street, Lancaster LA1 1RE — MB BS Lond. 1998.

ORR, Jane Elizabeth Keppel, Maj. RAMC Retd. Upper Gordon Road Surgery, 37 Upper Gordon Road, Camberley GU15 2HJ Tel: 01276 26424 Fax: 01276 63486; Selhurst, 119 Gordon Road, Camberley GU15 2JQ Tel: 01276 22584 Fax: 01276 502873 — MB BS Lond. 1974 (St. Mary's) MRCS Eng. LRCP Lond. 1974; DRCOG 1980. Staff Grade Psychiat. Broadmoor Hosp. Specialty: Gen. Pract. Prev: Clin. Asst. (Colposcopy) Frimley Pk. Hosp. Camberley; Cadets' Med. Off. Roy. Milit. Acad. Sandhurst; Clincal Med. Off. (Family Plann.) Surrey HA.

ORR, Jean Forbes Moonrakers, Forest Road, Binfield, Bracknell RG42 4HB — MB ChB Ed. 1957; DA Eng. 1963.

ORR, John Anthony 428 Lanark Road, Colinton, Edinburgh EH13 0LT — MB ChB Aberd. 1998.

ORR, John Douglas Gilbert Road Medical Group, 39 Gilbert Road, Bucksburn, Aberdeen AB21 9AN Tel: 01224 712138 Fax: 01224 712239; 15 Glenhome Walk, Dyce, Aberdeen AB21 7FJ Tel: 01224 722801 Email: d.orr@easynet.co.uk — MB ChB Ed. 1969; BSc (Med. Sci.) Ed. 1966; DObst RCOG 1971; MRCP (UK) 1973; FPA 1975; MRCGP 1975; Dip. Sports Med. Scotl. 1992; Primary Care Certificate in Homeopathy 1996; FRCGP 2002. GP; Sen. Lect. (Gen. Pract.). Specialty: Rheumatol.; Sports Med. Prev: Regist. (Gen. Med.) Foresterhill & Assoc. Hosps. Aberd.; Ho. Phys. Milesmark Hosp. Dunfermline; Ho. Surg. Bangour Gen. Hosp. W. Lothian.

ORR, Mr John Douglas Royal Hospital for Sick Children, Sciennes Road, Edinburgh EH9 1LF Tel: 0131 536 0667 Fax: 0131 536 0666 Email: john.orr@luht.scot.nhs.uk — MB ChB St. And. 1969; FRCS Ed. 1975; CCST (Gen. Surg.) 1981; CCST (Paed. Surg) 1983; MBA Stirling 1998; FRCGP 2003. Cons. Paediat. Surg. Roy. Hosp. Sick Childr. Edin.; Chairm., Intercollegiate Comm. for Basic Surgic. Train.; Assoc. Med. Director Univ. Hosps. Div.,LHB; Vice Pres. Roy. Coll. of Surgeons of Edin.; Chairm. SAC in Paediatric Surg. Specialty: Paediat. Surg. Socs: Scott. Comm. for Hosp. Med. Serv.s (Treas.); Brit. Asscoiation of Med. Managers (BAMM).; Brit. Asscoiation of Paediatric Surg. Prev: Sen. Regist. (Surg.) Roy. Hosp. for Sick Childr. Edin.; Sen. Regist. (Paediat. Surg.) Hosp. for Sick Childr Gt. Ormond St.; Lond.; Sen. Regist. (Surg.) Aberd. Roy. Infirm.

ORR, Katherine Elizabeth Freeman Hospital, Freeman Road, High Heaton, Newcastle upon Tyne NE7 7DN Tel: 0191 284 3111 — MB ChB Bristol 1985; FRCPath; MRCPath 1991. Cons. Med. Microbiol. Freeman Hosp. Newc. u. Tyne. Specialty: Med. Microbiol.

ORR, Keith Matthew Meadowbank Health Centre, 3 Salmon Inn Road, Falkirk FK2 0XF Tel: 01324 715753 Fax: 01324 717565 — MB ChB Glas. 1985.

ORR, Mr Kenneth Gibson (retired) 1 Avonbrook Gardens, Mountsandel Road, Coleraine BT52 1SS Tel: 028 7034 2355 — MB BCh BAO Belf. 1949 (Belf) FRCS Ed. 1956. Prev: Cons. Surg. Mid-Ulster Hosp. Magherafelt.

ORR, Lesley Ann Accident & Emergency Dept, Hairmyres Hosp, Eaglesham Road, East Kilbride, Glasgow G75 8RG Tel: 01355 220292; 6 Lochend Road, Bearsden, Glasgow G61 1DU — MB ChB Dundee 1983; DA (UK) 1987. Staff Grade (A & E), Hairmyres Hosp., E. Kilbride. Specialty: Accid. & Emerg. Prev: Regist. (Anaesth.) Law Hosp. Carluke; SHO (Surg.) Vict. Infirm. Glas.; SHO (A & E) Glas. Roy. Infirm.

ORR, Miss Linda Elizabeth 62 Seahill Road, Holywood BT18 0DW Tel: 028 9042 2648 — MB ChB Bristol 1991; FRSM; BSc (Hons.) Bristol 1986; Dip. App. Basic Sci. RCS Eng. 1997; FRCS (Eng) 1999. SPR SW Region Otolaryngol. Specialty: Otolaryngol. Socs: Wom. in Surg. Train.; Roy. Soc. Med. Prev: SHO Ent, Roy. Hosp. HASLAR; Med. Off. Roy. Army Med. Corps; SHO (Burno & Plastics) Frenchay Hosp. Bristol.

ORR, Malcolm John 150 Chesterholm, Sandsfield Park, Carlisle CA2 7XY — MB ChB Dund. 1998.

ORR, Margaret Jane Parklands Surgery, 4 Parklands Road, Chichester PO19 3DT Tel: 01243 782819/786827 — BM (Hons.) Soton. 1979; DRCOG 1982; DCH RCP Lond. 1983; MRCGP 1986.

ORR, Mr Mark Monro (retired) Department of Surgery, Horton General Hospital Oxford Radcliffe Trust, Oxford Road, Banbury OX16 9AL Tel: 01295 229206 Fax: 01295 229271; Motte Hollow, Ratley, Banbury OX15 6DT Tel: 01295 670364 — MB BS Lond. 1962 (St. Bart.) BSc (Physiol.) Lond. 1959; FRCS Eng. 1969. Prev: Lect. (Surg.) St. Bart. Hosp. Lond.

ORR, Martin James 9 Lamond Place, Aberdeen AB25 3UT — MB ChB Glas. 1997.

ORR, Michael William Isham House, St. Andrew's Group of Hospitals, Billing Road, Northampton NN1 2DG Tel: 01604 616188 Email: michaelworr@aol.com — MD Malta 1967; BSc Oxf. 1971, BA 1969; DPM Eng. 1973; FRCPsych 1987, M 1974; DM Oxf. 1981. Specialty: Gen. Psychiat.; Intens. Care. Socs: Roy. Coll. of Psychiatrists; Roy. Soc. of Med. Prev: Dist. Clin. Tutor Oxon. HA; Lect. Univ. Dept. Psychiat. Warneford; Hosp. Oxf.; Research Fell. Clin. Psychopharmacol. Univ. Dept. & MRC; Unit of Clin. Pharmacol. Radcliffe Infirm. Oxf.

ORR, Mr Neil Wallace Morison (retired) 45 Lexden Road, Colchester CO3 3PY Tel: 01206 573854 — (Camb. & St. Thos.) MA Camb. 1957, MD 1963, MChir 1966, MB 1957, BChir 1956; FRCS Eng. 1966. Prev: Cons. Surg. Colchester Gen. Hosp.

ORR, Pauline Ann The Health Centre, Loftus Hill, Sedbergh LA10 5RX Tel: 01539 620218 Fax: 01539 620265; Farley Croft, Joss Lane, Sedbergh LA10 5AS Tel: 01539 621496 — MB ChB Aberd. 1972; Fam. Planning Certif. 1975; DCH Eng. 1975; MRCGP 1976; Dip. Pract. Dermat. Wales 1990; Dip. Ther. Newc. 1995. GP Sedbergh, Cumbria; Med. Mem. Indep. Tribunal Serv. Specialty: Gen. Pract. Prev: GP Morecambe; SHO (Gen. Med.) Roy. Lancaster Infirm.; SHO (O & G) Dudley Rd. Hosp. Birm.

ORR, Peter Kenneth 21 Durham Road, Bishop Auckland DL14 7HU — MB BS Newc. 1980; FRCR 1987. Cons. Radiol. Bishop Auckland Gen. Hosp. Specialty: Radiol.

ORR, Mr Peter Stewart — MB ChB Glas. 1967; DObst RCOG 1969; FRCS Glas. 1973; MPhil (Law & Ethics in Med.) Glas. 1994. Cons. (Urol.) Monklands, Hosp. Specialty: Urol. Socs: BMA; Brit. Assn. of Urological Surg.s; Scottish Medico-Legal Soc. Prev: Sen. Regist. (Urol.) Glas. Roy. Infirm.; Ho. Off. (Surg.) Vict. Infirm. Glas.; Ho. Off. (Med.) South. Gen. Hosp. Glas.

ORR, Raymond Michael 83 Mount Annan Dr, Kingspark, Glasgow G44 4RX — MB ChB Glas. 1997.

ORR, Richard Burnet Faris Eldon Health Clinic, 12 Torquay Road, Newton Abbot TQ12 1AH Tel: 01626 205400 Fax: 01626 205402 — MB BS Lond. 1959 (St. Thos.) MRCS Eng. LRCP Lond. 1959; DPM Eng. 1968; MRCPsych 1972. Cons. S. Devon Healthcare Trust; Civil. Cons. Psychiat., Roy. Navy. Specialty: Gen. Psychiat. Prev: Ho. Phys. St. Thos. Hosp. Lond.; Resid. in Med. New York Univ., U.S.A.; Sen. Regist. Profess. Unit, Warneford Hosp. Oxf.

ORR, Robert Lindsay 76 Jackson Avenue, Mickleover, Derby DE3 9AT — MB ChB Leic. 1995.

ORR, Robin Gooch 9 Pointers Hill, Westcott, Dorking RH4 3PF Tel: 01306 888596 — MB BS Lond. 1953 (Guy's) LMSSA Lond. 1953; DObst RCOG 1955; DPH Lond. 1956; DIH Eng. 1957; MFOM RCP Lond. 1978. Specialty: Occupat. Health. Socs: BMA. Prev: Resid. Obst., Ho. Phys., Asst. Ho. Surg. & Outpats. Off. Guy's Hosp. Lond.

ORR, Roslyn Denise 133 Mountsandel Road, Coleraine BT52 1TA — MB BS Newc. 1995.

ORR, Thomas Andrew Linlithgow Health Centre, 288 High Street, Linlithgow EH49 7ER Tel: 01506 670027; Bonnytounside, Linlithgow EH49 7RQ Tel: 01506 845237 — MB ChB Ed. 1973; DObst RCOG 1975.

ORR, Valerie Anne Randerston, Kings Barns, St Andrews KY16 8QE Tel: 01333 450462 — MB ChB Aberd. 1996.

ORR, William Graham The Health Centre, Loftus Hill, Sedbergh LA10 5RX — MB BS Lond. 1967 (St. Mary's) MRCGP 1976. Locum GP; Med. Mem. Appeals Tribunal Serv. Specialty: Gen. Pract. Socs: Roy. Soc. Med. Prev: GP Morecambe.

ORR, William Peter Department of Cardiology, Royal Berkshire Hospital NHS Trust, London Road, Reading RG1 5AN Tel: 0118 963 6695 Fax: 0118 963 6622 Email: william.orr@rbbh-tr.nhs.uk; BUPA Dunedin Hospital, 16 Bath Road, Reading RG1 6NB Tel: 0118 955-3458 Fax: 0118 955-3478 Email: adamssu@bupa.com — MB BS Lond. 1989 (Lond. Hosp. Med. Coll.) MRCP (UK) 1993. Cons. Cardiol. Roy. Berks. Hosp. NHS Trust, Reading, Berks. Specialty: Gen. Med.; Cardiol. Special Interest: Coronary Artery Dis., AF, Syncope, Heart Failure. Prev: Interventional Cardiol. Fell.. Green La. Hosp., Auckland, NZ.; Specialist Regist. Cardiol. John Radcliffe Hosp. Oxf.; BHF Jun. Research Fell., Dept of Cardiovasc. Med., Univ. of Oxf.

ORR, Mr William Stephen Michael Yarm Medical Centre, 1 Worsall Road, Yarm TS15 9DD Tel: 01642 786422 Fax: 01642 785617; The Old School, Crathorne, Yarm TS15 0BA — MB BCh BAO Dub. 1974; BA (Hons.) Dub. 1971, MB BCh BAO 1974; FRCSI 1978; MRCGP 1984; DRCOG 1985. Prev: Clin. Research Fell. Roy. Vict. Hosp. Belf.

ORRELL, David Howard (retired) Royal Lancaster Infirmary, Lancaster LA1 4RP Tel: 01524 65944; Yew Tree Cottage, Selby Lane, Melling, Carnforth LA6 2RA — MB BChir Camb. 1962 (Camb. & St. Bart.) BA Camb. 1958, MA, MB 1962, BChir 1961; FRCP Lond. 1992, M 1964; FRCPath 1987, M 1970. Cons. Chem. Path. Roy. Lancaster Infirm. Prev: Cons. Chem. Path. Roy. Lancaster Infirm.

ORRELL, Jonathan Martin 12 Coldharbour, Chickerell, Weymouth DT3 4BG; Abbey Manor Surgery, Abbey Village Centre, Abbey Manor Park, Yeovil BA21 3TL Tel: 01305 33434 — MB BS Lond. 1985; DRCOG 1989; MRCGP 1990. Socs: Christ. Med. Fellowsh.; Caring Professions Concern. Prev: Trainee GP Som. VTS.

ORRELL, Judith Clare 11 Beechwood Drive, Ormskirk L39 3NU Tel: 01695 574477; 63 Ash Close, Appley Bridge, Wigan WN6 9HU Tel: 0125 725 4695 — MB ChB Manch. 1988. Trainee GP Wrexham Maelor Hosp.

ORRELL, Julian Maxwell Department of Pathology, Ipswich Hospital NHS Trust, Ipswich IP4 5PD Tel: 01473 703359 — MB ChB Manch. 1985; MRCPath 1992; BSc Manch. 1982, MD Manch. 1994. Cons. Histopath. Ipswich Hosp. NHS Trust. Specialty: Histopath. Prev: Lect. & Hon. Sen. Regist. (Path.) Ninewells Hosp. & Med. Sch. Dundee; Regist. (Histopath.) Ninewells Hosp. Med. Sch. Dundee; Regist. (Path. Biochem.) West. Infirm. Glas.

ORRELL, Martin John (retired) 7 Brunel Drive, Weymouth DT3 6NU Tel: 01305 834049 Fax: 08700 940045 Email: orrellhq@globalnet.co.uk — (Westm.) MB BChir Camb. 1960; MA Camb. 1960; DObst RCOG 1961; MRCGP 1967. Prev: GP Weymouth.

ORRELL, Martin William Princess Alexandra Hospital, Harlow CM20 1QX Tel: 01279 827260 Fax: 01279 454018 Email: m.orrell@ucl.ac.uk; 27 Wickfield Avenue, Christchurch BH23 1JB — BM BS Nottm. 1982; BMedSci (Hons.) Nottm. 1980; MRCPsych. 1989; PhD Lond. 1994. Reader (Psychiat. of Ageing) Univ. Coll. Lond.; Hon. Cons. Psychiat. of Elderly Princess Alexandra Hosp. Harlow; Edr. Internat. Jl. Aging & Ment. Health. Specialty: Geriat. Psychiat. Socs: Eur. Assn. Sci. Eds. Prev: Sen. Regist. Maudsley Hosp. Lond.; Research Regist. Inst. Psychiat. Maudsley Hosp.

ORRELL, Mary Gillian (retired) Wick House, 17 Well Cross, Edith Weston, Oakham LE15 8HG Tel: 01780 720196 — MB BChir Camb. 1955 (Camb. & St. Thos.) MA Camb. 1956; DObst RCOG 1957. Prev: Med. Adviser DSS.

ORRELL, Richard William Department of Neurology, Royal Free Hospital, Pond Street, London NW3 2QG Tel: 020 7830 2387 Fax: 020 7472 6829 Email: r.orrell@rfc.ucl.ac.uk — MB ChB Manch. 1982; DCH RCP Lond. 1984; MRCP (UK) 1987; BSc (Hons. Physiol.) Manch. 1979, MD 1996; FRCP UK 2002. Sen. Lect. (Clin. Neurosci.s) Roy. Free &Univ. Coll. Med. Sch., Lond.; Nat. Hosp. For Neurol. & Neurosurg.; Cons. Neurologist Roy. Free Hosp. Lond.; Cons. Neurologist Qu. Eliz. Hosp. Welwyn Garden City. Specialty: Neurol. Prev: Sen. Regist. (Neurol.) Hammersmith Hosp. & Char. Cross Hosp. Lond.; Hon. Lect. Acad. Unit. Neurosci. Char. Cross & Westm. Med. Sch. Univ. Lond.; Vis. Prof. MRC Trav. Fell. (Neurol.) Univ. Rochester Med. Center NY, USA.

ORRIDGE, Howard William St John's Group Practice, 1 Greenfield Lane, Balby, Doncaster DN4 0TH Tel: 01302 854521 Fax: 01302 310823; Stonecross Cottage, Wadworth Hall Lane, Wadworth, Doncaster DN11 9BH — MB BS Lond. 1981.

ORRITT, Sterry Gordon Charles Medical Centre, 1 Rawling Road, Gateshead NE8 4QS Tel: 0191 477 2180 — (Newcastle Upon Tyne) MB BS Newc. 1986; DA (UK) 1989; DRCOG 1991; MRCGP 1993.

ORSI, Claudia Rosa — MB BS 1990; BSc Lond. 1987; DCH RCP Lond. 1992; MRCGP 1995. GP Retainer Rickmansworth Herts. Prev: Trainee GP/SHO St. Mary's Hosp. Lond. VTS.

ORTEGA, Luis Salvador 274 West Way, Broadstone BH18 9LL — LMS U Autonoma Bilbao 1988.

ORTEGA SIPAN, Anna Maria Royal Hospital for Sick Children, 129 Drumchapel Road, Glasgow G15 6PX — LMS U Autonoma Barcelona 1992.

ORTEU, Catherine Helene Dermatology Department, Clinic 6, Royal Free Hospital, Pond Street, London NW3 2QG Email: cate.orteu@royalfree.nhs.uk; 94 Eton Rise, Eton College Road, London NW3 2DB — MB BS Lond. 1987 (Royal London) BSc Lond. 1984; MRCP (UK) 1992; MD Lond. 1999. Cons. & Hon. Sen. Lect. Dermat., Roy. Free Hosp., Lond. Specialty: Dermat. Socs: Brit. Assn. Dermat.; Soc. Clinique Française; Brit. Soc. for Investigative Dermat. Prev: Hon. Sen. Regist. (Dermat) & Clin. Research Fell. Acad. Dept. Med. Roy. Free Hosp. Sch. of Med. Lond.; Regist. (Dermat.) Roy. Free Hosp. Lond.; Regist. Rotat. (Hosp. Med.) & SHO Lond. Hosp. Whitechapel.

ORTH, Astrid 75 Highcliffe Road, Sheffield S11 7LP — State Exam Med Munich 1988; State Exam Med Technical Univ. Munich 1988. Regist. (Paediat.) Sheff. Prev: SHO King's Mill Hosp. Mansfield.

ORTON, Caroline Jane Cookridge Hospital, Hospital Lane, Cookridge, Leeds LS16 6QB Tel: 0113 392 4035 Fax: 0113 392 4072 Email: jane.orton@leedsth.nhs.uk — MB ChB Sheff. 1982; MRCPsych 1988; FRCR 1994. Cons. (Clin. Oncol.) Cookridge Hosp. Leeds; Counc. Mem. of Brit. Gyn. Cancer Soc. 2000. Specialty: Oncol. Socs: Brit. Gyn. Cancer Soc. - Counc. Mem. Prev: Specialist Regist. (Clin. Oncol.) Christie Hosp. Manch.; Clin. Research Fell. Paterson Inst. Cancer Research Manch.; Regist. (Clin. Oncol.) Newc.

ORTON, Christine Margaret Park View Surgery, Haverflatts Lane, Milnthorpe LA7 7PS Tel: 015395 63327 Fax: 015395 64059; Stoneleigh Surg., Police Square, Milntnonee Tel: 01639 663307; Brookside Cottage, Over Kellet, Carnforth LA6 1BS — MB ChB Dundee 1987; BSc Sheff. 1983. Specialty: Gen. Pract.; Palliat. Med. Prev: Trainee GP Stoneleigh Surg. Milnthorpe; SHO (A & E & Psychiat.) Lancaster.

ORTON, Mr Clive Ian BUPA Hospital, Russell Road, Whalley Range, Manchester M16 8AJ Tel: 0161 861 0553 Fax: 0161 226 9014 Email: clive@cliveorton.com — MB BS Lond. 1967 (Univ. Coll. Hosp.) BDS Lond. 1962; MRCS Eng. LRCP Lond. 1967; FDS RCS Eng. 1969; FRCS Eng. 1972. Pres. of the Brit. Assn. of Aesthetic Plastic Surg.s. Specialty: Plastic Surg. Socs: Brit. Assn. Plastic Surg.; Brit Assn. Of Aesthetic Plastic Surg.; Internat. Soc. Of Aesthetic Plastic Surg. Prev: Cons. Plastic Surg. at the Christie Hosp. and the Univ. Hosp. of S. Manch.

ORTON, David Arnold The Laurels CMHC, C/o Newton Abbot Hospital, 62 East Street, Newton Abbot TQ12 4PT Tel: 01626 357335 Fax: 01626 357338 — MB ChB Birm. 1970; MRCP (UK) 1974; MRCPsych 1982. Cons. Psychiat. S. Devon Healthcare Trust; Vis. Cons. The Priory N. Lond.. Specialty: Gen. Psychiat. Prev: Cons. Psychiat. W. Herts. Community (NHS) Trust; Sen. Regist. Princess Margt. Migraine Clinic & Hon. Lect. (Clin. Pharmacol.) St. Bart. Hosp. Lond.; Regist. (Psychiat.) Northwich Pk. & Shenley Hosps.

ORTON, David Ian Amersham Hospital, Department of Dermatology, Whielden Street, Amersham HP7 0JD Tel: 01494 734613 Fax: 01494 734662; 56 Cuckoo Hill Drive, Pinner HA5 3PJ — MB BS Lond. 1988 (Char. Cross & Westm.) BSc (Hons.) Lond. 1985; MRCP (UK) 1992. Cons. Dermatol. Amersham Hosp.; Cons. (Dermatology) Wycombe Hosp.; Cons. (Dermatology) Stoke Mandeville Hosp. Specialty: Dermat. Socs: Brit. Assn. Dermatol.; Europ. Soc. Contact Dermatitis; Brit. Soc. Allergy & Clin. Immunol. Prev: SpR Dermat. Rotat., Roy. Free Hosp. Lond. & Lond. Hosp.

ORTON, Dean Wells (retired) Mayfield, Ullesthorpe Road, Bitteswell, Lutterworth LE17 4SD — MRCS Eng. LRCP Lond. 1950 (Ed.) DObst RCOG 1952. Prev: SHO (Surg.) Bolton Roy. Infirm.

ORTON, Edward Maurice 109 Lords' View, St John's Wood Road, London NW8 7HG Tel: 020 7289 1786 — (Camb. & Char. Cross) MRCS Eng. LRCP Lond. 1950; BA Camb. 1947, MA 1950, MB BChir 1952. Prev: Med. Off. Tesco Stores Ltd. & Dentsply Ltd.; Ho. Phys. Char. Cross Hosp. Unit, Mt. Vernon Hosp. N.wood.

ORTON, Julian Jasper Soring Street Surgery, Bourne Hall Health Centre, Ewell, Epsom KT17 1TG Tel: 020 8394 1362 Fax: 020 8394 8650 — MB ChB Manch. 1986; MRCP (UK) 1990; DRCOG 1992. Specialty: Gen. Pract. Prev: SHO (Paediat.) Epsom Gen. Hosp.; Regist. (Psychiat.) Priory Hosp. Roehampton; Trainee GP Fetcham, Surrey VTS.

ORTON, Katharine Anne The Surgery, Broomfields, Hatfield Heath, Bishop's Stortford CM22 7EH Tel: 01279 730616 Fax: 01279 730408; Matching Parsonage Farm, Newmans End, Matching, Harlow CM17 0QX Tel: 01279 731536 — MB BS Lond. 1978 (Charing Cross Hospital Medical School) DRCOG 1980; DCH RCP Lond. 1981; MRCGP 1982; Dip. Addic. Behaviour Lond. 1994; FRCGP 2003. F/T Princip. in G.P at Broomfield N.Health; Community Specialist (NEMHPT) N. Essex Ment. Health NHS Partnership Trust. Socs: Fell.Roy. Soc. Med.; GP Tutor UCL & Roy. Free.

ORTON, Peggy Kathleen Lillian (retired) Oakwood, North Road, Chideock, Bridport DT6 6LE Tel: 01297 489742 — MRCS Eng. LRCP Lond. 1943 (Roy. Free) DLO Eng. 1947; FRCS Eng. 1955. Prev: Cons. Otolaryngol. Qu. Mary's Hosp. Childr., St. Helier Hosp. Carshalton, S. Lond. Hosp. Wom. & Eliz. Garrett Anderson Hosp. Lond.

ORTON, Peter Kenneth The Surgery, Broomfields, Hatfield Heath, Bishop's Stortford CM22 7EH Tel: 01279 730616 Fax: 01279 730408; Matching Parsonage Farm, Newmans End, Matching, Harlow CM17 0QX Tel: 01279 731536 — MB BS Lond. 1980 (Char. Cross) MRCS Eng. LRCP Lond. 1980; DRCOG 1984; Cert. Family Plann. JCC 1984; FRCGP 1995, M 1985; MMedSc Leeds 1986; DFFP 1996; Cert. Av. Med. 1996. GP Princip.; Sen. Lect. (Postgrad. Med.) Centre for Continuing Educat. Bath Univ.; Sen. Lect. Inst. of Gen. Pract. Exeter. Specialty: Gen. Pract. Socs: Fell. Roy. Soc. Med. (Ex-Pres. Gen. Pract. Sect.).

ORTON, William Taylor (retired) 145 Thornton Road, Cambridge CB3 0NE Tel: 01223 277511 — MB BCh BAO Belf. 1948; DPH Belf. 1951; MFPHM 1974. Hon. Sec. Inst. Sports Med. Lond. Prev: Dist. Community Phys. Haringey Health Dist.

ORUGUN, Enoch Oluwambe — MB BS Lagos 1979 (Univ. Of Lagos Nigeria) MRCPI 1987; MSc Aberd. 1989; FRCP Lond. 1999; FRCPI 2002. Cons. Phys. (Geriatric Med.) N. Cumbria NHS Trust Whitehaven. Special Interest: Clin. Pharmacol.; Health Servs. Research. Socs: Brit. Geriat. Soc.; Brit. Assn. of Stroke Physicians; BMA. Prev: Regist. (Gen. Med.) Whitehaven; Regist. (Gen. Med.) Stracatard Hosp Brechin.; Lect. Univ. Coll. Hosp. Lond.

ORWIN, John Michael (retired) 73 Albany Mansions, Albert Bridge Road, London SW11 4PQ — MB ChB Ed. 1963; DA Eng. 1965; FRCA 1968; FFPM RCP (UK) 1990. Centre Dir. Marion Merrell Dow Research & Developm. Centre. Prev: Managing Dir. & Vice Pres. Global Clin. Research Marion Merrell Dow Inc. Kansas City, USA.

OSAKWE, Edwin Aniamaka 10 Jeymer Avenue, London NW2 4PL — MB BS Lond. 1998.

OSBORN, Mr David Eric The Dower House, Vicarage Lane, Barkby, Leicester LE7 — MRCS Eng. LRCP Lond. 1968 (Char. Cross) MS Lond. 1979, MB BS 1968; FRCS Eng. 1974. Cons. Urol. Leic. Gen. Hosp. Specialty: Urol. Prev: Sen. Regist. (Urol.) Withington & Christie Hosps. Manch.; Regist. (Urol. & Transpl.) Hammersmith Hosp. Lond.; Lect. in Physiol. Char. Cross Hosp. Med. Sch. Lond.

OSBORN, David Philip John University College London (Hampstead Campus), University Department of Mental Health Sciences, Rowland Hill Street, London NW3 2PF Tel: 020 7794 0500 Email: d.osborn@medsch.ucl.ac.uk — MB BS Lond. 1993; BA. Cantab. 1990; MRC Psych 1997; MA Cantab. 1998; MSc (Epidemiol. Distinc.) MSC Lond 2000; PhD (Psychiat.) Univ. Coll. Lond. 2004. Sen. Lect. & Hon. Cons. Adult Psychiat. UCL Lond. Specialty: Gen. Psychiat. Special Interest: Physical health of people with Ment. health problems. Socs: BMA; RCPsych; ILTM. Prev: Lect. (Psychiat.) Roy. Free Hosp. Lond.; Hon. Specialist Regist. (Roy. Free Hosp. Lond); Regist. (Psychiat.) Roy. Free Hosp. Lond.

OSBORN, Donna Michelle 77 Goodrich Road, London SE22 0EQ — MB BS Lond. 1998.

OSBORN, Frances Ann 56 Thornyville Villas, Oreston, Plymouth PL9 7LD Tel: 01752 406595 — BM Soton. 1987. SHO (Anaesth.) Torbay Hosp. Prev: SHO (Obsts. & Gyn.) S. Glam. HA; Ho. Phys. St.

Marys Hosp. Newport I. of Wight; Ho. Surg. Cumbld. Infirm. Carlisle.

OSBORN, Gillian Rosemary King George Surgery, 135 High Street, Stevenage SG1 3HT Tel: 01438 361111 Fax: 01438 361227 — MB ChB Birm. 1967 (Birmingham) BSc Birm. 1965. Prev: GP Taunton; Ho. Surg. Childr. Hosp. Birm.; Ho. Phys. Dudley Rd. Hosp. Birm.

OSBORN, Helen Mary St James Surgery, Gains Lane, Devizes SN10 1QU Tel: 01380 722206 Fax: 01380 721552 — MB BS Lond. 1988; DRCOG 1992; MRCGP 1993.

OSBORN, Janet Anne Thorneloe Lodge Surgery, 29 Barbourne Road, Worcester WR1 1RU Tel: 01905 22445 Fax: 01905 610963; Pursers Orchard, Callow End, Worcester WR2 4TY Tel: 22445 — MB ChB Birm. 1963. Prev: Regist. Psychiat. Mabledon Hosp. Dartford.

OSBORN, Marian Lucy (retired) Weavers Hill House, Stoney Lane, Ashmore Green, Thatcham RG18 9HQ — MB BS Lond. 1955 (Roy. Free) Prev: Ho. Surg. & Sen. Cas. Off. Roy. Free Hosp. Lond..

OSBORN, Nicola Anne Pursers Orchard, Callow End, Worcester WR2 4UF — MB ChB Birm. 1988; ChB Birm. 1988.

OSBORN, Stephanie Victoria 25A Scotts Av, Bromley BR2 0LG — MB ChB Sheff. 1997.

OSBORN-SMITH, Erle Hamilton (retired) 5 Royal Walk, Ryde PO33 1NL Tel: 01983 563359 — (Guy's) LMSSA Lond. 1946 DPH Eng. 1957; MRCS Eng. LRCP Lond. 1958; MB BS Lond. 1959; Dip. Audiol. Univ. Manch. 1962; MFCM 1974. Prev: Sen. Med. Off. (Audiol.) E. Sussex AHA.

OSBORNE, Abraham Bertram (retired) 56/2 Spylaw Road, Edinburgh EH10 5BR Tel: 0131 337 2018 — (Ed.) MB ChB Ed. 1945. Prev: Med. Asst. in Psychiat. (Drug Addict) Guy's Hosp.

OSBORNE, Alice Jane — BM BS Nottm. 1993; DRCOG 1996; MRCGP 1997; DFFP 1997. GP Retainer. Specialty: Gen. Pract. Prev: GP Regist. Clevedon Health.

OSBORNE, Andrew William 25 Wellfield Road, Culchetch, Warrington WA3 4JR — MB ChB Sheff. 1987.

OSBORNE, Andrew William Howard 76 Vineyard Hill Road, London SW19 7JJ — MB BS Lond. 1991 (The London Hospital Medical College) FRCS Eng 1997. Specialty: Orthop.

OSBORNE, Mr Anthony Howard, Surg. Capt. RN Retd. Obsborne House, Brook Avenue, Warsash, Southampton SO31 9HP Tel: 01489 577652; 152 Harley Street, London W1N 1AH — (Guy's) MRCS Eng. LRCP Lond. 1967; FRCS Eng. 1976; FRCS Ed. 1976; MCh (Orthop.) Liverp. 1980; FRCS (Orthop.) Ed. 1980. Wessex Nuffield Hosp. E.leigh. Specialty: Orthop. Socs: Fell. Roy. Soc. Med.; Brit. Assn. Surg. Knee. Prev: Head (Orthop.) RNH Haslar Gosport.

OSBORNE, Bridget Virginia Llys Meddyg Surgery, Llys Meddyg, 23 Castle Street, Conwy LL32 8AY Tel: 01492 592424 Fax: 01492 593068 — MB BS Lond. 1980 (Roy. Free) MRCP (UK) 1983; MRCGP 1987. Assoc. GP Conwy Retainer Scheme.

OSBORNE, Caroline Julie Orwell Medical Practice, Loch Leven Health Centre, Kinross — MB ChB Aberd. 1994 (Aberdeen) DRCOG 1996; DFFP 1996; MRCGP. 1998. GP Loch Leven Health Centre Kinross Scotl. Prev: GP Dollar Health Centre Clackmannansh. 2000-2004.

OSBORNE, Caroline Louise Elizabeth Homeleigh Cottage, Guineaford, Barnstaple EX31 4EA — MB BS Lond. 1996.

OSBORNE, Christopher Derek Ian (retired) Nuttall Farmhouse, The Vale, Frostenden, Beccles NR34 7HZ — (Univ. Coll. Hosp.) MB BS Lond. 1966; MRCS Eng. LRCP Lond. 1966; DObst RCOG 1968. Prev: Ho. Surg. W. Norwich Hosp.

OSBORNE, Christopher John 10 Danesboro Road, Bridgwater TA6 7LR — MB ChB Manch. 1980.

OSBORNE, Clifford Ernest The Health Centre, 55 High Street, Great Wakering, Southend-on-Sea SS3 0EF Tel: 01702 218678 Fax: 01702 577853; 17 Plymtree, Thorpe Bay, Southend-on-Sea SS1 3RA Tel: 01702 586934 — LRCPI & LM, LRSCI & LM 1970; LRCPI & LM, LRCSI & LM 1970. Prev: Ho. Phys. & Ho. Surg. Qu. Mary's Hosp. Sidcup.

OSBORNE, David Bruce Rowan (retired) Westacott House, Goodleigh, Barnstaple EX32 7NF Tel: 01271 323200 — MB Camb. 1955, BChir 1954; DObst RCOG 1956.

OSBORNE, David Carl Ashworth Street Surgery, 85 Spotland Road, Rochdale OL12 6RT Tel: 01706 44582 Fax: 01706 346767; 47 Bleakholt Road, Turn Village, Ramsbottom, Bury BL0 0RU — MB ChB Manch. 1992; BSc (Med Sci.) St. And. 1989; MB ChB St. Manch. 1992. GP Rochdale. Lancs. Specialty: Gen. Pract.

OSBORNE, David John 3 Graigola Road, Glais, Swansea SA7 9HS Tel: 01792 845312 — MB BS Lond. 1967 (Guy's) MRCS Eng. LRCP Lond. 1967; DMJ Soc. Apoth. Lond. 1980. Med. Off. Clydach War Memor. Hosp; HM Coroner for Co. W. Glam.

OSBORNE, David Michael 90 Livingstone Road, Hove BN3 3WL — MB ChB Liverp. 1993.

OSBORNE, Mr David Robert Ladywell House, Ladywell Lane, Great Baddow, Chelmsford CM2 7AE — MRCS Eng. LRCP Lond. 1968 (Roy. Free) MS Lond. 1983, MB BS 1968; FRCS Eng. 1974. Cons. Surg. Basildon & Orsett Hosps. Specialty: Gen. Surg. Prev: Lect. Surg. Roy. Free Hosp. Med. Sch. Lond.; Surg. Regist. Roy. Free Hosp. Lond. Surg. Regist. Cheltenham & Gloucester Health Dists.

OSBORNE, Elaine Marion (retired) 19 Alnwick Road, Newton Hall, Durham DH1 5NL Tel: 0191 386 1337 — MB ChB Leeds 1947; DObst RCOG 1948; DPH Leeds 1961; DCH Eng. 1963; MFCM 1974. Prev: Cons. Phys. Sedgefield Dist. Counc.

OSBORNE, Elizabeth Sara Hopwood Medical Centre, 1-3 Walton Street, Hopwood, Heywood OL10 2BS Tel: 01706 369886 Fax: 01706 627619 — MB ChB Manch. 1992 (Manchester) MRCGP; BSc (Med. Sci.) St. And. 1989. GP Princip. & GP Trainer. Specialty: Gen. Pract. Socs: BMA; SPA; RCGP.

OSBORNE, Mr Eric Alexander (retired) Thorterburn Farm, nr. Neilston, Glasgow G78 3AX Tel: 0141 585222; (cons. rooms) The Langside Clinic, Bon Secours Hospital, 36A Mansionhouse Road, Glasgow G41 3DW — MB ChB Glas. 1960; DObst RCOG 1962; FRCS Ed. 1968; FRCS Glas. 1968. Prev: Ho. Phys. Stobhill Gen. Hosp. Glas.

OSBORNE, Fiona Lesley 47 Fredrick Road, Selly Oak, Birmingham B16 1NZ — MB ChB Birm. 1998; ChB Birm. 1998.

OSBORNE, Genevieve Emily Norah St Mary's Hospital, Department of Dermatology, Praed Street, London W2 1NY — BM Soton. 1992; MRCP. Cons. Dermat. St Mary's Hosp. Lond.

OSBORNE, Mr Geoffrey Vaughan (retired) 26 Waterloo Road, Southport PR8 2NF Tel: 01704 65215 — MB ChB Liverp. 1940; MCh Orth. Liverp. 1947, MB ChB 1940; FRCS Ed. 1946; FRCS Eng. 1973. Cons. Emerit. & Orthop. Surg., Roy. Liverp. Hosp. & Southport Gen. Hosp.; Hon. Research Fell. Sch. Engin. Liverp. John Mores Univ. Prev: Lect. (Orthop. Surg.) Univ. Liverp.

OSBORNE, Joanne 187 Battenhall Road, Worcester WR5 2BU — MB BS Lond. 1990. Regist. (O & G) NE Thames RHA. Specialty: Obst. & Gyn.

OSBORNE, John Antony Bro-Morganning NHS Trust, Princess of Wales Hospital, Bridgend; Diamond House, Westgate, Cowbridge CF72 8SH Tel: 07968 141164 — MB BS Lond. 1988; BSc (Psych.) Lond. 1985; FRCA 1996. Cons. Anaesth. Specialty: Anaesth. Socs: BMA; Fell. Roy. Coll. Anaesths.; Assn. Anaesths. Prev: Regist. (Cardiol. & Renal Med.) Wellington, NZ; SHO (Anaesth.) Gloucester Roy. Hosp.

OSBORNE, Mr John Leslie 212-214 Great Portland Street, London W1W 5QN Tel: 020 7387 7055 Fax: 020 7387 7066 Email: johnosborneobgyn@doctors.org.uk; 17 Grove Park Gardens, Chiswick, London W4 3RY Tel: 020 8995 0019 — MB BS Lond. 1966 (Lond. Hosp.) FRCOG 1985, M 1973. Cons. Obst., Gynaecologist and Uro-gynaecologist, Univ. Coll. Hosp, Lond. Specialty: Obst. & Gyn. Socs: Internat. Continence Soc.; Roy. Soc. Med..; Assoc. Mem. Brit. Assn. Urological Surg. Prev: Cons. Obst. & Gynaecologist to Qu. Charlotte's Hosp. & the Hosp. Forwonien; Sen. Regist. & Lect. Inst. O & G Qu. Charlotte's & Chelsea Hosps. Wom.; Research Asst. & Hon. Sen. Regist. Urodynamic Unit Middlx. Hosp.

OSBORNE, Professor John Paul Royal United Hospital, Combe Park, Bath BA1 3NG Tel: 01225 824218 Fax: 01225 824212 — MB BS Lond. 1971 (St. Thos.) DObst RCOG 1973; MRCP (UK) 1974; DCH Eng. 1974; MD Lond. 1980; FRCP Lond. 1989. Cons. Paediat. Roy. United Hosp. Bath; Hon. Prof. Univ. Bath. Specialty: Paediat. Socs: Brit. Paediat. Neurol. Assn.; Fell. Roy. Coll. Paediat. and Child. Health. Prev: Sen. Regist. (Paediat.) Roy. Hosp. Sick Childr. Bristol; Fell. (Neurol.) Hosp. Sick Childr. Toronto, Canada; Regist. (Paediat.) St. Thos. Hosp. Lond.

OSBORNE, Mr Jonathan Edward C/O ENT Department, Glan Clwyd Hospital, Bodelwyddan, Rhyl Tel: 01745 534233 Fax: 01745 534160 Email: jon.osborne@cd-tr.wales.nhs.uk; Tyddyn Ucha, Glan Conwy, Colwyn Bay LL28 5PN — MB BS Lond. 1978 (Middlx.

Hosp. Med. Sch.) FRCS Ed. 1985; FRCS Eng. 1985. Cons. ENT Surg., Glan Clwyd Hosp. Bodelwyddan. Specialty: Otorhinolaryngol. Socs: Sect. Otol. & Laryngol.; Roy. Soc. Med.; Treas. Welsh Assn. Otoloryngol. Prev: Sen. Regist. (ENT) Ninewells Hosp. Dundee & N. Riding Infirm. Middlesbrough; Med. Off. Save The Childr. Fund, Karamoja, Uganda.

OSBORNE, Joy Elizabeth Department of Dermatology, Leicester Royal Infirmary, Infirmary Square, Leicester LE1 5WW Tel: 0116 258 5762; 32 Church Lane, Ratcliffe-on-the-Wreake, Leicester LE7 4SF — BM BS Nottm. 1978; MRCGP 1982. Assoc. Specialist Dermat. Leicester Roy. Infirm. NHS Trust. Specialty: Dermat.

OSBORNE, Julie Elaine — MB BS Lond. 1986; MA Camb. 1987; DRCOG 1989; MRCGP (Distinc.) 1990. Specialty: Gen. Pract. Prev: Trainee GP Derby VTS; Dist. Med. Off. Mansa, Zambia (VSO).

OSBORNE, Kathleen Anne 158 Lindisfarne Road, Durham DH1 5YX — MB BS Lond. 1994.

OSBORNE, Keith Norman Alexander Southern General Hospital, 1345 Govan Road, Glasgow G51 4TF Tel: 0141 201 1100 Email: keith.osborne@sgh.scot.nhs.uk — MB ChB Glas. 1985; BSc (Hons.) Glas. 1983; MRCP (UK) 1988; FRCR 1991. Cons. (Radiol.) South. Gen. Hosp. Glas. Specialty: Radiol. Special Interest: CT; MRI. Socs: Roy. Coll. of Radiologists; Roy. Coll. Of Phys. Surg. Glas.; Brit. Soc. of Interventional Radiol. Prev: Cons. (Radiol.) Ayr Hosp.; Sen. Regist. (Radiol.) Roy. Infirm. Glas.; Sen. Ho. Off. (Gen. Med.) W. Infirm. Glas.

OSBORNE, Margaret Anne (retired) Wildacrres, Consall, Wetley Rocks, Stoke-on-Trent ST9 0AH — MB ChB Birm. 1963. Prev: GP Principle, Eccleshall.

OSBORNE, Mr Martin John Warwick Hospital, Lakin Road, Warwick CV34 5BW Tel: 01926 495321 Fax: 01926 482602 Email: martin.osbourne@swh.nhs.uk — MB BS Lond. 1982 (Middlx.) BA Oxf. 1979; FRCS Ed. 1986; FRCS Eng. 1988; FRCS (Gen.) 1998. Cons. Gen. & Colorectal Surg. Warwick Hosp. Warwick. Specialty: Gen. Surg. Special Interest: Coloproctology. Socs: Association of Coloproctology of GB & Ireland; Association of Surgeons of GB & Ireland. Prev: Sen. Regist. Rotat. (Gen. Surg.) Roy. Free & Whittington Hosps. Lond., Chase Farm Hosp. Middlx. & Sir Chas. Gairdner Hosp. Perth, W. Austral.; Vis. Regist. (Gen. Surg.) Perth West. Australia.

OSBORNE, Melanie Ann Withington Hospital, Nell lane, Manchester M20 2LR — MB ChB Leic. 1982; MRCP (UK) 1986; DA (UK) 1988; FCAnaesth 1991. Cons. Anaesth. & ICU Lancs. Specialty: Anaesth. Socs: RCP Edin.; Intens. Care Soc.; Assn. Anaesth. Prev: Sen. Regist. (Anaesth.) N. West. Region; Regist. (Anaesth.) Manch. Roy. Infirm. & Wigan Roy. Albert Edwd. Infirm.; Regist. (Gen. Med.) N. Manch. Gen. Hosp.

OSBORNE, Melanie Elizabeth 7 Silver Street — MB BS Lond. 1988; BSc (Hons.) Lond. 1985; MRCP (UK) 1992; FRCR 1997. Cons. Clin. Oncologist Roy. Devon & Exeter Hosp. Specialty: Oncol.; Radiother. Prev: Cons. Clin. Oncologist, Mt. Vernon Hosp. Northwood.

OSBORNE, Melvyn Ambrose University Health Service, 2 Claremont Place, Sheffield S10 2TB Tel: 0114 222 2100 Fax: 0114 222 2123 — MB ChB Sheff. 1969; DCH RCPS Glas. 1971; DObst RCOG 1973; Cert Family Plann. RCOG RCGP & Family Plann Assn. 1976; MRCGP 1981. Med. Off. Univ. Sheff. Specialty: Dermat. Prev: SHO (Obst.) North. Gen. Hosp. Sheff.; SHO (Paediat.) Hull Roy. Infirm.; Ho. Surg. Sheff. Roy. Hosp.

OSBORNE, Nigel Jonathan Russell First Floor Flat, 11 Lansdown Place, Clifton, Bristol BS8 3AF — BM BS Nottm. 1993 (Univ. Nottm.) MRCP (UK) 1996. S. W. Deanery Calman Paediatri Specialist Regist. Specialty: Paediat. Prev: SHO Rotat. (Paediat.) Bristol; SHO (A & E) Bristol; Ho. Off. (Med.) Qu. Med. Centre Nottm.

OSBORNE, Nigel William Anstey Surgery, 21A The Nook, Anstey, Leicester LE7 7AZ Tel: 0116 236 2531 Fax: 0116 235 7867 — MB ChB Leic. 1982; DCH RCP Lond. 1984; DRCOG 1985; MRCGP 1986. Clin. Asst. Minor Accid. Dept. Gen. Hosp. LoughBoro.

OSBORNE, Pamela Agnew (retired) Rosewood, Marley Common, Haslemere GU27 3PU — MB ChB Birm. 1947. Prev: Med. Off. S.W. Surrey HA.

OSBORNE, Patricia Mary (retired) Greenend Lodge, Ochtertyre, Crieff PH7 4LD Tel: 01764 652935 — MB ChB Liverp. 1959; MSc (Comm. Med.) Manch. 1980. Prev: Cons. Pub. Health Med. Tayside HB.

OSBORNE, Paul Benjamin Church Street Surgery, Church Street, Starcross, Exeter EX6 8PZ Tel: 01626 890368 Fax: 01626 891330; 4 Westwood, Starcross, Exeter EX6 8RW Tel: 01626 890515 — MB Camb. 1974; BChir 1973; DCH Eng. 1976; MRCGP 1980.

OSBORNE, Penelope Pauline Greyswood Practice, 238 Mitcham Lane, London SW16 6NT Tel: 020 8769 0845/8363 Fax: 020 8677 2960; 101 Nimrod Road, London SW16 6TH — MB BS Lond. 1989 (St. George's) BSc (1st cl. Hons.) Lond. 1986; DRCOG 1992; DFFP 1993; MRCGP 1995. Prev: Trainee GP St. Helier Hosp. Carshalton VTS; GP Asst. Wrythe Green Surg. Carshalton.

OSBORNE, Richard John Dorset Cancer Centre, Poole Hospital, Longfleet Road, Poole BH15 2JB; The Engine House, Quarleston Farm, Clenston Road Winterborne Stickland, Blandford Forum DT11 0NP — MD Manch. 1988; MB ChB 1979; MRCP (UK) 1982; FRCP 1995. Cons Med Oncol. Dorset Cancer Centre. Specialty: Oncol. Prev: NCI-EORTC Vis. Research Fell. NCI-Navy Med. Oncol. Br. Nat. Cancer Inst. Maryland, USA.; Univ Lect Addenbrookes Hosp Camb.

OSBORNE, Sally — MB BS Lond. 1997. GP. Specialty: Gen. Pract.

OSBORNE, Sally Frances 18 Sunningdale, Bristol BS8 2NF — MB ChB Bristol 1998.

OSBORNE, Sarah Ann Institute of Psychiatry, De Crespigny Park, London SE5 8AF — MB BS Lond. 1990 (Royal Free Hospital School of Medicine) Clin. Researcher and Hon. Staff Grade Psychiat., Inst. of Psychiat., Lond. Specialty: Gen. Psychiat. Socs: Brit. Med. Assn.; Med. Protec. Soc. Prev: Regist. (Psychiat.) St Bart. Hosp. Lond.

OSBORNE, Simon Christopher Pollokshaws Doctors Centre, 26 Wellgreen, Glasgow G43 1RR Tel: 0141 649 2836 Fax: 0141 649 5238; 24 Marlborough Avenue, Broomhill, Glasgow G11 7BW Tel: 0141 334 4096 — MB ChB Glas. 1982; BSc (Med. Sci.) St. And. 1979; MRCGP 1986; Dip FMS 2002.

OSBORNE, Stuart Anthony 8 Wyvis Avenue, Bearsden, Glasgow G61 4RD — MB ChB Glas. 1995.

OSBORNE, Wendy Louise Department of Haematology, Royal Victoria Infirmary, Queen Victoria Road, Newcastle upon Tyne — MB BS Newc. 1998; MB BS Newc 1998; MB BS Newcaste 1998; MRCP 2001.

OSBOROUGH, Fiona Kings Avenue Surgery, 23 Kings Avenue, Buckhurst Hill IG9 5LP Tel: 020 8504 0122 Fax: 020 8559 2984 — MB BCh Belf. 1974. Specialty: Gen. Pract.; Family Plann. & Reproduc. Health.

OSBOURNE, Garrick Knox Hairmyres Hospital, Eaglesham Road, East Kilbride, Glasgow G75 8RG Tel: 01355 585098 Fax: 01355 684607 Email: garryosbourne@thedoctor.co.uk; 1 Avenel Crescent, Strathaven ML10 6JF Tel: 01357 520862 — MB ChB Glas. 1972; FRCOG 1990, M 1977. Cons. (O & G) Hairmyres Hosp., E. Kilbride and Wishaw Gen. Hosp. Specialty: Obst. & Gyn. Prev: Sen. Regist. (O & G) Ninewells Hosp. Dundee; Regist. (O & G) Glas. Roy. Infirm., Glas. Roy. & Rutherglen; Matern. Hosps. & Roy. Samarit. Hosp. Glas.

OSCIER, David Graham 11 Littledown Avenue, Queens Park, Bournemouth BH7 7AT — MB BChir Camb. 1974; MA Camb. 1974; MRCP (UK) 1976; FRCP Lond. 1990; FRCPath 1991. Cons. Haemat. Roy. Bournemouth Hosp.; Hon. Clin. Sen. Lect. Univ. Soton. Specialty: Haematology. Prev: Research Fell. MRC Leukaemia Unit Roy. Postgrad. Med. Sch. Lond.; Regist. (Haemat.) Hammersmith Hosp. Lond.; SHO (Path.) Westm. Hosp. Lond.

OSEI, Edward King George Hospital, Barley Lane, Goodmayes, Ilford IG3 8YB Tel: 020 8983 8000; 47 Sylvan Avenue, Emerson Park, Hornchurch RM11 2PW Tel: 01708 449759 — MB ChB Ghana 1976; MRCOG 1981; MFFP 1995. Cons. O & G Redbridge Health Care Essex. Specialty: Obst. & Gyn. Socs: Brit. Med. Ultrasound Soc. & BMA. Prev: Sen. Specialist K. Khalid Hosp. Hail, Saudi Arabia; Regist. (O & G) Barking Hosp.; Lect. (O & G) Univ. Bristol.

OSEI-BONSU, Michael Ampadu 72 Broadash, Greystoke Gardens, Jesmond, Newcastle upon Tyne NE2 1PZ — BChir Camb. 1991.

OSEI-FRIMPONG, Samuel 21 Clwydian Park Crescent, St Asaph LL17 0BJ — MB ChB Ghana 1976; FFA RCSI 1985. Specialty: Anaesth.

OSEN, Hyman Emmanuel 41 Cedra Court, Cazenove Road, London N16 6AT — MRCS Eng. LRCP Lond. 1934 (St. Bart.)

OSEN, Julian Sinclair 10 Courtland Drive, Chigwell IG7 6PN — MB BS Lond. 1998.

OSEN, Melvyn Alan 10 Courtland Drive, Chigwell IG7 6PN — MRCS Eng. LRCP Lond. 1962 (Lond. Hosp. & Camb.) MA Camb. 1962, MB BChir 1968; DMedRehab RCP Lond. 1984. Socs: BMA. Prev: SHO Wanstead Hosp.; Ho. Surg. Lond. Hosp.; Ho. Phys. Mile End. Hosp.

OSGOOD, Vicky Mary Holmleigh, Solomon's Lane, Shirrell Heath, Southampton SO32 2HU — MB BS Lond. 1977; MRCOG 1983; FRCOG 2002. Cons. Obst. Portsmouth Hosps. NHS Trust; Dir. Med. Educat. Portsmouth Hosp. NHS Trust. Specialty: Obst. & Gyn.

OSHEA, Carmel Patricia Oakhill Health Centre, Oakhill Road, Surbiton KT6 6EN Tel: 020 8390 7839; 14 Westbank, Dorking RH4 3BZ Tel: 01306 883880 — MB BCh Wales 1990; MRCGP 1994. Specialty: Gen. Pract. Prev: SHO (Med.) E. Surrey Hosp. Redhill.

OSHO, Olushola Festus c/o Drive J. Ugbomba, 27 Wimpole St., London W1G 8GN — MB BS Benin 1978; MB BS Benin, Nigeria 1978; MRCPI 1985.

OSHODI, Mustafa Akanni Milson Road Health Centre, 1-13 Milson Road, London W14 0LJ Tel: 020 8846 6262 Fax: 020 8846 6239 — MB ChB Wales 1967; DTM & H Liverp. 1970; Fellow Medical Council (GP) Nigeria 1981; Fellow West Africa of Physician (GP) 1986; Dip. Primary Care Therapeutics Lond. 1999. Sen. Partner. Specialty: Gen. Pract. Socs: BMA; Nigeria Med. Assn.; RSM.

OSHODI, Mr Taohid Oladele Rochdale Road, Oldham OL1 2JH Email: taohid.oshodi@oldham-tr.nwest.nhs.uk; 6 Emsworth Dirve, Sale M33 3PR — MB BS Lagos 1983; FRCS Ed. 1990; FRCS 2000. Specialty: Gen. Surg. Socs: BMA; Vasc. Surg. Soc.; Assn. Surg. Prev: Roy. Lancaster Infirm. Lancaster.

OSHOWO, Mr Ayodele Oluwapelumi 26 Caversham Avenue, Sutton SM3 9AH — MB BS Ibadan 1986; FRCS Ed. 1995.

OSIFODUNRIN, Olanrewaju Olukayode Olatokunbo 5 Craigmount Hill, Edinburgh EH4 8DP — MB BCh BAO NUI 1984; LRCPI & LM, LRCSI & LM 1984.

OSINDERO, Adesola Olugbemiga Chells Way Surgery, 265 Chells Way, Stevenage SG2 0HN Tel: 01438 313001 Fax: 01438 362322 — MB BS Lond. 1983; MRCGP; T(GP) 1993.

OSLER, David Farnworth (retired) 7 Station Road, South Queensferry EH30 9HY Tel: 0131 331 1565 Fax: 0131 331 5783 — MB ChB Ed. 1961; DObst RCOG 1965. Prev: Ho. Phys. E. Gen. Hosp. Edin.

OSLER, Kay The Surgery, Main Street, Leiston IP16 4ES Tel: 01728 830526 Fax: 01728 832029 — MRCS Eng. LRCP Lond. 1973 (Roy. Free) MSc Univ. Lond. 1990, MB BS 1973; DRCOG 1978; MRCGP 1980.

OSMAN, Abd El Azim Abd El Monem City Way Surgery, 67 City Way, Rochester ME1 2AY Tel: 01634 843351 Fax: 01634 830421; Uplands, Gravelly Bottom Road, Kingswood, Maidstone ME17 3NS Tel: 01622 842066 Fax: 01622 842066 Email: azimosman@doctors.org.uk — MB BCh Egypt 1974 (Mansourah Univ. Egypt) GP Kent. Specialty: Gen. Pract.; Anaesth.

OSMAN, Aheed El-Toam Fawzi 26 Twmpath Lane, Gobowen, Oswestry SY10 7AQ — MB ChB Alexandria, Egypt 1982.

OSMAN, Ahmed El Murtada Department of Clinical Oncology, The Leicester Roayl Infirmary, NHS Trust, Infirmary Square, Leicester LE1 5WW — MB BS Khartoum 1979.

OSMAN, Bader El Din Ismail Abd El Meguid 68 Fishbourne Lane, Ryde PO33 4EX — MB BCh Cairo 1969.

OSMAN, Catriona Helen 7 Orchard Close, Monk Fryston, Leeds LS25 5EY — MB ChB Leeds 1987.

OSMAN, Elsir Mohamed 10 Osborn Gardens, Mill Hill, London NW7 1DY Tel: 020 8346 5858 — MB BS Khartoum 1978; MRCPI 1988. Cons. Phys. St. Albans & Hemel Hempstead NHS Trust. Specialty: Gen. Med. Socs: Roy. Soc. Med. Prev: Sen. Regist. Roy. Free Hosp. Lond.

OSMAN, Faizel 23 Deanston Croft, Coventry CV2 2NX — MB BCh Wales 1995.

OSMAN, Hamdy Mohamed 7 Cuckoo Close, Woolton, Liverpool L25 4UA — MB BCh Ain Shams 1962.

OSMAN, Inass Flat 2R, 8 Dunearn St., Glasgow G4 9EF — MB ChB Glas. 1998; MB ChB Glas 1998.

OSMAN, John Health & Safety Executive, Magdalen House, Stanley Precinct, Bootle L20 3QZ Tel: 0151 951 4000; 10 Suncroft Road, Heswall, Wirral CH60 1XZ — MB ChB Bristol 1973; MRCP (UK) 1976; Specialist Accreditation, Roy. Coll. Of Phys., 1984. Sen. Employm. Med. Adviser Health & Safety Exec. Epidemiol. & Med. Statistics Unit Bootle. Specialty: Epidemiol.

OSMAN, Khalid Hussein Elsayed All Saints Hospital, Flat 32 Mackenzie Court, Lodge Road, Hockley, Birmingham B18 5SD — MB BS Khartoum 1987; MRCP (UK) 1992.

OSMAN, Mohamed 195 Bath Road, Hounslow TW3 3BU Tel: 020 8570 6524 — MB BS Osmania 1946; DCH Eng. 1960; LMSSA Lond. 1965. Socs: BMA. Prev: Sen. Regist. Paediat. St. Helier Hosp.; Paediat. Regist. Hope Hosp. Manch. & Northampton Gen. Hosp.

OSMAN, Mohamed Ahmed 48 Ashcombe Gardens, Weston Super Mare BS23 2XD Tel: 01934 29233 — Ptychio Iatrikes Athens 1975.

OSMAN, Mr Monzir Khogali Crosshouse Hospital, Kilmarnock KA2 0BE Tel: 01563 577985 — MB BS Khartoum 1980; FRCS Glas. 1989; FRCS (Gen. Surg.) 2001. Staff Surg. Monklands Hosp. Airdrie. Specialty: Gen. Surg.

OSMAN, Mustafa 14 Azalea Road, Blackburn BB2 6JU — MB ChB Manch. 1993.

OSMAN, Noor Mahomed Omar (retired) Highfield, 139 The Avenue, Leigh WN7 1HR Tel: 01942 674158 — MB BS Karachi 1956 (Dow Med. Coll.)

OSMAN, Rabia 37 Arnold Gardens, London N13 5JE — MB BS Lond. 1996.

OSMAN, Tasneem 29 Galley Lane, Arkley, Barnet EN5 4AR — MB BS Lond. 1989; MRCGP 1994. Locum GP Barnet.

OSMAN, Zubeda Mattock Lane Health Centre, 78 Mattock Lane, London W13 9NZ Tel: 020 8567 8329; 280B Staines Road, Hounslow TW3 3LX Tel: 020 8570 1950/572 8610 — MB BS Hyberabad 1953 (Osmania Med. Coll. Hyderabad) DGO Hyberabad 1958; DObst 1960; MRCOG 1972. Specialty: Gen. Med. Prev: Hosp. Pract. (Gyn) Mt. Vernon Hosp. N.wood.

OSMOND, Alexander (retired) Pinetrees, 38 Willow Lane, Stanion, Kettering NN14 1DT Tel: 01536 443182 — MB BS Durh. 1956; DObst RCOG 1960; MRCGP 1965.

OSMOND, David Frederick Risca Surgery, St. Mary Street, Risca, Newport NP11 6YS Tel: 01633 612666; 3 Woodville Road, Newport NP20 4JB Tel: 01633 669000 — MB BCh Wales 1979; BA Camb. 1976. Socs: Roy. Coll. Gen. Practs.

OSMOND, Thomas George, MBE (retired) North Lodge, Lambourn, Newbury RG17 8XR Tel: 01488 71695 — MB BChir Camb. 1947 (St. Thos.) BA Camb. 1944; DObst RCOG 1952. JP.; Local Treasury Med. Off.; Div. Surg. St. John Ambul. Brig. Prev: Ho. Phys. St. Thos. Hosp. Lond. & Roy. Portsmouth Hosp.

OSMONT, Jonathan Mark, OSJ Halkett Place Surgery, 84 Halkett Place, St Helier, Jersey JE1 4XL Tel: 01534 736301 Fax: 01534 887793; La Rochelle, Route D'Ebenezer, Trinity, Jersey JE3 5DT Tel: 01534 862255 — MB BS Lond. 1973 (St. Bart.) DObst RCOG 1976. CMO St. John Ambul. Jersey. Socs: Jersey Med. Soc. Prev: Co. Surg. St. John Ambul. Jersey; SHO (Obst.) Redhill Gen. Hosp.; Ho. Surg. & Ho. Phys. Ards Hosp. Newtownards.

OSRIN, David 19 Bancroft Avenue, London N2 0AR — MB BChir Camb. 1990; MA Camb. 1990; MRCP RCP 1992; DTM & H 1997; MRCPCH 1999.

OSRIN, Ivan Mill Lane Medical Centre, 112 Mill Lane, London NW6 1XQ Tel: 020 7431 1588 Fax: 020 7431 8919 Email: ivan.osrin@gp-f83055.nhs.uk; 7 Albermarle Mansions, Heath Drive, London NW3 7TA Tel: 020 7435 2069 — MB ChB Stellenbosch 1964; BSc Stellenbosch 1960; DCH Eng. 1968.

OSSEI-GERNING, Nicholas 6 Harper Avenue, Idle, Bradford BD10 8NU — MB BS Lond. 1990.

OSSELTON, Michael Friarwood Surgery, Carleton Glen, Pontefract WF8 1SU Tel: 01977 703235 — MB ChB Leeds 1985; DRCOG 1989.

OSTBERG, Julia Elisabeth Department of Endocrinology, Middlesex Hospital, Mortimer Street, London W1N 8AA — MB BS Lond. 1996 (University College, London) BSc Hons. Lond. 1993; MRCP (UK) Part I 1998; MRCP (UK) Part 2. 1999. Specialty: Gen. Med.

OSTENFELD, Thor 15 Chamberlin Court, Westfield Lane, Cambridge CB4 3QX — MB ChB Dundee 1991; BSc (1st cl. Hons.) Pharmacol. Dund 1986; DA (UK) 1993; FRCA 1996. Wellcome Trust Clin. Research Fell. MRC Centre for Brain Repair Univ. of Camb.; Hon. Specialist Regist. (Anaesth.) Addenbrooke's Hosp. Camb. Specialty: Anaesth. Prev: Specialist Regist. (Anaesth.) PeterBoro. Dist. Hosps. Camb.; Regist. (Anaesth.) Addenbrooke's Hosp. & Papworth Hosp. Camb.; SHO (Anaesth.) W. Suff. Hosp. Bury St. Edmunds & Ashford Hosp. Middlx.

OSTERBERG, Mr Paul Harald (retired) 13 Ulsterville Avenue, Belfast BT9 Tel: 028 9066 7741; The Old Manse, Hillsborough BT26 6HW Tel: 028 9268 2226 — MB BCh BAO Dub. 1953; BA Dub. 1953; FRCSI 1959; FRCS Eng. 1961. Hon. Cons. Orthop. Surg. Roy. Vict. Hosp. Belf. & Musgrave Pk. Hosp. Belf. Prev: Vis. Prof. Surg. Pahlavi Univ. Iran.

OSTERLOH, Ian Howard Pfizer Central Research, Ramsgate Road, Sandwich CT13 9NJ Tel: 01304 648652 Fax: 01304 658143 — MB BS Lond. 1982 (Guy's Hospital) MSc Bristol 1976, BSc 1975; MRCP (UK) 1985. Global Candidate Team Ldr. Pfizer Centr. Research Sandwich Kent. Specialty: Pharmaceutical Medicine. Socs: Roy. Coll. Phys.; BMA; Internat. Soc. Impotence Research. Prev: Europ. Clin. Team Ldr. Pfizer Centr. Research Sandwich; Head of Phase 1 Operat. & Head Clin. Regulatory Affairs Pfizer Centr. Research Sandwich.

OSTERMANN, Maria Elisabeth Intensive Care Unit, Royal Brompton Hospital, Sydney St., London SW3 6NP — State Exam. Med. Gottingen 1990.

OSTICK, Mr David Graham Bridge House, Bolton Road, Bradshaw, Bolton BL2 3EU Tel: 01204 300214 — MB ChB Manch. 1966; FRCS Eng. 1973. Cons. (Gen. Surg.) Roy. Bolton Hosp. Specialty: Gen. Surg.

OSTICK, Susan The James Cochrane Practice, Maude Street, Kendal LA9 4QE Tel: 01539 722124 Fax: 01539 734995 — MB BS Lond. 1982 (St. Bart. Hosp. Med. Sch.) DRCOG 1984; Cert. Family Plann. RCOG & RCGP 1984. GP Kendal; Clin. Asst. (Psychiat.) Cumbria; Clinical Assistant (Surgery), Cumbria. Prev: Clin. Asst. (Obst. & Gyn. & Psychiat.) Cumbria.

OSTINS, Andrew William 4 Greenlands Way, Henbury, Bristol BS10 7PR; 62 Margards Lane, Verwood BH31 6JP — MB ChB Birm. 1974; DRCOG 1978; DTM & H 1991. Med. Miss. Hosp. de Kipushya. Specialty: Trop. Med. Socs: Roy. Soc. Trop. Med. & Hyg. & Christian Med. Fellowsh. Prev: GP Verwood.

OSTLE, Karen 242 Bream Close, off Ferry Lane, Tottenham, London N17 9DW — MB ChB Dundee 1989; DRCOG 1993; DFFP 1993; MRCGP 1995. Salaried GP. Prev: GP Lond.; Trainee GP E. Cumbria VTS.; Med. Adviser Benefits Agency Med. Servs.

OSTLE, Kirstin Elizabeth Randolph Medical Centre, 4 Green Lane, Datchet, Slough SL3 9EX Tel: 01753 541268 Fax: 01753 582324; Estcourt, 1 Clayhall Lane, Windsor SL4 2SW Tel: 01753 868283 — MB ChB Ed. 1986; DCH RCP Lond. 1989; DRCOG 1991; MRCGP 1992. GP Princip. Slough; Police Surg. Berks. Specialty: Gen. Pract. Socs: Windsor Med. Soc.; Forens. Div. Roy. Med. Soc. Prev: SHO (Med., Paediat. & O & G) Heatherwood Hosp. Ascot.

OSTLER, Alec Michael 4 Aspen Close, Bishopsmead, Tavistock PL19 9LN — MB BS Lond. 1998; MB BS Lond 1998.

OSTLER, Edward George 1 Queens Drive, Taunton TA1 4XW Tel: 01823 286244 — MB BS Lond. 1963 (King's Coll. Hosp.) MRCS Eng. LRCP Lond. 1963; DPM Eng. 1967; FRCPsych 1992, M 1972. Med. Dir. Som. Patner NHS & Social Care Trust. Specialty: Ment. Health. Socs: BMA. Prev: Cons. Child Psychiat. & Ment. Handicap Som. NHS Trust; Sen. Regist. Tone Vale Hosp. Taunton; Regist. Glenside Hosp. Bristol.

OSTLER, Kevin John Cavendish House, 18 Victoria Road S., Southsea PO5 2BZ Tel: 023 9229 1867 Fax: 023 9287 2932 Email: kevin.ostler@ports.nhs.uk — MB BS Lond. 1989; BSc (2nd cl. Hons.) Lond. 1986. Cons. (Adult Ment. Health), Portsmouth Health NHS Trust. Specialty: Gen. Psychiat. Socs: Roy. Coll. Psychiat. Prev: Clin. Research Fell. (Psychiat.) Roy S. Hants. Hosp. Soton.

OSTLER, Peter James 46 Cowper Road, Harpenden AL5 5NG — MB BS Lond. 1989; MRCP (UK) 1992; FRCR 1996. Cons., Clin. Onicologist, Mt. Vernon Hosp., Northwood Lond. Specialty: Oncol.

OSTLERE, Lucy Sinclair St Georges Hospital, Blackshaw Road, London SW17 0QT Tel: 020 8725 1996 Email: lucy.ostlrer@stgeorges.nhs.uk — MB BS Lond. 1986; FRCP; BSc (Hons) Lond. 1983; MB BS (Hons.) Lond. 1986; MRCP (UK) 1989; MD 1997. Cons. Dermat. St. Geo. Hosp. Lond & Kingston Hosp. Specialty: Dermat. Prev: Sen. Regist. (Dermat.) St. Geo. Hosp. Lond.; Regist. & SHO (Dermat.) Roy. Free Hosp. & Westm. Hosp. Lond.; Regist. (Med.) Northwick Pk. Hosp. Lond.

OSTLERE, Simon John Gordon Dept. of Radiology, Nuffield Orthopaedic Centre, Oxford OX3 7LD Tel: 01865 227512 Fax: 01865 227825 — MB BS Lond. 1979; MRCP (UK) 1983; FRCR 1988. Specialty: Radiol.

OSTOR, Andrew James Knowles Addenbrookes Hospital, Rheumatology Research Unit, Box 194, Cambridge CB2 2QQ Tel: 01223 217459 Fax: 01223 217838 Email: andrew.ostor@addenbrookes.nhs.uk — MB BS Monash 1993; FRACP Australia 2002. Locum Cons. Rheumatologist, Addenbrookes Hosp., Camb. Specialty: Rheumatol. Special Interest: Osteoporosis; Rheumatoid Arthritis; Soft Tissue Rheumatism. Prev: Research Fell. (Rheum.) Addenbrookes Hosp. Camb.

OSTROWSKI, Julian Leon Barnsley District General Hospital, Department of Pathology, Gawber Road, Barnsley S75 2EP Tel: 01226 730000 Fax: 012267300 00 Email: julian.ostrowski@bdgh-tr.trent.nhs.uk — MB ChB Sheff. 1988 (Univ. Sheff.) BMedSci Sheff. 1987; MRCPath 1998. Cons. Histopath./Cytopath., Barnsley Dist. Gen. Hosp. Specialty: Histopath. Prev: Kaberry Research Fell. Leeds NHS Trust; Regist. (Histopath.) Leeds Gen. Infirm.; Lect. (Histopath.) Univ. of Leeds.

OSTROWSKI, Marek Josef Department of Oncology, Norfolk & Norwich Hospital, Brunswick Road, Norwich NR1 3SR Tel: 01603 287225 Fax: 01603 287463 — MB ChB Birm. 1967; DMRT Eng. 1970; FRCR 1974. Cons. Radiother. & Oncol. Norf. & Norwich Health Care Trust; Hon. Cons. Radiother. & Oncol. Addenbrooke's Hosp. Camb. Specialty: Oncol.; Radiother. Socs: Brit. Inst. Radiol.

OSTROWSKI, Nigel Michael Jan Bangholm Medical Centre, 21-25 Bangholm Loan, Edinburgh EH5 3AH Tel: 0131 552 7676 — MB ChB Dundee 1977; DRCOG 1980; MRCGP 1981; DCH Eng. 1981. Princip. GP Edin.

OSU, Benjamin Asikadi 19 Fellpark Road, Manchester M23 0EX — State Exam Bologna 1984.

OSUAGWU, Fiona Ifeyinwa — MB BS Univ. Nigeria 1990; DFFP 1995; MRCGP 2004. GP Regist. Parkbury Ho. Surg. St Albans; Specialist Regist. in Obs. & Gyn., Lutton & Dunstable Hosp., Lewsey Rd., Luton. Specialty: Obst. & Gyn. Socs: Brit. Matern. & Fetal Med. Soc. Prev: Research Regist. (Obst.) Qu. Charlotte's & Chelsea Hosp. Lond.; SHO (Obst.) Qu. Charlotte's & Chelsea Hosp. Lond.; Sen. SHO (Obst.) Birm. Wom.'s Hosp.

OSUHOR, Professor Paul Chukwunyeike (retired) 11 Oulton Way, Oxton, Birkenhead CH43 0XH Tel: 0151 608 0358 — MB BS Durh. 1963; DPH Glas. 1970; MPH 1971; DIH Dund 1975; FFCM 1989, M 1982; FFPHM RCP (UK) 1989. Cons. Pub. Health Med. E. Lancs. HA. Prev: Prof. Community Health Univ. Benin & Cons. Community Phys. Univ. Benin Teach. Hosp. Benin City, Nigeria.

OSWAL, Mr Vasant Hansraj (retired) Far Shirby, Upleatham, Redcar TS11 8AG Tel: 01287 622000 Fax: 01287 625751 Email: voswal@aol.com — MB BS Poona 1960; DORL BOM 1961; MS Bombay 1963; DLO Eng. 1964; FRCS Ed. 1968. Hon. Cons. Ent. Surg. Cpt. James Cook Univ. Hosp. Middlesbrough, Cleveland.; Hon. Vis. Prof. & Head, ENT Dept. Deenath Mangeshkar Hosp. Pune, India. Prev: Cons. ENT Surg. S. Tees Acute Trust NHS Hosp.

OSWALD, George Anthony The Medical Specialist Group, Alexandra House,Ruette Braye,, St Peter Port, Guernsey GY1 3EX Tel: 01481 238565 Fax: 01481 237782; Les Messieres, Route De Pleinmont, Torteval, Guernsey GY8 0LP — MB BS Lond. 1977 (King's Coll. Hosp.) MRCP (UK) 1980; BSc (Hons.) Physiol. Lond. 1973, MD 1986; T(M) 1991; FRCP Lond. 1995. Phys. Princess Eliz. Hosp. Guernsey, CI. Specialty: Gen. Med.; Diabetes; Endocrinol.

OSWALD, Iain Henry St George 55 Dartmouth Park Road, London NW5 1SL; 24 Dartmouth Park Avenue, London NW5 1JN — MB ChB Bristol 1976; MRCPsych 1984; (Psychoanalyst) Mem. Brit. Psychanalytic Soc. 1993. Cons. Psychother. Watford Gen. Hosp.; Psychoanalyst Inst. Psychoanal. Lond. Specialty: Psychother.; Gen. Psychiat. Socs: Brit. Psychoanal. Soc.; Assn. PsychoAnalyt. Psychtherap.; Tavistock Soc. Psychotherap. Prev: Sen. Regist. (Psychother.) Tavistock Clin. Lond.; Regist. Rotat. (Psychiat.) Maudsley Hosp. Train. Scheme; Field Dr. Brit. Nepal Med. Trust East. Nepal.

OSWALD, Professor Ian The Birches, 41 St Ronan's Terrace, Innerleithen EH44 6RB Tel: 01896 830817 — BChir Camb. 1953 (Camb. & Bristol) BA (1st cl. Hons.) 1950. 1950; MB BChir Camb. 1954; MA Camb 1954; MD 1958; DPM Eng. 1961; DSc Ed. 1963; FRCPsych 1971. Emerit. Prof. Psychiat. Univ. Edin. Prev: Vis. Prof. (Psychiat.) Univ. W. Austral.; Lect. (Psychiat.) Univ. Edin.; Beit Memor. Fell. For Med. Research Univ. Oxf.

OSWALD, Janet Colinton Surgery, 296B Colinton Road, Edinburgh EH13 0LB Tel: 0131 441 4555 Fax: 0131 441 3963 — BSc (Med. Sci.) Ed. 1979, MB ChB 1982; DRCOG 1985; DCH RCPS Glas. 1985; MRCGP 1986; Dip. Rehab. Med. RCP Lond. 1988. GP Retainer Scheme for Wom. Doctors in Gen. Pract. Prev: Regist. (Rehabil. Med.) Astley Ainslie Hosp. Edin.

OSWALD, Neville Christopher, TD (retired) — MB BChir Camb. 1935 (Char. Cross) MRCS Eng. LRCP Lond. 1934; FRCP Lond. 1947, M 1935; MD Camb. 1946. Prev: Hon. Cons. St. Bart. Hosp. Lond., Brompton Hosp. Lond. & King Edwd. VII Hosp. Offs. Lond.

OSWALD, Professor Nigel Tatham Allan University of Teeside, Primary Care Resource & Development Centre, Grey Towers Ct., Stokesley Road, Middlesbrough TS7 0PN Tel: 01642 304146 Fax: 01642 304127 Email: nigel.oswald@tees.ac.uk; Hempsyke, Littlebeck Lane, Sneaton, Whitby YO22 5HY Tel: 01947 810302 Fax: 01947 810302 — MB BChir Camb. 1971; DObst RCOG 1973; FRCGP 1995, M 1977; MPhil Camb. 1985. Prof. Primary Care Univ. Teeside & Newc. Specialty: Gen. Pract. Prev: Lect. (Gen. Pract.) Univ. Camb.

OSWALD, Tamsin Fiona Bennett 40 Eastfield Road, Duston, Northampton NN5 6TQ — MB ChB Bristol 1998.

OTAKI, Alan Tadashi (retired) 63 Imperial Way, Chislehurst BR7 6JR Email: tadaki@doctors.net.uk — MB BS Lond. 1954 (St Geo.) FRCP Lond. 1972, M 1960; MD Lond. 1968. Prev: Cons. Phys., Clin. Tutor & Phys. Medway Gp. Hosps.

OTENG-NTIM, Eugene 4 Zair Court, Voltaire Road, London SW4 6DE; 22 Briar Walk, Edgware HA8 0TX Tel: 020 8959 4077 — MB BS Lond. 1991; MRCOG 1997. Spicialist Regist. O & G. Specialty: Obst. & Gyn. Socs: Roy. Coll. Obs. & Gyn.

OTIM-OYET, David Department of Oncology, Derbyshire Royal Infirmary, London Road, Derby DE1 2QY Tel: 01332 254843 Fax: 01332 254980; 12a Rachel Court, 30 Albion Road, Sutton SM2 5TF Tel: 01332 254843 Fax: 01332 254980 — MB ChB Makerere 1975 (Makerere University) FRCR 1986; T(R) (CO) 1991. Cons. Clin. Oncol., Derbysh. Roy. Infirm. Specialty: Oncol. Socs: Fell.Roy. Coll. Radiol.; BMA. Prev: Sen. Regist. (Radiother. & Oncol.) Roy. Marsden Hosp. Lond.; WHO Cons. Radiotherapist & Oncol. Zimbabwe Oncological Train. Project Harare; Hon. Lect. Univ. Zimbabwe Med. Sch.

OTIV, S Castlefields Health Centre, Chester Close, Castlefields, Runcorn WA7 2HY Tel: 01928 566671 Fax: 01928 581631 — BM BS Nottingham 1978; BM BS Nottingham 1978.

OTLET, Alan Benjamin, MBE (retired) 6 Hutton Close, Westbury on Trym, Bristol BS9 3PS Tel: 0117 968 7116 Email: otletab@aol.com — MB ChB Bristol 1952; FRCGP 1978, M 1966. Prev: GP Southmead Med. Centre Bristol.

OTLEY, Andrew John The Surgery, 1 Church Road, Mitcham CR4 3YU — MB BS Lond. 1993; BSc (Hons) Lond. 1990. GP Prinicipal. Prev: GP Asst. Mitcham Surrey.

OTO LLORENS, Meritxell 9 Park Avenue, Stirling FK8 2QR — LMS Barcelona 1992.

OTTEN, Katherine Anne 23 Ramsey Road, Sheffield S10 1LR — MB ChB Sheff. 1995.

OTTENSMEIER, Christian Hermann Heinrich Somers Cancer Sciences Building, Southampton General Hospital, CRC Wessex Oncology Unit, Tremona Road, Southampton SO16 6YD Tel: 02380 796184 Fax: 02380 795152 Email: cho@soton.ac.uk — State Exam Med Munster 1986; MD Munster 1988; PhD Univ of Southampton 1997. Sen. Lect. Med. Oncol. Southampton Univ. Hosp. Southampton. Specialty: Oncol.

OTTER, Alan Edwin Mytton Oak Medical Practice, Racecourse Lane, Shrewsbury SY3 5LZ Tel: 01743 362223 Fax: 01743 244 5811 — MB BS Lond. 1985; DCH RCP Lond. 1987; DRCOG 1988; MRCGP 1988.

OTTER, Mark Ian Royal Shrewsbury Hospital, Department of Histopathology, Mytton Oak Road, Shrewsbury SY3 8XQ Tel: 01743 261168 Fax: 01743 355963 — MB BCh Wales 1989; BSc (Hons.) Wales 1986; MRCPath 1997, D 1995. Cons. Histopath. Roy. Shrewsbury Hosp. Specialty: Histopath. Prev: Cons. Histopath. Wrexham Maelor Hosp.; Sen. Regist. (Histopath.) SW. Thames; Regist. (Histopath.) SW. Thames.

OTTERBURN, David Michael The Malthouse Surgery, The Charter, Abingdon OX14 3JY Tel: 01235 524001 Fax: 01235 532197; Thatched Cottage, 12 Kennel Lane, Steventon, Abingdon OX13 6SB Tel: 01235 834725 — MB BS Lond. 1973; Cert JCC Lond. 1976; MRCP (UK) 1977.

OTTEY, Dominic Sean 17 School Lane, Newbold, Coleorton, Leicester LE67 8PF — MB ChB Sheff. 1991.

OTTLEY, Geoffrey Bickersteth Penny's Hill Practice, St Mary's Road, Ferndown BH22 9HB Tel: 01202 897200 Fax: 01202 875553; Willowcombe, Keepers Lane, Stapehill, Wimborne BH21 7NE — MB BS Lond. 1978 (Char. Cross) MRCS Eng. LRCP Lond. 1978. Prev: SHO (Anaesth.) St. Richards Hosp. Chichester; SHO (Psychiat. & Dermat.) Char. Cross Hosp. Lond.; SHO (O & G) Roy. Sussex Co. Hosp. Brighton.

OTTLEY, Victoria Rachel 1 Augustus Gardens, Camberley GU15 1HL — MB ChB Bristol 1998.

OTTMAN, Simon Charles Carlton Gardens Surgery, 27 Carlton Gardens, Leeds LS7 1JL Tel: 0113 295 2678 Fax: 0113 295 2679; 4 Shadwell Park Avenue, Roundhay, Leeds LS17 8TL — MB ChB Leeds 1987; MRCGP 1994.

OTTO, Alison Dawn Roade Medical Centre, 16 London Road, Roade, Northampton NN7 2NN Tel: 01604 862218 Fax: 01604 862129 — BM Soton. 1983; DRCOG 1987; MRCGP 1989. GP Princip. N.ants.; Hosp. Practitioner (Gen. Med. & Gastroenterol.) Northampton Gen. Hosp. Specialty: Gastroenterol. Socs: Brit. Assn. Sport & Med.; Primary Care Soc. Gastroenterol. Prev: SHO (Geriat. & Gen. Med., Paediat. & O & G) Leic. Gen. & Leic. Roy. Infirm.; Ho. Off. (Surg.) Roy. Hants. Co. Hosp. Winchester; Ho. Off. (Med.) Soton Gen. Hosp.

OTTON, Sophie Helen 4 East Shrubbery, Redland, Bristol BS6 6SX — MB BChir Camb. 1993.

OTTY, Catherine Joy Donmall and Partners, 87 Albion Street, London SE16 7JX Tel: 020 7237 2092 Fax: 020 7231 1435; 57 Stradella Road, London SE24 9HL — MB BChir Camb. 1982; MA Camb. 1984; DRCOG 1985; DCH RCP Lond. 1986; Cert. Family Plann. JCC 1986; MRCGP 1987; T(GP) 1991. G.P. Princip. Prev: Trainee GP/SHO Addenbrooke's Hosp. Camb. VTS; Resid. Med. Off. P. Wales Childr. Hosp. Sydney, Austral.

OTUTEYE, Ernest Teye 28 Hollman Gardens, London SW16 3SJ Tel: 020 8679 0303 — MB ChB Ghana 1969 (Ghana Med. Sch.) MRCOG 1979; LRCP LRCS Ed. LRCPS Glas. 1980. Cons. O & G King Saudi Univ. Riyadh; Gyn. Fertil. & Endocrinol. Unit Lister Hosp. Lond. Specialty: Obst. & Gyn. Socs: Riyadh Perinatol. & Neonatol. Club. Prev: Sen. Med. Off. MoH Ghana; Vis. Cons. Gyn. & Regist. (O & G) Stobhill Hosp. Glas.

OUBRIDGE, John Victor The Spinney, Ramsey Road, St Ives, Huntingdon PE27 3TP Tel: 01480 492501 Fax: 01480 492504; Cross Keys, High St, Hemingford Abbots, Huntingdon PE28 9AE Tel: 01480 468600 — MB BChir Camb. 1965 (St. Thos.) FRCGP 1996, M 1977. Course Organiser Huntingdon VTS. Prev: SHO Yeovil Gen. Hosp.; SHO Warneford Hosp. Oxf.; Ho. Off. Warwick Hosp.

OUDEH, Bashier Ahmed Rashied Mousa c/o 40 High Street, Dysart, Kirkcaldy KY1 2UG Tel: 01592 53590 — MB BCh Ain Shams 1974; DObst RCPI 1983.

OUGH, Richard W Hardwicke Building, New Square, Lincolns Inn, London WC2A 3SB Tel: 0207 242 2523 — MB BS Lond. 1973 (St. Mary's Hosp. Lond.) MRCS Eng. LRCP Lond. 1972; LMCC 1975; Dip. Law City Univ. 1984; MA (Law) City Univ. 1986; MSc (Managem.) Lond. 1995. Barrister; Dep. Chairm. NHS Tribunal. Socs: Fell. Roy. Soc. Med. Prev: Sloan Fell. Lond. Business Sch.

OUGHTIBRIDGE, David Brenan (retired) 40 Woodland Drive, Sandal, Wakefield WF2 6DD Tel: 01924 256599 — MB ChB (Distinc. Surg.) Leeds 1961 (Leeds) Prev: GP New Southgate Surg. Wakefield.

OUGHTON, Nora Marion (retired) Southlands, Walgrave, Northampton NN6 9QN Tel: 01604 978 1255 — MB ChB Birm. 1941; DO Oxf. 1943.

OULD, Georgina Ann 10 Elgin Road, Lilliput, Poole BH14 8ER — MB BS Lond. 1990.

OUNSTED, Christopher Martin Abbey Medical Practice, Health Centre, Merstow Green, Evesham WR11 4BS Tel: 01386 76111 Fax: 01386 769515; Greylyn, Broadway Lane, Fladbury, Pershore WR10 2QF Tel: 01386 860363 Fax: 01386 861412 Email: martin@ounsted.co.uk — MB BS Lond. 1974 (Roy. Free) MRCS Eng. LRCP Lond. 1974; DRCOG 1980; MRCGP 1981. GP Evesham; Vice - Chairm. LMC. Specialty: Gen. Pract. Socs: BMA; Roy. Coll. Gen. Pract. Prev: SHO Rotat. (Med.) Stoke Mandeville Hosp. Aylesbury; Ho. Phys. Worthing Hosp.; Ho. Surg. Roy. Free Hosp. Lond.

OUNSTED, Jean Mary Winyates Health Centre, Winyates, Redditch B98 0NR Tel: 01527 525533 Fax: 01527 517969; Greylyn, Broadway Lane, Fladbury, Pershore WR10 2QF — MB BS Lond. 1974 (Roy. Free) MRCS Eng. LRCP Lond. 1974; DA Eng. 1976; DRCOG 1978; MRCGP 1980. Specialty: Gen. Pract. Prev: Clin. Med. Off. Hereford & Worcester HA; Trainee GP Aylesbury VTS; Ho. Phys. Roy. Free Hosp. Lond.

OUSEY, Tamsin Jane 1 Strode Cottages, Strode, Ivybridge PL21 0LY — MB BCh Wales 1997.

OUTAR, Kampta Persaud Orton Medical Practice, Orton Centre, Orton Goldhay, Peterborough PE2 5RQ Tel: 01733 238111 Fax: 01733 238236 — MB BCh BAO Dub. 1976.

OUTEN, Peter Ronald Avenue Road Surgery, 2 Avenue Road, Warley, Brentwood CM14 5EL Tel: 01277 212820 — MB BChir Camb. 1976; MA Camb. 1976; DCH Eng. 1978; DRCOG 1978; (PGCAE) Ang 2000. Primary Care Tutor Brentwood PCG. Socs: Primary Care Rheum. Soc. Prev: Clin. Asst. (Rheum.) Broomfield Hosp. Chelmsford.

OUTHOFF, Kim The Plough, 7 The Street, Wallington, Baldock SG7 6SW — MB ChB Cape Town 1991. Phys. Guy's Drug Research Unit Guy's Hosp. Lond. Specialty: Pharmaceutical Medicine.

OUTHWAITE, John Martin Nuffield Orthopaedic Centre, Windmill Road, Headington, Oxford OX3 7LD Tel: 01865 227462 Fax: 01865 227460 — BM BCh Oxf. 1978; FRCP; MRCP (UK) 1983. Cons. Phys., Musculoskeletal Rehabil., Nuffield Orthopaedic Centre Oxon; Cons. Orthopaedic Med., The Lister Hosp.; Cons. Orthopaedic Med., The Lond. Bridge Hosp.; Cons. Orthopaedic Med., The Wellington Hosp., Lond. Specialty: Rehabil. Med. Special Interest: Low Back Pain; Whiplash Injury; Work Related Upper limb Pains. Socs: BSRM; BSR; LCA. Prev: Sen. Regist. (Rheum.) NOC Oxon.

OUTRAM, Duncan Peter The Surgery, School Lane, Alembury, Huntingdon PE28 4EQ — BChir Camb. 1994; MA Camb. 1996; DRCOG 1997; DFFP 1997; MRCGP MA Camb. 1966, BChir 1964 1999. GP Princip.; Prescribing Lead Clinician Exec. Comm. Mem., Hunts. Primary Care Trust The Priory St. Ives Cambs. Specialty: Gen. Pract. Socs: BMA. Prev: GP Regist., Dr Rawinsm & Partners, Hunters Way, Huttingdon; VTS Hinchingbrooke Hosp., Huntingdon; SHO (Gen. Med.) Hinchingbrooke Hosp. Huntingdon.

OUTRAM, Matthew The Wagon House, Oxenford, Dowlish Wake, Ilminster TA19 0PP — MB BS Lond. 1998.

OUTRED, Robert The Woottons Surgery, Priory Lane, North Wooton, King's Lynn PE30 3PT Tel: 01553 631550 Fax: 01553 631011; 54 Pilot Street, King's Lynn PE30 1QL Tel: 01553 691425 — MB ChB Manch. 1980. Clin. Asst. (Psychiat.) King's Lynn Norf. Specialty: Gen. Psychiat.

OUTTRIM, Jane Elizabeth Nancy 80 Kirkstone Road, Walkley, Sheffield S6 2PP — MB ChB Sheff. 1996 (Sheffield) GP Regist. Rotherham. Specialty: Gen. Pract.

OUTWIN, Wendy Ruth The Park Surgery, 4 Alexandra Road, Great Yarmouth NR30 2HW Tel: 01493 855672 — MB ChB Birm. 1987; DRCOG 1990; MRCGP 1991. Gen. Pract. Principle.

OVENDEN, Lynn Anne The Surgery, 178 Musters Road, West Bridgford, Nottingham NG2 7AA Tel: 0115 981 4472 Fax: 0115 981 2812 — MB ChB Sheff. 1990.

OVENDEN, Penelope Anne Hawthorn Cotttage, Kingsland, Leominster HR6 9QN Tel: 01568 708568 — (St. Thos.) MB BS Lond. 1963. Clin. Asst. (Dermat.) Co. Hosp. Hereford. Prev: Ho. Surg. Peace Memor. Hosp. Watford; Ho. Phys. Shrodells Hosp. Watford.

OVENDEN, Richard Nicholas (retired) The Dairy, Eardisland, Leominster HR6 9BP Tel: 01568 708762 Fax: 01568 708449; 31 Broad Street, Ludlow, Ludlow SY8 1NJ Tel: 01544 388503 Email: nicholasovenden@aol.com — (St. Thos.) Advanced Train. Course (KCH) 1999; MB BS Lond. 1962; DObst RCOG 1964; Cert Av. Med. MoD (Air) & CAA 1978. Hon. Phys. Heref. Flying Club; Authorised Med. Examr. CAA; GP, Kingsland, Herefordshire. Prev: Med. Adviser H & W FHSA.

OVENS, Joyce Elizabeth Anne (retired) Weavers House, 20 Dam Hill, Shelley, Huddersfield HD8 8JH Tel: 01484 605496 — LRCP LRCS Ed. 1952; LRCP LRCS Ed. LRFPS Glas. 1952; DObst RCOG 1954. Prev: Clin. Asst. (Dermat.) Huddersfield Roy. Infirm.

OVENSTONE, Irene Margaret Kinnear (retired) 10 Moor Road, Calverton, Nottingham NG14 6FW Tel: 01158 477970 Fax: 01159 477975 — MB ChB St And. 1954; DPH St And. 1957; DPM Leeds 1963; MD (Commend.) Dundee 1972; MRCPsych 1973; FRCPsych 1979. Locum Cons. Psychiat., Nottm. Health Care Trust, Mansfield.; Emirit. Cons. Psychiat. (Geriat.) St Francis Unit City Hosp. Nottm. Prev: on Scientif. Staff & Hon. Sen. Regist. MRC Epidemiol. Unit Univ. Edin.

OVER, Dawn Carol 16 Dyrham, Harford Drive, Frenchay, Bristol BS16 1NW — MB BS Lond. 1982; FCAnaesth 1989. Specialty: Anaesth. Prev: Cons. Anaesth. Southmead Hosp. Bristol; Medico-legal Adviser, Med. Protec. Soc.

OVER, Jacqueline Mary Alton Health Centre, Anstey Road, Alton GU34 2QX Tel: 01420 542542 Fax: 01420 549466 — MB BCh Wales 1989 (UWCM) DCH 1992; MRCGP 1994; DFFP 1994.

OVER, Kathryn Elizabeth Flat 4, 1 Mossley Hill Drive, Liverpool L17 1AJ — MB ChB Liverp. 1989; MRCP (UK) 1993. Sen. Regist. (Rheum. & Gen. Med.) Roy. Liverp. Univ. Hosp. Trust.

OVERAL, Susan Gillian Collings Park Medical Centre, 57 Eggbuckland Road, Hartley, Plymouth PL3 5JR Tel: 01752 771500 Fax: 01752 769946; Appletree House, Back Road, Calstock PL18 9QL Tel: 01822 832961 Mob: 01822 832961 — MB BS Lond. 1979 (Guy's, London) BSc (Pharmacol., Hons.) Lond. 1974; MRCS Eng. LRCP Lond. 1977; MRCGP 1984. Princip. in Gen. Pract. Plymouth; Mem. S. W. Devon Local Med. Comm. Specialty: Gen. Pract. Socs: BMA; Roy. Coll. Gen. Pract. (Tamar Fac.); Fac. Fam. Plann. & Reproduc. Health Care.

OVERELL, James Richard 6 Rosslyn Terrace, Glasgow G12 9NB — MB ChB Ed. 1994.

OVEREND, Alison Jane Maryport Group Practice, Alneburgh House, Ewanrigg Road, Maryport CA15 8EL Tel: 01900 815544 Fax: 01900 816626; Swan Cottage, Hayton, Aspatria, Carlisle CA7 2PD Tel: 016973 20610 Fax: 016973 23456 Email: the_overend_practice@compuserve.com — MB ChB Bristol 1988; MA Oxf. 1979; DRCOG Lond. 1991; Dip. Primary Care Therap. Newc. 1995MRCGP 1992; Dip. Primary Care Therap. Newc. 1995; DFFP 1998. Specialty: Gen. Pract. Socs: BMA; Med. Wom. Federat.; Roy. Coll. Gen. Pract. Prev: Trainee GP Airedale VTS; Ho. Off. Southmead Hosp.; Ho. Off. West. Isles Hosp. Stornoway.

OVEREND, Gillian Sydney Ashcroft Surgery, 22 Sherwood Place, Undercliffe, Bradford BD2 3AG Tel: 01274 637076 Fax: 01274 626979; 22 Harbour Crescent, Wibsey, Bradford BD6 3QG — MB ChB Leeds 1976.

OVEREND, John Simpson Maghera Health Centre, 3 Church Street, Maghera BT46 5EA Tel: 028 7964 2579 Fax: 028 7964 3002 — MB BCh BAO Belf. 1976; FFA RCSI 1981; MRCGP 1982. Specialty: Anaesth.

OVERINGTON, Felicity Jane Square Medical Centre, High Street, Godalming GU7 1AZ Tel: 01483 419764 — MB BS Lond. 1988; MRCGP 1992. Prev: SHO (Cas.) St. Peters Hosp. Chertsey; Ho. Off. (Neurol./Gen. Med.) Roy. Surrey Hosp. Guildford; Ho. Off. (Urol./Gen. Surg.) W. Berks. HA.

OVERS, Karen GP Suite, Palmer Community Hospital, Jarrow NE32 3UX — MB BS Newc. 1980; Cert. Family Plann. JCC 1984; DRCOG 1984; MRCGP 1985. GP Jarrow.

OVERSHOTT, Ross Alexander St Benets, Belmont St, Tywardreath, Par PL24 2PP — MB ChB Birm. 1996; ChB Birm. 1996.

OVERSTALL, Peter Webb Age Care, County Hospital, Hereford HR1 2ER Tel: 01432 355444 Fax: 01432 274039; Little Cwm, Dulas, Hereford HR2 0HL — MB BS Lond. 1968 (St. Geo.) MRCP (UK) 1971; FRCP Lond. 1984. Cons. Geriat. Med. Hereford County. Hosp. Specialty: Care of the Elderly. Socs: Brit. Geriat. Soc.; Internat. Continence Soc. Prev: Cons. Geriat. Med. Univ. Coll. Hosp. Lond.; Sen. Regist. (Geriat.) Univ. Coll. Hosp. Lond. & Whittington Hosp.; Lond.

OVERTON, Caroline Elizabeth St Michael's Hospital & Bristol Royal Infirmary, Department of Obstetrics and Gynaecology, Southwell Street, Bristol BS2 8EG — MB BS Lond. 1987 (Roy. Free) MRCOG 1995; MD Lond. 1996. Cons. (Obst. & Gyn.) St Michael's Hosp. & Bristol Roy. Infirm.; Sen. Clin. Lect. Univ. Bristol. Specialty: Obst. & Gyn. Special Interest: Preceptor in Gyn. & Early Pregn. Ultrasound; Preceptor in Laparoscopic & Hysteroscopic Surg. Prev: Cons. (Obst. & Gyn.) Norf. & Norwich Univ. Hosp.; Regist. & Sen. Regist. Rotat. (Obst. & Gyn.) Addenbrooke's, Peterboro. & Norf. & Norwich Hosps.; Subspecialist Sen. Regist. in Reproductive Med. & Surg. Univ. Coll. Hosp. Lond.

OVERTON, Christopher 7 Butterbache Road, Huntington, Chester CH3 6BY Tel: 01244 310199 — MB ChB Liverp. 1982; Dip. Ven. Liverp. 1986; Cert. Family Plann. JCC 1986; MRCOG 1991. Regist. (O & G) Chester Roy. Infirm. Specialty: Obst. & Gyn. Prev: Regist. (O & G) Princess Margt. Hosp. Swindon.

OVERTON, Dennis James Holyoakes Farm, Holyoakes Lane, Hewell, Redditch B97 5SR — MB ChB Birm. 1985; ChB Birm. 1985; FRCA Lond. 1993. Cons. (Anaesth.) Worcester Roy. Hosp. Worcester. Specialty: Anaesth. Prev: Cons. (Anaesth.), Wycombe Gen. Hosp. High Wycombe, Buckshire.

OVERTON, John Geraint 6A Broomhill Gardens, Glasgow G11 7QD — BM Soton. 1987; MRCGP 1993; Dip. Palliat. Med. Wales 1997. Cons. in Palliat. Med., Salisbury Dist. Hosp. NHS Trust; Cons. in Palliat. Med., Soton. Univ. Hosps. NHS Trust, Countess Mt.batten Ho. Specialty: Palliat. Med. Prev: Specialist Regist., Palliat. Med., Soton. Univ. Hosp. NHS Trust; Regist. (Palliat. Med.) St. Josephs Lond.; SHO (Palliat. Med.) City Hosp. Nottm.

OVERTON, Marion Ruth Langley Health Centre, Common Road, Langley, Slough SL3 8LE Tel: 01753 544288; 8 Palmerston Avenue, Slough SL3 7PU Tel: 01753 572300 Fax: 01753 572300 — MB BS Lond. 1974; DCH Eng. 1977; MRCGP 1978; DRCOG 1978. Prev: Trainee GP Ascot VTS.

OVERTON, Mark John Porthcawl Group Practice, The Portway, Porthcawl CF36 3XB — MB ChB Ed. 1991.

OVERTON, Michael Andrew Young, Ellis and Overton, 41 David Place, St Helier JE2 4TE Tel: 01534 723318 Fax: 01534 611062; Kenricia, St. Peter's Valley, St Lawrence, Jersey JE3 4TE Tel: 01534 871440 — MB ChB Manch. 1980; DRCOG 1983. Prev: GP Manch.

OVERTON, Rachel Catherine 192 Scartho Road, Grimsby DN33 2BP — MB ChB Manch. 1985.

OVERTON, Robert David Charles The Keston House Medical Practice, 70 Brighton Road, Purley CR8 2LJ Tel: 020 8660 8292 Fax: 020 8763 2142 — MB BS Lond. 1988; DRCOG 1993. Specialty: Gen. Med.

OVERTON, Mr Timothy Graeme — MB BS Lond. 1986 (Westm.) MD 1999 (Univ. of Lond.); BSc (Immunol. & Physiol.) Lond. 1983; MRCGP 1990; DRCOG 1990; MRCOG 1994. Cons. (Fetal Med.) St Michael's Hosp. Bristol. Specialty: Obst. & Gyn. Socs: Blair Bell Res. Soc.; Brit. Matern. & Fetal Med. Soc.; Victor Bonney Soc. Prev: Cons. (Obst. & Gyn.), Subspecialist in Materno-Fetal Med., Norf. & Norwich Hosp.; Sen. Regist. (Materno-Fetal Med.) Qu. Charlottes & Chelsea Hosp. Lond.; Sen. Regist. (Obst. & Gyn.) Rosie Matern. Unit Camb.

OVERY, Meriel Kate Dujardin School Lane Surgery, Thetford IP24 2AG Email: m.sykes@tinyonline.co.uk; Rymer Lodge, Barnham, Thetford IP24 2PP Email: m.sykes@tinyonline.co.uk — BM BS Nottm. 1991 (Nottingham) MRCGP 2000. p/t GP Princip. Sch. La. Surg., Thetford, Norf. Specialty: Gen. Med. Prev: Ho. Phys. Pembury Hosp. Tunbridge Wells; Ho. Surg. Qu. Mary's Hosp. Sidcup.; VTS Trainee, N.er Staffs. 1992-1995.

OVERY, Richard Douglas Mulbarton Surgery, The Common, Mulbarton, Norwich NR14 8JG Tel: 01508 570212 Fax: 01508 570042; Corporation Farm House, Wymondham Road, Hethel, Norwich NR14 8EU Tel: 01953 607779 — MB ChB Leeds 1979; DCH RCP Lond. 1984; MRCGP 1986.

OVIS, Simeon (retired) Spa Road Surgery, Spa Road East, Llandrindod Wells LD1 5ES Tel: 01597 824291 / 842292 Fax: 01597 824503 — MB BS Lond. 1957 (St. Mary's) MRCS Eng. LRCP Lond. 1957. Prev: Gen. Practitioner, Llandrindod Wells.

OW, Kevin Khai Huat 14B Highnam Crescent Road, Sheffield S10 1BZ — MB ChB Sheff. 1998.

OWA, Mr Anthony Oloruntoba Flat 30, 133 East India Dock Road, London E14 6DE — MB BS Benin 1987; FRCS Ed. 1993.

OWEN, Ailwen Meinir Llanishen Court Surgery, Llanishen Court, Llanishen, Cardiff CF14 5YU Tel: 02920 757025 Fax: 02920 747931; 12 Cae Garw, Thornhill, Cardiff CF14 9DX Tel: 02920 522924 — MB BCh Wales 1977 (Univ. Hosp. of Wales) G.P. Princip.

OWEN, Mr Alan Ernest (retired) 4 Russell Field, Shrewsbury SY3 9AY Tel: 01743 231980 — MB BCh Wales 1963 (Cardiff) FRCOG 1983, M 1970; FRCS Ed. 1974. Prev: Cons. O & G Roy. Shrewsbury Hosp. Trust.

OWEN, Alexander Guy Roger — MB BCh Wales 1997 (Cardiff) BSc Lond. 1991. GP Princip. Portland Pract. & Hatherley Surg. Cheltenham. Prev: GP Regist. Overton Pk. Surg. Cheltenham; SHO O & G Cheltenham Gen. Hosp.; SHO Paediat. Cheltenham Gen. Hosp.

OWEN, Amanda Mehefin Mayday University Hospital, London Road, Thornton Heath, Croydon CR7 7YE; 3 Chase Ley Street, Limehouse, London E14 7LX Tel: 020 7265 8258 — MRCS Eng. LRCP Lond. 1978 (Guy's) Assoc. Specialist (Liaison Psychiat.) Mayday Hosp. Thornton Heath. Specialty: Gen. Psychiat. Socs: BMA; Med. Wom. Federat. Prev: Clin. Asst. (Psychiat.) E. Ham Day Hosp.; Regist. & SHO Guy's & Bexley Hosps. Lond.

OWEN, Andrew Nunnery Fields Hospital, Nunnery Fields, Canterbury CT1 3LP — MB BChir Camb. 1985.

OWEN, Andrew John 4 Wentworth Park Avenue, Birmingham B17 9QU — MB ChB Birm. 1992.

OWEN, Angela Christine St. Tydfils Hospital, Merthyr Tydfil CF47 0SJ — MB BCh Wales 1979; MRCPsych 1984. St. Tydfils Hospital, Merthyr Tydfil. Specialty: Geriat. Psychiat. Prev: Sen. Regist. (Psychiat.) Cefn Coed Hosp. Swansea; Hon. Sen. Research Regist., Regist. (Psychiat.) & SHO WhitCh. Hosp. Cardiff; Cons. Psychiat. Old Age Bryntirion Hosp. Llanelli.

OWEN, Annaliese Catherine 61 Warwick Street, Oxford OX4 1SZ — MB BS Lond. 1993.

OWEN, Annalise Park House, Nursery Road, Huntingdon PE29 3RJ Tel: 01480 415357 Fax: 01480 415363 Email: annalise.owen@hinchingbrooke.nhs.uk — BSc, MBChB 1992 (Stellenbosch) Cons. (Psychiat. Geriat.) Cambs. & P'boro. Ment. Health Partnership NHS Trust. Specialty: Geriat. Psychiat.

OWEN, Mr Anthony Wynn Michael Carton 21 Hale Road, Hale, Liverpool L24 5RB Tel: 0151 425 2288 — MB ChB Liverp. 1968; BSc (Hons.) Liverp. 1965; FRCS Eng. 1973; FRCS Ed. 1973. Lect. Surg. Univ. Hosp. S. Manch. Socs: BMA. Prev: Surg. Regist. Liverp. RHB & Chester Roy. Infirm.; Lect. Surg. Roy. Infirm. Edin.

OWEN, Brian Clifford Mountain View, Penrhos Road, Bangor LL57 2NA Tel: 01248 351127 Fax: 01248 371101 — MB BCh Wales 1980; BSc Cardiff 1977; DRCOG 1983; MRCGP 1984; AFOM RCP Lond. 1988; MFOM 1994. Cons. (Occupat. Health) Bangor. Specialty: Occupat. Health.

OWEN, Buddug, OBE (retired) Bwthyn, Cwm Road, Rhuallt, St Asaph LL17 0TP Tel: 01745 584446 — (Cardiff) BSc Wales 1946; MB BCh Wales 1949; DA Eng. 1954; FFA RCS Eng. 1970. Trustee Museum of Med. & Health, Wales. Prev: Med. Off. (Complaints) Wales.

OWEN, Caroline Megan 12 Whitecroft Lane, Mellor, Blackburn BB2 7HA — MB ChB Bristol 1993; MRCP (UK) 1996. Specialist Regist. (Dermat.) Lancaster Roy. Infirm. & Hope Hosp. Salford Manch. Specialty: Dermat.

OWEN, Colin Griffith The Surgery, Swan Barton, Sherston, Malmesbury Tel: 01666 840270 — MRCS Eng. LRCP Lond. 1953 (St. Mary's) Prev: Clin. Asst. (Orthop.) Ormskirk & Dist. Gen. Hosp.; Ho. Surg. Orthop. Dept. St. Mary's Hosp. Lond.; Ho. Phys. Roy. Edwd. Infirm. Wigan.

OWEN, Mr David Ainslie 229 Coppermill Road, Wraysbury, Staines TW19 5NW Tel: 0128 125405 — MRCS Eng. LRCP Lond. 1962 (St. Thos.) MB Camb. 1963, BChir 1962; DO Eng. 1967; FRCS Ed. 1970; FRCS Eng. 1971. Socs: BMA.

OWEN, Lord David Anthony Llewellyn, PC, CH (retired) House of Lords, London SW1A 0PW Tel: 020 7787 2751 Fax: 01442 876108 Email: lordowen@nildram.co.uk; 78 Narrow Street, Limehouse, London E14 8BP — (St. Thos.) MA, MB Camb. 1963, BChir 1962. Chairm. Global Natural Energy; Chairm. Yukos International B.V.; Dir. Abbott Laborat.; Fell. Sidney Sussex Coll. Camb. Prev: EU Chairm. Internat. Conf. on Former Yugoslavia.

OWEN, David Christopher 30 The Parade, Roath, Cardiff CF24 3AD — MB BCh Wales 1984.

OWEN, David John Currie Road Health Centre, Currie Road, Galashiels TD1 2UA; Galashiels Health Centre Tel: 01896 661355 Fax: 01896 661357; Fernlea, Ormiston Terrace, Melrose TD6 9SP Tel: 01896 822537 — MB ChB Ed. 1976; MRCGP 1982; DRCOG 1983.
OWEN, David Kenny Bradford House, 106 Stockbridge Road, Winchester SO22 6RL Tel: 01962 856310 — MB BS Lond. 1982; MRCS Eng LRCP Lond. 1982; FFHom 1983. Specialty: Homeop. Med.
OWEN, David Norman Howell (retired) Bryn-y-mor, Fishguard SA65 Tel: 01348 872214 — MB BChir Camb. 1952 (Camb. & Guy's) MA; MRCS Eng. LRCP Lond. 1949; DObst RCOG 1954; MRCGP 1962; DA Eng. 1968. Prev: Ho. Surg., Ho. Phys. & Paediat. Resid. Pembury Hosp. (Guy's Sector).
OWEN, David Roy (retired) The Old Vicarage, Soulbury, Leighton Buzzard LU7 0BX Tel: 01525 270305 Email: drowen@doctors.org.uk — MRCS Eng. LRCP Lond. 1957 (Char. Cross) DLO Eng. 1961; DObst RCOG 1962. Honoarary Cons., The Gt. West. Hosp., Swindon. Prev: GP Leighton Buzzard.
OWEN, Mr Dewi Wyn (retired) 9 Dolgwili Road, Carmarthen SA31 2AE Tel: 01267 235965 — MB ChB Liverp. 1957; MRCS Eng. LRCP Lond. 1957; FRCS Eng. 1965. Manager, Ment. Health Act Appeals Panel (Ment. Illness) Pembrokesh. NHS Trust Gen. Hosp. Fishguard Rd. Haverford W. Pembrokesh.; Mem. Carmarthen/Dihefwr C.H.C. Prev: Sen. Med. Off. Welsh Office Cardiff.
OWEN, Diane 54 Glantawe Park, Ystradgynlais, Swansea SA9 1AE — MB BCh Wales 1994.
OWEN, Dulcie Ann Lenthall (retired) 4 Cloutman's Lane, Braunton EX33 1NG Tel: 01271 890228 — MB BS Lond. 1955 (St. Mary's)
OWEN, Mr Edwin Nicholas (retired) 18 Kenton Drive, Shrewsbury SY2 6TH Tel: 01743 235858 — (Liverp.) MB ChB Liverp. 1938; MRCS Eng. LRCP Lond. 1938; DLO Eng. 1946; FRCS Eng. 1949. Prev: Cons. ENT Shrewsbury Gp. Hosps.
OWEN, Elin Gwarcwm Bach, 18 Heol Ffynnon Asa, Eglwysbach, Colwyn Bay LL28 5BL — MB BCh Wales 1997.
OWEN, Elizabeth Jane Dept O&G, West Middlesex University Hospital Trust, Twickenham Road, Isleworth TW7 6AF Tel: 020 8565 5117 — MB BS Lond. 1980 (Royal Free Hospital) MRCOG 1986; MD Lond. 1993; FRCOG 1998. Cons. O & G W. Middlx. Univ. Hosp. Trust Isleworth; Director (Clinical Studies) Imperial Coll. Lond. Specialty: Obst. & Gyn.; Family Plann. & Reproduc. Health. Socs: (Counc.) Roy. Soc. Med.; Brit. Fertil. Soc.; Brit. Menopause Soc. Prev: Sen. Regist. (O & G) St. Mary's Hosp. Lond.; Research Regist. (Gyn. Endocrinol.) Middlx. Hosp. Lond.; Regist. (Obst & Gyn.) Univ. Coll. Hosp. Lond.
OWEN, Mr Eoghan Ronan Thomas Carton Pipers Hollow, Forest Road, Horsham RH12 4HL Tel: 01403 242904 Fax: 01403 248773 Email: owen@uk-consultants.co.uk; Brookfield House, 21 Hale Road, Hale, Liverpool L24 5RB Tel: 0151 425 2288 — MB ChB Liverp. 1978; FRCS Ed. 1984; FRCSI 1984. Cons. Surg. Gen. & Gastrointestinal Surg. Surrey & Sussex NHS Trust. Specialty: Gen. Surg. Socs: Fell. New York Acad. Sci.; Surg. Research Soc. Prev: Resid. Surg. Off. St. Mark's Hosp. Lond.; Sen. Regist. St. Mary's & Hammersmith Hosps. Lond.; Regist. (Surg.) Northwick Pk. Hosp. & Clin. Research Centre Harrow.
OWEN, Garth Buchanan (retired) 26 Links Road, Romiley, Stockport SK6 4HU Tel: 0161 494 1416 Fax: 0161 494 1416 Email: owen@romiley26.fsnet.co.uk — MB ChB Manch. 1952. Prev: Gen. Practioner.
OWEN, Gerallt 10 Firgrove Corner, Wrexham LL12 7UF Tel: 01978 359219; Block D, 26 Wetherby Road, Harrogate HG2 7SA — MB ChB Liverp. 1990; MRCP (UK) 1995. Regist. (c/o Elderly) Harrogate & St. Jas. Hosps. Leeds. Specialty: Care of the Elderly. Socs: BMA; Brit. Geriat. Soc. Prev: Regist. (Med.) Glan Clwyd Hosp. Rhyl; SHO (Nephrol.) Roy. Liverp. Univ. Hosp.
OWEN, Gerwyn Portishead Health Centre, Victoria Square, Portishead, Bristol BS20 6AQ Tel: 01275 847474 Fax: 01275 817516; The Orchard, Sheepway, Portbury, Bristol BS20 7TE Tel: 01275 848346 — MB ChB Bristol 1984; BSc (Hons.) Bristol 1981, MB ChB 1984; DRCOG 1986; MRCGP 1994. Specialty: Obst. & Gyn. Prev: SHO (Paediat.) Bristol Childr. Hosp.; SHO (Gen. Med.) Frenchay Hosp. Bristol; SHO (Obst.) Bristol Matern. Hosp.
OWEN, Glyn Ward Bryn-yr-Ashwrn, Llanrhaeadr, Denbigh LL16 4PH — BM Soton. 1993.
OWEN, Griffith Tudor Penychen, Chwilog, Pwllheli LL53 6HJ — MRCS Eng. LRCP Lond. 1979 (Guy's) Prev: SHO (A & E) Guy's Hosp. Lond.; Ho. Surg. Guy's Hosp. Lond.; Ho. Phys. Harefield Hosp. Middlx.
OWEN, Gwen Ellis (retired) Gwenarth, 184 Hale Road, Hale, Altrincham WA15 8SQ Tel: 0161 928 1321 — MB ChB Liverp. 1948. SCMO S. Manch. HA.
OWEN, Gwyneth c/o Department of Paediatrics, West Wales General Hospital, Dolgwili Road, Carmarthen SA31 2AF — MB BCh Wales 1979; FRCPCH; DCH RCP Lond. 1981; MRCP (UK) 1984. Cons. Paediat. W. Wales Gen. Hosp. Carmarthen. Specialty: Paediat.
OWEN, Miss Gwyneth Olwen Lincoln Country Hospital, Greetwell Road, Lincoln LN2 5QY Tel: 01522 512512 — MB BS Lond. 1982 (The Lond. Hosp. Med. Coll.) FRCS Ed. 1987; FRCS Eng. (Orl.) 1990; Master of Surger, Univ. of Bath. 1994. Specialty: Otolaryngol.
OWEN, Gwynfryn Anwyl (retired) 11 Peters Way, Knebworth SG3 6HP Tel: 01438 812864 — MRCS Eng. LRCP Lond. 1939; DTM & H Eng. 1949.
OWEN, Harriet Alice 50 Hillside Crescent, Harrow HA2 0QX — MB BS Lond. 1998; MB BS Lond 1998.
OWEN, Ian Glyn Pemberton Primary Care Resource Centre, Sherwood Drive, Pemberton, Wigan WN5 9QX Tel: 01942 775880 Fax: 01942 775882; Kinnaird House, Curtis St, Pemberton, Wigan WN5 9LB Tel: 01942 222304 — LMSSA Lond. 1990; MRCGP 1994; DRCOG 1994.
OWEN, Ivor Tudor, Squadron Ldr. RAF Med. Br. Retd. Royal Lancaster Infirmary, OH Department, Ashton Road, Lancaster LA1 4RP Tel: 01524 583218 Email: ivor.owen@mbht.nhs.uk; 35 Lindbergh Avenue, Lancaster LA1 5FR Fax: 01524 581550 Email: ivorowen@doctors.org.uk — MB ChB Birm. 1986; DRCOG 1991; DCH RCP Lond. 1991; T (GP) 1992; DFFP 1994; MRCGP 1994; DAvMed FOM RCP Lond. 1995; D Occ Med. RCP Lond. 1996; AFOM, RCP Lond. 2001; MSc (Occ Med) Manch. 2004; MFOM RCP Lond. 2004. Cons. Occupat. Phys. Morecambe Bay Hosps. NHS Trust; Occupat. Phys. (Aviat. Med.) Roy. Preston Hosp. & BAE Systems Warton. Specialty: Occupat. Health; Aviat. Med.; Gen. Pract. Socs: Inst. Occupat. Safety & Health (MIOSH); Roy. Inst. Public Health (FRIPH); Soc. Occupat. Med. (North W. Exec. Comm. Mem.). Prev: Chief Med. Off. BAE Systems Warton Unit; RAF Sen. Med. Off. RAF Decimomannu; Emirates Airline Clinic Doctor, Dubai.
OWEN, Mr James Edward 61 Warwick Street, Oxford OX4 1SZ — BChir Camb. 1992; MA 1994 Camb.; BA Camb. 1990; FRCS Eng. 1997. Specialist Regist. Orthop. Oxf. Regional Train. Program. Specialty: Trauma & Orthop. Surg.; Orthop. Socs: Assoc. Mem. BOA; Fell.of Roy. Coll. Of Surg.s of Eng.
OWEN, Lt. Col. Jeremy Peter, Lt.-Col. — MB ChB Birm. 1985; MFOM RCP Lond. 1996, AFOM 1992; MMedSc (Occupat. Health) Birm. 1994. Cons. (Occupat. Med.) & Med. Off. RAMC. Specialty: Occupat. Health. Socs: Soc. Occupat. Med. Prev: Med. Off. Brit. Antarctic Survey.
OWEN, Joanne Alison 5 Fairview Place, Danestone, Aberdeen AB22 8ZJ — MB ChB Aberd. 1997.
***OWEN, Joanne Claire** 2 Furzehatt Villas, Plymstock, Plymouth PL9 9HB — BM BS Nottm. 1998; BM BS Nottm 1998. SHO in A & E, Chesterfield Roy. Hosp. Chesterfield. Specialty: Accid. & Emerg. Prev: PRHO in Med., Qu.'s Med. Centre, Nottm.
OWEN, John Douglas, MBE (retired) 8 Achnacone Drive, Colchester CO4 5AZ — MB BChir Camb. 1959 (Westm.) MA, MB Camb. 1959, BChir 1958; MRCS Eng. LRCP Lond. 1958; DObst RCOG 1960. Prev: Ho. Surg. Gordon Hosp. Lond.
OWEN, John Hughes c/o Cossham Hospital, Lodge Road, Kingswood, Bristol BS15 1LQ Tel: 0117 967 1661 — MB ChB Bristol 1982; MRCPsych 1987. Cons. Psychiat. Cossham Hosp. Kingswood Bristol. Specialty: Gen. Psychiat. Prev: Regist. (Psychiat.) Glenside Hosp. Stapleton, Bristol; Psychiat. Crisis Interven. Team Melbourne, Austral.; Lect. (Ment. Health) Univ. Bristol.
OWEN, Professor John Joseph Thomas Department of Anatomy, The Medical School, Edgbaston, Birmingham B15 2TT Tel: 0121 414 6812 Fax: 0121 414 6815 — (Liverp.) BSc Liverp. 1955, MD 1963, MB ChB 1959; MA Oxf. 1964; FRS 1988. Sands Cox Prof. Anat. Med. Sch. Univ. Birm. Specialty: Immunol. Prev: Prof.

Anat. Med. Sch. Univ. Newc.; Fell. St. Cross Coll. Oxf.; Lect. Univ. Oxf.

OWEN, John Philip Glannrafon Surgery, Glannrafon, Amlwch LL68 9AG Tel: 01407 830878 Fax: 01407 832512 — MB ChB Liverp. 1974; MRCP (UK) 1977.

OWEN, John Robson (retired) Little Donnings, Prinsted, Emsworth PO10 8HS Tel: 01243 373021 — (Birm.) MB ChB Birm. 1952. Prev: G.P. 1955-1995.

OWEN, John Roger 81 Painswick Road, Cheltenham GL50 2EX — MB BS Lond. 1971; FRCR 1977; FRCP (UK) 1998. Cons. Clin. Oncol. Cheltenham Gen. Hosp. Specialty: Oncol.; Radiol. Prev: Sen. Regist. (Radiother.) Roy. Marsden Hosp. Lond.; Regist. (Radiother.) Hammersmith Hosp. Lond.; Ho. Surg. Lond. Hosp.

OWEN, John Tudor (retired) 6 Eresby House, Rutland Gate, London SW7 1BG — MB BS Lond. 1948.

OWEN, Jonathan Richard Bower Offerton Health Centre, Offerton Lane, Stockport SK2 5AR Tel: 0161 480 0324; 105 Overdale Road, Romiley, Stockport SK6 3JB — MB ChB Manch. 1982 (Manchester) DCH RCP Lond. 1987; MRCGP 1990; T(G) 1992. GP Princip. Specialty: Gen. Pract. Prev: SHO (A & E Psychiat. & ENT) Tameside Gen. Hosp. Ashton u Lyne.

OWEN, Joyce Mary (retired) 11 Rotherwood Close, Mill Road, Bebington, Wirral CH63 5RG — MB ChB Liverp. 1938; DObst RCOG 1942. Mem. Liverp. Med. Inst. Prev: Res. Med. Off. Alder Hey Childr. Hosp. Liverp.

OWEN, Julie Clare 28 Sandbanks Road, Lower Parkstone, Poole BH14 8BU — MB ChB Liverp. 1996.

OWEN, Katharine Ruth 19 Tetbury Grove, Birmingham B31 5RB — MB ChB Birm. 1992.

OWEN, Katherine Clare 4 Wentworth Park Avenue, Birmingham B17 9QU — MB ChB Birm. 1993.

OWEN, Kathryn Ruth 13 Hart Road, Manchester M14 7LD — MB ChB Manch. 1991.

OWEN, Keith Rysseldene Surgery, 98 Conway Road, Colwyn Bay LL29 7LE Tel: 01492 532807 Fax: 01492 534846 — MB BCh Wales 1977; DRCOG 1980.

OWEN, Kelyth Lloyd South Lawn, Moorend Park Road, Cheltenham Tel: 01242 522764 — MRCS Eng. LRCP Lond. 1948 (Univ. Coll. Hosp.) FFA RCS Eng. 1954. Cons. Anaesth. Cheltenham & Gloucester Health Dists. Specialty: Anaesth. Socs: Assn. Anaesth.; S.W. Soc. Anaesths. Prev: Regist. & Sen. Regist. (Anaesth.) Cardiff Roy. Infirm.; RAMC, Clin. Off. Anaesth. Hong Kong.

OWEN, Mr Kenneth (retired) Hillside Farm, Adlestrop, Moreton-in-Marsh GL56 0YR Tel: 01608 658277 Fax: 01608 659170 Email: keno@adleside.u-net.com — (St. Mary's) MB BS Lond. 1944; MRCS Eng. LRCP Lond. 1944; FRCS Eng. 1950; MS Lond. 1957. p/t Cons. Surg. St. Mary's Hosp. Lond.; Cons. Urol. St. Peter's & St. Paul's Hosps. Lond. & King Edwd. VII Hosp Offs Lond. Prev: Research Asst. Harvard Univ.

OWEN, Louise Sarah Isobel 29 Avenue Rise, Bushey, Watford WD23 3AS — MB ChB Bristol 1996. SpR Paediat. Specialty: Paediat. Socs: BMA. Prev: Ho. Off. (Med.) Exeter; Ho. Off. (Surg.) Bristol.

OWEN, Lysa Edith Accident & Emergency Department, Ninewells Hospital and Medical School, Dundee DD1 9SY Tel: 01382 660111; 43 Hyndford Street, Dundee DD2 1HX Email: lysa@balny.org — MB ChB Dundee 1992; MFAEM 2003. Specialist Regist. (A & E) Dundee. Specialty: Accid. & Emerg.

OWEN, Maldwyn Henry Dean Cross Surgery, 21 Radford Park Road, Plymstock, Plymouth PL9 9DL Tel: 01752 404743; Old Staddon Farm, Staddon Heights, Plymstock, Plymouth PS9 9SP Tel: 01752 404775 — MB Camb. 1975; MA; BChir 1974; DObst RCOG 1976; MRCGP 1980.

OWEN, Marie Elizabeth Paediatric Department, Gloucestershire Royal Hospital, Great Western Road, Gloucester GL1 3NN Tel: 01452 528555; 81 Painswick Road, Cheltenham GL50 2EX Tel: 01242 522501 — MB BS Lond. 1972; DCH Eng. 1978. Clin. Asst. (Paediat.) Gloucester Roy. Hosp. Specialty: Paediat. Prev: Regist. (Paediat.) Whittington Hosp. Lond.; SHO (Paediat.) Univ. Coll. Hosp. Lond.

OWEN, Mark Julian 1 The Park, London W5 5NE — MB BS Lond. 1982; MSc Lond. 1975, BSc (Engineering) 1974, MB BS 1982.

OWEN, Mary 32 St Albans Road, Edinburgh EH9 2LU Tel: 0131 667 2222 — MB BCh Wales 1962 (Cardiff) DA Eng. 1965. Clin. Asst. Colposcopy Clinic Edin. Roy. Infirm. Specialty: Anaesth. Prev: Regist. (Anaesth.) SE RHB Scotl.

OWEN, Mererid Market Street Surgery, 3-5 Market Street, Caernarfon LL55 1RT Tel: 01286 673224 Fax: 01286 676405 — MB BCh Wales 1985.

OWEN, Mervyn Edwards 3 Market Street, Caernarfon LL55 1RT Tel: 01286 673224; Bryn Rhug, England Road N., Caernarfon LL55 1HS Tel: 01286 671122 — LRCPI & LM, LRSCI & LM 1957; Mem. BMA; LRCPI & LM, LRCSI & LM 1957; DObst RCOG 1965. Prev: Ho. Phys. Lincoln Co. Hosp.; Ho. Surg. City Hosp. Nottm.; Obst. Ho. Off. St. David's Hosp. Bangor.

OWEN, Professor Michael John Cardiff University, School of Medicine, Department of Psychological Medicine, Heath Park, Cardiff CF14 4XN Tel: 029 2074 3248 Fax: 029 2074 6554 Email: owenmj@cf.ac.uk — MB ChB Birm. 1983; PhD Birm. 1982, BSc 1977; FRCPsych 1997, M 1987; F.Med.Sci. 1999. Prof. & Head (Psychol. Med.) Sch. of Med.; Hon. Cons. Psychiat. Univ. Hosp. Wales, Cardiff & Vale Health Care Trust. Specialty: Gen. Psychiat. Socs: (Pres.) Internat. Soc. Psychiat. Genetics; Amer. Soc. Human Genetics; Acad. Med. Sci. Prev: MRC Research Fell. (Biochem. & Molecular Genetics) St Mary's Hosp. Med. Sch. Lond.; Hon. Lect. Inst. Psychiat. Lond.

OWEN, Michael Robert Director of Public Health, North & East Devon Health Authority, Dean Clarke House, Southern Hay East, Exeter EX1 1PQ Tel: 01392 207380 Fax: 01392 207377 — MB BCh BAO Dub. 1972 (Univ. Dub. Trinity Coll.) DCH Eng. 1974; MRCGP 1976; DObst RCOG 1976; MSc Lond. 1981, MD 1983; FFPHM RCP (UK) 1995. Dir. Pub. Health N. & E. Devon HA; Hon. Sen. Lect. Postgrad. Med. Sch. Univ. Exeter. Specialty: Pub. Health Med. Prev: Cons. Pub. Health Med. Exeter HA & SW RHA; Sen. Med. Adviser Overseas Developm. Admin.; Princip. in Gen. Pract. Weston Super Mare.

OWEN, Neil Macarthur Deerness Park Medical Centre, Suffolk Street, Sunderland SR2 8AD Tel: 0191 567 0961; Seaforth, 35B Sea View Road, Grangetown, Sunderland SR2 7UP Tel: 0191 514 0527 — MB ChB Glas. 1980.

OWEN, Neil Trevor Poyntz St Lawrence's Hospital, Boundary Road, Bodmin PL31 2QT Tel: 01208 251318 — MB ChB Ed. 1985; MRCPsych 1991. Cons. Psychiat. (Gen. Adult) Cornw. Healthcare Trust. Specialty: Gen. Psychiat. Prev: Sen. Regist. Rotat. Wessex Region; Research Fell. (Psychiat.) Roy. Edin. Hosp.; Regist. (Psychiat.) Ailsa Hosp. Ayr.

OWEN, Mr Nicholas John 58 Parliament Hill, London NW3 2TL — BM BCh Oxf. 1988 (Oxford) BA (Hons.) Camb. 1985; FRCS Eng. 1992; FRCR 1998. Regist. (Radiol.) Roy. Lond. Hosp., GP Regist. Specialty: Radiol. Prev: Regist. (Surg., Urol. & Emerg. Med.) Monash Med. Centre Melbourne, Austral.; SHO (Surg. & Urol.) Reading Hosps.

OWEN, Norman Charles Watkin (retired) 11 Prestwick Drive, Blundellsands, Liverpool L23 7XB Tel: 0151 924 1574 — MB ChB Liverp. 1948; MRCS Eng. LRCP Lond. 1949. Prev: Resid. Asst. Med. Off. Walton Hosp. Liverp.

OWEN, Mr Owen Elias (retired) Bryn Meurig, Bethesda, Bangor LL57 4YW Tel: 01248 600322 — MB ChB Ed. 1946 (Univ. Ed.) FRCS Eng. 1953. Prev: Consult. in Gen. Surg. Gwynedd HA.

OWEN, Penelope Ann Heald Green Health Centre, Heald Green, Stockport; Beech Trylls, Trouthall Lane, Plumley, Knutsford WA16 0UN — BM Soton. 1986; DRCOG 1989. Specialty: Gen. Pract. Prev: SHO (Geriat. Med.) Portsmouth; Trainee GP Havant & Baddesley; SHO (O & G) Princess Anne Hosp. Soton.

OWEN, Penelope Judith Dawn 13 Highland Close, Cymdda, Sarn, Bridgend CF32 9SB — MB BCh Wales 1997. SHO (Med.) P. Chas. Hosp. Merthyr. Specialty: Gen. Med. Prev: Ho. Off. (Med.) P. Philip Hosp. Llanelli; Ho. Off. (Neurosurg.) Univ. Hosp. Wales; Ho. Off. (Gen. Surg.) Llandough Hosp.

OWEN, Mr Peter Julian 32 Vale Road, Claygate, Esher KT10 0NJ Tel: 01372 802726 Email: jules@csi.com — MB BChir Camb. 1990 (Cambridge) MA Camb. 1990; FRCS Ed. 1994; FRCS (TRODRTH) 1999. Specialist Regist. (Orthop. Surg.) SW Thames. Specialty: Orthop. Socs: BOA, Assoc. Mem.; BOTA Mem.; Fell. RCS (Ed.). Prev: Fell. in Orthop., Sunnybrook Heatlh Sci. Centre, Toronto, Ontario,

Canada; Fell. (Callotasis) Robt. Jones & Agnes Hunt Orthop. Hosp. Oswestry.

OWEN, Philip Princess Royal Maternity Hospital and Stobhill, General Hospital, Glasgow G21 3UW Tel: 0141 201 3432 Email: philipowen1@hotmail.com; 12 Craigievar Place, Newton Mearns, Glasgow G77 6YE — MB BCh Wales 1985; MRCOG 1990; MD Wales 1998; DFM 2000. Cons. (O & G) The Princess Roy. Matern. Unit and Stophill Hosp. Glas. Specialty: Obst. & Gyn. Special Interest: Obstetric Ultrasound. Socs: RCOG Council 2002. Prev: Clin. Lect. & Hon. Sen. Regist. Ninewells Hosp. Dundee; Research Fell. (O & G) Ninewells Hosp. Dundee.

OWEN, Rachel Anne 148 Lords Street, Cadishead, Manchester M44 5YB — MB ChB Manch. 1998.

OWEN, Rhian Elin Y Bwthyn Newydd, Princess of Wales Hospital, Bridgend CF31 1RQ Tel: 0292 084 2972 Email: rhian.owen@bromor-tr.wales.nhs.uk — MB BCh Wales 1974 (Welsh National School of Medicine) MRCP (UK) 1980; Dip. Palliat. Med. Wales 1992; FRCP Lond. 1996. Macmillan Cons. Palliat. Med. Bro Morganncog NHS Trust. Socs: Brit. Geriat. Soc. (Sec. Welsh Br.); Rhondda Med. Soc. (Ex-Pres.); Fell. RSM. Prev: Sen. Med. Off. Welsh Off. Cardiff; Cons. Phys. (Geriat. Med.) Dewi Sant Hosp. Pontypridd; Cons. Phys. (Geriat. Med.) Tan Tock Seng Hosp., Singapore.

OWEN, Rhodri Wyn Bodnant Surgery, Menai Avenue, Bangor LL57 2HH Tel: 01248 364567 Fax: 01248 370654 — MB BCh Wales 1978; MRCS Eng. LRCP Lond. 1978; DRCOG 1982.

OWEN, Rhys Prys The Health Centre, Bridge Street, Thorne, Doncaster DN8 5QH Tel: 01405 812121 Fax: 01405 741059 — MB ChB Leeds 1969.

OWEN, Professor Robert, OBE Bryn Celyn, 41 Pwllycrochan Avenue, Colwyn Bay LL29 7BW Tel: 01492 533432 — MB BS Lond. 1946 (Guy's) FRCS Eng. 1951; MCh Orth. Liverp. 1953. Emerit. Prof. Surg. Univ. Liverp. (Orthopaedic). Specialty: Orthop. Socs: Fell. Brit. Orthop. Assn.; (Ex-Pres.) Brit. Scoliosis Soc.; Counc. RCS Eng. Prev: Cons. Orthop. Surg. Robt. Jones & Agnes Hunt Orthop. Hosp. Oswestry; Sen. Orthop. Regist. Liverp. United Hosps.; Squadron Ldr. RAFVR Med. Serv.

OWEN, Robert Andrew Department of Histopathology & Cytopathology, Whipps Cross Hospital, Whipps Cross Road, Leytonstone, London E11 1NR Tel: 020 8539 5522 — MB BChir Camb. 1980 (St. Geo.) MRCPath 1989. Cons. Histopath. & Cytopath. Whipps Cross Hosp. Lond. Specialty: Histopath.

OWEN, Robert Arwyn (retired) Meadowbank, Greenfield Lane, Rowton, Chester CH3 6AU — MB BCh Wales 1953; BSc Wales 1950; DMRD Liverp. 1959; DMRD Eng. 1959; FRCP Ed. 1977, M 1962; FRCR 1962; FFR 1962. Prev: Cons. Radiol. Chester HA.

OWEN, Robert Elwy (retired) Cornel Penypentre, Llanfihangel Talyllyn, Brecon LD3 7TG Tel: 01874 658432 — (Guy's) MB BS Lond. 1957; MRCS Eng. LRCP Lond. 1957; LMSSA Lond. 1957; DPM Eng. 1964. Prev: Asst. Psychiat. Mid Wales Hosp. Talgarth.

OWEN, Robert Elwyn (retired) The Lugger, 21 Beach Road, Cemaes Bay LL67 0ES — MB BS Lond. 1976; BA Oxf. 1973; MRCGP 1981. Prev: GP Amlwch.

OWEN, Robert Thomas Southern Derbyshire Mental Health (NHS) Trust, Derby City General Hospital, Psychiatric Unit, Uttoxeter Road, Derby DE22 3NE Tel: 01332 625587 — MB ChB Liverp. 1973; MRCPsych 1979. Cons. Psychiat. Derby City Gen. Hosp. Specialty: Gen. Psychiat. Prev: Cons. Psychiat. Pastures Hosp. Derby.

OWEN, Mr Robin Arthur (retired) Twitten End, Bickley Park Road, Bromley BR1 2AY Tel: 020 8467 4660 — MB BChir Camb. 1954 (King's Coll. Hosp.) DO Eng. 1957; FRCS Eng. 1960; MD Camb. 1965; FCOphth 1991. Prev: Cons. Ophth. Dartford, Sidcup, Lewisham Childr. & FarnBoro. Hosps.

OWEN, Robin Dylan 52 North Eastern Road, Thorne, Doncaster DN8 4AW — MB ChB Manch. 1998.

OWEN, Roger Graham HMDS Laboratory, Leeds General Infirmary, Great George St., Leeds LS1 3EX Tel: 0113 392 6285 Fax: 0113 392 6286 Email: rgowen@hmds.org.uk — MB BCh Wales 1988; BSc Wales 1985; MRCP (UK) 1991; MD 1999; MRCPath 1999. Cons. Haematologist, Leeds Teachg. Hosps. NHS Trust. Specialty: Haematology. Prev: Research Fell. (Haemat.) Leeds Gen. Infirm.; Regist. (Haemat.) Leeds Hosps.; SHO Cardiff. Roy. Infirm. & Leeds Gen. Infirm.

OWEN, Ronald, OBE (retired) Oakengates, 24 Greenway, Harpenden AL5 1NQ Tel: 015827 715501 — MB ChB Liverp. 1953; CChem; DIH Soc. Apoth. Lond. 1961, DMJ (Clin.) 1964; FFOM RCP Lond. 1982, MFOM 1978; FRSC 1987. Prev: Cons. to Trades Union Congr.

OWEN, Rosalind Janet 51 Stonehill, Street BA16 0PG Tel: 01458 443098 — MB ChB Manch. 1967; MFFP 1993. SCMO (Family Plann.) Taunton Deane PCT; Mem. UK Family Plann. Research Network Exeter Univ. Specialty: Family Plann. & Reproduc. Health. Prev: Asst. (Family Plann. & Well Wom.) Vine Surg. St.

OWEN, Ruth (retired) 17 Devonhurst Place, Heathfield Terrace, London W4 4JB Tel: 020 8995 3228 Email: sg.owen@clara.co.uk; 17 Devonhurst Place, Heathfield Terrace, London Tel: 020 8995 3228 Email: sg.owen@clara.co.uk — (University of Pennsylvania School of Medicine) MD Univ. Pennsylvania 1955; LMSSA Lond. 1957; FRCA Eng. 1972. Prev: Cons. Anaesth. Ealing Hosp. Lond.

OWEN, Ruth Diana Child Health Department, Isaac Maddox House, Shrub Hill Road, Worcester WR4 9RW Tel: 01905 763333; Dovecote House, Charlton, Pershore WR10 3LL Tel: 01386 860712 — MB ChB Liverp. 1967; DCH Eng. 1971; DCCH RCP Ed. 1985; DCP Warwick 1985. SCMO Worcs. Community Healthcare Trust. Specialty: Audiol. Med. Socs: Fac. Comm. Health; Brit. Assn. Community Drs in Audiol.

OWEN, Samantha Jane 28 Stafford Road, Bloxwich, Walsall WS3 3NL — MB ChB Birm. 1997.

OWEN, Samuel Griffith, CBE (retired) Flat 17, 9 Devonhurst Place, Heathfield Terrace, London W4 4JB Tel: 020 8995 3228 Email: sg.owen@clara.co.uk — (Newc. upon Tyne) MB BS Durh. 1948; FRCP Lond. 1965, M 1951; MD Durh. 1955. Prev: Second Sec. Med. Research Counc.

OWEN, Sandra 40 Parkhill Road, Bexley DA5 1HU Tel: 01322 522056 — MB BS Lond. 1966 (St. Mary's) MRCS Eng. LRCP Lond. 1966.

OWEN, Sandra Jayne 35 Ty Wern Avenue, Rhiwbina, Cardiff CF14 6AW — MB BCh Wales 1993.

OWEN, Stephen William 19 Greengates Crescent, Neston, South Wirral CH64 0XH — MB BS Liverp. 1993.

OWEN, Susan Judith The Marches Medical Practice, Mill Lane Surgery, 46 Mill Lane, Buckley CH7 3HB Tel: 01244 550939; 9 Lumley Road, Chester CH2 2AQ Tel: 01244 390230 Fax: 01244 390230 — MB BS Newc. 1975; DRCOG 1978; MRCGP 1979.

OWEN, Terry Wawn Street Surgery, Wawn Street, South Shields NE33 4DX Tel: 0191 454 0421 Fax: 0191 454 9428; 7 Blagdon Avenue, South Shields NE34 0SG — MB BS Newc. 1980; DRCOG 1983; MRCGP 1984.

OWEN, Thomas Emlyn (retired) Tygarn, 96 Farrar Road, Bangor LL57 2DU Tel: 01248 353108 — MB BS Lond. 1945 (Lond. Hosp.) MRCP Lond. 1951; FRCP Lond. 1978; MRCS Eng. LRCP Lond. 1945. Prev: Cons. Phys. (Geriat. Med.) Gwynedd HA.

OWEN, Thomas Peter (retired) Trevaunance, Whitchurch, Tavistock PL19 9DD — MRCS Eng. LRCP Lond. 1963 (St. Mary's) MA Camb. 1959, MB BChir 1964; DA Eng. 1966; DObst RCOG 1967; DCH Eng. 1968. Prev: SHO Childr. Hosp. Sydenham.

OWEN, Timothy Clive Ethel Street Surgery, 88/90 Ethel Street, Benwell, Newcastle upon Tyne NE4 8QA Tel: 0191 219 5456 Fax: 0191 226 0300; 1 Lesbury Road, Heaton, Newcastle upon Tyne NE6 5LB Tel: 0191 265 8898 — MB BS Lond. 1979; DRCOG 1981; MRCGP 1983.

OWEN, Mr Timothy David 49 Chillingham Drive, Chester-le-Street DH2 3TJ Tel: 029 2061 1565 — MB BCh Wales 1986; FRCS Eng. 1990; FRCS Orth. 1995. Sen. Regist. (Orthop. Surg.) N. RHA. Specialty: Orthop. Prev: Regist. (Orthop Surg.) North. RHA; Regist. Rotat. (Surg.) Cardiff.

OWEN, Tracy Amanda 85 Hermitage, Culcavy, Hillsborough BT26 6RJ — MB BCh BAO Belf. 1993. Specialty: Pub. Health Med.

OWEN, Trefor John 3 Market Street, Caernarfon LL55 1RT Tel: 01286 673224; Tyn y Coed, Caeathro, Caernarfon LL55 2TA Tel: 01286 671166 — MB BS Lond. 1959 (St. Geo.) MRCS Eng. LRCP Lond. 1959; DA Eng. 1965; FFA RCS Eng. 1972. Hosp. Pract. (Anaesth.) Gwynedd HA; Med. Off. Ferodo Ltd. Caernarvon. Specialty: Anaesth. Prev: Regist. (Anaesth.) Caernarvon & Anglesey Gen. Hosp. Bangor; Sen. Resid. (Anaesth.) Peter Bent Brigham Hosp. Boston, Mass.; Ho. Surg. St. Geo. Hosp. Lond.

OWEN, Tudor 10 Marine Road, Llandudno LL30 3NA Tel: 01492 541018 — MB ChB Liverp. 1955. Prev: GP Conwy N. Wales; Regist. (Paediat.) St. David's Hosp. Bangor; Ho. Phys. & Ho. Surg. Whiston Hosp.

OWEN, Victoria Jane 6 Ninelands Spur, Garfath, Leeds LS25 1NH Tel: 01132 866799 — MB ChB Dundee 1994; Bmsc Dund 1994; DRCOG 1998; MRCGP 1998.

OWEN, Wanda Irena St George Health Centre, Bellevue Road, St. George, Bristol BS5 7PH Tel: 0117 961 2161 Fax: 0117 961 8761; 17 Normanton Road, Clifton, Bristol BS8 2TY Tel: 0117 973 2433 — MB ChB Bristol 1981 (Univ. Bristol) MRCGP 1986. Specialty: Paediat. Prev: Clin. Asst. (Ment. Handicap) Phoenix Trust Bristol.

OWEN, Wendy Ann 32 North Park, Eltham, London SE9 5AP — MB BS Lond. 1968 (Middlx.) MRCS Eng. LRCP Lond. 1968. Clin. Asst. Oesoph. Laborat. St Thomas' Hosp. Lond. Prev: Ho. Phys. St. Mary Abbot's Hosp. Kensington; Ho. Surg. Middlx. Hosp. Lond.; Asst. Lect. Bland-Sutton Inst. Path. Middlx. Hosp. Med. Sch. Lond.

OWEN, Wendy Anne Lanceburn Health Centre, Clarendon Surgery, Churchill Way, Salford M6 5AU Tel: 0161 736 4529 Fax: 0161 736 2724; 42 Lombard Grove, Fallowfield, Manchester M14 6AN — MB ChB Manch. 1985; DRCOG 1989; MRCGP 1990.

OWEN, William Glyn (retired) 4 Cooper Hill Close, Walton-le-Dale, Preston PR5 4BE — (UCH London) MB BS Lond. 1952; FRCPath 1982, M 1966.

OWEN, William Lewis (retired) Glennydd, Llanbedrog, Pwllheli LL53 7PG Tel: 01758 740009 — MB ChB Liverp. 1947; MRCGP 1965. Prev: GP Llyn.

OWEN, Yvonne Eleanor Mary The Wolds Practice, Tetford, Horncastle LN9 6QP Tel: 01507 533133 Fax: 01507 533489; Langton Hill Farm, Langton Hill, Horncastle LN9 5JP — BM BS Nottm. 1985; Dip. IMC RCS Ed. 1991. Prev: Trainee GP Lincoln VTS.

OWEN-JONES, Jane Louise Horfield Health Centre, Lockleaze Road, Horfield, Bristol BS7 9RR Tel: 0117 969 5391; 91 Coombe Lane, Westbury on Trym, Bristol BS9 2AR — MB ChB Bristol 1979; BA (Hons.) Bristol 1971, MB ChB 1979; DRCOG 1985; MRCGP 1987.

OWEN-JONES, Josephine Margaret Sarah Abbey Meads Medical Practice, Elstree Way, Swindon SN25 4YZ Tel: 01793 709100; Hollyhock Cottage, Union St, Ramsbury, Marlborough SN8 2PR Tel: 01672 520649 — MB BS Lond. 1976 (Roy. Free) MRCS Eng. LRCP Lond. 1976; DRCOG 1979; MRCGP 1982; MSc (Univ. Westminster) 1999.

OWEN-JONES, Rodney James Ferguson Ramsbury Surgery, High Street, Ramsbury, Marlborough SN8 2QT Tel: 01672 520366 Fax: 01672 520180; Hollyhock Cottage, Union St, Ramsbury, Marlborough SN8 2PR Tel: 01672 520649 — MB BS Lond. 1977 (Roy. Free) MRCS Eng. LRCP Lond. 1977; MRCGP 1982; DRCOG 1982. Prev: Clin. Asst. (Rheum.) Princess Margt. Hosp. Swindon; Ho. Surg. Kent & Canterbury Hosp.; Ho. Phys. I. of Thanet Dist. Hosp. Ramsgate.

OWEN-REECE, Mr Aneurin Roy (retired) Hunters Cottage, Houghton, Stockbridge SO20 6LW Tel: 01794 388 8375 — MB BS Lond. 1960 (King's Coll. Hosp.) MRCS Eng. LRCP Lond. 1960; FRCS Eng. 1964. Prev: Regional Med. Off. DSS Birm.

OWEN-REECE, Huw 7A Clarendon Gardens, London W9 1AY Tel: 020 7286 2971 Email: ricz@yesmate.com — MB BS Lond. 1988 (St. Mary's Hosp.) BSc Lond. 1985, MBBS (Hons. Clin. Pharm.) 1988; FRCA 1994. Cons. In Anaesthetics and Intens. Care, Roy. Lond. Hosp., Lond., E1 1BB. Specialty: Anaesth. Socs: Intens. Care Soc.; Anaesthetic Research Soc. Prev: Lect. (Paediat.) UCL, Lond.; SHO (Intens. Care) Nat. Hosp. for Neurol. & Neurosurg. Lond.; SHO (Anaesth.) Centr. Middlx. Hosp. Lond.

OWEN-SMITH, Angela Mary (retired) Richmond House, 3 Old Houghton Road, Hartford, Huntingdon PE29 1YB Tel: 01480 458678 Fax: 01480 458678 — MB BS Lond. 1962 (Univ. Coll. Hosp.) MRCS Eng. LRCP Lond. 1962; DCH Eng. 1970; FRCPCH 1997. Prev: Cons. Community Paediat. Hinchingbrooke Healthcare NHS Trust.

OWEN-SMITH, Mr Bertram (retired) Awelon, Pentregat, Plwmp, Llandysul SA44 6HN Tel: 01239 654202 — MB BS Lond. 1950 (Westm.) MRCS Eng. LRCP Lond. 1950; FRCS Eng. 1955. Prev: Hon. Cons. Plast. & Reconstruc. Surg. Harare, Zimbabwe.

OWEN-SMITH, Brian David 48 Westgate, Chichester PO19 3EU Tel: 01243 786688 Fax: 01243 786688 — MB BChir Camb. 1963 (Guy's) MRCS Eng. LRCP Lond. 1963; DPhysMed Eng. 1970; MRCP (U.K.) 1970; FRCP Lond. 1984. Cons. (Rheum. & Rehabil.) & Med. Dir. Donald Wilson Ho. Roy. W. Sussex Hosp. (St. Richard's) Chichester; Mem. Vis. Staff King Edwd. VII Hosp. Midhurst. Specialty: Rehabil. Med.; Rheumatol. Socs: Hunt. Soc.; Fell Roy. Soc. Med; Heberd. Soc. Prev: Sen. Regist. Roy. Nat. Hosp. Rheum. Dis. Bath & Hon. Lect. Clin.; Pharmacol. Univ. Bath; Lilly Fell. in Clin. Pharmacol. Indiana Univ. Sch. Med., U.S.A.

OWEN-SMITH, Mr Michael Stephen (retired) Richmond House, 3 Old Houghton Road, Hartford, Huntingdon PE29 1YB Tel: 01480 458678 Fax: 01480 458678 — MS BS Lond. 1962 (Univ. Coll. Hosp.) MRCS Eng. LRCP Lond. 1962; FRCS Ed. 1965; FRCS Eng. 1966; MS Lond. 1971; MA Camb. 1987; MD (hons. causa) Linkoping 1993. Prev: Cons. Surg., Cromwell Clinic, Huntingdon.

OWEN-SMITH, Oliver Gregory Stephen The Spinney, 19 St Johns Avenue, Kidderminster DY11 6AU Tel: 015262 865363 — MB BS Lond. 1988. Cons. Anaesth. Roy. Orthopadic Hosp. Birm. Specialty: Anaesth. Prev: Specialist Regist. in Anaesth. Leicester.

OWEN-SMITH, Richard John 20 The Russetts, Wakefield WF2 6JF — MB ChB Leeds 1993.

OWEN-SMITH, Victoria Helen Stockport Primary Care Trust, Regent House, Heaton Lane, Stockport SK4 1BS Tel: 0161 426 5094 Email: vicci@nhs.net — MB BS Lond. 1986 (Roy. Free) DCH RCP Lond. 1988; MRCGP 1990; DRCOG 1990; MPH 1999; MFPH 2002. p/t Cons. in Pub. Health. Specialty: Pub. Health Med.

OWENS, Alan Stephen 29 Hollocombe Road, West Derby, Liverpool L12 0RW — MB ChB Liverp. 1994.

OWENS, Catherine Mary 13 Eyot Gardens, London W6 9TN Tel: 020 8748 6729 Email: owensc@gosh.nhs.uk — MB BS Lond. 1984; BSc (Hons.) Lond. 1981, MB BS 1984; MRCP (UK) 1987; FRCR 1991. Cons. Radiologist and Clin. Director, Gt. Ormond St. Hosp., Lond. Specialty: Radiol. Socs: BMA. Prev: Fell. (Diag. Radiol.) HSC Toronto, Canada; Sen. Regist. (Diag. Radiol.) Middlx. & Univ. Coll. Hosps. Lond.; Regist. (Diag. Radiol.) Roy. Free Hosp. Lond.

OWENS, Christopher Thomas 7 Berkeley Road, Talbot Woods, Bournemouth BH3 7JL Tel: 01202 529606 Fax: 01202 242986 Email: 106515.3374@compuserve.com — MB BCh BAO NUI 1982 (University of Cork National University of Ireland) DCM Beijing 1998. GP Traditional Chinese Med.; Gerson Ther. Practitioner. Specialty: Gen. Pract.; Rheumatol. Socs: Primary Care Rheum. Soc.; Brit. Hyperlipid. Assn.; Chinese Med. Assn. Prev: Chef de Clinique Med. Hopital Ambroise Pare Paris.

OWENS, Christopher William Instone Dept. of Clinical Phaumacology, UCL School of Medicine, 5 University Street, London WC1E Tel: 020 7387 9300 Ext: 8339 Email: c.owens@ucl.ac.uk; 24 Pembridge Mews, London W11 3EQ — MB BS Lond. 1969 (Univ. Coll. Hosp.) BSc Wales 1961; PhD Lond. 1965, MB BS (Hons. Med.) 1969; MRCP (UK) 1971; FRCP Lond. 1989; FFPM RCP (UK) 1993. Sen. Clin. Lect. (Clin. Pharmacol.) & Hon. Cons. Univ. Coll. Hosp. Lond. Specialty: Pharmacology. Prev: Lect. (Clin. Med.) & Ho. Phys. Med. Unit Univ. Coll. Hosp. Lond.; SHO Hammersmith Hosp.

OWENS, Colum Gerard 11 Strandview Street, Belfast BT9 5FF — MB BCh Belf. 1998; MB BCh Belf 1998.

OWENS, Daniel Francis 16 Buckmaster Road, London SW11 1EN — MB BS Tasmania 1987.

OWENS, David Ysbyty Gwynedd, Penrhos Road, Bangor LL57 2PW Tel: 01248 384326 — MB ChB (1st Class Hons.) Liverp. 1967; MRCP (UK) 1970; MD Liverp. 1975; FRCP Lond. 1984. Cons. Phys. N. Wales NHS Trust Bangor; Hon. Sen. Lect. Univ. Wales Bangor. Specialty: Gastroenterol. Socs: Brit. Soc. Gastroenterol. Prev: Cons. Phys. Walton Hosp. Liverp.; Regist. (Med.) Roy. Free Hosp. Lond.; Wellcome Research Fell. Liverp. Univ.

OWENS, Professor David Griffith Cunningham The University Division of Psychiatry, Kennedy Tower, Royal Edinburgh Hospital, Morningside Park, Edinburgh EH10 Tel: 0131 537 6262 Fax: 0131 537 6291 Email: david.owens@ed.ac.uk — MD Glas. 1986 (Univ. Glas.) MB ChB Glas 1972; MRCP (U.K.) 1975; FRCPsych. 1989, M 1976; FRCP 1988. Prof. of Clin. Psychiat., Univ. Edin. & Hon. Cons. Psychiat. Roy. Edin. Hosp. Specialty: Gen. Psychiat. Prev: Sen. Lect. (Psychiat.) Univ. Edin. & Hon. Cons. Psychiat. Roy. Edin. Hosp.; Cons. Psychiat. Northwick Pk. Hosp. Harrow; Mem. Scientif. Staff MRC.

OWENS, Professor David Raymond, CBE Cardiff University, Diabetes Research Unit, 1st Floor Academic Centre, Llandough Hospital, Penlan Road, Penarth CF64 2XX Email: owensdr@cf.ac.uk; 220 Cyncoed Road, Cyncoed, Cardiff CF23 6RS — MB BCh Wales 1966 (Cardiff) FRCP; MD Wales 1985; CBiol 1993, MIBiol 1986; MRCP (UK) 1994; FIBiol 1995. Cons. Diabetologist; Prof. Specialty: Diabetes; Endocrinol. Socs: Fell. Roy. Soc. Med.; Brit. Pharm. Soc. Prev: Sen. Lect. (Med.) Univ. Wales Coll. Med. Cardiff; Lect. (Med.) Univ. Wales Coll. Med. Cardiff; Head Cardiovasc. & Metab. Research Ciba-Geigy Basle, Switz.

OWENS, David Wallace Division of Psychiatry, University of Leeds School of Medicine, 15 Hyde Terrace, Leeds LS2 9LT — MB ChB Leeds 1979; MRCPsych 1983; BSc (Psychol.) Leeds 1976, MD 1990. Sen. Lect. (Psychiat.) Univ. Leeds; Hon. Cons. Psychiat. Leeds Community & Ment. Health Servs. NHS Trust. Specialty: Gen. Psychiat. Prev: Lect. (Psychiat.) Univ. Leeds; Sen. Regist. (Psychiat.) Nottm. HA; Regist. (Psychiat.) Nottm. HA.

OWENS, Eifion Pryce 11 Windsor Road, Radyr, Cardiff CF15 8BQ Tel: 029 2084 2596 — MB ChB Birm. 1967; DPM Eng. 1971; FRCPsych 1993, M 1973. Clin. Lect. & Cons. (Psychiat.) Univ. Manch. Specialty: Alcohol & Substance Misuse. Socs: Roy. Coll. Psychiat. (Subst. Misuse Sect.); Soc. for Addic. Prev: Research Assoc. & Lect. (Psychiat.) Univ. Manch.; Sen. Regist. (Psychiat.) Univ. Hosp. S. Manch.

OWENS, Miss Elisabeth Joy Clare 36 Spring View Road, Sheffield S10 1LS Tel: 0114 268 0018 — MB ChB Sheff. 1997. Pre-Registration Ho. Off. Surg. N. Gen. Hosp. Sheff. Specialty: Gen. Surg.

OWENS, Gareth Wyn Bron Seiont Surgery, Bron Seiont, Segontium Terrace, Caernarfon LL55 2PH Tel: 01286 672236 Fax: 01286 676404; Y Gilfach, 4 Pen y Bryn, Caernarfon LL55 2YT Tel: 01286 673095 — MB BCh Wales 1977 (University Hospital Wales Cardiff) MRCGP 1988.

OWENS, Geraint Griffith 66 Ffordd Glyn, Coed y Glyn, Wrexham LL13 7QW — BM BCh Wales 1970; DCH Eng. 1972; MRCP (UK) 1975; FRCP Lond. 1992; FRCPCH 1997. Paediat. Maelor Hosp. Wrexham. Specialty: Paediat.

OWENS, Hazel Suzanne 19 Shaw Road, Royton, Oldham OL2 6DA — MB ChB Manch. 1998.

OWENS, Jane Mary The Surgery, Dedham Road, Ardleigh, Colchester CO7 7LD Tel: 01206 230224 Fax: 01206 231602 — MB BS Lond. 1980; BSc Lond. 1977; DRCOG 1983; MRCGP 1984.

OWENS, Jennifer Lindsay 40 Poll Hill Road, Wirral CH60 7SW — MB ChB Liverp. 1996.

OWENS, John 56 Trumpington Street, Cambridge CB2 1RG Tel: 01223 61611 Fax: 01223 356837; 11 Clarendon Road, Cambridge CB2 2BH Tel: 01223 62760 — MB BS London 1959 (St. Bart.) DCH Eng. 1962; MRCGP 1975. Med. Adviser Camb. Univ. Press; Med. Off. Electronic Indust. Camb.; Hon. Med. Off. Camb. Univ. Rugby Club & Tennis Club; Clin. Teach. Fac. Clin. Med. Univ. Camb. Socs: Pres. Camb. Med. Soc.

OWENS, John 2 Hollyfield Drive, Sutton Coldfield B75 7SF — MB ChB Glas. 1951 (Univ. Glas.) DPM Eng. 1957. Socs: Fell. Roy. Soc. Med.; Roy. Med. Psych. Assn.

OWENS, John Raymond Macclesfield DGH, Victoria Rd, Macclesfield SK10 3BL Tel: 01625 661301 Fax: 01625 663055 Email: jowens@echeshire-tr.nwest.nhs.uk; 44 Ryles Park Road, Macclesfield SK11 8AH Tel: 01625 262335 — MB ChB Manch. 1969; DCH Eng. 1972; FRCP Lond. 1994; Dip. Hlth Mgt. Keele 1995; FRCPCH 1997. Cons. Paediat. Macclesfield Dist. Specialty: Community Child Health. Socs: Brit. Assn. Community Child Health; Manch. Med. Soc. Prev: SCMO Liverp. AHA; Lect. (Child Health) Univ. Liverp.; Med. Superintendent Hôpital Yoseki, Zaire.

OWENS, Julie Fleming Noffield Unit, Burdon Terrace, Jesmond, Newcastle upon Tyne NE2 3AE — MB BS Newc. 1992; MRCPsych 1997. Specialist Child & Adolesc. Psychiat.; Specialist Regist. (Child & Adolesc. Psychiat.) Newc. Specialty: Child & Adolesc. Psychiat. Socs: Roy. Coll. Psychiat.

OWENS, Kelly Elizabeth 23 Clayford Cr, Liverpool L14 1PE — MB ChB Leeds 1997.

OWENS, Lucy Alexandra Apsley House, Thicket Grove, Maidenhead SL6 4LW — MB ChB Bristol 1997.

OWENS, Owen Joseph David BUPA Hospital Harpenden, Ambrose Lane, Harpenden AL5 4BP Tel: 01582 763191 Fax: 01582 712312; 12 Birch Way, Harpenden AL5 5TP Tel: 01582 760045 — MB BCh BAO NUI 1980 (Ireland) LRCPI & LM, LRCSI & LM 1980; DCH NUI 1983; MRCOG 1986; MRCPI 1988; MD Dub. 1991. Cons. O & G Luton & Dunstable NHS Trust. Specialty: Obst. & Gyn. Socs: Brit. Soc. Colpos. & Cerv. Path.; Brit. Gyn. Cancer Soc. Prev: Sen. Regist. (O & G) Gtr. Glas. HB; Hon. Regist. Gtr. Glas. HB; Clin. Research Fell. (Biochem.) Glas. Univ.

OWENS, Patricia Margaret Clinical Skills Resource, 2nd Floor E Block Centre, Old Infirmary, 70 Pembroke Place, Liverpool L69 3EF Tel: 0151 794 8235 Email: p.owens@liv.ac.uk — MB ChB Ed. 1979; FRCGP 1998. Director. Clin. Skills Resource Centre. Univ. of Liverp. Prev: Princip. In Gen. Pract. Lache Health Centre Chester.

OWENS, Paul James 12 Broughton Gardens, Ravenhill Road, Belfast BT6 0BB — MB BCh BAO Belf. 1996.

OWENS, Rachel Elizabeth 220 Cyncoed Road, Cardiff CF23 6RS — MB BCh Wales 1997.

OWENS, Rebecca Wynne 220 Cyncoed Road, Cyncoed, Cardiff CF23 6RS — BM Soton. 1996.

OWENS, Stephen 64 Archway Road, Huyton, Liverpool L36 9XE — MB ChB Ed. 1998.

OWENS, Valerie Barbara 12 Birch Close, Oxton, Prenton, Wirral CH43 5XE — MB ChB Manch. 1986. Staff Phys. (Medicine for the Elderly) Wirral Hosp. NHS Trust. Specialty: Care of the Elderly. Prev: Clin. Asst. (Med. for Elderly) St. Catherine Hosp. Birkenhead.

OWENS, Mr William Andrew James Cook University Hospital, Department of Cardiothoracic Surgery, Marton Road, Middlesbrough TS4 3BW Tel: 01642 854728 Fax: 01642 854613 — MB BCh BAO (Hons.) Belf. 1990; FRCS Eng. 1994; FRCSI 1994. Cons. Cardiothoracic Surg. & Clin. Director James Cook Univ. Hosp. Middlesbrough. Specialty: Cardiothoracic Surg.

OWER, David Cheyne, TD (retired) 94 Coombe Lane W., Kingston upon Thames KT2 7DB Tel: 020 8942 8552 — (King's Coll. Hosp.) MB BS Lond. 1954; DObst RCOG 1959; FFPHM 1983, M 1976. Lt.-Col. RAMC (TA). Prev: Sen. PMO Dept. Health & Social Security.

OWERS, Deborah Louise 5 Menlo Close, Oxton, Birkenhead CH43 9YD — MB BS Lond. 1985 (St. Mary's) SHO (Paediat.) Centr. Middlx. Hosp. Lond. Prev: Trainee GP Lond.; SHO (O & G) Hillingdon Hosp. Lond.; SHO (Geriat. Med.) Moriston Hosp, Swansea.

OWERS, Fred Max 5 Menlo Close, Birkenhead CH43 9YD Tel: 0151 652 2939 — MB BS Lond. 1952 (St. Mary's) Socs: (Pres.) Birkenhead Med. Soc. Prev: Clin. Asst. Ment. Handicap Wirral HA; Med. Off. Mobil Oil Co.; SHO (Med.) Walton Hosp. Liverp.

OWERS, Russell Cameron, Lt.-Col. RAMC Willoughby Road, Larkhill, Salisbury SP4 8QY Tel: 01980 845423 Fax: 01980 845056 — MB BS Lond. 1987; MA Camb. 1987, BA 1983; DRCOG 1992; MRCGP 1993. GP Trainer. Prev: Med. Off. SHAPE BFPO 26 (1997-2000); RMO 2 LI BFPO 22 (1994-1997); RMO 1 R.Irish BFPO 53 (1993-1994).

OWINO, Walter Edwin Jason 235 Hampden Way, Southgate, London N14 7LD Tel: 020 8368 4157 Fax: 020 8368 7192 — MB ChB Nairobi 1976; DPM Eng. 1979; MRCPsych 1981; FRCPsych 2002.

OWSTON, Ethel Winifred Wells (retired) Afton Cottage, Berks Hill, Chorleywood, Rickmansworth WD3 5AJ Tel: 01923 283708 — (Sheff.) MB ChB Sheff. 1943; DObst RCOG 1949. Prev: Med. Off. Family Plann. Assn. Caryl Thomas Clinic Harrow.

OWUSU-AGYEI, Peter Yaw Peterborough Hospitals NHS Trust, Edith Cavell Hospital, Bretton Gate PE3 9GZ; 27 Hospital Close, Evington, Leicester LE5 4WP — MB ChB Ghana 1982; MRCP (UK) 1993; FRCP, CCST 2003. Cons. Phys., Dept. of Med. for the elderly, P'boro. Hosps., NHS Trust, P'boro. Specialty: Gen. Med.; Care of the Elderly. Special Interest: Stroke. Socs: Brit. Geriat. Soc.; Brit. Med. Assn. Prev: Sen. Regist., Gen. & Geriat. Med., Leicester Hosps.; Regist. (Gen. Med. & Gastroenterol.) Mersey Regional Health Auth.; Regist. (Gen. Med.) W. Suff. Hosp.

OWUSUANSA, Ntow 3 Royal Lodge Gardens, Purdysburn Road, Belfast BT8 7YS — Lekarz Warsaw 1970.

OXBORROW, Neil Jeffrey 14 Lidgett Park Grove, Leeds LS8 1HW — MB ChB (Hons) Leeds 1991; BSc (Hons) Leeds 1988; MD Leeds 2002; FRCS (Tr. & Orth.) 2002. Fell. Spinal Surg. Manch. Socs: BOA; BOTA; BSS.

OXBORROW, Susan Mary Prentice Building, Langdon Hospital, Dawlish EX7 0NR — MB BS Lond. 1985; DTM & H RCP Lond.

1992. Specialty: Forens. Psychiat. Prev: Asst. Dir. Lepra Eval. Project Chilumba, Malawi; Regist. (Genitourin. Med.) Bristol Roy. Infirm.; SHO (Med.) Roy. Devon & Exeter Hosp.

OXBURY, John Michael (retired) Felstead House, 23 Banbury Road, Oxford OX2 6NX Tel: 01865 558532 Fax: 01865 558532 — MB BChir Camb. 1964 (Camb. & Lond. Hosp.) MA, PhD Camb. 1962, MB 1964, BChir 1963; MRCP (U.K.) 1970; MA Oxf. 1972; FRCP Lond. 1979. Cons. Neurol. (Private Practioner Only) at The Cromwell Hosp., Lond. SW5 0TU and The Acland Hosp., Oxf. OX2 6NX; Hon. Consg. NeUrol. to the Oxf. Radcliffe Hosp.s. Prev: Ment. Health Research Fund Sen. Research Fell. & Hon. Sen. Regist. (Neurol.) United Oxf. Hosps.

OXBY, Alison Diane — MB BS Lond. 1989; MRCGP 1994. Specialty: Family Plann. & Reproduc. Health; Gen. Pract. Prev: Civil. Med. Practitioner; Lead Clinician, Reproductive and Sexual Health, Northumbria NHS Trust; Locum Gen. Practitioner, Seaton Hirst Primary Care Centre, Ashington.

OXBY, Claire Louise Squirrel Walk, Winder, Frizington CA26 3UH — MB ChB Manch. 1995.

OXENBURY, Julia Lynne Woodbridge Hill Surgery, 1 Deerbarn Road, Guildford GU2 8YB Tel: 01483 562230 Fax: 01483 452442; Hillerton House, Chandlers Lane, Yateley GU46 7SR Tel: 01252 860637 — MB BS Lond. 1978; DCH RCP Lond. 1982; MRCGP 1983; DRCOG 1983; FRCGP 1997; M.Med. Dund. 1998. GP Tutor Frimley Pk. Hosp.

OXENHAM, Helen Caroline Cardiology New Royal Infirmary, Little France Cresent, Edinburgh — MB ChB Ed. 1989; MRCP (Ed.) 1992. SHO (Gen. Med.) Lothian HB; Specialist Regist. (Cardiol.) Western Gen. Hosp. Edin. Specialty: Cardiol. Prev: Staff Grade (Cardiol.) Roy. Infirm. Edin.; Ho. Off. & SHO (Renal) Roy. Infirm. Edin.

OXFORD, Peter Christopher Jude Doctors Surgery, 2 Danson Crescent, Welling DA16 2AT Tel: 020 8303 4204 Fax: 020 8298 1192; 12 Avery Hill Road, New Eltham, London SE9 2BD Tel: 020 8850 1804 Fax: 020 8850 4993 — MB BS Newc. 1981 (Newcastle uponTyne) DRCOG 1984.

OXLEY, Charles Falcon Sterry Attleborough Surgeries (Station Road), Station Road, Attleborough NR17 2AS Tel: 01953 452394 Fax: 01953 453569 — MB BS Lond. 1968 (St. Thos.) MRCS Eng. LRCP Lond. 1968; DObst RCOG 1971. Prev: Sen. Ho. Surg. Norf. & Norwich Hosp.; Ho. Surg. St. Thos. Hosp. Lond.

OXLEY, Jolyon Rawson 21 Station Road, Geldeston, Beccles NR34 0HS Tel: 01508 518136 Email: contact@ncssd.org.uk — MB BChir Camb. 1972 (Univ. Camb. & St. Bart. Hosp. Lond.) MRCS Eng. LRCP Lond. 1971; MA Camb. 1973; MRCP (UK) 1973; FRCP Lond. 1991. Advisor Acad. of Med. Sciences' Mentoring Scheme for Clin. Scientists; Hon. Sec., Nat. Counselling Serv. for Sick Doctors (NCSSD). Special Interest: Health support and mentoring for doctors; Med. Educat.; Personal and professional career developm. for doctors. Prev: Sec. Standing Comm. Postgrad. Med. & Dent. Educat. (SCOPME) (1990-1999); Exec. Director, Acad. of Med. Sci. 1999-2000; Med. Direct. Nat. Soc. for Epilepsy (1979-1988).

OXLEY, Jon Dept of Cellular Pathology, Southmead Hospital, Westbury-on-Trym, Bristol BS10 5NB Tel: 0117 959 5623 Fax: 0117 959 0191 Email: jon.oxley@bristol.ac.uk — MB BS Lond. 1993 (St. Bartholomews, Lond.) BSc Lond. 1990; Mem. Roy. Coll. Pathologists 2000; MD Lond. 2000; Dip. Dermatopathology, RCPath 2001. Consultant (Histopath.) Southmead Hosp. Bristol. Specialty: Histopath. Special Interest: Dermatopathology; Uropathology. Prev: Specialist Regist. (Histopath) Brist. Roy. Infirm.; Regist. (Histopath.) Southmead Hosp. Bristol; SHO (Histopath.) UMDS Lond.

OXLEY, Vernon Ernest Pathology Laboratory, Princess Alexandra Hospital, Hamstel Road, Harlow CM20 1QX Tel: 01279 827035 Fax: 01279 416846 — MB BS Newc. 1970 (Newcastle-upon-Tyne) MRCP (U.K.) 1974; MRCPath 1979. Cons. Haemat. Princess Alexandra Hosp. Harlow. Specialty: Haematology. Prev: Sen. Regist. (Haemat.) Roy. Infirm. Bristol; Regist. (Haemat.) Lond. Hosp.; Regist. (Paediat. & Gen. Med.) St. Margts. Hosp. Epping.

OXTOBY, John William Chy An Drea, Moss Hill, Stockton Brook, Stoke-on-Trent ST9 9NW — MB ChB Ed. 1984; MRCP (UK) 1990.

OXTOBY, Julie Dawn Chy-an-Drea, Moss Hill, Stockton Brook, Stoke-on-Trent ST9 9NW — BM Soton. 1988.

OXTOBY, Sarah Jane Leatside Surgery, Babbage Road, Totnes TQ9 5JA — BM Soton. 1993; DRCOG; DFFP.

OXYNOS, Costas 12 Ridgway Gardens, Lymm WA13 0HQ; 1 Arch Makarios Are C, Flat 104, Aglanjia 2107, Nicosia, Cyprus — MB BS Lond. 1994. SHO (Med.) Whithington Hosp. Manch. Prev: SHO (Med. & Cardiol.) Chase Farm Hosp. Lond.; SHO (c/o Elderly) Enfield Community Care Trust & Chase Farm Hosp.; Ho. Off. (Surg. & Med.) King's Coll. Hosp. Lond.

OYAIDE, Onajite Mavis 41 Old Farm Road, Birmingham B33 9HH Tel: 0121 784 5403 Fax: 0121 784 5403 — MB ChB Liverp. 1997. SHO Merseyside Paediat. Roatation Scheme. Aug 1998 - Aug 2000. Specialty: Paediat. Prev: Pre-Regist. Ho. Off., Fazakerley Hosp., Aintree.

OYEBODE, Babatunde Oyedeji Springfield Hospital, 61 Glenburnie Road, London SW17 7DJ Tel: 020 8682 6381 Fax: 020 8682 6434 — MB BS Benin, Nigeria 1980; MRCPsych 1987; Dip. Criminol. Lond. 1991; MPhil Ed. 1993; FRCPsych 2004. Cons. Forens. Psychiat. S. W. Lond. & St. Geo. Ment. Health NHS Trust; Hon. Sen. Lect. St. Geo. Hosp. Med. Sch. Univ. Lond. Specialty: Forens. Psychiat. Prev: Sen. Regist. Rotat. (Forens. Psychiat.) Maudsley Hosp.; Sen. Regist. Rotat. (Psychiat.) North. Region; Regist. & SHO (Psychiat.) Roy. Edin. Hosp.

OYEBODE, Professor Oluwafemi Akinwunmi Queen Elizabeth Psychiatric Hospital, Mindelsohn Way, Edgbaston, Birmingham B15 2QZ Tel: 0121 627 2999 Fax: 0121 627 2855 — MB BS Ibadan 1977 (Ibadan, Nigeria) FRCPsych 1996, M 1983; MD Newc. 1989; T(Psych) 1991; PhD Wales 1998. Cons. Psychiat. Qu. Eliz. Psychiat. Hosp. Birm.; Med. Dir.; Prof. Univ. Birm. Specialty: Gen. Psychiat. Socs: Fell. Roy. Soc. Med.; Birm. Med. Inst. Prev: Sen. Clin. Lect. Univ. of Birm.; Cons. Psychiat. John Conolly Hosp. Birm.; Sen. Regist. Roy. Vict. Infirm. Newc. u. Tyne.

OYEDIRAN, Muriel Ayodeji Flat 9, The Grange, The Knoll, Ealing, London W13 8JJ — MB BS Lond. 1965; MRCS Eng. LRCP Lond. 1965.

OYELEYE, Mr Abiola Olatunbosun c/o Eye Department, James Paget Hospital, Lowestoft Road, Gorleston, Great Yarmouth NR31 6LA Tel: 01493 452648; 55 Gainsborough Drive, Gunton, Lowestoft NR32 4NJ Tel: 01502 518752 — MB BS Lagos, Nigeria 1987; FRCOphth 1994. Staff Grade (Ophth.) James Paget Hosp. Gt. Yarmouth. Specialty: Ophth. Prev: Regist. (Ophth.) Roy. Infirm. Edin.; SHO Worthing Hosp.; SHO (Ophth.) E. Surrey Hosp.

OYESANYA, Olufunso Abiodun 16 Dunster Way, Harrow HA2 9PN — MB BS Ibadan 1979; MRCOG 1988; FICS 1990.

OYSTON, Mr John Kenneth (retired) 7 Heath Gardens, Halifax HX3 0BD Tel: 01422 363272 — MB BS Durh. 1948; FRCS Eng. 1955. Prev: Cons. Orthop. Surg. RAF & Halifax Roy. Infirm.

OYSTON, Margaret Greville (retired) 11 Alexandra Road, Epsom KT17 4BH Tel: 01327 23005 — MB BS Lond. 1948 (King's Coll. Hosp.) MRCS Eng. LRCP Lond. 1948; DObst RCOG 1949.

OZA, Amit Manulal Department of Medical Oncology, St. Bartholomew's Hospital, London EC1A 7BE Tel: 020 7601 7462; 14 Broadmead Road, Woodford Green IG8 0AY — MB BS Lond. 1983 (St. Bart.) BSc (Hons.) Lond. 1980, MB BS 1983; MRCP (UK) 1986. ICRF Research Fell./Hon. Sen. Regist. (Med. Oncol.) St. Bart. Hosp. Lond. Specialty: Oncol. Prev: Regist. (Med.) Whipps Cross Hosp. Lond.; Resid. Med. Off. Nat. Heart Hosp. Lond.; SHO (Med. Rotat.) Churchill Hosp. & Radcliffe Infirm. Oxf.

OZA, Nandu Health Care Complex, 52 Low Moor Road, Kirkby in Ashfield, Nottingham NG17 3EE Tel: 01623 752312 Fax: 01623 723700; 5 Sheepwalk Lane, Ravenhead, Nottingham NG15 9FD Tel: 01623 793223 — MB BS Bombay 1966 (Grant Med. Coll.) BSc Bombay 1960; DA Eng. 1970. Clin. Asst. (Anaesth.) Mansfield Gp. of Hosps. Specialty: Anaesth. Prev: Regist. (Anaesth.) Mansfield & Dist. Hosp.; SHO (Anaesth.) Sheff. RHB; SHO (Cas.) Chesterfield Roy. Hosp.

OZA, Piush Health Care Complex, 52 Low Moor Road, Kirkby in Ashfield, Nottingham NG17 3EE Tel: 01623 752312 Fax: 01623 723700 — MB ChB Leic. 1984; DRCOG 1988.

OZCAN, Kamile 32 Howard Road, London N16 8PU — BM BS Nottm. 1994.

OZDEMIR, Joanne Brywffynon Child & Family Centre, Pontypridd; 17 Heol Fair, Llandaf, Cardiff CF5 2EE — MB BCh Wales 1989; MRCPsych 1998. Specialist Regist.In Child & Adolesc. Psychiat. Univ. of Wales Coll. of Med. Specialty: Child & Adolesc. Psychiat. Socs: Mem. Roy. Coll. of Psychiat.s.

OZUA, Christopher Irabor 12 Miller Road, Chalk, Gravesend DA12 4TP — MB BS Benin 1988 (Benin, Nigeria) SHO (Psychiat.) Greenwich Dist. Hosp. Lond. Specialty: Obst. & Gyn.; Gen. Pract. Prev: Med. Off. The Chaucer Hosp. Canterbury; SHO (O & G) Harold Wood Hosp. Romford; SHO (O & G) Doncaster Roy. Infirm. Doncaster.

OZUA, Peter Osezua Basildon University Hospital, Cellular Pathology Department, Nethermayne, Basildon SS16 5NL Tel: 01268 598219 Fax: 01268 598210 Email: peter.ozua@btuh.nhs.uk; Morningside, 42 Sylvan Avenue, Emerson Park, Hornchurch RM11 2PW Tel: 01708 469668 Fax: 01708 479502 Email: osezua@aol.com — MB BS Benin, Nigeria 1982; DipRCPath 1997; MRCPath 1998. Cons. (Histopath.) Basildon Univ. Hosp. Specialty: Histopath. Socs: Brit. Div. of Internat. Acad. of Pathologists; Europ. Soc. of Path.; Path. Soc. of Gt. Britain & Irel. Prev: Cons. (Histopath.) Luton & Dunstable Hosp. Luton; Specialist Regist. (Histopath.) Univ. Coll. Hosp. UCH Lond.; Specialist Regist. Whittington Hosp. Lond.

PABARI, Deepak 490 Summerwood Road, Isleworth TW7 7QZ — BM Soton. 1996.

PABBINEEDI, Raghunath 33 Twmpath, Oswestry SY10 7AQ — MB BS Andhra 1980.

PABLA, Herbel Singh Bulwell Health Centre, Main Street, Bulwell, Nottingham NG6 8QJ Tel: 0115 977 1181 Fax: 0115 977 1377; 18 Cheviot Road, Long Eaton, Nottingham NG10 4FU Tel: 0115 946 1154 — MB ChB Manch. 1983 (Manchester) DA (UK) 1986; DRCOG 1988; MRCGP 1989. GP Partner; Clin. Asst. (Anaesth.) 1990. Specialty: Anaesth. Prev: SHO (Anaesth.) Nottm. HA; SHO (Cas.) N. West. RHA; Ho. (Surg.) Bolton HA.

PACE, Helen Elizabeth Lepton Surgery, Highgate Lane, Lepton, Huddersfield HD8 0HH Tel: 01484 606161; 15 Bilwell, Long Crendon, Aylesbury HP18 9AD — MB ChB Leeds 1980. Clin. Asst., Accid. and Emerg., Bradford Roy. Infirm.

PACE, Ian Gerard Bourne Galletly Practice Team, 40 North Road, Bourne PE10 9BT Tel: 01778 562200 Fax: 01778 562207 — MB ChB Birm. 1985; BSc (Physiol. Sci.) Birm. 1982; DCH RCP Lond. 1991; DRCOG 1992. Prev: Dep. Station Med. Off. RAF Cranwell; SHO (Psychiat.) RAF Hosp. Ely VTS; SHO (O & G) Hinchingbrooke Hosp.

PACE, Jacqueline Elizabeth St Albans City Hospital, Waverley Road, St Albans AL3 5PN Tel: 01727 897624 — MB BS Lond. 1981; FRCP (UK) 1999. Cons. Phys. (Elderly) Hemel Hempstead & St Albans City Hosps. Specialty: Gen. Med.

PACE, Nicholas Adrian Department of Anaesthesia, Western Infirmary, Glasgow G12 Tel: 0141 339 2000 — MB ChB Glas. 1982; MRCP Ed. 1989; FRCA. 1989; MPhil Glas. 1992. Cons. Anaesth. West. Infirm. Glas.; Hon. Sen. Lect. Specialty: Anaesth. Prev: Vis. Asst. Prof. Univ. Texas 1991-92.

PACE, Richard Francis Everett 17 Walpole Road, Teddington TW11 8PJ — MB BS Lond. 1991.

PACE, Thomas, MBE, OStJ Central Surgery, Sussex Road, Gorleston-on-Sea, Great Yarmouth NR31 6QB Tel: 01493 414141 Fax: 01493 656253; Acornfield, Back Lane, Lound, Lowestoft NR32 5NE — MB ChB Sheff. 1970; MRCGP 1976; DIH Eng. 1981; MSc (Occupat. Med.) 1981; FFOM RCP Lond. 1994, MFOM 1984, AFOM 1981. Dir. N. Sea Med. Centre. Specialty: Occupat. Health. Prev: Surg. Cdr. RN.

PACE, Thomas Anastasi, OBE, Col. late RAMC Retd. 28 Cochrane Close, Cochrane St, London NW8 7NS Tel: 020 7722 2387 — MD Malta 1937 (Royal University of Malta) BSc Malta 1934, MD 1937; DPH Eng. 1952. Specialty: Pub. Health Med. Socs: BMA; Harv. Soc. Prev: Med. Off. i/c Med. Centre MOD(A) Whitehall; Chief Med. Off. SHAPE; Chief Med. Off. United Nations Force in Cyprus.

PACE-BALZAN, Mr Albert St. John's Hospital, Wood St., Chelmsford CM2 9BG Tel: 012405 440761; Canonfylde, Porters Hall Road, Stebbing, Dunmow CM6 3TB — MRCS Eng. LRCP Lond. 1977; FRCS Eng. 1981; T(S) 1991. Cons. Surg. (ENT) Mid-Essex Hosps. NHS Trust. Specialty: Otolaryngol.

PACEY, Simon Christopher — MB BS Lond. 1998.

PACHMAYR, Henry K (retired) 17 Provost Road, London NW3 4ST Tel: 020 7722 5093 — MB BCh Wales 1954 (Cardiff) Prev: Ho. Off. (O & G) Roy. United Hosp. & St. Martin's Hosp. Bath.

PACHMAYR, John (retired) 17 Provost Road, London NW3 4ST Tel: 020 7722 0561; (resid.) 17 Provost Road, London NW3 4ST Tel: 020 7722 0561 — (Guy's) MB BS Lond. 1951; MRCS Eng. LRCP Lond. 1951.

PACIFICO, Marc Dominic Flat 12, Stone House, 9 Weymouth St., London W1W 6DB — MB BS Lond. 1997.

PACIOREK, Paulina Mary X-Ray Department, William Harvey Hospital, Kennington Road, Ashford TN24 0LZ Tel: 01233 633331 Fax: 01233 616123 Email: paulina.paciorek@ekht.nhs.uk — MB BS Lond. 1976 (St. Geo.) MRCOG; MRCS Eng. LRCP Lond. 1976; DMRD Eng. 1983; FRCR 1983. Cons. Radiol. Nuclear Med. S.E. Kent HA. Specialty: Radiol. Prev: Sen. Regist. (Radiol.) Leic. Roy. Infirm.

PACK, Gordon James (retired) River Mead, Wherwell, Andover SP11 7JS Tel: 01264 860500 — (Univ. Coll. Hosp.) MB BS Lond. 1947; DObst RCOG 1952. Prev: Ho. Phys. Roy. North. Hosp.

PACK, Helen Margaret High Street Surgery, 15 High Street, Overton, Wrexham LL13 0ED Tel: 01978 710666 Fax: 01978 710494 (Call before faxing); Fairfield, 32 Salop Road, Overton-on-Dee, Wrexham LL13 0EH Tel: 01978 710595 — MB ChB Liverp. 1982; DA (UK) 1987.

PACK, Mr Mowafaq Yousif Abdul-Maseeh 19 Northfield Avenue, Sudbrook, Lincoln LN2 2FB Tel: 01522 595752 Email: pack@otago.co.uk; 19 Northfield Avenue, Sudbrook, Lincoln LN2 2FB — MB ChB Mosul 1976; MB ChB Mosul, Iraq 1976; FRCS Glas. 1989. Assoc. Specialist (Orthop.) Co. Hosp. Lincoln. Specialty: Orthop. Socs: BOA; Soc. of Hand Surg.; BMA. Prev: Regist. (Plastic Surg.) Univ. Coll. Hosp. Lond.

PACK, Susan Frances Hadwen Medical Practice, Glevum Way Surgery, Abbeydale, Gloucester GL4 4BL Tel: 01452 529933; Holcombe Farm Stable, Painswick, Stroud GL6 6RG — MB BS Lond. 1975; DRCOG 1977; MRCP (UK) 1978; MRCGP 1984.

PACKARD, Mr Richard Bruce Selig Princess Christian's Hospital, 12 Clarence Road, Windsor SL4 5AG Tel: 01753 853121 Fax: 01753 831185; 96 Harley Street, London W1N 1AF Tel: 020 7935 9555 — MD Lond. 1979 (Middlx. Hosp.) MB BS 1970; DO RCS Lond. 1975; FRCS Eng. 1977; FRCOphth. 1990. Cons. Ophth. Surg. P. Chas. Eye Unit King Edwd. VII Hosp. Windsor. Specialty: Ophth. Socs: Internat. Mem. Amer. Acad. Ophth.; Amer. Soc. Cataract & Refractive Surg. Prev: Sen. Regist. Char. Cross Hosp. Lond.; Resid. Surg. Off. Moorfields Eye Hosp. Lond.

PACKARD, Robert Spencer 20 Quick Road, London W4 2BU Tel: 020 8994 6003 Fax: 0870 054 8199 Email: home@bobp.co.uk — MB BS Sydney 1951; FRACP 1965, M 1955; FFPM RCP (UK) 1989. Cons. Pharmaceut. Phys. Specialty: Pharmaceutical Medicine. Socs: Fell. Roy. Soc. Med. Prev: Med. Dir. Pfizer Ltd. Sandwich; Phys. Roy. P. Alfred Hosp. Sydney, Austral.; Med. Dir. Pfizer Asia.

PACKE, Geoffrey Edward Department of Medicine, Newham General Hospital, Glen Road, Plaistow, London E13 8SL Tel: 020 7476 4000 Fax: 020 7363 8081 — MD Liverp. 1989; MB CHB 1978; MRCP (UK) 1981; FRCP 1998. Cons. Phys. Thoracic & Gen. Med. Newham Gen. Hosp. Lond. Specialty: Respirat. Med.; Gen. Med. Socs: Brit. Thorac. Soc. Prev: Sen. Regist. (Thorac. Med.) Aberd. Hosps.; Tutor (Thorac. Med.) Cardiothorac. Inst. & Brompton Hosp.

PACKE, Rosemary Irene (retired) 43A Mount Hermon Road, Woking GU22 7UN Tel: 01483 772662 — (King's Coll. Hosp.) MRCS Eng. LRCP Lond. 1942; MB BS Lond. 1943; DCH Eng. 1949. Prev: Asst. Med. Off. Surrey CC.

PACKER, Claire Nancy — BM BS Nottm. 1983; BMedSci Nottm. 1981; DCH RCP Lond. 1986; MFPHM RCP (UK) 1994. Sen. Lect. (Pub. Health) Univ. Birm. Specialty: Pub. Health Med. Prev: Sen. Regist. (Pub. Health) N. Worcs. HA; Trainee GP Coventy VTS.

PACKER, Mr Gregory John Department of Orthopaedic Surgery, Southend District General Hospital, Prittlewell Chase, Westcliff on Sea SS0 0RY — MB BS Lond. 1983; FRCS Ed. 1988; FRCS (Orth.) 1994. Cons. Orthop. Surg. Southend Health Care NHS Trust. Specialty: Orthop.

PACKER, John Michael Valentine (retired) 15 Tothill, Shipton under Wychwood, Chipping Norton OX7 6BX Tel: 01993 831113 — MB ChB Bristol 1954 (Aberd. & Bristol) DPH Liverp. 1958; FFPHM 1981, M 1974. Prev: Cons. Pub. Health Med. (Epidemiol. & Environm. Health) Salford HA.

PACKER, Paul Frederick Church Farm, Church Lane, Brigsley, Grimsby DN37 0RH — MB BS (Hons.) Newc. 1965; DMRD Eng. 1970; FFR 1972; FRCR 1975. Cons. Radiol. St Hugys Hosp. Grimsby. Specialty: Radiol. Prev: Cons. (Radiol.) Riyadh Milit. Hosp.; Cons. Radiol. Newc. Gen. Hosp. & Clin. Lect. (Radiol.) Univ. Newc.; Cons. Radiol. Grimsby HA.

PACKER, Timothy Francis 7 Newton House, Newton St Cyres, Exeter EX5 5BL Tel: 01392 851377 — MB BChir Camb. 1975; BA Camb. 1972, MB BChir 1975; MRCPsych 1982. Cons. Psychiat. Exeter HA. Specialty: Gen. Psychiat.

PACKHAM, Bruce Anthony Woodgate and Packham, Fairfield Surgery, High Street, Etchingham TN19 7EU Tel: 01435 882306 Fax: 01435 882064; 18 Wedderburn Road, Willingdon, Eastbourne BN20 9EB Tel: 01323 502035 Fax: 01323 502035 — MB BS Lond. 1980 (King's Coll.) DRCOG 1983. GP Burwash, E. Sussex. Specialty: Accid. & Emerg.; Ophth. Socs: E.bourne Med. Soc. Prev: Dir. Med. Affairs Rorer Health Care Eastbourne; GP Eastbourne; Trainee GP Eastbourne AHA.

PACKHAM, Christopher John Nottingham City PCT, Standard Court, 1 Park Row, Nottingham NG1 6GN Tel: 0115 912 3344 Fax: 0115 912 3300 Email: chris.packham@nottingham.ac.uk/ chris.packham@nottinghamcity-pct.nhs.uk — BM BS (Hons) Nottm. 1981; BMedSci 1979; MRCP (UK) 1984; MRCGP 1986; DRCOG 1986; DCH Lond. 1986; MMedSci Nottm. 1991; DFFP 1993; MFPHM RCP (UK) 1994; FRCP 2001; DM Nottm. 2002; FFPH 2002. Director of Pub. Health Nottm. City PCT; Assoc. GP Nottm; Cons. Sen. Lect. (Pub. Health Med.)Nottm. Univ. Med. Sch. Specialty: Pub. Health Med.; Gen. Pract. Socs: Nottm. M-C Soc. Prev: Special Clin. Lect. Nottm. Univ. Med. Sch.; GP Nottm; SHO (Med.) Freeman Hosp. Newc.

PACKHAM, Gavin Bruce Central Buchan Medical Group, The Surgery, School Street, Fraserburgh AB43 6NE Tel: 01771 653205 Fax: 01771 653294 — MB ChB Aberd. 1988; MRCGP 1992.

PACKHAM, Iain Nicholas 7 Priorswood, Compton, Guildford GU3 1DS — BM BS Nottm. 1996.

PACKHAM, Jonathan Charles 28 Silvermead, Worming Hall, Thame, Aylesbury HP18 9JS — BM Soton. 1991; MRCP (UK) 1994. Specialist Regist. (Rheumatol.) Wexham Pk. Hosp. Slough. Specialty: Rehabil. Med.; Rheumatol. Socs: Brit. Soc. Rheum.; BMA; Brit. Soc. Med. (Coun. Young Mem.s Rep. Rheumatol. & Rehabil.).

PACKHAM, Roger Nigel 42 Nairn Road, Canford Cliffs, Poole BH13 7NH — MB BS Lond. 1972 (St. Bart.) MRCS Eng. LRCP Lond. 1971; FFA RCS Eng. 1978. Cons. Anaesth. Poole Hosp. NHS Trust.; Med. Dir. Poole Hosps. NHS Trust. Specialty: Anaesth.

PACSOO, Tokefat Christian 77 Moor Park Drive, Addingham, Ilkley LS29 0PU Tel: 01943 830670 — MB ChB Aberd. 1962; DMRD Eng. 1969.

PACTOR, Ronald (retired) 19 Coudray Road, Hesketh Park, Southport PR9 9NL Tel: 01704 537579 — MB ChB Liverp. 1959.

PACYNKO, Michael Kazimierz Meltham Village Surgery, Parkin Lane, Meltham, Huddersfield HD7 3BJ Tel: 01484 850638 Fax: 01484 854891 — MB ChB Leeds 1985.

PADDAY, Ruth The Medical Centre, 24-28 Lower Northam Road, Hedge End, Southampton SO30 4FQ Tel: 01483 785722 Fax: 01486 799414 Email: drpadday@gp-J82089.nhs.uk; Yarrawonga, Brook Lane, Botley, Southampton SO30 2ER Tel: 01489 782783 Fax: 01489 796791 Email: ruthpadday@btopenworld.com — BM Soton. 1979; DCH RCPS Glas. 1984; DRACOG 1985. Teenage Drop-in Centre, Hedge End. Specialty: Paediat. Prev: GP Perth, W. Austral.; Regist. (Paediat.) Sydney & Perth, Austral.

PADDISON, David John (retired) Field Close, Joiners Road, Linton, Cambridge CB1 6NP Tel: 01223 893222 — MB BS Lond. 1946 (Char. Cross) MRCS Eng. LRCP Lond. 1939. Prev: Ho. Surg. (ENT) Char. Cross Hosp.

PADDLE, John Stewart 2 Hast Hill House, Baston Manor Road, Keston BR2 7AH Tel: 020 8462 7575 — BA, MB Camb. 1959, BChir 1958; FFA RCS Eng. 1965. Private Pract. Specialist (Anaesth.). Specialty: Anaesth. Prev: Cons. Anaesth. Guy's Hosp. Lond.; Sen. Regist. Anaesth. St. Thos. Hosp. Lond.; Regist. Anaesth. Soton. Hosp. Gp. & Hosp. Sick Childr. Gt.

PADDLE, Jonathan James 2 Hast Hill, Baston Manor Road, Keston BR2 7AH — MB BS Lond. 1989 (Guy's Hospital) MRCP (UK) 1994; FRCA 1997. Specialist Regist. (Anaesth.) S. Western Deanery Derriford Hosp. Plymouth. Specialty: Anaesth.

PADDOCK, Pamela Mary (retired) 113 Park Hall Road, Walsall WS5 3HS Tel: 01922 625726 — MB ChB Birm. 1950; FRCA Eng. 1958. Prev: Cons. Anaesth. Sandwell AHA & Midl. Centre for Neurosurg. Smethwick.

PADDON, Alexander James The Rectory, Weybourne, Holt NR25 7SY Tel: 01263 70268 — MB BS Lond. 1991; BSc (Hons.) Lond. 1988.

PADDON, Angela Margaret 3 Kelston Cottages, Little Bedwyn, Marlborough SN8 3JL — MB BS Lond. 1994.

PADEL, Adam Frederick Stoke Mandeville Hospital, Department of Cellular Pathology, Aylesbury HP21 8AL Tel: 01296 315000 Ext: 6572 Email: Adam.Padel@smh.nhs.uk — MB BS Lond. 1983 (King's College, London) BSc Lond. 1980; MRCPath 1991; FRCPath, 1999. Cons. Histopath. Stoke Mandeville Hosp. Aylesbury. Specialty: Histopath. Prev: Sen. Regist. (Histopath. & Cytol.) & Regist. (Histopath.) John Radcliffe Hosp. Oxf. & Northampton Gen. Hosp.; Regist. & SHO (Path.) Wycombe Gen. Hosp. High Wycombe.

PADFIELD, Adrian 351 Fulwood Road, Sheffield S10 3BQ Email: a.padfield@sheffield.ac.uk — (St. Bart.) MB BS Lond. 1961; DA Eng. 1963; FRCA Eng. 1968. Emerit. Cons. Anaesth. Centr. Sheff. Univ. Hosps. NHS Trust; Hon. Clin. Lect. Univ. Sheff. Specialty: Anaesth. Socs: Fell. Roy. Soc. Med. (Ex-Pres. Sect. Anaesth.); Assn. Anaesth. Of Gt. Brit. & Ire.; (Ex-Pres.) Assn. Dent. Anaesth. Prev: Sen. Regist. (Anaesth.) United Bristol Hosps. & SW RHB; Regist. (Anaesth.) Roy. Free Hosp. Lond.; SHO (Anaesth.) St. Bart. Hosp. Lond.

PADFIELD, Charles James Henry Department of Histopathology, University Hospital, Queens Medical Centre, Nottingham NG7 2UH Tel: 01159709270 Fax: 0115 970 9759 — MB ChB Manch. 1977; FRCS Eng. 1982; MRCPath 1989. Cons. Fetal & Neonat. Path. Univ. Hosp. Qu. Med. Centre Nottm. Specialty: Histopath. Prev: Sen. Regist. Rotat. (Histopath.) Bristol.

PADFIELD, Hazel Jean Lawn Farm, Straight Lane, Staunton, Gloucester GL19 3NX Tel: 01452 840371 Fax: 01452 840371 — MB BS Newc. 1971. Clin. Med. Off. (Community Child Health) Glos. Specialty: Community Child Health.

PADFIELD, Nicholas Leonard Lister Hospital, Room 8 Lister House, Chelsea Bridge Road, London SW1W 8RH Tel: 020 7730 4706 Email: padfin@atlas.co.uk; 49 Smith Street, London SW3 4EP — MB BS Lond. 1976; FFA RCS Eng. 1981. p/t Cons. Anaesth. St Thos. Hosp. Lond. Specialty: Anaesth. Special Interest: Interven. Pain Managem.; Neuromodulation. Socs: Pain Soc.; Internat. Assn. Study of Pain; Assn. Anaesth. GB & Irel. Prev: Cons. Anaesth. Brook Gen. Hosp. & Greenwich Dist. Hosp. Lond.

PADFIELD, Nigel Norton Whitley Okethampton Medical Centre, East Street, Okehampton EX20 1AY Tel: 01837 52233; Upperton, Drewstrignton, Exeter EX6 6PY Tel: 01647 281660 Email: BNMTNP@aol.com — (St. Mary's) BChir Camb. 1970, MB 1971; DCH RCP Lond. 1972; MRCP (UK) 1974. GP Okehampton Devon. Prev: Primary Health Care Adviser Actionaid Lond.; GP Thame.

PADFIELD, Paul Lynch 2/3 Albyn place, Edinburgh EH2 4NG Tel: 0131 226 1770/0131 537 1716 Fax: 0131 537 1037 — MB BCh Wales 1970 (Cardiff) MRCP (UK) 1973; FRCP Ed. 1983; MBA 2001. Cons. Phys. in Endocrinol. & Gen. Med. West. Gen. Hosp. Edin.; Reader. (Med.) Univ. Edin.; Assoc. Med. Director, Lothian Univ. Hosp.s NHS Trust. Specialty: Endocrinol. Socs: Endocrine Soc. USA & Internat. Soc. Hypertens.

PADGET, Kenneth Isaac (retired) 6 Glade Close, Burton Latimer, Kettering NN15 5YG — MB BS Lond. 1949 (St. Thos.) FRCGP 1982, M 1953. Prev: Ho. Surg. St. Peter's Hosp. Chertsey.

PADGHAM, Katharine Lindsay Flat 2/R, 21 Hayburn Crescent, Glasgow G11 5AY Tel: 0141 339 6604; The Old Farm House, Norton, Sutton Scotney, Winchester SO21 3NE Tel: 01962 760383 — MB ChB Glas. 1997. SHO (Med.) Gartnaval Gen. & Western Infirm. Glas. Specialty: Gen. Med.

PADGHAM, Michael Richard John Charles The Old Farmhouse, Norton, Sutton Scotney, Winchester SO21 3NE Tel: 01962 760236 — MB BS Lond. 1965 (Lond. Hosp.) MRCS Eng. LRCP Lond. 1965; DO Eng. 1968. Specialty: Ophth.

PADGHAM, Mr Nigel David ENT Department, Kent & Canterbury Hospitals NHS Trust, Ethelbert Road, Canterbury CT1 3NG Tel: 01227 766877; Rayham Farm, Rayham Road, Whitstable CT5 3DZ — MB ChB Leic. 1981 (Leicester Univ. Med. Sch.) FRCS Ed. 1987; FRCS Eng. 1988. Cons. ENT Surg. E. Kent Hosp.s NHS Trust.

Specialty: Otorhinolaryngol. Socs: Roy. Soc. Med.; Scott. Ocologol. Soc.

PADHANI, Anwar Roshanali Mount Vernon Hospital, Rickmansworth Road, Northwood HA6 2RN Tel: 01923 844353 Fax: 01923 844600 — MB BS Mysore 1985; LRCP LRCS Ed. LRCPS Glas. 1984; MRCP (UK) 1987; FRCR 1991; FRCP Lond. 2004. Cons. (Radiol.) and Clin. Lead in MRI, Mt. Vernon Hosp. Lond.; Cons. (Radiol.), The Lond. Clinic, Devonshire Pl. Lond. Specialty: Radiol. Special Interest: cancer imaging;MRI; spiral CT; chest diseases. Prev: Sen. Regist. (Radiol.) Guy's Hosp. Lond.; Regist. (Radiol.) Addenbrooke's Hosp. Camb.; Fellowship (Chest Radiol.) John Hopkins Hosp. Baltimore, USA.

PADKIN, Andrew John Royal United Hospital, Combe Park, Bath BA1 3NG — MB ChB Bristol 1990; BSc (Mech. Engin.) Bristol 1984; MRCP (UK) 1993. Cons. Anaesth., Roy. United Hosp., Bath. Specialty: Anaesth. Prev: Specialist Regist. Rotat. (Anaesth.) Treliske Hosp. Truro; SHO Rotat. (Anaesth.) Nottm.; SHO Rotat. (Med.) Qu. Med. Centre Nottm.

PADLEY, Noel Richard Oak Walk House, Oak Walk, Hythe CT21 5DN — MB ChB Birm. 1968; FRCPath 1986, M 1974. Med. Director E. Kent Hosps. NHS Trust. Specialty: Histopath. Prev: Cons. Histopath. SE Kent Health Dist.

PADLEY, Robert George The Surgery, Traingate, Kirton Lindsey, Gainsborough DN21 4DQ Tel: 01652 648214 Fax: 01652 648398; Glentworth Cliff House, Glentworth, Gainsborough DN21 5DA Email: robert.padley@virgin.net — MB ChB Sheff. 1989 (Sheffield) DRCOG 1993; MRCGP 1993; Cert. Family Plann. JCC 1993. Socs: BMA; RCGP. Prev: Trainee GP/SHO Scunthorpe VTS.

PADLEY, Simon Peter Gale Radiology Department, 369 Fulham Road, London SW10 9NH Tel: 020 8746 8580 Fax: 020 8746 8588 Email: s.padley@ic.ac.uk — MB BS Lond. 1984; BSc Lond. 1981; MRCP (UK) 1987; FRCR Lond. 1990; FRCP 1996. Serv. Director and Cons. Radiologist; Cons. Radiol. Roy. Brompton Hosp. Lond. Specialty: Radiol. Socs: RCR; BIR. Prev: Sen. Regist. (Radiol.) Westm. Hosp. & Roy. Brompton Nat. Heart & Lung Inst. Lond.; Regist. (Radiol.) Addenbrooke's Hosp. Camb.

PADLEY, Timothy James Dean Cross Surgery, 21 Radford Park Road, Plymstock, Plymouth PL9 9DL Tel: 01752 404743 — BM BCh Oxf. 1985; MA Oxf. 1987; DRCOG 1989; DA (UK) 1991. Specialty: Anaesth. Prev: Trainee GP/SHO (Anaesth.) Plymouth VTS.

PADMA, Kumari Walderslade Medical Centre, Princes Avenue, Chatham ME5 7PQ Tel: 01636 668160 — MB BS Bangalore 1972; LLM 2001. GP Princip. Specialty: Medico Legal.

PADMAKUMAR, Kadukkavil Whiston Hospital, Prescot L35 5DR Tel: 0151 426 1600 Fax: 0151 430 1892 Email: bpadmakuma@aol.com — MB BS Madras 1984; MRCP (UK) 1989. Cons. Gastroenterol. Roy. Bolton Hosp. Specialty: Gen. Med.; Gastroenterol. Prev: Cons. Phys. Whitston Hosp.

PADMANABHAN, Hariharan (retired) Apple Tree Barn, Woodhouse Road, Todmorden OL14 5RJ — MB BS Nagpur 1956; DA Eng. 1963; Dip. Amer. Bd. Anaesth. 1963; FFA RCS Eng. 1967. Prev: Cons. Anaesth. Rochdale NHS Trust.

PADMANABHAN, Margaret Helen (retired) Apple Tree Barn, Woodhouse Road, Todmorden OL14 5RJ — MB ChB Manch. 1960; MRCOG 1967, DObst 1964. Prev: Lect. (O & G) Radcliffe Infirm. Oxf. & Milnrow Health Centre.

PADMANABHAN, Neal Department of Medicine & Therapeutics, Gardiner Institute, Western Infirmary, Dumbarton Road, Glasgow G11 6NT — BM BCh Oxf. 1993.

PADMANATHAN, Chinnathambi King George Hospital, Barley Lane, Goodmayes, Ilford IG3 8YB Tel: 020 8983 8000; Aruna, 15A Manor Road, Chigwell IG7 5PF Tel: 020 8505 9306 — MB BS Ceylon 1963 (Colombo) DMRD Eng. 1974; FRCR 1975. Cons. Radiol. King Geo. Hosp. Ilford & Barking Hosp. Specialty: Radiol.

PADMASRI, Poonati 18 Sydney Road, Woolaton, Nottingham NG8 1LH — MB BS Osmania U 1988; MRCOG 1994. Post-grad. Stud. Univ. Nottm. Specialty: Obst. & Gyn. Socs: Med. Soc.; BMA. Prev: Regist. Rotat. (O & G) N.W. RHA.

PADMORE, Susan Jane 4 Strathmore Drive, Kirklevington, Yarm TS15 9NS Tel: 01642 785311 — MB ChB Birm. 1971; DA Eng. 1973. Clin. Asst. (Anaesth.) N. Tees Gen. Hosp. Stockton. Specialty: Anaesth. Prev: Regist. Rotat. (Anaesth.) Birm. Accid. Hosp. & Selly Oak Hosp. Birm.; SHO (Anaesth.) & Ho. Surg. Selly Oak Hosp. Birm.

PADWELL, Malcolm Anthony (retired) 15 Airedale Quay, Rodley, Leeds LS13 1NZ Tel: 0113 255 0379 Email: malc@mpadwell.freeserve.co.uk — MB ChB Leeds 1963; DObst RCOG 1965; Dip. Psychoth. 1983. Course Organiser Leeds VTS.

PADWICK, Malcolm Lynn Watford General Hospital, Vicarage Road, Watford WD1 8HP Tel: 01923 244366; BUPA Bushey Hospital, Heathbourne Road, Bushey, Watford WD1 1RD Tel: 020 8950 9090 — MB BS Lond. 1980 (Kings College London) LMSSA Lond. 1980; T(OG) 1991; MD Lond. 1995. Cons. O & G Watford Gen. Hosp. & Mt. Vernon Hosp. Specialty: Obst. & Gyn. Socs: Brit. Gyn. Oncol. Soc.; Internat. Soc. Gyn. Endoscopy; Brit. Soc. Colpos. & Cerv. Path.

PAES, Anthony Rabi Huddersfield Royal Infirmary, Acre Street, Lindley, Huddersfield HD3 3EA Tel: 01484 342700 — MB BS Lond. 1978 (Lond. Hosp.) FRCR 1987, ; MRCP (UK) 1982. Cons. (Radiol.) Huddersfield Roy. Infirm.; Nat. Clin. Assessm. Auth. (Assessor); Roy. Coll. of Radiologists Serv. Review Comm. Specialty: Radiol. Special Interest: Musculoskeletal and Chest Radiol. Socs: Brit. Soc. of Skeletal Radiol.; Magnetic Resonance Radiologists Assn. Prev: Regist. & Sen. Regist. (Radiol.) Soton. Gen. Hosp.

PAES, Paul Vincent 18 Roseworth Crescent, Newcastle upon Tyne NE3 1NR — MB BS Newc. 1997.

PAES, Mr Trevor Rudrah Franco The Hillingdon Hospital, Pield Heath Road, Uxbridge UB8 3NN Tel: 01895 238282 — MRCS Eng. LRCP Lond. 1978 (Bart's) BSc Lond. 1973, MB BS 1978; FRCS Eng. 1982; MS Lond. 1989. Cons. (Surg.) Hillingdon & Mt. Vernon NHS Trust; Hon. Cons. (Surg.) Harefield Hosp. NHS Trust; Hon. Sen. Lec. Surg. Imperial coll. Specialty: Gen. Surg. Socs: Vasc. Surg. Soc. UK; Assn. Roy. Coll. Sci. Prev: Lect. in Surg. Kings Coll. Hosp.; Hon. Surg. of St Barts Hosp.

PAFFENHOLZ, Michael c/o 117 Waverley Road, Harrow HA2 9RQ — State Exam Med Bonn 1993.

PAFFEY, Mark David 201 Chelmsford Road, Shenfield, Brentwood CM15 8SA — MB ChB Sheff. 1998.

PAFFORD, Marguerite — MB ChB Leeds 1977; MRCPsych 1984. Cons. Psychiat. Specialty: Gen. Psychiat. Prev: Cons. Psychiat. S. Bucks. NHS Trust.

PAGADALA, Vasundhara The Surgery, 24 High Street, Colliers Wood, London SW19 2AE Tel: 020 8542 1483 — MB BS Andhra 1962; DObst RCPI 1970. GP; Sessional Med. Assessor to the Benebits Agency.

PAGAN, Francis Stephen (retired) — (St. Bart.) MB BChir Camb. 1968; MA Camb. 1972; FRCPath 1987, M 1975. Cons. Microbiol. Darlington Memor. Hosp. Prev: Lect. (Bact.) Middlx. Hosp. Med. Sch. Lond.

PAGAN, William Hugh (retired) The Homestead, Holton, Halesworth IP19 8PN Tel: 01986 872342 — MB BS Lond. 1961; DObst RCOG 1963; DA Eng. 1964. Prev: GP Clin. Asst. St. Bart. Hosp. Lond.

PAGANO, Kristin Christiania, Arkesden, Saffron Walden CB11 4EY — MB BS Lond. 1982 (Guy's) DRCOG 1993; MFPM RCP (UK) 1993. Sen. Med. Adviser Cilaq Ltd. High Wycombe Bucks. Specialty: Pharmaceutical Medicine. Prev: Clin. Pharmacol. Beechams Research Div. Betchworth.

PAGDIN, George Hockley (retired) 29 Cranford Drive, Owlthorpe, Sheffield S20 6RP — MB ChB Sheff. 1949; FRCGP 1994, M 1968; MD Sheff. 1992.

PAGDIN, Judith Claire Church Grange Health Centre, Bramblys Drive, Basingstoke RG21 8QN Tel: 01256 329021 Fax: 01256 817466 — BM Soton. 1981; MRCGP 1985; DRCOG 1985. Socs: BMA. Prev: Trainee GP/SHO Basingstoke Dist. Hosp.VTS; Ho. Off. (Med.) West. Hosp. Soton.; Ho. Off. (Surg.) Basingstoke Dist. Hosp.

PAGE, Mr Albert Brian 4 Old Fort, Helens Bay, Bangor BT19 1LL — MD Belf. 1988; MB BCh BAO 1974; DRCOG 1978; MRCGP 1981; FRCS Ed. 1984. Cons. Ophth. Roy. Vict. Hosp. Belf. Specialty: Ophth.

PAGE, Alison Jane West Midlands Radiology Rotation City Hospital NHS Trust, Dudley Road, Winson Green, Birmingham B18 7QH Tel: 0121 554 3801 — MB ChB Birm. 1992 (Univ. of Birm. Med. Sch.) BSc (Hons.) (Med. Biochem.) Birm. 1989; MRCP (UK) 1995; FRCR 1999. Specialty: Radiol.

PAGE, Andrew Clive Department of Radiology, Royal Hampshire County Hospital, Romsey Road, Winchester SO22 5DG — MB BS Lond. 1981 (King's Coll.) FRCR 1988. Cons. Roy. Hants. Co. Hosp.

Winchester. Specialty: Radiol. Socs: Roy. Coll. of Radiologists; BSIR; CIRSE. Prev: Sen. Regist. Kings Coll. Hosp. Lond.; Regist. Dept. Radiol. Freedom Fields Hosp. Plymouth.; SHO (Med.) North. Gen. Hosp. Sheff.

PAGE, Anthony Dane Garth, Furness General Hospital, Dalton Lane, Barrow-in-Furness LA14 4LF — MB ChB Leeds 1980; MRCPsych 1984. Cons. Psychiat. Furness Gen. Hosp. Barrow-in-Furness. Specialty: Gen. Psychiat.

PAGE, Antony John Frederick Norfolk & Norwich University Hospital, Department of Cardiology, Colney Lane, Norwich NR4 7UY Tel: 01603 287516 Fax: 01603 287494 Email: tony.page@nnuh.nhs.uk; The Chestnuts, 215 Unthank Road, Norwich NR2 2PH Tel: 01603 250011 Fax: 01603 453191 Email: a.j.f.page@btinternet.com — MB BS Lond. 1971 (Lond. Hosp.) MRCP (UK) 1974; FRCP Lond. 1992. Cons. & Cardiol. Norf. & Norwich Univ. Hosp. Specialty: Cardiol. Socs: Brit. Cardiac Soc.; Brit. Pacing and Electrophysiology Group. Prev: Lect. (Cardiol.) Brit. Heart Foundat. Univ. Birm.

PAGE, Arthur Reginald Webster Testvale Surgery, 12 Salisbury Road, Totton, Southampton SO40 3PY; Forelands, Woodlands Drive, Woodlands, Southampton SO40 7HW — MB BS Lond. 1952 (St. Bart.) MRCGP 1967. Admiralty Surg & Agent. Socs: Soton. Med. Soc. Prev: Ho. Surg. & Ho. Phys. Norf. & Norwich Hosp.; Ho. Surg. (O & G) Gen. Hosp. Soton.

PAGE, Barbara Elizabeth Abbots Cross Medical Practice, 92 Doagh Road, Newtownabbey BT37 9QW; 15 Lenamore Avenue, Jordanstown, Newtownabbey BT37 0PF — MB BCh BAO Belf. 1981; DRCOG 1984; MRCGP 1985.

PAGE, Barnaby Mills Winterwood, Nyetimber Copse, West Chiltington, Pulborough RH20 2NE — MB ChB Manch. 1998.

PAGE, Carol Susan 4 Bonhard Road, Scone, Perth PH2 6QL — MB ChB Dundee 1979; MRCPsych Lond. 1990.

PAGE, Carolyn Jane Hathaway Surgery, 32 New Road, Chippenham SN15 1HR Tel: 01249 447766 Fax: 01249 443948; Godley's Farm House, Avon, Chippenham SN15 4LS — MB BS Lond. 1961.

PAGE, Christopher Murray Temple Fortune Health Centre, 23 Temple Fortune Lane, London NW11 7TE Tel: 020 8458 4431 Fax: 020 8731 8257; 32 Wordsworth Walk, London NW11 6AU Tel: 020 8455 2785 — MB BS Lond. 1971; MRCP (UK) 1975; FRCP 2000. Prev: Sen. Lect. (Primary Care & Pub. Health) Roy. Free Hosp. Lond.; Research Fell. & Hon. Sen. Regist. St. Mary's Hosp. Lond. & Cas. Med. Off. Middlx. Hosp. Lond.

PAGE, Elizabeth Anne 38 Fielding Street, Kennington, London SE17 3HD — LMSSA Lond. 1978.

PAGE, Fiona Cameron The Royal Oldham Hospital, Rochdale Road, Oldham OL1 2JH — MB ChB Manch. 1981; BSc St. And. 1979; DRCOG 1984; MRCGP 1985; MFOM RCP Lond. 1991, AFOM 1989; DFFP 1993; FFOM 1998. Cons. Occupat. Health Roy. Oldham Hosp. Specialty: Occupat. Health.

PAGE, Frances Mary Larman 15 Sherwood Street, Whetstone, London N20 0NB — MB BS Lond. 1992 (Univ. College and Middlesex Hospital Medical School London) BSc Lond. 1989; DA 1996. Specialist Regist. Rotat. N. Lond. Specialty: Anaesth.

PAGE, Frank Bernard Tower House Medical Centre, Stockway South, Nailsea, Bristol BS48 2XX Tel: 01275 866700 Fax: 01275 866711; Rosedale, 108 Station Road, Nailsea, Bristol BS48 1TB Tel: 01275 852723 — MB BS Lond. 1968 (Lond. Hosp.) DTM & H Liverp. 1970; DA Eng. 1970; MRCGP 1981; TM 1998. G.P. Specialty: Gen. Pract. Socs: Christ. Med. Fellowsh. Prev: Med. Dir. Med. Asst. Program Inc. Afghanistan Project.

PAGE, Graham Wallace (retired) 9 Nightingale Lane, Beechwood Gardens, Coventry CV5 6AY Tel: 024 7667 3125 Fax: 024 7667 3125 — MB BChir Camb. 1948 (Camb. & St. Bart) MRCGP 1966. Prev: Unit. Gen. Manager/Specialist in Comm. Med. N. Warks. HA.

PAGE, Gregory Christopher Thomas Skewen Medical Centre, Queens Road, Skewen, Neath SA10 6UL Tel: 01792 812316 Fax: 01792 323208 — MB BCh Wales 1979.

PAGE, Hilary 43 Slayleigh Lane, Sheffield S10 3RG Tel: 0114 230 7826 — MD (Distinc.) Leeds 1992, MB ChB 1970; DObst RCOG 1973; MRCGP 1978; MFPHM RCP (UK) 1987; FFPHM RCP (UK) 1997. Ass. Dir. (Pub. Health) Trent Regional Office NHS Exec.; Hon. Sen. Lect. Sheff. Univ. Med. Sch. Specialty: Pub. Health Med. Socs: Nat. Assn. Family Plann. Doctors & BMA. Prev: Lect. (Epidemiol.) Sheff. Univ. Med. Sch.; Dir. (Pub. Health) Doncaster.

PAGE, Ian John (retired) Royal Lancaster Infirmary, Ashton Road, Lancaster LA1 4RP Tel: 01524 65944 Fax: 01524 583585 — MB BS Lond. 1979 (Guy's Hosp.) MRCS Eng. LRCP Lond. 1978; MRCOG 1985; T(OG) 1991; FRCDG 1998. Cons. O & G Roy. Lancaster Infirm. & Westmorland Gen. Hosp. Kendal. Prev: Cons. O & G Army Med. Servs.

PAGE, James Martin The Village Green Surgery, The Green, Wallsend NE28 6BB Tel: 0191 295 8500 Fax: 0191 295 8519 — MB BCh BAO Belf. 1978; DRCOG 1981; MRCGP 1982. GP Trainer.

PAGE, Janet Elizabeth 7 Hurstfield, Hayes Park, Bromley BR2 9BB — MB BS Lond. 1959 (Roy. Free) MRCS Eng. LRCP Lond. 1959; DA Eng. 1961. Clin. Asst. (Rhesus Immunisation) Lewisham Hosp. Socs: Fac. Anaesth. RCS Eng. Prev: Clin. Asst. (Anaesth.) Dreadnought & Greenwich Dist. Hosps.; Regist. (Anaesth.) Qu. Mary's Hosp. Sidcup; SHO (Anaesth.) Bromley Hosp.

PAGE, Janet Elizabeth Medical Protection Society, 33 Cavendish Square, London W1G 0PS Tel: 020 7399 1327 Fax: 020 7399 1301 Email: janet.page@mps.org.uk; Coniston, 29 Westward Ho, Abbotswood, Guildford GU1 1UU Tel: 01483 453138 Email: drjanet.page@ntlworld.com — MB BS Lond. 1982 (St. Mary's) BSc (Hons.) Lond. 1979; MRCP (UK) 1985; FRCR 1988. Medico Legal Adviser. Specialty: Radiol.; Medico Legal. Socs: BMA. Prev: Cons. Diagn. Radiol. E. Surrey Hosp. Redhill/18116; Cons. Radiologist, Surrey & Sussex Healthcare NHS Trust, Redhill.

PAGE, Jason McKinley 18 Wingrove Avenue, Newcastle upon Tyne NE4 9AL Tel: 0191 245 1489 — MB BS Newc. 1995. SHO Paediat, N. Shields. Specialty: Gen. Pract. Prev: SHO Psychiat. Tranwell Unit AE Gateshead; SHO O & G Ashington; SHO A&E RVI & NGH, Newc.

PAGE, Jennifer Margaret 8 The Squirrels, Belmont Hill, London SE13 5DR — MB BS Lond. 1985.

PAGE, Joanne Maria Hook and Hartley Wintney Medical Partnership, 1 Chapter Terrace, Hartley Wintney, Hook RG27 8QJ Tel: 01252 842087 Fax: 01252 843145; 51 Longbridge Road, Bramley, Tadley RG26 5AN Tel: 01256 881231 — MB ChB Manch. 1988; Cert. Family Plann. JCC 1994; DRCOG 1994; MRCGP 1996. GP Princip. Prev: Trainee GP Bramblys Grange Surg. Basingstoke; Ho. Surg. ChristCh. HA, NZ; Ho. Phys. & Ho. Surg. Vict. Hosp. Blackpool.

PAGE, Professor John Graham Accident & Emergency Department, Aberdeen Royal Infirmary, Aberdeen AB25 2ZN Tel: 01224 681818 Fax: 01224 840718 Email: g.page@abdn.ac.uk; 16 Kingswood Avenue, Kingswells, Aberdeen AB15 8AE Tel: 01224 742945 Fax: 01224 742945 — (Aberd.) FFOM 1998 RCP Lond.; MB ChB Aberd. 1968; FRCS Ed. 1972; ChM Aberd. 1977; FFAEM 1993. Cons. A & E Aberd. Roy. Hosps. NHS Trust; Hon. Prof. Emerg. Med. Robt. Gordon Univ. Aberd.; Hon. Sen. Lect. (Surg.) Univ. Aberd. Specialty: Accid. & Emerg. Socs: Eur. Undersea Biomed. Soc.; BMA. Prev: Regist. (Surg.) Grampian HB; Research Fell. Harvard Univ. Boston, USA; Terminable Lect. (Path.) Aberd. Univ.

PAGE, John Patrick Anthony, Col. late RAMC Princes Street Surgery, Princes Street, Thurso KW14 7DH Tel: 01847 893154 Email: jpapage99@hotmail.com — MB Camb. 1962 (Camb. & St. Bart.) BChir 1961; DTM & H RCP Lond. 1964; T(GP) 1991. GP Thurso. Socs: BMA; Caius Coll. Med. Soc. Prev: Staff Phys. NW AFH Tabuk, Saudi Arabia; Regtl. Med. Off. Blues & Roy.s; Specialist Dermat. Qu. Alexandra Milit. Hosp.

PAGE, Julian (Surgery) 30 Bradshaw Brow, Bradshaw, Bolton BL2 3DH Tel: 01204 302212; 6 Holkar Meadows, Bromley Cross, Bolton BL7 9NA Tel: 01204 592653 — MB ChB Manch. 1984; DRCOG 1987; MRCGP 1989; D.Occ Med 1997; FRCGP 1997. Course Organisor, Wigan and Bolton VTS Research Fellow. Prev: GP Tutor Bolton; Med. Off. Hick Hargreaves & Beliot Walmsley Ltd.; Fell. Summative Assessm.

PAGE, Katharine Isabel Claremont House, Regional Department of Psychotherapy, Off Framlington Place, Newcastle upon Tyne NE2 4AA Tel: 0191 282 4547 Fax: 0191 282 4542 Email: claremonthouse@nmht.nhs.uk — MB BS Lond. 1986 (Guy's) BCP Accredit.; MRCPsych 1993; NEATPP 2003. Cons. (Psychother.) Regional Dept. Psychother. Newc. u. Tyne.

PAGE, Kathleen Margaret The White Cottage, 39 Blackbrook Park Avenue, Fareham PO15 5JN Tel: 01329 280455 — (Roy. Free) MB BS Lond. 1964; MRCS Eng. LRCP Lond. 1964; DObst RCOG 1966; DA Eng. 1967; DCH Eng. 1969. Hosp. Pract. (Anaesth.) Hants. Specialty: Anaesth. Socs: BMA. Prev: GP Lee-on-the-Solent; Ho. Phys. Roy. Free Hosp. Lawn Rd.; Ho. Surg. St. Mary Abbott's Hosp. Kensington.

PAGE, Kevin Barry Department of Clinical Chemistry, Royal Hallamshire Hospital, Glossop Road, Sheffield S10 2JF Tel: 0114 271 2787 Email: kevin.page@sth.nhs.uk; 5 Rowell Cottages, Rowell Lane, Loxley, Sheffield S6 6SH — MB BS Lond. (King's Coll. Hosp. Med. Sch.) 1983 (Kings Coll. Hosp. Med. Sch.) MRCPath 1996; M. Ed. (Sheff. Univ.) 2000. Assoc. Specialist (Chem. Pathol.) Sheff. Teachg. Hosp. NHS Trust. Specialty: Chem. Path. Socs: Nutrit. Soc.

PAGE, Kim Elizabeth Rampton Hospital, Retford, Nottingham DN22 0PD Tel: 01777 248321 — MB ChB Birm. 1984; MRCPsych 1993. Cons Forens. Psychiat. Rampton Hosp. Retford Notts. Specialty: Forens. Psychiat. Socs: BMA. Prev: Regist. (Psychiat.) Mapperley Hosp. Nottm.; SHO (Med.) Kings Mill Hosp. Sutton-in-Ashfield; Sen Regis Forens. Psychiat. Trent scheme.

PAGE, Louise Jessamy Lambley Lane Surgery, 6 Lambley Lane, Burton Joyce, Nottingham NG14 3GW — MB ChB Leic. 1996; MRCGP. GP Registr., Nottm. VTS. Specialty: Gen. Med.

PAGE, Margaret Jane Claremont Bank Surgery, Claremont Bank, Shrewsbury SY1 1RL Tel: 01743 357355 — MB BS Lond. 1980 (Middlx. Hosp.) MRCGP 1984; DRCOG 1985; DA (UK) 1987. Specialty: Gen. Pract.; Gen. Psychiat. Prev: Trainee GP/SHO (O & G, Med. & Anaesth.) Salop. HA VTS; Regist. Anaesthetia.

PAGE, Mary Elizabeth The Health Centre, Church Road, Thornton-Cleveleys; Five Gables, 67 Moorland Road, Poulton-le-Fylde FY6 7ER Tel: 01253 899449 — MB ChB Manch. 1979.

PAGE, Mervyn James (retired) 12 Trossachs Drive, Bath BA2 6RP Tel: 01225 421171 — MB ChB Bristol 1954; DCH Eng. 1958; DObst RCOG 1960. Prev: Sen. Res. Off. Bristol Matern. Hosp.

PAGE, Michael Clayton Medicines Control Agency, Room 1322, Market Towers, 1 Nine Elms Lane, London SW8 5NQ Tel: 020 7273 0529 Fax: 020 7273 0195; Little Orchard, Chiltern Road, Peppard, Henley-on-Thames RG9 5LP Tel: 01189 722576 — MB BS Lond. 1974 (St. Bart.) MRCP (UK) 1980. Sen. Med. Off. Meds. Control Agency. Specialty: Pharmaceutical Medicine; Rheumatol. Prev: Med. Dir. Fournier Pharmaceut. Ltd.

PAGE, Michael Denyer Solstice, Millcroft Court, St Mary Church, Cowbridge CF7 7LH — MD Wales 1991; MB BCh 1980; MRCP (UK) 1984; FRCP 1998. Cons. Phys. Roy. Glam. Hosp. Specialty: Gen. Med.; Endocrinol.; Diabetes. Prev: Sen. Regist. (Med.) Leeds.

PAGE, Michael James Scott Mount View Practice, London Street Medical Centre, London Street, Fleetwood FY7 6HD Tel: 01253 873312 Fax: 01253 873130; Flat 7, Bleasdale Court, Queens Terrace, Fleetwood FY7 6DP Tel: 07971 452856 — MB ChB Dundee 1975; MRCGP 1980. Clin. Asst. EMI Unit Fleetwood Hosp.; Police Surg. to N. Fylde.

PAGE, Michael McBean The Manor Hospital, Walsall W52 9PS Tel: 01922 721172; 532 City Road, Edgbaston, Birmingham B17 8LN Tel: 0121 434 5516 Fax: 0121 434 5516 Email: michaelpg@aol.com — MB BChir Camb. 1969; FRCP Lond. 1988, M 1972; MD Camb. 1981. Locum Cons. Phys. Manor Hosp. Walsall. Specialty: Diabetes; Gen. Med. Socs: Brit. Diabetic Assn. Prev: Cons. Phys. Selly Oak Hosp. Birm.; Sen. Regist. (Med.) Nottm. Gen. Hosp.; Regist. (Diabetes) King's Coll. Hosp. Lond.

PAGE, Nicholas Goodwin Richardson 15 Basil Mansions, Basil St., London SW3 1AP Tel: 020 7589 4780 Fax: 020 7581 0244 Email: nicdoc@aol.com; 72 Rodenhurst Road, London SW4 8AR — MB BS Lond. 1972 (Westm.) MRCP (UK) 1976; FRCP Lond. 1998. Private Med. Pract. Socs: Med Soc. Lond.; Chelsea Clin. Soc. Prev: Resid. Fell. (Neurol.) Nat. Hosp. Lond.; Regist. (Med.) St. Thos. Hosp. & Westm. Hosp. Lond.

PAGE, Nicholas Philip Freeman Ludlow Hill Surgery, 152 Melton Road, West Bridgford, Nottingham NG2 6ER Tel: 0115 945 2656 Fax: 0115 923 5166 — (Guys) BSc (Hons.) Lond. 1980, MB BS 1983; DCH RCP Lond. 1988; DRCOG 1988; MRCGP 1989.

PAGE, Mr Nigel Eric 5 The Rise, Southill, Weymouth DT4 0TD — MB ChB Birm. 1977; FRCS Ed. 1983. Specialty: Neurosurg.

PAGE, Nigel Geoffrey Sandwell Health NHS Trust, Lyndon, West Bromwich B71 4HJ — MB ChB Birm 1992; BSc (1st cl. Hons.) Pharmacol. Birm. 1989; MRCP (UK) 1995. Cons. Geriat., Sandwell Healthcare NHS Trust W. Bromwich. Specialty: Care of the Elderly; Gen. Med.

PAGE, Renee Claire Lesley Department of Diabetes, Nottingham City Hospital, Hucknall Road, Nottingham NG5 1PB — MB ChB Manch. 1983; BSc Med. Sci. (St. And.) 1980; MB ChB (Hons.) Manch. 1983; MRCP (UK) 1986. Cons. Phys. Specialty: Gen. Med. Prev: Regist. Radcliffe Infirm. Oxf. RHA.

PAGE, Mr Richard Denyer The Cardiothoracic Centre, Thomas Drive, Liverpool L14 3PE; 25 Barton Heys Road, Formby, Liverpool L37 2EY — MB ChB Liverp. 1982 (Liverpool) FRCS Ed. 1987; FRCS (Cth.) 1993; ChM Liverp. 1994. Cons. Cardiothoracic Surg. Cardiothoracic Centre Liverp. Specialty: Cardiothoracic Surg. Socs: Soc. Cardiothoracic Surg. GB & Irel. Prev: Sen. Regist. (Cardiothoracic Surg.) Cardiothoracic Centre Liverp.; Regist. (Cardiothoracic Surg.) Broadgreen Hosp. Liverp.; Fell. (Cardiac Surg.) Harvard Med. Sch., Boston, USA.

PAGE, Richard James Holsworthy Medical Centre, Dobles Lane, Holsworthy EX22 6GH Tel: 01409 253692 Fax: 01409 254184; Sunnymeade, 6 Holnicote Road, Bude EX23 8EJ Tel: 01288 354464 — MB ChB Bristol 1975; DRCOG 1976; MRCGP 1980. GP Trainer Holsworthy. Specialty: Gen. Pract. Prev: Med. Off. I/C Amalo Refugee Camp Somalia.; Trainee GP Barnstaple VTS; SHO (Anaesth.) Roy. Devon & Exeter Hosp.

PAGE, Mr Richard John Page and Partners, Health Centre, Church Street, Stoke-on-Trent ST7 8EW Tel: 01782 721345 Fax: 01782 723808; Park Lane Farm, Park Lane, Audley, Stoke-on-Trent ST7 8HP — MB ChB Birm. 1981 (University of Birmingham) FRCS Ed. 1986; MRCGP 1990. GP Princip.; Police Surg. Staffs. Police Force; Clin. Asst. in Gastroenterol.; Clin. Asst. in Orthop. Specialty: Gen. Pract.; Gastroenterol.; Orthop.

PAGE, Richard Louis St James's University Hospital, Beckett St., Leeds LS9 7TF Tel: 0113 243 3144; Leeds Chest Clinic, 74 new Briggate, Leeds LS1 6PH Tel: 0113 2951153 — MB BS Lond. 1967 (Middlx.) MRCS Eng. LRCP Lond. 1967; MRCP (U.K.) 1970; DM Nottm. 1978; FRCP Lond. 1986; MFOM RCP Lond. 1988. Cons. Phys. St. Jas. Univ. Hosp. Leeds. Specialty: Respirat. Med. Special Interest: Occupational Lung Dis. Socs: Brit. Thorac. Soc.; Soc. Occupat. Med. Prev: Sen. Regist. (Med.) Addenbrooke's Hosp. Camb.; MRC Fell. Med. Unit Nottm. Univ.; Regist. (Med.) Middlx. Hosp. Lond.

PAGE, Richard Mackay Yealm Medical Centre, Market St., Yealmpton, Plymouth PL8 2EA Tel: 01752 880392; Little Copse, New Road, Yealmpton, Plymouth PL8 2HH — MRCS Eng. LRCP Lond. 1969 (St. Bart.) DA Eng. 1975; DRCOG 1977. Specialty: Anaesth. Socs: Chairm. Plymouth LMC. Prev: Clin. Asst. Anaesth. Dept. Reinford Hosp. Plymouth.

PAGE, Mr Richard Samuel — MB BS Tasmania 1989 (Univ. Tasmania) BMedSci. Tasmania 1985; FRACS (Pt 1) 1995; FRACS (orth) 2000. Cons. Ortho. Surg. Geelong Hosp. Vic. Aus.; Orthopaedic Surg., Surg LCDR, RANR; Roy. Austral. Naval Reserves; Chairm. Barwon Orthopaedic Research Unit Geelong. Specialty: Orthop. Socs: Fell. of Roy. Austral. Coll. of Surg.s; Assoc. Mem. Austral. Orthop. Assn.; Austral. Milit. Med. Assn. Prev: Upper Limb Fell., Wrightington Hosp., Lancs., UK; Cons. Orthopaedic Surg. Roy. Hosp. Haslar & Portsmouth Hosp.; Sen. Regist. & Fell. Orthopeaduc Trauma Unit, Roy. Inif. Edin.

PAGE, Robert Edward Northern General Hospital, Department of Plastic Surgery, Herries Road, Sheffield S5 7AU Tel: 0114 271 4560 Fax: 0114 271 5294 Email: moira.irving@sth.nhs.uk — MB ChB Leeds 1970. Specialty: Plastic Surg.

PAGE, Ronald Mallis The Health Centre, Victoria Road, Leven KY8 4ET Tel: 01333 425656 Fax: 01333 422249 — MB ChB Ed. 1978; BSc 1975; DRCOG 1981; MRCGP (Distinc.) 1982. Syntex Award Research in Gen. Pract.-Highlands & Is.s.

PAGE, Rosemary Beatrice (retired) Ardnamurchan, Thirlby, Thirsk YO7 2DJ Tel: 01845 597602 — MB Camb. 1972; BChir 1971.

PAGE, Mrs Rosemary Fiona McLeish Witley Surgery, Wheeler Lane, Witley, Godalming GU8 5QR Tel: 01428 682218 Fax: 01428 685790; Fernside Cottage, Brook Road, Wormley, Godalming GU8 5UA Tel: 0142 684291 — MB BS Lond. 1959 (St. Mary's) DObst RCOG 1961. Prev: Clin. Asst. (Cas.) Roy. Surrey Co. Hosp. Guildford.; Ho. Phys. & Ho. Surg. Roy. Hants. Co. Hosp. Winchester; Ho. Off. (Obst & Gyn.) St. Luke's Hosp. Guildford.

PAGE, Simon John The Lennard Surgery, 1-3 Lewis Road, Bishopsworth, Bristol BS13 7JD Tel: 0117 964 0900 Fax: 0117 987 3227 — MB ChB Bristol 1975; MRCGP 1981. GP Princip. Bristol. Prev: Lead Gp Bristol S. Locality Commissioning; Clin. Asst. (ENT) Weston Gen. Hosp.; Clin. Teach. (Gen. Pract. & Child Health) Bristol Univ.

PAGE, Simon Richard Department of Diabetes, Endocrinology and Metabolism, University Hospital, Nottingham NG7 2UH Tel: 0115 924 9924 Fax: 0115 970 1080 — MB ChB Bristol 1982; MB ChB (Hons.) Bristol 1982; MRCP (UK) 1985; MD Bristol 1991; FRCP UK 1999. Cons. Phys. Univ. Hosp. Nottm. Specialty: Diabetes; Endocrinol. Prev: Sen. Regist. (Med., Diabetes & Endocrinol.) Nottm. & Derby Hosps.; Clin. Research Fell. Univ. Lond. St. Geo. Hosp. Med. Sch.; Regist. (Med.) St. Geo. Hosp. Lond.

PAGE, Valerie Joan 24 Grosvenor Avenue, Newcastle upon Tyne NE2 2NP — MB ChB Manch. 1982.

PAGE, William 4 Glebe Manor, Anahilt, Hillsborough BT26 6NS — MB BCh BAO Belf. 1976; DMRD Eng. 1982; FRCR 1983. Cons. (Radiol.) Belvoir Pk. & Foster Green. Hosps. Belf. & Lagan Valley Lisburn. Specialty: Radiol.

PAGET, Cecil John Hayward (retired) Coombe Rise, 34 The Drive, Wallington SM6 9LX Tel: 020 8647 8084 — MB BChir Camb. 1945 (St. Bart) Prev: Hon. Med. Off. Carshalton, Beddington & Wallington Memor. Hosp.

PAGET, Jacques Pierre Malezieux (retired) 15 Bladon Close, London Road, Guildford GU1 1TY Tel: 01483 571421 — (Lille) MD Lille, France 1949; Lic. New Brunswick Med. Bd. 1961; Cert. Pathol, Canada 1961; Lic. Newfld. Med. Bd. 1968; DPH Bristol 1969.

PAGET, Richard Ian James North Ladbrook Hall, Penn Lane, Tanworth-in-Arden, Solihull B94 5HJ — MB ChB Birm. 1993.

PAGET, Richard James (retired) Glebe Farm House, Harthill, Sheffield S26 7YG — MB ChB Bristol 1963; BSc (Hons.) Bristol 1960; MB ChB (Hons.) 1963; MIBiol 1976; MRCGP 1977. Prev: SHO Cardiff Roy. Infirm.

PAGET, Sally Elizabeth Roebuck House, High Street, Hastings TN34 3ES Tel: 01424 420378 Fax: 01424 452824; 12 High Wickham, Hastings TN35 5PB Tel: 01424 714369 — MB BS Lond. 1981 (Guy's) MRCP (UK) 1984; MRCGP 1987.

PAGET, Seaton Chamberlain Roebuck House Surgery, High St., Hastings TN34 3EY Tel: 01424 420378 — MB BS Lond. 1951 (Guy's) MRCS Eng. LRCP Lond. 1951; DObst RCOG 1957.

PAGET, Timothy David 55 St Cross Road, Winchester SO23 9RE — MB BS Lond. 1990; T(GP) 1994; Dip. Pharma. Med. 1997; MFPM 2002. Consultant Pharmaceutical Physician. Specialty: Pharmaceutical Medicine.

PAGLIERO, Mr Keith Michael Low Water, 36 Countess Wear Road, Exeter EX2 6LR Tel: 01392 877520 Fax: 01392 877520 Email: michael.pagliero@virgin.net — MB BS Lond. 1962 (Guy's) MRCS Eng. LRCP Lond. 1962; FRCS Eng. 1967. Indep. Cons. Thoracic Surg. Devon; Hon. Research Fell. Surgic. Oncol. Exeter Univ. Postgrad. Med. Sch. Specialty: Cardiothoracic Surg. Socs: (Ex. Chairm.) Nat. Assn. Clin. Tutors; Soc. Thoracic & Cardiovasc. Surgs. Prev: Cons. Thoracic Surg. Roy. Devon & Exeter Hosp., N. Devon Infirm. & Torbay Hosps.; Dir. Educat. & Thoracic Surg. King Fahad Armed Forces Hosp. Jeddah; Sen. Regist. (Thoracic Surg.) Hammersmith & Guy's Hosps. Lond.

PAGLIUCA, Antonio Department of Haematological Medicine, King's College Hospital, Denmark Hill, London SE5 9RS Tel: 020 7346 3709 Fax: 020 7346 3514 Email: antonio.pagliuca@kcl.ac.uk — MB BS Lond. 1983 (King's Coll. Lond.) MA Camb. 1984; MRCP (UK) 1986; MRCPath 1992; FRCPath 2000. Cons. Haemat. King's Coll. Hosp. Lond.; Hon. Sen. Lect., Kings Coll. Hosp.; Clin. Director Specialist Med. Specialty: Haematology. Special Interest: Bone marrow Transplantation. Socs: Brit. Soc. of Haematol.; Amer. Soc. Haemat.; Europ. Gp. For Bone marrow transplantation. Prev: Lect. (Haemat.) King's Coll. Sch. Med. & Dent.; SHO (Neurol.) Nat. Hosp. Nerv. Dis. Lond.; SHO (Med.) St. Geo. & Roy. Marsden Hosps. Lond.

PAGNI, Paul Anthony McKenzie House Surgery, Kendal Road, Hartlepool TS25 1QU Tel: 01429 233611 Fax: 01429 297713 — MB BCh BAO NUI 1983.

PAHAL, Gurmit Singh 27 Campbell Road, Gravesend DA11 0JZ — MB BS Lond. 1994.

PAHOR, Mr Ahmes Labib ENT Department, City Hospital NHS Trust, Dudley Road, PO Box 293, Birmingham B18 7QH Tel: 0121 507 4559 Fax: 0121 507 4557 — MB BCh Cairo 1964 (Kasr Al-Aini Med. Sch. Cairo) DLO Cairo 1966; DMSc (Path.) Ain Shams 1968; FRCS Ed. 1974; FICS Fellow International College of Surgeons, USA 1977; Specialist Accredit. (ENT) RCS Ed. 1977; MRCS Eng. LRCP Lond. 1978; MA Cairo 1986; DHMSA Soc. Apoth. Lond. 1994. Cons. Surg. ENT City Hosp. Trust Birm., Sandwell NHS Trust, W. Bromwich; Hon. Sen. Clin. Lect. Univ. Birm.; Cert. Special Traing. Otolaryngol. (Europ. Union) 1995. Specialty: Otolaryngol. Socs: Midl. Inst. Otol. (Hon. Libr.); Irish OtoLaryngol. Soc.; Brit. Soc. For the Hist. Of ENT (Hon. Sec.). Prev: Regist. Roy. Vict. Hosp. Belf.; Sen. Regist. Qu. Eliz. Hosp. Birm. & Walsgrave Hosp. Coventry, Roy. Infirm. Stoke-on-Trent.

PAHWA, Balram Krishan 10 Leicester Road, Wanstead, London E11 2DP Tel: 020 8989 3224; 320 Commercial Road, London E1 2PY — MB BS Rajasthan 1957 (Sawai Man Singh Med. Coll. Jaipur) Prev: Regist. W. Ham Chest Clinic Plaistow; Regist. Med. Post-Grad. Med. Inst. Chandigarh.

PAHWA, Mr Mahendra Kumar Goldthorn Medical Centre, 130a Park Street South, Off Goldthorn Hill, Wolverhampton WV2 3JF Tel: 01902 339283 Fax: 01902 339283 — MB BS Vikram 1963; MS Delhi 1970.

PAI, Mr Ballambettu Yogish (retired) The Avenue, Linthorpe, Middlesbrough TS5 6 — MB BS Madras 1954 (Christian Med. Coll. Vellore) MS Madras 1958, MB BS 1954; FRCS Eng. 1960; FRCS Ed. 1960. Prev: Cons. Orthop. Surg. S. & N. Tees Health Auths.

PAI, Elfreeda D'Souza 7 Daubeney Gate, Shenley Church End, Milton Keynes MK5 6EH — MB BS Mysore 1978; DCH Dub. 1981; LRCP LRCS Ed. LRCPS Glas. 1984.

PAI, Haridas Upendra Shafton Lane Surgery, 20A Shafton Lane, Holbeck, Leeds LS11 9RE Tel: 0113 295 4393 Fax: 0113 295 4390 — MB BS Mysore 1974. GP Leeds.

PAI, Mr Karkala Purushotham Department of General Surgery, The General Hospital, St Helier, Jersey JE2 3QS Tel: 01534 622000 Fax: 01534 622880 Email: purshot@hotmail.com; 126/A, Road 4, West Nehrunagar, Secunderabad, Andhra Pradesh 500026, India Tel: 780 1523 — MB BS Osmania 1983; FRCS Ed. 1988. Ass. Staff Grade (Gen. Surg.), Gen. Hosp., St.Helier, Jersey. Specialty: Gen. Surg. Prev: Regist. (Gen. Surg.) St. Helier Jersey.; Vis. Regist. (Gen. & Vasc. Surg.) N. Staffs. HA; Regist. (Gen. Surg.) Princess Roy. Hosp. Telford & Burton Gp Hosps.

PAI, Kasturi Ganesh Atkinson Health Centre, Market Street, Barrow-in-Furness LA14 2LR Tel: 01229 821669 — MB BS Mysore 1970. GP Barrow-in-Furness.

PAI, Mr Keshav Shrinivas Gudgeheath Lane Surgery, 187 Gudgeheath Lane, Fareham PO15 6QA Tel: 01329 280887 Fax: 01329 231321; High Pines, 30 Milvil Road, Lee-on-the-Solent PO13 9LX Tel: 01705 551700 — MB BS Karnatak 1965 (Karnatak Med. Coll. Hubli) FRCS Ed. 1970. Hosp. Pract. (Gen. Surg.) Hants. AHA (T).

PAI, Manoj Sanathan Pai and Dillon, Tile Hill Primary Health Care, Jardine Crescent, Coventry CV4 9PN Tel: 024 7646 0800 Fax: 024 7646 7512 — MB BS Bombay 1980.

PAI, Ramanath Umanath Sutherland Road Surgery, 44 Sutherland Road, Plymouth PL4 6BN Tel: 01752 662992 Fax: 01752 265538; 78 Windermere Crescent, Derriford, Plymouth PL6 5HX Tel: 01752 705702 Fax: 01752 265538 — MB BS Mysore 1966 (Kasturba Med. Coll.) DA Eng. 1972. Specialty: Gastroenterol.; Anaesth. Socs: MDU. Prev: Regist. (Anaesth.) Canad. Red Cross Hosp. Taplow, Bucks.; Clin. Asst. (Anaesth.) Bronglais Gen. Hosp. Aberystwyth, Dyfed.

PAI, Shailaja Manoj 42 Glasshouse Lane, Kenilworth CV8 2AJ — MB BS Bombay 1979; FRCS Ed. 1986.

PAI, Srinivas Hemachandra 24 Brookhus Farm Road, Walmley, Sutton Coldfield B76 1QP Tel: 0121 240 4818; 140 Coleshill Road, Hodge Hill, Birmingham B36 8AD Tel: 0121 776 6444 Fax: 0121 688 4544 — MB BS Mysore 1966 (Kasthurba Med. Coll. Manipal.) DTM & H Liverp. 1972. Princip. GP. Specialty: Dermat. Prev: Med. Regist. St. Mary's Hosp. Isle of Wight; Med. Regist. Southport Infirm.

***PAI, Sripat Kasturi** — MB BS Newc. 1998; MB BS Newc 1998.

PAI, Mr Vittaldas Panemangalore c/o 65 Herdman Close, Liverpool L25 2XS Tel: 0151 488 0181 — MB BS Mysore 1984; DO RCS Eng. 1990; FCOphth. 1991; FRCS (Ophth.) Ed. 1991. Socs:

UK Intraocular Implant Soc.; N. Eng. Ophth. Soc. Prev: Regist. Rotat. (Ophth.) Yorks. Train. Scheme.

PAICE, Brian Joseph Kenmure Medical Practice, 7 Springfield Road, Bishopbriggs, Glasgow G64 1PJ Tel: 0141 772 6309; 46 Fernlea, Bearsden, Glasgow G61 1NB Tel: 0141 772 6309 — MB ChB Glas. 1976; MRCP (UK) 1980; MRCGP 1984; FRCP Ed. 1992; FRCP Glas 1998.

PAICE, Elisabeth Willemien London Postgraduate, Medical and Dental Education, 20 Guilford St, London WC1N 1DZ Tel: 020 7692 3355 Fax: 020 7692 3396 — (Westm.) MRCS Eng. LRCP Lond. 1970; MB BCh BAO Dub. 1970; MRCP (UK) 1972; FRCP Lond. 1989; Dip. Med. Ed. Dund 1994; MA Dublin Univ. 1995. Dean Dir. Postgrad. Med. & Dent. Educat., Lond.; Vis. Prof., Fac. of Clin. Sci. Univ. Coll. Lond. Specialty: Rehabil. Med.; Rheumatol. Socs: Brit. Soc. Rheum.; Counc. Nat. Assn. Clin. Tutors (NACT); Counc. Assn. Study of Med. Educat. (ASME). Prev: Cons. Rheum. Whittington Hosp.; Sen. Regist. (Rheum.) Univ. Coll. Hosp.; Sen. Regist. (Rheum.) Stoke Mandeville Hosp.

PAIGE, David Geoffrey Dermatology Department, Royal London Hospital, Whitechapel, London E1 1BB Tel: 020 7377 7383 Fax: 020 7377 7383 — MB BS Lond. 1986; MA Camb. 1987; FRCP (UK) 2000. Cons. Dermat. Roy. Lond. Hosp. & St. Bart. Hosp. Lond. Specialty: Dermat. Prev: Sen. Regist. (Dermat.) Bristol Roy. Infirm.; Clin. Research Fell. (Dermat.) Hosp. for Sick Childr. Gt. Ormond St. Lond.; Regist. (Dermat.) St. Mary's Hosp. Lond.

PAIGE, Graham John Balmore Park Surgery, 59A Hemdean Road, Caversham, Reading RG4 7SS Tel: 0118 947 1455 Fax: 0118 946 1766 — MB BS Lond. 1984; DRCOG 1987; MRCGP 1989.

PAIGE, Helen Curtis House, Tokers Green Lane, Kidmore End, Reading RG4 9AY — MB BS Lond. 1986; DRCOG 1989; MRCP 1991.

PAIGE, Peter George Mount Street Surgery, 69 Mount Street, Coventry CV5 8DE Tel: 024 7667 2277 Fax: 024 7671 7352; 3 Bransford Avenue, Cannon Park, Coventry CV4 7EP Tel: 024 76 412594 — MB ChB Birm. 1979 (Oxford/Birmingham) MA Oxf. 1981; DRCOG 1981; FRCGP 1995, M 1983. Prev: Clin. Asst. (Psychiat.) Walsgrave Ment. Health Unit Coventry; Trainee GP Swindon VTS.

PAILTHORPE, Mr Charles Andrew Royal Berkshire Hospital, London Road, Reading RG1 5AN — MB ChB Birm. 1977; FRCS Ed. 1985. Cons. Orthop. Surg. Roy. Berks. Hosp. Reading. Specialty: Orthop.

PAILTHORPE, David Bruce Leonard (retired) North Cottage, Raughmere Drive, Lavant, Chichester PO18 0AB — MB BS Lond. 1944 (Middlx.) MRCS Eng. LRCP Lond. 1944. Prev: Regist. (Med.) & Ho. Phys. Mt. Vernon Hosp. N.wood.

PAIN, Amiya Kumar 2 Burleigh Avenue, Blackfen, Sidcup DA15 8QA Tel: 020 8859 1315 — MB BS Calcutta 1958 (Calcutta Med. Coll.) MRCP (U.K.) 1974. Lect. Infec. Dis. Guy's Hosp. & King's Coll. Hosp. Lond.; Cons. Phys. Hither Green & Guy's Hosps. Lond. Specialty: Gen. Med. Socs: Brit. Soc. Study Infec. Prev: Sen. Regist. (Infec. Dis.) St. Ann's Gen. Hosp. Lond.; Regist. (Med. Unit) Hosp. Trop. Dis. & Univ. Coll. Hosp. Lond.; Med. Regist. Dreadnought Seamen's Hosp. Greenwich.

PAIN, Ashley Nigel The Hoppit Surgery, Butts Lane, Danbury, Chelmsford CM3 4NP Tel: 01245 222518 Fax: 01245 222116; 85 Main Street, Danbury, Chelmsford CM3 4DJ Tel: 01245 225882 — MB ChB Leeds 1980; DRCOG 1986. GP Danbury; Mem. BASICS. Socs: Chelmsford Med. Soc.

PAIN, Mr James Andrew Poole Hospital NHS Trust, Longfleet Road, Poole BH15 2JB Tel: 01202 442951 Email: jamespain@poole.nhs.uk; Stourbank House, Old Ham Lane, Little Canford, Wimborne BH21 7LB Tel: 01202 872782 Fax: 01202 890158 — MB BS Lond. 1978 (Guy's Hosp.) MRCS Eng. LRCP Lond. 1978; FRCS Ed. 1981; FRCS Eng. 1981; BSc Lond. 1975, MS 1986. Cons. Surg. Poole Gen. Hosp. NHS Trust; Vis. Surg. Vict. Hosp. Wimborne. Specialty: Gen. Surg. Special Interest: Breast; Melanoma; Pancreatico-Biliary. Socs: Brit. Assn. Surg. Oncol.; Brit. Soc. Gastroenterol.; The Assn. of Surg. of Gt. Britain & Irel. Prev: Registar (Surg.) St. Geo.'s. Hosp. Lond.; Sen. Registar (Surg.) King's Coll. Hosp. Lond.

PAIN, Simon John Seafield House, Brantham, Manningtree CO11 1PT — MB BChir Camb. 1992.

PAIN, Vivian Maureen Huntsmans House, Kennel Lane, Billericay CM12 9RT Tel: 01277 658411 — MB BS Lond. 1963 (St. Bart.) MRCS Eng. LRCP Lond. 1963; DCH Eng. 1965. Sen. Regist. Nuffield Hearing & Speech Centre Roy. Nat. ENT Hosp.; Sen. Med. Off. (Audiol.) Redbridge & Waltham Forest AHA. Socs: BMA. Prev: Regist. (Paediat.) Hillingdon Hosp. Uxbridge; Ho. Off. Qu. Eliz. Hosp. Childr. Lond.

PAINE, Sir Christopher Hammon Kings Farm, Withypool, Minehead TA24 7RE Tel: 01643 831381 Fax: 01643 831508 — BM BCh Oxf. 1961 (Oxf. & St. Bart.) BSc, MA Oxf. 1961; MRCP Lond. 1964; DMRT Eng. 1967; FFR 1969; FRCR 1975; FRCP Lond. 1976; DM 1981. Trustee The Lond. Clinic; Mem. Med. Advisery Bd. Internat. Hosp.s Gp.; Past Pres. BMA (2001-02); Non Exec. Director Medicsight PLC. Specialty: Oncol. Socs: (Past-Pres.) Roy. Soc. of Med.; (Past-Pres.) BMA. Prev: Pres. Roy. Coll. of Radiologists (1992-95); Med. Director Advisery Comm. on Distinc. Awards (1994-99); Pres. Roy. Soc. of Med. (1996-98).

PAINE, David Leon Stanley Orchard Paddock, Bugbrooke, Northampton NN7 3QR Tel: 01604 832256 Fax: 01604 832256 — MB ChB Manch. 1961 (Manch.) Dip. Med. Acup. Member British Medical Acupuncture Society; MRCGP 1972; Dip. Ac. Beijing 1980; MF Hom. London 1990. Cons. in Acupunc. and Homeopathy and other Complementary Therapies. Specialty: Homeop. Med. Socs: Fac. Homoeop.; Brit. Med. Acupunct. Soc.; Brit. Soc. Med. & Dent. Hypn. Prev: GP; Hon. Cons. Acupunc. Abingdon Pain Relief Clinic Oxf.; SHO (Thoracic Surg. & Chest Dis.) Baguley Hosp. Manch.

PAINE, David Stevens 42 Newton Road, Cambridge CB2 2AL Tel: 01223 353300 — MB BChir Camb. 1948 (Middlx.) MA (Hons.) Camb. 1952, BA (Hons.) 1946, MB Bchir 1948; DPM Lond. 1966; MRC Psych 1972. Psychiat. Adviser Camb. Marriage Guid. Counc.; Hon. Asst. Psychiat. Addenbrooke's Hosp. Camb. Prev: Regist. Netherne Hosp. Coulsdon; Res. Med. Off. St. And. Hosp. Dollis Hill; Sen. Regist. Fulbourn & Addenbrooke's Hosps. Camb.

PAINE, Douglas Harold Davey Aragon, 34 Dudsbury Road, Ferndown BH22 8RE Tel: 01202 861137 — MB BS Lond. 1943 (Middlx.) MRCS Eng. LRCP Lond. 1944; DPM Eng. 1948; MRCPsych 1971. Cons. Psychiat. & Phys. Supt. Tatchbury Mt. Hosp. Calmore. Specialty: Gen. Psychiat. Socs: Fell. Roy. Soc. Med. Prev: Cons. Psychiat. & Med. Supt. St. Margt. Hosp. Birm.; Sen. Phys. Botleys Pk. Hosp. Chertsey; Regist. (Med.) Middlx. Hosp.

PAINE, Peter Andrew 974A Garratt Lane, Tooting, London SW17 0ND Tel: 020 8767 7261 — MB BS Lond. 1996 (St. Geo.) BSc 1993. Specialty: Gen. Med.

PAINE, Timothy Frank The Family Practice, Western College, Cotham Road, Bristol BS6 6DF Tel: 0117 946 6455 Fax: 0117 946 6410; 13 Limerick Road, Bristol BS6 7DY Tel: 0117 924 5332 — MB BChir Camb. 1966 (Camb. & Lond. Hosp.) BA Camb. 1962; MRCP Lond. 1968; FRCGP 1986, M 1976. Specialty: Rehabil. Med.; Rheumatol. Socs: (Vice-Pres.) Nat. Assn. Pat. Participation. Prev: Hosp. Pract. (Rheum.) Univ. Bristol; GP Clin. Tutor Bristol Roy. Infirm.; Assoc. Adviser (Gen. Pract.) Univ. Bristol.

PAINTER, Andrew Neil Station Road Surgery, 46 Station Road, New Barnet, Barnet EN5 1QH Tel: 020 8441 4425 Fax: 020 8441 4957 — MB BS Lond. 1984. Trainee GP Barnet Gen. Hosp. VTS. Prev: Ho. Surg. Friarage Hosp. Northallerton; Ho. Phys. Chase Farm Hosp. Enfield.

PAINTER, Daniel John 10 Woodcroft Drive, Wirral CH61 6XJ — MB BS Lond. 1993.

PAINTER, Gillian Elizabeth Audiology Department, Moss Side Health Centre, Monton St., Manchester M14 4GP Tel: 0161 232 4214 Fax: 0161 232 4210; 108 Wythenshawe Road, Northenden, Manchester M23 0PA Tel: 0114 2307119/0161 998 9688 — MB BS Lond. 1973 (St. Mary's) DObst RCOG 1975; MSc (Audiol. Med.) Manch. 1990; FRCPCH 1996. Cons. Community Paediat. (Audiol.) Centr. Manc. Primary Care NHS Trust. Specialty: Audiol. Med. Socs: Brit Assn Of Community Doctors in Audiol.; Brit. Assn. Of Audiological Phys.s; Brit,. Assn. Of Community Child Health. Prev: SCMO (Audiol.) Mancunian Community Health NHS Trust; SCMO N. Manch. HA; Clin. Med. Off. (Child Health) Manch. HA.

PAINTER, Michael John Infection Control And Surveilance Unit, Gateway House, Picadilly Approach, Manchester M60 7LP Tel: 0161 236 2400 — MB BS Lond. 1973 (St. Mary's) MSc Manch. 1983; MFCM 1985; FFPHM RCP (UK) 1993. Cons. Communicable Dis. Control Manch. Specialty: Pub. Health Med. Socs: Fell. Manch. Med.

Soc. Prev: Sen. Regist. (Community Med.) N. West. RHA; SCMO & Assoc. Dir. Treloar Haemophilia Centre Alton.

PAINTER, Patricia (retired) 13 Springcroft Avenue, London N2 9JH — MB BS Lond. 1954 (Roy. Free) MRCS Eng. LRCP Lond. 1954; DA Eng. 1956; FFA RCS Eng. 1958. Prev: Cons. Anaesth. Eliz. G. Anderson & Soho Hosp. for Wom. Lond.

PAINTIN, Mr David Bernard (retired) Whitecroft, Broombarn Lane, Prestwood, Great Missenden HP16 9JD — MB ChB Bristol 1954; MRCOG 1960; FRCOG 1972; FFFP (Hon.) 1993. Prev: Emerit. Reader Obst. & Gyn. Imperial Coll. Sch. Med. St. Mary's Lond.

PAIRAUDEAU, Peter William Hull Royal Infirmary, Anlaby Road, Hull HU3 2JZ Tel: 01482 328541 6 — MB ChB Bristol 1980; MRCP (UK) 1984. Cons. Paediat. Roy. Hull Hosp. NHS Trust. Specialty: Paediat.

PAIS, Victor 26 Avenue Clamart, Scunthorpe DN15 8EQ — MB BS Mysore 1973.

PAIS, Winston Alexis Treetops, 17 Wilmerhatch Lane, Epsom KT18 7EQ — MB ChB East Africa 1967 (Makerere Univ. Coll. Kampala) FFA RCS Eng. 1974. Cons. Anaesth. Epsom Dist. Hosp. Specialty: Anaesth. Prev: Rotating Sen. Regist. (Anaesth.) Brighton & Guy's Hosps.

PAISEY, Richard Bayley Torbay Hospital, Lawes Bridge, Torquay TQ2 7AA Tel: 01803 64567; Whitehill House, 18 Whitehill Road, Highweek, Newton Abbot TQ12 6PR — MD Bristol 1981 (Guy's Hospital) MB Camb. 1974, BChir 1973; MRCP (UK) 1975; FRCP (UK) 1992. Cons. Phys. & Endocrinol. Torbay Dist. Hosp. Specialty: Endocrinol.; Diabetes. Socs: Brit. Diabetic Assn.; Eur. Assn. Study Diabetes. Prev: Lect. (Med.) Univ. of Bristol; Regist. (Med.) Northwick Pk. Hosp.; SHO (Med.) Soton. Gen. Hosp.

PAISH, Nicholas Robert, Squadron Ldr. RAF Med. Br. RAF Centre of Aviation Medicine, RAF Henlow SG16 6DL — MB BS Lond. 1988 (UCL) DCCH RCP Ed. 1992; MRCGP 1994; Dip Av Med 2000. Lect. Aviat. Med. Train. Wing.

PAISLEY, Andrew Charles East Quay Medical Centre, East Quay, Bridgwater TA6 5YB Tel: 01278 444666 — MB ChB Bristol 1988; PhD Bristol 1982, MB ChB 1988; T(GP) 1994. Trainee GP Bridgwater.

PAISLEY, Miss Anna Mary 15 Alnwickhill Park, Liberton, Edinburgh EH16 6UH — BM BCh Oxf. 1993 (Oxford) MA Oxford; FRCS (Ed.) 1998. Res. Fell. (Gen. Surg.) Roy. Infirm. Edin. Specialty: Gen. Surg. Prev: SHO (Basic Surg. Train. Scheme) SE Scotl.

PAISLEY, Jane Menzies 62 Stanford Avenue, Brighton BN1 6FD Tel: 01273 553837 — MB ChB Sheff. 1984; MRCP (UK) 1991. Cons. in Med. for the elderly. Specialty: Care of the Elderly.

PAISLEY, Jennifer Ann Dromore Doctors' Surgery, 50 Gallows Street, Dromore BT25 1BD Tel: 028 9269 2758; 9 Barronstown Court, Barronstown Road, Dromore BT25 1FB Tel: 01846 699454 — MB BCh BAO Belf. 1987; DRCOG 1991; MRCGP 1991; DMH Belf. 1992. Socs: BMA; RCGP. Prev: Trainee GP HillsBoro., Co. Down; SHO Lagan Valley Hosp. Lisburn & Belvoir Pk. Hosp. Belf.

PAISLEY, Jonathan MacGregor Glenwood Health Centre, Napier Road, Glenrothes KY6 1HL Tel: 01592 611171 Fax: 01592 611931 — MB ChB Ed. 1984; DObst Auckland 1988; MRCGP 1989. Clin. Asst. - Culposcopy; Clin., Forth Pk. Hosp., Kirkialoy.

PAISLEY, Thomas Allan 16 Branning Court, Kirkcaldy KY1 2PD — MB ChB Glas. 1974.

PAJOVIC, Slav Barton Surgery, Barton Terrace, Dawlish EX7 9QH Tel: 01626 888877 Fax: 01626 888360; Larkbeare Farm, Mamhead, Kenton, Exeter EX6 8HQ Tel: 01626 866297 — MB BS Lond. 1979 (Middlx.) MRCGP 1983.

PAJWANI, Kishor Shamlal Sydenham House, Monkswick Road, Harlow CM20 3NT Tel: 01279 424075 Fax: 01279 423936; 17 Walbrook, Woodford Road, South Woodford, London E18 2EG Tel: 020 8989 4456 — MB BS Karnatak 1959; BSc (Hons.) Bombay 1952; LMSSA Lond. 1965. Hon. Adviser (Gen. Pract. Study) Kasturba Med. Coll. Manipal, India. Prev: Regist. (Chest Dis.) Kelling Hosp. Holt; Regist. (Geriat.) N.gate Hosp. Gt. Yarmouth; Ho. Surg. Dreadnought Seamens Hosp. Greenwich.

PAKARIAN, Bouzourgmehr Farzin 27 Greenlaw Court, 1A Mount Park Road, London W5 2RX — MB ChB Leic. 1988.

PAKENHAM, Ralph William Medical Centre, 12 High Street, Fochabers IV32 7EP Tel: 01343 820247 Fax: 01343 820132 — MRCS Eng. LRCP Lond. 1975.

PAKENHAM-WALSH, Neil Martin International Network for the Availability of Scientific Publications, 58 St Aldates, Oxford OX1 1ST Email: health@inasp.info; International Network for the Availability of Scientific Publications, 27 Park End St., Oxford OX1 1HU Tel: 01865 249909 Fax: 01865 251060 Email: inasp-health@gn.apc.org — MB BS Lond. 1983; DRCOG 1986; DCH 1988.

PAKOULAS, Ms Christina Anthoula Emily (retired) 17 Homefield Road, Radlett WD7 8PX — MB BS Lond. 1984 (Charing Cross Hospital Medical School) BSc (Hons.) Basic Med. Scs. & Physiol. Lond. 1981; FRCS Ed. (Ophth.) 1991. Prev: Specialist Regist. (Ophth.) Moorfields Eye Hosp. Lond.

PAKTSUN, Lam Wai-Ping 8 Rose Court, Sherwood Road, Harrow HA2 8UU — MB BS Ceylon 1964; DA Eng. 1976. Assoc. Specialist (Anaesth.) Mid Essex HA. Prev: Regist. (Anaesth.) Joyce Green Hosp. Dartford; Regist. (Anaesth.) Chelmsford Health Dist.

PAL, Abani Kumar (retired) Shanti, 27 Plastirion Avenue, Prestatyn LL19 9DU — (R.G. Kar Med. Coll.) MB BS Calcutta 1958; MB BS Calcutta 1958; FICS 1988; FFAEM 1993. Cons. A & E Dept. Glan Clwyd Hosp. Rhyl. Prev: Resid. St. Vincent's Hosp. New York City, USA.

PAL, Ajita c/o Dr G. S. Pal, Horsham Hospital, Hurst Road, Horsham RH12 2DR — MRCS Eng. LRCP Lond. 1980.

PAL, Babi Rani 19 Warrington Close, Foxhollies Meadow, Walmley, Sutton Coldfield B76 2BL — MB ChB Glas. 1984; MRCP (UK) 1988. SHO (Neonat.) St. Mary's Hosp. Manch.

PAL, Badal Department of Rheumatology, R10H4, Withington Hospital, Manchester M20 2LR Tel: 0161 611 4283 Fax: 0161 445 5631 Email: badal.pal@smuht.nwest.nhs.uk; 7 Poolcroft, The Nurseries, Sale Moor, Manchester M33 2LF Tel: 0161 973 6304 Fax: 0161 445 5631 Email: bpal@fs1.with.man.ac.uk — MB BS Calcutta 1975; MRCP (UK) 1979; MD Newc. 1988; FRCP Lond. 1996; FRCP Ed. 1998. Cons. Rheum. & Withington Hosp. Manch.; Hon. Lect. (Rheum.) Univ. Manch. Specialty: Rheumatol. Socs: BMA; Brit. Soc. Rheum.; FRCP Lond. Edin. Prev: Sen. Regist. Roy. Vict. Infirm. Newc. & Durh.; Regist. (Med.) Wythenshawe Hosp. Manch.

PAL, Cauvery — MB BS Lond. 1996 (UMDS, Guy's & St. Thos.) BSc Lond. 1993; MRPCH 2000. Specialist Regist. Paediat. N. Middlx. Univ. Hosp. Lond. Specialty: Paediat.

PAL, Chhabi Rani 16 Chaldon Green, Lychpit, Basingstoke RG24 8YS Tel: 01256 471979 — MB BS Lond. 1985; BSc Lond. 1982, MB BS 1985; MRCP (UK) 1988. Sen. Regist. (Radiol.) John Radcliffe Hosp. Oxf. Specialty: Radiol.

PAL, Mr Dharam 1 Killowen Avenue, Northolt UB5 4QT — MB BS Delhi 1968 (Maulana Azad Med. Coll.) FRCS Glas. 1983. SHO (Gen. Surg.) Warrington Infirm.

PAL, Guru Saday c/o Dr P. Dasgupta, 54 Abbotts Park Road, London E10 6HX — MB BS Calcutta 1974 (Calcutta Med. Coll.) MRCP (UK) 1983. Regist. (Haemat.) Clatterbridge Hosp. Wirral. Specialty: Haematology. Prev: Regist. (Gen. Med.) War Memor. Hosp. Wrexham; Regist. (Geriat. Med.) Leicester Gen. Hosp.; SHO (Gen. Med.) Dewsbury Gen. Hosp.

PAL, Madhu 1 Killowen Avenue, Northolt UB5 4QT Tel: 020 8864 7141 — MB BS Rajasthan 1974 (Ravinder Nath Tagore Med. Coll. Udaipur) DRCOG 1984; DObst RCPI 1984. SHO (O & G) Chorley Dist. Hosp.

PAL, Paragprasun Group Practice Surgery, 33 Newton Road, Great Barr, Birmingham B43 6AA Tel: 0121 357 1690 Fax: 0121 357 4253 — MB BS Calcutta 1976; MB BS Calcutta 1976.

PAL, Prasanta Kumar 91 Mossfield Road, Kings Heath, Birmingham B14 7JE Tel: 0121 444 2242; 48 Sellywick Drive, Selly Park, Birmingham B29 7JH Tel: 0121 414 1987 — (Calcutta) MB BS Calcutta 1959; DA Delhi 1964; FFA RCSI 1974. Indep. Pract. Cons. Anaesth. W. Midl. Specialty: Anaesth. Socs: Assn. Anaesths. Prev: Cons. Anaesth. North. RHA; Regist. (Anaesth.) Roy. Vict. Hosp. Belf.; Sen. Regist. (Anaesth.) Belf. City Hosp.

PAL, Rama Six Dials Surgery, 130-131 St. Marys Road, Southampton SO14 0BB Tel: 023 8033 5151 Fax: 023 8033 9677 — (Culcutta) MB BS Calcutta 1974. GP Soton.

PAL, Sandip Kumar 1 Vale Court, The Vale, Stock, Ingatestone CM4 9PX — MB BS Delhi 1977.

PAL, Santosh Kumar 65 Disraeli Road, London E7 9JU Tel: 020 8534 4388 Fax: 0208 5344388 — MB BS Calcutta 1963 (Med. Coll. Calcutta) BSc Calcutta 1954. MQPM Appeals Serv. Lord Chancellors Dept Lond; Locum. GP Upton La. Med. Centre, Forest

Gate Lond. E7 9PB. Specialty: Rehabil. Med.; Rheumatol. Socs: Companion Fell. BOA; Soc. Occupat. Med. Lond.; Fell. Hunt. Soc. Prev: Exam. Med. Off. Disablem. Servs. Auth.; Med. Off. i/c Balham & Kingston Appliances Centres DHSS; Med. Off. Limb-Fitting Centre Qu. Mary's Hosp. Roehampton.

PAL, Saphal Kanti Royton Medical Centre, Rochdale Road, Royton, Oldham OL2 5QB Tel: 0161 624 4857 Fax: 0161 628 5010 — MB BS Calcutta 1965.

PAL, Sheena The Health Centre, Whyteman's Brae, Kirkcaldy KY1 2NA Tel: 01592 640600 Fax: 01592 641462.

PAL, Sipra Brinnington Road Surgery, 30-32 Brinnington Road, Stockport SK1 2EX Tel: 0161 480 4164 Fax: 0161 476 1996.

PAL, Uday 3 Index Drive, Dunstable LU6 3TU — MB BS Calcutta 1969.

PALACCI, Alain Edward The Surgery, 22 Castelnau, Barnes, London SW13 9RU Tel: 020 8748 7574 Fax: 020 8563 8821 — MB BS Lond. 1986. Assoc. Specialist Diabetic Unit Qu. Mary Hosp. Roehampton; Chairm. Therap. Comm. Richmond PCG.

PALACE, Jacqueline Ann Clinical Neurology, Radcliffe Infirmary, Woodstock Road, Oxford OX2 6HE Tel: 01865 224310 Fax: 01865 790493 — BM Soton. 1983; MRCP (UK) 1986; DM 1992. Cons. (Neurol.) Oxf. RHA. Specialty: Neurol.

PALANIAPPAN, Rudrapathy Consultant in Audiological Medicine, Royal National Throat & Nose & Ear Hospital, Gray's Inn Road, London WC1X 8DA Tel: 020 7915 1559 Fax: 020 7915 1483 — MB BS Madras 1986 (Jawaharlal Insitutue of Post-graduate Medical Education & Research) DLO Madras 1985; PLAB, UK 1990; DLO Eng. 1991; FRCS Edin. 1995. Cons Audiologist Phys. Roy. Nat. Throat,Nose & Ear Hosp., Gray's Inn Rd. Lond.; Hon. Sen. Lect., Univ. Coll. Lond. Specialty: Audiol. Med. Socs: Brit. Soc. Audiol.; RCS Edin.; BMA. Prev: Locum Cons., RTNE Hosp., Lond.; Locum Cons., GOSH for Childr., Lond.; Sen. Regist., St. Georges' Hosp., Lond.

PALANIAPPAN, Selambaram Moorfield Road Health Centre, 2 Moorfield Road, Enfield EN3 5PS Tel: 020 8804 1522 Fax: 020 8443 1465 — MB BS Ceylon 1968; DCH Ceylon 1974; MRCOG 1980. GP Enfield. Specialty: Gen. Pract. Socs: BMA. Prev: Regional Co-ordinator Rural Health Support Project Sudan (USAID Project).

PALAZZO, Mr Francesco Fausto Department of Endocrine Surgery, Timone Hospital, Marseille, France — State Exam Med Bari 1992; FRCS Eng. 1997; FRSCI 1997; MS Lond. 2002. Specialty: Gen. Surg. Socs: Internat. Assn. of Endocrine Surgeons; Assn. of Surgeons of Gt. Britain and Irel.; Brit. Assn. of Endocrine Surgeons. Prev: TS Reeve Fell. in Endocrine Surg., Roy. N. Shore, Sydney, Australia; SpR Endocrine Surg., John Radcliffe Hosp., Oxf.

PALAZZO, Mark George Anthony Division of Clinical Care Medicine, Charing Cross Hospital, Fulham Palace Road, London W6 8RF — MB ChB Bristol 1975; MRCP (UK) 1978; FFA RCS Eng. 1982; MD Bristol 1989; FRCP Lond. 1995. Dir. (Intens. Care) Char. Cross Hosp. Lond. Specialty: Intens. Care.

PALCHAUDHURI, Mihir Ranjan Crosshouse Hospital, Kilmarnock KA2 0BE — MB BS Calcutta 1972; MD All India Med. Scs. 1977; MRCP UK 1983. Cons. Phys. (Geriat. Med.) Ayrsh. & Arran Acute Hosps. NHS Trust. Specialty: Gen. Med. Prev: Locum Cons. Phys. Roy. Free Hosp. Lond.; Cons. Phys. (Gen. Med.) Saudi Arabia; Regist. (Gen. Med.) St Ann's Hosp. Lond.

PALCZYNSKI, Stephen Hunter Newlands Medical Centre, Borough Road, Middlesbrough TS1 3RX Tel: 01642 247401 Fax: 01642 223803; 106 Low Lane, Middlesbrough TS5 8EB Tel: 01642 593657 — MB BS Newc. 1969; DObst RCOG 1972; DCH RCPS Glas. 1973; MRCGP 1974; FRCGP 1997. Princip. in Pract.; Year Tutor & Course Organiser Cleveland VTS; Trainer (Gen. Pract.) Cleveland. Specialty: Child & Adolesc. Psychiat. Socs: BMA & Med. Defence Union; Exec. Comm. Middlesbrough PCT. Prev: Hosp. Pract. (Child & Family Psychiat.) N. Tees Gen. Hosp. Stockton-on-Tees; Police Surg. Cleveland Constab.; Trainee GP Newc. VTS.

PALEJWALA, Altaf Ali 27 Cherry Vale, Liverpool L25 5PX — MB ChB Liverp. 1991. Specialist Regist., Gastroenterol.

PALEY, Helen Walnut Lodge Surgery, Walnut Road, Chelston, Torquay TQ2 6HP Tel: 01803 605359 Fax: 01803 605772; Venton Lodge, Dartington, Totnes TQ9 6DP Tel: 01364 73382 — MB BS Newc. 1988 (New. u. Tyne) DRCOG 1992; MRCGP 1993. Prev: GP Newc.

PALEY, Judith Dorothy 11 Rodgersfield, Langho, Blackburn BB6 8HB — MB ChB Aberd. 1995.

PALEY, Mark Robert Department of Radiology, Frimley Park Hospital, Portsmouth Road, Frimley, Camberley GU16 7UJ Tel: 01276 604370 Fax: 01276 604546; 9 Portside, Brighton Marina Village, Brighton BN2 5UW Tel: 01273 605806 Email: paleym@globalnet.co.uk — BM BCh Oxf. 1988 (Oxford) BA Oxf. 1985, BM BCh 1988; FRCR 1995. Cons. Radiol. Frimley Pk. Hosp. Surrey; Hon. Cons. Radiol. KCH Lond. Specialty: Radiol. Socs: Fell. Roy. Coll. Radiol.; Radiol. Soc. N. Amer. Prev: Fell. (Body Imaging & MRI) Univ. of Florida Gainesville USA; Sen. Regist. (Radiol.) King's Coll. Hosp. Lond.

PALEY, Martin Douglas 11 Rogersfield, Langho, Blackburn BB6 8HB — MB ChB Aberd. 1997.

PALEY, Mr William George (retired) 11 Rogers Field, Langho, Blackburn BB6 8HB Tel: 01254 240124 — MB ChB Ed. 1958; FRCS Ed. 1967; FRCS Eng. 1969. Prev: Cons. Surg. (Gen. & Vasc. Surg.) Blackburn & Dist. Gp. Hosps.

PALFERMAN, Thomas George Yeovil District Hospital, Higher Kingston, Yeovil BA21 4AT Tel: 01935 384302 Fax: 01935 384302 Email: palft@est.nhs.uk — MB BS Lond. 1971 (Char. Cross) MRCS Eng. LRCP Lond. 1971; DCH Eng. 1974; DObst RCOG 1974; MRCP (UK) 1977; FRCP Lond. 1992. Cons. Phys. & Rheum. Yeovil Dist. Hosp. Som.; Scientif. Adviser Nat. Osteoporosis Soc.; Expert Advisor to NICE; Chair Clin. Affairs Comm. No. of Council & Exec of Brit. Soc for Rheum. Treasurer Authority & Alliance. Specialty: Rheumatol. Socs: MRCP Exam. RCP Lond.; Fell. Roy. Soc. Med. (Counc. Sect. Rheum.); (Counc.) Brit. Soc. Rheum. (Pres-Elect.). Prev: Sen. Regist. Rotat. (Gen. Med. & Rheum.) St. Bart. Hosp. Lond.; Regist. (Rheum.) St. Thos. Hosp. Lond.; Regist. (Med. & Neurol.) Westm. Hosp. Lond.

PALFRAMAN, Anthony Heathgate Surgery, The Street, Poringland, Norwich NR14 7JT Tel: 01508 494343; 120 The St, Rockland St. Mary, Norwich NR14 7HQ Tel: 01508 537190 — MB BS Lond. 1979; DRCOG 1987; MRCGP 1988. Prev: Med. Regist. Roy. Cornw. Hosps.

PALFREEMAN, Adrian John The Cottage, Caldecott, Cheveston, Wellingborough NN9 6AR Tel: 01933 460807 Fax: 01933 460807 — MB ChB Sheff. 1985; FRCPI 2002. Cons. (Genitourin. Med.) PeterBoro. Dist. Hosp.; Clin. Tutor PeterBoro. Dist. Hosp. Specialty: Genitourinary Medicine. Socs: Assn. Genitourin. Med.; Council Med. Soc. Study VD; Brit. HIV Assn. Prev: Sen. Regist. (Genitourin. Med.) Leicester Roy. Infirm.; Regist. (Genitourin. Med. & HIV) Westm. Hosp. Lond.; SHO Rotat. (Med.) Leicester Gp. Hosps.

PALFREEMAN, Roger Adam Olive House, Black Lane, Loxley, Sheffield S6 6SE Tel: 0114 234 3082 — MB ChB Sheff. 1997.

PALFREMAN, Timothy Mark 4 Loudhams Road, Little Chalfront, Amersham HP7 9NY — MB BS Lond. 1996.

PALFREY, Alec John 146 Hurlingham Road, London SW6 3NG Tel: 020 7736 2013 — (Univ. Coll. Hosp.) MB BChir Camb. 1951; MA Camb. 1950, MD 1975. Emerit. Reader (Func.al Morphol.) Char. Cross & Westm. Med. Sch. Lond. Specialty: Anat. Socs: FRMS; Anat. Soc.; Brit. Assn. Clin. Anat. Prev: Sen. Lect. (Anat.) & Dir. Electron Microscope Unit Arthritis Rheum Counc. St. Thos. Hosp. Lond.; Lect. (Anat.) Univ. Coll., Ibadan.

PALFREY, Mr Edward Leslie Hinton Shepp House, Hamlash Lane, Frensham, Farnham GU10 3AU Tel: 01252 793481 Fax: 01252 793481 — MB BChir Camb. 1977 (St. Mary's) MA, MB Camb. 1977, BChir 1976; FRCS Eng. 1980; FRCS Ed. 1980. Cons. Urol. Frimley Pk. Hosp. Surrey; Hon. Cons. Urol. Guy's & St. Thos. Hosp. Lond.; Med. Dir., Frimley Pk. Hosp. NHS Trust. Specialty: Urol. Socs: Brit. Assn. Urol. Surg.; BSFE; BAUS - Sect. of Oncol. Prev: Sen. Regist. (Urol.) St. Thos. Hosp. Lond.; Asst. Dir. Lithotripter Centr. St. Thos. Hosp. Lond.; Research Fell. St. Thos. Hosp. Lond.

PALFREY, Penelope Ann (retired) 4 Sheaf Cottages, Weston Green, Thames Ditton KT7 0JR Tel: 020 8398 9209 — MB BChir Camb. 1951 (St. Thos.) BA Cantab 1948; BA Camb. 1951. Prev: Research Asst. (Anat.) Univ. Coll. Ibadan.

PALIA, Satnam Singh (retired) — MB BS Guru Nanak Dev 1976 (Med. Coll. Amritsar, India) Cert. Med. & Law; DPM Eng. 1980; FRCPsych 1996, M 1981. Consultant Psychiatrist, Adult Psychiatry, Princess of Wales Hospital, Bridgend; Assoc. Director, Ment. Health Servs. (Sessional). Prev: Cons. Psychiat. Old Age, Pontypridd 1999-2002.

PALIN, Alastair Noel c/o The Ross Clinic, Royal Cornhill Hospital, Aberdeen AB25 2ZF — MB ChB Aberd. 1982; MRCPsych 1987. Cons. Gen. Adult Psychiat. Grampian HB. Specialty: Gen. Psychiat. Prev: Sen. Regist. (Psychiat.) Grampian HB; Regist. (Psychiat.) Lothian HB.

PALIN, Christopher Garden Flat, 15 Kitto Road, London SE14 5TW — MB ChB Birm. 1987.

PALIN, Christopher Anthony 19 Rylett Crescent, London W12 9RP — MB BS Lond. 1996.

PALIN, Donald John St Budeaux Health Centre, Stirling Road, St. Budeaux, Plymouth PL5 1PL Tel: 01752 361010 Fax: 01752 350675; 387 Fort Austin Avenue, Eggbuckland, Plymouth PL6 5TG Tel: 01752 788640 — MB BS Lond. 1972 (Guy's Hospital) MRCS Eng. LRCP Lond. 1973. Prev: SHO (Paediat.) St. Richards Hosp. Chichester; SHO (O & G) Lewisham Hosp. Lond.

PALIN, Iain Stuart Clarendon Medical, 35 Northland Avenue, Londonderry BT48 7JW Tel: 028 7126 5391 Fax: 028 7126 5932 — MB ChB Ed. 1973; BSc (Hons.) Ed. 1970, MB ChB 1973. Prev: Regist. (Med.) Raigmore Hosp. Inverness; SHO (Med.) Roy Infirm. Edin.

PALIN, Jonathan Ashley Broomwood Road Surgery, 41 Broomwood Road, St Paul's Cray, Orpington BR5 2JP Tel: 01689 832454 Fax: 01689 826165; 13 Henham Gardens, East Peckham, Tonbridge TN12 5PD Tel: 01622 871176 — MB ChB Sheff. 1989; DRCOG 1994; MRCGP 1996.

PALIN, Peter Haydn 17 Rowland Lane, Thornton-Cleveleys FY5 2QX — MB ChB St. And. 1965; DA Eng. 1968; FFA RCS Eng. 1969. Cons. (Anaesth.) Vict. Hosp. Blackpool. Specialty: Anaesth.

PALIN, Richard David 6 Morland Avenue, Leicester LE2 2PE — MB ChB Leic. 1991.

PALIN, Stephen John 19 Pencae, Llandegfan, Menai Bridge LL59 5TT — MB ChB Liverp. 1996.

PALIN, Suzanne Lydia Dept. Of Medicine, Univ. Of Birmingham, Queen Elizabeth Hospital, Edgbaston, Birmingham B15 Email: S.L.Palin@bham.ac.uk — MB ChB Birm. 1994; MRCP 1998; MD Birm. 2003. Special Interest: diabetes and Endocrinol.

PALIT, Arabinda 'Hillside', Cox Hill, Narberth SA67 8EH Tel: 01834860268 — MB BS Calcutta 1960 (N.R.S. Med. Coll.) DCH Eng. 1964; FRCP Ed. 1983, M 1967. Cons. Paediat. Withybush Gen. Hosp. HaverfordW.. Specialty: Paediat.

PALIT, Jayanta Department of Rheumatology, Basildon Hospital, Basildon SS16 5NL Tel: 01268 593397 Fax: 01268 593799; Department of Rheumatology, Orsett Hospital, Orsett, Grays RM16 3EU Tel: 01268 552267 Fax: 01268 592318 — MB BS Calcutta 1971; MD All India Inst. Med. Scs. New Delhi 1976; MRCP (UK) 1982; FRCP Lond. 1997. Cons. Rheum. Basildon Hosp. & Orsett Hosp. Specialty: Rheumatol. Socs: Brit. Soc. for Rheum. (B.S.R). Prev: Sen. Regist. (Rheum.) Withington Gen. Hosp. & Manch. Roy. Infirm.; Clin. Research Fell. (Rheum.) N. Gen. Univ. Edin.; Sen. Resid. (Rheum.) Dalhousie Univ. Halifax, Nova Scotia.

PALIT, Sanjit Lynwood Medical Centre, Lynwood Drive, 2A-6 Collier Row, Romford RM5 3QL Tel: 01708 743244 Fax: 01708 736783 — MB BS Calcutta 1976; LRCP LRCS Ed. LRCPS Glas. 1986.

PALIT, Tarun Department of Anaesthetics, Pilgrim Hospital, Sibsey Road, Boston PE21 9QS Tel: 01205 364801 Fax: 01205 442076 — MB BS Mithila U, India 1981; MD (Anaesth.) Patna Univ. 1990; FFARCS (Irel.) 1998. Staff Grade (Anaesth.) Pilgrim Hosp. Boston. Specialty: Anaesth. Socs: BMA. Prev: Vis. Regist. (Anaesth.) Pilgrim Hosp. Boston; SHO (Anaesth. & IC) Pilgrim Hosp. Boston; SHO (Anaesth. & Intens.. Care) Geo. Eliot Hosp. Nuneaton & Kettering Gen. Hosp.

PALIWALA, Abdulali Hasanali Potter Street, Harlow CM17 9BG; Osler House, Potter St, Harlow CM17 9BQ Tel: 01279 422664 Fax: 01279 422576 — MB BS Lond. 1968 (Univ. Coll. Hosp.) MRCS Eng. LRCP Lond. 1968; DCH Eng. 1971; MRCP (UK) 1974; FRCGP 1996, M 1979. Specialty: Gen. Pract. Prev: Course Organiser W. Essex GP VTS; Examr. MRCGP; Regist. (Paediat.) Qu. Mary's Hosp. Childr. Carshalton.

PALL, Abeed Ahmed 132 Hook rise N., Surbiton KT6 7JU — MB ChB Dundee 1984.

PALL, Joginder The Surgery, Tinchbourne Street, Dudley DY1 1RH Tel: 01384 235540 Fax: 01384 458135; The Old Vicarage House, Vicarage Lane, Pensnett, Brierley Hill DY5 4JH Tel: 01384 262929 — MB BS Punjab 1968 (Govt. Med. Coll. Patiala) MB BS Punjabi 1968.

PALL, Navnit Kaur The Smethwick Medical Centre, Regent Street, Smethwick, Warley B66 3BQ — (Medical College, Lohrak, India) MB BS Maharshi Dayanand 1982; MB BS Maharshi Dayanand 1982; MRCS Eng. LRCP London 1991.

PALLAN, Arvind 2 Derby Road, Bramcote, Nottingham NG9 3BA — MB ChB Birm. 1997.

PALLAN, Joginder Pal 2 Derby Road, Bramcote, Nottingham NG9 3BA Tel: 0115 925 4674 — MB ChB Manch. 1966; DMRD Eng. 1972; FRCR 1976. Cons. Radiol. Derby City Gen. Hosp. Specialty: Radiol. Prev: Sen. Regist. & Regist. Gen. & City Hosps. Nottm.; SHO Roy. Manch. Childr. Hosp.

PALLANT, Eirwen Anne 56 Pickurst Lane, Bromley BR2 7JF; 45 Ravenswood crescent, West Wickham BR4 0JH — MB ChB Leeds 1986; BSc (Hons.) Physiol. Leeds 1983; DTM & H RCP Lond. 1992; MRCGP Lond. 1993. Med. Off. Salvation Army Hosp. Chikankata, Mazabuka, Zambia. Specialty: Gen. Pract.

PALLANT, Julia Madeleine Alexandra Surgery, 2 Wellington Avenue, Aldershot GU11 1SD Tel: 01252 332210 Fax: 01252 312490; 45 Bridgefield, Farnham GU9 8AW — MB ChB Birm. 1981; DCH RCP Lond. 1984; DRCOG 1985; MRCGP 1986.

PALLAWELA, Mr Gunasiri D S Pallawela and Partners, Belmont Health Centre, 516 Kenton Lane, Kenton, Harrow HA3 7LT Tel: 020 8863 6863 Fax: 020 8863 9815; Red House, 188 Headstone Lane, North Harrow, Harrow HA2 6LY Tel: 020 8907 6046 — MB BS Ceylon 1957 (Colombo) FRCS Ed. 1968. Police Surg. Metrop. Police.

PALLECAROS, Anna Sotira 30 Rollscourt Avenue, Herne Hill, London SE24 0EA — MB BS Lond. 1988; BSc (Hist. of Med.) Lond. 1985; MRCP (UK) 1991; DTM & H RCP Lond. 1992; Cert. Family Plann. JCC 1993. Sen. Regist. (GUM & HIV) St. Mary's Hosp. Lond. Specialty: Genitourinary Medicine. Socs: Hellenic Med. Soc.; Med. Soc. Study VD. Prev: Clin. Research Fell. (Genitourin. Med.) St. Mary's Hosp. Lond.; Regist. Univ. Coll. Hosp. Sexual Health Clinic. Lond.

PALLETT, Ann Patricia Public Health Laboratory Service, Level B, South Laboratory Block, Southampton General Hospital, Southampton SO16 6YD Tel: 023 8079 6408 — MB BS Lond. 1978 (University College Hospital London) FRCPath; BSc (1st cl. Hons.) Lond. 1975; MRCPath 1986. Cons. Med. Microbiol. Soton. & SW Hants. AHA. Specialty: Med. Microbiol. Prev: Sen. Regist. (Med. Microbiol.) Rotat. St. Richards Hosp. Chichester & St. Geo. Hosp. Lond; Regist. (Med. Microbiol.) Westm. Hosp. Lond.

PALLETT, Joan Lesley 9 The Glebe, Church Road, Copthorne, Crawley RH10 3RP Tel: 01342 713756 — MB BS Lond. 1967 (Univ. Coll. Hosp.) DA Eng. 1969; FFA RCS Eng. 1972; Dip. Pharma. Med. RCP Lond. 1993; FFPM RCP(UK) 2001. Sen. Med. Assessor Medicines Control Agency UK. Specialty: Pharmaceutical Medicine. Prev: Med. Adviser, Novartis Consumer Health; Assoc. Specialist (Anaesth.) Qu. Vict. Hosp. E. Grinstead.; Sen. Clin. Phys. Bibra Internat. Carshalton.

PALLETT, Joyce Mary (retired) 36 Majorfield Road, Topsham, Exeter EX3 0ES — MB BS Lond. 1955 (Univ. Coll. Hosp.) DObst RCOG 1958; DPM Eng. 1971; MRCPsych 1972. Prev: Cons. Psychiat. Centr. Hosp. Warwick.

PALLIS, Doros John 191A Bravington Road, Maida Vale, London W9 3AR Tel: 0208 9687883 — Ptychio Iatrikes (Distinc.) Athens 1964; DPM Eng. 1968; Dip. Psychother. Aberd. 1970; FRCPsych 1994, M 1973; MD (Commendat.) Aberd. 1977; Cert. Neuropsychiat. 1979. Cons. Psychiat. Med. Mem., Ment. Health Review Tribunal. Specialty: Gen. Psychiat. Prev: Scientif. Off. MRC Clin. Psychiat. Unit; Sen. Regist. Graylingwell Hosp. Chichester; Scientif. Dir. Dept. Social Psychiat. Inst. Child Health Athens.

PALLISTER, Deirdre Heather 4 King Edward Close, Christ's Hospital, Horsham RH13 0LX Tel: 01403 267159 — MB BS Lond. 1983. SCMO & Breast Phys. Jarvis Breast Screening Centre Guildford. Specialty: Orthop. Prev: Med. Off. (Orthop.) King Edwd. VII Hosp. Midhurst; Sen. Regist. (Pub. Health Med.) W. Midl. RHA.

PALLISTER, Ian 4 St. Margaret's Road, Whitchurch, Cardiff CF14 7AA Email: ianpallister@hotmail.com — MB BS Newc. 1989; FRCS (Eng) 1993; MMedSci Birm. 1995. Specialty: Trauma & Orthop. Surg.

PALLISTER, Michael Alan, Air Commodore RAF Med. Br. (retired) Abbascombe Barn, Lily Lane, Templecombe BA8 0HN Tel: 01963

371163 — MRCS Eng. LRCP Lond. 1955 (Camb. & St. Thos.) BChir 1955, MB 1956; DTM & H Liverp. 1958; DPH Lond. 1963; DIH Eng. 1963; MRCGP 1975; MFOM RCP Lond. 1981; FFCM RCP (UK) 1989; MA Contab. 1992. Station Commdr. Princess Alexandra Hosp. RAF Wroughton; Cons. Community Med. RAF.

PALLISTER, William Knott (retired) 21 Denewood Road, Highgate, London N6 4AQ Tel: 020 8340 8438; (resid.), 21 Denewood Road, Highgate, London N6 4AQ Tel: 020 8340 8438 — (King's Coll. Lond. & Westm.) MB BS Lond. 1949; DA Eng. 1951; FFA RCS Eng. 1955; DHMSA Lond. 1978. Emerit. Cons. Anaesth. Middlx. Hosp. & Hosp. Wom. Soho; Hon. Sen. Lect. Univ. Coll. & Middlx. Sch. Med.; Emerit. Hon. Cons. Anaesth. Hosp. St. John & Eliz. Prev: Jt. Sen. Regist. (Anaesth.) Brompton Hosp. Dis. Chest & Westm. Hosp. Lond.

PALLOT, Doreen Betty (retired) 36 Parkway, Welwyn Garden City AL8 6HQ Tel: 01707 323115 — MB BS Lond. 1949 (King's Coll. Lond. & W. Lond.) MRCS Eng. LRCP Lond. 1949; DA Eng. 1952; FFA RCS Eng. 1955. Hon. Cons. Anaesth. Roy. Nat. Throat, Nose & Ear Hosp, & Moorfields Eye Hosp. Prev: Regist. (Anaesth.) Hosp. Sick Childr. Gt. Ormond St.

PALMER, Mr Alan (retired) 7 Wise Close, Beverley HU17 9GR Tel: 01482 873867 Fax: 01482 873867 — (Guy's) MB BS Lond. 1964; MRCS Eng. LRCP Lond. 1964; DObst RCOG 1967; FRCOG 1985, M 1972. Prev: Cons. O & G Hull Health Dist.

PALMER, Alan Charles HMS Herald BFPO 296 — MB ChB Leic. 1990.

PALMER, Alastair Anderson Teviot Medical Practice, Hawick Health Centre, Teviot Road, Hawick TD9 9DT Tel: 01450 370999 Fax: 01450 371025; Newmill House, Hawick TD9 9UQ — MB ChB Glas. 1982.

PALMER, Alison Rachel Boundary House Medical Centre, 462 Northenden Road, Sale M33 2RH — MB ChB Birm. 1995 (Birmingham) DCH Lond. 1998; DRCOG Lond. 1998; MRCGP Lond. 1999; DFFP Lond. 1999. GP Chesh. Specialty: Gen. Pract.

PALMER, Andrew Barlborough Medical Practice, The Old Malthouse, 7 Worksop Road, Barlborough, Chesterfield S43 4TY Tel: 01246 819994 — MB ChB Leic. 1984; MRCGP 1988; DRCOG 1988. GP Chesterfield.

PALMER, Andrew Bernard David St. Mary's Hospital, Renal Unit, Praed St., Paddington, London W2 1NY Tel: 020 7886 1615 Fax: 020 7402 7784; Studd Cottage, Bedmond Road, Abbots Langley WD5 0QE — MB BS Lond. 1980; MRCP (UK) 1984; FRCP (UK) 1997. Cons. Nephrol. St. Mary's Hosp. Lond.; Hon. Cons. Nephrol. Centr. Middlx. Hosp. & Northwick Pk. Hosp. Specialty: Nephrol. Socs: Renal Assn.; Brit. Transpl. Soc. Prev: Sen. Regist. (Nephrol.) St. Mary's Hosp. Lond.; Regist. (Nephrol.) Kings Coll. Hosp. Lond.

PALMER, Ann Patricia Dartford, Gravesham & Swanley PCT, Gravesend & North Kent Hospital, Bath Street, Gravesend DA11 0DG — MD Ed. 1989; MB ChB 1969; MSc (Community Med.) Lond. Sch. Hyg. & Trop. Med. 1983; FFPHM RCP (UK) 1992; MBA 1995. Cons. (Public Health Med.) Dartford Gravesham & Swanley PCT; Hon. Sen. Res. Fell. Centre for Health Servs. Studies Univ. of Kent; Med. Ref. Medway Crematorium. Specialty: Pub. Health Med. Socs: Soc. Social Med.; Inst. Health Servs. Man. Prev: Sen. Research Fell. Health Servs. Research Unit Univ. Kent & Canterbury; SCM Medway HA; Regist. (Community Med.) N.W. Thames RHA.

PALMER, Bernard Kevin (retired) Brent Knoll, Glasllwch Lane, Newport NP20 3PR — MB ChB Bristol 1955; DObst RCOG 1957; MRCGP 1963. Prev: Clin. Asst. (Obst.) Gen. Pract. Matern. Unit Roy. Gwent Hosp. Newport.

PALMER, Mr Bernard Victor Lister Hospital, Coreys Mill Lane, Stevenage Tel: 01438 781106; Southacre, 39 Pasture Road, Letchworth SG6 3LR Tel: 01462 683064 Email: bernardpalmer@ntlworld.com — MB BChir Camb. 1970 (Camb. & Lond. Hosp.) MA Camb. 1970; MRCP UK 1972; FRCS Eng. 1974; MChir Camb. 1981. Cons. Gen. Surg. Lister Hosp. Stevenage. Specialty: Gen. Surg.; Gastroenterol. Special Interest: Breast Diseases; Coloproctology. Socs: Christ. Med. Fellowsh.; Brit. Assn. Surg. Oncol.; B.M.A. Prev: Sen. Regist. (Surg.) Roy. Marsden Hosp. & King's Coll. Hosp. Lond.; Regist. (Surg.) Whipps Cross Hosp. & St. Bart. Hosp. Lond.

PALMER, Beverley Ann — MB BS Lond. 1997. SHO (Med.). Specialty: Gen. Med.

PALMER, Bryan Mark The Central Practice Fareham Health Centre, Osborn Road, Fareham PO16 7ER Tel: 01329 823456 — (Bristol) MB ChB Bristol 1993; DGM RCP Lond. 1996; DRCOG 1998; MRCGP 1998. GP Princip. Prev: SHO (Geriat.) Whipps Cross Hosp. Lond.; Trainee GP Taunton Som. VTS; Ho. Off. (Surg.) MusGr. Pk. Hosp. Taunton.

PALMER, Celia Department of Occupational Health & Safety, King's College Healthcare NHS Trust, King's College Hospital, Denmark Hill, London SE5 9RS Tel: 020 7346 3387 / 3511 Fax: 020 7346 3261; 2 Horseshoe Wharf Apartments, Clink Street, London SE1 9FE Tel: 020 7378 0637 Fax: 020 7401 9158 — MB BS Lond. 1966 (Roy. Lond. Hosp.) MRCS Eng. LRCP Lond. 1966; DA Eng. 1968; AFOM RCP Lond. 1987. Staff Grade Ocupational Phys.; Hon. Occupat. Phys. St. Luke's Hosp. Fitzroy Sq. Lond. Specialty: Occupat. Health. Socs: Soc. Occupat. Med.; Roy. Soc. Med.; Dir. Soc. Relief of Widows & Orphans of Med. Men. Prev: Sen. Occupat. Phys. BMI Health Servs.; Occupat. Phys. Marks & Spencer plc Lond.; Med. Dir. Harlow Indust. Health Serv.

PALMER, Charles Rupert, TD Huntsland Barn, Crawley Down, Crawley RH10 4HB Tel: 01342 712313 Fax: 01342 712313 — MRCS Eng. LRCP Lond. 1944 (St. Thos.) Hon. Med. Off. Qu. Vict. Hosp. E. Grinstead. Specialty: Gen. Med. Socs: Fell. Hunt. Soc. & Roy. Soc. Med. (Mem. Sect. Gen. Pract.).; Fell. Sy. Benevolent Med. Soc. Prev: Ho. Surg. Orthop. Dept. Roy. Vict. & W. Hants. Hosp. Bournemouth; Ho. Surg. Plastic Surg. & Maxillo-Facial Centre, Qu. Vict. Hosp. E.; Grinstead; Maj. RAMC TA (Sussex Yeomanry).

PALMER, Cheryl Anne 51 Priorswood, Thorpe Mamott, Norwich NR8 6FW Tel: 01603 864202 — BM BCh Oxf. 1997; MA Camb. 1994. SHO (Gen. Med.) Norf. & Norwich Hosp. Specialty: Gen. Med. Prev: PRHO (Gen. Surg.) Roy. Surrey Co. Hosp. Guildford Surrey; PRHO (Gen. Med.) Northampton Gen. Hosp.; Sen. Ho. Off. Qu. Eliz. Hosp. Kings Lynn.

PALMER, Christopher Douglas 151 Ecclesall Road S., Sheffield S11 9PJ Tel: 0114 235 2115 — MB BS Newc. 1990; FRCA 1996. Specialist Regist. Rotat. (Anaesth.) Sheff. Specialty: Intens. Care. Socs: BMA; MRCAnaesth.; Train. Mem. Assn. Anaesth. Prev: SHO (Anaesth.) Chesterfield & N. Derbysh. Roy. Infirm.; SHO (Anaesth.) North. Gen. Hosp. Sheff. & Rotherham Dist. Gen. Hosp.

PALMER, Mr Colin Attwell Lynch (retired) Rose Cottage, Whirlow Lane, Sheffield S11 9QF Tel: 0114 236 3773 — MB BS Lond. 1952 (St. Bart.) DO Eng. 1957; FRCS Ed. 1962; FRCS Eng. 1962. Prev: Hon. Clin. Lect. (Ophth.) Univ. Sheff.

PALMER, Daniel Harrison 29 Chevril Court, Wickersley, Rotherham S66 2BN — MB ChB Birm. 1995; ChB Birm. 1995.

PALMER, David Allan The Medical Centre, Forest Gate Road, Corby NN17 1TR Tel: 01536 202507 Fax: 01536 206099 — BM BS Nottm. 1980 (Nottingham) BMedSci Nottm. 1978; DRCOG 1982; Cert. Family Plann. JCC 1983; MRCGP 1984. Police Surg. 1998. Socs: Roy. Coll. Gen. Pract.; Assn. Police Surg. Prev: Trainee GP Lincoln VTS; Ho. Off. Derby City Hosp.

PALMER, David Jonathan Lloyd 8 Chestnut Grove, Penkridge, Stafford ST19 5LX — MB ChB Birm. 1989.

PALMER, Didier Jon Wilfred 24 Maitland Street, Cardiff CF14 3JU — MB BCh Wales 1987.

PALMER, Edward Gray The Surgery, 71 The Avenue, Wivenhoe, Colchester CO7 9PP Tel: 01206 824447 Fax: 01206 827973 — MB BS Lond. 1954 (Guy's) MRCS Eng. LRCP Lond. 1954; DObst RCOG 1957. Socs: BMA.

PALMER, Eileen Mary Workington Infirmary, Infirmary Road, Workington CA14 2UN — MB ChB Leeds 1979; BSc (1st cl. Hons.) Leeds 1976; DRCOG 1984; MRCGP 1985; Dip. Palliat. Med. Wales 1992; Cert. In Med. Edu. Newcastle 1998. Med.Dir. W. Cumbria Hospice at home; Cons Palliat. Med W Cumbria. Specialty: Palliat. Med. Prev: Med. Dir. P. of Wales Hospice Pontefract; GP Leeds; SHO (Med.) Wharfedale Gen. Hosp. Otley.

PALMER, Elizabeth Ann 12 Brookvale Road, Highfield, Southampton SO17 1QP — MB BS Lond. 1977; MRCGP 1981; DRCOG 1983. GP Soton.

PALMER, Elizabeth Nina Edith Garden Flat, 11 Manby Road, Malvern WR14 3BD — MB ChB Birm 1992.

PALMER, Graham Robert Stockton Heath Medical Centre, The Forge, London Road, Warrington WA4 6HJ Tel: 01925 604427 Fax:

01925 210501; 5 Teddington Close, Appleton, Warrington WA4 5QG — MB ChB Manch. 1983.

PALMER, Harry James Graham Northfields, Jericho St., Thorverton, Exeter EX5 5PA — MB BS Lond. 1950 (St. Mary's) MRCS Eng. LRCP Lond. 1950.

PALMER, Helen Elizabeth Selly Oak Hospital, Department of Ophthalmology, Raddlebarn Road, Birmingham B29 6JD — MB BS Lond. 1988; FRCS Ed. 1993. Prev: Regist. (Ophth.) St Thos. Hosp. Lond.

PALMER, Helen Margaret South Tyneside Health Care Trust, Palmer Community Hospital, Wear St., Jarrow NE32 3UX Tel: 0191 451 6031 Fax: 0191 451 6000; 2 Coalburns Cottages, Coalburns, Greenside, Ryton NE40 4JN Tel: 0191 413 1211 — MB BS Newc. 1980; MRCP (UK) (Paediat.) 1985; DTM & H Liverp. 1989. Cons. Community Paediat. S. Tyneside Health Care Trust. Specialty: Community Child Health. Prev: Sen. Regist. (Community Paediat.) Community Unit Newc. Gen. Hosp.

PALMER, Mr James David Derriford Hospital, Plymouth PL6 8DH Tel: 01752 792542 Fax: 01752 763395 — MB BS Lond. 1985 (Lond. Hosp.) FRCS Ed. 1989; FRCS (SN) 1996; MS Soton. 1998. Cons. Neurosurg. Deffiford Hosp. Plymouth. Specialty: Neurosurg. Socs: Soc. Brit. Neurol. Surg.; Examr. Europe Bd. Europe Assoc. NeuroSurgic. Soc. Prev: Cons. Neurosurg. & Clin. Sen. Lect. Inst. Neurol. Nat. Hosp. Neurol. & Neurosurg. Lond.; Sen. Regist. (Neurosurg.) South. Gen. Hosp. Glas.; Regist. (Neurosurg.) Wessex. Neuro Centre Soton.

PALMER, Mr James Gordon Cumberland Infirmary, Carlisle CA2 7HY Tel: 01228 23444 — MB BS Lond. 1973 (Lond. Hosp. Med. Coll.) FRCS Eng. 1978; MS Lond. 1989. Cons. Surg. Cumbld. Infirm. Carlisle; Hon. Lect. (Surg.) Univ. Newc. Specialty: Gen. Surg. Socs: (Counc.) Assn. Coloproctol. Prev: Research Fell. (Surg.) Univ. Michigan, USA; Clin. Fell. ICRF Colorectal Cancer Unit St. Mark's Hosp. Lond.; Resid. Surg. Off. St. Mark's Hosp. Lond.

PALMER, James Hector MacGowan Hope Hospital, Stott Lane, Salford M6 8HD Tel: 0161 787 5107 Email: james.palmer@srht.nhs.uk — MB ChB Manch. 1986 (St Andrews & Manchester) BSc (Med. Sci.) St. And. 1983; FRCA 1992. Cons. Anaesth.Hope Hosp. Specialty: Anaesth. Socs: Assn. Anaesth.& Manch. Med. Soc.; Difficult Airway Soc.; William Scott Memor. Soc. Prev: Cons (Anaesth.) Dumfries & Galloway RI.; Locum Cons. (Anaesth.) Hope Hosp. Salford; Cons. (Anaesth.) SE Queensland Australia.

PALMER, Joanne Victoria Preston Mill, Wensley Station, Leyburn DL8 4AG — MB BS Lond. 1992.

PALMER, Mr John Hendley Plastic & Reconstructive Surgery Unit, Royal Devon & Exeter Healthcare NHS Trust, Barrack Road, Exeter EX2 5DW; 8 Lyndhurst Road, Exeter EX2 4PA Tel: 01392 437138 — MB BS Lond. 1976; FRCS Eng. 1981; T(S) 1991. Cons. Plastic Surg. Devon, Exeter & Som. HAs. Specialty: Plastic Surg. Special Interest: Breast Reconstruction; Hypospadia; Oculoplastic. Socs: BMA; Brit. Assn. Plastic Surg.; (Counc.) Brit. Assn. Aesthetic Plastic Surgs. Prev: Cons. Plastic Surg. Bradford NHS Trust; Sen. Regist. Rotat. Leeds & Bradford; Regist. (Plastic Surg.) Edin.

PALMER, Mr John Herbert Medway Hospital, Windmill Road, Gillingham ME7 5NY; 1 King Edward Road, Rochester ME1 1UA Tel: 01634 407198 Fax: 01634 833771 — MB ChB Ed. 1970; FRCS Ed. 1976. Cons. Urol. Medway Maritini Hosp. Gillingham. Specialty: Urol. Prev: Sen. Regist. (Urol.) Roy. Hallamsh. Hosp. Sheff.; Regist. St. Paul's Hosp. Lond.; Research Fell. Inst. Urol. Lond.

PALMER, Jonathan Charles Netherwood, Southwater, Horsham RH13 9DB Tel: 01403 733233 — MB BS Lond. 1980 (Guy's) MRCS Eng. LRCP Lond. 1979.

PALMER, Joseph Maximiar c/o Mrs Teresa McCann, Lower Corr, Dungannon BT71 6HQ — MB BCh BAO Belf. 1992.

PALMER, Judith Angela (retired) School Health Service, Park Cottage, The Main Drive, Bootham Park, Bootham, York YO30 7BY; 20 Bedern, York YO1 7LP Tel: 01904 637629 — MB ChB Bristol 1971; DCH Eng. 1974. Clin. Med. Off. (Child Health) York Health NHS Trust. Prev: Princip. GP York.

PALMER, Julia Claire Woodland Centre, Hillingdon Hospital, Uxbridge UB8 3NN Tel: 01895 279969 Fax: 01895 279918 Email: julia.palmer@152.hillingh-tr.nthames.nhs.uk — MB BChir Camb. 1981; MA, BA Camb. 1978; MRCPsych 1987. Cons. Old Age Psychiat. Hillingdon Hosp. Uxbridge. Specialty: Geriat. Psychiat. Prev: Sen. Regist. (Psychiat.) St. Geo. Hosp. Lond.

PALMER, Julia Elizabeth 39 Broadway, Pontypool NP4 6HW — MB BCh Wales 1996.

PALMER, Karen Susan Community Mental Health Team, Inchkeith House, 137 Leith Walk, Edinburgh EH6 8NP Tel: 0131 537 4530 — MB ChB Glas. 1987 (Glasgow) BSc Aberd. 1982; MRCPsych 1992. Staff Grade (Psychiat.) Roy. Edin. Hosp. Specialty: Gen. Psychiat. Prev: Experienced SHO in Psychiat. (Retainer Scheme) Roy. Edin. Hosp.; Clin. Asst. (Learning Disabilities) Gogarburn, Edin.; Regist. Rotat. (Psychiat.) Greater Glas. Health Bd. Parkhead Hosp. Glas.

PALMER, Katherine Sarah Old Vicarage W., Castle Bank, Stafford ST16 1DJ; North Staffordford Hospital City General, London Road, Stoke-on-Trent ST4 6SD Tel: 01782 552445 — FRCPCH; BM BS Nottm. 1985; MRCP (UK) 1989; DM Nottm. 1994. Cons. Paediat. (Neonat.) N. Staffs. Hosp. NHS Trust. Specialty: Paediat.; Neonat.

PALMER, Keith Trevor MRC Environmental Epidemiology Unit, University of Southampton, Southampton General Hospital, Southampton SO16 6YD Tel: 023 8077 7624 Fax: 023 8070 4021; 12 Brookvale Road, Highfield, Southampton SO17 1QP — BM BCh Oxf. 1981 (DM Oxf. Univ.) MA Oxf. 1981; DRCOG 1984; MRCGP (Distinc.) 1986; Cert. Family Plann. JCC 1986; MFOM RCP Lond. 1994; FFOM RCP Lond. 1998. Clin. Scientist (Occupat. & Environm. Epidemiol.) MRC & Hon. Cons. Occupat. Health Phys. Soton. Univ. Hosps. NHS Trust; Director of CPD, Fac. Occupat. Med. Specialty: Occupat. Health. Prev: Employm. Med. Adviser Health & Safety Exec.; Asst. Regist. Fac. Occupat. Med.

PALMER, Kelvin Raymond 7 Abbotsfield Park, Edinburgh EH10 5DX; GI Unit, Western General Hospital, Edinburgh EH4 2XU Tel: 0131 537 1007 — MD Sheff. 1981 (Sheffield) MB ChB 1974; MRCP (UK) 1977; FRCP (Ed.) 1987; FRCP 2000. Cons. Gastroenterol. Western Gen. Hosp. Edin.; Assoc. Postgrad. Dean, S.E. Scotl. Specialty: Gastroenterol. Socs: Brit. Soc. Gastroenterol.

PALMER, Lindsay Anne Lambgates Doctors Surgery, 1-5 Lambgates, Hadfield, Glossop SK13 1AW Tel: 01457 869090 Fax: 01457 857367; 18 Hollybank, Manor Croft, Glossop SK13 8TS Tel: 01457 852397 — MB ChB Manch. 1989 (Manchester) BSc (Hons.) Anat. Manch. 1986; Cert. Family Plann. JCC 1991; DCH RCP Lond. 1992; MRCGP 1993; DRCOG 1993. Prev: SHO (A & E) Withington & Wythenshawe Hosp.; Trainee GP Bramhall Health Centre Chesh.; SHO (O & G, Geriat., Paediat. & Psychiat.) Stepping Hill Hosp. Stockport.

PALMER, Lyndon John (retired) Littlefield, Webbs Green, Soberton, Southampton SO32 3PY Tel: 01489 877174 — MB BS Lond. 1966 (St. Geo.) MRCS Eng. LRCP Lond. 1966; DObst RCOG 1968. Prev: SHO (Midw. & Gyn.) Soton. Gen. Hosp.

PALMER, Margaret Anne The Oaklands Practice, Yateley Medical Centre, Oaklands, Yateley GU46 7LS Tel: 01252 872333 Fax: 01252 890084; 32 Masefield Gardens, Crowthorne RG45 7QS — MB ChB Manch. 1974.

PALMER, Mark Antony Lofthouse Surgery, 2 Church Farm Close, Lofthouse, Wakefield WF3 3SA Tel: 01924 822273 Fax: 01924 825168 — MB ChB Leeds 1990 (University of Leeds) T(GP) 1994; DFFP 1994. GP. Specialty: Gen. Pract.

PALMER, Michael Ian 6 Brettenham Road, Hitcham, Ipswich IP7 7NT — MB BS Lond. 1993.

PALMER, Michael John The Surgery, Station Road, East Looe, Looe PL13 1HA Tel: 01503 263195; Teghyjy, Brentfields, Polperro, Looe PL13 2JJ Tel: 01503 272426 Fax: 01503 272426 — MRCS Eng. LRCP Lond. 1972 (Sheff.) DObst RCOG 1975; MRCGP 1983; MFFP 1995. Local Med. Off. Civil Serv. Dept. (Looe Dist.); CMO (Family Plann.) Liskeard. Specialty: Gen. Pract.

PALMER, Michael Kenneth Department Diagnostic Imaging, St Helier Hospital, Wrythe Lane, Carshalton SM5 1AA Tel: 0208 296 2426 — MB ChB Ed. 1974; FRCR 1982. Cons. Radiol. St. Helier Hosp. Carshalton. Prev: Sen. Regist. (Radiol.) St. Geo. Hosp. Lond.; Ho. Surg. (Thoracic Surg.) Roy. Infirm. Edin.; Sen. Ho. Phys. (Gen. Med.) N. Middlx. Hosp. Lond.

PALMER, Michael Sydney Morton (retired) 24 Matham Road, East Molesey KT8 0SU Tel: 020 8979 1872 — (Guy's) MB BChir Camb. 1941; MD Camb. 1949. Prev: Cons. Phys. Roy. Free Hosp. Lond.

PALMER, Natalie Jane — MB ChB Liverp. 1998.

PALMER, Neil Ingamells The Old School House, Bramcote Lane, Wollaton, Nottingham NG8 2ND — MB BS Lond. 1969 (St. Thos.) FFA RCS Eng. 1974. Cons. Anaesth. Univ. Hosp. Nottm. Specialty: Anaesth. Prev: Sen. Regist. (Anaesth.) St. Thos. Hosp. Lond.; Regist. Dept. Anaesth. Hosp. Sick Childr. Gt. Ormond St. Lond.; Regist. Dept. Anaesth. Lond. Hosp.

PALMER, Nigel William Park Grove Surgery, 94 Park Grove, Barnsley S70 1QE Tel: 01226 282345 — MB ChB Sheff. 1986.

PALMER, Pauline Anne 3 Amersham Court, Woodside Road, Amersham HF6 6AG Tel: 01494 432940 — MB BChir Camb. 1993 (St. Andrews/Camb.) BSc (Hons.) St. And 1991; DCH Lond. 1998; DFFP (RCOG) 1998. Clin. Research Phys. Berks. Specialty: Gen. Pract. Prev: Northumbria Vocational Train. Scheme Newc. u. Tyne.

PALMER, Rachel Mary Radbrook Green Surgery, Bank Farm Road, Shrewsbury SY3 6DU Tel: 01743 231816 Fax: 01743 344099 — MB ChB Birm. 1981; MA Camb. 1982, BA (Hons.) 1978; DCH RCP Lond. 1984; DRCOG 1985; MRCGP 1986. GP. Specialty: Gen. Pract.

PALMER, Richard Holden, OStJ (retired) Sideways, 48 Station Road, Herne Bay CT6 5QH Tel: 01227 363595 — (Royal College of Surgeons Dublin) LRCPI & LM, LRCSI & LM 1959. Prev: Ho. Surg. (Obst.) I. of Thanet Gen. Hosps.

PALMER, Richard Mark Lisburn Health Centre, Linenhall St., Lisburn BT28 1LU Tel: 01846 603088; 6 Sequoia Park, Lambeg, Lisburn BT27 4SJ Tel: 01846 604390 — MB ChB Manch. 1988; DMH (Distinc.) Belf. 1990; DCH Dub. 1991; MRCGP 1992; Cert. Family Plann. JCC 1992; DRCOG 1993. Prev: Trainee GP Lisburn; SHO (O & G & Med.) Lagan Valley Hosp.; SHO (ENT) Roy. Vict. Hosp.

PALMER, Robert George Birmingham, Heartlands & Solihull NHS Trust (Teaching), Solihull Hospital, Lode Lane, Solihull B91 2JL — MB BS Lond. 1976 (Guy's) MRCS Eng. LRCP Lond. 1976; MRCP (UK) 1978; MA Oxf. 1977, DM 1985; DM DM Oxon 1985; FRCP 1995; MBA 1995. Cons. Phys. and Rheum.; Assoc. Postgrad. Dean W. Midl.s; Sen. Clin. Lect. (Univ. of Birm.). Specialty: Gen. Med.; Rheumatol. Prev: Clin. Sci. Clin. Med. Research Centre & Northwick Pk. Hosp. Harrow; Cons. Rheumatologist Dudley Rd. Hosp. Birm.

PALMER, Robert Julian Department of Anaesthetics, Queen Alexandra Hospital, Cosham, Portsmouth PO6 3LY; Tower Cottage, 67 Links Lane, Rowlands Castle PO9 6AF — MB BS Lond. 1968; MRCS Eng. LRCP Lond. 1968; FFA RCS Eng. 1974. Cons. Anaesth. Portsmouth & SE Hants. Specialty: Anaesth. Prev: Staff. Anaesth. Worcester Memor. Hosp., USA.

PALMER, Roger David 482 Bideford Green, Leighton Buzzard LU7 7TZ Tel: 01525 378526 Fax: 01525 378526 — BChir Camb. 1993; BSc (Hons.) St. And. 1991; MB BCh Camb. 1993; MRCP (UK) 1999; MRCPCH 2001. SpR (Paediat.) Addenbrooke's Hosp. Camb. East. Deanery Regist. Rotat. Specialty: Paediat. Prev: Sen. SHO (Paediat.) Dryburn Hosp. Durh.; SHO Rotat. (Paediat.) Newc. Centr.

PALMER, Roy Alan — (St. And.) MB ChB St. And. 1972. Sen. Med. Off. Carlisle Racecourse. Prev: SHO (Geriat.) Roy. Vict. Hosp. Dundee; SHO (O & G) Dundee Roy. Infirm.; SHO (Dermat.) Dundee Roy. Infirm.

PALMER, Roy Newberry HM Coroner's Court, Barclay Road, Croydon CR9 3NE Tel: 020 8681 5019 Fax: 020 8686 3491 Email: londoncoroner@aol.com; 2 Horseshoe Wharf Apartments, 6 Clink Street, London SE1 9FE Tel: 020 7378 0637 — MB BS Lond. 1968 (Roy. Lond. Hosp.) MRCS Eng. LRCP Lond. 1968; DObst RCOG 1970; LLB Lond. 1974; Barrister at Law Middle Temple 1977. HM Coroner for the South. Dist. of Gtr. Lond.; Governor Expert Witness Inst.; Dep. Coroner, City of Lond.; President, Society for Relief of Widows and Orphans of Medical Men (A charity founded 1788). Specialty: Medico Legal. Socs: S. E. Eng. Coroners Soc. (Pres. to 06/2005); The Coroner's Soc. of Eng. & Wales; Medico-Legal Soc. (Coun. Mem.). Prev: GP Herts.; Sec. & Med. Dir. Med. Protec. Soc.; Dep. Coroner Greater Lond, Western District.

PALMER, Ruth Bridget Manor Farm House, Manor Farm Drive, Sutton Benger, Chippenham SN15 4RW — MB BS Lond. 1986; MRCGP 1991; DRCOG 1991.

PALMER, Sarah Catherine Dr Dow and Partners, 87-89 Prince of Wales Road, London NW5 3NT; 21a Burma Road, Stoke Newington, London N16 9BH — MB BS London 1991 (St. Bartholomews) Member Royal College of General Practioners London 1998. GP Princip. Socs: Roy. Coll. Gen. Pract.

PALMER, Sharon Manor Oak Surgery, Horebeech Lane, Horam, Heathfield TN21 0DS Tel: 01435 812116 Fax: 01435 813737; 1 Tate House, Sandy Lane, Mayfield TN20 6UF Tel: 01435 874711 — MB BS Lond. 1986 (St. Thos.) MRCGP 1990. Prev: SHO (A & E Geriat.Paediat. & O & G) Qu. Marys Hosp. Sidcup; Ho. Phys. Poole Gen. Hosp.; Ho. Surg. St. Thos. Hosp. Lond.

PALMER, Mr Simon Hastings Farthings, The Thatchway, Rustington, Littlehampton BN16 2BN — MB BS Lond. 1990; FRCS Eng. 1994; FRCS (Tr & Orth) 2000. Specialty: Orthop. Socs: BOA; Brit. Orthop. Trainee Assn.; Brit. Trauma Soc. Prev: Research Regist. (Orthop. & Trauma) Bath; Hon. Res. Fell. Bath Univ.; Specialist Regist. Oxf. Rotat.

PALMER, Stephen John Broomfield Hospital, Court Road, Broomfield, Chelmsford CM1 7ET Tel: 01245 514825 — MB BS Lond. 1990 (St. Thomas's) FRCS 1994; FRCS (Tr. & Orth.) 1999. Cons. Orthopaedic Surg., specialising in knees.

PALMER, Stephen John The Fairfield Centre, Fairfield Grove, Charlton, London SE7 8TX Tel: 020 8858 5738 Fax: 020 8305 3005 — MB BS Lond. 1976 (St. Thos.) DRCOG 1980; DCH Eng. 1980; MRCGP 1981. GP Charlton Lond. Specialty: Gen. Pract. Prev: GP VTS Greenwich Lond.; Ho. Surg. Qu. Alexandra Hosp. Cosham; Ho. Phys. Worthing Gen. Hosp.

PALMER, Professor Stephen Royston Department of Epidermiolgy and Public Health, University of Wales, College of Medicine, Heath Park, Cardiff CF14 4XN Tel: 029 2074 2321 — MB BChir Camb. 1976; MA Camb. 1976; FFCM 1987, M 1980; FRCP 1999. Dir. Welsh Combined Centres for Pub. Health Univ. Wales Coll. Med.; Head of Dept. of Epidemiol. & Pub. Health; Mansel Talbot Prof. of Epidemiol. & Pub. Health. Specialty: Epidemiol. Prev: Sen. Regist. Communicable Dis. Surveillance Centre; Lect. (Community Med.) St. Thos. Hosp. Med. Sch. Lond.; Ho. Phys. King's Coll. Hosp. Lond.

PALMER, Timothy Allan Dunorlan Medical Group, 64 Pembury Road, Tonbridge TN9 2JG Tel: 01732 352907 Fax: 01732 367408 — MB BS Lond. 1982 (Guy's Hosp. Lond.) BSc Lond. 1979; DRCOG 1986; DMJ 2000. GP; Med. Off. Kent Sch. RFU; Princip. Forens. Med. Examr., Kent Police Auth., Tonbridge. Specialty: Gen. Pract.; Medico Legal. Socs: Assn. Police Surg. Prev: Police Surg. Kent Police Auth. (Sevenoaks); Trainee GP Tunbridge Wells VTS.

PALMER, Timothy James Dun Macbeth, 14 Auldcastle Road, Inverness IV2 3PZ — MB BS Lond. 1978 (Guy's) BSc Lond. 1975, MB BS 1978; MRCP (UK) 1982; MRCPath 1985. Cons. Histopath/Cytopath Raigmore Hosp. Inverness. Specialty: Histopath. Prev: Sen. Lect./Hon. Cons. Histopath./Cytopath. Guy's Hosp. Med. Sch., Guy's & Lewisham Hosps.; Lect. (Histopath.) United Med. & Dent. Sch. Guy's Hosp. Lond.; Sen. Regist. (Histopath.) Guy's & Lewisham Hosps.

PALMER, Valerie Frances Dalston Medical Group, Townhead Road, Dalston, Carlisle CA5 7PZ Tel: 01228 710451 Fax: 01228 711898 — BM BCh Oxf. 1976; MA (Physiol.) Oxf. 1977; MRCGP 1984. Specialty: Gen. Pract. Prev: GP Lond.

PALMER, William Coningsby (retired) 2 Quarry Hill Lane, Wetherby LS22 6RY Tel: 01937 584755 — LRCP LRCS Ed. LRFPS Glas. 1947.

PALMIER, Beryl Mary 115 Epsom Road, Sutton SM3 9EY Tel: 020 8644 7718 — MB ChB Birm. 1948; MRCS Eng. LRCP Lond. 1948; MRCOG 1955; DCH Eng. 1956. Prev: Regist. O & G Whittington Hosp.; Ho. Phys. Southmead Hosp. Bristol; Cas. Off. Birm. Gen. Hosp.

PALMIERI, Carlo 5 Silverton Road, London W6 9NY — MB BS Lond. 1994 (Char. Cross & Westm.) BSc (1st cl. Hons.) Lond. 1991; MRCP (UK) 1997. SpR Med. Oncol. Hammersmith Hosp. NHS Trust. Specialty: Oncol. Prev: Clin. Research Fell. & Hon. Regist. (Med. Oncol.) Imperial Coll. Sch. Of Med., Lond. & Hammersmith Hosps. NHS Trust; SHO Med. Roy. Lond. Hosp.; SHO Med. Oncol. St. Bart. Hosp.

PALMOWSKI, Bogdan Maciej 6 Lane Ends, Hibson Road, Nelson BB9 0PX — LMSSA Lond. 1992.

PALOMBO, Andrew Stewart Larachan, 7 Dochfour Drive, Inverness IV3 5EB — MB ChB Aberd. 1996.

PALSINGH, Jasbinder Flat 1, 76 Portland Road, Edgbaston, Birmingham B16 9QU — MB ChB Dundee 1988.

PALTA, Narinder Singh (retired) York District Hospital, Wigginton Road, York YO31 8HE Tel: 01904 631313; 53 Askham Lane,

Acomb, York YO24 3HB Tel: 01904 798344 — MB BS Punjab 1959 (Govt. Med. Coll. Patiala) MB BS Punjab (India) 1959; MRCP (UK) 1971; FRCP Lond. 1991. Prev: Cons. Phys. York Dist. Hosp.

PALUCH, Nicholas Anthony Fleetwood La Gallie, Rue de la Gallie, St Peter Port, Guernsey GY7 9ED Tel: 01481 264242 — (Univ. Coll. Hosp.) BSc (Hons.) 1976; MB BS 1979; DRCOG 1982; DCH RCP Lond. 1982; MRCGP 1985; DPD Wales 1991. GP St. Peters, Guernsey.

PALUMBO, Luigina 6 Dundas St. West, Saltburn-by-the-Sea TS12 1BL Tel: 01287 622207 Fax: 01287 623803; Beechwood, Victoria Terrace, Saltburn-by-the-Sea TS12 1HN Tel: 01287 622822 — MB BS Nottm. 1982; BMedSci Nottm. 1980, MB BS 1982; MRCP (UK) 1985; DRCOG 1990; MRCGP 1992. Princip. Gen. Pract. Prev: Regist. (Med.) Sheff.; SHO (Obst. & Gyn.) S. Cleveland Hosp.

PAMBAKIAN, Alidz Lucy Marina 41 Southdown Avenue, London W7 2AG — MB BS Lond. 1991.

PAMBAKIAN, Hosep 41 Southdown Avenue, Boston Manor, London W7 2AG — MB BS Lond. 1956; MRCS Eng. LRCP Lond. 1956; LMSSA Lond. 1956.

PAMBAKIAN, Nazaret Haig Crown Street Surgery, 2 Lombard Court, Crown Street, Acton, London W3 8SA Tel: 020 8992 1963 — MB BS Lond. 1984; DRCOG 1987; MRCGP 1995. Specialty: Gen. Pract.

PAMBAKIAN, Samuel 41 Southdown Avenue, London W7 2AG — MB BS Lond. 1989.

PAMBAKIAN, Yvonne Emma Louise Arpi 5 Holders Hill Avenue, London NW4 1EN — MB BS Lond. 1993. SHO (Paediat.) Barnet Gen. Hosp. Specialty: Paediat. Prev: SHO (O & G) Edgware Gen. Hosp.; SHO (Orthop. & A & E) Barnet Gen. Hosp.

PAMPEL, Maralyn Marcia Bacon Lane Surgery, 11 Bacon Lane, Edgware HA8 5AT Tel: 020 8952 5073/7876 — MB BS Lond. 1974 (King's Coll. Hosp.) MRCGP 1995. GP Trainer Edgware & Barnet VTS. Prev: SHO (Paediat.) Sydenham Childr. Hosp. Lond.; SHO (O & G) Barnet Gen. Hosp.; SHO (Orthop. & Cas.) Barnet Gen. Hosp.

PAMPHILON, Derwood Harold National Blood Service, Bristol Centre, Bristol BS10 5ND Tel: 0117 991 2096 Fax: 0117 991 2002 Email: derwood.pamphilon@nbs.nhs.uk — MB BS Bristol 1974 (London) MB BS Lond. 1974; MRCPath 1984; MD Bristol 1991; FRCPath 1996; MRCPCH 1998. Cons. Haemat. Nat. Blood Serv.; Cons. & Sen. Clin. Lect. (Haemat.) Bristol Roy. Hosp. Sick Childr. Specialty: Haematology. Prev: Sen. Regist. Immunohaemat. Southmead Hosp. Bristol.; Regist. (Haemat.) Gen. Infirm. & St. Jas. Univ. Hosp. Leeds.

PAMPIGLIONE, Julian Sheridan The Bournemouth Nuffield Hospital, 67 Lansdowne Road, Bournemouth BH1 1RW Tel: 01202 292234 Fax: 01202 317848; 93 Canford Cliffs, Poole BH13 7EP — MB BS Lond. 1980 (Lond. Hosp.) MRCOG 1986; T(OG) 1992; MD Lond. 1992; FRCOG 1998. Cons. O & G Roy. Bournemouth Gen. Hosp.; Cons. Obst. & Gyn. Poole Gen. Hosp.; Jt. Director, Dorset InFertil. Serv.s. Specialty: Obst. & Gyn. Prev: Sen. Regist. (Human Reproduc. & Obst.) Princess Anne Hosp. Soton.; Clin. Research Fell. Assisted Conception Unit King's Coll. Hosp. Lond.; SHO (Neonatol.) John Radcliffe Hosp. Oxf.

PANACER, Davinder Singh St Matthews Medical Centre, Prince Phillip House, Malabar Road, Leicester LE1 2NZ; 10 Waveney Rise, Oadby, Leicester LE2 4GG — BM BS Nottm. 1988 (Nott.) BMedSci. Nottm. 1986; DRCOG 1993; DCCH 1993; DFFP 1994; MRCGP 1994. GP. Specialty: Gen. Pract. Prev: Trainee GP Centr. Birm. VTS.

PANAGAMUWA, Channa Sanjeewa Bandara 57A Frederick Road, Selly Oak, Birmingham B29 6NX — MB ChB Sheff. 1998.

PANAGEA, Stavroula Elias c/o Microbiology Department, North Manchester General Hospital, Central Drive, Crumpsall, Manchester M8 5RL — Ptychio Iatrikes Athens 1990.

PANAGIOTOPOULOS, Ioannis Hermes Lodge, 14 Apple Way, Chelmsford CM2 9HX Tel: 01245 443379 Email: yiannispvascular@aol.com — Ptychio Iatrikes Thessalonika 1981.

PANAHLOO, Arshia Ali St George's Hospital, Department of Endocrinology & Diabetes, Blackshaw Road, London SW17 0QT Tel: 020 8725 3902 Email: arshia.panahloo@stgeorges.nhs.uk — MB BS Lond. 1986 (St. Thos.) MRCP (UK) 1989; MD Lond. 1998; FRCP 2003. Cons. Phys. (Diabetes & Endoc.) St. Geo.'s Hosp. Lond. Specialty: Diabetes; Endocrinol.; Gen. Med. Socs: Brit. Endoc. Soc.; Eur. Assoc. for the Study of Diabetes; Diabetes UK. Prev: Sen. Regist. (Endocrinol. & Diabetes) Hammersmith Hosp. Lond.; Clin. Lect. (Med.) Whittington Hosp. Lond.; Regist. (Gen. Med.) St. Albans City Hosp. & St. Mary's Hosp. Lond.

PANAHY, Mr Cambyse 6 Kingsmead Court, Avenue Road, Highgate, London N6 5DU Tel: 020 8341 4938 — (Bristol) MB ChB Bristol 1959; FRCS Ed. 1966; FRCS Eng. 1967. Specialty: Gen. Surg. Socs: Fell. Roy. Soc. Med. Prev: Assoc. Prof. Surg. Nat. Univ. Iran; Lect. Surg. Unit Lond. Hosp.; Surg. Regist. City Hosp. Stoke on Trent.

PANAKIS, Niki 33 Ethelburt Avenue, Southampton SO16 3DG — BM BS Nottm. 1994.

PANANGHAT, Tony Paul 2 Knights Close, Thornton-Cleveleys FY5 3BF — MB BS Bangalor 1971; MB BS Bangalore 1971.

PANARESE, Alessandro Dept of Ent., Royal Hallamshire Hospital, Sheffield S10 2JF; 75 Highcliffe Road, Sheffield S11 7LP — State Exam Milan 1986. Specialist Regist., Dept of Ent. Roy. Hallamshire Hosp. Sheff.

PANAY, Nicholas Queen Charcotte's Hospital, Du Lane Rd, London W12 0HS Tel: 020 8383 5313 Fax: 020 8383 3521; 1 Shaftesbury Road, Richmond TW9 2TD Tel: 0973 543657 — MB BS Lond. 1988 (UCL/Middlesex) BSc (Hons.) Lond. 1985; MRCOG 1994; MFFP 1996. Cons. Obst. & Gyn.; Specialist Reproductive Med. Specialty: Obst. & Gyn. Special Interest: Reproductive Med. Socs: Roy. Soc. Med.; Med. Defence Union; Med. Sickness Soc. Prev: Regist. Rotat. (O & G) Guy's Hosp. Lond. & Lewisham; SHO (Perinatol.) St. Mary's Hosp.; SHO (Gyn.) Univ. Coll. Hosp.

PANAYI, Professor Gabriel Stavros Guy's, King's, St Thomas' School of Medicine, Guys Hospital, London SE1 9RT Email: gabriel.panayi@kcl.ac.uk — (Univ. Camb. & St. Mary's Hosp. Lond.) MB BChir Camb. 1966; MD Camb. 1971; MRCP (UK) 1972; FRCP Lond. 1982; ScD Camb. 1991. ARC Prof. (Rheum.) King's Coll. Lond.; Hon. Cons. Rheum. Guy's & St. Thos. Hosp. Trust Lond. Specialty: Rheumatol. Special Interest: Connective Tissue Diseases; Gen. Rheum.; Inflammatory Jt. Diseases. Socs: (Counc.) Brit. Soc. for Rheum.; Brit. Soc. Immunol.; Roy. Soc. Med. Prev: ARC Prof. (Rheum.) United Med.& Dent. Schs. Lond.; MRC Jun. Research Fell. Wright-Fleming Inst. & Kennedy Inst. Rheum. Lond.; Arthritis & Rheum. Counc. Research Fell. Dis. Unit North. Gen.

PANAYIDES, Socrates Mathew (retired) Chartham Surgery, Parish Road, Chartham, Canterbury CT4 7JU Tel: 01227 738224; The White Lodge, 2 Abbots Barton Walk, Canterbury CT1 3AX Tel: 01227 768246 — LMSSA Lond. 1972 (Athens) Med. Dipl. Athens 1965. Prev: Regist. (Thoracic Surg.) Roy. Infirm. Edin.

PANAYIOTOU, Barnabas Nicos Department of Geriatrics, City General Hospital, Newcastle-under-Lyme ST4 6QG Tel: 01782 715444 Fax: 01782 747319 — BM BS Nottm. 1983; BMedSci (Hons.) Nottm. 1981; MRCP (UK) 1988; MD (Keale) 1999; FRCP (London) 2000. Cons. Phys. & Geriat. City Gen. Hosp. Stoke-on-Trent; Hon. Sen. Clin. Lect. Keele Univ. Specialty: Care of the Elderly. Socs: BMA & Brit. Geriat. Soc.; Med. Res. Soc. Prev: Sen. Regist. (Gen. Med.) City Gen. Hosp. Stoke-on-Trent; Sen. Regist. (Geriat.) Manor Hosp. Walsall; Clin. Research Fell & Hon. Regist. (Med. Elderly) Leicester Gen. Hosp.

PANCH, Gnanie Whittington Hospital, Highgate Hill, London N19 5NF Tel: 020 7272 3070 Fax: 020 7288 5417 — MB BS Sri Lanka 1974 (Colombo (SRI Lanka)) MRCS Eng. LRCP Lond. 1981; FRCA 1986. Cons. (Anaesth.) Whittington Hosp. Lond. Specialty: Anaesth. Socs: MRCAnaesth. & Pain Soc.; Assn. of Anaesth. Prev: Sen. Regist. in anE.hesia UCH; Clin. Asst. (Anaesth.) Univ. Coll. Hosp. Lond.; Regist. (Anaesth.) Centr. Middlx. & Northwick Pk. Hosp.

PANCHAM, Prem Kumar (retired) Aldersyde, 26 Rotchell Park, Dumfries DG2 7RH Tel: 01387 254541 — (Nagpur) MB BS Nagpur 1959; DOMS Punjab 1960; MS (Ophth.) Lucknow 1963; FICS 1967. Prev: Ophth. Med. Pract. Med. Free Lance.

PANCHARATNAM, Mr Manoah Dhyanchand West Hertfordshire NHS Trust, Hillfield Road, Hemel Hempstead HP2 4AD Tel: 01727 897147 Fax: 01727 897606 Email: manopanch@doctors.org.uk; 71 West Common, Harpenden AL5 2LD Tel: 01582 460281 Fax: 01582 761512 — MB BS Madras 1974 (Jawaharlal Inst. Med. Educat. Pondicherry) FRCS Ed. 1977; T(S) 1991. Cons. Urol. W. Herts NHS Trust. Specialty: Urol. Special Interest: Radical Cystectomy and Orthotopic Bladder Reconstuction/Radical Prostatectomy/Paediatric Urol. Socs: Brit. Assn. Urol. Surgs.; BAUS Oncol.; BMA. Prev: Cons.

& Head Unit Urol. King Faisal Hosp. Taif, Saudi Arabia; Regist. & Cons. Gen. Surg. & Urol. King Geo. Hosp. Greenwich; Sen. Regist. (Urol.) St. Peters Gp. Inst. Urol.

PANCHAUD, Marcus Laurence Thomas Haslemere Health Centre, Church Lane, Haslemere GU27 2BQ Tel: 01483 783023 Fax: 01428 645065 — MB BS Lond. 1987; DRCOG 1991; MRCGP 1992.

PANCHOLI, Prakash Spinney Hill Medical Centre, 143 St. Saviours Road, Leicester LE5 3HX Tel: 0116 251 7870 — MB ChB Leic. 1983; DRCOG 1986. Professional Exec. Comm. Mem. Of Eastern Leicester PCT.

PANDA, Jitendra Kumar 26 Cotton Close, Broadstone BH18 9AJ — (S.C.B. Med. Coll. Cuttack) BSc (Hons.) Utkal 1966; MB BS Utkal 1973; MD (Obst. & Gyn.) Chandigarh 1976; MRCOG 1984; FRCOG 1998. Specialist O & G Poole Hosp. NHS Trust Dorset; Regist. (Obst. & Gyn.) Southport Gen. Infirm. Specialty: Obst. & Gyn. Socs: Roy. Coll. Obst. & Gyn. Lond.; Med. Protec. Soc.; BMA. Prev: Regist. (O & G) St. David's Hosp. Bangor & Fazakerley Hosp. Liverp.; Regist. (O & G) St. James Univ. Hosp. Leeds; Regist. (O & G) Soton. Gen. Infirm.

PANDA, Veena Pani 26 Cotton Close, Broadstone BH18 9AJ — MB BS Ravishankar U, India 1986.

PANDAY, Sheila 18 Stour Court, Stour St., Canterbury CT1 2PG — MB BCh BAO NUI 1993; LRCPS 1993.

PANDAY, Sohrab Lincoln Road Practice, 63 Lincoln Road, Peterborough PE1 2SF Tel: 01733 565511 Fax: 01733 569230; 12 Livermore Green, Peterborough PE4 5DG — MB ChB Manch. 1984 (Manchester) BSc Manch. 1982; MRCP (UK) 1987; DCH RCP Lond. 1989; MRCGP 1992. Specialty: Gen. Pract. Socs: BMA; RCGP; RCP. Prev: Tutor Paediat. St. Jas. Univ. Hosp.; Trainee GP Leeds.

PANDE, Ira Rheumatology Department, City Hospital & Queens Medical Centre, Nottingham Tel: 01159 627 697 Fax: 01159 627 709 — MB BS Lucknow 1986; MD, India 1990; PhD, London 2000. Cons. Rheum., City Hosp., Nottm.; Cons. Rheum., Queens Hosp. Centre, Nottm. Specialty: Rheumatol. Special Interest: Connective Tissue Dis.; Inflammatory Arthritics; Osteoporosis. Socs: IRA; BSR; RCP.

PANDE, Kanan Spring Bank Group Practice, 168 Spring Bank, Hull HU3 1QW; Spring Bank Group Practice, Walseley House, 168 Spring Bank, Hull HU3 1QW — MB BS Delhi 1984; MRCOG 1992; MRCGP 1997. GP Princip. Specialty: Gen. Pract.

PANDE, Mr Milind 33 Woodfield Crescent, London W5 1PD — MB BS Delhi 1981; FRCS Glas. 1989; FCOphth 1989. Regist. Hull Roy. Infirm.

PANDE, Salil Kumar 18 Barnhurst Close, Childwall, Liverpool L16 7QT Tel: 0151 722 0872 Fax: 0151 280 7794 — MB BS Lond. 1996 (Univ. Coll. Hosp.) GP Regist. Liverp.

PANDE, Sandeep Kumar Longcroft Clinic, 5 Woodmansterne Lane, Banstead SM7 3HH — MB BS Lond. 1991 (University College and Middlesex Hospital Medical School) MRCGP 1995; DCH RCP Lond. 1995. GP Princip.; Forens. Med. Examr. Socs: Roy. Soc. Med.; Assn. of Police Surg.

PANDE, Shiv Kumar, MBE Dr S K Pande, 14 North View, Edge Hill, Liverpool L7 8TS Tel: 0151 709 3779 Fax: 0151 475 3353; 18 Barnhurst Close, Childwall, Liverpool L16 7QT Tel: 0151 722 0872 Fax: 0151 280 7794 — (M.G.M. Med. Coll. Indore) MB BS Vikram 1962; MS Indore 1965; MRCGP 1996; FRCGP 2003. GP/Presenter of TV Progr. Aap Kaa Hak; JP. Socs: Fell. Fac. Community Med.; Fell. Roy. Inst. Pub. Health & Hyg.; Fell. Overseas Doctors Assn. Prev: Regist. (Surg.) Lond. Chest Hosp., Roy. Liverp. Childr. Hosp. & Fazakerley Hosp. Liverp.

PANDE, Shyam Kumar (retired) 3 Sayers Close, Harlington, Doncaster DN5 7JA Tel: 01709 893066 — MB BS Nagpur 1956; DPH Eng. 1968; MFCM 1974. Prev: SCMO (Child Health) Doncaster HA.

PANDEY, Manish Flat 4, 34-35 Newman St., London W1T 1PZ — BChir Camb. 1992.

PANDEY, Surendra Kumar Department of Child Health, Stanley Health Centre, Stanley DH9 0XE Tel: 01207 214857 Fax: 01207 214800 — MB BS Patna 1974 (P. Wales Med. Coll. Patna) FRCP 1997 Lond.; MRCPI 1982; FRCPCH 1997. Cons. Paediat. Community Child Health Derwentside, Co. Durh. Hosp. Dryburn Hosp. Durh. Specialty: Paediat.

PANDEY, Vikas Anand 10 Garth Edge, Whitworth, Rochdale OL12 8EH — MB ChB Liverp. 1998.

PANDHER, Baltej Singh 7 Kelso Mews, Caversham Park, Reading RG4 6RJ — MB BS Lond. 1997 (Roy. Free Hosp. Sch. of Med.) SHO (A & E) Lister Hosp. Stevenage. Specialty: Accid. & Emerg. Prev: PRHO Orthop. Surg. Lister Hosp.; PRHO Md. Basildon, Thurrock NHS Trust.

PANDHER, Gurpreet Kaur 6 St Mary's Road, Heckford Park, Poole BH15 2LH Tel: 01202 673588 — MB BS Lond. 1990 (King's Coll. Sch. Med. & Dent.) MRCOG 1996. Specialist Regist. (O & G) Princess Anne Hosp. Soton. Specialty: Obst. & Gyn.

PANDHER, Kulwant Singh Kidlington Health Centre, Exeter Close, Oxford Road, Kidlington OX5 1AP Tel: 01865 841941 — MRCS Eng. LRCP Lond. 1981; MB ChB Liverp. 1981. Research Regist. Nuffield Laborat. Ophth. Oxf. Univ. Specialty: Gen. Pract. Socs: Fell. Roy. Soc. Med.

PANDIS, Vasilios Department of Orthopaedics, York Hill NHS Trust, Yorkhill, Glasgow G3 8SJ — Ptychio Iatrikes Athens 1986.

PANDIT, Adam Nisar 51 Langley Road, Watford WD17 4PB — MB BS Lond. 1998.

PANDIT, Anita 60 Ripplevale Grove, London N1 1HT Tel: 020 7700 6735 — MD Bombay 1986 (Grant Medical, Bombay) MBBS 1984; MRCP I 1991. Specialty: Respirat. Med.

PANDIT, Jaideep Jagdeesh Nuffield dept of Anaesthetics, John Radcliffe Hosp, Oxford OX3 9AJ — BM BCh Oxf. 1988; DPhil Oxf. 1993, BA 1985; FRCA 1995. Lect. (Med.) St. John's Coll. Oxf. & cons. (Anaesth.) Nuffield Dept. Anaesth. Oxf.; Assessor Final Honour Sch. Physiol. Univ. Oxf. Specialty: Anaesth. Socs: Sen. Common Room Corpus Christie Coll. Oxf.; BMA; Internat. Anaesthetic research centre. Prev: Wellcome Trust Research Fell. Univ. Oxf.; ass pro anE.hetics.uni Michigan.

PANDIT, Mr Jyotin Chittaranjan Bristol Eye Hospital, Lower Maudlin St., Bristol BS1 2LX Tel: 0117 923 0060 Fax: 0117 928 4686; 29 Vernon Avenue, Handsworth Wood, Birmingham B20 1DD Tel: 0121 554 1629 — MB BCh Wales 1988; FRCS Ed. 1993. Specialist Regist. (Ophth.) Bristol Eye Hosp.; Clin. Lect. Univ. Bristol. Specialty: Ophth. Socs: BMA; Roy. Soc. Med.; Internat. Mem.-in-Train. Amer. Acad. Ophth. Prev: Specialist Regist. (Ophth.) REI Plymouth; Research Regist. Nuffield Laborat. of Ophth. Oxf.; Regist. (Ophth.) Torbay Hosp.

PANDIT, Nisar Ahmad Springfield, 51 Langley Road, Watford WD17 4PB Tel: 01923 32056 — MB BS Punjab 1959 (King Edwd. VII Med. Coll. Lahore) MB BS Punjab (Pakistan) 1959; FRCP Lond. 1985, M 1968. Cons. Phys. Dept. Rheum. & Neurol. Rehabil. Watford Gen. Hosp. & Garston Manor Med. Rehabil. Centre. Specialty: Gen. Med. Prev: Sen. Regist. (Rheum. & Rehabil.) & Regist. Dept. Neurol. Middlx.; Hosp. Lond.; Sen. Regist. (Gen. Med. & Neurol.) W. Lond. Hosp.

PANDIT, Mr Ranjeet Jagdeesh Royal Victoria Infirmatory, Newcastle upon Tyne NE1 4LP — BM BCh Oxf. 1990; BA (Hons.) Physiol. Oxf. 1987; MRCP (UK) 1993; FRCOphth 1998. Cons. Med. Ophth. Roy. Vict. Infirm. Newc. Upon Tyne. Specialty: Ophth. Prev: SHO (Ophth.) Gt. Ormond St. Hosp. Lond.; SHO (Ophth.) Radcliffe Infirm. Oxf.; SHO (Ophth.) Roy. Berks. Hosp. Reading.

PANDIT, Mr Sharad Shripadrao Highgate Medical Centre, 1 Brinklow Tower, Upper Highgate Street, Birmingham B12 0XT Tel: 0121 440 3605 Fax: 0121 440 5063; 290 Lordswood Road, Hasborne, Birmingham B17 8AN Tel: 0121 420 2525 — MB BS Poona 1971; FRCS Glas. 1981. GP. Specialty: Orthop. Socs: BMA; LMC Birm.; ODA.

PANDIT, Suchitra Narayan c/o Mr Laxman Pankhaniya, 704 Leyton High Road, London E10 6JP — MB BS Nagpur, India 1984.

PANDIT, Versha 48 Charter Avenue, Ilford IG2 7AB — MB ChB Dundee 1994.

PANDITA-GUNAWARDENA, Nandin Daya 132 Foxley Lane, Purley CR8 3NE Tel: 020 8660 7404 Fax: 020 8660 6491 — MB BS Ceylon 1965 (Colombo) MRCP (UK) 1973; FRCP Lond. 1995. Cons. Phys. (Geriat. Med.) Hither Green Hosp. & Lewisham Hosp. Lond.; Hon. Sen. Lect. UMDS Guy's & St. Thos. Hosp. Lond. Specialty: Gen. Med. Prev: Sen. Regist. (Geriat. Med.) W. Middlx. Hosp. Isleworth & St. Mary's Hosp. Lond.; Regist. (Geriat.) St. Helier Hosp. Carshalton & W. Middlx. Hosp.

PANDITA-GUNAWARDENA, Vijitha Ranjanikanthi (retired) Beechcroft Living Skills Resource Centre, 120 Victoria Road, Horley

RH6 7AB Tel: 01293 821183 Fax: 01293 822536; 132 Foxley Lane, Purley CR8 3NE Tel: 020 8660 7404 Fax: 020 8660 6491 — (Colombo) MB BS Ceylon 1965; DPM Eng. 1971; FRCPsych 1996, M 1972. Cons. Psychiat. Surrey Oaklands NHS Trust; Dep. Med. Director, Surrey Oaklands NHS Trust. Prev: Cons. Psychiat. Netherne Hosp. Coulsdon.

PANDOLFI, Andrew Lawrence The Surgery, Baird Road, Ratho, Newbridge EH28 8RA Tel: 0131 333 1062 — MB ChB Glas. 1973; DObst RCOG 1975; Cert. Family Plann. JCC 1980. Socs: BMA. Prev: Ho. Phys. & Ho. Surg. Roy. Infirm. Stirling; Govt. Med. Off. Malawi; GP Arbroath.

PANDOR, Shamin Banu South Street Surgeries, 83 South St., Bishop's Stortford CM23 3AP — MB ChB Leic. 1990.

PANDYA, Darshna 6 Styles Way, Beckenham BR3 3AJ — MB BS Lond. 1989; T(GP) 1993.

PANDYA, Hemendra Kashinath Wyken Medical Centre, Brixham Drive, Coventry CV2 3LB Tel: 024 7668 9149 Fax: 024 7666 5151 — MB BS Saurashtra 1972.

PANDYA, Hitesh Champaklal 21 Raine Way, Oadby, Leicester LE2 4UB Email: hp28@leicester.ac.uk — MB ChB Glas. 1987; MD Lond.; MRCP (UK) Paediat. 1993. Cons. (Paediat.) Respiratry Med. Intens. Care & ECMO. Specialty: Paediat. Socs: Brit. Paediat. Soc.; RCPCH; BMA. Prev: Clin. Regist. Univ. of Leicester; Research Regist. St. Thomas's Hosp. Lond.

PANDYA, Jayshree 324 Thorold Road, Ilford IG1 4HD Tel: 020 8262 6312 — MB BS Lond. 1988 (Royal Free Medical School) BSc BPharm. (Hons.) CNAA 1982. Specialist Regist. Paediat. Oncol., St Bart./Roy. Lond. Hosp. Specialty: Paediat.

PANDYA, Jyotindra Keshavlal Laurence House, 107 Philip Lane, Tottenham, London N15 4JR; 101 Osidge Lane, Southgate, London N14 5JL Tel: 020 8361 6898 — MB BS Gujarat 1973; FRCGP; DFFP 1994; MRCGP 1994. Mem. LMC. Specialty: Gen. Med.

PANDYA, Lalit 9 Partridge Close, Leegomery, Telford TF1 6WF Tel: 01952 223600 Email: lalit1000@hotmail.com — MB BS Indore 1978 (MGM Med. Coll. INDIA) MSc (Biochem.) Indore 1971, MD (Gen. Med.) 1981, MB BS 1978; MRCP (UK) 1985; MRCPI 1985. Staff Grade (Phys. in Med.) Telford. Specialty: Gen. Med. Prev: Sen. Regist. (Med.) King Khalid Univ. Hosp. Saudi Arabia.

PANDYA, Mr Mukesh Dalpatbhai The Surgery, 48 Harrow View, Harrow HA1 1RQ Tel: 020 8427 7172 Fax: 020 8424 9375 — MB BS Gujarat 1973; FRCS Ed. 1983.

PANDYA, Mr Pranav Department of Fetal Medicine, Obstetric Hospital, Huntley St., London WC1E 6AU Tel: 020 7387 9300 Email: pranav.pandya@uclh.org — MB BS Lond. 1988 (University College Hospital) BSc (Hons.) Lond. 1985; MRCOG 1997; MD Univ. Of Lond. 1999. Specialist Regist. (O & G) Univ. Coll. Hosp. Lond. & Cons. In Fetal Med. & Obst. Specialty: Obst. & Gyn. Socs: Roy. Soc. Med.; BMA. Prev: Research Fell. (Fetal Med.) King's Coll. Hosp. Lond.; SHO (O & G) St. Mary's Hosp. Lond.; SHO (A & E) Univ. Coll. Hosp. Lond.

PANDYA, Rajesh Parmanand East Park Road Medical Centre, 264 East Park Road, Leicester LE5 5FD Tel: 0116 273 7700 Fax: 0116 273 5872 — MB BS Saurashtra 1986; MRCS Eng. LRCP Lond. 1992; DFFP 1994; DRCOG 1994; MRCGP 1996. Gen. Practioner; Hosp. Pract. Glenfield Gen. Hosp. Leicester. Specialty: Gen. Pract. Socs: Fell.of Roy. Soc. of Med. Prev: Trainee GP Leics.; SMC, Paeds, Rugby; SMC, MBSQ gynae, Leicester Hosp.

PANDYA, Ramchandra Jatashankar (retired) 18 Peel Place, Clayhall Avenue, Ilford IG5 0PS Tel: 020 8551 5062 Fax: 020 8551 5062 — MB BS Gujarat 1956 (B.J. Med. Coll. & Civil Hosp. Ahmedabad) Prev: SHO (Cas.) E. Ham Memor. Hosp. Lond.

PANESAR, Bhupinder Singh Southern General Hospital, 1345 Govan Road, Glasgow G51 4TF — MB ChB Glasg. 1986.

PANESAR, Harminder Singh 82 Dale Street, Chatham ME4 6QG — MB BS Lond. 1996.

PANESAR, Mr Kanwar Jit Singh, OBE Altnagelvin Area Hospital, Glenshane Road, Londonderry BT47 6SB Tel: 028 71345171 Fax: 028 71296136 Email: kpanesar@alt.n-i.nhs.uk; Hinton House, 1 Clooney Park West, Londonderry BT47 6LA Tel: 028 7134 3935 Fax: 028 7134 3935 — MB BS Panjab (India) 1965 (Med. Coll. Amritsar) FRCS Ed. 1972; FRCS Eng. 1972; MRCS Eng. LRCP Lond. 1974; FRCSI 1994. Cons. Surg. Altnagelvin Hosp. Lond.derry.; Hon. Assoc. Clin. Prof., Surg., Internat. Sch. of Med. Specialty: Gen. Surg. Special Interest: Laparoscopic Surg.; Paediatric Surg.; Upper GI & Hepatobiliary Surg. Socs: Gen. Med. Counc.; Brit. Med. Assn.; Assn. of Surgeons, Gt. Britain & Irel.

PANESAR, Ravinder Singh 8 Wolds Drive, Orpington BR6 8NS — LMSSA Lond. 1979 (Glancy) MB BS Guru Nanak 1973. CMP RAF MoD Lond. Prev: CMP RAF Biggin Hill; Vocational Train. in Gen. Pract. Lond.; SHO (Surg.) Whittington Hosp. Lond.

PANESAR, Satwant Kaur 39 Castleknowe Gardens, Carluke ML8 5UX — MB ChB Glas. 1992; MRCGP; Dip Dermat Glas. Specialty: Dermat.

PANEZAI, Mr Amir Mohammad 51 Newton Garth, Leeds LS7 4HG Tel: 0113 262 1779 — MB BS Karachi 1973; FRCS Glas. 1990; FRCSI 1990.

PANEZAI, Mr Jamil Ur Rehman 25 Helensburgh Close, Pogmoor Road, Barnsley S75 2EU — MB BS Karachi 1974; FRCS Ed. 1992.

PANG, Alison 42 Buttermere Court, Boundary Road, London NW8 6NR — MB ChB Bristol 1995.

PANG, Hin Tat 8 Colson Road, Loughton IG10 3RN — MB BS Lond. 1986; MRCPsych 1993. Assoc. Prof. Dept. Psychiat. Chinese Univ. Hong Kong. Specialty: Gen. Psychiat. Prev: Regist. (Psychiat.) NW Thames Regional Train. Scheme.

PANG, Kwok-Ki 3 Clarke Avenue, Nottingham NG5 8DL — BM BS Nottm. 1990; BMedSci Nottm. 1988; MRCPI 1995. Regist. (Paediat. Intens. Care) Birm. Childr. Hosp. Specialty: Paediat.

PANG, Lillian Shu Chao (retired) 175 Salmon Street, Kingsbury, London NW9 8NE Tel: 020 8205 5442 — MD Shanghai 1941 (Wom. Christian Med. Coll. Shanghai) BSc, MD Women's Christian Med. Coll. Shanghai 1941; PhD Leeds 1957; FRCPath 1976, M 1964; LAH Dub. 1968. Histopath. Imperial Cancer Research Fund. Prev: Chief Resid. Margt. Williamson Hosp. Shanghai.

PANG, Lyndon 16 The Beeches, Liverpool L18 3LT — MB ChB Liverp. 1991.

PANG, Pauline 146 Adventurers Quay, Butetown, Cardiff CF10 4NR — MB BCh Wales 1998; DRCOG 2002; MRCGP 2004.

PANGAYATSELVAN, Mr Thiyagarajah Orthopaedic Department, East Surrey Hospital, Canada Avenue, Redhill RH1 5RH Tel: 01737 768511; 58 Smitham Downs Road, Purley CR8 4NF Tel: 020 8660 1714 — MB BS Peradeniya 1979; LRCP LRCS Ed. LRCPS Glas. 1985; FRCS Ed. 1985; MSc (Orthop.) Lond. 1987; FRCS (Orthop.) Ed. 1990. Cons. Trauma & Orthop. Surg. E. Surrey Hosp. Redhill. Specialty: Orthop. Socs: Fell. BOA. Prev: Assoc. Specialist (Orthop.) New E. Surrey Hosp. Redhill; Regist. (Orthop.) N. Middlx. Hosp. Lond. & Memor. Hosp. Darlington.

PANHWAR, Ghylam-Mustafa College Road Surgery, 4-6 College Road, Woking GU22 8BT Tel: 01483 771309; Goldsworth Park Health Centre, Denton Way, Woking Tel: 01483 770355 — MRCS Eng. LRCP Lond. 1980 (Liaquat Med. Coll.) MB BS Sind, Pakistan 1959; DCMT . Lond. 1968. Prev: SHO (Cas. & Orthop.) Bridgend Gen. Hosp. Mem Roy. Soc. Trop. Med.; SHO (Gen. Surg. & Cas.) Waveney Hosp. Ballymena; SHO (Thoracic Surg. & Cardiac Surg.) Frenchay Hosp. Bristol.

PANIGRAHI, Hari North Manchester General Hospital, Delaunays Road, Manchester M8 6RB Tel: 0161 720 2884 Fax: 0161 720 2886 Email: hari.panigrahi@mail.nmanhc-tr.nwest.nhs.uk — MB BS Calcutta 1971; D.Bact; MD; FRCPath. Cons. (Microbiol. & Infect. Control). Specialty: Med. Microbiol. Special Interest: Antimicrobial Ther.

PANIGRAHI, Krishna Donald Wilde Medical Centre, 283 Rochdale Road, Oldham OL1 2HG Tel: 0161 652 3184 Fax: 0161 620 2101 — MB BS Calcutta 1972; MB BS Calcutta 1972.

PANIGRAHI, Padmalochan The Surgery, 70 Winslow Drive, Immingham, Grimsby DN40 2DL Tel: 01469 574197 Fax: 01469 574198 — MRCS Eng. LRCP Lond. 1979 (Burla Med. Coll. Orissa) MB BS Utkal India 1965; DTM & H Lond. 1968; Dip Ven. Liverp. 1969; DCH RCPSI 1972. GP Grimsby. Prev: Regist. (Paediat.) York Dist. Hosp.; Regist. (Psychiat.) Hartwood Hosp. Shotts; SHO (Paediat.) Seacroft Hosp. Leeds.

PANIKKAR, Apsara 8A Collingwood Terrace, Newcastle upon Tyne NE2 2JP — MB BS Newc. 1991.

PANIKKAR, Jane Bromiley, Clayton-Le-Dale, Blackburn BB1 9EG — MB ChB Sheff. 1989; MRCOG 1985; MD Sheff. 2000. Cons. (O & G) Shrewsbury. Specialty: Obst. & Gyn. Prev: Specialist Regist. (O & G) N. Trent.

PANIKKAR, Krishna Kumar Department of Anaesthetics, Stoke Man Deville Hospital, Mandeville Road, Aylesbury HP21 8AL Tel:

01296 315000 — MB BS Lond. 1987; FRCA 1994. Cons. (Anaesth. & Intens. Care) Stoke Mandeville Hosp. Aylesbury. Specialty: Anaesth. Prev: Sen. Regist. Hammersmith Hosp. Lond.; Lect. (Anaesth.) Chelsea & Westm. Hosp. Lond.; Regist. Roy. Free Hosp. & Whittington Hosp. Lond.

PANIKKER, Narayana Ravindra Heath Lane Hopsital, Heath Lane, Sandwell, West Bromwich B71 2BQ Tel: 0121 5537676 Fax: 0121 8073229; 6 Canberra Crescent, Meir Park, Longton, Stoke-on-Trent ST3 7RA — MB ChB Ed. 1976 (Univ. Ed.) BSc (Med. Sci.) Ed. 1973; MRCP (UK) 1983; MRCPsych 1990; DPM RCPSI 1990. Specialist Regist., Psychiat. of Learning Disabil., W. Midl.s Rotary. Specialty: Gen. Psychiat. Socs: Brit. Soc. Rehabil. Med.; Brit. Inst. Learning Disabil.; Soc. Clin. Psychiats. Prev: Sen. Regist. (Rehabil. Med.) Soton. & Salisbury; Sen. Med. Off. (Brain Injury) Roy. Hosp. & Home Putney, Lond.; Regist. (Psychiat.) Pk.head, Duke St. & Gartloch Hosps. Glas.

PANIKKER, Sujatha Division of Bacteriology, University of Manchester, Clinical Sciences Building, Royal Infirmary, Oxford Road, Manchester M13 9WL Tel: 0161 276 8828 Fax: 0161 276 8826; 1 Grangelands, Macclesfield SK10 4AB Tel: 01625 266716 — MB BS Kerala 1963 (Trivandrum Med. Coll.) DTM & H Ed. 1964; MSc Ed. 1967. Lect. (Bact.) Univ. Manch. Med. Sch. Specialty: Med. Microbiol. Prev: Regist. (Pub. Health) Laborat. Serv. Manch.

PANIS, Egidius Anna Hubertus 49 Trenchard Avenue, Stafford ST16 3RD — Artsexamen Utrecht 1989.

PANJA, Ayan Sarasija The Greens Medical Practice, 96 Umfreville Road, London N4 1TL Tel: 020 8374 0707 — MB BS Lond. 1999 (Imp. Coll.) DRCOG 2001; DFFP 2002; MRCGP 2003. GP Princip. The Greens Med. Pract. (www.greensmedicalpractice.co.uk); GP Tutor Roy. Free/UCL Med. Sch. Specialty: Gen. Pract. Special Interest: Med. NLP; Writing; Men's Health. Socs: Soc. Med. Writers; Soc. Med. NLP. Prev: GP The Medici Pract. Luton; GP Regist. Aston Clinton Surg. Bucks.; VTS SHO (Med.) Stoke Mandeville Hosp. Aylesbury.

PANJA, Kishan Kumar The Surgery, 4 Cross Street, Leicester LE4 5BA Tel: 0116 268 1242; 11 Grenfell Road, Stoneygate, Leicester LE2 2PA Tel: 0116 270 5099 — MB BS Calcutta 1970 (R.G. Kar Med. Coll.)

PANJA, Mr Sanat Kumar Claude Nicol Centre, Royal Sussex County Hospital, Brighton BN2 5BE Tel: 01273 664717 Fax: 01273 664720; 135 Shirley Drive, Hove BN3 6UJ Tel: 01273 551530 Fax: 01273 551530 — MB BS Calcutta 1967 (Med. Coll. Calcutta) DGO Calcutta 1969; FRCOG 1989, M 1973; FRCS Ed. 1976. Cons. Roy. Sussex Co. Hosp. Brighton. Specialty: Genitourinary Medicine. Prev: Sen. Regist. Cardiff Roy. Infirm.

PANJA, Shuba Rani Victoria Road Surgery, 27 Victoria Road, Horwich, Bolton BL6 5NA Tel: 01204 467197 — MB ChB Manch. 1979. GP Horwich.

PANJWANI, Suresh 18 Chailey Av, Enfield EN1 3LY — MB BS Delhi 1978; LRCP LRCS Ed. LRCPS Glas. 1986; MRCS Eng. LRCP Lond. 1986; DGM RCP Lond. 1988; T(GP) 1991. Regist. (Geriat. Med.) St. Michael's Hosp. Enfield. Specialty: Care of the Elderly. Prev: SHO (Gen. Med.) Chingford Hosp.; SHO (A & E) Mt. Vernon Hosp. Northwood; SHO (Geriat.) N. Devon Dist. Hosp. Barnstaple.

PANKHANIA, Ajay Chhaganlal 40 Cambridge Close, Hounslow TW4 7BG — MB ChB Manch. 1996.

PANKHANIA, Bharat 38 Pantiles Close, St. John's, Woking GU21 1PT Tel: 01483 724028 Fax: 01483 837080 Email: bharat999@netscape.net; 83 Evington Drive, Leicester LE5 5PG Tel: 01483 724028 — MB BCh Wales 1985 (Univ. Wales Coll. Med.) MRCGP 1989; DGM RCP Lond. 1990; DCH RCP Lond. 1992; MFPHM Lond. 1999. Communicable Dis. Control, Wilts. Health Auth. Specialty: Pub. Health Med. Prev: Sen. Regist. (Pub. Health Med.) S. Thames RHA.

PANKHANIA, Rajesh The Harlequin Surgery, 160 Shard End Crescent, Shard End, Birmingham B34 7BP Tel: 0121 747 8291 Fax: 0121 749 5497 — MB ChB Birm. 1991; ChB Birm. 1991; MRCGP 1995.

PANKHURST, Maria-Teresa Anne 3 Copley Park, London SW16 3DE — MB BS Lond. 1996.

PANNELL, Bryony Mary Burnet Hillfoot, Byfield Road, Priors Marston, Southam CV47 7RP — MB ChB Aberd. 1981; Dip. Community Paediat. Warwick 1987. Asst. GP Byfield, N.ants.; Gen. Pract. Specialty: Gen. Pract.

PANNETT, Richard Neil Yare Medical Practice, 202 Thorpe Road, Norwich NR1 1TJ Tel: 01603 437559 Email: richard.pannett@nhs.net — MB ChB Manch. 1973; DRCOG 1978; DCH RCP Lond. 1979. Specialty: Gen. Pract.

PANNIKER, Clare Bernadette (retired) Chase View, Hilltop Drive, Oughtibridge, Sheffield S35 0AX Tel: 0116 286 3065 — LRCPI & LM, LRSCI & LM 1960. Prev: GP Sheff.

PANNIKER, Richard Michael Wadsley Bridge Medical Centre, 103 Halifax Road, Sheffield S6 1LA Tel: 0114 234 5025 — MB BS Lond. 1983 (St. Mary's) DRCOG 1986; MRCGP 1989. Prev: Trainee GP Bradford VTS; Ho. Phys. Bradford Roy. Infirm.; Ho. Surg. Derbysh. Roy. Infirm.

PANNU, Gurprit Singh 1 Forge Lane, Crawley RH10 1QS — BChir Camb. 1992.

PANNU, Harpreet Singh 236 Queens Road, Leicester LE2 3FT — MB ChB Leic. 1994.

PANNU, Upkar Singh Bensham Family Practice, 1 Sidney Grove, Bensham, Gateshead NE8 2XB Tel: 0191 477 1554 — MB BS Durh. 1963.

PANOS, George Zenon 75 Eyre Court, Finchley Road, St John's Wood, London NW8 9TX Tel: 020 7722 3700 — Ptychio Iatrikes Athens 1983; BSc Salford 1978. Specialty: Gen. Med.

PANOS, Marios Zenon 75 Eyre Court, Finchley Road, London NW8 9TX Email: marzepanos@aol.com — MB BS Lond. 1981 (Middlx.) MRCP (UK) 1984; BSc Lond. 1976, MD 1990; FRCP Lond. 1998. Private Pract.; Med. Regist., St. Stephen's Hosp., Lond. Specialty: Gen. Med.; Gastroenterol. Socs: Brit. Soc. Gastroenterol.; Amer. Gastroenterol. Assn.; Europ. Assn. Of study of the Liver. Prev: Cons. Phys. (Med & Gastroenterol.) Roy. Berks Hosp. Reading; Lect. & Hon. Sen. Regist. (Med. & Gastroenterol.) Qu. Eliz. Hosp. & E. Birm. Hosp.; Clin. Research Fell. Liver Unit King's Coll. Hosp. Lond.

PANOSKALTSIS, Theodoros Department of Obstetrics & Gynaecology, Hammersmith Hospital-Queen Charlotte's Hosp., Du Cane Road, London W12 0HS; 5 Portobello Mews, London W11 3DQ — Ptychio Iatrikes Athens 1987. Sen. Regist. (O & G). Specialty: Obst. & Gyn. Socs: MRCOG.

PANSARI, Natwar Gopal Doctors Surgery, Short Street, Brownhills, Walsall WS8 6AD Tel: 01543 373222 Fax: 01543 454640 — MB BS Indore 1971.

PANTAZIS, Andreas 82 Clarence Road, London N22 8PW — BM Soton. 1992 (Southampton University) BSc Soton. 1991; MRCP (UK) 1996; DRCOG 1999; DFFP 2001. Specialty: Gen. Pract. Prev: SHO Renal Med., St. Mary's, Paddington; SHO, Gen. Med., Soton. Gen. Hosp.; GP (VTS) Hinchingbrooke NHS Trust.

PANTELIDES, Michalakis Leonida 2 Farrer Road, Longsight, Manchester M13 0QX — MB ChB Manch. 1979. SHO (Surg. Rotat.) Manch. Roy. Infirm.

PANTER, Simon James 35 Crowles Road, Mirfield WF14 9PJ — MB ChB Ed. 1994 (Edinburgh) BSc (Hons.) Ed. 1992; MRCP 1997. Specialist Regist. (Gastroenterol.) Northern Deanery Based S. Cleveland. Specialty: Gastroenterol. Prev: SHO Respirat. Unit Freeman Newc.; SHO GI RVI Newc.; SHO Neuro RVI Newc.

PANTIN, Charles Frank Alcock University Hospital of North Staffordshire, Directorate of Respiratory Medicine, Newcastle Road, Stoke-on-Trent ST4 6QG Tel: 01782 552329 Fax: 01782 552323 Email: charles.pantin@uhns.nhs.uk — MB BS Lond. 1977 (St Bartholomews Hospital, University of London) PhD, MA Camb. 1972; MRCP (UK) 1980; FRCP Lond. 1993. Cons. Phys. Univ. Hosp. of N. Staffs.; Sen. Lect. (Postgrad. Med.) Keele Univ. Specialty: Respirat. Med. Prev: Sen. Regist. Brompton & Westm. Hosps. Lond.

PANTIN, Priscilla Leslie 9 Coalecroft Road, London SW15 6LW — BM BCh Oxf. 1970; DA Eng. 1972; FFA RCS Eng. 1976. Cons. Anaesth. Centr. Middlx. Hosp. Lond. Specialty: Anaesth.

PANTING, Gerard Patrick The Medical Protection Society, 33 Cavendish Square, London W1M 0PS Tel: 020 7399 1300 Fax: 020 7399 1301; Waters Green, Marshalls Heath Lane, Wheatampstead, St Albans AL48HJ Tel: 01582 831664 — MB BS Lond. 1976 (Char. Cross) MRCS Eng. LRCP Lond. 1976; DRCOG 1981; DCH RCP Lond. 1982; MRCGP 1985; DMJ Soc. Apoth. Lond. 1987; MA (Med. Ethics & Law) Lond. 1992. Communications & Policy Dir. Specialty: Forens. Path. Prev: Dep. Police Surg. St. Albans & Hemel Hempstead; Course Organiser & Trainer St Albans GP VTS.

PANTING, Jonathan Rory MR Unit, Royal Brompton Hospital, Sydney St., London SW3 6NP Tel: 020 8898 7239 Fax: 020 8351

8816; 57 Powder Mill Lane, Twickenham TW2 6EF — BSc (1st cl. Hons.) St. And. 1985; MB BChir Camb. 1989; DTM & H RCP Lond. 1990; MRCP (UK) 1992. Clin. Research Fell. MR Unit Roy. Brompton Hosp. Lond. Specialty: Cardiol.; Gen. Med. Socs: Stud. Mem. Internat. Soc. Magnetic Resonance in Med.; Soc. Cardiovasc. Magnetic Resonance. Prev: SHO Rotat. (Med.) E. Birm. Hosp.; Regist. Rotat. (Cardiol.) Hull.

PANTING, Kim 2 Blacon Farm Cottages, Snitterfield Lane, Warwick CV35 8JJ Tel: 017889 730336; 2 Blacon Farm Cottages, Snitterfield Lane, Warwick CV35 8HH Tel: 01789 730336 — MB ChB Birm. 1987; DRCOG 1992; MRCGP 1995. Gen. Practitioner. Prev: Locum Gen. Practitioner.

PANTLIN, Adrian William Llanarth Court, Llanarth, Raglan NP15 2YD Tel: 01873 840555 Fax: 01873 840591 — MB ChB Bristol 1971; MRCPsych 1975. Cons. Psychiat. Llanarth Ct. Raglan Gwent. Specialty: Ment. Health; Psychother.; Forens. Psychiat. Socs: Assoc. Mem. Gp. Anal. Soc. Lond. Prev: Cons. Psychiat. Basildon & Thurrock HA; Sen. Regist. N.W. Thames RHA; Sen. Regist. Uffculme Clinic Birm.

PANTO, Philip Nigel Department of Radiology, Kings Mill Hospital, Mansfield Road, Sutton-in-Ashfield NG17 4JL Tel: 01623 622515; 30 Summercourt Drive, Ravenshead, Nottingham NG15 9FT Tel: 01623 484186 — MB BS Lond. 1979 (King's Coll. Hosp.); BM Oxf. 1975; MA Oxf. 1979; FRCR 1986. Cons. Diag. Radiol. N. Notts. HA. Specialty: Radiol. Socs: Brit. Nuclear Med. Soc.; Brit. Soc. Interven. Radiol.; Cardiovasc. & Interven. Radiol. Soc. of Europe. Prev: Sen. Regist. (Diag. Radiol.) Nottm. Hosps.; SHO (Cardiol. & Gen. Med.) Kent & Canterbury Hosp.; SHO (Neurol. Surg.) Radcliffe Infirm. Oxf.

PANTON, David John Kelseys Doctors Surgery, Mill Road, Liss GU33 7AZ Tel: 01730 892184 Fax: 01730 893634; The Old Rectory, West Liss, Liss GU33 6JU Tel: 01730 892366 — MB BS Lond. 1974 (Lond. Hosp.) DRCOG 1979. GP Staff Petersfield Hosp. Prev: Ho. Phys. & Ho. Surg. St. Stephen's Hosp. Lond.; Maj. RAMC.

PANTON, Heather Maureen (retired) 36 Lulworth Lodge, Palatine Rd, Southport PR8 2BS — MB ChB Manch. 1951; DObst RCOG 1953; FRCOG 1974, M 1960; FRCS Ed. 1965. Prev: Cons. Gyn. St. Helens & Knowsley DHA.

PANTON, Ian Robert Oakmeadow Surgery, 87 Tatlow Road, Glenfield, Leicester LE3 8NF Tel: 0116 287 7911 — MB Camb. 1978 (St. Geo.) BA Camb. 1974, MB 1978, BChir 1977; DRCOG 1980; MRCGP 1982.

PANTON, Nicholas Timothy MacIver Gervis Road Surgery, 14 Gervis Road, Bournemouth BH1 3EG Tel: 01202 293418 Fax: 01202 317866; 20 St. Leonard's Road, Charminster, Bournemouth BH8 8QN Tel: 01202 527761 Fax: 01202 549370 — MB BS Lond. 1972 (Westm.) ILTM; MRCS Eng.; LRCP Lond. 1972; Dobst RCOG 1975; DA Eng. 1976; MRCGP 1981. GP Bournemouth; Course Organiser Dorset VTS. Socs: BMA.

PANTON, Sally Meadowbrook, 4 Flagshaw Lane, Kirk Langley, Derby DE6 4NW — MB ChB Ed. 1977 (Edinburgh) MRCGP 1981; DRCOG 1981; DCCH RCGP 1992. Clin. Med. Off. (Child Health) Derby. Specialty: Community Child Health.

PANTON, Susanna The Surgery, 107 Weoley Castle Road, Weoley Castle, Birmingham B29 5QD Tel: 0121 427 1530 — MB BS Lond. 1988; MRCGP 1993.

PANTRIDGE, Professor James Francis, CBE, MC (retired) Woodlands Corcreeny, Hillsborough BT26 6EH Tel: 01846 689976 Fax: 01846 689807 — MD Belf. 1946 (Queens Univ Belfast) MB BCh BAO (Hons.) 1939; FRCP Lond. 1962, M 1947; Hon. FRCPI 1970; Hon. DSc Ulster 1981, Hon. DSc Open 1981. Prev: Phys. Roy. Vict. Hosp. Belf.

PAO, Caroline Shien-Lan Flat 4, 81 Alderney St., London SW1V 4HF — MB BS Lond. 1991.

PAO, David Shien Phen Mei-Lan, 5 Rosebriars, Esher KT10 9NN — MB BS Lond. 1994.

PAOLONI, Claudia Christina Erika — MB BS Lond. 1991; BSc (Hons.) Lond. 1988; FRCA 1997. Cons. (Anaesth.) Bristol Roy. Infirm. Specialty: Anaesth. Special Interest: Cardiothoracic. Socs: Brit. Med. Assn.; Eur. Acad. Anaesth. Prev: Specialist Regist. (Anaesth.) Soton.; Med. Off. Roy. Flying Doctor Serv., Australia; SHO (Med.) Soton.

PAPACHRYSOSTOMOU EVGENIKOS, Maria Gastrointestinal Unit, Western General Hospital, Crewe Road S., Edinburgh EH4 2XU Tel: 0131 537 1756 Fax: 0131 336 4492 Email: mpapachrysostomou@ed.ac.uk; 17 Barnton Park Avenue, Edinburgh EH4 6ES Tel: 0131 336 4492 — Vrach Rostov Med. Inst. 1984 (Rostov Med. Institute and Edinburgh University) MD Rostov Med. Inst. 1984; PhD (Med.) Ed. 1992. Staff Gastroenterol. Western Gen. Hosp. Edin. Specialty: Gastroenterol.; Gen. Med.; Immunol. Socs: Caledonian Soc. Gastroenterol.; Eur. Soc. Gastroenterol. & Hepatol.; Assoc. of Coloproct. Gt. Brit. & Ire. Prev: Lect. (Med.) Univ. of Edin. Western Gen. Hosp.

PAPACONSTANTINOU, Helen Inverclyde Royal Hospital, Larkfield Road, Greenock PA16 0XN Tel: 01475 633777; 2 Shields, Bridesmill Road, Lochwinnoch PA12 4HL — FRCP Glasgow 2002; Ptychio Iatrikes Athens 1984. Consultant Cardiologist. Specialty: Cardiol.; Gen. Med.

PAPACOSTOPOULOS, Demetrios 41 Northumberland Road, Bristol BS6 7BA — Ptychio Iatrikes Athens 1962; PhD Bristol 1982.

PAPADAKIS, Mr Antonios c/o Urology Department, Ealing Hospital, Uxbridge Road, Southall UB1 3HW; 5 Broadway Close, Urmston, Manchester M41 7NR — Ptychio Iatrikes Athens 1986; FRCS Ed. 1994. SHO Rotat. (Surg.) Whiston Hosp. Prescot; Mem. Bristol Urol. Inst. Specialty: Urol. Socs: Hellenic Med. Soc. Prev: SHO (Urol. & Surg.) Dist. Gen. Hosp. Glan Clwyd; SHO (Surg.) Vict. Hopsp. Blackburn.

PAPADOPOULOS, Andreas John 5 The Murreys, Barnettwood Lane, Ashtead KT21 2LU — MB BS Lond. 1990.

PAPADOPOULOU, Anthie Maria First Floor Flat, 16 Crossfield Road, London NW3 4NT — MB BS Lond. 1998.

PAPAGEORGHIOU, Aris Theodosis 4 Portland Buildings, Sheffield S6 3DZ — MB ChB Sheff. 1996.

PAPAGEORGIOU, George Labros 17 Tedworth Green, Leicester LE4 2NG — Ptychio Iatrikes Athens 1978.

PAPAGIANNOPOULOS, Mr Konstantinos Leeds General Infirmary, Department of Cardiothoracic Surgery, Jubilee Building, Level D, Room 196, Great George Street, Leeds LS1 3EX Tel: 0113 392 5194 Fax: 0113 392 8436 Email: kpapagiannopoulos@yahoo.com — Ptychio Iatrikes Crete 1990. Cons. Leeds Teaching Hosps. NHS Trust. Specialty: Cardiothoracic Surg. Special Interest: Pectus deformity; Chest Wall Resections; Lung Cancer. Socs: Europ. Assn. of Cardiothoracic Surgeons; Europ. Assn. of Thoracic Surgeons; Soc. of Cardiothoracic Surgeons of Gt. Britain and Irel.

PAPAKOSTAS, Pavlos 169A Grey Turner House, Du Cane Road, London W12 0UA — Ptychio Iatrikes Athens 1979.

PAPAMICHAEL, Demetrios Flat 16, Cedarland Court, 1A Roland Gardens, London SW7 3RW Tel: 020 7460 6491 — MB BS Lond. 1988 (Char Cross & Westm.) MRCP (UK) 1992. Specialist Regist. (Med. Oncol.) & Clin. Research Fell. ICRF Dept. Med. Oncol. St. Bart. Hosp. Lond. Specialty: Oncol.

PAPANASTASSIOU, Mr Varnavas Department of Neurosurgery, Institute of Neurological Sciences, The Southern General Hospital, Glasgow G51 4TF Tel: 0141 201 2107 Fax: 0141 201 2995 Email: vp7s@clinmed.gla.ac.uk — MB ChB Manch. 1985; FRCS Eng. 1989; FRCS Ed. 1989; MD Manch. 1994; FRCS (SN) 1995; CCST (Neurosurg.) UK 1997. Sen. Lect. & Cons. Neurosurg. Inst. Neurol. Sc. Glasg. Specialty: Neurosurg. Socs: SBNS; Hellenic Med. Soc.; EANO. Prev: Sen. Regist. (Neurosurg.) Radcliffe Infirm. Oxf.; Regist. (Neurosurg.) Radcliffe Infirm. Oxf.; Clin. Research Fell. Imperial Cancer Research Fund Frenchay Hosp. Bristol.

PAPAPANAGIOTOU, George 35 Elmwood Road, London SE24 9NS — Ptychio Iatrikes Athens 1981.

PAPAS, Kyvelie 91 Westbourne Terrace, London W2 6QT Tel: 020 7262 5600 Email: kyvelie@aol.com — MD Athens 1969; FRCPCH; MB 1954; LAH Dub. 1964. SCMO W. Lambeth HA. Socs: ACPP. Prev: Deptm. Med. Off. Lond. Boro. Haringey.

PAPASAVVAS, Georghios Kyriacos Department Rheumatology, Royal Sussex County Hospital, Eastern Road, Brighton BN2 5BE Tel: 01273 696955 Fax: 01273 673466 — MB BS Lond. 1980 (Lond. Hosp.) MRCP (UK) 1983; FRCP 1997. Cons. Rheum. Roy. Sussex Co. Hosp. Specialty: Rheumatol. Socs: Brit. Soc. Rheum. Prev: Sen. Regist. (Rheum. & Rehabil.) King's Coll. Hosp. Lond.; Regist. (Rheum.) Middlx. Hosp.

PAPASIOPOULOS, Sophie West Middlesex University Hospital, Isleworth TW7 6AF Tel: 020 8560 2121 — Ptychion Iatzikis Thessaloniki 1963; DA Eng. 1970; FRCAI 1971; FRCA Eng. 1972;

MD Athens 1975. Cons. Anaesth. W. Middlx. Univ. Hosp. Isleworth. Specialty: Anaesth.

PAPASTATHIS, Dimitrios ENT Department, Royal Hallamshire County Hospital, Winchester SO22 5DG — Ptychio Iatrikes Athens 1972.

PAPAYANNAKOS, Efthimios 2 Gilston Road, London SW10 9SL — Ptychio Iatrikes Athens 1957.

PAPE, Mrs Sarah Amanda — MB ChB Leeds 1982; FRCS Ed. 1987; FRCS (Plast) Ed. 1994. Cons. Plastic Surg. Roy. Vict. Infirm. Newc. u. Tyne; Med. Director, Laser Care Clinics, Newc. upon Tyne. Specialty: Plastic Surg. Socs: Brit. Burns Assn.; Brit. Skin Laser Study Gp.; Assn. for the study of Med. Educat. Prev: Sen. Regist. (Plastic Surg.) Newc. Teach. Hosp. Newc.; Regist. (Plastic Surg.) Whiston Hosp. Merseyside; Regist. & SHO Postgrad. Train Scheme (Surg.) St. Jas. Hosp. Leeds.

PAPEE, Eva (retired) 28 Grasmere Avenue, London W3 6JU Tel: 020 8992 3875 Fax: 020 8248 8284 — Lekarz Katowice 1960 (Silesian Med. Acad. Katowice) Dip. Anaesth. Katowice 1963. Prev: Clin. Asst. (Anaesth.) Edgware Gen. Hosp.

PAPENFUS, Carolyn Barbara 3 Aubrey Close, Marlborough SN8 1TS — LRCP LRCS Ed. LRCPS Glas. 1988; MB ChB Zimbabwe 1985; MRCP (UK) 1991; MRCGP 1993.

PAPINI, Mr Remo Pio Giuseppe Plastic Surgery Department, University Hospital Birmingham NHS Trust, Selly Oak Hospital, Raddlebarn Road, Birmingham B24 6JD Tel: 0121 627 8784 Fax: 0121 627 8782; 29 Hallcroft Way, Knowle, Solihull B93 9ET — MB BS Lond. 1984 (Royal Free Hosp. Sch. Of Med.) FRCS Ed. 1990; FRCS (Plast) Ed. 1998. Cons. (Plastic & Burns Surg.). Specialty: Plastic Surg. Socs: Brit. Burn Assoc.; Internat. Soc. For Burn Injury; Brit. Assoc. of Plastic Surgs. Prev: Burns Fell. Roy. Perth Hosp. Perth, Western Australia; Sen. Regist. (Plastic Surg.) Whiston Hosp. Merseyside; Regist. (Plastic Surg.) Newc. u. Tyne.

PAPOUCHADO, Mark 14 York Place, Clifton, Bristol BS8 1AH — MB BChir Camb. 1976 (Camb. & Char. Cross) BA Camb. 1972, MA, MB 1976, BChir 1975; DA Eng. 1978; MRCP (UK) 1982. Cons. Cardiol. Frenchay Hosp. Bristol. Specialty: Cardiol. Prev: Sen. Research Regist. (Cardiol.) Bristol Roy. Infirm.; Regist. (Cardiol.) Bristol Roy. Infirm.; Regist. (Med.) King Edwd. VII Hosp. Windsor.

PAPPACHAN, Vithayathil John Fence Houses Surgery, Gill CrescentN., Fence House, Houghton-le-Spring DH4 6DW Tel: 0191 385 2508 — MB BChir Camb. 1991.

PAPPIN, Catherine Jane Eileen Wessex Fertility Clinic, 72-76 Anglesea Road, Southampton SO15 5QS; 7 Pointout Road, Southampton SO16 7DL — MB BS Lond. 1996 (Guys & St Thos.) DFFP 1998; MRCOG 2003. IVF Clin. Fell., Wessex Fertil., Soton. Socs: BMA; MDU. Prev: SpR, Wessex Obst. and Gyn., N. Hants. Hosp., Basingstoke; SpR, Wessex Obst. and Gyn., Roy. Hants. Co. Hosp., Winchester; SpR, Wessex Obst. and Gyn., St. Mary's Hosp., Portsmouth.

PAPPIN, John Christopher Anaesthetic Department, Torbay Hospital, Lawes Bridge, Torquay TQ2 7AA Tel: 01803 654310 Fax: 01803 654312; Netherlee, Roundham Avenue, Paignton TQ4 6DE Tel: 01803 551430 Email: jcpappin@hotmail.com — MB BS Lond. 1967 (Middlx.) MRCS Eng. LRCP Lond. 1967; FFA RCS Eng. 1972. Cons. Anaesth. Torbay Hosp. Specialty: Anaesth. Socs: BMA; Assn. Of Anaesth.s; S. W. Soc. Of Anaesth. Prev: Sen. Regist. Rotat. Avon AHA (T) & S. West. RHA; Regist. (Anaesth.) Frenchay Hosp. Bristol; Regist. Chelmsford Gp. Hosps.

PAPWORTH, George William John (retired) 12 Queens Road, Weston Super Mare BS23 2LQ Tel: 01934 624729 Fax: 01934 625845 Email: george-linda@westondoc.freeserve.co.uk — MB ChB Leeds 1968. Director. Weston Primary Care Co-Operat.; Audit Assessor Area Health Auth. Prev: Sen. Partner, Graham Rd Surg., Weston Super Mare.

PAPWORTH, James Edward John 12 Queens Road, Weston Super Mare BS23 2LQ — MB ChB Leeds 1994.

PAPWORTH-SMITH, John William c/o Occupational Health Service, University Road, University of Leeds, Leeds LS2 9JT Tel: 0113 233 2997 Fax: 0113 233 2997 — MB ChB Leeds 1976; BSc (Physiol.) Leeds 1973; DRCOG 1982; DCH RCP Lond. 1983; MRCGP 1983; Dip. Pract. Dermat. Wales 1991; Dip. Occupat. Med. 1996. Med. Off. Univ. Leeds. Specialty: Occupat. Health.

PARAB, Suresh Bhikaji Woodlands View, Hedl Eglwys, Pen-y-Fai, Bridgend CF31 4LY — MB BS Vikram 1961.

PARADINAS, Professor Fernando Juan (retired) Histopathology Department, Charing Cross Hospital, Fulham Palace Road, London W6 8RF Tel: 020 8846 7142 Fax: 020 8846 7139; 54 Eton Court, Eton Avenue, London NW3 3HJ Tel: 020 7722 8585 — LRCP LRCS Ed. LRCPS Glas. 1965 (Madrid Univ.) LMS Madrid 1962; FRCPath 1983, M 1971; MRCR 1994. Prev: Emerit. Prof. Imperial Coll. Sch. Med.

PARAMAGNANAM, Nalliah Chestnut Green Surgery, 27 Chestnut Green, Upper Cwmbran, Cwmbran NP44 5TH Tel: 01633 482248 Fax: 01633 484228; 2 Meyricks, Coed Eva, Cwmbran NP44 6TU — MB BS Ceylon 1962 (Colombo) Specialty: Gen. Pract.

PARAMANATHAN, Kanjana 31 Manor Road N., Birmingham B16 9JS — MB BS Ceylon 1976 (Colombo) LRCP LRCS Ed. LRCPS Glas. 1981. Regist. (Anaesth.) Geo. Eliot Hosp. Nuneaton. Specialty: Anaesth. Prev: SHO (Anaesth.) St. Margts. Hosp. Epping; SHO (Anaesth.) Good Hope Gen. Hosp. Sutton Coldfield; SHO (Anaesth.) Roy. Hosp. Wolverhampton.

PARAMANATHAN, Nirmala Dept of Surgery, Royal Hampshire County Hospital, Romsey Road, Winchester SO22 5DG Tel: 01962 863535 — MRCS Eng. LRCP Lond. 1987; FRCS Glas. 1996. Staff Grade (Gen. Surg.) Roy. Hamp. Co. Hosp. Winchester. Specialty: Gen. Surg. Prev: Regist. (Gen. Surg.) Roy. Hamp. Co. Hosp. Winchester; SHO (Gen. Surg.) Southend Gen. Hosp.; SHO (Gen. Surg.) Co. Hosp. Lincoln.

PARAMANATHAN, Sivapragasam 31 Manor Road N., Birmingham B16 9JS — MB BS Ceylon 1973 (Univ. Ceylon) LRCP LRCS Ed. LRCPS Glas. 1981. SHO (O & G) Hosp. of St. Cross Rugby. Prev: SHO (O & G) Wordsley Hosp. Stourbridge.

PARAMANATHAN, Veluppillai Otterfield Road Medical Centre, 25 Otterfield Road, Yiewsley, West Drayton UB7 8PE Tel: 01895 422611 Fax: 01895 431309; 11 Pastures Mead, Hillingdon, Uxbridge UB10 9PU — (University of Sri Lanka) DFFP (1992); MB BS Ceylon 1970; T(GP) 1991. GP.

PARAMESHWAR, Karat Jayan Transplant Unit, Papworth Hospital, Papworth Everard, Cambridge CB3 8RE Tel: 01480 830541 — MD All India Med. Scs. 1981; MB BS Madras 1977; MD (Med.) All India Med. Scs. 1981; MRCP (UK) 1984; MPhil Lond. 1992. Cons. Transpl. Cardiol. Papworth Hosp. Specialty: Cardiol. Socs: Brit. Cardiac Soc.; Internat. Soc. of Heart and Lung Transpl.ation. Prev: Regist. (Cardiol.) Roy. Brompton & Nat. Heart & Lung Hosps. Lond.; Regist. (Med. & Cardiol.) Hillingdon Hosp. Uxbridge; Regist. (Gen. Med.) Bedford Gen. Hosp.

PARAMESWARAN, Raghavannair 25 Whitemeadows, Darlington DL3 8SR Tel: 01642 813166 — MD Panjab 1970 (Trivandrum Med. Coll.) MB BS Kerala 1968; MD (Rad.) Panjab India 1970; FRCR 1979. Cons. (Neuroradiol.) S. Tees HA, Middlesbrough Gen. & S. Cleveland. Specialty: Radiol. Socs: Brit. Soc. Neuroradiol. Prev: Sen. Regist. (Neuroradiol.) Regional Neurol. Centre Newc.; Regist. (Radiol.) & Sen. Regist. (Radiol.) Roy. Vict. Infirm. & Hosp.

PARAMESWARAN, Shanthy Santhanayagi Paediatric Department, Wexham Park Hospital, Slough SL2 4HL Tel: 01753 633 737/01753 638 685 Fax: 01753 638 373 — MB BS Ceylon 1966; MRCPsych 1978; T(Psychiat) 1991; FRC(Psy) 2004. Cons., Child/Adolescent Psychiat., Berks. Health Care Trust, Berks.; Examr., Diploma in Child Health; Med. Mem., Ment. health Review Tribunal. Specialty: Child & Adolesc. Psychiat. Special Interest: Chronic Physical Illness; Disaster- War Related; Parental Ment. Illness & Effect on Childr. Socs: Roy. Coll. of Psychiat.; Sri Lanka Trauma Gp., UK Br. Prev: Cons., Child/Adolescent Psychiat., Basildon/ Grays Essex; Specialist Regist., St Georges Med. Sch.

PARAMESWARAN, Umadevi The Wandle Surgery, 161 Wandle Road, Morden SM4 6AA Tel: 020 8648 1877 Fax: 020 8648 4737 — MB BS Peradeniya, Sri Lanka 1982.

PARAMOTHAYAN, Brinda Navaluxmi Glenlyn Medical Centre, 115 Molesey Park Road, East Molesey KT8 0JX Tel: 020 8979 3253 Fax: 020 8941 7914 — MB ChB Liverp. 1992; BSc (Hons.) Physiol. Liverp. 1989. SHO Rotat. (O & G, Palliat. Med., Radiat. Oncol., Paediat. & Psychogeriat.) Wessex RHA VTS.

PARAMOTHAYAN, Niranjala Shanthimanoharie The Lighthouse, 47 Banstead Road S., Sutton SM2 5LG — MB BS Lond. 1993 (St. Bartholomew's) BSc Birm. 1984; PhD Camb. 1987; MRCP (UK) 1996. Locum Cons. Phys. (Respirat. & Gen. Med.) St. Geo.'s. Specialty: Respirat. Med.; Gen. Med. Socs: Roy. Coll. Phys.; Brit. Thorac. Soc.; BMA.

PARANJAPE, Ruchira Nitin 30 Silverwood Close, Brackley Road, Beckenham BR3 1RN — MB BS Lond. 1996.

PARANJOTHY, Chellatturai Eric Moore Health Centre, Tanners Lane, Warrington WA2 7LY Tel: 01925 411210 Fax: 01925 632868; 18 Norlands Lane, Rainhill, Prescot L35 6NR Tel: 0151 289 8905 — MB BS Ceylon 1962. Specialty: Gen. Pract. Socs: BMA; ODA.

PARANJOTHY, Renuka 3 Cedar Walk, Osborn Park, Welwyn Garden City AL7 1HQ — MB ChB Manch. 1995.

PARANJOTHY, Shantini Horton General Hospital NHS Trust, Banbury OX16 9BR — MB BCh Wales 1995.

PARAPIA, Liakatali Gulamhussein Habib Dept. of Haemat., Bradford Royal Infirmary, Duckworth Lane, Bradford BD9 6RJ Tel: 01274 364203 Fax: 01274 364681; Farnhill, Kelcliffe Lane, Guiseley, Leeds LS20 9DE Tel: 01943 877282 Fax: 01274 364681 — MB BCh Wales 1974 (Univ. Coll. Cardiff, Welsh Nat. Sch. Med.) MRCP (UK) 1978; MRCPath. 1981; FRCPath 1991; FRCP Lond. 1992; FRCP Ed. 1992. Cons. Haematolgy Bradford Roy. Infirm. Hosps.; Hon. Cons. Leeds Teachg. Hosp.; Dir. Pathol. Yorks. Clinic Bradford; Operat. Med. Dir. Bradford. Specialty: Haematology. Special Interest: Coagulation; Oncology. Socs: Brit. Soc. Haemat.; Roy. Microscopical Soc.; Brit. Med. Assn. Prev: Sen. Regist. (Haemat.) Leeds AHA.

PARARAJASINGAM, Ravi 22 Lutterworth Road, Leicester LE2 8PE — MB ChB Leic. 1991. SHO (A & E Med.) Northampton Gen. Hosp. Specialty: Accid. & Emerg. Socs: BMA & Med. Protec. Soc. Prev: Demonst. (Anat.) St. Bart. Hosp. Lond.; Ho. Off. (Gen. Surg.) Leics. Gen. Hosp.

PARASHAR, Mr Karan Children's Hospital, Steelhouse Lane, Birmingham B4 6NH Tel: 0121 333 8082 Email: karan.parashar@bhamchildrens.wmids.nhs.uk; 145 Moor Green Lane, Moseley, Birmingham B13 8NT — MB BS Poona 1978; MB BS Poona, India 1978; FRCS Glas. 1983; FRCS Ed. 1987; FRCS (Paediat.) 1994. Cons. Paediat. Surg. The Childr. Hosp. Birm. Specialty: Paediat. Surg.

PARASHCHAK, Myroslav Roman Longford Street Surgery, Longford Street, Heywood OL10 4NH Tel: 01706 621417 Fax: 01706 622915; Hawthorn House, White Horse Meadows, Broad Lane, Rochdale OL16 4PU Tel: 01706 712746 Email: mpdoc@zen.co.uk — MB ChB Manch. 1979 (St And. & Manch.) BSc (Med. Sci.) St And. 1976; MRCP (UK) 1983; DRCOG 1984; MRCGP 1985. Specialty: Cardiol.

PARASKEVA, Paraskevas Antonios 27 Crown Street, Harrow HA2 0HX — MB BS Lond. 1994.

PARASKEVAIDES, Mr Eftis Costas Hinchingbrooke Hospital, Hinchingbrooke Park, Huntingdon PE29 6NT Tel: 01480 416416; Clyde Farm, Silver St, Godmanchester, Huntingdon PE29 2LF — MB ChB Manch. 1980; BSc Manch. 1977, MB ChB 1980; FRCS Glas. 1986; FRCS Ed. 1987; MRCOG 1990; MRCPI 1993. Cons. O & G Hinchingbrooke Hosp. Huntingdon. Specialty: Obst. & Gyn. Socs: Manch. Med. Soc. (Surgic. Div.); E. Anglia Obst. & Gyn. Soc. Prev: Lect. (O & G) Roy. Coll. Surg. Irel. Rotunda Hosp. Dub.

PARASURAM, Pothina c/o Mr M. N. Patrudu, 52 Mellanear Road, Hayle TR27 4QT — MB BS Andhra 1974.

PARBHOO, Ishverlal 57-59 East Dulwich Road, London SE22 9AP Tel: 020 8693 3047 — LRCPI & LM, LRSCI & LM 1953 (RCSI) LRCPI & LM, LRCSI & LM 1953. Prev: SHMO (Cas. & Orthop.) Roy. Infirm. Blackburn; Regist. Vict. Hosp. Burnley & Reedyford Memor. Hosp. Nelson.

PARBHOO, Krishnapathee 57-59 East Dulwich Road, London SE22 9AP Tel: 020 8693 3047 — LRCPI & LM, LRSCI & LM 1953 (RCSI) LRCPI & LM, LRCSI & LM 1953; DA Eng. 1957. Prev: Regist. (Anaesth.) Blackburn Hosp. Gp.; SHO (Cas.) Pub. Disp. & Hosp. Leeds; SHO (Anaesth.) Colchester Hosp. Gp.

PARBHOO, Pravinkumar Hurrilal The Paagon Suite, Wexham Park Hospital, Wexham St., Slough SL2 4HL — MB ChB Natal 1975.

PARBHOO, Rakesh Green Lanes Surgery, 939 Green Lanes, London N21 2PB — MB BS Lond. 1991 (UCL & Middlx.) MRCP 1997; DCH 2000; MRCGP 2000. Special Interest: Integated Med.

PARBHOO, Mr Santilal Parag Hospital of St John & St Elizabeth, Brampton House, 60 Grove End Road, St John's Wood, London NW8 9NH Tel: 020 7266 4272 Fax: 020 7289 8349 Email: spparbhoo@doctors.org.uk; Royal Free Hospital, Cancerkin Centre, Pond Street, London NW3 2QG Tel: 020 7830 2323 Fax: 020 7830 2324; 6 Woodberry Way, London N12 0HG Tel: 020 8445 0348 Fax: 020 8445 0348 Email: spparbhoo@doctors.org.uk — MB ChB Cape Town 1960; PhD (Surgic. Sci.) Belf. 1967; FRCS Eng. 1967. Cons. Surg. (Breast) Hosp. of St John & St Eliz. Lond.; Hon. Cons. Surg. Roy. Free Hosp.; Med. Director, Cancerkin; Chairm. Cancerkin Trust. Specialty: Gen. Surg. Special Interest: Breast Cancer; Lymphoedema. Socs: Fell. Assn. Surgs.; Brit. Assn. Surg. Oncol.; Internat. Soc. Of Lymphology. Prev: Cons. Surg. (Gen. & Breast Surg.) Roy. Free Hosp. Lond.; Cons. Sen. Lect. Roy Free Hosp. Med. Sch. Lond.; Vis. Prof. Univ. Amman (1983), Capetown (1987) & Cairo (1989).

PARBROOK, Evelyn Ogilvie (retired) Kinord, 7 Buchanan St., Milngavie, Glasgow G62 8DB — MB ChB Aberd. 1964; BSc Aberd. 1962. Prev: GP Glas.

PARCHURE, Nikhil Queen Mary's Hospital, Frognal Avenue, Sidcup DA14 6LT Tel: 020 8302 2678 Ext: 2998 Fax: 020 8308 5418 — MB BS Jiwaji 1987; MD Gwalior; MRCP (UK) 1994. Cons. Cardiol., Qu. Mary's Hosp., Sidcup; Vis. Cons. Cardiol., St Thomas' Hosp., Lond. Specialty: Cardiol. Special Interest: Interventional Cardiol.; Pacing; TOE.

PARDHANANI, Gianni Boehringer Ingelheim, Ellesfield Ave, Bracknell RG12 8YS Email: gpardhanani@doctors.org.uk — MB BS Lond. 1997 (Camb. & St. Geo's.) BA Camb. 1994; MB BS (Hons.) Lond. 1997; MA Camb. 1998.

PARDOE, Celia Anne Bridge Cottage Surgery, 41 High Street, Welwyn AL6 9EF Tel: 01438 715044 Fax: 01438 714013; 15 Sherrardspark Road, Welwyn Garden City AL8 7JW Tel: 01707 331746 — MB ChB Liverp. 1978 (Liverpool) Cert. Family Plann. JCC 1981; DRCOG 1981; DCH RCP Lond. 1982; MRCGP 1983. GP Trainer; Acupunc. Qu. Eliz. II Hosp. Pain Clinic. Specialty: Gen. Pract. Socs: BMA; Brit. Med. Acupunct. Assn. Prev: Regist. (Pub. Health) N. Herts. HA; GP Alderley Edge Chesh.; GP Huyton Liverp.

PARDOE, Helen Dorothy — MB ChB Ed. 1989 (Edinburgh) FRCS Ed. 1993; MSc 1996. Specialty: Gen. Surg.

PARDOE, Ian Stuart The Old Priory Surgery, 319 Vicarage Road, Kings Heath, Birmingham B14 7NN Tel: 0121 444 1120 — MB ChB Birm. 1985; MRCGP 1990; Dip. Med. Acupunc 1996. Socs: Accred. Mem. Brit. Med. Acupunc. Soc.

PARDOE, James Leslie (retired) Church Cottage, Church Road N., Portishead, Bristol BS20 6PS Tel: 01275 848249 — MB ChB Bristol 1942.

PARDOE, Robin Francis Carcroft Health Centre, Chestnut Avenue, Carcroft, Doncaster DN6 8AG Tel: 01302 723510; 91 Tenterbank Lane, Adwick-Le-Street, Doncaster DN6 — MB ChB Sheff. 1969. Specialty: Dermat.

PARDOE, Roger Braddy (retired) Innisfree, 79 Nore Road, Portishead, Bristol BS20 6JZ Tel: 01275 849497 — MB BS Lond. 1953 (St. Mary's) MRCS Eng. LRCP Lond. 1953; DObst RCOG 1956.

PARDOE, Timothy Hugh Old Hall Grounds Health Centre, Old Hall Grounds, Cowbridge CF71 7AH Tel: 01446 772383 Fax: 01446 774022 — MB BCh Wales 1978; MRCP (UK) 1981.

PARDOE, Timothy Savile The Stennack Surgery, The Old Stennack School, St Ives TR26 1RU Tel: 01736 796413 Fax: 01736 796245 — MB ChB Bristol 1972. GP Princip.

PARDY, Mr Bruce James 144 Harley Street, London W1G 7LD Tel: 020 7935 0023 Fax: 020 7376 9708 Email: vascularsurgery@brucepardy.com; 49 Abingdon Villas, Kensington, London W8 6XA Tel: 020 7937 3417 Fax: 020 7376 9708 — MB ChB Otago 1963; BMedSc NZ 1961; ChM Otago 1980, MB ChB 1963; FRACS 1969; FRCS Eng. 1973. Special Interest: Aortic Aneurysm; Deep Vein Thrombosis; Venous Surg. Socs: Med. Soc. Lond.; Eur. Vasc. Soc.; Assn. of Surgeons of Gt. Britain & Irel. Prev: Sen. Regist. (Gen. Surg.) St. Mary's Hosp. Lond.; Cons. Surg. Newnham Healthcare NHS Trust.

PARDY, Karen 11 Maes Y Briallu, Morganstown, Cardiff CF15 8FA — MB BCh Wales 1997.

PAREKH, Shanti — MB BS Bombay 1973; FRCS Eng. 1981. Specialty: Gen. Pract.

PAREKH, Vistasp Jal The Surgery, 212 Richmond Road, Kingston upon Thames KT2 5HF Tel: 020 8546 0400 Fax: 020 8974 5771 — MB BS Bombay 1973 (Grant Med. Coll.) MS Bombay 1978. Prev: Trainee GP Chessington Surrey; SHO (O & G) St. Helier Hosp. Carshalton; SHO (Paediat.) Qu. Mary's Hosp. Carshalton.

PAREMAIN, Mr Guy Perry Royal Surrey County Hospital, Egerton Road, Guildford GU2 7XX Tel: 01483 571122 Ext: 4217 Fax: 01483 406 782 Email: guy.paremain@virgin.net — MB BS Lond. 1985; FRCS Lond. 1991; FRCS (Orth) 1997. Cons. (Orthop. Surg.) Roy. Surrey Co. Hosp. Guildford. Specialty: Trauma & Orthop. Surg. Special Interest: Lower Limb Jt. Replacement; Lumbar Spine. Socs: British Orthopaedic Association; British Association of Spinal Surgeons.

PAREMAIN, Tessa Jane 10 High Path Road, Merrow, Guildford GU1 2QG — MB BS Lond. 1991.

PARFITT, Mr Andrew 22 Dulais Road, Seven Sisters, Neath SA10 9EL — MB BS Lond. 1990; DRCOG 1993; FRCS Eng. 1995; FFAEM 2001; MA Ed. 2001. Cons. St Thos. Hosp. Lond. Specialty: Accid. & Emerg.

PARFITT, Caroline Jane Health Centre, Old Street, Clevedon BS21 6DG Tel: 01275 335534 — MB BS Lond. 1987; T(GP) 1991; DRCOG 1991; MRCGP 1992; Dip. Community Paediat. Warwick 1994. Specialty: Gen. Pract. Prev: Clin. Med. Off. Community Child Health Kidderminster; Trainee GP Brighton VTS.

PARFITT, Catharine Jane Littlewick Medical Centre, 42 Nottingham Road, Ilkeston DE7 5PR Tel: 0115 932 5229 Fax: 0115 932 5413; 133 Parkside, Wollaton, Nottingham NG8 2NL Tel: 0115 916 3627 — (St. Bart.) MRCS Eng. LRCP Lond. 1970; MB BS Lond. 1970; DTM & H Liverp. 1974; DCH Eng. 1975; MRCGP 1978. Socs: BMA; Nottm. M-C Soc. Prev: Trainee GP Bristol VTS; Med. Off Wusasa Hosp. Zaria, Nigeria; Ho. Phys. & Ho. Surg. Hillingdon Hosp. Uxbridge.

PARFITT, Graham George 44 Mantilla Drive, Styvechale Grange, Coventry CV3 6LQ — MRCS Eng. LRCP Lond. 1966 (Guy's) BSc Physiol. Lond. 1963. Clin. Asst. in Ophth. Warneford Hosp. Leamington Spa. Socs: Leamington Med. Soc. Prev: Ho. Surg., Ho. Phys. & Ho. Surg. (O & G) Warneford Hosp.

PARFITT, Jeremy 60 Devonshire Road, Harrow HA1 4LR — MB BS Lond. 1994 (St Marys) BSc Lond. 1991; FRCS (Eng.) 1999. SpR (Gen. Surg.) N. W. Thames; Vasc. SHO St Marys Hosp. Lond. Prev: SHO (Gen. Surg.) Hammersmith Hosp. Lond.

PARFITT, Julia Carolyn Royal Hampshire County Hosp., Romsey Road, Winchester SO22 5DG Tel: 01962 863535; 39 Hocombe Road, Chandlers Ford, Hants, Eastleigh SO53 5SP Email: parfittjulia@hotmail.com — BM Soton. 1986; DA (UK) 1989; FRCA 1995. Staff Grade(Anaesth.) RHCH Winchester. Specialty: Anaesth. Prev: Specialist Regist. Yr3 Winchester(Wessex RHA); Regist. (Anaesth.) Wessex RHA.; SHO (Anaesth. & Med.) Portsmouth & SE Hants. HA.

PARFITT, Matthew David Harrey Group Practice, 13-15 Russell Avenue, St Albans AL3 5HB — MB BS Lond. 1996; BSc Lond. 1992. SHO (Med.). Specialty: Gen. Med.

PARFITT, Ronald (retired) 165 Shirley Church Road, Croydon CR0 5AJ Tel: 020 8777 4746 — MRCS Eng. LRCP Lond. 1939 (Guy's) LDS RCS Eng. 1936; DMRT Eng. 1949; FFR 1958; FRCR 1975. Prev: Cons. (Radiother.) St. Thos. Hosp. Lond.

PARFITT, Vernon John Consultant Physician, Diabetes and Endocrinology, Diabetes and Endocrinology Service, Gloucestershire Royal Hospital, Great Western Road, Gloucester GL1 3NN Tel: 01452 394758 Fax: 01452 394755 — MB ChB Bristol 1983; MRCP (UK) 1987; MD Bristol 1994. Cons. Phys. (Diabetes & Endocrinol.). Specialty: Gen. Med.; Diabetes; Endocrinol. Socs: Clin. Mem. BDA; Brit. Hyperlipid. Assn.; Med. Res. Soc. Prev: Sen. Regist. Rotat. (Gen. Med., Diabetes & Endocrinol.) Soton. & Bath; Lect. (Med.) Bristol Univ. & Southmead Hosp.; Research Regist. (Med.) Univ. Bristol.

PARFREY, Helen 1 Archerfield Road, Liverpool L18 7HS Tel: 0151 724 3867 — BM BCh Oxf. 1993; MA Oxf. 1996; MRCP (UK) 1996. Specialist Regist. (Gen. Med. & Respirat.) Camb. Specialty: Respirat. Med.

PARGE, Frauke Maria Elizabeth 101A High Street, Waddesdon, Aylesbury HP18 0JE Tel: 01296 651282 — State Exam Med. Essen 1989. SHO (Neonat.) John Radcliffe Hosp. Headington Oxon. Specialty: Paediat. Prev: SHO High Wycombe Gen. Hosp.; Ho. Off. Mandeville Hosp. Aylesbury.

PARGETER, Jane Margaret Walton and Partners, West Street Surgery, 12 West Street, Chipping Norton OX7 5AA Tel: 01608 642529 Fax: 01608 645066; Easter Cottage, Southrop Road, Hook Norton, Banbury OX15 5PP — MB BS Lond. 1986; DCH RCP Lond. 1990; DGM RCP Lond. 1991; MRCGP 1992.

PARHAM, Andrew Leonard West End Medical Centre, 102 Stockport Road, Ashton-under-Lyne OL7 0LH Tel: 0161 339 5488 Fax: 0161 330 0945; Charity Farm, Millcroft Lane, Delph, Oldham OL3 5UX — MB ChB Manch. 1988; MRCGP 1992. Specialty: Gen. Pract.

PARHAM, Andrew Leslie Scott Veterans Agency, Norcross, Blackpool FY2 0WP Tel: 01253 332440 Email: Andylsparham@aol.com — BM BCh Oxf. 1975; BA (Animal Physiol.) Oxf. 1971; MA Oxf. 1975. Med. Adviser Veterans Agency. Specialty: Civil Serv. Prev: Sen. Med. Adviser War Pens. Agency Blackpool; Med. Adviser War Pens. Agency.

PARHAM, David McCausland Department of Pathology, Royal Bournemouth Hospital, Castle Lane E., Bournemouth BH7 7DW Tel: 01202 704832 Fax: 01202 704 833 — MB ChB Dundee 1983; BMSc (Hons.) Dund 1980, MD 1990; MRCPath 1990. Cons. Path. Roy. Bournemouth Hosp. Specialty: Histopath. Prev: Lect. & Hon. Sen. Regist. (Path.) Ninewells Hosp. Dundee; Regist. (Path.) Ninewells Hosp. Dundee; Ho. Off. Edin. Roy. Infirm.

PARIENTE, David 152 Harley Street, London W1G 7LH Tel: 020 7935 2477 Fax: 020 8455 2883 Email: parientedoc@lineone.net — (University of Aberdeen) MB ChB Aberd. 1967; MRCPsych 1974; DPM Eng. 1974; FRCPsych 1998. Cons. Adult Gen. Psychiat. Barnet - Enfield & Haringay Ment. Health. Specialty: Gen. Psychiat. Socs: Soc. Clin. Psychiats.; Acad. Experts; Soc. Expert Witnesses. Prev: Sen. Regist. Napsbury Hosp.; Hon. Clin. Asst. Univ. Coll. Hosp. Lond.; Cons. Psychiat. Nassbury. Hosp. Lond.

PARIENTE, Laura Sands End Health Clinic, 170 Wandsworth Bridge Road, London SW6 2UQ — MD Bordeaux 2001. Asst. Salaried GP.

PARIHAR, P David Medical Centre, 274 Barlow Moor Road, Chorlton, Manchester M21 8HA Tel: 0161 881 1681 Fax: 0161 860 7071 — MB BS delhi 1973; MB BS Delhi 1973.

PARIHAR, S S David Medical Centre, 274 Barlow Moor Road, Chorlton, Manchester M21 8HA Tel: 0161 881 1681 Fax: 0161 860 7071 — MB BS Kanpur 1973; MB BS kanpur 1973.

PARIKH, Mr Aashish Madhusudan 73 The Vale, London NW11 8TJ — MB BS Gujarat 1986; FRCS Eng. 1989; FRCS Ed. 1989.

PARIKH, Ami 3 Cringleford Chase, Norwich NR4 7RS — BM Soton. 1992.

PARIKH, Mr Balkrishna Kantilal High Bank, Addersgate Lane, Shibden, Halifax HX3 7TD Tel: 01422 205687 — MB BS Karnatak 1959 (Kasturba Med. Coll. Mangalore) FRCS Eng. 1964. Cons. Surg. A & E Dept. Roy. Halifax Infirm. Specialty: Accid. & Emerg.

PARIKH, Camilla Room 917, Market Towers, 1 Nine Elms Lane, London SW8 5NQ Tel: 020 7273 0374 Fax: 020 7273 0554 — MB BS Lond. 1982 (Westminster Medical School) MSc Lond. 1991, MB BS 1982; MRCPsych 1989. Sen. Med. Off. Dept. of Health. Prev: Regist. (Pub. Health Med.) SE Thames RHA; Regist. (Psychiat.) Westm. & Char. Cross Hosp. Lond.

PARIKH, Mr Daxesh Harivadan The Birmingham Childrens Hospital, Dept. of Paediatric Surgery, Steelhouse Lane, Birmingham B4 6MH Tel: 0121 333 9999; 57 Moorcroft Road, Birmingham B13 8LT — MB BS Bombay 1980 (Bombay Univ.) FRCS Glas. 1988; FRCS (Paed.) 1994; MD Bris 1994. Cons. (Paediat. Surg.) Birm. Childr.'s Hosp. Specialty: Paediat. Surg. Socs: Brit. Assn. Paediat. Surg.; BMA. Prev: Sen. Regist. (Paediat. Surg.) Roy. Liverp. Childr. Hosp. Alder Hey.; Research Fell. (Paediat. Surg.) Univ. Liverp. Roy. Liverp. Childr. Hosp.; Regist. (Paediat. Surg. & Urol.) Alder Hey Childr. Hosp. Liverp.

PARIKH, Harshad Shantilal Potteries Medical Centre, Beverley Drive, Bentilee, Stoke-on-Trent ST2 0JG Tel: 01782 208755 — MB BS Gujarat 1971; MB BS Gujarat 1971.

PARIKH, Jitinkumar Kanchanlal The Surgery, 9 Beaconsfield Road, Brighton BN1 4QH Tel: 01273 698666 Fax: 01273 672742 — MB BS Bombay 1952. GP Brighton.

PARIKH, Jyoti 15 Rayleas Close, London SE18 3JN; 15 Rayleas Close, London SE18 3JN — (Cambridge and Oxford) BM BCh Oxf. 1997; MA (Hons.) Cantab. 1998. SHO Med. Rotat. St Thomas' Hosp. Lond. Specialty: Gen. Med. Socs: BMA.

PARIKH, Ketankumar Satishchandra 12 Stangate, Royal St., London SE1 7EQ — MB BS Bombay 1988.

PARIKH, Nalin Sakerlal (Surgery), 12 Movers Lane, Barking IG11 7UN Tel: 020 8594 4700 — MB BS Bombay 1955.

PARIKH, Paresh 223 Styal Road, Heald Green, Stockport SK8 3UA Tel: 09058 582748 — MB ChB Leeds 1996. Specialty: Gen. Pract.

PARIKH, Rajesh Kantilal Ashfield Road Surgery, 70 Ashfield Road, Blackpool FY2 0DJ Tel: 01253 357739 Fax: 01253 596161 — MB BS Saurashtra 1975 (M.P. Shah Med. Coll. Jamnagar) Clin. Asst. (Anaesth.) Vict. Hosp. Blackpool; Med. Off. Trinity Hospice in the Fylde. Prev: Regist. (Anaesth.) & SHO (A & E & O & G) Sunderland Dist. Gen. Hosp.

PARIKH, Ranjit Kantilal (retired) 62 Stokiemuir Avenue, Bearsden, Glasgow G61 3LX Tel: 0141 942 3925 — MB BS Bombay 1960 (Grant Med. Coll.) DObst RCOG 1964; FFA RCSI 1970; FFA RCS Eng. 1971. Prev: Cons. Anaesth. Stobhill Gen. Hosp. Glas.

PARIKH, Rashmikant Vadilal Norfolk Street Surgery, 40 Norfolk Street, Glossop SK13 7QU Tel: 01457 864984 Fax: 01457 860966; Lee Mount, Marple Road, Charlesworth, Broadbottom, Hyde SK13 5DA — MB BS Bombay 1960; DLO Eng. 1965; DA Eng. 1968. Prev: Regist. (ENT) Salford Hosp. Gp. & Angus Gp. Hosp.; SHO (Anaesth.) Salford Gp. Hosp.

PARIKH, Renuka Amulakhray Flat 17, Harwood Court, Harwood Road, Heaton Mersey, Stockport SK4 3BE — MB BS Saurashtra 1971 (M.P. Shah Med. Coll. Jamnagar)

PARIS, Mr Andrew Martin Ingledew, OStJ The London Independent Hospital, 1 Beaumont Square, Stepney Green, London E1 4NL Tel: 020 7702 8818 Fax: 020 7702 8868; The Royal London Hospital, Whitechapel, London E1 1BB Tel: 020 7377 7262 Fax: 020 7377 7292 — MB BS Lond. 1964 (Lond. Hosp.) MRCS Eng. LRCP Lond. 1964; DObst RCOG 1966; FRCS Eng. 1971. Cons. Urol. Surg. Roy. Lond. Hosp. & St. Barts. Hosp.; Clin. Dir. Specialist Surg. Roy. Hosp. Trust. Specialty: Urol. Socs: Fell. Roy. Soc. Med. (Vice Pres. Counc. Sect. Urol.); Brit. Assn. Urol. Surgs.; Brit. Assn. Transpl. Surgs. Prev: Hon. Cons. Surg. Urol. Ital. Hosp. Lond.; Res. Surgic. Off. St. Peter's Hosps. Lond.; Sen. Regist. (Urol.) Lond. Hosp.

PARIS, James Alexander Gordon Blackburn & Darwen PCT, Guide Business Centre, School Lane, Blackburn BB1 2QH Tel: 01254 267047 Fax: 01254 267009 — MB BS Lond. 1969 (Univ. Coll. Hosp.) MRCP (UK) 1973; MFPHM RCP (UK) 1993. Director (Pub. Health) Blackburn & Darwen PCT. Specialty: Pub. Health Med. Prev: Cons. (Pub. Health Med.) & Head of Clin. Governance Bury & Rochdale HA; Hon. Sen. Lect. Univ. of Centr. Lancs. Postgrad. Med. & Health Sch.; GP Birm.

PARIS, Simon Tancred Flat 115, Bishops Mansions, Bishops Park Road, London SW6 6DY Tel: 020 7736 9912 — MB BS Lond. 1990; BSc (Hons.) Lond. 1987, MB BS 1990. SHO (Anaesth.) Guy's Hosp. Lond. Specialty: Anaesth. Socs: BMA; Assn. Anaesth. Gt. Brit. & Irel.

PARISH, Mr Christopher (retired) Church Farm, Boxworth, Cambridge CB3 8LZ Tel: 01954 267267; R3, Garden Court, Sidney Sussex College, Cambridge CB2 3HU Tel: 01223 338854 Fax: 01223 338884 — MB ChB Manch. 1940; BSc Manch. 1937; MB ChB (Distinc. Surg.) 1940; FRCS Eng. 1948; MA Camb. 1956; FSA 1965; FFPHM 1983. Fell. Sidney Sussex Coll. Camb. Prev: Postgrad. Dean Fac. Clin. Med. Univ. Camb.

PARISH, James Gordon (retired) Red Rocks, Perth Road, Stanley, Perth PH1 4NF Tel: 01738 828313 Fax: 01738 828313 — MB ChB Ed. 1947 (Univ. Ed.) DPhysMed. Eng. 1952; MD Ed. 1957; Cert Physical Med. RCPS Canada 1961; FRCP Canada 1972. Prev: Cons. Phys. (Rheum. & Rehabil.) Colchester Health Dist.

PARISH, Stephen Peter Edward School House Surgery, Hertford Road, Brighton BN1 7GF Tel: 01273 551031 Fax: 01273 382036 — MB BS Lond. 1980. Specialty: Gen. Pract. Socs: Brighton & Hove Med. Soc.; BMA. Prev: GP Swindon.

PARK, Adrian John Dept of Chemical Pathology, Charing Cross Hospital, Hammersmith, London W6 8RF; 10 Clare Avenue, Wokingham RG40 1EB — MB BS Lond. 1993.

PARK, Mr Alan John 45 Sharman Close, Stoke-on-Trent ST4 7LS — MB ChB Glas. 1988; FRCS Glas. 1994. Regist. Rotat. (Plastic Surg.) W. Midl. Specialty: Plastic Surg. Prev: SHO (Plastic Surg.) Addenbrooke's Hosp. Camb. & St. John's Hosp. Livingston; SHO Rotat. (Surg.) St. John's Hosp. Livingstone, Bangor & West. Gen. Hosp. Edin.

PARK, Alison Victoria Health Centre, Meddygfa, Betws-y-Coed LL24 0BB Tel: 01690 710205 Fax: 01690 710051; The Cottage, Bunbury Common, Tarporley CW6 9QE Tel: 01829 261141 — MB ChB Liverp. 1971; MRCGP 1994. Specialty: Gen. Pract. Prev: VTS GI Cruise Organiser Clan Clwyd N. Wales.

PARK, Alistair James Oakhill Medical Practice, Dronfield S18 2FA Tel: 01246 412073 Fax: 01246 291904; 11 Meadowbank Avenue, Sheffield S7 1PB — MB ChB Sheff. 1988; MRCGP 1994. GP Bd. Mem. N. E. Derbysh. PCG.

PARK, Anne Elizabeth 6 Lower Brook Street, Oswestry SY11 2HJ Tel: 01691 655844; Plas Wilmot, Weston Lane, Oswestry SY11 2BB Tel: 01691 653615 — MB ChB Aberd. 1959; DObst RCOG 1961.

PARK, Miss Caroline Ann Birmingham Heartlands Hospital, Emergency Department, Bordesley Green East, Birmingham B9 5SS Tel: 0121 424 1257 Fax: 0121 424 0260 Email: caroline.park@heartsol.wmids.nhs.uk — MB ChB Birm. 1987 (Birmingham) FRCS Eng. 1992; FFAEM 1996. p/t Cons. in Emerg. Med. Specialty: Accid. & Emerg.; Emergency Medicine. Socs: BAEM.

PARK, Christine Mary 7 Burnside Road, Largs KA30 9BX — MB ChB Glas. 1994.

PARK, Daniel Paul Buttery Lodge, Kynnersley, Telford TF6 6DX — BChir Camb. 1996.

PARK, David John 2 Dunbar Avenue, Coatbridge ML5 5QJ — MB ChB Glas. 1975.

PARK, David Maxwell 11 Winton Lodge, Imperial Avenue, Westcliff on Sea SS0 8NF Tel: 01702 347467 Mob: 07860 407627 Email: parkdm@aol.com — BM BCh Oxf. 1965 (Oxf. Univ.) MA Oxf. 1965; FRCP Lond. 1986, M 1969. Cons. Neurol. Barts & Lond NHS Trust Southend Health Care. Specialty: Neurol. Socs: Fell. Roy. Soc. Med.; Med. Soc. Lond.; Assn. Brit. Neurol. Prev: Sen. Regist. (Neurol.) Char. Cross Hosp. Lond.; Research Fell. & Regist. (Neurol.) Univ. Glas.

PARK, David Samuel (retired) Yew Cottage, 34A Carrowdore Road, Greyabbey, Newtownards BT22 2LX Tel: 01247 788625 — MB BCh BAO Belf. 1959; DObst RCOG 1961; DCH Eng. 1962. Prev: Ho. Off. Roy. Vict. & Roy. Matern. Hosps. Belf. & Roy. Belf. Hosp. Sick Childr.

PARK, Deryn Joyce The Richmond Practice, Health Centre, Dean Road, Bo'ness EH51 0DH Tel: 01506 822665 Fax: 01506 825939; 14 Grahams Dyke Road, Bo'ness EH51 9EG Tel: 01506 824383 — MB ChB Ed. 1970. GP. Socs: BMA.

PARK, Emily Stevenson Flat 1, 15 Grand Avenue, Hove BN3 2NG Tel: 01273 734460 Fax: 01273 734460 — MB ChB Aberd. 1942. JP. Socs: Brighton & Sussex M-C Soc. Prev: Ho. Surg. Aberd. Roy. Infirm., Aberd. Matern. Hosp. & Roy. Sussex Co. Hosp. Brighton.

PARK, Emma Jane 21 Cloverhill Park, Belfast BT4 2JW — MB ChB Sheff. 1997.

PARK, George Edwin The Health Centre, North Road, Stokesley, Middlesbrough TS9 5DY Tel: 01642 710748 Fax: 01642 713037 — MB BS Newc. 1977; DRCOG 1980; MRCGP 1981. GP Stokesley.

PARK, Gilbert Lindsay (retired) Barnetts Ridge, Barnetts Hill, Peasmarsh, Rye TN31 6YJ Tel: 01797 230852 — (Roy. Colls. Ed.) LRCP LRCS Ed. LRFPS Glas. 1946. Hon. Phys. Roy. Scott. Corp. Lond.; Scientif. Adviser The Humane Research Trust Bramhall, Stockport. Prev: Regist. Roy. Infirm. Edin.

PARK, Gilbert Richard, TD Addenbrookes Hospital, Box 17, Hills Road, Cambridge CB2 2QQ Tel: 01223 217433 Fax: 01223 217898; Malyons, 15 High Green, Great Shelford, Cambridge CB2 5EG — MB ChB Ed. 1974; Honary Degree DMedSci Pleven; FFA RCS Eng. 1978; MA Camb. 1987; BSc (Med. Sci.) Ed. 1971, MD 1991; MD Edinburgh 1991. Cons. Anaesth. & Intens. Care Addenbrooke's Hosp. Camb. Specialty: Intens. Care; Anaesth. Socs: Intens. Care Soc. Prev: Vis. Prof. Duke Univ. 1995.

PARK, Helen Loreen 40 Chesterfield Road S., Mansfield NG19 7AQ — MB BS Newc. 1996.

PARK, Helen Murray Old Mill Surgery, 100 Old Mill Road, Uddingston, Glasgow G71 7JB; 11 Main Street, Uddingston, Glasgow G71 7HD Tel: 01698 817219 — MB ChB Glas. 1977. GP Uddingston.

PARK, Hilda Gillian Janet 10 Vestry Mews, Vestry Road, Camberwell, London SE5 8NS — MB BCh Wales 1977.

PARK, James David Department of Anaesthetics, South Cleveland Hospital, Marton Road, Middlesbrough TS4 3BW Tel: 01642 850850 Fax: 01642 854613 — MB ChB Aberd. 1985. Cons.

Cardiothoracic Anaesth. S. Cleveland Hosp. Middlesbrough. Specialty: Anaesth.; Intens. Care.

PARK, John The Richmond Practice, Health Centre, Dean Road, Bo'ness EH51 0DH Tel: 01506 822665 Fax: 01506 825939 — MB ChB Ed. 1970; FRCGP; FRCP Ed.; MRCP (U.K.) 1973; MRCGP 1982.

PARK, John Michael William Cloneen, 11 Belfast Road, Newtownards BT23 4BJ Tel: 01247 816449 — MB BCh BAO Belf. 1965 (Qu. Univ. Belf.) FRCOG 1986, M 1971, DObst 1967. Cons. O & G Ards & Bangor Hosps. Specialty: Obst. & Gyn. Socs: Ulster Obst. & Gyn. Soc.

PARK, Keith Charles Health Centre, Green Lane, Corwen LL21 0DN Tel: 01490 412362 Fax: 01490 412970; Trawscoed Bach, Maerdy, Corwen LL21 0PD Tel: 01490 81472 — MB ChB Liverp. 1971. Prev: MoH Tristan Da Cunha.

PARK, Kenneth George Marquis Aberdeen Royal Infirmary, Foresterhill, Aberdeen AB25 2ZN — MB ChB Ed. 1982; FRCS. Specialty: Gen. Surg.

PARK, Kirsten Anne 21 Main Street, Dalrymple, Ayr KA6 6DF — MB ChB Glas. 1976.

PARK, Lindsay Marian Eglinton Street Surgery, 16 Eglinton Street, Irvine KA12 8AS Tel: 01294 279178 Fax: 01294 313095; 13 Craven Grove, Stanecastle Village, South Stanecastle, Irvine KA11 1RY — MB ChB Aberd. 1984; DRCOG 1989. Prev: Trainee GP Aviemore; SHO (Paediat.) Dist. Gen. Hosp. Grimsby; SHO (A & E & Psychiat.) N. Tees Hosp. Stockton.

PARK, Margaret Joan Queen Margaret Hospital NHS Trust, Whitefield Road, Dunfermline KY12 0SU Tel: 01383 623623; Gowanbrae House, 120 Garvock Hill, Dunfermline KY11 4JY Tel: 01383 729957 — MB ChB Ed. 1971; DObst RCOG 1973; DO Eng. 1978. Staff Grade (Ophth.) Qu. Margt. Hosp. NHS Trust Dunfermline. Specialty: Ophth.

PARK, Pauline Mary Bell 42 Granville Park, Aughton, Ormskirk L39 5DU — MB ChB Liverp. 1956.

PARK, Philip Wesley 20 The Crest, Hillcrest, Whitehaven CA28 6TJ — MB ChB Leeds 1993.

PARK, Rebecca Jane Warneford Hospital, Oxford Adult Eating Disorders Service, Roosevelt Drive, Oxford OX3 7JX Tel: 01865 226988 Email: rebecca.park@psychiatry.ox.ac.uk — MB ChB Bristol 1990; BSc Bristol 1987; MRCPsych 1995; PhD 2002. Cons. Psychiat. Oxon. Ment. Healthcare Trust; Res. Assoc. (Devel. Psychiat.) Univ. of Camb.; Hon. Cons. (Child & Adolesc. Psychiat.) BrooksiDE CFC & Lifespan NHS Trust. Specialty: Child & Adolesc. Psychiat. Socs: ACPP; Assoc. of Cognitive Analytic Therapists; Assoc. of Infant Ment. Health. Prev: Regist. (Psychiat.) Roy. Edin. Hosp.; SHO (Psychiat.) Roy. Edin. Hosp.; SHO (Paediat.) Alder Hey Hosp. Liverp.

PARK, Richard Hammond Reid Southend General Hospital NHS Trust, 1345 Govan Road, Glasgow G51 4TF Tel: 0141 201 1100; 1 Melford Avenue, Glasgow G46 6NA Tel: 0141 638 0273 — MD Glas. 1992; FRCP Glas. and Edin.; MB ChB 1979; MRCP (UK) 1983. Cons. Phys. & Gastroenterol. South. Gen. Hosp. NHS Trust; Hon. Clin. Sen. Lect. Glas. Univ. Specialty: Gen. Med.; Gastroenterol. Socs: Brit. Soc. Gastroenterol.

PARK, Richard Montgomery Clinical Oncology, Belvoir Park Hospital, Hospital Road, Belfast BT8 6HD; 14Kilmakee Park, Gilnahirk, Belfast BT5 7QY Tel: 01232 794809 Email: richardpark@kilmakee.fsnet.co.uk — MB BCh BAO Belf. 1996; MRCP Edinburgh 2000. Specialist Regist., Clin. Oncol., Belvoir Pk. Hosp. Specialty: Gen. Med.; Oncol.

PARK, Robert Robert Park, Warrington Hospital NHS Trust, Lovely Lane, Warrington; 112 Moor Drive, Crosby, Liverpool L23 2UT — MRCS Eng. LRCP Lond. 1973; DObst. RCOG 1975; FFA RCSI 1980. Cons. Anaesth., Warrington Hosp. NHS Trust. Specialty: Anaesth. Socs: BMA; Assn. Anaesth.; The Pain Soc.

PARK, Robert Riverside Medical Practice, Roushill, Shrewsbury SY1 1PQ Tel: 01743 352371 Fax: 01743 340269 — MB ChB Liverp. 1972; MRCS Eng. LRCP Lond. 1972; DObst. Univ. Auckland 1976.

PARK, Robert Hood Wright (retired) 4 The Paddock, Dirleton EH39 5AD Tel: 01620 850686 — MB ChB Ed. 1957 (Edinburgh University) DA Eng. 1962; FRCA 1968. Prev: Cons. Anaesth. Roy. Infirm. Edin. NHS Trust.

PARK, Robert Wilson George Street Surgery, 99 George Street, Dumfries DG1 1DS Tel: 01387 253333 Fax: 01387 253301; 99 George Street, Dumfries DG1 1DS Tel: profess. 53333 — MB ChB Glas. 1982; DRCOG; MRCGP 1986. Prev: Trainee GP Dumfries VTS; Ho. Phys. Stirling Roy. Infirm.; Ho. Surg. Vict. Infirm. Glas.

PARK, Soo-Mi Cambridge Instsitute for Medical Research, Box 139, Lab 4.36, Addenbrooke's Hospital, Cambridge CB2 2XY Tel: 01223 762618/9 — MB BS Lond. 1994 (King's Coll. Sch. Of Med. & Dent.) BSc Lond. 1991; MRCP (UK) 1997. Hon. Clin. Fell. (Endocrinol. & Diabetes) Univ. of Camb. Specialty: Endocrinol.; Diabetes. Prev: LAT (Gen. Med. / Endocrinol. & Diabetes; SHO (Gen. Med.); HO.

PARK, Stewart Bertrand Geoffrey University Department of Psychiatry, Duncan MacMillan House, Porchester Road, Nottingham NG3 6AA Tel: 0115 969 1300 — BM BCh Oxf. 1986; MRCP (UK) 1989; MRCPsych 1992. Sen. Lect. (Psychiat.) Univ. Nottm. Specialty: Gen. Psychiat. Prev: Wellcome Train. Fell. MRC Clin. Psychopharmacol. Unit Littlemore Hosp. Oxf.; SHO & Regist. Rotat. (Psychiat.) Oxf.; Regist. (Med.) Princess Margt. Hosp. Swindon.

PARK, Thomas (retired) Drumshiel, Thornhill DG3 5DW Tel: 01848 330513 — MB ChB Glas. 1952. Prev: GP Thornhill.

PARK, Thomas Harling (retired) Redlands, The Green, Acomb, York YO19 5XP Tel: 01904 798686 & 798329 — MB ChB Ed. 1945.

PARK, Wallace Galloway Meadowside, Cove Road, Silverdale, Carnforth LA5 0SQ Tel: 01524 701770 — (Ed.) MB ChB Ed. 1969; FFA RCS Eng. 1975. Cons. (Anaesth.) Morcambe Bay NHS Trust. Specialty: Anaesth. Prev: Sen. Regist. (Anaesth.) S. West. RHA.

PARK, William Douglas Station Road Surgery, 2 Station Road, Prestwick KA9 1AQ Tel: 01292 671444 Fax: 01292 678023 — MB ChB Glas. 1983; MRCP (UK) 1986; MRCGP 1988; FRCP Glas. 2000. Specialty: Gastroenterol.

PARKAR, Hasratali Bhaudin 144-50 High Road, Willesden, London NW10 2PT Tel: 020 8459 5550; 28 Bromefield, Stanmore HA7 1AE — MB BS Newc. 1984; MRCGP 1990. Mem. Brent & Harrow LMC. Socs: Brent & Harrow Med. Audit Advis. Gp. Prev: SHO (A & E) Roy. Vict. Infirm. Newc.; SHO (O & G) Newc. Gen. Hosp.; Ho. Phys. & Ho. Surg. Freeman Hosp. Newc u. Tyne.

PARKAR, Washik 89 Moorfield, Salford M6 7GD — MB ChB Liverp. 1992.

PARKASH, Vijay Kumari 20 Leila Parnell Close, Victoria Way, London SE7 7TD — MB BS Lond. 1988; MRCPsych 1995.

PARKE, Mr Roger Christopher Regional Disablement Services, Musgrave Park Hospital, Stockman's Lane, Belfast BT9 7JB Tel: 028 9066 9501 Fax: 028 9068 3662 Email: roger.parke@greenpark.n-i.nhs.uk; 3 Tudor Park, Holywood BT18 0NX Tel: 028 9042 3140 Fax: 028 9042 3140 — MB BCh BAO Belf. 1970 (Qu. Univ. Belf.) FRCSI 1975; FRCS Ed. 1976. Cons. Rehabil. Med./ Green Pk. Healthcare Trust, Musgrave Pk. Hosp, Belf. Specialty: Rehabil. Med. Socs: Internat. Soc. Prosth.s & Orthotics; Brit. Soc. Rehabil. Med.; Brit. Orthopaedic Assn. Prev: Cons. Prosth. Surg. Musgrave Pk. Hosp. Belf.

PARKE, Roger Jeremy Greville 27 Oak Tree Drive, Aller Park, Newton Abbot TQ12 4NN — MB BS Lond. 1979.

PARKE, Simon Charles 8 Kensington Gate, Belfast BT5 6PF Tel: 028 9070 5805 — MB ChB Ed. 1993; MRCP (UK) 1997. SHO (Paediat. Oncol. & Haemat.) Gt. Ormond St. Hosp. Lond.; Specialist Regist. Paediat. Birm. Heartlands Hosp. Specialty: Paediat. Prev: SHO (Paediat.) Roy. Berks. Hosp. Reading & John Radcliffe Hosp. Oxf.; Ho. Off. (Med.) Falkirk & Dist. Roy. Infirm.; Ho. Off. (Surg.) St. John's Hosp. Livingstone.

PARKE, Timothy John Department of Anaesthetics, Royal Berkshire Hospital, London Road, Reading RG1 5AN Tel: 01734 875111 — MB ChB Bristol 1980; MRCP (UK) 1985; FFA RCS Eng. 1986; MRCGP 1989; DRCOG 1989. Cons. Anaesth. Roy. Berks. Hosp. Reading. Specialty: Anaesth. Socs: Intens. Care Soc. Prev: Sen. Regist. (Anaesth.) Bristol Roy. Infirm.

PARKE, Timothy Robert James Accident & Emergency Department, Southern General Hospital, 1345 Govan Road, Glasgow G51 4TF Tel: 0141 201 1100 Fax: 0141 201 2997 — MB ChB Ed. 1986; MRCP (UK) 1989; DA (UK) 1995; FFAEM 1996. Cons. A & E & Intens. Care South. Gen. Hosp. Glas. Specialty: Accid. & Emerg. Socs: Intens. Care Soc.; Brit. Assn. Emerg. Med. Prev: Sen. Regist. (A & E & ITU) West. Infirm. Glas.; Regist. (A & E) Roy. Infirm. Edin.

PARKEN, Douglas Stuart (retired) Cascais Haven, 32B Lulworth Road, Birkdale, Southport PR8 2BQ — (St. Mary's) MB BS Lond. 1948; MRCS Eng. LRCP Lond. 1948; DCH Eng. 1950; DPH Liverp. 1954; FFCM 1976, M 1974. Prev: Area Med. Off. Lancs. AHA.

PARKEN, Helen Frances Mary Potter Health Centre, Gregory Boulevard, Hyson Green, Nottingham NG7 5HY Tel: 0115 942 0330; 115 Melton Road, West Bridgford, Nottingham NG2 6ET — MB BS Lond. 1975 (St. Mary's) MRCS Eng. LRCP Lond. 1975; MRCP (UK) 1979.

PARKEN, Paul Nicholas Stuart Clifton Medical Centre, 571 Farnborough Road, Clifton, Nottingham NG11 9DN Tel: 0115 921 1288; 115 Melton Road, West Bridgford, Nottingham NG2 6ET — MRCS Eng. LRCP Lond. 1978 (St. Mary's)

PARKER, Alasdair Patrick John Child Development Centre, Box 107, Addenbrooke's Hospital, Cambridge CB1 1EZ Tel: 01223 311947 Email: alasdair.parker@addenbrookes.nhs.uk — MB BS Lond. 1987; MRCP (UK) 1990; MD Lond. 2000. Cons. Paediatric NeUrol., Addenbrookes Hosp., Camb. Specialty: Paediat. Prev: Co-ordinator Médècins Sans Frontiérès, Vietnam; SHO (Paediat.) Bristol & Brighton Childr. Hosp.; Regist., Cray's Hosp.

PARKER, Alfred Patrick The Surgery, 5 Enys Road, Eastbourne BN21 2DQ Tel: 01323 410088 Fax: 01323 644638 — MB BS Lond. 1977; Cert. Family Plann. JCC 1979. Socs: BMA (Sec. E.bourne Div.). Prev: SHO (O & G) Roy. Sussex Co. Hosp. Brighton; Ho. Off. (Gen. Med.) St. Mary's Hosp. Eastbourne; Ho. Off. Gen. Surg. (ENT & Orthop.) N. Middlx. Hosp. Lond.

PARKER, Alistair Cameron (retired) Upton Farm, Gate House Lane, Framfield TA22 5RS — MB ChB Ed. 1967; PhD Ed. 1976, BSc 1964; FRCPath. 1988, M 1977; FRCP Ed. 1979. Prev: Cons. Haemat. Roy. Infirm. Edin.

PARKER, Andrew Frank (retired) 14 Hobgate, Acomb, York YO24 4HF Tel: 01904 798850 — (Leeds) MRCS Eng. LRCP Lond. 1957; DPH Leeds 1967; DIH Soc. Apoth. Lond. 1972; FFOM RCP Lond. 1988, MFOM 1978. Prev: Sen. Regional Med. Off. BT plc NE Eng.

PARKER, Andrew John 2 West Lawn, Sunderland SR2 7HW — MB BS Lond. 1992.

PARKER, Mr Andrew John Department of Otolaryngology, Royal Hallamshire Hospital, Sheffield S10 2JF — MB ChB Leeds 1981; DLO RCS Eng. 1985; FRCS Ed 1986; FRCS Eng 1987; ChM Bristol 1991. Cons. Otolaryngol. Head & Neck Surg. United Sheff. Hosp.; Sen. Lect. Univ. Sheff. Specialty: Otorhinolaryngol. Socs: Otorhinolaryngological Research Soc.; Europ. Gp. for Func.al Laryngeal Surg.; Ct. of Examiners at the Roy. Coll. of Surgeons of Eng. Prev: Sen. Regist. (ENT) Sheff. United Hosps; Research Fell. (ENT) Bristol Roy. Infirm.; Regist. (ENT) Bristol & Bath Hosps.

PARKER, Angela Mary Torrington Park Health Centre, Torrington Park, North Finchley, London N12 9SS; 203 Holders Hill Road, London NW7 1ND — MB BS Lond. 1974 (Univ. Coll. Hosp.) BSc Lond. 1971; DCH Eng. 1978; DRCOG 1979; MRCGP 1979; DFP RHC RCOG 1993. Specialty: Dermat. Socs: Primary Care Dermatol. Soc.; NAFPD. Prev: SHO (Med.) Whittington Hosp. Lond.; Trainee GP Barnet VTS.

PARKER, Ann (retired) South View, School Lane, Offley, Hitchin SG5 3AZ — MB BS Lond. 1960; MRCS Eng. LRCP Lond. 1960; FRCOG 1980, M 1967, DObst 1962. Prev: Cons. (O & G) Lister & N. Herts. Gp. Hosps.

PARKER, Ann, OBE 17 Derwen Deg close, Govilon, Abergavenny NP7 9RJ Tel: 01873 830336; 17 Derwen Deg close, Govilon, Abergavenny NP7 9RJ Tel: 01873 830336 — MB BS Lond. 1963 (Guy's) MRCS Eng. LRCP Lond. 1963. Cons. psychosexual Med. Gwent healthcare NHS trust. Specialty: Psychosexual Med.; Family Plann. & Reproduc. Health. Socs: Inst. Psychosexual Med.; Fac. Fam. Plann. & Reproduc. Health Care. Prev: Cons. Reproductive & Sexual Health Gwent Community NHS Trust; Clin. Dir. (Family Plann. & Sexual Health) Community Unit Gwent AHA; SCMO Gwent AHA.

PARKER, Mrs Ann Gwillim (retired) The Firs, Firs Road, Duxmere, Ross-on-Wye HR9 5BH Tel: 01989 563995 Fax: 01989 563995 — (Univ. Coll. Hosp.) BM BCh Oxf. 1953; BA Oxf. 1953. Prev: Med. Off. Family Plann. Gloucester Health Dist.

PARKER, Anne Naomi Department Haematology, Glasgow Royal Infirmary, Castle St., Glasgow G4 0SF Tel: 0141 211 4672 Fax: 0141 552 8196 — MB ChB Bristol 1987 (Univ. Bristol) BSc (Hons.) Biochem. Bristol 1984; MRCP (UK) 1991; MRCP MRCPATH 1997; MD MD Bristol 1998; FRCP UK 2001. Cons. haematologist; honary Sen. Lect. Univ. of Glas.; Cons. Haematologist, Health Care Internat., Glas. Specialty: Haematology. Prev: Clin. Research Fell. Beatson Inst. Cancer Research; Regist. (Haemat.) Leicester Roy. Infirm.; Sen. Lect., Haemat., W. of Scotl.

PARKER, Anthony Leonard (retired) South Lodge, Pease Pottage, Crawley RH11 9AR Tel: 01293 542008 — MB ChB Birm. 1955; DPM Eng. 1962; FRCPsych. 1983, M 1971. Prev: Cons. Psychiat. Crawley Hosp.

PARKER, Anthony Philip 16 Swathwick Close, Wingerworth, Chesterfield S42 6UA — MB ChB Birm. 1991; DCH RCP Lond. 1994; MRCGP 1995. Specialty: Gastroenterol.

PARKER, Barbara Doherty (retired) 52B Linden Road, Bournville, Birmingham B30 1JU Tel: 0121 472 2344 — MB BS Lond. 1942 (Roy. Free) MRCS Eng. LRCP Lond. 1942; DA Eng. 1947; FFA RCS Eng. 1954. Prev: Cons. Anaesth. Birm. Regional Plastic Surg. Unit Wordsley.

PARKER, Barbara Louise Guidepost Health Centre, North Parade, Guidepost, Choppington NE62 5RA Tel: 01670 822071 Fax: 01670 531068 Email: blp888@hotmail.com — MB BS Newc. 1978 (Newcastle) Cert. Family Plann. JCC 1980; MRCGP 1982.

PARKER, Mr Barrie Charles Epsom General Hospital, South West London Elective Orthopaedic Centre, Dorking Road, Epsom KT18 7EG; Delaval, Furzefield, Oxshott, Leatherhead KT22 0UR Email: bparker@uk-consultants.co.uk — MB BS Lond. 1965 (Char. Cross) FRCS Eng. 1970. Cons. Orthop. Surg. Specialty: Orthop. Socs: Fell. (Mem. Counc & Hon. Treas.) BOA; Roy. Soc. Med.; Brit. Hip Soc. Prev: Cons. Orthop. Surg. Kingston Hosp.; Sen. Regist. (Orthop.) Char. Cross Hosp. & Roy. Nat. Orthop. Hosp.; Clin. Tutor Kingston Hosp.

PARKER, Brenda 378 Kilmarnock Road, Glasgow G43 2DH — MB ChB Liverp. 1952; DPH 1957.

PARKER, Carl David McKenzie House Surgery, Kendal Road, Hartlepool TS25 1QU Tel: 01429 233611 Fax: 01429 297713; Cross Keys Farm, Borrowby, Thirsk YO7 4QY — MB BS Lond. 1987; DRCOG 1991; Section 12 Approved 1996. Police Surg. N. Yorks. Police; Commissioning Lead, Hartlepool PCT.

PARKER, Catherine Sian McKenzie House Surgery, Kendal Road, Hartlepool TS25 1QU — MB BS Lond. 1990.

PARKER, Charles Marcus The Surgery, Long Street, Topcliffe, Thirsk YO7 3RP Tel: 01845 577297 Fax: 01845 577128; Jubilee House, Long St., Topcliffe, Thirsk YO7 3RL Tel: 01845 577980 Fax: 01845 577140 Email: charles.parker@lineone.net — MB BS Lond. 1987. Dir. N. Yorks. Emerg. Doctors York.

PARKER, Christopher Charles — BM BCh Oxf. 1989; BA Camb. 1986; MRCP (UK) 1992; FRCR 1996; MD 2000. Sen. Lect. Clin. Oncol., Inst. Cancer Research. Specialty: Oncol.; Radiother. Prev: Regist. (Clin. Oncol.) Roy. Marsden Hosp. Lond.

PARKER, Mr Christopher John Yeovil District Hospital, Higher Kingston, Yeovil BA21 4AT Tel: 01935 384345 Fax: 01935 384643 — MB BS Lond. 1979 (Guy's Hospital Medical School) FRCS Ed. 1984; FRCS Eng. 1985; FRCS (Urol.) 1993. Cons. Urol. (Urol.) E. Som. NHS Trust Yeovil. Specialty: Urol. Prev: Sen. Regist. St. Peter's Hosp. & Inst. Urol. Lond.; Cons. Urol. Yeovil Dist. Hosp. Yeovil & Yeatman Hosp. Sherborne; Med. Directort, E. Somerster NHS Trust, Yeovil.

PARKER, Christopher John Richard Royal Liverpool University Hospital, Department of Anaesthesia, 12th Floor, Prescot Street, Liverpool L7 8XP — MD Liverp. 1991; MRCS Eng. LRCP Lond. 1979; MA Camb. 1980, MB BChir 1980; FRCA 1984; LLB Liverp. 2003. Cons. Anaesth. Roy. Liverp. & Broadgreen Univ. Hosp. Trust Liverp. Specialty: Anaesth.

PARKER, Christopher Paul 18 Eight Street, Birkenshaw, Tannochside, Larkhall — MB ChB Aberd. 1994.

PARKER, Christopher Richard The Lindley Group Practice, 62 Acre Street, Lindley, Huddersfield HD3 3DY Tel: 01484 342190 — MB ChB Leeds 1984.

PARKER, Claire Elizabeth 6 Apsley Road, Oxford OX2 7QY — MB BChir Camb. 1980; DRCOG 1982; MRCGP 1983; DPhil 1994.

PARKER, Claire Ruth 76 Pant-y-Celyn Road, Llandough, Penarth CF64 2PH — MB BCh Wales 1994.

PARKER, Clare Luise 35 Redgrave Close, St. James Village, Gateshead NE8 3JD — MB BS Lond. 1993; DRCOG 1996; MRCGP 1998; MRCS Ed. 2002.

PARKER, Clare Rhian 128 Pembroke Road, Canton, Cardiff CF5 1QQ — MB BCh Wales 1998; MRCP UK 2001.
PARKER, Mr Clive (retired) 2 West Lawn, Ashbrooke, Sunderland SR2 7HW — MB ChB Ed. 1957; FRCS Eng. 1966. Cons. Urol. Surg. Sunderland Gp. Hosps.
PARKER, Colin Ernest 59 Clinton Lane, Kenilworth CV8 1AS Tel: 01926 54852 — MB BS Lond. 1969 (Univ. Coll. Hosp.) MRCS Eng. LRCP Lond. 1969; DObst RCOG 1972. Clin. Asst. (Dermat.). Socs: Midl. Dermatol. Soc. Prev: Ho. Surg. & Ho. Phys. Basingstoke & Dist. Hosp.; Ho. Off. Paediat. Gulson Hosp. Coventry; SHO Obst. N. Tees. Gen. Hosp. Stockton on Tees.
PARKER, Cornelle Ruth Airedale General Hospital, Skipton Road, Steeton, Keighley BD20 6TD Tel: 01535 652511 — MB ChB Liverp. 1988; MRCP (UK) 1993; DM Nottm. 2000; FRCP Ed. 2004. Cons. Phys. (Diabetes & Endocrinol.) Airedale Gen. Hosp. Keighley; Hon. Sen. Lect., Univ. of Leeds. Specialty: Endocrinol.; Diabetes; Gen. Med. Special Interest: Diabetes in Pregn.; Diabetic Nephropathy; Metab. Bone Dis. Prev: Specialist Regist. (Diabetes & Endocrinol.) Nottm.; SHO (Med.) Soton.
PARKER, Mr David Alan Derbyshire Royal Infirmary, London Road, Derby DE1 2QY Tel: 01332 254654 Fax: 01332 254054 Email: sue.wright@sdah-tr.trent.nhs.uk — MB BChir Camb. 1980; BA Camb. 1978, MA 1982; FRCS Ed. 1985. Serv. Dir. for Surg. Derby Roy. Infirm. Specialty: Otorhinolaryngol. Special Interest: Otology; Paediatric ENT; Rhinology. Prev: Cons. ENT Derby Roy. Infirm.; Sen. Regist. (ENT) W. Midl. Train. Scheme.
PARKER, David Allan Wrexham Maelor Hospital, Croesnewydd Road, Wrexham LL13 7TD Tel: 01978 291100; Ty'r Graig, Ruthin Road, Bwlchgwyn, Wrexham LL11 5UT Tel: 01978 750620 — MB ChB Birm. 1979; MRCP (UK) 1982; FRCR 1986. Cons. (Radiol.) Wrexham Maelor NHS Trust. Specialty: Radiol.; Nuclear Med.
PARKER, David James Barton Surgery, 1 Edmunds Close, Barton Court Avenue, New Milton BH25 7EN Tel: 01425 620830 Fax: 01425 629812; 87 Barton Court Avenue, Barton on Sea, New Milton BH28 7ET Tel: 01425 638101 — MB BCh BAO Dub. 1971; MB BCh BAO Dub 1971; MRCGP 1976.
PARKER, David Leonard Berinsfield Health Centre, Fane Drive, Berinsfield, Wallingford OX10 7NE Tel: 01865 340558 Fax: 01865 341973; 26 Manor Farm Road, Dorchester-on-Thames, Wallingford OX10 7HZ Tel: 01865 340402 — MB BChir Camb. 1965 (Cambridge & St. Thomas' Hospital) MA, MB Camb. 1965, BChir 1964; DObst RCOG 1967; DA Eng. 1968; FRCGP 1997, M 1976. Clin. Asst. (Anaesth.) Oxon. DHA (T). Prev: Med. Off. Uganda Govt., Fort Portal; Cas. Off. St. Thos. Hosp. Lond.; Ho. Surg. & Ho. Phys. St. Mary's Hosp. Portsmouth.
PARKER, David Robert Department of Gastroenterology, Weston General Hospital, Grange Road, Uphill, Weston Super Mare BS23 4TQ — MB BCh Wales 1986; BSc (Hons.) Wales 1983; MRCP (UK) 1989; MD Bristol 1996; FRCP Lond 1999. Cons. Phys. & Gastroenterol. Weston Gen. Hosp. Weston-Super-Mare; Sen. Clin. Lect. Univ. of Bristol. Specialty: Gen. Med.; Gastroenterol. Socs: Brit. Soc. Gastroenterol.; The Physiological Soc. Prev: Sen. Regist. (Gen. Med. & Gastroenterol.) Singleton & Morriston Hosps. Swansea; Research Fell. Bristol Roy. Infirm.; Regist. (Gen. Med. & Gastroenterol.) Bristol Roy. Infirm.
PARKER, Deborah Ann Norwood Medical Centre, 360 Herries Road, Sheffield S5 7HD Tel: 0114 242 6208 Fax: 0114 261 9243 — MB ChB Manch. 1992; BSc (Physiol.) Manch. 1989; DRCOG 1995. Partern Sheff. Norwood Med. Centre. Specialty: Gen. Pract. Socs: BMA; Roy. Coll. Gen. Pract. Prev: Trainee GP Sheff. VTS.
PARKER, Deborah Francine (retired) Jubilee House, Long Street, Topcliffe, Thirsk YO7 3RL — MB BS Lond. 1988; BSc Lond. 1985.
PARKER, Dennis 29 St Paul's Square, York YO24 4BD Tel: 01904 620871 — MB BS Newc. 1969; BSc (Anat., Hons.) Newc. 1966; DPhil Oxf. 1973; MRCP (UK) 1976; FRCP Lond. 1991. Cons. Phys. (Oncol.) Bradford Roy. Infirm. & St. Luke's Hosp. Bradford; Hon. Sen. Lect. Univ. Bradford. Specialty: Oncol. Prev: Sen. Regist. (Med.) Chapel Allerton Hosp. Leeds; Gordon Hamilton Fairley Fell. (Med. Oncol.) St. Bart. Hosp. Lond.; Regist. (Med.) Ninewells Hosp. Dundee.
PARKER, Dennis Mackinder, MBE (retired) — (Leeds) MB ChB Leeds 1953; MRCGP 1963. GP Sheff. Prev: GP Sheff.
PARKER, Mr Edward John Colton (retired) Tudor Lodge, Churchill, Kidderminster DY10 3LX Tel: 01562 700710 — MB BChir Camb. 1967 (Camb. & Lond. Hosp.) MA Camb. 1969, BA 1963; FRCS Eng. 1971; MRCGP 1977. Prev: SHO Roy. Nat. Orthop. Hosp. Stanmore.
PARKER, Elizabeth Mary — MB Camb. 1980; BA Camb. 1976, BChir 1979; MRCPsych 1983. Cons. Psychiat. S. Lond. & Maudsley NHS Trust; Sen. Lect. GKT Lond. Specialty: Gen. Psychiat. Prev: Cons. Psychiat. Springfield Hosp. Lond.; Sen. Regist. (Psychiat.) Guy's Hosp. Lond.; Regist. (Psychiat.) Guy's Hosp. Lond.
PARKER, Felicity Anne Riverside Surgery, Le Molay Littry Way, Bovey Tacey, Newton Abbot TQ13 9QP Tel: 01626 832666 — MB ChB Manch. 1982; MRCGP 1986.
PARKER, Francis Bruce Wyndham, MBE (retired) 2 Tilsley Road, Chipping Norton OX7 5JA Tel: 01608 642822 Fax: 01608 642822 — (Birm.) MB ChB Birm. 1954; DObst RCOG 1956; DCH Eng. 1958. Prev: Med. Off. Chipping Norton War Memor. Hosp. & Kingham Hill Sch.
PARKER, George Talbot 168 Spring Bank, Hull HU3 1QW; 247 Northgate, Cottingham HU16 5RL — MRCS Eng. LRCP Lond. 1956 (Leeds)
PARKER, Glynn North Trent Medical Audiology, Royal Hallamshire Hospital, Glossop Road, Sheffield S10 2JF; The Old Rectory, Churchtown, Darley Dale, Matlock DE4 2GL — MB ChB Leeds 1981; DCH RCP Lond. 1983; MRCP (UK) 1985; MSc Manchester 1999. Cons. Audiological Phys.; Cons. Audiological Phys. Childr.s Audiol.,Chesterfield. Specialty: Audiol. Med. Prev: Clin. Med. Off. (Child Health) N. Derbysh.; Asst. GP Rotherham; Sen. Regist. (Audiol. Med.) Roy. Hallamsh. Hosp. Sheff.
PARKER, Gordon Occupational Health Dept., Royal Preston Hospital, Sharoe Green Lane, Preston PR2 9HT Email: gordon.parker2@doctors.org.uk — MB ChB Sheff. 1979; MA Camb. 1980; MRCGP 1984; MFOM 1993; FFOM RCP Lond. 1998. Cons. Occupational Phys. Lancs. Teachg. Hosps. NHS Trust; Hon. Lect. (Occupat. Med.) Univ. Manch. Specialty: Occupat. Health. Prev: Head of Health & Safety Servs. & Univ. Occupat. Phys. Univ. Manch.; Group Medical Adviser, Ranks Hovis McDougall.
PARKER, Graham The Archways Surgery, 86 Stockport Road, Romiley, Stockport SK6 3AA Tel: 0161 494 5337 Fax: 0161 406 7884 — BM BS Nottingham 1989; BMedSci Nottm 1987; MRCGP 1994; Post Graduate Certificate in GP University of Central Lancashire 1998. Specialty: Gen. Pract. Prev: Trainee GP Stockport VTS.
PARKER, Graham David Colne Medical Centre, 40 Station Road, Brightlingsea, Colchester CO7 0DT Tel: 01206 302522 Fax: 01206 305131 — MB BS Lond. 1976.
PARKER, Graham Stuart Marsh Medical Practice, Keeling Street, North Somercotes, Louth LN11 7QU — MB BS Lond. 1980; DRCOG 1983.
PARKER, Harold Gordon (retired) Pont-Ar-Dulas, Llanafan Fawr, Builth Wells LD2 3LW Tel: 01591 620300 — (Birm.) MB ChB Birm. 1946. Prev: Ho. Surg. Qu. Eliz. Hosp. Birm. & Birm. Matern. Hosp.
PARKER, Helen 16 Swinburne House, Roman Road, London E2 0HJ — MB BS Lond. 1998.
PARKER, Hilary Honley Surgery, Marsh Gardens, Honley, Huddersfield HD9 6AG Tel: 01484 303366 Fax: 01484 303365 — MB ChB Birm. 1971.
PARKER, Ian 10 Allanton Road, Bonkle, Wishaw ML2 9QF Tel: 01698 384183 — MB ChB Ed. 1972; DMRD Eng. 1978; FRCR 1980. Cons. Radiol St. John's Hosp. Howden Livingstone. Specialty: Nuclear Med. Prev: Cons. Radiol. Bangour Gen. Hosp. Broxburn.
PARKER, Ian Richard Green End Surgery, 58 Green End, Comberton, Cambridge CB3 7DY Tel: 01223 262500 Fax: 01223 264401 — MB BChir Camb. 1978; MSc E. Anglia 1976; DRCOG 1981; MRCGP 1982. Specialty: Accid. & Emerg.
PARKER, Ian Wyndham 4 Collice Street, Islip, Kidlington OX5 2TB — MB BS Lond. 1986; MRCGP 1993.
PARKER, James Barry 45 Hillpark Avenue, Edinburgh EH4 7AH Tel: 0131 336 3181 — MB ChB Ed. 1985; MRCGP 1989; DCCH RCP Ed. 1989. GP Edin.
PARKER, James Desmond Amylin Pharmaceuticals Inc., Magdalen Centre, Oxford Science Park, Oxford OX4 4GA Tel: 01865 784094 Fax: 01865 787901 — MB ChB Glas. 1979; MRCP (UK) 1982; MFPM RCP(UK) 1990. Sen. Med. Dir. Europe; Hon. Cons. Guys Hosp. Lond. Specialty: Pharmaceutical Medicine; Rheumatol. Prev: Sen. Regist. Rheum. Nuffield Orthop. Hosp. Oxf.

PARKER, Jan Ceridwen 59 Oakwood Road, Henleaze, Bristol BS9 4NT — BM Soton. 1996.

PARKER, Jane Elizabeth 158 Barton Road, Luton LU3 2BE Tel: 01582 591360 — MB BS Lond. 1989; MRCP (UK) 1992. Regist. (Haemat.) Pembury Hosp. Tunbridge Wells & Kings Coll. Hosp. Lond. Specialty: Haematology. Prev: SHO (Med.) S. Warks. Hosp.; SHO (Cas.) Cheltenham Gen. Hosp.; Ho. Phys. Ipswich Hosp.

PARKER, Jean Helen St Johns Medical Centre, 287A Lewisham Way, London SE4 1XF — MRCS Eng. LRCP Lond. 1974 (St. Bart.) BPharm (Hons.) Lond. 1969, MB BS 1974; DRCOG 1977; DCH RCP Lond. 1986; MRCGP 1987. Specialty: Obst. & Gyn. Prev: Trainee GP Lewisham VTS; Med. Off. Lond. Brook Advis. Centres for Young People.; SHO (Paediat.) Sydenham Childr. Hosp.

PARKER, Jeremy Russell 28 Sunningvale Avenue, Biggin Hill, Westerham TN16 3BU Tel: 01959 571525 — MB BS Lond. 1991 (King's Coll. Hosp.) FRCS Eng. 1996. Specialist Regist. Roy. Lond. Hosp. Rotat. Specialty: Orthop.

PARKER, Joanne Louise 20 Wentworth Crescent, Mayals, Swansea SA3 5HT — MB BCh Wales 1998.

PARKER, John Worden Medical Centre, West Paddock, Leyland, Preston PR25 1HR Tel: 01772 423555 Fax: 01772 623878; 119 Worden Lane, Leyland PR25 3BD Tel: 01772 436930 — MB ChB Manch. 1977; BSc Med. Sci St. And.1974.

PARKER, John Anthony Richard (retired) Blue Gates, 2 Nayland Road, Mile End, Colchester CO4 5EG Tel: 01206 577510 — MB BS Lond. 1947 (Guy's) DA Eng. 1953. Prev: GP & Asst. Anaesth. Colchester.

PARKER, John Charles 61 Bold Lane, Aughton, Ormskirk L39 6SG — MB ChB Sheff. 1993.

PARKER, John Howard Knight (retired) Pound Cottage, Pound Lane, Martock TA12 6LU Tel: 01935 823650 — (Bristol) MB ChB Bristol 1945; DObst RCOG 1948. Prev: Ho. Surg. & Res. Obst. Off. Southmead Hosp. Bristol.

PARKER, John Lauchlan Wilson County Hospital, Greetwell Road, Lincoln LN2 5QY Tel: 01522 573359; Torridon, 1 Cliff Avenue, Nettleham, Lincoln LN2 2PU Tel: 01522 750746 — (Glas.) MB ChB Glas. 1967; MRCP (UK) 1972; FRCP Ed. 1981; FRCP Glas. 1985. United Lincs. Hosps. NHS Trust, Co. Hosp., Lincoln LN2 5QY, Cons. Phys. with interest in Diabetes & Endrocrinology. Specialty: Gen. Med. Socs: BMA; Lincoln Med. Soc.; Assn. Of Brit. Clin. Diabetologists. Prev: Cons. Phys. St. Geo. Hosp. Lincoln; Sen. Regist. (Gen. Med.) Gartnavel Gen. Hosp. Glas. & Roy. Infirm. Glas.; Regist. (Gen. Med. & Endocrinol.) West. Infirm. Glas.

PARKER, John Lee 11 Thurcaston Lane, Rothley, Leicester LE7 7LF — MB BS Lond. 1993.

PARKER, John Stephen Morrill Street Health Centre, Holderness Road, Hull HU9 2LJ Tel: 01482 320046; 1 Herne View, Beverley HU17 — MB ChB Leeds 1979; DCH RCP Lond. 1982; MRCGP 1983; DRCOG 1983. Socs: Brit. Soc. Med. Dent. Hypn.

PARKER, Jonathan Chester 17 Paddockfields, Old Basing, Basingstoke RG24 7DB Tel: 01256 26460 — (St. Mary's) MB BS Lond. 1963; MRCS Eng. LRCP Lond. 1963; DMRD Eng. 1968; FFR 1970; FRCR 1975. Cons. Radiol. Basingstoke & Dist. Gen. Hosp. Specialty: Radiol. Prev: Sen. Regist. Univ. Coll. Hosp. Lond. & Hosp. Sick Childr. Gt. Ormond; St.; SHO West. Hosp. Fulham.

PARKER, Joyce Mary (retired) The Hollies, Florida St., Castle Cary BA7 7AE Tel: 01963 50709 — MRCS Eng. LRCP Lond. 1949 (Roy. Free)

PARKER, Judith Alison The Lindley Group Practice, 62 Acre Street, Lindley, Huddersfield HD3 3DY Tel: 01484 342191 — MB ChB Leeds 1984; MB ChB Leeds l984.

PARKER, Julie Woodlands, 5A Condover Park, Condover, Shrewsbury SY5 7DU — MB ChB Liverp. 1981.

PARKER, Julie Long Fox Unit, Weston General Hospital, Grange Road, Uphill, Weston Super Mare BS23 4TQ Tel: 01934 647064 Fax: 01934 643061 — BM BCh Oxf. 1978; BA Camb. 1975; MRCPsych. 1982; MSc Bristol 1988. Cons., Old Age Psychiat., N. Som. Specialty: Geriat. Psychiat. Special Interest: Old Age Med.

PARKER, Julius Clifford 3 Norden Meadows, Altwood Road, Maidenhead SL6 4SB — MB ChB Leic. 1988; BA Oxf. 1983; DRCOG 1991; T(GP) 1992; MRCGP 1992. Lect. (Child Health) Brit. Coll. of Naturopathy & Osteop. Socs: BMA. Prev: SHO (Community Paediat.) Banbury; Trainee GP N.ants. VTS.

PARKER, Lewis (retired) 3 Dovercourt Avenue, Heaton Mersey, Stockport SK4 3QB — BM BCh Oxf. 1944; MA Oxf. 1945, BM BCh 1944; FRCPath 1966. Hon. Cons. Microbiol. N. Manch. Gen. Hosp. Prev: Cons. Microbiol. N. Manch. Gen. Hosp.

PARKER, Linda Stella The Old Penny School House, St Johns Road, St Leonards-on-Sea TN37 6ET — MB BChir Camb. 1989 (Univ. Camb. Clin. Sch.) MA Camb. 1990, BA (Hons.) 1986; ECFMG Cert. 1989; DRCOG 1995; DFFP 1995. GP Regist. Jenner Hse. Old Harlow. Specialty: Gen. Pract. Prev: SHO (A & E Psychiat. & O & G) Princess Alexandra Hosp. Harlow.

PARKER, Lisa Belinda 38 Crescent Avenue, Hornchurch RM12 4ED — MB BS Lond. 1992.

PARKER, Luke Robert Cowdy Close Farm Surgery, 47 Victoria Road, Warmley, Bristol BS30 5JZ Tel: 0117 932 2108 Fax: 0117 987 3977 Email: luke.parker@gp-l81050.nhs.uk — MB BS Lond. 1985; BSc Lond. 1982; DGM RCP Lond. 1989; DCH RCP Lond. 1991; MRCGP 1993. Specialty: Gen. Pract. Prev: Trainee GP Avon VTS.

PARKER, Margaret Beryl (retired) 68 Ladies Mile Road, Patcham, Brighton BN1 8TD Tel: 01273 555791 — MB ChB Birm. 1939 (Birm) DPH Eng. 1948; MFCM 1974. Prev: Sen. Med. Off. (Child Health) Brighton Health Dist.

PARKER, Marler Thomas (retired) 9 Sunrise at Frognal House, Frognal Avenue, Sidcup DA14 6LF Tel: 0208 269 9404 — MD Camb. 1956 (Camb. & Char. Cross) MB BChir 1937; Dip. Bact. Lond 1939; FRCPath 1964. Prev: Dir. Cross Infec. Ref. Laborat. Colindale, Manch. Regional Pub.

PARKER, Martyn John 113 Cumberland House, St Mary's Court, Peterborough PE1 1UN Tel: 01733 569945 — MB ChB Birm. 1979; DRCOG 1983; DCH RCP Lond. 1984; FRCS Ed. (A&E) 1987; FRCS Ed. (Gen.) 1988; MD Birm. 1995. Research Fell. (Orthop.) PeterBoro. Dist. Hosp. Specialty: Orthop. Prev: Research Regist. (Orthop.) P.boro. Dist. Hosp.

PARKER, Matthew Richard 18 Laburnum Road, Chorley PR6 7BG — MB ChB Leeds 1998.

PARKER, Melanie Hearing Assessment Centre, Children's Hospital, Paul O'Gorman Building, Upper Maudlin Street, Bristol BS2 8BJ Tel: 0117 342 8350 Email: melanie.parker@ubht.swest.nhs.uk — MB BCh Wales 1980 (Welsh Nat. Sch. Med.) DCCH 1988; MRCP Ed. 1994. Staff Grade (Comm. Paediat.) United Bristol Healthcare Trust, Bris.; Mem. Autism Assessm. Team; Chair of Social & Communication Advis. Panel. Socs: BASPCAN; BACCH; BACDA. Prev: Flexible Regist. (Paediat.) Southmead Hosp. Bristol; Clin. Med. Off. Fife HB.

PARKER, Mr Michael Christopher Owen Darent Valley Hospital, Darenth Wood Road, Dartford DA2 8DA Tel: 01322 428100 Fax: 01322 428635 Email: mike.parker@dag-tr.sthames.nhs.uk; Darenth Vicarage Hill, Westerham TN16 1TL Tel: 01959 564743 Fax: 01959 561209 Email: mikesurg@aol.com — MB BS Lond. 1973 (Westm.) BSc (Hons.) Lond. 1970; MRCS Eng. LRCP Lond. 1973; FRCS Eng. 1980; FRCS Ed. 1980. Cons. Surg. Laparascopic & Colorectal, Darent Valley Hosp. Specialty: Gen. Surg. Socs: Founder Mem. Assn. Colproctol. GB & Irel.; Fell. Roy. Soc. Med. (Pres. of Surg. Sect.); Counc. Mem. Assn. Encoscopic Surgeons of GB and Ire. Prev: Lect. & Sen. Regist. (Surg.) St. Geo. Hosp. Lond.; Regist. (Surg.) St. Geo. & St. Jas. Hosp. Lond.; Sen. Regist., S.W. Thames.

PARKER, Michael Donovan (retired) Thornbers, Slaidburn Road, Waddington, Clitheroe BB7 3JJ Tel: 01200 425318 Email: parkerm@beeb.net — MB ChB Birm. 1953; DObst RCOG 1954; DCH Eng. 1958; FRCGP 1985, M 1966. Prev: Ho. Phys. Childr. Hosp. Birm.

PARKER, Michael James North Trent Clinical Genetics Service, Sheffield Children's NHS Trust, Blue Wing, Western Bank, Sheffield S10 2TH Tel: 0114 271 7025; 4 Behay Gardens, Staythorpe, Newark NG23 5RL Email: mick@doctors.org.uk — MB ChB Leeds 1992; BSc Leeds 1990; MRCP (Paediat.) 1995; MD 1999. Consultant Clinical Geneticist. Specialty: Genetics. Prev: Specialist Regist.

PARKER, Michael Julian Reid Altnagelvin Area Hospital, Londonderry BT47 6SB; Ashton Lodge, 1 Rosswater, Limavady Road, Londonderry BT47 6YR — MD Belf. 1988; MB BCh BAO 1980; MRCOG 1985, D 1982; FRCOG 1999. Cons. Obst. & Gyn. Specialty: Obst. & Gyn.

PARKER, Michael Rowland 2 Ashdown Road, Heaton Moor, Stockport SK4 4JN — MB ChB Liverp. 1994.

PARKER, Myrtle Lee (retired) Ger-y-Plas, Talybont SY24 5HJ Tel: 01970 832449 — MB BS Lond. 1953 (Char. Cross) Prev: GP.

PARKER, Nicola Jane Main Road Surgery, 173 Main Road, Sundridge, Sevenoaks TN14 6EH Tel: 01959 562531; Winterton Surgery, Russell House, Westerham TN16 1RB — MB ChB Birm. 1986; DRCOG 1989; DCH RCP Lond. 1990.

PARKER, Norman Eric Whittington Hospital, Highgate Hill, London N19 5NF Tel: 020 7288 5437 Fax: 020 7288 3485 Email: norman.parker@whittington.nhs.uk; 2A, Ashfield Road, Southgate, London N14 7JY — MB BS Lond. 1974 (Univ. Coll. Hosp.) MRCP (UK) 1976; FRCPath 1993, M 1981; FRCP Lond. 1993. Cons. Haemat. Whittington Hosp. Lond. Specialty: Haematology. Socs: Brit. Soc. Haematol. Prev: Lect. (Clin. Haemat.) Univ. Coll. Hosp. Med. Sch. Lond.; Med. Director Whittington NHS Trust.

PARKER, Patricia Mary The Dial House, Frensham, Farnham GU10 3AZ Tel: 01252 794249 — MB BS Lond. 1969.

PARKER, Patrick William McLean Crossways, Chagford, Newton Abbot TQ13 8DA Tel: 01647 432430 — MB BS Lond. 1961; DObst RCOG 1963. Prev: SHO (Obst.) St. Mary's Hosp. Kettering; Ho. Surg. Kettering Gen. Hosp.; Ho. Phys. Middlx. Hosp.

PARKER, Mr Paul Jeremy 18 Lancedean Road, Beflast, Milnthorpe BT6 9QP — MB BCh BAO Belf. 1985 (Queen's Univ. Belfast) Dip. IMC RCS Ed. 1990; FRCS Ed. 1992; FRCS (Orth) 1997. Cons. Orthop. Surg. Friarage Hosp. N. Allerton; ATLS Co-Dir. AO Instruc. Specialty: Trauma & Orthop. Surg. Socs: Orthop. Dangerous Sports Soc. Prev: Osteoarticular Research Fell. Univ. Edin. Med. Sch.; Sen. Regist. (Orthop. & Traumatol.) Roy. Infirm. Edin.; Fell. (Orthop. Trauma) R. Adams Cowley Shock-Trauma Center Baltimore MD, USA.

PARKER, Richard Henry Oxlade (retired) The Firs, Firs Road, Ross-on-Wye HR9 5BH Tel: 01989 563995 — BM BCh Oxf. 1953 (Oxf. & Middlx.) BSc Oxf.; DObst RCOG 1956; DA Eng. 1970; MRCGP 1972. Med. Adviserr Ldr.ship trust, Ross On Wye. Prev: GP Ross-on-Wye.

PARKER, Richard Hugh c/ The Manager, National Westminster Bank, 22 George St., Richmond TW9 1JW — MB BChir Camb. 1981; MA, MB Camb. 1981, BChir 1980; DRCOG 1986; DCH RCP Lond. 1986; MRCGP 1988. Prev: Trainee GP Greenwich VTS; Med. Off. Brit. Antarctic Survey.

PARKER, Richard Lewis Edward South Ham House, 96 Paddock Road, Basingstoke RG22 6RL Tel: 01256 324666 Fax: 01256 810849; 7 Litton Gardens, Oakley, Basingstoke RG23 7JS — MB BS Lond. 1990. Specialty: Gen. Pract.

PARKER, Robert Bunten (retired) 9 Tudor Way, Murton, Swansea SA3 3AZ Tel: 01792 234664 — MB BS Lond. 1953 (St. Bart.) MRCS Eng. LRCP Lond. 1952.

PARKER, Robert Stansfeld 9 Rowton Grange Road, Chapel-en-le Frith, High Peak SK23 0LA Tel: 01298 812686 Fax: 01298 815287 — MB ChB Manch. 1960; DObst RCOG 1964. Forens. Med. Examr. Derbysh. Constab.; Co. Path. High Peak Derbysh. Socs: BMA; Assn. Police Surg. Prev: Resid. (Clin. Path.) Bolton Roy. Infirm.; Ho. Off. (O & G) Bolton Dist. Gen. Hosp.; Ho. Off. (Surg.) Salford Roy. Hosp.

PARKER, Rodney Kevan Hassard Bushey Health Centre, London Road, Bushey, Watford WD23 2NN Tel: 01923 225224 Fax: 01923 213270; Oundle, 46 Little Bushey Lane, Bushey Heath, Watford WD23 4RN Tel: 020 8950 1013 Fax: 020 8950 1013 — MB ChB Bristol 1959; DObst RCOG 1961; MRCGP 1977. Prev: Ho. Surg. (Obst.) Bristol Matern. Hosp.

PARKER, Roger The Health Centre, Doctor Lane, Mirfield WF14 8DU Tel: 01924 495721 Fax: 01924 480605; Pinfold Lodge, Pinfold Lane, Mirfield WF14 9HZ Tel: 01924 495549 — MB ChB Leeds 1969. Specialty: Dermat. Socs: Hudds. Med. Soc. Prev: SHO (O & G), Ho. Phys. (Med. & Dermat.) & Ho. Surg. (Surg. & ENT) Staincliffe Gen. Hsop. Dewsbury.

PARKER, Roger Durnal Lloyd (retired) 24 Argarmeols Road, Formby, Liverpool L37 7DA — MB ChB Liverp. 1960; DObst RCOG 1962. Prev: Ho. Surg. & Ho. Phys. David Lewis North. Hosp. Liverp.

PARKER, Roger John (retired) 17 Derwen Deg Close, Govilon, Abergavenny NP7 9RJ Tel: 01873 830336 — (Guy's) MRCS Eng. LRCP Lond. 1964; DMRD Eng. 1967. Cons. Radiol. P. Chas. Hosp. Merthyr Tydfil. Prev: Sen Regist. (Radiol) Bristol Roy. Infirm.

PARKER, Mr Ronald William Davenport Consulting Rooms, 5 Davenport Road, Coventry CV5 6QA — MB ChB Birm. 1963; FRCS Ed. 1968; FRCS Eng. 1969. Governor Warks. Private Hosp.; Cons. Gen. Surg. Walsgrave Hosp. Coventry. Specialty: Gen. Surg. Socs: Chairm. Brit. Assn. Med. Managers; BMA & Brit. Assn. Surg. Oncol. Prev: Sen. Regist. Qu. Eliz. Hosp. Birm. & Selly Oak Hosp. Birm.

PARKER, Sally Elizabeth 6 Kempe's Close, Long Ashton, Bristol BS41 9ER Tel: 01275 392016 — BM Soton. 1986; DCH RCP Lond. 1992; FRCA 1994. Specialist Regist. (Anaesth.) St. Geo.s Hosp. Lond. Specialty: Anaesth. Prev: Attend. (Pediatric Anesthesia) Childr.s Hosp. & Regional Med. Center Seattle, USA; Fell. (Paediat. Anaesth.) Hosp. Sick Childr. Toronto, Canada; Regist. (Anaesth.) Torbay Hosp. Torquay & Derriford Hosp. Plymouth.

PARKER, Sara Louise Ashford Public Health Laboratory, William Harvey Hospital, Willesborough, Ashford TN24 0LZ Tel: 01233 635731 Fax: 01233 643432; Stede Court, Stede Hill, Harrietsham, Maidstone ME17 1NR Tel: 01622 850944 — MB BS Lond. 1986; MSc (Med. Microbiol.) Lond. 1993; MRCPath 1998. Cons. (Med. Microbiol.) Ashford Pub. Health Laborat. William Harvey Hosp. Specialty: Med. Microbiol. Prev: Sen. Regist. (Med. Microbiol.) Ashford Pub. Health Laborat. William Harvey Hosp.; Sen. Regist. (Med. Microbiol.) St. Geo. Hosp. Lond.

PARKER, Sarah Caroline Barrow Health Centre, 27 High Street, Barrow on Soar, Loughborough LE12 8PY Tel: 01509 413525 Fax: 01509 620664; Glebe Farm, 1 Main St, Hoby, Melton Mowbray LE14 3DT Tel: 01664 434263 Fax: 01664 434147 — MB BS Lond. 1982 (St. Mary's)

PARKER, Sheena Stevenson 2 Regent Terrace, Edinburgh EH7 5BN Tel: 0131 556 7164 — MB ChB Ed. 1967; Dip Soc Med Ed. 1974; MFPHM 1995; MFPHM RCP (UK) 1995; FFPHM 1998; FRCP Ed 1998. Dir. Pub. Health, W. Sussex Health Auth. Specialty: Pub. Health Med. Prev: Cons. Pub. Health Med. Lothian HB.; Unit Gen. Manager Lothian HB.; Specialist (Community Med.) Lothian HB.

PARKER, Sheila Margaret Pasture Wood, Crawley Down, Crawley RH10 4LL Tel: 01342 2870 — MRCS Eng. LRCP Lond. 1946 (Roy. Free) FFA RCS Eng. 1956. Cons. Anaesth. Dudley & Stourbridge Hosp. Gp. Specialty: Anaesth. Prev: Sen. Anaesth. Regist. United Birm. Hosps. & Regional Thoracic; Centres.

PARKER, Sheila Morgan (retired) 2 Tilsley Road, Chipping Norton OX7 5JA Tel: 01608 642822 — MB ChB Birm. 1953; FFA RCS Eng. 1956; DA Eng. 1956. Med. Off. Chipping Norton War Memor. Hosp. Prev: Regist. (Anaesth.), Ho. Phys. & Ho. Surg. Qu. Eliz. Hosp. Birm.

PARKER, Sidney James 85 Old Kilmore Road, Moira, Craigavon BT67 0NA Tel: 01846 611278; 52 Main Street, Moira, Craigavon BT67 0LQ Tel: 01846 611278 — MB BCh BAO Belf. 1978; DRCOG 1980; MRCGP 1982; DGM RCP Lond. 1985.

PARKER, Mr Stephen John University Hospital, Cifford Bridge Road, Coventry CV2 2DX Tel: 024 7653 8879 Fax: 024 7660 4431 — MB BS Lond. 1988 (St Geo.) BSc Lond. 1985; FRCS Eng. 1994; FRCS Ed. 1994; MS Soton. 1999; FRCS (Gen. Surg.) 2001. Cons. Breast & Gen. Paediat. Surg. Univ. Hosps. Coventry & Warks. NHS Trust. Specialty: Gen. Surg. Special Interest: Oncoplastic Breast Surgery; Paediatric Surgery.

PARKER, Steven John The Surgery, Revelstoke Way, Rise Park, Nottingham NG14 7DW — MB ChB Manch. 1983; DRCOG 1989; MRCGP 1989; DGM RCP Lond. 1993. Socs: Nottm. Medico-Chirurgical Soc.

PARKER, Stuart James 69 Lakin Drive, Barry CF62 8AH Tel: 01446 735282 — MB BCh Wales 1966 (Cardiff) DObst RCOG 1968; DCH Eng. 1968; MRCGP 1974; DMJ (Clin.) Soc. Apoth. Lond. 1981; BA (Hons.) Open 1989. Med. Adviser SEMA Med. Servs. Caridff. Specialty: Disabil. Med. Prev: Princip. GP Barry; Gen. Med. Off. Uganda.

PARKER, Stuart Samuel Ireland (retired) 25 Burnside Place, Larkhall ML9 2EQ Tel: 01698 882724 Email: stuartparker@larkhall.demon.co.uk — (Glasgow University) MB ChB Glas. 1958; MB ChB Glas. 1958; DObst RCOG 1960; DObst RCOG 1960.

PARKER, Susan Clare Department of Dermatology, West Middlesex University Hospital, Twickenham Rd, Isleworth TW7 6AF Tel: 020 8321 5473 — MB BChir Camb. 1980 (St. Thos.) MA Camb. 1981; MRCP (UK) 1983; FRCP (Uk) 1999. Cons. Dermat. W.

Middlx. Univ. Hosps. & Chelsea and Westm. Hosp. Specialty: Dermat. Prev: Sen. Regist. St. Johns Dermat. Centre St. Thos. Hosp. Lond.; Regist. (Dermat.) St. Thos. Hosp. Lond.; Regist. Dermat. Roy. Vict. Infirm. Newc.

PARKER, Susan Patricia 89 Preston New Road, Marton, Blackpool FY3 9ND — BM BCh Oxf. 1991; BA Oxf. 1988; DA (UK) 1993; DCH RCP Lond. 1995; DRCOG 1996. GP/Regist. Cawley Rd. Med. Centre, Chichester.

PARKER, Susan Woodward Oak House, 42 Glenferness Avenue, Bournemouth BH3 7ET — MB BS West. Austral. 1983; MPsych (Clin.) 1973. Assoc. Specialist (Endocrinol.) Roy. Bournemouth Hosp.; Psychosexual Med. Specialist Dorset Healthcare Trust. Specialty: Endocrinol. Socs: Fell. Roy. Soc. Med.; BPS; BMA. Prev: Sen. Clin. Psychol. West. Austral. Pub. Serv. Bd.; Trainee GP Dorset.

PARKER, Thomas Frederick James 17 Dingle Road, Abergavenny NP7 7AR Tel: 01873 3395 — MB ChB Bristol 1954; DA Eng. 1957; FFA RCS Eng. 1966. Specialty: Anaesth.

PARKER, Timothy Guy Church Stretton Medical Centre, Church Stretton SY6 6BL Tel: 01694 722127; Fairway, 6 Windle Hill, Church Stretton SY6 7AP — MB ChB Birm. 1984; ChB Birm. 1984; DRCOG 1989. GP Ch. Stretton Shrops. Prev: Trainee GP Sandwell Dist. Gen. Hosp. VTS.

PARKER, Tom James 2 Ashdown Road, Stockport SK4 4JN — MB ChB Leeds 1993.

PARKER, Valerie Anne Newpark Surgery, Talbot Green, Pontyclun CF72 8AJ Tel: 01443 224213 — MB BS Newc. 1981 (Univ. Newc. u. Tyne) MRCGP 1987. Clin. Asst. in Diabetes Roy. Glamorgn Hosp. Prev: SHO (O & G) E. Glam. Gen. Hosp. Pontypridd; SHO (Haemat.) Roy. Infirm. Sunderland; Ho. Off. (Gen. Surg. & Gen. Med.) Newc. Gen. Hosp.

PARKER, Vernon Lester The Family Surgery, 7 High St, Green St Green, Orpington BR6 6BG Tel: 01689 850231 Fax: 01689 857122 Email: vernon.parker@gp-g84009.nhs.uk — MB BS Lond. 1983.

PARKER, Vivienne (retired) 3 Meadowgate, Tallington Road, Bainton, Stamford PE9 3AS Tel: 01780 740700 Fax: 01780 740700 — MB ChB Leeds 1966; DObst RCPI 1969; FFCM RCP (UK) 1989, M 1982; FFPHM RCP (UK) 1989. Prev: Dir. Pub. Health NW Anglia Health Commiss.

PARKER, William Arthur (retired) 44 Kenilworth Road, Bridge of Allan, Stirling FK9 4RP Tel: 01786 833342 — (Glasgow) MB BCh MB BCh 1941; MRCP MRCP (uk) 1962 1962; FRCP FRCP Glas 1967 1967. Prev: Cons. Phys. Stirling Roy. Infirm.

PARKER, William Neil Baron (retired) 67 Victoria Drive, Bognor Regis PO21 2TD Tel: 01243 823538 — (Camb. & Guy's) MA Camb. 1969, MB BChir 1952; MRCS Eng. LRCP Lond. 1952; DObst RCOG 1954. Prev: GP Bognor Regis.

PARKER, Yvette-Marie Anne Department of Child & Adolescent Psychiatry, Larkby Young Persons Unit, Victoria Park Road, Exeter EX2 4NU Email: juli.colley@devonptnrs.nhs.uk — MB ChB Leeds 1977; MRCGP (Distinc.) 1984; MRCPsych 1986.

PARKER-WILLIAMS, Edward John St George's Hospital Medical School, Cranmer Terrace, London SW17 0RE Tel: 020 8725 5446 Fax: 020 8725 0245 — MB BS Lond. 1957 (Middlx.) FRCPath 1988. Sen. Lect. & Cons. Haemat. St Geo. Hosp. Med. Sch. Lond. (Emerit.); Dir. UKNEQAS, Gen. Haemat. Specialty: Haematology. Prev: Cons. Haemat. & Sen. Lect. Centr. Middlx. Hosp. Lond.; Lect. (Haemat.) Middlx. Hosp. Med. Sch. Lond.; Sen. Regist. Hammersmith Hosp. Lond.

PARKES, Adrian John 21 Merridale Avenue, Wolverhampton WV3 9RE Tel: 01902 772070 — MB ChB Birm. 1986.

PARKES, Alan Walton Adlerwood Precinct Surgery, 8 Alderwood Precinct, Northway, Sedgley, Dudley DY3 3QY Tel: 01902 85180/880825; (Surgery) 8 Alderwood Precinct, Dudley DY3 3QY Tel: 0190 735180 — MB ChB Birm. 1955; BDS 1964.

PARKES, Andrew Michael Hackenthorpe Medical Centre, Main Street, Hackenthorpe, Sheffield S12 4LA Fax: 0114 251 0539 — MB ChB Sheff. 1984.

PARKES, Andrew William 15 Wellington Road, Lancaster LA1 4DN — MB BS Newc. 1998.

PARKES, Carol Ann Surrey and Sussex Strategic Health Authority, York House, Massetts Road, Horley Tel: 01293 778899 — MB BS Lond. 1985; MSc Lond. 1990, MB BS 1985; MFPHM RCP (UK) 1994. Cons. in Pub. Health Med.

PARKES, Colin Murray, OBE — (Westm.) MB BS Lond. 1951; DPM Eng. 1959; MD Lond. 1962; FRCPsych 1975, M 1971. Hon. Cons. Psychiat. St. Christopher's Hospice Sydenham & St. Josephs Hospice. Specialty: Gen. Psychiat.; Palliat. Med. Socs: Fell. Roy. Coll. Psychiat.; Roy. Soc. Med. Prev: Sen. Lect. Lond. Hosp. Med. Coll.; Mem. Research Staff Tavistock Inst. Human Relats. Lond.; Mem. Scientif. Staff, MRC Social Psychiat. Unit & Regist. Maudsley Hosp. Lond.

PARKES, Eric Charles Williams (retired) 18 Park Drive, Grimsby DN32 0EF Tel: 01472 322140/01472 78478 — MB ChB Birm. 1940. Prev: Ho. Surg. Selly Oak Hosp. Birm.

PARKES, Gary The Limes Surgery, 8-14 Limes Court, Hoddesdon EN11 8EP Tel: 01992 464533 Fax: 01992 470729 — MB ChB Manch. 1980; MRCGP 1985; DRCOG 1985; DCH RCP Lond. 1985. GP & Surg. Amp-Pipal Hosp. Kathmandu, Nepal; Princip. Gen. Pract. Hoddesdon. Prev: Trainee GP Eastbourne.

PARKES, Georgina 7 Falcon Way, Colindale, London NW9 5DT Tel: 020 8203 4387 — MB BS Lond. 1994 (Royal Free Hospital School of Medicine) Specialty: Gen. Psychiat.; Gen. Pract. Socs: MPS.

PARKES, Howard Guy, MBE (retired) The Old Orchard, Broad Green, Broadwas-on-Tyne, Worcester WR6 5NW Tel: 01866 821118 Email: guy.parkes@virgin.net — (Birm.) MB ChB Birm. 1953; FFOM RCP Lond. 1981 MFOM 1978. Prev: Med. Dir. Brit. Rubber Manufacturers' Assn. Ltd.

PARKES, Isobel Rose Park Lane Surgery, 2 Park Lane, Allestree, Derby DE22 2DS Tel: 01332 552461 Fax: 01332 541500; Ivy Bank House, Old Hillcliff Lane, Turnditch, Belper DE36 2EA Email: isobel@parkes2.fsnet.co.uk — BM BS Nottm. 1991; BMedSci. (Hons.) Nottm. 1989; MRCP (UK) 1996. GP, Pk. La. Surg. Derby. Specialty: Dermat. Prev: GP Regist. Derby VTS.

PARKES, Janet 17 Poplar Drive, Barnt Green, Birmingham B45 8NQ — MB ChB Manch. 1964.

PARKES, John David 2 Boakes Meadow, Shoreham, Sevenoaks TN14 7SH Tel: 01959 523732 Fax: 020 7703 9989 — MD Camb. 1964; MB 1960, BChir 1959; FRCP Lond. 1976, M 1961. Prof. Clin. Neurol. Univ. Dept. Neurol. Inst. Psychiat. & Kings Coll.; Hosp. Lond. Hon. Cons. Neurol. Maudsley Hosp. & KCH Lond. Specialty: Neurol. Prev: Reader Neurol. Univ. Dept. Neurol. Inst. Psychiat. & King's Coll. Hosp. Lond.; Acad. Regist. Nat. Hosp. Nerv. Dis. Qu. Sq. Lond.

PARKES, John Graham (retired) 62 Hammersmith Road, Aberdeen AB10 6ND — (Guy's) MB BS Lond. 1955; MRCS Eng. LRCP Lond. 1955; MRCGP 1970; DCH Eng. 1970. Prev: Ho. Surg. ENT Dept. & Ho. Phys. Childr. Dept. Guy's Hosp.

PARKES, Julian David The Health Centre, Alfred Squire Road, Wednesfield, Wolverhampton WV11 1XU Tel: 01902 575033 Fax: 01902 575013 — MB ChB Birm. 1984; DRCOG 1987; MRCGP 1989.

PARKES, Karen Nina Edwana, Woodland Way, Maidstone ME14 2EY — MB ChB Otago 1989.

PARKES, Miles Addenbrooke's Hospital, Hills Road, Cambridge CB2 2QQ Tel: 01223 216389 Fax: 01223 596213 Email: miles.parkes@addenbrookes.nhs.uk — MB BS Lond. 1990; BA Oxf. 1987; MRCP UK 1993; DM Oxf. 2000. Cons. Gastroenterol. Specialty: Gastroenterol. Special Interest: Inflammatory Bowel Disease. Prev: MRC Clin. Train. Fell. Nuffield Dept. Med. Gastroenterol. Unit. Radcliffe Infirm. Oxf.; Regist. (Med. & Gastroenterol.) John Radcliffe Hosp. Oxf.

PARKES, Neal Richard Quine Newmarket Medical Practice, 153 Newmarket, Louth LW11 9EH Tel: 01507 603121 Fax: 01507 605916; The Old Vicarage, School Lane, Hainton, Market Rasen LN8 6LW — MB BS Lond. 1993 (Royal Free Lond.) DFFP 1996; MRCGP 1997. GP Princip.; CMO (Fam. Plg.) Race Course Doctor. Specialty: Gen. Pract.

PARKES, Norman McNeill 1A Lynors Avenue, Strood, Rochester ME2 3NQ Tel: 01634 711463 — MB BCh BAO Dub. 1948 (TC Dub.) BA Dub. 1945, MB BCh BAO 1948; LAH Dub. 1948. Prev: Cas. Off. & Ho. Phys. St. Bart. Hosp. Rochester.

PARKES, Peter William Joseph (retired) Turvy House, Holner, Hereford HR1 1LH Tel: 01432 358811 — MRCS Eng. LRCP Lond. 1938 (Bristol & W. Lond.) Med. Off. Bristol Prison.; Phys. Bristol Homoeop. Hosp. Prev: Ho. Phys.Homeopath Hosp. Bristol.

PARKES, Robin Trevor The Surgery, St. Peters Close, Cowfold, Horsham RH13 8DN Tel: 01403 864204 Fax: 01403 864408 — MB BS Lond. 1969 (Middlx.)

PARKES, Stephen John 21 Hightrees Road, Copt Heath, Knowle, Solihull B93 9PR — MB ChB Sheff. 1979; MRCGP 1984; DCH RCP Lond. 1984. GP Solihull.

PARKES, Thomas Alan Whitehouse (retired) Willow Cottage, Willow Green, Martley, Worcester WR6 6PT Tel: 01886 821332 — (Birm.) MB ChB Birm. 1945; DA Eng. 1963. Prev: GP Sutton Coldfield.

PARKES, William Raymond, OBE (retired) Pixham Firs Cottage, Pixham Lane, Dorking RH4 1PH — (Liverp.) MB ChB Liverp. 1948 Kanthack Medal (Path.); MD Liverp. 1956; FRCP Ed. 1976, M 1959; DIH Soc. Apoth. Lond. 1962; FFOM RCP Lond. 1983, MFOM 1979. Hon. Clin. Lect. Prof. Unit Dept. Med. Nat. Heart & Lung Inst. Univ. Lond. Prev: Phys. (Respirat. Dis.) DSS Med. Bd.ing Centre Lond.

PARKES BOWEN, Malcolm David Marston (retired) The Manor House, 63 Anstey Lane, Thurcaston, Leicester LE7 7JB Tel: 0116 236 2434 Email: davidpb@netlineuk.net — MB BChir Camb. 1948 (Guy's & Camb.) MRCS Eng. LRCP Lond. 1948; FRCGP 1979, M 1960. Prev: Clin. Asst. (Phys. Med.) Leicester Roy. Infirm.

PARKHOUSE, Duncan Anthony Francis Harlidge, Maj. 26 Alsue Road, Deepant, Camberley GU16 6SS — MB BS Lond. 1991 (Univ. Coll. Hosp. Lond.) BSc (Hons) 1989; FRCA 1998. Specialist Regist. (Anaesth.) Milit. Specialty: Anaesth.

PARKHOUSE, Helen 149 Harley Street, London W1G 6DE Tel: 020 7935 8391 Fax: 020 7935 8391 Email: h.parkhouse@thelondonclinic.co.uk — MB ChB Birm. 1978; FRCS Eng. 1982; FRCS (Urol.) 1989; FEBU 1992. Cons. (Urol.) Benenden Hosp., Cranbrook, Kent. Specialty: Urol. Special Interest: Female and Reconstruc. Urol. Socs: Brit. Assn. Urol. Surgs.; Amer. Acad. of Pediatrics; Societe Internationale d'Urologie. Prev: Cons. Urol. Hillingdon & Mt. Vernon Hosps.; Sen. Lect. (Urol.) St. Thos. Hosp. Lond.; Sen. Regist. (Urol.) St. Bart. Hosp. Lond.

PARKHOUSE, James (retired) 3 Mallory Close, New Earswick, York YO32 4DL Tel: 01904 767558 — MB ChB Liverp. 1950; DA Eng. 1952; FFA RCS Eng. 1954; MD Liverp. 1955; MA Oxf. 1960; MSc Manch. 1974. Prev: Cons. Med. Careers Research Gp. Oxf.

PARKHOUSE, Mr Nicholas Queen Victoria Hospital, East Grinstead RH19 3DZ Tel: 01342 410210 Email: davidpb@supanet.com; 149 Harley Street, London W1N 2DE Tel: 020 7224 0864 — MB BS Lond. 1981; MA Oxf. 1985, BA 1978; FRCS Eng. 1985; DM Oxf. 1990; MCh Oxf. 1991. Cons. Plastic Surg. Qu. Vict. Hosp. E. Grinstead; Dir. McIndoe Burn Centre; Hon. Cons. St. Luke's Hosp. for Clergy Lond. Specialty: Plastic Surg. Socs: Fell. Med. Soc. Lond.; Fell. Chelsea Clin. Soc. Prev: Cons. Plastic Surg. Mt. Vernon Hosp. Northwood Middlx.; Sen. Regist. (Plastic Surg.) Qu. Vict. Hosp. E. Grinstead; Clin. Lect. (Surg.) Studies Middlx. Hosp. Lond.

PARKIANATHAN, Mr Visuvanather George Eliot Hospital, College Street, Nuneaton CV10 7DJ Tel: 024 7635 1351; 19 Norwich Close, Nuneaton CV11 6GF Tel: 024 7632 6625 — MB BS Sri Lanka 1973; FRCS Glas. 1985; FRCS Ed. 1985; FRCS (Gen.) 2000. Assoc. Specialist Geo. Eliot Hosp. Nuneaton. Specialty: Gen. Surg. Prev: Staff Surg. Geo. Eliot Hosp. Nuneaton; Regist. (Gen. Surg.) Geo. Eliot Hosp. Nuneaton.

PARKIN, Andrew Westcotes House, Westcotes Drive, Leicester LE3 0QU Tel: 0116 225 2900 Fax: 0116 225 2899 — BM BS Nottm. 1985; BMedSci Nottm. 1983; MRCPsych 1990. Sen. Lect. & Hon. Cons. Child & Adolesc. Psychiat. Leicester. Specialty: Child & Adolesc. Psychiat. Prev: Clin. Research Fell. & Hon. Sen. Regist. (Child & Adolesc. Psychiat.) Univ. Leicester; Sen. Regist. (Child & Adolesc. Psychiat.) Leicester & Trent RHA; Regist. & SHO (Psychiat.) Nottm. HA.

PARKIN, Andrew John The Surgeries, Lombard Street, Newark NG24 1XG Tel: 01636 702363 Fax: 01636 613037; The Old Rectory, Gainsborough Road, Winthorpe, Newark NG24 2NN Tel: 01636 703197 — BChir Camb. 1976; BChir 1976, MB Camb. 1977; MRCP (UK) 1979; MRCGP 1990. GP Trainer Centr. Notts. VTS.

PARKIN, Anne Elizabeth Newland Group Medical Practice, 239-243 Newland Avenue, Hull HU5 2EJ Tel: 01482 448456 Fax: 01482 441302; 63 Canada Drive, Cottingham HU16 5EH — MB ChB Dundee 1975; DRCOG 1989. Continuing Med. Educat. Tutor Postgrad. Centre Hull.

PARKIN, Mr Benjamin Thomas 107 Sandbanks Road, Poole BH14 8BT — BM Soton. 1989; FRCOphth 1995; MD Bristol 2001. Consult. Opthamologist and oculoplastic Surgeon, Royal Bournemouth Hospital, Bournemouth BH7 7DW. Specialty: Ophth.

PARKIN, Brian Derek Health Care Group, Rohais Health Centre, Rohais, St Peter Port, Guernsey GY1 1FF Tel: 01481 723322 Fax: 01481 725200 Email: bparkin56@hotmail.com; Le Vau Des Velines, Les Effards, St Sampsons, Guernsey GY2 4US Tel: 01481 52275 Fax: 01481 302275 — MB BS Lond. 1981 (Lond. Hosp.) BSc Lond. 1978; MRCP (UK) 1984; MRCGP 1987; DRCOG 1987; Cert. Family Plann. JCC 1987. Mem. Med. Staff Princess Eliz. Hosp. Guernsey; Dep. Med. Off. of Health Guernsey. Specialty: Gen. Med. Prev: Regist. Whipps Cross Hosp. Lond.; SHO Northwick Pk. Hosp. Harrow.; SHO Manch. Roy. Infirm.

PARKIN, David Emrys Department of Gynaecology, Aberdeen Royal Infirmary, Aberdeen Tel: 01224 681818; Western Cottage, Crathes, Banchory, Aberdeen AB31 6LA Tel: 01330 844753 — MD Manch. 1988; MB ChB 1978; MRCOG 1985; FRCOG 1998. Cons. (Gynae. Oncologist) Aberd. Roy. Infirm.; Clin. Sen. Lect. (Obst. & Gyn.) Univ. Aberd. Specialty: Obst. & Gyn. Prev: Regist. (O & G) Stobhill Hosp. Glas.; Sen. Regist. N. Staffs. Matern. Hosp.; Cons. O & G Aberd. Matern. Hosp. & Aberd. Roy. Infirm.

PARKIN, Geoffrey James Scott 8 Wedgewood Grove, Roundhay, Leeds LS8 1EG — MB ChB (Hons.) Leeds 1967; BSc (1st. cl. Hons. Anat.) Leeds 1964; DMRD Eng. 1970; FFR 1972; FRCR 1975. Cons. Radiol. United Leeds Teachg. Hosps. NHS Trust; Sen. Clin. Lect. (Diag. Radiol.) Univ. Leeds. Specialty: Radiol. Prev: Cons. Radiol. St. James Univ. Hosp. Leeds.

PARKIN, Gillian Harrogate District Hospital, Lancaster Park Road, Harrogate HG1 7SX Tel: 01423 885959; 1 Green Way, Rossett Green, Harrogate HG2 9LR — MB BS Newc. 1980; FFA RCSI 1989. Cons. (Anaesth.) Specialty: ICU Harrogate Dist. Hosp. Harrogate. Specialty: Anaesth. Prev: Flexible Trainee Yorks. Region.

PARKIN, Gordon Tallyn The Surgery, 12 Victoria Road South, Southsea PO5 2BZ Tel: 023 9282 3857; 86 Bowes Hill, Rowlands Castle PO9 6BS — MB BS Lond. 1977; DRCOG 1981; MRCGP 1981.

PARKIN, Ian Geoffrey Department of Anatomy, Downing Street, Cambridge CB2 3DY Tel: 01223 339333 Email: igp20@mole.bio.cam.ac.uk — MB ChB Aberd. 1975. Clin. Anat. Univ. Camb. Specialty: Anat. Socs: Fell. Brit. Assn. Clin. Anat. Prev: Sen. Lect. (Anat.) Birm. Univ.

PARKIN, Jacqueline Mary Department of Immunology, St. Bartholomew's Hospital Medical College, London EC1A 7BE Tel: 020 7601 8428 Fax: 020 7600 3839 — MB BS Lond. 1981; MRCP (UK) 1988; PhD Lond. 1990; FRCP (UK) 1996. Sen. Lect. & Hon. Cons. Clin. Immunol. St. Bartholomews & the Roy. Lond Hosp Sch of Med & Dent.; Assoc. Director, St. Bart's. & The Lond. Med. & Dent. Edu. Dept.; Chair, Nth. Thames Specialist Train. Comm. in Immunol. Specialty: Immunol.; HIV Med.; Infec. Dis. Prev: Sen. Regist. (Clin. Immunol.) St. Mary's Hosp. Med. Sch. Lond.; Wellcome Research Fell. (Immunol.) St. Mary's Hosp. Med. Sch. Lond.

PARKIN, Jeffrey (retired) Rose Bank, 132 Chester Road, Northwich CW8 4AN — MB ChB Manch. 1953.

PARKIN, John 31 Brandling Place S., Newcastle upon Tyne NE2 4RU — MB BS Lond. 1994.

PARKIN, John Lewis Branston Surgery, Station Road, Branston, Lincoln LN4 1LH Tel: 01522 793081 Fax: 01522 793562 — MB BCh Witwatersrand 1982.

PARKIN, John Whitehouse 12 Hawkesford Close, Sutton Coldfield B74 2TR — MB ChB Birm. 1950; MRCS Eng. LRCP Lond. 1950; DObst RCOG 1955. Prev: Ho. Phys. Birm. Gen. Hosp. & Birm. Childrs. Hosp.; Capt. RAMC.; Capt. RAMC; Clin. Asst. (A & E) Gen. Hosp. Birm. Clin. Asst. A & E Dept. Gen. Hosp. Birm.

PARKIN, Jon Richard Institute of Psychiatry, De Crespigny Park, Denmark Hill, London SE5 8AF Tel: 020 7919 3365 Fax: 020 7703 5796 — MB ChB Aberd. 1985; MRCPsych 1991. Clin. Research Worker & Hon. Sen. Regist. (Psychiat.) Inst. Psychiat. Lond. Specialty: Gen. Psychiat. Prev: Trainee GP Aberd.; Aberd. Psychait. Train. Scheme.

PARKIN, Louise Healthcare Group, Rohais, St Peter Port, Guernsey Tel: 01481 723322 Fax: 01481 725200 — MB ChB Manch. 1983. Specialty: Gen. Pract.; Family Plann. & Reproduc. Health.

PARKIN, Michael Gerard St Peters Hill Surgery, 15 St. Peters Hill, Grantham NG31 6QA Tel: 01476 590009 Fax: 01476 570898; Ironstone Cottage, Stroxton, Grantham NG33 5DA Fax: 01476 570898 — BM BS Nottm. 1987; BMedSci Nottm. 1985; MRCGP 1992.

PARKIN, Norman Derek Sycamores, Church Road, Freiston, Boston PE22 0NX Tel: 01205 760590 — MB BS Lond. 1958 (King's Coll. Hosp.) MRCS Eng. LRCP Lond. 1958; DCP Lond 1968; FRCPath 1986, M 1973. Cons. Microbiol. Pilgrim Hosp. Boston S. Lincs. HA. Specialty: Med. Microbiol. Socs: Brit. Soc. Antimicrobial. Chemotherap. Hosp. Infec. Soc. Prev: Cons. Microbiol. Inst. Pathol. & Trop. Med. RAF Halton; Wing Cdr. RAF Med. Br.

PARKIN, Richard Anthony The Health Centre, Byland Road, Skelton-in-Cleveland, Saltburn-by-the-Sea TS12 2NN Tel: 01287 650430 Fax: 01287 651268; 17 Upleatham Village, Redcar TS11 8AG Tel: 01287 624225 — MB BS Durh. 1965; DObst RCOG 1973; MRCGP 1974. Prev: Nuffield Research Fell. (Adverse Drug Reactions) Shotley Bridge Hosp. Consett; Regist. (Gen. Med.) Shotley Bridge Hosp.

PARKIN, Robert Tallyn (retired) Driftway House, Mill Lane, Langstone, Havant PO9 1RX Tel: 02392 450741 — MB BS Lond. 1943 (Guy's) MRCS Eng. LRCP Lond. 1943; MRCP Lond. 1949. Prev: Maj. RAMC.

PARKIN, Roger Downend The Medical Centre, Beech Grove, Sherburn-in-Elmet, Leeds LS25 6ED Tel: 01977 682208/682974 — MB ChB Leeds 1970; DObst RCOG 1972; FRCGP 1986, M 1976. Specialty: Gen. Pract. Socs: York Med. Soc. Prev: Chairm. Educat. Subcomm. Yorks. Fac. Bd. RCGP.

PARKIN, Simon Graham Musgrove Park Hospital, Department of Neurology, Taunton — MB ChB Ed. 1993. Specialty: Neurol.

PARKIN, Timothy Limes Medical Centre, Limes Avenue, Alfreton DE55 7DW Tel: 01773 833133 Fax: 01773 836099; Rough Close Farm, High Oredish, Ashover, Chesterfield S45 0JX Tel: 01629 580980 Fax: 01629 580980 Email: tparkin489@aol.com — MB ChB Sheff. 1989; DRCOG 1993; MRCGP 1994; DFFP 1994. GP Princip.; Med. Adviser Carlton TV (Peak Pract.); Clin. Asst. in Learning Disabilities S. Derbysh. Socs: BMA (Pl. of Work Accred. Represen.). Prev: Trainee GP Chesterfield VTS; Clin. Med. Off. (Family Plann.) N. Derbysh.

PARKINS, Anthony Christopher Westbrook Medical Centre, 301 Westbrook Centre, Westbrook, Warrington WA5 5UF Tel: 01925 232706; 15 Hunts Field Close, Lymm WA13 0SS Tel: 01925 213359 Email: antonpark@aol.com — MB BS Lond. 1988 (Charing Cross and Westminster London) BSc Lond. 1986; MRCP (UK) 1993; DRCOG 1994. Gen. Practitioner, W.brook Med. Centre, Warrington; Clin. Asst., Cardiol., Halton Hosp., Runcorn. Specialty: Gen. Pract.

PARKINS, David Redvers James Cons. in Accident & Emergency Medicine, Wanbeck Gen. Hospital, Woodhorn Road, Ashington NE63 9JJ Fax: 0191 569 9215 — MB BS Newc. 1985; BDS Newc. 1980; FDS RCS Eng. 1989; MRCGP 1994; Dip. IMC RCS Ed. 1996; FRCS Ed. 1998; FIMC RCS Ed. 2001. Cons in Accid. & Emerg. Wasnbeck Gen Hosp N.umberland; Pre-Hosp. Immediate Care (BMJ); Mem. BASICS Exec. Counc.; Northumbria E. Ambul. Serv.; Clin. Advis. Gp.; Dir. Educat. BASICS. Specialty: Accid. & Emerg. Socs: Brit. Assn. Immed. Care; Brit. Assn. Accid. & Emerg. Med.; RCS Ed, Fac. of Pre-Hosp. Care. Prev: Cons. A & E Med. City Hosp. Sunderland NHS Trust; Hon. Surg. Newc. Gen. Hosp.; Hon. Phys. Roy. Vict. Infirm. Newc.

PARKINS, Joanne 5 Saxilby Drive, Whitebridge Park, Gosforth, Newcastle upon Tyne NE3 5LS — MB BS Newc. 1986; BMedSc Newc. 1983. Regist. N. RHA. Specialty: Anaesth. Socs: Brit. Med. Assoc. & Assn. Anaesth. Gt. Brit. & Irel. Prev: Ho. Surg. Newc. Gen. Hosp.; Ho. Phys. Roy. Vict. Infirm Newc.

PARKINS, Kathryn Jane Eaton Road, West Derby, Liverpool L12 2AP; 15 Hunts Field Close, Lymm WA13 0SS Tel: 01925 754 087 Email: kateparkins@aol.com — MB BS Lond. 1988 (Charing Cross and Westminster London) MRCPI 1995. p/t Specialist Regist.(Paediat. Intens. Care) Roy. Liverp. Children's Hosp. Alder Hey. Specialty: Paediat. Socs: Paediatric Intens. Care Soc. Prev: Specialist Regist. (Paediat. IC) Roy. Manch. Childr.s Hosp. Manch.; Specialist Regist. (Paediatric Intens. Care), Roy. Liverp. Childr.'s Hosp., Eaton Rd., Liverp. L12 2AP; Specialist Regist. (Paediat.) S. Manch. Univ. Hosps. (Wythenshawe).

PARKINS, Robert Anthony (retired) 26 Chadwick Place, Long Ditton, Surbiton KT6 5RE Tel: 020 8224 6168 Fax: 020 8255 0766 — MB BS Lond. 1950 (Char. Cross) MB BS (Hons.) Lond. 1950; FRCP Lond. 1971, M 1955; MD Lond. 1962. Hon. Cons. Phys. Gen. Med. & Gastroenterol. Char. Cross Hosp. Lond. Prev: Lect. (Med.) Univ. Washington, Seattle.

PARKINSON, Adrian Michael Dr A.M Parkinson & Partners, Station View Health Centre, Southfield Road, Hinckley LE10 1UA Tel: 01455 635362 Fax: 01455 619797; 5 Castlemaine Drive, Hinckley LE10 1RY — MB BS Lond. 1976 (Lond. Hosp.) DCH Eng. 1980; DRCOG 1981; MRCGP 1981.

PARKINSON, Bryan Francis The Medical Centre, 4 Craven Avenue, Thornton, Bradford BD13 3LG Tel: 01274 832110/834387 Fax: 01274 831694 — MB ChB Manch. 1975; BSc Manch. 1972, MB ChB 1975; DRCOG 1978.

PARKINSON, Craig 42 Dovecote Green, Westbrook, Warrington WA5 7XH Tel: 01925 710026 — MB ChB Liverp. 1992 (Liverpool) MRCP (UK) 1996. Specialist Regist. in Diabetes & Endocrinol. & Gen. Med., Manch.; Specialist Regist., Stepping Hill Hosp. Specialty: Diabetes; Endocrinol.; Gen. Med. Socs: BMA; Brit. Diabetic Assn.; N. W. Endocrine Soc. Prev: Specialist Regist., Trafford DGM; SHO, Trafford DGM; Sen. Ho. Off. Countess of Chester Hosp.

PARKINSON, Cyril Derek 19 The Gables, Baildon, Shipley BD17 6DG — MB ChB Leeds 1985 (Univ. Leeds) DRCOG 1988.

PARKINSON, David Richard Nelson Health Centre, Cecil Street, North Shields NE29 0DZ Tel: 0191 257 1204/4001 Fax: 0191 258 7191; 53 Earnshaw Way, Whitley Bay NE25 9UL — MB BS Newc. 1976; MRCGP 1980.

PARKINSON, David William Lakeside Surgery, Lakeside Road, Lymm, Warrington WA13 0QE Tel: 0161 941 6950 — MB ChB Liverp. 1968; DCH RCP Lond. 1972; DRCOG 1973. Clin. Med. Off. Lymm.

PARKINSON, Derek John Department of Obstetrics & Gynaecology, Welsh Nat. School of Medicine, Heath Park, Cardiff CF14 4XN — MB ChB Liverp. 1975; MRCOG 1980. Lect. (O & G) Welsh Nat. Sch. Med. Cardiff. Socs: N. Eng. Obst. & Gyn. Soc. Prev: Regist. (O & G) Mill Rd. Natern. Hosp. Liverp. & Liverp.; Matern. Hosp.

PARKINSON, Geoffrey Hope, Maj. RAMC (retired) Spout Hill, Kilmington, Axminster EX13 7RW Tel: 01297 32263 — MB BChir Camb. 1941 (Camb. & Lond. Hosp.) MA Camb. 1941. Prev: Ho. Phys. & Ho. Surg. Lond. Hosp.

PARKINSON, Gillian Nelson Health Centre, Cecil Street, North Shields NE29 0DZ Tel: 0191 257 1204/4001 Fax: 0191 258 7191 — MB BS Newcastle 1978; MB BS Newc. 1978. GP N. Shields, Tyne & Wear.

PARKINSON, Graeme Francis Lytham Road Surgery, 352 Lytham Road, Blackpool FY4 1DW Tel: 01253 402546 Fax: 01253 349637 — MB ChB Manch. 1980; DRCOG 1983.

PARKINSON, Heidi Samantha Blackwoods Medical Centre, 8 Station Road, Muirhead, Glasgow G69 9EE — MB ChB Glas. 1993; DRCOG; MRCGP. GP Glas.; Clin. Asst.; Breast hys. Socs: MRCGP.

PARKINSON, Helen The Surgery, Astonia House, High Street, Baldock SG7 6BP Tel: 01462 892458 Fax: 01462 490821; 63 Norton Road, Letchworth SG6 1AD Tel: 01462 482840 — MB BChir Camb. 1983; MA Camb. 1984; DA (UK) 1985; DRCOG 1990; MRCGP 1992. GP Princip. Specialty: Gen. Pract. Prev: Doctor Brit. Embassy Sofia, Bulgaria; GP Asst. Birchwood Surg. Letchworth; SHO (A & E & c/o the Elderly & O & G) Lister Hosp. Stevenage.

PARKINSON, Helen Mary 30 Mill Brow, Marple Bridge, Stockport SK6 5LW — MB ChB Leic. 1982.

PARKINSON, Ian Mark 113 Byrons Lane, Macclesfield SK11 7JS — MB ChB Ed. 1996.

PARKINSON, Jeremy Charles Ellis (retired) Blencathra, 3 Belfield Park Drive, Weymouth DT4 9RB Tel: 01305 784118 — MB ChB Birm. 1959; MRCS Eng. LRCP Lond. 1959; DObst RCOG 1962. Prev: GP Weymouth.

PARKINSON, Joanne Maria Teresa Bristol Oncology Centre, Horfield Road, Bristol BS2 8ED Tel: 0117 923 0000; Flat 2, 68 Pembroke Road, Clifton, Bristol BS8 3ED Tel: 0117 973 5115 — MB BS Lond. 1989 (Univ. Coll. & The Middx Sch. Of Med. Lond.)

MRCP (UK) 1995. Specialist Regist. (Clin. Oncol.) Bristol Oncol. Centre. Specialty: Oncol.; Radiother.

PARKINSON, John David Hayes Barton, Totteridge Lane, Totteridge, London N20 Tel: 020 8445 0475; Strathyre, Boat of Garten PH24 3BP — MB ChB Aberd. 1962. Prev: Clin. Asst. Finchley Memor. Hosp.; Paediat. Inverness Hosps.; Ho. Surg. & Ho. Phys. Woodend Hosp. Aberd.

PARKINSON, Karin Ann (retired) 11 Dinorben Avenue, Fleet GU52 7SQ Tel: 01252 622982 — (Queens, Belfast) MB BCh BAO Belf. 1960. Prev: Staff Grade (Paediat.) Loddon NHS Trust Basingstoke.

PARKINSON, Kenneth Brook Medical Centre, 98 Chell Heath Road, Bradeley, Stoke-on-Trent ST6 7NN Tel: 01782 838355 Fax: 01782 836245; Squirrels Hollow, Church Lane, Endon, Stoke-on-Trent ST9 9HF — MB ChB Manch. 1982; BSc Med. Sci. St. And. 1979.

PARKINSON, Margaret Constance Rockefeller Building, University College Hospital Medical School, University St., London WC1E 6JJ — MRCS Eng. LRCP Lond. 1966 (Roy. Free) BSc (Hons.) Lond. 1963; MD 1978, MB BS 1966; FRCPath 1986, M 1973. Cons. & Hon. Sen. Lect. (Histopath.) St. Peter's Hosp. & Inst. Urol. At UCL Hosp.s Trust; Hon. Lect. Roy. Free Hosp. Lond. Prev: Sen. Lect. (Foren. Path.) Guy's Hosp. Lond.; Sen. Regist. (Histopath.) Centr. Middlx. Hosp. Lond. & Middlx. Hosp. Lond.

PARKINSON, Mary Vere, OBE (retired) 205 Braemor Road, Calne SN11 9EA Tel: 01249 816127 — MB BCh BAO Dub. 1952 (T.C. Dub.) MRCGP 1978. Prev: Civil. Med. Pract. RAF Hullavington.

PARKINSON, Mr Michael John Rose Cottage, Waldringfield, Woodbridge IP12 4QX Tel: 0147336 697 — BM BCh Oxf. 1960; MA, BM BCh Oxf. 1960; DO Eng. 1963; FRCS Ed. 1968. Cons. Ophth. Surg. Ipswich & E. Suff. Hosp. Specialty: Ophth. Prev: Sen. Regist. Birm. & Midl. Eye Hosp. Regist. Ophth. Norf. & Norwich; Hosp.

PARKINSON, Michael John Offerton Health Centre, 10 Offerton Lane, Offerton, Stockport SK2 5AR Tel: 0161 480 0324 — MB ChB Leic. 1982.

PARKINSON, Michael Stuart Northamptonshire Heartlands PCT, Department of Community Paediatrics, St Mary's Hospital, Kettering NN15 7PW Tel: 01536 410141; Quarrybank House, 95 Parkview, Kettering Road, Moulton, Northampton NN3 7UZ Tel: 01604 645029 Email: parkinsn@qbh.u-net.com — MB ChB Manch. 1964 (Manchester University) DObst RCOG 1967; DCH Eng. 1968; MRCPCH 1997. Assoc. Specialist Dept Community Paediat., Kettering; Med. Adviser Adoption/Fostering Northants SC and H, Kettering. Specialty: Community Child Health; Paediat. Socs: BMA, Mem. Prev: GP Northampton; Regist. (Paediat. & Infec. Dis.) Northampton Gen. Hosp.; Ho. Phys. & Ho. Surg. St. Geo. Hosp. Lincoln.

PARKINSON, Rachel Janet The Barn, Higher Mithian Farm, Mithian Downs, St Agnes TR5 0PY — BM BS Nottm. 1995.

PARKINSON, Richard John 68 Station Road, Alsager, Stoke-on-Trent ST7 2PD — BM BS Nottm. 1995.

PARKINSON, Mr Richard Wellesley Orthopaedic Department, Arrowe Park Hospital, Arrowe Park Road, Upton, Wirral CH49 5PE Tel: 0151 604 7023 Fax: 0151 604 7078 — MB ChB Manch. 1981; FRCS Glas. 1985; FRCS Ed. 1985; FRCS (Orth.) 1992. Cons. Orthop. Surg. Arrowe Pk. & Clatterbridge Hosps. Specialty: Orthop.; Trauma & Orthop. Surg. Socs: BOA; Brit. Assoc. for Surg. of the Knee (BASK); BMA. Prev: Sen. Regist. (Orthop. Surg.) Wrightington Hosp.; Vis. Fell. Austin Hosp. Melbourne, Austral.; Sen. Regist. Roy. Preston Hosp.

PARKINSON, Shelagh Ann St Francis' Hospital, Private Bag 11, Katete, Zambia Tel: 06 252278 Fax: 06 252278 — MB BS Lond. 1986 (St. Bart. Hosp. Med. Coll.) MRCP (UK) 1994. Sen. Regist. (Paediat.) N. & Yorks. RHA; Paediat. St Francis' Mission Hosp. Katete, Zambia. Specialty: Paediat. Prev: Regist. (Paediat.) Roy. Manch. Childr. Hosp. Pendlebury; Regist. (Paediat.) Burnley Gen. Hosp. & Fairfield Gen. Hosp. Bury; SHO (Paediat.) Qu. Charlotte's Hosp. Lond.

PARKINSON, Simon John St Stephens Surgery, Adelaide Street, Redditch B97 4AL Tel: 01527 65444 Fax: 01527 69218 — MB ChB Birm. 1982 (Birmingham) DRCOG 1985; MRCGP 1986; DFFD 1986. Sec. Worcs. Local Med. Comm.

PARKS, Lady Caroline Jean Whitefriars, Dunwich, Saxmundham IP17 3DW — MB BS Lond. 1954 (St. Bart.)

PARKS, Lorraine 25 Hampton Manor, Belfast BT7 3EL — MB BCh BAO Belf. 1991 (Queens University Belfast) FFARCSI, Dub 1997. Specialist Regist. (Anaesth.) Roy. Gp. of Hosps. Specialty: Anaesth.

PARKS, Robert John 142 Park Road, Timperley, Altrincham WA15 6TQ — MB BS Lond. 1987; BSc (Hons.) Glas. 1980; DRCOG 1993.

PARKS, Roger Guy Merchiston Surgery, Highworth Road, Swindon SN3 4BF Tel: 01793 823307 Fax: 01793 820923 — MB ChB Bristol 1969.

PARKS, Mr Rowan Wesley Univ. Dept. of Clin. and Surgic. Sci. (Surg.), Royal Infirmary of Edinburgh, 51 Little France Crescent, Edinburgh EH16 4SA Tel: 0131 242 3616 Fax: 0131 242 3617 Email: r.w.parks@ed.ac.uk — MB BCh BAO Belf. 1989; FRCSI 1993; MD Belf. 1997; FRCS Ed. 2001. Sen. Lect. in Surg. and Hon. Cons. Surg. Specialty: Gen. Surg. Socs: Assn. of Surgeons of Gt. Britain and Irel.; Assn. of Upper Gastrointestinal Surgeons; Internat. Hepato-Biliary Assn. Prev: Specialist Regist., North. Irleand Higher Surgic. Train. Scheme.

PARKS, Sharmila 5 Cheswick Drive, Gosforth, Newcastle upon Tyne NE3 5DF — MB ChB Sheff. 1995. SHO Rotat. (Anaesth.) Traom/ Wansbeck DGN; SHO (Gen. Med.) Wansbeck DGN; SHO (Anaesth.) Freeman Hosp. Specialty: Anaesth. Prev: SHO (A & E) Hallamsh. Hosp.

PARKS, Mr Thomas George Department of Surgery, Belfast City Hospital, Lisburn Road, Belfast BT9 7AX Tel: 028 9032 9241 Fax: 028 9032 6614; 6 Malone View Road, Belfast BT9 5PH Tel: 028 9061 5013 — MB BCh BAO Belf. 1959 (Qu. Univ. Belf.) FRCS Ed. 1963; Mch 1966; FRCS Glas. 1981; FRCSI 1983. Prof. Surg. Sc. Qu. Univ. Belf.; Cons. Surg. E. Health & Social Servs. Bd. Specialty: Gastroenterol. Socs: Surg. Research Soc.; ((Ex-Pres.) Assn. Surgs. Prev: Sen. Regist. Roy. Vict. Hosp. Belf., St. Marks Hosp. Lond. & Lond.; Hosp.

PARKS, Yvonne Alyson Child Health, Temple Ward, St. Martins Hospital, Littlebourne Road, Canterbury CT1 1TD Tel: 01227 812009 Fax: 01227 812002; 105A London Road, River, Dover CT16 3AA — MB ChB Birm. 1980; MRCP (UK) 1983; MD Leic. 1991; FRCPCH 1997. Cons. Paediat. (Community) E. Kent Community Trust. Specialty: Community Child Health. Prev: Sen. Regist. (Community Paediat.) Canterbury; Clin. Med. Off. Canterbury & Thanet HA; Clin. Research Fell. (Child Health) Leicester Univ.

PARKYN, Theresa Mary Department of Paediatrics, Royal Devon & Exeter Hospital, Exeter; East Exstowe, Starcross, Exeter EX6 8PD — MB BS Lond. 1968 (Roy. Free) MRCS Eng. LRCP Lond. 1968. Clin. Asst. (Paediat.) Roy. Devon & Exeter Hosp.; Asst. Specialist Paediat. Oncol. Roy. Devon & Exeter Hosp. Specialty: Paediat. Prev: SHO (Med. & Paediat.) & Ho. Phys. Lister Hosp. Hitchin; Ho. Surg. Hampstead Gen. Hosp.

PARLE, Hilary Jane Elizabeth Jiggins Lane Surgery, 17 Jiggins Lane, Bartley Green, Birmingham B32 3LE Tel: 0121 477 7272 Fax: 0121 478 4319 — MB ChB Birmingham 1978; MB ChB Birmingham 1978.

PARLE, James Vivian Jiggins Lane Medical Centre, 17 Jiggins Lane, Bartley Green, Birmingham B32 3LE Tel: 0121 477 7272 Fax: 0121 478 4319; 7 Harrisons Road, Edgbaston, Birmingham B15 3QR — MB ChB Birm. 1978; DRCOG 1981; MRCGP 1982. Sen. Lect. (Gen. Pract.) Univ. Birm.

PARMAR, Bina 74 Parkfield Avenue, Harrow HA2 6NP — MB BS Lond. 1998.

PARMAR, Dipak Navnitlal Specialist Registrar, Department of Opthalmology, Moorfields Eye Hospital, 162 City Road, London EC1V 2PD — MB BS Lond. 1993; BSc (Hons.) Lond. 1991.

PARMAR, Hansraj Ravji Newbury Park Health Centre, Newbury Park Health Centre, 40 Perrymans Farm Road, Ilford IG2 7LE Tel: 020 554 1094 Fax: 020 518 5911 — MB BS Andhra 1969 (Andhra Med. Coll. Visakhapatnam) MRCP (UK) 1978. Senoir Partner Newbury Gp. Pract. Prev: Ho. Off Irwin Hosp. Jamnagar, India & Newsham Gen. Hosp. Liverp.; SHO (Med.) Newsham Gen. Hosp. Liverp.

PARMAR, Mr Harishbhai Queen Elizabeth II Hospital, Howlands, Welwyn Garden City AL7 4HQ Tel: 01707 365267 Fax: 01707 385244; 5 Connaught Road, St Albans AL3 5RX — MB BS Lond. 1982 (Char. Cross Med. Sch.) BSc (Hons.) Lond. 1979; FRCS Ed.

1986; FRCS (Orth.) 1995; FRCS Eng 1998. Cons. Orthop. Surg. Qu. Eliz. II Hosp. Welwyn Garden City; Roy. Coll. of Surgeons Tutor. Specialty: Orthop. Special Interest: degenerative Disease in Young Adults; Lower Limb Surgery; Sports Injuries. Socs: Fell. BOA; Brit. Orthop. Research Soc.; RSM. Prev: Sen. Regist. (Orthop. Surg.) Roy. Nat. Orthop. Hosp. Stanmore; Lect. & Wishbone Research Fell. Univ. Leicester; Regist. (Orthop.) Leics. HA.

PARMAR, Harsukh 4 Kitson Road, Camberwell, London SE5 7LF Tel: 020 7701 5106 — MB ChB Aberd. 1980. Research Regist. (Oncol.) Char. Cross & Westm. Hosp. Med. Sch. Lond. Specialty: Oncol. Socs: Brit. Oncol. Assn.; Amer. Assn. of Cancer Research. Prev: Asst. Lect. (Med. Oncol.) St. Bart. Hosp. Med. Coll. Lond.; SHO (Gen. Med.) St. Bart. Hosp. Rochester; SHO (Med.) Medway Hosp. Gillingham.

PARMAR, Hitendra Parshottambhai 14 Kedleston Road, Evington, Leicester LE5 5HU — MB BS Lond. 1994.

PARMAR, Mr Jitendra Maganlal Department of Cardiothoracic Surgery, North Staffordshire Hospitals, Royal Infirmary, Princes Road, Stoke-on-Trent ST4 7LN Tel: 01782 554865 Fax: 01782 554830 — MB ChB Birm. 1977; BSc Birm. 1974; FRCS Eng. 1982. Cons. Cardiothoracic Surg. N. Staffs. Roy. Infirm. Stoke-on-Trent. Specialty: Cardiothoracic Surg. Prev: Sen. Regist. (Cardiothoracic Surg.) W. Midl. RHA; Lect. (Anat.) Univ. Birm.; Regist. (Cardiothoracic & Gen. Surg.) W. Midl. RHA.

PARMAR, Kantilal Bhagoobhai Whitehall Road Surgery, 1 Whitehall Road, Rugby CV21 3AE Tel: 01788 561319 Fax: 01788 553762; 1 Whitehall Road, Rugby CV21 3AE Tel: 01788 561319 — MB BS Gujarat 1964 (B.J. Med. Coll. Ahmedabad) GP Rugby; Clin. Asst. (Rheum.) St. Cross Hosp. Rugby; Med. Off. Fam. Plann. Clinic Rugby Area Health Office. Prev: SHO & Ho. Surg. (Obst.& Gyn.) St. Mary's Hosp. HarBoro. Magna; Ho. Surg. & Ho. Phys. Hosp. St. Cross Rugby.

PARMAR, Mahesh Chhabildas Cheltenham General Hospital, Department of Anaesthetics, Sandford Road GL53 7AN Tel: 01242 274143 Email: maresh.parmar@glos.nhs.uk — MB BS Lond. 1988; BSc (Hons.) Lond. 1985; MRCP (UK) 1992; FRCA 1994. Cons. Anaesth., Cheltenham Gen. Hosp. Specialty: Anaesth.; Intens. Care. Socs: BMA; RCA; AA. Prev: SHO (Anaesth.) Soton.; SHO (Anaesth., ITU & Gen. Med.) Chichester; Regist. (Specialist) Soton. Gen. & Salisbury Dist. Gen. Hosp.

PARMAR, Pravinbhai Prahladbhai Bankfield Surgery, 15 Huddersfield Road, Elland HX5 9BA — MB ChB Manch. 1978. GP Elland.

PARMAR, Mrs Samyukta 5 Naill Close, Agustus Road, Edgbaston, Birmingham B15 3LU Tel: 0121 454 7818 — MB BS Mysore 1958. Mem. Birm. Med. Inst. Prev: Ho. Off. (Surg.) Selly Oak Hosp. Birm.; SHO Highcroft Hall Hosp. Birm.; Regist. (Psychiat.) Hollymoor Hosp. Birm.

PARMAR, Sanjay Jayanti Brownlow Medical Centre, 140-142 Brownlow Road, New Southgate, London N11 2BD — MB BS Lond. 1991; BSc (Hons.) Radiol. Sci. Lond. 1988; DFFP 1994; DRCOG 1994; MRCGP 1996; DPD 1998. Woodgrange Med. Pract., 40 Woodgrange Rd., Forest Gate, Lond. E7 0QH Tel: 020 8250 7585 Fax: 020 8250 7587. Specialty: Gen. Pract. Prev: SHO (Med.) Basildon Dist. Gen. Hosp.; SHO (Paediat.) Princess Alexandra Hosp. Harlow.; Trainee GP Lond.

PARMAR, Satyesh Chimanlal 27 Belfry Way, Edwalton, Nottingham NG12 4FA — BM BS Nottm. 1995; BChD Leeds 1986; FDS RCS Eng. 1990; BMedSci Nottm. 1993; FRCS 1997. Specialist Regist. (Oral & Maxillofacial Surg.) Trent Region. Specialty: Oral & Maxillofacial Surg. Prev: SHO (Gen. Surg.) Trent Region; SHO (Orthop.) Trent Region; SHO (A & E) Trent Region.

PARMAR, Tajinder Singh 11 Talbot Road, Smethwick, Smethwick B66 4DX — MB BS Lond. 1994.

PARMENTER, John Grantley 15 Eirene Terrace, Pill, Bristol BS20 0ET Tel: 01275 372137 — MB ChB Bristol 1962.

PARNABY-PRICE, Adrian Ocular Immunology Group, Rayne Institute, St Thomas' Hospital, Lambeth Palace Road, London SE1 7EH Tel: 020 7928 9292 ext 6414; 39 The Hawthorns, Charvil, Reading RG10 9TS — MB BChir Camb. 1987; MA, MB BChir Camb. 1987; FRCS Ed. 1992. Fell. cular immunol. St. Thos. Hosp. Lond. Specialty: Ophth.

PARNACOTT, Sarah Margaret Ashgate Hospice, Ashgate Road, Old Brampton, Chesterfield S42 73E Tel: 01246 568801 Fax: 01246 569043 Email: sarah.parnacott@ashgatehospice.nhs.uk — MB ChB Sheff. 1989; BMedSci (Hons.) Sheff. 1988; MRCP (UK) 1994. Cons. (Palliat. Med.) Ashgate Hospice, Chesterfield. Specialty: Palliat. Med. Prev: Specialist Regist. (Palliat. Med.) Weston Pk. Hosp. & St. Lukes Hospice Sheff.; Regist. (Clin. Oncol.) Weston Pk. Hosp. Sheff.; SHO Med. Rotat., Dundee.

PARNAIK, Vijaykumar G Castle Practice, 2 Hawthorne Road, Castle Bromwich, Birmingham B36 0HH Tel: 0121 747 2422 Fax: 0121 749 1196 — MB BS Poona 1966; MB BS Poona 1966.

PARNELL, Adrian Paul Good Hope Hospital, Radiology Department, Rectory Road, Sutton Coldfield B75 7RR Tel: 0121 378 2211 Email: adrian.parnell@goodhope.nhs.uk — MB ChB Manch. 1978; BSc Manch. 1975; MRCP (UK) 1982; FRCR 1985; FRCP 2001. Cons. Radiologist Good Hope Hosp. Sutton Cold Field; Assoc. Med. Director Good Hope Hosp. Sutton Cold Field. Specialty: Radiol. Special Interest: Gastroenterol.; Gyn. Socs: West Midlands Association of Radiologists; Midlands Gastroenterological Society. Prev: Sen. Regist. (Radiol.) N. RHA.

PARNELL, Caroline Emma The Old Vicarage, Pennington, Ulverston LA12 7NY — MB BS Lond. 1996.

PARNELL, Cathryn Rooley Lane Medical Centre, Rooley Lane, Bradford BD4 7SS Tel: 01274 770777 — MB ChB Leeds 1975; DRCOG 1978. GP Bradford.

PARNELL, Christopher John 83 St Margaret's Street, Rochester ME1 3BJ — MB BS Lond. 1975 (Univ. Coll. Hosp.) MRCS Eng. LRCP Lond. 1975; FFA RCS Eng. 1981; T(Anaesth.) 1991. Clin. Dir. (Anaesth. & Intens. Care) Medway NHS Trust Gillingham. Specialty: Anaesth. Prev: Cons. & Sen. Lect. Anaesth. & Resusc. RAMC.

PARNELL, Mr Edward John Princess Royal Hospital, Lewes Road, Haywards Heath RH16 4EX Tel: 01444 441881; Kemps House, East Chiltington, Lewes BN7 3QT Tel: 01273 891143 Fax: 01273 891143 — MB BS Lond. 1978; FRCS Ed. 1984. Cons. Orthop. Surg. Princess Roy. Hosp. Haywards Heath; cons. Orthopaedic surge, Qu. Vic Hosp, E.Grinstead. Specialty: Orthop. Socs: Fell. BOA; Mem. RSM; Mem. BORS.

PARNELL, Katherine Elizabeth The Surgery, 1 Streatfield Road, Harrow HA3 9BP Tel: 020 8907 0381 Fax: 020 8909 2134; Highcroft, Brookshill, Harrow HA3 6RW Tel: 020 8385 7397 — MB BS Lond. 1992 (Roy. Lond. Hosp.) DCH RCP Lond. 1994; DRCOG 1995; MRCGP (Distinc.) 1996.

PARNELL, Nicholas David Jeffrey Princess Royal Hospital, Haywards Heath RH16 4EX — MB BS Lond. 1989.

PARNELL, Stephen John Moss Grove Surgery, 15 Moss Grove, Kingswinford DY6 9HS Tel: 01384 277377 Fax: 01384 402329; Pound Cottage, 8 School Road, Himley, Dudley DY3 4LG Tel: 01902 326112 Email: drsparnell@aol.com — MB ChB Birm. 1978; DCH RCP Lond. 1981; MRCGP 1982; DRCOG 1982. Hosp. Pract. (Diabetes) Corbett Hosp. Stourbridge.

PARNHAM, Alan 91 Kendon Drive, Manor Farm, Southmead, Bristol BS10 5BU — MB BS Lond. 1985.

PARNHAM-COPE, Delia Anne A & E Department, A & E Department, Great Western Road, Gloucester GL1 3NN — MB BS Lond. 1990; BSc Lond. 1987; MB BS (Lond.) 1990; DRCOG 1992; DGM RCP Lond. 1993; FRCS Ed. 1997. Cons. A & E Med. Roy. Gloucs. Hosp. Specialty: Accid. & Emerg. Socs: Med. Protec. Soc.

PARR, Alison Marie Bolton Hospice, Queens Park Street, Bolton BL1 4QT Tel: 01204 364375 Fax: 01204 313163 Email: drparr@boltonhospice.org — MB BS Newc. 1992 (Newc. Upon Tyne) MRCP (UK) 1995; MSc Oncology, University of Manchester 1999. Cons. (Palliat. Med.) Roy. Bolton Hosp. & Bolton Hospice. Specialty: Palliat. Med. Socs: Jun. Mem. NW Pall. Care Phys. Grp.; Assoc. of Pall. Med.; Fell. Roy. Soc. of Med. Prev: Specialist Regist. (Med. Oncol.) Christie Hosp. Manch.; SHO (Palliat. Care) St. Ann's Hospice Manch.; SHO Rotat. (Med.) N. Manch. Gen. Hosp.

PARR, Mr David Caffrey Home Layne, Annington Road, Steyning BN44 3WA Tel: 01903 812505 — MB Camb. 1966 (Camb. & St. Bart.) MA Camb. 1968, MB 1966, BChir 1965; FRCS Ed. 1971; FRCS Eng. 1972. Cons. Surg. Worthing HA. Specialty: Gen. Surg.; Urol. Prev: Sen. Regist. (Gen. Surg. & Urol.) Nottm. Hosp. & Derby Roy. Infirm.; Demonst. (Anat.) Univ. Camb.; Ho. Surg. & Jun. Surg. Regist. St. Bart. Hosp. Lond.

PARR, Gwendolen Doris (retired) Lordings, Station Road, Pulborough RH20 1AH Tel: 01798 872872 Email: 75337.2252@compuserve.com — MB BChir Camb. 1961 (Univ.

Coll. Hosp.) Dip. Pharm. Med. RCP (UK) 1983; FFPHM RCP (UK) 1993, M 1991. Prev: Head Pharma Policy & Head Drug Monitoring Dept. Ciba Pharmaceut. Horsham.

PARR, Jeremy Ross 29 Hambalt Road, London SW4 9EA — MB ChB Leic. 1996.

PARR, John Henry South Tyneside District Hospital, Harton Lane, South Shields NE34 0PL Tel: 0191 454 8888 — MB ChB Liverp. 1974; MRCP (UK) 1979; MD Liverp. 1989; FRCP Lond. 1994; MRCP Ed. 2001. Cons. Phys. S. Tyneside Healthcare Trust. Specialty: Gen. Med.; Diabetes; Endocrinol. Socs: Soc. Endocrinol.; Diabetes UK. Prev: Lect. (Diabetes & Endocrinol.) Centr. Middlx. Hosp. & St. Mary's Hosp. Med. Sch. Lond.; Regist. (Med.) N. Middlx. Hosp. Lond., Chester City Hosp. & St. Catherine's Hosp. Birkenhead.

PARR, Linda Susan Adcroft Surgery, Prospect Place, Trowbridge BA14 8QA Tel: 01225 755878 Fax: 01225 775445 Email: linda.parr@gp-j83016.nhs.uk; Mistletoe Cottage, 24 High St, Steeple Ashton, Trowbridge BA14 6EL — MB BS Lond. 1975 (St. Mary's) FRCOG 1995, M 1980, D 1977. Specialty: Obst. & Gyn.

PARR, Margaret Ann (retired) Wigan & Bolton Health Authority, Bryan House, 61 Standishgate, Wigan WN1 1AH Tel: 01942 822843; 22 Parkway, Shevington Moor, Wigan WN6 0SJ Tel: 01257 424168 — MB ChB Sheff. 1966; DObst RCOG 1970; DCH Eng. 1970; MSc (Community Med.) Manch. 1979; MFCM 1980. Prev: Ho. Off. Chesterfield Roy. Hosp.

PARR, Michael Joseph Anthony Stockland, Beechen Cliff Road, Bath BA2 4QR — MB BS Lond. 1983; DA (UK) 1986; MRCP (UK) 1987; FRCA 1989.

PARR, Mr Nigel John Wirral Trust Hospital, Upton, Wirral Tel: 0151 678 5111; Centaur House, 33 Tower Road N., Heswall, Wirral CH60 6RS Tel: 0151 342 6100 Fax: 01513426100 Email: nigelparr@lineone.net — MD Liverp. 1989; MB ChB 1980; FRCS (Urol.) Ed. 1984. Cons. Urol. Wirral Trust Hosp. Specialty: Urol. Socs: Brit. Assn. Urol. Soc.; Am. Urol. Assn.; Brit. Soc. Endocrinol. Prev: Sen. Regist. West. Gen. Hosp. Edin.; Lect. (Urol.) Scott. Lithotriptor Centre Edin.

PARR, Penelope Jane Ladybridge Surgery, 10-12 Broadgate, Ladybridge, Bolton BL3 4PZ Tel: 01204 653267 Fax: 01204 665350 — MB ChB Leeds 1988; DRCOG 1991; MRCGP 1992. Specialty: Gen. Pract. Socs: BMA; Bolton Med. Soc. Prev: Trainee GP Bolton; SHO Wigan HA VTS.; Clin. Asst. Bolton Hospice.

PARR, Robert Thornton (retired) The Barn House, Broughton, Stockbridge SO20 8AA Tel: 01794 301401 — MB BS Durh. 1947; MRCS Eng. LRCP Lond. 1947; DObst RCOG 1952.

PARR, Stephen Matthew 35 Alder Lane, Balsall Common, Coventry CV7 7DZ — BM Soton. 1982; FRCA 1989. Cons. Anasethetist, Heartlands & Solihull Hosp. Specialty: Anaesth.

PARR-BURMAN, Stephen John North Shore Surgery, 95-99 Holmfield Road, Blackpool FY2 9RS Tel: 01253 593971 Fax: 01253 596039; Norwood, 15 Lockwood Avenue, Poulton-le-Fylde FY6 7AB Tel: 01253 899328 — MB ChB Dundee 1982; DCH RCP Lond. 1984; DRCOG 1988; MRCGP 1989. GP; Dir. of Ltd. Company specialising in Medico-legal Pract.; Medico-legal expert witness. Specialty: Gen. Pract. Socs: Soc. Occup. Med.; Inst. Expert Witnesses; Brit. Acupunc. Soc.

PARRACK, Stella Margaret (retired) Willow Bank, Blendellsands Road W., Blundellsands, Liverpool L23 6TE Tel: 0151 924 8499 Email: stella_parrack@doctors.org.uk; Willow Bank, Blundellsands Road W., Blundellsands, Liverpool L23 6TE Tel: 0151 924 8499 — MB ChB Manch. 1957; DObst RCOG 1959. Locum GP. Prev: GP Liverp.

PARRATT, David (retired) 91 Strathern Road, Broughty Ferry, Dundee DD5 1JT Tel: 01382 477305 — MD Dundee 1977; MB ChB St. And. 1969; FRCPath 1988, M 1975.

PARRATT, Jennifer Ruth 47 Brookside Glen, Chesterfield S40 3PG — MB ChB Liverp. 1990; BSc Liverp. 1987; MD Liverp. 1997; MRCOG 2001. Specialty: Obst. & Gyn. Socs: BMA. Prev: SHO (O & G) Arrowe Pk. Hosp.; SHO (O & G) Liverp. O & G Trust.

PARRATT, Jon Taunton Road Medical Centre, 12-16 Taunton Road, Bridgwater TA6 3LS Tel: 01278 720000 Fax: 01278 423691 — MB ChB Birm. 1985; MRCGP 1990. Prev: Trainee GP Taunton VTS.

PARRIS, Michael Paul 223 Croxted Road, London SE21 8NL — MB BS Lond. 1996.

PARRIS, Robert Crahamel Medical Practice, Crahamel House, 1 Duhamel Place, St Helier JE2 4TP Tel: 01534 735419/735742 — MB BS Lond. 1995; BSc (Hons.) Clin. Sciences, Lond. 1994; LocInt 1998; DFFP 1998; DRCOG 1998; DCH 1999; MRCGP 2000. GP, Crahamel Med. Pract., St Helier, Jersey.

PARRIS-PIPER, Timothy William 24 Church Street, Boughton Monchelsea, Maidstone ME17 4HW — MB BS Lond. 1992 (St George's London) MRCA 1997. Specialist Regist. (Anaesth.) N. Thames E. Specialty: Anaesth. Socs: Assn. Anaesthes.; BMA. Prev: SHO (Anaesth.) Addenbrooke's Hosp. Camb.; SHO (Anaesth.) PeterBoro. Dist. Gen.

PARRISH, David John Dawley Medical Practice, Dawley, Telford TF4 3AL Tel: 01952 505213 Fax: 01952 503089; 31 Church Road, Lilleshall, Newport TF10 9HE Tel: 01952 505213 — MB ChB Birm. 1982.

PARRISH, Frances Mary (retired) Ashdown Cottage, Tanyard Lane, Danehill, Haywards Heath RH17 7JW — (Ed.) MB ChB Ed. 1968; DObst RCOG 1970; MRCP (UK) 1974. Prev: Staff Grade Paediat. Chailey Heritage Clin. Servs.

PARRISH, Frank John Old Fleet, Grimsby DN37 9RT — MB ChB Leeds 1987; FRCR 1996. Fell. (Radiol.) & Clin. Assoc. Lect. Univ. Queensland, Austral. Specialty: Radiol. Prev: Sen. Regist. (Radiol.) North. Train. Scheme.

PARRISH, Jane Endellion, 36 Callington Road, Saltash PL12 6DY — MB BCh Wales 1974.

PARRISH, John Anthony (retired) Kingsmead, 47 The Ridge, Purley CR8 3PF Tel: 020 8660 8317 — MB BS Lond. 1951 (St. Bart.) MRCS Eng. LRCP Lond. 1951; FRCP Lond. 1973, M 1957; MD Lond. 1964. Emerit. Cons. Phys. Mayday Hosp. Croydon; Chief Med. Off. Woolwich Life Assur. Soc. Prev: Cons. Phys. Shirley Oaks Hosp. Croydon.

PARRISH, John Richard The Surgery, 212 Richmond Road, Kingston upon Thames KT2 5HF Tel: 020 8546 0400 Fax: 020 8974 5771; 27 Turner Road, New Malden KT3 5NL — MCRS Eng. LRCP Lond. 1983; DRCOG 1986; DCH RCP Lond. 1988; MRCGP 1988. Clin. Asst. (Ophth.) Kingston Hosp. Prev: Trainee GP Croydon; SHO (Geriat.) Qu. Hosp. Croydon; SHO (O & G) & (Paediat.) Mayday Hosp. Croydon.

PARRISH, Mark McKenzie, Surg. Lt.-Cdr. RN Flat 7, Bramley House, Crescent Road, Gosport PO12 2DJ — MB ChB Birm. 1983; MRCGP 1991. DPMO HMS Neptune. Specialty: Cardiol. Prev: SMO HMS Kutnabul Sydney, Austral.; Trainee GP/SHO (Med.) RN Hosp. Haslar.

PARRISH, Richard William Endellion, 36 Callington Road, Saltash PL12 6DY — MB BCh Wales 1974; MRCP (UK) 1978; FRCR 1988.

PARROTT, Charles Edward Merrymead, Stanford-on-Soar, Loughborough LE12 5QL — MB ChB Birm. 1994; ChB Birm. 1994.

PARROTT, David (retired) 29 West Tytherley, Salisbury SP5 1NF Tel: 01794 40621 — (Guy's) MB BS Lond. 1956; MRCS Eng. LRCP Lond. 1956; DObst RCOG 1963; DPhil Med. (SA) 1982; FFPM RCP (UK) 1989. Med. Dir. (Europe) Syntex Research Palo Alto, USA. Prev: Gen. Duties Med. Off. HM Overseas Civil Serv., Nigeria.

PARROTT, David Robert John (retired) North Edge, 18 Whidborne Avenue, Torquay TQ1 2PQ Tel: 01803 212309 — MB BS Lond. 1956 (Middlx.) DObst RCOG 1959. Prev: Ho. Phys. & Ho. Surg. Mt. Vernon Hosp. Northwood.

PARROTT, Janet Mary Bracton Centre, Bracton Lane, Dartford DA2 7AF — MB ChB Manch. 1976; BSc (Hons.) St. And. 1973; FRCPsych. 1993, M 1981; Dip. Criminol Lond. 1983. Cons. Psychiat. Bracton Centre, Oxleas NHS Trust; Hon. Lect. Guy's Hosp. Lond. Specialty: Forens. Psychiat. Prev: Sen. Regist. & Regist. Bethlem Roy. & Maudsley Hosps. Lond.

PARROTT, Jeffrey Peter Stanley Eastville Health Centre, East Park, Bristol BS5 6YA Tel: 0117 951 1261 Fax: 0117 935 5056 — MB ChB Bristol 1981.

PARROTT, Mr Neil Raymond Department of Surgery, Manchester Royal Infirmary, Oxford Road, Manchester M13 9WL Tel: 0161 276 8531 Fax: 0161 273 4530 Email: neil.parrott@cmmc.nhs.uk; 43 Hazlewood Road, Wilmslow SK9 2QA Tel: 01625 539582 Email: n.parrott@virgin.net — MB BS Newc. 1978; FRCS Ed. 1983; FRCS Eng. 1984; MD Newc. 1989. Cons. Gen., Endocrine and Transpl. Surg., Manch. Roy. Infirm.; Clin. Manager of Transplantation Manch. Roy. Infirm. Specialty: Gen. Surg.; Transpl. Surg.; Endocrinol. Socs: Brit. Assn. Of Endocrine Surg.; Am. Assn. Of Tranpl. Surg.s;

Brit. Transpl. Soc. Prev: Asst. (Surg.) Univ. Newc.; Hon. Research Assoc. (Surg.) Univ. Newc.

PARROTT, Rachel Janet Eaglescliffe Health Centre, Sunningdale Drive, Eaglescliffe, Stockton-on-Tees TS16 9EA Tel: 01642 780113 Fax: 01642 791020; Swiss Cottage, 21 The Green, Romanby, Northallerton DL7 8NL Tel: 01609 776467 — MB ChB Bristol 1986; DRCOG 1988; MRCGP 1991; T(GP) 1991. GP Asst. N. Region Retainer Scheme. Socs: Christian Med. Fellowsh.; Christians in Caring Professions. Prev: Trainee GP Northallerton VTS.

PARROTT, Richard Humphrey (retired) Blackdown Cottage, Lerryn, Lostwithiel PL22 0NW Tel: 01208 873828 Email: rhparrott@doctors.org.uk — MB BS Lond. 1960 (Lond. Hosp.) DObst RCOG 1963; FRCGP 1981. Prev: GP St. Germans.

PARRY, Alan Charles 206 Queen's Court, Ramsey IM8 1LG — MB BS Durh. 1945; LRCP LRCS Ed. LRFPS Glas. 1945.

PARRY, Alison James House Doctors Surgery, Maryport Street, Usk NP15 1AB Tel: 01291 672633 Fax: 01291 672631 — BM Soton. 1993 (Southampton) DFFP 1995; DRCOG 1996; MRCGP 1997. GP Partner The Surg. James Ho. Usk. Specialty: Gen. Pract. Prev: SHO (Psychiat.) St. Jas. Hosp. Posrtsmouth; SHO (Paediat.) Jersey Gen. Hosp., CI; SHO (O & G) St. Mary's Hosp. Portsmouth.

PARRY, Alister Richard John 421 Mile End Road, London E3 4PB — MB BS Lond. 1989.

PARRY, Allyson Margaret Morgan 22 Skene Close, Headington, Oxford OX3 7XQ — MB ChB Birm. 1995; ChB Birm. 1995.

PARRY, Alwyn Llewelyn Llanberis Surgery, High Street, Llanberis, Caernarfon LL55 4SU Tel: 01286 870634 Fax: 01286 871722 — MB BCh Wales 1988. Socs: Welsh Med. Soc.; Arfon Med. Soc. Prev: Trainee GP Bodannt Bangor.

PARRY, Mr Andrew David James Cook University Hospital, Marton Road, Middlesbrough TS4 3BW; The Cottage, Entwistle Hall Lane, Entwistle, Bolton BL7 0LR — MB ChB Bristol 1987; FRCS Eng. 1992. Specialty: Gen. Surg. Prev: Tutor (Surg.) Withington Hosp. Manch.

PARRY, Mr Andrew John Bristol Royal Hospital for Sick Children, Department of Paediatric Cardiac Surgery, Upper Maudlin Street, Bristol BS2 8BJ Tel: 0117 342 8854 — BM BCh Oxf. 1985; MA Oxf. 1986; FRCS Eng. 1990; FRCS (CTH) Eng. 1995; FECTS 2003. Cons. (Paediat. Cardiac Surg.) Bristol Roy. Hosp. Sick Childr.; Hon. Sen. Lect. Inst. Child Health Univ. Bristol. Specialty: Cardiothoracic Surg. Socs: Soc. Cardiothoracic Surg. GB & Irel.; Europ. Assn. Cardiothoracic Surg. Prev: Asst. Prof. (Paediat. Cardiac Surg.) Univ. Calif. San Francisco USA; Fell. (Paediat. Cardiac Surg.) Univ. Calif. San Francisco; Sen. Regist. (Cardiothoracic Surg.) Oxf. Heart Centre.

PARRY, Angela Karen Woodlands Surgery, Woodlands, Shadsworth Road, Blackburn BB1 2HR Tel: 01254 665664 Fax: 01254 695883; 69 Highercroft Road, Lower Darwen, Darwen BB3 0QT Tel: 01254 694633 — MB ChB Manch. 1987; BSc (Med. Sci.) St. And. 1985; MRCGP 1992; DMJ 2003.

PARRY, Anthea Catherine Hillingdon Hospital, Pield Heath Road, Hillingdon, Uxbridge UB8 3NN Tel: 01895 238282; 23 Homefield Road, Chiswick, London W4 2LW Fax: 01895 279454 — MB BS Lond. 1981; MRCP UK 1984; FRCP 2000. Cons. Phys. (c/o Elderly) Hillingdon Hosp. Uxbridge. Specialty: Care of the Elderly. Prev: Sen. Regist. St. Geo. Hosp. Lond.

PARRY, Celia Rosamund 8 Dovepoint Road, Meols, Wirral CH47 6AR — MB ChB Liverp. 1971.

PARRY, Christine Susan Spring Hall Group Practice, Spring Hall Medical Centre, Spring Hall Lane, Halifax HX1 4JG Tel: 01422 349501 Fax: 01422 323091; 112 Huddersfield Road, Brighouse HD6 3RH — MB ChB Aberd. 1978; MRCGP 1982. Socs: BMA.

PARRY, Christopher Adrian, Surg. Lt. RN 7 Vernon Close, Gosport PO12 3NU Tel: 023 9258 1100 — MB BS Lond. 1993; BSc (Hons.) Cell Path. Lond. 1987. Med. Off. RN.

PARRY, Christopher Martin Nuffield Department of Clinical Medicine, Level 5, John Radcliffe Hospital, Headington, Oxford OX3 9DU — MB BChir Camb. 1984; MA Camb. 1984; MRCP (UK) 1987; MRCPath 1993. Clin. Microbiol. John Radcliffe Hosp. Oxf. Specialty: Med. Microbiol. Prev: Lect. (Microbiol.) Roy. Liverp. Hosp.

PARRY, Christopher William Kickham Badcocks Farmhouse, Easthorpe Road, Colchester CO5 9EZ Tel: 01206 211 245 Fax: 01206 211 245 — MB BS Lond. 1984 (St. Bartholomew's Hospital) DRCOG 1990; LF Hon. University fo Glasgow 1999.

PARRY, Claire Louise 44 Mitford Road, London N19 4HL — MB BS Lond. 1985 (St. Thos. Hosp.) MRCGP 1996. GP.

PARRY, Dafydd Emyr Grovehurst, Middle Lane, Denbigh LL16 3UW — MRCS Eng. LRCP Lond. 1990.

PARRY, David (retired) Greyholme, West Road, Nottage Village, Porthcawl CF36 3SS Tel: 01656 784211 Fax: 01656 786828 Email: davidparry@dsl.pipex.com — (Cardiff) MB BCh Wales 1962; DCH Eng. 1964; DObst RCOG 1965; DPH Manch. 1968; FRCGP 1980, M 1971; Dip. Pract. Dermat. Wales 1989. Clin. Complaints Adviser MDU. Prev: Princip. GP.

PARRY, David Gareth West Kirby Health Centre, Grange Road, Wirral CH48 4HZ Tel: 0151 625 9171 Fax: 0151 625 9171; 8 Dovepoint Road, Meols, Wirral CH47 6AR — MB ChB Liverp. 1971. Hon. Med. Adviser (RNLI Hoylake Offshore Station & RNLI W. Kirby Inshore Station).

PARRY, David Gratton Cross Street Health Centre, Cross Street, Dudley DY1 1RN Tel: 01384 459044 Fax: 01384 232467; 4 Station Drive, Hagley, Stourbridge DY9 0NX Tel: 01562 886129 — MB BS Lond. 1982 (Guy's) DRCOG 1985; MRCGP 1986; DCH RCP Lond. 1986. Prev: Trainee GP Doncaster VTS; Ho. Phys. Roy. Cornw. Hosp.; Ho. Surg. Worcester Roy. Infirm.

PARRY, David Hugh Bryniau, Llangoed, Beaumaris LL58 8ND Tel: 0124 878269 — MB BS Lond. 1969 (St. Geo.) MRCPath 1977. Cons. Haemat. Gwynedd Hosp. Bangor. Specialty: Haematology. Prev: Lect. (Haemat.) Welsh Nat. Sch. Med. Cardiff.

PARRY, David Lewis Clarence House, Rhyl LL18 6BY Tel: 01745 350980 Fax: 01745 353293; Tan yr Onnen, Waen, St Asaph LL17 0DU Tel: 01745 583821 — MB ChB Liverp. 1958. Clin. Asst. (Geriat.) Roy. Alexandra Hosp. Rhyl. Socs: Assoc. Mem. RCGP & Mem. BMA. Prev: Ho. Phys. & Ho. Surg. Alexandra Hosp. Rhyl; Ho. Surg. H.M. Stanley Hosp. St. Asaph.

PARRY, David Lloyd Thr Belgravia Surgery, 26 Eccleston Street, Belgravia, London SW1W 9PY Tel: 020 7590 8000 Fax: 020 7590 8010 Email: david.parry@nhs.net — MB ChB Birm. 1984. GP. Prev: Ho. Off. (Med.) Sandwell Dist. Gen. Hosp.; Ho. Off. (Surg.) Good Hope Hosp.; Trainee GP Sandwell VTS.

PARRY, Deborah Elizabeth Albert Road Surgery, Albert Road, Penarth CF64 1BX Tel: 029 2070 5884 Fax: 029 2071 1735 — MB BS Lond. 1985; Cert. Family Plann. JCC 1987; DRCOG 1989; MFFP 1993. Clin. Asst. (Cytol.).

PARRY, Deborah Margaret Elizabeth House Surgery, 515 Limpsfield Road, Warlingham CR6 9LF Tel: 01883 625262 — MB BS Lond. 1990 (Middlesex Hospital) BSc Lond. 1987; DGM RCP Lond. 1993; DRCOG 1993; DFFP 1994; MRCGP 1994. Asst. GP Warlingham, Surrey; Community Med. Off. Family Plann. Specialty: Gen. Pract.

PARRY, Delyth Meredydd Oak Vale Medical Centre, 158-160 Edge Lane Drive, Liverpool L13 4AQ Tel: 0151 259 1551 Fax: 0151 252 1121; 18 Brentwood Ave, Aigburth, Liverpool L17 4LD Tel: 0151 727 2635 — MB BCh Wales 1989; BSc 1986; MRCGP 1996. GP Princip. Oakdale Med. Centre, L'pool; Clin. Asst. in Drug Dependency. Specialty: Alcohol & Substance Misuse.

PARRY, Duncan John 5 Ashfield Park, Leeds LS6 2QT — MB ChB Sheff. 1993.

PARRY, Dylan Clwyd Meddygfa Cadwgan, 11 Bodelwyddan Avenue, Old Colwyn, Conwy LL29 9NP Tel: 01492 515410 — MB BCh Wales 1994; DRCOG; MRCGP; DFFP; BSc (Hons.) Wales 1991. GP Princip. Specialty: Gen. Pract.

PARRY, Mr Edgar Williams (retired) Brynteg Cottage, Brynteg Lane, Llandegfan, Menai Bridge LL59 5NU Tel: 01248 714612 — MB ChB Liverp. 1943; FRCS Ed. 1949; ChM Liverp. 1953; FRCS Eng. 1955. Prev: Cons. Surg. Broadgreen Hosp. Liverp.

PARRY, Ednyfed Wyn (retired) Department of Human Anatomy & Cell Biology, The University, PO Box 147, Liverpool L69 3BX; 12 Isallt Park, Trearddur Bay, Holyhead LL65 2US — MB ChB Liverp. 1962; MB ChB (Hons.) Liverp. 1962; MD Liverp. 1967; FRCPath 1991. Prev: Sen. Lect. (Histol.) Univ. Liverp.

PARRY, Edward Elwyn Corwen House Surgery, Corwen House, Market Place, Caernarfon LL54 6NN Tel: 01286 880336 Fax: 01286 881500 — MB ChB Liverp. 1973; DObst RCOG 1975; DCH Eng. 1977; MRCGP 1978.

PARRY, Eileen Jennifer Tameside General Hospital, Fountain Street, Ashton-under-Lyne OL6 9RW — MB ChB Liverp. 1988; BSc Liverp. 1985; BSc (Hons.) Liverp. 1985, MB ChB 1988; MRCP (UK)

1991. p/t Cons. (Dermat.) Tameside Gen. Hosp. Lancs.; Cons. Dermat. Hope Hosp. Dermat. Centre Salford; Cons. Dermat. Christie Hosp. Manch. Specialty: Dermat. Special Interest: Cutaneous Lymphoma.

PARRY, Emyr Hafod, Ruthin Roadd, Denbigh LL16 3EU — MB ChB Manch. 1962; MRCS Eng. LRCP Lond. 1962; MRCOG 1967. Specialty: Obst. & Gyn.

PARRY, Enid Brynteg Cottage, Brynteg Lane, Llandegfan, Menai Bridge LL59 5NU Tel: 01248 714612 — MB ChB Liverp. 1948; CPH 1949. Clin. Med. Off. Gwynedd HA. Socs: BMA. Prev: Clin. Med. Off. Sefton HA; Sch. Med. Off. Pub. Health Dept. Bristol; Med. Off. Rochester State Hosp. Minn., USA.

PARRY, Gareth Freeman Hospital, Department of Cardiac Transplantation, Newcastle upon Tyne NE7 7DN Tel: 0191 233 6161 Fax: 0191 223 1152 Email: gareth.parry@nuth.nhs.uk; 20 Foxhills Covert, Fellside Park, Whickham, Newcastle upon Tyne NE16 5TN Tel: 0191 488 0487 — MB BCh Wales 1981; MRCP (UK) 1985; FRCP Ed 1998. Consult. Phys Cardiac Transpl. Specialty: Cardiol. Socs: Brit. Cardiac Soc.; Internat. Soc. for Heart and Lung Transplantation. Prev: Regist. (Cardiol.) Freeman Hosp. Newc.; Regional Research Regist. Profess. Cardiol. Unit Freeman Hosp. Newc.; Assoc. Specialist Cardiac Transpl. Freeman Hosp. Newc. u. Tyne.

PARRY, Gareth Michael Horsman's Place Surgery, Instone Road, Dartford DA1 2JP Tel: 01322 01322 228363; Copthorne, Ash Road Hartley, Longfield DA3 8EY Tel: 01474 708906 Email: gareth@parryfy.demon.co.uk — MB BS Lond. 1981 (Guy's) BSc Lond. 1978; MRCGP 1985; DRCOG 1985; MSc 2000. Prev: GP Tutor Dartford & Gravesham Dist.

PARRY, Mr Gareth Wyn Thoracic Surgical Unit, Norfolk & Norwich University Hospital, Colney Lane, Norwich NR4 7UZ Tel: 01603 286396 Fax: 01603 287882 Email: wyn.parry@nnuh.nhs.uk — MB BCh Wales 1984; BSc Wales 1981, MB BCh 1984; FRCS Eng. 1989; FRCS (C/th) 1996. Cons. (Thoracic Sug.) Norf. & Norwich Univ. Hosp. Norwich; Med. Dir. (Clin. Gov), Norf. and Norwich Univ. Hosp.; Hon. Sen. Lect., UEA Sch. of Med.; Mem. of the Ct. of Examr.s Roy. Coll. Of Surg. Eng. Specialty: Cardiothoracic Surg. Socs: Pres. Norwich Div. BMA. Prev: Cons. (Cardiothoracic Surg.)Freeman Hosp. Newc. upon Tyne; Sen. Regist. (Cardiothoracic Surg.) Glenfield Hosp. Leicester; Sen. Regist. (Cardiothoracic Surg.) N. Gen. Hosp. Sheff.

PARRY, George Robert Oak Vale Medical Centre, 158-160 Edge Lane Drive, Liverpool L13 4AQ Tel: 0151 259 1551 Fax: 0151 252 1121; 6 Sandhurst, Blundellsands Road E., Liverpool L23 8UJ — MB ChB Liverp. 1978; DCH RCPSI 1981; DRCOG 1981; MRCGP 1982. Phys. (Occupat. Health) NW Water & Evans Meds.

PARRY, Harry Vaughan (retired) 9 Avondale Road, St Leonards-on-Sea TN38 0SA — BM BCh Oxf. 1957 (Oxf. & Univ. Coll. Hosp.) BA 1953, BSc 1956, BM BCh 1957; DObst RCOG 1960. Prev: Ho. Phys. Univ. Coll. Hosp.

PARRY, Heather Mary Anaesthetic Department, Watford General Hospital, Vicarage Road, Watford WD18 0HB Tel: 01923 217604; Greenways, 33 Orchard Close, Cassiobury, Watford WD17 3DU Tel: 01923 228942 — MB ChB Bristol 1974; FFA RCS Eng. 1979. Cons. Anaesth. Watford Gen. Hosp. Specialty: Anaesth. Prev: Sen. Regist. (Anaesth.) St. Geo. Hosp. Lond. & Hosp. Sick Childr. Gt.; Ormond St.; SHO (Anaesth.) Chester Roy. Infirm.

PARRY, Helen Stephanie Ribbleton Medical Centre, 243 Ribbleton Avenue, Preston PR2 6RD Tel: 01772 792512 — MB ChB Birm. 1977; MRCGP 1982.

PARRY, Hilary Rosamund 6 Upper Belmont Road, Bishopston, Bristol BS7 9DQ Tel: 0117 942 2873 — MB BS Lond. 1990 (Med. Coll. St. Bart. Hosp. Lond.) BA (Hons.) Oxf. 1984; DRCOG 1993; MRCGP 1994.

PARRY, Hugh Evan (retired) 21 Rose Place, Aughton, Ormskirk L39 4UJ Tel: 01695 421154 — (St. Bart.) MRCS Eng. LRCP Lond. 1944; DCH Eng. 1945; MB BS Lond. 1945; FRCP Lond. 1974, M 1951. Prev: Cons. Phys. (Infec. Dis.) Fazakerley Hosp. Liverp.

PARRY, Hugh Francis Danewell House, The Borough, Downton, Salisbury SP5 3LT — MB BS Lond. 1972 (Guy's) MRCS Eng. LRCP Lond. 1972; MRCPath 1981. Cons. Haemat. Gen. Infirm. Salisbury; Clin. Tutor, Salisbury HA. Specialty: Haematology. Socs: Brit. Soc. Haemat.; Assn. Clin. Path. Prev: Sen. Regist. (Haemat.) St. Thos. Hosp. Lond.; Jules Thorn Research Fell. & Hon. Sen. Regist. Univ. Coll. Hosp.; Lond.; Regist. (Clin. Path.) Univ. Coll. Hosp. Lond.

PARRY, Huw Cambria Surgery, Ucheldre Avenue, Holyhead LL65 1RA Tel: 01407 762735; Tyn Pwll, Bodedern, Holyhead LL65 3PB — MB ChB Leeds 1982; BSc (Hons.) Pharmacol. Leeds 1979.

PARRY, Huw David Greyholme, West Rd, Nottage Village, Porthcawl CF36 3SS — MB BCh Wales 1996.

PARRY, James Charles 1 Rectory Close, Sutton-cum-Duckmanton, Chesterfield S44 5JT — MB ChB Sheff. 1978.

PARRY, James Dennis (retired) (Surgery), Margaret St., Ammanford SA18 2TJ; Glyndwr, 21 Newtown, Pen y Banc, Ammanford SA18 3TE Tel: 01269 593033 — MB ChB Sheff. 1952; DObst RCOG 1956. Prev: Treas. Med. Off. & Med. Examr. Dept. Educat. & Civil Serv. Comms. BritTelecom.

PARRY, Jayne Morgan 17 Sandiway, Shrewsbury SY3 9BN — MB ChB Birm. 1993; ChB Birm. 1993.

PARRY, Jean Corfield (retired) Bridge House, Rowton Bridge Road, Christleton, Chester CH3 7BD Tel: 01244 332066 — MB ChB Liverp. 1943. Prev: Med. Off. Chesh. HA.

PARRY, Jennifer Imogen Bennets End Surgery, Gatecroft, Hemel Hempstead HP3 9LY — MB BS Lond. 1985; MRCP (UK) 1988; DCH RCP Lond. 1990; DRCOG 1991. Prev: Trainee GP/SHO St. Albans City Hosp.

PARRY, Rev. John Edward (retired) 3 Portlands, Oxford Road, Gerrards Cross SL9 7RH Tel: 01753 481559 Email: john@parry-haughton.freeserve.co.uk — MB ChB Manch. 1947; DTM & H Liverp. 1953. Prev: Med. Supt. Livingstone Hosp., Zambia.

PARRY, John Gareth Greyholme, West Road, Nottage, Porthcawl CF36 3SS — BM Soton. 1992.

PARRY, John Hilary Holycroft Surgery, The Health Centre, Oakworth Road, Keighley BD21 1SA Tel: 01535 602010 Fax: 01535 691313; Spring House, 157 Keighley Road, Cowling, Keighley BD22 0AH Tel: 01535 635510 — MB BChir Camb. 1981; MA Camb. 1982; DRCOG 1983; MRCGP 1985. Prev: Med. Off. Sue Ryder Home Oxenhope; Trainee GP Camb. VTS; SHO (Radiother.) Addenbrooke's Hosp. Camb.

PARRY, John Morton (retired) Waterside Cottage, Tyrley Wharf, Market Drayton TF9 2AH Tel: 01630 654228 — (Middlx.) MB BS Lond. 1962; MRCS Eng. LRCP Lond. 1962; DObst RCOG 1965. Prev: Late GP Rainham, Kent.

PARRY, Mr John Rhys Williams Department of Urology, Ipswich Hospital NHS Trust, Heath Road, Ipswich IP6 9BT Tel: 01473 703534 Fax: 01473 703528 Email: jrwparry@hotmail.com — MB BS Lond. 1976 (St. Bart.) MRCS Eng. LRCP Lond. 1976; FRCS Ed. 1982. p/t Cons. (Urol.) Ipswich Hosp. NHS Trust. Specialty: Urol. Special Interest: Renal / Bladder Cancer; Unrinary Incontinence; Urological Oncology. Socs: RSM; BMA; BAUS. Prev: Sen. Regist. in Urol., Guys Hosp.; Sen. Regist. in Urol., Brighton Hosp.; Regist. in Urol., Inst. of Urol.

PARRY, John Stephen Westcotes Health Centre, Fosse Road South, Leicester LE3 0LP Tel: 0116 254 8568 — MB BCh Wales 1968.

PARRY, Jonathan Edward Parry, The Surgery, Spring Wells, Sleaford NG34 0QQ Tel: 01529 240234 Fax: 01529 240520; Westhill House, Hangman's Lane, Stainfield, Bourne PE10 0RS Tel: 01778 570888 Fax: 01778 570478 — MB BS Lond. 1982 (Lond. Hosp.) DGM RCP Lond. 1986; MRCGP 1986. Dep. Police Surg. Sleaford; St John Ambul., Bourne, Med. Off.; Lincs. Integrated Volun. Emerg. Serv.; Gen. Practitioner Trainer.

PARRY, Joseph Jones Evergreen, Gannock Park W., Deganwy, Conwy LL31 9HQ Tel: 01492 583338 — MB BS Lond. 1953 (St. Geo.) MRCS Eng. LRCP Lond. 1953. Prev: Squadron Ldr. RAF Med. Br.; Ho. Surg. & Ho. Phys. Mayday Hosp. Croydon.

PARRY, Keith Teasdale Forest Gate Surgery, Hazel Farm Road, Totton, Southampton SO40 8WU Tel: 023 8066 3839 Fax: 023 8066 7090 — MB ChB Manchester 1971; MB ChB Manch. 1971. GP Soton.

PARRY, Kenneth Michael, OBE (retired) 9 Moray Place, Edinburgh EH3 6DS Tel: 0131 226 3054 — MB ChB Bristol 1956; DCH Eng. 1961; FRCP Ed. 1973, M 1970; FFPHM 1974; FRCGP 1982, M 1976. Prev: Sec. Scott. Counc. Postgrad. Med. Educat. & UK Conf. Postgrad. Med. Deans.

PARRY, Llewellen Graham Mill Road Surgery, Mill Road, Market Rasen LN8 3BP Tel: 01673 843556 Fax: 01673 844388; The Water Mill, Middle Rasen, Market Rasen LN8 3TY — MRCS Eng. LRCP Lond. 1965 (Guy's) Prev: SHO (Surg.) St. Mary's Hosp. Eastbourne; Regist. (O & G) Pembury Hosp. Tunbridge Wells.

PARRY, Mair Lleifior, Y Felinheli LL56 4QF — MB BCh Wales 1991.

PARRY, Margaret Olwen Lloyd Student Health Service, 25 Belgrave Road, Bristol BS8 2AA Tel: 0117 973 7716 Fax: 0117 970 6804; 5 Pembroke Vale, Clifton, Bristol BS8 3DN — MB BS Lond. 1962 (St. Mary's) MRCS Eng. LRCP Lond. 1962. JP; Med. Off. Bristol Univ. Stud. Health Serv. Prev: Ho. Surg. Surgic. Unit & Med. Outpat. Asst. St. Mary's Hosp. Lond.; Ho. Phys. King Edwd. Memor. Hosp. Ealing.

PARRY, Marianne Isabelle 14 Cae Gwyn, Caernarfon LL55 1LL; 35 Primrose Hill, Chalcot Square, London NW1 8YP — MB ChB Manch. 1994; DTM & H 1997. Prev: Ho. Off. (Surg.) Macclesfield Dist. Gen. Hosp.; Ho. Off. (Med.) N. Manch. Dist. Gen. Hosp.

PARRY, Mark Stephen Doncaster Drug Team, 37 Thorne Road, Doncaster DN1 2EZ — MB ChB Sheff. 1986; MRCPsych 2000. Locum Cons. Psychiat. in Subst. Misuse. Specialty: Gen. Psychiat. Socs: Brit. Med. Assn.; Soc. for the Study of Addic. Prev: Specialist Regist. in Psychiat. Community Health Sheff. NHS Trust, Sheff.; Trainee GP Bassetlaw VTS; SHO Psychiat., Sheff. & N.Trent.

PARRY, Martin Gratton The Royal Sussx County Hospital, Eastern Road, Brighton BN2 5BE Tel: 01273 696955 — MB BS Lond. 1989 (Guy's Hospital Medical School) BSc (Hons.) Lond. 1987, MB BS 1989; FRCA 1995. Cons. (Anaesth.). Specialty: Anaesth. Socs: Roy. Soc. Med.; Difficult Airway Soc.; Assn. Paed. Anaesth. Prev: Clin. Fell. The Hosp. For Sick Childr., Toronto, Canada; Specialist Regist. (Anaesth.) Middlx. Hosp. & The Hosp. for Sick Childr. Gt. Ormond St. Lond.

PARRY, Mary Wyn (retired) 97 Long Road, Cambridge CB2 2HE Tel: 01223 501487 — (W. Lond.) MRCS Eng. LRCP Lond. 1958; DObst RCOG 1960. Med. Off. Hinchinbrooke Trust Huntingdon Cambs. Prev: Med. Off. Hinchinbrooke Trust Huntingdon Cambs.

PARRY, Michael Richard Hexham General Hospital, Hexham NE46 1QJ; Bank House, Shield Court, Hexham NE46 1RA — MB ChB Ed. 1978; BSc (Med. Sci.) Ed. 1975, MB ChB 1978; MRCPsych 1984. Cons. Psychiat. Hexham Gen. Hosp. Hexham N.d.; Hon. Clin. Lect. (Psychiat.) Univ. Newc. Specialty: Gen. Psychiat. Prev: Sen. Regist. (Psychiat.) Roy. Vic. Infirm. Newc.; Sen. Regist. (Psychiat.) Newc. Gen. Hosp.; Regist. (Psychiat.) Roy. Edin. Hosp.

PARRY, Nicholas Sebastian 40 Elm Grove, Didsbury, Manchester M20 6PN — MB ChB Manch. 1990; FRCA 1997. Specialty: Anaesth.

PARRY, Patricia Anne Portway Surgery, 1 The Portway, Porthcawl CF36 3XB Tel: 01656 304204 Fax: 01656 772605; Greyholme, West Road, Nottage, Porthcawl CF36 3SS Tel: 01656 784211 Fax: 01656 786828 — MB BCh Wales 1965 (Cardiff)

PARRY, Peter Gratton (retired) Llannerch, Morfa Bychan Road, Porthmadog LL49 9UR Tel: 01766 512921 — MB BS Lond. 1959 (Guy's) MRCS Eng. LRCP Lond. 1958. Prev: GP Porthmadog & Dist.

PARRY, Richard John 31 Mornington Terrace, London NW1 7RS — MB BS Lond. 1998.

PARRY, Richard Tonson Ribbleton Medical Centre, 243, Ribbleton Avenue,, Preston PR2 6RD Tel: 01772 792512; 229 Garstang Road,, Fulwood, Preston PR2 8XE — MB ChB Manch. 1977; DRCOG 1979; MRCGP 1981. GP Preston; Med. Director, Heartbeat (Cardiac Rehab. Charity).

PARRY, Robert Langhorne 74 Trafalgar Road, Birkdale, Southport PR8 2NJ Tel: 01704 562712 — MB ChB Liverp. 1979; MRCP (UK) 1986; FRCR 1990. Cons. Vasc. Radiol. Southport Dist. Gen. Hosp. Specialty: Radiol. Prev: Merck Lect. (Cardiovasc. Radiol.) Univ. Bristol; Sen. Regist. (Radiol.) Univ. Hosp. Wales Cardiff.

PARRY, Robin Llanberis Surgery, High Street, Llanberis, Caernarfon LL55 4SU Tel: 01286 870634 Fax: 01286 871722; Rhiwerfa, Frongoch, Llanberis, Caernarfon LL55 4LE Tel: 012486 872211 — MB ChB Manch. 1984; DRCOG 1987; MRCGP 1988. Socs: BMA; Cadeirydd Cymdeithas Feddygol Arfon. Prev: Trainee GP Gwynedd VTS.

PARRY, Robin Geoffrey 13 Lingwood Road, Great Sankey, Warrington WA5 3EN — MB ChB Leeds 1989.

PARRY, Rosemary Margaret Whiteparish Surgery, Common Road, Whiteparish, Salisbury SP5 2SU Tel: 01794 884269 Fax: 01794 884109; Danewell House, 130 The Borough, Downton, Salisbury SP5 3LT Tel: 01725 20425 — MB BS Lond. 1972 (Guy's) MRCS Eng. LRCP Lond. 1972; DCH Eng. 1974; DObst RCOG 1974. Hon. Clin. Teach. Univ. Soton.; GP Trainer. Prev: SHO (Paediat.) Qu. Eliz. Hosp. Childr. Lond.; SHO (O & G) FarnBoro. Hosp. Kent; Ho. Phys. Hither Green Hosp.

PARRY, Sally Davina — MB BS Lond. 1993 (Univ. Coll. & Middlx. Sch. Med.) BPharm (Hons.) Lond. 1987; MRCP 1996; MD Newc. 2002. Cons. Phys.; Specialist Regist., S. Thames (G(I)M and Gastroenterol.) Guys and St Thomas' Lond.; T&RF, N. Tyneside Hosp. Specialty: Gastroenterol.; Gen. Med. Prev: Kings Liver Unit, Lond.; SpR Kings Coll., London; Roy. Sussex Co., Brighton; Kent & Sussex, Tunbridge Wells; SHO QMC Nottm.

PARRY, Steve Wayne c/o Ward 13 Office, Freeman Hospital, Newcastle upon Tyne NE7 7DN; 45 Lonsdale Road, Stamford PE9 2RW — MB BS Newc. 1991.

PARRY, Tom Evelyn (retired) Awelon, Pen-y-Turnpike, Dinas Powys CF64 4HG Tel: 029 2051 2338 Fax: 029 2076 2208 — MB ChB Manch. 1941; MRCS Eng. LRCP Lond. 1941; FRCP Lond. 1974, M 1950; FRCPath 1963. Hon. Cons. Haemat. S. Glam. HA (T); Hon. Vice-Pres. Leukaemia Research Appeal for Wales; Recognised Clin. Teach. (Haemat.) Univ. Wales Coll. Med. Cardiff. Prev: Cons. Haemat. S. Glam. HA (T).

PARRY, Tomos Health Services Centre, Wynne Road, Blaenau Ffestiniog LL41 3DW Tel: 01766 830205 Fax: 01766 831121; Afallon, Holyhead Road, Menai Bridge LL59 5RH Tel: 712633 — MB BCh Wales 1983. Trainee GP/SHO Gwynedd HA VTS. Socs: BMA; Med. Defence Union. Prev: Ho. Phys. & Ho. Surg. Llandudno Gen. Hosp.

PARRY, William Gwyn Wakefield Llys Meddyg, Pen-y-Groes, Caernarfon LL54 6HD Tel: 01286 207 — MB ChB Liverp. 1952.

PARRY DAVIES, Miss Michaela Frances Department of Plastic Surgery, Aberdeen Royal Infirmary, Foresterhill, Aberdeen AB25 2ZN — MB BS Lond. 1982 (Univ. Coll. Lond.) FRCS Lond. 1986; FRCS (Plast.) 1996. Cons. (Plastic Surg.). Specialty: Plastic Surg.

PARRY-JONES, Adrian Tegfan, Llandegfan, Menai Bridge LL59 5PY — MB ChB Manch. 1998.

PARRY-JONES, Alexander Jack Duncan 57 Scholars Road, London SW12 0PF — MB BS Lond. 1992 (UCMSM) MRCP (Lond.) 1995; FRCA (Lond.) 1998. Specialist Regist., Anaesth., N. Thames. Specialty: Anaesth.

PARRY-JONES, Charles Edward Ty Bodafon, Mynydd Bodafon, Llanerchymedd LL71 8BN — MB ChB Ed. 1993.

PARRY-JONES, Gareth Bron Seiont Surgery, Bron Seiont, Segontium Terrace, Caernarfon LL55 2PH Tel: 01286 672236 Fax: 01286 676404; Bryn Eglwys, Caeathro, Caernarfon LL55 2TA Tel: 01286 671195 — MB ChB Liverp. 1975; DRCOG 1978; FRCGP 1991, M 1979; DFFP 1993; MSc (Med. Educat.) Wales 1996. Sen. Lect. & Assoc. Adviser (Gen. Pract.) Gwynedd; Clin. Asst. MacMillan Terminal Care Unit; Examr. RCGP. Socs: (Chairm.) Welsh Med. Soc.; FRCGP. Prev: Trainee GP Gwynedd VTS; Ho. Surg. Univ. Hosp. Wales; Ho. Phys. (Paediat.) Llandough Hosp. Cardiff.

PARRY-JONES, John (retired) Bodynys Penrodyn, Valley, Holyhead LL65 3BE Tel: 01407 741118 — BSc Wales 1949; MRCS Eng. LRCP Lond. 1954.

PARRY-JONES, Mary (retired) Bodynys, Penrodyn, Valley, Holyhead LL65 3BE Tel: 01407 741118 — (Lond. Sch. Med. Wom.) MRCS Eng. LRCP Lond. 1945; DPH Eng. 1949.

PARRY-JONES, Nicholas Owen Douglas Grove Surgery, Douglas Grove, Witham CM8 1TE Tel: 01376 512827 Fax: 01376 502463 — MB BChir Camb. 1970 (Camb. & St. Thos.) MRCP (UK) 1975; DRCOG 1979. Prev: Sen. Lect. (Gen. Pract.) UMDS & Hon. Cons. Guy's & St. Thos. Hosps. Lond.

PARRY-JONES, Nilima Dept. Of Academic Haematology, Royal Marsden Hospital, 203 Fulham Road, London SW3 6JJ — MB BS Lond. 1992 (Univ. Coll. & Middlx.) MRCP (UK) 1995; DRCPath 2001. Clin. Research Fell., Dept. Of Acad. Haemat. Roy. Marsden Hosp. Inst. of Cancer Research, Lond. Sw3. Specialty: Haematology.

PARRY-JONES, Owen Charles Craigle, Beach Road, Benllech, Tyn-y-Gongl LL74 8SW Tel: 01248 853853 — LRCPI & LM, LRSCI & LM 1958 (RCSI) LRCPI & LM, LRCSI & LM 1958; LM Coombe 1960; MICGP 1986. Med. Off. advising allocation of Pub. housing to Conwy, Gwynedd & Ynys Mon Co. Counc.s; Anglesey Co. Surg. St. John's Ambul.; Hon. Med. Off. Moelfre Lifeboat; Chief MO Anglesey Motor Racing Circuit. Socs: BASICS. Prev: Clin. Asst. (Geriat.) Gwynedd AHA; Sen. Res. Paediatr. Rotunda Hosp. Dub.; Clin. Clerk Coombe Lying-in Hosp. Dub.

PARRY-MORTON, Monica 11 Maynard Court, Llandaff, Cardiff CF5 2LS Tel: 029 2056 9106 — MB BCh Wales 1941 (Cardiff) BSc, MB BCh Wales 1941. Clin. Med. Off. Mid Glam. AHA.

PARRY OKEDEN, Peter Christopher Uvedale Pemberley Avenue Surgery, 32 Pemberley Avenue, Bedford MK40 2LA Tel: 01234 351051 Fax: 01234 349246; 38 Kimbolton Avenue, Bedford MK40 3AA Tel: 01234 344148 — MB ChB Sheff. 1979; DRCOG 1982; MRCGP 1984. Chairm. Bedford PCG. Prev: Trainee GP Bedford VTS; Ho. Surg. & Ho. Phys. Rotherham Dist. Gen. Hosp.

PARRY-SMITH, Hywel John Meddygfa Surgery, Meddygfa Rhydbach, Botwnnog, Pwllheli LL53 8RE Tel: 01758 730266 Fax: 01758 730307; 8 Glyn y Mor, Llanbedrog, Pwllheli LL53 7NW — MB BS Lond. 1979 (Middlesex Hospital Medical School) DRCOG 1982; MRCGP 1985. Prev: Ho. Surg. Harefield Hosp. Ho. Phys. Cent. Middlx. Hosp. Lond.

PARRY-WILLIAMS, Ann Wyn Cadwgan Surgery, 11 Bodelwyddan Avenue, Old Colwyn, Colwyn Bay LL29 9NP Tel: 01492 515410 Fax: 01492 513270 — MB ChB Liverp. 1982; BSc Liverp. 1977; DRCOG 1985.

PARRY-WILLIAMS, Henry Wyn (retired) The Randolph Medical Centre, Green Lane, Datchet, Slough SL3 9EX Tel: 01753 41268 Fax: 01753 582324; Longacre, Slough Road, Datchet, Slough SL3 9AP Tel: 01753 542538 — (Univ. Coll. Hosp.) MB Camb. 1956, BChir 1955; MA Camb. 1956; DObst RCOG 1957. Prev: Ho. Off. (Med. & Surg.) Univ. Coll. Hosp.

PARSHALL, Alice Margaret Gordon Hospital, Bloomberg St., London SW1 Tel: 020 8746 8000; 55 Bridge View, London W6 9DD — PhD Lond. 1983; MRCPsych 1990. Cons. Psychiat. S. Marylebone & Gordon Hosp. Lond. Specialty: Gen. Psychiat. Prev: Sen. Regist. & Regist. (Psychiat.) Maudsley Hosp. Lond.; SHO (Rheum.) Hammersmith Hosp. Lond.

PARSLEW, Richard Anthony Gerard 10C Link, Royal Liverpool University Hospital, Prescot Street, Liverpool L7 8XP Tel: 0151 706 3477; Norwood, 26 Merrilocks Road, Blundellsands, Liverpool L23 6UN Tel: 0151 932 9023 — MB ChB Liverp. 1990 (Liverpool) MRCP (UK) 1993. Cons. Dermatol. Roy. Liverp. Hosp. & Alder Hey Roy. Liverp.. Specialty: Dermat. Socs: MDU; Brit. Assn. Dermat..; Brit. Soc. for Investigative Dermat. Prev: Sen. Regist. (Dermat.) Roy. Liverp. Univ. Hosp.; Regist. (Dermat.) Roy. Liverp. Hosp.; SHO (Med.) Roy. Liverp. Hosp.

PARSLEY, John Flat 5, 31 Sussex Square, Brighton BN2 5AB — BM Soton. 1984.

PARSLOE, Justin Bruce Kingsley St Annes Group Practice, 161 Station Road, Herne Bay CT6 5NF Tel: 01227 742226 Fax: 01227 741439; 11 Seymour Close, Herne Bay CT6 7AS — MB BS Lond. 1984; DRCOG 1988; MRCGP 1989. Prev: Trainee GP S. Warks. VTS.

PARSLOE, Malcolm Richard Justin Department of Anaesthesia, Leeds General Infirmary, Great George St., Leeds LS1 3EX Tel: 0113 392 6672 Fax: 0113 392 2645; 22 Elmete Avenue, Oakwood, Leeds LS8 2QN Tel: 0113 293 1625 — MB ChB Manch. 1981 (Manchester) FFA RCS Eng. 1986. Cons. Anaesth. Leeds Gen. Infirm. Specialty: Anaesth. Prev: Sen. Regist. (Anaesth.) North. RHA; Regist. (Anaesth.) St. Jas. Univ. Hosp. Leeds; SHO (Paediat. & Anaesth.) Warwick Hosp.

PARSON, Alison Mary Yule Lytham Road Surgery, 2A Lytham Road, Fulwood, Preston PR2 8JB Tel: 01772 716033 Fax: 01772 715445 — MB ChB Manch. 1976; DRCOG 1980; MRCGP 1981. Gen. Practitioner; Clin. Asst. Paediat.; Roy. Preston Hosp., Preston, Lancs. Prev: Ho. Off. Blackpool Vict. Hosp.; SHO (Paediat.) Hull Roy. Infirm. & (Neonat. Paediat.) St. Mary's; Hosp. Manch.

PARSON, Andrew Francis Chislehurst Medical Practice, 42 High Street, Chislehurst BR7 5AQ Tel: 020 8467 5551 Fax: 020 8468 7658 — MB ChB Liverp. 1988; DRCOG 1992; MRCGP 1993.

PARSONAGE, Maurice John (retired) BUPA Hospital Leeds, Jackson Avenue, Roundhay, Leeds LS8 1NT Tel: 0113 269 3939 Fax: 0113 268 1340; 2 Cornwall Close, Harrogate HG1 2NY Tel: 01423 565310 — MB ChB Manch. 1939; BSc Manch. 1936; MRCS Eng. LRCP Lond. 1940; DCH Eng. 1940; FRCP Lond. 1959, M 1945. Indep. Cons. BUPA Hosp. Leeds; Mem. Hon. Med. Advis. Panel Driving & Disorders of The New System (Dept. of Transport); Med. Adviser Brit. Epilepsy Assn. Prev: Cons. Phys. (Neurol.) & Phys. (Electroenceph.) Gen. Infirm. Leeds.

PARSONAGE, Sarah Madeleine Cornerstones, Broughton Hackett, Worcester WR7 4BA — BM BS Nottm. 1989; BMedSci 1987; FRCS Glas. 1997; FRCR 2000. Cons. (Radiol.) Worcs. Roy. Hosp. NHS Trust. Specialty: Radiol.

PARSONAGE, William Anthony The Cottage, 2 Cross Lane Head, Bridgnorth WV16 4SJ — BM BS Nottm. 1991.

PARSONS, Adrian Priory Medical Centre Partnership, Cape Road, Warwick CV34 4JP Tel: 01926 494411 Fax: 01926 402394; 2 Verden Avenue, Warwick CV34 6RX — BM BCh Oxf. 1989; BA Oxf. 1986; MRCGP 1994.

PARSONS, Anthony David Hospital of St Cross, Barby Road, Rugby CV22 5PX Tel: 01788 545208 Fax: 02476 524311 Email: anthony.parsons@uhcw.nhs.uk; Warwick Medical School, Gibbet Hill Site, University of Warwick, Coventry CV4 7AL Tel: 024 7652 2913 — MB BS Lond. 1971 (King's Coll. Hosp.) FRCOG 1990, M 1978; MA Wales 1989; MFFP 1993; FRIPHH 2001. Cons. (Gynaecology) Univ. Hosps. of Coventry and Warks. NHS Trust; Sen. Lect. (Gyn.) Warwick Med. Sch. Specialty: Obst. & Gyn.; Family Plann. & Reproduc. Health; Gynaecology. Socs: Fell. Roy. Soc. Med.; (Ex-Chairm.) Brit. Menopause Soc. Prev: Lect. (O & G) Birm. Univ.; Sen. Regist. (O & G) Stoke-on-Trent; Regist. (Psychiat.) King's Coll. Hosp. Lond.

PARSONS, Anthony Stephen Brynderwen Surgery, Crickhowell Road, St. Mellons, Cardiff CF3 0EF Tel: 029 2079 9921 Fax: 029 2077 7740 — MB BCh Wales 1968.

PARSONS, Beate Elisabeth Annick West Riding, Billingham, Newport PO30 3HE Tel: 01983 721804 — State Exam Med Aachen 1989; State Exam Med. Aachen 1989.

PARSONS, Benedicte Lawrence West Oak Surgery, 319 Westdale Lane, Mapperley, Nottingham NG3 6EW Tel: 0115 952 5320 Fax: 0115 952 5321 — MB BS Lond. 1976 (UCL) DRCOG 1979; MRCGP 1980.

PARSONS, Carol Ruth The Health Centre, Rikenel, The Park, Gloucester GL1 1XR Tel: 01452 891110 Fax: 01452 891111; Health Centre, Rikenel, The Park, Gloucester GL1 1XR Tel: 01452 891110 — MB ChB Liverp. 1978; MRCGP 1982.

PARSONS, Charles Anthony (retired) Woodford House, Knightwick, Worcester WR6 5PH Tel: 01886 821630 — MB ChB Birm. 1948; MRCS Eng. LRCP Lond. 1948; MRCGP 1960. Prev: GP Kt.wick, Worcs.

PARSONS, Christopher John The Meeting House, New Road, Flaxley, Newnham GL14 1JS Tel: 01594 544566 — MB ChB Birm. 1971; FLCOM 1980; DMS Med. Soc. Apoth. Lond. 1993. Indep. Specialist (Musculoskeletal Med.) Mitcheldean, Glos. Socs: (Pres.) Brit. Osteop. Assn.; Brit. Inst. Musculoskel. Med.; Med. Acupunct. Soc.

PARSONS, Claire Elizabeth Mary Oakhill Medical practice, Oakhill Road, Dronfield S18 2EJ Tel: 01246 296900; 39 Smithywood Crescent, Woodseats, Sheffield S8 0NT Tel: 0114 258 8454 — MB ChB Sheff. 1982. GP. Prev: Trainee GP Chesterfield VTS; Clin. Asst. Breast Clinic Chesterfield & N. Derbysh. Roy. Hosp.

PARSONS, David Leslie Thomas St. John's Medical Centre, 287A Lewisham Way, London SE4 1XF; Two Ridges, Summerhill, Chislehurst BR7 5NY Tel: 020 8467 4099 Fax: 020 8467 1944 — MB ChB St. And. 1957; MRCGP 1966. Socs: Worshipful Soc. of Apoth.; (Chairm.) Benefits Agency Sessional Docs. Assn. Prev: Resid. Obst. Off. Matern. Hosp. Cheltenham; Resid. Therap. Unit. Maryfield Hosp. Dundee; Resid. (Surg. & Gyn. Units) Gen. Infirm. S.port.

PARSONS, Dennis Shirley Merton College, Oxford OX4 Tel: 01865 276310 Fax: 01865 276361; 27A Norham Road, Oxford OX2 6SQ Tel: 01865 557637 — BM BCh Oxf. 1942; BA Oxf. 1939, MA 1946, DM 1950. Emerit. Reader (Physiol. Biochem.) Oxf; Fell. Merton Coll. Oxf.; Mem. Edit. Bd. Biomembranes Reviews. Socs: Physiol. Soc. Prev: Chairm. Europ. Ed. Bd. Physiol. Rev.; Mem. Edit. Bd. Biochim. Biophys. Acta.; Hon. Maj. RAMC.

PARSONS, Mr Derek Walter 10 Harley Street, London W1G 9PF Tel: 020 7436 5252; Meon House, Meon Close, Tadworth KT20 5DJ Tel: 01737 813762 — MB BS Lond. 1957 (Univ. Coll. Hosp.) FRCS Eng. 1963. Hon. Cons. Orthop. St. Anthony's Hosp. Cheam; Cons. Orthopaedic Surg. St Helier and Epsom Hosp.s Trust.

Specialty: Orthop. Socs: Fell. Roy. Soc. Med. & BOA; SICOT; Brit. Hip Soc.,Europ. Hip Soc. Prev: Sen. Regist. (Orthop.) Roy. Nat. Orthop. Hosp. Lond.; John Marshall Fell. Univ. Coll. Hosp. Med. Sch.

PARSONS, Mr Donald Colin Stuart Top Farm House, Shrubbery Lane, Wilden, Bedford MK44 2PH Tel: 01234 792064 Fax: 01234 792322 — (St. Mary's) MRCS Eng. LRCP Lond. 1966; MB BS MB BS Lond. 1966 1966; FRCS Eng. 1971; MS Lond. 1978. Cons. Surg. (Vasc. Surg.) Bedford Hosp. NHS Trust; Recognised Clin. Teach. Sch. Clin. Med. Addenbrooke's Hosp. Camb.; Chairm. N. Beds. Hospice Care; Examr. Ct. of RCS Eng. Specialty: Gen. Surg. Socs: Assn. Surg.; Vasc. Surgic. Soc. GB & Irel. Prev: Sen. Regist. (Surg.) & Research Regist. St. Mary's Hosp. Lond.; Regist. (Vasc. Surg.) Chelmsford Gp. Hosps.; Regist. (Surg.) Lewisham Hosp.

PARSONS, Emma Jane 68 Wallingford Avenue, London W10 6PY — MB ChB Dundee 1995.

PARSONS, Gary John The Health Centre, Worcester Street, Stourport-on-Severn DY13 8EH Tel: 01299 827141 Fax: 01299 879074 — MB ChB Birm. 1980; MRCP (UK) 1983; MRCGP 1986.

PARSONS, Gary Jonathan — MB ChB Liverp. 1983 (Liverpool) DRCOG 1986. GP & Medico-Legal Expert. Special Interest: Medico-Legal Expert.

PARSONS, Gillian Mary Bacon Lane Surgery, 11 Bacon Lane, Edgware HA8 5AT Tel: 020 8952 5073/7876 — MB BS Lond. 1989; DRCOG 1991; DCH RCP Lond. 1992; MA Camb. 1994; MRCGP (Distinc.) 1994. Socs: BMA. Prev: Trainee GP Barnet.

PARSONS, Helena Kate 233 Carter Knowle Road, Sheffield S11 9FW — MB ChB Sheff. 1995. SHO (Gen. Med.) Chesterfield Roy. Hosp. Specialty: Gen. Med.

PARSONS, Mr Howard Michael (retired) 22 Manor Way, South Croydon CR2 7BR Tel: 020 8686 2121 — (Univ. Coll. Hosp.) MRCS Eng. LRCP Lond. 1942; DLO Eng. 1949; FRCS Eng. 1956. Prev: Cons. ENT Surg. Croydon HA.

PARSONS, Jean Mary (retired) 68A St Wilfred's Road, West Hallam, Derby DE7 6HH Tel: 0115 932 0340 — MB ChB Ed. 1957; FRCGP 1992, M 1972. Prev: GP Ilkeston.

PARSONS, John Arthur (retired) West Billingham Farm, Chillerton, Newport PO30 3HE — MB BS Lond. 1964 (Westm.) MRCS Eng. LRCP Lond. 1964; DObst RCOG 1966; MRCP (U.K.) 1971; FRCP Lond. 1986. Prev: Cons. Rheum. I. of Wight AHA.

PARSONS, John Bruce (retired) 59 Bleadon Hill, Weston Super Mare BS24 9JW — MB BS Lond. 1950 (Guy's) MB BS (Hnrs.) Lond. 1950; MRCS Eng. LRCP Lond. 1950; FFA RCS Eng. 1962. Prev: Cons. Anaesth. Weston-Super-Mare Gen. Hosp.

PARSONS, John Howard Assisted Conception Unit, King's College Hospital, Denmark Hill, London SE5 8RX Tel: 020 7274 3242 — MB ChB Dundee 1970; MRCOG 1979; DA Eng. 1979. Sen. Lect. (O & G) King's Coll Sch. Med. & Dent. Lond. Prev: Regist. (O & G) Hammersmith Hosp. Lond.; Regist. (O & G) Roy. Hants Co. Hosp. Winchester; Gen. Med. Off. Malawi Govt.

PARSONS, John Whitehill (retired) 9 The Paddocks, Ramsbury, Marlborough SN8 2QF — LRCP LRCS Ed. 1952 (Roy. Colls. Ed.) LRCP LRCS Ed. LRFPS Glas. 1952; DTM & H Eng. 1962; DPH Lond. 1963; DIH Soc. Apoth. Lond. 1963; FFCM 1983, M 1974. Prev: Director of Pub. Health, Swindon HA.

PARSONS, Jonathan Michael Ashbery House, Main St., Wighill, Tadcaster LS24 8BQ — MB BS Lond. 1981; MRCP (UK) 1985; FRCP Lond. 1995. Cons. Paediat. Cardiol. Killingbeck Hosp. Lond. Specialty: Cardiol. Prev: Sen. Regist. (Paediat. Cardiol.) Killingbeck Hosp. Leeds; Research Fell. Dept. Paediat. Cardiol. Guy's Hosp. Lond.; Regist. (Cardiol., Thoracic Med.) Harefield Hosp.

PARSONS, Judith Mollie 8 Lon-Ysgubor, Cardiff CF14 6SG — MB ChB Leic. 1992.

PARSONS, Mr Keith Francis Royal Liverpool and Broadgreen University Hospitals NHS Trust, Prescot Street, Liverpool L7 8XP Tel: 0151 706 2000 Fax: 0151 706 5310 Email: parsons_keith@hotmail.com; Roscoe House, 27 Rodney Street, Liverpool L37 7BN Tel: 0151 709 2003 — (Liverp.) MB ChB Liverp. 1970; FRCS Ed. 1975; FRCS Eng. 1975. Cons. Urol. (Surg.) Roy. Liverp. & Broadgreen Univ. Hosp. NHS Trust. Specialty: Urol. Special Interest: Reconstruction; Stone Disease; Urooncology. Socs: Fell. Roy. Soc. Med; Brit. Assn. Urol. Surgs.; Liverp. Med. Inst. Prev: Chief Exec., the Roy. Liverp. and BRd. Green NHS Trust.

PARSONS, Kenneth Charles (retired) Trevonny, Eastfield Road, Ross-on-Wye HR9 5JZ Tel: 01989 562091 — MB BCh Wales 1952 (Cardiff) BSc Wales 1952; DObst RCOG 1954.

PARSONS, Linda Marguerite Neurology Department, St. Albans City Hospital, Waverley Road, St Albans AL3 5PN — MB ChB Sheff. 1973 (Sheffield) MRCP (UK) 1977; MD Sheff. 1983; FRCP UK 2000. Cons. Neurol. St. Albans Hemel Hempstead & Roy. Free Hosps.; Assoc. Specialist (Neurol.) Luton & Dunstable Hosp. Specialty: Neurol. Socs: Fell. Roy. Soc. Med.; Assn. Brit. Neurol.; BMA. Prev: Sen. Regist. (Neurol.) St. Mary's Hosp. Lond.; Sen. Research Fell. Neurovirol. Unit & Hon. Clin. Asst. (Neurol.) St. Thos. Hosp. Lond.; Regist. (Neurol.) Dudley Rd. Hosp. Birm.

PARSONS, Malcolm (retired) 1 Ancaster View, Leeds LS16 5HR — MB BChir Camb. 1958 (Univ. Coll. Hosp.) MA Camb. 1957; FRCP Lond. 1978, M 1963. Prev: Cons. Neurol. Gen. Infirm. Leeds.

PARSONS, Maria Andrea 92 Salop Road, London E17 7HT — MB BS Lond. 1990.

PARSONS, Marjorie (retired) 11 Breary Court, Breary Lane, Bramhope, Leeds LS16 9LB Tel: 0113 284 2211 — MB ChB Leeds 1943. Prev: Med. Off. Leeds AHA.

PARSONS, Matthew St John 144 Wyndcliffe Road, Charlton, London SE7 7LF Tel: 020 7346 3377 Fax: 07771 879066 — MB ChB Bristol 1993; DFFP 1997; CCST (Ons & Gynae) 2003. Cons. Obst. Urogynaecologist Birm. Women's Hosp.; Urogynaecology Fell. King's Coll. Hosp. Specialty: Obst. & Gyn. Prev: Specialist Regist. (O & G) NE Thames Deanery Lond.

PARSONS, Michael Andrew Royal Hallamshire Hospital, Ophthalmic Sciences Unit, Glossop Road, Sheffield S10 2JF Tel: 0114 271 2745 Fax: 0114 276 6381 Email: andy.parsons@sth.nhs.uk — MB ChB Sheff. 1974; FRCPath 1982. Sen. Lect. & Hon. Cons. Ophth. Path. Univ. Sheff. & Roy. Hallamsh. Hosp. Sheff.; Dir. Ophth. Sci. Unit Univ. Sheff. Specialty: Histopath. Special Interest: Child Abuse/Forensic Ophth. Path.; Ocular Oncol.; Trauma. Socs: Eur. Ophth. Path. Soc.; Brit. Assn. Ocular Path.; Assn Clin. Path. Prev: Sen. Lect. & Hon. Cons. Path. Univ. Sheff. & Roy. Hallamsh. Hosp. Sheff.

PARSONS, Michael Hume 7 Swanage Road, Lee-on-the-Solent PO13 9JW Tel: 023 9255 3525 — BM BCh Oxf. 1957; MA Oxf. 1958; DObst RCOG 1959. Prev: GP Gosport; Hosp. Pract. (Psychiat.) St. Jas. Hosp. Portsmouth.; Surg. Lt.-Cdr. RN.

PARSONS, Patricia Ann Cellular Pathology Department, Uited Lincolnshire Hospitals NHS Trusts, Lincoln County Hospital, Lincoln LN2 5QY Tel: 01522 512512 Ext: 2707 Fax: 01909 502462; Park Farm, 45 Main St, Hayton, Retford DN22 9LF — MB BS Lond. 1982; PhD Lond. 1974, BSc 1970, MB BS 1982; MRCPath 1993. Cons. Histopath. & Cytopathologist United Lincs. Hopsitals NHS Trust Lincoln. Specialty: Histopath. Prev: Sen. Regist. (Cytol. & Histopath.) St. Stephens & Char. Cross Hosp. Lond.; Regist. (Histopath.) Westm. Hosp. Lond.; Cons. Histopath & CytoPath. Bassetlaw Dist. Gen. Hosp. Worksop. Notts.

PARSONS, Paul William 30 Warkworth Close, Banbury OX16 1BD — MB ChB Birm. 1991; DRCOG 1998; DFFP 1998. GP Non-Princip., Banbury, Oxon. Specialty: Gen. Pract. Prev: GP Trainee Banbury VTS.

PARSONS, Peter Henry Irving (retired) 103 Park Road, Brentwood CM14 4TT Tel: 01277 210569 — MB BS Lond. 1956 (Univ. Coll. Hosp.) LMSSA Lond. 1950; MRCS Eng. LRCP Lond. 1955. Assoc. Specialist Nat. Blood Transfus. Centre Brentwood. Prev: Regist. (Surg.) Lambeth Hosp.

PARSONS, Richard Simon (retired) — (Oxf.) BM BCh Oxf. 1968; MA Camb. 1969; MA Oxf. 1969; FFA RCS Eng. 1973. Cons. Anaesth. Guy's Hosp. Lond. Prev: Sen. Regist. (Anaesth.) Westm. Hosp. Lond.

PARSONS, Samantha Louise 41 De Burgh Street, Cardiff CF11 6LB — MB BS Lond. 1998.

PARSONS, Samuel Joseph 4 St Johns Row, Long Wittenham, Abingdon OX14 4QG — MB BS Lond. 1997.

PARSONS, Sarah Aerona (retired) Trevonny, Eastfield Road, Ross-on-Wye HR9 5JZ Tel: 01989 562091 — MB BCh Wales 1948 (Cardiff) BSc Wales 1948. JP.

PARSONS, Sarah Luise Foley Chrisp Street Health Centre, 100 Chrisp Street, Poplar, London E14 6PG — MB BS Lond. 1977; MRCGP 2002.

PARSONS, Mr Simon Leslie Nottingham City Hospital, Hucknall Road, Nottingham NG5 1PB — BM BS Nottm. 1989; FRCS Eng. 1993; MD Nottm. 1996; FRCS (Gen. Surg.) 2000. Cons. Gen. & Gastro-oesophogeal Surg. Nottm. Specialty: Gen. Surg. Socs: Brit. Assn. Surgic. Oncol.; Assn. of Surgeons of GB & Irel.; Assn. of Upper Gastro-intestinal Surgeons.

PARSONS, Mr Stephen Wyndham c/o Department of Orthopaedics, Royal Cornwall Hospital, Infirmary Hill, Truro TR1 2HZ; The Beeches, Greensplatt, Perranwell Station, Truro TR3 7LZ Tel: 01872 74242 — MB BS Lond. 1979 (Middlx. Hosp. Med. Sch.) FRCS Eng. 1984; FRCS Ed. 1984. Cons. Orthop. Surg. Roy. Cornw. Hosps. Trust. Specialty: Orthop. Socs: Fell. BOA; Brit. Childr. Orthop. Surg. Soc.; (Ex-Pres.) Brit. Orthop. Foot Surg. Soc. Prev: Lect. (Orthop. Surg.) Univ. Soton.

PARSONS, Vincent John Hope Hospital, Eccles Old Road, Salford M6 8HD — MB BCh BAO NUI 1986; MRCPI 1989; FRCR 1993; FFR RCSI 1993. Sen. Regist. Manch. Specialty: Radiol. Socs: BMA. Prev: Regist. (Radiol.) Manch.

PART, Maiu Part, Maiu St Francis, Great Doward, Ross-on-Wye HR9 6DY Tel: 01600 890026 — (Bristol) MB ChB Bristol 1964; Cert. Family Plann. JCC 1974. Specialty: Family Plann. & Reproduc. Health.

PARTHA, Jagadish Staploe Medical Centre, Brewhouse Lane, Soham, Ely CB7 5JD Tel: 01353 624123 Fax: 01353 624203; 5 The Birches, Townsend, Soham, Ely CB7 5FH — MB BS Mysore 1973.

PARTHASARADHI, Karri 10 Jonquil Way, Colchester CO4 5UW — MB BS Andhra 1972.

PARTHASARATHY, Doralsamy Front Street Surgery, 16 Front Street, Annfield Plain, Stanley DH9 8HY Tel: 01207 281888 — MB BS Madras 1975; MB BS 1975 Madras; LMSSA Lond 1989. GP Stanley, Co. Durh.

PARTHASARATHY, Mallika Front Street Surgery, 16 Front Street, Annfield Plain, Stanley DH9 8HY Tel: 01207 231112 — MB BS Madras 1975; MB BS 1975 Madras; LMSSA Lond 1989. GP Stanley, Co. Durh.

PARTHASARATHY, Pobbathi Balaramaiah Chesterfield & North Derbyshire Royal Hospital, Orthopaedics Department, Calow, Chesterfield S44 5BL — MB BS Bangalor 1974; MB BS Bangalore 1974.

PARTHIPAN, Kanthapillai 49 Haverford Way, Edgware HA8 6DJ — LMSSA Lond. 1993. Specialty: Respirat. Med.; General Internal Medicine.

PARTINGTON, Andrew Lamond Cottage, Over Kellet, Carnforth LA6 1DN Tel: 01524 734565 — MB ChB Leeds 1989; DRCOG 1992; DFFP 1993; MRCGP 1993. Prev: Trainee GP/SHO Bolton AHA VTS; Ho. Off. (Med.) Bolton Gen. Hosp.; Ho. Off. (Surg.) Bolton Roy. Infirm.

PARTINGTON, Andrew Gareth Chy-an-Bron, St Tudy, Bodmin PL30 3NH — BM BCh Oxf. 1981; MA Camb. 1978; MRCGP 1986; DRCOG 1986. GP St. Columb Maj..

PARTINGTON, Christopher Terence The Medical Centre, Forest Gate Road, Corby NN17 1TR — MB ChB Leic. 1990; DRCOG 1995; DMJ (Clin) 2000. GP; Police Surg. Leics.; Police Surg. N.ants. Specialty: Obst. & Gyn. Socs: BMA & Assn. Police Surgs. Prev: Trainee GP Leicester VTS.

PARTINGTON, Colin Kjeld, Squadron Ldr. RAF Med. Br. Retd. Department of Obstetrics & Gynaecology, St. John's Hospital, Wood Street, Chelmsford CM2 9BG Tel: 01245 513047 Mob: 07881 826701 — MB BS Lond. 1975 (Westm. Hosp. Sch. of Med., Univ. of Lond.) MRCOG 1983; MD Lond. 1992. Cons. O & G Mid Essex NHS Hosps. Trust. Specialty: Obst. & Gyn. Special Interest: Colposcopy; Gen. Obst. & Gyn. Socs: Brit. Gyn. Cancer Soc.; Brit. Soc. Gyn. Endoscopy; Brit Soc. Colp & Cervical Path. (BSCCP). Prev: Sen. Regist. (O & G) Inst. O & G Hammersmith Hosp. Lond.; Regist. (O & G) Centr. Middlx. Hosp. Lond.; Sen. Specialist (O & G) RAF Med. Br.

PARTINGTON, Eileen Patricia Port Isaac Practice, Hillson Close, Port Isaac PL29 3TR; Chy-an-Bron, St Tudy, Bodmin PL30 3NH — MB ChB Bristol 1982; DRCOG 1985; MRCGP 1986. GP Asst. Prev: GP Trainee Plymouth HA VTS.; Ho. Phys. Plymouth HA; Ho. Surg. Plymouth HA.

PARTINGTON, Francis Ian (retired) High Bank, 183 Havant Road, Drayton, Portsmouth PO6 1EE Tel: 023 9237 5450 — (St. Geo.) MB BS Lond. 1952; MRCS Eng. LRCP Lond. 1952; DObst RCOG 1954. Prev: Med. Examr. Roy. Lond. Mutual Insur. Soc. & Other Insur. Cos.

PARTINGTON, Jane Rebecca 2 The Old Bobbin Mill, Wray, Lancaster LA2 8QR — BM BS Nottm. 1997.

PARTINGTON, John Stanley The New City Medical Centre, Tatham Street, Hendon, Sunderland SR1 2QB Tel: 0191 567 5571 — MB BS Newc. 1987.

PARTINGTON, Michael James Hope House, Anstey, Buntingford SG9 0BP — MB ChB Otago 1984.

PARTINGTON, Mr Paul Francis Wansbeck General Hospital, Woodhorn Lane, Ashington NE63 9JJ Tel: 01670 529672 Fax: 01670529656; 8 McCracken Close, Gosforth, Newcastle upon Tyne NE3 2DW Tel: 0191 217 1768 Fax: 0191 217 1768 — MB BS Newc. 1987 (Univ. of Newc upon Tyne) FRCS Eng. 1992; FRCS (Orth) 1997. Cons. (Orthop. Surg.) Ashington, N.umberland. Specialty: Trauma & Orthop. Surg. Prev: Sen. Regist. (Orthop. Surg.) Newc.; Clin. Fell. Lower Limb Reconstruction Univ. Hosp. Lond. Ont. Canada.

PARTINGTON, Robert John 33 Camm Street, Walkley, Sheffield S6 3TR — MB ChB Sheff. 1994.

PARTINGTON, Susan Isabel Perrancoomb House, Perrancoomb, Perranporth TR6 0HZ — MB BS Lond. 1974. Clin. Med. Off. Child Health Cornw. & I. of Scilly AHA. Prev: Ho. Phys. & Ho. Surg. Cornw. & I. of Scilly AHA.

PARTLETT, Polly 4 Westbridge Road, Launceston PL15 8HS — MB BS Lond. 1998 (Char. Cross & Westm.) SHO Surgic. Rotat., Kingston Hosp., Surrey. Specialty: Gen. Surg. Prev: POHO, Surg. & Orthop., Kingston Hosp., Surrey; PRHO, Rheum. & Endocrinol. with Gen. Med., Char. Cross Hosp., Lond.

PARTON, Andrew Brian The Surgery, 2 Mark Street, Rochdale OL12 9BE Tel: 01204 884873 — MB ChB Liverp. 1992; BSc (Molecular Biol.) Liverp. 1987, MB ChB 1992; DCH 1997; DFFP 1998; DRCOG 1998; MRCGP (merit) 1999. SHO (A & E) Roy. Liverp. Hosp. & Demonst. (Anat.) Liverp. Univ. Specialty: Gen. Pract. Prev: GP VTS Bury. Lancs.

PARTON, Elizabeth Querida 31 Ambleside Avenue, London SW16 1QE — MB BS Lond. 1980. Dept. Forens. Gyn. Caldecot Centre Kings Coll. Hosp. Lond.; Dept. Community Gyanecology S. W. Lond. Consultants Trust.

PARTON, Jeremy (retired) 200 Victoria Road, Wargrave, Reading RG10 8AJ — (Middlx.) MB BS Lond. 1958; MRCGP 1981; Dip. Palliat. Med. Wales 1996. Prev: Assoc. Specialist (Palliat. Med.) Sue Ryder Home Nettlebed Oxon.

PARTON, John Bayard (retired) The Hollies, Higher St., Norton Sub Hamdon, Stoke-sub-Hamdon TA14 6SN Tel: 01935 881445 — (St. Mary's) MB BS Lond. 1950; MRCS Eng. LRCP Lond. 1950; DO Eng. 1958. Prev: Clin. Asst. Ashford Hosp. Middlx. & Char. Cross Hosp. Lond.

PARTON, Matthew James Department of Neurology, King's College Hospital, London SE5 8AF — BChir Camb. 1992.

PARTON, Michael James West Kirby Health Centre, The Concourse, West Kirby, Wirral CH48 4HZ — MB ChB Liverp. 1993 (L'pool) BSc Liverpl 1990; DLO RCS (Eng) 1999; DRCOG 2000. Specialty: Otorhinolaryngol.

PARTON, Simon Dominic 99 Hassett Road, London E9 5SL — MB BS Lond. 1995.

PARTRIDGE, Mr Alan Bernard (retired) 55 Hipwell Court, Olney MK46 5QB — MB ChB Ed. 1952; BA Nat. Sc. Trip. Camb. 1946, MA 1952; DMRD Eng. 1967. Prev: Radiol. Christian Med. Coll. Hosp. Vellore, S. India.

PARTRIDGE, Barbara Winifred Mary (retired) Cheriton, Redcliffe Road, Torquay TQ1 4QG Tel: 01803 329998 — MB BCh BAO Dub. 1952 (T.C. Dub.) MA Dub. 1954, MD 1961. Assoc. Specialist (A & E) Torbay Hosp. Prev: SHO (Phys.) Torbay Hosp. Torquay.

PARTRIDGE, Brian Edward Cobbs Garden Surgery, West Street, Olney MK46 5QG Tel: 01234 711344; 12 St. Josephs Close, Olney MK46 5HD Tel: 01234 712583 — MB ChB Leic. 1983; DRCOG 1986. Prev: Trainee GP Kettering VTS.

PARTRIDGE, Carolyn — MB BCh Wales 1995 (Univ. Wales Coll. Med. Cardiff) BMedSc (Path. Sci.) Wales 1994; Dip. Biomed. Methods Wales 1997. Staff Grade (Psychiat.) Lidttlecourt/Belmont Ho. Burnham-on-Sea. Specialty: Gen. Psychiat. Prev: CMO (Psychiat.) Littlecourt/Belmont Ho., Burnham-on-Sea; CMO (Psychiat.) Priory Pk., Wells; Ho. Off. (Surg.) Univ. Hosp. Wales Cardiff.

PARTRIDGE, Carolyn Rosemary-Anne Wellington House Practice, Wades Field, Stratton Rd, Princes Risborough HP27 9AX Tel: 01844 344281 Fax: 01844 274719; 1 Upper Ashlyns Road, Berkhamsted HP4 3BW Tel: 01442 864582 — MB BChir Camb. 1973 (Camb. & Newc.) BA Camb. 1969; MB (conferred) 1972; MRCP (UK) 1975. Clin. Asst. (Rheum.) Watford Gen. Hosp. Specialty: Rheumatol.

PARTRIDGE, Christiaan James The Health Centre, Castleton Way, Eye IP23 7DD Tel: 01379 870689 Fax: 01379 871182; 29 Windgap Lane, Haughley, Stowmarket IP14 3PB — MB ChB Dund. 1998; DCH 2001; DRCOG Lond. 2001; MRCGP 2002. GP Princip. Specialty: Gen. Pract. Special Interest: Sexual Health.

PARTRIDGE, Craig Andrew 23 Barnes Avenue, Stockport SK4 4DR — MB ChB Leeds 1994.

PARTRIDGE, David Ralph 45 Pembroke Road, Clifton, Bristol BS8 3BE — MB ChB Bristol 1982; BSc Psychol. Bristol 1979, MB ChB 1982; DRCOG 1985; MRCGP 1986. Prev: Trainee GP Avon VTS.

PARTRIDGE, Edward Deverall Pentlands Cottage, High Road, Chipstead, Coulsdon CR5 3SB — MB ChB Birm. 1996; ChB Birm. 1996.

PARTRIDGE, Elspeth Murray Macclesfield District General Hospital, Victoria Road, Macclesfield SK10 3BL — MB ChB Glas. 1985; MRCP (UK) 1988; FRCR 1992. Cons. Radiol. E. Chesh. NHS Trust. Specialty: Radiol. Prev: Sen. Regist. (Radiol.) Mersey RHA.

PARTRIDGE, Fiona Jane Hedges Medical Centre, Pasley Road, Eyres Monsell, Leicester LE2 9BU Tel: 0116 225 1277 — MB ChB Leic. 1994; MA Cantab. GP Princip., The Hedges Med. Centre, Leicester. Specialty: Gen. Pract.; Genitourinary Medicine; Infec. Dis. Prev: SHO (Ophth.) Leicester Roy. Infirm.

PARTRIDGE, Gerald William Holycroft Surgery, The Health Centre, Oakworth Road, Keighley BD21 1SA Tel: 020 7941 1831 Fax: 020 7941 1830 — BM BCh Oxf. 1976 (Oxford) MA Oxf. 1976; MRCGP 1982. Cardiac NSF Lead, Airedale Primary Care Trust. Socs: BMA; Primary Care Cardiovasc. Soc.; Christian Med. Fell. Prev: Trainee GP Kettering VTS; Regist. (Path.) Radcliffe Infirm. Oxf.; Ho. Phys. & Ho. Surg. Gen. Infirm. Leeds.

PARTRIDGE, James William (retired) 85 Willes Road, Leamington Spa CV31 1BS Tel: 01926 427452 — MB BChir Camb. 1962 (Middlx.) DObst RCOG 1963; DCH Eng. 1963; FRCP Lond. 1982, M 1965; MA Camb. 1967. Prev: Cons. Paediat. S. Warks. Hosp. Gp.

PARTRIDGE, John Upper Green Road, St. Helens, Ryde PO33 1UG Tel: 01983 872772; 49 Foreland Road, Bembridge PO35 5XN — MB ChB Bristol 1977; DRCOG 1979; FRCGP 2000; MSc Principal in Gen. Practice 2001. Princip. in Gen. Pract.

PARTRIDGE, John Barry Department of Radiology, Harefield Hospital, Harefield, Uxbridge UB9 6JH Tel: 01895 828628 Fax: 01895 828590 — (UCHMS London) MB BS Lond. 1969; FFR 1974; FRCR 1975; FRACR 1984; FRCP 1998. Cons. Cardiothoracic Radiol. Harefield Hosp. Middlx. Specialty: Radiol. Socs: Cardiac Radiol. Gp. RCR; Cardiac Soc.; Brit. Soc. Echocardiogr. Prev: Assoc. Prof. Radiol. Univ. Queensland, Austral.; Specialist Cardiac Radiol. P. Chas. Hosp. Brisbane, Austral.; Cardiac Radiol. Killingbeck Hosp. Leeds.

PARTRIDGE, Mr John Philip (retired) Tawton House, Bishop's Tawton, Barnstaple EX32 0DB — MB BS Lond. 1944 (St. Mary's) MRCS Eng. LRCP Lond. 1943; FRCS Eng. 1951. Prev: Cons. Surg. N. Devon Dist. Hosp. Barnstaple.

PARTRIDGE, Jonathan Miles Flat 1F1, 27 Montague St., Edinburgh EH8 9QT — MB ChB Ed. 1996.

PARTRIDGE, Professor Martyn Richard Charing Cross Hospital, Charing Cross Campus, Department of Respiratory Medicine Imperial College London, Fulham Palace Road, London W6 8RP Tel: 020 8846 7181 Fax: 020 8846 7999 Email: m.partridge@imperial.ac.uk; Westfields, 4 Westfield, Loughton IG10 4EB Tel: 020 8502 1156 Email: Martyn.Partridge@btinternet.com — MB ChB Manch. 1972; MRCP (UK) 1975; MD Manch. 1980; FRCP Lond. 1989. Prof. of Respiratory Med. Imperial Coll. Lond. & Hon. Cons. Phys. Char. Cross Hosp. Lond. (Hammersmith Hosps. NHS Trust); Chief Med. Adviser Nat. Asthma Campaign; Chairman Trustees Nat. Resp. Training Centre; Mem Specialist Advis. Comm. in Respirat. Med. Specialty: Respirat. Med. Prev: Cons. Phys. Whipps Cross Hosp. Lond.; Sen. Regist. (Med.) Lond. Chest. & Univ. Coll. Hosps. Lond.; Regist. Hammersmith Hosp. Lond.

PARTRIDGE, Rena Elizabeth (retired) 55 Hipwell Court, Olney MK46 5QB Tel: 01234 240018 — MB ChB Ed. 1952; DObst RCOG 1955. Prev: Family Plann. Off. Christian Med. Coll. Hosp. Vellore, S. India.

PARTRIDGE, Richard Francis c/o Duchess of Kent House, 22 Liebenrood Road, Reading RG30 2DX — BM BS Nottm. 1998; BMedSci Nottm. 1996; MRCP 2001.

PARTRIDGE, Mr Richard James 23 Middle Bourne Lane, Farnham GU10 3NH Tel: 01252 719244 Fax: 01252 719244 — MB BS Lond. 1978 (St.Geo.) FRCS Ed. 1983; FFAEM 1993. Cons. A & E Med., Frimley Pk. Hosp. Surrey; Lect. (Orthop. & Rheum.) Brit. Sch. Osteop. Lond. Specialty: Accid. & Emerg.; Sports Med. Special Interest: Surgical Dermatology.

PARTRIDGE, Sally Joy The Limes Surgery, 172 High Street, Lye, Stourbridge DY9 8LL Tel: 01384 422234 — MB ChB Birm. 1983; MB ChB (Hons.) Birm. 1983; DRCOG 1986; MRCGP 1987; DCH 1988. GP Stourbridge. Prev: Trainee GP E. Birm. Hosp. VTS.

PARTRIDGE, Samuel James 134 Broadoak Road, Langford, Bristol BS40 5HB Tel: 01934 853381 — MB ChB Bristol 1996; MRCP (UK); DRCOG. GP Regist. Specialty: Gen. Med.

PARTRIDGE, Sarah Elizabeth Clinical Oncology, Charing Cross Hospital, Fulham Palace Road, London W6 8RF Tel: 0208 8461234 — FRCR 1998; MB BS UMDS Lond. 1990; MRCP (UK) 1994. Specialty: Oncol.; Radiother. Socs: Assoc. Mem. Roy. Soc. Med. Prev: SHO (Gen. Med.) Chelsea & Westm. Hosp. Lond.; SHO (Med.) Watford Gen. Hosp.; Ho. Surg. Qu. Alexandra Hosp. Portsmouth.

PARTRIDGE, Susan Marie Dept. of Pathology, Furness General Hospital, Dalton Lane, Barrow-in-Furness LA14 4LF Tel: 01229 491022 Fax: 01229 491044 — MB ChB Leic. 1987; BSc (Hons) Med. Sci. Leic 1984; MRCPath 2000. Cons. Microbiol., Furness Gen. Hosp. Specialty: Med. Microbiol. Prev: SHO (Microbiol.) Qu. Med. Centre Nottm.; Regist./Specialist Regist. (Microbiol.) Sheff. Teachg. Hosps.

PARTRIDGE, Suzanne Brough and South Cave Medical Practice, 4 Centurion Way, Brough HU15 1AY Tel: 01482 658446 Fax: 01482 665090 — BM BS Nottm. 1993; BMedSci Nottm. 1991; DRCOG Lond. 1997; MRCGP Lond. 1997. GP Princip. Hull. Specialty: Gen. Pract.

PARTRIDGE, Thomas Murray Upton Group Practice, 32 Ford Road, Wirral CH49 0TF Tel: 0151 677 0486 Fax: 0151 604 0635; 26 Croome Drive, West Kirby, Wirral CH48 8AH — MB ChB Ed. 1985; MRCGP 1992.

PARUMS, Dinah Velta The Keysmith,, High Street, Boxworth, Cambridge CB3 8LY Tel: 01954267738 Fax: 01954 267738 Email: dvp@dinahmac.demon.co.uk — BM BCh Oxf. 1983 (Camb. & Oxf.) PhD Camb 1987, MA 1984, BA 1980; MRCPath 1992; FCCP 1998; FRCPath 1999. Cancer Clin. Expert - Histopath., Astrazeneca UK. Specialty: Histopath. Special Interest: Cardiovascular; Oncology; Pulmonary. Socs: Path. Soc. of Gt. Britain and Irel.; Internat. Acad. of Path. Prev: Cons. Cardiothoracic Path. Freeman Hosp. Newc.; Sen. Lect. & Cons. (Histopath.) Roy. Postgrad. Med. Sch. Hammersmith Hosp. Lond.; Clin. Tutor, Clin. Lect. & Hon. Sen. Regist. Nuffield Dept. Path. John Radcliffe Hosp. Oxf.

PARVATHAM, Krishnamurty Edward St Hospital, Edward Street, West Bromwich P70 8NL Tel: 0121 553 7676 Email: kparvatham@yahoo.co.uk — MB BS Andhra 1962. Assoc. Specialist (Psychiat. Geriat.) Edwd. St Hosp. W. Bromwich. Specialty: Geriat. Psychiat.

PARVEEN, Shada Shane Maybury Surgery, Alpha Road, Maybury, Woking GU22 8HF Tel: 01483 728757 Fax: 01483 729169 — MB BS Lond. 1982 (Charing Cross Hosp. Med. Sch.) Specialty: Gen. Pract. Socs: BMA.

PARVIN, Mr Simon Dudley Royal Bournemouth Hospital, Castle Lane East, Bournemouth BH7 7DW Tel: 01202 704621 Fax: 01202 704622 Email: simon.parvin@rbch.nhs.uk; 12 Spencer Road, Canford Cliffs, Poole BH13 7EU Tel: 01202 709626 Fax: 01202 709693 — MD Leic. 1988; MB BS Lond. 1975; FRCS Ed. 1980; FRCS Eng. 1981. Cons. Gen. & Vasc. Surg. Bournemouth & Poole Hosps. Specialty: Gen. Surg. Prev: Lect./Hon. Sen. Regist. Leic. Univ.

PARVIS, Alexander Home (retired) 954 Chelsea Cloisters, Sloane Avenue, London SW3 3EU — MRCS Eng. LRCP Lond. 1947 (Guy's) BA, MD Amer. Univ. Beirut 1941; DOMS Eng. 1949. Prev: Cons. Lect. (Ophth.) City Univ. Lond.

PARWAIZ, Mr Khalid Hinchingbrooke Hospital, Department of Urology, Huntingdon PE29 6JB Email: kparwciz0108@yahoo.co.uk — MB BS Patna 1986 (Patna.med.Coll) FRCS Ed. 1991; Dip. Urol. 1994. Staff Urol. Hinchingbrooke Hosp. Huntingdon; Cons. Vasectomy Clinic Cromwell Clinic Huntingdon. Specialty: Urol. Special Interest: Andrology; Endo-Urology. Socs: MDU.
PARWAIZ, Paul Ratby Surgery, 122-124 Station Road, Ratby, Leicester LE6 0JP — MRCS Eng. LRCP Lond. 1979 (Manch.)
PARWANI, Mr Ghanshyam Shivaldas 64 Kingsway, Gillingham ME7 3BD — MB BS Nagpur 1956 (Nagpur Med. Coll.) FRCS Eng. 1966. Cons. Rehabil. Med. Disabil. Servs. Centre Harold Wood Hosp. Romford. Socs: Fell. Brit. Soc. Orthop. Assn.; Internat. Soc. Prosth.s & Orthotics. Prev: Ho. Surg. Safdarjung Hosp. New Delhi, India; Regist. (Orthop.) Notley Orthop. Centre Braintree; Regist. (Surg.) NE Essex HA.
PARYS, Mr Bohdan Tadeusz Department of Urology, Rotherham District General Hospital, Moorgate Road, Rotherham S60 2UD Tel: 01709 304061 Fax: 01709 307193 Email: parys.sec@rothgen.nhs.uk; 3 Castle Dyke Mews, Ringinglow Road, Sheffield S11 7TA — MB BS Lond. 1979 (Roy. Free) FRCS Ed. 1985; ChM Liverp. 1990; FRCS (Urol.) 1993. Cons. Urol. Rotherham Dist. Gen. Hosp. Specialty: Urol. Socs: Brit. Assn. Urol. Surgs.; BMA; Internat. Continence Soc. Prev: Sen. Regist. (Urol.) Roy. Hallamsh. Hosp. Sheff.; Regist. (Urol.) Roy. Preston Hosp.; Research Fell. (Urol.) Roy. Liverp. Hosp.
PASAPULA, Chadra Seker 5 Dickens Close, Cheshunt, Waltham Cross EN7 6BG — MB BS Lond. 1996.
PASCALL, Caroline Margaret Emma 46 Brandon Village, Brandon, Durham DH7 8SU — MB BS Lond. 1983; MRCGP 1988.
PASCALL, Mr Charles Richard Williton and Watchet Surgeries, Robert Street, Williton, Taunton TA4 4QE Tel: 01984 632701 Fax: 01984 633933; Heddon House, Crowcombe, Taunton TA4 4BJ — MB BS Lond. 1974; FRCS Eng. 1979. Clin. Asst. Gen. Surg. Som. HA. Prev: Surgic. Regist. Norwich HA.
PASCALL, Emma Jane Heddon House, Crowcombe, Taunton TA4 4BJ Tel: 01984 618642 — MB ChB Liverp. 1978; FFA RCS Eng. 1987. Assoc. Specialist (Anaesth.) Taunton & Som. NHS Trust. Specialty: Anaesth.
PASCALL, Mr Keith Gardner (retired) Wiverton House, Plympton, Plymouth PL7 5AA Tel: 01752 337276 — (Guy's) LMSSA Lond. 1937; MB BS Lond. 1938; FRCS Ed. 1946. Prev: Sen. Cas. Off. Plymouth Gen. Hosp.
PASCALL, Nicola Jayne — BM Soton. 1997.
PASCALL, Olive Joyce The Glade, Grindley Bank, Mickle Trafford, Chester CH2 4EQ — MB BCh BAO NUI 1947; DA Eng. 1956. Med. Off. Blood Transfus. Serv. Mersey RHA; Sessional Med. Off. Chesh. HA. Prev: Sessional Med. Off. Sheff. Blood Transfus. Serv.; Regist. (Anaesth.) N. Sheff. Gen. Hosp.
PASCOE, Karen Frances 28 Heol Y Foel, Llawtwit Fardre, Pontypridd CF38 2EQ — MB ChB Liverp. 1988; MRCGP 1992. GP Retainer Scheme M. Glam.
PASCOE, Keith Laurence Crown Medical Practice, Tamworth Health Centre, Upper Gungate, Tamworth B79 7EA Tel: 01827 58728 Fax: 01827 63873 — MB BCh Wales 1973.
PASCOE, R J M Belgrave Medical Centre, 22 Asline Road, Sheffield S2 4UJ Tel: 0114 255 1184.
PASH, Jonathan David — MB ChB Dundee 1993.
PASH, Raphael (retired) 31 Tormead Road, Guildford GU1 2JA Tel: 01483 838290 — MB BCh Wales 1957; DA Eng. 1966.
PASHA, Mahmood Seymour Grove Health Centre, 70 Seymour Grove, Old Trafford, Manchester M16 0LW; 381 Wilbraham Road, Whalley Range, Manchester M16 8NG Tel: 0161 881 0171 — MB BS Karachi 1960 (Dow Med. Coll.) BSc. Punjab 1955; DIH Eng. 1974. Socs: Fell. Manch. Med. Soc. Prev: SHO Memor. Hosp. Darlington; Asst. Resid. Med. Off. Salford Roy. Hosp.
PASHA, Mohamed Abdulla (retired) 31 Willingale Way, Thorpe Bay, Southend-on-Sea SS1 3SN Tel: 01702 586610 — MB BS Andhra 1953; FRCP Glas. 1979, M 1965. Cons. Phys. (Geriat.) Southend-on-Sea Hosp. Gp. Prev: Med. Asst. Chest Unit, Southend-on-Sea Hosp. Gp.
PASHA, Nadeem Dean 536 Chelsea Cloisters, Sloane Avenue, London SW3 3EH Email: pdean121@aol.com — MB BS Lond. 1993. Cosmetic Doctor with special interest in gynaecolgy, anti-ageing & sports medicine; Chief Med. Director C B Health Los Angeles USA; Med. Cons. to several eminent healthcare organisations in Europe & USA advising on FDA protocols. Socs: Brit. Assn. Cosmetic Doctors.
PASHANKAR, Dinesh Shrikrishna 6 Amity Road, London E15 4AT — MB BS Poona 1987; MRCP (UK) 1993.
PASHANKAR, Farzana Dinesh 6 Amity Road, London E15 4AT — MB BS Poona 1989.
PASHBY, Mr Nigel Lowthrop Northgate, Church St., Uttoxeter ST14 8AG Tel: 01889 562010 — MB BS Lond. 1969 (Roy. Free) MRCS Eng. LRCP Lond. 1969; FRCS Eng. 1977. GP Uttoxeter. Prev: Research Fell. Dept. Surg. Univ. Hosp. Wales Card.; Regist. (Surg.) Bristol Roy. Infirm.
PASHLEY, Camilla Elizabeth Headcorn Surgery, Headcorn; Stream Barn, Golford Road, Cranbrook TN17 3NT Tel: 01580 713423 — BM BS Nottm. 1986; MRCGP 1991; DRCOG 1991. GP. Specialty: Gen. Pract. Prev: GP Princip.; Regist. (Palliat. Med.) Princess Alice Hospice Esher.
PASHLEY, Julia Kathryn 2 Chestnut Spinney, Droitwich WR9 7QD — MB BS Lond. 1993.
PASI, Kanwal Chandra 2 Castel Close, Seabridge, Newcastle ST5 3EG — MB BS Punjab 1954; DPH Leeds 1965. Prev: GP Stoke-on-Trent; PMO Lond. Boro Havering; Admin. Med. Off. City of Birm.
PASI, Kanwal John Division of Haematology, University of Leicester, Leicester Royal Infirmary, Leicester LE2 7LX Tel: 0116 252 3256 Email: jp69@le.ac.uk/kjp@rfhsm.ac.uk — MB ChB Birm. 1983; MRCP (UK) 1986; MRCPath 1993; PhD Birm. 1994; FRCPCH 1997; FRCP Lond. 1998; FRCPath 2001. Prof. of Haemat., Univ. of Leicester, Hon. Cons., Univ. Hosp. of Leicester NHS Trust. Specialty: Haematology. Prev: Lect. (Haemat.) Roy. Free Hosp. Lond.; Research Fell. (Haemat.) Childr. Hosp. Birm.; Con. Haemat. & Hon Gen. Lect. Roy. Free Hosp. Lond.
PASKA, Lubomyr Mychajlo 11 Lucknow Street, Rochdale OL11 1RH — MB BS Lond. 1990; BSc (Hons.) Lond. 1984, MB BS 1990. SHO (Gen. Med.) Maidsstone Hosp. Barming. Prev: SHO (Geriat. Med.) Qu. Mary Univ. Hosp. Lond.; SHO (A & E) Ashford Hosp. Middlx.
PASKIN, Donald George (retired) Chestnut Tree Cottage, Whitegate, Northwich CW8 2BY — MRCS Eng. LRCP Lond. 1956; DObst RCOG 1958. Prev: GP N.wich.
PASKINS, Mr John Roderick 17 Birchwood Dell, Doncaster DN4 6SY — MB BS Lond. 1972 (Char. Cross) FRCS Eng. 1977. Cons. A & E Med., Doncaster Roy. Infirm. Specialty: Accid. & Emerg. Socs: Cas. Surgs. Assn. Prev: Sen. Regist. (A & E Med.) Roy. Hallamshire Hosp. Sheff.; Research Fell. Paediat. Surg. St. Thos. Hosp. Lond.; Regist. (Surg.) St. Thos. Hosp. Lond.
PASSANI, Stefano Little Blakes, South View Road, Danbury, Chelmsford CM3 4DX — State Exam Rome 1978; Stat Exam Rome 1978.
PASSANT, Colin Charles Windhill Green Medical Centre, 2 Thackley Old Road, Shipley BD18 1QB Tel: 01274 584223 Fax: 01274 530182 — MB ChB Leeds 1985; DRCOG 1988; MRCGP 1990. Socs: Brit. Med. Acupunct. Soc. Prev: Ho. Phys. & Ho. Surg. Airedale Gen. Hosp. Keighley.
PASSANT, Wendy Sharon Grey Haigh Hall Medical Centre, Haigh Hall Road, Greengates, Bradford BD10 9AZ Tel: 01274 613326 — (Leeds) BSc (Hons.) Leeds 1982; MB ChB Leeds 1985; DCH RCP Lond. 1989; DRCOG 1990. GP Principle.
PASSI, Man Mohan Lal Leicester Street Medical Centre, Leicester Street, Wolverhampton WV6 0PS Tel: 01902 24118; 16 Showell Lane, Wolverhampton WV4 4UA Tel: 01902 58846 — MB BS Rajasthan 1957; DPH Calcutta 1960; DIH Eng. 1964; DTM & H Lond 1964.
PASSI, Uma 16 Showell Lane, Wolverhampton WV4 4UA Tel: 01902 58846 — MB BS Punjab 1961; MB BS Punjab (India) 1961; DObst RCOG 1964; DA Eng. 1964.
PASSI, Vimmi 16 Showell Lane, Wolverhampton WV4 4UA — MB BCh Wales 1995.
PASSMORE, Anthony Peter 108 Malone Road, Belfast BT9 5HP Tel: 02890 272158 Fax: 02890 325839 Email: p.passmore@qub.ac.uk; 108 Malone Road, Belfast BT9 5HP Tel: 02890 272158 Fax: 02890 325839 Email: p.passmore@qub.ac.uk — MB BCh Belf. 1981; FRCP (Lond. 1995, Glas. 1996); BSc Physiol. (1st cl. Hons.) Belf. 1978, MD 1987, MB BCh BAO 1981; MRCP (UK) 1984. Sen. Lect. Dept. Geriat. Med., Qu.s Univ. Belf.;

Cons. Phys. Specialty: Care of the Elderly. Socs: Mem. Brit. Geriatics Soc.; Mem. Brit. Hypertens. Soc.; Fell. Ulster Med. Soc. Prev: Sen. Regist. Dept. Therap. & Clin. Pharmacol. Qu. Univ. Belf.

PASSMORE, Kirsty Emma 36 Avon Way, Portishead, Bristol BS20 6JQ — MB ChB Leeds 1996.

PASSMORE, Sarah Jane Hospital for Sick Children, Gt Ormond Street, London WC1N Tel: 020 7405 9200 x0112 Fax: 020 7813 8588 Email: jane@ccrg.ox.ac.uk — MB BS Newc. 1984 (Newcastle Upon Tyne) MRCP (UK) 1987; DCH RCP Lond. 1989. Cons. Paediatric Oncologist; Snr Regist..Childh. Cancer Research Grp Oxford. Specialty: Paediat. Special Interest: Paediatric Myelodysplasia & JMML. Socs: UKCCSG (United Kingdom Childhood Cancer Study Group). Prev: Clin. Research Fell. (Haemat. & Oncol.) Hosp. for Sick Childr. Gt. Ormond St. Lond.; Regist. (Paediat.) Roy. Devon & Exeter Hosp. & Southmead Hosp.

PASTERSKI, Jerzy Kazimierz — Lekarz Warsaw 1969; MRCPsych. 1979; T(Psych.) 1991; FRCPsych 1998. Med. Dir., Altrincham Priory Hosp., Chesh. Specialty: Gen. Psychiat. Special Interest: Biopolar disorder. Prev: Cons. Psychiat.. Trafford Area Health Auth., Manch.

PASTOR, Thomas Greenacres & Homefield, Homefield Road, Worthing BN11 2HS Tel: 01903 212206 Fax: 01903 218799; Goring Hall Hospital, Bodiam Avenue, Goring-by-Sea, Worthing BN12 5AT Tel: 01903 506699 Fax: 01903 700782 — MB BS Lond. 1968 (Univ. Coll. Hosp.) MRCS Eng. LRCP Lond. 1968; DPM Eng. 1974; MRCPsych 1975. Cons. Psychiat. (Psychother.) Worthing Priority Care NHS Trust. Specialty: Gen. Psychiat. Socs: Fell. Roy. Soc. Med.; BMA. Prev: Lect. (Psychiat.) Univ. Lond. & Hon. Sen. Regist. St. Mary's Hosp. Lond.; Regist. (Psychiat.) Roy. Free Hosp. Friern Hosp.; SHO Univ. Coll. Hosp. Lond.

PASUPATHY, Amirtha 26 Lapstone Gardens, Harrow HA3 0ED — MB BS Peradeniya, Sri Lanka 1983.

PASUPATHY, Dharmintra Flat 1, Block 10, Wilsford Green, Oakhill Drive, Edgbaston, Birmingham B15 3UG; Flat 1, Block 10,, Wilsford Green, Oakhill Drive, Edgbaston, Birmingham B15 3UG — MB ChB Liverp. 1997; MBGB Liverpool 1997.

PASUPATHY RAJAH, Sathasivam The Haven, Wrotham Road, Hook Green, Meopham, Gravesend DA13 0HX Tel: 01474 812287 — MB BS Ceylon 1955 (Colombo) DCH Ceylon 1967; DPM Eng. 1973.

PASVOL, Professor Geoffrey Imperial College School of Medicine, Infection & Tropical Medicine Unit, Northwick Park Hospital, Harrow HA1 3UJ Tel: 020 8869 2831/2 Fax: 020 8869 2836 Email: g.pasvol@ic.ac.uk; 85 Fordington Road, Highgate, London N6 4TH Tel: 020 8444 7784 — MB ChB Cape Town 1972 (Univ. Cape Town) MRCP (UK) 1975; MA Oxf. 1987, DPhil 1978; FRCP Lond. 1990; FRCP Ed. 1996. Prof. Infec. Dis. & Trop. Med. Imperial Coll. Sch. Med. Harrow; Hon Cons in Infec dis & Trop Med N.W. Lond. Hosp.s Trust & St Mary's Hosp.; Hon Prof. Kings Coll. Lond. Specialty: Infec. Dis. Socs: Fell. RCP; Fell. Roy. Soc. Trop. Med. & Hyg.; Assn. Phys. Prev: Wellcome Sen. Lect. & Dep. Univ. Med. Off. Univ. Oxf.; Clin. Lect. (Trop. Med.) Nuffield Dept. Med. John Radcliffe Hosp. Oxf.; Research Stud. Nuffield Dept. Med. Radcliffe Infirm. Oxf.

PASZKOWSKA, Kazimiera Netheravon Road Surgery, 29 Netheravon Road, Chiswick, London W4 2NA Tel: 020 8994 2506 — LRCPI & LM, LRSCI & LM 1957; LRCPI & LM, LRCSI & LM 1957. Socs: BMA. Prev: Ho. Phys. St. Leonard's Hosp.; SHO Cas. & Orthop. Roy. Hosp. Richmond; SHO Anaesth. W. Middlx. Hosp. Isleworth.

PATALAY, Mr Tuljaram The Surgery, 62 Church Street, Edmonton, London N9 9PA — MB BS Osmania 1967 (Osmania Med. Coll.) FRCS Ed. 1974. Socs: Med. Defence Union.

PATANKAR, Mr Roy Suneel Vasudev University Surgical Unit, F Level, Southampton General Hospital, Southampton SO16 6YD — MB BS Bombay 1988; FRCS Glas. 1993; FRCS Ed. 1993.

PATANWALA, Saifuddin Kamruddin 11 Southlands Gardens, Morton, Gainsborough DN21 3EX Tel: 01427 610071 — MB BS Rajasthan 1971 (R.N.T. Med. Coll. Udaipur) MRCPI 1981; FRCP (I) 1998. Assoc. Specialist (Geriat & Gen. Med.) Lincoln Co. Hosp. Specialty: Care of the Elderly; Diabetes; Gen. Med. Socs: Lincoln Med. Soc.; BMA; Brit. Geriat. Soc. Prev: Assoc. Specialist (Geriat. & Gen. Med.) John Coupland Hosp. GainsBoro. & Co. Hosp. Lincoln; SCMO (Geriat. & Gen. Med.) John Coupland Hosp. GainsBoro.; Regist. (Geriat. & Gen. Med.) Pilgrim Hosp. Boston.

PATCH, David William Michael Dept of surgery,9th floor, Royal Free Hospital, Pond St., London NW3 2QG Tel: 020 7794 4688 — MB BS Lond. 1987; FRCP 2002. Cons. & Hon. Sen. Lect. Dept of Liver transplantation and Hepato. Med. Specialty: Gen. Med.; Gastroenterol.

PATCHETT, Douglas Robert, MC (retired) 58 Regency House, Newbold Terrace, Leamington Spa CV32 4HD Tel: 01926 423679 — (St. Mary's) MRCS Eng. LRCP Lond. 1944. Prev: Capt. RAMC.

PATCHETT, Ian Douglas Groby Road Medical Centre, 9 Groby Road, Leicester LE3 9ED Tel: 0116 253 8185 — MB ChB Leic. 1984; DRCOG 1988; MRCGP 1989. GP Leics.

PATCHETT, Paul Anthony Waterloo House Surgery, Waterloo House, 42-44 Wellington Street, Millom LA18 4DE Tel: 01229 772123 — MB ChB Bristol 1975; MRCP (UK) 1979; MRCGP 1984.

PATE, Elizabeth Gilmore 13 Laurel Avenue, Lenzie, Glasgow G66 4RX — MB ChB Glas. 1960; DCH RCPS Glas. 1964; DPH Glas. 1969.

PATEL, Aarron Neil Annie Prendergast Health Centre, Ashton Gardens, Chadwell Heath, Romford RM6 6RT — MB BS Lond. 1995.

PATEL, Abdul Rahim Ahmed Queen Elizabeth Psychiatric Hospital, Mindlesohn Way, Edgbaston, Birmingham B15 2QZ Tel: 0121 678 2027 Fax: 0121 678 2075; 5 Fitzroy Avenue, Harborne, Birmingham B17 8RL — MB ChB Zambia 1982 (University of Zambia) MSc Clin. Trop. Med. Lond. 1985; MRCPsych 1992. Cons. (Old Age Psychiat.), Qu. Eliz. Psychiatric Hosp. Specialty: Geriat. Psychiat. Prev: Sen. Regist. (Old Age Psychiat.) W. Midl. RHA.; Regist. Birm. Train. Scheme.

PATEL, Abhilash 3 Fugelmere Close, Harborne, Birmingham B17 8SE Tel: 0121 429 2488 — MB BS Newc. 1974 (Univ. Newc. u. Tyne) FFA RCS Eng. 1978. Cons. Anaesth. Univ. Hosp. Birm. NHS Trust & Sandwell NHS Trust. Specialty: Anaesth. Prev: Sen. Regist. (Anaesth.) W. Midl. RHA; Regist. & SHO (Anaesth.) Notts. AHA (T).

PATEL, Alberta Elizabeth 119 Chester Road, St.ly, Sutton Coldfield B74 2HE Tel: 0121 353 1888; 96 Chester Road N., Sutton Coldfield B73 6SL — MB BCh BAO Belf. 1957; DObst RCOG 1960. Socs: Med. Wom. Federat. (Hon. Br. Sec. Birm. & W. Midl.).

PATEL, Alka Manish 114 Francklyn Gardens, Edgware HA8 8SA Tel: 020 8958 3657 Fax: 020 8357 3471 Email: dralka@hotmail.com — MB BS Lond. 1995 (UMDS) DFFP 1997; DRCOG 1997; DCH 1998.

PATEL, Allison 5 Betony Walk, Haverhill CB9 7YA — MB BCh BAO NUI 1991; LRCPSI 1991; MRCOG 1997. Regist. (O & G) P'boro. Dist. Hosp., Cambs; Regist. (O & G). Specialty: Obst. & Gyn. Prev: Regist. (O & G) Whipps Cross Hosp. Lond.; Regist. (Obst. & Gyn.) Homerton Hosp. Lond.; Regist. (O & G) Princess Alex Andra Hosp., Harlaw.

PATEL, Alpa Mohanbhai 70 Lawn Street, Bolton BL1 3AY — MB ChB Manch. 1998.

PATEL, Alpesh 7 Lens Road, London E7 8PU — MB ChB Manch. 1992; BSc (Hons.) Manch. 1989; DCH RCP Lond. 1994; MRCGP 1997. Princip. GP Loughton Health Centre. Specialty: Gen. Pract.

PATEL, Ambalal Shankerlal The Surgery, Station Road, Shotton Colliery, Durham DH6 2JL Tel: 0191 526 5913 Fax: 0191 526 2651; Peterlee Health Centre, Peterlee SR8 1AD Tel: 0191 586 7414 — MB BS Gujarat 1973 (B.J. Med. Coll. Ahmedabad) Cert. Family Plann. JCC 1977; DObst RCPI 1979. Prev: Regist. (O & G) Gen. Hosp. Bishop Auckland, Middlesbrough Matern. Hosp. & Middlesbrough Gen. Hosp.; SHO (Obst.) Craigtoun Matern. Hosp. St. And.; SHO (O & G) North. Gen. Hosp. Sheff.

PATEL, Mr Ameet Ghanshyam Dept. of Surgery, King's College Hospital, Denmark Hill, London SE5 9RS Tel: 020 7346 3065 Fax: 020 7346 3438 Email: agp@ameet.dircon.co.uk — MB BS Lond. 1985 (St. George's Hosp. Med. Sch. Lond.) FRCS Ed. 1991; FRCS (Eng) 1992; MS 1999. Cons. (Surg.) King's Coll. Hosp. Lond. Specialty: Gen. Surg.

PATEL, Amish 19a Birch Park, Harrow HA3 6SP — MB ChB Manch. 1996. SHO (Gen. Med.) Rotat. Roy. Berksh. & Battle NHS Trust. Specialty: Gen. Med. Socs: MDU; BMA. Prev: Ho. Off. Roy. Preston Hosp. Lancs.

PATEL, Amish 12 Belvoir Close, Oadby, Leicester LE2 4SG Tel: 0116 271 9295 — MB BS Lond. 1998 (St Geo.) SHO (A&E) St.

Geo.'s Hosp. Lond. Specialty: Accid. & Emerg. Prev: Ho. Off. (Surg.) PeterBoro. Dist. Hosp. Cambs.; Ho. Off. (Med.) St. Geo.'s Hosp.

PATEL, Mr Amratlal Norfolk & Norwich University Hospital, Colney Lane, Norwich NR4 7UY Tel: 01603 286711 Fax: 01603 287160; 77 Newmarket Road, Norwich NR2 2HW Tel: 01603 763645 Fax: 01603 763645 — MB ChB Sheff. 1976; FRCS Eng. 1981. Cons. Orthop. Surg. & Specialist Trauma & Shoulder Disorders Norf. & Norwich Univ. Hosp. (since 1992). Specialty: Orthop. Socs: Brit. Trauma Soc.; Brit. Shoulder & Elbow Soc.; Brit. Limb Reconstruction Soc. Prev: Sen. Regist. SW Thames Region Train. Scheme; Clin. Fell. (Trauma) Sunnybrook Med. Centre Toronto, Canada; Regist. St. Geo. Hosp. Lond.

PATEL, Angela 1 Ennerdale Close, Huntingdon PE29 6UU — MB ChB Liverp. 1993.

PATEL, Anil Royal National Throat Nose and Ear Hospital, Grays Inn Road, London WC1X 8DA Tel: 020 7915 1669 Fax: 020 7278 3018 — MB BS Lond. 1991 (University College and Middlesex School of Medicine(London University)) FRCA 1995. Cons. Anaesth., The Roy. Nat. Throat, Nose & Ear Hosp., Lond.; Hon. Sen. Roy. Fre & Univ. Coll. Med. Sch., UCL. Specialty: Anaesth. Socs: Difficult Airway Soc. Prev: research fell., Paediat. IC Unit, Guy's Hosp.; Sen. Regist., Anaesth. Dept., Guy's Hosp.; Regist. Rotat. (Anaesth.) Qu. Vict. Hosp. E. Grinstead.

PATEL, Anilkumar Maganbhai 224 Balgores Lane, Romford RM2 6BS — MRCS Eng. LRCP Lond. 1991.

PATEL, Anita 12 Pinewood Drive, Potters Bar EN6 2BD — MB BCh Wales 1993.

PATEL, Anita — MB BS Lond. 1997. GP. Specialty: Gen. Pract.

PATEL, Anita Givindji 21 Farrans Court, Northwick Avenue, Harrow HA3 0AT — MB ChB Glas. 1986.

PATEL, Anjana 20 Brecknock Road, London N7 0DD — MB BS Lond. 1993.

PATEL, Anuj Wentworth Medical Practice, 38 Wentworth Avenue, Finchley Central, London N3 1YL Tel: 020 8346 1242 Fax: 020 8343 3614 — MB BS Lond. 1993.

PATEL, Mr Anup Department of Urology, St Mary's Hospital, Praed Street, London W2 1NY Tel: 020 886 1006/1033 Fax: 0207 7886 1546 — MB BS Lond. 1983 (St. Bart.) BSc (1st cl. Hons.) Lond. 1980; FRCS Eng. 1987; ECFMG 1993; MS 1994; (Urol.) FRCS 1994. Cons Urological Surg St Mary's Hosp Lond. Specialty: Urol. Special Interest: Endourology & endo-oncology; New technologies in urologic endo-oncology; Prostate Cancer. Socs: Full mem BAUS; Full Mem EAU; Corr. Mem AUA. Prev: Clin Instruc. in EndoUrol. & Urological Oncol. UCLA Calif.

PATEL, Anup Madhusudan 5 Broadcroft Avenue, Stanmore HA7 1NT Tel: 020 8357 5858 — MB BS Lond. 1993 (UMDS of Guy's and St. Thomas's Hosps.) MRCGP 1998. Princip. in Gen. Pract. Specialty: Gen. Pract. Socs: BMA & Med. Defence Union. Prev: SHO (Palliat. Care & A & E) N. Lond. Hospice; Trainee GP/SHO (O & G) Edgware.

PATEL, Arati Bhavesh Lawnside, St. Georges Road, Bickley, Bromley BR1 2LB Tel: 020 8467 6094 — MB ChB Sheff. 1990; DFFP 1994; T(GP) 1995. Trainee GP Lewisham & N. Southwark HA VTS. Prev: Ho. Off. Qu. Mary's Hosp. Sidcup; Ho. Off. Joyce Green Hosp. Dartford.

PATEL, Arti Manaharlal Sandy Health Centre Medical Practice, Northcroft, Sandy SG19 1JP; 10 Park Court, Sandy SG19 1NP — MB ChB Glasg. 1986. GP Princip. Sandy Health Centre Med. Pract. Specialty: Paediat.

PATEL, Aruna Ramanbhai St James House Surgery, County Court Road, King's Lynn PE30 5SY Tel: 01553 774221 Fax: 01553 692181 — MB BCh BAO NUI 1981; LRCPI & LM, LRCSI & LM 1981.

PATEL, Arunbhai Bhagwanbhai Health Centre, Wardles Lane, Great Wyrley, Walsall WS6 6EW Tel: 01922 411948 Fax: 01922 412994 — MB BS Gujarat 1971.

PATEL, Arvind Chhotu c/o Boydens Estate Agents, Aston House, 57-59 Crouch St., Colchester CO3 3EL — MB ChB Bristol 1975; DRCOG 1978; MRCGP 1979. Princip. Med. Off. (Communicable Dis.) Dept. Health, Wellington, NZ. Socs: Roy. NZ Coll. GP's & NZ Coll. Community Med.

PATEL, Arvind Manibhai (retired) Haematology Department, New Cross Hospital, Wolverhampton WV10 0QP Tel: 01902 307999 Fax: 01902 643104 — (Assam Med. Coll.) MB BS Gauhati 1965; FRCPath 1984, M, 1972. Cons. Haemat. New Cross Hosp. Wolverhampton. Prev: Demonst. (Path.) King's Coll. Hosp. Med. Sch. Lond.

PATEL, Ashok Nanubhai Deepdale Road Healthcare Centre, Deepdale Road, Preston PR1 5AF Tel: 01772 655533 Fax: 01772 653414; 7 Langport Close, Fulwood, Preston PR2 9FE — MB ChB Manch. 1983; MRCGP 1990.

PATEL, Ashokkumar Gordhanbhai Bedford Hospital, Weller Wing, Bedford MK42 PDJ Tel: 01234 355122 Fax: 01234 792279; 26 Aubreys, Letchworth SG6 3TZ Tel: 01462 676714 Fax: 01462 638513 — MB BS Baroda 1976 (Baroda, India) DPM Eng. 1981; FRCPsych 1997, M 1983. Cons. Psychiat. Bedford Hosp.; Clin. Dir. (Ment. Health) Bedford Hosp. Specialty: Gen. Psychiat. Prev: Sen. Regist. St. Bernards Hosp. S.all; Regist. & SHO Rotat. (Psychiat.) Char. Cross Hosp. Lond.; Clin. Tutor (Psychiat.) Fairfield Hosp.

PATEL, Ashokkumar Ramanbhai 50 Sheffield Drive, Lea, Preston PR2 1TS — MB ChB Manch. 1994.

PATEL, Ashvinkumar Raojibhai Leicester Road Surgery, 57 Leicester Road, Bedworth, Nuneaton CV12 8AB Tel: 024 7631 2288 Fax: 024 7631 3502; 5 Mill Close, Nuneaton CV11 6QD Tel: 01203 642009 — (Med. Coll. Baroda) MB BS Baroda 1968; DTM & H Liverp. 1971; DCH RCPSI 1972; Cert. Family Plann. JCC 1974. Sch. Med. Off. Exhall Grange Sch. for Handicap. Childr. Coventry. Socs: Dent. & Hypnotic Assn.

PATEL, Ashwin Mukesh 230 Turncroft Lane, Stockport SK1 4AX — MB ChB Manch. 1994.

PATEL, Mr Ashwinkumar Rambhai Preston Medical Centre, 23 Preston Road, Wembley HA9 8JZ Tel: 020 8904 3263; 11 Ford End, Denham Village, Uxbridge UB9 5AL — MB BS Bombay 1972; MB BS Bombay 1970; FRCS Ed. 1979; FRCS Eng. 1979. Specialty: Sports Med.

PATEL, Atulkumar The Health Centre, Gibson Lane, Kippax, Leeds LS25 7JN Tel: 0113 287 0870 Fax: 0113 232 0746; 3 The Coppice, Sherburn-in-Elmet, Leeds LS25 6LU — MB ChB Manch. 1985; Cert. Family Plann. JCC 1989; DRCOG 1989. GP N. Yorks.; Hosp. Pract. Endoscopy Unit St. Jas. Univ. Hosp. Leeds. Specialty: Gastroenterol.

PATEL, Avni 22B Crookham Road, London SW6 4EQ; Flat 3, 14 Brunswick Terrace, Hove BN3 1HL Tel: 01273 823304 — MB BS Lond. 1994 (King's Sch. Of Med. & Dent.) DRCOG 1998; MRCGP 1998.

PATEL, Azad Jashbhai St Giles Surgery, 40 St. Giles Road, London SE5 7RF Tel: 020 7252 5936; 38a Stanley Avenue, Beckenham BR3 6PX Tel: 020 8658 3944 — MB BS Gujarat 1973 (B.J. Med. Coll. Ahmedabad)

PATEL, Bachubhai Bhogilal 39 The Paddocks, Wembley HA9 9HG — MB BS Saurashtra 1971.

PATEL, Bakula 15 Albert Promenade, Loughborough LE11 1RB — MB ChB Leic. 1995.

PATEL, Bela 23 The Dene, Wembley HA9 7QS — MB BCh Wales 1989; DRCOG 1993; MRCGP 1994. Specialty: Gen. Pract.

PATEL, Bhanukumar Ambalal 3 Downs Walk, Peacehaven BN10 7SN — MB BS Indore 1973.

PATEL, Bharat Radiology Department, Swansea NHS Trust, Singleton Hospital, Sketty, Swansea SA2 8QA Tel: 01792 285431 Fax: 01792 286090 Email: bharat.patel@swansea-tr.wales.nhs.uk; Inshallah, Bishopston Road, Bishopston, Swansea SA3 3EW — MB BCh Wales 1981 (Welsh National School of Medicine) FRCR 1987; Dip Health Managem 1998. Cons. (Diagnostic Radiol.) Singleton Hosp. Swansea; Sen. Clin. Tutor Swansea Clin. Sch.; Coll. Tutor - Roy. Coll. of Radiologists. Specialty: Radiol. Prev: Clinical Director (Radiology) 1994-2001.

PATEL, Bharat Chunibhai 21 Compton Close, London NW11 8SX Tel: 020 7267 2868 — MB BS Lond. 1992. SHO (Geriat.) St Helier Hosp. Carshalton. Prev: SHO (A & E) E. Surrey Hosp. Redhill.

PATEL, Bharatkumar Chimanbhai PHLS Collaborating Centre, Department of Microbiology, North Middlesex University Hospital, Sterling Way, London N18 1QX Tel: 020 8887 2472 Fax: 020 8887 4227 — MB BS Lond. 1980; MSc Lond. 1992; MRCPath 1993. Cons. Med. microbiologist Med. microBiol. Pub. health Laborat. Serv..Lond. Specialty: Med. Microbiol. Socs: Hosp. Infec. Soc.; Brit. Soc. Antimicrob. Chemother.; Assn. Med. Microbiol. Prev: Cons. Med. Microbiol. Pub. Health Laborat. Serv. Ashford; Sen. Regist. Pub. Health Laborat. Serv. Centr. Middlx. Hosp.; Regist. & Hon. Asst. Lect. (Med. Microbiol.) King's Coll. Hosp. Lond.

PATEL, Bharatkumar Popatlal Star Lane Medical Centre, 121 Star Lane, London E16 4QH Tel: 0207 476 4862; 131 Prince Regent Lane, Plaistow, London E13 8RY Tel: 020 7476 1964 — MB BS Baroda 1973 (Med. Coll. Baroda) Specialty: Gen. Pract.

PATEL, Bhasker Chunibhai 134 Bath Road, Hounslow TW3 3ET Tel: 0208 570 9609 Fax: 0208 572 0935 — MB BS Gujarat 1977; MRCS Eng. LRCP Lond. 1980; MRCOG 1983. Specialty: Obst. & Gyn. Socs: Roy. Coll. of Obst. & Gynae.

PATEL, Bhavesh Kantibhai The Surgery, 188 Ann Street, London SE18 7LU Tel: 020 8854 6444 Fax: 020 8855 7656; Lawnside, St. Georges Road, Bickley, Bromley BR1 2LB Tel: 020 8467 6094 — MB ChB Sheff. 1989; T(GP) 1993; DFFP 1993. Trainee GP Qu. Mary's Hosp. Sidcup VTS. Prev: Ho. Off. (Med.) Bassettlaw Dist. Gen. Hosp.; Ho. Off. Joyce Green Hosp. Dartford.

PATEL, Bhavesh Sarajchandra 13 Triumph Road, Glenfield, Leicester LE3 8FR — MB BS Lond. 1997.

PATEL, Bhupen Motibhai The Surgery, 54 Thorne Road, Doncaster DN1 2JP Tel: 01302 361222; 34 Cantley Lane, Bessacarr, Doncaster DN4 6ND Tel: 01302 538478 — MB ChB Manch. 1983; DRCOG 1987; MRCGP 1989.

PATEL, Bhupendra Dahyabhai Longton Health Centre, Drayton Road, Longton, Stoke-on-Trent ST3 1EQ Tel: 01782 332176 Fax: 01782 598602 — MB BS Gujarat 1965; MB BS Gujarat 1965.

PATEL, Bhupendra Purshottam Charnwood Health Centre, 1 Spinney Hill Road, Leicester LE5 3GH Tel: 0116 262 5102; 12 Belvoir Close, Oadby, Leicester LE2 4SG — MB BS Calcutta 1966 (Calcutta Nat. Med. Coll.)

PATEL, Bhupendra Ramanlal 24 Stockport Road, Streatham Vale, London SW16 5XF Tel: 020 8764 5709 — MB BS Bombay 1969 (T.N. Med. Coll. Bombay)

PATEL, Bhupendra T The Dowlais Medical Practice, Ivor Street, Dowlais, Merthyr Tydfil CF48 3LU Tel: 01685 721400 Fax: 01685 375287.

PATEL, Bijesh Drs Coll, Patel and Kanani, Family Doctor Unit, 92 Bath Road, Hounslow TW3 3LN Tel: 020 8577 9555 Fax: 020 8570 2266; Orchard Lodge, 88 Sandy Lane, Teddington TW11 0DF — MB ChB Dundee 1985 (Univ. of Dundee) BMSc (Hons.) 1982; DRCOG 1987; MRCGP 1989. GP Tutor Char. Cross Hosp. Prev: Trainee GP Croydon; SHO (A & E, O & G, Geriat. & Rheum.) Mayday Hosp. Croydon.

PATEL, Bina 36 Longaford Way, Hutton Mount, Brentwood CM13 2LT — BM Soton. 1990. Cons. Phys. Specialty: Gen. Med. Socs: Amer. Coll. Phys. Prev: Resid. (Internal Med.) Temple Univ. & Hahnemann Univ. Philadelphia, USA; Ho. Surg. Univ. Soton.

PATEL, Binit Ramnik 40 Avondale Road, Benfleet SS7 1EJ — MB ChB Manch. 1996.

PATEL, Bipen Dahyabhai 8 Bilberry Close, Leicester LE3 2JA — MB BS Lond. 1992; BSc (Hons.) Human Physiol. Lond. 1989; MRCP (UK) 1996; MPhil Epidemiology, Univ. of Cambridge 2001. Health Serv. Research fell. Inst. Of Pub. Health, Forvic Uni. Site Hills Rd Camb.; Hon. SpR (Resp. Med.) Addenbrookes Hosp. Camb. Specialty: Respirat. Med.; Gen. Med. Socs: Brit. Thorac. Soc. Prev: Specialist Regist. (Respirat. Med.) Southmead Hosp. Bristol; SpR (Resp. Med.) Roy. Devon & Exeter Hosp. Exeter.; SpR Respiratory Med. Cheltenham Gen. Hosp.

PATEL, Bipin Bhikhabhai Watling Vale Medical Centre, Burchard Crescent, Shenley Church End, Milton Keynes MK5 6EY Tel: 01908 501177 Fax: 01908 504916; 6 Stonegate, Bancroft, Milton Keynes MK13 0PX — MB BCh Wales 1982; DRCOG 1985; DCH RCP Lond. 1986; MRCGP 1987; MRCP (UK) 1993. Specialty: Accid. & Emerg. Prev: Trainee GP/SHO Milton Keynes Hosp.; SHO (Anaesth.) E. Birm. Hosp.; Ho. Off. Univ. Hosp. Wales Cardiff.

PATEL, Bipinchandra Oakham Surgery, 213 Regent Road, Tividale, Oldbury B69 1RZ Tel: 01384 252274 Fax: 01348 240088; 55 The Broadway, Dudley DY1 4AP — MB BCh Wales 1978.

PATEL, Bipinchandra Naginbhai The Sorrels Surgery, 7 The Sorrels, Stanford-le-Hope SS17 7DZ Tel: 01375 671344 Fax: 01375 676913 — MB BS Bombay 1969 (Seth G.S. Med. Coll. Bombay) DObst. RCOG 1974; Cert. FPA 1974. Med. Off. Basildon Family Plann. Clin.

PATEL, Biral Pratap 66 Somerset Street, Kingsdown, Bristol BS2 8NB — MB ChB Bristol 1995.

PATEL, Chaitanya, CBE Priory Group, Priory House, Randalls Way, Leatherhead KT22 7TP Tel: 01372 860403 Fax: 01372 860402 Email: chaipatel@priorygroup.com — BM Soton. 1979; FRCP (UK) 1999. Chief Exec, Priory Group. Socs: Brit. Geriat.Soc. Prev: Chief Exec. Westm. Healthcare Grp.; Chairm. And Chief Exec. Ct. Cavendish Gp. plc Lond.; Chief Exec., Care 1st Gp.

PATEL, Mrs Chandra Vinodchandra The Surgery, 117 Knypersley Road, Norton-in-the-Moors, Stoke-on-Trent ST6 8JA Tel: 01782 545728 Fax: 01782 570069; Sanmay, Basnetts Wood, Endon, Stoke-on-Trent ST9 9DQ Tel: 01782 504403 — MB BS Gujarat 1964 (B.J. Med. Coll. Ahmedabad) DGO Gujarat 1965; DA Eng. 1966.

PATEL, Chandrakant Great Barr Group Practice, 912 Walsall Road, Great Barr, Birmingham B42 1TG Tel: 0121 357 1250 Fax: 0121 358 4857 — MB BCh Wales 1986. Specialty: Anaesth. Socs: Birm. Med. Inst.

PATEL, Chandrakant Bhailal Bhai Medical Centre, Chatsworth Road, Chesterfield S40 Tel: 01246 568065; 173 Old Road, Brampton, Chesterfield S40 3QL Tel: 01246 206341 — MB ChB Manch. 1963. Prev: Ho. Off. (Surg.) Pk. Hosp. Davyhulme; SHO (Anaesth.) City Gen. Hosp. Stoke-on-Trent.

PATEL, Chandrakant Jashbhai The Cottage Surgery, 179 South Coast Road, Peacehaven BN10 8NR Tel: 01273 581629 Fax: 01273 584648 — MB BS Gujarat 1967.

PATEL, Chandrakant Prabhudas Patel's Surgery, 90-92 Malvern Road, Gillingham ME7 4BB Tel: 01634 578333 Fax: 01634 852581 — MB BS Bombay 1963.

PATEL, Chandrakant Rambhai London Road Surgery, 519 London Road, Thornton Heath CR7 6AR Tel: 020 8684 2161; Westdean, 5 Downsway, Sanderstead, South Croydon CR2 0JB — MB BCh Wales 1972 (University of Wales) Dip Therp 1998. GP Tutor St. Geo. Hosp. Med. Sch. Lond. Socs: BMA. Prev: Trainee GP Hackney VTS; Ho. Phys. (Med.) Singleton Hosp. Swansea; Ho. Surg. E. Glam. Gen. Hosp. Pontypridd.

PATEL, Chandrakant Ranchhodbhai Pickhurst Surgery, 56 Pickhurst Lane, Bromley BR2 7JF Tel: 020 8462 2880 Fax: 020 8462 9581; Manraj, 19 Pk Avenue, Farnbrorough Park, Orpington BR6 8LJ Tel: 01689 855312 — MB ChB East Africa 1964 (Makerere Med. Sch.) MRCP (UK) 1972.

PATEL, Chandrakant Shankerbhai 13-16 Brondesbury Road, London NW6 6BX; 112 Princess Avenue, Palmers Green, London N13 6HD — MB BS Baroda 1975. Staff Grade Psychiat. CNWL Ment. Health NHS Trust Lond. Prev: Staff Grade Psychiat. NW Lond. Ment. Health NHS Trust Lond.; Regist. (Psychiat.) Wexham Pk. Hosp. Slough.

PATEL, Chandresh Ratilal Woodlands Surgery, 301 New Town Road, Bedworth, Nuneaton CV12 0AJ Tel: 024 7649 0909 — MB BS Baroda 1971.

PATEL, Chandresh Thakorbhai 165 Woodmansterne Road, London SW16 5UB — MB BCh Wales 1990.

PATEL, Chandubhai Bhailalbhai 51 Newdene Avenue, Northolt UB5 5JE — MB BS Gujarat 1961.

PATEL, Chetan Kantibhai Oxford Eye Hospital, Radcliffe Infirmary, Oxford OX2 9AN — MB BS Lond. 1988 (Lond. Hosp. Med. Coll.) BSc (Hons.) Lond. 1987; FRCOphth 1993. Cons. Ophth. Surg. Oxf. Eye Hosp. Specialty: Ophth. Prev: Research Regist. Cataract Research Unit Oxf. Eye Hosp.; SHO Rotat. (Ophth.) St. Geo. Hosp., E. Surrey Hosp. & Worthing Dist. Gen. Hosp.; SHO (Neurosurg.) Brook Gen. Hosp.

PATEL, Chetankumar 57 Burnley Road, London NW10 1EE Tel: 0976 620973 — MB BS Lond. 1992. Specialty: Anaesth.

PATEL, Miss Daksha 57 Redcar Road, Broomhill, Sheffield S10 1EX Tel: 0114 266 8589 — MB ChB Sheff. 1985; MRCOG 1990; MD Sheff. Univ. 1999. Cons. Gyn. Specialty: Obst. & Gyn. Special Interest: Minimal Access Surg.; Urogynecology. Prev: Sen. Lect., Obst. & Gyn., Sheff. Univ.; Sen. Regist. N. W. Region; Research Regist., Sheff. Univ.

PATEL, Davandra North West Regional Health Authority, Manchester M20 2PL; 25 Truro Drive, Sale M33 5DF — MB ChB Manch. 1986; DA (UK) 1988; FRCA 1991. Sen. Regist. (Anaesth.) NW RHA Manch. Specialty: Anaesth. Socs: Train. Mem. Assn. AnE.h.; Manch. Med. Soc. Prev: Instruc. (Anesthesiol.) Univ. Michigan Ann Arbor, USA.

PATEL, Dayavanti Shashikant The Surgery, 1A Oak Road, Canvey Island SS8 7AX Tel: 01268 692211 — MB BS Gujarat 1968

(B.J. Med. Coll. Ahmedabad) Med. Off. Family Plann. Clinics Essex AHA.

PATEL, Deepal Arunbhai 115 Hatherton Road, Cannock WS11 1HH — MB BS Lond. 1997.

PATEL, Deven Jashbhai Barnet General Hospital, Wellhouse Lane, Barnet EN5 3DY Tel: 020 8216 5455 Fax: 020 8216 4228 Email: deven.patel@bcf.nhs.uk — MB BS Lond. 1985 (The Middlx. Hosp. Med. Sch.) Cons. Cardiol.; Cons. Cardiol., The Roy. Free Hosp. Lond.; Cons. Cardiol., Chase Farm Hosp., Enfield; Cons. Cardiol., The Wellington Hosp., Lond.; Cons. Cardiol., BUPA Hosp., Bushey, Watford. Specialty: Cardiol. Special Interest: Coronary Heart disease; Interventional cardiology. Socs: Brit. Cardiac Soc.; Brit. Cardiac Interven. Soc. Prev: Regist. (Cardiol.) Roy. Brompton Nat. Heart & Lung Hosp. Lond.; Sen. Regist. (Cardiol.) Harefield Hosp. Middlx.

PATEL, Devyani Ramubhai Dartmouth Medical Centre, 1 Richard St., West Bromwich B70 9JL Tel: 0121 553 1144 Fax: 0121 580 1914; Central Clinic, Horseley Road, Tipton DY4 7NB Tel: 0121 557 4377 — MB BS Gujarat 1966 (B.J. Med. Coll. Ahmedabad) LM Rotunda 1969; DGO Dub. 1969. Med. Off. Family Plann. Assn. Birm. Prev: SHO (Gyn. & Obst.) Leicester Gen. Hosp.

PATEL, Dharmesh Paradise Medical Centre, Broad Street, Coventry CV6 5BG Tel: 024 7668 9343 Fax: 024 7663 8733 — MB ChB Leic. 1994.

PATEL, Dharmesh 20 Windermere Street, Castle Gardens, Leicester LE2 7GT — MB ChB Manch. 1995.

PATEL, Dheeren 1 Crossway, Raynes Park, London SW20 9JA Tel: 020 8543 1059 — BM Soton. 1987; DRCOG 1991; Cert. Family Plann. JCC 1991. Prev: SHO (Paediat.) Soton. Gen. Hosp.; SHO (Geriat. Med.) Univ. Coll. Hosp. Lond.; SHO (A & E) Epsom Dist. Hosp.

PATEL, Dhruva Doncaster Drive Surgery, 45 Doncaster Drive, Northolt UB5 4AT Tel: 020 8864 8133; 6 Thomas A Beckett Close, Wembley HA0 2SH — MB ChB Aberd. 1990 (Univ. Aberd.) MRCGP 1994. Specialty: Gen. Pract.

PATEL, Dilip Kumar Bhikhabhai Royal Infirmary of Edinburgh, Department of Radiology, 51 Little France Crescent, Old Dalkeith Road, Edinburgh EH16 4SA Tel: 0131 242 3734 Fax: 0131 242 3736 — MB BS Newc. 1988; BMedSc (Hons.) Newc. 1985; MRCP (UK) 1991; FRCR 1996. Cons. Radiol., Roy. Infirm. of Edinb.; Hon. Clin. Sen. Lect., Univ. of Edin. Specialty: Radiol. Special Interest: Cross Sectional Imaging; Radionuclide. Socs: Radiological Soc. of N. America; Scott. Radiological Soc. Prev: Sen. Regist. (Radiol.) Edin. Hosps. Train. Progr.; Regist. (Radiol.) West. Austral. Train. Progr. & (Med.) Fremantle Hosp., Austral.; SHO Rotat. (Med.) Newc. HA.

PATEL, Dilip Kumar Chhotabhai Civic Medical Centre, 18 Bethecar Road, Harrow HA1 1SE Tel: 020 8427 9445 Fax: 020 8424 0652; 3 Arnside Gardens, Wembley HA9 8TJ Tel: 020 8908 21444 — MB BCh BAO NUI 1984; LRCPSI 1984.

PATEL, Dilip Kumar Kunverji MT Vernon Hospital, NorthWood — MB ChB Bristol 1978 (Univ. of Bristol) FFARCS 1982. Cons. Anaesth. Mt. Vernon Hosp. Trust Middlx. Specialty: Anaesth. Special Interest: Burns ITU; Paediatric Anaesth. Socs: Assn. Anaesth. & Intens. Care Soc.; The Intens. Care Soc. Prev: Sen. Regist. Middlx. Hosp. Lond.

PATEL, Dilip Maganlal — MB ChB Manch. 1994 (The Victoria University of Manchester) DRCOG 1996; DCH RCP Lond. 1996; MRCGP 1998; DFFP 1998. GP Princip. Greenford. Specialty: Gen. Pract. Prev: GP Locum Preston; SHO (Paediat.) & Ho. Off. (Gen. Surg. & Urol.) Roy. Preston Hosp.; SHO (A & E) Roy. Preston Hosp.

PATEL, Dilipkumar Chaturbhai 21 Knights Manor Way, Dartford DA1 5SB — MB BS Ranchi 1980; LMSSA Lond. 1989.

PATEL, Dinesh Kumar Kantibhai The Consulting Rooms, Oxhey Drive, South Oxhey, Watford WD19 7RU Tel: 020 8428 2292; 3 Holbein Gate, Eastglade, Northwood HA6 3SH — MB BS Banaras Hindu 1973 (Inst. Med. Sc. Varanasi) Prev: SHO (Med., A & E & Orthop.) Hertford Co. Hosp.

PATEL, Dineshchandra Broadway Surgery, 2 Broadway, Fulwood, Preston PR2 9TH Tel: 01772 717261 Fax: 01772 787652 — MB ChB Manch. 1984; DCH RCP Lond. 1988; MRCGP 1990; DRCOG 1990. Occupat. Health Off. Preston; Represen. Lancs. LMC; NW Lorg Represen.; EMCS Nat. User Gp. Comm. Mem.; Edr. EMCS NUG. Specialty: Gen. Pract. Socs: Subfac. Represen. Roy. Coll. Gen. Pract. Prev: Trainee GP Preston VTS.

PATEL, Dinkerrai Purshottamdass Health Centre, Lake Lock Road, Stanley, Wakefield WF3 4HS Tel: 01924 822328 Fax: 01924 870052 — MB BS Bombay 1967. GP Wakefield, W. Yorks.

PATEL, Dipak 5 Charles Road, London E7 8PT — MB ChB Liverp. 1992; DCH; DTM & H; DRCOG.

PATEL, Dipesh Chandrakant Imperial College, Department of Metabolic Medicine, St. Mary's Hospital, 2nd floor Mint Wing, Praed Street W2 1NY Tel: 020 7886 6120 — MB BS Lond. 1998; BSc 1995; MRCP 2001.

PATEL, Dipti UMDS/Guys & St Thomas' NHS Trust, Lambeth Palace Road, London SE1 7EH — MB BS Lond. 1989; DRCOG 1992; MRCGP 1993; Dip. Occ. Med. RCP Lond. 1997. Lect. (Occupat. Health) UMDS Guys & St. Thomas' NHS Trust Lond. Specialty: Occupat. Health. Prev: Med. Adviser to the Foreign & Commonw. Office Lond.

PATEL, Ela Dayalji Park Surgery, 278 Stratford Road, Shirley, Solihull B90 3AF Tel: 0121 241 1700 Fax: 0121 241 1710 — MB ChB Leic. 1983.

PATEL, Falgun 219 Charlton Road, Harrow HA3 9HT — MB ChB Manch. 1992.

PATEL, Geeta Devi Salisbury Road Surgery, 1 Salisbury Road, Seven Kings, Ilford IG3 8BG Tel: 020 8590 1143 Fax: 020 8599 7162 — MB BCh Wales 1989; BSc (Hons.) Wales 1989. Specialty: Gen. Pract. Socs: Roy. Coll. Gen. Pract. Prev: Trainee GP Harlow; SHO (O & G, Med. & c/o Elderly)) Harlow; SHO (A & E) St. Margt. Hosp. Epping.

PATEL, Geeta Harendra Patel, Latimer Health Centre, 4 Homerton Terrace, off Morning Lane, Hackney, London E9 6RT Tel: 020 8985 2249 Fax: 020 8985 7333; Rosedene, 4 Mellish Gardens, Woodford Green IG8 0BH — MB BS Rajasthan 1979. GP; Clin. Asst. Psychiat. Homerton Hosp. Specialty: Gen. Psychiat. Prev: Regist. (Psychiat.) Claybury Hosp. Woodbridge Essex & Warley Hosp. Brentwood.

PATEL, Ghanashyambhai Umedbhai Meersbrook Medical Centre, 243-245 Chesterfield Road, Sheffield S8 0RT Tel: 0114 258 3997 — MB BS Jiwaji 1972 (Gajra Raja Med. Coll. Gwalior)

PATEL, Ghanshyam Maganbhai 57 Woodfield Road, Oadby, Leicester LE2 4HQ — MB BS Gujarat 1969.

PATEL, Girishchandra Keshavlal 22 Church View, Roger Lane, Rd. 1, Laleston, Bridgend CF32 0HF Tel: 01656 659745; 83 Tremains Court, Brackla, Bridgend CF31 2SS Tel: 01656 669519 — MB BS Baroda 1969 (Med. Coll. Baroda) DTCD Wales 1972. Regist. (Geriat. Med.) Bridgend Gen. Hosp. Specialty: Care of the Elderly. Socs: Brit. Tuberc. & Thoracic Assn. & BMA.

PATEL, Gokul Maganlal Tawe Medical Centre, 6 Thomas Street, St. Thomas, Swansea SA1 8AT Tel: 01792 650400 Fax: 01792 464914; St Davids Medical Centre, Caldicot Close, Winchwen, Swansea SA1 7HT Tel: 01792 702700 — MB ChB Wales 1979 (Cardiff) MRCGP 1983.

PATEL, Govindbhai Ranchhodbhai 99 Whiteacre Road, Ashton-under-Lyne OL6 9PJ Tel: 0161 339 2034 — MB BS Bombay 1963 (Grant Med. Coll.) Trainee Gen. Pract. Manch. Vocational Train. Scheme.

PATEL, Gulam Ahmed Abdulla Musa Flat 7, 55 Woodville Gardens, London W5 2LN — MB BS Lond. 1987.

PATEL, Gunvantbhai Jashubhai Department of Orthopaedics, Queen Margaret Hospital, Dunfermline KY12 0SU Tel: 01383 623623 — MB BS S. Gujarat 1973; FRCS Glas. 1987. Staff Grade (Orthop. Surg.) Qu. Margt. Hosp. Dunfermline. Specialty: Orthop.

PATEL, Gunvantrai Dalabhai Petworth Drive Medical Centre, 5 Petworth Drive, Leicester LE3 9RF Tel: 0116 255 0030 — MB BS Bombay 1974.

PATEL, H R Seabank Road Surgery, 213/215 Seabank Road, Wallasey CH45 1HE Tel: 0151 630 6577 Fax: 0151 639 7477.

PATEL, Hamina Jayantibhai — MB BCh Wales 1990 (University of Wales, College of Medicine) MRCPI 1995; MSc Glasgow 1998. Clin. Research Phys., Lond. Specialty: Gen. Med.; Pharmaceutical Medicine. Prev: Regist. (Pharmacol. & Gen. Med.) Univ. Coll. Hosp. Lond.

PATEL, Hansa Thakor 1 Banckside, Hartley, Longfield DA3 7RD — MB BS Bombay 1970 (Grant Med. Coll.) DA Eng. 1972; FFA RCSI 1976. Cons. Anaesth. Dartford & Gravesham Health Dist. Specialty: Anaesth. Prev: Sen. Regist. (Anaesth.) Guy's Hosp. Lond.

PATEL, Hansa Thakor Darent Valley Hospital, Darenth Wood Road, Dartford DA2 8DA Tel: 01322 428100 Ext: 8648 — (Grant) MB BS Bombay 1970; DA 1972; FFARCSI 1974. Cons. Anaesth. Specialty: Vasc. Med. Socs: Vascular; Obstetric; Pain. Prev: College Tutor.

PATEL, Harendra Gordhanbhai Patel, Latimer Health Centre, 4 Homerton Terrace, off Morning Lane, Hackney, London E9 6RT Tel: 020 8985 2249 Fax: 020 8985 7333; Rosedene, 4 Mellish Gardens, Woodford Green IG8 0BH — MB BS Baroda 1978; MRCS Eng. LRCP Lond. 1984. GP. Specialty: Obst. & Gyn. Prev: Princip. GP Redbridge.

PATEL, Harikrishna Purushottamdas 3 Ashleigh Court, Preston PR2 9WU — MB BS Gujarat 1958 (B.J. Med. Coll. Ahmedabad) DPH Eng. 1962; MFCM 1974; FFCM 1981. Specialist Community Med. Preston HA. Prev: Area SCM Acute & Scientif. Servs. Blackburn; Princip. Ahmadu Bello Univ. Med. Auxil. Train. Sch. Kaduna, Nigeria; PMO Min. of Health & Social Welf. Kano State, Nigeria.

PATEL, Harischandra Chimanbhai Ore Clinic, Old London Road, Hastings TN35 5BH Tel: 01424 448410; 40 Bowmans Drive, Battle TN33 0LU Tel: 01424 775245 — MB BS Mysore 1981; MRCOG 1988; Dip GU Med Lond. 1990; MFFP 1995. Cons. Genitourin. Med. Hastings & Eastbourne. Specialty: Genitourinary Medicine. Socs: BMA; Soc. Study of VD. Prev: Sen. Regist. (Genitourin. Med.) Roy. Lond. Hosp.; Regist. (Genitourin. Med.) St. Geo. & St. Helier Hosp. Lond.; Regist. (O & G) Hope Hosp. Salford & Rochford Gen. Hosp.

PATEL, Harshadaben Maheshkumar Westbury Medical Centre, 205 Westbury Avenue, Wood Green, London N22 6RX Tel: 020 8888 3021 Fax: 020 8888 6898 — MB BS Saurashtra 1974 (M. P. Shah Medical College Jamnagar, India) Specialty: Gen. Pract.

PATEL, Harshadrao Dahyabhai Lynwood Medical Centre, Lynwood Drive, 2A-6 Collier Row, Romford RM5 3QL Tel: 01708 743244 Fax: 01708 736783 — MB BS Gujarat 1968 (B.J. Med. Coll. Ahmedabad)

PATEL, Mr Hashumati Dajibhai Laxman 14 Evans Close, Tipton DY4 8BG — MB ChB Aberd. 1989; FRCS Ed. 1995.

PATEL, Hasmukh Rambhai Darent Valley Hospital, Dartford DA2 8ND Tel: 01322 428100 Ext: 8221 Fax: 01322 428231; Freeby, The Green, Sidcup DA14 6BS Tel: 020 8302 7400 Fax: 020 8302 7400 Email: hrzp@hotmail.com — (King's Coll. Hosp.) MB BS Lond. 1967; MRCS Eng. LRCP Lond. 1967; DCH Eng. 1970; MRCP (UK) 1972; FRCP Ed. 1985; FRCP Lond. 1986; FRCPCH 1997. Cons. Paediat. Darent Valley hosp., Dartford, Kent. Specialty: Paediat. Socs: Pres., N. W. Kent Med. Assoc. Prev: Chairm. Specialist Train. Comm. Paediat. S. Thames RHA; Postgrad. Assoc. Dean. S. Thames RHA; Sen. Regist., Regist. & SHO (Paediat.) King's Coll. Hosp. Lond.

PATEL, Hasmukh Shivabhai St Bartholomews Surgery, 292A Barking Road, London E6 3BA Tel: 020 8472 0669/1077 Fax: 020 8471 9122 — MB BS Gujarat 1973 (B.J. Med. Coll. Ahmedabad) Ho. Surg. OldCh. Hosp. Romford.

PATEL, Heather Frances Capelfield Surgery, Elm Road, Claygate, Esher KT10 0EH Tel: 01372 462501 Fax: 01372 470258; The Thatched House, Manor Way, Oxshott, Leatherhead KT22 0HU Tel: 01372 843995 — BM Soton. 1982; DRCOG 1984; MRCGP 1986. Socs: Bd. Mem. E. Elmbridge PCG (Vice Chairm.).

PATEL, Heena The Surgery, 577 Carlton Road, Nottingham NG3 7AF Tel: 0115 958 0415 Fax: 0115 950 9245 — BM BS Nottm. 1980 (Univ. Nottm. Med. Sch.) BMedSci Nottm. 1978; DCH RCP Lond. 1984; DRCOG 1985; MRCGP 1987. Tutorsh. Nottm. Med. Sch.; Clin. Asst. Asian Diabetes Nottm. City Hosp. Specialty: Diabetes; Paediat.

PATEL, Heman Kumar Bhanubhai 113 Godfrey House, Bath St., London EC1V 9ET — MB BS Lond. 1996.

PATEL, Hemantkumar 20 Eastmead Avenue, Greenford UB6 9RB — MB BS Lond. 1988 (St. Georges) DRCOG 1992; MRCGP 1994. GP Princip.

PATEL, Hemlata 36 Lamorrey Close, Sidcup DA15 8BA — MB BS Rajasthan 1973.

PATEL, Hemlata Bharatkumar 228 Watford Road, Harrow HA1 3TY — MB BS Baroda 1979. Gen. Practitioner, Primary Care Lond. Specialty: Gen. Pract.

PATEL, Hemlata Shantuprasai The Warren Medical Practice, The Warren, Uxbridge Road, Hayes UB4 0SF Tel: 020 8573 2476/1781 Fax: 020 8561 3461; 5 Sandy Lodge Lane, Moor Park, Northwood HA6 2JA Tel: 01923 829276 Fax: 01923 823063 — MB BS Baroda 1972 (Baroda Med. Coll.) DA Eng. 1975. GP.

PATEL, Himanshu 3 Windermere Close, Dartford DA1 2TX — MB BCh Wales 1991; MRPharmS; Dip Pharm Med.

PATEL, Himanshu Jairamdas 21 Blakes Avenue, New Malden KT3 6RJ — MB BS Lond. 1994.

PATEL, Himanshu Jayantilal Myatts Field Health Centre, Patmos Road, London SW9 7RX Tel: 020 7411 3573 Fax: 020 7411 3583 — MB BS Lond. 1983; DRCOG 1987. Clin. Asst. (Dermat.) KCH Lond. Prev: SHO (A & E) N. Middlx. Hosp. Lond.; SHO (Psychiat.) E. Glam. Gen. Hosp.; SHO (Paediat.) P. Chas. Hosp. Merthyr Tydfil.

PATEL, Hiren Chandrakant 22 Alliance Court, Hills Road, Cambridge CB1 7XE — MB ChB Sheff. 1995.

PATEL, Hitendra Ramesh Himanshu School of Surgical Sciences, The Medical School, Framlington Place, Newcastle upon Tyne NE2 4HH Tel: 0191 232 5131 Fax: 0191 222 8514 — MB ChB Dundee 1992; BMSc (Hons.) Dund 1990. Med. Research Counc. Clin. Train. Fell. (Surg.) Univ. Newc. Specialty: Gen. Surg. Socs: Fell. Roy. Microscopical Soc.

PATEL, Hitesh 50 Blenheim Gardens, Wembley HA9 7NP; 56 Intwood Road, Cringlefield, Norwich NR4 6TH — MB ChB Aberd. 1982; MRCP (UK) 1988; MRCGP 1993; DRCOG 1993.

PATEL, Hitesh 40 Rissington Avenue, Selly Oak, Birmingham B29 7SX — MB BCh BAO Dub. 1992.

PATEL, Mr Hitesh 1 Steele Road, London W4 5AE Tel: 020 8746 8231 Email: hitesh.patel@ic.ac.uk — MB ChB Liverp. 1994 (University Liverpool Medical School) FRCS (Eng) 1998. Res. Fell. (Surg.) Acad. Surg. Chelsea & Westminster Hosp. Lond. Specialty: Gen. Surg. Prev: SHO (Surg.) Chelsea & Westm. Hosp. Lond.; SHO (Surg.) Watford Gen. Hosp.; Demonst. (Anat.) Char. Cross & Westm. Med. Sch.

PATEL, Indira Ghanshyam Melbourne Road Medical Centre, 47 Melbourne Road, Leicester LE2 0GT Tel: 0116 255 9869 — MB BS Gujarat 1969.

PATEL, Indravadan Purshottamdas, MBE (Surgery), 85/87 Acton Lane, Harlesden, London NW10 8UT Tel: 020 8961 1183 Fax: 020 8961 4785; 113 Green Lane, Stanmore HA7 3AD — MB BS Gujarat 1965 (B.J. Med. Coll. Ahmedabad) DLO Eng. 1976. ENT Surg. Lond. Hosp.; ENT Surg. Northwick Pk. Hosp. Wembley Hosp. Socs: Brit. Otol. Soc. & BMA. Prev: Regist. (ENT) Lewisham Hosp. Lond.; Regist. (ENT), Ho. Surg. & Ho. Phys. Mulago Hosp. Kampala, Uganda.

PATEL, Irem Suzan Queen Mary's Hospital, Sidcup DA14 6LT Tel: 020 8302 2678 Email: rkpandisp@aol.com; 190 Farnaby Road, Bromley BR2 0BB Tel: 020 8290 6932 — MB BS Lond. 1994 (University College and Middlesex) MRCP (UK) 1997. Specialist Regist. (Respir. Med.) SE Thames. Specialty: Respirat. Med. Socs: Brit Thoracic Soc.; SE Thames Thoracic Soc.; Lond. Int. Care Grp.

PATEL, J D The Surgery, 94 Highbury Park, London N5 2XE Tel: 020 7226 5360 — MB BS Bombay 1969; DRCOG London 1975.

PATEL, Jagdish Babubhai Priory Lodge, 72 Grosvenor Way, Barton Seagrave, Kettering NN15 6TZ — MB BS Gujarat 1965 (B.J. Med. Coll. Ahmedabad) DLO 1968. Socs: BMA. Prev: Regist. (ENT) Kettering Gen. Hosp.; SHO Oldham Roy. Infirm. & W. Kent Gen. Hosp. Maidstone.

PATEL, Jagdishchandra Maganbhai Park House Surgery, 2 St. Georges Road, Stoke, Coventry CV1 2DL Tel: 024 7622 4438 — MB BS Baroda 1968; FRCOG 1974. GP. Specialty: Gen. Pract.

PATEL, Jagdishchandra Nagjibhai 1 Whitehall Road, Rugby CV21 3AE Tel: 01788 561319 — MB BS Gujarat 1968 (B.J. Med. Coll. Ahmedabad) DA Gujarat 1970; MD (Anaesth.) Gujarat 1972. Prev: Regist. (Anaesth.) Gen. Hosp. Northampton; SHO (Anaesth.) Princess Margt. Hosp. Swindon & Ashton-under-Lyne Gen. Hosp.

PATEL, Jai Vinodray St James's University Hospital, Department of Radiology, Beckett Street, Leeds LS9 7TF Tel: 0113 206 4047 Email: jai.patel@leedsth.nhs.uk; Email: jai@jvpatel.freeserve.co.uk — MB ChB Manch. 1990 (Univ. Manch.) MRCP (UK) 1994; FRCR 1998. Cons. radiologist. Specialty: Radiol. Special Interest: Vasc. Radiol. Socs: Roy. Coll. of Radiologist.

PATEL, Jaikrishna Rambhai Dhulabhai 14 Northwick Park Road, Harrow HA1 2NU — MB BS Lond. 1986; BSc (Hons.) Lond. 1983; MB BS (Hons.) Lond. 1986; MRCP (UK) 1989. Dir. Diabetes & Metabol. SmithKline Beecham Philadelphia. Specialty:

Pharmaceutical Medicine. Prev: Regist. (Med.) King's Coll. Hosp. Lond.; SHO (Gen. Med.) St. Bart. Hosp. Lond.; Ho. Phys. Med. Profess. Unit St. Bart. Hosp. Lond.

PATEL, Jatin Kumar Vishnooprasad Melbourne Road Surgery, 71 Melbourne Road, Leicester LE2 0GU Tel: 0116 253 9479 Fax: 0116 242 5602; 25 Carisbrooke Avenue, South Knighton, Leicester LE2 3PA Tel: 0116 270 3792 — MB ChB Leeds 1983; Cert. Family Plann. JCC 1986; MRCGP 1987; DRCOG 1988. Specialty: Gen. Med. Prev: Intern. Psychiat. Med. Coll. Georgia Augusta, USA; Trainee GP Leicester VTS; SHO (Psychiat. & O & G) ScarBoro. HA.

PATEL, Jayantibhai Ashabhai Thorns Road Surgery, 43 Thorns Road, Quarry Bank, Brierley Hill DY5 2JS Tel: 01384 77524 Fax: 01384 486540; 10 Ironbridge Walk, Pedmore, Stourbridge DY9 0SF Tel: 01562 886465 — (M.G.M. Med. Coll. Indore) MB BS Indore 1966. GP.

PATEL, Jayesh Purushottamdas A & E Department, Southampton General Hospital, Tremona Road, Southampton SO16 6YD — LRCP LRCS Ed. 1983; LRCP LRCS Ed. LRCPS Glas. 1983.

PATEL, Jayesh Rajnikant Ambalal 34 Fairview Road, Istead Rise, Gravesend DA13 9DR Tel: 01474 355331 — MB ChB Sheff. 1982. Specialty: Gen. Pract.

PATEL, Jayeshkumar Slab Cottage, 11 Old Cottage Close, West Wellow, Romsey SO51 6RL Tel: 01794 324154 — MB BS Lond. 1987 (St. Geo. Hosp. Lond.) BSc Lond. 1984; DCH 1990; MRCP Lond. 1991. Paediat. Neurol. Sen. Regist. Soton. Gen. Hosp. Soton. Specialty: Paediat. Neurol. Socs: Neonat. Soc.; MRCPCH.

PATEL, Jayshree Narrendra Dudley Park Medical Centre, 28 Dudley Park Road, Acocks Green, Birmingham B27 6QR Tel: 0121 706 0072 Fax: 0121 707 0418 — MB BS Bombay 1974; DRCOG 1976.

PATEL, Jigisha 38 St Mary's Road, London E13 9AD — MB BS Lond. 1991.

PATEL, Jignesh Indravadan 113 Green Lane, Stanmore HA7 3AD Tel: 020 8854 9922 Fax: 020 8961 4785 — MB BS Lond. 1993; BSc Lond. 1990. Demonst. (Anat.) Char. Cross & Westm. Med. Sch. Lond. Prev: SHO (Cas.) & Ho. Off. (Med.) Char. Cross Hosp. Lond.; Ho. Off. (Surg.) W. Middlx. Univ. Hosp.

PATEL, Mr Jignesh Vinodrai Department of Orthopaedics, Kings College Hospital, Denmark Hill, London SE5 9RS — BM Soton. 1991 (Southampton) FRCSI 1994; FRCS Eng. 1996; FRCS (Tr & Orth) 2000. Specialist Regist. (Orthop.) Chelsea & Westm. Hosp. Lond. Specialty: Orthop. Prev: SHO (Plastics) Char. Cross Hosp. Lond.; SHO (Orthop.) Chelsea & Westm. Hosp. Lond. & Addenbrooke's NHS Trust Camb.

PATEL, Jitendra 38 Deptford Broadway, Deptford, London SE8 4PQ — MB ChB Sheff. 1980.

PATEL, Jitendra 23 Colin Drive, Colindale, London NW9 6ES — BM Soton. 1980.

PATEL, Jitendra Ishwarbhai c/o D. M. Patel, 17 Watford Road, Wembley HA0 3ET — MB BS Gujarat 1969.

PATEL, Jyotsana Suresh The Surgery, 1 Uxendon Crescent, Wembley HA9 9TW Tel: 020 8904 3883 Fax: 020 8904 3899 — MB BS Baroda 1978; MRCS Eng. LRCP Lond. 1980; DRCOG 1982; MRCGP 1983; Dip Chinese Med Bejing 1999.

PATEL, Kalpana Lallubhai 2 Berners Road, London N22 5NE — MB BS Lond. 1997.

PATEL, Kalpana Prakash Wallasey Crescent Practice, 1 Wallasey Crescent, Ickenham, Uxbridge UB10 8SA Tel: 01895 674156 Fax: 01895 623334 — MB BS Bombay 1974; MB BS Bombay 1974.

PATEL, Mr Kalpesh Santuram Department of Otolaryngology - Head & Neck Surgery, St. Mary's Hospital, Praed St., London W2 1NY Tel: 020 7886 2151 Fax: 020 1886 1847 — (St. Bart.) BSc (Hons.) Lond. 1981; MB BS Lond. 1984; FRCS Eng. (Orl.) 1989; FRCS (Orl.) 1994. Cons. ENT Surg. St. Mary's Hosp. Lond. Specialty: Otorhinolaryngol. Socs: Fell. Roy. Soc. Med.; Am. Acad. Otolaryngol - Head & Neck Surg.; Europ. Acad. Facial Surg. Prev: Sen. Regist. Rotat. (ENT Surg.) St. Mary's Hosp. & Roy. Marsden Hosp. Lond.; Regist. (ENT & Plastics) King's Coll. Hosp. Lond.; Demonst. Univ. St. And. Fife.

PATEL, Kamal Chelsea & Westminster Hospital, Fulham Road, London SW10 9NH; 23 Bernard Street, St Albans AL3 5QW Tel: 01727 811287 — MB BS Lond. 1990; MRCP (UK) 1993. Regist. (Paediat.) Chelsea & Westm. Hosp. Lond. Specialty: Paediat. Prev: Regist. Watford Gen. Hosp.; SHO (Paediat.) St. Jas. Univ. Hosp. Leeds; SHO (O & G) St. Peter's NHS Trust Chertsey.

PATEL, Kamini 28A Milton Avenue, London N6 5QE — MB BS Lond. 1983.

PATEL, Kanak Kumar The Stables, Old Vicarage Lane, Monk Fryston, Leeds LS25 5EA — MB ChB Manch. 1997; BDS 1987; FDS RCPS 1991; FRCSI (Gen) 1999. Specialist Regist. Oral & Maxillofacial Surg. Specialty: Gen. Surg.; Oral & Maxillofacial Surg. Socs: BMA; RCS (Glas.); RCSI. Prev: SHO (Gen. Surg.); Ho. Off. (Surg.); Ho. Off. (Med.).

PATEL, Kantibhai Maganbhai The Surgery, 47 Boundaries Road, Balham, London SW12 8EU Tel: 020 8673 1476; 7 Willows Avenue, Morden SM4 5SG Tel: 020 8648 6354 — (Grant Med. Coll.) MB BS Bombay 1956; DCH Eng. 1958; MRCS Eng. LRCP Lond. 1958; DTM & H Eng. 1958; MRCP Glas. 1960; MRCP Ed. 1961; FRCP Ed. 1994; FRCP Ed 1995. Prev: Sen. Lect. & Cons. Phys. Makerere Med. Sch. Mulago Hosp. Kampala, Uganda.

PATEL, Kantilal Chhaganbhai Littleover Medical Centre, 640 Burton Road, Littleover, Derby DE23 6EL Tel: 01332 207100 Fax: 01332 342680; 640 Burton Road, Littleover, Derby DE23 6EL Tel: 01332 44441 — MB BS Banaras 1971; DObst. RCPI 1977. Socs: Derby Med. Soc.

PATEL, Kantilal Motibhai (retired) 42 Buckhurst Way, Buckhurst Hill IG9 6HJ — MB BS Bombay 1951 (Grant Med. Coll.) MRCGP 1962.

PATEL, Kantilal Rambhai Department of Respiratory Medicine, Gartnavel General Hospital, Glasgow G12 0YN Tel: 0141 211 3000; 9 Lomond Place, Linburn, Erskine PA8 6AP Tel: 0141 812 4569 — MB BS Bombay 1967 (Grant Med. Coll.) MCPS Bombay 1967; PhD Glas. 1976; FRCP Glas. 1980; FRCP Lond. 1985. Cons. Phys. Respirat. Med. & Gartnavel Gen. Hosp. Glas.; Hon. Clin. Sen. Lect. (Med.) Univ. Glas. Specialty: Respirat. Med. Socs: Brit. Thorac. Soc. & Scott. Thoracic Soc.; Amer. Thoracic Soc.; Europ. Thoracic Soc. Prev: Sen. Regist. (Gen. Med. & Respirat. Dis.) Greater Glas. Health Bd.; Research Fell. & Regist. (Respirat. Dis.) West. Infirm. Glas.

PATEL, Kantilal Raojibhai Royton Medical Centre, Market Street, Royton, Oldham OL25 5QA Tel: 0161 652 6336 Fax: 0161 620 3986; 182 Castleton Road, Royton, Oldham OL2 6UP Tel: 0161 652 5486 — MB BS Bombay 1963 (Grant Med. Coll.) DTM & H Liverp. 1967; MRCP Glas. 1969; MRCGP 1978. Specialty: Care of the Elderly. Socs: BMA & Cardiol. Soc. India. Prev: Clin. Asst. (Geriat.) Tameside Gen. Hosp.; Regist. (Med.) Cheltenham Gen. Hosp.; Med. Adviser Sandoz (India) Ltd. Bombay.

PATEL, Kanubhai Mangalbhai Patel and Partners, Thornley Road Surgery, Thornley Road, Durham DH6 3NR Tel: 01429 820233 Fax: 01429 823667 — MB BS Baroda 1969.

PATEL, Karen Elizabeth Lime Tree Surgery, Lime Tree Avenue, Findon Valley, Worthing BN14 0DL Tel: 01903 264101 Fax: 01903 695494; 7 Longlands Glade, Charmandean, Worthing BN14 9NR Tel: 01903 232246 — MB ChB Leic. 1987; DRCOG 1991. GP.

PATEL, Kashyap Bhogilal 3 Ashleigh Court, Fulwood, Preston PR2 9WU — MB BS Gujarat 1984; MB BS Gujarat India 1984.

PATEL, Kaushik Ramanbhai Kingston Hospital, Galsworth Road, Kingston upon Thames KT2 7QB Tel: 020 8934 2515 Fax: 020 8934 3288 Email: kaushik@doctors.org.uk — MB ChB Sheff. 1987; BMedSci Sheff. 1986; MRCPath 1994. Cons. (Histopath. & Cytol.). Specialty: Histopath. Prev: Sen. Regist. (Histopath.) Leeds Gen. Infirm.; Regist. (Histopath.) Watford Gen. Hosp.; SHO (Clin. Path.) Roy. Hallamsh. Hosp. Sheff.

PATEL, Kersasp Rustomji (retired) 57 Butt Lane, Farnley, Leeds LS12 5AY Tel: 0113 263 1815 — MB BS Bombay 1952 (Seth. G.S. Med. Coll.) DTM & H Eng. 1955. Prev: Regist. (Med.) Kilton Hosp. Worksop & Beckett Hosp. Barnsley.

PATEL, Ketan Central Park Surgery, Balfour Street, Leyland, Preston PR25 2TD Tel: 01772 451940 Fax: 01772 623885 — MB ChB Bristol 1989.

PATEL, Ketan Chandubhai 279 Main Road, Sidcup DA14 6QL — MB BS Lond. 1994.

PATEL, Ketankumar Jerambhai Alastair Ross Health Centre, Breightmet Fold Lane, Breightmet, Bolton BL2 6NT — MB ChB Manch. 1991 (Manchester) DRCOG 1994; MRCGP 1995. General Practitioner Bolton. Specialty: Gen. Pract. Prev: Trainee GP/SHO Rochdale VTS.

PATEL, Khalid Ismail 59 Chaucer Road, London E7 9LZ — LMSSA Lond. 1996.

PATEL, Kinnari 104 High Moor Crescent, Moortown, Leeds LS17 6DZ — MB ChB Bristol 1990 (Bristol University) MRCP (UK) Roy. Coll. Of Physcians 1996. SpR Med. Oncol., Cookridge Hosp. Leeds.

PATEL, Kiranbhai Chhaganbhai University Hospital Birminghm, Department of Cardiology, Metchley Lane, Edgbaston, Birmingham Tel: 0121 472 1311; 19 Rowley View, West Bromwich B70 8QR — MB BChir Camb. 1994; BA (Hons.) Cantab 1991; MA Camb. 1995; MRCP Lond. 1997; PhD Bristol 2002. SpR (Cardiol) Univ. Hosp. Birm. Specialty: Cardiol.; Gen. Med. Special Interest: Heart Failure; Transpl.; Device Therap. Socs: BMA; Chairm. S. Asian Health Foundat. UK; Trainees Comm., Roy. Coll. Of Phys. Prev: SpR In Cardiol., Bristol Roy. Infirm.; SHO (Cardiol.) Bristol Infirm.; SHO (Gen. Med., Rheum., Therap. & c/o Elderly) Bristol Infirm.

PATEL, Kiritkumar Punjabhai Springfield Unit, City General Hospital, Stoke-on-Trent ST4 6QG Tel: 01782 553585 Fax: 01782 553587 Email: kiritp.patel@ncsh-tr.wmids.nhs.uk — MB BS Baroda 1967 (Baroda Med. Coll.) MRCP (UK) 1973; FRCP Lond. 1988. Cons. Phys. Gen./Geriat. Med. City Gen. Hosp. Stoke-on-Trent. Specialty: Gen. Med.; Care of the Elderly. Special Interest: Parkinsons Disease. Socs: Brit. Geriat. Soc.; W. Midlands Physicians Assn.

PATEL, Kirti 14 Whitton Avenue E., Greenford UB6 0PU — MB BS Lond. 1994.

PATEL, Kirtikbhai Amratlal 79 Belmont Road, Penn, Wolverhampton WV4 5UE — MB ChB Manch. 1993 (Manchester) FRCS Ed 1997; FRCS 1997. Specialty: Gen. Surg.

PATEL, Kishor Kantilal 25 Churchfields Road, Wednesbury WS10 9DX — MB BCh Wales 1994.

PATEL, Krutika 3 Freeman Street, Coventry CV6 5FF — MB ChB Leic. 1993.

PATEL, Lalitkumar Chaturbhai Patel, Brocklebank Health Centre, 249 Garrett Lane, London SW18 4UE Tel: 020 8870 1341; Triangle Surgery, Unit 3, Triangle House, 2 Broomhill Road, London SW18 4HX Tel: 020 8874 1700 Fax: 020 8870 7695 — MB BS Baroda 1957; DTM & H Eng. 1959; DObst & DGO Dub. 1960; LM Rotunda 1960.

PATEL, Lata Manojkumar Lynwood Medical Centre, Lynwood Drive, 2A-6 Collier Row, Romford RM5 3QL Tel: 01708 743244 Fax: 01708 736783 — MB BS Saurashtra 1977. Specialty: Geriat. Psychiat.

PATEL, Leena Department of Child Health, Booth Hall Children's Hospital, Manchester M9 7AA Tel: 0161 795 7000 Fax: 0161 740 6239 — MB BS Gujarat 1982 (V.S. Municipal medical School, Ahmedabad, India) MD Gujarat 1985; MRCP (UK) 1989; MHPE (Maastricht) 1996; MD (Manchester) 1998. Sen. Lect. (Child Health) & Hon. Cons. Paediat. Manch. Childr.s Hosp. Specialty: Paediat. Prev: Regist. (Paediat.) Hammersmith Hosp. & Hillingdon Hosp. Lond.; Lect. (Child Health) Booth Hall Childr. Hosp. Manch.

PATEL, Lily Sashikant Chichester Road, Romiley, Stockport SK6 4QR.

PATEL, Madhu Ganeshbhai The Surgery, 44 Broadway, Twydall, Gillingham ME8 6BD Tel: 01634 231364 — LRCP LRCS Ed. 1981 (M.P. Shah Med. Coll. Jamnagar) MB BS Saurashrta 1976; LRCP LRCS Ed. LRCPS Glas. 1981; MRCGP 1984. GP Gillingham.

PATEL, Madhumita The Park Practice, 113 Anerley Road, Anerley, London SE20 — MB BCh Wales 1992; MRCGP 1996.

PATEL, Maganlal Popatlal Ledbury, 10 Cannon Close, Coventry CV4 7AS — MB ChB Sheff. 1959; DMRD Ed. 1966. Regist. Edin. Roy. Infirm. & Sen. Regist. Aberd. Roy. Infirm.; Cons. Radiol. Walsgrave Hosp. NHS Trust. Specialty: Radiol. Special Interest: Nuclear Med. (Radio-Isotope Scanning). Socs: BMA (Chairm. Coventry Div.); RCR; ODA (Exec. Comm. Coventry Div.). Prev: Sen. Regist. (Radiol.) Roy. Infirm. Aberd.; SHO (Radiodiag.) Roy. Hosp. Edin.; Med. Off. Mulago Hosp. Kampala, Uganda.

PATEL, Mahendra Shay Lane Medical Centre, Shay Lane, Hale, Altrincham WA15 8NZ Tel: 0161 980 3835 Fax: 0161 903 9848; 6 Oldbrook Fold, Wood Lane, Timperley, Altrincham WA15 7PA — MB ChB Manch. 1984; DRCOG 1987; MRCGP (Distinc.) 1988; DCH RCP Lond. 1988.

PATEL, Mahendra Maganbhai Lamorna Surgery, 55A Thomas Drive, Gravesend DA12 5PZ Tel: 01474 363217 Fax: 01474 353746; Southlands, 363 Singlewell Road, Gravesend DA11 7RL Tel: 01474 363217 Fax: 01474 353746 — (Med. Coll. Baroda) MB BS Baroda 1969. Hosp. Pract. (Geriat. Med.) Gravesend Hosp., Gravesend. Specialty: Care of the Elderly. Socs: BMA. Prev: Ho. Off. (Med. & Surg.) Mulago Hosp. Kampala, Uganda.

PATEL, Mahendrakumar Chimanbhai Hartington Street Surgery, 28-30 Hartington Street, Barrow-in-Furness LA14 5SL Tel: 01229 870170 Fax: 01229 834677 — MB BS Bombay 1971. GP Barrow-in-Furness, Cumbria.

PATEL, Maheskumar Ramanlal 266 Lea Bridge Road, Leyton, London E10 7LD Tel: 020 8539 1221 — MB BS Saurashtra Univ. 1975. GP. Specialty: Gen. Pract.

PATEL, Mamta 1/R 50 Kelbourne Street, Glasgow G20 8PR — MB ChB Glas. 1993.

PATEL, Manashkumar 23 Freeman Road N., Leicester LE5 4NB — MB BCh Wales 1984; FRCA. 1990. Sen. Regist. (Anaesth.) Char. Cross Hosp. Lond. Specialty: Anaesth. Prev: Research Regist. Middlx. Hosp. Lond.

PATEL, Maneesh Chandrakant Department of Radiology, Charing Cross Hospital, Fulham Palace Road, London W6 8RF Tel: 020 8846 1835 Fax: 020 8383 0111 Email: mcpatel@hhnt.org — MB BS Lond. 1990. Cons. Neuroradiologist.

PATEL, Mr Maneklal Bhaktibhai 30 Tranmere Road, London SW18 3QQ — MB BS Bombay 1968 (Grant Med. Coll.) MS Bombay 1971, MB BS 1968; DO RCPSI 1974; DO Eng. 1974. Regist. (Ophth.) Roy. Surrey Co. Hosp. Guildford. Specialty: Ophth.

PATEL, Manibhai Hirabhai 19 Westminster Drive, London N13 4NT — MB BS India 1960; LAH; LM Dub. 1963.

PATEL, Manish — MB ChB Glas. 1997.

PATEL, Manu Khandubhai Longshoot Health Centre, Scholes, Wigan WN1 3NH Tel: 01942 242610 Fax: 01942 826612 — MB ChB Manch. 1976.

PATEL, Manubhai Kevaldas Neasden Medical Centre, 21 Tanfield Avenue, London NW2 7SA Tel: 020 8450 2834 Fax: 020 8452 4324; 63 Alicia Gardens, Harrow HA3 8JB Tel: 020 8907 9698 — MB BS Bombay 1968 (Grant Med. Coll.) Specialty: Gen. Pract.

PATEL, Mayank Bhaskar Rao 126 Kingston Road, New Malden KT3 3ND — BM Soton. 1995.

PATEL, Meeta — BM BS (Hons.) Nottm. 1998; BMedSci 1996. Specialty: Gen. Med.

PATEL, Minal Myra 13 Powis Gardens, London NW11 8HH — MB BCh BAO NUI 1984; LRCPSI 1984; MRCGP 1991. Specialty: Palliat. Med.

PATEL, Minesh 19 Rowsley Street, Leicester LE5 5JN — MB ChB Birm. 1994; ChB Birm. 1994.

PATEL, Minesh Kumar — MB BS Lond. 1991; MRCGP.

PATEL, Minoti Kalpesh Station Road Surgery, 46 Station Road, New Barnet, Barnet EN5 1QH Tel: 020 8441 4425 Fax: 020 8441 4957; 3 Gatcombe Way, Barnet EN4 9TT Tel: 020 8441 9630 — MB BS Baroda 1982.

PATEL, Mohamed Salim Ahmed Carmondean Medical Group, Carmondean Health Centre, Livingston EH54 8PY Tel: 01506 430031 Fax: 01506 432775; Roshni, 11 Northwood Park, Livingston EH54 8BD Tel: 01506 415591 — MB ChB Glas. 1973.

PATEL, Mohammed Yahya — MB BS Sind 1962 (Liaqat Med. Coll. Hyderabad) Prev: Sen. Ho. Surg. St. Mary Abbot's Hosp. Lond., Roy. North. Hosp. Lond. & St. And. Hosp. Dollis Hill.

PATEL, Motilal Rambhai Abercynon Health Centre, Abercynon, Mountain Ash CF45 4SU Tel: 01443 740447 Fax: 01443 740228; The Grove, 1 Aberfrwdd Road, Caegarw, Mountain Ash CF45 4DD Tel: 01443 478087 — MB BS Bombay 1972 (Seth G.S. Med. Coll.) Dip. Pract. Dermat. Wales 1991. Specialty: Dermat. Prev: Clin. Asst. (Dermat.) Aberdare Gen. Hosp.; SHO (Paediat. & Obst.) E. Glam. Hosp.; SHO (Dermat. & O & G) E. Glam. Hosp.

PATEL, Mukesh 16 Westwood Lane, Welling DA16 2HE — MB BCh Wales 1983; DRCOG 1987; MRCGP 1988.

PATEL, Mukesh Kantilal 35 Shale Street, Bilston WV14 0HF — MB BS Lond. 1996.

PATEL, Mukesh Narendra Vine House Surgery, Vine Street, Grantham NG31 6RQ Tel: 01476 576851 Fax: 01476 591732; Waltham House, 34 Swinegate, Grantham NG31 6RL Email: mukesh@freecard.co.uk — MB ChB Glas. 1979. Specialty: Anaesth.

Prev: Regist. Rotat. (Anaesth.) Liverp. HA; SHO (Anaesth.) Walton Hosp. Liverp.; SHO (Anaesth.) Roy. Liverp. Hosp.

PATEL, Mukundchandra Kanubhai Westbury Medical Centre, 205 Westbury Avenue, Wood Green, London N22 6RX Tel: 020 8888 3021 Fax: 020 8888 6898; Westbury Medical Centre Tel: 020 8445 8733 Fax: 020 8888 6898 — MB BS Rajasthan 1971 (S.P. Med. Coll. Bikaner)

PATEL, Mumtaz 141 Sharoe Green Lane, Fulwood, Preston PR2 8HE Tel: 01772 787786; 141 Sharoe Green Lane, Fulwood, Preston PR2 8HE Tel: 01772 787786 — MRCP 2000; MB ChB (Hons) Manch. 1996 (Manch.) SHO (Med. Rotat.) Leeds Gen. Infirm. Leeds. Specialty: Cardiol. Socs: Med. Sickness Soc.; MDU; BMA. Prev: SHO (Cardiothoracic Med. Rotat.) Wythenshawe Hosp. Manch.; Ho. Off. (Renal / Gen. Med.) Manch. Roy. Infirm.; Ho. Off. (Urol. / Vasc. Surg.) Manch. Roy. Infirm.

PATEL, Mumuksh Bhupendra The Surgery, 1 Glebe St., Chiswick, London W4 2BD Tel: 020 8747 4800 Fax: 020 8995 4388; 322 Goldhawk Road, Stamford Brook, London W6 0XF Tel: 020 8563 1863 — MB ChB Manch. 1992 (Manchester) GP. Specialty: Gen. Pract.; Acupunc. Prev: GP Assit. Chiswick; GP Private GP Clinic Stamford Hosp. Lond. W6.

PATEL, N M Langbank Medical Centre, Broad lane, Norris Green, Liverpool L11 1AD Tel: 0151 226 1976 Fax: 0151 270 2873; 18a Druids Cross Road, Calderstones, Liverpool L18 3HW Tel: 0151 428 9119 — M.B.B.S. (MRM Medical College, Gulbarga) MBBS 1978; (Scottish Cojoint Board) LRCP, LRCS, LRCPSS 1982; RCOG 1982. GP Principle, Liverp. FMSA; Wavertree Lodge, Clin. Asst. in Learning Disabil. & Challenging Behaviour organisation, Liverp. Health Auth. Socs: BMA; Overseas Doctors Assoc.; Med. Protec. Soc. Prev: Colposcopy (Clin. Asst.) '87-'01, Whiston Hosp. Prescott.

PATEL, Mrs Nalini 40 Whitgift Avenue, South Croydon CR2 6AY Tel: 020 8688 6975 — MB BS Gujarat 1973.

PATEL, Narendra Whinshiels, Main Road, Wrinehill, Crewe CW3 9BJ — MB ChB Manch. 1981. GP Crewe.

PATEL, Narendrakumar Babubhai Birkenbrae, Spoutwells, Dunkeld PH8 0AZ — MB ChB St. And. 1964; MRCOG 1969; FRCOG 1988.

PATEL, Naresh Ambalal Patel and Partners, Broom Lane Medical Centre, 70 Broom Lane, Rotherham S60 3EW Tel: 01709 364470 Fax: 01709 820009; 4 Newman Court, Moorgate, Rotherham S60 3JA Tel: 01709 366294 — MB BS Bombay 1977 (Topiwala Nat. Med. Coll. Bombay) MRCS Eng. LRCP Lond. 1978. GP Tutor Med. Stud. Sheff. Med. Sch. Prev: Trainee GP Rotherham VTS; SHO (Thoracic Med.) Milford Chest Hosp. Godalming; Ho. Off. (Gen. Med.) Staincliffe Gen. Hosp. Dewsbury.

PATEL, Mr Natwarlal Gangjibhai Oxford Road Surgery, 292 Oxford Road, Reading RG30 1AD Tel: 0118 957 4614 Fax: 0118 959 5486 — MB BS Bombay 1956; DLO RCS Eng. 1958; FRCS Ed. 1960.

PATEL, Natwarlal Shivabhai 19 Dewhurst Road, London W14 0ET Tel: 020 7603 2103 Fax: 020 7603 2103 — (Roy. Lond. Hosp.) MB BS Gujarat 1960; DMJ Soc. Apoth. Lond. 1965; PhD Lond. 1972. State Forens. Path. & Hon. Lect. Lusaka, Zambia. Specialty: Gen. Pract. Socs: Brit. Acad. Forens. Med.; Assn. Police Surg. Prev: Sen. Lect. & Forens. Path. The Lond. Hosp. Med. Coll.; Lect. & Asst. Forens. Path. The Lond. Hosp. Med. Coll.; Regist. (Path.) Moorgate Gen. Hosp. Rotherham.

PATEL, Navnitbhai Hargovindbhai Southey Green Medical Centre, 281 Southey Green Road, Sheffield S5 7QB Tel: 0114 232 6401 Fax: 0114 285 4402 — MB BS Baroda 1973.

PATEL, Nayan 48 Ragburn Road, Sidcup DA15 8RB — MB BS Lond. 1993.

PATEL, Nayana Pravin 507 Kenton Road, Harrow HA3 0UL — MB BS Gujarat 1973; DGO 1976.

PATEL, Neelanjana Kantilal 9 Lomond Place, Linburn, Erskine PA8 6AP Tel: 0141 812 4569 — MB BS Bombay 1967 (Grant Med. Coll.) Prev: Regist. (O & G) Redland Hosp. Glas.

PATEL, Neera Kanubhai Department of Histopathology, Royal Sussex County Hospital, Eastern Road, Brighton BN2 5BE Tel: 01273 664502 Fax: 01273 664412 — MB BS Lond. 1990 (Univ. Coll. Hosp.) BSc (Hons.) Lond. 1987; DRCPath 1995; MRCPath 1997. Cons. (Histopath. & Cytopath.) Roy. Sussx Co. Hosp. Brighton. Specialty: Histopath. Prev: Lect. & Hon. Sen. Regist. (Histopath. & Cytopath.) St. Thos. Hosp. Lond.

PATEL, Neeta 37c Elm Park Road, London N3 1EG — MB ChB Manch. 1992.

PATEL, Neil Dinesh 20 Sycamore Tree Close, Radyr, Cardiff CF15 8RT — MB BS Lond. 1994.

PATEL, Nikhil Raman Eastbourne District Hospital, Kings Drive, Eastbourne BN20 7AF — MB BS Lond. 1989; MRCP Lond. 1992; FRCP 2003. Cons. Cardiol., Eastbourne Dist. Hosp.; Hon. Cons., Guys and St Thomas' Hosp., Lond. Specialty: Cardiol. Special Interest: Acute Coronary Syndrome; Complex Pacing; Echocardiography. Prev: Regist. (Cardiol.) Guy's Hosp. Lond.

PATEL, Nikunj Kantilal 4 Streatham Vale, London SW16 5TE; 205 Westway, Raynes Park, London SW20 9LW Tel: 020 8542 1580 — MB BS Lond. 1994 (Charing Cross and Westerminster) BSc Lond. 1991; FRCS 1998. Specialty: Gen. Surg.

PATEL, Nila Dilip The Village Surgery, Worle, Hill Road East, Worle, Weston Super Mare BS22 9HF Tel: 01934 516671 Fax: 01934 520664 — MB BS Mysore 1977; LRCP LRCS Ed. LRCPS Glas. 1982.

PATEL, Nilam 2 Sandringham Park, Swansea Vale, Swansea SA6 8QD Tel: 01792 761349 Fax: 01792 761104 — MB BCh Wales 1981; MRCGP 1986. Med. Adviser Dept. Transport Swansea.

PATEL, Nilesh Rajnikant North Brink Practice, 7 North Brink, Wisbech PE13 1JR Tel: 01945 585121 Fax: 01945 476423; 55 Clarkson Avenue, Wisbech PE13 2EH — MB BCh BAO NUI 1980 (Royal College of Surgeons in Ireland) DRCOG 1986; MRCGP 1986; FRCGP 2003. GP N. Brink Pract., Wisbech.

PATEL, Nilesh Ravji 38 Dale Avenue, Edgware HA8 6AE; 29 Fairway Avenue, Kingsbury, London NW9 0ET Tel: 020 8206 0066 — MB BS Lond. 1997. Ho. Off. (Med. & Surg.); SHO (A & E). Specialty: Accid. & Emerg. Socs: BMA; MDU.

PATEL, Nilkanth Princess Alexandra Hospital, Department of Anaesthetics, Hamstel Road, Harlow CM20 1QX — MB BS Ibadan 1978; FFARCSI 1986. Cons. Anaesth. Princess Alexandra Hosp. Harlow. Specialty: Anaesth. Special Interest: Acute Pain Management; Obstetric Anaesthesia. Prev: Sen. Regist. (Anaesth.) St Jas. Univ. & Leeds Gen. Infirm.

PATEL, Mr Nimesh Narendra — MB ChB Manch. 1992 (Manchester) FRCS 1997. Specialty: Otorhinolaryngol.

PATEL, Nina Rasikbhai 93 Michleham Down, London N12 7JL — MB BS Lond. 1991.

PATEL, Niranjana Ramanlal 14 Sinclair Grove, Golders Green, London NW11 9JG Tel: 020 8455 0430 — MB BS Rajasthan 1973 (S.M.S. Med. Coll. Jaipur) Ho. Off. Dept. Gen. Med. & Chest Unit Bangour Gen. Hosp. Broxburn.

PATEL, Niranjanbhai Ratilal The Surgery, 27 Burges Road, East Ham, London E6 2BJ Tel: 020 8472 0421 Fax: 020 8552 9912; 34 Hillington Gardens, Woodford Green IG8 8QT Tel: 020 8550 3413 Fax: 020 8550 3413 — MB BS Lond. 1977 (London Hospital Medical College) Specialty: Family Plann. & Reproduc. Health.

PATEL, Nishal Basildon Hospital, Nether Mayne, Basildon SS16 5NL — MB BS Lond. 1998.

PATEL, Nitesh 5 Nutfield Road, Thornton Heath, Croydon CR7 7DP — MB ChB Manch. 1994.

PATEL, Mr Nitin Kumar Ratilal 50 Hillside Court, Gledhow Lane, Leeds LS7 4NJ — MB BCh Wales 1987; FRCS Eng. 1992. Sen. Regist. (Neurosurg.) Frenchay Hosp. Bristol. Specialty: Neurosurg. Socs: MDU. Prev: SHO Rotat. (Surg.) St. Jas. Hosp. Leeds; SHO (Neurosurg.) Hope Hosp. Salford; Ho. Off. (Gen. Med. & Neurol.) Singleton Hosp. Swansea.

PATEL, Or Timeer Shantilal 102 Sidcup High Street, Sidcup DA14 6DS — MB BS Lond. 1996.

PATEL, Pankaj Stoney Stanton Medical Centre, 475 Stoney Stanton Road, Coventry CV6 5EA Tel: 024 7688 8484 Fax: 024 7658 1247; 23 Cotswold Drive, Finham, Coventry CV3 6EZ Tel: 024 76 690588 — BM Soton. 1983.

PATEL, Parag Wolverhampton Road Surgery, 13 Wolverhampton Road, Stafford ST17 4BP Tel: 01785 258161 Fax: 01785 224140 — MB BS Lond. 1989.

PATEL, Parimal Rushey Mead Health Centre, 8 Lockerbie Walk, Leicester LE4 7ZX Tel: 0116 266 9616; 5 Southland Road, South Knighton, Leicester LE2 3RJ — MB ChB Manch. 1986.

PATEL, Parindkumar Bipinchandra 17 Orchard Rise, Ruislip HA4 7LR Tel: 0410 597320 — MB BS Lond. 1995 (St George's) SHO (Surg.) Mayday Univ. Hosp. Specialty: Anaesth.; Intens. Care.

Socs: MDU. Prev: SHO (Med.) St Geo.'s Hosp.; SHO (Med.) Frimley Pk. Hosp.; SHO (Anaesth.) Mt. Vernon Hosp.

PATEL, Paritosh Chandubhai 43 Fircroft Road, London SW17 7PR — MB BS Lond. 1994.

PATEL, Pinakin Bhanubhai 21 Tylers Court, Vicars Bridge Close, Alperton, Wembley HA0 1XT — MB BS Lond. 1989.

PATEL, Mr Piyush Jashbhai 11 Dalton Road, Earlsdon, Coventry CV5 6PB Tel: 024 76 677444 Fax: 024 76 691436 — MB BChir (Distinc. Surg.) Camb. 1980 (Univ. of Camb.) MA (Hons.) Camb. 1981, BA (Hons.) 1977; FRCS Ed. 1987; FRCS Eng. 1987. Cons. ENT Surg. Walsgrave Hosp. NHS Trust Coventry. Specialty: Otolaryngol. Prev: Sen. Regist. (ENT Surg.) W. Midl. Otolaryngol. Train. Scheme.

PATEL, Poulam Manubhai ICRF Cancer Medicine Research Unit, St. James University Hospital, Leeds LS9 7TF — MB BS Lond. 1983; MRCP (UK) 1989; PhD Lond. 1994. ICRF Sen. Clin. Scientist & Hon. Cons. Med. Oncol. St. Jas. Univ. Hosp. Leeds. Specialty: Oncol. Prev: ICRF Clin. Research Scientist & Hon. Sen. Regist. St. Jas. Univ. Hosp. Leeds; CRC Clin. Research Fell. Inst. Cancer Research Chester Beaty Laborat. Lond.; Regist. (Med.) Mayday Hosp. Croydon.

PATEL, Prabhudas Govindbhai 193 Chase Side, London N14 5JB — MB ChB Makerere 1966.

PATEL, Pradeepkumar Chimanbhai (Patrick) The Surgery, 1 Tollington Court, Tollington Park, London N4 3QT Tel: 020 7272 2121 Fax: 020 7561 1901; 3 Neeld Crescent, Wembley HA9 6LW Tel: 020 8903 4501 Fax: 020 8903 5397 — MB BS Bombay 1975 (Topiwala National Medical College Bombay University India) MRCS Eng. LRCP Lond. 1980; ECFMG 1980. GP Princip. Specialty: Gen. Pract. Socs: Camden & Islington Local Med. Comm., Med. Audit Advisery Gp. & Primary Care Educat. Bd. Commiss.ing Sub-Gp.; BMA. Prev: Clin. Asst. in the c/o the Elderly Geo. Eliot Hosp. Nuneaton Warks; Trainee GP Manch.; Hosp. posts.

PATEL, Pradipkumar Rambhai Ealing Hospital, Radiology Department, Uxbridge Road, Southall UB1 3HW Tel: 020 8967 5373; 34 High Drive, New Malden KT3 3UG Tel: 020 8949 9202 — MB BCh Wales 1977 (University of Wales Cardiff) FRCR 1982; DMRD 1982. Cons. Radiol. Ealing Hosp. Middlx. & Hon. Clin. Sen. Lect. Imperial Coll. Lond. Specialty: Radiol. Prev: Cons. Radiol. Ealing Hosp. Lond.; Sen. Regist. & Regist. (Radiol.) St. Mary's Hosp. Lond. W2; SHO (Paediat.) King's Coll. Hosp. Lond.

PATEL, Prafulchandra 31 Leven Close, Chandlers Ford, Eastleigh SO53 4SH — MB ChB Manch. 1986; MRCP (UK) 1990; MD Manch. 1995. Cons. Gastroenterol. & Hon. Sen. Lect. Soton. Univ. Hosp. Trust. Specialty: Gastroenterol. Socs: Brit. Soc. Gastroenterol.; RCP.

PATEL, Prafulchandra Chimanbhai Charnwood Health Centre, 1 Spinney Hill Road, Leicester LE5 3GH; 37 Carisbrooke Gardens, Leicester LE2 3PR — MB ChB Glas. 1970; MRCP (UK) 1974.

PATEL, Prafulchandra Chunibhai Rectory Park Drive Surgery, 6 Rectory Park Drive, Pitsea, Basildon SS13 3DW Tel: 01268 552999 Fax: 01268 559986 — MB BS Bombay 1972.

PATEL, Prafulchandra Jashbhai (retired) 167 Ellesmere Road, London NW10 1LG Tel: 020 8208 0188 — MB BS Gujarat 1965. Clin. Med. Off. Enfield HA.

PATEL, Prafull Ambalal 63 Belvoir Drive, Loughborough LE11 2SN Tel: 01509 236906 — MB BS Bombay 1952 (Seth G.S. Med. Coll.)

PATEL, Mr Pravin Chaturbhai 507 Kenton Road, Harrow HA3 0UL — MB BS Gujarat 1973; FRCS Ed. 1980.

PATEL, Pravina Kantilal Littleover Medical Centre, 640 Burton Road, Littleover, Derby DE23 6EL Tel: 01332 207100 Fax: 01332 342680 — MB BS Poona 1973 (B.J. Med. Coll.) DO RCPSI 1977.

PATEL, Pravinbhai Kantilal 9 Athlone Road, Walsall WS5 3QU Tel: 01922 29395; 291 Walsall Road, West Bromwich B71 3LN Tel: 0121 588 2286 — MB BS Baroda 1968 (Med. Coll. Baroda) GP W. Midl.

PATEL, Pravinkumar Maganbhai The Surgery, 24 Suttons Avenue, Hornchurch RM12 4LF Tel: 01708 442711 Fax: 01708 471756 — MB BS Bombay 1980; MB BS Bombay 1980; MRCS Eng. LRCP Lond. London 1989.

PATEL, Mr Prem Swaroop 9 Hanging Water Close, Sheffield S11 7FH — MB BS Jabalpur 1979; MS Jabalpur 1982, MB BS 1979; FRCS Ed. 1985.

PATEL, Priti City of London Migraine Clinic, 22 Charterhouse Square, London EC1M 6DX — MB ChB Dundee 1988; DA (UK) 1993. Specialty: Gen. Med. Socs: BMA; IMS. Prev: Regist.(Anaesth.) NE Thames Regional Plastics Burns Unit St. And. Hosp. Billericay,Essex; SHO (Anaesth.) Leicester Teachg. Hosps.

PATEL, Priti Islington Child & Family Consultation Service, Northern Health Centre, 580 Holloway Road, London N7 — MB BS Lond. 1992 (King's Coll.) BSc Lond. 1988; MRCPsych 1996. Cons. Child & Adolesc. Psychiat., Islington Child & Family Consultation Serv. Specialty: Child & Adolesc. Psychiat.

PATEL, Punambhai Somabhai 7 Coape Road, Stockwood, Bristol BS14 8TN — MB BS Bombay 1955 (Grant Med. Coll.)

PATEL, R S Holmlands Medical Centre, 16-20 Holmlands Drive, Oxton, Birkenhead CH43 0TX Tel: 0151 608 7750 Fax: 0151 608 0989.

PATEL, Mr Rahmikant Haridas CARE, Victoria Park, 108 -112 Daisybank Road, Manchester M14 5QH Tel: 0161 257 3799 Fax: 0161 224 4283; Ashtree Cottage, South Hill Avenue, Harrow HA1 3PA Tel: 020 8864 2400 — MB BS Baroda 1975; MRCOG 1983; FRCOG 1999. CARE, The Alexandra Hosp. Cons. Gynaecologist/Reproductive Med. Vict. Pk. 108-112 Daisybank Toad, Manch. M14 5QH. Specialty: Obst. & Gyn. Socs: BMA; Brit. Menopause Soc.; BSPOGA. Prev: Clin. research Fell. & Hon. Regist. St Geo.'s Hosp. Lond.; Med. Off. & Research Lect. (O & G) St Geo.'s Hosp. Lond.; Assoc. Specialist (Obst.& Gyn.) St Geo.'s Hosp. Lond.

PATEL, Rahul Vinayak 16 Endcliffe Hall Avenue, Sheffield S10 3EL — MB BS Lond. 1998.

PATEL, Mr Rajan Shashi 22 Stormont Road, London N6 4NL — MB ChB Glas. 1995; MRCS Glas. 1998. SHO (Gen. Surg.) Vict. Roy. Infirm. NHS Trust Glas. Specialty: Otorhinolaryngol. Socs: BMA.

PATEL, Mr Rajankumar Consultant Surgeon, Department of Surgery, Russells Hall Hospital, Dudley DY1 2HQ Tel: 01384 244021 Email: r.patel@dgoh.nhs.uk; 90 Fitzroy Avenue, Harborne, Birmingham B17 8RQ Email: rajtpatel@ed.com — MB BCh Wales 1984 (Cardiff) FRCS Eng. 1989; MD Birm. 1995; FRCS (Gen) 1997. Cons. Gen. & Vasc. Surg., Dudley. Specialty: Gen. Surg. Special Interest: Colorectal Surg.; Vasc. Surg. Prev: Sen. Regist. (Gen. Surg.) Good Hope Hosp. Birm.; Sen. Regist. (Gen. Surg.) City Hosp. Birm.; Sen. Regist. (Rotating), W. Midlands.

PATEL, Rajen — MB BS Lond. 1993; BSc (Hons.) Lond. 1990. SHO (Med.) Hastings & Rotherham NHS Trust. Specialty: Gen. Med.

PATEL, Rajendra Melbourne Road Surgery, 71 Melbourne Road, Leicester LE2 0GU Tel: 0116 253 9479 Fax: 0116 242 5602 — MB ChB Manch. 1977. Prev: Princip. GP Leic.; SHO (O & G) Tameside Matern. Hosp.; SHO (Orthop./A & E) Leicester Roy. Infirm.

PATEL, Rajendra Bhailalbhai The Health Centre, Trenchard Avenue, Thornaby, Stockton-on-Tees TS17 0DD Tel: 01642 762636 Fax: 01642 766464; 26 Church Lane, Middleton Saint George, Darlington DL2 1DF Tel: 01325 333179 — MB BS Saurashtra 1980. Specialty: Gen. Pract.

PATEL, Rajendra Nagindas 6 Wedgwood Way, London SE19 3ES — MB BS Lond. 1987; DCH RCP Lond. 1991.

PATEL, Rajesh The Brooke Surgery, 20 Market Street, Hyde SK14 1AT Tel: 0161 368 3312 Fax: 0161 368 5670 Email: patel@which.net — MB ChB Manch. 1985; MRCGP 1992; Dip. Pract. Dermat. Wales 1996. p/t Gen. Med. Practitioner; PEC Chair Tameside & Glossop PCT. Special Interest: Primary Care Dermat. Socs: Primary Care Dermat. Soc.

PATEL, Rajesh Bhailalbhai The Fullwell Avenue Surgery, 272 Fullwell Avenue, Clayhall, Ilford IG5 0SB Tel: 020 8550 9988 Fax: 020 8550 1241; 96 Cheriton Avenue, Clayhall, Ilford IG5 0QL Tel: 020 8551 1586 — MB BS Mysore 1979; MRCS Eng. LRCP Lond. 1981. GP Ilford. Prev: SHO (O & G, A & E Radiother. & Oncol.) Redbridge & Waltham Forest HA.

PATEL, Rajesh Manubhai Bethnal Green Health Centre, 60 Florida Street, London E2 6LL Tel: 020 7739 4837 Fax: 020 7729 2190 — MB BS Lond. 1979 (King's Coll.) BSc (Physiol.) Lond. 1976, MB BS 1979.

PATEL, Rajesh Rasikbhai Manchester Road Surgery, 57 Manchester Road, Southport PR9 9BN Tel: 01704 532314 Fax: 01704 539740; 46 Cambridge Road, Southport PR9 9PP — MB BS Newc. 1985; DRCOG 1988; MRCGP 1989; FRCGP 1999. Civic Serv. Clin. Local Med. Off. S.port. Prev: SHO Geriat. Southport & Formby

Dist. Gen. Hosp.; Trainee GP Southport; SHO (Geriat. & A & E) Middlesbrough.

PATEL, Rajnika Niranjan 94 Mackenzie Road, London N7 8RE — MB BS Baroda 1972.

PATEL, Rajnikant Bhanabhai Bourne Galletly Practice Team, 40 North Road, Bourne PE10 9BT Tel: 01778 562200 Fax: 01778 562207; 79 West Road, Bourne PE10 9PX — MB BCh Wales 1977; DRCOG 1982; Dip. Pract. Dermat. Wales 1992. GP Bourne. Prev: Trainee GP P'boro. VTS; Ho. Surg., Surg. Unit Univ. Hosp. Cardiff; Ho. Off. (Med.) War Memor. & Maelor Hosps. Wrexham.

PATEL, Rajnikant Jorabhai Department of Radiology, George Eliot Hospital, Nuneaton CV10 7DJ Tel: 024 7686 5391 Fax: 024 7686 5095; 29 Norwich Close, Nuneaton CV11 6GF Tel: 024 7686 5164 — (Med. Coll. Baroda) MB BS Baroda 1970; MS Univ. Barado 1974; DMRD Liverp. 1978; FFR RCSI 1981. Cons. Radiol Geo. Eliot. Hosp. Nuneaton NHS Trust. Specialty: Radiol. Socs: Roy. Coll. Radiol.; BMA. Prev: Sen. Cons. Roy. Hosp.; Cons. Radiol. MOH Muscat Sultanate of Oman; Sen. Regist. Walton Hosp. Liverp.

PATEL, Rajnikant Manibhai Heath View Practice, Glascote Health Centre, Caledonian, Tamworth B77 2ED Tel: 01827 281000 Fax: 01827 262048; 5 Blackdown, Wilnecote, Tamworth B77 4JQ Tel: 01827 895462 — (Gandhi Med. Coll. Bhopal) MB BS Vikram 1969.

PATEL, Rajnikant Shambhubhai Town Surgery, Baxter Lane, Loughborough LE11 1TT Tel: 01509 268060 Fax: 01509 216146; 283 Forest Road, Loughborough LE11 3HT — MB BS Bombay 1973.

PATEL, Rakesh 19 Hodgson Street, Darwen BB3 2DS — MB ChB Manch. 1991.

PATEL, Rakesh 135 Somerton Road, Breightmet, Bolton BL2 6LW — MB ChB Sheff. 1996.

PATEL, Ramanbhai Vaghajibhai The Health Centre, Wallsgreen Road, Cardenden, Lochgelly KY5 0JE Tel: 01592 722443 Fax: 01592 721679 — MB BS Bombay 1941. GP Lochgelly, Fife.

PATEL, Ramanlal Gopalji Royal Manchester Chilren's Hospital, Hospital Road, Swinton, Manchester M27 4HA — MB BS Bombay 1966 (Grant Med. Coll.) DCH Eng. 1968; MRCP (UK) 1971; FRCP Lond. 1984. Cons. Paediat. Cardiol. Roy. Manch. Childr. Hosp. Pendlebury & Wythenshawe Hosp. Manch. Specialty: Cardiol. Socs: Brit. Paediat. Assn. & Brit. Cardiac Soc. Prev: Staff Cardiol. Hosp. Sick Childr. Toronto Canada & Asst. Prof.; Paediat. Univ. Toronto; Sen. Regist. Hosp. Sick Childr. Lond.

PATEL, Ramesh Walsgrave Hospital, Coventry CV2 2DX; The North Lodge, Coventry Road, Berkswell, Coventry CV7 7AZ — MB ChB Sheff. 1980; FRCS (Ed.) 1985; MD 1994; FRCS (CTh) 1994. Regist. (Cardiothorocic Surg.) Harefield Hosp.; Research Fell. Rayne Inst. St. Ths. Hosp.; Sen. Regist. Qu. Eliz. Hosp. Birm.; Sen. Regist. Birm. Childr. Hosp.; Sen. Regist. Birm. Heartlands Hosp. Specialty: Cardiothoracic Surg. Socs: Fell. Roy. Coll. Surgs. Edin.; Soc. Cardiothorocic Surgs. GB.

PATEL, Ramesh Chandra Paston Health Centre, Chadburn, Peterborough PE4 7DH Tel: 01733 572584 Fax: 01733 328131; 18 Lakeside, Werrington, Peterborough PE4 6QZ Tel: 01733 578288 Fax: 01733 578288 — MB BS Lond. 1976 (St. Mary's) MRCS Eng. LRCP Lond. 1976; MRCGP 1980. Prev: Trainee GP Dudley VTS; Ho. Surg. & Ho. Phys. Roy. Hosp. Wolverhampton.

PATEL, Ramesh Dhanjibhai 22 Rowbank Way, Loughborough LE11 4AJ Email: spiderram@hotmail.com — BM BS Nottm. 1994; BMedSci Nottm. 1992.

PATEL, Ramesh Govindji St George's Medical Centre, Field Road, New Brighton, Wallasey CH45 5LN Tel: 0151 630 2080 Fax: 0151 637 0370 — MB BS Gujarat 1971.

PATEL, Rameshbhai Ramubhai The Health Centre, Main Road, Radcliffe-on-Trent, Nottingham NG12 2GD Tel: 0115 933 3737 — MB BS Lond. 1984 (Royal Free Hospital) MRCP (UK) 1987; DCH RCP Lond. 1989; MRCGP 1989. GP Trainer Nottm. VTS. Prev: Trainee GP Nottm. VTS.

PATEL, Rameshchandra Ashabhai 32 Baldwyns Park, Bexley, Dartford DA5 2BA Tel: 01322 529026; 32 Baldwyns Park, Bexley DA5 2BA Tel: 01322 529026 Fax: 01322 529026 — (Amritsar) MFFP 1994 Lond.; MB BS Punjab (India) 1962; DA Eng. 1967; DObst RCOG 1967. Clin. Asst. Chistlehurst; Family Plann. Instruc. Doctor. Specialty: Family Plann. & Reproduc. Health. Socs: BMA; Med. & Dent. Assn. Prev: Clin. Asst. W. Hill Hosp. Dartford & Clin. Med. Off. FPC Memor. Hosp.; Med. Off. Kenya Govt.; SHO (Anaesth.) Essex Co. Hosp. Colchester.

PATEL, Rameshchandra Chhotabhai Ascot Medical Centre, 690 Osmaston Road, Derby DE24 8GT Tel: 01332 348845; 163 Pastures Hill, Littleover, Derby DE23 7AZ — MB BS Bombay 1971.

PATEL, Rameshchandra Harmanbhai Patel and Partners, 4 Bedford Street, Bletchley, Milton Keynes MK2 2TX Tel: 01908 377101 Fax: 01908 645903; 7 Carnoustie Grove, Bletchley, Milton Keynes MK3 7RP — MB ChB Manch. 1974.

PATEL, Rameshchandra Maganbhai Stroud Avenue, 250 Stroud Avenue, Willenhall WV12 3DA Tel: 01902 609500 Fax: 01902 603625; 233 Stroud Avenue, Willenhall WV12 4DA — MB BS Bombay 1965. Specialty: Dermat. Socs: BMA; ODA; MDU. Prev: Clin Dermat New Cross Hosp Wolverhampton.

PATEL, Rameshchandra Nathabhai East Park Road Medical Centre, 264 East Park Road, Leicester LE5 5FD Tel: 0116 273 7700; 10 Campbell Avenue, Thurmaston, Leicester LE4 8HB Tel: 0116 25100 — MB BS Baroda 1964.

PATEL, Ramilaben Ramanlal Chorlton Health Centre, 1 Nicolas Road, Chorlton, Manchester M21 9NJ Tel: 0161 881 7941 Fax: 0161 861 7567; 2 Rowantree Drive, Brooklands, Sale M33 3PA — MB BS Baroda 1966; DRCOG 1968; MRCOG 1974. Prev: GP Greenford; Train. GP Birm.; Regist. (O & G) Dudley Rd. Hosp. Birm.

PATEL, Ramnik Mathurbhai Rushbottom Lane Surgery, 91 Rushbottom Lane, Benfleet SS7 4EA Tel: 01268 754311 Fax: 01268 795150; 40 Avondale Road, Benfleet SS7 1EJ Tel: 01268 755150 Fax: 01268 795150 — (Med. Coll. Baroda) MB BS Baroda 1969. SHO (Gen. Med. & O & G) Hallam Hosp. W. Bromwich. Specialty: Family Plann. & Reproduc. Health. Prev: Ho. Off. (Gen. Surg. & Med.) Kenyatta Nat. Teachg. Hosp. Nairobi, Kenya; Med. Adviser SW Essex Adopt. Panel.

PATEL, Ramubhai Mitthalbhai Dartmouth Medical Centre, 1 Richard Street, West Bromwich B70 9JL Tel: 0121 553 1144 Fax: 0121 580 1914; Central Clinic, Horseley Road, Tipton DY4 7NB Tel: 0121 557 4377 — MB BS Gujarat 1964 (B.J. Med. Coll. Ahmedabad) DTM & H Liverp. 1972. Prev: Regist. Summerfield Hosp. Birm.; SHO Maelor Gen. Hosp. Wrexham & Dudley Rd. Hosp. Birm.

PATEL, Rasiklal Somabhai 93 Michelham Down, London N12 7JL — MB BS Bombay 1954 (Grant Med. Coll.) Specialty: Gen. Pract.

PATEL, Ravindrabhai 7 Chelsea Close, Worcester Park KT4 7SF — MB BS Lond. 1988.

PATEL, Rayhana — MB ChB Manch. 1998.

PATEL, Rekha Dhirubhai 23 Geneva Drive, Newcastle ST5 2QQ Tel: 01782 622650 — MB BS Mysore 1972 (Kasturba Med. Coll. Mangalore) DA Eng. 1975; FFA RCSI 1977. Cons. Anaesth. Wolverhampton DHA. Specialty: Anaesth. Prev: Sen. Regist. (Anaesth.) Birm. AHA (T).

PATEL, Rekha Kantilal Compton Health Centre, High St., Shaw, Oldham; Shawdale, Castleton Road, Royton, Oldham OL2 6UP — MB BS Bombay 1964 (Grant Med. Coll.) DObst RCOG 1967. Prev: SCMO Rochdale AHA; SHO (O & G) Ashton-under-Lyne Gen. Hosp.; Deptm. Med. Off. Essex CC.

PATEL, Rita Mohanbhai 70 Lawn Street, Bolton BL1 3AY — MB ChB Manch. 1996.

PATEL, Roger Nagindas 7 Chaston Road, Great Shelford, Cambridge CB2 5AS — MB BChir Camb. 1995; MRCP (UK) 1999. Specialist Regist. (Radiol.) Camb. Rotat.

PATEL, Roshni Raman 36 Meadow Brook Road, Birmingham B31 1NE — MB ChB Bristol 1995.

PATEL, Rupal 24 Whitebridge Parkway, Newcastle upon Tyne NE3 5LU — MB ChB Dundee 1996; MRCPCH. Specialty: Paediat.

PATEL, Ruth Shahani 51 Heybridge Drive, Ilford IG6 1PE — MB BS Lond. 1993; DRCOG Lond. 1996. GP Regist. Specialty: Gen. Pract. Prev: GP Trainee.

PATEL, Sameer 9 Lomond Place, Erskine PA8 6AP — MB ChB Glas. 1995.

PATEL, Samir 147 Turner Road, Edgware HA8 6AS — BM Soton. 1993; (American Board of Internal Medicine 2000); MRCP 1997. Regist. Elderly Care Barnet Hosp.; Fell. in Pulm. and Critical Care Med., Yale Univ. Connecticut, USA. Specialty: Care of the Elderly. Socs: Assoc. Mem. Amer. Coll. of Chest Phys.s.

PATEL, Samir Niranjan Pavilion Practice, 9 Brighton Terrace, London SW9 8DJ Tel: 020 7274 9252 Fax: 020 7274 0740 — MB BS Lond. 1988.

PATEL, Sandip 204 Whitehall Road, Leeds LS12 4AR — MB BS Lond. 1994.

PATEL, Sangeeta Balham Park Surgery, 92 Balham Park Road, London SW12 8EA Tel: 020 8767 8828 Fax: 020 8682 1736 — MB BS Lond. 1986 (Kings College Hosp. School of Med.) DRCOG 1990; MRCGP (Distinc.) 1990; MA (Med. Anthropology) 1997. GP Princip.; Clin. Lect. (Gen. Pract.) St. Geo. Hosp. Med. Sch. Lond.

PATEL, Sangita 4 Hatherleigh Road, Leicester LE5 5NR — MB ChB Sheff. 1990.

PATEL, Sanjay 19 Courtleigh Avenue, Barnet EN4 0HT — MB ChB Manch. 1988; DRCOG 1991; MRCGP 1992.

PATEL, Sanjay 208 Church Hill Road, Barnet EN4 8PP — MB BS Lond. 1998.

PATEL, Sanjay Kumar Sanderson and Partners, Adan House Surgery, St. Andrews Lane, Spennymoor DL16 6QA Tel: 01388 817777 Fax: 01388 811700 — MB ChB Leeds 1986; DRCOG 1991; DCCH RCGP 1991; MRCGP 1992. GP. Specialty: Palliat. Med. Socs: BMA.

PATEL, Sanjay Vinod Sanmay, Basnetts Wood, Endon, Stoke-on-Trent ST9 9DQ Fax: 01782 570069 — BM BS Nottm. 1995; BMedSci Nottm. 1993. Demonst. (Biomed. Sci.) & SHO (Ophth.) Sheff. Univ. & Roy. Hallamsh. Hosp. Specialty: Ophth.

PATEL, Sanjaykumar 42 Sheridan Street, Walsall WS2 9QX — MB ChB Leeds 1993.

PATEL, Sanjeev Rasikbhai Department of Rheumatology, St. Helier Hospital, Carshalton SM5 1AA Tel: 020 8296 2473; 24 Haverhill Road, London SW12 0HA — BM Soton. 1984 (Univ. Soton.) MRCP (UK) 1989; DM Nottm. 1995. Cons. Phys. & Rheum. St. Helier Hosp. Carshalton; Sen. Lect. (Rheum.) St. Helier Hosp. Carshalton. Specialty: Rehabil. Med., Rheumatol. Socs: Brit. Soc. Rheum. Prev: Sen. Regist. (Med. & Rheum.) St. Geo. Hosp. Lond.

PATEL, Sanjiv Shashikant 60 Park Avenue, Mitcham CR4 2EN — MB BS Lond. 1990 (Guy's Hosp. Med. Sch. Lond.) MRCP (UK) 1993; MRCGP 1998. GP Princip., Lond. Prev: Resid. Internal Med. Cleveland Clinic Foundat. Ohio, USA; SHO (Med.) Crawley Hosp.; GP Regist. Lond.

PATEL, Sarad Kumar — MB BS Lond. 1975 (Guy's) Locum GP Leics.; Out of Hours doctor with MRHDOC,Market Harborough,Leics. Specialty: Gen. Pract. Prev: Locum Gen. Practitioner Birm. & W. Midlands; Gen. Practitioner,Opotiki Health Centre,Opotiki,New Zealand.

PATEL, Sarit Amritlal St Katharine Docks Practice, 12-14 Nightingale House, 50 Thomas More Street, London E1 9UA — MB BS Lond. 1991; DRCOG Lond. 1997.

PATEL, Satish Manibhai London Road Practice, 172 London Road, Reading RG1 3PA Tel: 0118 926 4992 Fax: 0118 926 3231; 5 Whitley Wood Road, Reading RG2 8HX Tel: 01734 311377 — MB BS All India Inst. 1969 (All India Inst. Med. Scs. New Delhi) MB BS All India Inst. Med. Scs. 1969.

PATEL, Satiskumar Purshotamdas 4 Willcox Drive, Melton Mowbray LE13 1HH — MB ChB Leeds 1994.

PATEL, Shailesh Jayantilal 1 Troutbeck Road, Gatley, Cheadle SK8 4RP — MB ChB Manch. 1982.

PATEL, Shailesh Somabhai Saffron Lane Health Centre, 612 Saffron Lane, Leicester LE2 6TD Tel: 0116 291 1212 Fax: 0116 291 0300; 49 Spon Lane, Grendon, Atherstone CV9 2PD Tel: 01827 714035 — MB ChB Glas. 1981 (Univ. Glas.) DA (UK) 1984; DRCOG 1986. Prev: SHO (Anaesth.) Geo. Eliot Hosp. Nuneaton; SHO (O & G & A & E) Bedford Gen. Hosp.

PATEL, Mr Shaileshkumar Bhailalbhai 36 Doyle Gardens, Kensal Rise, London NW10 3DA — MB BS Lond. 1985; BSc (Hons.) Lond. 1982, MB BS 1985; FRCS Eng. 1990; FRCS Ed. 1990. Research Fell. (Paediat. Surg.) St. Thos. Hosp. Lond. Specialty: Paediat. Surg. Prev: Regist. (Paediat. Surg.) St. Thos. Hosp. Lond.; Regist. (Gen. Surg.) St. Mary's Hosp. Lond.; Regist. (Gen. Surg.) Hillingdon Hosp. Middlx.

PATEL, Shalini Narendra c/o The Osteopathic Surgery, Worton Hall, Worton Road, Isleworth TW7 6ER; 73 Constance Road, Whitton, Twickenham TW2 7HX — MB BS Lond. 1996 (St. George's Hosp. Med. Sch.) BSc Lond. 1995; DRCOG 1999. GP VTS, St. Peter's Hosp. Chertsey. Specialty: Gen. Pract. Prev: Ho. Off. (Med.) Luton & Dunstable Hosp.; Ho. Off. (Surg.) St. Peter's Hosp. Chertsey.

PATEL, Shamima (retired) 107 Drewstead Road, London SW16 1AD Tel: 020 8769 7359 — MB ChB Sheff. 1949.

PATEL, Shantilal Devshibhai 172 Wandsworth Bridge Road, London SW6 2UQ — MB BS Gujarat 1977; LRCP LRCS Ed. LRCPS Glas. 1983. GP Lond.

PATEL, Shashikant Haribhai (retired) Oak Road Surgery, 1 Oak Road, Canvey Island SS8 7AX Tel: 01268 692211; 55 Leigh Road, Canvey Island SS8 0AW — MB BS Poona 1966 (B.J. Med. Coll. Poona)

PATEL, Shashikant Jethabhai 60 Park Avenue, Mitcham CR4 2EN Tel: 020 8640 4984 — MB BS Bombay 1964.

PATEL, Shashikant Ratilal Penvale Park Medical Centre, Hardwick Road, East Hunsbury, Northampton NN4 0GP Tel: 01604 700660 Fax: 01604 700772; 15 Rixon Close, Western Favell, Northampton NN3 3PF Tel: 01604 404843 — MB BS Calicut 1976; DA Eng. 1981; DRCOG 1987.

PATEL, Sheena 75 Moorcroft Road, Moseley, Birmingham B13 8LS Tel: 0121 449 2105; Cambridge University Department of Anatomy, Downing St, Cambridge CB2 3DY — BChir Camb. 1996 (Downing College Cambridge University) MB Camb. 1996; MA Camb. 1998. Anat. Demonst. Camb. Univ.; Resid. Med. Off. The Evelyn Hosp. Camb. Specialty: Anat. Prev: Ho. Phys. Bedford Hosp.; Ho. Surg. Norf. & Norwich Hosp.

PATEL, Sheetal Thakor 1 Banckside, Hartley, Longfield DA3 7RD Tel: 01474 705644 Email: sheetal50@hotmail.com — MB BS Lond. 1997.

PATEL, Sheila (retired) 173 Old Road, Brampton, Chesterfield S40 3QL Tel: 01246 206341 — MB ChB Manch. 1963. SCMO (Audiol.) N. Derbysh. Health Auth.

PATEL, Shetal 44 Dudley Avenue, Kenton, Harrow HA3 8SS — MB ChB Manch. 1990.

PATEL, Shirish Chunibhai Mill Road Surgery, Mill Road, Pontnewynydd, Pontypool NP4 6NG Tel: 01495 757575 Fax: 01495 758402 — MB BS Bombay 1973.

PATEL, Shobana 51 Dalkeith Grove, Stanmore HA7 4SQ Tel: 020 8958 5982 — MB BS Gujarat 1974; MB BS Gujarat India 1974; FRCA 1994.

PATEL, Shobhana Oxford Road Surgery, 292 Oxford Road, Reading RG30 1AD Tel: 0118 957 4614 Fax: 0118 959 5486 — MB BS Delhi 1972.

PATEL, Shruti Devyani 27 St Michael's Hill, Kingstown, Bristol BS2 8DZ — MB ChB Bristol 1993.

PATEL, Shveta Thakorlal Princess Margaret Hospital, Perth, Australia Tel: 020 8882 0974 — MB BS Lond. 1990; DCH RCP Lond. 1994; DRCOG 1995. Specialty: Gen. Pract. Socs: Med. Protec. Soc. Prev: GP/Regist. Forest Rd. Health Centre Edmonton; Trainee GP/SHO (Psychiat.) Enfield HA.

PATEL, Siddharth Ramkrishna Oxnead, Marsham Way, Gerrards Cross SL9 8AW Tel: 01753 882492 Email: sidrpatel@aol.com — MB BS Gujarat 1964 (B.J. Med. Coll. Ahmedabad) DMRD Eng. 1972. Cons. Radiol. Ashford Hosp. Middlx. Specialty: Radiol. Prev: Sen. Regist. (Diag. Radiol.) Windsor Gp. Hosps. & Northwick Pk. Hosp.; Harrow; Trainee Regist. (Radiol.) Roy. Free Hosp. Lond.

PATEL, Smita Chimanbhai Suthergrey House Surgery, 37A St. Johns Road, Watford WD17 1LS — MB BS Lond. 1985 (St. Georges Hosp. Med. Sch. Lond.) DRCOG 1990; MRCGP 1992. Prev: Trainee GP Belmont Health Centre Harrow; SHO (Obst.) Basildon Hosp.; SHO (A & E & Paediat. Southend Hosp.

PATEL, Smitaben Yashwantbhai 62 Foxbourne Road, London SW17 8EW — MB BS Lond. 1994.

PATEL, Smruti High Peak, Rownhams Lane, Rownhams, Southampton SO16 8AR — BM Soton. 1991.

PATEL, Sneha Narsing — MB BS Lond. 1993 (Roy. Free Hosp. Lond.) DTM & H UK 1997; MRCPath (Part 1) UK 1997; MSc UK 1997; MRCP UK 1997. Specialty: Gen. Med.; Infec. Dis.; Med. Microbiol.

PATEL, Snehlata Mukundchandra St Johns Villas Surgery, 16 St Johns Villas, Friern Barnet Road, London N11 3BU Tel: 020 8368 1707; 16 St. John's Villas, Friern Barnet Road, London N11 3BU Tel: 020 8368 1707 — MB BS Gujarat 1972 (B.J. Med. Coll. Ahmedabad)

PATEL, Soonie Rameshchandra 73 Warlingham Road, Thornton Heath, Croydon CR7 7DF — MB ChB Leeds 1994.

PATEL, Subhash Chandrakant The Surgery, Welbeck Street, Creswell, Worksop S80 4HA Tel: 01909 721206; The Stables, Old Hall Lane, Whitwell, Worksop S80 4QX — MB ChB Glas. 1980; DCH RCP Lond. 1986; DRCOG 1987.

PATEL, Sujal Suryakant 13 Badgers Holt, Oadby, Leicester LE2 5PU — MB ChB Leeds 1995.

PATEL, Sumitraben Mukundbhai 16 Timber Pond Road, London SE16 6AG — MB BS Gujarat 1970.

PATEL, Sundeept 78 Butler Road, Harrow HA1 4DR — MB BS Lond. 1991.

PATEL, Sundip Jagdishchandra 1 Marshfield Drive, Coventry CV4 7ER — MB BCh Wales 1992 (Univ. Wales Coll. Med.) MRCP (UK) 1996. Specialist Regist. Cardio. S. Thames. Specialty: Cardiol. Prev: Clin. Research Fell. Blood Pressure Unit St Geo.s Hosp.; SHO Med. Rotat. Leicester.

PATEL, Surendra Ambalal The Surgery, 86 Audley Road, Hendon, London NW4 3HB Tel: 020 8203 5150 Fax: 020 8202 5682 — MB BS Gujarat 1969.

PATEL, Surendra Purshottam 39 Winchester Way, Ashby-de-la-Zouch LE65 2NR Tel: 01530 411064 — MB BS Gujarat 1970 (B.J. Med. Coll. Ahmedabad) GP Midway & Ch. Greasley. Prev: Med. Off. Homa Bay Dist. Hosp. Kenya; Med. Off. Kapsabet Dist. Hosp. Kenya; Clin. Asst. Groby Rd. Hosp. Leicester.

PATEL, Suresh Kanubhai The Surgery, 11-13 Charlton Road, Blackheath, London SE3 7HB Tel: 020 8858 2632 Fax: 020 8293 9286 — MB BS Bombay 1975; MB BS Bombay 1975.

PATEL, Suresh Kumar 38 Mollison Way, Edgware HA8 5QW — MB BCh Wales 1992 (Univ. Wales) BSc (Hons) (Anat.) 1989; FRCS Ed. 1996; FRCS (Oto) 1998. Specialist Regist.Oxf. Region; SHO ENT Roy. Nat. Throat, Nose & Ear Hosp. W. Midl. Gen. Surg. Rotat.; SHO St Mary's Hosp.; SHO St Bart's Hosp.; LAT Spr Bristol & S.W. Eng. Specialty: Otorhinolaryngol.

PATEL, Suresh Madhavlal Wenlock Street Surgery, 40 Wenlock Street, Luton LU2 0NN Tel: 01582 27094 — MB BS Gujarat 1962 (B.J. Med. Coll. Ahmedabad)

PATEL, Sureshchandra Rambhai The Health Centre, High Street, Arnold, Nottingham NG5 7BQ Tel: 0115 926 7257 Fax: 0115 956 3232 — MB BS Newc. 1969; DCH Eng. 1972; DObst RCOG 1973.

PATEL, Sushila Deveshi 2 Cedar Tree Drive, off Copse Hill, Wimbledon, London SW20 — MB BS Calcutta 1966 (R.G. Kar Med. Coll.) DObst RCOG 1970. Med. Off. (Community Med.) Wandsworth & Merton HAs.

PATEL, Swati South Ham House, 96 Paddock Road, Basingstoke RG22 6RL Tel: 01256 324666 Fax: 01256 810849; Malabar House, 2 The Baredown, Nately Scures, Hook RG27 9JT Tel: 01256 763702 Fax: 01256 760274 — BM Soton. 1980; DRCOG 1984. GP Basingstoke. Prev: Trainee GP Overton VTS; SHO (Psychiat.) Basingstoke Dist. Hosp.; SHO (Med. & O & G) Basingstoke Dist. Hosp.

PATEL, Tapin Barindra Devoran Lime Grove, London N20 8PU — MB BS Lond. 1996.

PATEL, Tarangini Purushottam Whitehill House Surgery, 1 Crayford Road, Crayford, Dartford DA1 4AN Tel: 01322 225603 Fax: 01322 293244 — MB BS Baroda 1971.

PATEL, Thakor Dahyabhai Kent House Surgery, 36 Station Road, Longfield DA3 7QD Tel: 01474 703550; 1 Banckside, Hartley, Longfield DA3 7RD Tel: 01474 705644 — MB BS Baroda 1963 (Med. Coll. Baroda) MRCOG 1971. Specialty: Gen. Pract.; Obst. & Gyn. Socs: MDU.

PATEL, Thakorlal Bhailalbhai — MB BS Bombay 1963 (Grant Med. Coll.) Mem. of Lions Club of Enfield. Socs: BMA.

PATEL, Trilok Bercharbhai Craven Road Medical Centre, 60 Craven Road, Leeds LS6 2RX Tel: 0113 295 3530 Fax: 0113 295 3542 — MB ChB Leeds 1973; DRCOG RCOG 1975; MRCGP Royal College of General Practioners 1981. GP Leeds; GP Trauma.

PATEL, Uday Department of Radiology, St. George's Hospital, Blackshaw Road, London SW17 0QT Tel: 020 8725 1481 Fax: 020 8725 2936; 6 Fontarabia Road, London SW11 5PF — MB ChB Dundee 1982; MRCP (UK) 1985; FRCR 1992. Cons. & Hon. Sen. Lect. St. Geo. Hosp. Lond. Specialty: Radiol. Prev: Fell. (Interven. Radiol.) Univ. Texas Med. Br., USA; Sen. Regist. (Radiol.) Middlx. Hosp. Lond.; Hon. Regist. Univ. Dept. Med. Glas. Roy. Infirm.

PATEL, V R Southey Green Medical Centre, 281 Southey Green Road, Sheffield S5 7QB Tel: 0114 232 6401 Fax: 0114 285 4402.

PATEL, Valabh Shambhubhai Patel, Erith Health Centre, Queen Street, Erith DA8 1TT Tel: 01322 330283 Fax: 01322 351504; 11 Lansdown Road, Sidcup DA14 4EF Tel: 020 8300 6217 — MB BS Bombay 1973 (Topiwala Nat. Med. Coll. Bombay India) DRCOG 1976. Specialty: Gen. Pract.

PATEL, Venita 8 The Mews, Hitchen Hatch Lane, Sevenoaks TN13 3BQ — MB BS Lond. 1993; DRCOG 1995; MRCPCH 1998. SHO (Paediat.) St. Geo. Hosp. Lond.; Specialist Regist. (Community Paediat.) Lambeth PCT and St Thomas' Hosp. Specialty: Paediat. Prev: SHO (A & E) Kingston Gen. Hosp.; SHO (O & G) Newham Gen. Hosp.

PATEL, Vijaychandra Jashbhai Annie Prendergast Health Centre, Ashton Gardens, Romford RM6 6RT Tel: 020 8590 1461 Fax: 020 8597 7819 — MB BS Lond. 1989; MRCGP 1993.

PATEL, Vijaykumar Maganbhai 224 Balgores Lane, Gidea Park, Romford RM2 6BS — MB BS Baroda 1981; MRCS Eng. LRCP Lond. 1988.

PATEL, Vikesh 7 Gatley Drive, Guildford GU4 7JJ — MB ChB Dundee 1998.

PATEL, Vimla Harikrishna 3 Ashleigh Court, Fulwood, Preston PR2 9WU — MB BS Gujarat 1960.

PATEL, Vinaben 19 Factory Street, Loughborough LE11 1AL — MB ChB Birm. 1992; DRCOG 1995; MRCGP 1996. Specialty: Gen. Pract.

PATEL, Vinaykumar 1 Poynton Close, Grappenhall, Warrington WA4 2NG — MB ChB Liverp. 1993.

PATEL, Vinod Kumar 30 Newstead Drive, Bolton BL3 3RE — MB BS Lond. 1995.

PATEL, Mr Vinod Shamalji (retired) White Gables, Kitnocks Hill, Curdridge, Southampton SO32 2HJ Tel: 01489 781789 — (G.S. Med. Coll.) MB BS Bombay 1952; FRCS Eng. 1965; FRCS Ed. 1965. Cons. Rehabil. Med. St. Mary's Hosp. Portsmouth. Prev: Sen. Med. Off. DHSS.

PATEL, Vinodkumar Natubhai Manor House Health Centre, Manor Lane, Feltham TW13 4JQ Tel: 020 8321 3737 Fax: 020 8321 3739 — MB BS Saurashtra 1973.

PATEL, Vinodray Chaturbhai 1 Oaks Avenue, London SE19 1QY — MB BS Poona 1969 (B.J. Med. Coll.) Assoc. RCGP. Socs: BMA. Prev: Intern (Paediat.) New Mulago Hosp. Kampala, Uganda; Intern (Surg.) Jinja Hosp., Uganda; SHO Pumwani Matern. Hosp. Nairobi, Kenya.

PATEL, Vinubhai Natubhai (retired) 11 Moorlands View, Bolton BL3 3TN Tel: 01204 64957 — MB BS Indore 1974 (M.G.M. Med. Coll.) BSc Vikram 1961. Prev: GP Asst. Essex.

PATEL, Vipin Family Doctor Unit Surgery, 92 Bath Road, Hounslow TW3 3LN Tel: 020 8577 9666 Fax: 020 8577 0692; 8 Kingsbridge Road, Norwood Green, Southall UB2 5RT Tel: 020 8574 5683 — BM BS Nottm. 1975; DRCOG 1977. Specialty: Obst. & Gyn.; Paediat.

PATEL, Vipinchandra Chhotabhai Water Lane Surgery, 48 Brixton Water Lane, London SW2 1QE Tel: 020 7274 1521 Fax: 020 7738 3258 — LRCPI & LM, LRSCI & LM 1969; LRCPI & LM, LRCSI & LM 1969.

PATEL, Vipul 145 Kingston Road, Teddington TW11 9JP; Flat 6, 75 Ravenhurst Road, Harborne, Birmingham B17 9SR Tel: 0121 427 4887 — BM Soton. 1992; MRCP (UK) 1997. Specialist Regist. Diagnostic Radio. W. Midl. Rotat. Birm. Specialty: Radiol.

PATEL, Mr Vipul Ramubhai Epsom & St Helier NHS Trust, Wrythe Lane, London Road, Carshalton CM5 1AA Tel: 0208 296 2374 Fax: 0208 288 1838 Email: vipulpatel@stanthonys.og.uk — MB BS Gujarat 1986 (Municip. Med. Coll. Ahmedabad India) MS (Orth.) Gujarat 1988; FRCS Eng. 1991; FRCS (Orth) Lond. 1998. Cons. Orthopaedic Surg. Epsom & St Helier Univ. Hosps. NHS Trust; Cons. Orthopaedic Surg. St Anthony's Hosp. N. Cheam Surrey, Parksie Hosp. Wimbledon. Specialty: Orthop. Special Interest: Shoulder & Knee Surg. Socs: British Orthpaedic Association; British Trauma Association; MPS. Prev: Cons. Orthopaedic Surg. St Richards Hosp. Chichester; Sen. Regist. (Orthop.) St. Geo. Hosp. Lond.; Research Fell. Univ. of Maryland Baltimore.

PATEL, Vishnubhai Rambhai Melbourne Road Surgery, 71 Melbourne Road, Leicester LE2 0GU Tel: 0116 253 9479 Fax: 0116 242 5602; (branch Surgery), 24 Moira St., Leicester LE4 6FL Tel:

0116 266 5384 — MB BS Bombay 1958 (Grant Med. Coll.) Socs: BMA & LM Soc.; Med. Protec. Soc.

PATEL, Yajurbala Sharadchandra 47 Shirley Hills Road, Croydon CR0 5HQ Tel: 020 8654 5075 — MB BS Bombay 1967 (Grant Med. Coll.) DA Eng. 1972. Prev: SHO (Anaesth.) Cumbld. Infirm. Carlisle; SHO (Anaesth.) Roy. Surrey Co. Hosp. Guildford; Regist. (Anaesth.) Bolingbroke Hosp. Lond.

PATEL, Yakub Valibhai Suleman Slaithwaite Road Surgery, 140 Slaithwaite Road, Thornhill Lees, Dewsbury WF12 9DW Tel: 01924 461369 — MB ChB Leeds 1978 (Leeds Un) BSc (Hon.) Leeds 1975. GP Dewsbury. Specialty: Dermat.

PATEL, Yashvant Ashabhai New Medical Centre, Main Road, Highley, Bridgnorth WV16 6HG Tel: 01746 861572 Fax: 01746 862295 — MB BS Baroda 1969.

PATEL, Yusuf Ahmed Llysmeddyg Surgery, Dew Road, Sandfields Estate, Port Talbot SA12 7HE Tel: 01639 871039 Fax: 01639 898616 — MB ChB Zambia 1974; BSc Zambia 1971; MRCOG 1981. Princip. Gen. Pract.; Clin. Asst. (Ophth.) Neath & Port Talbot Hosp.; Police Surg. S. Wales Constab. Specialty: Obst. & Gyn. Socs: BMA; Med. Protec. Soc.; (Sec.) Overseas Doctors Assn. Prev: Lect. (O & G) Sch. of Med. Univ. Teachg. Hosp. Lusara, Zambia; Clin. Asst. (Colposcopy & Ophth.) Neath Gen. Hosp.; Med. Adviser (Palliat. Care) Iechyd Morgannwg Health Swansea.

PATEL, Yusuf Ismail Woodgrange Medical Practice, 40 Woodgrange Road, Forest Gate, London E7 0QH Tel: 020 8250 7585 — MB ChB Sheff. 1984; MRCGP 1988.

PATEL, Zaki 5 The Dene, Beardwood, Blackburn BB2 7QS — MB ChB Aberd. 1998.

PATEMAN, Jane Ann Brighton General Hospital, Elm Grove, Brighton BN2 3EW Tel: 01273 696955; Silverthorn, Minsted, Midhurst GU29 0JH — MB BS Lond. 1982; DA Eng. 1985; FFA RCS Eng. 1987. Cons. Anaesth. Brighton Health Care Trust. Specialty: Anaesth. Prev: Vis. Asst. Prof. Anesthesiol. Univ Maryland, Baltimore, USA; Sen. Regist. (Anaesth.) St. Thos. Hosp. Lond.

PATEMAN, Myrtle Thelma Chattis Hill, Moulsham Thrift, Chelmsford CM2 8BP — MB BS Calcutta 1951; DObst RCOG 1954. Prev: Regist. (O & G) OldCh. Hosp. Romford; Ho. Surg. Eliz. G. Anderson Hosp.; Ho. Phys. Rush Green Hosp. Romford.

PATEMAN, Sally Elizabeth (retired) Craig y Trwyn, Wattsville, Cross Keys, Newport NP11 7QW Tel: 01495 273045 Fax: 01495 270370 — MRCS Eng. LRCP Lond. 1966 (Roy. Free) Cert. Family Plann. JCC 1976. GP Gwent; Police Surg. Gwent. Prev: SCMO (Geriat., Young Chronic Sick & Renal Dialysis) Gwent HA.

PATERSON, Abigail Ann — MB ChB Dundee 1996 (Univ. of Dundee) DFFP 1998; DRCOG 1999; MRCGP 2000. GP - Love Road Group Prac. 2001-. Specialty: Gen. Pract. Prev: SHO (Infec. Dis.s) GP Train. Scheme; SHO (O & G) GP Train. Scheme; SHO (Med.) GP Train. Scheme.

PATERSON, Aileen Margaret Elizabeth Milngavie Road Surgery, 85 Milngavie Road, Bearsden, Glasgow G61 2DN Tel: 0141 211 5621 Fax: 0141 211 5625 — MB ChB Glas. 1983; DRCOG 1986; MRCGP 1987. Socs: Roy. Coll. Gen. Pract.

PATERSON, Mr Alastair Glen Department of Surgery, West Cornwall Hospital, St Clare St., Penzance TR18 2PF Tel: 01736 62382 Fax: 01736 50134; St. Loy Farm, St. Buryan, Penzance TR19 6DH Tel: 01736 810430 — MB ChB Ed. 1972; FRCS Ed. 1977; BSc (Med. Sci.) Ed. 1969, MD 1988. Cons. Surg. W. Cornw. Hosp. Penzance & Dir. Mermaid Centre Roy. Cornw. Hosps. Trust Treliske. Specialty: Gen. Surg. Socs: Brit. Assn. Surgic. Oncol.; Surgic. Research Soc.; Assn. Surg. GB & Irel. Prev: Cons. Surg. CrossHo. Hosp. Kilmarnock; Sen. Regist. (Surg.) Univ. Hosp. Wales Cardiff & Roy. Marsden Hosp. Lond.; Research Fell. Univ. Dept. Surg. Welsh Nat. Sch. Med. Cardiff.

PATERSON, Alexander Southside Surgery, 17 Bernard Terrace, Edinburgh EH8 9NU Tel: 0131 667 2240 — MB ChB Dundee 1978; MRCGP 1983.

PATERSON, Mr Alexander Dumgoyach House, Blanefield, Glasgow G63 9AJ Email: PatersonAlistair@aol.com — MB ChB Glas. 1940 (Univ. Glas.) FRFPS Glas. 1947; FRCS Glas. 1962. Cons. Neurosurg. Glas. & W. Scotl. Neurosurg. Unit, Killearn Hosp.; W. Infirm. Glas. & South. Gen. Hosp. Glas. Specialty: Neurosurg. Socs: Soc. Brit. Neurol. Surgs. Prev: 1st Asst. Neurosurg. Dept. St. Geo. Hosp. Lond.; Neurosurg. Fell. Montreal Neurol. Inst. & Montreal Gen. Hosp.; Regist. Hosp. Nerv. Dis. Qu. Sq. Lond.

PATERSON, Alexander MacGregor St Thomas Surgery, Rifleman Lane, St. Thomas Green, Haverfordwest SA61 1QX Tel: 01437 762162 Fax: 01437 776811 — MB ChB Aberd. 1987. Specialty: Occupat. Health.

PATERSON, Alistair Graham Friary Surgery, Queens Road, Richmond DL10 4UJ Tel: 01748 822306 Fax: 01748 850356 — MB ChB Aberd. 1978; MRCGP 1984. Prev: Maj. RAMC.

PATERSON, Andrew David North End House, Hutton Rudby, Yarm TS15 0DG Tel: 01642 700056 — BM BCh Oxf. 1975 (King's Coll. Hosp.) MA Oxf. 1976, BM BCh 1975; MRCP (UK) 1978; FRCP Lond. 1994; FRCP Ed. 1997. Cons. Phys. & Nephrol. S. Cleveland Hosp. Middlesbrough. Specialty: Gen. Med.; Nephrol. Socs: Renal Assn. Prev: Sen. Regist. (Nephrol.) City Hosp. Nottm.; Regist. (Med.) Hallamsh. Hosp. Sheff.; Epidemiol. WHO Smallpox Eradicat. Progr. Bangladesh.

PATERSON, Andrew James The Surgery, Park Lane, Stubbington, Fareham PO14 2JP Tel: 01329 664231 Fax: 01329 664958 — MB BChir Camb. 1983 (Middlx.) MA Camb. 1983; DRCOG 1985; MRCGP 1986. Gen. Practitioner, Pk. La. Surg., Stubbington, Fareham; GP Bd. Mem., Fareham PCG. Specialty: Gen. Pract. Prev: Trainee GP Portsmouth VTS; SHO (Paediat.) Soton Gen. Hosp.; SHO (Geriat.) Upton Hosp. Slough.

PATERSON, Anne Radiology Department, Royal Belfast Hospital for Sick Children, 180 Falls Road, Belfast BT12 6BE Tel: 028 9089 4963 Fax: 028 9031 3789 Email: anne.paterson@royalhospitals.n-i.nhs.uk; 21 Downview Road, Greenisland, Carrickfergus BT38 8YA Email: anniep@csi.com — MB BS Lond. 1990 (St. Bartholomew's Hospital) MRCP (UK) 1993; FRCR 1997. Cons. (Paediat. Radiol.) Roy. Belf. Hosp. For Sick Childr. Specialty: Radiol. Socs: Eur. Soc. Of Paed. Radiol.; Radiol. Soc. of N. Amer.; British Society of Paediatric Radiology. Prev: Specialist Regist. (Radiol.) Roy. Vict. Hosp. Belf.; Fell. Sect. of Pediatric Radiol. Duke Univ. Med. Center Durh. NC 27710, USA.

PATERSON, Mr Anthony William Southwaite House, Southwaite, Carlisle CA4 0ER — MRCS Eng. LRCP Lond. 1987; BDS Ed. 1977; FDS RCS Ed. 1981; DOrth. 1982; FRCS Ed. 1991. Sen. Regist. (Maxillofacial Surg.) Roy. Lond. Hosp. Trust.

PATERSON, Barbara Ann 119 Newark Avenue, Peterborough PE1 4NL Tel: 01733 343658; 4/260 Casuarina Drive, Nightcliff, Darwin NT 0810, Australia Tel: 00 61 0889 480221 Email: barbara.paterson@nt.gov.au — MB ChB Manch. 1984; DCH RCP Lond. 1986; DGM RCP Lond. 1987; DRCOG 1989; MRCGP 1990; T(GP) 1991; MPH NSW Austral. 1995; FAFPHM 1995. Specialist (Pub. Health Med.) Matern. & Child Health Policy. Specialty: Gen. Pract. Socs: BMA; Austral. Med. Assn.; Fell. Austral. Fac. Pub. Health Med. Prev: Dist. Med. Off. Territory Health Servs. Austral.

PATERSON, Miss Catherine Margaret St Mary's Hospital NHS Trust, Praed Street, London W2 1NY Tel: 020 7886 1959 Email: kate.paterson@st-marys.nhs.uk — MB BS Lond. 1975 (Roy. Free) MFFP; MRCS Eng. LRCP Lond. 1975; MRCOG 1986; MFFP 1993. Cons. Community Gyn. & Reproduc. Health Care St Mary's Hosp. NHS Trust Lond.; Forens. Med. Examr. Metrop. Police Lond. Specialty: Obst. & Gyn. Special Interest: Fertil. Control. Socs: Fell. Roy. Soc. Med.; Lond. Soc. Famil Plann. Doctors. Prev: Regist. Ipswich Hosp. Suff.; Research Fell. (Perinatal Epidemiol.) St. Mary's Hosp. Med. Sch. Lond.

PATERSON, Charlotte Frances MRC Health Services Research Collaboration, Department of Social Medicine, University of Bristol, Canynge Hall, Whiteladies Road, Bristol BS8 2PR Tel: 0117 973 4672 Email: c.paterson@bristol.ac.uk; Top Flat, 13 York Place, Bristol BS8 1AH Tel: 0117 973 4672 Email: c.paterson@dial.pipex.com — MB ChB Bristol 1972; DObst RCOG 1975; MRCGP 1978; MSc Lond. 1995. Research Fell. Self Employed. Specialty: Research.

PATERSON, Mrs Christina Craig Christie (retired) Watsonhead Cottage, Newmains, Wishaw ML2 9PL Tel: 01698 382487 — (Univ. Glas.) MB ChB Glas. 1941. Prev: Late. Med. Asst. Motherwell & Hamilton Geriat. Serv.

PATERSON, Cordelia Lynn Reevy Hill Health Centre, 50 Reevy Road West, Buttershaw, Bradford BD6 3LT Tel: 01274 691098 Fax: 01274 694008 — MB BS Lond. 1981.

PATERSON, David Alexander Department of Pathology, Weston General Hospital, Grange Road, Uphill, Weston Super Mare BS23 4TQ — MB ChB Manch. 1983; BSc (Hons.) St And. 1980;

MRCPath 1990. Cons. Histopath. Weston Area Health Trust Weston Gen. Hosp. Weston-Super-Mare. Specialty: Histopath. Prev: Lect. (Histopath.) Univ. Edin.; Demonst. (Histopath.) Brist. Roy. Infirm.; SHO (Path.) Southmead Hosp. Bristol.

PATERSON, David Hood (retired) 14 Landsborough Drive, Kilmarnock KA3 1RY Tel: 01563 522282 — MB ChB Glas. 1948 (Univ. Glas.) DObst RCOG 1955; DPH 1956; MFCM 1972. Prev: SCM Ayrsh. & Arran Health Bd.

PATERSON, Douglas Robert 6B Castle Terrace, Edinburgh EH1 2DP; Medical Flats, St. George's Hospital, Morpeth NE61 2NU Tel: 01670 512121 — MB ChB Ed. 1996 (Edin. Univ.) BSc 1994. SHO (Psychiat. Rotat.) St. Geo.'s Hosp. S. Tyneside Area. Specialty: Gen. Psychiat. Prev: SHO (Infec. Dis.s) Kirkaldy; SHO (Oncol.) Edin.; SHO (Med.) Dumfermline.

PATERSON, Miss Elfriede Katherine Jessie (retired) Wood End, Labour-in-Vain Road, Wrotham, Sevenoaks TN15 7NY Tel: 01732 822465 — (Lond. Sch. Med. Wom.) MRCS Eng. LRCP Lond. 1938. Prev: Deptm. Med. Off. Kent CC.

PATERSON, Elizabeth Ann 600 Old Chester Road, Birkenhead CH42 4NW — MB ChB Manch. 1997.

PATERSON, Eric Horsburgh (retired) Glenview, 38 Station Road, Carluke ML8 5AD Tel: 01555 751311 — MB ChB Glas. 1956. Prev: GP Carluke.

PATERSON, Evelyn Jean (retired) The Ochils, Brimstage Road, Heswall, Wirral CH60 1XA Tel: 0151 342 3184 — MB ChB St. And. 1949; FRCPath 1971. Prev: Cons. Path. Clatterbridge Hosp. Bebington.

PATERSON, Mr Fergus William Nigel Cromwell Hospital, Cromwell Road, London SW5 0TU Tel: 020 7460 5914 Fax: 020 7460 5709 Email: fergus.paterson@knee-surgery.co.uk — MB BS Lond. 1971 (St Mary's) FRCS Ed. 1976; FRCS Eng. 1977. Hon. Cons. Orthop. Surg. W. Middlx. Univ. Hosp. Trust Isleworth; Hon. Lect., Imperial Coll., Lond. Specialty: Orthop. Socs: Fell. BOA; Roy. Soc. Med. Prev: Clin. Lect. Inst. Orthop. Lond.; Sen. Regist. Roy. Nat. Orthop. Hosp. Lond.

PATERSON, Fiona Campbell Ailsa Hospital, Dalmellington Road, Ayr KA6 6AB Tel: 01292 610556; 10 Beechwood Paddock, Loans, Troon KA10 7LX Tel: 01292 311209 — MB ChB Glas. 1985. Staff Grade (Psychiat. Old Age) Ailsa Hosp. Ayr. Specialty: Geriat. Psychiat. Prev: GP Dukes Rd. Troon; Trainee GP Alloway Pl. Ayr; SHO (Psychiat. & O & G) CrossHo. Hosp.

PATERSON, Francis Lyle (retired) Willowbrae, Alexandra Terrace, Forres IV36 1DL Tel: 01309672355 — LRCP LRCS Ed. 1945 (Anderson Coll. Glas.) LRCP LRCS Ed. LRFPS Glas. 1945.

PATERSON, Fraser Neil Grove House Surgery, 80 Pryors Lane, Rose Green, Bognor Regis PO21 4JB Tel: 01243 265222/266413 Fax: 01243 268693 — MB BS Lond. 1987; DRCOG 1991.

PATERSON, Gavin William Hausen 4 Westfield Road, Ayr KA7 2XN Tel: 0292 268096 — MB ChB Glas. 1943.

PATERSON, Gordon Murray Charles McDonald, RD Bridge House, Linlithgow Bridge, Linlithgow EH49 7PX Tel: 01506 840530 Email: gordon.paterson@nda.ox.ac.uk — MB ChB Ed. 1959; FRCA 1964. Cons. Anaesth. Oxf. Radcliffe NHS Trust. Specialty: Anaesth.

PATERSON, Hamish Robert 34 Sandringham Road, South Gosforth, Newcastle upon Tyne NE3 1PY — MB BS Newc. 1985.

PATERSON, Hugh Mackenzie Dept of General Surgery, Stirling Royal Infirmary, Stirling FR8 2AU; 27 Bredero Drive, Ellon AB41 9QF — MB ChB Aberd. 1994. SHO Dept. Gen. Surg. Stirling Roy. Infirm.

PATERSON, Mr Iain MacKenzie Frimley Park Hospital NHS Trust, Portsmouth Road, Frimley, Camberley GU16 7UJ Tel: 01276 604588; Sherwood, 14 Middle Avenue, Farnham GU9 8JL Tel: 01252 711201 Fax: 01252 712580 — MB ChB Aberd. 1976; FRCS 1980; PhD Aberd. 1984. Cons. Surg. Frimley Pk. Hosp. Surrey. Specialty: Gen. Surg. Socs: Fell. Assoc. Surg.s GB & Irel.; Brit. Soc. Gastroenterol.; Assn. Upper G.I. Surg. Prev: Vis. Prof. Univ. Hong Kong 1997; Sen. Registar (Surgury) St. Geo.'s Hosp. Lond.; Clin. Fell. Univ. Hong Kong.

PATERSON, Iain Wallace 1 Arlington Road, Eastbourne BN21 7DH Tel: 01323 727531 Fax: 01323 417085 — MB BS Lond. 1965 (St. Mary's) MRCS Eng. LRCP Lond. 1965; DObst RCOG 1967; MRCGP 1982. Med. Off. Chaseley Home for Disabled Servicemen & Eastbourne Coll. Art & Technol.; Chairm. Trustees Seadoc. Doctors Co-op.. Prev: Ho. Surg. St. Mary's Hosp. Lond.; Ho. Phys. & Ho. Surg. (O & G) Paddington Gen. Hosp.

PATERSON, Ian Charles 21 The Green, Ingham, Lincoln LN1 2XT Tel: 01522 730545 — MB ChB Manch. 1968; BSc (Hons.), MB ChB Manch. 1968; MRCP (UK) 1972; FRCP Eng. 1988; FRCP Ed. 1988. Cons. Phys. (s/i Respirat. Dis.) N. Lincs. (Lincoln) Dist. Specialty: Gen. Med. Socs: Brit. Thorac. Assn. Prev: Regist. (Respirat. Dis.) North. Gen. Hosp. Edin.; Sen. Regist. (Gen. Med.) N. Lothian Health Dist.; Ho. Surg. & Ho. Phys. Manch. Roy. Infirm.

PATERSON, Ian Gavin — MB BS Lond. 1986; MA Camb. 1983; FRCA 1992. Cons. Anaesth. N. Gen. Hosp. Sheff. Specialty: Anaesth. Prev: Sen. Regist. Rotat. (Anaesth.) UCL; Regist. Rotat. (Anaesth.) Char. Cross Hosp. Lond.; SHO (Anaesth.) St Geo. Hosp. Lond.

PATERSON, Irene Dalkeith Road Medical Practice, 145 Dalkeith Road, Edinburgh EH16 5HQ Tel: 0131 667 1289; 26 Danube Street, Edinburgh EH4 1NT Tel: 0131 332 0370 — MB BS Lond. 1977; MRCP (UK) 1981; DRCOG 1981; MRCGP 1982; Dip. Thev. 1998. Teachg. Med. Stud.s (Univ. of Edin.). Specialty: Gen. Pract.

PATERSON, Jacqueline Anne 125 Craigleith Road, Edinburgh EH4 2EH — MB ChB Manch. 1987; BSc St. And. 1984; MRCP (UK) 1993. Sen. Regist. (Genitourin. Med.) Edin. Roy. Infirm. Specialty: Genitourinary Medicine.

PATERSON, James Alexander (retired) Abbotts Barton Home, 40 Worthy Road, Winchester SO23 7HB — MB ChB Ed. 1944 (Univ. Ed.) Prev: GP Winchester.

PATERSON, Jeremy Robert Mount Chambers Surgery, 92 Coggeshall Road, Braintree CM7 9BY Tel: 01376 553415 Fax: 01376 552451; Winnipeg, Church Road, Gosfield, Halstead CO9 1TL Tel: 01787 472514 — MB BS Lond. 1976 (Guy's) MRCS Eng. LRCP Lond. 1976; DCH Eng. 1979; DRCOG 1979; MRCGP 1980. Prev: Trainee GP Worthing VTS; Ho. Phys. & Ho. Surg. Greenwich Dist. Hosp. Lond.

PATERSON, Joan Catherine 13 Craigstewart Crescent, Alloway, Ayr KA7 4DB Tel: 01292 443484 — MB ChB Glas. 1964.

PATERSON, Joan Patricia The Surgery, Northwick Road, Pilning, Bristol BS35 4JF Tel: 01454 632393 — MB ChB Aberd. 1973.

PATERSON, Joan Sheila Dept of Medical Genetics, Box 134, Addenbrookes NHS Trust, Hills Road, Cambridge CB2 2QQ Tel: 01223 216446 — MB ChB Glas. 1983; BSc (Hons.) (Genetics) Glas. 1980; MRCP (UK) (Paediat.) 1988. Cons. (Clinical Genetics) Addenbrookes NHS Trust. Specialty: Genetics. Prev: Cons. (Clin. Genetics) NW Lond. NHS Trust; Regist. (Med. Genetics) Roy. Hosp. Sick Childr., Glas.

PATERSON, John Gordon (retired) Hansy House, Parkhill, Lumphanan, Banchory AB31 4RN Tel: 01339 883376 Fax: 01339 883376 Email: gordon@gpaterson6.freeserve.co.uk — MB ChB Ed. 1965; DObst RCOG 1968; Dip. Community Med. Ed. 1975; FFCM 1986, M 1977; FRCP Ed. 1994. Prev: GP.

PATERSON, John Gray (retired) Thorncliffe, Tighnabruaich PA21 2DU Tel: 0170 0811 387 — (Glas.) MB ChB Glas. 1961; DMRD Eng. 1967; FFR 1972; FRCR 1975. Prev: Cons. Radiol. Roy. Alexandra Infirm. Paisley.

PATERSON, John Kirkpatrick (retired) 1 rue du Castellas, 13640, La Roque D'Anthéron, France Tel: 0033 442 505776 Fax: 0033 442 505688 Email: john.paterson@tps.fr; The Old Dairy, Dullingham, Newmarket CB8 9UP — MB BS Lond. 1950 (St. Thomas' Hosp.) MRCGP 1956. Prev: Chairm. Scientif. Advis. Comm. Federat. Internat. Médecine Manuelle.

PATERSON, Mr John Mark Hamilton — MB BS Lond. 1977 (Middlesex Hosp) FRCS Eng. 1982. Cons. Paediatric Orthopaedic Surg., Barts and The Lond. NHS Trust Lond. Specialty: Orthop. Special Interest: Cerebral Palsy; Neuromuscular Surg. Socs: Brit. Soc. for Surg. in Cerebral Palsy; Brit. Soc. for Childrens Orthopaedic Surg.; Brit. Orthopaedic Assn. Prev: Sen. Regist. (Orthop.) Lond. Hosp. & Roy. Nat. Orthop. Hosp. Lond.; Regist. (Orthop.) Portsmouth & Alton.

PATERSON, John Thomson 33 Newton Road, Great Barr, Birmingham B43 6AA Tel: 0121 357 1690 Fax: 0121 357 4253; 62 Charlemont Road, Walsall WS5 3NQ Tel: 01922 26780 — (Aberd.) MB ChB Aberd. 1963; DObst RCOG 1966.

PATERSON, John William Links Medical Centre, 4 Hermitage Place, Edinburgh EH6 8BW Tel: 0131 554 1036 Fax: 0131 555 3995 — MB ChB Aberd. 1980 (Aberdeen) DRCOG 1982; DCH RCP Glas. 1984; MRCGP 1985. Lect. (Gen. Pract.) Univ. Edin.

PATERSON, Joseph Dunbar (retired) 77 Greenbank Crescent, Morningside, Edinburgh EH10 5TB Tel: 0131 447 1515 — MB ChB Glas. 1946 (Univ. Glas.) Prev: Med. Dir. M.M.R.U. Manch. Regional Health Bd.

PATERSON, Katherine Elizabeth Katherine Paterson Mhordon, St James Place, Inverurie AB51 3UB Tel: 01467 622566 Email: katherine@doctors.org.uk — MB ChB Glas. 1998. SHO (Med.) Kingston-upon-Thames, Lond.

PATERSON, Kenneth Ross Diabetes Centre, Royal Infirmary, Castle St., Glasgow G4 0SF Tel: 0141 211 4745 Fax: 0141 800 1971 Email: ken.paterson@northglasgow.scot.nhs.uk; Strathcashel, Lochlibo Road, Uplawmoor, Glasgow G78 4AA Tel: 01505 850344 Email: ken.mairi@dial.pipex.com — MB ChB Glas. 1977; MRCP (UK) 1980; FRCP Glas. 1989; FRCP Ed. 1990; FFPM 2002. Cons. Phys. Roy. Infirm. Glas. Specialty: Gen. Med.; Diabetes. Socs: Vice-Chair, Scott. Medicines Consortium. Prev: Sen. Regist. (Gen. Med.) Roy. Infirm. & South. Gen. Hosp. Glas.; Regist. (Gen. Med.) Roy. Infirm. Glas. & Roy. Alexandra Infirm. Paisley.

PATERSON, Laura Margaret — MB ChB Bristol 1994; MRCGP 1999. Gen. Pract. Principle Nailsea. Specialty: Gen. Pract. Socs: BMA.

PATERSON, Lorraine Mary (retired) Ansonhill House, Crossgates, Cowdenbeath KY4 8HA Tel: 01863 610146 — MB ChB Ed. 1948.

PATERSON, Louise Charlotte The Health Centre, Station Approach, Bradford-on-Avon BA15 1DQ Tel: 01225 866611 — MB BS Lond. 1993; MRCGP; DRCOG.

PATERSON, Margaret Tran Department of Community Child Health, Ayrshire Central Hospital, Irvine KA12 8SS Tel: 01294 323441 Email: Margaret.Paterson@aapct.scot.nhs.uk; 10 Machrie Place, Kilwinning KA13 6RW Tel: 01294 554393 — MB ChB Glas. 1971; BSc Glas. 1967; DFFP 1995. Staff Grade (Community Child Health) Ayrsh. Centr. Hosp. Irvine. Specialty: Community Child Health; Family Plann. & Reproduc. Health. Prev: Regist. (Clin. Biochem.) Roy. Hosp. Sick Childr. Glas.

PATERSON, Margarita Mary Frances 16 Devonshire Road, Sheffield S17 3NT — MB BS Lond. 1989; MRCP (UK) 1994; DRCOG 1995.

PATERSON, Mark Anthony 72 Middlebeck Drive, Arnold, Nottingham NG5 8AF — MB BS Lond. 1996.

PATERSON, Mark Eian Oak Lodge Surgery, 32 Miller Street, Hamilton ML3 7EN Tel: 01698 282350 Fax: 01698 282502 — MB ChB Glas. 1983; DRCOG 1987; MRCGP 1988. GP Lanarksh.

PATERSON, Mary Tregelles 50 South Grove House, Highgate, London N6 6LR Tel: 020 8340 3818 — MB BS Lond. 1932 (Char. Cross) DPH Eng. 1940. Socs: Fell. Roy. Soc. Med. Prev: Dep. MoH City Westm.; Asst. MoH Boro St. Pancras; Asst. Phys. Roy. Edin. Hosp.

PATERSON, Mr Maurice Peacock Longwood House, The Bath Clinic, Claverton Down Road, Bath BA2 7BR Tel: 01225 835555 — MB BCh Witwatersrand 1978 (Univ. Witwatersrand) FCS (Orthop.) S. Afr. 1987; FRCS Ed. (Orthop.) 1989. Cons. Orthop. Surg.Royal United Hospital Bath Clinic. Specialty: Orthop. Socs: Brit. Soc. Surg. Hand; Brit. Scoliosis Soc.; Brit. Orthop. Assn.

PATERSON, Mr Michael Edward Lockhart West Lawn, 54 Clarendon Road, Fulwood, Sheffield S10 3TR Tel: 0114 230 8054 Fax: 0114 230 7871 Email: michael.paterson@btconnect.com — MD Birm. 1980; MB ChB 1971; FRCOG 1989, M 1977; FRCS Ed. 1981. Cons. (Obst. & Gyn.) Roy. Hallamshire Hosp. Sheff. Specialty: Obst. & Gyn. Socs: Brit. Gyn. Cancer Soc.; Gyn. Travellers; Brit. Med. Assn. Prev: Sen. Regist. Rotat. (Obst. & Gyn.) Bradford & Leeds; Regist. Birm. & Midl. Hosp. Wom.; Regist. (Surg.) United Birm. Hosps.

PATERSON, Patricia Mary Margaret Orr (retired) 14 Dick Place, Edinburgh EH9 2JL Tel: 0131 667 1245 — M.B., Ch.B. Ed. 1945.

PATERSON, Peter Monklands Hospital, Department of Anaesthesia, Monkscourt Avenue, Airdrie ML6 0JS Tel: 01236 748748 Fax: 01236 756211 Email: peter.paterson@laht.scot.nhs.uk — MB ChB Glas. 1971 (Univ of Glasgow) DObst RCOG 1974; FFA RCS Eng. 1977; FRCA 1992. Cons. Anaesth. Monklands Hosp. Airdrie. Specialty: Anaesth.; Intens. Care. Special Interest: Intens. Care. Socs: Association of Anaesthetists of GB & Ireland; Scottish Society of Anaesthetists; Glasgow & West of Scotland Society of Anaesthetists. Prev: GP Airdrie; Sen. Regist. West. Infirm. Glas.; Sen. Regist. Roy. Infirm. Glas.

PATERSON, Mr Peter John Nuffield McAlpin Clinic, 25 Beaconsfield Road, Glasgow G12 0PJ Tel: 0141 334 9441; Ross Hall Hospital, 221 Crookston Road, Glasgow G52 3NQ — MB ChB Liverp. 1969; FRCS Eng. 1974. Cons. Urol. Glas. Roy. Infirm.; Hon. Sen. Lect. (Urol.) Univ. Glas. Specialty: Urol. Prev: Sen. Regist. (Urol.) Glas. Roy. Infirm.

PATERSON, Rhona Anton Aldershot Health Centre, Wellington Avenue, Aldershot GU11 1PA Tel: 01252 24577; 19 Church Road W., Farnborough GU14 6QG Tel: 01252 517001 — MB BS Lond. 1985; DGM RCP Lond. 1987; DCH RCP Lond. 1990; MRCGP 1994.

PATERSON, Richard Graham The Croft Surgery, Barnham Road, Eastergate, Chichester PO20 3RP — MB BS Lond. 1990; BSc 1987; MRCGP 1994.

PATERSON, Robert Alexander Harcourt Queensway Clinic, 226 Queensway, Bletchley, Milton Keynes MK2 2TE Tel: 01908 643200 Fax: 01908 368943 — BM BCh Oxf. 1968; MA Oxf. 1968; MRCPsych 1980. Cons. Community Ment. Health Team Bletchley. Specialty: Gen. Psychiat. Prev: Sen. Regist. (Psychiat.) Oxf. Rotat Train. Scheme; Regist. (Psychiat.) St. John's Hosp. Stone; Med. Off. Brit. Antarctic Survey.

PATERSON, Robert Craig (retired) 32A Bellerue Crescent, Ayr KA7 2DR Tel: 01292 288128 — MB ChB Glas. 1955.

PATERSON, Robert Euan Govan Health Centre, 5 Drumoyne Road, Glasgow G51 4BJ Tel: 0141 531 8490 Fax: 0141 531 8487; 467 Kilmarnock Road, Glasgow G43 2TJ — MB ChB Glas. 1981; DRCOG 1984; MRCGP 1985.

PATERSON, Robert James Rosebank Surgery, 153B Stroud Road, Gloucester GL1 5JQ Tel: 01452 522767; Lealands, 2 Kenilworth Avenue, Gloucester GL2 0QJ Tel: 01452 306651 — MB ChB Birm. 1970; DCH Eng. 1972. Prev: SHO (Paediat.) E. Birm. Hosp.; SHO (Psychiat.) Coney Hill Hosp. Gloucester; Ho. Phys. (Paediat.) Birm. Childr. Hosp.

PATERSON, Mr Robert William Walker 13 Craigstewart Crescent, Alloway, Ayr KA7 4DB Tel: 01292 443484 — MB ChB Glas. 1962; DObst RCOG 1964; DO Eng. 1965; FRCS Ed. 1968. Cons. Ophth. Heathfield Hosp. Ayr. Specialty: Ophth.

PATERSON, Roger Wellwood St Margarets Health Centre, St. Margaret's Drive, Auchterarder PH3 1JH — MB ChB Glas. 1984 (Glasgow) MRCGP 1992. GP Princip.; GP Trainer.

PATERSON, Ross Lindsey 2 Corstorphine Hill Crescent, Edinburgh EH12 6LH — MB ChB Aberd. 1994.

PATERSON, Samuel Muir 22 Silverknowes Drive, Edinburgh EH4 5LQ — MB ChB Ed. 1969; MRCGP 1975.

PATERSON, Sarah Llywela Susan (retired) 10 Lyndhurst Drive, Hale, Altrincham WA15 8EA — MB ChB Leeds 1948. Prev: Jun. Anaesth. Off. Leeds Gen. Infirm.

***PATERSON, Stuart** Fkat 9, 2 Fotheringay Road, Glasgow G41 4LW — MB ChB Glas. 1998; BSc (Hons) 1996; MRCP 2001.

PATERSON, Terence Andrew The Surgery, Northwick Road, Pilning, Bristol BS35 4JF Tel: 01454 632393 — MB ChB Aberd. 1972; DA Eng. 1974; DObst. RCOG 1975; FRACGP 1978; MRCGP 1994.

PATERSON, Thomas Macilvean (retired) Ty-Bach, Moreton Avenue, Newcastle ST5 4DE Tel: 01782 641444 — (Univ. Glas.) MB ChB Glas. 1942; BSc Glas. 1939, MD 1949; FRCGP 1978, M 1953. Prev: Hsopital Practitioner, Diabetic Clinic, Nth. Staffs. Hosp.

PATERSON, Walter Gouinlock (retired) Balchrystie House, Colinsburgh, Leven KY9 1HE Tel: 01333 340517 — MB ChB Ed. 1955; BA Oxon 1952; FRCS Ed. 1962; MRCOE 1962; FRCOE 1974.

PATERSON, Mr William David (retired) Black Hough Farm, Allimore Green, Haughton, Stafford ST18 9JG Tel: 01785 780599 — MB ChB St. And. 1945; FRCS Ed. 1948. Prev: Cons. ENT Surg. Mid. Staffs. HA.

PATERSON, William David Carolina, 56 Longlands Road, Carlisle CA3 9AE Tel: 01228 521166 — MB ChB Ed. 1967; DObst RCOG 1970; MRCP (UK) 1972; FRCP Ed. 1983; FRCP Lond. 1985. Cons. Dermat. N. Cumbria Health Distr. Carlisle. Specialty: Dermat. Socs: Brit. Assn. Dermat. & BMA. Prev: Sen. Regist. (Dermat.) Roy. Infirm. Edin.; Regist. (Med.) Chalmers Hosp. Edin.; Ho. Surg. Bellshill Matern. Hosp.

PATERSON, Mr William Ian (retired) Craig Dhu, North Queensferry, Inverkeithing KY11 Tel: 01383 2647 — MB ChB Ed. 1938; FRCS Ed. 1946. Adviser (Orthop.) El Fateh Hosp. Tripoli. Prev:

Cons. Orthop. Surg. Princess Margt. Rose Orthop. Hosp. Edin., Vict. Hosp. Kirkcaldy & Dunfermline & W. Fife Hosp.

PATERSON-BROWN, June, CBE (retired) Norwood, Roadhead, Hawick TD9 7HP Tel: 01450 372352 Fax: 01450 379697 Email: pbnorwood@btinternet.com — (Edinburgh University) MB ChB Ed. 1955. Lord Lt Roxburgh Ettrick & Lauderdale. Prev: Med. Off. Family Plann. & Well Woman Clinics Borders HB.

PATERSON-BROWN, Peter Neville (retired) Norwood, Hawick TD9 7HP Tel: 01450 372352 Fax: 01450 379697 Email: pbnorwood@btinternet.com — MB ChB Ed. 1955; DObst RCOG 1958. Prev: Dir. Childr. Hospice Assn. Scotl.

PATERSON-BROWN, Sara Queen Charlottes & Chelsea Hospital, Ducane Rd, London W12 0NN Tel: 020 8383 1000 Fax: 020 8383 3419; 24 Mount Park Crescent, London W5 2RN — MB BChir Camb. 1984; FRCS Eng. 1988; MRCOG 1990; FRCOG 2003. Cons. O & G Qu. Charlottes & Chelsea Hosp. Lond. Specialty: Obst. & Gyn. Socs: RSM. Prev: Sen. Regist. (O & G) Qu. Charlottes & Chelsea Hosp. Lond.; Regist. (O & G) Ashford Middlx. & St. Thos. Hosp. Lond.; SHO (Gyn.) Qu. Charlotte's & Chelsea Hosps.

PATERSON-BROWN, Sheila Philomena Princess Alexandra Eye Pavillion, Edinburgh EH3 9YW Tel: 0131 536 1000 Fax: 0131 536 1001 — MB BS Lond. 1982 (St. Mary's Hosp. Med. Sch.) MRCP (UK) 1985; DRCOG 1986; MRCGP 1987. Clin. Asst. (Ophth.) Princess Alexandra Eye Pavil. Edin. Specialty: Ophth. Prev: GP Lond.; GP Hong Kong; Trainee GP Yateley VTS.

PATERSON-BROWN, Mr Simon Department of Surgery, Royal Infirmary, 51 Little France Crescent, Old Dalkeith Road, Edinburgh EH16 4SA Tel: 0131 536 1000 Ext: 23645 Fax: 0131 242 3664 Email: tricia.kelly@luht.scot.nhs.uk — MB BS Lond. 1982 (St Mary's Hospital London) FRCS Eng. 1986; FRCS Ed. 1986; MPhil Lond. 1989, MS 1993. Cons. Surg. Roy. Infirm. Edin.; Clin. Director Gen., Vasc. and Urological Surg.; Hon. Sen. Lect. Univ. Edin. Specialty: Gen. Surg.; Gastroenterol. Special Interest: Emerg. Surg.; Surgic. Train. and Assessm. Socs: Assn. Surg.; Assn. of Upper Gastrointestinal Surgeons. Prev: Sen. Lect. (Surg.) St Mary's Hosp. Lond.; Lead Clinician, Gen. surg.; Sen. Regist. (Surg.) Hammersmith & St Mary's Hosp. Lond.

PATEY, David Geoffrey Hamilton, TD 1 Bures House, Nayland Road, Bures CO8 5BX Tel: 01787 227096 — (Oxf. & Middlx.) BM BCh Oxf. 1952; MA Oxf. 1952; DPH Eng. 1960; FFCM 1980, M 1974. Prev: Co. MOH W. Suff.; PMO W. Sussex CC.

PATEY, George Laurence Thomas Macnamara 29 Conisboro Avenue, Caversham, Reading RG4 7JE — LMSSA Lond. 1943 (Oxf.) MA Oxon. 1943, BM BCh 1948.

PATEY, Rona Elizabeth Department of Anaesthetics, Aberdeen Royal Infirmary, Foresterhill, Aberdeen AB25 2ZN Tel: 01224 681818 Fax: 01224 685307; 61 Gray St, Aberdeen AB10 6JD — MB ChB Aberd. 1982. Cons. Anaesth. Aberd. Roy. Infirm. Specialty: Anaesth.; Intens. Care.

PATHAK, Binay Kumar Wollaton Vale Health Centre, Wollaton Vale, Nottingham NG8 2GR Tel: 0115 928 1151 Fax: 0115 928 8703 — MRCGP (Assam Med. Coll. Dibrugarh) MBE; MB BS. GP Wollaton Vale Health Centre, Wollaton. Prev: Regist. (Gen. Med.) & Resid. SHO (Paediat.) City Hosp. Chester; Regist. (Geriat. Med.) W. Chesh. Hosp. Chester.

PATHAK, Catherine Anne 11 Northfield Crescent, Beeston, Nottingham NG9 5GR — MB ChB Sheff. 1995.

PATHAK, Mrs Madhu Lata Rush Green Medical Centre, 261 Dagenham Road, Romford RM7 0XR Tel: 01708 728261 Fax: 01708 722645; 84 Parkway, Gidea Park, Romford RM2 5PL Tel: 01708 726835 Fax: 01708 722645 — MB BS Aligarh 1967 (J.L.N. Med. Coll. Aligarh) DTM & H Liverp. 1969; DA Eng. 1973; DCH Eng. 1974; LMSSA Lond. 1979; MRCGP 1986; Dip. Law 1996. GP; Trainer (Gen. Pract.) Romford; Sec. LMC. Socs: BMA. Prev: Regist. (Paediat.) OldCh. Hosp. Romford & Rush Green Hosp. Romford.

PATHAK, Nisha Dattatray 52 Lake Avenue, Walsall WS5 3PA — MB BS Baroda 1973.

PATHAK, Pankaj 17 Hill Field, Oadby, Leicester LE2 4RW — MB BS Punjab, Pakistan 1976; MChOrth Liverp. 1993.

PATHAK, Pransanta Kumar Caerphilly District Miners Hospital, Martin's Road, Caerphilly CF8 2WN — MB BS Calcutta 1971.

PATHAK, Mr Pratap Narayan (rooms), 41 The Downs, Altrincham WA14 2QG Tel: 0161 928 0611; 19 The Avenue, Sale M33 4PB Tel: 0161 969 6311 — MB BS Vikram 1961 (Gandhi Med. Coll. Bhopal) MRCS Eng. LRCP Lond. 1966; DLO Eng. 1968; FRCS Ed. 1968. Specialty: Otolaryngol. Socs: N. Eng. Otolaryngol. Soc. & Roy. Soc. Med. Prev: Cons. Surg. (Otolaryngol.) Trafford Gen. Hosp. Davyhulme; Sen. Regist. (ENT Surg.) Newc. Gen. Hosp.

PATHAK, Prem Lata Wilmslow Road Medical Centre, 156 Wilmslow Road, Rusholme, Manchester M14 5LQ Tel: 0161 224 2452 Fax: 0161 248 9261 — MB BS Delhi 1961 (Lady Hardinge Med. Coll.) DObst RCOG 1967. Prev: SHO (O & G) Newc. Gen. Hosp.

PATHAK, Priscilla Lotha 17 Hill Field, Oadby, Leicester LE2 4RW — MB BS Delhi 1983.

PATHAK, Sanjeev Kumar 85 Oak Lane, West Bromwich B70 8PR — MB ChB Leic. 1994. SHO (Orthop.) Roy. Urthopaedic Hosp. Prev: SHO (Urol.) Roy. Preson Hosp.; Prosector Anat. Oxf. Univ.; SHO (A & E) Solihull Hosp.

PATHAK, Miss Smriti 101 Fishponds Road, London SW17 7LL Tel: 020 8672 5626; 101 Fishponds Road, London SW17 7LL Tel: 020 8672 5626 — MB BS Lond. 1996 (UMDS of Guy's and St. Thomas' Hosp.) BSc (Hons.) Lond. 1993. SHO (Med.) City Gen. Hosp. Stoke-on Trent. Specialty: Gen. Med. Socs: MDU; BMA. Prev: Cas. SHO St. Geo.'s Hosp. Lond. f/t; Surg. Ho. Off. Feb-Aug 1997; Med. Ho. Off. Aug-Feb 1996-7.

PATHAK, Suresh Kumar Rush Green Medical Centre, 261 Dagenham Road, Romford RM7 0XR Tel: 01708 728261 Fax: 01708 722645; 84 Parkway, Gidea Park, Romford RM2 5PL Tel: 01708 726835 Fax: 01708 722645 — MB BS Vikram 1963 (G.R. Med. Coll. Gwalior) DObst RCPI 1969; DFFM 1998. Trainer, Tutor (Gen. Pract.) Med. Sch. Lond. Specialty: Gen. Pract. Socs: Balint's Soc.; GP Writers Assn.; Fell. Roy. Soc. Med. Prev: SHO Waterford Matern. Hosp. Waterford & Pinderfields Gen. Hosp. Wakefield; Med. Off. Tuberc. Hosp. Hathras, India.

PATHAN, Abdul Hafiz 83 Lynmouth Avenue, Enfield EN1 2LS — MB ChB Aberd. 1985. Specialty: Accid. & Emerg.

PATHAN, Mohammed Aslam Longford Medical Centre, 18a Sydnall Road, Coventry CV6 6BW Tel: 024 7664 4123 Fax: 024 7636 3157 — MB BS Peshawar 1966.

PATHAN, Nazima Paediatric Intensive Care Unit, Great Ormond Street Hospital, London WC1 Tel: 020 7405 9200; Apartment 3.G., The Ziggurat, 60-66 Saffron Hill, London EC1 — MB BS Lond. 1993; BSc Lond. 1990; MRCP (UK) 1996. Paediatric Intens. Care Regist., Gt. Ormond St. Hosp.; Hon. Clin. Research Fell., Imperial Coll. Lond. Specialty: Paediat. Prev: Specialist Regist. (Paediat.) Northwick Pk. Hosp.; SHO (Neonates) John Radcliffe Hosp. Oxf.; SHO (Paediat.) John Radcliffe Hosp. Oxf.

PATHANSALI, Rohan 83 Seaford Road, London W13 9HS — MB BS Lond. 1988; MRCP (UK) 1992.

PATHARE, Soumitra Ramesh Academic Unit of Psychiatry, North Wing 4th Floor, St Thomas Hospital, London SE1 Tel: 020 7928 9292 Fax: 020 7633 0061; 403 City View, 463 Bethnal Green Road, London E2 9QH Tel: 020 7739 5028 — MB BS Bombay 1988 (Seth G.S. Med. Coll. Bombay India) DPM Bomaby 1990; MD Bombay 1991; MRCPsych 1994. Wellcome Research Fell. (Psychiat.) UMDS (Guy's & St. Thos.). Specialty: Gen. Psychiat. Prev: Research Assoc. & Regist. (Psychiat.) UMDS.

PATHINAYAKE, Bethmage Dona Achirawathie Chulakantha 19 Milton Road, Sutton Courtenay, Abingdon OX14 4BP Tel: 01235 848375 — MB BS Colombo 1986 (University of Columbo Sri Lanka) MRCP (UK) 1994; MRCGP 1997. Specialty: Gen. Pract. Prev: GP Regist. Ch. St. Pract. Wantage; SHO (Gen. Paediat.) Princess Margt. Hosp. Swindon; SHO (O & G) Hoxton Gen. Hosp. Banbury.

PATHIRANA, Chandrawansa Kankanamge 225 Hoo Road, Kidderminster DY10 1LT Tel: 01562 639189 Email: pathick@hotmail.com — MB BS Ceylon 1968; MRCPI 1981. Staff Phys. (Gen. Med. & Geriat.) Gen. Hosp. Kidderminster. Specialty: Gen. Med.; Diabetes; Rehabil. Med.

PATHMABASKARAN, Selvaranee 63 Fishponds Road, Tooting Broadway, London SW17 7LH — MRCS Eng. LRCP Lond. 1987; MB BS Colombo, Sri Lanka 1983.

PATHMADEVA, Chryshanthi 6 Buriton Road, Harestock, Winchester SO22 6HX Tel: 01962 880770; Connaught House, 63B Romsey Road, Winchester SO22 5DE Tel: 01962 825128 Fax: 01962 840912 — MB BS Sri Lanka 1972; MRCPsych 1988. SCMO (Psychiat.) Connaught Ho. Day Hosp. Winchester. Specialty: Gen. Psychiat. Prev: Regist. (Psychiat.) Pk. Prewett Hosp. Basingstoke.

PATHMADEVA, Thiraviyam Wesley 6 Buriton Road, Harestock, Winchester SO22 6HX Tel: 01962 880770 — MB BS Sri Lanka 1973. Assoc. Specialist St. Jas. Hosp. Portsmouth. Specialty: Geriat. Psychiat.

PATHMANABAN, Praveen 36 Upton Gardens, Worthing BN13 1DA — MB BCh Wales 1993.

PATHMANANDAM, Hemachandran 50 Old Park Ridings, London N21 2ES — MB BS Lond. 1997.

PATHMANATHAN, Ishwara Kumar 14 Grafton Close, Worcester Park KT4 7JY — MB BS Lond. 1989.

PATHMANATHAN, Ravi Kumar Department of Cardiology, Leicester General Hospital, Gwendolen Road, Leicester LE5 4PW Tel: 0116 258 4436; Four Gables, 33 Elms Road, Stoneygate, Leicester LE2 3JD — MB BS Newc. 1989 (Newcastle-Upon-Tyne) MRCP (UK) 1992. Cons. Cardiol., Leicester. Specialty: Cardiol.

PATHMANATHAN, Sironmany 70 Kirkcroft, Wiggington, York YO32 2GH Tel: 01904 762329 — MB BS Sri Lanka 1966. SHO (Psychiat.) Hartlepool Gen. Hosp. Cleveland; Staff Grade (Psychiat.), Malton; Staff Grade (Psychiat.), Whitby & ScarBoro. Specialty: Geriat. Psychiat. Prev: SHO (O & G) York. Dist. Gen. Hosp. & Barnsley Dist. Hosp.; Unified SHO S. Tyneside NHS Rotatational Scheme.

PATHMANATHAN, Yoshana Flat 12, Mellior Court, 79 Shepherds Hill, London N6 5RQ — MB BS Lond. 1983.

PATHY, Damian John Gallwey Cathays Surgery, 137 Cathays Terrace, Cardiff CF24 4HU Tel: 029 2022 0878 Fax: 029 2038 8771 — MB BS Lond. 1987 (St. Bartholomew's) MRCP (UK) 1991; MRCGP 1994. Specialty: Gen. Pract. Prev: Regist. (Dermat.) Skin Hosp. Birm.; SHO Rotat. (Med.) MusGr. Pk. Hosp. Taunton; Ho. Off. (Cardiol. & Gen. Med.) St Bart. Hosp. Lond.

PATHY, Professor Mohan Sankar John, OBE — (King's Coll. Hosp.) MRCS Eng. LRCP Lond. 1948; FRCP Ed. 1968, M 1957; FRCP Lond. 1973, M 1960; FRCP Glas. 1997. Prof. Emerit. Univ. Wales; Health Research & Developm. Assoc., Cardiff. Specialty: Care of the Elderly. Socs: BMA; Brit. Geriat. Soc.; Amer. Geriat. Soc. Prev: Prof. Geriat. Med. Univ. Wales Coll. Med. Cardiff; Cons. Phys. (Geriat. Med.) Univ. Hosp. Wales Cardiff; Ho. Phys. King's Coll. Hosp. Lond.

PATI, Jhumur 1 Aldridge Walk, Southgate, London N14 6AF Tel: 020 7601 8387 — MB BS Dacca 1985; FRCS Eng. 1992; FRCS Ed. 1992.

PATI, Upendra Mohan 147 Liverpool Road, Birkdale, Southport PR8 4NT — MB BS Utkal 1963 (S.C.B. Med. Coll. Cuttack) FRCP Glas. 1986, M 1966; MRCGP 1975. Mem. Southport & Formby HA. Socs: BMA (Pres. Sefton Div.). Prev: Med. Regist. Southport Gen. Infirm.; Neurol. Regist. Walton Hosp. Liverp.

PATIENCE, Lesley Anne Dryden Cottage, Robert St., Stonehaven AB3 — MB ChB Aberd. 1980.

PATIENT, Miss Charlotte Jane Addenbrookes Hospital, Hills Road, Cambridge CB2 2QQ; 3 Coniston Road, Cambridge CB1 7BZ — MB BS Lond. 1991; MRCOG 1996. Specialist Regist. (O & G) Camb. Specialty: Obst. & Gyn.

PATIENT, David Neil 114 Lower Ham Road, Kingston upon Thames KT2 5BD — MB BS Lond. 1981; MRCP (UK) 1986; DRCOG 1988; MRCGP 1996; Dip. Occ. Med. RCP Lond. 1997.

PATIENT, Dennis Willoughby (retired) 8 Chattis Hill, Spitfire Lane, Stockbridge SO20 6JS Tel: 01264 810779 — (Westm.) MB BS Lond. 1957; MRCS Eng. LRCP Lond. 1957; DObst RCOG 1959; DA Eng. 1964. Prev: GP Heathcote Med. Centre Tadworth Surrey 1978-95.

PATIENT, Peter Stuart Anaesthetics Department, Colchester General Hospital, Turner Road, Colchester CO4 5JL — MB BS Lond. 1986; BSc Lond. 1983; DRCOG 1991; FRCA 1996. Cons. (Anaesth.) Colchester Gen. Hosp. Specialty: Anaesth. Special Interest: Vasc. Prev: Specialist Regist. Rotat. (anaseth.) UCLH & Roy. Free; Regist. Rotat. (Anaesth.) UCLH.

PATIENT, Mr Stafford Mortimer (retired) 24 Park Road, Ipswich IP1 3SU Tel: 01473 250728 — MB BS Lond. 1960 (Guys) MRCS Eng. LRCP Lond. 1960; FRCOG 1979, M 1966, DObst 1962; DCH Eng. 1963; FRCS Ed. 1968. Prev: Cons. O & G Ipswich Hosp.

PATIL, Dilip Bhimagouda Department of Obstetrics & Gynaecology, James Paget Hospital, Great Yarmouth NR31 6LA; 10 Diana Way, Caister on Sea, Great Yarmouth NR30 5TP Tel: 01493 377060 Fax: 01493 377060 Email: dilippatil@compuserve.com — MB BS Karnatak 1982; MRCOG 1992. Assoc. Specialist (O & G) Jas. Paget Hosp. Gt. Yarmouth. Specialty: Obst. & Gyn. Prev: Regist. (Obst.) Roy. Lond. Hosp.; Regist. (O & G) Shotley Bridge Gen. Hosp. Consett; SHO (Fertil. Regulat.) Newc. Gen. Hosp. Newc. u. Tyne.

PATIL, Mr Krishnaji Pandurang c/o Department of Urology, St Peters Hospital, Guildford Road, Chertsey KT16 0PZ — MB BS Bombay 1978; FRCS Ed. 1992.

PATINIOTT, Anthony Kieron Birchwood Medical Centre, 15 Benson Road, Birchwood, Warrington WA3 7PJ; 8 Barns Place, Halebarns, Altrincham WA15 0HP — MB ChB Birm. 1995; DRCOG 1999; MRCGP (Distinc.) 1999. GP Warrington.

PATINIOTT, Francis Joseph Birchwood Medical Centre, 15 Benson Road, Birchwood, Warrington WA3 7PJ Tel: 01925 823502 Fax: 01925 852422; Mosswood, 15 Castleway, Hale Barns, Altrincham WA15 0AD Tel: 0161 980 5507 — MRCS Eng. LRCP Lond. 1962 (Manch.) DObst RCOG 1965. Prev: Regist. (O & G) Stepping Hill Hosp. Stockport; SHO (Paediat.) Birch Hill Hosp. Rochdale; Ho. Surg. Pk. Hosp. Davyhulme.

PATKAR, Ashwin Anand 17 Perryford Drive, Solihull B91 3XE — MB BS Bombay 1988; MRCPsych 1993.

PATMORE, Jane Elizabeth 3 Thornleys, Cherry Burton, Beverley HU17 7SJ — BM BS Nottm. 1989; MRCP (UK) 1992; CCST (Endocrinol. & Diabetes & Gen. Med.) 2003. Cons. Diabetologist. Hull Roy. Infirm. Specialty: Diabetes; Endocrinol. Socs: BDA; Soc. Edocrinol. Prev: Specialist Regist. Yorks. Rotat. Flexible Train.; Regist. (Chem. Path.) St. Jas. Univ. Hosp. Leeds; SHO (Gen. Med.) Harrogate Dist. Hosp.

PATMORE, Russell David department of Haematology, Hull Royal infirmary, Anlaby rd, Hull HU3 2JZ Tel: 01482 607742 Fax: 01482 607739; 3 Thornleys, Cherry Burton, Beverley HU17 7SJ Tel: 01964 550007 — BM BS Nottm. 1989; MRCP (UK) 1992; MRCPath 1997. Cons. hamatology Hull & E Yorks. Hosp. NHS trust Hull. Specialty: Haematology. Socs: Brit. Soc. Haematol. Prev: Cons. (Haematol.) Roy. Hull Hosp. Hull; Regist. (Haemat.) Yorks. RHA.

PATMORE, Susan Jane Harriet 5 Cavendish Place, Cavendish Crescent S., The Park, Nottingham NG7 1ED — BM Soton. 1996. SHO (Surg.) Rotat. QMC Nottm.

PATNAIK, Sharmistha Brookeside House, Brookside Cottages, Ashbrooke Road, Sunderland SR2 7HQ — MB BS Utka 1969.

PATNAIK, Surya Narayan The New City Medical Centre, Tatham Street, Hendon, Sunderland SR1 2QB Tel: 0191 567 5571 — LRCP LRCS Ed. 1980; MB BS Sambalpur 1969; LRCP LRCS Ed. LRCPS Glas. 1980.

PATODI, Mamta c/o Drive K.C. Jain, 24 Redlake Drive, Stourbridge DY9 0RX — LMSSA Lond. 1986.

PATODI, Sanat Kumar Keynell Covert Surgery, 33 Keynell Covert, Kings Norton, Birmingham B30 3QT Tel: 0121 458 2619 Fax: 0121 459 9640 — MB BS Indore 1971; MB BS Indore 1971.

PATON, Alastair George Peter (retired) Ben Ard, The Mount, Peebles EH45 9EX Tel: 01721 720098; Ben Ard, The Mount, Peebles EH45 9EX Tel: 01721 20098 — MB ChB Ed. 1954 (Edin.) DObst RCOG 1960.

PATON, Alexander (retired) 16 Hammer Lane, Warborough, Oxford OX10 7DJ Tel: 01865 859932 — MB BS Lond. 1947 (St Thos.) MD Lond. 1958; MRCS Eng. LRCP Lond. 1947; FRCP Lond. 1967; MRCP Lond. 1951. Prev: Postgrad. Med. Dean NE Thames RHA.

PATON, Alexander Campbell Kingfisher Surgery, 26 Elthorne Way, Newport Pagnell MK16 0JR Tel: 01908 618265 Fax: 01908 01908 217804 — MB ChB Glas. 1973; MRCP (UK) 1975. Dep. Coroner Beds.

PATON, Andrew Lindsay Dalton Square Surgery, 8 Dalton Square, Lancaster LA1 1PN Tel: 01524 842200; 11 Eden Park, Lancaster LA1 4SJ Tel: 01524 39633 — MB ChB Ed. 1979; MA Oxf. 1982; DRCOG 1982; MRCGP 1983.

PATON, Andrew Nicholas Compass House Medical Centres, 25 Bolton Street, Brixham TQ5 9BZ Tel: 01803 855897 Fax: 01803 855613; 1 The Drive, Upton Manor, Brixham TQ5 9RA Tel: 01803 851494 Email: drpaton@aol.com — MB ChB Bristol 1981; DCH RCPS Glas. 1985; MRCGP (Distinc.) 1987.

PATON, David (retired) Purbeck Lodge, 48 Britwell Road, Burnham, Slough SL1 8DE Tel: 01628 604993 — MB ChB Glas. 1938. Prev: Clin. Asst. Co. Lanark Matern. Hosp. Bellshill.

PATON, Mr David Frederic (retired) Grove Cottage, Sidestrand Road, Southrepps, Norwich NR11 8XB Tel: 01263 833540 Fax: 01263 833540 — MB ChB Cape Town 1958; FRCS Ed. 1964; FRCS Eng. 1965. Prev: Prof. (Orthop. Surg.) Head Dept. Orthop. Surg. Univ. Cape Town.

PATON, David Hill Tryst Medical Centre, 431 King Street, Stenhousemuir, Larbert FK5 4HT Tel: 01324 551555 Fax: 01324 551925; Muirlands, 69 Bellsdyke Road, Larbert FK5 4EQ Tel: 01324 557584 — MB ChB Ed. 1974; BSc Ed. 1971, MB ChB 1974; DObst RCOG 1976; MRCGP 1978.

PATON, Douglas Henry Hay War Memorial Health Centre, Crickhowell NP8 1AG Tel: 01873 810255 — MB ChB Ed. 1983; DCH RCPS Glas. 1989; MRCGP 1990. Prev: Trainee GP Gwent VTS.

PATON, Maj-Gen Douglas Stuart, CBE, CStJ, Maj.-Gen. late RAMC (retired) Brampton, Springfield Road, Camberley GU15 1AB Tel: 01276 63669 — (Bristol) MB ChB Bristol 1951; FFCM 1982, M 1974; FFPHM 1989. Prev: Hon. Phys. to HM the Qn.

PATON, Edward Robert Ley, Col. late RAMC Retd. (retired) 7/5 Fountainhall Road, Edinburgh EH9 2NL — MB ChB St. And. 1956; DTM & H Eng. 1963; DCH Eng. 1970; MRCGP 1974. Prev: Clin. Med. Off. Lothian Health Bd. 1986-2002.

PATON, Gerald Maybole Health Centre and Day Hospital, 6 High Street, Maybole KA19 7BY Tel: 01655 882278 Fax: 01655 889616 — MB ChB Glas. 1982.

PATON, Mr Iain Campbell Cruachan, 1A Dennistoun Road, Langbank, Port Glasgow PA14 6XH — MB ChB Glas. 1972; FRCS Ed. 1978. Cons. ENT Surg. Roy. Alex. Hosp. Paisley & Inverclyde Roy. Hosp. Greenock. Specialty: Otolaryngol. Special Interest: Otology; Rhinology. Prev: Sen. Regist. Leeds.

PATON, Irene Kennedy (retired) 14 James Watt Road, Milngavie, Glasgow G62 7JY Tel: 0141 956 3802 — MB ChB Glas. 1965; DCH RCPS Glas. 1967.

PATON, James Stewart Henry Yewlands, Crundalls Lane, Bewdley DY12 1ND — BM BCh Oxf. 1973; MA. Prev: Med. Off. Tugela Ferry Hosp., S. Africa; Ho. Phys. Amersham Hosp.; Ho. Surg. Churchill Hosp. Oxf.

PATON, James Young Department of Child Health, Royal Hospital for Sick Children, Yorkhill, Glasgow G3 8SJ Tel: 0141 201 0238 Fax: 0141 209 0387 Email: j.y.paton@clinmed.gla.ac.uk — MB ChB (Hons.) Glas. 1977; BSc (Hons.) Glas. 1973; MRCP (UK) 1979; DCH Eng. 1979; MD Leic. 1987; FRCP Glas. 1995. Reader, Paediatric Resperatory Dis. and Hon. Cons. Paediat., Yorkhill NHS Trust, Glas. Specialty: Paediat. Socs: American Thoracic Soc.; Eur. Respirat. Soc.; Brit. Thorac. Soc. Prev: Sen. Regist. Roy. Hosp. Sick Childr. Glas.; MRC Trav. Fell. Childr. Hosp. Los Angeles, USA.

PATON, Janet Forth View Practice, Dean Road, Bo'ness EH51 0DQ Tel: 01506 822466 Fax: 01506 826216; 28 Linlithgow Road, Bo'ness EH51 0DN Tel: 01506 822418 — MB ChB Ed. 1977 (University of Edinburgh) MRCGP 1981.

PATON, Nicholas Iain James 34 Dundonald Road, London SW19 3QN — MB BChir Camb. 1989; MA Camb. 1990, MB BChir 1989; MRCP (UK) 1993. Specialty: Infec. Dis.

PATON, Richard Stewart The Hawthorns, Stonepit Lane, Inkberrow, Worcester WR7 4ED Tel: 01386 792784 Fax: 01386 792637 — MB ChB Glas. 1967. GP Princip. The Hawthorns PMS Pilot, Inkberrow, Worcs WR7 4ED; Pharamacological Research & Medico-Legal Cons. Specialty: Gen. Pract.

PATON, Robert Colin Milton Keynes General Hospital NHS Trust, Eaglestone, Milton Keynes MK6 5LD Tel: 01908 243006; 7 Dene Close, Aspley Hill, Woburn Sands, Milton Keynes MK17 8NL — MD Ed. 1983; MB ChB 1972; MRCP (UK) 1974; FRCP Ed. 1986; FRCP Lond. 1989. Cons. Phys. Milton Keynes Gen. Hosp. Specialty: Gen. Med.; Diabetes; Endocrinol. Prev: Lect. Med. Univ. Leeds.

PATON, Robert Hamish 8 Lime Street, Ossett, Wakefield — MB ChB Sheff. 1985; DCH RCP Lond. 1987; FRCA 1994. Specialty: Anaesth.

PATON, Robert McCracken (retired) 5 Monks Road, Airdrie ML6 9QW Tel: 01236 762322 — MB ChB Glas. 1929. Prev: Ho. Surg. Clayton Hosp. Wakefield.

PATON, Mr Robin William Blackburn Royal Infirmary, Bolton Road, Blackburn BB2 3LR Tel: 01254 263 555 Ext: 4165 — MB ChB Glas. 1980; FRCS Ed. 1984; FRCS Glas. 1985; FRCS (Orth.) Ed. 1989. Cons. Orthop. Surg. Blackburn Roy. Infirm.; Hon. Clin. Lect. Univ. of Manch. 1997. Specialty: Orthop.; Trauma & Orthop. Surg. Special Interest: Adult Knee Surg.; Childrens Orthopaedic Surg. Socs: Sec. Childr.'s Orthop. Gp. NW & Merseyside. Prev: Sen. Regist. (Orthop. Surg.) North. West. Region.

PATRE, Pamela — MB BS Lond. 1998.

PATRICK, Alan William Royal Infirmary of Birmingham, 51 Little France Crescent, Edinburgh E16 4SA Tel: 0131 536 1000 Fax: 0131 242 1485 Email: alan.patrick@luht.scot.nhs.uk; 50 Braid Road, Edinburgh EH10 6AL Tel: 0131 447 9402 — MB ChB Ed. 1981 (Edinburgh) MRCP (UK) 1984; MD Ed. 1994; FRCP Ed. 1996. Cons. Phys. (Diabetes & Endocrinol.) Roy. Infirm. Edin. Specialty: Diabetes; Endocrinol.; Gen. Med.

PATRICK, Andrew Godson 35 Norwood Avenue, Alloa FK10 2BY Tel: 01259 724198 — MB ChB Glas. 1960.

PATRICK, David Hexham General Hospital,, Hexham NE46 1QJ; 9 Green Close, Stannington, Morpeth NE61 6PE — MB BS Newc. 1974; BSc Newc. 1971, MB BS 1974; DMRD Eng. 1980; FRCR 1981. Cons. Radiologist Hexham Gen. Hosp., Hexham, N.umberland; Cons. Radiol., Wansbew Gen. Hosp., Ashington, N.umberland. Specialty: Radiol.

PATRICK, David Anthony — BM BS Nottm. 1996. SpR (Anaesth.) Mersey Region. Specialty: Anaesth. Prev: SHO (Anaesth.) Derby City Hosp.; SHO (A & E) Chorley & S. Ribble Hosp.; SHO (Paediat.) Roy. Preston Hosp.

PATRICK, Elizabeth Anne Shenton Sunnyside Surgery, 4 Sunnyside Road, Clevedon BS21 7TA Tel: 01275 873588 Fax: 01275 341381 Email: elizabethpatrick@gp-l81102.nhs.uk — MB ChB Leic. 1982 (Leicester) DRCOG 1985; MRCGP 1986; DCH RCP Lond. 1986; D.Occ.Med London 2000. Specialty: Gen. Pract.; Occupat. Health. Prev: Trainee GP Leics. VTS; SHO (Geriat. Ophth. Cas.) Leic. HA.

PATRICK, Emma May — MB BS Lond. 1998.

PATRICK, Guy Michael IBAH (UK), Wessex Business Centre, Bumpers Farm, Chippenham SN14 6NQ Tel: 01249 440727 Fax: 01249 463004 — MB ChB Bristol 1984; BSc Bristol 1981; MRCP UK 1990. Pharmacutical Phys. Specialty: Pharmaceutical Medicine; Nephrol. Prev: Cons. Nephrol.

PATRICK, Ian Thomas, OStJ (retired) Ochiltree, Merse Way, Kippford, Dalbeattie DG5 4LH — MB ChB Glas. 1948 (Univ. Glas.) Prev: Co. Surg. St. John Ambul. Brig.

PATRICK, James Alexander Directorate of Anaesthesia, Glasgow Royal Infirmary, Glasgow G4 0SF Tel: 0141 211 4620/1 Fax: 0141 211 4622 — MB ChB Glas. 1981; BSc Glas. 1976; FRCA 1986. Cons. Anaesth. Glas. Roy. Infirm. Specialty: Anaesth. Prev: Sen. Regist. (Anaesth.) St. Thos. Hosp. Lond.; Regist. (Anaesth.) Glas. Roy. Infirm.; SHO (Anaesth.) Roy. Infirm. Edin.

PATRICK, Janet Frances Royal Oldham Hospital, Rochdale Road, Oldham OL1 2JH — MB ChB Sheff. 1975; BSc Ed. 1969; MRCOG 1983. Cons. O & G Roy. Oldham Hosp. Lancs. Specialty: Obst. & Gyn.

PATRICK, Janice Station Approach Health Centre, Station Approach, Bradford-on-Avon BA15 1DQ Tel: 01225 866611 — MB BS Newc. 1988; DRCOG 1991; MRCGP 1992; Dip. Ther. Wales 1998.

PATRICK, Jenneth Mary Witton Street Surgery, 162 Witton Street, Northwich CW9 5QU Tel: 01606 42007 Fax: 01606 350659; Barberry Cottage, Mill Lane, Cuddington, Northwich CW8 2TA — MB ChB Manch. 1982. Prev: SHO (A & E) Stockport Infirm.; SHO (Psychiat.) Univ. Hosp. S. Manch.; SHO/Trainee GP Bolton Gen. Hosp. VTS.

PATRICK, Mr John Howard 27 Kennedy Road, Shrewsbury SY3 7AB — MB BS Lond. 1966 (St. Thos.) FRCS Eng. 1972. Dir. ORLAU & Cons. Orthop. Surg. Robt. Jones & Agnes Hunt Hosp. Oswestry. Specialty: Orthop. Socs: Fell. BOA; Fell. Roy. coll. Surgs. Prev: Sen. Lect. (Orthop. Surg.) Univ. Liverp.; Specialist (Surg.) RAF Med. Br.; Chief Asst. (Orthop. Surg.) St. Thos. Hosp. Lond.

PATRICK, Kathryn Antoinette — MB ChB Birm. 1998.

PATRICK, Kevin, Capt. Anaesth. Department, Royal Hospital Hasler, Gosport PO12 2AA; The Cottage, Cairnbulg Castle, Fraserburgh AB43 8TN — MB ChB Aberd. 1996. SHO (Anaesth.) Roy. Hosp. Hasler, Gosport. Specialty: Anaesth. Prev: Regt.. Med. Off. Med. Centre QRH Catterick Garrison.

PATRICK, Mark Ronald Department of Anaesthesia, Wythenshawe Hospital, Southmoor Road, Manchester M23 9LT Tel: 0161 291 5710 Fax: 0161 291 5709; Lindow Cottage, 65

Racecourse Road, Wilmslow SK9 5LJ Tel: 01625 522499 — MB BS Lond. 1976 (St. Bart.) BSc Lond. 1973; FRCA 1981. Cons. Anaesth. Wythenshawe Hosp. Manch.; Hon. Clin. Lect. Univ. Manch. Specialty: Anaesth. Socs: BMA & Assn. Anaesth.; Assn. Cardiothoracic Anaesth. Prev: Sen. Regist. (Anaesth.) Lond. Hosp.; Regist. (Anaesth.) Hosp. Sick Childr. Lond. & St. Bart. Hosp. Lond.

PATRICK, Matthew Paul Hugh Adult Department, Tavistock and Portman NHS Trust, 120 Belsize Lane, London NW3 5BA Tel: 020 7435 7111 Fax: 020 7447 3745 — MB BS Lond. 1985 (Roy. Lond. Hosp.) BSc (1st cl. Hons.) Lond. 1982; MRCPsych 1990. Cons. Psychother. Tavistock & Portman NHS Trust Lond. Specialty: Psychother. Socs: Full. Mem. Brit. Psychoanalyt. Soc. Prev: MRC Train. Fell. Univ. Coll. Lond.; Hon. Sen. Regist. (Psychother.) Tavistock Clinic Lond.; Regist. (Psychiat.) Maudsley & Bethlem Roy. Hosp. Lond.

PATRICK, Paul Richard Patrick and Partners, Rise Park Surgery, Revelstoke Way, Nottingham NG5 5EB Tel: 0115 927 2525 Fax: 0115 979 7056; George's Hill House, George's Hill, Arnold, Nottingham NG5 8PU Tel: 0115 920 7795 — BM BS Nottm. 1976; BMedSci Nottm. 1974; DRCOG 1979. Hosp. Pract. (Disabil. Med.) City Hosp. Nottm.; Clin. Tutor (Gen. Pract.) Univ. Nottm. Specialty: Obst. & Gyn.

PATRICK, Mr Robert Kenneth 9 Heatherstones, Queens Gate, Halifax HX3 0DH — MB BS Sydney 1968; FRCS Ed. 1973.

PATRICK, Sharon (retired) Public Health Laboratory, Salisbury District Hospital, Salisbury SP2 8BJ — MB ChB Sheff. 1970; Dip. Bact. Manch. 1976; FRCPath 1989, M 1977. Prev: Dir. & Cons. Med. Microbiol. Pub. Health Laborat. Salisbury.

PATRICK, Mr William John Ainslie Dept of Paediatric Pathology, Yorkhill NHS Trust, Yorkhill, Glasgow G3 8SJ Tel: 0141 201 0401 Fax: 0141 201 0397 — MB ChB Glas. 1962; FRCS Eng. 1970; FRCS Ed. 1970; FRCPath 1990, M 1978. Cons. Path. Roy. Hosp. Sick Childr. Glas.; Hon. Clin. Sen. Lect. Univ. Glas.; cons and Gardiner lec. Roy.hosp.sick.childr.glas. Specialty: Paediat. Socs: Paediat. Path. Soc.; Brit. & Irish Paediat. Path. Assn. Prev: Sen. Regist. Path. Roy. Hosp. Sick Childr. Edin.

PATROCLOU, Aristotelis c/o Mr. A. Pickles, 69 Lewsey Road, Luton LU4 0EN — MD Liege 1985. Specialty: Obst. & Gyn.

PATRONI, Bruno Flat 4, 51 St James Road, Sutton SM1 2TG — MB BS West. Austral. 1984.

PATRUDU, Mr Makena Narasimha St Michael's Hospital, 4 Trelissick Road, Hayle TR27 4HY Tel: 01736 753234; 52 Mellanear Road, Hayle TR27 4QT — (Andhra Med. Coll.) MB BS Andhra 1970; FRCS Ed. 1985. Assoc. Specialist (Surg.) St. Michael's Hosp. Hayle. Specialty: Gen. Surg.

PATSALIDES, Mr Christodoulos Theodosiou Knee Research Room, 4th Floor, Musculoskeletal Science, UCD Building, Royal Liverpool University Hospital, Liverpool L69 3GA Tel: 0151 706 4126 Fax: 0151 706 5815; Flat 10, 2 Strathmore Road, Newsham Park, Liverpool L6 7UD Tel: 0151 281 4645 — MB ChB Leic. 1994; FRCS (I) Dubl. 1998. Clin. Res. Asst., Roy. L'pool & Braodgreen Hosps Knee Serv., L'pool. Specialty: Orthop.

PATSIOS, Demetris Andrea 68 Green Bridges, Headington, Oxford OX3 8PL — BM BCh Oxf. 1994.

PATTANAYAK, Mr Kalidas 25 Valley View Road, Rochester ME1 3PB Tel: 01634 826289 — MB BS Calcutta 1967 (Sir Nilratan Sircar Med. Coll.) FRCS Eng. 1978. Specialty: Gen. Surg.; Urol. Socs: Fell. Roy. Soc. Med.; Fell. Assn. Surgs. India; Assoc.Mem.Brit.Assoc.s.Urol.Surg. Prev: Cons. Surg. & Chief Surg. P. Salman Hosp. Riyadh, Saudi Arabia; Regist. (Surg.) Friarage Hosp. Northallerton; Surg. Specialist Calcutta Nat. Med. Coll. Hosp., India.

PATTANI, Shriti Mansukh Occupational Health Department, North West London NHS Trust, Watford Rd, Harrow — MB ChB Leic. 1991; BSc, MRCGP,DRCOG,MFOM.

PATTANI, Sumitra Kanjibhai Church Lane Surgery, 282 Church Lane, London NW9 8BU Tel: 020 82000077 Fax: 020 82005999 — MB BS Bombay 1964; DCH Lond. 1982. Specialty: Family Plann. & Reproduc. Health.

PATTAR, Subhas Mahadev 23 Pickering Close, Leicester LE4 6ER — MB BS Karnatak 1974.

PATTARA, Alexander Joseph The Surgery, High Road, Horndon-on-the-Hill, Stanford-le-Hope SS17 8LB Tel: 01375 642362 Fax: 01375 641747 — MB BS Mysore 1972. Specialty: Diabetes.

PATTEKAR, Bhanuvilas Digamber Orthopaedic Department, Queen Elizabeth Hospital, Sheriff Hill, Gateshead NE9 6SX Tel: 0191 482 0000; 1 Brenkley Court, Seaton Burn, Newcastle upon Tyne NE13 6DR Tel: 0191 236 7375 Fax: 0191 403 2833 — MB BS Jabalpur 1971. Assoc. Specialist (Orthop.) Qu. Eliz. Hosp. Tyne & Wear. Specialty: Orthop. Prev: Regist. (Orthop.) CrossHo. Hosp. Kilmarnock, StoneHo. Hosp. & Kilmarnock Infirm.; Regist. Ayr Hosp.

PATTEKAR, Jyotsna Bhanuvilas Perrins and Partners, Trinity Medical Centre, New George Street, South Shields NE33 5DU Tel: 0191 454 7775 — MB BS Univ. Marathwada 1971; MB BS Univ. Marathwada India 1971; DObst RCPI 1980. GP (Long Term Locum) Gateshead, Tyne & Wear. Specialty: Obst. & Gyn. Prev: Regist. (O & G) Ayrsh. Centr. Hosp. Irvine; SHO (Gyn.) Cross Hse. Hosp. Kilmarnock; SHO (Paediat.) Seafield Childr. Hosp. Ayr.

PATTEN, John Philip (retired) Pelham, Mead Road, Hindhead GU26 6SG Tel: 01428 604975 Fax: 01428 607085 — MB BS Lond. 1960 (Westm.) BSc Lond. 1957; FRCP Lond. 1979, M 1964. Private Pract. Prev: Hon. Cons. Neurol. King Edwd. VII Hosp. Midhurst.

PATTEN, Maria Juliette 21 Gosling Grove, Downley, High Wycombe HP13 5YS — MB BS Lond. 1991.

PATTEN, Mark Thomas Luton & Dunstable, Hosp., Lewsey Road, Luton LU4 0DZ Tel: 01582 497230; 8 High Ash Road, Wheathampstead, St Albans AL4 8DY Tel: 01582 833038 — MB ChB Glas. 1988; FRCA 1994. Cons. (Instensive Care & Anaesth.) Luton & Dunstable Hosp. Specialty: Intens. Care. Prev: Sen. Regist. (Anaesth.) NW RHA; Clin. Fell. (Intens. Care) Academisch Ziekenhuis Groningen, Netherlands; Regist. Rotat. (Anaesth.) NW RHA.

PATTEN, Michael Gordon Banks Medical Centre, 272 Wimborne Road, Bournemouth BH3 7AT; 272 Wimborne Road, Winton, Bournemouth BH3 7AT Tel: 01202 512549 — BM Soton. 1980; DRCOG 1984; MRCGP 1985. Princip. GP Bournemouth. Prev: SHO (Med. & Oncol.) Roy. Marsden Hosp. Sutton; SHO (Med. & O & G) Bedford Gen. Hosp.

PATTEN, Piers Edward Major 121 Blenheim Crescent, London W11 2EQ — MB ChB Bristol 1997; BSc (Hons.) Bristol 1994.

PATTEN, Timothy James Cheviot Road Surgery, 1 Cheviot Road, Millbrook, Southampton SO16 4AH Tel: 023 8077 3174 Fax: 023 8070 2748 — MB BS Lond. 1983 (Oxford St. Mary's Paddington) MA Oxf. 1979; MRCGP 1987; DRCOG 1987. Sen. Lect., Primary Care, Univ. of Southampton. Specialty: Gen. Pract. Prev: Trainee GP Som. HA VTS.

PATTERSON, Agnes Campbell Woodlands, Inverdale, Aviemore PH22 1QH — MB ChB Ed. 1961.

PATTERSON, Aileen Dept of Pathology, Hinchingbrooke NHS Trust, Hinchingbrooke Park, Huntingdon PE29 6NT Tel: 01480 416150 Fax: 01480 416527 — MB BS Lond. 1981 (Roy. Free) MRCPath 1993; FRCPath 2001. Cons. (Path.) Hinchingbrooke Hosp. Huntingdon. Specialty: Histopath.

PATTERSON, Mr Alan (retired) Blythe Wood Lodge, Lady Alice Drive, Blythe Lane, Ormskirk L40 5UD — MB ChB Liverp. 1956; MD Liverp. 1960; DO Eng. 1962; FRCS Eng. 1965; FRCOphth 1989. Cons. Ophth. Liverp. HA (T). Prev: Sen. Regist. Lond. Hosp.

PATTERSON, Alison Sandra 328 Stranmillis Road, Belfast BT9 5EB — MB BCh BAO Belf. 1994.

PATTERSON, Andrew Barry Burnside, 12 Ballynahinch Road, Dromore BT25 1DJ; 106 Hillsborough Road, Dromore, Down, Dromore BT25 1QW Tel: 01846 693876 Fax: 01846 693876 — MB BCh BAO Belf. 1995 (Quenn's Univ. Belf.) Specialty: Orthop.

PATTERSON, Angus James 11 Lenamore Avenue, Newtownabbey BT37 0PF — MB BCh BAO Belf. 1988; MRCP Glas. 1991. Regist. (Clin. Oncol.) Belvoir Pk. Hosp. Belf. Specialty: Oncol.; Radiother.

PATTERSON, Anne Elizabeth Jane Sth. Ken, & Chelsea Mental Hlth. Centre, 1 Nightingale Place, London SW10 9NG Tel: 020 8846 6051 Fax: 020 8237 5282 — MB ChB Manch. 1985; MRCPSych 1991. Cons. Psychiat. in Psychother., Chelsea & West. Hosp., Lond. Specialty: Psychother. Prev: Sen. Regist. (Psychother.) Glas.

PATTERSON, Brian George Portglenone Health Centre, 17 Townhill Road, Portglenone, Ballymena BT44 8AD Tel: 028 2582 1551 Fax: 028 2582 2539; Stoneleigh House, 20 Largy Road, Portglenone, Ballymena BT44 8BX Tel: 01266 821263 Fax: 01266 822539 — MB BCh BAO Belf. 1977; DRCOG 1979; MRCGP 1985. Socs: BMA.

PATTERSON, Carole Anne Whitley Vicarage, Hexham NE46 2LA — MB BS Newc. 1990.

PATTERSON, Cathryn Emma 5 Strandview Street, Belfast BT9 5FF — MB BCh BAO Belf. 1995. SpR Geriat. Med. Belf. City Hosp. Prev: SHO Rotat. (Med.) Belf. City Hosp.

PATTERSON, Christopher John Care of the Elderly Department, St. Luke's Hospital, Little Horton Lane, Bradford BD5 0NA Tel: 01274 365148 — MB ChB Leeds 1990; BSc 1987; MRCP (UK) 1993. Specialty: Care of the Elderly.

PATTERSON, Colin Brunswick House Medical Group, 1 Brunswick Street, Carlisle CA1 1ED Tel: 01228 515808 Fax: 01228 593048 — MB BCh BAO Belf. 1986.

PATTERSON, Damian David Lister Abbey View Medical Centre, Shaftesbury SP7 8DH Tel: 01747 856700 Fax: 01747 856701 — MB BS Lond. 1992 (St Geo.) BSc (Hons.) Lond. 1989; MRCP UK 1996; DFFP 2000; MRCGP 2001. GP Dorset; Clin. Asst. (Diabetes) Dorset Co. Hosp. Dorchester. Specialty: Gen. Pract.; Diabetes. Prev: GP Trainee Dorchester; Clin. Research Fell. (Liver Unit) King's Coll. Hosp. Lond.; SHO (Med.) Derriford Hosp. Plymouth.

PATTERSON, Daniel Mark 8 David Close, Aylesbury HP21 9XF — MB BS Lond. 1996.

PATTERSON, David Llewhelin Hood Department of Cardiovascular Medicine, Whittington Hospital, Highgate Hill, London N19 5NF Tel: 020 7288 5292 Fax: 020 7288 5010 Email: d.patterson@ucl.ac.uk; 25 South Villas, Camden Town, London NW1 9BT Tel: 020 7267 2394 Fax: 0870 054 3737 — (Univ. Coll. Hosp.) MB BS Lond. 1965; MRCS Eng. LRCP Lond. 1965; FRCP Lond. 1980, M 1969; MD Lond. 1973. Cons. Phys. & Cardiol. Whittington Hosp. & Univ. Coll. Lond. Hosps.; Vice-Dean Whittington Campus, Roy. Free & Univ. Coll. Sch. of Med., UCL. Specialty: Cardiol. Socs: Brit. Cardiac Soc.; Brit. Med. Informat. Soc.; Europ. Soc. Cardiol. Prev: Sen. Regist. Roy. Free Hosp. Lond.; Regist. Nat. Heart Hosp. Lond.; Regist. Univ. Coll. Hosp. Lond.

PATTERSON, David Robert Main Street Surgery, 29 Main Street, Eglinton, Londonderry BT47 3AB Tel: 028 7181 0252 Fax: 028 7181 1347 — MB BCh BAO Belf. 1985; MRCGP 1990.

PATTERSON, Diana Georgina, OBE Shaftesbury Square Hospital, 116-120 Great Victoria St., Belfast BT2 7BG Tel: 01232 329808 Fax: 01232 312208 — MB BCh BAO Belf. 1977 (Queen's University Belfast) MRC Psych 1981; MD Belf. 1983; FRCPsych 1996. Cons. Psychiat. Shaftesbury Sq. Hosp. Belf.; Hon. Lect. Qu. Univ. Belf. Specialty: Alcohol & Substance Misuse.

PATTERSON, Donald Howard (Surgery) 6 East Mount Road, York YO2 2DB; 100 Tadcaster Road, Dringhouses, York YO24 1LT — MB ChB Leeds 1968; DCH Eng. 1970; DObst. RCOG 1975. Prev: Med. Dir. Brit. Nepal Med. Trust; Princip. Gen. Pract. Watton; Regist. (Paediat.) St. John's Hosp. Chelmsford.

PATTERSON, Edna Rosemary Ellen 16 Pen y Ffordd, St Clears, Carmarthen SA33 4DX Tel: 01994 230799 Email: rosemary.patterson@virgin.net — MB BCh BAO Belf. 1979 (Qu. Univ. Belf.) DA (UK) 1986; Dip. Occ Med 1996. Med. Adviser (DVLA Swansea). Specialty: Civil Serv.

PATTERSON, Eleanor Jill Handforth Health Centre, Handforth, Wilmslow SK9 3HL Tel: 01625 529421 Fax: 01625 536560; Parkend, Bradford Lane, Nether Alderly, Macclesfield SK10 4TR — MB ChB Manch. 1974; DCH Eng. 1976; DRCOG 1977. Princip. GP.

PATTERSON, George Charles Cardiac Catheterisation Unit, Royal Victoria Hospital, Belfast BT12 6BA — MD Belf. 1955; PhD Belf. 1968, MD 1955, MB BCh BAO 1950. Cons. Cardiol. Roy. Vict. Hosp. Belf. Specialty: Cardiol.

PATTERSON, Gillian Mary 3 Cumberland Avenue, Basingstoke RG22 4BG — MB ChB Bristol 1980; Cert. Family Plann. JCC 1985; T(GP) 1991. Asst. GP Basingstoke; Community Med. Off. (Family Plann.) Loddon Trust Basingstoke. Specialty: Gen. Pract.

PATTERSON, Gordon Joseph 2A Grey Point, Helen's Bay, Bangor BT19 1LE — MB BCh BAO Belf. 1979; MRCGP 1983; AFOM RCP Lond. 1992. Med. Off. Civil Serv. Occupat. Health Serv. Specialty: Civil Serv.; Occupat. Health. Socs: Soc. Occupat. Med. Prev: GP Co. Fermanagh; GP Bournemouth.

PATTERSON, Helen 4 Hartington Road, North Shields NE30 3SA — BM BCh Oxf. 1986; MRCP (UK) 1989. CRC Clin. Research Fell. Inst. Cancer Research Sutton. Specialty: Gen. Med.

PATTERSON, Jacoby Vivien Mary 42 Springfield Road, Windsor SL4 3PQ — MB BChir Camb. 1988; MA Camb. 1989; MFPHM 1995; MD 2002. Research Cons. Specialty: Pub. Health Med. Prev: Sen. Regist. (Pub. Health Med.) Oxf. HA.; Regist. (Pub. Health Med.) Berks. HA; SHO (Radiother.) Roy. Berks. Hosp. Reading.

PATTERSON, James Alexander 95 Cinderhill Lane, Scholar Green, Stoke-on-Trent ST7 3HR — MB ChB Dundee 1984. Prev: Trainee GP Pathhead Midlothian; SHO (O & G) East. Gen. Hosp. Edin.; SHO (Paediat.) Falkirk & Dist. Roy. Infirm.

PATTERSON, James Fleming (retired) Heron's Hill, Cherry Lane, Great Bridgeford, Stafford ST18 9SL Tel: 01785 282749 — MB ChB Glas. 1946 (Univ. Glas.) DCH Eng. 1956. Assoc. Specialist Paediat. Stafford Dist. Gen. Hosp. Prev: ass specialist paediat Stafford Gen. Hosp.

PATTERSON, Janet Allison Littlemore Hospital, Sandford Road, Oxford OX4 4XN Tel: 01865 455805 Fax: 01865 455805 — MB ChB Manch. 1984; MRCPsych 1991. Cons. (Psychiat.) Oxf. Ment. Health Care NHS Trust. Specialty: Gen. Psychiat. Socs: Roy. Coll. Psychiat. Prev: Sen. Regist. (Gen. Psychiat.) Oxf. & Anglia RHA; Sen. Regist. & Regist. (Psychiat.) N. W. RHA; Staff (Psychiat.) N. Mersey Community Trust.

PATTERSON, Joan Elizabeth 18 Braehead Terrace, Milltimber AB13 0ED — MB ChB Aberd. 1990.

PATTERSON, John Kenneth 19 Glennor Crescent, Carryduff, Belfast BT8 8HW — BChir Camb. 1996.

PATTERSON, John Lonsdale (retired) 8 Blackshaw Drive, Westbrook, Warrington WA5 8XT Tel: 01925 264599 — MB ChB Glas. 1948 (Univ. Glas.) DPH Liverp. 1954. Prev: Div. MOH Runcorn.

PATTERSON, John Simon Zeneca Pharmaceuticals, Alderley House, Alderley Park, Macclesfield SK10 4TF Tel: 01625 582828; Park End, Bradford Lane, Nether Alderley, Macclesfield SK10 4TR — MB ChB Manch. 1971; FFPM RCP (UK) 1990; FRCP 1997. Territorial Business Dir. Zeneca Pharmaceut. Macclesfield. Specialty: Pharmaceutical Medicine. Prev: Internat. Med. Dir. Zeneca Phamaceut. Macclesfield; Vice Pres. Clin. & Med. Affairs ICI Americas Wilmington Del., USA; Head of Med. Research Dept. ICI Pharmaceut. Div. Macclesfield.

PATTERSON, Julie Anne Wilsden Medical Practice, Health Centre, Townfield, Wilsden, Bradford BD15 0HT Tel: 01535 273227 Fax: 01535 274860 — MB ChB Leeds 1990; DRCOG 1992. Specialty: Gen. Pract.

PATTERSON, Keith Graham Department of Haematology, University College Hospital, Gower St., London WC1E 6AU — MB BS Lond. 1972; MRCS Eng. LRCP Lond. 1972; MRCP (UK) 1976; FRCPath 1995, M 1979; FRCP Lond. 1995. Cons. Haemat. Univ. Coll. Hosp. Lond. Specialty: Haematology. Prev: Sen. Lect. & Hon. Cons. Haemat. Middlx. Hosp. Lond. & Univ. Coll Hosp. Lond.

PATTERSON, Laura Claire — MB ChB Bristol 1994; DCH 1996; DFFP 1997; MRCGP 1998. Locum GP. Specialty: Gen. Pract.

PATTERSON, Linda Joyce, OBE Commission for Health Improvement, Finsbury Tower, 103-5 Bunhill Row, London EC1Y 8TG Tel: 020 7448 9263 Email: linda.patterson@chi.nhs.uk; Knott Hall, Charlestown, Hebden Bridge HX7 6PE Tel: 01422 845390 Email: l.patterson@zen.co.uk — MB BS Lond. 1975 (London) MRCP (UK) 1979; FRCP Ed. 1991; FRCP Lond. 1993. p/t Med. Director Commiss. for Health Improvement; Clin. Lect. Univ. Manch. Specialty: Gen. Med.; Care of the Elderly. Special Interest: Med. leadership; Quality improvement in healthcare. Socs: British Geriatrics Society; British Association of Medical Managers; Royal Society of Medicine. Prev: Cons. Phys. (Gen. and Geriat. Med.), Burnley Health Care NHS Trust; Asst. Prof. Univ. Sashatchewan, Canada; Sen. Regist. (Gen. & Geriat. Med.) Univ. Hosp. S. Manch.

PATTERSON, Lindsey Jane 7 Holbeck Avenue, Healey, Rochdale OL12 6DN — MB ChB Leeds 1990; FRCA 1996. Regist. Rotat. (Anaesth.) Cardiff. Specialty: Anaesth. Prev: SHO (Paediat.) St Mary's Hosp. Lond.; SHO (Anaesth.) Bradford Hosps. NHS Trust.

PATTERSON, Malcolm David Torrington Health Centre, New Road, Torrington EX38 8EL Tel: 01805 622247 Fax: 01805 625083 — MB BS Lond. 1980; DA Eng. 1983; MRCGP 1987.

PATTERSON, Mr Marc Henry Princess Royal Hospital, Lewes Road, Haywards Heath RH16 4EX Tel: 01444 441881; Ladywell, Black Hill, Haywards Heath RH16 2HE Tel: 01444 483097 — MB BS Lond. 1977 (King's Coll.) Associate King's College 1977; FRCS Eng. 1981. Cons. Trauma & Orthop. Surg. Princess Roy. Hosp. Haywards Heath; Examr., Roy. Coll. of Surg.s of Eng. Specialty:

Orthop. Socs: Fell. BOA; S.I.C.O.T.; Expert Witness Inst. Prev: Sen. Regist. (Orthop.) St. Mary's Hosp. Lond.; Microsurg. Research Fell. Univ. Singapore; Regist. (Orthop.) St. Geo. Hosp. Lond.

PATTERSON, Marion Ruth 6 Parkwood, Lisburn BT27 4EE — MB BCh BAO Belf. 1939. Prev: Cas. Off. Altnagelvin Hosp.; Res. Med. Off. Musgrave Clinic Belf; GP Asst. Cas. Off. Ulster Hosp. Dundonald.

PATTERSON, Mark Jonathan Lister Department of Haematology, Leighton Hospital, Crewe CW1 4QJ Tel: 01270 612345 Fax: 01270 250639 Email: mark.patterson@mcht.nhs.uk; Wolverton Manor, Shorwell, Newport PO30 3JS Tel: 01983 740609 Fax: 01983 740977 Email: markl.patterson@btinternet.com — MB BS Lond 1959 (St Barts) MB BS Lond. 1959; MRCS Eng. LRCP Lond. 1959; MRCP (UK) 1963. Cons. Haemat. Leighton Hosp. Crewe & Hon. Cons. (Haematol.) Manch. Roy. Infirm. Specialty: Haematology.

PATTERSON, Mark Simon 43 Ware Road, Hoddesdon EN11 9AB — MB BS Lond. 1991.

PATTERSON, Michael Campbell (retired) 44 Gipsy Lane, Earley, Reading RG6 7HD Tel: 01189 264141 Email: emanvee@fish.co.uk — (Middlx.) MB BS Lond. 1958; DRCOG 1962; DTM & H Eng. 1968. Director of Health Progr. of the African Ch., Argentine Chaco, Argentina. Prev: SHO (Med.) Ipswich & E. Suff. Hosp.

PATTERSON, Paul Robindra Nath 92 Leechmere Road, Sunderland SR2 9NF — MB BS Lond. 1994.

PATTERSON, Rebekah Dean Pool House Cottage, Ellerton, Newport TF10 8AW — MB ChB Manch. 1986. Trainee GP Stafford VTS; Clin. Asst. (Psychogeriat.) St. Geo. Hosp. Stafford. Specialty: Geriat. Psychiat.

PATTERSON, Robert Charles Elan Medical Services Ltd, The Davenhill Centre, Parkhaven Trust, Liverpool Road South, Maghull, Liverpool L31 8BL; 44 Granville Park, Aughton, Ormskirk L39 5DU — MB ChB Liverp. 1986.

PATTERSON, Robert Neil 91 Tadworth, Bangor BT19 7WG Tel: 01247 464601 — MB BCh BAO Belf. 1996.

PATTERSON, Ronald Springburn Health Centre, 200 Springburn Way, Glasgow G21 1TR Tel: 0141 531 9660 Fax: 0141 531 9666 — MB ChB Glas. 1965. Specialty: Gen. Pract. Prev: SHO (Gen. Surg. & Urol.) & Ho. Off. (Gen. Surg.) Vict. Infirm. Glas.; Ho. Phys. Stobhill Hosp. Glas.

PATTERSON, Samuel Clive Alexander 14 Richmond Av., Lisburn BT28 2DL — MB BCh BAO Belf. 1991.

PATTERSON, Stephen — MB ChB Leeds 1989.

PATTERSON, Sybil Margaret (retired) 36 Meadow Lane, Beadnell, Chathill NE67 5AJ Tel: 01665 720769 — MB BS Durh. 1943 (Newc.) Prev: Med. Off. Dept. Health & Social Security.

PATTERSON, Mr Thomas John Starling (retired) 80 St Bernard's Road, Oxford OX2 6EJ Tel: 01865 553892 — (Camb. & St. Thos.) MRCS Eng. LRCP Lond. 1944; MD Camb. 1960, MChir 1967, MA, MB BChir 1945; FRCS Eng. 1951; DM Oxf. 1965. Prev: Clin. Lect. in Plastic Surg. Univ. Oxf.

PATTERSON, Victor Howard 58 Lisnabreeny Road E., Belfast BT6 9SS — MB BChir Camb. 1973; MRCP (UK) 1974; FRCP Lond. 1990. Cons. Neurol. Roy. Vict. Hosp. Belf. Specialty: Neurol. Prev: MDA Clin. Fell. Washington Univ. Sch. Med., USA; Sheldon Clin. Research Fell. & Regist. (Neurol.) N. Staffs. Hosp. Centre Stoke-on-Trent.

PATTERSON, William James Lothian NHS Board, Deaconess House, 148 Pleasance, Edinburgh EH8 9RS Tel: 0131 536 9186 Fax: 0131 536 9164 — MB BCh BAO Belf. 1983; DGM RCP Lond. 1986; DCH Dub. 1986; DRCOG 1986; MRCGP 1987; MPH 1989; MFPHM RCP (UK) 1992; FFPHM RCP (UK) 1998. Cons. Pub. Health Med. N. Yorks. HA. Specialty: Pub. Health Med.

PATTERSON, William Michael Potter Sherwood, Hengist Road, Westgate, Margate Tel: 01843 32175 — MRCS Eng. LRCP Lond. 1961 (Guy's) MB Camb. 1962, BChir 1961; FRCOG 1979, M 1966, DObst 1963. Cons. Gyn. & Obst. Canterbury & I. of Thanet Gps. Hosps. Specialty: Obst. & Gyn. Socs: Fell. Roy. Soc. Med. Prev: Sen. Regist. (O & G) Guy's Hosp. Lond.; Resid. Med. Off. Qu. Charlotte's Matern. Hosp. Lond.; Regist. (O & G) Addenbrookes Hosp. Camb.

PATTERSON, William Rodney Maurice 44 Knockdarragh Park, Lisburn BT28 2XZ — MB BCh BAO Belf. 1996.

PATTINSON, Brian Pattinson Clinic, The Forge, 37 Red Lion St., Richmond TW9 1RJ Tel: 020 8332 6184 Fax: 020 8332 0424; East Sheen, London SW14 8BE Tel: 020 8878 5611 — Dip Med Ac; MB BS Durh. 1962; LRCP LRCS Ed. LRCPS Glas. 1964; MLCOM 1973; DObst RCOG 1973; DMS Med. Soc. Apoth. Lond. 1994. Specialist in Musculo-Skeletal Med. Pattinson Clinic, Richmond-upon-Thames.

PATTINSON, Catherine Pamela Central Clinic, Victoria Place, Carlisle CA1 1HP; Linden House, Plumpton, Penrith CA11 9PA — MB BS Newc. 1978. Staff Grade Community Paediat. Eden Valley Primary Care Trust. Specialty: Community Child Health. Prev: Clin. Med. Off. E. Cumbria HA.

PATTINSON, Christopher John 16 Woodcote Park Road, Epsom KT18 7EX Tel: 01372 812985 — MB BChir Camb. 1954 (Guy's) MA, MB Camb. 1954, BChir 1953; DPM Eng. 1963; MRCPsych 1971. Cons. Psychiat. Private Pract. Specialty: Gen. Psychiat. Socs: Brit. Soc. Med. & Dent. Hypn. Metrop. & S. (Gen. Comm. Mem.). Prev: Cons. Psychiat. W. Lambeth HA; Ho. Off. Guy's Hosp.; SHO Guy's-Maudsley Neurosurg. Unit Lond.

PATTINSON, Jonathan Kyle Larch Corner, Ballinger Road, South Heath, Great Missenden HP16 9QJ — MB BS Lond. 1981.

PATTINSON, Kyle Thomas Shane Ridgens Farm, Mynthurst, Leigh, Reigate RH2 8RJ — BM Soton. 1993.

PATTINSON, Maureen Frances (retired) Azes Cottage, Atherington, Umberleigh EX37 9HY Tel: 01769 60730 — LRCP LRCS Ed. 1951 (Roy. Colls. Ed.) LRCP LRCS Ed. LRFPS Glas. 1951. JP. Prev: Squadron Ldr. RAF Med. Br.

PATTISON, Mr Andrew 77 London Road, Shrewsbury SY2 6PQ Tel: 01743 366230 — MB ChB Birm. 1972; BSc Birm. 1969, MB ChB 1972; FRCS Eng. 1977; MRCGP 1982.

PATTISON, Andrew Christopher 16 Newton Drive, Wakefield WF1 3HZ — MB ChB Leeds 1993.

PATTISON, Mr Charles William 42 Wimpole Street, London W1G 8YF Tel: 020 7486 7416 Fax: 020 7487 2569 — MB ChB Birm. 1980; FRCS Eng. 1984; FRCS Ed. 1984. Clin. Lect. (Cardiac Surg.) Nat. Heart & Lung Inst. Lond.; Fell. & Mem. Scientif. Counc. Internat. Coll. Angiol. NY. Specialty: Cardiothoracic Surg. Socs: Brit. Cardiac Soc.; Soc. Cardiothoracic Surgs.; Amer. Assn. Thoracic Surg. Prev: Cons. Cardiothoracic Surg. Univ. Coll. Hosps. Lond.; Sen. Regist. (Cariothoracic Surg.) Nat. Heart & Chest Hosp.; Regist. (Cardiothoracic Surg.) Harefield Hosp. & St. Thos. Hosp. Lond.

PATTISON, Denise Carol Belvedere Medical Centre, 15 Albert Road, Belvedere DA17 5LP Tel: 01322 446700; 65 Whitworth Road, Woolwich, London SE18 3QG Tel: 020 8854 8520 — MB BS Lond. 1987 (King's College Medical School London) GP. Specialty: Gen. Pract. Prev: Trainee GP Lond. VTS.

PATTISON, Mr Giles Thomas Ridley Department of Orthopaedics & Trauma, Yeovil District Hospital, Higher Kingston, Yeovil BA21 4AT Tel: 01935 75122; Farndon Thatch, Puckington, Ilminster TA19 9JA Tel: 01460 57392 — MB BS Lond. 1991; FRCS Ed 1996. Specialist Regist., Trauma & Orthop. Bristol & S.W. Rotat. Specialty: Trauma & Orthop. Surg. Socs: BOTA. Prev: SHO (Orthop.) Southmead Hosp.; SHO (Orthop.) Taunton & Som. Hosp.; SHO (Orthop.) Frenchay Hosp. Bristol.

PATTISON, Helen Fiona Rose Holding, Latteridge Road, Iron Acton, Bristol BS37 9TW — MB ChB Birm. 1985.

PATTISON, Ian 86 Horsley Hill Road, South Shields NE33 3EP — MB BS Newc. 1996.

PATTISON, James Michael Guy's Hospital, Renal Unit, 6th Floor, New Guy's House, St Thomas Street, London SE1 9RT Tel: 020 7188 5663 Fax: 020 7188 5692 Email: james.pattison@gstt.sthames.nhs.uk — BM BCh Oxf. 1987; BA Oxf. 1984; MRCP (UK) 1990; DM Oxf. 1996; FRCP 2000. Cons. Nephrol. Renal Unit Guys' Hosp. Lond. Specialty: Nephrol. Socs: Renal Assn.; Brit. Transpl. Soc. Prev: Sen. Regist. & Regist. (Renal) Guy's Hosp. Lond.; Research Fell. Stanford Univ. Calif., USA; SHO Brompton & Hammersmith Hosps. Lond.

PATTISON, Jill 57 Esmond Road, London W4 1JG — MB BS Lond. 1983; DA (UK) 1985; FFA RCS Eng. 1988. Cons. Anaesth. & ITU Heatherwood Hosp. Ascot & Wexham Pk. Hosp. Specialty: Anaesth. Socs: Roy. Soc. Med. & Intens. Care Soc. Prev: Sen. Regist. (Anaesth.) Westm. & Char. Cross Hosp. Lond.; Regist. (Anaesth.) St. Mary's Hosp. Lond.; SHO (Anaesth. & ITU) Middlx. Hosp. Lond.

PATTISON, Professor Sir John Ridley Director of Research & Development, Department of Health, Richmond House, 79 Whitehall, London SW1A 2NS Tel: 020 7210 5556 Fax: 020 7210 5868 Email: john.pattison@doh.gsi.gov.uk — (Oxf. Univ. & Middx. Hosp. Med. Sch.) BM BCh Oxf. 1968; FRCPath 1989, M 1975; BA

Oxf. 1964, BSc 1967, DM 1975; F.Med.Sci. 1998. Dir.Research & Developm., Dept. of Health; Prof. Med. Microbiol. UCL (on secondment to Dept. of Health); Hon. Cons. UCL Hosps. NHS Trust. Specialty: Virology. Prev: Prof. Med. Microbiol. King's Coll. Hosp. Med. Sch. Lond.; Hon. Cons. Camberwell HA.

PATTISON, Philip Brian HM Prison Service HQ, Cleland House, Page St., London SW1P 4LN — MB BS Lond. 1961; MRCS Eng. LRCP Lond. 1960; DRCOG 1962. Health Care Adviser Directorate of Operats. (N.) Prison Serv. HQ.

PATTISON, Roderick Brown Muiredge Surgery, Merlin Crescent, Buckhaven, Leven KY8 1HJ Tel: 01592 713299 Fax: 01592 715728; 71 Alexandra Street, Kirkcaldy KY1 1HH Tel: 01592 200474 — MB ChB Aberd. 1989; MRCGP 1995; DFFP 1995; DRCOG 1995. Trainee GP/SHO (Geriat.) Vict. Hosp. Kirkcaldy. Socs: BMA. Prev: SHO (Psychiat.) Vict. Hosp. Kirkcaldy; Trainee GP Glenrothes; SHO (Clin. Path.) Nat. Hosp. Neurol. & Neurosurg.

PATTISON, Sophie Harriet Ground Floor Flat, 21 Trelawney Rd, Bristol BS6 6DX — MB ChB Bristol 1997.

PATTISSON, Mr Patrick Henry (retired) Chesterfield, 32 Broad Lane, Hampton TW12 3AZ Tel: 020 8979 5409 — MB BS Lond. 1957 (St. Geo.) FRCS Ed. 1966; FRCS Eng. 1967. Prev: Cons. Surg. W. Middlx. Univ. Hosp. Isleworth.

PATTISSON, Peter Richard Merriman, OBE (retired) Waterfield House Surgery, 186 Henwood Green Road, Pembury, Tunbridge Wells TN2 4LR Tel: 01892 825488; Russets Woodlands, Pembury, Tunbridge Wells TN2 4AZ Tel: 01892 824872 — (St Georges Lond) MB Camb. 1964, BChir 1963. Prev: Med. Off. Save The Childr. Fund Masan, Korea.

PATTMAN, Mary Geraldine Denton Park Medical Group, Denton Park Centre, West Denton Way, Newcastle upon Tyne NE5 2QZ Tel: 0191 267 2751 Fax: 0191 264 1588; Balnakeil, 9 Westfield, Gosforth, Newcastle upon Tyne NE3 4YE Tel: 0191 285 3049 — MB ChB Glas. 1973; DObst RCOG 1975; DFFP 1994; Dip. Ther. Newc. 1995. Specialty: Gen. Pract.

PATTNI, Bhikhu Ladhabhai The Surgery, 1222 Coventry Road, Hay Mills, Birmingham B25 8BY Tel: 0121 772 1898 Fax: 0121 608 1222 — MB ChB Nairobi 1979; LMSSA 1984; DRCOG 1989.

PATTNI, Tejal Ashvin 15 Glebe Road, London N3 2BA — MB BS Lond. 1998.

PATTON, Alexandra Park Road Surgery, 37 Park Road, Teddington TW11 0AU Tel: 020 8977 5481 — MB BChir Camb. 1993 (Cambridge University) DCH 1995; DRCOG 1996; MRCGP 1997. GP Partner. Specialty: Gen. Pract.

PATTON, David Thomas Carrick Brae, 146 Gilford Road, Portadown, Craigavon BT63 5LD — MB BCh BAO Belf. 1946.

PATTON, Mr David William, TD Penmaen Cottage, Penmaen, Swansea SA3 2HH Tel: 01792 371607 Fax: 01792 371605 Email: dwpatton@btinternet.com — (Guy's) BDS Dundee 1969; FDS RCS Eng. 1975; FDS RCPS Glas. 1975; MB BS Lond. 1980; FRCS Ed. 1985. Cons. Maxillofacial Surg. Morriston Hosp. Swansea; Hon. Sen. Lect. (Maxillofacial Surg.) Sch. Postgrad. Studies in Med. & Healthcare Swansea; Hon. Civil. Cons. Oral & Maxillofacial Surg. to the Army. Specialty: Oral & Maxillofacial Surg. Socs: Fell. Brit. Assn. Oral & Maxillofacial Surg.; BMA; British Dental Assoc. Prev: Sen. Regist. (Maxillofacial Surg.) Canniesburn Hosp. Glas.

PATTON, Hugh Fergus 4 The Dell, Fulbeck, Morpeth NE61 3JY Tel: 01670 515782 Fax: 01670 515782 Email: hf.mpatton@talk21.com — MB BCh BAO Dub. 1974 (TC Dub.) MA Dub. 1977, BA, MB BCh BAO 1974; MICGP 1984. Forens. Med. Examr. Northumbria Police. Prev: Capt. RAMC; Ho. Off. Roy. City of Dub. Hosp.; GP.

PATTON, Hugh Henry Terence 39 Dromore Road, Hillsborough BT26 6HU — MB BCh BAO Belf. 1981; MB BCh Belf. 1981.

PATTON, John Terence, RD 23 Anson Road, Victoria Park, Manchester M14 5BZ Tel: 0161 224 0006; Fallows Hall, Chelford, Macclesfield SK10 4SZ Tel: 01625 861252 — MRCS Eng. LRCP Lond. 1951 (Liverp.) DMRD Eng. 1959; FFR 1963; FRCR 1975; Hon. FRCP Ed. 1984. Hon. Cons. Manch. Roy. Infirm.; Hon. Lect. (Radiol.) Univ. Manch.; Chairm. Armed Servs. Cons. Approval Bd. (Radiol.). Specialty: Radiol. Socs: Fell. Manch. Med. Soc. Prev: Cons. Radiol. to RN; Cons. i/c (Radiol.) Manch. Roy. Infirm.; Ed. Brit. Jl. Radiol.

PATTON, Lara 23 Rosepark, Belfast BT5 7RG — MB BCh BAO Belf. 1993.

PATTON, Margaret 146 Gilford Road, Portadown, Craigavon BT63 5LD — MB BS Lond. 1949.

PATTON, Melanie Kay West Bar Surgery, 1 West Bar Street, Banbury OX16 9SF Tel: 01295 256261 Fax: 01295 756848; Oakleigh, Weeping Cross, Bodicote, Banbury OX15 4ED — MB ChB Sheff. 1984; DTM & H Liverp. 1988; MRCGP 1989.

PATTON, Professor Michael Alexander St. Georges Hospital Medical School, Cranmer Terrace, London SW17 0RE Tel: 020 8725 5335 Fax: 020 8725 3444 — MB ChB Ed. 1974; MA Camb. 1975; MSc (Human Genetics) Ed. 1976; DCH Eng. 1977; MRCP (UK) 1979; FRCP Lond. 1993; FRCPCH 1997. Cons. & Prof. (Med. Genetics) St. Geo. Hosp. Med. Sch. Lond.; Med. Dir. Birth Defects Foundat.; Cons. Clin. Geneticist TDL Genetics; Pres., Med. Genetics, Roy. Soc. of Med. Specialty: Genetics. Socs: Fell. Roy. Soc. Med.; Brit Soc human genetics; Expert Witness Inst. Prev: Chairm. Ethics Comm. RCPCH 2002-04; Insp. Human Fertilization & Embryol. Auth.; Pres. Jenner Soc. 1997-1998.

PATTON, Michael Sean 7 Dukes Lane, Ballykelly, Limavady BT49 9JT — MB ChB Aberd. 1997.

PATTON, Michelle The Village Surgery, Dudley Lane, Cramlington NE23 6US Tel: 01670 712821; 4 The Dell, Fulbeck, Morpeth NE61 3JY Tel: 01670 515782 Fax: 01670 515782 — MB BS Lond. 1989. Priciple Gen. Practioner; Clin. Asst. (Psychogerat.), St Geo. Hosp.,Morpeth.; Dep. (Forens. Med. Examr.), Northumbria Police. Specialty: Gen. Pract.; Geriat. Psychiat. Socs: MRCQP; Assoc.s of Police Surg.s.

PATTON, Niall 6 Rossbay, Waterside, Londonderry BT47 6JF — MB ChB Manch. 1996. SHO (Opthal.) Roy. Eye Hosp. Manch. Specialty: Ophth.

PATTON, Nicholas David The Surgery, 9 Albion Street, Brighton BN2 9PS Tel: 01273 601122/601344/01322 428100 Ext: 8221 — MB BS Lond. 1979; DRCOG 1984; MRCGP 1989.

PATTON, Stephen Nadim 90 Lisnafin Park, Strabane BT82 9DH — MB BCh Belf. 1996 (Queen's University Belfast) DRCOG. SHO (Psychiat.) Mater Hosp. Belf. Specialty: Gen. Pract. Prev: A & E; O & G.

PATTON, William Collim 23 Rosepark, Dundonald, Belfast BT5 7RG — MB BCh BAO Belf. 1966 (Qu. Univ. Belf.) BSc (Hons.) Belf. 1963, MB BCh BAO 1966; FRCPsych 1974. Cons. Psychiat. Downsh. Hosp. Downpatrick. Specialty: Gen. Psychiat.

PATTOO, Bashir Ahmad Bollington Road Surgery, 126 Bollington Road, Ancoats, Manchester M40 7HD Tel: 0161 205 2979 Fax: 0161 205 6368 — MB BS Kashmir 1974.

PATTRICK, Martin Graham 83 Barkers Lane, Sale M33 6SH — MB ChB Bristol 1981; BSc (Cellular Path.) Bristol 1978, MB ChB 1981; MCRP (UK) 1983. Clin. Research Fell. & Hon. Regist. (Rheumat.) Nottm. HA; Cons. in Acute Med. and Rheum. Special Interest: Chronic Fatigue, Lupus, Fibromyalgia. Socs: Brit. Soc. Rheumat. Prev: SHO (Med.) & Regist. N. Staffs. HA; Ho. Off. Bristol & Weston HA.

PATUCK, David Fram Summervale Medical Centre, Wharf Lane, Ilminster TA19 0DT Tel: 01460 52354 Email: david.patuck@summervaleilm.nhs.uk; Chatsworth, Broadway Road, Broadway, Ilminster TA19 9RX Tel: 01460 52088 Email: david@patucks.co.uk — MB BS Lond. 1975; MRCS Eng. LRCP Lond. 1974; DRCOG 1980. Specialty: Gen. Pract. Prev: Med. Off. Brit. Antarctic Survey.

PATUCK, Dina Rowantree House, Robinson Lane, Woodmancote, Cirencester GL7 7EN Tel: 01285 831700 — MB BS Lond. 1950 (Roy. Free) MRCS Eng. LRCP Lond. 1949; DCH Eng. 1952; DObst RCOG 1954. Regist. (Paediat.) King Edwd. VII Hosp. Windsor. Specialty: Paediat. Prev: Ho. Phys. Roy. Free Hosp.; Ho. Surg. (O & G) Canad. Red Cross Memor. Hosp. Taplow.

PATUCK, Fram (retired) Rowantree House, Robinson Lane, Woodmancote, Cirencester GL7 7EN Tel: 01285 831700 — MRCS Eng. LRCP Lond. 1946 (St. Bart.) FRCGP 1989, M 1977; Assoc. Fac. Occupat. Med. RCP Lond. 1980. Prev: Surg. S. Div. Metrop. Police.

PATUCK, Julie Frances North Street Surgery, 22 North Street, Ilminster TA19 0DG Tel: 01460 52284; Chatsworth, Broadway Road, Broadway, Ilminster TA19 9RX Tel: 01460 52088 — MB ChB Liverp. 1977; DRCOG 1980; MRCGP 1981. Specialty: Gen. Pract.

PATWALA, D Y Church Road Medical Centre, 64 Church Road, Bebington, Wirral CH63 3EY — MB BS 1972 (Topiwala National Medical School) DGO, DFP.

PATWARDHAN, Kiran 1 West Kensington Court, Edith Villas, London W14 9AA — MB BS Nagpur 1986; MRCP (UK) 1994.

PAUFFLEY, John Hamilton (retired) Pengymill, Chignal St James, Chelmsford CM1 4TZ Tel: 01245 440515 — MRCS Eng. LRCP Lond. 1949 (Lond. Hosp.) DObst RCOG 1954. Prev: Ho. Phys. Poplar Hosp.

PAUL, Mr Alan Burnett Pyrah Department of Urology, St James' Univ.Hosp., Beckett St., Leeds LSG 7TF Tel: 0113 206 4949 Email: alan.paul@leedsth.nhs.uk — MB ChB Ed. 1985 (Edinburgh) FRCS Ed. 1990; FRCS Ed (Urol.) 1998; MD (Edin.) 1999. Cons. Urological Surg., St James, Leeds. Specialty: Urol. Socs: BMA; Assoc. Mem. BAUS. Prev: Clin. Research Fell. Nuffield Transpl. Unit West. Gen. Hosp. Edin.; Sen. Regist. Withington Hosp. Manch.

PAUL, Amal Chandra 4 Bayswater Row, Leeds LS8 5LH — MB ChB Leeds 1994.

PAUL, Anindita 40 Alton Road, Birmingham B29 7DU — MB ChB Birm. 1992.

PAUL, Mr Ashok Samuel 9 Tilby Close, Urmston, Manchester M41 6JN — MB BS Madras 1983; FRCS Ed. 1987.

PAUL, Beverley Bassetlaw Hospital, Kilton, Worksop S81 0BD Tel: 01909 500990 Fax: 01909 502462 Email: beverley.paul@nhs.net; Stonebeck, Low St, Carlton in Lindrick, Worksop S81 9EJ Tel: 01909 730284 Email: bevpaul@lineone.net — MB BS Lond. 1973 (Univ. Lond.) MRCS Eng. LRCP Lond. 1973; FRCPath 1995, M 1983; T(Path.) 1991. Cons. Haemat.Doncaster & Bassetlaw Hosps. NHS Trust. Specialty: Haematology. Socs: Brit. Soc. Haematol.; Brit. Blood Transfus. Soc.; Eur. Haematol. Assn. Prev: Lect. (Haemat.) Univ. Zimbabwe; Sen. Regist. (Haemat.) North. RHA.

PAUL, Carolyn Ann 167 Moss Lane, Bramhall, Stockport SK7 1BG — MB ChB Manch. 1994.

PAUL, Carolyn Patricia 5A Gerrard Road, London N1 8AY — MB BS Lond. 1988; MRCOG 1994. Specialty: Obst. & Gyn.

PAUL, Clive Conrad The Old Rectory Surgery, 18 Castle Street, Saffron Walden CB10 1BP Tel: 01799 522327 Fax: 01799 525436 — MB BS Lond. 1980 (Guys) BSc Lond. 1976; MRCS Eng. LRCP Lond. 1979; DRCOG 1988; MRCGP 1988. Specialty: Gen. Pract.

PAUL, David Hendrie Greencroft Medical Centre (South), Greencroft Wynd, Annan DG12 6GS Tel: 01461 202244 Fax: 01461 205401; 63 Hecklegirth, Annan DG12 6HL — MB ChB St. And. 1971; DObst RCOG 1973; MRCGP 1983. Socs: BMA. Prev: Gen. Med. Off. Nchanga Consolidated Copper Mines Hosp. Kitwe, Zambia; SHO (Paediat.) Perth Roy. Infirm.; SHO (O & G) West. Gen. Hosp. Edin.

PAUL, Derek Lindsay 28 Birkdale Crescent, Dullatur, Glasgow G68 0JZ Tel: 0141 722078 — MB ChB Ed. 1980; FRCA 1986. Cons. Cardiothoracic Anaesth. Roy. Infirm. Glas. Specialty: Anaesth. Socs: Assn. Anaesth. Prev: Sen. Regist. (Anaesth.) West. Infirm. Glas.; Astra Research Fell. (Anaesth.) Roy. Infirm. Edin.

PAUL, Eric Andre Albert Salisbury Road Surgery, 1 Salisbury Road, Seven Kings, Ilford IG3 8BG Tel: 020 8597 0924 Fax: 020 8598 8254 — Artsexamen Amsterdam 1986; T(GP) 1992. Specialty: Gen. Pract.

PAUL, Euan Hector Menzies 12 Market Street, Chipping Norton OX7 5NQ Tel: 01608 645566 Fax: 01608 645300 Email: cosic@btinternet.com — MB BS Lond. 1960 (St. Thos.) DObst RCOG 1962; FFOM RCPI 1984; FFOM RCP Lond. 1996. Scientif. Adviser COSIC; Cons. Occupat. Health & Safety Oxon. Specialty: Occupat. Health. Socs: Fell. Roy. Soc. Med.; SOM; BMA. Prev: Dir. Health, Safety & Risk Managem. Europe; Ho. Phys. & Ho. Surg. Kent & Canterbury Hosp.; Ho. Surg. (Obst.) St. Mary's Matern. Hosp. W. Croydon.

PAUL, Gideon Andrew 23c Lyme Street, London NW1 0EE — MB BS Lond. 1998; MRCP UK 2001.

PAUL, Hans-Joerg Health Centre, East St., Thame OX9 3JZ; 14 Onslow Drive, Thame OX9 3YX — State Exam Med Freiburg 1990; State Exam Med. Freiburg 1990; MD Freiburg 1990; MRCP (UK) 1993; DRCOG 1997. GP Regist. Thame VTS. Specialty: Gen. Pract. Prev: Sen. Regist. (Radiol.) West. Infirm. Glas.; SHO (Gen. Med.) Roy. Alexandra Hosp. Paisley.

PAUL, Heather Elizabeth (retired) 63 Hecklegirth, Annan DG12 6HL — MB ChB Ed. 1970; DObst RCOG 1972; DCH RCPS Glas. 1972. Prev: Staff Grade (Geriat.) Dumfries & Galloway Roy. Infirm.

PAUL, Helga Judith — MB BS Lond. 1987; DRCOG 1995; Cert. Prescribed Experience. 1995. Locum GP. Specialty: Gen. Pract.; Care of the Elderly. Prev: Regist. (c/o the Elderly) Kent & Canterbury Hosp. Canterbury.; SHO (Med.) Kent & Canterbury Hosp.; SHO (A & E) Wexham Pk. Hosp. Slough.

PAUL, Henryck Marian Pawel (retired) 23 Windermere Road, Bolton Le Sands, Carnforth LA5 8LL Tel: 01524 824071 — MB BS Lond. 1964 (Westm.) MRCS Eng. LRCP Lond. 1964. Prev: Ho. Surg. (Orthop.) Qu. Mary's Hosp. Roehampton.

PAUL, Ian Robert Coniston Medical Practice, The Parade, Coniston Road, Patchway, Bristol BS34 5TF Tel: 0117 969 2508 Fax: 0117 969 0456 — MB BCh BAO Belf. 1985; DRCOG 1989; MRCGP 1992. GP, Coniston Med. Pract., Bristol.

PAUL, Israel Pep (retired) 26 Seagry Road, London E11 2NH Tel: 020 8989 0741 — (Ed.) MB ChB Ed. 1938. Prev: Ho. Surg. Roy. Infirm. Oldham.

PAUL, James Rupert 23 Vineyard Hill Road, London SW19 7JL Email: jamespaul@compuserve.com — MB BS Lond. 1994 (RFHSM London) BSc Lond. 1992; MRCP 1998. SHO (Med.). Specialty: Palliat. Med. Socs: Mem. Christian Med. Fell.ship.

PAUL, Mrs Jill Barns Street Surgery, 3 Barns Street, Ayr KA7 1XB Tel: 01292 281439 Fax: 01292 288268; 2 Inverkar Road, Ayr KA7 2JT Tel: 01292 263669 — MB ChB Glas. 1988 (Glasgow) DRCOG 1991; MRCGP 1992. GP Princip. Specialty: Gen. Pract. Prev: Trainee GP Ayr; SHO (Geriat.) Vict. Hosp. Glas.; SHO (Psychiat.) Levendale Hosp. Glas.

PAUL, John Royal Sussex County Hospital, Department of Microbiology & Infectious Diseases, Eastern Road, Brighton BN2 5BE Tel: 01273 696955 Ext: 4596 Email: john.paul@bsuh.nhs.uk; Downsflint, High Street, Upper Beeding, Steyning BN44 3WN — MB ChB Birm. 1985; FRCPath; BSc Birm. 1982; MSc Lond. 1990; MD Birm 1999. Cons. Microbiol. Brighton & Sussex Univ. Hosps. NHS Trust. Specialty: Med. Microbiol. Special Interest: Med. Entomology. Socs: Fell. Roy. Soc. Trop. Med. & Hyg. Prev: Sen. Regist. John Radcliffe Hosp. Oxf.; Microbiol. Wellcome Trust Research Laborats., Nairobi.

PAUL, Kusem 8 Sequoia Park, Pinner HA5 4BS — MB BS Lond. 1983.

PAUL, Leela Department of Psychiatry, Ashford Hospital, Ashford TW15 3AA Tel: 01784 884488; 18 Parkland Grove, Ashford TW15 2JW Tel: 01784 255540 — (Trivandrum) MB BS Kerala 1968; DRCOG 1975; DPM Eng. 1980. Assoc. Specialist (Psychiat.) Ashford Hosp. Specialty: Gen. Psychiat. Prev: SHO (O & G) Grantham & Kesteven Hosp.; SHO (Psychiat.) St. Mary's Hosp. ScarBoro.; CL. Asst. Psychiat. Ashford Hosp.

PAUL, Mark Nicholas Watersmeet House, Yarde, Williton, Taunton TA4 4HW — MB BS Lond. 1997.

PAUL, Martin Bedgrove Surgery, Brentwood Way, Aylesbury HP21 7TL Tel: 01296 330330 Fax: 01296 399179; 5 Orchard Way, Botolph Claydon, Buckingham MK18 2NG — MB BS Lond. 1971; DCH Eng. 1976; DRCOG 1977; MRCGP 1983. GP Aylesbury; Course Organiser Aylesbury VTS. Specialty: Gastroenterol. Socs: Roy. Coll. GPs. Prev: Chairm. of Aylesbury GP fundholding forum.

PAUL, Matthew Leon Henry The New Surgery, Lindo Close, Chesham HP5 2JN Tel: 01494 782262; 13 Chartridge Lane, Chesham HP5 2JJ Tel: 01494 793284 — MB BS Lond. 1990 (King's College Hospital) BSc Lond. 1985, MB BS 1990. Prev: Ho. Surg. (Cardiothoracic & Gen. Surg.) & Ho. Phys. (Oncol. & Gen. Med.) KCH Lond.

PAUL, Meenu 56 Goodman Park, Slough SL2 5NN — MB BS Lond. 1996.

PAUL, Michael General Medical Clinics PLC, 2-3 Salisbury Court, London EC4Y 8AA Tel: 020 7427 0605 Fax: 020 7427 0608 Email: michael.paul@genmed.org.uk — MB ChB Manch. 1972 (St And. & Manch.) DObst RCOG 1975; MRCGP 1977. Med. Dir. Gen. Med. Clinics. Specialty: Gen. Pract. Socs: Fell. Roy. Soc. Med. Prev: GP Sunninghill Ascot; Clin. Asst. Infertil. Clinic Heatherwood Hosp. Ascot; Med. Off. Priory Convent Ascot.

PAUL, Milena Mary (retired) 1 Greenacres, Tettenhall, Wolverhampton WV6 8SR Tel: 01902 753284 — MRCS Eng. LRCP Lond. 1976 (Masaryk Univ. Brno) DA Eng. 1972. Prev: Clin. Asst. (Anaesth.) Walsall Gen. Hosp.

PAUL, Narinder Radiology Department, Bradford Royal Infirmary, Duckworth Lane, Bradford BD9 6RJ — BM Soton. 1987; MRCP

(UK) 1991; FRCR 1994. Cons. Radiol. St. Jas. Univ. Hosp. Leeds. Specialty: Radiol. Prev: Regist. (Radiol.) Freeman Hosp. Newc.; SHO (Renal & Respirat. Med., Neurol. & A & E) Soton.

PAUL, Natasha Kamaljeet 245 Popes Lane, London W5 4NH — MB BS Lond. 1993.

PAUL, Neil Robin 21 Portland Close, Hazel Grove, Stockport SK7 5HF — MB ChB Manch. 1994.

PAUL, Nigel Croyard Road Surgery, Croyard Road, Beauly IV4 7DT Tel: 01463 782794 Fax: 01463 782111 — MB ChB Aberd. 1984. Prev: SHO (O & G) Falkirk Roy. Infirm.

PAUL, Pallipurathukaren Joseph 110 Ecclesfield Road, Eccleston, St Helens WA10 5ND — MB BS Andhra 1968 (Kakinada Med. Coll.) MRCP (UK) 1977. Cons. (Geriat. Med.) St. Helens Hosp. Specialty: Care of the Elderly. Prev: Regist. (Gen. Med.) King's Mill Hosp. Sutton-in-Ashfield.

PAUL, Mr Prasanta Kumar 72 Windmill Avenue, St Albans AL4 9SN Tel: 01727 762291 — MRCS Eng. LRCP Lond. 1987; FRCS Glas. 1995. Regist. (Trauma & Orthop. Surg.) Hemel Hempstead Gen. Hosp. Herts. Specialty: Orthop. Socs: BMA; Assn. Surg. Train. Prev: Regist. (Gen. Surg.) Milton Keynes Gen. Hosp.; Ho. Off. (Gen. Surg.) Ormskirk & Dist. Gen. Hosp.

PAUL, Raymond Thomas — MB BCh Belf. 1998.

PAUL, Rini 252 Boundary Road, Wood Green, London N22 6AJ — MB BS Lond. 1997; MRCGP; DFFP; DRCOG.

PAUL, Roger Graham The Park Surgery, 375 Chepstow Road, Newport NP19 8XR Tel: 01633 277333 Fax: 01633 279078 — MB BS Lond. 1971; MRCS Eng. LRCP Lond. 1970.

PAUL, Sheila Sarah The Misbourne Surgery, Church Lane, Chalfont St Peter, Gerrards Cross SL9 9RR Tel: 01753 891010; 40 Batchelors Way, Amersham HP7 9AJ Tel: 01494 434718 — MB ChB Manch. 1975; DRCOG 1977; ATLS 1983 & 1995; Section 12 approved 1998; DMJ 1999; DAB 2002. Police Surg. Thames Valley Police; Med. Off. Community Drug & Alcohol Team Aylesbury. Socs: Assn. Police Surg.; Fell. Roy. Soc. Med.; Brit. Acad. Forens. Sci. Prev: Gen. Phys. US Army Hosp. Frankfurt, W. Germany.

PAUL, Simon Neil Mayday Hospital, Croydon CR7 7YE — MB BS Lond. 1994 (Univ. Coll. Lond. Med. Sch.) BSc Kingston 1996; MRCP (UK) 1998. Specialty: Gen. Med.

PAUL, Mr Sudhansu Bhusan (retired) 70 Abinger Avenue, Cheam, Sutton SM2 7LW — MB BS Calcutta 1955; FRCS Eng. 1969. Prev: Assoc. Specialist (Orthop.) SW Thames Regional Auth.

PAUL, Mr Surendramohan Chandpal Hinchingbrooke Hospital, Hinchingbrooke Park, Huntingdon PE29 6NT — MRCS Eng. LRCP Lond. 1974 (Cambridge) MB Camb. 1976, BChir 1975; FRCS Ed. 1979. Staff Grade Surg., Dept. of Gen. Surg.,Hitchingbrooke Hosp., Huntingdon. Specialty: Paediat. Surg.; Cardiothoracic Surg.; Gen. Surg. Special Interest: Critical care; Liver Injuries; Oesophagal cancer. Socs: Camb. Univ. Med. Soc.; Former Edr. Sri Lanka Coll. of Surgeons; Former Counc. Mem. Sri Lanka Med. Assn. Prev: Cons. Surg. Teachg. Hosp., Ragama, Sri Lanka; Resid. Surg. Nat. Hosp. of Sri Lanka; Cons. Surg., Teachg. Hosp. Kurunegala, Sri Lanka.

PAUL CHOUDHURY, Saumitra Kumar Bell House Medical Centre, 163 Dunstable Road, Luton LU1 1BW Tel: 01582 23553; 3 Ambrose Lane, Harpenden AL5 4AU — MB BS Dacca 1975; DLO RCS Eng. 1984. Clin. Dir. GP Liaison Luton & Dunstable Hosp. NHS Trust (Exec. Bd.); Clin. Asst. (Gen. Psychiat.); Exec. Mem. of Luton Teachg.; PCT. Specialty: Gen. Psychiat.

PAULDING, Elizabeth Anne The Alton Practice, 208 Roehampton Lane, London SW15 4LE Tel: 020 8788 4844 Fax: 020 8788 4844; 8 Stuart Road, London SW19 8DH Tel: 020 8946 8495 — MB BCh BAO Dub. 1964. Socs: BMA.

PAULEAU, Anne Essex Lodge, 94 Greengate Street, Plaistow, London E13 0AS Tel: 020 8472 4888 Fax: 020 8472 5777 Email: anne.pauleau@gp-f84052.nhs.uk — MB BS Lond. 1986; MRCGP 1992; DRCOG 1993. Hon. Clin. Lect. Dept. Gen. Pract. & Primary Care Qu. Mary & Westfield Coll. Specialty: Gen. Pract. Prev: Clin. Lect Qu. Mary Westfield Coll.

PAULEAU, Nitza Francoise 56A Cleveden Drive, Glasgow G12 0NX — MB BS Lond. 1958; MRCS Eng. LRCP Lond. 1958.

PAULI, Helen Mary Triangle Cottage, Englishcombe, Bath BA2 9DU Tel: 01225 311134 — MB BChir Camb. 1990; MA Camb. 1989; DRCOG 1993; MRCGP 1995. GP Princip. Bath. Specialty: Gen. Pract. Prev: Asst. GP Bath; Trainee GP/SHO Bath HA; Ho. Off. (Surg.) Swindon HA.

PAULIN, Mary Neilson Macqueen 41D Sans Souce Park, Belfast BT9 5BZ Tel: 028 665864 — MB BCh BAO Belf. 1941 (Qu. Univ. Belf.) DPH Eng. 1946. Prev: Asst. MOH Co. Antrim.; Hon. Clin Asst. Fertil. Clinic Samarit. Hosp. Belf.; Asst. MoH Lees.

PAULLEY, Jean Susan 25 Clarksfield Street, Clarksfield, Oldham OL4 3AW — MB ChB Manch. 1968. Clin. Med. Off. Oldham HA. Specialty: Community Child Health.

PAULLEY, John Wylmer (retired) Sufolk Nuffield Hospital at Christchurch Park, 57 Fonnereau Rd, Ipswich IP1 3JN Tel: 01473 623771; Cross Keys, Stoke-by-Nayland, Colchester CO6 4QU Tel: 01206 262598 — MB BS Lond. 1940 (Middlx.) MRCS Eng. LRCP Lond. 1939; FRCP Lond. 1959, M 1941; MD Lond. 1944. Will. Edmunds' Clin. Research Fell. RCP. Prev: Cons. Phys. Ipswich Health Dist.

PAULUS, Ulrike Staff Residence, Monkland District General Hospital, Monkscourt Avenue, Airdrie ML6 0JS — State Exam Med Kiel 1992.

PAUN, Sadguna Manharlal Arcadian Gardens Surgery, 1 Arcadian Gardens, Bowes Park, London N22 5AB; 15A Eversleigh Road, New Barnet, Barnet EN5 1NE — MB BS Gujarat 1965 (B.J. Med. Coll. Ahmedabad) DGO 1967. GP Lond. Prev: Res. SHO Obst. Bearstead Hosp. Stoke Newington.

PAUN, Santdeep Harilal 4 Sudbury Court Drive, Harrow HA1 3TA — MB BS Lond. 1991. Specialty: Otolaryngol.

PAVAR, Jayashri Sreenivasarao Boundfield Medical Centre, 103 Boundfield Road, London SE6 1PG Tel: 020 8697 2920; 2 Silverdale Drive, Mottingham, London SE9 4DH Tel: 020 8851 2259 — MB BS Marathwada 1974 (Avramgabad India) DA (UK) 1978; DO RCPSI 1980. GP; Ophth. Med. Pract. Lond. Specialty: Gen. Med. Socs: Med. Protec. Soc. Prev: Regist./SHO (Ophth.) Arrowe Pk. Hosp. Wirral; SHO (Ophth.) Lister Hosp. Stevenage & Whipps Cross Hosp. Lond.; SHO (Anaesth.) St. Mary's Hosp. Lond.

PAVELEY, William Frederick (retired) Edina Cottage, Main St., Wilson, Melbourne, Derby DE73 1AD Tel: 01332 864717 — MB ChB Ed. 1952; DObst RCOG 1955.

PAVESI, Lucy Anne Proctor & Gamble (Technical Centres) Limited, Rusham Park Technical Centre, Whitehall Lane, Egham TW20 9NW Tel: 01784 474346 Fax: 01784 498787 Email: pavesi.l@pg.com — MB BChir Camb. 1991 (Camb. Univ. Roy. Free Hosp. Lond.) MFPM; MA Camb. 1992; Dip. Pharm. Med. 1997. Med. Adviser Procter & Gamble (Technical Centres) Ltd. Specialty: Pharmaceutical Medicine. Socs: Assoc. Mem., faculity of pharmaceltical Med. Prev: Clin. Research Phys. Roche Products Ltd. Welwyn Garden City; SHO (Cas.) Lister Hosp. Stevenage; SHO (Med. for Elderly) Hemel Hempstead Hosp.

PAVEY, Ina Shelagh Joan Moor Park Surgery, 49 Garstang Road, Preston PR1 1LB Tel: 01772 252077 Fax: 01772 885451; Bridge House, Knowle Green, Longridge, Preston PR3 2YN Tel: 01254 878235 — MB BS Lond. 1968 (Lond. Hosp.) Prev: Ho. Surg. & Ho. Phys. Roy. Vict. Hosp. Folkestone.

PAVEY, Kevin Michael Francis Gordon Stonebridge Surgery, Preston Road, Longridge, Preston PR3 3AP Tel: 01204 390938 Fax: 01204 390141 — MB BS Lond. 1968 (Lond. Hosp.) MRCGP 1977. Prev: SHO (O & G), SHO (Paediat.) & SHO Emerg. & Accid. Dept.; Preston Roy. Infirm.

PAVEY, Susan Kate 64 Manor Road, Barnet EN5 2LG Tel: 020 8449 1805 — MB ChB Glas. 1994; BA (Hons.) Medieval & Modern Hist. Birm. 1986. SHO (Emerg.) Roy. Perth Hosp. Perth, W. Austral. Specialty: Accid. & Emerg. Prev: Ho. Off. Dumfries & Galloway Roy. Infirm.

PAVIER, Peter Colin (retired) The Health Centre, High Street, Arnold, Nottingham NG5 7BQ Tel: 0115 926 7257 — MB BS Lond. 1960.

***PAVIOUR, Dominic Curtis** — MB BS Lond. 1998; MB BS Lond 1998.

PAVIS, Hilary Margaret Nightingale Macmillan Unit, 117a London Road, Derby DE1 2QS — BM BCh Oxf. 1982; MA Oxf. 1983; DRCOG 1991; MRCGP 1995. Specialty: Palliat. Med. Prev: SHO (Psychiat.) Fulbourn Hosp. Camb.; SHO (Gen. Med.) Roy. Sussex Co. Hosp.; Ho. Off. Nuffield (Surg.) John Radcliffe Hosp. Oxf.

PAVITT, Jane Anne Orchard Medical Practice, Orchard Street, Ipswich IP4 2PU Tel: 01473 213261 — MB BS Lond. 1976; DCH Eng. 1978.

PAVLIDIS, Sotira 12 Saundersfoot Way, Oakwood, Derby DE21 2RH — (Faculty of Medicine - University of Brussels) Dip Trop. Med. Univ. Antwerpen (Belgium) 1980; MD Brussels 1980. Specialty: Gen. Pract.; Geriat. Psychiat.

PAVLOU, Mr Criton 48 Wimpole Street, London W1G 8SF Tel: 020 7935 7886 Fax: 020 7935 7886; Manor Lodge, 37 College Road, London SE21 7BA — MB BS Lond. 1963 (Middlx.) FRCOG 1991, M 1970; FRCS Ed. 1973. Indep. O & G Lond. Specialty: Obst. & Gyn. Socs: Fell. Roy. Soc. Med.; BMA. Prev: SHO & Regist. (O & G) Hammersmith Hosp. Lond.; Hon. Sen.Lecturer(O&G) Qu. Charlotte Hosp. Lond.

PAVLOU, Philip Theoklis 23 Woodcote Close, Enfield EN3 4NZ — MB BS Lond. 1998.

PAVLOU, Stelios Chase Farm Hospital NHS Trust, The Ridgeway, Enfield EN2 8JL Tel: 020 8366 6600; 13 Bancroft Avenue, East Finchley, London N2 0AR Tel: 020 8340 0777 — Ptychio Iatrikes Athens 1976; T(Anaes.) 1994. Cons. Anaesth. Chase Farm Hosp. NHS Trust. Specialty: Anaesth. Socs: Assn. Anaesth.; Obst. Anaesth. Assn.; BMA.

PAVORD, Ian Douglas Glenfield Hospital NHS Trust, Groby Road, Leicester LE3 9QP Tel: 0116 287 1471 Fax: 0116 236 7768; 17 Maplewell Road, Woodhouse Eaves, Loughborough LE12 8RG Tel: 01509 890927 Email: ian.pavord@uhl-tr.nhs.uk — MB BS Lond. 1984 (Westm.) MRCP (UK) 1987; DM Nottm. 1992; FRCP FRCP Lond 2000. Cons. Phys. Glenfield Hosp. Leicester; Hon. Reader Univ. Leics. Specialty: Respirat. Med.; Gen. Med. Prev: Lect. & Hon. Sen. Regist. (Respirat. Med.) City Hosp. Nottm.; Clin. Fell. St. Josephs Hosp. McMaster Univ. Hamilton, Canada; Research Fell. (Respirat. Med.) City Hosp. Nottm.

PAVORD, Susannah Ruth Department of Haematology, Leicester Royal Infirmary, Leicester LE1 5WW — MB ChB Leic. 1988; MRCP (UK) 1991; MRCPath 1997; FRCP 2003. Cons. (Haemat.) & Sen. Lect. In Med. Educ. Specialty: Haematology. Socs: Brit. Soc. Homeo. & Throm.; Brit. Soc. Haematol. Prev: Clin. Fell. McMasters Univ. Hamilton, Ontario, Canada; Regist. (Haemat.) Leicester Roy. Infirm.; SHO Rotat. (Med.) Leicester Hosps.

PAVY, Corinne Rose 17 Circus, Bath BA1 2ET — BM Soton. 1994.

PAW, Henry Gee Wai 17 Mander Way, Cambridge CB1 7SF Tel: 01223 411806 — (Newc.-u-Tyne) BPharm (1st cl.) Cardiff 1984; MRPharmS 1985; MB BS Newc. 1990; DA (UK) 1992; FRCA 1994. Specialist Regist. (Anaesth.) Norf. & Norwich Hosp. Specialty: Anaesth. Prev: Regist. (Anaesth.) Addenbrooke's, Papworth & P'boro. Dist. Hosp.; Specialist Regist. (Anaesth.) Jas. Paget Hosp. Gt. Yarmouth.

PAW, Jayantilal Devji Pleck Health Centre, 16 Oxford Street, Pleck, Walsall WS2 9HY Tel: 01922 647660 Fax: 01922 629251; Jay Nivas, 123 Longwood Road, Aldridge, Walsall WS9 0TB Tel: 01922 629251 Fax: 01922 633397 — MB BS Poona 1960 (B.J. Med. Coll.) Prev: Police Surg. Walsall; Med. Off. Govt. Hosps. Uganda.; Police Surg. Uganda Govt.

PAW, Rajan Chimanlal 54 Eastlands Road, Birmingham B13 9RG — MB ChB Birm. 1997. Specialty: Anaesth.

PAWA, Chandra Mohan Fieldway Surgery, 15A Danebury, New Addington, Croydon CR0 9EU Tel: 01689 84166 Fax: 01689 800643; 7 Pampisford Road, Purley CR8 2NG Tel: 020 8660 0641 Fax: 01689 800643 — MB BS Lucknow 1965 (G.S.V.M. Med. Coll. Kanpur) MSc (Gen. Pract.) Lond. 1991. Clin. Asst. (Diabetes & Endocrinol.) St. Hellier Hosp. Carshalton. Prev: Regist. (Med.) Markfield Hosp.; SHO & Regist. (Gen. Med.) Kilton Hosp. Worksop.

PAWADE, Mr Ashwinikumar Madhukar The Red Lodge, Abbots Leigh Road, Leigh Woods, Bristol BS8 3PX Tel: 0117 973 3473 — MB BS Nagpur 1978; FRCS Ed. 1987. Cons. Paediat. (Cardiac Surg.) Roy. Bristol Hosp. for Sick Childr.; Cons. Cardiac Surg. Bristol Roy. Infirm.; Cons. & Sen. Lect. (Surg.) Univ. Bristol. Specialty: Cardiothoracic Surg. Prev: Dep. Dir. Vict.n Paediat. Cardiac Surgic. Unit Roy. Childr. Hosp. Melbourne, Austral.

PAWAR, Jo Eluned 5 Stanley Pl, Cadoxton, Neath SA10 8BE — MB ChB Birm. 1997.

PAWAROO, Lalldhar Pawaroo and Partners, The Old Forge Surgery, Pallion Pk, Sunderland SR4 6QE Tel: 0191 510 9393 Fax: 0191 510 9595; 1 Nookside, Grindon, Sunderland SR4 8PH Tel: 0191 528 55320 — MB ChB Glas. 1969.

PAWLEY, Ann Frances Shepherd Spring Medical Centre, Cricketers Way, Andover SP10 5DE Tel: 01264 361126 Fax: 01264 350138 — MB ChB Bristol 1985; MRCGP 1990; DRCOG 1992. Prev: Trainee GP Nailsworth Glos.

PAWLEY, Jeremy John 12 Spinney Drive, Great Shelford, Cambridge CB2 5LY; Flat 5, 9 Kingston Hill, Kingston upon Thames KT2 7PN Tel: 020 8541 1474 — MB BS Lond. 1991 (King's College School of Medicine and Dentistry) DRCOG 1996; MRCGP 1997.

PAWLEY, Martin Kenneth Hereford County Hospital, Union Walk, Hereford HR1 2ER Tel: 029 2084 3140 — MB BCh Wales 1980 (Welsh Nat. Sch. of Med. Cardiff) Specialty: Care of the Elderly.

PAWLEY, Susannah Elisabeth 21 Cobbold Av, Eastbourne BN21 1UY — BM Soton. 1997.

PAWLIKOWSKI, Teresa Rosalia Barbara 2 Scarsdale Place, London W8 5SX Tel: 020 7938 1885; 6 Poplar Grove, London W6 7RE — MB BS Lond. 1978 (Univ. Coll. Hosp.) BSc, MB BS Lond. 1978. Sen. Lect. (Dept. Primary Care & Pop. Scis.) Roy. Free & Univ. Coll. Med. Sch. Lond. Specialty: Gen. Pract.

PAWLOWICZ, Anna Queen Elizabeth Hospital, Gayton Road, King's Lynn PE30 4ET Tel: 01553 613712 Fax: 01553 613984 — Lekarz Warsaw 1985; MRCP (UK) 1995; FRCP 2000. Cons. Gen. Med. with an interest in Respirat. Med. Specialty: Gen. Med.; Respirat. Med. Socs: BMA; E. Angl. Thoracic Soc.

PAWLOWSKA, Elzbieta St Johns Medical Centre, 287A Lewisham Way, London SE4 1XF — MRCS Eng. LRCP Lond. 1985; DRCOG 1989.

PAWSEY, Stephen David 21 The Orchard, Virginia Water GU25 4DT — MB BS Lond. 1988; FRCA 1993. Clin. Research Phys. Upjohn Laborat. Europe. Specialty: Pharmaceutical Medicine. Prev: Regist. Rotat. (Anaesth.) NE Thames Region; SHO (Anaesth.) St. Mary's Hosp. Lond.

PAWSON, Margaret Elizabeth (retired) 3 St John's Ave, Filey YO14 9AZ Tel: 01723 513042 — MB ChB Ed. 1959; LRCP LRCS Ed. LRFPS Glas. 1959; DObst RCOG 1961. Prev: Med. Off. Kalyani Hosp. (Ch. of S. India) Mylapore, India.

PAWSON, Michael Edward (retired) Braywood House, Drift Road, Windsor SL4 4RR Tel: 01344 882670 Email: mike.pawson.@virgin.net — (St. Thos.) MB BS Lond. 1962; MRCS Eng. LRCP Lond. 1962; DObst RCOG 1964; FRCOG 1983, M 1970. Prev: Cons. Chelsea & Westm. Hosp. Lond.

PAWSON, Rachel NBS Oxford Centre, John Radcliffe Hospital, Headington, Oxford OX3 9BQ Tel: 01865 447576 Fax: 01865 447957 Email: rachel.pawson@nbs.nhs.uk — MB BS Lond. 1988 (King's College Hospital London) BSc (Hons.) Lond. 1985; MRCP (UK) 1991; MRCPath 1998; MD 1998. Cons. (Haemat.), Nat. Blood Serv. & John Radcliffe Hosp., Oxf. Specialty: Haematology.

PAWSON, Robert Hugh Belford Medical Practice, The Belford Health Centre, Croftfield, Belford NE70 7ER Tel: 01668 213738 Fax: 01668 213072; Redeford, South Road, Belford NE70 7DP Tel: 01668 213384 — MB ChB St. And. 1970; DObst RCOG 1972; MRCGP 1974.

PAWSON, Roger Michael Mitchell and Partners, The Park Surgery, Old Tetbury Road, Cirencester GL7 1UX Tel: 01285 654733 Fax: 01285 641408 — BM BCh Oxf. 1977. GP Cirencester; Clin. Asst. in Psychiat. & Old Age Psychiat. Specialty: Gen. Psychiat. Prev: Trainee GP Swindon VTS; Ho. Phys. Radcliffe Infirm. & Churchill Hosp. Oxf.

PAWULSKI, Yvonne Maria 10 Hudsons, Tadworth KT20 5TZ — MB BS Lond. 1986. SHO (ENT) Wexham Pk. Hosp. Slough.

PAXTON, Adam Guy North Hykeham Health Centre, Moor Lane, North Hykeham, Lincoln LN6 9BA Tel: 01522 682848 Fax: 01522 697930; 9 Thurlby Road, Bassingham, Lincoln LN5 9LG — MB ChB Leic. 1983. Specialty: Gen. Pract.

PAXTON, Ann Margaret (retired) Birchwood Cottage, Birchwood, Chard TA20 3QH — MB BS Lond. 1962 (St. Geo.) MRCS Eng. LRCP Lond. 1962; MRCPath 1970. Prev: Cons. Haemat. E. Surrey & Mid Downs HA's., St. Bart. Hosp. Lond. & Oncol. Unit. Hackney Hosp.

PAXTON, Christopher Patrick Charles Courtside Surgery, Kennedy Way, Yate, Bristol BS37 4DQ Tel: 01454 313874 Fax: 01454 327110; Coppinhall, 23 Church Lane, Old Sodbury, Bristol BS37 6NB — MB BS Lond. 1979 (St. Mary's Hosp. Lond.) DRCOG 1983; LFHom. 1998.

PAXTON, George Clifford Wards Medical Practice, 25 Dundonald Road, Kilmarnock KA1 1RU Tel: 01563 526514 Fax: 01563 573558 — MB ChB Glas. 1990; DFFP 1993; DRCOG 1994; MRCGP 1994. Specialty: Gen. Psychiat. Socs: BMA. Prev: Trainee GP Lanarksh.

PAXTON, Jane Ralston 4 Seaford Street, Kilmarnock KA1 2DA Tel: 01563 33911 — MB ChB Glas. 1992; BSc (1st cl. Hons.) Pharmacol. Glas. 1989, MB ChB 1992. SHO (Histopath.) Stobhill Hosp. Glas. Specialty: Histopath. Prev: Ho. Off. (Surg. & Med.) Paisley Roy. Alexandra Hosp. & Glas. Roy. Infirm.

PAXTON, Lionel Douglas Dept. of Clinical Anaesthesia, Royal Victoria Hospital, Grosvenor Road, Belfast BT12 6BA Tel: 01232 240503 Fax: 01232 325725; 12 Waterloo Road, Lisburn BT27 5NW — MB ChB Zimbabwe 1984; LRCP LRCS Ed. LRCPS Glas. 1986; FFA RCSI 1992. Cons. (Cardio thoracic anaesth.). Specialty: Anaesth.

PAXTON, Michael John The Penryn Surgery, Saracen Way, Penryn TR10 8HX Tel: 01326 372502 Fax: 01326 378126; Chy Worval, Old Tram Road, Devoran, Truro TR3 6NF Tel: 01872 863950 — MB Camb. 1974 (Camb. & Middlx.) BChir 1973. Prev: SHO (O & G) & SHO (A & E) Ipswich Hosp.

PAXTON, Paul James Lensfield Medical Practice, 48 Lensfield Road, Cambridge CB2 1EH Tel: 01223 352779 Fax: 01223 566930 — MB ChB Birm 1975; DRCOG 1977; MRCGP 1979. Course Organiser Addenbrooke's Hosp. VTS Scheme.

PAXTON, Ross Meuros (retired) Caradon Villa, Downgate, Upton Cross, Liskeard PL14 5AJ; 35 Lakeview Drive, Tamerton Foliot, Plymouth PL5 4LW — MB BS Lond. 1967; DMRD Eng. 1971; FFR 1974; FRCR 1975. Prev: Cons. Neuroradiol. Plymouth Hosps. NHS Trust.

PAY, Charlotte Louise Hode Oast, Hode Lane, Patrixbourne, Canterbury CT4 5DH — MB BS Lond. 1996.

PAY, Jennifer Anne (retired) Hode Oast House, Hode Lane, Patrixbourne, Canterbury CT4 5DH — MB BS Lond. 1967 (Char. Cross) MRCS Eng. LRCP Lond. 1967. Prev: Clin. Asst. (Ophth.) Kent & Canterbury Hosp.

PAY, Rachel Karen 4 Patcham Grange, Grangeways, Brighton BN1 8UR — MB BS Lond. 1998.

PAYAN, José d'Aumale Cottages, 19 The Embankment, Twickenham TW1 3DU Tel: 020 8892 9231 — MB BS Lond. 1956 (Guy's) MRCP (UK) 1961; FRCP Lond. 1980. Emerit. Cons. Clin. Neurophysiol. Guy's Hosp. Lond. Specialty: Clin. Neurophysiol. Socs: Fell. Roy. Soc. Med.; Assn. Brit. Neurol. Prev: Sen. Regist. (Clin. Neurophysiol.) Nat. Hosp. Nerv. Dis. Qu. Sq.; Regist. (EMG) RigsHosp.et, Copenhagen; Fell. (Neurol.) Stanford Univ., USA.

PAYKEL, Professor Eugene Stern Department of Psychiatry, University of Cambridge, Douglas House, 18e Trumpington Road, Cambridge CB2 1AH Tel: 01223 741930 Fax: 01223 741924 Email: esp10@cam.ac.uk — MB ChB Otago 1956; FRCP Ed. 1978, M 1960; FRCP Lond. 1977, M 1961; DPM Lond. 1965; MD Otago 1971; FRCPsych 1977, M 1971; MA Camb. 1986, MD 1988; F Med Sci 1998. Emeritus Prof. Psychiat. Univ. Camb.; Fell. Gonville & Caius Coll.; Edr. Psychol. Med. Specialty: Gen. Psychiat. Prev: Prof. Psychiat. St. Geo. Hosp. Med. Sch. (Univ. Lond.); Vice-Pres. RCPsych.

PAYLER, David Kingsley (retired) The Court Road Surgery, Court Road, Malvern WR14 3BL Tel: 01684 573161 Fax: 01684 561593; Ham Court, Longdon Heath, Upton-upon-Severn, Worcester WR8 0QZ Tel: 01684 592065 — MB BS Lond. 1959 (Guy's) MRCS Eng. LRCP Lond. 1959; DObst RCOG 1964. Hosp. Pract. (Surg.) Worcester Roy. Infirm.; Med. Off. Malvern Coll.

PAYLING, Sandra Mary The Surgery, Bach Victoria Terrace, Thiochly, Newcastle upon Tyne NE18 0PF Tel: 0191 267 4005; 17 Algernon Terrace, Wylam NE41 8AX Tel: 01661 85281 — MB BS Durh. 1964 (Newc.) Socs: BMA. Prev: Ho. Off. (Paediat.) & Ho. Off. (Gen. Med.) Newc. Gen. Hosp.; Med. Off. Stud. Health Serv. Newc. Univ.

PAYMASTER, Nalin Jagmohandas (retired) — MB BS Bombay 1955 (G.S. Med. Coll. Bombay) DA Bombay 1958; DA Eng. 1960; FRCA Eng. 1961. Prev: Cons. Anaesth. Wirral Hosp. NHS Trust Mersey RHA.

PAYNE, Alison Judith Department of Orthopaedics, Royal Hallamshire Hospital, Sheffield S10 Tel: 0114 271 1900; 71 Southgrove Road, Sheffield S10 2NP — MB ChB Sheff. 1995 (Univ. Sheff.) BSc (Hons.) Pharmacol. & Chem. Sheff. 1989; MB ChB (Hons.) Med. Sheff. 1995. SHO (Orthop. & Trauma) Roy. Hallamsh. Hosp. Sheff. Specialty: Orthop.

PAYNE, Andrew John Broadmoor Hospital, Crowthorne RG45 7EG Tel: 01344 773111 — MB BS Lond. 1984; BSc Lond. 1981; MRCP (UK) 1988; MRCPsych 1991. Clin. Director & Cons. Forens. Psychiat. Broadmoor Hosp. Specialty: Forens. Psychiat. Prev: Sen. Regist. & Regist. (Forens. Psychiat.) Roy. Bethlem & Maudsley Hosp. Lond.; SHO Rotat. (Med.) Walsgrave Hosp. Coventry.

PAYNE, Arthur Dudley, SBStJ (retired) Randwick, Amroth, Narberth SA67 8NQ — (St. Bart.) MA Camb. 1942, MB BChir. 1940; MRCS Eng. LRCP Lond. 1943. Prev: Capt. RAMC (Mentioned in Despatches).

PAYNE, Brian Victor Norfolk & Norwich University Hospital, Colney Lane, Norwich NR4 7UY Tel: 01603 288000 Email: brian.payne@nnuh.nhs.uk; 15 Wentworth Green, Norwich NR4 6AE Tel: 01603 452393 — MB BChir Camb. 1970 (Camb. & Middlx.) MRCP (UK) 1974; FRCP Lond. 1989. Cons. Phys. the Elderly Norf. & Norwich Univ. Hosp NHS Trust. Specialty: Care of the Elderly. Socs: Brit. Geriat. Soc. Prev: Sen. Regist. (Geriat. Med.) Chesterton Hosp. Camb.

PAYNE, Miss Caroline Elizabeth 22 Barnhill, Pinner HA5 2SX — MB BS Lond. 1994 (Guy's & St. Thos.) BSc (Hons.) Lond. 1989; FRCS (Eng) 1998. Specialty: Plastic Surg.

PAYNE, Christopher James Irving South Gloucestershire Primary Care Trust, 1 Monarch Court, Emerald Business Park, Emersons' Green, Bristol BS16 7FH Tel: 0117 330 2433 — MB ChB Bristol 1978; MRCGP 1982; MPH Wales 1998; MFPHM 2000. Director of Pub. Health, S. Gloucestershire PCT. Specialty: Pub. Health Med. Prev: Cons. in Pub. Health Med., Avon Health Auth.

PAYNE, Christopher Oliver Bermondsey and Lansdowne Medical Centre, The Surgery, Decima Street, London SE1 4QX Tel: 020 7407 0752 Fax: 020 7378 8209; 90 Kidbrooke Park Road, Blackheath, London SE3 0DX — MB BS Lond. 1963 (King's Coll. Hosp.) MRCS Eng. LRCP Lond. 1963; MRCP (UK) 1971. Specialty: Gen. Med. Socs: W. Kent M-C Soc.; BMA. Prev: Dir. Community Health Servs. Lewisham & N. Southwark HA; Cons. Phys. The Christian Hosp. Shiraz, Iran; Med. Specialist RAF Hosp. Nocton Hall.

PAYNE, Christopher Robert Consulting Suite, Alexandra Hospital, Mill Lane, Cheadle SK8 2PX Tel: 0161 428 3656 Fax: 0161 282 5005; Ramillies, 2 Marlborough Road, Bowdon, Altrincham WA14 2RT Tel: 0161 928 0177 Fax: 0161 331 6401 — MB ChB Manch. 1971; DObst RCOG 1975; MRCP (UK) 1976; FRCP Lond. 1992. Cons. Phys. Tameside Gen. Hosp., Ashton-under-Lyne. Specialty: Gen. Med.; Respirat. Med. Socs: Brit. Thorac. Soc.; BMA. Prev: Sen. Regist. (Med.) Manch. Roy. Infirm.; Sen. Regist. (Med.) Withington Hosp. Manch.; Regist. (Med.) Brompton Hosp. Lond.

PAYNE, Clare Elisabeth Butlers Farm, Chittlehamholt, Umberleigh EX37 9NT — MB BChir Camb. 1985 (Univ. & Westm. Hosp. Camb.) SCMO Family Plann. N. Devon PCT. Specialty: Genitourinary Medicine.

PAYNE, David Anthony 4 Murrayfield, Bamford, Rochdale OL11 5UQ — MB ChB Leic. 1994.

PAYNE, David John Downsway Medical Practice, Shorne Village Surgery, Crown Lane, Shorne, Gravesend DA12 3DY Tel: 01474 822037/01474 824419; 11 Millfield Drive, Northfleet, Gravesend DA11 8BH — MB BS Lond. 1988; DRCOG 1990; MRCGP 1992.

PAYNE, Donald Neil Russell 23 Patience Road, London SW11 2PY Tel: 020 7585 1789 — MB BChir Camb. 1990 (Univ. Camb. & Lond. Hosp. Med. Coll.) BA (Hons.) Camb. 1987; MRCP (UK) 1993; MRCPCH 2000. Clin. Research Fell., Roy. Brompton Hosp. Specialty: Paediat. Prev: Specialist Regist. (Paediat.) Roy. Brompton Hosp. Lond.

PAYNE, Elizabeth Mary Margaret (retired) 23 Blenheim Road, Penylan, Cardiff CF23 5DS Tel: 029 2021 4067 — MB BCh Wales 1950 (Welsh Nat. Sch. Med. Cardiff) BSc Wales 1947.

PAYNE, Elizabeth Susan Princess of Wales Womens Unit, Birmingham Heartlands Hospital, Bordesley Green E., Birmingham B9 5SS Tel: 0121 685 5951 — MD Birm. 1991 (Birmingham) MB ChB 1977; MRCOG 1983; FRCOG 1997. Cons. O & G Birm. Heartlands Hosp. Specialty: Obst. & Gyn. Socs: Brit. Menopause Soc.; Brit. Fertililty Soc.; Brit. Soc. paediatric and Adolesc. Gyn. Prev: Cons. O & G; City Hosp. NHS Trust 1990-1995.

PAYNE, Elspeth Margaret Conroy 17 Deanburn Road, Linlithgow EH49 6EY — MB ChB Glas. 1997.

PAYNE, Eric Eustace 23 Blenheim Road, Penylan, Cardiff CF23 5DS Tel: 029 2021 4067 — MB BCh Wales 1953 (Welsh Nat. Sch. Med. Cardiff) BSc Wales 1950, MD 1958. Indep. Med. Pract. Cardiff; Research Investig. Cardiff; Hon. Med. Off. Cardiff Inst. Blind; Hon. Curator Museum Hist. Med. UWCM. Specialty: Neuropath. Socs: Cardiff Med. Soc. Prev: Sen. Lect. (Path.) Welsh Nat. Sch. Med. Cardiff.

PAYNE, Fiona Beverley Dept. Of Cellular Path., Southmead Hosp., Westbury-on-Trym, Bristol BS10 5NB — MB ChB Bristol 1988; DRCPath 1993; MRCPath 1999. Cons. Cellular Pathologist. Specialty: Pathology, General. Prev: Regist. (Histopath.) Leics. Roy. Infirm.; Clin. Research Fell. (Path.) St Michael's Hosp. Bristol.

PAYNE, Fiona Margaret The Surgery, 327D Upper Richmond Road, London SW15 6SU Tel: 020 8788 6002 Fax: 020 8789 8568 — MB BS Lond. 1989 (St. Thomas's Hosp.) Specialty: Gen. Pract.

PAYNE, Geoffrey Paul Ingleby The New Surgery, Lindo Close, Chesham HP5 2JN Tel: 01494 782262; Winstons, Weedon Hill, Hyde Heath, Amersham HP6 5RN — BM BCh Oxf. 1975; MA Oxf. 1975; MRCP (UK) 1977; DCH Eng. 1978; DRCOG 1979; MRCGP 1979; FRCGP 2002; FRCP Lond. 2002. GP; Med. Adviser, Bucks HA. Socs: Fell.Roy. Soc. of Med.; PEC, Chiltern & South Bucks PCT. Prev: Bd. Mem. Chiltern PCG.

PAYNE, George Stuart Alford Medical Practice, 2 Gordon Road, Alford AB33 8AL Tel: 019755 62253 Fax: 019755 62613; Callater, Kingsfield, Alford AB33 8HN Tel: 019755 62976 — MB ChB Aberd. 1976; DRCOG 1980; MRCGP 1982.

PAYNE, Gillian Elizabeth Doncaster Royal Infirmary, Armthorpe Lane, Doncaster DN2 5LZ Tel: 01302 366666; 6 Oaklands, Warning Tongue Lane, Bessacarr, Doncaster DN4 6XW — MB ChB Leeds 1987 (Univ. Leeds) MD Leic. 1996; FRCP 2002. Cons. Gen. Phys. (Cardiol.) Doncaster Roy. Infirm. Specialty: Cardiol. Prev: Research Regist. (Cardiol.) Glenfield Hosp. Leicester.

PAYNE, Graham Spencer Yeovil District Hospital, Higher Kingston, Yeovil BA21 4AT — MB ChB Bristol 1974.

PAYNE, Heather Ann 117 Aveling Park Road, Walthamstow, London E17 4NS Tel: 020 8527 4071 — MB BS Lond. 1983 (St. Mary's Hospital Medical School) FRCR; MRCP (UK) 1988. Cons. (Clin. Oncoloy) The Middlx. Hosp. Lond. Specialty: Oncol. Prev: Sen. Regist. (Clin. Oncol.) The Middlx. Hosp. Lond.; Sen. Regist. Mt. Vernon Hosp.

PAYNE, Mr Ian William (retired) Swallow Cottage, Teigngrace, Newton Abbot TQ12 6QW — MB ChB Manch. 1946; DOMS Eng. 1949; FRCS Eng. 1953. Prev: Surg. Roy. Eye Infirm. Plymouth.

PAYNE, Jacqueline Dorfold Cottage, Wrexham Road, Acton, Nantwich CW5 8LP — MB BCh BAO NUI 1980; FFA RCS Eng. 1987. Specialty: Anaesth.

PAYNE, Jacqueline Station House Surgery, Station Road, Kendal LA9 6SA Tel: 01539 722660 Fax: 01539 734845 — MB BS Newc. 1986; Cert. Family Plann. JCC 1990; MRCGP 1990; DRCOG 1990.

PAYNE, Jacqueline Mary Pound House Surgery, 8 The Green, Wooburn Green, High Wycombe HP10 0EE; 70 Westwood Drive, Little Chalfont, Amersham HP6 6RW — MB BS Lond. 1989; BSc (Hons.) Lond. 1986; DCH RCP Lond. 1992; DRCOG 1993; MRCGP 1993.

PAYNE, Professor James Patrick, OStJ 36 Raymond Road, Wimbledon, London SW19 4AP Tel: 020 8946 8456 — (Ed.) MB ChB Ed. 1946; DA Eng. 1951; FFA RCS Eng. 1954; MD (Hon. Causa) Uppsala 1984; DSc (Med.) Lond. 1988; FRCA 1992. Emerit. Prof. Anaesth. RCS Eng.; Emerit. Prof. Anaesth. Univ. Lond. (Lond. Hosp. Med. Coll.); Hon. Cons. Anaesth. Lond. Hosp. & St. Peter's Hosps. Lond. Specialty: Anaesth. Socs: Fell BMA (Ex-Chairm. Merton & Sutton Div.); Hon. Mem. (Ex-Vice Pres.) Assn. Anaesth.; Liveryman Soc. Apoth. Lond. Prev: Lect. (Anaesth.) Postgrad. Med. Sch.; Research Asst. (Anaesth.) Univ. Manch.; Sen. Regist. (Anaesth.) Roy. Infirm. Edin.

PAYNE, Mr John Gordon 90 Sloane Street, London SW1X 9PQ Tel: 020 7259 6308 Fax: 020 7235 7233; 19 Bramerton Street, London SW3 5JS Tel: 020 7352 7555 Fax: 020 7352 7111 Email: johngordon.payne@virgin.net — MB BS Lond. 1968 (Guy's) MRCS Eng. LRCP Lond. 1968; FRCS Eng. 1974; MD Lond. 1976. Cons. Surg. Qu. Mary's Sidcup NHS Trust; Hon. Surg. Tutor Imperial Coll. Lond.; Regional Specialty Advis. (Gen. Surg.) RCS; Mem. Intercollegiate Bd. Gen. Surg. Specialty: Gen. Surg. Special Interest: Colorectal Surg.; Endocrine Surg.; Paediatric Surg. Socs: Fell. Assn. Surg. GB & Irel.; ACPGBI; RSM Sect. Surg. (Past-Pres. Sect. Surg.). Prev: Assoc. Staff Surg. (Colon & Rectal Dis.) Ochsner Med. Inst. New Orleans; Sen. Regist. (Surg.) St. Mark's Hosp. & Guy's Hosp. Lond.

PAYNE, John Halliday Rowland Monnow St, Monmouth NP25 3EQ Tel: 01600 713811; Ingleside, Lone Lane, Penallt, Monmouth NP25 4AJ Tel: 01600 712170 — MB BS Lond. 1972 (St. Bart.) MRCS Eng. 1972; LRCP Lond. 1972; MRCS Eng. LRCP Lond. 1972; DCH Eng. 1977; DCH Eng. 1977; MRCGP 1978; MRACGP 1978; Diploma in Therapeutics 2002; Certificate in the Management of Drug Misuse 2002. Clin. Asst. (Geriat.) Bridges Day Hosp. Monmouth.

PAYNE, John Martin Victor Barton House Surgery, Barton House, Beaminster DT8 3EQ Tel: 01308 862233 Fax: 01308 863785 — MB BS Lond. 1978; MRCP (UK) 1981; MRCGP 1986.

PAYNE, John Nicholas (Nick) North Eastern Derbyshire Primary Care Trust, Block C, St Mary's Court, St Mary's Gate, Chesterfield S41 7TD Tel: 01246 551158 Fax: 01246 544620 Email: nick.payne@nederbypct.nhs.uk — BM BCh Oxf. 1977 (Oxford) MA Camb. 1978; FFA RCS Eng. 1981; PhD Sheff. 1987; FFPHM RCP (UK) 1998. Director Pub. Health NE. Derbysh. PCT; Hon. Sen. Lect. Sch. Health & Related Research Univ. Sheff. Specialty: Pub. Health Med. Prev: Dep. Director Pub. Health Med. Sheff. HA; Cons. Pub. Health Med. Sheff. HA; Regist. (Pub. Health Med.) Trent RHA.

PAYNE, John Stiling The Avenue Surgery, 14 The Avenue, Warminster BA12 9AA Tel: 01985 846224; 87 Boreham Road, Warminster BA12 9JX Tel: 01985 214030 — MB ChB Bristol 1971; DObst RCOG 1973. Prev: SHO (Psychiat.) Barrow Hosp. Bristol; Obst. Ho. Off. Southmead Gen. Hosp. Bristol.

PAYNE, Jonathan Frank Anaesthetic Department, Norfolk & Norwich Hospital, Brunswick Road, Norwich NR1 3RS Tel: 01603 287086 — MB BS Lond. 1987; FRCA 1991. Cons. Anaesth. Norf. & Norwich Hosp. Specialty: Anaesth. Prev: SR (Anaesth.) Birm. Sch. Anaesth.; Clin. Fell. (Anaesth.) Childr. Hosp. Birm.; Regist. (Anaesth.) Kingston Hosp. Surrey & St. Geo. Hosp. Lond.

PAYNE, Julia Helen Cheshire & Wirral Partnership NHS Trust, Clatterbridge Hospital, Bebington, Wirral CH63 4JY — BM BS Nottm. 1992. Consultant Old Age Psychiatry; Specialist Regist. Hon. Mersey Deanery. Specialty: Geriat. Psychiat. Prev: Clin. Lect. (Old Age Psychiat.) Univ. of L'pool.

PAYNE, Leonard Robert (retired) 125D Beechwood Avenue, Coventry CV5 6FQ Tel: 024 7667 2406 Fax: 024 7667 2406 — MB ChB St. And. 1957.

PAYNE, Margaret Anne Breast Screening Office, Wycombe Hospital, Queen Alexandra Road, High Wycombe HP11 2TT Tel: 01494 425689; Winstons, Weedon Hill, Hyde Heath, Amersham HP6 5RN Tel: 01494 783167 — BM BCh Oxf. 1975; MA Oxf. 1975; DRCOG 1977; DCH Eng. 1978. Assoc. Specialist (Breast Screening & Fam. Plg.) S. Bucks. HNS Trust, High Wycombe. Specialty: Family Plann. & Reproduc. Health. Prev: Clin. Med. Off. (Child Health) High Wycombe; SCMO & Clin. Co-ordinator Breast Screening Serv. S. Bucks. NHS Trust High Wycombe.

PAYNE, Mrs Margaret Catherine (retired) Barnstones, Old Seaview Lane, Seaview PO34 5BJ — (Royal Free Hospital) MB BS Lond. 1940; MRCS Eng. LRCP Lond. 1940.

PAYNE, Mark Nicholas 104A Bellingdon Road, Chesham HP5 2HF Tel: 01494 785525 — MB BS Lond. 1984; MRCP (UK) 1988. Regist. (Cardiol.) Birm. Heartlands Hosp. Specialty: Cardiol. Prev: Regist. (Med. & Cardiol.) Selly Oak Hosp. Birm.

PAYNE, Martin Richard Department of Anaesthetics, Cumberland Infirmary, Carlisle CA2 7HY Tel: 01228 814196 — MB ChB Bristol 1977; FFA RCS Eng. 1982; DTM & H Eng. 1987. Cons. Cumbld. Infirm. Carlisle. Specialty: Anaesth. Socs: Eur. Soc. Regional Anaesth. Prev: Sen. Regist. Roy. Infirm. Edin.; Specialist Med. Off. (Anaesth.) Angau Memor. Hosp. Lae Papua New Guinea; Regist. (Anaesth.) Univ. Hosp. Wales, Cardiff & W.mead Centre, NSW Australia.

PAYNE, Mary Rosalind — MB ChB Dundee 1980; MRCGP 1987; MPhil (Med. Law) Glas. 2002. Freelance GP since 1999 Scotl., New Zealand.

PAYNE, Michael James Butlers Farm, Chittlehamholt, Umberleigh EX37 9NT — MB BS Lond. 1985.

PAYNE, Mr Michael John, Col. late RAMC Retd. Tiree Cottage, West Ridge, Hogs Back, Seale, Farnham GU10 1JU Tel: 01252

782014 Fax: 01252 782014 — MB BS Lond. 1966 (Westm.) MRCS Eng. LRCP Lond. 1966; FRCS Ed. 1973; Dip. IMC RCS Ed. 1995. Cons. Gen. Surg. King. Edwd. VII Hosp. Midhurst. Specialty: Gen. Surg. Special Interest: Breast Surg. Socs: Fell. Assn. Surgs.; Milit. Surg. Soc.; BASO.

PAYNE, Michael Lawrence Harborne Medical Practice, 4 York Street, Harborne, Birmingham B17 0HG Tel: 0121 427 5246 — MB ChB Manch. 1979; MRCGP 1983.

PAYNE, Michael Robert 409 City View House, 463 Bethnal Green Road, London E2 9QY Tel: 020 7729 4979 — MB BS Lond. 1990; MRCPsych 1995. Specialist Regist. St Clements Hosp. Lond. Specialty: Gen. Psychiat.; Geriat. Psychiat.

PAYNE, N M The Surgery, Southview Lodge, South View, Bromley BR1 3DR Tel: 020 8460 1932 Fax: 020 8323 1423.

PAYNE, Nicholas David Gerhard 57A Constantine Road, London NW3 2LP Tel: 020 7482 7122 Fax: 020 7482 7122 — MB BS Lond. 1993 (Roy. Free Hosp. Sch. Med.) Staff Grade (A & E) Lister Hosp. Stevenage. Specialty: Accid. & Emerg.

PAYNE, Nigel Edric Sven 10 Justice Avenue, Saltford, Bristol BS31 3DR — MB BS Lond. 1985; FCAnaesth 1990. Cons. (Anaesth.) Guildford Roy Surrey Co. Hosp. Specialty: Anaesth. Socs: Fell. Roy. Coll. Anaesths.

PAYNE, Paul Anthony Gullock Gloucester Road Medical Centre, Tramway House, 1A Church Road, Horfield, Bristol BS7 8SA Tel: 0117 949 7774 Fax: 0117 949 7730; The South Barn, Lower Almondsbury, Bristol BS32 4EF Tel: 01454 615553 — MB BS Lond. 1969 (St. Bart.) MRCS Eng. LRCP Lond. 1969; DO Eng. 1972. Police Surg.; Hosp. Pract. Bristol Eye Hosp. Specialty: Ophth. Prev: SHO Croydon Eye Unit; Ho. Surg., Ho. Phys. & Cas. Off. Bethnal Green Hosp. Lond.

PAYNE, Mr Peter Russell (retired) The Hampshire Clinic, Basing Road, Basing, Basingstoke RG24 7AL Tel: 01256 57111 Fax: 01256 397517; Glendevon, Nateley Scures, Basingstoke RG27 9JS Tel: 01256 762661 — (TC Dub.) MB BCh BAO Dub. 1954; FRCS Ed. 1959; FRCOG 1979, M 1966. Prev: Cons. Gyn. Hants. Clinic Basingstoke.

PAYNE, Reginald Brian (retired) 50 North Park Avenue, Leeds LS8 1EY Tel: 0113 266 1577 Email: rbrianpayne@doctors.org.uk — MB BCh Wales 1954; MD Wales 1963; FRCPath 1977, M 1965; PhD Leeds 1970. Prev: Cons. Chem. Path. St. Jas. Univ. Hosp. Leeds.

PAYNE, Reuben Frederick (retired) Huxtable Farm, West Buckland, Barnstaple EX32 0SR Tel: 0159 86 254 — MRCS Eng. LRCP Lond. 1945 (Char. Cross) BA Camb. 1942; DTM & H Eng. 1952. Prev: Assoc. Specialist Accid. Dept. N. Devon Dist. Hosp. Barnstaple.

PAYNE, Mr Richard Frederick Barford Cliff Cottage, Barford Lane, Downton, Salisbury SP5 3QF Tel: 01725 512449 — MB BS Lond. 1993; BSc Lond. 1990, MB BS 1993; FRCS Lond. 1997; MS Lond. 2002.

PAYNE, Richard Wyman (retired) 22 Silverwell Park, Modbury, Ivybridge PL21 0RJ Tel: 01548 831053 — MB BChir Camb. 1954 (Camb. & St. Thos.) MA Camb. 1955, BA (Hons.) 1951, MD 1960; FRCPath 1973, M 1963; FRCP Glas. 1977, M 1974. Prev: Cons. Haemat. Worcester Roy. Infirm. & Vict. Infirm. Glas.

PAYNE, Roger John Ward End Medical Centre, 794A Washwood Heath Road, Ward End, Birmingham B8 2JN Tel: 0121 327 1049 Fax: 0121 327 0964; 5 Anton Drive, Walmley, Sutton Coldfield B76 1XQ — MB ChB Birm. 1981; DRCOG 1983; Cert. FPA 1983; MRCGP 1985. Socs: BMA & Med. Defence Union. Prev: Trainee GP Birm.

PAYNE, Ronald John Top Flat Left, 318 Queen St., Broughty Ferry, Dundee DD5 2HQ — MB ChB Dundee 1990.

PAYNE, Sandra Anne National Public Health Service (North Wales), Preswylfa, Hendy Road, Mold CH7 1PZ Tel: 01352 700227; Whiteacres, Llanelian Heights, Colwyn Bay LL29 8YB Email: sandrapayne@fsmail.net — MB BS Lond. 1977 (Guy's Hospital Medical School) MRCS Eng. LRCP Lond. 1977; MFPHM 1990; FFPHM 2000. Regional Director of Public Health; Hon. Sen. Lect. Univ. Bangor. Specialty: Pub. Health Med. Special Interest: Health Promotion; Health Protec. Prev: Sen. Registar (Community Med.) Clwyd HA; Sen. Clin. Med. Off. (Child Health) Clwyd HA; Director of Public Health, North Wales Health Authority.

PAYNE, Simon David Plymouth Assertive Outreach Service, Riverview, Mount Gould Hospital, Plymouth PL4 7QD — MB ChB Leic. 1981; MRCPsych 1988. Cons. (Psychiat.) AOS Plymouth. Specialty: Gen. Psychiat. Prev: Cons. Psychiat. Rehabil. & Community Care Nottm. Healthcare Unit Mapperley Hosp.; Sen. Regist. (Adult Psychiat.) Nottm. VTS.

PAYNE, Mr Simon David William Ealing Hospital, A/E Department, Uxbridge RD, Southall UB1 3HW; 28 Emanuel Avenue, Acton, London W3 6JJ — MB BS Lond. 1978 (Middlx. Hosp. Med. Sch.) FRCS Ed. 1983; FRCS Eng. 1984; LLM Wales 1992; FFAEM 1995. Cons. & Clin. Dir. A & E Ealing Hosp. Lond. Specialty: Accid. & Emerg.; Medico Legal. Special Interest: Foot Surg. Socs: Cardiff Med. Soc. - Mem.; Roy. Soc. Med. - Mem.; Medico-Legal Soc. - Mem. Prev: Hon. Sen. Lect. in A/E Med. Imperial Coll. Med. Sch. Lond.; Cons. A & E Roy. Hants. Co. Hosp. Winchester; Sen. Regist. Rotat. (A & E) Basingstoke, Portsmouth & Soton.

PAYNE, Simon Nicholas Lester Department of Pathology, University Medical Buildings, Foresterhill, Aberdeen AB25 2ZD Tel: 01224 681818 Fax: 01224 633002; 6H Belgrave Terrace, Aberdeen AB25 2NS Tel: 01224 658534 — MB ChB Aberd. 1991; BMedBiol. (Hons.) Aberd. 1988; MRCPath (UK) 1999. Cons. (Histopath./Cytopath.) Aberd. Specialty: Histopath. Prev: Specialist Regist. (Path.) Aberd.; SHO & Hon. Lect. (Path.) Univ. Aberd.; Research Fell. (Path.) Univ. Aberd.

PAYNE, Mr Stephen Richard Anson Medical Centre, 23 Anson Road, Victoria Park, Manchester M14 5BZ Tel: 0161 248 2010 Fax: 0161 276 4221 Email: stevepayne.urol@btinternet.com; 21 Ollerbarrow Road, Hale, Altrincham WA15 9PP Tel: 0161 941 1267 Fax: 0161 941 1267 — MB BS Lond. 1977 (Roy. Free) FRCS Eng. 1981; MS Lond. 1987; FEBU 1992. Cons. Urol. Centr. Manch.and Manch. Childr. Hosp. Univ. Trust, Manch. Royal Infirm, & St. Marys Hosp. Manch; Hon. Clin. Lect. (Urol.) Univ. Manch. Specialty: Urol. Socs: Brit. Assn. Urol. Surgs.- Counc. Mem. 2001-2004; BAUS Urolink Chairman; Intercollegiate Bd. Memb 2003-2008. Prev: Sen. Registar (Urol.) St. Mary's Hosp. Portsmouth; Lect. (Percutaneous Renal Surg.) Inst. Urol. Univ. Lond.; RSO St. Peter's Hosp. Lond.

PAYNE, Susan Ann 43 Brompton Place, Tredegar NP22 4NF — MB BCh Wales 1976.

PAYNE, Thomas Christopher 103 Sidney Grove, Newcastle upon Tyne NE4 5PE — MB BS Newc. 1993.

PAYNE, William Nigel (retired) Wareham Health Centre, Streche Road, Wareham BH20 4PG Tel: 01929 553444 Fax: 01929 550703 — MB BS Lond. 1962 (Univ. Coll. Hosp.) MRCS Eng. LRCP Lond. 1962. Prev: Ho. Surg. (O & G), Ho. Surg. & Ho. Phys. Dorset Co. Hosp.

PAYNE-JAMES, John Jason 19 Speldhurst Road, London E9 7EH Tel: 07956 960304 Fax: 01621 772200 Email: jasonpaynejames@aol.com; Forensic Health Services Ltd, 100 Station Road, Leigh-on-sea SS9 1SU Tel: 01702 711140 Fax: 01702 711153 Email: office@forensic-healthcare.com — MB BS Lond. 1980 (Roy. Lond. Hosp.) FRCS Ed. 1985; FRCS Eng. 1986; RNutr 1989; LLM 1995; DFM 2000. p/t Cons. Forens. Phys.; Extern. Cons., Nat. Injuries Database & Nat. Crime & Operations Fac.; Med. Edr. and author; Forens. Med. Examr., Metrop. Police Serv., City of Lond. Police; Endoscopist/Gastroenterologist Queensway Surg. Southend-on-Sea; Registered Nutritionist; Dir. Forens. Healthcare Serv.s Ltd.; Edr. Jl. Clin. Forens. Med. Specialty: Medico Legal; Gastroenterol.; Forensic and MedicoLegal. Socs: Fell. Roy. Soc. Med.; Forens. Sci. Soc.; Assn. of Forens. Physicians. Prev: Regist. (A & E) Whipps Cross Hosp. Lond.; Regist. Rotat. (Surg.) Roy. Free, Whittington, Roy. Northern & Westminster Hosps. Lond.; Lect. & Demonst. (Anat.) Roy. Lond. Hosp. Med. Coll.

PAYNTER, Arthur Stephen Central Clinic, 50 Victoria Place, Carlisle CA1 1HP Tel: 01228 603274 Fax: 01228 603201; 26 Tullie Street, Carlisle CA1 2BA Tel: 01228 819318 — MB BS Madras 1971 (Christian Med. Coll. Vellore) DCH RCPS Glas. 1974; FRCP 1997. Cons. Paediat. (Community Child Health) N. Lakeland Health Care. Specialty: Community Child Health. Socs: FRCP; FRCPCh. Prev: Cons. Paediat. (Community Child Health) W. Cumbria Health Care; Cons. Paediat. (Community Child Health) NW Durh. HA; Cons. Paediat. to Govt. Solomon Is.s.

PAYNTER, Helen Elizabeth Gloucestershire Royal Hospital, Great Western Road, Gloucester GL1 3NN Tel: 01452 528555; 47 Fabian Drive, Stoke Gifford, Bristol BS34 8XL Tel: 0117 969 9263 Email:

hep@paynter1.demon.co.uk — MB ChB Bristol 1992; DRCOG 1994; MRCP (UK) 1996. Specialist Regist. (Renal/Gen. Med.) Gloucestershire Roy. Hosp. Specialty: Nephrol.

PAYNTON, David John Bath Lodge Practice, Bitterne Health Centre, Commercial Street, Southampton SO18 6BT; 210 Bridge Road, Sarisbury Green, Southampton SO31 7ED Tel: 0148 95 573049 — MB ChB Manch. 1975; DRCOG 1978; DCH Eng. 1979; FRCGP 1994, M 1980. Chair of Exec. Comm., Soton. City Primary Care Trust.

PAYTON, Colin David Royal United Occupational Health & Safety, Royal United Hospital, Combe Park, Bath BA1 3NG Tel: 01225 824064 Fax: 01225 825427 Email: colin.payton@ruh-bath.swest.nhs.uk — MB ChB Manch. 1977; MRCP (UK) 1982; FRCP Glas. 1994; MFOM RCP Lond. 1994. Cons. Occupat. Phys. Roy. United Occupat. Health & Safety Bath; Clin. Dir. Occupat. Health & Safety Roy. United Hosp. Bath. Specialty: Occupat. Health. Socs: Soc. Occupat. Med.; Assn. NHS Occupat. Phys. Prev: Sen. Regist. Leicester Roy. Infirm.

PEACE, Julian Miles Valley Medical Centre, Johnson Street, Stocksbridge, Sheffield S36 1BX — MB ChB Sheff. 1990; BMedSci Sheff. 1987; (Dip. Practical Dermat.) Cardiff 2000.

PEACE, Mr Peter Kirkby Frere House, Kenwyn, Truro TR1 3DR — MB BS Lond. 1966 (Guy's) BSc (Hons. Anat.) Lond. 1963; MRCS Eng. LRCP Lond. 1966; FRCS Eng. 1972. Cons. Surg. (Orthop. & Trauma) Roy. Cornw. Hosps. Trust. Specialty: Orthop. Socs: Fell. BOA; BMA. Prev: Ho. Phys. Guy's Hosp. Lond.; Jun. Lect. (Anat.) Guy's Hosp. Med. Sch.; Sen. Regist. Princess Eliz. Orthop. Hosp. Exeter.

PEACE, Mr Richard Henry Nightingale Surgery, Greatwell Drive, Cupernham Lane, Romsey SO51 7QN Tel: 01794 517878 Fax: 01794 514236; The Well House, Canada Road, West Wellow, Romsey SO51 6DE Tel: 01794 322970 — MB BS Lond. 1976; MRCS Eng. LRCP Lond. 1975; FRCS Eng. 1981.

PEACE, Savita 13 Pondcroft Road, Knebworth SG3 6DB Email: savpeace@hotmail.com — MB ChB Liverp. 1996.

PEACEY, Mrs Jean Menzies 46 Riverside Court, Nine Elms Lane, London SW8 5BY Tel: 020 7627 2818 Fax: 020 7627 2818; The Old Grain House, 27 High St, Bourn, Cambridge CB3 7SQ Fax: 01954 718310 — (St. Bart.) MB BS Lond. 1957; MRCGP 1968. Prev: Sen. Med. Off. MoD; Ho. Surg. King Geo. Hosp. Ilford; Ho. Phys. St. And. Hosp. Bow.

PEACEY, Steven Raymond Department of Endocrinology and Diabetes, Bradford Teaching Hospitals NHS Trust, Duckworth Lane, Bradford BD9 6RJ Tel: 01274 382019 — MB ChB Leeds 1985; MRCP (UK) l988; MD Sheff. 1998; FRCP 2003. Cons. (Endocrinol. & Diabetes) Bradford Hosps. NHS Trust Bradford. Specialty: Endocrinol.; Diabetes; Gen. Med. Socs: Soc. Endocrinol.; Roy. Coll. Phys. Lond.; Endocrine Soc. USA. Prev: Sen. Regist. (Endocrinol. & Diabetes) Christie Hosp. Manch.; Lect. & Research Fell. (Endocrinol. & Diabetes) Univ. Sheff.; Regist. (Endocrinol.) Leeds Gen. Infirm.

PEACH, Mr Alfred Nowell Hamilton (retired) 124 Brighton Road, Horsham RH13 6EY Tel: 01403 262573 — MB ChB Bristol 1937; FRCS Eng. 1948. Prev: Surg. Horsham Hosp.

PEACH, Mr Barry Griffith Skyrme (retired) Cranford House, 244 Clifton Drive Sth., Lytham St Annes FY8 1NH Tel: 01253 726203 — MB ChB Birm. 1959; FRCS Ed. 1968; MChOrth Liverp. 1970. Prev: Cons. Surg. (Orthop.) Blackpool Health Dist.

PEACH, Christopher John David The Surgery, 77 Thurleigh Road, Balham, London SW12 8TZ Tel: 020 8675 3521 Fax: 020 8675 3800 — MB BS Lond. 1974 (Char. Cross) MSc (Community Med.) 1983; MRCGP 1984. GP Battersea Lond.; Chief Med. Off. Gesa Asst.ance (UK) Lond. Socs: Chairm. Brit. Aeromed. Pract. Assn. Prev: Regist. (Community Med.) S.W. Thames RHA; Regist. (Gen. Med.) Princess Margt. Hosp. Nassau, Bahamas.

PEACH, Fiona Jane Cross Plain Surgery, 84 Bulford Road, Durrington, Salisbury SP4 8DH Tel: 01980 652221; 4 Heath Road, Salisbury SP2 9JS — BM Soton. 1986; MRCGP 1991. Specialty: Gen. Pract. Prev: Trainee GP Salisbury VTS.

PEACH, Ian David (Surgery), Recreation Drive, Billinge, Wigan WN5 7LY Tel: 01744 892205 — MB ChB Manch. 1990; MRCGP 1994.

PEACH, Rosalind Margaret (retired) Cranford House, 244 Clifton Drive S., Lytham St Annes FY8 1NH Tel: 01253 726203 — (Ed.) MB ChB Ed. 1960; DA Eng. 1963; MFFP 1994. Locum Med. Off. Family Plann. Prev: SCMO (Family Plann.) Blackpool, Wyre & Community Health Servs. NHS Trust.

PEACHEY, Geoffrey Robert Weybridge Health Centre, Minorca Road, Weybridge KT13 8DU Tel: 01932 853366 Fax: 01932 844902; Waverley Lodge, Elgin Road, Weybridge KT13 8SN — MB BS Lond. 1958 (Guy's) MRCS Eng. LRCP Lond. 1958. Prev: Res. Med. Off. Nuffield Ho., Guy's Hosp.; Res. (Obst.) & Asst. Ho. Phys. & Ho. Surg. Guy's Hosp. Lond.

PEACHEY, Jean Aylott (retired) 3 Kingslake, Kings Road, Cranleigh GU6 7JQ Tel: 01483 277939 — MB BS Lond. 1957 (King's Coll. Hosp.) MRCS Eng. LRCP Lond. 1957; DO Eng. 1959. Prev: Assoc. Specialist (Ophth.) Qu. Eliz. II Hosp. Welwyn Gdn. City.

PEACHEY, Robin David Gordon (retired) Litfield House, 1 Litfield Place, Clifton Down, Bristol BS8 3LS Tel: 0117 973 1323; Blue Lodge, Abson, Wick, Bristol BS30 5TX Tel: 0117 937 2401 — MB BS Lond. 1956 (St. Thos.) BSc (Anat.) Lond. 1953, MD 1972, MB BS 1956; FRCP Lond. 1975, M 1958. Prev: Cons. Dermat. Bristol Roy. Infirm. & Frenchay Hosp. Bristol.

PEACHEY, Ronald Sidney (retired) 3 Kingslake, Kings Road, Cranleigh GU6 7JQ Tel: 01483 277939 — MRCS Eng. LRCP Lond. 1956 (King's Coll. Hosp.) BSc (1st cl. Hons.) Lond. 1950, MB BS 1956; DObst RCOG 1958; FFA RCS Eng. 1967. Prev: Cons. Anaesth. Qu. Eliz. II Hosp. Welwyn Garden City.

PEACHEY, Timothy David Dept of Anaesthesia, The Royal Free Hospital, Pond Street, London NW3 2QP Tel: 0207 794 0500 Ext: 6503 Fax: 0207 830 2245 Email: tim.peachey@rfh.nthames.nhs.uk — MB BS Lond. 1983 (King's college Hospital) FFA RCS Eng. 1988. Cons. Anaesth. Roy. Free Hosp. Lond. Specialty: Anaesth.; Intens. Care.

PEACOCK, Professor Andrew John Scottish Pulmonary Vascular Unit, Department Respiratory Medicine, Western Infirmary, Glasgow G11 6NT Tel: 0141 211 6327 Fax: 0141 211 6334; 6 Roman Road, Bearsden, Glasgow G61 2SW — MB BS Lond. 1973 (St. Bart.) BSc (Hons.) Lond. 1971; MRCP (UK) 1976; MPhil Camb. 1978, MD 1984; FRCP Glas. 1994; FRCP Lond. 1995. Director, Scott. Pulm. Vasc. Unit; Vis. Sci. Nat. Heart & Lung Inst.; Respirat. Research Fellowship. Specialty: Respirat. Med. Socs: Assn. Phys. Of Gt. Britain & Irel.; Amer. thoracic Soc.; Europ. thoracic Soc. Prev: Cons. Phys. (Respirat. Med.) West. Infirm. Glas.; Sen. Regist. (Thoracic Med.) Soton. Hosps.; Vis. Scientist Cardiovasc. Pulm. Research Laborat. Denver, Colorado.

PEACOCK, Brian Silver Street Surgery, 26 Silver Street, Great Barford, Bedford MK44 3HX Tel: 01234 870325 Fax: 01234 871323 — MB BS Lond. 1983 (St. Mary's) DRCOG 1988. Prev: SHO (Paediat., O & G & Orthop.) Bedford Gen. Hosp.

PEACOCK, Christine Elizabeth (retired) Bliss Cottage, Hentland, Ross-on-Wye HR9 6LP Tel: 01989 730427 Fax: 01298 815506 Email: chrispeacock@doctors.org.uk — MB ChB Manch. 1962; BSc (1st cl. Hons.) Physiol. Manch. 1962; MB ChB Manch. 1980; DRCOG 1982; MFCH 1990. Prev: Sen. Med. Off. i/c Stud. Health Centre Manch.

PEACOCK, Clare Top Flat, 50 Gloucester St., Pimlico, London SW1V 4EH — MB BS Lond. 1989; MRCP (UK) 1993. Regist. (Radiol.) Soton. Gen. Hosp. Specialty: Radiol. Prev: Regist. (ITU) Roy. N.shore Hosp. Sydney, Austral.; Acting Regist. (Cardiol. & Chest) Roy. Sussex Co. Hosp.; SHO Rotat. (A & E & Med.) Roy. Sussex Co. Hosp.

PEACOCK, David MDP Practice, 44 High Street, Portaferry, Newtownards BT22 1QT Tel: 028 9128 420 Fax: 028 4272 9834 — MB BCh BAO Belf. 1972; DObst RCOG 1974; MRCGP 1976.

PEACOCK, Gillian Frances The Old Manor, Ubley, Bristol BS40 6PJ — MB ChB Bristol 1952.

PEACOCK, Ian Castle House, 2 Castle Hill, Duffield, Belper DE56 4EA Tel: 01332 842663 Fax: 01332 843075 Email: ip@btinternet.com — MB BChir Camb. 1974; MD Camb. 1985; FRCP Lond. 1994. Specialty: Gen. Med.; Diabetes; Endocrinol. Prev: Cons. Phys. (Diabetes) Derbysh. Roy. Infirm.; Research Fell. (Diabetes) & Regist. (Med.) Univ. Hosp. Nottm.; Sen. Regist. (Med.) Nottm. City Hosp.

PEACOCK, Joanna Elizabeth Margaret The Surgery, 75 Bank St., Alexandria G83 0NB Tel: 01389 752626 Fax: 01389 752169; 25 Mansewood Drive, Dumbarton G82 3EU Tel: 01389 767174 — MB ChB Glas. 1956. Prev: Med. Miss. Duncan Hosp. Raxaul India; SHO (Surg.) Vale of Leven Hosp. Alexandria.

PEACOCK, John Stable Fold Surgery, Church St., Westhoughton, Bolton BL5 3SF Tel: 01942 813678 Fax: 01942 812028; Blythewood, 13 Towncroft Lane, Heaton, Bolton BL1 5EW Tel: 01204 847626 — MB ChB Sheff. 1966; DObst RCOG 1968.

PEACOCK, John Edward Department of Anaesthetics, C Floor, Royal Hallamshire Hospital, Glossop Road, Sheffield S10 2JF Tel: 0114 271 2494 Fax: 0114 279 8314 Email: john.peacock@sth.nhs.uk; 10 Crimicar Lane, Fulwood, Sheffield S10 4FB — MB ChB Sheff. 1979; FRCA 1985. Cons. Anaesth. Roy. Hallamsh. Hosp. Sheff. Specialty: Anaesth. Socs: Soc. Intravenous Anaesth. (UK). Prev: Sen. Lect. (Anaesth.) Univ. Sheff.

PEACOCK, Kate Elizabeth 124 Broadway N., Walsall WS1 2QE — MB ChB Bristol 1993.

PEACOCK, Kim Field House Medical Centre, 13 Dudley Street, Grimsby DN31 2AE Tel: 01472 350327; 12 Dudley Street, Grimsby DN31 2AB Tel: 01472 50327 — MB ChB Sheff. 1974; DRCOG 1976.

PEACOCK, Matthew Lockhart (retired) 25 Mansewood Drive, Dumbarton G82 3EU Tel: 01389 767174 — MB ChB Glas. 1956. Prev: GP Alexandria.

PEACOCK, Sharon Jayne Nyfield Department of Pathology & Baderology, Level 4 Academic Block, John Radcliffe Hospital, Oxford OX3 9DU Tel: 01865 741166 — BM Soton. 1988; MRCP (UK) 1991; DTM & H RCP Lond. 1994; MSc Lond. 1994; BA (Open) 1995; MRCPath 1997. Univ. Lect. & Hon. Cons. (MicroBiol.). Specialty: Med. Microbiol. Prev: Wellcome Research Fell. & Hon. Sen. Regist. (Microbiol.) John Radcliffe Hosp. Oxf.; Regist. (Microbiol.) John Radcliffe Hosp. Oxf.; SHO (Med.) John Radcliffe Hosp. Oxf., Whittington Hosp. Lond. & Roy. Sussex Co. Hosp. Brighton.

PEACOCK, Simon Gregory Leeds Student Medical Practice, 4 Blenheim Court Walk, Leeds LS2 9AE Tel: 0113 295 4488 — MB ChB Leeds 1989; MRCGP 1993.

PEACOCK, Stephen Richard The Surgery, Woden Road, Wolverhampton WV10 0BD Tel: 01902 454242 Fax: 01902 352438 — BM Soton. 1982. Specialty: Gen. Pract.

PEACOCK, Timothy Edward The Old Vicarage, Easthall Road, North Kelsey, Market Rasen LN7 6HA — MB ChB Manch. 1997.

PEACOCK, Timothy Guy Meadowcroft Surgery, Jackson Road, Aylesbury HP19 9EX Tel: 01296 425775 Fax: 01296 330324; 4 Spenser Road, Aylesbury HP21 7LR Tel: 01296 81364 — MB ChB Bristol 1979; MRCGP 1985; DRCOG 1987. Prev: Surg. Lt. RN.

PEACOCK, Vanessa Anne 70 Rannoch Drive, Mansfield NG19 6QX — MB BS Newc. 1992.

PEAD, Michael Elliott 70 Putnoe Street, Bedford MK41 8HL — MB BS Lond. 1986. Specialty: Anaesth.

PEAKE, David Ronald Queen Elizabeth Hospital, Edgbaston, Birmingham B15 2TH Tel: 0121 697 8350 — MB ChB Liverp. 1984; MRCP (UK) 1989; FRCR 1994. Cons. Clin. Oncologist, Qu. Eliz. Hosp., Birm. Specialty: Oncol.; Radiother. Prev: Regist. (Med.) Roy. Liverp. Hosp.; Regist. (Med.) Arrowe Pk. Hosp. Wirral Merseyside.; Regist. (Radiotherap. & Oncol.) Clatterbridge Hosp. Merseyside.

PEAKE, Michael David Respiratory Medicine Unit, Glenfield Hospital, Groby Rd, Leicester LE3 9QP Tel: 0116 250 2610 Fax: 0116 250 2415 Email: mick.peake@uhl-tr.nhs.uk; 6 Riverside Mews, Wanlip, Leicester LE7 4PH — MB ChB Birm. 1973; MRCP (UK) 1976; FRCP Lond. 1990. Cons. Phys. Glenfield Hosp, Leicester; Lead clinician for lung cancer; assoc director, CEEU, Roy. Coll. of Phys.s of Lond.; Nat. Lead Clinician for Lung Cancer, Cancer Servs. Collaborative. Specialty: Respirat. Med. Special Interest: Lung Cancer and Mesothelioma. Socs: Med. Research Soc.; Eur. Respirat. Soc.; International Association Study of Lung Cancer. Prev: Peel Trust Research Fell. Johns Hopkins Hosp. Baltimore, USA; Lect. & MRC Research Fell. Profess. Med. Unit Univ. Sheff.; Cons. Phys. Pontefract Gen. Infirm.

PEAKMAN, David John 16 Rectory Terrace, Gosforth, Newcastle upon Tyne NE3 1YB Tel: 0191 213 2863 Email: dj@peakman.com — MB BS Lond. 1979 (Univ. Coll. Hosp.) BSc (Hons.) Lond. 1976; FRCR 1986; MS Newc. 1994. Cons. Radiol. Qu. Eliz. Hosp. Gateshead; Hon. Lect. Med. Sch. Newc. Specialty: Radiol.

PEAKMAN, Mark 12 Ferndene Road, London SE24 0AQ — MB BS Lond. 1984 (Univ. Lond.) MSc Lond. 1988, BSc 1981, MB BS 1984; MRCPath 1992; PhD 1993. Lect. (Immunol.) & Hon. Sen. Regist. (Immunol.) King's Coll. Sch. Med. Dent. Specialty: Immunol. Prev: Wellcome Research Train. Fell. & Hon. Sen. Regist. (Immunol.) King's Coll. Hosp. Lond.

PEARCE, Adrian Colven Department of Anaesthetics, Guy's Hospital, London SE1 9RT — MB BChir Camb. 1976; MA, MB Camb. 1976, BChir 1975; FFA RCS Eng. 1980; MRCP (UK) 1981. Cons. Anaesth. Guy's Hosp., Lond. Specialty: Anaesth.

PEARCE, Alan John (retired) — MB ChB Birm. 1945; MRCS Eng. LRCP Lond. 1945; FRCGP 1970, M 1953. Prev: Clin. Asst. Migraine Clinic Birm. & Midl. Eye Hosp.

PEARCE, Alan John Seaforth Farm Surgery, Vicarage Lane, Hailsham BN27 1BH Tel: 01323 848494 Fax: 01323 849316 — MB BS Lond. 1984; DRCOG 1987; DCH RCP Lond. 1988; MRCGP 1988; Dip. IMC RCS Ed. 1995. Specialty: Gen. Pract.

PEARCE, Alison Virginia 44 Bettwys-y-Coed Road, Cardiff CF23 6PL — BM Soton. 1989; MRCP (UK) 1994.

PEARCE, Andrew Francis Bissett Lydbrook Health Centre, Lydbrook GL17 9LG Tel: 01594 860219 Fax: 01594 860987 — MB BS London 1974; MB BS 1974 Lond. GP Lydbrook, Glos.

PEARCE, Anthony John (retired) 22 Park Road, Wollaston, Stourbridge DY8 3QX Tel: 01384 392723 — (Birm.) MB ChB Birm. 1951; DObst RCOG 1958. Prev: Ho. Surg. (O & G) Ronkswood Hosp. Worcester.

PEARCE, Callum Bruce 31 Orchards Way, Highfield, Southampton SO17 1RF — MB ChB Liverp. 1992.

PEARCE, Caroline Elizabeth — MB ChB Sheff. 1998.

PEARCE, Catherine Rebecca 33 Forest Drive West, London E11 1JZ — MB BS Lond. 1998.

PEARCE, Christopher Jon West Cottage, Grandon Lodge, South Holmwood, Dorking RH5 4LT — MB ChB Manch. 1998.

PEARCE, Christopher Patrick Reepham Surgery, Smugglers Lane, Reepham, Norwich NR10 4QT Tel: 01603 870271 Fax: 01603 872995 — MB BChir Camb. 1989.

PEARCE, Daniel Jon — BM Soton. 1997; MRCPsych 2003.

PEARCE, Daryl Elizabeth 51 Middle Park Road, Birmingham B29 4BH Tel: 0121 475 3600 — MB BS Lond. 1991; BDS Birm. 1981; BSc (Hons.) Lond. 1988; DFFP 1995; MRCGP 1995. Specialty: Gen. Pract.

PEARCE, David Nigel The Laurels CMHL, Newton Abbot Hospital, 62 East Street, Newton Abbot TQ12 4PT — MB BCh Wales 1986. Staff Grade (Psychiat.) Newton Abbot Hosp. Specialty: Gen. Psychiat. Prev: SHO Rainhill Hosp. Prescot; Ho. Off. Ysbyty Gwynedd; Ho. Off. Ysbyty Glan Clwyd.

PEARCE, Douglas John (retired) The Old Vicarage, Forest Park Road, Brockenhurst SO42 7SW Tel: 01590 622001 — MB BS Lond. 1950 (Westm.) MRCS Eng. LRCP Lond. 1950; DA Eng. 1952; FFA RCS Eng. 1954. Prev: Cons. Anaesth. Soton. & SW Hants. Health Dist.(T).

PEARCE, Drusilla Ann Bromley NHS Trust, Orpington Hospital, Sevenoaks Road, Orpington BR6 9JU Tel: 01689 815100 Fax: 01689 815285; Coldharbour, Bletchingley, Redhill RH1 4NA Tel: 01883 742685 Fax: 01883 743661 — MB BS Lond. 1971 (King's Coll. Hosp.) BSc (Pharmacol.) Lond. 1968, MB BS 1971; FRCR 1977. Clin. Dir. - diagnostic imaging; Cons. Radiol. Bromley HA. Specialty: Radiol. Prev: Sen. Cons. Dept. Diag. Radiol. Riyadh & Al Khari Hosp. Progr. Saudi Arabia; Sen. Regist. (Radiol.) King's Coll. Hosp. Lond.

PEARCE, Florence Muriel (retired) 30 Dulwich Common, London SE21 7EX Tel: 020 8693 4189 — MB BS Lond. 1946 (W. Lond.)

PEARCE, Gillian 10 Kings Hill Fields, Wednesbury WS10 9JF — BM BCh Oxf. 1997; BSc (Hons.) CNAA 1980; Fell Roy Astronom Soc. 1981; PhD Keele Univ. 1983; BSc (Hons.) Wolverhampton 1994. Ho. Off. (Med.) Wordsley Hosp. Stourbridge; SHO (Orthop.) Princess Roy. Hosp. Telford, Shrops. Specialty: Orthop. Socs: Med. Protec. Soc. Prev: Res. Fell. (Astrophysics) Univ. Wolverhampton 1992-1999; Lect. & Atlas Research Fell. (Astrophysics) Oxf. Univ. 1987-1992, 1993; Vis. Res. Fells. GSFC/NASA 1991, Univ. Glas. 1992.

PEARCE, Hilary Lockhart — MB ChB Dundee 1997. SHO3 (Paed) Roy. Hosp. For Sick Childr. Edin. Specialty: Paediat. Prev: SHO (Paed) Yorkhill Hosp. Glas.

PEARCE, Mr Ian 7 Brockholes, Simmondley, Glossop SK13 6YT Tel: 0411 696217 — BM BS Nottm. 1993 (Univ. of Nottm.) BMedSci (Hons.) 1991; FRCS Glas. 1997. Specialist Regist. Rotat.

Urol. Manch. Specialty: Urol. Socs: Roy. Soc. Med.; Assn. Surg. Train.

PEARCE, James Frederick (retired) Bryony Cottage, New House Lane, Poslingford, Clare, Sudbury CO10 8QX Tel: 01787 278624 — MB BS Lond. 1954 (St. Bart.) DPM 1963; BSc (1st cl. Hons.) Lond. 1951, MD 1964; MRCPsych 1972. Prev: Cons. Psychiat. Home Office Prison Dept.

PEARCE, Jennifer Jane Sunbury Health Centre Group Practice, Green Street, Sunbury-on-Thames TW16 6RH Tel: 01932 713399 Fax: 01932 713354; 181 French Street, Sunbury-on-Thames TW16 5JY — MB BS Lond. 1974 (Middlesex) MRCP (UK) 1976.

PEARCE, Professor John Barber 4 Knighton Drive, Leicester LE2 3HB Tel: 0116 2929055 Fax: 0116 2929055 — (Univ. Coll. Hosp.) MB BS Lond. 1965; DCH RCP Lond. 1968; MRCP (UK) 1970; FRCPsych 1984, M 1973; MPhil Lond. 1974; FRCP Lond. 1991. Prof. Child & Adolesc. Psychiat. Nottm. Univ. Specialty: Child & Adolesc. Psychiat. Prev: Cons. Child & Adolesc. Psychiat. Guy's Hosp. Lond.; Sen. Regist. Maudsley Hosp. Lond.; Regist. (Paediat.) St. Bart. Hosp. Lond.

PEARCE, John Leonard — MB BS Lond. 1967 (St. Thos.) DCH Eng. 1969; FRACP 1976; FRCP Lond. 1993; FRCPCH 1999. Cons. (Paediat.) E. Berks. Health Dist. Specialty: Paediat. Socs: Brit. Paediat. Assn. Prev: Cons. Paediat. Taranaki Hosp. Bd., NZ; Sen. Regist. (Paediat.) ChristCh. Pub. Hosp., NZ; Resid. Hosp. Sick Childr. Toronto, Canada.

PEARCE, John Macfarlane Church Street Surgery, 30 Church Street, Dunoon PA23 8BG Tel: 01369 703482/702772 Fax: 01369 704502; Lochview, sandbank, Dunoon PA23 8QH Tel: 01369 706241 — MB ChB Manch. 1979. Prev: Trainee GP Paisley VTS.

PEARCE, John Michael Schofield 304 Beverley Road, Anlaby, Hull HU10 7BG Tel: 01482 654165 Fax: 01482 654165 Email: jmspearce@freenet.co.uk — MB ChB Leeds 1959; MB ChB (Hons.) Leeds 1959; FRCP Lond. 1975, M 1962; MD Leeds 1965. Emerit. Cons. Neurol. Hull. Specialty: Neurol. Socs: Assn. Brit. Neurol. (Ex. Counc.); (Exec Comm.) Assn. Phys.; (Pres. Counc.) N. Eng. Neurol. Assn. Prev: Sen. Regist. (Neurol.) Gen. Infirm. Leeds; Fulbright Trav. Fell. (Neurol.) Mass. Gen. Hosp. Boston, USA; Clin. Research Fell. & Regist. (Neurol.) Regional Neurol. Centre Newc.

PEARCE, Jonathan Christopher The Surgery, Stone Drive, Colwall, Malvern WR13 6QJ Tel: 01684 540323; Woostock, Walwyn Road, Upper Colwall, Malvern WR13 6PR Tel: 01684 541144 — MB ChB Birm. 1981; DA Eng. 1983; DRCOG 1985. Prev: SHO (O & G) Worcs.; SHO (Anaesth.) Shrewsbury; SHO (Med.) Abergavenny.

PEARCE, Mr Jonathan Gale St. Sampsons Medical Centre, Grandes Maison Road, St Sampsons, Guernsey GY2 4JS Tel: 01481 45915 — MB ChB Zimbabwe 1983; LRCP LRCS Ed. LRCPS Glas. 1983; FRCS Glas. 1990; Dip MS Med 2002.

PEARCE, Juliet Anne 50 Cottonmill Lane, St Albans AL1 2BB MB BS Lond. 1993.

PEARCE, Katherine Anne — BM BCh Oxf. 1988; MRCGP 1994.

PEARCE, Katherine Jane Dr Conrad & Partners, Willow Surgery, Coronation Road, Downend, Bristol BS16 Tel: 0117 956 2979/0117 970 9500 — BM Soton. 1989. GP Retainer, Willow Surg., Coronation Rd. Specialty: Gen. Pract. Prev: SHO (Paediat.) Southmead Hosp. Bristol; SHO (Psychiat.) Southmead Hosp. Bristol; SHO (O & G) Fairfield Hosp. Bury.

PEARCE, Keith William Hamilton Road Surgery, 201 Hamilton Road, Felixstowe IP11 7DT Tel: 01394 283197 Fax: 01394 270304 — MB BS Lond. 1982.

PEARCE, Mark Quentin 42 Dorchester Road, Tolpuddle, Dorchester DT2 — MB BS Lond. 1991.

PEARCE, Mary-Jane The Fulbrook Centre, Churchill Hospital, Old Road, Headington, Oxford OX3 7JU Tel: 01865 223840 Fax: 01865 223829; 72 Lonsdale Road, Oxford OX2 7EP — BM BS Nottm. 1976; BMedSci Nottm. 1974; MRCGP 1980; MRCPsych 1983; FRCPsych 2001. Cons. Psychiat. Oxf. Ment. Healthcare Trust. Specialty: Geriat. Psychiat. Prev: Cons. Psychiat. Oxf. HA.

PEARCE, Meryn McLachlan (retired) 23 Carnethy Avenue, Edinburgh EH13 0DL Tel: 0131 441 2142 — MB ChB Ed. 1961; DCH Eng. 1963. Prev: Clin. Med. Off. Edin. Sick Childr. Hosp. Trust.

PEARCE, Michael John — MB ChB Leic. 1998.

PEARCE, Neil William Southampton General Hospital, Department of Surgery, E Level, West Wing, Southampton SO16 6YD Tel: 023 8079 6977; The Lichen, Newport Lane, Braishfield, Romsey SO51 0PL Tel: 01794 368351 — BM Soton. 1990; FRCS Eng. 1995; DM Soton. 2004. Specialist Regist. (Gen. Surg.) Wessex Rotat.; Cons. Gen. Surg. Soton. Gen. Hosp. Specialty: Gen. Surg. Special Interest: HPB Surg.

PEARCE, Nicholas Ricardo Sunbury Health Centre Group Practice, Green Street, Sunbury-on-Thames TW16 6RH Tel: 01932 713399 Fax: 01932 713354; 181 French Street, Sunbury-on-Thames TW16 5JY — MB BS Lond. 1976; BSc Cardiff 1970.

PEARCE, Paula Ann 5 Churchmere Drive, Crewe CW1 4SN — BM BS Nottm. 1992.

PEARCE, Richard Jack Ivry Street Medical Practice, 5 Ivry Street, Ipswich IP1 3QW Tel: 01473 254718 Fax: 01473 287790 — MB BS Lond. 1972 (King's Coll. Hosp.) DObst RCOG 1974. Prev: SHO (Paediat.), (Cas.) & (O & G) Ipswich Hosp.

PEARCE, Robert Handel (retired) 32 Gloster Gardens, Wellesbourne, Warwick CV35 9TQ — (Lond. Hosp.) MRCS Eng. LRCP Lond. 1960; MB BS Lond. 1961; MRCGP 1976; Dip. Pract. Dermat. Wales 1991; DFFP 1994. Prev: Med. Off. Myton Hamlet Hospice Warwick.

PEARCE, Robert Leslie Vernon (retired) Dorincourt, 51 The Glade, Leatherhead KT22 9TB Tel: 01372 453559 — (Westm.) MB BS Lond. 1956; MRCS Eng. LRCP Lond. 1956; DCH RCP Lond. 1960; FRCPC 1971. Prev: Regist. (Med.) Stoke Mandeville Hosp.

PEARCE, Ruth Elizabeth Dale End Surgery, Danby, Whitby YO21 2JE Tel: 01287 660739 Fax: 01287 660069 — MB BS Lond. 1986; DRCOG 1991; Dip Therap. Newc. 2000. GP Princip. Danby Whitby. Prev: GP Train. Scheme Harrogate Healthcare Trust; Ho. Off. (Med.) Bedford Gen. Hosp.; SHO (Med.) S. Cleveland Hosp. Middlesbrough.

PEARCE, Sarah Jane 9 Almoner's Barn, Durham DH1 3TZ Tel: 0191 383 2469 Fax: 0191 383 9859 — MB ChB Cape Town 1967; MRCP (UK) 1970; FRCP Lond. 1985; Cert. of Med. Educat. Newc. 2000. Cons. Gen. Med. & Respirat., Dis. Univ. Hosp. of N. Durh.; Hon. Clin. Sen. Lect. Univ. Newc. Specialty: Respirat. Med. Socs: Europ. Respiratoy Soc.; Roy. Soc. of Med.; Brit. Thorac. Soc. Prev: Sen. Regist. (Med.) Newc. AHA (T); Regist. (Med.) Southmead Hosp. Bristol; Regist. Chest Unit City Hosp. Edin.

PEARCE, Sarah Nicole Palace Flop House, Manor Farm, Chillington, Ilminster TA19 0PU Tel: 01460 52646 Fax: 01460 52646 — MB ChB Bristol 1994. SHO Barley Wood Alcohol & Drug Rehabil. Centre, Bristol. Specialty: Alcohol & Substance Misuse.

PEARCE, Simon Henry Schofield Endocrine Unit, Royal Victoria Infirmary, Newcastle upon Tyne NE1 4LP — MB BS Newc. 1989; MB BS (1st cl. Hons.) Newc. 1989; MRCP (UK) 1992; MD 1998. Senior Lecturer in Endocrinology, Honorary Consultant Physician, University of Newcastle. Specialty: Endocrinol. Socs: Soc. Endocrinol.; Bone & Tooth Soc.; Amer. Soc. Bone & Mineral Research. Prev: MRC Train. Fell. Roy. Postgrad. Med. Sch. Lond.; Regional Regist. Rotat. (Diabetes & Endocrinol.) North. Region; Advanced Research Fell & Hon. Sen. Regist. (Med.) Univ. Newc. u. Tyne.

PEARCE, Stephen Dept. of Psychiatry, Royal Southants Hospital, Brintons Terrace, Southampton SO14 0YG — MB ChB Manch. 1990; BSc St. And. 1987; MRCP (UK) 1993; MRCPsych 1996.

PEARCE, Sushmita 8 Whinney Lane, Langho, Blackburn BB6 8DC; 6 Rider Road, Hillsborough, Sheffield S6 2LH Tel: 0114 234 9618 — BM BS Nottm. 1993; BMedSci (Hons.) Nottm. 1991; MRCP (UK) 1997. Specialty: Endocrinol.

PEARCE, Thomas Trien Surgery, Trien, Carbost, Isle of Skye IV47 8ST Tel: 01478 640202 Fax: 01478 640464 — MB ChB Manch. 1972. Prev: Med. Off. Brit. Antarctic Survey 1974-75; Chief Med. Off. Govt. Med. Dept. Falkland Is.

PEARCE, Vanessa Lynne Churchside Medical Practice, Wood Street, Mansfield NG18 1QB Tel: 01623 622541 Fax: 01623 423821; The Beeches, Main St, Eakring, Newark NG22 0DD — MB ChB Leeds 1989; DRCOG 1992; DFFP 1994; MRCGP 1994.

PEARCE, Vaughan Roy Royal Devon & Exeter Hospital (Wonford), Barrack Road, Exeter EX2 5DW — MRCS Eng. LRCP Lond. 1972 (St Mary's Hospital) BSc Lond. 1969, MB BS 1972; MRCP (UK) 1975; FRCP Lond. 1989. Cons. Phys. Roy. Devon & Exeter Hosp. (Wonford). Specialty: Gen. Med.; Care of the Elderly. Prev: Sen. Regist. Chesterton Hosp. Camb.

PEARCE, Walter Brian (retired) West Hill House, Blunsdon, Swindon SN26 7BN Tel: 01793 721218 — MB BS Lond. 1959 (Guy's) MRCS Eng. LRCP Lond. 1959; DObst RCOG 1963. Prev: Clin. Asst. (Obst.) Princess Marg. Hosp. Swindon.

PEARCY, Patricia Alison Mary — MB BS Durh. 1960; DObst RCOG 1961; DPH Newc. 1968. Prev: Sen. Research Asst. Dept. Midw. & Gyn. Univ. Newc.

PEARCY, Richard Malcolm 1 Winchcombe Road, Frampton Cotterell, Bristol BS36 2AG Tel: 01454 773102 — MB BS (Hons.) Lond. 1993 (St Geo.) BSc (Hons.) Lond. 1990; FRCS Eng. 1997; FRCS Ed. 1997; FRCSI 1997; MD Bristol 2003. BAUS Sen. Clin. Fell. in Andrology. Specialty: Urol. Prev: Specialist Regist. (Urol.) SW Region; Research Regist. (Urol. Surg.) Taunton; SHO Rotat. (Surg.) Bristol.

PEARD, Mary Catherine (retired) 2 Squires Close, Crawley Down, Crawley RH10 4JQ Tel: 01342 712540 — MB BS Lond. 1952 (Roy. Free) FRCP Lond.; FRCPCH. Prev: Cons. Paediat. Crawley & Redhill Hosps.

PEARL, Bradley Andrew The Foreland Medical Centre, 188 Walmer Road, London W11 4EP Tel: 020 7727 2604 Fax: 020 7792 1261; 47 Vespan Road, London W12 9QG — MB BS Lond. 1983; BSc Lond. 1980, MB BS 1983; DRCOG 1985; MRCGP 1987. Specialty: Gen. Psychiat.; HIV Med.; Palliat. Med.

PEARL, Robert Ashley — BM Soton. 1998.

PEARL, Stephanie Ann 8 Culcabock Road, Inverness IV2 3XQ — MB ChB Glas. 1997; BA (Oxon) 1987; DRCOG 1999. GP Train. Scheme, Highlands,. Specialty: Gen. Pract.

PEARLGOOD, Morris, SBStJ 40 Westmount Road, Eltham Park, London SE9 1JE Email: mpearlgood@doctors.net.uk; 40 Westmount Road, Eltham Park, London Tel: 020 8850 2870 Email: mpearlgood@doctors.net. Uk — MB ChB Sheff. 1962; DObst RCOG 1964; MRCGP 1972. p/t Indep. Cons., Med. Adviser Non-Princip. GP; Cons. Med. Adviser to Bexley, Bromley & Greenwich HA and Bexley PCT; Med. Mem. of Appeals Tribunals; Med. Adviser Publishing. Specialty: Psychother.; Obst. & Gyn.; Med. Publishing. Prev: Gp. Med. Edr. Modern Med. Gp. UK; Hosp. Pract. (Psychiat.) FarnBoro. Hosp. Kent; Ho. Surg. & Ho. Phys. City Gen. Hosp. Sheff.

PEARLMAN, Juliet Ann 29 Firbeck Road, Bramham, Wetherby LS23 6NE — MB ChB Leeds 1983; MRCGP 1987; DRCOG 1987; AFOM RCP Lond. 1993. Dep. Force Med. Off. W. Yorks. Police. Specialty: Occupat. Health.

PEARMAIN, Brendan Michael Paul 20 Scratton Road, Southend-on-Sea SS1 1EN — MB BS Lond. 1994.

PEARMAN, Mr Kenneth ENT Department, Birmingham Heartlands Hopsital, Bordeslet Green East, Birmingham B9 5SS Tel: 0121 4242351; 33 Rollswood Drive, Solihull B91 1NL Tel: 0121 7044429 Email: k@pearman.demon.co.uk — MB BS Lond. 1970 (Roy. Free) MRCS Eng. LRCP Lond. 1970; FRCS Eng. 1975. Cons. ENT Surg. Birm. Heartlands & Solihull Hosp. Trust, Childr. Hosp. Birm. Specialty: Otorhinolaryngol. Socs: Roy. Soc. Med. & Brit. Assn. Paediat. Otorhinlaryng.

PEARS, Carl Richard Hereward Medical Centre, Exeter Street, Bourne PE10 9NJ Tel: 01778 393 399 Fax: 01778 391 715 — MB BS Lond. 1990 (St. George's Hospital Medical School) MRCGP 1995; DFFP 1995. GP Partner; GP Trainer. Specialty: Gen. Pract. Prev: GP The Doctors Ltd. Napier, Hawkes Bay, New Zealand; Duke of Cornw. Spinal Injuries Unit Salisbury; GP VTS Gr. Ho. Surg. & Salisbury Dist. Hosp.

PEARS, Jane Reedsford, Mindrum TD12 4QQ — MB ChB Manch. 1996.

PEARS, John Stuart Medical Research Department, Zeneca Pharmaceuticals, Mereside, Macclesfield SK10 4TG Tel: 01625 515617 Fax: 01625 585626; 17 Hall Road, Wilmslow SK9 5BN Tel: 01625 524453 — MB ChB Ed. 1983; MRCP (UK) 1987; MD Ed. 1993; Dip. Pharm. Med. RCP (UK) 1994. Med. Advisor Zeneca Pharmaceut. Macclesfield.; Clin. Asst. Manch. Diabetes Centre. Specialty: Pharmaceutical Medicine. Prev: Dep. Dir. Drug Developm. (Scotl.) Ltd.; Novo Research Fell. (Diabetic) Ninewells Hosp. Dundee; Regist. (Med. & Endocrinol.) Ninewells Hosp. Dundee.

PEARS, Peter Edwin Hazelwood, 27 Parkfield Road, Coleshill, Birmingham B46 3LD Tel: 01675 463165 — MB ChB Dundee 1972; DObst RCOG 1974; MRCGP 1977. Med. Adviser (Adoptions) Father Hudson's Soc. Birm. Specialty: Gen. Pract. Socs: Birm. & Midl. Med. Inst. Prev: SHO (Paediat.) Maelor Gen. Hosp. Wrexham; SHO (O & G) Norf. & Norwich Hosp. Norwich; Ho. Surg. & Ho. Phys. Bridge of Earn Hosp.

PEARSALL, Fiona Jean Burns Directorate of Anaesthesia, Royal Infirmary, Castle St., Glasgow G4 0SF — MB ChB Glas. 1986; FRCA 1991; MSc (Med. Sci.) Glas. 1993. Cons. (Anaesth.) Roy. Infirm. Glas.; Hon. Sen. Clin. Lect. Glas. Univ. Specialty: Anaesth. Socs: GMC (Counc. Mem.); BMA; Assn. Anaesths. Prev: Sen. Regist. (Anaesth.) Glas. Roy. Infirm.; Research Regist. (Anaesth.) West. Infirm. Glas.; Regist. (Anaesth.) Vict. Infirm. Glas.

PEARSALL, Robert William Harold 54 Newark Drive, Pollokshields, Glasgow G41 4PX — MB ChB Glas. 1988.

PEARSE, Andrew John — MB ChB Manch. 1998.

PEARSE, Dorothy Jill 98 Marsh Lane, Stanmore HA7 4HP Tel: 020 8954 4075 — MB BS Lond. 1949 (King's Coll. Hosp.) MRCS Eng. LRCP Lond. 1949.

PEARSE, Hazel Anne 82 Bolingbroke Road, Cleethorpes DN35 0HQ — MB ChB Leeds 1994.

PEARSE, Helen Roxane Amherst Medical Practice, 21 St. Botolphs Road, Sevenoaks TN13 3AQ Tel: 01732 459255 Fax: 01732 450751 — MB BCh Witwatersrand 1991 (Univ. Witwatersrand) DCH RCP Lond. 1996; MRCGP, UK 1998. Socs: Med. Protec. Soc.; BMA.

PEARSE, Henry Arthur Chernocke Caen Health Centre, Braunton EX33 1LR Tel: 01271 812005; Fullabrook Mill, Little Comfort, Braunton EX33 2NJ Tel: 0127 814735 — (Birm.) BSc Physiol. (1st cl. Hons.) Birm. 1985; MB ChB Birm. 1988; DCH Otago 1992; MRCGP 1998. GP Braunton N. Devon. Specialty: Paediat. Prev: Govt. Med. Off. (Police & Prisons) Bermuda; SHO (Paediat.) Poole Gen. Hosp.; Regist. (Paediat.) Wellington NZ.

PEARSE, Mr Michael Department Orthopaedic Surgery, Central Middlesex Hospital, Acton Lane, Park Royal, London NW10 7NS Tel: 020 8453 2423 Fax: 020 8453 2579 Email: m.pearse@ic.ac.uk; Department of Orthopaediac Surgery, Charing Cross Hospital, Fulham Palace Road, London W6 8RF Tel: 020 8846 1473 — MB ChB Leic. 1984; FRCS Ed. 1988; FRCS (Orth.) 1993. Sen. Lect. (Orthop. Surg.) Hammersmith Hosps. Trust; Vis. Asst. Prof. Univ. Texas Med. Sch. Houston, USA 1995; Hon. Cons. Centr. Middlx. Hosp. Lond. Specialty: Trauma & Orthop. Surg. Socs: Assoc. Mem. BOA; Brit. Orthop. Research Soc. Prev: Sen. Regist. Rotat. (Orthop.) Bristol, Frenchay & Plymouth Hosps.; Clin. Research Fell. (Arthritis & Rheum. Counc.) Univ. Dept. Orthop. Surg. Bristol Roy. Infirm.; Regist. (Orthop.) Princess Eliz. Orthop. Hosp.

PEARSE, Patricia Alcyone Everson Highgate Group Practice, 44 North Hill, London N6 4QA Tel: 020 8348 6628 — MB BS Lond. 1973; DCH Eng. 1978. GP Highgate.

PEARSE, Richard Granville The Jessop Wing, Sheff. Teachg. Hosps. NHS Trust, Sheffield S10 2SF Tel: 0114 226 8000; Bourne House, 49 Westbourne Road, Sheffield S10 2QT Tel: 0114 268 3027 Fax: 0114 267 1300 Email: rgpearse@hotmail.com — MB BChir Camb. 1969 (St. Thos.) MA Camb. 1970; FRCP Lond. 1988, M 1974. Cons. Neonat. Paediat. Jessop Wing, Sheff. Teachg. Hosps. NHS Trust. Specialty: Neonat. Prev: Lect. (Paediat.) & Hon. Sen. Regist. St. Thos. Hosp. Lond.; Fell. (Paediat. Cardiol.) Hosp. Sick Childr. Toronto, Canada.; Chef De Clin. Neonat. Unit, Acad. Hosp. Rotterdam, Netherlands.

PEARSE, Rupert Mark Flamstead House, Flamstead, St Albans AL3 8BZ — MB BS Lond. 1996.

PEARSE, Sonja Blyton Ciba-Geigy Pharmaceuticals, Wimblehurst Road, Horsham RH12 5AB Tel: 01403 272827; 14 The Murreys, Barnett Wood Lane, Ashtead KT21 2LU Tel: 01372 278530 — MB BCh Wales 1968 (Cardiff) FFA RCS Eng. 1975; MFPM RCP (UK) 1989; FFPM 1992. Head Clin. Drug Safety & Pharmacoepidemiol. Ciba-Geigy Pharmaceut. Horsham. Specialty: Pharmaceutical Medicine. Socs: Fell. Roy. Soc. Med.; Assn. Anaesth. Prev: Dir. Clin. Research (UK & Eire) Cyanamid Internat. Research Centre Richmond; Research Phys. Dept. Internat. Clin. Research Warner Lambert-Pk.e Davis Pontypool; Sen. Regist. (Anaesth.) Qu. Eliz. Hosp. Birm.

PEARSE-DANKER, Steven Christian The Surgery, 9 Ebdon Road, Worle, Weston Super Mare BS22 6UB Tel: 01934 514145 Fax: 01934 521345 — MB BS Lond. 1982.

PEARSON, Alan Ernest Gerald (retired) 29 Birchwood Road, Parkstone, Poole BH14 9NW — MB BChir Camb. 1977 (Camb. & St. Bart.) MA Camb. 1954, BA (Nat. Sc. Trip.) 1952; PhD Lond. 1959. Prev: Assoc. Specialist (Psychiat.) Alderney Hosp. Dorset.

PEARSON, Alison Jane Derwent House Surgery, Derwent House, Wakefield Road, Cockermouth CA13 0HZ Tel: 01900 822345 Fax: 01900 828469 — MB ChB Sheff. 1988; DRCOG; DFFP. GP. Specialty: Gen. Pract. Prev: Trainee GP Cumbria FHSA.

PEARSON, Andrew David Chest Department, 1st Floor Lambeth Wing, Guy's & St Thomas Hospital Trust, Lambeth Palace Road, London SE1 7EH Tel: 020 7922 8046 Fax: 020 7620 2596 — BM BCh Oxf. 1968 (Oxf. & Lond. Hosp.) BA, BM BCh Oxf. 1968; Dip Bact Lond. 1972. Cons. Communicable Dis. Control for Lambeth Lond.; Infect. Control Doctor St. Thos. Hosp. Lond.; Sec. PHLS AIDS Co-ordinating Comm. Specialty: Med. Microbiol. Socs: Amer. Soc. Microbiol. & Brit. Soc. Study Infec. Prev: Dir. Soton. Pub. Health Laborat.; Hon. Clin. Sen. Lect. Soton Univ.; Hon. Cons. Microbiol. Soton & S.W. Hants. HA.

PEARSON, Professor Andrew David John Sir James Spencer Institute of Child Health, Royal Victoria Infirmary, Queen Victoria Road, Newcastle upon Tyne NE1 4LP Tel: 0191 202 3036 Fax: 0191 202 3060 Email: a.d.j.pearson@ncl.ac.uk; 2 Queensway, Ponteland, Newcastle upon Tyne NE20 9RZ — MD Newc. 1989; MB BS (1st Cl. Hons.) 1977; MRCP (UK) 1979; DCH Eng. 1980; FRCP Lond. 1992; FRCPCH 1996. Prof. Paediat. Oncol. Univ. Newc.; Hon. Cons. Child Health Roy. Vict. Infirm. Newc. Specialty: Paediat. Socs: Internat. Soc. Paediat. Oncol. & UK Childr. Cancer Study Gp.; Eur. Neuroblastoma Study Gp. Prev: Sen. Lect. & Lect. (Paediat. Oncol.) Univ. Newc.; Hon. Sen. Regist. (Paediat.) Dept. Child Health Roy. Vict. Infirm. Newc.; Lilly Internat. Med. Research Counc. Trav. fell. Univ. Minnesota, USA.

PEARSON, Andrew James Department of Radiology, Borders General Hospital, Melrose TD6 9BS Tel: 01896 826423 Fax: 01896 826438; Birchdale, Boleside, Galashiels TD1 3NV Tel: 01896 758317 — MB ChB Glas. 1979; FRCR 1987. Cons. Radiol., Borders Gen. Hosp., Melrose. Specialty: Radiol.; Nuclear Med. Socs: Brit. Nuclear Med. Soc.; Eur. Assn. Nuclear Med.; Soc. Nuclear Med. Prev: Sen. Regist. (Radiol.) Manch. Teach. Hosps.; Regist. West. Infirm., Glas.

PEARSON, Andrew Robert — MB BChir Camb. 1989 (Camb. & St. Mary's) MA Camb. 1989; MRCP (UK) 1993; FRCOphth 1996. Cons. (Ophth.) Roy. Berks. Hosp. Reading and King Edwd. VII Hosp. Windsor. Specialty: Ophth. Prev: Specialist Regist. (Ophth.) Leicester Roy. Infirm.

PEARSON, Anne Rachel Newtyle Farmhouse, Drums of Foveran, Ellon AB41 6AS — MB ChB Aberd. 1987; BA York 1978; MRCGP 1991. GP Retainer Scheme Ellon. Prev: Trainee GP Aberd. VTS.

PEARSON, Anthony John Fairway Surgery, 475 Bordesley Green East, Yardley, Birmingham B33 8PP Tel: 0121 783 2125 Fax: 0121 785 0416; Willowbrook Barn, Preston Fields Lane, Lowsonford, Solihull B95 5EZ — MB ChB Birm. 1971; Dip. Occ. Med. 1995. Specialty: Gen. Pract.; Occupat. Health.

PEARSON, Anthony John Grayhurst Barnet General Hospital, Wellhouse Lane, Barnet EN5 3DJ — MRCS Eng. LRCP Lond. 1966; MB Camb. 1967, BChir 1966; MRCP Lond. 1969. Cons. Phys. Barnet Gen. Hosp. Specialty: Gen. Med.

PEARSON, Audrey Vilma Ann 49 High Bannerdown, Batheaston, Bath BA1 7JZ Tel: 01225 858293 Email: pearson@bannerdown.fsnet.co.uk — MRCS Eng. LRCP Lond. 1969; MFHom Lond. 1989; Dip Med Acupunct (BMAS) 1995. p/t Indep. Pract. Homoeopathy & Acupunc. Specialty: Homeop. Med.; Acupunc. Special Interest: Nutrition. Socs: Fac. Homoeop.; Accred. Mem. Brit. Med. Acupunc. Soc.; The Clinical Soc. of Bath. Prev: GP Bath.; Homoeop. Phys. Roy. Lond. Homeop. Hosp.

PEARSON, Benedict Joseph 29 Horton Street, Lincoln LN2 5NG Tel: 01522 511704 — MB BS Lond. 1993.

PEARSON, Beryl Coline Low Lickbarrow Farm, Lickbarrow Close, Heathwaite, Windermere LA23 2NF — MB ChB Liverp. 1949; DCH Eng. 1951. Prev: Ho. Surg. Profess. Unit Broadgreen Hosp. Liverp.; Paediat. Ho. Phys. Taunton & Som. Hosp.; Ho. Surg. O & G Chester City Hosp.

PEARSON, C Michael G Ash Cottage, Farley Common, Westerham TN16 1UB Tel: 01959 65347 — MB BS Lond. 1946 (Guy's) Prev: Ho. Phys. Childr. Dept. Pembury Hosp.; Res. Med. Off. Qu. Eliz. Hosp. Childr. Shadwell.

PEARSON, Mr Charles Justly Probyn, Surg. Capt. RN Retd. Northernhay, Pathfields, Townstal, Dartmouth EX39 2HL — (St. Thos.) MRCS Eng. LRCP Lond. 1932; FRCS Ed. 1935. Prev: Ho. Surg. & Cas. Off. St. Thos. Hosp.

PEARSON, Christine Freya Rodwell, East Dean Road, Lockerley, Romsey SO51 0JQ — MB BS Lond. 1995.

PEARSON, Christopher Alan Robert Stirchley Medical Practice, Stirchley Health Centre, Stirchley, Telford TF3 1FB Tel: 01952 660444 Fax: 01952 415139 — MB ChB Sheff. 1982; DRCOG 1985; MRCGP 1986.

PEARSON, Christopher Almack Aldershot Health Centre, Wellington Avenue, Aldershot GU11 1PA Tel: 01252 324577 Fax: 01252 324861; Lorien, 1 Highlands Close, Shortheath, Farnham GU9 8SP Tel: 01252 24577 — MB BS Lond. 1971 (Middlx.) Specialty: Gen. Pract.

PEARSON, Clive Henry Crown House Surgery, Chapelgate, Retford DN22 6NX Tel: 01777 703672 Fax: 01777 710534 — MB ChB Sheff. 1979.

PEARSON, Daphne Mary (retired) Camelot, 21 The Ridgway, Sutton SM2 5JX Tel: 020 8642 4770 — (Char. Cross) MB BS Lond. 1966; MRCS Eng. LRCP Lond. 1966. Prev: Community Paediat. (SCMO) Richmond, Twickenham & Roehampton.

PEARSON, David Anthony Woolpit Health Centre, Heath Road, Woolpit, Bury St Edmunds IP30 9QU Tel: 01359 240298 Fax: 01359 241975 — (Middlx.) MA, MB BChir Camb. 1980; DRCOG 1982; DCH RCP Lond. 1984; MRCGP 1986; Cert. Av. Med. 1990; MSc 1999. Socs: BMA.

PEARSON, David Charles (retired) Woodland Cottage, Eggerslack, Grange-over-Sands LA11 6EX — MB ChB Birm. 1955; DObst RCOG 1957; FFA RCS Eng. 1964. Prev: Cons. Anaesth. W. Birm. Health Dist.

PEARSON, David Gerald Roger Doctors Surgery, Salisbury Road, Southsea PO4 9QX Tel: 023 9273 1458 — MB BS Lond. 1977 (Univ. Coll. Hosp.) BSc (Pharmacol.) Lond. 1974; DRCOG 1979; MRCGP 1982; Dip. Occ. Med. 1997. Socs: Soc. Occupat. Med.

PEARSON, David John Royd House, 224 Hale Road, Hale, Altrincham WA15 8EB Tel: 0161 998 1999/0161 946 1697 Email: david@allergy.uk.com — MB BS Lond. 1968 (St. Geo.) MRCS Eng. LRCP Lond. 1968; MRCP (UK) 1972; PhD Manch. 1976; FRCP Lond. 1987. Cons. Phys. Univ. Hosp. S. Manch. Specialty: Gen. Med. Socs: Brit. Soc. Allergy & Clin. Immunol.; Eur. Acad. Allergy & Clin. Immunol.; Amer. Acad. Asthma, Allergy & Clin. Immunol. Prev: Sen. Lect. (Med.) Univ. Manch.; Vis. Scientist Nat. Occupat. Safety & Health Pub. Health Serv.; Asst. Prof. (Med.) W. Virginia Univ.

PEARSON, David John Fisher Medical Centre, Millfields, Coach Street, Skipton BD23 1EU — MB ChB Ed. 1988; BA Camb. 1982; MRCGP 1993. Prev: GP/SHO (Gen. Med.) Airedale Gen. Hosp. VTS.

PEARSON, Deborah Christine Johnson & Johnson PRD, 50-100 Holmers Farm Way, High Wycombe HP12 4DP Tel: 01494 658098 — BM BCh Oxf. 1986; MA Camb. 1987; Dip. Pharm. Med. RCP (UK) 1991. Specialty: Pharmaceutical Medicine. Socs: Fac. Pharmaceut. Med.

PEARSON, Deborah Jane Compton Hospice, 4 Compton Road West, Wolverhampton WV3 9DH — MB ChB Birm. 1984; MRCGP 1988. Med. Dir. Compton Hospice Wolverhampton. Specialty: Palliat. Med. Prev: GP Bushbury Wolverhampton; SHO (A & E) Roy. Hosp. Wolverhampton; SHO (Paediat. & O & G) New Cross Hosp. Wolverhampton.

PEARSON, Derek Thomas (retired) 9 Lowther Glen, Eamont Bridge, Penrith CA10 2BP Email: dtpearson@dsl.pipex.com — MB BS Durh. 1959; FRCP Lond. 1976, M 1962; FRCA Eng. 1964. Prev: Cons. Anaesth. Regional Cardiothoracic Centre Freeman Hosp. Newc.

PEARSON, Donald 62 Park Road, Hale, Altrincham WA15 9LR Tel 0161 980 2237 — MD Liverp. 1969; MB ChB 1960; FRCP Lond. 1978, M 1964. Cons. Phys. Warrington Hosp. NHS Trust; Sen. Regist. (Med.) Liverp. Roy. Infirm. Specialty: Gen. Med. Socs: BMA & Liverp. Med. Inst. Prev: Regist. (Med.) Walton Hosp. Liverp. & Vict. Centr. Hosp. Wallasey; Ho. Surg. Mill Rd. Matern. Hosp. Liverp.

PEARSON, Donald William MacIntyre Diabetic Clinic, Woolmanhill, Aberdeen Royal Infirmary, Gampian University Hospitals NHS Trust, Aberdeen Tel: 01224 681818 Fax: 01224 681818; 19 Corunna Place, Aberdeen AB23 8DA Tel: 01224 702463 — MB ChB Glas. 1976; BSc (Hons.) Glas. 1972; FRCP Glas. 1988; FRCP Ed. 1990. Cons. Phys. (With s/i in Diabetes

Mellitus) Aberd. Teach. Hosps.; Clin. Sen. Lect. Univ. Aberd. Specialty: Diabetes; Gen. Med. Socs: Scott. Soc. Phys.; Brit. Diabetic Assn.; Diabetic Pregn. study Gp. of EASD. Prev: Sen. Regist. (Gen. Med.) (With s/i in Endocrinol. & Diabetes) Aberd. Teach. Hosps.; Lect. (Med.) Univ. Aberd.; Regist. (Gen. Med.) Glas. Roy. Infirm.

PEARSON, Dorothy (retired) 5 Meadowfields, Whaley Bridge, High Peak SK23 7AX Tel: 01663 732570 Fax: 01663 732570 — MB ChB Manch. 1948; DMRT Eng. 1951; FFR 1958; FRCR 1975. Prev: Cons. Radiotherap. Christie Hosp. & Holt Radium Inst. Manch.

PEARSON, Elaine Janet Stoneleigh Surgery, Police Square, Milnthorpe LA7 7PW Tel: 015395 63307; 12 Chestnut Way, Milnthorpe LA7 7RB — MB ChB Manch. 1983; MRCP (UK) 1986; DRCOG 1989; MRCGP 1990.

PEARSON, Elizabeth Margaret 355 Harrogate Road, Leeds LS17 6PZ Tel: 0113 268 0066 Fax: 0113 288 8643 — MB BS Lond. 1973 (Lond. Hosp.) DCH Eng. 1976; DRCOG 1976; MRCGP 1980. Specialty: Gen. Pract. Prev: Trainee GP Nottm. VTS; SHO Wom. Hosp. Nottm.; SHO (Paediat.) Childr. Hosp. Nottm.

PEARSON, Ewan Robert 2 St Johns Close, East Grinstead RH19 3YR — BChir Camb. 1995.

PEARSON, Gale Adrian Birmingham Childrens Hospital, Steelhouse Lane, Birmingham B4 6NH; 205 Northfield Road, Kings Norton, Birmingham B30 1EA — MB BS Newc. 1985; MRCP (UK) 1990; FRCPCH 1997. Cons. Paediat. Intensivist Birm. Childr. Hosp.; Hon. Sen. Lect. Dept. of Anaesth. & Int. Care, Birm. Univ. Specialty: Paediat.; Intens. Care. Socs: Chairm. PICS; PRS; ICS. Prev: Chief Regist. PICU Roy. Childr. Melbourne, Austral.; ECMO Fell. Leicester Univ.

PEARSON, George Halley (retired) Hadrian, 34 High West Road, Crook DL15 9NS Tel: 01388 762552 — MB ChB Ed. 1943 (Univ. Ed.) Prev: Ho. Surg. OldCh. Co. Hosp. Romford.

PEARSON, Gillian Charlotte Osteoporosis Research Unit, Southampton General Hospital, Southampton SO16 6YD Tel: 023 8079 4857 Fax: 023 8079 8505 — MB ChB Bristol 1977; MF Hom Lond. 1997. Research Fell. (Osteoporosis Research Unit) Soton. Gen. Hosp.; Homeopathic Physician, Winch. Homeopathic. Pract. Specialty: Rehabil. Med.; Rheumatol.; Homeop. Med. Prev: GP VTS; Med. Off. RAMC.

PEARSON, Gillian Lesley 2 Queensway, Ponteland, Newcastle upon Tyne NE20 9RZ — MB BS Newc. 1976; MRCGP 1980. Salaried Asst. GP Morpeth (Associate Specialist Rhuematology). Specialty: Rehabil. Med.; Rheumatol. Prev: Regist. Dept. Radiother. Newc. Gen. Hosp.; GP Wom. Retainer Scheme Morpeth.

PEARSON, Gordon Horden Group Practice, The Surgery, Sunderland Road, Peterlee SR8 4QP Tel: 0191 586 4210 Fax: 0191 587 0700; 37 Elsdon Close, Peterlee SR8 1NE — MB ChB Ed. 1977 (Edinburgh) MRCGP 1981; DRCOG 1981. Specialty: Gen. Pract.

PEARSON, Mr Henry James Diana Princess of Wales Hospital, Scartho Road, Grimsby DN33 2BA Tel: 01472 874 111 — MB BS London 1974 (Middlx.) FRCS 1978; MD Leic. 1987. Cons. Surg. (Gen., Breast & Colorectal); Hon. Sen. Lect., Sheff. Med. Sch.; Chairm., Humber & Yorks. Coast, Colorectal Cancer Network. Specialty: Gen. Surg. Socs: Roy. Coll. of Surg., Eng.; Assn. of Surg. of Gt. Britain & Irel.; Assn. of Coloproctology of Gt. Britain and Irel.

PEARSON, Ian Barrie (retired) 94 Tamworth Drive, Fleet GU51 2UP — MB ChB Sheff. 1965; MD Sheff. 1965; DPM Eng. 1967; MRCPsych 1971. Cons. Psychiat. Dumfries & Galloway HB., Crichton Roy. Hosp. Prev: Head of Clin. Research, Roche Products Ltd.

PEARSON, Ian Christopher 21 The Ridgeway, Sutton SM2 5JX — MB BS Lond. 1996.

PEARSON, James Francis (retired) 14 Sherborne Avenue, Cyncoed, Cardiff CF23 6SJ Tel: 029 2075 2909 Fax: 029 2075 3050 — MB BS Lond. 1960 (Char. Cross) DObst RCOG 1963; FRCOG 1978, M 1965; MD Lond. 1973. Prev: Sen. Regist. (O & G) United Birm. Hosps. & Birm. RHB.

PEARSON, James Gordon Royal Crescent Surgery, 11 Royal Crescent, Cheltenham GL50 3DA Tel: 01242 580248 Fax: 01242 253618; Quintain, Old Mansion Drive, Prestbury, Cheltenham GL52 3AS Tel: 01242 580198 — MB BS Lond. 1971 (Roy. Free) MRCS Eng. LRCP Lond. 1971. Med. Off. Cheltenham Coll.; Med. Off. Cheltenham Tour AFC; Clin. Asst. in Psychiat. (Learning Disabilities).

PEARSON, Joanna Mary 31 Pennine Walk, Tunbridge Wells TN2 3NW — MB BS Lond. 1991 (University College and Middlesex School of Medicine London) BSc Lond. 1982; Dip. Dietetics Lond. 1983; DRCOG 1994; MRCGP 1996; DFFP 1996; DPD 1999. Specialty: Gen. Pract. Prev: Vocationally Trained Assoc. W. Kent; GP/Regist. Tunbridge Wells VTS.

PEARSON, Mr John Brian (retired) Copthall Green House, Upshire, Waltham Abbey EN9 3SZ Tel: 01992 711273 Email: upshirepearson@yahoo.co.uk; Copthall Green House, Upshire, Waltham Abbey EN9 3SZ Tel: 01992 711273 Email: kerner@btinternet.com/upshirepearson@yahoo.co.uk — MB ChB Birm. 1953; DObst RCOG 1955; FRCS Eng. 1961; FACS 1977. Cons. Surg. Redbridge Dist. HA. Prev: Sen. Surg. Regist. United Birm. Hosps.

PEARSON, John Dale West Cairn, The Shore, Hest Bank, Lancaster LA2 6HW — MB ChB Liverp. 1964; DTM & H 1965; MRCP (U.K.) 1970. Cons. Phys. Roy. Lancaster Infirm., Lancaster Moor & Kendal Hosps. Specialty: Gen. Med. Socs: Fell. RCP Lond.; Brit. Geriat. Soc. Prev: Sen. Regist. Liverp. Regional Hosp. Bd.; Regist. United Liverp. Hosp.

PEARSON, John Gilbert Havelock 10 Morley Road, Twickenham TW1 2HF — MRCS Eng. LRCP Lond. 1974; BSc Lond. 1972, MB BS 1975.

PEARSON, John Michael Henry (retired) 3 Swan Cottage, Asthall Leigh, Witney OX29 9PZ Tel: 01993 878384 — (St. Bart.) BM BCh Oxf. 1955; FRCP Lond. 1981, M 1963; DM Oxf. 1975. Prev: Mem. Scientif. Staff Med. Research Counc.

PEARSON, John Robert Centre Surgery, Health Centre, Hill St., Hinckley LE10 1DS Tel: 01455 632277 — MRCS Eng. LRCP Lond. 1963.

PEARSON, Mr John Roy (retired) 66 Arthur Road, Edgbaston, Birmingham B15 2UW — MB ChB Birm. 1950; FRCS Eng. 1958; FRCS Ed. 1958. Prev: Cons. Surg. (Orthop.) Birm. Gen. Hosp. & Roy. Orthop. Hosp. Birm.

PEARSON, Jonathan Mark Department of Pathology, Royal Bolton Hospital, Minerva Road, Farnworth, Bolton BL4 0JR Tel: 01204 390534 — MB ChB Manch. 1985; BSc (Hons.) Manch. 1982; MB ChB (Hons.) Manch. 1985; MRCPath 1992; FRCPath 2000. Cons. Histopath. Roy. Bolton Hosp. Specialty: Histopath.

PEARSON, Joseph Robert 14 Sherborne Avenue, Cyncoed, Cardiff CF23 6SJ Tel: 029 2075 2909 — MB BCh Wales 1995 (UWCM) MRCGP 2002; DFFP 2002. Free Lance GP. Specialty: Anaesth. Socs: MPS; MSS. Prev: Cardiff-Llandough Hosp.

PEARSON, Julia Melissa Nelson Health Centre, Leeds Road, Nelson BB9 9TG Tel: 01282 698036; Acorn House, Lanehouse, Trawden, Colne BB88SN — MB BS Lond. 1983; DRCOG 1987; DCH 1988.

PEARSON, Julie Claire Belves, The Chantry, Rooksbridge, Axbridge BS26 2TR — MB ChB Liverp. 1998.

PEARSON, Kathleen Marianne (retired) Mellor's Wing, Plumtree, Heversham, Milnthorpe LA7 7RS Tel: 01539 563121 — MB ChB Liverp. 1936; FRCGP 1971, M 1953. Prev: Med. Off. Family Plann. Assn.

PEARSON, Mr Kenneth William 29 Knowsley Street, Bury BL9 0ST Tel: 0161 797 9771 — MD Manch. 1974; MB ChB 1964; DObst RCOG 1966; FRCS Ed. 1970; FRCS Eng. 1972. Cons. Gen. Surg. Bury AHA. Specialty: Gen. Surg. Socs: Fell. Manch. Med. Soc. Prev: Sen. Surg. Regist. Manch. AHA (T).

PEARSON, Kiri Joanne 1 Drakes Meadow, Cheriton Fitzpaine, Crediton EX17 4HU Tel: 01363 866305 Fax: 01363 866305 — MB ChB Ed. 1998; MRCS (A & E) Edin. 2001.

PEARSON, Lezli Ann The Stewart Medical Centre, 15 Hartington Road, Buxton SK17 6JP Tel: 01298 22338 Fax: 01298 72678 — MB BS Lond. 1984. Trainee GP Hillingdon Hosp. VTS. Prev: SHO (Orthop.) Kingston & Esher HA; Ho. Off. (Med. & Surg.) W. Cumbria HA.

PEARSON, Linda Claire 4 The Fairways, Leamington Spa CV32 6PR — MB ChB Manch. 1987; DA (UK) 1992. Staff Grade Anaesth. Warwick Hosp. Specialty: Anaesth. Prev: SHO (Anaesth.) Oldham Hosp.

PEARSON, Lorraine Crescent Villa, Crescent St., Cottingham HU16 5QS — MB ChB Manch. 1982.

PEARSON, Lucy Samantha Farthings, Park Road, Slinfold, Horsham RH13 7SD — MB ChB Leic. 1993. SHO (Nephrol.)

Leicester Gen. Hosp. Specialty: Gen. Med. Prev: SHO (A & E) Selly Oak Hosp.; Ho. Off. (Med.) Leicester Roy. Hosp.; Ho. Off. (Surg.) Geo. Eliot Hosp. Nuneaton.

PEARSON, Margaret (retired) 82 Harrison Gardens, Edinburgh EH11 1SB — MB ChB Ed. 1947 (Univ. Ed.) MB ChB (Hnrs.) Ed. 1947. Prev: Med. Asst. (Path.) Bangour Gen. Hosp. Broxburn.

PEARSON, Margaret Joan Beechgrove, Strachan, Banchory AB31 6NL Tel: 01330 822072 — MB ChB Aberd. 1991.

PEARSON, Mark Joseph 41 Alderbrook Road, Solihull B91 1NW — MB ChB Birm. 1979; MA Camb. 1980; MRCPsych 1983; MSc (Psychother.) Warwick 1986.

PEARSON, Maurice Robert Wick Medical Centre, Martha Terrace, Wick KW1 5EL Tel: 01955 605885 Fax: 01955 602434; 22 Port Dunbar, Port Dunbar, Wick KW1 4JJ Tel: 01955 602450 Fax: 01955 606637 Email: mrpwick@aol.com — (Durh.) BSc Durham. 1962; MB BS Durh. 1965. Specialty: Gen. Pract. Socs: BMA. Prev: Regist. Gen. Med. Qu. Eliz. Hosp. Gateshead; SHO Artific. Kidney Unit, & Ho. Surg. & Ho. Phys. Roy. Vict. Infirm. Newc.

PEARSON, Michael Carden (retired) Bleak House, Horsted Keynes, Haywards Heath RH17 7ED — MB BChir Camb. 1963 (Camb. & Guy's) MA Camb. 1963; MRCP Lond. 1967; DMRD Eng. 1969; FFR 1971; FRCR 1975; MSc (Med.) Lond. 1993; FRCP Lond. 1994. Prev: Cons. Radiol. Lond. Chest Hosp. Roy. Hosps. NHS Trust & Roy. Brompton & Nat. Heart Hosps.

PEARSON, Michael David 23 Bladon Way, Haverhill CB9 0AB Tel: 01440 705299 — MB ChB Sheff. 1966. Occupat. Health Phys.; Police Surg. Prev: Ho. Surg. St. Luke's Matern. Hosp. Bradford & Roy. Infirm. Sheff.; Ho. Phys. Nottm. Gen. Hosp.; Home Off. Prison Med. Off.

PEARSON, Michael George Aintree Chest Centre, University Hospital, Aintree, Longmoor Lane, Liverpool L9 7AL Tel: 0151 529 3857 Fax: 0151 529 2873 — MB BChir Camb. 1976; MA Camb. 1976; MRCP (UK) 1978; FRCP Lond. 1991. Cons. Phys. Aintree Chest Centre Univ. Hosp., Aintree, Liverp.; Dir. Clin. Effectiveness & Eval. Unit of RCP Lond.; Vis. Prof. Univ. Salford. Specialty: Respirat. Med.; Gen. Med. Socs: Brit. Thorac. Soc.; Amer. Thoracic Soc.; Eur. Respirat. Soc. Prev: Hon. Lect. (Med.) Univ. Liverp.; Clin. Research Fell. Univ. of W. Ontario & Lond., Canada; Sen. Regist. Rotat. (Gen. & Respirat. Med.) Mersey RHA.

PEARSON, Michael John 11 Millholme Close, Southam, Leamington Spa CV47 1FQ — MB ChB Birm. 1982; MRCOG 1988; MD Birm. 1995. Cons. O & G S. Warks. Hosps. NHS Trust. Specialty: Obst. & Gyn.

PEARSON, Michael Lawrence 5 Woodland Place, Bathwick Hill, Bath BA2 6EH; 15 Choir Green, Knaphill, Woking GU21 2NQ — MB BS Lond. 1989. Trainee GP St. John's Health Centre Woking.

PEARSON, Mr Morton Gilmour (retired) 27 Bryanston Drive, Dollar FK14 7EF Tel: 01259 742444 — MB ChB Ed. 1941; FRCOG 1963, M 1950; FRCS Ed. 1953. Prev: Cons. O & G Roy. Infirm. Edin., Simpson Memor. Matern. Pavil. Edin. & Scott. Borders Hosp. Gp.

PEARSON, Nanette Mirrington Family Planning Office, Bodwrdda, St David's Road, Caernarfon LL55 1EL Tel: 01286 684015; Pant Hywel, Llandegfan, Menai Bridge LL59 5SB — MB BS Lond. 1971 (Middlx.) DObst RCOG 1973; DCH Eng. 1974; DFFP 2001. Locum Sen. Clin. Med. Off. (Family Planning) N. W. Wales NHS Trust; CMO (Family Planning) Conwy & Denbighsh. NHS Trust. Prev: Med. Off. (Community Med.) Gwynedd Health Auth.; Regist. (Paediat.) W. Middlx. Hosp. Isleworth; Lond.

PEARSON, Nicholas David Kings Park Hospital, Gloucester Road, Bournemouth BH7 6JE Tel: 01202 303757 — MB BS Lond. 1977; MRCPsych 1987. Cons. Psychiat. (Old Age Psychiat.) Kings Pk. Hosp., Bournemouth. Specialty: Geriat. Psychiat. Prev: Cons. Psychiat. (Old Age Psychiat.) Oakley Hse. Bungalow.

PEARSON, Nicola Jane Somerset Health Authority, Wellsprings Road, Taunton TA2 7PQ; The Anchorage, Othery, Bridgwater TA7 0PY Tel: 01823 698036 — MB BS Lond. 1986 (Lond. Hosp. Med. Coll.) MFPHM RCP (UK) 1995. Cons. (Pub. Health Med.) Som. HA. Specialty: Pub. Health Med. Prev: Lect. (Epidemiol. & Pub. Health Med.) Dept. Social Med. Bristol Univ.

PEARSON, Nigel Ian Campbell — MB ChB Bristol 1987; Cert. Equiv Experience; DCH RCPS Glas. 1990; DTM & H Liverp. 1991. Locum Gen. Practitioner, Oxf.; Freelance Cons. in Health Care in Poor, deprived and conflict areas; Cons. assignments with Oxfam IRC Medair ECO Refugees Internat. Specialty: Gen. Pract. Prev: Trainee GP I. of Mull; SHO (Paediat. & O & G) Boston.; Dist. Med. Off. Health Dist. of Boga, DR Congo.

PEARSON, Nina Rosemary Saltaire Medical Centre, Richmond Road, Saltaire, Shipley BD18 4RX Tel: 01274 593101; 7 Bramham Drive, Baildon, Shipley BD17 6SZ — MB BS Newc. 1983; DRCOG 1986; MRCGP 1987; Cert. Family Plann. JCC 1987. GP Shipley Retainer Scheme. Prev: Trainee GP Harrogate VTS.

PEARSON, Owen Rhys 5 Bryneglwys Gardens, Porthcawl CF36 5PR — MB BCh Wales 1997.

PEARSON, Patricia Frithwood Surgery, 45 Tanglewood Way, Bussage, Stroud GL6 8DE Tel: 01453 884646 Fax: 01453 731302; Rectory Barn, Bisley, Stroud GL6 7AD Tel: 01452 770707 — MB BS Durh. 1967 (King's Coll. Newc.) MRCGP 1977. Prev: Clin. Asst. (Gyn.) Gloucester Roy. Hosp.

PEARSON, Patrick Joseph Thomas Longcroft Clinic, 5 Woodmansterne Lane, Banstead SM7 3HH Tel: 01737 359332 Fax: 01737 370835; Myrtle Cottage, 20 Myrtle Road, Sutton SM1 4BX Tel: 020 8643 8680 — MB BChir Camb. 1979 (Kings Coll. Hosp.) MA Camb. 1978; DRCOG 1982; MRCGP (Distinc.) 1984. Dep. Police Surg. Epsom; Med. Adviser Catholic Childr. Adoption Soc. Socs: BMA; Sutton Med. Soc. Prev: Trainee GP Croydon VTS; SHO (A & E) Kingston Hosp.; Ho. Surg. King's Coll. Hosp. Lond.

PEARSON, Paul (retired) Low Lickbarrow Farm, Lickbarrow Close, Heathwaite, Windermere LA23 2NF; Low Lickbarrow Farm, Lickbarrow Close, Heathwaite, Windermere LA23 2NF — MRCS Eng. LRCP Lond. 1949; MRCGP 1962; DA Eng. 1963; DObst RCOG 1964. Prev: Ho. Surg. Liverp. Stanley Hosp.

PEARSON, Randall Murray Gloynes, Capt. RAMC Retd. 83 Church Walk, Atherstone CV9 1PS Tel: 01827 712070 Email: randall.pearson@ntlworld.com — MB BS Lond. 1975 (Lond. Hosp.) FFA RCS Eng. 1984. Cons. Anaesth. Geo. Eliot Hosp. Nuneaton. Specialty: Anaesth. Socs: BMA & Assn. Anaesths. Gt. Brit. & Irel.; Fell. Roy. Soc. Med.; Obst. Anaesth. Assn. Prev: Cons. Anaesth. Burton-on-Trent; Sen. Regist. (Anaesth.) Nottm. & E. Midl. Higher Profess. Train. Scheme; Regist. (Anaesth.) Norf. & Norwich Hosp.

PEARSON, Richard Alan 17 Shillingford Drive, Stoke-on-Trent ST4 8YG — MB ChB Manch. 1990.

PEARSON, Richard Francis (retired) 78 Woodside Avenue, Muswell Hill, London N10 3HY Tel: 020 8883 1965 — MRCS Eng. LRCP Lond. 1947 (Camb. & Univ. Coll. Hosp.) MA Camb. 1947, MB BChir 1952. Prev: Ho. Phys. Hope Hosp. Salford.

PEARSON, Richard Martin St Bartholomew's & the Royal London School of Medicine & Dentistry, Charterhouse Square, London EC1M 6BQ Tel: 020 7882 3411 Fax: 020 7882 3408; 152 Harley Street, London W1N 1HH Tel: 020 7935 3834 Fax: 020 7354 1501 Email: richard.pearson@which.com — MB BChir Camb. 1968 (Camb. & St. Mary's) MA, MB Camb. 1968, BChir 1967; FRCP (UK) 1996, MRCP 1970. Cons. Phys. Harold Wood & Oldchurdh Hosp. Romford & Sen. Lect. Clin. Pharmacol. St. Bart. Hosp. Lond. Specialty: Gen. Med.; Pharmacology; Vasc. Med. Socs: Fell. Roy. Soc. Med.; Brit. Pharm. Soc.; BMA. Prev: Cons. Phys. Nottm. AHA.; Sen. Regist. (Med.) Roy. Free Hosp. Lond.; Research Fell. Roy. Postgrad. Med. Sch. Hammersmith Hosp. Lond.

PEARSON, Robert (retired) Hauxwell Grange, Marwood, Barnard Castle DL12 8QU Tel: 01833 695022 — MB ChB Bristol 1970; MSc Bristol 1970, BSc (Physiol.) 1966; MRCP (UK) 1974; DObst RCOG 1976. Prev: Director of Med. Affairs, GlaxoSmithKline UK Ltd, Uxbridge.

PEARSON, Mr Robert Charles Department of Surgery, Manchester Royal Infirmary, Ocford Road, Manchester M13 9WL Tel: 0161 276 4250 Fax: 0161 276 4530 Email: bob.pearson@cmmc.nhs.uk; 55 Bramhall Park Road, Bramhall, Stockport SK7 3NA — MB ChB Manch. 1978 (Manchester) BSc And. 1975; FRCS Eng. 1983; MD Manch. 1989. Cons. Surg. Manch. Roy. Infirm.; Clin. Head of Div. of Surg., Manch. Roy. Infirm.; Progr. Director and Chair of STSC, N. W. Specialty: Gen. Surg. Special Interest: Colorectal Surg. Socs: Assn. of Surgeons of Gt. Britain and Irel.; Assn. of Coloproctology of Gt. Britain and Irel.

PEARSON, Robert Edmund Moresdale Lane Surgery, 95 Moresdale Lane, Leeds LS14 6GG Tel: 0113 295 1200 Fax: 0113 295 1210 — MB ChB Manch. 1981; BSc Manch. 1979; DGM RCP Lond. 1986; DRCOG 1986; MRCGP 1989; Adv Professional Dip (Mentoring) LMU 1997. Specialty: Care of the Elderly. Prev: SHO

(Orthop.) Pontefract Gen. Infirm.; SHO (O & G) Huddersfield Roy. Infirm.; SHO (Gen. Med.) Bury Gen. Hosp.

PEARSON, Robert Henry Dept. of Radiology, Perth Royal Infirmary, Perth PH1 1NX — MB ChB Manch. 1988; BSc MedSci St. Andrews. 1985; MRCP (UK) 1992; FRCR 1998; MD Aberdeen 2000. Cons. (Radiol.) Perth Roy. Infirm. Perth. Specialty: Radiol.

PEARSON, Robin Lochrie Elgin Medical Centre, 10 Victoria Crescent, Elgin IV30 1RQ Tel: 01343 547512 Fax: 01343 546781; The Grange, 14 Seafield Crescent, Elgin IV30 1RE Tel: 01343 542146 — MB ChB Glas. 1976; DRCOG 1978; MRCGP 1985.

PEARSON, Roger Hardacre (retired) Lowther Medical Centre, 1 Castle Meadows, Whitehaven CA28 7RG Tel: 01946 692241 Fax: 01946 590617; 17 Eden Drive, Moresby Parks, Whitehaven CA28 8XA Tel: 01946 694494 Fax: 01946 590617 — MB BS Durh. 1964. Prev: SHO Sunderland Matern. Hosp.

PEARSON, Ronald Carl Alan 12 Kingswood Avenue, Newcastle upon Tyne NE2 3NS — BM BCh Oxf. 1980; BA Oxf. 1974; DPhil Oxf. 1980; MA Oxf. 1984. Prof. Neurosci. Dept. Biomed. Sci. Univ. Sheff. Prev: Lect. (Anat.) St. Mary's Hosp. Med. Sch. Lond.; Wellcome Trust Research Fell. (Ment. Health); Demonst. (Human Anat.) Univ. Oxf.

PEARSON, Ronald Norman Bosmere Medical Practice, PO Box 41, Civic Centre Road, Havant PO9 2AJ Tel: 023 9245 1300 Fax: 023 9249 2524; Applegarth, Church Lane, Hayling Island PO11 0SB Tel: 023 9246 3565 — MB BS Lond. 1964 (Guy's) MRCS Eng. LRCP Lond. 1964; DObst RCOG 1967. Hosp. Pract. (Geniourin. Med.) St. Mary's Hosp. Portsmouth. Specialty: Genitourinary Medicine. Socs: BMA. Prev: Ho. Phys. & Ho. Surg. Roy. Sussex Co. Hosp. Brighton; Ho. Surg. (Obst.) Brighton Gen. Hosp.; Med. Off. King Edwd. VII Memor. Hosp. Bermuda.

PEARSON, Rowan Elisabeth — MB ChB Leeds 1986; MRCPsych 1991. Assoc. Specialist in Perinatal Psychiat. Leeds Parent and Child Unit. Specialty: Gen. Psychiat. Prev: Staff Grade Malham Hse. Day Hosp. Leeds CMH Trust.

PEARSON, Mr Russell Vaughan Southend General Hospital, Ophthalmology Department, Prittlewell Chase, Southend-on-Sea SS0 0RY Tel: 01702 435555; 59 Priests Lane, Shenfield, Brentwood CM15 8BX Tel: 01277 214577 Fax: 01277 848580 Email: russell.pearson1@virgin.net — MB BS Lond. 1980 (Lond. Hosp.) BSc (Physiol) Lond. 1977; MRCP (UK) 1985; FRCS Eng. 1986; FRCOphth. 1989. Cons. Ophth. Surg. Southend Health Care Trust and Basildon & Orsett Hosp. Specialty: Ophth. Socs: Fell. Roy. Soc. Med.; Oxf. Ophth. Congr.; Euro. Soc. Of Cataract & Refractive Surg.s. Prev: Sen. Regist. (Ophth.) Lond. & Moorfield Eye Hosps. Lond.; Resid. Regist. (Surg.) Moorfields Eye Hosp. Lond.; SHO (Ophth.) West. Ophth. & Char. Cross Hosps. Lond.

PEARSON, Ruth Hutchison Dept of Radiology, Kingston Hospital, Galsworthy Road, Kingston upon Thames KT2 7QB Tel: 020 8789 6611; Queen Mary's Hospital, London SW15 5PN Tel: 0208 355 2030; Jasmine House, 190 New King's Road, London SW6 4NF Tel: 020 7731 0818 — MB BCh BAO Dub. 1973 (TC Dub.) BA Dub. 1971; DMRD Eng. 1977; FRCR 1978. Cons. Radiol. Kingston Hospital. Specialty: Radiol. Prev: Sen. Regist. Radiol. Hammersmith Hosp. Lond.

PEARSON, Sally Anne Department of Ultrasound, Derriford Hospital, Derriford, Plymouth PL6 8DH; Langston, Kingston, Kingsbridge TQ7 4HB Tel: 01548 810234 Fax: 01548 810453 — MB BS Lond. 1972 (Roy. Free) MRCS Eng. LRCP Lond. 1972; DObst RCOG 1974. Assoc. Specialist Radiol. (Ultrasound) Derriford Hosp. Plymouth. Specialty: Radiol. Socs: Plymouth Med. Soc.; Brit. Med. Ultrasound Soc.

PEARSON, Sally Elizabeth Gloucestershire Hospitals NHS Trust, 1 College Lawn, Cheltenham GL53 7AG Tel: 08454 222860 — MB ChB Leeds 1984; MPH Leeds 1989; MFPHM RCP (UK) 1991; FFPHM RCP (UK) 1997. Specialty: Pub. Health Med. Prev: Dir. Pub. Health Glos. HA; Cons. Pub. Health Med. Wakefield & Pontefract HA.

PEARSON, Sally Jane Ardnagrask Mains, Muir of Ord IV6 7TW — MB ChB Aberd. 1993; MRCGP 2002.

PEARSON, Sandra Wessex Deanery, Highcroft, Romsey Road, Winchester SO22 5EY Tel: 01962 863511 — MB ChB Leeds 1981; MRCPsych. 1998. Specialist Regist. (Psychiat.) Wessex Rotat. Specialty: Gen. Psychiat. Prev: Staff Grade (Psychiat.) Alderney Hosp. Poole; Regist. (Psychiat.) St. Ann's Hosp. Poole.

PEARSON, Sarah Laneside, West Bradford Rd, Waddington, Clitheroe BB7 3JE — MB ChB Birm. 1997.

PEARSON, Sheila Elizabeth Cumberland Infirmary, Carlisle CA2 7HY — MB BS Newc. 1981 (Newcastle upon Tyne) MRCOG 1987; FRCOG 1999. Cons. O & G Carlisle Hosps. Specialty: Obst. & Gyn.

PEARSON, Sheila Hamilton Crawford (retired) Askernish, 45 Polmaise Road, Stirling FK7 9JH — MB ChB Glas. 1964.

PEARSON, Stanley Barwis Department of Respiratory Medicine, Leeds general infirmary, Great George Street, Leeds LS1 3EX Tel: 0113 392 2891 Fax: 0113 392 6316 Email: stan.pearson@leedsth.nhs.uk; 14 Charville Gardens, Leeds LS17 8JL Email: mail@stanley-pearson.co.uk — (Lond. Hosp.) DPhil Oxf. 1971, MA 1972, BA (1st Cl. Hons.) 1968, DM 1990, BM BCh; Oxf. 1974; MRCP (UK) 1976; FRCP Lond. 1988. Cons. Phys. Leeds Gen. Infirm.; Sen. Clin. Lect., Univ. of Leeds. Specialty: Respirat. Med.; Gen. Med. Socs: Brit. Thorac. Soc. & Europ. Respirat. Soc. Prev: Sen. Regist. (Gen. & Thoracic Med.) Hants. AHA; Regist. (Gen. Med.) Nottm. City Hosp.; SHO (Gen. Med.) Univ. Med. Unit. Nottm. Gen. Hosp.

PEARSON, Susan Grace Leeds BAMS, Government Buildings, Otley Road, Leeds LS16 5PU Tel: 0113 230 9247; 10 Summerhill Gardens, Roundhay, Leeds LS8 2EL — MB ChB Leeds 1970. Specialty: Civil Serv. Socs: BMA. Prev: Clin. Med. Off. Leeds AHA (T); Ho. Phys. St. Jas. Hosp. Leeds; Ho. Surg. Seacroft Hosp. Leeds.

PEARSON, Susan Lynn West Wing, Esk Medical Centre, Ladywell Way, Musselburgh EH21 6AB Tel: 0131 665 2594 Fax: 0131 665 2428; Old Bank House, 18 Hillhead, Bonnyrigg EH19 2JG Tel: 0131 660 3407 — MB ChB Ed. 1986; DRCOG 1989.

PEARSON, Professor Thomas Claud Department of Haematology, St Thomas Hospital, London SE1 7EH Tel: 020 7928 9292 Fax: 020 7928 5698 — (Char. Cross) MD Lond. 1977, MB BS 1966; MRCS Eng. LRCP Lond. 1966; FRCPath 1989, M 1977; MRCP Lond. 1997. Prof. Haemat. The Guy's, King's Coll. & St. Thomas' Hosps.' Med. & Dent. Sch.; Hon. Cons. Haemat. Guy's & St. Thos. Trust. Specialty: Haematology.

PEARSON, Thomas Eric Mellows, Brayton Lane, Selby YO8 9DZ — MB BS Lond. 1992.

PEARSON, Timothy Friary Surgery, Queens Road, Richmond DL10 4UJ Tel: 01748 822306 Fax: 01748 850356 — MB ChB Sheff. 1990.

PEARSON, Timothy John Holmside Medical Group, 142 Armstrong Road, Benwell, Newcastle upon Tyne NE4 8QB Tel: 0191 273 4009 Fax: 0191 273 2745 — MB BS Newc. 1981.

PEARSON, Veronica Ashville Medical Centre, 430 Doncaster Road, Barnsley S70 3RJ Tel: 01226 282280 Fax: 01226 216002 — MB ChB Leeds 1976.

PEARSON, Veronica (retired) 21 Orrin Close, York YO24 2RA Tel: 01904 708521 — (Camb. & St. Thos.) BA (Nat. Sc. Trip. Pts. I & II Path.) Camb. 1952; MB BChir Camb. 1955; DObst RCOG 1957; DCH Eng. 1958; MFFP 1993. Prev: GP Pontefract.

PEARSON, Virginia Alison Hardy — MB BChir Camb. 1985; MA Oxf. 1985, BA 1981; DRCOG 1987; MRCGP 1988; DCH RCP Lond. 1988; MFPHM RCP (UK) 1993; FFPHM 2000. Chief Exec., S. Som. Primary Care Trust. Specialty: Pub. Health Med.

PEARSON, William John Christopher (retired) 110 Station Road, Mickleover, Derby DE3 9FP Tel: 01332 512646 — MB BCh BAO Dub. 1952 (T.C. Dub.) BA Dub. 1949, MB BCh BAO 1952.

PEARSONS, David Ernest (retired) 37 Chadwick Road, Westcliff on Sea SS0 8LD Tel: 01702 353551 — MB BS Lond. 1953 (St. Bart.) Mem. (Ex-Chairm.) Essex Local Med. Comm.; Mem. Family Plann. Pract. Prev: Ho. Surg. & Ho. Phys. Rochford Gen. Hosp.

PEARSTON, Gordon James Walker Medical Group, Church Walk, Walker, Newcastle upon Tyne NE6 3BS Tel: 0191 220 5905 Fax: 0191 220 5904; 14 Woodlands, Gosforth, Newcastle upon Tyne NE3 4YL Tel: 0191 284 7363 — MB ChB Ed. 1979; BSc Ed. 1976, MB ChB 1979; DRCOG 1982; MRCGP 1983. Specialty: Gen. Pract.

PEARSTON, Mary Kathleen 14 Woodlands, Gosforth, Newcastle upon Tyne NE3 4YL Tel: 0191 284 7363 Email: mkpearston@aol.com — MB BS Lond. 1981 (University College London) BSc Lond. 1978; MRCGP 1987. Princip. (Gen. Med.). Specialty: Gen. Pract.

PEART, Charlotte Louise Maryfield Medical Centre, 9 Morgan Street, Dundee DD4 6QE Tel: 01382 462292; 28 Cortachy Crescent,

Balgillo Park, Dundee DD5 3BF Email: charlotte1972@hotmail.com — MB ChB Dundee 1996; DFFP; MRCGP Edinburgh 2000. Specialty: Gen. Pract. Prev: GP Regist. Maryfield Health Centre, Dundee; GP Princip., Abbey Health Centre, Pract. 3, Arbroam.

PEART, Emma Jane Felix House Surgery, Middleton Lane, Middleton St. George, Darlington DL2 1AE Tel: 01325 332235 Fax: 01325 333626 — BM BS Nottm. 1991; BMedSci Nottm. 1989; DCH RCP Lond. 1994. GP Regist. Darlington.

PEART, Ian 1 Birkdale Close, Huyton with Roby, Liverpool L36 4QW Tel: 0151 449 1401 — MB ChB Manch. 1976; MRCP (UK) 1979. Cons. Paediat. Cardiol. Roy. Liverp. Childr. Hosp. Specialty: Cardiol. Prev: Sen. Regist. (Paediat. Cardiol.) Freeman Hosp. Newc.; Nat. Heart Research Fund Research Fell. (Cardiol.) Roy. Vict. Infirm. Newc.; Regist. (Cardiol.) Regional Cardiothoracic Centre Freeman.

PEART, Sir (William) Stanley (retired) 17 Highgate Close, Highgate, London N6 4SD Tel: 020 8341 3111 Fax: 020 8341 3111 — (St. Mary's) FRS; MB BS (Hons.) Lond. 1945; FRCP Lond. 1958, M 1946; MD Lond. 1949. Prev: Prof. Med. St. Mary's Hosp. Lond.

PEASE, Colin Thomas Leeds General Infirmary, Great George St., Leeds LS1 3EX; 4 Lancaster Road, Harrogate HG2 0EZ — MB BS Lond. 1976; MRCP (UK) 1979; MD Lond. 1988; FRCP Lond. 1995. Cons. Rheum. Leeds Gen. Infirm.; Sen. Clin. Lect. (Rheum.) Univ. Leeds. Specialty: Gen. Med.; Rheumatol. Socs: Brit. Soc. Rheum. Prev: Cons. Roy. Bath Hosp. Harrogate; Sen. Regist. Rotat. (Rheum. & Gen. Med.) Char. Cross Hosp.; Research Regist. Bone & Jt. Research Unit Lond. Hosp.

PEASE, Elizabeth Hamilton Errol Kingsley, 64 Woodford Road, Bramhall, Stockport SK7 1PA; Department Reproductive Medicine, St. Mary's Hospital, Hathersage Road, Manchester M13 0JH Tel: 0161 276 6494 Fax: 0161 224 0957 — MB ChB Manch. 1972; FRCS Ed. 1978; FRCOG 1994, M 1978. Cons. (Reproductive Med.) St. Mary's Hosp. Manch.; Insp. Human Fertilisation & Embyology Auth. Lond. Specialty: Obst. & Gyn. Prev: Mem. Brit. Fertil. Soc.; Mem. Brit. Andrology Soc.

PEASE, Mr Hon William Simon (retired) 45 Elizabeth Court, 47 Milmans Street, London SW10 0DA Tel: 020 7351 0954 — MB BS Lond. 1956 (St. Thos.) MA Oxf. 1957; FRCS Eng. 1960. Prev: Cons. ENT Surg. Centr. Middlx., Northwick Pk. Wembley & Acton Hosps.

PEASE, James Jonathan 10 Headlands, Kettering NN15 7HP Tel: 01536 518022 Fax: 01536 517002 — (Middlx.) MB BS Lond. 1970; FRCPsych 1993, M 1976. Cons. Child Family Psychiat. N.hamptonshire Health Care NHS Trust. Specialty: Child & Adolesc. Psychiat. Prev: Sen. Regist. (Child Psychiat.) Cambs. AHA (T).

PEASE, John Clifford (retired) The Ark, Church St., Wells-next-the-Sea NR23 1JB Tel: 01328 710605 — BM BCh Oxf. 1941 (Oxf. & Middlx.) FRCP Lond. 1970, M 1948; DM Oxf. 1950. Prev: Emerit. Cons. Phys. Centr. Notts. (Mansfield) Health Dist.

PEASE, Nicola Jane Frances 23 Station Road, Llanfennech, Llanelli SA14 8UD — MB BCh Wales 1992.

PEASEGOOD, Joanna Aislinn 27 Keele Road, Newcastle ST5 2JT — MB ChB Ed. 1998.

PEASTON, Michael John Thorpe (retired) Wheatmill House, 7 New Wood Lane, Blakedown, Kidderminster DY10 3LD — MB ChB Liverp. 1959; FRCP Glas. 1979, M 1964; PhD Liverp. 1967; FRCP Lond. 1981, M 1968. Prev: Cons. Phys. Countess of Chester Hosp.

PEAT, Clive Cecil 36 Glebe Road, Sheffield S10 1FB — MB ChB Sheff. 1960.

PEAT, Irene Mary The Leicester Royal Infirmary, Leicester LE1 5WW — MB BS Lond. 1975 (Univ. Coll. Hosp.) MRCP (UK) 1978; FRCR 1983; FRCP Lond. 1994. Cons. Clin. Oncol. Leicester Roy. Infirm. Specialty: Oncol.; Radiother. Prev: Sen. Regist. (Radiother. & Oncol.) Qu. Eliz. Hosp. Edgbaston Birm.; Regist. (Radiother. & Oncol.) Churchill Hosp. Oxf.; Lect. (Med. Oncol.) Westm. Med. Sch. Lond.;330.

PEAT, Janet 36 Glebe Road, Broomhill, Sheffield S10 1FB — MB ChB Sheff. 1962.

PEAT, Judith Mary Glen Farm, Church Hill, Honiton EX14 9TE — MB BS Lond. 1975; MRCP (UK) 1979.

PEAT, Meryl Lesley 25 Granby Road, Edinburgh EH16 5NP Tel: 0131 667 7983 — BM BS Nottm. 1989; MRCGP 1995.

PEAT, Michael John 10 Prospect Drive, Hest Bank, Lancaster LA2 6HX — MB ChB Leic. 1983.

PEAT, Susan Joan 29 Museum House, Roman Road, London E2 0JA — MB BS Lond. 1982; BSc Lond. 1979; FFA RCS Eng. 1986. Specialty: Anaesth.

PEATFIELD, Richard Crompton 23 Mount Park Road, Ealing, London W5 2RS — MB BChir Camb. 1973 (Middlx.) MA Camb. 1974; MRCP (UK) 1976; MD Camb. 1982; FRCP Lond. 1995. Cons. Neurol. Char. Cross Hosp. Lond. & Mt. Vernon Hosp. Northwood; Cons. Neurologist, Mt. Vernon and Harefield Hosps. Specialty: Neurol. Special Interest: Headache. Socs: Fell. Roy. Soc. Med.; Internat. Headache Soc. Prev: Sen. Regist. (Neurol.) Leeds & Wakefield Hosps.; Research Fell. (Neurol.) Char. Cross Hosp. Lond.; Regist. (Med.) Centr. Middlx. Hosp. Lond.

PEATMAN, Suzanne Jane 9 Claremont Street, Newcastle upon Tyne NE2 4AH — MB BS Newc. 1992 (Newcastle upon Tyne) BA (Hons.) Newc 1985. Specialist Regist. (O & G) Northern Deanery. Specialty: Obst. & Gyn.

PEATTIE, Alison Brunton Long House, Countess of Chester NHS Trust, Liverpool Road, Chester CH2 1UL Tel: 01244 365 012 Email: alison.peattie@coch.nhs.uk; Penketh House, Church Lane, Neston, South Wirral CH64 9UU Email: peattiebushby@compuserve.com — MB ChB Glas. 1978 (Univ. Glas.) MRCOG 1983. Cons. O & G, Countess of Chester NHS Trust. Specialty: Obst. & Gyn. Special Interest: Urogynecology. Socs: Brit. Soc. of Urogynecology; Brit. Soc. of Paediat. & Adolesc. Gyn. Prev: Sen. Lect. (O & G & Gyn. Urol.) St. Geo. Hosp. Med. Sch. Lond.; Lect. (O & G) St. Geo. Hosp. Med. Sch. Lond. & St. Helier Hosp. Carshalton.

PEBERDY, Mary (retired) Norney Cottage, Whittingham, Alnwick NE66 4UP Tel: 01665 574268 — MRCS Eng. LRCP Lond. 1939 (Univ. Coll. Hosp.) Prev: Lect. (Family Plann.) Univ. Newc.

PEBERDY, Robert John Walton Grove Surgery, Walton Grove, Aylesbury HP21 7SU Tel: 01296 82554; 3 First Court, Aylesbury Road, Bierton, Aylesbury HP22 5AY — MB BChir Camb. 1963 (Middlx.) BA, MB BChir Camb. 1963. Socs: BMA. Prev: Ho. Surg. Middlx. Hosp. Lond.; Ho. Phys. Bolingbroke Hosp. Lond.

PEBERDY, Roger Michael (retired) Wistley, 79 Corbett Avenue, Droitwich WR9 7BH Tel: 01905 772847 — MB ChB Birm. 1962; DA Eng. 1965. Prev: GP Droitwich Spa.

PECCHIA, Kiersten Antoinette — MB BS Lond. 1998.

PECHAL, Arthur James, Surg. Cdr. RN 9A Catsfield Road, Fareham PO15 5QP Tel: 01329 43752 — MB BS Lond. 1958 (Roy. Free) MRCS Eng. LRCP Lond. 1958; DTM & H Eng. 1965; DO Eng. 1970. Ophth. Specialist RN Hosp. Haslar. Socs: S. West. Ophth. Soc. Prev: PMO HMS St. Angelo & Ophth. Specialist RN Hosp. Imtarfa, Malta; Ophth. Specialist RN Hosp. Plymouth; Dep. PMO HMS Nelson Portsmouth.

PECHAN, Jiri — MUDr Prague 1982; LRCP LRCS Ed. LRCPS Glas. 1985; DRCOG 1988. GP Chigwell. Specialty: Gen. Pract. Socs: BMA; Ilford Med. Soc.

PECK, Anthony Wilson (retired) Pavilion End, Bickley Park Road, Bromley BR1 2AT Tel: 020 8467 1406 — (Middlx.) PhD Lond. 1967, BSc (1st cl. Hons.) 1955; MB BS Lond. (Distinc. Med., Path. & Therap. Univ. Medal) Lond. 1958; MRCP (UK) 1963; FRCP Lond. 1981; FFPM RCP (UK) 1992. Prev: Sen. Med. Off. Med. Control Agency.

PECK, Audrey Barbara The Surgery, 139 Valley Road, London SW16 2XT Tel: 020 8769 2566 Fax: 020 8769 5301 — MB BChir Camb. 1982; MA 1983; DRCOG 1985; MRCGP 1986. Princip. GP Streatham.

PECK, Barbara Wendy Upton Medical Partnership, 18 Sussex Place, Slough SL1 1NS Tel: 01753 522713 Fax: 01753 552790; Greenacres, Bracken Close, Farnham Common, Slough SL2 3JP — MB BS Lond. 1982; DRCOG 1985; MRCGP 1988.

PECK, David John — MB BS Lond. 1985 (St Bartholomews) FRCA 1993. Locum Cons. Specialty: Anaesth.; Plastic Surg.; Paediat. Prev: Cons. (Anaesth.) St Andrews Centre Broomfield Hosp. Essex; Sen. Regist. Rotat. (Anaesth.) Roy. Free Hosp. NHS Trust; Pre-Fellowsh. Regist. (Cardiothoracic Anaesth.) Gree La. Hosp. Auckland, NZ.

PECK, John Derek Weston (retired) Bilboa House, Dulverton TA22 9DW Tel: 01398 23475 — MB BS Lond. 1953 (St. Mary's) MRCS Eng. LRCP Lond. 1953; DObst RCOG 1955; DCH Eng. 1958. Prev: Med. Regist. Weymouth & Dist. Hosp.

PECK, John Eric (retired) Rivendell, Halifax Road, Todmorden OL14 6DW Tel: 01706 810619 — (Char. Cross) MB BS Lond.

1961; FRCOG 1982, M 1969, DObst 1964. Prev: Cons. (O & G) Halifax Gen. Hosp. & Halifax Roy. Infirm.

PECK, Marcus John Edwards 51 Dukes Avenue, Theydon Bois, Epping CM16 7HQ — MB BS Lond. 1998.

PECK, Mark Andrew 2 Antoinette Court, Abbots Langley WD5 0QL — MB BS Lond. 1982.

PECK, Richard Wilson Eli Lilly & Co Ltd, Earl Wood Manor, Sunninghill Road, Windlesham GU20 6PH Tel: 01276 483000 — MB BChir Camb. 1985; MA Camb. 1986; MRCP (UK) 1987; FPM 2000. Dir. Europ. Exploratory Med. Eli Lilly. Specialty: Pharmacology. Socs: Brit. Pharm. Soc.; (Comm.) Assn. Human Pharmacol. in Pharmaceut. Industry. Prev: Gp. Dir. (Clin. Pharmacol.) SmithKline Beecham Pharmaceut.; Sen. Clin. Pharmacol. Research & Developm. Glaxo Wellcome; Regist. (Med.) Leic. Roy. Infirm.

PECK, Robert James Royal Hallamshire Hospital, Glossop Road, Sheffield S10 2JF Tel: 0114 276 6222; 1 Stone Delf, Fulwood, Sheffield S10 3QX — MB BS Lond. 1980 (Guy's) BSc Lond. 1977, MB BS 1980; FRCR 1986. Cons. (Radiol.) Sheff. HA. Specialty: Radiol. Prev: Lect. (Radiol.) Chinese Univ., Hong Kong; Sen. Regist. (Radiol.) Trent RHA; Regist. (Radiol.) Sheff. HA.

PECK, Rodney Miles D3 Monument Mansions, Wigan Lane, Wigan WN1 2LE — LAH Dub. 1949.

PECK, Sibel Private GP Services, Springfield Hospital, Lawn Lane, Chelmsford CM1 7GU Tel: 01245 234000 Fax: 01245 234107 — MB BS Lond. 1988 (Univ. Lond. Med. Sch. St Bart.) DRCOG 1991; DCH RCP Lond. 1992; MRCGP 1993. Private GP - set up own Pract. Specialty: Gen. Pract. Prev: Trainee GP Leicester VTS; Trainee GP Surrey VTS.

PECKAR, Mr Clive Orde Warrington Hospital NHS Trust, Lovely Lane, Warrington WA5 1QG Tel: 01925 662188 Fax: 01925 662395; BUPA North Cheshire Hospital, Fir Tree Close, Stretton, Warrington WA4 4LU Tel: 01925 265000 Fax: 01925 215038 — MRCS Eng. LRCP Lond. 1971 (St. Thos.) DO Eng. 1974; FRCS Eng. 1979; MSc Oxf. 1983; FRCOphth 1989; FRCS Ed. 2000. Cons. Ophth. Surg. Warrington Hosp. NHS Trust; Edr. Cataract & Refractive Surg. Eurotimes. Specialty: Ophth. Socs: Fell. Coll. Ophth. And Fell. Roy. Coll. of Surg.s, Edin.; Internat. Intraocular Implant Club.; Pub.ations Comm. And Director of Surgic. Skills Train. Europ. Soc. Cat. & Ref. Surg. Prev: Sen. Regist. St. Pauls Eye Hosp. Liverp.; Sen. Research Regist. Oxf. Univ. & Oxf. Eye Hosp.; Regist. Manch. Roy. Eye Hosp.

PECKETT, Mr William Robert Charles 29 Sherbrooke Road, London SW6 7QJ; Bosky Barn, Church Lane, Ripe, Lewes BN8 6AS Tel: 01323 811839 — (Uniersity College & Middlesex Hospital Medical School) MB BS Lond. 1991. Specialist Regist. Trauma & Orthop. S. E. Thames Rotat. Specialty: Trauma & Orthop. Surg.

PECKHAM, Professor Catherine Stevenson, CBE Centre for Paediatric Epidemiology & Biostatics, The Institute of Child Health, 30 Guildford St., London WC1N 1EH Fax: 020 7242 2723 Email: c.peckham@ich.ucl.ac.uk — MB BS Lond. 1960 (University College Hospital, London) MRCS Eng. LRCP Lond. 1960; MFPHM 1973; FFCM 1980, M 1974; MD Lond. 1975; FRCP Lond. 1988; Hon. FRCPath 1991; Hon. FRCOG 1994; FRCPCH 1997. Prof. Paediat. Epidemiol. Inst. of Child Health Lond. & Hon. Cons. Hosp. for Sick Childr. Gt. Ormond St. Lond.; Hon. Cons. Community Med. (Epidemiol.) PHLS (Communicable Dis. Surveillance Centre. Specialty: Epidemiol.; Paediat.; Infec. Dis. Socs: Founder Mem. of Acad. of Med. Sci.s. Prev: Reader (Community Med.) & Hon Cons. Char. Cross Hosp. Lond.; Sen. Med. Research Off. Nat. Childr. Bureau.

PECKHAM, Clare Louise 3 Ashley Gardens, Eastleigh SO53 2JH Tel: 023 8026 5954; 50 Marcliffe Road, Wadsley, Sheffield S6 4AG Tel: 0114 233 7907 — MB BS Lond. 1989 (Char. Cross & Westm. Med. Sch.) DCH RCP Lond. 1993; MRCPI 1996; MRCPCH 1996. Specialist Regist. Rotat. (Paediat.) Sheff. Childr. Hosp. Specialty: Paediat. Prev: SHO (Paediat. Cardiol.) Alder Hey Liverp.; SHO (Neonat.) St. Geo. Hosp. Lond.; SHO (Paediat.) Kingston Hosp. Surrey.

PECKHAM, Daniel Gavin Seacroft Hospital, Leeds Teaching Hospitals NHS Trust, Adult Cystic Fibrosis Unit, York Road, Leeds LS14 6UH Tel: 0113 2063323; St James's University Hospital , Leeds Teaching Hospitals NHS Trust, Beckett Street, Leeds LS9 7TF — MB BS Lond. 1987 (Char. Cross) FRCP; MRCP (UK) 1991; DM Nottm. 1994. Cons. Phys. Respirat. & Cystic Fibrosis St James Univ. Hosp. & Seacroft Hosp. Specialty: Respirat. Med.; Gen. Med.; Cystic Fibrosis.

PECKHAM, Fiona Claire Burton Croft Surgery, 5 Burton Crescent, Leeds LS6 4DN Tel: 0113 274 4777 Fax: 0113 230 4219 — MB BS Lond. 1986 (Lond. Med. Coll. & St Bart.) DCH RCP Lond. 1990. Specialty: Community Child Health.

PECKHAM, Professor Sir Michael John School of Public Policy, University College London, 29 Tavistock Square, London WC1H 9EZ Tel: 020 7679 4966 Fax: 020 7679 4969 Email: spp@ucl.ac.uk — MB BChir Camb. 1960 (Univ. Coll. Lond. Med. Sch.) MD Camb. 1969; FRCP Lond. 1986, M 1974; FRCR 1975; FRCPath 1991; FRCS 1996. Dir. Sch. Pub. Policy Univ. Coll. Lond. Specialty: Oncol. Prev: Dir. Research Developm. NHS DoH; Dir. Brit. Postgrad. Med. Federat.

PECKHAM, Mr Timothy James — MB BS Newc. 1984 (Newc. u. Tyne) BMedSc Newc. 1981; FRCS Eng. 1990; FRCS (Orth.) 1996. Cons. Orthop. Surg. Basildon & Thurrock Gen. Hosps. NHS Trust. Specialty: Trauma & Orthop. Surg. Socs: Fell. BOA; Fell. Roy. Soc. Med.; Brit. Elbow & Shoulder Soc. Prev: Sen. Regist. Rotat. (Orthop.) Guy's & St. Thos. Hosp. Lond.; Regist. Rotat. (Orthop.) King's Coll. Hosp. Lond.; Shoulder Fell., Guy's Hosp. Lond.

PECKITT, Gavin Beattie Clifton Lane Health Centre, Clifton Lane, Doncaster Road, Rotherham S65 1DU Tel: 01709 382315 Fax: 01709 512646 — MB ChB Aberd. 1973; DObst RCOG 1975. Clin. Asst. (ENT Surg.) Rotherham Dist. Gen. Hosp. Prev: SHO Aberd. Matern. Hosp.; Ho. Off. Aberd. Roy. Infirm.

PECKITT, Kenneth 7 Herringthorpe Avenue, Rotherham S65 3AA — MB ChB Manch. 1998.

PECKITT, Mr Ninian Spenceley St. Chad's House, Hooton Pagnell, Doncaster DN5 7BW Tel: 01977 644535 Fax: 01977 644535 Email: nspeckitt@maxfac.com — MB ChB Sheff. 1979; BDS Ed. 1974; MRCS Eng. LRCP Lond. 1979; FRCS Ed. 1984; FFD RCSI 1986; FDS RCS Eng. 1987. Director Nat. Centre for Aesthetic Facial and Oral Surg. www.maxfac.com. Specialty: Oral & Maxillofacial Surg. Special Interest: Platelet Rich Plasma; Reconstruc. Maxillofacial Surg.; Facial Trauma. Socs: BMA; BAOMS. Prev: Cons. Oral & Maxillofacial Surg. Pk. Hill Hosp. Thorne Rd. Doncaster; Cosmetic Facial Surg. Birkdale Clinics Rotherham & Liverp.; Dir. ComputerGen Implants Ltd.

PEDDER, Claire Elizabeth Eyre Medical Practice, 31 Eyre Crescent, Edinburgh EH3 5EU Tel: 0131 556 8842; 23 Edinburgh Road, Musselburgh EH21 6EA — MB ChB Ed. 1990 (Edinburgh) BSc (Med. Sci.) Hons. Ed. 1989; DRCOG 1994; MRCGP 1996. GP Princip.; Clin. Asst. Cardiol., Roy. Infirm. Edin.

PEDDER, Gillian Helen 45 Stonnall Road, Aldridge, Walsall WS9 8JZ Tel: 01922 454355 — MB ChB Leeds 1993. Specialty: Paediat. Dent.

PEDDER, Jonathan Richard (retired) 26 Alwyne Road, London N1 2HN Tel: 020 7226 3807 — (Oxf. & Middlx.) BM BCh Oxf. 1961; MA Oxf. 1961; FRCP Lond. 1992, M 1965; DPM Lond. 1967; FRCPsych 1979, M 1971. Prev: Cons. Psychother. Bethlem Roy. & Maudsley Hosps.

PEDDER, Samantha Jane 6 Providence Court, Morley, Leeds LS27 9RP — BSc (Hons.) Anat. & Human Biol. Liverp. 1989, MB ChB 1992. SHO (Anat.) NHS Trust, Aintree Walton Hosp. & Fazakerley Hosp. Liverp.

PEDDI, Nagabhushanam Choudary 15 Stowe Close, Liverpool L25 7YE — MB ChB Ed. 1998.

PEDDI, V Belle Vale Health Centre, Hedgefield Road, Liverpool L25 2XE Tel: 0151 487 0514 Fax: 0151 488 6601.

PEDDIE, Mary Margaret The Wallace Medical Centre, 254 Thornhill Road, Falkirk FK2 7AZ Tel: 01324 622826 Fax: 01324 633447; 8 Greenhorn's Well Drive, Falkirk FK1 5HJ — MB ChB Glas. 1979; DRCOG 1981; MRCGP 1984. GP Falkirk.

PEDEN, Carol Jane Royal United Hospital, Bath BA1 3NG Tel: 01225 428331 — MB ChB Ed. 1983; FRCA 1988; MD Ed. 1996. Cons. Anaesth. & Intens. Care Roy. United Hosp. Bath; Primary Fell. Examr., Roy. Col. Of Anaesth.s; Course Organiser, Bristol/Bath Primary Fellowship Course. Specialty: Anaesth. Prev: Lect. (Anaesth.) Bristol Roy. Infirm.; Hon. Sen. Regist. & MRC Research Fell. Hammersmith Hosp. Lond.

PEDEN, Karen Irene Sunnyside Royal Hospital, Montrose DP10 9JP — MB ChB Aberd. 1989 (Aberdeen University) MRCGP

1995; DRCOG 1995. Specialty: Alcohol & Substance Misuse; Gen. Pract.

PEDEN, Norman Robert Falkirk & District Royal Infirmary, Major's Loan, Falkirk FK1 5QE Tel: 01324 616128 Fax: 01324 616020 — MB BChir Camb. 1976 (Middlesex hospital) MA, MB Camb. 1976, BChir 1975; MRCP (UK) 1977; FRCP Ed. 1988. Cons. Phys. Falkirk & Dist. Roy. Infirm.; Hon. Sen. Lect. Dept. of Postgrad. Med. University of Glas. Specialty: Gen. Med. Socs: Brit. Diabetic Assn.; Brit. Thyroid Assn.; Caledonian Soc. Endrocrinol. Prev: Lect. (Pharmacol./Ther.) Univ. Dundee & Hon. Sen. Regist. (Gen. Med.) Ninewells Hosp. Dundee; Registar (Gen. Med.) Ninewells Hosp. & Med. Sch. Dundee; Chief Resid. (Endocrinol. Metab.) Univ., Ottawa.

PEDEN, Thomas Craig (retired) 202 Glasgow Road, Paisley PA1 3LS Tel: 0141 889 9040 — MB ChB Glas. 1951.

PEDERSEN, David Lawrence (retired) The Knoll House, Hinksey Hill, Oxford OX1 5BN Tel: 01865 735345 Fax: 01865 327660 — MB BS Lond. 1950 (St. Bart.) MRCS Eng. LRCP Lond. 1950; MRCGP 1968. Prev: Hosp. Pract. (ENT) Orsett Hosp.

PEDERSEN, Sarah Wendy Child & Adolescent Mental Health Service, Newtown Centre, Nursery Road, Huntingdon PE29 3RJ Tel: 01480 415331 Fax: 01480 415393 — MB BS Lond. 1979 (St. Mary's) MRCPsych 1983. Cons. Child & Adolesc. Psychiat. Hinchingbrooke Hosp. Huntingdon. Specialty: Child & Adolesc. Psychiat. Prev: Sen. Regist. (Child & Adolesc. Psychiat.) Camb. HA.

PEDLER, Stephen John 12 Rudby Close, Whitebridge Park, Gosforth, Newcastle upon Tyne NE3 5JF — MB ChB Bristol 1978; MRCPath 1984. Cons. (Microbiol.) Roy. Vict. Infirm. Newc. u. Tyne. Specialty: Med. Microbiol. Socs: BMA & Brit. Soc. Antimicrobial Chemother. Prev: Sen. Regist. (Microbiol.) Roy. Vict. Infirm. Newc.; Regist. (Microbiol.) Bristol Roy. Infirm.

PEDLEY, David Keith 3 Higher Tunsteads, Greenfield, Oldham OL3 7NX Tel: 01457 875259 Fax: 0161 343 2716; Blafrual House, Lod Backello, Ancterhouse, Dundee DD30Qy Tel: 0131 662 0021 Fax: 01382 320430 — MB ChB Dundee 1994; MRCP (UK) 1997. SHO (A & E) St. Johns Hosp. Ed.; SHO III A & E Nimbercus Hosp. Specialty: Accid. & Emerg.; Intens. Care. Socs: MRCP (Ed.); Assoc. Mem. of Brit. Assoc. of Accid. & Emerg. Med. Prev: SHO (A & E) Dundee Roy. Infirm.; SHO (Orthop.) Edin. Roy. Infirm.; SHO (Med.) Ninewells Hosp. Dundee.

PEDLEY, Ian David 334 Stainbeck Road, Chapel Allerton, Leeds LS7 3PP Tel: 0113 294 0771 — MB ChB Leeds 1990; BSc Chem. Path. (Hons.) Leeds 1987; MRCP (UK) 1994. Regist. (Clin. Oncol.) Yorks. Regional Cancer Centre Cookridge Hosp. Leeds. Specialty: Oncol.; Radiother.

PEDLEY, Julian Eric Medical Protection Society, 33 Cavendish Square, London W1G 0PS Tel: 020 7399 1300 Fax: 020 7399 1301; 4 Andrewes Croft, Marsh Drive, Great Linford, Milton Keynes MK14 5HP Tel: 01908 660706 Email: julian_pedley@tinyworld.co.uk — MB BS Lond. 1967 (Middlx.) MB Lond. 1967; DTM & H Liverp. 1968; DTPH 1970; MSc (Social Med.) Lond. 1976; FFPHM 1987, M 1979. Medico-Legal Advis. (Internat. Div.) Med. Protec. Soc. Lond.; Chairm. Willen Hospice Counc. of Managem. Milton Keynes. Specialty: Pub. Health Med. Socs: Medico-Legal Soc.; IAPOS; Roy. Soc. Med. Prev: Chief Exec. Bucks. HA; Dist. Gen. Manager & Dir. Pub. Health Milton Keynes HA; Sen. Med. Off., Commonw. Developm. Corp. Swaziland.

PEDLOW, Paula Leslie Department of Child & Family Mental Health, Homoeopathic Hospital, 41 Church Road, Tunbridge Wells TN1 1JU Tel: 01892 522598 Fax: 01892 532629 — MB BS Newc. 1970; MRCPsych 1978. Cons. Child Psychiat. & Clin. Dir. Child & Adol. Ment. Health Serv. W. Kent NHS & Social Care Trust. Specialty: Child & Adolesc. Psychiat. Prev: Cons. Child Psychiat. & Med. Dir. Hastings & Rother NHS Trust; Sen. Regist. (Child Psychiat.) W. Midl. RHA; Cons. Child Psychiat. & Clin. Dir. Child & Family Servs. Invicta Community Care NHS Trust.

PEDLOW, Mr Peter Robert Bradley (retired) c/o Pinehill Hospital, Benslow Lane, Hitchin SG4 9QZ Tel: 01462 422822 — MB BCh BAO Belf. 1954; FRCOG 1975, M 1960, DObst 1956; FRCS Ed. 1963; FRCS Glas. 1963. Prev: Cons. Gyn. Pinehill Hosp. Hitchin.

PEDRAZZINI, Anne Elizabeth Bedford House Clinic, Havelock Place, Shelton, Stoke-on-Trent ST1 4PR Tel: 01782 425012 Fax: 01782 425006; Fig Tree House, 15 Sandy Lane, Newcastle ST5 0LX Tel: 01782 613830 — MB ChB Birm. 1963; DObst RCOG 1965. SCMO Family Plann. (Community Med. & Sexual & Reproduc. Med.) N. Staffs. HA. Specialty: Family Plann. & Reproduc. Health; Psychosexual Med.; Obst. & Gyn. Socs: Assoc. Mem. Inst. Psychosexual Med; Assn. Marital & Sexual Therapists; Assoc. Mem. Inst. Psycho-Sexual Med. Prev: Med. Off. (Community Med.) N. Staffs. Health Dist.; Clin. Asst. (Dermat.) Mid. Staffs. Health Dist.

PEDRAZZINI, Sarah-Louise 44 Eason Drive, Abingdon OX14 3YD — MB BCh Wales 1997. SHO (A&E) Morriston Hosp. Swansea. Specialty: Accid. & Emerg. Prev: Ho. Off. (Gen. Med.) Princess of Wales Hosp. Bridgend; Ho. Off. (Gen. Surg.) Singleton Hosp. Swansea.

PEEBLES, Charles Robert 16 Cherville Street, Romsey SO51 8FD — MB BS Lond. 1990.

PEEBLES, Donald Mark 25 Finsen Road, London SE5 9AX — MB BS Lond. 1986.

PEEBLES, Douglas James (retired) 101 Plaistow Lane, Bromley BR1 3AR Tel: 020 8460 0871 — MB BS Lond. 1959 (St. Bart.) DObst RCOG 1962; FFA RCS Eng. 1965. Cons. Anaesth. Sydenham Childr. Hosp. & Bromley Hosp. Gp. Prev: Sen. Regist. Dept. Anaesth. Lond. Hosp.

PEEBLES, Jennifer Payne (retired) The Bell Tower, Old Kingsdown House, Upper Street, Deal CT14 8EU; 14 Riverbank, East Molesey KT8 9BH — MB BS Lond. 1960 (Guy's) MB BS (Hons.) Distinc. Midw. & Gyn.) Lond. 1960; MRCS Eng. LRCP Lond. 1960; DObst RCOG 1962. Prev: Med. Off. Pilgrims Canterbury Hospice.

PEEBLES, Margaret Kerr 36 Crieff Road, Perth PH1 2RS — MB ChB Ed. 1988.

PEEBLES, Mary Anne Clark Durrockstock, 8 Castle Terrace, Ullapool IV26 2XD — MB ChB Glas. 1947 (Univ. Glas.)

PEEBLES, Robert Anthony, RD (retired) The Bell Tower, Old Kingsdown House, Upper Street, Kingsdown, Deal CT14 8EU; 14 Riverbank, East Molesey KT8 9BH — MRCS Eng. LRCP Lond. 1961 (Guy's) MB BS Lond. 1961, BDS 1957; FDS RCS Eng. 1964. Prev: Cons. Oral & Maxillofacial Surg. Kingston & NW Surrey Hosp. Gps.

PEEBLES-BROWN, Anne Elizabeth Mayday University Hospital, Mayday Road, Croydon CR7 7YE Tel: 020 8401 3266 — MB ChB Glas. 1976; DRCOG 1978; FFA RCS Eng. 1980. Cons. Anaesth. Mayday Univ. Hosp. Croydon. Specialty: Anaesth.

PEEBLES BROWN, David (retired) 8 St. Marys Close, Hessle HU3 0HJ — MB ChB Glas. 1972; DObst RCOG 1975; MRCGP 1977. Prev: Gen. Practitioner, Hessle, E. Yorks.

PEEBLES BROWN, Doris Agnes Rothery (retired) 18 The Chestnuts, Winscombe BS25 1LD Tel: 01934 844377 — (Univ. Glas.) MB ChB Glas. 1943. Prev: Clin. Med. Off. Chesh. Co. Counc.

PEECOCK, Fiona Patricia Mary 563 Felixstowe Road, Ipswich IP3 8TE — MB BS Newc. 1982; DRCOG 1986. Prev: Ho. Off. (Med.) Preston Hosp. N. Shields; Ho. Off. (Surg.) S. Shields Gen. Hosp.

PEEDELL, Clive 1 Sweetmans Road, Oxford OX2 9BA — BM Soton. 1995.

PEEK, Brenda Mains of Melginch Farmhouse, Balbeggie, Perth PH2 6HJ Tel: 01821 640528 — MB ChB Dundee 1978; MRCGP 1986; MSc Birmingham 2001. Staff Grade Oncologist Beatson Oncol. Centre Glas. Specialty: Gen. Med.

PEEK, Mr Giles John ECMO Office, Glenfield Hospital, Leicester LE3 9QP Tel: 0116 256 3256 Email: ycq57@dial.pipex.com — MB BS Lond. 1990 (Kings Coll. Hosp.) FRCS Eng. 1994; MD Leic. 1998; FRCS (CTh) Intercollegiate Speciality Bd. 2002. Cons. in Cardiothoracic Surg. & ECMO. Specialty: Cardiothoracic Surg. Special Interest: ECMO, Paediatric Cardiac & Thoracic Surg. Socs: BMA; Soc. Of Cardiothoracic Surg. of GB & Irel. Prev: Lect. (Cardiac Surg.) Univ.of Leic.; Hon. Specialist Regist. (Cardio-Thoracic Surg.); Specialist Regist. (Cardio-Thoracic Surg.) Trent Rotat.

PEEK, Ian Maurice (retired) Daleham Practice, 5 Daleham Gardens, London NW3 5BY Tel: 020 7530 2510 Fax: 020 7530 2511; 4 Holly Terrace, 89 Highgate West Hill, London N6 6LU — MB BS Lond. 1966 (St. Bart.) MRCS Eng. LRCP Lond. 1966; DObst RCOG 1968; DCH Eng. 1971; MRCGP 1976. Prev: Regtl. Med. Off. 4th Bn. Roy. Green Jackets (T & AVR).

PEEK, William Henry Yew Tree, Lymington Road, Milford on Sea, Lymington, Southampton SO4 0QL — MRCS Eng. LRCP Lond. 1939 (Westm.) FRCOG 1963, M 1948. Prev: Res. Obst. Asst. Westm. Hosp.; Med. Off. RAFVR 1940-5; Obstetr. & Gynaecol. Walsall Gp. Hosps.

PEEL, Andrew James Headwell House, Headwell Lane, Saxton, Tadcaster LS24 9PX; Medical Centre, Beech Grove, Sherburn in Elmet, Leeds LS25 6ED — BM BS Nottm. 1988.

PEEL, Mr Anthony Lawrence Geoffrey 77 Junction Road, Norton, Stockton-on-Tees TS20 1PU Tel: 01642 554354 — MB Camb. 1966 (St. Thos.) MChir Camb. 1977, MB 1966, BChir 1965; FRCS Ed. 1969; FRCS Eng. 1970. Cons. Surg. N. Tees Dist. Gen. Hosp. Stockton-on-Tees. Specialty: Gen. Surg. Prev: Sen. Regist. (Surg.) St. Thos. Hosp. Lond.

PEEL, Darryl Michael Cutlers Hill Surgery, Bunsey Rd, Halesworth IP19 8SG Tel: 01986 874618; Threeways, Cookley, Halesworth IP19 9AT — MB ChB Sheff. 1986.

PEEL, David Jonathan Dean Lane Family Practice, 1 Dean Lane, Bedminster, Bristol BS3 1DE Tel: 0117 966 3149 Fax: 0117 953 0699 — MB BS Lond. 1992.

PEEL, Edwin Timothy North Tyneside General Hospital, North Shields NE29 8NH Tel: 0191 293 2722 Fax: 0191 293 2722 — MB BS Lond. 1974 (UCHMS) BSc (Hons.) Lond. 1971; FRCP (Lond.) 1992, M 1977. Cons. Phys. (Gen. & Respirat. Med. & Palliat. Med.) N. Tyneside Gen. Hosp. Specialty: Respirat. Med.; Palliat. Med. Socs: Brit. Thorac. Soc. Assoc. Palliat. Med. Prev: Sen. Regist. (Respirat. Med.) Gwent & S. Glam. HA; Regist. Dept. Respirat. Med. & Chest Unit City Hosp. Edin.; Regist. Newc. AHA (T).

PEEL, Elizabeth Mary The Surgery, 46 Stewkley Road, Wing, Leighton Buzzard LU7 0NE Tel: 01296 688949 Fax: 01296 682250 — MB BS Lond. 1989; MRCGP 1993. Socs: BMA.

PEEL, George William Bryan (retired) Haygrove House, Roman Lane, Bridgwater TA6 7JB Tel: 01278 423044 — MB ChB Bristol 1950; DObst RCOG 1951. Prev: O & G RAMC.

PEEL, Sir John, KCVO (retired) 11 Harnwood Road, Salisbury SP2 8DD Tel: 01722 334892 — BM BCh Oxf 1932 (Oxf. & King's Coll. Hosp.) MRCS Eng. FRCP Lond. 1930; FRCP Lond. 1971; Hon. DSc Birm. 1972; Hon. DM Soton. 1974; Hon. DCh Newc. 1980; Hon. FRCOG 1989; BA (1st cl. Hons. Nat. Sc.) Oxf. 1928, MA 1932; FRCS Eng. 1933; FRCOG 1944; Hon. FRCS Canada 1967; Hon. FCM (S. Afr.) 1968; Hon. FACS 1970; Hon. MMSA Lond. 1970; Hon. FACOG 1971. Consg. O & G Surg. King's Coll. Hosp. Lond.; Emerit. Lect. KCH Med. Sch. Prev: Surg. Gyn. to HM The Qu.

PEEL, Juliet Margaret School House, Hassop, Bakewell DE45 1NT Tel: 01629 640324 Fax: 01629 640324 Email: pjpeel@onetel.com — MB BS Lond. 1966 (Middlx.) DObst RCOG 1968; MFFP 1992. p/t Coloscopy Pract. Jessop Wing Hallamshire Hosp. Sheff. Teachg. Hosp. Trust; Fam. Plann. SCMO High Peek & Dales PCT; Cervical Screening Co-ordinator Chesterfield PCT. Specialty: Obst. & Gyn. Prev: SHO (O & G) North. Gen. Hosp. Sheff.; SCMO (Colposcopy) Rotherham Gen. Hosp. Trust.

PEEL, Mr Kenneth Roger — MB ChB Leeds 1958; DObst RCOG 1960; FRCS Ed. 1965; FRCOG 1977, M 1965. Cons. (Gyn.) Nuffield Hosp. Leeds. Specialty: Obst. & Gyn. Socs: BMA; Soc. Apoth. Lond. Prev: Se. Aclin. Lect. (Obst. & Gyn.) Uni. Leeds; Hon. Cons. (Gyn.) Regional RadiopTher. Centre Cookridge Hosp. Leeds.; (Gyn. Surg.) Leeds Gen. Infirm.

PEEL, Michael John (retired) Millstone, Mill Lane, St Ippolyts, Hitchin SG4 7NN Tel: 01462 459748 — MB BChir Camb. 1950 (St. Mary's) MA, MB BChir Camb. 1950.

PEEL, Michael Robert Occupational Health Department, St. Thomas Hospital, London SE1 7EH Tel: 020 7928 9292; Flat 3, 47 Pembridge Villas, London W11 3EP — MB BS Lond. 1978 (St. Mary's) MRCGP 1984; MFOM RCP Lond. 1989. Sen. Lect. (Occupat. Med.) UMDS Guy's & St. Thos. Hosps.; Med. Adviser Hse. of Parliament; Sen. Med. Examr. Med. Fundat. Specialty: Occupat. Health. Socs: Fell. Roy. Soc. Med.; Soc. Occupat. Med. Prev: Sen. Manager Health, Safety & Welf. Brit. Telecom Internat.; Med. Off. Brit. Airways Med. Serv.

PEEL, Nicola Frances Anne Northern General Hospital, Herries Road, Sheffield S5 7AU Tel: 0114 226 6044 Email: nicola.peel@sth.nhs.uk — BM BS Nottm. 1984; BMedSci Nottm. 1982; DM 1984; MRCP (UK) 1988. Cons., Metab. Bone Med.; Hon. Sen. Clin. Lect. Specialty: Rheumatol. Socs: Bone and Tooth Soc.; Brit. Soc. for Rheum.; Amer. Soc. for Bone and Mineral Research. Prev: Regist. (Gen. Med.) Roy. Hallamsh. Hosp. Sheff.; SHO (Gen. Med.) Chesterfield Roy. Hosp.; SHO (Rheum. & Gen. Med.) Harold Wood Hosp.

PEEL, Philip Hedley 3 Brancepeth Close, Durham DH1 5XL — MB ChB Leeds 1988.

PEEL, Robert Kemsley 116 Moor Lane, York YO24 2QY — MB BS Lond. 1994.

PEEL, Robert Nigel (retired) 116 Moor Lane, Dringhouses, York YO24 2QY Tel: 01904 704375 — (Char. Cross) MB BS Lond. 1964; FRCPath 1983, M 1971. Prev: Cons. Med. Microbiol. & Dir. Regional Pub. Health Laborat. Leeds.

PEEL, Sheelagh Patricia (retired) Hollybank, Ward Lane, Higher Disley, Stockport SK12 2BZ Tel: 01663 762253 Fax: 01663 762253 — (Liverp.) MB ChB Liverp. 1955; DPH Liverp. 1962; MFPHM RCP (UK) 1974. Prev: SCMO Stockport DHA.

PEEL, Stephen 5 Cousins Grove, Southsea PO4 9RP Tel: 023 9273 2043 — MB BS Durh. 1942. Prev: Asst. Res. Med. Off. Roy. Vict. Infirm. Newc.; Surg. Lt. RNVR 1943-7; Med. Off. H.M. Prison Portsmouth.

PEELING, Audrey Margaret (retired) 17 Stow Park Circle, Newport NP20 4HF Tel: 01633 255463 Fax: 01633 223357 Email: ampeeling@aol.com — MB BS Lond. 1955 (Lond. Hosp.) DA Eng. 1958; FFA RCS Eng. 1960. Prev: Cons. Anaesth. S. Gwent Health Dist.

PEER, Emily Jane 2 Scotsmansfield, Burway Road, Church Stretton SY6 6DP Tel: 01694 722437 — BM BS Nottm. 1991; BMedSci Nottm. 1989; DFFP 1997; MRCGP 1997; DRCOG 1997. GP Retainer Mytton Oak Surg. Shrewsbury; Clin. Asst., Rehabillitation Med., Shrewsbury Hosp. Specialty: Gen. Pract. Socs: BMA & Med. Defence Union. Prev: SHO (Paediat.) Roy. Shrewsbury Hosp.; Sen. Med. Off. Proserpine Hosp. N. Queensland, Austral.; Locum GP.

PEER, Rachel Margaret Wasen Hill, Evesham Road, Binton, Stratford-upon-Avon CV37 9UD — MB BS Lond. 1975; FFA RCS Eng. 1979. Assoc. Specialist (Anaesth.) Warwick Hosp. Specialty: Anaesth.

PEEREBOOM, Jeffery Mark Flat 2, Girdlestone Close, Headington, Oxford OX3 7NS — MB BS Queensland 1985.

PEERMAHOMED, Rafic Conifers Resource Centre, Church Road, Caterham CR3 5RA Tel: 01883 347373 Fax: 01883 346492; 57 Mulgrave Road, Sutton SM2 6LR Tel: 020 8661 9285 — MB BS Osmania 1966 (Gandhi Med. Coll. Hyderabad) DPM RCPSI 1973; MRCPsych 1974. Cons. Psychiat. E. Surrey Learning Disabil. Ment. Health Serv. NHS Trust Redhill, Surrey. Specialty: Gen. Psychiat. Prev: Med. Asst. (Psychiat.) Tooting Bec. Hosp. Lond.; Regist. (Psychiat.) Clifton Hosp. York.

PEERS, Christina Maria — MFFP; MB BS Lond. 1983; DRCOG 1986; Cert. Family Plann. JCC. 1986. Cons. (Family Plann. & Reprod. Healthcare). Specialty: Family Plann. & Reproduc. Health. Prev: GP Cuckfield Sussex VTS; Med. Off. St. Catherines Hospice Crawley.

PEERS, Lesley Anne 121 Brookhouse Hill, Fulwood, Sheffield S10 3TE — MB ChB Sheff. 1996.

PEET, Andrew Charles Birmingham Childrens Hospital, Steelhouse Lane, Birmingham B4 6NH; 82 Underdale Road, Shrewsbury SY2 5EE Tel: 01743 340038 Fax: 01743 340038 — MB BS Lond. 1994 (St Georges London) MRCP UK 1998. Specialist Regist., Birm. Childr.s Hosp., Birm. Specialty: Paediat.

PEET, Angela Suzanne 27 Park Avenue, Barbourne, Worcester WR3 7AJ Tel: 01905 612371 — MB BS Lond. 1993 (Royal London) FRCS (A&E) 1998. Specialty: Accid. & Emerg.

PEET, Eleanor Joan Robertson Penarth Health Centre, Stanwell Road, Penarth CF64 3XE Tel: 029 2071 1216; 47 Clive Place, Penarth CF64 1AX Tel: 01222 711216 — MB ChB Manch. 1977; DRCOG 1979; MRCGP 1981.

PEET, John Spencer Lethbridge Farmhouse, Lovacott, Newton Tracey, Barnstaple EX31 3PY — MB BS Lond. 1954.

***PEET, Julia Anne** Le Chene, Forest, Guernsey GY8 0BB — MB BS Lond. 1969; MRCS Eng. LRCP Lond. 1969.

PEET, Katharine Mary Skrine (retired) 4 Stephen Road, Headington, Oxford OX3 9AY Tel: 01865 761763 — BM BCh Oxf. 1948; MA Oxf. 1949; MRCP Lond. 1953. Cons. Phys. Younger Disabled Churchill Hosp. & Migraine Clinic Dept. Neurol. Radcliffe Infirm. Oxf. Prev: Med. Asst. (Physical. Med.) Rivermead Hosp. Oxf.

PEET, Professor Malcolm Swallownest Court Hospital, Aughton Rd, Swallownest, Sheffield S26 4TH Tel: 0114 287 2570 Fax: 0114 287 9147 Email: malcolmpeet@yahoo.com — MB ChB Leeds 1968; BSc (Physiol.) Leeds 1965, MB ChB 1968; DPM Eng. 1972;

FRCPsych 1990, M 1973. Prof. Assoc., Sheff. Univ. Specialty: Gen. Psychiat. Prev: Med. Adviser (Clin. Research) ICI Pharmaceuts. Div. Alderley Edge; Med. Adviser Med. Unit. Organon Oss, Holland.; Cons. Psychiat. Scarsdale Hosp. Chesterfield.

PEET, Mrs Suzanne Elizabeth Ethel (retired) Flat 4, Shaftesbury House,, Trinity St., London SE1 4JF Tel: 020 7407 5158 — MB BS Lond. 1965 (Guy's) MRCS Eng. LRCP Lond. 1965. Prev: Clin. Asst. Dept. Occupat. Health Univ. Coll. Hosp. Lond.

PEET, Mr Timothy Nigel Dexter (retired) Le Chene, Forest, Guernsey GY8 0BB — (Guy's) MB BS Lond. 1965; MRCS Eng. LRCP Lond. 1965; FRCS Eng. 1973. Prev: Cons. Surg. Princess Eliz. Hosp. Guernsey.

PEFFERS, Gillian Mary — MB BS Newc. 1986 (Newcastle upon Tyne) DRCOG 1993; DFFP 1995.

PEGG, Mr Christopher Arthur Sunley The Convent Hospital, 748 Mansfield Road, Woodthorpe, Nottingham NG5 3FZ Tel: 0115 920 9209 Fax: 0115 967 3005 — MB BS Lond. 1962 (St. Thos.) FRCS Eng. 1967; ChM Aberd. 1969. Cons. Gen. Surg. Nottm. Univ. Hosp. & Gen. Hosp. Nottm. Specialty: Gen. Surg. Socs: Fell. Assn. Surgs.; Thyroid Club & Europ. Thyroid Assn. Prev: Sen. Regist. (Surg.) Roy. Infirm. Aberd.; Sen. Surg. Cas. Off. & Ho. Surg. Profess. Unit, St. Thos. Hosp. Lond.

PEGG, Professor David Edward Medical Cryobiol. Unit, Department Biology, University of York, Heslington, York YO10 5DD Tel: 01904 328716 Fax: 01904 328715 Email: dep1@york.ac.uk; 10 St. Paul's Square, Holgate, York YO24 4BD Tel: 01904 630751 — MD Lond. 1963 (Westm.) MB BS 1956; MRCPath. 1968. Dir. Med. Crybiol. Unit. Specialty: Blood Transfus. Socs: Fell. Roy. Soc. Med.; Brit. Transpl. Soc. Prev: Dir. E. Anglian Regional Tissue Bank; Head, MRC Med. Cryobiol. Gp. Douglas Ho. Camb.; Research Haemat. Westm. Med. Sch. Lond.

PEGG, Mr Derek Jonathan Leighton Hospital, Middlewich Road, Crewe CW1 4QJ Email: derek.pegg@mcht.nhs.uk — MB BS Lond. 1984 (Westm.) FRCS Ed. 1989; FRCS (Orth.) 1996. Cons. Orthop. Surg. Leighton Hosp. Crewe, Chesh. Specialty: Trauma & Orthop. Surg.; Orthop.

PEGG, Elizabeth Margaret (retired) Holden Cottage, 2 West St., Withycombe, Minehead TA24 6PX Tel: 01984 640781 — (Univ. Coll. Lond. & W. Lond. Hosp.) MRCS Eng. LRCP Lond. 1951; DObst RCOG 1954. Prev: Regist. (O & G) Eliz. G. Anderson Hosp. Lond.

PEGG, Graham Charles Whiteladies Health Centre, Whatley Road, Clifton, Bristol BS8 2PU Tel: 0117 973 1201 Fax: 0117 946 7031; 17 Downs Cote View, Westbury-on-Trym, Bristol BS9 3TU Tel: 0117 962 1513 — MB ChB Bristol 1970. Prev: SHO (Gen. Surg.) Bristol Homoeop. Hosp.; SHO (Neurosurg.) Frenchay Hosp. Bristol; SHO (Orthop. Surg.) Winford Orthop. Hosp.

PEGG, John Gordon (retired) Sunnyside, Venn Ottery, Ottery St Mary EX11 1RX Tel: 01404 812166 — MB BS Lond. 1959 (St. Thos.) DObst RCOG 1969.

PEGG, Michael Stuart Newstead, 3 Canons Close, Radlett WD7 7ER — MB BS Lond. 1972 (Westm.) BSc Lond. 1969; MRCS Eng. LRCP Lond. 1972; DObst RCOG 1974; FFA RCS Eng. 1977; LLM Wales. 1995. Cons. Anaesth. Roy. Free Hosp. Lond.; Hon. Sen. Lect. Roy. Free Hosp. Med. Sch. Lond.; Hon. Cons. Anaesth. St. Lukes Hosp. for Clergy. Specialty: Anaesth. Socs: Assn. Anaesths.; BMA. Prev: Sen. Regist. (Anaesth.) St. Geo. Hosp. Lond.; Staff Anaesth. Univ. Amsterdam & Willhelmina Hosp. Amsterdam Holland; Regist. (Anaesth.) King's Coll. Hosp. Lond.

PEGG, Rachel Lisa 3 East Lane Cottages, East Lane, Shipton By Beningbrough, York YO30 1AJ Email: rachel_pegg@hotmail.com — MB BS Lond. 1992 (King's College London) MRCP (Paed.) UK 1997. Specialty: Paediat.

PEGG, Stephen Mark 8 Davan Place, Broughty Ferry, Dundee DD5 3HG — MB ChB Dundee 1989.

PEGGE, Nicholas Christopher University of Wales College of Medicine, Dept. of Cardiology, Heath Park, Cardiff CF14 4XN Tel: 029 2074 7747 Fax: 029 2074 3500; Bryher, 39 Village Farm, Bonvilston, Vale of Glamorgan, Cardiff CF5 6TY Tel: 01446 781553 — MB BS Lond. 1993 (Jesus Coll. Camb. & St. Thos. Hosp. Lond.) MA Camb. 1990; MRCP (UK) 1996. Regist. (Cardiol.) Univ. Hosp. of Wales Cardiff. Specialty: Cardiol. Prev: Regist. (Cardiol.) Morriston Hosp. Swansea; Regist. (Cardiol.) Singleton Hosp. Swansea.

PEGGIE, David Anderson Reform Street Health Centre, Reform Street, Beith KA15 2AE Tel: 01505 502888 Fax: 01505 504151; 1 Whitelea Crescent, Kilmacolm PA13 4JP Tel: 01505 873776 Email: david.peggie@virgin.net — MB ChB Ed. 1978; DRCOG 1981. GP Princip. Beith; Occupat. Health Med. Off. N. Ayrsh. & Arran NHS Trust; Police Surg. Ayrsh. Specialty: Gen. Pract.

PEGGS, Karl Stuart 20 Upper Hollis, Great Missenden HP16 9HP — BM BCh Oxf. 1991.

PEGMAN, Amanda Jane 9 The Chase, Rickleton, Washington NE38 9DX — BM BCh Oxf. 1988.

PEGRUM, Anthony Charles — MB BS Lond. 1993 (St. Geo. Hosp. Med. Sch.) BSc Lond. 1990; FRCA (UK) 2000. GP Registrar, York.

PEGRUM, Helen Louise 11 Barley Mead, Warfield, Bracknell RG42 3SA — MB BS Lond. 1989; DCH RCP Lond. 1992; DRCOG 1993; MRCGP 1995. Specialty: Palliat. Med.

PEI, Kee Cheong Benjamin 15 Holmdene Avenue, London NW7 2LY — MB ChB Glas. 1990.

PEI, Yuk Man Debra 15 Holmdene Avenue, London NW7 2LY — MB ChB Bristol 1992.

PEI YAW LIANG, Gordon 15 Holmdene Avenue, Mill Hill, London NW7 2LY Tel: 020 8959 4792 Fax: 020 8906 0598 — MB BS Hong Kong 1959; DTM & H RCP Lond. 1996. Specialty: Trop. Med.

PEILE, Professor Edward Basil Warwick Medical School, University of Warwick, Coventry CV4 7AL Email: ed.peile@warwick.ac.uk; Chiltern Waters, 1 Stablebridge Road, Aston Clinton, Aylesbury HP22 5ND — MB BS Lond. 1975 (Middlx.) MRCS Eng. LRCP Lond. 1975; DRCOG 1978; DCH Eng. 1978; MRCGP 1980; MRCP (UK) 1981; FRCGP 1993; MRCPCH 1997; FRCP 1999; EdD (Oxf.) 2003. Director of Medical Education. Specialty: Paediat.; Educat. Special Interest: Interproffessional Educat. Prev: Educational Adviser, Oxf. Postgrad. Med. and Dent. Educat.; Partner, Aston Clinton Surg., Aston Clinton Bucks; Hon. Sen. Clin. Lect. Unversity of Oxf.

PEIRCE, Clive Ronald Glendevon Medical Centre, Carlton Place, Teignmouth TQ14 8AB Tel: 01626 770955; Little Court, Shaldon Road, Combeinteignhead, Newton Abbot TQ12 4RR — MB ChB Dundee 1989; MRCGP 1994; DFFP 1995; DGM RCP Lond. 1995. Specialty: Gen. Pract.

PEIRCE, Kate Sarah 79 Lauriston Road, London E9 7HJ — MB BS Lond. 1994.

PEIRCE, Nicholas Sheridan 51 Kelly Street, London NW1 8PG — BM BS Nottm. 1988.

PEIRIS, Mr Collin Sweithin Linton (retired) 6 Argyle Road, Southport PR9 9LH Tel: 01704 532123 — MB BS Ceylon 1952; DO Eng. 1957; FRCS Ed. 1963. Prev: Cons. Ophth. Surg. Southport & Formby Dist. Gen. Hosp. & Ormskirk & Dist. Gen. Hosp.

PEIRIS, Jeffrey Gordon Christopher 31 Oakfield Avenue, Kenton, Harrow HA3 8TH Tel: 020 8907 0606 — MB BS Ceylon 1959; DCH Ceylon 1967. Clin. Med. Off. Brent & Harrow AHA.

PEIRIS, Lokukankanamge Heshanth Sandun 69 Shirley Park Road, Addiscombe, Croydon CR0 7EW — MB BS Lond. 1996.

PEIRIS, Mathew Laith Quintus 6 Langworth Close, Dartford DA2 7ET — MB BS Ceylon 1968; MRCP (UK) 1977; T(GP) 1991.

PEISACH, Carole Melanie Torrington Park Group Practice, 16 Torrington Park, North Finchley, London N12 9SS Tel: 020 8445 7622/4127 — MB ChB Cape Town 1989; DCH Lond. 1994; MRCGP Lond. 1995. GP Princip. Lond.; Clin. Asst. Gyn. Specialty: Obst. & Gyn.

PEJOVIC, Ivan 128 Barrowgate Road, London W4 4QP — (Sarajevo) Lekar Sarajevo, Yugoslavia 1964.

PEKTAS, Tevfik 143 Conisborough Crescent, Catford, London SE6 2SQ; 29 Gilbert Close, Shooters Hill, London SE18 4PT — LMSSA Lond. 1972; DCH RCPS Glas. 1970. Clin. Med. Off. (Child Health) Bromley Primary Care Trust Lond. Socs: Med. Protec. Soc. Prev: Clin. Med. Off. (Child Health) Optimum Health Servs. Lond.

PELEKOUDA, Eleni Queens Hospital, Block B Flat B, Belvedere Road, Burton-on-Trent DE13 0RB — Ptychio Iatrikes Thessalonika 1991.

PELEKOUDAS, Nicolaos 11 Belsize Road, London NW6 4RX — Ptychio Iatrikes Athens 1990.

PELENDRIDES, Helen Wood Green Surgery, 22 Cheshire Road, London N22 8JJ Tel: 020 8888 8378 Fax: 020 8888 8364 Email: helen.pelendrides@gp-e83005.nhs.uk; 112 Creighton Avenue,

London N2 9BJ — MB BS Lond. 1984 (Guy's Hospital London) DRCOG 1988.

PELFRENE, Eric 255 Kennington Road, London SE11 6BY — MD Ghent 1983; T(M) 1994.

PELHAM, Anne 230 Jesmond Dene Road, Jesmond, Newcastle upon Tyne NE2 2JU — MB ChB Aberd. 1986; MRCGP 1990; Dipl Cognitive Therapy 2000. Specialist Regist., Northern Region. Specialty: Palliat. Med.

PELL, Heather (retired) 23 Parkgate, Blackheath, London SE3 9XF — (Lond. Hosp.) MB BS Lond. 1960; MRCS Eng. LRCP Lond. 1960.

PELL, Jill Patricia Department Public Health, Greater Glasgow Health Board, Dalian House, 350 St Vincents St., Glasgow G3 8YU Tel: 0141 201 4544 Fax: 0141 201 4949 — MB ChB Ed. 1987; MSc Ed. 1994, MB ChB Ed. 1987; DCH Glas. 1989; MRCGP 1991; MFPHM RCP (UK) 1995; MD ed 1999. Cons. Pub. Health Med. Greater Glas. HB; Reader (cardiol) Univ. Glas.full time. Specialty: Pub. Health Med. Prev: Sen. Regist. (Pub. Health) Glas.; Research Fell. (Health Servs.) Univ. Edininburgh; GP Trainee, Fife.

PELL, Judith Barbara West Hayes Lodge, Sarum Road, Winchester SO22 5EZ — BM Soton. 1981; MRCGP 1985; MFFP 1993; MFFP 1993. Asst. GP, Southampton. Specialty: Family Plann. & Reproduc. Health. Socs: Fac. Fam. Plann. & Reproduc. Health Care. Prev: GP Winchester.

PELL, Mr Rodney Lang — MB BS Lond. 1961 (Lond. Hosp.) Cert. T.A. (1993); BSc (Hons.) Lond. 1958; MRCS Eng. LRCP Lond. 1961; FRCSI 1969. Cons. Orthop. Surg. Chaucer Hosp. Canterbury, Kent.; Cons. Othop. Surg. The Spencer Wing, Qu. Eliz. the Qu. Mother Hosp. Margate, Kent. Specialty: Trauma & Orthop. Surg.; Orthop.; Sports Med. Socs: Fell. BOA; Fell. Roy. Soc. Med.; Acad. Experts. Prev: Cons. Orthop. Surg. City & E. Lond. HA; Regist. St. Bart. Hosp. Lond.; Regist. (Orthop.) Guy's Hosp. Lond.

PELL-ILDERTON, Richard (retired) The New House, Ryme Intrinseca, Sherborne DT9 6JX — MB ChB Manch. 1953; DPath Eng. 1961; FRCPath 1973, M 1963. Prev: Cons. Path. N. Manch. Gen. Hosp.

PELLEGRINI, Arthur Vincent 87 Larkfield Road, Liverpool L17 9PS — MB ChB Liverp. 1980.

PELLER, Sally Elizabeth Collurian, Gilly Lane, Whitecross, Penzance TR20 8BZ Tel: 01736 740441 Fax: 01736 740441 — MB ChB Bristol 1982; MRCGP 1989. GP Locum, Cornw. Specialty: Gen. Pract. Socs: BMA; RCGP. Prev: GP Regist. Cornw. VTS; Staff Grade (A & E) GTruro Cornw.; GP Regist. Soton. VTS.

PELLING, Marc Xavier 46 Aberdeen Gardens, London NW6 3QA — MB ChB Bristol 1984.

PELLOW, Roy John Newman, MC (retired) 32 Lansdowne Road, Luton LU3 1EE Tel: 01582 731700 — MB BS Lond. 1943 (St. Mary's) MRCS Eng. LRCP Lond. 1941.

PELLUET, Emma Jane 10 Roland Mews, London E1 3JT; 12 The Windmills, Broomfield Hospital, Chelmsford CM1 7ET — MB BS Lond. 1996.

PELLY, Hugh John Wordsworth Dean Lane Surgery, Dean Lane, Sixpenny Handley, Salisbury SP5 5PA Tel: 01725 552500 Fax: 01725 552029; Doves Meadow Surgery, Broadchalke, Salisbury SP5 5EL Tel: 01722 780282 Fax: 01722 780041 — MB BS Lond. 1969 (Middlx.) DCH Eng. 1971; MRCGP 1980; FRCGP 2000. Socs: Expert Witness Inst.; Brit. Inst. Manip. Med. Prev: Clin. Asst. (Rheumatol.) Salisbury Gen. Hosp.; Med. Off. Brit. Nepal Med. Trust; Resid. Med. Off. Middlx. Hosp. Lond.

PELLY, Michael Eliot Chelsea & Westminster Hospital, 369 Fulham Road, London SW10 9NH Tel: 0208 746 8071/ 8057 Fax: 0208 746 8554 Email: m.pelly@imperial.ac.uk — MB BS Lond. 1978 (St. Mary's) MRCP (UK) 1980; MRCGP 1986; DTM & H RCP Lond. 1987; MSc (Clin. Trop. Med.) Lond. 1987; FRCP UK 1997. Cons. Phys. Chelsea & Westm.Hosp. Lond.; Hon. Sen. Lect. Imperial Coll. Sch. of Med.; Sen. Med. Cons.(Volun.) Internat. Federat. of Red Cross & Red Cresc. Societies. Specialty: Gen. Med.; Care of the Elderly. Special Interest: Humanitarian Aid; Med. for the Elderly; Stroke. Socs: Soc. of Apoth.; Roy. Soc. of Trop. Med. and Hyg.; Huntarian Society. Prev: Med. Adviser Med. Emerg. Relief Internat.

PELOSI, Anthony Joseph Department of Psychiatry, Hairmyres Hospital, East Kilbridge, Glasgow G75 8RG Tel: 0135 572620 Fax: 0135 572615 Email: anthonypelosi@compuserve.com — MB ChB Glas. 1977; MRCP (UK) 1980; MRCPsych 1985; MSc (Epidemiol.) Lond. 1987; FRCP Glas. 1992. Specialty: Gen. Psychiat.; Epidemiol.

PELTA, David Elliott Queensway Surgery, 75 Queensway, Southend-on-Sea SS1 2AB Tel: 01702 463333 Fax: 01702 603026 — MB ChB Bristol 1973; DCH Eng. 1975; MRCP (UK) 1976; MRCGP 1977.

PELTON, Christopher Ian Wellington Health Centre, Chapel Lane, Wellington, Telford TF1 1PZ Tel: 01952 242304; Hillside, 13 Princes End, Lawley bank, Telford TF4 2JN Tel: 01952 630108 — MB BS Lond. 1978 (Middlesex) FFA RCS Eng. 1982; MRCGP 1985; DRCOG 1987. Specialty: Anaesth. Prev: Regist. (Anaesth.) Univ. Hosp. Wales Cardiff; Sen. Med. Off. Jane Furse Hosp. Lebowa S. Afr.

PELTON, Jane — MB ChB Birm. 1980; DRCOG 1982. Princip. in Gen. Pract., Telford. Prev: GP Telford; Med. Off. Jane Furse Memor. Hosp. Lebowa, S. Afr.; Trainee GP Cardiff VTS.

PEMBERTON, Colin James (retired) 8 Gleneagles Road, Heald Green, Cheadle SK8 3EL Tel: 0161 491 6953 — MB ChB Manch. 1964; MRCS Eng. LRCP Lond. 1966; DA Eng. 1968; FFA RCS Eng. 1971. Cons. Anaesth. Stockport NHS Trust. Prev: Sen. Regist. (Anaesth.) United Manch. Hosps. & Manch. RHB.

PEMBERTON, David Almond (retired) 16 High Street, Dunblane FK15 0AD Tel: 01786 822927 — MB ChB Ed. 1961; DPM Eng. 1965; MRCPsych 1972. Prev: Cons. & Unit Med. Manager Bellsdyke Hosp. Larbert.

PEMBERTON, Mr David John Royal Glamorgan Hospital, Pontyclun CF72 8XR Tel: 01443 443576 — MB BCh Wales 1984 (Welsh Nat. Sch. Med.) FRCS Ed. 1988; FRCS (Orth.) 1992. Cons. Orthop. Surg.Roy. Glam. NHS Trust. Specialty: Orthop. Socs: BASK; BOSTA. Prev: Sen. Regist. (Orthop. Surg.) Cardiff Roy. Infirm.; Lect. (Orthop. Surg.) Univ. Wales Coll. Med.

PEMBERTON, Derek John Circuit Lane Surgery, 53 Circuit Lane, Reading RG30 3AN Tel: 0118 958 2537 Fax: 0118 957 6115 — MB BCh Wales 1983; DA (UK) 1986; MRCGP 1989.

PEMBERTON, Douglas Pye Apartment 4, The Empire, Grand Parade, Bath BA2 4DF — (Camb. & Royal Lond. Hosp.) BA Camb. 1956; MRCS Eng. LRCP Lond. 1961. Life Insur. Med. Examr. Socs: BMA. Prev: Sen. Med. Off. ADMA-OPCO Med. Dept. Das Is., Abu Dhabi, UAE; Dist. Med. Off. Long Is., Bahamas; MOH Elgin N. Dakota, USA.

PEMBERTON, Elaine (retired) 118 Main Road, Ravenshead, Nottingham NG15 9GW — MB ChB Ed. 1967. SCMO (Family Plann.) Nottm. HA (T); Sen. Clin. Med. Off. Centr. Notts. HA.

PEMBERTON, James 18 Village Way, Dulwich, London SE21 7AN Tel: 020 7737 2220 — MRCS Eng. LRCP Lond. 1967 (St. Bart.) BSc Lond. 1963, MB BS 1967; MRCP (U.K.) 1971; DMRD Eng. 1972; FFR 1974; FRCR 1975. Cons. (Diag. Radiol.) St. Thos. Hosp. Lond. Specialty: Radiol. Prev: Jun. Regist. (Med.) & Regist. (Diag. Radiol.) St. Bart. Hosp. Lond.; Sen. Regist. (Diag. Radiol.) King's Coll. Hosp. Lond.

PEMBERTON, James Anthony 161 Osborne Road, West Jesmond, Newcastle upon Tyne NE2 3JT — MB BS Newc. 1996.

PEMBERTON, Janet Mary Scunthorpe Community Healthcare Trust, Brumby Hospital, Scunthorpe DN16 1QQ Tel: 01724 290068 — (King's Coll. Hosp.) MB BS Lond. 1970. SCMO Scunthorpe Community Healthcare Trust. Specialty: Community Child Health; Paediat. Cardiol. Prev: Ho. Phys. Belgrave Hosp. Childr.; Ho. Surg. (Gen. Surg.) Wythenshawe Hosp. Manch.

PEMBERTON, John Central Surgery, King St., Barton-upon-Humber DN18 5ER Tel: 01652 635435 Fax: 01652 636122 — MB BS Lond. 1969 (King's Coll. Hosp.) BDS Lond. 1964; FDS RCS Eng. 1972. Prev: Lect. (Oral Med.) Univ. Manch.; Ho. Surg. (ENT) Kings Coll. Hosp. Lond.; Ho. Phys. Belgrave Hosp. Childr. Lond.

PEMBERTON, John (retired) Iona, Cannonfields, Hathersage, Hope Valley S32 1AG — (Univ. Coll. Hosp.) MB BS Lond. 1936; MRCS Eng. LRCP Lond. 1936; MD Lond. 1940; FRCP Lond. 1964, M 1941; DPH Leeds 1956; FFCM 1974; FFCMI 1976. Emerit. Prof. Social & Preven. Med., Qu. Univ. Belf. Prev: Cons. Social & Preven. Med. Roy. Vict. Hosp. Belf.

PEMBERTON, Laura Shelley 79 1/L Lumsden Street, Yorkhill, Glasgow G3 8RH — MB ChB Glas. 1996.

PEMBERTON, Michael Neal University Dental Hospital of Manchester, Manchester M15 6FH — MB ChB Sheff. 1995. Cons. Oral Med. Univ. Dent. Hosp. Manch.

PEMBERTON, Nicholas Charles 528 Upper Brentwood Road, Romford RM2 6HX — MB BS Lond. 1995.

PEMBERTON, Philippa Louise 18 Village Way, London SE21 7AN — MB BS Lond. 1993.

PEMBERTON, Phillip Edward Portishead Health Centre, Victoria Square, Portishead, Bristol BS20 6AQ Tel: 01275 847474 Fax: 01275 817516 Email: ppemberton@cix.co.uk — MB ChB Bristol 1978; MRCOG 1984; MRCGP 1994. Course Organiser, Bristol Vocational Train. Scheme.

PEMBERTON, Mr Richard Mark Queen Alexandra Hospital, Cosham, Portsmouth PO6 3LY Tel: 023 92 286000 — MB BS Lond. 1986 (Kings College Hospital) BA Camb. 1982; MA Camb. 1985; FRCS Eng. 1990; MS (Gen.) 1998. Cons. Vasc. Srugeon Portsmouth Hosps. Specialty: Gen. Surg.

PEMBLETON, Alec 14c St Bridge Street, Liverpool L8 7PL — MB ChB Liverp. 1996.

PEMBREY, John Seymour The Surgery, 48 Mulgrave Road, Belmont, Sutton SM2 6LX Tel: 020 8642 2050 Fax: 020 8643 6264 Email: john.pembrey@nhs.net.co.uk; 50 Mulgrave Road, Sutton SM2 6LX Tel: 020 8643 3596 Email: pembrey@blueyonder.co.uk — MB BS Lond. 1966 (St. Bart.) MRCS Eng. LRCP Lond. 1966; DCH Eng. 1968; DObst RCOG 1969; MRCGP 1974. Socs: BMA; Sutton Med. Soc. Prev: SHO (Paediat.) Sydenham Childr. Hosp.; Ho. Surg. Metrop. Hosp. Lond.; Ho. Off. (Obst.) St. Bart. Hosp. Lond.

PEMBREY, Rachel Lisa Birchwood, 2 College Road, Upper Beeding, Steyning BN44 3TB; Birchwood, 2 College Road, Upper Beeding, Steyning BN44 3TB — MB BS Lond. 1998 (St. George's Hosp. Med Sch.) MB BS Lond 1998. SHO (A&E) St. Richard's Hosp. Chichester, W. Sussex. Specialty: Accid. & Emerg. Prev: Ho. Off. (Med.) Princess Roy. Hosp. Hayward's Heath; Ho. Off. (Surg.) St. Richard's Hosp. Chichester, W. Sussex.

PEMBRIDGE, Bette Theresa Marcham Road Family Health Centre, Marcham Road, Abingdon OX14 1BT Tel: 01235 522602 Fax: 01235 534605 Email: bette.pembridge@gp-k84041.nhs.uk; Sutton Wick Barn, Sutton Wick, Drayton, Abingdon OX14 4HJ Tel: 01235 559291 — MB BS Lond. 1974 (Roy. Free) MRCS Eng. LRCP Lond. 1974; DRCOG 1977; DCH Eng. 1978; T(GP) 1991; MRCGP 1992. Gen. Practitioner Princip.

PEMBRIDGE, Jonathan Mark Maesmarchog House, Cross Inn, Llantrisant, Pontyclun CF7 8PF — MB BCh Wales 1994.

PEMBROKE, Andrew Charles 28 Dartford Road, Sevenoaks TN13 3TQ Tel: 01732 450197 — MB BChir Camb. 1971 (St. Bart.) MA Camb. 1972; MRCP (UK) 1974; FRCP Lond. 1988. Cons. Dermat. Bromley Hosps. NHS Trust. Specialty: Dermat. Prev: Cons. Dermat. King's Coll. Hosp. Lond.; Sen. Regist. (Dermat.) King's Coll. Hosp. Lond.; Regist. (Dermat.) Lond. Hosp.

PENA, Mr Milton Arquimides Tameside General Hospital, Fountain St., Ashton-under-Lyne OL6 9RW Tel: 0161 331 6768 Fax: 0161 331 6300; Ribbleton House, 30 Crow Lane W., Newton-le-Willows WA12 9YG Tel: 01925 226122 — Medico Cirujano Chile 1973; FRCS Ed. 1984; T(S) 1991. Cons. Orthop. Surg. Tameside Gen. Hosp. Specialty: Orthop. Prev: Sen. Regist. (Orthop.) Wrightington Hosp., Manch Roy. Infirm. & Hope Hosp. Salford.

PENCHEON, David Charles 51 Mill Road, Lode, Cambridge CB5 9EN — BM BCh Oxf. 1982.

PENCHEON, Pamela Edna (retired) — (Leeds) MB ChB Leeds 1952; DPM Eng. 1966; MRCPsych 1972. Prev: Cons. Psychiat. (Adult Psychiat.) Roy. Cornw. Hosp. Truro.

PENDER, James Blackwoods Medical Centre, 8 Station Road, Muirhead, Glasgow G69 9EE Tel: 0141 779 2228 Fax: 0141 779 3225 — MB ChB Glas. 1972.

PENDERED, Lucy Frances The Crown Medical Centre, Venture Way, Taunton TA2 8QY Tel: 01823 282151 Fax: 01823 326755 — MB ChB Bristol 1985; F.P. Cert 1989; DRCOG 1989; T(GP) 1990; MRCGP 1990. Partner.

PENDLEBURY, Donald Granville (retired) Southern Pines, Little London Road, Horam, Heathfield TN21 0BD Tel: 01435 812300 — MB BS Lond. 1959; DPM Eng. 1962; MRCPsych 1971. Prev: Cons. Psychiat. Hellingly Hosp. Hailsham.

PENDLEBURY, Sarah Tamsin 5 Ferry Road, Marston, Oxford OX3 0ET Tel: 01865 721344 Fax: 01865 221122; Oxford Centre for Functional Magnetic, John Radcliffe Hospital, Oxford OX3 9DU Tel: 01865 222738 Fax: 01865 221122 — (Univ. Camb. & Univ. Oxf.) BM BCh Oxf. 1992; MA Camb. 1993; MRCP (UK) 1995. Clin. Research Fell. & Hon. Regist. (Neurol.) Oxf. Specialty: Neurol. Prev: SHO (Neurol.) Radcliffe Infirm.; Clin. Attaché (Respirat. Med.) Centre Hosp.ie Universitaire de Grenoble, France; SHO (Intens. Care) Roy. Sussex Co. Hosp. Brighton.

PENDLETON, Adrian 82 Willowvale Gardens, Belfast BT11 9JW — MB BCh BAO Belf. 1993.

PENDLETON, Ann Pia Mary Mount Pleasant Practice, Tempest Way, Chepstow NP16 5XR Tel: 01291 636500 Fax: 01291 636518 — MB BCh BAO NUI 1982; MRCGP 1991.

PENDLETON, Neil 43 Elmswood Road, Liverpool L17 0DH — MB ChB Liverp. 1985.

PENDLINGTON, Matthew, TD 49 Cannock Road, New Invention, Willenhall WV12 5SA Tel: 01922 76477 Fax: 01922 476477 — (Birm.) MB ChB Birm. 1957. Prev: Ho. Surg. Gen. Hosp. Birm.; Ho. Phys. & Sen. Ho. Surg. O & G Dryburn Hosp. Durh.

PENDOWER, Mr John Edward Hicks (retired) Rosemary, Promenade de Verdun, Purley CR8 3LN Tel: 020 8660 8949 — MB BS Lond. 1950 (King's Coll. Lond. & Char. Cross) MRCS Eng. LRCP Lond. 1950; FRCS Eng. 1955. Barrister-at-Law Inner Temple 1972. Prev: Dean Char. Cross & Westm. Med. Sch.

PENDRIGH, David Croll (retired) 24 Scarbrough Avenue, Skegness PE25 2SY Tel: 01754 3050 — MB ChB Glas. 1949. Prev: Anaesth. Skegness & Dist. Hosp.

PENDRY, Katherine Royal Albert Edward Infirmary., Wigan Lane, Wigan WN1 2NN — MB ChB Bristol 1983; MRCP (UK) 1986; MRCPath 1991; FRCP 1999; FRCPath 2000. Cons. Haemat. Wrightington, Wigan & Leigh Health Serv. NHS Trust. Specialty: Haematology. Prev: Cons. Haemat. Bury Health Care NHS Trust; Cons Haemat. BUPA Healthcare NHS Trust; Sen. Regist. (Haemat.) N. West. RHA.

PENFIELD, Beverley South Woodford Health Centre, 114 High Road, London E18 2QS; 14 Chester Road, Chigwell IG7 6AJ Tel: 020 8500 7018 — MB BS Lond. 1982; DA Eng. 1985. GP Princip.; Family Plann. Doctor Chigwell. Prev: Trainee GP Epping VTS; SHO (O & G/Anaesth.) Whipps Cross Hosp. Lond.

PENFOLD, Bernard Mark 45 Fairways Drive, Blackwell, Bromsgrove B60 1BB — MB ChB Liverp. 1972; MRCS Eng. LRCP Lond. 1972; DObst RCOG 1975; DDAM 2000. Med. Adviser, Med. Servs., SEMA Gp., Birm. Specialty: Disabil. Med.; Respirat. Med.; Occupat. Health. Socs: Soc. Occupat. Med.

PENFOLD, Mr Christopher Neil Glan Clwyd Hospital, Rhyl LL18 5UJ Tel: 01745 583910; Tyddyn Llan, Corwen LL21 9SL Tel: 01824 750472 Email: cnp@globalnet.co.uk — MB BS Lond. 1988; BDS 1978; FDS RCS Ed. 1982; FRCS Ed. 1991. Cons. Oral & Maxillofacial Surg., Glan Clwyd Hosp. Specialty: Oral & Maxillofacial Surg. Socs: Fell. Brit. Assoc. Oral & Maxillofacial Surg.s; Craniofacial Soc.; Brit. Assn. Head & Neck Oncol. Prev: Regist. (Oral & Maxillofacial Surg.) Southampton Gen. Hosp.; Sen. Regist. KCH Lond.; Sen. Regist., Qu. Vict. Hosp., E. Grinstead.

PENFOLD, Grace Kent The Nest, Higher Porthpean, St Austell PL26 6AY — MB BS Lond. 1963 (Univ. Coll. Hosp.)

PENFOLD, Helen Margaret Waterlooville Health Centre, Dryden Close, Waterlooville PO7 6AL Tel: 02392 257321 Fax: 02392 230739 — MB ChB Sheff. 1976; DRCOG 1978; MRCP (UK) 1980; MFFP 1993.

PENFOLD, Hilary Anne Wootton Medical Centre, 36-38 High Street, Wootton, Northampton NN4 6LW Tel: 01604 709933 Fax: 01604 709944; Harlestone House Lodge, Church Lane, Lower Harlestone, Northampton NN7 4EN — MB ChB Sheff. 1987; DRCOG 1991.

PENFOLD, Jason John 350 Scalby Road, Scarborough YO12 6ED — MB BS Lond. 1996.

PENFOLD, Nigel William Department of Anaesthesia, West Suffolk Hospital, Hardwick Lane, Bury St Edmunds IP33 2QZ Tel: 01284 713330 Fax: 01284 713100; St. Helier, Bury Road, Kentford, Newmarket CB8 7PT Tel: 01638 750269 Fax: 01638 555124 Email: nigelwpenfold@aol.com — MB BS Lond. 1980 (St. Bart.) FFA RCS Eng. 1985. Cons. Anaesth. W. Suff. Hosp. Bury St. Edmunds; Regional Adviser (Anglia) Roy. Collaege of Anaesth.s. Specialty: Anaesth. Socs: Assn. Anaesth.; Obst. Anaesth. Assn.; Brit. Assn. Day Surg. Prev: Sen. Regist. Rotat. (Anaesth.) E. Anglian HA; Regist. (Anaesth.) Char. Cross & Brompton Hosps. Lond.; Ho. Surg. St. Bart. Hosp. Lond.

PENFOLD, Susan Elizabeth Handsworth Wood Medical Centre, 110 Church Lane, Handsworth Wood, Birmingham B20 2ES Tel: 0121 523 7117 Fax: 0121 554 2406; 35 Lee Crescent, Edgbaston,

Birmingham B15 2BJ — BM Soton. 1987; MRCGP 1991. Specialty: Endocrinol. Socs: Comm. Mem. Birm. Med. Inst.

PENGE, Daniela Joy 14 Strathblaine Road, London SW11 1RJ Tel: 020 7228 0726 — MB BS Lond. 1992. GP Regist. W. Middlx. Hosp. Lond. Specialty: Gen. Pract. Prev: SHO (Generam Med.) King's Coll. Hosp. Lond.

PENGELLY, Mr Andrew William (retired) Fieldgate House, Hollington, Woolton Hill, Newbury RG20 9XR Tel: 01635 254429 Fax: 01635 253741 Email: awp@ab12.demon.co.uk — (Oxf. & Middlx.) BM BCh Oxf. 1968; MA Oxf. 1968; FRCS Eng. 1974; FEBU 1989. Prev: Cons. Urol. & Med. Exec. Dir. Roy. Berks. & Battle Hosps. NHS Trust Reading.

PENGELLY, Charles Desmond Ross (cons. rooms), 60 Manchester Road, Altrincham WA14 4PJ Tel: 0161 928 2833; Flat 10, Inglewood, St Margaret's Road, Bowdon, Altrincham WA14 2AP Tel: 0161 928 6781 — MB ChB Bristol 1946; FRCP Ed. 1969, M 1952; FRCP Lond. 1968, M 1954; MD Bristol 1959; FRCP Glas. 1986, M 1984. Hon. Cons. Phys. Altrincham Gen. Hosp., St Anne's Hosp. Bowdon & Trafford Gen. Hosp. Davyhulme; Examr. PLAB. Specialty: Gen. Med.; Haematology. Socs: Fell. Roy. Soc. Med.; Fell. Manch. Med. Soc.; Hon. Mem. Nat. Assn. Clin. Tutors. Prev: Univ. Manch. Postgrad. Tutor Altrincham; Sen. Regist. (Med.) Manch. RHB, Manch. Roy. Infirm. & W. Cornw. Clin. Area.

PENIKET, Andrew James Water Works Cottage, Simons Lane, Shipton-under-Wychwood, Chipping Norton OX7 6DH — MB BChir Camb. 1992.

PENIKET, John Bernard 11 The Avenue, Churchdown, Gloucester GL3 2HB Tel: 01452 713727 Fax: 01452 713727 Email: jpeniket@compuserve.com — (King's Coll. Hosp.) MRCS Eng. LRCP Lond. 1965; MB BChir Camb. 1966; DObst RCOG 1967; MRCP Lond. 1969; MRCGP 1981. Med. Adviser Med. Servs. by Sema. Specialty: Disabil. Med. Prev: Med. Servs. Manager Benefits Agency; GP Gloucester; Research Asst. (Cardiac) Radcliffe Infirm. Oxf.

PENKETH, Andrea Regan Lea Roscalen, 19 Eldorado Road, Cheltenham GL50 2PU — MB BS Lond. 1977 (St. Mary's) MRCP (UK) 1980; BSc Lond. 1974, MD 1984; T(M) 1991. Cons. Phys. Cheltenham Gen. Hosp. Specialty: Respirat. Med. Prev: Cons. Phys. Worcester Roy. Infirm.; Lect. (Thoracic Med.) Cardiothoracic Inst. Lond.; SHO (Med.) Hammersmith Hosp. Lond.

PENKETH, Richard John Anderson Department of O & G, UHW, Cardiff CF4 4XW Tel: 02920 744390 Email: pat.mannder@cardiffandvale.wales.nhs.uk — MB BS Lond. 1980 (Univ. Coll. Hosp.) BSc (Human Genetics) Lond. 1977, MB BS 1980; MRCOG 1991; MD 1996. Cons. (O & G); Hon. Cons. Gwent NHS Trust; Hon. Cons. Pembrokeshire & Devon NHS Trust; Hon. Cons. Mid Wales NHS Trust. Specialty: Obst. & Gyn. Special Interest: Minimal Access Surg.; Pelvic Pain; Premenstral Syndrome. Socs: British Society for Gynaecological Endoscopy; International Society for Gynaecological Endoscopy; British Fertility Society. Prev: Lect. (O & G) Birm. Womens Hosp.

PENKETHMAN, Andrew John Felixstowe Road Surgery, 235 Felixstowe Road, Ipswich IP3 9BN Tel: 01473 719112; 14 Borrowdale Avenue, Ipswich IP4 2TN Tel: 01473 251260 — MB BS Lond. 1980; DRCOG 1983; MRCGP 1984.

PENLINGTON, Elizabeth Ruth (retired) 2 Leighton Close, Gibbet Hill, Coventry CV4 7AE Tel: 024 7641 9707 Email: napierpenlington@compuserve.com — MB BCh Wales 1959 (Cardiff) MFCH 1989. Bishop's Represen. for Child Protec. (Coventry Diocese). Prev: Princip. Clin. Med. Off. (Child Health I/c Child Protec.) Coventry Health Care NHS Trust.

PENLINGTON, (Gilbert) Napier (retired) 2 Leighton Close, Gibbet Hill, Coventry CV4 7AE Tel: 024 7641 9707 — MB Camb. 1954 (Camb. & Middlx.) BChir 1953; DA Eng. 1961; DObst RCOG 1961; FFA RCS Eng. 1965. Prev: Cons. Anaesth. Regional Cardiothoracic Unit Walsgrave Hosp. Coventry.

PENMAN, Mr David Gerard Fetal Medicine Unit, Medway Maritime Hospital, Windmill Road, Gillingham ME7 5NY Tel: 01634 825110 Email: penman@ndirect.co.uk — MB BS Lond. 1984 (St. Thos.) MRCOG 1993. Cons. In O & G, Specialist in Fetal Med., Fetal Med. Unit, Medway Maritime Hosp.; Hon. Cons. Harris Birthright Centre KCH Lond. Specialty: Obst. & Gyn. Socs: Milit. Surg. Soc.; Brit. Matern. & Fetal Med. Soc.; Brit. Med. Ultrasound Soc. Prev: Cons. (Matern. & Foetal Med.) All St.s Hosp. Chatham; Sen. Regist. (Matern. & Foetal Med.) St. Michael's Hosp. Bristol; Regist. Rotat. (O & G) St. Geo.'s Hosp. Lond.

PENMAN, Edward Hugh Giles The Old House, Baschurch Road, Bomere Heath, Shrewsbury SY4 3PN Email: ed@ehgp.com — (Roy. Free) MB BS Lond. 1990; DCH RCP Lond. 1993; DRCOG 1994; DFFP 1995; MRCGP 1996. Specialty: Gen. Pract.

PENMAN, Hugh Gerard (retired) Kaduna, Lyons Road, Slinfold, Horsham RH13 7QS — (St. Thos.) MB BChir Camb. 1953; MRCP Lond. 1955; DTM & H Eng. 1960; FRCPath 1975, M 1963; MA Camb. 1954, MD 1966. Prev: Cons. Path. Histopath. & Clin. Dir. (Path.) Crawley Hosp. Path. Lagos &Kaduna, Nigeria Cons. Path. Queen Alexandra Hosp,Portsm. Cons. Histop.& Sen. Lect. Uni. Otago Med. Sch. NZ Sen. Cons. Dept. Path., Riyahd/Al Khapq Hosps.(Crawley secondment).

PENMAN, Ian Douglas 4 Howe Park, Edinburgh EH10 7HF — MB ChB Glas. 1988; MRCP (UK) 1991; BSc (Hons.) Glas. 1986, MD 1995. Cons. Gastroenterol. West. Gen. Hosp. Edin.; Sen. Lect. Univ. Edin. 1997-. Specialty: Gastroenterol. Socs: Brit. Soc. Gastroenterol. Prev: Advanced Fell. (Med.) Univ. S. Carolina USA; Sen. Regist. & Regist. (Med. & Gastroenterol.) West. Gen. Hosp. Edin.; Research Fell. (Gastroenterol.) West. Infirm. Glas.

PENMAN, Robert Anthony East Parade Surgery, East Parade, Harrogate HG1 5LW Tel: 01423 566574 Fax: 01423 568015 — MB ChB Leeds 1983; BSc (Hons.) Biochem. Leeds 1980; DRCOG 1986; DCH RCP Lond. 1987; MRCGP 1988. Prev: Trainee GP Harrogate VTS; Ho. Off. (Surg.) St. James Hosp. Leeds; Ho. Off. (Med.) Huddersfield Roy. Infirm.

PENMAN, Walter Andrew (retired) 3 St Cuthberts Avenue, Dumfries DG2 7NZ Tel: 01387 254584 — MB ChB Edinburgh 1950 (Ed.) MB ChB Ed. 1950; FRCP Ed. 1971, M 1958. Prev: Cons. Phys. Dumfries & Galloway Health Bd.

PENN, Adrian Falklands Surgery, Falkland Way, Bradwell, Great Yarmouth NR31 8RW Tel: 01493 442233 — MB BS Lond. 1982.

PENN, Christopher Robert Howard (retired) Sprey House, 1 Holcombe Road, Teignmouth TQ14 8UP Tel: 01626 778448 — MB BChir Camb. 1965 (Camb. & Lond. Hosp.) MA Camb. 1965; DMRT Eng. 1970; FFR 1972; FRCR 1975. Prev: Sen. Cons. Clin. Oncol., Roy. Devon, Exeter & Torbay Hosps.

PENN, Michael Anthony Southbourne Surgery, 17 Beaufort Road, Southbourne, Bournemouth BH6 5BF Tel: 01202 427878 Fax: 01202 430730 — (St. Mary's) LMSSA Lond. 1961; MB BS Lond. 1964; MRCOG 1969. Prev: SHO (Gyn.) Jessop. Hosp. Wom. Sheff. Regist. (O & G) Roy. Vict. Hosp. Bournemouth; Ho. Surg. King Edwd. VII Hosp. Windsor.

PENN, Naomi Kathryn Shaftesbury Medical Centre, 480 Harehills Lane, Leeds LS9 6DE Tel: 0113 248 5631 Fax: 0113 235 0658; Dale Brow, Breary Lane E., Bramhope, Leeds LS16 9ET Tel: 0113 267 2959 — MB ChB Leeds 1983; MRCGP 1987; DRCOG 1988.

PENN, Neil David St. James University Hospital, Beckett St., Leeds LS9 7TF; Dale Brow, Breary Lane E., Bramhope, Leeds LS16 9FT Tel: 0113 267 2959 — MB ChB Leeds 1982; MRCP (UK) 1985. Cons. Phys. Med. for Elderly St. Jas. Univ. Hosp. Leeds. Specialty: Care of the Elderly.

PENN, Raymond George (retired) 5 Springfield Crescent, Sherborne DT9 6DN — MB BCh Wales 1956; DHMSA Soc. Apoth. Lond. 1978; MD Wales 1982. Prev: Dept of Health.

PENN, Zoe Jillian Chelsea & Westminster Hospital, 369 Fulham Road, London SW10 9NM Tel: 020 8846 7902 Fax: 020 8846 7998; 3 Walerand Road, London SE13 7PE Tel: 020 8318 4950 — MB BS Lond. 1982 (Westm.) MRCOG 1986; MD Lond. 1997. Cons. Obst. Chelsea & Westm. Hosp. Lond. Specialty: Obst. & Gyn. Prev: Research Regist. (Obst.) Char. Cross & Westm. Med. Sch. W. Lond. Hosp.; Regist. (O & G) Westm. Hosp. Lond. & Barnet Gen. Hosp.; SHO (Surg.) Roy. Marsden Hosp. Lond.

PENNA, Leonie Kay St. Helier Hospital, Carshalton SM5 1AA Tel: 020 8296 2985; 81 Upland Road, Sutton SM2 5JA — MB BS Lond. 1986; MRCOG 1993. Cons. Obst., St. Helier Hosp., Carshalton, Surrey. Specialty: Obst. & Gyn. Prev: Lect. (O & G) St. Geo. Hosp. Lond.

PENNANT-LEWIS, Rhian Anaesthetic Department, Ysbyty Gwynedd, Bangor LL57 2PW Tel: 01248 384185 Fax: 01248 384920 Email: rhian.lewis@nww-tr.wales.nhs.uk; 7 Tyin y Cae, Llanfairpwllgwyngyll LL61 6UX Tel: 01248 715925 — MB ChB Manch. 1982; FFA RCS Eng. 1987. Cons. Anaesth. Ysbyty Gwynedd

Bangor. Specialty: Anaesth. Special Interest: Chronic Pain. Prev: Sen. Regist. (Anaesth.) Addenbrooke's Hosp. Camb.; Regist. (Anaesth.) Leicester Roy. Infirm.; Lect. (Anaesth.) Roy. Hallamsh. Hosp. Sheff.

PENNEFATHER, Marguerite Eleanor (retired) Church Gate, Church Lane, Northiam, Rye TN31 6NN Tel: 01797 253341 — (Bristol) MB ChB Bristol 1953; DObst RCOG 1956. Prev: Med. Asst. (Geriat.) The Irvine Unit, Bexhill.

PENNELL, Angela Mary Taverham Surgery, Sandy Lane, Taverham, Norwich NR8 6JR Tel: 01603 867481 Fax: 01603 740670 — MB ChB Birm. 1970.

PENNELL, Professor Dudley John Cardiovasc. Magnetic Resonance Unit, Royal Brompton Hospital, Sydney St., London SW3 6NP Tel: 020 7351 8810 Fax: 020 7351 8816 Email: d.pennell@ic.ac.uk — MB BChir Camb. 1983 (St. Thos.) MB BChir (Distinc. Med.) Camb. 1983; FRCP 1997, M 1986; MA Camb. 1983, BA 1980, MD 1992; FESC 1996; FACC 1996. Prof. Cardiology & Hon. Cons. Roy. Brompton Hosp.; Dir. Clin. Cardiovasc. MR. Specialty: Cardiol.; Nuclear Med.; Radiol. Socs: Ex-Pres. Soc. Cardiovasc. MR; Ex-Chairm., Euro. Soc. Of Cardiol. Working Grp. On CMR; Ex-Chairm., Study Grp. On CMR of the Internat. Soc. Of MR in Med. Prev: Lect. Roy. Brompton Nat. Heart & Lung Hosp. Lond.; Regist. (Med. & Cardiol.) St. Thos. Hosp. Lond.; SHO (Med.) Hammersmith & St. Thos. Hosps. Lond.

PENNELL, Ian Philip — MB ChB Manch. 1980; BSc Manch. 1977; MRCPsych 1985. Cons. Psychiat. Worcs. Gloucestershire partnership NHS Trust. Specialty: Gen. Psychiat. Prev: Sen. Regist. (Psychiat.) Warneford Hosp. Oxf.

PENNELL, Simon Craigen Southbourne Surgery, 17 Beaufort Road, Southbourne, Bournemouth BH6 5BF Tel: 01202 427878 Fax: 01202 430730 — BM Soton. 1981; DA (UK) 1986. Prev: SHO Rotat. (Surg.) Roy. Hants. Co. Hosp. Winchester; Ho. Surg. Roy. Vict. Hosp. Bournemouth; Ho. Phys. Poole Gen. Hosp. Dorset.

PENNELLS, Robert Arthur Pennells and Partners, Gosport Health Centre, Bury Road, Gosport PO12 3PN Tel: 023 9258 3344 Fax: 023 9260 2704; Bury Cottage, 79 Bury Road, Gosport PO12 3PR Tel: 02392 523510 — MB BS Lond. 1971 (St. Mary's) DObst RCOG 1975. GP Gosport. Prev: Regist. (Anaesth.) Hillingdon Hosp. Uxbridge; Regist. (Paediat.) Palmerston N. Hosp., N.Z.

PENNEY, Adrian Peter St John School House Lane Surgery, School House Lane, Bishops Castle SY9 5BP Tel: 01588 632285 — MB BS Lond. 1980; MRCS Eng. LRCP Lond. 1980.

PENNEY, Basil Francis Carmel Surgery, Nunnery Lane, Darlington DL3 8SQ Tel: 01325 463149; 3 Glenfield Road, Darlington DL3 8DZ — MB BCh BAO Dub. 1982; DCH RCPSI 1985; MRCGP 1986; DObst RCPI 1986.

PENNEY, Christopher Charles 42 Langton Way, Blackheath, London SE3 7TJ — MA Camb. 1969, MB 1967, BChir 1966; MRCP (U.K.) 1970; DMRD Eng. 1972; FFR 1974; FRCR 1975; FRCP Lond. 1986. Cons. Neuroradiol. Kings Coll. Hosp. Lond. Specialty: Radiol.

PENNEY, David James 17 Broadway, Wheathampstead, St Albans AL4 8LW — MB BS Lond. 1993.

PENNEY, Gerald Norman St John (retired) Black Lion House, Bishops Castle SY9 5BS Tel: 01588 638128 — MB BChir Camb. 1950 (Guy's) MA Camb. 1951; DCH Eng. 1954; DRCOG 1976; FRCGP 1987, M 1977. Prev: Admiralty Surg. & Agent.

PENNEY, Gillian Constance Knapperna House, Udny, Ellon AB41 6SA — MD Ed. 1981; MB ChB 1975; MRCOG 1980; MFFP 1993. Sen. Regist. (Community Gyn.) Aberd. Roy. Infirm. Specialty: Obst. & Gyn.

PENNEY, Michael David Royal Gwent Hospital, Department of Clinical Biochemistry, Newport NP20 2UB — MB BS Lond. 1975 (Middlx.) BSc (Hons.) Birm. 1970; FRCPath 1991, M 1981; MD Lond. 1985. Cons. Chem. Path. Roy. Gwent. Hosp. Newport; Clin. Teach. Univ. Hosp. Wales Cardiff; Hon. Cons. Chem. Path. Bristol Roy. Infirm. Specialty: Biochem. Special Interest: Disorders of Salt & Water Metab. Socs: BMA; Assn. Clin. Biochem.; Assn. Clin. Path. Prev: Dir. (Path.) Gwent Healthcare Trust; Sen. Regist. (Chem. Path.) Leeds Gen. Infirm.; Regist. (Path.) Bristol Roy. Infirm.

PENNEY, Oliver James St John The Surgery, Staunton-on-Wye, Hereford HR4 7LT Tel: 01981 500227 Fax: 01981 500603 — MB BS Lond. 1983 (Guy's) DRCOG 1985; DCH RCP Lond. 1988; MRCGP 1988. Prev: Med. Off. I/c Raihu Hosp., Aitape, Papua New Guinea.

PENNEY, Rachel Marion The Surgery, Gadbridge Road, Weobley, Hereford HR4 8SN; Castle Farm, Kinnersley, Hereford HR3 6QB — BM Soton. 1983; DCH 1985; DRCOG 1987; MRCGP 1988. p/t GP Principal. Prev: Med. Off. Raihu Hosp.,Aitape Papua New Guinea.

PENNEY, Richard John Cwmavon Health Centre, Cwmavon, Port Talbot SA12 9PY Tel: 01639 896244 Fax: 01639 895183 — MB BChir Camb. 1991 (Princip. (General Practice)) MRCGP 1995; T(GP) 1995. Specialty: Gen. Pract. Prev: Trainee GP/SHO Rotat. Neath Gen. Hosp. W. Glam. HA VTS; Ho. Off. (Med.) Hull Roy. Infirm.; Ho. Off. (Surg.) Castle Hill Hosp. Cottingham.

PENNEY, Sarah Christine 45 Springkell Drive, Pollokshields, Glasgow G41 4EZ Tel: 0141 427 2023 — MB ChB Glas. 1976; MRCGP 1983. Staff Grade (Gastroenterol.) Glas.

PENNEY, Tony Martin Linden Medical Group, Linden Medical Centre, Linden Avenue, Kettering NN15 7NX Fax: 01536 415930 — MB BS Lond. 1984 (Roy. Free Sch. of Med.) DRCOG 1987. Prev: Ho. Off. Luton & Dunstable Hosp.; Ho. Off. Roy. Free Hosp. Lond.; Trainee GP Luton & Dunstable Hosp. VTS.

PENNI, Mr Ack Nichodemus Department of ENT, District General Hospital, Warrington WA5 1QG Tel: 01925 35911; 36 Reaper Close, Great Sankey, Warrington WA5 1DX Tel: 01925 416762 Fax: 01925 416762 — MB ChB Ghana 1978; FRCS Ed. 1990; DLO RCS Eng. 1994. Specialty: Otorhinolaryngol.

PENNIE, Mr Bruce Hamilton Orthopaedic Department, University Hospital Aintree, Longmoor Lane, Liverpool L9 7AL Tel: 0151 529 2547 Fax: 0151 529 2549 — MB ChB Ed. 1980; FRCS Ed. 1984; MCh (Orthop.) Liverp. 1987. Cons. Orthop. Surg. Aintree Hosp.s, NHS Trust. Specialty: Orthop. Socs: BOA; Brit. Assn. of Spinal Surg.s. Prev: Sen. Regist. (Orthop. Surg.) Roy. Liverp. Hosp.; SHO (Accid & Emerg. & Orthop.) Walton Hosp. Liverp.; Ho. Off. (Med.) Bangour Hosp. W. Lothian.

PENNIE, Donald Durance (retired) 24 Turfbeg Avenue, Forfar DD8 3LL Tel: 01307 462592 — MB ChB Aberd. 1942; MRCGP 1958. Prev: RAMC.

PENNING-ROWSELL, Virginia Wintringham Dept. of Anaesthesia, Bristol Royal Infirmary, Bristol BS2 8HW Tel: 0117 928 2163; Corners, Stone Allerton, Axbridge BS26 2NW Tel: 01934 712567 — MB BS Lond. 1968 (Univ. Coll. Hosp.) FFA RCS Eng. 1972. Cons. Anaesth. United Bristol Hosps. Trust. Specialty: Anaesth. Prev: Sen. Regist. (Anaesth.) Bristol Weston, Southmead & Frenchay HAs; Sen. Regist. (Anaesth.) Addenbrooke's Hosp. Camb.; Regist. (Anaesth.) Guy's Hosp. Lond.

PENNINGTON, Elizabeth Rebecca Moorside Surgery, 1 Thornbridge Mews, Bradford BD2 3BL Tel: 01274 626691 — MB ChB Leeds 1989; MRCGP 1994.

PENNINGTON, George William (retired) Sullane, Eaton Hill, Baslow, Bakewell DE45 1SB Tel: 01246 582212 — MB ChB Liverp. 1956; MRCS Eng. LRCP Lond. 1956; MD Liverp. 1959; MSc Calif. 1961; MA Dub. 1962; FRCPath 1973, M 1963; FRCOG 1987. Prev: Cons. Chem. Path. Jessop Hosp. Wom. & Sheff. HA.

PENNINGTON, Jonathan Mark 192 Maney Hill Road, Sutton Coldfield B72 1JX Email: john.pennington@xtra.co.nz; 4 Swansea Street, Khandallah, Wellington, New Zealand Email: john.pennington@xtra.co.nz — MB ChB Liverp. 1993. Specialty: Orthop.

PENNINGTON, Sarah Helen 311 Tag La, Ingol, Preston PR2 3XA — MB ChB Manch. 1997.

PENNINGTON, Sheila Jane 6 Berkley Crescent, Birmingham B13 9YD — MB ChB Birm. 1985; BSc (Hons.) Birm. 1982, MB ChB 1985; DRCOG 1987. Trainee GP Wolverhampton VTS.

PENNINGTON, Sylvia Elizabeth Forest Hall Medical Centre, Station Road, Forest Hall, Newcastle upon Tyne NE12 9BQ Tel: 0191 266 5823 — MB ChB Sheffield 1974; MB ChB Sheff 1974. GP Newc.

PENNINGTON, Professor Thomas Hugh Department of Medical Microbiology, Medical School Buildings, Foresterhill, Aberdeen AB25 2ZD Tel: 01224 681818 Fax: 01224 685604 — MB BS Lond. 1962 (St. Thos.) PhD Lond. 1967; FRCPath 1990, M 1978. Prof. Bact. Univ. Aberd.; Hon. Cons. (Bact.) Grampian HB. Specialty: Med. Microbiol. Prev: Sen. Lect. Dept. Virol. Univ. Glas.; Lect. (Bact.) St. Thos. Hosp. Med. Sch. Lond; Project Assoc. Univ. Wisconsin Med. Sch. Madison, USA.

PENNOCK, Charles Anthony (retired) Warners Cottage, Chewton Keynsham, Bristol BS31 2SU Tel: 01179 862320 Email:

charles.pennock@btinternet.com — (Bristol) BSc Bristol 1968, MD 1973, MB ChB 1962; FRCPath 1982, M 1970; FRCPCH 1998. Prev: Cons. Paediat. Chem. Path. United Bristol Hosps. Trust & Southmead Hosp. Trust.

PENNOCK, Helen Claire 32 Nash Lane, Belbroughton, Stourbridge DY9 9SW — MB ChB Manch. 1989.

PENNOCK, Philip Francis Louis The Bull Ring Surgery, 5 The Bull Ring, St. John's, Worcester WR2 5AA Tel: 01905 422883 Fax: 01905 423639; The Barley House, Clevelode Farm, Clevelode, Malvern WR13 6PD Tel: 01684 311201 Fax: 01684 311975 Email: ppennock@aol.com — MB BS Lond. 1980 (Barts) BA Oxf. 1975; DRCOG 1984; Dip. Occupational Medicine 1999.

PENNY, Elizabeth Philomena Cardiff & Vale NHS Trust, Child Health Directorate, Childrens Centre, St Davids Hospital, Conbridge Road East, Canton, Cardiff CF11 9XB Tel: 029 2053 6610 — MB BCh BAO NUI 1976 (Cork) DCH Eng. 1979; MPH Wales 1995; Dip. POS. Lond. 2000. Cons. Community Paediat. Cardiff and Vale NHS Trust. Specialty: Community Child Health. Socs: Fell. Roy. Coll. Paediat. & Child Health; Welsh Paediat. Soc.; Brit. Assn. Community Child Health. Prev: Project Ldr. Audit of Cerebral Palsy for Childr. in Wales; SCMO (Child Health) S. Glam. AHA; SHO (Paediat.) Morriston Hosp. Swansea.

PENNY, Emma Clare Berkeley Place Surgery, 11 High Street, Cheltenham GL52 6DA Tel: 01242 513975; 11 Pirton Meadow, Churchdown, Gloucester GL3 2RW — MB BS Lond. 1989; BSc Lond. 1986; DCH RCPS Glas. 1992; DFFP 1994; MRCGP 1994.

PENNY, James Leith (retired) Hazelburn, 13 Orchard Park, Crieff PH7 3ES — MB ChB St. And. 1958; DObst RCOG 1960.

PENNY, Judith Margaret Bruntsfield Medical Practice, 11 Forbes Road, Edinburgh EH10 4EY Tel: 01506 871403; 124 Viewforth, Edinburgh EH10 4LN — MB ChB Ed. 1986; DObst RCOG 1988; MRCGP 1991; DCH RCP Ed. 1992. Partner Gen. Pract. W. Calder. Prev: Trainee GP Edin.

PENNY, Lisa Antonia Robin House, Garden Close La., Newbury RG14 6PP — MB ChB Bristol 1995.

PENNY, Philip Trevor Overton House, West Monkton, Taunton TA2 8RA Tel: 01823 413013 Fax: 01823 413707 Email: pennyswims@hotmail.com — MB BS Lond. 1956 (Univ. Coll. Hosp.) MRCS Eng. LRCP Lond 1956; AFOM RCP Lond 1983. Dir. S. West. Indust. Med. Servs. SWIMs; Med. Adviser Inst. Swimming Teachs. & Coaches & ASA (Amateur Swimming Assn.); HM (Dep.) Coroner W. Som. Specialty: Occupat. Health. Socs: Soc. Occupat. Med.; Assn. Local Auth. Med. Advisors.; Royal Society of Medicine Fellowship. Prev: Occupat. Phys. Weston Area Health Trust and Royal Cornwall Hospital, Truro; Occupational Physisian, Taunton & Som. Hosps.

PENNY, Ronald Maxwell (retired) Pennys, Cutlers Green, Thaxted, Dunmow CM6 2PZ Tel: 01371 831166 — MRCS Eng. LRCP Lond. 1946 (Oxf. & Middlx.) MRCGP 1970. Prev: Res. Med. Off. St. Mary's Hosp. Eastbourne.

PENNY, William John Department of Cardiology, University of Wales College of Medicine, Heath Park, Cardiff CF14 4XN Tel: 029 2074 7747 Fax: 029 2074 5360 — MB BCh BAO NUI 1976 (Cork) MRCP (UK) 1980; MD NUI 1984; FRCP Lond. 1995. Cons. Cardiol. Cardiff & Wales NHS Trust. Specialty: Cardiol. Prev: Lect. (Cardiol.) Univ. Wales Coll. Med.; Cardiol. Fell. Mayo Clinic Rochester MN, USA; Regist. (Cardiol.) Lond. Chest Hosp.

PENNYCOOK, Alan Gordon Arrowe Park Hospital, Upton, Wirral CH49 5PE Tel: 0151 604 7080 Fax: 0151 604 7114 — MB ChB Glas. 1980; FRCS Glas. 1989; FFAEM 1994. Cons. Accid. and Emerg., Wirral Hosps. NHS Trust, Birkenhead. Specialty: Accid. & Emerg. Special Interest: Resussitation; Trauma. Socs: BAEM; Roy. Soc. of Med. Prev: Cons. Accid. and Emerg., Warrington Hosps. NHS Trust.

PENNYCOOK, Julie Alison 364 Glasgow Road, Ralston, Paisley PA1 3BQ — MB ChB Glas. 1990.

PENRICE, Gillian Mary — MB ChB Glas. 1986; DRCOG 1990; MRCGP 1990; MPH 1999; MFPHM 2002.

PENRICE, Juliet Mellanby The Neonatal Unit Chelsea & Westminster Hospital, 369 Fulham Road, London SW10 9NH — MB BChir Camb. 1989; MA Camb. 1985; MRCP (UK) 1992. Cons. (Neonat. Paediat.) Chelsea & Westminster Hosp. Lond. Specialty: Neonat. Socs: RCPCH; Eur. Soc. Of Paed. Res.; Perinatal Soc. Of Aust. & NZ.

PENRICE, Miss Lisa Margaret 185 Coombe Lane, London SW20 0RG — MB ChB Manch. 1988.

PENROSE, Gaynor Louise 4 Green Row, Machen, Caerphilly CF83 8NU — MB BCh Wales 1994 (Univ. Wales) DCH 1996; DRCOG 1997; MRCGP 1998. GP. Specialty: Gen. Pract.

PENROSE, Mr Joscelyn Hugh (retired) Glebe Field, 21 St Michael's Road, Claverdon, Warwick CV35 8NT Tel: 01926 842802 — (Camb. & St. Thos.) MB BChir Camb. 1939; MA Camb. 1939; MRCS Eng. LRCP Lond. 1939; FRCS Eng. 1946. Prev: Cons. Orthop. Surg. Coventry Hosp. Gp. & Warks. Orthop. Hosp. Coleshill.

PENROSE, Richard James Jackson 16 The Orangery, Ham, Richmond TW10 7HJ Tel: 020 8392 4297 — MB BS Lond. 1966 (Char. Cross) MRCS Eng. LRCP Lond. 1966; DPM Eng. 1970; MRCPsych 1973. Cons. Psychiat. The Priory Hosp. Roehampton Lond. Specialty: Gen. Psychiat. Socs: Brit. Assn. Of PscyhoPharmacol. Prev: Cons. Psychiat. Epsom Gen. Hosp. Surrey.; Cons. Psychiat. St. Geo. & Springfield Hosps. Lond.; Sen. Regist. (Psychiat.) St. Geo. Hosp. Lond.

PENRY, Elizabeth Margaret Forsythe (retired) Brincliffe, 20 Westbury Lane, Coombe Dingle, Bristol BS9 2PE Tel: 0117 968 1471 — MB ChB Bristol 1956; DCH Eng. 1958; DObst RCOG 1959. Prev: SCMO (Paediat. & Audiol.) United Bristol Hosp. Trust.

PENRY, John Bernard (retired) Brincliffe, 20 Westbury Lane, Coombe Dingle, Bristol BS9 2PE Tel: 0117 968 1471 — MB BCh Wales 1957 (Cardiff) DMRD Eng. 1961; FFR 1964; FRCR 1975. Prev: Cons. Radiol. Southmead Hosp. & Ham Green Hosp. Bristol.

PENRY, Karen Sian Plas Bryn Y Mor, Bryn Y Mor Road, Aberystwyth SY23 2HY Tel: 01970 627871 — BM Soton. 1986 (Southampton) DCH RCP Lond. 1990; MRCGP 1991; DRCOG 1991; PGCME Cardiff 2001. Specialty: Gen. Pract.

PENSTON, James Geoffrey Mary 8 West Field Garth, Ealand, Scunthorpe DN17 4JR; Scunthorpe General Hospital, Cliff Gardens, Scunthorpe DN15 7BH — MB BS Lond. 1975. Cons. (Phys./Gastroenterol.) Scunthorpe & Goole NHS Trust. Specialty: Gastroenterol.

PENTECOST, Mr Alan Frederick (retired) 24 Bower Mount Road, Maidstone ME16 8AU — MB BS Lond. 1962 (St. Mary's) MRCS Eng. LRCP Lond. 1962; FRCOG 1982 M 1969; FRCS Ed. 1970. Cons. (O & G) Maidstone Hosp.

PENTECOST, Professor Brian Leonard, OBE 37 Farquhar Road, Edgbaston, Birmingham B15 3RA Tel: 0121 454 1287 Email: bpentecost@supanet.com — (St. Mary's) MB BS (Hons. Med. & Path.) Lond. 1957; FRCP Lond. 1971, M 1959; MD Lond. 1965; Hon DSc (Aston) 1998. Emerit. Prof. Med. Univ. Birm. Specialty: Cardiol. Socs: Fell. Europ. Soc. Cardiol.; Brit. Cardiac Soc. & Assn. of Phys. Prev: Med. Dir. Brit. Heart Foundat.; Linacre Fell. Roy. Coll. Phys. Lond.; Cons. Phys. United Birm. Hosps.

PENTER, Gail Radiology Department, Warwick Hospital, Lakin Road, Warwick CV34 5BW Tel: 01926 495321 — MB BCh Wales 1980; FRCR 1986. Cons. Radiol. Warwick Hosp. & Stratford u. Avon Hosp. Specialty: Radiol. Prev: Sen. Regist. (Radiol.) W. Mldl. RHA.

PENTLAND, Brian Lothian Primary Care Trust, Astley Ainslie Hospital, Grange Loan, Edinburgh EH9 2HL Tel: 0131 537 9039 Fax: 0131 537 9030 — MB ChB Ed. 1974 (Edinburgh) BSc Ed. 1972; MRCP (UK) 1978; FRCP Ed. 1986. Cons. Neurol. (Rehabil. Med.) & Clin. Dir. Astley Ainslie Hosp. Edin.; Dip. Europ. Bd. Phys. Med. & Rehabil. Specialty: Neurol.; Rehabil. Med. Socs: Assn. Brit. Neurols.; Hon. Fell. Roy. Coll. Speech & Language Therapists; Brit. Soc. Rehabil. Med. Prev: Lect. (Med. Neurol.) Roy. Infirm. Edin.; Regist. King's Cross Hosp. Dundee; SHO North. Gen. Hosp. Edin.

PENTLOW, Mr Barry Dennis Consulting Rooms, The Glen Hospital, Bristol BS6 7JJ Tel: 0117 973 2562; 36 Great Brockeridge, Bristol BS9 3TZ Tel: 0117 962 1166 — MB BS Lond. 1968; MRCS Eng. LRCP Lond. 1968; FRCS Eng. 1974. Cons. Surg. Southmead Hosp. Bristol. Specialty: Gen. Surg.; Transpl. Surg. Prev: Sen. Lect. (Surg.) Univ. Bristol & Hon. Cons. Surg. Southmead Hosp. Bristol; Lect. (Surg.) Univ. Camb. & Hon. Sen. Regist. Addenbrookes Hosp. Camb.

PENTNEY, Millicent Joy (retired) 4 Cokers Lane, Dulwich, London SE21 8NF Tel: 020 8670 7355 — MB BS Lond. 1952 (Guy's) Prev: Assoc. Specialist (Psychiat.) Bexley Hosp. Kent.

PENWARDEN, David Brian The Surgery, Marlpits Lane, Honiton EX14 ZNY Tel: 01404 41141 Fax: 01404 46621; The Surgery,

Marlpits Road, Honiton EX14 2DD Tel: 01404 41141 Fax: 01406 46621 — MB BS Lond. 1970 (Westm.) MRCS Eng. LRCP Lond. 1970; DObst RCOG 1973; MRCGP 1976.

PEOPLES, Joseph Anthony 28 Henstead Road, Southampton SO15 2DD — MB BS Lond. 1994; BSc (Hons.) Lond. 1990, MB BS 1994. Specialty: Accid. & Emerg.

PEOPLES, Sharon 13 Beach Road, Whitehead, Carrickfergus BT38 9QS — MB ChB Ed. 1996.

PEPE, Gloria Brookvale Adolesent Services, 30 Brookvale Road, Southampton SO17 1QR Tel: 023 8058 6154; 18 Stoke Road, Winchester SO23 7ET Tel: 01962 862122 Fax: 01962 622533 — State Exam Rome 1981 (La Sapienza University of Rome) Dip. Specialist Psychiat. Rome 1985. Sen. Regist. (Child & Adolesc. Psychiat.) Soton. Specialty: Child & Adolesc. Psychiat.; Gen. Psychiat. Socs: Mem. Italian Med. Soc. UK; Mem. Brit Assn. Psychopharmacol.; Mem. Assn. Child Psychol. & Psychiatr. Prev: Clin. Asst. Clinica Belvedere Montello Rome; Regist. (Psychiat.) St. Jas. Hosp. Portsmouth; Regist. (Psychiat.) Pk. Prewitt Hosp. Basingstoke.

PEPERA, Theodora Audrey Ansoma c/o MSL (UK) Ltd., 16 Victoria Way, Burgess Hill RH15 1NF — MB BS Lond. 1987 (Roy. Free Hosp. Sch. Med. Univ. Lond.) MRCOG 1996. Regist. (O & G) Roy. Free Hosp. Lond. Specialty: Obst. & Gyn. Prev: SHO (Obst.) St. Mary's Hosp. Lond.; SHO (Gyn.) Leicester Gen. Hosp.; SHO (Genitourin. Med.) Guy's Hosp. Lond.

PEPKE-ZABA, Joanna Wanda Chest Medical Unit, Papworth Hospital, Papworth Everard, Cambridge CB3 8RE Tel: 01480 830541; 56 Melvin Way, Histon, Cambridge CB4 9HY Tel: 01223 503770 — MB BS Warsaw 1977; PhD Warsaw 1995. SpR (Gen. (Internal) Med. & Resp. Med.) Papworth Hosp. Camb. Specialty: Respirat. Med. Socs: Brit. Thoracic Soc. Prev: Assoc. Specialist (Resp. Med.) Papworth Hosp. Camb.; Regist. (Chest Med.) Papworth & Addenbrooke's Hosps. Camb.

PEPPER, Anne Vivienne Norah Hedon Group Practice, 4 Market Hill, Hedon, Hull HU12 8JD Tel: 01482 899111 Fax: 01482 890967 — MRCS Eng. LRCP Lond. 1970 (Roy. Free)

PEPPER, Bryan James (retired) Heavitree Health Centre, South Lawn Terrace, Heavitree, Exeter EX1 2RX Tel: 01392 211511 Fax: 01392 499451 — MB ChB Birm. 1964. Med. Off. Dept. Educat. Univ. Exeter.

PEPPER, Christopher Bryan Dept of Cardiology, G Floor, Leeds General Infirmary, Leeds LS1 3EX Tel: 0113 392 2463 Fax: 0113 392 3981 Email: chris.pepper@leedsth.nhs.uk — MB ChB Birm. 1989 (Birmingham University Medical School) BSc (Hons.) Birm. 1986; MRCP (UK) 1992; MD 1997. Cons. Cardiol., Leeds Nuffield Hosp. Specialty: Cardiol. Socs: Brit. Cardiac Soc.; Brit. Pacing & Electrophysiocology Group. Prev: Research Fell. & Hon. Regist. (Cardiol.) Univ. Wales Coll. Med.; SHO (Med. Cardiol.) Glas. Roy. Infirm.; SHO (Med.) Sandwell Hosp. W. Bromwich.

PEPPER, Gregory James Amberley, 89 High St., Sidford, Sidmouth EX10 9SA — MB BS Lond. 1984; DCH RCP Lond. 1987; DRCOG 1988; MRCGP 1989.

PEPPER, Helen Mary Hetton Group Practice, Hetton Medical Centre, Francis Way, Hetton-le-Hole, Houghton-le-Spring DH5 9EZ Tel: 0191 526 1177 Fax: 0191 517 3859; 176 Burnpark Road, Houghton-le-Spring DH4 5DH — MB BS Newc. 1971; DCH RCPS Glas. 1974; MRCPsych 1978.

PEPPER, John Mark 23 Belvidere Road, Shrewsbury SY2 5LS — MB ChB Sheff. 1990; BMedSci Sheff. 1990; DRCOG 1993; DFFP 1994; MRCGP 1994. Specialty: Gen. Pract.

PEPPER, Jonathan Mark Carriage House, Carriage Drive, Frodsham, Warrington WA6 6EB — BM BS Nottm. 1989.

PEPPER, Michael Bernard (retired) The Birches, 115 Station Road, Hugglescote, Coalville, Leicester LE67 2GB Tel: 01530 35397 — MB BS Lond. 1954 (St. Thos.) DPH Bristol 1966; MFCM 1974. Prev: Med. Off. DHSS.

PEPPER, Sarah Helen 52 Apsley Road, Bristol BS8 2ST — MB ChB Bristol 1993.

PEPPER, Susan Jane — MB ChB Ed. 1987; MRCGP 1992.

PEPPERCORN, Miss Penelope Delia MRI, North Hampshire Hospital, Aldermaston Road, Basingstoke RG9 4NA Tel: 01256 842600 Email: delia.peppercorn@nhht.nhs.uk — MB ChB Birm. 1988 (Birmingham) FRCR; MRCP. p/t Cons. Radiologist, MRI N. Hants. Hosp., Basignstoke.

PEPPERELL, Irene Avondale Medical Practice, Strathaven Health Centre, The Ward, Strathaven ML10 6AS Tel: 01357 529595 Fax: 01357 529494 — MB ChB Glas. 1975.

PEPPERELL, Justin Charles Thane The Old Bakery, 51 Castle St., Nether Stowey, Bridgwater TA5 1LW — MB BChir Camb. 1992; MA Camb. 1992, MB BChir 1992. Specialist Regist. (Respir. Med.) SW Rotat. Specialty: Respirat. Med.; Gen. Med. Socs: Brit. Thoracic Soc.

PEPPERMAN, Mark Andrew Pepperman and Partners, The Cottons, Meadow Lane, Wellingborough NN9 6YA Tel: 01933 623327 Fax: 01933 623370 — MRCS Eng. LRCP Lond. 1975 (King's Coll. Hosp.) BSc (Hons.) (Physiol.) Lond. 1972, MB BS 1975; DRCOG 1979; DMedLaw 1995. GP Raunds. Specialty: Gen. Pract. Socs: Fell. Roy. Soc. Med. Prev: SHO (Communicable & Trop. Dis.) E. Birm. Hosp.; SHO Metab. & Renal Unit E. Birm. Hosp.; Ho. Off. Liver Unit King's Coll. Hosp. Lond.

PEPPERMAN, Michael Leon Leicester Royal Infirmary, University Hospitals of Leicester NHS Trust, Infirmary Close, Leicester LE1 5WW Tel: 0116 254 1414 Fax: 0116 258 6474 Email: m.pepperman@btinternet.com; Farcroft, Links Road, Kirby Muxloe, Leicester LE9 2BP Tel: 0116 239 3048 — BSc (Anat., Hons.) Birm. 1965; MRCS Eng. LRCP Lond. 1968; MB ChB Birm. 1968; FFA RCS Eng. 1972. Cons. Anaesth. Leicester Roy. Infirm. NHS Trust; Nat. Clin. Lead - Med., NHS Modernisation Agency Critical Care Progr. Specialty: Anaesth.; Intens. Care. Prev: Cons. Anaesth. Princess Margt. Hosp. Nassau, Bahamas; Sen. Regist. (Anaesth.) Wolverhampton Gp. Hosps. & United Birm. Hosps.

PEPPIATT, Roger Dartford West Health Centre, Tower Road, Dartford DA1 2HA Tel: 01322 228032/223960 — MB BS Lond. 1974 (St. Bart.) MB BS (Hons.) Lond. 1974; MRCP (UK) 1976; MRCGP 1978; DCH RCP Lond. 1978; Dip. Palliat. Med. Wales 1994. Trainer (Gen. Pract.) Joyce Green Hosp. Dartford; Clin. Asst. Lions Hospice N.fleet. Specialty: Palliat. Med. Socs: Fell.Roy.Soc.Med. Prev: Tutor (Gen. Pract.) Dartford; Trainee GP Univ. Exeter VTS; Sen. Med. Off. Nixon Memor. Hosp., Segbwema, Sierra Leone.

PEPPIATT, Timothy Neil 2 Leys Avenue, Cambridge CB4 2AW — BM Soton. 1990.

PEPYS, Elizabeth Olga Department of Medicine, Royal Free & University College Medical School, Rowland Hill St., London NW3 2PF Tel: 020 7433 2801 Fax: 020 7433 2803 Email: m.pepys@rfc.ucl.ac.uk; 22 Wildwood Road, London NW11 6TE — BM BCh Oxf. 1968 (Univ. Coll. Hosp.) MA Oxf. 1968. p/t Clin.Asst. Allergy Roy. Free. Univ. Coll. Med. Sch.Lond. Specialty: Allergy. Socs: Brit. Soc. Allergy & Clin. Immunol. Prev: Res. Fell. Roy. Post-Grad. Med. Sch. Lond; Ho. Phys. Med. Unit Univ. Coll. Hosp. Lond.; Jun. Asst. Path. Camb. Univ.

PEPYS, Professor Mark Brian Department of Medicine, Royal Free & University College Medical School, Rowland Hill St, London NW3 2PF Tel: 020 7433 2801 Fax: 020 7433 2803 Email: m.pepys@rfc.ucl.ac.uk; 22 Wildwood Road, London NW11 6TE Tel: 020 8455 9387 — MB BChir Camb. 1968 (Univ. Coll. Hosp.) MA Camb. 1968; MRCP (UK) 1970; FRCPath 1991, M 1981; FRCP Lond. 1981; PhD Camb. 1974, MD 1982; FRS 1998; F Med Sci 1998. Prof. and Head of Med., Roy. Free Campus, RFUCMS, Lond. Specialty: Gen. Med.; Immunol. Special Interest: Acute phase proteins; Amyloidosis; C-reactive protein. Socs: Hon. Mem. Assoc. of Phys.; Founder Fell. Acad. of Med. Sci.; Fell. of the Roy. Soc. Prev: Prof. of Immunol. Med., Roy. Postgratuate Med. Sch., Hammersmith Hosp., Lond., 1977-1999.

PEPYS, Miriam Elizabeth 22 Wildwood Road, London NW11 6TE — MB BS Lond. 1998.

PERAHIA, David Gunther Sam 56 Harthall Lane, Kings Langley WD4 8JH Tel: 01923 268437 — MB BS Lond. 1992; BSc (Hons.) Lond. 1989, MB BS 1992.

PERAVALI, Mr Buddhababu 26 Wharncliffe Close, Hadfield, Hyde SK13 1QE; 26 Wharncliffe CloseTameside General Hospital, Fountain St, Ashton-under-Lyne OL6 9RW — MB BS Sri Venkateswara 1976; FRCS Glas. 1983.

PERCHARD, Stanley Drelaud 2 Edwards Cottages, Compton avenue, London N1 2XL Tel: 020 7226 2478 — MB BS Lond. 1940 (Univ. Coll. Hosp.) MRCS Eng. LRCP Lond. 1939; FRCOG 1963, M 1948; MD Lond. 1951. Emerit. Cons. O & G Lond. Hosp. Specialty: Obst. & Gyn. Socs: BMA; Liveryman Soc. Apoth.; Fell.Munterian Soc.

Prev: Examr. Univ. Lond. RCOG & RCS; Cons. O & G Lond. Hosp.; Cons. Gyn. Guy's Health Dist.

PERCIVAL, Professor Alan (retired) 3 Coudray Road, Southport PR9 9NL Tel: 01704 534530 — (Oxf. & St. Mary's) BM BCh MA Oxf. 1958; MRCPath 1970. Prev: Emerit. Prof. Clin. Bact. Univ. Liverp.

PERCIVAL, Elisabeth Jane 6 Regent Close, Wilmslow SK9 6LF — BM BS Nottm. 1996.

PERCIVAL, Geoffrey Nigel The Surgery, White Cliff Mill Street, Blandford Forum DT11 7DQ Tel: 01258 452501 Fax: 01258 455675; Cob Cottage, Tarrant Gunville, Blandford Forum DT11 8JR — MB ChB Birm. 1981; DRCOG 1984; DCH RCP Lond. 1985; DA (UK) 1988.

PERCIVAL, George Oliver 18 Orchard Close, Roughton, Norwich NR11 8SR — MRCS Eng. LRCP Lond. 1964.

PERCIVAL, Helen Jane Saxoncross Surgery, 97 Derby Road, Stapleford, Nottingham NG9 7AT Tel: 0115 939 2444 — BM BS Nottm. 1982; BMedSci (Hons.) Nottm. 1980. BUPA Screening Doctor Phoenix Pk. Nottm. Specialty: Gen. Pract. Prev: GP Stapleford, Nottm.

PERCIVAL, Mr Hubert George 94 Islip Road, Oxford OX2 7SW — MB ChB Birm. 1962; MRCS LRCP Lond. 1962; FRCS Eng. 1976. Specialty: Civil Serv.

PERCIVAL, Ian Duncan Cleveland House, 16 Spital Terrace, Gainsborough DN21 2HE Tel: 01427 613158 Fax: 01427 616644 — MB ChB Sheff. 1990.

PERCIVAL, Ingrid Monica 3 Hill Rise, Twyford, Winchester SO21 1QH — BM BS Nottm. 1990; DRCOG 1995. Trainee GP Roy. Hants. Co. Hosp. Winchester. Specialty: Gen. Pract. Prev: Trainee GP Winchester VTS.

PERCIVAL, Mr Nicholas John Department of Plastic Surgery, Charing Cross Hospital, Fulham Palace Road, London W6 8RF Tel: 020 8846 1234 Fax: 020 8846 1719 Email: nperc@aol.com — MB BS Lond. 1977 (Univ. Coll. Hosp. Lond.) FRCS Eng. 1984. Cons. Plastic Surg., Char. Cross Hosp., Lond.; Private Pract., Cosmetic Surg., 55 Harley St., Lond. Specialty: Plastic Surg. Special Interest: Cosmetic Surgery; hand Surgery. Socs: Brit. Assn. Plastic Surg.; Brit. Assn. Aesthetic Plastic Surgs.; Brit. Soc. Surg. Hand. Prev: Sen. Regist. (Plastic Surg.) Edin.; Regist. (Plastic Surg.) Chepstow; Lect. (Anat.) Stanford Univ. Med. Sch. Calif., USA.

PERCIVAL, Richard Newland Avenue Surgery, 129 Newland Avenue, Hull HU5 2ES Tel: 01482 343671 Fax: 01482 448839; 249 Willerby Road, Hull HU5 5HH Tel: 01482 353671 — MB ChB Manch. 1978. Specialty: Gen. Pract.

PERCIVAL, Richard Edward The Medical Centre, 24-28 Lower Northam Road, Hedge End, Southampton SO30 4FQ Tel: 01962 713668 — BM Soton. 1990; DRCOG 1995; MRCGP 1996. GP Hants. Specialty: Gen. Pract. Prev: Trainee GP Twyford, Hants.

PERCIVAL, Robert Kirkhall Surgery, 4 Alexandra Avenue, Prestwick KA9 1AW Tel: 01292 476626 Fax: 01292 678022; 17 Trinity, 35 Lynedoch St, Glasgow G3 — MB ChB Glas. 1977; MRCGP 1981. Specialty: Care of the Elderly.

PERCIVAL, Mr Stanley Piers Bassnett The Manor House, Hutton Buscel, Scarborough YO13 9LL Tel: 01723 862811 — (St. Thos.) MA Camb. 1964, MB 1962, BChir 1961; DO Eng. 1964; DObst RCOG 1964; FRCS Eng. 1970; FRCOphth 1989. Cons. Ophth. Surg. Specialty: Ophth. Socs: (Ex-Pres.) UK Intraocular Implant Soc.; Internat. Intraocular Implant Club; (Ex-Pres.) N. Eng. Ophth. Soc. Prev: Cons. Ophth. Surg. ScarBoro. Health Care Trust; Sen. Regist. Birm. & Midl. Eye Hosp.; Ho. Surg. (Ophth.) St. Thos. Hosp. Lond.

PERCY, Mr Anthony John Leahy (retired) Tadhurst, Hill Brow, Bickley, Bromley BR1 2PQ Tel: 020 8460 6513 Fax: 020 8460 6513 — MB BS Lond. 1965 (Westm.) MRCS Eng. LRCP Lond. 1964; DObst RCOG 1966; FRCS Ed. 1972; FRCS Eng. 1973. Prev: Cons. Orthop. Surg. Qu. Mary's Hosp. Sidcup.

PERCY, Catherine Mary The New Surgery, The Nap, Kings Langley WD4 8ET; Cottingham Farm, Flaunden Lane, Bovingdon, Hemel Hempstead HP3 0PD — MB BS Lond. 1975 (Royal Free Hospital School of Medicine) MRCS Eng. LRCP Lond. 1975; DCH Eng. 1977. Asst. GP Kings Langley Herts.; Clin. Asst. (Orthop.) Hemel Hempstead Hosp. Specialty: Gen. Pract.; Orthop. Prev: Regist. (Paediat.) Stobhill Hosp. Glas.

PERCY, David Bryden NHSU, 40 Eastbourne Terrace, London W2 3QR Tel: 020 7725 2745 Fax: 020 7725 2741 Email: dpercy@doh.gov.uk; 10 Nightingale Close, Winchester SO22 5QA Tel: 01962 877962 Email: dandgpercy@aol.com — MB BS Lond. 1972 (Roy. Free) FRCGP 1995, M 1976. Head of Special Projects. Special Interest: Educat. Socs: Guild Psychother. Prev: Trainee GP Soton. VTS; GP Princip. Soton.; Assoc. Postgrad. Dean Winchester.

PERCY-ROBB, Professor Iain Walter Medical Education Unit, 11 Southpark Terrace, Glasgow G12 8LG Tel: 0141 339 8855 Fax: 0141 330 2776 Email: iwpr1h@clinmed.gla.ac.uk — MB ChB Ed. 1959 (Edin.) DObst RCOG 1962; PhD Ed. 1968; FRCPath 1980, M 1972; FRCP Ed. 1980, M 1976. Prof. Path. Biochem. Univ. Glas.; Assoc. Dean of Med. Educat. Glas. Med. Sch; Cons. Biochem. Gtr. Glas. HB. Specialty: Chem. Path. Socs: Brit. Soc. Gastroenterol. & Assn. Clin. Biochems. Prev: Reader Clin. Chem. Univ. Edin.

PEREGRINE, Anthony David Llynfi Surgery, Llynfi Road, Maesteg CF34 9DT Tel: 01656 732115 Fax: 01656 864451 — MB BCh Wales 1970.

PEREIRA, Albert Anthony Lazarus Moreton Medical Centre, 27 Upton Road, Wirral CH46 0PE Tel: 0151 677 2327 Fax: 0151 677 8181 — MB ChB Liverp. 1991 (Liverpool) DRCOG 1995; MRCGP 1997. Communication Skills Tutor Univ. of Liverp.; Higher Professional Educat. Tutor, Wirral. Specialty: Gen. Pract. Prev: Trainee GP Birkenhead; SHO (Paediat.) Wirral NHS Trust.

PEREIRA, Anthony Chrysoligo 122 South Parkside Drive, West Derby, Liverpool L12 8RP — MB BChir Camb. 1992; MA Camb. 1993, BA (Hons.) 1989; MRCP (UK) 1994. Lect. (Clin. Neurosci.) St. Geo. Hosp. Med. Sch. Lond.; Hon. Regist. (Neurol.) Atkinson Morley's Hosp. Lond. Specialty: Gen. Med.; Neurol. Prev: SHO (Med.) Qu. Med. Centre Nottm.; Cas. Off. Char. Cross Hosp. Lond.; Ho. Phys. Qu. Eliz. II Hosp. Welwyn Gdn. City.

PEREIRA, Bernadette Livramenta Sandra 80 Norbury Crescent, Norbury, London SW16 4LA Tel: 020 8764 8348 Email: bernadettep@iname.com — LRCP LRCS LRCPS Ed., Glas. 1998 (St Geo.) Specialty: Gen. Surg. Prev: Ho. Off. (Gen. Surg.) St. Geo.'s Hosp. Lond.; Ho. Off. (Med.) Princess Roy. Hosp. Haywards Heath, W. Sussex.

PEREIRA, Celina Maria The Health Centre, Laindon, Basildon SS15 5TR Tel: 01268 546411 Fax: 01268 491248 — MB BS Lond. 1987; MA Camb. 1988; DCH RCP Lond. 1991; MRCGP 1994. GP Laindon. Specialty: Community Child Health. Prev: Trainee GP Frimley Pk. Hosp. Camberley VTS.

PEREIRA, Daphne Teresa Maria Rm 109 Albert Bridge House, Bridge Street, Manchester M60 9DA Tel: 0161 831 2094 — MB ChB Manch. 1973; MRCGP 1985; DMRO 1985; AFOM RCP Lond. 1995; MSc Occupat. Health Sciences Manchester 1997. Med. Adviser Schlumbergersema Med. Serv.s. Specialty: Occupat. Health; Gen. Pract. Socs: Fell. Manch. Med. Soc.; Manch. & Dist. Medico-Legal Soc. Prev: Regist. (Radiother. & Oncol.) Christie Hosp. Manch.; Regist. (Gen. Med.) Wythenshawe Hosp. Manch.; SHO (Cardiothoracic Med.) Wythenshawe Hosp. Manch.

PEREIRA, Diana Aldina St Philomena (retired) 17 Hayes Gardens, Hayes, Bromley BR2 7DQ — MB BCh BAO NUI 1961 (Galway) DCH Eng. 1964; DPH Eng. 1965. Prev: Med. Off. Nairobi City Counc.

PEREIRA, Edgar Paul (retired) 142 Wricklemarsh Road, Kidbrooke, London SE3 8DR Tel: 020 8319 2029 — MRCS Eng. LRCP Lond. 1960 (Madras & W. Lond.) DObst RCOG 1963. Prev: Capt. IMS, Staff Capt. to Dir.-Gen.

PEREIRA, Eric Denzil (retired) 36 Linden Way, Boston PE21 9DS — MB BS Lond. 1969 (Char. Cross) MRCS Eng. LRCP Lond. 1969; DObst 1971; FRCOG 1993, M 1977. Prev: Cons. O & G Vict. Hosp. Mahe, Seychelles.

PEREIRA, Mr Jerome Harry James Paget Hospital, Lowestoft Road, Gorleston on Sea, Great Yarmouth NR31 6LA Tel: 01493 452452 Fax: 01493 452666 Email: jerome.pereira@jpaget.nhs.uk; Fir House, Priory Road, St. Olaves, Great Yarmouth NR31 9HQ — MB BS Madras 1976 (Stanley Med. Coll. Madras) FRCS Ed. 1983; MD Univ. East Angl. 2000. Cons. (Surg.) James Paget Hosp.; Hon. Sen. Lect. Univ. of E. Anglia, Norwich. Specialty: Gen. Surg. Socs: Fell. Assoc. of Surgs. Of GB & Ire.; Brit. Assn. Surg. Oncol.; Med. Protec. Soc. Prev: Sen. Regist. (Gen. Surg.) Luton & Dunstable Hosp.; Hon. Sen. Regist. (Plastic Surg.) Qu. Vict. Hosp.; Bern. Surg. Res. Fell. Roy. Coll. Of Surgs. of Eng.

PEREIRA, Joaquim Matthew Da Santana 4 All Hallows Road, London N17 7AD — MB ChB Aberd. 1992.

PEREIRA, Mr John Anthony Anmaryn, Luxford Road, Crowborough TN6 2PP Email: johnpereira@compuserve.com — MB BS Lond. 1991 (Guy's Hosp. Lond.) FRCS (Eng) 1994. Specialist Regist. (Plastic & Reconstruc. Surg.) Pan-Thames Rotat. Specialty: Plastic Surg. Socs: Roy. Soc. Med.; Brit. Assoc. of Plastic Surg.

PEREIRA, John Reginald 31 Parkfield Road S., Didsbury, Manchester M20 6DH — MB BS Bombay 1941 (Grant Med. Coll.)

PEREIRA, Mr Jose Filomeno (retired) Lark Lodge, The Street, Fornham St Martin, Bury St Edmunds IP31 1SW — MB BS Bombay 1955 (Grant Med. Coll. Bombay) DO Eng. 1960; FRCS Ed. 1966. Prev: Cons. Ophth. Surg. W. Suff. Hosp. Gp.

PEREIRA, Madhu Leon Blackfriars, 64 St. Giles', Oxford OX1 3LY — MB ChB Leeds 1997.

PEREIRA, Nigel Hugh Tapton Heights, 29 Taptonville Road, Broomhill, Sheffield S10 5BQ — MB ChB Sheff. 1975; FFA RCS Eng. 1979. Cons. Anaesth. Sheff. Childr. Hosp. Specialty: Anaesth.

PEREIRA, Noel Bertram Michael Mount Chambers Surgery, 92 Coggeshall Road, Braintree CM7 9BY Tel: 01376 553415 Fax: 01376 552451 — (Guy's) MB BS Lond. 1969; MRCS Eng. LRCP Lond. 1969; DObst RCOG 1973.

PEREIRA, Raul Scott Immunology Department, Northwick Park Hospital, Watford Road, Harrow HA1 3UJ Tel: 020 8869 2120; Yacht Lilian, 3 Ducks Walk, Twickenham TW1 2DD Tel: 020 8892 5086 Fax: 020 8255 9494 — (Oxf.) MB BChir Camb. 1973; MA Camb. 1973; FRCPath 1993, M 1981; PhD Lond. 1985. Cons Immunol, NW Lond. Hosp.s Trust; Cons Immunol, The Doctors Laborat., Lond.; Hon. Cons. Immunol, Roy. Brompton Hosp Lond. Specialty: Immunol. Socs: Fell. Roy. Soc. Med.; Assn. Clin. Path.; Brit Soc for allergy & Clin. Immunol. Prev: Sen Cons Immuno Imperial Coll; Cons. Immunol. St. Helier Hosp. Carshalton & Sen. Lect. (Immunol.) St. Geo. Hosp. Med. Sch. Lond.; Research Sen. Regist. W. Middlx. Univ. Hosp.

PEREIRA, Stephen Maxim — MB BS Bombay 1986; DPM 1987, MD 1989 Bombay; BCPsych Lond. 1992; MRCPysch 1993; MSc Lond. 1995. Lead Cons. Psychiat. Pathways PICU Goodmayes Hosp. Essex; Hon. Sen. Lect. (Psychiat.) United Med. & Dent. Sch., Guys Hosp.; Hon. Fell., Nat. Inst. of Ment. Health, Eng. Specialty: Gen. Psychiat. Socs: Med. Defense Union; Fellow, Royal Society of Medicine; Elected Fell., The Roy. Coll. of Psychiatrists. Prev: Cons. Psychiat., Greenwich Dist. Hosp., Lond.

PEREIRA, Stephen Paul Institute of Hepatology, University College London Medical School, 69-75 Chenies Mews, London WC1E 6HX Tel: 020 7679 6510 Fax: 020 7380 6405 Email: stephen.pereira@uclh.ac.uk; Flat 1, 12 Mecklenburgh Square, London WC1N 2AD Tel: 020 7833 3934 — MB BS New South Wales 1989 (Univ. of NSW) BMedSc NSW 1987; MRCP (UK) 1991; DGM RCP Lond. 1991; PhD Lond. 2002; FRCP Lond. 2003. Sen. Lect. in Hepat. and Gastroenterol.; Hon. Cons., Univ. Coll. Lond. Hosps. NHS Trust; Hon. Cons., Gt. Ormond St. Hosp. for Childr. Specialty: Gastroenterol. Special Interest: Edoscopil Ultrasound; ERCP; Hepatic and Pancreatic Malignancy. Socs: Amer. Assoc. for the study of Liver Dis.s; Amer. Society for Gastro. Eniouscopy; Roy. Coll. of Physicians. Prev: Sen. Regist. Univ. Hosp. Lewisham, Lond.; Regist. (Liver Transpl.) King's Coll. Hosp.; Research Fell. (Gastroenterol.) Guy's Hosp. Lond.

PEREPECZKO, Biruta 2 Braemar Mansions, Cornwall Gardens, London SW7 4AF Tel: 020 7937 7969 — MD Warsaw 1937.

PERERA, A D The Surgery, 123 Towncourt Lane, Petts Wood, Orpington BR5 1EL Tel: 01689 821551 Fax: 01689 818692.

PERERA, Antony Nihal Ranjit Chesterfield Royal Hospital, Calow, Chesterfield S44 5BL Tel: 01246 277271; 102 Morland View Road, Walton, Chesterfield S40 3DF Tel: 01246 276683 — (University of Sri Lanka Colombo Faculty) MB BS Sri Lanka 1972; DCH RCPSI 1987. Trust Paediat. Specialty: Community Child Health; Paediat. Socs: BMA. Prev: Regist. (Paediat.) Geo. Eliot Hosp. Nuneaton; Staff Grade (Paediat.) Grimsby NHS Trust.

PERERA, Balasooriyage Leelananda 11 Bidle Grove, Wigmore Gardens, Water Lane, West Bromwich B71 3SF — MB BS Ceylon 1968; DPM 1981. Prev: Regist. (Psychiat.) Arrowe Pk. Hosp. Upton & Clatterbridge Hosp Bebington; Regist. Dist. Gen. Hosp. Bangor.

PERERA, Mr Bodiyabaduge Sumith Felix Highview, 22A Fenton Road, Redhill RH1 4BN — MB BS Colombo 1983; MRCOphth 1991; FRCS Ed. 1993. Assoc. Specialist (Ophth.) E. Surrey Hosp. Redhill. Prev: Assoc. Specialist (Ophth.) RN Hosp. Haslar Gosport.

PERERA, Christopher Nihal 25 Bron y Nant, Croesnewydd Road, Wrexham LL13 7TX — Vrach People's Freindship, U Moscow 1988; Vrach People's Freindship U, Moscow 1988; FFARCSI Dub. 1996; DA (UK) 1997. Specialist Regist. (Anaesth.) All Wales Higher Train. Prog. Cardiff. Specialty: Anaesth. Socs: Fac. Anaesth. Coll. Surgs. Dub. Irel.; Vasc. Anaesth. Soc. UK. Prev: Staff Grade (Anaesth.) Scunthorpe Gen. Hosp.

PERERA, Cuthbert Aelian Maurice Top Flat, 9 Wolseley Road, London N8 8RR — MB BS Ceylon 1959.

PERERA, Devamullage Devapriya Tikakarsiri 2 Woodend Close, St Johns Hill Road, Woking GU21 7RJ — MB BS Ceylon 1958.

PERERA, Devi Chandra Thavapalan and Partners, 55 Little Heath Road, Bexleyheath DA7 5HL Tel: 01322 430129 Fax: 01322 440949 — MB BS Sri Lanka 1974; MRCS Eng. LRCP Lond. London 1980; MRCP UK 1982.

PERERA, Dona Marina Dilukshi Manchester Cytology Centre, Christie Hospital NHS Trust, Kinnaird Road, Withington, Manchester Tel: 0161 446 3656; 3 Clarence Park, Blackburn BB2 7FA Tel: 01254 681997 — MB BS Colombo 1979; DRCPath 1995, MRCPath 1989; MSc (Cytol.) Lond. 1994; FRCPath 1997. Cons. Cytopath. Christie Hosp. NHS Trust Manch. Socs: Brit. Soc. Clin. Cytol. Prev: Sen. Regist. NW RHA & W. Midl. HA; Regist. Wigan Infirm.

PERERA, Gayathri Kanchania — BM BCh Oxf. 1997; BA Oxf. 1994; MRCP UK 2000; MA Oxf. 2002. Specialty: Dermat.

PERERA, Gerard Sheran George Stuart Montague Health Centre, Oakenhurst Road, Blackburn BB2 1PP Tel: 01254 263631; 3 Clarence Park, Berardwood, Blackburn BB2 7FA — MB BS Colombo 1980; MRCP (UK) 1985; DCH RCP Lond. 1985. Cons. Paediat. Community Child Health Blackburn, Hyndburn & Ribble Valley NHS Trust. Specialty: Community Child Health. Prev: Sen. Train. Post (Community Paediat.) Smallwood Health Centre Redditch; Regist. (Paediat.) Roy. Manch. Childr. Hosp., Glas. Roy. Matern. Hosp.& Roy. Hosp. Sick Childr. Glas.

PERERA, Gunatungamudalige Leslie Senarath St. Mary's Hospital, London Road, Kettering NN15 7PW Tel: 01536 410141 Fax: 01536 493244; 41 Hall Close, Kettering NN15 7LQ Tel: 01536 392580 — MB BS Ceylon 1966; MRCP (UK) 1978. Assoc. Specialist St. Mary's Hosp. Kettering. Specialty: Care of the Elderly. Socs: Sri Lanka Coll. Phys.; Sri Lanka Med. Assn. Prev: Cons. Phys. DoH, Sri Lanka.

PERERA, Hasitha Roshal Flat 11, Grove Court, Rampley Lane, Little Paxton, St Neots, Huntingdon PE19 6PQ — MB ChB Leic. 1998; DRCOG 2002.

PERERA, Herath Muditanselage Gnana 16 Fairway, Whitestone, Nuneaton CV11 6NP — Vrach Moscow 1974; Vrach 2nd Moscow Med. Inst. 1974.

PERERA, Hewage Don Padmasiri Wijeratne 8 Sudley Grange, North Sudley Road, Liverpool L17 6DY — MB BS Sri Lanka 1978.

PERERA, Irma Marie Frances 44 Sigrist Square, Kingston upon Thames KT2 6JT — MB BS Sri Lanka 1973.

PERERA, Mr John Kenneth Percival (retired) 10 Brickwall Green, Sefton Village, Liverpool L29 9AF Tel: 0151 531 9407 — MB BChir Camb. 1947 (Camb. & Manch.) MA Camb. 1959, BA (Hons.) 1944; FRCOG 1968, M 1956; FRCS Ed. 1959. Prev: Cons. O & G N. Liverp. Hosp. Gp.

PERERA, Lokuwattage Deepal Senarath Flat 14 The Grange, Ivy Road, Macclesfield SK11 8NA Tel: 01625 438023 Email: deepal_perera@hotmail.com — MB BS Colombo 1992; DCH; MRCPCH; MRCP; MD (Paediat.). SHO (Paediat.).

PERERA, Mahesh Jude Department of Obstetrics & Gynaecology, Glasgow Royal Infirmary, Castle Street, Glasgow Tel: 0141 211 5132 Email: mahesh.perera@northglasgow.scot.nhs.uk; Ross Hall Hospital, 221 Crookston Road, Glasgow G52 3NQ Tel: 0141 810 3151; 100 Fernlea,, Bearsden, Glasgow G61 1NB Tel: 0141 570 1391 — MB ChB Ed. 1992 (Univ. Ed.) BSc Sri Lanka 1989; DFFP 1996; MRCOG 2000. Cons. (O & G). Specialty: Obst. & Gyn. Special Interest: Urogynaecology, Pelvic Floor Dysfunction, Menopause. Socs: BMA; Royal College of Obstetrics and Gynaecology; Catholic doctors guild. Prev: SHO (Oncol.) Beatson Oncol. Centre Glas.; SHO (Gyn.) Stobhill Gen. Hosp. & West. Infirm. Glas.; SHO (O & G) Qu. Mothers Hosp. Glas.

PERERA, Panawalage George Alfred Alexander 59 Nicola Close, South Croydon CR2 6NA Tel: 020 8688 6510 — MB BS Ceylon 1963; DPM Eng. 1972; MRCPsych 1973.

PERERA, Panawalage Suraj Alfred 59 Nicola Close, South Croydon CR2 6NA — BM BCh Oxf. 1996.

PERERA, Mr Peter Hemelge Meary Arnott ENT Depart. Farnborough Hospital, Farnborough Common, Orpington BR6 8ND — MB BS Sri Lanka 1973; MRCS Eng. LRCP Lond. 1979; FRCS Ed. 1986. Assoc. Specialist (ENT Surg.) Bromley HA.

PERERA, Preethi 22 Clareville Road, Orpington BR5 1RS — MB BCh Wales 1989.

PERERA, Rohan Chandra 18 Eland Road, London SW11 5JY — MB BS Lond. 1994.

PERERA, Rohanta Kumar Netherton Health Centre, Halesowen Road, Dudley DY2 9PU Tel: 01384 254935 Fax: 01384 242468; 69 Greyhound Lane, Norton, Stourbridge DY8 3AD — MB ChB Bristol 1984; BSc (Hons.) Bristol 1979, MB ChB 1984. Prev: SHO (Dermat.) Falmouth Hosp.; SHO (Geriat. & A & E) Bristol & Weston HA.

PERERA, Saman Devapriya Southend Hospital, Prittlewell Chase, Westcliff on Sea SS0 0RY Tel: 01702 348911 — MB BS Newc. 1982; FRCR 1988; DMRD Aberd. 1988. Cons. Radiol. Southend Hosp. Westcliff-on-Sea. Specialty: Radiol. Prev: Sen. Regist. (Diag. Radiol.) Roy. Hallamsh. Hosp. Sheff.; Regist. (Diag. Radiol.) Aberd. Roy. Infirm.; SHO (A & E & Neurosurg.) Middlesbrough Gen. Hosp.

PERERA, Samantha Rovina 104a Highbury Park, London N5 2XE — MB ChB Bristol 1993.

PERERA, Sattambiralalage Anthony Michael Nirdosh 35 Farthing Court, Graham Street, Birmingham B1 3JR — MB ChB Birm. 1995; ChB Birm. 1995.

PERERA, Senerath Jayanthi Department of Paediatrics, Southend Health Care NHS Trust, Southend Hospital, Prittlewell Chase, Westcliff on Sea SS0 0RY — MB BS Peradeniya, Sri Lanka 1982.

PERERA, Shamira Asith — MB BS Lond. 1997.

PERERA, Shyam Divaka 10 Chalmers Road, Cambridge CB1 3SX — BChir Camb. 1995.

PERERA, Srimathie Therese Benodini 126 Wandle Road, Morden SM4 6AE — MB BS Ceylon 1970 (Colombo) Regist. Manor Hosp. Epsom.

PERERA, Sunimalee Himalika Bernadine 13 Dalcross Road, Hounslow TW4 7RA — MB BS Lond. 1994.

PERERA, Weditantirige Nihal Ranjit 16 Fairway, Whitestone, Nuneaton CV11 6NP Tel: 024 7632 5489 — MRCS Eng. LRCP Lond. 1978; MRCP (UK) 1984; FRCP Lond. 1998. Cons. Phys. c/o Elderly ScarBoro. Hosp. Specialty: Care of the Elderly; Gen. Med. Prev: Lect. & Hon. Sen. Regist. (c/o the Elderly) King's Coll. Hosp. Lond.

PERERA, Wijesinghe Aratchige Titus Edward 48 Uplands Way, London N21 1DT — MB BS Ceylon 1962.

PEREZ, Adrian Apple Tree House, Butcher's Lane, Boughton, Northampton NN2 8SL — LMS Madrid 1967; DPM Eng. 1976; MRCPsych 1977. Cons. Psychiat. St. Crispin & Northampton Gen. Hosps.; Vis. Cons. St. And. Hosp. N.ampton. Specialty: Gen. Psychiat. Prev: Regist. (Psychiat.) Acad. Dept. Newc.; Sen. Regist. (Psychiat.) South. Gen. Hosp. Glas.

PEREZ, Mr Joseph Valentine Mark — MB BS Lond. 1987 (Guy's Hospital) FRCS Ed. 1993; FRCS (Tr & Orth) 1999; CCST 2002. Cons. Hand and Orthopaedic Surg., Northwick Pk. Hosp., Lond. Specialty: Orthop. Socs: Brit. Soc. for Sugery of the Hand; Brit. Elbow and Shoulder Soc.; Brit. Orthopaedic Assn.

PEREZ, Lisa Anne 11 Coda Avenue, Bishopthorpe, York YO23 2SE — BM Soton. 1995.

PEREZ-AVILA, Mr Carlos Arturo, OBE Accident & Emergency Department, Royal Sussex County Hospital, Brighton Tel: 01273 696955 — DMed El Salvador 1970 (Univ. El Salvador) FRCS Ed. 1981; FRCS Eng. 1994; FFAEM 1994. Cons. A & E Roy. Sussex Co. Hosp. Brighton. Specialty: Accid. & Emerg. Socs: Brit. Assn. for Accid. & Emerg. Med. Prev: Sen. Regist. (A & E) Plymouth HD.

PEREZ-CAJARAVILLE, Juan Jesus Department of Anaesthesia, Royal Preston Hospital, Sharoe Green Lane, Fulwood, Preston PR2 9HT Tel: 01772 716565 — Licenciated in Med. & Surg. Pamplona 1991.

PEREZ CELORRIO, Inigo Dept of Stroke Medicine, Guy;s King's & St Thomas's School of Medicine, London SE5 9PJ; Crysie Cottage, Stanton, Ashbourne DE6 2DA — LMS Basque Provinces 1986. Research. Fell. Dept. Stroke. Med. Guy's. King's & St Thomas's. Sch. Med. Lond.

PEREZ DE ALBENIZ, Alberto Javier Caludon Centre, Clifford Bridge Road, Walsgrave, Coventry CV2 2TE Tel: 024 7660 2020 — LMS Basque Provinces 1987; MRCPsych 1994. Cons. Psychi. In Psychother., Coventry, W Midl.s. Specialty: Psychother. Socs: Inst. Gp. Anal.; Soc Psychoth. Research; Internat. Attachment Network. Prev: Sen. Regist. (Psychother.) W. Midl. Scheme.

PEREZ-MORALES, Maria de las Mercedes CDU, 40 Upton Road, Norwich NR4 7PA — LMS Zaragoza 1986; BSc Zaragoza 1987; DCH Lond. 1997; MSc Audiol. 2000. Specialty: Paediat.

PEREZ TERUEL, Maria Isabel 20 Florence Road, West Bridgford, Nottingham NG2 5HR — LMS Navarre 1987.

PERHAM, Elizabeth Greystone, Milnthorpe LA7 7QW — MB ChB Liverp. 1952.

PERHAM, Timothy Geoffrey Maslen Baccamore, Sparkwell, Plymouth PL7 5DF Tel: 01752 837404 — MB ChB Bristol 1966; MB ChB (Hons.) Bristol 1966; DObst RCOG 1968; FRCP Lond. 1986, M 1971; DCH Eng. 1973. Cons. Paediat. Plymouth Gen. Hosp.; OCC Lect. (Social Studies) Plymouth Univ.; Hon. Tutor (Child Health) Guy's Hosp. Lond. Specialty: Paediat. Socs: Brit. Paediat. Assn. & Plymouth Med. Soc. Prev: Regist. (Paediat.) Plymouth Gen. Hosp. & United Bristol Hosps.; Sen. Regist. (Med. Paediat.) Hosp. Sick Childr. Gt. Ormond St. Lond.; Regist. (Med.) Frenchay Hosp. Bristol.

PERIAPPURAM, Mathew John Radcliffe Hospital, Headley Way, Headington, Oxford OX3 9DU Tel: 01865 741166; 64 Ivy Lane, Headington, Oxford OX3 9DY Tel: 01865 220786 — MB BS Kerala 1980; DCH RPCSI 1985. Regist. (Paediat.) John Radcliffe Hosp. Oxf. Prev: Regist. (Paediat.) Milton Keynes Gen. Hosp.

PERIASAMY, Mr Paramasivan 20 Salt Market Place, Glasgow G1 5NF Tel: 0141 552 6610 — MB BS Madras 1986; FRCS Ed. 1990; FRCS Glas. 1991.

PERIES, Aubrey Cromwell Hospital, Cromwell Road, London SW5 0TU Tel: 020 7460 2000 Fax: 020 7460 5555; Chanterelle, Hook Heath Gardens, Woking GU22 0QG Tel: 01483 730022 Fax: 01483 730022 — MB BS Lond. 1976 (St. Bart. Hosp. Med. Coll. Lond.) BSc Biochem. Lond. 1970; MRCS Eng. LRCP Lond. 1976; DCH RCP Lond. 1991. Gen. Phys. Cromwell Hosp. Lond.; Hon. Regist. (Paediat.) Nat. Heart & Lung Hosp. Brompton. Specialty: Paediat. Socs: Fell. Roy. Soc. Med.; Roy. Coll. Of Paediat. & Child Health; Internat. Coll. of Paediat., Child & Adolesc. Care. Prev: Med. Off. (Paediat.) Cromwell Hosp. Lond.; Regist. (Paediat.) Frimley Pk. Hosp. Surrey (SW AHA).

PERINGER, Jane Elizabeth 35 Josephine Avenue, London SW2 2JY Email: janeperinger@f2s.com — MB BS Lond. 1978; BA Camb. 1975; MRCPsych 1982. Indep. Psychoanal. Lond. Specialty: Psychother. Socs: Mem. Brit. Psychoanal. Soc. Prev: Sen. Regist. (Child Psychiat.) St. Mary's Hosp. Lond.; Regist. Child Guid. Train. Centre Lond.; Regist. (Psychiat.) Middlx. Hosp. Lond.

PERINI, Anthony Francis Northgate & Prudhoe NHS Trust, Northgate Hospital, Morpeth NE61 3BP Tel: 01670 394070 Fax: 01670 394004 — MB BS Newc. 1980 (Newc. u. Tyne) MRCPsych 1985; MSc Lond. 1997. Med. Dir. & Cons. Psychiat. (Learning Disabil.) N.gate & Prudhoe NHS Trust. Specialty: Ment. Health. Socs: Brit. Neuropsychiat. Assn. Prev: Cons. Psychiat. & Clin. Dir. (Learn. Disabil.) Rampton Hosp.; Sen. Regist. (Ment. Handicap) N.gate Hosp.; Clin. Research Fell. Brain Metab Unit, Edin. Univ.

PERINPANAYAGAM, Kulenthiran Savunthararaj (retired) 72 Fordwych Road, London NW2 3TH Tel: 020 8452 3489 Fax: 020 7813 5723 Email: southyperin@compuserve.com — MB BS Ceylon 1961; DPM Eng. 1967; MRCPsych 1972. Cons. Psychiat. & Chief Exec. Sheperd's Youth Trust; Vis. Cons. Grovelands Priory Hosp. Lond. N14. Prev: Cons. (Psychiat.) & Med. Dir. Brookside Young People's.

PERINPANAYAGAM, Ruth Manorangitham 72 Fordwych Road, London NW2 3TH Tel: 020 8452 3489 — MB BS Ceylon 1959; DPath Eng. 1967; MRCPath 1970. Cons. (Microbiol.) Merton, Sutton & Wandsworth AHA (T). Specialty: Med. Microbiol. Socs: Assn. Clin. Pathols. Prev: Rotat. Sen. Regist. (Microbiol.) Univ. Coll. Hosp. Lond. & Whittington Hosp. Lond. & Edgware Gen. Hosp. & St. Mary's Hosp. Lond.; Regist. (Microbiol.) Hammersmith Hosp. Lond.

PERISELNERIS, Savirimuthu Rayappu Beach Road Surgery, 15 Beach Road, Lowestoft NR32 1EA Tel: 01502 572000 Fax: 01502 508892 — MB BS Sri Lanka 1976; MRCS Eng. LRCP Lond. 1988. Trainee GP RavensCt. Surg. Barry S. Glam. VTS. Socs: Med. Defence Union. Prev: SHO (Paediat.) Manor Hosp. Walsall; SHO (O & G & Anaesth.) Pontefract Gen. Infirm.; SHO (Gyn.) Walsgrave Hosp. Coventry.

PERIYASAMY, Thiyagarajah Om Sai Clinic, 248 Earls Court Road, London SW5 9AD Tel: 020 7935 1455 Fax: 020 7370 7497 — MB BS Sri Lanka 1973; MB BS Sri Lanka 1973.

PERKIN, George David Charing Cross Hospital, Regional Neurosciences Unit, Fulham Palace Road, London W6 8RF Tel: 020 8846 1153 Fax: 020 8846 7487 Email: d.perkin@ic.ac.uk; 80 Chestnut Road, West Norwood, London SE27 9LE Tel: 020 8761 5110 — MB BChir Camb. 1967 (Camb. & King's Coll. Hosp.) MRCS Eng. LRCP Lond. 1966; FRCP Lond. 1985, M 1969. p/t Cons. Neurol. Char. Cross Hosp. Lond.; Cons. Neurol. Maidenhead Hosp. Specialty: Neurol. Prev: Sen. Regist. (Neurol.) Maida Vale & Univ. Coll. Hosps.; Regist. Nat. Hosp. Nerv. Dis. Qu. Sq.; Ho. Phys. & Ho. Surg. King's Coll. Hosp. Lond.

PERKIN, Michael Richard 26 Barrington Road, Carshalton, Sutton SM3 9PP — MB BS Lond. 1993; BSc (Hons.) Lond. 1990; MB BS (Hons.) Lond. 1993; MRCP (UK) 1996; MRCPCH 1997. Specialist Regist. (Paediat.) St. Heliers Hosp. Carshalton, Lond. Specialty: Paediat. Prev: SHO (Paediat. Oncol.) Gt. Ormond St. Hosp.

PERKINS, Adrian Dryland Surgery, 1 Field Street, Kettering NN16 8JZ Tel: 01536 518951 Fax: 01536 486200 — MB ChB Leeds 1990; MRCGP 1994. Prev: GP Asst. Bradford; Trainee GP Harrogate VTS.

PERKINS, Andrew Stuart Road Surgery, Stuart Road, Pontefract WF8 4PQ Tel: 01977 703437 Fax: 01977 602334; Chestnut Avenue, Boston Spa, Wetherby LS23 6EE Tel: 01937 849804 — MB BS Lond. 1983 (Lond. Hosp.) DRCOG 1986; MSc (Gen. Pract.) Lond. 1993. Prev: Trainee GP Medway VTS.

PERKINS, Andrew Leonard c/o 71 Basing Way, London N3 3BP — MB BS Lond. 1977; DRCOG 1979; DO RCPSI 1985; MCOphth 1989.

PERKINS, Anne Marie Yorwerth The Clift Surgery, Minchens Lane, Bramley, Tadley RG26 5BH Tel: 01256 881228 — MB BS Lond. 1983 (St. Geo. Hosp.) DCH RCP Lond. 1990; DFFP 1995; MRCGP 1996. Specialty: Gen. Pract. Socs: RCGP (Fac. Family Plann.). Prev: Volunteer GP Romania; SHO (O & G) Roy. Shrewsbury Hosp.

PERKINS, Brian 21 Cherry Tree Avenue, Farnworth, Bolton BL4 9SB — BM BCh Oxf. 1993.

PERKINS, Carol Ann 28-30 Kings Road, Harrogate HG1 5JP; Ceylon House, 11 Robert St, Harrogate HG1 1HP Tel: 01423 521733 — MB ChB Leeds 1985; DRCOG 1987; T(GP) 1991.

PERKINS, Mr Charles Shepherd Department of Maxillofacial Surgery, Cheltenham General Hospital, Sandford Road, Cheltenham GL53 7AN Tel: 08454 222222 — BM Soton. 1989; BDS Liverp. 1980; FDS RCS 1984; (Oral Surg./Oral Med.) RCSI 1985; FRCS Ed. 1993. Cons. Oral & Maxillofacial Surg. Cheltenham Gen. & Glos. Roy. Hosps. Specialty: Oral & Maxillofacial Surg. Socs: BMA; Fell. Brit. Assoc. Oral & Maxillofacial Surg.; Eur. Assoc. Craniomaxillofacial Surg. Prev: Sen. Regist. (Oral & Maxillofacial Surg.) Cheltenham Gen., Gloucester Roy & John Radcliffe Hosp. Oxf.; Regist. (Oral & Maxillofacial Surg.) Soton. Gen. Hosp. & Odstock Hosp. Salisbury; SHO (Gen. Surg.) Qu. Alexandra Hosp. Portsmouth.

PERKINS, Colin Michael Zeneca Pharmaceuticals, Alderley Park, Macclesfield SK10 4TG Tel: 01625 515997 Fax: 01625 512406 — MD Leeds 1983; MB ChB 1974; MRCP (UK) 1977; FRCP Ed. 1988; FFPM 1990. Gp. Manager Regulatory Strategy Zeneca Pharmaceuts. Alderley Pk. Socs: Brit. Inst. Regulatory Affairs. Prev: MRC Clin. Scientist (Med.) Univ. Oxf.; Research Fell. (Med.) Univ. Leeds.

PERKINS, Elizabeth Lilian Madeleine (retired) Thorpe Lee, Denne Park, Horsham RH13 7AY Tel: 01403 252186 — MB BS Lond. 1953; DObst RCOG 1955; DA Eng. 1957.

PERKINS, Hugh David (retired) 199 East Dulwich Grove, London SE22 8SY — MB BS Lond. 1962 (St. Mary's) FFA RCS Eng. 1967. Prev: Retd. Cons. Anaesth. Greenwich Health Dist.

PERKINS, Hywel Hopcyn Bowen (retired) Netherdon, 3 Beech Walk, Ewell, Epsom KT17 1PU — LMSSA Lond. 1948 (Guy's) Prev: Resid. Med. Off. & Regist. (Cas.) Sutton & Cheam Gen. Hosp.

PERKINS, Jane Deborah Alison Toddington Medical Centre, Luton Road, Toddington, Dunstable LU5 6DE Tel: 01525 872222 Fax: 01525 876711; St. Andrews, Pk Road, Toddington, Dunstable LU5 6AB — MB BS Lond. 1980; DRCOG 1982.

PERKINS, Jennifer Anne 8 Brunstath Close, Barnston, Wirral CH60 1UH — MB ChB Liverp. 1994 (Liverpool) DRCOG. Specialty: Paediat. Dent.

PERKINS, Jeremy Mark Michael 3 Ribblesdale, Whitby, Ellesmere Port, South Wirral CH65 6RF — MB ChB Liverp. 1994.

PERKINS, Mr Jeremy Michael Towers Department of Vascular Surgery, Level 6, The John Radcliffe, Oxford OX3 9DU Tel: 01865 221288 Fax: 01865 221117 Email: jeremy.perkins@orth.nhs.uk — MB ChB Bristol 1988 (Univ. of Bristol) FRCS Eng. 1992; MD Bristol 1998. Cons. Vascular Surg., Oxford Radcliffe Hosp. NHS Trust, Oxford. Specialty: Gen. Surg. Socs: Vascular Surgical Soc. Of GB & I; Euro. Soc of Vascular & Endovascular Surg.; Assoc. of Surg. Of GB & I.

PERKINS, John Hilmar Church Street Surgery, Church Street, Starcross, Exeter EX6 8PZ Tel: 01626 890368 Fax: 01626 891330 — MB BS Lond. 1982; MRCGP 1987. GP. Exeter.

PERKINS, Katrina Mary Gibbs Marsh Farm, Stalbridge, Sturminster Newton DT10 2RU Tel: 01963 362655 Fax: 01963 362655 Email: perkins@gibbsmarsh.freeserve.co.uk — MB ChB Bristol 1998.

PERKINS, Marian Joan Park Hospital, Headington, Oxford OX3 1LQ — MB BS Lond. 1981; BSc (Hons.) Anat. Lond 1978, MB BS 1981; MRCP (UK) 1984; MRCPsych 1988. Drummond Prize Biochem. 1977.

PERKINS, Peter Doré Southbourne Surgery, 17 Beaufort Road, Southbourne, Bournemouth BH6 5BF Tel: 01202 427878 Fax: 01202 430730 Email: postmaster@gp-j81059.nhs.uk — MB BS Lond. 1977 (Westm.) MRCS Eng. LRCP Lond. 1977; Cert. Family Plann. JCC 1978; DRCOG 1979; MRCGP 1981; Dip Ad. Educat. Soton 1986. GP Southbourne Surg. Bournemouth; Chairm. Dept. of Minimally Invasive Gen. Pract.; Clin. Tutor Univ. Soton.; Clin. Pract. (Accid.) Bournemouth Gen. Hosp.; Pres. Bournemouth and ChristCh. Br. of the Roy. Coll. of Midw. Specialty: Gen. Med. Socs: Fell. of the Roy. Soc. of Med. Prev: SHO & Ho. Phys. (O & G) Roy. Vict. Hosp. Boscombe, Bournemouth; Ho. Surg. Qu. Mary's Hosp. Roehampton.

PERKINS, Peter John Veor Surgery, South Terrace, Camborne TR14 8SN Fax: 01209 886569; Walpole Cottage, South Tehidy, Camborne TR14 0HU — MB BS Lond. 1978 (Lond. Hosp.) DRCOG 1982.

PERKINS, Peter Paul 58 Eaton Crescent, Swansea SA1 4QN — MB BCh Wales 1996.

PERKINS, Philip James 8 Ivelbury Close, Buckden, St Neots, Huntingdon PE19 5XE — MB BS Lond. 1985.

PERKINS, Rosslyn Mary 301 Kingston Road, Wimbledon Chase, London SW20 8LB Tel: 020 8296 8154 — BM Soton. 1995; DCH 1999. SHO (GP Train. Scheme) Roy. Surrey Co. Hosp. Guildford. Specialty: Gen. Pract. Socs: MPS; BMA. Prev: SHO (A & E) Roy. Berks. Hosp. Reading.

PERKINS, Russell James Kevin Dept of Anaesthesia, Booth Hall Childrens Hospital, Blackley, Manchester — MB BS Lond. 1988; DA (UK) 1990; FRCA 1994. Cons. Manch. Childr. Hosp. NHS Trust. Specialty: Anaesth. Prev: Sen. Regist. NW Region; Research Fell. Hope Hosp. Salford; Anaesth. NW Regional Train. Scheme.

PERKINS, Sarah Louise Eaton Wood Medical Centre, 1128 Tyburn Road, Erdington, Birmingham B24 0SY Tel: 0121 373 0959 Fax: 0121 350 2719; 4 Shottery Close, Walmley, Sutton Coldfield B76 2WS Tel: 0121 313 1466 — MB ChB Birm. 1981 (Birmingham) MRCGP 1985; DRCOG 1985. GP; Hon. Clin. Lect. Dept Gen. Pract. Birm. Med. Sch.

PERKINS, Scott Marcus 1 Osprey Close, Worcester WR2 4BX — MB ChB Manch. 1997.

PERKINS, Susanne Alderton Health Centre, Alderton, Woodbridge IP12 3DA — BM Soton. 1988.

PERKINS, Vincent Dumfries & Galloway NHS Trust, Anaesthetic Department, Dumfries DG1 4AP Email: v.perkins@dgri.scot.nhs.uk — MB ChB Aberd. 1987; FRCA 1994. Cons. Anaesth. Dumfries & Galloway NHS Trust. Specialty: Anaesth.; Intens. Care. Socs: BMA.

Prev: Sen. Regist. Rotat. (Anaesth.) Cardiff; Regist. Rotat. (Anaesth.) Cardiff; SHO (Med. & Cas.) ChristCh., NZ.

PERKINS, William Department of Dematology & Dermatologic Surgery, The University Hospital, Nottingham NG7 2UH; The Manor House, Old Main Road, Bulcote, Nottingham NG14 5GU — MB BS Newc. 1984; FRCP (UK) 2000. Cons. Dermat. Qu. Med. Centre Nottm. Specialty: Dermat. Socs: Brit. Assn. Dermat. Prev: Cutaneous Surg. Fell. Univ. Minnesota, USA; Sen. Regist. Soton. Univ. Hosps. Trust.

PERKS, Alan Station Drive Surgery, Station Drive, Ludlow SY8 2AB Tel: 01584 8724461; Hills Farm, Middleton, Ludlow SY8 3DY — MB BS Lond. 1985; DRCOG 1988; MRACGP 1991. Prev: GP Queensland, Australia.

PERKS, Mr Anthony Graeme Bowman Nottingham City Hospital, Department of Plastic & Reconstructive Surgery, Nottingham NG5 1PB Tel: 0115 969 1169 Ext: 46428 Fax: 0115 962 7939 — MB BS Lond. 1979 (King's Coll. Hosp. Lond.) FRCS Eng. 1984; FRACS 1991; FRCS (Plast) 1994. Cons. (Plastic & Reconstruc. Surg.) Nottm. City Hosp. Specialty: Plastic Surg. Socs: Nat. Comm. Mem. Brit. Assn. Head & Neck Oncologists; Brit. Assn. Surg. Oncol.; Brit. Assn. Aesthetic Plastic Surgs. Prev: Cons. (Plastic & Reconstruc. Surg.) City Hosp. & Qu. Med. Centre Nottm.; Cons. (Plastic & Reconstruc. Surg.) The Pk. Hosp. Nottm.; Cons. (Plastic & Reconstruc. Surg.) King's Mill Hosp. Manfield.

PERKS, Barbara Mary Helena Hunningham Meadows, Long Itchington Road, Hunningham, Leamington Spa CV33 9EN Tel: 01926 633318 — MB ChB Birm. 1969. Cons. Anaesth. S. Warks. Community Dent. Serv.; Clin. Asst. (Anaesth.) Birm. Heartland Hosp. Specialty: Anaesth. Prev: Regist. (Anaesth.) United Birm. Hosps.

PERKS, Christian Edward Pershore Health Centre, Priest Lane, Pershore WR10 1RD Tel: 01386 502030 Fax: 01386 502058 — MB BChir Camb. 1989; MA Camb. 1990.

PERKS, Geoffrey Thomas (retired) The Grange Coach House, Yarm Lane, Great Ayton, Middlesbrough TS9 6PJ Tel: 01642 722595 — MB BS Durh. 1955.

PERKS, Janet Mary North Road West Medical Centre, 167 North Road West, Plymouth PL1 5BZ Tel: 01752 662780 Fax: 01752 254541; 7 Thorn Park, Mannamead, Plymouth PL3 4TG Tel: 01752 266078 — MB ChB Birm. 1976; DRCOG 1978; MRCGP 1980.

PERKS, John Stewart (retired) Hunningham Meadows, Long Itchington Road, Hunningham, Leamington Spa CV33 9EN Tel: 01926 633318 — MB ChB Birm. 1969; FFA RCS Eng. 1974. Cons. Anaesth. Coventry AHA.

PERKS, Mr Nigel Francis 58 Royal Hill, Greenwich, London SE10 8RT Tel: 020 8691 3183 — MB BS Newc. 1982; MRCOG 1988; FRCOG 2000. Cons. O & G Greenwich Dist. Hosp. Lond.; Cons. Reproductive Med. & Asst.ed Conception St. Bart Hosp. Lond. Specialty: Obst. & Gyn. Socs: Brit. Fertil. Soc.; Treas. & Sec. Forum for Qual. in Healthcare; Acad. Bd., Roy.Soc. Of Med.

PERKS, Richard Henry George (retired) 18 St Peters Close, Church Lane, Goodworth Clatford, Andover SP11 7SF Tel: 01264 354680 — (Oxf. & St. Thos.) BM BCh Oxf. 1952; MA Oxf. 1952; MRCGP 1963. Prev: Cas. Off. & Ho. Surg. St. Thos. Hosp.

PERKS, Warren Hamilton 25 Ridgebourne Road, Shrewsbury SY3 9AA Tel: 01743 232028 Fax: 01743 357652 Email: wazperks@hotmail.com — MB ChB Manch. 1971; MRCP (UK) 1975; MD Manch. 1980; FRCP Ed. 1989; FRCP Lond. 1990. Cons. Phys. Roy. Shrewsbury Hosp. Specialty: Gen. Med. Socs: Brit. Thorac. Soc.; Eur. Sch. Respirat. Med. Prev: Cons. (Phys.) Princess Roy. Hosp. Telford; Research Regist. Brompton Hosp.; Regist. (Neurol.) Manch. Roy. Infirm.

PERLIK-KOLACKI, Danuta Bozena Bredon Avenue Surgery, 232 Bredon Avenue, Binley, Coventry CV3 2FD Tel: 02476 447139 Fax: 02476 431839; 7A St. Martins Road, Finham, Coventry CV3 6ET Tel: 024 76 411148 Fax: 02476 412 — (Poznan) Med. Dipl. Poznan 1963; LAH Dub. 1970. Socs: BMA. Prev: SHO (Med. & Geriat.) Horton Gen. Hosp. Banbury; SHO (Med. & O & G) New Cross Hosp. Wolverhampton.; SHO (Med. & Chest), Creation Hosp., Northampton.

PERLMAN, Francesca Jane Andrea 8 Sutton Lane, Banstead SM7 3QP — MB BS Lond. 1989; MRCGP 1994. Prev: GP Lambeth, Southwark & Lewisham; Trainee GP Kent VTS.

PERLOW, Bernard Woolf (retired) 17 Hillcrest Gardens, Finchley, London N3 3EY Tel: 020 8349 9913 — MRCS Eng. LRCP Lond. 1946 (Lond. Hosp.) Prev: Capt. RAMC.

PERN, Peter Oliphant (retired) Woodside House, Cromarty IV11 8XU — MB ChB Ed. 1970; BSc (Med. Sci.) Ed. 1967; DIH Soc. Apoth. Lond. 1977; AFOM RCP Lond. 1981; MFOM RCP Lond. 1984; FRCP Ed. 1986; FFOM RCP Lond. 1994.

PERRAUDEAU, Mohini Kamala 102 Lavenham Road, London SW18 5HF — MB BS Lond. 1990; BSc Lond. 1987, MB BS 1990; MRCP (UK) 1993. Regist. (Rheum.) Hammersmith Hosp. Lond. Specialty: Rehabil. Med.; Rheumatol. Prev: Regist. (Gen. Med.) Wrexham Pk. Trust; SHO (Renal Med.) St. Mary's Hosp. Lond.; SHO Hammersmith Hosp. Lond.

PERREN, John Frederick (retired) 1 Graysfield, Welwyn Garden City AL7 4BL — MB BS Lond. 1953 (Char. Cross) DObst RCOG 1958; D.Occ.Med. RCP Lond. 1996. Prev: GP Force Med. Off. Herts. Constab. Welwyn Gdn. City.

PERREN, Timothy John CRUK Clinical Centre in Leeds, Cancer Research Building, St James' University Hospital, Beckett Street, Leeds LS9 7TF Tel: 0113 206 4670 Fax: 0113 242 9886 Email: t.j.perren@leeds.ac.uk — MB BS Lond. 1978 (Char. Cross) MRCS Eng. LRCP Lond. 1978; MRCP (UK) 1982; MD Lond. 1990; FRCP Lond. 1995. Hon. Sen. Lect. & Cons. Med. Oncol. CRUK Clin. Centre in Leeds Univ. Leeds & St. Jas. Univ. Hosp. NHS Trust Leeds; Chair of Jt. Speciality Comm. for Med. Oncol. at the Roy. Coll. of Physicians; Speciality Lead (Gyn. cancer) Leeds Cancer Centre. Specialty: Oncol. Special Interest: Clin. trials in, & Chemother. for Breast cancer & Gyn. cancers. Prev: Sen. Lect. In Med. Oncol., Leeds Univ.; Research Fell. (Med. Oncol.) Qu. Eliz. Hosp. Birm.; Regist. & SHO (Gen. Med.) N. Staffs. Hosp. Centre Stoke-on-Trent.

PERRETT, Andrew Gordon — MB BCh Camb. 1993; DRCOG; MRCGP; ACLS.

PERRETT, Anthony David (retired) 22 St Johns Terrace, Devoran, Truro TR3 6NE Tel: 01872 863358 — (Otago) MB ChB Otago 1958; FRCP Lond. 1979, M 1965; MD Otago 1968. Prev: Cons. Phys. Roy. Cornw. Hosp. Treliske.

PERRETT, Conal Martin 31 Shelwood Road, Brentwood CM14 6AD — MB ChB Bristol 1996.

PERRETT, Jennifer Margaret 22 St Johns Terrace, Devoran, Truro TR3 6NE Tel: 01872 863358 — MRCS Eng. LRCP Lond. 1969 (Guy's.) DA Eng. 1971. Clin. Asst. (Ophth.) Roy. Cornw. Hosps. Trust. Specialty: Ophth.

PERRETT, Kevin 53 Endowood Road, Millhouses, Sheffield S7 2LY Tel: 0114 236 5973 Email: kevinperrett@hotmail.com — MB ChB Sheff. 1985; MRCGP 1990; T(GP) 1991; MFPHM 1997. Cons. In Communicable Dis. Control/Pub. Health Protec. Agency. Specialty: Pub. Health Med. Socs: BMA; Fac. Publ. Health Med.; Soc. Social Med. Prev: Sen. Regist. (Pub. Health Med.) Trent RHA.

PERRICONE, Vittorio Blackpool Victoria Hospital, Whinney Heys Road, Blackpool FY3 8NR; 25 Infirmary Road, Blackburn BB2 3LP — State Exam Palermo 1992.

PERRIN, Clifford Edwin 344 Seafront, Hayling Island PO11 0BA Tel: 023 9246 8041 — MB BS Lond. 1958 (St Thos.)

PERRIN, Felicity Margaret Roche 19 Sidney Square, London E1 2EY — MB BS Lond. 1994.

PERRIN, Janet Anne 21 Alexandra Road, Gloucester GL1 3DR Tel: 01452 539116 — MB ChB Birm. 1959; MRCS Eng. LRCP Lond. 1959. Sen. Clin. Med. Off. (Psychosexual Med.) S. Worcs. Community Trust & S. Gloucestershire PCT. Specialty: Psychosexual Med. Socs: BMA; Inst. Psychosexual Med. Prev: Clin. Asst. (Orthop.) Gloucester Roy. Hosp.; GP Glos.; Ho. Surg. Gen. Hosp. Birm.

PERRIN, John (retired) Woodmans, Copthorne, Crawley RH10 3JU — MB BChir Camb. 1941 (Camb. & Lond. Hosp.) MRCP Lond. 1948; MD Camb. 1952. Cons. Immunol. Lond. Hosp. Prev: Asst. Dir. Clin. Laborats. Lond. Hosp.

PERRIN, John Eric (retired) 21 Alexandra Road, Gloucester GL1 3DR Tel: 01452 539116 — MB ChB Birm. 1959; MRCS Eng. LRCP Lond. 1959; DObst RCOG 1964; FRCGP 1985, M 1968. Prev: GP Gloucester.

PERRIN, Mandy Elizabeth 6 Norwood Gardens, Belfast BT4 2DX — MB ChB Birm 1992. SpR (Anaesth.) Nottm. Specialty: Anaesth.

PERRIN, Peter Francis 22 Eastway, Maghull, Liverpool L31 6BR — MB ChB Liverp. 1985.

PERRIN, Sarah Margaret 13 Larkfield Close, Caerleon, Newport NP18 3EX — MB ChB Bristol 1996.

PERRIN, Val Lawrence 13 Pettitts Lane, Dry Drayton, Cambridge CB3 8BT Email: val.perrin@dial.pipex.com — MB BS Lond. 1972 (St. Geo.) BSc Lond. 1969; MFPM 1992. Cons. Pharmaceut. Med. Camb. Specialty: Pharmaceutical Medicine. Prev: Sen. Research Phys. Glaxo Gp. Research Ltd. Greenford; GP Camb.; Med. Off. i/c Port Saunders Community Health Centre Newfld.

PERRINS, Mr David John Dyson (retired) 7 Fairlawn Wharf, East St Helen Street, Abingdon OX14 5ED Tel: 01235 521592 Email: david.perrins@talk21.com — MD Camb. 1973; FRCS Ed. 1958; FRCS Eng. 1960. Prev: Hon. Med. Adviser Federat. Multiple Sclerosis Treatm. Centres.

PERRINS, Edward John Department of Cardiology, The General Infirmary, Great George St., Leeds LS1 3EX Tel: 0113 392 2650 Fax: 0113 392 6343 — MB ChB Leeds 1975; MB ChB (Hons.) Leeds 1975; MRCP (UK) 1977; FACC 1983; BSc (Anat.) (1st cl. Hons.) Leeds 1972, MD 1985; FRCP Lond. 1989. Cons. Cardiol. Gen. Infirm. Leeds. Specialty: Cardiol. Socs: Brit. Cardiac Soc.; Pres. Brit. Card. Interven. Soc. 1996-2000. Prev: Pres. Soc. Cardiol. Technicians; Sec. Brit. Pacing Gp.

PERRINS, John Kenneth Perrins and Partners, Trinity Medical Centre, New George Street, South Shields NE33 5DU Tel: 0191 454 7775 Fax: 0191 454 6787; Shanklin, 20 Underhill Road, Cleadon Village, Sunderland SR6 7RS — MB BS Newc. 1981 (Newcastle upon Tyne) MRCGP 1985; MRCP (UK) 1988.

PERRIS, Allison Jane — MB ChB Leeds 1998.

PERRIS, Thomas Michael 97 Lichfield Road, Sutton Coldfield B74 2RR — MB ChB Bristol 1993.

PERRISS, Brian William Department of Anaesthetics, Royal Devon & Exeter Hospital, Barrack Road, Exeter EX2 5DW Tel: 01392 402474; Lyneham Farm, Chudleigh, Newton Abbot TQ13 0EH Tel: 01626 854513 — MB BS Lond. 1963 (St. Bart.) BSc (Hons.) Lond. 1959, MB BS 1963; DA Eng. 1965; FFA RCS Eng. 1968. Cons. Anaesth. Roy. Devon & Exeter Hosps. Specialty: Anaesth. Socs: BMA & Soc. Anaesth. SW Region. Prev: Sen. Regist. (Anaesth.) S.W. RHA & United Bristol Hosps.; Sen. Clin. Fell. Univ. Colorado, Denver, USA; Regist. (Anaesth.) United Bristol Hosps.

PERRISS, Richard William 6 Windsor Court, South Gosforth, Newcastle upon Tyne NE3 1YN — MB ChB Sheff. 1993. Demonst. (Anat.) Univ. of Newc. Upon Tyne. Specialty: Anat. Prev: SHO (Surg.) Darlington Memor. Hosp.; SHO (ENT) Freeman Hosp. Newc.; SHO (Cardiothoracic) North. Gen. Hosp. Sheff.

PERRITT, Simon Jeremy 2 French Street, Widnes WA8 0BT — MB ChB Liverp. 1996.

PERRONS, Anthony John Tigh Nan Sgeiran, Isle of Islay PA49 7UN — MB ChB Birm. 1959.

PERROS, Petros Endocrine Unit, Level 6, Freeman Hospital, Freeman Road, Newcastle upon Tyne NE7 7DN Tel: 0191 284 3111 Fax: 0191 213 1968 — MB BS Newc. 1983; MRCP (UK) 1986; BSc (Hons.) 1978, MD 1992; FRCP 2000. Cons. Phys. (Endocrinol.) Freeman Hosp. Newc. u. Tyne; Hon. Sen. Lect. Newc. Univ. Specialty: Endocrinol.

PERROTT, Barry David (retired) Flat 4, 18 Campden Hill Gardens, London W8 — MRCS Eng. LRCP Lond. 1961 (Westm.) Prev: Ho. Surg. Westm. Hosp.

PERROTT, Charles Stephen Halse Road Health Centre, Halse Road, Brackley NN13 6EJ Tel: 01280 703460; The Old Stone House, Greatworth, Banbury OX17 2DZ — MB BS Lond. 1987; DCH RCP Lond. 1989; MRCGP 1992. Prev: Trainee GP Banbury VTS; SHO (A & E) Gen. Hosp. St. Helier, Jersey; Ho. Surg. Roy. Free Hosp. Lond.

PERRY, Aideen Dorothy Campbell (retired) Manor Cottage, Kingstone, Ilminster TA19 0NS — MB ChB Liverp. 1961; DObst RCOG 1964; DCH Eng. 1966; MRCP (U.K.) 1972.

PERRY, Alastair James House Doctors Surgery, Maryport Street, Usk NP15 1AB Tel: 01291 672633 Fax: 01291 672631; Tyn-y-Caeau Farm, Llangibby, Usk NP15 1PS Tel: 01291 2888 — (National University of Ireland University College Galloav) MB BCh BAO NUI 1958. Med. Off. HM Prison & HM Young Offenders Inst. Usk. Socs: BMA. Prev: Med. Off. Balfour Beatty (Overseas) Ltd. W. Pakistan; Regist. (Path.) Roy. North. Hosp. & Char. Cross Hosp. Lond.

PERRY, Amanda Ruth Department of Academic Haematology, Institute of Cancer Research, Cotswold Road, Sutton SM2 5NG Tel: 020 8643 8901; 195C Camberwell Grove, London SE5 8JU Tel: 020 7924 0497 — BM BCh Oxf. 1990; MRCP (UK) 1993; Dip. RCPath 1996. Specialty: Haematology.

PERRY, Andrew John Warwick House Medical Centre, Holway Green, Upper Holway Road, Taunton TA1 2YJ Tel: 01823 282147 Fax: 01823 338181; Orchard Cottage, Nailsbourne, Taunton TA2 8AG Tel: 01823 451415 Email: harris.perry@which.net — MB BS Lond. 1985 (Char. Cross) BSc Lond. 1982; DA (UK) 1987; DCH RCP Lond. 1989; MRCGP 1990; DRCOG 1990. Hosp. Practitioner (Anaesth.) MusGr. Pk. Hosp. Taunton. Specialty: Gen. Pract.

PERRY, Mr Andrew Richard 108 Faraday Road, London SW19 8PB — MB BS Lond. 1992; BSc Lond. 1989; FRCS Eng. 1997; FRCS Ed. 1997; FRCS Tr & Orth. 2001. Locum Cons. Orth. Surg. Frimley Pk. Hosp. Specialty: Orthop. Socs: BOA; Brit. Orthop. Train. Assn. Prev: Specialist Regist. Rotat. (Orthop.) S. W. Thames; SHO (Plastics & Reconstruc. Surg.) Qu. Mary's Roehampton; SHO (A & E) St. Thos. Hosp. Lond.

PERRY, Anne Catherine Psychotherapy Department, 50-52 Clifden Road, Hackney, London E5 0LJ Tel: 020 8510 8242 — MB BS Lond. 1991 (Univ. Lond. & St. Geo. Hosp. Med. Sch.) MRCPsych 1995; Dip. Cog Therapy Oxf. 1998. Specialty: Psychother.; Gen. Psychiat. Prev: Sen. Regist. (Behavioural & Cognitive Psychother.) Springfield Hosp. Lond.

PERRY, Anthony Treetops, Penycoedcae, Pontypridd CF37 1PY Tel: 01443 402448; 5 Tythebarn Lane, Dicken's Heath, Solihull B90 1RN Tel: 0121 745 2556 — BM BS Nottm. 1993; BMedSci (Hons.) 1991; FRCS Glas. 1997; FRCS Ed. 1997. Specialist Regist. (Gen. Surg.) W. Midl. Rotat. Specialty: Gen. Surg. Prev: Sen. SHO Gen. Surg. Birm. Heartlands & Solihill Trust.

PERRY, Catherine Ann Grace The Brant Road Surgery, 291 Brant Road, Lincoln LN5 9AB Tel: 01522 722853 Fax: 01522 722195 — BM BS Nottm. 1989; BMedSci Nottm. 1987; MRCGP 1993; DRCOG 1993. GP Princip. Lincoln. Prev: Lincoln VTS.

PERRY, Lady (Catherine Hilda) Glenholm, 2 Cramond Road S., Davidsons Mains, Edinburgh EH4 6AD — MB ChB Ed. 1970. Socs: Med. Wom. Federat. & Cas. Surgs. Assn. Prev: Regist. (A & E) Northampton Gen. Hosp.; Med. Off. (Gen. Surg. & Traum. & Orthop. Surg.) Stoke; Mandeville Hosp.; Ho. Off. Stoke Mandeville Hosp.

PERRY, Charles Lyn, SJM (retired) Windrush, 39 Haven Road, Haverfordwest SA61 1DU Tel: 01437 762973 — MB BCh Wales 1949 (Cardiff) BSc Wales 1944; DObst RCOG 1954; MRCGP 1960. Prev: GP HaverfordW.

PERRY, Christopher Michael 2 Woodhall Avenue, London SE21 7HL Tel: 020 7351 4173 — (King's Coll. Lond. & St. Geo.) MB BS Lond. 1969; FRCOG 1989, M 1976. Cons. Gyn. St. Helier NHS Trust & Roy. Marsden Hosp. Lond.; Edit. Bd. Mem. of Cytopathol. Specialty: Obst. & Gyn. Socs: Brit. Soc. Colpos. & Cerv. Path. Prev: Sen. Regist. St. Helier Hosp. Carshalton & Roy. Marsden Hosp.; Regist. (O & G) St. Helier Hosp. Carshalton; Ho. Surg. Surgic. Unit & Regist. (O & G) St. Geo. Hosp. Lond.

PERRY, Colin Graham 1/R 103 Woodford Street, Shawlands, Glasgow G41 3HW — MB ChB Glas. 1991; MCP (UK) 1995. Specialist Regist. (Diabetics/Endocrinol.) Glas. Specialty: Diabetes.

PERRY, David James Haemophilia Centre & Haemostasis Unit, Royal Free & University Colege Medical School, Royal Free Campus, Rowland Hill Street, London NW3 2PF; 17 Long Road, Cambridge CB2 2PP Tel: 01223 244299 — MB ChB Ed. 1978; BSc Edin. 1975; MB ChB Edin. 1978; MRCP Roy. Coll. Of Physicians (UK) 1980; MRCPath Roy. Coll. Of Pathologists 1985; MD Edin. 1992; PhD Camb. 1993; FRCPath Roy. Coll. Of Pathologists 1995. Sen. Hon. / Hon. Cons., Haemostasis & Thrombosis, London. Specialty: Haematology. Prev: Lect. (Molecular Haemat.) Wellcome Trust.

PERRY, David William 20 Ufton Close, Shirley, Solihull B90 3SB — MB ChB Birm. 1987.

PERRY, Mr Dexter Royal Bournmouth Hospital, Castle Lane East, Bournemouth BH7 7DW Tel: 01202 303626 Email: dexterperry@yahoo.co.uk — BM Soton. 1991; FRCS Eng. 1995. Cons. (Gen. Surg.) Roy. Bournmouth Hosp. Specialty: Gen. Surg. Special Interest: Breast; Surgic. Oncol. Prev: Specialist Regist. (Gen. Surg.) Qu. Alexandra Hosp. Ports.; Specialist Regist. (Gen. Surg.) I. of Wight Health Care Trust St. Mary's Hosp. Newport.

PERRY, Diana Parsonage House, 17 Orlingbury Road, Pytchley, Kettering NN14 1ET — MB BS Lond. 1964 (King's Coll. Hosp.) MRCS Eng. LRCP Lond. 1964; DObst RCOG 1966; DCH Eng. 1967.

PERRY, Duncan Ross Alastair Tyn-Y-Caeau Farm, Llanbadoc, Usk NP15 1PS — MB BS Lond. 1994.

PERRY, Eileen Elizabeth (retired) Movilla House Nursing Home, 51 Movilla Road, Newtownards BT23 8RG Tel: 028 9182 6390 — (Qu. Univ. Belf.) MB BCh BAO Belf. 1937; DPH 1939; DObst RCOG 1942; DCH Eng. 1946; MFCM 1974. Prev: Div. Med. Off. Antrim Co. Health Comm.

PERRY, Elizabeth Mary Cornerstone Surgery, 469 Chorley Old Road, Bolton BL1 6AH Tel: 01204 495426 Fax: 01204 497423 — MB ChB Liverp. 1983.

PERRY, Eugene Philip Scarborough Hospital, Woodlands Drive, Scarborough YO12 6QL — MB ChB Leic. 1980. Specialty: Gen. Surg.

PERRY, Fiona Mary The Surgery, 138 Beaconsfield Villas, Brighton BN1 6HQ Tel: 01273 552212/555401 Fax: 01273 271148; Bankside, Ditchling Common, Burgess Hill RH15 0SJ Tel: 01444 233307 — MB BS Lond. 1981 (Roy. Free)

PERRY, Geoffrey Lawrence Bloomfield, Yarmouth Road, Hales, Norwich NR14 6AB — MB BS Lond. 1990.

PERRY, Huw Miles 4 St Anne's Court, Talgarn, Pontyclun CF72 9HH — MB BS Lond. 1985.

PERRY, Ian Charles Old Farm House, Grateley, Andover SP11 8JR Tel: 0126 488 9659 Fax: 0126 488 9639 Email: ian@ianperry.com; 19 Cliveden Place, London SW1W 8HD Tel: 020 7730 8045 Fax: 020 7730 1985 — MB BS Lond. 1963 (Guy's) MRCS Eng. LRCP Lond. 1963; DAvMed RCP Lond. 1968; MFOM RCP Lond. 1979. Cons. Occupat. Med. Various Cos.; Authorised Sen. Med. Examr. Civil Aviat. Auth. (UK), Federal Aviat. Agency (USA) & Other Foreign Aviat. Auths.; Med. Cons. to Various Airlines & Companies; Med. Cons. Brit. Helicopter Advis. Bd. & IAOPA; Sen. Cons. Avimed Ltd. & TIAMC & HAS; Cons. (Occup. Med.) Winchester & Eversleigh NHS; UK Home Office Referree & SMP. Specialty: Occupat. Health; Aviat. Med.; Trop. Med. Socs: FRAeS; FICM; FIOSH. Prev: Master of Guild. Air Pilots & Air Navigators; Maj. RAMC, Sen. Med. Off. & Aviat. Med. Adviser RAMC & Army Air Corps; UK Delegate NATO Agard Aerospace Med. Panel.

PERRY, James Herbert (retired) 2 Combe Street Lane, Yeovil BA21 3PB Tel: 01935 475504 — (Bristol) MB ChB Bristol 1953; DObst RCOG 1960. Prev: Sen. Res. Off. Bristol Matern. Hosp.

PERRY, Jane Elizabeth 11 Cherry Gardens, Sawbridgeworth CM21 9DW — MB BS Lond. 1988.

PERRY, Jeremy David Department of Rheumatology, Barts. & The London NHS Trust, Royal London Hospital, Mile End, Bancroft Road, London E1 4DG Tel: 020 7377 7859 Fax: 020 7377 7801 — MB BS Lond. 1970 (Middlx.) Acad. Dip. Biochem. Univ. Lond. 1967; MRCP (UK) 1973; FRCP Lond. 1986. Cons. Rheumatologist, Barts and the Lond. Trust, Roy. Lon. Hosp.; Cons. Adviser Crystal Palace Nat. Sports Centre; Hon. Sen. Lect. Lond. Hosp. Med. Coll., Q.M.W.. Lond. Sch. Med. & Dent Teach. Univ. Lond. Specialty: Rheumatol. Socs: Brit. Soc. Rheum.; Roy. Soc. Med. (Comm. Mem. Sect. Sports Med.); Brit. Assn. Sport & Med. Prev: Cons. Rheum. Newham Health Care; Sen. Regist. (Rheum.) Colchester and P. Of Wales Hosp.; Regist.&SHO (Med.) Lond. Hosp.

PERRY, John Fraser Unit 8, Torbay Hospital, Newton Road, Torquay TQ2 7AA — MB ChB New Zealand 1995.

PERRY, John Reginald (retired) 49 New Wokingham Road, Crowthorne RG45 6JG Tel: 01344 774210 — MB ChB Birm. 1959; DObst RCOG 1961; DCH Eng. 1963. Prev: Med. Off. Wellington Coll.

PERRY, John Rodham Nuffield Road Medical Centre, Nuffield Road, Chesterton, Cambridge CB4 1GL Tel: 01223 423424 Fax: 01223 566450 — MB BCh Wales 1970 (Welsh National School of Medicine) DObst RCOG 1973; FRCGP 1987, M 1974; MSc 1998. Dir. (Studies in Gen. Pract.) Univ. Camb.

PERRY, Jonathan James Dilston Mill House, Corbridge NE45 5QZ — MB BS Lond. 1997.

PERRY, Jonathan Neil, Surg. Cdr. RN Department of Radiology, Derriford Hospital, Derriford Road, Plymouth PL6 8DH Tel: 01752 763297; Westlake Brake, Renny Road, Down Thomas, Plymouth PL9 0BG — MB ChB Birm. 1984; FRCR 1994. Cons. Radiol. Derriford Hosp. Plymouth. Specialty: Radiol. Prev: Med. Off. HMS Revenge.

PERRY, Joseph John 2 Adenburgh Drive, Attenborough, Nottingham NG9 6AZ — MB ChB Birm. 1948; MRCGP 1961; DA Eng. 1969. Prev: Ho. Phys. Gen. Hosp. Birm.

PERRY, Keith Alan Worcester Street Surgery, 24 Worcester Street, Stourbridge DY8 1AW Tel: 01384 371616 — MB ChB Birm. 1961; DObst RCOG 1963. Socs: BMA. Prev: Clin. Asst. (Ophth.) Corbett Hosp. Stourbridge; Clin. Asst. Birm. & Midl. Eye Hosp.; Ho. Phys. & Ho. Surg. Corbett Hosp. Stourbridge.

PERRY, Louise Jane Department of Histopathology, Wexham Park Hospital, Wexham Street, Slough SL2 4HL — MB BS Lond. 1987; JCPTGP 1991; MSc (Distinc. Experim. Path. & Toxicol.) Lond. 1993; MRCPath 2000. Specialty: Histopath.

PERRY, Mark Stephen The Robert Darbishire Practice, Rusholme Health Centre, Walmer Street, Manchester M14 5NP Tel: 0161 225 6699 Fax: 0161 248 4580 — MB ChB Leeds 1979. Specialty: Alcohol & Substance Misuse.

PERRY, Mark Stephen 38 Mount Street, Aberdeen AB25 2QT — MB ChB Aberd. 1997.

PERRY, Mrs Mary Elisabeth Rhael Windrush, 39 Haven Road, Haverfordwest SA61 1DU Tel: 01437 762973 — MRCS Eng. LRCP Lond. 1952 (Cardiff) JP. Specialty: Family Plann. & Reproduc. Health. Prev: Med. Advisor to Schs. & Clin. Med. Off. Pembrokesh. HA.

PERRY, Matthew Giles Bampton Surgery, Landells, Bampton OX18 2LJ Tel: 01993 850257; Blackthorn Cottage, Queen St, Bampton OX18 2LP — MB BS Lond. 1973 (Univ. Coll. Hosp.) BSc (Genetics) Lond. 1970, MB BS 1973; DObst RCOG 1975. Prev: SHO (A & E) & SHO (O & G) Princess Margt. Hosp.; Swindon; Ho. Surg. Bolingbroke Hosp. Lond.

PERRY, Matthew Robert The Surgery, Shaw Lane, Albrighton, Wolverhampton WV7 3DT Tel: 0190 722 2301 Fax: 01902 373807; Cloverleigh, Shaw Lane, Albrighton, Wolverhampton WV7 3DT — MB ChB Birm. 1982; DRCOG 1985; MRCGP 1986; MSc Warwick University Primary Care Management 1998. Chair S. E. Shrops. PCG.

PERRY, Mr Michael John Maxillofacial Unit, North Staffs NHS Trust, COPD, Hartshill Road, Stoke-on-Trent ST4 7PA Tel: 91782 554696 — MB ChB Leeds 1988; BSc Leeds 1985; BChD Leeds 1993; FDS Lond. 1995; FRCS Eng. 1995; FRCS (OMFS) Middlesborough 2001. Cons. Maxillofacial Surg. N. Staff NHS Trust Stoke-on-Trent; SHO Neurosurg., Leeds Gen. Infirm.; SHO Accid. and Emerg. Med., SJUH Leeds. Specialty: Oral & Maxillofacial Surg. Prev: SHO (Oral Surg.) Sunderland Dist. Gen. Hosp.; SHO (Gen. Surg. & Orthop.) York Dist. Gen. Hosp.; SpR Maxillofacial Surg. S. Thames.

PERRY, Nicholas David 13 Aylmer House, Eastney St., London SE10 9NU — MB BS Lond. 1992.

PERRY, Nicholas Keith 27 Lansdown Park, Lansdown, Bath BA1 5TG — BM BS Nottm. 1982.

PERRY, Nicholas Mark St Bartholomey's Hospital, Breast Assessment Centre, West Smithfield, London EC1A 7BE Tel: 020 7601 8074; 10 Cloncurry Street, London SW6 6DS — (St. Bart.) MB BS Lond. 1975; FRCS Eng. 1980; FRCR 1984. Cons. Radiol. St Bart. Hosp. Lond.; Clin. Dir.Centr. & E. Lond. Breast Screening Progr. Specialty: Radiol. Prev: Sen. Regist. (Radiol.) St. Bart. Hosp. Lond.; Quality Assur. Manager N. Thames Breast Screening Progr.; Cons. Europ. Commiss. Europe. Against Cancer Breast Screening Progr.

PERRY, Nicola Ground Floor Flat, 22 Steerforth St., London SW18 9HE — MB ChB Bristol 1996.

PERRY, Nigel Farningham Surgery, Braeside, Gorse Hill, Farningham, Dartford DA4 0JU Tel: 01322 862110 Fax: 01322 862991; 19 Eardley Road, Sevenoaks TN13 1XX Tel: 01732 458443 Email: drnperry@aol.com — MB ChB Cape Town 1976; BSc Cape Town 1971. Asst. Med. Adviser Nuclear Electric plc & Magnox Electric; Apptd. Dr under ionizing Radiat. Regulat.s. Specialty: Gen. Med.

PERRY, Professor Philip Michael (retired) Queen Alexandra Hospital, Cosham, Portsmouth PO6 3LY Tel: 023 92 286000 — (St. Bart.) MB BS Lond. 1962; FRCS Eng. 1968; MS Lond. 1974. Cons. Surg. Qu. Alexandra Hosp. Portsmouth; Vis. Prof. Postgrad. Med. Fac. Univ. Portsmouth; Cons. Surg. Portsmouth & SE Hants. Health

Dist.; Arris & Gale Lect. & Erasmus Wilson Demonst. RCS Eng; Hon Cons. jure. Prev: Lect. (Surg.) Unit St. Bart. Hosp. Lond.

***PERRY, Rachel Elizabeth** 1 Bowling Leys, Middleton, Milton Keynes MK10 9BD Tel: 01908 395235 Fax: 01908 395235 — MB BS Lond. 1998 (RFHSM) MB BS Lond 1998. SHO (Cas.) Northampton Gen. Hosp. Specialty: Accid. & Emerg. Socs: RSM.

PERRY, Rachel Kitrick Kaye 23 Barnfield Road, Petersfield GU31 4DQ; 7 Clare Lawn Avenue, East Sheen, London SW14 8BH Tel: 020 8876 8883 Email: neil@perry10.freeserve.co.uk — BChir Camb. 1994; MRCP 1998. Specialist Regist. (Clin. Oncol.) Roy. Marsden NHS Trust, Lond. Specialty: Oncol. Prev: SHO (Gen. Med.) Kent & Canterbury NHS Trust; Locum Regist. (c/o Elderly) St. Chas. Hosp. Lond.

PERRY, Raphael Adam Cardiothoracic Centre Liverpool NHS Trust, Thomas Drive, Broadgreen, Liverpool L14 3PE Tel: 0151 293 2399 Fax: 0151 293 2429 Email: raphael.perry@ctc.nhs.uk — BM BS Nottm. 1980; DM Nottm. 1990, BMedSci 1978; MRCP (UK) 1984; FACC 1993; FRCP Lond. 1995. Cons. Cardiol. Cardiothoracic Centre Liverp.; Clin. Director Cardiol. Specialty: Cardiol. Socs: Brit. Cardiac Soc.; Brit. Cardiovasc. Interven. Soc. Prev: Postgrad. Clin. Tutor & Clin. Lect. (Med.) Cardiothoracic Centre Liverp.; Sen. Regist. (Cardiol.) Regional Adult Cardiothoracic Unit Broadgreen Hosp. Liverp.; Brit. Heart Foundat. Research Fell. Deptartment Cardiovasc. Med. Qu. Eliz. Hosp. Birm.

PERRY, Rebecca Jane 11 St Tristan Close, Locks Heath, Southampton SO31 6XR Tel: 01489 576828 — MB ChB Glas. 1994; MRCP Glasgow 1998. SpR (Paediat. Med.) Roy.Hosp. For Sick Children. Specialty: Paediat. Socs: Roy. Coll. Phys.s and Surg. Glas.; RCPCH. Prev: SHO (Paediat. Med.) Roy. Hosp. For Sick Childr., Glas.; SHO (Paediat. Med.) Roy. Alexandra Hosp.; SHO (Paediat. Med.) Roy. Hosp. Sick Childr. Glas.

PERRY, Richard James 20C Queensdown Road, London E5 8NN — MB BS Lond. 1990; MRCP (UK) 1994.

PERRY, Richard John Parkside Family Practice, Green Road Surgery, 224 Wokingham Road, Reading RG6 1JT Tel: 0118 966 3366 Fax: 0118 926 3269; 3 Knossington Close, Lower Earley, Reading RG6 4EU — MB BS Lond. 1996.

PERRY, Richard Jolyon Doctor's Mess, Level 3, John Radcliffe Hospital, Headley Way, Oxford OX3 9DU Tel: 01865 741166; 8 Pembroke Court, Rectory Road, Oxford OX4 1BY Tel: 01865 721830 — BM BCh Oxf. 1993; PhD Camb. 1991; MA Oxf. 1993. SHO Rotat. (Gen. Med.) Oxf. Radcliffe NHS Trust. Specialty: Gen. Med. Prev: Ho. Phys. John Radcliffe Hosp. Oxf.; Ho. Surg. Wycombe Gen. Hosp. High Wycombe.

PERRY, Professor Robert Henry Newcastle General Hospital, Neuropathology Department, Westgate Road, Newcastle upon Tyne NE4 6BE Tel: 0191 256 3684 Fax: 0191 256 3196 Email: robert.perry@ncl.ac.uk; Dilston Mill House, Corbridge NE45 5QZ Tel: 01434 632308 Email: r@perry.net — MB ChB St. And. 1969 (St Andrews) MRCP (UK) 1972; MRCPath 1978; FRCPath 1990; FRCP Ed. 1992; FRCP Lond. 1993; DSc Newc. 1993. Cons. Neuropath. Newc. upon Tyne Hosps. NHS Trust; Prof. Neuropath. Newc. Univ.; Clin. Scientist Developm. in Brain Ageing. Specialty: Neuropath. Special Interest: Dementia. Socs: Brit. Neuropath. Soc.

PERRY, Roger Malcolm The Redwell Medical Centre, 1 Turner Road, Wellingborough NN8 4UT Tel: 01933 400777 Fax: 01933 671959 — MB ChB Birm. 1977; MRCGP 1981.

PERRY, Samantha Frances 7 Turnberry Road, Glasgow G11 5AF — BM BS Nottm. 1988; MRCP (UK) 1991. Regist. (A & E) West. Infirm. Glas. Specialty: Accid. & Emerg. Socs: BMA; Brit. Accid. & Emerg. Med. Soc. Prev: SHO (A & E) CrossHo. Kilmarnock; SHO (A & E & Clin. Pharmacol.) Glas. Roy. Infirm.

PERRY, Shona Catriona 14 Chatelherault Avenue, Cambuslang, Glasgow G72 8BJ — MB ChB Aberd. 1997.

PERRY, Mr Stephen Robert Kidderminster Hospital, Bewdley Road, Kidderminster DY11 6RJ Tel: 01562 823424; Hillhampton farmhouse, Hillhampton lane, Great Willy, Worcester WR6 6DV — MB BChir Camb. 1983; MA Camb. 1980; DO RCS Lond. 1986; FRCS Ed. 1989; FCOphth 1989. Worcester Acute Hosp.s NHS Trust. Specialty: Ophth. Socs: Roy. Soc. Med.; Midl. Ophth. Soc. Prev: Fell. Oculoplastic & Orbital Surg. Univ. Brit. Columbia; Sen. Regist. (Ophth.) Bristol Eye Hosp.

PERRY-KEENE, Gillian Heather Prices Mill Surgery, New Market Road, Nailsworth, Stroud GL6 0DQ Tel: 01453 832424 Fax: 01453 833833; Street Farm Cottage, 22 The St, Uley, Dursley GL11 5TB — MB BS Lond. 1968 (Univ. Coll. Hosp.) MRCS Eng. LRCP Lond. 1968. Dep. Police Surg. Glos. Constab. Specialty: Community Child Health. Socs: Assn. Police Surg.; Fell. Roy. Soc. Med. Prev: Dep. Police Surg. Glos. Constab.; Clin. Asst. (Geriat.) Qu.s Hosp. Cirencester; Ho. Off. (Surg. & Phys.) Cirencester Memor. Hosp.

PERRYER, Carolyn Jane Delapre Medical Centre, Gloucester Avenue, Northampton NN4 8QF Tel: 01604 761713 Fax: 01604 708589; 1 High Street, Greens Norton, Towcester NN12 8BA Tel: 01327 353681 — MRCS Eng. LRCP Lond. 1984 (Char. Cross) T(GP) 1991.

PERRYER, Susan Elizabeth Summertown Group Practice, 160 Banbury Road, Oxford OX2 7BS Tel: 01865 515552 Fax: 01865 311237; 7 Walton Crescent, Oxford OX1 2JG Tel: 01865 522416 — MB BS Lond. 1983; MRCP (UK) 1987.

PERSAD, Mr Krishna Flat 65, Queens Court, Queensway, London W2 4QW Tel: 020 7727 4309 — MB ChB St. And. 1967; FRCS Ed. 1974; MRCOG 1976. Locum Cons. Specialty: Obst. & Gyn.

PERSAD, Mr Rajendra Asita Rajkrishna Department of Urology, Bristol Royal Infirmary, Bristol BS2 8HW Tel: 0117 928 3509 Fax: 0117 928 3505 Email: raj.persad@ubht.swest.nhs.uk; 10 Clifton Park Road, Bristol BS8 3HL Tel: 0117 377 7173 Fax: 01275 846 117 — MB BS Lond. 1983 (Univ. Coll. Hosp.) FRCS Eng. 1987; ChM Bristol 1993; FEBU 1994; FRCS (Urol.) 1994. Cons. Urol. Surg. & Surg. Uro-Oncol. Bristol Roy. Infirm.; Sen. Clin. Lect. Univ. Bristol; Hon. Assoc. Prof. of Med. Univ. Pittsburgh. Specialty: Urol. Socs: Roy. Soc. Med.; Brit. Assn. Urol. Surg.; Brit. Prostate Gp. Exec. Mem. Prev: Regist. Rotat. (Gen. Surg.) Guy's Hosp. Lond. & Kent & Sussex Hosp.; SHO (Surg.) Frenchay & Southmead HA; Ho. Phys. (Gen. Med. & Gastroenterol.) Northwick Pk. Hosp.

PERSAUD, Janki London Road Surgery, 64 London Road, Wickford SS12 0AH Tel: 01268 765533 Fax: 01268 570762 — MB ChB Dundee 1982.

PERSAUD, Mark Christopher Insurance Medical Services, Unit 8 Cambridge Court, 210 Shepherds Bush Road, London W6 7NL — MB BS Lond. 1990.

PERSAUD, Rajendra Dhwarka Westways, 49 St James Road, Croydon CR9 2UR Tel: 020 8700 8512 Fax: 020 8700 8504; The Maudsley Hospital, Denmark Hill, London SE5 Tel: 020 7703 6333 — MB BS Lond. 1986 (Univ. Coll. Lond.) BSc Lond 1983; DHMSA Soc. Apoth. 1988; Dip. Phil 1990; MRCPsych 1990; MPhil Lond 1991; Dip Hlth Econ 1994; MSc City 1995. Cons. Psychiat. Bethlem Roy. & Maudsley Hosps. Lond.; Research Worker Inst. Neurol. Univ. Lond.; Fell. Univ. Coll. Lond.; Resid. Doctor TV Programs; Vis. Prof. Gresham Coll.; Columnist for Hosp. Doctor. Specialty: Gen. Psychiat. Socs: Fell. Worshipful Soc. Apoth.; Fell. Roy. Soc. Med.; Aristotlean Soc. Prev: Regist. & SHO Bethlem Roy. & Maudsley Hosps.; Research Schol. John Hopkins Hosp., USA; Post Doctoral Fell. Johns Hopkins Hosp. USA (1990).

PERSAUD, Ricardo Abraham Petember 50 Waller Road, Telegraph Hill, London SE14 5LA — MB BS Lond. 1996 (Univ. Coll. Lond. Med. Sch.) MPHIL Lond. 1994; MRCS (Eng.) 2000; CBiol (EU) 2001; MIBiol (UK) 2001; DOHNS (Eng.) 2003. Lond. ENT SHO Rotat.; ENT SpR Rotat. N. Thames Lond.; S. Thames Basic Surg. Rotat.; Orthop. SHO, Joyce Green Hosp. Dartford Kent; Gen. Surg. SHO, Mayday Hosp. Mayday Rd. Surrey; Neurosurg. SHO, KCH Lond. Socs: Grad. Mem. Inst. Biol. Lond.; Middlx. Hosp. Med. Soc. Prev: Surg. Ho. Off. Whittington Hosp. Lond.; Med. Ho. Off. N. Middlx. Hosp. Lond.

PERSEY, Alexander (retired) 62 Stanton Road, Sandiacre, Nottingham NG10 5EL Tel: 0115 939 7356 — MB BS Lond. 1944; DObst 1949, (Middlx.); Mem. Coll. GP; MRCS Eng. LRCP Lond. 1944; MRCOG 1952. Prev: Surg. Lt. RNVR.

PERSEY, Dorothy Joyce (retired) 62 Stanton Road, Sandiacre, Nottingham NG10 5EL Tel: 0115 939 7356 — MB ChB Bristol 1945; DCH Eng. 1950; DObst RCOG 1952. Prev: Asst. Matern. & Child Welf. Off. & Sch. Med. Off. Derbysh. CC.

PERSHAD, Dharam Ram 19 Nelwyn Avenue, Emerson Park, Hornchurch RM11 2PY Tel: 01708 447250 — MB BS Osmania 1951; DTM & H Liverp. 1952; LMSSA Lond. 1958; MRCGP 1968. GP Rainham; Clin. Asst. Romford Chest Clinics. Prev: Med. Off. Highwood Hosp. Brentwood & Harold Wood Hosp.; Regist. (Med.) Warrington Gen. Hosp.; Clin. Asst. Brentwood & Newham Chest Clinics.

PERSHAD, Nirvisha — MB ChB Glas. 1998.

PERSOFF, David Asher 152 Harley Street, London W1G 1HH Tel: 020 8202 8877 Email: dpersoff@aol.com; dr.dap@doctors.net.uk; 5 Raleigh Close, London NW4 2SX Tel: 020 8202 6161 — (Lond. Hosp.) MSc Lond. 1959, BSc 1955, MB BS 1961; FRCP Lond. 1982, M 1969. Hon. Cons. Phys. Newham HA (Retd.). Specialty: Gen. Med.; Diabetes; Medico Legal. Socs: Fell. Roy. Soc. Med. Prev: Cons. Phys. St. And.& Newham Dist. Gen. Hosps. Lond.; Lect (Med.) Univ. Lond.; Cons. Phys. Poplar Hosp. Lond.

PERTHEN, Katharine Sarah 21 Corbison Close, Warwick CV34 5EZ — MB ChB Liverp. 1997. Whiston Hosp. Prescot, Merseyside. Specialty: Gen. Med.

PERTWEE, Richard The Heathfield Surgery, 96-98 High Street, Heathfield TN21 8JD Tel: 01435 864999 Fax: 01435 867449 — MB BS Lond. 1998. GP E. Sussex.

PERUMAINAR, Manohara 3 Paddock Rise, Beechwood, Runcorn WA7 3HL Tel: 01928 715531 — MB BS Ceylon 1972; DGM RCP Lond. 1990; LMSSA Lond. 1990.

PERUMAL, Joseph Remy Ayam (retired) Flat 5, 64 Sinclair Rd, West Kensington, London W14 0NT — MB BS Ceylon 1963 (Colombo) MRCP (UK) 1974; FRCP Lond. 1991; FACP 1998. Locum Cons. Rheumatologist, Surrey & Sussex Healthcare NHS Trust. Prev: Cons. Rheum. & Gen. Med. Scunthorpe & Goole Hosps. Trust.

PERUMALPILLAI, Mr Ravi Gnanasundaram The John Radcliffe Hospital, Headley Way, Headington, Oxford OX3 9DU — MB BS Lond. 1974 (Middlx.) FRCS Ed. 1979; FRCS Eng. 1979. Cons. Cardiothoracic Surg. John Radcliffe Hosp. Oxf. Specialty: Cardiothoracic Surg. Prev: Sen. Regist. (Cardiothoracic Surg.) Brompton Nat. Heart & Chest Hosp. Lond.; Regist. Rotat. (Surg.) Middlx. Hosp. Lond.; Regist. (Cardiothoracic Surg.) Harefield & Brompton Hosps.

PERVAIZ, Mr Khalid Queen Marys hospital, Sidcup DA16 8LT Tel: 020 8302 2678 Fax: 020 8308 3041 — MB BS Karachi 1984 (Dow Med. Coll. Karachi) FRCS Ed. 1994; FFAEM 1998. Cons.A & E Med. Qu. Marys Hosp., Sidcup. Specialty: Accid. & Emerg. Socs: Mem. Specialist Train. Comm. A & E Med.. S Thames. Prev: Sen. Regist. A+E Med. Basildon; Sen. Regist. A+E Med. Roy. Free Hosp.; Sen. Regist. A+E Med. OldCh. Hosp.

PERVAIZ KHAN, Nasir 13 Seafield Terrace, South Shields NE33 2NP; 19-N Gulberg II, Lahore, Pakistan Tel: 878967 — MB BS Sind 1964; MB BS Lond. 1974; DO RCS Eng. 1974; FRCOphth 1990, M 1989. Assoc. Eye Specialist Sunderland Eye Infirm. Prev: Sen. Regist. (Ophth.) Punjab Med. Coll. Pakistan; Asst. Prof. Ophth. King Edwd. Med. Coll. & Postgrad. Med. Inst. Lahore, Pakistan.

PERVEZ, Mujeeb Department of Paediatrics, Pilgrim Hospital, Silisey Road, Boston Tel: 01205 364801 Email: mujeeb.pervez@ulh.nhs.uk — (King Edward Medical College, Pakistan) MRCP; MRCPCH; MB BS Pakistan 1989. Cons. Paediatrician. Specialty: Paediat. Prev: Junior Doctor in Paediatrics.

PESKETT, David John Peskett, 38 Old Shoreham Road, Lancing BN15 0QT Tel: 01903 754358 — MB BS Lond. 1976; DRCOG 1978; DCH Eng. 1979; MRCGP 1980. GP Lancing. Prev: Trainee GP Chelmsford VTS; Ho. Phys. Qu. Mary's Hosp. Stratford; Ho. Surg. Lond. Hosp. (Mile End).

PESKETT, Sheila Anne 137 Priests Lane, Shenfield, Brentwood CM15 8HJ Tel: 01277 223010 Fax: 0374 595735 — (St. Mary's) MA Oxf. 1974, BA 1966, BM BCh 1969; FRCP (UK) 1990, M 1975. Cons. (Rheum. & Rehabil.) Mid Essex Health Dist. Specialty: Rehabil. Med.; Rheumatol. Socs: Brit. Assn. Rheum.; Roy. Soc. Med.; Brit. Assn. Rehabil. Med. Prev: Sen. Regist. (Rheum.) Middlx. Hosp. Lond.

PESTELL, Anne Main Street Surgery, 45 Main Street, Willerby, Hull HU10 6BY Tel: 01482 652652 — MB BS Newc. 1983.

PESTON, Samantha Aydit 48 The Reddings, London NW7 4JR — MB ChB Manch. 1997.

PESTRIDGE, Andrew David 8 Charlton House Court, Charlton Marshall, Blandford Forum DT11 9NT — BM Soton. 1993.

PETANGODA, Gamini Dogsthorpe Medical Centre, Poplar Avenue, Peterborough PE1 4QF — (Univ. of Ceylon) MB BS (Ceylon) 1972. GP Princip., P'boro. Specialty: Gen. Pract.

PETCH, Edward William Adrian West London Mental Health NHS Trust, The Three Bridges Unit, Uxbridge Road, Southall UB1 3EU Tel: 020 8354 8874 Fax: 020 8354 8877 Email: edward.petch@wlmht.nhs.uk — MB BS Lond. 1990 (Royal Free Hospital School of Medicine) MSc Lond. 1995; MRCPsych 1995; DFP 1997; Dip.Criminol. Lond. 1999. Cons. (Foren. Psychiat.) W. Lond. Ment. Health NHS Trust, Lond. Specialty: Forens. Psychiat. Prev: Sen. Regist. (Forens. Psychiat.) Maudsley Hosp. Lond.

PETCH, Michael Charles, OBE Cardiac Unit, Papworth Hospital, Cambridge CB3 8RE Tel: 01480 364351 Fax: 01223 302858; 20 Brookside, Cambridge CB2 1JQ Tel: 01223 365226 Fax: 01223 302858 — MB BChir Camb. 1965 (St. Thos.) FRCP Lond. 1980, M 1967; MA Camb. 1966, MD 1977. Cons. Cardiol. Papworth Hosp. NHS Trust; Assoc. Lect. Camb. Univ. Specialty: Cardiol. Socs: Fell. Europ. Soc. Cardiol.; Fell. Amer. Coll. Cardiol.; Brit. Cardiac Soc. Prev: Sen. Regist. (Med.) Nat. Heart Hosp. Lond.; Regist. (Med.) & Ho. Phys. St. Thos. Hosp. Lond.

PETCHEY, David Rodney (retired) 151 Ellesmere Road, Shrewsbury SY1 2RA Tel: 01743 241754 Email: david@petcheyd.fsnet.co.uk — MB ChB Manch. 1959. Prev: GP Shrewsbury.

PETER, Antonypillai Manuelpillai Willesden Medical Centre, 144-150 High Road, London NW10 2PJ Tel: 020 8459 5550 Fax: 020 8451 7268 — MB BS Sri Lanka 1973; MRCOG 1985.

PETER, Beverly Maralyn — MB BS Lond. 1974 (Westm.) MRCS Eng. LRCP Lond. 1974; DRCOG 1976; DCH Eng. 1977; MRCGP 1980. Assoc. GP Northwick Pk. Hosp. Harrow; Tutor (Gen. Pract.) UCL Sch. Med.; Mem. Harrow Area Child Protec. Comm.; Facilitator (Gen. Pract.) Imperial Coll. Sch. of Med.; Sen. Lect. Imperial Coll. Fac. of Med. Prev: Trainee GP Northwick Pk. (Harrow) VTS; Ho. Phys. Westm. Hosp. Lond.; Ho. Surg. St. Luke's Hosp. Guildford.

PETER, Judith 21 Langley Avenue, Surbiton KT6 6QN — State Exam Med. Munich 1987.

PETER, Justin Luke Timothy Millway Medical Practice, Hartley Avenue, Mill Hill, London NW7 2HX Tel: 020 8959 0888 Fax: 020 8959 7050 — MB BS Lond. 1992; BSc BioMedSci. (1st cl. Hons.) Lond. 1989.

PETER, Leonard Harold The Medical Centre, 45 Enderley Road, Harrow Weald, Harrow HA3 5HF Tel: 020 8863 3333 Fax: 020 8901 3307 Email: leonard.peter@gp-e84009.nhs.uk — MB BS Lond. 1974 (King's Coll. Hosp.) DCH Eng. 1976; DRCOG 1977; MRCGP 1978. Prev: Trainee GP Northwick Pk. Hosp. VTS; Ho. Phys. King's Coll. Hosp. Lond.; Ho. Surg. Roy. Surrey Co. Hosp. Guildford.

PETER, Michael William Littlebury Medical Centre, Fishpond Lane, Holbeach, Spalding PE12 7DE Tel: 01775 22231/22054 — MB BS Lond. 1967 (King's Coll. Hosp.) Socs: BMA. Prev: Med. Off. RAF; Ho. Phys. Gen. Med. Freedom Fields Hosp. Plymouth; Ho. Surg. (Ophth.) King's Coll. Hosp. Lond.

PETER, Thankamma 16 Chestnut Avenue, Langley, Slough SL3 7DE — MB BS Kerala 1976.

PETERKIN, Conon William Grant (retired) 44 Brechin Road, Kirriemuir DD8 4DD Tel: 01575 575232 Fax: 01575 57239 — (Ed.) MB ChB Ed. 1967; DObst RCOG 1970; MRCGP 1978. Prev: Ho. Off. Roy. Infirm. Edin.

PETERKIN, Douglas Brock, MBE (retired) — (Ed.) MB ChB Ed. 1937; MD (Commend.) Ed. 1947; MRCGP 1962. Prev: Ho. Phys. Profess. Unit West. Gen. Hosp. Edin.

PETERKIN, Gordon Stuart David Grampian Primary Care NHS Trust, Summerfield House, Eday Road, Aberdeen AB15 6RE Tel: 01224 558578 Email: gordon.peterkin@gpct.grampian.scot.nhs.uk; Thistle Croft, Carseburm, Forfar DD8 3NJ Tel: 01307 463556 — MB ChB Glas. 1971; MRCP (U.K.) 1974; MRCGP 1977; FRCGP 1997; FRCP 2000. Med. Director Graupiam Primary Care Trust; Hon.Sen.Lect. dept of GP,Univ. of Aberd. Socs: Scott. Assoc of Community Hosps,Comm. Mem. (Past Secy).

PETERS, Professor Adrien Michael Addenbrooke's Hospital, Department of Nuclear Medicine, Hills Road, Cambridge CB2 2QQ Tel: 01223 217147 Fax: 01223 586671 Email: michael.peters@addenbrookes.nhs.uk; 32 Station Road, Waterbeach, Cambridge CB5 9HT — MB ChB Liverp. 1970; MD Liverp. 1974; FRCPath 1996, M 1984; BSc (Physiol.) Lond. 1967, MSc (Nuclear Med.) 1987; MRCP (UK) 1993; FRCR 1995; FRCP 1997; FMedSci 2002; MA Cantabury 2002. Nuclear Med., Camb. Univ. Specialty: Nuclear Med. Socs: Hon. Mem. Brit. Inst. Radiol.; Brit. Nuclear Med. Soc.; Soc. Nuclear Med. Prev: Prof. Diagn. Radiol. Hammersmith Hosp. Lond.; Prof.(Diagn. Radiol.) Imperial Coll. Med. Sch.

PETERS, Alexander John (retired) 7 New Edinburgh Road, Uddingston, Glasgow G71 6BT Tel: 01698 813662 — MB ChB

Glas. 1956; DPH Glas. 1965. Sen. Med. Off. Sch. Health Serv. Gtr. Glas. HB.

PETERS, Anthony Russell (retired) William Budd Health Centre, Leinster Avenue, Bristol BS4 1NL Tel: 0117 963 6201; 5 The Orchard, Upper Stanton Drew, Bristol BS39 4DS Tel: 01275 332741 Fax: 01275 332741 Email: russ.peters@ukgateway.net — MB ChB Bristol 1965.

PETERS, Antoinette Jeyarahini 9 Burdett Avenue, London SW20 0ST Tel: 020 8241 8715 — MB BS Ceylon 1966; DPM Eng. 1978. Staff (Psychiat.) W. Pk. Hosp. Adult Psychiat. Springfield Hosp. Old Age Psychiat. Specialty: Gen. Psychiat.

PETERS, Barry Stephen Harrison Wing, St. Thomas' Hospital, Lambeth Palace Road, London SE1 7EH Tel: 020 7928 9292 Fax: 020 7922 8291 Email: barry.peters@gstt.sthames.nhs.uk — MD Lond. 1994 (St. Bartholomew's) MB BS 1979; MRCP (UK) 1985; FRCP Lond. 1998. Sen. Lect & Hon. Cons. (Genitourin. Med. & HIV) GKT Med. Sch. Specialty: Genitourinary Medicine; HIV Med. Socs: Med. Soc. Study VD; Assn. Genitourin. Med.; Exec. Mem. Brit. HIV Assn. Prev: Lect. (Genitourin. Med. & Communicable Dis.) St Mary's Hosp. Lond.

PETERS, Catherine Jane 39 Willifield Way, London NW11 7XU — MB BS Lond. 1994.

PETERS, Catherine Jane 37 Blake Hill Crescent, Lilliput, Poole BH14 8QP — MB ChB Birm. 1995; ChB Birm. 1995.

PETERS, Charles Douglas, VRD 34 Combe Road, Combe Down, Bath BA2 5HY Tel: 01225 833605 Email: cdpeters@ukhome.net — (Char. Cross) MB BS Lond. 1949; MRCS Eng. LRCP Lond. 1949; DObst RCOG 1954. Specialty: Gen. Pract. Prev: Hon. Phys. to HM the Qu.; Surg. Capt. RNR; Asst. Cas. Off. & Ho. Phys. Char Cross Hosp. Lond.

PETERS, Colin 18 Wemyss Drive, Blackwood, Cumbernauld, Glasgow G68 9NP — MB ChB Glas. 1998; MB ChB Glas 1998.

PETERS, Colin George Anaesthetic Department, New Cross Hospital, Wolverhampton WV10 0QP Tel: 01902 307999 — MB ChB Manch. 1973; FFA RCS Eng. 1977. Cons. Anaesth. Wolverhampton AHA; Dir. Wolverhampton Pain Relief Clinic. Specialty: Anaesth. Socs: Assn. Anaesth.; The Pain Soc. Prev: Sen. Regist. (Anaesth.) Sheff. Higher Prof. Train. Scheme; Regist. (Anaesth.) Bristol Gen. Profess. Train. Scheme; SHO (Anaesth.) Salford AHA.

PETERS, David Marylebone Health Centre, 17 Marylebone Road, London NW1 5LT — MB ChB Manch. 1971 (Manchester) Sen. Lect. (Community Care Primary Health) Univ. of Westminster; Dir. Complementary Ther. Unit Marylebone Health Centre. Specialty: Homeop. Med.; Gen. Pract. Socs: Fac. Homoeop.; Brit. Holistic Med. Assn. Prev: Sen. Research Fell St Mary's Waites Project; Lect. (Gen. Pract.) St Mary's.

PETERS, David John, RD Avisford Medical Group, North End Road, Yapton, Arundel BN18 0DU Tel: 01243 551321 Fax: 01243 555101 — MB BChir Camb. 1968 (Camb. & Guy's) MA, BChir 1967; MRCS Eng. LRCP Lond. 1967; DObst RCOG 1971. Med. Off. Ford Prison. Socs: Anglo-German Med. Soc. Prev: SHO (Cas.) St. Richard's Hosp. Chichester; Ho. Surg. (Thoracic Med.) Guy's Hosp.; Ho. Phys. Addenbrooke's Hosp. Camb.

PETERS, Professor Sir David Keith University of Cambridge School of Clinical Medicine, Addenbrooke's Hospital, Hills Road, Cambridge CB2 2SP Tel: 01223 336738 Fax: 01223 336721 — MB BCh Wales 1961; MRCP (UK) 1964; FRCP Lond. 1975; FRCPath 1991; FRCP Ed. 1995; FRS 1995. Regius Prof. of Physic Univ. Camb.; Hon. Cons. Phys. Addenbrooke's Hosp. Camb. Specialty: Gen. Med. Prev: Prof. Med. Roy. Postgrad. Med. Sch. Hammersmith Hosp. Lond.; Reader (Med.) Roy. Postgrad. Med. Sch. Lond.; Lect. (Med.) & Hon. Cons. Phys. Roy. Postgrad. Med. Sch. Hammersmith Hosp. Lond.

PETERS, Diogu Arulanandam (retired) 9 Burdett Avenue, London SW20 0ST Tel: 020 8241 8715 — MB BS Ceylon 1954; DPM Eng. 1966; MRCPsych 1972. Prev: Cons. Psychiat. Health Serv. Sri Lanka.

PETERS, Edward John The Surgery, 148 Forton Road, Gosport PO12 3HH Tel: 023 9258 3333 Fax: 023 9260 1107 — MB BS Lond. 1977; MRCS Eng. LRCP Lond. 1977; DRCOG 1981; MRCGP 1987. GP Gosport.

PETERS, Elizabeth Eileen (retired) 67 Tor Bryan, Ingatestone CM4 9HN Tel: 01277 353998 Fax: 01277 355497 — MB ChB Glas. 1960; FRCPath 1991, M 1979. Prev: Cons. Histopath. & Cytol. Basildon & Southend Hosps.

PETERS, Eric (retired) Leacroft, 19 St John's Road, Stafford ST17 9AS Tel: 01785 223516 Fax: 01785 223516 — (Birm.) MB ChB Birm. 1955. Prev: GP Stafford.

PETERS, Esmeralda Margery 60 Audley Road, London NW4 3HB — MB BS Lond. 1993; DRCOG; DFFP.

PETERS, Francesca Hedda — MB ChB Liverp. 1997.

PETERS, Gerald 65 Thames Drive, Leigh-on-Sea SS9 2XQ — MB BS Lond. 1971 (Guy's) MRCS Eng. LRCP Lond. 1971; DObst RCOG 1973. Prev: SHO (Path.) & Ho. Surg. Greenwich Dist. Hosp.; Ho. Surg. (O & G) Glos. Roy. Hosp.

PETERS, Graeme Kearley Clare House Practice, Clare House Surgery, Newport Street, Tiverton EX16 6NJ Tel: 01884 252337 Fax: 01884 254401; The Old Vicarage, Cove, Tiverton EX16 7RX Tel: 01398 331859 Email: graeme.peters@btinternet.com — MB ChB Bristol 1977; MRCP (UK) 1981; MRCGP 1988; DRCOG 1988. Princip. in Gen. Pract. Clare Ho. Tiverton; Hosp. Practitioner Gen. Med. Tiverton & Dist. Hosp.; Med. Off. Blundell's Sch. Tiverton; Endoscopist Tiverton & Distmct Hosp. Socs: Roy. Coll. Phys.; Med. Off.s Sch.s Assn.; Devon & Exeter Med. Soc.

PETERS, Helen 107 Egerton Street, Wallasey CH45 2LS — MB ChB Birm. 1992.

PETERS, Henry Gordon The Medical Centre, Bulford, Wellington TA21 8PW Tel: 01823 663551 Fax: 01823 660650; Burts House, Wellington TA21 9PG Tel: 01823 662820 — MB BS Lond. 1960 (Univ. Coll. Hosp.) BSc (Anat.) Lond. 1956; MRCS Eng. LRCP Lond. 1960; MRCGP 1978. Specialty: Gen. Pract.

PETERS, Janet Anne 67 Falcon Court, Edinburgh EH10 4AG Tel: 0131 447 6531 — MB ChB Ed. 1959; DObst RCOG 1962; DCH Eng. 1962; MFCM 1974. SCMO S. W. Edin. Lothian Health Bd. Prev: SCMO Forth Valley Health Bd.

PETERS, Jean Mair 22 Mustow Place, London SW6 4EL — (Welsh Nat. Sch. Med.) MB BCh Wales 1961; MRCS Eng. LRCP Lond. 1962; DO Eng. 1975; MCOphth 1990. Med. Pract. (Ophth.) Surrey; Med. Pract. (Ophth.) Surrey. Specialty: Ophth. Socs: Med. Contact Lens & Ocular Surface Assn. Prev: Assoc. Specialist (Ophth.) West. Eye Hosp. & St. Mary's Hosp. Lond.; Assoc. Specialist Char. Cross Hosp. Lond.; Clin. Asst. Cardiff Roy. Infirm. & Birm. & Midl. Eye Hosp.

PETERS, Joanne West Street Surgery, 89 West Street, Dunstable LU6 1SF Tel: 01582 664401 Fax: 01582 475766 — MB BS Newc. 1981; DRCOG 1984; MRCGP 1985; DFFP 1993.

PETERS, John Gerard 31 Acres Lane, Stalybridge SK15 2JR — MB BCh BAO NUI 1987; LRCPSI 1987.

PETERS, Mr John Leslie Department of Urology, Whipps Cross Hospital, Whipps Cross Road, London E11 1NR Tel: 0208 535 6725 — MB BS Lond. 1991 (Charing Cross & Westminster Medical School) BSc Lond. 1988; FRCS Eng. 1995; FRCS (Urol.) 2001. Consultant Urologist, Whipps Cross University Hospital; Specialist Regist. Inst. of Urol., Middlx. Hosp., Lond. Specialty: Urol. Socs: RSM; EAU; BAUS. Prev: Regist. (Urol. & Gen. Surg.) W. Middlx. Univ. Hosp. Lond.

PETERS, John Redmond Department of Medicine, University Hospital of Wales, Heath Park, Cardiff CF14 4XW Tel: 029 2074 2344 Fax: 029 2074 4581; 24 Ty Draw Road, Roath Park, Cardiff CF23 5HB Tel: 029 2049 6410 — MB BCh Wales 1972; BSc (1st cl. Hons.) Wales 1969, MD 1980, MB BCh 1972; MRCP (UK) 1974; FRCP Lond. 1989. Cons. Phys. Univ. Hosp. Wales Cardiff. Specialty: Gen. Med. Prev: Lect. (Med.) Welsh Nat. Sch. Med. Card.; Wellcome Research Fell. & Hon. Sen. Regist. MRC Unit Dept. Clin. Pharmacol. Radcliffe Infirm. Oxf.

PETERS, Jonathan Tadley Medical Partnership, Holmwood Health Centre, Franklin Avenue, Tadley RG26 4ER Tel: 0118 981 6661; Hedgerows, 1B Church Road, Tadley, Basingstoke RG26 3AU — BM Soton. 1983; MRCGP 1987; DRCOG 1987; AFOM 2001. Gen. Practitioner; Occupational hys.

PETERS, Mr Joseph Lennox Highfield, Little Widbury Lane, Ware SG12 7AU Tel: 01920 466349 Fax: 01920 486783 Email: josephpeters@btinternet.com — MB BS Lond. 1969 (Univ. Coll. Hosp.) BSc (Hons. Physiol.) Lond. 1967; FRCS Eng. 1975. p/t Cons. Surg., The Princess Alexandra Hosp., Harlow, Essex. Specialty: Gen. Surg. Special Interest: Design, innovation and Developm. of safer Clin. devices and infusion systems. Socs: Fell. Roy. Soc. Med.; Fell.

Assn. of Surg.s; Fell. Assn. of Colo-Proctol. of Gt. Britain and Irel. Prev: Resid. Asst. Surg. Univ. Coll. Hosp. Lond.; Sen. Surg. Regist. Middx. Hosp. Lond.; Resid. Surg. Off. Brompton Hosp. Lond.

PETERS, Julia Jane Courtyard Surgery, London Road, Horsham RH12 1AT Tel: 01403 253100 Fax: 01403 267480 — MB BS Lond. 1974.

PETERS, Lesley Anne Drugs North W., Mental Health Services of Salford, Bury New Road, Prestwich, Manchester M25 3BL Tel: 0161 772 3694 Fax: 0161 772 3595 — MB ChB Ed. 1989 (Edinburgh) Clin. Res. Fell. Specialty: Alcohol & Substance Misuse.

PETERS, Margaret Wallace (retired) Leacroft, 19 St Johns Road, Rowley Park, Stafford ST17 9AS Tel: 01785 223516 — MB ChB Birm. 1955; DA Eng. 1966. Prev: Benefits Agency Med. Servs.

PETERS, Mark John 55 Battlefield Road, St Albans AL1 4DB — MB ChB Bristol 1989.

PETERS, Martin Godfrey (retired) Basildon & Thurrock Occupational Health Service, Basildon Hospital, Nethermayne, Basildon SS16 5NL Tel: 01268 280585 Fax: 01268 534127; 16 The Belvedere, Burnham-on-Crouch CM0 8AW Tel: 01621 783175 Fax: 01621 783175 — MB BS Lond. 1959 (St. Geo.) MRCS Eng. LRCP Lond. 1959; DObst RCOG 1960; FFOM RCP Lond. 1995. Dir. Basildon & Thurrock Dept. Occupat. Health & Safety; JP.; Med. Off. Various Ltd. Companies; Occupat. Health Adviser MGP Consults. Ltd. Lond.; Hon. Lect. (Occupat. Health) Barking Coll. Technol. Prev: Employm. Med. Adviser EMAS.

PETERS, Martin John 204 Yoxall Road, Shirley, Solihull B90 3RN — MB BS West Indies 1987; MRCP (UK) 1994.

PETERS, Michael David 111 Adelaide Road, London NW3 — MB BS Lond. 1974.

PETERS, Nicholas John Monrad 69 Bury Road, Gosport PO12 3PR Tel: 02392 580363; 70 Newtown Road, Warsash, Southampton SO31 9GB Tel: 01489 573360 — BM Soton. 1978; DFFP 1995. GP. Prev: Trainee GP Is. of Thanet VTS; SHO Rotat. (Surg.) Yeovil Dist. Hosp.; Ho. Surg. & Ho. Phys. Soton. Gen. Hosp.

PETERS, Nicholas Simon St Marys hospital, Praed St, London W2 1NY Tel: 020 7886 2468 Fax: 020 7886 1763 Email: n.peters@ic.ac.uk — MD Lond. 1994; MB BS 1984; MRCP (UK) 1987; FRCP FRCP 1999 1999. Prof. of Cardiol. St Marys Hosp. Lond.; Adj Prof. of Pharmacol., Columbia Univ., New York USA. Specialty: Cardiol.

PETERS, Norman (retired) — MB BS Lond. 1958 (St. Geo.) MRCS Eng. LRCP Lond. 1958; FRCP Lond. 1977, M 1963. Cons. Phys. Chase Farm Hosp. Enfield. Prev: Sen. Regist. (Med.) & Ho. Phys. St. Geo. Hosp. Lond.

PETERS, Roderick Michael 55 Clancarty Road, Fulham, London SW6 3AH Tel: 020 7736 7256 Fax: 020 7736 7256; Weavers, Ewhurst Green, Cranleigh GU6 7RR Tel: 01483 278481 Fax: 020 7736 7256 — (St. Geo.) MB BS Lond. 1966; MRCS Eng. LRCP Lond. 1966; MRCP (UK) 1970; MSc (Occupat. Med.) Lond. 1978. Specialty: Psychother. Prev: Specialist Phys. Brunei Shell Petroleum Ltd., Brunei.

PETERS, Samuel Boyd Ian Charles Cottage Hospital, The Health Centre, Castle Road East, Grantown-on-Spey PH26 3HR Tel: 01479 872484 Fax: 01479 873503; Clachnastrone, Old Spey Bridge, Grantown-on-Spey PH26 3NQ Tel: 01479 873700 — MB BCh BAO Belf. 1988; MRCGP 1992. Specialty: Gen. Pract.

PETERS, Seija Erica Basement Flat, 44 Queens Park, Royal Crescent, Glasgow G44 8DD Tel: 0141 423 0985 Mob: 079005 03840 — MB ChB Glas. 1993.

PETERS, Sharon Elizabeth Hobs Moat Medical Centre, Ulleries Road, Solihull B92 8ED Tel: 0121 742 5517 Fax: 0121 743 4217; 5 Naseby Road, Solihull B91 2DR Tel: 0121 705 6843 — BM Soton 1984; DCH RCP Lond. 1986; DRCOG 1987; MRCGP 1988. Prev: Asst. GP Birm. Doctors Retainer Scheme; Trainee GP Wythall; SHO (O & G) Selly Oak Hosp. Birm.

PETERS, Sheila Anne St Mary's Hospital, Milton Rd, Portsmouth PO3 6AD Tel: 02392 866102 Fax: 02392 866101 — BM Soton. 1983; MRCP (UK) 1988; FRCPCH (UK) 1999. Cons. Paediat. St. Mary's Hosp. Portsmouth. Specialty: Paediat. Prev: Sen. Regist. St. Mary's Hosp. Portsmouth.

PETERS, Stephen Academic Department of Psychiatry, Northern General Hospital, Herries Road, Sheffield S5 7AU Tel: 0114 226 1517; Oakwood, Lincoln Road, East Markham, Newark NG22 0SW — MB BS Lond. 1988; MRCPsych 1993. Sen. Lect. (Psychiat.) Sheff. Univ.; Hon. Cons. Psychiat. Bassetlaw Hosp. Notts. Specialty: Gen. Psychiat.

PETERS, Professor Timothy John Department of Clinical Biochemistry, Kings College School of Medicine, Bessemer Road, London SE5 9PJ Tel: 020 7346 3008 Fax: 020 7737 7434 — MB ChB (Hons) St. And. 1964 (Univ. of St Andrews, Scotl.) MSc St. And. 1967; FRCP Ed. 1981, M 1967; FRCP Lond. 1976, M 1968; PhD. Lond. 1971; FRCPath 1984, M 1980; DSc St. And. 1986. Prof. Clin. Biochem. King's Coll. Lond. - Assoc. Dean for Flexible Train. Lond. And Kent, Surrey and Sussex Deaneries; Cons. Chem. Path. & Phys. KCH Lond. Specialty: Chem. Path. Socs: Counc. Mem. & Trustee Sir Richard Stapley Educat. Trust; Chairm. and Trustee, Area Concern; Assn. Phys. Med. Research Soc. Prev: Sen. Lect. & Reader Roy. Postgrad. Med. Sch. Lond.; MRC Trav. Research Fell. The Rockefeller Univ. New York City, USA; Head Div. Clin. Cell. Biol. MRC Clin. Research Centre Harrow.

PETERS, Timothy Malcolm West Middlesex University Hospital NHS Trust, Twickenham Road, Isleworth TW7 6AF Tel: 020 8565 5826; 85 Hamlet Gardens, London W6 0SX Tel: 020 8741 2447 Email: tim.peters@btinternet.com — MB BS Lond. 1985 (Westminster) MA Camb. 1982; DA (UK) 1988; DCH RCP Lond. 1989; MRCGP 1990; FRCA 1994. Cons. (Anaesth. & ITU) W. Middlx. Hosp. Lond. Specialty: Anaesth.; Intens. Care. Socs: Assn. Anaesth.s; Eur. Soc. Regional Anaesth.; Intens. Care Soc. Prev: Sen. Regist. Rotat. (Anaesth.) Roy. Free Hosp. Lond.; Regist. (Anaesth.) Walsgrave Hosp. Coventry; Med. Off. Roy. Flying Doctor Serv. Broken Hill, Austral.

PETERS, Professor Wallace Northwick Park Institute for Medical Research, Centre for Tropical Antiprotozoal Chemotherapy, Y Block, Watford Road, Harrow HA1 3UJ Tel: 0208 869 3292 Fax: 0208 422 7136 Email: w.peters@ic.ac.uk — (St. Bart.) MB BS (Hons.) Lond. 1947; MRCS Eng. LRCP Lond. 1948; DTM & H Eng. 1950; MD 1966; M 1973; DSc Lond. 1976; FRCP Lond. 1978. p/t Dir. Centre Trop. Antiprot. Chemo; Hon. Prof. Res. Fellow, Imperial Coll. 2000; Emerit. Prof. Med. Protozool. Univ. Lond. 1989 & Prof. 1979. Specialty: Trop. Med. Special Interest: Med. parasitology. Socs: Fell.. Roy. Soc. Med.; Fell. (Ex-Pres.) Roy. Soc. Trop. Med. Hyg.; BMA. Prev: Walter Myers Prof. Parasitol. Univ. Liverp.; Dean Liverp. Sch. Trop. Med.; Sen. Malariol. Territory of Papua & New Guinea.

PETERS, William Martin Department of Pathology, District General Hospital, Scartho Road, Grimsby DN33 2BA Tel: 01472 874111 Fax: 01472 875333 Email: martin.peters@nlg.nhs.uk — MB ChB Sheff. 1977 (Sheffield) MRC Pathology 1985; FRCPath 1995. Cons. Histopath. Grimsby Dist. Gen. Hosp. Specialty: Histopath. Prev: Sen. Regist. (Histopath.) Yorks. RHA.

PETERSEN, Lorraine Anne 3 Alowick Drive, Maidenhead SL6 4JQ — BM BCh Oxf. 1996.

PETERSEN, Mark Erik Victor c/o Ward 13 Cardiology Office, Gloucester Royal Hospital, Great Western Road, Gloucester GL1 3NN Tel: 01452 528555; The Manor, Aston-on-Carrant, Tewkesbury GL20 8HL — MB BS Lond. 1984; MB BS (Hons.) Lond. 1984; MRCP (UK) 1987. Cons. Phys. (Cardiol.) Glouc. Roy. NHS Trust. Specialty: Cardiol.

PETERSON, Angus Cameron (retired) Dunham Cottage, 3 Blidworth Lodge, Rigg Lane, Mansfield NG21 0NX Tel: 01623 797145 — MB ChB Manch. 1958; DA Eng. 1962; FFA RCS Eng. 1965. Prev: Cons. Anaesth. N. (Manch.) Health Dist.

PETERSON, David Bernard Luton & Dunstable Hospital NHS Trust, Lewsey Road, Luton LU4 0DZ Tel: 01582 491122 — MB BChir Camb. 1975 (Middlx.) MRCP (UK) 1978; MA Camb. 1976, MD 1990; FRCP 1998. Cons. Phys. (Gen. Med. & Diabetes) Luton & Dunstable Hosp.; Clin. Director of Med. Specialty: Diabetes. Prev: Sen. Regist. Rotat. (Gen. Med.) St. Geo. Hosp. Lond.; MRC Train. Fell. & Hon. Sen. Regist. Oxf. HA; Regist. (Med.) Centr. Middlx. Hosp. Lond.

PETERSON, Mr David Charles Department of Neurosurgery, Charing Cross Hospital, Fulham Palace Road, London W8 8RF Tel: 020 8846 1186 Fax: 020 8383 0321 Email: dpeterson@hhnt.org — MB BS Lond. 1985; BSc Lond. 1982; FRCS Eng. 1989; FRCS (SN) 1994. Cons. Neurosurg. Char. Cross Hosp. & Chelsea & Westm. Hosp.; Hon. Sen. Lect., Imperial Colllege Sch. of Med., Lond.; Hon. Cons. Neurosurg., Chelsea and Westm. Hosp. Lond. Specialty: Neurosurg.

PETERSON, David John Maxwell Eynsham Medical Group, Eynsham Medical Centre, Conduit Lane, Witney OX29 4QB Tel: 01865 881206 Fax: 01865 881342; The Shrubbery, 26 High St, Eynsham, Witney OX29 4HB — (Roy. Free) MB BS Lond. 1969; MRCS Eng. LRCP Lond. 1969; MRCGP 1986. Med. Off. Boggles Racing Club. Prev: Sen. Resid. Med. Off. Roy. Free Hosp. Lond.; Resid. Amer. Hosp. Paris, France.

PETERSON, Mark Maple House, 7 College Avenue, Leicester LE2 0JF; 23 Whitewell Drive, Upton, Wirral CH49 4PE — MB ChB Leic. 1991.

PETERSON, Sarah Elizabeth — MB BS Newc. 1998.

PETERSON, Mr Stephen 25 Ridgway Road, Kettering NN15 5AQ — MB ChB Liverp. 1981; FRCS Ed. 1985; FRCR 1992. Sen. Regist. (Radiol.) N. Staffs. Hosp. & Roy. Shrewsbury Hosp. Specialty: Radiol.

PETHEN, Samantha 11 Poolmans Road, Windsor SL4 4PB — BM Soton. 1996.

PETHER, John Victor Sebastian (retired) The Old School, Church Lane, Kingston St Mary, Taunton TA2 8HR Tel: 01823 451311 — BM BCh Oxf. 1959; MA Oxf. 1959; DTM & H Eng. 1963; Dip. Bact. Lond 1966; FRCPath 1979, M 1967. Prev: Dir. Pub. Health Laborat. Taunton.

PETHERAM, Christine Dorothy Five Lanes Farmhouse, Rhiwderin, Newport NP1 9RQ — MB BCh Wales 1970.

PETHERBRIDGE, Sean Paul 26 Cliff Road, Welton, Lincoln LN2 3JJ Tel: 0410 407902 — MB BS Lond. 1997 (St George's Hosp. Med. Sch.) Psychiat. SHO, Coventry. Specialty: Gen. Psychiat. Socs: BMA; MDU. Prev: A & E SHO, Kings Lynn.

PETHERICK, Colin Samuel 13 Beverley Close, Newtownards BT23 7FN — MB BCh BAO Belf. 1994; BDS Belf. 1983.

PETILLON, Claudia Maria 4 Station Street, Kibworth Beauchamp, Leicester LE8 0LN — BM BS Nottm. 1997.

PETIT, Christopher Gerard Curzon The Mill House, Buxted, Uckfield TN22 4DP Tel: 01826 733620 — MB BCh BAO Dub. 1955 (T.C. Dub.) LM Rotunda 1956.

PETKOVA, Dimitrina Kostova — State Exam Med Higher Med. Inst. Varna 1985. Cons. Phys. (Respirat. Med.) Good Hope Hosp. Sutton Coldfield. Specialty: Gen. Med.; Respirat. Med. Special Interest: Interstitial Lung Diseases; Lung Cancer.

PETO, Professor Timothy Edward Alexander Nuffield Department Medicine, John Radcliffe Hospital, Headington, Oxford OX3 9DU Tel: 01865 220154 Fax: 01865 222962 Email: tim.peto@ndm.ox.ac.uk — BM BCh Oxf. 1977 (Oxford) DPhil Oxf. 1974, MA, BM BCh 1977; MRCP (UK) 1978; FRCP Lond. 1992; FRCPath 2000. Cons. Phys. Infec. Dis. Nuffield Dept. Med. John Radcliffe Hosp. Oxf.; Prof. (Med.); Sec. MRC AIDS Therap. Trials Comm.; Chairm., interDept.al Acad. unit of Infec. Dis.s and microBiol. Specialty: Infec. Dis.; Gen. Med.; HIV Med. Socs: Brit. Infec. Soc.; Fell. Roy. Soc. Trop. Med.; Ass. Of Phys.s. Prev: Clin. Lect. Nuffield Dept. Med. John Radcliffe Hosp. Oxf.; MRC Train. Fell. & Wellcome Fell. Nuffield Dept. Med. Oxf.; SHO (Med.) Hammersmith Hosp. Lond.

***PETO, Ms Tunde** Moorfields Eye Hospital, 162 City Road, London EC1V 2PD Email: tunde.peto@moorfields.nhs.uk — MD Szeged 1990 (Albert Srent-Gyorgyi Med. Sch.) PhD NSW, Australia; Master of Heart Educat. (Hungary) 1991. Fell. Moorfields Eye Hosp. Lond.

PETRI, Gianfranco John James Paget Hospital, Lowestoft Road, Gorleston, Great Yarmouth NR31 6LA Tel: 01493 452699 Fax: 01493 452066 Email: john.petri@jpaget.nhs.uk — State Exam Naples 1981; Specialist (Orthop.) Univ. Naples 1987; D.U. Hand & Upper Limb Surg Paris 1994. Cons. Orthop. Surg. James Paget Healthcare NHS Trust; Clin. Dir. Specialty: Orthop. Socs: Fell. BOA; A. O. Alumni; BMA. Prev: Cons. Orthop. Surg. Centre Hosp.ier de Macon, France.

PETRI, Michael Philip 28 Burlington Road, Swanage BH19 1LT Tel: 01929 425464 — MB BS Lond. 1977 (Char. Cross) MRCS Eng. LRCP Lond. 1977; MRCP (UK) 1980; FRCP Ed. 1993. Specialty: Gen. Med. Prev: Cons. Phys. Poole Gen. Hosp.; Sen. Regist. (Gen. Med. & Geriat. Med.) Bath; Regist. (Cardiol. & Med.) Birm. Gen. Hosp.

PETRICCIONE DI VADI, Pierluigi University Hospital Lewisham, Lewisham High St., London SE13 6LH Tel: 020 8690 9127 Fax: 020 8333 3248 — State Exam Naples 1978; Post Graduate Degree Endocrinology Naples 1981; Post Graduate training in Anaesthetic and Intensive Care Naples 1991. Cons. in Pain Managem. Unit Lewisham Hosp., Lond.; Hon. Cons., Dept. of Anaesth., Guy's & St Thos. Hosp. Trust, Lond. Specialty: Palliat. Med. Socs: Europ. Acad. Anaesth.; Internat. Soc. Study Pain; Assn. Palliat. Med. Prev: Med. Advisor Europ. Research & Developm. Procter & Gamble Pharmaceut.; Locum Cons. Pain Relief Unit Guy's Hosp. Lond.; Regist. (Anaesth. & Intens. Care) A. Cardarelli Hosp. Naples, Italy.

PETRIDES, Simon Peter Blackberry Orthopaedic Clinic, Blackberry Court, Walnut Tree, Milton Keynes MK7 7PB Tel: 01908 604666 Fax: 01908 692711 Email: info@boc.powernet.co.uk — MB BS Lond. 1985; Dip. Osteop 1988; Dip. Sports Med. Soc. Apoth Lond. 1991. Dir. Milton Keynes Sports Injury Clinic & Blackberry Orthop. Clinic. Specialty: Sports Med. Socs: Coun.lor Brit. Inst. Musculoskeletal Med.; Brit. Assn. Sport & Med.; Gen. Counc. & Register Osteop. Prev: Treas. Soc. Orthop. Med.; Med. Off. Everest Marathon.

PETRIE, Alan James 11 South Street, Greenock PA16 8TZ — MB ChB Glas. 1994.

PETRIE, Alison Margaret North Berwick Health Centre, 54 St Baldreds Road, North Berwick EH49 4PU — BM BS Nottm. 1989; DCH RCP Lond. 1991; MRCGP 1994.

PETRIE, Allyson Marie 11 South Street, Greenock PA16 8TZ — MB ChB Glas. 1992. Specialty: Paediat.; Neonat.

PETRIE, Colin James Sauchur Garden Cottage, Wadeslea, Elie, Leven KY9 1EA — MB ChB Aberd. 1997.

PETRIE, Gavin Ross Chest Unit, Ward 16, Victoria Hospital, Mayfield Road, Kirkcaldy KY2 5AH Tel: 01592 643355 Fax: 01592 648047; Mol Hall, Dewars Mill, St Andrews KY16 9TY — MB ChB Aberd. 1971; MRCGP UK 1974; FRCP Ed. 1985; FRCP 1991. Cons. Chest. Phys. Vict. Hosp. Kirkcaldy Fife. Specialty: Gen. Med. Socs: BTS; ATS; ERS. Prev: Research Fell. in Med. Aberd. Univ.; Regist. (Respirat. Dis.) S. Lothian Health Dist.; Sen. Regist. Glas. Roy. Infirm.

PETRIE, Gillian Alison Flat 2nd Left, 13 Naseby Avenue, Broomhill, Glasgow G11 7JQ — MB ChB Glas. 1996.

PETRIE, Graham Maxwell (retired) College Farmhouse, 2 Balsham Road, Fulbourn, Cambridge CB1 5BZ Tel: 01223 881429 — MB BChir Camb. 1956 (Camb. & St. Mary's) MRCS Eng. LRCP Lond. 1955; DObst RCOG 1959; DPM Eng. 1970; FRCPsych 1983, M 1972. Prev: Cons. Psychiat. Addenbrooke's Hosp. Camb.

PETRIE, Henry Peterson Surrey Lodge Practice, 11 Anson Road, Victoria Park, Manchester M14 5BY Tel: 0161 224 2471 Fax: 0161 257 2264 — MB ChB Leic. 1984; DRCOG 1987.

PETRIE, John Ross University Department of Medicine & Therapeutics, Gardiner Institute, Western Infirmary, Glasgow G11 6NT Tel: 0141 211 2000 Fax: 0141 339 2800 Email: jrpls@clinmed.gla.ac.uk; 24 Station Road, Bearsden, Glasgow G61 4AL Tel: 0141 942 9523 — MB ChB Ed. 1989; BSc (Ed) 1987; MRCP (UK) 1992; PhD (Glasgow) 1997. Lect. (Diabetes & Endocrinol.) & Hon. Specialist Regist. Univ. Glas. Specialty: Endocrinol.; Diabetes. Socs: Chairm. Brit. Hypertens. Research Gp. Prev: Clin. Research Fell. (Med. & Therap.) Univ. Glas.; Brit. Heart Foundat. Jun. Research Fell.

PETRIE, Kathryn (retired) College Farmhouse, Balsham Road, Fulbourn, Cambridge CB1 5BZ Tel: 01223 881429 — (St. Mary's) MB BS Lond. 1955. Prev: Clin. Asst. (Ophth.) Addenbrooke's Hosp. Camb.

PETRIE, Margaret Xanthe Patricia (retired) 126 Desswood Place, Aberdeen AB15 4DQ Tel: 01224 640537 — FRCP Edin.; MB ChB Aberd. 1964. Prev: Regist. Gastroenterol. Research Project Foresterhill & Assoc. Hosps. Gp.

PETRIE, Mark Colquhoun 126 Desswood Place, Aberdeen AB15 4DQ — MB ChB Ed. 1993.

PETRIE, Nicola Clare First Floor Flat, 3 Vyvyan Terrace, Clifton, Bristol BS8 3DF Tel: 0117 974 1403 — MB ChB Bristol 1997. Ho. Off. (Gen. Med.) Southmead Hosp. Bristol. Specialty: Gen. Med. Prev: Ho. Off. (Gen. Surg.) Torbay Hosp. Torquay.

PETRIE, Paula Jane Bolton Hospitals, Mineria Road, Farnworth, Bolton BL4 0JR Tel: 01204 390390; 14 Copperfields, Chew Moor, Lostock, Bolton BL6 4HZ — MB ChB Ed. 1993 (Edinburgh) MRCP Ed 1996. Staff Grade Stroke, Bolton Hosps., Bolton. Specialty: Gen. Med. Prev: Lect. Geriat.s, Hope, Manch.; Specialist Regist. Geriat. Hope, Manch.

PETRIE, Rachel Xanthe Ann Department of Psychiatry, University of Dundee, Ninewells Hospital, Dundee DD1 9SY Tel: 01382

660111 Ext: 33111 Fax: 01382 633923; Northwest Cottages, Middlebank Farm, Westown, Perth PH2 7SX Tel: 01828 686769 — MB ChB Ed. 1991 (Edinburgh Univ.) BSc (Hons.) Psychol. Ed. 1989; MRCPsych 1996. Sim Research Fell. (Psychiat.) Univ. Dundee. Specialty: Gen. Psychiat. Prev: Regist. Tayside Psychiat. Train. Scheme.

PETRIE, Robert Alexander Neill, TD (Surgery) Walpole Court, 1A Park Road, Wallington SM6 8AW Tel: 020 8647 4485 — MRCS Eng. LRCP Lond. 1952 (Camb. & King's Coll. Hosp.) MA, MB BChir Camb. 1957. Maj. RAMC (V). Prev: Ho. Surg. (ENT) King's Coll. Hosp.

PETRIE, Sheena Edwards (retired) 4 Transy Place, Dunfermline KY12 7QN Tel: 01383 723622 — MB ChB Ed. 1962; DObst RCOG 1965; MFFP 1993. SCMO (Family Plann.) Fife HB. Prev: SHO (O & G) Roy. Infirm. Edin.

PETROPOULOS, Maria-Christina — MB BS Lond. 1990 (St. Geo. Hosp. Med. Sch.) DCH RCP Lond. 1992; MRCP (UK) 1995; MSc (Distinc.) Lond. 2002. Specialist Regist. Community Paediat., Chelsea and Westminster Hosp., Lond.; Specialist Regist. (Paediat.) Northwick Pk. Hosp. (1998-1999). Specialty: Paediat. Special Interest: Ambulatory Paediat. Socs: Roy. Coll. of Paedatrics and Child Health (RCPCH); Brit. Assn. of Community Child Health (BACCH). Prev: Specialist Regist. Neurol./NeuroDisabil., Gt. Ormond St. Hosp., Lond. (1999-2001; Regist (Paediat.) Roy. Free Hosp (1996-1998); SHO (Neonat.) St. Geo. Hosp. Lond. (1995).

PETROS, Andranick Joseph Paediatric Intensive Care Unit, Great Ormond Street Hospital, London WC1N 3JH — MB BS Lond. 1979 (Middlx.) FRCP uk 1998. Cons. Paediatric Intens. Care, Gt. Ormond St. Specialty: Anaesth.

PETROU, Petros Panoyiotis Crowndale Road Surgery, 53 Crowndale Road, London NW1 1TU Tel: 020 7387 7762 — MB ChB Leeds 1972. Prev: Ho. Phys. (Gen. Med.) & Ho. Surg. Pontefract Gen. Infirm.

PETT, Raymond John (retired) Wisteria Lodge, 15 Millbourn Close, Winsley, Bradford-on-Avon BA15 2NN Tel: 01225 723477 — MB BS Lond. 1951 (St. Mary's) MRCS Eng. LRCP Lond. 1951; DObst RCOG 1952; DCH Eng. 1955; MRCGP 1963.

PETT, Simon The Surgery, Grove Street, Petworth GU28 0LP Tel: 01798 342248 Fax: 01798 343987 — MB BS Lond. 1977 (Middlx. Hosp.) MRCP (UK) 1980; DCH RCP Lond. 1981; DTM & H Lond 1981; DRCOG 1983; MRCGP 1989. Socs: Fell. Roy. Soc. Trop. Med. & Hyg.; Fell. Roy. Soc. Med. Prev: Research Fell. (Liver Dis. Childr.) King's Coll. Hosp. Lond.; Perinatal Research Fell. Hammersmith Hosp. Lond.; SHO (Med. & Neurol.) Soton. Gen. Hosp.

PETT, Stephen Jonathan Dental Surgery, 31 Bridge Avenue, Hammersmith, London W6 9JA Tel: 020 8748 5246 Fax: 020 8748 5248 — MB BS Lond. 1984.

PETTENGELL, Ruth St George's Hospital Medical School, Department of Haematology, Cranmer Terrace, London SW17 0RE Tel: 020 8725 3829 Fax: 020 8725 1199 Email: rpetteng@sghms.ac.uk — MB ChB Otago 1983; BSc Vict. Austral. 1979; FRACP 1991; PhD Manch. 1994. Sen. Lect. (Haemat.) & Hon. Cons. (Oncol.) St Geo. Hosp. Med. Sch. Lond. Specialty: Oncol. Special Interest: Immunother.; Lymphoma. Socs: Amer. Assn. Cancer Research (AACR); NZ Med. Assn.; Brit. Assn. Cancer Research (BACR). Prev: Sen. Research Fell. (Jas. Ewing Dept. of Developm. Haematopoiesis) Memor. Sloan-Kettering Cancer Centre NY USA; Clin. Research Fell. & Hon. Regist. Christie Hosp. Univ. Manch.; Specialist Regist. (Clin. Oncol.) Unv. Hosp. Auckland NZ.

PETTER, John Roger Coles Lane Health Centre, Coles Lane, Linton, Cambridge CB1 6JS Tel: 01223 891456 Fax: 01223 890033 — MB BChir Camb. 1987 (Univ. Camb.) MA Camb. 1989; DGM RCP Lond. 1991; MRCGP 1992; DRCOG 1992.

PETTERSON, Diane Margaret Consett Medical Centre, Station Yard, Consett DH8 5YA Tel: 01207 216116 Fax: 01207 216119 — MB ChB Liverp. 1987; Cert. Family Plann. JCC 1990; DRCOG 1990.

PETTERSON, Jane Anne — MB BCh Wales 1991; MRCGP 1995; FRCA 2002. SpR Anaesth. Newport. Specialty: Anaesth.

PETTERSON, Louise Elaine 2nd Floor, East Wing, Homerton Hospital, Homerton Row, London E9 6SR Tel: 020 8510 8297 Fax: 020 8510 8716 — MB BS Monash 1978 (Univ. Monash) DPM Eng. 1983; MRCPsych 1984. Cons. Rehabil. Psychiat. E. Lond. & The city Ment. health Serv.s NHS trust. Specialty: Gen. Psychiat. Prev: Cons. Psychiat. South. Psychiat. Servs. Network & Heatherton Hosp. Vict., Austral.

PETTERSON, Timothy University Hospital of North Durham, Durham DH1 5TW; Acorn Cottage, Iveston, Consett DH8 7TL — MB ChB Liverp. 1986; BSc (Hons.) Liverp. 1982; MRCP (UK) 1991; MD Manch. 1995. Specialty: Care of the Elderly. Socs: Brit. Geriat. Soc. Prev: Clin. Research Fell. (Geriat. Med.) Univ. Manch. Hope Hosp.

PETTERSSON, Mr Bo Adrian Tanglewood, 15 Green Bank, Off Eaton Road, Chester CH4 7EH Tel: 01244 671902 Fax: 01244 681499 — Med Lic Lund 1973 (Lund Univ. Sweden) Med. Dr. Karolinska Inst. Sweden; Med Kand. Lund. 1968. Cons. Urol. Specialty: Urol. Socs: Brit. Assn. Urol. Surg.; Eur. Assn. Urol.; Amer. Urological Assoc. Prev: Attend. Urol. New Eng. Med. Center, Boston; Asst. Prof. Tuft's Med. Sch. Boston.

PETTIFER, Brenda Jane Pettifer and Mok, Colville Health Centre, 51 Kensington Park Road, London W11 1PA Tel: 020 7727 4592 Fax: 020 7221 4613 — (Roy. Free) MB BS Lond. 1969; MRCS Eng. LRCP Lond. 1969. Lect. (Gen. Pract.) Imperial Coll. Socs: RSM. Prev: Ho. Phys. (Endocrinol.) Roy. Free Hosp. Lond. (New End Br.); Ho. Phys. Roy. Free Hosp. Lond. (Lawn Rd. Br.); Ho. Surg. Whipps Cross Hosp. Lond.

PETTIFER, Claudia Fenella 18 Bassett Close, Bassett, Southampton SO16 7PE Tel: 023 8076 8470 — BM Soton. 1985; DFFP 1993.

PETTIFER, Matthew William Coquet Medical Group, Amble Health Centre, Percy Drive, Morpeth NE65 0HD Tel: 01665 710481 Fax: 01665 713031; Togston House, North Togston, Morpeth NE65 0HR Tel: 01665 710145 — MB BS Newc. 1989; MRCGP 1993.

PETTIFORD, Geoffrey Hugh — MB Camb. 1966 (Guy's) BChir 1965.

PETTIGREW, Mr Alastair Morrison ENT Department, Royal Infirmary, Stirling FK8 2AU Tel: 01786 434000 — MB ChB Glas. 1968; FRCS Ed. 1973. Cons. Otolaryngol. Stirling Roy. Infirm. Specialty: Otolaryngol.

PETTIGREW, Anna Frances Springburn Health Centre, 200 Springburn Way, Glasgow G21 1TR Tel: 0141 531 9611 Fax: 0141 531 6706; 617 Kilmarnock Road, Glasgow G43 2TH — MB ChB Glas. 1975; BSc (Hons. Biochem.) Glas. 1972, MB ChB 1975. Specialty: Gen. Med. Prev: Clin. Asst. (Haemat. & Oncol.) Roy. Hosp. Sick Childr. Glas.

PETTIGREW, Anne Margaret Ardgowan Medical Practice, 2 Finnart Street, Greenock PA16 8HW Tel: 01475 888155 Fax: 01475 785060 — MB ChB Glas. 1974; MFFP 1994; MFHom 1997; MSc Oxon 2003. GP NHS Private Homoep. Pract. Specialty: Family Plann. & Reproduc. Health; Homeop. Med. Prev: Trainee GP Kilbride VTS; SHO Rotat. (Med.) Gartnavel Gen. Hosp. Glas. & West. Infirm. Glas.; Ho. Off. Roy. Hosp. Sick Childr. Glas.

PETTIGREW, Mr Gavin 41 Southbrae Drive, Jordanhill, Glasgow G13 1PU — MB ChB Glas. 1990; FRCS Glas. 1994.

PETTIGREW, Naomi Margaret Elizabeth Eckford Cottage, 38 Broomieknowe, Lasswade EH18 1LN — MB ChB Manch. 1986.

PETTIGREW, Rachel Alyson Assisted Conception Unit, Department of Obstetrics and Gynaecology, St Thomas Hospital, Lambeth Palace Road, London SE1 7EH Tel: 020 7928 9292 ext 2773 Fax: 020 7633 0152 — MB ChB Birm. 1992. Research Assoc. Reproductive Med. O & G St. Thos. Hosp. Lond. Specialty: Obst. & Gyn.

PETTIGREW, Richard Christopher Bruce (retired) 5 Edale Avenue, Haslingden, Rossendale BB4 6QL — (Sheff.) MB ChB Sheff. 1966; DObst RCOG 1968. Clin. Asst. in Rheum. & Rehabil. Med., Burnley Gen. Hosp., Burnley; Clin. Asst. in Rheum., Dept. of Rheum., Rochdale Infirm., Rochdale. Prev: Regist. (Psychiat.) Burnley Gen. Hosp.

PETTINGALE, Keith William Department of Health Care for the Elderly, GKT School of medicine, Kings College Hospital (Dulwich), East Dulwich Grove, London SE22 8PT Tel: 020 7346 6077 Fax: 020 7346 6476 Email: keith.pettingale@kcl.ac.uk; 32 Buckingham Close, Orpington BR5 1SA — MB BS Lond. 1964 (King's Coll. Hosp.) MRCS Eng. LRCP Lond. 1964; FRCP Lond. 1980, M 1966; MD Lond. 1971. Guy's, Kings and St Thomas's (GKT) Sch. of Med.; Hon. Cons. Phys. KCH Lond. Specialty: Gen. Med.; Care of the Elderly; Oncol. Socs: Assn. Palliat. Med.; Brit. Geriat. Soc.;

Me.Brit.Psycho.Ssocial.Oncolog.Soc. Prev: Director of underGrad. studios kings Coll. Med. 95/98; Med. Dir. MacMillan Continuing Care Team Camberwell HA; Vis. Prof. Lund Univ. (Sweden) 1994.

PETTINGER, Andrew John Catherine House Surgery, New Walk, The Plains, Totnes TQ9 5HA Tel: 01803 862073 Fax: 01803 862056; Watsons, Belsford, Haberton, Totnes TQ9 7SP Tel: 01803 863687 — BM Soton. 1987. GP.

PETTINGER, Graham Devonshire Green Medical Centre, 126 Devonshire Street, Sheffield S3 7SF Tel: 0114 272 1626; 73 Hallam Grange Crescent, Fulwood, Sheffield S10 4BB — MB ChB Sheff. 1984.

PETTINGER, Mrs Rachel Bluebell Medical Centre, 356 Bluebell Road, Sheffield S5 6BS Tel: 0114 242 1406 Fax: 0114 261 8074 — MB ChB Sheff. 1986.

PETTIT, Andrew Ian 103 Knighton Church Road, Leicester LE2 3JN — MB ChB Leic. 1994; MRCP 1998. Clin. Res. Fell. (Med. & Therap.) Univ. of Leic. Specialty: Pharmacology.

PETTIT, Barry The Upper Surgery, 27 Lemon Street, Truro TR1 2NW Tel: 01872 274931 Fax: 01872 260339; Summerville, Crescent Road, Truro TR1 3EP Tel: 01872 73222 — MB ChB Bristol 1969; DObst RCOG 1971; DA Eng. 1972. Hosp. Pract. (Gastrointestinal Endoscopy) Roy. Cornw. Hosp. Truro. Prev: SHO (Anaesth. & Obst.) Treliske Hosp. Truro; Ho. Phys. Torbay Hosp. Torquay.

PETTIT, Derek Richard Poole Hospital NHS Trust, Dorset Breast Screening Unit, Longfleet Road, Poole BH15 2JB/01202 665511 — MB ChB Birm. 1973; BSc (Anat. 1st Cl. Hons.) Birm. 1969; DRCOG 1977; Cert. JCC Lond. 1978; MRCP UK 1990; DFFP 1994. Staff Breast Phys. Dorset Cancer Centre. Specialty: Radiol.; Oncol. Socs: Brit. Soc. Colpos. & Cerv. Path.; BMA; Roy. Soc. Med. Prev: GP Princip. Droitwich Worcs.; Regist. (Gen. Med.) Hollymoor Hosp. Birm.; SHO (Accid. & Emerg., Paediat., Med.) Birm. AHA & Worcs. AHA.

PETTIT, Elizabeth Kirsty Fishponds Health Centre, Beechwood road, Fishponds, Bristol BS16 3TD — MB ChB Leic. 1993; DRCOG 1997; MRCGP 1998. GP Princip. Specialty: Gen. Pract.

PETTIT, James David — MB ChB Leeds 1997.

PETTIT, John Gregory Gable House, 46 High Street, Malmesbury SN16 9AT Tel: 01666 825825; Pinkney Cottage, Pinkney, Malmesbury SN16 0NZ — BM Soton. 1987 (Univ. Soton.) MRCGP 1993. Specialty: Gen. Psychiat.

PETTIT, Katrina Erica Olivia 1 Claremont Street, Spital Tongues, Newcastle upon Tyne NE2 4AH — MB BS Newc. 1996.

PETTIT, Mark Linthorpe Road Surgery, 378 Linthorpe Road, Middlesbrough TS5 6HA Tel: 01642 817166 Fax: 01642 824094; Millfield House, Little Ayton Lane, Middlesbrough TS9 6HU — (Edinburgh) MB ChB Ed. 1968; DObst RCOG 1970.

PETTIT, Philippa Clare The Tolsey Surgery, High Street, Sherston, Malmesbury SN16 0LQ Tel: 01666 840270 Fax: 01666 841074 — BM Soton. 1987 (Southampton) DRCOG 1990; MRCGP 1993.

PETTIT, Mr Stephen Harold Dept. of Surgery, Victoria Hospital NHS Trust, Whinney Heys Road, Blackpool FY3 8NR Tel: 01253 303564; 1 The Oaks, St. Michaels, Preston PR3 0TF — MB ChB Manch. 1976 (Manchester and Oxford) MA Oxf. 1977; DRCOG 1978; FRCS Eng. 1981; FRCS Ed. 1981; ChM 1986. Cons. Gen. Surg. Vict. Hosp. Blackpool & Lytham Hosp. Specialty: Gen. Surg. Prev: Sen. Regist. (Gen. Surg.) Manch. Roy. Infirm., Withington Hosp. Manch.& Hope Hosp. Salford.; Huntarian Prof. Surgery 1986.

PETTIT, William John Peel Hall Medical Centre, 2 Bleak Hey Road, Peel Hall, Manchester M22 5ES — MB ChB Manch. 1973; DObst RCOG 1975; MRCGP 1977; FRCGP 1991.

PETTITT, Andrew Royston Department of Haematology, Royal Liverpool University Hospital, Prescot St., Liverpool L7 8XP Tel: 0151 706 4343 Fax: 0151 706 5810 Email: andrew.pettitt@rlbuh-tr.nwest.nhs.uk — MB BChir Camb. 1989; BA Camb. 1986; MRCP (UK) 1991; MRCPath 2000; PhD 2000. Sen. Lect. & Hon. Cons. (Haemat.) Roy. Liverp. Univ. Hosp. Specialty: Haematology. Prev: Regist. (Haemat.) Roy. Liverp. Univ. Hosp.; Lect. & Hon. Sen. Regist. (Haemat.) Roy. Liverp. Univ. Hosp.

PETTMAN, Jean Calvert (retired) 107 Northampton Road, Kettering NN15 7JY Tel: 01536 485799 — (Durh.) MB BS Durh. 1955.

PETTMAN, Sarah Barbara Bedford Road Surgery, 273 Bedford Road, Kempston, Bedford MK42 8QD Tel: 01234 852222 Fax: 01234 843558 — BM BCh Oxf. 1987; DRCOG 1991; MRCGP 1992.

PETTS, Alison Louise — MB BS Newc. 1998.

PETTY, Mr Alfred Holdsworth (retired) 7 Elmfield Park, Newcastle upon Tyne NE3 4UX Tel: 0191 285 1706 Email: ahv@onyxnet.co.uk — MB BS Durh. 1948; FRCS Eng. 1958. Prev: Cons. Surg. Newc. Gen. Hosp.

PETTY, Daniel Robert 15 Beech Hill, Hexham NE46 3AD — MB ChB Birm. 1994; ChB Birm. 1994.

PETTY, David John Health Centre, Eaton Place, Bingham, Nottingham NG13 8BE Tel: 01949 837338; Thoroton Road, Thoroton, Nottingham NG13 9DT — BM BS Nottm. 1984; BDS Lond. 1976; LDS RCS Eng. 1977. Prev: SHO Odstock Hosp. Salisbury; Ho. Surg. Salisbury Gen. Infirm.; Ho. Phys. York Dist. Hosp.

PETTY, Hugh Richard 32 Weymouth Street, London W1G 7BU Tel: 020 7352 6351 Fax: 020 7637 2019 — MB BChir Camb. 1965 (Camb. & St. Bart.) BChir 1964; MRCS Eng. LRCP Lond. 1964. Med. Dir. The Wellman Clinic Lond. Prev: Med. Adviser Roy. Commonw. Soc., Blick Internat. & other Cos.; Regist. & Resid. Med. Off. (Gen. Med. & Neurol.) Gen. Hosp. Rochford; Ho. Phys. St. Bart. Hosp. Lond.

PETTY, Jane Windhill Green Medical Centre, 2 Thackley Old Road, Shipley BD18 1QB Tel: 01274 584223 Fax: 01274 530182 — MB ChB Leeds 1990; BSc (Hons.) Physiol. Lond. 1985; DRCOG 1994; DFFP 1994; MRCGP 1995. Neurol. Clin. Asst. Socs: BMA; Roy. Coll. Obst. & Gyn.; Roy. Coll. GP's.

PETTY, Laurence Gilbert 5 Hardy Road, Blackheath, London SE3 7NS — MB BS Lond. 1964.

PETTY, Martyn Glyn David Victoria Surgery, 5 Victoria Road, Holyhead LL65 1UD; Clydfan, Gorad Road, Valley, Holyhead LL65 3AT Tel: 01407 740706 — MB ChB Manch. 1986; BSc (Physiol.) Manch. 1982; MB ChB Hons. Manch. 1986; Cert. Family Plann. JCC 1989; DRCOG 1989.

PETTY, Melanie Joanne 145 Birmingham Road, Wylde Green, Sutton Coldfield B72 1LX — MB BS Lond. 1996.

PETTY, Richard Kenneth Holdsworth Institute of Neurological Science, Southern General Hospital, Glasgow G51 4TF Tel: 0141 201 1100 — MB BS Newc. 1978; MRCP (UK) 1980; MD Newc. 1989; FRCP 1999. Cons. Neurol. South. Gen. Hosp. Glas. Specialty: Neurol. Socs: Assn. Brit. Neurol.; World Muscle Soc. Prev: Lect. (Neurol. & Neurovirol.) Univ. Glas.

PETTY, Russell David Department of Medicinal Theraputics (oncology), University of Aberdeen, Institute of Medical Sciences, Foresterhill, Aberdeen AB25 2ZN — MB ChB Dundee 1996; BMSc (Hons.) Dundee 1993; MRCP (UK) 2000.

PETTY, William Harry 123 Church Road, Worle, Weston Super Mare BS22 9EL — MRCS Eng. LRCP Lond. 1942 (Guy's & Camb.) MA Camb. 1942. Prev: Asst. Surg. Regist. St. Bart Hosp. Rochester; Dep. Res. Surg. Off. King Edwd. Memor. Hosp. Ealing; Ho. Surg. Co. Hosp. Dartford.

PETZOLD, Axel Institute of Neurology, Department of Neuroimmunology, Queen Square, London WC1N 3BG Tel: 020 7837 3611 Ext: 4202 Fax: 020 7837 8553 Email: a.petzold@ion.ucl.ac.uk — State Exam Med Freiburg 1996; MD (Hons.) Freiburg 1998; PhD UCL 2003; CCST (Neurol.) 2004. Clin. Fell.(Neurocritical Care) Nat. Hosp. for Neurol. & Neurosurg. Care. Specialty: Neurol. Special Interest: Neuroimmunology; Neurocritical Care. Prev: Clin. Asst. Insitute of Neurol. Lond.

PEUTHERER, John Forrest Department of Mewdical Microbiology, Medical School, Teviot Place, Edinburgh EH8 9AG Tel: 0131 650 3159 Fax: 0131 650 6531; 44 Bridge Road, Edinburgh EH13 0LQ Tel: 0131 441 1201 — MD Ed. 1975; BSc Ed. 1957, MD 1975, MB ChB 1962; FRCPath 1986, M 1975; FRCP Ed. 1988 M 1986. Hon. Cons., Head of Dept. & Sen. Lect. Med. Microbiol. Edin. Univ. Med. Sch.

PEUTRELL, Jane Margaret 48 Victoria Crescent Road, Glasgow G12 9DE; Department of Anaesthetics, Royal Hospital For Sick Children, Yorkshill NHS Trust, Dalnair St., Glasgow G3 8SJ Tel: 0141 201 0000 Fax: 0141 201 0821 — MB BS Newc. 1982; MRCP (UK) 1985; DA (UK) 1986; FCAnaesth. 1989; FRCP Ed 1998. Cons. Paediat. Anaesth. Roy. Hosp. for Sick Childr. Yorkshill NHS Trust, Glas. Specialty: Paediat.

PEVELER, Professor Robert Charles University Mental Health Group, Royal South Hants Hospital, Brinitons Terrace, Southampton SO14 0YG Tel: 023 8082 5533 Fax: 023 8023 4243 — BM BCh Oxf. 1982 (Univ. Oxf.) MA Oxf. 1980, DPhil 1980; FRCPsych 1998. Prof. & Cons. (Psychiat.) Univ. Dept. Psychiat. Soton.; Hon. Cons. W. Hants. NHS Trust. Specialty: Gen. Psychiat. Prev: Clin. Lect. (Psychiat.) Univ. Dept. Psychiat. Oxf.; Wellcome Trust Research Fell. Univ. Dept. Psychiat. Oxf.; Regist. & SHO (Psychiat.) Oxf. HA.

PEVERLEY, Martin Christopher 63 Castledene Court, South Gosforth, Newcastle upon Tyne NE3 1NZ — MB BS Newc. 1989.

PEXTON, Nigel Frederick Williamwood Practice, Williamwood Medical Centre, 85 Seres Road, Glasgow G76 7NW Tel: 0141 638 7984 Fax: 0141 638 8827 — MB ChB Glas. 1985; DRCOG 1988; MRCGP 1990.

PEYMAN, Michael Anthony 37B New Cavendish Street, Marylebone, London W1G 8JR Tel: 020 7735 7128; 36 Cleaver Street, Kennington, North Lambeth, London SE11 4DP Tel: 020 7735 7128 — BM BCh Oxf. 1948 (Oxf. & St Thos.) MA Oxf. 1950; MRCP Lond. 1950; DM Oxf. 1957. Socs: Fell. Roy. Soc. Med. Prev: Med. Adviser Brit. Home Stores Ltd; Clin. Asst. Med. Profess. Unit & Sen. Regist. (Med.) Char. Cross Hosp.; Evans Med. Research Fell. New Eng. Center Hosp. Boston, USA.

PEYSER, Edith Erna Charlotte (retired) Woodrow, Asheldon Road, Wellswood, Torquay TQ1 2QN Tel: 01803 299551 — Staatsexamen Univ. Berlin 1934.

PEYTON, Henry Newnham 10 Manor Road, Ipswich IP4 2UX Tel: 01473 57842 — MRCS Eng. LRCP Lond. 1939 (St. Bart.) Prev: Resid. W. Herts. Hosp.; Ho. Surg. King Edwd. Memor. Hosp. Ealing; RAMC 1940-46.

PEYTON, Mr James William Rodney, TD Beechlyn Court, Ballynorthland Park, Dungannon BT71 6DY Tel: 02887 727134 Fax: 02887 724255 Email: rpeyton@rpeyton.demon.co.uk — MB BCh BAO Belf. 1973 (Queen's University, Belfast) MRCP (UK) 1975; FRCS Ed. 1978; BSc (Hons.) Belf. 1970, MD 1982; FRCSI 1993; MSc Cardiff 1995; FRCS Eng. 1996; FRCP Lond. 1997; PGDL Guildford 1999. Cons. Surg. Craigavon Area Hosp. N. Irel.; Princip. Tutor (Fac. Development)/Educ. Adviser RCS Eng. Specialty: Gen. Surg.; Trauma & Orthop. Surg. Prev: Cons. Surg. S. Tyrone Hosp. Dungannon.

PEYTON, Patricia Anne Hospital Hill Surgery, 7 Izatt Avenue, Dunfermline KY11 3BA Tel: 01383 731721 Fax: 01383 623352 — MB ChB Ed. 1973.

PEYTON-JONES, Benjamin 37 Swallowfields, Totnes TQ9 5LB — MB ChB Leic. 1996. SHO (O & G) Bath. Specialty: Obst. & Gyn.

PEZESHGI, Djallilah Sadri 6 Roman Road, Bearsden, Glasgow G61 2SW — MRCS Eng. LRCP Lond. 1973 (St. Bart.) BA (Hon) Lond. 1984, MB BS 1974; DRCOG 1978. Prev: GP Soton.

PFANG, Jennifer Anne PO Box 900, Norwich NR2 3ER — MB BS Lond. 1988.

PFEFFER, Jeremy Michael 97 Harley Street, London W1N 1DF Tel: 020 7935 3878 Fax: 020 7935 3865; 84 Southover, London N12 7HD Tel: 020 8446 4475 — MB BS Lond. 1971 (Univ. Coll. Hosp.) BSc (Hons. Biochem.) Lond. 1968; MRCP (UK) 1974; FRCPsych 1988, M 1977; FRCP Lond. 1990. Cons. Psychiat. & Hon. Sen. Lect. The Roy. Brompton Hosp. Specialty: Gen. Psychiat. Socs: Fell. Roy. Soc. Med. Prev: Sen. Regist. (Psychiat.) The Maudsley Hosp. Lond.; Regist. (Chest Med.) Papworth Hosp. Camb.; Ho. Surg. Univ. Coll. Hosp. Lond.

PFEIFER, Christine Zdenka Drs COTTERELL,PFEIFFER & PTNRS, College Way Surgery, Comeytrowe Centre, Taunton TA1 4TY Tel: 01823 259333 Fax: 01823 259336; Park Gate House, Ash Priors, Taunton TA4 3NF Tel: 01823 432122 — (St. Geo.) MB BS Lond. 1970; DObst RCOG 1972; DCH Eng. 1974; Cert. JCC Lond. 1976; MRCGP 1977. Family Plann. Doctor Som. HA. Prev: GP Nottm.; SHO (Obst.) Roy. Berks. Hosp. Reading; SHO (Anaesth.) Frenchay Hosp. Bristol.

PFEIFER, Peter Michael Anaesthetic Department, Robert Jones Agnes Hunt Orthopaedic Hospital, Oswestry SY10 7AG Tel: 01691 404000 Fax: 01691 404068; Ochr, The Llawnt, Rhydycroesau, Oswestry SY10 7HY — MB BS Lond. 1978 (St. Bart.) PhD (Biochem.) Liverp. 1969, BSc (Hons.) 1966; FFA RCS Eng. 1984. Cons. Anaesth. Robt. Jones & Agnes Hunt. Orthop. Hosp. Specialty: Anaesth. Socs: Soc. for Computing & Technol. in Anaesth.; Free Radical Soc.; Brit. Soc. of Orthopaedic Anaesth.s. Prev: Research fell. Oklahoma Med. Research Foundat. Oklahoma City, USA.

PFEIFFER, U Meldrum, Vitty and Pfeiffer, 40-42 Kingsway, Waterloo, Liverpool L22 4RQ Tel: 0151 928 8800 Fax: 0151 928 3775 Email: upfeiffer@rcsed.ac.uk — State Exam Med., Bonn 1981 (Guy's) MD (Bonn) 1984; FRCS (Ed.) 1988; MRCGP 1994; DFFP 1995; Regis. Spec. in Gen. Surg. 1996. GP Princip.; Hon. Consul Federal Republic of Germany in Liverp. Specialty: Gen. Pract.; Gen. Surg.

PFLANZ, Sebastian The Clinic, Mill Isle, Craignair Street, Dalbeattie DG5 4HE Tel: 01556 610331 — MB ChB Aberd. 1988; BMedBiol. 1986; MRCP (UK) 1992; DRCOG 1994. Specialty: Endocrinol. Prev: Regist. (Med.) Dundee; SHO (Med.) Aberd.

PFLEIDERER, Mr Andrew Garth Edith Cavell Hospital, Bretton Gate, Peterborough PE3 9GZ Tel: 01733 875511 Email: agpfleiderer@doctors.org.uk — FRCS (E) 1983; FRCS Glas. 1980; MB BS Lond. 1977; FRCS (Ed) 1982. Cons. Otolaryngol. Head, Neck & Thyroid Surg., P'boro. NHS Trust. Specialty: Otorhinolaryngol.

PHADKE, Anil Sriram Bryncelyn Clinic Premises, Bryncelyn, Nelson, Treharris CF46 6HL Tel: 01443 450340 Fax: 01443 453127 — MB BS Calcutta 1966 (Nat. Med. Coll. Calcutta) BA Open Univ. 1991. Specialty: Accid. & Emerg.

PHADNIS, Sunil Gangadhar 26 The Bourne, London N14 6QS — MB BS Poona 1975.

PHALKE, Indrajit Madhavarao (retired) North Hampshire Hospitals NHS Trust, Aldermaston Road, Basingstoke RG24 9NA; Anantpat, 18 Colton Road, Shrivenham, Swindon SN6 8AZ Tel: 01793 782786 — MB BS Agra 1956; DMRE Vikram 1959; DMRD Eng. 1965. Prev: Cons. Radiol. Princess Margt. Hosp. Swindon.

PHALP, Charles George Anderson Rother House Medical Centre, Alcester Road, Stratford-upon-Avon CV37 6PP Tel: 01789 269386 Fax: 01789 298742; Cherry Tree Cottage, Loxley, Warwick CV35 9JS Tel: 01789 842902 — MB ChB Birm. 1972; DObst RCOG 1974; MMedSci Birm. 1994. Chairm. Warks. LMC. Socs: Roy. Soc. Med. Prev: Chairm. Warks. Health Auth. Strategy Comm.

PHAN, Phuong-Anh Thi 40 Kelly Street, London NW1 8PH — MB BS Lond. 1997.

PHANJOO, Andre Ludovic 29 Blacket Place, Edinburgh EH9 1RJ Tel: 0131 667 9809 Fax: 0131 537 6112 — MB ChB Ed. 1966; DPM Ed. 1969; FRCPsych 1984, M 1972. Cons. Psychiat. Roy. Edin. Hosp.; Clin. Dir. (c/o the Elderly) Roy. Edin. Hosp.; Hon. Sen. Lect. Fac. Med. Univ. Edin. Specialty: Geriat. Psychiat.; Psychosexual Med.

PHARAOH, Alice Mary The Old Dispensary, 32 East Borough, Wimborne BH21 1PL Tel: 01202 880786 Fax: 01202 880736; Corfe Cottage, Broadmoor Road, Corfe Mullen, Wimborne BH21 3RB Tel: 01202 693215 — MB BS Lond. 1972 (St. Geo.) Cert. Family Plann. Clin. Asst. Wimborne Community Hosp. Socs: BMA; LMC. Prev: Clin. Asst. Lipid Clinic & Diabetic Clinic; Mem. PCG.

PHARAOH, Amy Jane 15 Grantchester Street, Newnham, Cambridge CB3 9HY — BM BS Nottm. 1998; MRCP UK; BMedSci Nottm. 1998.

PHARAOH, James Mark Hadleigh House, 20 Kirkway, Broadstone BH18 8EE Tel: 01202 692268 Fax: 01202 658954; Corfe Cottage, Broadmoor Road, Corfe Mullen, Wimborne BH21 3RB Tel: 01202 693215 — MB BS Lond. 1971 (St. Geo.) DObst RCOG 1973; DA Eng. 1974.

PHARE, Alexis Jonathon Longacre, Compton, Paignton TQ3 1TD — MB BCh Wales 1996.

PHAROAH, Fiona Margaret Lifespan Healthcare NHS Trust, Block 14, The Ida Darwin Hospital, Fulbourn, Cambridge CB1 5EE Tel: 01223 884243; c/o 11 Fawley Road, Allerton, Liverpool L18 9TE — MB ChB Manch. 1991; MRCPsych; MA Camb. 1986. Specialist Regist. (Gen. Psychiat.). Specialty: Gen. Psychiat. Prev: Regist. Rotat. Broadmoor Hosp. Crowthorne; Regits. (Psychiat) Warneford Hosp.; SHO (Psychiat.) Fairmile Hosp. Oxon.

PHAROAH, Paul David Peter Strangeways Research Laboratories, Worts Causeway, Cambridge CB1 8RN Tel: 01223 740166 Email: paul.pharoah@srl.cam.ac.uk; 71 Hinton Avenue, Cambridge CB1 7AR — BM BCh Oxf. 1986; MA (CAMB) 1986; MRCP (UK) 1990; DPH (CAMB) 1993; MFPHM RCP (UK) 1995; PhD (CAMB) 2000. Cancer Research UK, Sen. Clin. Research Fell. & Hon. Cons. Pub. Health. Specialty: Epidemiol.; Pub. Health Med.

PHAROAH, Professor Peter Oswald Derrick (retired) Department of Public Health, University of Liverpool, Liverpool

L69 3GB Tel: 0151 794 5577 Fax: 0151 794 5272 Email: p.o.d.pharoah@liverpool.ac.uk; 11 Fawley Road, Liverpool L18 9TE Tel: 0151 724 4896 — (St. Mary's) MB BS Lond. 1958; MRCS Eng. LRCP Lond. 1958; MSc Lond. 1974, BSc 1955, MD 1972; FFPHM 1980; FRCPCH 1997; FRCP 1997. Emeri. Prof. Pub. Health Univ. Liverp. Prev: Prof. Pub. Health Univ. Liverp.

PHATAK, Mr Prabhakar Shankar (retired) 2 Longlands Park Crescent, Sidcup DA15 7NE Tel: 020 8302 1535 — (Nagpur) MB BS Nagpur 1960; FRCS Eng. 1967.

PHAURE, Trevor Albert Joseph (retired) Ivanhoe, New Road, Timsbury, Romsey SO51 0NH Tel: 01794 368385 — (St Bart.) MB BS Lond. 1963; FRCPath 1984, M 1972. Prev: Cons. Haemat. Mid. Staffs. HA.

PHEAR, David Norman (retired) West Common, Redbourn, St Albans AL3 7DY Tel: 01582 792 430 — MB BChir Camb. 1949 (Middlx.) Nat. Sc. Trip. cl. 1 Pts. 1 & 2; MD Camb. 1956, MA 1949; FRCP Lond 1973, M 1954; FRACP 1972, M 1961. Prev: Cons. Phys. St. Albans City Hosp. & Qu. Eliz. II Hosp. Welwyn Gdn. City.

PHEAR, Rita Winifred (retired) West Common, Redbourn, St Albans AL3 7DY Tel: 01582 792 430 — MB BS Lond. 1953 (Roy. Free) MRCS Eng. LRCP Lond. 1953; DCH Eng. 1955; FRCOG 1976, M 1959, DObst 1956. Prev: Cons. O & G St. Albans City Hosp.

PHEARA, Jezziniah c/o Anaesthetics Department, Darlington Memorial Hospital NHS Trust, Hollyhurst Road, Darlington DL3 6HX — MB ChB Stellenbosch 1994.

PHEBY, Derek Francis Henry University of the West of England, Unit of Applied Epidemiology, Frenchay Campus, Coldharbour Lane, Bristol BS16 1QY Tel: 0117 344 3912 Fax: 0117 344 3940 Email: derek.pheby@uwe.ac.uk; Plaishetts House, Hadspen, Castle Cary BA7 7LR — MB BS Lond. 1969 (St Thos.) BSc Lond. 1966; MRCS Eng. LRCP Lond. 1969; DObst RCOG 1973; MPhil York 1983; MFPHM 1986; LLM 1992. Dir. Unit Applied Epidemiol. Univ. W. Eng. Specialty: Epidemiol. Socs: Medicolegal Soc; Melvyn Ramsey Soc. Prev: Dir. Cancer Epidemiol. Unit Univ. Bristol; Cons. Pub. Health Med. Gloucester HA; Sen. Regist. (Community Med.) Wessex RHA.

PHEILS, Mr Peter John Oaktree House, 36 Callis Court Road, Broadstairs CT10 3AG Tel: 01843 863170 Fax: 01843 602343 — MB BS Lond. 1968 (St. Thos.) FRCS Eng. 1973; MS Lond. 1981. Cons. Gen. Surg. E. Kent Hosp.Trust. Specialty: Gen. Surg. Socs: Fell. Assn. Surgs.; Fell. Roy. Soc. Med.; Brit. Assn. Surg. Oncol. Prev: Sen. Regist. (Gen. Surg.) St. Bart. Hosp. Lond.; Lect. (Surg.) St. Thos. Hosp. Lond.; Regist. (Surg.) Brighton & High Wycombe Health Dists.

PHELAN, Aideen Elizabeth 47 Albany Road, New Malden KT3 3NY — MB BCh BAO NUI 1991.

PHELAN, Declan Richard Statham Grove Surgery, Statham Grove, London N16 9DP Tel: 020 7254 4327 Fax: 020 7241 4098; 68 Malvern Road, Hackney, London E8 3LJ Email: dphelan@doctors.org.uk — MB BCh BAO NUI 1983 (UCD) DCH NUI 1985; DObst. RCPI 1987; MRCGP 1988. Specialty: Gen. Pract.

PHELAN, Francis Joseph Department of Elderly Medicine, Seacroft Hospital, Leeds LS14 Tel: 0113 264 8164; 17 Kingscroft Gardens, Moortown, Leeds LS17 6PB Tel: 0113 216 5791 — BM Soton. 1991; MSc Cork 1984; MRCP (UK) 1996. Specialty: Care of the Elderly.

PHELAN, Lorna Karen 137 Sandy Lane S., Wallington SM6 9NW — BM BS Nottm. 1992.

PHELAN, Margaret Sarah 19 Asmara Road, London NW2 3SS — MB BCh BAO NUI 1976; MRCPI 1980; DMRD Eng. 1980; FRCR 1981. Cons. Radiol. The Chelsea & Westm. Hosp. Lond. Specialty: Radiol.

PHELAN, Martin Richard 148 Harley Street, London W1G 6DH Tel: 020 7935 3356 Fax: 020 7224 0557 — MB BChir Camb. 1980 (Addenbrooke's & Univ. Coll. Hosp. Lond.) BDS Lond. 1963; DOrth 1969; FDS RCS Eng. 1970; LMSSA Lond. 1977; MLCOM 1987. Specialist Orthop. & Sports Med. Lond. And Psychosocratic Med.; Medico-Legal Expert Witness; Sen. Mem. Clare Coll. Camb. Specialty: Orthop.

PHELAN, Mary Bernadette 35 Park Road, London W4 3EY — MB BS Lond. 1964; MRCS Eng. LRCP Lond. 1964.

PHELAN, Michael Boland 53 Great Cumberland Place, London W1H 7LH Tel: 020 7723 6482 — MB BS Lond. 1962 (St. Mary's) MRCS Eng. LRCP Lond. 1962; LAH Dub. 1963; AMQ 1964; DTM & H Liverp. 1965. Socs: BMA; Chelsea Clin. Soc.; Med. Soc. Lond. Prev: Resid. Fell. Geo.town Univ. Hosp. Washington, USA; Ho. Surg. (Orthop.) St. Mary's Hosp.; Ho. Phys. Rochford Gen. Hosp.

PHELAN, Michael Cornelius Dept. of Psychiatry, Charing Cross Hospital, Fulham Palace Road, London W6 8RF — MB BS Lond. 1984; BSc (Psychol.) Lond. 1981, MB BS 1984. Cons. (Psychiat.) Char. Cross Hosp. Specialty: Gen. Psychiat.

PHELAN, Mr Peter Stephen Sunderland Eye Infirmary, Queen Alexandra Road, Sunderland SR2 9HP Tel: 0191 569 9068 Fax: 0191 569 9060; BUPA Hospital Washington, Picktree Lane, Rickleton, Washington NE38 9JZ; 13 Ashwood Terrace, Thornhill, Sunderland SR2 7NB Tel: 0191 567 6901 Email: psphelan@doctors.org.uk — MB BCh BAO NUI 1979 (Univ. Coll. Galway) DO RCPSI 1984; FCOphth 1986; FRCS Ed. (Ophth.) 1987. Cons. Ophth. Sunderland Eye Infirm.; Dir. Glaucoma Resource Dept. Sunderland Eye Infirm. Specialty: Ophth. Special Interest: Glaucoma; High Volume Cataract Surg. Socs: MDU; N. Eng. Med. Soc. Prev: Regist. (Ophth.) Roy. Free Hosp. Lond.; Clin. Tutor (Ophth.) UCC; Sen. Regist. (Ophth.) Univ. Coll. Hosp. & Moorfield Eye Hosp. Lond.

PHELLAS, Andrew The Cambridge Medical Group, 10A Cambridge Road, Linthorpe, Middlesbrough TS5 5NN Tel: 01642 851177 Fax: 01642 851176 — MB ChB Ed. 1984; MRCGP 1989; DRCOG 1989.

PHELLAS, Anne Jacqueline Linthorpe Road Surgery, 378 Linthorpe Road, Middlesbrough TS5 6HA Tel: 01642 817166 Fax: 01642 824094 — MB BS Lond. 1986; BSc Lond. 1983, MB BS 1986; MRCGP 1990; DRCOG 1990.

PHELLAS, Georgina Doris (retired) 10 Fern Drive, Magherafelt BT45 5HZ Tel: 028 796 32965 — MB BCh BAO Belf. 1954; DA Eng. 1958.

PHELLAS, Paul Medical Group Practice, Fairhill, Magherafelt, Londonderry Tel: 01648 32621; 10 Fern Drive, Magherafelt BT45 5HZ Tel: 01648 32965 — MB ChB Ed. 1957; DObst RCOG 1959.

PHELLAS, Renos (retired) 67 Paddock Road, London NW2 7DH Tel: 020 8452 7916 — MB ChB Ed. 1952. Prev: Dir. Surg. Unit. St. And. Clinic Famagusta.

PHELPS, Miss Fiona Avrille The Surgery, 20 New Street, Lord Harris Square, Port of Spain, West Indies Tel: 627 2466 Fax: 627 8231; 12 Rossdale Road, Putney, London SW15 1AD Tel: 020 8789 7895 — MB BS West Indies 1988; MRCOG 1995. Regional Regist. (Obst. & Gyn.) SW Thames RHA. Specialty: Obst. & Gyn. Prev: Regist. Qu. Charlotte's Hosp., Univ. Coll. Hosp. & St. Geo. Hosp. Med. Sch. Lond.

PHELPS, Richard Grenville 22 Argyle Court, Edinburgh EH15 2QD — MB BChir Camb. 1986.

PHELPS, Mr Simon Richard 42 Station Road, Alvechurch, Birmingham B48 7SD — MB BS Lond. 1986 (Charing Cross Hospital) FRCS Ed. 1991. Fell. (Paediat. IC) Roy. Manch. Childr.s Hosp. Specialty: Paediat. Surg.

PHELPS, Susan Vicky Health Centre, High Street, Bedworth, Nuneaton CV12 8NQ Tel: 024 7631 5432 Fax: 024 7631 0038; Doric House, Main Street, Easenhall, Rugby CV23 0JA Tel: 01788 832347 — MB BS Lond. 1969 (Char. Cross) MRCS Eng. LRCP Lond. 1969.

PHELPS, Thelma Marjorie (retired) 3 Bromley Road, West Bridgford, Nottingham NG2 7AP Tel: 0115 981 0563 — MB BS Lond. 1946 (Lond. Sch. Med. Wom.) MRCS Eng. LRCP Lond. 1945; DPH Bristol 1970; MFCM 1974; MFPHM 1990. Prev: Cons. Pub. Health Nottm.

PHEMISTER, John Clark Belaire, Chagford, Newton Abbot TQ13 8AT Tel: 01647 432477 — MB ChB Ed. 1946; FRCP Ed. 1972, M 1954. Socs: Assn. Brit. Neurol. Prev: Cons. Neurol. Centr. Middlx. Hosp., Hillingdon Hosp. & Wexham Pk. Hosp. Slough; Surg. Antarctic Whaling Expedit.; Clin. Tutor Roy. Infirm. Edin.

PHIBBS, Peter Alban Thorburn 27 The Square, Latimer, Chesham HP5 1TY — MB BChir Camb. 1938 (St. Thos.) MRCS Eng. LRCP Lond. 1937. Surg. Lt.-Cdr. RNVR. Prev: Regist. (Med.) King Geo. Hosp. Ilford; Ho. Phys. Roy. North. Hosp.; Ho. Surg. W. Lond. Hosp.

PHILBIN, John Christopher Whaddon House Surgery, 221 Whaddon Way, Bletchley, Milton Keynes MK3 7EA Tel: 01908 373058 Fax: 01908 630076 — MB BCh Wales 1980; DRCOG 1985; DCH RCP Lond. 1986.

PHILBIN, Karen Hilary 12 Great Brickhill Lane, Little Brickhill, Milton Keynes MK17 9NW — MB BCh Wales 1980.
PHILIP, Colin John Drs Philip, Sharkey, Manley and Croft, The Stennack Surgery, The Old Stennack School, St Ives TR26 1RU Tel: 01736 795237 Fax: 01736 795362; Booby's Castle, Nancledra, Penzance TR20 8NE — MB ChB Bristol 1978; DRCOG 1980; MRCGP 1983.
PHILIP, Dawn Barn Brae, Dalcross, Inverness IV2 7JH — MB ChB Aberd. 1987; MRCGP 1992. SHO (Obst.& Gyn.) St. Richard's Hosp. Chichester.
PHILIP, George Department of Histopathology, Royal Sussex County Hospital, Brighton BN2 5BE — BM BCh 1970 (Oxf. & Univ. Coll. Hosp.) MA Oxf. 1970; MRCPath 1977. Cons. Path. Brighton & Sussex Univ. Hosps. Specialty: Histopath. Prev: Cons. Path. St Helier Hosp., Surrey.
PHILIP, George Eugene Newton Medical Centre, 14/18 Newton Road, London W2 5LT Tel: 020 7229 4578 — MB ChB Ed. 1960. Socs: Fell. BMA.
PHILIP, Ian Grant (retired) 1 Orchard Road, Maldon CM9 6EW Tel: 01621 841560 Fax: 01621 841560 Email: iph6789582@aol.com — (Glas.) MB ChB Glas. 1957; DObst RCOG 1959. Prev: Ho. Phys. Univ. Med. Unit, Stobhill Hosp. Glas.
PHILIP, Professor James Fiddes (retired) Broomhill, Lumphanan, Banchory AB31 4QH Tel: 013398 83672 — (Aberd.) ChM (Hons.) Aberd. 1937, MB ChB 1933; FRCS Ed. 1938. Hon. Cons. Malig. Dis. Grampian HB. Prev: Clin. Dir. Roxburghe Hse. Milltimber.
PHILIP, Mr John Pennine Screening Programme, Trinity Road, Bradford BD5 0JX Tel: 01274 365521 Fax: 01274 727322 — MB BS Madras 1972 (Jawaharlal Inst. Postgrad. Med. Educat. Pondicherry) FRCS Ed. 1976; PhD Leeds 1985. Clin. Dir. DHSS Breast Screening Progr. Bradford; Surg. Breast Screen. & Advis. Centre. Specialty: Gen. Surg. Socs: BASO. Prev: Clin. Research Fell. Breast Unit St. Lukes Hosp. Huddersfield; Med. Off. Nigeria; Regist. Gen. Hosp. Nottm.
PHILIP, John Murray Ure (retired) Penlan, Holm Farm Road, Catrine, Mauchline KA5 6TA — (Univ. Ed.) MB ChB Ed. 1945; DTM & H Ed. 1949. Prev: Princip., Gen. Pract., Catrine.
PHILIP, Lynne Liberton Medical Group, 65 Liberton Gardens, Edinburgh EH16 6JT Tel: 0131 664 3050 Fax: 0131 692 1952 — MB ChB Aberd. 1982; MRCGP 1987.
PHILIP, Mary Frances (retired) 3 Ferguson Gardens, Musselburgh EH21 6XF Tel: 0131 653 2310 Email: jamesandmary.philip@virgin.net — (Cape Town Uni., Ed. University) MB ChB Ed. 1958; MRCPsych 1980. Prev: Cons. Psychiat. Gogarburn Hosp. Edin.
PHILIP, Mr Peter Forbes (retired) Toldrum Cottage, Winksley, Ripon HG4 3PG Tel: 01765 658650 Email: jandpphilip@toldrumcottage.fsnet.co.uk — (King's Coll. Lond. & Char. Cross) MB BS Lond. 1945; FRCS Eng. 1948; MS Lond. 1953. Prev: Cons. Urol. Char. Cross Hosp. Lond. & Roy. Masonic Hosp.
PHILIP, Rebecca Anne 12 Burnet Place, Aberdeen AB24 4QD — MB ChB Aberd. 1991; MRCGP 1995; MRCPsych. 1997. Specialist Regist. (Child & Adolesc. Psychiat.) Aberd. Roy. Hosps. NHS Trust Aberd. Specialty: Child & Adolesc. Psychiat.; Gen. Psychiat. Prev: Trainee GP Grampian HB VTS.; SHO (Psychiat.) Grampian Health Care Aberd.
PHILIP, Valerie Jane 23 New Road, Ham, Richmond TW10 7HZ — MB ChB Bristol 1976; DRCOG 1979; DCH Eng. 1980.
PHILIP, William James Unwin 12 Burnett Place, Kittybrewster, Aberdeen AB24 4QD Tel: 01224 492038 — MB ChB Aberd. 1990; MRCP (UK) 1993. Clin. Research Fell. & Hon. Regist. (Cardiol.) Aberd. Roy. Infirm. Specialty: Cardiol.
PHILIP, William Marshall 4 Carpenter Road, Edgbaston, Birmingham B15 2JT Tel: 0121 454 3981 — MB BS Lond. 1938 (Guy's) MRCS Eng. LRCP Lond. 1936; FRCP Lond. 1975, M 1939. Hon. Cons. Phys. Birm. HA. Specialty: Gen. Med. Prev: Cons. Phys. E. Birm. Gen. Hosp.; Squadron Ldr. RAFVR; Ho. Phys. Brompton Hosp. & Guy's Hosp.
PHILIPP, Mr Elliot Elias (retired) 166 Rivermead Court, Ranelagh Gardens, London SW6 3SF Tel: 020 7736 2851 Fax: 020 7736 2851 — MB BChir Camb. 1947 (Cambridge & Middlesex Hospital) MRCS Eng. LRCP Lond. 1939; BA Camb. 1936, MA 1942; FRCOG 1962, M 1947; FRCS Eng. 1951. Hon. Cons. Obst. & Gyn. City Lond. Matern. Hosp., Whittington & Roy. N. Hosps Lond; Hon. Cons. Gyn. French Disp. Lond. Prev: Cons. O & G OldCh. Hosp. Romford.
PHILIPP, Robin Department of Occupational Medicine, Bristol Royal Infirmary, Bristol BS2 8HW Tel: 0117 928 2223 Fax: 0117 928 3840 — MB ChB Otago 1968; DPH Bristol 1974; DCH Eng. 1974; DIH Dund 1976; MFCMI 1977; MSc Bristol 1979; FFOM RCP Lond. 1991, MFOM, 1984, AFOM 1979; MCCM (NZ) 1980; FAFPHM 1994, FFPHM RCP (UK) 1990, M 1985; FRCP Lond. 1999. Cons. Occupat. Phys. United Bristol NHS Health Care Trust; Hon. Sen. Lect. Occupat. & Pub. Health Med. Univ. Bristol. Specialty: Occupat. Health; Pub. Health Med. Prev: Vis. Lect. (Environm. Epidemiol.) Wellington Clin. Sch. Univ. Otago; Regist. (Med.) Wellington Pub. Hosp., NZ; Dir. WHO Collaborating Centre for Environm. Health Promotion & Ecology Univ Bristol.
PHILIPPIDIS, Pandelis 277 Otley Road, Leeds LS16 5LN — MB ChB Ed. 1994.
PHILIPPOU, George Nicolaou 1 Bury Hall Villas, Great Cambridge Road, London N9 9LE Tel: 020 8360 0319 — State Exam. Med. Sofia 1969.
PHILIPPSON, Margaret Elizabeth Anne Longrove Surgery, 70 Union Street, Barnet EN5 4HT Tel: 020 8441 9440/9563 Fax: 020 8441 4037 — (Guy's) MB BS Lond. 1976; DRCOG 1980. Clin. Asst. (Genitourin. Med.) Barnet. Specialty: Gen. Pract. Prev: Prinicip. GP Broxbourne, Herts; Med. Off. Turks & Caicos Isles; Trainee GP Tunbridge Wells VTS.
PHILIPS, Barbara Janet Department of Anaesthetics (Intensive Care), St George's Hospital Medical School, Cranmer Terrace, Tooting, London SW17 0RE Email: bphilips@sghms.ac.uk — MB BS Lond. 1988; FRCA Lond. 1993; MD Lond. 1999. Sen. Lect. Intens. Care Med. St Geo. Hosp. Med. Sch. Lond. Specialty: Anaesth. Socs: Europ. Intens. Care Soc.; Europ. Shock Soc.; Intens. Care Soc. Prev: Specialist Regist. Intens. Care Roy. Infirm. Edin.; Sen. Regist. Anaesth. Roy. Infirm. Edin.; Clin. Research Fell. Liver Transpl. Serv. Roy. Infirm. Edin.
PHILIPS, Frances Katharine Shieldaig, La Rocque, Grouville JE3 9FD Tel: 01534 854149 — MB ChB Glas. 1954; DObst RCOG 1957.
PHILIPSON, Gavin Patrick 29 Westgate, Leslie, Glenrothes KY6 3LR — MB ChB Ed. 1992.
PHILIPSON, Mr John Anthony Moore (retired) Clifton Farm House, Pullover Road, West Lynn, King's Lynn PE34 3LS Tel: 01553 775619 Fax: 01553 775619 — MB BChir Camb. 1963 (Camb. & Westm.) MB Camb. 1963, BChir 1962; MRCS Eng. LRCP Lond. 1962; MA Camb. 1963; FRCS Ed. 1969. Prev: Sen. Cons. Orthop. The Qu. Eliz. Hosp., King's Lynn.
PHILIPSON, Mark Robert — MB ChB Leeds 1998.
PHILIPSON, Richard Simon GSK R&D Ltd, New Frontiers Science Park, Third Avenue, Harlow CM19 5AW Tel: 01279 644731 Fax: 01279 646697 Email: Richard_S_Philipson@gsk.com; 98 North End, Bassingbourn, Royston SG8 5PD — MB BS Lond. 1988 (Middlx. Hosp. Med. Sch.) BSc Lond. 1985; MRCP (UK) 1992; MRCGP 1994; T(GP) 1995; MFPM 2002. Clin. Pharmacol.
PHILIPSZ, Mary Louise Wellwood House, Saline, Dunfermline KY12 9TD — MB ChB Glas. 1993.
PHILLIMORE, Catherine Elizabeth 26 Welland Way, Oakham LE15 6SL — MB BS Lond. 1994; BSc Lond. 1991.
PHILLIPPS, Mr James John Singleton Hospital, Sketty, Swansea SA2 8QA; Tawel Fryn, Cae Mansel Road, Gowerton, Swansea SA4 3HN — MB BS Lond. 1977; FRCS Eng. 1983. Cons. Surg. ENT W. Glam HA. Specialty: Otolaryngol. Prev: Sen. Regist. (ENT) Soton. Gen. Hosp.
PHILLIPS, Adrian Wilkin Wolverhampton Health Authority, Loncston House, Chapel Ash, Wolverhampton WU3 OXE — MB ChB Birm. 1985; MRCP (UK) 1990; MFPHM 1997. Specialty: Pub. Health Med. Prev: Sen. Regist. (Pub. Health Med.) NHS Exec. W. Midl.; Regist. (Med.) Goodhope Hosp. Sutton Coldfield.
PHILLIPS, Alan Hewett (retired) Myrtle Bank, Allt-yr-Yn Avenue, Newport NP20 5DE Tel: 01633 263546 — MB BS Lond. 1949 (Guy's) MRCS Eng. LRCP Lond. 1949; FFA RCS Eng. 1956. Cons. Anaesth. Roy. Gwent Hosp. Newport. Prev: Sen. Regist. & Regist. Dept. Anaesth. Roy. Infirm. Cardiff.
PHILLIPS, Aled Myrddin Llysgwyn, Cellan, Lampeter SA48 8HY — MB BCh Wales 1994.

PHILLIPS, Aled Owain Institute of Nephrology, Cardiff Royal Infirmary, Cardiff Tel: 029 2049 2233 Fax: 029 2045 3643 Email: phillipsao@cf.ac.uk; 3 Cyncoed Avenue, Cyncoed, Cardiff CF23 6ST — MB BCh Wales 1986; BSc Wales 1983; MRCP (UK) 1989; MD Wales 1995. Sen. Lect. (Nephrol.) Cardiff Roy. Infirm.; Research Fell. Inst. Nephrol. Cardiff Roy. Infirm.; Hon. Cons. Nephrologist/Gen. Phys. Specialty: Nephrol.; Gen. Med. Socs: Renal Assn.; Amer. Soc. Nephrol. Prev: Sen. Regist. (Renal & Gen. Med.) Cardiff Roy. Infirm.; Regist. (Renal) Dulwich Hosp. Lond.; Regist. & SHO Rotat. (Med.) S. Glam. HA.

PHILLIPS, Alexander Blackwood Riverside Medical Centre, Victoria Road, Walton-le-Dale, Preston PR5 4AY Tel: 01772 556703 — MB ChB Dundee 1975; DRCOG 1978.

PHILLIPS, Andrea Jayne 49 Demesne Furze, Headington, Oxford OX3 7XG Tel: 01865 741142 — MB BS Lond. 1989; BSc Lond. 1986; MRCP (UK) 1992; FRCR 1996. Specialist Regist. (Radiol.) John Radcliffe Hosp. Oxf. Specialty: Radiol. Prev: SHO (Cardiol.) Roy. Brompton Nat. Heart & Lung Hosp. Lond.; SHO (Med. & Infec. Dis.) Northwick Pk. Hosp. Harrow.

PHILLIPS, Andrew Alexander 25 Littleton Close, Kenilworth CV8 2WA — MB ChB Aberd. 1981; FCAnaesth. 1990. Cons. Anaesth. Walsgrave Hosps. NHS Trust. Specialty: Anaesth.

PHILLIPS, Andrew Jonathan Department of Anaesthetics, New Cross Hospital, Wolverhampton WV10 0QP Tel: 01902 307999 — MB BS Lond. 1980; BSc Lond. 1977; FRCA 1985. Cons. Anaesth. New Cross Hosp. Wolverhampton. Specialty: Anaesth.

PHILLIPS, Mr Andrew Mark — MB BChir Camb. 1989; FRCS Eng. 1993. Cons. (Orthop.) King's Coll. Hosp. Lond. Specialty: Orthop. Special Interest: Hand Surg.; Limb Reconstruction. Prev: Specialist Regist. (Orthop.) King's Coll. Hosp. Lond.

PHILLIPS, Ann Allister Southfields Group Practice, 7 Revelstoke Road, London SW18 5NJ Tel: 020 8947 0061 Fax: 020 8944 8694; 1 Grangemuir, 2 Southside Common, Wimbledon, London SW19 4TG Tel: 020 8946 1446 — MB BS Lond. 1965 (St. George's Hospital) MRCS Eng. LRCP Lond. 1965. Specialty: Respirat. Med. Prev: Sch. Med. Off. St. Paul's Girls' Sch. Lond.; Clin. Asst. (Chest Med.) St. Geo. Hosp. Lond.

PHILLIPS, Ann Elizabeth Margaret Tal-y-Coed Court, Monmouth NP25 5HR Tel: 01600 85272 — MB BCh Wales 1955.

PHILLIPS, Anne Fiona The Glebeland Surgery, The Glebe, Belbroughton, Stourbridge DY9 9TH Tel: 01562 730303 Fax: 01562 731220; 67 Love Lane, Stourbridge DY8 2DZ — MB ChB Birm. 1987.

PHILLIPS, Anne Frances Crookes Valley Medical Centre, 1 Barber Rd, Sheffield S10 1EA Tel: 0114 266 0703/02920 747747 Fax: 0114 267 8354; 33 Cliffe Road, Walkley, Sheffield S6 5DR Tel: 0114 233 8529 — MB ChB Birm 1953 (Birm.) Asst. GP Crookes Valley Med. Centre Sheff. Specialty: Gen. Pract. Socs: BMA & Christian Med. Fellowsh. Prev: Med. Adviser Benefits Agency Med. Servs.; Dir. of Diocesan Med. Servs. Diocese on the Niger; Med. Supt. Iyi Enu Hosp. Onitsha, Nigeria.

PHILLIPS, Anne Sarah Department of Aneasthetics, Royal Hospitals Trust, Grosvenor Road, Belfast BT12 6BA Tel: 01232 240503; 364 Beersbridge Road, Belfast BT5 5DZ — MD Belf. 1993; MB BCh BAO 1984; DA (UK) 1987; FFA RCSI 1988. Specialty: Anaesth.

PHILLIPS, Anthony Graham Skylarks, Hutton Village, Guisborough TS14 8EP — MB BS Lond. 1984; MA Camb. 1985; DCH RCP Lond. 1987; MRCOG 1994. Cons. Obst. & Gynaecologist James Cook Univ. Hosp. Middlesbrough. Specialty: Obst. & Gyn. Prev: Trainee GP Kingston Hosp. Surrey.

PHILLIPS, Arnold Morley (retired) 74 Chaffers Mead, Ashtead KT21 1NH Tel: 01372 272567 — MB ChB Ed. 1937 (Univ. Ed.) DA Eng. 1962.

PHILLIPS, Barbara Elizabeth Child Development Centre, Heath Lane, Hemel Hempstead HP1 1TT Tel: 01442 232022; 51 Watling Street, St Albans AL1 2QF Tel: 01727 831481 — MB ChB Bristol 1974. Specialty: Psychosexual Med.; Family Plann. & Reproduc. Health. Socs: Inst. Psychosexual Med.

PHILLIPS, Barbara Helen (retired) 7 Bathwick Hill, Bath BA2 6EW — MB BS Lond. 1955 (Univ. Coll. Hosp.) MRCS Eng. LRCP Lond. 1954.

PHILLIPS, Barbara May Alder Hey Children's Hospital, Eaton Road, Liverpool L12 2AP Tel: 0151 228 4811 Fax: 0151 252 5033 — MB ChB Birm. 1969; MRCP (UK) 1973; FRCP Lond. 1990; FFAEM 1993; FRCPCH 1997. Cons. Paediat. (A & E Med.) Alder Hey Childr. Hosp. & Manch. Roy. Infirm.; Chairm. Paediat. Life Support Comm. of Rususcitation Counc. UK; Chairm. Europ. Resusc. Counc. PLS Comm.; Chairm. APLS Working Party. Specialty: Paediat. Socs: Chairm. Brit. Paediat. A & E Gp.; Fell. Fac. A & E Med. (Exam. Comm.). Prev: Cons. Paediat. A & E Med. Booth Hall Childr. Hosp. Manch.

PHILLIPS, Berkeley Simon 15 Rhodes Drive, Bury BL9 8NH — MB BS Lond. 1993.

PHILLIPS, Brenda Joyce Liverpool Women's Hospital NHS Trust, Crown Street, Liverpool L8 7SS Tel: 0151 708 9988 — MB ChB Ghana 1979 (Univ. of Ghana, Legon) FFA RCS Eng. 1987. Cons. Anaesth. Liverp. Women's Hosp., Liverp.; Cons. Anaesth. Roy. Liverp. & Broadgreen Univ. Hospital Trust, Liverp. Specialty: Anaesth. Special Interest: Obst.; Vasc. Socs: Liverpool Society of Anaesthetists; Obstetric Anaesthetists Association; Association of Anaesthetists of GB & Ireland.

PHILLIPS, Brian Lester David Murray House, 5 Vandon Street, London SW1H 0AL Tel: 020 7593 5300 Fax: 020 7593 5301; 5 White Orchards, London N20 8AQ — BM BCh Oxf. 1954 (Oxf. & Roy. Free) BA (Hons.) Oxf. 1951; MA Oxf. 1956; DObst RCOG 1959; AFOM RCP Lond. 1979; T(GP) 1991. Occupat. Health Phys. BMI Health Servs. Specialty: Occupat. Health. Socs: Soc. Occupat. Med. Prev: Occupat. Health Phys. Glaxo Holdings plc; Resid. Med. Off. Matern. Hosp. Beckenham; SHO (Paediat.) Memor. Hosp. P'boro.

PHILLIPS, Brian Morgan (retired) Waitawhiti, Nicholston, Gower, Swansea Tel: 01792 371633 — (St. Geo.) MB BS Lond. 1958; MRCS Eng. LRCP Lond. 1958; FRCP Lond. 1974, M 1960. Prev: Cons. Neurol. Glantawe Hosp. Gp. & Morriston Hosp.

PHILLIPS, Professor Calbert Inglis 5 Braid Mount Crest, Edinburgh EH10 6JN — MB ChB Aberd. 1946; DPH Ed. 1950; DO Eng. 1953; FRCS Eng. 1955; MD Aberd. 1957; PhD Bristol 1961; MSc Manch. 1969; FRCS Ed. 1973; Hon. FBOA 1975; FRCOphth 1993. Emerit. Prof. Edin. Specialty: Ophth.; Genetics. Prev: Prof. Ophth. Univ. Edin. & Hon. Cons. Ophth. Surg. Roy. Infirm. Edin.; Prof. Ophth. Univ. Manch. & Hon. Cons. Ophth. Surg. Univ. Manch.; Cons. Surg. St. Geo. Hosp. Lond.

PHILLIPS, Catherine Jane Cheslyn, Barlaston, Stoke-on-Trent ST12 9DE — BM BS Nottm. 1990.

PHILLIPS, Charles Edward William Pfitzer Limited, Walton Oaks, Dorking Road, Tadworth KT20 7NT Email: charles.phillips@pfizer.com — MB BS Lond. 1992; MRCP 1996; MFPM 2001. Category Medical Manager, Pfiezer. Specialty: Pharmaceutical Medicine. Prev: Sen. Med. Adviser, Sanofi-Synthelabo, Guildford; Research Regist., Roy. Sussex Co. Hosp.; Ho. Off. St. Thos. Hosp. Lond.

PHILLIPS, Charles Russell (retired) Millennium Medical Centre, 121 Weoley Castle Road, Weoley Castle, Birmingham B29 5QD Tel: 0121 427 5201 Fax: 0121 427 5052; 7 Beaks Hill Road, Kings Norton, Birmingham B38 8BJ Tel: 0121 433 5818 — MB ChB Birm. 1958; DObst RCOG 1961. Prev: Ho. Surg. & Ho. Phys. Dudley Rd. Hosp. Birm.

PHILLIPS, Charles William Derek (retired) Ebbor House, Barrack Hill, Hythe CT21 4BY Tel: 01303 267884 Email: zoe@ebbor.freeserve.co.uk — MB BCh BAO Belf. 1956; FRCGP 1981, M 1972.

PHILLIPS, Christian Guy Hambro 2 Cricket Close, Crawley, Winchester SO21 2PX — BM Soton. 1995.

PHILLIPS, Mr Christopher Edward A&E Department, University Hospital of North Durham, North Road, Durham DH1 5TW Tel: 0191 333 2081 — MB BS Newc. 1986; FRCS Ed. 1991; FFAEM 1996. Cons. in Accid. and Emerg., Univ. Hosp. of Durh. Specialty: Accid. & Emerg.

PHILLIPS, Christopher John 34 Rotherwick Road, London NW11 7DA Tel: 020 8455 2421 — MB BS Lond. 1974 (Univ. Coll. Hosp. Lond.) MRCPsych Lond. 1986. Vis. Cons. Rhodes Farm Clinic Lond.; Vis. Cons. Harrow Sch. Middx. Specialty: Child & Adolesc. Psychiat.; Psychother.

PHILLIPS, Christopher John Department of Radiology, Alexandra Hospital, Woodrow Drive, Redditch B60 4BX — MB ChB Leeds 1980; FRCR 1989; MBA Keel University 1999. Cons. Radiol. Alexandra Hosp. Redditch. Specialty: Radiol.; Oncol. Special Interest:

Cross Sectional. Prev: Cons. Radiol. Qu. Eliz. Hosp. Lond.; Sen. Regist. (Radiol.) King's Coll. Hosp. Lond.

PHILLIPS, Claire Patricia 5 Chestnut Rise, Droxford, Southampton SO32 3NY — MB BS Lond. 1988.

PHILLIPS, Clare Frances Macmillan Palliative Care Team, Barts and The London NHS Trust, St. Bartholomew's Hospital, West Smithfield, London EC1A 7BE — MB BS Lond. 1984; BSc (Hons.) Lond. 1981, MB BS 1984. Macmillan Palliat. Care Team Barts and The Lond. NHS Trust St. Bartholomew Hosp. W. Smithfield Lond.

PHILLIPS, Clive William Eveswell Surgery, 254 Chepstow Road, Newport NP19 8NL Tel: 01633 277494 Fax: 01633 290709 — MB BCh Wales 1983; DA (UK) 1985; DRCOG 1987; MRCGP 1988.

PHILLIPS, Corrin Jane Kinnen Dell, Bathgate EH48 4NJ — MB ChB Manch. 1995.

PHILLIPS, Mrs Cynthia Mary 10 Hawkswell Gardens, Oxford OX2 7EX — BM BCh Oxf. 1943 (Oxf. & Univ. Coll. Hosp.) MA, BM BCh Oxf. 1943.

PHILLIPS, David 2 Mereworth Cottages, Lower Cousley Wood, Wadhurst TN5 6EZ — MB BS Lond. 1977.

PHILLIPS, Mr David Esmond Consultant ENT/Head & Neck Surgeon, Warwick Hospital, Lakin Road, Warwick CV34 5BW Tel: 01926 495321 Ext: 4620 Fax: 01926 482607 Email: david.phillips@swh.nhs; Struan, 47 Kenilworth Road, Leamington Spa CV32 6JJ Email: david.phillips@surh.nhs.uk — MB BS Lond. 1982 (Lond. Hosp.) FRCS Ed. 1988; FRCS Eng. 1989. Cons. ENT Surg. Warwick Hosp. Specialty: Otorhinolaryngol. Socs: Brit. Assn. of Otorhino Head & Neck Surgeons; Roy. Soc. Med.; Brit. Rhinological Soc. Prev: Hon. Cons. ENT Roy. Liverp. Univ. Hosp. & Aintree Hosp.; Sen. Lect. (ENT) Univ. Liverp.; Sen. Regist. (ENT) Roy. Liverp. Univ. Trust. Hosp.

PHILLIPS, Professor David Ivor Wyn MRC Environmental Epidemiology Unit, Southampton General Hospital, Tremona Road, Southampton SO16 6YD Tel: 02380 777624 Fax: 02380 704021 Email: diwp@mrc.soton.ac.uk — MB BChir Camb. 1978; MA Camb. 1978; MRCP (UK) 1979; MSc Lond. 1981; PhD Soton. 1985; FRCP (Lond) 1997. Prof. of Endocrine and Metab. Proramming, MRC Environ Epidemiol Unit, Univ. of Southampton; Hon. Cons. Phys. Soton Univ. Hosp. NHS Trust. Specialty: Gen. Med. Socs: Endocrine Soc.; Brit. Diabetes Assn.; Brit. Endocrine Soc. Prev: Lect. (Med.) Univ. Wales Coll. Med.; Wellcome Research Fell. (Clin. Epidemiol.) Univ. Soton.

PHILLIPS, David Llewellyn Caldicot Medical Group, Gray Hill Surgery, Woodstock Way, Caldicot, Newport NP26 4DB Tel: 01291 420282 Fax: 01291 425853; Brookside, Well Lane, Llanvair Discoed, Chepstow NP16 6LP Tel: 01633 400669 — MB BS Lond. 1974 (Kings Coll. Hosp.) PhD Lond. 1970, BSc (Hons.) 1964, MB BS 1974. Princip. Gen. Pract. Caldicot. Prev: Ho. Phys. & Regist. King's Coll. Hosp. Lond.; Lect. (Physiol.) Kings Coll. Lond.

PHILLIPS, David Lynn The Surgery, 75 Longridge Avenue, Saltdean, Brighton BN2 8LA Tel: 01273 305723 Fax: 01273 300962; The Farriers, Mill Lane, Rodmell, Lewes BN7 3HS Tel: 01273 475241 Fax: 01273 477823 Email: rnlidoc@aol.com — MRCS Eng. LRCP Lond. 1974. Hon. Med. Adviser Brighton Lifeboat. Specialty: Gen. Pract.

PHILLIPS, David Wyndham Dr Graetz and Partners, Queen Anne Street, Shelton, Stoke-on-Trent ST4 2EQ Tel: 01782 848642 Fax: 01782 747617; Alpine View, Stone Road, Hill Chorlton, Newcastle ST5 5DR Tel: 01782 680709 Email: 100025.660@compuserve.com — MB ChB Liverp. 1978.

PHILLIPS, Deborah Clare St. Peter's Lodge, 18 1/2 Eastgate, Lincoln LN2 4AA — MB ChB Leeds 1976; FFA RCS Eng. 1980. Specialty: Anaesth.

PHILLIPS, Deborah Joan 12 Crown Mews, Ock St., Abingdon OX14 5DS Tel: 01235 536822 — BM BS Nottm. 1994; FRCS Ed. 1994. Regist. (Gen. Surg.) John Radcliffe Hosp. Oxf. Specialty: Gen. Surg. Prev: SHO (Gen. Surg.) Derriford Hosp. Plymouth & Cheltenham Gen. Hosp.; SHO (Orthop. & ITU) Derriford Hosp. Plymouth; SHO (Orthop. & A & E) & Ho. Off. (Surg.) Qu. Med. Centre Nottm.

PHILLIPS, Diana Margaret Worcestershire Acute Hospitals NHS Trust, Worcestershire Royal Hospital, Charles Hasting Way, Worcester WR5 1DD Tel: 01905 763333; Letts Mill, Hollowfields Road, Hanbury, Redditch B96 6TG Email: diphillips007@aol.com — MB ChB Liverp. 1971; FRCA 1981. p/t Cons. Anaesth. Specialty: Anaesth. Prev: Sen. Regist. Nuffield Dept. Anaesth. Oxf.

PHILLIPS, Diane Heather c/o The Manager, Natwest Bank Plc, PO Box 306, 36 Earlsdon St, Coventry CV3 5ZZ — MB BS Lond. 1985; DA RCA 1987.

PHILLIPS, Donald Leslie (retired) Stock Lodge, Stock, Ingatestone CM4 9BS Tel: 01277 840546 Fax: 01277 841050 — (Middlx.) FRCR 1975; FRCOG 1978. Prev: Cons. Radiotherap. Southend Hosp.

PHILLIPS, Mr Douglas George 42 Over Lane, Almondsbury, Bristol BS32 4BW — MB ChB N.Z. 1935 (Otago) FRCS Eng. 1939. Socs: Soc. Brit. Neurol. Surgs. Prev: Surg. i/c S.W. Regional Neurosurg. Unit Bristol; Clin. Lect. (Neurosurg.) Univ. Bristol; Chief Asst. Neurosurg. Dept. Lond. Hosp.

PHILLIPS, Dylan Gwynne Leyshon Elms Medical Practice, 5 Stewart Road, Harpenden AL5 4QA Tel: 01582 769393 Fax: 01582 461735; 24 Amenbury Lane, Harpenden AL5 2DF — MB BS Lond. 1981 (St. Marys) BSc (Hons.) Lond. 1978; DRCOG 1985; DFFP 1993. Socs: BMA. Prev: Trainee GP Frimley Pk. Hosp. VTS.; Ho. Phys. Profess. Med. Unit St. Mary's Hosp. Lond. W2; Ho. Surg. St. Mary's Hosp. Lond. W2.

PHILLIPS, Edward Hamilton Dalrymple (retired) Herne Cottage, Smuggler's Way, The Sands, Farnham GU10 1NA Tel: 01252 782850 — MRCS Eng. LRCP Lond. 1935 (Camb. & St. Bart .) BA Camb. 1932; DA Eng. 1945. Prev: Maj. RAMC, Specialist Anaesth.

PHILLIPS, Eileen Blossom Field House, 53 Knowsley Road, Wilpshire, Blackburn BB1 9PN — MB ChB Ed. 1959.

PHILLIPS, Eileen Margaret — MB BS Lond. 1966 (St. Bart.) BSc (Hons. Pharmacol.) Lond. 1970, MD 1975, MB BS 1966; FRCP Lond. 1985, M 1969; BSc (Hons. Pharmacol.) 1970; MD 1975. Cons. Phys. Gastroenterol. E. Surrey Hosp. Surrey Sussex Healthcare Trust; Chairm., STC G(1)M, S. Thames. Specialty: Gastroenterol. Socs: Fell. Roy. Soc. Med.; Brit. Soc. Gastroenterol.; BMA. Prev: Sen. Regist. (Med.) St. Geo. Hosp. Lond.; MRC Clin. Research Fell. & Hon. Assoc. Chief Asst. St. Bart. Hosp. Lond.

PHILLIPS, Elfyn Arfon 32 Melyd Avenue, Johnstown, Wrexham LL14 2TB — MB ChB Liverp. 1994.

PHILLIPS, Elizabeth Mary Gibbon The Liver Unit, Freeman Hospital, Newcastle upon Tyne NE7 7DN; 132 Kenton Lane, Gosforth, Newcastle upon Tyne NE3 3QE — MB BS Newc. 1986; BMedSc Newc. 1983; MRCP (UK) 1989. Sen. Regist. (Med.) Freeman Hosp. Newc. u. Tyne. Specialty: Gastroenterol. Prev: Research Regist. (Med.) Univ. Newc.; Regist. (Med.) Ashington Gen. Hosp. N.d.

PHILLIPS, Ernest Prabhu Kumar Trent View Medical Practice, 45 Trent View, Keadby, Scunthorpe DN17 3DR Tel: 01724 782209 Fax: 01724 784472; 9 Acer Grove, Silica Lodge, Scunthorpe DN17 2AJ — MB BS Osmania 1965 (Osmania Med. Coll. Hyderabad)

PHILLIPS, Gareth Huw Department of Anaesthetics, Princess Royal Hospital, Telford Tel: 01952 641222 Ext: 4522 — MB ChB Bristol 1980; FRCA London 1985. Cons. Anaesth., Princess Roy. Hosp., Telford. Specialty: Anaesth.; Paediat.; Orthop. Socs: BMA; HCSA; AAGBI. Prev: Sen. Regist., Univ. Hosp. of Wales, Cardiff; Assoc. Prof., Univ. of W. Texas, Lubbock, Texas; Regist., Univ. Hosp. of Wales, Cardiff.

PHILLIPS, Gareth Rhys The Rogerstone Practice, Chapel Wood, Western Valley Road, Newport NP10 9DU Tel: 01752 763789 — MB BCh Wales 1988; BPharm (Hons.) 1979; MRPharms 1980; DPD 1992. GP Princip. Socs: Roy. Pharmaceut. Soc. Gt. Brit.

PHILLIPS, Geoffrey 7 Garth Drive, Calderstones, Liverpool L18 6HN — MB BCh Wales 1976; MRCP (UK) 1978; FRCP Lond. 1993. Cons. Geriat. Broadgreen Hosp. Liverp. Specialty: Care of the Elderly. Prev: Sen. Regist. (Geriat. Med.) Newsham Gen. Hosp. Liverp.; Regist. (Med.) Broadgreen Hosp. Liverp.; Ho. Phys. Llandough Hosp. Penarth.

PHILLIPS, George Bevan 104 Belgrave Road, Loughor, Swansea SA4 6RE Tel: 01792 2218 — MB BS Lond. 1956 (St. Geo.) MRCS Eng. LRCP Lond. 1955. Anaesth. Glantawe, Hosp. Gp.; Med. Off. Bowden Engin. Co. (LLa.lly); Apptd. Fact. Doctor. Socs: BMA. Prev: Ho. Surg., Ho. Phys. & Ho. Off. Anaesth. Roy. Hosp. Wolverhampton.

PHILLIPS, Gerrard David Dorset County Hospital, Williams Avenue, Dorchester DT1 2JY — MB BS Lond. 1978; MA Oxf. 1975; LMSSA Lond. 1978; MRCP (UK) 1982; DM Soton. 1991; FRCP 1998. Cons. Thoracic & Gen. Med. W. Dorset Gen. Hosps. NHS

Trust. Specialty: Respirat. Med. Socs: SAC Respirat. Med.; Brit. Thorac. Soc.; Chairm. Educat. and Train. Comm. Prev: Sen. Regist. (Thoracic & Gen. Med.) Brompton Hosp. St. Geo. Hosp. Lond.; Clin. Research Fell. Soton. Univ.; Regist. (Med.) Roy. Vict. Hosp. Boscombe & Westm. Hosp. Lond.

PHILLIPS, Glenys 22 Downham Chase, Timperley, Altrincham WA15 7TJ — MB BCh Wales 1968; FFA RCS Eng. 1972. Cons. Anaesth. Wythenshawe Hosp. Manch. Specialty: Anaesth.

PHILLIPS, Glyn Michael Greenhills Health Centre, 20 Greenhills Square, East Kilbride, Glasgow G75 8TT Tel: 01355 236331 Fax: 01355 234977; 36 Queensberry Avenue, Clarkston, Glasgow G76 7DU — MB ChB Leeds 1980 (Univ. Leeds) MRCGP 1986; DRCOG 1988. Prev: Med. Off. HMS Revenge (S); SHO (A & E) RN Hosp. Plymouth; SHO (Dermat.) South. Gen. Hosp. Glas.

PHILLIPS, Gwen Elizabeth Hodgson Oxford Road Medical Centre, 25 Oxford Road, Burnley BB11 3BB Tel: 01282 423603 Fax: 01282 832827; Meadow Bank, 7 Watt St, Burnley BB12 8AA Tel: 01282 426716 — MB BS Newc. 1980; BA (Hons.) Camb. 1977. Prev: Clin. Med. Off. (Family Plann.) Burnley, Pendle & Rossendale HA.

PHILLIPS, Gwyn William (retired) Maes-yr-Afon, Felindre Road, Pencoed, Bridgend CF35 5PB Tel: 01656 860998 — MB BCh Wales 1962 (Welsh Nat. Sch. Med.) DObst RCOG 1969. Prev: Research Schol. (Pharmacol.) Welsh. Nat. Sch. Med. Cardiff.

PHILLIPS, Hamish Andrew Dept. of Clinical Oncology, Western General Hospital, Edinburgh EH4 2XU Tel: 0131 537 1000 — MB BChir Camb. 1986; BSc (Hons.) St. And. 1984; MRCP (UK) 1990; MSc (Clin. Oncol.) Ed. 1993; FRCR 1995; MD Edin. 1998. Cons. (Clin. Oncol.) W. Gen. Hosp. Edin. Specialty: Oncol. Prev: Sen. Regist. (Clin. Oncol.) West. Gen. Hosp. Edin.; Clin. Research Fell. (Clin. Oncol.) West. Gen. Hosp. Edin.; Regist. (Clin. Oncol.) West. Gen. Hosp. Edin.

PHILLIPS, Helen Claire Langholm Health Centre, Langholm, Langholm DG13 0LR; Arresgill Farm, Langholm DG13 0LR — MB ChB Manch. 1989; DCH 1991; MRCGP 1996. GP Princip. Langholm. Specialty: Gen. Pract. Socs: RCGP.

PHILLIPS, Helen Margaret Burney Street Practice, 48 Burney Street, Greenwich, London SE10 8EX Tel: 020 8858 0631 Fax: 020 8293 9616; 6 The Orchard, Blackheath, London SE3 0QS Tel: 020 8297 1600 Fax: 020 8297 1684 Email: helen@phillipsfamily.u-net.com — MB BS Lond. 1988; DCH RCP Lond. 1991; DRCOG 1992; MRCGP 1994. Specialty: Gen. Psychiat.; Obst. & Gyn.; Paediat.

PHILLIPS, Helen Victoria 53 Tottehale Close, North Baddesley, Southampton SO52 9NQ Tel: 023 8073 3490 — MB ChB Birm. 1995; DRCOG 1997; Dip. Fac. Family Planning 1998; MRCGP 1999. GP Retainer. Specialty: Gen. Pract. Prev: GP; GP Regist. Soton.; GP Locum.

PHILLIPS, Mr Hugh — MB BS Lond. 1964 (St. Bart.) BSc (Hons.) Lond. 1961; FRCS Eng. 1970. p/t Cons. Orthop. Surg., Norf. & Norwich NHS Health Care Trust; Vice Pres., Roy. Coll. of Surgeons; Hon. Sen. Lect., Univ. of E. Anglia. Specialty: Orthop. Special Interest: Jt. Replacement. Socs: Fell. BOA; Roy. Soc. Med.; Brit. Hip Soc. Prev: Past Chairm. Specialist Adv. Comm. Orthop. Surg 1995-1997; Pres. Brit. Orthopaedic Assn. 1999-2000; Pres. Brit. Hip Soc. 1998-2000.

PHILLIPS, Iain Geoffrey Wincanton Health Centre, Carrington Way, Wincanton BA9 9JY Tel: 01963 32000 Fax: 01963 32146 Email: dr.phillips@wincantonhc.nhs.uk — MB BS Lond. 1985 (Charing Cross and Westminster) MRCGP 1990. Specialty: Gen. Pract.

PHILLIPS, Professor Ian (retired) — (Camb. & St. Thos.) MB BChir Camb. 1961; MA Camb. 1962, MD 1966; FRCPath 1981, M 1969; FRCP Lond. 1983, M 1978; FFPHM RCP (UK) 1997. Emerit. Prof. Med. Microbiol. United. Med. & Dent. Schs. Guy's & St. Thos. Hosp. Lond.; Emerit. Hon. Cons. Bacteriol. Guy's & St. Thos. Hosp. Lond. Prev: Lect. (Med. Microbiol.) Makerere Univ. Coll. Kampala, Uganda.

PHILLIPS, James Neil Janssen-Cilag Ltd, PO Box 79, Saunderton, High Wycombe HP14 4HJ — MB ChB Bristol 1988; MBA Lond. 1991; MRCGP 1994; DFFP 1994. Specialty: Gen. Pract. Prev: Non-Exec. Dir. W. Sussex DHA.

PHILLIPS, James Ronald Nigel Consultant Physician, Queen Elizabeth Hospital, Gayton Road, King's Lynn PE30 4ET Tel: 01553 613895 Fax: 01553 613900 — MB BS Lond. 1989 (Char. Cross & Westm.) MRCP (UK) 1993. Cons. Phys. (Gen. Med.) c/o the Elderly. Specialty: Gen. Med.; Care of the Elderly. Prev: Sen. Regist. (Gen. Med. & Elderly Care) Chelsea & West. Hosp. Lond.; Sen. Regist. (Gen. Med. & Elderly Care) Lister Hosp. Stevenage.

PHILLIPS, James William 32 Villiers Road, Woodthorpe, Nottingham NG5 4FB — MB BS Newc. 1996.

PHILLIPS, Jane Hilary 95 Park Avenue, Ruislip HA4 7UL — MB ChB Leic. 1996.

PHILLIPS, Jason — MB BCh Wales 1992.

PHILLIPS, Jean Dorothy (retired) Bryn Hyfryd, Rhydwyn, Holyhead LL65 4ED Tel: 01407 730744 — (Liverp.) MB ChB Liverp. 1951. Prev: SCMO Community Child Health Serv. Liverp. HA.

PHILLIPS, Jeannette Veronica Constantia, 18 Mill Road, Rochester ME2 3BT — MB BS Lond. 1980; MRCP (UK) 1987; MRCPsych 1994.

PHILLIPS, Jeffrey Alan James Princess Alexandre Hospital, Harlow CM20 1QX — MB BS Lond. 1990 (St. Mary's Hosp. Med. Sch.) BSc Lond. 1987; FRCA 1996. Cons. In Intens. Care & Anaesthetics. Specialty: Anaesth.; Intens. Care. Prev: SHO (Anaesth.) St. Bart. Hosp., Homerton Hosp. Lond. & Hillingdon Hosp. Middx.; Specialist Regist. Rotat. (Anaesth.) UCH & Middlx. Hosps. Lond.

PHILLIPS, Jeremy Keith The Surgery, Lorne Street, Lochgilphead PA31 8LU Tel: 01546 602921 Fax: 01546 606735 — MRCS Eng. LRCP Lond. 1984; DRCOG 1988; MRCGP 1990.

PHILLIPS, John 26 Buckingham Terrace, Edinburgh EH4 3AE — MB ChB Ed. 1975; MRCGP 1979.

PHILLIPS, John Andrew (retired) 60 Old Rossorry Road, Enniskillen BT74 7LF Tel: 028 6632 9359 Email: john@thephillipses.fsnet.co.uk — MB ChB Ed. 1962; DCH Glas. 1964; DRCOG Lond. 1965; MRCP (UK) 1971; MSc Lond. 1992; FRCP Lond. 1992; FRCP Ed. 1995; FRCPCH 1996. Prev: Paediat. Erne Hosp. Enniskillen.

PHILLIPS, Mr John Barrie (cons. rooms), 7 Greenhill Court, 25B Green Lane, Northwood HA6 2UZ Tel: 01923 826948; 15 Hill Crescent, Totteridge, London N20 8HB Tel: 020 8445 0932 Fax: 020 8445 8499 — (Univ. Coll. Lond. & Univ. Coll. Hosp.) MB BS Lond. 1959; MRCS Eng. LRCP Lond. 1960; FRCS Eng. 1965. Northwood Pinner Dist. Hosp. & St. Vincent's Orthop. Hosp. Pinner; Assoc. Cons. Roy. Masonic Hosp. Lond; Hon. Cons. Orthop. Surg. Roy. Masonic Sch. Girls & Merchant Taylors Sch. Boys Northwood. Specialty: Orthop. Socs: Fell. Roy. Soc. Med. & BOA. Prev: Cons. Orthop. Surg. Mt. Vernon Hosp. N.wood, Harefield Hosp.; Sen. Regist. (Orthop.) Roy. Free Hosp. Lond. & Windsor Gp. Hosps.; Regist. Roy. Nat. Orthop. Hosp.

PHILLIPS, John Dale The Burnham Surgery, Foundry Lane, Burnham-on-Crouch CM0 8SJ Tel: 01621 782054 Fax: 01621 785592; 33 Maple Way, Burnham-on-Crouch CM0 8DF — MB BS Lond. 1963 (St. Bart.) MRCS Eng. LRCP Lond. 1963; DObst RCOG 1966; MRCGP 1976. Socs: BMA (Clin. Ecology Gp.) & Brit. Soc. Med. & Dent. Hypn. Prev: Obst. Ho. Off. Forest Gate Hosp.; SHO (Neurol. & Chest Dis.) Whipps Cross Hosp. Lond.; SHO (Psychiat.) Claybury Hosp. Woodford Bridge.

PHILLIPS, Mr John Edward 32 Dalhousie Terrace, Edinburgh EH10 5PD Tel: 0131 447 3334 — MB ChB Liverp. 1973; FRCS Ed. 1979. Cons. Orthop. Surg. Borders Gen. Hosp. Melrose. Specialty: Orthop. Prev: Sen. Regist. Lothian Health Bd; Lect. Univ. Edin.; Cons. Orthop. Surg. Khoula Hosp. Muscat, Oman.

PHILLIPS, John Ernest (retired) Hawkes Barn, Hawkes Lane, Bracon Ash, Norwich NR14 8EW Tel: 01508 578576 Fax: 01508 578576 — MB BCh Wales 1959; DPM Eng. 1965; CRCP Canada 1968; FRCPsych 1987, M 1971. Prev: Cons. Psychiat. S. Devon Health Care Trust & Exe Vale Hosp. Exminster.

PHILLIPS, John Gareth Maxillo-Facial Unit, Glan Clwyd Hospital, Bodelwyddan, Rhyl LL18 5UJ Tel: 01745 534309 Fax: 01745 534296; 81 Marine Drive, Colwyn Bay LL28 4HT — MB ChB Bristol 1980; LDS Durham 1962; FDS RCPS Glas. 1973; FFD RCSI 1974; FDS RCS Eng. 1974; MRCS Eng. LRCP Lond. 1981. Cons. Maxillo-facial Unit Glan Clwyd Hosp. Bodelwyddan. Specialty: Oral & Maxillofacial Surg.

PHILLIPS, John Jeffery (retired) 102 Harewood Avenue, Bournemouth BH7 6NS Tel: 01202 394919 — MB ChB Leeds 1941; MFCM 1974. Prev: Sen. Med. Off. E. Dorset Health Dist.

PHILLIPS, John Kendrick Field House, 53 Knowsley Road, Wilpshire, Blackburn BB1 9PN — MB ChB Ed. 1957.

PHILLIPS, John Michael (retired) 4 Ashlar Court, Marlborough Road, Swindon SN3 1QW Tel: 01793 527844 — MB BS Lond. 1957 (St. Thos.) BSc Lond. 1954, MB BS 1957. Prev: GP Swindon.

PHILLIPS, John Norman 2 Kitcat Terrace, London E3 2SA — LMSSA Lond. 1947 (Lond. Hosp.)

PHILLIPS, John Peter Keith Avondale Health Centre, Avondale St., Bolton BL1 4JP Fax: 01204 493751; 8 Grasmere Avenue, Whitefield, Manchester M45 7GN — MB ChB Manch. 1982. Specialty: Gen. Pract.

PHILLIPS, Julia Katharine Haematology Department, Royal Hallamshire Hospital, Glossop Road, Sheffield S10 2JF Tel: 0114 271 1900; 57 Evelyn Road, Crookes, Sheffield S10 5FE Tel: 0114 268 7397 — (Liverp.) MB ChB Liverp. 1981; MRCP (UK) 1985; MD Liverp. 1996; MRCPath 1997. Sen. Regist. (Haemat.) Sheff. Train. Scheme. Specialty: Haematology. Prev: Lect. & Hon. Sen. Regist. (Haemat.) St. Thos. Hosp. Lond.; Regist. (Haemat.) Roy. Liverp. Hosp. & Broadgreen Hosp. Liverp.; Research Fell. & Hon. Sen. Regist. (Haemat.) Roy. Liverp. Hosp.

PHILLIPS, Julia Margaret (retired) 87 Mayals Avenue, Mayals, Swansea SA3 5DD — MB ChB Birm. 1964.

PHILLIPS, June (retired) 15 Greenhill Road, Liverpool L18 6JJ Tel: 0151 724 1940 — MB ChB Liverp. 1956; DPH Liverp. 1959; FFPHM RCP (UK) 1982, M 1974. Prev: Dir. Pub. Health Liverp. HA.

PHILLIPS, Karl 10 Islay Drive, Newton Mearns, Glasgow G77 6UD — MB ChB Dundee 1981; BMSc (Hons.) Dund 1978, MB ChB 1981; MRCPsych 1985. Cons. Psychiat. Dykebar Hosp. Paisley. Specialty: Geriat. Psychiat. Prev: Sen. Regist. Gtr. Glas. HB; Research Regist. Crighton Roy. Hosp. Dumfries; Regist. (Psychiat.) Roy. Dundee Liff Hosp.

PHILLIPS, Katherine Gemma Peacock Farmhouse, 29 Main St., Kirby Bellars, Melton Mowbray LE14 2EA — BM BS Nottm. 1993.

PHILLIPS, Kay Anne Pensby Walk Practice, 8 Pensby Walk, Miles Platting, Manchester M40 8GN Tel: 0161 205 2867 Fax: 0161 205 2972 — MB ChB Manch. 1990.

PHILLIPS, Kenneth David 10 Harley Street, London W1G 9PF Tel: 020 8868 0338; 47 Azalea Walk, Pinner HA5 2EH Tel: 020 8868 7426 Fax: 020 8868 9273 Email: k.d.phillips@which.net — MB BS Lond. 1954. Private Practitioner (Psychother.) Lond. Specialty: Psychother. Special Interest: Adult ADHD; Post Abortion/Miscarriage Trauma. Socs: Brit. Soc. Med. & Dent. Hypn.; Brit. Soc. Experim. & Clin. Hypn.

PHILLIPS, Kevin Willow Tree Lodge, 9 Grosvenor Place, Beverley HU17 8LY — MB ChB Leeds 1986; MRCOG 1991. Cons. (British Soc. of Gyn. Endoscopy) Castlehill Hosp. Cotttingham. Specialty: Obst. & Gyn. Socs: Glas. Obst. & Gyn. Soc. Prev: Sen. Regist. (O & G) Glas. Roy. Infirm Glas.; Regist. (O & G) Ayrsh. Centr. Hosp. & Qu. Mother's Hosp. Glas.; Regist. (O & G) ChristCh. Wom. Hosp., NZ.

PHILLIPS, Laurence (Surgery), 266 Lea Bridge Road, London E10 Tel: 020 8539 1221; 194 Clarence Gate Gardens, Glentworth St., London NW1 6AU Tel: 020 7723 5439 — MRCS Eng. LRCP Lond. 1947 (Middlx.) Socs: Local Med. Comm. Co. Lond. Prev: Clin. Asst. (Gyn.) Hackney Hosp.

PHILLIPS, Leighton John Brockencote, Chaddesley Corbett, Kidderminster DY10 4PT — MB ChB Leic. 1996.

PHILLIPS, Lesley Jane City Way Surgery, 67 City Way, Rochester ME1 2AY Tel: 01634 843351 Fax: 01634 830421 — MB BS Lond. 1986; DRCOG 1988. Prev: Trainee GP Dartford & Gravesham VTS.

PHILLIPS, Louise Angela 325 Boldmere Road, Sutton Coldfield B73 5HQ — MB ChB Manch. 1997 (Manchester) Alder Hey Childr.s Hosp. Liverp. Specialty: Paediat.

PHILLIPS, Malcolm Edward Charing Cross Hospital, Fulham Palace Road, London W6 8RF Tel: 020 8846 7591 Fax: 020 8846 7589 Email: mphillipsesher@aol.com — MB BS Lond. 1964 (Char. Cross) MRCS Eng. LRCP Lond. 1964; MRCP (UK) 1970; MD Lond. 1979; FRCP Lond. 1986. Cons. Phys. & Nephrol. Char. Cross Hosp. Lond.; Hon. Cons. Nephrol. Chelsea & Westm. Hosp. Lond.; Hon. Cons. Phys. & Nephrol. W. Middlx. Univ. Hosp. Isleworth. Specialty: Nephrol.; Gen. Med. Prev: Lect., Hon. Sen. Regist. & Regist. (Med.) Char. Cross Hosp. Lond.; Wellcome Research Fell. (Nephrol.) Univ. Naples, Italy.

PHILLIPS, Malcolm John (retired) Luffield Cottage, Rumwell, Taunton TA4 1EJ Tel: 01823 461509 — MB ChB Sheff. 1954; DCP Lond 1960; FRCPath 1976, M 1964; DTM & H Eng. 1964. Hons. Cons. Clin. Haemat. Taunton & Som. Hosp. NHS Trust; Clin. Tutor Univ. Bristol; Research Fell. Univ. Exeter. Prev: Ho. Phys. Profess. Med. & Cardiol. Units City Gen. Hosp. Sheff.

PHILLIPS, Malcolm Kenneth Crawcrook Medical Centre, Back Chamberlain Street, Crawcrook, Ryton NE40 4TZ Tel: 0191 413 2243 Fax: 0191 413 8098; Tynedale, 53 Woodcroft Road, Wylam NE41 8DH Tel: 01661 852546 — MB BS Newc. 1970; MRCGP 1974. Prev: Trainee GP VTS.

PHILLIPS, Margaret Frances Pulmonary & Rehabilitation Research Group, University Clinical Department at Aintree, University Hospital Aintree, Liverpool L9 7AL Tel: 0151 529 2946 Fax: 0151 529 2931 — MB BCh Wales 1989 (Univ. Wales Coll. Med.) BSc (Hons.) Physiol. Wales 1986; MRCP 1992. Hon. Specialist Regist. (Rehabil. Med.) Fazakerley Hosp. Liverp.; Lect. (Med. Rehabil.) Univ. of Liverp. Specialty: Rehabil. Med. Socs: Brit. Soc. Rehabil. Med.; Soc. for Research in Rehabil.; World Muscle Soc. Prev: Research Fell. Inst. Med. Genetics Univ. Wales Coll. Med.; SHO (A & E) Sandwell Dist. Gen. Hosp. W. Bromwich; SHO (Med.) Dudley Rd. Hosp. Birm. & Roy. Gwent Hosp. Newport.

PHILLIPS, Marie Gabrielle Anne Medical Microbiology, Ninewells Hospital, Dundee DD1 9SY Tel: 01382 633183 Email: gabby.phillips@tuht.scot.nhs.uk — MB BS Lond. 1981; MRCPath 1988. Cons. Microbiol. Ninewells Hosp. & Med. Sch. Dundee. Specialty: Med. Microbiol.; Virology; Infec. Dis. Socs: HIS; AMM; BSAC. Prev: Sen. Regist. & Hon. Lect. Ninewells Hosp. & Med. Sch. Dundee.

PHILLIPS, Mark Anthony Thomas 69 Walter Street, Stockton-on-Tees TS18 3PP — MB ChB Sheff. 1995.

PHILLIPS, Mark Christopher Read Bird-in-Eye Surgery, Uckfield Community Hospital, Framfield Road, Uckfield TN22 5AW Tel: 01825 763196; Delgany, Belmont Road, Uckfield TN22 1BP Tel: 01825 763191 — MB BS Lond. 1973 (St. Bart.) Clin. Asst. Uckfield Hosp. Prev: SHO (Orthop.) Barnet Gen. Hosp.; Ho. Phys. & Ho. Surg. Orpington Hosp.

PHILLIPS, Mark Leslie Clifford The Health Centre, Charles Street, Langholm DG13 0JY; Arresgill Farm, Langholm DG13 0LR — MB ChB Liverp. 1988 (Univ. Liverp.) MRCGP 1992; DTM & H Liverp. 1993. SHO (Orthop. & Trauma) Lancaster; Resid. Med. Off. Chatham Is. NZ. Specialty: Gen. Pract. Prev: Trainee GP Lancaster VTS; Ho. Phys. & Ho. Surg. Ormskirk Dist. Gen. Hosp.

PHILLIPS, Martin The Newbridge Surgery, 255 Tettenhall Road, Wolverhampton WV6 0ED Tel: 01902 751420 Fax: 01902 747936 — MB BS Lond. 1977 (St. Mary's) DA (UK) 1985. Specialty: Anaesth.

PHILLIPS, Martin Geoffrey Dept. of Gastroenterology, University Hospital Lewisham, Lewisham High St., London SE13 6LH; 14 Camborne Road, Southfields, London SW18 4BJ — MB BS Lond. 1991 (St Mary's Hospital) BSc Lond. 1988; MRCP (UK) 1994. Specialty: Gen. Med.; Gastroenterol.; Intens. Care. Socs: Asst. Sec. BMA; BASL. Prev: Regist. (Hepatol.) Inst. Of Liver Studies, King's Coll. Hosp. Lond.; Regist. (Gastrol.) Roy. Surrey Co. Hosp. Guildford; SHO (Gen. Med.) Addenbrooke's Hosp. Camb.

PHILLIPS, Martin Ronald James Street Practice, 4 James Street, Crossgar, Downpatrick BT30 9JU — MB BCh BAO Belf. 1967.

PHILLIPS, Mary (retired) 1 Briarwood Road, Woodbridge IP12 4DQ — MB BS Lond. 1964 (St. Bart.) DObst RCOG 1966.

PHILLIPS, Mary Gordon (retired) Southwood, Gordon Road, Horsham RH12 2EF Tel: 01403 52894 — (Roy. Free) MB BS Lond. 1945.

PHILLIPS, Mary Louise — MB BChir Camb. 1990 (Cambridge) MA Camb. 1990, BA 1986; MSc Keele 1989; MRCPsych 1994; MD Camb. 2000. Prof. Inst. of Psychiat. Lond.; Hon. Cons. Psychiat., Maudsley Hosp. Specialty: Gen. Psychiat. Prev: Hon. Lect. Inst. of Psychiat. Lond.; Clin. Lect. Inst. of Psychiat. Lond.; Hon Sen. Lect.. Inst. of Psychiatary Lond.

PHILLIPS, Mr Michael John Mailpoint 67, Southampton General Hospital, Southampton SO16 6YD Tel: 02380 798802 Email: michael.phillips@suht.swest.nhs.uk — BM Soton. 1986; FRCS Eng. 1990; FRCS (Gen. Sug.) 1998; MS Southampton 1998. Cons. Vasc. & Gen. Surg., Soton. Univ. NHS Trust; Surgic. Tutor, Soton. Specialty: Gen. Surg. Socs: VSS GB & Ire.; Assn. of Surg.s; Europ.

Soc. Vasc. Surg. Prev: Regist. (Gen. Surg.)Wessex Rotat.; Vasc. Research Fell. Thrombosis Research Inst. Lond.; Vasc. Fell., Roy. Adelaide Hosp.

PHILLIPS, Michelle Elaine 22 Bramley Road, Bramhall, Stockport SK7 2DP — MB BS Lond. 1993.

PHILLIPS, Morley Clayton Owen (retired) Pendragon, Station Hill, Lelant, St Ives TR26 3DJ Tel: 01736 752282 — (St. Mary's) MA Camb. 1955; MRCS Eng. LRCP Lond. 1960; MB BS Lond. 1961; DObst RCOG 1962. Prev: Ho. Surg. Surgic. Unit St. Mary's Hosp. Lond.

PHILLIPS, Nansi Eluned Local Health Partnerships NHS Trust, Elm Street Clinic, Elm St., Ipswich IP1 1HB Tel: 01473 275200 Email: nansi@copthall.freeserve.co.uk; Great Copt Hall, Bildeston, Ipswich IP7 7BH — MB BCh Wales 1975; DCH Eng. 1978; FRCPCH 1997. Cons. Community Child Health (Audiol.), L.H.P. NHS Trust, Ipswich. Specialty: Paediat. Prev: SCMO (Child Health) E. Suff. HA.

PHILLIPS, Naomi Noble Vinayakumar Radford Health Centre, Ilkeston Road, Nottingham NG7 3GW Tel: 0115 979 1313 Fax: 0115 979 1470 — MB BS Osmania 1971 (Gandhi Med. Coll. Hyderabad) DObst RCOG 1974. Prev: SHO (O & G) Doncaster Roy. Infirm. & Nottm. Hosp. Wom.

PHILLIPS, Mr Nicholas Ian Department of Neurosurgery, Leeds General Infirmary, Great George St., Leeds LS1 3EX — MB ChB Ed. 1988; BSc Leeds 1980; PhD Lond. 1983; FRCS Eng. 1992; FRCS (SN) 1996. SHO Rotat. (Surg.) Leeds Gen. Infirm.; Regist. (Neurosurg.) Qu. Med. Centre Nottm.; Cons. Neurosurg. Leeds Gen. Infirm. Specialty: Neurosurg. Prev: SHO (Cas.) Manch. Roy. Infirm.; Ho. Phys. Edin. Roy. Infirm.

PHILLIPS, Noble Vinaya-Kumar 14 Pavillion Road, Bestwood Lodge, Nottingham NG5 8NL Tel: 0115 202077; (Surgery) 112 Graylands Road, Bilborough, Nottingham NG8 4FD Tel: 0115 929 2358 — MB BS Osmania 1969 (Osmania Med. Coll. Hyderabad & India) DA Eng. 1975. Prev: Regist. (Anaesth.) Nottm. City Hosp.

PHILLIPS, Patricia Coulson The Keston House Medical Practice, 70 Brighton Road, Purley CR8 2LJ Tel: 020 8660 8292 Fax: 020 8763 2142 — MB BS Lond. 1974.

PHILLIPS, Paul David Scarborough Hospital, Scarborough YO12 6QL; 4 Welbourn Drive, Seamer, Scarborough YO12 4RP — MB ChB Leeds 1993. GP/Regist. ScarBoro. VTS. Specialty: Gen. Pract.

PHILLIPS, Penelope Kate 9 Witham Lodge, Witham CM8 1HG — BM Soton. 1991.

PHILLIPS, Peter Alan Ipswich Hospital, Department of Medicine for the Elderly, Heath Road Wing, Ipswich IP4 5PD Tel: 01473 704134 Fax: 01473 704166 Email: peter.phillips@ipswichhospital.nhs.uk; 118 Constable Road, Ipswich IP4 2XA Tel: 01473 401184 Fax: 01473 704166 — MB BS Queensland 1974; MB BS (1st cl. Hons.) Queensland 1974; FRCP Lond. 1995. Cons. Phys. (Geriat. Med + Gen. Med..) Ipswich Hosp.; Lead Clinician, Dept. of Med. for the Elderly, Ipswich Hosp. Specialty: Care of the Elderly; Gen. Med. Socs: Brit. Assn. of Stroke Physicians; Brit. Geriat. Soc. Prev: Dir. Geriat. Med. P. Chas. Hosp. Brisbane, Austral.

PHILLIPS, Peter David — MB BS Lond. 1976 (St Mary's) BSc (Biochem.) Birm. 1967; FRCA Lond. 1981. Cons. Anaesth. Norwich. Specialty: Anaesth.

PHILLIPS, Peter Gerard 67 Penwinnick Road, St Austell PL25 5DS Email: peter_phillips@sandwich.pfizer.com — MB BS Lond. 1993. Specialty: Respirat. Med.; Gen. Med.

PHILLIPS, Peter James Giffords Primary Care Centre, Spa Road, Melksham SN12 7EA Tel: 01225 703370; Giffords, Lowbourne, Melksham Tel: 01225 703320 — MB ChB Bristol 1974; DRCOG 1979; DCH Eng. 1980; MRCGP 1981. Gen. Med. Pract. Melksham.

PHILLIPS, Peter Rolleston Pendyffryn Medical Group, Ffordd Pendyffryn, Prestatyn LL19 9DH Tel: 01745 886444 Fax: 01745 889831 — MB ChB Manch. 1981; BSc (Med. Sci.) St. And. 1978. Specialty: Gen. Pract.

PHILLIPS, Philippa Margaret 76 Ormiston Road, Greenwich, London SE10 0LN Tel: 020 8853 4009 — BM BCh Oxf. 1987; MA Camb. 1988; MCOphth 1990; FRCOphth 1994. Clin. Asst. Qu. Mary's Hosp. Lond. Specialty: Ophth. Prev: Regist. (Ophth.) Greenwich Dist. Hosp. Lond.; Research Fell. (Ophth.) Roy. Free Hosp. Lond.; SHO (Ophth.) Roy. Free Hosp. Lond.

PHILLIPS, Rachel Rhodes 144 Walton Street, Oxford OX1 2HG Email: rachelrp@aol.com — MB ChB Leeds 1982 (Univ. Leeds) DCH RCP Lond. 1984; MRCP (UK) 1986; FRCR 1990. Cons. Radiol. The Churchill Hosp. Oxford. Specialty: Radiol. Socs: Radiol. Soc. N. Amer.; Brit. Soc. Skeletal Radiol.; NW Soc. Paediat. Radiol. (USA, Canad). Prev: Cons. Radiol. Whittington Hosp. Lond.; Hon. Sen. Lect. Dept. Med. Imaging UCL; Mem. Standing Comm. Mems. RCP.

PHILLIPS, Rhodri Linkwood, Hornbeam Lane, London E4 7QT — MB BCh Wales 1992.

PHILLIPS, Richard Charles Saxonbrook Medical, Maidenbower Square, Crawley RH10 7QH Tel: 01293450400 Fax: 01293 450401 Email: richard@saxonbrook.co.uk; 156 Buckswood Drive, Crawley RH11 8JF Tel: 01293 513317 — MB BS Lond. 1972 (St. Geo.) DObst RCOG 1975; Cert FPA 1976; MRCGP 1976. Sen. Partner Saxonbrook Med.; Med. Off. to Fire Brig. Specialty: Gen. Pract.; Occupat. Health. Prev: Trainee GP Mid-Sussex VTS; Ho. Phys. Good Hope Hosp. Sutton Coldfield; Ho. Surg. Cuckfield Hosp.

PHILLIPS, Richard John Maxwell The Goffin Consultancy Ltd., The Riding House, Bossingham Rd., Stelling Minnis, Keighley CT4 6AZ Tel: 01227 709220 Fax: 01227 709220; Riding House, Bossingham Road, Stelling Minnis, Canterbury CT4 6AZ Tel: 01227 709618 Email: richard_jm.phillips@virgin.net — MB BS Lond. 1980 (St. Mary's Hospital Medical School) DPM Eng. 1987; MFPM RCP (UK) 1990; MBA Kingston 1991. Princip. & Managing Dir.; Hon. Sen. Lect. Dept. Managem. Univ. St. And. Specialty: Pharmaceutical Medicine. Socs: Brit. Soc. Antimicrob. Chemother.; Health Economic Study Gp.; Brit. Assn. Pharm. Phys. Prev: Head of Outcomes Research Pfizer Ltd. Sandwich Kent; Gp. Med. Adviser Pfizer Ltd. Sandwich Kent; SHO (Anaesth.) Dewsbury Gen. Hosp. & Wakefield HA.

PHILLIPS, Richard John Wyndham The New Surgery, Linom Road, Clapham, London SW4 7PB Tel: 020 7274 4220 Fax: 020 7737 0205 — BM BCh Oxf. 1978; MA Camb. 1980; MRCP (UK) 1985. Sen. Lect. (Gen. Pract.) UMDS. Prev: Brit. Heart Foundat. Research Fell. (Cardiovasc. Med.) St. Geo. Hosp. Med. Sch. Lond.

PHILLIPS, Richard Kenneth (retired) 4 Channel View, Penarth CF64 5DQ Tel: 029 2070 9437 — MRCS Eng. LRCP Lond. 1941 (Univ. Coll. Hosp., Lond.) DIH Eng. 1950. Prev: Sen. Med. Off. David Brown Corp.

PHILLIPS, Mr Robert Sneddon (retired) 11 St John Street, Manchester M3 4DW Tel: 0161 832 9999 Fax: 0161 834 7855; 3 Milverton Drive, Bramhall, Stockport SK7 1EY Tel: 0161 440 8037 — MB ChB Ed. 1956; FRCS Ed. 1959; FRCS Eng. 1991. Prev: Cons. Orthop. Surg. N. Manch. Health Dist.

PHILLIPS, Robert Stephen — BM BCh Oxf. 1997.

PHILLIPS, Professor Robin Kenneth Stewart St Marks Hospital, Harrow HA1 3UJ Tel: 020 8235 4251 Fax: 020 8235 4277 Email: marie.gun@cancer.org.uk — MB BS Lond. 1975 (Roy. Free) FRCS Eng. 1979; MS Lond. 1985. p/t Cons. Surg. St. Marks Hosp. Lond.; Cons. Surg. Cancer Research UK; Hon. Prof. (Colorectal Surg.) Imperial Coll. Lond.; Civil. Cons. (Colorectal Surg.) Roy. Navy. Specialty: Gen. Surg. Special Interest: Colorectal Surg.; Inherited Colectoral Cancer. Socs: FRSM; Assn. Coloproct.Counc. mem for NW Thames; Pres. Brit Colostomy Assoc. Prev: CRC Research Fell. & Hon. Sen. Regist. (Surg.) Large Bowel Cancer Project St. Mary's Hosp. Lond.; Dir. Thames Region Polyposis Registry; Cons. Surg. Homerton Hosp. Lond.

PHILLIPS, Mr Rodney (retired) 16 Old Hall Road, Whitefield, Manchester M45 7QW Tel: 0161 740 7824 — MB ChB Manch. 1961; MRCS Eng. LRCP Lond. 1961; FRCS Eng. 1967. Prev: Sen. Regist. Welsh Hosp. Bd. & United Cardiff Hosps.

PHILLIPS, Professor Rodney Ernest Nuffield Department of Clinical Medicine, John Radcliffe Hospital, Headington, Oxford OX3 9DU Tel: 01865 221478 Fax: 01865 220993 — MD Oxf. 1987; MB BS Melbourne 1976; FRACP 1983; MD Melbourne 1987; MA Ox. 1995; FRCP 1995. Prof. of Med. Univ. Oxf.; Prof.ial Fell. Wolfson Coll. Oxf.; Hon. Cons. Phys. Oxon. Radcliffe Churchill Trust. Specialty: Gen. Med. Prev: Clin. Reader (Clin. Med.) Univ. Oxf.; Wellcome Trust Sen. Clin. Research Fell.; Wellcome Lect. (Trop. Med.) John Radcliffe Hosp. Oxf.

PHILLIPS, Rosalind Alethea (retired) Cheslyn, Barlaston, Stoke-on-Trent ST12 9DE Tel: 01782 372638 — MB BS Lond. 1952 (Char. Cross) DObst RCOG 1954; DCH Eng. 1955. Prev: Clin. Asst. (Cardiac) City Gen. Hosp. Stoke-on-Trent.

PHILLIPS, Rosemary Helen Princess Alexandra Hospital, Hamstel Road, Harlow CM20 1QX Tel: 01279 827821 — MB BS Lond. 1990 (St. Mary's Hosp. Med. Sch. Lond.) BSc Lond. 1987; MRCP (UK) 1993. Cons. Gastroenterol. and Gen. Med. Specialty: Gastroenterol.; Gen. Med. Special Interest: Nutrit. Prev: SpR (Gastro) Middlx. Hosp., Lond.; SpR (Gastro), Princess Alexandra Hospital, Harlow, Essex; SpR (Gastro), Royal London Hospital, London.

PHILLIPS, Roy Percy, VRD (retired) 51 Church Road, Whitchurch, Cardiff CF14 2DY Tel: 029 2062 5300 — (Cardiff) BSc Wales 1948, MB BCh 1951; MRCGP 1962. Prev: Ho. Surg. & SHO (Paediat.) Llandough Hosp.

PHILLIPS, Russell Langley 15 Underne Avenue, London N14 7ND — MB BS Lond. 1997 (Royal Free)

PHILLIPS, Mr Russell Picton Department of Ophthalmology, Arrowe Park Hospial, Upton, Wirral CH49 5PE Tel: 0151 604 7193; Redstones, Redstones Farm, Arrowe Brook Lane, Wirral CH49 3NY Tel: 0151 677 9545 — MB ChB Birm. 1982; MD Birm. 1982; DO RCS Eng. 1986; FRCS (Ophth.) Ed. 1987; FCOphth 1988. Cons. Wirral Hosps. Trust; Hon. Lect. Univ. Liverp.; Hon. Research Assoc. Univ. Aberd. Specialty: Ophth. Prev: Sen. Regist. (Ophth.) Aberd. Roy. Infirm.; Regist. (Ophth.) Aberd. Roy. Infirm.; SHO (Ophth.) Birm & Midl. Eye Hosp.

PHILLIPS, Samuel Graham (retired) 98 Stafford Road, Bloxwich, Walsall WS3 3PA Tel: 01922 476670 — MB ChB Birm. 1948; DTM & H Eng. 1955; DObst RCOG 1958; DPH Glas. 1961; FFPHM 1983, M 1974. Prev: Cons. Pub. Health Med. Wolverhampton HA.

PHILLIPS, Sara Dawn 15 Rhodes Drive, Sunnybank, Bury BL9 8NH — BChir Camb. 1996.

PHILLIPS, Sarah Louise Orthopaedic Department, King's College Hospital, Denmark Hill, London SE5 9RS Fax: 01752 345443; 69B Shoorers Hill Road, Blackheath, London SE3 7HU Tel: 01423 781618/020 8853 4847 Email: slphillips@btinternet.com — MB BS Lond. 1986; BSc Lond. 1983; FRCS Eng. 1991; FRCS (Orth.) 1997. Cons. Orthop. Surg. King's Coll. Hosp. Specialty: Trauma & Orthop. Surg. Prev: Sen. Regist. Rotat. (Orthop.) King's Coll. Hosp.

PHILLIPS, Sharon Louise The Oakwood Surgery, Masham Road, Cantley, Doncaster DN4 6BU Tel: 01302 537611 Fax: 01302 371804 — MB ChB Sheff. 1988; DRCOG 1992; MRCGP 1992. Prev: Trainee GP/SHO Doncaster Roy. Infirm. VTS; Ho. Phys. Doncaster Roy. Infirm.; Ho. Surg. (Orthop.) North. Gen. Hosp. Sheff.

PHILLIPS, Sheelagh Helen 13 Westbourne Crescent, Bearsden, Glasgow G61 — MB BCh BAO Dub. 1970; DObst RCOG 1972; DCH RCPS Glas. 1974; DPH Glas. 1974. Assoc. Specialist (Community Paediatrics) Yorkhill NHS Trust. Prev: Clin. Med. Off. Gtr. Glas. Health Bd. (2); Mem. Wom. Doctors Retainer Scheme Gtr. Glas. Health Bd.; Clin. Med. Off. Gtr. Glas. Health Bd. (1).

PHILLIPS, Sian 10 Hanbury Close, Whitchurch, Cardiff CF14 2TB Tel: 029 2052 1048; Department of Radiology, University Hospital of Wales, Heath Park, Cardiff CF4 4XN Tel: 029 2074 7747 Email: phillipss1@cardiff.ac.uk — MB BCh Wales 1989 (University of Wales College of Medicine) MRCP (UK) 1993; FRCR 1998. Specialist Regist. (Radiol.). Specialty: Radiol.

PHILLIPS, Sian Eleri Briton Ferry Health Centre, Hunter Street, Briton Ferry, Neath SA11 5SF Tel: 01639 812270 Fax: 01639 813019; 3 Llys Hebog, Birchgrove, Swansea SA7 9PY Tel: 01792 814813 — MB BCh Wales 1987; MRCGP 1991. Princip. in Gen. Pract.

PHILLIPS, Simon Jeremy Church Holding, Etchilhampton, Devizes SN10 3JL Tel: 01380 860291 — (St. Bart.) MRCS Eng. LRCP Lond. 1966; MB BS Lond. 1966; DObst RCOG 1968; DCH Eng. 1970; MPhil Bath 1990. Hon. Co-Dir. Inst. Refugee Healthcare Studies PG Med. Sch., Univ. of Bath. Specialty: Educat.; Research. Socs: Clin. Soc. Bath. Prev: Phys. Devizes & Dist. Hosp.; Research Regist. (Neonat. Paediat.) & SHO (Paediat.) Roy. Berks. Hosp. Reading; SHO (Obst.) Battle Hosp. Reading.

PHILLIPS, Simon Marcus The Paddocks, 50 Bristol Road, Frenchay, Bristol BS16 1LQ — MB BChir Camb. 1994 (Univ. of Cambridge) FRCS (Eng) 1997; MA Oxon. 1998. Specialist Regist. (Gen. Surg.) NW Thames. Specialty: Gen. Surg.

PHILLIPS, Simon Robert Thatchers' Court, Traps Lane, New Malden KT3 4SQ Tel: 020 8949 1705 Fax: 020 8942 3545 — MB BS Lond. 1998 (Imperial Coll.) PRHO (Surg.) Colchester Gen Hosp. Essex. Prev: PRHO (Med.) Poole Hosp. Dorset.

PHILLIPS, Sophie Anne Queen Alexandra Hospital, Cosham, Portsmouth PO6 3LY — BM Soton. 1990; FRCS Eng. 1994; FRCS (Trauma & Orthopaedics) 1999. Consultant Orthopaedic Surgeon. Specialty: Gen. Surg.

PHILLIPS, Spencer Lea Bridge Road Surgery, 266 Lea Bridge Road, Leyton, London E10 7LD Tel: 020 8539 1221 Fax: 020 8539 2303 — MB BS Lond. 1978; MRCS Eng. LRCP Lond. 1977.

PHILLIPS, Stephen John 47 Oakwood Drive, Clydach, Swansea SA8 4DF — MB BCh Wales 1996.

PHILLIPS, Stephen Walter Pewsey Surgery, High Street, Pewsey SN9 5AQ Tel: 01672 563511 Fax: 01672 563004; Bield House, Church Road, Woodborough, Pewsey SN9 5PH Tel: 01672 851564 — MB BS Lond. 1975; MRCS Eng. LRCP Lond. 1975; DRCOG 1979; MRCGP 1980.

PHILLIPS, Susan 12 Lymister Avenue, Rotherham S60 3DD — MB ChB Sheff. 1975; MRCPsych 1981. Sen. Regist. Brighton Clinic Newc. Gen. Hosp.; Cons. Psycho. Geriat. Kingsway Hosp. Derby. Specialty: Care of the Elderly. Prev: Sen. Regist. Doncaster Roy. Infirm.; Regist. Sheff. HA; Hon. Sec. Coll. Trainee Comm. Roy. Coll. Psychiat.

PHILLIPS, Susan Elizabeth Caldicot Medical Group, Gray Hill Surgery, Woodstock Way, Caldicot, Newport NP26 4DB Tel: 01291 420282 Fax: 01291 425853; Brookside, Well Lane, Llanfair Discoed, Chepstow NP16 6LP Tel: 01633 400669 — (Roy. Free) MB BS Lond. 1970; MRCS Eng. LRCP Lond. 1970; DCH RCP Lond. 1972; DObst RCOG 1973. GP.

PHILLIPS, Suzanne The Surgery, Station Road, Great Massingham, King's Lynn PE32 2JQ — MB BS Lond. 1992 (Royal Free Hospital) DRCOG 1996; MRCGP 1997. Asst. GP. Specialty: Gen. Pract.

PHILLIPS, Suzanne Mary 130a Upper Westwood, Bradford-on-Avon BA15 2DE — MB BS Lond. 1998 (St. George's) BSc Lond. 1995; MRCP Uk 2003. Specialty: Diabetes; Endocrinol.

PHILLIPS, Tania 16 Thornhill Road, Uxbridge UB10 8SF — BM Soton. 1994.

PHILLIPS, Thomas (retired) 41 Bentinck Drive, Troon KA10 6HY Tel: 01292 314468 — MB BCh BAO Belf. 1948; DTM & H Eng. 1963. Prev: Med. Off. Unit 2 Ayrsh. & Arran HB.

PHILLIPS, Thomas John (retired) The Croft, 8 Clifford Road, Ilkley LS29 0AL Tel: 01943 608536 — MB ChB Leeds 1959; DObst RCOG 1962; FRCOG 1981, M 1968; T(OG) 1991. Cons. Gyn. Yorks. Clinic Bingley, W. Yorks. Prev: Cons. O & G Airedale Gen. Hosp. Steeton.

PHILLIPS, Toby Teresa Bloomer (retired) Tilt Cottage, 6 Tilt Road, Cobham KT11 3EZ Tel: 01932 863354 — MB ChB St. And. 1958. Immunol. Community Child Health. Prev: Clin. Med. Off. Croydon Community Health Trust & Ealing, Hammersmith & Hounslow HA.

PHILLIPS, Trevor John Graham (retired) 2 Blenheim Gardens, Sanderstead, South Croydon CR2 9AA Tel: 020 8657 2960 — MB BS Ceylon 1952; DCH Eng. 1958; FRFPS Glas. 1961; MRCP Glas. 1962; MFOM RCP Lond. 1980. Prev: Princip. Med. Off. (Pneumoconiosis) DHSS Lond.

PHILLIPS, Ugo Neil (retired) 8 Strensham Court Mews, Strensham, Worcester WR8 9LR Tel: 01684 299560 Email: neil27@supanet.com — MB ChB Sheff. 1955; DObst RCOG 1956; MRCGP 1965. Prev: Sen. Team Phys. Eng. Football Team.

PHILLIPS, Ugo Neil (retired) 8 Strensham Court Mews, Russell Drive, Strensham, Worcester WR8 9LR Tel: 01684 299560 Email: neil27@supanet.com — MB ChB Sheff 1955 (Sheff.) MB ChB Sheff. 1955; Obst. RCOG Lond. 1956. Chairm. The Fitness League Surrey. Prev: Chief. Exec. S. Worcs. Community NHS Trust.

PHILLIPS, Vivian John Muirwood, Green Lane, Pangbourne RG8 7BG Tel: 0118 984 2957 Fax: 0118 984 2022 Email: viv.phillips@medicalis.co.uk — MB ChB Bristol 1971; MRCS Eng. LRCP Lond. 1970; DObst RCOG 1973; DIH Eng. 1978; MFPM RCP (UK) 1989; AFOM RCP Lond. 1989; FFPM RCP (UK) 1993; MBA 1999. Healthcare Cons. Specialty: Pharmaceutical Medicine. Special Interest: Female Health; Diabetes Mellitus. Socs: BMA; Fell Fac. Pharm. Med. Roy. Coll. Phys. Prev: Managing Dir. Med. Monitoring & Research Ltd. Hertford; Med. Dir. Wyeth Laborat. Ltd. & Wyeth Research (UK) Ltd.; Pres. Clin. Strategic Cons. Gp. Kern McNeill Internat.

PHILLIPS, Wayne Stephen Double Helix Development, 66-70 Baker Street, London W1U 7DJ Tel: 020 7299 9830 Fax: 020 7935

3889 Email: wphillips@doublehelixdevelopment.co.uk — MB ChB Liverp. 1976; Dip. Pharm. Med. RCP Lond. 1981; FFPM 1992, M 1990; MIBiol 1992, C 1992. Man. Dir. Double Helix. Specialty: Pharmaceutical Medicine. Socs: Fell. Fac. Pharmaceutical Phys.s; Fell. Roy. Soc. Med.; (Ex-Chairm.) Brit. Assn. Pharmaceut. Phys. Prev: Europ. Med. Dir. Genentech; Med. Dir. Sandoz Pharmaceut. Frimley Surrey; Head Clin. Med. Beecham Pharmaceut. UK Ltd.

PHILLIPS, Wendy Susan 47 Annesley Road, Sheffield S8 7SD — MB ChB Sheff. 1982.

PHILLIPS, William Denstone Powell Perth Royal Infirmary, Department Obstetrics & Gynaecology, Perth PH1 1NA Tel: 01738 623311 Fax: 01738 473545 Email: denny.phillips@tuht.scot.nhs.uk; Greylag House, Forteviot, Perth PH2 9BT Tel: 01764 684245 Email: dennyp@onetel.net.uk — MB BCh Wales 1971; DObst RCOG 1974; FRCOG 1989, M 1976. Cons. (Obst. & Gyn.) Perth Roy. Infirm. Scotland. Specialty: Obst. & Gyn. Special Interest: Colposcopy; Minimum Access Surg. Socs: BSCCP; BSGE; TENS. Prev: Clin. Fell. Foetal Monitoring Unit Univ. Brit. Columbia, Vancouver; Regist. Univ. Hosp. Wales Cardiff; Lect. (O & G) Aberd. Univ.

PHILLIPS, William John Oakfields, 50 Winterbourne Road, Solihull B91 1LX — MB ChB Birm. 1971.

PHILLIPS, William Roger Spence Group Practice, Westcliffe House, 48-50 Logan Road, Bristol BS7 8DR Tel: 0117 944 0701 — MB ChB Bristol 1968; DObst RCOG 1971; DMJ(Clin) Soc. Apoth. Lond. 1986.

PHILLIPS-HUGHES, Jane Radiology Department, John Radcliffe Hospital, Headington, Oxford OX3 9DU Tel: 01865 220814 Fax: 01865 220801 Email: jane.phillips-hughes@crh.anglox.nhs.uk — MB BCh Wales 1986; MRCP (UK) 1989; FRCR 1992. Cons. Radiol. John Radcliffe Hosp. Oxf. Specialty: Radiol. Special Interest: Endoscopy; Interventional Radiol. Socs: Brit. Soc. Interven. Radiol.; Cardiovasc. & Interven. Radiol. Soc. of Europe; Europ. Soc. of Gastrointestinal and Abdom. Radiol. Prev: Lect. (Diagn. Radiol.) & Sen. Regist. (Radiol.) Univ. Hosp. Wales Cardiff; SHO (Gen. Med.) Roy. Gwent Hosp. Newport Gwent.

PHILLIPSON, Mr Andrew Peter Forest Way, Waste Lane, Kelsall, Tarporley CW6 0PE Email: andyphilipson@aol.com — MB ChB Liverp. 1985; FRCS Eng. 1989; FRCS (Orth.) 1995. Cons. Orthop. & Trauma. Specialty: Orthop. Socs: Brit. Orthop. Assn.; BASK (Brit. Assn. Knee Surg).

PHILLIPSON, Elizabeth Mary The Old Rectory, Chapel Lane, Costock, Loughborough LE12 6UY — MB BS Lond. 1969; MRCS Eng. LRCP Lond. 1969.

PHILLPOTS, Stacey 1 Silverdale Croft, Ecclesall, Sheffield S11 9JP Tel: 0114 220 8266 Email: randsbin@senet.com.au — MB ChB Leic. 1988; DFFP. GP Adelaide; Wom. Health & Family Plann. S. Australia. Specialty: Gen. Pract.; Family Plann. & Reproduc. Health. Socs: Roy. Coll. Gen. Pract.; Fell. Roy. Austral. Coll. Gen. Practitioners.

PHILP, Mr Bruce Malcolm 12 Windermere Road, Northfields, Ealing, London W5 4TD — BM BCh Oxf. 1987; FRCSI 1992.

PHILP, Professor Ian Northern General Hospital, Sheffield S5 7AU Tel: 0114 243 4343; 24 Sterndale Road, Sheffield S7 2LB — MD Ed. 1991; MB ChB 1981; FRCP Ed. 1993; T(M) 1993. Prof. Healthcare for the Elderly N. Gen. Hosp. Sheff.; Hon. Cons. Phys. N. Gen. Hosp. Sheff. Specialty: Care of the Elderly. Socs: Brit. Geriat. Soc.; Brit. Soc. Gerontol. Prev: Sen. Lect. (Geriat. Med.) Soton. Gen. Hosp.; Sen. Regist. (Geriat. Med.) Roy. Vict. Hosp. Dundee.

PHILP, Lawrence Douglas The Rookery, 15 Scotby Village, Scotby, Carlisle CA4 8BS Tel: 01228 513554; The Rookery, 15 Scotby Village, Scotby, Carlisle CA4 8BS Tel: 01228 513554 — MB ChB Ed. 1940; DMRD 1948. Specialty: Radiol. Prev: Cons. Radiol. Diag. Special Area Cumbld. & N. W.mld.; Sen. Regist. (Radiol.) Salford Hosp. Gp.; Maj. RAMC.

PHILP, Margaret Ruth Jessamine Cottage, Bowling Bank, Wrexham LL13 9RL Tel: 01978 661619 Fax: 01978 661619 — MB BS Lond. 1966; MRCS Eng. LRCP Lond. 1966; DObst RCOG 1968; DFFP 1995. Specialty: Palliat. Med.

PHILP, Marie Christine 17 Kelfield Avenue, Harborne, Birmingham B17 0QN — MB ChB Birm. 1998.

PHILP, Mr Nigel Hastings New Cross Hospital, Wolverhampton WV10 0QP Tel: 01902 642822; Quartford Wood House, Chapel Lane, Quatford, Bridgnorth WW15 6QH Tel: 01746 763132 — MB ChB Liverp. 1970 (Liverpool) DRCOG; FRCS Ed. 1976; FRCS Eng. 1976. Cons. Urol. New Cross Hosp. Wolverhampton. Specialty: Urol. Socs: Brit. Assn. Urol. Surg. Prev: Research Regist. (Urol./Spinal Injs.) Lodge Moor Hosp. Sheff.; Regist. (Urol.) Roy. Hallamsh. Hosp. Sheff.; Sen. Regist. (Urol.) St. James Hosp. Leeds.

PHILP, Mr Timothy 30 Cleveland Road, South Woodford, London E18 2AL Tel: 020 8530 4917 Fax: 020 8530 4917 Email: timphilp@uk-consultants.co.uk — MB BChir Camb. 1973 (Camb. & St. Thos. Hosp. Med. Sch.) FRCS Eng. 1979; MA Camb. 1974, MChir 1987. Cons. Urol. Whipps Cross Hosp. Lond.; Cons. Urol. St. Peters. Hosp. & Middlx. Hosp. Lond. Specialty: Urol. Socs: Fell. Roy. Soc. Med.; Brit. Assn. Urol. Surgs.; Corr. Mem. Amer. Urol. Assn. Prev: Sen. Regist. (Urol.) St. Peter's Gp. Hosps. Lond.; Research Regist. (Urol.) Radcliffe Infirm. Oxf.; Regist. (Urol.) Whittington Hosp. Lond.

PHILPOT, Kate Anne Hillcroft, Hillcourt Road, Cheltenham GL52 3JL — MB ChB Birm. 1994; ChB Birm. 1994.

PHILPOT, Michael Peter Department of Mental Health of Older Adults, Maudsley Hospital, Denmark Hill, London SE5 8AZ Tel: 020 7919 2193 — MB BS Lond. 1978 (Univ. Coll. Hosp.) BSc Lond. 1975; MRCPsych 1983; FRCPsych 1998. Cons. & Hon. Sen. Lect. (Old Age Psychiat.) Maudsley Hosp. Lond. Specialty: Geriat. Psychiat. Socs: Europ. Assoc. for Geriat. Psychiat. (Sec.). Prev: Cons. & Sen. Lect. (PsychoGeriat.s) Lewisham & Guy's Ment. Health NHS Trust; Registar Bethlem Roy. & Maudsley Hosp. Lond.; Clin. Lect. Inst. Psychiat. Lond.

PHILPOTT, Bruce (retired) Honeywood, 12 Kingswood Firs, Grayshott, Hindhead GU26 6EU Tel: 01428 604712 — MB BS Lond. 1956 (Char. Cross) MRCS Eng. LRCP Lond. 1956; DA Eng. 1958; FFA RCS Eng. 1964; FRCA 1992. Cons. Anaesth. King Edwd. VII Hosp. Midhurst & Mt. Alvernia Hosp. Guildford; Emerit. Cons. Anaesth. Roy. Surrey Co. Hosp. Guildford. Prev: Cons. Anaesth. King Edwd. VII Hosp. Midhurst & Mt. Alvernia Hosp. Guildford.

PHILPOTT, Carl Martin Leicester Royal Infirmary, Infirmary Square, Leicester LE1 5WW Tel: 0116 254 1414 Fax: 0116 258 6082 — MB ChB Leic. 1998; MRCS; DLO; RCS (Eng) 2001; RCS (Eng) 2002. Clinical Research Fellow (Registrar Level). Specialty: Otorhinolaryngol.

PHILPOTT, David Neil Homecroft Surgery, Voguebeloth, Illogan, Redruth TR16 4ET Fax: 01209 842027/01209 842707 — MB ChB Birm. 1976; BSc (Hons.) Birm. 1973; MRCGP 1984.

PHILPOTT, Graham John 1 Parsonage Cottage, The Street, High Easter, Chelmsford CM1 4QS — MB BS Lond. 1983; DRCOG 1987; FRCA 1993. Cons. Anaesth. Broomfield & St. Johns Hosps. Chelmsford. Specialty: Anaesth.

PHILPOTT, Hedley Guy Dalkeith Medical Centre, 24-26 St Andrew Street, Dalkeith EH22 1AP Tel: 0131 561 5500 Fax: 0131 561 5555; Leadburnlea, Leadburn, West Linton EH46 7BE — MB ChB Dundee 1984; BSc Physiol. Newc. 1977; PhD Physiol. Dundee 1980. Prev: Rotat. SHO (Med.) Leeds Gen. Infirm.

PHILPOTT, Jonathan Mark The Cottage, Wyatts Green Road, Doddinghurst, Brentwood CM15 0PT — MB BS Lond. 1994.

PHILPOTT, Maurice George (retired) 4 Crofter's Drive, Thwaite St., Cottingham HU16 4SD Tel: 01482 876606 — MB BS Lond. 1943 (St. Barts.) MRCS Eng. LRCP Lond. 1943; DCH Eng. 1944; FRCP Lond. 1971, M 1946; MD Lond. 1952; FRCPCH 1997. Prev: Cons. Paediat. Hull & E. Yorks. Health Dists.

PHILPOTT, Megan Elizabeth — BM Soton. 1997.

PHILPOTT, Megan Jane Grovehurst Surgery, Grovehurst Road, Kemsley, Sittingbourne ME10 2ST Tel: 01795 430444 Fax: 01795 410539 — MB ChB Birm. 1983; BSc Birm. 1980; DRCOG 1987. MacMillan GP Facilitator, Swale PCT.

PHILPOTT, Nicola Jane Dept. of Haemotology, Ealing Hospital NHS Trust, Uxbridge Rd, Southall UB1 3HW Tel: 020 8967 5432 — BM BCh Oxf. 1988; BA (Hons.) Oxf. 1985; MRCP (UK) 1991; DM Oxf. 1997; MRCPath 1999; FRCP 2003. Cons. Haemotol. Ealing Hosp. NHS Trust Middx. Specialty: Haematology. Socs: BMA; BSH; UK Myeloma Forum. Prev: LRF Research Fell. St. Geo. Hosp. Med. Sch. Lond.; Regist. Rotat. (Haemat.) SW Thames RHA; SHO Rotat. (Med.) St. Geo. Hosp. Lond.

PHILPOTT, Robert Martin Sir Douglas Crawford Unit, Park Avenue, Liverpool L18 8BU Tel: 0151 724 2335 — MB BS Lond. 1968 (King's Coll. Hosp.) MRCS Eng. LRCP Lond. 1968; MRCPsych 1973; FRCPsych 1985. Cons. Psychiat. Old Age N. Mersey Community NHS Trust; Dir. Age Concern Liverp.; Med. Dir. N.

Mersey Community Trust; Chairm. Dist. Med. Advis. Comm. Liverp. Dist. HA; Trustee Health Advisery Serv. Specialty: Geriat. Psychiat. Socs: Liverp. Med. Inst.; BMA; Brit. Geriat. Soc. Prev: Cons. Psychiat. Airedale Gen. Hosp.; Sen. Regist. Maudsley Hosp. Lond.

PHILPOTT, Ruth Grace Edith Worcestershire Specialist Childrens Service, Isaac Maddox House, Shrub Hill Road, Worcester WR4 9RW Tel: 01905 681560; 17 Shrubbery Avenue, Worcester WR1 1QN Tel: 01905 613545 — MB ChB Bristol 1968; MSc (Child Health). SCMO (Community Health) S. Worcs. Community Trust. Specialty: Community Child Health. Prev: Med. Off. VOM Plateau State MoH, Nigeria.

PHILPOTT-HOWARD, John Nigel GKST School Medicine, Department of Infection, Bessemer Road, London SE5 9PJ Tel: 020 7346 3213 Fax: 020 7346 3404 Email: john.philpott-howard@kcl.ac.uk — MB BCh Wales 1977 (Welsh Nat. Sch. of Med.) MRCPath 1983; Dip. Clin. Microbiol. Lond. 1983. Sen. Lect. & Cons. in Med. Microbiol., Guys, Kings, & St. Thomas' Sch. of Med., Lond. Specialty: Med. Microbiol. Socs: Brit. Infec. Soc.; Brit. Soc. For Antimicrobial Chemother.; Am. Soc. For Microbio. Prev: Lect. (Med. Microbiol.) Lond. Hosp. Med. Coll.

PHIMESTER, Mary Eryl Tynemouth Medical Practice, Tynemouth Road, Tottenham, London N15 4RH Tel: 020 8275 4062 Fax: 020 8275 4120; The Old Vicarage, Blanche Lane, South Mimms EN6 3PE Tel: 01707 651717 — MB BS Lond. 1977 (St. Mary's) DRCOG 1979; MRCGP 1982. Prev: Trainee GP Watford VTS.

PHIN, Nicholas Fulton 3 Woodlands, Escrick, York YO19 6LU — MB ChB Glas. 1981 (Glasgow) MFPHM RCP (UK) 1991; LLM (Legal of Aspects Med.) Wales 1996; FFPHM RCP (UK) 1998. Dir. Pub. Health Dwfed Powys HA. Specialty: Pub. Health Med. Socs: Vice-Chairm. Bolam Soc. Prev: Dir. Pub. Health & Plann. United Health Grimsby & Scunthorpe HA; Dir. Pub. Health Grimsby HA; Sen. Regist. (Pub. Health Med.) Yorks. RHA.

PHIPP, Laura Helen — MB BS Lond. 1993 (Roy. Free Hosp. Lond.) FRCS Eng. 1997. Specialist Regist. (Gen. Surg.) Leeds. Specialty: Gen. Surg. Prev: SpR Gen. Surg., York Dist. Hosp.; SpR Gen. Surg., Harrowgate Dist. Hosp.; SpR Gen. Surg., Dewsbury Dist. Hosp.

PHIPPS, Mr Alan Roderick Pinderfields General Hospital, Aberford Road, Wakefield WF1 4DG Tel: 01924 201688 Fax: 01924 814938; 7 Lowther Avenue, Garforth, Leeds LS25 1EP Tel: 0113 287 5489 Fax: 0113 287 5489 Email: arphipps@aol.com — BM BCh Oxf. 1978; MA Camb. 1976; FRCS Ed. 1983; FRCS (Plast) 1995. Cons. Plastic Surg. Pinderfields & Pontefract Hosp. NHS Trust. Specialty: Plastic Surg. Socs: Brit. Assn. Plast. Surgs.; Brit. Assn. Aesthetic Plastic Surgs.; Brit. Burns Assn. Prev: Sen. Regist. (Plastic Surg.) St. Thos. Hosp. Lond.; Regist. (Plastic Surg.) Qu. Mary's Hosp. Roehampton & W. Midl. Regional Burns Unit.

PHIPPS, Alleyne Elizabeth — MB ChB Liverp. 1987; DFFP 1993; MRCGP 1994. Long-term GP Locum. S. Wales. Specialty: Gen. Pract. Socs: MPS; RCGP; BMA. Prev: GP Asst., Lond.; G Locum; Trainee GP Kilburn Pk. Med. Centre Lond.

PHIPPS, Andrew John Hundens Lane Resource Centre, Hundens Lane, Darlington DL1 1DT Tel: 0191 383 1036 — MB BS Lond. 1980; DRCOG 1983; MRCGP 1984; MRCPsych 1998. Cons. in Old Age Psychiat. (Darlington/Teesdale). Specialty: Gen. Psychiat.

PHIPPS, Barbara Mary 2 Killaire Road, Carnalea, Bangor BT19 1EY — BM BS Nottm. 1997.

PHIPPS, Claire Kathleen Louise Thrum Mill Farm, Rothbury, Morpeth NE65 7XH — MB BS Lond. 1992.

PHIPPS, Jeremy Simon Key The Deepings Practice, Godsey Lane, Market Deeping, Peterborough PE6 8DD Tel: 01778 579000 Fax: 01778 579009 — MB BChir Camb. 1986; BA Oxf. 1984; MRCGP 1992.

PHIPPS, Jonathan Andrew 299 Green Lane, Norbury, London SW16 3LU — MB BS Lond. 1975; FFA RCS Eng. 1979. Specialty: Anaesth.

PHIPPS, Kathryn 16 St Andrews Avenue, Ashton, Preston PR2 1JN Tel: 01772 732494 — BM Soton. 1985; DRCOG 1988; MRCGP 1990. Med. Off. Preston. Prev: Trainee GP/SHO (O & G) Sharoe Green Hosp. Fulwood VTS; Trainee GP Lancs. Family Plann. Comm.

PHIPPS, Kevin Nigel Orchard Medical Practice, Innisdoon, Mansfield NG19 7AE Tel: 01623 400100 Fax: 01623 400101; 3 Pool Meadow, Colwick, Nottingham NG4 2DF — BM BS Nottm. 1985 (Nottingham) BMedSci Nottm. 1983. Specialty: Gen. Pract.

PHIPPS, Madeleine Elizabeth 11 Wilson Closse, Willesborough, Ashford TN24 0HX — MB BS Lond. 1991; BSc Lond. 1988, MB BS 1991. Specialty: Anaesth.

PHIRI, Duke Edward Dalliance 43 Boundary Lane, Howlands, Welwyn Garden City AL7 4EG — MB ChB Univ. Zambia 1982; MRCPI 1994.

PHIZACKERLEY, Patrick John Ruthven 365A Woodstock Road, Oxford OX2 8AA — BM BCh Oxf. 1952.

PHIZACKLEA, Sheila Fairfield Surgery, Station Road, Flookburgh, Grange-over-Sands LA11 7JY Tel: 015395 58307 Fax: 015395 58442 Email: shielaphizacklea@angelfire.com; Allithwaite Lodge, Allithwaite, Grange-over-Sands LA11 7RJ Tel: 015395 33422 Fax: 015395 33882 — MB BS Lond. 1973 (Middlx.) DObst RCOG 1975; DCH Eng. 1976. Chair Med. Audit Advis. Gp. Morecambe Bay HA. Specialty: Gen. Pract. Prev: GP Barrow-in-Furness.

PHONGSATHORN, Virach East Surrey Hospital, Canada Avenue, Redhill RH1 5RH Tel: 01737 768511 — MB BS Mahidol, Thailand 1976; MRCP (UK) 1980; FRCP 1998. Cons. Elderly Med. E. Surrey Hosp.; Lead clinician in Med. Surrey & Sussex healthcare NHS Trust. Specialty: Care of the Elderly. Prev: Sen. Regist. (Geriat. Med.) Whittington Hosp. Lond.

PHORNNARIT, Jedth 81 Crane Court, Gurnell Grove, London W13 0AQ — MB BCh Wales 1994.

PHOTIOU, Mr Sophocles Photiou and Partners, 1 Warren Road, Blundellsands, Liverpool L23 6TZ Tel: 0151 924 6464 Fax: 0151 932 0663; 14 Heatherways, Formby, Liverpool L37 7HL — MB ChB Aberd. 1971; MB ChB Aberd. 1971; FRCS Ed. 1978; MRCGP 1982; DRCOG 1983.

PHOTOS, Elias Turnpike Lane Surgery, 114 Turnpike Lane, London N8 0PH — MRCS Eng. LRCP Lond. 1977. Prev: Regist. Whipps Cross Hosp. Lond.

PHULL, Elizabeth Anne Elmbark Group, Foresthill Health Centre, Westburn Rd, Aberdeen AB25 2AY Tel: 01224 696949 — MB BS Lond. 1990; DRCOG 1992; DCH RCP Lond. 1993; MRCGP 1994.

PHULL, Perminder Singh Gastroenterology Unit, Aberdeen Royal Infirmary, Foresterhill, Aberdeen AB25 2ZN Tel: 01224 681818 Fax: 01224 840711 — MB BS Lond. 1984 (Guy's Hosp. Med. Sch.) MRCP (UK) 1991; MD Lond. 1997. Cons. (Phys. & Gastrol.) Aberd. Roy. Infirm.; Hon. Sen. Clin. Lect. Aberd. Univ. Med. Sch. Specialty: Gastroenterol.; Gen. Med. Socs: Brit. Soc. Gastroenterol. Prev: Sen. Regist. & Hon. Clin. Lect. Aberd. Roy. Infrim.; Clin. Research Fell. (Gastroenterol.) Northwick Pk. Hosp. Harrow.

PHYTHIAN-ADAMS, Julia Mary 24 Oakbrook Road, Sheffield S11 7EA Email: julia@p-a.1to1.org; 88 Howard Road, Clarendon Park, Leicester LE2 1XH — MB ChB Sheff. 1991; MRCGP 1997. Asylum Seeker Health, Sheffield. Specialty: Gen. Pract. Socs: BMA; Med. Protec. Soc. Prev: Darnall Community Health Sheff. - GP Salaried to S.-E. PCT Sheff.; SHO (O & G) Chesterfield & N. Derbysh. Roy. Hosp.; Trainee GP Chesterfield.

PHYU PHYU, Dr Paediatric Department, North Tees General Hospital, Stockton-on-Tees TS19 8PE Tel: 01642 617617; 3 Bulmer Close, Yarm TS15 9UX Tel: 01642 898230 — MB BS Med. Inst. (I) Rangoon 1982; MRCP (UK) 1994. Regist. (Paediat.) N. Tees Gen. Hosp. Stockton-on-Tees. Specialty: Paediat. Prev: SHO N. Tees Gen. Hosp. Stockton-on-Tees; SHO S. Cleveland Hosp. & Middlesbrough Gen. Hosp.

PIACHAUD, Michael James Henry Medical Foundation, 111 Iseldon Road, London N7 7JW Tel: 0207 697 7222 Email: m.piachaud@ic.ac.uk — BM BCh Oxf. 1973; MRCPsych 1978; FRCPsych 1996. Cons. Psychiat., Harperbury Hosp.; Hon. Sen. Lect. St. Mary's Hosp. Lond.; Psychiat. at the Med. Foundat. Specialty: Ment. Health. Special Interest: Psychosocial Consequences of war.

PIACHAUD, Mr Raoul Alfred (retired) 18 Princes Avenue, London N10 3LR — MRCS Eng. LRCP Lond. 1934; FRCS Eng. 1942. Prev: Surg. Newc. Gen. Hosp.

PICARD, John James 36 Castlebar Road, London W5 2DD Email: john.picard@bigfoot.com — BM BCh Oxf. 1995. Cons. Anaes. Char. Cross Hosp.

***PICARDO, Karen Joanna Maria** — MB ChB Bristol 1998; DCH 2002; DRCOG 2003; DFFP 2003.

PICARDO, Luciano 38 Victoria Road, Whalley Range, Manchester M16 8DP — MB ChB Manch. 1987.

PICCAVER, James George The Barley Close, Butts Road, Ashover, Chesterfield S45 0AY Tel: 01246 590230 — MB ChB Birm. 1945; MRCS Eng. LRCP Lond. 1945. Socs: Derby Med. Soc; BMA.

PICCHIONI, Mark Michael Section of Neuroimaging, Institute of Psychiatry, De Crespigny Park, London SE5 8AF — MB BS Lond. 1992; MRCP 1995; MRCPsych 1999.

PICCINELLI, Katherine Jane 32 Russet Way, Melbourn, Royston SG8 6HE Tel: 01763 261386; 32 Russet Way, Melbourn, Royston SG8 6HE Tel: 01763 261386 — MB BS Lond. 1997 (UCLMS) SHO (Paediat.) King's Lynn & Wisbech NHS Trust, Norf. Specialty: Paediat. Prev: PRHO (Surg.) Darlington Memor. Hosp., Co. Durh.; PRHO (Med.) Lister Hosp. Stevenage.

PICCINI, Paola Hammersmith Hospital, MRC Clinical Sciences Centre, Du Cane Road, London W12 0NN Tel: 020 8383 3773 Fax: 020 8383 2029; 11A Addison Grove, Chiswick, London W4 1EP — State DMS Pisa 1985; MD; PhD. Regist. (Neurol.) Hammersmith Hosp. Lond.; Sen. Lect. & Cons (Neurol.) Hammersmith Hosp. Lond. Specialty: Neurol.

PICK, Frederick Walter (retired) 18 St Marys Avenue, Gosport PO12 2HX — MB BS Lond. 1959 (Univ. Coll. Hosp.) DMRD Eng. 1971; FFR 1973; FRCR 1975. Cons. Radiol. MoD. Prev: Cons. radiologist Min. of defence.

PICK, James Timothy Hessel (retired) 25 Victoria Road, Barnsley S70 2BE Tel: 01226 206532 — MB BChir Camb. 1952 (Camb. & Leeds) MA Camb., MB BChir. 1952. JP. Prev: SHO (O & G) St. Helen Hosp. Barnsley.

PICK, Michael John (retired) — MB BS Lond. 1969; MRCS Eng. LRCP Lond. 1969; FCAnaesth. 1973. Cons. Anaesth. Medway NHS Trust. Prev: Cons. Anaesth. Benenden Hosp. Kent.

PICK, Michael John — MB BS Lond. 1986 (Oxford/UCH/Middlesex) MA Oxf. 1988, BA 1983; DCH RCP Lond. 1988; DRCOG 1990; MRCGP 1990. GP Partner Ramsgate; Med. Adviser Air Atlanta/Avia Serv.s; Clin. Asst. in Ocupational Health Kent and Canterbury Hosp. Specialty: Gen. Pract.; Occupat. Health. Socs: RCGP; Primary Care Dermatol. Soc.; Soc. Occupat. Med. Prev: Trainee GP Ipswich VTS; Ho. Off. (Med.) Chase Farm Hosp. Enfield; Ho. Off. (Surgic. & Orthop.) NW Herts. HA.

PICK, Stephen Grovelands Medical Centre, 701 Oxford Road, Reading RG30 1HG Tel: 0118 958 2525 Fax: 0118 950 9284; 100 Oaktree Road, Tilehurst, Reading RG31 6JY — MB BS Lond. 1973; DObst RCOG 1975; Cert JCC Lond. 1976; MRCGP 1977. Prev: Trainee Gen. Pract. Reading Vocational Train. Scheme.

PICKARD, Mr Brian Harold Cromwell Hospital, Cromwell Road, London SW5 0TU; 19 Waltham Way, Frinton-on-Sea CO13 9JE Tel: 01255 674808 Fax: 01255 674808 — (Guy's) LMSSA Lond. 1945; MB BS Lond. 1946; DLO Eng. 1947; FRCS Eng. 1954. Hon. Cons. ENT Surg. St. Geo., Moorfields Eye Hosp. & Dispensaire Français Lond.; Authorised Med. Examr. for Civil Aviat. Auth.; Vis. Cons. Is. of St. Helena. Specialty: Otorhinolaryngol.; Aviat. Med. Socs: Fell. Roy. Soc. Med.; (Ex-Pres.) Brit. Med. Pilots Assn.; Fell. Roy. Aeronautical Soc. Prev: Sen. Regist. ENT Dept. King's Coll. Hosp., Nat. Hosp. Nerv. Dis. Qu. Sq. & Hosp. Sick Childr. Gt. Ormond St. Lond.

PICKARD, Cecil (retired) Anston House, 30 Strathern Road, Dundee DD5 1PN — MD Leeds 1952; BSc Leeds 1936, MD 1952, MB ChB 1939; DMRD Eng. 1946; MRCP Ed. 1966.

PICKARD, Christine Alice Margaret Regents Park Medical Centre, Cumberland Market, London NW1 3RH Tel: 020 7387 4576; Springfield, Barnoldswick, Colne BB8 7EA Tel: 01282 3348 — MB ChB Liverp. 1962. Prev: Ho. Surg. Ho. Phys. Whiston Gen. Hosp. Prescot.

PICKARD, Grant Alexander 81 Hollow Road, Anstey, Leicester LE7 7FR — MB ChB Leeds 1996.

PICKARD, Professor John Douglas Department of Neurosurgery, Addenbrooke's Hospital, Hill Road, Cambridge CB2 2QQ Tel: 01223 336946 — MB BChir Camb. 1971 (Camb. & King's Coll. Hosp.) FRCS Ed. 1974; MA Camb. 1970, MChir (Distinc.) 1981; FRCS Lond. 1989; T(S) 1991; Fmed.Sci. 1998. Prof. Neurosurg. & Cons. Neurosurg. Addenbrooke's Hosp. Camb. Specialty: Neurosurg. Socs: (Counc.) Soc. Brit. Neurol. Surg.; (Counc.)Academy of Medical Sciences. Prev: Prof. Clin. Neurol. Sci. & Cons. Neurosurg. Wessex Neurol. Centre Soton.; Lect. (Neurosurg.) Inst. Neurol. Scs. Glas.; Research Fell. (Neurosurg.) Hosp. Univ. Pennsylvania Philadelphia, USA.

PICKARD, John Gimson Beaumont Villa Surgery, 23 Beaumont Road, Plymouth PL4 9BL Tel: 01752 663776 Fax: 01752 261520; Prospect Farm, Latchley, Gunnislake PL18 9AX Tel: 01822 832008 — MB BChir Camb. 1978; MA, MB Camb. 1979, BChir 1978; DMRT 1985; MRCGP 1987. Clin. Asst. (Radiother.) Plymouth Gen. Hosp. Prev: SHO (A & E) & Regist. (Radiother.) Plymouth Gen. Hosp.; SHO (Gen. Med.) Univ. Hosp. Nottm.

PICKARD, Mr Malcolm Alexander Dunn Carolside Medical Centre, 1 Carolside Gardens, Clarkston, Glasgow G76 7BX Tel: 0141 644 3511 Fax: 0141 644 5525 — MB ChB Glas. 1981; FRCS Glas. 1985.

PICKARD, Marjorie Annette Dingly Dell, 2 Liquorstane, Falkland, Cupar KY15 7DQ Tel: 01337 857297 — MB ChB St. And. 1972.

PICKARD, Richard James Beechcroft Cottage, School Lane, Baslow, Bakewell DE45 1RZ — BM Soton. 1993.

PICKARD, Mr Robert Gordon Wishaw General Hospital, 50 Netherton Street, Wishaw ML2 0DP — MB ChB Camb. 1963 (Camb. & St. Bart.) MA, MB Camb. 1964, MChir 1976, MB ChB 1963; MRCP Lond. 1965; FRCS Eng. 1967. Cons. Surg. Law Hosp. Carluke. Specialty: Gen. Surg. Prev: Surgic. 1st. Asst. St. Geo. Hosp. Lond.; Surg. Regist. Chester Roy. Infirm.; Ho. Surg. Birm. Accid. Hosp.

PICKARD, Robert Stephen Freeman Hospital, Freeman Road, High Heaton, Newcastle upon Tyne NE7 7DN Email: robert.pickard@nuth.northy.nhs.uk; 66 Brockmer House, Crowder Street, London E1 0BJ — MB BS Lond. 1984. Clin. Urol. Freeman Hosp. Newc. u. Tyne.

PICKARD, Sally Juliet Basement Flat, 81 Pepys Road, London SE14 5SE — MB BS Lond. 1992.

PICKARD, Mr Simon John Benchmark Cottage, Marchanley, Shrewsbury SY4 5LQ — MB BS Lond. 1992 (CXWMS) FRCS 1997. Regist. (Ortho) Stoke Oswestry Rotat. Specialty: Trauma & Orthop. Surg.

PICKARD, Timothy Martin (retired) Tennyson House Surgery, 20 Merlin Place, Chelmsford CM1 4HW Tel: 01245 260459 Fax: 01245 344287; 6 Fanners Green, Great Waltham, Chelmsford CM3 1EA — MB BChir Camb. 1970; MA, MB BChir Camb. 1970; DObst RCOG 1973.

PICKARD, William Russell Allerton, 8 Orleans Avenue, Jordanhill, Glasgow G14 9LA Tel: 0141 959 3575; Department of Radiology, Victoria Infirmary NHS Trust, Langside Road, Glasgow G42 9TY Tel: 0141 201 5556 Fax: 0141 201 5497 — MB ChB Glas. 1976 (Glasgow) FRCS Glas. 1980; FRCR 1990. Cons. Radiol. Vict. Infirm. Glas. Specialty: Radiol. Prev: Sen. Regist. (Radiol.) Glas. Roy. Infirm.

PICKARD-MICHELS, Patricia Michele Helene Bench Mark Cottage, Rookery Lane, Marchamley, Shrewsbury SY4 5LQ; Bench Mark Cottage, Rookery Lane, Marchamley, Shrewsbury SY4 5LQ — MB BS Lond. 1992. GP - work in local Pract. as locum Curr.ing. Specialty: Gen. Pract.; Obst. & Gyn. Socs: MDU. Prev: SHO O & G; GP Regist.

PICKAVANCE, Gillian The Newbridge Surgery, 255 Tettenhall Road, Wolverhampton WV6 0ED Tel: 01902 751420 Fax: 01902 747936; Holly Tree Cottage, Tong, Shifnal TF11 8PW Tel: 01902 375179 — (Birmingham) MB ChB Birm. 1990; DRCOG 1992; DCH RCP Lond. 1993; DFFP 1993; MRCGP 1994. Specialty: Obst. & Gyn.

PICKEN, Gary The Ipswich Hospital, Heath Road, Ipswich IP4 5PD Tel: 01473 712233 Fax: 01473 703400 — MB ChB Bristol 1985; MRCP (UK) 1989; FRCR 1991. Cons. Radiol. Ipswich Hosp., E. Suff. Specialty: Radiol. Prev: Sen. Regist. (Radiol.) Addenbrooke's Hosp. Cambs.; Cons. Radicol. Wellington Hosp. NZ.

PICKEN, Sheila Dialysis Unit, Addenbrookes Hospital, Hills Road, Cambridge CB2 2QQ Tel: 01223 217832; 3 Lansdowne Road, Cambridge CB3 0EU — MB ChB Ed. 1967; DCH Eng. 1971; MRCP (UK) 1972. Clin. Asst. (Dialysis Unit) Addenbrooke's Hosp. Camb.; Med. Adviser Adoption Panel Adopt Anglia (CORAM). Specialty: Nephrol. Socs: Med. Wom.'s Federat. Prev: Regist. (Med) Deaconess Hosp. Edin.; Resid. (Paediat.) Janeway Child Health Centre, St. John's, Newfld.

PICKENS, Peter Tudor (retired) 20 Eldon Grove, Hartlepool TS26 9LY — BM BCh Oxf. 1954 (King's Coll. Hosp.) FRCP Lond. 1977, M 1960. Prev: Cons. Phys. Hartlepool Health Dist.

PICKENS, Samuel 7 Crowtrees Grove, Roughlee, Nelson BB9 6NE — MB ChB Ed. 1966; MRCP (UK) 1971; FRCP Ed. 1985; FRCP Lond. 1994. Cons. Phys. Burnley Gen. Hosp. Specialty: Gen. Med.

Prev: Sen. Regist. (Diabetic Outpat. & Gen. Med.) Edin. Roy. Infirm.; Sen. Regist. (Communicable Dis.) City Hosp. Edin.

PICKERELL, Lindsay Mark Warren The Bull Ring Surgery, 5 The Bull Ring, St. John's, Worcester WR2 5AA Tel: 01905 422883 Fax: 01905 423639 — MB ChB Bristol 1986. Specialty: Infec. Dis.

PICKERING, Annette Mary Avenue Road Surgery, 3 Avenue Road, Dorridge, Solihull B93 8LH Tel: 01564 776262 Fax: 01564 779599 — MB BS Lond. 1983; DRCOG 1987. Retainer Scheme Croydon HA. Socs: BMA. Prev: Trainee GP/SHO St. Geo. Hosp. Lond. VTS.

PICKERING, Mr Anthony 18 The Bryn, Sketty, Swansea SA2 8DD Tel: 01792 299384 — MB ChB Ed. 1965; BSc (Hons. Physiol.) Ed. 1962, MB ChB 1965; DO Eng. 1968; FRCS Ed. 1969. Cons. Ophth. Singleton Hosp. Swansea. Specialty: Ophth. Prev: Ho. Surg. & Ho. Phys. Roy. Infirm. Edin.

PICKERING, Anthony Edward 38B Rowallan Road, Fulham, London SW6 6AG — MB ChB Birm. 1994; PHD Birm. 1993, BSc (Hons.) Physiol. 1988. SHO (Anaesth.) Roy. Free Hosp. Lond. Specialty: Anaesth.

PICKERING, Anthony Jean-Marie Coutin Orchard Lane Surgery, Orchard Lane, Denton, Northampton NN7 1HT Tel: 01604 890313 Fax: 01604 890143 — BM BCh Oxf. 1980; MA, DPhil. Oxf. 1978. Prev: Tutor (Gen. Pract.) Northampton.

PICKERING, Arthur Holmes Hambro Lodge, 141 Slough Road, Datchet, Slough SL3 9AE Tel: 01753 547707 Fax: 01753 547707 — (St. Mary's) MB BS Lond. 1960; DObst RCOG 1965; CIH Dund 1973; Specialist Accredit. (Occupat. Med.) JCHMT 1980; FFOM RCP Lond. 1991, MFOM 1981. JP Slough; Mem. Med. Appeal Tribunal; Cons. Occupational Health Phys. Roy. Natioanl Orthopaedic Hosp. Stanmore. Specialty: Occupat. Health. Socs: Hon. Mem. Soc. Occupat. Health Phys. of Nigeria; Liveryman Worshipful Soc. Apoth. Lond.; Fell. Roy. Inst. Pub. Health. Prev: Regional Med. Dir. Gulf Oil Co. & Chevron Corpn. E. Hemisphere Lond.; Ho. Off. (Surg. & Cas.) & Admitting Off. Paddington Gen. Hosp.; Med. Off. Unilever & United Afr. Co. Cameroons & Nigeria.

PICKERING, Brian James Seaford Health Centre, Dane Road, Seaford BN25 1DH Tel: 01323 490022 Fax: 01323 492156 — MB BS Lond. 1975 (King's Coll. Hosp.) DRCOG 1978; Cert. Family Plann. JCC 1980; DCH Eng. 1980.

PICKERING, Catherine Patricia Northcote Surgery, 2 Victoria Circus, Glasgow G12 9LD Tel: 0141 339 3211 Fax: 0141 357 4480; 7 Cleveden Crescent, Glasgow G12 0PD Tel: 0141 357 0743 — MB ChB Glas. 1984; MRCGP 1989. Prev: GP Aberd.

PICKERING, Professor Charles Anthony Cary Department of Thoracic Medicine, Northwest Lung Centre, Wythenshaw Hospital, Manchester M23 9LT Tel: 0161 946 2832; 10 The Mount, Church St, Altrincham WA14 4DX — MRCS Eng. LRCP Lond. 1966; MB BS Lond. 1966; MRCP (UK) 1970; DIH Eng. 1976; FFOM RCP Lond. 1991, MFOM 1981; FRCP Lond. 1987. Cons. Thoracic Phys. Wythenshawe Hosp. & Withington Hosp. Manch. Specialty: Gen. Med. Prev: Sen. Regist. Brompton & Westm. Hosps. Lond.

PICKERING, Derek Frank — MB ChB Sheff. 1979; DRCOG 1982; DCH RCP Lond. 1983; MRCGP 1983; AFOM RCP Lond. 1987. Med. Off. Sheff. Univ. Health Serv.; Occupat. Health Phys. Sheff. Univ. Specialty: Gen. Pract.

PICKERING, Elspeth Evelyn Sketty, Swansea SA2 8DD — MB ChB Birm. 1998.

PICKERING, Frederick Charles 53 Cronk Ny Greiney, Tromode Park, Douglas IM2 5LW Tel: 01624 663746 — MB BS Durham 1951. Med. Dir. Rheum. Dis. Foundat. (UK); Med. Dir. Avondale Clinic I. of Man. Prev: Med. Off. Winthrop Laborat.; SHO Guy's & Maudsley Hosps. Neurosurg. Units Lond.; Ho. Surg. Roy. Vict. Infirm. Newc. upon Tyne.

PICKERING, Frederick Charles Sanofi Winthrop Ltd., Edgefield Avenue, Newcastle upon Tyne NE3 3TT Tel: 0191 250 0471 Fax: 0191 213 3129 Email: oh@sanpd.onyxnet.co.uk; 18 Glastonbury Grove, Newcastle upon Tyne NE2 2HA Tel: 0191 281 5177 — MB BS Newc. 1969; DIH Eng. 1978. Gp. Occupat. Phys. Sanofi Winthrop Ltd. Specialty: Occupat. Health. Socs: Fac. Occupat. Med. Prev: Sen Occupat. Phys. Sterling Winthrop Gp.

PICKERING, Geraldine Bowland Road, 52 Bowland Road, Baguley, Manchester M23 1JX Tel: 0161 998 2014 Fax: 0161 945 6354; 10 The Mount, Church St, Altrincham WA14 4DX — MB BS Lond. 1965 (St. Mary's) MRCS Eng. LRCP Lond. 1965; DObst RCOG 1967; DPH NUI 1968.

PICKERING, Ian Frederick 64 Hartley Avenue, Woodhouse, Leeds LS6 2LP — MB ChB Leeds 1998.

PICKERING, John Gilbert (retired) 38 West Street, Reigate RH2 9BX — MB BChir Camb. 1968 (Camb. & Guy's) B.Chir 1967; MRCS Eng. LRCP Lond. 1967; MB Camb. 1968; MA Camb. 1968; MRCP (UK) 1971; DObst RCOG 1975. Prev: Ho. Phys. (Neurol.) Guy's Hosp.

PICKERING, Margaret Ann 5 The Pastures, Narborough, Leicester LE19 3DT Tel: 0116 286 7557 — MB ChB Manch. 1973. Med. Adviser, SEMA Gp. Med. Servs.

PICKERING, Mary Evelyn Anne Clavell Shovers Green House, Wadhurst TN5 7JY — MB BS Durh. 1962 (Newc.) Specialty: Community Child Health. Socs: BMA. Prev: Community Med. Off. (Community Health Servs.) CrowBoro. & Eastbourne HA; Sch. Med. Off. Heref. & Worcs. AHA & Hexham; Clin. Asst. (Med.) Roy. Vict. Infirm. Newc.

PICKERING, Matthew Caleb Dept. of Rheumatology, Hammersmith Hospital, London W12 0NN — MB BS Lond. 1992. Specialty: Rheumatol.

PICKERING, Nigel The Medical Centre, Cranwell Road, Driffield YO25 6UH Tel: 01377 253334 Fax: 01377 241728; 37 St. Johns Road, Driffield YO25 6RS Tel: 01377 256741 — MB BS Lond. 1982.

PICKERING, Nigel John Gable House, 46 High Street, Malmesbury SN16 9AT Tel: 01666 825825 — BM BCh Oxf. 1982; BA Oxf. 1979; DRCOG 1985; MRCGP 1987.

PICKERING, Rachel Anna 224 Ashenden, Deacon Way, London SE17 1UB — MB BS Lond. 1998.

PICKERING, Robert Spencer The Avenue Surgery, 71 The Avenue, Wivenhoe, Colchester CO7 9PP Tel: 01206 824447 Fax: 01206 827973 — MB BS Lond. 1987. Prev: SHO (O & G) Essex. Co. Hosp. Colchester; SHO (Gen. Med.) Severalls Hosp. Colchester; SHO (Geriat. Med.) St. Mary's Hosp. Colchester.

PICKERING, Mr Simon Anthony William 3 Henry Road, West Bridgford, Nottingham NG2 7NA — MB ChB Birm. 1993; BSc 1990; FRCS Eng. 1998.

PICKERING, Veronica Ridingleaze Medical Centre, Ridingleaze, Bristol BS11 0QE Tel: 0117 982 2693 Fax: 0117 938 1707; 243 Canford Lane, Westbury-on-Trym, Bristol BS9 3PD — MB ChB Birm. 1992.

PICKERING, William Graham 7 Moor Place, Gosforth, Newcastle upon Tyne NE3 4AL Tel: 01590 616322/0191 284 2259 — MB BS Lond. 1973 (King's Coll. Hosp.) DCH Eng. 1975; MRCP (UK) 1976; DRCOG 1980; MRCGP 1981; AFOM RCP Lond. 1985. Specialty: Gen. Med.; Paediat.; Medico Legal.

PICKERING, Zoe Gail 123 Moyallan Road, Portadown, Craigavon BT63 5JY — MB BCh Belf. 1998.

PICKERING-PICK, Margaret Elizabeth (retired) 35 Battlefield Road, St Albans AL1 4DB Tel: 01727 860651 — MB BS Lond. 1954 (St. Bart.) DA Eng. 1958; FFA RCS Eng. 1963. Prev: Cons. Anaesth. St. Albans City Hosp. & Hemel Hempstead Gen. Hosp.

PICKERSGILL, Andrew Stepping Hill Hospital, Poplar Grove, Stockport SK2 7JE Tel: 0161 483 1010 Fax: 0161 456 3726 Email: andypick@aol.com — MB ChB Liverp. 1989; MRCOG 1994; MD Manch. 1999. Cons. Obst. & Gynaecologist,Stepping Hill Hosp., Poplar Gr., Stockport; Cons. Buxton Cottage Hosp. Buxton; Cons. Alexandra Hosp. Cheadle; Cons. BUPA Regency Hosp. Macclesfield. Special Interest: Laparoscopic & Hysteroscopic Suregery; Endometriosis. Socs: BFS; ASRM; BSGE. Prev: Lect. (O & G) Univ.of Manch; Specialist Regist. (O & G).

PICKERSGILL, David Eric Birchwood Surgery, Park Lane, North Walsham NR28 0BQ Tel: 01692 402035 Fax: 01692 500367 — MB ChB Bristol 1969; DObst RCOG 1971. Socs: Gen. Med. Servs. Comm.; (Mem. Counc.) BMA. Prev: Regist. (Gen. Med. & Dis. Chest.) & SHO (Orthop.) Worcester Roy. Infirm.; Ho. Off. Southmead Hosp. Bristol.

PICKERSGILL, David Eric Upper Snape Farm, Sowerby Bridge HX6 1PB — MB ChB Leeds 1981.

PICKERSGILL, Hilary Beryl Birchwood Surgery, Park Lane, North Walsham NR28 0BQ Tel: 01692 402035 Fax: 01692 500367 — MB ChB Bristol 1964. Prev: SHO (Cas. & Anaesth.) Southmead Hosp. Bristol; Demonst. (Anat.) Univ. Bristol.

PICKERSGILL, Trevor Paul University Hospital of Wales, Heath Park, Cardiff CF14 4XW Email: trevor.pickersgill@cardiffandvale.wales.nhs.uk — MB BCh Wales 1991 (Univ. Wales Coll. Med.) MRCP (UK) 1994. Cons. (Neurol.) Univ. Hosp. Wales; Cons. (Neurol.) Univ. Hosp. of Wales and Roy. Glam. Hosp. Specialty: Neurol. Special Interest: Multiple Sclerosis; Headache; Obstetric Neurol. Socs: Brit. Soc. Rehabil. Med.; Assn. of Brit. Neurologists; Brit. Assn. for the Study of Headache. Prev: SpR, Univ. Hosp. Wales, Roy. Gwent Hosp. & Rookwood Hosp.; Specialist Regist. (Neurol.) Morriston Hosp. Swansea; Research Fell. (Neurol.) Univ. of Wales Coll. of Med.

PICKETT, Denise Ada Disability Benefits Centre, Government Buildings, Flowers Hill, Bristol BS4 5LA Tel: 0117 971 8343 Fax: 0117 971 8482; Cotswold, 19A Pedlars Grove, Frome BA11 2SL Tel: 01373 451650 — MB BS Newc. 1971; DMRD Eng. 1975; MBA Birm. 1995. Area Med. Adviser Benefits Agency Med. Servs. Bristol; Tutor Open Univ. Specialty: Civil Serv. Prev: GP N.d.; Regist. (Radiol.), Ho. Phys. & Ho. Surg. Roy. Vict. Infirm. Newc.; SHO (Med.) Newc. Gen. Hosp.

PICKETT, Liza Clare The Portmill Surgery, 114 Queen Street, Hitchin SG4 9TH Tel: 01462 434246; 3 Pullman Drive, Hitchin SG4 0ED — BM BCh Oxf. 1986; MA Camb. 1987; DRCOG 1990; MRCGP 1990; DCH RCP Lond. 1991. GP. Specialty: Gen. Pract.; Diabetes; Paediat. Prev: Clin. Med. Off. (Paediat.) Worthing HA; Lister Hosp. Stevenage VTS.

PICKETT, Margaret Elizabeth Jacqueline Knightswood Clinic, 129 Knightswood Road, Glasgow G13 2XF Tel: 0141 211 9069; The Hollow, 22 Kirkhouse Road, Blanefield, Glasgow G63 9BX — MB ChB Glas. 1982; MRCPsych 1988. Cons. Adolesc. Psychiat. Gtr. Glas. Primary Care NHS Trust. Specialty: Child & Adolesc. Psychiat.

PICKETT, Thomas Mark Department of Renal Medicine, Gloucestershire Royal Hospital, Great Western Road, Gloucester GL1 3NN Tel: 08454 226299 — MB BS Lond. 1986 (Univ. of Camb., Univ. Coll., Lond.) MA Camb. 1987; MRCP (UK) 1990. Cons. Phys., Gloucestershire Hosps. NHS Trust, Gloucester. Specialty: Nephrol.; Gen. Med. Socs: Renal Assn.; DGH Nephrologists Soc.; Soc. for Acute Med. Prev: SpR (Nephrol) Lister Hospital, Stevenage; Train. Fell. Nat. Kidney Research Fund St. Thomas's Hosp. Lond.; Regist. (Gen. Med.) Worthing Hosp.

PICKFORD, Mr Ian Roger 6 Marchmont Terrace, Glasgow G12 9LS Tel: 0141 357 3804 Fax: 0141 357 3804 — MB ChB Leeds 1975; BSc (Physiol.) Leeds 1972; FRCS Eng. 1981; PhD Lond. 1988. Cons. Gen. & Colorectal Surg. Vict. Infirm.; Hon. Sen. Lect. (Surg.) Glas. Univ.; Assoc. Scientist Beatson Inst. Cancer Research Glas. Specialty: Gen. Surg. Socs: Med. & Dent. Defence Union Scotl. Prev: Lect. (Surg.) Glas. Roy. Infirm.; Clin. Research Fell. Imperial Cancer Research Fund Lond.

PICKFORD, Mr Mark Ashton The Queen Victoria Hospital NHS Trust, Holtye Road, East Grinstead RH19 3DZ Email: pickford@picky.demon.co.uk — MB BS Lond. 1983 (King Coll. Hosp. Med. Sch.) FRCS Eng. 1987; MS 1991; FRCS (Plast.) 1995. Cons. Plastic & Hand Surg. Qu. Vict. Hosp. E. Grinstead. Specialty: Plastic Surg. Socs: Brit. Soc. Surg. Hand; Brit. Assn. Plastic Surg. Prev: Hand Surg. Fell. Christine M. Kleinet Inst. Hand & Microsurg. Louisville Kentucky, USA; Sen. Regist. Plastic Surg. Qu. Vict. Hosp.; Regist. Plastic Surg. Cannierbum Hosp. Glas.

PICKFORD, Roger Baron Nevill Hall Hospital, X-Ray Department, Beacon Road, Abergavenny NP7 7EG Tel: 01873 732460 — MB ChB Birm. 1970; DMRD 1973; FRCR 1974. Cons. Radiol. Specialty: Radiol. Special Interest: Chest Disease; Echocardiology; Paediatrics.

PICKHAVER, Kathleen Mary Ground Floor Flat, 49 Thornby Road, London E5 9QL — MB BS Lond. 1988.

PICKIN, Christine Anne 20 Windsor Road, Levenshulme, Manchester M19 2EB — MB ChB Liverp. 1982.

PICKIN, David Mark Medical Care Research Unit, Regent Court, 30 Regent St., Sheffield S1 4DA Fax: 0114 222 0749 — MB ChB Bristol 1986 (Bris.) DRCOG 1989; DCH RCP Lond. 1989; MRCGP 1991; MFPHM 1996. Clin. Sen. Lect. in Health Serv. Research, Med. Care Research Unit, Sch. Of Health & related Research, Sheff. Univ.; Hon. Cons. In Pub. Health Med., Nth Derbysh. Health Auth. Chesterfield. Specialty: Pub. Health Med. Prev: MRC Special Train. Research Fell. (Pub. Health Med.) Univ. Sheff.; Sen. Regist. (Pub. Health Med.) NHS Exec. Trent.

PICKIN, Jacqueline Heidi Oxshott Medical Centre, Holtwood Road, Oxshott, Leatherhead KT22 0QJ Tel: 01372 844000; 126 Woodlands Road, Little Bookham, Leatherhead KT23 4HJ Fax: 01372 453151 — MB ChB Ed. 1974; MRCP (UK) 1978. Specialty: Gen. Pract.

PICKIN, John Michael Brook Mill Medical Centre, College Street, Leigh WN7 2RB Tel: 0161 973 1036 — MB BS Lond. 1977. GP Manch.

PICKIN, Margaret Claire Keresley Road, 2 Keresley Road, Coventry CV6 2JD Tel: 024 7633 2628 Fax: 024 7633 1326 — MB ChB Liverp. 1981; BSc (Hons.) Biochem. Liverp. 1973; MFHom 1998. Specialty: Gen. Pract.; Homeop. Med.

PICKIN, Richard Brian Upton Group Practice, 32 Ford Road, Wirral CH49 0TF Tel: 0151 677 0486 Fax: 0151 604 0635 — MB ChB Liverp. 1972; MRCGP 1976.

PICKLES, Basil George (retired) High Bank, 3 Darnley Drive, Southborough, Tunbridge Wells TN4 0TH Tel: 01892 28385 — MB BS Lond. 1947 (King's Coll. Hosp.) MRCS Eng. LRCP Lond. 1947; FRCOG 1970, M 1953; MMSA Lond. 1956. Cons. O & G Tunbridge Wells Health Dist. Examr. Centr.; Surg. Lt.-Cdr. RNR.; Midw. Bd. & RCOG Capt. RAMC. Prev: Sen. Regist. (O & G) King's Coll. Hosp. Lond.

PICKLES, Bryan Christopher Beaumont (retired) 41 Walsall Road, Little Aston, Sutton Coldfield B74 3BA Tel: 0121 353 1547 — MB ChB Birm. 1957; MRCS Eng. LRCP Lond. 1957; DObst RCOG 1959. Indep. GP Sutton Coldfield.

PICKLES, Clive John Kings Mill Centre, Mansfield Road, Sutton-in-Ashfield NG17 4NA; Stud Farm, Hardstoft, Pilsley, Chesterfield S45 8AE Tel: 01773 875994 — MB ChB Manch. 1976. Cons. O & G Kingsmill Hosp. Sutton-in-Ashfield. Specialty: Obst. & Gyn. Socs: Roy. Coll. Obst. & Gyns. Prev: Sen. Regist. (O & G) Univ. Hosp. Nottm.; Research Fell. (O & G) Univ. Hosp. Nottm.; Regist. (O & G) Univ. Hosp. Nottm. & Burnley Gen. Hosp.

PICKLES, Edward James William Westbury Cottage, Panarama Drive, Ilkley LS29 9RA — MB ChB Dundee 1996.

PICKLES, Hilary Glen 3 Ducks Walk, Twickenham TW1 2DD Tel: 020 8892 5086 — MB BChir Camb. 1973; MA Camb. 1972; MRCP (UK) 1974; PhD Lond. 1978; FRCP 1997; MFPHM 1998; FFPHM 2002. Dir. (Pub. Health & Health Strategy) Hillingdon PCT. Specialty: Pub. Health Med. Prev: Princip. Med. Off. Dept. Health, Elephant & Castle Lond.; MRC Fell. Clin. Pharmacol. St. Bart. Hosp. Med. Coll. & Nat. Hosp. Lond.; Teachg. Fell. Dept. Pharmacol. Lond. Sch. Pharmacy.

PICKLES, Joanna — BM BCh Oxf. 1995; MRCP 1998. Research Fell. Brit. Lung Foundat. Specialty: Respirat. Med. Special Interest: Respiritory Med.

PICKLES, Mr John Michael Luton and Dunstable Hospital, Dunstable Road, Luton LU4 0DZ; Topstreet Farm House, Crabtree Lane, Harpenden AL5 5NU — MB ChB Dundee 1976; FRCS Ed. 1982; FRCS Eng. 1984. Cons. Otolaryngol. Luton & Dunstable Hosp. Specialty: Otolaryngol. Socs: Brit. Assn. Otolaryngol.; Brit. Voice Assn. Prev: Sen. Regist. Yorks. RHA.

PICKLES, John Stephen Health Centre, Holme Lane, Cross Hills, Keighley BD20 7LG Tel: 01535 632147 Fax: 01535 637576; The Barn, Glusburn Moor, Keighley BD20 8DY Tel: 01535 635717 Fax: 01535 637576 — MB BS Newc. 1972; MRCGP 1976. Med. Off. Malsis Preparatory Sch. Socs: Keighley & Dist. Med. Soc. Prev: Trainee GP Airedale VTS.

PICKLES, Lisa Jane The Old Vicarage, Moorbottom Lane, Greetland, Halifax HX4 8PZ — MB BS Newc. 1987; T(GP) 1991; MRCGP 1991.

PICKLES, Margaret Muriel (retired) Chaucer's House, Woodstock OX20 1SP Tel: 01993 811244 — BM BCh Oxf. 1939 (Oxf. & Univ. Coll. Hosp.) DM Oxf. 1947, MA 1939; FRCPath 1970. Prev: Cons. Path. AHA (T).

PICKLES, Richard Mark Plas y Bryn Surgery, Chapel Street, Wrexham LL13 7DD Tel: 01978 351308 Fax: 01978 312324 — MRCS Eng. LRCP Lond. 1968 (Guy's)

PICKLES, Roger Llewellyn Silverdale Medical Centre, Mount Avenue, Heswall, Wirral CH60 4RH Tel: 0151 342 6128 Fax: 0151 342 2435 — MB ChB Liverp. 1976.

PICKLES, Stanley Thomas (retired) Pengwerne, St. Nicholas Close, Penn Hill, Yeovil BA20 1SB Tel: 01935 475866 — (Camb. &

Lond. Hosp.) MB BChir Camb. 1950; MLCOM 1963. Prev: Med. Off. Summerlands Hosp. Yeovil.

PICKLES, Valerie Ann Park Lane House Medical Centre, 187 Park Lane, Macclesfield SK11 6UD Tel: 01625 422893 Fax: 01625 424870 — MB ChB Aberd. 1989; BSc Aberd. 1984. Princip. GP. Specialty: Gen. Pract. Socs: RCGP.

PICKLES, Victoria Marylin CLarendon Wing, Leeds General Infirmary, Leeds LS2 9NS — MB ChB Leeds 1994.

PICKRELL, Morgan David Birchend Farmhouse, Ockeridge, Wichenford, Worcester WR6 6YR Tel: 01886 888414 Email: d.pickrell@ukonline.co.uk — MB BS Lond. 1975 (Univ. Coll. Hosp.) DRCOG 1980; MRCOG 1983; FRCOG 2000. Cons. O & G Worcester Roy. Infirm. Specialty: Obst. & Gyn. Prev: Sen. Regist. (O & G) Birm. Matern. Hosp.

PICKSTOCK, Colette Cecilia, OStJ, Surg. Lt.-Cdr. RN Retd. (retired) 35 Portsdown Avenue, Drayton, Portsmouth PO6 1EL Tel: 023 9221 9084 Fax: 023 9264 9004 — (Liverp.) MB ChB Liverp. 1957; DObst RCOG 1960; FRCS Ed. 1964. Cons. Forens. Gyn. MoD. Prev: Clin. Asst. (Orthop.) Qu. Alexandra Hosp. Cosham.

PICKTHALL, Pamela Dorothy, Wing Cdr. RAF Med. Br. Retd. Medical Centre, Buckley Barracks, Stanton St Quintin, Chippenham SN14 6BT Tel: 01666 508906 Fax: 01666 508905; Glebelands, Easton Town, Sherston, Malmesbury SN16 0LS Tel: 01666 841072 — MB ChB Manch. 1974 (Manchester) DA Eng. 1979. Civil. Med. Practitioner Med. Centre Buckley Barracks, Chippenham. Specialty: Gen. Pract. Prev: GP Rowden Surg. Chippenham; Med. Off. RAF.

PICKUP, Anthony John The Old Chapel, Drury Lane, Mortimer, Reading RG7 2JN Tel: 0118 933 2135 Fax: 0118 933 1273 — MRCS Eng. LRCP Lond. 1973 (Guy's) BSc (1st cl. Hons. Physics appl. Med.) Lond. 1970; FFPM RCP (UK) 1995. Med. Director Merck Pharmaceut. Specialty: Cardiol. Socs: Fell. Roy. Soc. Med. Prev: Med. Dir. Otsuka Pharmaceut. Co. Ltd.; Med. Dir. Abbott Laborat.

PICKUP, John Christopher 60 Dorrington Court, South Norwood Hill, London SE25 6BG Tel: 020 8771 1963 — BM BCh Oxf. 1974; DPhil, MA Oxf. 1972, BM BCh 1974. Hon. Lect. Unit Metab. Med. Guy's Hosp. Lond.; Asst. Endocrine Physiol. & Pharmacol. Laborat. Nat. Inst. Med Research Lond. Prev: SHO (Endocrinol. & Gen. Med.) Hammersmith Hosp. Lond.; Ho. Surg. Northampton Gen. Hosp.; Ho. Phys. Radcliffe Infirm. Oxf.

PICKVANCE, Nicholas John Warner Lambert, Lambert Court, Chestnut Avenue, Eastleigh SO53 3ZQ Tel: 023 8062 8625 Fax: 023 8062 9726; Littlewood House, Cowesfield, Whiteparish, Salisbury SP5 2RB Tel: 01794 884783 — MB ChB Bristol 1972; MRCP (UK) 1977; FRCP (UK) 1998. Vice Pres. R&D Warner Lambert Consumer Health. Specialty: Pharmaceutical Medicine.

PICKWORTH, Anthony James Department of Anaesthetics, The Great Western Hospital, Marlborough Road, Swindon SN3 6BB Tel: 01793 604020 Fax: 01793 604512 — BM BCh Oxf. 1987; MA Camb. 1988; MRCP (UK) 1992; FRCA 1993. Cons. Anaesth. & Inten. Care, Princess Margt. Hosp. Swindon. Specialty: Anaesth. Prev: Sen. Regist. Rotat. (Anaesth.) Addenbrooke's Hosp. & W. Suff. Hosp. Bury St. Edmunds; Regist. Rotat. (Anaesth.) Addenbrooke's Hosp. Camb. & Heath Rd. Hosp. Ipswich; SHO (Anaesth.) City Gen. Hosp. Stoke-on-Trent.

PICKWORTH, David Christopher The Darley Dale Medical Centre, Two Dales, Darley Dale, Matlock DE4 3FD Tel: 01629 733205; Clevedon House, Brookleton, Youlgrave, Bakewell — MB BS Newc. 1973; DObst RCOG 1976; MRCGP 1977. Princip. in Gen. Pract.; Clin. Asst. Psychiat. of Learning Disabil.; Clin. Asst. in Elderly Med.; PCG Bd. Mem.

PICKWORTH, Frederick Edward Norfolk & Norwich University Hospital, Colney Lane, Norwich NR4 7UZ Tel: 01603 286737 Fax: 01603 286088 Email: fred.pickworth@nnuh.nhs.uk — LMSSA Lond. 1983 (Cambridge) MA Camb. 1984, MB BChir 1983; MRCP (UK) 1987; FRCR 1992. Cons. Radiol. Norf. & Norwich Health Care NHS Trust.; Hon. Cons. Jas. Paget Hosp. NHS Trust. Specialty: Radiol. Prev: Sen. Regist. (Radiol.) Mersey RHA.

PICKWORTH, Frederick John (retired) The Coach House, 10 Cherry Hill Road, Barnt Green, Birmingham B45 8LJ Tel: 0121 445 3066 Email: johnpickworth@b-g.demon.co.uk — MB ChB Birm. 1956 (Bimingham) DObst RCOG 1959. Prev: GP Worcs.

PICKWORTH, Julia Christine Pinfold Lane Surgery, 40 Pinfold Lane, Butterknowle, Bishop Auckland DL13 5NU Tel: 01388 718230 Fax: 01388 718808 — MB BS Newcastle 1975; MB BS Ncle 1975. GP Bishop Auckland, Co. Durh.

PICKWORTH, Kenneth Hart (retired) 41 Woodside, Barnard Castle DL12 8DZ Tel: 01833 638398 — (Durh.) MB BS Durh. 1944; MRCGP 1960.

PICKWORTH, Michael John Wylie 18 Clifford Close, Droitwich, Worcester WR9 8UT — MB ChB Birm. 1993; ChB Birm. 1993; MB Ch.B Birm. 1993; DCH 1996. GP Locum; GP Princip., Corbett Med. Pract., Droitwich, Worcester. Specialty: Gen. Pract. Prev: GP Regist. Lowesmoor Med. Centre, Worcester; Worcester Roy. Infirm. GP VTS.

PICKWORTH, Richard William Alderman Jack Cohen Health Centre, Springwell Road, Sunderland SR3 4HG Tel: 0191 528 2727 Fax: 0191 528 3262; 13 Thornhill Terrace, Sunderland SR2 7JL — MB ChB Leeds 1978.

PICKWORTH, Sarah Anne Margaret 13 Pevensey Road, Worthing BN11 5NP Tel: 01903502220 Fax: 01903502220; 13 Pevensey Road, Worthing BN11 5NP Tel: 01903502220 Fax: 01903502220 — (Char. Cross & Westm.) Cert Prescribed Exp; BSc. (1st cl. Hons.) Nutrit. & Basic. Med. Sc. Lond. 1987; MB BS Lond. 1990; DFFP 1997; PHEC 1997; DTM & H 1999. MB BS Lond. 1990. Specialty: Gen. Pract. Socs: BMA; Roy. Soc. Hyg. And Trop. Med.

PICKWORTH, Sheila Mary (retired) The Coach House, 10 Cherry Hill Road, Barnt Green, Birmingham B45 8LJ Tel: 0121 445 3066 — MB BS Lond. 1956 (Roy. Free) MRCS Eng. LRCP Lond. 1956. Prev: Clin. Asst. (Gen. Med.) BromsGr. Gen. Hosp.

PICOZZI, Mr Gerard Louis 8 Muir Street, Coatbridge ML5 1NH — MB ChB Glas. 1974; FRCS Glas. 1980.

PICOZZI, Joan 8 Muir Street, Coatbridge ML5 1NH — MB ChB Glas. 1974. Clin. Asst. Diabetes Opd Glas. Roy. Infirm. Specialty: Diabetes.

PICTON, Catherine Ellison The Medical Centre, 6 The Green, West Drayton UB7 7PJ Tel: 01895 442026 Fax: 01895 430753; Fortune Gate, Manor Crescent, Seer Green, Beaconsfield HP9 2QX — MB ChB Dundee 1983; BSc Leeds 1973; DRCOG 1986; DCH RCP Lond. 1989.

PICTON, June Margaret Winslade, Lower Priory, Milford Haven SA73 3UB — MB BS Lond. 1981; MRCGP, MSc; MRCS Eng. LRCP Lond. 1981; DRCOG 1983.

PICTON, Paul — MB ChB Sheff. 1993 (Sheff. Univ. Med. Sch.) BMedSci Sheff. 1990; MRCP (UK) 1996; FRCA 2000. SpR Anaesthetics Wessex. Specialty: Anaesth.

PICTON, Susan Vanessa Department of Paediatric Oncology, Childrens Day Hospital, St. James Hospital, Beckett Street, Leeds LS9 7TF Tel: 0113 206 4985 Fax: 0113 247 0248 Email: susan.picton@leedsh.nhs.uk; 37 Gledhow Wood Road, Leeds LS8 4BZ — BM BS Nottm. 1986; BMedSci. Nottm. 1984; MRCP (UK) 1990; FRCPCH Lond. 1996. Cons. Paediat. Oncol. St. Jas. Univ. Hosp. NHS Trust Leeds. Specialty: Paediat. Socs: UK Childrens Cancer Study Gp.; RCPCH. Prev: Lect. (Paediat. Oncol.) Manch. Univ. & Roy. Manch. Childr. Hosp.; Regist. (Paediat.) Qu. Pk. Hosp. Blackburn.

PICTON, Thomas Andrew — MB BS Lond. 1994; MRCPsych.

PICTON-JONES, Evan Ceredig Fountain Hill, Eglwyswrw, Crymych SA41 3RY — MB BCh Wales 1995.

PICTON-JONES, Jennifer (retired) 12 Shirley Avenue, Cheam, Sutton SM2 7QR Tel: 020 8642 2760 — MB BS Lond. 1962 (Roy. Free) MRCS Eng. LRCP Lond. 1962; DPM Eng. 1966; FRCPsych 1985, M 1972; T(Psych.) 1991. Prev: Med. Dir. Croydon Ment. Health Serv.

PICTON-ROBINSON, Ian 43 Valley View, Market Drayton TF9 1EA Tel: 01630 654300 — (St. Thos.) BSc (Anat.) Lond. 1960; MB BS Lond. 1963; DIH Soc. Apoth. Lond. 1968; FFOM Lond. 1992. Independent Occupational Physician. Specialty: Occupat. Health. Prev: Regional Med. Off. Austin-Rover Ltd.; SHO St. Matthew's Hosp. Burntwood.; Sen. Med. Off. Jaguar Cars Ltd.

PICTS, Alexandra Claire 65 Shakespeare Road, St Ives, Huntingdon PE27 6TT Tel: 01480 468369 — MB ChB Bristol 1996 (Univ. of Bris.) SHO (Surgic. Rotat.) Roy. Sussx Co. Hosp. Brighton. Prev: Demonst. (Anat.) Roy. Free Med. Sch.; SHO (Orthop.) Soton. Gen. Hosp.; SHO (A&E) Western Gen. Hosp.

PIDD, Sally Anne Victoria House, Thornton Road, Morecambe LA4 5NN Tel: 01524 400445 Fax: 01524 400357 — MB ChB Birm. 1972; FRCPsych 1991, M 1976. Cons. Psychiat. Morecambe Bay PCT. Specialty: Gen. Psychiat. Prev: Sen. Regist. (Psychother.)

Whittingham Hosp. Preston; Sen. Regist. (Psychiat.) Lancaster Moor Hosp.; Research Fell. Dept. Psychiat. Univ. Birm.

PIDGEON, Colleen Alison Sandhurst Group Practice, 72 Yorktown Road, Sandhurst GU47 9BT Tel: 01252 872455 Fax: 01252 872456 — MB BCh Wales 1976; BSc Bristol 1973; DCH Eng. 1979; DRCOG 1979; MRCGP 1982.

PIDGEON, Nigel David New Hall Lane Practice, The Health Centre, Geoffrey Street, Preston PR1 5NE Tel: 01772 401730 Fax: 01772 401731; Jonah House, 19 Sheraton Park, Ingol, Preston PR2 7AZ Tel: 01772 727094 — MB BS Lond. 1978 (Char. Cross) MRCS Eng. LRCP Lond. 1978; DRCOG 1984; MRCGP 1985. Hosp. Pract. (Gastroenterol.) Roy. Preston Hosp. Specialty: Gen. Pract.; Gastroenterol. Socs: Christ. Med. Fellowsh.

PIDSLEY, Charles Godfrey Laurence Bridge Surgery, St Peters Street, Stapenhill, Burton-on-Trent DE15 9AW Tel: 01283 563451 Fax: 01283 500896; 46 Meadow View, Rolleston on Trent, Burton-on-Trent DE13 9AN — MB BS Lond. 1982; DRCOG 1986; MRCGP 1987.

PIDSLEY, Godfrey Kenneth (retired) Tanglewood, Elmbridge, Droitwich WR9 0DA Tel: 01299 851667 — MB BS Lond. 1954 (Middlx.) Prev: Ho. Off. (Cas.) Mt. Vernon Hosp. Northwood Middlx.

PIECHOWSKI, Leszek Dryland Surgery, 1 Field Street, Kettering NN16 8JZ Tel: 01536 518951 Fax: 01536 486200 — MB BS Lond. 1980; Primary FRCS London 1982; Cert Family Plann 1985; MRCGP 1989. Chairm. Kettering PCG; Northamptonshire eartlands PCT Lead Clinician. Prev: Regist. (Geriat. & Gen. Med.) Upton Hosp. Slough; SHO (Paediat.) Wexham Pk. Hosp. Slough; SHO (A & E) St. Geo. Hosp. Tooting.

PIENAAR, Georg Frederick 22 Tylsworth Close, Amersham HP6 5DF — MB ChB Orange Free State 1995.

PIEPER, Hans The Surgery, 3 Racecourse Road, Ayr KA7 2DF Tel: 01292 886622; 53 Ottoline Drive, Troon KA10 7AN — State Exam Med Hanover 1984; MD Hanover 1986; DA (UK) 1990; MRCGP 1994. GP Principal. Specialty: Rehabil. Med.; Rheumatol. Prev: Staff Grade (A & E) The Ayr Hosp.; Trainee GP Salen Isle of Mull; Sen. Anaesth. Ahli Hosp. Gaza, Israeli Occupied Territories.

PIERCE, Agnes Main (retired) 11 Roseacre, West Kirby, Wirral CH48 5JW — MB ChB Ed. 1952. Cons. Child Abuse Merseyside Police Auth. Prev: Med. Off. (Paediat.) Alder Hey Hosp. Liverp.

PIERCE, Alison Agnes Bootham Park Hospital, Bootham, York YO30 7BY Tel: 01904 454072 — MB ChB Ed. 1984; BSc (Hons.) Ed. 1982; MRCPsych 1991. Specialist Regist. Old Age Psychiat. Bootham Pk. Hosp., York. Specialty: Geriat. Psychiat. Prev: Staff Grade Psychiat. Springwood Community Unit for the Eldrly, Malton, NY; Staff Grade Psychiat. ScarsBoro. & NE Yorks. Health Care.; Regist. (Psychiat.) Roy. Edin. & Assoc. Hosp. Edin.

PIERCE, Elsbeth Wyn Bron-y-Fedw, 6 Llysgwyn, Caernarfon LL55 1EN — MB ChB Liverp. 1985.

PIERCE, Emma Louise 38 Cleveland Road, Brighton BN1 6FG — BM Soton. 1996.

PIERCE, Jonathan Mark Thomas Southampton General Hospital, Anaesthetic Department, MP24, Southampton SO16 6YD Tel: 023 8079 6135 Fax: 023 8079 4348 — BM Soton. 1981; MRCP (UK) 1985; DA (UK) 1986; FFA RCS Eng. 1988. Cons. Cardiac Anaesth. Soton. Gen. Hosp. Soton. Specialty: Anaesth. Special Interest: Cardiac Anasthesia (Adult & Paediatric); Cardiothractic Intens. Care. Socs: Assn.of Cardiothoracic Anaesth. Prev: Sen. Regist. (Anaesth.) Soton. & Portsmouth Hosps.; Fell. (Cardiothoracic Anaesth.) Groningen, Netherlands.

PIERCE, Julie Francis Flat B, 34 Hans Road, London SW3 1RW — MB BS Lond. 1991.

PIERCE, Mary Bridget (retired) 8 Eliot Place, London SE3 0QL Tel: 020 8852 4423 Mob: 07774 759213 Email: yof30@uk.uumail.com — MB BChir Camb. 1978; LMSSA Lond. 1977; MRCGP 1982; MD Lond. 1997. p/t Sen. Lect. (Gen. Pract.) Univ. of Warwick. Prev: Lect. (Gen. Pract.) UMDS Lond.

PIERCE-WILLIAMS, Gwyn Clarence House, 14 Russell Road, Rhyl LL18 3BY Tel: 01745 350680 Fax: 01745 353293; Brithdir, 24 Bryntirion Avenue, Rhyl LL18 3NP — MB ChB Liverp. 1977; DRCOG 1980; MRCGP 1981; DFFP 1994.

PIERCY, Melanie Louise Royal Devon & Exeter Hospital, Barrack Road, Exeter EX2 5DW — MB ChB Bristol 1994.

PIERCY, Norman MacLennan (retired) Shandon, 4 Rosehill, Montrose DD10 8RZ Tel: 01674 673665 — (St. And.) MB ChB St. And. 1952; MRCGP 1968; DObst RCOG 1970. Prev: GP Montrose.

PIERECHOD, Bogdan Antony Nova Scotia Medical Centre, Leeds Road, Allerton Bywater, Castleford WF10 2DP — MB ChB Leeds 1975.

PIERIDES, Marios Capio Nightingale Hospital, Edward House, 7 Lisson Grove, London NW1 6SH Tel: 020 7535 7901 Fax: 020 7724 8115 Email: kelly.riley@capio.co.uk — MB BCh Witwatersrand 1982; BA S. Africa 1984; MRCPsych 1993. Cons. Psychiat. Capio Nightingale Hosp. Lond. Specialty: Gen. Psychiat. Socs: Indep. Doctors Forum. Prev: Cons. Psychiat. S. Lond. & Maudsley NHS Trust; Sen. Regist. Guy's & St Thos. Hosp. Lond.

PIERINI, Stephen Victor — BM BCh Oxf. 1997; MRCP; MA; MRCGP. Specialty: Gen. Med.

PIERIS, Malwattage Janaka Asitha 11 Linley Court, Rouse Gardens, London SE21 8AQ — MB BS Lond. 1994.

PIERONI, Joyce Elaine Shaftesbury Medical Centre, 480 Harehills Lane, Leeds LS9 6DE Tel: 0113 248 5631 Fax: 0113 235 0658 — MB ChB Leeds 1984; DRCOG 1987; MRCGP 1988.

PIERPOINT, Steven Hill and Partners, 36 Belmont Hill, London SE13 5AY Tel: 020 8852 8357 Fax: 020 8297 2011 — BM Soton. 1984; MRCGP.

PIERRE, Sylvan Lyndon 14 Teynton Terrace, London N17 7PZ — MB BS West Indies 1988.

PIERREPOINT, Marcus John Department of Child Health, University Hospital Wales, Heath Park, Cardiff CF14 4XW — MB BCh Wales 1991 (UWCM) MRCPCH; MRCP (UK) 1995. Res. Fell. (Cystic Fibrosis) UWCM. Specialty: Paediat. Socs: MDU. Prev: SHO (Cardiopulm. Med.) S. Glam. HA; Specialist Regist. (Paediat.) Mid Glam.; SHO (Paediat.) UHW Cardiff.

PIERREPOINT, Susan Elizabeth The Park Canol Group Practice, Park Canol Surgery, Central Park, Pontypridd CF38 1RJ Tel: 01443 203414 Fax: 01443 218218; The Blackthorns, Chapel Lane, Upper Church Village, Pontypridd CF38 1EE Tel: 01443 202312 — MB ChB Liverp. 1962; MB ChB (Hons.) Liverp. 1962; DObst RCOG 1964.

PIERRO, Mr Agostino Department of Paediatric Surgery, Institute of Child Health & Great Ormond Street Hospital NHS Trust, 30 Guildford St., London WC1N 1EH Tel: 020 7905 2175 Fax: 020 7404 6181 Email: a.pierro@ich.ucl.ac.uk; 80 Etheldene Avenue, London N10 3QB Tel: 020 8444 8605 — State Exam Rome 1978; FRCS Ed.; FRCS Engl. Prof. of Paediat. Surg.; Hon. Cons. in Paediat. Surg. UCL. Specialty: Paediat. Surg. Socs: Counc. Mem. Brit. Assn. of Paed. Surgs.; Canad. Assn. of Paed. Surg.; Clin. Nutrit. & Metabol. Gp. (Chairm.). Prev: Cons. Paediat. Surg. & Reader Lond.; Cons. & Sen. Lect. Paediat. Surg. Liverp. Alderhey Hosp.

PIERRY, Adrian Arrau Cardiff Road Medical Centre, 31 Cardiff Road, Llandaff, Cardiff CF5 2DP Tel: 029 2057 6675 Fax: 029 2057 5367; Coast Guard Cottage, 2 Marine Parade, Penarth CF64 3BE Tel: 029 2070 4609 — MRCS Eng. LRCP Lond. 1975 (Univ. Chile) Medico Cirujano Chile 1970; MRCPI 1978; MRCGP 1983; DRCOG 1983. Clin. Tutor Univ. Wales Sch. Med. Specialty: Gen. Pract. Prev: Trainee GP Cardiff VTS; Regist. (Med.) Glas. Roy. Infirm.; SHO Regist. (Med.) Hope Hosp.

PIERSON, Janet Gagnon Byways, South Harting, Petersfield GU31 5PH — BM Soton. 1979; DCH RCP Lond. 1984; MRCGP 1984; AFOM Lond. 1996. Occupational Health Phys. Specialty: Occupat. Health. Socs: BMA; SOM. Prev: GP Portsmouth.

PIERZCHNIAK, Piotr 8 Medgbury Road, Swindon SN1 2AS — MB BS Lond. 1987; MRCPsych 1992.

PIESOWICZ, Alina Teresa (retired) 78 Grosvenor Avenue, Carshalton SM5 3EP Tel: 020 8647 2917 — (Guy's) MB BS Lond. 1958; MRCS Eng. LRCP Lond. 1958; DCH Eng. 1960; FRCP Lond. 1979, M 1961; FRCPCH 1997. Prev: Cons. Paediatr. Qu. Mary's Hosp. Childr. & St. Helier Hosp. Carshalton.

PIETRONI, Mark Arthur Charles Lamb Hospital, Po Parbntipur, Dist. Dinajpur 5250, Dinajpur, Bangladesh Tel: 00 880 552 69011 Email: lamb@citechco.net; 54 Medway Road, London E3 5BY Tel: 020 8980 3969 — MB BChir Camb. 1992 (Lond.) MA Camb. 1992; MRCP (UK) 1994; DTM & H RCP Lond. 1996; MA (Open Univ.) 1997. Med. Cons. Lamb Hosp. TB Control Progr.; Chief Dept. of Med. Lamb Hosp. Specialty: Trop. Med.; Gen. Med.; Respirat. Med. Socs: BMA; Christ. Med. Fellowsh. Prev: Regist. (Infec. Dis. &

Trop. Med.) Northwick Pk. Hosp.; Regist. (Chest Med.) Northwick Pk. Hosp.; SHO (Med.) & Ho. Phys. OldCh. Hosp.

PIETRONI, Raymond Allan Yves Princess Street Group Practice, 2 Princess Street, London SE1 6JP Tel: 020 7928 0253 Fax: 020 7261 9804 — MRCS Eng. LRCP Lond. 1964 (Guy's) BSc (Anat.) Lond. 1962, MB BS 1965; DCH Eng. 1968; MRCGP 1970. GP Princess St. Gp. Pract.; Sen. Lect. (Gen. Pract.) United Med. & Dent. Sch. Lond. Univ.; Med. Adviser Ch. Eng. Childr. Soc. Socs: BMA. Prev: SHO (Chest) Whittington Hosp. Lond.; Ho. Surg. & Cas. Off. & Ho. Phys. Guy's Hosp. Lond.

PIETRONI, Roger Gabriel Ealing Park Health Centre, 195A South Ealing Road, Ealing, London W5 4RH Tel: 020 8758 0570 Fax: 020 8560 5182; 2 Layer Gardens, London W3 9PR Tel: 020 8992 4362 — MB BS Lond. 1972 (Guy's Hospital) MRCS Eng. LRCP Lond. 1972; FRCGP 1992, M 1976; Dip. Med. Educat. Dund 1989; MMed. Dundee 1992. GP; Sen. Teachg. Fell. Imperial Coll. Sch. of Med. Prev: Assn. Adiviser Gen. Pract. NW Thames; RCGP Schering Schol.ship 1987; Course Organiser VTS Ealing Hosp.

PIETRONI, Teresa Lesley Chrisp Street Health Centre, 100 Chrisp St., London E14 6PG Tel: 020 7515 4860; 54 Medway Road, London E3 5BY Tel: 020 8980 3969 — MB BChir Camb. 1992; MA Camb. 1992; DRCOG 1994; MRCGP 1996. Specialty: Gen. Psychiat. Prev: Trainee GP/SHO Roy. Lond. Hosp. VTS.

PIGGOT, Mr Thomas Alan, TD (retired) Ardlui, 3 Osbaldeston Gardens, Gosforth, Newcastle upon Tyne NE3 4JE Tel: 0191 285 8934 — MB BCh BAO Belf. 1953 (Qu. Univ. Belf.) FRCS Ed. 1961. Prev: Sen. Regist. (Plastic Surg.) Wythenshawe Hosp. Manch.

PIGGOTT, Andrea Grosvenor Medical Centre, Grosvenor Street, Crewe CW1 3HB Tel: 01270 256348 Fax: 01270 250786; 56 Millbeck Close, Weston, Crewe CW2 5LR — MB ChB Liverp. 1986; MRCGP 1990.

PIGGOTT, Mr Harry (retired) Orchard House, 28 Bradshaw Drive, Holbrook, Belper DE56 0SZ — (Camb. & St. Thos.) MB BChir Camb. 1948; FRCS Eng. 1955. Hon. Cons. Orthop. Surg. United Birm. Hosps., Roy. Orthop. Hosp. Birm. & Midl. Centre For Neurosurg. & Neurol. Smethwick. Prev: Sen. Regist. (Orthop.) Middlx. Hosp. Lond.

PIGGOTT, Rosemary Margaret Moorland Practice Centre, Regent St., Leek ST13 6LU — MB ChB Birm. 1983; MRCPsych 1987. GP Retainer Scheme Leek, Staffs. Prev: Clin. Med. Off. (Community Paediat.) Stoke-on-Trent; Clin. Asst. (Psychiat.) Parent & Baby Unit Stoke-on-Trent; Regist. (Psychiat.) N. Staffs. VTS.

PIGGOTT, Susanna Elizabeth — MB ChB Birm. 1980; FRCA 1987. Specialty: Anaesth.

PIGOTT, Ailie Elizabeth Amilla House, Windmill Lane, Wheatley, Oxford OX33 1TA — MB BS Lond. 1998.

PIGOTT, Brian (retired) 20 Beaufort Close, Lynden Gate, Putney Heath, London SW15 3TL Tel: 020 8789 2513 Fax: 020 8789 2513 — BM BCh Oxf. 1952 (Oxf. & Guy's) BA Oxf. 1949. Prev: Regist. (Med.) & Ho. Phys. Guy's Hosp. Lond.

PIGOTT, Mr Humphrey William Shilton (retired) The Stone House, Felsham Road, Cockfields, Bury St Edmunds IP30 0AB Tel: 01284 828727 — MRCS Eng. LRCP Lond. 1962 (Middlx.) BA Camb. 1959, MB 1963, BChir 1962; FRCS Eng. 1967. Prev: Regist. (Surg.) Middlx. Hosp. Lond.

PIGOTT, Jacqueline Dawn 17 Burnaby Gardens, London W4 3DR — MB BChir Camb. 1988; MA Camb. 1989.

PIGOTT, Jean Lesley Child and Family Department, Tavistock Clinic, 120 Belsize Lane, London NW3 5BA Tel: 020 7435 7111 — MB BS Lond. 1985 (University College Hospital (London)) PhD Lond. 1981, BA 1977; DCH RCP Lond. 1989; MRCPsych. 1991. Cons. in Child & Adolesc. Psychiat. Tavistock & Portman NHS Trust & Clin. Dir. Tavistock Munrae Young Family Centre. Specialty: Child & Adolesc. Psychiat. Socs: RCPsych - ACPP. Prev: Sen. Regist. Rotat. (Child & Adolesc. Psychiat.) Tavistock & Portman NHS Trust.

PIGOTT, Julia Elizabeth M Brennan and Partners, Captain French Lane Surgery, Kendal LA9 4HR Tel: 01539 720241 Fax: 01539 725084 — MB ChB Manch. 1982; BSc (Hons.) Manch. 1979; MRCGP 1986. Med. Off. Family Plann. & Police Surg. Kendal.

PIGOTT, Katharine Hamilton Royal Free Hospital, Pond St., London NW3 2QG Tel: 020 7830 2169 Fax: 020 7830 2968 — MB BS Lond. 1985 (Middlesex hospital) FRCP (UK); MRCP (UK) 1988; FRCR 1992; MD MD 1995. Cons. (Clin. Oncol.) Roy. Free Hosp. Lond. Specialty: Oncol. Prev: Sen. Regist. (Radiother.) Mt. Vernon Hosp.

PIGOTT, Nicholas Brian Great Ormond Street Hospital for Children NHS Trust, Great Ormond Street, London WC1N 3JH Tel: 020 7405 9200 Fax: 020 7829 8673 Email: pigotn@gosh.nhs.uk — MB BS Lond. 1984 (St. Thos. Hosp. Med. Sch. Lond.) MRCPI 1994; MRCPCH 1996. Cons. Paediatric Intens. Care, Gt. Ormond St. Hosp. for Childr., Lond.. Specialty: Paediat.; Intens. Care. Socs: Med. Protec. Soc.; MRCPCH; Paediat. Intens. Care Soc.

PIGOTT, Peter Vilven Fairhurst, Peppard Common, Henley-on-Thames RG9 — MB BChir Camb. 1959 (St. Thos.) MA Camb. 1959; DO Eng. 1961. Med. Dir. YRCR Ltd. Henley-on-Thames. Socs: Fell. Roy. Soc. Med.; BMA. Prev: Specialist (Ophth.) Brit. Milit. Hosp. Dhekelia, Cyprus; Regist. (Ophth.) Aylesbury & High Wycombe Hosps.; Ho. Surg. (Ophth.) St. Thos. Hosp. Lond.

PIGOTT, Stephen Christopher Merchiston Surgery, Highworth Road, Swindon SN3 4BF Tel: 01793 823307 Fax: 01793 820923 — MB BS Lond. 1974; MRCS Eng. LRCP Lond. 1974; GP(T) 1978. Lect. & Course Organiser Sch. Postgrad. Med. Univ. Bath. Socs: Med. Equestrian Assn.

PIGOTT, Susan Jane Plymyard Avenue Surgery, 170 Plymyard Avenue, Eastham, Wirral CH62 8EH Tel: 0151 327 1391 — BM BS Nottm. 1984; BMedSci Nottm. 1982, BM BS 1984; MRCGP 1990; DRCOG 1990. Prev: Trainee GP Nottm. VTS.

PIGOTT, Tara Grace 9 Woodland Avenue, Hemel Hempstead HP1 1RG — MB BS Lond. 1991. Trainee GP Carlisle VTS.

PIGOTT, Mr Timothy John Drummond The Walton Centre for Neurology and Neurosurgery, Rice Lane, Liverpool L9 1AE Tel: 0151 525 3611 — MB ChB Birm. 1982; FRCS Eng. 1986; DM Nottm. 1990; FRCS (SN) 1992. Cons. Neurosurg. Walton Centre Neurol. & Neurosurg. Liverp. Specialty: Neurosurg. Prev: Sen. Regist. (Neurosurg.) Gen. Infirm. Leeds; Regist. (Neurosurg.) Qu. Med. Centre Nottm.; Stanhope Research Fell. (Neurosurg.) S. Derbysh. HA.

PIHLENS, Hugh Lynton Hungerford Surgery, The Croft, Hungerford RG17 0HY Tel: 01488 682507 Fax: 01488 681018; Canver House, 2 Canal Walk, Hungerford RG17 0EQ — MB BS Lond. 1971 (Roy. Free) MRCS Eng. LRCP Lond. 1971.

PIILBERG, Olaf (retired) 4 Withers Road, Worcester WR2 4AG Tel: 01905 424246 — Med. Dip. Tartu 1941.

PIKE, Alison Anne Southmead Hospital, Westbury-on-Trym, Bristol BS10 5NB Tel: 0117 959 5325 Fax: 0117 959 5324 — MB BS Lond. 1984; DCH RCP Lond. 1986; MRCP (UK) 1988; MD 1997. p/t Cons. (Neonatol.) Southmead Hosp. Bristol. Specialty: Neonat.

PIKE, Alison Carol Newton Heath HC, 2 Old Church St, Newton Heath, Manchester M40 2JF Tel: 0161 684 9696 — MB BS Lond. 1988; MRCP (UK) 1993. Sen. Regist. Rotat. (Paediat. & Community Paediat.) Roy. Manch. Childr. Hosp. Specialty: Community Child Health. Prev: Regist. Rotat. (Paediat.) Roy. Manch. Childr. Hosp.; Clin. Med. Off. (Paediat.) Leicester; SHO (Paediat.) Birm. Childr. Hosp.

PIKE, Brian Richard Bishopgate Medical Centre, 178 Newgate Street, Bishop Auckland DL14 7EJ Tel: 01388 603983 Fax: 01388 607782; The Old Vicarage, Kingsway, Bishop Auckland DL14 7JN Tel: 01388 608191 — MB BS Newc. 1968; DObst RCOG 1970; MRCGP 1972. Trainer (Gen. Pract.) & Hosp. Pract. (Geriat.) Bishop Auckland. Specialty: Orthop. Socs: BMA. Prev: GP, New Zealand; Med. Off. W. Austral. Govt.; Ho. Off. Roy Vict. Infirm. Newc.

PIKE, Catherine Provan (retired) Blatchfeld, Littleford Lane, Blackheath, Guildford GU4 8QY Tel: 01483 892358 — MB ChB Glas. 1943. Prev: Cons. Histopath. (Cytopath.) S.W. Surrey Health Dist.

PIKE, Eileen Elizabeth Radiology Department, Bishop Auckland General Hospital, Cockton Hill Road, Bishop Auckland DL14 6AD; The Old Vicarage, Kingsway, Bishop Auckland DL14 7JN — MB BS Newc. 1970; DObst RCOG 1972; FRCR 1985. Cons. Radiol. Gateshead Hosps. NHS Trust. Specialty: Radiol. Prev: Cons. Radiol. Darlington Memor. Hosp.

PIKE, Helen Sarah — MB ChB Manch. 1998; DFFP; DRCOG; MRCGP 2002.

PIKE, Mr Jeremy Martin Frimley Park Hospital, Portsmouth Road, Frimley, Camberley GU16 7UJ Tel: 01276 604456 Fax: 01276 604457; 4 Lakeside Grange, Weybridge KT13 9ZE Tel: 01932 821362 — BM Soton. 1984; FRCS Eng. 1990; FRCS (Orth.) 1995.

Cons. Orthop. Frimley Pk. Hosp. Camberley. Specialty: Orthop. Prev: Sen. Regist. (Orthop.) St. Geo. Hosp. Lond.

PIKE, John Kingswood Health Centre, Alma Road, Kingswood, Bristol BS15 4EJ Tel: 0117 961 1774 Fax: 0117 947 8969; 17 Kennington Avenue, Bishopston, Bristol BS7 9EU Tel: 0117 944 4084 — MB BS Lond. 1987; Cert. Family Plann. JCC 1990; MRCGP 1991. Specialty: Gen. Pract. Socs: BMA; Med. Protec. Soc. Prev: Trainee GP Dorset; SHO (O & G, Gen. Med. & A & E) W. Dorset Hosps.

PIKE, John Lindsay The Warren, 17 Meadowfield Road, Stocksfield NE43 7PY — MB ChB Leeds 1995; MRCP 1999; FRCA 2002. Specialty: Anaesth.

PIKE, Jonathan Maxwell 23 High Street, Alconbury, Huntingdon PE28 4DS — BM BS Nottm. 1991. Prev: Ho. Off. (Med.) St. Geo. Hosp. Lincoln; Ho. Off. (Surg.) MusGr. Pk. Hosp. Taunton.

PIKE, Katherine Claire West Suffolk Hospital, Hardwick Lane, Bury St Edmunds IP33 2QZ — BM BCh Oxf. 1998. SHO (Paediat.) W. Suff. Hosp. Bury St. Edmunds. Specialty: Paediat. Socs: BMA; MDU.

PIKE, Lawrence Charles James Street Family Practice, 49 James Street, Louth LN11 0JN Tel: 01507 611122 Fax: 01507 610435; High Bridge House, High Bridge Road, Alvingham, Louth LN11 0QE Tel: 01507 327875 — MB ChB Birm. 1980; MRCGP 1985.

PIKE, Michael Graham John Radcliffe Hospital, Oxford OX3 9DU — MB BS Lond. 1977 (Guy's) MA Oxf. 1971; MRCS Eng. LRCP Lond. 1977; MRCP (UK) 1981; MD Lond. 1989; FRCPCH 1997. Cons. Paediat. Neurol. Oxf. Radcliffe Hosp.; Hon. Sen. Clin. Lect. (Paediat.) Univ. of Oxf. Specialty: Paediat. Neurol. Socs: Brit. Paediat. Neurol. Assn. Prev: Sen. Regist. (Paediat. Neurol. & Neurodevelopm. Paediat.) Hosp. Sick Childr. Gt. Ormond St. Lond.; Fell. (Paediat. Neurol.) BC Childr. Hosp. Vancouver, BC, Canada.

PIKE, Shaun Hugo Elgar House Surgery, Church Road, Redditch B97 4AB Tel: 01527 69261 Fax: 01527 596856 — MB ChB Birm. 1984. GP Redditch.

PIKE, Stephen Charles Selden Medical Centre, 6 Selden Road, Worthing BN11 2LL Tel: 01903 234962 — MB BS Lond. 1986 (St. Geo. Hosp. Med. Sch. Lond.) DCH RCP Lond. 1989; DRCOG 1990; MRCGP 1991; DFFP 1994; Dip. Ther. 1998. GP Worthing. Specialty: Gen. Pract. Prev: Trainee GP/SHO (Psychiat.) Medway VTS.

PIKE, Warwick John, Air Vice-Marshal RAF Med. Br. Director General Medical Services (Royal Air Force), HQ Personnel and Training Command, Royal Air Force Innsworth, Gloucester GL3 1EZ Tel: 01452 712612 — (Guy's) MB BS Lond. 1968; MRCS Eng. LRCP Lond. 1968; DObst RCOG 1975; MRCGP 1975; DAvMed Eng. 1979; MFOM RCP 1992, AFOM 1981; MSc Lond. 1988. Dir. Gen. Med. Servs. RAF. Specialty: Occupat. Health; Aviat. Med.; Gen. Pract. Socs: Soc. Occupat. Med.; Fell. Roy. Soc. of Med. Prev: Dir. Personnel & Servs. Defence Secondary Care Agency; Dir. Med. Personnel RAF; Command. Off. Princess Mary's RAF Hosp., Akrotiri.

PILAPITIYA, Rahula Bandara Ashburne Medical Centre, 74-75 Toward Road, Sunderland SR2 8JG Tel: 0191 567 4397 Fax: 0191 567 1035; 2 Seaton Park, Seaham SR7 0HH Tel: 0191 581 8705 — Vrach 2nd Moscow Med. Inst. USSR 1971 (2nd Moscow State Pyzogovs Med. Inst.) DA Eng. 1980; DRCOG 1981; Cert. Prescribed Equiv. Exp. JCPTGP 1983; Cert. Family Plann. JCC 1984. Staff Grade (Anaesth.) City Hosps. Sunderland. Specialty: Diabetes; Cardiol.; Neurol. Socs: Obst. Anaesth. Assn. Prev: Trainee GP Som.; Trainee GP Newc. VTS; Regist. & Clin. Asst. (Anaesth.) Som. AHA.

PILBROW, Lisa Katharine 56 Copthall Lane, Chalfont St Peter, Gerrards Cross SL9 0DJ — MB BS Lond. 1991.

PILCH, David John Fuller The Blofield Surgery, Plantation Road, Blofield, Norwich NR13 4PL Tel: 01603 712337 Fax: 01603 712899 — BM BCh Oxf. 1974.

PILCHER, Christopher John Chatsworth Road Medical Centre, Chatsworth Road, Brampton, Chesterfield S40 3PY Tel: 01246 568065 Fax: 01246 567116 — MB ChB Sheff. 1981; DRCOG 1985.

PILCHER, David Vytas 15 Roebuck Lane, Rochester ME1 1UE Tel: 01634 832509 — MB BS Lond. 1993 (Camb. Univ. & Royal Lond. Hosp. Med. Sch.) MRCP 1996. Specialty: Gen. Med.; Respirat. Med.; Intens. Care.

PILCHER, James Martin 7 St Nicholas Mansions, Trinity Crescent, London SW17 7AF — MB BS Lond. 1990.

PILCHER, Mr Richard, Air Commodore RAF Dent. Br. c/o National Westminster Bank plc, PO Box 2DG, 208 Picadilly, London W1A 2DG; 14 Westwell Court, Castle Dene, South Gosforth, Newcastle upon Tyne NE3 1YY Tel: 0191 285 2667 — LMSSA Lond. 1993 (University College and Middlesex Hospital London) BSc (Hons.) Dund 1977, BDS 1981; FDS RCPS Glas. 1987; FRCS Glas. 1998. Staff Grade (Oral & Maxillofacial Surg.) Newc. Gen. Hosp. Specialty: Oral & Maxillofacial Surg. Socs: Brit. Assn. Oral & Maxillofacial Surg.; BMA; Med. Protec. Soc. Prev: Specialist Regist. Rotat. (Oral & Maxillofacial Surg.); Sen. Specialist (Oral Surg.) Camb. Milit. Hosp. Aldershot.; Specialist (Oral Surg.) Brit. Milit. Hosp. Munster, Germany.

PILE, Horace Francis (retired) 104 Summercourt Way, Brixham TQ5 0RB Tel: 01803 852857; 104 Summercourt way, Brixham TQ5 0RB Tel: 01803 852857 — MB BS Lond. 1950 (Guy's) MRCS Eng. LRCP Lond. 1950.

PILE, Nicholas Richard Phoenix Surgery, 33 Bell Lane, Burham, Rochester ME1 3SX Tel: 01634 367982 Fax: 01634 864513 — MB BS Lond. 1982 (Roy. Free) DCH RCP Lond. 1985; MRCGP 1988; DRCOG 1988. Specialty: Gen. Pract.

PILGRIM, Jane Moreton Lodge, Farmhouse, Culworth, Banbury OX17 2HL — MB BS Lond. 1970 (St. Bart.) MRCS Eng. LRCP Lond. 1970; FFA RCS Eng. 1978; MRCGP 1981; DRCOG 1982. Specialty: Anaesth.

PILGRIM, John Anthony Department of Psychiatry, Doncaster Royal Infirmary, Armthorpe Road, Doncaster DN2 5LT Tel: 01302 366666 Fax: 01302 761317 Email: john.pilgrim@dsh.nhs.uk — MB BS Lond. 1986 (University college London) MA (Hons.) St And. 1980; MRCPsych 1990. Cons. Psychiat. Doncaster Roy. Infirm. Specialty: Gen. Psychiat. Socs: MRCPsych. Prev: Sen. Regist. Bethlem & Maudsley Hosp. Lond.

PILGRIM, Lisa Louisa Pilgrims Rest, Sudbury Road, Bures CO8 5JL — MB ChB Leeds 1988.

PILKINGTON, Adele IOM, 8 Roxburgh Place, Edinburgh EH8 9SU Tel: 0131 667 5131; 120 Candlemakers Park, Edinburgh EH17 8TL — MB BS Lond. 1985; DA (UK) 1987; DCH RCP Lond. 1988; Cert. Family Plann. JCC 1989; DRCOG 1989; MRCGP 1990; MFOM RCP Lond. 1996. Cons. Occupat. Phys. Inst. Occupat. Med. Edin. Specialty: Occupat. Health. Prev: Occupat. Phys. Inst. Occupat. Med. Edin.; Sen. Regist. (Occupat. Med.) IBH Company Health Ltd. & Blackpool Vict. Hosp. & Community Trusts; Asst. Med. Edr. The Practitioner.

PILKINGTON, Anna Clare 24 Holly Road, London E8 3XP; 35 Balfour Road, London N5 2HB — MB BS Lond. 1981.

PILKINGTON, Barbara Susan 1 Claddach Carinish, Lochmaddy HS6 5HP Tel: 01876 580218 — MB BS Lond. 1982; BSc Lond. 1979, MB BS 1982; MRCGP 1986.

PILKINGTON, Carole Elaine 2 Beeches Close, Marton Road, Gargrave, Skipton BD23 3NL — MB ChB Manch. 1986.

PILKINGTON, Clare Joanne Westgate Practice, Greenhill Health Centre, Church Street, Lichfield WS13 6JL Tel: 01543 414311 Fax: 01543 256364; 14 Rock Farm Road, Whittington, Lichfield WS14 9LZ — MB BS Lond. 1987.

PILKINGTON, Clarissa Anne Department of Rheumatology, Middlesex Hospital, Tottenham St., London W1 Tel: 020 7636 8333; 23 Sulgrave Road, London W6 7RD — MB BS Lond. 1984; BSc Lond. 1981; MRCP (UK) 1989. Specialty: Paediat. Prev: Cons. (Adolesc. & Paediatric Rheumatology); Hon. Sen. Lect. at ICH, VCL.

PILKINGTON, Edward Michael (retired) 3 Bellsmeadow, necton, Swaffham PE37 8NE Tel: 01760 721355 Fax: 01760 720924 Email: empilkington@necton.fsbusiness.co.uk — MB BS Lond. 1953 (Middlx.) MRCS Eng. LRCP Lond. 1952; DObst RCOG 1955.

PILKINGTON, George Anthony 19 Pine Walk, Great Bookham, Leatherhead KT23 4AS Tel: 01372 459235 — MB ChB Bristol 1951. Socs: (Ex-Pres.) Epsom Med. Soc.

PILKINGTON, Guy Stephen Cruddas Park Surgery, 178 Westmoreland Road, Newcastle upon Tyne NE4 7JT Tel: 0191 226 1414 — MB BS Newc. 1983; BA Oxf. 1980; MRCP (UK) 1986; MRCGP 1989. Prev: Trainee GP N.d. VTS; SHO (Med. & Geriat.) Newc. Gen. Hosp.; SHO (Med.) Shotley Bridge Gen. Hosp. Consett.

PILKINGTON, Harriet 9 Avoca Road, Tooting Bec, London SW17 8SQ — MRCS Eng. LRCP Lond. 1978. Clin. Asst. GU Med. Specialty: Genitourinary Medicine; Psychother.

PILKINGTON, Pamela (retired) 16 Lichfield Road, Kew, Richmond TW9 3JR Tel: 020 8940 0369 — MB BS Lond. 1951 (St Geo.) MRCPsych 1977. Prev: Cons. Psychiat. Long. Gr. Hosp. Epsom.

PILKINGTON, Miss Rachel Sarah 6 Brabham Mews, Swinton, Manchester M27 0HH Tel: 0161 728 3486 — MB ChB Manch. 1991 (Manchester) FRCS Ed. 1996. Specialist Regist. A & E Med. Manch. Deanery; Forens. Police Surg. Greater Manch. Police. Specialty: Accid. & Emerg. Prev: Research Fell. Min. of Defence.

PILKINGTON, Sophie Anne Oaklands, Backwoods Close, Lindfield, Haywards Heath RH16 2EG — BM BCh Oxf. 1996.

PILKINGTON, Thomas Roger Edward 16 Lichfield Road, Kew, Richmond TW9 3JR Tel: 020 8940 0369 — MB BS Lond. 1945 (Middlx.) MRCP Lond. 1946; MD Lond. 1949; FRCP Lond. 1965. Prof. Emerit. Med. St. Geo. Hosp. Med. Sch. Lond.

PILL, Stephen Howard Christopher Health Centre, Old Street, Clevedon BS21 6DG Tel: 01275 871454; 5 Canowie Road, Redland, Bristol BS6 7HP Tel: 0117 973 9501 Email: pill@btinternet.com — MB ChB Bristol 1980; DRCOG 1985; DCH RCP Lond. 1985; MRCGP 1989; MSc Bristol 1990. Cons. Med. Electronic Data Interchange. Socs: RCGP Represent. RCGP/GMSC Jt. Computing Gp.; RCGP Represent. MIG(Med. Informat. Gp.). Prev: GP Melbourne; SHO Bristol VTS.

PILLAI, Aravind 246 Chiswick Village, London W4 3DF — MB BS Lond. 1997.

PILLAI, Chittaranjan Narayana Plains View Surgery, 57 Plains Road, Mapperley, Nottingham NG3 5LB Tel: 0115 962 1717 Email: chic.pillai@gp-c84115.nhs.uk — MB BS Lond. 1976 (King's Coll. Hosp. & Guy's) DCH Eng. 1979; FRCGP 1994, M 1982; Dip Med Educat Nottm. 2005. Trainer (GP) Nottm. VTS.; G. P. Adviser, PostGrad. Dept. Nottm. Univ. Med. Sch.; Exec. Comm. Mem., Gedling PCT. Prev: SHO Univ. Hosp. Nottm. & Hammersmith Hosp. Lond.; Ho. Off. King's Coll. Hosp. Lond.; Course Organiser Nottm. VTS.

PILLAI, Joseph Arulappa Calnwood Court, Calnwood Road, Luton LU4 0LX Tel: 01582 709153 Fax: 01582 709164 — MB BS Ceylon 1971.

PILLAI, Mr Kanapathipillai Oppilamani Boundary House Surgery, 459 Hertford Road, Edmonton, London N9 7DU Tel: 020 8804 2190; 123 Fitzjohn Avenue, Barnet EN5 2HR Tel: 020 8441 8748 — MB BS Ceylon 1973; FRCS Eng. 1982; DRCOG 1987; MRCGP 1989.

PILLAI, Mary Bernadette St. Paul's Wing, Cheltenham General Hospital, Cheltenham GL53 7AN Tel: 08454 222222 Fax: 08454 222337; Glenfall Lodge, Mill Lane, Charlton Kings, Cheltenham GL54 4EP Tel: 01242 578453 Fax: 01242 269528 — MB ChB Bristol 1980; MRCP (UK) 1985; DCH RCP Lond. 1985; MRCOG 1987; MD Bristol 1992. Cons. O & G Cheltenham Gen. Hosp. Specialty: Obst. & Gyn. Prev: Cons. O & G (Fetal Med.) St. Michael's Hosp. Bristol; Perinatal Fell. Wom. Hosp. Winnipeg, Canada; Sen. Regist. (O & G) Glos. Roy. Hosp.

PILLAI, Padmanabha Madhav (retired) 17 Union Way, Witney OX28 6HD Tel: 01993 779088 — MB BS Lucknow 1952 (King Geo. Med. Coll. Lucknow) DTM & H Calcutta 1954; DCH Eng. 1962. Prev: Regist. (Paediat.) Roy. Manch. Childr. Hosp.

PILLAI, Sarah Watson 459 Hertford Road, Edmonton, London N9 7DW Tel: 020 8804 2190; 123 Fitzjohn Avenue, Barnet EN5 2HR Tel: 020 8441 8748 — MB BS Lond. 1984 (Middlx. Hosp.) DFFP; BA Open 1992. Lead. Sen. CMO (Fam. Plann.) Barnet Primary Care Trust; GP Asst.; Clin. Asst. GUM. Specialty: Family Plann. & Reproduc. Health.

PILLAI, Mr Sivathanu Subramania 27 Longmeadows, East Herrington, Sunderland SR3 3SB — (Madras Med. Coll.) MB BS Madras 1950; FRCS Ed. 1959; FRCS Eng. 1962. Cons. Surg. (ENT) N. RHA.

PILLAI, Sunil Kumar — MB BS Lond. 1998.

PILLAY, Deenan Regional Virus Laboratory, Birmingham Heartlands Hospital, Bordesley Green East, Bordesley Green, Birmingham B9 5SS — MB BS Newc. 1987; BSc (1st. cl. Hons.) Biochem. Lond. 1979; PhD Sheff. 1982; MRCPath 1993. Cons. Virol. Birm. Pub. Health Laborat. Birm. Heartlands Hosp. Specialty: Med. Microbiol.; Virology. Prev: Lect. & Hon. Sen. Regist. (Virol.) Div. Communicable Dis. Roy. Free Hosp. Sch. Med. Lond.; Research Fell. (Med. & Path.) Univ. Calif., San Diego, USA; Asst. Lect. & Hon. Regist. (Virol.) UMDS Guys & St. Thos. Hosp. Lond.

PILLAY, Mr Jayapragassen Govindasamy Accident & Emergency Department, County Hospital, Greetwell Road, Lincoln LN2 5QY Tel: 01522 512512; Stonegarth, Northgate, Lincoln LN2 1QT — MB ChB Glas. 1977; FRCS Glas. 1981; FFAEM 1995. Cons. A & E Dept. Co. Hosp. Lincoln. Specialty: Accid. & Emerg.

PILLAYE, Jayshree Health Education Authority, Hamilton House, Habledon Place, London WC1H 9TX Tel: 020 7413 1915 Fax: 020 7413 0342; 1 Tudor House, Pinner Hill Road, Pinner HA5 3RY Tel: 020 8429 2344 — MB ChB Natal 1972; DA Hamburg 1979; Cert. Family Plann. JCC 1984; Cert. Internat. Studies Lond. 1986; MSc Lond. Sch. Economics 1990; DFFP 1993. Sen. Med. Off. (Pub. Health) Health Educat. Auth. Specialty: Pub. Health Med. Socs: Fell. Roy. Soc. Med.; Med. Soc. Study VD. Prev: GP Lond.; SHO (O & G) K. Edwd. VII Hosp. Durban, S. Afr.; Anaesth. Allgemeines Krankenhaus, Hamburg.

PILLEY, Christine Helen Frances 20 Colbourne Road, Hove BN3 1TB — MB ChB Birm. 1991; ChB Birm. 1991.

PILLING, Adrian Charles Kensington Group Practice, Kensington Road, Douglas IM1 3PF Tel: 01624 676774 Fax: 01624 614668 — MB BS Lond. 1972 (St. Mary's) MRCS Eng. LRCP Lond. 1972; DObst RCOG 1975; MRCGP 1979. Prev: Sen. Med. Off. Station Med. Centre RAF Henlow. Sqdn. Ldr. RAF Med.; Br.

PILLING, David John Cleveleys Health Centre, Kelso Avenue, Thornton-Cleveleys FY5 3LF Tel: 01253 823215 Fax: 01253 860640 — MB ChB Liverp. 1974; DObst RCOG 1976. Prev: Trainee GP Blackpool VTS; SHO (O & G) St. Catherine's Hosp. Birkenhead; Ho. Phys. & Ho. Surg. Whiston Hosp. Prescot.

PILLING, David William 20 Riverside, West Kirby, Wirral CH48 3JB Tel: 0151 625 1011 — MB ChB Liverp. 1970 (Liverpool) DCH Eng. 1972; DMRD Eng. 1974; FRCR 1975; FRCPCH 1997. Cons. Radiol. Alder Hey Childr. Hosp. & Liverp. Wom.s Hosp. Specialty: Radiol. Prev: Cons. Radiol. Broadgreen & Alder Hey Childr. Hosp.; Sen. Regist. (Radiol.) Sheff. AHA; Regist. (Radiol.) United Sheff. Hosps.

PILLING, Gillian Mary Elizabeth Dalton Square Surgery, 8 Dalton Square, Lancaster LA1 1PP Tel: 01524 842200; 6 Wyresdale Gardens, Wyresdale Road, Lancaster LA1 3FA Tel: 01524 382856 — MB BS Lond. 1974.

PILLING, John Barry Sutton Lodge, 15 Ipswich Road, Norwich NR2 2LN Tel: 01603 610249 Fax: 01603 610249 — MB BS Lond. 1966 (St. Bart.) MRCS Eng. LRCP Lond. 1966; MRCP (U.K.) 1970; FRCP Lond. 1984. Cons. Neurol. Norf. & Norwich Hosp. & Addenbrooke's Hosp. Camb. Specialty: Neurol. Prev: Sen. Regist. (Neurol.) Nat. Hosp. Nerv. Dis. & St. Bart. Hosp. Lond.; Regist. (Neurol.) Addenbrooke's Hosp. Camb.

PILLING, John Richard Norfolk & Norwich University Hospital NHS Trust, Colney Lane, Norwich NR4 7UY Tel: 01603 286086 Email: john.pilling@nnuh.nhs.uk; 10 Old Grove Court, Catton Grove Road, Norwich NR3 3NL — BM BCh Oxf. 1972; MA Oxf. 1973; DCH Eng. 1974; FRCR 1978. Cons. (Radiol.) Norf. & Norwich Hosp. Norwich. Specialty: Radiol. Prev: Sen. Regist. (Diag. Radiol.) Addenbrooke's Hosp. Camb.; Regist. (Diag. Radiol.) Addenbrooke's Hosp. Camb.; SHO (Paediat. Med.) Childr. Hosp. Sheff.

PILLING, Keith James Occhea Ltd, Occupational Health Services, Stafford Road, Solihull B90 4JJ Tel: 0121 627 4359 Fax: 0121 627 4354 Email: info@occhea.com; 32 Oldway Drive, Solihull B91 3HP Tel: 0121 247 5569 — MB BCh Wales 1982; BSc Wales 1977; FFOM RCP Lond. 1995, MFOM 1992, AFOM 1988; Spec. Accredit. Occupat. Med. JCHMT 1992. Man. Dir. Occhea Ltd.; Hon. Sen. Clin. Lect. Inst. Occupat. Health Birm. Specialty: Occupat. Health. Prev: Dir. Health & Safety Rover Gp. Ltd; Chief Med. Off. UK Atomic Energy Auth.

PILLING, Patricia Jane Penny's Hill Practice, St Mary's Road, Ferndown BH22 9HB Tel: 01202 897200 Fax: 01202 877753 — MB ChB Liverp. 1977; DRCOG 1979.

PILLINGER, John Edward Terence Highcliffe Medical Centre, 248 Lymington Road, Highcliffe, Christchurch BH23 5ET Tel: 01425 272203 Fax: 01425 271086; 1 Howe Close, Mudeford, Christchurch BH23 3JA — MB ChB Liverp. 1982; DRCOG 1984. Specialty: Respirat. Med. Prev: Trainee GP/SHO W. Lancs. HA VTS; Ho. Off. Roy. Liverp. Hosp.

PILLITTERI, Angelo John 157 Clare Road, Maidenhead SL6 4DL — MB ChB Liverp. 1990.

PILLOW, Joan Rosalie (retired) Brookview, Riverside Road, West Moors, Ferndown BH22 0LQ Tel: 01202 875660 — MRCS Eng. LRCP Lond. 1936 (Roy. Free)

PILLOW, Stephen John Civic Medical Centre, Civic Way, Bebington, Wirral CH63 7RX Tel: 0151 645 6936 Fax: 0151 643 1698; Fieldside Cottage, 38 Spital Road, Spital, Wirral CH63 9JF Tel: 0151 334 6318 — MB ChB Leeds 1972; MRCGP 1976; DObst RCOG 1976. Hospice Practitioner St. John's Hospice Wirral. Prev: Trainee GP Doncaster VTS.

PILPEL, James Malcolm The New Surgery, Old Road, Tean, Stoke-on-Trent ST10 4EG Tel: 01538 722323 Fax: 01538 722215 — BM BS Nottm. 1976; BMedSci Nottm. 1974, BM BS 1976; DCH Eng. 1979; Cert FPA. 1980; DRCOG 1980; DA Eng. 1983.

PILPEL, Pamela Jean The Firs, Firbob Lane, Hollington, Stoke-on-Trent ST10 4HT — BMedSci Nottm. 1974, BM BS 1976; Cert. Family Plann. JCC 1979; DCH RCP Lond. 1983. Clin. Med. Off. N. Staffs. HA.

PILSTON, Matthew John 15 Prebend Street, Islington, London N1 8PF Tel: 020 7226 9090 — BM Soton. 1986.

PILSWORTH, Roy (retired) 8 Sidwell Park, South Benfleet, Benfleet SS7 1LQ Tel: 01268 754822 — MB BS Lond. 1943 (St. Mary's) MRCS Eng., LRCP Lond. 1942; MD Lond. 1951, MB BS 1943, Dipl. Bact. (Distinc.) 1947.

PILTON, Donald William (retired) St. Michael's Surgery, Walwyn Close, Twerton, Bath BA2 1ER Tel: 01225 428277 — MB ChB Bristol 1959. Prev: Clin. Asst. in Orthop. Roy. United Hosp. Bath.

PILZ, Daniela Theresa Institute of Medical Genetics, University Hospital of Wales, Cardiff CF14 4XW Email: daniela.pilz@cardiffandvale.wales.nhs.uk — State Exam Med Hannover 1986 (Medizinische Mochschule, Hannover, Germ.) State Exam Med. Hannover 1986; MRCP (UK) 1990; MD 1997; FRCP 2003. Cons. (Med. Genetics) Inst. Med. Genetics. Univ. Hosp. Wales Cardiff. Specialty: Genetics.

PIM, Arthur Joseph (retired) Vane House, Nuffield, Henley-on-Thames RG9 5RT Tel: 01491 641444 — MB BS Lond. 1958 (St. Thos.) DObst RCOG 1960. Coroner Reading.

PIMBLETT, John Hugh Sutcliffe Apple Tree Cottage, Sutton Marsh, Cross Keys, Hereford HR1 3NL Tel: 01432 72523 — MB BS Durh. 1960; DObst RCOG 1963; DA Eng. 1965; BA Open 1985.

PIMENTA, Darren Joseph 19 Blackberry Walk, Lychpit, Basingstoke RG24 8SN — MB ChB Aberd. 1995.

PIMENTA, Neale Gerard Horsman's Place Surgery, Instone Road, Dartford DA1 2JP Tel: 01322 228363/277444 — BM Soton. 1985; Cert. Family Plann. JCC 1987; MRCGP 1989. Specialty: Dermat. Socs: BMA & Med. Protec. Soc. Prev: Trainee GP E. Dorset VTS; Ho. Phys. & Ho. Surg. Roy. Vict. Hosp. Bournemouth.

PIMENTA, Susan Mary Horsman's Place Surgery, Instone Road, Dartford DA1 2JP Tel: 01322 228363/277444 — BM Soton. 1986; DCH RCP Lond. 1988; Cert. Family Plann. JCC 1990; DRCOG 1991. Socs: Med. Protec. Soc.

PIMLEY, Kenneth Gordon (retired) Flat 63 St. Marys Mews, 1 Fernlea Avenue, Ferndown BH22 8HF — MB ChB Aberd. 1946. Prev: Cons. Psychiat. Cranage Hall Hosp. Crewe.

PIMLEY, Mrs Sheila King (retired) Ben Shiel, 1 Gordon St., Fochabers IV32 7DL Tel: 01343 821396 — (Dundee) MB ChB St. And. 1955. Prev: Assoc. Specialist (Child & Family Psychiat.) Bilbohall Hosp. Elgin.

PIMM, James Tait Brookside Group Practice, Brookside Close, Gipsy Lane, Earley, Reading RG6 7HG Tel: 0118 966 9222 Fax: 0118 935 3174; 66 Beech Lane, Earley, Reading RG6 5QA Tel: 0118 986 3073 — MB ChB Univ. Zimbabwe 1981 (Godfrey Huggins) LRCP LRCS Ed. LRCPS Glas. 1981; MRCGP 1989. Gen. Pract.; Lord Harris Ct. Med. Off. - c/o the Elderly; Dir. Ask Your Doctor Ltd 2003.

PIMM, John Borstal Cottage, 138 Borstal Road, Rochester ME1 3BB Tel: 01634 42323 — MB BS Lond. 1957 (Lond. Hosp.) Prev: SHO Lond. Hosp.; Gen. Med. Off. South. Rhodesia; Sen. Med. Off. North. Rhodesia.

PIMM, Jonathan 138 Borstal Road, Rochester ME1 3BB — MB BS Lond. 1987.

PIMM, Mr Lionel Henry (retired) Barken Cottage, Courtlands Lane, Bower Ashton, Bristol BS3 2JS Tel: 0117 909 9397 — MB BS Lond. 1945 (St. Mary's) FRCS Eng. 1952. Prev: Cons. Orthop. Surg. Ipswich Hosp. & Suff. AHA.

PIMM, Michael Henry James The Cedars Surgery, 87 New Bristol Road, Worle, Weston Super Mare BS22 6AJ Tel: 01934 515878 Fax: 01934 520263; 42 Uphill Road S., Weston Super Mare BS23 4SQ Tel: 01934 413407 — MB ChB Bristol 1982; DCH RCP Lond. 1985; Cert. Family Plann. JCC 1985; DRCOG 1985; MRCGP 1986. Prev: Trainee GP Rugby VTS.

PINCH, Edward Thomas 1 Tor Close, Hartley, Plymouth PL3 5TH Tel: 01752 705372 — MB BS Lond. 1994. SHO (ENT) St Michaels Hosp. Bristol.

PINCHBECK, Frank Walter Sleaford Road Surgery, 1 Sleaford Road, Heckington, Sleaford NG34 9QP Tel: 01529 460213 Fax: 01529 460087; 12 Houldon Way, Hockington, Sleaford NG34 9TY Tel: 01529 460600 — MB ChB Sheff. 1960.

PINCHEN, Christopher John The Surgery, Margaret Street, Thaxted, Dunmow CM6 2QN Tel: 01371 830213 Fax: 01371 831278 — MB BS Lond. 1978 (St. Bart.) BSc (Pharm.) CNAA 1969; MPS 1970; MRCS Eng. LRCP Lond. 1978; DRCOG 1981. GP Thaxted.; CMP 33 Eng Regt. (EOD) Wimbish; HSE Approved Diving Doctor. Prev: GP Trainee Addenbrooke's Hosp. Camb. VTS.; Ho. Phys. OldCh. Hosp. Romford; Ho. Surg. Hackney Hosp. Lond.

PINCHES, Claire Elaine Elm Lane Surgery, 104 Elm Lane, Sheffield S5 7TW Tel: 0114 245 6994 Fax: 0114 257 1260 — MB ChB Bristol 1986; DRCOG 1988; DGM RCP Lond. 1989; MRCGP 1990; DCH RCP Lond. 1991. GP Princip. Prev: SHO (Paediat.) Rotherham Dist. Gen. Hosp.; Trainee GP Bristol VTS.

PINCHES, Patricia Joyce Elizabeth Faringdon Health Centre, Coxwell Road, Faringdon SN7 7ED Tel: 01367 242388 Fax: 01367 243394; April Cottage, 32C London St, Faringdon SN7 7AA Tel: 01367 243316 — (St. And.) MB ChB St. And. 1961. Clin. Asst. Paediat.Oncol.P.ss Margt. Hosp. Swindon Wilts.

PINCHES, Robert Smythe Marcham Road Family Health Centre, Abingdon OX14 1BT Tel: 01235 522602 — MB ChB St. And. 1961; DObst RCOG 1971; MRCGP 1975. Socs: Medico-Legal Soc.

PINCHIN, Roberta Mary Erasmus Paynesfield House, Tatsfield, Westerham TN16 2BQ Tel: 01959 541212 — MB BS Lond. 1970; FFA RCS Eng. 1974; T(Anaesth.) 1991. Cons. Anaesth. Bromley Hosps. NHS Trust. Specialty: Anaesth. Prev: Cons. Anaesth. Barnet Gen. Hosp.; Sen. Regist. (Anaesth.) Barnet Gen. Hosp. & Roy. Free Hosp. Lond.; Regist. (Anaesth.) Westm. Hosp. Lond.

PINCHING, Professor Anthony John Peninsula Medical School, Knowledge Spa, Royal Cornwall Hospital, Truro TR1 3DH Tel: 01872 256402 Fax: 01872 256401 Email: anthony.pinching@pms.ac.uk; 22 Cuckoo Hill Road, Pinner HA5 1AY — BM BCh Oxf. 1973 (Oxford University) MA Oxf. 1973, DPhil 1972, BA 1968; MRCP (UK) 1976; FRCP Lond. 1986. Assoc. Dean for Cornw. & Prof. Peninsula Med. Sch. Truro. Specialty: Immunol.; HIV Med. Prev: Prof. Immunol. St. Bart. & Roy. Lond. Sch. Med. & Dent., Qu. Mary & Westfield Coll. Lond.; Reader & Hon. Cons. Clin. Immunol. St. Mary's Hosp. Med. Sch. Lond.; Sen. Regist. (Med.) Hammersmith Hosp. Lond.

PINCHING, John Hillbury House, Wells Tel: 01749 3356 — MRCS Eng. LRCP Lond. 1942 (Oxf. & Guy's) BM BCh Oxon. 1942; MRCPLond. 1948. Clin. Asst. (Med.) Bath Gp. Hosps. Prev: Res. Med. Off. St. Cross Hosp. Rugby; Asst. Med. Off. Co. Hosp. FarnBoro..

PINCHING, Nicola Jane Adelaide Street Health Centre, Norwich NR2 5DL Tel: 01603 625015 — MB ChB Leic. 1990; MRCGP 1996. GP Asst. Specialty: Gen. Pract.

PINCOTT, Richard Glynne Sway Road Surgery, 65 Sway Road, Morriston, Swansea SA6 6JA Tel: 01792 773150 / 771392 Fax: 01792 790880 — MB BS Lond. 1971 (King's Coll. Hosp.) DCH Eng. 1974.

PINDER, Alison Orchard Cottage, Cranford Way, Highfield, Southampton SO17 1RN — MB BS Lond. 1975 (St. Bart.) DRCOG 1978.

PINDER, Amanda Jane 28 Elm Tree Close, Colton, Leeds LS15 9JE Email: drajppig@aol.com — MB ChB Leeds 1994; BSc (Chem. Path.) Leeds 1991. Specialist Regist. (Anaesth.) N. & W. Yorks. Specialty: Anaesth. Socs: Assn. Anaesth. Prev: Clin. Fell. (NeuroIC) Leeds Gen. Infirm.; SHO (Anaesth.) Dewsbury Dist. Hosp.; SHO (Anaesth.) Pontefract Gen. Infirm.

PINDER, Carole Ann Ferrybridge Medical Centre, 8-10 High Street, Ferrybridge, Knottingley WF11 8NQ Tel: 01977 672109 Fax: 01977 671107; Manor Grange, Church St, Brotherton, Knottingley

WF11 9HE — MB ChB Leeds 1975; DOCC Med 1997. Dr Capinder, GP Ferrybridge Med. Centre, 8-10 High St., Ferrybridge, Knottingley WF11 8NQ; Med. Adviser Pioneer Electronics Castleford; Med. Adviser Monkhill Confectionery Pontefract, Dunhill Haribo (Pontefract) Ltd; Med. Adviser, Monkhill Confectionery, York; Med. Adviser Constar, Sherburn in Elmet. Specialty: Gen. Pract. Socs: Soc. Occupat. Med. Prev: SHO (Paediat., A & E & O & G) Pontefract Gen. Infirm.

PINDER, Christopher Gerard 31 Chichele Road, Oxted RH8 0AE — MB BS Lond. 1975 (Guy's) FRCR Lond. 1983. Cons. Radiol. Qu. Mary's Hosp. Sidcup. Specialty: Radiol.

PINDER, Colin Anthony Frederick Wirral Neurological Rehabilitation Unit, Clatterbridge Hospitall, Wirral CH63 4JY Fax: 0151 483 7790 Email: colin.pinder@whnt.nhs.uk — MB ChB Leeds 1988; MRCP (UK) 1994; MD Leeds 2002. Cons. in Neurol. Rehabil., Walton Centre for Neurol. and Neurosurg., Liverp. Specialty: Rehabil. Med.

PINDER, Darren Kenneth The Holmes, Ryarsh, West Malling ME19 5LQ — BChir Camb. 1992.

PINDER, David Charles Woking PCT, Villa 22, Bournewood House, Guildford Road, Chertsey KT16 0QA; 31 Grasmere Road, Lightwater GU18 5TG Tel: 01276 476721 — MB BChir Camb. 1969; MA Camb. 1970; DPH Manch. 1972; BA Open 1975; FFPHM RCP (UK) 1995, M 1977. Cons. Pub. Health Med. W Surrey DHA. Specialty: Pub. Health Med. Prev: SCM (Informat. & Primary Care) Leics. HA & (Informat. & Research) Mersey RHA; Med. Off. DHSS.

PINDER, Gillian Anne 6 St Helens Grove, Wakefield WF2 6RR — MB ChB Birm. 1979; MFCM 1988; MFPHM RCP (UK) 1990. Cons. Pub. Health Med. Wakefield HA. Specialty: Pub. Health Med. Prev: Sen. Regist. (Community Med.) Yorks. RHA; Trainee GP East. Dist. Wakefield AHA.

PINDER, Gordon Whittaker (retired) Moor Garth, Hutton-le-Hole, York YO62 6UA Tel: 01751 417581 — MRCS Eng. LRCP Lond. 1940 (Camb. & Guy's) BA Camb. 1937; DObst RCOG 1948. Prev: Lt.-Col. RAMC 1942-46.

PINDER, Ian Fred Manor Grange, Church Lane, Brotherton, Knottingley WF11 9HE Tel: 01977 676777 Fax: 01977 673111 — MB ChB Leeds 1975; MRCP (UK) 1979; AFOM 1999. Occupat. Phys. Covance, Harrogate; Internat. Speciality Chem. Ltd, Scott. & Newc. Breweries, Regromac Indep. Media, Nestle UK. Specialty: Occupat. Health. Socs: Soc. Occupat. Med.; Chairm. Yorks. Grp. Prev: CMO Courage Ltd.

PINDER, Mr Ian Maurice Newcastle Nuffield Hospital, Clayton Road, Jesmond, Newcastle upon Tyne NE2 1JP; 126 Darras Road, Newcastle upon Tyne NE20 9PG — MB ChB Sheff. 1961; FRCS Ed. 1966. Cons. (Orthop.) Surg. Newc. Nuffield Hosp. Specialty: Orthop. Prev: Cons. (Orthop.) Surg. Newc. AHA (T).

PINDER, Joe Rawdon Sycamore House, High St., Barmby-on-the-March, Goole DN14 7HU — MB ChB Leeds 1993.

PINDER, Mary 97 Kingsmead Road, London SW2 3HZ — MB BS Lond. 1982.

PINDER, Norman Richard Pond Farm, Kirby Bedon, Norwich NR14 7DY — MB BS Lond. 1972 (Guy's) MSc (Community Med.) Lond. 1988, MB BS 1972; DObst RCOG 1975; MFPHM RCP (UK) 1991; FFPHM 1998. Head of Clin. Governance & Dep. Clin. Dir. Norf. Suff. & Cambs. SHA. Specialty: Pub. Health Med. Prev: Cons. Pub. Health Med. E. Norf. Health Auth.; Dir. Community Med. Grenfell Regional Health Serv. Newfld., Canada.

PINDER, Sarah Elizabeth Addenbrooke's Hospital, Department of Histopathology, Box 235, Hills Road, Cambridge CB2 2QQ — MB ChB Manch. 1986; FRCPath 2001. Cons. Breast Pathologist. Specialty: Histopath. Special Interest: Breast Path. Prev: Sen. Lect. & Hon. Cons. Univ. of Nottm.; Clin. Research Fell. & Hon. Sen. Regist. City Hosp. Nottm.

PINDER, Sarah Jane 15 Mill Street, Warwick CV34 4HB — BChir Camb. 1992.

PINDER, Stephen Paul Hetherington — MB BS Lond. 1976; DAvMed FOM RCP Lond. 1990; D.Occ.Med. RCP Lond. 1996.

PINDOLIA, Narendra Kumar Station View Medical Centre, 29A Escomb Road, Bishop Auckland DL14 6AB Tel: 01388 663539 Fax: 01388 601847 — MB BS Lond. 1983; MRCGP 1988.

PINE, Isabel Mary (retired) 22 Norfolk Street, Southsea PO5 4DS — (Roy. Free) FRIPHH; MB BS Lond. 1950; DPH Eng. 1965; MFCM 1974; MFPHM 1989. Prev: Sen. Med. Off. Portsmouth & SE Hants. Health Dist.

PINE, Mr Richard Campbell 21 Hatherden Avenue, Lower Parkstone, Poole BH14 0PJ — MB BS Lond. 1966 (St. Bart.) MRCS Eng. LRCP Lond. 1965; LMSSA Lond. 1971; FRCS Ed. 1980; FRCS Glas. 1980. Surg. Roy. Fleet Auxil. Prev: Ho. Surg. Roy. Vict. Hosp. Bournemouth; SHO (Gen. Surg.) Roy. Berks. Hosp. Reading; Demonst. (Anat.) Roy. Free Hosp. Sch. Med.

PINFOLD, Terence James 4 Southwood Close, Kingswinford DY6 8JL — MB ChB Birm. 1961. Cons. (Accid. Emerg.) Dudley & Stourbridge AHA. Specialty: Accid. & Emerg. Socs: Fell. Brit. Orthop. Assn. Prev: Med. Asst. (Trauma & Orthop.) Dudley & Stourbridge AHA.

PING, Emma Claire — MB ChB Sheff. 1998.

PINGREE, Brian James William, RD Institute of Naval Medicine, Alverstoke, Gosport PO12 2DL; Long Durford, Upper Durford Wood, Petersfield GU31 5AW — MB ChB Bristol 1968; BSc (Engin.) Bristol 1960, MB ChB 1968; MSc (Bioeng.) Strathclyde 1974; DAvMed. FOM RCP Lond. 1982; MFOM RCP Lond. 1983. Sen. Med. Off. Submarine Med. Inst. Naval Med. Gosport. Socs: Soc. Occupat. Med. Prev: Sen. Med. Off. (Environm. Med.) Inst. Naval Med. Alverstoke; Princip. Med. Off. Clyde Submarine Base; Head of Human Factors Inst. Naval Med. Alverstoke.

PINHEIRO, Neville Leslie Acreswood Surgery, 5 Acreswood Close, Coppull, Chorley PR7 5EJ Tel: 01257 793578 Fax: 01257 794005 — MRCS Eng. LRCP Lond. 1976 (Navarra, Spain) LSM Spain 1973.

PINHORN, Anja 19 Marston Lane, Rolleston-on-Dove, Burton-on-Trent DE13 9BH — MB BS Lond. 1989; BSc Lond. 1986, MB BS 1989. SHO Rotat. (Med.) St. Mary's Hosp. Lond.

PINION, Sheena Barbara Forth Park Maternity Hospital, Bennochy Road, Kirkcaldy KY2 5RA Tel: 01592 643355 — MB ChB Ed. 1981; MRCOG 1988; FRCS Glas. 1990; MD (Ed) 1997. Cons. O & G Forth Pk. Matern. Hosp. Kirkcaldy. Specialty: Obst. & Gyn. Prev: Sen. Regist. (O & G) Dundee; Research Fell. (Gyn.) Univ. Aberd.; Regist. (O & G) Glas.

PINK, Edith Jean (retired) 10 Balgove Avenue, Gauldry, Newport-on-Tay DD6 8SQ — MB ChB St. And. 1955 (St. And. & Dundee) DA Eng. 1960; FRCP Canada 1973. Prev: Cons. Anaesth. Monklands Dist. Gen. Hosp. Coatbridge.

***PINK, Edward** 24 Lawrence Road, Biggleswade SG18 0LS — MB ChB Birm. 1998; ChB Birm. 1998.

PINK, Quintin James (retired) Hawthorn Cottage, East Farndon, Market Harborough LE16 9SH Tel: 01858 467717 — MB Camb. 1974, BChir 1973. Prev: GP Market HarBoro. Leics.

PINKER, Sir George Douglas, KCVO (retired) — MB BS Lond. 1947 (St. Mary's) DObst 1949; FRCOG 1964, M 1954; FRCS Ed. 1957; Hon. FRCSI 1988; Hon. FRACOG 1989; FRCS 1989; Hon. FACOG 1990. Cons. Gyn. Surg. & Obst. St. Mary's Hosp., Samarit. Hosp. Lond. & King Edwd. VII Hosp. for Offs.; Hon. Cons. Roy. Wom. Hosp. Melbourne, Austral.; Examr. FRCS Ed.; Examr. (Obst. & Gyn.) Univs. Camb., Birm., Glas., Lond., Dub. & Dundee. Prev: Pres. Roy. Soc. Med. 1992-1994 & RCOG 1987-1990 (Vice-Pres. 1980).

PINKERTON, Amanda Louise Lubards Lodge Farm, Ranreth Lane, Rayleigh SS6 — MB ChB Leeds 1996.

PINKERTON, Professor Charles Ross Children's Department, Royal Marsden NHS Trust, Downs Road, Sutton SM2 5PT Tel: 020 8661 3498 Fax: 020 8770 7168 Email: rossp@icr.ac.uk — MB BCh BAO Belf. 1974; DCH RCPSI 1978; FRCPI (Paediat.) 1979, M 1979; MD (Hons.) Belf. 1981; FRCPCH 1997. Prof. Paediat. Oncol. Roy. Marsden Hosp. & Inst. Cancer Research Lond. Specialty: Oncol.; Paediat.

PINKERTON, Florence (retired) 41C Sans Souci Park, Belfast BT9 5QZ Tel: 02890 682956 — MB BCh BAO Belf. 1945. Prev: Clin. Med. Off. (Community Health) Clinic EHSSB.

PINKERTON, George Eustace, MC (retired) 17 Church Lane, Upwood, Huntingdon PE26 2QF Tel: 01487 813946 — MB BChir Camb. 1941 (Lond. Hosp.) BA Camb. 1938, MB BChir 1941. Prev: Capt. RAMC.

PINKERTON, Ian Watt, OBE, OStJ, TD (retired) 10 Langside Drive, Comrie, Crieff PH6 2HR Tel: 01764 670578 — MB ChB Glas. 1951; FRFPS Glas. 1957; FRCP Ed. 1979, M 1960; FRCP Glas. 1970. Hon. Lect. (Infec. Dis.) Univ. Glas. Prev: Cons. Phys. Dept. Infec. Dis. Ruchill Hosp. Glas.

PINKERTON, (Isabella) Madeleine (retired) 64 Portsmouth Road, Surbiton KT6 4HT Tel: 020 8399 0067 — MB BCh Wales 1944 (Cardiff) DPH Lond. 1949; FFOM RCP Lond. 1978. Prev: Gp. Med. Adviser Marks & Spencer Ltd.

PINKERTON, John Henry McKnight, CBE (retired) 41c Sans Souci Park, Belfast BT9 5QZ Tel: 02890 682956 — MB BCh BAO Belf. 1943; MD Belf. 1948; FRCOG 1960, M 1950; FRCPI 1977, M 1974; DSc Hon. NUI 1986. Prev: Emerit. Prof. Midw. & Gyn. Qu. Univ. Belf.

PINKERTON, Rachel Mariama 15 Colenso Pde, Belfast BT9 5AN — MB BCh BAO Belf. 1997.

PINKERTON, Stuart Melvyn Old Barn House, Nomansland Farm, Wheathampstead, St Albans AL4 8EY Tel: 01582 831029 Fax: 01582 834965 Email: stuart@pinkertonhealthcare.com — MB ChB Liverp. 1979; Cert. Family Plann. JCC 1982; Cert. Prescribed Equiv. Exp. JCPTGP 1982; Dip. Pharm. Med. RCP (UK) 1985; MFPM RCP (UK) 1989; FFPM RCP (UK) 1997. Chairm. Europ. Healthcare. Burson- Marsteller; Hon. Clin. Asst. (Cardiol.) St. Albans City Hosp. Specialty: Pharmaceutical Medicine. Socs: BMA; FFPM. Prev: Med. Dir. Roche Products Ltd. Welwyn Gdn. City; Med. Dir. Syntex UK & Scand.; Head Europ. Clin. Research Syntex Internat.

PINKEY, Basil 2 Edith Marriage House, 5 Cambridge Road, Colchester CO3 3NS — MB BCh BAO Belf. 1959; MRCP (UK) 1969.

PINKHAM, Kathryn Louise 1 Dehewydd Isaf, Llantwit Fardre, Pontypridd CF38 2EX — MB BCh Wales 1992.

PINKNEY, Jonathan Henley — MB BS Lond. 1985 (Char. Cross & Westm.) BSc Lond. 1982; MRCP (UK) 1988; MD Lond. 1997. Sen. Lect. In Endocrinol. and Diabetes, Univ. of Liverp. and Aintree Hosps. NHS Trust; Hon. Cons. Phys. in Endocrinol. and Diabetes, Univ. of Liverp. and Aintree Hosps. NHS Trust. Specialty: Diabetes; Endocrinol.; Gen. Med. Special Interest: neuroendocrinology; Obesity. Socs: Brit. Endocrine Soc.; Diabetes UK; Amer. Diabetes Assn. Prev: Research Fell. Univ. Coll. Lond. Sch. Med.; Lect. (Med.) Univ. Bristol; Vis. Fell. Louisiana State Univ.

PINKNEY, Moira Ann 7 George Frost Close, Ipswich IP4 2UG Tel: 01473 252798 — MB ChB Bristol 1973; DCH Eng. 1975; DObst RCOG 1975; MRCP (UK) 1978; DGM RCP Lond. 1985; MRCGP 1990. Cons. community Paediat..local health partnerships trust Ipswich; GP Ipswich. Specialty: Community Child Health; Gen. Pract. Prev: Sen. Regist. (Community Paediats.) Allington NHS Trust Ipswich; Regist. (Med.) Norf. & Norwich Hosp.; SHO Rotat. (Med.) Oxon. AHA (T).

PINNELL, Jeremy Robert 28 Bedford Close, Kettering NN15 6TQ Tel: 01536 723976 — MB ChB Leeds 1994. SHO (Anaesth.). Specialty: Anaesth.

PINNER, Gillian Tracy Dencourt, London rd, Newark, Nottingham NG7 2UH Tel: 01636 685948 Fax: 0115 942 3618 — MB BS Lond. 1989 (Kings College Hospital London) MSc Lond. 1994; MRCPsych 1995. Cons. old age Psychiat., Centr. Nottm. Health Care Trust; acedemic Cons.. Old age psychiarty. Specialty: Geriat. Psychiat. Socs: Roy. Coll. Psychiat. Prev: Lect. & Hon. Sen. Regist. (Old Age Psychiat.) Univ. Hosp. Nottm.; Research Assoc. (Psychiat.) UMDS.; Regist. Bexley Hosp. Oxleas NHS Trust.

PINNER-HARTH, Johanna A (retired) 29 Thanet Lodge, Mapesbury Road, London NW2 4JA Tel: 020 8459 6776 — MD Vienna 1931. Prev: Regist. Qu.'s Hosp. Croydon.

PINNEY, Deborah Elizabeth — BM Soton. 1988.

PINNEY, Sally Ann Elthorne Park Surgery, 106 Elthorne Park Road, Hanwell, London W7 2JJ — MB BS Lond. 1984 (Charing Cross Hospital) BSc (Hons.) Anat. Lond. 1981; DRCOG 1987; Cert. Family Plann. JCC 1987. GP Princip.

PINNINGTON, Julie 10 Peacock Drive, Bottisham, Cambridge CB5 9EF Tel: 01223 812595 — BChir Camb. 1994.

PINNINGTON, Susan Osborne Road Surgery, 17 Osborne Road, Newcastle upon Tyne NE2 2AH Tel: 0191 281 4588 Fax: 0191 212 0379 — MB BS Lond. 1993 (Univ. Coll. & Middx Sch. Med.) BSc Lond. 1977; MRCGP 1997; DRCOG 1998. GP. Specialty: Gen. Pract.

PINNOCK, Colin Andrew 8 Pear tree way, Church Lane, Wychbold, Worcester WR9 7SW — MB BS Lond. 1977; FFA RCS Eng. 1982. Cons. Anaesth. Alexandra Hosp. Redditch. Specialty: Anaesth. Prev: Cons. Anaesth. BromsGr. & Redditch Dist. Gen. Hosp.

PINNOCK, Eileen Mary (retired) Meadow Rise, Atch Lench, Evesham WR11 5SP Tel: 01386 870718 — (Birm.) MB ChB Birm. 1947. Prev: Med. Asst. (Anaesth.) Worcester Roy. Infirm.

PINNOCK, Hilary Joan Whitstable Health Centre, Harbour Street, Whitstable CT5 1BZ Tel: 01277 594400 Fax: 01277 771474 — MB ChB Leeds 1974; MRCGP 1982. Princip. in Gen. Practise, Whitstable Med. Pracrise; Course Organiser Primary Focus; Clin. research Fell.ship, Dept of Gen. Practise& Primary core; Aberd. Uni. Specialty: Respirat. Med.; Gen. Pract. Special Interest: Practical Train. in asthma and COPD for primary care professionals; Primary care research in Respirat. Med. Socs: Brit. Thorac. Soc.; Comm. Mem. GP Airways grp; Internat. Primary Care Respiratary grp. Prev: GP Prestwich Manch. & Burgess Hill W. Sussex; SHO (Gen. Med.) Salford AHA.

PINNOCK, Malcolm Raymond (retired) Meadow Rise, Atch Lench, Evesham WR11 4SW Tel: 01386 870718 — MB ChB Aberd. 1950. Prev: Princip. in Gen. Pract., Worcs.

PINNOCK, Roger Graham North Street Surgery, 28 North Street, Ashford TN24 8JR Tel: 01233 661133 Fax: 01233 662727; Yew Tree House, Westwell Leacon, Charing, Ashford TN27 0EE Tel: 01233 712840 — MB BS Lond. 1974 (St Mary's) Cert. Family Plann. JCC 1984. Chairm. E. Kent MAAG. Prev: Clin. Asst. (Dermat.) William Harvey Hosp.

PINSENT, Susan Elizabeth Mallett Higher Ludbrook, Ermington, Ivybridge PL21 0LL — MB ChB Liverp. 1978; DRCOG 1980; DA Eng. 1982.

PINSON, Kenneth Donovan — MB ChB Manch. 1949.

PINTO, Alan Lawrence Premkumar Wigan & Leigh Health Services NHS Trust, Royal Albert Edward Infirmary, Wigan Lane, Wigan WN1 2NN; 50 Bempton Road, St. Michaels Wood, Liverpool L17 5BB Tel: 0151 727 0820 Email: alanpinto@lineone.net — MB BS Bangalor 1980 (St. John's Med. Coll. Bangalore) MB BS Bangalore 1980; FRCPS Glas. 1992; FFAEM 1997. Cons. (A&E). Specialty: Accid. & Emerg.

PINTO, Mr Anthony Phillip Rozario 125 Carshalton Park Road, Carshalton SM5 3SJ — MB BS Bombay 1940; MS Bombay 1943, MB BS 1940; FRCS Ed. 1946; FRCS Eng. 1946.

PINTO, Ashwin Arnold Victoria Cottage, High Street, Chinnor OX39 4DH — BM BCh Oxf. 1992; D. PHIL (2000); MRCP (UK) 1995.

PINTO, Mr Domingos Joseph Diago Teodoro, OBE 89 Kevlin Road, Coolnagard, Omagh BT78 1PQ Tel: 028 8224 6854 — (Lond. Hosp.) MRCS Eng. LRCP Lond. 1962; MB BS Lond. 1962; FRCS Ed. 1966; FRCS Eng. 1967; MS Lond. 1970; FRCSI 1996. Cons. Surg. Tyrone Co. Hosp. Specialty: Gen. Surg. Socs: Fell. Assn. Surgs.; Fell. Assn. Upper G.I. Surg. Prev: Scientif. Asst. & Hon. Cons. Med. Research Counc.; Regist. Rotat. (Surg.) Middlx. Hosp. Lond.; Sen. Lect. Makerere Univ. Kampala, Uganda.

PINTO, Robin Trevor 354 Old Bedford Road, Luton LU2 7BS Tel: 01582 31065 — LMSSA Lond. 1967; MRCP Glas. 1966; MPhil (Psychiat.) Lond. 1970; FRCPsych. 1984, M 1972. Cons. Psychiat. Luton & Dunstable Hosp. Specialty: Gen. Psychiat.; Forens. Psychiat. Socs: Fell. Roy. Soc. Med. Prev: Sen. Regist. Bethlem Roy. & Maudsley Hosps.; Med. Regist. King's Lynn Gen. Hosp.

PINTO, Stella Matilda Cradley Road Surgery, 62 Cradley Road, Cradley Heath, Warley B64 6AG Fax: 01934 612813 — MB ChB Birm. 1987; DCH RCP Lond. 1989; DRCOG 1991; MRCGP 1992. Specialty: Dermat.

PINTO, Sunil Christopher 354 Old Bedford Road, Luton LU2 7BS — MB BS Lond. 1989; DRCOG 1992; DCH RCP Lond. 1993.

PINTO, Tara (retired) Homestead, 18 Cambridge Road, Linthorpe, Middlesbrough TS5 5NN — MB BS Vikram 1961 (Mahatma Gandhi Memor. Med. Coll. Indore) MRCOG 1965.

PINTO, Thelma Queen Elizebeth Hospital, Stadium Road, Woolwich, London SE18 4QH Tel: 020 8836 5656 — MB BS Lond. 1977; MRCP (UK) 1980; FRCPath 1995. Cons. (Histopath.) Qu. Eliz. Hosp., Woolwich, Lond. Specialty: Histopath.

PINTO, Zoe Anne Penshurst Gardens Surgery, 39 Penshurst Gardens, Edgware HA8 9TN Tel: 020 8958 3141 Fax: 020 8905 4638; 2 Stoneyfields Gardens, Edgware HA8 9SP — MB ChB Bristol 1983; DRCOG 1987; MRCGP 1988.

PIOTROWICZ, Andrzej Jan Krzysztof 133 Whitaker Road, Derby DE23 6AQ — MB ChB Bristol 1989; BSc Bristol 1986, MB ChB

1989; MRCP (UK) 1992. Regist. (Gen. Med.) Guy's Hosp. Lond. Specialty: Gen. Med.

PIOTROWICZ, Andrzej Leszek Maria (retired) 133 Whitaker Road, Derby DE23 6AQ — MB BCh BAO NUI 1956; DMRD Eng. 1965; FFR 1968. Cons. Radiol. Derby Hosp. Gp. Prev: Regist. Dept. Radiol. United Sheff. Hosps.

PIOTROWSKI, Anthony George The Surgery, 232-234 Milton Road, Weston Super Mare BS22 8AG Tel: 01934 625022 Fax: 01934 612470; 7 Highpath, Wellington TA21 8NH — MB BS Lond. 1991 (St. George's HMS Lond.) Specialty: Gen. Pract.

PIPE, Mr Norman Geoffrey James Huntersfield, Highlands Road, Reigate RH2 0LA Tel: 01737 244029 Fax: 01737 226267 — MB BS Lond. 1969 (Char. Cross) MRCS Eng. LRCP Lond. 1968; FRCOG 1987, M 1973, DObst 1971. Cons. O & G Surrey & Sussex Healthcare NHS Trust. Specialty: Obst. & Gyn. Socs: Brit. Soc. Colpos. & Cerv. Path.; BMA; Blair Bell Res. Soc. Prev: Sen. Regist. (O & G) Guy's Hosp. Lond. & Farnbororough Hosp. Kent; Regist. (O & G) Luton & Dunstable & Hammersmith Hosps.

PIPE, Roderic Alan The Priory Ticehurst House, Ticehurst, Wadhurst TN5 7HU Tel: 01580 200391; 2 Riverview Road, London W4 3QH Tel: 020 8995 9265 — MB ChB Ed. 1984; MRCPsych 1989. Cons. Psychiat. (Child & Adolesc. Psychiat.), The Priory Ticehurst Ho. Socs: Assn. Child Psychol. & Psychiat.; Assn. for Profess. in Servs. for Adolesc.; Roy. Coll. Psychiat. Prev: Sen. Regist. (Child & Adolesc. Psychiat.) Bethlem & Maudsley Hosps. Lond.; Regist. & SHO (Psychiat.) St. Geo. Hosp. Lond.; Cons. Psychiat. (Child & Adolesc. Psychiat.) Bethlem & Maudsley NHS Trust Lond.

PIPER, Anthony Richard Rose Dean Surgery, 8 Dean Street, Liskeard PL14 4AQ Tel: 01579 343133 — MB BS Lond. 1967 (Char. Cross) MRCS Eng. LRCP Lond. 1967; DObst RCOG 1969; DA Eng. 1971; MRCGP 1980.

PIPER, Edward John Sanofi-aventis, 1 Onslow Gardens, Guildford GU1 4YS Tel: 01483 505515 — MB BS Lond. 1995; MFPM; MRCGP; DCH; BSc; DRCOG. Sen. Med. Adviser Sanofi-aventis. Special Interest: Diabetes.

PIPER, Mr Ian Hedley Orthopaedic Department, Barnsley General Hospital, Gawber Road, Barnsley S75 2EP Tel: 01226 777741 Fax: 01226 380470; Week Cottage, Week Hill, Notton, Dartmouth TQ6 0JT Tel: 01226 380180 Fax: 01226 380470 — MB BS Lond. 1968 (St Thomas's, London) AFPM CSPQ 1981, Canada; MRCS Eng. LRCP Lond. 1968; FRCS Eng. 1974; LRCP Canada 1978. Cons. Orthop. Surg. Barnsley Dist. Gen. Hosp. Specialty: Orthop. Socs: Brit. Orthop. Assn.; BMA; BESS. Prev: Staff Surg. Santa Cabrini Hosp. Montreal, Quebec; Staff Surg. Omineca Clin, Vanderhoof, Brit. Columbia.

PIPER, Julia Alison Beech House, 3 Knighton Grange Road, Stoneygate, Leicester LE2 2LF Tel: 01162 700373 Fax: 01162 701660 Email: drjpiper@btinternet.com; 3 Knighton Grange Road, Stoneygate, Leicester LE2 2LF Tel: 0116 270 0373 Fax: 0116 270 1660 Email: drjpiper@btinternet.com — BM BS Nottm. 1980 (Nottingham) BMedSci Nottm. 1978; Cert. FPA 1984; MRCGP 1984; DFFP 2000; Dip Occ Med 2001. Private GP, Stoneygate, Leicester; Private GP Leicester. Specialty: Gen. Pract.; Acupunc.; Hypnother. Socs: BMA (Brit. Med. Assn.); RCGP (Roy. Coll. of GPs); BMAS (Brit. Med. Acupunc. Soc.). Prev: GP Chorleywood; Screening Clinic Dr. Bupa Hosps., Bushey & Harpenden; GP Oadby, Leicester.

PIPER, Mark Patrick Peter 13 Westley Avenue, Whitley Bay NE26 4NW — MB ChB Ed. 1988 (Univ. Ed.) BSc (Med. Sci.) Hons. Ed. 1986; FRCA 1996. Specialty: Anaesth.

PIPER, Mary Prison Health, Department of Health, Wellington House, 133-155 Waterloo Road, London SE1 Tel: 020 7972 4952 — MB BS Lond. 1971; MRCS Eng. LRCP Lond. 1971; MRCP (UK) 1974; FRCP Lond. 1986; MSc Lond. 1993; MFPHM RCP (UK) 1995. Sen. Pub. Health Adviser, Prison Health, Dept. of Health. Specialty: Care of the Elderly. Prev: Lect. (Geriat. Med.) Univ. Coll. Hosp. Lond.; Sen. Regist. (Geriat. Med.) Northwick Pk. Hosp. Harrow.; Cons. (Geriat. Med.) Northwick Pk. Hosp. Harrow.

PIPER, Mary Evelyn, Maj. RAMC Department of Psychiatry, Mrs Tidworth, Delhi Barracks, Tidworth SP9 — LMSSA Lond. 1978; MRCPsych 1983. Cons. Psychiat. Dept. Psychiat. Delhi Barracks Tidworth. Specialty: Gen. Psychiat.

PIPER, Philippa Claire The Medical Centre, Greystone House, 99 Station Road, Redhill RH1 1EB — MB ChB Manch. 1978; DFFP. Trainee GP Cleveland VTS. Specialty: Gen. Pract. Prev: SHO (Paediat.) Booth Hall Childr. Hosp. N. Manch.; Ho. Off. (Med.) Hope Hosp. Salford; Ho. Off. (Surg.) Chester Roy. Infirm.

PIPER, Rosalind Olivia Jane Bramblecote, 42 Tupwood Lane, Caterham CR3 6DP — MB BS Lond. 1996.

PIPER, Sally Joanne Corial, Northlands Road, Warnham, Horsham RH12 3SQ — MB BS Lond. 1989; DRCOG 1991; MRCGP 1993.

PIPER, Simon Austen Road Surgery, 1 Austen Road, Guildford GU1 3NW Tel: 01483 564578 Fax: 01483 505368 — MB BS Lond. 1977 (St Marys) Med. Off. Probation Hostels Guildford. Specialty: Gen. Pract. Socs: Soc. Occup. Med.

PIPKIN, Christopher, Surg. Capt. RN HQ Defence Medical Education & Training Agency, Fort Blockhouse, Gosport PO12 2AB Tel: 023 9276 5621 Email: chris.pipkin@fbigs.mod.uk — MB BS Lond. 1982 (Univ. Coll. Hosp.) Dip. Clin. Microbiol. Lond 1991; MRCPath 1992; FRCPath 2000. Staff Officer Medical Commitments. Specialty: Med. Microbiol. Prev: Hon. Sen. Regist. (Microbiol.) Roy. Lond. Hosp.; Sen. Regist. (Microbiol.) Pub. Health Laborat. St. Mary's Hosp. Portsmouth; Trainee (Path.) RN Hosp. Haslar.

PIPON, Madeleine Louise 3 Shakespeare Road, London W7 1LT — MB BS Lond. 1994.

PIPPARD, Kathleen Marjorie (retired) 9 Princes Avenue, Woodford Green IG8 0LL — MB ChB Birm. 1943; MFFP 1993. Prev: Med. Off. Family Plann. Clinics W. Essex & E. Herts HAs.

PIPPARD, Professor Martin John Ninewells Hospital & Medical School, Division of Pathology and Neuroscience, Dundee DD1 9SY Tel: 01382 660111 Ext: 33113 Fax: 01382 633952 Email: martin.j.pippard@tuht.scot.nhs.uk — MB ChB Birm. 1972; BSc Birmingham 1969; FRCP Lond 1988; FRCPath 1994; FRCP Ed 1998. Profess. Haemat. Univ. Dundee & Cons. Haemat. Ninewells Hosp. & Med. Sch. Dundee. Specialty: Haematology. Socs: Brit. Soc. Haematol.; Assn. Clin. Path.; Amer. Soc. Hemat. Prev: Cons. Haemat. Northwick Pk. Hosp. & Clin. Research Centre Harrow Middlx.; Research Fell. & Clin. Lect. Nuffield Dept. Clin. Med. John Radcliffe Hosp. Oxf.; Sen. Fell. Div. Hemat. Dept. Med. Univ. Washington, USA.

PIPPEN, Catherine Ann Rhoda The White House, 103 Cyncoed Road, Cardiff CF23 6AD Tel: 029 2075 1750 — MB BCh Wales 1956 (Cardiff) MRCP Ed. 1968. Cons. Phys. (Geriat. Med.) S. Glam. AHA (T). Specialty: Gen. Med. Socs: Brit. Geriat. Soc. & Cardiff Med. Soc. Prev: Sen. Regist. (Geriat. Med.) St. David's Hosp. Cardiff; Regist. (Gen. Med.) Cardiff Roy. Infirm.

PIPPET, Diana June 18A Monalla Road, Ballinamallard, Enniskillen BT94 2GS Tel: 01365 324377 — (St. Bart.) MB BS Lond. 1954; DCH Eng. 1956.

PIQUERAS ARENAS, Ana Isabel Department of Nephrology, Birmingham Children's Hospital, Ladywood Middleway, Birmingham B16 8ET — LMS Valencia 1988.

PIRA, Almas Mocha Parade Surgery, 4-5 Mocha Parade, Salford M7 1QE Tel: 0161 839 2721 Fax: 0161 819 1191.

PIRACHA, Arshid The Surgery, Exchange Road, Alrewas, Burton-on-Trent DE13 7AS; 66 Chads Road, Derby DE23 6RQ — MB ChB Manch. 1985.

PIRES, Philip (retired) 12 Woodside Close, Tolworth, Surbiton KT5 9JU Tel: 020 8241 4987 — LAH Dub. 1961. Prev: Med. Asst. Manor Hosp. Epsom.

PIRIE, Alexander McKenzie Birmingham Women's Hospital, Metchley Park Road, Edgbaston, Birmingham B15 2TG Tel: 0121 627 2672 Email: a.m.pirie@bham.ac.uk — MB ChB Ed. 1989; BSc (Hons.) Ed.; DRCOG 1993; MRCP (UK) 1993; DFFP 1995; MRCOG (Commend.) 1998; FRCP Ed. 2002. Cons. (Obst. & Gyn.) & Hon. Sen. Lect. Univ. Birm.; Private Pract. The Priory Hosp. Birm. Specialty: Obst. & Gyn. Special Interest: Epilepsy & Neurol. disorders in Pregn.; Matern. Med., obstetric ultrasound; Thyroid disorders, Diabetes, Hypertens., HIV in Pregn. Socs: Brit. Matern. & Fetal Med. Soc.; Brit. Assn. of Perinatal Med. Prev: Teachg. hosp. posts in Edin., Glas., Dundee, Cardiff, Soton.

PIRIE, Antoinette 188A Sutherland Avenue, London W9 1HR — MB BS Lond. 1981; MA Oxf. 1982, BA 1978; MRCOG 1989; MBA Warwick 1990. Med. Dir. W. Herts NHS Trust. Specialty: Pub. Health Med.; Obst. & Gyn. Prev: Med. Dir. Mt. Vernan & Watford NHS Hosps Trust.

PIRIE, Catherine Mary Royal Aberdeen Children's Hospital, Department of Community Child Health, Westburn Road, Aberdeen AB25 2ZG — MB ChB Aberd. 1972. Staff Grade. Specialty:

Community Child Health. Prev: Clin. Med. Off. Grampian Healthcare NHS Trust; Ho. Phys. Woodend Gen. Hosp. Aberd. & Roy. Aberd. Childr. Hosp.; Ho. Surg. Aberd. Roy. Infirm.

PIRIE, Keith The Surgery, Mackenzie Avenue, Auchenblae, Laurencekirk AB30 1XU Tel: 01561 320202 Fax: 01561 320774 — MB ChB Aberd. 1981.

PIRIE, Lesley Kathryn Ian Charles Cottage Hospital, The Health Centre, Castle Road East, Grantown-on-Spey PH26 3HR Tel: 01479 872484 Fax: 01479 873503 — MB BCh BAO Dub. 1982; MB BCh Dub. 1982; MRCGP 1986. Prev: Trainee GP Renfrewsh. VTS.

PIRIE, Linda Ellen Farriers House, 35 Main St., Middleton, Market Harborough LE16 8YU Tel: 01536 771140 — MB BS Lond. 1983; LLB (Hons.) Leics. 1994. Indep. Med. Practitioner. Specialty: Psychother. Socs: Brit. Soc. Med. & Dent. Hypn. Prev: Sen. Regist. (Histopath.) Lewisham Hosp. & Guy's Hosp. Lond.; Regist. & SHO (Histopath.) Roy. Free Hosp. Lond.

PIRIS, Juan Department of Cellular Pathology, John Radcliffe Hospital, Headington, Oxford OX3 9DU — LMS Spain 1972 (Univ. Navarra) DPhil Oxf. 1975; FRCPath 1991, M 1979; MBA Ed. 1996. Cons Gastrointestinal and Liver Pathologist. Specialty: Pathology, General. Socs: Assn. Clin. Path.; Brit. Soc. of Gastroenterol.; Brit. Div. of Internat. Acad. of Path. Prev: Sen. Lect. (Path.) Univ. Edin; Clin. Lect. & Hon. Sen. Regist. Nuffield Dept. Univ. Oxf.; Ho. Off. Clinica Univ. Pamplona, Navarra, Spain.

PIRIS, Monica 2F2 13 Brunsfield Avenue, Edinburgh EH10 4EL — MB ChB Ed. 1998. PRHO (Surg.) Edin. Roy. Infirm. Prev: PRHO (Med.) Edin. Roy. Infirm.

PIRMOHAMED, Professor Munir University of Liverpool, Department of Pharmacology & Therapeutics, PO Box 147, Liverpool L69 3BX Tel: 0151 794 5549 Fax: 0151 794 5540 Email: munirp@liv.ac.uk — MB ChB (Hons.) Liverp. 1985; MRCP (UK) 1988; PhD Liverp. 1993; FRCP Edin. 1999; FRCP London 2000; FBPharmacolS 2004. Prof. od Clin. Pharmacol. Liverp. Univ.; Hon. Cons. Phys. Roy. Liverp. & Broadgreen Univ. Hosp. Trust. Specialty: Gen. Med.; Pharmacology. Socs: Brit. Pharmacological Soc.; Med. Research Soc.; Fac. of PostGrad. Med. Prev: Lect. (Clin. Pharmacol). Liverp. Univ.; MRC Train. Fell. (Pharmacol.) Liverp. Univ.; Regist. (Gen. Med.) Hope Hosp. Manch.

PIRRET, Marie Frances Park Surgery, Baker Street, Glasgow G41 3YE Tel: 0141 632 0203 Fax: 0141 636 5349 — MB ChB Glas. 1975; DCH RCPS Glas. 1977.

PIRRIE, Augusta Jane 15 Onslow Road, Burwood Park, Walton-on-Thames KT12 5BB — MB BS Lond. 1966; MRCS Eng. LRCP Lond. 1966; DCH RCP Lond. 1983.

PIRRIE, John Miller (retired) Conlig, Copt Hill, Danbury, Chelmsford CM3 4NN — MB BS Lond. 1954 (St. Thos.) MRCS Eng. LRCP Lond. 1950.

PIRWANY, Imran Rahmetullah Queen Mothers Hospital, Yorkhill, Glasgow G3 8SJ Tel: 0141 201 0000 Fax: 0141 357 3610 Email: ipirwany@hotmail.com; Flat PF1, 3 Marchmont St, Edinburgh EH9 1EJ Tel: 0131 228 8635 Fax: 0131 228 8635 Email: ipirwany@compuserve.com — MB BS Karachi 1986 (University of Karachi) MFFP 1994; MRCOG 1994. Sen. Regist. (Obsterics & Gyn.) Qu. Marys Hosp. Yorkhil. Specialty: Obst. & Gyn. Socs: Glas. Obst. Soc.; Ed. Obst. Soc.; Munroe Kerr Soc. Prev: Clin. Research Fell. Univ. of Glas.; Career Regist. Edin. Roy. Infirm. & Simpson Memor. Hosp. Edin.; Regist. Southmead Hosp. Bristol.

PIRZADA, Aslam Fiaz 10 Lancia Crescent, Bracebridge Heath, Lincoln LN4 2QN — MB BS Lond. 1997.

PIRZADA, Mr Badr-ul-Islam St. Catherine Surgery, 19 St Catherines, Lincoln LN5 8LW Tel: 01522 20389; 10 Lancia Crescent, Bracebridge Heath, Lincoln LN4 2QN Tel: 01522 524326 — MB BS Punjab 1950 (King Edwd. Med. Coll. Lahore) MB BS Punjab (Pakistan) 1950; FRFPS Glas. 1960; FRCS Glas. 1962; FRCS Ed. 1966; FRCGP 1989, M 1976; MRCGP 1976. Med. Off. Smith Clayton Forge GKN Lincoln; Clin. Tutor (Gen. Pract.) N. Lincs. HA; Sec. N. Lincs. Gen. Practs. Comm. Specialty: Occupat. Health. Socs: Fell. Roy. Soc. Med.; Lincs. LMC; Trent Regional Med. Comm. Prev: Sen. Regist. (Surg.) Co. Hosp. Lincoln; Regist. (Orthop.) Brighton & Lewes Hosp. Gp. & Halifax Roy. Infirm.

PIRZADA, Omar Masood 10 Lancia Crescent, Bracebridge Heath, Lincoln LN4 2QN — MB BS Lond. 1993.

PISKOROWSKYJ, Nicola 19 Bryngwili Road, Pontardulais, Swansea SA4 0XB — MB BCh Wales 1988.

PITALIA, Mr Anil Kumar 34 Haydock Park Gardens, Newton-le-Willows WA12 0JF — MB ChB Manch. 1992 (Manchester) BSc Hons 1990; FRCS Ed 1997. Specialty: Ophth.

PITALIA, Pyare Lal 34 Haydock Park Gardens, Newton-le-Willows WA12 0JF — MB BS Vikram 1961 (Gandhi Med. Coll. Bhopal)

PITALIA, Sanjay Kumar Wigan Road Surgery, 120 Wigan Road, Ashton-in-Makerfield, Wigan WN4 9ST Tel: 01942 727325 Fax: 01942 709081 — MB ChB Manch. 1983 (Manchester) DRCOG 1985; DCH RCPS Glas. 1986; MRCGP 1987. Chairm. Ashton PLC. Specialty: Cardiol.; Pharmacology; Pharmaceutical Medicine.

PITALIA, Shikha The Bowery Medical Centre, Elephant Lane, St Helens WA9 5PR Tel: 01744 816837 Fax: 01744 850800; Lakeview, 28 Willow Bank, Newton-le-Willows WA12 0DQ — MB ChB Manch. 1987 (Lond.) MRCGP 1991. Specialty: Gen. Pract.

PITCHER, Christopher Sotheby (retired) Rother View, 24 Military Road, Rye TN31 7NY Tel: 01797 226015 Fax: 01797 226015 — (Middlx.) DM Oxf. 1963, BM BCh 1950; DPath Eng. 1960; FRCPath 1974. Prev: Cons. Haematol. Stoke Mandeville Hosp. Aylesbury.

PITCHER, David Corbett Reid 144 Harley Street, London W1N 1AH Tel: 020 7935 0023; 37 The Croft, Barnet EN5 2TN Tel: 020 8440 0100 — (Westm.) MB BS Lond. 1965; MRCS Eng. LRCP Lond. 1965; DPM Eng. 1969; MPhil (Psychiat.) Lond. 1971; FRCPsych 1979, M 1972. Hon. Cons. Psychiat. Roy. Free Hosps. Lond. Specialty: Gen. Psychiat.; Forens. Psychiat. Socs: Fell. Roy. Soc. Med.; Brit. Acad. Forens. Sci.; Medico-Legal Soc. Prev: Regist. Bethlem & Maudsley Hosps.; Sen. Lect. (Psychiat.) Roy. Free Hosp. Sch. Med. Lond.

PITCHER, David William Worcestershire Royal Hospital, Charles Hastings Way, Worcester WR5 1DD Tel: 01905 763333; BMI The Droitwich Spa Hospital, St Andrew's Road, Droitwich WR9 8DN; 17 Teasel Way, Claines, Worcester WR3 7LD Tel: 01905 755484 Fax: 01905 458496 Email: davidpitcher@btinternet.com — MB BS Lond. 1973 (St. Geo.) MD Lond. 1986; FRCP Lond. 1991. Cons. Cardiol., Worcs. Acute Hosps., NHS Trust. Specialty: Cardiol. Special Interest: Arrhythmia, Pacing, Echocardiography, Heart Failure; Resusc. and Resusc. Train.; Med. Educat. Socs: Hon. Sec. Resusc. Counc. (UK); Heart Rhythm UK; Brit. Cardiac Soc. Prev: Cons. Cardiol. Co. Hosp. Hereford.

PITCHER, Maxton Charles Leighton Northwick Park Hospital, Dept. of Gastroenterology, Watford Road, Harrow HA1 3UJ Tel: 020 8869 2628 Fax: 020 8869 2626 — BM BCh Oxf. 1988; MRCP (UK) 1991; MA Camb. 1989, BA (Hons.) 1985, MD 1996; FRCP Lond. 2002. Cons. (Phys. & Gastro.) Northwick Pk. & St. Mark's Hosp. Harrow. Specialty: Gastroenterol.; Gen. Med. Socs: Brit. Soc. Gastroenterol.

PITCHER, Robert William Department Path., Royal Cornwall Hospital (Treliske), Truro TR1 3LJ — MB ChB Bristol 1977.

PITCHES, David William 26 Springbridge Road, Manchester M16 8PW Email: dwp@ukgateway.net — MB BS Lond. 1997 (King's Coll. Lond.) AKC 1994; BSc 1994; DCH 1999; MSc 2002; DFPH 2002. Specialist Regist. (Pub. Health) Birm. Specialty: Pub. Health Med. Special Interest: Transport and health. Socs: Diplomate of the Faculty of Public Health; Christian Medical Fellowship. Prev: SHO (Palliat. Med.) Mildmay Hosp. Lond.; SHO (c/o the Elderly) Qu. Hosp. Burton-on-Trent; SHO (Paediat.) Good Hope Hosp. Sutton Coldfield.

PITCHFORTH, Anthony Edmund Brvaich Bhan, Aberfeldy Tel: 01887 820 213 — MB BS Durh. 1964; DObst RCOG 1970; DCH RCPS Glas. 1970; DTM & H Liverpool 2001. p/t GP.

PITHER, Charles Edward St. Thomas' Hospital, London SE1 7EH Tel: 020 792208107 Fax: 020 7922 8229 Email: charles.pither@gstt.sthames.nhs.uk; 20 Corkran Road, Surbiton KT6 6PN Tel: 020 8225 0911 Fax: 020 8225 0939 Email: cpither@doctors.org.uk — MB BS Lond. 1977 (St. Thos.) FFA RCS Lond. 1982. Cons. In Pain Med. St. Thos. Hosp. Lond.; Med. Dir.; Pain Managem. Progr. Bronnllys Hosp. Brecon Powys. Specialty: Anaesth. Socs: Fell. Med. Soc. Lond.; Eur. Soc. Regional Anaesth.; Internat. Assn. Study of Pain. Prev: Sen. Regist. (Anaesth.) St. Thos. Hosp. Lond.; Fell. (Regional Anaesth. & Pain Control) Univ. Cincinnati Med. Centre Ohio, USA.

PITHIE, Alan David Brownler Centre Infection Service, Gartnavel General Hospital, Great Western Road, Glasgow G12 0YN — MB ChB Dundee 1993; MD Dundee 1993, BMsc (Hons.) 1979; MB ChB

Dundee 1982; MRCP (UK) 1985; DTM & H RCP Lond. 1988. Cons. Phys. (Gen. Med. & Infec.s Dis.s) Glasglow. Specialty: Infec. Dis.

PITKEATHLY, Denis Aitken (retired) 4C Victoria Square, Mearnskirk Road, Newton Mearns, Glasgow G77 5TD Tel: 0141 616 3421 — MB ChB St. And. 1957; FRCP Ed. 1972, M 1962; FRCP Glas. 1972, M 1962. Med. Off.. Appeals Serv.. Glas. Prev: Cons. Phys. South. Gen. Hosp. Glas.

PITKEATHLY, Isabella Gilmour (retired) Govan Health Centre, 295 Langlands Road, Glasgow G51 4BJ; 4C Victoria Square, Mearnskirk Road, Newton Mearns, Glasgow G77 5TD — MB ChB Glas. 1960; DObst RCOG 1962. Prev: Asst. Div. Med. Off. Lancs. CC.

PITKEATHLY, William Thomas Nigel 10 Huntsmans Gate, Burntwood, Walsall WS7 9LL — MB ChB St. And. 1967.

PITKIN, Andrew David Institute of Naval Medicine, Alverstoke, Gosport PO12 2DL Tel: 023 9276 8026 Fax: 023 9250 4823; 61 Village Road, Alverstoke, Gosport PO12 2LE Tel: 023 9252 4879 Email: apitkin@cix.compulink.co.uk — MB BS Lond. 1990; MRCP (UK) 1994. Civil. Med. Pract. (Undersea Med.) Inst. Naval Med. Gosport, Hants. Specialty: Gen. Med. Socs: Undersea & Hyperbaric Med. Soc.

PITKIN, Joan Directorate of Obstetrics & Gynaecology, Northwick Park & St. Marks Hospital, Watford Road, Harrow HA1 3UJ Tel: 0208 869 2863 Fax: 0208 869 2864 — MB BS Lond. 1976 (Royal Free) MRCS Eng. LRCP Lond. 1976; FRCS Ed. 1982; MRCOG 1985. p/t Cons.Gynaecologist, with speical interet in Urol., Nothwick Pk. and St. Marks Hosp., Harrow, Middlx.; Hon. Sen. Clin. Lect., Faculity of Med., Imperial Coll., Lond.; Vis. Lect., in Gyn. Specialty: Obst. & Gyn. Socs: Fell. Roy. Soc. Med.; Internat. Continence Soc.; Amer. Menopause Soc,Euro Menopause Soc,Internat. Menopause Soc. Prev: Hon. Lect. & Sen. Regist. (O & G) Char. Cross & Westm. Hosp. Lond.; Regist. (O & G) Roy. Free Hosp. Lond.; Regist. (Surg.) Brook Gen. Hosp. Lond.

PITKIN, Lisa Jane Stoke Road Farm, Stoke Road, Newton Longville, Milton Keynes MK17 0BQ — MB BS Lond. 1994.

PITMAN, Ian John 4 Brook Place, Cwm, Ebbw Vale NP23 7QZ — MB BCh Wales 1994.

PITMAN, Jane Chaddlewood Surgery, 128 Bellingham Crescent, Plympton, Plymouth PL7 2QP — MB BS Lond. 1992 (King's Coll. Lond.) DRCOG 1996. Specialty: Gen. Pract.

PITMAN, Marianne Alice 60 Bishops Road, Cleeve, Bristol BS49 4NG — MB BCh Wales 1968; FRCOG 1993, M 1974, DObst 1970; FFPHM RCP (UK) 1994, M 1980; T(PHM) 1991; MFFP 1996. Locum Family Plann. CMO UBHT, N. Bristol Trust. Specialty: Family Plann. & Reproduc. Health. Prev: Cons.Health.Pub.Med.NHSE S & W. Regional Off; Sen. Regist. (Community Med.) SE Thames RHA; Regist. (Community Med.) S. West. RHA.

PITMAN, Mr Martyn Clive The Royal Hampshire County Hospital, Winchester & Eastleigh Healthcare NHS Trust, Romsey Road, Winchester SO22 5DG Tel: 01962 825 162; 10 Long Barrow Close, South Wonston, Winchester SO21 3ED Tel: 01962 889421 Fax: 01962 889421 — MB BS Lond. 1991 (Char. Cross & Westm. Med. Sch.) BSc (Hons.) Physiol. Lond. 1988; MRCOG 2001. Cons. Obst. & Gynaecologist Roy. Hants. Co. Hosp. Winchester. Specialty: Obst. & Gyn. Socs: BMA; MDU. Prev: Specialist Regist. (O & G) Soton. Univ. Hosp. NHS Trust; Specialist Regist. (O & G) Wessex Regional Rotat.; Research Fell. & Hon. Regist. (O & G) Chelsea & Westm. Hosp. Lond.

PITMAN, Richard Hugh 27 Lemon Street, Truro TR1 2LS — MB ChB Bristol 1960; DObst RCOG 1964.

PITSIAELI, Andreas Plisi Heathcote Medical Centre, Heathcote, Tadworth KT20 5TH Tel: 01737 360202; 43 Chequers Lane, Walton on the Hill, Tadworth KT20 7SF — MB BS Lond. 1988 (Char. Cross & Westm. Med. Sch. Lond.) BSc Lond. 1985; DRCOG 1992; MRCGP 1992. Prev: SHO (Gen. Med.) Qu. Mary's Univ. Hosp. Lond.

PITT, Angela Elizabeth Rylett Road Surgery, 45A Rylett Road, Shepherds Bush, London W12 9ST Tel: 020 8749 7863 Fax: 020 8743 5161 — MB BS Lond. 1984; DGM RCP Lond. 1986; DRCOG 1987. Prev: Trainee GP Lond.; SHO (O & G) W. Middlx. Univ. Hosp. Isleworth; SHO (Geriat., Cas. & Paediat.) W. Middlx. Univ. Hosp. Isleworth.

PITT, Bronwen Mary Melbourne House Surgery, 12 Napier Court, Queensland Crescent, Chelmsford CM1 2ED Tel: 01245 354370 Fax: 01245 344476; Pipers Farm, Good Easter, Chelmsford CM1 4RL — MB BCh Wales 1987; DRCOG 1990.

PITT, Deborah June Gabalfa Community Clinic, 213 North Road, Cardiff CF14 3AG Tel: 029 2069 3941 Fax: 029 2062 7954; 10 Erw'r Delyn Close, Penarth CF64 2TU Tel: 029 2071 1762 — MB BS Lond. 1972 (St. George's Hospital London) Dip. (Psychol Med.) Wales. Staff Grade Psychiat. Specialty: Gen. Psychiat. Socs: BMA; Christ. Med. Fellowsh. Prev: SHO Rotat. (Psychiat.) Gwent; SHO Rotat. (Psychiat.) S. Glam.; SHO Rotat. (Psychiat.) Mid Glam.

PITT, Miss Elspeth Sheena A&E Department, Aberdeen Royal Infirmary, Foresthill, Aberdeen AB25 2ZN Tel: 01224 681818; 14 Leddach Gardens, Westhill AB32 6FX — MB ChB Aberd. 1992; DRCOG 1995; MRCGP 1996; Dip. IMC RCS Ed 1998; FRCS (Ed) A&E 1998. Specialist Regist. (A&E). Specialty: Accid. & Emerg.

PITT, Frances Ann South Leicestershire PCT, The Rosings, Forest Road, Narborough, Leicester LE19 3EG Tel: 0116 286 4042 Email: fran.pitt@slpct.nhs.uk; 44 Bannercross Road, Sheffield S11 9HR — MB ChB Sheff. 1978; MFPHM RCP (UK) 1991; FFPH (UK) 2002. Director of Pub. Health S. Leics. PCT; Cons. Pub. Health Med. Sheff. Health. Specialty: Pub. Health Med. Socs: Fac. Pub. Health Med. Prev: Cons. Pub. Health Med. Barnsley HA; Sen. Regist. (Pub. Health Med.) Trent RHA; Regist. (Anaesth.) Doncaster Roy. Infirm.

PITT, Giles Hugh Townsend House Medical Centre, 49 Harepath Road, Seaton EX12 2RY Tel: 01297 20616 Fax: 01297 20810 — BM BCh Oxf. 1982; Cert. Family Plann. JCC 1986; MA Camb. 1986; DObst. Otago 1987; FRCGP (FBA) 2000. Princip. in GP.

PITT, Ian Victor Street Surgery, Victor Street, Shirley, Southampton SO15 5SY Tel: 023 8077 4781 Fax: 023 8039 0680; 360 Winchester Road, Shirley, Southampton SO16 6TW — MB Camb. 1975; BChir 1974; MRCGP 1979. Prev: Med. Off. Kapsowar Hosp. Kenya.

PITT, Jacqueline Mary JA - Rose, Post Office Rd, Toft Monks, Beccles NR34 0EH Tel: 01502 677342 — MB BS Lond. 1965 (St Bart.) DObst RCOG 1967. Specialty: Obst. & Gyn.

PITT, Mr James Ipswich Hospital, Heath Road, Ipswich IP4 5PD Tel: 01473 703755 Email: james.pitt@ipswitchhospital.nhs.uk — MB BS Lond. 1989 (Lond. Hosp.) FRCS Eng. 1994; MSc (Hons.) Lond. 1996; FRCS (Gen. Surg.) 2000. Cons. (Gen. Surg.) Ipswich Hosp.; Cons. (Gen. Surg.) Ipswich Nuffield Hosp. Specialty: Gen. Surg. Special Interest: Colorectal. Socs: Roy. Soc. Med.; Hunt. Soc.; Livesyman Soc. of Apoth. Prev: Research Fell. Univ. Coll. Hosp. Lond.; Specialist Regist. (Gen. Surg.) Char. Cross Hosp.; Specialist Regist. St. Mary's Hosp.

PITT, John Brian Mount Oriel Medical Centre, 2 Mount Oriel, Belfast BT8 7HR Tel: 028 9070 1653; 23 Glencregagh Road, Belfast BT8 6FZ Tel: 01232 799241 — MB BCh BAO Belf. 1963 (Qu. Univ. Belf.) MB BCh BAO (Hons.) Belf. 1963; DObst RCOG 1967; MRCGP 1971. Prev: Resid. Med. Off. Belf. City Hosp.; SHO Roy. Vict. Hosp. Belf.

PITT, Mark Adrian Department of Histopathology, Royal Preston Hospital, Sharoe Green Lane North, Fulwood, Preston PR2 9HT Tel: 01772 710148 — MB ChB Manch. 1986; BSc Manch. 1983; MRCPath 1993. Cons. Histopath. Roy. Preston Hosp. Specialty: Histopath.

PITT, Matthew Carey Department of Clinical Neurophysiology, The Hospital for Children, Great Ormond St., London WC1N 3JH Tel: 020 7405 9200; St Maximin, Blakes Lane, East Clandon, Guildford GU4 7RR — MD Camb. 1989; MB 1978, BChir 1977; FRCP (UK) 1997. Cons. Clin. Neurophysiol. Hosp. Sick Childr. Gt. Ormond St. Lond. Specialty: Clin. Neurophysiol.

PITT, Michael Peter Ian Hob Cottage, Wheeley Road, Alvechurch, Birmingham B48 7DD — MB ChB Birm. 1990; ChB Birm. 1990.

PITT, Nicola Sara 30 Damer Gardens, Henley-on-Thames RG9 1HX — MB ChB Sheff. 1987. Prev: Jun. Ho. Off. (Gen. Surg.) W. Cornw. Hosp. Penzance; Jun. Ho. Off. (Gen. Med.) N. Devon Dist. Hosp. Barnstaple.

PITT, Pauline Isobel Orpington Hospital, Rheumatology Department, Bromley Hospitals NHS Trust, Orpington BR6 8JG Tel: 01689 865239 Fax: 01689 805148 — MB BS Lond. 1975 (Univ. Coll. Lond.) FRCP; MD Lond. 1989. Cons. (Rheum.) Bromley Hosp. NHS Trust. Specialty: Rheumatol. Socs: Brit. Soc. of Rheum. Prev: Sen. Regist. (Rheum. & Rehabil.) King's Coll. Hosp. Lond.

PITT, Mr Peter Clive Crawford, TD Garnish Hall, Margaret Roding, Dunmow CM6 1QL Tel: 01245 231209 Fax: 01245 231224

Email: peter@garnishhall.fsnet.co.uk — MB BS Lond. 1957 (Guy's) MRCS Eng. LRCP Lond. 1957; DTM & H Eng. 1960; MRCP Ed. 1961; FRCS Ed. 1963; FRCS Eng. 1964; FRCP Ed 1998. Specialty: Gen. Surg. Socs: Fell. Roy. Soc. Med.; Hunt Soc. Prev: Cons. Gen. Surg. Havering Hosps. Romford; Sen. Regist. (Surg.) Guy's Hosp. Lond. & Chase Farm Hosp. Enfield; Maj. RAMC Sen. Surg. Specialist.

PITT, Shaun Michael 515A Clifton Drive N., Lytham St Annes FY8 2QX — MB BS Lond. 1994.

PITT, William Henry Paisley Road West Surgery, 1600 Paisley Road West, Glasgow G52 Tel: 0141 882 4567 Fax: 0141 882 4548; 6 Lednock Road, Cardonald, Glasgow G52 2SJ Tel: 0141 882 2245 — MB ChB Glas. 1960. Specialty: Gen. Pract.; Aviat. Med. Socs: BMA; Scott. Assn. Auth. Med. Examr.s Aviat.

PITTAM, Joan Kathryn Templehill Surgery, 23 Templehill, Troon KA10 6BQ Tel: 01292 312012 Fax: 01292 317594; 52 Wilson Avenue, Troon KA10 7AJ — MB ChB Manch. 1972. GP Templehill Troon. Prev: Ho. Surg. & Ho. Phys. Manch. Roy. Infirm.; SHO (Psychiat.) Univ. Hosp. S. Manch.

PITTAM, Mr Michael Robert Luton & Dunstable Hospital, Lewsey Road, Luton LU4 0DZ Tel: 01582 497097 Fax: 01582 497176; Vicarage Cottage, Valley Road, Studham, Dunstable LU6 2NN Tel: 01582 872264 Fax: 01582 873843 — MB Camb. 1973; FRCS Eng. 1977; MA Camb. 1973, MChir 1986. Cons. Gen. Breast & Vasc. Surg. Luton & Dunstable Hosp. Specialty: Gen. Surg. Prev: Sen. Regist. (Surg.) Westm. Hosp. Lond.; Vandervell Research Fell. & Lect. (Surg.) Inst. Cancer Research Lond.; Regist. (Surg.) St. Jas. Hosp. Leeds.

PITTARD, Alison Jane General Intensive Care Unit, The General Infirmary at Leeds, Great George St., Leeds LS1 3EX Tel: 0113 392 6672 Email: alison.pittard@leedsth.nhs.uk — MB ChB Leeds 1988; FRCA Lond. 1993; MD (Leeds) 1998. Cons. (Int. Care) The Gen. Infirm. at Leeds. Specialty: Anaesth. Prev: Sen. Regist. (Anaesth.) St. Jas. Univ. Hosp. Trust Leeds.; Research Fell. (Intens. Care) Leeds; Regist. (Anaesth.) Yorks.

PITTARD, John Barry Chertsey Lane Surgery, 5 Chertsey Lane, Staines TW18 3JH Tel: 01784 454164 Fax: 01784 464360 — BM BCh Oxf. 1972; BSc (1st cl. Hons.) Newc. 1969; MSc (Social Med.) Lond. 1978. Hosp. Pract. (Cardiol.) St. Peter's Hosp. Chertsey; CMD/Stroke Lead, N. Surrey PCT. Specialty: Cardiol. Socs: Sec. Primary Care Cardiovasc. Soc. Prev: Sen. Regist. (Community Med.) Oxf. AHA (T) & Lond. Sch. Hyg. & Trop. Med.; SHO (Med.) Hammersmith Hosp. Lond.

PITTAWAY, Andrew John 48 Sandrock Drive, Bessacarr, Doncaster DN4 6DT — BM BS Nottm. 1991; FRCA 1998. Specialty: Anaesth.

PITTMAN, James Alexander Leader The Old Rectory, Poyntington, Sherborne DT9 4LF — MB BS Lond. 1992; BSc (Hons.) Lond. 1989, MB BS 1992.

PITTS, Christopher Mark 33 Wyston Brook, Hilton, Derby DE65 5JB — MB BS Lond. 1998.

PITTS, Isabella Deri, Maj. RAMC(V) Queens Corner Surgery, 1 New Queen Street, Scarborough YO12 7HL Tel: 01723 378078 Fax: 01723 378010 — State DMS Siena 1968 (Pisa & Siena) State Exam Siena 1968; RCGP Dip. Drug Addic. 2002. GP. Specialty: Alcohol & Substance Misuse. Socs: BMA & Med. Defence Union. Prev: Clin. Asst. (Dermat. & A & E) ScarBoro. Hosp.

PITTS, John Elliot (retired) Stable Cottage, School Road, Bursledon, Southampton SO31 8BW Tel: 023 8040 2433 — MB BChir Camb. 1946 (Middlx.)

PITTS, John Richard The Red Practice, Waterside Health Centre, Beaulieu Road, Hythe SO45 5WX Tel: 023 8084 5955; 31 Sir Christopher Court, Hythe, Southampton SO45 6JR Tel: 023 8084 7155 — MB BS Lond. 1973; BSc (Hons.) Lond. 1970; MRCP (UK) 1975; MRCGP 1979; MSc (Med. Educat.) Cardiff 1991. Assoc. Adviser Wessex; Edr., "Educat. for Primary Care". Prev: Ho. Surg. Univ. Coll. Hosp. Lond.; SHO (Med.) & Ho. Phys. Whittington Hosp. Lond.

PITTS, Jonathan Edward 34 Adam Close, St Leonards-on-Sea TN38 9QW Tel: 01424 758289 Fax: 01424 757086 — MB BS Lond. 1993 (Char. Cross & Westm.) Staff Grade (Cardiol.) Conquest Hosp. Hastings. Specialty: Cardiol. Special Interest: Chest Pain Clinics. Socs: Fell. Roy. Soc. Med. Prev: Staff Grade Phys. (Emerg. Med. Assessm.) Unit Llandough Hosp. Penarth; Regist. (Emerg. Admissions) William Harvey Hosp. Ashford; SHO (Gen. Med.) S. Kent Hosps.

PITTS, Sarah 18 Hart Street, Lenton, Nottingham NG7 1SF — BM BS Nottm. 1996.

PITTS CRICK, Jonathan Charles Department of Cardiology, Bristol Royal Infirmary, Marlborough St., Bristol BS2 8HW Tel: 0117 928 2664 Fax: 0117 928 2666; Burnett House, Burnett, Bristol BS31 2TF Tel: 0117 986 0242 — MRCS Eng. LRCP Lond. 1973 (King's Coll. Hosp.) MRCP (UK) 1979; DPhil Sussex 1984; FRCP Lond. 1994. Cons. Cardiol. Bristol Roy. Infirm.; Hon. Clin. Lect. (Med.) Univ. Bristol. Specialty: Cardiol. Socs: Brit. Cardiac Soc. & Brit. Cardiovasc. Interven. Soc. Prev: Sen. Regist. (Cardiol.) Hammersmith Hosp. Lond.; Regist. (Cardiol.) Guy's Hosp. Lond.; Hon. Regist. (Cardiol.) Roy. Sussex Co. Hosp. Brighton.

PITTS-TUCKER, Thomas John Pershore Health Centre, Priest Lane, Pershore WR10 1RD Tel: 01386 502030 Fax: 01386 502058 — BM BCh Oxf. 1978; MRCP (UK) 1980; DRCOG 1980; MRCGP 1982; DCH RCP Lond. 1983; MMedSci Birm. 1996.

PIYARISI, Mr Dadallage Lalitha 33 Ripley Road, Ilford IG3 9HA — MB BS Peradeniya, Sri Lanka 1980; FRCS Ed. 1991.

PIYASENA, Chandrani 191 Bishopsford Road, Morden SM4 6BH Tel: 020 8648 3187 Fax: 020 8440 3157; 33 Shirley Avenue, Cheam, Sutton SM2 7QS — MB BS Sri Lanka 1972 (Colombo) MRCS Eng. LRCP Lond. 1976; DRCOG 1977. GP Morden. Specialty: Gen. Pract. Prev: SHO (O & G) Merton, Sutton & Wandsworth AHA (T); Ho. Off. (Gyn.) Merton, Sutton & Wandsworth AHA (T); Ho. Off. (Gyn.) Barnet AHA.

PIZEY, Mr Noel Cyril Douglas Horsecombe House, Shepherd's Walk, Bath BA2 5QU Tel: 01225 833510 — MB BS Lond. 1947 (St. Thos.) MRCS Eng. LRCP Lond. 1946; FRCS Eng. 1950; DMRT Eng. 1963; FFR 1966. Cons. Radiotherap. Radiother. Centre Bristol & Roy. United Hosp. Bath. Socs: Assn. Head & Neck Oncol.; Brit. Inst. Radiol. Prev: Sen. Regist. Dept. Radiother. Addenbrooke's Hosp. Camb.; Research Asst. Dept. Radiother. & Sen. Surg. Regist. St. Thos. Hosp.; Lond.

PIZURA, Volodimir Alexander Chancellor House Surgery, 6 Shinfield Road, Reading RG2 7BW Tel: 0118 931 0006 Fax: 0118 975 7194 — MB BS Lond. 1983 (St. Geo.) BSc Lond. 1980, MB BS 1983; MRCGP 1988; DRCOG 1990. Specialty: Anat. Socs: Pharmaceut. Soc. Prev: GP Crowthorne; Regist. (Psychiat.) Fairmile Hosp.; Med. Off. Jane Furze Hosp., Africa.

PLAAT, Felicity Sarah Department of Anaesthesia, Queen Charlotte's and Chelsea Hospital, Du Cane Road, London W12 0HS Tel: 020 8383 3991 Fax: 020 8838 5373 Email: fplaat@hhnt.org; 34 Aubert Park, London N5 1TU Tel: 020 7354 5252 — MB BS Lond. 1985 (Middlesex Hospital) BA Camb. 1981; FRCA 1994. Lead Cons. Anaesth. Qu. Charlotte's & Chelsea Hosp.; Coll. Tutor. Specialty: Anaesth. Socs: Assn. Anaesth.; Obst. Anaesth. Assn.; BMA. Prev: Sen. Regist. Rotat. (Anaesth.) Hammersmith Hosp. Lond.

PLACE, Collin (retired) The Coppice, The Green, Thornborough, Buckingham MK18 2DL Tel: 01280 812514 Fax: 01280 813796 — MB ChB St. And. 1963; DObst RCOG 1965. Prev: Princip. GP, Verney Cl. Family Pract., Buckingham.

PLACE, Gregory Francis Ashfield House, Forest Road, Annesley Woodhouse, Kirkby in Ashfield, Nottingham NG17 9JB Tel: 01623 752295/153 — MB BChir Camb. 1984. LMC Chairm., N. Nottm. LMC Chairm. N. Nottm. LMC LMC Chairm.

PLACE, Professor Maurice Child, Adolescent & Family Psychiatry Department, Sunderland General Hospital, Sunderland SR4 7TP Tel: 0191 569 9026 Email: maurice.place@unn.ac.uk — MD Newc. 1988; MB BS Newc. 1975; FRCPsych 1994, M 1979; LLB Univ Northumbria 1995. Cons. Child & Adolesc. Psychiat. Sunderland Gen. Hosp.; Prof. Child & Family Psychiat. Univ. of Northumbria at Newc. Specialty: Child & Adolesc. Psychiat. Socs: Assn. Child Psychol Psychiat.; Fell. Child Psychiat. Research Soc. Prev: Med. Dir. of City Hosps Sunderland; Sen. Regist. (Psychiat.) Newc. Teach. Hosp.; Research Assoc. Human Developm. Unit Newc. Univ.

PLACZEK, Monica Maria Crinkle Cottage, 9 The Green, Silverdale, Carnforth LA5 0TJ Tel: 0524 701318 — MB ChB Manch. 1973; DRCOG 1976; DCH Eng. 1976; FRCP (UK) 1979; FRCPCH 1995. Cons. Paediat. Lancaster HA & N. RHA. Specialty: Paediat.

PLAGARO COWEE, Samantha 84 East Street, Littlehampton BN17 6AN — LMS La Laguna 1993. SHO (A & E) Roy. Gwent

Hosp., Gwent, Newport. Specialty: Accid. & Emerg. Prev: SHO (Gen. Surg.); SHO (Urol.); SHO (A & E).

PLAHA, Mr Harbhajan Singh Oldchurch Hospital, Waterloo Road, Romford RM7 0BE Tel: 01708 708041 Fax: 01708 708041 — MB BS Bombay 1973; MS Bombay 1975; FRCS Ed. 1979 FCPS Bombay 1975; FRCS Eng. 1979; FRCS Ed. (Orth.) 1983. Cons. Orthop. Surg. Specialty: Orthop. Special Interest: Lower Limb Primary & Revision Surg. Prev: Tutor (Gen. Surg.) Lokmanya Tilak Municip. Med. Coll. Univ. Bombay; Sen. Regist. (Gen. Surg.) Topiwala Nat. Med. Coll. Univ. Bombay; Regist. (Orthop. Surg.) Ealing Hosp. Southall.

PLAIL, Mr Roger Oliver East Sussex NHS Trust, Conquest Hospital, The Ridge, St Leonards-on-Sea TN37 4RD Tel: 01424 755255 Fax: 01424 758115 Email: roger.plail@esht.nhs.uk — MB BS Lond. 1976; BSc Lond. 1973, MS 1990, MB BS 1976; FRCS Eng. 1981. Cons. Urol. Conquest Hosp. St. Leonards-on-Sea. Specialty: Urol. Special Interest: Erectile Dysfunction; Female Incontinence; Oncology. Socs: RSM; BAUS; Roy. Coll. of Surgeons. Prev: Sen. Regist. (Urol.) Roy. Marsden Hosp. Lond.

PLANA VIVES, Fausto 11 Lock Chase, London SE3 9HB — LMS Barcelona 1982.

PLANCHE, Timothy David 4 Warren Road, Banstead SM7 1LA — MB BS Lond. 1991.

PLANE, Andrew Raymond Portsdown Group Practice, Crookhorn Lane, Waterlooville PO7 5XP Tel: 023 9226 3078 Fax: 023 9223 0316; 15 Magdala Road, Cosham, Portsmouth PO6 2QG Tel: 02392 380694 — MB BS Lond. 1987 (Univ. Coll. Lond.) BSc (Physiol.) Lond. 1980; MRCGP 1991; DRCOG 1991; Cert. Family Plann. JCC 1991; DGM RCP Lond. 1994; DCH RCP Lond. 1994. GP Princip.; Clin. Asst. (Elderly Med.) Hants.; Hosp. Practitioner, Elderly Med., Qu. Alexandra and St Mary's Hosp., Portsmouth. Specialty: Care of the Elderly. Prev: Trainee GP Petersfield Hants.; SHO (Elderly Med.) Portsmouth; SHO (Paediat.) Jersey.

PLANT, Alan Russell House Surgery, Bakers Way, Codsall, Wolverhampton WV8 1HD Tel: 01902 842488; Moleshill, Mill Lane, Codsall, Wolverhampton WV8 1EG Tel: 01902 843819 — MB ChB Birm. 1964; MRCS Eng. LRCP Lond. 1964; DA Eng. 1967. Prev: Clin. Asst. Anaesth. Wolverhampton HA; SHO (Anaesth. & O & G) Walsall Hosp. Gp.

PLANT, Arthur Maxwell (retired) Tanglewood, Summerhill, Kingswinford DY6 9JG Tel: 01384 274060 — MB ChB Edin. 1941; MB ChB (Edin.) 1941. Prev: Ship's Surg. Merchant Navy 1942-46.

PLANT, Berwyn (retired) 22 Lancaster Way, Scalby, Scarborough YO13 0QH Tel: 01723 370928 Email: plantmed@aol.com — MRCS Eng. LRCP Lond. 1949 (Guy's) MRCGP 1966. Prev: Regist. Gen. Surg. Hull 'A' Hosp. Gp.

PLANT, Gillian Dorne Smith and Partners, South Park Surgery, 250 Park Lane, Macclesfield SK11 8AD Tel: 01625 422249 Fax: 01625 502169; Golden Slack Farm, Wincle SK11 0QL — MB ChB Manch. 1979 (Manchester) DRCOG 1982; FRCGP 1994, M 1983; DCCH Ed. 1986. hpe Tutor, Macclesfield (2001-). Socs: Fell. Manch. Med. Soc. Prev: GP Postrad. Tutor Macclesfield 1991-1998; Trainee GP Bramhall Health Centre Stockport FPC; SHO GP VTS Stockport HA.

PLANT, Gordon Terence The National Hospital for Neurology and Neurosurgery, Box 93, Queen Square, London WC1N 3BG Tel: 020 7837 3611 Ext: 3852 Fax: 020 7829 8720 Email: gordon.plant@uclh.org — MB BChir Camb. 1978 (Camb. & St. Thos.) MRCP (UK) 1979; MA Camb. 1978, MD 1986; FRCP Lond. 1993; FRCOphth Lond. 2005. Cons. Phys. Nat. Hosp. for Neurol. & Neurosurg. Lond.; Serv. Director Neuro-ophthalmology Moorfields Eye Hosp.; Cons. (Neurol.) St. Thos. Hosp. & Moorfields Eye Hosp. Lond.; Hon. Cons. (Neurol.) St Lukes Hosp. Lond.; Hon. Sec. Lect. Guys, Kings, St Thomas, Med. Sch. Lond.; Hon. Sen.lct Univ. Coll. Lond. Specialty: Neurol.; Ophth. Special Interest: Visual disorders due to Neurol. Dis. Socs: Eur. Neurol. Soc.; Amer. Assn. for the Advancem. of Sci.; Inst. for Cognitive Sci. Prev: Sen. Regist. Middlx. & Univ. Coll. Hosps. Lond.; Wellcome Research Assoc. Physiol. Laborat. Camb.; MRC Trav. Fell. Smith-Kettlewell Eye Research Inst., San Francisco.

PLANT, Graham Richard Tudor Department of Radiology, North Hampshire Hospital, Basingstoke RG24 9NA Tel: 01256 313477 Fax: 01256 314773 Email: graham.plant@nhht.nhs.uk — MB BS Lond. 1978 (Westm.) MRCS Eng. LRCP Lond. 1977; FRCR 1986. Cons. (Radiol.) N. Hants. Hosp. Specialty: Radiol. Special Interest: Vena cava filtration; Vasc. Interven.; IT in Med. Socs: Brit. Inst. Radiol.; Fell. Cardiovasc. Interven. Radiol. Soc. Europ.; Brit. Soc. Interven. Radiol. Prev: Sen. Registar (Radiol.) Westm., Brompton & Roy. Marsden Hosps. Lond.

PLANT, Ian David Connaught House, 63B Romsey Road, Winchester SO22 5DE — MB ChB Liverp. 1967; DPM Eng. 1972; FRCPsych 1991, M 1973; LMCC 1986; FRCPC 1987. Cons. Psychiat. Roy. Hants. Co. Hosp. Winchester; Cons. Psychiat. Marchwood Priory Hosp. Soton. Specialty: Gen. Psychiat. Prev: Sen. Regist. (Psychiat.) Profess. Unit Knowle Hosp. Fareham; Specialist in Psychiat. RAMC; Ho. Off. Clatterbridge Hosp. Bebington & Ashford Hosp., Middlx.

PLANT, Irene Mary South Staffords. Healthcare NHS Trust, Greenhill Health Centre, Church St, Lichfield WS13 6JL Tel: 01543 414311; Wellcroft, Stanley, Stoke-on-Trent ST9 9LX Tel: 01782 502693 — MB ChB Liverp. 1968; DRCOG 1970; DCH RCP Lond. 1971; MSc (Primary Med. Care) Keele 1995. Cons. Community Paediat. (Lichfield). Specialty: Community Child Health. Socs: Roy. Coll. Paediat. & Child Health; MRCPCH; Fac. Community Health. Prev: SCMO (Community Paediat.) Stoke on Trent.

PLANT, Lee Anthony 231A Manchester Road W., Little Hulton, Manchester M38 9XD — MB ChB Birm. 1997.

PLANT, Marilyn Jane The Surgery, 1 Glebe Road, Barnes, London SW13 0DR Tel: 020 8748 1065 Fax: 020 8741 8665 — MB BChir Camb. 1977; MPhil Camb. 1983, MA 1978; MRCP (UK) 1980; DRCOG 1985; MRCGP 1988.

PLANT, Michael James Department of Rhematology, University Hospital Wales, Cardiff CF4 4XW Tel: 029 2074 2346; 4 Egerton Walk, Dodleston, Chester CH4 9NS Tel: 01244 660052 — MB BS Lond. 1984; MA Camb. 1984; MRCP (UK) 1987; MD Lond. 1996. Sen. Regist. (Rheum.) Univ. Hosp. Wales Cardiff & Wrexham Maelor Hosp. Specialty: Gen. Med. Prev: Regist. (Rheum.) Staffs. Rheum. Centre Stoke-on-Trent; Regist. (Diag. Radiol.) Manch. Roy. Infirm.; Regist. (Med.) Char. Cross Hosp. Lond.

PLANT, Nicholas Anthony The Surgery, Summerhill, Kingswinford DY6 9JG; Carr House, 32 Moss Grove, Kingswinford DY6 9HU — MB ChB Birm. 1974. Chairm. Duvky S. Primary Care Gp., Paryton's Ho., Ridge Hill, Brievley Hill Rd., Stowbridge, W. Midl.s, DY8 5ST. Prev: Sen. Ho. Surg. (O & G) New Cross Hosp. Wolverhampton; Ho. Phys. Roy. Hosp. Wolverhampton; Ho. Surg. Dept. Urol. Qu. Eliz. Hosp. Birm.

PLANT, Nicholas David Royal Manchester Children's Hospital, Hospital Road, Pendlebury, Manchester M27 4HA Tel: 0161 727 2162 — MB BCh Wales 1984 (Welsh National School of Medicine) FRCPCH; MRCP (UK) 1988; FRCP 2000. Cons. Paediatric Nephrologist Roy. Manch. Children's Hosp. Specialty: Paediat.

PLANT, Patricia Anne 3 Wintney Close, Harborne, Birmingham B17 8SQ — MB ChB Bristol 1963. Specialty: Family Plann. & Reproduc. Health.

PLANT, Paul Keith 5 Sandhill Drive, Leeds LS17 8DU — BM BS Nottm. 1990; MRCP 1993. Specialty: Gen. Med.; Respirat. Med.

PLANT, Sara Jane Withymoor Surgery, Turners Lane, Brierley Hill DY9 2PG Tel: 01384 366740 Fax: 01384 350444; Prospect House, 17 Birmingham Road, Blakedown, Kidderminster DY10 3JD — MB ChB Birm. 1993; DRCOG 1997; DFFP 1997. Salaried GP, PMS Pilot, Withymoor Surg., Brierley Hill; CMO Family Plann., Dudley Priority Community NHS Trust, W. Mids. Specialty: Family Plann. & Reproduc. Health; Ment. Health; Genitourinary Medicine. Prev: SHO (A & E) Russells Hall Hosp. Dudley.; GP Partner, Aston Univ. Health Centre, Birm.; Asst. GP Worcs.

PLANT, Simon Haddon Lyle and Partners, The Surgery, 4 Silverdale Road, Burgess Hill RH15 0EF Tel: 01444 233450 Fax: 01444 230412 — MB BS Lond. 1991 (King's Coll. Hosp. Lond.) BSc (Hons.) Lond. 1987; DCH RCP Lond. 1995.

PLANT, William David Department of Renal Medicine, Royal Infirmary of Edinburgh, Lauriston Place, Edinburgh EH3 9YW Tel: 0131 536 2281 Fax: 0131 536 1441; 19A Blackford Road, Grange, Edinburgh EH9 2DT Tel: 0131 447 0791 — MB BCh BAO NUI 1985 (Cork, Ireland) BSc (Hons.) NUI 1982; MB BCh BAO (Hons.) NUI 1985; MRCPI 1988; FRCP FRCP Edinburgh 1999 1999. Cons. renal Phys. Roy. Infirm. of Edin.; Hon. Sen. Lect. (Med.) Univ. Edin. Specialty: Nephrol. Socs: Scott. Renal Assn.; Eur. Soc. Philosophy in Med. & Health Care; Renal Assn. Prev: Sen. Regist. (Renal Med.)

Roy. Infirm. Edinbugh; Regist. (Renal Med.) Roy. Infirm. Edin.; Regist. (Nephrol. & Gen. Med.) Cork Univ. Hosp.

PLANTEVIN, Odile Marie Emma Paule (retired) 23 Broom Park, Teddington TW11 9RS Tel: 020 8943 0412 — (Manch.) MB ChB Manch. 1951; DA Eng. 1955; FFA RCS Eng. 1958. Prev: Cons. Anaesth. St. Thos. Hosp. Lond.

PLATER, Marianne Elaine 8 Hillside Road, Marlow SL7 3JY; 27 Charles Road, Cowes PO31 8HG — MB ChB Liverp. 1988; MRCP (UK) 1991. Specialist Regist. (Gen. Med. & c/o the Elderly). Specialty: Care of the Elderly; Gen. Med. Socs: Brit. Geriat. Soc.

PLATFORD, Joan Camphill, Japonica Lane, Willen Park S., Milton Keynes MK15 9JY Tel: 01908 235505 — MB ChB Bristol 1983.

PLATMAN, Andrew Maurice Sydenham Green Group Practice, 26 Holmshaw Close, London SE26 4TH Tel: 020 8676 8836 Fax: 020 7771 4710; 203 Lennard Road, Beckenham BR3 1QN Tel: 020 8659 1990 — MB BChir Camb. 1977 (Camb. & King's Coll. Hosp.) MA Camb. 1978; MRCP (UK) 1980; MRCGP 1983.

PLATT, Mr Alastair James 17 The Mount, Wrenthorpe, Wakefield WF2 0NZ — BM BCh Oxf. 1989; FRCS Eng. 1993. Specialist Regist. (Plastic Surg.) Yorks. Specialty: Plastic Surg.

PLATT, Celia Lesley Willenhall Medical Centre, Croft Street, Willenhall WV13 2DR Tel: 01902 600833 — MB ChB Sheff. 1959. GP Willenhall. Socs: BMA. Prev: SHO (Cas.) Clatterbridge Hosp. Bebington.

PLATT, Craig Charles Department of Pathology, Birmingham Women's Health Care NHS Trust, Metchley Park Road, Birmingham B15 2TG; 8 Romford Meadow, Eccleshall, Stafford ST21 6SP — MB ChB Leic. 1984; MRCPath 1993. Specialty: Histopath. Socs: Paediat. Path. Soc.

PLATT, Graham Norris Road Surgery, 356 Norris Road, Sale M33 2RL Tel: 0161 962 5464 — MB BCh Wales 1981; BSc Wales 1978, MB BCH 1981; MRCGP 1986. Specialty: Gen. Pract.

PLATT, Hugh Shuter, TD, OStJ, OBE Royal College of Pathologists, 2 Carlton House Terrace, London SW1Y 5AF Tel: 020 7451 6758; 6 Rewland Drive, Winchester SO22 6PA Tel: 01962 881050 — MB BS (Hons. Surg.) Lond. 1958 (Univ. Coll. Hosp.) BSc Lond. 1955, MD 1970; FRCPath (Hon.) 1986; FRCOphth 1999; FRCP 2001. p/t Dir. of Studies RCPath; Scientif. Fell. Zool. Soc. Lond. Specialty: Chem. Path. Socs: Fell. Roy. Soc. Med.; BMA; Scientif. Fell. Zool. Soc. Lond. Prev: PostGrad Dean (Wessex); Hon. Sen. Clin. Lect. Soton Med. Sch.; Hon. Phys. to HM the Qu.

PLATT, Ian Thomas Skellern and Partners, Bridport Medical Centre, North Allington, Bridport DT6 5DU Tel: 01308 421109 Fax: 01308 420869 — BM Soton. 1990; BSc Durham 1986; MRCGP 1995. GP Trainee GP W. Dorset Gen. Hosps. NHS Trust.

PLATT, John Old School Medical Centre, School Lane, Greenhill, Sheffield S8 7RL Tel: 0114 237 8866 Fax: 0114 237 3400 — MB ChB Sheff. 1974.

PLATT, John Stephen West Middlesex University Hospital NHS Trust, Twickenham Road, Isleworth TW7 6AF Tel: 020 8565 5449 Fax: 020 8565 5318 Email: maria.classick@wmuh-tr.nthames.nhs.uk — MB BChir Camb. 1980 (St Catharines College Cambridge and Middlesex Hosp. Med. Sch) MA Camb. 1979; MB Camb 1979, BChir 1980; MRCP (UK) 1982; FRCP Lond. 1996. Cons. Phys. (c/o the Elderly & Gen. Med.) W. Middlx. Univ. Hosp. NHS Trust. Specialty: Care of the Elderly; Gen. Med.; Brit. Geriat. Soc. Regional sec 94-97 & Brit. Geriat. Soc. Counc. Represen. for N. W. Thames 2000. Prev: Sen. Regist. (Geriat. Med.) North. Gen. Hosp. Sheff. & Barnsley Dist. Gen. Hosp.; Regist. (Geriat. Med.) Char. Cross Hosp. Lond.; Regist. (Gen. Med.) Greenwich Dist. Hosp. Lond.

PLATT, Julie Elizabeth — MB BS Newc. 1997.

PLATT, Kaye Alison 66 Fairlawn Road, Tadley, Basingstoke RG26 3SP — MB BCh (Hons.) Wales 1990; MRCP (UK) 1993; FRCR 1999. Cons. Radiologist John Radcliffe Hosp. Oxf. Specialty: Radiol. Prev: Specialist Regist. (Radiol.) Univ. Coll. Lond. Hosp. Trust; Research Regist. (Med.) Univ. Wales Coll. Med. Cardiff.; SHO (Gen. Med.) Princess of Wales Hosp. Bridgend.

PLATT, Mark Richard 49 Cherville Street, Romsey SO51 8FB — MB BChir Camb. 1982; MA Camb. 1982; FFA RCS 1987. Cons. Anaesth. Soton. Gen. Hosp. Specialty: Anaesth. Prev: Sen. Regist. (Anaesth.) Soton. Univ. Hosp.

PLATT, Mark Robson South Sefton Child and Family Services, Empire House, 138-148 Linacre Road, Litherland, Liverpool L21 8JU Tel: 0151 285 6500 Fax: 0151 285 6503 — MB BS Lond. 1981; MA Oxf. 1985; MRCPsych 1986. Cons. Child & Adolesc. Psychiat. Roy. Liverp. Childr.s NHS Trust, Liverp. Specialty: Child & Adolesc. Psychiat.

PLATT, Mary Jane Department of Public Health, University of Liverpool, Whelan Building Quadrangle, Liverpool L69 3GB Tel: 0151 794 5580 Fax: 0151 794 5588 Email: mjplatt@liv.ac.uk — MB BS Lond. 1982 (Char. Cross Hosp. Med. Sch.) MPH John Hopkins Univ. Baltimore; MRCGP 1985; DRCOG 1987; MFPHM RCP (UK) 1995; FRCPCH 1997. Sen. Lect. (Pub. Health Med.) Univ. Liverp. Specialty: Pub. Health Med. Prev: Sen. Regist. (Pub. Health Med.) Mersey Region; Post Doctoral Fell. John Hopkins Univ. Sch. Hyg. & Pub. Health Baltimore, USA; Trainee GP Swindon & Cirencester VTS.

PLATT, Michael William St Mary's Hospital, Department of Anaesthetics, Praed Street, London W2 1NY Tel: 020 7725 6216 Fax: 020 7725 6425 — MB BS West. Austral. 1977; FRCA 1988. Cons. Anaesth. & Pain St. Mary's Hosp. Trust Lond.; Lead Clinician Pain Servs.; Hon. Sen. Lect. (Anaesth.) Imperial Coll. of Sci., Technol. & Med. Lond. Specialty: Anaesth. Special Interest: Pain Med.; Neuropathic Pain; Cardiothoracic Anaesth. Socs: Roy. Soc. Med. (Anaesth. Sect.); Assn. Anaesth.; Pain Soc. Prev: Sen. Lect. (Anaesth.) St. Mary's Hosp. Med. Sch., Imperial Coll. Sci., Technol. & Med. Lond.

PLATT, Philip Neil 31 Mitchell Avenue, Jesmond, Newcastle upon Tyne NE2 3JY — MD Birm. 1988; MB ChB Birm. 1976; MRCP (UK) 1980; FRCP Lond. 1992. Cons. Rheum. Freeman Hosp. Trust; Hon. Lect. (Med.) Univ. Newc. Specialty: Rehabil. Med.; Rheumatol. Prev: Cons. Rheum. Roy. Vict. Infirm. Newc.

PLATT, Rosemary 34 Blackroot Road, Four Oaks, Sutton Coldfield B74 2QP — MB ChB Manch. 1974; DCH Eng 1976; DRCOG 1977; MRCGP 1979.

PLATT, Sarah Gillian Selly Park Surgery, 2 Reaview Drive, Pershore Road, Birmingham B29 7NT Tel: 0121 472 0187 Fax: 0121 472 4181; 49 Moor Green Lane, Moseley, Birmingham B13 8NE Tel: 0121 449 2764 — MB ChB Birm. 1975. Post Grad. Tutor Birm. Med. Inst. Specialty: Gen. Pract. Socs: Birm. Med. Inst.

PLATT, Simon Robert 67 Lake View, Edgware HA8 7SA — MB ChB Bristol 1993.

PLATT, Tracey Louise Clifton Applewood, Alleyns Lane, Cookham-Dean, Maidenhead SL6 9AD — MB BS Lond. 1998.

PLATTEN, Harriet Maud Jenny Charles Hicks Centre, 75 Ermine Street, Huntingdon PE29 3EZ Tel: 01480 453038 Fax: 01480 434104; 13 Hawkes End, Brampton, Huntingdon PE28 4TW Tel: 01480 453978 Fax: 01480 453978 — MB ChB Bristol 1976; MRCGP 1982. Hosp. Practitioner (Rheum.) Hinchingbrooke Hosp. Huntingdon.

PLATTEN, Michael Cotterell Elm Rise, 46 High St., Finstock, Chipping Norton OX7 3DW — MB ChB Birm. 1942; MA Camb.

PLATTS, Alan Samuel Gregory Helsby Street Medical Centre, 2 Helsby Street, Warrington WA1 3AW Tel: 01925 637304 Fax: 01925 570430; 2 Stoneacre Gardens, Appleton, Warrington WA4 5ET Email: ap@appleton.demon.co.uk — MB ChB Manch. 1980; BSc St. And. 1977; DRCOG 1984. Trainer (Gen. Pract.) Warrington.

PLATTS, Amanda Jill Parkbury House Surgery, St Peters Street, St Albans AL1 3HD Tel: 01727 851589; 60 Worley Road, St Albans AL3 5NN Tel: 01727 832046 — MB BS Lond. 1977 (Roy. Free) MRCP (UK) 1982; MRCGP 1996; FRCP 2001; FRCGP 2002. Assoc. Dean Lond. Deanery; Assoc. Director East. Deanery. Prev: Course Organiser NW Herts. Train. Scheme.

PLATTS, Mr Andrew Duncan Royal Free Hampstead NHS Trust, Radiology Department, Pond Street, London NW3 2QG Tel: 020 7830 2013 Fax: 020 7830 2969 Email: andrew.platts@royalfree.nhs.uk; 60 Worley Road, St Albans AL3 5NN Tel: 01727 832046 — MB BS Lond. 1977; FRCS Ed. 1981; FRCS Eng. 1981; FRCR 1985. Cons. Neuroradiol. Roy. Free Hampstead NHS Trust; Hon. Sen. Lect. Roy. Free and Univ. Coll. Med. Sch. Specialty: Radiol.

PLATTS, Anthony John (retired) 9 Blackley Close, Watford WD17 4TE Tel: 01923 243394 — (St. Mary's) MB BS Lond. 1952; MRCS Eng. LRCP Lond. 1952; DObst RCOG 1958. Prev: Ho. Surg. St. Mary's Hosp. (Harrow Rd. Br.) & Camb. Matern. Hosp.

PLATTS, Brian William, TD Park Cottage, Nottingham Road, Southwell NG25 0LG Tel: 01636 812587 Fax: 01636 812587

Email: drbrianplatts@hotmail.com; Park Cottage, Nottingham Road, Southwell NG25 0LG Tel: 01636 812587 — MB ChB Manch. 1975; MRCGP 1979; DIH Eng. 1981; FFOM RCP Lond. 1995, MFOM 1984, AFOM 1982. Indep. Cons. Occ. Phys. Specialty: Occupat. Health. Socs: (Ex-Chairm. Sec. & Treas.) Soc. Occupat. Med. (E. Midl. Gp.); Ex-Treas. Assn. NHS Occupat. Phys. (Ex-Chairm. Educat. Comm.). Prev: Regional Med. Off. Brit. Gas E. Midl.; Employm. Med. Adviser Health & Safety Exec. Nottm.; Med. Off. Brit. Steel Sheff.

PLATTS, Christopher Hanson The Medical Centre, King George Dock, Hull HU9 5PQ Tel: 01482 712113 Fax: 01482 704373; 5 Driffield Road, Beverley HU17 7LP Tel: 01482 882304 Fax: 01482 882304 — MB ChB Leeds 1964; DObst RCOG 1967; MRCGP 1971. p/t Med. Off. Assn. Brit. Ports Hull. Specialty: Occupat. Health. Prev: GP Princip. Beverley; SHO (O & G) Westwood Hosp. Beverley; Ho. Phys., Ho. Surg. & Ho. Off. (Paediat. & Dermat.) St Jas. Hosp. Leeds.

PLATTS, Hazel Florence Mary Ashworth Street Surgery, 85 Spotland Road, Rochdale OL12 6RT Tel: 01706 44582 Fax: 01706 346767; Buckley Hill House, Buckley Hill Lane, Milnrow, Rochdale OL16 4BU — MB ChB Manch. 1978; MRCGP 1982.

PLATTS, Hilary Adele Selsey Medical Centre, High Street, Selsey, Chichester PO20 0QG Tel: 01243 604321/602261 Fax: 01243 607996; 19 Bonnar Road, Selsey, Chichester PO20 9AT — MB ChB Leic. 1982; BSc Leic. 1980; DRCOG 1989. GP Princip. Chichester; Med. Off. (Family Plann.) Chichester; Hosp. Practitioner, Breast Clinic. Specialty: Family Plann. & Reproduc. Health.

PLATTS, Julia Karen 8 Farmhouse Mews, Wrexham LL13 9SX — MB BS Lond. 1989; MRCP (UK) 1993. Specialist Regist. Rotat. (Diabetes & Endocrinol.) Wrexham Maelor Hosp. Specialty: Diabetes; Endocrinol.

PLATTS, Karena Anne The Surgery, High Street, Epworth, Doncaster DN9 1EP Tel: 01427 872232 Fax: 01427 874944 — MB ChB Sheff. 1983 (Sheffield) DRCOG 1987; MRCGP 1987; MFFP 1993; Dip. Genitourin. 1996; Dip Pract Derm 2003. GP Doncaster. Prev: Mem. Humberside MAAG; Clin. Asst. (Genitourin. Med.).

PLATTS, Margaret Machon (retired) 47 Coldwell Lane, Sheffield S10 5TJ Tel: 0114 230 7300 Email: margaret@platts2307.freeserve.co.uk — (Sheff.) MB ChB Sheff. 1948; FRCP Lond. 1971, M 1950; DObst RCOG 1950; BSc Sheff. 1947, MD (Commend.) 1957. Prev: Cons. Phys. Lodge Moor Hosp. & Roy. Hallamsh. Hosp. Sheff.

PLATTS, Marina Margaret — MB ChB Glas. 1993; MRCPI 1998. Specialist Regist. Rehabil. Med. Southern Gen. Hosp. Glas. Specialty: Rehabil. Med.

PLATTS, Paul Health Centre, Blaby Road, Wigston, Leicester — BM BS Nottm. 1975; MRCGP 1980.

PLATTS, Sydney Herbert Bingley (retired) 16 Pannal Avenue, Harrogate HG3 1JR — MRCS Eng. LRCP Lond. 1932 (Camb.) MB Camb. 1937, BChir 1932.

PLATTS, Timothy Simon Castleton Health Centre, 2 Elizabeth Street, Castleton, Rochdale OL11 3HY Tel: 01706 658905 Fax: 01706 343990; Buckley Hill House, Buckley Hill Lane, Milnrow, Rochdale OL16 4BU — MB ChB Manch. 1978; MRCGP 1982.

PLAUT, Mr Gustav S, TD (retired) 18 North Mill Place, Mill Chase, Halstead CO9 2FA Tel: 01787 478114 — MB BChir Camb. 1947 (Camb. & Lond. Hosp.) MA Camb. 1947; FRCS Ed. 1954; FRCS Eng. 1955; FRCGP 1980, M 1965. Prev: GP Lond.

PLAXTON, Michael Robert Kirby (retired) Dean's Orchard, Angel Lane, Mere, Warminster BA12 6DH Tel: 01747 860523 — MB BChir Camb. 1954 (Camb. & Middlx.) BA, MB BChir Camb. 1954; DObst RCOG 1958.

PLAYER, David Arnott (retired) 7 Ann Street, Edinburgh EH4 1PL Tel: 0131 332 1088 — MB ChB Glas. 1950; DPH Glas. 1959; DPM RCPSI 1965; FRCPsych 1981, M 1972; FFCM 1978, M 1974; FRCP Ed 1979, M 1977; MA (Hons.) 1995. Prev: Chairm. Pub. Health Alliance.

PLAYER, Mark Hort Patwell Lane Surgery, Patwell Lane, Bruton BA10 0EG Tel: 01749 812310 Fax: 01749 812938; Bird's Hill Farm, Upton Noble, Shepton Mallet BA4 6AP Tel: 0174 985244 — MB BS Lond. 1980 (St. Mary's) BSc (Hons.) Leeds 1974; DRCOG 1984; MRCGP 1986. Specialty: Gen. Pract. Socs: BMA. Prev: Regist. (Med.) Wexham Pk. Hosp. Slough; SHO (Paediat. & O & G) Hillingdon Hosp. Uxbridge; Ho. Surg. St. Mary's Hosp. Lond.

PLAYER, Peter Val North Ridge Medical Practice, North Ridge, Rye Road, Cranbrook TN18 4EX Tel: 01580 753935 Fax: 01580 754452; Keeper's Cottage, Hastings Road, Flimwell, Wadhurst TN5 7PR Tel: 01580 879503 Fax: 01580 879640 — MB BS Lond. 1975 (Middlx.) BSc (Hons. Ecological Sc.) Ed. 1970; DRCOG 1978. Socs: Weald & Marsh Med. Soc. Prev: SHO (Otolaryng.) Cheltenham Gen. Hosp.; SHO (Paediat.) St. Mary's Hosp. Lond.; Ho. Phys. Centr Middlx. Hosp.

PLAYFAIR, Christopher James Adam Practice, Upton Health Centre, Blandford Road North, Poole BH16 5PW Tel: 01202 632764; Siyabonga, 69 Kingland Road, Poole BH15 1TN — BM Soton. 1978; DO RCS Eng. 1986; MRCGP 1988. GP Princip.; Clin. Asst. Opthalmology Roy. Bournmouth Hosp. Castle La. Bournemouth. Specialty: Ophth.

PLAYFAIR, James Ronald St James Surgery, 6 Northampton Buildings, Bath BA1 2SR Tel: 01225 422911 Fax: 01225 428398; 13 Bathwick Hill, Bath BA2 6EW Tel: 012255 462105 — MB BS Lond. 1977 (Lond. Hosp. Lond. Univ.) DRCOG 1979; MRCGP 1982. GP Princip. Prev: SHO (Radiotherap. & Oncol.) Addenbrooke's Hosp. Camb.; Ho. Phys. Lond. Hosp.; Ho. Surg. Epsom Dist. Hosp.

PLAYFER, Jeremy Robin Embleton, 59 Brimstage Road, Hewswall, Wirral CH60 1XE — MB ChB Liverp. 1970; MRCP (UK) 1974; MD Liverp. 1977; FRCP Lond. 1988. Cons. Phys. Roy. Liverp. Hosp.; Clin. Lect. Univ. Liverp. Specialty: Gen. Med. Socs: (Treas.) Brit. Geriat. Soc. Prev: Sen. Regist. Cowley Rd. Hosp. Oxf.; Research Fell. (Med.) Univ. Liverp.; Regist. (Med.) Liverp. RHB.

PLAYFOR, Bridget Emma 21 Hawkshead Drive, Knowle, Solihull B93 9QE — MB BS Lond. 1992.

PLAYFOR, Stephen Derek 27 Mounthouse Road, Freshfield, Liverpool L37 3LA — MB BS Lond. 1991.

PLAYFORD, Edith Diane National Hospital for Neurology and Neurosurgery, Queen Square, London WC1N 3BG Tel: 020 7837 3611 Ext: 3166 Fax: 020 7813 0924 — MD Lond. 1994; MB BS 1984; MRCP (UK) 1987. Cons. Neurologist, UCLH Trust. Specialty: Neurol. Prev: Lect. (Neurol.) Nat. Hosp. for Neurol. & Neurosurg. Lond.; Regist. Nat. Hosp. for Neurol. & Neurosurg. Lond.; Regist. (Med.) Atkinson Morley Hosp. Lond.

PLAYFORD, Vanda Jane Gill Street Health Centre, 11 Gill Street, London E14 8HQ Tel: 020 7515 2211; 145 Glenarm Road, London E5 0NB Tel: 020 8985 6506 Fax: 020 8985 6506 — MB BS Lond. 1982; MA Derby 1996. Lect. Gen. Pract. 1997-. Specialty: Gen. Pract. Socs: Med. Practs. Union (MSF Br.).

PLAYFORTH, Mr Michael John Accident and Emergency Department, Pontefract General Infirmary, Friarwood Lane, Pontefract WF8 1PL Tel: 01977 600600 Fax: 01977 606909 Email: micheal.playforth@panp-tr.northy.nhs.uk — MB ChB Leeds 1976; FRCS Ed. 1984; MD Leeds 1988; FFAEM 1993. Cons. A & E Pontefract Gen. Infirm. Specialty: Accid. & Emerg.

PLEASANCE, Clive Martin Whiteway, 2 Ryecroft Road, Heswall, Wirral CH60 1XB — MB ChB Liverp. 1979; DCH NUI 1981; DRCOG 1981.

PLEASANT, Elizabeth Ann St. Gerardines, Lossiemouth IV31 6RD Tel: 0134 381 2055 — MB BS Lond. 1955; MRCS Eng. LRCP Lond. 1955.

PLEDGE, Simon David Department of Clinical Oncology, Weston Park Hospital, Whitham Road, Sheffield S10 2SJ — BM BCh Oxf. 1988; MA Oxf. 1985, BM BCh 1988; MRCP (UK) 1992; FRCR 1998. Cons. Clin. Oncol., Weston Pk. Hosp. Specialty: Oncol.; Radiother. Socs: UKCCSA (full). Prev: Research Fell. Paterson Inst. for Cancer Research; Regist. (Clin. Oncol.) City Hosp. Nottm.; Lect. & Hon. Sen. Regist. Univ. Sheff..

PLEDGER, Herbert Gordon (retired) Oaktree Cottage, Mitford, Morpeth NE61 3PN Tel: 01670 513339 — MD Newc. 1964 (Durh.) MB BS Durh. 1953; FFA RCS Eng. 1960; FFCM 1986, M 1982. Prev: Dist. Med. Off. Newc. HA.

PLEMING, Aled Wyn Bryn Hafod, Pen-y-Berth, Llanfairpwllgwyngyll LL61 5YT — MB BS Lond. 1989.

PLENDERLEITH, Anne Caroline Hay Kinning Park Medical Centre, 42 Admiral Street, Glasgow G41 1HU Tel: 0141 429 0913 Fax: 0141 429 8491; 17 Rowan Road, Glasgow G41 5BZ — MB ChB Glas. 1977.

PLENDERLEITH, John Louie Western Infirmary, Glasgow G11 6NT; 17 Rowan Road, Glasgow G41 5BZ — MB ChB Ed.

1979; BSc Ed. 1976; FFA RCS Eng. 1984. Cons. Anaesth. (Intens. Care) West. Infirm. Glas. Specialty: Intens. Care.

PLENDERLEITH, Mark Flat 12, 27 Demesne Road, Whalley Range, Manchester M16 8HJ — MB ChB Manch. 1988.

PLENDERLEITH, Stephen James Countess House, Moorgreen Hospital, Botley Road, Southampton Email: steve.plenderleith@sht.swest.nhs.uk — MB ChB Liverp. 1991; MRCGP 1997; Dip Palliat Med 2000. Sen. Med. Off. (Pall. Care) St. Rocco's Hospice, Warrington. Specialty: Palliat. Med.

PLENTY, David Ronald Lake Road Health Centre, Nutfield Place, Portsmouth PO1 4JT Tel: 023 9282 1201 Fax: 023 9287 5658 — BM Soton. 1980; BSc Manch. 1974; DRCOG 1984; MRCGP 1984.

PLESTER, George Leonard Abbotsford, 9 Briars Close, Hinckley Road, Nuneaton CV11 Tel: 024 7638 4073 — LRCP LRCS Ed. 1944; LRCP LRCS Ed. LRFPS Glas. 1944; AFOM RCP Lond. 1981. Med. Off. Occupat. Health Dept. Nuneaton (N. Warks.) Health Dist.; Med. Advis. to Various Local Firms. Socs: Med.-Leg. Soc. Prev: Sen. Med. Off. E. Gen. Hosp. Edin.; Res. Surg. Off. Gen. Infirm. Burton-on-Trent.

PLETTS, Robert Charles White Wings, 4 Broadsands Road, Paignton TQ4 6JY — MB BS Lond. 1975; BSc Bristol 1969; MRCS Eng. LRCP Lond. 1975; DIP IMC RCS Ed. 1991; FFAEM 1993. Assoc. Specialist (A & E) Torbay Hosp. Specialty: Accid. & Emerg.

PLEVRIS, Ioannis 50 Gogarloch Syke, Edinburgh EH12 9JB — Ptychio Iatrikes Athens 1983; MRCP (UK) 1993.

PLEWES, Mr Jeremy John Lawrence The Royal Orthopaedic Hospital, Northfield, Birmingham B31 2AP Tel: 0121 685 4026; Selvas Cottage, Withybed Green, Alvechurch, Birmingham B48 7PR Tel: 0121 445 1624 — MA Oxf. 1964 (Oxford/Middlx.) FRCS Lond. 1970. p/t Cons. Orthop. Surg. Roy. Orthop. Hosp. Birm.; Progr. Director, W. Midlands Orthopaedic Train. Progamme (Birmingham). Specialty: Orthop. Prev: Cons. Orthop. Surg., Univ. Hosp., Birm.

PLEWS, David Julian Market Surgery, Warehouse Lane, Wath-On-Dearne, Rotherham S63 7RA Tel: 01709 877524 Fax: 01709 875089 — MB ChB Leeds 1982; Cert. Family Plann. JCC 1986; MRCGP 1986; FRCGP 2002.

PLEWS, Dianne Elaine 9/5 Great King Street, Edinburgh EH3 6QW — MB ChB Ed. 1992; MRCP 1996. Specialist Regist. (Blook Transfus.) Scott. Nat. Blood Transfus. Serv. Specialty: Haematology.

PLEWS, Normana Rose Imphal, 3 Banks Howe, Onchan, Douglas IM3 2EN Tel: 01624 629247 — MB ChB Glas. 1942. Prev: Med. Off. E.M.S. Hosp. StoneHo.; Ho. Phys. Roy. Infirm. Glas.; Ho. Surg. Vict. Infirm. Glas.

PLEYDELL-PEARCE, Julian St John North Hampshire Hospital, Department of Child Health, Aldermaston Road, Basingstoke RG24 9NA Tel: 01256 314725 Fax: 01256 314796 Email: julian.pleydell-pearce@nhht.nhs.uk — MB ChB Bristol 1990; BA (Hons.) Lond. 1976; MRCS Eng. LRCP Lond. 1990; MRCP (UK) 1995; FRCPCH 1999. Cons. Paediat. Specialty: Paediat. Special Interest: Med. Educat.; Oncol.; Rheum. Socs: BMA; Brit. Paediat. Assn. Prev: Sen. Regist. (Paediat.) Musgr. Pk. Hosp. Taunton; Regist. (Paediat.) Musgr. Pk. Hosp. Taunton; SHO (Paediat.) Bristol Roy. Hosp. Sick Childr.

PLIETH, Charlotte E.A.C. Boga, Dem. Rep. of Congo, PO Box 21285, Nairobi, Kenya; Downs Cottage, Rivar Road, Shalbourne, Marlborough SN8 3QE Tel: 01672 870514 — State Exam Med Kiel 1989; State Exam Med. Kiel 1989.

PLIMMER, Anna Louise 97 Gladstone Road, London SW19 1QR — MB BS Lond. 1993 (Univ. Lond.) SHO (Gen. Med. & Geriat.) E. Surrey Hosp. Redhill. Prev: SHO (Cas.) Ashford Hosp. Middlx.; Ho. Off. (Med.) W. Middlx. Hosp.; Ho. Off. (Surg.) Frimley Pk. Hosp. Surrey.

PLIMMER, Wendy Nicola 2 Herbert Villa, Pelham Road, London SW19 1NW — MB BS Lond. 1992; FRCA 2000.

PLINT, Simon John Beaumont Street Surgery, 19 Beaumont Street, Oxford OX1 2NA Tel: 01865 240501 Fax: 01865 240503; 16 Farndon Road, Oxford OX2 6RT — MB BS Lond. 1984; MA (Mod. & Medieval Langs.) Camb. 1981; DCH RCP Lond. 1986; MRCGP 1988; DRCOG 1989. Assoc. Adviser Gen. Pract. Oxf. PGMDE. Prev: Med. Off. Oxf. Univ. Rugby Football Club; Course Organiser Oxf. Sub-Regional GP VTS.

PLOTNEK, Jonothan Stuart Field House Medical Centre, 13 Dudley Street, Grimsby DN31 2AE Tel: 01472 350327; Greenways, 10 Park Drive, Grimsby DN32 0EF — MB ChB Leeds 1982; Cert. Developm. Paediat. Leeds 1985.

PLOWMAN, Margaret Anne (retired) The Health Centre, 80 Knaresborough Road, Harrogate HG2 7LU Tel: 01423 557200 Fax: 01423 557201; 17 Boroughbridge Road, Knaresborough HG5 0LX Tel: 01423 862958 Fax: 01423 862958 — MB ChB Sheff. 1967.

PLOWMAN, Patricia Elizabeth (retired) Fiveacres, Browning Hill Green, Baughurst, Basingstoke RG26 5JZ Tel: 01734 816172 — MB BS Lond. 1966 (Roy. Free) MRCS Eng. LRCP Lond. 1966; FFA RCS Eng. 1970. Prev: Cons. Anaesth. Basingstoke Dist. Hosp.

PLOWMAN, Piers Nicholas 14 Harmont House, 20 Harley Street, London W1G 9PH Tel: 020 7631 1632 Fax: 020 7323 3487; 101 Barnsbury Street, Islington, London N1 1EP Tel: 020 7607 5307 Fax: 020 7323 3487 — MB BChir (Hons.) Camb. 1974; MRCP (UK) 1976; FRCR 1980; MD Camb. 1980; FRCP Lond. 1989. Cons. Phys. Radiother. & Oncol. St. Bart. Hosp. (Head) & Hosp. for Sick Childr. Lond.; Hon. Sen. Lect. Inst. Child Health Lond. Specialty: Oncol.; Radiother.

PLOWMAN, Raymond Albert (retired) 4 Rectory Garth, Hemsworth, Pontefract WF9 4NB Tel: 01977 611298 — (Leeds) MB ChB Leeds 1959; DPM Eng. 1963; MRCPsych 1993. Prev: Sen. Regist. & Regist. (Psychiat.) St. Jas. Hosp. Leeds.

PLOWS, Charles David (retired) 31 Roman Lane, Little Aston, Sutton Coldfield B74 3AE Tel: 0121 353 2243 — MB BChir Camb. 1958 (Westm.) MB BChir Camb. 1957; MA Camb. 1958; Dip. Bact. Lond 1965; FRCPath 1980, M 1968. Cons. Microbiol. Good Hope Dist. Gen. Hosp. Sutton Coldfield. Prev: Sen. Bacteriol. Pub. Health Laborat. Serv. Sheff.

PLOYE, Philippe Maurice (retired) 45A Beauchamp Road, East Molesey KT8 0PA Tel: 020 8979 9181 — MD Montpellier 1941; FRCPsych 1978, M 1972. Prev: Hon. & Cons. Psychother. Cassel Hosp. Ham Common.

PLUCK, Judith Catherine Broomfields, Hatfield Heath, Chelmsford CM3 7EH Tel: 01279 730616; 4 Snows Court, Great Waltham, Chelmsford CM3 1DE Tel: 01245 360145 — MB BS Lond. 1987; BPharm (Hons.) Bradford 1979. GP Hatfield Heath. Socs: MRCP; Roy. Plann. Soc.

PLUCK, Nigel David 29 Barn Close, Oxford OX2 9JP — BM BCh Oxf. 1985; MA, DPhil, BM BCh Oxf. 1985.

PLUGGE, Emma Harriet 75 Boyne Road, Lewisham, London SE13 5AN Tel: 020 8318 6018 — MB BChir Camb. 1991; MA Camb. 1991; DTM & H 1992. Regist. (Pub. Health Med.) W. Sussex. Specialty: Pub. Health Med.

PLUMB, Mr Andrew Philip Eastbourne DGH, Kings Drive, Eastbourne BN21 2UD Tel: 01323 417400 — MB BS Lond. 1977 (Guy's) MRCS Eng. LRCP Lond. 1977; DO Eng. 1980; FRCS Eng. 1983; FCOphth 1988. Cons. Ophth. Surg. Eastbourne HA. Specialty: Ophth. Special Interest: Medical Retina; Paediatric Ophthalmology; Refractive and Corneal Surgery. Prev: Sen. Regist. (Ophth.) Univ. Coll. Hosp., Roy. Free Hosp. Lond. & Moorfield Hosp. Lond.; Regist. (Ophth.) St. Thos. Hosp. Lond.

PLUMB, Elizabeth Anne Dennis and Partners, The Medical Centre, Folly Lane, Warrington WA5 0LU Tel: 01925 417247 Fax: 01925 444319; 7 Caversham Close, Appleton, Warrington WA4 5JX Tel: 01925 860167 — MB ChB Manch. 1982.

PLUMB, John Martin Tudor Gate Surgery, Tudor Street, Abergavenny NP7 5DL Tel: 01873 855991 Fax: 01873 850162 — MB BS Lond. 1969 (Westm.) MRCS Eng. LRCP Lond. 1969; MRCP (U.K.) 1973; MRCGP 1982. Prev: Ho. Phys. St. Stephen's Hosp. Lond.; Sen. Ho. Phys. Nevill Hall Hosp. Abergavenny; Med. Off. Nchanga Consolidated Copper Mines Ltd. Konkola, Zambia.

PLUMB, Marjory Ernestine (retired) Claremont, 2 Woodland Avenue, Leighton Buzzard LU7 3JW Tel: 01525 373165 — MB BS Lond. 1956 (St. Bart.) DCH Eng. 1960. Prev: GP Tring Herts.

PLUMB, Stephen Argyle Street Surgery, 141 Argyle Street, Heywood OL10 3SD Tel: 01706 366135 Fax: 01706 627706 — BM BCh Oxf. 1973; MA Oxf., BM BCh 1973; DObst RCOG 1976; MRCGP 1980.

PLUMLEY, Michael Hugh Department of Anaesthetics, Queen Elizabeth Hospital, Gayton Road, King's Lynn PE30 4ET Tel: 01553 766266; Bridge House, Winch Road, Gayton, King's Lynn PE32 1QP — MB BS Lond. 1975 (St Marys) BA Oxf. 1972; FFARCS Eng. 1982. Cons. Anaesth. W. Norf. & Wisbech HAs. Specialty: Anaesth. Socs: Intens. Care Soc.; Fell. Roy. Soc. Med.; Assn. Anaesth. Prev:

Sen. Regist. (Anaesth.) Westm. Hosp. & W.m. Childr. Hosp. Lond.; Clin. Fell. Roy. Vict. Hosp., Montreal; Clin. Fell. Montreal Childr. Hosp. Quebec, Canada.

PLUMLEY, Mr Peter Francis (retired) 20 Tobago, West Parade, Bexhill-on-Sea TN39 3YB Tel: 01424 213618 — MB BChir Camb. 1952 (Middlx.) MChir Camb. 1967, MA, MB BChir 1952; FRCS Eng. 1958. Prev: Cons. Gen. Surg. Roy. E. Sussex & St. Helen's Hosps. Hastings & Bexhill Hosp.

PLUMLEY, Susan Mary Putneymead Medical Centre, 350 Upper Richmond Road, London SW15 6TL Tel: 020 8788 0686; 1 St. Margaret's Crescent, London SW15 6HL — MB BS Lond. 1982; DRCOG 1987; MRCGP 1988.

PLUMLEY, Thomas Alfred (retired) Mill Villa, Millfield, Willingham, Cambridge CB4 5HD Tel: 01954 261210 — MB BS Lond. 1951 (St. Mary's) DPH Lond. 1954; MRCS Eng. LRCP Lond. 1955; DObst RCOG 1955; MFCM 1972; AFOM 1978. Prev: Employm. Med. Adviser Health & Safety Exec.

PLUMMER, Christopher John Wansbeck General Hospital, Wood Horn Lane, Ashington NE63 9JJ Tel: 01670 521212 Fax: 01670 529452 Email: c.j.plummer@ncl.ac.uk — BM BCh Oxf. 1992; BSc Bristol 1986; PhD Bristol 1989; MRCP UK 1995. Cons. Cardiol. Northumbria Healthcare NHS Trust; Hon. Cons. Freeman Hosp. Newc. Upon Tyne; Hon. Clin. Lect. Univ. of Newc. Upon Tyne. Specialty: Cardiol. Socs: Brit. Cardiac Soc. (Mem.); Britsh Pacing & Electrophysiol. Gp. (Mem.). Prev: Specialsist Regist. (Cardiol.) N. Deanery; Regist. (Acad. Cardiol.) Freeman Hosp. Newc.; SHO Rotat. (Med.) Newc. u. Tyne.

PLUMMER, Elizabeth Ruth Northern Centre for Cancer Treatment, Newcastle General Hospital, Westgate Road, Newcastle upon Tyne NE4 6BE Tel: 0191 233 6161 Email: e.r.plummer@ncl.ac.uk — BM BCh Oxf. 1992; DPhil Oxf. 1989; MA Camb. 1990; MRCP (UK) 1995; MD Newc. 2004. Sen. Lect. in Med. Oncol., North. Inst. for Cancer Research. Specialty: Oncol. Prev: Clin. Lect. in Med. Oncol., Univ. of Newc.; Specialist Regist. (Med. Oncol.) Newc. u. Tyne; Research Regist. (Med. Oncol.) Newc.

PLUMMER, Hugh Exwick Surgery, New Valley Road, Exwick, Exeter EX4 2AD Tel: 01392 70063; Orchard View, Kenn, Exeter EX6 7UH Tel: 01392 833033 — BM Soton. 1979; BSc Soton. 1966; PhD Lond. 1969; DRCOG 1983; MRCGP 1984. Prev: Princip. GP Exeter.

PLUMMER, Richard Bruce Leys House, Bridge St., Great Kimble, Aylesbury HP17 9TW Tel: 01844 346532 Fax: 01844 346532 Email: richardbplummer@aol.com — (Guy's) MRCS Eng. LRCP Lond. 1969; DObst RCOG 1972; FRCA Eng 1975. Cons. Anaesth. Stoke Mandeville Hosp. Aylesbury. Specialty: Anaesth. Prev: Sen. Regist. (Anaesth.) Guy's Health Dist. (T) & Brighton Health Dist.

PLUMMER, Sarah Jane Grove Cottage, Siginstone, Cowbridge CF71 7LP Tel: 01446 775492; Spindrift, 10 Smugglers Close, Old Hunstanton, Hunstanton PE36 6JU Tel: 01485 533953 — MB BS Lond. 1990; DA (UK) 1992; FRCA 1995. Regist. (Anaesth.) Univ. Hosp. Wales Cardiff. Specialty: Anaesth. Socs: Fell. Roy. Coll. Anaesth.; Assn. Anaesth. Prev: SHO (Neonates) Exeter; SHO (Anaesth.) Bristol Roy. Infirm. & Worthing Gen. Hosp.

PLUMMER, William Philip East Kent Community Alcolol Service, Mount Zeehan Unit, St. Martin's Hospital, Little Bourne Road, Canterbury CT1 1TD Tel: 01227 761310 Fax: 01227 463254 — MB BS Lond. 1980 (St. Thomas' Hospital Medical School) BSc Lond. 1977; BSc Lond. 1977, MB BS 1980; MRCGP 1985; DRCOG 1986; MRCPsych 1990. Cons. Psychiat. E. Kent Community NHS Trust; Hon. Sen. Lect. (Psychiat) KIMHS Univ. of Kent at Canterbury. Specialty: Alcohol & Substance Misuse; Gen. Psychiat. Prev: Sen. Regist. (Psychiat.) UMDS SE Thames RHA; Regist. (Psychiat.) Guy's Hosp. Lond.; GP Herne Bay.

PLUMMER, Yvonne Myra 122 Maltby Drive, Enfield EN1 4EN Tel: 020 8804 7336 — MB BS Lond. 1979 (Roy. Free) MRCS Eng. LRCP Lond. 1977; DRCOG 1993; DFFP 1993. Assoc. Specialist (Gyn.) Homerton Hosp. NHS Trust. Specialty: Obst. & Gyn.; Family Plann. & Reproduc. Health; Genitourinary Medicine. Socs: Fell. Roy. Soc. Med. Prev: Clin. Asst. (Gyn.) Homerton Hosp. NHS Trust; Regist. (O & G) N. Middlx. Hosp. Lond.; Regist. (O & G) St. Jas. & St. Geo. Hosp. Lond.

PLUMMERIDGE, Martin James Lung Research Group, University of Bristol, Medical School Unit, Southmead Hospital, Westbury on Trym, Bristol BS10 5NB Tel: 0117 959 5156; 13 Apsley Road, Clifton, Bristol BS8 2SH Tel: 0117 973 3440 — MB ChB Bristol 1990; MRCP (UK) 1994. Clin. Research Fell. Lung Research Gp. Univ. Bristol. Specialty: Respirat. Med. Prev: Regist. (Thoracic Med.) Roy. United Hosp. Bath; Regist. (Gen. & Thoracic Med.) Princess Margt. Hosp. Swindon & Salisbury Dist. Hosp.; Regist. (Gen. & Thoracic Med.) Gold Coast Hosp. Queensland.

PLUMPTON, Frederic Salkeld (retired) 241 Wishing Tree Road, St Leonards-on-Sea TN38 9LA Tel: 01424 854077 Fax: 01424 854077 — (Oxf. & Lond. Hosp.) BM BCh Oxf. 1958; MA Oxf. 1958; DObst RCOG 1960; DA Eng. 1964; FFA RCS Eng. 1965. Hon. Cons. Anaesth. Hastings Hosp. Gp.; Vice-Pres. St. Michael's Hospice Hastings. Prev: Examr. FFA RCS Eng.

PLUMPTON, Helen Patricia The Surgery, 24 Albert Road, Bexhill-on-Sea TN40 1DG Tel: 01424 730456/734430 Fax: 01424 225615 — MB ChB Manch. 1991 (St. Andrews & Manchester) BSc St. And. 1988; DRCOG 1994; MRCGP 1995. Specialty: Gen. Pract. Prev: Trainee GP/SHO Roy. Lancs. Infirm.

PLUMPTRE, Aubrey Martin Macdonald (retired) Ragdon Cottage, Ragdon, Church Stretton SY6 7EY — MB BS Lond. 1957 (St. Bart.) DObst RCOG 1959; Cert. Family Plann. JCC 1975. Prev: GP Soton.

***PLUMTREE, Jane Rebecca** 19 Hazon Way, Epsom KT19 8HD Tel: 01372 812038; 19 Hazon Way, Epsom KT19 8HD Tel: 01372 812038 — MB ChB Leeds 1998. SHO (A&E). Specialty: Accid. & Emerg. Prev: Ho. Off. (Gen. Surg.); Ho. Off. (Gen. Med.).

PLUNKETT, Ciaran Nial 30 The Ridgeway, London N11 3LJ Tel: 020 8368 4433 — MB BCh BAO NUI 1959.

PLUNKETT, Gerald Barry (retired) 3 St Mark's Place, The Mall, Armagh BT61 9BH — (Univ. Coll. Dub.) MB BCh BAO NUI 1951; FRCPI 1969, M 1958; DPM TCDI 1961; FRCPsych 1991. Prev: Cons. Psychiat. St. Luke's Hosp. Armagh.

PLUNKETT, Michael Charles Academic Department of Paediatrics, City General Hospital, Stoke-on-Trent ST4 6QG Tel: 01782 552663 Fax: 01782 713946 Email: MCPlunkett@aol.com — BM Soton. 1987; MRCPI 1993. Specialist Regist. (Paediat.) N. Staffs. Hosp. NHS Trust Stoke-on-Trent. Specialty: Paediat.

PLUNKETT, Simon Gerald 4 The Square, Lymm WA13 0HX — MB ChB Aberd. 1989.

PLUNKETT, Timothy Andrew ICRF Clinical Oncology Unit, Guy's Hospital, London SE1 9RT — MB BS Lond. 1992 (Guy's Hosp.) BSc (Hons.) Lond. 1989; MRCP (UK) 1995. ICRF Clin. Research Fell. Guy's Hosp. Lond. Specialty: Oncol.

PLUNKETT, Trevor George Yare Valley Medical Practice, 202 Thorpe Road, Norwich NR1 1TJ Tel: 01603 437559 Fax: 01603 701773; 13 South Avenue, Thorpe St. Andrew, Norwich NR7 0EY Tel: 01603 435622 — (Ed.) MB ChB Ed. 1961. Specialty: Rheumatol. Socs: Brit. Soc. Rheum.; Fell. Roy.Soc.Med.

PLUSA, Mr Stefan Murray Dept. of Surgery, Royal Victoria Infirmary, Newcastle upon Tyne NE1 4LP Tel: 0191 282 4744 — MB ChB Leeds 1984; FRCS Ed. 1989; FRCS Eng. 1989; FRCS (Gen) 1997. Cons. (Colorectal Surg.) Roy. Vict. Infirm. Newc. Upon Tyne. Specialty: Gen. Surg. Socs: Surg. Research Soc. & Nutrit. Soc.; Brit Soc. Of Castroent.; Assoc. of Coleproct. Prev: Lect. & Sen. Regist. (Surg.) Roy. Vict. Infirm. Newc.; Research Regist. (Surg.) St. Jas. Univ. Hosp. Leeds; Regist. (Transpl. & Urol.) St. Mary's Hosp. Portsmouth.

PLYMING, Annabelle Virginia Louise The Rooksdown Practice, Mill Road, Rooksdown, Basingstoke RG24 9SP Tel: 01256 399710 Fax: 01256 399733 — MB ChB Ed. 1997 (Edin.)

POBERESKIN, Mr Louis Howard Derriford Hospital, Department of Neurosurgery, Plymouth PL6 8DH Tel: 01752 792539 Fax: 01752 763395 Email: louis.pobereskin@phnt.swest.nhs.uk — MD Case Western Reserve 1970; FRCS Ed. (SN) 1987. Cons. Neurosurg. Specialty: Neurosurg. Special Interest: Lumbar Spine; Pituitary Surg. Socs: Soc. Brit. Neurol. Surg.

POBLETE GRIBBELL, Maria Ximena Northwick Park Hospital, Watford Road, Harrow HA1 3UJ — MRCS Eng. LRCP Lond. 1981; DCH RCP Lond. 1985; MSc (Community Paediat.) Lond. 1991; MRCP (UK) 1995. Cons. Paediat. Northwick Pk. Hosp. Harrow. Specialty: Paediat. Prev: Sen. Regist. (Community Paediat.) Optimum NHS Trust; Clin. Med . Off, City & Hackney Hlth. Auth.; Clin. Res. Fell., Behavioural Sci., Inst. Child Hlth.

POCHA, Meher Jehangir The Child Development Centre, Hill Rise, Kempston, Bedford MK42 7EB Tel: 01234 310278 Fax: 01234

310277; Homefield, 3 Baldock Road, Letchworth SG6 3LB Tel: 01462 686987 — MB BS Bombay 1971 (Grant Med. Coll.) DCH CPS Bombay 1972; MD (Paediat.) Bombay 1974; MRCP (UK) 1977. Cons. Paediat. Child Developm. Centre Bedford & Bedford Hosp. Specialty: Paediat. Socs: EACD; EPNS; BPNA. Prev: SCMO (Child Health) Parkside HA; Regist. (Paediat.) Alder Hey Childr. Hosp. Liverp.; Research Fell. Inst. Child Health & Hon. Clin. Asst. Gt. Ormond St. Hosp. Lond.

POCKLINGTON, Anthony Geoffrey 25 Clifton Road, Heaton Moor, Stockport SK4 4DD — MB ChB Manch. 1968; DObst RCOG 1971; FFA RCS Eng. 1977. Specialty: Anaesth.

POCKLINGTON, Susan Lynne Imperial Surgery, 49 Imperial Road, Exmouth EX8 1DQ — MB ChB Leeds 1969; MRCGP 1978. Socs: BMA. Prev: Regist. (Anaesth.) United Birm. Hosps.; Ho. Surg., Ho. Phys. & SHO (Anaesth.) Corbett Hosp. Stourbridge.

POCKNEY, Peter Graham 23 Greville Road, Southampton SO15 5AW — MB BS Lond. 1996.

POCOCK, Christopher Francis Elliott 34 Longridge House, Falmouth Road, London SE1 6QN Email: c.pocock@ic.ac.uk — MB BS Lond. 1987; MRCP (UK) 1991; PhD Lond. 1995; Dip. RCPath 1998. Allogeneic BMT Coordinator, Hammersmith Hosp. Lond. Specialty: Haematology. Prev: Clin. Research Fell. & Hon. Lect. (Haemat.) Roy. Lond. Trust Whitechapel.

POCOCK, David Ian Gordon 66A Station Approach, South Ruislip, Ruislip HA4 6SA — MB BS Lond. 1996.

POCOCK, Jessica Dept. of Ophthalmology, King's College Hospital, London SE5 9RS Tel: 020 7346 1523; 111 Babington Road, Streatham, London SW16 6AN Tel: 020 8769 3194 — MB ChB Bristol 1971; BSc (Anat.) Bristol 1967; MRCOphth 1994. Assoc. Specialist (Ophth.) King's Coll. Hosp. Lond. Specialty: Ophth. Prev: Clin. Asst. (Ophth.) King's Coll., St. Geo. Hosp. & Roy. Hosp. for Neurodisabil. Lond.; Clin. Asst. Bristol Eye Hosp.; Lect. (Anat.) St. Geo. Hosp. Med. Sch. Lond.

POCOCK, Kenneth Norman Johnston, OStJ Ridge Cottage, 305 Luton Road, Harpenden AL5 3LW Tel: 01582 461624 — (Camb. & Bristol) MA Camb. 1953, BA, MB BChir 1949; MRCS Eng. LRCP Lond. 1949; DIH Soc. Apoth. Lond. 1955; CPH Eng. 1955; MFOM RCP Lond. 1978. Specialty: Occupat. Health. Socs: Fell. Roy. Soc. Med.; Soc. Occupat. Med. Prev: Chief Med. Off. Vauxhall Motors Ltd.; Squadron Ldr. RAF Med. Br.; Area Commr. St. John Ambul. Brig.

POCOCK, Marilyn Ann Josephine Royal Devon & Exeter Hospital, Exeter; Chilton, Bickleigh, Tiverton EX16 8RT — MB ChB Manch. 1970; MRCP (UK) 1977; FRCPath 1992, M 1981; FRCP Lond. 1996; BA (Hons) 1997. Cons. Haemat. Roy. Devon & Exeter Hosp. Specialty: Haematology. Socs: Brit. Soc. Haematol. Prev: Cons. Haemat. Cheltenham Gen. Hosp.; Leukaemia Research Fund Fell. 1982/84; Lect. & Sen. Regist. (Haemat.) King's Coll. Hosp. Lond.

POCOCK, Mr Richard Duncan Royal Devon & Exeter Hospital, Barrack Road, Exeter EX5 2DW Tel: 01392 402133 Email: rdp@quadrant1.u-net.com; Chilton, Cadeleigh, Tiverton EX16 8RT — MB ChB Bristol 1973; FRCS Eng. 1978. Specialty: Urol. Prev: Sen. Regist. (Urol.) Bristol Roy. Infirm. & Southmead Hosp. Bristol.; Regist. St. Geo. Hosp. Lond.; Regist. St. Jas. Hosp. Lond.

POCOCK, Mr Timothy John Wellesley Hospital, Eastern Avenue, Southend-on-Sea SS2 4XH Tel: 01702 258262 Fax: 01702 258262 — MB ChB Bristol 1971; MRCOG 1978, DObst 1975; FRCS Ed. 1979; FRCOG 1995. Cons. O & G Southend Gen. Hosps. Specialty: Obst. & Gyn. Socs: Roy. Coll. Obitetrician Gynaecologist; Roy. Coll. Med.; Brit. Soc. Colposcopy Clin. Path. Prev: Sen. Regist. (O & G) Westm. Hosp. Lond.; SHO (Obst.), SHO (Paediat.) & SHO (Surg.) Avon AHA (T).

PODD, Mr Timothy James Radiotherapy Department, Newcastle General Hospital, Westgate Road, Newcastle upon Tyne NE4 6BE — MB BChir Camb. 1982; MA Oxf. 1984; FRCS Ed. 1987; FRCS Eng. 1987; FRCR 1992. Cons. Clin. Oncol. Newc. Gen. Hosp. Specialty: Oncol.; Radiother. Prev: Sen. Regist. (Radiother.) Newc. Gen. Hosp.; Regist. Rotat. Poole Gen. Hosp.; Regist. (Radiol. & Oncol.) Roy. S. Hants. Hosp.

PODDAR, Mohan Lal 25 Sandringham Avenue, Newton Mearns, Glasgow G77 5DU — MB BS Bihar 1954 (Darbhanga Med. Coll. Bihar) DTM & H Calcutta 1956; DCH RCPS Glas. 1965; MRCGP 1972. Socs: BMA.

PODDAR, Subhashish 35 Delafield Road, Abergavenny NP7 7AW — MB BCh Wales 1988.

PODICHETTY, Madhavi West Berkshire Psychotherapy Service, 53-55 Argyle Road, Reading RG1 7YL Email: meddypodichetty@doctors.org.uk — MB ChB Manch. 1991; BSc St And. 1988; MRCPsych 1997. Specialty: Psychother.

PODKOLINSKI, Marek Thomas Endless Street Surgery, 72 Endless Street, Salisbury SP1 3UH Tel: 01722 336441 Fax: 01722 410319 — MB BS Lond. 1974.

PODMORE, Mr Malcolm Dennis North Devon District Hospital, Raleigh Park, Barnstaple EX31 4JB Tel: 01271 322491 Email: malcolm@sussie106.freeserve.co.uk; Lower Upcott, Stowford, Umberleigh EX37 9RX Tel: 01769 540083 — MB BS Lond. 1987 (Middlesex Hospital) BSc (Hons.) Lond. 1984; FRCS Eng. 1992; FRCS (Orth) 2001. Hon. Cons. Orthopaedic Surg. Roy. Devon & Exeter Hosp. Devon. Specialty: Orthop.; Trauma & Orthop. Surg. Special Interest: Hip & Knee Surg., Arthroscopy, Lumbar Spine Problems.

POELS, Peter John Sandpitts, Heathstock, Stockland, Honiton EX14 9EX — MRCS Eng. LRCP Lond. 1942 (St. Thos.) Prev: ENT & Gyn. Ho. Surg. St. Thos. Hosp.

POEPPINGHAUS, Vanessa Jane Ida Department of Accident & Emergency, Ysbyty Gwynedd, Bangor LL57 2PW Tel: 01248 384384 Fax: 01248 384936; Mefus, Glyn Garth, Menai Bridge LL59 5PF Tel: 01248 712365 — MB BCh Wales 1984; BSc (Hons.) St. And. 1980. Assoc. Specialist (A & E) Ysbyty Gwynedd Bangor.; Community Med. Off. Wom. & Childs. Health; Police Surg. N. Wales Police. Specialty: Accid. & Emerg. Prev: Trainee GP Cardiff VTS; SHO (Psychiat.) Ysbyty Gwynedd Bangor; SHO (O & G) Univ. Coll. Wales Cardiff.

POGMORE, Mr John Richard, Wing Cdr. RAF Med. Br. Retd. The Birmingham Womens Hospital, Edgbaston, Birmingham B15 2TG Tel: 0121 6074711 Fax: 0121 627 2667 Email: john.pogmore@bwhet.nhs.uk — (St. Bart.) MB BS Lond. 1965; MRCS Eng. LRCP Lond. 1965; DObst 1970; FRCOG 1988, M 1975. p/t Cons. Gynaecologist Birm. Wom. Healthcare NHS Trust. Specialty: Gynaecology. Socs: BMOGS; LOGS; BSCCP. Prev: Cons. O & G RAF Hosp. Wroughton; Hon. Lect. & Sen. Regist. (O & G) Nottm. City Hosp.; Resid. Surg. Off. Hosp. Wom. Soho Sq. Lond.

POGREL, Graham Philip Waterloo House Surgery, Waterloo House, 42-44 Wellington Street, Millom LA18 4DE Tel: 01229 772123 Fax: 01229 771300; 1 Low Beck Stones, The Green, Millom LA18 5HZ Tel: 01229 773144 — MB ChB Liverp. 1971; MRCS Eng. LRCP Lond. 1971; DObst RCOG 1973; DCH Eng. 1973; MRCGP 1975; FRCGP 2000; Cert in Medical Education (Durham) 2000. Socs: RCGP; BMA. Prev: Police Surg. Cumbria; Course Organiser SW Cumbria VTS 1982-1988; SHO (Med.) Liverp. Roy. Infirm.

POGSON, Caroline Jane 30 Ross Road, Wallington SM6 8QR — MB BS Lond. 1991.

POGSON, David Graeme Anaesthetic Department, Singleton Hospital, Swansea SA2 8QA Tel: 01792 205666; Manor Cottage, Thorpe Bassett, Rillington, Malton YO17 8LU — MB BCh Wales 1992. SHO (Anaesth.) Singleton Hosp. Swansea. Specialty: Anaesth. Socs: BMA; Med. Protec. Soc.; Assn. Anaesth. Prev: SHO (Med.) Roy. Gwent Hosp.

POGUE, Laura Jane Justine Lancaster House, 22-26 North Road, St Helens Wa10 2TL — MB ChB Liverp. 1993; DCH Lond. 1996; MRCGP Lond. 1997; DFFP Liverp. 1997.

POH, Choo Hean 33 Meadowlands, Jordanstown, Newtownabbey BT37 0UR — MB BCh BAO Belf. 1996.

POHL, Debbie Susan 9 Woodland Avenue, Leicester LE2 3HG — MB ChB Leic. 1998.

POHL, Jurgen Ernst Friedrich (retired) 9 Woodland Avenue, Stoneygate, Leicester LE2 3HG Tel: 0116 270 8129 — (Melbourne) BSc Melbourne 1955, MB BS 1959; FRCP Lond. 1979, M 1964. Prev: Lect. (Therap.) Univ. Manch.

POHL, Keith Richard Erik Newcomen Centre, Guy's Hospital, London Bridge, London SE1 9RT Tel: 020 7955 4270 Fax: 020 7955 4950 Email: keith.pohla@gstl.sthame.nhs.uk; 7 Oakley Avenue, Ealing, London W5 3SA Tel: 020 8992 7366 — (Royal Free Hospital London) BSc (Basic Med. Sci.) Lond., MB BS 1981; DCH RCP Lond. 1983; MRCP (UK) 1985; FRCPCH 1997. Cons. Paediat. Neurol. Guy's & St. Thos. Trust Lond. Specialty: Paediat.

Neurol. Prev: Sen. Regist. (Paediat.) Univ. Coll. Hosp. Lond.; Fell. & Regist. (Neurol.) Brit. Columbia's Childr. Hosp., Vancouver & Hosp. Sick Childr. Lond.

POINTEN, Emma Juliet 21 Nayland Croft, Birmingham B28 0QH — MB ChB Manch. 1995.

POINTING, Teresa Dawn Westfield Surgery, Waterford Park, Radstock, Bath BA3 3UJ Tel: 01761 463333; 7 Sarabeth Drive, Tunley, Bath BA2 0EA — MB BS Lond. 1987. GP Princip.; Clin. Asst. (Psychiat.) Barrow Hosp. Bristol. Specialty: Gen. Pract.; Geriat. Psychiat. Prev: GP Bonnybrigg, Midlothian.

POINTON, Andrew David University Laboratory of Physiology, Parks Road, Oxford OX1 3PT Tel: 01865 272500 — MB BS Lond. 1992; BA (Hons.) Oxf. 1989. MRC Clin. Train. Fell. Neurophysiol.

POINTON, Gweneth Irene (retired) — MRCS Eng. LRCP Lond. 1953 (St. Bart.) FRCGP 1981, M 1962.

POIRIER, Mr Henry, TD (retired) Hangerlea, Stansted Road, Bishop's Stortford CM23 2DA Tel: 01279 835880/020 7017 5274 Fax: 01279 835880 — MB BS Lond. 1954 (St. Bart.) FRCS Eng. 1960. Hon. Cons. Orthop. Surg. Herts. & Essex Hosp. Bishop's Stortford & Princess Alexandra Hosp. Harlow; Cons. Orthop. Surg. Rivers Hosp. Sawbridgeworth. Prev: Regist. Roy. Nat. Orthop. Hosp. & St. Bart. Hosp. Lond.

POKINSKYJ, Stefanie Katrina Longford Street Surgery, Longford Street, Heywood OL10 4NH Tel: 01706 621417 Fax: 01706 622915 — MB BCh Wales 1979; DRCOG 1982; MRCGP 1983. Clin. Asst. (Psychiat.) Prestwich.

POKORNY, Michael Robert Mullhampton Cottage, Mullhampton Cottage, Upton Bishop, Ross-on-Wye HR9 7UE Tel: 01989 780 395 Email: mrp@mpokorny.freeserve.co.uk — (Sheff.) MB ChB Sheff. 1961; DPM Eng. 1966; FRCPsych 1994, M 1972. Various Locums,Adult Psychiatry. Specialty: Psychother. Special Interest: Couples. Socs: Hon. Mem. Assn. Grp. & Individual Psychother. Prev: Cons. Psychiat. Prestwood Lodge Sch. Bucks. CC.; Hon Cons Psychiat. Lond centre for Psychother.

POLACARZ, Stephen Victor Department of Pathology, Withybush General Hospital, Fishguard, Haverfordwest SA61 2PZ Tel: 01437 773269 Fax: 01437 773549 Email: stephen.polacarz@pdt-tr.wales.nhs.uk — MB ChB Sheff. 1981; BSc (Hons.) Hull 1973; PhD Lond. 1984; MRCPath 1991; FRCPath 1999. Cons. Histopath. Withybush Gen. Hosp. HaverfordW.. Specialty: Histopath. Socs: Brit. Soc. Clin. Cytol.; Assn. Clin. Path.; Internat. Acad. Path. Prev: Lect. (Path.) Univ. Sheff. Med. Sch.

POLACK, Clare 224 Hills Road, Cambridge CB2 2QE Tel: 01223 247661 — MB BS Newc. 1994 (Univ. Newc.) BSc Ed. 1989; MRCP 1997; MRCGP 1998, DTM&H 1998. GP Edinburgh. Specialty: Gen. Pract. Prev: SHO (Med.) N. Tyneside Gen. Hosp. Tyne & Wear.

POLAK, Adolf (retired) The Old Rectory, Bidbury Lane, Havant PO9 3JG — (Univ. Coll. Hosp.) MD Camb. 1955, MB BChir 1949; FRCP Lond. 1970, M 1953. Prof. Renal Med. Soton Univ. Prev: Cons. Phys. Wessex Regional Renal Unit.

POLAK, Gerard Jan Anton HMYOI Glen Parva, Tigers Road, Wigston LE18 4TN Tel: 0116 264 3101 Fax: 0116 264 3000 — Artsexamen Amsterdam 1982 (University Vrye Amsterdam) Dip. Addic. Behaviour Lond. 1996. Med. Off. HMYOI Glen Parva Wigston. Specialty: Gen. Psychiat.; Forens. Psychiat. Prev: Med. Off. HMP Hull; Staff Psychiat. (Psychiat. for Deaf People) Whittingham Hosp. Preston; Regist. (Psychiat.) De La Pole Hosp. Hull.

POLAK, Louisa North Hill Surgery, 18 North Hill, Colchester CO1 1DZ Tel: 01206 578070 Fax: 01206 769880; The Latch, Church St, Boxted, Colchester CO4 5SX — BM BCh Oxf. 1979; MRCP (UK) (Paediat.) 1982; DRCOG 1982. GP Colchester.

POLAKOFF, Sheila (retired) 31 Templemead Close, Gordon Avenue, Stanmore HA7 3RG — MB BCh BAO Dub. 1948; MD Dub. 1971.

POLAND, Karen Monica 1 Millbrook Drive, Ballynahinch BT24 8HQ — MB BCh BAO Belf. 1996.

POLANI, Professor Paul E Division of Medical & Molecular Genetics, Paediatric Research Unit, Prince Philip Research Laboratories, Guy's Hospital, London SE1 9RT Tel: 020 7955 4456 Fax: 020 7955 4644; Little Meadow, Clandon Road, West Clandon, Guildford GU4 7TL Tel: 01483 222436 — MD Pisa 1938 (Siena & Pisa, Italy) DCH Eng. 1945; FRCP Lond. 1961, M 1948; FRS 1973; FRCOG 1979; FRCPath 1985; FRCPI 1989; FRCPCH 1997. Geneticist Paediat. Research Unit Div. Med. Molec. Genetics UMDS, Guy's & St. Thos. Hosps. Lond.; Emerit. Prof. Paediat. Research Lond.; Hon. Fell. Guy's St. Thos. & King's Coll., Fell. King's Coll., Lond. Specialty: Genetics; Paediat.; Neurol. Socs: Genet. Soc.; Clin. Genetics Soc.; Assn. Brit. Neurol. Prev: Vis. Prof. (Human Genetics & Developm.) Coll. of Phys. & Surg. Columbia Univ., New York; Dir. Paediat. Research Unit Guys Hosp. Med. Sch. & SE Thames Regional Genetics Centre; P. Phillip Prof. Paediat. Research & Hon. Childr. Phys. Guy's Hosp. Lond. & Geneticist Guy's Hosp. & Med. Sch., Lond.

POLANSKA, Antonina Isabella 6 Revell Road, Kingston upon Thames KT1 3SW — MB ChB Glas. 1965; MSc (Biochem.) Lond. 1976; MRCPath 1977. Cons. Chem. Path. Qu. Mary's Hosp. Lond. Specialty: Chem. Path. Socs: BMA & Assn. Clin. Biochems. Prev: Rotat. Sen. Regist. (Chem. Path.) Roy. Free Hosp. Lond. & W. Middlx.; Hosp. Isleworth; Regist. (Path.) Dept. Chem. Path. & Metab. Unit Roy. Infirm. Liverp.

POLE, Deborah Mary Bodmin Road Health Centre, Bodmin Road, Sale M33 5JH Tel: 0161 962 4625 Fax: 0161 905 3317 Email: rich.debs@dial.pipex.com — MB ChB Manch. 1994 (St. Andrews and Manchester) BSc St. And. 1991; MRCP Lond. 1996; MRCGP Lond. 1999. GP Bodmin Rd. Surg., Sale. Specialty: Gen. Pract. Socs: RCGP. Prev: SHO (Chest Med.) Wythenshawe Hosp. Manch.; Ho. Off. (Surg.) Blackpool Vict. Hosp.; Ho. Off. (Med.) Withington Hosp. Manch.

POLE, Indira Blackwoods Medical Centre, 8 Station Road, Muirhead, Glasgow G69 9EE Tel: 0141 779 2228 Fax: 0141 779 3225; 11A Fraser Gardens, Kirkintilloch, Glasgow G66 1DB — MB BS Bombay 1974 (Grant Med. Coll.) FFA RCS Eng. 1980; FFA RCSI 1980.

POLE, Pamela Margaret 7 Hadfield Cross, Hadfield, Glossop, Hyde SK13 1NT — MB ChB Manch. 1991.

POLEY, Bryan Anthony (retired) 6 Grosvenor Avenue, Torquay TQ2 7LA — MB ChB Bristol 1955; DA Eng. 1958; FFA RCS Eng. 1963. Prev: Cons. Anaesth. Torbay Hosp. Gp.

POLGE, Christopher Mark Roysia Surgery, Burns Road, Royston SG8 5PT Tel: 01763 243166 Fax: 01763 245315 — MB ChB Bristol 1983.

POLIAKOFF, Lucinda Jane 3 Waverley Road, Norwich NR4 6SG — MB BChir Camb. 1982; DRCOG 1984.

POLIHILL, Sara Louise Flat L, 90 Warwick Square, London SW1V 2AJ — BM Soton. 1996.

POLITO, Thomas Charles The Garden Flat, 16 York Place, Harrogate HG1 1HL — MB ChB Sheff. 1995. GP Regist. Harrogate. Specialty: Gen. Pract. Prev: Ho. Off. (Med.) Bassetlaw Hosp. Worksop; Ho. Off. (Gen. Surg.) Norf. & Norwich Hosp.

POLKEY, Anne Elizabeth 121 Court Lane, London SE21 7EE — MB ChB Leeds 1990.

POLKEY, Professor Charles Edward Dept. of Neurosurgery, King's College Hospital, Denmark Hill, London SE5 9RS; 121 Court Lane, Dulwich, London SE21 7EE — MD Bristol 1968; BSc Bristol 1960, MD 1968, MB ChB 1963; FRCS Eng. 1971. Prof. Of Func.al Neurosurg. GKST Sch. of Med.; Hon. Cons. Neurosurg. King's Healthcare Trust. Specialty: Neurosurg. Socs: Soc. Brit. Neurol. Surgs.; Europ.Soc. Funct. Neurosurg. Prev: Sen. Regist. Neurosurg. Unit Maudsley Hosp. Lond.; MRC Jun. Research Fell. Dept. Physiol. Univ. Bristol.; Cons. Neurosurg. Guy's Hosp. & Bethlem Roy. Hosp. & Maudsley Hosp. Lond.

POLKEY, Michael Iain Respiratory Muscle Laboratory, Department of Thoracic Medicine, King's College School of Medicine, Bessemer Road, London SE5 9PJ Tel: 020 7346 4493 Fax: 020 7346 3589; 23 Ashmead Road, Deptford, London SE8 4DY — MB ChB Bristol 1988; MRCP (UK) 1991; PhD Lond. 1998. Specialist Regist. (Thoracic & Gen. Med.) King's Coll. Hosp. Lond.; Hon. Regist. Roy. Brompton Hosp. Specialty: Respirat. Med.; Gen. Med. Socs: Brit. Thorac. Soc.; Eur. Respirat. Soc.; Amer. Thoracic Soc. Prev: Lect. (Med.) King's Coll. Sch. Med. & Dent.; Regist. (Med.) Guy's Hosp. Lond.; SHO Rotat. (Med.) Middlx. Hosp. Lond.

POLKINGHORN, Andrew The Verwood Surgery, 54 Manor Road, Verwood BH31 7PY Tel: 01202 825353 Fax: 01202 829697 — BM Soton. 1992; MRCGP Lond. 1997 - RCGP; DCH RCP Lond. 1996; DRCOG Lond. 1997; DFFP Lond. 1997. GP Princip., Sandy & Partners, Verwood. Specialty: Gen. Pract.

POLKINGHORN, Claire Louise Hunter 2 Bassett Crescent W., Southampton SO16 7DZ — BM Soton. 1994.

POLKINGHORN, David Gareth Market Surgery, Warehouse Lane, Wath-On-Dearne, Rotherham S63 7RA Tel: 01709 877524; Woodfalls, 14 New Road, Wath-upon-Dearne, Rotherham S63 7LQ Tel: 01709 877900 — BM Soton. 1978; MRCGP 1982. GP Princip.; GP Tutor Continuing Professional Developm. Socs: BMA & Soc. Med. & Dent. Hypn. Prev: GP Trainee Rotherham; Ho. Phys. Gen. Hosp. Poole Dorset; Ho. Surg. Roy. S. Hants. Hosp. Soton.

POLKINGHORNE, Kevan Roy 109A Chiswick High Road, Chiswick, London W4 2ED — MB ChB Auckland 1994.

POLKINHORN, John Skewes Dr Polkinhorn and Partners, The Surgery, Boyden Close, Nunnery Green, Wickhambrook, Newmarket CB8 8XU Tel: 01440 820140 Fax: 01440 823809; Jack's Cottage, Ousden, Newmarket CB8 8TN Tel: 01638 500483 — MB BChir Camb. 1972 (Guy's) MB Camb. 1972, BChir 1971; DObst RCOG 1974; DCH Eng. 1975; MRCGP 1976; FRCGP 1999.

POLKINHORN, Mary Ethna Newmarket Road Surgery, 125 Newmarket Road, Cambridge CB5 8HA Tel: 01223 364116 Fax: 01223 366088; Jack's Cottage, Ousden, Newmarket CB8 8TN Tel: 01638 500483 — (King's Coll. Hosp.) MB Camb. 1974, BChir 1973; MRCGP 1986.

POLL, David James Riversdale Surgery, 59 Bridge Street, Belper DE56 1AY Tel: 0177 382 2386 — MB BS Lond. 1980; BSc (Hons.) Immunol. Lond. 1977, MB BS 1980; DRCOG 1983; Cert. Family Plann. JCC 1985; MRCGP 1986. GP Belper, Derbysh.

POLLACK, Jonathan Stockbridge Village Health Centre, The Withens, Liverpool L28 1NL; 33 Rockbourne Avenue, Liverpool L25 4TQ Tel: 0151 428 1007 — MB BS Newc. 1969; DObst RCOG 1972; MRCGP 1975.

POLLAK, Thomas Edward 30 Thames Rise, Kettering NN16 9JL — MB ChB Sheff. 1976.

POLLARD, Alfred James Department Radiology, Stepping Hill Hospital, Stockport SK2 7JE; 41 Sevenoaks Avenue, Heaton Moor, Stockport SK4 4AU — MB ChB Manch. 1974; FRCR 1982. Cons. Radiol. Stockport HA. Specialty: Radiol.

POLLARD, Andrew John John Radcliffe Hospital , University of Oxford, Department of Paediatrics, Oxford OX3 9DU Tel: 01865 221060 Fax: 01865 221060 Email: andrew.pollard@paediatrics.ox.ac.uk — MB BS Lond. 1989 (St. Bart's Med. Sch. Lond.) BSc Lond. 1986; MRCP (UK) 1993; MRCPCH 1996; DIC Imperial Coll. 1999; PhD Lond. 1999. Sen. Lect. in Paediat. Infec.s Dis.s, Univ. of Oxf., Oxf.; Hon. Cons. Paediat., Univ. of Oxf., Oxf. Specialty: Paediat. Prev: SpR (Paed. Int. Care) St. Mary's Hosp. Lond.; Action Research Train. Fell. & Hon. NHS Regist. (Paediat. Infec. Dis.) St. Mary's Hosp. Lond.; Regist. (Paed. Infec. Dis.) St. Mary's Hosp. Lond.

POLLARD, Andrew Michael — MB ChB Leeds 1998; MRCP.

POLLARD, Professor Brian James Department of Anaesthesia, Manchester Royal Infirmary, Oxford Road, Manchester M13 9WL Tel: 0161 276 8650 Fax: 0161 273 5685 Email: brian.pollard@man.ac.uk — MB ChB Sheff. 1977 (Sheffield) BPharm Lond. 1971; FFA RCS Eng. 1981; MD Sheff. 1992. Prof. Anaesth. Univ. Manch.; Hon. Cons. Anaesth. Manch. Roy. Infirm. & UHSM; Edr.in Chief, Europ. Jl. Anaesthsiol. Specialty: Anaesth. Socs: Amer. Soc. af Anesthesiologists; Anaesth. Res. Soc.; Assn. Anaesth. GB & Irel. Prev: Sen. Lect. (Anaesth.) Univ. Manch.; Edr. Curr. Anaesth. & Critical Care.

POLLARD, Brian John Wycliffe Surgery, Elliott Road, Prince Rock, Plymouth PL4 9NH Tel: 01752 660648 Fax: 01752 261468 — MB ChB Birm. 1977.

POLLARD, Brian John (retired) Mullion Court, Linton Hill, Linton, Maidstone ME17 4AP Tel: 01622 743330 — (Univ. Coll. Hosp.) MB BS Lond. 1954; MRCGP 1977.

POLLARD, Claire Elizabeth 1b Greenbank Road, Sefton Park, Liverpool L18 1HG Tel: 0151 733 3224 Fax: 0151 522 1121 — MB ChB Liverp. 1990; DRCOG 1993; MRCGP (Distinc.) 1996. GP Princip. Liverp.

POLLARD, Corinna Mary 49 Selcroft Road, Purley CR8 1AJ — MB BS Lond. 1974; MRCP (UK) 1979; FRCPath 1996, M 1983; FRCP Lond. 1995. Cons. Haemat. Mayday Hosp. Croydon. Specialty: Haematology. Socs: Brit. Soc. Haematol. Prev: Sen. Regist. (Haemat.) St. Geo. Hosp. Lond.

POLLARD, David Edward — MB ChB Sheff. 1994.

POLLARD, Hugh Charles 64 The Brow, Widley, Waterlooville PO7 5DA Tel: 023 92 321184 — (St. Mary's Hospital Medical School London) MB BS Lond. 1986; DRCOG 1991. Specialty: Gen. Pract.

POLLARD, Ilene Isabel (retired) Broadgate, Storrs Park, Bowness on Windermere, Windermere LA23 3LT Tel: 015394 43097 — (Leeds) MB ChB Leeds 1948.

POLLARD, John Geoffrey 2 Fore Street, Hessenford, Torpoint PL11 3HP — MB ChB Bristol 1987.

POLLARD, Mr John Patrick Horton Hospital, Oxford Road, Banbury OX16 9AL Tel: 01295 275500 Fax: 01295 229055; Berry Hill House, Berry Hill Road, Adderbury, Banbury OX17 3HF Tel: 01295 810534 — MB BChir Camb. 1969; FRCS Eng. 1973; MA 1967, MChir Camb. 1983. Cons. Orthop. Surg. Horton Hosp., Oxf. Radcliffe NHS Trust. Specialty: Orthop. Socs: Fell. BOA. Prev: Sen. Regist. (Orthop. Surg.) Middlx. Hosp., Centr. Middlx. Hosp. & Roy. Nat. Orthop. Hosp.; Regist. (Orthop. Surg.) Bath Health Dist.

POLLARD, Kenneth Philip South Tyneside District Hospital, Harton Lane, South Shields NE34 0PL Tel: 0191 454 8888 — MB ChB Sheff. 1977; FRCPath 1996. Cons. Path., S. Tyneside Dist. Hosp. Specialty: Histopath.

POLLARD, Maria Ann Western Road Surgery, 41 Western Road, Billericay CM12 9DX Tel: 01277 658117 Fax: 01277 658119 — MB BS Lond. 1986.

POLLARD, Martin, Squadron Ldr. RAF Med. Br. Retd. High Street Surgery, High Street, Willingham by Stow, Gainsborough DN21 5JZ Tel: 01427 788277 Fax: 01427 787630; Heywoods House, Willingham Road, Kexby, Gainsborough DN21 5ND — MB BS Lond. 1971; MRCGP 1977 (Lond. Hosp.); MRCS Eng. LRCP Lond. 1971. GP Willingham. Prev: Sen. Med. Off. RAF Marham; Sen. Med. Off. Episkopi Garrison, Cyprus.

POLLARD, Michael Fallon and Partners, 1 Houghton Lane, Shevington, Wigan WN6 8ET Tel: 01257 253311 Fax: 01257 251081 — MB ChB Manch. 1986; BSc (Hons.) Physiol. Manch. 1983; DRCOG 1989; MRCGP 1990; T(GP) 1991. Scheme Organiser Wigan VTS. Specialty: Gen. Pract. Prev: Trainee GP Bolton VTS; SHO (Med. & Paediat.) Wigan Infirm.; SHO (O & G) Billinge Hosp.

POLLARD, Neil Adrian The Hops, 9 Leys Farm, Tarrington, Hereford HR1 4EX — MB BS Lond. 1984; MRCP (UK) 1990.

POLLARD, Rachel Clare Nuffield Department of Anaesthetics, John Radcliff Hospital, Headley Way, Oxford OX3 9DZ Email: rcpollard@btopenwold.com — MB BChir Camb. 1988; DA (UK) 1990; FRCA 1993. Cons. (Anaesth.) John Radcliffe Hosp. Oxf. Specialty: Anaesth. Prev: Regist. Rotat. (Anaesth.) Centr. Birm. Hosp.; SHO (Anaesth.) Leicester Gen. Hosp.; SHO (A & E & Cardiothoracic Surg.) Leicester.

POLLARD, Richard Charles Hayward (retired) 102 Looseleigh Lane, Crownhill, Plymouth PL6 5HH Tel: 01752 774033 — (Char. Cross) MB BS Lond. 1959. Prev: GP Plymouth.

POLLARD, Mr Roy North Tyneside General Hospital, North Shields NE29 8NH Tel: 0191 596660 Fax: 0191 293 2578; 5 Camp Terrace, North Shields NE29 0NE Tel: 0191 259 5823 Fax: 0191 280 1113 — MB ChB Leeds 1961; FRCS Ed. 1968; FRCS (Eng) 1996. Cons. Surg. N. Tyneside Dist. Gen. Hosp. N. Shields. Specialty: Gen. Surg. Prev: Sen. Regist. (Surg.) Guy's Hosp. Lond.

POLLARD, Stella Marguerite 69 Forest Lane, Kirklevington, Yarm TS15 9NE Tel: 01642 780941 — BChir Camb. 1969 (Camb. & St. Geo.) MB; MRCPath 1987, M 1975. Cons. Histopath. & Cytol. Univ. Hosp. Of N. Tees, Stockton On Tees. Specialty: Histopath. Prev: Lect. in Path. Univ. Nottm.; Regist. (Path.) Radcliffe Infirm. Oxf.; Ho. Phys. St. Geo. Hosp. Lond.

POLLARD, Mr Stephen Geoffrey St James's University Hospital, Department of Surgery, Beckett Street, Leeds LS9 7TF Tel: 0113 243 3144; Lime Kiln House, Woodhall, Linton, Wetherby LS22 4HZ Tel: 01937 587706 — MB BS Lond. 1981; BSc Lond. 1978; FRCS Lond. 1986; MA Camb. 1993; MS Lond. 1994. Cons. Surg. St Jas. Univ. Hosp. Leeds; Vis. Asst. Prof. Surg. Indianapolis Univ. Hosp. USA; Regent & Ethicon Trav. Schol. 1990. Specialty: Gen. Surg.; Transpl. Surg. Prev: Clin. Lect. & Sen. Regist. (Surg.) Addenbrooke's Hosp. Camb.; E. Anglian Research Fell.; Regist. Rotat. Addenbrookes Hosp. Camb.

POLLARD, Valerie Audrey Clipstone Health Centre, First Avenue, Clipstone, Mansfield NG21 9DA Tel: 01623 626132 Fax: 01623 420578 — MB ChB Sheff. 1980; DRCOG 1984. Exec. Comm. Mem. Newark & Sherwood PCT.

POLLARD, William Anton 3 The Mews, Shincliffe Vill., Durham DH1 2YH — MB BS Newc. 1980; BMedSc (Hons.) Newc. 1977, MB BS 1980. Socs: Fell. Roy. Soc. Med.; (Treas.) Durh. Clin. Soc. Prev: Demonst. (Histopath.) Roy. Vict. Infirm. Newc.; Ho. Phys. Roy. Vict. Infirm. Newc.; Ho. Surg. Hexham Gen. Hosp. N.d.

POLLEN, Roseanna Mary Bethnal Green Health Centre, 60 Florida Street, London E2 6LL Tel: 020 7739 4837 Fax: 020 7729 2190; 62 Malvern Road, London E2 3LJ — MB BS Lond. 1979 (St. Bartholomew's Hospital) MRCGP 1984; MSc BEcon Lond. 1995. Socs: Inst. Psychosexual Med. Prev: Trainee GP Whipps Cross Hosp. Lond. VTS.

POLLER, David Nigel Department of Histopathology, Queen Alexandra Hospital, Cosham, Portsmouth PO6 3LY Tel: 023 92 286000 Fax: 023 92 286493 — MB ChB Liverp. 1984; MRCPath 1994; MD 2000. Cons. Histopath. Portsmouth Acute Hosps. NHS Trust; Hon. Reader in Path., Univ. of Portsmouth. Specialty: Histopath.

POLLER, Professor Leon School of Biological Sciences, Stopford Building, The university of Manchester, Oxford Road, Manchester M13 9PT Tel: 0161 275 5316 Fax: 0161 275 5316 Email: ecaa@man.ac.uk — MB ChB Manch. 1951; MRCS Eng. LRCP Lond. 1951; DSc Manch. 1980, MD 1957; FRCPath 1973, M 1964. Co-ordinator EC Concerted Action on Anticoagulation of the E.C. (Hon.); Hon. Prof. Univ. Manch.1989-; ACCP Consensus 1982 to date. Specialty: Haematology. Socs: Internat. Soc. Haematol.; Internat. Soc. Thrombosis & Haemostasis. Prev: Mem. Counc. ICSH/ICTH Expert Panel on APTT Standardisation; Dir. Nat. (UK) Ref. Laborat. Anticoagulant Reagents & Contr. (WHO Centre) & Haemat. Withington Hosp. Manch.; Co-Chairm. Standardisation Subcomm. ISHT Anticoagulant Contr.

POLLET, Mr John Eugene Halton General Hospital, Hospital Way, Runcorn WA7 2DA Tel: 01928 714567 Fax: 01928 753440 — MB ChB Aberd. 1972; PhD Aberd. 1984, MD 1985, BMedBiol 1968, MB ChB 1972; FRCS Ed. 1977. Cons. Surg. Halton Hosp. Mersey RHA. Specialty: Gen. Surg. Prev: Regist. & Sen. Regist. (Gen. Surg.) Grampian HB; Lect. (Path.) Univ. Dundee.

POLLET, Sheena Margaret Thorn Road Clinic, Thorn Road, Runcorn WA7 5HQ Tel: 01928 575073 Fax: 01928 576969; Cherry Tree Farm, Bushells Lane, Kingswood, Frodsham WA6 6HX Tel: 01928 740296 — MB ChB Aberd. 1972 (Aberdeen) BMedBiol (Hons.) Aberd. 1969; MRCPsych 1979; Dip. Psychother. Aberd. 1983; FRCPsych 1997. Cons. Psychother. Halton Gen. Hosp. NHS Trust; Assoc. Mem. Brit. Psychoanalytic Soc. Specialty: Psychother. Socs: Merseyside Psychother. Inst. Prev: Lect. & Acad. Tutor (Psychother.) Liverp.

POLLING, Michael Roy James Street Surgery, 2 James Street, Boston PE21 8RD Tel: 01205 362556 Fax: 01205 359050 — MB ChB Leeds 1970; MRCS Eng. LRCP Lond. 1970; MRCGP 1977; MLCOM 1981. Socs: Brit. Osteop. Assn.; Soc. Orthop. Med.; Brit. Med. & Dent. Hypn. Soc.

POLLINGTON, Bruce Ian Marsham Street Surgery, 1 Marsham Street, Maidstone ME14 1EW Tel: 01622 752615/756129 — MB ChB Manch. 1992.

POLLINGTON, Graham David Auchtermuchty Health Centre, 12 Carswell Wynd, Auchtermuchty, Cupar KY14 7AW Tel: 01337 828262 Fax: 01337 828986; Taybank, Cupar Road, Cupar KY14 Tel: 01337 840541 — MB ChB Dundee 1990. Clin. Asst. (A & E) Qu. Margt. NHS Trust Dunfermline. Specialty: Gen. Pract. Prev: SHO (A & E Gen. Med. & Palliat. Care) Qu. Margt. NHS Trust Dunfermline.

POLLITT, Geoffrey (retired) c/o Lloyds Bank, 14 Church St., Sheffield S1 1HP; 79A Atherstone Road, Measham, Swadlincote DE12 7EG Tel: 01530 272266 — (Camb. & Univ. Coll. Hosp.) MRCS Eng. LRCP Lond. 1945; DPM Eng. 1958; DMJ (Clin.) Soc. Apoth. Lond. 1966; FRCPsych 1979, M 1971. Prev: Surg. Cdr. RN.

POLLITT, Michael John Kensey — MB BCh Wales 1997.

POLLITT, Norman Travers (retired) 18 Curzon Place, Eastcote, Pinner HA5 2TQ Tel: 020 8868 4082 Email: ntp@waitrose.com — (St. Mary's) MB BS Lond. 1952; MRCS Eng. LRCP Lond. 1952; MRCGP 1961. Prev: Phys. BUPA Med. Centre Lond. & Bushey.

POLLITT, Peter Geoffrey Harris Tomlin (retired) Sharrow, Bidford Road, Cleeve Prior, Evesham WR11 8LQ — MB ChB Birm. 1944. Prev: Med. Asst. (A & E) Walsall Gen. Hosp.

POLLITT, William Alfred (retired) Touchstone, Greenfields Lane, Rowton, Chester CH3 6AU Tel: 01244 335689 — MRCS Eng. LRCP Lond. 1950; DPH Liverp. 1953; FFCM 1978, M 1974. Prev: Dist. Med. Off. Chester HA.

POLLITT, Yvonne S. A. F. E. Family Planning Office, Seventrees Clinic, Baring St., Greenbank, Plymouth PL4 8NF Tel: 01753 389531; Langmans Quarry, West Buckland, Thurlestone, Kingsbridge TQ7 3AG Tel: 01548 561713 — (Middlx.) MB BS Lond. 1964; MRCS Eng. LRCP Lond. 1964; MFFP 1993. Med. Head (Family Plann. & Wom. Health Servs.) Plymouth Community Servs. NHS Trust. Specialty: Family Plann. & Reproduc. Health. Prev: Clin. Asst. (Genitourin. Med.) Freedom Fields Hosp. Plymouth; Clin. Asst (Ultrasound) Plymouth Hosps. Trust.

POLLITZER, Melanie Paediatric Department, Royal Berkshire Hospital, Reading RG1 5AN Tel: 0118 9877993 Fax: 0118 9878383 Email: mjpollitzer@doctors.org.uk; Bear Place Farm, Hare Hatch, Reading RG10 9TA Tel: 0118 940 3016 Fax: 0118 940 4487 Email: bearplacefarm@compuserve.com — MB BS Lond. 1973 (Roy. Free Hosp. Lond.) DCH Eng. 1976. p/t Assoc. Specialist (Paediat.) Roy. Berks. Hosp. Reading. Specialty: Paediat. Socs: MRCPCH; Neonat. Soc.; Royal Society of Medicine.

POLLOCK, Mr Alan Victor (retired) Scarborough Hospital, Scarborough YO12 6QL Tel: 01723 368111 Fax: 01723 501692 — MB ChB Cape Town 1943; FRCS Eng. 1948; FRCS Ed. 1984. Edr. Curr. Opinion in Surg. Infects.; Edr. Bd. Europ. Jl. Surg. Prev: Hon. Cons. Surg. ScarBoro. Hosp.

POLLOCK, Alexander Chapman Health Centre, Deanfoot Road, West Linton EH46 7EX Tel: 01968 660808 Fax: 01968 660856; Corra Linn, Medwyn Road, West Linton EH46 7HA Fax: 01968 660856 — MB ChB Glas. 1970; MRCGP 1986; MPhil Glas. 2003. JP.

***POLLOCK, Alison Ann** Stobhill Hospital, 133 Balornock Road, Glasgow G21 3UW Tel: 0141 201 3000; 1 Fern Avenue, Lenzie, Glasgow G66 4LE Tel: 0141 776 1072 — MB ChB Manch. 1998 (St. Andrew's / Manch.) BSc Ed. 1996; MB ChB Manch 1998. Jun. Ho. Off. (Med.) Stubhill Hosp. Glas. Specialty: Gen. Med. Prev: Jun. Ho. Off. (Urol.) B'burn RI; Jun. Ho. Off. (Surg.) B'burn RI.

POLLOCK, Professor Allyson Mary Public Health Policy Unit, School of Public Policy, University College, London WC1H 9QU; 21 Rutland Street, Edinburgh EH1 2AE — MB ChB Dundee 1983; BSc (Hons.) Dundee 1979; MSc Lond. 1988; MFPHM RCP (UK) 1990; FFPHM (UK) 1996. Dir. Research & Development, UCLH. Specialty: Pub. Health Med. Prev: Cons. & Sen. Lect. St. Geo. Med. Sch. Lond.

POLLOCK, Angus James Elliot (retired) Belwood, 3 Seacroft Square, Skegness PE25 3AQ Tel: 01754 767433 — MB ChB Glas. 1949. Prev: Ho. Surg. Roy. Infirm. Glas. & City Matern. Hosp. Carlisle.

POLLOCK, Anne Maclean Dunblane Medical Practice, Health Centre, Well Place, Dunblane FK15 9BQ Tel: 01786 822595 Fax: 01786 825298 — MB ChB Glas. 1969; DObst RCOG 1971; MFFP 1993. Princip. GP DunbLa..

POLLOCK, Anthony Louis Park Grove Surgery, 94 Park Grove, Barnsley S70 1QE Tel: 01226 282345 — MB ChB Manchester 1977; MB ChB Manch. 1977. GP Barnsley, S. Yorks.

POLLOCK, Bruce James 96 Moor Lane, Rickmansworth WD3 1LQ — MB BS Lond. 1991.

POLLOCK, Catherine Louise Mountsandel Surgery, 4 Mountsandel Road, Coleraine BT52 1JB Tel: 028 7034 2650 Fax: 028 7032 1000; Macleary Lodge, 9 Macleary Road, Coleraine BT51 3QX — MB BCh BAO Belf. 1983; DRCOG 1986; MRCGP 1988. Prev: Clin. Med. Off. Lisburn Health Centre; Trainee GP Ballymena Health Centre VTS.

POLLOCK, Christopher George Holme Farm, Rowley, Little Weighton, Cottingham HU20 3XR Tel: 01482 843578 — MB ChB Ed. 1976; FFA RCS Eng. 1981. Cons. Anaesth. Hull & E. Yorks. Dist. Specialty: Anaesth.

POLLOCK, Colin Thomas Stephen Wakefield Health Authority, White Rose House, West Parade, Wakefield WF1 1LT Tel: 01924 213041 Email: colin.pollock@gw.wakeha.northy.nhs.uk; 15 Holray Park, Carlton, Goole DN14 9QP Tel: 01405 860607 Email: pollock1@which.net — MB BChir Camb. 1982; BA Camb. 1980, MB BChir 1982; DRCOG 1985; MRCGP 1986; MPH Leeds 1991; MFPHM 1993. Med. Dir. (Pub. Health) White Rose Hse. Wakefield. Specialty: Pub. Health Med.

POLLOCK, Mr David (retired) The Ridge, 26 Radbrook Road, Shrewsbury SY3 9BE Tel: 01743 344397 Email: davjan@zoom.co.uk — (Glas.) MB ChB Glas. 1957; FRCS Glas. 1964; FRCS Ed. 1965; FRCS Eng. 1992. Prev: Sen. Regist. (Surg.) Glas. Roy. Infirm.

POLLOCK, David Josephus Ratmoyle, 96 Moor Lane, Rickmansworth WD3 1LQ Tel: 01923 72361 — MB ChB Liverp. 1956; BSc (Hons.) Liverp. 1953, MB ChB 1956; FRCPath 1977, M 1965. Sen. Lect. Path. Inst. Lond. Hosp. Socs: Fell. Roy. Soc. Med. Prev: Sen. Regist. Dept. Histopath. & Regist. Path. Dept. W. Middlx. Hosp.; Isleworth; Regist. Dept. Morbid Anat. Postgrad. Med. Sch. Lond.

POLLOCK, Deborah Marion Pynes Farmhouse, Pitney, Langport TA10 9AG — MB BChir Camb. 1962 (St. Bart.) DO RCPSI 1976; FRCS Ed. 1979. Specialty: Ophth. Prev: Assoc. Specialist (Ophth.) N. Irel. Hosp. Auth.; Regist. St. Geo. Hosp. Lond.; Ho. Phys. & Ho. Surg. Barnet Gen. Hosp.

POLLOCK, Elaine Elizabeth Clarkston Manse, Forrest St., Airdrie ML6 7BE — MB ChB Glas. 1983; MRCGP 1987. GP Glas. Prev: Clin. Asst. (Colposcopy) Glas. Roy. Infirm.

POLLOCK, Estella Gertrude (retired) 7 Greenacre Walk, Southgate, London N14 7DB Tel: 020 8886 0157 — MB BS Lond. 1947 (Roy. Free) DCH Eng. 1954. Prev: SCMO Enfield DHA.

POLLOCK, Evelyn Marian Margaret Hailsham Chambers, 4 Paper Buildings, Temple, London EC4Y 9AH Tel: 0207 643 5000 Fax: 0207 353 5778; 21 Thomas More House, Barbican, London EC2Y 8BT Tel: 020 7638 0023 — MB ChB Ed. 1978; FFA RCS Eng. 1983; BSc Ed. 1975, MD 1991. Dep. Coroner Lond. S. Dist.; Barrister at Law Inner Temple Lond. Specialty: Anaesth. Socs: BMA; Medico-Legal Soc. Prev: Sen. Regist. (Anaesth.) West. Infirm. Glas.; Clin. Fell. (Critical Care Med.) Hosp. for Sick Childr. Toronto, Canada; Regist. (Anaesth.) Glas. Roy. Infirm.

POLLOCK, Geoffrey George (retired) 10 Dunstall Road, Wimbledon, London SW20 0HR Tel: 020 8946 9879 — MB BS Lond. 1955 (Lond. Hosp.) MRCS Eng. LRCP Lond. 1955; DObst RCOG 1957; DA Eng. 1966; MRCP Lond. 1968; FFA RCS Eng. 1971; FRCGP 1983. Prev: GP Wimbledon.

POLLOCK, George Tullo University of Birmingham, Department of Public Health & Epidemiology, Edgbaston, Birmingham B15 2TT Tel: 0121 414 3163 Fax: 0121 414 7878 Email: g.t.pollock.1@bham.ac.uk — MB ChB Aberd. 1953; DPH Aberd. 1957; MFCM RCP (UK) 1974; FFCM RCP (UK) 1981; FFPHM RCP (UK) 1989; MD Birm. 1999. p/t Hon. Sen. Clin. Lect. (Pub. Health Med.) Univ. Birm. Specialty: Pub. Health Med. Socs: Fell. Roy. Soc. Med.; BMA; Green Coll. Soc. Oxf. (Ex-Vis. Schol.). Prev: Vis. Lect. (Pub. Health) Univ. Malta; Cons. Epidemiol. PHLS Communicable Dis. Surveillance Centre; Dir. Pub. Health Coventry HA.

POLLOCK, Henry Bernard (retired) 23 Coach Road, Warton, Carnforth LA5 9PR Tel: 01524 735181 — MB BS Lond. 1952 (King's Coll. Hosp. Lond.) DObst RCOG 1954. Prev: GP (Sen. Partner) Morecambe.

POLLOCK, Ian Chase Farm Hospital, The Ridgeway, Enfield EN2 8JL Tel: 020 8967 5902 Fax: 020 8367 3577 Email: childhealth@chasefarmhospital.org.uk — MB BS Lond. 1976 (Lond. Hosp.) DRCOG 1979; DCH Eng. 1981; MRCP 1982; FRCPCH 1997. Cons. Paediat. Chase Farm Hosp. Enfield; Charm of Paediative & Clin. Managem. Gp. Specialty: Paediat. Socs: Brit. Soc. Allergy & Clin. Immunol.; BMA. Prev: Sen. Regist. (Paediat.) St. Geo. Hosp. Lond.; Research Fell. Cardiothoracic Inst. Lond.; Regist. (Paediat.) St. Mary's Hosp. Lond.

POLLOCK, Ilse c/o Stewart, 22 Watling House, 4 Woolwich Common, London SE18 4HP — LRCP Ed. 1954; LRCP Ed. LRCS Ed. LRFPS Glas. 1954.

POLLOCK, Mr James Campbell Shaw 60 Balshagray Drive, Glasgow G11 7BZ Tel: 0141 339 3944 — MB ChB Glas. 1972; FRCS Glas. 1976; FRCS Canada 1979. Cons. Cardiac Surg. Roy. Hosp. Sick Childr. Glas. & Glas. Roy. Specialty: Cardiothoracic Surg. Prev: Sen. Resid. & Fell. Dept. Cardiac Surg. Univ. Toronto; Regist. Glas. Roy. Infirm.; Resid. (Gen. Surg.) St. Luke's Hosp. New York City, U.S.A.

POLLOCK, Janet Elizabeth Bloomfield Medical Centre, 118/120 Bloomfield Road, Blackpool FY1 6JW Tel: 01253 344123 Fax: 01253 349696; 242 Clifton Drive S., St Annes, Lytham St Annes FY8 1NH Tel: 01253 723759 — MB ChB Glas. 1985 (Glasgow) DCH RCPS Glas. 1988; DRCOG 1988; MRCGP 1989.

POLLOCK, Janet Somerville Shaw Girthill Farm, Warlock Road, Bridge of Weir PA11 3SR — MB ChB Glas. 1976; FFA RCS Eng. 1982. Specialty: Anaesth.

POLLOCK, Joan Margaret Macpherson Airdrie Health Centre, Monkscourt Avenue, Airdrie ML6 0JU Tel: 01236 769388 — MB ChB Glas. 1961. Socs: BMA.

POLLOCK, John Alan Morden Lodge, Lion Road, Bexleyheath DA6 8PE Tel: 020 8303 2121 — MB BS Lond. 1954 (Guy's) Prev: Asst. Ho. Surg. Guy's Hosp.; Ho. Phys. Glos. Roy. Infirm. Gloucester; Ho. Phys. Roy. Infirm. Glouc.

POLLOCK, John Alexander Russell (retired) Leckonby Lodge, Blackpool Old Road, Little Eccleston, Preston PR3 0YQ — MB BCh BAO Dub. 1953 (TC Dub.)

POLLOCK, Mr John Graham (retired) Nuffield and Ross Hall Hospitals, Glasgow G12 0PJ Tel: 0141 334 9441/810 3151; Waringfield, 18 Ralston Rd, Bearsden, Glasgow G61 3BA Tel: 0141 942 5407 Fax: 0141 9425407 — (Glas.) MB ChB Glas. 1958; FRCS Ed. 1965; FRCS Glas. 1965. Cons. Surg. Glas. Prev: Research Regist. (Surg.) West. Infirm. Glas.

POLLOCK, John Graham 5 Imperial Avenue, Beeston, Nottingham NG9 1EZ Tel: 0115 922 9011 — BM BCh Oxf. 1992; MA (Med. Sci.) Camb. 1989; MRCP (UK) 1995; FRCR 1998. Regist. (Radiol.) Qu. Med. Centre Nottm. Specialty: Radiol. Prev: SHO (Gen. Med.) Qu. Med. Centre Nottm.; Ho. Off. (Med.) John Radcliffe Hosp. Oxf.; Ho. Off. (Surg.) Roy. United Hosp. Bath.

POLLOCK, Mr Jonathan Robert Department of Neurology, OldChurch Hospital, Romford RM7 0BE Tel: 01708 708 318 Fax: 01708 732184 Email: jonathan.pollock@btopenworld.com — BM BCh Oxf. 1990; MA Camb. 1991; FRCS Ed. 1994; FRCS Ed. (Surg. Neurol.) 2000. Cons. Neurosurg., Barking, Havering & Redbridge Hosps. NHS Trust; Hon. Cons. Neurosurg., Basildon Univ. Hosp. Specialty: Neurosurg. Special Interest: Pituitary; Skull Base; Spinal. Socs: Soc. of Brit. Neurol. Surg.; Congr. of Neurol. Surg.; The Pituitary Soc. Prev: Specialist Regist., N. Thames Train., Rotat.

POLLOCK, Karin Janet St. James Surgery, Bath BA1 2SR Tel: 01225 422911; 106 Newbridge Hill, Bath BA1 3QB Tel: 01225 330728 — MB BCh Wales 1977.

POLLOCK, Keith Douglas Windsor House Surgery, 2 Corporation Street, Morley, Leeds LS27 9NB Tel: 0113 252 5223 Fax: 0113 238 1262 — MB ChB Leeds 1982.

POLLOCK, Kenneth McKenzie 122 Kelvinhaugh St., Yorkhill, Glasgow G3 8PP — MB ChB Glas. 1993; FRCA 1999. Specialist Regist. Anaesthetics West. Inf. Glas.

POLLOCK, Lucy Elizabeth Department of Histopathology, Kings College Hospital, Denmark Hill, London SE5 9RS — MB BS Lond. 1983; BA Oxf. 1980; MRCPath 1992. Cons. Histopath. Kings Coll. Hosp. Lond. Specialty: Histopath.

POLLOCK, Lucy Mary Musgrove Park Hospital, Taunton TA1 5DA — MB BChir Camb. 1991 (Trinity Coll. Camb.) MRCP Lond. Specialty: Care of the Elderly.

POLLOCK, Marian Ruth The Old Schoolhouse, Station Road, Hatton, Peterhead AB42 7RX — MB ChB Aberd. 1991. SHO (Ophth.) Wolverhampton Eye Infirm.

POLLOCK, Myra Welsh West Linton Health Centre, Deanfoot Road, West Linton EH46 7EX Tel: 01968 660808 — MB ChB Glas. 1970. Princip. GP W. Linton Med. Pract. Prev: Princip. GP Penicuik Med. Pract.; Jun. Ho. Off. (Med. & Surg.) Stirling Roy. Infirm.; Jun. Ho. Off. (O & G) Stobhill Hosp. Glas.

POLLOCK, Nigel Charles Omagh Health Centre, Mountjoy Road, Omagh BT79 7BA Tel: 028 8224 3521 — MB BCh BAO Belf. 1980; DRCOG 1983.

POLLOCK, Richard Sayles St George's Surgery, 46A Preston New Road, Blackburn BB2 6AH Tel: 01254 53791 Fax: 01254 697221 Email: deanl.millican@virgin.net — MB ChB Manch. 1982; BSc St. And. 1979; DRCOG 1985; MRCGP 1986; Cert. Family Plann. JCC 1988. Lead GP for Ment. Health & Commissioning Blackburn with Darwen Primary Care Trust. Prev: Ho. Phys. & Ho. Surg. Noble's Isle of Man Hosp.; SHO GP VTS Blackburn, Hyndburn & Ribble Valley HA; SHO (Psychiat.) Qu. Pk. Hosp. Blackburn.

POLLOCK, Ronald Matthew MPA Health Strategy & Planning Ltd, 105-111 Euston Street, London NW1 2EW Tel: 020 7388 2454 Fax: 020 7387 2320 Email: mpahealth@philippank.com; 2 Basildon Court, 28 Devonshire Street, London W1G 6PP — MB BChir Camb. 1957 (Middlx.) MA; FFPH 1977, M 1972. Director MPA Health

Strategy & Plann. Specialty: Pub. Health Med.; Epidemiol. Socs: Fell.Roy. Soc. of Med.; Pres. Sect. of Epidemiol. & Pub. Health. Prev: Regional Med. Off. & Dir. Pub. Health Med. Oxf. RHA; Surg. Regist. Roy. North. Infirm. Inverness.; Director Health Services Research.

POLLOCK, Ruth (retired) 23 Coach Road, Warton, Carnforth LA5 9PR Tel: 01524 735181 — MB ChB St. And. 1957. Prev: SCMO (Child Health) Lancs. AHA.

POLLOCK, Stephen Swinnerton Department of Neurosciences, Ethelbert Road, Canterbury CT1 3LP Tel: 01227 866489 Fax: 01227 783048 — MB BS Lond. 1973 (Royal Free) MRCS Eng. LRCP Lond. 1973; MRCP (UK) 1976; MD Lond. 1985; FRCP Lond. 1993. Cons. (Neurol.) Kent & Canterbury Acute Hosp. NHS Trust & Regional Neurosci.s Unit King's Coll. Hosp. Healthcare Trust Lond.; Honorary Senior Lecturer, University of London. Specialty: Neurol.; Vasc. Med. Socs: Fell. Roy. Soc. Med.; Coun. Stroke Assoc.; BMA. Prev: Sen. Regist. (Neurol.) Manch. Roy. Infirm.; Research Asst. (Neurol.) Middlx. Hosp. Lond.; Regist. (Neurol. Sci.s) Roy. Free Hosp. Lond.

POLLOCK, William Cockenzie & Port Seton Health Centre, Avenue Road, Cockenzie, Prestonpans EH32 0JL Tel: 01875 812998 Fax: 01875 814421 — MB ChB Ed. 1970; DObst RCOG 1972.

POLLOCK, Mr William Somerville Thomson Blackpool Victoria Hospital, Whinney Heys Road, Blackpool FY3 8NR Tel: 01253 300000 — MB ChB Glas. 1985; MRCP (UK) 1989; FRCS Glas. 1991. Cons. Ophth. Surg. Blackpool Vict. Hosp. Specialty: Ophth. Prev: Sen. Regist. Rotat. Sunderland, MiddlesBoro. & Newc.; Regist. Rotat. (Ophth.) St. Thos. Hosp. Lond. & Brighton & Canterbury Hosps.; SHO Rotat. (Ophth.) Bristol Eye Hosp.

POLLOK, Arthur (retired) Wellwood, Scott St., Galashiels TD1 1DU Tel: 01896 753487 — LRCP LRCS Ed. LRFPS Glas. 1950 (St. Mungo's Coll. Glas.) MRCGP 1965. Prev: Hosp. Pract. (Geriat.) Borders Gen. Hosp. Melrose.

POLLOK, Richard Charles Goodall St Georges Hospital, Department of Gastroenterology, Blackshaw Road, London SW17 0QT Tel: 020 8725 1206 Email: rpollok@sghms.ac.uk; Parkside Hospital, 53 Parkside, Wimbledon, London SW19 Tel: 020 8355 2229 — MB BS Lond. 1989 (St Bartholomews Hosp. Med. Sch.) BSc Lond. 1987; DTM & H Liverp. 1991; MRCP (UK) 1992; PhD 2002. Cons. (Gastroenterol.) & Hon. Sen. Lect. St Geo. Hosp. Lond. Specialty: Gastroenterol. Special Interest: Inflammatory Bowel Dis.; GI Infec.; IBS. Socs: RCP. Prev: Res. Fell. (Gastro.) Wellcome Trust, St. Bart's Hosp. Lond.; Regist. (Gastroenterol.) Qu. Mary's Hosp. Lond.; Regist. (Gastroenterol. & HIV Med.) Chelsea & Westm. Hosp. Lond.

POLLOK, William Mowat Aberfoyle Medical Centre, Main Street, Aberfoyle, Stirling FK8 3UX Tel: 01877 382421 Fax: 01877 382718 — MB ChB Glas. 1970.

POLMEAR, Andrew Fraser 20 Sackville Road, Hove BN3 3FF Tel: 01273 778585; 9 Powis Square, Brighton BN1 3HH Tel: 01273 328085 — MB BChir Camb. 1971 (St. Geo.) MRCS Eng. LRCP Lond. 1971; MRCP (UK) 1973; DObst RCOG 1973; FRCGP 1993, M 1978. Prev: Sen. Med. Off. United Christian Hosp., Hong Kong.; SHO St. Geo. Hosp. Lond.; Ho. Off. Roy. Hants. Co. Hosp. Winchester.

POLNAY, Janet Carole (retired) 41A Valley Road, West Bridgford, Nottingham NG2 6HG Tel: 0115 923 3718 Fax: 0115 974 3666 Email: janetpolnay@hotmail.com — MB BS Lond. 1975 (Lond. Hosp. & St Mary's) BSc (Hons.) Lond. 1972; MA Leics. 1999. p/t Assoc. Specialist in Paediat. (Cystic Fibrosis & Child Protec.) & named Doctor in Child Protec., Notts. City Hosp. NHS Trust. Prev: Sen. Doctor Child Protec. (Primary Care) Nottm. Community NHS Trust.

POLNAY, Professor Leon Division of Child Health, School of Human Development, Floor E East Block, Hospital Queens Medical Centre, Nottingham NG7 2UH Tel: 0115 970 9255 Fax: 0115 970 9382 Email: leon.polnay@nottingham.ac.uk; 41A Valley Road, West Bridgford, Nottingham NG2 6HG Fax: 0115 974 3666 Email: leon.polnay@nottingham.ac.uk — MB BS Lond. 1971 (Lond. Hosp.) BSc Lond. 1968; MRCP (UK) 1974; DCH Eng. 1974; DObst RCOG 1975; FRCP Lond. 1988; FRCPCH 1997. Prof. (Community Paediat.) Univ. Nottm. Specialty: Community Child Health. Socs: Fell. Brit. Assn. Comm. Child Health; RCP Lond.; Roy. Coll. Paediat. & Child Health. Prev: Clin. Med. Off. S. Hammersmith Health Dist.; Hon. Lect. (Paediat.) Char. Cross Hosp. Med. Sch.; SHO (Paediat.) W. Middlx. Hosp. Isleworth.

POLSON, David William Hope Hospital, Eccles Old Road, Salford M6 8HD Tel: 0161 789 7373 Fax: 0161 787 5475; 31 New Forest Road, Manchester M23 9JT Tel: 0161 969 2057 — MB BS Lond. 1980 (St. Mary's) MRCOG 1987; MD Lond. 1990. Cons. (O & G) Salford Roy. Hosps NHS Trust, Salford. Specialty: Obst. & Gyn. Socs: Brit. Fertil. Soc.; ESHRE. Prev: Sen. Regist. (O & G) Manch.; Clin. Research Fell. Monash Med. Centre, Australia; SHO (Obst.& Gyn.) St. Mary's & Qu. Charlotte's Hosps. Lond.

POLSON, Gertrude Mary (retired) 16 Tewit Well Road, Harrogate HG2 8JE Tel: 01423 503434 — (Leeds) BSc (Hons.) Leeds 1947; MB ChB Leeds 1950; DObst RCOG 1953; MFCM RCP (UK) 1974. Prev: SCMO Harrogate HA.

POLSON, Hamish William Morrison Leith Mount, 46 Ferry Road, Edinburgh EH6 4AE Tel: 0131 554 0558 Fax: 0131 555 6911; 16 Blinkbonny Terrace, Edinburgh EH4 3NA Tel: 0131 332 3227 — MB ChB Ed. 1962; DObst RCOG 1965. Socs: BMA & Soc. Occupat. Med.

POLSON, Rex James Solihull Hospital, Lode Lane, Solihull B91 2JL Tel: 0121 424 4549 Fax: 0121 424 5548 — (St. Mary's) MB BS Lond. 1979; MRCP (UK) 1983; BSc Lond. 1976, MD 1990; FRCP Lond. 1996; LLM 2003. Cons. Phys. (Gastroenterol.) Birm. Heartlands & Solihull NhS Trust; Hon. Sen. Clin. Lect., Univ. of Birm. Specialty: Gastroenterol.; Gen. Med. Socs: Brit. Soc. Gastroenterol.; Brit. Ass. Study Liver.; Fell. of Roy. Coll. of Phys.s. Prev: Sen. Regist. Rotat. (Gen. Med. & Gastroenterol.) Centr. Middlx. Hosp. & St. Mary's Hosp. Lond.; Clin. Research Fell. (Liver Unit) King's Coll. Hosp. Lond.; SHO & Regist. Rotat. (Med.) Lond. Hosp.

POLSON, Richard Gordon Osborn Clinic, Osborn Road, Fareham PO16 7ES Tel: 01329 288331 — MB BS Lond. 1982; MRCPsych 1989. Cons. Psychiat. Portsmouth Healthcare Trust. Specialty: Gen. Psychiat. Prev: Sen. Regist. (Psychiat.) St. Jas. Hosp. Portsmouth; Regist. (Psychiat.) Friern Hosp. Lond.

POLTOCK, Tracy Louise 1 Manor House Lane, Yardley, Birmingham B26 1PE Tel: 0121 743 2273 Fax: 0121 722 2037; 14 Swinbrook Way, Shirley, Solihull B90 3LZ — MB ChB Sheff. 1986. Socs: BMA. Prev: Trainee GP/SHO Mold VTS; SHO (Psychiat.) Arrowe Pk. Hosp.; SHO (O & G) Wrexham Maelor Hosp.

POLWIN, Philip John Stephen The Surgery, Roman Way, Billingshurst RH14 9QZ Tel: 01403 782931 Fax: 01403 785505 — MB BS Lond. 1978; Cert. Family Plann. JCC 1982; DRCOG 1982; Cert. Aviation Med. 1993. Prev: Trainee GP Portsmouth VTS; SHO (A & E) Qu. Alexandra Hosp. Portsmouth; Ho. Surg. Qu. Mary's Hosp. for the E. End Lond.

POLWIN, Stephen John Sidney, RD (retired) 18 Lower Bere Wood, Waterlooville PO7 7NQ — MB BCh Wales 1950 (Cardiff & Roy. Lond. Hosp.) Cert Contracep. & Family Plann. RCOG; BSc Wales 1947; DObst RCOG 1952; MRCGP 1974; RCGP & Family Plann. Assn. 1975. Prev: Princip. GP Waterlooville.

POLYCHRONIS, Andreas Guy's Hospital, London SE1 9RT Tel: 020 7955 5000; 277 Camberwell New Road, London SE5 0TF — MB BCh Wales 1995. SHO (Gen. Med.) Guy's Hosp. Lond. Specialty: Gen. Med.

POMERANCE, Ariela (retired) 42 Davenham Avenue, Northwood HA6 3HQ Tel: 01923 22773 — MRCS Eng. LRCP Lond. 1951 (Roy. Free) MD Lond. 1958, MB BS 1951; MRCPath 1970. Cons. Histopath. Harefield & Mt. Vernon Laborat. N.wood.

POMEROY, Ann 10 Tivoli Road, Cheltenham GL50 2TG Tel: 01242 233168 Fax: 01242 255658 — MB BS Lond. 1972 (St. Mary's) MRCS Eng. LRCP Lond. 1972. Assoc. Specialist (Dermat.) Gloucester Roy. Hosp., Cheltenham Gen. Hosp. & Stroud Gen. Hosp. Specialty: Dermat.

POMEROY, Richard Thomas, MBE The Medical Centre, Craig Croft, Chelmsley Wood, Birmingham B37 7TR Tel: 0121 770 5656 Fax: 0121 779 5619; 22 The Cricketers, Meriden Road, Hampton in Arden, Solihull B92 6BT Tel: 01675 443663 Fax: 0121 779 5619 — MB BCh BAO NUI 1965; DObst RCOG 1966; FRCGP 1987, M 1973. Specialty: Aviat. Med. Socs: BMA. Prev: Ho. Off. Gen. Hosp. Stratford-on-Avon & Manor Matern. Hosp. Walsall.

POMEROY, William Shubrook The Oaks, Nightingale Way, Swanley BR8 7UP Tel: 01322 668775 Fax: 01322 668010 — MB ChB 1975 (UCT Cape Town, South Africa) DCH London; MRCGP UK. GP. Specialty: Gen. Pract. Socs: BMA.

POMFRET, Steven Mark The Knoll Surgery, 46 High Street, Frodsham, Warrington WA6 7HF Tel: 01928 733249 Fax: 01928

739367; 29 Ashlands, Frodsham, Warrington WA6 6RG — BM Soton. 1987; MRCGP 1991; DRCOG 1991.

POMIRSKA, Maria Bernadeta 61 Lower Redland Road, Redland, Bristol BS6 6SR — MB ChB Birm. 1982.

POMPA, Peter Anthony Philip (retired) 5 Haslar Crescent, Waterlooville PO7 6DB — (King's Coll. Hosp.) MB BS Lond. 1954; MRCS Eng. LRCP Lond. 1954; DObst. RCOG 1956; DA Eng. 1957; MRCGP 1965. Prev: Dep. Med. Dir. Lederle Laborats.

POMPHREY, Elizabeth O'Hara Trust Research Office, 4th Floor, Queen Elizabeth Building, 10 Alexandra Parade, Royal Infirmary, Glasgow G31 2ER Tel: 0141 211 4587 Fax: 0141 553 2558; The Gardeners House, Formakin, Bishopton PA7 5NX — MB ChB Glas. 1963; DObst RCOG 1965. Research & Developm. Manager Glas. Roy. Infirm. NHS & Univ. Trust. Prev: Clin. Research Fell. (Path., Biochem. & Med. Cardiol.) Univ. Glas.; Clin. Research Asst. (Cardiol.) Univ. Glas.; Med. Off. (Cytol.) Gtr. Glas. HB.

POMSON, Hyman Robert 38 South Grove House, South Grove, London N6 6LR — MB BS Lond. 1940 (Char. Cross) Prev: Ho. Surg. Char. Cross Hosp. & Bolingbroke Hosp. Lond.; Res. Surg. Off. P. of Wales Hosp. Plymouth.

PONCIA, James Robert 15 Durham Road, London N2 9DP — MB ChB Birm. 1994.

POND, John Bellingham (retired) Dromore, 10 Granville Road, Walmer, Deal CT14 7LU Tel: 01304 372977 — MB BChir Camb. 1955 (Camb. & Guy's) MRCS Eng. LRCP Lond. 1954; MA Camb. 1955; DObst RCOG 1957. Prev: Clin. Asst. (Orthop.) Kent & Canterbury Hosp. & Vict. Hosp. Deal.

POND, Margaret Helen (retired) 38 Strand Court, The Strand, Topsham, Exeter EX3 0AZ Tel: 01392 873189 — (Camb. & King's Coll. Hosp.) MB BChir Camb. 1945; MRCS Eng. LRCP Lond. 1946; MA Camb. 1946, MD 1953. Prev: Clin. Asst. (Diabetic) King's Coll. Hosp. Lond.

POND, Michael Neil Lynfield, 9 Malvern Road, Chellow Dene, Bradford BD9 6AR — MB BS Lond. 1986; MA Camb. 1987, BA 1983; MRCP (UK) 1990. Regist. (Chest Med.) Glenfield Hosp. Leicester. Specialty: Respirat. Med. Socs: Brit. Thorac. Soc. Prev: Clin. Fell. Adult Cystic Fibrosis Unit Seacroft Hosp. Leeds.

PONDA, Bipin Gatubhai (retired) 32 Beeston Drive, Winsford CW7 1ER Tel: 01606 861201 Email: bsponda@hotmail.com — MB BS Bombay 1960 (Grant Med. Coll. Bombay) DTM & H Liverp. 1963. Private Pratise; GP Locum work. Prev: Regist. (Med.) S. Chesh. Hosp. Gp.

PONDER, Professor Bruce Anthony John Department of Oncology, Addenbrooke's Hospital, Hills Road, Cambridge CB2 2QQ Tel: 01223 336900 Fax: 01223 336902 Email: bajp@mole.bio.cam.ac.uk; 43 High Street, Cottenham, Cambridge CB4 8SA Tel: 01954 252163 Fax: 01954 252103 — MB Camb. 1969 (Camb. & St. Thos.) MB BChir Camb. 1969; MA Camb. 1972; PhD Lond. 1977; FRCP 1988; FMedSci 1998; FRS 2001; FRCPath 2001. CRC Prof. Clin. Oncol. Univ. Camb.; Fell. Jesus Coll. Camb.; Hon. Cons. Phys. Addenbrooke's Hosp. Camb.; Co-Dir. Strangeways Research Laborat.; Dir. Cancer Research UK Human Cancer Genetics Research Gp.; Gibb Fell. Specialty: Oncol. Socs: (Ex-Treas.) Brit. Assn. Cancer Research; Fell. Acad. Med. Sc.; Amer. Soc. Human Genetics. Prev: Prof. Human Cancer Genetics Univ. Camb.; Head Sect. Human Cancer Genetics Inst. Cancer Research; Reader (Human Cancer Genetics) Univ. Lond.

PONNAMPALAM, Joanna Sharmila 4 Whitehall Road, Sittingbourne ME10 4HB — MB BS Lond. 1994.

PONNAMPALAM, Mr Mark Saundarasingam PO Box 35257, London E1 7WE — (St. Bart. Hosp. Med. Coll.) MB BS Lond. 1960; FRCS Ed. 1971; FRCS Eng. 1972; LMCC 1974; FRCSC 1974. GP Non-Princip.; Specialist Cert. (Gen. Surg.) RCSC; Assoc. Internat. Federat. Surg. Coll. Specialty: Gen. Pract. Socs: FICS. Prev: Regist. Rotat. (Surg.) North. Irel. Hosps. Auth.; Sen. Resid. Westm. Hosp. Ontario, Canada; Ho. Surg. St. John's Hosp. Chelmsford.

PONNAMPALAVANAR, Anusha 26 Chepstow Rise, Croydon CR0 5JB — MB BS Lond. 1996.

PONNAPPA, Muruvanda Aiyappa Yiewsley Health Centre, 20 High St., Yiewsley, West Drayton UB7 8DP — MB BS Mysore 1964.

PONSFORD, Joan Margaret (retired) 17 Buttsfield Lane, E. Hoathly, Lewes BN8 6EE Tel: 0182 584615 — LRCP LRCS Ed. 1949 (Roy. Colls. Ed.) LRCP LRCS Ed. LRFPS Glas. 1949; DObst RCOG 1952; DPH Lond. 1961. Clin. Med. Off. E. Herts. AHA. Prev: SHO Pk. Hosp. Davyhulme.

PONSFORD, John Richard c/o C5 Ward, Walsgrave Hospital, Coventry — MB BS Lond. 1969 (St. Geo.) BSc (Physiol.) Lond. 1965, MB BS 1969; FRCP Lond. 1987. Cons. Neurol. Coventry & Warks. HAs. Specialty: Neurol. Prev: Sen. Regist. (Neurol.) St. Mary's Hosp. Lond. & Nat. Hosp. Lond.

PONSFORD, John Steel 17 Crowsnest Lane, Boorley Green, Botley, Southampton SO32 2DD — MB BS Lond. 1974 (Middlx.) DRCOG 1977; MRCGP 1978.

PONSONBY, Christine Elizabeth The Manor Street Surgery, Manor Street, Berkhamsted HP4 2DL Tel: 01442 875935; Street Farm, Bovingdon, Hemel Hempstead HP3 0JR Tel: 01442 834149 — MB BS Lond. 1968 (St Thomas Hosp. Med. Sch.) DCH Eng. 1973; MRCP (UK) 1973; MRCGP 1986. Specialty: Diabetes. Prev: Ho. Phys. St. Thos. Hosp. Lond.; SHO Wexham Pk. Hosp.

PONSONBY, William John Carleton — MB ChB Birm. 1986; MRCGP 1991; MBA Durham Univ. 1997; AFOM 2002; FRIPH 2002. Team Ldr. Occupational Health Shell UK Ltd; Internat. Med. Support OMS Baku. Specialty: Gen. Pract.; Occupat. Health. Socs: BMA; RIPH Fell.; Fac. of Occupat.al Med. (Assoc.). Prev: Med. Director Med. Serv.s CIS Region, Internat. SOS; Gen. Manager Med. Operat.s Azerbaijan.

PONTE, Jose Castelhano Department of Anaesthesia, GKST School of Medicine & Dentistry, Denmark Hill, London SE5 9RS Tel: 020 7346 3358 Fax: 020 7346 3632 — Lic Med Lisbon 1967 (Lisbon, Portugal) Lic. Med. Lisbon 1967; DIC Lond. 1971; PhD Bristol 1973; FFA RCS Eng. 1979. Sen. Lect., Cons. & Dep. Head Anaesth. GKST Sch. Med. & Dent. Lond. Specialty: Anaesth. Socs: Roy. Coll. Anaesth.; Physiol. Soc.; Europ. Acad. Anaesthesiol.

PONTEFRACT, Carolyn Ann Grove Hill Medical Centre, Kilbride Court, Hemel Hempstead HP2 6AD Tel: 01442 212038; 16 Alzey Gardens, Harpenden AL5 5SZ Tel: 01582 768912 — BM BS Nottm. 1988; DGM RCP Lond. 1990; MRCGP 1992.

PONTEFRACT, David Robert 4 The Woodlands, Eccleston Park, Prescot L34 2TN — MB ChB Ed. 1996.

PONTEFRACT, Lesley Gorton Road Family Surgery, 306 Gorton Road, Reddish, Stockport SK5 6RN Tel: 0161 432 1235 Fax: 0161 442 2495 — MB ChB Manch. 1982; DRCOG 1986; MRCGP 1986. Prev: SHO (O & G, Psychiat. & Paediat.) Tameside Gen. Hosp. Ashton-under-Lyne.

PONTIN, Mr Alan Roger c/o 18 Whychford Drive, Sawbridgeworth CM21 0HA — MB ChB Birm. 1968; FRCS Ed. 1973.

PONTIN, Alyson Jane The Minster Practice, Cabourne Court, Cabourne Avenue, Lincoln LN2 2JP Tel: 01522 568838 Fax: 01522 546740; Gilcrest, 32 Washdyke Lane, Nettleham, Lincoln LN2 2PY Tel: 01522 595698 — MB BS Lond. 1981 (Roy. Free Hosp. Lond.) MRCGP 1985; DRCOG 1985; FRCGP 1999; DFFP 2000.

PONTIN, Mark John 26 Hermitage Woods Crescent, Woking GU21 8UE — MB BS Lond. 1994.

PONTON, Alastair William Gordon Heatherview Medical Centre, Alder Road, Parkstone, Poole BH12 4AY Tel: 01202 743678 Fax: 01202 739960 — MB ChB Leic. 1985.

PONTY, Ralph Churchman's Farm, Inworth, Tiptree, Colchester CO5 9SP — MB BS Lond. 1965; MRCS Eng. LRCP Lond. 1965.

POOBALASINGAM, Nagalingam 61 Oakleigh Park N., Whetstone, London N20 9AT Tel: 020 8445 7924 — MB BS Ceylon 1964 (Univ. Sri Lanka) FRCA 1971; DA Eng. 1971. Cons. Anaesth. N. Middlx. Hosp. Specialty: Anaesth. Prev: Cons. Anaesth. Haringey Dist. Hosp. (N. Middlx., St. Ann's & P. of Wales Hosps.); Sen. Regist. Research Dept. Anaesth. Roy. Coll. Surg. Eng. & Whittington Hosp.

POOK, Asha 16 Granville Avenue, Oadby, Leicester LE2 5FL — MB BS Lond. 1995 (King's Coll. Sch. Med.) BSc (Hons.) Lond. 1991. Prev: Ho. Surg. King's Coll. Hosp. Lond.; Ho. Phys. Bromley Hosp.

POOK, Clifford Wilford Pantiles, Raglan NP15 2YE — MB BS Lond. 1954; MRCS Eng. LRCP Lond. 1954; DObst RCOG 1957.

POOK, John Anthony Ronald 18 Cedars Road, Beckenham BR3 4JF — MB BS Lond. 1970; MRCS Eng. LRCP Lond. 1970; DA Eng. 1972; FFA RCS Eng. 1974. Specialty: Anaesth.

POOL, Mr Christopher John Fenton Cherrywynd House, High St., Ballinger, Great Missenden HP16 9LF Tel: 01494 837254 —

MB BS Lond. 1960 (Lond. Hosp.) MRCS Eng. LRCP Lond. 1960; DObst RCOG 1963; FRCS Eng. 1968. Specialty: Orthop.

POOL, Richard John Greenfield Surgery, 1 Claremont Avenue, Woking GU22 7SF Tel: 01483 771171; Lindsay Cottage, Guildford Road, Woking GU22 7UT Tel: 0148 62 768545 — MB BS Lond. 1984; DRCOG 1987. GP Woking. Prev: Trainee GP W. Dorset HA.; Ho. Off. Med. Roy. Sussex Co. Hosp.; Ho. Off. Surg. N. Devon Dist. Hosp.

POOL, Richard William 14 Lambert Road, Grimsby DN32 0HT — MB BS Lond. 1991.

POOL, Roger Watson Brig Royd Surgery, Brig Royd, Ripponden, Sowerby Bridge HX6 4AN Tel: 01422 822209; Little Merrybent Farm, Ripponden, Sowerby Bridge HX6 4NH — MB ChB Leeds 1976; MRCP (UK) 1979; MRCGP 1983.

POOL, Mr Rowan Donald The Orthopaedic Centre, Woking Nuffield Hospital, Shores Road, Woking GU21 4BY Tel: 01483 768 051; The Windsor Orthopaedic Clinic, Phoenix House, Nightingale Walk, Windsor Tel: 01753 868 622; The Willows, 32 Allen House Park, Hook Heath, Woking GU22 0DB Tel: 01483 730795 — MB ChB Leeds 1974; FRCS Eng. 1980. Cons. Traum. & Orthop. Surg. Specialty: Trauma & Orthop. Surg. Socs: Brit. Limb Reconstruc. Soc. Prev: Sen. Regist. (Orthop.) St. Geo. Hosp. Lond.

***POOLE, Abigail Elizabeth** 33 Parkwood Drive, Rawstenstall, Rossendale BB4 6RP; 3 Cottingham, Kettering General Hospital, Rothwell Raod, Kettering NN16 8UZ Tel: 01536 492000 — MB ChB Leic. 1998; BSc Leic. 1995; MB ChB Leic 1998. Kettering VTS.

POOLE, Alan Julian Sanford House, Rock Hill, Wrantage, Taunton TA3 6DW — MB BS Lond. 1961 (Lond. Hosp.) BSc Lond. 1957, MB BS 1961; MRCP Lond. 1966; DPM Eng. 1971; FRCPsych 1984, M 1972. Prev: Ho. Phys. Med. Unit Lond. Hosp.; Ho. Phys. Endocrine Unit Hammersmith Hosp. & Postgrad. Med. Sch.; Lond.

POOLE, Alexander Geoffrey Bruce (retired) Ednam East Mill, Kelso TD5 7QB Tel: 01573 224000 Fax: 01573 226288 Email: poole@scotborders.co.uk; Nether Woodside, Kelso TD5 7SP Tel: 01573 224000 Fax: 01573 226288 Email: poole@scottishborders.co.uk — (Ed.) MB ChB Ed. 1947; MRCGP 1956; DA Eng. 1969.

POOLE, Bernard Joseph Branton House, North Road, Hembsy, Great Yarmouth NR29 4LR — MB BS Lond. 1954.

POOLE, Charles Jonathan Mortiboy Health Centre, Cross St., Dudley DY1 1RN Tel: 01384 366423; Hunters Rise, Holy Cross Green, Clent, Stourbridge DY9 0HG Tel: 01562 730804 — MB BS Lond. 1978 (Westm.) AKC 1975; MRCP (UK) 1981; MD Lond. 1988; FFOM RCP Lond. 1996, MFOM 1992, AFOM 1989; FRCP Lond. 1995. Cons. Occupat. Phys. DudleyBeacon & Castle NHS Trust; Hon. Reader in Occupat. Med. Univ. of Wolverhampton. Specialty: Occupat. Health. Socs: Soc. Occup. Med.; Assn. NHS Occupat.al Phys.; Assn. Local Auth. Med. Advisors. Prev: Sen. Occupat. Phys. Rover Gp. Birm.; Occupat. Phys. Brit. Steel W. Midl.; Research Fell. (Med.) Westminster Hosp. Lond.

POOLE, Christopher John CRC Institute for Cancer Studies, The Medical School, University Hospital Birmingham, Birmingham B15 2TH Tel: 0121 472 4311 Fax: 0121 414 3700; 112 Oxford Road, Moseley, Birmingham B13 9SQ Tel: 0121 449 3784 — MB BChir Camb. 1979 (King's Coll. Hosp.) MA Camb. 1980, BA (Med. Sci.) 1976; MRCP (UK) 1983; FRCP 2001. Macmillan Sen. Lect. (Med. Oncol.) Qu. Eliz. Hosp. & City Hosp. Birm. Specialty: Oncol. Socs: Brit. Assn. for Cancer Res.; Assn. Cancer Phys.; Am. Soc. Clin. Onc. Prev: CRC Clin. Research Fell. Beatson Inst. Glas. & ICRF Research Fell. St. Bart. Hosp. Lond.; Regist. (Med.) St. Thos. Hosp. Lond.; SHO (Med.) Roy. Marsden Hosp. Sutton.

POOLE, David The Hurley Clinic, Ebenezer House, Kennington Lane, London SE11 4HJ Tel: 020 7735 7918 Fax: 020 7587 5296 — MB ChB Ed. 1967. GP Hurley Clin. Lond.

POOLE, David Robert Scarborough Hospital, Woodlands Drive, Scarborough YO12 6QL — MB BS Newc. 1971; FRCOG 1991, M 1977. Cons. (O & G); Med. Dir. Specialty: Obst. & Gyn.

POOLE, Elman William 18 Victoria Road, Oxford OX2 7QD Tel: 01865 59489 — MB ChB New Zealand 1950 (Otago) FRCP Ed. 1965, M 1956; DPM Eng. 1957; MRCPsych 1972. Cons. Clin. Neurophysiol. Oxf. HA & RHA; Clin. Lect. (Neurol.) Univ. Oxf. Specialty: Neurol. Prev: Lect. Inst. Psychiat. Lond.; Rockefeller Trav. Fell. 1960-61; Regist. Nat. Hosp. Nerv. Dis. Qu. Sq. Lond.

POOLE, Gillian Gwyneth Ty Croes, Llanymynech SY22 6ER Tel: 01691 830872 Fax: 01691 839202 — MB BCh Wales 1962; DCH Eng. 1964; DObst RCOG 1964. Clin. Asst. (Rheum.) Robt. Jones & Agnes Hunt Orthop. & Dist. Hosp. Oswestry. Prev: Regist. (Obst.) Sorrento Matern. Hosp. Birm.; Ho. Off. United Cardiff Hosps.

POOLE, Graham White (retired) Mayflower Waters, Beacon Lane, Kingswear, Dartmouth TQ6 0BU Tel: 01803 752738 — MB ChB Birm. 1944 (Birmingham) MB ChB (Distinc. Med. Paediat. & Midw.) Birm; MRCS Eng. LRCP Lond. 1944; FRCP Lond. 1976, M 1949. Prev: Cons. Phys. Respirat. Dis. & Sen. Lect. Hammersmith Hosp. & Roy. Postgrad. Med. Sch.

POOLE, Jacqueline St. Nicholas Hospital, Department of Forensic Psychiatry, Jubilee Road, Newcastle upon Tyne NE3 3XT — MB BS Lond. 1986.

POOLE, Jill (retired) Mayflower Waters, Beacon Lane, Kingswear, Dartmouth TQ6 0BU Tel: 01803 752738 — MB ChB Birm. 1949; MRCS Eng. LRCP Lond. 1949; DCH . Lond. 1952.

POOLE, Kingsley Kahlil Arun, The Close, Ashington, Pulborough RH20 3LJ — BM BCh Oxf. 1996.

POOLE, Norman Alan

POOLE, Norman Walter — MB ChB Glas. 1969; MRCGP 1977. Prev: Research Fell. Dept. Gen. Pract. Univ. Glas.

POOLE, Pauline Marcia (retired) Fairy's Oak, 19 Pentre Close, Ashton, Chester CH3 8BR — MB BCh BAO Dub. 1950 (T.C. Dub.) Dip. Bact. Lond 1954; MA, MD Dub. 1961; FRCPath 1972, M 1963. Prev: Dir. Pub. Health Laborat. Chester.

POOLE, Rebecca Anne 5 The Budding, Stroud GL5 1XU Tel: 01453 759363 Email: rebecca.poole@bigfoot.com; 5 The Budding,, Stroud GL5 1XU Tel: 01453 759363 — MB ChB Ed. 1994 (Edinburgh) Specialty: Gen. Pract.

POOLE, Richard Roy Graydon Richardson Road Surgery, 56 Richardson Road, East Bergholt, Colchester CO7 6RR Tel: 01206 298272 Fax: 01206 299010; The Beeches, Gaston St, E. Bergholt, Colchester CO7 6SD — MB ChB Dundee 1973; BSc St. And. 1969; DObst RCOG 1975.

POOLE, Robert Godfree Mersey Care NHS Trust, Windsor House, 40 Upper Parliament Street, Liverpool L8 7LF Tel: 0151 250 5322 — MB BS Lond. 1980 (St. Geo. Hosp. Lond.) FRCPsych 1997, M 1984. Cons. Psychiat. N. Mersey Community (NHS) Trust; Hon. Clin. Lect. (Psychiat.) Univ. Liverp. Specialty: Gen. Psychiat. Prev: Sen. Regist. (Psychiat.) Oxf. RHA; Regist. (Psychiat.) St. Geo. Hosp. Lond.

POOLE, Robin Geoffrey 34 Selwyn Dr, Broadstairs CT10 2SW — MB ChB Birm. 1997.

POOLE, Simon Benedict Firs House Surgery, Station Road, Impington, Cambridge CB4 9NP Tel: 01223 234286 Fax: 01223 235931 — MB BS Lond. 1987.

POOLE, Mr Thomas Robert Guimaraes Frimley Park Hospital NHS Trust, Portsmouth Road GU16 7UJ — MB BS Lond. 1992 (St Mary's) BSc Lond. 1991; FRCOphth 1997. Cons. Ophth. Surg. Specialty: Ophth. Socs: Amer. Acad. of Ophth.; UKISCRS; ESCRS. Prev: Cornea, Extern. Dis., Cataract & Refractive Surg. Fell., Moorfields Eye Hosp.; Specialist Regist. Ophth. St Thomas Hosp. Lond.; Ophth. Kilimanjaro Christian Med. Centre Tanzania.

POOLE, Thomas Williams (retired) Conifers, 13 Wealden Way, Haywards Heath RH16 4AF Tel: 01444 450877 — LRCP LRCS Ed. 1945 (Anderson & St. Mungo's Colls. Glas.) LRCP&S Glas. 1945; MFOM RCP Lond. 1983. Prev: Chief Med. Off. P & O Steam Navigation Co.

POOLE-WILSON, Professor Philip Alexander National Heart & Lung Institute, Imperial College Faculty of Medicine, Dovehouse Street, London SW3 6LY Tel: 020 7351 8179 Fax: 020 7351 8113 Email: p.poole-wilson@imperial.ac.uk; 174 Burbage Road, Dulwich Village, London SE21 7AG Tel: 020 7274 6742 — (Camb. & St. Thos.) MB BChir Camb. 1968; MRCP (UK) 1970; MA Camb. 1991, BA 1969, MD 1975; FRCP Lond. 1983; FESC 1988; FACC 1992; F Med Sci 1998. Brit. Heart Foundat. Simon Marks Prof. of Cardiol.; Hon. Cons. Phys. Roy. Brompton Nat. Heart & Lung Hosp.; Simon Marks Brit. Heart Foundat. Prof. Cardiol. Nat. Heart & Lung Inst. Imperial Coll; Chair of Cardiovascular Science, Nat. Heart and Lung Inst. Specialty: Cardiol. Socs: (Pres.) Europ. Soc. Cardiol. 1994-1996; Pres. Elect World Heart Federat. 2003-2005; Counc. of the Roy. Coll. and Physicians 1997-2000. Prev: Lect. (Med.) St. Thos. Hosp. Lond.; Regist. St. Thos. Hosp. Lond.; SHO St. Thos., Brompton & Hammersmith Hosps. Lond.

POOLER, Alan Francis William Marshall (retired) 7 Priory Gardens, Old Basing, Basingstoke RG24 7DS Tel: 01256 462332; Orchard Farm, Stokeinteignhead, Newton Abbot TQ12 4QL Tel: 01626 872474 Email: coby.pooler@virgin.net — MB BS Lond. 1953 (St. Mary's) MRCS Eng. LRCP Lond. 1953; FCP(SA) 1968; MRCP (UK) 1972; FRCP Lond. 1982. Prev: Cons. Phys. (Geriat Med.) Basingstoke Dist. Hosp.

POOLEY, Andrew Stuart Department of Obstetrics and Gynaecology, Kingston Hospital, Galsworthy Road, Kingston upon Thames KT2 7QB Tel: 020 8546 7711 — MB BS Lond. 1987 (St. George's Hosp. Lond.) MRCOG 1993. Cons. (O & G) Kingston Healthcare Trust, Surrey. Specialty: Obst. & Gyn. Special Interest: Endometriosis; Minimal Access Surgery. Socs: BMA; Brit. Soc. CCP; RSM.

POOLEY, Mr Joseph 12 Darras Road, Ponteland, Newcastle upon Tyne NE20 9PA — MD Newc. 1983; MB BS 1971; FRCS Eng. 1977. Brit. Orthop. Research Soc. Pres. Medal 1982; Cons. & Sen. Lect. Orthop. Surg. Univ. Newc. upon Tyne. Specialty: Orthop. Prev: Sen. Regist. Orthop. Surg. North. RHA; Lect. (Orthop. Surg.) Univ. Newc. upon Tyne; Ho. Surg. & Ho. Phys. Roy. Vict. Infirm. Newc.

POOLEY, Simon Francis Lambert Medical Centre, 2 Chapel Street, Thirsk YO7 1LU Tel: 01845 523157 Fax: 01845 524508; Village Farm, Little Thirkleby, Thirkleby, Thirsk YO7 2AZ Tel: 01845 501539 — BM BS Nottm. 1981; BMedSci Nottm. 1979, BM BS 1981; DRCOG 1987; MRCGP 1987.

POOLOGANATHAN, Saravanamuthu Rush Green Medical Centre, 261 Dagenham Road, Romford RM7 0XR Tel: 01708 740730 Fax: 01708 725388 — MB BS Sri Lanka 1978; MRCS (Eng.); Dip Immediate Care RCS Ed. 1988; LRCP Lond. 1988; FRCS Ed. 1989. GP Princip. Prev: Dep. Doctor Health Call Ltd. Leigh-on-Sea.

POON, Choong Leng Royal Albert Edward Infirmary, Department of Radiology, Wigan Lane, Wigan WN1 2NN Tel: 01942 822407 Fax: 01942 822402 Email: Choong.Poon@wwl.nhs.uk — MB ChB Manch. 1984; BSc St. And. 1981; MRCP (UK) 1990; FRCR 1994. Cons. Radiol. Roy. Albert Edw. Infirm. Wigan. Specialty: Radiol. Socs: Brit. Soc. Interven. Radiol.; Radiol. Soc. N. Amer.; Cardiovasc. & Interven. Radiol. Soc. Europe. Prev: Sen. Regist. & Regist (Diagn. Radiol.) N. West. RHA; Regist. (Gen. Med. & Diabetol.) Wythenshawe Hosp. Manch.; Regist. & SHO (Gen. Med.) Stepping Hill Hosp. Stockport.

POON, Fat Wui Glasgow Royal Infirmary, Glasgow G4 0SF; 60 Colonsay Drive, Newton Mearns, Glasgow G77 6TY — MB ChB (Commend.) Aberd. 1979; FRCS Glas. 1984; FRCR 1988; MBA 1996. Specialty: Radiol.

POON, Jasmine Hei-Wan 38 Heron Drive, Lenton, Nottingham NG7 2DE — BM BS Nottm. 1998.

POON, Karen — BM BS Nottm. 1998.

POON, Pui Yee Alice Anaesthetic Department, Harrogate District Hospital, Harrogate HG2 7SX — MB ChB Leeds 1986; DA (UK) 1988; FRCA 1998. Cons. Anaesth. Specialty: Anaesth. Socs: Fell. Roy. Coll. Anaesths.; Obst. Anaesth.s Assn. Prev: Specialist Regist. (Anaesth.) S. Thames W. Region.

POONAWALA, Mr Shabbir Saleh Royal Liverpool University Hospital, Prescot Street, Liverpool L7 8XP Tel: 0151 7063452 Email: shabbirsp@hotmail.com — MB BS Bombay 1985 (Grant Medical College, Bombay) FRCS Glas. 1992. Specialty: Gen. Surg.

POONI, Jagtar Singh Royal Wolverhampton NHS Trust, Wednesfield, Wolverhampton Tel: 01902 307999 — MB ChB Manch. 1986; BSc (Hons) Manch. 1983; MRCP (UK) 1990; FRCA 1993; FRCP 2003. Cons. Anaesth. & Intens. Care Med. Specialty: Anaesth. Special Interest: Intens. Care. Socs: Assn. Anaesth.; Gp. Anaesth. in Train. (GAT Comm.). Prev: Regist. (Anaesth.) N. Staffs. NHS Trust Stoke-on-Trent, Princess Roy. Hosp. Telford & Roy. Shrewsbury Hosp.; SHO (Anaesth.) Countess of Chester Hosp.; SHO (A & E) Hope Hosp, Salford.

POOR, Stephen Hedrick 1st Floor Flat, 36 Rainville Road, London W6 9HA — MB BS Lond. 1996.

POORE, Peter David Reading Green Farm House, Denham, Eye IP21 5DH — MB BS Lond. 1964; DCH RCP Lond. 1970; DTM & H Liverp. 1978.

POORNAN, Annamalai Mudaliar Cauveri, Springhill Lane, Lower Penn, Wolverhampton WV4 Tel: 01902 34821 — MB BS Madras 1949 (Madras Med. Coll.) Prev: Ho. Off. Govt. Gen. Hosp. Madras; Med. Off. IAMC; SHO Childr. Hosp. Nottm.

POOTS, David Frederick John 8 St Michael's Road, Farnborough GU14 8NE — MB BS Lond. 1987.

POOTS, Eileen Dorothy Miriam Helena (retired) 4 Abercorn Park, Hillsborough BT26 6HA Tel: 028 9268 2024 — MB BCh BAO Belf. 1948 (Qu. Univ. Belf.) Prev: Regist. Perivale Matern. Hosp. Middlx.

POOTS, Gwendoline Gladys Lowry Kilsorrel, Rew Lane, Summersdale, Chichester PO19 5QH — MB BCh BAO Dub. 1949.

POOTS, Samuel James Staines Health Centre, Knowle Green, Kingston Road, Staines TW18 1AJ — MB BCh BAO Dub. 1946 (TC Dub.)

POOTS, Stephen Allan Mourne Family Surgery, Mourne Hospital, Newry Street, Newry BT34 4DN — MB BCh BAO Belf. 1981; DRCOG 1983; MRCGP 1985.

POPAT, Jayantilal Thakarshi Station Road Surgery, 42 Station Road, London NW4 3SU Tel: 020 8202 3733 Fax: 020 8203 8096 — MB BS Baroda 1969. Socs: BMA.

POPAT, Ramniklal Thakarshi Tynemouth Medical Practice, 24 Tynemouth Road, Tottenham, London N15 4RH Tel: 020 8275 4062 Fax: 020 8275 4120 — MB BS Baroda 1972.

POPAT, Sanjaykumar Batuklal Institute of Cancer Research, Haddow Laboratories, 15 Cotswold Road, Sutton SM2 5NG Tel: 020 8722 4113 Fax: 020 8643 0257 — MB BS Lond. 1994 (United Medical and Dental Schools) BSc (Hons.) Lond. 1991; MB BS (Hons.) Lond. 1994; MRCP (UK) 1997. Clin. Res. Fell. (Cancer Genetics) Inst. Of Cancer Res./ Roy. Marsden NHS Trust, Sutton. Specialty: Oncol.; Gen. Med.; Genetics. Prev: SHO (Gen. Med.) Lewisham Hosp.; SHO (Med. Oncol.) Roy. Masden Hosp.; SHO (Chest/ICU) Roy. Brompton Hosp.

POPAT, Uday Rameshchandra 10 Glebe Road, Finchley, London N3 2AX — MB BS Bombay 1986; MRCP (UK) 1991.

POPAT-HADDEN, Alpha Olympia — MB ChB Aberd. 1988; FRCS Edin. 1995. Specialty: Plastic Surg.

POPE, Mr Alvan John, TD Hillingdon Hospital, Pield Heath Road, Uxbridge UB8 3NN Tel: 01895 279698 Fax: 01895 279890 Email: alvan.pope@thh.nhs.uk; Yarra House, 73 Camp Road, Gerrards Cross SL9 7PF Tel: 01753 893068 Email: ajpope@compuserve.com — MB BS Lond. 1980 (Middlx.) BSc Lond. 1977; FRCS Eng. 1985; MD Lond. 1992; FRCS (Urol.) 1994. Cons. Urol. Char. Cross & Hillingdon Hosps. Specialty: Urol. Socs: Brit. Assn. Urol. Surg. Prev: Sen. Regist. (Urol.) St. Peters Hosp. Lond.; Research Regist. Inst. Urol. Lond.; RSO St. Peter's Hosps. Lond.

POPE, Mr David Charles Quarter Jack Surgery, Rodways Corner, Wimborne BH21 1AP Tel: 01202 882112 Fax: 01202 882368; Huish House, Winterborne Zelston, Blandford Forum DT11 9ES Tel: 01929 459461 — MB BS Lond. 1967 (St. Bart.) MRCS Eng. LRCP Lond. 1967; FRCS Eng. 1972. Clin. Dir. & Surg. Off. Vict. Hosp. Wimborne. Specialty: Gen. Surg. Socs: (Comm.) Community Hosp. Assn. Prev: Regist. (Surg.) Poole Gen. Hosp. & St. Bart. Hosp. Lond.; Resid. Surg. Off. (Thoracic Surg.) Brompton Hosp. Lond.

POPE, David Graham La Solaize, Rue Du Craslin, St Peter, Jersey JE3 7YN Tel: 01534 36301 — MB ChB Bristol 1970. Prev: SHO Obst. Bristol Matern. Hosp.

POPE, Dean Granville West End Medical Practice, 21 Chester Street, Edinburgh EH3 7RF Tel: 0131 225 5220 Fax: 0131 226 1910; 10d Abbotsford Crescent, Edinburgh EH4 5DY Tel: 0131 332 8480 — MB ChB Ed. 1986; DRCOG 1990; MRCGP 1990. Prev: Trainee GP Cumbria VTS.

POPE, Professor Francis Michael Division of Life Sciences, King's College London, Franklin Wilkins Building, 150 Stamford Street, London SE1 9NN; 91 Marsh Road, Pinner HA5 5PA — MB BCh Wales 1963 (Welsh Nat. Sch. Med.) FRCP Glas. 1981, M 1967; FRCP Lond. 1981, M 1968; MRCP Ed. 1968; MD Wales 1974; FRCP Ed. 1994. Cons. Dermatol. W. Middlx. Univ. Hosp.& Chelsea & Westm. Hosp. (Nov 2001); Hon. Cons. Clin. Genetics Inst. Med. Genetics UHW Cardiff; Vis. Prof. Connective Tissue Matrix Genetics, Kings Coll. Lond.; Hon. Head Connective Tissue Genetics Gp. Div. Life Sci. Kings Coll. Lond. (Nov 2001). Specialty: Dermat.; Genetics. Socs: Assn. Phys.; Brit. Assn. Dermat.; Amer. Soc. of Human Genetics. Prev: Hon. Cons. Clin. Genetics Addenbrooke's Hosp. Camb.; Hon. Cons. Phys. Div. of Clin. Sci. & MRC Clin. Research

Centre & Northwick Pk. Hosp.; Hon. Sen. Lect. & Cons. Dermat. Inst. Dermat. & St. John's Hosp. Dis. Skin. Lond.

POPE, Mr Ian Michael 16 Merlin Gardens, Brickhill, Bedford MK41 7HL — BM BCh Oxf. 1991; BA (Hons.) Camb. 1988; FRCS Ed. 1995. Specialist Regist. (Gen. Surg.) S. E. Scot. Higher Surg. Train. Rotat. Edin. Specialty: Gen. Surg. Socs: Brit. Assn. Surg. Oncol. Prev: Research Fell. (Surg.) Univ. Liverp.; SHO (Gen. Surg.) Roy. Liverp. Univ. Hosp.

POPE, Isabel Joy Kildonan House, Ramsbottom Road, Horwich, Bolton BL6 5NW Tel: 01204 468161 Fax: 01204 698186; 10 Ansdell Road, Horwich, Bolton BL6 7HL — MB ChB Manch. 1979; DRCOG 1981; DTM & H Liverp. 1985; DCH RCPS Glas. 1985; MRCGP 1985.

POPE, Joanna Brownfield Wyndhams, Quarry Lane, Chicksgrove, Tisbury, Salisbury SP3 6LY — MB ChB Ed. 1996.

POPE, John Alfred ffitch Essex Way Surgery, 34 Essex Way, Benfleet SS7 1LT Tel: 01268 792203 Fax: 01268 759495 — MB BS Lond. 1960 (St. Bart.) DObst RCOG 1962.

POPE, John David Kitson The Monklands, Seafield Road, Bilston EH25 9RP Tel: 0131 440 2399 Email: jdkpope@yahoo.co.uk — MB ChB St. And. 1965 (Dundee) FFA RCS Eng. 1972; DA Eng. 1972. Specialty: Anaesth.

POPE, Laysan Edward Roy 18 Bury Street, Norwich NR2 2DN — MB BS Lond. 1996.

POPE, Mark Edward 59 Sunray Avenue, London SE24 9PX — MB BS Lond. 1994.

POPE, Mary Halcyon Meredith Marcham Health Centre, Marcham Road, Abingdon OX14 1BT Tel: 01235 522602; 16 Bostock Road, Abingdon OX14 1DW Tel: 01235 532120 — BM BCh Oxf. 1990; MRCGP 1995. Specialty: Gen. Pract. Prev: Trainee GP Abingdon; SHO (O & G) Princess Margt. Hosp. Swindon.

POPE, Rachel Trixie Herschel Medical Centre, 45 Osborne Street, Slough SL1 1TT — MB BS Lond. 1984 (Middlx. Hosp.) DCH RCP Lond. 1986; DRCOG 1987; MRCGP 1988. Prev: GP Lond.; Clin. Med. Off. W. Lambeth HA; Trainee GP/SHO Qu. Eliz. II Hosp. Welwyn Gdn. City VTS.

POPE, Richard Martin Airedale General Hospital, Skipton Road, Steeton, Keighley BD20 6TD Tel: 01535 652511 — MB BCh Wales 1981; MD Wales 1990; FRCP 1997. Medical Director, Cons. Phys. (Diabetes & Endocrinol.) Airedale Gen. Hosp. Specialty: Endocrinol. Prev: Lect. (Med.) Univ. Leeds; MRC Train. Fell. King's Coll. Hosp. Lond. & Cardiff HA.

POPE, Romney Jane Elliott 2 Bradiston Road, London W9 3HN — MB BS Lond. 1994.

POPE, Mr Stephen John 53 Disraeli Road, Ealing, London W5 5HS — MB BS Lond. 1989 (London Hospital Medical College) BSc (Hons.) Lond. 1986; FRCSI 1993; FRCS Eng. 1994; FRCS (Tr & Orth) 1998. Specialty: Orthop.

POPE, Stephen Paul The Bishop's Cottage, Church Hill, Crayke, York YO61 4TA — MB ChB Liverp. 1973; FFA RCS Eng. 1980; MRCGP 1988; DRCOG 1988; T(GP) 1991. GP Asst. (p/t) Derwent Surg. Multon. Prev: Staff Phys. (Palliat. Med.) St. Gemma's Hospice Leeds; GP Benfleet; Regist. (Anaesth.) Broadgreen Hosp. Liverp.

POPE, Miss Vanessa 28 Carrwood Road, Wilmslow SK9 5DL — MB BS Lond. 1993 (Univ. Coll. & Middlx. Lond.) BSc (Hons.) Lond. 1990; FRCS Eng. 1997. Specialist Regist. Gen. Surg., Manch. Specialty: Gen. Surg. Prev: Sen. SHO (Surg.) Bolton; Sen. SHO (Surg.) Shrewsbury; SHO Rotat. (Surg.) Leic.

POPELY, Claire Sarah 14 Harrod Dr, Southport PR8 2HA — MB BS Newc. 1997.

POPERT, John Bransford House, Bransford, Worcester WR6 5JL Tel: 01886 832373 — MB BS Lond. 1948 (St. Bart.) FRCP Lond. 1973, M 1956; MD Lond. 1962. Hon. Cons. Phys. Worcester Roy. Infirm.; Hon. Cons. Rheum. Roy. Orthop. Hosp.Birm. Specialty: Rehabil. Med.; Rheumatol. Socs: Brit. Soc. Rheum.; Midl.s Rheum. Soc. Prev: Lect. & Asst. Dir. Clin. Sect. Rheum. Research Clinic Manch. Univ.; Hon. Cons. Phys. Manch. Roy. Infirm.

POPERT, Mr Richard John Mackay Peter Department of Urology, King's College Hospital, Denmark Hill, London SE5 Tel: 020 7274 6222; Flat 1, 22 Grove Park, Camberwell, London SE5 8LH Tel: 020 7733 4859 — MB BS Lond. 1985; FRCS Eng. 1989; FRCS Ed. 1989. Research Regist. (Urol.) King's Coll. Hosp. Lond. Specialty: Urol. Socs: Fell. Roy. Soc. Med.; Assoc. Mem. BAUS. Prev: Regist. (Urol.) King's Coll. Hosp. Lond.; Regist. (Gen. Surg.) Qu. Alexandra Hosp. Portsmouth; Demonst. (Anat.) Camb. Univ.

POPERT, Sheila Jane Bransford House, Bransford Court Lane, Bransford, Worcester WR6 5JL Tel: 01886 832373 — MRCS Eng. LRCP Lond. 1985; BDS (Hons.) Lond. 1980. Cons. (Palliat. Medicine) St Richards Hospice Worcester; Cons. (Palliat. Medicine) Worcester Roy. Hosp. Specialty: Palliat. Med. Prev: Med. Dir. St. Raphael's Hospice Sutton.; Cons. (Palliat. Med.) St. Christopher's Hospice, Sydenham; Cons. (Pall. Med.) Mayday Univ. Hosp. Croydon.

POPHAM, Carolyn Mary 25 Grosvenor Crescent Mews, London SW1X 7EX Email: carpop@btopenworld.com — BM (Hons.) Soton. 1978.

POPHAM, Philip Andrew Bryan Dept of Anaesthesia, Addenbrookes' Hospital, Hills Road, Cambridge CB2 2QQ — MB BS Lond. 1982; FFA RCS 1987; BSc (Hons.) Lond. 1979, MD 1992. Cons. Anaesth. Addenbrooke's Hosp. Camb. Specialty: Anaesth. Socs: BMA; (Treas.) E. Anglian Obst. Anaesth. Gp.; Assn. Anaesth. Prev: Staff Specialist (Anaesth.) Roy. Woms. Hosp. Melbourne, Austral.; Sen. Regist. (Anaesth.) Addenbrooke's Hosp. Camb.; Sir Jules Thorn Research Fell. (Physiol.) St. Thos. Hosp. Lond.

POPLAR, Christopher Charles Edward 36 Bowers Park Drive, Woolwell, Plymouth PL6 7SK Email: popsincycle@yahoo.co.uk — BM Soton. 1997; DRCOG 2003.

POPLE, Andrew Robert Wordsworth Health Centre, 19 Wordsworth Avenue, Manor Park, London E12 6SU Tel: 020 8548 5960 Fax: 020 8548 5983; 8 The Vale, Woodford Green IG8 9BT — MB BS Lond. 1986. Prev: SHO (Psychiat.) Goodmayes Hosp.; SHO (O & G & A & E) Newham Gen. Hosp.; SHO (Paediat.) Newham Gen. Hosp.

POPLE, Mr Ian Kenneth Frenchay Hospital, Frenchay Park Road, Frenchay, Bristol BS16 1LE Tel: 0117 975 3960 Email: ikpople@hotmail.com; 49A Shirehampton Road, Stoke Bishop, Bristol BS9 2DN Tel: 0117 968 7026 — MB ChB Sheff. 1983; FRCS Eng. 1987; ECFMG Cert. 1992; MD Sheff. 1992; FRCS (SN) 1993; Fell Paedc Neurosurg Univ Tennessee USA 1995. Cons. Neurosurg. Frenchay Hosp. Bristol. Specialty: Neurosurg. Socs: Soc. Brit. Neurolog. Surg.; Soc. for Research into Hydrocephalus & Spina Bifida; Brit. Paediat. Neurosurg. Gp. Prev: Sen. Registar & Registar (Neurosurg.) Frenchay Hosp. Bristol; Registar (Neurosurg.) Hosp. Sick Childr. Gt. Ormond St. Lond.; SHO (Neurosurg.) Leeds Gen. Infirm.

POPLETT, Neil David Charing Surgery, Charing, Ashford TN27 0HZ Tel: 01233 714141 Fax: 01233 713782 — MB BS Lond. 1990 (Univ. Lond.) DRCOG 1993 or 94; BSc Lond. 1987, MB BS 1990; MRCGP 1995. SHO (O & G) Pembury Hosp. Tonbridge. Prev: SHO (A & E) Kent & Canterbury Hosps.; SHO (Geriat. & Paediat.) William Harvey Hosp. Ashford; Ho. Off. (Med. & Surg.) Maidstone Hosp. Kent.

POPLI, Sanjeev c/o Mapledown, Little Windmill Hill, Chipperfield, Kings Langley WD4 9DG — MB ChB Liverp. 1991; DRCOG 1996. Specialty: Gen. Pract.

POPOV, Alain 39 Berwick Chase, Peterlee SR8 1NQ — MB ChB Manch. 1997.

POPOVIC, Sara Brighton House, 14 Droitwich Road, Worcester WR3 7LJ — MB BS Lond. 1991.

POPPER, Stefan Leopold 8 Colwick Park Close, Colwick, Nottingham NG4 2DZ Tel: 0115 987 9002 — BM BS Nottm. 1981; BMedSci Nottm. 1979, BM BS 1981.

POPPLE, Anthony Willis Green Head House, 37 The Green, Dalston, Carlisle CA5 7QD — MB BS Lond. 1969; BSc, MB BS Lond. 1969; MRCPath 1978. Cons. (Histopath.) Cumbld. Infirm. Carlisle. Specialty: Histopath.

POPPLE, Mark David Hollies Medical Practice, Tamworth Health Centre, Upper Gungate, Tamworth B79 7EA Tel: 01827 68511 Fax: 01827 51163; Wigginton Lodge, Wigginton Road, Tamworth B79 8RH Tel: 01827 62808 — MB BS Lond. 1982. Prev: Regist. (A & E) Derbysh. Roy. Infirm.; Trainee GP Tamworth.

POPPLESTONE, Gaynor Anne Swallowfield Medical Practice, Swallowfield RG7 1QY — MB ChB Liverp. 1986 (Liverpool) DCH RCP Lond. 1994; MRCGP 1995. Gen. Practitioner, Swallowfield Med. Pract.

POPPLESTONE, Mark — MB ChB Liverp. 1983; MB ChB Liverpool 1983; AFOM RCP Lond 1992; MFOM (RCP) London 1998. Cons.

Occupat. Phys. Brit. Airways. Specialty: Occupat. Health. Prev: Occupat. Phys., Nestlé Rowntree, York; Med. Off. Brit. Steel Scunthorpe.

POPPLETON, John Frank (retired) 6 Graham Close, Paradise, Scarborough YO11 1RU Tel: 01723 373143 — MB ChB Leeds 1955; AFOM RCP Lond. 1983. Prev: Occupat. Phys. McCain Foods (GB) plc.

POPPLEWELL, Julie Ann Coppers, Temple Grafton, Alcester B49 6NR — MB ChB Birm. 1975; DRCOG 1978.

POPPLEWELL, Martin Coppers, Temple Grafton, Alcester B49 6NR — MB ChB Birm. 1975; DRCOG 1978; DA Eng. 1980.

PORCHERET, Mark Ernest Paul The John Kelso Practice, Park Medical Centre, Ball Haye Road, Leek ST13 6QR Tel: 01538 399007 Fax: 01538 370014 — MB BS Lond. 1978; DCH RCP Lond. 1982; DRCOG 1983; FRCGP 2001.

PORCHEROT, Roger Charles Crahamel Medical Practice, Crahamel House, 1 Duhamel Place, St Helier JE2 4TP; Le Flieurion, Rue de L'Eglise, St John, Jersey JE3 4BA Tel: 01534 864625 Fax: 01534 864834 — MB BS Lond. 1967 (St Bart.) MRCS Eng. LRCP Lond. 1967; BA O.U. 1997. Prev: Ho. Surg. St. Bart. Hosp. Lond.; Ho. Phys. Brook Hosp. Lond.; Ho. Surg. Woolwich Memor. Hosp.

PORCZYNSKA, Krystyna Regina 4 Thomas Telford Basin, Piccadilly Village, Manchester M1 2NH — MB ChB Manch. 1989. Clin. Asst. (Haemat.) Bolton Gen. Hosp. Specialty: Haematology.

PORCZYNSKA, Wladyslawa Irena 24 Argyle Road, Wolverhampton WV2 4NY — MB ChB Manch. 1987.

PORE, Padmaja Suhas 7 Kernel Close, Littleover, Derby DE23 3SA — MB BS Bombay 1977; MRCPI 1995.

POROOHAN, Rowshanak — MB ChB Sheff. 1998.

PORRITT, Andrea Janice 110 Hazelhurst Road, Worsley, Manchester M28 2SP — MB ChB Ed. 1989.

PORRU, Daniele Department of Urology, Gartnavel General Hospital, 1053 Great Western Road, Glasgow G12 0YN — State DMS Cagliari 1992; T(S) 1994.

***PORT, Ann** 30 Sandmoor Green, Leeds LS17 7SB — MB BCh Wales 1985.

PORTANIER, John (retired) 10 Vivian House, Seven Sisters Road, London N4 1QZ Tel: 020 7503 9836 — LM Rotunda 1938; PhC Malta 1933, MD 1937.

PORTAS, Charles David Wrington Vale Medical Practice, Station Road, Wrington, Bristol BS40 5NG Tel: 01934 862532 Fax: 01934 863568 — BSc Wales 1977; MB BCh 1984; DRCOG 1987; DCH RCP Lond. 1987; MRCGP 1988. GP Bristol. Prev: Trainee GP Dept. Gen. Pract. Univ. Wales Coll. of Med. Cardiff; SHO (Paediat.) Gwent HA; SHO (O & G & Geriat. Med.) S. Glam. HA.

PORTAS-DOMINGUEZ, Luis-Carlos 8 College Road, London SW19 2BS — State Exam Med. Tubingen 1990.

PORTCH, Hilary Ruth Royal Cornwall Hospital NHS Trust, Truro TR1 3LJ Tel: 01872 250000 — BM Soton. 1988; DRCOG 1993; DFFP 1995; MRCGP 1996. Staff Grade Cardiol., Roy. Cornw. Hosp. Specialty: Gen. Pract.; Cardiol. Socs: Brit. Soc. Of Endocardiography; Brit. Med. Assn.; Primary Care Cardiovasc. Soc. Prev: Clin. Asst. (Cardiol.); Clin. Asst. Cardiol., Brit. Roy. Infirm.

PORTE, Aileen McKenzie 3 Crosshill Road, Strathaven ML10 6DS Tel: 01357 522464 — MB ChB Glas. 1990; MRCGP 1994. Prev: Trainee GP Lanarksh.

PORTE, Mr Hubert Eran (retired) Springwood Cottage, Shenmore, Madley, Hereford HR2 9NX Tel: 01981 250561 — MB ChB Manch. 1960; FRCS Ed. 1964; DLO Eng. 1967. Prev: Cons. ENT Surg. Lincs AHA.

PORTE, Mr Michael Eran 179 Mountview Road, Stroud Green, London N4 4JT — MB BS Lond. 1982; BSc Lond. 1979, MB BS 1982; FRCS Eng. 1986.

PORTELLY, John Edward (retired) 169 Coombe Lane, West Wimbledon, London SW20 0QX Tel: 020 8946 7006 — MB BChir Camb. 1957 (St. Bart. & W. Lond. Hosp.) MA Camb. 1952; LMSSA Lond. 1952. Prev: SHO (Surg.) S. Devon & E. Cornw. Hosp.

PORTELLY, John Patrick The Ross Practice, Keats House, Bush Fair, Harlow CM18 6LY Tel: 01279 692747 Fax: 01279 692737 — MB BS Lond. 1982 (Royal London Hospital) MRCGP 1986; DRCOG 1986. Gen. Practitioner. Specialty: Paediat. Socs: BMA. Prev: Trainee GP Harold Wood Hosp. VTS.

PORTEOUS, Alexander Calvert (retired) Quantocks, 81 Church Road, Ryde PO33 4PZ Tel: 01983 882840 — MB BS Lond. 1947 (St. Mary's) MRCS Eng. LRCP Lond. 1942. Prev: Postgrad. Regist. (Med.) St. Mary's Hosp.

PORTEOUS, Mr Colin Royal Alexander Hospital, Corsebow Road, Paisley Tel: 01415 804 518 Fax: 01415 804 572 — MB ChB Aberd. 1980; FRCS Glas.; MD Aberd. Specialty: Gen. Surg. Special Interest: Colorectal. Socs: The Assn. of Coloproctology of Gt. Britain and Irel.; The Assn. of Surg. of Gt. Britain and Irel.

PORTEOUS, Colin Ross (retired) The Glebe, 200 Prescot Road, Aughton, Ormskirk L39 5AG Tel: 0695 423771; The Glebe, 200 Prescot Road, Aughton, Ormskirk L39 5AG Tel: 0695 423771 — MB ChB Liverp. 1953; FRCOG 1975, M 1961, DObst 1958. Cons. O & G Ormskirk & Dist. Gen. Hosp. Prev: Lect. Obst. Univ. Liverp.

PORTEOUS, David John Fishponds Health Centre, Beechwood Road, Fishponds, Bristol BS16 3TD Tel: 0117 908 2365 Fax: 0117 908 2377; 10 Marlfield, Pensby, Wirral CH61 1AJ — MB BS Lond. 1991; BSc (Hons) Lond. 1988.

PORTEOUS, Elizabeth Mary Ellen 16 Overton Drive, West Kilbride KA23 9LH Tel: 01294 823134 — MB ChB Ed. 1977.

PORTEOUS, George Alexander Lockerbie Medical Practice, Victoria Gardens, Lockerbie DG11 2BJ Tel: 01576 203665 Fax: 01576 202773; Janalla, Cargenbridge, Dumfries DG2 8LW Tel: 01387 264042 — MB ChB Glas. 1990 (University of Glasgow) Specialty: Gen. Pract.

PORTEOUS, Gordon Sloane 16 Overton Drive, West Kilbride KA23 9LH Tel: 01294 823134 — MB ChB Ed. 1976. GP Ardrossan.

PORTEOUS, Ian Brenton (retired) 79 Woodlands Road, Shotley Bridge, Consett DH8 0DT Tel: 01207 503063 — MB BS Durh. 1952; DPath Eng. 1961; MRCPath 1964. Prev: Cons. Path. NW Durh. Hosp. Gp.

PORTEOUS, Jean Margaret (retired) 140 Hamilton Place, Aberdeen AB15 5BB Tel: 01224 50110 — MB ChB Liverp. 1949. Med. Off. N.E. Scotl. Transfus. Centre Aberd. Prev: Ho. Phys. & Ho. Surg. Vict. Hosp. Burnley.

PORTEOUS, John Patrick Joseph Littlemount Lodge, Maguiresbridge, Enniskillen BT94 4RS Tel: 013655 31876 — MB BCh BAO Belf. 1984; DGM RCP Lond. 1986. Primary Care Cons. Gen. Pract. Drumham Health Centre Lisnaskea. Socs: W.ern Local Med. Comm.; Centr. Serv.s Agency Med. Comm. (Mem.); W.ern Area Med. Adv. Comm. (Vice Chairm.). Prev: SHO (O & G) Route Hosp. Ballymoney; SHO (Med.) Altnagelvin Area Hosp. Londonderry; SHO (Psychiat.) Tyrone & Fermanagh Hosp. Omagh.

PORTEOUS, Lorna Anderson 6 Denecroft, Wylam NE41 8DE — MB ChB Ed. 1987; DCH RCP Lond. 1990; MRCGP 1991; DRCOG 1991.

PORTEOUS, Margaret Ann Eastham Group Practice, Treetops PHCC, Bridle Road, Bromborough, Wirral CH62 6EE — MB ChB Ed. 1983; MRCGP 1988.

PORTEOUS, Mary Elizabeth Muir Clinical Genetics Service, Western General Hospital, Crewe Road, Edinburgh EH4 2XU Tel: 0131 651 1012 Fax: 0131 651 1013 Email: mary.porteous@ed.ac.uk — MB ChB Manch. 1983; MSc Clin. Genetics Glas. 1988; MRCP (UK) 1989; MD Manch. 1992; FRCP Ed 1999. Cons. Clin. Geneticist Western Gen. Hosp. Edin.; Sen. Lect. (Clin. Genetics) Univ. Edin. Specialty: Genetics.

PORTEOUS, Mr Matthew John Le Fanu West Suffolk Hospital, Hardwick Lane, Bury St Edmunds IP33 2QZ Tel: 01284 713334 Email: matthew.porteous@wsh.nhs.uk — MB BS Lond. 1982 (London Hospital) FRCS Eng. 1986; FRCS (Orth.) 1992. Cons. (Orthop. Surg.) W. Suff. Hosp. Bury St Edmunds. Specialty: Trauma & Orthop. Surg. Socs: Fell. BOA; Brit. Hip Soc.; AOUK. Prev: Cons. (Orthop. Surg.) King's Coll. Hosp. Lond.

PORTEOUS, Michael Belgrave Medical Centre, 22 Asline Road, Sheffield S2 4UJ Tel: 0114 255 1184 — MB ChB Sheff. 1964; DObst RCOG 1968.

PORTEOUS, Myfanwy Rhiwen Hughes The Glebe, 200 Prescot Road, Aughton, Ormskirk L39 5AG — MB ChB Liverp. 1949; DPH 1956.

PORTEOUS, Patrick Joseph (retired) Castlebalfour, Lisnaskea, Enniskillen BT92 0LT Tel: 028 6772 1800 — MB BCh BAO NUI 1947 (Univ. Coll. Dub.) FRCGP 1982, M 1961. Prev: Med. Off. Gen. Med. Servs. Bd. Dub.

PORTEOUS, Robert (retired) 4 Merchants Quay, Bristol BS1 4RL — MB BS Lond. 1955 (Middlx.) FFA RCS Eng. 1961. Prev: Cons. Anaesth. Swindon & MarlBoro. NHS Trust.

***PORTER-BROWN, Benjamin Gareth** 19 Cheriton Place, Westbury-on-Trym, Bristol BS9 4AW — MB BS Lond. 1998; MB BS Lond 1998.

PORTER, Ada Margaret Grange Road Surgery, Dudley DY1 2AW Tel: 01384 255387/252095 Fax: 01384 242109; 17 Foley Road, Pedmore, Stourbridge DY9 0RT — MB ChB Birm. 1958; DObst RCOG 1961.

PORTER, Alan Newtown Surgery, Park Street, Newtown SY16 1EF Tel: 01686 626221/626224 Fax: 01686 622610 — MB ChB Glas. 1982.

PORTER, Alan Michael Woodward (retired) Redcrest, Heath Rise, Camberley GU15 2ER Email: aporter@talk21.com — MB BS Lond. 1954 (St. Thos.) MD Lond. 1968; PhD Lond. 1996.

PORTER, Alexandra Fiona 9 Heol Y Brenin, Penarth CF64 3HR Tel: 029 2035 0123 Email: fiporter@aol.com — MB BCh Wales 1997. GP Regist. Bridgend S. Wales. Specialty: Gen. Pract.

PORTER, Amber Durdana Woolsthorpe Surgery, Main Street, Woolsthorpe, By Belvoir, Grantham NG32 1LX Tel: 01476 870166 Fax: 01476 870560 — MB BS Punjab 1968 (Fatima Jinnah Med. Coll. Lahore) MB BS Punjab (Pakistan) 1968; DCH Eng. 1972.

PORTER, Andrew John Carlton Street Surgery, Carlton Street, Horninglow, Burton-on-Trent DE13 0TE Tel: 01283 511387 Fax: 01283 517174; 181 Horninglow Street, Burton-on-Trent DE14 1NU Tel: 01283 63561 — MB BS Lond. 1974.

PORTER, Andrew John 6 Abbey Crescent, Beauchief, Sheffield S7 2QX — MB BS Newc. 1996.

PORTER, Anita — MB BS Lond. 1991 (St. Geo. Hosp.) DRCORG 1995; MRCGP Lond. 1999. Salaried GP. Specialty: Gen. Pract.

PORTER, Barbara Helen Temple Cowley Health Centre, Templar House, Temple Road, Oxford OX4 2HL Tel: 01865 777024 Fax: 01865 777548; Green Glades, 3 bayswater farm Road, Headington, Oxford OX3 8BX — MB ChB Ed. 1987; MRCGP 1996. Gen. Practitioner Temple Cowley Med. Gp., Oxf. Specialty: Diabetes. Socs: BMA; Christian Med. Fell.ship; Med. Wom.s Federat., Treas., Oxf. Br. Prev: Trainee GP Edin.; SHO (O & G) East. Gen. Hosp. Edin.; SHO (Geriat.) Roy. Vict. Hosp. Edin.

PORTER, Mr Bertram Butterworth (retired) Glebe House, Tweedsmuir, Biggar ML12 6QP Tel: 01899 880204 — MB ChB (Hnrs.) Ed. 1958 (Ed.) FRCS Eng. 1963. Med. Mem. Appeals Serv.s (Scotl. Region). Prev: on Scientif. Staff MRC Clin. Research Centre Harrow & Hon. Cons.

PORTER, Bryan John Guardian Medical Centre, Guardian St., Warrington WA5 1UD Tel: 01925 650226 — MB ChB Sheff. 1959; DTM & H Eng. 1962; DObst RCOG 1966.

PORTER, Charles Andrew 18 Chequers Park, Wye, Ashford TN25 5BB — MB BS Lond. 1961 (Middlx.) MRCS Eng. LRCP Lond. 1961; DObst RCOG 1963; MRCP Lond. 1969. Cons. Paediat. S.E. Kent, & Canterbury & Thanet Health Dist. Specialty: Paediat. Prev: Resid. (Paediat.) Bellevue Hosp. New York City; Regist. Renal Unit Roy. Sussex Hosp. Brighton; Ho. Surg. Whittington Hosp. Lond.

PORTER, Charlotte Lawson House, Sawley, Clitheroe BB7 4NJ — MB BS Lond. 1988.

PORTER, Clement Ian (retired) Elm Cottage, Little Burstead, Billericay CM12 9TJ Tel: 01277 623054 — MRCS Eng. LRCP Lond. 1960. Prev: GP Billericay.

PORTER, Crispin Jon, Maj. The Royal Bristol Hospital for Children, Paul O'Gorman Building, Upper Maudlin Street, Bristol BS2 8BJ — MB ChB Dundee 1994. Specialist Regist. Paediatric Ememrgency Med. Specialty: Accid. & Emerg. Socs: BASICS; BAEM; BAETA. Prev: RMO Belf.; RMO Cyprus; SHO (Med.) Frimley Pk.

PORTER, Mr Daniel Edward Department of Orthopaedic Surgery, New Royal Infirmary of Edinburgh, Little France, Edinburgh EH16 4SN Tel: 0131 242 3508 — MB ChB Ed. 1989; BSc Ed. 1987; FRCS Ed. 1994; MD Ed. 1995; FRCS Glas. 1995; FRCS (Tr + Orth) 2000. Snr Lect. & Hon. Cons. (Orthop. Surg.) Ed. Infirm. Specialty: Orthop. Prev: Regist. (Orthop.) Lothian HB.; Research Fell. (Surg.) MRC Unit of Human Genetics West. Gen. Hosp. Edin.; Clin. Lect. (Orthop. Surg.) Univ. Oxf.

PORTER, David CCVTM, Churchill Hospital, Old Road, Headington, Oxford OX3 7LJ Tel: 01865 857419 — MB BS Lond 1998 (The Roy. Lond. & St Bart.) BA (Hons) Oxf 1995; MRCPCH 2002. Clin. Research Fell. Specialty: Paediat. Socs: Mem. Roy. Coll. Paediat. & Child Health. Prev: Specialist Regist. Paediat. Birm. City Hosp.; SHO. (Paediat.) Birm. Child. Hosp.

PORTER, Mr David Geoffrey Department of Neurosurgery, Frenchay Hospital, Frenchay Park Road, Bristol BS16 1LE Tel: 0117 975 3959 Fax: 0117 970 1161 — MB BS Lond. 1987 (Royal Free) FRCS 1992; FRCS (SN) 1997. Cons. (Neurosurg.) Frenchay Bristol. Specialty: Neurosurg. Socs: SBNS; MPS. Prev: Sen. Regist. (Neurosurg.) Leeds Gen. Infirm.; Research Regist. Inst. Neurol. Qu. Sq.; Regist. (Neurosurg.) Roy. Free & Char. Cross.

PORTER, David Ian (retired) Hospital of St Cross, Barby Road, Rugby CV22 5PX Tel: 01788 545196 Fax: 01788 561561; 60 Stanley Road, Hillmorton, Rugby CV21 3UE Tel: 01788 543803 Fax: 01788 543803 — MB BS Lond. 1958 (Lond. Hosp.) FRCP Lond. 1984, M 1962. Prev: Cons. Dermat. Hosp. St. Cross Rugby.

PORTER, Mr Derek Spencer London Independent Hospital, Beaumont Square, London E1 4NL Tel: 020 7790 0990 Fax: 020 7795 0112; 31 Redburn Street, London SW3 4DA Tel: 020 7351 3090 — (St. Thos.) MB BS Lond. 1954; FRCS Eng. 1963. Specialty: Trauma & Orthop. Surg.; Medico Legal. Socs: Fell. BOA. Prev: Cons. Orthop. & Trauma Surg. Greenwich Dist. HA; Sen. Regist. (Orthop.) King's Coll. Hosp. Lond.; Regist. (Orthop.) Rowley Bristow Orthop. Hosp.

PORTER, Duncan Roderick Gartnavel General Hospital, 1053 Great Western Road, Glasgow G12 0YN Tel: 0141 211 3262 — BM BCh Oxf. 1985; MRCP (UK) 1988. Cons. Rheum. Gartnavel Gen. Hosp. Glas. Specialty: Gen. Med.

PORTER, Edward Joseph Brian 89 Elers Road, Ealing, London W13 9QE — MRCS Eng. LRCP Lond. 1976; BSc Lond. 1972, MB BS 1976; FFA RCS Eng. 1980. Specialty: Anaesth.

PORTER, Edward Robert 10 Lethbridge Park, Bishops Lydeard, Taunton TA4 3QU — MB BS Lond. 1998; MB BS Lond 1998.

PORTER, Elizabeth 146 Maidstone Road, Borough Green, Sevenoaks TN15 8HQ; 2/2 Iiseggielea Road, Jordanhill, Glasgow G13 1XJ Tel: 0141 954 8317 — MB ChB Glas. 1996.

PORTER, Fiona Vivien Charing Cross Hospital, Fulham Palace Road, London W6 8RF Tel: 020 8846 1234 Fax: 020 8846 1111 Email: fporter@hhnt.org; 94 Broom Park, Broom Road, Teddington TW11 9RR — MB BS Lond. 1993 (Univ. Coll. & Middlx. Sch. Med.) BSc (Hons.) Lond. 1990; FRCA 1998. Cons. Anaethetist Char. Cross Hosp. Lond. Specialty: Anaesth. Socs: Roy. Coll. Anaesth.; BMA; Assn. Anaesth. Prev: Specialist Regist. (Anaesth.)Roy. Brompton and Harefield NHS Trust, Lond.; Specialist Regist. (Anaesth.) Roy. Marsden Hosp., Lond.; Specialist Regist. (Anaesth.) Roy. Nat. Throat, Nose and Ear Hosp. Lond..

PORTER, Frederick John The Health Centre, Linenhall St., Lisburn BT28 1LU Tel: 01846 666266; 611 Kensington Gardens, Hillsborough BT26 6HP Tel: 01846 682766 — MB BCh BAO Belf. 1965; FRCGP 1990, M 1973. Hosp. Pract. E. Health & Social Serv. Bd.

PORTER, Frederick Nelson The Croft, 95 Manthorpe Road, Grantham NG31 8DE Tel: 01476 564204 — MB ChB Sheff. 1970; MRCS Eng. LRCP Lond. 1970; DCH Eng. 1973; MRCP (UK) 1975; Post Grad Cert.Managem. 1994; FRCP Lond. 1994; FRCPCH 1996; MSc 1999. Cons. Paediat. Child Developm. Centre Nottm. City Hosp. Specialty: Paediat. Socs: Collegiate Mem. RCP Edin.; Fell.Roy.Coll.Paediat.Child Health; BMA. Prev: Lect. (Child Health) Univ. Aberd.; Sen. Regist. (Paediat.) Waikato Hosp. Hamilton, NZ; Cons. Paediat. Grantham & Kesteven Gen.

PORTER, Gareth James Richard 77 Galwally Avenue, Belfast BT8 7AJ — MB ChB Bristol 1996.

PORTER, Geoffrey Duncan Gaston Wood, Upper Wyke, St Mary Bourne, Andover SP11 6EA — MB ChB Ed. 1957. Prev: Ho. Surg. Addenbrooke's Hosp. Camb.; Ho. Phys. & Ho. Surg. (Obst.) St. Mary's Hosp. Portsmouth.

PORTER, George Robert York Road, Green Hammerton, York YO26 8BN Tel: 01423 330030 Fax: 01423 331433; Mosswood House, Crayke, York YO61 4TQ Tel: 01347 822228 — MRCS Eng. LRCP Lond. 1968 (Univ. Coll. Hosp.) Hon. Med. Off. York City AFC; Examr. in 1st Aid for St. John Ambul. Socs: Roy. Soc. Med.; York Med. Soc. Pres. 2001-2002. Prev: Med. Off. Whixley Hosp. York; Dep. Med. Off. HMP Full Sutton; SHO Lond. Hosp.

PORTER, Mr Graham Charles 1a Briarfield Road, Heswall, Wirral CH60 2TH — MB BS Lond. 1990; BSc Lond. 1987; FRCS (CSiG)

Eng. 1995; FRCS (Oto.) Eng. 1996; FRCS (ORL-HNS) 2001. Specialist Regist. (OtoLaryngol.) Mersey Region. Specialty: Otorhinolaryngol.

PORTER, Mr Graham Peter Frome Farm, West Stafford, Dorchester DT2 8AA Tel: 01305 266872 — MB BS Newc. 1973; BSc (Hons.) Newc. 1970; FRCS Ed. 1978; DO RCS Eng. 1978; FRCOphth 1989. Cons. Ophth. W. Dorset Gen. Hosp. Trust Dorchester. Specialty: Ophth. Socs: S.. Ophth. Soc. & Oxf. Congr. Ophth. Prev: Sen. Regist. Addenbrooke's Hosp. Camb. & Norf. & Norwich Hosp.; Specialist Ophth. Groote Schuur Hosp. Cape Town, S. Afr.

PORTER, Guy Greig Parrot Brow, Woodside Lane, Conoley, Keighley BD20 8PE Tel: 01535 634541 — MB BS Lond. 1978; MRCP (UK) 1982; FRCR 1988. Cons. Radiol. Airedale Gen. Hosp. Keighley. Specialty: Radiol. Prev: Asst. Prof. Radiol. Univ. Miami Florida, USA; Sen. Regist. (Radiol.) St. Jas. Hosp. Leeds.

PORTER, Gwenda Elizabeth Department of Anaesthesia, Norfolk and Norwich University Hospital, Colney Lane, Norwich NR4 7UY Tel: 01603 286286 Fax: 01603 287886 Email: gwen.porter@nnuh.nhs.uk — MB BS Newc. 1977; FFA RCS Eng. 1982. Cons. Anaesth. Norf. & Norwich Hosp. Specialty: Anaesth.

PORTER, Helen 69 Fitzgerald House, 169 East India Dock Road, London E14 0HH — MB BS Lond. 1990.

PORTER, Helen Jane Leicester Royal Infirmary, Department of Histopathology, Sandringham Building Level 3, Leicester LE1 5WW Tel: 0116 258 6589 Fax: 0116 258 6585 — MD Manch. 1990; FRCPath; MB ChB 1981. Cons. Perinatal Pathologist Leicester Roy. Infirm. Specialty: Histopath.; Paediat. Prev: Cons. Sen. Lect. Perinatal Path. Univ. Bristol.; Sen. Regist. (Histopath.) Leicester Roy. Infirm.

PORTER, Helen Patricia 52 Warmington Road, Birmingham B26 3SY — MB ChB Leeds 1996.

PORTER, Ian Alexander (retired) Byethorn, Abergeldie Road, Ballater AB35 5RR — MB ChB Glas. 1945 (Univ. Glas.) MD Glas. 1960; FRCPath 1973, M 1963. Prev: Cons. Bact. & Cons. i/c Admin. Regional Laborat. City Hosp. Aberd.

PORTER, Ian John 36 Downend Park, Horfield, Bristol BS7 9PU — MB ChB Bristol 1984; MRCPsych 1992. Regist. (Psychiat.) Blackberry Hosp. Bristol. Specialty: Gen. Psychiat. Prev: SHO (Psychiat.) Glenside Hosp. Bristol; SHO (ENT & A & E) Southmead Hosp. Bristol; SHO Whakatane Hosp., New Zealand.

PORTER, Jacqueline Sarah Department Anaesthetics, St. Thomas' Hospital, London SE1 7EH Tel: 020 7928 9292 Email: jackie.porter@gstt.sthames.nhs.uk — MB BS Lond. 1987 (Univ. Coll. Hosp.) FRCA 1993; MD Lond. 2001. Cons. (Anaesth.) St Thos. Hosp. Lond. Specialty: Anaesth. Prev: Sen. Regist. St. Thos. Hosp. Lond.

PORTER, James Harrison Lawson House, Bolton-by-Bowland Road, Clitheroe BB7 4NJ — MB BS Lond. 1992.

PORTER, Jane Kreewood, Vicarage Road, Whaddon, Milton Keynes MK17 0LU Tel: 01908 501709 — MB ChB Liverp. 1967; FFA RCS Eng. 1973. Cons. Anaesth. Milton Keynes Hosp. Specialty: Anaesth. Socs: Assn. Anaesths.; Obst. Anaesth. Assn. Prev: Sen. Regist. (Anaesth.) Nuffield Dept. Anaesth. John Radcliffe Hosp. Oxf.; Sen. Regist. (Anaesth.) St. Geo. Hosp. Lond.; Regist. (Anaesth.) Kingston-upon-Thames Hosp. & Centr. Middlx. Hosp. Lond.

PORTER, Miss Janet Elizabeth 114 Woodside, Leigh-on-Sea SS9 4RB Tel: 01702 421704 Fax: 01702 421661 Email: j.porter@doctors.org.uk — MB BChir Camb. 1972 (Westm.) MA Camb. 1968; FRCS Eng. 1977; FFAEM 1991. Sen. Lect. (Med. Educat.) St Geo. Hosp. Med. Sch. Lond.; Medico-legal Cons.; Cons. (Accid. & Emerg.) Princess Alexandra Hosp. Harlow. Specialty: Accid. & Emerg.; Sports Med.; Medico Legal. Prev: Cons. (Accid. & Emerg.) Southend Hosp.

PORTER, Jayne Margaret 52 Stoneypath, Londonderry BT47 2AF — MB BCh BAO Belf. 1986.

PORTER, Joanna Catherine Laboratory of Molecular Cell Biology, University College, Gower Street, London WC1E 6BT Tel: 020 7679 7911 Fax: 020 7679 7805 Email: joanna.porter@ucl.ac.uk; 114 Hemingford Road, London N1 1DE — BM BCh Oxf. 1988 (Oxford University) MA Camb. 1989; MRCP (UK) 1991; PhD Lond. 1998. Wellcome Advanced Clin. Fell.; Hon. Cons. in Thoracic and Gen. Med. UCH; Hon. Sen. Lect. in Med., UCL. Specialty: Respirat. Med.; Gen. Med.; Intens. Care. Special Interest: Cell Biol. Prev: ICRF Clin. Fell. ICRF Lond.; MRC Train. Fell. ICRF Lond.; Regist. (Intens. Care) St. Geo. Hosp. Lond.

PORTER, Joanne Norma Chorlton Fold Farm, Rocky Lane, Monton, Eccles, Manchester M30 9NA — MB BS Lond. 1987; MRCP (UK) 1990. Regist. (Gen. Med. & Cardiol.) West. Gen. Hosp. Edin. Specialty: Cardiol.

PORTER, John David The Surgery, Station Lane, Farnsfield, Newark NG22 8LA Tel: 01623 882289 Fax: 01623 882286; 117 Station Lane, Farnsfield, Newark NG22 8LB Tel: 01636 883126 — BMedSci (Hons.) Nottm. 1979, BM BS 1981; DCH RCP Lond. 1984; MRCGP 1985. Specialty: Gen. Med.

PORTER, John David Henley 17 Rigault Road, London SW6 4JJ — MB BS Lond. 1977 (King's Coll. Hosp.) DA Eng. 1980; MRCP (UK) 1982; DCH RCP 1982; MPH Harvard 1984; MFPHM 1988. Sen. Lect. (Clin. Sci.) Lond. Sch. Hyg. & Trop. Med.; Cons. Epidemiol. Communicable Dis. Surveillance Centre Lond. Specialty: Pub. Health Med. Prev: Sen. Regist. (Communicable Dis.) Surveillance Centre Lond.; SHO (Neonat. Paediat.) Qu. Charlottes Hosp. Lond.; Epidemic Intellig. Serv. Off. Centers for Dis. Control Atlanta, USA.

PORTER, John Francis Hugh The Cripps Health Centre, University Park, Nottingham NG7 2QW Tel: 0115 950 1654 — MB ChB Leic. 1987; MRCGP 1991; DRCOG 1991; MSc (Travel Medicine) Glasgow University 1999. Socs: MRCGP; Mem. of Internat. Travel Med.; Mem. of Brit. Travel Health Assn.

PORTER, Mr John Michael Plastic Surgery Unit, Sandwell General Hospital, Lyndon, West Bromwich B71 4HJ Tel: 0121 607 3355 Fax: 0121 607 3355 Email: benara.rahman@swbh.nhs.uk — MB BS Lond. 1969 (King's Coll. Lond. & King's Coll. Hosp.) AKC 1969; MRCS Eng. LRCP Lond. 1969; FRCS Eng. 1974; MS Soton. 1988. Cons. Plastic Surg., Sandwell Gen. Hosp. Specialty: Plastic Surg. Socs: Brit. Assn. of Aesthetic Plastic Surgeons; Academy of Expert Witnesses. Prev: SHO (Plastic Surg.) Odstock Hosp. Salisbury; Regist. (Plastic Surg.) Odstock Hosp. Salisbury; Hon. Regist. (Plastic Surg.) Odstock Hosp. Salisbury.

PORTER, Jonathan Mark University Hospitals Coventry and Warwickshire NHS Trust, Walsgrave, Coventry CV2 2DX Tel: 024 7660 2020 Email: mark.porter@uhcw.nhs.uk; 6 Broadsword Way, Burbage, Hinckley LE10 2QL Tel: 01455 611345 Fax: 087 0137 6261 Email: mark@porter.uk.com — MB ChB Leic. 1989; BSc Leic. 1983; FRCA 1994; Dip. ATLS RCS Eng. 1996. Cons. Anaesth. with s/i in Obstetric Anaesth. Univ. Hosp.s Coventry & Warks. NHS Trust. Coventry. Specialty: Anaesth. Special Interest: Obstetric Anaesth. Socs: Obst. Anaesth. Assn.; Assn. Anaesth. GB & Irel.; BMA (former Chairm., Jun. Doctor Comm.; Mem., Centr. Cons.s & Specialists Comm.). Prev: Specialist Regist. (Anaesth.) Coventry Sch. of Anaesth.; SHO (A & E & Intens. Care) Derbysh. Roy. Infirm.; SHO (Anaesth.) P'boro. Dist. Hosp. & Leicester Gp. Hosps.

PORTER, Kamilla Kiron — MB BS Lond. 1996 (Univ. Coll. Hosp.) BSc Lond. 1993; MRCP (UK) Part 1 1998; MRCP (UK) Part II 1999; DCH 1999. GP Kent. Specialty: Gen. Pract. Socs: BMA. Prev: GP Regist. Holland Pk. Surg. Lond.; SHO (Psychiat.) Gordon Hosp. Lond.; SpR (Radiol) Chelsea & Westm. Hosp. Lond.

PORTER, Kathryn 108 Pembroke Road, Clifton, Bristol BS8 3EW — MB ChB Liverp. 1991; MRCP (UK) 1995; DCH RCP Lond. 1996. Specialty: Gen. Pract.

PORTER, Mr Keith Macdonald Longfield Cottage, Rowney Green, Alvechurch, Birmingham B48 7RB Tel: 0121 445 1921 Fax: 0121 627 8075 Email: keith.porter@uhb.nhs.uk — MB BS Lond. 1974; FRCS Eng. 1978; Dip. IMC RCS Ed. 1992; FRCS Ed. 1998. Cons. Trauma Surg. Univ. Hosp. Birm. NHS Trust; Med. Director W. Midlands Care Team Bolton; Chairm. Trauma Care Charity Lond. Specialty: Trauma & Orthop. Surg. Special Interest: Sport Injuries; Trauma. Socs: British Trauma Society; British Orthopaedic Association. Prev: Cons. Trauma & Orthop. Surg. Birm. Accid. Hosp.; Sen. Regist. & Regist. (Orthop.) Roy. Orthop. Hosp. Birm.; Surg. Regist. Roy. Hosp. Wolverhampton.

PORTER, Professor Kendrick Arthur Reynolds Barn, Burys Bank Road, Thatcham RG19 8DD Tel: 01635 31839 Fax: 01635 33793 — (St. Mary's) MB BS Lond. 1948; MRCS Eng. LRCP Lond. 1948; DSc Lond. 1961, MD 1953; FRCPath 1972. Emerit. Prof. Path. Imperial Coll. Sch of Med. At St Mary's, Univ. Lond.; Vis. Prof. Path. Univ. Pittsburgh Sch. Med.; Hon. Cons. Path. St. Mary's Hosp. Lond. Specialty: Histopath. Socs: Path. Soc.; Transpl. Soc. Prev: Research

Fell. Harvard Med. Sch.; Brit. Postgrad. Med. Federat. Trav. Fell.; Fulbright Fellowship.

PORTER, Kevin Greaves Garforth Medical Centre, Church Lane, Garforth, Leeds LS25 1ER Tel: 0113 286 5311 Fax: 0113 281 2679 — MB ChB Leeds 1974; DObst RCOG 1976.

PORTER, Lissy Woodspring Community Mental Health Centre, Marine Hill House, Marine Hill, Clevedon BS21 7PW Tel: 01275 341811; The Old Court House, 2 Hallen Road, Henbury, Bristol BS10 7QX Tel: 0117 377 4718 — MD Aarhus 1983. Staff Grade Psychiat. Woodspring Community Ment. Health Centre. Specialty: Gen. Psychiat. Prev: Clin. Asst. (Psychiat.) Southmead Hosp. Bristol.

PORTER, Lynn Joyce Weavers Lane Surgery, 1 Weavers Lane, Whitburn, Bathgate EH47 0SD Tel: 01501 740297 Fax: 01501 744302; 4 Kettilstoun Mains, Linlithgow EH49 6SN — MB ChB Aberd. 1980; MRCGP 1984.

PORTER, Mark Christopher Milsom Locking Hill Surgery, Stroud GL5 1UY Tel: 01453 764222 Fax: 01453 756278 Email: drmarkp@aol.com — MB BS Lond. 1986 (Westminster Hospital) DA (UK) 1989; DCH RCP Lond. 1990. GP Stroud.; Med. Broadcaster & Med. Jl.ist. Specialty: Gen. Pract.

PORTER, Martin Herdman (retired) Undercliffe, Pilgrims Way, Lenham, Maidstone ME17 2HA Tel: 01622 858788 — MB BS Lond. 1967 (Middlx.) DObst RCOG 1969; MRCGP 1977. Prev: SHO (Obst. & Med.) Orsett Hosp.

PORTER, Mr Martin John Worcestershire Royal Hospital, Charles Hastings Way, Worcester WR5 1DD Tel: 01905 760887 — BM BCh Oxf. 1984; FRCS Eng. 1989; FRCS (Orl.) 1994; MD 1997. Cons. (ENT) Worcs. Roy. Infirm. Specialty: Otolaryngol. Special Interest: Rhinology. Socs: BAOHNS; BRS. Prev: Head & Neck Fell. Green La. Hosp. Auckland, NZ; Hon. Lect. Chinese Univ. Hong Kong.

PORTER, Mr Martyn Lonsdale Wrightington Hospital for Joint Disease, Hall Lane, Appley Bridge, Wigan WN6 9EP Tel: 01257 256288 Fax: 01257 256291 — MB ChB Manch. 1979; FRCS Ed. 1983; FRCS Ed. (Orth.) 1989. Cons. Orthop. Surg. Hip Centre Wrightington Hosp.; Hon. Sen. Research Fell. (Med. Biophysics) Manch.; Hon. Sen. Lect. Univ. of Centr. Lancs. Specialty: Orthop. Special Interest: Primary & Revision Knees & Hips. Socs: BOA Counc. Mem. 2001-2003; Brit. Hip Soc.; B.A.S.K. Prev: Cons. Orthop. Roy. Preston Hosp.; Sen. Regist. (Orthop.) NW RHA; Tutor (Orthop. Surg.) Univ. Manch.

PORTER, Matthew Charles Bromley Crossroads Medical Practice, Lincoln Road, Moore Lane, North Hykeham, Lincoln LN6 8NH Tel: 01522 682848 — MB ChB Sheff. 1994; DFFP London 1998; DRCOG London 1999. GP Princip. Specialty: Gen. Pract.

PORTER, Mr Michael Francis (retired) 30 Anstruther Road, Edgbaston, Birmingham B15 3NW Tel: 0121 684 6644 Fax: 0121 684 6644 — MB BS Lond. 1953; MRCS Eng. LRCP Lond. 1953; FRCS Ed. 1960. Prev: Cons. Orthop. Surg. E. Birm. Hosp. & Birm. Accid. Hosp.

PORTER, Moira Elaine 8 Moorfoot Way, Baljaffray, Bearsden, Glasgow G61 4RL — MB ChB Glas. 1984; MB ChB Glas. l984; DRCOG 1986; MRCGP 1988. Trainee GP Glas. VTS. Specialty: Dermat. Prev: Regist. (Dermat.) Inverclyde Hosp. Greenock.

PORTER, Mr Nigel Harry (retired) (cons. rooms), 98 The Drive, Hove BN3 6GP Tel: 01273 731807 Fax: 01273 723105; Manning's Farm, Edburton, Henfield BN5 9LJ Tel: 01903 813055 — MB BS Lond. 1949 (Guy's) LMSSA Lond. 1949; FRCS Eng. 1954. Prev: Sen. Regist. (Surg.), Out-pat. Off. & Ho. Surg. Guy's Hosp. Lond.

PORTER, Patricia Jacqueline Regents Park Surgery, Park Street, Shirley, Southampton SO16 4RJ Tel: 023 8078 3618 Fax: 023 8070 3103; Little Elcombes, Elcombes Close, Lyndhurst SO43 7BB — BM Soton. 1982; BSc (Psych.) Durham. 1974.

PORTER, Mr Richard (retired) 11 Graham Park Road, Gosforth, Newcastle upon Tyne NE3 4BH Tel: 0191 285 7500 — MB BS Durh. 1964 (Newc.) DO Eng. 1968; FRCS Eng. 1970; FRCOphth 1989. Prev: Clin. Asst. Moorfields Eye Hosp. Lond.

PORTER, Richard Howell John Elliott Unit, Department of Psychiatry, Birch Hill Hospital, Rochdale OL12 9QB — MB ChB Manch. 1982; MRCPsych 1986; MSc (Psychiat.) Manch. 1991. Cons. Ment. Illness Rochdale Healthcare Trust. Specialty: Gen. Psychiat. Prev: Sen. Regist. (Psychiat.) NW RHA.

PORTER, Richard James Royal United Hospital, Combe Park, Bath BA1 3NG Tel: 01225 824657 Fax: 01225 825077; Weston Lea, Weston Park, Bath BA1 4AL Tel: 01225 425618 Fax: 01225 429223 Email: rjporter@community.co.uk — BM BCh Oxf. 1977 (Oxford) MA Oxf. MSc Oxf. 1977; MRCOG 1983; FRCOG 1998. Cons. O & G Roy. United Hosp. NHS Trust & Wilts. Health Care NHS Trust; Clin. director Matern. Serv.s Wilts. Healthcare trust; Hon. Sen. Lect. Soton. & Bristol Univs. Specialty: Obst. & Gyn. Socs: Roy. Soc. Med.; Chairm., Assn. for community based Matern. care. Prev: Sen. Regist. (O & G) St. Mary's Hosp. Lond. & Rosie Matern. Hosp. Camb.; Med. Dir. Wilts. Health Care NHS Trust:.

PORTER, Professor Richard William 34 Bawtry Road, Doncaster DN4 7AZ Tel: 01302 538888 — MB ChB Ed. 1958; DObst RCOG 1961; FRCS Ed. 1961; FRCS Eng. 1966; MD Ed. 1981; DSc Ed. 2001. 1st Syme Prof. RCS Ed. Specialty: Orthop. Socs: (Pres.) Back Pain Research Soc.; (Counc.) Brit. Orthop. Assn.; Soc. Clin. Anatomists. Prev: Prof. Sir Harry Platt Chair of Orthop. Surg. of Aberd.; Dir. Educat./Train. RCS Ed.; Prof. Orthop. Aberd. Univ.

PORTER, Ruth (retired) Pittville Lodge Cottage, 39 Malden Road, Cheltenham GL52 2BU — (Ed.) MB ChB Ed. 1948; DCH Eng. 1951; FRCP Lond. 1973, M 1958; FRCPsych 1980, M 1974. Prev: Psychotherapist (Old Age Psychiat.) Roy. Free Hosp. & St. Chas. Hosp. Lond.

PORTER, Sally-Anne Mary Department of Addictive Behaviour, St. Georges Hospital Medical School, London SW17 0RE — MB BS Lond. 1987; MRCPsych 1991. Sen. Lect. & Hon. Cons. Psychiat. St. Geo. Hosp. Med. Sch. Lond. Specialty: Alcohol & Substance Misuse. Prev: Sen. Regist. (Addic. Behaviour) St. Geo. Hosp. Med. Sch. Lond.

PORTER, Stephen O'Neill 65 Pinner Road, Northwood HAG 1QN Email: steveporter@hotmail.com — MB BS Lond. 1992 (St. Geo. Hosp.) BSc Lond. 1991; MRCOG 2001. Specialist Regist. (O & G) NW Thames Rotat. Specialty: Obst. & Gyn. Socs: Blair-Bell research Soc.; Roy. Soc. of Med. Prev: SPR (O & G) Qu. Charlottes & Chelsea Hosps.; SPR (O & G) W.ford Gen. Hosp.; Clin. Research Fell. Roy. Free Hosp.

PORTER, Professor Stephen Ross Department of Oral Medicine,, Eastman Dental Institute, 256 Gray's Inn Road, London WC1X 8LD Tel: 020 7915 1197 Fax: 020 7915 2341 — MB ChB Bristol 1991; BSc Glas. 1979, BDS 1982; FDS RCS Eng. 1987; FDS RCS Ed. 1987; PhD Bristol 1987, MD 1993. Prof. (Oral Med.) Eastman Dent. Inst. for Oral Health Care Scis. & Univ. Coll., Lond. Specialty: Oral & Maxillofacial Surg.; Oral Medicine. Special Interest: non-surgical Managem. of Dis. or the oral mucosa and salivary glands. Socs: Brit. Soc. for Oral Med.; Europ. Acad. of Oral Med.

PORTER, Steven Michael Grove House Surgery, 102 Albert Street, Ventnor PO38 1EU Tel: 01983 852427 — MB ChB Bristol 1985; DRCOG 1988; MRCGP 1989. GP Gr. Ho. Surg., Ventnor. Prev: Trainee GP Bristol.

PORTER, Stuart William 23 Blucher Street, Ashton-under-Lyne OL7 9NG — MB ChB Sheff. 1996.

PORTER, Ms Susan MD Alexandra Hospital, Woodrow Drive, Redditch B98 7UB Tel: 01527 503030; Ingeva, Tutnall Lane, Tutnall, Bromsgrove B60 1NA — MB BS Lond. 1976 (Westm.) FRCOphth; BSc (Hons.) Lond. 1973; DO Eng. 1981; FRCS Eng. 1982. Cons. Ophth. Surg. Alexandra Hosp. Redditch. Specialty: Ophth. Prev: Sen. Regist. St. Paul's Eye Hosp. Liverp.

PORTER, Suzanne, Surg. Lt. RN 3A Rutland Lane, Sale M33 2GG Tel: 0161 969 1631 Fax: 0161 969 1631 — MB ChB Manch. 1995; BSc (Med. Sci.) St. And. 1993. SHO Higher Med. Train. RN; SHO HMS Neptune FasLa. Scotl.; SHO Roy. Hosp. Hasler, Gosport, Hants. Socs: Life Mem. Bute Med. Soc. (St. And.). Prev: SHO (A & E) R Hosp. Haslar; Ho. Off. (Surg.) RN Hosp. Haslar; Ho. Off. (Med.) Blackpool Vict. Hosp.

PORTER, Suzanne Maria Bootham Park Hospital, York YO30 7BY; 134 Glen Road, Oadby, Leicester LE2 4RF — MB ChB Birm. 1991; MRC Psych. Specialist Regist. (Old Age Psychiat.) Bootham Pk. Hosp. York. (p/t). Specialty: Geriat. Psychiat.

PORTER, Timothy Aberhoyw Farmhouse, Cyffredin Lane, Llangynidr, Crickhowell NP8 1LR — MB BS Lond. 1988.

PORTER, William Aubrey Blackwood 17 Foley Road, Stourbridge DY9 0RT — MB ChB Manch. 1986.

PORTER, William Davis (retired) 19 Annadale Avenue, Belfast BT7 3JJ Tel: 028 9064 3441 — (Belf.) LAH Dub. 1953. Prev: Sen. Med. Off. Somme Hosp. Belf.

PORTER, William Morier Gloucestershire Royal Hospital, Department of Dermatology, Great Western Road, Gloucester GL1 3NN Tel: 08454 225584 Fax: 01452 395583 Email: william.porter@gloucr-tr.swest.nhs.uk — MB BS Lond. 1992 (St Mary's) BSc 1989; MRCP 1996. Cons. Dematol. Glous. & Cheltenham. Specialty: Dermat. Special Interest: Male Genital; Paediat.; Skin Surg. Socs: Brit. Assn. Dermatol.; Dowling Club; St John's Dermatol. Soc. Prev: SHO Rotat. St Mary's Hosp. Med.; SHO (ITU, A & E & Orthop.) Roy. Sussex Co. Hosp. Brighton; REG (OERM) St. Mary's, Chelsea & Westminster & Char. Cross Hosp.s.

PORTERFIELD, Alexandra June (retired) The Little Manor House, 9 Manor Close, Tunbridge Wells TN4 8YB Tel: 01892 528261 — MB ChB Liverp. 1965; FFA RCS Eng. 1968. Prev: Cons. Anaesth. Kent & Sussex Weald Trust.

PORTERFIELD, James Stuart (retired) Green Valleys, Goodleigh, Barnstaple EX32 7NH Tel: 01271 345325 Fax: 01271 345325 Email: porterfield@sosi.net — (Liverp.) MB ChB Liverp. 1947; MRCS Eng. LRCP Lond. 1947; MD Liverp. 1949. Emerit. Fell. Wadham Coll. Oxf. Prev: Reader (Bacteriol.) Sir William Dunn Sch. Path. Univ. Oxf.

PORTERFIELD, John Arnold (retired) 4 Princes Close, Berkhamsted HP4 1JS Tel: 01442 876697 — MB BChir Camb. 1963; MA, MB Camb. 1963, BChir 1962.

PORTERFIELD, Philip Norman Stannery Surgery, Abbey Rise, Whitchurch, Tavistock PL19 9BB Tel: 01822 613517 Fax: 01822 618294 — MB BS Lond. 1975.

PORTERGILL, Nicola Clare The Surgery, Great Lumley, Chester-le-Street DH3 4LE Tel: 01474 770 6473/0191 388 5600 Fax: 01474 705279 — MB BS Newc. 1990.

PORTMANN, Professor Bernard Claude Institute of Liver Studies, King's College Hospital, Denmark Hill, London SE5 9RS Tel: 020 7346 3734 Fax: 020 7346 3125 Email: bernard.portmann@kcl.ac.uk — MD Geneva 1972; Dip Federal Switzerland 1966; FRCPath 1989, M 1977. Cons. & Prof. (Histopath.) Inst. Liver Studies King's Coll. Hosp. Lond.; Prof. Hepatopathol. Lond. Univ. 1997. Specialty: Histopath.; Gastroenterol. Socs: Brit. Soc. Gastroenterol.; Path. Soc.; Internat. Acad. Pathol. Prev: 1st Asst. (Histopath.) Univ. Hosp., Geneva; Research (Histopath.) Clin. Asst. Liver Unit King's Coll. Hosp. Lond.

PORTNOY, Amanda Elizabeth Ilkeston Health Centre, South Street, Ilkeston DE7 5PZ Tel: 0115 932 2933 — MB ChB Leic. 1982; AKC; BSc Lond. 1976; DRCOG 1986. GP Princip.; Clin. Asst. (Dermat.) Nottm.; CME Course Organiser Nottm. Specialty: Dermat.

PORTNOY, Benjamin, TD (retired) Forest Lodge, Bollinway Hale, Altrincham WA15 0NZ Tel: 0161 980 2307 — (Manch. & San Francisco) Dichinson Travelling Scholar 1938-39, Univ. California, San Francisco; MB ChB (Distinc.) Pharmacol. Path. Med. Manch. 1936; MD Manch. 1938; FRCP Lond. 1976, M 1945; PhD New York 1951. JP.; Hon. Cons. Phys. Manch. & Salford Hosp. Skin Dis.; Clin. Lect. (Dermat.) Univ. Manch. 1960; Mem. Gray's Inn. Prev: Chief Med. Asst. (Clin. Investigs. & Research) Manch. Univ. & Infirm.

PORTNOY, David 42 Nottingham Road, Ilkeston DE7 5RE Tel: 0115 932 5229 Fax: 0115 932 5413 — MB ChB Leic. 1982; BSc Lond. 1976; AKC 1976; DA (UK) 1986; DRCOG 1987; MRCGP 1988.

PORTO, Luiz Otavio da Rocha 102 Ramillies Road, Bedford Park, Chiswick, London W4 1JA — Medico Gama Filho 1976; DMR (RCP UK) 1983. Clin. Asst. St. Mary's NHS Trust Lond.; Dir. PCL UK. Specialty: Pharmaceutical Medicine. Socs: Fell. Roy. Soc. Med.; Fac. Pharmaceut. Med. Prev: Dir. Clin. Research & Developm. Antisoma plc; Head Clin. Developm. Bayer plc; Regist. (Med.) King's Coll. Hosp. Lond.

PORTSMOUTH, Owen Henry Donald 12 Paddock Drive, Dorridge, Solihull B93 8BZ Tel: 01564 775032 — (St. Thos.) MB BS Lond. 1953; DTM & H Eng. 1956; FRCP Ed. 1971, M 1960; FRCP Lond. 1977, M 1960; MA Keele 1993. Hon. Sen. Clin. Lect. (Biomed. Ethics) Univ. Birm.; Hon. Cons. Phys. (Geriat. & Gen. Med.) Birm. Heartlands & Solihull NHS Trust (Teachg.); Pres. W. Midl. Inst. Geriat. Med. & Gerontol. Specialty: Care of the Elderly. Socs: Fell. Roy. Soc. Trop. Med. & Hyg.; Brit. Geriat. Soc.; Fell.Roy.Soc.Med. Prev: Cons. Phys. (Geriat.) E. Birm. Hosp. & Solihull HA; Specialist (Med.) Kenya.

PORTSMOUTH, Simon David 20 Falmer Road, London N15 5BA Tel: 020 8800 4164 — MB ChB Sheff. 1992.

PORTWOOD, John Keith (retired) 105 Lansdown Road, Gloucester GL1 3JF Tel: 01452 527116 Email: kasomitrice@onetel.net — MB ChB Birm. 1961; DObst RCOG 1964. Prev: GP Gloucester.

PORTWOOD, Mrs Rosemary (retired) 3 Belmont Villas, The Avenue, Truro TR1 1HS Tel: 01872 273856 — (Univ. Coll. Hosp.) MB BS Lond. 1954; MFFP 1993. SCMO (Instruc.) St. Austell, Truro & Bodmin Family Plann. Clinics & Cervical Cytol. Clinics Cornw. HA.

POSKITT, Elizabeth Margaret Embree, OBE (retired) International Nutrition Group, London School of Hygiene & Tropical Medicine, 49-51 Bedford Square, London WC1B 3DP Tel: 020 7299 4688 — MB Camb. 1964; BChir 1963; FRCP Lond. 1980, M 1966; FRCPCH 1997. Hon. Sen. Lect. Int. Nutrit. Gp. Lond. Prev: Head of Station, MRC Dunn Nutrit. Gp., Keneba, Banjul, The Gambia.

POSKITT, Mr Keith Richard Department of Surgery, Cheltenham General Hospital, Sandford Road, Cheltenham GL54 7AN Tel: 01242 222222 — MB ChB Sheff. 1977; FRCS Eng. 1981; MD Sheff. 1988. Cons. Gen. Vasc. Surg. Cheltenham Gen. Hosp. Specialty: Gen. Surg. Socs: Surgic. Research Soc.; Vasc. Surgic. Soc. GB & Irel.; BMA. Prev: Sen. Regist (Gen. Surg.) Bristol Roy. Infirm. & Southmead Hosp. Bristol; Regist. (Gen. Surg.) Char. Cross Hosp. Lond.; Regist. Rotat. (Gen. Surg.) Roy. Hallamsh. Hosp. Sheff.

POSKITT, Vivienne Jayne 149 Knighton Field Road E., Leicester LE2 6DR — MB ChB Leic. 1993.

POSNER, Brian Hyman (retired) 39 Moor Crescent, Gosforth, Newcastle upon Tyne NE3 4AQ Tel: 0191 213 1166 Fax: 0191 213 1166 — (Durham University) MB BS Durh. 1957; MRCGP 1965. Med. Adviser Univ. Sunderland. Prev: GP Sunderland.

POSNER, John 95 Copers Cope Road, Beckenham BR3 1NY Tel: 020 8650 7521 Fax: 020 8325 8856 — MB BS Lond. 1974; PhD Lond. 1971, BSc (Hons.) 1968; MRCP (UK) 1976; FRCP Lond. 1991; FFPM RCP (UK) 1995. Med. Dir. BIOS Ltd. Surrey; Hon. Sen. Lect. (Med.) Kings Coll. Sch. Med. & Dent. Lond. Specialty: Pharmacology. Socs: Brit. Pharm. Soc. Prev: Dir. Clin Pharmacol. Studies Glaxo Wellcome Unit Northwick Pk. Hosp.

POSNER, Nicholas Charles Parkway Medical Centre, 2 Frenton Close, Chapel House Estate, Newcastle upon Tyne NE5 1EH Tel: 0191 267 1313 Fax: 0191 229 0630 — MB ChB Leeds 1990; DRCOG 1993; DFFP 1994; MRCGP 1994. GP Newc.u.Tyne. Specialty: Gen. Pract. Prev: Trainee GP Northumbria VTS; Ho. Off. Airedale Hosp. W. Yorks.

POSNER, Philip Joseph James Wigg Group Practice, Kentish Town Health Centre, 2 Bartholomew Road, London NW5 2AJ Tel: 020 7530 4747 Fax: 020 7530 4750 — MB ChB Leeds 1987; DRCOG 1990; MRCGP 1991; DFFP 1993. Specialty: Gen. Pract. Socs: BMA. Prev: Trainee GP ScarBoro. Hosp. VTS.; SHO (Palliat. Med.) Edenhall Hospice; SHO (Geriat.) St. Albans City Hosp.

POSTINGS, Samantha Jane 8 White's Meadow, Ranton, Stafford ST18 9JB Tel: 01785 282444; 8 White's Meadow, Ranton, Stafford ST18 9JB Tel: 01785 282444 — MB ChB Leeds 1990. Staff Grade (Paediat.) Shrops. Community NHS Trust Shrewsbury. Specialty: Community Child Health.

POSTLETHWAITE, Dennis Leslie (retired) Lyndene, 15 Highbury Avenue, Springwell, Gateshead NE9 7PX Tel: 0191 416 3315 Fax: 0191 416 3315 — (King's Coll.) MB BS Durh. 1948; MRCS Eng. LRCP Lond. 1948. Prev: Flight Lt. RAF Med. Br.

POSTLETHWAITE, Mr John Crispian North London Nuffield Hospital, Cavell Drive, Uplands Park Road, Enfield EN2 7PR Tel: 020 8366 2122; Hollybush, Hammonds Lane, Sandridge, St Albans AL4 9BG Email: john.pos@tinyworld.co.uk — (St. Mary's) MB BS Lond. 1963; MRCS Eng. LRCP Lond. 1963; FRCS Ed. 1969; FRCS Eng. 1971. Specialty: Gen. Surg. Special Interest: Gall Bladder Surg. Prev: Cons. Surg. Barnet Gen. Hosp.; Sen. Regist. (Surg.) Roy. Free Hosp. Lond.; Regist. (Surg.) St. Mary's Hosp. Lond.

POSTLETHWAITE, Mr Keith Roy Maxillofacial Unit, Newcastle general Hospital, Wsetgate Road, Newcastle upon Tyne NE4 6BE Tel: 0191 236 3157 Fax: 01434 633998 Email: keith.postlethwaite@onetel.net.uk — MB ChB Birm. 1982; BDS; FDS RCS Eng. 1977; FRCS Ed. 1987. Cons. Oral & Maxillofacial Surg. Newc. Gen. Hosp. Westgate Rd. Newc. u. Tyne; Hon. Clin. Lect. Univ. Newc. Specialty: Oral & Maxillofacial Surg. Prev: Sen. Regist. (Oral & Maxillofacial Surg.) Clwyd HA; Regist. (Oral & Maxillofacial Surg.) Roy. Surrey Co. Hosp.

POSTLETHWAITE, Robert Joseph Royal Manchester Childrens Hospital, Hospital Road, Pendlebury, Manchester M27 4HA — MB ChB Manch. 1970; MRCP (UK) 1973; FRCP Lond. 1988. Cons. Paediat. Nephrol. Roy. Manch. Childr. Hosp.; Hon. Lect. (Child Health) Univ. Manch. Specialty: Paediat. Prev: Lect. (Child Health) Univ. Manch.; Regist. Hammersmith Hosp. Lond. & Booth Hall Childr. Hosp. Manch.

POSTLETHWAITE, Professor Roy (retired) 6 Rendcomb Drive, Cirencester GL7 1YN Tel: 01285 885345 — MB ChB Manch. 1954; BSc (Hons. Physiol.) Manch. 1951, MD (Gold Medal) 1959; FRCPath 1973, M 1963. Prev: Personal Chair Virol. Univ. Aberd.

POSTON, Bernard Leslie The Hazeldene Medical Centre, 97 Moston Lane East, New Moston, Manchester M40 3HD Tel: 0161 681 7287 Fax: 0161 681 7438; 73 Bishops Road, Prestwich, Manchester M25 0AS Tel: 0161 773 1008 Fax: 0161 773 1008 — MB ChB Manch. 1956; MRCGP 1976. Prev: Ho. Phys. & Cas. Off. Crumpsall Hosp. Manch.; Ho. Surg. Ancoats Hosp. Manch.

POSTON, Mr Graeme John University Hospital Aintree, Lower Lane, Liverpool L9 7AL Tel: 0151 525 5980 Fax: 0151 706 5827 Email: GRAEME.POSTON@aht.nwest.nhs.uk/ graemeposton@blueyonder.co.uk; Royal Liverpool University Hospital, Prescot Street, Liverpool L7 8XP Tel: 0151 706 3484 — MB BS Lond. 1979 (Univ. Lond. & St. Geo. Hosp. Med. Sch.) FRCS Eng. 1984; FRCS Ed. 1984; MS Lond. 1988. Cons. Surg. Univ. Hosp. Aintree; Lect. (Surg.) Univ. Liverp.; Edit. Bd. Europ. Jl. Surg. Oncol. Specialty: Gen. Surg. Special Interest: Hepato Biliary Surg.; Hernia Surg. Socs: Internat. Hepato Pancreato Biliary Assn.; Assn. of Upper G.I. Surgeons; Assn. of Surgeons. Prev: Cons. Surg. Roy. Liverp. Univ. Hosp.; Lect. (Surg.) St. Mary's Hosp. Med. Sch. Univ. Lond.; Instruc. (Surg.) Univ. Texas Med. Br. Galveston, Texas.

POSTON, Robert Nigel King's College London, Centre for Cardiovascular Biology Medicine, New Hunt's House, Guy's Hospital Campus, London SE1 1UL Tel: 020 7848 6232 Fax: 020 7848 6220 Email: robin@poston.eurobell.co.uk; 11 Marlborough Crescent, Riverhead, Sevenoaks TN13 2HH Tel: 01732 454575 Email: poston@eclipse.co.uk — (Middlx.) MD Camb. 1981, MB 1970, BChir 1969; FRCPath 1994, M 1981. Sen. Lect. (Immunopath.) Kings coll Lond Guy's Hosp. Lond.; Hon. Cons. (Immunol.) Guy's & St Thos. Hosp. Trust. Specialty: Immunol.; Pathology, General. Socs: Roy. Soc. Med.; Path. Soc.; Brit. Soc. Immunol. Prev: Lect. (Path.) Guy's Hosp. Med. Sch.; Brit. Heart Foundat. Jun. Research Fell.; Research Assoc. (Immunol.) Middlx. Hosp. Med. Sch.

POSTON, Rosemary Anne — MB BS Lond. 1972 (Middlx.) MRCGP 1984. Prev: Princip. GP Melbourne, Derbysh. & Oadby, Leics.

POTAMITIS, Theodoros 26 Cedar Road, Dudley DY1 4HW — MB ChB Leic. 1987; FCOphth. 1992. Specialty: Ophth.

POTDAR, Mr Nandkishore Purushottam Department of Surgery, Grantham & Kesteven General Hospital, 101 Manthorpe Road, Grantham NG31 8DG — MB BS Bombay 1978; FRCSI 1982.

POTE, Allan Herbert 3 Ripplevale Grove, London N1 1HS Tel: 020 7607 2629 — MB BS Lond. 1944 (Lond. Hosp.) LMSSA Lond. 1944. Hon. Lect. in Gen. Pract. Univ. Coll. Hosp. Med. Sch. Prev: Asst. Chest Phys. Walthamstow Chest Clinic; Asst. Med. Off. Whipps Cross Hosp.; Graded Chest Phys. RAMC.

POTE, Francis William (retired) Cornheys Farm, Wash, Chapel en le Frith, High Peak SK23 0QW — MRCS Eng. LRCP Lond. 1939 (Char. Cross) Prev: Med. Admin. War on Want.

POTE, Jonathan Lamington, 32 Willoway Lane, Braunton EX33 1BS Tel: 01271 814412; Lamington, 32 Willoway Lane, Braunton EX33 1BS Tel: 01271 814412 — MB BS Lond. 1972 (Char. Cross Hosp.) BSc (Human Physiol.) Lond. 1969; MRCS Eng. LRCP Lond. 1972; MRCGP 1982; Dip. IMC RCS Ed. 1993. Med. Off. AeroMed. Evac. 4626 (Aeromed Evac) Squadron, R Aux AF, Roy. Air Force Lyneham, Wilts. Specialty: Aviat. Med. Prev: GP Braunton; Regist. (Gen. Orthop. & Cardiothoracic Surg.) Roy. Brisbane Hosp., Austral.

POTELIAKHOFF, Alexander (retired) Sudbury, 16B Prince Arthur Road, London NW3 6AY Tel: 0207 435 1872 — MB BS Lond. 1941 (Westm.) MRCS Eng. LRCP Lond. 1941; MRCP Lond. 1947; MD Lond. 1949. Prev: Sen. Regist. (Med.) St. Mary Abbots Hosp. Lond.

POTHANIKAT, Mr George South Tyrone Hospital, Dungannon BT71 4AU Tel: 018657 22821; 8 Viewfort, Killymeal Road, Dungannon BT71 6LP Tel: 018687 26428 — State DMS Padua 1965; BSc Madras 1958; FRCSI 1985. Assoc. Specialist (Gen. Surg.) S. Tyrone Hosp. Specialty: Gastroenterol.

POTHANIKAT, Mary George Waveney Hospital, Cushendall Road, Ballymena BT43 6HH Tel: 028 2565 3377; 8 Viewfort, Killymeal Road, Dungannon BT71 6LP — State DMS Padua 1966; BSc Mysore 1959; LM 1975; DGO TC Dub. 1976.

POTHECARY, Ian Colin 31 Hurst Avenue, Horsham RH12 2EL — MB BS Lond. 1998.

POTIPHAR, Darren Wayne, Surg. Lt. RN 8 Southways, Stubbington, Fareham PO14 2AG Tel: 01329 668039 — MB ChB Liverp. 1993. Med. Off. HMS Collingwood. Specialty: Gen. Pract. Prev: Med. Off. HMS Drake; Mixed Module SHO RNH Haslar; Med. Off. HMS Glas. & RNAS Culdrose.

POTLURI, Mr Bernard Shaw Princess Alexandra Hospital, Hamstel Road, Harlow CM20 1QX Tel: 01279 444445 Fax: 01279 827092 Email: potluri@doctors.org.uk — MB BS Andhra 1977; MS Andhra 1981; FRCS 1989; Dip. Urol. Lond 1991. Cons. Urological Surg., Princess Alexandra Hosp., Harlow; Cons. Urological Surg., Rwers Hosp., Sawbridgeworth, Herts. Specialty: Urol. Socs: Brit. Assn. Urol. Surgs. & BMA; Life Mem. Assn. Surg. India; Eur. Assn. of Urol. Prev: Cons. Urol. Princess Alexandra Hosp. Harlow; Cons. Urol. Hairmyres Hosp. E. Kilbride.

POTOKAR, John Piers — MB ChB Birm. 1987; MRCPsych 1991; MD Bristol 2000. Hon. Cons. In Liaison Psychi. Bristol Roy. Infirm. Specialty: Gen. Psychiat. Socs: Coll. Internat. Neuropsychopharmacologicum; Brit. Assn. For Psychopharm. Prev: Lect., Div. of Psychiat. Bristol Univ.; Hon. Sen. Regist. (Psychopharmacol.) Bristol Roy. Infirm.

POTOKAR, Mr Thomas Stephen No 3, Vyvyan Terrace, Clifton, Bristol BS8 — MB ChB Birm. 1988; DTM & H Liverp. 1989; DA (UK) 1992; FRCS Ed. 1995.

POTRYKUS, Michael The Tollerton Surgery, 5-7 Hambleton View, Tollerton, York YO61 1QW Tel: 01347 838231 Fax: 01347 838699; 26 Mallison Hill Drive, Easinghold, York YO61 3RY Tel: 01347 821505 — MB ChB Ed. 1981; BSc Ed. 1979; MRCGP 1985; DRCOG 1985. Bd. Mem. York PCG. Prev: Trainee GP Northallerton VTS.

POTTAGE, Anthony (retired) 14 Caiystane Hill, Edinburgh EH10 6SL Tel: 0131 445 1351 Fax: 0131 445 3456 Email: tpottage@tiscali.co.uk — MB ChB Ed. 1972; MRCP (UK) 1975; FRCP Ed. 1985; FFPM RCP (UK) 1989. Prev: Vice Pres. R&D Admin. Astra Zeneca Sweden.

POTTER, Alexander Wilson Clydebank Health Centre , Red Wing, Kilbowie Road, Clydebank G81 2TQ Tel: 0141 531 6475 Fax: 0141 531 6478; 19 Campbell Drive, Bearsden, Glasgow G61 4NF Tel: 0141 942 8366 Email: alexwpotter@hotmail.com — MB ChB Glas. 1982 (Glasgow) DRCOG 1985; MRCGP 1986. GP Princip.; GP Trainer. Specialty: Gen. Pract.

POTTER, Alice Naghlia 64 Ryecroft Road, London SW16 3EH — LRCPI & LM, LRSCI & LM 1956 (RCSI) LRCPI & LM, LRCSI & LM 1956. Princip. Phys. (Child Health) Richmond Twickenham & Roehampton HA. Specialty: Paediat.; Neurol. Socs: Brit. Paediat. Assn. & Fac. Community Health of Soc. Community Med. Prev: SCMO (Community Health) Merton, Sutton & Wandsworth; AHA (T); Hon. Clin. Asst. (Child Health) King's Health Dist. (T).

POTTER, Andrew Boyce North Road West Medical Centre, 167 North Road West, Plymouth PL1 5BZ Tel: 01752 662780 Fax: 01752 254541 — MB ChB Bristol 1989; DRCOG 1992; Dip. IMC RCS Ed. 1993; DFFP 1995; MRCGP 1995.

POTTER, Andrew Robert, MBE 7 St Peter's Close, Goodworth Clatford, Andover SP11 7SF; BP 924, Parakou, Benin Tel: 229 61 11 09 Fax: 229 61 08 91 Email: postmast@parakou.sim.org — MB BChir Camb. 1975 (Cambridge University and Westminster Medical School) MA Camb. 1976; DRCOG 1979; DA Eng. 1980; Cert. JCC Lond. 1980; MRCGP 1981; DO RCPSI 1985; MRCOphth 1988; DTM & H Liverp. 1989. Ophth. Hopital St. Jean De Dieu Boko. Parakou, Benin; Vis. Ophth. Hosps. In Benin, Burkina Faso & Niger. Specialty: Ophth. Socs: BMA. Prev: Ophth. Centre Hosp.ier, Abomey, Benin.

POTTER, Christopher John Frederick (retired) 45 Seabrook Road, Hythe CT21 5LX Tel: 01303 267116 Fax: 01303 267116 — MA, MB BChir Camb. 1955; DA Eng. 1958; FFA RCS Eng. 1963. Cons. Anaesth. SE Kent NHS Trust. Prev: Sen. Regist. St. Mary's Hosp. Lond.

POTTER, Mr David Northern General Hospital, Herries Road, Sheffield S5 7AU Tel: 0114 243 4343; 4 Holt House Grove, Millhouses, Sheffield S7 2QG — MB ChB Sheff. 1990; FRCS Eng. 1999. Cons. Orthopaedic Surgery, Sheff. Teaching Hosp. Specialty: Orthop. Socs: Assoc. Mem. BOA; BESS; BOTA. Prev: Regist. (Orthop. Surg.) Rotherham Dist. Gen. Hosp.; Specialist Regist. (Orthop. Surg.) Barnsley Dist. Gen. Hosp.; Specialist Regist. (Orthop. Surg.) N. Gen. Hosp.

POTTER, Dennis Ralph (retired) 64 Ryecroft Road, London SW16 3EH — MB BS Lond. 1957 (King's Coll. Hosp.) MRCS Eng. LRCP Lond. 1957; FFA RCS Eng. 1964. Prev: Cons. Anaesth. King's Coll. Hosp. Lond.

POTTER, Frances Aileen (retired) 63 Polwarth Road, Brunton Park, Newcastle upon Tyne NE3 5NE Tel: 0191 236 2059 — MB ChB Manch. 1941; BSc Manch. 1938, MB ChB 1941; DCH Eng. 1947. Prev: Sen. Med. Off. Family Plann. N. Tyneside AHA.

POTTER, Francis Anthony 17 Shaws Drive, Wirral CH47 5AP — MB ChB Manch. 1983.

POTTER, Geoffrey James Arthur The Surgery, Denmark Street, Darlington DL3 0PD Tel: 01325 460731 Fax: 01325 362183; 17 Abercorn Court, High Grange, Darlington DL3 0GF Tel: 01325 361309 — MB ChB Leeds 1980; DRCOG 1983; MRCGP 1984; Dip. Med. Educat. 1995. Course Trainer, Cleveland VTS.

POTTER, Gillian Margaret NHS Lothian University Hospitals Division, The Royal Infirmary of Edinburgh, 51 Little France Cresent, Old Dalkeith Road, Edinburgh EH16 4SA Tel: 0131 242 3700 Email: potter22@hotmail.com — MB ChB Ed. 1998; BSc (Hons); BSc (Hons. Med. Sci.) Ed. 1995; MRCP 2001. Specialist Regist. Radiol. Specialty: Respirat. Med.

POTTER, Heather Christine Skewen Medical Centre, Queens Road, Skewen, Neath SA10 6UL Tel: 01792 812316 Fax: 01792 323208; 68 Derwen Fawr Road, Derwen Fawr, Swansea SA2 8AQ Tel: 01792 203440 — MB ChB Manch. 1985; MRCGP 1991.

POTTER, Helen Louise Zoe 14 Gallacher Way, Saltash PL12 4UT — MB BS Lond. 1997.

POTTER, Hilary Anne Furnace House Surgery, St Andrews Road, Carmarthen SA31 1EX Tel: 01267 236616 Fax: 01267 222673; Y Wern, Capel Dewi, Carmarthen SA32 8AY Tel: 01267 290084 — MB BCh Wales 1978 (Welsh Nat. Sch. Med.) DCH RCP Lond. 1983.

POTTER, Jacobus Louw (retired) 40A Morningside Park, Edinburgh EH10 5HA Tel: 0131 447 8467 — MB ChB Ed. 1948 (Univ. Ed.) FRCP Ed. 1971, M 1953. Prev: Exec. Dean Fac. Med. Univ. Edin.

POTTER, Janette Marie 25 Penrith Avenue, Giffnock, Glasgow G46 6LU — MB ChB Glas. 1985; FRCP Glas.; MRCP (UK) 1989. Cons. Phys. Med. for Elderly & Stroke Vict. Infirm. Glas.; Hon. Clin. Sen. Lect. Glas. Univ.; Hosp. sub dean Vict. Infirm. Glas. Specialty: Gen. Med.

POTTER, Jeanette Dawn Francesca 71 Moira Road, Cricklewood, London NW2 6TB — MB BS Lond. 1993; MRCP London 1996. Specialist Regist. Palliat. Med., N. Thames Rotat.

POTTER, Jennifer Gae Psychotheraphy Department, Lower Gnd. Floor, Adamson Centre, Sth. Wing, Block 8, St. Thomas's Hospital, Lambeth Palace Road, London SE1 7EH Tel: 0207 928 9292 Ext: 2272 Fax: 0207 960 5663 Email: jenny.potter@slam.nhs.uk — MB ChB Cape Town 1977; BSc Natal 1972; MRCPsych 1982; MSc (Group Analysis) Birkbeck, University of London 2002; TQAP(Tavistock Qualification in Adult Psychotheraphy) 2003; BCP Register 2003. p/t Cons. Psychotherapist St. Thomas's Hosp. Lond. Specialty: Psychother. Prev: SHO. & Reg. (Psychiat.) Roy. Beth. & Maudsley Hosps. Lond.; Sen. Reg. Tavistock Clinic (Psychoth.) Tavistock & Portman NHS Trust; Sen. Reg. Cassel Hosp. (Psychoth.) Riverside NHS Trust Lond.

POTTER, Mr John 1 Greystoke Park, Gosforth, Newcastle upon Tyne NE3 2DZ — MB BS Durh. 1938; FRCS Ed. 1942. Socs: Brit. Assn. Plastic Surg. Prev: Plastic Surg. Teesside, Darlington & Northallerton Hosp. Gps.; Plastic Surg. Shotley Bridge Hosp. & Newc. Gen. Hosp.; Maj. RAMC. Surg. Specialist.

POTTER, Professor John Francis University Department of Medicine for the Elderly, The Glenfield Trust Hospital, Groby Road, Leicester LE3 9QP Tel: 0116 256 3365 Fax: 0116 232 2976 Email: jp34@le.ac.uk — BM BS Nottm. 1976; DM Nottm. 1989, BM BS 1976; MRCP (UK) 1979; FRCP Lond. 1992. Prof. Med. for Elderly. Univ. Leicester; Frohlich Vis. Prof. Roy. Soc. Med. Specialty: Gen. Med. Socs: Internat. Soc. Hypertens.; Exec. Comm. Mem. Brit. Hypertens. Soc.; Assn. Phys.

POTTER, John Maclaren — BM BCh Oxf. 1988; FRCS (Urol); MA Camb. Cons. Urol. Northampton Gen. Hosp. Specialty: Urol. Prev: SHO Urol. Battle Hosp. Reading; SpR Urol. The Roy. Free Hosp. Lond.; Spr Middlx. Hosp. Lond.

POTTER, John Michael — MB ChB Dundee 1997.

POTTER, John Richard Crisop Woodford Surgery, 29-31 Chantry Lane, Grimsby DN31 2LL Tel: 01472 342325 Fax: 01472 251739; 2 Devonshire Avenue, Grimsby DN32 0BW Tel: 01472 276228 Email: 101623.2123@compuserve.com — MB ChB Sheff. 1980; FRCGP 1996, M 1984. Course Organiser N. Lincs. VTS.

POTTER, Jonathan Martin Kent and Canterbury Hospital, Canterbury CT1 3NG Tel: 01227 766877; Tyler Hall, Summer Lane, Tyler Hill, Canterbury CT2 9NJ Tel: 01227 471682 — BM BCh Oxf. 1973 (St Thomas') DM Oxf. 1983; FRCP (UK) 1992. Cons. Phys. (Geriat. Med.) Kent & Canterbury Hosp.; Hon. Sen. Research Fell. Centre for Health Serv. Studies Univ.of Kent; Hon. Sen. Lect. Kent Inst. of Health & Med. Scis.; Assoc. Director, Clin. Effectivness and Eval. Unit, Roy. Coll. of Phys.s, Lond. Specialty: Care of the Elderly. Socs: Brit. Geriat. Soc. Prev: Sen. Regist. (Gen. & Geriat. Med.) Roy. Hallamsh. Hosp. & Nether Edge Hosp. Sheff.; Radcliffe Trav. Fell. N.W.. Univ. Med. Center, USA.

POTTER, Mr Mark Adrian 33 Muir Wood Drive, Currie EH14 5EZ — MB ChB Ed. 1990; FRCS Eng. 1994.

POTTER, Michael Neil Department of Haematology, Royal Free Hospital School of Medicine, Rowland Hill St., London NW3 2PF Tel: 020 7794 0500 Fax: 020 7794 0645; 141 North Hill, Highgate, London N6 4DP Tel: 020 8348 4040 — MB BS Lond. 1984 (Univ. Camb., Univ. Lond. & Middlx. Hosp.) MA Camb. 1984; MRCP (UK) 1987; PhD Bristol 1993; MRCPath 1993. Cons. & Sen. Lect. (Haemat.) Roy. Free Hosp NHS Trust & Roy. Free & Univ coll med sch Lond.; Hon Cons (Haemat) Gt Ormond St. Hosp for Childr. NHS Trust. Specialty: Haematology. Socs: ASH; BSH; (Sec.) Brit. Soc. Blood & Marrow Transpl. Prev: Cons. & Sen. Lect. (Haemat. & Bone Marrow Transpl.) United Bristol Healthcare Trust & Univ. Bristol; Sen. Regist. (Haemat.) Yorks. RHA; Research Regist. (Paediat. Haemat.) Bristol Childr. Hosp. & Bristol Univ. Med. Sch.

POTTER, Neil David Mowbray Marden Medical Centre, Church Green, Marden, Tonbridge TN12 9HP Tel: 01622 831257 Fax: 01622 832840; 1A Mill Bank, Headcorn, Ashford TN27 9QX Tel: 01622 891971 Fax: 01622 891971 — MB BChir Camb. 1991 (Cambridge) MA Camb. 1992; DCH RCP Lond. 1993; MRCGP 1995; DFFP 1996. GT Princip. Specialty: Gen. Pract. Socs: (Founder Mem.) Maidstone Area New Genuinely Young Principles and Recent Train.s Soc. Prev: Trainee GP Maidstone VTS; SHO Nat. Wom. Hosp. Auckland, NZ.

POTTER, Patricia Eustace (retired) Holywell Hospital, Steeple Road, Antrim BT41 2RJ; 39 Osborne Park, Belfast BT9 6JP — MB BCh BAO Belf. 1959 (Qu. Univ. Belf.) BSc Belf. 1956, MB BCh BAO 1959; DPM RCPSI 1963; MRCPsych 1972. Prev: Cons. Psychiat. Holywell Hosp. Antrim.

POTTER, Robert Graham Department of Child & Family Psychiatry, Royal United Hospital, Bath BA1 3NG Tel: 01225 825075 Fax: 01225 825076; Abbey View House, Abbey View, Bath BA2 6DG Tel: 01225 333774 Email: bob.potter@argonet.co.uk — MB ChB Bristol 1971; MRCPsych 1975. Cons. Child Psychiat. Roy. United Hosp. Bath. Specialty: Child & Adolesc. Psychiat. Socs: Assn. Psychiat. Study Adolesc.; Assn. Child Psychol. & Psychiat. Prev: Sen. Regist. (Child & Adolsc. Psychiat.) Warneford & Pk. Hosp. Oxf.; Sen. Regist. (Psychiat.) Profess. Dept. Psychiat. Warneford Hosp. Oxf.

POTTER, Robert John 68 Derwen Fawr Road, Sketty, Swansea SA2 8AQ — MB ChB Manch. 1985.

POTTER, Russell Shaw 47 Earls Way, Ayr KA7 4HQ — MB ChB Glas. 1994. Dir. Medic8.com. Specialty: Anaesth.

POTTER, Samantha Margaret Balmore Park Surgery, 59A Hemdean Road, Caversham, Reading RG4 7SS — MB BS Lond. 1991; BSc (Med. Microbiol.) Lond. 1988; DRCOG 1995; DFFP 1996; MRCGP 1996. GP Princip., Balmore Pk. Surg. Prev: SHO (Cas.) Chase Farm Hosp. Enfield; GP Regist. Wycombe VTS.

POTTER, Sara Maureen (retired) Honey House, Lodes Lane, Kingston St Mary, Taunton TA2 8HU — MB BCh Wales 1944; LM Rotunda 1947. Prev: Ho. Surg. Roy. W. Sussex Hosp. Chichester & Roy. Surrey Co. Hosp.

POTTER, Sarah Frances Kelso Medical Group Practice, Health Centre, Inch Road, Kelso TD5 7JP Tel: 01573 224424 Fax: 01573 226388; Ferneyhill Cottage, Kelso TD5 7SU — MB ChB Ed. 1990.

POTTER, Stephen Mark 3 Halterburn Close, Kingsmere, Gosforth, Newcastle upon Tyne NE3 4YT — MB ChB Ed. 1994.

POTTER, Susan Jane Moss Grove Surgery, 15 Moss Grove, Kingswinford DY8 3AS — BM BS Nottm. 1989; DRCOG 1992; Dip Eur Hum (Open) Dip Lit (Open) BA (Hons) (Open) 2003. Socs: Roy. Coll. Gen. Pract.

POTTER, Tanya Buchanan 1 Margaret Street, Derby DE1 3FE — MB ChB Sheff. 1994.

POTTER, Vanessa Alice Joyce — MB ChB Birm. 1992; MRCP; PhD.

POTTER, Vanessa Jane Faversham Health Centre, Bank St., Faversham ME13 8QR Tel: 01795 562011; Tyler Hall, Tyler Hill, Canterbury CT2 9NJ Tel: 01227 471682 — MB BS Lond. 1974 (St. Thomas's Hosp. Med. Sch.) DRCOG 1988. GP. Specialty: Gen. Pract.

POTTERTON, Amanda Jane Department of Radiology, Royal Victoria Infirmary, Newcastle upon Tyne NE1 4LP Tel: 0191 282 4431 — MB BS Newc. 1985 (Newcastle) MRCP (UK) 1989; FRCR 1992. Cons. Diagnostic Radiol. Newc. Hosps. NHS Trust; Cons. radiologist.Breast screening & Assessm. centre,Qu. Eliz. Hosp. Specialty: Radiol. Prev: Sen. Regist. (Diag. Radiol.) North. RHA Newc. u Tyne; Regist. (Gen. Med.) Gateshead HA; SHO (Gen. Med.) Sunderland HA.

POTTERTON, Karen Louise Woodlands Health Centre, Paddock Wood, Tonbridge TN12 6AX Tel: 01892 833331 Fax: 01892 838269 — MB BS Lond. 1992.

POTTINGER, Gillian Ruth — BM BCh Oxf. 1996 (Oxford University) BA Oxf. 1993; MRCS (Lond.) 2000. GP. Specialty: Gen. Surg. Prev: SHO Rotat. (Surg.).

POTTS, Mr David John c/o Accident & Emergency Department, Wycombe General Hospital, High Wycombe HP11 2TT Tel: 01494 425318 — MB BCh Wales 1981; BSc (Hons.) Anat. Wales 1978; FRCS Eng. 1987. Cons. A & E Wycombe Gen. Hosp. Specialty: Accid. & Emerg.

POTTS, Donald Agar c/o The Old New House, Avon Dassett, Leamington Spa; 1228 Kensington Road, Calgary Alb. T2N 4PQ, Canada — MRCS Eng. LRCP Lond. 1953; MD Alberta 1958. Asst. Prof. Univ. of Calgary Med. Sch.; Chief of Staff Sarcee Auxil. Hosp. Calgary Alta; Med. Dir. Bowcrest Nursing Home Calgary Alta. Prev: Chief of Staff Col. Belcher Hosp. Calgary.

POTTS, Elizabeth Deirdre Ann Pinderfields General Hospital, West Cottage Aberford Road, Wakefield WF1 4TU; Oakwood Lodge, 6 Park Avenue, Leeds LS8 2JH — MB BCh BAO Belf. 1972; DObst RCOG 1974; MRCP (UK) 1976; FRCP Lond. 1993. Cons. Dermat. Pinderfields Gen. Hosp. Specialty: Dermat.; DVMAT.

POTTS, Mr Hamish Elder 132 Bentinck Drive, Troon KA10 6JB Tel: 01292 318789; The Ayr Hospital, Dalmellington Road, Ayr KA6 6DX — MB ChB Glas. 1976; BSc Glas. 1970; FRCS Glas. 1984; FRCS Ed. (Orth.) 1990. Cons. Orthop. Surg. The Ayr Hosp. Specialty: Orthop. Socs: Fell. BOA. Prev: Sen. Regist. Edin.; Surg. Lt. RN.

POTTS, Jane Jason 27 Murray Road, Northwood HA6 2YP Tel: 01923 825318 — MB ChB Leeds 1971; DObst RCOG 1976. Psychiat. Hounslow & Spelthorne AHA.

POTTS, Lindsay Fraser Raigmore Hospital, Inverness IV2 3UJ Tel: 01463 704000 Fax: 01463 705460 Email: lindsay.potts@haht.scot.nhs.uk; Hillside, Upper Myrltefield, Nairnside, Inverness IV2 5BX — MB ChB Ed. 1985; BSc Physiol. Ed. 1983; FRCP Edin. 2001. Cons. (Phys.) Raigmore Hosp. Inverness. Specialty: Gastroenterol.; Gen. Med. Special Interest: Luminal Gastroenterol. Socs: BMA; Roy. Soc. Med.; RCP (Edin). Prev: Regist. (Geriat.) Edin.

POTTS, Mrs Lorna Anne Village Green Surgery, The Green, Wallsend NE28 6BB Tel: 0191 262 3252 Fax: 0191 263 4260; 5 Beverley Park, Monkseaton, Whitley Bay NE25 8JL — MB BS Durh. 1959. Prev: Ho. Phys. Sunderland Roy. Infirm.; Ho. Off. (Paediat.) Sunderland Child. Hosp.

POTTS, Mary Anne 1 Chapel Row, Sandhutton, Thirsk YO7 4RW Tel: 01845 587333 — MB ChB Cape Town 1978. GP Trainee.

POTTS, Michael 10 Highbury, Newcastle upon Tyne NE2 3DX — MB BS Newc. 1985; FRCS Glas. 1995; FFAEM (UK) 1999. Specialty: Accid. & Emerg.

POTTS, Mr Michael John Private Rooms, 2 Clifton Park, Clifton, Bristol BS8 3BS Tel: 0117 906 4215 Fax: 0117 973 0887; 192 Stoke Lane, Westbury on Trym, Bristol BS9 3RU Tel: 0117 968 7550 — MB ChB Bristol 1981; BSc (Hons. Physics) Bristol 1973; PhD Bristol 1979; FRCS (Ophth.) Eng. 1986; FRCOphth 1989. Cons. Ophth. Bristol Eye Hosp. Specialty: Ophth. Socs: Europ. Soc. Plastic. & Reconstruc. Surg. Prev: Oculoplastic Fell. Moorfields Eye Hosp. Lond.; Sen. Regist. Moorfields Eye Hosp. Lond.; Regist. (Ophth.) Bristol & Weston HA.

POTTS, Nicolette Jane 12 Holt Park Gardens, Leeds LS16 7RB — MB ChB Leic. 1994; MRCGP; DPhil; MPH.

POTTS, Roger Karl Shadwell Medical Centre, 137 Shadwell Lane, Leeds LS17 8AE Tel: 0113 293 9999 Fax: 0113 248 5888 — MB BS Lond. 1972 (King's College Hospital Medical School London) MRCS Eng. LRCP Lond. 1972. Specialty: Gen. Pract.

POTTS, Stephen Graham Royal Infirmary of Edinburgh, Edinburgh EH16 4SA Tel: 0131 242 1398 Fax: 0131 242 1393 Email: psychmed.rie@luht.scot.nhs.uk — BM BCh Oxf. 1982; MA Camb. 1985, BA 1979; MRCPsych 1990. Cons. Liaison Psychiat. (Psychol. Med.) Roy. Infirm. Edin. Specialty: Gen. Psychiat. Socs: Roy. Coll. Psychiat. Prev: Regist. (Psychiat.) Maudsley Hosp. Lond.; Sen.Regist. (Psychiat.) Roy. Edin. Hosp.; Hon.Sen.Regist. (Psychiat.) & Research Fell.Unov.Edin.

POTTS, Stephen Randolph Royal Belfast Hospital For Sick Children, 180 Falls Road, Belfast BT12 6BE Tel: 028 9063 2000 Fax: 028 9063 2921 Email: denise.slevin@royalhospitals.n-i.nhs.uk — MB BCh BAO Belfast; FRCSI. Cons. Paediatric Surg., Roy. Belf. Hosp. for Sick Childr. Specialty: Paediat. Surg. Socs: Brit. Assn. of Paediatric Surgeons; Brit. Assn. of Endoscopic Surgeons (Paeds); Internat. Paediatric Endoscopic Gp.

POTTS, Timothy Marc Victoria Surgery, Victoria Road, Rhymney NP22 5NU Tel: 01685 840614 Fax: 01685 843770; Wenallt Fach, Gilwern, Abergavenny NP7 0HP Tel: 01873 832221 — MB BCh Wales 1986 (University of Wales) BDS Wales 1977; FDS RCS Eng. 1982; DCH RCP Lond. 1988; Dip. IMC RCS Ed. 1989; MRCGP 1993. Med. Off. Longtown Mt.ain Rescue Team; Mem. Mid. Glam. Emerg. Doctor Serv. Socs: Brit. Assn. Immed. Care Schemes. Prev: Trainee GP N. Gwent VTS; Regist. (Oral & Dent. Surg.) Bristol Dent. Hosp.

POTTS, Wendy Ann 53 Parkway, New Mills, High Peak SK22 4DU — MB ChB Ed. 1992.

POTU, Mr Prabhakar Hadleigh, Rolvenden Road, Benenden, Cranbrook TN17 4EH — MB BS Osmania 1970; DO RCPSI 1978; FRCS Ed. 1988; FRCOphth 1989.

POTWORSKA-SILLITOE, Krystyna Maria (retired) 6 Fullbrooks Avenue, Worcester Park KT4 7PE — MB ChB Silesia 1959; LAH Dub. 1964.

POULDEN, Mr Mark Alan 9 Dysgwylfa, Sketty, Swansea SA2 9BG Tel: 01792 207458 — MB BCh Wales 1992; FRCSI 1997. Specialist Regist. All Wales A & E Team. Specialty: Accid. & Emerg. Prev: SHO (A & E) Morriston Hosp. Swansea.

POULIER, Robin Arcot Ilkley Health Centre, Springs Lane, Ilkley LS29 8TQ; 53 Ben Rhydding Road, Ilkley LS29 8RN — MB BS Newc. 1980; Cert. Family Plann. RCOG & RCGP 1982; DRCOG 1983; DCCH RCGP & FCM 1984; MRCGP 1984; Dip. Palliat. Med. Wales 1992. Med. Off. Marie Curie Cancer Care Ilkley. Specialty: Palliat. Med. Prev: Trainee GP N.ld. VTS; Ho. Phys. Freeman Hosp. Newc.; Ho. Surg. Sunderland Roy. Infirm.

POULLIS, Andrew Patroclos 61 Moring Road, London SW17 8DN — MB BS Lond. 1994; BSc 1991; MRCP 1997; MD 2003. Specialty: Gastroenterol.; Gen. Med.

POULSEN, Helle 10 Parkside, High St., Worthing BN11 1NB — MD Copenhagen 1983.

POULSEN-HANSEN, Alfred Gerhardt (retired) 24 Noel Road, London N1 8HA Tel: 020 7226 8037 — MD Copenhagen 1941; DTM & H Liverp. 1948; DPH Lond. 1952; MFCM 1974. Prev: Dep. MOH Harlow & Epping UDCs & Epping & Ongar RDC & Asst. Co. Med. Off. Essex CC.

POULSOM, William John High Walls, Over Court, Over La., Almondsbury, Bristol BS32 4DG — MB BS Lond. 1966; MRCS Eng. LRCP Lond. 1966; DObst RCOG 1969; DPH Bristol 1972; MFCM 1979.

POULSON, Arabella Valentine 46 Ross Street, Cambridge CB1 3BX — MB BS Lond. 1989; FRCOphth 1995. Specialty: Ophth.

POULTER, Andrea Elizabeth 20 Manse Road, Newtownards BT23 4TP — MB BCh BAO Belf. 1996 (Qus. Univ. Belf.) Med. SHO Antrim Area Hosp. Antrim, N. Irel. Socs: BMA.

POULTER, Professor Neil Reginald Imperial College School of Medicine, St Mary's Campus, Cardiovascular Studies Unit, Department Clinical Pharmacology, London W2 1PG Tel: 020 7594 3445/6 Fax: 020 7594 3411 Email: n.poulter@imperial.ac.uk — MB BS Lond. 1975; MRCS Eng. LRCP Lond. 1974; MRCP (UK) 1977; MSc Lond. 1986; FRCP Lond. 1994. Prof. Preven. Cardiovasc. Med. Imperial Coll. Lond.; Hon. Cons. Peart- Rose (Hypertens.) Clinic. St. Mary's Hosp. Lond. Specialty: Vasc. Med.; Epidemiol. Special Interest: Assn. Between Birthweight and Hypertens.; Investig. & Managem. of Hypertens. & Dyslipidaemia; The Effects of Oestrogen/ Progesterone & CND in the 3rd World. Socs: Pres. Brit. Hypertens. Soc.; Member of BHF Primary Prevention commitee; FRCP. Prev: Reader in Clin. Epidem. Univ. Coll. Lond. Med. Sch.; Sen. Lect. In Clin. Epidem. Univ. Coll. Lond. Med. Sch.; Dir. Cardiovasc. Studies Unit Dept. of Clin. Pharm. & Therap.

POULTER, Simon David Anaesthetic Department, Princess of Wales Hospital, Coity Road, Bridgend CF31 1RQ Tel: 01656 752361 — MB BCh Wales 1990 (Univ. Wales Coll. Med. Cardiff) FRCA 1996. Cons. Anaesth., BRO Morgannwg NHS Trust. Specialty: Anaesth. Socs: Brit. Ophth. Anaesth. Soc.; Soc. for Computing and Technol. in Anaesth.; Assn. of Anaesthestists of Gt. Britain & Irel. Prev: Specialist Regist. (Anaesth.) Roy. Gwent Hosp.

POULTNEY, Joanne Michelle 56 Cole Bank Road, Hall Green, Birmingham B28 8EY — MB ChB Leic. 1996.

POULTON, Brodyn Bryant Norfolk & Norwich Hospital, Brunswick Rd, Norwich NR1 3SR; Corner House, Plump Road, Tharston, Norwich NR15 2YR — MB ChB Cape Town 1989; FRCA 1994. Cons. (Anaesth.) Norf. & Norwich Hosp. Specialty: Anaesth.

POULTON, David John Adeline Road Surgery, 4 Adeline Road, Boscombe, Bournemouth BH5 1EF Tel: 01202 309421 Fax: 01202 304893; 12 Leicester Road, Poole BH13 6BZ Tel: 01202 760054 — MB ChB Liverp. 1975; MRCGP 1979; DRCOG 1979. Police Surg. Bournemouth. Prev: Clin. Asst. Cardiol. Roy. Bournmouth Hosp.

POULTON, Joanna University of Oxford, Nuffield Department of Obstetrics & Gynaecology, John Radcliffe Hospital, Headington, Oxford OX3 9DU Tel: 01865 221227 Fax: 01865 769141 Email: joanna.poulton@obs-gyn.ox.ac.uk — BM BCh Oxf. 1979; MRCP (UK) 1982; DM Oxf. 1991. Univ. Research Fell. (Roy. Soc.) (Paediat.) Univ. Oxf.; Hon. Cons. (Mitochondrial Genetics) Oxf.; Convenor Mitochondrial Workshop for the Europ. Neuromuscular Centre; Hon. Readership in Mitochondrial Genetics, Univ. of Oxf.; Prof. (Mitochondrial Genetics). Specialty: Paediat.; Genetics. Socs: BPA; Clin. Genetics Soc. Prev: Wellcome Sen. Research Fell. in Clin. Sc.; Action Research Train. Fellowship (Paediat.) Univ. Oxf.; Regist. (Paediat.) Birm. Childr. Hosp.

POULTON, Julian Walker 32 Springbank Gardens, Lymm WA13 9GR — MB ChB Liverp. 1998; DCH 2003.

POULTON, Mary Bernadette 30 Bowater Place, London SE3 8ST — MB BS Lond. 1992 (King's Coll. Lond.) MRCP (UK) 1996; Dip GU Med. Soc Apoth 1997; DFFP 1998. Cons. (GUM/HIV) Newham Gen. Hosp. Specialty: Genitourinary Medicine. Socs: MSSVD; BHIVA. Prev: SHO (Immunol. & HIV) St. Bart. Hosp. Lond.; SHO (Genitourin. Med.) Char. Cross Hosp. Lond.; SHO (Paediat.) Greenwich Hosp.

POULTON, Susan Elizabeth Dept of Elderly Medicine, Queen Alexandra Hospital, Cosham, Portsmouth PO6 3LY Tel: 023 9228 6423 Fax: 02392200381 — BM Soton. 1983; MRCP (UK) 1986; DRCOG 1989. Cons. (Geriat. Med.) Qu. Alexandra Hosp. Portsmouth. Specialty: Care of the Elderly. Prev: Sen. Regist. (Geriat. Med.) Soton. Gen. Hosp.; Sen. Regist. (Geriat. Med.) Qu. Alexandra Hosp. Portsmouth; Regist. & SHO (Med.) Qu. Alexandra & St. Mary's Hosps. Portsmouth.

POUNCEY, Catherine Margaret Godwin The Surgery, Malthouse Meadows, Portesham, Weymouth DT3 4NS Tel: 01305 871468 Fax: 01305 871977; Bridehead, Littlebredy, Dorchester DT2 9JA Tel: 01308 482232 — MB BS Lond. 1972 (King's Coll. Hosp.) DObst RCOG 1974; MRCP (UK) 1975; DCH Eng. 1975. Specialty: Gen. Pract. Prev: Sen. Regist. & Regist. (Paediat.) Horton Gen. Hosp. Banbury; Regist. (Paediat.) Soton. Gen. Hosp.

POUNCEY, David Anthony Columba Godwin Marlow and Partners, The Surgery, Bell Lane, Stroud GL6 9JF Tel: 01453 883793 Fax: 01453 731670; 18 Rodborough Avenue, Stroud GL5 3RS — MB BS Lond. 1983; MA Camb. 1984, BA 1980; DRCOG 1986; MRCGP 1987; DTM & H Lond. 1988.

POUND, Neil 3 Regency Close, Littleover, Derby DE23 1TR Tel: 01332 776488 — BM BS Nottm. 1990. Specialty: Gen. Pract.

POUND, Susan Elizabeth 17 Corrennie Gardens, Edinburgh EH10 6DG Tel: 0131 447 0044 — MB ChB Ed. 1986; BSc (Med. Sci.) Ed. 1984; MRCP (UK) 1989; MD Ed. 1994. Cons. Phys. (Gen. Med. & c/o Elderly) Qu. Margt. Hosp. Dunfermline. Specialty: Gen. Med. Prev: Sen. Regist. (Geriat. & Gen. Med.) St. John's Hosp. Livingston; MRC Clin. Train. Fell. MRC Human Genetics Unit West. Gen. Hosp. Edin.; Regist. (Gen. Med.) Roy. Infirm. Edin.

POUNDALL, Clare Elise 16 Ralliwood Road, Ashtead KT21 1DE Tel: 01372 275160 — MB BCh BAO NUI 1952 (Univ. Coll. Dub.) DObst RCOG 1954. Socs: Brit. Assn. Dermat. Prev: Assoc. Specialist (Dermat.) Roy. Surrey Co. Hosp. Guildford & Nelson Hosp. Lond.

POUNDER, Derek 79 Bowes Hill, Rowlands Castle PO9 6BS Tel: 023 9241 2437 Fax: 023 9241 2437 — MB ChB Dundee 1973; DA Eng. 1977; FFA RCS Eng. 1979. Cons. (Anaesth.) Portsmouth Hosps. Acute Unit Trust. Specialty: Anaesth. Prev: Sen. Regist. (Anaesth.) Soton. & Portsmouth Hosps.; Regist. (Anaesth.) Addenbrooke's & Papworth Hosps. Camb.

POUNDER, Fiona Alison 23 Wellcroft Close, Wheatley Hills, Doncaster DN2 5RU; Morton Grange, The Avenue, Morton, Lincoln LN6 9HW — MB ChB Sheff. 1986. Trainee GP/SHO (Med.) Doncaster Roy. Infirm.

POUNDER, Leanne Wye Valley Surgery, 2A Desborough Avenue, High Wycombe HP11 2RN — BM BS Nottm. 1996; DRCOG 1999; DFFP 2000; MRCGP 2000. GP Princip. High Wycombe; Clin. Asst. (Palliat. Care) Sue Ryder Home, Nettlebed, Henley-on-Thames. Specialty: Gen. Pract.; Palliat. Med.

POUNDER, Professor Robert Roy Edward Centre for Gastroenterology (10th floor), Royal Free and University College Medical School, Rowland Hill St., London NW3 2PF Tel: 020 7830 2243 Fax: 020 7431 5261 Email: r.pounder@rfc.ucl.ac.uk — MB BChir Camb. 1969 (Camb. & Guy's) BA Camb. 1966, MD 1977, MA 1970; MRCP (UK) 1971; FRCP Lond. 1984; DSc (Med.) Lond. 1992. Prof. Med. Roy. Free & Univ. Coll. Med. Sch. of Univ. Med. Coll. Lond. - Vice-Pres., Roy. Coll. of Phys., Lond.; Co-Edr. Alimentary Pharmacol. & Therap.; Hon. Cons. Phys. & Gastroenterol. Roy. Free Hosp. Lond.; Co-Edr., GastroHep.com. Specialty: Gastroenterol. Socs: Brit. Soc. Gastroenterol.; Amer. Gastroenterol. Assn.; Amer. College Gastroenterol. Prev: Sen. Regist. (Med.) St. Thos. Hosp. Lond.; Sen. Regist. (Gastroenterol.) Centr. Middlx. Hosp. Lond.; SHO (Gastroenterol.) Hammersmith Hosp.

POUNDER, Ronald The Pease Way Medical Centre, 2 Pease Way, Newton Aycliffe DL5 5NH Tel: 01325 301888 — MB BS Newc. 1983; MRCGP 1987.

POUNDS, Frances Jessie (retired) Fairlic House, 2 -6 Uppington Road, West Norwood, London SE27 0RP Tel: 020 8693 8396 — MD Lond. 1943 (Roy. Free) MB BS 1938; MRCP Lond. 1942. Prev: Med. Off. Resid. Staff Health Serv. King's Coll. Hosp. Lond.

POUNSFORD, John Christopher Frenchay Day Hospital, Frenchay, Bristol BS16 1LE Tel: 0117 970 1212 Fax: 0117 970 2290; 1 Knoll Hill, Stoke Bishop, Bristol BS9 1QY Tel: 0117 968 4934 — MB BS Lond. 1975 (Westm.) MRCS Eng. LRCP Lond. 1975; MRCP (UK) 1978; MD Lond. 1986; FRCP Lond. 1994. Cons. Phys. Frenchay Hosp. Bristol; Sen. Clin. Lect. Univ. Bristol. Specialty: Care of the Elderly. Socs: Brit. Geriat. Soc. & Brit. Thoracic Soc. Prev: Cons. Sen. Lect. (Med.) Univ. Bristol; Regist. & Research Fell. St. Geo. Hosp. Lond.; Ho. Phys. & Ho. Surg. Westm. Hosp. Lond.

POUNTAIN, Gillian Diane Hinchingbrooke Hospital, Hinchingbrooke Park, Huntingdon PE29 6NT Tel: 01480 416416; 13 Church Street, Bourn, Cambridge CB3 7SJ — MB BS Lond. 1976 (University College Hosp London) BSc (Pharmacol.) Lond. 1973; MRCP (UK) 1980; MD Lond. 1995; FRCP 1999. Specialty: Rheumatol. Socs: Paediatric E Anglian Rheum Soc. (Chair.); Brit. Soc. for Rheum.; Brit. Paediatric RheumGp. Prev: Sen. Regist. (Rheum.) Addenbrooke's Hosp. Camb.; Regist. (Rheum.) Manch. Roy. Infirm.; Regist. (Rheum.) Canad. Red Cross Memor. Hosp. Taplow.

POUNTNEY, Alison Mary Claremont Surgery, Wilderness Medical Centre, 2 Cookham Road, Maidenhead SL6 8AN Tel: 01628 673033; Bishops Farm Lodge, Oakley Green Road, Windsor SL4 4PY — MB BS Lond. 1981 (Univ. Coll.) BSc Lond. 1978, MB BS 1981;

DRCOG 1984. Prev: SHO (A & E) Wexham Pk. Hosp. Slough; SHO (O & G) Heatherwood Hosp. Ascot; SHO (Anaesth.) E. Berks. HA.

POUNTNEY, Andrew James 2 Pitchstone Court, Farnley, Leeds LS12 5SZ — MB ChB (Hons.) Leeds 1998; MRCP. SHO A& E at IGI. Specialty: Accid. & Emerg. Socs: MPS. Prev: PRHO in Med. at Harrogate Dist.; PRHO in Surg. at St. James, Leeds.

POURAMINI, Morteza The Body Sculpture Clinic, 54A Pennhill Avenue, Poole BH14 9NA Tel: 01202 737274 Fax: 01202 737444 — MD Tehran 1966 (Tehran Med. Univ.) OB Gyn UK 1976. Cons. "Cosmetic Surg."; Med. Dir. Of Body Sculpture Clinic, Dorset UK. Specialty: Obst. & Gyn. Socs: Fell. Europ. Acad. Cosmetic Surg.; Amer. Acad. of Cosmetic Surg.; Internat. Soc. Of Lipos. Surg.

POURGHAZI, Saied 34 Montague Street, Glasgow G4 9HX — MB ChB Glas. 1992.

POURGOURIDES, Christina Kyriacou Sutton South CMHT, Chiltern Wing, Sutton Hospital, Cotswold Road, Sutton SM2 5NF Tel: 0208 296 4239 Fax: 0208 642 7503 — MB ChB Birm. 1989; MRC Psych 1994. Specialty: Gen. Psychiat.

POURGOURIDES, Effie Kyriacou Garden Flat, 5 Gladwyn Road, Putney, London SW15 1JY — MB ChB Birm. 1992; MBChB (Hons.) 1992; MRCP (UK) 1996. Specialist Regist. in Haemat. Specialty: Haematology.

POURIA, Shideh GRT School of Medicine, Department of Renal Medicine, Weston Education Centre, 10 Cutcombe Road, London SE5 9RJ — MB BS Lond. 1991; MRCP 1994. Specialist Regist. (Nephrology) King's Coll. Lond. Specialty: Nephrol.

POUYA, Amitis 17 Argie Gardens, Leeds LS4 2JL — MB ChB Aberd. 1992.

POVEDANO CANIZARES, Cristobal Eduardo 6 Victoria Crescent, Ashton Road, Lancaster LA1 5FD — LMS Cordoba 1991.

POVER, Andrew Benedict Town House, Station Road, Madeley, Crewe CW3 9PW — MB ChB Dundee 1992.

POVEY, Jane Margaret Mytton Oak Surgery, Racecourse Lane, Shrewsbury SY1 1RL Tel: 01743 362223; The Lodge, Boreton, Cross Houses, Shrewsbury SY5 6HJ — MB BS Lond. 1991 (St. Bart.) DFFP 1994; DRCOG 1995; T(GP 1996. GP Retainer. Specialty: Gen. Pract. Prev: SHO (O & G) Northampton Hosp.; SHO (A & E) Bendigo Base Hosp. Vict., Australia; SHO (Paediat.) Princess Roy. Hosp. Telford.

POVEY, Janet Rowan The Haybarn, Home Farm Court, Holdenby, Northampton NN6 8EE Tel: 01604 770124 Fax: 01604 770124 — MB ChB Liverp. 1982. Med. Director SR Pharma Ltd. Specialty: Pharmaceutical Medicine. Prev: Cons. Mapleleaf Assocs. Ltd.; Med. Affairs Manager Lederle Laborat. Gosport; Med. Dir. Pasteur Merieux MSD Ltd.

POVEY, John Sullivan (retired) Martlets, Westerland, Marldon, Paignton TQ3 1RR Tel: 01803 557054 — MRCS Eng. LRCP Lond. 1957 (Roy. Free) DObst RCOG 1959; MRCGP 1965. Prev: GP Paignton.

POVEY, Julian David Pontesbury Medical Practice, Pontesbury, Shrewsbury SY5 0RF Email: julian.povey@gp-m82030.nhs.uk — (St. Bart.) MB BS Lond. 1991; Cert. Prescribed Equiv. Exp. JCPTGP 1996; MRCGP 1996; DFFP 1996. Specialty: Gen. Pract. Prev: SHO (Paediat.) Princess Roy. Hosp. Telford; SHO (A & E) Milton Keynes Hosp.; SHO (Med.) Echuca Hosp. Vict., Austral.

POVEY, Margaret Susan 20 Church Lane, Cheddington, Leighton Buzzard LU7 0RU — MD Camb. 1977 (Camb. & Univ. Coll. Hosp.) MB BChir 1967; DTM & H Liverp. 1968. Prof. of Human Genetics Univ. Coll. Lond.. Prev: Scientif. Staff MRC Unit Galton Laborat. Univ. Coll. Lond.

POVEY, Mr Robert William, CStJ (retired) Heath Rise, 48 Horncastle Road, Woodhall Spa LN10 6UZ Tel: 01526 53379 — MB BS Lond. 1945 (Westm.) MRCS Eng. LRCP Lond. 1945; FRCS Eng. 1953. Prev: Cons. Adviser Orthop. Surg. RAF.

POVEY, William Peter (retired) The Gables, 153 Chester Road, Grappenhall, Warrington WA4 2SB — MRCS Eng. LRCP Lond. 1961 (Manch.) DObst RCOG 1966; DPH Liverp. 1968; FFCM 1979, M 1972; MSc Manch. 1982; FFPHM RCP (UK) 1990. NSM Assoc. Priest, All St.s Ch., Daresbury, Chesh.; Hon. Cons. Pub. Health Med. Wigan & Bolton HA. Prev: Dir. Pub. Health Centr. M/C HA.

POVLSEN, Professor Bo Guy's Hospital, St. Thomas Street, London SE1 9RT Tel: 0207 955 5000 Ext: 5607 — MD Copenhagen 1984 (Copenhagen 1984) PhD Sweden 1994; Assoc. Professor 1998. Cons. Orthop. Guy's & St. Thos. Hosps. NHS Trust. Specialty: Trauma & Orthop. Surg.; Plastic Surg. Socs: Brit. Elbow & Shoulder Soc.; Brit. Soc. Surg. Hand; Brit. Orthop. Assn. Prev: Cons. & Trainee Hand Surg. Univ. Hosp. Linköping, Sweden; Fell. (Microsurg.) St. Jas. Univ. Hosp. Leeds.

POW, Arthur Alexander (retired) 45 Esplanade, Greenock PA16 7RY Tel: 01475 20977 — MB ChB Glas. 1940 (Univ. Glas.) Prev: Maj. RAMC, TA.

POW, Colin Edward Lindsay 134 Newton Street, Greenock PA16 8SJ — MB ChB Aberd. 1997.

POWAR, Michael Paramjit 10 Vanilla and Sesame Court, Curlew Street, London SE1 2NN — BM BS Nottm. 1997.

POWAR, Motilal R Porth Farm Surgery, Porth Street, Porth CF39 9RR Tel: 01443 682579 Fax: 01443 683667.

POWELL, Adele Patricia South Uist Medical Practice, The Surgery, Daliburgh, Lochboisdale HS8 5SS Tel: 01878 700302 Fax: 01878 700675; 26 Aldwickbury Crescent, Harpenden AL5 5RR Tel: 015827 64513 — MRCS Eng. LRCP Lond. 1966 (Liverp.) FRCSI 1978. Princip. GP Lochboisdale, I. of S. Uist. Specialty: Gen. Pract.; Gen. Surg. Socs: BMA. Prev: Sen. Surg. Resid. (A & E) Univ. Hosp. Jamaica; Regist. (Surg.) Belf. VTS; Ho. Surg. United Liverp. Hosp.

POWELL, Alexandra 81 Ardwyn, Cardiff CF14 7HE — MB ChB Bristol 1995.

POWELL, Andrew Philip Park Medical Centre, 2 Park Road, West Kirby, Wirral CH48 4DW Tel: 0151 625 6128; 32 Beacon Drive, West Kirby, Wirral CH48 7ED — MB BChir Camb. 1985; MA Camb. 1987, MB BChir 1985; Cert. Family Plann. JCC 1989. Prev: Trainee GP N. Staffs. Hosp. Centre; Ho. Phys. & Ho. Surg. N. Staffs. Hosp. Centre.

POWELL, Andrew Stephen The Warneford Hospital, Warneford Lane, Headington, Oxford OX3 7JX Tel: 01865 226330 Fax: 01865 226507 — MB BChir Camb. 1970 (St. Thos.) MA Camb. 1972; MRCP (UK) 1972; FRCPsych 1988, M 1975. Cons. Psychother. & Hon. Sen. Lect. Univ. Oxf. Specialty: Psychother. Socs: Assoc. Mem. Brit. Assn. Psychother.; Inst. Gp. Anal.; Brit. Psychodrama Assn. & Mem. Inst. Gp. Anal. Prev: Cons. & Head Psychother. St. Geo. Hosp. Lond.; Sen. Lect. (Psychiat.) St. Geo. Med. Sch. Lond.; Sen. Regist. (Psychother.) Maudsley & Bethlem Roy. Hosps. Lond.

POWELL, Anna Louise Hendy, Church St., Addingham, Ilkley LS29 0QS — BM BS Nottm. 1991.

POWELL, Anthony Richard 210 Liverpool Road, Reading RG1 3PJ — MB BS Lond. 1991.

POWELL, Arnold 5 Canons Close, London N2 0BH Tel: 020 7624 4414 — MB ChB Sheff. 1957; MRCS Eng. LRCP Lond. 1958.

POWELL, Mr Barry Willoughby Eric Merrick 51 George's Hospital, Blackshaw Road, London SW17 0QT Tel: 020 8672 1255 Fax: 020 8725 2416 Email: bpowell@sghms.ac.uk; Baronsmead, Pachesham Park, Leatherhead KT22 0DJ Tel: 01372 844419 Fax: 01372 844742 Email: bpowell@sghms.ac.uk — MB BCh BAO Dub. 1978 (Dublin University) FRCS Ed. 1984; MA Dub. 1992, MCh 1992. Cons. Burns, Plastic & Reconstruc. Surg. St. Geo. Hosp. Lond.; Represen. on Plastic Surg. STC Pan Thames; Regional Adviser Plastic Surg. S. Thames Deanery & KSS Deanery; Examr. Specialist Fellowship plastic Surg. Specialty: Plastic Surg. Socs: Brit. Assn. Plastic Surg.; Brit. Assn. Aesthetic Plastic Surgs.; Brit. Assn. Tissue Banks.

POWELL, Benedict Walter (retired) The Willows, Theberton, Leiston IP16 4SF Tel: 01728 830588 — MB BChir Camb. 1939 (St. Thos.) MRCS Eng., LRCP Lond. 1939; FRCP Lond. 1970, M 1946; DCH Eng. 1947. Prev: Cons. Paediat. P'boro. Area.

POWELL, Bruce Patrick 218 Chippinghouse Road, Nether Edge, Sheffield S7 1DR Tel: 0114 255 6371 — MB BS Lond. 1991 (Royal Free) MRCP Lond. 1997. Specialist Regist. (Nephrol.) Northern Gen. Hosp. Sheff. Specialty: Nephrol.; Gen. Med. Socs: Roy. Coll Phys.

POWELL, Catherine Georgina Bransom 3 Parfrey Street, London W6 9EW Tel: 020 8741 9278; Efford Farm, Yealmpton, Plymouth PL8 2LB Tel: 01752 881387 — MB BS Lond. 1988 (Char. Cross & Westm. Hosp. Lond.) FRCA 1991. Specialist Regist. Rotat. (Anaesth.) SW Region. Specialty: Anaesth.

POWELL, Catherine Margaret 28 Quentin Road, London SE13 5DF Tel: 020 8318 4462; 8 Harboro Road, Sale M33 5AB Tel: 0161 973 3295 — MB BS Lond. 1993; BSc (Human Genetics & Basic Med. Scis.) Lond. 1991. SHO (GUM) St. Thomas Hosp. Specialty: Paediat. Prev: SHO (Paediat. Rotat.) Kingston Hosp. & Guy's Hosp.; SHO (Paediat.) Greenwich Dist. Hosp.; SHO (Neurol. & Rheum.) Roy. Surrey Co. Hosp. Guildford.

POWELL, Catherine Riva Orpington Hospital, The Peter Samman Dermatology Unit, Sevenoaks Road, Orpington BR6 9JU Tel: 01689 865261 — MB BS (Hons.) Lond. 1979. Assoc. Specialist (Dermat.). Specialty: Dermat. Prev: Staff Grade (Dermat.) Qu. Eliz. Healthcare Trust.

POWELL, Charles Edward Adam Practice, Upton Health Centre, Blandford Road North, Poole BH16 5PW Tel: 01202 622339 — BM Soton. 1987; MRCGP 1992; DCH RCP Lond. 1992. Hosp. Practitioner (Paediat.) Poole.

POWELL, Christopher Duncan New Hayesbank Surgery, Cemetery Lane, Kennington, Ashford TN24 9JZ Tel: 01233 624642 Fax: 01233 637304; 127 Lakemead, Ashford TN23 4XZ — MB ChB Manch. 1981.

POWELL, Mr Christopher Stephen Department of Urology, Countess of Chester Hospital, Liverpool Road, Chester CH2 1UL Tel: 01244 366588 Fax: 01244 366587 — MB BS Lond. 1975; MRCS Eng. LRCP Lond. 1975; FRCS Eng. 1979. Cons. Urol. Surg. Countess of Chester Hosp. Specialty: Urol. Socs: Brit. Prostate Gp.; Brit. Assn. Urol. Surgs. Prev: Cons. Urol. Surg. Leighton Hosp. Crewe; Sen. Regist. (Urol.) Swansea & Cardiff Gp. Hosps.; Research Regist. (Urol. & Transpl.) Roy. Hallamsh. Hosp. Sheff.

POWELL, Claire Elaine Wallis and Partners, The Health Centre, 5 Stanmore Road, Stevenage SG1 3QA Tel: 01438 313223 Fax: 01438 749734 — MB BS Lond. 1981 (Westm.) BSc Lond. 1978, MB BS 1981; DRCOG 1987. GP Lond. Prev: Trainee GP Sheff. VTS; Regist. (Anaesth.) Glos. Roy. Hosp.

POWELL, Colin Victor Eric Knowles House Farm, Hollin Lane, Sutton, Macclesfield SK11 0HR — MB ChB Manch. 1984; DCH RCP Lond. 1987; MRCP (UK) 1989. Hon. Regist. Research Fell. (Respirat.) Univ. Sheff. Specialty: Epidemiol. Prev: Tutor (Child Health) Univ. Manch.; SHO (Paediat.) Wythenshawe Hosp. Manch.; SHO (Paediat.) Booth Hall Childr. Hosp. Manch.

POWELL, David (retired) Piranhuthlant, Hatches Green, Gunnislake PL18 9BX — MB BS Lond. 1956 (Middlx.) EMP Benefits Agency. Prev: Princip. in Gen. Pract., Plympton Health Centre, Plympotn, Devon.

POWELL, David Edward Baden 7 Maes Baynglas, Peniels, Carmarthen SA32 7HF Tel: 01267 221198; Maesmor, 4 West Farm Close, Ogmore-by-Sea, Bridgend CF32 0PT — MB ChB Ed. 1952; FRCP Lond. 1981, M 1955; MD (Commend.) Ed. 1959; FRCPath 1974, M 1963; MA Wales 1992. Cons. Pathologist; Chairm. Panel D Bro Taf LREC Cardiff. Specialty: Pathology, General; Haematology; Forens. Path. Special Interest: Forens. Path. Socs: Path. Soc.; BMA. Prev: Cons. Path. Mid Glam. AHA; Sen. Regist. (Path.) United Bristol Hosps.; Asst. Lect. (Path. & Bact.) Welsh Nat. Sch. Med. Cardiff.

POWELL, David Fred Three Villages Medical Practice, Audnam Lodge, Wordsley, Stourbridge DY8 4AL Tel: 01384 395054 Fax: 01384 390969; 16 Dark Lane, Kinver, Stourbridge DY7 6JB Tel: 01384 873761 — MB BS Newc. 1968.

POWELL, David Howel Thomas Eastleigh Surgery, Station Road, Westbury BA13 3JD Tel: 01373 822807 Fax: 01373 828904 — MB BS Lond. 1981 (St. Bart.) MRCGP 1986. Prev: Trainee GP Hythe Med. Centre Soton.; SHO (O & G) St. Geo. Hosp. Lond.; SHO (Med.) Soton. Gen. Hosp.

POWELL, David Jolyan Stroud Whittington Road Surgery, 9 Whittington Road, Norton, Stourbridge DY8 3DB Tel: 01384 393120 Fax: 01384 353636; 2 Riverside Court, Caunsall, Kidderminster DY11 5YW — MB BS Lond. 1974 (St. Thos. Hosp. Lond.) Prev: Trainee GP Torquay VTS; SHO (O & G) Torbay Hosp. Torquay; Ho. Surg. (ENT) St. Thos. Hosp. Lond.

POWELL, David Lewis 21 Elizabeth Crescent, Queens Park, Chester CH4 7AY Tel: 01244 679236 — MB BS Lond. 1961 (Char. Cross) DObst RCOG 1964; FFA RCS Eng. 1970. Cons. Anaesth. Chester Roy. Infirm.; Clin. Tutor Chester HA. Specialty: Anaesth. Socs: Assn. Anaesths. Prev: Maj. RAMC T & AVR; Sen. Regist. United Liverp. & Liverp. Regional Hosps.; Lect. Dept. Anaesth. Univ. Liverp.

POWELL, Eileen Felvus Ladyfield, CAMHS, Glencare Road, Dumfries DG1 4TE Tel: 01387 244327 Fax: 01387 244337 — MB ChB Glas. 1974; MRCPsych 1980. Cons. Psychiat. Child Psychiat. & Learning Disabilitiy Dumfries & Galloway HB. Specialty: Child & Adolesc. Psychiat. Prev: Cons. (Child & Adolesc. Psychiat.) Forth Valley HB.

POWELL, Elizabeth Anne Crinnis, 3 Woodland Avenue, Teignmouth TQ14 8UU Tel: 01626 775328 — MB BS Lond. 1982; Cert. Family Plann. JCC 1985; DRCOG 1985; MRCGP 1986. Clin. Med. Off. (Family Plann.) Devon. Prev: GP St. Austell; Trainee GP N. Devon Dist. Hosp. Barnstaple VTS; SHO Worcester Eye Hosp.

POWELL, Elizabeth Jane 2 Caraway Drive, Meanwood, Leeds LS6 4RX — MB ChB Leeds 1998.

POWELL, Florence Mary Noreen Burn Brae Surgery, Hencotes, Hexham NE46 2ED Tel: 01434 603627 Fax: 01434 606373 — MB ChB Leeds 1980; DCH RCP Lond. 1983; DRCOG 1983; MRCGP 1984. Partner Burn Brae Med. Gp. Hencotes Hexham. Specialty: Gen. Pract. Socs: RCGP; Fac. Fam. Plann. & Reproduc. Health Care. Prev: Trainee GP Wakefield VTS; Partner Almondbury Huddersfield W. Yorks.; Partner Middlestown W. Yorks.

POWELL, Francis Iorwerth 249 Cwmamman Road, Garnant, Ammanford SA18 1LS Tel: 01269 822115 — (Cardiff) BSc Wales 1944; MB BCh Wales 1947; DMJ (Clin.) Soc. Apoth. Lond. 1970. Specialty: Forens. Path.; Gen. Pract. Socs: BMA; Assn. Police Surg. Prev: Clin. Asst. Amman Valley Hosp. Glanamman.; Regist. (Orthop. & Fract.) Roy. Infirm. Cardiff; Asst. Surg. Off. Accid. Unit St. David's Hosp. Cardiff.

POWELL, Frederic James (retired) Summerfield Lodge, Compton Chamberlayne, Salisbury SP3 5DB Tel: 01722 714705 — (St. Bart.) MRCS Eng. LRCP Lond. 1948; MB BS Lond. 1949; DObst RCOG 1952; FRCGP 1988, M 1960. Prev: Gp Shaftesbury.

POWELL, Gareth John 31 Upper Simpson Street, Crosshouse Hospital, Kilmarnock KA2 0BE Tel: 01563 521133; Ty'r Capel, Bishops Frome, Worcester WR6 5AS Tel: 01885 490316 — MB ChB Dundee 1994. SHO (O & G) CrossHo. Hosp. Kilmarnock. Specialty: Obst. & Gyn. Prev: SHO (Paediat.) Ayr Hosp.; SHO (A & E) Darlington Memor. Hosp.; Ho. Off. (Gen. Surg.) S. Cleveland Hosp. Middlesbrough.

POWELL, Glyn Douglas, TD (retired) 35 Cavendish Avenue, Dore, Sheffield S17 3NJ Tel: 0114 236 3578 — MB BCh Wales 1944 (Cardiff) BSc Wales 1941; FRCPath 1975, M 1963. Maj. RAMC, TARO. Prev: Cons. Path. Rotherham Dist. Gen. Hosp.

POWELL, Guy Alan Cowslip Farm, Devizes Road, Salisbury SP2 7NB — BM Soton. 1989.

POWELL, Hazel Department Cardiothoracic Anaesthesia, Freeman Hospital, High Henton, Newcastle upon Tyne NE7 7DN Tel: 0191 284 3111 Ext: 26488 Fax: 0191 223 1175 Email: hazel.powell@tfh.nuth.northy.nhs.uk — MB BS Lond. 1980; FFA RCS Eng. 1987. Cons. (Anaesth.) Freeman Hosp. Newc. upon Tyne. Specialty: Anaesth. Socs: Assn. of Anaesth.s; Assn. of Cardiothoracic Anaesth.s; Intens. Care Soc. Prev: Sen. Regist. (Anaesth.) Hammersmith Hosp. Lond.; Regist. (Anaesth.) Harefield Hosp.; Regist. (Anaesth.) Univ. Hosp. Nottm. & Northampton Gen. Hosp.

POWELL, Hazel Morag Pangbourne Medical Practice, The Boat House Surgery, Whitchurch Road, Pangbourne, Reading RG8 7DP Tel: 0118 984 2234 Fax: 0118 984 3022; Rickstools, Manor Farm Lane, Tidmarsh, Reading RG8 8EX Tel: 01189 843129 — MB BS Lond. 1972 (Guy's) MRCS Eng. LRCP Lond. 1972; DObst RCOG 1974; MRCGP 1983.

POWELL, Helen Kathleen Roma Ballaloch, Nethermill Road, Lochmaben, Lockerbie DG11 1QA — MB BCh BAO NUI 1965; DA Eng. 1969; Cert. Prescribed Equiv. Exp. JCPTGP 1981. Community Med. Off. E. Cumbria HA. Prev: Anaesth. Regist. Dumfries & Galloway Roy. Infirm.; Med. Off. Blood Transf. Serv.

POWELL, Mr Henry Denis Whitwell (retired) Old Fox Cottage, Heath End Road, Great Kingshill, High Wycombe HP15 6HS Tel: 01494 713176 — MB ChB Ed. 1944 (Camb. Edin.) MA Camb. 1945; FRCS Eng. 1953. Prev: Cons. Surg. Orthop. High Wycombe & Amersham Dist.

POWELL, Howell William Robert — MB BS Lond. 1998; MRCP 2001. Clin. Research Fell. (Neurol.) Insituite of Neurol. Lond. Specialty: Neurol. Socs: MPS; BMA. Prev: SHO Nat. Hosp. Neurol. & Neurosurg.; SHO (Gen. Med.) N. Middlx. Hosp.; SHO (A&E) St Thomas' Hosp.

POWELL, Hugh Benedict Bockhampton Road Surgery, Bockhampton Road, Lambourn, Hungerford RG17 8PS Tel: 01488 71715 Fax: 01488 73569; The Old Vicarage, Eastbury, Hungerford RG17 7JN Tel: 01488 71407 — MB BChir Camb. 1979; DCH Eng. 1981; DRCOG 1983; MRCGP 1984.

POWELL, James Francis Department of Anaesthesia, Royal Cornwall Hospital, Treliske, Truro TR1 3LJ Tel: 01872 253133 Fax: 01872 252480 Email: james.powell@rcht.cornwall.nhs.uk; Kerthen Wood Farm House, Townshend, Hayle TR27 6AH Tel: 01736 851001 — MB BS Lond. 1980 (Univ. Lond. & Guy's Hosp.) DRCOG 1983; DA (UK) 1987; FRCA 1991. Cons. Anaesth. Roy. Cornw. Hosp. Teliske Truro. Specialty: Anaesth. Socs: BMA; Europ. Soc. of Regional Anaesth.; Brit. Assn. of Day Surg. Prev: Sen. Regist. (Anaesth.) Qu. Eliz. Hosp. Kings Lynn; Sen. Regist. (Anaesth.) Addenbrooke's Hosp. Camb.

POWELL, James Hugo Peplow Royal Surrey County Hospital, Egerton Road, Guildford GU2 7XX Tel: 01483 571122 Fax: 01483 302683 Email: hugopowell@royalsurrey.nhs.uk — MRCS Eng. LRCP Lond. 1982; MA Camb. 1983, MB BChir 1982; MRCP (UK) 1987; FRCP 1999. Cons. Phys. Geriat. Med. Roy. Surrey Co. Hosp. Guildford. Specialty: Care of the Elderly; Gen. Med. Socs: Brit. Geriat.s Soc. (Counc. Mem. & Hon. Sec. SW Thames Regional Br.); Fell.and Coll. tutor Roy. Coll. Phys. Prev: Sen. Regist. (Geriat. Med.) St. Geo. Hosp. Lond.

POWELL, James John 2/2, 10 Sandbank Street, Glasgow G20 0PJ — MB ChB Glas. 1994.

POWELL, James Rees Redwood, Lisvane Road, Llanishen, Cardiff CF14 0SD Tel: 02920 752212 — MB BS Lond. 2001. Sen. Ho. Off. (Cardiol.) P. Chas. Hosp. Specialty: Gen. Med.

POWELL, James Shanklin Hoveton & Wroxham Medical Centre, Stalham Road, Hoveton, Norwich NR12 8DU Tel: 01603 782155 Fax: 01603 782189 — MB ChB Ed. 1970; MRCGP 1976. Prev: Surg. Lt. RN.

POWELL, Jean Charlotte Milngavie Road Surgery, 85 Milngavie Road, Bearsden, Glasgow G61 2DN Tel: 0141 211 5621 Fax: 0141 211 5625 — MB ChB Glas. 1979; DRCOG 1981; MRCGP 1983. Specialty: Diabetes; Paediat.; Gastroenterol.

POWELL, Jennifer Jean Department of Dermatology, North Hampshire Hospital, Aldermaston Road, Basingstoke RG24 9NA Tel: 01256 314784 Email: jenny.powell@nhht.nhs.uk; The Old Vicarage, Eastbury, Newbury RG17 7JN Tel: 01488 71407 — MB BS Lond. 1979 (St. Thos.) BA Oxf. (Hons.) 1976; MRCP (UK) 1982. Cons. Dermatol., N. Hants. Hosps.; Hon. Cons. Dermatol., The Churchill, Oxf. Specialty: Dermat. Special Interest: genital Dermatome; Paediatrics. Socs: Brit. Assn. Dermatol.; Dowling Club; RSM. Prev: Specialist Regist. (Dermat.) Oxf. Radcliffe Hosps.

POWELL, Jennifer Margaret 4 Langbank Rise, Kilmacolm PA13 4LF — MB ChB Glas. 1994.

POWELL, Joan Veronica Tudor Cottage, The Street, South Stoke, Reading RG8 0JS Tel: 01491 874113 — MB BS Lond. 1942 (Lond. Sch. Med. Wom.) MRCS Eng. LRCP Lond. 1942. Clin. Asst. (Accid. Dept.) Orpington Hosp.; Med. Off. Family Plann. Clinic Bromley AHA & Tunbridge Wells Health Dist. Prev: Ho. Surg. Roy. Free Hosp.; Ho. Phys. & Ho. Surg. Chester City Hosp.; Res. Obst. Off. St. Helier's Hosp. Carshalton.

POWELL, John Antony Buckinghamshire Health Authority, Aylesbury HP19 8ET; Haining Chace, Brockenhurst Road, Ascot SL5 9HB — (Univ. Camb.) BA (Hons.) Camb. 1990; MB BChir Camb. 1992; MA Camb. 1994; MRCPsych 1997. Regist. Rotat. (Psychiat.) Oxf. Regional Train. Scheme. Specialty: Pub. Health Med. Prev: SHO (Psychiat.) Oxf. Train. Scheme; SHO (Old Age Psychiat.) Northwick Pk. Hosp.

POWELL, Mr John Michael Orthopaedic Department, Ipswich Hospital, Heath Road, Ipswich IP4 5PD Tel: 01473 702032 Fax: 01473 702032 — MB BS Lond. 1977 (St. Bart.) FRCS Eng. 1981. Cons. Orthop. Surg. Ipswich Hosp. Specialty: Orthop.; Trauma & Orthop. Surg.; Orthop. Socs: Brit. Orthop. Spinal Soc.; Brit. Orthop. Assn.; Brit. Assn. of Spinal Surg.s. Prev: Clin. Research Fell. Univ., Toronto; Spinal Research Fell. WCB Rehabil. Centre, Toronto; Sen. Regist. Rotat. (Orthop. Surg.) St. Bart. Hosp. Lond.

POWELL, John Nevill 17 Gloucester Road, Almondsbury, Bristol BS32 4HD Tel: 01454 613027 — (Guy's) MRCS Eng. LRCP Lond. 1958; MB BChir Camb. 1960; DA Eng. 1961; FFA RCS Eng. 1963. Emerit. Cons. Anaesth. Southmead Health Servs. NHS Trust. Specialty: Anaesth. Socs: Assn. Anaesths.; (Ex-Pres.) Soc. Anaesth. SW Region. Prev: Instruc. (Anaesth.) Univ. Colorado Med. Center Denver, USA; Cons. Sen. Lect. (Anaesth.) Univ. Bristol.; Cons. Anaesth. Southmead Health Servs. NHS Trust.

POWELL, John Owen James 24 Gladstone Street, Skipton BD23 1PT — MB ChB Bristol 1990; MRCP (UK) 1993. Trainee GP Skipton. Specialty: Neurol. Prev: SHO (Med.) Morriston Hosp. Swansea; Regist. (Radiol.) St. Jas. Hosp. Leeds; Ho. Phys. Ham Green Hosp.

POWELL, Karen Josephine 76 Buxton Street, London E1 5AT — MB BS Lond. 1987.

POWELL, Katayoun Yasamin 2 Curzon Mews, Wilmslow SK9 5JN; 30 Spruce Avenue, Loughborough LE11 2QW — BM BS Nottm. 1990; BMedSci. (Hons.) Nottm. 1988, BM BS 1990; MRCGP 1994. Asst. Gen. Pract. LoughBoro. Leics. Specialty: Gen. Pract.

POWELL, Katharine Ursula Ley The Cottage, Thorpe Lane, Trimley St Martin, Felixstowe IP11 0RZ Tel: 01394 273688 — MB BS Lond. 1977 (Roy. Free) MRCS Eng. LRCP Lond. 1977; DCH Lond. 1980; DRCOG 1981; MRCGP 1981. Clin. Research Asst. (Gastroenterol. & Neurol.) Ipswich Hosp.; Assoc. specialist (Rheum. & Neurol.) Ipswich Hosp. Specialty: Gastroenterol.; Hypnother.; Neurol. Socs: Brit. Soc. Gastroenterol.

POWELL, Kelly Damask 20A St Anne's Road, Barnes, London SW13 9LJ Tel: 020 8878 1647 — MB BS Lond. 1990 (Charing Cross & Westminster) DRCOG 1995; MRCGP 1995; MSc Public Health (Lond.), 1998; MFPHM (P. I) 1998. Regist. (Pub. Health Med.) W. Surrey Health Auth. Specialty: Pub. Health Med.; Gen. Pract. Prev: SHO (A & E) Char. Cross Hosp. Lond.; GP Train.

POWELL, Mrs Lilian Jean 4 Watts Close, High Cross, Newport NP10 0DW; J Bwythan Bach, 4 Watts Close, Rogerstone, Newport NP10 0DW — MB BCh Wales 1950 (Cardiff) BSc Wales 1950; DObst RCOG 1966; DPH Bristol 1968; MFCM RCP (UK) 1974. Med. Off. Welsh Office Cardiff. Socs: Fell. Soc. Community Med.; BMA. Prev: Ho. Off. St. David's Hosp. Cardiff; Ho. Surg. O & G Cardiff Roy. Infirm.; Dist. MOH Magor & St. Mellons RD & Risca & Bedwas & Machen UDs.

POWELL, Louise Ann Kennedy Way Surgery, Kennedy Way, Yate, Bristol BS37 4AA Tel: 01454 313849 Fax: 01454 329039 — MB ChB Birm. 1989; MRCGP 1993.

POWELL, Mair Medicines & Healthcare Products Regulatory Agency, Market Towers, 1 Nine Elms Lane, London SW8 5NQ Tel: 020 7084 2486 Fax: 020 7084 2170 Email: mair.powell@mhra.gsi.gov.uk — MB BS Lond. 1980; MB BS (Hons.) Lond. 1980; MRCP (UK) 1984; FRCPath 1997, M 1988; MSc (Med. Microbiol.) Lond. 1987, MD 1989; FRCP 2003. Sen. Med. Assessor MHRA. Specialty: Med. Microbiol. Prev: Sen. Assoc. Med. Dir. Pfizer Incorp. New York, USA; Assoc. Med. Dir. Lederle Internat. Wayne, New Jersey, USA; Sen. Lect. (Med. Microbiol.) Lond. Hosp. Med. Coll.

POWELL, Marie Jose Endless Street Surgery, 72 Endless Street, Salisbury SP1 3UH Tel: 01722 336441 Fax: 01722 410319 — BM (Hons.) Soton. 1991. SHO (Geriat.) Odstock Hosp. Salisbury. Prev: Ho. Off. Roy. S. Hants. Hosp. Soton.; Ho. Off. Poole Gen. Hosp.

POWELL, Martin Barry Manor Brook Medical Centre, 117 Brook Lane, London SE3 0EN Tel: 020 8856 5678 Fax: 020 8856 8632; The Chimes, Felix Manor, Old Perry St, Chislehurst BR7 6PL Tel: 020 8295 0868 Fax: 020 8856 8632 Email: martin@the-chimes.freeserve.co.uk — MB BChir Camb. 1978 (Gonville and Caius College Cambridge) MA, MB Camb. 1978, BChir 1977; DRCOG 1980. GP Bexley & Greenwich HA. Socs: W. Kent Medico-Chirurgical Soc. (Past Pres. 2003-2004). Prev: Trainee GP Greenwich & Brook Hosps. VTS; Employm. Med. Off. DoH Attendance & Disabil. Living Allowance Units.; Ho. Surg. Brook Hosp. Lond.

POWELL, Mr Martin Charles Consultant Obstetrician and Gynaecologist, East Block, Queens Medical Centre, Nottingham NG8 2UH Tel: 0115 924 9924 Ext: 44872 — MB ChB Sheff. 1978; FRCS Ed. 1984; MRCOG 1989; DM Nottm. 1990. Cons. O & G Qu. Med. Centre Nottm. Specialty: Obst. & Gyn.

POWELL, Melanie Estelle Barrington Department of Radiotherapy, St Bartholomews Hospital, London EC1 7BE Tel: 020 7601 8353 — MB BS Lond. 1986; MRCP (UK) 1989; FRCR 1994; MD Lond. 1998. Cons. Clin. Oncol. St. Bart's. Hosp. Lond. Specialty: Oncol. Prev: Clin. Research Fell. Marie Curie Research Wing Mt. Vernon Hosp.; Regist. (Radiother. & Oncol.) Roy. Marsden Hosp.

POWELL, Michael Allan Rysseldene Surgery, 98 Conway Road, Colwyn Bay LL29 7LE Tel: 01492 532807 Fax: 01492 534846 — MB BS Newc. 1971; DObst RCOG 1973; MRCGP 1975.

POWELL, Michael Edward Arthur (retired) 37 Ridgeway Road, Redhill RH1 6PQ Tel: 01737 763991 — MD Lond. 1969 (King's Coll. Hosp.) MB BS 1952; FRCPath 1972, M 1964. Prev: Cons. (Histopath.) Kingston Hosp. Surrey.

POWELL, Michael Francis 4 Balfour Close, Little Thornton, Thornton-Cleveleys FY5 5AY — MB ChB Liverp. 1984.

POWELL, Michael Leonard (retired) c/o The Royal Bank of Scotland, 1 Market Place, Poulton-le-Fylde, Blackpool FY1 1LE — MRCS Eng. LRCP Lond. 1962; Cert. Av. Med. 1982.

POWELL, Michael Pearce Pangbourne Medical Practice, The Boat House Surgery, Whitchurch Road, Pangbourne, Reading RG8 7DP Tel: 0118 984 2234 Fax: 0118 984 3022; Rickstools, Manor Farm Lane, Tidmarsh, Reading RG8 8EX Tel: 01723 573129 — MB BS Lond. 1972; MRCS Eng. LRCP Lond. 1972; DObst. RCOG 1974. GP Reading. Prev: SHO (Obst.) St. Helier Hosp. Carshalton; SHO (Paediat.) Auckland Hosp. Bd., N.Z.

POWELL, Mr Michael Peter National Hospital for Neurology & Neurosurgery, Queen Square, London WC1N 3BG Tel: 020 7837 3611 Fax: 020 7833 8658; 66 The Avenue, London NW6 7NP — MB BS Lond. 1975; MA Oxf. 1988, BA 1972; FRCS Eng. 1980. Cons. Neurosurg. Nat. Hosp. Neurol. & Neurosurg. UCLH (Trust) & Roy. Nat. Orthop. Hosp. Trust; Hon. Cons. Neurosurg. & Roy. Free Hosp. Trust, St. Luke's Hosp. for Clergy, Whittingtoin Hosp & K Edwd VII Hosp for Offs; Hon. Cons. Surg. St. Thos. Hosp. Lond.; Civil. Adviser (Neurosurg.) RAF. Specialty: Neurosurg.

POWELL, Niels Department of Radiology, Morriston Hospital NHS Trust, Swansea SA6 6NL Tel: 01792 703139 Fax: 01792 703139 Email: niels.powell@swansea-tr.eales.nhs.uk; 121 Summerland Lane, Caswell, Swansea SA3 4RS — MB BCh Wales 1974 (Welsh Nat. Sch. Med.) DCH Eng. 1976; DMRD Eng. 1982; FRCR 1983. Cons. Neuroradiol. Morriston Hosp. Swansea. Specialty: Radiol. Socs: BNSR; RSNA; HCSA. Prev: Cons. Radiol. W. Glam. HA; Sen. Regist. (Radiol.) S. Glam. HA.

POWELL, Olive Joyce Hawthorn Drive Surgery, 206 Hawthorn Drive, Ipswich IP2 0QQ Tel: 01473 685070 Fax: 01473 688707; Appletree Cottage, The St, Harkstead, Ipswich IP9 1BN Tel: 01473 328678 — MB BS Lond. 1970 (Univ. Coll. Hosp.) DObst RCOG 1972; MRCP (UK) 1973. Prev: Regist. (Rheum.) Roy. Free Hosp. Lond.

POWELL, Patricia Copeland (retired) Knowles House, Hollin Lane, Sutton, Macclesfield SK11 0HR Tel: 01260 252334 — MB BS Durh. 1956 (Durham) Prev: Research Asst. (Paediat. Nephrol.) Roy. Manch. Childr. Hosp.

POWELL, Paula Marie Bridge Road Surgery, 30 Bridge Road, Litherland, Liverpool L18 5EG Tel: 0151 949 0249 — MB BS Lond. 1989; MRCGP 1993.

POWELL, Peter David (retired) Cwmbach Lodge, Glasbury-on-Wye, Hereford HR3 5LT Tel: 01497 847218 — MB ChB Ed. 1951. Prev: SHO & Ho. Phys. Gen. Hosp. Grimsby.

POWELL, Peter David Ahern (retired) The Old Barn, Whiteshill Common, Hambrook, Bristol BS16 1SN Tel: 0117 956 5760 — MB BS Lond. 1956 (St. Mary's) Prev: Sen. Cas. Off. & SHO (Surg.) Bristol Roy. Infirm.

POWELL, Peter John Royal Bolton Hospital Email: peter.powell@boltonh-tr.nwest.nhs.uk — MB BChir Camb. 1984 (Cambridge and The London) MA, BChir Camb. 1983, MB 1984; MRCP (UK) 1986; FRCPCH 1997; FRCP 1998. Cons. Paediat. Bolton Gen. Hosp.; Clin. Dir. Dept. of Child Health; Hon. Lect. Univ. of Manch. Med. Sch. Specialty: Paediat. Special Interest: Chronic Health Problems and Liaison with CAMHS. Socs: Neonat. Soc. & Manch. Paediat. Club; NORPEG; BAPM. Prev: Sen. Regist. (Paedait.) NW RHA; Research Fell. (Paediat.) Hope Hosp. Salford & Univ. Camb.

POWELL, Mr Philip Hugh 38 Rectory Road, Gosforth, Newcastle upon Tyne NE3 1XP — MD Bristol 1981; MB ChB 1973; FRCS Eng. 1977. Cons. (Urol.) Freeman Hosp. Newc. Specialty: Urol.

POWELL, Reginald Maldwyn (retired) The Coach House, Legsheath Lane, East Grinstead RH19 4JW — MRCS Eng. LRCP Lond. 1946 (Univ. Coll. Hosp.) MRCGP 1962. Prev: Ho. Surg. Univ. Coll. Hosp. Lond.

POWELL, Professor Richard John Queen's Medical Centre, Clinical Immunology Unit, Derby Road, Nottingham NG7 2UH Tel: 0115 970 9130 Fax: 0115 970 9919 Email: richard.powell@nottingham.ac.uk — MB BS Lond. 1971 (Char. Cross) MRCS Eng. LRCP Lond. 1971; MRCP (UK) 1974; FRCP Lond. 1992; DM Nottm 1994; FRCPath Lond. 2000. Prof. of Clin. Immunol. & Allergy & Cons. Qu. Med. Centre Nottm.; Reader Univ. Med. Sch. Specialty: Immunol.; Allergy. Special Interest: Allergy. Socs: Int. Mem. American Acad. Allergy & Imuology; Int. Fellow American Coll. Rheumathology; Council member Britsh Soc Allergy & Clin. Imuology. Prev: Sen. Lect. Univ. Med. Sch.

POWELL, Robin Barrington Park Royal Centre for Mental Health, Central Middlesex Hospital, Acton Lane, London NW10 7NS Tel: 020 8453 2780 Fax: 020 8961 6339 Email: robin.powell@dial.pipex.com — MB BS Lond. 1984 (Westminster) MRCPsych 1989; MSc Lond. 1992. p/t Cons. Old Age Psychiat. Centre Middlsex Hosp. Lond.; Hon. Sen. Lect. Imperial Coll. Sch. of Med. Specialty: Geriat. Psychiat.; Gen. Psychiat. Prev: Sen. Regist. (Psychiat.) Maudsley Hosp. Lond.; Regist. Rotat. (Psychiat.) Roy. Free Hosp. Lond.

POWELL, Sarah Lucy 82 Park Lea, East Herrington, Sunderland SR3 3SZ — MB BS Newc. 1991.

POWELL, Sharon Jeanne The Medical Centre, Kingston Avenue, East Horsley, Leatherhead KT24 6QT — MB BCh Witwatersrand 1989; MRCGP (UK) 1995. GP Associate. Specialty: Gen. Pract.

POWELL, Sheila Margaret Churchill Hospital, Department of Dermatology, Oxford OX3 7LJ Tel: 01865 228205; 3 Morlands, East Hanney, Wantage OX12 0JW Tel: 01235 868518 Fax: 01865 228260 — MB BS Lond. 1965 (Roy. Free) MRCS Eng. LRCP Lond. 1965; FRCP Lond. 1993. Cons. (Dermat.) Oxford Radciffe NHS Trust. Specialty: Dermat. Special Interest: Contact Dermatitis. Socs: BMA & Brit. Contact Dermat. Gp.; Eur. Soc. Contact Dermat. Prev: Lect. (Community Med.) Univ. Sheff.; SHO (Med.) Lusaka Centr. Hosp., Zambia; Ho. Phys. Hampstead Gen. Hosp.

POWELL, Simon Nicholas 153 Melrose Avenue, Wimbledon Park, London SW19 8AU — MB BS Lond. 1981; BA Oxf. 1976; MRCP (UK) 1985; FRCR 1988. Clin. Scientist Inst. Cancer Research Lond.; Hon. Sen. Regist. Roy. Marsden Hosp.

POWELL, Stephen Mark John 49 Woollin Crescent, Tingley, Wakefield WF3 1ET — MB ChB Leeds 1989.

POWELL, Stephen William Wellington Road Surgery, Wellington Road, Newport TF10 7HG Tel: 01952 811677 Fax: 01952 825981; The Brook Cottage, Longford, Newport TF10 8LS Tel: 01952 825544 — MB BS Lond. 1982 (St. Bart.) DCH RCP Lond. 1984; MRCGP 1986; DRCOG 1986. Prev: Trainee GP Stafford VTS; SHO (Psychiat.) Lister Hosp. Stevenage.

POWELL, Teyrnon Glyn Paediatric Department, Ysbyty Gwynedd, Bangor LL57 2PW Tel: 01248 384125 Fax: 01248 370629; Tyddyn Eden, Benllech, Tyn-y-Gongl LL74 8RU Tel: 01248 851006 Email: tgp@doctors.org.uk — MB BChir Camb. 1975 (Lond.) DCH Eng. 1976; MA Camb. 1975, MD 1987; FRCP 1997; FRCPCH 1997. Cons. Paediat. Ysbyty Gwynedd Bangor. Specialty: Paediat. Prev: Cons. Paediat. Neath Gen. Hosp. W. Glam.; Regist. (Paediat.) Melbourne, Austral.; Sen. Regist. (Paediat.) Manch.

POWELL, Thomas Paul Stansfield (retired) Bryn Eryl, Bryn Goodman, Ruthin LL15 1EL Tel: 01824 703199 — (Leeds) MB ChB Leeds 1950; MRCS Eng. LRCP Lond. 1952; FRCPsych 1980, M 1952; DPM Eng. 1959. Prev: Cons. Psychiat. N. Wales Hosp. Denbigh.

POWELL, Trevor Adrian St Bartholomews Surgery, 292A Barking Road, London E6 3BA Tel: 020 8472 0669/1077 Fax: 020 8471 9122 — MB Camb. 1976; BChir 1975; MRCGP 1980; DRCOG 1980.

POWELL, William Malcolm Court View Surgery, Rosemary Street, Mansfield NG19 6AB Tel: 01623 623600 Fax: 01623 635460 — MB ChB Sheff. 1974 (Sheffield) Dip. Pract. Dermat. Wales 1991.

POWELL-BRETT, Christopher Francis 3 Basil Street, London SW3 1AU Tel: 020 7235 6642 Fax: 020 7235 6052; 13 Alderney Street, London SW1V 4ES Tel: 020 7834 1118 — MB BS Lond. 1966 (St. Thos.) MRCS Eng. LRCP Lond. 1966; DObst RCOG 1968; MFOM RCP Lond. 1980. Med. Examr. United Nations in Gt. Brit.; Med. Adviser Jaine Spencer Ch. and transmitter Computer. Socs: Med. Soc. Lond.; Chelsea Clin. Soc.; Skane Med. Soc.

POWELL-JACKSON, John David Newick, Edward Road, St Cross, Winchester SO23 9RB — MB BChir Camb. 1967 (Camb. & Guy's) MD Camb. 1977, MA, MB 1967, BChir 1966; MRCS Eng. 1966; LRCP Lond. 1967; FRCP Lond. 1983, M 1969. Cons. Phys. Roy. Hants. Co. Hosp. Winchester. Specialty: Gen. Med. Socs: Internat.

Soc. Hypertens; Brit. Cardiac Soc. Prev: Ho. Phys. & Sen. Regist. (Med.) Guy's Hosp. Lond.; Clin. Research Fell. MRC Blood Pressure Unit Westm. Infirm. Glas.

POWELL-JACKSON, Mary Ann Newick, Edward Road, St Cross, Winchester SO23 9RB — MB BS Lond. 1966 (St. Geo.) MRCS Eng. LRCP Lond. 1966; FFA RCS Eng. 1971. Clin. Asst. (Anaesth.) Basingstoke Dist. Hosp. Specialty: Anaesth. Prev: Anaesth. Sen. Regist. St. Geo. Hosp. Lond.; Anaesth. Regist. St. Geo. Hosp. Lond.; Ho. Surg. St. Geo. Hosp. Lond.

POWELL-JACKSON, Paul Richard Maidstone & Tunbridge Wells NHS Trust, The Maidstone Hospital, Hermitage Lane, Maidstone ME16 9QQ Tel: 01622 224642 Fax: 01622 224865 — MB BChir Camb. 1973 (Guy's) MRCP (UK) 1975; MA Camb. 1970, BA (Hons.) 1969, MD 1985; FRCP Lond. 1994. Cons. Phys. & Gastroenterol. Maidstone & Tunbridge Wells NHS Trust. Specialty: Gastroenterol. Special Interest: Gastro-oesophageal Reflux; Inflammatory Bowel Dis. Socs: Brit. Soc. Gastroenterol.

POWELL-TUCK, Professor Jeremy St Bart. & The Royal London. Hospital School of Med. & Dent., Turner St., London E1 2AD Tel: 020 7426 5603 Fax: 020 7377 7790 Email: j.powell-tuck@qmul.ac.uk; 9 Horbury Crescent, London W11 3NF — (Birm.) MD Birm. 1980, MB ChB 1970; MRCP (UK) 1973; FRCP Lond. 1992. Prof. Clin. Nutrit., Cons. Gastroenterologist, Lond. Hosp. & St. Bart. Hosp. Med. Colls.; Hon. Cons. Phys. Barts & the Lond. NHS Trust. Specialty: Gastroenterol. Socs: RSM; ESPEN; BAPEN. Prev: Sen. Regist. (Med.) Char. Cross, Westm. & W. Middlx. Hosps. Lond.; Wellcome Research Fell. (Clin. Nutrit & Metab. Unit) Lond. Sch. Hyg. & Trop. Med.; Research Fell. & Hon. Sen. Regist. St. Mark's Hosp. Lond.

POWER, Aidan Colman Pfizer Central Research, Sandwich CT13 9NJ Tel: 01304 648140 Fax: 01304 655614; 4 Oaks Park, Rough Common, Canterbury CT2 9DP — MB BCh BAO NUI 1984; MRCPsych 1989; MSc History of Sci. & Med. Lond. 1991. Pharmaceut. Phys. Pfizer Centr. Research Sandwich Kent. Specialty: Pharmaceutical Medicine.

POWER, Andrew Primary Care Trust HQ, Garhavel Royal Hospital, 1055 Great Western Road, Glasgow G12 0XH Tel: 0141 211 0327 Fax: 0141 211 3826 Email: powera@netscape.net — MB ChB Glas. 1988; BSc (Hons.) Glas. 1985; DRCOG 1991; MRCGP 1992; Dip. Therap. Wales 1997. Asst. Med. Prescribing Adviser Gtr. Glas. HB. Prev: GP Glas.; SHO (Psychiat.) Levendale Hosp. Glas.; SHO (O & G) Rutherglen Matern. Hosp. Glas.

POWER, Andrew Patrick Whitkirk Medical Centre, 9A Austhorpe View, Leeds LS15 8NN — MB ChB Leeds 1985.

POWER, Anthony Lyn 27 Rhyd-y-Defaid Drive, Derwen Fawr, Sketty, Swansea SA2 8AJ Tel: 01792 299760 — MB BCh Wales 1969; FFR 1974; FRCR 1975. Clin. Dir. (Radiol.) Singleton Hosp. Swansea; Cons. Radiol. Swansea NHS Trust. Specialty: Radiol. Socs: BMA. Prev: Cons. Radiol. W. Glam. AHA; Sen. Regist. & Trainee Regist. (Radiodiag.) Univ. Hosp. of Wales; SHO (Cardiothoracic Med.) Sully Hosp.

POWER, Mr Brian John Department of Ophthalmology, Dumfries and Galloway Royal Infirmary, Dumfries DG1 4AP — MB BS Lond. 1970; DO Eng. 1974; FRCS Eng. 1978. Specialty: Ophth.

POWER, Bryan Edward Victoria House Surgery, 228 Dewsbury Road, Leeds LS11 6HQ Tel: 0113 270 4754 Fax: 0113 272 0561 — MB BCh BAO NUI 1982.

POWER, Christine Anne Cottage Farm, Main St., Keyham, Leicester LE7 9JQ — MB BS Lond. 1980; DA (UK) 1988. Clin. Asst. (Anaesth.) Glenfield Hosp. Leicester. Specialty: Anaesth. Prev: SHO (Anaesth.) Roy. Devon & Exeter Hosp.; Regist. (Microbiol.) Kingston Hosp. Kingston upon Thames; Trainee GP Exeter VTS.

POWER, Dominic Michael 14 Thoday Street, Cambridge CB1 3AS — BChir Camb. 1994.

POWER, Eileen Laura (retired) 10 Johnson Mansions, Queen's Club Gardens, London W14 9SJ Tel: 020 7385 0155 — MB BCh BAO NUI 1942; LAH Dub. 1951; MPSI 1952; DPH Eng. 1961; MFCM 1974. PMO King's Health Dist. (T). Prev: Ho. Phys. St. Vincent's Hosp. Dub. & Alder Hey Childr. Hosp. Liverp.

POWER, Francis John Upper Portclew House, Freshwater East, Pembroke SA71 5LA Tel: 01646 672661 — MB BCh Wales 1971; MRCGP 1976.

POWER, Jacqueline Anne Susan Silverdale, Fieldhouse Lane, Hepscott, Morpeth NE61 6LT — MB BS Newc. 1990; MRCGP 1994. Community Doctor Child & Adolesc. Ment. Health City Health Trust Newc. Specialty: Child & Adolesc. Psychiat.

POWER, Jennifer Susan Fiona 3 West View, Wylam NE41 8DT — MB ChB Manch. 1993; MA (Medieval Archaeology) Univ. Lond. 1984, BA (Modern Hist.) 1983.

POWER, Joanna 25 Yeoman's Row, London SW3 2AL — BM BCh Oxf. 1991.

POWER, Mr John Washington 130 Harley Street, London W1N 1AH Tel: 020 7235 2190 Fax: 020 7460 0985 — MB BS Sydney 1959; FRCS Eng. 1964; FRCS Ed. 1964. Cons. Orthop. Cromwell Hosp. Lond.; Cons. Repatriation Dept. Austral. Specialty: Orthop. Socs: Fell. Austral. Orthop. Assn.; Roy. Soc. Med.; Internat. Coll. Surgs. (Ex-Pres. Austral.). Prev: Governor & Mem. Nominating Comm. Represen. WHO; Princip. OMAES Pty Ltd. Sydney, Austral.; Cons. Harley St. Clinic Lond.

POWER, Kenneth John Ronald Fisher Department of Anaesthesia, Poole Hospital NHS Trust, Longfleet Road, Poole BH15 2JB Tel: 01202 442443; 23 Penn Hill Avenue, Parkstone, Poole BH14 9LU — BM Soton. 1980; MRCP (UK) 1983; FFA (RCS Eng.) 1986. Cons. Anaesth. & Intens. Care Poole Gen. Hosp. Specialty: Anaesth.; Intens. Care. Prev: Sen. Regist. (Anaesth.) Roy. United Hosp. Bath.

POWER, Lucy Mary Department of Psychiatry, East Wing, Homerton Hospital, Homerton Road, Hackney, London E9 6SR — BChir Camb. 1990. SHO Barts and The Homerton Psychiat. Train. Rotat. Specialty: Gen. Psychiat.

POWER, Michael James Patrick Department Elderly Medicine, Ulster Hospital, Dundonald, Belfast BT16 1RH Tel: 028 9048 4511 Ext: 2845 Fax: 028 9055 0415 Email: michael.power@ucht.n-i.nhs.uk — MB BCh BAO NUI 1979 (Nat. Univ. Ire. Galway) MRCPI 1982; MRCP UK 1983; FRCPI 1994; FRCP Ed. 1994; FRCP (L) 1997. Cons. Phys. Dept. Elderly Med. Ulster Hosp. Specialty: Care of the Elderly. Special Interest: Hypertens.; Stroke Dis.

POWER, Michael Patrick Waterfoot Health Centre, Cowpe Road, Waterfoot, Rossendale BB4 7DN Tel: 01706 215178 — MB ChB Manch. 1988.

POWER, Neil Richard 52 Noblehill Avenue, Dumfries DG1 3HX — MB ChB Glas. 1993.

POWER, Norman Athol Mill Pond House, Iping, Midhurst GU29 0PE Tel: 01730 812970 — MRCS Eng. LRCP Lond. 1950; LDS RCS Eng. 1941.

POWER, Peter Colin (retired) 91 Cottage Grove, Southsea PO5 1EH Tel: 023 9287 2490 — MB ChB Bristol 1959; DObst RCOG 1966; (MLCOM) (Mem. Of London college of osteopathic med.) 1988.

POWER, Mr Richard Anthony Department of Orthopaedic Surgery, Glenfield Hospital, Groby Road, Leicester LE3 9QP Tel: 0116 256 3440; Cottage Farm, Main St, Keysham, Leicester LE3 9JQ Tel: 0116 259 5263 — MB BS Lond. 1980; FRCS Ed. 1986; FRCS (Orth.) 1993. Cons. Orthop. Glenfield Hosp. & Leicester Roy. Infirm. Specialty: Orthop.

POWER, Richard John 79 Gallys Road, Windsor SL4 5QS — MB ChB Sheff. 1992.

POWER, Sharon Jane Department of Anaesthetics, Queen Elizabeth Hospital, Stadium Road, Woolwich, London SE18 4QH; The Knoll, 17 Kidbrooke Grove, Blackheath, London SE3 0LE — MB BS Lond. 1976; FFA RCS Eng. 1982. Cons. Anaesth. Qu. Eliz. Hosp. NHS Trust. Specialty: Anaesth.

POWER-BREEN, Patricia Anne 3 Hillview Avenue, George Town, Dumfries DG1 4DX — MB BCh BAO NUI 1976; MRCGP 1984. Clin. Asst. (Psychogeriat.) Crichton Roy. Hosp. Dumfries. Specialty: Geriat. Psychiat. Prev: Clin. Asst. (ENT) Dumfries & Galloway Roy. Infirm. Dumfries; Clin. Asst. (Ophth.) Edin. Roy. Infirm.; Asst. GP Kerry, Eire.

POWERS, Anthony Michael (retired) Fairway House, Mossley Court, Hawarden, Deeside CH5 3DQ Tel: 01244 539517 — MB ChB Liverp. 1971; DA Eng. 1977.

POWERS, David Samuel 14 Meadowbrook Court, Stone ST15 8LX Tel: 01785 286115 — MB ChB Dundee 1996.

POWERS, Lynette Ann The Gainsborough Practice, Warfield Medical Centre, 1 County Lane, Whitegrove, Bracknell RG42 3JP Tel: 01344 428742 Fax: 01344 428743 — BM BCh Wales 1982.

POWERS, Michael John Clerksroom, Equity House, Blackbrook Park Avenue, Taunton TA1 2PX Tel: 0845 083 3000 Fax: 0845 083 3001 Email: powersqc@medneg.co.uk; Flat 2, 21 Old Buildings,

Lincoln's Inn, London WC2A 3UP Tel: 0207 405 6965 — MB BS Lond. 1972 (Middlx.) BSc Lond. 1969; DA Eng. 1975. Queen's Counsel, London. Specialty: Medico Legal. Special Interest: Obst. & Anaesth. Socs: Medico-Legal Soc.; Roy. Soc. Med.; Soc. Of Doctors in Law. Prev: Regist. (Anaesth.) Northwick Pk. Hosp. Harrow; Ho. Surg. (O & G) Middlx. Hosp. Lond.; Ho. Phys. (Gen. Med.) Roy. S. Hants. Hosp. Soton.

POWERSMITH, Parsley Sheena Mary St. James University Hospital, Beckett St., Leeds LS9 7TF Tel: 0113 243 3144 — MRCS Eng. LRCP Lond. 1981; MRCPsych 1985; Dip. Clin. Hypn. Sheff. 1991. Cons. Psychiat. & Sen. Clin. Lect. St. Jas. Univ. Hosp. & Univ. Leeds. Specialty: Gen. Psychiat. Socs: BMA.

POWICK, Dawn Rose Inverbeg, Pinkham, Cleobury Mortimer, Kidderminster DY14 8QE Tel: 01299 271181 — MB ChB Birm. 1985; ChB Birm. 1985.

POWIS, Mr Mark Robert Flat 1, 47 Gondar Gardens, London NW6 1EP Tel: 020 7433 1456 — MB BS Lond. 1987 (St. Mary's Hosp. Med. Sch.) BSc (Hons.) Lond. 1984; FRCS Eng. 1992; FRCS FRCS(PAED.SURG)1999 1999. Specialist Regist. Paediat. Surg. Roy. Lond. Hosp. Specialty: Paediat. Surg. Socs: Fell. Roy. Soc. Med.; Assoc. Mem. Brit. Assn. Paediat. Surgs.; Brit. Assn. Paediatric Endoscopic Surg. Prev: SPR Paediatric Surg..Gt Ormond St Hosp; SPR Paediatric Surg.. Kings Coll. Hosp; SPR Paediatric Surg.. Qu. Eliz. Hosp.

POWIS, Martin David Meadowside Family Health Centre, 30 Winchcombe Road, Solihull B92 8PJ Tel: 0121 743 2560/742 5666 Fax: 0121 743 4216; 218 Stoney Lane, Yardley, Birmingham B25 8YJ Tel: 0121 783 4584 Fax: 0121 783 4584 — MB ChB Birm. 1976 (Birmingham) DRCOG 1978; MRCGP 1980; DFFR 1998; MSc (Community Gyn. & Reproductive Healthcare) 2002; Dip.Ther. 2002. Undergrad. Tutor Birm. Univ. Prev: SHO (O & G) Solihull Hosp.; SHO (Infect. Dis.) E. Birm. Hosp.; Ho. Off. (Radiother.) Qu. Eliz. Hosp. Birm.

POWIS, Rachel Anne 40 Greatwood Terrace, Topsham, Exeter EX3 0EB Tel: 01392 877685 — MB BS Lond. 1993 (St Georges Hospital) Specialty: Gen. Med.

POWIS, Professor Stephen Huw Centre for Nephrology, Royal Free & University College Medical School, Rowland Hill St., London NW3 2PF Tel: 020 7830 2695 Fax: 020 7830 2125 Email: powis@rfhsm.ac.uk — BM BCh Oxf. 1985; BSc (Hons.) Glas. 1981; MRCP (UK) 1988; PhD Univ. Lond. 1995; FRCP 1998. Prof. (Renal Med.) Roy. Free Hosp. Sch. Med. Lond. Specialty: Nephrol. Socs: Renal Assn. (Exec. Comm. 1998-2001); Brit. Transpl. Soc.; Brit. Soc. Immunol. Prev: Sen. Lect. (Renal Med.) Guy's Hosp. Lond.; Regist. (Renal Med.) Guy's Hosp. Lond.

POWLES, Allan Badgett Jubilee Farm, Fen Road, Washingborough, Lincoln LN4 1AE Tel: 01522 793620 — MB BS Lond. 1974; FFA RCSI 1977; FFA RCS Eng. 1978. Cons. Anaesth. Lincoln Co. Hosp. Specialty: Anaesth.

POWLES, Anne Veronica St. Mary's Hospital, Praed St., London W2 2NY Tel: 020 7725 1194; St. Ibbs Bush, St. Ippolytts, Hitchin SG4 7NL Tel: 01462 457956 — MB ChB Aberd. 1972; MD Aberd. 1989; FRCP Lond. 1995. Cons. Dermat. St. Mary's Hosp. & Centr. Middlx. Hosp. Lond. Specialty: Dermat. Prev: Sen. Regist. (Dermat.) St. Mary's Hosp. Lond.

POWLES, Mr David Pritchard Lister Hospital, Coreys Mill Lane, Stevenage SG1 4AB Tel: 01438 314333 Fax: 01438 781274; St. Ibbs Bush, St. Ippolyts, Hitchin SG4 7NL Tel: 01462 457956 — MD Queen's Univ. Kingston, Canada 1973 (Qu. Univ., Canada) BSc McGill 1969; FRCS Eng. 1978. Cons. Orthop. Surg. Lister Hosp. Stevenage. Specialty: Orthop. Socs: Fell. BOA; Brit. Assn. Surg. Knee; Eur. Soc. Knee Surg. Sports Med. Arthroscopy. Prev: Sen. Regist. (Orthop.) King's Coll. Hosp. Lond.

POWLES, Mr James Watson Green Hedges, Coulsdon Lane, Coulsdon CR5 3QL Tel: 01737 556352 — MB BS Lond. 1994 (St.Bart's, Lond.) BSc (Hons) 1991; FRCS (Eng) 1998. SHO (Otoaryn.) Radcliffe Infirm. Oxf. Specialty: Otolaryngol.

POWLES, John William Department of Public Health and Primary Care, Institute of Public Health, Robinson Way, Cambridge CB2 2SR Tel: 01223 330310 Fax: 01223 330330 Email: jwp11@cam.ac.uk; 164 Gwydir Street, Cambridge CB1 2LW Tel: 01223 740245 — MB BS Sydney 1968; FFPHM RCP (UK) 1987, M 1974; MA Camb. 1997. Univ. Lect. (Pub. Health Med.) Univ. Camb.; Hon. Cons. Pub. Health Med. Camb. Specialty: Pub. Health Med.; Epidemiol. Socs: Internat. Epidemiol. Assn.; Soc. for Epidemiological Research; Soc. for Social Med. Prev: Lect., Dept. of Social and Preven. Med., Monash Med. Sch., Melbourne, Australia, 1975-1991.

POWLES, Professor Raymond Leonard Little Garratts, 19 Garratts Lane, Banstead SM7 2EA Tel: 01737 353632; The Royal Marsden Hospital, Downs Road, Sutton SM2 5PT Tel: 020 8770 1027 — (St. Bart.) MB BS Lond. 1964; FRCP Lond. 1980, M 1968; BSc (Special) Lond. 1961, MD 1976; FRCPath Lond. 1993. Head & Prof. Haematological Oncol. i/c Leukaemia & Myeloma Units & Cons. Phys. Roy. Marsden Hosp. Sutton; Mem. Med. Research Counc. Working Party on Adult Leukaemia. Specialty: Gen. Med. Socs: (Advis. Comm.) Internat. Bone Marrow Transpl. Registry; Internat. Soc. Experim. Haematol.; Amer. Soc. Haemat. Prev: Imperial Cancer Research Fund. Sen. Scientif. Off. St. Bart. Hosp. Lond.; Ho. Phys. St. Bart. Hosp. Lond.; Ho. Phys. Brompton Hosp. Lond.

POWLES, Professor Trevor James, CBE Parkside Oncology Clinic, 49 Parkside, Wimbledon, London SW19 5NF Tel: 0208 2473384 Fax: 0208 2473385 Email: amccabe@parkside-hospital.co.uk; Green Hedges, Coulsdon Lane, Chipstead, Coulsdon CR5 3QL Tel: 01737 556352 — (St. Bart.) MRCS Eng. LRCP Lond. 1964; PhD Lond. 1975, BSc 1961, MB BS 1964; MRCP (UK) 1969; FRCP Lond. 1983; Specialist Accredit. (Gen. Med. & Med. Oncol.) RCP Lond. 1983. Lead Clinician & Breast Oncologist, Parkside Oncology Clinic; Head Breast Unit Roy. Marsden Hosp, 1994-; Med. Director.Common Cancers Div.,Roy. Marsden Hosp.; Prof. (Breast Oncol.) Inst. Cancer Research Lond. 1998-. Specialty: Oncol. Socs: Soc. Endocrinol.; Brit. Breast Gp.; Assn. Cancer Phys. Prev: Sen. Lect. (Med.) & Hon. Cons. Phys. Roy. Marsden Hosp. & St. Geo. Hosp. Lond.; MRC Clin. Research Fell. Chester Beatty Research Inst. Lond.; Ho. Phys. Hammersmith Hosp. Lond.

POWLEY, Elaine The Kirkbymoorside Surgery, Tinley Garth, Kirkbymoorside, York YO62 6AR Tel: 01751 431254 Fax: 01751 432980; Lund Head, Skiplam, Nawton, York YO62 7RH Tel: 01751 431249 Fax: 01751 432980 — MB ChB Bristol 1968; DPM Leeds 1971. Course Organiser Postgrad. Centre & Gen. Hosp. ScarBoro. VTS. Prev: Clin. Asst. (Child & Adolesc. Psychiat.) Clifton Hosp. York; Regist. (Psychiat.) York Hosps.; Ho. Off. (Obst.) Matern. Hosp. Fulford.

POWLEY, Mr John Michael (retired) 18 Compton Drive, Eastbourne BN20 8BX Tel: 01323 727520 — MB BS Lond. 1951 (King's Coll. Hosp.) MRCS Eng. LRCP Lond. 1951; FRCS Eng. 1958. Prev: Cons. Surg. Eastbourne Health Dist.

POWLEY, Mr Philip Harold (retired) 47 Corby Avenue, Swindon SN3 1PS Tel: 01793 536570 — MB BS Lond. 1958 (St. Thos.) FRCS Ed. 1962; FRCS Eng. 1962. Prev: Cons. Surg. Swindon Dist. Hosps.

POWLS, David Andrew Princess Royal Maternity, 16 Alexandra Parade, Glasgow G31 2ER Tel: 0141 211 5400 Email: powlsa@northglasgow.scot.nhs.uk — MB BCh Wales 1986; MRCP Ed. 1991; MD (Univ. Liverp.) 1997. Cons. Neonatologist. Prev: Research Regist. (Child Health) Liverp. Univ.

POWLSON, Mark Medicines Control Agency, Room 1202 Market Towers, 1 Nine Elms Lane, London SW8 5NQ Tel: 020 7273 0908 Email: mark.powlson@mca.gov.uk; Vellum Lodge, 2A Read Road, Ashtead KT21 2HS — MB BS Lond. 1983 (Guy's) BSc (Hons.) Lond. 1979; MRCS Eng. LRCP Lond. 1982. Editorial & Pub.ations Co-ordinator, MCA. Specialty: Gen. Med. Socs: Fell. Roy. Soc. Med.; Fell. Roy. Soc. Arts; Eur. Assn. Sci. Edr.s. Prev: Head, Med. Edit Unit DoH; Asst. Edr. The Lancet; Regist. (Med.) Roy. Shrewsbury Hosp.

POWNALL, Christine Catherine Graham (retired) — MB ChB Ed. 1952 (Edinburgh) Prev: Ho. Surg. Simpson Matern. Hosp. Edin.

POWNALL, Mr Philip John 22 Bottom O'Th Moor, Horwich, Bolton BL6 6QF Tel: 01204 669096 — MB ChB Manch. 1961; FRCS Ed. 1971; FRCS Eng. 1972. Cons. Orthop. Surg. Bolton Gp. Hosps. Socs: Fell. Manch. Med. Soc. Prev: Tutor/ Hon. Sen. Regist. (Orthop. Surg.) Univ. Leeds.

POWNER, Helen Ruth 3 Grange Crescent, Bridgend CF35 5HP — MB ChB Birm. 1989.

POWNEY, Alan (retired) 4 The Barn, Garden Farm, Chester-le-Street DH2 3RD Tel: 0191 387 3251; 1B Mantis Seaview, Yeriskipou, Paphos 8201, Cyprus Tel: 357 6 260 161 — MB BS Durh. 1958; MB BS Durh., 1958.

POWRIE, James Kenneth Diabetes & Endocrine Unit, Thoma Guy House, St Thomas St., London SE1 9RT Tel: 020 7955 5000 Fax: 020 7955 2121 Email: jake.powrie@kcl.ac.uk — MB ChB Aberd. 1982; BMedBiol Aberdeen 1979; MB ChB Aberdeen 1982; MRCP (UK) 1986; MD Aberdeen 1992; FRCP Ed 1999; FRCP Lond. 2000. Cons. Phys. & Hon. Sen. Lect. (Gen. Med., Diabetes & Endocrinol.) Guy's & St. Thos. NHS Trust Lond. Specialty: Diabetes; Endocrinol.; Gen. Med. Socs: Brit. Diabetic Assn.; Brit. Endocrine Soc.; Roy. Soc. Med. Prev: Lect. (Med.) St. Thos. Hosp. Lond.; Research Fell. (Clin.) St. Thos. Hosp. Lond.; Regist. (Med.) Aberd. Roy. Infirm.

POWRIE, Suzanne Elizabeth 21 Chipstead Street, Fulham, London SW6 3SR Tel: 020 7731 5697 — MRCS Eng. LRCP Lond. 1967 (Sheff.) DA Eng. 1969; FFA RACS 1972; FFA RCS Eng. 1974. Cons. (Anaesth.) Moorfields Eye Hosp. Lond. Specialty: Anaesth. Socs: Assn. Anaesths. Prev: Sen. Regist. (Anaesth.) Hammersmith Hosp. Lond.; Regist. (Anaesth.) Brompton Hosp. Lond. & Roy. Wom. Hosp. Melb.; Australia.

POWROZNYK, Arsenyj Vasyl Volodyslav Department of Anaesthesia, St Thomas' Hospital, Lambeth Palace Road, London SE1 7EH Tel: 020 7928 9292 Ext: 2353 Fax: 020 7960 5615 — MB BS Lond. 1986 (Charing Cross Hospital Medical School) MA Camb. 1987, BA 1983; DA (UK) 1988; FRCA 1993. Cons. Anaesth. St. Thomas' Hosp. Lond. Specialty: Anaesth. Socs: Assn. Anaesth.; Eur. Assn. Cardiothoracic Anaesth.; Assn. Cardiothoracic Anaesth. (UK). Prev: Sen. Regist. (Cardiothoracic Anaesth.) Roy. Brompton Hosp. Lond.; Sen. Regist. (Anaesth.) St. Thomas' Hosp. Lond.; Clin. Fell. (Caerdiothoracic Anaesth.) Papworth Hosp. Camb.

POXON, Ian Mark — MB ChB Sheff. 1992; FRCA Lond. 2000. Specialist Regist. (Anaesth.) W. Midl. Higher Specialist Train. Scheme, Staffs. Specialty: Anaesth.

POYNER, Amy Louise — MB BS Lond. 1998.

POYNER, Fiona Elizabeth Accident and Emergency Department, Northampton General Hospital Trust, Cliftonville, Northampton NN1 5BD Tel: 01604 634700 Fax: 01604 545615 — MB BCh Oxf. 1986; FFAEM; MRCP (UK) 1992; FRCP 2003. Cons. A & E Northampton Gen. Hosp. Trust. Specialty: Accid. & Emerg.

POYNER, John Gerard St Annes Road East, 24 St. Annes Road East, Lytham St Annes FY8 1UR Tel: 01253 722121 Fax: 01253 781121; 42 St Annes Road E., St Annes, Lytham St Annes FY8 1UR Tel: 01253 722121 — MB ChB Manch. 1981; MRCGP 1985; DRCOG 1986. Specialty: Gen. Med.

POYNER, Thomas Francis Queens Park Medical Centre, Farrer Street, Stockton-on-Tees TS18 2AW Tel: 01642 679681 Fax: 01642 677124 Email: thomas.poyner@nhs.net — MB BS Lond. 1974 (Roy. Free) MRCS Eng. LRCP Lond. 1974; DRCOG 1978; MRCGP 1978; MRCP (UK) 1981; Dip. Pract. Dermat. (Merit) Wales 1993; FRCP Lond. 2001; FRCP Glas. 2002. Hosp. Practitioner; Hon. Lect. Univ. of Durh. Specialty: Pharmacology. Socs: Edit. Bd. Dermat. Pract.; (Vice Chairm.) Primary Care Dermat. Soc.; Mem. of the Assur. Med. Soc.

POYNOR, Margaret Ursula 586 Chorley New Road, Bolton BL6 4DW — MB BS Lond. 1975 (Guy's) MRCS Eng. LRCP Lond. 1975; DRCOG 1977; DCH Eng. 1978; MRCP (UK) 1980. Cons. Community Paediat. Bolton HA. Specialty: Paediat.

***POYNTER SMITH, Paul Nicholas** Pinewood, Hannington Rd, Hannington, Tadley RG26 5TW — MB BS Lond. 1997 (UMDS - Guy's and St Thomas') SHO AEE, St Thomas' Hosp., Lond. Specialty: Accid. & Emerg. Prev: Ho. Off. Surg., St Thomas' Hosp.; Ho. Off. Gen. Med., Salisbury Dist. Hosp.

POYNTON, Amanda Mary Rawnsley Building, Manchester Royal Infirmary, Oxford Road, Manchester M13 9BX Tel: 0161 276 5354 — MB BS Lond. 1981; MA Oxf. 1984, BA (Physiol. Sci.) 1978; MRCPsych 1985. Cons. Psychiat. Manch. Roy. Infirm. Specialty: Gen. Psychiat. Prev: Cons. Psychiat. & Sen. Lect. Guy's Hosp. Lond.; Lect. (Biol. Psychiat.) United Med. & Dent. Sch. Lond.; Regist. Rotat. (Psychiat.) Guy's Hosp. Lond.

POYNTON, Christopher Hilton University Hospital of Wales, Department of Haematology, Heath Park, Cardiff CF14 4XN Tel: 02920 742654 Fax: 02920 743895 Email: poynton@cardiff.ac.uk; 47 Stanhope Road, Croydon CR0 5NS — BM BCh Oxf. 1974 (Oxford) MRCP (UK) 1979; MRCPath 1986; DM Oxf. 1991; FRCP Lond. 1995; FRCPath 1997; FRCP Ed 1999. Sen. Lect. & Hon. Cons. Haemat. Univ. Hosp. Wales Cardiff; State of Texas Med. License (Hemat. & Oncol.). Specialty: Haematology. Socs: Amer. Soc. Haemat.; Internat. Soc. Hemat. & Graft Engin.; Brit. Soc. Haematol.

POYSER, John Tramways Medical Centre, 54a Holme Lane, Sheffield S6 4JQ Tel: 0114 233 9462; Newstead, 76 Langsett Avenue, Sheffield S6 4AA — MB ChB Sheff. 1976; MPhil. Sheff. 1995. Chair Sheff. W. PCG; Lect. (GP) Univ. Sheff. Specialty: Gen. Pract.

POZNIAK, Anton Louis HIV Unit Chelsea and Westminster Hospital NHS Trust, 369 Fulham Road, London SW10 9NH Tel: 020 8746 5620 Fax: 020 8746 5628 Email: anton.pozniak@chelwest.nhs.uk — MB ChB Bristol 1979 (University of Bristol) MRCP (UK) 1982; MD Bristol 1994; FRCP Lond. 1996. Cons. Phys. GUM/HIV Chelsea & Westminster Hosp. NHS Trust; Hon. Sen. Lect. Imperial Coll. Lond. Specialty: Gen. Med.; HIV Med.; Genitourinary Medicine. Socs: Brit. Thorac. Soc.; Brit. HIV Assn.; BASSH. Prev: Sen. Lect. Kings Coll. Sch. Med.; Lect. Acad. Dept. Genitourin. Med. Middlx. Hosp.; Lect. (Med.) Univ. Zimbabwe.

POZO, Mr Joseph Louis The Royal United Hospital, Combe Park, Bath BA1 3NG Tel: 01225 824426 Email: louis.pozo@ruh-bath.swest.nhs.uk; The Royal National Hospital for Rheumatic Diseases, Upper Borough Walls, Bath BA1 1RL — BM BCh Oxf. 1974; MA Oxf. 1974; FRCS Eng. 1980. Cons. Orthop. Surg. Roy. United Hosp. Bath.; Cons. Orthopaedic Surg., Roy. Nat. Hosp. for Rheumatic Diseases, Bath. Specialty: Trauma & Orthop. Surg. Special Interest: Arthroscopy; Surgery of the Knee. Socs: Fell. BOA; Brit. Assn. Surg. Knee; Eur. Soc. Sports Traumatol. Knee Surg. & Arthroscopy. Prev: Sen. Regist. (Orthop. Rotat.) Univ. Coll. Hosp. & Westm. Hosp. Lond.

POZYCZKA, Teofil Andrzej (Andrew) The Poppins, Thrigby Rd, Filby, Great Yarmouth NR29 3HJ — MB BS Lond. 1971 (Westm.) MRCOG 1980, DObst RCOG 1973; FRCOG 1997. Cons. O & G James Paget Healthcare NHS Trust, Gt. Yarmouth; Clin. Director Wom. and Childhealth Directorate James Paget Healthcare NHS Trust. Specialty: Obst. & Gyn. Special Interest: Hysteroscopic Surg.; Endometrial Ablations; Vaginal Hysterectomy; Minimal invasive Surg. Socs: Brit. Med. Assn.; Brit. Soc. for Colposcopy and Cervical Path. Prev: RAF Med. Br. Wg. Cdr. (Ret'd) - Cons. O & G; Hon. Lect. Nuffield Dept. O & G John Radcliffe Hosp. Oxf.

POZZI, Marco 16 College Road, Liverpool L23 0RW — State Exam Milan 1981 (Univ. Milan) Cons. Cardiac Surg. Roy. Liverp. Childr. Hosp.; Clin. Lect. Univ. Liverp. Specialty: Cardiothoracic Surg. Socs: Eur. Soc. Cardiothorac. Surg.; Brit. Paediat. Cardiac Assn.; Soc. Cardiothoracic Surgs. GB.

POZZILLI, Paolo Department of Diabetes & Metabolism, St. Bartholomew's Hospital, West Smithfield, London EC1A 7BE Tel: 020 7601 7454 Fax: 020 7601 7449 Email: p.p.pozzilli@qmul.ac.uk — State Exam Rome 1976 (Univ. Rome) Dip. Endocrinol. Univ. Lond. 1979. Prof. of Clin. research St. Bartholomews Hosp. Lond.; Prof. Endocrinol. & Metab. Dis.s, Univ. Campus Biomedico, Rome 2001. Specialty: Endocrinol. Socs: Fell.Roy. Soc. Med.; Fell.Int. Diabetes Federatation.; Eur. Assn. Study Diabetes. Prev: Wellcome Foundat. Fell. 1980; Juvenile Diabetes Foundat. Fell. (USA) 1983; Sen. Investigator, Asst. Prof., Univ. of Rome "La Sapienza".

POZZONI, Lynda Suzanne 19 Bowness Avenue, Southfront, Southport PR8 3QP — MB BS Lond. 1995.

PRABHAKAR, Deepak Trilok Chand Prestwich Health Centre, Fairfax Road, Prestwich, Manchester M25 1BT Tel: 0161 773 2483 Fax: 0161 773 9218; Branch Surgery, The Uplands, Whitefield Health Centre, Bury New Road, Whitefield, Manchester M45 8GH Tel: 0161 796 2296 — MB BS Poona 1972 (Armed Forces Med. Coll.) DA Eng. 1976. Prev: Regist. (Anaesth.) Bury Gen. Hosp.; SHO (Anaesth.) Bury Gen. Hosp.

PRABHAKARAN, Narayanan Cambridge House, 124 Werrington Road, Bucknall, Stoke-on-Trent ST2 9AJ Tel: 01782 219075 Fax: 01782 279047 — MB BS Kerala 1971; MB BS Kerala 1971.

PRABHAKARAN, Unniparambath Pattaveettil Pontynewynydd Clinic, Mill Road, Pontynewynydd, Pontypool NP4 6NG Tel: 01495 752115 — MB BS Kerala 1974 (Med. Coll. Trivandrum) MRCGP 1983; MFHom 1985; MSc (Med. Sci.) Gen. Pract. 1985; MLCOM 1987. RCGP/Syntex Fellowship Rheum. 1981; Univ. Glas. Fellowship 1982; RCGP Fac. Tutor; Sen. Lect. in Gen. Pract. Socs: RCGP Research Sec.

PRABHU, Manur Radhakrishna Kildean Day Hospital, Drip Road, Stirling FK8 1RW Tel: 01786 458607 Fax: 01786 458605 — MB

BS Madras 1971 (Jawaharlal Inst. Postgrad. Med. Educat Pondicherry) DPM Leeds 1976; MRCPsych 1980. Cons. Psychiat.Forth Valley Primary CareHealthcare NHS Trust. Specialty: Gen. Psychiat. Prev: Regist. (Psychiat.) Middlx. Hosp. Lond. & Gtr. Glas. HB.

PRABHU, Matti Achuth (retired) 6 St James Mount, Rainhill, Prescot L35 0QU Tel: 0151 426 4332 — MB BS Dibrugarh 1971; MB BS Dibrugarh, India 1971. Assoc. Specialist. Prev: Clin. Asst. A & E Warrington NHS Trust Hosp.

PRABHU, Mudar Anantha Rampton Hospital, Retford DN22 0PD Tel: 01777 248321 Email: maprabhu@aol.com — MB BS Bangalor 1970 (Bangalore Med. Coll.) MB BS Bangalore 1970. Assoc. Specialist (Primary Care); Hosp. Practitioner (GUM). Specialty: Gen. Psychiat. Prev: GP Derby.

PRABHU, Palimar Umesh Fairfield General Hospital, Rochdale Old Road, Jerico, Bury BL9 7TD Tel: 0161 705 3755 Email: umesh.prabhu@pat.nhs.uk — MB BS Mysore 1980; DCH Mysore; DCH RCP Lond.; FRCPCH. Cons. (Paediat.); Clin. Dir. NHS Professional; Advis Nat. Clin. Assessment Auth. (NCAA). Specialty: Paediat. Special Interest: Allergy; Asthma; Infection. Socs: Indian Paediat. Assn. Prev: Med. Dir. Bury NHS Trust; Bd. Mem. Nat. Pat. Safety Agency.

PRABHU, Mrs Poornima Shrinivas Ashok East Glamorgan General Hospital, Church Village, Pontypridd CF38 1AB Tel: 01443 204242; 4 Clos Darran Las, Cardiff Road, Creigiau, Cardiff CF15 9SL Tel: 01222 892525 — MB BS Bombay 1979; DObst RCPI 1981; MRCOG 1986. Clin. Med. Off. Community Family Plann. & RHC; Clin. Asst. (Obst. & Gyn.). Specialty: Family Plann. & Reproduc. Health; Obst. & Gyn.; Gen. Pract.

PRABHU, Suman Longshoot Health Centre, Scholes, Wigan WN1 3NH — MB ChB Manch. 1996 (Manchester) DRCOG 1998; DCH 1999. GP Principal. Specialty: Gen. Pract.

PRABHU, Usha Achuth 6 St James Mount, Rainhill, Prescot L35 0QU Tel: 0151 426 4332 — Vrach People's Friendship U. Moscow 1972 (People's Friendship U.) DCH Eng. 1979; MRCOG 1981; MFFP 1993; FRCOG 1996. SCMO (Wom. Health) N. Mersey Community NHS Trust. Specialty: Family Plann. & Reproduc. Health; Obst. & Gyn. Socs: Med. Protec. Soc.; BMA. Prev: Clin. Med. Off. (Childhealth) St Helens & Knowsley HA; Regist. (O & G) Warrington Dist. Gen. Hosp.; SHO & Regist. (O & G) Halifax Gen. Hosp.

PRABHU, Mr Vithaldas Ramchandra (retired) Galleries Health Centre, Washington Centre, Washington NE38 7NQ Tel: 0191 416 6130 Fax: 0191 416 6344 — MB BS Karnatak 1962 (Kasturba Med. Coll. Mangalore) MS Bombay 1969; FRCS Ed. 1975.

PRABHU-KHANOLKAR, Mr Sudhir Dinkar 12 Fairlie, E. Kilbridge, Glasgow G74 4SE; 109 Calderbraes Avenue, Uddingston, Glasgow G71 6ES Tel: 0141 818724 — MB BS Poona 1971 (B.J. Med. Coll.) FRCS Glas. 1978. Regist. (Gen. Surg.) Roy. Alex. Hosp. Paisley; Regist. (Gen. Surg.) Vict. Infirm. Glas; Regist. (Paediat. Surg.) Roy. Hosp. Sick Childr. Glas. Specialty: Gen. Surg.

PRABHU-PALAV, Sarojini Sharad 50 Rodney Road, Wanstead, London E11 2DE Tel: 020 8989 1009 Fax: 020 8989 1009 — MB BS Bombay 1959. Specialty: Obst. & Gyn.; Gen. Pract. Special Interest: Complementary Med.; Homeopathy.

PRACH, Andrzej Tomasz Monklands Hospital, Monkscourt Avenue, Airdrie ML6 0JS Tel: 01236 748748 Fax: 01236 760015 — MB ChB Glas. 1987; BSc (Pharmacol.) Ed. 1982; MRCPI 1993. Cons. Phys. & Gastroenterol., Monklands Hosp., Airdrie. Specialty: Gastroenterol.; Gen. Med. Prev: Specialist Regist. (Med. & Gastroenterol.), Ninewells Hosp. & Med. Sch., Dundee; Clin. Research Fell. (Gastroenterol.) Ninewells Hosp. & Med. Sch. Dundee.; SHO (Gen. Med. & Gastroenterol.) Stobhill Gen. Hosp. Glas.

PRACY, John Paul Myles 98 Liverpool Road, Islington, London N1 0RE; 98 Liverpool Road, London N1 0RE — MB BS Lond. 1987; FRCPS Glas. 1992.

PRACY, Mr Robert (retired) Ginkgo House, New Road, Moreton-in-Marsh GL56 0AS Tel: 01608 650740 Fax: 01608 651893 Email: robert.pracy@btopenworld.com — (St. Bart.) MRCS Eng. LRCP Lond. 1944; MPhil Lond. 1984, MB BS 1945; FRCS Eng. 1953; Hon. FRCSI 1983. Mem. & Chairm. (Med.) Pension Appeals Tribunals. Prev: Dean Inst. Laryngol. & Otol. Lond.

PRADEEP KUMAR, Narasimhan 236 Nottingham Road, Burton Joyce, Nottingham NG14 5BD — MB BS Madras 1986.

PRADHAN, Abhay Madhav Pradhan and Partners, Traps Hill Surgery, 25 Traps Hill, Loughton IG10 1SZ Tel: 020 8508 4403 Fax: 020 8508 7269 — MB BS Poona 1974 (Armed Forces Medical College) DA (UK) 1980; DRCOG 1985.

PRADHAN, Mr Chandra Bahadur 3 Regent Close, Edgbaston, Birmingham — MB BS India 1975 (All India Institute of Medical Sciences, New Delhi) FRCSI 1985; MCh (Ortho) L'pool 1990. Staff Grade (Orthop.) Roy. Orthop. Hosp. NHS Trust, Birm.; Staff Grade (Orthop. Surg.). Specialty: Orthop. Socs: BMA; BOA; Life Mem. Nepal Med. Coun. Prev: Cons. Orthop. Surg. Birm. Nuffield Hosp. Birm.; Assoc. Prof. & Head of Dept. of Orthop., Tribhuvan Univ. Teachg. Hosp. Kathmandu, Nepal.

PRADHAN, Mr Keshav Tularam 121 Old Road, Neath SA11 2DF Tel: 01639 631929; 6 The Avenue, Eagles Bush Valley, Neath SA11 2FD Tel: 01639 631929 — MB BS Marathwada 1970; FRCS Ed. 1987; FRCS Glas. 1987. Staff Grade (Gen. Surg.) Singleton Hosp. NHS Trust Swansea. Specialty: Gen. Surg.

PRADHAN, Mr Nitin Shripad 22 Church Road, Wootton, Ryde PO33 4PX — MB BS Bombay 1976; MS Bombay 1980, MB BS 1976; FRCS Ed. 1984.

PRADHAN, Rizwan Mohamedtaki High Street Surgery, 301 High Street, Epping CM16 4DA Tel: 01992 572012 Fax: 01992 572956; 1 Wedgwood Close, Theydon Grove, Epping CM16 4QD Tel: 01992 575064 — MB BS Lond. 1983; DRCOG 1987; MRCGP 1988.

PRADHAN, Shubhra 2 Dunlin Cl, Rochdale OL11 5PZ — MB ChB Manch. 1997.

PRADHAN, Vijaykumar Shyamsunder Newham General Hospital, Glen Road, Plaistow, London E13 8SL Tel: 020 7476 4000; 39 The Drive, Loughton IG10 1HB — MB BS Jabalpur 1961; DA Bombay 1964; FFA RCS Eng. 1970. Cons. Anaesth. Newham Gen. Hosp. Specialty: Anaesth. Socs: Research Soc. Anaesth. Prev: Sen. Regist. Whittington Hosp. Lond.; Sen. Regist. (Research) Roy. Coll. Surgs. Lond.; Regist. (Anaesth.) Roy. Infirm. & Canniesburn Hosp. Glas.

PRAGNELL, Anthony Arthur (Surgery), Charing Surgery, Charing, Ashford TN27 0HZ Tel: 01233 713782; Stonebridge Green House, Egerton, Ashford TN27 9AP Tel: 01233 756216 — (Char. Cross) MB BS Lond. 1962; DObst RCOG 1964.

PRAHALIAS, Andreas Aggelos 32 Rodenhurst Road, London SW4 8AR — Ptychio Iatrikes Crete 1990.

PRAIN, John Henry, TD (retired) Ruadhchre, Longforgan, Dundee Tel: 01382 360308 — (St. And.) MD (Commend. & Silver Medal) St. And. 1950, MB ChB; FRCPath 1963. Cons. Pathol. Perth City & Co. Hosp. Gp.; Lect. in Path. Univ. Dundee. Prev: JP.

PRAIS, Lesley Birmingham Skin Centre, City Hospital, Dudley Road, Birmingham B15 5TS; 64 Arthur Road, Edgbaston, Birmingham B15 2UW Tel: 0121 454 1049 — MB ChB Birm. 1976; D.Occ.Med. RCP Lond. 1996. Staff Grade (Dermat.) Skin Centre, City Hosp. Birm. Specialty: Dermat.; Occupat. Health. Prev: Clin. Asst. (Occupat. Dermat.) Birm. Skin Hosp.; SCMO (Community Health) Centr. Birm. HA.

PRAIS, Susan Sarah 4 Heath Drive, Hampstead, London NW3 7SY — MB ChB Glas. 1969; Cert FPA 1971.

PRAJAPATI, Chandravadan Laxmanlal East Surrey Hospital, Canada Avenue, Redhill RH1 5RH Tel: 01737 768511; 2 Taunton Close, Poundhill, Crawley RH10 7XT Tel: 01293 889058 — MB BS Saurashtra 1978; MRCPI 1991; FRCP UK 2004. Cons. Phys. (Gen./Elderly Med.) E. Surrey Hosp. Redhill. Specialty: Gen. Med. Socs: Brit. Diabetic Assn.; Geriat. Soc.; BMA. Prev: Sen. Regist. Rotat. (Gen. /Elderly Med.) Guy's Hosp. Lond.; Sen. Regist. Rotat. (Gen./Elderly Med.) Brighton Health Care; Regist. Rotat. (Gen. Med., Diabetes & Endocrinol.) Broadgreen Hosp. Liverp.

PRAJAPATI, Devant Pradhan and Partners, Traps Hill Surgery, 25 Traps Hill, Loughton IG10 1SZ Tel: 020 8508 4403 Fax: 020 8508 7269; 51 Fontayne Avenue, Chigwell IG7 5HD — MB BS Lond. 1994 (St. Bartholomew's) DFFP 1998. GP Loughton, Essex. Specialty: Gen. Pract. Socs: Assoc. Mem. Roy. Coll. Gen. Pract.; MDU; BMA. Prev: GP Regist. Gen. Pract. Romford Essex; SHO (Psychiat.) Warley Hosp. Essex; SHO (Paediat.) Old Ch. Hosp. Romford.

PRAKASAM, Stanley Francis Reginald 15 Hallamshire Road, Sheffield S10 4FN — MB BS Madras 1961; DTM & H (RCP Lond.) 1964; DCH (RCP Lond.) 1980.

PRAKASH, Mr Dhruva Hairmyres Hospital, East Kilbride, Glasgow G75 8RG Tel: 01355 585000 Email: letitia.evans@lanarkshire.scot.nhs.uk — MB BS Madras 1967; FRCS Ed. 1973; MS Madras 1970, MCh (Cardiothoracic) 1976. Cons. Thoracic Surg. Hairmyres Hosp. Glas. & Crosshouse Hosp. Ayrsh.; Hon. Sen. Lect. In Thoracic Surg., Univ. of Glas.; Vis. Thor. Surg., Cross Ho. Hosp., Kilmarnock; Coll. Tutor Roy. Coll. Surg. Scotl. Specialty: Cardiothoracic Surg. Socs: Scott. Thoracic Soc.; Assn. Cardiothoracic Surg. GB & Irel.; Eur. Assn. Cardiothoracic Surg. Prev: Hon. Sen. Regist. Frenchay Hosp. Bristol; Sen. Regist. (Cardiothoracic Surg.) Roy. Vict. Hosp. Belf.; Clin. Research Fell. Oesoph. Func. Laborat. Toronto Gen. Hosp. Canada.

PRAKASH, Halahally Channaiah Harrogate General Hospital, Harrogate HG2 7ND Tel: 01423 885959; 14 Masham Road, Harrogate HG2 8QF — MB BS Karnatak 1975. Sen. Staff Anaesth. Harrogate Gen. Hosp. N. Yorks. Specialty: Anaesth.

PRAKASH, Hari Victoria Hospital, Blackpool FY3 8NR Tel: 01253 300000 — MB BS Delhi 1977 (Maluna Azad) DA Eng. 1982. Specialty: Anaesth.

PRAKASH, Mr Kudigae Gurappagowda Meddygfa Penygroes, Bridge Street, Penygroes, Llanelli SA14 7RP Tel: 01269 831193 Fax: 01269 832116 — MB BS Mysore 1970 (Kasturba Med. Coll.) MS Mysore 1974, MB BS 1970; FRCS Ed. 1978.

PRAKASH, Nandhini Govinda 2 Langdale Avenue, Rochdale OL16 4SA — MB BS Madras 1981; MRCPI 1990.

PRAKASH, Mr Om Dilkush, 73 Ringwood Road, Luton LU2 7BG; 25 Gadebridge Road, Hemel Hempstead HP1 3DT Tel: 61820 — MB BS Agra 1968 (S.N. Med. Coll. Agra) MS Agra 1971, MB BS 1968; DO Eng. 1972.

PRAKASH, Swatantra Devi (retired) 11 Bracewell Avenue, Greenford UB6 7QU Tel: 020 8903 4325 Fax: 020 8204 0721 — MB BS Lucknow 1951; DRCOG Lond. 1962; DCH Lond. 1962.

PRAKASH, Mr Udai 20 Colliston Drive, Balgillo Road, Broughty Ferry, Dundee DD5 3TL Tel: 01382 779253 — MB BS Gulbarga 1990; FRCS Ed. 1994; FRCS Eng. 1994. Specialist Regist. (Orthop.) Dundee Roy. Infirm.; Hon. Clin. Tutor (Orthops. & Trauma) Univ. Dundee. Specialty: Orthop. Prev: SHO (Plastic Surg.) St. John's Hosp. Livingston.

PRAKASH, Vineet 36 Hallamshire Road, Sheffield S10 4FP — MB ChB Leeds 1995.

PRAKASH-BABU, Pandichary Chandra Westfield Medical Centre, 2 St Martin's Terrace, Chapeltown Road, Leeds LS7 4JB Tel: 0113 295 4750 Fax: 0113 295 4755 — MB BS Calcutta 1974. GP Leeds.

PRAMANIK, Amit Ladywell Building, Hope Hospital, Stott Lane, Salford M6 8HD — MB BS Calcutta 1982; MRCP (UK) 1992.

PRAMANIK, K Hornspit Medical Centre, Hornspit Lane, Liverpool L12 5LT Tel: 0151 256 5755.

PRAMANIK, P The Surgery, 142 Marshland Road, Moorends, Doncaster DN8 4SU Tel: 01405 740094 Fax: 01405 741063 — MB BS Calcutta 1972; MB BS Calcutta 1972.

PRANCE, Sarah Elizabeth Department of General Surgery, Derriford Hospital, Derriford Road, Plymouth PL6 8DH — MB BS Lond. 1993 (St George's Hospital Medical School) BA Univ. Rochester, USA 1988. Specialty: Gen. Surg.

PRANGNELL, Dennis Roy Glendale, Broadholme Road, Saxilby, Lincoln LN1 2NE Tel: 01522 703844 Fax: 01522 703844 — MB ChB Birm. 1971; FRCPath 1983, M 1977. Cons. Haemat. Lincoln Co. Hosp. Specialty: Haematology.

PRANK, Christopher John Brockwell Medical Group, Brockwell Centre, Northumbrian Road, Cramlington NE23 1XZ Tel: 01670 392700 — MB BChir Camb. 1989; MA Camb. 1989; DRCOG 1991; MRCGP 1994. Princip. in Gen. Pract., Brockwell Med. Gp., Cramlington. Prev: SHO (A & E Med.) Kettering Gen. Hosp.

PRANKERD, Thomas Arthur John (retired) 6 Stinsford House, Stinsford, Dorchester DT2 8PT Email: prankerd@abbaslake.freeserve.co.uk — MB BS Lond. 1947 (St. Bart.) MRCS Eng. LRCP Lond. 1947; MD (Gold Medal) Lond. 1949; FRCP Lond. 1962, M 1951. Prev: Dean & Prof. Clin. Haemat. Univ. Coll. Hosp. Med. Sch. & Hon. Cons.

PRASAD, Amoolya Kumar 63 Bloxwich Road, Willenhall WV13 1AZ Tel: 01902 608838 Fax: 01902 604866 Email: amooly@aol.com — MB ChB Manch. 1982 (Manchester University) GP Willenhall W. Midl. Socs: Brit. Med. Acupunct. Soc.; Birm. Med. Inst.; Primary Care Spec. Gp. of Brit. Computer Soc. Prev: MRC Research Stud.ship (Physiol.) Univ. Manch. 1983-4; SHO (Geriat. Med.) Burnley, Pendle & Rossendale HA; SHO (A & E) Bury HA.

PRASAD, Arjun The Health Centre, Welbeck Street, Castleford WF10 1DP Tel: 01977 465777 Fax: 01977 519342; 1 Dale View, Pontefract WF8 3SE Tel: 01977 600258 — MB BS Bihar 1966 (Darbhanga Med. Coll.) Clin. Asst. Castleford & Normanton Dist. Hosp. Prev: Regist. (Psychiat. & Ment. Handicap) Stanley Royd & Field Head Hosps. Wakefield; SHO (Psychiat.) Fairfield Gen. Hosp. Bury.

PRASAD, Avinashi Clarendon Park Road Health Centre, 296 Clarendon Park Road, Leicester LE2 3AG Tel: 0116 270 5049 — MB ChB Leic. 1981 (Leicester) ECFMG Cert. 1984; DRCOG 1985. GP Leics. Specialty: Cardiol.

PRASAD, Birendra Belle Isle Medical Centre, Middleton Road, Leeds LS10 3DZ Tel: 0113 270 9139 Fax: 0113 270 9139 — MB BS Prasad 1963; MB BS Patna 1963. GP Leeds.

PRASAD, Brij Kishore Ridge Lea Hospital, Quernmore Road, Lancaster LA1 3JT — MB BS Patna 1962; T(Psych) 1991.

PRASAD, Jwala The Surgery, 137 Straight Road, Harold Hill, Romford RM3 7JJ Tel: 01708 343281 Fax: 01708 345386 — MB BS Patna 1962 (P. of Wales Med. Coll. Hosp. Patna, India)

PRASAD, Kalyanaraman Hallam Street Hospital, Hallam St., West Bromwich B71 4NH Tel: 0121 607 3911 Fax: 0121 607 3901 — MB BS Osmania 1973; Dip. Psychiat. W. Indies 1977; DM (Psychiat.) Univ. W. Indies 1980; MRCPsych 2001. Cons. Psychiat. Sandwell Ment. Health & Social Care Trust. Specialty: Gen. Psychiat. Socs: BMA; Med. Protec. Soc.; Brit. Indian Psychiat.s Assn. Prev: Cons. (Psychiat.) All St.s Hosp. Birm.; Assoc. Specialist Fairfield Hosp. Hitchin; Resid. Psychiat. Tobago, W. Indies.

PRASAD, Kolanu Venkateshwara Friarage Hospital, Department of Pathology, Northallerton DL6 1JG Tel: 01609 764210 Fax: 01609 764632 Email: kolanu.prasad@stees.nhs.uk — MB BS Poona 1979; MD (Path.) Madras Univ. 1982; MRCPath 1988; FRCPath 1997. Cons. Histopath. S. Tees Hosps. NHS Trust; Hons. Cons. (Histopath.) York Hosps.; Hon. Sen. Lect. Leeds Univ. Specialty: Histopath. Socs: Assn. Clin. Path.; Internat. Acad. Path. (Brit. Div.).

PRASAD, Mr Krishna Korlakunta Consultant Urologist, George Eliot Hospital, College Street, Nuneaton CV10 7DJ Tel: 024 7635 1351 Email: kkprasad@nhs.net — MB BS (India) FRCS Ed.; FRCSI. Consultant Urologist, George Eliot Hospital, Nuneaton; Consultant Urologist, Hospital of St. Cross, Rugby. Specialty: Urol. Socs: AUA; EAU; BAUS.

PRASAD, Kumar Tripurari Prasad, Blackford, Commander and Ormiunu, 6 Dyas Road, Great Barr, Birmingham B44 8SF Tel: 0121 373 1885 — MB BS Patna 1974.

PRASAD, Mr Mangalore Govinda Consultant Orthopaedic Surgeon, North Tyneside Hospital, Rake Cane, North Shields NE29 8NH; 28 Queensway, Ponteland, Newcastle upon Tyne NE20 9RZ Tel: 01661 821329 — MB BS Mysore 1981; FRCS Glas. 1989; FRCS (Orthop.) 1998. Specialty: Trauma & Orthop. Surg. Prev: Cons. Orthopaedic Surg., Qu. Eliz. Hosp., Gateshead.

PRASAD, N Stockbridge Lane Surgery, 45 Stockbridge Lane, Huyton, Liverpool L36 3SA Tel: 0151 489 2888.

PRASAD, Neelam Newbridges, Off Birkdale Way, Newbridge Road, Hull HU9 2BH Fax: 01482 336916; 1 Barleycorn Close, Pindersheath, Wakefield WF1 4TD Tel: 01924 379334 Fax: 01924 211418 — MB BS Patna 1978; LRCP LRCS Ed. LRCPS Glas. 1985; DFFP 1993; DPM 1997. Specialty: Alcohol & Substance Misuse; Gen. Psychiat. Socs: Affil. Mem. Roy. Coll. Psychiat. 1995; BMA; Med. Protec. Soc. Prev: Cons. Psychiat. Hull & Holderness Community Health NHS Trust; Regist. (Psychiat.) Wakefield HA.

PRASAD, Neeraj Jasmine Cottages, High St., Church Eaton, Stafford ST20 0AG — MB ChB Dundee 1988.

PRASAD, Patricia Margaret Brunswick Health Centre, 139/140 St Helen's Road, Swansea SA1 4DE; 22 Chestnut Avenue, West Cross, Swansea SA3 5NL — MB BCh Wales 1985; MRCGP 1989; DRCOG 1990.

PRASAD, Pradip Nath 33 Croydon Road, London SE20 7TJ Tel: 020 8778 5135; 11 Bucknall Way, Beckenham BR3 3XL Tel: 0208 650 1726 — MB BS Bihar 1958 (Darbhanga Med. Coll.) BSc Bihar 1953; MD Delhi 1961; MRCP (UK) 1970; FRCP Ed. 1990. Princip. GP Bromley Family Pract. Comm. Specialty: Cardiol.; Respirat. Med.

Prev: Med. Specialist Safdarjang Hosp. New Delhi, India; Asst. Prof. Med. Univ. Mosul, Iraq; Assoc. Prof. Med. Univ. Benghazi, Libya.
PRASAD, Priyajit Pines, Westbourne Road, Edgbaston, Birmingham B15 3TR — MB BS Lond. 1994.
PRASAD, Punam 25 Poppleton Road, West Ardsley, Wakefield WF3 1UX — MB ChB Manch. 1995.
PRASAD, Raghavan Shankar NICU, Harold Wood Hospital, Gubbins Lane, Harold Wood, Romford RM3 0BE Tel: 01708 746090 Fax: 01708 708374 — MB BS Mysore 1978; MRCP (UK) 1989; T(M) (Paed.) 1995. Cons. Paediat. (Neonat.) Harold Wood Hosp. Essex. Specialty: Paediat.
PRASAD, Raghureshwar The Surgery, 74 Brooksbys Walk, London E9 6DA Tel: 020 020 8985 2797 Fax: 020 8985 0999; 30A Grove Park, Wanstead, London E11 2DL Tel: 020 8989 5637 — MD Bihar 1965 (P. of Wales Med. Coll. Patna) MB BS 1960; MB BS Bihar 1960; MRCGP 1972. Specialty: Occupat. Health. Socs: Med. Protec. Soc.
PRASAD, Mr Rajendra 3 Orchard Court, Royal National Orthopaedic Hospital, Brockley Hill, Stanmore HA7 4LP — MB BS Ranchi 1980; FRCS Glas. 1983.
PRASAD, Rajendra Consultant Anaesthetist, West Wales General Hospital, Carmarthen SA31 2AF Tel: 01267 227075 — MB BS Bihar 1973 (New Delhi) MD India 1990; T(GP) 1991; FRCA Lond. 1996; FFARCSI Dublin 1996. Cons. Anaesth. & Specialist in chronic pain. Specialty: Anaesth. Socs: Pain Soc.
PRASAD, Ramesh Chander Kings Road Medical Centre, 73 Kings Road, North Ormesby, Middlesbrough TS3 6HA Tel: 01642 244766 Fax: 01642 246243 — MB BS Osmania 1973 (Osmania Med. Coll. Hyderabad) GP Middlesbrough.
PRASAD, Ranjit Pendeford Health Centre, Whitburn Close, Wolverhampton WV9 5NJ Tel: 01902 781728 Fax: 01902 781728; 10 Elviron Drive, Tettenhall, Wolverhampton WV6 8SZ — MB BS Patna 1967 (P.W. Med. Coll.) DTM & H Bihar 1975. Prev: Trainee GP Neath; SHO (Chest Dis. & Geriat.) Mt. Pleasant Hosp. Chepstow; SHO (Geriat. Med.) Withybush Hosp. HaverfordW..
PRASAD, Mr Roopendra Kumar Lostock Hall Medical Centre, 410 Leyland Road, Lostock Hall, Preston PR5 5SA; Rulyn House, Parkside Drive, Whittle le Woods, Chorley PR6 7PL — (P. of Wales Med. Coll.) MB BS Patna 1965; MS Patna 1968; FRCS Glas. 1971; FRCGP 2001. GP. Socs: BMA (Gen. Med. Servs.) (Counc. Mem. BMA); Preston Medico Ethical Soc.; BMA Counc. Prev: Chairm. S. Lancs. LMC; Chairm. NW Regional Med. Comm.; Regist. (Cardiothoracic Surg.) Trafford AHA.
PRASAD, Sachida Nand The Surgery, 40-42 Brooke Road, London N16 7LR — MB BS Ranchi 1966.
PRASAD, Sanjay 18 Acland Crescent, Camberwell, London SE5 8EQ — MB BCh Wales 1990.
PRASAD, Sheo Narayan 25 Poppleton Road, Tingley, Wakefield WF3 1UX — MB BS Patna 1963.
PRASAD, Shyam King's College Hospital, Denmark Hill, London SE5; 398 Tempest Road, Chew Moor, Bolton BL6 4HL — MB BS Lond. 1994; MA Oxf. 1995. SHO (Med.) King's Coll. Hosp. Lond.
PRASAD, Mr Somdutt Wirral Hospital, Arrowe Park Road, Upton, Wirral CH49 5PE Tel: 0151 604 7193 Fax: 0151 604 7152 Email: sprasad@rcsed.ac.uk; BUPA Murrayfield Hospital, Holmwood Drive, Thingwall, Wirral CH61 4JY — MB BS Calcutta 1990; MS (Ophth.) 1993; FRCS (Ophth.) Ed. 1994. Cons. Ophth. Wirral Hosp. NHS Trust; Cons. Ophth. BUPA Murrayfield Hosp. Wirral. Specialty: Ophth. Special Interest: Cataract Surg., retinal Surg., diabetic eye Dis. Socs: Europ. Soc. Cataract & Refractive Surg.; Amer. Soc. Retina Specialists; Amer. Acad. Ophth. Prev: Clin. Lect. Univ. Sheff. & Hon. Specialist Regist. Roy. Hallamsh. Hosp. Sheff.; Retinal Fell. Arrow Pk. Hosp. Wirral; Fell (Diabetic Eye Dis.) Arrow Pk. Hosp. Wirral.
PRASAD, Sudama Rosemary Surgery, 2 Rosemary Avenue, Finchley, London N3 2QN Tel: 020 8346 1997; 42 Bancroft Avenue, London N2 0AS — MB BS Patna 1966.
PRASAD, Suyash Cromwell Hospital, Cromwell Road, London SW5 0ST Tel: 07775 705217 Email: suyashprasad@hotmail.com — MB BS Newc. 1993 (newcastle-upon-Tyne) MRCP; MRCPCH. Clin. Med. Off. Pediatric Intens. Care, Cromwell Hosp. Lond.; Clin. Research Phys., Pediatrics, Eli Lilly and Co. Specialty: Paediat. Prev: Specialist Regist., Pediatrics, Childrens Hosp. at Westmead, Sydney, Australia.
PRASAD, T St James Health Centre, 29 Great George Square, Liverpool L1 5DZ Tel: 0151 709 1120.
PRASAD, Usha Kumari 25 Poppleton Road, Tingley, Wakefield WF3 1UX — MB ChB Leeds 1994.
PRASAD, Vineet 1 Dale View, Pontefract WF8 3SE — MB ChB Leeds 1995.
PRASAD, Mr Vireshwar 4 The Causeway, London N2 0PR — MB BS Patna 1980; FRCS Glas. 1988.
PRASAD, Vishal 35 Poplar Avenue, Newton Mearns, Glasgow G77 5QZ — MB ChB Manch. 1996.
PRASAD, Yadu Nandan Kelvin Grove Surgery, Kelvin Grove, Wombwell, Barnsley S73 0DL Tel: 01226 752361 Fax: 01226 341577; 2 Upper Hoyland Road, Hoyland, Barnsley S74 9NJ Tel: 01226 742302 Fax: 01226 742302 — MB BS Bihar 1965 (Darbhanga Med. Coll.) Clin. Asst. Family Plann. Clinic Barnsley. Socs: BMA & Overseas Doctors Assn. Prev: Med. Pract. & Hosp. Pract. (ENT) Barnsley Gen. Hosp.
PRASAD RAO, Mr Garikapati St. Paul's Eye Unit, Royal Liverpool Hospital, Prescot St., Liverpool L7 8XP Tel: 0151 706 2000 Fax: 0151 706 5861; 16 Newbury Close, Widnes WA8 9YX Tel: 0151 495 3078 — MB BS Osmania 1982 (Gandhi Med. Coll., A.P. India) MS (Ophth.) Osmania 1987; FCOphth 1991; FRCS Ed. 1991. Sen. Regist. (Ophth.) St. Paul's Eye Unit Roy. Liverp. Hosp. Specialty: Ophth. Socs: Med. Protec. Soc.; Assn. Research in Vision & Ophth. Prev: Dir. (Primary Care in Ophth.) Liverp.
PRASAD REDDY, Kasu 85A Thealby Gardens, Doncaster DN4 7EQ — MB BS Andhra 1974.
PRASAI, Mr Janak Keshar 7 Valley Prospect, Newark NG24 4QH — MB BS Calcutta 1973; MS Chandigarh 1977; FRCS Ed. 1980.
PRASEEDOM, Mr Raaj Kumar Box 201, Addenbrooke's Hospital, Cambridge CB2 2QQ Email: praseedom@ntlworld.com; 26 The Croft, Fulbourn, Cambridge CB1 5DR Tel: 01223 880062 Email: rpraseedom@aol.com — MB BS Kerala 1988 (Trivandrum, India) FRCS; MS Kerala 1991; FRCS Ed. 1993. Cons. Surg. HPB Surg. & Liver Transplantation Addenbrooke's Hosp. Camb.; Cons. Surg. HPB - Gen. Surg. BUPA LEA Hosp. Camb. Specialty: Gen. Surg.; Transpl. Surg. Special Interest: Surg. for Pancreatic Cancer & Hepatobiliary Cancer. Socs: IHPBA; AUGIS; BTS. Prev: Specialist Regist. (Transpl. Surg.) Addenbrooke's Hosp. Camb.; Specialist Regist. (Gen. Surg.) Roy. Infirm. Edin.; Specialist Regist. (Gen. Surg.) Qu. Margt. Dunfermline.
PRASHAR, Sanjeev 15 Gurney Road, Northolt UB5 6LJ — MB ChB Manch. 1986.
PRASHARA, Krishan Gopal (retired) 8 Acacia Close, Green Acres, Greasby, Wirral CH49 3QE Tel: 0151 678 1752 — MB BS Nagpur 1962 (Med. Coll. Nagpur) DPH Eng. 1969.
PRASHER, Verinder Paul Department of Psychiatry, Queen Elizabeth Psychiatric Hospital, Birmingham B15 2QZ Tel: 0121 627 2840 Fax: 0121 627 2832 — MB ChB Birm. 1985; MRCPsych 1990; MMedSc Birm. 1992; MD Birm. 1994. Sen. Clin. Lect. (Learning Disabil.) Qu. Eliz. Psychiat. Hosp. Birm. Specialty: Gen. Psychiat.
PRASHNER, Philip Louis (retired) Loughton Health Centre, The Drive, Loughton IG10 1HW Tel: 020 8508 8117 Fax: 020 8508 7895 — (Middlx.) MB BS Lond. 1963; DObst RCOG 1968. Therapist Sexual Dysfunc. Clinic Holly Hse. Hosp. Buckhurst Hill, Loughton HC Loughton. Prev: Regist. (Psychiat.) Claybury Hosp. Woodford.
PRATAP, Bhoom Raj 38 Crewe Road, Alsager, Stoke-on-Trent ST7 3DD — MB BS Osmania 1954; DCH Eng. 1957.
PRATAP, Ravi (retired) 1 Pine View, Ashgate, Chesterfield S40 4DN Tel: 01246 234224 — MB BS Lucknow 1960 (King Geo. Med. Coll.)
PRATAP, Rohit 249 Court Road, London SE9 4TQ — MB BS Lond. 1996.
PRATAP VARMA, Mr Medavaram Jagdish Clifton House Medical Centre, 263-265 Beverley Road, Hull HU5 2ST Tel: 01482 341423 Fax: 01482 449373; 5 Feren's Gardens, Park Lane, Cottingham HU16 5SP Tel: 01482 842675 Fax: 01482 842675 — MB BS Osmania 1965 (Osmania Med. Coll. Hyderabad) MS Osmania 1973. Clin. Assit. Cardio Thorach Surg. Castle Hill Hosp. Cottingham Clin. Assis. Orthop. Surg. Both at Castle Hill Hosp. Cottingham. Specialty: Cardiothoracic Surg. Socs: BMA.

PRATHIBHA, Bandipalyam Vamanarao 45 Bron-y-nant, Maelor Hospital Residences, Croesnewydd Road, Wrexham LL13 7TZ — MB BS Bangalor 1985; MB BS Bangalore 1985.

PRATLEY, Jonathan Spring Gardens Health Centre, Providence Street, Worcester WR1 2BS Tel: 01905 681681 Fax: 01905 681699; 92 Hallow Road, Worcester WR2 6BY Tel: 01905 428929 — MB ChB Leeds 1975. Princip. GP Worcester. Prev: SHO (Paediat. & Neonates) Southmead Hosp. Bristol; SHO (Paediat.) Battledown Hosp. Cheltenham.

PRATT, Albert Edward (retired) Hawthorns, 8 Mill Road, Swanland, North Ferriby HU14 3PL Tel: 01482 632264 — MB BS Lond. 1960 (Char. Cross) DMRD Eng. 1964; FFR 1972; FRCR 1975. Med. Sch., Char. Cross Hosp. Prev: Sen. Regist. (Radiodiag.) St. Mary's Hosp. Lond.

PRATT, Barbara Anne (retired) Greenlands, Chorley Hall Lane, Alderley Edge SK9 7UL Tel: 01625 583397 — MB ChB Manch. 1953; DObst RCOG 1954; DA Eng. 1956. Prev: Anaesth. Crew & Macclesfield DHA.

PRATT, Charles William McElroy Huntington House, Huntington Lane, Hereford HR4 7RA Tel: 01432 350927 — (Manch.) MB ChB Manch. 1949; MA Camb. 1953; MD Manch. 1 9641. Prev: Lect. (Anat.) Camb.; Fell. & Dir. of Studies in Med. Pembroke Coll. Camb.; Vis. Assoc. Prof. Univs. Illinois & Calif., USA.

PRATT, Charlotte Frances Wilson Care of Elderly Department, St. Andrews Hospital, Devons Road, London E3 3NT — MB BS Lond. 1985; BSc Lond. Psychol. 1982; MRCP (UK) 1988; FRCP (UK) 2000. Cons. Geriat. Newham Healthcare NHS Trust Lond. Special Interest: Orthogeriatrics. Socs: Brit. Geriat. Soc.; Roy. Soc. Med. Prev: Sen. Regist. UCH & Whittington Hosps. Lond.; Lect. & Hon. Sen. Regist. St. Geo. Hosp. Med. Sch. Lond.; Regist. (Med.) Centr. Middlx. Hosp.

PRATT, Clarence Lucan Gray, OBE Far End, Chideock, Bridport DT6 6JW Tel: 01297 89300 — MD Liverp. 1931; MA Liverp. 1936, MSc 1933, MD 1931, MB ChB 1929; MA Camb. 1946. Fell. Christ's Coll. Socs: Physiol. Soc. Prev: Lect. Physiol. Univ. Camb.; Sen. Lect. Physiol. St. Thos. Hosp.; Med. Off. i/c RN Physiol. Laborat. Alverstoke.

PRATT, Mr Clive Alan Department of Maxillo-Facial Surgery, Kettering General Hospital, Rothwell Road, Kettering NN16 8UZ — MB BS Lond. 1990; MB BS (Hons.) Lond. 1990, BDS (Hons.) 1983, BSc (Hons.) Med. Sci. &; Anat. 1980; FDS RCS Eng. 1990; FRCS Ed. 1993. Specialty: Accid. & Emerg.

PRATT, Clive Ian Medical Specialists Group Guernsey, Alexandra House, Les Friteaux, St Martin's, Guernsey GY1 1XE Tel: 01481 38565; La Marcherie, La Villette, St. Martins, Guernsey GY4 6QG Tel: 01481 37344 — BM BCh Oxf. 1974; DRCOG 1978; DCH Eng. 1979; MRCGP 1979; FFA RCS Eng. 1982. Specialty: Anaesth.

PRATT, Mr David BUPA Hospital, Roundhay Hall, Jackson Avenue, Leeds LS8 Tel: 0113 269 3939; 101 Southway, Horsforth, Leeds LS18 5RW Tel: 0113 258 4561 — MB ChB Leeds 1951; BSc (1st cl. Hons. Anat.) Leeds 1951; MB ChB (1st cl. Hons.) Leeds 1954; FRCS Eng. 1962. Cons. Surg. St. Jas. Hosp. & Chapel Allerton Hosp. Leeds; Tutor (Clin. Surg.) Univ. Leeds. Socs: Vasc. Surg. Soc.; Trav. Surg. Soc. GB & N. Irel.

PRATT, David Alastair Hayman (retired) St. Andrews Lodge, 51 The Avenue, Fareham PO14 1PF Tel: 01329 284443 — MB BS Lond. 1957 (King's Coll. Hosp.) BSc St. And. 1951; MRCS Eng. LRCP Lond. 1956; FRCPath 1978, M 1966. Prev: Head Path. Dept. Glaxo Gp. Research Ltd. Ware.

PRATT, David Anthony 110 Cofton Road, Birmingham B31 3QR — MB BS Lond. 1994.

PRATT, David George St. Stephen's Surgery, St. Stephen's Green, Canterbury CT2 7JT Tel: 01227 454085; Glebe House, St. Stephen's Green, Canterbury CT2 7JT Tel: 01227 760667 — MB BS Lond. 1964 (St. Thos.) DObst RCOG 1973. Prev: Regist. (Cardiac) & Ho. Phys. & Ho. Surg. Profess. Surgic. Unit St. Thos. Hosp. Lond.; Regist. (Med.) Peace Memor. Hosp. Watford.

PRATT, Donald Reginald Winton Health Centre, Alma Road, Bournemouth BH9 1BP Tel: 01202 519311; Church Cottage, Burton Green, Christchurch BH23 7JN Tel: 474144 — MB ChB Aberd. 1954; MA Aberd. 1949, MB ChB 1954; DObst RCOG 1958. Clin. Asst. (A & E) Bournemouth Gen. Hosp. Specialty: Accid. & Emerg.

PRATT, Edward John 26 Salterns Road, Lower Parkstone, Poole BH14 8BJ — BM Soton. 1992; BSc (Hons.) Soton. 1991; MRCP (UK) 1996. Regist. (Med.) Roy. Bournemouth Gen. Hosp. Specialty: Diabetes; Endocrinol.; Gen. Med. Socs: BMA. Prev: SHO (Med.) Roy. Bournemouth Gen. Hosp.

PRATT, Giles Castlegate surgery, 42 Castle Street, Hereford SG14 1HH Tel: 01992 589928 Fax: 01992 501430 — MB BS Lond. 1995. GP. Specialty: Gen. Pract.

PRATT, Guy Edward Dickens 73 Widney Lane, Solihull B91 3LJ — MB BChir Camb. 1989; MRCP (UK) 1993; DRCPath 1995; MD 2000; MRCPath 2000. Regist. (Haemat.) Mersey RHA.; Regist. (Haemat.) Yorks. RHA; Sen. Lect. Univ. of Birm.; Hon. Cons. (Haemat.) Birm. Heartlands & Solihull NHS Trust. Specialty: Haematology.

PRATT, Helenor Ferguson (retired) Town Farm, West St, Marlow SL7 2BP Tel: 01628 483896 — MB ChB Ed. 1946; DCH Eng. 1951. Prev: Regist. Hosp. Sick Childr. Gt. Ormond St. Lond.

PRATT, Joyce Diana 110 Cofton Road, West Heath, Birmingham B31 3QR — MB BS Lond. 1987.

PRATT, Julian Charles (retired) Flat D, 74 Eccleston Sqaure, London SW1V 1PJ Email: julian@wholesystems.co.uk — BM BCh Oxf. 1973 (Univ. Coll. Hosp.) DRCOG 1978; MRCP (UK) 1980; MRCGP 1982. PPG Partnership. Prev: GP Heeley Green.

PRATT, Michael Alexander North Wing, Denburn Health Centre, Rosemount Viaduct, Aberdeen AB25 1QB Tel: 01224 643333/642757 Fax: 01224 404989; 9 Abbotshall Crescent, Cults, Aberdeen AB15 9JQ — MB ChB Aberd. 1967; MRCP (UK) 1972; FRCP Ed. 1989.

PRATT, Noel James 8 Bluebell Crescent, Norwich NR4 7LE Tel: 01603 452851 — MRCS Eng. LRCP Lond. 1940 (Univ. Coll. Hosp.) FFHom 1983, M 1956. Prev: Regist. Jenny Lind Hosp. Childr. Norwich; Flight Lt. RAFVR; Resid. Med. Off. Weir Hosp. Balham.

PRATT, Oliver William 12 The Shroggs, Steeton, Keighley BD20 6TG — MB BS Newc. 1994.

PRATT, Paul Geoffrey Radiology Department, Mid Essex Hospital Services NHS Trust, Broomfield Court, Pudding Wood Lane, Broomfield, Chelmsford CM1 7WE Tel: 01245 514771 Fax: 01245 514979 Email: geoff.pratt@meht.nsh.uk — MB BCh Zimbabwe 1984; MRCP Lond. 1990; FRCR Lond. 1993. Clin. Director in Radiol., Broomfield Hosp., Chelmsford; Cons. Radiologist, Springfield Hosp., Chelmsford. Specialty: Radiol. Socs: RCR; BMA; BIR. Prev: SR in Radiol. at the Roy. Lond. Hosp.

PRATT, Peter Leslie Greenwood Farm, Ham, West Wittering, Chichester PO20 7NX Tel: 01243 641046 — (King's Coll. Hosp.) LMSSA Lond. 1956.

PRATT, Mr Roland Kristian 51 Hartburn Avenue, Stockton-on-Tees TS18 4ES — MB BChir Camb. 1991; MA Camb. 1991; FRCS Eng. 1995. Specialist Regist., Orthop., Northern Deanery. Specialty: Orthop.

PRATT, Stanley Dennington (retired) Greenlands, Chorley Hall Lane, Alderley Edge SK9 7UL Tel: 01625 583397 — MB ChB Manch. 1948; DA Eng. 1953; MRCGP 1962. Prev: Princip. GP Chelford.

PRATT, Stephen Francis The Portland Practice, St Paul's Medical Centre, 121 Swindon Road, Cheltenham GL50 4DP Tel: 01242 707792; Tall Trees, 8 Shrublands, Charlton Kings, Cheltenham GL53 0ND — MB ChB Bristol 1977; DRCOG 1982; MRCGP 1983. Specialty: Gen. Med. Prev: GP Postgrad. Clin. Tutor Cheltenham HA.

PRATT, Steven Cedars Surgery, 8 Cookham Road, Maidenhead SL6 8AJ Tel: 01628 620458 — MB BS Lond. 1974 (St. Geo.) MB BS (Distinc. Path. & Therap.) Lond. 1983; MRCP (UK) 1986; DRCOG 1987; Cert. Family Plann. JCC 1987; MRCGP 1988; MSc (Pub. Health) Lond. 1993. Specialty: Gen. Pract. Socs: Windsor Med. Soc. Prev: Sen. Regist. (Pub. Health Med.) Anglia & Oxf. RHA; Regist. (Med.) Ealing Hosp. Lond.; SHO (Med.) St. Geo. Hosp. Lond.

PRATT, Tunde Sekweyama and Pratt, 10 Trafalgar Avenue, London SE15 6NR Tel: 020 7703 9271 Fax: 020 7252 7209 — MB BS Lond. 1978; MRCS Eng. LRCP Lond. 1977.

PRATT, William Robert Essex County Hospital, Lexden Road, Colchester CO3 3NB Tel: 01206744582 Fax: 01206 744739; 162 Maldon Road, Colchester CO3 3AY Tel: 01206 541246 — MB BS Lond. 1972 (King's Coll. Hosp.) MRCP (UK) 1975; FRCR 1979. Cons. Radiother. & Oncol. Essex Co. Hosp. Colchester. Specialty: Oncol. Prev: Sen. Regist. (Radiother.) Middlx. Hosp. Lond.; Regist. (Radiother.) Roy. Marsden Hosp. Sutton; SHO (Gen. Med.) Qu. Mary's Hosp. Roehampton.

PREBBLE, Sylvia Ethel (retired) 18 Greysfield Flats, Ferma Lane, Great Barrow, Chester CH3 7HU Tel: 01829 741767 — (Liverp.) MRCS Eng. LRCP Lond. 1952; DObst RCOG 1954. Prev: Asst. Specialist (O & G) Chester City Hosp., Chester Roy. Infirm. & New Matern. Unit Chester.

PRECIOUS, Sheila Helen West Cumberland Hospital, Whitehaven CA28 8JG Tel: 01946 693181 — MB ChB Manch. 1978; MRCP (UK) 1982; FRCP (UK) 1997; FRCPCH 1997. Cons. Paediat. W. Cumbria Health Care. Specialty: Paediat.

PREECE, Arthur Patrick James (retired) The Old Buck, Church Lane, Sedgeford, Hunstanton PE36 5NA Tel: 01485 570905 Fax: 01485 570891 — (St. Thos.) MA, MB Camb. 1965, BChir 1964; DObst RCOG 1966. Prev: GP Fakenham.

PREECE, John Fryer (retired) Cliff House, Yealm Road, Newton Ferrers, Plymouth PL8 1BN — (Cambridge/St Bartholomew's Hospital) MA Camb. 1949; MB BChir Camb. 1952; DObst RCOG 1954; MRCGP 1995. Cons. Ed. Health Serv. Computing Magazine. Prev: Edr. Pract. Computing Magazine.

PREECE, John Mark Yew Tree Cottage, Tredunnock, Usk NP15 1LY Tel: 01633 450464 Email: mark@preecem.demon.co.uk — MB BS Lond. 1983 (King's Coll.) BSc (Hons.) Lond. 1979; FRCS (Otol.) Eng. 1990. Cons. ENT Roy. Gwent Hosp. Newport. Specialty: Otolaryngol. Prev: Sen. Regist. & Regist (ENT) Univ. Hosp. Wales; SHO (ENT) Gt. Ormond St. Hosp. Lond.; SHO (ENT) Radcliffe Infirm. Oxf.

PREECE, Michael Andrew Institute of Child Health, 30 Guildford St., London WC1 Tel: 020 7242 9789 — MRCS Eng. LRCP Lond. 1967 (Guy's) MSc (Statistics) Lond. 1977, MD 1976, MB BS 1967; DCH Eng. 1969; MRCP (U.K.) 1971; FRCP Lond. 1982. Prof. (Child Health & Growth) Inst. Child Health Lond.; Hon. Cons. Phys. Hosp. Sick Childr. Gt. Ormond St. Specialty: Gen. Med. Socs: Fell. Roy. Soc. Med. FSS. Prev: Reader (Child Health & Growth) Inst. Child Health Lond.; Research Fell. Middlx. Hosp. Med. Sch. Lond.

PREECE, Mr Paul Edward clinical Skill Centre, Ninewells Hospital & Medical School, Dundee DD1 9SY Tel: 01382 660111 Fax: 01382 641795; 11 Marchfield Road, Dundee DD2 1JG Tel: 01382 668126 — MB BCh Wales 1966; FRCS Ed. 1972; FRCS Eng. 1974; MD Wales 1983. Hon.Sen.Lect.Centre.Med.Ed.; Edit. Bd. Europ. Jl. Surgic. Oncol.; Mem. Brit. Breast Gp. Specialty: Gen. Surg. Socs: BMA; Surgic. Research Soc.; Brit. Assn. Surgic. Oncol. Prev: SHO Accid. Serv. Radcliffe Infirm. Oxf.; Research Regist. Univ. Hosp. Wales; Lect. Univ. Dept. Surg. Welsh Nat. Sch. Med. Cardiff.

PREECE, Philip Milburn Chesterfield & North Derbyshire Royal Hospital NHS Trust, Chesterfield S44 5BL Tel: 01246 277271 Ext: 3141/2508 — MB ChB (Edinburgh) MRCP; MD; DRCOG 1977; FRCPCH 1980. Cons. Paediat. Chesterfield & N. Derbysh. Roy. Hosp. Specialty: Paediat. Socs: FRCPCH.

PREECE, Richard Mark Astrazeneca, Alderley Park, Macclesfield SK10 4TF Tel: 01625 513276 Fax: 01625 513527 Email: richard.preece@astrazeneca.com; 14 The Crescent, Mottram St. Andrew, Macclesfield SK10 4QW — MB ChB Manch. 1987 (Manch. Univ.) MFOM RCP, Lond. 1998. Occupat. Phys.Astrazeneca. Specialty: Occupat. Health. Prev: Regist. (Occupat. Med.) HM Naval Base Clyde; Regist. (Diving Med.) Inst. Naval Med. Gosport; Regist. (Occupat. Med.) Naval Base Devonport.

PREES, Karen Adele Batheaston Medical Centre, Coalpit Road, Bath BA1 7NP Tel: 01225 858686 — MB ChB Bristol 1989; DRCOG 1992. Specialty: Gen. Pract. Prev: Trainee GP Box Surg. Wilts.; SHO (Paediat., Geriat., O & G & A & E) Roy. United Hosp. Bath.

PREJBISZ, Jan Wojciech Southend Hospital, Prittlewell Chase, Westcliff on Sea SS0 0RY Tel: 01702 345555 Fax: 01702 226145 Email: jprejbisz@southend.nhs.uk — Lekarz Warsaw 1977; DMRT 1989. Ass. Spec., Clin. Oncol., Cancer Centre, Southend Hosp. NHS Trust. Specialty: Oncol.; Genitourinary Medicine. Socs: Roy. Coll. Radiol. Prev: SHO (Radiother. & Oncol.) Christie Hosp. Manch.; Clin. Research Regist. (Radiother. & Oncol.) Roy. Lond. Hosp.; Staff Grade (Radiother. & Oncol.) Southend Health Care NHS Trust.

PRELEVIC, Gordana Department of Endocrinology, The Royal Free Hospital, Pond Street, London NW3 2QG Tel: 020 7794 0500 Fax: 020 7380 2416 Email: g.prelevic@ucl.ac.uk; Flat 2, 20 Crossfield Road, London NW3 4NT Tel: 020 7433 1337 Fax: 020 7813 6233 — MD Belgrade 1971; MSc Belgrade 1978; DSc Belgrade 1985; FRCP (Lond.) 1995. Sen. Lect. & Hon. Cons. Reproductive Med. Roy. Free & Univ. Coll. Med. Sch. Lond.; Prof. (Med.) Belgrade Univ. Sch. of Med. Yugoslavia. Specialty: Endocrinol. Socs: RSM; Soc. Endocrinol.; Amer. Endocrine Soc. Prev: Cons. (Endocrinol.) Zvezdara Univ. Med. Centre Belgrade Yugoslavia; Head of Dept. (Endocrinol.) Zvezdara Univ. Med. Centre Belgrade Yugoslavia.

PREM, Alan Govindan 64 London Road, Wickford SS12 0AN Tel: 01268 765533; 35 Riverside Walk, Wickford SS12 0DU Tel: 01268 560521 — MB BS Madras 1960 (Stanley Med. Coll.) Prev: Regist. (Paediat.) St. John's Hosp. Chelmsford; SHO (Paediat.) Roy. Vict. Infirm. Newc.; Regist. (Med.) Newc. Gen. Hosp.

PREM, Daniel Matthew — BM BS Nottm. 1997; DRCOG 2000; MRCGP 2001.

PREM SWARUP, Mr Immaraju Joel Department of Accident & Emergency, Basildon Hospital, Basildon SS16 5NL Tel: 01268 533911 — MB BS Sri Venkatatewara 1979; FRCS Glas. 1988. Staff Grade Doctor Basildon Hosp. Specialty: Accid. & Emerg. Prev: Regist. (Surg.) Bromley Hosp.

PREMACHANDRA, Mr Don Jayantha James Paget Hospital, Great Yarmouth NR31 6LA Tel: 01493 452452; Asconia, Gunton Cliff, Lowestoft NR32 4PF Tel: 01502 585779 Fax: 01502 585779 — MB BS Ceylon 1975; FRCS Ed. 1984; DLO RCS Eng. 1984. Cons. ENT Surg. James Paget Hosp. Gt. Yarmouth & Norf. & Norwich Hosp.; Hon. Sen. Lect. Univ. E. Anglia. Specialty: Otorhinolaryngol. Socs: BMA; Med. Protec. Soc.; Roy. Soc. Med. Prev: Research Fell. Blood McIndoe Centre for Research; Sen. Regist. (ENT) Kent & Sussex Hosp. Tunbridge Wells; Regist. (ENT) Metrop. ENT Hosps. Lond.

PREMACHANDRAN, Sandrasekeram 1 Callow Field, Purley CR8 4DU — MB BS Sri Lanka 1983; MRCS Eng. LRCP Lond. 1987; FRCP Ed. 1992. Career Regist. (A & E) Mayday Univ. Hosp. Surrey. Specialty: Accid. & Emerg. Prev: Critial Care Fell. Trauma Centre N. Staffs. Hosp. Stoke-on-Trent; Regist. (Surg.) Altnagelvin Area Hosp. Londonderry; Regist. (Surg.) Whiteabbey Hosp. Belf.

PREMARATNE, Robolge Vijayalakshmi The Medical Centre, Gun Lane, Strood, Rochester ME2 4UW Tel: 01634 720220 — MB BS Peradeniya 1979; MRCP (UK) 1986; MRCS Eng. LRCP Lond. 1986.

PREMAWARDHANA, Lakdasa Devananda Kuvera Ellawela 19 Coedyafarn, Lisvane, Cardiff CF4 5RQ; 9 Timothy Rees Close, Cardiff CF5 2RH — MB BS Ceylon 1975; MRCP (UK) 1982.

PREMCHAND, Vattakkatt Balakrishnan Ellergreen, 3 Willoughby Close, Kings Coughton, Alcester B49 5QJ — MB BS Kerala 1987; MRCP (UK) 1994.

PREMKUMAR, Chittor Shadaksharam Solva Surgery, Cysgod-Yr-Eglwys, Solva, Haverfordwest SA62 6TW Tel: 01437 721306 Fax: 01437 720046 — MB BS Madras 1974; FRCSI 1984; FRCS Glas. 1985; FRCS Ed. 1985; Dip Therapeutics 2000.

PREMKUMAR, Gopalakrishna 9 Coggles Causeway, Bourne PE10 9LN Tel: 01778 421623 — (Madurai) MD (Paediat.) Madras 1974, MB BS 1966; DCH Madras 1969; DCH Eng. 1979. SCMO N. Lincs. HA.

PREMNATH, Pankaj White Cliffs Medical Centre, 143 Folkestone Road, Dover CT17 9SG Tel: 01304 216224 — (Armed Forces Medical College, Pouna, India) MB BS. Gen. Pract. Princip. Socs: LMC; PCG.

PREMNATH, Ramal White Cliffs Medical Centre, 143 Folkestone Road, Dover CT17 9SG Tel: 01304 201705 — MB BS Bhopal 1980; DA Roy. Coll. Anaesth. Lond.; LMSSA Lond. 1983. Gen. Med. Practitioner. Specialty: Anaesth.; Family Plann. & Reproduc. Health; Gen. Med.

PREMPEH, Thomas Bonsu 40 Greenfield Gardens, London NW2 1HX — MB ChB Aberd. 1966; MRCP (U.K.) 1972.

PREMRAJ, Koppada 5 'Toulouse', Brooklands Road, Sale M33 3QH Tel: 0161 973 4647 — MB BS Osmania U, India 1978; DLO, London 1994. Clin. Asst. (ENT), Warrington Dist. Gen. Hosp., Lovely La., Warrington, Chesh. Specialty: Otolaryngol.

PREMRAJ, Kumudini c/o Dr T. George, 82 Mellor Brow, Mellor, Blackburn BB2 7EX — MB BS Madras 1980; FRCA 1994.

PREMSEKAR, Rajasekaran 3 Partridge Road, Parkhurst Estate, Newport PO30 5NS — MB BS Madras 1988; MRCPI 1995.

PRENDERGAST, Anne Elizabeth Muirhouse Medical Group, 1 Muirhouse Avenue, Edinburgh EH4 4PL Tel: 0131 332 2201; 83 Dundas Street, Edinburgh EH3 6SD Tel: 0131 556 3983 — BM BS Nottm. 1987 (Nottingham) BMedSci Nottm. 1985; DRCOG 1990; DCH RCP Lond. 1991; MRCGP 1992. GP Retainee.

PRENDERGAST, Bernard David Department of Cardiology, North West Regional Cardiothoracic Centre, Wythenshawe Hospital, Manchester M23 9LT Fax: 0044 161 291 2389 Email: bernard.prendergast@smuht.nwest.nhs.uk — BM BS Nottm. 1987 (Univ. Nottm.) BMedSci Nottm. 1985; MRCP (UK) 1990; DM 1998. Cons. Cardiol. Wythenshawe Hosp. Manch., UK. Specialty: Cardiol. Special Interest: Ischaemic & Valvular Heart Dis.; Coronary Interven., Valve Dis. Socs: Scott. Cardiac Soc.; Brit. Cardiovasc. Interven. Soc.; Brit. Soc. of Echocardiography. Prev: BHF Jun. Research Fell. (Cardiol.) Univ. Wales Coll. of Med. Cardiff; Regist. (Cardiol.) Univ. Hosp. Wales Cardiff; Regist. (Gen. Med.) Soton. & Salisbury Gen. Hosps.

PRENDERGAST, Mr Brian Cathcart House, New Lane, Beal, Goole DN14 0RN Tel: 0197 676570 — BSc Liverp. l982; MB ChB Liverp. 1987; FRCS Ed. 1993. Regist. (Cardiothoracic Surg.) Edin. Specialty: Cardiothoracic Surg. Prev: Research Fell. (Transpl. & Cardiac) Sheff.; SHO Rotat. (Surg.) Pontefract.

PRENDERGAST, Colm Michael Lister Hospital, Stevenage SG1 4AB Tel: 01438 314333 Fax: 01438 781176; 83 Station Road, Harpenden AL5 4RL Tel: 01582 761947 — MB BCh BAO Dub. 1980; MA Dub. 1981; MRCP (UK) 1985; FRCR 1989. Cons. Radiol. Lister Hosp. Stevenage.; Med. Dir. E &N Herts NHS Trust. Specialty: Radiol. Prev: Sen. Regist. (Radiol.) Westm., Brompton & Roy. Marsden Hosps. Lond.; Regist. (Radiol.) Westm. Hosp. Lond.

PRENDERGAST, Jayne Mary 22 Frenchmans Close, Toddington, Dunstable LU5 6BD — MB BCh BAO NUI 1992.

PRENDERGAST, Kenneth Francis 88 Landor Road, London SW9 9PE — MB BCh BAO Dub. 1979; BDentSc Dub. 1983; FDS RCS Eng. 1990.

PRENDERGAST, Marie Theresa Anne 20 Devonshire Avenue, Dartford DA1 3DW — MB ChB Liverp. 1990. Trainee GP/SHO (A & E) Qu. Mary's. Hosp. Carshalton VTS. Specialty: Dermat.

PRENDERGAST, Mary Carmel Medical Centre, High Street, Ruabon, Wrexham LL14 6NH — MB BCh BAO NUI 1979 (Galway) DCH Univ. Coll. Dub. 1984; D Obst. Univ. Coll. Dub. 1985; MRCGP 1989.

PRENDERGAST, Michael Birmingham Childrens Hospital, Steelhouse Lane, Birmingham B4 6NH Tel: 0121 333 9181 — MB BS Lond. 1972 (St. Thomas' Univ. Lond.) DCH Eng. 1974; FRCP 1997, MRCP 1975; FRCPCH 1997, MRCPsych 1980; T(Psych) 1991; FRCPsych 1997. Cons. (Child Psychiat.) Birm. Childr.s Hosp. Specialty: Child & Adolesc. Psychiat.; Paediat. Neurol. Socs: Brit. Paediat. Neurol. Assn.; Brit. Neuropsychiat. Assn.; Paediatric Psychopharmacology Gp. Prev: Cons. (Child Psychiat.) Hosp. Sick Childr. Gt. Ormond St. Lond.; Clin. Lect. (Child Adolesc. Psychiat.) Maudsley Hosp. & Inst. Psychiat. Lond.; Cons. (Child & Adolesc. Psychiat.) Prudhoe Hosp.

PRENDIVILLE, Joseph Aloysius 48A Prince of Wales Mansions, Prince of Wales Drive, Battersea, London SW11 4BH Tel: 020 7720 2803 Email: josprend@dircon.co.uk — MB BCh BAO NUI 1984; MRCP (UK) 1988; PhD Manch. 1993. Cons. (Med. Oncol.) Guy's & St Thomas'Hosp Lond. Specialty: Oncol. Prev: Research Regist. (Med. Oncol.) Christie Hosp. Manch.; Sen. Regist. (Med.) Roy. Marsden Hosp. Lond.

PRENTICE, Andrew Department of Obst. & Gyn., Rosie Maternity Hospital, Robinson Way, Cambridge CB2 2SW Tel: 01223 336876 Fax: 01223 215327 Email: ap128@mole.bio.cam.ac.uk; 20 Rotherwick Way, Cambridge CB1 8RX — MB ChB Glas. 1983; BSc Glas. 1980; MRCOG 1988; MD Newc. 1992; MA Camb. 1994. Sen. Lect., Univ. of Camb. Specialty: Obst. & Gyn. Socs: BMA; Europ. Soc. of Embryology and Human Reprodich; World Endonetriosis Soc. Prev: Univ. Lect., Hon. Cons., Univ Camb.; Clin. Lect. Univ. Camb.; Research Assoc. Univ. Newc.

PRENTICE, Colin Richard Murray (retired) 3 Manor House, Thorner, Leeds LS14 3EQ; 3 Manor House, Thorner, Leeds LS14 3EQ Tel: 0113 892502 Email: profprentice@yahoo.com — MD Camb. 1970 (Westm.) MB BChir 1959; DTM & H Eng. 1961; FRCP Lond. 1977, M 1964; FRCP Glas. 1977, M 1974. Emerit. Prof. Of Med., Univ. Leeds. Prev: Reader & Hon. Cons. Phys. (Med.) Roy. Infirm. Glas.

PRENTICE, Professor Hugh Grant Pharmion Ltd, Maclintock Building, Granta Park, Great Abington, Cambridge CB1 6GX Email: gprentice@pharmion.com; 28 Church Road, Wimbledon, London SW19 5DH Tel: 020 8946 9181 Fax: 020 8946 9181 — MB BS Lond. 1968 (St Geo.) MRCP (UK) 1972; FRCPath 1988, M 1976; FRCP Lond. 1984. Med. Advis. Pharmion Corp.; Emerit. Prof. of Haematological-Oncology Univ. Coll. Lond. Specialty: Haematology. Special Interest: Bone Marrow Transplantation; Leukaemia/Lymphoma Treatm. Socs: Internat. Soc. Experim. Haemat.; Brit. Soc. Haematol.; Amer. Soc. Haemat. Prev: Sen. Regist. St. Geo. Hosp. Lond. & Roy. Marsden Hosp. Lond. & Sutton; Regist. West. Gen. Hosp. Edin.; Head (Haemat.) Roy. Free Campus Roy. Free & Univ. Coll. Lond.

PRENTICE, Ian James 34 Ash Grove, Kirklevington, Yarm TS15 9NQ — MB ChB Sheff. 1996.

PRENTICE, Janet Mary (retired) 5 Borage close, Pontprennau, Cardiff CF23 8SJ — MB ChB Leic. 1983; DRCOG 1987; DTM & H Liverp. 1988; DFPH. Prev: Sen. Regist. (Pub. Health Med.) Wessex RHA.

PRENTICE, Lesley-Ann Valleyfield Health Centre, Chapel Street, High Valleyfield, Dunfermline KY12 8SJ Tel: 01383 880511 Fax: 01383 881848 — MB ChB Leeds 1986.

PRENTICE, Malcolm George — MB BS Lond. 1974 (King's College Hospital) BSc (Hons.) Pharmacol. Lond. 1971; MRCP (UK) 1978; FRCP Lond. 1994. Cons. Phys. (Gen. Med., Endocrinol. & Diabetes) Mayday Univ. Hosp. Croydon; Hon. Cons. St. Geo. Hosp. Lond.; Clin. Teach. UCL. Specialty: Endocrinol.; Gen. Med.; Diabetes. Special Interest: Radioactive Iodine Ther.; Thyroid Ultrasound and Biopsy. Socs: Brit Med Ultrasound soc; Brit. Thyroid Assn. (Sec. 1996-2002); Soc. Endocrinol. Prev: Sen. Regist. (Med. Diabetes & Endocrinol.) Middlx. Hosp. Lond.; Regist. (Med.) Char. Cross Hosp. Lond.; Ho. Phys. King's Coll. Hosp. Gp. Lond.

PRENTICE, Matthew Grant 2 Woodlands Road, Surbiton KT6 6PS — MB ChB Bristol 1998.

PRENTICE, Michael Charles 5 Lingmell Dene, Coundon, Bishop Auckland DL14 8QX — MB ChB Leic. 1989; DRCOG 1994; DFFP 1994; MRCGP 1995. SHO (A & E) Stockton-on-Tees. Socs: BMA; PHCSG. Prev: Trainee GP P'boro. VTS; Ho. Off. (Surg. & Orthop.) Leics. HA; Ho. Off. (Med.) P'boro.

PRENTICE, Neil Paterson Murray Royal Hospital, Perth PH2 7BH Tel: 01738 621151 Fax: 01738 440431; 26 Hillpark Terrace, Wormit, Newport-on-Tay DD6 8PN — MB ChB Dundee 1985; MRCPsych 1991. Sen. Lect. old age Psychiat. Murray Roy. Hosp. Specialty: Geriat. Psychiat. Prev: SHO (Psychiat.) Roy. Edin. Hosp.; Ho. Off. (Surg.) Stracathro Hosp. Brechin; Ho. Off. (Med.) Falkirk & Dist. Roy. Infirm.

PRENTICE, Patricia Ann 2 Woodlands Road, Surbiton KT6 6PS Tel: 020 8390 7445 — MB BS Lond. 1968 (St. Geo.) DO Eng. 1979. Assoc. Specialist (Ophth.) Roy. Eye Unit Kingston Hosp. Socs: Coll. Ophth.

PRENTICE, Robert Thomson West (retired) 7 Kings Park, Torrance, Glasgow G64 4DX Tel: 01360 620204 Email: roy@twprentice.freeserve.co.uk — (Glas.) BSc (Hons.) Glas. 1958; MB ChB (Commend.) Glas. 1961; FRCP Glas. 1982, M 1965. Prev: Princip. in Gen. Pract. 68/97, Glas.

PRENTICE, Wendy Mary Marie Wrie Centre, Marie Wrie Drive, Newcastle upon Tyne NE4 6SS — MB BS Newc. 1992 (Newc. Upon Tyne) MRCP (UK). Specialist Regist. (Palliat. Med.) Newc. Specialty: Palliat. Med. Socs: MRCP Lond.

PRESCOTT, Professor Laurence Francis (retired) Redfern, 24 Colinton Road, Edinburgh EH10 5EQ Tel: 0131 447 2571 — MB BChir Camb. 1960 (Camb. & Middlx.) MA Camb. 1960, MD 1968; FRCP Ed. 1970, M 1968; FRSE 1988; FFPM RCP (UK) 1990; FRCP Lond. 1991; DCPSA 1998. p/t Emerit. Prof. Clin. Pharmacol. Edin. Univ. Prev: on Staff Roy. Infirm. Edin.

PRESCOTT, Mr Mark Vincent Royal Shrewsbury Hospital, Mytton Oak Road, Shrewsbury SY3 8XQ Tel: 01743 261000; Willow Brook, Church Road, Meole Brace, Shrewsbury SY3 9HQ Tel: 01743 249637 — MB ChB Dundee 1973; FRCS Ed. 1979. Cons. A & E Med. Roy. Shrewsbury Hosp. Specialty: Accid. & Emerg. Socs: Fell. Fac. Accid. & Emerg. Med.; Brit. Assn. Accid. & Emerg. Med. Prev: Cons. N. Staffs. Hosp. NHS Trust; Cons. A & E Med. Roy. Shrewsbury & Telford Hosps.; Sen. Clin. Lect., Dept. Orthop. s, Keel Univ.

PRESCOTT, Mary Cordelia Nuclear Medicine Department, Manchester Royal Infirmary, Oxford Road, Manchester M13 9WL Tel: 0161 276 4780 — MB ChB Manch. 1975; MD Manch. 1982; MRCP 1999; FRCR 2001. Cons. Nuclear Med. Manch. Roy. Infirm.

Specialty: Nuclear Med. Socs: Brit. Nuclear Med. Soc.; Eur. Assn. Nuclear Med.; Brit. Inst. Radiol. Prev: Research Asst. Nuclear Med. Manch. Roy. Infirm.

PRESCOTT, Richard John Department of Histopathology, Blackburn Royal Infirmary, Bolton Road, Blackburn BB2 3LR Tel: 01254 678300; 24 The Dene, Blackburn BB2 7QS Tel: 01254 690953 — MB ChB Manch. 1983; MRCPath 1992. Cons. (Histopathoogy) Blackburn Roy. Infirm. Specialty: Histopath. Prev: Sen. Regist. (Histopath.) Hope Hosp. Manch.

PRESCOTT, Richard William George 18 Blaidwood Drive, Durham DH1 3TD — MB BS (Hons.) Newc. 1977; MRCP (UK) 1979; MD Newc. 1983; FRCP Ed. 1990; FRCP Lond. 1992; MBA Dunelm 1995. Cons. Phys. (Special Responsibil. for Elderly) Bishop Auckland Gen. Hosp. Specialty: Care of the Elderly.

PRESCOTT, Mr Stephen c/o Department of Urology, St. James' Hospital, Beckett St., Leeds LS9 7TF Tel: 0113 206 5495 Fax: 0113 206 4920; Anscot House, Brackenthwaite Lane, Pannal, Harrogate HG3 1PJ Tel: 01423 872172 Fax: 01423 872172 — MB ChB Manch. 1981; FRCS Ed. 1986; MD Manch. 1990; FRCS (Urol.) 1993. Cons. Urol. St. Jas. Univ. Hosp. & Gen. Infirm. Leeds. Specialty: Urol. Socs: Brit. Assn. Urol. Surgs. Prev: Sen. Lect. (Urol.) Univ. Edin. & West. Gen. Hosp. Edin.

PRESHAW, Colin Taylor Roy. Scot. Nat. Hospital, Old Denny Road,, Larbert FK5 4SD Tel: 01325 570700 Fax: 01324 563788; 2 Allander Avenue, Bardowie, Milngavie, Glasgow G62 6EU — MB ChB Aberd. 1967; DPM Ed. & Glas. 1970; MRCPsych 1973. Specialty: Ment. Health.

PRESHAW, John Mulligan Kilmeny Surgery, 50 Ashbourne Road, Keighley BD21 1LA Tel: 01535 606415 Fax: 01535 669895 — (Leeds) MB ChB Leeds 1969; MRCGP 1978. GP Specialist in Dermat. Socs: Keighley & Dist. Med. Soc.; BMA. Prev: Regist. (Med.) Airedale Gen. Hosp. Keighley; Ho. Surg. & Ho. Off. (Med.) Chapel Allerton Hosp. Leeds.

PRESKEY, Mark Stephen Waterloo Road Surgery, 178 Waterloo Road, Blackpool FY4 3AD Tel: 01253 348619 Fax: 01253 404330 — BSc (Hons.) Lond. 1980; MB BS Lond. 1983; DGM RCP Lond. 1985; DRCOG 1986; DCH RCP Lond. 1987; MRCGP 1987. Prev: Trainee GP Ulverston VTS.

PRESLEY, Robert Anatomy Department, University of Wales, Cardiff CF1 3YF Tel: 029 2087 4000; La Frenaie, Bryn Rhedyn Close, Llanfrechfa, Cwmbran NP44 8UB Tel: 01633 482856 — MB BChir Camb. 1963 (Univ. Coll. Hosp.) MB Camb. 1964, MA, BChir 1963. Sen. Lect. (Anat.) Univ. Coll. Cardiff. Specialty: Anat. Socs: Fell. Zool. Soc. Lond.; FLS. Prev: Ho. Phys. Paediat. Unit Univ. Coll. Hosp. Lond.; Ho. Surg. (Orthop.) W. Middlx. Hosp. Isleworth; Univ. Demonst. (Anat.) & Fell. Emmanuel Coll. Univ. Camb.

PRESS, Anthony Martin Doctors Surgery, Great Melton Road, Hethersett, Norwich NR9 3AB Tel: 01603 810250 Fax: 01603 812402 — MB BS Lond. 1978 (Char. Cross) MA Camb. 1979, BA 1975; MRCS Eng. LRCP Lond. 1978; DA Eng. 1981; DRCOG 1983; MRCGP (Distinc.) 1986; Dip. IMC RCS Ed. 1991. Princip. (GP); Med. Adviser to Fitness Express. Prev: Trainee GP Norwich VTS; SHO (Anaesth.) Norf. & Norwich Hosp.; Ho. Off. (Med.) Char. Cross Hosp. Lond.

PRESS, Christopher Martin 99 Highfield Lane, Southampton SO17 1NN Email: martin.press@royalfree.nhs.uk — MB BChir Camb. 1968 (Univ. Coll. Hosp. Cambridge) MA Camb. 1969; MRCP (UK) 1971; MSc Lond. 1972; FRCP Lond. 1996. Cons. Phys. & Hon. Sen. Lect. Roy. Free Hosp. & Med. Sch. Lond. Specialty: Diabetes; Endocrinol. Socs: RSM (Sec. Sect. for Transpl.ation); EASD (Sec., Study Gp. on Insulin Pumps and Pancreatic Transpl.s. '97-'01). Prev: Asst. Prof. Med. & Paediat. Yale Univ. Sch. of Med. New Haven CT, USA; Lect. (Metab. Med.) Soton. Univ.; Regist. (Med.) Hammersmith Hosp. Lond.

PRESS, James David 87 Gorsty Lane, Hereford HR1 1UN — MB BS Lond. 1994.

PRESS, John Randolph 9A Magheralave Road, Lisburn BT28 3BE — MB BCh BAO Dub. 1960. Cons. Path. Inst. Forens. Med. Belf. Specialty: Forens. Path.

PRESSLER, Janice Mary Greenmount Medical Centre, 9 Brandlesholme Road, Greenmount, Bury BL8 4DR Tel: 01204 883375 Fax: 01204 887431; 11 Henwick Hall Avenue, Ramsbottom, Bury BL0 9YH Tel: 01706 825448 — MB ChB Sheff. 1979; MRCGP 1983.

PRESSLEY, Kieran Joseph Totley Rise Medical Centre, 96 Baslow Road, Sheffield S17 4DQ Tel: 0114 236 5450 Fax: 0114 262 0942 Email: senlac@doctors.org.uk — MB ChB Manch. 1978 (Manchester) DA 1981; DRCOG 1982; MRCGP 1986; Dip. Ther. Wales Coll Med 1998. Specialty: Gen. Pract.

PRESTON, Alan Eley Botolph House, Botolph Claydon, Winslow, Buckingham MK18 2LR Tel: 0129 671 4555 Fax: 0129 671 4806 — BM BCh Oxf. 1944; BM BCh Oxon. 1944; FRCPath 1971, M 1963. Socs: Brit. Soc. Haematol. & Assn. Clin. Path.

PRESTON, Andrew Paul Doctors Surgery, Salisbury Road, Southsea PO4 9QX Tel: 023 9273 1458; 95 Festing Grove, Southsea PO4 9QE — MB BS Lond. 1977 (Univ. Coll. Hosp.) BA Oxf. 1974; DRCOG 1980; MRCGP 1981. Prev: GP Bromley.

PRESTON, Bryan John 124 Parkside, Wollaton, Nottingham NG8 2NP Tel: 0115 928 3650 — MB BS Lond. 1961; MRCS Eng. LRCP Lond. 1961; FRCS Ed. 1967; DMRD Eng. 1969; FFR 1971; FRCR 1975. Cons. (Diag. Radiol.) Nottm. Univ. Gp. Hosps. Specialty: Radiol. Socs: Brit. Inst. Radiol. & Internat. Skeletal Soc.; Europ. Soc. of Skeletal Radiologist. Prev: Sen. Regist. (Diag. Radiol.) St. Mary's Hosp. Lond.; SHO N. Middlx. Hosp. Lond.; Ho. Surg. St. Mary's Hosp. Paddington.

PRESTON, Catherine Wray 39 Boulevard, Weston Super Mare BS23 1PF Tel: 01934 624242; Church Farm, The Bury, Locking, Weston Super Mare BS24 8BZ Tel: 01934 823468 — MB ChB Bristol 1972.

PRESTON, Clive Ian 64 Inverleith Row, Edinburgh EH3 5PX Tel: 0131 551 1919 — MB ChB Ed. 1977 (Univ. Edin.) BSc (Hons.) Ed. 1974; DMRT Ed. 1985; FRCR 1988. Specialty: Palliat. Med. Prev: Cons. Radiother. & Oncol. Princess Roy. Hosp. Hull; Sen. Regist. (Radiother. & Oncol.) Velindre Hosp. Cardiff; Regist. (Radiat. Oncol.) West. Gen. Hosp. Edin.

PRESTON, David Michael Princess Alexandra Hospital, Hamstel Road, Harlow CM20 1QX Tel: 01279 444455; Amwellbury House, Walnut Tree Walk, Great Amwell, Ware SG12 9RD Tel: 01920 462108 Fax: 01920 485190 Email: dmpreston@compuserve.com — MB BS Lond. 1974 (Guy's) MRCS Eng. LRCP Lond. 1974; MRCP (UK) 1977; MD Lond. 1985; T(M) 1991; FRCP Lond. 1993. Cons. Gastroenterol. Princess Alexandra NHS Trust. Specialty: Gastroenterol. Special Interest: ERCP; Inflammatory Bowel Dis.; Irritable Bowel Syndrome. Socs: Brit. Soc. Gastroenterol.; Brit. Soc. Med. & Dent. Hypn. Prev: Cons. Phys. Louth Co. & Lincoln Co. Hosps. & Postgrad. Tutor Louth Co. Hosp.; Sen. Regist. (Med.) John Radcliffe Hosp. Oxf.; Research Fell. St. Mark's Hosp. Lond.

PRESTON, Denys Wallwork (retired) 15 Parkstone Lane, Worsley, Manchester M28 2PW Tel: 0161 793 4914 — (Manch.) MB ChB Manch. 1951; DPH Manch. 1958; MFCM 1974.

PRESTON, Elizabeth Mary Aintree Hospitals NHS Trust, University Hospital Aintree, Longmoor Lane, Liverpool L9 7AL Tel: 0151 529 2231 Fax: 0151 529 3286 Email: elizabeth.preston@aht.nwest.nhs.uk; Jack Leg Farm, Cranes Lane, Lathom, Ormskirk L40 5UJ Tel: 01695 575026 Fax: 01695 571032 Email: elizabethmpreston@hotmail.com — MB ChB Liverp. 1968; FFA RCSI 1971. Med. Dir. Aintree Hosps. NHS Trust, Liverp.; Cons. Anaesth. Aintree Hosp. NHS Trust Liverp. Specialty: Anaesth. Socs: Brit. Assn. Anaesth.; Liverp. Inst.; Brit. Assn. of Med. Managers. Prev: Sen. Registar (Anaesth.) BRd.green, Alder Hey & Walton Hosps. Liverp.; Registar (Anaesth.) Walton Hosp. Liverp.; SHO (Anaesth.) David Lewis Northern Hosp. Liverp.

PRESTON, Professor Francis Eric Department of Haematology, Royal Hallamshire Hospital, Sheffield S10 2JF Tel: 0114 273 9107 Fax: 0114 275 6126; 7 Broomhall Road, Sheffield S10 2DN — MD Liverp. 1970; MB ChB 1963; FRCPath 1982, M 1970; FRCP Lond. 1992. Prof. Haemat. Univ. Sheff. & Hallamsh. Hosp. Sheff.; Dir. Sheff. Ref. Haemophilia Centre. Socs: (Pres.) Brit. Soc. Haemostasis & Thrombosis. Prev: Reader & Cons. Haemat. Univ. Sheff. & Hallamsh. Hosp. Sheff.

PRESTON, Helen Sarah 518 Chatsworth Road, Chesterfield S40 3BA — MB ChB Leic. 1996.

PRESTON, Hilary Gay Loddon NHS Trust, North Hampshire Hospital, Basingstoke RG24 9NA; Summerdown House, Malshanger, Basingstoke RG23 7ES — MB BS Lond. 1968; FRIPHH; MRCS Eng. LRCP Lond. 1968; DObst RCOG 1970. Staff Grade Paediat. (Community Child Health) Basingstoke & N. Hants. HA. Specialty:

Community Child Health. Socs: Assoc. Mem. BPA; Fac. Comm. Health.

PRESTON, James William Peter West Colonnade, Euston Station, London NW1 2HS Tel: 020 7506 5900 Fax: 020 7506 5901 Email: prestonj@BUPA.com — MB BCh Wales 1991 (University of Wales) MRCGP 1998; DoccMed 2003. Specialist Regist., Occupational Med., BUPA Wellness, Lond. Specialty: Occupat. Health. Socs: Soc. of Occupational Med. Prev: Occupational Phys., Occupational Med., BUPA Wellness, Lond.

PRESTON, Jane Thomas 458 Unthank Road, Norwich NR4 7QJ — MB ChB Aberd. 1984; BMedBiol Aberd. 1981; MRCOG 1989. Cons. James Paget Hosp. Gorleston-on-Sea Norf. Specialty: Obst. & Gyn. Prev: Sen. Regist. Norf. & Norwich Hosp.; Research Regist. (O & G) Addenbrooke's Hosp. Camb.; Regist. (Obst.) Qu. Mother's Hosp. Glas.

PRESTON, Jennifer Ann Helen 19 Raw Nock Road, Huddersfield HD3 3UX — MB ChB Sheff. 1998.

PRESTON, Joanne Elizabeth 31 Crosswood Crescent, Balerno EH14 7LX — MB ChB Glas. 1994.

PRESTON, John Grainger Group Practice Surgery, Middle Chare, Chester-le-Street DH3 3QD Tel: 0191 388 4857 Fax: 0191 388 7448; 28 Denwick Close, Chester-le-Street DH2 3TL Tel: 0191 389 2479 — MB BS Newc. 1983; MRCGP 1987. Chairm. of Durh. & Chester-le-St. Community Alliance.

PRESTON, Katherine Elaine Botolph House, Botolph Claydon, Buckingham MK18 2LR — MB BCh Wales 1998.

PRESTON, Mark Richard Preston and Austin, Killingworth Health Centre, Citadel East, Killingworth, Newcastle upon Tyne NE12 6UR — MB BS Newc. 1984; DRCOG 1987; MRCGP 1988; Cert. Family Plann. 1988; DFFP 2000. GP Killingworth.; Police Surg./Forens. Med. Examr.

PRESTON, Michelle Joanne Barnfield, Main St., Bishampton, Pershore WR10 2NH — MB ChB Bristol 1997.

PRESTON, Morag Samantha 52 Stanford Hall Crescent, Ramsbottom, Bury BL0 9FD — MB ChB Manch. 1993; DFFP; MRCOG.

PRESTON, Noel Wallace (retired) 36 Queen's Drive, Heaton Mersey, Stockport SK4 3JW Tel: 0161 432 2870 — (Manch.) MD Manch. 1954, MB ChB 1946; LRCP LRCS Ed. LRFPS Glas. 1947; Dp. Bact. Manch. 1950; FRCPath 1971, M 1963. WHO Expert Advis. Panel on Bacterial Dis.; Hon. Fell. Microbial Immunol. Univ. Manch. Prev: Dir. WHO Pertussis Ref. Laborat. Univ. Manch.

PRESTON, Penelope East Street Surgery, 6-7 East Street, Ware SG12 9HJ Tel: 01920 468777 Fax: 01920 484892.

PRESTON, Penelope Jane — MB ChB Manch. 1989.

PRESTON, Peter George 74 Eaton Road, Norwich NR4 6PR — MB ChB Ed. 1976; BSc Ed. 1973, MB ChB 1976; MRCP (UK) 1978; FRCR 1984. Cons. Radiol.(Norf. & Norwich Univ. Hosp.) Norwich. Specialty: Radiol. Prev: Sen. Regist. (Radiol.) Lothian Health Bd.

PRESTON, Roger Clifford The Surgery, 6 Longton Grove Road, Weston Super Mare BS23 1LT Tel: 01934 628 118/ Fax: 01934 645893; Church Farm, The Bury, Locking, Weston Super Mare BS24 8BZ — MB ChB Bristol 1969; DObst RCOG 1971. GP Weston-Super-Mare. Prev: SHO Gen. Pract. Train. Scheme Roy. Hosp. Wolverhampton; Ho. Phys. Ham Green Hosp. Bristol; Ho. Surg. Cossham Hosp. Bristol.

PRESTON, Mr Shaun Ralph Division of Surgery, Level 8, Clinical Sciences Building, St Jame's Univesity Hospital, Leeds LS9 7TF Tel: 0113 206 5282 Fax: 0113 244 9618; 12 Brookfield Place, Headingley, Leeds LS6 4EH — MB ChB Leeds 1990; BSc (Hons.) Leeds 1987; MD Leeds 1997. Lect. (Surg.) Univ. Div. Of Surg., St James Univ. Hosp. Leeds; Hon. Specialist Regist. Specialty: Gen. Surg.

PRESTON, Stanley David Grosvenor Street Surgery, 4 Grosvenor Street, St Helier, Jersey JE1 4HB Tel: 01534 30541 Fax: 01534 887948; Hautes Murailles, Rue de Samares, St Clement, Jersey JE2 6LS Tel: 01534 53229 — MB ChB Aberd. 1960; MB ChB (Commend.) Aberd. 1960.

PRESTON, Thomas Russell (retired) Priorsford, Vetch Park, Haddington EH41 3LH Tel: 0162 082 2634 — MB ChB Ed. 1948.

PRESTON, Mr Timothy Russell (retired) 72 Rodney Street, Liverpool L1 9AF Tel: 0151 709 5644 Fax: 01695 571032; Jack Leg Farm, Cranes Lane, Lathom, Ormskirk L40 5UJ Tel: 01695 575026 Fax: 01695 571032 Email: timothypreston@hotmail.com — MB BChir Camb. 1957 (Char. Cross) MA Camb. 1969, BA 1957; FRCS Ed. 1965; FRCS Eng. 1965. InDepend. Med. appeals tribunal Serv. Liverp. Prev: Cons. Gen. Surg. Whiston Hosp. & St. Helens Hosp.

PRESTON, Wilfrid Edwin Bentley Rose Cottage, Wroxham Road, Coltishall, Norwich NR12 7AE — MB BS Lond. 1950 (Middlx.) DObst RCOG 1954. Socs: BMA & Norwich M-C Soc. Prev: Ho. Surg. Jenny Lind Childr. Hosp. & Norf. & Norwich Hosp.; Ho. Phys. Roy. S. Hants. Hosp. Soton.

PRESTON-WHYTE, Margaret Elan Department of General Practice and Primary Healthcare, University of Leicester, Leicester Gen Hospital, Gwendolen Road, Leicester LE5 4PW Tel: 0116 258 4078 Fax: 0116 258 4982; 3 The Poplars, Billesdon, Leicester LE7 9AT Tel: 0116 259 6636 — MB BCh Wales 1961; DA Eng. 1966; FRCGP 1983, M 1976. Lect. (Gen. Pract. & Primary Health Care) Univ. Leicester. Specialty: Gen. Pract. Socs: Assn. Univ. Depts. Gen. Pract.; Leic. Med. Soc. Prev: GP Leicester; SHO MRC Pneumoconiosis Research Unit Llandough Hosp. Cardiff; Regist. (Anaesth.) Groote Schuur Hosp. Cape Town, S. Afr.

PRESTWICH, Heather Rachel Bennett Street Surgery, Stretford, Manchester M32 8SG Tel: 0161 865 1100; 13 River Street, Wilmslow SK9 4AB Tel: 01625 520078 — MB ChB Manch. 1988; DCH RCP Lond. 1992; DRCOG 1993; MRCGP 1994. GP Princip. Stretford Manch. Prev: Asst. GP Macclesfield.

PRESTWICH, Nichola Claire The Grange Medical Centre, 99 York Road, Leeds LS14 6NX Tel: 0113 295 1801 — MB BS Lond. 1998 (St Mary's Hosp.) BSc (Hons.) Lond. 1995. Salaried GP. Specialty: Gen. Pract.

PRESTWICH, Robin James Daniel — BM BCh Oxf. 1998.

PRESTWOOD, John Michael Brecon, 26 St Aubins Park, Hayling Island PO11 0HQ — MB ChB Bristol 1965. Prev: GP Hayling Is.

PRETLOVE, Samantha Jane 160 Tiverton Road, Selly Oak, Birmingham B29 6BU — MB ChB Birm. 1996; ChB Birm. 1996.

PRETORIUS, Marina 73 Manor Road, Scarborough YO12 7RT — MB ChB Pretoria 1990.

PRETSELL, Alexander Ogilvy 17 Law Road, North Berwick EH39 4PT; Seaview, 17 Law Road, North Berwick EH39 4PT Tel: 01620 2766 — MB ChB Ed. 1964; DObst RCOG 1967.

PRETTEJOHN, Edward Joseph Tucker (retired) Kings Gatchell Cottage, Gatchell Green, Trull, Taunton TA3 7ER Tel: 01823 338041 — (Lond. Hosp.) MRCS Eng., LRCP Lond. 1942; MB BChir Camb. 1943; FRCP Lond. 1974, M 1948. Prev: Cons. Dermatol. Taunton & Bridgwater Hosps.

PRETTY, Madeline Ann Dipple Medical Centre, South Wing, Wickford Avenue, Pitsea, Basildon SS13 3HQ Tel: 01268 553321 Fax: 01268 556231; 24 The Finches, Thundersley, Benfleet SS7 3LR Tel: 01268 775356 — MB BS Lond. 1967 (Roy. Free) Prev: Regist. (Surg.) S. Lond. Hosp. Wom.; Cas. Off. Roy. Free Hosp. Lond.

PRETTYMAN, Richard John Bennion Centre, Groby Road, Leicester LE3 9DZ Tel: 0116 250 2752 Fax: 0116 250 2770 Email: pd12@le.ac.uk — MB ChB Leic. 1985; DGM RCP Lond. 1987; DRCOG 1988; MRCGP 1990; MRCPsych 1992. Sen. Lect. (Old Age Psychiat.) Univ. Leicester. Specialty: Geriat. Psychiat. Socs: Brit. Geriat. Soc.; Brit. Neuropsychiat. Assn.; Brit. Neurosci. Assn. Prev: Lect. (Health c/o Elderly) Univ. Nottm. Med. Sch.; Regist. (Psychiat.) Leicester; Trainee GP Leicester VTS.

PREVETT, Martin Charles Wessex Neurological Centre, Southampton General Hospital, Southampton Tel: 023 8079 4793 — BM Soton. 1987 (Univ. Soton.) MRCP (UK) 1990; DM Soton. 1995; FRCP 2002. Cons. (Neurol.) Wessex Neurol. Centre Soton. Specialty: Neurol. Socs: Counc. Clin. Neurosci.s Sect. Prev: Sen. Regist. (Neurol.) Nat. Hosp. Neurol. & Neurosurg. Lond. & St. Mary's Hosp. Lond.; Regist. & SHO (Neurol.) Nat. Hosp. Neurol. & Neurosurg. Lond.; Research Regist. (Neurol.) Hammersmith Hosp. Lond.

PREZIOSI, Josef John 57/6 Holland Park, London W11 3RS — MRCS Eng. LRCP Lond. 1981.

PRIAULX, Mr Le-Roy Yeovil General Hospital, Yeovil BA22 4AT; Rowe Croft, Rimpton, Yeovil BA22 8AD Tel: 01935 850321 — MB ChB Liverp. 1961; MRCS Eng. LRCP Lond. 1961; FRCS Eng. 1967; MChOrth Liverp. 1969. Prev: Cons. Orthop. Surg. Yeovil Dist. Hosp.

PRICE, Adam Stainton Portscatho Surgery, Gerrans Hill, Portscatho, Truro TR2 5EE Tel: 01872 580345 Fax: 01872 580788 — MB BChir Camb. 1975; MA Camb. 1972; FRCGP 1993, M

1980. Course Organiser (Gen. Pract.) Cornw. VTS Scheme Postgrad. Centre Treliske Hosp. Truro.

PRICE, Mr Alan John The Alexandra Hospital, Woodrow Drive, Redditch B98 7UB Tel: 01527 503030; Vicarage House, Himbleton, Droitwich WR9 7LE Tel: 01905 391404 — MB BS Lond. 1969 (Univ. Coll. Hosp.) FRCS Ed. 1975; T(S) 1991. Cons. Orthop. & Traum. Surg. Alexandra Healthcare Trust Redditch, Worcs. Specialty: Trauma & Orthop. Surg. Socs: Fell. BOA; Brit. Assn. Surg. Knee. Prev: Sen. Regist. (Orthop.) King's Coll. Hosp. Lond.; Regist. (Gen. Surg.) Roy. E. Sussex & St. Helens Hosps. Hastings & Bexhill Hosp.

PRICE, Alan Richard West Kirby Health Centre, Grange Road, Wirral CH48 4HZ Tel: 0151 625 9171 Fax: 0151 625 9171 — MB ChB Liverp. 1968. GP Hoylake.

PRICE, Alison Nicola Clare Blackbrook Surgery, Lisieux Way, Taunton TA1 2LB Tel: 01823 259444 Fax: 01823 322715; West Lodge, Pitminster, Taunton TA3 7AZ Tel: 01823 421396 — MB BS Lond. 1977; DRCOG 1980.

PRICE, Professor Allan Edinburgh Cancer Centre, Western General Hospital, Edinburgh EH4 2XU Tel: 0131 537 2205 Fax: 0131 537 2240 Email: aprice@staffmail.ed.ac.uk — MB BCh Wales 1980; MRCP (UK) 1984; DMRT Ed. 1986; FRCR 1988; PhD Lond. 1992; FRCP Ed. 1997. Cons. (Clin. Oncol.) NHS Lothian. Specialty: Oncol.; Radiother.

PRICE, Althea Grace Hill Brow Surgery, Long Croft, Staincross, Barnsley S75 6FH Tel: 01226 383131; 62 Huddersfield Road, Barnsley S75 1DR Tel: 01226 206205 Fax: 01226 380100 — MB BS Lond. 1951 (Roy. Free) DCH Eng. 1953; MRCP Lond. 1954. Prev: SHO Roy. United Hosp. Bath.; Ho. Phys. Roy. Free Hosp. & Hosp. Sick Childr. Gt. Ormond St.

PRICE, Andrea Louise — MB ChB Birm. 1998.

PRICE, Andrew Frederick 6 Saxilby Drive, Whitebridge Park, Gosforth, Newcastle upon Tyne NE3 5LS Tel: 0191 284 0606 — MB BS Newc. 1984; MRCGP 1988; DRCOG 1988. Prev: SHO (Obst.) Qu. Eliz. Hosp. Gateshead; Trainee GP N.d. VTS; SHO (Med.) Preston Hosp. N. Shields.

PRICE, Mr Andrew James 81 Warwick Street, Oxford OX4 1SZ — MB BChir Camb. 1993 (Camb. & St. Thos. Hosp.) BA Camb. 1989; FRCS Eng. 1996. SHO (Orthop.) Northwick Pk. Hosp. Harrow; Specialist Regist. (Orthop.) Oxf. Rotat. Specialty: Orthop. Socs: BMA; BOA.

PRICE, Andrew Jonathan — MB ChB Glas. 1998.

PRICE, Andrew Richard — MB ChB Leeds 1981; MRCPsych 1986. Cons. in Child and Adolesc. Psychiat., CAMHS, Eastbourne & Co. NHS Trust. Specialty: Child & Adolesc. Psychiat. Prev: Sen. Regist. (Child & Adoles. Psychiat.) Soton. Child Guid. Clinic.; Clin. Director CAMHS, Eastbourne and Co. Healthcare Trust.

PRICE, Ann 45 Heol Maendy, North Cornelly, Bridgend CF33 4DF — MB ChB Bristol 1993.

PRICE, Professor Ashley Beresford 40 Cleveland Road, Ealing, London W13 8AL Tel: 020 8998 6208 Fax: 020 8864 1933 — BM BCh Oxf. 1964; FRCPath 1984. Cons. Histopath. Northwick Pk. & St. Mark's NHS Trust. Specialty: Histopath. Prev: Research Fell. & Hon. Sen. Regist. St. Mark's Hosp. Lond.; Sen. Regist. (Path.) St. Mary's Hosp. Portsmouth & St. Thos. Hosp. Lond.

PRICE, Audrey Joyce Nadine (retired) Little Manor, Church Lane, Burghfield, Reading RG30 3TG Tel: 0118 983 2569 Email: aud@ajprice.fsnet.co.uk — (St. Bart.) MB BS Lond. 1957; MRCS Eng. LRCP Lond. 1957; DObst RCOG Lond. 1960. Prev: Ho. Phys. Southlands Hosp. Shoreham-by-Sea.

PRICE, Mr Barrie Anthony, Lt.-Col. RAMC Frimley Park Hospital NHS Trust, Portsmouth Road, Frimley, Camberley GU16 7UJ Tel: 01276 604772 Fax: 01276 604019; 7 Minorca Avenue, Deepcut, Camberley GU16 6TT Tel: 01252 837432 Fax: 01252 837432 Email: barriep@aol.com — MB BS Lond. 1977 (Guy's) MRCS Eng. LRCP Lond. 1977; FRCS Ed. 1981; FRCS Eng. 1981; MS Lond. 1987, MD 1995. Cons. Vasc. Surg. Frimley Pk. Hosp. NHS Trust. Specialty: Gen. Surg.; Vasc. Med. Socs: Surgic. Research Soc.; Vasc. Surg. Soc. Gt. Brit. & Irel. Prev: Cons. Surg. Musgrave Pk. Hosp. BFPO 801; Cons. Surg. Princess Mary's RAF Hosp. RAF Akrotiri, BFPO 57; Hon. Sen. Regist. (Surg.) St. Bart. Hosp. Lond.

PRICE, Carol Ann Kingsnorth Medical Centre, Ashford Road, Kingsnorth, Ashford TN23 3ED Tel: 01233 610140 — MB BCh BAO Dub. 1977 (Trinity College, Dublin) GP.

PRICE, Catherine Mary Child Development Centre, Leicester Royal Infirmary, Leicester LE1 5WW; 59 Gartree Road, Oadby, Leicester LE2 2FD — MB BS Lond. 1971; MRCP (UK) 1978. Clin. Asst. (Paediat.) Leicester Roy. Infirm. Specialty: Paediat. Neurol.; Paediat.

PRICE, Christopher Gerard Adrian Bristol Oncology Centre, Horfield Road, Bristol BS2 8ED Tel: 0117 928 2238 Fax: 0117 928 2027 Email: chris.price@ubht.swest.nhs.uk; 13 Woodhill Road, Portishead, Bristol BS20 8ED Email: portprice@supanet.com — MB BS Lond. 1981 (King's Coll. Hosp.) BSc (Pharmacol.) Lond. 1978; MRCP (UK) 1984; MD Lond. 1993. Cons. Med. Oncol. Bristol Oncol. Centre Bristol Roy. Infirm. Specialty: Oncol. Prev: Sen. Regist. (Med. Oncol.) Soton. Univ. Hosps.; ICRF Research Fell. (Med. Oncol.) St. Bart. Hosp. Lond.; Ho. Phys. Liver Unit King's Coll. Hosp. Lond.

PRICE, Christopher John Little Maristone, 53 Western Avenue, Glasllwch, Newport NP20 3SN — MB BCh Wales 1985.

PRICE, Christopher Patrick Joseph Old Hall, Little Plumstead Hospital, Norwich NR13 5EW Tel: 01603 711401 — MB ChB Bristol 1979; MRCGP 1984. CEO, NORWICH PCT. Specialty: Pub. Health Med.; Gen. Pract. Prev: CEO Norwich City pcg; Regist. (Pub. Health Med.) Trent RHA.; GP LoughBoro. Univ.

PRICE, Mr Colin NHS Centre for Coding & Classification, Woodgate, Loughborough LE11 3SD Tel: 01509 211411; 317 Beacon Road, Loughborough LE11 2RA — MB ChB Manch. 1978; BSc Manch. 1976; FRCS Eng. 1982; MPhil Sheff. 1996. Sen. Med. Coding Cons. NHS CCC LoughBoro. Socs: BMA; Manch. Med. Soc.; Amer. Med. Informatics Assn. Prev: Regist. (Surg.) N. Manch. Roy. HA; Lect. (Anat.) Univ. Manch.; Ho. Phys. Preston Roy. Infirm.

PRICE, David Alun Chatsworth Road Medical Centre, Chatsworth Road, Brampton, Chesterfield S40 3PY Tel: 01246 568065 Fax: 01246 567116; The Old Rectory, 408 Chatsworth Road, Chesterfield S40 3BQ Tel: 01246 205900 Email: alun@doctor.gp — MB ChB Dundee 1980. Clin. Asst. (Pychogeriats.) Walton Hosp. Chesterfield.

PRICE, David Anthony Royal Manchester Children's Hospital, Pendlebury, Manchester M27 4HA Tel: 0161 794 4696; Woodside, 2 Ringley Road, Whitefield, Manchester M45 7LB — BM BCh Oxf. 1967; MA Oxf. 1967; FRCP (UK) 1983, M 1970; FRCPCH 1997. Sen. Lect. (Child Health) Manch. Univ.; Hon. Cons. Roy. Manch. Childr. Pendlebury. Specialty: Paediat. Prev: Ho. Off. (Med. & Surg.) Radcliffe Infirm. Oxf.; Research Fell. Sophia Kinderziekenhuis, Rotterdam.

PRICE, David Ashley Pine View, Cwm Crawnon Road, Llangynidr, Crickhowell NP8 1LS — MB ChB Sheff. 1995; MRCP II 1998. SHO (MicroBiol.). Specialty: Med. Microbiol. Prev: SHO (Gen. Med.).

PRICE, David Barry The Surgery, London Lighthouse, 111-117 Lancaster Road, London W11 1QT Tel: 020 7792 1200 — MB ChB Dundee 1988; MRCGP 1992. Princip. Med. Off. Lond. LightHo. (Centre for HIV & AIDS). Specialty: Gen. Psychiat.

PRICE, David Brendan Thorpe Wood Surgery, 140 Woodside Road, Norwich NR7 9QL Tel: 01603 701477 Fax: 01603 701512 — MB Camb. 1985; BChir 1984. Hon. Sen. Lect. Univ. of E. Anglia; Nat. Comm. of GPIAG. Prev: Course Organiser Norwich VTS.

PRICE, David Brian, OBE (retired) 22 Bryntyrion Hill, Bridgend CF31 4DA — MB BCh Wales 1945 (Cardiff) DObst RCOG 1949; MRCGP 1962. Regist. Obst. St. Davids Hosp. Cardiff. Prev: Maj. RAMC.

PRICE, David Elwyn Morriston Hospital, Swansea SA6 6NL Tel: 01792 703182 — MD Camb. 1990; MB BChir 1979; MRCP (UK) 1982; FRCP Lond. 1997. Cons. Gen. Med., Endocrinol. & Diabetes Morriston Hosp. Swansea; Sen. Lect. Univ. Wales. Swansea. Specialty: Gen. Med.; Diabetes; Endocrinol. Socs: Diabetes UK; Brit. Endocrine Soc. Prev: Sen. Regist. (Gen. Med., Endocrinol. & Diabetes) Leicester Roy. Infirm.; Research Fell. (Med.) Univ. Leeds; Regist. (Med.) Gen. Infirm. Leeds.

PRICE, David Gareth Royal Well Surgery, St Pauls Medical Centre, 121 Swindon Road, Cheltenham GL50 4DP; 75 Shaw Green Lane, Prestbury, Cheltenham GL52 3BS — MB BS Lond. 1974 (Lond. Hosp.) BSc (Physiol.) Lond. 1971; DCH Eng. 1980.

PRICE, David Glynne (retired) The Little Manor, Church Lane, Burghfield, Reading RG30 3TG Tel: 0118 983 2569 Email: aud@ajprice.fsnet.co.uk — (St. Thos.) MB BS Lond. 1948; MRCS Eng. LRCP Lond. 1948; DObst RCOG 1953; DA Eng. 1959; FFA RCS Eng. 1965. Prev: Cons. Anaesth. Roy. Berks. Hosp. Reading.

PRICE, David John Wishing Gate, Mount Road, Bebington, Wirral CH63 6HB — BM BS Nottm. 1988; MRCGP 1993; DCH RCP Lond. 1993.

PRICE, David John 82 Gravelly Bank, Lightwood, Stoke-on-Trent ST3 7EF Fax: 01782 316102 Email: davej.price@btopenworld.com; 82 Gravelly Bank, Lightwood, Stoke-on-Trent ST3 7EF Fax: 01782 316102 — MB ChB Sheff. 1965; D.Occ. Med. RCP Lond. 1995. Med. Off. various companies; Project Lead for Integration, N. Staffs. Urgent Care. Socs: Soc. Occupat. Med. Prev: SHO (O & G) City Gen. Hosp. Stoke-on-Trent; Ho. Off. (Gen. Med., Dermat. & Gen. Surg.) N. Staffs. Roy. Infirm.; Chairm. Centr. Stoke PCG.

PRICE, David K Dept of Community Psychiatry, HMS Drake, HMNB Devonport, Plymouth PL2 2BG — MB BS London 1974 (St Bartholomews Hospital Medical School) MRCPsych 1986. Cons.Psychiat., MOD UK (RN) Plymouth. Specialty: Gen. Psychiat.; Medico Legal. Prev: Cons. Psychiat., Cornw. Health Care Trust; Surg. Cdr., Head of Community Psychiat., Plymouth; Cons. Psychiat., Community Alcohol Serv., plymouth Community Trust.

PRICE, David Malcolm Charlotte Keel Health Centre, Seymour Road, Easton, Bristol BS5 0UA Tel: 0117 951 2244 Fax: 0117 935 4447; 18 Maurice Road, St Andrews, Bristol BS6 5BZ Tel: 0117 942 1616 — MB BS Newc. 1979; DCH RCP Lond. 1981; DRCOG 1984; MRCGP 1986.

PRICE, Dennis Thornton (retired) 14 Hurstlea Court, Alderley Edge SK9 7QF Tel: 01625 590450 — MB ChB Manch. 1961; DObst RCOG 1963; MRCGP 1974. Prev: GP Wilmslow.

PRICE, Dora Elizabeth 35 Alleyn Road, West Dulwich, London SE21 8AD — (Lond. Sch. Med. Wom.) M.B., B.S. Lond. 1930. Prev: Asst. Med. Off. Grosvenor Sanat. Ashford; Ho. Surg. Roy. Vict. Hosp. Folkestone; Res. Med. Off. Childr. Hosp. Hampstead.

PRICE, Doris May Clewett (retired) 19 Oaklands Park, Bishop's Stortford CM23 2BY Tel: 01279 652629 — MB ChB Birm. 1953; DO Eng. 1956; FRCS Ed. (Ophth.) 1963; FRCS Eng. (Ophth.) 1963; FCOphth 1988. Prev: Cons. Ophth. Surg. W. Essex & E. Herts. HAs.

PRICE, Douglas James (retired) Box Cottage, Balls Cross, Petworth GU28 9JS Tel: 01403 820302 — (Univ. Coll. Hosp.) MB BS Lond. 1949; FRCGP 1974, M 1957. Prev: Postgrad. Adviser Gen. Pract (SW Thames Region) Brit. Postgrad. Med. Federat. Univ. Lond.

PRICE, Mr Edgar Charles Vincent, TD (retired) The Old Rectory, Skirpenbeck, York YO41 1HF Tel: 01759 371465 Email: edgar.price@breathemail.net — MB BS Lond. 1952 (Middlx.) MRCS Eng. LRCP Lond. 1952; FRCS Ed. 1962; FRCS Eng. 1990. Prev: Cons. Orthop. Surg. York Hosp. Gp.

PRICE, Edith Patricia (retired) Tircwm, Leigh Road, Pontypool NP4 8HY — MB BCh Wales 1959 (Waks welsh national school of medicine) DObst RCOG 1961. Prev: SCMO (Child Health) Gwent DHA.

PRICE, Edward David Peregrine Corinthian Surgery, St Paul's Medical Centre, 121 Swindon Road, Cheltenham GL50 4DP Tel: 01242 707777 Fax: 01242 707776; Dowdeswell House, Dowdeswell, Cheltenham GL54 4LX Tel: 01242 820993 — MB BS Lond. 1967 (St. Geo.) LRCP Lond. 1967; MRCS Eng. 1967; DObst RCOG 1969. Med. Off. Cheltenham Coll. Specialty: Gen. Med. Prev: Ho. Off. (Med.) Cheltenham Gen. Hosp.; Ho. Surg. St. Geo. Hosp. Lond.; Ho. Off. (Obst.) Cheltenham Matern. Hosp.

PRICE, Eifion Wyn Anaesthetic Department, Royal Bolton Hospital, Minerva Road, Farnworth, Bolton BL4 0JR Tel: 01204 390762 Email: wyn.price@breathemail.net — MB BS Lond. 1990; FRCA 1996. Cons. Anaesth. Roy. Bolton Hosp. Specialty: Anaesth.; Intens. Care. Prev: Specialist Regist. (Anaesth.) N. W. Region.

PRICE, Elinor Myles Morland House Surgery, 2 London Road, Wheatley, Oxford OX33 1YJ Tel: 01865 872448 Fax: 01865 874158; Alan Court, Mill Lane, Old Marston, Oxford OX3 0PY — MB BS Lond. 1972 (Univ. Coll. Hosp.) MRCGP 1979. Prev: Ho. Phys. Med. Unit Univ. Coll. Hosp. Lond.; Ho. Phys. Endocrine Unit Roy. Free Hosp. Lond.

PRICE, Elizabeth Helen 48 Middleway, London NW11 6SG — (Westm.) MB BS Lond. 1967; MRCS Eng. LRCP Lond. 1967; DCH Eng. 1969; MRCPath 1975; FRCPath 1988. Cons. Med. Microbiol. Roy. Lond. Hosp. Whitechapel Lond. Specialty: Med. Microbiol.; Virology. Prev: Cons. Med. Microbiol. Qu. Eliz. Hosp. for Childr. & Hosp. for Childr. Gt. Ormond St. Lond.; Sen. Lect. (Microbiol.) Qu. Eliz. Hosp. Childr. Lond. & Inst. Child Health Lond.

PRICE, Elizabeth Jayne Great Western Hospital, Marlborough Road, Swindon SN3 6BB Tel: 01793 604317 Fax: 01793 604387 — MB BCh Wales 1987 (Univ. Wales Coll. Med.) MRCP (UK) 1990; MD Wales 1997; FRCP 2002. Cons. Rheumatologist Gt. W.. Hosp. Swindon. Specialty: Rheumatol. Prev: Cons. Rheum. Princess Margt. Hosp. Swindon; Sen. Regist. (Rheum. & Gen. Med.) Char. Cross. Hosp. Lond.; Research Regist. Kennedy Inst. Rheum. Lond.

PRICE, Elizabeth Mary (retired) Pear Tree Cottage, Hewelsfield, Lydney GL15 6UU — MB ChB Manch. 1953; DObst RCOG 1955; DCH Eng. 1956.

PRICE, Emily Eileen (retired) Merry Piece, Oxford Road, Woodstock, Oxford OX20 1QW — MB BCh Wales 1956 (Cardiff)

PRICE, Mrs Erika Burscough Health Centre, Stanley Court, Lord Street, Burscough, Ormskirk L40 4LA Tel: 01704 892229; 63 Harridge Lane, Scarisbrick, Ormskirk L40 8HD — MB ChB Manch. 1971.

PRICE, Felicity Margaret Spring Hall Group Practice, Spring Hall Medical Centre, Spring Hall Lane, Halifax HX1 4JG Tel: 01422 349501 Fax: 01422 323091 — BM BS Nottm. 1989.

PRICE, Fiona Jane The Coach House, Crawford Park, Perth Road, Dunblane FK15 0HA Tel: 01786 825045 — MB ChB Glas. 1989.

PRICE, Frances Mary Reepham Surgery, Smugglers Lane, Reepham, Norwich NR10 4QT Tel: 01263 733693 — MB ChB Manch. 1977; MRCGP 1988. Prev: Med. Miss. Segbwema Sierra Leone.

PRICE, Gail Victoria Pencoed and Llanharan Medical Centres, Heol-yr-Onnen, Pencoed, Bridgend CF35 5PF Tel: 01656 860270 Fax: 01656 861228; Haulfa, 7 Rogers Lane, Laleston, Bridgend CF32 0LB Tel: 01656 638753 — MB BCh Wales 1988 (Univ. Wales Coll. Med.) BA (Hons.) Wales 1983.

PRICE, Gary 16 Carr Close, Liverpool L11 4UA — MB ChB Liverp. 1996.

PRICE, Mr Gavin Fontaine Watson 11 Ganaway Drive, Whiterock, Killinchy, Newtownards BT23 6QT — MB BCh BAO Belf. 1967; FRCS Ed. 1973. Orthop. Surg. Altnagelvin Hosp. Lond.derry. Prev: Princip. Orthop. Surg. & Sen. Lect. Univ. Natal, S. Africa.

PRICE, Geoffrey John Royal Sussex County Hospital, Main X-Ray Department, Eastern Road, Brighton BN2 5BE Tel: 01273 696955 — MB ChB Sheff. 1978; FRCR 1988. Cons. Radiol. Main X-Ray Dept. Roy. Sussex Co. Hosp. Brighton. Specialty: Radiol.

PRICE, Gillian — MB BS Lond. 1996 (St Bart.) MRCPsych 2001.

PRICE, Gillian Mary Cramond Surgery, 2 Cramond Glebe Road, Edinburgh EH4 6NS Tel: 0131 336 5432 Fax: 0131 336 2203; Basement Flat, 104 St. Stephens St., Edinburgh EH3 5AQ Tel: 0131 225 3595 — MB ChB Ed. 1987 (Edinburgh) BSc Med. Sci. (Hons.) Ed. 1985.

PRICE, Graham Anthony Roscoe Paston Surgery, 9-11 Park Lane, North Walsham NR28 0BQ Tel: 01692 403015 Fax: 01692 500619 Email: grahamprice@nhs.net — MB BCh Wales 1972; MRCP (UK) 1975; MRCGP 1978; DRCOG 1978; DFFP 1993. Mem. Med. Staff N. Walsham War Memor. Cottage Hosp.; Hosp. Pract. (Dermat.) Cromer Hosp. & Norwich & Norf. Univ. Hosp. Specialty: Gen. Pract. Prev: Regist. (Dermat.) Liverp. Roy. Infirm.; Ho. Off. Univ. Hosp. of Wales Cardiff.

PRICE, Graham David Lewis Takeda Europe R&D ltd., Savannah House, 11 Charles II St., London SW1Y 4QU; 131 Saltram Crescent, Maida Vale, London W9 3JT Tel: 020 8960 8420 Fax: 020 8964 2845 — MB BS Lond. 1991; BSc (Hons.) Lond. 1989; DRCOG 1994; DFFP 1995; DFPM 2000; MFPM 2002. Med. Man. Takeda Res. & Dev. Europe. Lond.; Mem. Osler Club Lond. Specialty: Pharmaceutical Medicine. Socs: Roy. Soc. Med. Prev: Pharmaceut. Phys. Servier Laborats. Ltd., Paris; SHO (O & G) Roy. Free Hosp. Lond. & St. Mary's Hosp. Lond.; SHO (Med.) Centr. Middlx. Hosp. Lond.

PRICE, Grant Crichton 3FL, 37 Arden St., Edinburgh EH9 1BS — MB ChB Manch. 1995.

PRICE, Harold 47 Oakleigh Park N., London N20 9AT — MB ChB Bristol 1953; DCH Eng. 1955. Barrister-at-Law Lincoln's Inn 1967; Retd. HM Coroner.

PRICE, Hazel Margaret (retired) Vue De La Saline, Petit Val, Alderney GY9 3UX — MB BS Lond. 1955 (Roy. Free) DA Eng. 1959; DMRD Eng. 1973; FRCR 1978. Prev: Cons. Radiol. Univ. Hosp. Nottm.

PRICE, Heather Mary Rea Kidlington Health Centre, Exeter Close, Kidlington OX5 1AP — BM Soton. 1991; MRCGP 1995. GP. Specialty: Palliat. Med. Prev: Trainee GP Reading; SHO (Paediat., Rheum., Gen. Med. & O & G) Basingstoke Dist. Hosp.

PRICE, Helen Louise Great Western Hospital, Marlborough Road, Swindon SN3 6BB Tel: 01793 604925 Fax: 01793 604962 Email: helen.price@smnhst.swest.nhs.uk — MD New York 1982; BSc Yale 1978. p/t Cons. Paediat. Gt. West. Hosp. Swindon. Specialty: Paediat. Socs: BMA; Fell. Roy. Coll. Paediat. & Child Health; Fell. Amer. Acad. Pediatrics. Prev: Cons. Paediat. Lewisham Hosp. Lond.; Sen. Regist. (Paediat.) Kings Coll. Hosp. Lond.

PRICE, Helen Louise Sadlers End, 52 Sadlers Way, Ringmer, Lewes BN8 5HG — MB BS Lond. 1996.

PRICE, Helen Samantha 10 Manchester Road, Knutsford WA16 0NT — MB ChB Bristol 1989; Cert. Family Plann. JCC 1993; DRCOG 1993; MRCOG 1995. Med. Adviser Zeneca Pharmaceuts. Chesh. Specialty: Pharmaceutical Medicine. Prev: Trainee GP Wycombe Gen. Hosp. VTS; SHO (O & G) Macclesfield Dist. Gen. Hosp.

PRICE, Hugh Francis (retired) 15 Castle Hill, Duffield, Derby DE56 4EA Tel: 01332 840115 — (St. Thos.) MB BS Lond. 1955. Prev: Asst. Med. Off. Babington Hosp. Belper.

PRICE, Isabel Mary Shirvell (retired) Bright's Orchard, Hole-in-the-Wall, Ross-on-Wye HR9 7JW Tel: 01989 565804 Fax: 01989 565804 — MB ChB 1960 (Bristol) DObst RCOG 1962; DCH Eng. 1967; MFCM RCP (UK) 1974; FRCPCH 1997. SCMO Hereford Community Health Trust. Prev: Cons. Pub. Health Med. Mid Downs HA.

PRICE, Jacqueline Frances 4 Strathalmond Road, Edinburgh EH4 8AD; 107 Candlemaker's Park, Edinburgh EH17 8TL — MB ChB Ed. 1992; BSc Ed. 1990. Clin. Lect. Dept. of Pub. Health Sci.s Univ. Edin.; Hon. Specialist Regist. (Pub. Health Med.) Lothian Health Edin. Specialty: Pub. Health Med.; Epidemiol. Socs: Soc. Social Med. Prev: Clin. Research Fell. Epidemiol. Wolfson Unit for Preven. of Peripheral Vasc. Dis. Univ. Edin.; SHO (Gen. Med.) St. John's Hosp. at Howden Livingston.

PRICE, James David Sabrina House, 98 Abingdon Road, Grandpoint, Oxford OX1 4PX Tel: 01865 727770; Radcliffe Infirmary, Woodstock Road, Oxford OX2 6HE — BM BCh Oxf. 1991; BSc (Hons.) Bristol 1988; MRCP (UK) 1994. Res. Fell. (Clin. Gerat.) Radcliffe Infirm. Oxf. Specialty: Gen. Med. Prev: Specialist Regist. (Gen. Med. & Geratology) Radcliffe Infirm. Oxf.; SHO Rotat. (Gen. Med.) Gen. Infirm. Leeds; Ho. Surg. Nuffield Dept. Surg. John Radcliffe Hosp. Oxf.

PRICE, James Michael Parklands Surgery, 4 Parklands Road, Chichester PO19 3DT Tel: 01243 782819/786827 — MB BChir Camb. 1984 (Camb. & St. Thos.) MA Camb. 1985; MRCP (UK) 1989; DRCOG 1991; MRCGP 1992; T(GP) 1992; DFFP 1993; Dip Health Mgt Keele 2000. p/t Princip. in GP; Clin. Governance Lead, West. Sussex PCT; Sen. Lect. in Primary Care, Univ. of Brighton; GP Tutor, Chichester. Specialty: Gen. Pract.; Educat. Special Interest: Med. Educat. Socs: ASME; Complexity in Primary Care; SAPC.

PRICE, Jane Rosalyn Westbury House, Belmont St., Bognor Regis PO21 1LE — BM BChir Camb. 1969 (Camb. & Middlx.) MA Camb. 1969; DObst RCOG 1973. Clin. Asst. Regis Day Hosp. Bognor Regis. & St Richards Hosp. Chichester. Specialty: Care of the Elderly. Prev: Princip. Rochdale Gp. Pract. Lond.

PRICE, Jean 12 Woodview Close,, Bassett, Southampton SO16 3PZ — (Durh.) MB BS Durh. 1966; DObst RCOG 1969; DPH Bristol 1971; DPM Eng. 1974; FRCPCH 1996. Cons. Community Paediat.; Forens. Examr. Specialty: Paediat. Socs: BACCH; PCAIG (Exec. Comm. Mem.); CCP, Chairm. CPIG. Prev: SCMO Southmead HA; Sen. Regist. (Child Psychiat.) Bristol Childr. Hosp.; Regist. (Gen. Med.) Jersey Gp. Hosps.

PRICE, John David Springhead Medical Centre, 376 Willerby Road, Hull HU5 5JT Tel: 01482 352263 Fax: 01482 352480 — LRCPI & LM, LRSCI & LM 1968. Chairm. Exec. Comm. W. Hull Primary Care Trust. Socs: Brit. Soc. Gastroenterol. Prev: Ho. Phys. & Ho. Surg. Mercer's Hosp. Dub.; SHO Hull Matern. Hosp.

PRICE, John David 144 Harley Street, London W1G 7LD Tel: 020 7935 0023 Fax: 020 7935 5972; 30 The Drive, Hove BN3 3JD Tel: 01273 778123 Mob: 07956 597177 — MB BS Lond. 1958 (Westm.) MRCS Eng. LRCP Lond. 1958; DObst RCOG 1960; Dip Pharm Med RCP (UK) 1977. Cons. Specialty: Orthop. Special Interest: Cervical Spondylosis. Socs: Fell. Roy. Soc. Med.; Brit. Assn. Manip. Med.; Primary Care Soc. Prev: Med. Dir. Beecham Pharmaceut. Lond.; Med. Dir. Clin. Research Glaxo Laborats. Greenford; Assoc. Cons. Char. Cross Hosp. Lond.

PRICE, Professor John Frederick Department of Child Health, King's College Hospital, London SE5 9RS Tel: 020 7326 3562; 119 Dacre Park, London SE13 5BZ Tel: 020 8318 5450 — MB BChir Camb. 1970 (Camb. & Guy's) MA, MB Camb. 1970, MD 1986, BChir 1969; FRCP Lond. 1985, M 1972; DCH Eng. 1973. Prof. Paediat. Respirology & Cons. Paediat. King's Coll. Hosp. Lond.; Prof. Paediat. Respirology King's Coll. Sch. Med. Lond. Specialty: Paediat. Socs: (Counc.) Brit. Thoracic Soc. & Europ. Respirat. Soc. Prev: Ho. Phys. Brompton Hosp. Lond.; Regist. Hosp. Sick Childr. Gt. Ormond St.; MRC Research Fell. Inst. Child Health Lond.

PRICE, John Hardy (retired) Pear Tree Cottage, Hewelsfield, Lydney GL15 6UU — MB ChB Manch. 1953; FRCGP 1977, M 1962. Prev: Hon. Sen. Clin. Lect. Univ. Birm.

PRICE, John Hazlett Department of Gynaecology, Belfast City Hospital, Lisburn Road, Belfast BT9 7AB Tel: 01232 263810 Fax: 01232 263953 — MD Belf. 1989; MB BCh BAO Belf. 1977; MRCOG 1982, D 1979; FRCOG 1995. Cons. O & G Belf. City Hosp.; Hon sen Lec Qu.s Univ Belf. Specialty: Obst. & Gyn. Socs: Brit. Gyn. Cancer Soc. (Counc. Mem.); BSCCP; Irish Gyn. Oncol. Soc. (Ulster Represent.).

PRICE, Mr John Jeffrey The Yorkshire Clinic, Bradford Road, Bingley BD16 1TW — MB ChB (Hons.) Leeds 1965; MRCP Lond. 1968; FRCS Eng. 1971; FRCP 1999. Cons. (Gen. Surg.) Bradford Hosps. Specialty: Gen. Surg.

PRICE, Mr John Lawrence, TD (retired) 70 Brackenrig Crescent, Eaglesham, Glasgow G76 0HF Tel: 0141 644 3395 — MB ChB Glas. 1956; FRCOG 1980, M 1966, DObst 1960; FRCS Ed. 1972. Prev: Cons. Lanarksh. Area Health Bd.

PRICE, John Lewis, OBE, RD (retired) 1 Little Warren Close, Guildford GU4 8PW Tel: 01483 563868 — MB BS Lond. 1950 (Lond. Hosp.) DMRD Eng. 1961; FRCR 1963. Prev: Profess. Fell. Radiol. Dept. Phys. Univ. Surrey.

PRICE, John Scott Odintune Place, Plumpton, Lewes BN7 3AN Tel: 01273 890362 Fax: 01273 890614 Email: johnscottprice@hotmail.com — BM BCh Oxf. 1958 (St Bart.) DPM Lond. 1965; DM Oxf. 1969; FRCPsych 1979, M 1971; MRCP Lond. 1973; T(Psych) 1991. Cons. Psychiat. Milton Keynes Health Dist. Specialty: Gen. Psychiat. Socs: Chairm. Sect. on Psychother., World Psychiatric Assn. Prev: Cons. Psychiat. Northwick Pk. Hosp. & Clin. Research Centre Harrow; Mem. Scientif. Staff MRC Psychiat. Genetics Unit Inst. Psychiat.; Sen. Lect. (Psychol. Med.) Univ. Newc.

PRICE, John Stephen 74 Madison Springs, Madison CT 06443, USA — MB ChB Ed. 1983; BSc (Hons.) Ed. 1980; PhD Camb. 1990. Vice-Pres. Risk Eval. & Documentation, Safety & Risk Managem. Pfizer Inc New Lond. CT USA. Prev: Sen. Director and Global Head Clin. Regulatory Submissions Grp. Centr. Res.; Sen. Clin. Submissions Manager Pfizer Centr. Research; Head Clin. Eval. Unit, Med. Centre Agency, DOH.

PRICE, Jonathan Neil Moat House, Crescent Road, Ivybridge PL21 0BP — BM Soton. 1992.

PRICE, Jonathan Paul David Osborne Practice Surgery, 25 Osborne Road, Southsea PO5 3ND Tel: 023 9282 1371 — BMSc Nottm. 1983, BM BS 1985; DRCOG 1988; MRCGP 1989; DCH RCP Lond. 1990; D.Occ.Med. 2000. Prev: Trainee GP Portsmouth; SHO Portsmouth VTS; Ho. Off. Univ. Hosp. Nottm.

PRICE, Jonathan Raymond University of Oxford, Department of Psychiatry, The Warneford Hospital, Oxford OX3 7JX Tel: 01865 226 467 Fax: 01865 793101 Email: jonathan.price@psych.ox.ac.uk — BM BCh Oxf. 1991; MA Camb. 1992; MRCPsych 1995; MSc (Evidence Based Healthcare) Oxf. 1999; Dip. Cognitive Ther, Oxf. 1999; Dip in Learning & Teaching of Higher Education, Oxford 2001; DPhil Oxf. 2003. Clin. Tutor in Psychiat. Specialty: Gen. Psychiat. Special Interest: Evidence-based Med.; Gen. Hosp. Psychiat.; Managem. of Depression. Socs: Assn. of Univ. Teachers of Psychiat.; Higher Educat. Acad. Prev: MRC Fell. Health Servs. Research; Univ. Oxf. 97-2001; Regist. Rotat. (Psychiat.) Oxf. Train. Scheme; SHO (Oncol.) Qu. Eliz. Hosp. Birm.

PRICE, Judith-Ann Wharton Health Centre, Greville Drive, Winsford CW7 3EP Tel: 01606 861220 Fax: 01606 863354; 87

Chester Road, Winsford CW7 2NG — MB ChB Manch. 1987; BSc 1984; DRCOG 1989. Socs: Roy. Coll. Gen. Pract.

PRICE, Julie Pield Heath Road, Uxbridge UB8 3NN Tel: 01895 279889 Fax: 01895 279444 — MB BS Lond. 1978 (King's Coll. Hosp.) BSc Lond. 1975; FRCOG 1997. Cons. O & G Hillingdon Hosp. Uxbridge. Specialty: Obst. & Gyn. Prev: Sen. Regist. & Lect. (O & G) Char. Cross Hosp. Lond.; Regist. & Lect. (O & G) St. Thos. Hosp. Lond.

PRICE, Katherine Jean 8 Woodvale Road, Sheffield S10 3EX — MB ChB Sheff. 1979; DCH RCP Lond. 1983; MRCP (Paediat.) (UK) 1985. Cons. Paediat. N. Gen. Hosp. Sheff. & Sheff. Childr. Hosp. Specialty: Paediat.; Diabetes. Prev: Sen. Regist. (Paediat.) Roy. Devon & Exeter Hosp.; SHO (Paediat.) & (Med.) Exeter HA; Med. Off. Kwa Zulu Rep. S. Afr.

PRICE, Kathryn Anne 3 Thornholme Road, Sunderland SR2 7QF — MB ChB Liverp. 1978; FFA RCS Eng. 1983. Cons. (Anaesth.) Newc. Gen. Hosp. Specialty: Anaesth. Socs: Dep. Regional Adviser (Anaesth.) North. Region; Counc., SEA UK. Prev: Cons. (Anaesth.) Sunderland DGH; Sen. Regist. & Regist. (Anaesth.) Newc. HA; Clin. Research Fell. (Neurosurg.) Newc. HA.

PRICE, Keith Gerrard University Health Centre, University of York, Heslington, York YO10 5DD Tel: 01904 430000 — MB ChB Liverp. 1974.

PRICE, Laura Claire 9 Wellgarth Road, London NW11 7HP — MB ChB Bristol 1998.

PRICE, Leonie Jones The Surgery, Bennett St., Stretford, Manchester M32 8SG Tel: 0161 865 1100 Fax: 0161 865 7710 — MB BCh Wales 1992 (Univ. of Wales Coll. Of Med.) MRCGP 1996. Specialty: Gen. Pract.

PRICE, Lindsay James Roscoe Bangor Medical Centre, Bryn Hydd, Holyhead Road, Bangor LL57 2EE Tel: 01248 372373 Fax: 01248 372244 — MB BS Newc. 1974. Specialty: Gen. Pract.

PRICE, Lisa Jane — MB BCh Wales 1998.

PRICE, Lois Emilie Noble Brewery Cottage, South Stoke, Bath BA2 7DL Tel: 01225 832122 — MB ChB Manch. 1943; DCH Eng. 1948; DPM Eng. 1968; MRCPsych 1973. Assoc. Specialist Dept. Ment. Health Bristol. Socs: Roy. Med.-Psych. Assn. Prev: SHO Dept. Ment. Health Bristol Roy. Infirm.; Regist. (Psychiat.) Bath Clin. Area; Ho. Phys. Booth Hall Childr. Hosp. Manch.

PRICE, Lynfa The Surgery, 30 Old Road West, Gravesend DA11 0LL Tel: 01474 352075/567799 Fax: 01474 333952 Email: lynfaprice@hotmail.com — MB BCh Wales 1968.

PRICE, Margaret Louise Brighton General Hospital, Elm Grove, Brighton BN2 3EW Tel: 01273 696955 Fax: 01273 665025 — BM BCh Oxf. 1973; MRCP (UK) 1977; FRCP Lond. 1992. Cons. Dermatol. Brighton & Sussex University Hospitals Trust; Hon. Lect. Brighton Univ. Specialty: Dermat. Socs: Roy. Soc. Med. (Dermatol. Sect.); Brit. Assn. Dermatol.; President B&D. Prev: Sen. Registar Guy's Hosp. & Brighton HA.

PRICE, Margaret Mary Park Road Health Centre, Park Road, Radyr, Cardiff CF15 8DF Tel: 029 2084 2767 Fax: 029 2084 2507; 23 Lon Y Fro, Pentyrch, Cardiff CF15 9TE — MB BCh Wales 1978; MRCGP 1982. Specialty: Gen. Pract.

PRICE, Mark 2 Greenlawns, Cardiff CF23 6AW — BM Soton. 1997.

PRICE, Mark Alexander 86 Angus Street, Cardiff CF24 3LX — MB BCh Wales 1988.

PRICE, Martin Laurence 54 Eland Road, London SW11 5JY — MB BS Lond. 1980; BSc (cl. 2 Hons.) Lond. 1978; FFA RCS Eng. 1984. Cons. Anaesth. St. Mary's Hosp. Lond. Specialty: Anaesth. Prev: Sen. Regist. St. Geo. Hosp. Lond.; Regist. Qu. Charlottes Matern. Hosp. Lond.; Regist. (Anaesth.) King's Coll. Hosp. Lond.

PRICE, Mary (retired) Leith Mount, 46 Ferry Road, Edinburgh EH6 4AE Tel: 0131 554 0558 Fax: 0131 555 6911; 4 Strathalmond Road, Edinburgh EH4 8AD Tel: 0131 339 2129 — MB BCh Wales 1955 (Cardiff) BSc Wales 1952; DCH Eng. 1957. Prev: Asst. Med. Off. Pub. Health Dept. City Edin. SHO (Paediat.) Llandough.

PRICE, Melinda Ann Meddygfa'r Llan, Church Surgery, Portland Street, Aberystwyth SY23 2DX — MB BCh Wales 1984; DRCOG 1987; AFOM 2001. Clin. Assit. Ocupational Health, Bronglais Hosp. Aberystwyth. Prev: Trainee GP Aberystwyth VTS.

PRICE, Michael Price and Partners, The Surgery, Park Road, Holbeach, Spalding PE12 7EE Tel: 01406 423288 Fax: 01406 426284 — MB ChB St. And. 1965.

PRICE, Michael Ernest Reepham Surgery, Smugglers Lane, Reepham, Norwich NR10 4QT Tel: 01603 870271 Fax: 01603 872995 — MB BS Lond. 1977; MA Camb. 1979; MRCP (UK) 1980; MRCGP 1988. GP Princip.(1986) & GP Trainer. Prev: Regist. (Med.) W. Norwich Hosp.; Med. Miss. Segbwena, Sierra Leone.

PRICE, Michael Gregory (retired) Windrush, Cocklawelva, Rock, Wadebridge PL27 6LW Tel: 01208 863622 — (St. Bart) BSc (Hons. Physiol.) Lond. 1949, MB BS 1952; DObst RCOG 1956; MRCGP 1965. Prev: Sen. Ho. Phys. St. Bart. Hosp. Lond.

PRICE, Michael John Moat House, Crescent Road, Ivybridge PL21 0BP — MB BS Lond. 1965 (Univ. Coll. Hosp.) DPM Eng. 1971; MRCPsych 1972. Cons. Psychiat. of Old Age Cotehele Unit Mt. Gould Hosp. Plymouth. Specialty: Geriat. Psychiat. Prev: Sen. Regist. (Psychiat.) Barrow & United Bristol Hosps.; Regist. (Geriat.) Qu. Alexandra & St. Mary's Hosps. Portsmouth; Regist. (Psychiat.) St. Francis Hosp. Haywards Heath.

PRICE, Michael Leslie Hulbert, Price, Hulbert and Davies, Laurel Bank Surgery, Old Hall Street, Malpas SY14 8PS Tel: 01948 860205 Fax: 01948 860142; Rock Cottage, Sarn, Threapwood, Malpas SY14 7LN Tel: 01948 770329 — MB ChB Bristol 1972; DRCOG 1977.

PRICE, Mitchel The Limes Surgery, 172 High Street, Lye, Stourbridge DY9 8LL Tel: 01384 422234 — MB ChB Birm. 1986.

PRICE, Mr Neil Morriston Hospital, Department of Trauma and Orthopaedics, Morriston, Swansea SA6 6NL Tel: 01792 703090 — BM BCh Oxf. 1987; MA Camb. 1988; FRCS Eng. 1992; FRCS (Orth) 1997. Cons. Orthopaedic Surg., Swansea NHS Trust; Sen. Clin. Tutor, Swansea Clin. Sch. Specialty: Trauma & Orthop. Surg. Prev: Clin. Orthopaedic Fell., Gt. Ormond St. Hosp., Lond. and Roy. Nat. Orthopaedic Hosp., Lond.

PRICE, Mr Nicholas Charles (cons. rooms), Lansdown Lodge, Lansdown Road, Cheltenham GL51 6QL Tel: 01242 522475 Fax: 01242 253816 Email: nick@lansdownlodge.co.uk; Church Farm House, Mill Street, Prestbury, Cheltenham GL52 3BG — MB BS Lond. 1978 (Westm.) BSc Lond. 1975; FRCS Eng. 1985; FCOphth 1989; T(Ophth.) 1991. Cons. Ophth. E. Gloucester NHS Trust. Specialty: Ophth. Socs: BMA; Roy. Soc. of Med.; SWOS (Hon. Sec). Prev: Sen. Regist. Oxf. Eye Hosp.; Resid. Surg. Off. Moorfields Eye Hosp. Lond.; SHO (Ophth.) West. Ophth. Hosp. Lond.

PRICE, Nicholas Henley Upper Royd House Farm, Black Moor Road, Oxenhope, Keighley BD22 9ST — MB ChB Leeds 1986.

PRICE, Mr Nicholas James Wolverhampton & Midland Counties Eye Infirmary, Compton Road, Wolverhampton WV3 9QR Tel: 01902 307999 Fax: 01902 645018 — MB BS Lond. 1979 (St Thos.) MA Camb. 1978; FRCS Eng. 1986; FRCOphth 1988. Cons. Ophth. Wolverhampton & Midl. Co. Eye Infirm. & Stafford Gen. Hosp.; Cons. Ophth. Wolverhampton Nuffield Hosp. Specialty: Ophth. Prev: Sen. Regist. Wolverhampton, Stoke, Birm. & Moorfields, Lond.

PRICE, Nicholas Martin St Thomas' Hospital, Department of Infection, Lambeth Palace Road, London SE1 7EH — MB ChB Birm. 1991; BSc Birm. 1988; MRCP (UK) 1994; DTM & H Lond. 1995. Cons. Phys. Dept of Infec. St Thomas' Hosp. Lond. Specialty: Infec. Dis.; General (Internal) Medicine. Socs: Roy. Soc. of Trop. Med. and Hyg. Prev: Med. Research Coun. Fell., Dept. of Infect. Dis., Imperial Coll. Sch. of Med. Hammersmith Hosp. Lond.; Regist. Hammersmith Hosp.

PRICE, Nicolette Sian 239 Botley Road, Burridge, Southampton SO31 1BJ — MB BS Lond. 1993. Trainee GP/SHO (Adult Med.) Roy. Oldham Hosp. Lancs. Prev: SHO (A & E) Roy. Oldham Hosp.

PRICE, Nigel Carsley Poole Road Medical Centre, 7 Poole Road, Bournemouth BH2 5QR; 33 Compton Avenue, Lilliput, Poole BH14 8PU Tel: 01202 701127 — (Roy. Free Hosp. Sch. Med.) MB BS Lond. 1984; MRCGP 1988; DRCOG 1989. Princip. GP Bournmouth. Specialty: Cardiol.; Sports Med. Prev: SHO (O & G) St. Mary's Hosp. I. of Wight; SHO (Paediat.) Chase Farm Hosp. Enfield; SHO (Geriat.) Whipps Cross Hosp. Lond.

PRICE, Mrs Patricia Emily (retired) 17 Bay Court, Cliff Road, Falmouth TR11 4NP Tel: 01326 319260 — (Ed.) MB ChB Ed. 1951; DObst RCOG 1953. Prev: Occupat. Health Solihull MB Counc.

PRICE, Professor Patricia Mary Christie Hospital, Academic Department of Radiation Oncology, University of Manchester, Manchester M20 4BX Tel: 0161 446 8003 Fax: 0161 446 8111 Email: anne.mason@man.ac.uk — MB BChir Camb. 1981; MRCP (UK) 1984; FRCR 1987; MA Camb. 1982, MD 1991; FRCP Lond.

1995. Ralston Paterson Prof of Radiat. Oncol. & Head of Acad. Dept of Radiat. Oncol. & Hon Cons. Clin. Oncologist, Christie Hosp.; Head CR UK PET Research Gp.; Vis. Hon. Profess. Research Fell. Imperial Coll. Sch. of Med. Lond.; Hon. Cons. in Clin. Oncol. Hammersmith Hosp. Lond.; MRC Cyclotron Unit Hammersmith Hosp. Lond.; Director of Wolfson Molecular Imaging Centre. Specialty: Oncol.; Radiother. Special Interest: Molecular Imaging. Socs: Pres. Of Brit. Oncol. Assn. 2002/2004. Prev: Reader (Clin. Oncol.)& Head of Sect. of Cancer Therap., Imp. Coll. Sch Med. & Cons. Hammersmith Hosp ., St. Mary's Hosp. & Ealing Hosp. Lond.; Clin. Scientist & Hon. Sen. Regist. Inst. Cancer Research & Roy. Marsden Hosp. Sutton; Regist. (Radiother.) Roy. Marsden Hosp. Lond.

PRICE, Paul Anthony 33 Gloucester Street, Cirencester GL7 2DJ Tel: 01285 654524 Fax: 01285 654524 — MB BS Lond. 1973 (University College Hospital Medical School) BSc (Hons.) Pharmacol. Lond. 1970; FRCP Lond. 1993. Cons. Phys. & Endocrinol. Swindon & MarlBoro. Hosps. NHS Trust. Specialty: Gen. Med.; Endocrinol.; Diabetes. Socs: Diabetes UK; Soc. Endocrinol. Prev: Sen. Regist. (Med.) St. Geo. Hosp. Lond.; Hon. Lect. (Endocrinol.) St. Bart. Hosp. Lond.; Regist. (Gen. Med.) Univ. Coll. Hosp. Lond.

PRICE, Paul Terence Manor Street Surgery, Manor Street, Ruskington, Sleaford NG34 9EN Tel: 01526 832204 — MB BS Lond. 1980 (Univ. Coll. Hosp.) Prev: Trainee GP Kings Lynn VTS; Ho. Off. (Cardiorespirat. Med.) Pilgrim Hosp. Boston; Ho. Surg. Lincoln Co. Hosp.

PRICE, Pauline Muriel The Dekeyser Group Practice, The Fountain Medical Centre, Little Fountain, Leeds LS27 9EN Tel: 0113 295 1600 Fax: 0113 238 1901; Westwood, Pk Avenue, Morley, Leeds LS27 0JW Tel: 0113 252 8849 — MB ChB Leeds 1969; MMedSci (Gen. Pract.) Leeds 1985. Specialty: Homeop. Med.

PRICE, Peter Harry Woodlands, Preston Road, Lonsonford, Solihull B95 5EY — MB ChB Birm. 1962.

PRICE, Rhys Michael John The Surgery, Parkwood Drive, Warners End, Hemel Hempstead HP1 2LD Tel: 01442 250117 Fax: 01442 256185; 38 Oakwood, Berkhamsted HP4 3NQ Tel: 01442 866871 — MB BChir Camb. 1969 (Camb. & Middlx.) MB Camb. 1969, BChir 1968; MA Camb. 1969; FRCGP 1984, M 1976. Mem. Edit. Bd. RCGP. Socs: BMA.

PRICE, Richard Alan 587 Lichfield Road, Sutton Coldfield B74 4EG — MB BS Lond. 1990.

PRICE, Richard Edward The Health Centre, Magna Lane, Dalton, Rotherham S65 4HH Tel: 01709 850229; Silverdale, 234 Doncaster Road, Thrybergh, Rotherham S65 4NU — MB BS Lond. 1954 (Univ. Coll. Hosp.)

PRICE, Richard John Department of Anaesthetics, Gowtnavel Hospital, Glasgow G11 0VN — MB ChB Aberd. 1998; BSc (Hons. Med. Sci.) Aberd. 1996; Dip. RCS Ed 2003; FRCA 2004.

PRICE, Richard Norman Orchard Lodge, Cranleigh Road, Ewhurst, Cranleigh GU6 7RJ — MB BChir Camb. 1989; MA Camb. 1990; MRCP (UK) 1993; MD 2000; MRCPath (UK) 2001.

PRICE, Richard Vaughan Rydal, 375 High Road, Woodford Green IG8 9QJ Tel: 020 8504 0532 Fax: 020 8559 1503; 5 High Road, Buckhurst Hill IG9 5HT Fax: 020 8559 1503 — MB BS Lond. 1983.

PRICE, Robert 43 Crossfield Drive, Worsley, Manchester M28 2QQ — MB ChB Manch. 1950. Clin. Asst. Bridgwater Hosp. Patricroft. Socs: Fell. Manch. Med. Soc.; Manch. Med. Engineer. Soc.

PRICE, Robert Kimberley 12 Fitzjames Avenue, Croydon CR0 5DH — MB BS Lond. 1993; MRCS Edin. 2001.

PRICE, Rodney Bernard Four Gables, 5 Ferry Lane, Hook, Goole DN14 5NZ — Artsexamen Maastricht 1983.

PRICE, Roger John Anthony Pinfold Medical Practice, The Health Centre, Pinfold Gate, Loughborough LE11 1DQ Tel: 01509 263753 Fax: 01509 264124 — MB BS Lond. 1975; MRCS Eng. LRCP Lond. 1975; DRCOG 1979; MRCGP 1979. GP Adviser, S. Trent Dearery.

PRICE, Rosemary May Blackburn Street Health Centre, Blackburn Street, Radcliffe, Manchester M26 1WS; 2 Ringley Road, Whitefield, Manchester M45 7LB — BM BCh Oxf. 1967; DFFP 1993.

PRICE, Mr Rupert Francis Old Bank House, 18 Hillhead, Bonnyrigg EH19 2JG — MB ChB Ed. 1990; PhD Ed. 1991, BSc (Hons.) 1985, MB ChB 1990; FRCS Ed. 1995. SHO (Surg.) SE Scotl. Train. Scheme. Specialty: Gen. Surg.

PRICE, Russell John 9 Beaufort Close, Oadby, Leicester LE2 4TP — MB BS Queensland 1983.

PRICE, Sarah Ann (retired) New House Surgery, 142A South Street, Dorking RH4 2QR Tel: 01306 881313 Fax: 01306 877305; Keepers Cottage, Wellhouse Lane, Betchworth RH3 7HH — (Guy's) MB BS Lond. 1964; MRCS Eng. LRCP Lond. 1964. Prev: Clin. Med. Off. E. Surrey AHA.

PRICE, Sarah Margaret Holmside Medical Group, 142 Armstrong Road, Benwell, Newcastle upon Tyne NE4 8QB Tel: 0191 273 4009 Fax: 0191 273 2745; 6 Saxilby Drive, Gosforth, Newcastle upon Tyne NE3 5LS Tel: 0191 284 0606 — MB BS Newc. 1984; DRCOG 1986; MRCGP 1988. GP Newc. Prev: SHO (Med.) Hexham Gen. Hosp.; SHO (Obst.) Newc. Gen. Hosp.; Trainee GP N.d. VTS.

PRICE, Sarah Penelope Top Floor Flat, 106 Hampton Road, Bristol BS6 6JD — MB ChB Birm. 1992.

PRICE, Septimus Harold Mervyn White Gates, 66 The Drive, Harefield Place, Uxbridge UB10 8AQ Tel: 01895 33782 — MB BS Lond. 1947 (Westm.) MRCS Eng. LRCP Lond. 1939; DObst RCOG 1948. Prev: Ho. Surg. & Cas. Off. Connaught Hosp. Walthamstow; Ho. Phys. Staines EMS Hosp.

PRICE, Sian Elen 69 Ridding Close, Southampton SO15 5PN; 69 Ridding Close, Shirley, Southampton SO15 5PN — MB BS Lond. 1988; AKC 1985; BSc (Hons.) Lond. 1985, MB BS 1988; MRCP (UK) 1991. Specialty: Neurol.

PRICE, Simon David St Julians Medical Centre, 13A Stafford Road, Newport NP19 7DQ Tel: 01633 251304 Fax: 01633 221977; 11 Alwyn Close, Rogerstone, Newport NP10 9HW Tel: 01633 893649 — MB BCh Wales 1980; MB BCh Wales. 1980; DRCOG 1982; Cert. Family Plann. JCC 1983; MRCGP 1986. Socs: BMA.

PRICE, Mr Stephen John 41 Rayfield, Epping CM16 5AD Tel: 01992 576864 — MB BS Lond. 1994 (St. Barts. Hosp. Med. Coll.) BSc (Hons.) Lond. 1991; FRCS Eng. 1998. Specialist Regist., Dep. Neurosurg., Addenbrooke's Hosp., Camb. Specialty: Neurosurg. Prev: Specialist Regist. (Neurosurg.) OldCh. Hosp. Romford; SHO Neurosurg. Addenbrookes; SHO Neurosurg. Qu. Med. Centre Nottm.

PRICE, Stephen Rhys Exmouth Health Centre, Claremont Grove, Exmouth EX8 2JF Tel: 01395 273001 Fax: 01395 273771 — MB ChB Bristol 1972; BSc (Hons., Biochem.) Bristol 1969, MB ChB 1972; DRCOG 1977; DA Eng. 1978; MRCGP 1982.

PRICE, Stephen Rowland Department of Clinical Biochemistry, Wycombe General Hospital, High Wycombe HP11 2TT Tel: 01494 425244 Fax: 01494 425220; Chiltern Retreat, Queens Road, Princes Risborough HP27 0JR Tel: 01844 342018 — MB ChB Birm. 1979 (Birmingham) MRCPath 1988; FRCPath 1998. Cons. Chem. Path. Wycombe Gen. Hosp. Specialty: Chem. Path. Prev: Sen. Regist. (Chem. PAth.) Oxf. HA.; Regist. (Chem. Path.) W. Midl. RHA.

PRICE, Stephen Vincent, Flight Lt. RAF Med. Br. (retired) West Street Surgery, 89 West St., Dunstable LU6 1SF Tel: 01582 664401 Fax: 01582 475766; 90 Merthyr Mawr Road, Bridgend CF31 3NS Tel: 01656 658797 Fax: 01656 658797 — MB BS Lond. 1990 (Kings Coll. Hosp.) Cert. Av. Med. 1991; DCCH RCP Ed. 1993; DRCOG 1995; DFFP 1995; T(GP) 1995; MRCGP 1996. GP W. St. Surg. Dunstable. Prev: Family Care Med. Serv. Brisband Australia.

PRICE, Susan Margaret Child Health Directorate, Northampton General Hospital NHS Trust, Cliftonville, Northampton NN1 5BD Tel: 01604 544638 Fax: 01604 545988 Email: sue.price@ngh.nhs.uk — MB ChB Manch. 1982; MRCP (UK) 1985; Dip Clin Genetics 1992; FRCP (UK) 2002. Cons. (Clin. Genetics) Northampton Gen. Hosp. NHS Trust. Specialty: Genetics. Socs: Brit Soc of Human Genetics. Prev: Regist. & Sen. Regist. (Clin. Genetics) Leicester Roy. Infirm.; Regist. (Paediat.) Roy. Infirm. Leicester.

PRICE, Susan Mary Carlisle House Surgery, 53 Lagland Street, Poole BH15 1QD Tel: 01202 672534; 169 Albian Way, Verwood BH31 7LT — MB ChB Birm 1992; DRCOG 1994; DCH RCP Lond. 1996. GP Retainer, Dorset.

PRICE, Susanna 7 Canada Rise, Market Lavington, Devizes SN10 4AD — MB BS Lond. 1990.

PRICE, Sydney Lionel The Surgery, 75 Gloucester Place, London W1H 3PF Tel: 020 7935 4153; F1, 133-135 Park Road, The Beverley, London NW8 7JB Tel: 020 7586 2759 — MB BS Lond. 1956 (King's Coll. Hosp.) MRCS Eng. LRCP Lond. 1956. Specialty: Rehabil. Med.; Rheumatol. Socs: Brit. Assn. Manip. Med.; Assoc. Mem. Brit. Assn. Rheum. & Rehabil. Prev: Clin. Asst. (Physical Med.) Guy's Hosp. Lond.; Ho. Phys. & Ho. Surg. Mayday Hosp. Croydon.

PRICE, Thomas Cannock Chase Hospital, Brunswick Road, Cannock WS11 2XY Tel: 01543 576451 Fax: 01543 576455;

Fielden House, Stowe Lane, Stowe-by-Chartley, Stafford ST18 0NA Tel: 01889 270962 Fax: 01889 271588 Email: thomas.price@btinternet.com — BM BCh Oxf. 1973 (Univ. Coll. Hosp.) MA, BM BCh Oxf. 1973; MRCP (UK) 1977; FRCP Lond. 1992. Cons. Rheum. Mid. Staffs. Hosps. Specialty: Rheumatol. Prev: Sen. Regist. Middlx. Hosp., Northwick Pk. Hosp. & Roy. Nat. Orthop. Hosp. Lond.

PRICE, Thomas George (retired) — MB ChB Liverp. 1959; FRCOG 1985, M 1970, DObst 1962. Prev: Locum Work.

PRICE, Thomas Matthew Dodds 57 Cambridge Road, London SW20 0PX — MB BS Lond. 1996.

PRICE, Thomas Michael Lloyd (retired) Hobbs Cottage, Piltdown, Uckfield TN22 3XB Tel: 01825 722028 — MRCS Eng. LRCP Lond. 1939 (Guy's) MD Lond. 1948, MB BS 1939; FRCP Lond. 1963, M 1947. Prev: Cons. Phys. Lewisham Hosp. & St. Nicholas' Hosp. Plumstead.

PRICE, Thomas Richard 5 North Several, Orchard Drive, London SE3 0QR — MB BS Lond. 1976; PhD Lond. 1974, BSc 1968, MB BS 1976; MRCP (UK) 1979.

PRICE, Thomas Richard Hughes Jesmond Clinic, 48 Osborne Road, Jesmond, Newcastle upon Tyne NE2 2AL Tel: 0191 281 4060 Fax: 0191 281 0231; 32 Waterbury Road, Brunton Park, Newcastle upon Tyne NE3 5AJ Tel: 0191 217 0365 — BMedSci Nottm. 1984; MB BS Nottm. 1986; DCH RCP Lond. 1990; MRCGP 1992. Lect. (Gen. Pract.) Univ. Newc. u. Tyne. Prev: Trainee GP VTS.

PRICE, Thomas Waldron Beacon Surgery, Beacon Road, Crowborough TN6 1AF Tel: 01892 652233 Fax: 01892 668840; The Dog House, Hankham, Eastbourne BN2X 5AY — MB BS Lond. 1965 (Middlx.) MRCS Eng. 1965, LRCP Lond. 1966; DA Eng. 1971; DObst RCOG 1973. Prev: Ho. Phys. Middlx. Hosp.; Ho. Surg. Centr. Middlx. Hosp.

PRICE, Thomas Wentworth (retired) Long Acre, Yawl Uplyme, Lyme Regis DT7 3XA Tel: 01297 443214 — BM BCh Oxf. 1945; BA, BM BCh Oxf. 1945. Prev: GP S.sea.

PRICE, Mrs Vanessa Hinchingbrooke Hospital, Hinchingbrooke Park, Huntingdon PE29 6NT Tel: 01480 416416 — MB BS Lond. 1967 (Middlx.) DA Eng. 1969; FFA RCS Eng. 1973. Specialty: Anaesth. Socs: Assn. Anaesths. Gt. Brit. & Irel.; Pain Soc. (uk chapter). Prev: Sen. Regist. (Anaesth.) Addenbrookes Hosp. Camb.; Sen. Regist. (Anaesth.) Roy. Free Hosp. Lond.; Regist. (Anaesth.) Middlx. Hosp. Lond.

PRICE, Victoria Jane — MB ChB Manch. 1998 (Manchester) MB ChB Manch 1998; DRCOG 2001. GP Regist., Alderley Edge. Specialty: Gen. Pract. Prev: SHO Obs & Gynae. Arrowe Pk. Hosp. Wirral; SHO Paediat. Arrowe Pk. Hosp. Wirral; SHO Medine, Arrowe Pk. Hosp. Wirral.

PRICE, Victoria Juliette 62 Llanrhos Road, Penrhyn Bay, Llandudno LL30 3HY — MB ChB Ed. 1998.

PRICE, Walter John (retired) Tor Cragg, Slade Lane, Kiln Bank, Riddlesden, Keighley BD20 5DT — MB ChB Leeds 1954; FFA RCS Eng. 1965. Prev: Cons. Anaesth. Bradford Trust Hosps.

PRICE, Walter Rostron Regis Medical Centre, Darby Street, Rowley Regis, Warley B65 0BA Tel: 0121 559 3957 Fax: 0121 502 9117; 31 Whitehall Road, Pedmore, Stourbridge DY8 2JT Tel: 01384 394544 — MB ChB Birm. 1974; PhD Liverp. 1965, BSc (Hons.) 1962; MB ChB (Hons.) Birm. 1974; DRCOG 1977; Cert. Family Plann. JCC 1978; MRCGP 1980. Hosp. Pract. (Gastroenterol.) Russells Hall Hosp. Dudley. Prev: Clin. Asst. (Gastroenterol.) Wordsley Hosp. Stourbridge & Russells Hall Hosp. Dudley.

PRICE, William Henry (retired) 4 Strathalmond Road, Barnton, Edinburgh EH4 8AD Tel: 0131 339 2129 Fax: 0131 476 3432 Email: drwhprice@aol.com — MB BCh Wales 1955 (Cardiff) BSc Wales 1952; FRCP Ed. 1972, M 1962. Hon. Fell. Molecular & Clin. Med. Univ. Edin. Prev: Sen. Lect. (Med.) Univ. Dept. Med. West. Gen. Hosp. Edin.

PRICE, William James Pembroke Mere Surgery, Dark Lane, Mere, Warminster BA12 6DT Tel: 01747 860001 Fax: 01747 860119; Apple Tree Cottage, Huntingford, Gillingham SP8 5QQ Tel: 01747 861233 — MB BS Lond. 1979; MRCP (UK) 1982; MRCGP 1987. Clin. Asst. Diabetic Clinic Salisbury Dist. Hosp. Specialty: Gen. Med. Prev: Regist. Rotat. (Med.) Salisbury & Soton.; SHO (Paediat.) St. Richard's Hosp. Chichester; SHO Rotat. (Med.) Bath.

PRICE-JONES, Jonathan Christian Oxford Street Surgery, Oxford Street, Aberaeron SA46 0JB Tel: 01545 570273 Fax: 01545 571625 — MB BCh Wales 1985. Specialty: Gen. Med.

PRICE-THOMAS, Simon Phillip, Maj. RAMC Broadgate Frm., Cookbury, Holsworthy EX22 7YG; 39 Blenheim Park, Aldershot GU11 2HS Tel: 01252 324270 — MB ChB Aberd. 1988; DRCOG 1994; MRCGP 1995. GP Aldershot. Specialty: Gen. Pract.

PRICE WILLIAMS, Deborah Anne The Child Development Centre, The Hillingdon Hospital, Pield Heath Road, Uxbridge UB8 3NN Tel: 01895 279395 Fax: 01895 279299 — MB BCh Wales 1981; Cert. Family Plann. JCC 1988; MSc Warwick 1997. Assoc. Specialist Community Child Health Hillingdon PCT; Med. Adviser to Lond. Boro. of Hillingdon. Specialty: Community Child Health. Socs: Assoc. Mem. RCPCH. Prev: Clin. Med. Off. (Child Health) Richmond & Roehampton HA; Ho. Phys. (Med./Geriat./Cardiol.) Cardiff Roy. Infirm. & Univ. Hosp. Wales Cardiff; Ho. Surg. (Surg.) Mt. Vernon Hosp. Northwood Middlx.

PRICE-WILLIAMS, Ruth Dorothy 3 Hawtrey Drive, Ruislip HA4 8QW Tel: 01895 673722 — MB ChB Bristol 1954. Med. Off. C.D.T. Fountains Mill, Uxbridge. Prev: Div. Surg. St. John's Ambul.; GP Fell. HIV Med. Hillingdon HA; Vis. Med. Off. Hillingdon.

PRICHARD, Mr Andrew John Norman Head & Neck Centre, Royal Shrewsbury Hospital, Mytton Oak Road, Shrewsbury SY3 8AX — MB BS Lond. 1983 (UCH) FRCS Ed. 1989; Intercollegiate FRCS (ORL) 1992. Cons. (Otolaryngol.) Shrewsbury. Specialty: Otolaryngol. Prev: Sen. Regist. (Otolaryngol.) Freeman Hosp. Newc.; Regist. (Otolaryng.) Leic. Roy. Infirm.; SHO (Otolaryng.) Roy. Surrey Co. Hosp. Guildford.

PRICHARD, Professor Brian Norman Christopher, CBE Clinical Pharmacology Centre, University College, 5 University Street, London WC1E 6JJ Fax: 020 7691 2838; 24 Lyford Road, Wandsworth Common, London SW18 3LG Tel: 020 8870 3066 — MB BS Lond. 1958 (St. Geo.) MSc Lond. 1954, BSc 1953; MRCS Eng. LRCP Lond. 1957; FRCP Lond. 1977, M 1966; FFPM RCP (UK) 1989; FESC 1996; FACC 1997. Prof. Clin. Pharmacol. Univ. Coll. & Middlx. Sch. Med.; Cons. Phys. Univ. Coll. Hosp. Lond. Specialty: Gen. Med. Socs: Assn. Phys.; Internat. Soc. Hypertens.; Brit. Pharm. Soc. Prev: Regist. (Med.) St. Geo. Hosp. Lond.; Reader & Sen. Lect. (Clin. Pharmacol.) Univ. Coll. Hosp. Med. Sch. Lond.

PRICHARD, David Robert North West Wales NHS Trust, Ysbyty Gwynedd, Bangor LL57 2PW — MB ChB Ed. 1973; MRCP (UK) 1976; FRCP Lond. 1994; Dip. Health Care Law 1997. Exec. Med. Director, Hon. Sen. Lect., Univ. of Wales, Bangor; Cons. Phys., Med. for the Elderly. Specialty: Gen. Med.

PRICHARD, Jonathan Edgar Birchgrove Surgery, 104 Caerphilly Road, Cardiff CF14 4AG Tel: 029 2052 2344 Fax: 029 2052 2487 — MB BCh Wales 1981; DRCOG 1983.

PRICHARD, Owain Merfyn Tristan, Penrhyndeudraeth LL48 6AY Tel: 01766 77304 — MB ChB Ed. 1936 (Univ. Ed.) Med. Off. Brony-Garth Chronic Sick Hosp. Penrhyndeudraeth. Prev: Ho. Phys. Roy. United Hosp. Bath; Ho. Surg. Princess Beatrice Hosp. Lond.; Sen. Ho. Surg. Caern. & Anglesey Infirm. Bangor.

PRICKETT, Frances Mary Emma Room 2 Staff Corridor, Llandough Hospital, Penlan Road, Llandough, Penarth CF64 1XX — MB ChB Leic. 1988; DCH RCP Lond. 1991. Prev: Trainee GP Oxf. VTS; Ho. Off. (Med.) P'boro; Ho. Off. (Gyn. & Surg.) Leicester.

PRIDDLE, Deborah Jane Drumchapel Health Centre, 80/90 Kinfauns Drive, Glasgow G15 7TS Tel: 0141 211 6110; 3 Sanda Street, North Kelvinside, Glasgow G20 8PU Tel: 0141 946 2933 — MB ChB Glas. 1981. Specialty: Gen. Pract. Socs: Assoc. Mem. Roy. Coll. Gen. Pract.

PRIDDLE, Evelyn Susan (retired) 99 Westmoreland Road, Bromley BR2 0TQ Tel: 020 8464 8040 — BM BCh Oxf. 1961 (St. Bart.) DCH Eng. 1965; MFFP 1993. Asst. Dir. (Community Med. Servs.) Ravensbourne NHS Trust.

PRIDDY, Alvan Robert Adrian The North West London Hospitals NHS Trust, Northwick Park Hospital, Watford Road, Harrow HA1 3RX Tel: 020 8864 3232 Fax: 020 8869 2864 Email: alvanpriddy@nwlh.nhs.uk — MB ChB Manch. 1983; MRCOG 1989; MD Manch. 1992; FRCOG 2002. Cons. O & G Northwick Pk. Hosp.; Dep. Clin. Director; lead Clinician in Gyanecology, Risk Managem.; Cons. Obst. and Gynaecologist, The Clementine Churchill Hosp., Harrow. Specialty: Obst. & Gyn. Socs: Brit. Fertil. Soc.; Brit. Soc. Gyn. Endoscopy; BMA. Prev: Sen. Regist. (O & G) Hammersmith

Hosp. & Northwick Pk. Hosp. Lond.; Regist. (O & G) Roy. Oldham Hosp., St. Mary's Hosp. Manch & Fairfield Gen. Hosp. Bury; Research Fell. (O & G) Withington Hosp. Manch.

PRIDDY, Ronald Joseph 4 Hanover Court, Bishop Auckland DL14 6EG — MB BS Lond. 1962 (Lond. Hosp.) LMSSA Lond. 1958; DTM & H RCP Lond. 1969. Prev: Maj. RAMC; Ho. Surg. Mile End Hosp. Lond.; Ho. Phys. St. Albans City Hosp.

PRIDE, Andrew John — MB BS Lond. 1976 (Roy. Free) MRCS Eng. LRCP Lond. 1976; DRCOG 1980. GP Berkhamstead. Prev: Trainee GP/SHO (Paediat.) Qu. Mary's Hosp. Lond. VTS; SHO (Obst.) Profess. Unit O & G Westm. Hosp. Lond.; SHO (Psychiat.) Westm. Hosp. Lond.

PRIDE, Neil Blair (retired) 49 Ranelagh Road, London W5 5RP Tel: 020 8567 2705 Email: m.pride@imperial.ac.uk; 49 Ranelagh Road, London W5 5RP — (Camb. & St. Mary's) MB BChir Camb. 1956; FRCP Lond. 1974, M 1959; MD Camb. 1968. Prev: Prof. Emerit. Respirat. Med. Imperial Coll. Sch. Med.

PRIDEAUX, Christopher Patrick Bushloe End Surgery, 48 Bushloe End, Wigston LE18 2BA — MB BS Lond. 1977 (Westm.)

PRIDEAUX, Cyril Frank Gifford Flat One, 11A Greenhill, Weymouth DT4 7SW Tel: 01305 750924 — MB BS Lond. 1950 (St. Thos.) MRCS Eng. LRCP Lond. 1944; DA Eng. 1949; FFA RCS Eng. 1954. Emerit. Cons. Anaesth. Chichester Health Dist. Specialty: Anaesth. Prev: Sen. Cons. Anaesth. Chichester & Graylingwell Hosp. Gp. & King Edwd. VII Hosp. Midhurst; Sen. Regist. (Anaesth.) Univ. Coll. Hosp.

PRIDGEON, Jennie Madeline 68 Spur Hill Avenue, Poole BH14 9PL — MB ChB Dundee 1994.

PRIDIE, Angus Kenneth 9 The Grove, Monkseaton, Whitley Bay NE25 8BH Tel: 0191 289 1239 Email: anguspridie@yahoo.com — MB ChB Bristol 1968; DObst RCOG 1970; DA Eng. 1971; FFA RCS Eng. 1973. Cons Anaeth. Newc. Hosp. Trust. Specialty: Anaesth. Special Interest: Pain Relief. Socs: Assn. of Anaesthetists; Europ. Assn. Of Regional Anaesth.; North. Regional Pain Gp. Prev: Sen. Regist. Anaesth. Newc. Univ. Hosp. Gp.; Cons. (Anaesth.) Freeman Hosp. Newc.

PRIDIE, Joanna Mary (retired) 58 St John's Road, Clifton, Bristol BS8 2HG — MRCS Eng. LRCP Lond. 1931 (King's Coll.) Prev: Ho. Surg. King's Coll. Hosp.

PRIEST, Alison Vanessa 12 Linksway, Gatley, Cheadle SK8 4LB Tel: 0161 428 6160 — MB ChB Bristol 1992; DRCOG 1996. SHO (Surg.) ChristCh. Hosp., NZ. Specialty: Gen. Pract. Prev: SHO Bristol Matern. Hosp.; SHO (Psychiat.) Southmead Hosp. Bristol; SHO (Paediat.) Tameside Hosp. Manch.

PRIEST, Martin Stuart Padstow Medical Centre, Boyd Avenue, Padstow PL28 8ER Tel: 01637 880359; Little Tregustick, Withiel, Bodmin PL30 5NG Tel: 01208 815948 — BM BS Nottm. 1987; MRCP (UK) 1991; DRCOG 1993; MRCGP 1995. Princip.

PRIEST, Matthew 23 Woodlands Gate, Glasgow G46 7SS — MB ChB Birm. 1993; MRCP UK 1997.

PRIEST, Oliver Hartwell Melrose, 3 Argyle Rd, Whitby YO21 3HS — MB ChB Manch. 1996.

PRIEST, Mrs Pamela (retired) Old Manor Farmhouse, Hewish, Crewkerne TA18 8QT — MRCS Eng. LRCP Lond. 1951; DPM Durham. 1960.

PRIEST, Peter James 7 Kinlock Drive, Heaton, Bolton BL1 4LZ — MB ChB Sheff. 1986; MRCGP 1990; DRCOG 1990.

PRIEST, Professor Robert George 29 Old Slade Lane, Richings Park, Iver SL0 9DY Tel: 01753 653178 — (Univ. Coll. Hosp.) MB BS Lond. 1956; DPM Eng. 1963; FRCP Ed. 1974, M 1964; MD Lond. 1970; FRCPsych 1974, M 1971; T(Psych) 1991. Prof. Emerit. Univ. Lond.; Prof. Psychiat. Imperial Coll. Sch. Med. St. Mary's Hosp. Specialty: Gen. Psychiat.; Gen. Pract.; Gen. Med. Socs: Fell. Roy. Coll. Psychiat.; Hon. Corr. Fell. Amer. Psychiat. Assn.; Hon. Corr. Fell. Assn. Francaise de Psychiatrie. Prev: Regist. Roy. Coll. Psychiat.; Sen. Lect. St. Geo. Hosp. Med. Sch. Lond.; Vis. Lect. Univ. Chicago.

PRIEST, Timothy David INPUT Pain Management Unit, St. Thomas's Hospital, London SE1 7EH Tel: 020 7922 8107 Fax: 020 7922 8229; 34 Thames Drive, Ruislip HA4 7AY Tel: 01895 633848 — MB BS Lond. 1990 (Univ. Coll. & Middlx. Hosp.) PhD Glas. 1983; MA Oxf. 1984; FRCA 1995. Clin. Fell. (Pain Managem.) St. Thomas's Hosp. Lond. Specialty: Anaesth. Socs: Fell. Roy. Coll. Of Anaesth.; The Pain Soc.; Int. Assn. Study of Pain. Prev: Specialist Regist. Rotat. (Anaesth.) St. Mary's Hosp. Lond.

PRIESTLEY, Anne Catherine Crawcrook Surgery, Crawcrook, Ryton NE40 4TZ; Craigmont, Barlow, Blaydon-on-Tyne NE21 6JT — MB BS Newc. 1972; MRCP (UK) 1975. Prev: Regist. (Gen. Med.) Newc. Gen. Hosp.; SHO (Gen. Med.) Newc. Gen. Hosp.; Ho. Surg. Hexham Gen. Hosp.

PRIESTLEY, Betty Leila (retired) 3A Eastbury Avenue, Northwood HA6 3LB Tel: 01923 840889 — MB BS Lond. 1958 (Roy. Free) MRCS Eng. LRCP Lond. 1958; FRCP Lond. 1977, M 1961; DCH Eng. 1963; FRCPCH 1997. Prev: Hon. Cons. Paediat. Sheff. Childrs. Hosp.

PRIESTLEY, Cecilia Juliette Fiona Department of Genitourinary Medicine, Weymouth Community Hospital, Melcombe Avenue, Weymouth DT4 7TB Tel: 01305 762682 Fax: 01305 762695 Email: cecilia.priestley@wdgh.nhs.uk — MB ChB Sheff. 1985; MRCP (UK) 1990; FRCP (London) 2000. Cons. (Genitour. Med.) W. Dorset Gen. Hosps. NHS Trust Weymouth. Specialty: Genitourinary Medicine. Socs: MSSVD; AGUM. Prev: Sen. Regist. (Genitourin. Med.) Roy. Hallamsh. Hosp. Sheff.; Regist. (Genitourin. Med.) Stoke-on-Trent; Regist. (Gen. Med.) Macclesfield Dist. Gen. Hosp. & Walton Hosp. Liverp.

PRIESTLEY, Colin Thomas Penketh Health Centre, Honiton Way, Penketh, Warrington WA5 2EY Tel: 01925 725644 Fax: 01925 791017 — MB ChB Ed. 1974.

PRIESTLEY, Edward (retired) 195 Highfield Road, South Shore, Blackpool FY4 3NS; Flat 7, St John's Wood, 2 Clifton Drive, Lytham St Annes FY8 5PF Tel: 01253 730686 — (Manch.) MB ChB Manch. 1946.

PRIESTLEY, George Shearer 10 Dryden Avenue, Cheadle SK8 2AW Tel: 0161 491 3720 Fax: 0870 055 9647 Email: george@maddys.demon.co.uk — MB ChB Manch. 1985; MRCP (UK) 1992; DA (UK) 1992; FRCA 1993. Cons. (Int. Care & Anaesth.) York Dist. Hosp. Specialty: Intens. Care; Anaesth. Socs: Intens. Care Soc. & Assn. Anaesth.; Europ. Soc. of Intens. Care Med. Prev: Specialist Regist. (Anaesth.) Soton. Gen. Hosp.

PRIESTLEY, Hugh Stephen Abbotsbury Road Surgery, 24 Abbotsbury Road, Weymouth DT4 0AE Tel: 01305 786257 — MB BS Lond. 1983 (Westminster)

PRIESTLEY, Kim Anita Solihull Hospital, Lode Lane, Solihull B91 2JL Tel: 0121 424 4368 — MB ChB Leic. 1982; MRCP (UK) 1985. Cons. Phys. (Cardiol.) Solihull Hosp. W. Midl. Specialty: Cardiol.

PRIESTLEY, Martin Benjamin Perth Royal Infirmary, Jeanfield Road, Perth PH1 1NX Tel: 01738 473637 — MB ChB St And. 1969; DObst RCOG 1971. Staff Grade Phys. (Hon.) Acute Med.

PRIESTLEY, Nicholas (retired) 111 Burges Road, Thorpe Bay, Southend-on-Sea SS1 3JL Tel: 01702 588585 — MB ChB Leeds 1963.

PRIESTLEY, Veronica Ruth The Grove Medical Centre, Church Road, Egham TW20 9QJ Tel: 01784 433159 Fax: 01784 477208; 46 Northcroft Road, Englefield Green, Egham TW20 0EA — MB ChB Sheff. 1984; MRCGP 1994.

PRIESTMAN, John Frederick Walter Health Services Centre, Shelley Lane, Kirkburton, Huddersfield HD8 0SJ Tel: 01484 602040 Fax: 01484 602012; 18 Cleveland Way, Shelley, Huddersfield HD8 8NQ Email: 100717.3066@compuserve.com — MB ChB Leeds 1978; MRCGP 1982. Trainer Huddersfield VTS; Examg. Med. Pract. for Benefits Agency. Specialty: Gen. Pract. Socs: BMA; Hudds. Med. Soc.; Brit. Med. & Dent. Hypn. Soc. Prev: Trainee GP Huddersfield VTS; Ho. Phys. Leeds Gen. Infirm.; Ho. Surg. Clayton Hosp. Wakefield.

PRIESTMAN, Samuel (retired) 5 Church Street, Woolley, Bath BA1 8AS Tel: 01225 858075 — (Camb. & St. Geo.) BChir Camb. 1955; MA MB Camb. 1956; DObst RCOG 1957; MRCGP 1966. Prev: Princip. GP Bath.

PRIESTMAN, William Steven — MB ChB Leic. 1998.

PRIGG, Nicholas James 501 Crewe Road, Wistaston, Crewe CW2 6QP Tel: 01270 567250 Fax: 01270 665829 — MB ChB Birm. 1996; ChB Birm. 1996; MRCPCH 2001. Gen. Practitioner, salaried, Wistaston Shavington Med. Pract., Crewe.

PRIGMORE, Gerrard Timothy Camarthen Road Health Centre, Carmarthen Road, Cross Hands, Llanelli SA14 6SU Tel: 01269 831091 — MB BCh Wales 1991; MRCGP 1996; DFFP 2002.

PRIMAVESI, Richard John Paediatric Consulting Suite, 234 Great Portland St., London W1W 5QT Tel: 020 7390 8355 Fax: 020 7390 8356 Email: primadoc@easynet.co.uk; 11 Devonshire Place 1, London W1G 6HT Tel: 0207 224 4668 Fax: 0207 224 5008 Email: richard@primadoc.co.uk — MB BS Lond. 1974 (Roy. Lond.) FRCP (1997); MRCP (UK) 1980; FRCP (CH) 1998. Cons. Paediat. The Portland Hosp. Gt. Portland St. Lond. Specialty: Paediat. Special Interest: Allergy; Immunisation; Infec. Dis. Socs: Roy. Soc. Med.; Internat. Diabetes Federat. Prev: Cons. Paediat. N. Hants. Hosp. Basingstoke.

PRIMAVESI, Sarah Margaret Mitchell Road Surgery, 9 Mitchell Road, Canferd Heath, Poole BH17 8UE Tel: 01202 672474 Fax: 01202 660926 — MB BS Lond. 1978; MRCS Eng. LRCP Lond. 1978; DRCOG 1981. Gen. Practitioner.

PRIME, Alison Judith 1E Urquhart Street, Aberdeen AB24 5PL Tel: 01224 635826 — MB ChB Aberd. 1993. Specialty: Gen. Pract.

PRIME, Carl Francis 35 Steel Road, Birmingham B31 2RQ — MB Camb. 1976; BChir 1975.

PRIME, Katarina Petia 88 Tooting Bec Road, Balham High Rd, London SW17 8BE — MB ChB Manch. 1996; BSc (Hons. Med. Microbiol.) Manch. 1993. SHO GU Med., Mortimer Market Centre, ULL.; SpR GU Med., Mortimer Market Centre, UCH. Prev: SHO (Med.) N.Middlx. Hosp. Sterling Way Edmunton Lond.; PRHO Surg. Mayday Hosp. Thornton Heath; PRHO Med./Infec. Dis. N. Manch. Gen. Hosp.

PRIMHAK, Robert Anthony Sheffield Children's Hospital, Western Bank, Sheffield S10 2TH Tel: 0114 271 7585 Fax: 0114 273 0522 Email: r.a.primhak@sheffield.ac.uk; 45 Whiteley Wood Road, Sheffield S11 7FF — MD Sheff. 1986 (King's Coll. Hosp.) MB BS Lond. 1975; MRCP (UK) 1980; FRCP Lond. 1993; FRCPCH (UK) 1997. Sen. Lect. (Paediat.) Univ. Sheff. Specialty: Paediat. Socs: Eur. Respirat. Soc.; Brit. Thorac. Soc. Prev: Sen. Lect. (Child Health) Univ., Papua New Guinea.

PRIMROSE, David Alexander Anderson (retired) 26 Garngaber Avenue, Lenzie, Glasgow G66 4LL Tel: 0141 776 1600 — MB ChB Glas. 1951; MRCGP 1958; MD Glas. 1966; FRCPsych 1974, M 1971; FRCP Glas. 1978, M 1975. Hon. Sec. Internat. Assn. Scientif. Study Ment. Defic. Prev: Phys. Supt. Roy. Scott. Nat. Hosp. Larbert.

PRIMROSE, Evangelene Daphne S&E Belfast H+SS Trust, Holywood Arches Health Centre, Westminster Avenue North, Belfast BT4 1QQ Tel: 01232 563318 Fax: 01232 563327 Email: daphne.primrose@sebt.n-i.nhs.uk; 23 Station Road, Craigavad, Holywood BT18 0BP — MB BCh BAO Belf. 1982; MRCP (UK) 1985; MD Belf. 1992. Cons. (Paediat.) S&E Belf. H+SS Trust, Belf.; Cons. (Paediat.) Ulster Comm. & Hosps. Trust, Belf. Specialty: Paediat. Socs: Brit. Paediat. Assn.; BACCH; UPS.

PRIMROSE, Professor John Neil Southampton General Hospital, University Surgical Unit, Level F, Centre Block, Southampton SO16 6YD Tel: 023 8079 6144 — MB ChB (Hons.) Glas. 1977; FRCS Glas. 1981; MD Glas. 1984. Prof. & Cons. Surg. Soton. Gen. Hosp. Specialty: Gen. Surg. Prev: Cons. Surg. & Sen. Lect. St. Jas. Hosp. Leeds; Lect. & Sen. Regist. (Surg.) Leeds Gen. Infirm.; Regist. (Surg.) Glas. Roy. Infirm.

PRIMROSE, Kathleen Mary 14 Cousins Grove, Southsea PO4 9RP — MB BS Lond. 1976 (Roy. Free) MRCS Eng. LRCP Lond. 1976; DRCOG 1978; MRCGP 1981. Prev: Ho. Surg. Roy. Portsmouth Hosp.; Ho. Phys. Qu. Alex. Hosp. Portsmouth.

PRIMROSE, Pauline Ann Brooklea Health Centre, Wick Road, Brislington, Bristol BS4 4HU Tel: 0117 971 1211 Fax: 0117 972 3370 — (Bristol) MB ChB Bristol 1962; DObst RCOG 1964.

PRIMROSE, Mr William John 59 Richmond Court, Lisburn BT27 4QX — MB BCh BAO Belf. 1977; FRCSI 1981. Cons. Roy. Vict. Hosp. Belf. Specialty: Otolaryngol.

PRIMROSE, William Robertson Woodend Hospital, Aberdeen AB15 6XS Tel: 01224 681818 Fax: 01224 556339; 41 Richmondhill Road, Aberdeen AB15 5EQ Tel: 01224 311276 — MB ChB Aberd. 1976; BMedBiol. Aberd. 1973; MRCP (UK) 1978; DObst Otago 1980; MRCGP 1981; FRCP Glas. 1990; FRCP Edin 1999. Cons. Phys. (Geriat. Med.) Woodend Hosp. Aberd. Specialty: Care of the Elderly. Socs: Brit. Geriat. Soc. Prev: Sen. Regist. (Geriat. & Gen. Med.) City Hosp. Edin.; Regist. (Respirat. Med. & Infec. Dis.) King's Cross Hosp. Dundee; SHO Regist. (Gen. Med.) South. Gen. Hosp. Glas.

PRINCE, Arthur Wilfred The Park Surgery, 116 Kings Road, Herne Bay CT6 5RE Tel: 01227 742200 Fax: 01227 742277 — MB BS Newc. 1969; DObst RCOG 1971; MRCGP (Distinc. & Fraser Rose Gold Medal) 1973; Cert. Family Plann. JCC 1976. Postgrad. Teach. (Gen. Pract.) SE Thames RHA; Port Med. Insp. H. M. Immigr. Serv. Socs: Beckett Med. Soc. Prev: Trainee GP Newc. Univ. VTS; Postgrad. Teach. (Gen. Pract.) North. RHA.

PRINCE, Carolyn Ann Heston Health Centre, Cranford Lane, Heston, Hounslow TW5 9ER Tel: 020 8321 3400 Fax: 020 8321 3413; 45 Dene Avenue, Hounslow TW3 3AQ — MB ChB Leic. 1988; BSc (1st cl. Hons.) Leic. 1985; DFFP 1993. Clin. Med. Off. (Houns. HA) Wom.s Servs. Specialty: Pub. Health Med.; Family Plann. & Reproduc. Health. Prev: SHO (Gen. Med.) Ealing Hosp.; SHO (Chem. Path. & Research) Char. Cross Hosp. Lond.; Ho. Phys. (Coronary Care) Leicester Roy. Infirm.

PRINCE, Clive Benjamin Bewdley Medical Centre, Dog Lane, Bewdley DY12 2EG Tel: 01299 402157 Fax: 01299 404364; The Stables, Park Farm, Ribbesford, Bewdley DY12 2TW Tel: 01295 402 157 Email: clive.prince@gp-m81057.nhs.uk — MB ChB Birm. 1979; DRCOG 1982; Cert. Family Plann. JCC 1982; DCH RCP Lond. 1983; MRCGP 1984. p/t Tutor Wyre Forest Primary Care Trust; NPfIT - Diabetes Implementation Expert Refer. Gp: NWWM cluster; Hon. GP Tutor; Summative Assessm. Examr. Specialty: Diabetes; Gen. Pract. Socs: Primary Care Spec. Gp. of Brit. Computer Soc. Prev: Examr. (Gen. Pract.) Birm. Med. Sch.; Computer Manager Wyre Forest Primary Care Centre; Lead Partner Advanced Train. Pract.

PRINCE, George Harrald Abingdon Family Health Centre, 361/365 Queens Drive, Liverpool L4 8SJ Tel: 0151 525 1298 — MB ChB Liverp. 1958.

PRINCE, Graham David Jersey General Hospital, St Helier, Jersey JE1 3QS Tel: 01534 622492 Fax: 01534 617245; Hamilton House, Le Chemin Des Hautes Croix, Trinity, Jersey JE3 5DT Email: gdprince@iti.net — MB BS Lond. 1977; DRCOG 1979; FFA RCS Eng. 1983. Cons. Anaesth. Jersey Gen. Hosp. Specialty: Anaesth. Prev: Sen. Regist. (Anaesth.) Newc. HA.

PRINCE, Heather Gail 6 Chartwell Grove, Nottingham NG3 5RD; Oakbank, 6 Chartwell Grove, Mapporley Plains, Nottingham NG3 5RD — MB ChB Liverp. 1972; FRCS Eng. 1978. Cons. spinal Surg..Univ. Hosp. Nottm. Specialty: Orthop. Socs: BMA, BOA. Prev: Cons. Orthop. Kingsmill Hosp. Mansfield & Univ. Hosp. Nottm.; Sen. Lect. (Orthop. & Accid. Surg.) Univ. Nottm. Harlow Wood Orthop. Hosp. & Mansfield Gen. Hosp.; Hon. Cons. Mansfield & Dist. Gen. Hosp., Harlow Wood Orthop. Hosp. & Univ. Hosp. Nottm.

PRINCE, John Anthony Tower Medical Centre, 129 Cannon Street Road, London E1 2LX Tel: 020 7488 4240 Fax: 020 7702 2443 — BM BCh Oxf. 1966; MA, BM BCh Oxf. 1966; DIH 1981; MRCGP 1981; MFOM RCP Lond. 1985, A 1981; DFFP 1984. Exam. Med. Off. DSS; Local Med. Off. Civil Serv. OHS. Specialty: Gen. Med. Socs: BMA & Soc. Occupat. Med. Prev: Occupat. Phys. Tower Hamlets DHA & Cons. to Lond. Boro. Tower Hamlets & Dockland Developm.; Ho. Surg. St. Thos. Hosp. Lond.; Mem. GP Tower Hamlets HA.

PRINCE, Karen Laura 8 South Morton Street, Joppa, Edinburgh EH15 2NB — MB ChB Ed. 1979; BA Oxf. 1976; MRCGP 1983; MRCP (UK) 1983.

PRINCE, Martin Ivor 48 Alwinton Terrace, Gosforth, Newcastle upon Tyne NE3 1UD Tel: 0191 284 5022 — BM BS Nottm. 1992; BMedSci Nottm. 1990; MRCP (UK) 1995. Regist. (Gostroenteral.) Freeman Hosp. Newc. Specialty: Gastroenterol. Prev: Regist. (Gen. Med.) N. Tyneside Dist. Gen. Hosp.

PRINCE, Martin James Flat 3, 43 Granville Park, London SE13 7DY — MB BChir Camb. 1984.

PRINCE, Michael Fred Charles (retired) Tan Yr Allt, Cefn Canol, Rhydycroesau, Oswestry SY10 7PS — MB ChB Birm. 1959; DObst RCOG 1965. Med. Off. Benefits Agency Birm. Disablem. Centre. Prev: GP Handsworth Birm.

PRINCE, Sarah 2 West End Av, Guisborough TS14 6NP — MB ChB Birm. 1997.

PRINCE, Simon Richard The Surgery, High Street, Lowestoft NR32 1JE Tel: 01502 589151 Fax: 01502 566719 — MB BS Lond. 1982 (Univ. Coll. Hosp.) BSc Pharmacol. Lond. 1978, MB BS 1982; MRC Psych 1988; DRCOG 1989; MRCGP 1990. Socs: Princip. Fell. Roy. Soc. Med. Prev: SHO Rotat. (Med.) Univ. Coll. Hosp.; Ho. Surg. St. Pancras Hosp. Lond.; Ho Phys. Harefield Hosp.

PRINCE, William Tom 18 St Albans Avenue, Weybridge KT13 8EN — MB BChir Camb. 1980; PhD Camb. 1971 MA 1970, BA 1967; Dip. Pharm. Med. RCP (UK) 1987. Dir. Clin. Graduation Acad. Therap. Chelsea & Westm. Hosp. Lond.; Mem. Fac. Pharmaceut. Med. Specialty: Pharmaceutical Medicine. Socs: Fell. Roy. Soc. Med.; Brit. Pharm. Soc.; Soc. Pharmaceut. Med. Prev: Phys. i/c Clin. Pharmacol. SmithKline Beecham Pharmaceut.

PRINCEWILL, Opribo Mpakaboari Orthopaedic Department, Newham General Hospital, Glen Road, Plaistow, London E13 8SL; 6 Stanmore House, Smedley Street, Union Grove, London SW8 2QT — MB BS Ibadan 1979 (IBADAN) MBBS IBADAN 1979; FRCS England 1992; FRCS Edinburgh 1992. Orthopaedic Regist., Newham Gen. Hosp., Plaistow. Specialty: Trauma & Orthop. Surg. Socs: BOA; BMA. Prev: Dept. of Orthop., Stepping Hill Hosital, Stockport.

PRING, Christopher Michael 22 Tinwell Road, Stamford PE9 2SD — MB BChir Camb. 1994; FRCS (Gen.) 1998.

PRING, Mr David James The Princess Elizabeth Hospital, Le Vauquiedor, St Martin's, Guernsey GY4 6UU Tel: 01481 725241; The Medical Specialist Group, PO Box 113, Alexandra House, Les Frieteaux, St Martins, Guernsey GY1 3EX Tel: 01481 38565 Fax: 01481 37782 Email: davidp@medspec.demon.co.uk — MB BS Newc. 1974; FRCS Eng. 1979; FRCS Ed. 1979. Cons. Orthop. Guernsey Med. Specialist Gp. Specialty: Orthop. Prev: Sen. Regist. (Orthop.) Roy. Nat. Orthop. Hosp. Lond.; Regist. (Orthop.) Hammersmith Postgrad. Hosp.; Surg. Leprosy Mission Asia.

PRING, David William Department of Obstetrics and Gynaecology, York District Hospital, York YO31 8HE Tel: 01904 631313 Fax: 01904 726880; The Old Vicarage, Main Street, Wilberfoss, York YO41 5NN Email: dr@pring.net — MB BS Lond. 1975 (Lond. Hosp.) BSc (Hons.) Lond. 1971; DRCOG 1978; FRCOG 1994, M 1981. Cons. Gyn. & Obst. York Dist. Hosp. Specialty: Obst. & Gyn. Socs: Fell. Med. Soc. Lond.; York Med. Soc.; Ospreys Gyn. Soc. Prev: Sen. Regist. (O & G) St. Bart. Hosp. Lond.; Regist. (O & G) St. Mary's Hosp. Lond.; SHO (Obst.) Qu. Charlotte's Hosp. Wom.

PRING, John Ernest 5 Lidden Road, Penzance TR18 4PG; West Cornwall Hospital, St. Clare St, Penzance TR18 2PF — MB BS Lond. 1971 (Lond. Hosp.) MRCS Eng. LRCP Lond. 1971; DObst RCOG 1974; DA Eng. 1975; FFA RCS Eng. 1978. Cons. Anaesth. Cornw. & Isles of Scilly HA. Specialty: Anaesth. Socs: Assn. Anaesths. Prev: Sen. Regist. Withington Hosp. Manch.; Res. Accouch. & SHO (Anaesth.) Lond. Hosp.

PRING, Rachel Caroline — MB BS Lond. 1998.

PRINGLE, Adam James Lawley Medical Practice, Lawley, Telford TF4 2LL Tel: 01952 560011 Fax: 01952 501502 — MB ChB Birm. 1990; DRCOG 1993; DCH RCPS Glas. 1995; MRCGP 1996; Dip Occ Med 2000. GP Princip.; Occupat. Health Med. Adviser. Specialty: Gen. Pract.

PRINGLE, Alexander (retired) 17 Crescent Road, Chingford, London E4 6AT Tel: 020 8529 4402 — (Glas.) BSc (Hons.) Glas. 1952, MB ChB (Commend.) 1955; FRFPS Glas. 1959; MRCP Ed. 1960; FRCP Lond. 1975, M 1961; FRCP Glas. 1968; FRCP Ed. 1994. Prev: Cons. Phys. N. Middlx. Hosp.

PRINGLE, Alexander Ferguson The Cannons, Fisher St., Methil, Leven KY8 3HE Tel: 01333 426083; The Paddock, Main St, Upper Largo, Leven KY8 6EW Tel: 0133 336707 — MB ChB Aberd. 1960. Specialty: Care of the Elderly.

PRINGLE, Edward, TD (retired) Kingswood, McBean Road, Wolverhampton WV6 0JQ Tel: 01902 751661 — MB BChir Camb. 1946 (Lond. Hosp.) MRCGP; MRCS Eng., LRCP Lond. 1942; BA Camb. 1939, MA, MB BChir 1946; DCH Eng. 1948. Prev: Ho. Phys. Lond. Hosp.

***PRINGLE, Edward Marc** 54 Cayser Drive, Kingswood, Maidstone ME17 3QD — BM BCh Oxf. 1998; BM BCh Oxf 1998. Specialty: Gen. Med.

PRINGLE, Gordon Mitchell Benreary Surgery, Seaview Place, Buckie AB56 1JT Tel: 01542 831555 Fax: 01542 835799 — MB ChB Glas. 1976; DRCOG 1978; MRCGP 1980.

PRINGLE, Jane Karen Waterlooville Health Centre, Dryden Close, Waterlooville PO7 6AL Tel: 023 9225 7321; 3 Abbotts Way, Highfield, Southampton SO17 1QU — MB BCh BAO Belf. 1982; DCH RCP Lond. 1985; MRCGP 1986; DRCOG 1986.

PRINGLE, Jean Anne Smellie Morbid Anatomy Department, Institute of Orthopaedics, Royal National Orthopaedic Hospital, Brockley Hill, Stanmore HA7 4LP Tel: 020 8954 5908 Fax: 020 8954 5908; 17 Crescent Road, Chingford, London E4 6AT Tel: 020 8529 4402 — MB ChB Glas. 1959; FRCS 1995. Sen. Lect., Hon. Cons. & Head Dept. (Morbid Anat.) Inst. Orthop. Lond.; Pathol. Lond. Bone & Soft Tissue Tumour Serv. Specialty: Histopath. Socs: Internat. Skeletal Soc.; Eur. Musculoskeletal Oncol. Soc.; Nat. Bone Tumour Panel (Sec.).

PRINGLE, Jean Rosemary Carmondean Medical Group, Carmondean Health Centre, Livingston EH54 8PY — MB ChB Glas. 1981; DRCOG 1984; MFHom 1988.

PRINGLE, Jonathan James Austen Shirley Avenue Surgery, 1 Shirley Avenue, Shirley, Southampton SO15 5RP Tel: 023 8077 3258/1356 Fax: 023 8070 3078; 3 Abbotts Way, Highfield, Southampton SO17 1QU Tel: 02380 558688 Fax: 01703 558688 — MB BS Lond. 1980 (Guy's Hospital Medical School) DCH Otago 1983; MRCP (UK) 1985; DRCOG 1986; MRCGP 1987.

PRINGLE, Keith Holmcroft Surgery, Holmcroft Road, Stafford ST16 1JG Tel: 01785 242172 — BM BCh Oxf. 1978; BA Oxf. 1975.

PRINGLE, Mary Willows Brook, Llangoed, Beaumaris LL58 8NY — MB BS Lond. 1943 (King's Coll. Lond.) BSc (Physiol.) 1939; MRCS Eng. LRCP Lond. 1942; DCH Eng. 1948. Prev: Regist. (Med.) Whiston Hosp.; Capt. RAMC.

PRINGLE, Professor Michael Alexander Leary Collingham Health Centre, High Street, Collingham, Newark NG23 7LB Tel: 01636 892156 Fax: 01636 893391; Department of General Practice, Queens Medical Centre, Nottingham NG7 2UH Tel: 0115 970 9391 Fax: 0115 970 9389 Email: mike.pringle@nottingham.ac.uk — MB BS Lond. 1973 (Guy's) MRCS Eng. LRCP Lond 1973; DRCOG 1977; MRCGP 1978; MD Lond. 1987; FRCGP 1989. Prof. Gen. Pract. Univ. Nottm. Specialty: Gen. Pract.

PRINGLE, Mr Michael Blair Queen Alexandra Hospital, Cosham, Portsmouth PO6 3LY Tel: 023 92 379451 — MB BS Lond. 1983 (St. Geo. Hosp. Med. Sch.) FRCS Eng. 1988; FRCS (Orl.) Eng. 1990; FRCS (Orl.) 1994. Cons. ENT Qu. Alexandra Hosp. Portsmouth; Hon. Cons. ENT Soton. Gen. Hosp.; Cons. ENT S. Eng. Cochear Implant Centre Soton. Specialty: Otorhinolaryngol.

PRINGLE, Mr Robert Greig Burnell House, 82 Berwick Road, Shrewsbury SY1 2NF Tel: 01743 353012 — MB ChB New Zealand 1960; FRCS Eng. 1966. Surg. (Orthop.) in Medicolegal Pract. Specialty: Trauma & Orthop. Surg.; Medico Legal. Prev: Indep. Cons. Orthop. Surg. Shrops.; Cons. Orthop. Surg. Robt. Jones & Agnes Hunt Orthop. Hosp. Oswestry & Roy. Shrewsbury Hosp.; Cons. Orthop. Midl. Spinal Injuries Centre Robt. Jones & Agnes Hunt Orthop. Hosp.

PRINGLE, Mr Robert Macaulay (retired) 15 Lenzie Road, Stepps, Glasgow G33 6DU — MB ChB Aberd. 1964; FRCS Ed. 1971. Prev: Cons. Orthop. Surg. Monklands Dist. Gen. Hosp. Airdrie.

PRINGLE, Stewart 8 Woodend Drive, Glasgow G13 1QS Email: 100724.2333@compuserve.com — MB ChB Glas. 1983; BSc Glas. 1981; MRCGP 1988; MRCOG 1994. Specialist Regist. (O & G) Southern Gen. Hosp. Glas. Specialty: Obst. & Gyn. Prev: Career Regist. (O & G) Stirling Roy. Infirm.; Regist. (O & G) Stobhill Hosp. & Roy. Matern. Hosp. Glas.; SHO (Obst.) Qu. Mother's Hosp. Glas.

PRINGLE, Stuart David Ninewells Hospital & Medical School, Department of Cardiology, Dundee DD1 9SY Tel: 01382 632263; Bankview, Main St, Longforgan, Dundee DD2 5EW — MB ChB Dundee 1979; MRCP (UK) 1983; MD Dundee 1990; FRCP Glas. 1994; FRCP Ed. 1996. Cons. Cardiol. & Hon.Prof. Ninewells Hosp. & Med. Sch. Dundee. Specialty: Cardiol. Socs: Brit. Cardiac Soc.; Scot. Cardiac Soc.; Brit. Soc. Of Echocardiography. Prev: Sen. Lect. Ninewells Hosp. Dundee; Sen. Regist. (Cardiol.) Roy. Infirm. Edin.; Regist. (Cardiol.) Glas. Roy. Infirm.

PRINGLE, Terence Harold Cardiac Department, Ninewells Hospital, Dundee DD1 9SY Tel: 01382 60111; Balnagar, Tealing, Dundee DD4 0QZ Tel: 01382 380463 — MB BCh BAO Dub. 1972 (TC Dub.) FRCPI 1989, M 1975; MD Dub. 1987; FRCP Ed. 1992. Cons. Cardiol. Ninewells Hosp. Dundee; Hon. Sen. Lect. (Med.) Univ. Dundee. Specialty: Cardiol. Prev: Sen. Regist. (Gen. Med.) Belf. City Hosp. & Roy. Vict. Hosp. Belf.; Regist. (Cardiol.) Roy. Infirm. Glas.

PRINGLE, Victoria Alexandra — MB ChB Aberd. 1993; Dip FP 1996; DRCOG 1996; MRCGP 1998.

PRINJA, Aparna Flat 1, 14 Carols Place, London W1Y 5AG — MB BS Lond. 1992 (St. Thos. UMDS) SHO (Paediat.) Chelsea & Westminster Hosp. Lond. Specialty: Paediat.

PRINN, Mr Michael George (retired) Four Seasons, Brockley Grove, Hutton Mount, Brentwood CM13 2JJ Tel: 01277 219698 Fax: 01277 219698 — MB BS Lond. 1961 (Lond. Hosp.) MRCS Eng. LRCP Lond. 1961; DObst RCOG 1964; FRCS Eng. 1966. Prev: Cons. Gen. Surg. Harold Wood Hosp. & Brentwood Hosp. Gp.

PRINSEN, Agatha Krista Elisabet 84 Malmesbury Road, Southampton SO15 5FQ — Artsexamen Nijmegen 1993.

PRINSLEY, Mr Peter Richard 26 Eaton Road, Norwich NR4 6PZ — MB ChB Sheff. 1982; BMedSci Sheff. 1981; FRCS Ed. 1987; FRCS Eng. 1989. Cons. ENT Surg. Norf. & Norwich Hosp. & Jas. Paget Hosp. Gt. Yarmouth Norf. Specialty: Otolaryngol. Prev: Sen. Regist. (ENT Surg.) Yorks. Region; Regist. (ENT Surg.) Barnet Gen. Hosp. & Roy. Free Hosp.

PRINTER, Keki Dinshaw, Col. late RAMC Retd. (retired) 13 Deben Crescent, Greenmeadow, Swindon SN25 3QB — MB BS Bombay 1952 (Grant Med. Coll. Bombay) DObst 1955; FRCOG 1974, M 1959. Prev: Cons. Gyn. & Obst. & Command Cons. BAOR BMH Rinteln, BFPO 29.

PRIOR, Alison Department of Gastroenterology, Norfolk and Norwich University Hospital NHS Trust, Colney Lane, Norwich NR4 7UY; Hackford Hall, Reepham, Norwich NR10 4RL — MB ChB Manch. 1981; MRCP (UK) 1984; BSc Manch. 1978, MD 1990; FRCP 1999. Cons. Phys. (Gastroenterol.) Norf. & Norwich Univ. Hosp. NHS Trust, Norwich. Specialty: Gastroenterol. Prev: Sen. Regist. Rotat. E. Anglia; Lect. (Med.) Univ. Hosp. S. Manch.

PRIOR, Mr Andrew John — MB ChB Birm. 1987; BSc (Hons.) Birm. 1984; FRCS Eng. 1992; FRCS Ed. 1992; FRCS (ORL-HNS) 1998. Cons. ENT Surg., Bromley Hosps., NHS Trust, Kent. Specialty: Otorhinolaryngol. Special Interest: Rhinology. Socs: Roy. Soc. of Med.; Brit. Assn. of Otorhinolaryngol., Head & Neck Surg.; Otorhinolaryngol. Research Soc. Prev: Sen. Regist., Roy. Nat. Throat, Nose and Ear Hosp., Lond.

PRIOR, Andrew Ronald John, MBE, Wing Cdr. RAF Med. Br. Prior Data Sciences Ltd, 12 Pondtaic Road, Fleet GU51 3JW Tel: 01252 819959 — MB BS Lond. 1978; PhD Lond. 1992, BSc 1974, MB BS 1978. Specialty: Aviat. Med.

PRIOR, Carolyn Ann Woodlands Surgery, 146 Halfway Street, Sidcup DA15 8DF Tel: 0208 300 1680 — MB ChB Birm. 1987 (Birmingham) MRCGP 1991; DRCOG 1991. GP Woodlands Surg. Sidcup. Prev: GP Harrow; Trainee GP Rotat. E. Birm.

PRIOR, Eileen Mary (retired) 23 Eaton Court, Augusta St., Grimsby DN34 4UD Tel: 01472 343748 — MRCS Eng. LRCP Lond. 1942. Prev: Asst. Med. Off. Grimsby.

PRIOR, Gethin Thomas James Bryntirion Surgery, Cardiff Road, Bargoed CF81 8NN Tel: 01443 830796 Fax: 01443 835962 — MB BS Lond. 1990 (UCH Lond.) BSc Lond. 1987. Specialty: Gen. Pract. Prev: SHO Salisbury VTS.

PRIOR, John Gareth Winfield Hospital, Tewkesbury Road, Gloucester GL2 9WH Tel: 01452 331111 Fax: 01452 331200 Email: drjohnprior@compuserve.com; Stonecourt, Stone, Berkeley GL13 9JY Tel: 01454 260964 Email: drjohnprior@compuserve.com — MB BChir Camb. 1975 (Univ. Camb. & Guy's Hosp. Lond.) MA MB BChir (Hons.) Camb. 1974; MRCP (UK) 1976; MD Camb. 1984; FRCP Lond. 1994. Cons. Phys. (Thoracic & Gen. Med.) Glos. Roy. NHS Trust. Specialty: Gen. Med.; Respirat. Med.; Medico Legal. Socs: Brit. Thorac. Soc.; Eur. Respirat. Soc.; Amer. Thoracic Soc. Prev: Sen. Regist. (Thoracic & Gen. Med.) Guy's Hosp. Lond.; Sir Philip Oppenheimer Research Fell. (Med.) Guys Hosp. Lond.; Ho. Phys. Brompton Hosp. Lond.

PRIOR, Kate Rebecca Edna Jane 1 Highbridge Court, Farrow Lane, London SE14 5EB — MB BS Lond. 1996.

PRIOR, Katherine Moncrieffe 9 Goose Pasture, Yarm TS15 9EP — MB BS Newc. 1997.

PRIOR, Keith Sidney, Air Commodore RAF Med. Br. (retired) Tanpenygarnedd, Penybontfawr, Oswestry SY10 0PE — MB BS Lond. 1966 (St. Thos.) MRCS Eng. LRCP Lond. 1966; FRCGP 1981, M 1971; DAvMed Eng. 1977; MFOM RCP Lond. 1981. Prev: Princip. Adviser (Gen. Pract.) RAF.

PRIOR, Michael Bushmead Avenue Medical Centre, 21 Bushmead Avenue, Bedford MK40 3QJ Tel: 01234 267797 Fax: 01234 269649; 21 Bushmead Avenue, Bedford MK40 3QJ Tel: 01234 267797 — MB BS Lond. 1970 (St Georges) MRCS Eng. LRCP Lond. 1970.

PRIOR, Natasha Giselle 10 Appletree Close, Oxford OX4 7GP — MB BS Lond. 1998; BSc (Hons.) 1995.

PRIOR, Pamela Frances Department of Clinical Neurophysiology, St. Barts Hospital, West Smithfield, London EC1A 7BE Tel: 020 7601 8859 Fax: 020 7601 7875 — MD Lond. 1972 (Lond. Hosp.) MB BS 1958; MRCP (UK) 1985; FRCP Lond. 1990. Cons. Clin. Neurophysiol. St. Bart. Hosp. Lond. Specialty: Clin. Neurophysiol. Socs: Fell. Roy. Soc. Med.; Brit. Soc. Clin. Neurophysiol. Prev: Extern. Staff MRC Laborats. Carshalton; Med. Asst. EEG Dept. Lond. Hosp.; Ho. Surg. Roy. Devon & Exeter Hosp.

PRIOR, Roderick Clive Glendower Road Surgery, 54 Glendower Road, Peverell, Plymouth PL3 4LD Tel: 01752 673336 Fax: 01752 267130 — MB ChB Manch. 1977; BSc (Med. Sci.) St. And. 1974. Specialty: Cardiol. Prev: SHO (Anaesth.) Hope Hosp. Salford; SHO (Psychiat.) Prestwich Hosp. Manch.; SHO (Obst.) Hope Hosp. Salford.

PRIOR, Mr Roger James Yew Hedge House, Child Okeford, Blandford Forum DT11 8EF — MB BS Lond. 1970 (Char. Cross) MRCS Eng. LRCP Lond. 1970; FRCS Eng. 1975; MRCP (UK) 1977; MRCGP 1983.

PRIOR, Tova Two Elms, Chobham Road, Knaphill, Woking GU21 2QF — MB BS Lond. 1990.

PRISCOTT, Robin Beverley, MBE (retired) 67 St Mark Drive, Colchester CO4 4LP Tel: 01206 842338 Fax: 01206 842338 — MB BS Lond. 1960 (St. Bart.) Prev: Med. Dir. Dr Ghassan N. Pharaon Gen. Hosp., Jeddah, KSA.

PRISK, Adrian John Central Milton Keynes Medical, 1 North Sixth Street, Saxon Gate West, Milton Keynes MK9 2NR Tel: 01908 605775 Fax: 01908 676752 — MB BS Lond. 1972 (Guy's) MRCS Eng. LRCP Lond. 1972; DObst RCOG 1975; MRCGP 1976. Prev: Princip. GP LoW.oft; Trainee GP Livingston VTS.

PRITCHARD, Adrian John 21 Stuart Way, Market Drayton TF9 3TT — BM BS Nottm. 1994.

PRITCHARD, Ann Strawberry Place Surgery, 5 Strawberry Place, Morriston, Swansea SA6 7AQ Tel: 01792 522526 Fax: 01792 411020 — MB BS Lond. 1987 (St George's London)

PRITCHARD, Caroline Anne 10 Wingrave Road, London W6 9HF — MB BS Lond. 1994; MA Camb. 1995. Prev: Ho. Phys. St. Richards Hosp. Chichester; Ho. Surg. Char. Cross Lond.

PRITCHARD, David Arnold Rees (retired) 12 Gerddi Menai, Bangor Road, Caernarfon LL55 1LN — MRCS Eng. LRCP Lond. 1935 (Liverp.) Prev: Anaesth. Caern. & Anglesey Hosp. Gp.

PRITCHARD, David Mark Liverpool University, Department of Medicine, 5th Floor UCD Building, Daulby Street, Liverpool L69 3GA Tel: 0151 794 5772 Fax: 0151 794 6825 — MB ChB (Hons.) Manch. 1991; BSc (Hons.) Manch. 1988; MRCP (UK) 1994; PhD Manch. 1999. Sen. Lect. / Hon. Cons. Liverp. Univ. and Roy. Liverp. Univ. Hosp. Specialty: Gastroenterol. Special Interest: Hypergastrinaemia, gastric carcinoids. Socs: Brit. Soc. of Gastroenterol. Prev: Clin. lecturer/honorary SpR Liverp. Univ. and Roy. Liverp. Univ. Hosp.; Specialist Regist. (Gen. Med./Gastro.) Roy. Preston Hosp. Preston on NW Rotat.; MRC Clin. Train. Fell. Manch. Univ.

PRITCHARD, Deborah Susan 6 The Old Drive, Welwyn Garden City AL8 6TB Tel: 01707 321297 — MB BS Lond. 1987; DCH RCP Lond. 1989. Clin. Med. Off. E. Herts. Hosp. Specialty: Community Child Health.

PRITCHARD, Dewi Bryn — MB BCh Wales 1992 (Cardiff) BMedSci (Hons.) Wales 1992; MSc Wales 1998. Specialist Regist. Roy. Free Hosp. Rotat. St Ann's Hosp. Lond. Specialty: Geriat. Psychiat. Socs: Roy. Coll. Psychiats.

PRITCHARD, Emma Louise 59 Mooreland Road, Bromley BR1 3RD — MB ChB Birm. 1997. Specialty: Paediat.

PRITCHARD, Gillian Pleiad Ltd, Balmoral Suite, Royal British House, Leonard Street, Perth PH2 8HA; Hope Villa, 236 Couper Angus Road, Muirhead of Liff, Dundee DD2 5QN Tel: 01382 580129 — MB ChB Liverp. 1985; MSc Aberd. 1989; MRCP (UK) 1992; AFPM RCP Lond. 1995; MBA Dundee 1998. Clin. Project Manager Pleiad Ltd Perth. Specialty: Pharmaceutical Medicine. Prev: Clin. Project Manager Pfizer Centr. Research.; Asst. Med. Dir. Scotia Pharmaceut. Ltd. Stirling; Dep. Med. Dir. Drug Developm. (Scotl.) Ltd. Dundee.

PRITCHARD, Mr Graham Arthur Department of Surgery, Princess of Wales Hospital, Coity Road, Bridgend CF31 1RQ Tel: 01656 752752 Fax: 01656 752593; Caegarw, Court Colman, Bridgend CF31 4NG — BM BS Nottm. 1979; BMedSci (Hons.) Nottm. 1977; FRCS Eng. 1983; DM Nottm. 1989. Cons. Surg. Gen. Surg. & Gastroenterol. Princess of Wales Hosp. Bridgend. Specialty: Gen. Surg. Socs: Assn. Surg.; Assn. Coloproctol.; Assn. Endoscopic Surgs. Prev: Sen. Regist. (Gen. Surg.) Singleton Hosp. Swansea; Research Fell. (Surg.) Univ. Wales Coll. Med. Cardiff; Regist. (Surg.) Glam. & Gwent HAs.

PRITCHARD, Mr Graham Cleverly (retired) Shawkbottom Cottage, Cumdivock, Dalston, Carlisle CA5 7JH Tel: 01228 710854 Email: pritchard@cumdivock.fsnet.co.uk — MB BChir Camb. 1939 (Camb. & King's Coll. Hosp.) DOMS Eng. 1942; FRCS Eng. 1953. Prev: Cons. Ophth. Surg. King's Coll. Hosp. & Kensington, Chelsea & Westm. AHA (T).

PRITCHARD, Guy Marcus 3 Towers Close, Poynton, Stockport SK12 1DH — MB ChB Birm. 1996.

PRITCHARD, Gwenda Rosamond Grace (retired) Church Court, Hillside, Tingewick, Buckingham MK18 4QY Tel: 01280 848265 — MB BS Lond. 1963 (Roy. Free) DRCOG 1965. Clin. Asst. (Genitourin. Med.) Radcliffe Infirm. Oxf. & Milton Keynes Hosp. Prev: Clin. Asst. (Genitourin. Med.) Radcliffe Infirm. Oxf. & Milton Keynes Hosp.

PRITCHARD, Harri Robert Owen Siop Isaf, Tudweiliog, Pwllheli LL53 8NF — MB BCh Wales 1994; BSc (Hons.) Wales 1991, MB BCh 1994.

PRITCHARD, Hefin Wyn Hove Medical Centre, West Way, Hove BN3 8LD Tel: 01273 430088 Fax: 01273 430172; 22 Tivoli Road, Brighton BN1 5BH Tel: 01273 5559473 — MB BS Lond. 1979. Socs: Soc. Apoth. Lond.; Sussex M-C Soc.

PRITCHARD, Hugh Malcolm Clarence House, 14 Russell Road, Rhyl LL18 3BY Tel: 01745 350680 Fax: 01745 353293; White Lodge, 35 Brighton Road, Rhyl LL18 3HL — MB ChB Manch. 1974; DRCOG 1977.

PRITCHARD, Ian Paul Birbeck Medical Group, Penrith Health Centre, Bridge Lane, Penrith CA11 8HW Tel: 01768 245200 Fax: 01768 245295 — MB BS Lond. 1986; DRCOG 1991; DCCH RCP Ed. 1992; DCH RCP Lond. 1992; MRCGP 1993; DA (UK) 1997. GP. Specialty: Gen. Pract. Prev: SHO (Anaesth.) Cumbld. Infirm.; Dist. Med. Off. Forteau, Canada.

PRITCHARD, Jane Department of Clinical Neuroscience, Guy's King's & St. Thomas' School of Medicine, Hodgkin Builiding, Guy's Hospital, London SE1 1UL Tel: 020 7848 6126 Fax: 020 7848 6123 Email: jane.pritchard@kcl.ac.uk — BM BCh Oxf. 1993; BA Camb. 1990; MRCP (UK) 1996. MRC Fell., Dept of NeuroImmunol., Guy's, King's & St Thomas' Sch. of Med. Specialty: Neurol. Socs: Roy. Coll. Phys. (UK) 1996; Assoc. Mem. Assn. Brit. Neurol. Prev: Specialist Regist. (Neurol.) Ninewells Hosp., Dundee.

PRITCHARD, Jillian Margaret Huntersfield, Highlands Road, Reigate RH2 0LA Tel: 01737 244029 — BM BCh Oxf. 1975; MA Oxf. 1976; MRCOG 1982, D 1977; DCH Eng. 1979; FRCOG 2003. Cons. Genitourin. Med. St. Peter's Hosp. Chertsey. Specialty: Genitourinary Medicine. Socs: BMA; Med. Soc. Study VD; AGUM. Prev: Sen. Regist. (Genitourin. Med.) St. Mary's Hosp. Lond.

PRITCHARD, John Arthur Wyndrush, Newlands Road, Leominster HR6 8PS Tel: 01568 613586 — BM Soton. 1987; MRCP (UK) 1991. SHO (O & G) Taunton & Som. Hosp. Prev: SHO (,Med.) St. Mary's Hosp. Portsmouth.

PRITCHARD, John Guthrie (retired) 15 Monastery Street, Canterbury CT1 1NJ — LMSSA Lond. 1956 (St. Mary's) MD Lond. 1968, MB BS 1958. Prev: Cons. Phys. (Geriat. Med.) St. Lukes Hosp. Huddersfield.

PRITCHARD, Jonathan Institute of Child Health, Guilford St., London WC1N 1EH Tel: 020 7242 9782 Fax: 020 7404 6181; 12 Richborne Terrace, London SW8 1AU Tel: 020 7582 4582 — (Camb. & St. Thos.) MB BChir Camb. 1967; BA Camb. 1967; FRCP Lond. 1981, M 1970. Sen. Lect. (Paediat. Oncol.) Inst. Child Health & Cons. Hosp. for Childr. Gt. Ormond St. Lond.; Vis. Prof. Paediat. Perth, W Australia 1999 & MacDonald Orator; Vis. Prof. Paediat. Delhi, Chandigarh 1993. Specialty: Oncol.; Paediat. Socs: Hon. Fell. Amer. Acad. Pediat.; Fell. Roy. Coll. Paeds. & Child Health; Amer. Soc. Clin. Oncol. Prev: Leukaemia Research Fell. (Haemat.) Univ. Liverp.; MRC Trav. Fell. Childr. Hosp. Boston, USA 1974-5; (Founder) Cons. Oncol. Unit Gt. Ormond St. Hosp. Lond. 1978-98.

PRITCHARD, Kathryn Amelia Bideford Medical Centre, Abbotsham Road, Bideford EX39 3AF Tel: 01237 476363 Fax: 01237 423351; Gables, First Raleigh, Bideford EX39 3NJ — MB BS Lond. 1983; MRCGP 1987; DGM RCP Lond. 1987. GP Bideford.

PRITCHARD, Keith (retired) 2 Honeythorn Close, Hempsted, Gloucester GL2 5LU Tel: 01452 303018 — MB BS Lond. 1956 (St. Mary's) LMSSA Lond. 1956. Prev: GP Gloucester.

PRITCHARD, Lucinda Jane Humphris (retired) South Point, Berkeley Road, Cirencester GL7 1TY Tel: 01285 652260 — MRCS Eng. LRCP Lond. 1965. Prev: Med. Dir. of Prospect Hospice Swindon.

PRITCHARD, Mr Mark Gawain St. Anns, Charles St., Tredegar NP22 4AF — MB BS Lond. 1992; FRCS (Eng.) 1996. Specialist Regist. (Trauma & Orthop.) W. Midl. Deanery. Specialty: Trauma & Orthop. Surg.

PRITCHARD, Michael Hugo Department of Rheumatology, University Hospital of Wales, Heath Park, Cardiff CF14 4XW Tel: 029 2074 2626 Fax: 029 2074 4388; East Barn, White Farm, Leckwith, Cardiff CF11 8AS Tel: 029 2051 4753 Fax: 01222 744388 — MB BCh BAO Belf. 1970; BA Oxf. 1964; FRCP Lond. 1988. Cons. Rheumat. Univ. Hosp. Wales Cardiff. Specialty: Rehabil. Med.; Rheumatol.

PRITCHARD, Michael John 3 Great Spilmans, London SE22 8SZ — (St. Thos.) MB BChir Camb. 1953; FRCP Lond. 1977, M 1958; DPM Lond. 1961; FRCPsych 1974, M 1971. Emerit. Reader (Psychiat.) United Med. & Dent. Sch. Guy's & St. Thos. Hosp. Lond. Specialty: Gen. Psychiat. Prev: Reader (Psychiat.) United Med. & Dent. Sch. Guy's & St. Thos. Hosp. Lond.; Sen. Lect. & Asst. Dir. (Psychiat.) Lond. Hosp. Med. Coll.; Sen. Regist. Maudsley Hosp. Lond.

PRITCHARD, Nicholas Charles Bromley Moorfields Eye Hospital, City Road, London EC1V 2PD Tel: 020 7253 3411 — MB BS Lond. 1989 (St. Mary's Hosp. Lond.) BSc Lond. 1988; FRCA 1995. Cons. Anaesth., Moorfields Eye Hosp., Lond. Specialty: Anaesth. Socs: Anaesth. Assn.; Brit. Ophth. Anaesthetic Soc. Prev: Sen. Regist. (Anaesth.) Hammersmith Hosp.; Regist. (Anaesth.) Marsden & Hammersmith Hosp. Lond.; SHO (Anaesth.) Hammersmith Hosp. & St. Mary's Hosp. Lond.

PRITCHARD, Nicola Louise 19 Orwell Drive, Didcot OX11 7RX Tel: 01235 819246 Email: nl.pritchard@tiscali.co.uk — BM BS Nottm. 1994; BMedSci Nottm. 1992. Specialist Regist. Oxford Rotat. (Paediat.). Specialty: Paediat. Socs: RCPCH. Prev: Ho. Off. (Med.) St. Geo. Hosp. Lincoln; Ho. Off. (Surg.) Furness Gen. Hosp.; SHO (Paediat.) City Gen. Hosp. Stoke-on-Trent.

PRITCHARD, Peter Michael Maddock (retired) 31 Martins Lane, Dorchester-on-Thames, Wallingford OX10 7JF Tel: 01865 340008 Fax: 01865 341593 — MB BChir Camb. 1942 (St. Thos.) MA Camb. 1942; DCH Eng. 1947; FRCGP 1978, M 1957. Sen. Med. Adviser Advanced Computation Laborat. Cancer Research UK; Hon. Sec. UK - Nordic Med. Educat. Trust. Prev: Regist. (Paediat.) Univ. Coll. Hosp. Lond.

PRITCHARD, Philip Leslie James The Culverhay Surgery, Culverhay, Wotton-under-Edge GL12 7LS Tel: 01453 843252 — MB BS London 1982; MB BS 1982 Lond; MRCS Eng LRCP Lond 1981. GP Wotton-under-Edge, Glos.

PRITCHARD, Richard Michael Shotton Lane Surgery, 38 Shotton Lane, Shotton, Deeside CH5 1QW Tel: 01244 812094 Fax: 01244 811728 — MB ChB Liverp. 1972; DObst RCOG 1974.

PRITCHARD, Robert Ifor Siop Isaf, Tudweiliog, Pwllheli LL53 8NF Tel: 01758 770277; Siop Isaf, Tudweiliog, Pwllheli LL53 8NF Tel: 01758 770277 — MB ChB Liverp. 1967.

PRITCHARD, Stephen John Rozel, Arleston Hill, Telford TF1 2JY — MB BS Lond. 1987.

PRITCHARD, Stephen Robert Ty'r Felin Surgery, Cecil Road, Gorseinon, Swansea SA4 4BY Tel: 01792 898844 — MB BCh Wales 1974.

PRITCHARD, Susan Ann 18 The Street, Cherhill, Calne SN11 8XP — MB ChB Sheff. 1989.

PRITCHARD, Terence Rodney The Surgery, 30 Westfield Road, Acocks Green, Birmingham B27 7TL Tel: 0121 706 5131 Fax: 0121 706 7593 — MB ChB Birm. 1976; BSc Aston 1967.

PRITCHARD, Violet Gladys (retired) Taintree House, Heathfield Road, Audlem, Crewe CW3 0AU Tel: 01270 811833 — MB BS Lond. 1953 (London Hospital Medical College) MRCS Eng. LRCP Lond. 1953; DCH Eng. 1956. Prev: SCMO Crewe HA.

PRITCHARD-HOWARTH, Martin Roy 26 Ford Road, Upton, Wirral CH49 0TF — MB ChB Liverp. 1993 (Liverpool) BSc Liverp. 1990; MRCP (UK) 1997. Acting Cons. Geriat. Med. Roy. Liverp. & Broadgreen Univ. Hosp. NHS Trust Liverp. Specialty: Care of the Elderly. Prev: Specialist Regist. Arrowe Pk. Hosp.

PRITCHARD-JONES, Kathryn Royal Marsden Hospital, Department of Paediatric Oncology, Downs Road, Sutton SM2 5PT Tel: 020 8642 6011 Fax: 020 8661 3617 Email: kpj@icr.ac.uk — BM BCh Oxf. 1983; MA Oxf. 1984; MRCP (UK) 1986; PhD CNAA 1992; FRPCH 1997; FRCP Ed. 1998. Cancer Research UK Sen. Lect. & Hon. Cons. Paediat. Oncol. Inst. Cancer Research Roy. Marsden Hosp. Sutton. Specialty: Oncol.

PRITCHARD JONES, Rowan Oliver 7 The Firs, Chester Rd, Whitchurch SY13 1NL — MB ChB Bristol 1997.

PRITCHETT, Andrew Harold James New Hall Lane Practice, The Health Centre, Geoffrey Street, Preston PR1 5NE Tel: 01772 401730 Fax: 01772 401731; 10 Sharoe Green Park, Fulwood, Preston PR2 8HW — MB BS Lond. 1974; DRCOG 1977; MRCGP 1979.

PRITCHETT, Mr Christopher Julian Ellengowam, Preston Park, North Shields NE29 9JL — MB ChB Bristol 1974; BSc Bristol 1971; FRCS Eng. 1978; MD Bristol 1983. Cons. Gen. Surg. S. Shields Gen. Hosp. Specialty: Gen. Surg. Prev: Lect. Univ. Hong. Kong.

PRITCHETT, Jane Kathleen — MB BCh Wales 1998. Specialty: Gen. Surg. Prev: Pre-Regist. Ho. Off. (Gen. Surg.) P. Philip Hosp. Llanelli; Pre-Reg. Ho. Off. (Gen Med.) P. Chas. Hosp. Merthyr Tydfil.

PRITLOVE, Janice Carlton Gardens Surgery, 27 Carlton Gardens, Leeds LS7 1JL Tel: 0113 295 2678 Fax: 0113 295 2679; 9 West Pasture Close, Horsforth, Leeds LS18 5PB Tel: 0113 258 0116 — MB ChB Manch. 1971; MRCGP 1975.

PRITTY, Mr Paul Edmund Accident & Emergency Department, Derbyshire Royal Infirmary NHS Trust, London Road, Derby DE1 2QY Tel: 01332 254925 Email: paul.pritty@sdah-tr.trent.nhs.uk — MB Camb. 1971 (St. George's London) MB BChir Camb. 1971; FRCS Eng. 1978; FFAEM 1994. Cons. Accid. Roy. Infirm. Derby.; Train. Progr. Director (A & E), Trent. Specialty: Accid. & Emerg. Prev: Ass Post Grad. Dean mid Trent; Sen. Regist. (Accid.) Univ. Hosp. Nottm.; Regist. (Accid.) Chester Hosp.

PRIVETT, James Thomas John 4 Windmill Croft, Windmill Hill, Cubbington, Leamington Spa CV32 7JU — MB ChB Bristol 1964; DMRD Eng. 1971; FFR 1973.

PRIVONITZ, Dorothea Magdalena Little Harwood Health Centre, Plane Tree Road, Blackburn BB1 6PH Tel: 01254 580931 Fax: 01254 695794 — State Exam Med Mainz 1987; State Exam Med Mainz 1987.

PRIYADARSHI, Saket 7 Parklands, Broxburn EH52 5RB — MB ChB Glas. 1994.

PRIYADHARSHAN, Rajasingham Bennochy Medical Centre, 65 Bennochy Road, Kirkcaldy KY2 5RB Tel: 01592 263332 Fax: 01592 207599 — MB BS Peradeniya 1985. GP Kirkcaldy, Fife.

PROBERT, Christopher Simon John Rose Holding, Latteridge Road, Iron Acton, Bristol BS37 9TW — MB ChB Birm. 1985; MRCP (UK) 1988.

PROBERT, Clive Barrington (retired) Redlam Surgery, 62 Redlam, Blackburn BB2 1UW Tel: 01254 260051 Fax: 01254 691937; Bentham Road Health Centre, Bentham Road, Blackburn BB2 4QD Tel: 01254 209918 — MB ChB Liverp. 1962. Prev: Med. Adviser Akzo-Nobel Ltd., St. Regis Paper Company, SCA Ltd. & Secto Ltd Blackburn.

PROBERT, Doris Evelyn (retired) 33 Cefn Coed Avenue, Cyncoed, Cardiff CF23 6HF Tel: 029 2075 9764 — MB ChB Manch. 1959; Cert FPA 1963. Prev: Clin. Med. Off. S. Glam. AHA (T).

PROBERT, Joanne Lisa 15 Sunningdale, Clifton, Bristol BS8 2NF — MB ChB Bristol 1998.

PROBERT, Mr John Llewellyn — BM BS Nottm. 1991 (Univ. Nottm.) BMedSci (Hons.) Nottm. 1989; FRCS Ed. 1995; FRCS UROL 2001. Specialist Regist. (Urol.) Bristol; Tutor (Surg.) Univ. Bristol. Specialty: Urol. Socs: Brit. Assoc. of Urological Surgs. Prev: Specialist Regist. (Urol.) Roy. Cornw. Hosp. Truro; Research Regist. (Urol.) Southmead Hosp. Bristol & Bristol Roy. Infirm.; SHO (Urol.) Weston Gen. Hosp.

PROBERT, Winifred Evelyn (retired) 14 Llandaff Close, Penarth CF64 3JH — MRCS Eng. LRCP Lond. 1926 (Westm.) DPH Eng. 1928. Prev: Asst. MOH Aberdare & Mt.ain Ash Div. & Mon. Co. & Co. BreCons.

PROBST, Avalon Fey The Accident & Emergency Department, Charing Cross Hospital, Fulham Palace Road, London W6 Tel: 020 846 1008 — MB BS Lond. 1990.

PROBY, Charlotte Mary Centre for Cutaneous Research, St Bartholomews & Royal London School of Med. & Dentistry, 2 Newark St., London E1 2AT Tel: 020 78827160 Ext: 7173 Fax: 020 78827171 Email: charlotte.proby@cancer.org.uk — MB BS Lond. 1982; BA Oxf. 1979; MRCP (UK) 1986. Sen. Lect. (Hon. Cons.) (Dermat.) St Bart. & The Roy. Lond. Sch. of Med. & Dent., Qu. Mary & Westfield Coll. Lond. Specialty: Dermat. Socs: Fell. Roy. Soc. Med. (Sect. of Dermat.); Brit. Assn. Dermat.; Brit. Soc. Investig. Dermat. Prev: Sen. Regist. (Dermat.) St John's Inst. Dermat. St Thomas' Hosp. Lond.; Wellcome Research Fell. Experimen. Dermatol. Lond. Hosp.; Regist. (Dermatol.) St. Geo. Hosp. Lond.

PROCTER, Andrew William Rawnsley Building, Manchester Royal Infirmary, Oxford Road, Manchester M13 9BX — MB BS Lond. 1981; PhD Lond. 1992, MB BS 1981; MA Camb. 1982; MRCPsych 1985; FRCPsych 2000. Cons. Psychiat. Manch. Roy. Infirm. & Hon. Clin. Sen. Lect. Univ. Manch. Specialty: Gen. Psychiat. Prev: Sen. Lect. (Psychiat.) United. Med. & Dent. Sch. Guy's Hosp. Lond.

PROCTER, Ann Marie 12 Windermere Avenue, Roath Park, Cardiff CF23 5PQ — MB BCh Wales 1985; MRCP (UK) 1990.

PROCTER, Anne Elisabeth X-Ray Department, Northern General Hospital, Herries Road, Sheffield S5 7AU Tel: 0114 243 4343 — MB ChB Sheff. 1979; FRCR 1986. Cons. Diag. Radiol. N. Gen. Hosp. NHS Trust Sheff. Specialty: Radiol.

PROCTER, Claire Nicola Netherhouses, Rochester, Newcastle upon Tyne NE19 1RX Tel: 01830 20411 — MB BS Newc. 1983. Specialty: Gen. Psychiat.

PROCTER, David Brian, Squadron Ldr. RAF Med. Br. — MB BCh Wales 1990; MRCGP 1995; DRCOG 1995; DFFP 1995; Dip Theraputic (HWCM) 1998; L/A Vesectory 2004. GP Aldermoor Surg. Soton. Prev: Dep. Sen. Med. Off. RAF Laarbruch; SHO (Psychiat.) Princess Alexandra Hosp. Wroughton; SHO (O & G) Roy. United Hosp. Bath.

PROCTER, Denis 15 Ilton Garth, Clifton, York YO30 4XJ Tel: 01904 693240 — (Liverp. & Cardiff) LMSSA Lond. 1955; MRCS Eng. LRCP Lond. 1957; DA Eng. 1958; DPM Eng. 1964; FRANZCP 1983, M 1968; MRCPsych 1973. Hon. Cons. (Psychiat.) Birch Hill Hosp. Rochdale. Specialty: Gen. Psychiat. Prev: Cons. (Psychiat.) Birch Hill Hosp. Rochdale.

PROCTER, Elizabeth Ann Canada House, Barnsole Road, Gillingham ME7 4JL Tel: 01634 583000 Fax: 01634 583048 — MB ChB Bristol 1976; BSc (Hons.) Psychol. Bristol 1973; MMedSci Leeds 1994; MRCPsych 1994. Cons. Child Adolesc. Psychiat., Canada Ho., Gillingham. Specialty: Child & Adolesc. Psychiat.

PROCTER, Gillian Sarah Ropery Road Surgery, 2A Ropery Road, Gainsborough DN21 2NL Tel: 01427 612895 Fax: 01427 811763 — MB ChB Manch. 1980; DFFP. RCOG 1995; Dip. Occ. Med. Manch. 1996; L.F.Hom 1998. Socs: Soc. Occupat. Med.; Roy. Soc. Med.

PROCTER, Heather Mary Clarendon Medical Practice, Clarendon Street, Hyde SK14 2AQ Tel: 0161 368 5224 Fax: 0161 368 4767 — MB ChB Leeds 1981; DLO RCS Eng. 1986; MRCGP 1994; MFFP 1994. Clin. Asst. (ENT) Tameside Gen. Hosp. Prev: Trainee GP HildenBoro..

PROCTER, James Jason 29 Parkland Terrace, Meanwood, Leeds LS6 4PW — MB ChB Leeds 1998.

PROCTER, Julian Christopher Hollies Surgery, 83 Birch Lane, Dukinfield SK16 4AJ Tel: 0161 330 2039 Fax: 0161 330 5149; 440 Huddersfield Road, Carrbrook, Stalybridge SK15 3JP — MB ChB Liverp. 1981.

PROCTER, Laura 78 Southborough Road, Bickley, Bromley BR1 2EN — MB BS Lond. 1981.

PROCTER, Malcolm Scott The Surgery, 1 Crawley Lane, Pound Hill, Crawley RH10 7DX Tel: 01293 549916 Fax: 01293 615382 — MB BS Lond. 1983; DRCOG 1987; MRCGP 1988.

PROCTER, Robbyn Simone A&E, Wronswood Branch, Newtown Road, Worcester WR1; 21 Himbleton Road, St Johns, Worcester WR2 6BA Tel: 01905 428450 — BM Nottm. 1991; DCH; DRCOG; DFFP; BM BS Nottm. 1991. Sen. Trust Dr. (A&E). Specialty: Accid. & Emerg. Prev: GP Locum Worcester; Worcester VTS Scheme.

PROCTOR, Andrew James Hill House, Melbury Rd, Newcastle upon Tyne NE7 7DE — BM BS Nottm. 1997.

PROCTOR, David Wilson Howeburn, Auchattie, Banchory AB31 6PT Tel: 0133 022205 — MB ChB Aberd. 1961; DObst RCOG 1963; FFA RCS Eng. 1968. Anaesth. Regist. Aberd. Roy. Infirm. Specialty: Anaesth. Prev: Med. Regist. Aberd. Roy. Infirm.

PROCTOR, Mr Edward The Cottage, Penbidwal Lane, Pandy, Abergavenny NP7 8EA Tel: 01873 890269 — (Westm.) BA Keele 1954; MB BS Lond. 1960; MRCS Eng. LRCP Lond. 1960; MD Lond. 1974; FRCS Eng. 1986. Linder Foundat. Research Fell. RCS Unit Biophysics Inst. Child Health Lond. Specialty: Neurol. Socs: BMA; Roy. Soc. Med. Prev: Surg. Research Fell. (Thoracic Surg.) Guy's Hosp. Lond.; Ho. Surg. & Ho. Phys. St. Chas. Hosp. Lond.

PROCTOR, Edward Andrew (retired) Elm Tree Farm, Grove, Canterbury CT3 4BN Tel: 01227 722280 — MB BS Lond. 1968 (Roy. Free) MRCS Eng. LRCP Lond. 1967; FFA RCS Eng. 1976. Prev: Anaesth. Canterbury & Thanet Health Auth.

PROCTOR, Gillian 22 Sunniside Drive, South Shields NE34 8DH — MB ChB Glas. 1997.

PROCTOR, Harold Leslie, RD (retired) Rosecroft, Furzeley Corner, Denmead, Waterlooville PO7 6TS Tel: 023922 262192 — (Leeds) MB ChB Leeds 1959. Prev: Ho. Surg. (Obst.) St. Mary's Hosp. Portsmouth.

PROCTOR, Mr Henry (retired) 7 Tudor Grove, Sutton Coldfield B74 2LL Tel: 0121 353 9855 — MB BS Durh. 1938 (Durh. & St. Bart.) FRCS Ed. 1948. Hon. Cons. Birm. AHA (T). Prev: Cons. Surg. Birm. Accid. Hosp.

PROCTOR, Iain Lochee Health Centre, 1 Marshall Street, Lochee, Dundee DD2 3BR Tel: 01382 611283 Fax: 01382 624480 — MB BCh BAO Belf. 1988 (Qu. Univ. Belf.) DRCOG 1991; MRCGP 1993. GP Lochee Health Centre Dundee. Specialty: Gen. Pract. Socs: MDDUS. Prev: Locum GP; Staff Grade (Med.) Coleraine Hosp.; SHO (Paediat. & Med.) Coleraine Hosp.

PROCTOR, Ian Reginald Davidson (retired) Terwwnnack, Budock Vean Lane, Mawnan Smith, Falmouth TR11 5LH Tel: 01326 250253 Fax: 01326 250253 — (Camb. & St. Bart.) BA Camb. 1944; MB BChir Camb. 1947; MRCS Eng. LRCP Lond. 1947; MRCGP 1957. Prev: Flight Lt. RAFVR 1947-50.

PROCTOR, Janet Louise Chapel Lane Surgery, 13 Chapel Lane, Formby, Liverpool L37 4DT; Alt Road, Hightown, Liverpool L38 3RH — MB ChB Liverp. 1988.

PROCTOR, John Charles Christopher Stag Medical Centre, 162 Wickersley Road, Rotherham S60 4JW Tel: 01709 379285 Fax: 01709 820431 — MB ChB Sheff. 1982 (Sheffield) DRCOG 1986. Hosp. Practitioner, Dermat. Rotherham Gen. Hosp., Rotherham. Prev: SHO (Med.) Roy. Hallamsh. Hosp. Sheff.; SHO (O & G) Nether Edge Hosp. Sheff.; SHO (Paediat. & A & E) Childr. Hosp. Sheff.

PROCTOR, Mr Mark Timothy Kingston General Hospital, Galsworthy Road, Kingston upon Thames KT2 7QB Tel: 020 8546 7711 — MB BS Lond. 1983; MA Camb. 1984; FRCS Eng. 1987; FRCS (Orth.) 1994. Cons. Orthop. Surg. Qu. Mary's Hosp. Lond. Specialty: Orthop. Socs: Assoc. Mem. Brit. Orthopaedic Assn.; Roy. Soc. Med.; Brit. Elbow & Shoulder Soc. Prev: Sen. Regist. & Regist. (Orthop.) Roy. Lond. Hosp. & Roy. Nat. Orthop. Hosp. Stanmore.

PROCTOR, Martyn Charles Davidson Lemon Street Surgery, 18 Lemon Street, Truro TR1 2LZ Tel: 01872 273133 Fax: 01872 260900; Boscolla Farm, Kenwyn, Truro TR4 9EB Tel: 01872 264268 Fax: 01872 260900 — MB BS Lond. 1976 (St. Bart.) MRCS Eng. LRCP Lond. 1976; DRCOG 1979; Cert. Family Plann. JCC 1979; D.Occ.Med. RCP Lond. 1996. Med. Off. Truro High Sch. For Girls. Specialty: Care of the Elderly; Occupat. Health. Socs: BMA; Soc. Occupat. Med. Prev: Trainee GP Cornw. & Is. Scilly VTS.

PROCTOR, Robin David — BM BCh Oxf. 1999; DFFP; MRCP; DRCOG; MA; MRCGP. GP; Expedition Med. Off.; Clin. Asst. (A & E).

PROCTOR, Shirley Joyce Rennet Alloa Health Centre, Marshill, Alloa FK10 1AQ Tel: 01259 216476 — MB ChB Aberd. 1987.

PROCTOR, Stephen Clifford Clarendon Medical Practice, Clarendon Street, Hyde SK14 2AQ Tel: 0161 368 5224 Fax: 0161 366 6303 — MB ChB Sheff. 1979; DObst RCOG 1982. Prev: GP Doncaster VTS; Ho. Off. (Med.) Lodge Moor Hosp. Sheff.; Ho. Off. (Surg.) Lincoln Co. Hosp.

PROCTOR, Professor Stephen John Academic Haematology, Medical School, Framlington Place, Newcastle upon Tyne NE2 4HH; Hill House, Melbury Road, Newcastle upon Tyne NE7 7DE — (University Newcastle upon Tyne) MB BS Newc. 1970; MRCP (UK) 1973; FRCPath 1989, M 1978; FRCP Lond. 1985. Prof. Haemat. Med. Roy. Vict. Infirm. Newc.; Head Acad. Haem. Newc. Uni. Specialty: Haematology. Prev: Dir. Leukaemia Research Fund Remission Unit.; Head of Sch. - Clin. & Laborat. Scis.

PROCTOR, Susan Elizabeth St. George's Hospital, Morpeth NE61 2NU Tel: 01670 512121 — MB BS Newc. 1970; FRCPsych 1996, M 1979. Cons. Psychiat. St. Geo. Hosp. Morpeth. Specialty: Gen. Psychiat. Prev: Sen. Regist. (Psychiat.) Newc. Gen. Hosp.

PROCTOR, Thomas Augustus Pugh (retired) 11 Oakhill Drive, Prestatyn LL19 9PU Tel: 0174 562522 — LMSSA Lond. 1928 (Birm)

PRODHAN, Chitta Ranjan 2 Greenstone Place, Dundee DD2 4XB Tel: 01382 641725 — MB BS Calcutta 1957 (R.G. Kar Med. Coll.)

PRODHAN, Masud Salam Gloucester House Medical Centre, 17 Station Road, Urmston, Manchester M41 9JS Tel: 0161 748 7115 Fax: 0161 749 8032; Pinecroft, 38 Gibwood Road, Northenden, Manchester M22 4BS Tel: 0161 998 2451 — MB ChB Manch. 1992; MRCGP 1996. GP Princip. Urmston; GP Locum. Socs: BMA; (Dep. Chairm.) Gt.er Manch. Locum Gp. Prev: SHO (Psychogeriat.) Roy. Oldham Hosp. Trust; GP/Regist. Brooklands Med. Pract. Manch.

PRODROMOU, Salima — MB BS Lond. 1993 (University College London) DRCOG 1996; DCH 1996. Specialty: Gen. Pract. Socs: Roy. Coll. Gen. Pract.

PROFFITT, Catherine Mary St Michaels Surgery, Walwyn Close, Twerton-on-Avon, Bath BA2 1ER Tel: 01225 428277 Fax: 01225 338484 — BM BS Nottm. 1978; DCH RCP Lond. 1983; MRCGP 1983; DRCOG 1984; MFFP 1996.

PROFFITT, Dorothy 229 Leesons Hill, Chislehurst BR7 6QJ Tel: 01689 818277; 84 Long Lane, Grays RM16 2PL Tel: 01375 384246 — MCRS Eng. LRCP Lond. 1983 (Sheffield) DCH RCP Lond. 1987. Staff Grade (Paediat.) Greenwich Healthcare Trust. Specialty: Community Child Health. Socs: BACDA; Assoc. of Brit. Paed. Soc. For CME; BACCH (Comm. CH). Prev: Clin. Med. Off. Optimum Trust Lond.; Clin. Med. Off. & Trainee Clin. Med. Off. Basildon & Thurrock HA; Ho. Off. Grimsby HA.

PROKOP, Renate 82 Ninian Road, Roath Park, Cardiff CF23 5EP — MB BCh Wales 1996.

PROKOP, Stanislaw (retired) 16 Camborne Road, Sutton SM2 6RH Tel: 020 8642 4602 — MB BS Lond. 1975 (St. Bart.) BSc (Hons.) (Pharmacol.) Lond. 1972, MB BS 1975; MRCPsych 1980. Prev: Cons. Child & Adolesc. Psychiat. Croydon Child Guid. Clinic.

PROLL, Sabine Accident & Emergency Department, Charing Cross Hospital, Fulham Palace Road, London W6 8RF; Flat 8, Lister Court, Pasteur Close, London NW9 5HZ — State Exam Med Aachen 1993.

PRONER, Barry David 83 Strand-on-the-Green, London W4 3PU Tel: 020 8995 8319 Fax: 020 8995 8319 Email: barry.proner@blueyonder.co.uk — MD Wayne State 1967 (Wayne State Univ. Detroit) Adult Psychia. & Child Psychia. Qualifications Harvard Med. Sch.; BA Cornell 1962. Indep. Jungian Psychoanal. Adults & Childr. Lond.; Co-Dir. Child Analytic Train. Soc. Analyt. Psychol.; Train. Analyst Soc. Analyt. Psychol. (Adult & Child Anal.); Train. Therapist. Brit. Assn. Psychother. & Lond. Centre for; Psychother. Prev: Med. Dir. C.G. Jung Childr. Clinic; Cons. Child Psychiat. Hounslow Child Guid. Clin.; Clin. Asst. (Child & Family Psychiat.) W. Lond. & Char. Cross Hosps.

PRONGER, Elizabeth Ann 13 Ashburnham Road, Hastings TN35 5JN — MB BS Lond. 1996.

PROOPS, Mr David William Department of Otolarygoscopy, Queen Elizabeth Hospital, University Hospital Birmingham, Edgbaston, Birmingham B15 2TH Tel: 0121 627 2296 Fax: 0121 627 2296 Email: david.proops@uhb.nhs.uk — MB ChB Birm. 1975 (Birmingham) BDS (Hons.) Birm. 1969; FRCS Eng. 1980. Cons. ENT Surg. Qu. Eliz. Hosp. & Childr. Hosp. Birm.; President British Ass Otolaryngology, Head & Neck Surg RCS. Specialty: Otolaryngol. Socs: BMA; RSM; MID. Prev: Pres. Sect. of Otol. Roy. Soc. of Med.

PROPHET, Lynne Elizabeth 3 Dalrymple Place, Dundee DD2 2DN Tel: 01382 566679 Email: lyprop@aol.com — MB ChB Ed. 1992; BSc (Med. Sci) Hons. Human Genetics Ed. 1991. NCCG Anaesthetics

Borders Gen. Hosp. Melrose. Specialty: Anaesth. Prev: SHO (Anaesth.) Vict. Hosp. Kirkcaldy; SHO (Med.) Qu. Margt. Hosp. Dunfermline; SHO (Med.) West. Gen. Hosp. & Renal Unit Roy. Infirm. Edin.

PROPHET, Michael John (retired) Rose Cottage, Camp Road, Oldbury on Severn, Bristol BS35 1PR Tel: 01454 411154 Fax: 01454 411154 — MB BS Lond. 1955 (King's Coll. Hosp.) MRCS Eng. LRCP Lond. 1955. Prev: Sen. Med. Off. Dept. Health & Social Security.

PROPPER, David John Department of Medical Oncology, St. Bart's. Hospital, London EC1A 7BE Tel: 020 7601 7460 — MB ChB Liverp. 1982; MRCP (UK) 1985; MD Aberd. 1993. Cons. Med. Onc. St. Bart's. Hosp. Lond. Specialty: Oncol. Prev: ICRF Sen. Regist. (Med. Oncol.) Churchill Hosp. Oxf.; MRC Clin. Research Fell. Univ. Aberd.; Sen. Regist. Research Unit Univ. Leeds.

PROSSER, Barbara Mary (retired) 85 Winterbourne Close, Hastings TN34 1XQ Tel: 01424 425134 — MB BChir Camb. 1951 (Camb. & Roy. Free) MRCS Eng. LRCP Lond. 1948. Prev: SCMO Hastings HA.

PROSSER, Dacre John Herbert (retired) The Vinery, The Hill, Swanton Abbott, Norwich NR10 5EA Tel: 01692 538458 — MRCS Eng. LRCP Lond. 1955 (St. Geo.) MB Camb. 1955, BChir 1954; DObst RCOG 1960. Prev: Ho. Surg. St. Geo. Hosp. Lond.

PROSSER, David Keith Lloyd Maudsley Hospital, Denmark Hill, London SE5 — MB BChir Camb. 1989; MRCS Eng LRCP Lond. 1988.

PROSSER, Donald Ivor (retired) Flat 1, Mystole House, Chartham, Canterbury — MB BS Lond. 1961 (St. Bart.) FRCP Lond. 1984, M 1968. Cons. Phys. (Renal & Gen. Med.) Kent & Canterbury Hosp. Prev: Lect. (Med.) Westm. Hosp. Lond.

PROSSER, Elizabeth Joan Shrubbery Avenue Surgery, 13 Shrubbery Avenue, Worcester WR1 1QN Tel: 01905 22888 — MB BS Lond. 1962 (Char. Cross) DObst RCOG 1964; MFFP 1993. Sen. Clin. Med. Off. (Family Plann.) Worcester Community Trust; Clin. Asst. Worcester Dist. Hosp. Trust. Specialty: Family Plann. & Reproduc. Health. Socs: Midl. Ophth. Soc.; W Midl. Menopause Soc. Prev: Med. Off.(Family Plann.) Cardiff; SHO (O & G) Centr. Middlx. Hosp. Lond.

PROSSER, Gareth Harding 79 Three Acres Lane, Dickens Heath, Solihull B90 1NZ — MB ChB Manch. 1994; FRCS.

PROSSER, John Allen Croft House, 32 Albany Terrace, Worcester WR1 3DY Tel: 01905 20387 Fax: 01905 20387; Croft house, 32 Albany Terrace, Worcester WR1 3DY Tel: 01905 20387 Fax: 01905 20387 — MB BS Lond. 1963 (Char. Cross) DA Eng. 1965; FFA RCS Eng. 1967. Cons. Anaesth. Worcester Roy. Infirm.; Curator of Med. museum, Worcester. Specialty: Anaesth. Socs: Assn. Anaesths.

PROSSER, John Keith, MBE The Surgery, 6 College Road, Eastbourne BN21 4HY Tel: 01323 735044 Fax: 01323 417705; 15 Milton Crescent, Eastbourne BN21 1SP Tel: 01323 639881 — MB ChB Ed. 1968; DTM & H Ed. 1970; MRCGP 1982. GP. Prev: Regional Med. Off. S.A.M.S. Paraguay, S. America.

PROSSER, Jonathan George Stenson Osborn Clinic, Osborn Road, Fareham PO16 7ES Tel: 01329 822220 — MB BS Newc. 1988 (Newcastle) MRCPsych 1993; CCST Child & Adol. Psychiat 1998. Cons. (Child & Adol. Psychiat.) Fareham & Gosport, Hants. Specialty: Child & Adolesc. Psychiat.; Psychother. Prev: Sen. Regist. Rotat. (Child Psychiat.) Newc.

PROSSER, Lyn Julia Upwell Street Surgery, 93 Upwell Street, Sheffield S4 8AN Tel: 0114 261 8608 — MB ChB Sheff. 1981.

PROSSER, Oswald Andrew (retired) Hazeldene, 103 Hardhorn Road, Poulton-le-Fylde FY6 8AY — MB BCh Witwatersrand 1950; BSc Witwatersrand 1941; DCH Eng. 1953; DPH Eng. 1966. Prev: PMO DHSS.

PROSSER, Patricia Delphine Nuffield Health Centre, Welch Way, Witney OX28 6JQ Tel: 01993 703641 — MB BCh BAO Dub. 1975; DCH 1979; DObst RCPI 1980; MRCOG 1982; MRCGP 1983; MFFP 1993. Prev: Med. Off. Donald Fraser Hosp. Rep. Venda, N. Transvaal, S. Africa; Ho. Off. Nat. Childr. Hosp. Dub.; Ho. Off. Rotunda Hosp. Dub.

PROSSER, Ruth Ellen 13 Twyford Abbey Road, London NW10 7HH — MB BS Lond. 1992. SHO (A & E) St. Richard's Hosp. Chichester W. Sussex. Specialty: Accid. & Emerg. Prev: Ho. Off. (Surg.) St. Richard's Hosp. Chichester; Ho. Off. (Med.) Worthing Dist. Hosp.

PROSSER, Susan Elizabeth Abbey Medical Centre, 42 Station Road, Kenilworth CV8 1JD Tel: 01926 852576 Fax: 01926 851746 — MB BCh Wales 1982.

PROSSER, Yvonne Ingrid Jennifer Cherry Hayes, Newtown Road, Awbridge, Romsey SO51 0GG — MB BS Lond. 1989 (Charing Cross & Westminster) T(GP) 1994; MRCGP 1994. GP, Twyford, Hants.

PROSSOR, John Eckford 173 Ashley Road, Parkstone, Poole BH14 9DL; The Croft, 5 Ravine Road, Canford Cliffs, Poole BH13 7HS — MB ChB Leic. 1984; DCH RCP Lond. 1986; DRCOG 1987; MRCGP 1989.

PROTHERO, David Priory Hospital North London The Bourne, Southgate, London N14 6RA Tel: 020 8882 8191 Fax: 020 8447 8138; Four Elms, Spring Lane, Lower Ufford, Woodbridge IP13 6EF — MB BS Lond. 1960 (Univ. Coll. Hosp.) MRCS Eng. LRCP Lond. 1960; DPM Eng. 1964; FRCPsych 1985, M 1971. Cons. Psychiat. Priory Hosp. N. Lond. Specialty: Gen. Psychiat. Prev: Cons. Psychiat. Claybury Hosp. & St. Margt. Hosp. Epping.

PROTHERO, Joanna Dawn 71 Durham Road, Rainham, Gillingham ME8 0JJ — BM Soton. 1995.

PROTHEROE, Andrew Simon 7 Falcon Close, Otley LS21 3EG — MB BS Lond. 1990; MRCP (UK) 1994. SHO (Med.) King's Coll. Hosp. Lond.

PROTHEROE, Clement Keith Armada Surgery, 28 Oxford Place, Plymouth PL1 5AJ Tel: 01752 665805 Fax: 01752 220056; Little Court, St. Ive, Liskeard PL14 3ND Tel: 01579 362509 — MB ChB Bristol 1956. Prev: Ho. Surg. Cossham Hosp. Kingswood; Ho. Phys. Scott Isolat. Hosp. Plymouth.

PROTHEROE, Colin (retired) 20 Adeline Gardens, Kenton, Newcastle upon Tyne NE3 4JQ Tel: 0191 285 3080 — (Sheff.) MD Sheff. 1965, MB ChB 1953; MRCS Eng. LRCP Lond. 1953; DPM Durham. 1959; FRCP Ed. 1973, M 1960; FRCPsych 1974, M 1972. Prev: Cons. Psychiat. Newc. HA.

PROTHEROE, David Trevelyan Long Barn, Charlton, Kilmersdon, Bath BA3 5TN Tel: 01761 32326 — BM BCh Oxf. 1963; MA Oxf., BM BCh 1963; FFA RCS Eng. 1969. Cons. Anaesth. Bath Clin. Area. Specialty: Anaesth.

PROTHEROE, Dinah Elizabeth Drumhar Health Centre, North Methven St., Perth PH1 5PD Tel: 01738 564215 Fax: 01738 444410/01738 564293 Email: dinah.protheroe@tuht.scot.nhs.uk; Bellfield, Dalguise, Dunkeld PH8 0JU Tel: 01350 727380 Fax: 01350 727453 — (Univ. Camb. Girton Coll. & Univ. Oxf. Med. Sch.) MB BChir (Cantab); MA Camb. 1975; MB BChir Camb. 1975; DRCOG 1977; MRCP (UK) 1978; DCH RCP Lond. 1979; Cert. Prescribed Equiv. Exp. JCPTGP 1990; FRCPCH 1997. Cons. Community Paediat. Tayside Univ. Hosp.s NHS Trust; Med. Adviser, Perth & Kinross Fostering and Permanence Panel. Specialty: Community Child Health; Paediat. Special Interest: Child Protec. Prev: SCMO Perth & Kinross Healthcare NHS Trust; Assoc. GP Hong Kong.

PROTHEROE, Joanne Brier Cottage, 15 Arthog Road, Hale, Altrincham WA15 0NA Tel: 0161 980 2864 — MB ChB Bristol 1991; DFFP 1993; MRCGP 1997. MRC Research Traiing Fdellow, NPCRDC, Williamson Building, Univ. of Manch.; GP Sessions, Rusholne, Health Centre, Manch. Specialty: Gen. Pract.; Research. Socs: Brit. Med. Assn.; Assn. of Univ. Dept.s of Gen. Pract. Prev: SHO (O & G) Derriford Hosp. Plymouth; GP Retainer-Hanham Bristol.

PROTHEROE, Mr Keith (retired) 13 Arden Drive, Giffnock, Glasgow G46 7AF Tel: 0141 638 4185 — (Ed.) MB ChB Ed. 1956; FRCS Ed. 1964. Prev: Cons. Orthop. Surg. Glas. Roy. Infirm.

PROTHEROE, Mark Christopher Nettleham Medical Practice, 14 Lodge Lane, Nettleham, Lincoln LN2 2RS Tel: 01522 751717 Fax: 01522 754474 — BM Soton. 1991; BSc Wales 1986; DFFP 1996. GP Princip. Nettleham. Specialty: Gen. Pract. Socs: BMA; Soc. Wessex Grad.s; Christ. Med. Fellowsh. (Regional Represen.). Prev: SHO (O & G) Roy. Bournemouth Hosp.; SHO (Paediat. & ENT) Poole Gen. Hosp.; SHO (Palliat. Care & Rheum.) ChristCh. Hosp. Dorset.

PROTHEROE, Rachel Elizabeth — MB BS Lond. 1998.

PROTHEROE, Richard Trevelyan Intensive Care Unit, Hope Hospital, Stott Lane, Salford M6 8HD Tel: 0161 789 7373 Email: richard.protheroe@srht.nhs.uk; Brier Cottage, 15 Arthog Road, Hale, Altrincham WA15 0NA Tel: 0161 980 2864 — MB BS Lond. 1988 (St Thomas') MRCS Eng LRCP Lond. 1988; MRCP (UK) 1993; DA

(UK) 1995; FRCA 1996. Cons. Anaesth. With interest in Critical Care, Hope Hosp. Salford. Specialty: Anaesth.; Intens. Care. Socs: BMA; Assn. Anaesth.; Intens. Care Soc. Prev: Sen. Clin. Fell. In Anaesth. Bristol Roy. Infirm..; Sen. Regist. ICU, Roy. Adelaide Hosp. Adelaide, S.Australia; Specialist Regist. Rotat. (Anaesth.) Bristol.

PROTHEROE, Roger Henry Bertram (retired) 4 Riverside Drive, Solihull B91 3HH — (Camb. & Westm.) MA, MD Camb. 1956, MB BChir 1947; FRCPath 1972, M 1964. Prev: Cons. Pathol. E. Birm. & Solihull Hosps.

PROTHEROE, Susan Alison Boultham Park Medical Practice, Boultham Park Road, Lincoln LN6 7SS Tel: 01522 874444 Fax: 01522 874466 — (Univ. Soton.) BM Soton 1984; DRCOG 1988. GP Partner. Specialty: Alcohol & Substance Misuse. Socs: BMA; Christ. Med. Fellowsh. Prev: Staff Psychiat. Addic. Serv. E. Dorset; Regist. (Psychiat.) St. Ann's Hosp. Poole; Trainee GP/SHO Highcliffe & Poole Gen. Hosp.

PROTOPAPAS, Michael dept of anaesthetics, Darent Valley hospital, Darenthwood road, Dartford DA2 8DA Tel: 01322 428100 Fax: 01322 428652 — MB BS Lond. 1988 (St Marys Hospital medical school) BSc Lond. 1985; DA (UK) 1990; FRCA 1993. Cons. Anaesth. Specialty: Anaesth.; Intens. Care. Socs: BMA; FRCA; AAGBI. Prev: Sen. Regist. ITU Guys Hosp.; Specialist Regist. (spr) anaesthetics UCH/Roy. free Rotat.; Regist. anaesthetics Guys Hosp. Lonodn.

PROUD, Mr George (retired) Newcastle Nuffield Hospital, Clayton Road, Newcastle upon Tyne NE2 1JP Tel: 0191 281 6131; Cartref, Marchburn Lane, Riding Mill NE44 6DN Tel: 01434 682393 Fax: 01434 682781 Email: george@g-proud-frcs.demon.co.uk — MB BS Newc. 1971; BDS Durham. 1966; FRCS Eng. 1976; MD Newc. 1980; FRCS Ed 2000. p/t Member Medical Reference Panel Department of Trade & Industry for Vibration White Finger; Sen. Lect. (Surg.) Newc. Univ.; Mem. Fac. Occ. Health Working Party Hand-Arm Vibration Syndrome; Mem. HSE Workshop Hand Arm Vibration Syndrome; Ct. Examr. RCS Eng.; Regional Adviser RCS Eng.; Mem. Train. Bd. & the Hosp. Recognition Comm. RCS. Prev: Cons. Surg. (Endocrine & Vasc. Surg.) Newc. AHA (T).

PROUD, Rena Danae (retired) 1 Kidbrooke Gardens, London SE3 0PD — MB BS Lond. 1957 (Roy. Free) DPM Eng. 1963; MRCPsych 1973. Cons. Psychiat. Greenwich Dist. Hosp.

PROUDFOOT, Alexander Thompson (retired) 8 Mortonhall Park Avenue, Edinburgh EH17 8BP Tel: 0131 664 3942 — MB ChB Ed. 1962; BSc (Hons.) Ed. 1959; FRCP Ed. 1974, M 1965; FRCP Lond. 1994. Cons. Phys. Roy. Infirm. Edin.; Dir. Scott. Poisons Informat. Bureau.

PROUDFOOT, David James Hillbank Health Centre, Flat 1A, 1 Constitution Street, Dundee DD3 6NF Tel: 01382 221976 Fax: 01382 201980; 1 Glamis Terrace, Dundee DD2 1NA — MB ChB Dundee 1983; DRCOG 1986.

PROUDFOOT, Elizabeth McGruther (retired) 21 Inverary Terrace, Dundee DD3 6BR Tel: 01382 224490 — MB ChB Glas. 1948 (Univ. Glas.) Prev: Princip. GP Tayside HB.

PROUDFOOT, Frederick Buchan (retired) 21 Inverary Terrace, Dundee DD3 6BR Tel: 01382 224490 — MD Glas. 1979 (Univ. Glas.) MB ChB 1947; FRCGP 1981, M 1967. Prev: Princip. GP Tayside HB.

PROUDFOOT, Michael Crawford Hospital Hill Surgery, 7 Izatt Avenue, Dunfermline KY11 3BA Tel: 01383 731721 Fax: 01383 623352; Fernbank, 2 Bruccharen Road, Limekilns, Dunfermline KY11 3YZ — MB ChB Dundee 1976.

PROUDFOOT, Ronald Thomas Calabar, Pica, Workington CA14 4PZ — MB ChB Glas. 1974; FFA RCSI 1980. Specialty: Anaesth.

PROUDLOVE, Derek Allan Psychological Services Dept., Mulberry House, Alder Hey Hospital, Eaton road, Liverpool L12 2AP Tel: 0151 252 5586 Email: derek.proudlove@rlch-tr.nwest.nhs.uk — MB ChB Leeds 1988; MRCPsych 1994; MA Sheff. 1995. Cons child & Adolesc. Psychiat. Specialty: Child & Adolesc. Psychiat. Prev: Sen. Regist. Rotat. (Child & Adolesc. Psychiat.) Sheff.

PROUDLOVE, Robert Forth View Practice, Dean Road, Bo'ness EH51 0DQ Tel: 01506 822466 Fax: 01506 826216; 47 Green Tree Lane, Bo'ness EH51 0PH — MB ChB Manch. 1978; MRCGP 1982.

PROUSE, Peter Joseph The North Hampshire Hospital, Aldermaston Road, Basingstoke RG24 9NA Tel: 01256 313644 Fax: 01256 313645 Email: drpeter.prouse@nhht.nhs.uk — MB BS Melbourne 1974; FRACP 1985; MD Melbourne 1987; FRCP 1992. Cons. (Rheum.) N. Hants. Hosp. Basingstoke. Specialty: Rheumatol. Special Interest: Inflammatory Polyarthritis & Paediatric Rheumatology; Metabolic Bone Disease. Socs: Amer. Coll. Rheum.; Brit. Soc. Rheum. Prev: Sen. Regist. & Hon. Scientif. Worker Northwick Pk. Hosp. & CRC Harrow.

PROUT, Elizabeth Jane (retired) Whitehaven, Bissoe Road, Carnon Downs, Truro TR3 6JA Tel: 01872 863015 — MB BS Lond. 1959 (Univ. Coll. Hosp.) BSc Lond. 1956; DCH Eng. 1962. Prev: Research Regist. (Hypertens.) Roy. Cornw. Hosp. Truro.

PROUT, Mr Jeremy Robert 27B The Ridgeway, Enfield EN2 8PB — MB BS (Distinc. Path & Surg.) Lond. 1991 (Middlx. Hosp. Med. Sch.) BSc (1st. cl. Hons. Pharmacol.) Lond. 1988; MRCP (UK) 1995; FRCS Eng. 1996; FRCA 2000. Specialty: Anaesth. Prev: SHO (Cardiothoracic Surg.) Roy. Brompton Hosp. Lond.; SHO Rotat. (Surg.) St. Mary's Hosp. Lond.; Ho. Surg. Middlx. Hosp. & Univ. Coll. Hosp. Lond.

PROUT, John Warwick, CStJ (retired) 9 Crownfields, Sevenoaks TN13 1EF Tel: 01732 454768 — MRCS Eng. LRCP Lond. 1953 (Liverp.) DIH Eng. 1965; MFOM RCP Lond. 1978. Prev: Sen. Med. Off. Ford Motor Co. Warley.

PROUT, Rachel 22 Ermin Close, Baydon, Marlborough SN8 2JQ — MB ChB Bristol 1998.

PROUT, Mr William Geoffrey The White Cottage, 39 Blackbrook Park Avenue, Fareham PO15 5JN Tel: 01329 280455 Fax: 01329 280455 — (St. Thos.) MB BS Lond. 1961; FRCS Eng. 1965. Cons. Surg. Portsmouth Hosp. Gp. Specialty: Gen. Surg. Socs: Fell. Roy. Soc. Med. Prev: Sen. Surg. Regist. St. Thos. Hosp. Lond.; Surg. Regist. Wolverhampton Hosp. Gp.; Ho. Surg. Renal Unit Roy. Postgrad. Med. Sch. Lond.

PROVAN, Alison Anne Community Child Health Offices, Aros, Lochgilphead Tel: 01546 2323; Ashfield Old School House, Achnamara, Lochgilphead PA31 8PT Tel: 01546 850245 Fax: 01546 850302 — MB ChB Leic. 1982. Staff Grade (Comm. Child Health) Aros Lochgilphead. Prev: Clin. Asst. (Psychiat.) Argyll & Bute Hosp. Lochgilphead.

PROVAN, Andrew Benjamin Haematology Department, Royal United Hospital, Bath BA1 3NG Tel: 01225 428331 Fax: 01225 461044; 79 Roselands Gardens, Highfield, Southampton SO17 1QJ Tel: 01703 550262 — MB ChB Leic. 1984; BSc Leic. 1979; MRCP (UK) 1988; MRCPath 1992. Sen. Regist. (Haemat.) Roy. S. Hants. Hosp. Soton. Specialty: Haematology. Prev: LRF Research Fell. Roy. S. Hants. Hosp. Soton.; Regist. (Haemat.) Stobhill Hosp. Glas.; Regist. (Med.) Bradford Roy. Infirm. Bradford.

PROVAN, Christopher David Elmbank Group, Foresterhill Health Centre, Westburn Road, Aberdeen AB25 2AY Tel: 01224 696949 Fax: 01224 691650; 32 Burns Road, Aberdeen AB15 4NS Tel: 01224 317644 — MB ChB Aberd. 1989. Specialty: Gen. Pract. Socs: Roy. Coll. Gen. Pract. Prev: Trainee GP Aberd. VTS; Ho. Off. (Surg.) Aberd. Roy. Infirm.; Ho. Off. (Geriat.) Woodend Gen. Hosp. Aberd.

PROVAN, David Hart (retired) 66 St Michaels Drive, Cupar KY15 5BS — MB ChB St. And. 1944; DMRD Eng. 1958. Prev: Cons. Radiol. E. Surrey HA.

PROVAN, Janice 32 Burns Road, Aberdeen AB15 4NS — MB ChB Dundee 1984; FRCS Glas. 1992. Staff Grade Surg. (ENT) Aberd. Roy. Infirm. Specialty: Otorhinolaryngol.

PROVERBS, Allan Graham (retired) 28 Beechwood Crescent, Chandlers Ford, Eastleigh SO53 5PA — MB ChB Ed. 1935. Prev: Ho. Phys. & Ho. Surg. St. Luke's Hosp. Bradford.

PROVOST, Gillian Claire Vineyard Hill Road Surgery, 67 Vineyard Hill Road, London SW19 7JL Tel: 020 8947 2579 — MB BS Lond. 1978; BSc (2nd cl. Hons.) Immunol. Lond. 1978, MB BS 1981; DRCOG 1987; MRCGP 1988.

PROWSE, Alan David 46 Badingham Drive, Leatherhead KT22 9HA Tel: 01372 373798 — MB BCh Wales 1956 (Cardiff) BSc Wales 1952; DObst RCOG 1957. Med. Adviser Lond. Country Bus Serv. Ltd., Lond. Links, Speed Link, Rawlinson, Hunter & Silvertech Ltd; Med. Examr. Min of Transport. Specialty: Occupat. Health. Socs: Soc. Occupat. Med.; BMA. Prev: Ho. Phys. Bridgend Gen. Hosp.; Ho. Surg. (O & G) Neath Gen. Hosp.

PROWSE, Graham David Windsor The Limes Medical Centre, 65 Leicester Road, Narborough, Leicester LE9 5DU — MB BS Lond. 1979 (Westm.) MA Camb. 1980, BA 1976; DRCOG 1981; MRCGP

1983. GP Leicester; GP Trainer Leicester VTS; Clin. Teach. Leicester Univ. Med. Sch.; Clin. Asst. UHL Breast Care Centre; Forens. Med. Examr. Leics. Police. Socs: Leic. Med. Soc.; SW Leicester GP Gp.; Anplo French Med. Soc. Prev: SHO Leicester Roy. Infirm.; SHO Geo. Eliot Hosp. Nuneaton; Ho. Off. St. Stephens Hosp. Chelsea & Walsgrave Hosp. Coventry.

PROWSE, Keith 540 Etruria Road, Basford, Newcastle ST5 0SX Tel: 01782 614419 Fax: 01782 630270 — MB ChB Birm. 1962; MRCS Eng. LRCP Lond. 1962; FRCP Lond. 1979, M 1966; BSc Birm. 1959, MD 1971. Private Pract. Specialty: Respirat. Med. Special Interest: Occupational Lung Dis. Socs: Eur. Respirat. Soc.; (Chairm. & Pres.) Brit. Thoracic Soc.; (Pres.) Eur. Bd. Pnenmology. Prev: Cons. Phys. (Respirat. Med.) N. Staffs Hosp. Stoke-on-Trent; Dir. RCP Int'l. Office.; Med. Dir. N. Staffs. Hosp.

PROWSE, Margaret Judith (retired) 46 Badingham Drive, Leatherhead KT22 9HA Tel: 01372 373798 — MB BCh Wales 1955 (Cardiff) BSc Wales 1952, MB BCh 1955. Prev: Clin. Asst. (Psychiat.) W. Pk. Hosp. Epsom.

PROWSE, Roger Beresford (retired) 1 The Orchard, South St., Uley, Dursley GL11 5ST — MB BChir Camb. 1950; DObst RCOG 1952.

PRUDHAM, Roger Christopher Fairfield General Hospital, Rochdale Old Road, Bury BL9 7TD Tel: 0161 778 2648 Fax: 0161 788 2642 Email: roger.prudham@pat.nhs.uk — MB BS Lond. 1992 (St. Bartholomew's Hosp. Med. Coll.) MRCP (UK) 1995. Specialty: Gastroenterol.; Gen. Med. Special Interest: Colonoscopy; Health Informatics. Socs: Manch. Med. Soc.; N. of Eng. Gastroenterol. Soc.; Brit. Soc. Gastroenterol. Prev: Regist. (Gastroenterol. & Gen. Med.) Hope Hosp. Salford; Cons. Gastroenterologist Pennine Acute Hosps. NHS Trust Bury.

PRUDHOE, Kenneth Glenpark Medical Centre, Ravensorth Road, Dunston, Gateshead NE11 9AD Tel: 0191 460 4300/0191 461 0106 Email: kenneth.prudhoe@nhs.net — MB BS Newc. 1979 (Newcastle upon Tyne) PhD Newc. 1971, BSc 1968; FRCGP 1991, M 1983; AFOM RCP Lond. 1990; CChem MRSC 1991. Trainer (Gen. Pract.) Northumbria VTS; BMA Occupat. Health Advis. Comm. Specialty: Occupat. Health. Socs: RCGP (Mem. Counc.). Prev: Trainee GP N.d. VTS.

PRUDHOE, Rosemary Houghton Houghton Health Centre, Church Street, Houghton-le-Spring DH4 4DN Tel: 0191 584 2106 Fax: 0191 584 9493; 29 L'Arbre Crescent, Whickham, Newcastle upon Tyne NE16 5YQ Tel: 0191 488 6273 — MB BS Newc. 1974 (Newcastle-upon-Tyne) BSc Newc. 1971; MRCP (UK) 1977; MRCGP 1984. Princip. GP (Reduced Committment) Houghton-le-Spring; Clin. Asst. Bone Metab. Freeman Hosp. Newc.-upon-Tyne. Prev: GP Jarrow; Regist. (Gen. Pract.) Cruddas Pk. & Felling Northumbria VTS; Regist. (Paediat.) Newc. Gen. Hosp.

PRUDO-CHLEBOSZ, Raymond Richard Zbigniew 71 Shepherds Hill, London N6 5RE — MB BS Lond. 1970; MRCS Eng. LRCP Lond. 1969; MRCPsych 1973; FRCPC 1979. Dir. (Outpats. & Community Psychiat.) McMaster Univ. Med. Centre Hamilton Ontario, Canada; Prof. Dept. Psychiat. McMaster Univ. Hamilton Ontario, Canada. Prev: Sen. Regist. Bethlem Hosp. & Maudsley Hosps. Lond.

PRUNTY, Mark John 110 Bedford Avenue, Hayes UB4 0DU — MB ChB Leeds 1983.

PRUSS, Anthony Ewen 607 Green Lane, Goodmayes, Ilford IG3 9RN Tel: 020 8597 3054 — MB BS Lond. 1970; BSc Lond. 1967; MRCS Eng. LRCP Lond. 1970; AFOM RCP Lond. 1981. Gen. Practitioner; Princip. Forens. Med. Examr. Metrop. Police. Specialty: Forens. Path. Socs: Assn. Police Surg.; BMA. Prev: SHO (Gen. Med. & Paediat.) King Geo. Hosp. Ilford.

PRUSSIA, Celia Mary Hoseley Bank Cottage, Park Lane, Rossett, Wrexham LL12 0BL — MB ChB Liverp. 1967 (Liverpool) DA Eng. 1970; DPhysMed Eng. 1972; Dip. Psychother. 1994. Clin. Asst. Psychoth.Maelor Gen Hosp.Wrexham; Private Psychoth. BUPA Yale Hosp.Wrexham; Vol. Mem. Ethics Sub-committee Liverp. Psychother. Diploma Organisation. Specialty: Psychother. Socs: BMA. Prev: Vol. Counsellor. Stepping stones Wrexham.

PRVULOVICH, Elizabeth Mary Institute of Nuclear Medicine, Middlesex Hospital, London W1N 8AA Tel: 020 7380 9387 Fax: 020 7637 0578 Email: l.prvulovich@nucmed.ucl.ac.uk — MB ChB Manch. 1985; MD Manch. 1993; MSc (Nuclear Med.) Lond. 1995. p/t Cons. Phys. in Nuclear Med. Middlx. Hosp. Lond. Specialty: Cardiol. Socs: Brit. Cardiac Soc.; Amer. Soc. Nuclear Cardiol.; Soc. Of Nuclear Med. Prev: Sen. Regist. (Nuclear Med.) Middlx. Hosp. Lond.; Regist. (Cardiac & Research Cardiac) Kings Coll. Hosp. Lond.

PRYCE, Andrew Charles William Dinas Lane Medical Centre, 149 Dinas Lane, Huyton, Liverpool L36 2NW Tel: 0151 489 2298 — MB BS Lond. 1985. Prev: Trainee GP W. Suff. Hosp. Bury St. Edmunds VTS.

PRYCE, Damian William Taunton & Somerset Hospital, Musgrove Park, Taunton TA1 5DA Tel: 01823 342789 Fax: 01823 336877; Rooks House, Bishopswood, Chard TA20 3RZ — MB BS Lond. 1978 (St. Bart.) MA Camb. 1979; MRCP (UK) 1983; DIH 1988; MFOM RCP Lond. 1989; FRCP 1999. Cons. Dermat. Taunton & Som. NHS Trust. Specialty: Dermat. Prev: Sen. Regist. (Dermat.) Roy. Liverp. Hosp.; Occupat. Phys. BP Research; Hon. Clin. Asst. St. John's Hosp. for Dis. of Skin Lond.

PRYCE, Douglas Paul Beech Hurst, 28 Queens Road, Waterlooville PO7 7SB — MB BS Lond. 1968; MRCS Eng. LRCP Lond. 1968; MRCGP 1975; DRCOG 1981.

PRYCE, Elizabeth Mary — MB BS Lond. 1989 (Charing Cross and Westminster) BSc Pharm. Lond. 1986; MRCGP (Distinc.) 1994; DFFP 1994; DRCOG 1996. Specialty: Gen. Pract.

PRYCE, Heather Anne 14 Castlemaine Avenue, Ewell, Epsom KT17 2RA — MB BS Lond. 1981; BSc Lond. 1978; Cert. Family Plann. JCC 1984; DRCOG 1984; MRCGP 1986. Specialty: Family Plann. & Reproduc. Health.

PRYCE, Ivor Gwyndaf (retired) 5 The Close, Llanishen, Cardiff CF14 5NG — MB BS Lond. 1951 (Univ. Coll. Hosp.) MRCS Eng. LRCP Lond. 1951; DPM Eng. 1957; MD Lond. 1961; FRCPsych 1981, M 1971. Prev: Cons. Psychiat. WhitCh. Hosp. Cardiff.

PRYCE, John Charles The Surgery, Limes Avenue, Alfreton DE55 7DW Tel: 01773 832525 — MB BS Lond. 1983 (Univ. Coll. Hosp.) DRCOG 1987. Prev: Trainee GP Avon VTS; SHO (Orthop.) Qu. Eliz. II Hosp. Welwyn Garden City; Ho. Off. (Surg.) Northampton Gen. Hosp.

PRYCE, Linda Susan Moordown Medical Centre, 2A Redhill Crescent, Bournemouth BH9 2XF Tel: 01202 516139 Fax: 01202 548525 — MB ChB Bristol 1974. GP Bournemouth.

PRYCE, Rebekah Anne — BM BCh Oxf. 1998; MRCPCH; MA.

PRYCE-JONES, Elizabeth (retired) 73 Temple Sheen Road, London SW14 7RS Tel: 020 8876 5070 — MB ChB Leeds 1948 (Leeds Univ.) DCH RCP Lond. 1955; FRCPCH 1997. Prev: Cons. Clin. Asst. (Child Health) St. Geo. Hosp. Med. Sch. Lond.

PRYDAL, Jeremy Ikley Leicester Royal infirmary, Infirmary Square, Leicester LE1 5WW Tel: 0116 258 6964 Email: jip@elmc.demon.co.uk; Elm Cottage, Main Street, Keyham, Leicester LE7 9JQ Tel: 0116 259 5389 Fax: 01223 464969 Email: j.prydal@elmc.demon.co.uk — MB BS Lond. 1982; PhD Camb. 1991; FRCOphth 1993; MD Lond. 1995. Specialty: Ophth.

PRYDE, Alan Neil Morton Howe of Fife Medical Practice, 27 Commercial Road, Ladybank, Cupar KY15 7JS Tel: 01337 830765 Fax: 01337 831658 — MB ChB Ed. 1982 (Edinburgh) DRCOG 1986; MRCGP 1986. Clin. Asst. (A & E) Perth Roy. Infirm.; Med. Off. Knockhill Racing Circuit Fife.

PRYDE, Iain 29 Auchmithie Place, Finglassie, Glenrothes KY7 4TY — MB ChB Ed. 1996.

PRYDE, Louise Anne The Health Centre, 80 Main Street, Kelty KY4 0AE Tel: 01738 622293 — MB ChB Dundee 1989; MRCGP 1995. Med. Practitioner HMP Perth.

PRYER, Anthony Alastair Wells City Practice, 22 Chamberlain Street, Wells BA5 2PF Tel: 01749 673356 Fax: 01749 670031 — BM BCh Oxf. 1983; MA Camb. 1983; DRCOG 1986; MRCGP 1987; DCH RCP Lond. 1987. Prev: Trainee GP Bath VTS.

PRYER, Michael Phillip Lorimer Clarkson Surgery, De-Havilland Road, Wisbech PE13 3AN Tel: 01945 583133 Fax: 01945 464465 — MB BS Lond. 1980.

PRYKE, David Simon Ewart Churchfields Surgery, Recreation Road, Bromsgrove B61 8DT Tel: 01527 872163; Ingewood, 38 New Road, Bromsgrove B60 2JJ Tel: 01527 575610 — MB BS Lond. 1987; MRCGP 1994.

PRYKE, Gillian Rachel Winyates Health Centre, Winyates, Redditch B98 0NR Tel: 01527 525533 Fax: 01527 517969 — MB BS Lond. 1989; MRCGP 1994. Specialty: Gen. Pract.

PRYKE, Jason Russell 41B Echo Barn Lane, Wrecclesham, Farnham GU10 4NG — MB BS Lond. 1994 (London) DCH RCP

Lond. 1998; DRCOG Lond. 1999; MRCGP 2000. Specialty: Gen. Pract.

PRYLE, Belinda Jane Anaesthetic Department, Gloucestershire Royal Hospital, Gloucester GL1 3NN Tel: 01452 528555; 6 College Lawn, Cheltenham GL53 7AE Tel: 01452 864673 — MB BS Lond. 1983 (Middlx. Med. Sch.) FRCA 1990. Cons. Anaesth. Gloucester Roy. Hosp. Specialty: Anaesth. Socs: Pain Soc.; Assn. Anaesth.; Obst. Anaesth. Soc.

PRYN, Robert Brian The Surgery, Station Road, Great Massingham, King's Lynn PE32 2JQ Tel: 01485 518336 Fax: 01485 518725; Parsley Barn, Weasenham Road, Great Massingham, King's Lynn PE32 2EY Tel: 01485 520104 — MB BS Lond. 1980.

PRYN, Stephen John Sir Humphrey Davy Department Anaesthetics, Bristol Royal Infirmary, Bristol BS2 8HW Tel: 0117 928 2163 Fax: 0117 928 2098; 45 Logan Road, Bishopston, Bristol BS7 8DS Tel: 0117 924 7942 — (Cambridge University Addenbrookes Hospital) MB BChir Cam. 1981; MA Camb. 1983; DCH RCP Lond. 1985; ECFMG Cert. 1987; FFA RCS Eng. 1988. Cons. Anaesth. Bristol Roy. Infirm. Specialty: Anaesth.; Intens. Care. Prev: Sen. Regist. (Anaesth.) Oxf. RHA; Regist. (Anaesth.) S.ampton. Gen. Hosp.; Instruc. (Anaesth.) Univ. Michigan, USA.

PRYOR, Antony Damian 228 Olney Road, London SE17 3HU — MB BS Lond. 1987.

PRYOR, Mr Glyn Alan Edith Cavell Hospital, Orthopaedic Department, Bretton Gate, Peterborough PE3 9GZ Tel: 01733 875252 Fax: 01733 875172 Email: glyn.pryor@pbh-tr.nhs.uk; Eaglethorpe House, Eaglethorpe, Warmington, Peterborough PE8 6TJ — MB BS Lond. 1978 (Kings College Hospital) FRCS Eng. 1983; MS Lond. 1990. Cons. Orthop. Surg. Edith Cavell Hosp. P'boro.; Chairm., Secondary Care Forum of Nat. Osteoparosis Soc. Specialty: Orthop.; Trauma & Orthop. Surg. Special Interest: Hip Fractures; Osteoparosis Related Fractures; Primary and Revision Hip Arthroplasty. Socs: Fell. BOA. Prev: Sen. Regist. (Orthop.) Addenbrooke's Hosp. Camb.

PRYOR, Mr John Pembro The Lister Hospital, Chelsea Bridge Road, London SW1W 8RH Tel: 020 7730 3417 Fax: 020 7824 8867; The Beacon, Channel Way, Fairlight, Hastings TN35 4BP Tel: 01424 814945 — MB BS Lond. 1961 (King's Coll. Hosp.) AKC; MRCS Eng. LRCP Lond. 1961; FRCS Eng. 1967; MS Lond. 1971. Emerit. Reader Inst. Urol. Univ. Coll. Lond. Specialty: Urol. Socs: Past Pres. Europ. Soc. Impotence Research; (Ex-Chairm.) Europ. Assn. Gen. Microsurgs.; Europ. Assn. Genital Surgs. Prev: Cons. Uroandrol. King's Coll. & St. Peter's Hosps. Lond.; Dean Inst. Urol. Univ. Coll. Lond.; Pres. ESSIR.

PRYS-JONES, Oliver Edmund Plas Meddyg Surgery, Station Road, Ruthin LL15 1BP Tel: 01824 702255 Fax: 01824 707221 — MB ChB Liverp. 1987; BSc (Hons.) St. And. 1976; PhD Camb. 1982; MB ChB (Hons.) Liverp. 1987; DRCOG 1990; MRCGP 1992; T(GP) 1992. Socs: BMA. Prev: Trainee GP/SHO (Paediat. & O & G) Ysbyty Glan Clwyd Bodelwyddan VTS; Ho. Off. (Med. & Surg.) Broadgreen Hosp. Liverp.

PRYS-ROBERTS, Cedric Foxes Mead, Cleeve Hill Road, Cleeve, Bristol BS49 4PG Tel: 01934 834267 — MB BS Lond. 1959 (St. Bart.) DA Eng. 1962; FFA RCS Eng. 1964; PhD Leeds 1968; MA Oxf. 1967, DM 1975. Prof. Anaesth. Univ. Bristol; Hon. Cons. Anaesth. Bristol Roy. Infirm. & Bristol Roy. Hosp. Sick Childr; Edit. Bds. Brit. Jl. Anaesth., Europ. Jl. Anaesth. & Analgesia. Specialty: Anaesth. Socs: Anaesth. Research Soc. (Chairm.); Europ. Acad. Anaesth. (Senator). Prev: Clin. Reader Nuffield Dept. Anaesth. Univ. Oxf.; Prof. Anaesth. Univ. Calif. USA.; Research Fell. in Anaesth. Univ. Leeds.

PRYSE, Rebecca Diane North End Surgery, High Street, Buckingham MK18 1NU Tel: 01296 432742 Fax: 01296 398774; 12 Highfield Road, Winslow, Buckingham MK18 3DU Tel: 01296 712582 Email: drs.pryse@virgin.com — MB BS Lond. 1992 (UMDS Lond.) DCH RCP Lond. 1994; DRCOG 1995. GP. Specialty: Gen. Pract. Prev: GP/Regist. Sheff. VTS; Ho. Surg. Greenwich Dist. Hosp. Lond.; GP Asst.

PRZEMIOSLO, Robert Tadeusz Frenchay Hospital, Department of Gastroenterology, Frenchay Park Road, Bristol BS16 1LE Tel: 0117 975 3815 Email: robert.przemioslo@nbt.nhs.uk; The Barn House, Silver Street, Colerne, Chippenham SN14 8DY — MB BS Lond. 1988 (St Geo.) MRCP (UK) 1991; MD Lond. 1995; FRCP Lond. 2002. Cons. (Gastroenterol.) Frenchay Hosp. Bristol; Hon. Sen. Lect. Univ. Bristol. Specialty: Gastroenterol.; Gen. Med. Socs: Brit. Soc. Gastroenterol.; Cossham Med. Soc.; Amer. Gastroenterol. Assn. Prev: Sen. Regist. (Gastroenterol. & Hepatol.) Inst. Liver Studies King's Coll. Lond.; Hon. Sen. Regist. St Mark's Hosp. Harrow; Hon. Regist. (Gastroenterol.) Rayne Inst. St. Thos. Hosp.

PRZYSLO, Francis Richard Harley Street Medical Centre, Harley Street, Hanley, Stoke-on-Trent ST1 3RX Tel: 01782 212305 Fax: 01782 201326 — BM BS Nottm. 1980; DRCOG 1985; MRCGP 1989.

PSAILA, Bethan Flat 4, 176 Holland Road, Holland Park, London W14 8AH — MB BS Lond. 2003.

PSAILA, Mr Joseph Victor Doncaster Royal Infirmary, Armthorpe Road, Doncaster DN2 5TL Tel: 01302 366666; 7 St. Wilfrid's Road, Bessacarr, Doncaster DN4 6AA Fax: 01302 370610 — MD Malta 1971; FRCS Eng. 1976; MCH Wales 1981. Cons. Surg. Doncaster & Bassettlaw Hosp.s Trust; Lead Union Breast Serv., Doncaster & Bassett Law Hosp. Trust. Specialty: Gen. Surg.; Womens Health. Socs: Brit. Soc. & Assn. Surgs.; Brit. Assn. of Surgic. Encology. Prev: Lect. (Surg.) Welsh Nat. Sch. Med.; Research Off. (Clin. Surg.) Welsh Nat. Sch. Med. Cardiff; Regist. (Surg.) Univ. Hosp. Wales Cardiff.

PSIACHOU-LEONARD, Elene 79 Woolmer Gardens, Edgware HA8 8QH Tel: 020 8958 7491; 79 Woolmer Gardens, London HA8 8QH Email: epsiachou@hotmail.com — Ptychio Iatrikes Athens 1984 (Univ. Athens Sch. Med.) MRCPI 1996; MRCPCH 1997. Cons. (Paediat. Haemat. Oncol.) Agia Sophia Childr.'s Hosp. Athens Greece. Specialty: Paediat. Socs: Fell. Greek Paediat. Assn. (Athens Prefecture); SIOP; Brit. Soc. Haematol. Prev: SHO (Haemat. & Oncol.) Gt. Ormond St. Hosp. Lond.; Hon. Clin. Asst. (Paediat. Haemat. & Oncol.) Gt. Ormond St. Hosp. Lond.; SHO (Paediat.) St Geo. Hosp. Lond. & Westm. Childr. Hosp.

PSWARAYI, Ruveneko Zwirimumwoyo Tapiwa T 4 Romanny Road, West Norwood, London SE27 — MB BS Lond. 1980.

PUCCI, Martin John Ellon Group Practice, Health Centre, Schoolhill, Ellon AB41 9JH Tel: 01358 720333 Fax: 01358 721578 — MB ChB Aberd. 1979.

PUCKETT, John Rees Whitstable Health Centre, Harbour Street, Whitstable CT5 1BZ Tel: 01227 594400 Fax: 01227 771474; The Horseshoes, Share & Coulter Road, Chestfield, Whitstable CT5 3LE — (King's Coll. Hosp.) MB BS Lond. 1970; DObst RCOG 1974; DCH Eng. 1974; DA Eng. 1978. Prev: SHO (Paediat.) & SHO (Obst.) Kent & Canterbury Hosp.; SHO (Med. & Geriat.) Luton & Dunstable Hosp.

PUCKETT, Mark Anthony 43 East Wynd Road, Weymouth DT4 0RP — BM Soton. 1996.

PUDDY, Bernard Reginald Department of Anaesthasia, Royal Oldham Hospital, Rochdale Road, Oldham OL1 2JH — MB ChB Manch. 1963; DA Eng. 1967; FFA RCS Eng. 1969. Cons. Anaesth. Oldham AHA. Specialty: Anaesth. Prev: Asst. Resid. Surg. Off. & SHO Orthop. Dept. Salford Roy. Hosp.; Sen. Regist. Manch. Roy. Infirm.

PUDDY, Elizabeth Helen 2 Enfield Road, Eccles, Manchester M30 9NF — MB ChB Sheff. 1994.

PUDDY, Mark Richard Wargrave Surgery, Victoria Road, Wargrave, Reading RG10 8BP Tel: 0118 940 3939 Fax: 0118 940 1357; The Little House, 65 High St, Wargrave, Reading RG10 8BU Tel: 01189 402028 — BM BCh Oxf. 1985; BA Camb. 1982; MA Oxf. 1989, BM BCh 1985; DRCOG 1988; MRCGP 1989; DCH RCP Lond. 1989. Prev: Trainee GP Hereford VTS.

PUDDY, Victoria Fielding 2 Enfield Road, Eccles, Manchester M30 9NF — MB ChB Leic. 1992.

PUDNEY, Delia Mary 38 Caburn Heights, Southgate West, Crawley RH11 8QX — MB ChB Birm. 1997.

PUE, Philip Farfield Group Practice, St Andrew's Surgeries, West Lane, Keighley BD21 2LD Tel: 01535 607333 Fax: 01535 611818 — MB ChB Leeds 1983; DCH RCP Lond. 1986; MRCGP 1987; DRCOG 1987.

PUFFETT, Alison Ruth Invicta Community Care NHS Trust, Kingswood Mental Health Centre, 180-6 Union St., Maidstone ME14 1EY Tel: 01622 692686 — MB BS Lond. 1986; DRCOG 1988; MRCPsych 1992. Cons. (Psychiat.) W. Kent; Hon. Sen. Lect. Inst. Psychiat. Specialty: Gen. Psychiat. Prev: Sen. Regist. (Psychiat.) SE Thames Region.

PUGH, Alan Charles Old Road Surgery, Old Road, Abersychan, Pontypool NP4 7BH Tel: 01495 772239 Fax: 01495 773786;

Pentwyn Farm, Llanddewi Fach, Croesyceiliog, Cwmbran NP44 2DB Tel: 0163 333062 — MB ChB Sheff. 1958; MRCS Eng. LRCP Lond. 1958.

PUGH, Angela Mill Street Health Centre, Mill Street, Crewe CW2 7AQ Tel: 01270 212725 Fax: 01270 216323; Willow Farm, Whitehouse Lane, Nantwich CW5 6HQ — MB ChB Leeds 1971; DCH Eng. 1974; MRCGP 1988. Prev: Clin Asst. Crewe HA; Clin. Med. Off. Gtr. Glas. HB; SHO (Paediat. & Med.) Pontefract Gen. Infirm.

PUGH, Catrin Non 36 Cefn Coed Road, Cardiff CF23 6AR — BChir Camb. 1992.

***PUGH, Cerys Ann** 50 Lytton Road, Leicester LE2 1WJ — MB ChB Leic. 1998; MB ChB Leic 1998.

PUGH, Charles James The Forest Group Practice, The Surgery, Bury Road, Brandon IP27 0BU Tel: 01842 813353 Fax: 01842 815221; Hartley Place, Nursery Lane, Hockwold, Thetford IP26 4ND — MRCS Eng. LRCP Lond. 1975; BSc (Hons. Physiol.) Lond. 1972, MB BS 1975; DRCOG 1979.

PUGH, Charles Robert Hellesdon Hospital, Drayton High Road, Norwich NR6 5BE Tel: 01603 421487 — MB BS Lond. 1974 (St. Mary's) FRCPsych 1992, M 1978. Cons. Norf. Ment. Health Trust Norwich; Hon. Sen. Policy Adviser DOH; Hon. Sen. Lect. Univ. E. Anglia. Specialty: Gen. Psychiat. Prev: Hon. Sen. Lect. Univ. Coll. Lond.; Cons. Middlx. & St. Luke's Hosps. Lond.; Cons. Shenley Hosp. & Centr. Middlx. Hosp. Lond.

PUGH, Christopher Edward The Steadings, Laigh of Rossie, Whitemon Road, Dunning, Perth PH2 0QY — MB ChB Liverp. 1981; MRCS Eng. LRCP Lond. 1981; MFOM RCP Lond. 1990; Spec. Accredit. Occupat. Med. JCHMT 1991; FFOM 1999. Cons. (Occupat. Med.) Fife Healthcare NHS Trust; Med. Adviser Fife Counc. Specialty: Occupat. Health. Socs: Soc. Occupat. Med. Prev: Chief Med. Off. Translink Jt. Venture Channel Tunnel Construction.

PUGH, Professor Christopher William The Henry Wellcome Building for Genomic Medicine, Roosevelt Drive, Headington, Oxford OX3 7BN Tel: 01865 287669 Fax: 01865 287533 — (Oxf.) DPhil Oxf. 1981; MA 1981; BM BCh Oxf. 1985; MRCP (UK) 1990; FRCP 2000; FMedSci 2003. MRC Sen. Clin. Fell. Nuffield Dept. Clin. Med. & Hon. Cons. Renal Unit Oxf.; Prof. (Renal Med.) Univ. Oxf. Specialty: Nephrol. Socs: Brit. Med. Assn.; Renal Assn.; Assn. Physicians of Gt. Britain & Irel. Prev: MRC Train. Fell. Nuffield Dept. Clin. Med. & Hon. Sen. Regist. Renal Unit Oxf.; Regist. Nuffield Dept. Clin. Med. John Radcliffe Hosp. Oxf.; Deptm. Demonst. Sir William Dunn Sch. Path. Univ. Oxf.

PUGH, David Alexander Elstree Aeromedical Centre, Elstree Aerodrome, Borehamwood WD6 3AW Tel: 020 8953 1882 Fax: 020 8953 2775 Email: pughelstree@aol.com — MB BS Lond. 1972 (St. Bart.) MRCS Eng. LRCP Lond. 1972; Cert. JCC Lond. 1976; MRCGP 1979; Cert. Av Med. MoD (Air) CAA 1980. Authorised Med. Examr. Civil Aviat. Auth.; Private Gen. Pract.; Indust. Med. Off. Specialty: Aviat. Med.; Respirat. Med.; Ment. Health.

PUGH, David Henry Owen Royal Glamorgan Hospital, Llantrisant CF72 8XR Tel: 01443 443526; Wrangbrook, Lisvane Road, LLanishen, Cardiff CF14 0SE Tel: 01222 750263 — MB BCh Wales 1972; MRCOG 1980. Cons. O & G E. Glam. Gen. Hosp. Specialty: Obst. & Gyn. Prev: Sen. Regist. (O & G) Univ. Hosp. Wales Cardiff.; Sen. Regist. (O & G) Morriston Hosp. Swansea; Regist. (O & G) Univ. Hosp. Wales Cardiff.

PUGH, David Nicholas Edenkiln Surgery, 12 Dumbrock Road, Strathblane, Glasgow G63 9EG Tel: 01360 770340 Fax: 01360 771112 — MB ChB Glas. 1985; Dip Sp Med Scottish Royal Colls; DRCOG 1987. Specialty: Sports Med. Socs: Brit. Assoc. of Sports Med.

PUGH, David Robert (retired) 8 Parkmead, London SW15 5BS — MB BChir Camb. 1950; MA, MB BChir Camb. 1950. Prev: Ho. Surg. & Res. Obst. Guy's Hosp. Lond.

PUGH, Edwin John Wellhouse, East View, Sadberge, Darlington DL2 1SF Tel: 01325 333134 — MB BS Newc. 1977 (Newcastle upon Tyne) MRCGP 1984; MFCM 1986; MFPHM 1989; FFPHM 1994; Dip Palliat Med 1998. Cons. in Palliat. Med.; Tutor for Med. Educat. Progr. run by Postgrad. Inst. for Med. and Dent., Univ. of Newc. Specialty: Palliat. Med.; Educat. Prev: Dir. Pub. Health Co. Durh. HA; Cons. Epidemiol. & Specialist (Community Med.) N. RHA.; Med. Dir. & Cons. (Palliat. Med.).

PUGH, Elizabeth Wyn Nth. Manchester Gen. Hospital, Crumpsall, Manchester M8 5RL Tel: 0161 720 2038 Fax: 0161 720 2073 — MB BS Lond. 1967 (Roy. Free) MRCS Eng. LRCP Lond. 1967; FRCOG 1992, M 1971; FRCPsych 1996. Cons. Psychiat. N. Manch. HA.; Regional Adviser, RCPSYCH, N. Western Region. Specialty: Gen. Psychiat. Prev: Sen. Regist. & Regist. (Psychiat.) Manch.; Research Med. Off. Nuffield Inst. Oxf. Univ.

PUGH, Emma Caroline The Surgery, Margaret Street, Thaxted, Dunmow CM6 2QN Tel: 01371 830213 Fax: 01371 831278; The Old White Horse, High St, Great Chesterford, Saffron Walden CB10 1PL Tel: 01799 530450 — MB BChir (Bchir 1992, Mb 1993) Camb. 1993 (Qu. Coll. Camb. & Lond. Hosp. Med. Coll.) DRCOG 1994; DFFP 1995; DCH 1996; MRCGP 1997. GP Princip. The Surg. Margt. St. Thaxted, Essex. Specialty: Gen. Pract. Socs: Worshipful Soc. Apoth. Prev: Trainee GP/SHO Princess Alexdra Hosp. Harlow VTS; Ho. Off. (Gen. Surg.) Whipps Cross Hosp. Lond.; Ho. Off. (Gen. Med.) OldCh. Hosp. Romford.

PUGH, Geoffrey Hall Grove Surgery, 4 Hall Grove, Welwyn Garden City AL7 4PL Tel: 01707 328528 Fax: 01707 373139; 16 The Valley Green, Welwyn Garden City AL8 7DQ Tel: 01707 324760 — MB BS Lond. 1974 (King's Coll. Hosp.) BSc Lond. 1971; MRCGP 1979.

PUGH, Gilbert Geoffrey 44 Groombridge Road, Hackney, London E9 7DP — (Guy's) MB BS Lond. 1968; MRCS Eng. LRCP Lond. 1968. Psycho-Therap. Lond.; Clin. Asst. Psychotherap. King Geo. Hosp. Ilford. Specialty: Psychother. Prev: GP Princip.

PUGH, Gordon Cameron 129 Morningside Drive, Morningside, Edinburgh EH10 5NR — MB ChB Birm. 1975; BSc (1st cl. Hons.) CNAA 1970; DRCOG 1977; MRCGP 1979; DA (UK) 1980; FFA RCS Eng. 1984. Cons. Anaesth. City Hosp. Edin. Specialty: Anaesth.

PUGH, Hadyn William 273 London Road, Horns Cross, Dartford — LMSSA Lond. 1963.

PUGH, Helen Rosebank Medical Practice, Pointer Court, Ashton Road, Lancaster LA1 4JS Tel: 01524 842284; Ashcroft House, Ashton Road, Ashton-with-Stodday, Lancaster LA2 0AA Tel: 01524 35274 — MB ChB Manch. 1974; DRCOG 1977. GP Asst.; Occupat. Health Phys. Marks & Spencer; Health Screening Lanc. & Lakeland Nuffield Hosp.

PUGH, Helen Mary Bridge Lane Health Centre, 20 Bridge Lane, Battersea, London SW11 3AD Tel: 020 7585 1499 — MB BCh Wales 1979.

PUGH, James Kendrick, MC (retired) Cedar Lodge, Parc-yr-Irfon, Builth Wells LD2 3NG Tel: 01982 553286 — LRCP LRCS Ed. LRFPS Glas. 1940; MRCGP 1963.

PUGH, Jennifer Leslie (retired) 5 Steele's Road, London NW3 4SE Tel: 020 7586 0966 Fax: 020 7722 0571 Email: pughs@mikejenn.com — BM BCh Oxf. 1957 (Middlx.) MA Oxf. 1957; DA Eng. 1960; FFA RCS Eng. (Nuffield Prize) 1963. Prev: Hon. Cons. Anaesth. St. Luke's Hosp. for the Clergy Lond.

PUGH, Jill Kathryn St Margaret's Practices, 237 St. Margarets Road, Twickenham TW1 1NE Tel: 020 8892 1986 Fax: 020 8891 6466; 26 Cranes Park, Surbiton KT5 8AD Tel: 020 8399 8008 — MB BS Lond. 1977 (St. Mary's) MRCS Eng. LRCP Lond. 1977.

PUGH, Kathryn Elizabeth Gordon Hospital, Bloomburg Street, London SW1V 2RH Tel: 020 8746 8714; 4 Village Way, London SE21 7AW Tel: 0207 274 6208 Email: kate.pugh@nhs.uk — MB BS Newc. 1985; BMedSci Newc. 1982; MRCPsych 1989. Cons. Psychiat. in Psychother., Lond. Hosp., BKCW Ment. Health Trust. Specialty: Psychother. Socs: Roy. Coll. Psychiat. (Psychother. Sect.). Prev: Clin. Research Fell. Char. Cross & Westm. Med. Sch. Lond.; Regist. Rotat. (Psychiat.) St. Geo. Hosp. Lond.; Sen Regis Psychother. Maudsley Hosp Lond.

PUGH, Kim Childrens Services, South Durham NHS Trust, Escombe Road Health Centre, Bishop Auckland DL14 6AB; Well House, Sadberge, Darlington DL2 1SF — MB BS Newc. 1978; MRCPsych 1986; DCCH RCP Ed. 1994; MMedSci Leeds 1998. Staff Grade (Comm. Paeds) Part0Time. Specialty: Community Child Health.

PUGH, Laura Joan Loveday 93 Westhill Road, Birmingham B38 8SX — MB ChB Birm. 1988; MRCGP 1993.

PUGH, Mark David 47 Old Hall Drive, Ashton-in-Makefield, Wigan WN4 9NA — MB ChB Leeds 1992.

PUGH, Mark Timothy St. Mary's Hospital, Department of Rheumatology, Newport PO30 5TG Tel: 01983 534909 Fax: 01983 534872 Email: mark.pugh@iow.nhs.uk; 1, Westhill Road, Shanklin

PO37 6PT Tel: 01983 534909 — MB BCh BAO NUI 1985; LRCSI, LRCPI, DTM RCSI 1985; DCH NUI 1986; MRCPI 1990; MD 1996; FRCPI 2004. Cons. Rheumatologist St Mary's Hosp. Newport IoW. Specialty: Rheumatol. Special Interest: Connective Tissue Dis.; Inflammatory Arthritis; Osteoporosis. Socs: Brit. Soc. Rheum.; BMA; Amer. Coll. of Rheum. Prev: Cons. & Hon. Sen. Lect. Birm. Heartlands & Solihull NHS Trust (Teachg.) Birm.

PUGH, Mr Michael Arthur, AE St. Luke's Hosp. For the Clergy, Fitzroy Square, London W1T 6AH Tel: 01923 856200 Fax: 01923 857962 Email: pughs@mikejenn.com; 5 Steele's Road, Hampstead, London NW3 4SE Tel: 020 7586 0966 Fax: 020 7722 0571 Email: pughs@mikejenn.com — (St. Bart.) MB BS Lond. 1953; FRCOG 1971, M 1959; FRCS Eng. 1962. p/t Emerit. Cons. (Gynaecology) UCL Hosp. & Whittington Hosp.; Hon. Sen. Lect. ULC Hosps (O&G); Emerit. Cons. UCL Hosps. & Whittington Hosp. The Hosp. For Wom., Soho; Hon. Cons. Gynaeolgist St Lukes Hosp. for the Clergy, Lond. Specialty: Obst. & Gyn. Socs: Fell. Roy. Soc. Med.; Ct. Assoc. Soc. Apoth. Master 1997-8; Counc. Med. Soc. Lond. Prev: Sen. Regist. (O & G) Radcliffe Infirm. Oxf.; Examr. (O & G) ConJt. Bd., Univ. Lond. Soc. Apoth. & RCOG; Demonst. (Anat.) St. Bart. Hosp. Med. Coll.

PUGH, Peter John Frimley Park Hospital, Portsmouth Road, Frimley, Camberley GU16 7UJ Tel: 01276 692777; Westbury Cottage, Westbury, Sherborne DT9 3EL — MB BS Lond. 1994. SHO (A & E) Frimley Pk. Hosp. Surrey. Specialty: Accid. & Emerg. Prev: Ho. Off. (Med.) Kent & Canterbury Hosp.; Ho. Off. (Surg.) Frimley Pk. Hosp. Surrey.

PUGH, Richard James 33A St Winifreds Road, Biggin Hill, Westerham TN16 3HP — MB ChB Bristol 1997.

PUGH, Richard John Philip (retired) Thirley Cottage, Harwood Dale, Scarborough YO13 0DP — MB ChB Birm. 1944; MRCS Eng. LRCP Lond. 1944; DCH Eng. 1945; FRCP Lond. 1971, M 1946. Prev: Cons. (Paediat.) Hull & Beverley HAs.

PUGH, Richard Nicholas Hinsley 18 Bluebell Drive, Newcastle ST5 3UD Tel: 01782 617634 Fax: 01782 627441 — MB BChir Camb. 1971 (Camb. & King's Coll. Hosp.) MRCP (UK) 1974; DTM & H Liverp. 1975; FRCP Lond. 1992; MA Camb. 1971, MD 1992; MFPHM RCP (UK) 1994; FFPHM RCP (UK) 1999. Cons Pub. health med & communicable Dis. control Walsall HA W. Midl.s NHS. Specialty: Epidemiol.; Pub. Health Med.; Infec. Dis. Socs: Fell. Roy. Soc. Hyg. & Trop. Med.; BMA; Internat. Soc. Infec. Dis. Prev: Assoc prof. Fac. Med. & Health Sci. UAE Univ. Al Ain United Arab Emirates; Lect. (Clin. Epidemiol.) Liverp. Sch. Trop. Med. (seconded Nigeria & Malawi); SHO Chest Clinic Roy. Postgrad. Med. Sch. Hammersmith Hosp. Lond.

PUGH, Robert Eric Willow Farm, Whitehouse Lane, Nantwich CW5 6HQ Email: pughre@aol.com — MB ChB Leeds 1971 (Leeds University) FRCPCH; MRCP (UK) 1974; FRCP Lond. 1991. Cons. Paediat. Leighton Hosp. Crewe; Hon. Clin. Lect. (Child Health) Univ. Liverp. Specialty: Paediat. Socs: Brit. Paediat.y Assoc. Prev: Sen. Regist. & Honoray Tutor Child Health Roy. Liverp. Childr.'s Hosp.; Regist. Dept. Child Health Roy. Hosp. Sick Childr. Glas.; Fell. Roy. Coll. of Paediat. & Child Health.

PUGH, Roderick Morris Portland Road Surgery, 31 Portland Road, Kilmarnock KA1 2DJ Tel: 01563 522118 Fax: 01563 573562; 9 Howard Street, Kilmarnock KA1 2BP — MB ChB Glas. 1979; DRCOG 1982; MRCGP 1983.

PUGH, Rosamund Joy Macmillan Unit, Christchurch Hospital, Fairmile Road, Christchurch BH23 2JX Tel: 01202 705208 Fax: 01202 705213 — MB BS Lond. 1986; MRCGP 1992. Cons. (Palliat. Med.) Bournemouth & ChristCh. Hosps. NHS Trust. Specialty: Palliat. Med. Prev: Sen. Regist. (Palliat. Med.) Poole Hosp. NHS Trust & Roy. Bournemouth & ChristCh. Hosps. NHS Trust.; Trainee GP Crawley; SHO (Palliat. Care) St. Catherine's Hosp. Crawley.

PUGH, Sara Ellis Department of Medicine, Sunderland Royal Hospital, Sunderland SR4 7TP; Linwood, Ashbrooke Range, Sunderland SR2 9BP — MB BCh Wales 1974; MD Wales 1990, MB BCh 1974; MRCP (UK) 1977; FRCP Ed. 1994; FRCP Lond. 1995. Cons. Cardiol. & Phys.City Hosps Sunderland. Specialty: Cardiol. Socs: Brit. Cardiac Soc. Prev: Lect. & Hon. Sen. Regist. (Med. Cardiol.) Char. Cross Hosp. Med. Sch.; Clin. Research Asst. (Clin. Pharmacol.) Oxf.; Regist. (Cardiol.) Univ. Hosp. Wales Card.

PUGH, Simon Francis 10 Coniger Road, Fulham, London SW6 3TA — MB BS Lond. 1969; MRCP (UK) 1974.

PUGH, Stephen Charles Department of Aanesthetics, University Hospital of Wales, Heath Park, Cardiff CF14 4XW Tel: 029 2074 3107 — MB BS Lond. 1983; DA (UK) 1988; FRCA 1992. Cons. Anaesth. Univ. Hosp. Wales Cardiff. Specialty: Anaesth. Prev: Sen. Regist. (Anaesth.) Guy's Hosp. Lond.

PUGH, Stirling Taunton & Somerset NHS Hospital Trust, Musgrove Park Hospital, Taunton Tel: 01823 342720 Fax: 01823 342721; Croft Orchard, Curry Mallet, Taunton TA3 6TD — MRCS Eng. LRCP Lond. 1979; MRCP (UK) 1982; PhD Lond. 1989; FRCP (Eng) 1999. Clin. Dir. Med. Directorate Taunton & Som. NHS Hosp. Trust. Specialty: Gastroenterol. Socs: Brit. Soc. Gastroenterol. Prev: Sen. Regist. (Gen. Med.) Univ. Hosp. Wales Cardiff; Regist. (Gen. Med.) Whittington Hosp. Lond.; Cons. Phys. Gastroenterol. Taunton & Som. NHS Hosp. Trust.

PUGH, Venn Tannahill (retired) 49 Parc-Yr-Yrfon, Builth Wells LD2 3NG Tel: 01982 552220 — MB ChB Ed. 1941. Prev: Ho. Surg. Derby Roy. Infirm.

PUGH, Victor William 9 Knighton Road, Leicester LE2 3HL Tel: 0116 706994; Department of Pathology, Royal Infirmary, Leicester LE1 5WW Tel: 0116 541414 — MRCS Eng. LRCP Lond. 1943 (Lond. Hosp.) MD Lond. 1951, MB BS 1947; FRCPath 1963. Cons. Pathol. Leicester Area Path. Serv. Leicester Roy. Infirm.; Home Office Path.; Clin. Teach. Fac. Med. Univ. Leicester. Specialty: Pathology, General. Socs: Fell. Med. Soc. Lond.; Assn. Clin. Pathols. Prev: Asst. Pathol. Gp. Laborat. Mile End Hosp.; Supernum. Regist. Dept. Path. Lond. Hosp.; Surg. Lt. RNVR.

PUGH, Wendy Anne Berwyn House Surgery, 13 Shrubbery Avenue, Worcester WR1 1QW Tel: 01905 22888 Fax: 01905 617352; Saint Hill, Northwick Close, Worcester WR3 7EF — MB ChB Birm. 1981; DRCOG 1984; MRCGP 1986.

PUGH WILLIAMS, Sally 34 Millfield Drive, Cowbridge CF71 7BR — MB BCh Wales 1978; AFOM; FRCP (UK) 1998. Occupat. Health Phys. INCO (Ewgre) Clydach, Swansea. Specialty: Occupat. Health. Prev: SHO (Cardiac) Riyadh Milit. Hosp. Saudi Arabia; Regist. Rotat. (Med.) S. Glam. AHA (T)/Mid Glam. AHA.

PUGHE, Christopher Thomas 3 Hockenhull Lane, Tarvin, Chester CH3 8LA — MB ChB Manch. 1995.

PUGSLEY, Angela Denise Lyme Valley Medical Centre, Lyme Valley Road, Newcastle ST5 3TF Tel: 01782 615367 Fax: 01782 713355 — BM Soton. 1986; T(GP) 1991. Specialty: Gen. Pract.

PUGSLEY, Mr Wilfred Bernard The Cardiothoracic Unit, Millenium Wing, The Royal Sussex County Hospital, Brighton BN2 5BE Tel: 01273 696955 Email: wpugsley@hotmail.com — MB BS Lond. 1978 (Cambridge St Mary's) BA Camb. 1975; FRCS Ed. 1983. Cons. Cardiothoracic Surg. The Roy. Sussex Co. Hosp. Brighton; Squadron Ldr., Cons. Surg. R. Aux. A.F. Specialty: Cardiothoracic Surg. Socs: Of the Soc. Of Cardiothoracic Surg.s of GB. & Irel.; Roy. Soc. Med. Prev: Cons. Cardiothoracic Surg. UCLH Middlx. Hosp. Lond.; Sen. Regist. (Cardiothoracic Surg.) Lond. Chest & Nat. Heart Hosps.; BHF Research Fell. Middlx. Hosp. 1987-88.

PUJARA, Manpreet Singh Wrythe Green Surgery, Wrythe Lane, Carshalton SM5 2RE Tel: 020 8669 3232/1717 Fax: 020 8773 2524 — BM Soton. 1984 (Univ. Soton.) DRCOG 1988; MRCGP 1989. Mem. EMIS Nat. User Gp. (Vice-Chairm. & Conf. Chair). Specialty: Gen. Med. Socs: Sutton & Dist. Med. Soc. Prev: Trainee GP St. Helier VTS.

PULESTON, Brenda Mary (retired) 21 Beaver Close, Winterbourne, Bristol BS36 1QU Tel: 01454 772720 — (St. Bart.) MB BS Lond. 1964; MRCS Eng. LRCP Lond. 1964; Cert. Family Plann. JCC 1970; DO Eng. 1979. Prev: Clin. Asst. Soton. Eye Hosp.

PULESTON, Joanne Mary 23 St Lawrence Forstal, Canterbury CT1 3PA — MB BS Lond. 1992.

PULESTON, Richard Lewellyn Birmingham Childrens Hospital, Ladywood Middleway, Five Ways, Birmingham B4 6 Tel: 0121 454 4851; 40 Witherford Way, Selly Oak, Birmingham B29 4AX — MB ChB Birm. 1992; DCH RCP Lond. 1995; MRCGP 1996. SHO (Paediat.) Birm. Childr. Hosp. Specialty: Paediat. Prev: Trainee GP/SHO (Paediat.) Birm.

PULFORD, Elizabeth Claire Bolingbroke Hospital, Wandsworth, London SW11; 16 Russell Close, London W4 2NU — MB ChB Manch. 1990; BA (Cantab) 1987; MRCP 1993. Specialist Regist.

(Geriat. Med.). Specialty: Care of the Elderly; Gen. Med. Socs: Brit Thor. Soc.; Brit. Geriat. Soc.

PULHAM, Nicola Lesley The Orchard Medical Centre, Heath Road, Coxheath, Maidstone ME17 4PL Tel: 01622 744994 Fax: 01622 741162; Durrants House, West St, Hunton, Maidstone ME15 0RY — MB BS Lond. 1987.

PULLAN, Alistair David Furlong Medical Centre, Furlong Road, Tunstall, Stoke-on-Trent ST6 5UD Tel: 01782 577388 Fax: 01782 838610; 38 Saint Georges Avenue N., Wolstanton, Newcastle ST5 8DF — MB ChB Aberd. 1985; DRCOG 1989; MRCGP 1990.

PULLAN, Cedric William Alderson (retired) Borden Wood Lodge, Milland, Liphook GU30 7JY Tel: 01428 741369 — MRCS Eng. LRCP Lond. 1945 (Camb. & St. Thos.) MA, MB BChir Camb. 1946. Prev: Med. Off. RAF.

PULLAN, Constance Ruth 186 High Road, Chilwell, Nottingham NG9 5BB — MB BS Newc. 1970; MRCP (UK) 1973; MD Newc. 1985. Cons. Community Paediat. Nottm. HA. Specialty: Paediat. Prev: Sen. Regist. (Child Health) Univ. Hosp. Nottm.; Sen. Resid. Assoc. (Virol. & Child Health) Roy. Vict. Infirm. Newc.; Regist. (Paediat.) Newc. Gen. Hosp.

PULLAN, Mr David Mark Cardiothoracic Centre, Thomas Drive, Liverpool L14 3PE Tel: 0151 228 1616 Email: mark.pullen@ctc.nhs.uk — MB BS Lond. 1988; FRCS Eng. 1992; FRCS Ed. 1992; FRCS (CTh) 1999. Cons. Cardiac Surg., The Cardiothoracic Centre, Liverp. Specialty: Cardiothoracic Surg. Prev: SHO (Cardiothoracic Surg.) Leeds Gen. Infirm.; SpR (Cardio Thoracic Surg.) Liverpool CTC.

PULLAN, David Sebastian Bratby The Thatched Cottage, Binsted, Arundel BN18 0LQ — MB BS Lond. 1993; MRCGP.

PULLAN, Mr Rupert Derek Torbay Hospital, Lawes Bridge, Torquay TQ2 7AA Tel: 01803 654982 Fax: 01803 654996 Email: rupert.pullan@nhs.net — BM BCh Oxf. 1984 (University of Oxford) FRCS Ed. 1989; FRCS Eng. 1989; MA Oxf. 1987, DM 1994; FRCS (Gen. Surg.) 1996. Cons. Gen. & Colorectal Surg. Torbay Hosp. Torquay. Specialty: Gen. Surg. Socs: Assn. of ColoProctol. of GB & Irel.; Assn. of Surg.s of GB & Irel. Prev: Sen. Regist. (Colorectal Surg.) Singleton Hosp. Swansea; Sen. Regist. Rotat. (Gen. Surg.) Ysbyty Gwynedd Bangor; Hunt Prof. RCS Eng.

PULLAPERUMA, Sunil Palitha 4 Curtis Drive, London W3 6YL — MB BS Colombo 1980; MRCPI 1990.

PULLAR, Thomas Ninewells Hospital Medical School, Dundee DD1 9SY Tel: 01382 60111 — MB ChB Glas. 1978; MRCP (UK) 1980; MD Glas. 1986; FRCP Glas. 1992; FRCP ED. 1992. Cons. Phys. (Rheum.) Dundee Teach. Hosp. NHS Trust; Mem. Edit. Bd. Brit. Jl. Rheum.; Regional Adviser Tayside Roy. coll of Phys.s of Edin. Specialty: Gen. Med.; Rheumatol. Socs: Brit. Soc. Rheum. Prev: Sen. Lect. (Clin. Pharmaol.) & Hon. Cons. Phys. (Med.) Gen. Infirm. Leeds; Lect. & Hon. Sen. Regist. (Clin. Pharmacol.) The Gen. Infirm. Leeds.; Regist. & SHO (Med. & Rheum.) Glas. Roy. Infirm.

PULLEN, Andrew John Flat 2, 324 Lordship Lane, London SE22 8LZ — MB BS Lond. 1998.

PULLEN, Brian Walter (retired) Brook House, Harlton Road, Little Eversden, Cambridge CB3 7HB Tel: 01223 262579 — MB BS Lond. 1961 (King's Coll. Hosp.) MRCS Eng. LRCP Lond. 1961; DObst RCOG 1965. Prev: Regist. (Gen. Med.) Plymouth Clin. Area.

PULLEN, Frances Jill Vauxhall Surgery, Vauxhall Lane, Chepstow NP16 5PZ Tel: 01291 623246 Fax: 01291 627975; New House, Garway Hill, Hereford HR2 8EZ Tel: 01981 240032 — (Birm.) MB ChB Birm. 1976; DA Eng. 1978. Specialty: Obst. & Gyn.

PULLEN, Geoffrey Peter (retired) Fairlight House, Brightwell-cum-Sotwell, Wallingford OX10 0RU — MB BChir Camb. 1972 (Camb. & Middlx.) MA, MB Camb. 1972, BChir 1971; MRCPsych 1975; DPM Eng. 1975. Prev: Clin. Dir., Dept. of Rehabil. & Forens. Servs. Oxf.

PULLEN, Herbert (retired) 8 Whitechapel Close, Leeds LS8 2PT Tel: 0113 232 3038 — MB ChB Ed. 1957; DTM & H. Eng. 1960; FRCP Ed. 1978, M 1964. Prev: Cons. Infec. Dis. Seacroft Hosp. Leeds.

PULLEN, Ian Michael Scottish Executive Health Department, St. Andrew's House, Regent Road, Edinburgh EH1 3DG Tel: 0131 244 2805 Email: ian.pullen@scotland.gsi.gov.uk; NHS Borders, Huntlyburn House, Melrose TD6 9BD Tel: 01896 827155 Fax: 01896 827154 Email: ian.pullen@borders.scot.nhs.uk — MB BS Lond. 1970 (Lond. Hosp .) FRCPsych 1990, M 1977. Principal Medical Officer (Mental Health),Scot Exec Health Dept, Edin; Consult. Psychiatrist,NHS Bord. Melrose; Cons. Psychiat. Borders Care Trust, Melrose. Specialty: Gen. Psychiat. Socs: Fell. Roy. Coll. Psychiat. Prev: GP Aylsham, Norf.; Cons. Psychiat. Roy. Edin. Hosp. & Hon. Sen. Lect. Univ. Edin.; Borders Primary Care NHS Trust,Melrose.

PULLEN, Joanna Eve Southbroom Surgery, 15 Estcourt Street, Devizes SN10 1LQ Tel: 01380 720909 — MB BS Lond. 1987 (St George's Hospital Medical School) BSc Lond. 1984; MRCGP 1992. Specialty: Gen. Pract.

PULLEN, Michael Dahlbom The Surgery, Stock Hill, Biggin Hill, Westerham TN16 3TJ; 6 Trinity Close, South Croydon CR2 0EP Tel: 020 8657 7344 — BSc (Hons. Physiol.) Lond. 1985, MB BS 1987; DA (UK) 1989; DGM RCP Lond. 1990; DCH RCP Lond. 1991; DRCOG 1992; DFFP 1993; MRCGP 1993. SHO Duke of Cornw. Spinal Injuries Unit Salisbury Dist. Hosp. Prev: SHO (Anaesth.) Greenwich Dist. Hosp.

PULLEN, Peter Horace (retired) 51 High Street, Dilton Marsh, Westbury BA13 4DW — MB BChir Camb. 1953 (St. Thos.) DObst RCOG 1954. Prev: Obst. Ho. Phys. Lambeth Hosp.

PULLETZ, Mark Christopher Karl 7 Longmoor Street, Poundbury, Dorchester DT1 3GN Tel: 01305 261485 — MB BS Lond. 1992 (UCMSM) BSc Lond. 1989; MRCP (UK) 1996; DCH RCP Lond. 1997. SHO (Anaesth.) Yeovil Hosp. NHS Trust Higher Kingston Yeovil. Specialty: Anaesth.

PULLEY, Melanie Susan 58A Longhill Road, Oringdean, Brighton BN2 7BE — MB ChB Liverp. 1975.

PULLIN, Allan Vincent (retired) 21 Walmoor Park, Sandy Lane, Chester CH3 5UT Tel: 01244 348846 Fax: 01244 351057 Email: allan.pullin@btinternet.com — MB ChB Liverp. 1961. Prev: GP Heath La. Med. Centre, Chester.

PULLIN, Jacqueline Anne Tarr House, Kingston St Mary, Taunton TA2 8HY — MB BS Lond. 1984 (Guy's) FCAnaesth. 1989. Assoc. Specialist (Aneas) Taunton & Som. Hosp. Specialty: Anaesth. Prev: Clin. Asst. Pain Relief Unit. King's Coll. Hosp. Lond.; Regist. (Anaesth.) King's Coll. Hosp. Lond.; SHO (Anaesth.) St. Thos. Hosp. Lond.

PULLINGER, Roland Hugh 19 Werter Road, Putney, London SW15 2LL Tel: 020 8788 0792 Email: rpullinger@btinternet.com — (St. Mary's) MRCS Eng. LRCP Lond. 1968; MB BS Lond. 1968; DObst RCOG 1970. p/t Freelance GP Locum; Health Screening Doctor, Parkside Hosp., Wimbledon. Specialty: Gen. Pract. Prev: SHO A & E Unit W. Middlx. Hosp. Isleworth; Ho. Phys. Hillingdon Hosp. Uxbridge; Ho. Surg. Profess. Surg. Unit St. Mary's Hosp. Lond.

PULLINGER, Stephen (Surgery), 15 Winters Lane, Long Bennington, Newark NG23 5DW Tel: 01400 281220 Fax: 01400 282551 — BM BS Nottm. 1983; BMedSci Nottm. 1981; DRCOG 1986; MRCGP 1988. Prev: Trainee GP Nottm. VTS.

PULLON, Hilary Ruth (retired) 18 Georges Wood Road, Brookmans Park, Hatfield AL9 7BT Tel: 01707 657437 — MB ChB Ed. 1949; DObst RCOG 1952. Prev: Ho. Phys. Barnet Gen. Hosp. & Brook Gen. Hosp. Lond.

PULLYBLANK, Miss Anne Marie — MB BS Lond. 1990; BSc (Hons.) Lond. 1990; FRCS Eng. 1995; MD Lond. 1998. Specialist Regist. S.W. Rotat. Specialty: Gen. Surg.

PULMAN, Nicholas Robert Long Lane Surgery, Beacon House, Long Lane, Coalville LE67 4DR Tel: 01530 831331 — MB ChB Leic. 1983; DRCOG 1983; MRCGP 1988.

PULSFORD, David Robert The Surgery, 9 Godstow Road, Abbey Wood, London SE2 9AT Tel: 020 8310 7066 Fax: 020 8311 8867 — MB BS Lond. 1970.

PULVERTAFT, Robert James Valentine, OBE (retired) Stapeley House, Presteigne Road, Knighton LD7 1HY — MD Camb. 1933 (Camb. & St. Thos.) MRCS Eng. LRCP Lond. 1923; FRCP Lond. 1938; FCPath 1963. Prev: Vis. Prof. Univ. Coll. Ibadan & Makerere Univ. Coll. Kampala Uganda.

PUMFORD, Neil Andrew Gallions, Wexham Springs, Wexham, Slough SL3 6RJ Fax: 01753 666204/01753 666223 Email: npumford@yahoo.co.uk — MB ChB Ed. 1988; MRCGP 1992; MBA 2000; MFPM 2002. Specialty: Pharmaceutical Medicine.

PUMFORD, Stanley (retired) 16 Hepburn Gardens, St Andrews KY16 9DD — MB BS Durh. 1964; BSc, MB BS Durh. 1964; DIH Soc. Apoth. Lond. 1971; MFOM RCP Lond. 1980. Prev: Med. Dir. E. Scotl. Occupat. Health Serv. Ltd.

PUMPHREY, Charles Walter St. Georges Hospital, London SW17 0QT Tel: 020 8672 1255 — BM BCh Oxf. 1973; MRCP (UK) 1976; DM Oxf. 1982; FRCP Lond. 1990. Cons. Cardiol. St. Geo. Hosp. Lond. Specialty: Cardiol. Prev: Sen. Regist. Lond. Hosp.; Regist. (Med.) Nat. Heart Hosp. Lond.; Brit. Amer. Travel. Fell. Mayo Clinic, USA.

PUMPHREY, Judith Harries 4 Portland Road, Bowdon, Altrincham WA14 2NY Tel: 0161 928 7334 — MB BS Lond. 1968 (St. Bart.) MRCS Eng. LRCP Lond. 1968; Cert. Family Plann. JCC 1974; MFFP 1993. SCMO (Adult Health inc. Family Plann. & Genitourin. Med.) Trafford HA & Univ. S. Manch. Withington Hosp. Specialty: Genitourinary Medicine. Prev: Ho. Surg. Whittington Hosp. Lond.; Ho. Phys. Qu. Mary's Hosp. for E. End Lond.

PUMPHREY, Richard Stephen Hugh Regional Immunology Service, St. Mary's Hospital, Manchester M13 0JH Tel: 0161 276 6452 Fax: 0161 276 6439 Email: richard.pumphrey@man.ac.uk — MB Camb. 1971 (St. Bart.) BChir 1970; FRCPath 1988, M 1976. Cons. Immunol. N. West. Regional Immunol. Serv. St. Mary's Hosp. Manch. Specialty: Immunol. Socs: Brit. Soc. Immunol.; Coun. Mem. Brit. Soc. Allergy & Clin. Immunol. Prev: Sen. Regist. (Clin. Immunol.) Glas. Roy. Infirm.; Asst. Pathol. Addenbrooke's Hosp. (Univ. Camb.).

PUNCH, David Michael The Surgery, 221 Whaddon Way, Bletchley, Milton Keynes MK3 7EA Tel: 01908 373058 Fax: 01908 630076; 22/24 The Green, Stoke Hammond, Milton Keynes MK17 9BX — MB BS Lond. 1978 (St. Geo.) Med. Dir. Bletchley Community Hosp. Milton Keynes.

PUNCHIHEWA, Veerasiri Gardiye Department of Anaesthesia, Basildon Hospital, Basildon SS16 5NL Tel: 01268 533911; 24 Crescent Drive, Shenfield, Brentwood CM15 8DS — MB BS Ceylon 1970 (Peradeniya) FFA RCS Eng. 1977. Cons. Anaesth. Basildon & Thurrock HA. Specialty: Anaesth. Socs: Assn. Anaesth.; Brit. Assn. Day Surg.; Sri-Lankan Doctors' Assn. Prev: St. Chas. Hosp. Lond.; Qu. Charhottes Hosp. Lond.; Sen. Regist. (Anaesth.) Hammersmith Hosp. Lond. & Odstock Hosp. Salisbury.

PUNDIT, Mahesh 13 Hartgrove Court, Elmwood Crescent, London NW9 0NN — MB BS Lond. 1984 (Char. Cross) Research Schol. (Anaesth.) Chicago, Ill., USA.

PUNJA, Ali Nazim The Surgery, 118/120 Stanford Avenue, Brighton BN1 6FE Tel: 01273 506361 Fax: 01273 552483 — MB BS Lond. 1989 (St. Thos.) DRCOG 1994; MRCGP 1994. GP Princip. Specialty: Gen. Pract. Prev: Trainee GP/SHO Brighton HA; SHO (A & E) St. Peters Hosp. Chertsey; Ho. Surg. (Surg. & Orthop.) St. Thos. Hosp. Lond.

PUNT, Mr Jonathan Arthur Gilbert P.O. Box 6016, Keyworth, Nottingham NG12 5RP Tel: 01509 880445 Fax: 01509 881955 — MB BS Lond. 1971 (Guy's) FRCS Eng. 1976; FRCPCH 1996. Cons. Paediat. Neurosurg. Specialty: Neurosurg. Socs: Fell. Roy. Soc. Med.; Soc. Brit. Neurol. Surgs.; Internat. Soc. for Paediat. Neurosurg. Prev: Sen. Lect. (Paediat. Neurosurg.) Univ. of Nottm; Cons. (Paediat. Neurosurg.) Univ. Of Nottm. & Leicester Roy. Infirm.; Sen. Regist. (Neurosurg.) Wessex Neurol. Centre Soton.

PUNT, Lydia Flat 9, Ivy Lane, Headington, Oxford OX3 9DT — MB ChB Stellenbosch 1992.

PUNTAMBEKAR, Sulabha (retired) Erinor, Gresham Avenue, Hartley, Longfield DA3 7BT — MB BS Bihar 1961 (Darbhanga Med. Coll.) MRCOG 1967, DObst 1965. Cons. (O & G) Dartford & Gravesham Health Dist. Prev: Clin. Asst. (O & G) Dartford & Gravesham Health Dist. & Medway.

PUNTER, Jale Psychotherapy Department, Villiers House, Tolworth Hospital, Red Lion Road, Surbiton KT6 7QU Tel: 020 8390 0102 Fax: 020 8390 3877 — BM Soton. 1986; MRCPsych 1991; MInst.GA 2000. p/t Cons. Psychiat. in Psychother., Tolworth Hosp., Surbiton, Surrey. Specialty: Psychother. Special Interest: Cross cultural psychtherapy. Prev: Sen. Regist. (Psychother.) St. Geo. Hosp. Lond.; Regist. (Psychiat.) & SHO Soton. Hosps.; SHO (Orthop., A & E, Neurol. & Neurosurg.) Soton. Gen. Hosp.

PUNTIS, John William Lambert The General Infirmary at Leeds, Room142, B Floor, Clarendon Wing, Belmont Grove, Leeds LS2 9NS Tel: 0113 392 3828 Fax: 0113 392 6048 Email: john.puntis@leedsth.nhs.uk — BM (Hons.) Soton. 1977; MRCP (UK) 1980; FRCP Lond. 1996; DM Soton. 1996; FRCPCH 1996. Sen. Lect. (Paediat. & Child Health) Univ. Leeds; Cons. Paediat. (Gastroenterol.) Leeds Gen. Infirm. Specialty: Paediat. Special Interest: Gastroenterol. & Nutrit. Socs: BSPGHAN; ESPGHAN; BAPEN. Prev: Lect. (Paediat. & Child Health) Univ. Birm.

PUNTIS, Mr Malcolm Colin Albert University Department of Surgery, University of Wales College of Medicine, Heath Park, Cardiff CF14 4XN Tel: 029 2074 3268 Fax: 029 2074 4709 — MB BCh Wales 1972; FRCS Ed. 1980; FRCS Eng. 1981; PhD Camb. 1981. Hon. Cons. Surg. & Sen. Lect. Univ. Hosp. Wales NHS Trust; Edr.-in-Chief Hepato-Pancreato-Biliary Surg. Jl. Specialty: Gen. Surg. Socs: Internat. Hepato-Pancreato-Biliary Assn.; Surgic. Research Soc.; Brit. Soc. Gastroenterol.

PUNUNGWE, Maryline 40 Foremark Close, Hainault, Ilford IG6 3HS — MB ChB Zimbabwe 1983. SHO (Psychiat.) Goodmays Hosp. Ilford.

PURANDARE, Mr Arunkumar Shantaram 3 Bakers Farm Road, Verwood, Wimborne BH21 6QF Tel: 01202 825197 — MB BS Bombay 1966 (Topiwala Nat. Med. Coll.) MS Bombay 1969; FRCS Ed. 1973; Dip. Med. Acupunc. BMAS 1997. Specialty: Gen. Surg. Socs: BMA; Brit. Blood Transfus. Soc. Prev: Regist. (Surg.) Doncaster Roy. Infirm.; Cook Co. Hosp. Chicago Illinois, USA; LTM Gen. Hosp. Bombay, India.

PURANIK, Ananth Southlands, Keycol Hospital, Newington, Sittingbourne ME9 8NG — MB BS Osmania 1981; MRCPsych 1988.

PURANIK, Mr Indudhar Northallerton Health Trust, Department of Orthopaedics, Friarage Hospital, Northallerton DL6 1SE Tel: 01609 779911 Fax: 01609 764638 — MB BS Mysore 1973 (Kasturba Med. Coll.) MS (Gen. Surg.) Karnatak 1976. Assoc. Specialist (Orthop.) Friarage Hosp. Northallerton. Specialty: Orthop. Prev: Trust Med. Off. (Orthop.); Regist. (Orthop.).

PURBACH, Mr Bodo Wrightington Hospital, Hall Lane, Appley Bridge, Wigan WN6 9EP Tel: 01252 256290 — State Exam Med Wurzburg 1991 (Wurzburg Univ.) MD. Cons. Trauma & Orthop. Surg. Wrightington, Wigan & Leigh NHS Trust. Specialty: Trauma & Orthop. Surg. Special Interest: Hip & Knee Primary & Revision Arthroplasty. Socs: Brit. Hip Soc.; John Charnley Research Inst.; John Charnley Low Friction Soc.

PURBEY, Badri Narayan The Park Canol Group Practice, Park Carnol Surgery, Central Park, Church Village, Pontypridd CF38 1RJ Tel: 01443 203414 Fax: 01443 218218; 3 Pen-y-Waun, Efailisaf, Pontypridd CF38 1AY Tel: 01443 201337 Fax: 01443 400283 — MB BS Bihar 1971 (Darbhanga Med. Coll. Laheriasarai) DCH Darbhanga 1974; DCH NUI 1979. GP Pontypridd. Prev: SHO (O & G) Gen. Hosp. Aberdare; SHO (Gen. Med.) Co. Hosp. HaverfordW.; SHO (Paediat.) Withybush Gen. Hosp. HaverfordW..

PURBICK, Andrew 1 Highfield Avenue, Alconbury Weston, Huntingdon PE28 4JS — MB BS Lond. 1996.

PURBRICK, Susan Attenborough Surgery, Bushey Health Centre, London Road, Bushey, Watford WD23 2NN Tel: 01923 231633 Fax: 01923 818594 Email: susan.purbrick@gp-e82124.nhs.uk; 84 Coldharbour Lane, Bushey WD23 4NX Tel: 020 8950 2989 Email: suepurbrick@yahoo.co.uk — MB ChB Liverp. 1974; DRCOG 1976; MRCGP 1980. Gen. Practitioner Bushey Health Centre, Bushey. Socs: W. Herts & Watford Med. Soc.

PURCE, Elizabeth Jill Ballymena Health Centre, Cushendall Road, Ballymena BT43 6HQ Tel: 028 2564 2181 Fax: 028 2565 8919; 3 Leighinmohr Avenue, Ballymena BT42 2AT — MB BCh BAO Belf. 1981; DRCOG 1984; MRCGP 1985.

PURCELL, Anna Marie Almaur, Grove Park, Pontnewydd, Cwmbran NP44 1RW — BM Soton. 1995.

PURCELL, Bernadette Louise Wiltshire Health Authority, Southgate House, Pans Lane, Devizes SN10 5EQ Tel: 01380 728899 Fax: 01380 722443; 2nd Floor Flat, 27 Park St, Bath BA1 2TF Email: blpurcell@breathe.co.uk — MB BS Lond. 1992 (Oxford and St Bartholomews Medical School London) BA Oxf. 1989; MRCP (UK) 1997; MSc 1998. Specialist Regist. (Pub. Health Med.) Wilts. HA. Specialty: Pub. Health Med.

PURCELL, Colin 7 Rosepark, Belfast BT5 7RG — MB BCh Belf. 1998.

PURCELL, Daniel Joseph (retired) 13 Windermere Road, West Wickham BR4 9AN Tel: 0208 776 2501 — (Univ. Coll. Dub.) MB BCh BAO NUI 1948 1948. Prev: GP, Thornton Heath, Surrey.

PURCELL, Graham Roger Gillies The Grange, Leigh, Sherborne DT9 6HL Tel: 01935 872404 — MB BChir Camb. 1970 (Camb. & St. Bart.) MA, MB Camb. 1970, BChir 1969; MRCS Eng. LRCP Lond. 1969; FFA RCS Eng. 1975. Cons. Anaesth. Yeovil Dist. Hosp.

Specialty: Anaesth. Prev: Sen. Regist. (Anaesth.) Soton., S.W. Hants Health Dist. & Westm. Hosp. Lond.; Regist. (Anaesth.) Hosp. Sick Childr. Lond. & Salisbury Gen. Hosp.

PURCELL, Ian Findlay Cardiac Medicine, National Heart and Lung Institute, Douehouse St., London SW3 6LY Tel: 020 7352 8121 Fax: 020 7823 3392 Email: i.purcell@ic.ac.uk — MB ChB Ed. 1990; BSc (Hons.) Ed. 1988, MB ChB (Hons.) 1990; MRCP (UK) 1993. Research Fell. (Cardiol.) Nat. Heart & Lung Inst. Specialty: Cardiol. Socs: Internat. Soc. Heart Research; Brit. Soc. Heart Failure. Prev: Regist. (Cardiol.) Freeman Hosp. Newc.; SHO Rotat. (Med.) Newc. HA; Regist. (Med. & Surg.) Roy. Infirm. Edin.

PURCELL, Patricia Mary Jennifer Ty Cymorth W. Wales Gen. Hosp., Carmarthenshire, NHS Trust, Carmarthen SA31 2AF Tel: 01267 227071 Fax: 01267 234071 Email: patpurcell@carmarthen.wales.nhs.uk; Ringing Stones, Mayals Road, Mayals, Swansea SA3 5DH Tel: 01792 405700 — BM Soton. 1985; BSc (Hons.) Soton. 1975; MSc Lond. 1977; Cert Family Planning JCC 1990; T(GP) 1990; MRCGP 1990; Dip Palliat Med 1993. Cons. (Palliat. Care) W. Wales Gen. Hosp., Carmarthenshire NHS Trust. Specialty: Palliat. Med. Socs: Assn. Palliat. Med.; Brit. Med. Assn.; Assn. of Palliat. Med. Prev: Conusltant in Palliat. Med., Pembrokesh. & Derwen NHS Trust; Regist. (LATS) Palliat. Med., TY Olwen, Swansea; Research & Regist., Palliat. Med., Marie Curie Centre, Cardiff.

PURCELL, Patrick (retired) 6 Coney Hill Road, West Wickham BR4 9BX — MB BCh BAO NUI 1948; DMRD Eng. 1951; DMRD Lond 1951. Cons. Radiol. Bromley, Beckenham & FarnBoro. Hosps. Prev: Regist. Char. Cross Hosp.

PURCELL, Patrick Francis 21a Old Bath Road, Sonning, Reading RG4 6SY Tel: 0118 969 8128 Fax: 0118 969 2672; Clarkes Hill, Rochestown, Republic of Ireland Tel: 00 353 21 489 3632 Fax: 00 353 21 489 3632 — MB BCh BAO NUI 1984 (Univ. Coll. Cork Med. Sch.) Locum Cons. Dept. Psych. Surrey Hants. Borders NHS Trust. Specialty: Gen. Psychiat. Prev: Intern. Cork Regional Hosp. Cork; Resid. Dept. Intern. Med. St. Luke's Roosevelt Hosp., Columbia Univ. Med. Sch. New York, USA.

PURCELL, Rodney Thomas Gordon and Partners, 1 North Street, Peterborough PE1 2RA Tel: 01733 312731 Fax: 01733 311447 — MB ChB Ed. 1972; DObst RCOG 1974; DA Eng. 1976; MRCGP 1987.

PURCELL, William Wadsley Hall, Hillsborough, Sheffield S6 4FD Tel: 0114 232 5767 — MB ChB Glas. 1964; DObst RCOG 1966. Socs: BMA. Prev: Ho. Off. (Med.) Glas. Roy. Infirm.; Ho. Off. (Surg.) E. Dist. Hosp. Glas.; Ho. Off. (Obst.) Robroyston Hosp. Glas.

PURCELL-JONES, Gari Department Anaesthesia General Hospital, Gloucester St., St Helier, Jersey JE2 3 Tel: 01534 622000 Fax: 01534 622633 Email: purcell-jones@jerseymail.co.uk; Les Prés, La Rue des Prés, St Lawrence, Jersey JE3 1EH Tel: 01534 862829 — MRCS Eng. LRCP Lond. 1977 (Char. Cross) BSc (Hons.) (Biochem.) Lond. 1974, MB BS 1977; MRCP (UK) 1981; FRCA Eng. 1984; FRCP UK 2000. Cons. Anaesth. & Pain Relief Gen. Hosp. St. Helier, Jersey. Specialty: Anaesth. Socs: Intractable Pain Soc.; Internat. Assn. Study of Pain. Prev: Sen. Regist. (Anaesth.) St. Thos. Hosp. Lond.; Regist. (Anaesth.) Hosp. Sick Childr. Lond.; Regist. (Anaesth.) St. Bart. Hosp. Lond.

PURCHAS, Madeleine Anne 65 Gipsy Lane, Wokingham RG40 2BW; Torvean, Kenwyn Road, Truro TR1 3SY — MB ChB Bristol 1993; MRCP 1998. SpR Roy. Cornw. Hosp. Truro. Specialty: Care of the Elderly. Socs: BMA; MDU; BGS.

PURCHAS, Simon Francis Uthnoe Veor, Churchtown, Perranuthnoe, Penzance TR20 9NH Tel: 01736 711487 — MB ChB Bristol 1993; BSc (Pharmacol.) Bristol 1990; MRCP (UK) 1997. SHO (A&E) Derriford Hosp. Plymouth. Specialty: Accid. & Emerg. Socs: BMA; MDU. Prev: SHO (O & G) Roy. United Hosp. Bath; SHO Anaesth. Roy. Cornw. Hosp. Truro, Cornw.; SHO (Gen. Med.) Kingston Hosp. Kingston upon Thames Surrey.

PURCHASE, Mrs Sheila Marshall (retired) 232 Dyke Road, Brighton BN1 5AE Tel: 01273 550039 — MB ChB Aberd. 1951; DObst RCOG 1954. Prev: Ho. Surg. Roy. Hosp. Sick Childr. Aberd. & Mothers' Hosp. Clapton.

PURCHES, Anthony Charles — MB BChir Camb. 1973 (Camb. & Lond. Hosp.) MA Camb. 1974 (Camb and London Hospital); DPM Eng. 1977; MRCPsych 1978. Cons. Psychiat. Mascalls Park, Brentwood & OldCh. Hosp. Romford. Specialty: Gen. Psychiat. Prev: Sen. Regist. Maudsley & St. Mary's Hosps. Lond.; Ho. Surg. (Urol.) & Regist. (Psychiat.) Lond. Hosp.; Ho. Phys. St. Martins Hosp. Bath.

PURDAY, Jonathan Paul Knowlfield, Exton Lane, Exton, Exeter EX3 0PP Tel: 01392 873762 Fax: 01392 402472 Email: jon.purday@doctors.org.uk — MB BS Lond. 1983 (St Mary's Hospital London) MRCP (UK) 1986; FRCA 1991. Cons. Anaesth. Roy. Devon & Exeter Hosp.; Lead Paediatric Anaesth. Specialty: Anaesth.; Intens. Care. Socs: BMA; Intens. Care Soc.; Assn. Anaesth. Prev: Sen. Regist. Rotat. (Anaesth.) Exeter & Bristol; Clin. Fell. (Paediat. Anaesth.) BC's Childr. Hosp. Vancouver BC, Canada; Regist. (Anaesth.) Guy's Hosp. Lond.

PURDIE, Alasdair Thomas Flat 2/1, 110 Brunswick St., Glasgow G1 1TF — MB ChB Aberd. 1990.

PURDIE, Anne Veronica St Lawrence Medical Centre, 4 Bocking End, Braintree CM7 9AA Tel: 01376 552474 Fax: 01376 552417 — MB BS Lond. 1985; DGM RCP Lond. 1987; DRCOG 1989; DCH RCP Lond. 1989; MRCGP 1990. Prev: Trainee GP Fulwell VTS.

PURDIE, Colin Alexander Department of Pathology, Ninewells Hospital and Medical School, Dundee DD1 9SY Tel: 01382 660111 Fax: 01382 640966 Email: colinp@tuht.scot.nhs.uk — MB ChB Ed. 1985 (Edinburgh University) PhD Ed. 1994, BSc (Hons.) Med. Sci. 1986, MB ChB 1985; MRCPath 1997. Cons. Histopath./cytopathologist Path. Dept. Dundee; Hon. Sen. Lect. Dept. of molecular and cellular Path. Dundee Univrdity. Specialty: Histopath. Socs: Roy. Soc. Pathol.; Pathol. Soc.; Assn. Clin. Pathol. Prev: Sen. Regist., Univ. Dept. of Path. Edin.; Career Regist. Glas. Roy. Infirm.; Regist. (Med.) Roy. Infirm. Edin.

PURDIE, Professor David Wilkie Edinburgh Osteoporosis Centre, 1 Wemyss Place, Edinburgh EH3 6DH Tel: 0131 2259949 Fax: 0845 1196050 Email: d.w.purdie@gloplus.com; Duncan's Land, 4 India Place, Edinburgh EH3 6EH Tel: 0131 2251199 Email: dwpurdie@ednet.co.uk — MB ChB Glas. 1969 (Univ. Glas.) M 1976; FRCOG 1988; MD Leeds 1990; FRCP Ed. 1997. Cons. Edin. Osteoporosis Centre; Scientif. Advis. Gp., Nat. Osteoporosis Soc.; Publications Committee, RCOG. Specialty: Osteop. Socs: Nat. Osteoporosis Soc.; Brit. Endocrine. Soc; Fell., Roy. Soc. Med. Prev: Prof. and Head of Clin. Research, Centre for Metab. Bone Dis., Hull Univ.; Hon. Cons. gynaecologist, Hull Royal Infirmary; Mem., Scientif. Advisory Gp., The Nat. Osteoporosis Soc.

PURDIE, Erica Margaret Gertrude Helen (retired) Shearwater, Popes Lane, Colyford, Colyton EX24 6QR Tel: 01297 553206 — MB BCh Wales 1941 (Cardiff) BSc Wales 1938; DObst RCOG 1943; MTh Lond. 1978, BD 1974. Prev: Resid. Surg. Off. St. Helier Co. Hosp. Carshalton.

PURDIE, Gregor Castle Douglas Medical Group, Castle Douglas Health Centre, Academy Sreett, Castle Douglas DG7 1EE Tel: 01556 503888 Fax: 01556 504302; The Auld Kirk, Hardgate, Haugh of Urr, Castle Douglas DG7 3LD Tel: 01556 660286 Fax: 01556 660415 — MB ChB Ed. 1978 (Edinburgh) DRCOG 1982. GP Adviser Dumfries & Galloway Health Bd.; Chairm. Scott. Area Med. Comms. Chairm. Gp. Socs: Sec. Dumfries & Galloway Local Med. Comm. Prev: Trainee GP Castle Douglas; SHO (O & G) Simpson Memor. Matern. Pavilion & Roy. Infirm. Edin.; Ho. Surg. & Ho. Phys. Dumfries & Galloway Roy. Infirm.

PURDIE, Helen Rose Mary North Street Medical Care, 274 North Street, Romford RM1 4QJ Tel: 01268 533911 — MB BS Lond. 1979 (Middlx.) DA Eng. 1981; DRCOG 1983; Dip. Pract. Dermat. Cardiff 1993; DFFP 2001. Assoc. Specialist (Dermat.) Basildon & Thurrock NHS Trust; GPwSI (Dermatology) Billericay, Brentwood & Wickford PCT; Honarary Teachg. Assoc. (Dermatology) Univ. of Wales Coll. of Med. Specialty: Dermat. Prev: GP Chelmsford; Examr. for Dip. In Practical Derm., Univ. of Wales Coll. Of Med.

PURDIE, Jane Ann Mills 22 Mansefield Avenue, Gambuslang, Glasgow G72 8NZ — MB ChB Glas. 1981; FFA RCSI 1986; FFA RCS Eng. 1987. Cons. Anaesth. Vict. Infirm. NHS Trust Glas. Specialty: Anaesth.

PURDIE, Niall Lachlan Lochindaal, Mary Avenue, Aberlour AB38 9QN — MB ChB Dundee 1991.

PURDOM, Deborah Jane Dept. of Nuclear Med, Glenfield Hospital, Groby Road, Leicester LE3 9QP Tel: 0116 287 1471; 27 Burton Street, Loughborough LE11 2DT Tel: 01504 219497 — BM BS Nottm. 1983; BMedSci Nottm. 1981. Med. Off. Specialty: Nuclear Med.

PURDUE, Basil Nigel Forensic Medicine Unit, Department of Pathology, University Medical School, Teviot Place, Edinburgh EH8 9AG Tel: 0131 650 4518 Fax: 0131 650 6529 — MB ChB Manch. 1976; BSc St. And. 1973; DMJ(Path) Soc. Apoth. Lond. 1985; FRCPath 1996, M 1986. Sen. Lect. (Forens. Med.) Univ. Edin. Specialty: Forens. Path. Socs: Brit. Assn. Forens. Med.; Medico-Legal Soc.; Brit. Acad. Forens. Sci. Prev: Sen. Lect. Univ. Dundee; Lect. (Forens. Med.) St. Thos. Hosp. Lond. & Univ. Leeds.

PURDY, Brian 42A Lee Park, Blackheath, London SE3 9HZ Tel: 020 8852 7168 — MB ChB Birm. 1953; DObst RCOG 1963; DPH (Distinc.) Lond. 1963. Prev: Princip. Med. Off. DHSS.

PURDY, David Robert Pepperman and Partners, The Cottons, Meadow Lane, Raunds, Wellingborough NN9 6UA Tel: 01933 623327 Fax: 01933 623370 — MB BS Lond. 1984; MSc Warwick; MRCGP Lond. 1988. Prev: SHO (Paediat. & Psych.) Joyce Green Hosp. Dartford; SHO (Infect. Dis.) Joyce Green Hosp. Dartford.

PURDY, Gerard Michael 5 Vicarage Gardens, Elloughton, Brough HU15 1JB — MB BCh BAO NUI 1982; FFA RCSI 1986; MRCP (UK) 1987.

PURDY, Robert Hedley Dykes Hall Medical Centre, 156 Dykes Hall Road, Sheffield S6 4GQ Tel: 0114 232 3236 — MRCS Eng. LRCP Lond. 1975; MRCGP 1979; DRCOG 1979; Cert JCC Lond. 1979.

PURDY, Sarah — MB BS Lond. 1987 (Med. Coll. St. Bart. Hosp.) BSc (Hons.) Lond. 1984; MRCGP (Distinc.) 1991; MPH Harvard Univ. 1996; MD London 1998. Hon. Sen. Lect..(Primary Health Care) Ubiv.Newc. Prev: Vis. Fell. Harvard Med. Sch.; Health Policy Analyst Jackson Hole Gp. USA; Trainee GP (Gen. Pract.) Exeter VTS.

PURDY, Vivienne Lesley Birbeck Medical Group, Penrith Health Centre, Bridge Lane, Penrith CA11 8HW; Boxwood House, Plumpton, Penrith CA11 9PA Tel: 01768 885100 — BM BS Nottm. 1990; BMedSci Nottm. 1988; DRCOG 1994; MRCGP 1996. GP Princip. Birbeck Med. GP Penrith. Specialty: Gen. Pract. Prev: Trainee GP/SHO (Med.) Cumbld. Infirm. Carlise; SHO (O & G) City Gen. Hosp. Carlise; SHO (Rheum., Paediat. & A & E) Cumbld. Infirm. Carlisle.

PUREWAL, Tejpal Singh Link 6Z, Royal Liverpool University Hospital, Prescott St., Liverpool L7 8XP Tel: 0151 706 3561 Fax: 0151 706 5928 — MB ChB Leeds 1987; BSc (Hons.) Physiol. 1984; MBChB (Hons.) 1987; MRCP (UK) 1990; MD (Leeds) 1999; FRCP (UK) 2000. Cons. Phys. (Diabetes & Endocrinol.) Roy. Liverp. Univ. Hosp.; Cons phys Liverp. Wom.s' Hosp. Specialty: Diabetes; Endocrinol.; Gen. Med. Prev: Sen. Regist. Roy. United Hosp. Bath; Regist. Roy. Vict. Infirm. Newc. u. Tyne; Research Fell. (Diabetic) Kings Coll. Hosp. Lond.

PURI, Basant Kumar MRI Unit, Imperial College School of Medicine, Hammersmith Hospital, Du Cane Road, London W12 0HS Fax: 020 8383 3038 Email: basant.puri@csc.mrc.ac.uk; 63 Caraway Road, Fulbourn, Cambridge CB1 5DU — MB BChir Camb. 1984; BA (Med. Sci. Tripos) Univ. of Camb. 1982; MA Camb. 1986; MRCPsych 1989; DipMath 1999; DipStat 2000; BSc (1st Class Hons.) Open Univ. 2000; PhD Neuroimaging (Imp. Coll. Lond.) 2001; MMath 2002. Prof. (Imaging and Psychiatry) Imperial Coll. Lond.; Prof. Experim. and Clin. Pharmacol., UHI; Hon. Cons. Dept. of Radiol. Hammersmith Hosp. Lond. Specialty: Gen. Psychiat.; Radiol.; Pharmacology. Socs: Roy. Coll. Psychiat. Prev: Sen. Research Fell. (Neuroimaging) Roy. Postgrad. Med. Sch. Univ. Lond.; Sen. Lect. (Neuroimaging); Sen. Clin. Scientist MRC Clin. Scis. Centre Hammersmith Hosp. Lond.

PURI, Shiela Clare St James's University Hospital, Regional Child Development Centre, Beckett Street, Leeds LS9 7TF Tel: 0113 206 4591 — MB BS Dehli 1989; MRCP; FRCPCH UK 1992. Cons. Paediat. (Neurodisabil. & Community Paediat.). Specialty: Paediat. Special Interest: Neurodisability. Socs: RCPCCH; BACCH; BPNA.

PURI, Sundeep c/o Three Trees, 202 College Road, Whalley Range, Manchester M16 0AA — MB ChB Manch. 1986.

PURITZ, Rupert 13 Clifton House Close, Clifton, Shefford SG17 5EQ Tel: 01462 812246 Fax: 01462 851858; 109 Station Road, Lower Stondon, Henlow SG16 6JJ Tel: 01462 850305 Fax: 01462 851858 — MB BS Lond. 1970 (Roy. Free) MRCS Eng. LRCP Lond. 1970; MRCP (UK) 1975. Prev: Research Regist. (Cardiol.) Roy. Sussex Co. Hosp. Brighton; Rotat. Regist. (Med.) King's Coll. Hosp. Lond.; Ho. Phys. Roy. Free Hosp. Lond.

PURKIS, Jethro John McDonald — MB ChB Birm. 1995.

PURKISS, Muriel Edith (retired) 23 St Agnes Close, Victoria Park Road, London E9 7HS Tel: 020 8533 5979 — MB BS Lond. 1954; MFCM 1983.

PURKISS, Ruth Heather 24 Manor Park, Bristol BS6 7HH — MB ChB Bristol 1987.

PURNACHANDRA RAO, Vuyyuru Rydal Mount, 30 Dinting Road, Glossop SK13 7DT — MB BS Andhra 1971.

PURNELL, David Dept. Pathology, UHL Leicester Royal Infimary, Infirmary Square, Leicester LE1 5WW Email: davep@doctors.org.uk — MB ChB Leic. 1996; BSc Sheff. 1991. Specialist Regist. (Histopath.) Leicester. Specialty: Histopath. Prev: SHO (Histopath.) Roy. Free Hosp. Lond.; Ho. Off. (Med.) Leicester Roy. Infirm.

PURNELL, Elizabeth Mary (retired) Carr Hill, Shawclough Road, Rochdale OL12 6LG; 10 Windmill End, Rothley, Leicester LE7 7RP Tel: 0116 230 2174 — MB BS Lond. 1959 (Char. Cross) BSc Lond. 1952, MB BS 1959.

PURNELL, Kenneth Leslie (retired) Treetops, Wiswell Lane, Whalley, Clitheroe BB7 9AF Tel: 01254 824524 — MB ChB Manch. 1950. Prev: GP Accrington.

PURNELL, Nicola Windsor Cottage, Windsor Lane, Little Kingshill, Great Missenden HP16 0DP — BM Soton. 1995.

PURNELL, Richard Mark 192 Adventurer's Quay, Cardiff Bay, Cardiff CF10 4NS — BM BS Nottm. 1998.

PURNELL, Robin John (retired) 6 Taylor Avenue, Cringleford, Norwich NR4 6XY Tel: 01603 454491 — (St. Thos.) MB BS Lond. 1959; FFA RCS Eng. 1963. Prev: Cons. & Sen. Regist. (Anaesth.) Norf. & Norwich Health Care NHS Trust.

PURNELL, Simon Leslie Ilkeston Health Centre, South Street, Ilkeston DE7 5PZ Tel: 0115 932 2968 Fax: 0115 944 2578 Email: simon.purnell@nhs.net — BM BCh Oxf. 1988; MA Camb. 1985; DCH RCP Lond. 1990; DRCOG 1991; MRCGP 1992. Specialty: Gen. Pract.

PURNELL-MULLICK, Samir 55 Arden Street, Coventry CV5 6FB — MB BS Lond. 1989; BSc Physiol. Lond. 1986; MRCP (UK) 1992. Regist. (Radiol.) Leicester Roy. Infirm. Specialty: Radiol.

PUROHIT, Nimischandra Natverlal 242 The Fairway, New Moston, Manchester M40 3NH — MB BS Baroda 1979; DPM RCPSI 1986; MRCPsych 1992.

PUROHIT, Shyamsundar Jagannath Spinney Hill Medical Centre, 143 St. Saviours Road, Leicester LE5 3HX Tel: 0116 251 7870 Fax: 0116 262 9816; 4 Meadowcourt Road, Oadby, Leicester LE2 2PB — MB BS Nagpur 1973 (Govt med Coll Nagdur) MD Nagpur 1978.

PURR, Julia Margaret Haigh and Partners, 11 Church Street, Harston, Cambridge CB2 5NP Tel: 01223 870250 Fax: 01223 872741; The Surgery, 11 Church St, Harston, Cambridge CB2 5NP Tel: 01223 870250 Fax: 01223 872741 — MB BChir Camb. 1981 (Camb. (New Hull and Addenbrookes)) MA Camb. 1981.

PURRY, Nigel Angold (retired) 17 Chewton Common Road, Highcliffe, Christchurch BH23 5LX — (Charing Cross Hospital) MB BS Lond. 1959; DObst RCOG 1961; FRCS Eng. 1970. Prev: Cons. Rehabil. Med. Roy. Bournemouth & ChristCh. Hosp. NHS Trust.

PURSER, John Hedley Springfield House, New Lane, Patricroft, Manchester M30 7JE; Woodend, 44 Woodstock Drive, Worsley, Manchester M28 2WW Tel: 0161 794 4540 — MB ChB Manch. 1976. Clin. Asst. (Plastic Surg.) Withington Hosp.; Clin. Asst. (Gastroenterol.) Hope Hosp. Specialty: Gastroenterol. Prev: SHO Rotat. (Surg.) Univ. Hosp. S. Manch.

PURSER, Mr Nicholas John Saltway Cottage, 28 Droitwich Road, Feckenham, Redditch B96 6HX — MB ChB Birm. 1990; FRCS Glas.; ChB Birm. 1990. Specialist Regist. (Gen. Surg.). Specialty: Gen. Surg.

PURSER, Paul Cyril Purser and Partners, Clee Medical Centre, 323 Grimsby Road, Cleethorpes DN35 7XE Tel: 01472 697257 Fax: 01472 690852; 16 Abbey Drive W., Grimsby DN32 0HH Tel: 01472 352541 Fax: 01472 352541 Email: paulpurser@aol.com — MB ChB Leeds 1976. Med. Dir. St Andrews Hospice, Peaks Ln. Grimsby, N E Lincs; Macmillan Lead G.P. In Palliat. Care. Specialty: Palliat. Med.

PURSNANI, Mr Kishore 23 Mimosa Close, Euxton, Chorley PR2 1BT Tel: 01257 265805 Email: kpursnani@aol.com — MB BS Bombay 1986. Specialist Regist. (Gen. Surg.) Lancs. Teachg. Hosps. NHS Trust. Specialty: Gen. Surg. Special Interest: Upper Gastrointestinal Surg.

PURSSELL, Neville Richard Paddington Green Health Centre, 4 Princess Louise Close, London W2 1LQ Tel: 020 7887 1600 Fax: 020 7887 1635 — MB BS Lond. 1989 (UMDS (Guys)) MA Camb. 1982; DCH RCP Lond. 1992; DRCOG 1992; MRCGP 1995. Specialty: Gen. Pract.

PURUSHOTHAM, Mr Anand David Cambridge Breast Unit, Addenbrookes Hospital, Cambridge CB2 2QQ Tel: 01223 586627 Fax: 01223 586932 — MB BS Madras 1982; FRCS Ed. 1987; MD Glas. 1992; FRCS (Gen.) 1995; FRCS Glasgow 1999; FRCS England 2001. Cons. Surg. Addenbrookes Hosp. Camb. Specialty: Gen. Surg. Special Interest: Breast Cancer.

PURUSHOTHAMAN, Hema Nandini — MB BS Lond. 1998 (Imperial Coll.) BSc Lond. 1995. Specialty: Paediat.

PURUSHOTHAMAN, Sunil — MB BS Lond. 1998.

PURUSHOTHMAN, Girija 4 Benrek Close, Ilford IG6 2QL — MB BS Madras, India 1991; MRCS Eng. LRCP Lond. 1989.

PURVES, Alistair Martin Kings College Hospital, Denmark Hill, London SE5 9RS Tel: 020 7346 5373 Email: alistair.purves@kingsch.nhs.uk — MB BChir Camb. 1981; MRCP (UK) 1985; MRCP Ed. 1987; MD Camb. 1994. Cons. Neurophysiol. Specialty: Clin. Physiol.; Clin. Neurophysiol. Special Interest: Pain. Prev: Sen. Regist. (Clin. Neurophysiol.) Hosp. for Childr. Gt. Ormond St. Lond.; Hon. Clin. Asst. (Clin. Neurophysiol.) Nat. Hosp. Neurol. & Neurosurg.Lond.

PURVES, Hilda Jean (retired) 7 Worcester Crescent, Clifton, Bristol BS8 3JA Tel: 0117 973 6129 — MB BS Lond. 1953. Clin. Med. Off. (Child Health) Avon AHA; Instruc. Doctor (Family Plann.) Bristol & Weston HAs. Prev: SCMO Family Plann. & reproductive health.

PURVES, Professor Ian Nicholas Sowerby Centre for Health Informatics at Newcastle, University of Newcastle, Newcastle upon Tyne NE4 6BE Tel: 0191 256 3141 Fax: 0191 256 3099 Email: ian.purves@ncl.ac.uk; 45 Western Way, Ponteland, Newcastle upon Tyne NE20 9AS — MB BS Newc. 1985; DCCH RCGP & FCM 1988; MRCGP 1989; DRCOG 1989; MD Newc. 1998. Head of Sowerby Centre for Health Informatics, Newc. Univ., Newc. u. Tyne; Prof. (Health Informatics) Newc. Univ. Specialty: Gen. Pract. Socs: BMA; RCOGP; Chair RCGP Health Informatics Task Gp. Prev: GP Blaydon; Trainee GP N.d. VTS.

PURVES, Jonathan David 199 Dowson Road, Hyde SK14 5BR Tel: 0161 368 1947; 199 Dowson Road, Hyde SK14 5BR Tel: 0161 368 1947 — MB ChB Birm. 1997. SHO (Psychiat.) GP Rotat. Dudley Gp. of Hosps. Specialty: Gen. Psychiat.

PURVIS, Christopher Raymond (retired) Purvis and Partners, The Hart Surgery, York Road, Henley-on-Thames RG9 2DR Tel: 01491 843200 Fax: 01491 411296; Highfield, 11 Rotherfield Road, Henley-on-Thames RG9 1NR Tel: 01491 579295 Fax: 01491 579295 — (St. Thos.) MRCS Eng. LRCP Lond. 1964. Prev: SHO (Obst.) Gen. Lying-In Hosp. Lond.

PURVIS, Diana Joan Avenue Medical Centre, Wentworth Avenue, Slough SL2 2DG Tel: 01753 524549 Fax: 01753 552537; 2 Rambler Close, Taplow, Maidenhead SL6 0JT — MB ChB Sheff. 1983 (Sheffield) DRCOG 1986; MRCGP 1987.

PURVIS, Jane Torridon, Barmoor Lane, Ryton NE40 3AA — MB BS Newc. 1976.

PURVIS, John Arthur Department of Cardiology, Altnagelvin Area Hospital, Glenshane Road, Londonderry BT47 6SB Tel: 01504 451711 Fax: 01504 311020; 2 Cross Na Downell Park, Greystone Road, Limavady BT49 0TP Tel: 015047 69113 — MB BCh BAO Belf. 1985; MRCP Glas. 1988; MD Belf. 1992; FRCP Glas. 1998. Cons. Phys. (Cardiol.) Altnagelvin Area Hosp. Specialty: Cardiol. Socs: Amer. Heart Assn. (Counc. Clin. Cardiol.); Internat. Soc. Fibrinolysis & Thrombolysis.; Brit. Cardiac Soc. Prev: Sen. Regist. (Cardiol.) Roy. Vict. Hosp. Belf.; Sen. Regist. (Med.) Ulster Hosp. Dundonald; Regist. (Cardiol.) Belf. City Hosp. Belf.

PURVIS, Mark Julian 17 Uppertown, Pxenhope, Keighley BD22 9LL — MB ChB Leeds 1984.

PURVIS, Richard John Childrens Centre, Damers Road, Dorchester DT1 2LB Tel: 01305 251150 Fax: 01305 254737; 2 Queens Avenue, Dorchester DT1 2EW Tel: 01305 262670 — MB ChB Ed. 1964; DCH Eng. 1966; FRCP Ed. 1983, M 1967; FRCP Lond. 1986. Cons. Paediat. W. Dorset Gen. Hosps. NHS Trust; Med. Dir. W.Dorset Gen. Hosps. NHS Trust. Specialty: Paediat. Prev: Lect. (Child Life & Health) Univ. Edin.; SHO (Paediat.) Edin. Roy. Infirm. & Internat. Grenfell Assn. St. Anthony, Newfld.

PURWAR, Rajiv 48 Goddington Lane, Orpington BR6 9DS Tel: 01689 26638 — MB BS Lond. 1983; BA Camb. 1980; DRCOG 1986; DCH RCP Lond. 1987; MRCGP 1987. Princip. GP Lond.

PURWAR, Simon 46 Addison Road, Hove BN3 1TP; 4 Nursery Gardens, Chislehurst BR7 5BW Tel: 020 8456 7925 — MB BS Lond. 1992; MA Oxf. 1989.

PURWAR, Vijay Station Road Surgery, 74 Station Road, West Wickham BR4 0PU Tel: 020 8777 8245 — MB ChB Bristol 1985; MRCGP 1989; DCH RCP Lond. 1990.

PUSAVAT, Lilian Tharntip Department of Psychiatry, West Middlxsex University Hospital, Twickenham Road, Isleworth TW7 6AF Tel: 020 8565 5178 — MB BS Hong Kong 1979; MRCPsych 1985. Cons. Psychiat. W. Middlx. Univ. Hosp. Specialty: Gen. Psychiat.

PUSEY, Professor Charles Dickson Renal Section, Division of Medicine, Faculty of Medicine, Imperial College London, Hammersmith Hospital, Du Cane Road, London W12 0NN Tel: 020 8383 3152 Fax: 020 8383 2062 Email: c.pusey@imperial.ac.uk — MB BChir Camb. 1972 (Guy's) BA Camb. 1969; MA 1973; MRCP (UK) 1974; MSc Lond. 1983; FRCP Lond. 1989; FRCPath Lond. 1997; FMedSci 2002; DSc Lond. 2002. Prof. (Med.) Imperial Coll. Lond.; Cons. Phys. Hammersmith Hosp. Lond. Specialty: Nephrol.; Gen. Med. Special Interest: Glomerulonephritis; Systemic Vasculities. Socs: Acad. of Med. Sci.; Renal Assn.; Assn. Phys. Prev: Reader (Renal Med.) & Sen. Lect. (Med.) Roy. Postgrad. Med. Sch. Lond.; Cons. Phys. Hammersmith Hosp. Lond.

PUSEY, Clare Tonna Hospital, Tonna, Neath SA11 3AX Fax: 01639 635404 — MB BCh Wales 1992 (University of Wales Cardiff) MRC Psych 1996. Staff Grade (Psychiat.) Tonna Hosp. Neath. Specialty: Geriat. Psychiat. Prev: Regist. (Psychiat.) Cefn Coed Hosp. Swansea; SHO (Med.) P. Philip Hosp. Llanelli; Ho. Off. (Med.) Princess of Wales Hosp. Bridgend.

PUSEY, Johanna Mary Mill Top Farm, Mill Lane, Goosnargh, Preston PR3 2JX — MB BS Lond. 1975 (Roy. Free) MRCS Eng. LRCP Lond. 1975.

PUSEY, Judith Mary Hassengate Medical Centre, Southend Road, Stanford-le-Hope SS17 0PH; 12 Appleby Drive, Laindon, Basildon SS16 6NU — MB BS Lond. 1970 (Lond. Hosp.) DObst RCOG 1972. Princip. GP Stanford le Hope. Prev: Lect. (Gen. Pract.) Welsh Nat. Sch. Med. Cardiff.

PUSEY, Mr Richard John, TD Basildon Hospital, Nether Mayne, Basildon SS16 5NL Tel: 01268 592284 — MB ChB Birm. 1970; FRCS Eng. 1975. Cons. Orthop. Surg. Basildon & Thurrock NHS Trust. Specialty: Orthop.; Trauma & Orthop. Surg. Socs: World Orthop. Concern. Prev: Sen. Regist. (Orthop.) Addenbrookes Hosp. Camb.; Regist. (Orthop.) St. Thos. Hosp. Lond.

PUSHPANATHAN, Mr Rajadurai Joseph 1 Elvington Gayton Road, King's Lynn PE30 4TB — MB BS Sri Lanka 1975; DO RCS Eng. 1984; LMSSA Lond. 1984; FRCS Glas. 1985; FCOphth 1989. Cons. Ophth. Qu. Eliz. Hosp. King's Lynn. Specialty: Ophth. Prev: Ass. Specialist Ophth.

PUSHPANGADAN, Majnu 2 Woodlands Court, Longwood Avenue, Bingley BD16 2SW — MB ChB Leeds 1990; MRCP (UK) 1994. Regist. (Gen. Med. & Med. for Elderly) Yorks. Prev: SHO Rotat. (Med.) Bradford.

PUSHPARAJAH, Christeta Ratnakumari Knoll Rise Surgery, 1 Knoll Rise, Orpington BR6 0EJ Tel: 01689 824563 Fax: 01689 820712 — MB BS Sri Lanka 1982.

PUSHPARAJAH, Savitha 91 Beeston Road, Dunkirk, Nottingham NG7 2JQ — BM BS Nottm. 1996.

PUSZET, Jozef (retired) Willowtree Bungalow, 19 Bicester Road, Long Crendon, Aylesbury HP18 9BP — MB BS Lond. 1962 (King's Coll. Hosp.) DObst 1964; FRCOG 1990, M 1975. Prev: Sen. Cons. O & G Sultan Qaboos Univ. Hosp. Muscat, Oman.

PUSZTAI, Edit Esther — MB ChB Glas. 1988 (Glasgow) MRCPsych 1993; Dip Cog Psych Dund 1997. Specialty: Gen. Psychiat.; Ment. Health; Psychother. Socs: BMA; Roy. Coll. Psychiat.; Brit. Assn. Cognitive and Behaviour Psychotherapists. Prev: SR Gen. Psychiat. and LD, Ment. Welf. Commiss., Edin.; SR Gen. Psychiat. and LD Strathlea Resource Centre, Kilmarnook; SR Gen. Psychiat. and LD, Roy. Scott. Nat. Hosps.

PUTMAN, Helen Rose 14 Belgrave Street, Ossett WF5 0AD — MB ChB Leeds 1985.

PUTNAM, Elizabeth Ann Druids, Chilworth Ring, Chilworth, Southampton SO16 7HW — MB ChB Birm. 1975; FFA RCS Eng. 1979. Cons. Anaesth. Soton. & S.W. Hants. Health Dist. Specialty: Anaesth. Prev: Sen. Regist. (Anaesth.) Soton. & S.W. Hants. Health Dist.; Regist. (Anaesth.) Soton. Gen. Hosp.; SHO (Anaesth.) Roy. Devon & Exeter Hosp. (Wonford) Exeter.

PUTNAM, Mr Graham Douglas Cumberland Infirmary, Newtown Road, Carlisle CA2 7HY; Grayson House, Great Salkeld, Penrith CA11 9NB Tel: 01768 898080 — MB BCh Wales 1988 (University of Wales College of Medicine) BDS 1980; FDS RCS Eng. 1983; FRCS Ed. 1991. Cons. Oral & Maxillofacial Surg. Carlisle Hosps. NHS Trust. Specialty: Oral & Maxillofacial Surg. Socs: Fell. Brit. Assn. Oral & Maxillofacial Surg. Prev: Sen. Regist. Bristol S.W. Regional HA; Regist. N.E. Rotat. Newc., Sunderland, Middlesbrough.

PUTRIS, Samera Haseeb Grosvenor Road Surgery, 23 Grosvenor Road, Muswell Hill, London N10 2DR Tel: 020 8883 5600 Fax: 020 8883 3324 — MB ChB Mosul, Iraq 1972; DObst; RCP (Ire) 1981; T(GP) 1991.

PUTT, Christopher Mark New Road Clinic, 114 New Road, Chingford, London E4 9SY Tel: 020 8524 8124 Fax: 020 8529 8655 — MB ChB Leeds 1983; DRCOG 1986; MRCGP 1988.

PUTTA GOWDA, Hethur M Dr H M Putta Gowda, 8 Cardiff Road, Newtown, Mountain Ash CF45 4EY Tel: 01443 476505 Fax: 01443 473219.

PUTTAGUNTA, Balaji Park Grove Surgery, 94 Park Grove, Barnsley S70 1QE Tel: 01226 282345 — LRCP LRCS Ed. 1980; LRCP LRCS Ed. LRCPS Glas. 1980.

PUTTER-LAREMAN, Suren — MB ChB Stellenbosch 1993. Specialist Regist. (Psychiat. Child & Adolesc.) Gartnaval Roy. Hosp. Glas. Specialty: Child & Adolesc. Psychiat.

PUTTERILL, Janet Sinclair 87B Sandpit Lane, St Albans AL1 4EY — MB ChB Stellenbosch 1993.

PUTTICK, Michael Ian 62 Saltram Crescent, London W9 3HR Tel: 020 8969 8482 Email: m.puttick@bigfoot.com — MB BS Lond. 1996 (St. Mary's Lond.) BSc 1995. SHO (A&E) St. Mary's Hosp. Leeds; Hon. Res. Fell. (Acad. Surg. Unit) St. Mary's Hosp. Lond. Specialty: Gen. Surg. Socs: Roy. Soc. Med.; St. Mary's Assn. Prev: Research Fell. St. Mary's Hosp. Lond.

PUTTICK, Nigel 10 The Dorkings, Great Broughton, Middlesbrough TS9 7NA — MB BChir Camb. 1978; MA Camb. 1979; Dip. Obst. Auckland 1980; FFA RCS Lond. 1983. Cons. Anaesth. James Cook Univ. Hosp. Middlesbrough. Specialty: Anaesth. Prev: Lect. Dept. Anaesth. Univ. Wales Coll. Med.

PUVANACHANDRA, Mr Kathir HM Stanley Hospital, Directorate on Ophthalmology, St Asaph LL17 0RS Tel: 01745 583275; Bryn Sai, 4 Hayden Close, Old Colwyn, Colwyn Bay LL29 9PB Tel: 01492 516510 — MB BS Ceylon 1971 (Colombo) DO Eng. 1981; FRCS Ed. 1981; FRCOphth. 1993. Cons. Ophth. HM Stanley Hosp. St. Asaph; Ext. Examr. FRCS Ophth. RCS Glas.; Pant 3 MRCOpyth. RCOphth. Chairm. Overseas Doctors Train. Comm. RCOphth. Specialty: Ophth. Prev: Hon. Lect. Univ. Glas. & Sen. Regist. (Ophth.) West. Infirm. Glas.

PUVANENDRAN, Kanagasabai 600 Rayleigh Road, Hutton, Brentwood CM13 1SG — MB BS Sri Lanka 1978; MRCP (UK) 1987.

PUVANENDRAN, Priyadharshini 9 Rochester Gardens, Croydon CR0 5NN — MB ChB Dundee 1993.

PUVANENDRAN-THOMAS, Rukshini 85B Walton Street, Oxford OX2 6EA — MB BS Singapore 1989.

PUVEENDRAN, Arulnandhy (retired) — MB BS Ceylon 1954 (Colombo) DLO Eng. 1973.

PUVI, Nirmalan Great Clacton Medical Partnership, 17 North Road, Clacton-on-Sea CO15 4DA Tel: 01255 224600 Fax: 01255 224617 — MB ChB Dundee 1993; DRCOG 1997. Principal in General Practice. Specialty: Gen. Pract. Prev: SHO (Opthalmol.)/ENT Furness Gen. Hosp.

PUVINATHAN, Himasalakumari The Surgery, 119 Northcote Road, Battersea, London SW11 6PW Tel: 020 7228 6762 — LMSSA Lond. 1995.

PUXLEY, Deborah Mollie 13 Cunningham Avenue, St Albans AL1 1JJ — MB ChB Liverp. 1996.

PUXON, Christine Margaret 19 Clarence Gate Gardens, Glentworth St., London NW1 6AY Tel: 020 7723 7922 Fax: 020 7258 2038 Email: margaretpuxon@aol.com — (Birm.) MRCS Eng. LRCP Lond. 1941; MB ChB (Hons.) Birm. 1942; FRCOG 1979, M 1946; MD (Obst.) Birm. 1947. Cons. Med. Legal Consult. Lond.; QC; Chairm. (Ethics Comm.) IVF Unit Lister Hosp. Socs: Fell. Roy. Soc. Med.; Medico-Legal Soc.; Soc. Of Doctors in Law (Chairm.). Prev: Crown Ct. Recorder; Dep. Circuit Judge; Regist. (Gyn.) Qu. Eliz. Hosp. Birm.

PUZEY, Angela Jane Southwell House Surgery, Southwell House, Back Lane, Rochford SS4 1AY Tel: 01702 545241 Fax: 01702 546390; The Old Post Office, Church End, Paglesham, Rochford SS4 2DJ — MB ChB Bristol 1965. Prev: Cas. Off., Ho. Surg. & Ho. Phys. Stratford-on-Avon Hosp.; Sch. Med. Off. Southend.

PUZEY, Susan Hermione 1 Hillfield Road, Redhill RH1 4AP Tel: 01737 763888 — MB BS Lond. 1984; DRCOG 1987; MRCGP 1988.

PYATT, Jason Robert Royal Liverpool & Broadgreen University Hospital NHS Trust, Prescot Street, Liverpool L7 8XP Tel: 0151 706 2000 Email: jason.pyatt@rlbuht.nhs.uk — MB ChB Manch. 1990; BSc Hons Manchester 1987; MRCP (UK) 1995. Specialist Regist. (Cardiol.) Mersey Deanery; Res. Fell. (Cardio.). Specialty: Cardiol. Prev: SHO (Med.) Hope Hosp. Salford; SHO (Med.) Wigan Infirm. Wigan.

PYATT, Richard Niel Kirkton Manor, The School House, Peebles EH45 9JN — MB BChir Camb. 1994.

PYCOCK, Christopher John Department Medicine, Worcester Royal Infirmary, Newtown Road, Worcester WR5 1JG Tel: 01905 763333 Fax: 01905 760373 — MB ChB Bristol 1985; BSc Soton. 1969; PhD CNAA 1972; DSc Bristol 1984; MRCP (UK) 1988; FRCP (UK) 1999. Cons. Phys. Worcester Roy. Infirm.; PostGrad. Clin. Tutor; Regional Coll. Tutor. Specialty: Gen. Med.; Care of the Elderly. Socs: Pharmacol. Soc.; BMA; Brit. Geriat. Soc. Prev: Lect. (Neuropharmacol.) Bristol; Res. Fell. Pk.inson's Dis. Soc.

PYCOCK, Julie Elizabeth Hackenthorpe Medical Centre, Main Street, Hackenthorpe, Sheffield S12 4LA Fax: 0114 251 0539 — MB ChB Sheff. 1984.

PYE, Eleanor Mary — MB ChB Leeds 1996. Specialty: Neurol.

PYE, Mr Geoffrey Weston General Hospital, Uphill, Weston Super Mare BS23 4TQ Tel: 01934 647175 Fax: 01934 647018 — BM Soton. 1981; BSc Leeds 1974; MSc Aberd. 1975; FRCS Ed. 1985; DM Nottm. 1988; FRCS 2001. Cons. Gen. & Colorectal Surg. Weston Area Health Trust. Specialty: Gen. Surg. Socs: Assn. Coloproctol.; Brit. Soc. Gastroenterol. Prev: Lect. (Surg.) Univ. Nottm.

PYE, Geoffrey Francis Calcot Medical Centre, Hampden Road, Chalfont St Peter, Gerrards Cross SL9 9SA Tel: 01753 887311 Fax: 01753 891933; Kersham House, Bridge Reeve, Chulmleigh EX18 7BD Tel: 01769 581241 — MB BChir Camb. 1963 (King's Coll. Hosp.) BA Camb. 1959; MRCGP 1978. Course Organiser i/c GP VTS Scheme Wycombe Dist.

PYE, Ian Frederick 3 Knighton Road, Stoneygate, Leicester LE2 3HL Tel: 0116 270 8536 — MD Camb. 1980, MB 1967; BChir 1966 (Camb. & Lond. Hosp.) DObst RCOG 1969; MRCP (U.K.) 1970; FRCP Lond. 1984. Cons. Neurol. Leicester Roy. Infirm. Specialty: Neurol. Socs: Mem. Assn. Brit. Neurol.; Midl.s Neurol. Soc. Prev: Sen. Regist. (Neurol.) Univ. Hosp. Wales Cardiff; Regist. (Neurol.) N. Staffs. Hosp. Centre Stoke-on-Trent; Ho. Surg. & Ho. Phys. Lond. Hosp.

PYE, Mr Jonathan Kellow Department of Surgery, Wrexham Maelor Hospital, Croesnewydd Road, Wrexham LL13 7TD; Claremont Cottage, 29 Stansty Road, Wrexham LL11 2HR — MB BS Lond. 1974; MRCS Eng. LRCP Lond. 1974; FRCS Eng. 1979; MS Lond. 1987; Cert. Higher Surg. Train. RCS Eng. 1988. Cons. Surg. Wrexham Maelor Hosp. Specialty: Gen. Surg.; Gastroenterol. Prev: Sen. Regist. (Surg.) S. Glam. & Clwyd HAs; 1 Year Secondment Qu. Mary Hosp. Hong Kong; Clin. Research Off. (Surg.) Univ. Wales Sch. Med.

PYE, Maryan Jennifer 2 Wingate Close, The Old Mill, Haslers Lane, Dunmow CM6 1XS Tel: 01371 767007 Fax: 01371 767008 Email: maryan.pye@utlesford-pct.nhs.uk; 2 Wingate Close, Trumpington, Cambridge CB2 2HW — (Char. Cross) MB BS Lond. 1970; MRCS Eng. LRCP Lond. 1970; DA Eng. 1972; MFCM RCP (UK) 1984; FFPHM RCP (UK) 1993, M 1989. Dir. Pub. Health, Utlesford PCT; Pub. Health Cons. ALPHA. Specialty: Pub. Health Med. Special Interest: Organiasation & Manag.; Primary Preven. Socs: Soc. Social Med.; Pub. Health & Primary Care Gp.; Inst.

Healthcare Man. Prev: Sen. Cons. Dearden Consg.; Cons.Pub.Health Med.NHSE-E.ern; Cons. Pub. Health Med. Camb. & Huntingdon Health Auth.

PYE, Maurice Anthony Matthew Department of Cardiology, York District Hospital, York YO31 8HE Tel: 01904 631313 — MD Wales 1992 (Cardiff) FRCP FRCP; BSc 1979; MB BCh 1982; MRCP (UK) 1985; FCP Lond. 1998. Cons. Cardiol. York Dist. Hosp. Specialty: Cardiol.; Gen. Med. Socs: York Med. Soc.; Brit. Cardiovasc. Interven. Soc.; Brit. Cardiac Soc. Prev: Sen. Regist. (Cardiol.) St. Geo. Hosp. Lond.; Brit. Heart Foundat. Research Fell. Roy. Infirm. Glas.; Regist. (Cardiol.) Roy. Infirm. Glas.

PYE, Richard James 2A Wingate Close, Trumpington, Cambridge CB2 2HW Tel: 01223 843373 Fax: 01223 847006 Email: rjpye@dial.pipex.com — (Char. Cross) MB BS Lond. 1969; MRCS Eng. LRCP Lond. 1969; MRCP (UK) 1973; MD Lond. 1979; MA Camb. 1982; FRCP Lond. 1989. Cons. Dermat. Addenbrooke's Hosp. Camb. Specialty: Dermat. Socs: Brit. Assn. Dermat.; Eur. Soc. Micrographic Surg.; Amer. Acad. of Dermat. Prev: Sen. Regist. & Tutor (Dermat.) St. John's Hosp. Dis. Skin Lond.; Regist. (Dermat.) Bristol Roy. Infirm.

PYGOTT, Yvette Marie The Surgery, 4 Stoke Road, Bishops Cleeve, Cheltenham GL52 8RP Tel: 01242 672007 — MB ChB Birm. 1988; DCH RCP Lond. 1992.

PYKE, Mark Richard 38 High Street, Milton Malsor, Northampton NN7 3AS — MB BS Lond. 1993; BSc (Physiol.) Lond. 1990, MB BS 1993. Specialist Regist. Bristol Sch. Of Anaesth. Specialty: Anaesth. Prev: SHO (A & E) Freemantle Hosp. Aust.; SHO Qu. Mary's Hosp. Roehampton; SHO King Edwd. vii Hosp. Midhurst.

PYKE, Mr Robert Consulting rooms, Three Shires Hospital, Northampton NN1 5DR — MB Camb. 1965; BChir 1964; FRCS Ed. 1969; FRCS Eng. (Orl.) 1971. Cons. (Otolaryngol.) BMI Three Shires InDepend. Hosp. Specialty: Otolaryngol. Prev: Sen. Regist. (Otolaryngol.) United Bristol Hosps.

PYLE, Elizabeth Joy 81 Penland Road, Haywards Heath RH16 1PJ Tel: 01444 416303 Email: h2@ejpyle.freeserve.co.uk — MB BS Lond. 1994 (Kings College London) DRCOG 1997; DFFP 1999. GP Regist, W. Sussx. Specialty: Gen. Pract. Prev: SHO (Psychiat.) Princess Roy. Hosp. Haywards Heath; SHO (Med.) Princess Roy. Hosp. Haywards Heath; SHO (A & E) Princess Roy. Hosp. Haywards Heath.

PYLE, Peter Owen (retired) Southlands, Hawkcombe Lane, Compton Abbas, Shaftesbury SP7 0NN Tel: 01747 811575 — (St. Thos.) MB BS Lond. 1955; DA Eng. 1957; FFA RCS Eng. 1966.

PYLE, Ronald Leslie Strathmore Surgery, 19 Jessie Street, Blairgowrie PH10 6BT Tel: 01250 872552 Fax: 01250 874504; Stapleton, Rosemount, Blairgowrie PH10 6LA Tel: 01250 87 2898 Fax: 01250 87 2898 — MB ChB Aberd. 1958; DObst RCOG 1960. Prev: Med. Off. Trucial Oman Scouts; Obst. Brit. Milit. Hosp. Taiping, Malaya.

PYLE, Simon John 23 Broad Lane, Wilmington, Dartford DA2 7AQ — MB BS Lond. 1980; DRCOG 1984.

PYLE, William Dryden Bayview Surgery, Bayview, Longhope, Stromness KW16 3NY Tel: 01856 701209 Fax: 01856 701224 — MB ChB Aberd. 1958; DObst RCOG 1962; MRCGP 1968. Socs: BMA. Prev: Ho. Surg. Roy. Infirm. Inverness; Ho. Surg. (Obst.) Aberd. Matern. Hosp.; Ho. Phys. (Paediat.) Roy. Hosp. Sick Childr. Glas.

PYM, Jenny (retired) 36 The Horsefair, Malmesbury SN16 0AP — MB ChB Bristol 1948; DObst RCOG 1954. Prev: Internat. Planned Parenth. Federat. Organiser Family Plann. Train.

PYMONT, Frederick Edward Medical Centre, Greenyard, Waltham Abbey EN9 1RD Tel: 01992 714088 Fax: 01992 763866; 162 Honey Lane, Waltham Abbey EN9 3BE Tel: 01992 711897 — MB BS Lond. 1968 (Roy. Lond. Hosp.)

PYNE, Andrew 7 Royal Chase, Tunbridge Wells TN4 8AX — BM Soton. 1980; FRCA 1984. Cons. Anaesth. Kent & Sussex Weald NHS Trust Tunbridge Wells. Specialty: Anaesth.

PYNE, Mr John Robin Stoke House, Stoke Holy Cross, 140 Norwich Road, Norwich NR14 8QJ Tel: 01508 493931 Email: john.pyne@lineone.net — (Char. Cross) MB BS Lond. 1965; MRCS Eng. LRCP Lond. 1965; DO Eng. 1969; FRCS Eng. 1971; FRCOphth 1991. Cons. Ophth. Norf. & Norwich Hosp. Specialty: Ophth. Socs: Fac. Ophth.; (Ex-Sec.) Norf. & Norwich M-C Soc. Prev: Sen. Regist. Lond. Hosp.; Sen. Lect. Moorfields Eye Hosp.; Ho. Phys. & Ho. Surg. Char. Cross Hosp.

PYNE, Tessa Mary 11 Muirfield Crescent, Gullane EH31 2HN Tel: 01620 842415 — MB BS Lond. 1975; MRCS Eng. LRCP Lond. 1975; DCH RCPS Glas. 1978; DRCOG 1982; MRCGP 1983; MFFP 1992; Dip. GU Med. 1996. GP Asst.; CMO Family Plann. Specialty: Gen. Pract.; Genitourinary Medicine; Family Plann. & Reproduc. Health.

PYONE PYONE MYINT, Dr 4 Eriksay Crescent, Newron Mearns, Glasgow G77 6XE — MB BS Med. 1978; MB BS Med. Inst (II) Rangoon 1978.

PYOTT, Jonathan James Aylesbury Vales Healthcare NHS Trust, Aylesbury HP 1EG; 85 St Andrews Crescent, Stratford-upon-Avon CV37 9RP — BM Soton. 1995. SHO Psych. Aylesbury Vale Healthcare NHS Trust.

PYPER, Andrew James Unthank Road Surgery, 38 Unthank Road, Norwich NR2 2RD Tel: 01603 766815; Oakmead, 7 Stratford Crescent, Norwich NR4 7SF — MB ChB Aberd. 1980; MRCGP 1987. Gen. Practitioner Norwich.

PYPER, Mr Patrick Charles Mid Ulster Hospital, Magherafelt BT45 5EX Tel: 028 7963 1031; 60 Coolshinney Road, Magherafelt BT45 5JF Tel: 028 7963 1628 Email: pyperpc@aol.com — MB BCh BAO Belf. 1975; FRCS Ed. 1980. Cons. Surg. Mid Ulster Hosp. Magherafelt. Specialty: Gen. Surg. Prev: Sen. Regist. Roy. Vict. Hosp. & City Hosp. Belf. & Roy. N. Shore Hosp Sydney, Austral.

PYPER, Mr Richard Julian David Department of Gynaecology, Worthing Hospital, Lyndhurst Road, Worthing BN11 2DH Tel: 01903 285193 Fax: 01903 285191 Email: richard.pyper@wash.nhs.uk — MB BChir Camb. 1978 (Camb. and The Middlx.) MA Camb. 1979; FRCS Ed. 1984; MRCOG 1987; FRCOG 1999. Cons. O & G Worthing Hosp., Worthing; Chairm., Labour Ward Standing Comm. Specialty: Obst. & Gyn. Socs: Brit. Soc. Gyn. Endoscopy; Brith. Soc. Of Urogynacology. Prev: Sen. Regist. (O & G) St. Bart. Hosp. & N. Middlx. Hosp. Lond.; Lect. (O & G) Guy's Hosp. United Med. & Dent. Sch. Lond.; Regist. (Gen. Surg. & Urol.) St. Mary's Hosp. Lond.

PYRAH, Roger Dale (retired) Raikes Head, 90 Raikes Road, Skipton BD23 1LU Tel: 01756 792642 — MB BChir Camb. 1961 (Middlx.) FRCPath 1980, M 1968. Prev: Cons. Histopath. Airedale Gen. Hosp. Keighley.

PYRGOS, Nicos Accident & Emergency Department, County Hospital, Lincoln LN2 5QY Tel: 01522 573382 Fax: 01522 560334; 52 Hawthorn Road, Reepham, Lincoln LN3 4DU Tel: 01522 595728 — Ptychio Iatrikes Athens 1966; Dip. Surg. DSS Athens 1973; FFAEM 1993. Cons. A & E Lincoln Co. Hosp. Specialty: Accid. & Emerg. Socs: Lincoln Med. Soc.

PYRGOS, Vassiliki 52 Hawthorn Road, Reepham, Lincoln LN3 4DU — Ptychio Iatrikes Athens 1966.

***PYSDEN, Karen Suzanne** Whitegate, Macclesfield Road, Alderley Edge SK9 7BH; Whitegate, Macclesfield Road, Alderley Edge SK9 7BH — MB ChB Sheff. 1998 (Univ. of Sheffield) MB ChB Sheff 1998. PRHO. Socs: BMA; MPS.

PYSZORA, Natalie Mary 94B Bourne Road, Bexley DA5 1LU — MB ChB Birm. 1993.

PYVES, Catherine Anne Corner House, Priory Gardens, Bridgend CF31 3LB — MB BS Lond. 1989.

QADAN, Hasan Muhammad Ahmad Dormers Wells Medical Centre, 128 Dormers Wells Lane, Southall UB1 3JB; 3 Crossmead Avenue, Greenford UB6 9TY Tel: 020 8813 1155 — (Istanbul) Specialist in Internal Med. Univ. of Istanbul; DFFP; MD Istanbul 1968. Princip. in Gen. Pract., Ealing, Hammersmith and Hounslow Health Auth., Southall Middlx. Specialty: Gen. Med. Socs: BMA (Hon. Sec. Ealing Div.).; Med. Protec. Soc. Prev: Regist. (Gen. Med.) N.gate Hosp. Gt. Yarmouth & Scunthorpe Gen. Hosp.; Regist. (Diag. Radiol.) Centr. Middlx. Hosp.

QADIR, Mr Abdul Aberdeen Royal Infirmary, Foresterhill, Aberdeen AB25 2ZN — MB BS Punjab 1982; FRCS Glas. 1988. Specialty: Gen. Surg.

QADIR, Mr Muhammad County Hospital, Louth LN11 9EU Tel: 01507 600100; 30 St. Mary's Park, Louth LN11 0EF Tel: 01507 608129 — MB BS Bangladesh 1968; FRCS Ed. 1982; FICS 1991. Assoc. Specialist Co. Hosp. Louth. Specialty: Orthop.

QADIRI, Mohammed Rida Radi Yeovil District Hospital, Higher Kingston, Yeovil BA21 4AT Tel: 01935 384878 Fax: 01935 384446

Email: qadim@est.nhs.uk; 21 Parkside Drive, Edgware HA8 8JU Tel: 020 8906 8854 Fax: 020 8906 8854 Email: mohammed@mrq@doctordoctor.co.uk — MB ChB Baghdad 1975; FRCP Lond; FRCP Lond.; MRCP (UK) 1980. Cons. Phys. Yeovil Dist. Hosp. Specialty: Gen. Med.; Care of the Elderly. Socs: Arab-African Soc. Gastroenterol. & Endoscopy; Brit. Geriat. Soc. Prev: Med. Specialist Ahmadi Hosp. Kuwait; Research Fell. Acad. Dept. Med. Roy. Free HSM Univ. Lond.

QADRI, A Q The Surgery, 157 Leytonstone Road, Stratford, London E15 1LH Tel: 020 8534 1026 Fax: 020 8534 4415 — MB BS Kashmir 1974; MB BS Kashmir 1974.

QAIYUM, Mansoor-Ui 1 Belgrave Road, Halesowen B62 9HA — MB ChB Leeds 1991.

QAMAR, Arshad c/o Mr Ali Noorani, 119 Clarancegate Gardens, Glentworth St., London NW1 6AL — MB BS Karachi, Pakistan 1986.

QAMAR-UZ-ZAMAN, S Sheffield Medical Centre, 21 Spital Street, Sheffield S3 9LB Tel: 0114 272 5552.

QAMRUDDIN, Ahmed Omer 63 Kestrel Park, Skelmersdale WN8 6TA — MB ChB Manch. 1992.

QAMRUDDIN, Mr Mohamed Ashurst Health Centre, Lulworth, Ashurst, Skelmersdale WN8 6QS Tel: 01695 732468 Fax: 01695 555365; 63 Kestrel Park, Ashurst, Skelmersdale WN8 6TA Tel: 01695 725887 Fax: 01695 725887 — MB BS Osmania 1965; FRCS Ed. 1972; MRCS Eng. LRCP Lond. 1973. GP Skelmersdale. Specialty: Dermat.; Gen. Med. Socs: Assoc. Mem. Fac. Homoeop. Prev: Cons. Surg. Gen. Hosp. Kabwe, Zambia; Sen. Regist. & Tutor (Surg.) Meath Hosp. Dub.

QARSHI, Ahmed Ali The Surgery, 46 Montague Street, Wakefield WF1 5BB Tel: 01924 251811 Fax: 01924 242140 — MB BS Bihar 1961. GP Wakefield, W. Yorks.

QASIM, Asif 1 Higher Downs, Bradford BD8 0NA — BChir Camb. 1995.

QASIM, Faieza Jabeen Renal Unit, Manchester Royal Infirmary, Oxford Street, Manchester M13 9WL Tel: 0161 276 4454 — LMSSA Lond. 1986 (Cambridge) PHD 1995 Camb.; BA (Hons.) Camb. 1983, MB BChir 1985; MRCP (UK) 1989. Sen. Regist. Camb. Specialty: Nephrol. Socs: Renal. Assn; Brit Soc Immunol; Brit. Implantation soc. Prev: Regist. Rotat. (Med.) Newc. u Tyne; SHO (Neurol.) Addenbrooke's Hosp. Camb.; SHO (Med.) Leeds Gen. Infirm.

QAYYUM, Abdul 16 Douglas Road, Ilford IG3 8UX — MB BS Punjab 1972; MRCPI 1989.

QAZI, Mr Abdul Aziz (retired) 2 Croft Gardens, Dalton-in-Furness LA15 8BS Tel: 01229 62157 — MB BS Punjab 1951; MB BS Punjab (Pakistan) 1951; FRCS Ed. 1960; FRCS Eng. 1965; MChOrth Liverp. 1968. Cons. Orthop. Surg. Barrow & Furness Dist. Hosps.

QAZI, Fazle Azim 1 Foxhome Close, Chislehurst BR7 5XT; 6 Woodplace, Chislehurst Road, Sidcup DA14 6BG Tel: 020 8300 9258 — MB BS Karachi 1962.

QAZI, Hamid Shafi (retired) 206 Roderick Avenue, Peacehaven, Newhaven BN10 8JG Tel: 01273 588300 — MB BS Punjab 1942 (King Edwd. Med. Coll. Lahore) MB BS Punjab (Pakistan) 1942; DPM Eng. 1973. Prev: Cons. Psychiat. Greenwich Health Dist.

QAZI, Nadeem Ahmad 308 Cavendish Road, London SW12 0PJ Tel: 020 8675 0506 Email: nqazi@hotmail.com — MB BS Lond. 1994 (Char. Cross & Westm. Med. Sch.) LRCP 1997; LRCS Ed. 1997; LRCPS 1997; DGM.Glas 1998. Clin. Research Fell & Hon Regist in HIV Med. Univ. Lond. Specialty: HIV Med. Prev: SHO. HIV/GUM, Chelsea & Westminster Hosp. Lond; SHO. Rotat.(Med.) Kings Coll. Hosp. Lond.

QAZI, Rafiz Ahmad Brierfield Health Centre, Arthur Street, Brierfield, Nelson BB9 5SQ Tel: 01282 615175 — MB BS Delhi 1968; MB BS Delhi 1968.

QAZI, Shahjehan 222 Brasenose Avenue, Gorleston-On-Sea, Great Yarmouth NR31 7ED — MB ChB Sheff. 1998.

QIDWAI, Aliya 51 The Grange, Woodham, Newton Aycliffe DL5 4SZ — MB BS Lond. 1992.

QIZILBASH, Nawab Academic Division of Geriatric Medicine, University of Oxford, Radcliffe Infirmary, Oxford OX2 6HE Tel: 01865 224975 Fax: 01865 224815 — MB ChB Manch. 1980; BSc St. And. 1977; MRCP (UK) 1983; MSc Lond. 1985; DPhil Oxf. 1988. Clin. Lect. (Geriat. Med.) Univ. Oxf. Prev: Wellcome Research Train. Fellowship Madrid; Regist. (Med.) Leeds Gen. Infirm.

QUABA, Mr Awf-Abdul-Rahman Ali BUPA Hospital, 122 Corstorphine Road, Edinburgh EH12 6UD Tel: 0131 334 0363 Fax: 0131 334 7338; Williamcraigs House, Linlithgow EH49 6QF Tel: 01506 846244 Fax: 01506 846244 — MB ChB Mosul 1973; FRCS Ed. 1979; FRCS Ed. (Plast) 1986. Cons. Plastic Surg. Lothian Plastic & Oral Surg. Serv. St. John's Hosp. Howden & Roy. Hosp. for Sick Childr. Edin. Specialty: Plastic Surg. Socs: Brit. Assn. Plastic Surg. & Brit. Assn. Aesth. Plastic Surg.; Brit. Soc. Surg. Hand. Prev: Sen. Regist. NE Thames Regional Centre Billericay; Regist. Lond. Hosp. Whitechapel; SHO St. Lawrence's Hosp. Chepstow.

QUABECK, Gabriele c/o Arno Klefisch, 108 Church Lane, Coventry CV2 4AJ — State Exam Med Frankfurt 1990.

QUADER, Keya 15 Sea Mills Lane, Bristol BS9 1DN Email: kquader@hotmail.com — BM BS Nottm. 1990 (Nottingham University) FFARCSI 1998. Specialist Regist. (Anaesth.) Newc.u.Tyne. Specialty: Anaesth.

QUADER, Mohammad Abdul 22 Wilton Drive, Darlington DL3 9PS Tel: 01325 351010 — MB BS Dacca 1964 (Chittagong Med. Coll.) DA Eng. 1970; FFA RCS Eng. 1972. Cons. Anaesth. Darlington Memor. Hosp. Specialty: Anaesth. Socs: Obst. Anaesth. Assn.; BMA; Assn. Anaesth.

QUADER, Syed Eqbal 1 Long Meadow, The Pippins, Moss Pit, Stafford ST17 9DP Tel: 01785 41265 — MB BS Osmania 1967; DPM Eng. 1972; MRCPsych 1974. Cons. Psychiat. (Adult) St. Geo. Hosp. Stafford. Specialty: Gen. Psychiat.

QUADHIR, Mohamed Jawfer Ahamed 104 (Top Left), Great Northern Road, Aberdeen AB24 3QB — MB ChB Aberd. 1994.

QUADRI, Amal Fatima — MB BS Lond. 1993 (Char. Cross & Westm.) SpR (Paediat.) John Radcliffe Hosp. Oxf. Specialty: Paediat. Prev: SHO (Paediat.) Centr. Middlx. Hosp. Lond.; SHO (Neonat. & Paediat.) St. Geo. Hosp. Lond.

QUADRI, F R Church Road Surgery, 296 Church Road, Northolt UB5 5AP Tel: 020 8248 2609 — MB BS Vikram 1962; MB BS Vikram 1962.

QUADRI, Syed Arif Lansbury Drive Practice, 166 Lansbury Drive, Hayes UB4 9NS Tel: 020 8848 3858 Fax: 020 8573 2082; 39 Sweetcroft Lane, Hillingdon, Uxbridge UB10 9LE — MB BS Bangalor 1967 (Bangalore) MB BS Bangalore 1967. Socs: BMA; Affil. RCPsych. Prev: Ho. Phys. (Gen. Med.) Manor Hosp. Walsall; Regist. & SHO (Psychiat.) Runwell Hosp. Wickford.

QUADRI, Mr Syed Arifulla 160 Manor Court Road, Nuneaton CV11 5HG — MRCS Eng. LRCP Lond. 1935; FRFPS Glas. 1938; FRCS Glas. 1962.

QUAGHEBEUR, Gerardine Marie-Marthe Department of Neuroradiology, Radcliffe Infirmary, Woodstock Road, Oxford OX2 6HE Tel: 01865 224512 Fax: 01865 224689 Email: gqbeur@doctors.org.uk; Conifer House, Lamborough Hill, Wooton, Oxford OX13 6BY Tel: 01865 736862 Fax: 01865 730760 — MB BCh Witwatersrand 1982; FRCS Ed. 1987; FRCS Eng. 1988; FRCR 1993. Cons. Neuroradiol. Radcliffe Infirm. Oxf. Specialty: Radiol. Prev: Sen. Regist. (Neuroradiol.) Nat. Hosp. Neurol. & Neurosurg. Lond.

QUAIFE, John Benenden Chest Hospital, Goddards Green Road, Benenden, Cranbrook TN17 4AX — MB BChir Camb. 1978. Cons. Anaesth. Benenden Hosp. Cranbrook. Specialty: Anaesth.

QUAILE, Mr Andrew Clare Park Hospital, Crondall Lane, Farnham GU10 5XX Tel: 01252 852572 Fax: 01252 852358 Email: andrew@spine-works.com; Greenhill Farm, Baltons Borough, Glastonbury BA6 8QE Tel: 01458 851023 Fax: 01458 851059 — MB BS Lond. 1978 (Char. Cross) MRCS Eng. LRCP Lond. 1979. Spinal Orthopaedic Surg. Specialty: Orthop. Socs: Brit. Orthop. Assn.; Brit. Assn. of Spinal Surgeons; Brit. Scoliosis Soc. Prev: Vis. Surg. (Orthop.) Roy. Brisbane, St. And., Holy Spirit & NW Private Hosps.; Lect. (Orthop. Surg.) Soton. Univ.; Specialist (Orthop. Surg.), Austral. Army.

QUAITE, Thomas James, TD Old Mill Surgery, Church Street, Newtownards BT23 4AS Tel: 028 9181 7239; 45 Ballyrainey Road, Newtownards BT23 5AD — MB BCh BAO Belf. 1969; DObst RCOG 1974; MRCGP 1977.

QUALTROUGH, John Edward Over Wyre Medical Centre, Wilkinson Way, Off Pilling Lane, Poulton-le-Fylde FY6 0EX Tel: 01253 810722 — MB ChB Manch. 1975.

QUAN, Virginia Anne 40 Rowfant Road, London SW17 7AS — MB BChir Camb. 1989; MRCP (UK) 1992; PhD (Lond.) 2000. Cons. Nephrologist St Helier Hosp. Specialty: Nephrol.; Gen. Med.

QUANSAH, Benjamin Bassaw Halbutt Surgery, 2 Halbutt Street, Dagenham RM9 5AS Tel: 020 8592 1544 Fax: 020 8596 9833 — Vrach Kiev Med Inst 1968; Dip. Practical Deramtology Univ. of Wales Med. School 1997. Specialty: Gen. Med.; Dermat.

QUANT, John Antony, Air Commodore RAF Med. Br. (retired) 54 Clay Lane, Wendover, Aylesbury HP22 6NS Tel: 01296 624714 — MRCS Eng. LRCP Lond. 1970 (Guy's) BDS Lond. 1957; FDS RCS Eng. 1963; MB BS Lond. 1971. Cons. Oral Surg. & Oral Med. BMH Rinteln. Prev: RAF Cons. Adviser (Oral Surg.) Princess Mary's RAF Hosp. Halton.

QUANTEN, Patrick Paul Leonard Eagle Medical Practice, Stefan House, Olivier St, Alderney, Guernsey GY9 3TD Tel: 01481 822494 Fax: 01481 823892 — MD Brussels 1983. Specialty: Gen. Med.

QUANTRILL, John (retired) The Furlong, Tinwell Road, Stamford PE9 2QQ Tel: 01780 763171 — (King's Coll. Hosp.) MB BS Lond. 1956; MRCS Eng. LRCP Lond. 1956; DObst RCOG 1958. Prev: GP Stamford.

QUANTRILL, Simon John 12 Hyndman Court, Sheader Drive, Salford M5 5BX — MB ChB Manch. 1989. SHO (Endocrinol. & Ment. Oncol.) Christie Hosp. Manch. Prev: SHO (Geriat. & Gen. Med.) Trafford Gen. Hosp. Manch.; Ho. Off. (Renal & Gen. Med.) Manch. Roy. Infirm.; Ho. Off. (Gen. Surg.) Birch Hill Hosp. Rochdale.

QUARCOO, Samuel Tetteh 125 Stratton Road, Brighouse HD6 3UA — MD; Lekar Nov Sad, Yugoslavia 1967. Hosp. Specialist O & G Kirkcaldy Fife. Specialty: Obst. & Gyn. Socs: BMA; Med. Protec. Soc. Prev: Regist.

QUARCOOPOME, Mr Wilfred Nii Sackey George Elliot Hospital, College Street, Nuneaton CV11 7DJ Tel: 02476 351351; 11 Abingdon Way, St. Nicholas Park Estate, Nuneaton CV11 6DX Tel: 024 7637 1230 — MB ChB Ghana 1975; FRCS Ed. 1984. Trauma & Orthop., Geo. Elliot Hosp. Specialty: Accid. & Emerg. Socs: BMA. Prev: Regist. (Trauma & Orthop.) Manor Hosp. Nuneaton.

QUARISHI, Nasir Ali 263 Greenford Road, Greenford UB6 8QZ — MB ChB Manch. 1996.

QUARMBY, Mr John Winston Derby Royal Infirmary, London Road, Derby DE1 2QY Tel: 01332 347141 Ext: 4392 Fax: 01332 254637 — MB BS Lond. 1987; FRCS Ed. Gen. Surg.; BSc Lond. 1984, MB BS 1987; FRCS Ed. 1992. Cons. (Vasc. & Gen. Surg.) South. Derbysh. Acute Hosps. NHS Trust. Specialty: Gen. Surg. Special Interest: Vasc. Surg. Prev: Regist. (Gen. Surg.) Worthing Gen. Hosp.; Regist. (Gen. Surg.) St. Geos. Hosp. Lond. & Epsom Dist. Hosp.; Regist. (Gen. Surg.) St. Thos. Hosp. Lond.

QUARRELL, Oliver William John Dept. Clinical Genetics, Sheffield Children's Hospital, Sheffield S10 2TH Tel: 0114 271 7025 Fax: 0114 273 7467 Email: oliver.quarrell@sch.nhs.uk; 68 Woodholm Road, Sheffield S11 9HT — MB BS Lond. 1980 (St. Mary's Hospital London) BSc Lond. 1977, MD 1988; FRCP Ed. 1993; FRCP Lond. 1994. Cons. Clin. Genetics Sheff. Childr.'s Hosp. Specialty: Genetics. Prev: Sen. Regist. (Med. Genetics) Univ. Hosp. Wales Cardiff.

QUARRY, Daniel Peter Crwys Road Medical Centre, 151 Crwys Road, Cathays, Cardiff CF24 4XT — MB BCh Wales 1989; DCH; DRCOG; MRCGP; DFFP.

QUARRY, Samantha Jayne Radyr Health Centre, Park Road, Radyr, Cardiff CF15 8DF Tel: 02920 842767 — MB ChB Birm. 1994; DRCOG Bristol 1997; DFFP 1999; MRCGP (Distinc.) (UK) 2000. p/t GP Principal, Radyr Health Centre, Park Road, Radyr, Cardiff. Specialty: Gen. Pract.; Family Plann. & Reproduc. Health. Socs: Med. Defence Union; BMA. Prev: GP Non Princip. S. Wales; Psychiat. Regist. Gold Coast Hosp. Qld. Austral.; SHO (Med.) Jersey Gen. Hosp.

QUARTERMAN, Elizabeth Ann 19 Langdale Crescent, Bexleyheath DA7 5DZ — MB BS Lond. 1989; BSc Lond. 1986, MB BS 1989. SHO (Cas.) Watford Gen. Hosp. Prev: SHO (O & G) QECH Blantyre Malawi; Ho. Phys. King Edwd. VII Hosp. Windsor; Ho. Surg. Watford Gen. Hosp.

QUARTEY, Mr Paul Kelvin Schering-Plough, Shire Park, Welwyn Garden City AL7 1TW Tel: 01707 363756 Fax: 01707 363763; Beech Cottage, 48 Langley Hill, Kings Langley WD4 9HE Tel: 01923 263338 Fax: 01707 363763 — MB ChB Univ. Ghana 1982; FRCS Ed. 1987; Dip. Pharm Med. RCP (UK) 1994. Med. Dir. Schering-Plough Welwyn Gdn. City. Specialty: Pharmaceutical Medicine. Socs: BMA & BRAPP. Prev: Head Clin. Research & Med. Advisor Schering-Plough; Regist. (Surg.) Leeds Gen. Infirm.

QUARTLEY, Roger Graham Stuart The White Rose Surgery, Exchange Street, South Elmsall, Pontefract WF9 2RD Tel: 01977 642412 Fax: 01977 641290 — MB ChB Sheff. 1984; DA (UK) 1987.

QUARTLY, Christopher Francis West Street Surgery, 89 West Street, Dunstable LU6 1SF Tel: 01582 664401 Email: cesar.rodriguez@tpct.scot.nhs.uk — MB BS Lond. 1982; DCH RCP Lond. 1983; DRCOG 1984; DMJ(Clin) Soc. Apoth. Lond. 1993. GP Dunstable.

QUARTSON, Joseph Kwamina Harrogate General Hospital, Knaresborough Road, Harrogate HG2 7NG — MB BS Lond. 1964.

QUASEM, Mohammad Abul — MB BS Dacca 1966 (Dacca Med. Coll.) Specialty: Family Planning; Gen. Med.; Gen. Pract. Socs: MDU. Prev: Regist. (Diag. Radiol.) Leicester Roy. Infirm.

QUASIM, Isma Flat 2/R, 74 Dundrennan Road, Glasgow G42 9SG — MB ChB Glas. 1990.

QUASIM, Mohammad South Hetton Surgery, Front Street, South Hetton, Durham DH6 2TH Tel: 0191 517 1055 Fax: 0191 526 0001 — MB BS Dacca 1963; DTM & H Liverp.

QUASIM, Mohammed 239 Lutterworth Road, Nuneaton CV11 6PX — MB BS Karachi 1958.

QUASIM, Mohammed Nayar Iqbal The Health Centre, Trenchard Avenue, Thornaby, Stockton-on-Tees TS17 0DD Tel: 0191 245 1488 Fax: 0191 245 1488 Email: nquasim@compuserve.com; Thornaby Healthcare Practice, The Health Centre, Trenchard Avenue, Thornaby, Stockton-on-Tees TS17 0DD Tel: 01642 762636 Fax: 01642 766464 — MB BS Newc. 1992; DRCOG 1995; DFFP 1995; MRCGP 1996. Specialty: Gen. Pract.

QUASIM, Seema — MB ChB (Hons.) Birm. 1999; BMedSc (Pharmacol.) 1996; MRCS Ed. 2002; MRCS Eng. 2002. SpR (Anaesth.) Warks. Sch. of Anaesth. Specialty: Anaesth. Socs: Roy. Coll. Anaesth.; Assn. Anaesth. GB & Irel.; Roy. Coll. of Surgeons of Edin. Prev: SHO (Anaesth.) Good Hope Hosp. Sutton Coldfield; SHO (Anaesth.) Heartlands & Solihull NHS Trust Birm.; SHO (Surgic. Rotat.) Sandwell & Birm.

QUASIM, Tara 39 Herries Road, Pollockshields, Glasgow G41 4AH — MB ChB Glas. 1994.

QUASTEL, Anthony Stephen 204-206 High Street, Bromley BR1 1PW Tel: 020 8464 4599 Fax: 020 8464 3471; Rome Cottage, Rome Road, New Romney TN28 8DN Tel: 01797 362493 Fax: 01797 973 1417 — MB BS Lond. 1980 (Middlx. Hosp.) Indep. GP Bromley Kent. Socs: Fell. Roy. Soc. Med. Prev: SHO (Psychiat.) Middlx. Hosp. Lond.; Ho. Phys. Benenden Chest Hosp.; Ho. Surg. Croydon Gen. Hosp.

***QUATAN, Nadine** Flat 50, Parkview Court, Broomhill Road, London SW18 4JG — MB BS Lond. 1998; MRCS Eng. 2000. Clin. Research Fell. in Urol., St. George's Hosp., Lond.; Ho. Physcan. Eastbourne Dist Hosp. Specialty: Gastroenterol.; Gen. Med. Prev: Ho. Surg. Whittington Hosp.

QUATAN, Mr Saadon Mohamad Hassan The Gables, Houghton Avenue, Hempstead, Gillingham ME7 3RY — MB ChB Baghdad 1961 (Coll. Med. Baghdad) FRCS Eng. 1974; MRCS Eng. LRCP Lond. 1978. Socs: BMA. Prev: Regist. (Gen. Surg.) & SHO (Gen. Surg.) St. Bart. Hosp. Rochester; SHO (Paediat. Surg.) Roy. Manch. Childr. Hosp. Pendlebury.

QUATE, Leza Zarrine 4 Harland Cottages, Glasgow G14 0AS — MB ChB Glas. 1997.

QUATTAINAH, Mohammed Anwar Flat 33, Windmill Court, Claremont Rd, Newcastle upon Tyne NE2 4BA — MB BS Newc. 1996.

QUAYLE, Mr Andrew John McMullan Church Street Surgery, Church Street, Martock TA12 6JL Tel: 01935 822541 — MB BChir Camb. 1978; MA Camb. 1978; FRCS Eng. 1982; MRCGP 1984. GP Princip., Ch. St. Surg., Martock. Specialty: Gen. Pract. Prev: Med. Off. Bethesda Hosp, Ubombo, Kwazulu; Regist. (Surg.) Edendale Hosp. Nr. Pietermaritzburg Kwazulu, S. Afr.

QUAYLE, Mr Anthony Robert Macclesfield District Hospital, Victoria Road, Macclesfield SK10 3BL Tel: 01625 421000 — MB ChB Sheff. 1975; ChM Sheff. 1987, MB ChB 1975; FRCS Eng. 1980. Cons. Gen. Surg. Macclesfield Dist. Gen. Hosp. Specialty: Gen. Surg. Prev: Lect. (Surg.) Roy. Hallamsh. Hosp. Sheff.

QUAYLE, Mr John Bryant The Shrewsbury and Telford NHS Trust, Royal Shrewsbury Hospital, Mytton Oak Road, Shrewsbury SY3 8XQ Tel: 01743 261000 Fax: 01743 261320 Email: john.quayle@rsh.nhs.uk; The River House, Isle Lane, Bicton, Shrewsbury SY3 8ED Tel: 01743 850646 Fax: 01743 850639 — MB BChir Camb. 1970 (St. Geo.) MS Camb. 1982, MB BChir 1970; FRCS Eng. 1974. Cons. Gen. & Colerectal Surg. Shrewsbury and Telford; Private Pract., Shrops. Nuffield Hosp., Shrewsbury; Private Pract., Apley Clinic, Princess Roy. Hosp., Telford. Specialty: Gen. Surg. Special Interest: Colorectal; Gallbladder; Hernia. Socs: Roy. Soc. Med. & Assn. of Surgs.; Assn. Coloproctol. Prev: Sen. Regist., St Georges Hosp., Lond.

QUAYLE, Susan Elizabeth Netherfield House, Station Road, Seghill, Cramlington NE23 7EF Tel: 0191 237 0643 Fax: 0191 237 1091 — MB BS Newc. 1983. GP Cramlington, N.d.

QUBATY, Mr Mohamed Abdul-Mageed Ground Floor, 25 Birchington Road, London NW6 4LL; 14 Berkeley Court, Neasden Lane, Neasden, London NW10 1PX Tel: 020 8450 4998 — MB BS Lond. 1979 (King's Coll. Hosp.) MRCS Eng. LRCP Lond. 1979; FRCS Ed. 1989. Sen. Lect. (Surg.) Univ. Sana'a & Cons. Surg. Sana'a Univ. Teach. Hosp. Specialty: Gen. Surg. Prev: Regist. (Gen. Surg.) Manor Hse. Hosp. Lond.; Regist. (Urol.) Broomfield Hosp. Chelmsford; Regist. (Surg.) Al-Gamhooriya Teach. Hosp. Univ. Aden.

QUDDUS, Siraj Fatima 1A Denison Road, Manchester M14 5PW — MB BS Punjab 1950; MB BS Punjab (Pakistan) 1950. Prev: Regist. ENT Manch. North. Hosp., Booth Hall Hosp. Manch. & Manch.; Vict. Memor. Jewish Hosp.

QUEEN, Jane Karen 11 Antonine Gate, Verulam, St Albans AL3 4JA — MB BS Lond. 1987; MRCP (UK) 1991.

QUEEN, Mr Kenneth Brodie Department of General Surgery & Urology, Nevill Hall Hospital, Brecon Road, Abergavenny NP7 7EG — MB ChB Glas. 1970; FRCS Ed. 1977; LLM Wales 2000. Specialty: Urol.

QUEENAN, Maria Bernadette The Old Beer House, Chilson, Chipping Norton OX7 3HU — BM BCh Oxf. 1987; BSc Lond. 1977; MSc York 1978. Regist. (A & E) St. Peters Hosp. Chertsey. Prev: SHO (A & E) Hammersmith Hosp. Lond.; Tutor (Surg.) Univ. Liverp.

QUEENAN, Paul John Princes Avenue Surgery, 137 Princes Avenue, Hull HU5 3HH Tel: 01482 342473 Fax: 01482 493382 — MB ChB Leeds 1986. GP Princip., 137 P.s Avenue, Hull; Clin. Asst. NeuroPhysiol., Hull Roy. Infirm., Hull.

QUEENBOROUGH, Robert Wigan and Bolton Health Authority, Bryan House, 61 Standishgate, Wigan WN1 1AH Tel: 01942 772763 Fax: 01942 496567 — MB ChB Birm. 1979; DRCOG 1983; MRCGP 1991; MHSM 1994. Med. Dir. Wigan & Bolton HA.

QUEIROZ, Jane Elizabeth 64 Woodhall Road, Wollaton, Nottingham NG8 1LE — MB ChB Birm. 1992. Staff Grade Community Paediat.

QUEK, Fui Mee 48 Mulgrove Road, Sutton SM2 6LX; 48 Mulgrove Road, Sutton SM2 6LX — MB BS Lond. 1988; DRCOG 1992. Managing Director Synergen Europe Ltd; GP. Specialty: Gen. Pract.

QUEK, Selina Li Gek The Orchard Surgery, Constable Road, St Ives, Huntingdon Tel: 01480 466611; 209 High Street, Chesterton, Cambridge CB4 1NL Tel: 01223 500851 — MB ChB Leic. 1987. Specialty: Gen. Pract.

QUEKETT, James Thomas Scott Rowcroft Medical Centre, Rowcroft Retreat, Stroud GL5 3BE Tel: 01453 764471 — MB ChB Bristol 1994; BSc Bristol 1991; DRCOG 1999; MRGCP 2000. GP Partner. Specialty: Anaesth. Prev: GP Regist. Rosebank Surg., Gloucester; SHO (Paediat.) Glos. Roy. Hosp.; SHO (Obst & Gyn.) Glos.Roy. Hosp.

QUENAULT, Sandra Lesley Mandalay Medical Centre, 933 Blackburn Road, Bolton BL1 7LR Tel: 01204 302228; Nabbs Cottage, Greens Arms Road, Turton BL7 0NF Tel: 01204 853502 — MB BS Lond. 1986 (Roy. Free Hosp. Sch. Med.) DCH RCP Lond. 1988; MRCGP 1990; DPM Cardiff 1997. GP. Specialty: Gen. Pract. Prev: Trainee GP Torbay Hosp. Torquay VTS.

QUENBY, Siobhan Mary Faculty of Medicine & Health Sciences, Division of Obstetrics & Gynaecology, Nottingham City Hospital, Hucknall Road, Nottingham NG5 1PB Tel: 0115 962 7914 Fax: 0115 962 7670 — (St. Bartholomew's) MD 1998 Liverpool; CCST 1998 St Bart; MB BS Lond. 1988; MRCOG 1994. Sen. Lect. Hon. Cons. Univ. Liverp. & Liverp. Wom. Hosp.; Lect. & Hon. Sen. Regist. Univ. Liverp. & Liverp. Wom. Hosp.; Sen Lect. Specialty: Obst. & Gyn. Prev: Regist. Rotat. (O & G) Merseyside Region.

QUERCI DELLA ROVERE, Mr Guidubaldo Royal Marsden Hospital NHS Trust (London & Surrey), Downs Road, Sutton SM2 5PT Tel: 020 8661 3118 Fax: 020 86613126; 12 Minehead Road, Streatham, London SW16 2AW Tel: 020 8677 7244 Fax: 020 8677 7244 Email: gquercidellarovere@doctors.org.uk — MD Padua 1971; State DMS 1976; FRCS Ed. 1981; FRCS Eng. 1982. Cons. Surg. Roy. Marsden Hosp. Lond. & Surrey. Specialty: Gen. Surg. Socs: Fell. Roy. Soc. Med.; Eur. Soc. Surg. Oncol.; Eur. Soc. Mastol. Prev: Clin. Asst. Breast Clinic St Margt. Hosp. Epping, Essex; Lect. (Gen. Surg.) Padua Univ.; Regist. (Gen. Surg.) Roy. Marsden Hosp. Lond.

QUEST, Laura Jane 6 Marlfield Lane, Barnston, Wirral CH61 1AJ — MB ChB Leeds 1986.

QUESTED, Digby John Warneford Hospital, Headington, Oxford OX3 7JX Tel: 01865 223703 Email: digby.quested@psych.ox.ac.uk — MB ChB Cape Town 1983; MRCPsych 1993; MD 2003.

QUIBELL, Ernest Philip, OBE (retired) 9 Adastra Avenue, Hassocks BN6 8DP Tel: 0179 183812 — MRCS Eng. LRCP Lond. 1937 (Camb. & St. Bart.) BA Camb.; DCH Eng. 1947. Med. Cons. Thalidomide Trust. Prev: Med. Adminis. & Cons. Paediatr. Chailey Heritage (Craft Sch. & Hosp.).

QUIBELL, Rachel Mary 39A Hencotes, Hexham NE46 2EW Tel: 01434 601494 — MB BS Newc. 1992; MRCGP 2000. SpR (Palliative Med.) St. Oswalds Hospice Newc. Specialty: Gen. Med. Prev: SHO (Gen. Med.) St. Oswalds Hospice Newc.-u-Tyne; SHO (Gen. Med.) Marie Curie Centre, Newc.-u-Tyne; SHO (Gen. Med.) Sunderland Dist. Gen. Hosp.

QUICK, Mr Clive Robert Groves Hinchingbrooke Hospital, Huntingdon PE29 6NT Tel: 01480 416008; Brooklyn, Holywell, Huntingdon PE27 4TG Tel: 01480 468177 Fax: 01480 460275 — MB BS Lond. 1969; BDS Lond. 1963; LDS 1963; FDS RCS Eng. 1966; MRCS Eng. LRCP Lond. 1969; FRCS Eng. 1973; MS Lond. 1982; MA Camb. 1994. Cons. Gen. & Vasc. Surg. Hinchingbrooke Hosp. Huntingdon & Addenbrooke's Hosp. Camb.; Course Organiser Camb. Anastomosis Workshop; Assoc. Lect. Univ. Camb. Specialty: Gen. Surg.; Vasc. Med. Socs: Fell. Assn. Surgs.; Vasc. Surg. Soc. Prev: Research Fell. (Biomed. Engin.) KCH Lond.; Sen. Regist. Leicester Gen. Hosp.; Regist. King's Coll. Hosp. Lond.

QUICK, David Gordon Chase 13 Cowper House, Browning St., London SE17 1DD Tel: 020 7708 2843 — MB BS Lond. 1990. SHO (Anaesth.) Lond. Specialty: Anaesth.

QUICK, Felicity Jane Chelsea and Westminster Hosp, Fulham Rd, London SW10; 31 Queensmill Road, Fulham, London SW6 6JP Tel: 020 7386 7935 — MB BS Lond. 1996; DCH, UMDS. Lond. 1997. Specialty: Gen. Pract.

QUICK, Sarah Jayne Bridge House, Shalford Road, Guildford GU4 8BL — BM BCh Oxf. 1991; MA Camb. 1994, BA 1988; DFFP 1995; DRCOG 1996; MRCGP 1996. p/t Clin. Asst. Drug & Alcohol; GP Locum. Specialty: Gen. Pract.; Alcohol & Substance Misuse.

QUIERY, Aidan Francis John Coleraine Health Centre, Castlerock Road, Coleraine BT51 3HP Tel: 028 7034 4834 Fax: 028 7035 8914; 12 Tullybeg Avenue, Coleraine BT51 3NG — MB BCh BAO Belf. 1979; DRCOG 1982. Hosp. Pract. (Genitourin. Med.) Coleraine Hosp. Co. Derry. Specialty: Genitourinary Medicine.

QUIGG, Jennifer Lucianne — MB ChB Ed. 1998.

QUIGLEY, Arthur James Rutherglen Health Centre, Stonelaw Road, Rutherglen, Glasgow G73 2PQ Tel: 0141 647 7171; 1 Thorn Drive, Burnside, Glasgow G73 4RH Tel: 0141 634 6114 — MB ChB Glas. 1958. Socs: BMA. Prev: Ho. Phys. Kilmarnock Infirm.; Ho. Surg. Glas. Roy. Infirm.

QUIGLEY, Brian Michael Riverside Practice, Upper Main Street, Strabane BT82 8AS Tel: 028 7138 4100 Fax: 028 7138 4115; Radharc na Finne, 83 Urney Road, Strabane BT82 9RT — MB BCh BAO NUI 1974 (Univ. Coll. Dub.) DRCOG 1977. Prev: SHO (Med.) West. Infirm. Glas.; SHO (Psychiat.) Leverndale Hosp. Glas.; Ho. Off. Altnagelvin Hosp. Lond.derry.

QUIGLEY, Mrs Bridget Mary Agnes (retired) The Knoll, Barmoor, Morpeth NE61 6LB Tel: 01670 512880 — MB BCh BAO NUI 1949 (Cork) DPM Eng. 1957. Prev: Cons. Psychiat. St. Geo. Hosp. Morpeth.

QUIGLEY, Catherine Sefton Health Authority, Burlington Hosue, Crosby Rd North, Waterloo, Liverpool L22 0QB Tel: 0151 478 1234

Fax: 0151 949 0799; 13 Crescent Road, Hale, Altrincham WA15 9NB — MB BCh BAO NUI 1980; MSc Manch. 1987; MFPHM 1989. Specialty: Pub. Health Med. Socs: Manch. Med. Soc. Prev: Cons. Communicable Dis. Control N. Chesh. HA & Wirral HA; Cons. Pub. Health Med. Salford & Trafford HA; Sen. Regist. (Pub. Health Med.) NW RHA.

QUIGLEY, Columba Sheila Mary Department of Medical Oncology, Barry Reed Laboratory, St Bartholomews Hospital, London EC1A 7BE; 7 Cleveland Gardens, Barnes, London SW13 0AE — MB BCh BAO NUI 1985; MRCP Lond. 1990. Clin. Research Fell. St. Bart. Hosp. Lond. Specialty: Palliat. Med. Prev: Sen. Regist. (Palliat. Med.) St. Barts. Hosp. Lond.; Regist. (Palliat. Med.) St. Christopher's Hospice Lond.; SHO (Oncol. & Palliat. Med.) Roy. Marsden Hosp. Sutton.

QUIGLEY, Conor Nial Department of Psychiatry, Lagan Valley Hospital, Lisburn — MB BCh BAO Belf. 1985; MRCGP 1989; MRCPsych 1992. Specialty: Gen. Psychiat.

QUIGLEY, David Gavin 64 Thornleigh Drive, Lisburn BT28 2DS — MB ChB Dundee 1996.

QUIGLEY, Ian Graeme 24 Jasper Road, London E16 3TR Tel: 020 7511 460 — MB BS Lond. 1989. SHO (Gen. Med.) OldCh. Hosp. Romford. Prev: Ho. Phys. (Oncol. & Haemat.) OldCh. Hosp. Romford; Ho. Surg. (Urol. & Orthop.) Newham Gen. Hosp. Plaistow.

QUIGLEY, Margaret Garden 7 The Hawthorns, Gullane EH31 2DZ Tel: 01620 843359 — MB ChB Aberd. 1944. Fell. Brit. Soc. Med. & Dent. Hypn.

QUIGLEY, Mary Concepta Birling Avenue Surgery, 3 Birling Avenue, Rainham, Gillingham ME8 7HB Tel: 01634 360390/361843 Fax: 01634 264061 — MB BCh BAO NUI 1976; DCH NUI 1978; MRCGP 1985. p/t GP, Kent. Socs: BMA.

QUIGLEY, Mary Martha The Royal Marsden Hospital, Downs Road, Sutton SM2 5PT; 17 Owen Mansions, Queens Club Gardens, London W14 9RS — MB BCh BAO NUI 1978; MRCP (UK) 1982; FFR RCSI 1986.

QUIGLEY, Michael Anthony The Brae, Craig Road, Rhonehouse, Castle Douglas DG7 1UB — MB ChB Ed. 1991.

QUIGLEY, Michele Paula 34 Thornleigh Road, Newcastle upon Tyne NE2 3ET — MB BS Newc. 1987.

QUIGLEY, Mr Peter James Laurence 3 Fernwood Grove, Hamsterley Mill, Rowlands Gill NE39 1HJ Tel: 01207 542723 — (Newc.) MB BS Newc. 1968; FRCS Ed. 1974; MRCGP 1978.

QUIGLEY, Philip Joseph Gerard 18 Castle Street, Newry BT34 2BY — MB BCh BAO NUI 1954; Dip. Amer. Bd. Path. 1961. Specialty: Forens. Path. Socs: Fell. Coll. Amer. Pathols.; Med. Soc. New Jersey. Prev: Clin. Asst. Prof. Path. New Jersey Coll. Med. & Dent. Newark, USA; Chief Med. Exam. (State Path.) State of Delaware, USA.; Path. & Dir. Laborat. Alexian Brothers Hosp. Eliz., USA.

QUILLIAM, Robert Paul New Elgin Practice, 44 Chippenham Road, London W9 2AF Tel: 020 7266 2431 Fax: 020 7289 6275 — MB BCh Wales 1976; BSc (Hons.) Wales 1973, MB BCh 1976; MRCGP 1982. Specialty: Palliat. Med. Prev: Regist. (Gastroenterol.) Lond. Hosp. Whitechapel; Regist. (Med.) Basildon Hosp.; SHO (Med.) Lond. Hosp. Whitechapel.

QUILLIAM, Steven Juan Castle Surgery, Kepwell Bank Top, Prudhoe NE42 5PW Tel: 01661 832209 Fax: 01661 836338; West House, Hagg Farm, Wylam NE41 8JY Tel: 01661 852187 — MB BS Newc. 1981; DRCOG 1984; MRCGP 1985. Clin. Asst. (Ment. Handicap) Prudhoe Hosp. N.d. Prev: Trainee GP N.d. VTS; SHO (Psychiat.) St. Mary's Hosp. Stannington.

QUILLIAM, Thomas Andrew — MB BS Lond. 1943 (Univ. Coll. Hosp.) MRCS Eng. LRCP Lond. 1943; DLO Eng. 1946; DSc Lond. 1983, PhD 1954. Research Fell. Centre for Neurosc. Univ. Coll. Lond.; Med. Dir. Charity Heart Haven Lond.; Hon. Lect. St. Mary's Hosp. Med. Sch. Lond. & Lond. Foot Hosp.; Hon. Assoc. Westm. Univ. Specialty: Anat.; Cardiol.; Oral & Maxillofacial Surg. Socs: Anat. Soc., Physiol. Soc. & Genetic Interest Gp.; Emerit. Mem. Amer. Assn. of Anatomists. Prev: Vis. Prof. Dept. Anat. Univ. Calif. Los Angeles, USA; Hon. Research Fell. Univ. Minn., USA; Trav. Fell. of Postgrad. Med. Federat., Univ. Lond.

QUILTY, Brian Michael 185 Henley Road, Caversham, Reading RG4 6LH — MB BS Lond. 1987; MRCP (UK) 1993.

QUIN, Leslie Murray Mearns Medical Centre, 30 maple Avenue, Newton Mearns, Glasgow G77 5BQ Tel: 0141 639 2753 Fax: 0141 616 2403 — MB ChB Glas. 1970; DObst RCOG 1972.

QUIN, Margaret Moira 3 Magpie Close, Ewshot, Farnham GU10 5TF — (Durh.) MB BS Durh. 1964; DObst RCOG 1966; DA Eng. 1969.

QUIN, Norman Edward, Col. late RAMC (retired) 3 Magpie Close, Ewshot, Farnham GU10 5TF — MB ChB Manch. 1949; MFCM 1974.

QUINBY, Mrs Janice Mary Freeman Hospital, High Heaton, Newcastle upon Tyne NE7 7DN Tel: 0191 233 6161 Email: janice.quinby@nuth.nhs.uk; Black Close House, Black Close Bank, Ashington NE63 8TF Tel: 01670 811480 — MB ChB Liverp. 1975 (Liverpool) FRCS Ed. 1981; FRCS Eng. 1982. Cons. Childr.s Orthop. Surg. Newc. Hosps. NHS Trust. Specialty: Orthop. Socs: Brit. Orthop. Assn.; Brit. Soc. Childr. Orthop. Surg.; Brit. Soc. of Surg. in Cerebral Palsy. Prev: Cons. Orthopaedic Surg., S. Tyneside Dist. Hosp., 1990-1996.

QUINBY, Richard Melville Black Close House, Black Close Bank, Ashington NE63 8TF Tel: 01670 811481 — MB BS Newc. 1981; BA (Hons) Lond. 1972; DCCH RCP Ed. 1984; MRCGP 1985; DRCOG 1985.

QUINCEY, Caroline Histopathy Dept, Barsley District Hospital NHS Trust, Gawber Rd, Barnsley S75 2EP; 146 Dobercroft Road, Sheffield S7 2LU — MB ChB Sheff. 1988; DRCPath 1993; MRCPath 1997. Cons.(Histopath.)and (Cytol.) Barsley Dist. Hosp. Specialty: Histopath. Prev: Sen. Regist. (Histopath.) Roy. Hallamsh. Hosp. Sheff.

QUINE, David Juan 122 Sandal Street, Manchester M40 7EF — MB ChB Manch 1997.

QUINE, Mary Amanda Queen Alexandra Hospital, Portsmouth PO6 3LY; 24 Queens Road, Waterlooville PO7 7SB — MB BS Lond. 1986 (St. Bartholomews Medical College) MRCP (UK) 1990; MD 1998. Cons. (Gastroenterol.) Qu. Alexandra Hosp. Portsmouth. Specialty: Gastroenterol. Prev: Regist. NW Thames HA; Research Fell. (Gastroenterol.) Roy. Coll. Surg. Lond.; Regist. (Med.) Frimley Pk. Hosp. Surrey.

QUINE, Mr Stuart Miles 23 Hollybush Road, Cyncoed, Cardiff CF23 6SY — BM BS Nottm. 1987; BMedSci (Hons.) Nottm. 1985; DRCOG 1991; FRCSI 1994; FRCS (Orl.) 1995. Cons. Univ. Hosp. Of Wales. Specialty: Otorhinolaryngol. Prev: Regist. (ENT Surg.) Univ. Hosp. Wales Cardiff.

QUINEY, Iain Donald Washington House Surgery, 77 Halse Road, Brackley NN13 6EQ Tel: 01280 702436 Fax: 01280 701805; Hill House, Wrightons Hill, Helmdon, Brackley NN13 5UF Tel: 01295 768168 — MB BS Lond. 1981; DA (UK) 1985.

QUINEY, Jeremy Roderick Department of Clinical Chemistry, St. Richards Hospital, Spitalfield Lane, Chichester PO19 6SE Tel: 01243 788122 — MB BS Lond. 1976; BSc Sussex 1971; MRCPath 1984. Cons. Path. St. Richard's Hosp. Chichester. Specialty: Chem. Path.

QUINEY, Marion Joan Gatehampton, Mill Lane, Gerrards Cross SL9 8AY — MB BS Lond. 1985; DRCOG 1989.

QUINEY, Nial Francis Gentils Farm, Lickfold, Petworth GU28 9EY Tel: 01798 860847 — MB BS Lond. 1985; BSc Lond. 1982; DRCOG 1987; DCH RCP Lond. 1989; FCAnaesth 1991. Cons. Anaesth. Surrey. Specialty: Anaesth. Prev: Sen. Regist. SW Regional Scheme.; Regist. Rotat. (Anaesth.) Bristol & Weston HA.

QUINEY, Mr Robert Edward 55 Harley Street, London W1N 1DD Tel: 020 7580 2426 Fax: 020 7436 1645; Russets, Orchehill Avenue, Gerrards Cross SL9 8QE Tel: 01753 891336 — MRCS Eng. LRCP Lond. 1980 (Char. Cross) BSc (Hons.) Lond. 1977, MB BS 1980; FRCS Eng. 1986; FRCS Ed. 1986; T(S) 1991. Cons. ENT Surg. Roy. Free Hosp. & Barnet & Edgware Hosp. Lond.; Sen. Lect. Roy. Free Hosp. Sch. Med. Specialty: Otolaryngol. Prev: Sen. Regist. (ENT Surg.) Roy. Sussex Co. Hosp. Brighton; Sen. Regist. (ENT) Roy. Nat. Throat, Nose & Ear Hosp. Lond.

QUINLAN, Jonathan Mark 122 Pound Road, East Peckham, Tonbridge TN12 5BL — MB ChB Bristol 1994.

QUINLAN, Margaret Helen Magda House Medical Centre, 257 Dialstone Lane, Great Moor, Stockport SK2 7NA Tel: 0161 483 3175 Fax: 0161 483 4992; Dover Beck House, 4 Parsonage Gardens, Marple, Stockport SK6 7NB — MB ChB Liverp. 1971; DObst RCOG 1973; Cert. Family Plann. JCC 1982. Specialty: Gen.

Pract. Socs: BMA. Prev: GP Nottm.; SHO City Hosp. Nottm.; Ho. Phys. & Ho. Surg. Broadgreen Hosp. Liverp.

QUINLAN, Mary Jane Dept. Of Anaesthetics, John Radcliffe Hospital, Headley Way, Oxford OX3 9DU — MB BS Lond. 1990 (St. Thos.) FRCA 1995. Cons. Anaesth., John Radcliffe Hosp., Oxf. Specialty: Anaesth.

QUINLAN, Mr Michael The Guest Hospital, Tipton Rd, Dudley DY1 4SE Tel: 01384 456111 Ext: 5811; Sandwell General Hospital, Lyndon, West Bromwich — MB ChB Sheff. 1984; FRCOphth; FRCS Glas. 1989; DO RCS Eng. 1989. Cons. Ophth. Dudley Gp. & Sandwell Healthcare, NHS Trust. Specialty: Ophth. Special Interest: Anterior Segment Disorders; Refractive Cataract Surg. Socs: Roy. Coll. of Ophth.; UMISCRS; MCLOSA. Prev: Specialist Regist. E. Anglian Rotat.; Regist. (Ophth.) W. Norwich Hosp.

QUINLAN, Raymond Michael Business Healthcare, The Occupational Health Centre, Leeming Lane S., Mansfield NG19 9AG Tel: 01623 657446 Fax: 01623 423378 Email: rq@business-healthcare.co.uk; 11 Badgers Chase, Retford DN22 6RX Tel: 01777 708393 Email: ray.quinlan@btopenworld.com — MB BCh BAO NUI 1986 (University College Dublin) BSc NUI 1981; MRCP (UK) 1989; DA (UK) 1991; MFOM RCP Lond. 1996, AFOM 1993; MIOSH 1999; FFOM RCP Lond. 2002. Med. Director Occupat. Med. Business Healthcare, Mansfield, WoodHo. Specialty: Occupat. Health. Socs: Brit. Occupat. Hyg. Soc.; Mem. Inst. Occup. safety & health; Soc. Occupat. Med. (Chairm. E. Midl. Gp.). Prev: Sen. Regist. (Occupat. Med.) Brit. Coal Corp. Mansfield WoodHo.; SHO (Gen. Med., Intens. Care & Anaesth.) Derbysh. Roy. Infirm.; Safety, Health & Environm. Manager & Occupat. Phys. Zeneca, Huddersfield Works.

QUINLIVAN, Rosaline Christina Mary Robert Jones & Agnes Hunt Orthopaedic NHS Trust, Gobowen, Oswestry SY10 7AG Tel: 01691 404047 Fax: 01691 404629 Email: ros.quinlivan@rjah.nhs.uk; The Children's Hospital, Department of Paediatric Neurology, Steelehouse Lane, Birmingham B4 6NH — MB BS Lond. 1985; BSc (Hons.) 1980; DCH Lond. 1989; MRCP UK) 1990; FRCPCH 1997; FRCP 2000. Cons. in Paediatric Neuromuscular Disorders RJAH and BCH. Specialty: Paediat. Socs: World Muscle Soc.; Brit. Paediatric Neurol. Assn.; Roy. Coll. of Paediat. and Child Health. Prev: Cons. in Paediat., Roy. Shrewsbury Hosp.; Lect. in Paediat., Guy's Hosp.; Lect. in Neuromuscular Disorders, Guy's Hosp.

QUINN, Andrew Charles 22 Mountford Close, Wellesbourne, Warwick CV35 9QQ — MB ChB Leeds 1995.

QUINN, Andrew James Royal Alexandra Hospital, Corsebar Road, Paisley PA2 9PN; 5 Newlands Road, Newlands, Glasgow G43 2JB — MB BCh BAO Belf. 1986; MRCOG 1991. Cons. Obst. Roy. Alexandra Hosp. Paisley. Specialty: Obst. & Gyn.

QUINN, Professor Anthony Gerard Experimental Medicine, Astrazeneca R+D, Bakewell Road, Loughborough LE11 5RH Tel: 44 1509 644109 Fax: 44 1509 645514; 7 Blacksmiths Close, Thrussington, Leicester LE7 4UJ — MB ChB (Commend) Dundee 1985; BMSc (1st cl. Hons. Gen. Path.) Dundee 1982; MRCP (UK) 1988; PhD Newc. 1995; FRCP London 2000. Global Clin. Expert, Experim. Med., R+D Astrazenenca PLC. Specialty: Dermat. Socs: Brit. Assn. Dermatol.; Brit. Soc. Investig. Dermat.; Roy. Soc. Med. Prev: Prof. of Dermat., Bart's & The Roy. Lond. Hosp.; MRC Trav. Fellowship UCSF, Calif.; MRC Train. Fell. Dept. Dermatol, NEWC.

QUINN, Audrey Catherine 28 Briar Road, Newlands, Glasgow G43 2TX — MB ChB Glas. 1987.

QUINN, Benedict Noel Eugene 50 Wallasey Vill., Wallasey Tel: 0151 691 2088 — MB BCh BAO NUI 1979.

QUINN, Christopher Anthony — MB BS Lond. 1991; BSc Biochem. Pharmacol. (Hons.) Glas. 1979; PhD Biochem. Lond. 1983. SHO (Paediat.) Roy. Liverp. Childr. Hosp. Alder Hey Liverp.; SHO Psychiat., Leverndale Hosp., Glas. Specialty: Paediat. Socs: BMA. Prev: SHO (Paediat.) Addenbrookes Hosp. Cambs.; SHO (Neonat.) Rosie Matern. Hosp. Camb.; SHO (Paediat.) Qu. Eliz. Hosp. King's Lynn.

QUINN, David Warwick 35 St John's Wood Terrace, London NW8 6JL — MB BS Lond. 1991.

QUINN, Deborah Catherine 54 Waveney Road, Harpenden AL5 4QY Tel: 01582 767794 — MB BS Lond. 1988 (Middlesex Hosp. Medical School) DCH RCP Lond. 1992; MRCGP 1994; DFFP 1994. Assoc. Specialist (Palliat. Med.) Isabel Hospice Welwyn Garden City. Specialty: Palliat. Med. Socs: BMA; Assn. Palliat. Med.

QUINN, Elizabeth Ann 62 Corrour Road, Glasgow G43 2ED — MB ChB Glas. 1986.

QUINN, Fiona Mary 44 King's Road, Belfast BT5 6JJ Tel: 01232 656335 — MB BCh BAO Belf. 1992 (Qu. Univ. Belf.) DCH RCPSI 1995; DRCOG 1995; MRCGP 1996; DFFP 1997. Specialty: Gen. Pract.

QUINN, Fiona Michele 44 Rathfriland Road, Newry BT34 1LD — MB BCh BAO Belf. 1992.

QUINN, Jean 84 Black Horse Hill, West Kirby, Wirral CH48 6DT Tel: 0151 625 9547 — MB ChB Liverp. 1970; MRCGP 1995; ILTM 2001; FRCGP 2001. Prev: Clin. Teach. Univ. Liverp.; Mem. FHSA; Chairm. Wirral LMC.

QUINN, Josiette Suzanne St. Georges Hospital, Newcastle, North Tyneside & Northumberland Mental Health NHS Trust, Morpeth NE61 2NU Tel: 01670 512121 — MB ChB Glas. 1984 (Glasgow) MRCPsych. 1989. Cons. Psychiat. St. Geo. Hosp. Morpeth. Specialty: Gen. Psychiat.; Rehabil. Med. Prev: Sen. Regist. St. Nicholas Hosp. Newc. u Tyne; Regist. Gartnaval Roy. Hosp. Gt. Glas. HB.

QUINN, Kathleen 24J Constitution Road, Dundee DD1 1LD — MB ChB Dundee 1978. SHO (Psychiat.) Roy. Dundee Liff Hosp.

QUINN, Kathleen Susan New Craigs Hospital, Inverness IV3 8NP Tel: 01463 242860 Ext: 3627; 6 Newtonhill, Lentran, Inverness IV3 8RN Tel: 01463 831364 — MB ChB Aberd. 1968; Dobst RCOG 1970; DCH Eng. 1971; MRCPsych 1980. Specialist Psychiat. (Ment. Health) Highland Communities NHS Trust. Specialty: Gen. Psychiat.

QUINN, Kealan Murray Straidarran House, Claudy, Londonderry BT47 4DB — MB ChB Ed. 1996.

QUINN, Louise Anne Lowther Unit, St Andrews Hospital, Billing Rd, Northampton NN1 5DG Tel: 01604 661000 — MB ChB Sheff. 1987; MRCPsych 1991. Cons. Child & Adolesc. Psychiat. St Andrews Hosp., N.ampton. Specialty: Child & Adolesc. Psychiat. Prev: Sen. Regist. Train. Scheme Wessex; Cons. Child & Adolesc. Psychiat. Hosp. Campus Milton Keynes.

QUINN, Mark Alexander Dept. (Rhemat.) Leeds General Infirmary, Great George Street, Leeds LS1 3EX Tel: 0113 392 6505 — MB ChB Manch. 1994; MRCP 1998. Lect. (Rheumat.); SDDD. Specialty: Gen. Med.; Rheumatol. Prev: Research Fell. (Rheumat.); Ho. Off. (Surg. & Med.) Macclesfield Dist. Gen. Hosp.; SHO (Gen. Med.).

QUINN, Martin John 6 Cavendish Gardens, Sneyd Park, Bristol BS9 1RQ — MB ChB Bristol 1980; MRCOG 1987; MD Bristol 1994. Sen. Regist. (O & G) Univ. Hosp. Wales NHS Trust. Specialty: Obst. & Gyn. Prev: Lect. (O & G) Univ. Bristol.

QUINN, Mary Bridget Diabetes and Endocrinology, 1771 Victoria Building, Leicester Royal Infirmary, Leicester LE1 5WW Tel: 0116 258 6182 — MB ChB Leic. 1986; BSc (1st cl. Hons.) Leic. 1984; Cert. Family Plann. JCC 1992; T(GP) 1992; DFFP 1996. Assoc. Specialist in Diabetes Leicester Roy. Infirm. Leicester. Specialty: Diabetes.

QUINN, Mary Clare — MB ChB Dundee 1985; DRCOG 1991; MRCGP 1992.

QUINN, Mary Gerardine Herrington Medical Centre, Philadelphia Lane, Houghton-le-Spring DH4 4LE Tel: 0191 584 2632; 130 Benfieldside Road, Blackhill, Consett DH8 0RT — MB ChB Leeds 1981. Specialty: Gen. Pract. Prev: Trainee GP Doncaster Roy. Infirm.; Ho. Phys. Leeds Gen. Infirm.; Ho. Surg. St. Jas. Hosp. Leeds.

QUINN, Mary Margaret Cornmarket Surgery, Newry Health Village, Monaghan, Newry BT35 6BW Tel: 028 3026 5838 Fax: 028 3026 6727; 55 Crieve Court, Rathfriland Road, Newry BT34 2PE — MB BCh BAO NUI 1983; DGM RCP Lond. 1986; DRCOG 1987; MRCGP 1988. Specialty: Family Plann. & Reproduc. Health. Prev: Trainee GP Sandhead VTS; Clin. Med. Off. (Child Health & Family Plann.) Lurgan Co. Armagh.

QUINN, Michael (retired) Highlands, 25 Sheeplands Lane, Sherborne DT9 4BW Tel: 01935 813427 — MB BCh BAO NUI 1952 (Univ. Coll. Dub.) LM Nat. Matern. Hosp. Dub. 1955; DPM Eng. 1962; MRCPsych 1971. Prev: Cons. Psychiat. (Ment. Handicap) Dorset AHA.

QUINN, Michael Francis 6 Greenan Road, Newry BT34 2PJ — MB BCh BAO Belf. 1995.

QUINN, Mr Michael Joseph 4 Breda Avenue, Belfast BT8 6JS — MB BCh BAO Belf. 1981; FRCSI 1994.

QUINN, Michelle Claire 74 Ash Grove, Wavertree, Liverpool L15 1ET — MB ChB Liverp. 1996.

QUINN, Professor Niall Patrick Institute of Neurology, Queen Square, London WC1N 3BG Tel: 020 7837 3611 Ext: 4253 Fax: 020 7676 2175 Email: n.quinn@ion.ucl.ac.uk — MB BChir Camb. 1974 (Lond. Hosp.) MA Camb. 1976, MD 1988; FRCP Lond. 1994. Prof. (Neurol) Inst. Neurol. Lond.; Hon. Cons. Neurol. Nat. Hosp. Neurol. & Neurosurg. & Gt. Ormond St. Hosp. for Childr. Lond. Specialty: Neurol. Socs: Corr. Fell. Amer. Acad. Neurol.; Corr. Mem. Amer. Neurol. Assn.; Mem. Assn. Brit. Neurol. Prev: Reader & Sen. Lect. (Neurol.) Inst. Neurol. Lond.; Lect. (Neurol.) King's Coll. Hosp. Med. Sch. Lond.; Med. Resid. Neurol. Serv. Hôp. de la Salpêtrière Paris.

QUINN, Nicholas David 28 Eskdale Road, Hartlepool TS25 4AU — MB BS Lond. 1992.

QUINN, Patrick Henry Martin Omagh Health Centre, Mountjoy Road, Omagh BT79 7BA Tel: 028 8224 3521 — MB BCh BAO Belf. 1989.

QUINN, Patrick McDara 6 Fairfield Close, Exmouth EX8 2BN — MB BCh BAO Dub. 1980; MRCPsych 1986. Cons. Psychi. Devon. Specialty: Gen. Psychiat. Prev: Sen. Regist. (Child & Adolesc. Psychiat.) Swindon.

QUINN, Philip Wyndham Blackburn Road Surgery, 257 Blackburn Road, Accrington BB5 0AL Tel: 01254 233048; High Lawn, Whins Lane, Read, Burnley BB12 7QY Tel: 01282 772802 — (Sheff.) Cert. Contracep. & Family Plann. RCOG & RCGP &; MRCS Eng. LRCP Lond. 1956; DObst RCOG 1957; MRCGP 1965; Cert FPA 1975; DFFP 1993. SCMO (Occupat. Health) Blackburn Health Dist.; Med. Dir. Communicare NHS Trust. Specialty: Pub. Health Med. Socs: Blackburn & Accrington Med. Soc. Prev: Mem. Dist. Managem. Team Blackburn Health Dist.; Chairm. E. Lancs. HC.

QUINN, Robert James Murray Straidarran House, Claudy, Londonderry BT47 4DB Email: rjmquinn@btinternet.com — (Belf.) MB BCh BAO Belf. 1970; DCH RCPS Glas. 1972; MRCP (UK) 1973; FRCP Glas. 1986; FRCP (Ed.) 1996; FRCP (Lon.) 1996; FRCP&CH 1997. Cons. Paediatr. Altnagelvin Hosp. Londonderry. Specialty: Paediat. Socs: Brit. Paediat. Assn. Prev: Sen. Regist. & Sen. Tutor (Paediat.) Roy. Belf. Hosp. Sick Childr.; Sen. Regist. (Paediat.) King Edwd. VIII Hosp. Durban, S. Africa & Ulster Hosp. Dundonald.

QUINN, Ruadhri Paul Newtownhamilton Health Centre, 2A Markethill Road, Newtownhamilton, Newry BT35 0BE Tel: 028 3087 8202/8223 Fax: 028 3087 9043 — MB BCh BAO Belf. 1989; DCH Dub. 1992; MRCGP 1995.

QUINN, Sally Jane Flat 4, 182 Drake St., Rochdale OL16 1UP — MB BS Newc. 1990.

QUINN, Siobhan Rosemarie 85 Baronscourt Road, Carryduff, Belfast BT8 8BQ — MB BCh BAO Belf. 1988; MB BCh BAO Belf. 1989.

QUINN, Mr Steven James Apt. 13, Scotia West, 5 Jardine Road, London E1W 3WA — MB BS Lond. 1987; FRCS Eng. 1992. Regist. (Otolaryngol.) Addenbrooke's Hosp. Camb. Specialty: Otolaryngol.

QUINN, Teresa Josephine Dalkeith Road Medical Practice, 145 Dalkeith Road, Edinburgh EH16 5HQ Tel: 0131 667 1289 — MB BCh BAO Belf. 1985 (Qu. Univ. Belf.) DGM Lond. 1987; MRCGP 1990. Specialty: Gen. Pract. Prev: Staff Grade & Clin. Med. Off. (Community Paediat.) Edin.; SHO (Rehabil. Med.) Astley Ainslie Hosp. Edin.; Trainee Community Paediat. Howden Health Centre Livingstone.

QUINN, Tiernan George (retired) Wardlaw, 81 Winshields, Cramlington NE23 6JD Tel: 01670 712020 — MB BS Durh. 1951. Prev: Ho. Surg. Princess Mary Matern. Hosp. Newc., Fleming Memor. Hosp. Sick Childr. & Roy. Vict. Infirm.

QUINN, Vincent Philip c/o Fr. B. Curley, 250 Chapel St., Salford M3 5LL — MB BCh BAO Dub. 1950; MA Dub. 1953, MB BCh BAO 1950. Prev: Community Med. Off. Salford.

QUINN, Mrs Zandra Elizabeth 1 Queen Ethelburga's Gardens, Harrogate HG3 2GF Tel: 01423 340470 — MB ChB Dund. 1995 (Dundee Univ.) BMSc (Hons. Forens. Med.) Dund. 1992; DFFP 1997; DRCOG RCObst&Gyn. 1997. GP Asst. Catterick Village Health Centre; Med. Off. Family Plann. Clin.; Forens. Med. Examr. N. Yorks. Police. Specialty: Paediat. Socs: BMA; Med. Sickness Soc. Prev: SHO (Paediat.) Harrogate Dist. Hosp.; SHO (A & E) Harrogate Dist. Hosp.; GP Regist. Leeds Rd. Surg. Harrogate.

QUINNELL, Anthony John Prestwich Hospital, Drugs North West BST MH Trust, Bury New Road, Manchester M25 3BL Tel: 0161 773 9121 Fax: 0161 772 3595; Bolton CDT, 26 Higher Bridge Street, Bolton BL1 2HA Tel: 01204 398520 — MB ChB Aberd. 1982 (Aberdeen) Assoc. Specialist (Drug Dependance) Bolton CDT. Specialty: Alcohol & Substance Misuse.

QUINNELL, Philip Meyrick Croft Surgery, Barnham Road, Eastergate, Chichester PO20 6RP Tel: 01243 543240 Fax: 01243 544862; Spitchwick, Church Lane, Oving, Chichester PO20 2DG Tel: 01243 779898 — MB BS Lond. 1965 (Lond. Hosp.) DObst RCOG 1967; DA (UK) 1968; LMCC 1979. Prev: Chairm. W. Sussex LMC.

QUINNELL, Mr Richard Charles Little Orchard, 2 Ashbourne Road, Kirk Langley, Derby DE6 4NS Tel: 01332 824408 — (Guy's.) MB BS Lond. 1969; MRCS Eng. LRCP Lond. 1969; FRCS Eng. 1975. Cons. Orthop. Surg. S. Derbysh. Gp. Hosps. Specialty: Orthop.

QUINNELL, Timothy George 19 Wenvoe Close, Cherry Hinton, Cambridge CB1 9JG Tel: 01223 243465 — MB BS Lond. 1993 (Lond. Hosp.) BSc (Hist. Med. & Basic Med. Scis.) Lond. 1990; MRCP (Lond.) 1997; FRACP (Australasia) 2001. Specialty: Gen. Med.; Respirat. Med. Special Interest: Sleep Med.

QUINTON, Anthony Arthur Greves Suite D, Metropolitan House, The Millfields,, Stonehouse, Plymouth PL1 3JX Tel: 01752 229116 Fax: 01752 269098; Higher Quither, Milton Abbot, Tavistock PL19 0PZ Tel: 01822 860284 — MRCS Eng. LRCP Lond. 1966; DAvMed Eng. 1976; AFOM DCP Lond. 1980. Occupat. Phys.; Authorised Med. Examr. Civil Aviat. Auth. Specialty: Trauma & Orthop. Surg. Socs: Soc. Occupat. Med. & Assn. Aviat. Med. Examrs.

QUINTON, Catherine Frances c/o Mr. R.F. Quinton, 21 The Warren, Carshalton SM5 4EQ — MB BS Lond. 1988; BSc Lond. 1985, MB BS 1988; MRCPsych 1993. Cons. Old Age Psychiat. Centr. Worthing Sussex. Specialty: Geriat. Psychiat.

QUINTON, Mr David Neil Accident & Emergency Department, Leicester Royal Infirmary, Infirmary Square, Leicester LE1 5WW Email: ismail@aljalili.com; 24 Church Lane, Thrussington, Leicester LE7 4TE — MB BS Lond. 1976 (Middlesex London) FRCS Ed. 1981. Cons. A & E Leicester Roy. Infirm. Specialty: Accid. & Emerg. Socs: Hand Soc. Gt. Brit.

QUINTON, Peter John Orchard House, Lower Fold, Dorrington, Shrewsbury SY5 7JG — MB Camb. 1968; BChir 1967.

QUINTON, Richard Royal Victoria Infirmary, Department of Endocrinology, Ward 23, Claremont Wing, Newcastle upon Tyne NE1 4LP Tel: 0191 282 4635 Fax: 0191 282 0129 Email: therese.collins@nuth.northy.nhs.uk — MB BChir Camb. 1988; MA Camb. 1989; MRCP (UK) 1992; MD Camb. 2000; FRCP 2003. Cons.(Endocrinol.) Roy. Vict. Infirm. Newc.; N.E. Regional Specialty Adviser (Endocrinol. & Diabetes); Sen. Lect. (Med.), Univ. of Newc., Newc.; N. E. Regional Progr. Director (Endocrinol. & Diabetes). Specialty: Endocrinol.; Gen. Med. Special Interest: Hypogonadism, Pituitary Dis., Gen. Endocrinol. Socs: Soc. Endocrinol.; Endocrine Soc.; Hosp. Cons. & Specialists Assn. Prev: Lect. & Hon.Sen. Regist. (Endocrinol); U.C.L. & Roy. Free Hosp. Med. Sch. Lond.

QUINTON-TULLOCH, John Charles Fremington Medical Centre, Barnstaple EX31 2NT Tel: 01271 376655; The Verne, Instow, Bideford EX39 4JX — MB ChB Bristol 1987.

QUIRK, Jennifer Anne Bromley Hosp, Cromwell Avenue, Bromley BR2 9AJ Tel: 020 8289 7000 — MB BS Western Australia 1981; FRACP 1989. Cons. (Neurol.) Bromley Hosp.; Hon. Cons. (Neurol.) KCL. Specialty: Neurol.; Clin. Neurophysiol. Socs: BMA; ABN; AAN.

QUIRKE, Professor Philip Division of Clinical Sciences, School of Medicine, Algernon Firth Institute of Pathology, Leeds LS2 9JT Tel: 0113 233 3412 Fax: 0113 233 3404 Email: philq@pathology.leeds.ac.uk; The Old Granary, Main St, Linton, Wetherby LS22 4HT Tel: 01937 587797 Fax: 01937 587797 Email: philip.quirke@cqw.net — BM Soton. 1980; PhD Leeds 1987; MRCPath 1988; FRCPath 1997. Prof. Univ. Leeds; Hon. Cons. & Head Histopath. & Molecular Path. Leeds Gen. Infirm. Teachg. Hosp NHS Trust. Specialty: Histopath.

QUIRKE, Richard Joseph Ty Morlais, Berry Square, Merthyr Tydfil CF48 3AL Tel: 01685 722782 Fax: 01685 722951 — MB BCh BAO NUI 1982.

QUIYUM, S A Handsworth Grange Medical Centre, 432 Handsworth Road, Sheffield S13 9BZ Tel: 0114 269 7505 Fax: 0114 269 8535.

QULI, Rachel Elizabeth — MB ChB Sheff. 1997.

QULI, Xavier Haider 13 Joinings Bank, Oldbury, Oldbury B68 8QJ — MB ChB Sheff. 1997.

QUORAISHI, Abu Hashem Muhammad Ali Haider Public Health Laboratory Service, Llandough Hospital & Community NHS Trust, Penlan Road, Penarth CF64 2XX Tel: 029 2071 5298 Fax: 029 2071 5134 Email: llanbact@celtic.co.uk — MB BS Dacca 1963 (Dacca Med. Coll.) MPhil Karachi 1966; Dip. Bact. (Distinc.) Manch. 1972; FRCPath 1988, M 1977. Cons. Med. Microbiol. S. Glam. AHA (T). Specialty: Med. Microbiol.

QURAISHI, Mohammad Aslam Castleton Road Surgery, 19-21 Castleton Road, Goodmayes, Ilford IG3 9QW Tel: 020 8599 9951 Fax: 020 8597 9974 — MB BS Karachi 1962 (Dow Med. Coll.) BSc Karachi 1955; DTM & H Eng. 1965. Prev: SHO (Paediat.) Univ. Hosp. S. Manch.; SHO (Gen. Med.) W. Wales Gen. Hosp. Carmarthen; Ho. Phys. St. Mary's Hosp. Plaistow.

QURAISHY, Anzar Uddin 7 Grand Drive, Leigh-on-Sea SS9 1BG — MB BS Karachi 1966. Specialty: Community Child Health.

QURAISHY, Ehsanullah Stepping Hill Hospital, Stockport SK2 7JE Tel: 0161 483 1010; 303 Bramhall Lane S., Bramhall, Stockport SK7 3DN Tel: 0161 439 5272 Fax: 0161 440 0189 — MB BS Lucknow 1977; BSc Gorakhpur 1961; MB BS Lucknow 1967; Dip. Dermat. Lond 1971; DPM Eng. 1975; MRCPsych 1976. Cons. Psychiat. Stepping Hill Hosp. Stockport. & Clin. Dir. Ment. Health. Specialty: Gen. Psychiat. Socs: BMA. Prev: Sen. Regist. (Psychiat.) Sefton & Roy. Liverp. Hosps.; Regist. (Psychiat.) Mid-Wales Hosp. Talgarth; Regist. (Dermatol.) Manch. & Salford Skin Hosps.

QURAISHY, Muhammad Muneer 20A Long Lane, Stanwell, Staines TW19 7AA — MB BS Karachi 1987; FCOphth 1991. Specialty: Cardiol.

QURASHI, Intikhab 241 Manchester Road, Bury BL9 9HJ — MB ChB Dundee 1996.

QURESHI, Aamir Mahmood c/o D.O.M.E. Office, Woodend Hospital, Eday Road, Aberdeen AB15 6JP; Woodbine Cottage, Grandholm Vill., Persley Den, Aberdeen AB22 8AJ — MB BS Karachi 1983; MRCP (UK) 1993. Regist. (Med. for Elderly) Woodend Hosp. Aberd. Specialty: Care of the Elderly. Socs: Brit. Geriat. Soc. Prev: Regist. (Geriat. & Gen. Med.) Maelor Gen. Hosp. Wrexham.; Regist. (Med.) Cumbld. Infirm. Carlisle; SHO (Gen. Med. & Elderly Care) Llandudno Gen. Hosp.

QURESHI, Akhtar Hussain 'Akhtar Lodge', 148 High Road, Chigwell IG7 5BQ Tel: 020 8501 0566 — MB BS Sind 1958 (Liaquat Med. Coll.) LRCP LRCS Ed. LRFPS Glas. 1962. Socs: Assoc. MRCGP.

QURESHI, Amer Mehmood 42 Ancaster Crescent, New Malden KT3 6BE — MB ChB Manch. 1993; BSc (Hons.) 1990; MRCP (UK) 1997. SHO (Anaesth.) St. Helier's Hosp. Carshalton. Specialty: Anaesth.

QURESHI, Amir Ali — MB BCh Wales 1997.

QURESHI, Anser Suhail Mid Essex Hospital Services NHS Trust, Broomfield Hospital, Court Road, Chelmsford CM1 7ET Email: anser.qureshi@meht.nhs.uk; 4 Redmayne Drive, Chelmsford CM2 9AG Email: anserqureshi@hotmail.com — MB BS Punjab 1984; MRCP (UK) 1994; CCST Gen. Med. & Geriat. Med. 1999; FRCP Lond. 2004. Cons. Gen. Med. c/o Elderly, Broomfield Hosp. Chelsford; SR. Med. Bedford Hosp.; SR. Med.c/o elderly Camb. Hosp.; Sen. Regist. Med. James Paget Hosp.Gt. Yarmonth. Specialty: Gen. Med.; Care of the Elderly. Special Interest: Parkinson's Dis.; Stroke Med. Socs: BMA; RCP; Brit. Geriat.s Soc. Prev: Regist. (Med. for Elderly) W. Norwich Hosp.; SHO (Cardiol.) Papworth Hosp. Huntingdon; SHO (Med. for Elderly & Gen. Med.) Bedford Gen. Hosp.

QURESHI, Ashfaq Husain St Catherine Surgery, 19 St. Catherines, Lincoln LN5 8LT Tel: 01522 871771 Fax: 01522 871773.

QURESHI, Asjid Iqbal 83 Ballards Road, London NW2 7UE — MB ChB Ed. 1992.

QURESHI, Ayesha Salma Springhill House, Springhill Lane, Lower Penn, Wolverhampton WV4 4TJ — MB ChB Birm. 1995; ChB Birm. 1995.

QURESHI, Bashir Ahmed Al-Bashir, 32 Legrace Avenue, Hounslow TW4 7RS Tel: 020 8570 4008 Fax: 020 8570 4008 Email: drbashirqureshi@hotmail.com — MB BS Punjab (Pakistan) 1961 (Nishtar Med. Coll., Multan) LMSSA 1970; DHMSA Lond. 1974; Cert. Family Plann. JCC 1974; LRCP LRCS Ed. LRCPS Glas. 1975; DCH RCPSI 1976; FRCGP 1984, M 1976; ECFMG Cert. 1976; AFOM RCP Lond. 1978; DPMSA Lond. 1980; MICGP 1984; MFFP 1993; Hon. M GP Sec. RSM 1998; Hon. FRSH 1998; MRCPCH 1998; Hon. MAPHA 1998. GP Hounslow W. Lond.; Civil. Med. Practitioner, Roy. Milit. Sch. of Music, Lond.; Expert Witness Transcultural Medico-Legal Cases; Regular Book Reviewer of Jl. Roy. Soc. Hlth.; URDU-English Translator. Specialty: Paediat.; Family Plann. & Reproduc. Health; Occupat. Health; Gen. Pract. Special Interest: Transcultural Med. Socs: FRSH (Ex-Vice Pres.); Mem. Ct. of Governor of Lond. Sch. of Trop. Med. & Hyg.; FRIPHH. Prev: Examr. Brit. Red Cross Soc. Ealing & Dep. Med. Adviser Lond. Br. Brit. Red. CrosS; Med. Off. W. Lond. Healthcare NHS Trust; SHO Nat. Hosp. Qu. Sq. Lond.

QURESHI, Mr Hamidullah Rotherham District General Hospital, Moorgate Road, Rotherham S60 2UD Tel: 01709 820000 Fax: 01709 824282 — MB BS Sind 1958 (Liaquat Med. Coll. Hyderabad) MB BS Sind. 1958; FRCS Ed. 1971; FRCS Eng. 1972; MRCS Eng. LRCP Lond. 1975. Cons. A & E Dept. Rotherham Hosp. Specialty: Accid. & Emerg. Prev: Regist. (Orthop.) Rotherham Hosp. & Roy. Orthop. Hosp. Birm.; Med. Off. Pakistan Army Med. Corps.

QURESHI, Idris Fouad 27 Lucknow Drive, Nottingham NG3 5EU — MB BS Lond. 1994.

QURESHI, Irum Flat 40, Block 3, 5 Beech Hill Road, Sheffield S10 2RA — MB ChB Sheff. 1995.

QURESHI, Isaque D'Almendra 26 Downhurst Avenue, London NW7 3QA — MB BS Lond. 1996.

QURESHI, Khalda Nasreen Maidstone Road Surgery, 262 Maidstone Road, Chatham ME4 6JL Tel: 01634 842093 Fax: 01634 842151; 71 College Avenue, Gillingham ME7 5HY Tel: 01634 578016 — MB ChB Manch. 1974; DRCOG 1976.

QURESHI, Khalida 43 Athol Road, Whalley Range, Manchester M16 8QW — MB BCh Wales 1977.

QURESHI, Mr Khaver Naseer 46 Harley Terrace, Gosforth, Newcastle upon Tyne NE3 1UL — MB BS Lond. 1992 (St. Bart.) BSc (Hons.) Lond. 1989; FRCS Eng. 1996. Clin. Research Assoc. (Surg.) Med. Sch. Univ. Newc. Specialty: Urol. Prev: SHO (Gen. Surg.) Wansbeck N.umberland; SHO (Urol.) Freeman Hosp. Newc.; SHO (Gen. Surg.) Walsgrave Hosp. Coventry.

QURESHI, Mahmooda 79 Carlton Mansions, Randolph Avenue, London W9 1NS — MB BS Lond. 1992.

QURESHI, Mansur (retired) 16 Broxholm Road, Heaton, Newcastle upon Tyne NE6 5RL Tel: 0191 265 4516 — MB BS Punjab 1962 (Nishtar Med. Coll. Multan) FRCPath 1984, M 1972. Cons. Haemat. Freeman Hosp. Newc. Prev: Sen. Regist. (Haemat.) Newc. Gen. Hosp.

QURESHI, Mariam Amatullah 10 Sefton Grove, Bradford BD2 4JW Tel: 01274 640931 — MB ChB Manch. 1993; DFFP 1995 RCOG; DRCOG 1996 RCOG; MRCGP RCGP 2002. Non Principal GP. Specialty: Gen. Pract. Prev: Gen. Pract. VTS; Centr. Manch. Healthcare Trust; GP Regist. The Gables Surg. Pudsey.

QURESHI, Mazhar Uddin 34 Greaves Road, Walsall WS5 3QG — MB BS Punjab 1967.

QURESHI, Mr Mohammad Akhtar Cromwell Hospital, Cromwell Road, London SW5 0UT Tel: 020 7460 5577 Fax: 020 7460 5709 Email: akhtarqureshi@cromwell-hospital.co.uk — MB BS Karachi 1964 (Dow Med. Coll.) FRCS Glas. 1975; SpR Orthop. & Trauma Surg.; BSc. Cons. Orthop. Surg. Cromwell & Ashtead Hosps. Specialty: Orthop. Socs: Fell. Brit. Orthop. Assn.; Int. Musculoskeletal Laser Soc. (IMLAS); AO. Alumni Switz. (Study of Internal Fixation). Prev: Cons. Orthop. & Traum. Surg. Qu. Eliz. Milit. Hosp. Lond.; Sen. Regist. (Orthop.) St. Mary's Hosp. Lond. W9; Regist. (Surg.) Qu. Mary's Hosp. Sidcup.

QURESHI, Mr Mohammad Iqbal Blackburn Street Health Centre, Blackburn Street, Radcliffe, Manchester M26 1WS; 51 Hillsborough Drive, Unsworth, Bury BL9 8LF Tel: 0161 766 6089 — MB BS Punjab 1965 (King Edwd. Med. Coll. Lahore) BSc Punjab (Pakistan) 1962, MB BS 1965; FRCS Glas. 1971. Mem. Bury LMC; Chairm. Bury Fund Holding Pract. Socs: Local BMA; Pres. Pakistan Med. Assn. (UK). Prev: Surg. Specialist Ahmadi Hosp. Kuwait, Gulf.

QURESHI, Mohammad Sarfraz Akhtar The Calderdale Royal Hospital, Dudwell Lane, Halifax HX3 0PW Tel: 01422 357171 Fax: 01422 380357 — (King Edwd. Med. Coll. Lahore) MB BS Punjab (Pakistan) 1964; DCH RCPS Glas. 1968; DCH Eng. 1970; MRCP (UK) 1971; FRCP Lond. 1987. Cons. Phys. Gastroenterol. Halifax Gen. Hosp.; Sen. Clin. Lect. Univ. of Leeds Sch. of Med.; Hon. Sec. / Treas., N. of Eng. Gastroenterol. Soc. Specialty: Gen. Med.; Gastroenterol. Socs: BMA; BSG; NEGS.

QURESHI, Mohammed Abdul Hai Oldhill Medical Centre, 19-21 Oldhill Street, London N16 6LD Tel: 020 8806 6993 Fax: 020 8806 6008; 95 Langford Court, London NW8 9DP Tel: 020 7266 3225 Fax: 020 7266 3225 — MB BS Osmania 1955. Vis. Prof. Surg. Univ. La Paz, Bolivia. Specialty: Accid. & Emerg.; Gen. Pract. Socs: Fell. Roy. Soc. Med.; BMA & German Med. Assn.; Assoc. Mem. Brit. Assn. Plastic Surgs. Prev: Sen. Cas. Off. Farnham Hosp. Surrey; JHMO Booth Hall Hosp. Manch.; SHO Salford Roy. Hosp.

QURESHI, Mohammed Tahir St Paul's Road Surgery, 50 St Paul's Road, Bradford BD8 7LP Tel: 01274 543684 Fax: 01274 487674; 50 St Paul's Road, Manningham, Bradford BD8 7LP Tel: 01274 543684 Fax: 01274 487674 — MB BS Karachi 1956 (Dow Med. Coll.)

QURESHI, Mohammed Zubair 97 Granson Way, Washingborough, Lincoln LN4 1HH Email: zqureshi@granson97.freeserve.co.uk — BM BS Nottm. 1997; BMedSci, Nottm, 1995. Specialty: Gen. Pract.

QURESHI, Muhammad Akram 46 Stonehall Avenue, Ilford IG1 3SH — MB BS Punjab 1961 (Nishtar Med. Coll.) MB BS Punjab Pakistan 1961; DA Eng. 1965; DRCOG 1967. Clin. Asst. (Anaesth.) Qu. Mary's Hosp. Lond. Socs: BMA. Prev: SHO (O & G) St. Mary's Hosp. Leeds; Regist. (Anaesth.) Preston Hall Hosp. Maidstone & W. Kent. Gen. Hosp.; Maidstone.

QURESHI, Muhammad Aslam 8 Watery Lane, Walsall WS1 4HS — MB BS Karachi 1986; MRCP (UK) 1993.

QURESHI, Muna Bashir 84 Turnpike Link, Parkhill, Croydon CR0 5NY — MB ChB Manch. 1996.

QURESHI, Munir-ud-Din Nelson Road Surgery, 126 Nelson Road, Gillingham ME7 4LL Tel: 01634 571740 Fax: 01634 575024; 3 Bellwood Court, St Mary Hoo, Rochester ME3 8RT Tel: 01634 271425 — (Nishtar Med. Coll. Multan) MB BS Punjab (Pakistan) 1964.

QURESHI, Nadeem Patrick and Partners, Rise Park Surgery, Revelstoke Way, Nottingham NG5 5EB Tel: 0115 927 2525 Fax: 0115 979 7056 — MB BS Lond. 1986. Lect. (Gen. Pract.) Qu.s Med. Centre Univ. Nott. Specialty: Gen. Pract.

QURESHI, Naeem Akhtar 58 New Way Road, London NW9 6PG — MB BS Punjab 1987; LRCP LRCS Ed. LRCPS Glas. 1994.

QURESHI, Mr Navid Sadiq 15 Birchlea, Altrincham WA15 8WF — MB BS Punjab 1977; FRCS Ed. 1987.

QURESHI, Nazar Mohammad G.P. Unit, Cromwell Hospital, Cromwell Road, London SW5 0TU Tel: 020 7460 5700 Mob: 07836680723 — MB BS Punjab 1955; DPath Eng. 1966. Gen. Phys. Lond.

QURESHI, Nubeel Rotherham General Hospital, Moorgate Road, Oakwood, Rotherham S60 2UD Tel: 01709 307168 Fax: 01709 307288 — MB BS Newc. 1989; MRCP (UK) 1993. Regist. (Gen. Med.) Doncaster. Specialty: Gen. Med.

QURESHI, Mr Rashid The Clementine Churchill Hospital, Sudbury Hill, Harrow HA1 3RX Tel: 020 8872 3872; Cessnock, Courtland Avenue, Mill Hill, London NW7 3BG Tel: 020 8906 3049 — MB BS Karachi 1964; FRCS Eng. 1970. Cons. Breast Surg. Breast Unit Edgware & Barnet Gen. Hosps.; Sen. Lect. Middlx. & UCH. Lond.; Surg. Tutor RCS Eng.; Lead Surg. N.Lond Breast Cancer Screening Unit. Specialty: Gen. Surg. Socs: Fell. Roy. Soc. Med.; Brit. Assn. Surg. Oncol (Regional Co-ordinator Breast Gp.); Assn. of Surg. of GB & Irel. Prev: Hon. Sen. Lect. Guy's Hosp. Lond.; Sen. Regist. Breast Unit Guy's Hosp. Lond.

QURESHI, Ruby Nazar Medical Practice, 153 Copenhagen Street, London N1 0SR Tel: 020 7833 4981 Fax: 020 7837 2197; 38 Aylmer Road, London N2 0BX Tel: 020 8348 8642 — MB BS Punjab 1956 (F.J. Med. Coll. Lahore) MB BS Punjab Pakistan 1956; DObst RCPI 1962; DA Eng. 1964 DGO Dub. 1962. GP Lond.

QURESHI, Sajid Ali 53 Muirhead Gardens, Perth PH1 1JR — MB BS Punjab, Pakistan 1979 (King Edwards Medical College Lahore, Pakistan) LMSSA Lond. 1985; FFARCSI 1992. Cons. Anaesth. King Fahd Milit. Med. Complex Dhahran, Saudi-Arabia; Cons. Intensivist, Dewsbury & Dist. Hosp. Specialty: Anaesth. Prev: Sen. Regist. (Anaesth.) Riyadh Milit. Hosp. Riyadh, Saudi Arabia; Regist. (Anaesth.) Roy. Free Hosp. Hampstead Lond.

QURESHI, Sardar Mohammad, MBE Sherwood Rise Surgery, 31 Nottingham Road, Sherwood, Nottingham NG7 7AD Tel: 0115 962 3080 Fax: 0115 985 6522; 27 Lucknow Drive, Mapperley Park, Nottingham NG3 5EU Tel: 0115 962 5706 Fax: 0115 962 5706 — MB BS Karachi 1965 (Dow Med. Coll.) DTM & H Liverp. 1968; Dip. Ven. Liverp. 1969. GP Nottm.; Edr. Medicos. Specialty: Genitourinary Medicine. Socs: Chairm. DADA; Dir. AAAP UK. Prev: Clin. Asst. Univ. Nottm. Med. Sch. Venereol. Dept. (Genitourin. Med.) City Hosp. Nottm.

QURESHI, Shabbeer Ahmad Somerset Medical Centre, 64 Somerset Road, Southall UB1 2TS Tel: 020 8578 1903 Fax: 020 8578 0292; 113 Sudbury Court Drive, Harrow HA1 3SS Tel: 020 8922 6282 — (Nishtar Medical College Pakistan) BSc Punjab 1965, MB BS 1972; DLO Eng. 1979; Cert. Av. Med. 1988. Indep. Med. Pract. Lond. Specialty: Otolaryngol. Prev: Regist. (ENT Surg.) Highlands Hosp. Lond.; Assoc. Specialist ENT Ealing Hosp. Middlx.

QURESHI, Shahida Munir Nelson Road Surgery, 126 Nelson Road, Gillingham ME7 4LL Tel: 01634 571740 Fax: 01634 575024; 3 Bellwood Court, St Mary Hoo, Rochester ME3 8RT Tel: 01634 271425 — MB BS Punjab 1964 (Nishtar Med. Coll. Multan & Fatima Jinnah Med. Coll. Lahore) MB BS Punjab (Pakistan) 1964.

QURESHI, Shakeel Ahmed Department of Paediatric Cardiology, Guy's Hospital, 11th Floor Guy's Tower, St Thomas St., London SE1 9RT Tel: 020 7955 4616 Fax: 020 7955 4614; 41 Beechwood Gardens, Clayhall, Ilford IG5 0AE Tel: 020 8252 0269 — MB ChB Manch. 1976; MRCP (UK) 1979; FRCP Lond. 1995; FRCPCH 1997. Cons. Paediat. Cardiol. Guy's Hosp. Lond. Specialty: Paediat. Cardiol. Socs: Brit. Paediat. Cardiac Soc.; Assn. Europ. Paediat. Cardiol.; Roy. Coll. Paediat. and Child Health. Prev: Cons. Paediat. Cardiol. & Sen. Regist. Roy. Liverp. Childr. Hosp.; Regist. (Cardiol.) Harefield Hosp. Harefield.

QURESHI, Shameem 3 Blackthorne Close, Solihull B91 1PF Tel: 0121 356 7310 — MD Osmania 1961 (Osmania Med. Coll. Hyderabad) MB BS 1955; DObst RCOG 1973.

QURESHI, Siddiqua 4 Wheat Knoll, Hayes Lane, Kenley CR8 5JT — MB BS Karachi 1964.

QURESHI, Sumbal 2 Vicarage Mews, Chelmsford CM2 8JW — MB ChB Birm. 1995; MRCP Lond. 1998.

QURESHI, Tahseen Iftikhar 76 Byrefield Road, Guildford GU2 9UA — MB BS Lond. 1992.

QURESHI, Tariq Mahmud Flat 19, Frans Hals Court, 87 Amsterdam Road, London E14 3UX — MB BS Lond. 1995.

QURESHI, Tipo Riaz 1 Howard Place, St Andrews KY16 9HL — MB BS Lond. 1996.

QURESHI, Zafar Ahmad Arthur Street Health Centre, Arthur Street, Brierfield, Nelson BB9 5SN Tel: 01282 615175; 35 Fairfield Drive, Burnley BB10 2PU — MB BS Karachi 1962 (Dow Med. Coll. Karachi) DCH Eng. 1967. Socs: BMA. Prev: Regist. (Gen. Med.) Altrincham Gen. Hosp.; Regist. (Paediat.) Childr. Hosp. Nottm.; SHO (Gen. Med.) Roy. Hosp. Sheff.

QURESHI, Zarrin The Garden Hospital, 46-50 Sunny Gdns. Road, London NW4 1RX Tel: 020 8457 4500; Cessnock, Courtlands Avenue, Mill Hill, London NW7 3BG Tel: 020 8906 1881 — MB BS Karachi 1964; BSc Karachi 1960; DA Eng. 1969; FFA RCS Eng. 1971. Cons. Anaesth. Barnet & Edgware Gen. Hosps. Specialty: Anaesth. Socs: Roy. Soc. Med.; Assn. Anaesth. Prev: Regist. (Anaesth.) Greenwich Dist. Hosp. Lond.

RAAFAT, Faro The Children's Hospital, Steelhouse Lane, Birmingham B4 6NH Tel: 0121 333 9836 Fax: 0121 333 9831 — MD Geneva 1968; MRCPath 1983. Cons. Histopath. Birm. Childr.s Hosp.; Hon. Sen. Lect. Birm. Univ. Specialty: Histopath.; Paediat. Socs: RCPath; Brit. Paediat. Assn.; Paediat. Path. Soc. Prev: Lect. Histopath. Gt. Ormond St. Lond.

RAAFAT, Laura 11 Ferndale Cl, Hagley, Stourbridge DY9 0QA — MB ChB Birm. 1997.

RAASHED, Muhammad Airedale General Hospital, Skipton Road, Steeton, Keighley BD20 6TD Tel: 01535 292064 Fax: 01535 292068 — MB BS Punjab 1986; MRCP (UK) 1994. Cons. Phys. (Gen. & Respirat. Med.). Specialty: Respirat. Med. Special Interest: COPD; Sleep Related Breathing Disorder; Ventilation. Prev: Locum Cons. Phys. New Cross Hosp. Wolverhampton.

RABAN, John Salisbury (retired) Woodcock Cottage, Woolhampton, Reading RG7 5QG Tel: 0118 971 3374 Fax: 0118 971 3374 — (Middlx.) MB BS Lond. 1955; DObst RCOG 1959. Prev: Ho. Surg. Bedford Gen. Hosp. & Mill Rd. Matern. Hosp. Camb.

RABB, Leigh Michael Heartlands Hospital NHS Trust, Birmingham B9 5SS Tel: 0121 424 2685 — MB BS Lond. 1975; MRCP (UK)

1978; MD 1986. (Community Paediat.) Northern Birm. Specialty: Paediat.

RABBANI, Abu Adib Mohamed Zille 54 Hallam Road, Rotherham S60 3DA — MB BS Bihar 1965 (Darbhanga Med. Coll.) DPM Eng. 1981. Assc. Specialist (Psychogeriat.) Rotherham Dist. Gen. Hosp. Prev: Clin. Asst. (Psychiat.) Rotherham Dist. Gen. Hosp.; Regist. (Psychiat.) Hartwood Hosp. Shotts.

RABBETT, Helen Louise Moorside Hall, Wyresdale Road, Lancaster LA1 3DY — MB ChB Manch. 1994.

RABBIN, David Cecil 55 Somerset Road, Wimbledon, London SW19 5HT — MB BS Lond. 1949 (Middlx.) MRCS Eng. LRCP Lond. 1949. Temple Frere Obst. Prize, Middlx. Hosp. Prev: Flight Lt. RAF Med. Br.; Ho. Phys. St. Stephen's & Gordon (Westm.) Hosps.

RABBITT, Caroline Jayne Groby Road Medical Centre, 9 Groby Road, Leicester LE3 9ED Tel: 0116 253 8185 — MB ChB Leic. 1984. Prev: Trainee GP Huntingdon HA VTS.

RABBS, Jonathan Mark 20 Colbourne Road, Hove BN3 1TB — MB ChB Birm. 1989.

RABETT, Robert John (retired) Parfitt House, 8 Hovells Lane, Northwold, Thetford IP26 5NA Tel: 01366 727050 — MRCS Eng. LRCP Lond. 1945 (St. Mary's) DObst RCOG 1950; MFOM RCP Lond. 1978. Prev: Med. Dir. Occupat. Health Centre Char. Cross. Hosp. NW Thames HA.

RABEY, Graham Peter 14 Auckland Road, Cambridge CB5 8DW — (Lond. Hosp.) BDS Sydney 1955; MB BS Lond. 1961; MRCS Eng. LRCP Lond. 1961; FRACDS 1966; PhD Manch. 1983. Cons. Clin. MorphAnal. Stoke Mandeville Hosp. Aylesbury. Socs: (Ex-Pres.) Craniofacial Soc. Prev: Vis. Prof. Plastic Surg. (Research) Univ. Pittsburgh, USA; Sen. Lect. (Anat.) Univ. Manch.; Lect. Human Morphol. Centre for MorphAnal. Dept. Human Morphol. Univ. Soton.

RABEY, Peter George Department of Anaesth., University Hospital Of Leicester, Leicester General Hospital, Gwerdoler Road, Leicester LE4 5PW Tel: 01664 258 4661 — MB ChB Aberd. 1984; FRCA 1991. Cons. Anaesth. Leicester Gen. Hosp. Specialty: Anaesth.

RABIE, Sabah Merzi Mahmoud Kidsgrove Medical Centre, Mount Road, Kidsgrove, Stoke-on-Trent ST7 4AY Tel: 01782 784221 Fax: 01782 781703 — MB ChB Alexandria 1972; MB ChB Alexandria 1972.

RABIN, Neil Keith 17 Widecombe Way, London N2 0HJ — MB BS Lond. 1996.

RABINDRA, Buwaneswary 14 Waverely Avenue, Sutton SM1 4JY — MB BS Ceylon 1975; DO RCS Eng. 1983; MRCS Eng. LRCP 1986.

RABINDRA-ANANDH, Ketheeswary Petersfield Surgery, 70 Petersfield Avenue, Harold Hill, Romford RM3 9PD Tel: 01708 343113 Fax: 01708 384672 — MB BS Sri Lanka 1978; MRCP (UK) 1985; LMSSA Lond. 1985; DMedRehab RCP Lond. 1987. Specialty: Care of the Elderly. Prev: Regist. (Geriat. Med.) Char. Cross Hosp. Lond.; Regist. (Gen. Med.) Highlands Hosp. Lond.; SHO (Med. & Geriat.) OldCh. Hosp. Romford & St. Geo. Hosp. Lond. HornCh.

RABINOWICZ, Nathan David Health Centre, Durrow, Portlaoise, County Laois, Republic of Ireland; 31 Sherwood Road, London NW4 1AE — MB BChir Camb. 1985; DRCOG 1987; DCH RCP Lond. 1990; MRCGP 1991. Prev: Trainee GP/SHO (Paediat.) Hillingdon Hosp. VTS; SHO (Geriat.) Manor Pk. Hosp.; SHO (Obst. & Gyn., Accid. & Emerg. & Orthop.) Roy. Sussex Co. Hosp.

RABSON, Doreen (retired) 7 Village Close, Belsize Lane, London NW3 5AH — MB BS Lond. 1956 (Westm.) MRCS Eng. LRCP Lond. 1956; DCH Eng. 1959. Sessional Med. Off. BUPA & DSS. Prev: Med. Adviser Dr. Barnardo's.

RABUSZKO, Julian Paul 31 Sussex Garden, East Dean, Eastbourne BN20 0JF Tel: 01323 422466 — MB BS Lond. 1989 (St. Georges Hosp. Med. Sch.) DRCOG 1996. Specialty: Ophth. Prev: VTS Eastbourne 1993-1996.

RABY, Christine Leahurst, Walton Hospital, Chesterfield S40 3HW Tel: 01246 515 915; 18 Newbold Avenue, Chesterfield S41 7AR — MB ChB Sheff. 1976. Clin. Asst. (Psychogeriat.) Walton Hosp. Chesterfield.

RABY, James Roger (retired) 90 Station Road, Scholar Green, Stoke-on-Trent ST7 3JW Tel: 01782 783905 — MB ChB Manch. 1952; DObst RCOG 1956. Prev: Ho. Off. N. Staffs. Roy. Infirm. & Glenroyd Matern. Hosp. Blackpool.

RABY, Michael Bruce The Health Clinic, Weeping Cross, Stafford ST17 0EG Tel: 01785 662505 Fax: 01785 661064; Woodgate, 66 Brocton Road, Milford, Stafford ST17 0UH Tel: 01785 661979 — MB ChB Manch. 1950 (Manchester) DObst RCOG 1956. Socs: Mid Slelp Med. Soc.

RABY, Paul Richard Ashcombe Barton, Ashcombe, Dawlish EX7 0QE — MB ChB Birm. 1978.

RACE, (Alice) Catherine (retired) 11 Colletts Close, Corfe Castle, Wareham BH20 5HG — MB BS Lond. 1968; MRCPath 1976. Prev: Assoc. Specialist (Haemat.) Poole Hosp.

RACE, John William (retired) 86 Chelmsford Road, Brentwood CM15 8RL Tel: 01227 218389 — (Lond. Hosp.) BSc (Hons.) Lond. 1959, MB BS 1962. Prev: GP.

RACE, Julian Hilton Hafan Wen Drug and Alcohol Treatment Unit, Watery Road, Wrexham LL13 7NQ Tel: 01978 313904 — MB ChB Liverp. 1980; MRCS Eng. LRCP Lond. 1980; Cert. Family Plann. JCC 1986; Cert. Prescribed Equiv. Exp. JCPTGP 1986; MRCGP 1988; MRCPsych 1990. Cons. Psychiat. (Addic.) Hafan Wen, Wrexham. Specialty: Gen. Psychiat.; Alcohol & Substance Misuse. Prev: Sen. Regist. (Psychiat.) N. Wales Hosp. Denbigh Clwyd.; Hon. Sen. Regist., Rhondda NHS Trust; Hon. Sen. Regist., Cardiff Community Drug Serv.

RACHED, Sami Toufic Ferryview Health Centre, 25 John Wilson Street, Woolwich, London SE18 6PZ Tel: 020 8319 5400 Fax: 020 8319 5404 — MB ChB Ain Shams 1977; MB BCh Ain Shams 1977; MRCS Eng. LRCP Lond. London 1981.

RACHMAN, Sandra Carole Fernlea Surgery, 114 High Road, London N15 6JR Tel: 020 8809 6445 Fax: 020 8800 4224 — MB ChB Bristol 1983; DTM & H RCP Lond. 1987. Socs: BMA; MPS. Prev: GP Forest Gate; Trainee GP Islington; SHO (Gyn.) Redruth Hosp. Cornw.

RACK, Philip Horsman (retired) Rivulet Court, High Street, Pateley Bridge, Harrogate HG3 5JU Tel: 01423 712684 — MB Camb. 1958 (Roy. Lond. Hosp.) MA Camb. 1957; DPM Eng. 1962; FRCPsych 1980, M 1971. Prev: Cons. Psychiat. Lynfield Mt. Hosp. & Bradford Roy. Infirm.

RACKHAM, Alison Joy 107 Chilternn Avenue, Bushey, Watford WD23 4QE — MB BS Lond. 1987; MRCGP 1992.

RACKHAM, Jonathan Paul Caldicot Medical Group, Gray Hill Surgery, Woodstock Way, Caldicot, Newport NP26 4DB Tel: 01291 420282 Fax: 01291 425853 — MB ChB Leeds 1991; DRCOG 1994; DCH RCP Lond. 1995; MRCGP 1995.

RACKHAM, Kenneth Thomas (retired) Pasley Road Health Centre, Pasley Road, Leicester LE2 9BU; 25 Monsell Drive, Leicester LE2 8PP Tel: 0116 233 7195/0116 2831 206 Email: rackham@mensell.co.uk — MB ChB Bristol 1957; DCH Eng. 1959. Prev: Med. Off. Duncan Hosp. Raxaul, Bihar.

RACKHAM, Mary Miles (retired) The Central Surgery, Oadby, Leicester LE2 5AA Tel: 0116 271 2175; 25 Monsell Drive, Leicester LE2 8PP Tel: 0116 283 1206 Fax: 0116 271 4015 — MB BS Lond. 1957 (Roy. Free) DObst RCOG 1959. Prev: Med. Off. (Community Med.) Leicester AHA (T).

RACKHAM, Oliver James Arrowe Park Hospital, Arrowe Park Road, Upton CH49 5PE Tel: 0151 678 5111 — MB BS Lond. 1994 (St Bart.) MA Camb. 1995, BA (Hons.) 1991; MRCPCH 1999. Specialist Regist. in Paediat., Mersey Deanery. Specialty: Paediat. Socs: RCPCH, Roy. Coll. of Paediat. and Child Health, Mem.

RACKSTRAW, Simon Andrew 28 Old Market Square, London E2 7PQ — MB BS Lond. 1994.

RACZKOWSKI, Richard Matthew Marchmont Surgery, 10 Warrender Park Terrace, Edinburgh EH9 1JA — Lekarz Krakow 1981; LEKARZ Krakow, Poland 1981.

RADCLIFFE, Mr Andrew Grieg Llandough Hospital, Cardiff & Vale NHS Trust, Penlan Road, Penarth CF64 2XX Tel: 029 2071 5416 Fax: 029 2071 5416 — MB BS Lond. 1971 (University College London) BSc (Hons.) Lond. 1968; MRCS Eng. LRCP Lond. 1971; FRCS Eng. 1976; MS Lond. 1984. Cons. Gen. Colorectal Surg, Llandough Hosp. Penarth, Vale of Gamorgan CF64 2XX Univ. Hosp. Of Wales; Hon. Sen. Lect Univ. of Wales Coll. of Med. Specialty: Gen. Surg. Socs: Counc. Assn. Surgs.; Mem. Ct. Examr.ss Roy. Coll. Surg. Eng.; Counc. Assn. Coloproc. GB & Irel. Prev: Lect. (Surg.) St. Mary's Hosp. Med. Sch. Lond.; Regist. (Surg.) Addenbrooke's Hosp. Camb.; Research Fell. Harvard Med. Sch.

RADCLIFFE, Deborah 8 East Downs Road, Cheadle Hulme, Cheadle SK8 5ES — MB ChB Liverp. 1982.

RADCLIFFE, Douglas William John (retired) Compton Lodge, Egerton Road, Kearnsey, Dover CT16 3AF Tel: 01304 822443 — MB BS Lond. 1937 (King's Coll. Hosp.) MRCS Eng. LRCP Lond. 1937; MRCGP 1963. Prev: Med. Off. Dover Harbour Bd.

RADCLIFFE, Gordon Glodwick Health Centre, Glodwick Road, Oldham OL4 1YN Tel: 0161 652 5311 — MB ChB Manch. 1961.

RADCLIFFE, Mr Graham Stuart — BM BCh Oxf. 1990 (Oxford) MA Camb. 1987; FRCS Eng. 1994; FRCS Orthop. & Trauma 2001. Specialist Regist. Yorks. Orthop. Rotat. Specialty: Orthop.

RADCLIFFE, Mr Grant Jeremy 135 Harley Street, London W1N 1DJ Tel: 020 7935 8827 Fax: 020 7224 0732 — MB BS Lond. 1970 (St. Bart.) MRCS Eng. LRCP Lond. 1970; FRCS Eng. 1977. Cons. Otolaryngol. Roy. Free, Edgware & Barnet Hosps. Specialty: Otorhinolaryngol. Socs: Brit. Assn. Otol.; Joseph Soc.; Fell. Roy. Soc. Med. - Counc. Sect. Gargngology & Rhinology. Prev: Sen. Regist. Rotat. Char. Cross Hosp.; Chief Resid. Head & Neck Profess. Unit Toronto Gen. Hosp. Canada; Regist. Rotat. Roy. Nat. Throat Nose & Ear Hosp. Lond.

RADCLIFFE, Hilary 4 Corner Green, Blackheath, London SE3 9JJ — MB Camb. 1977; BChir 1976; DRCOG 1980; DCH Eng. 1981; MRCGP 1981; MFFP 1993.

RADCLIFFE, John Colin Meadowlands Surgery, Newry Health Village, Monaghan Street, Newry BT35 6BW Tel: 028 3026 7534; 36 Greenan Lough Road, Newry BT34 2PX Tel: 016937 53348 — MB BCh BAO Belf. 1987; DRCOG 1989; MRCGP (Distinc.) 1991; DCH Dub. 1992. Prev: Trainee GP Armagh Health Centre.

RADCLIFFE, Keith William Department of GU Medicine, Whittall Street Clinic, Whittall St., Birmingham B4 6DH Tel: 0121 237 5719 Fax: 0121 237 5729 Email: keith.radcliffe@hobtpct.nhs.uk — MB BS Lond. 1983 (Kings) MA Camb. 1984, BA (Hons.) 1980; MB BS (Hons.) Lond. 1983; MRCP (UK) 1987; DFFP 1993; FRCP 1997. Cons. Genitourin. Heart of Birm. Teachg. Primary Care Trust; Hon. Cons. Univ. Hosp. Birm. NHS Trust; Hon. Sen. Lect. (Genitourin. Med.) Univ. Birm. Specialty: Genitourinary Medicine. Special Interest: HIV Infec. / AIDS. Socs: Brit. Assn. for Sexual Health and HIV; Internat. Union Against Sexually Transm. Infec.; Brit. HIV Assn. Prev: Sen. Regist. (Genitourin. Med.) Char. Cross Hosp. Lond.; Regist. (Genitourin. Med.) Middlx. Hosp. Lond.

RADCLIFFE, Marion Elaine Davenal House Surgery, 28 Birmingham Road, Bromsgrove B61 0DD Tel: 01527 872008; 49 Wellington Road, Bromsgrove B60 2AX — BM BS Nottm. 1985; BMedSci Nottm. 1983; MRCGP 1989; DRCOG 1989. Tutor (Gen. Pract.) BromsGr.

RADCLIFFE, Mark Harry 49 Poleacre Lane, Woodley, Stockport SK6 1PH — MB ChB Sheff. 1988.

RADCLIFFE, Michael John 1 Leigh Road, Southampton SO17 1EF Tel: 023 80557755 Fax: 023 80671677 Email: michael@radcliffe.net. Cons. (Allergy Med.) IOW Healthcare NHS Trust; Cons. (Allergy Med.) Roy. Free NHS Trust; Hon. Clin. Research Fell. Univ. Southampton. Specialty: Allergy. Special Interest: Food Allergy; Food Intolerance. Socs: Fell. Amer. Acad. Environm. Med.; Brit. Soc. Allergy & Clin. Immunol.; Brit. Soc. Allergy Nutritional & Environm. Med.

RADCLIFFE, Shirley Anne 10 Norland Square, London W11 4PX Tel: 020 7727 5501 — MB BS Lond. 1979 (Char. Cross) MRCGP 1984; LLB (Hons.) 1996. Socs: Medico-Legal Soc. Prev: GP 1984-1994 Lond.

RADCLIFFE, Mr Simon Neil 40 Brockholme Road, Liverpool L18 4QQ — MB ChB Liverp. 1986; FRCS Ed. 1991. Specialty: Trauma & Orthop. Surg.

RADCLYFFE, Vivian Gerald 77/9 Falmouth Road, Southwark, London SE1 4JW Tel: 020 7407 4101; 116 Wimbledon Hill Road, Wimbledon, London SW19 7QU Tel: 020 8946 6670 — MB BS Lond. 1948 (Middlx.) MRCGP 1965. Hon. Maj. RAMC.

RADEMAKER, Johan Willem Ringletts Farm, Whatlington Road, Battle TN33 0NA Tel: 01424 774349 — MB BCh BAO NUI 1983; LRCPI & LM, LRCSI & LM 1983; MRCP (UK) 1987. Cons. Phys. Gastroenterol. Conquest Hosp. The Ridge, St Leonards on Sea, E. Sussex. Specialty: Gen. Med. Socs: Nutrit. Soc.; Brit. Soc. Gastroenterol. Prev: Sen. Regist. (Med. Gastroenterol.) Roy. United Hosp. Bath; Regist. (Gen. Med & Gastroenterol.) Qu. Alexandria Hosp. Portsmouth & Soton Gen. Hosp.; Research Fell. McMaster Univ. Hamilton, Canada.

RADERSCHADT, Emma Louise Les Lohiers, La Grande Lande, St Saviours, Guernsey GY7 9YZ — MB BS Lond. 1996 (King's College School of Medicine & Dentistry London) BSc (Hons.) Lond. 1993. Specialty: Gen. Med. Socs: BMA. Prev: Pre-regist. Ho. Off. (Surg.) Conquest Hosp. St. Leonards-on-Sea; Pre-regist. Ho. Off. (Med.) Warwick Hosp.

RADFORD, Allan Philip (retired) Crossways Cottage, West Bagborough, Taunton TA4 3EG Tel: 01823 432526 — MB ChB Bristol 1944; DCH Eng. 1948. Prev: Capt. RAMC.

RADFORD, Anne Mary 1 Tanyfron Street, Llanllechid, Bangor LL57 3HL Email: anneradford@doctors.org.uk; 1 Tanyford Street, Llanllechid, Bangor LL57 3HL — MB BS Lond. 1984; BSc Lond. 1981; DRCOG 1989.

RADFORD, Bryan James (retired) Health Centre, Broadfield, Crawley Tel: 01293 531951; Foresters, Colgate, Horsham RH12 4SY — MB BS Lond. 1961 (St. Geo.) BSc Lond. 1958; MRCS Eng. LRCP Lond. 1961; DObst RCOG 1964. Prev: Ho. Phys. & Cas. Off. (Surgic.) St. Geo. Hosp. Lond.

RADFORD, Dominic Herwin 123 Alresford Road, Winchester SO23 0JZ — MB ChB Birm. 1996; ChB Birm. 1996.

RADFORD, Ian Stanley The Upper Surgery, 27 Lemon Street, Truro TR1 2LS Tel: 01872 274931 Fax: 01872 260339; Kernou Veor, Greenbottom, Truro TR4 8QH — MB BS Lond. 1978 (St. Thos.) DRCOG 1981.

RADFORD, Professor John Anthony CRC Department of Medical Oncology, Christie Hospital NHS Trust, Wilmslow Road, Manchester M20 4BX Tel: 0161 446 3753 Fax: 0161 446 3299 — MB ChB Sheff. 1978; MRCP (UK) 1982; MD Sheff. 1993; FRCP 1998. Prof. of Med. Oncol., Christie Hosp. NHS Trust Manch. Specialty: Oncol. Prev: Gordon Hamilton Fairley Fell. (Med. Oncol.) Christie Hosp. Manch.; Leukaemia Research Fund Fell. (Med. Oncol.) Christie Hosp. Manch.; Imperial Cancer Research Fund Fell. (Med. Oncol.) Guy's Hosp.Lond.

RADFORD, John Michael Chantrell 459 Whirlowdale Road, Sheffield S11 9NG — MB ChB Sheff. 1980; DRCOG 1985; MRCGP 1986.

RADFORD, Martin (retired) Wootton House, The Crescent, Romsey SO51 7NG Tel: 01794 515220 — MRCS Eng. LRCP Lond. 1966 (Univ. Coll. Hosp.) MD Lond. 1977, MB BS 1966; MRACP 1971; FRCP (UK) 1982, M 1971. Prev: Cons. Paediat.

RADFORD, Michael James 20 West End Gardens, Esher KT10 8LD; 4 The Green, Horspath, Oxford OX33 1RP Tel: 01865 876432 — MB BS Lond. 1992 (Charing Cross & Westminster) FRCS (Ed); FRCS; CCST 2003. Specialist Regist., Orthop. Rotat., Oxf.; Cons. Weston-Super-Mare Gen. Hosp. Specialty: Orthop. Socs: BOA; BOTA.

RADFORD, Nicola Margaret 4 Woodcote Green, Wallington SM6 9NN — MB ChB Bristol 1998.

RADFORD, Patrick Department of Anaesthesia, St. Helier Hospital, Wrythe Lane, Carshalton SM5 1AA Tel: 020 8296 2444 Fax: 020 8296 2951 — MB BS Lond. 1969 (Univ. Coll. Hosp.) DA Eng. 1971; FRCA 1975. Cons. Anaesth. Epsom and St Helier Univ. Hosps. NHS Trust; Sen. Lect. (Anaesth.) St. Geo. Hosp. Med. Sch.; Instruc. for ATLS, ALS and PALS. Specialty: Anaesth. Socs: Assn. Paediat. Anaesth.; Obst. Anaesth. Assn..; Resusc. Counc. Prev: Sen. Regist. (Anaesth.) St. Geo. Hosp. Lond. & Hosp. Sick Childr. Gt. Ormond St. Lond.

RADFORD, Mr Philip John Department of Trauma & Orthopaedics, University Hospital, Queen's Medical Centre, Nottingham NG7 2UH Tel: 0115 924 9924 Fax: 0115 919 4468 Email: pjradford@doctors.org.uk — BM BCh Oxf. 1983 (Oxford) MA Camb. 1984, BA 1980; FRCS Eng. 1988; FRCS (Orth.) 1993. Cons. Orthop. Surg. Univ. Hosp. Qu. Med. Centre Nottm. Cons. Trauma & Orthopaedic Surg., Uni Hosp., Qu.s Med. Centre, Notts. Specialty: Orthop.; Trauma & Orthop. Surg. Socs: Brit. Trauma Soc., Mem.; Skeletal Dyspasia Soc., Mem.; Brit. Med. Assn. Prev: Sen. Regist. & Regist. (Orthop.) Harlow Wood Hosp. & Nottm. Univ. Hosp.; Regist. (Surg.) Addenbrooke's Hosp. Camb.

RADFORD, Rafe The Coach House, Wren Park, Hitchin Road, Shefford SG17 5JD — BM Soton. 1984.

RADFORD, Raymond 509 Box Works, Worsley Street, Manchester M15 4LD — MB ChB Manch. 1990; MRCP; FRCOphth.

RADFORD, Raymond, CBE (retired) 3 Lakeside, Lee-on-the-Solent PO13 9AP Tel: 023 9255 1060 — MB BS Lond. 1955 (Univ. Coll. Hosp.) BSc (Physiol.) Lond. 1952; DA Eng. 1966; FFA RCS Eng. 1968. Prev: Med. Off. i/c & Cons. Anaesth. RN Hosp. Haslar.
RADFORD, Miss Rita Christine A & E Department, Princess Royal University Hospital, Farnborough Common, Orpington BR6 8ND Tel: 01869 863000 Email: rita.radford@bromleyhospitals.nhs.uk — MB BS Lond. 1967 (Guy's) MRCS Eng. LRCP Lond. 1967; FRCS Eng. 1972. Cons. in A & E Bromley Hosp. NHS Trust. Specialty: Accid. & Emerg. Prev: Surg. Regist. Guy's Hosp. Lond.; Res. Surg. Off. Bolingbroke Hosp. Lond.; SHO (A & E) FarnBoro. Hosp., Kent.
RADFORD, Rosemary Jane Emily (retired) 4 Westfield, Loughton IG10 4EB Tel: 020 8502 1156 — MB ChB Manch. 1972. Prev: Med. Off. Marks & Spencers Ltd., Lond.
RADFORD, Sean Richard 14 Parry Close, Southdown, Bath BA2 1JR Tel: 01225 471374 Email: sean@bladesys.demon.co.uk — MB BS Lond. 1995. Specialty: Urol. Prev: Surgic. SHO, Greenwich Dist. Hosp.
RADHA KRISHNA, Lalit Kumar Flat 201, Minster Court, Liverpool L7 3QH — MB ChB Liverp. 1995.
RADHAKRISHNA, Ganesh 69 Brampton Drive, Liverpool L8 7SU — MB ChB Liverp. 1998; MB ChB Liverp 1998.
RADHAKRISHNAN, Gopi Rampton Hospital, Retford DN22 0PD — MB BS Poona 1979; MRCPsych 1988. Lect. Dept. Psychol. Med. (Ment. Handicap) Univ. Wales Coll. of Med. Ely Hosp. Cardiff. Specialty: Ment. Health. Prev: Regist. (Psych.) Hensol Hosp. Pontyclun; Regist. (Psych.) St. Edwd.s Hosp. Leek.
RADHAKRISHNAN, Mr Subbiah 27 Streatfield Road, Kenton, Harrow HA3 9BP Tel: 020 8907 0038 — MB BS Madras 1984; BSc Madras 1977, MB BS 1984; FRCSI 1990.
RADHAKRISHNAN, Suganthamala St Georges Avenue, 21 St Georges Avenue, Southall UB1 1PZ Tel: 020 8813 8122 — LRCP LRCS Ed. 1978; LRCP LRCS Ed. LRCPS Glas. 1978.
RADHAKRISHNAN, Thambiah The Hamilton Practice, Keats House, Bush Fair, Harlow CM18 6LY Tel: 01279 692700 Fax: 01279 692719; 4 Arrow Head House, Hertfordshire & Essex Hospital, Haymeade Lane, Bishop's Stortford CM23 6NS — MB BS Sri Lanka 1981; MRCS Eng. LRCP Lond. 1988; DLO RCS Eng. 1990; T(GP) 1992; MRCGP 1992. Prev: Trainee GP Bolton; SHO (Plastic Surg., ENT & O & G) Manch.
RADIA, Deepti Himantlal Ranchhoddas 130 Harrowdene Road, Wembley HA0 2JF — MB BS Lond. 1992.
RADIA, Krishnakant Beaconsfield Road Surgery, 21 Beaconsfield Road, Hastings TN34 3TW Tel: 01424 422389 Fax: 01424 431500; Kebuca, Winchelsea Road, Guestling, Hastings TN35 4LW — MRCS Eng. LRCP Lond. 1977; DRCOG 1979; MRCGP 1981; MBA (Strategic Health Management)(Univ. of Kent) 2000.
RADIX, Joan Cecelia Agatha 41 Grosvenor Court, London E10 6RH — MB BCh BAO NUI 1968.
RADJA, Neelam Consultant Genitourinary Medicine, North Hampshire Hospitals NHS Trust, The North Hampshire Hospital, Aldermaston Road, Basingstoke RG24 9NA Email: neelam.radja@nhht.nhs.uk — MB BS Madras 1991. Cons. Genitourin. Med., HIV, N. Hants. Hosp. Trust, Basingstoke. Socs: The Brit. HIV Assn.; BASSH. Prev: Specialist Regist., Genitourin. Med., St Geo., Hosp., Lond.
RADLEY, David James Malvern Health Centre, Victoria Park Road, Malvern Link, Malvern WR14 2JY Tel: 01684 612703 Fax: 01684 612779 — MB BS Lond. 1976; MRCGP 1980; DRCOG 1980. Prev: GP Trainee Bath VTS; Ho. Surg. St. Bart. Hosp. Lond.; Ho. Phys. St. Richard's Hosp. Chichester.
RADLEY, Hazel Mary 67 Stumperlowe Crescent Road, Sheffield S10 3PR — MRCS Eng. LRCP Lond. 1959; MB Camb. 1960, BChir 1959.
RADLEY, Jacqueline Rita St. John's House, 28 Bromyard Road, Worcester WR2 5BU; 5 Lansdowne Court, Worcester WR3 8JE Tel: 01905 53989 — BSc Lond. 1986, MB BS 1988; DCH RCP Lond. 1992. Specialty: Haematology. Socs: BMA. Prev: Trainee GP Worcester; SHO (Paediat. & O & G) Worcester & Dist. HA.
RADLEY, Jane Monkton Hospital, Monkton Lane, Jarrow NE32 5NN Tel: 0191 451 6293 Email: jane.radley@nap.nhs.uk — MB ChB Leic. 1985; MRCGP 1990; MRCPsych 1994. Cons. in Learning Disabil. Psychiat. Specialty: Ment. Health. Special Interest: Autism; Learning Disabil. Psychiat. Prev: Sen. Regist. (Psychiat. of Learning Disabil.) N.gate Hosp. Morpeth.; Regist. (Psychiat.) Earl's Hse. Hosp. Durh.; Trainee GP Northumbria VTS.
RADLEY, Mr Stephen Christopher 21 Brighton Terrace Road, Crookes, Sheffield S10 1NT Tel: 0114 266 0445 — MB BS Lond. 1987; FRCS Ed. 1991; MRCOG 1993. Sen. Regist. (O & G) Jessop Hosp. Wom. Sheff. Specialty: Obst. & Gyn. Prev: Lect. (Urol.) North. Gen. Hosp. Sheff.; Regist. (O & G) Rotherham & North. Gen. Hosps. Sheff.; SHO (O & G) Jessop & North. Gen. Hosps. Sheff.
RADLEY, William Henry (retired) 96 Barnfield Wood Road, Park Langley, Beckenham BR3 6SX Tel: 020 8658 9398 — MB BCh BAO (1st Pl. & 1st Cl. Hnrs.Gold Medal) NUI 1949 (Cork) Prev: Med. Asst. Profess. Unit NUI.
RADLEY SMITH, Rosemary Claire Hill End Road, Harefield, Uxbridge UB9 6JH; Old Vicarage, Langrish, Petersfield GU32 1QY — MB BS Lond. 1963 (Roy. Free) MRCS Eng. LRCP Lond. 1963; FRCP Lond. 1980, M 1968; FRACP 1976; FRCPCH 1997. Cons. (Paediat. Cardiol.) Roy. Brompton & Harefield Hosp. Gt. Ormond St. Hosp.; Hon. Cons. Roy. Free Hosp. Specialty: Cardiol. Socs: Brit. Cardiac Soc. & Assn. Europ. Paediat. Cardiols.; Roy. Soc. Med. Prev: Ho. Phys. Roy. Free & Brompton Hosps. Lond.; Med. Regist. Roy. Melb. Hosp. Australia.
RADOMSKI, Jerzy Waclaw Child & Family Psychiatric Service, Ashvilla, Rauceby Hospital, Sleaford NG34 8PP — Lekarz Warsaw 1970.
RADSTONE, David John Weston Park Hospital, Whitham Road, Sheffield S10 2SJ Tel: 0114 226 5000 Fax: 0114 226 5512; 34 Riverdale Road, Sheffield S10 3FB Tel: 0114 266 1260 Fax: 0114 266 1260 — MB BS Lond. 1976 (Lond. Hosp.) BA (Hons.) Keele 1968; DMRT Eng. 1981; FRCR 1984. Cons. Radiother. & Oncol. Sheff. HA; Hon. Clin. Lect. Univ. Sheff.; Solicitor Supreme Ct. of Judicature Eng. 1971; Examr. Roy. Coll. of Radiols. Specialty: Oncol. Socs: Fell. Roy. Soc. Med.; Assn. Palliat. Care & Hospice Doctors. Prev: Sen. Regist. (Radiother. Oncol.) Oxf. RHA; Regist. (Radiother. & Oncol.) & Ho. Surg. Lond. Hosp.
RADULA SCOTT, Teodor (retired) 5 Knighton Road, Leicester LE2 3HL Tel: 0116 270 6891 — MB ChB Polish Sch. of Med. 1943 (Strasbourg & Polish Sch. of Med.) Prev: Ho. Surg. Whipps Cross Hosp.
RADVAN, Johannes Royal Bournemouth Hospital, Castle Lane East, Bournemouth BH7 7DW — BM BS Nottm. 1985; FRCP; MRCP Lond. 1988. Cons. Cardiol., Roy. Bournemouth Hosp. Specialty: Cardiol.
RADWAN, Raouf Radwan Mohamed Ibrahim 11 Cooden Drive, Bexhill-on-Sea TN39 3DB Tel: 01424 222932 — MB ChB Cairo 1962; DLO RCS Eng. 1974. Assoc. Specialist (ENT) Hastings HA.
RADWAY, Cecil John (retired) 10 Cottenham Place, Wimbledon, London SW20 0NF Tel: 020 8946 7846 — BM BCh Oxf. 1945 (Oxf. & Westm.) MA Oxf. 1945; DPH Lond. 1954; MFCM 1974. Prev: Area Specialist in Community Med. (Child Health) Surrey HA.
RADY, Mr Aly Mohamed (retired) Flat 8, Winn Court, Winn Road, Highfield, Southampton SO17 1UZ Tel: 023 8055 9631/ 02380 559631 — MRCS Eng. LRCP Lond. 1976; FRCS Glas. 1964; FRCSI 1965; FRCS Eng. 1966. Hon. Cons. (Gen. Surg.) Roy. S. Hants. Hosp. Soton. Prev: Chairm. Dept. Surg., Kuwait.
RADY, Neveen A Convent Garden Medical Centre, 47 Shorts Gardens, London WC2H 9AA Tel: 020 7379 7209 Fax: 020 7379 7224 — BM Soton. 1991 (Univ. Soton.) BSc (Hons.) Lond. 1987; DFFP 1993; T(GP) 1996. Specialty: Gen. Pract. Socs: Assoc. RCGP; BMA; MPS.
RAE, Alan Philip Department of Medical Cardiology, Royal Infirmary, Glasgow G31 2ER Tel: 0141 211 4000 Fax: 0141 211 1124 Email: apr3f@clinmed.gla.ac.uk; 11 Glasgow Road, Uddingston, Glasgow G71 7AU — MB ChB Glas. 1975; MRCP (UK) 1978; BSc (Hons.) Glas. 1971, MD 1987; FRCP Glas. 1988. Cons. Cardiol. Roy. Infirm. Glas. Specialty: Cardiol.
RAE, Alistair Sutherland Livingston (retired) 1 Collingwood Place, Barnhill, Dundee DD5 2UG — (Univ. Ed.) MD Ed. 1951, MB ChB 1935; DPH Ed. & Glas. 1938; DPM Eng. 1948.
RAE, Allan James Health Clinic, Main Street, Lennoxtown, Glasgow G66 7DD Tel: 01360 310357 Fax: 01360 311740; Faerie Neuk, Dunmore St., Balfrow, Glasgow G63 0PZ Tel: 01360 449277 — MB ChB Glas. 1962; LM Rotunda 1972. Prev: Ship's Surg. Blue Star Line; Med. Dir. Dubai Petroleum Co., Dubai; Head Med. Servs. SSC N.E. Nigeria, W. Afr.

RAE, Catherine Anne Kenilworth Medical Centre, 1 Kenilworth Court, Greenfields, Glasgow G67 1BP Tel: 01236 727816 Fax: 01236 726306 — MB ChB Aberd. 1987; MRCGP 1991.

RAE, Colin Kennedy The Surgery, 77 John Street, Stromness KW16 3AD — MB ChB Aberd. 1971; DA Eng. 1979. Specialty: Anaesth.

RAE, Colin Peter 11 Abbey Drive, Jordanhill, Glasgow G14 9JZ — MB ChB Glas. 1990; FRCA Lond. 1994. Cons. (Anaesth.) Glas. Roy. Infirm. Specialty: Anaesth. Prev: Specialist Regist. (Anaesth.) West. Infirm. Glas.

RAE, Mr David McGregor Ipswich Hospital, Heath Road, Ipswich IP4 5PD — MB BS Lond. 1986 (Westm.) FRCS Ed. 1990; FRCS Eng. 1991; MS Lond. 1996. Cons. Surg. (Gastrointestinal & Laparascopic Surg.) Ipswich Hosp. Trust. Specialty: Gen. Surg.

RAE, Diana Elizabeth Tonglewood, Pump Hollow Lane, Mansfield NG18 3DU; Tonglewood, Pump Hollow Lane, Mansfield NG18 3DU — (Charing Cross Hospital London) MBBS Lond. 1986; DRCOG Lond. 1990; FP Cert. Lond. 1990. GP Non-Princip. Locum; Clin. Asst. (Oncol.) Kingsmill Hosp. Mansfield. Specialty: Gen. Pract. Prev: Clin. Asst. (Diabetes) Doncaster Roy. Infirm.

RAE, George Beaumont Park Surgery, 35 Hepscott Drive, Beaumont Park, Whitley Bay NE25 9XJ Tel: 0191 251 4548 — MB ChB Ed. 1971; BSc 1968. Gen. Med. Servs. Comm. (N.ern Region) N. Tyneside; Sec. Local Med. Comm.

RAE, George Buik Lochee Health Centre, 1 Marshall St., Lochee, Dundee DD2 3BR Tel: 01382 611283 — MB ChB St. And. 1957.

RAE, Hazel Heather 70 Findhorn Place (2FL), The Grange, Edinburgh EH9 2NW — MB ChB Ed. 1994.

RAE, Helen Elizabeth 66 Parkside Drive, Watford WD17 3AX Tel: 01923 241601 — MB BS Lond. 1989 (St. Georges Hosp. Med. Sch.) MRCGP 1994.

RAE, Isobel Watson (retired) 55 Hamilton Drive, Elgin IV30 4NL Tel: 01343 542210 — (Aberd.) M.B., Ch.B. Aberd. 1944. Prev: Asst. Med. Off. Qu. Mary's Hosp. Childr. Carshalton, Gr. (Fev.).

RAE, Jacqueline Louise 10 Wirral Gardens, Wirral CH63 3BQ — MB ChB Sheff. 1995.

RAE, James Wright (retired) Screel House, Auchencairn, Castle Douglas DG7 1QL Tel: 01556 640220 — MD Ed. 1947 (Univ. Ed.) MD (Commend.) Ed. 1947, MB ChB 1936; FRCP Ed. 1952, M 1947. Prev: Hon. Cons. (Neurol.) Bradford HA.

RAE, Mr Paul Jonathan Braeside, Markland Hill, Bolton BL1 5AL — MB ChB Manch. 1980; FRCS Eng. 1984. Sen. Regist. (Orthop.) NW. Region. HA. Specialty: Orthop.

RAE, Peter Gordon (retired) 3 The Rowans, Ormskirk L39 6TD Tel: 01695 423518 — MB ChB Liverp. 1958; FRCOG 1981, M 1968, DObst. 1960. Prev: Dir. Med. Manpower Plann. Mersey RHA.

RAE, Mr Peter Scott 26 Craigstewart Crescent, Doonbank, Ayr KA7 4DB — MB ChB Glas. 1972; FRCS Glas. 1977. Cons. Orthop. Surg. Ayrsh. & Arran Health Bd. Specialty: Orthop. Socs: Fell. Brit. Orthop. Assn.; Assoc. Brit. Soc. Surg. of Hand.

RAE, Peter William Hamley Department of Clinical Biochemistry, Royal Infirmary, Little France Crescent, Edinburgh EH16 4SA Tel: 0131 2426853 Email: peter.rae@luht.scot.nhs.uk; Department of Clinical Biochemistry, Western General Hospital, Crewe Road, Edinburgh EH4 2XU Tel: 0131 537 1890 Fax: 0131 537 1023 — MB ChB Ed. 1984; BA Oxf. 1976; PhD Ed. 1979; MRCP (UK) 1987; MRCPath 1994; FRCP Ed. 1999. Cons. Clin. Biochem. Roayl Infirmary, Edin.; Hon. Sen. Lect. Univ. Edin.; Cons. Clin. Biochem. West. Gen. Hosp. Edin. Specialty: Biochem.

RAE, Ruth 11 Abbey Drive, Jordanhill, Glasgow G14 9JZ — MB ChB Glas. 1990; FRCA Lond. 1994. SpR (Anaesth.) Glas. Roy. Infirm. Specialty: Anaesth. Socs: Assn. Anaesth.; BMA; Scot. Soc. Anaesths. Prev: Career Regist. (Anaesth.) Glas. Roy. Infirm.; SHO (Anaesth.) West. Infirm. & Stobhill Hosp. Glas.; SHO (Geriat.) Lightburn Hosp. Glas.

RAE, Sarah Alison Bedford Hospital, Bedford MK42 9DL Tel: 01234 792259 Fax: 01234 792260; 12 Chaucer Road, Bedford MK40 2AJ Tel: 01234 217977 — MB BS Lond. 1975; MRCS Eng. LRCP Lond. 1975; MRCP (UK) 1978. Cons. & Sen. Lect. Rehabil. Med. & Rheum. Roy. Devon & Exeter Hosp. Specialty: Rehabil. Med.; Rheumatol. Prev: Sen. Regist. Rotat. (Gen. Med. & Geriat.) Roy. Devon & Exeter Hosp.; Regist. & Sen. Regist. (Rheum.) Kings Coll. Hosp. Lond.

RAE, Stewart (retired) Craiginch, Tidmarsh Village, Reading RG8 8ER Tel: 0118 984 2998 — MB ChB Ed. 1944; FRCP Ed. 1968, M 1949; FFCM 1976, M 1974. Prev: Med. Adviser Nat. Radiol. Protec. Bd. Harwell.

RAE, Susan Jane Postern Gate Surgery, Cinque Port St., Rye TN31 7AP Tel: 01797 223333 Fax: 01797 227464; The Coach House, Flackley Ash, Peasmarsh, Rye TN31 6YH — MB ChB Ed. 1982. Specialty: Cardiol.

RAE, Susan Marjorie 13 Newmills Crescent, Balerno EH14 5SX — MB ChB Ed. 1989.

RAEBURN, Andrew Lindsay 49 Hellath Wen, Nantwich CW5 7BB — MB ChB Glas. 1977; DRCOG 1980; MRCGP 1981.

RAEBURN, Dorothy June (retired) Gables, Courtmead Road, Cuckfield, Haywards Heath RH17 5LP Tel: 01444 417829 — MB BS Lond. 1953 (Guy's) MRCS Eng. LRCP Lond. 1953; FRCOG 1974, M 1958, DObst 1955; FRCS Eng. 1961. Prev: Cons. (O & G) RN Hosp. Gibraltar.

RAEBURN, Henry Brian (retired) 12 Willow Court, Pool in Wharefdale, Otley LS21 1RX Tel: 0113 284 2948 — (St. Geo.) MB BS Lond. 1958; MRCS Eng. LRCP Lond. 1958; MRCGP 1968. Prev: Med. Off. DHSS Leeds.

RAEBURN, Janine Ruth Flat 1, Palm Court, 11-13 Fellows Road, Chalk Farm, London NW3 3LT — MB BS Lond. 1994.

RAEBURN, Joanna Nest 31A Alleyn Park, Dulwich, London SE21 8AT — BM BCh Oxf. 1973 (Middlx.) MA Oxf. 1973; MFFP 1993; FRCP (Lond.) 1997. Assoc. Specialist (Diabetes) King's Coll. Hosp. Lond.; Sessional Clin. Med. Off. (Family Plann. & Instruc.) Lond. Specialty: Diabetes.

RAEBURN, Professor John Alexander, TD Centre for Medical Genetics, City Hospital, Hucknall Road, Nottingham NG5 1PB Tel: 0115 962 7712 Fax: 0115 962 7711; Tighlagan, 3 Grove Farm, Lambley Road, Lowdham, Nottingham NG14 7AY Tel: 0115 966 4793 — MB ChB Ed. 1964; PhD Ed. 1976, MB ChB 1964; FRCP Ed. 1976, M 1968. Prof. Clin. Genetics Univ. Nottm. Specialty: Genetics. Socs: Fell. Roy. Med. Soc. Edin.; Clin. Genetics Soc. Prev: Sen. Lect. (Human Genetics) Univ. Edin.; Lect. (Therap.) Univ. Edin.; Research Fell. Univ. Leiden.

RAEBURN, Rhona Margaret Auchinairn Road Surgery, 127/129 Auchinairn Road, Bishopbriggs, Glasgow G64 1NF Tel: 0141 772 1808 Fax: 0141 762 1274; 23 Kennedy Drive, Airdrie ML6 9AN — MB ChB Glas. 1977.

RAESIDE, David Alexander McMclands Hospital, McMcscourt Avenue, London SE26 6PL Tel: 01236 748748 Fax: 01236 713152 Email: david.raeside@laht.scot.nhs.uk — MB ChB Glas. 1986 (Glasgow) MRCP (UK) 1992; FRCP (UK) 1992. Cons. Physician Respiratory and GIM. Specialty: Respirat. Med. Prev: SHO (Respirat. Med.) Glas. Roy. Infirm.

RAESIDE, John Apsley Street Surgery, 14 Apsley Street, Glasgow G11 7SY Tel: 0141 339 2960; Tregileen, 73 South Mains Road, Milngavie, Glasgow G62 6DE Tel: 0141 956 6722 — MB ChB Glas. 1981; BSc (Hons. Pharamacol.) Glas. 1978; DRCOG 1989; MRCGP 1989; DFM Glas. 1992.

RAFF, Peter Franz 13B Scotland Street, Stornoway HS1 2JN — State Exam Med Tubingen 1977; MD Tubingen 1980.

RAFFAELLI, Professor Philip Iain, Surg. Cdr. RN SO1 (Med) (NATO), D.Med. Prog. & Plans, Room 8121, Main Building, MoD, Whitehall, London SW1A 2HB Tel: 020 7807 0365 Fax: 020 7807 8834 Email: dmedops@gtnet.gov.uk; 9 Thorndyke Court, Hatch End, Pinner HA5 4JB Tel: 020 8421 6370 Email: piraffaelli@raftaeth.softnet.co.uk — MB ChB Ed. 1979 (Edinburgh) BSc Ed. 1976; MRCGP 1984; MFOM RCP Lond. 1989, AFOM 1987; MSc (Occupat. Med.) Lond. 1987; FFOM 1997. Naval Med. Off. Med. Operats. & Plans (NATO) MoD; Prof. Naval Occupat. Med. Specialty: Occupat. Health. Socs: Fell. Roy. Soc. Med.; Soc. Occupat. Med. Prev: Submarine Flotilla Med. Off. & Cons. Occupat. Med. Northwood; Naval Med. Off. Health (Flag Off. Portsmouth) & Princip. Med. Off. HM Naval Base; Princip. Med. Off. HMS Neptune.

RAFFEEQ, Parakkal Mohommed PICU, City General Hospital, Stoke-on-Trent ST4 6OG — MB BS Madras 1988; MRCP (UK) 1993. Cons. Paediat., Intens. Care. Specialty: Paediat.

RAFFERTY, Ann Margaret North West Surrey Mental Health Partnership NHS Trust, Abraham Cowley Unit, Holloway Hill, Lyne, Chertsey KT16 0AE Tel: 01932 872010 — MB BS Lond. 1982 (Char. Cross) MRCPsych 1988. Assoc. Specialist (Gen. Psychiat.)

Abraham Cowley Unit Chertsey. Specialty: Gen. Psychiat. Prev: Staff Grade (Gen. Psychiat.) Abraham Cowley Unit Chertsey.

RAFFERTY, Ciaran Vincent 44 Watermill Avenue, Kirkintilloch, Glasgow G66 5QS — MB BCh BAO Belf. 1985; FFA RCSI 1989. Sen. Regist. (Anaesth.) WHSS Bd. Specialty: Anaesth. Prev: Research Fell. (Anaesth.) Univ. Glas.

RAFFERTY, Claire Marie 7 Spelga Av, Newcastle BT33 0DR — MB BCh BAO Belf. 1997.

RAFFERTY, Colm Gerard 67 Sandhurst Drive, Belfast BT9 5AZ — MB BCh BAO Belf. 1987. SHO (Med.) Moyle Hosp. Larne.

RAFFERTY, Mary Sheila 169 Ballycoan Road, Belfast BT8 8LN — MB BCh BAO Belf. 1985 (The Queen's University of Belfast) DRCOG 1988; MRCGP 1990.

RAFFERTY, Patrick Gerard 6 Rowlls Road, Kingston upon Thames KT1 3ET — MB BCh BAO NUI 1989.

RAFFERTY, Paul Dumfries & Galloway Royal Infirmary, Bankend Road, Dumfries DG1 4AP Tel: 01387 46246 — MB ChB Sheff. 1977; MRCP (UK) 1980; DM Soton. 1990; FRCP Ed. 1995. Cons. Phys. Dumfries & Galloway Roy. Infirm. Specialty: Respirat. Med. Prev: Sen. Regist. (Respirat. Med.) West. Infirm. Glas.

RAFFERTY, Rosemary 48 Riverdale Road, Sheffield S10 3FB — MB ChB Leic. 1985; DRCOG 1988; MRCGP 1990.

RAFFETY, Richard Charles The Surgery, Madam's Paddock, Chew Magna, Bristol BS40 8PP Tel: 01275 332420 Fax: 01275 333860 — MB BS Lond. 1971; MRCGP 1977.

RAFFLE, Angela Elizabeth — MB ChB Birm. 1980; BSc (Hons.) Birm. 1977; MFPHM 1989; FFPHM RCP (UK) 1996. Cons. Pub. Health Med. Avon HA. Specialty: Pub. Health Med.

RAFFLE, Edmund James (retired) 10 Skene Street, Broughty Ferry, Dundee DD5 3ET Tel: 01382 477080 — MB ChB Liverp. 1953; DCH Eng. 1955; FRCP Ed. 1971, M 1958. Cons. Dermatol. Tayside Health Bd. Prev: Sen. Regist. Dept. Dermat. Dundee Roy. Infirm.

RAFFLE, Jean Alison 153 Kew Road, Richmond TW9 2PN Tel: 020 8940 7727 — (Liverp.) MB ChB Liverp. 1950. Indep. Analytic Psycother. Richmond; Assoc. Mem. Lincoln Clinic & Centre for Psychother. Specialty: Pub. Health Med.; Psychother.

RAFFLES, Andrew Keith Mark Queen Elizabeth II Hospital, Child Health Directorate, Howlands, Welwyn Garden City AL7 4HQ Tel: 01707 365041 Fax: 01707 373357; Skimpans Farmhouse, Bulls Lane, North Mymms, Hatfield AL9 7PE Tel: 01707 271517 Email: rafflesdr@btinternet.com — MB BS Lond. 1978 (St. Mary's) DCH Eng. 1981; MRCP (UK) 1982; FRCP Lond. 1995. Cons. Gen. Paediat. NW Thames RHA. Specialty: Paediat. Socs: Roy. Coll. Paediat. & Child Health. Prev: Lect. & Sen. Regist. Jt. Acad. Dept. Child Health Qu. Eliz. Hosp. for Childr. Lond.; Sen. Regist. Roy. Alexandra Hosp. for Childr. Camperdown, Sydney, Austral.; Regist. (Paediat.) Hammersmith Hosp. Lond.

RAFI, Imran Longcroft Clinic, 5 Woodmansterne Lane, Banstead SM7 3HH Tel: 01293 883158 Fax: 01293 883158; 94 Worcester Road, Sutton SM2 6QJ Tel: 020 8661 7913 — MB BS Newc. 1988 (Newcastle upon Tyne) BSc (Hons.) Computer Sc. Newc. 1983, MB BS 1988; MRCPI 1997. Clin. Research Fell. Cancer Research Unit. Med. Sch. Univ. Newc. u Tyne. Specialty: Gen. Pract. Socs: Assoc. Mem. Roy. Coll. Gen. Pract. Prev: SHO (Oncol.) Roy. Marsden Hosp. Sutton.; SHO Med. Rotat. Newc. Teachg. Hosps.

RAFIEIZADEH, Mohammad Chelsea & Westminster Hospital, Drug Treatment Centre, London; 33 Barmouth Avenue, Greenford UB6 8JS Fax: 020 8846 6112 — MD Azarabadegan 1977. Staff Grade (Psychiat.) Chelsesa & Westm. Hosp. Lond. Specialty: Gen. Psychiat.

RAFIQ, Mohammed 53 St Oswalds Road, Birmingham B10 9RB — MB BS Newc. 1989; BSc (Hons.) Newc. 1984, MB BS 1989. Lect. (Anat.) Univ. Birm. Prev: Ho. Surg. Newc. Gen. Hosp.

RAFIQ, S S The Surgery, 162 Boleyn Road, London E7 9QJ Tel: 020 8503 5656 Fax: 020 8586 9028 — MB BS Karachi 1981; MB BS Karachi 1981.

RAFIQ, Mr Shahid Mentisbury, 25 Abbey Road, West Kirby, Wirral CH48 7EN — MB BS Punjab 1977; FRCS Glas. 1984.

RAFIQI, Mohamad Aslam (retired) 20 Batsford Close, Redditch B98 7TF Tel: 01527 853870 Fax: 01527 857581 — MB BS Punjab 1950 (King Edwd. Med. Coll. Lahore) MB BS Punjab (Pakistan) 1950. Med. Off. HMP Blakenhurst, Redditch. Prev: ed OH. Hosp Blakenhurst Redditch.

RAFIQUE, Abdul 16 Briarswood Close, Poundhill, Crawley RH10 7TJ Tel: 01293 883014 — MB BS Punjab 1964; MB BS Punjab (Pakistan) 1964; DA Eng. 1970. Assoc. Specialist (Anaesth.) Mid Downs & E. Surrey HAs. Prev: Intern Holy Family Hosp. Rawalpindi Pakistan; Res. Anaesth. Nelson Hosp. Lond.; Regist. (Anaesth.) Redhill & Netherne Hosp. Gp.

RAFIQUE, Arshad 85 Napier Street, Burton-on-Trent DE14 3LL — MB BS Lond. 1994.

RAFIQUE, Farooq 169 Finborough Road, London SW10 9AP — MB BS Lond. 1992; BSc (Hons.) Lond. 1989; DCH RCP Lond. 1994; MRCGP 1995; MRCP 1996; MBA (Insead) 2000. Prev: SHO (Med., Obst., Psychiat. & Paediat.) St. Mary's Hosp. Lond.

RAFIQUE, Mohammad Akkib 249 Hook Rise S., Tolworth, Surbiton KT6 7LT — MB BS Lond. 1998; MB BS Lond 1998.

RAFIQUE, Mustafa South Quay Surgery, 35-36 South Quay, Great Yarmouth NR30 2RG Tel: 01493 843196 — MB BS Dacca 1963; MB BS Dacca 1963.

RAFIQUE, Syed Firoz Alfred (retired) 19 Foreshore, London SE8 3AQ — MB BS Durh. 1959 (Newc.) Asst. to GP, Lond. Prev: Clin. Asst. (Dermat.) Greenwich Dist. Hosp. Lond.

RAFLA, Mary Bridge Health Centre, Patrixbourne Road, Bridge, Canterbury CT4 5BL — MB BCh BAO Dub. 1978; DCH Eng. 1980; DRCOG 1981; MRCGP 1982. Prev: GP Trainee Stirling; SHO (Med.), (Psychiat.) & (O & G) Crawley Hosp.

RAFLA, Nagy Marcos — MB ChB Alexandria 1974 (Univ. Alexandria) DObst RCPI 1981; MRCOG 1986; MObstG Liverp. 1988; T(OG) 1991. Cons. (O & G); Dist. Tutor Roy. Coll. of Obst.s & Gyn. Specialty: Obst. & Gyn. Socs: Beckett Med. Soc.; BMA; Brit. Ultrasound Soc. Prev: Dir. IVF unit at BMI Chaucer Hosp.; Sen. Regist. Univ. Coll. Hosp. Galway; Research Assoc. (O & G) Roy. Liverp. Hosp.

RAFTER, Martin James Shannon, Ty-Llwyd Road, Lisvane, Cardiff CF14 0SG — MB BCh BAO NUI 1945.

RAFTERY, Mr Andrew Thomas Sheffield Kidney Institute, Northern General Hospital, Herries Road, Sheffield S5 7AU Fax: 0114 256 2514; Carnbrea, 280 Ecclesall Road S., Sheffield S11 9PS — MB ChB (Hons) Leeds 1969; BSc (Hons.) Leeds 1966, MD 1973; FRCS Eng. 1976; FRCS Edin. 2000. Cons. Gen. Surg. & Transpl. N. Gen. Hosp. Sheff.; Mem. Ct. Examrs. RCS Eng.; Mem. Of Counc. RCS Eng.; Sub Dean for Admissions, Sheff. Med. Sch. Specialty: Gen. Surg.; Transpl. Surg. Socs: (Pres.) Counc. Brit. Assn. Clin. Anat.; Brit. Med. Assn.; Assn. of Surgeons. Prev: Cons. Gen. Surg. & Transpl. Addenbrooke's Hosp. Camb.; Lect. (Surg.) Manch. Roy. Infirm.; Regist. Rotat. (Surg.) Pontefract. Gen. Infirm.

RAFTERY, Martin John Renal Unit, The London Hospital, Whitechapel, London E1 1BB Tel: 020 7377 7368 Fax: 020 7377 7003 — MB BCh BAO NUI 1975; MRCPI 1977; MD 1987; FRCP (UK) 1995. Cons./Sen. Lect. Nephrol. Lond. Hosp. Specialty: Nephrol. Prev: Sen. Regist. Renal Unit Guy's Hosp. Lond.; Regist. (Nephrol./Transpl.) Roy. Free Hosp. Lond.; SHO (Chest Med.) Brompton Hosp. Lond.

RAFTERY, Patricia 7 Peel Moat Road, Heaton Moor, Stockport SK4 4PL — LRCPI & LM, LRSCI & LM 1964; LRCPI & LM, LRCSI & LM 1964.

RAFTERY, Stephen Mark Department of Anaesthesia, Whiston Hospital, Prescot L35 5DR — MB BCh BAO NUI 1983; FFA RCSI 1988. Cons. (Anaesth.) Whiston Hosp., Prescot. Specialty: Anaesth. Prev: Sen. Regist. (Anesth) S.W. RHA; Clin. Research Fell. Univ. Bristol.

RAGBIR, Mr Maniram Department of Plastic & Reconstructive Surgery, Royal Devon & Exeter Hospital (Wonford), Barrack Road, Exeter EX2 5DW Tel: 01392 411611; 102 Jerningham Junction Road, Charlieville Chaduanas, Trinidad & Tobago Tel: 00 1 809 6651732 — MB BS West Indies 1989; FRCS Glas. 1995. SHO (Plastic & Reconstruc Surg.) Roy. Devon & Exeter Hosp. Specialty: Plastic Surg. Prev: Welsh Regional Centre Burns & Plastic Surg. Morriston Hosp. Swansea.

RAGBIR, Rai 28 Earlsmead, Harrow HA2 8SP — MB BS West Indies 1990.

RAGGE, Nicola Karyn Western Eye Hospital, Marylebone Road, London NW1 5YE Tel: 020 7402 4211 Fax: 020 7723 8726; 37 Langdon Park Road, Highgate, London N6 5PT — BM BCh Oxf. 1984; MA Camb. 1985; MRCP (Paediat.) (UK) 1987; FRCOphth. 1989; DO 1989. Sen. Regist. (Ophth.) West. Eye Hosp. Lond.

Specialty: Ophth. Prev: Fell. (Paediat. & Developm. Ophth. & Molecular Genetics) Childr. Hosp. Los Angeles, Univ. South. Calif.; Fell. (Paediat. & Neuro-ophth.) Univ. Calif., San Francisco; Regist. (Ophth.) Bristol Eye Hosp.

RAGGOO, Michel David Richard Latchets, Hackford Road, Hardingham, Norwich NR9 4ED — BM BS Nottm. 1997.

RAGHAVAIAH, Lingi Setty Dunoon General Hospital, Dunoon PA23 7RL — MB BS Andhra 1973.

RAGHAVAN, Manoj 127 Westway, London SW20 9LT — MB BS Lond. 1994; MRCP; MRCPath.

RAGHAVAN, Shiverdorayi The Surgery, 177 Church Hill Road, Handsworth, Birmingham B20 3PX Tel: 0121 705 9139 — BM Soton. 1984; BSc (Hons.) E. Anglia 1979; MSc Newc. 1980. Trainee GP/SHO E. Birm. Hosp. VTS. Prev: SHO (Med. & Geriat.) Birm. HA.

RAGHAVENDRA, Kulkarni 15 Linnburn Terrace, Ardrossan KA22 8NR Tel: 01294 61509 — MB BS Karnatak 1964 (Karnatak Med. Coll. Hubli) DObst RCOG 1972.

RAGHAVJEE, Indira Vaghjee 10 Kensington Street, Leicester LE4 5GL — MB BS Bombay 1973.

RAGHEB, Essam Abdel Aziz HM Prison Bullingdon, PO Box 50, Bicester OX25 1WD Tel: 01869 353339 Fax: 01869 323029 — MB BCh Cairo 1972. Dir. Health Care HM Prison Bullingdon; Dip. Addic. Behaviour. Specialty: Gen. Psychiat.; Forens. Psychiat.; Disabil. Med. Prev: Head Med. Servs. HM Prison Stafford; Med. Off. HM Prison Birm.; Assoc. Specialist (Psychiat.) Bassetlaw Dist. Gen. Hosp. Worksop.

RAGHU, Mr Cheruvalli Gopalan General Hospital, St Helier, Jersey JE2 3QS — MB BS Ranchi 1982; FRCS Ed. 1991; FRCS Glas. 1991.

RAGHUNATH, Joanne Vernita 19 Pollards Hill E., London SW16 4UX — BM BS Nottm. 1998; BM BS Nottm 1998.

RAGHUNATH, Nigel John 20 Hitherfield Road, London SW16 2LN — MB BCh Wales 1996.

RAGHUNATHAN, Mr Krishnan 31 Millwood, Lisvane, Cardiff CF14 0TL Tel: 029 2075 2971 — MB BS Kerala 1960; FRCS Eng. 1970. Orthop. Consult. Caerphilly Hosp. Specialty: Orthop. Prev: Ho. Surg. Copthorne Hosp. Shrewsbury; Trauma Regist. E. Glam. Hosp. Ch. Village; Orthop. Regist. P. of Wales Hosp. Rhydlafar.

RAGHUPATI, Rajan Flat 26, Halliard Court, Barquentine Place, Cardiff CF10 4NJ — MB BCh Wales 1994.

RAGHUPATI RAJU, Alluri Sathyanarayana 34 Railton Avenue, Prescot L35 0QB — MB BS Andhra 1962.

RAGI, Elias Fouad Elias Royal Devon & Exeter Hospital, Exeter EX2 5DW Tel: 01392 402456 Fax: 01392 402721; 11 Lamacraft Drive, Exeter EX4 8QS Tel: 01392 426629 Fax: 01392 671282 Email: er@medix-uk.com — MB ChB Baghdad 1972; DPhil Oxf. 1986. Cons. Clin. Neurophysiol. Roy. Devon & Exeter Hosp. Specialty: Clin. Neurophysiol. Socs: Assn. of Brit. Clin. Neurophysiologists; Association of British Neurologists; Amer. Assn. of Electrodiagnostic Med.

RAGLAN, Mrs Ewa Maria Great Ormond Street Hospital for Children, Great Ormond Street, London WC1N 3JH Tel: 020 7829 7844 Email: raglane@gosh.nhs.uk; 172 Cottenham Park Road, London SW20 0SX Tel: 020 8947 2648 Fax: 020 7278 8041 — Med. Dipl. Warsaw 1973 (Med. Acad. Warsaw) Med. Dip. (Distinc.) Warsaw 1973; DLO Eng. 1975; MRCS Eng. LRCP Lond. 1978; FRCS Eng. (Orl.) 1981. Sen. Lect. (Audiological Med.) Inst. Laryngol. & Otol. Univ. Coll. Lond.; Cons. (Audiological Med.) St. Geos. Hosp. Lond.; Govenor Sch. for Deaf Oak Lodge Lond. & Med. Represent. to BAOL; MSc Audiological Med. Lond. Course Tutor; Expert witness in Audiological Med. Specialty: Audiol. Med. Socs: Fell. Roy. Soc. Med.; Ethics Coll. Roy. Free Hosp.; Brit. Soc. Audiol. Prev: Cons. Audiol. Phys. & Neurootol. St. Geo. Hosp. Lond.; Sen. Regist. (Audiol. Med.) Roy. Nat. Hosp. Neurol. Dis. Lond.; Regist. (ENT) St. Thos Hosp. Lond.

RAGOOWANSI, Rajesh Hiranand Flat 33, 35 Buckingham Gate, London SW1E 6PA — MB BS Lond. 1992.

RAGU, Mr Hiremagalur Keshavadas Sethuraghavan 5 The Birches, Townsend, Soham, Ely CB7 5FH — MB BS Karnatak 1986; FRCS Ed. 1993.

RAGUNATHAN, Pakiyaluxmi 17 Dale View, Ilkley LS29 9BP — MB BS Sri Lanka 1977.

RAGUPATHY, Markandu The Surgery, 80 Torridon Road, London SE6 1RA Tel: 020 8698 5281 Fax: 020 8695 1841 — MB BS Sri Lanka 1976; DPM Eng. 1983; MRCGP 1997; DFFP 1998. GP; Clin. Asst. (Psychiat.) FarnBoro. Hosp. Orpington. Specialty: Gen. Pract.; Geriat. Psychiat. Socs: Med. Inst. of Tamils; BMA; RCGP. Prev: Regist. (Psychiat.) FarnBoro. Hosp. Orpington.

RAHA, Arun Kumar The Medical Centre, 78 Oswald Road, Scunthorpe DN15 7PG Tel: 01724 843168 — MB BS Calcutta 1961.

RAHA, H D Wath Health Centre, 35 Church Street, Wath-On-Dearne, Rotherham S63 7RF Tel: 01709 873233 — MB BS Dacca 1973; MB BS Dacca 1973.

RAHA, Sandip Kumar Princess of Wales Hospital, Coity Road, Bridgend CF31 1RQ Tel: 01656 752746 Fax: 01656 752038 — MB BS Bhagalpur 1978 (Bhagalpur Med. Coll., India) BSc (Hons.) Ranchi 1971. Assoc. Specialist Dept. of Integrated Med. Bromorgannwg NHS Trust; Locum Cons. Phys. Bromorgannwg NHS Trust, Bridgend. Specialty: Gen. Med.; Gastroenterol.; Rehabil. Med. Special Interest: Parkinson's Dis. & Movement Disorder. Socs: Med. Soc. Bridgend; Soc. for Research & Rehabil.; Brit. Geriat. Soc. Prev: Sen. Clin. Med. Off. Princess of Wales, Bridgend; Regist. (Geriat.) Cardiff Roy. Infirm.; Regist. (Med.) Princess Roy. Hosp. Haywards Heath.

RAHAMIM, Yousif Hyperion, Seymour Road, Mannamead, Plymouth PL3 5AU Tel: 01752 225198 — MB ChB Iraq 1973. Cons. Thoracic Surg. Plymouth HA. Specialty: Cardiothoracic Surg. Prev: Assoc. Specialist (Thoracic Surg.) Plymouth HA.

RAHBER, Mohammad S Mabarak Health Centre, 8-12 Cannon Hill Road, Balsall Heath, Birmingham B12 9NN Tel: 0121 440 4666 Fax: 0121 446 5986 — MB BS Patna 1974; MB BS Patna 1974.

RAHEJA, Sunil Kumar West Middlesex Hospital, Top Floor, O Block, Twickenham Road, Isleworth, Twickenham TW7 6AF Tel: 020 8321 6873 Email: sunil.raheja@hounslowpct.nhs.uk — BM Soton. 1989; MRCPsych 1994. Consultant Psychiatrist Learning Disabilities. Prev: Regist. Rotat. (Psychiat.) Solent; SHO (Psychiat.) St. Jas. Hosp Portsmouth & Roy. S. Hants. Hosp. Soton.; Higher Psychiat. Train. in Learning Disabilities.

RAHEMTULLA, Aminmohamed Nuffield Department of Clinical Medicine, University of Oxford, John Radcliffe Hospital, Oxford OX3 9DU Tel: 01865 221347 Fax: 01865 221327; 21 Oakthorpe Road, Summertown, Oxford OX2 7BD — (Univ. Coll. Hosp.) BSc Lond. 1978; MB BS Lond. 1981; MRCP (UK) 1984; PhD Toronto 1994. Wellcome Sen. Clin. Research Fell. & Hon. Cons. Phys. John Radcliffe Hosp. Specialty: Haematology. Prev: Terry Fox Research Fell. Ontario Cancer Inst. Toronto, Canada; Regist. (Haemat.) Roy. Postgrad. Med. Sch. Hammersmith Hosp. Lond.

RAHI, Jugnoo Sangeeta Centre for Paediatric Epidemiology & Department of Ophthal., GOS NHS Trust, Institute of Child Health, London WC1N 1EH Tel: 020 7905 2250 — MB BS Lond. 1986; DCH RCP Lond. 1989; DO RCS Eng. 1990; FCOphth 1992; MSc (Epidemiol.) Lond. 1994; PhD, Epidiol. Univ. Lond. 1998. Clin. Sen. Lect., Ophth. Epidemiol., GOS Inst. Child Health & Inst. Ophth. Specialty: Epidemiol.; Ophth. Socs: Fell. Roy. Soc. Med.; BMA. Prev: Clin. Lect., Ophth. Epidemiol., GOS Inst. of Child Health & Inst. of Ophth.

RAHI, Mr Muhammad Asad East Lancashire NHS Hospital, Department of Surgery, Penine House, Casterton Avenue, Burnley BB10 2PQ Tel: 01282 474640 Fax: 01282 474124 — MB BS Punjab 1985; FRCS (Gen); Hon. MSc (Vasc.); BSc (Med); FRCSI. Cons. Vasc. Surg. E. Lancs. NHS Hosps. Lancs.; Cons. Vasc. Surg. Beardford Hosp. Blackburn, Highfield Hosp.; Cons. Vasc. Surg. Blackburn Roy. Infirm., Gisburn Pk. Hosp.,Burnley Gen. Hosp. Specialty: Surgery, Vascular. Special Interest: Carotid Surg.; Endovascular Surg. Socs: Vascular Society of GB & Ireland; European Society of Vascular & Endovascular Surgery; Association of Surgeons of GB & Ireland. Prev: Vasc. Research Fell. St Mary's Hosp. Lond.; Vasc. Specialist Regist. Univ. Hosp. of Wales Cardiff.

RAHI, Swarn Lata (retired) Flat 59, Anchorage Point, Westferry Road, London E14 8NF Tel: 020 7537 7500 — MB BS Bihar 1962 (Darbhanga Med. Coll.) MS (Ophth.) Bihar 1964; DO Eng. 1971; MRCPath 1987. Med. Off. Moorfields Eye Hosp. (City Rd. Br.) Lond.; Assoc. Specialist (Ophth.) OldCh. Hosp. Romford. Prev: Regist. (Ophth.) Inst. Ophth. Aligarh Univ. India.

RAHIL, Hussein Mohammad Old Whint Road Surgery, 21A Old Whint Road, Haydock, St Helens WA11 0DN Tel: 01744 612555 Fax: 01744 454619; 42 Avery Road, Haydock, St Helens

WA11 0XA Tel: 01744 616420 Fax: 01744 454619 — MB BCh Assuit, Egypt 1971 (Assuit Med. Sch.) DTM & H Liverp. 1983; DFFP 1995. Clin. Asst. (Psychiat.) Warrington HA. Prev: Resid. Surg. Milit. Hosp., Abu Dhabi; Med. Off. UNRWA, Lebanon; Regist. (Cardiothoracic Surg.) Roy. Hallamsh. Hosp. Sheff. & Walsgrave Hosp. Coventry.

RAHILLY, David Maurice (retired) The Old School House, Broadway, Ilminster TA19 9RE — MRCS Eng. LRCP Lond. 1947 (Guy's) Prev: Flight Lt. RAF Med. Br.

RAHILLY, Maeve Anne Pathology Dept, Victoria Hospital, Hayfield road, Kirkcaldy KY2 5AH — MB BCh BAO NUI 1987; MRCPath 1993; MD NUI 1995; Dip FM 2001. Cons. Histopath. Fife Acute Hosps. Trust. Specialty: Histopath. Prev: Sen. Regist. (Histopath.) Dept Path. Univ. Edin.; Cons. Histopath. N. Glas. Univ. Hosp. Trust.

RAHIM, Abdur Merthyr Tydfil Health Centre, Merthyr Tydfil CF47 0AY Tel: 01685 350035 Fax: 01685 723345 — MB BS Dacca 1967. GP Merthyr Tydfil.

RAHIM, Asad 29 Swanage Road, Small Heath, Birmingham B10 9ER — MB ChB Leeds 1991.

RAHIM, Mr Md Abdur District General Hospital, Lovely Lane, Warrington WA5 1QG Tel: 01925 35911 — MB BS Dacca 1968; FRCS Eng. 1981; FRCS Ed. 1981. Specialty: Gen. Surg.

RAHIM, Mohamed Hanif Curacao, Grifon Road, Chafford Hundred, Grays RM16 6NP Tel: 01375 482156 — MB BCh Wales 1990 (Univ. Wales Coll. Med.) Regist. (O & G) Whipps Cross Hosp. Lond. Specialty: Obst. & Gyn. Prev: Regist. (O & G) Southend; Regist. (O & G) Portsmouth; SHO (O & G) Portsmouth.

RAHIM, Mustafa Sherali Warren Medical Centre, Uxbridge Road, Hayes UB4 0SG Tel: 020 8573 1781 Fax: 020 8561 3461; 17 St. Edmunds Drive, Stanmore HA7 2AT Tel: 020 8930 4291 — MB ChB Makerere 1971; CHS (Harrow & Hillingdon); DFFP; Minor Surgery (Hillingdon); Cert. Equiv. Registration JCPT GP; DFFP (RCOG). GP, Warren Med. Centre, Hayes. Socs: BMA; MPS.

RAHIM, Naeed Sadrudin Whispering Oaks, Broaldlands Close, Calcot, Reading RG31 7RP — MB BCh Wales 1977; FRCR 1983.

RAHIM, Owais 84 York Avenue, Whalley Range, Manchester M16 0AG — MB BS Punjab 1990; MRCP (UK) 1994. Regist. (Gen. Med.) Middlx. Hosp. Lond. Specialty: Gen. Med. Prev: Regist. (Med.) Colchester Gen. Hosp.; SHO (Med.) Jas. Paget Hosp. Gt. Yarmouth.

RAHIM, Sleem 69 Benton Road, Ilford IG1 4AS — MB BS Lond. 1994.

RAHMAAN, Gillian 212 Swakeleys Road, Uxbridge UB10 8AY — MB BS Durh. 1962; MRCOG 1967, D 1964. Clin. Asst. (Obst.) Hillingdon Hosp. Uxbridge.

RAHMAN, Mr Abdul Panteg Health Centre, Kemys Street, Griffithstown, Pontypool NP4 5DJ Tel: 01495 763608 Fax: 01495 753925 — MB BS Punjab 1977; LMSSA 1990; MRCS 1990; LRCP 1990; FRCS Glas. 1993.

RAHMAN, Abdul Quader Mohammed Hamidir Clydebank Health Centre, Kilbowie Road, Clydebank G81 2TQ Tel: 0141 531 6400 Fax: 0141 531 6419; 17 Carse View Drive, Bearsden, Glasgow G61 3NJ — MB BS Dacca 1970. GP Clydebank, Dunbaronsh.

RAHMAN, Mr Abdur Pilgrim Hospital, Sibsey Road, Boston PE21 9QS — MB BS Peshawar 1965 (Khyber Med. Coll.) FRCS 1979; FRCOphth 1987. Cons. (Ophthal. Surg.) Pilgrim Hosp. Boston. Specialty: Ophth. Special Interest: Anterior segment; Diabetic Retinopathy. Socs: Roy. Coll. of Ophth.; United Kingdom & Irel. Soc. of Cataract & Refractive Surg.; Brit. Med. Assn. Prev: Sen. Regist., Birm. & Midl. Eye Hosp.

RAHMAN, Abu Bazal Mohammad Shamsur 49 South Park Avenue, Mansfield NG18 4PJ — MB BS Dacca 1958; DTM & H Eng. 1965; FRCP Ed. 1983, M 1969; MRCP (UK) 1970; FRCP Lond. 1994. Geriat. Centr. Notts. Healthcare NHS Trust. Specialty: Care of the Elderly. Socs: Brit. Geriat. Soc. & BMA. Prev: Sen. Regist. (Geriat.) St. Jas. Hosp. Leeds; Regist. (Gen. Med.) Sedgefield Gen. Hosp. Stockton-on-Tees; Med. Off. Govt. of North. Nigeria.

RAHMAN, Abu Faiz Mohammad Shafiqur (retired) 40 Highfield, Letchworth SG6 3PZ Tel: 01462 676235 — (Dacca Med. Coll.) MB BS Dacca 1956; DPH Punjab (Pakistan) 1961; DTM & H Eng. 1963; Dip. Bact. Manch. 1965; FRCPath 1980, M 1968; LMSSA Lond. 1969. Prev: Cons. Microbiol. Lister Hosp. Stevenage.

RAHMAN, Abu Fakhr Muhammad Mustafizur (retired) 27 Dunstarn Drive, Adel, Leeds LS16 8EH Tel: 0113 225 7048 — MB BS Dacca 1961 (Dhaka Med. Coll.) MB BS Dhaka 1961; DTM & H Ed. 1966. Prev: Assoc. Specialist (Geriat.) Leeds Gen. Infirm.

RAHMAN, Abu Saleh Mohammad Matinur The Surgery, Sundial Lane, Great Barr, Birmingham B43 6PA Tel: 0121 358 0082 — MB BS Dacca 1969 (Dacca Med. Coll.)

RAHMAN, Abu Taher Mohammed Latifur 61 Applegrove, Enfield EN1 3DA Tel: 020 8366 5248 — MB BS Rajshahi 1964; MB BS Rajshahi Bangladesh 1964.

RAHMAN, Mr Abu Zafar Mohammad Mafizur (retired) The Parc, Litchard Hill, Bridgend CF31 1QQ Tel: 01656 657734 — (Dhaka) MB BS Dhaka 1969; FRCS Ed. 1980. Cons. Gen. Surg. Ealing Hosp. Lond. Prev: Cons. Gen. Surg. Ealing Hosp. Lond.

RAHMAN, Abul Kalam Mohammed Raziur, TD Marshall Street Surgery, 45-46 Marshall Street, Smethwick B67 7NA Tel: 0121 558 4446 Fax: 0121 555 5832 — LRCP LRCS Ed. LRCS Glas. 1979; DRCOG Lond. 1981; DObst RCPI 1981; DTM & H Liverp. 1984; T(GP) 1991; DFFP 1995. GP; JP; Maj. RAMC (TA), 35 Roy. Signal Regt., Coventry & Birm.; RMO. Socs: BMA; Bangladesh Med. Assn.; MDU.

RAHMAN, Altaf-Ur (Surgery), 156 Crankhall Lane, Friar Park, Wednesbury WS10 0EB Tel: 0121 556 3412 — MB BS Peshawar 1964.

RAHMAN, Amina 24A Tutbury Avenue, Coventry CV4 7BJ — BM BS Nottm. 1997.

RAHMAN, Arindam Rafiqur The Surgery, 69 Water Lane, London E15 4NL; 97 Burges Road, East Ham, London E6 2BJ Tel: 020 8470 0853 — MB BS Dacca 1970. Specialty: Cardiol.

RAHMAN, Asia 49 South Park Avenue, Mansfield NG18 4PJ Tel: 01623 29716 — MB BS Dacca 1960 (Dacca Med. Coll.) DA Eng. 1970. Assoc. Specialist (Anaesth.) Kings Mill Hosp. Sutton-in-Ashfield. Socs: BMA. Prev: Clin. Asst. (Anaesth.) Mansfield Gp. Hosp.; Regist. (Anaesth.) Mansfield & Newark Health Dist.

RAHMAN, Faiza Amal 17 St Paul's Way, Finchley, London N3 2PP — MB BS Lond. 1984 (St. Thos.) MRCOG 1991. Regist. St. Bart. Hosp. Lond. Specialty: Obst. & Gyn. Prev: SHO (Obst.) Qu. Charlotte's Matern. Hosp. Lond.

RAHMAN, Faizur (retired) 58 Fountain Road, Birmingham B17 8NR Tel: 0121 429 9769 — MB BS Patna 1951; DTM Sch. Trop. Med. Calcutta 1953; TDD Calcutta 1955; DCH Eng. 1959; DPM Eng. 1968. Med. Pract. Addic. Unit All St.s Hosp. Birm. Prev: Sen. Med. Off. H.M. Prisons, Winson Green Birm.

RAHMAN, Farida Khatoon Health Promotion Centre, 57 Lady Margaret Road, Southall UB1 2PH Tel: 020 8547 5186; WAFA House, Hillcrest Waye, Gerrards Cross SL9 8DN — MB BS Dacca 1958 (Dacca Med. Coll.) DTM & H Eng. 1962; DObst RCOG 1965. Specialty: Anaesth.

RAHMAN, Farooq Ziaur 3 Brentfield Gardens, London NW2 1JP — MB BS Lond. 1997.

RAHMAN, Fauzia Staplegrove House, Berghers Hill, Woodburn Common, High Wycombe HP10 0JP — MB BS Lond. 1986; LMSSA Lond. 1985.

RAHMAN, Fawzia Rafat CHS NHS Trust Southern Derbyshire, Wilderslowe, 121 Osmastun Road, Derby DE1 2GA Tel: 01332 363371 — MB BS All India Inst. Med. Sci. 1977; MD MD (poc)All India Insitit Med Sc 1980; DCH, Lond. 1986; MRCP (UK) 1986; MRCS Eng. LRCP Lond. 1987. Cons., Pediatrician, Community Child Health, Community Health Servs. Trust, Southern Derbysh. Specialty: Paediat. Socs: FRCPCh; BACCH.

RAHMAN, Habib Ur Canvey Village Surgery, 391 Long Road, Canvey Island SS8 0JH Tel: 01268 510520 Fax: 01268 684083; 205 Long Road, Canvey Island SS8 0JE Tel: 01268 680947 — MB BS Punjab 1975; LRCP LRCS Ed. LRCPS Glas. 1982.

RAHMAN, Mr Habib Ur Orthopaedic Department, Birmingham Heartlands Hospital, Bordesley Green E., Birmingham B9 5SS — MB BS Punjab 1981; FRCSI 1987; FRCS (Orth.) 1995. Cons. Orthop. Surg. Birm. Heartlands Hosp. Specialty: Trauma & Orthop. Surg.

RAHMAN, Imran 318 Pershore Road, Edgbaston, Birmingham B5 7QY — MB BS Lond. 1998; MB BS Lond 1998.

RAHMAN, Jarjis Springfield House, New Lane, Patricroft, Manchester M30 7JE — MB BS Dacca 1962 (Dacca Med. Coll.) DTM & H Eng. 1966.

RAHMAN, Junia, Surg. Lt. RN 40 Highfield, Letchworth SG6 3PZ Tel: 01462 676235; 117 Myddleton Avenue, Green Lanes, London N4 2FP Tel: 020 8880 1539 — MB BS Lond. 1996 (King's College

London) PRHO (Surg.) Derriford Hosp. Plymouth; PRHO (Med.) RSCH Brighton. Socs: BMA; MDU; Roy. Naval Med. Soc.

RAHMAN, Kazi Ataur Hawthorns Medical Centre, 94 Lewisham Road, Smethwick, Warley B66 2DD Tel: 01505 613240 Fax: 0121 565 0293 — MB BS Dacca 1970; MB BS Dacca 1970. Specialty: Rheumatol.; Gen. Psychiat.; Anaesth.

RAHMAN, Khandaker Masihur Station Road Medical Centre, 53 Station Road, Brynamman, Ammanford SA18 1SH Tel: 01269 823210; 10 James Griffiths Road, Ammanford SA18 2AS Tel: 01269 592078 — MB BS Dacca 1958; MB BS (Hons.) Dacca 1958; MRCP (UK) 1970. Family Phys. Brynamman. Specialty: Gen. Pract. Prev: Med. Specialist Pakistan Army (1962-69).

RAHMAN, Khondker Mahfuzar 26 Ravensdale Gardens, Eccles, Manchester M30 9JD Tel: 0161 789 3649 — MB BS Dhaka 1961; FRCOG 1989, M 1972. Cons. O & G Ashton-Under-Lyne. Specialty: Obst. & Gyn.

RAHMAN, Mr Mahfuzer 27 Rodney Road, New Malden KT3 5AB Tel: 020 8949 5352 — FRCS Glas. 1981. Specialty: Orthop.

RAHMAN, Manibur 16 Sainfoin Road, London SW17 8EP Tel: 020 8672 5388 Email: t.rahman@ic.ac.uk — BM BCh Oxf. 1992; BA (Hons.) Physiol. Oxf. 1989; MA Physiol. Oxf. 1993; MRCP (UK) 1995; PhD Imp. Col. Lond. 2003. SpR Roy. Surrey County Hosp., Guildford. Specialty: Gastroenterol.; Gen. Med.; Intens. Care. Socs: Roy. Soc. Med. Prev: Research Fell. (Gastroenterol.) Hammersmith Hosp. Lond.; Regist. (Med.) Inst. Liver Studies King's Coll. Hosp. Lond.; Regist. (Med.) Medway Hosp. Gillingham, Kent.

RAHMAN, Mazin Khalid Abdul c/o Frimley Park Hospital, Portsmouth Road, Frimley, Camberley GU16 7UJ Tel: 01276 692777; 89 Thrale Road, London SW16 1NU — MB ChB Baghdad 1976; MRCOG 1990. Regist. (O & G) Frimley Pk. Hosp. Surrey. Specialty: Obst. & Gyn.

RAHMAN, Mobinur 178 Cropston Road, Anstey, Leicester LE7 7BN Tel: 0116 236 5174 — MB BS Dacca 1962; DPM Eng. 1973. Assoc. Specialist (Psychiat.) Rehab Services. Leicester.

RAHMAN, Mohamed Abdur Ashmore Park Clinic, Griffiths Drive, Ashmore Park, Wolverhampton WV11 2LH Tel: 01902 732442 Fax: 01902 729048; 18 Corfton Drive, Tettenhall, Wolverhampton WV6 8NR Tel: 01902 732442 Fax: 01902 729048 — MB BS Dacca 1962 (Dacca Med. Coll.) Socs: Fell. Overseas Doctors Assn.; BMA; Fell. Roy. Soc. Med. Lond.

RAHMAN, Mohamed Altafur Great Harwood Health Centre, Water Street, Great Harwood, Blackburn BB6 7QR Tel: 01254 886400 Fax: 01254 877360; The Bungalow, Mill Lane, Great Harwood, Blackburn BB6 7UQ Tel: 01254 885787 — LAH Dub. 1971. Div. Police Surg. Lancs.; Pres. Bangladesh Med. Assn. (UK). Specialty: Forens. Psychiat.

RAHMAN, Mohammad Balmoral Road Surgery, 12 Balmoral Road, Gillingham ME7 4PG Tel: 01634 854933 — MB BS Peshawar 1962.

RAHMAN, Mohammad Azizar The Surgery, 38-46 Bradley road, Patchway, Bristol BS34 5LD Tel: 0117 969 2040 Fax: 0117 947 0440 — MB BS Dacca 1959. Prev: Regist. Bristol Roy. Infirm.; Ho. Phys. Whittington Hosp. Lond.

RAHMAN, Mohammad Bazlur c/o Drive S.M.S. Rahman, 16 Lynwood Avenue, Lowton, Warrington WA3 1HJ Tel: 01942 6649 — MB BS Dacca 1963; BSc (Hons.) Dacca 1957, MB BS 1963; DTM & H Liverp. 1967. Regist. (O & G) Ayrsh. Gen. Hosp. Irvine. Specialty: Obst. & Gyn. Socs: BMA. Prev: SHO (Gyn.) Roy. Samarit. Hosp. Wom. Glas.; SHO (Obst.) Bellshill Matern. Hosp.; SHO (O & G) Falkirk & Dist. Roy. Infirm.

RAHMAN, Mohammad Khaledur Cross Lane Surgery, 148 Cross Lane, Prescot L35 5DU Tel: 0151 426 5345 Fax: 0151 426 6017 — MB BS Dacca 1963 (Dacca Med. Coll.) DTM & H Liverp. 1966.

RAHMAN, Mr Mohammad Lutfor The Exmoor Surgery, Exmoor Street, London W10 6DZ Tel: 01268 20772 — MB BS Dacca 1965; FRCS Ed. 1972.

RAHMAN, Mohammad Masudur Stanley Health Centre, Clifford Road, Stanley DH9 0XE Tel: 01207 232696 Fax: 01207 239066 — MB BS Dacca 1968. GP Stanley, Co. Durh.

RAHMAN, Mr Mohammad Matiur Department of Surgery, Erne Hospital, Enniskillen BT74 6AY — MB BS Dacca 1972; FRCSI 1990.

RAHMAN, Mohammad Shamsur 190 Maidstone Road, Rochester ME1 3EJ Tel: 01634 814368 — MB BS Dacca 1967.

RAHMAN, Mohammad Zalilur Lyndoch, Larch Avenue, Lenzie, Glasgow G66 4HT — MB BS Dacca 1957 (Dacca Med. Coll.) DTM & H Ed. 1969; FRCPsych 1986, M 1976. Cons. Psychiat. Gartnavel Roy. Hosp. Glas.; Hon. Sen. Clin. Lect. (Psychol. Med.) Univ. Glas. Specialty: Gen. Psychiat. Socs: Fell. Roy. Coll. Psychiat.; BMA. Prev: Cons. Psychiat. Gtr. Glas. HB.

RAHMAN, Mohammed Abbas Anisur Centre for Rheumatology, University College Hospitals NHS Trust, Arthur Stanley House, 40-50 Tottenham Street, London W1T 4NS Tel: 020 7380 9281 Fax: 020 7380 9278 Email: anisur.rahman@ucl.ac.uk — BM BCh Oxf. 1988 (Oxford) BA Oxf. 1985; MRCP (UK) 1991; PhD Lond. 1998. Senior Lecturer and Honorary Consultant in Rheumatology, UCLH Trust, London. Specialty: Rheumatol. Socs: Brit. Soc. for Rheum.; BMA. Prev: Regist. (Rheum.) Roy. Hosp. NHS Trust; Regist. (Rheum.), UCLU Trust; Wellcome Trust Fellow, UCL.

RAHMAN, Mohammed Arif-Ur 2 Blair Place, Kirkcaldy KY2 5SQ — MB ChB Dundee 1994.

RAHMAN, Mohammed Atiqur The Health Centre, Wallsgreen Road, Cardenden, Lochgelly KY5 0JE Tel: 01592 722441 — MB BS Dacca 1960. GP Lochgelly. Fife.

RAHMAN, Mohammed Fazlur Dewsbury District Hospital, Healds Road, Dewsbury WF13 4HS Tel: 01924 465105; Carr Lodge, Beckett Road, Dewsbury WF13 2DB — MB BS Rajshahi 1972. Specialty: Gen. Psychiat.

RAHMAN, Mohammed Haseebur Ashmore Park Clinic, Griffiths Drive, Ashmore Park, Wolverhampton WV11 2LH Tel: 01902 732442 Fax: 01902 729048 — MB ChB Dundee 1992.

RAHMAN, Mohammed Lutfor Exmoor Surgery, Exmoor St., North Kensington, London W10 6DZ Tel: 0208 962 4245 Fax: 020 8962 4252; 18 Chestnut Drive, Harrow HA3 7DJ Tel: 020 8954 3935 Fax: 020 8954 3935 — (Dacca Med. Coll.) MB BS Dacca 1969. Specialty: Gen. Pract. Socs: MDU.

RAHMAN, Muhammad Abdur Tonypandy Health Centre, Winton Field, Tonypandy CF40 2LE Tel: 01443 433284 Fax: 01443 436848 — MB BS Dacca 1960. GP Tonypandy, Mid Glam.

RAHMAN, Muhammad Khalilur Church Road Surgery, 113a Church Road, Burgess Hill RH15 9AA Tel: 01444 244294 — MB BS Karachi 1964. GP Burgess Hill, W. Sussex.

RAHMAN, Muhammad Mahbubur The Surgery, 482 Southend Road, Hornchurch RM12 5PA Tel: 01708 476036 Fax: 01708 471330 — MB BS Dacca, Bangladesh 1970.

RAHMAN, Muhammad Rezaur 62 St Michael's Avenue, Margate CT9 3UH — MB BS Karachi 1981; MRCP (UK) 1993; MRCPI 1993.

RAHMAN, Muhammad Shafiquer 5 Gosberton Road, London SW12 8LE Tel: 020 8673 5309 — MB BS Dacca 1958.

RAHMAN, Muhammed Maerdy Surgery, North Terrace, Maerdy, Ferndale CF43 4DD Tel: 01443 733202 Fax: 01443 733730.

RAHMAN, Mustafizur Blackburn Royal Infirmary, Department of Diagnostic Radiology, Infirmary Road, Blackburn BB2 2LR Tel: 01254 294213 — MB BS Dacca 1966; FRCS Ed. 1974; DMRD Eng. 1977; FRCR 1979. Cons. Radiol. E. Lancs. NHS Trust. Specialty: Radiol. Special Interest: Musculo Skeletal Radiol.; G.I. Radiol.; Vasc. and Interventional Radiol. Socs: Brit. Soc. Interven. Radiol.; CIRSE. Prev: Sen. Regist. (Radiol.) Manch. Roy. Infirm.; Regist. (Gen. Surg.) Burnley Gen. Hosp.

RAHMAN, Mustafizur Department of Microbiology, King's Mill Hospital, Sutton-in-Ashfield NG17 4JL Fax: 01623 672304 Email: m.rahman@sfh-tr.nhs.uk; 2 Chartwell Grove, Mapperley Plains, Nottingham NG3 5RD Tel: 0115 920 7403 — MB BS Dacca 1967 (Dacca Med. Coll.) Dip. Bact. Lond 1972; FRCPath 1987, M 1975. Cons. Med. Microbiol. King's Mill Hosp. Near Mansfield, Notts.; Hon. Clin. Teach. Nottm. Univ. Med. Sch. Nottm. Specialty: Med. Microbiol. Socs: Hosp. Infec. Soc.; Brit. Infec. Soc.; Brit. Soc. Antimicrob. Chem. Prev: Sen. Regist. (Microbiol.) St. Geo. Hosp. Lond.; Regist. (Path.) St. Bart. Hosp. Lond.; Demonst. (Path.) Mymensingh Med. Coll., Bangladesh.

RAHMAN, Nasima Akhtar The Parc, Litchard Hill, Bridgend CF31 1QQ Tel: 01656 657734 — MB BS Dacca 1969 (Dhaka Med. Coll.) DObst Dub. 1981. Locum Cons. (Psychiat.) Princess of Wales Hosp. Bridgend. Specialty: Gen. Psychiat. Prev: Clin. Asst. (Psychiat.) Glanrhyd Hosp. Bridgend; Clin. Asst. (O & G) Princess of Wales Hosp. Bridgend.

RAHMAN, Nurun Nahar 53 St James Road, Rainhill, Prescot L35 0PE — LMSSA Lond. 1993.

RAHMAN, Rezaur Medical Centre, 3 Strouts Place, London E2 7QU Tel: 020 7739 1972; 10 Forest Close, Snaresbrook, London E11 1PY Tel: 020 8989 1411 Fax: 020 7739 6906 — MB BS Dacca 1961 (Dacca Med. Coll.) DPM Eng. 1966; MRCPsych 1972; MRCS Eng. LRCP Lond. 1975. Prev: Asst. Prof. Psychiat. Med. Coll. & Hosp. Rajshahi, Bangladesh; Consult. Ment. Hosp. Pabna, Bangladesh.

RAHMAN, Sabera Nazneen 4 Sates Way, Bristol BS9 4SD — BM BCh Oxf. 1991; BA Oxf. 1988.

RAHMAN, Sadequr Flat 5, Queens Court, 6 Grove Park, London SE5 8LS — MB BS Lond. 1998; MB BS Lond 1998.

RAHMAN, Sally-Anne The Surgery, Sundial Lane, Great Barr, Birmingham B43 6PA Tel: 0121 358 0082 — BM BCh Oxf. 1970; MRCGP 1975.

RAHMAN, Samantha 14 Railey Mews, London NW5 2PA — MB BS Lond. 1993.

RAHMAN, Shabana 318 Pershore Road, Edgbaston, Birmingham B5 7QY Tel: 0121 440 8598 — MB ChB Sheff. 1996. Specialty: Gen. Pract. Socs: BMA; MDU.

RAHMAN, Shah Mohammed Lutfur 7 Begbie Road, Blackheath, London SE3 8BY Tel: 020 8856 2025 — MB BS Dacca 1959 (Dacca Med. Coll.) DLO Eng. 1979. Prev: Regist. (ENT) Walsall Gp. Hosps.

RAHMAN, Shah Mohammed Siddiqur Shalimar, 131 Stonecross Lane, Lowton, Warrington WA3 1JT — MB BS Dacca 1962.

RAHMAN, Shahidur Woodland Avenue Practice, 30 Woodland Avenue, Luton LU3 1RW — MB BS Lond. 1995; DCH Lond. 1999; DFFP Lond. 2000; MRCGP (Merit) Lond. 2001.

RAHMAN, Shaikh O Cwmaman Surgery, 6-14 Glanaman Road, Aberdare CF44 6HY Tel: 01685 873002 Fax: 01685 872179.

RAHMAN, Shakil Ur M Floor Reception, Respiratory Medicine, Royal Hallamshire Hospital, Glossop Road, Sheffield S10 2JF Tel: 01742 766222; 36 Timbercroft, Ewell, Epsom KT19 0TD — MB BS Karachi 1983; MRCP (UK) 1991. Lect. & Sen. Regist. (Gen. Med.) Roy. Hallamsh. & N. Gen. Hosp. Sheff. Specialty: Gen. Med. Prev: Regist. (Teach.) Sheff. Univ. Hosp.; Regist. Doncaster Roy. Infirm.

RAHMAN, Shamima BEM Unit, Institute of Child Health, 30 Guilford Street, London WC1N 1EH Tel: 020 7404 6191/020 7905 2134 Email: s.rahman@ich.ucl.ac.uk — BM BCh Oxf. 1988 (Oxford University) BA (Hons.) Oxf. 1985; MRCP (UK) 1991; PhD Lond. 2002. Clin. Lect. in Paediat. Metab. Med., Inst. of Child Health, Lond.; Hon. Specialist Regist. in Paediat. Metab. Med., Gt. Ormond St. Hosp., Lond. Specialty: Paediat. Socs: Roy. Coll. of Paediat. and Child Health; Roy. Coll. of Physicians (London); Soc. for Study of Inborn Errors of Metab. Prev: Regist. (Paediat.) John Radcliffe Hosp. Oxf. MRC Clin. Train. Fell. Inst. Child Health Lond. & Hon. Regist. Gt. Ormond St. Hosp. Childr. Lond.; Clin. Research Fell. Roy. Childr. Hosp. Melbourne, Austral.; Regist. (Paediat.) St. Mary's Hosp. Paddington.

RAHMAN, Shanim Ara 8 Willerby Drive, Whitebridge Park, Gosforth, Newcastle upon Tyne NE3 5LL — MB ChB Liverp. 1996.

RAHMAN, Mr Sheikh Mohammad Jamalur 2 Llandennis Road, Cardiff CF23 6EF Tel: 029 2074 7525 Fax: 01222 747525 — (Dacca Medical Coll.) MB BS Dacca 1968; DLO RCS Eng. 1978; FRCS Ed. 1986. Locum Cons. ENT. Specialty: Otorhinolaryngol.

RAHMAN, Shelley Louise Flat 116, Albany House, 41 Judd St., London WC1H 9QS — BChir Camb. 1994.

RAHMAN, Shewli 2 Glyncornel Close, Tonypandy CF40 2JT Tel: 01443 431045 — MB ChB Birm. 1993. SHO (Gen. Med.) Derby Roy. Infirm.

RAHMAN, Shupa Gitika 93 Boundary Road, London SW19 2DE — MB BS Lond. 1992.

RAHMAN, Snigdha 23 Byron Close, Ouston, Chester-le-Street DH2 1JR Tel: 0191 410 3901 — MB BS Dacca 1970.

RAHMAN, Tahmina 18 Fairlie Avenue, Mansfield NG19 6RH — MB ChB Ed. 1996.

RAHMAN, Tariq Akhtar Cecil Square Surgery, 1 Cecil Square, Margate CT9 1BD Tel: 01843 232222 Fax: 01843 232205 — MRCS Eng. LRCP Lond. 1981; MBBS; MRCS Eng LRCP Lond 1981.

RAHMAN, Tracey Showkatara 3 Knight Street, Didsbury, Manchester M20 6WG — MB ChB Manch. 1993.

RAHMAN, Waheed — MB BCh Wales 1997.

RAHMAN, Yorick 83 Ribblesdale Road, London SW16 6SF — MB BS Lond. 1991.

RAHMAN, Ziaur 187 Ecclesall Road S., Sheffield S11 9PN — MB BS Gauhati 1962 (Assam Med. Coll. Dibrugarh) DTM & H Eng. 1968; DTCD Wales 1970. Med. Advis. DHSS. Socs: Pneumoconiosis Med. Panel Sheff.; Trent Regional Thoracic Soc. & Occupat. Soc. Prev: Med. Off. DHSS; Med. Asst. Lodge Moor Hosp. Sheff. & Chest Clinic Roy. Infirm. Sheff.; SHO (Chest Med. & Gen. Med.) Lodge Moor Hosp. Sheff.

RAHMANI, Muhammad Javaid Hameed Conquest Hospital, St Leonards-on-Sea TN37 7RD Tel: 01424 757518 — MB BS 1986; MRCP UK 1995; CCST 2001. Cons. Phys. Gen. Int. Med.; Cons. Phys., Care for the Elderly, Conquest Hosp. Specialty: Vasc. Med.; Care of the Elderly; Vascular Neurology. Special Interest: Med. for the Elderly and Vasc. Neurol. Socs: BMA; GMC; BASP.

RAHMANIE, Nooria 7 Claydon House, Holders Hill Road, London NW4 1LS — MD Kabul 1971.

RAHMANOU, Philip PO Box 20, Altrincham WA14 1BJ — MB ChB Liverp. 1997.

RAHMAT POUR MONFARED, Marjan 28 Sand's Wharf, Ferryman Quay, London SW6 2UT — MB BS Lond. 1993 (King's Coll. Sch. Med. & Dent.) Socs: BMA; RSM.

RAHMATHUNISA, Abdul Azeez c/o B.S.A. Rahman, East International Ltd., 2nd Floor Langham House, Regent St., London W1R 5AL — MB BS Madras 1970.

RAHMATI, Margaret Anne — MB BChir Camb. 1993; MA Camb. 1995, BA 1991; MRCP (UK) 1996. Specialty: Nephrol.; Gen. Med. Prev: Specialist Regist. (Nephrol.) W Mid. Rotat.; Research Fell., Renal Research Inst., New York, USA.

RAHMATULLAH KHAN, Dr 51 Fair Cross Avenue, Barking IG11 8RD — MB BS Punjab 1961 (King Edwd. Med. Coll. Lahore) MB BS Punjab (Pakistan) 1961; FRCR 1975.

RAHUJA, Saika Parveen — MB ChB Liverp. 1993.

RAHUJA, Shabbir Ahmed S King's Medical Centre, 7 Kings Road, Old Trafford, Manchester M16 7RT Tel: 0161 226 1288 Fax: 0161 232 1575; 11 Rivers Hill, Gdns., Hale, Altrincham WA15 0AZ Tel: 0161 980 1993 — MB BS Punjab 1965 (Nishtar Med. Coll. Multan) BSc Karachi 1959; MB BS Punjab (Pakistan) 1965; DLO Eng. 1973. Gen. Med. Practitioner; Clin. Asst. ENT Dept. Wyntheshaw Hosp. Manch. Specialty: Otorhinolaryngol. Socs: Med. Protect. Soc.; Pakistan Med. Assn.; Sindhi Doctors Assn.

RAHUL, Chauhan Wexham Park Hospital, Wexham Street, Slough SL3 4HL Tel: 01753 633631 Fax: 01753 860879 — MB BS; FRCP; MRCP. Gen. Internal Med. Specialty: Gen. Med.; Care of the Elderly. Socs: MPS; GMC; HSCA.

RAI, Mr Amarjit Singh Norfolk & Norwich University Hospital, Department of Trauma & Orthopaedics, Colney Lane, Norwich NR4 7UY — BM Soton. 1990; FRCS (Orth). Cons. Orthop. & Spinal Surg. Norf. & Norwich Univ. Hosp. Specialty: Trauma & Orthop. Surg.

RAI, Ashok Worcester Royal Infirmary, Dept. of Rheumatology, Newtown Branch, Newtown Rd, Worcester WR5 1HN; Clearview, 1 Chiltern Close, Great Witley, Worcester WR6 6HL — MB ChB Birm. 1985; FRCP, LLM. Cons. Rheumatologist acute Worcs. NHS Trust. Specialty: Rheumatol. Socs: Fell.Roy. Soc. of Med.

RAI, Gurcharan Singh 22 Northwick Circus, Kenton, Harrow HA3 0DY — MD Newc. 1978 (Newcastle-upon-Tyne) MB BS 1971; MRCP (UK) 1974; MSc Lond. 1977; FRCP Lond. 1988. Cons. Phys. (Geriat. Med.) Whittington Hosp. Lond. Specialty: Care of the Elderly; Gen. Med. Socs: FRSM (Sec. of Sect. of Geriat.s & Gerontology); Brit. Geriat. Soc.; Amer. Geriat. Soc. Prev: Sen. Regist. (Geriat. Med.) Cambrigde; Sen. Research Fell. Universisty Newc.; Regist. Newc. Univ. Hosps.

RAI, Harinder Manor Hospital, Walsall Hospitals NHS Trust, Moat Road, Walsall WS2 9PS Tel: 01922 656875 Fax: 01922 656868 Email: h.rai@walsallhospitals. nhs.uk — MB ChB Manch. 1985 (Manchester) MRCP (UK) 1989; FRCR 1995. Cons. Radiologist, Manor Hosp., Walshall. Specialty: Radiol.

RAI, Harjeev Singh 18 Alum Cl, Coventry CV6 5TQ — MB BCh Wales 1997.

RAI, Harnek Singh 16 Warstone Terrace, Birmingham B21 9NE — MB ChB Dundee 1989.

RAI, Jagjit 62 Homeway Road, Leicester LE5 5RG — MB ChB Sheff. 1992.

RAI, Jagjit Singh 43 Avenue Road, Southall UB1 3BW — MB ChB Aberd. 1993.

RAI, Jasdev Singh 32 Manor Avenue, Hounslow TW4 7JL — MB ChB Liverp. 1979.

RAI, Jatinder 46 Ednam Road, Wolverhampton WV4 5BP — MB BS Lond. 1998; MB BS Lond 1998.

RAI, Kundadka Divaker Honicknowle Green Medical Centre, Guy Miles Way, Honicknowle Green, Plymouth PL5 3PY Tel: 01752 777207 Fax: 01752 775556; 91 Dunraven Drive, Derriford, Plymouth PL6 6AT — MB BS Mysore 1974 (Mysore Medical College)

RAI, Nalini Rai and Duke, Bingley Health Centre, Myrtle Place, Bingley BD16 2TL Tel: 01274 566617 Fax: 01274 772345; Fieldhead Barn, Street Lane, West Morton, Keighley BD20 5UP Tel: 01535 609696 — MB BS Delhi 1973 (Maulana Azad Med. Coll. New Delhi) DCH RCPS Glas. 1976. Clin. Asst. Bingley Hosp. Specialty: Paediat. Prev: Clin. Med. Off. Leeds AHA; Clin. Med. Off. N.ants. AHA.

RAI, Neerja 11 Chafinch Close, Scunthorpe DN15 8EL — MB BS Lucknow 1981 (King Geo. Med. Coll. Lucknow, India) MD India 1985; MRCOG 1993. Specialist Regist. (O & G) Hull Matern. & Princess Roy. Hosp. Hull. Specialty: Obst. & Gyn. Prev: Regist. (O & G) P. Chas. Hosp. Merthyr Tydfil; Regist. (O & G) Glas. Roy. Infirm.

RAI, Rajendra Singh 105 Highview Road, London W13 0HL — MB BS Lond. 1988; BSc (Hons.) Lond. 1985, MB BS 1988; MRCOG 1997. Sen. Lect. & Cons. Gynaecologist St Marys Hosp. Lond. Specialty: Obst. & Gyn. Prev: SHO (Gyn.) Samarit. Hosp. for Wom. Lond.; SHO (O & G) Lond. Hosp. Whitechapel; Ho. Phys. Med. Unit. St. Thos. Hosp. Lond.

RAI, Santoch Singh Dove House, 15 Bakery Drive, Stockton-on-Tees TS19 0SN — MB ChB Manch. 1987.

RAI, Satya Kumar 21 The Green, St Leonards-on-Sea TN38 0SU — MB BS Punjabi, India 1979.

RAI CHOUDHURY, Krishna Bransholme Health Centre, Goodhart Road, Bransholme, Hull HU7 4DW Tel: 01482 825496; 4 Pine Meadows, Kirkella, Hull HU10 7NS — MB BS Dacca 1975; DCH RCP Lond. 1981; DFFP 1997. Assoc. Community Paediat. Childr.'s Centre Hull. Specialty: Gen. Med. Socs: Hull Med. Soc. Prev: Clin. Med. Off. (Community Med.) Hull; Trainee GP Hull VTS; Regist. (Paediat.) Luton & Dunstable Hosps.

RAI CHOWDHURY, Saroj Lal 208 Mill Lane, Liverpool L15 8LJ — MB BS Calcutta 1952 (R.G. Kar Med. Coll.) MRCOG 1964.

***RAICAR, Sheila** 45 Corringham Road, Wembley HA9 9PX — MB BS Karachi 1961.

RAICHOUDHURY, Benjamin Sailen Kingsway Surgery, 37 The Kingsway, Swansea SA1 5LF — MB BCh Wales 1974; MRCGP 1978.

RAICHURA, Manilal Madhavji The Surgery, 95 Grasmere Avenue, Wembley HA9 8TF Tel: 020 8904 8045 Fax: 020 8908 5363; 13 Sidney Road, Harrow HA2 6QE — MB ChB Birm. 1963; MRCP (UK) 1971; LMCC Canada 1975.

RAICHURA, Naresh Hodnet Medical Centre, Drayton Road, Hodnet, Market Drayton TF9 3NF Tel: 0163 084230 Fax: 0163 084770; The Old Vicarage, Cheswardine, Market Drayton TF9 2RN Tel: 01630 685230 Fax: 01630 685770 — MB ChB Liverp. 1978; MSc Lond. 1985.

RAICHURA, Vijay Kumar University Medical Practice, 5 Pritchatts Road, Edgbaston, Birmingham B15 2SE Tel: 0121 687 3055 — MB BS Lond. 1982 (Guy's) MRCGP 1986; DRCOG 1986. Med. Off. Univ. Birm. Prev: Trainee GP St. Bart. Hosp. VTS; Ho. Phys. Guy's Hosp. Lond.

RAIJIWALA, Nipun Tarunkumar House F11, Residences, Princess of Wales Hospital, Coity Road, Bridgend CF31 1RQ; 50 Tremains Court, Brackla, Bridgend CF31 2SR — MB BCh BAO Belf. 1986.

RAIKES, Annette Sylvia (retired) 9 Wychwood Drive, Bournemouth BH2 6JG Tel: 01202 290777 — MRCS Eng. LRCP Lond. 1961; FRCP Lond. 1985, MRCP (UK) 1977. Prev: Cons. Paediat.

RAIL, John Frederick Whitburn (retired) 1 Ruston Avenue, Rustington, Littlehampton BN16 2AP Tel: 01903 786522 Email: johnrail@onetel.net.uk; 1 Ruston Avenue, Rustington, Littlehampton BN16 2AP Tel: 01903 786522 Fax: 01903 786522 — MRCS Eng. LRCP Lond. 1952 (King's Coll. Hosp.) Prev: Local Civil Serv. Med. Off.

RAILTON, Angela Department of Obstetrics and Gynaecology, Hope Hospital, Salford M6 — MD Cape Town 1988; MB BCh Wales 1977; MRCOG 1982; FRCOG 1995. Cons. O & G Hope Hosp. Salford. Specialty: Obst. & Gyn.

RAILTON, Mr Gilbert Taylor Kingston Hospital, Wolverton Avenue, Kingston upon Thames KT2 7QB Tel: 020 8546 7711; Bell House, Fairmile Pk Road, Cobham KT11 2PP — MB BCh Wales 1977; FRCS Eng. 1982. Cons. Orthop. Surg. Kingston. Specialty: Orthop. Prev: Sen. Regist. (Orthop.) Lond. Hosp. Whitechapel.

RAILTON, Katherine Louise 3 The Brackens, Locks Heath, Southampton SO31 6TU — MB BS Lond. 1997.

RAIMAN, Alistair Charles Northbourne Medical Centre, Eastern Avenue, Shoreham-by-Sea BN43 6PE Tel: 01273 464640 Fax: 01273 440913; 16 Windlesham Gardens, Shoreham-by-Sea BN43 5AD Tel: 01273 273748 — MB BS Lond. 1985 (The Royal London Hospital) BSc (Hons.) Lond. 1982, MB BS 1985; MRCGP 1989. Clin. Asst. DOME Worthing Hosp.; Med. Off. Brighton Hove Albion Football Club. Socs: BMA & Med. Protect. Soc.; Brit. Med. Acupunct. Soc. Prev: Occupat. Health Phys. Worthing Priority Care Hosp. Trust; GP Kawerau. NZ; GP Lond.

RAIMAN, John Draper The Health Centre, Handsworth Avenue, Highams Park, London E4 9PD Tel: 020 8527 0913; The Park House Surgery, 1 Cavendish Road, Highams Park, London E4 9NQ Tel: 020 8523 1401 — MB BS Lond. 1957 (Lond. Hosp.) DObst RCOG 1960; FRCGP 1985, M 1965. Course Organiser Whipps Cross VTS. Prev: Ho. Surg. & Ho. Phys. St. Mary's Hosp. Eastbourne; Cas. Off. & Sen. Ho. Off. (O & G) St. Margts. Hosp. Epping.

RAIMAN, Julian Andrew Jonathon 35 Castle Avenue, London E4 9PY — MB BS Lond. 1992; MRCP (Paediat.) Lond. 1996. Specialist Regist. (Paediat.) S. E. Thames Region. Specialty: Paediat. Socs: MRCPCH.

RAIMES, Mr Simon Aylwin Department of Surgery, Cumberland Infirmary, Carlisle CA2 7HY Tel: 01228 814144 Email: susan.pedrosa@ncumbria-acute.nhs.uk — MD Newc. 1990; FRCS Eng. 1983. Cons. Gen. Surg. & Gastroenterol. Cumbld. Infirm. Specialty: Gen. Surg. Socs: Brit. Soc. Gastroenterol.; Assn. Upper G.I. Surg.; Assn. of Surg.s of Gt. Britain and Irel. (Counc. Mem.). Prev: Sen. Regist. (Gen. Surg.) Freeman Hosp. Newc. u Tyne; Lect. (Surg.) Chinese Univ., Hong Kong.

RAIMONDO, Carmelo 32 Windmill Rise, Kingston upon Thames KT2 7TU — State Exam Bologna 1983.

RAINA, C P The Surgery, 57 Gladstone Avenue, Manor Park, London E12 7NR Tel: 020 8471 4764 Fax: 020 8472 3378 — MB BS Jammu & Kashmir 1972; MB BS Jammu & Kashmir 1972.

RAINBOW, Josephine Ruth 6 Monkton Way, Speen, Princes Risborough HP27 0RZ Tel: 01494 488658 — BM BCh Oxf. 1993; MRCP (Paeds.) Lond. 1996. Paediat. Regist. New Childr.'s Hosp. Sydney, Australia. Specialty: Paediat.

RAINE, Anne Ward 15, Medical Oncology Unit, Bradford Royal Infirmary, Bradford BD9 6RJ Tel: 01274 364095 Fax: 01274 366745; Cleughend, 1 The Bullfield, Harden, Bingley BD16 1HN Tel: 01535 272780 Fax: 01535 274699 — MB BS Newc. 1977; DRCOG 1980; MRCGP 1981; Dip. Palliat. Med. Wales 1997; Dip. Ethics of Cancer & Palliative Care, Keele Univ, 2001. Staff Grade in Oncol. Specialty: Palliat. Med.; Oncol. Prev: Staff Grade in Palliat. Care; GP.

RAINE, Cameron Plastic Surgery, Shotley Bridge Hospital, Consett DH9 0NB — MB ChB Ed. 1990. Specialty: Plastic Surg.

RAINE, Mr Christopher Howard Department of Otorhinolarynogology, Bradford Royal Infirmary, Duckworth Lane, Bradford BD9 6RJ Tel: 01274 542200 — MB BS Newc. 1976; BSc (Hons.) Newc. 1973, MB BS 1976; FRCS Eng. 1980; ChM Liverp. 1987. Cons. Otorhinolarynogology Bradford; Cons. Airedale Gen. Hosp., Steeton, Keighley. Specialty: Otorhinolaryngol. Special Interest: Coculear Implantation. Socs: Eurpoean Soc. of Paediatric Otolarynogology; British Association of Otolarynogology- Head & Neck Injury.

RAINE, Geoffrey James 24B Beaconsfield Road, Bexley DA5 2AE; 6 Apton Road, Bishop's Stortford CM23 3SN Tel: 01279 758574 — MB ChB Bristol 1984; FRCA 1993. Cons. Anaesth. Princess Alexandra Hosp. Harlow. Specialty: Anaesth. Socs: OAA; ICS; Assn. Anaesth.

RAINE, Mr George Edward Thompson 144 Harley Street, London W1G 7LE Tel: 020 7935 0023 Fax: 020 7935 5972; 32

Pelhams Walk, Esher KT10 8QD Tel: 01372 466656 Fax: 01372 470265 Email: georgeraine@paedic.demon.co.uk — (Camb. & St. Thos.) MB BChir Camb. 1958; MA Camb. 1959; FRCS Eng. 1966. Cons. Orthop. Surg. Teddington Memor. Hosp. & New Vict. Hosp. Kingston; Orthop. Adviser Various Sporting Bodies. Specialty: Orthop.; Trauma & Orthop. Surg. Socs: Fell. BOA; BOSTA; Fell. Roy. Soc. Med. Prev: Cons. Orthop. Surg. W. Middlx. Univ. Hosp.; Orthop. Adviser Ballet Rambert Sch.; Sen. Regist. (Orthop.) St. Geo. Hosp. Lond., Rowley Bristow Orthop. Hosp. Pyrford & Centre for Hip Surg. Wrightington.

RAINE, John (retired) Mar House, Arkendale, Knaresborough HG5 0RG — MB ChB Leeds 1953; MRCGP 1964. Prev: Ho. Surg. Gen. Infirm. Leeds.

RAINE, Joseph Dept Paediatrics, Whittington Hospital, Highgate Hill, London N19 — MB ChB Manch. 1983; DCH RCP Lond. 1986; MRCP (UK) 1986; MD Manch. 1995. Cons. Paediat. Whittington Hosp. Hon. Sen. Lect., Univ. Coll., Lond. Specialty: Paediat. Socs: Brit. Soc. of Paediatric Endocrinol. and Diabetes. Prev: Sen. Regist. (Paediat.) Addenbrooke's Hosp. Camb.; Cons. Paediat. Whipps Cross Hosp.; Research Fell., Nat. Heart & Lung Inst.

RAINE, June Munro 177 Hadham Road, Bishop's Stortford CM23 2QA — BM BCh Oxf. 1978; MA, MSc, BM BCh Oxf. 1978; MRCP (UK) 1980; MRCGP 1982; DRCOG 1982. Sen. Med. Off. Meds. Div. DoH Lond. Specialty: Civil Serv. Prev: GP Oxf.; Research Regist. (Endocrinol. & Metab.) John Radcliffe Hosp. Oxf.; SHO (Med.) John Radcliffe Hosp. Oxf.

RAINE, Nicola Meriel Noble 19 Beaumont St, Oxford OX1 2NA Tel: 01865 240501; 40 Ash Grove, Headington, Oxford OX3 9JL Tel: 01865 762458 — MB BS Lond. 1989; MA Oxf. 1990; FRCS Ed. 1994. GP Princip. Specialty: Gen. Pract.

RAINE, Mr Peter Alan Malden Royal Hospital for Sick Children, Yorkhill, Glasgow G3 8SJ Tel: 0141 201 0000 Fax: 0141 201 0865 Email: peter.raine@yorkhill.scot.nhs.uk; 5 Westbourne Drive, Bearsden, Glasgow G61 4BD Tel: 0141 942 8881 — MB BChir Cantab. 1967 (Camb. & St. Bart.) MA Cantab. 1967; FRCS Ed. 1973; FRCS Glas. 1983. Cons. Paediat. Surg. Roy. Hosp. Sick Childr. Glas.; Barclay Lect. (Paediat. Surg.) Univ. Glas. Specialty: Paediat. Surg. Socs: Brit. Assn. Paediat. Surg.; Brit. Soc. Paediat. Gastroenterol.; Craniofacial Soc. Prev: Regist. Roy. Childr. Hosp. Melbourne, Austral.; Lect. (Paediat. Surg.) Univ. Glas.; Regist. (Surg.) Lothian (Edin.) HB.

RAINE, Philip Mark (retired) 120 Grange Road, Wigston, Wigston LE18 1JJ — MB BCh Wales 1977; DRCOG 1979.

RAINE, Richard Andrew 64 Oakham Road, Harborne, Birmingham B17 9DG — MB ChB Birm. 1987.

RAINE, Rosalind Ann Health Services Research Unit, London School of Hygiene & Tropical Medicine, Keppel St., London WC1E 7HT Tel: 020 7927 2038 Fax: 020 7580 8183 Email: rosalind.raine@lshtm.ac.uk; 2 Upper Terrace, London NW3 6RH Tel: 020 7432 8107 — MB BS Lond. 1989 (University College London) BSc (1st cl. Hons.) Lond. 1986; MSc (Distinc.) Lond. 1994; MFPHM 1997. MRC Clinical Scientist/Senior Lecturer (Health Services Research) LSHTM, London; Hon. Cons. in Pub. Health, North East London, SHA. Specialty: Pub. Health Med.

RAINE, Wendy Jane Bailey D.C.F.P. Old Mill Studios, 187 Old Rutherglen Road, Gorbals, Glasgow G5 0RE Tel: 0141 300 6360 Fax: 0141 300 6399; 5 Westbourne Drive, Bearsden, Glasgow G61 4BD Tel: 0141 942 8881 — MB ChB Ed. 1970 (Edin.) BMedSci Ed. 1968; MRCPsych 1975. Cons. Child Psychiat. Yorkhill NHS Trust Glas. Specialty: Child & Adolesc. Psychiat. Prev: Cons. Child & Adolesc. Psychiat. Roy. Hosp. Sick Childr. Glas.; Sen. Regist. (Child & Family Psychiat.) Roy. Hosp. Sick Childr. Glas.; Regist. (Child Psychiat.) Roy. Childr. Hosp. Melbourne, Austral.

RAINE-FENNING, Nicholas John 10 Westfield Hall, Hagley Road, Edgbaston, Birmingham B16 9LG — MB ChB Birm. 1992.

RAINES, Julia Elizabeth 37 Regent Road, Horsforth, Leeds LS18 4NP — MB ChB Leeds 1988; MRCP (UK) 1991; MPH Leeds 1994. Specialty: Pub. Health Med.

RAINES, Mr Michael Francis Victoria Hospital, Department of Ophthalmology, Blackpool FY3 8NR Tel: 01253 303472 Fax: 01253 306743 Email: mfraines@cataractcentre.co.uk; 8 Church Road, Lytham St Annes FY8 5LH Tel: 01253 730302 Fax: 01253 730304 — MB ChB Sheff. 1980; DO RCS Eng. 1984; FRCS Ed. 1985; FRCOphth 1989. Cons. Ophth. Surg. Vict. Hosp. Blackpool; Hon. Sen. Lect., Univ. of Centr. Lancs., Preston. Specialty: Ophth. Socs: FRSM; U.K. & N. Ire. Soc. Of Cataract & Refractive Surg.; Amer. Acad. Of Opthalmology. Prev: Sen. Regist. (Ophth.) Birm. & Midl. Eye Hosp.

RAINES, Reginald John Hall 270 Woodchurch Road, Birkenhead CH43 5UU Tel: 0151 608 3475 Fax: 0151 608 9535; Point House, Ferry Lane, Sealand Road, Chester CH1 6QF Tel: 01244 372787 — MRCS Eng. LRCP Lond. 1950 (St. Bart.) Prev: Capt. RAMC TA.

RAINEY, Mr Albert Edmund Simpson Iorama, 3 Sandal Avenue, Sandal, Wakefield WF2 7LP Tel: 01924 56971 — MB BCh BAO Belf. 1960 (Qu. Univ. Belf.) FRCSI 1965; FRCS Ed. 1966. Cons. Orthop. Surg. Pinderfields Gen. Hosp. & Clayton Hosp. Wakefield. Specialty: Orthop. Socs: BMA; Brit. Orthop. Assn. Prev: Ho. Off. Roy. Vict. Hosp. Belf.; Orthop. Regist. Belf. City Hosp.; Sen. Orthop. Regist. Musgrave Pk. Hosp. Belf. & North. Irel. Orthop.

RAINEY, Andrew John Royal Sussex County Hospital, Brighton; 34 Sussex Square, Brighton BN2 5AD — MB BS Newc. 1984; BMedSc Newc. 1981; MRCPath 1995; FRCPath 2003. Cons. Histopath, Royal Sussex County Hosptial, Brighton. Specialty: Histopath. Prev: Cons. (Histopath.) Lister Hosp. Stevenage Herts; Sen. Regist. (Histopath.) Roy. Sussex Co. Hosp. Brighton; Sen. Regist. (Morbid Anat.) King's Coll. Hosp. Lond.

RAINEY, David Selbert Neillsbrook Road Surgery, 5 Neillsbrook Road, Randalstown, Antrim BT41 3AE Tel: 028 9447 2575 Fax: 028 9447 3653; Connors Wood, Randalstown, Antrim BT41 3LB — MB BCh BAO Belf. 1964; FRCGP 1986, M 1971; MICGP 1987.

RAINEY, Garrett John 5 Thornhill Malone, Belfast BT9 6SS — MB ChB Dund. 1998; MB ChB Dund 1998.

RAINEY, George Wesley Ballysillan Group Practice, 321 Ballysillan Road, Belfast BT14 6RD Tel: 028 9071 3689/7843 Fax: 028 9071 0626 — MB BCh BAO Belf. 1975.

RAINEY, Mr Henry Adrian Woodram Mead, Corfe, Taunton TA3 7AP — MB BCh BAO Belf. 1958; FRCSI 1967. Cons. Orthop. & Traum. Surg. Som. AHA. Specialty: Trauma & Orthop. Surg. Prev: Ho. Off. Belf. City Hosp.; Surg. Regist. Roy. Vict. Hosp. Belf.; Sen. Regist. Princess Eliz. Orthop. Hosp. Exeter.

RAINEY, Jill Catherine Anne 61 Shore Road, Greenisland, Carrickfergus BT38 8TZ — MB ChB Glas. 1995.

RAINEY, Lynne The Hemmel, Great Whittington, Newcastle upon Tyne NE19 2HP — MB ChB Dundee 1983; MRCP (UK) 1987. Specialty: Anaesth.

RAINEY, Mervyn Glenn Argyll & Clyde Acute Hospitals NHS Trust, Inverclyde Royal Hospital, Greenock PA16 0XN Tel: 01475 633777 Email: mg.rainey@vol.scot.nhs.uk — MB ChB Ed. 1982; MA Camb. 1983, BA 1979; MRCP (UK) 1987; MRCPath 1997. Cons. Haematologist, Argyll & Clyde Acute Hosps. NHS Trust. Specialty: Haematology. Prev: Sen. Regist. (Haemat.) Plymouth; Sen. Regist. (Haemat.) Bristol.; Research Fell. (Haemat.) Southmead Hosp. Bristol.

RAINEY, Norman Alexander Ballysillan Group Practice, 321 Ballysillan Road, Belfast BT14 6RD Tel: 028 9071 3689/7843 Fax: 028 9071 0626 — (Queen's Belfast) MB BCh BAO Belf. 1970.

RAINEY, Robert Stephen Chapman and Partners, 370-372 Cregagh Road, Belfast BT6 9EY Tel: 028 9049 2214 Fax: 028 9049 2214 — MB BCh BAO Belf. 1982; DCH Dub. 1984; DRCOG 1985; MRCGP 1986. GP Belf. Socs: BMA.

RAINEY, Veronica 50 Barnhill Road, Dumbarton G82 2SN — MB ChB Glas. 1998; MB ChB Glas 1998.

RAINFORD, Alison Beighton Health Centre, Queens Road, Beighton, Sheffield S20 1BJ Tel: 0114 269 5061; 25 Ranmoor Crescent, Sheffield S10 3GW Tel: 0114 230 7274 — MB ChB Sheff. 1986; DRCOG 1990; DCH RCP Lond. 1990; MRCGP 1993. Prev: SHO (Psychiat.) Derby Ment. Health Unit Pastures Hosp.; Trainee GP Retainer Scheme Bolsover.

RAINFORD, David John, MBE, OStJ, Air Commodore RAF Med. Scotsford Close, 23 Bates Lane, Weston Turville, Aylesbury HP22 5SL Tel: 0129 661 3707 Email: david@rainford.clara.net — MB BS Lond. 1969 (Char. Cross) MRCS Eng. LRCP Lond. 1969; MRCP (UK) 1972; FRCP Lond. 1985; FRAeS 1998; FFOM (Hon.) 1999. Cons. Phys. to UK Civil Aviat. Auth., Cons. Adviser in Med. to Roy. Air Force of Oman; Med. Adviser to Main Grants Comm. RAF Benevolent Fund. Specialty: Nephrol. Special Interest: Clin. Aviat. Med. Socs: Fell. Roy. Soc. Med.; Renal Assn.; Eur. Dialysis & Transpl. Assn. Prev: Chief Exec., Defence Secondary Care Agency;

Hon. Sen. Lect. (Renal. Med.) Roy. Postgrad. Med. Sch. Hammersmith Hosp.; Clin. Dir., Roy. Air Force.

RAINFORD, Frederick Alan (retired) 6 Victoria Road, Aughton, Ormskirk L39 5AU Tel: 01695 422931 — (Manch.) MB ChB Manch. 1947; MRCS Eng. LRCP Lond. 1948. Prev: Ho. Surg. (Orthop.) & Ho. Surg. Withington Hosp. Manch.

RAINFORD, Paul Jeremy Pilgrim Hospital, Sibsey Road, Boston PE21 9QS Tel: 01205 364801; 47 Spilsby Road, Boston PE21 9NX Tel: 01205 369873 — MB BS Lond. 1979; MRCPsych 1983. Cons. Psychiat. Pilgrim Hosp. Boston. Specialty: Gen. Psychiat.

RAINFORD, Peter Anthony Parkway Medical Centre, 2 Frenton Close, Chapel House Estate, Newcastle upon Tyne NE5 1EH Tel: 0191 267 1313 Fax: 0191 229 0630; 27 The Chesters, West Denton, Newcastle upon Tyne NE5 1AF Tel: 0191 267 9944 — MB ChB Liverp. 1960; DObst. RCOG 1965. Specialty: Obst. & Gyn. Prev: SHO (O & G) MusGr. Pk. Hosp. Taunton; SHO (Med.) Bridgwater & Dist. Hosp.; Ho. Phys. & Ho. Surg. David Lewis North. Hosp. Liverp.

RAINS, Professor Anthony John Harding, CBE 39A St.Cross Road, Winchester SO23 9PR Tel: 01962 869419 — (St. Mary's) MB BS Lond. 1943; MRCS Eng. LRCP Lond. 1943; FRCS Eng. 1948; MS Lond. 1952. Specialty: Gen. Surg. Prev: Edr. Jl. Roy. Soc. Med.; Prof. Surg. Char. Cross Hosp.; Asst. Dir. & Regional Postgrad. Dean SW Thames RHA.

RAINS, Kathleen Maude (Fawcitt) 12 Leegate Gardens, Heaton Mersey, Stockport SK4 3NR — MRCS Eng. LRCP Lond. 1942 (Manch.) DA Eng. 1945; FFA RCS Eng. 1954. Cons. Anaesth. N. Manch. Hosps. Specialty: Anaesth. Prev: Cons. Anaesth. Lancaster & Kendal Hosp. Gp.; Asst. Anaesth. S. Manch. Hosp. Gp.; Sen. Regist. Manch. Roy. Infirm.

RAINS, Simon George Harding Church Street Surgery, Church Street, Starcross, Exeter EX6 8PZ Tel: 01626 890368 Fax: 01626 891330 — MB BS Lond. 1979 (St. Thos.) BA (Hons.) Oxf. 1976; MRCP (UK) 1982; MRCGP 1988. Prev: Regist. (Gen. Med.) St. Mary's Hosp. Lond.; SHO (Gen. Med.) Taunton & Som. Hosps.; Ho. Surg. St. Thos. Hosp. Lond.

RAINSBURY, Mr Paul Albert BUPA Medical Director, IVF Unit, BUPA Roding Hospital, Roding Lane S., Ilford IG4 5PZ Tel: 020 8551 7107 Fax: 020 8551 7486; 2 Woodedge Close, Chingford, London E4 6BB Tel: 020 8523 9171 Fax: 020 8529 1109 — MB BCh BAO Dub. 1969 (TC Dub.) MA Dub. 1969; FRCOG 1990, M 1974. Med. Dir. (IVF) BUPA Roding Hosp., Ilford. Specialty: Family Plann. & Reproduc. Health. Socs: Fell. Roy. Soc. Med.; Brit. Fertil. Soc.; Eur. Soc. Human Reprod. & Embryol. Prev: Med. Dir. Hallam Med. Centre Lond.; Dep. Med. Dir. Bourn Hall Clinic Camb.; Cons. Gyn. Fertil. & IVF Unit Humana Hosp. Lond.

RAINSBURY, Mr Richard Myles Surgical Unit, Royal Hampshire County Hospital, Romsey Road, Winchester SO22 5DG Tel: 01962 825146 Fax: 01962 824640 Email: breastunit@weht.swest.nhs.uk; Bridge House, Twyford, Winchester SO21 1QF Tel: 01962 712145 Fax: 01962 712145 Email: rrainsbury@aol.com — MB BS Lond. 1974 (Univ. Collee Hosp. Med. Sch.) MS Lond. 1984, BSc (Hon. Pharmacol.) 1971; FRCS Eng. 1979. Cons. Gen. Surg. Roy. Hants. Co. Hosp. Winchester.; Hill Skills Tutor, Raven Dept. of Educat., Roy. Coll. of Surg.s of Eng., Lond. Specialty: Gen. Surg. Socs: Brit. Breast Gp.; Breast Specialty Gp. of Brit. Assn. of Surgic. Oncol.; Fell. Roy. Soc. of Med. Prev: Sen. Regist. St. Geo. Hosp. Lond.; Hon. Sen. Regist. Roy. Marsden Hosp. Sutton; Regist. (Surg.) St. Jas. Hosp. Lond.

RAINSBURY, Sherwood George William (retired) 225 Manchester New Road, Middleton, manchester M24 1JT — MRCS Eng. LRCP Lond. 1943 (Sheff.) Prev: Surg. Lt. RNVR.

RAISON, Helen Elizabeth Guildford — MB BS Newc. 1996; BSc Soton. 1989; PG Dip BA (dist.) Newc. 1999.

RAISON, John Charles Anthony (retired) 15 The Woodlands, Church Lane, Kings Worthy, Winchester SO23 7QQ Tel: 01962 885722 Email: jonrai@aol.com — (Camb. & Birm.) MB BChir Camb. 1950; MD Camb. 1963; ECFMG Cert. 1966; FFPHM 1987, M 1974; FFPHM 1989. Prev: Cons. Clin. Physiol. Birm. RHA (Intens. Care).

RAISTRICK, Duncan Stuart 19 Springfield Mount, Leeds LS2 9NG Tel: 0113 295 1305 Fax: 0113 295 2789 — MB ChB Leeds 1971; MB ChB Leeds. 1971; FRCPsych 1977; MPhil Lond. 1978. Cons. Psychiat. Leeds Addic. Unit; Cons. Adviser to the Chief Med. Off. (Alcohol Misuse); Assoc.Sen. Lect. Univ. of Leeds. Specialty: Alcohol & Substance Misuse; Gen. Psychiat. Socs: Soc. Study Addic. Alcohol & other Drugs.

RAISTRICK, Eleanor Ruth (retired) 8 Southfield Road, Westbury-on-Trym, Bristol BS9 3BH Tel: 0117 962 9242 — MB ChB Leeds 1943 (Lond. & Leeds) DObst RCOG 1948. Prev: Med. Asst. Bristol Eye Hosp.

RAIT, David Ernest University Medical Practice, University of Aberdeen, Block E, Taylor Buildings, Aberdeen AB24 3UB Tel: 01224 276655 Fax: 01224 272463 — MB ChB Aberd. 1977.

RAIT, Elizabeth Anne East Donnington Street Clinic, East Donnington Street, Darvel KA17 0JR Tel: 01560 320205 Fax: 01560 321643 — MB ChB Ed. 1984.

RAIT, Greta 23 Vesper Rise, Leeds LS5 3NJ — MB ChB Manch. 1991.

RAITHATHA, Hasmukh Haridas Doncaster Royal Infirmary, Armthrop Road, Doncaster DN2 5LT Tel: 01302 366666 Fax: 01302 320098; 6 Grange Road, Bessacarr, Doncaster DN4 6SA Tel: 01302 532788 — MRCS Eng. LRCP Lond. 1973 (Lond. Hosp.) FFA RCSI 1980; T(Anaesth.) 1991. Cons. (Anaesth.) Doncaster Roy. Infirm. Specialty: Anaesth. Socs: Coll. Tutor - The Roy. Coll. of Anaesthetics 1992-1998; Linkman - Assn. of Anaesthetics of G.B. & Irel. 1999-to date; Local Negotiating Chairm. - Doncaster & Bassetlaw Hosps. Prev: Sen. Regist. Sheff. Gp. of Hosps.; Regist. (Anaesth.) Roy. Cornw. Hosp. Truro; Ho. Phys. Lond. Hosp.

RAITHATHA, Meera Mahendra 59 Kensington Avenue, Watford WD18 7RZ Tel: 01923 240462 — MB ChB Bristol 1995. SHO Rotat. (Paediat.) Nottm. QMC. Specialty: Paediat. Prev: SHO (Paediat.) Smithmead Bristol Cheltenham.

RAITHATHA, Nitesh University of East Anglia Health Centre, University of East Anglia, Earlham Road, Norwich NR4 7TJ Tel: 01603 592172; Rivendell Cottage, The St, Colton, Norwich NR9 5AB — MB BS Lond. 1987; BSc Lond. 1984; MRCGP 1991; DRCOG 1991. Prev: Trainee GP Taunton VTS.

RAITHATHA, Raju — MB BS Lond. 1983 (St. Bart.) BSc (Immunol. Physiol.) Lond. 1980; LMSSA Lond. 1983; DRCOG 1986; LMCC 1990.

RAITT, David Gordon Directorate of Anaesthesia, Leicester General Hospital, Gwendolen Road, Leicester LE5 4PW — MB ChB Aberd. 1969; DA Eng. 1973; FFA RCS Eng. 1976. Cons. & Clin. Dir. (Anaesth.) Univ. Hosp.s of Leicester NHS Trust. Specialty: Anaesth. Prev: Sen. Specialist (Anaesth.) RAF Med. Br.; Med. Director, Leicester Gen. Hosp..

RAITT, Elspeth Jane 25 Harcourt Road, Altrincham WA14 1NR — MB ChB Leic. 1991; MRCGP 1996. GP Locum, Chesh. Specialty: Gen. Pract.

RAITT, George Price (retired) — MB ChB St. And. 1963; DObst RCOG 1965; MRCGP 1973. Mem. Cumbria LMC. Prev: GP Princip. Eden Med. Pract. Carlisle.

RAITT, Neil Woodroffe, Dixon and Raitt, Ravenswood Surgery, New Road, Forfar DD8 2AE Tel: 01307 463558 Fax: 01307 468900 — BM BS Nottm. 1988; DRCOG 1991; MRCGP 1992.

RAJ, Anita Aruna Dilmuir, Penstraze, Chasewater, Truro TR4 8PN — MB ChB Leeds 1996.

RAJ, Mr Dev Eye Department, Queen's Medical Centre, Derby Road, Nottingham NG7 2QH Tel: 0115 924 9924 Fax: 0115 970 4008; 5 Kindlewood Drive, Chilwell, Beeston, Nottingham NG9 6NE Tel: 0115 973 2288 Fax: 0115 973 2288 — MB BS Delhi 1972; FRCS Glas. 1980; FRCS Ed. 1980. Staff Grade (Ophth.) Qu. Med. Centre Nottm. Specialty: Ophth. Prev: Regist. Midl. Eye Hosp. Birm.

RAJ, Geeti Ramachandram 9 Elizabeth Road, Birmingham B13 8QH — MB ChB Leeds 1986; BSc (Hons.) Microbiol. Lond. 1981; DRCOG 1991; MRCGP 1999. Specialty: Gen. Pract.

RAJ, Inderjeet 32 Baylis Road, Slough SL1 3PJ Tel: 01753 538328 — MB BS Lond. 1993. SHO (Geriat. Med.) Hillingdon Hosp. Specialty: Gen. Psychiat.

RAJ, Latha St Martins Medical Centre, 21 Eastcote Road, Ruislip HA4 8BE Tel: 01895 632410 Fax: 01895 675058; 108 Aylesham Drive, Ickenham, Uxbridge UB10 8UD — MB BS Bangalor 1973 (Bangalore Med. Coll.) BSc Bangalore 1966, MB BS 1973. Specialty: Community Child Health. Socs: Med. Protec. Soc.

RAJ, Mani Whitfield Surgery, 123 Whitfield Drive, Dundee DD4 0DX Tel: 01382 508410 Fax: 01382 509808 — MB BS Osmania 1969. GP Dundee.

RAJ, Nag St Martins Medical Centre, 21 Eastcote Road, Ruislip HA4 8BE Tel: 01895 632410 Fax: 01895 675058; 108 Aylsham Drive, Ickenham, Uxbridge UB10 8UD Tel: 01895 637800 Fax: 01895 675058 — MB BS Bangalor 1967 (Bangalore Med. Coll.) MB BS Bangalore 1967. GP Princip. Specialty: Cardiol. Socs: Med. Protec. Soc.; MPS.

RAJ, Sanjay Prem Dilmuir, Penstraze, Chacewater, Truro TR4 8PN — MB BS Lond. 1998 (Roy. Free) MRCP UK. Specialty: Gen. Med.

RAJ, Shivanee Jayanthi 26 Stonor Road, London W14 8RZ Tel: 020 7371 6495 — MB BS Lond. 1993; BA Oxf. 1990. Specialty: Paediat.

RAJ, Sunita 23 Glebe Crescent, Rugby CV21 2HG — MB ChB Leeds 1997. SHO A & E, Dewsbury. Prev: SHO Med. For Elderly, Dewsbury; Ho. Off. (Surg.) ScarBoro.; Ho. Off. (Med.) Airedale.

RAJ, Suresh Kumar Union Hall Road Surgery, 55 Union Hall Road, Lemington, Newcastle upon Tyne NE15 8BP Tel: 0191 267 4894 — MB BS Agra 1965.

RAJ, Venkatachalum Babu 37 Orient Road, Salford M6 8LE Tel: 0161 789 3029 — MB BS Madras 1982; LMSSA Lond. 1988; MRCPI 1990; MRCP (UK) 1991; DRCOG 1994. Specialty: Gen. Med. Socs: Manch. Med. Soc.; BMA. Prev: Trainee GP Rotat. Liverp. VTS; Regist. (Geriat. Med.) Broadgreen Hosp. Liverp.

RAJA, Aman Ullah Khan The Park Lane Medical and Surgical Services, 625 Green Lane, Hornsey, London N8 0RE Tel: 01992 624732.

RAJA, Apoorvaa Surendra 3 Teasel Close, Narborough, Leicester LE19 3DZ — MB BS Lond. 1998; MB BS Lond 1998.

RAJA, Jowad Hussan 50 Gibson Road, Birmingham B20 3UE — MB ChB Ed. 1996.

RAJA, Mr Mohammad Ashraf Khan 6 Harman Drive, London NW2 2EB Email: rajamak@yahoo.com — MB BS Punjab 1984 (King Edward Medical College, Lahore, Pakistan) BSc Punjab 1981; FCPS Pakistan 1991; FRCSI 1991; FRCS Eng. 1992; MSc (Surg. Sci.) Lond. 1996; Dip. Med. Educat. (Gen. Surg.) 1998, (Med.) 1997; FRCS (Gen) 1998. Specialist Regist. (Gen. Surg.) St. Geo.'s Hosp. Lond. Specialty: Gen. Surg. Socs: Roy. Soc. Med.; ASME. Prev: Specialist Regist. Worthing Hosp.; Specialist Regist. St Peter's Hosp. Chertsey; Research Fell. Univ. of Lond.

RAJA, Rakesh Forge Cottage, The Street, Horringer, Bury St Edmunds IP29 5RY — MB ChB Birm. 1992; BSc (Hons.) Med. Biochem. Birm. 1989; MRCP UK 1998; MRCGP 1999. Gp, Sudbury, Suff.; Pharmaceutical Cons.

RAJA, Rameshchandra Shamalji Radiology Department, Rochdale Infirmary, Whitehall Street, Rochdale OL12 0NB; 7 Beaumonds Way, Bamford, Rochdale OL11 5NL Tel: 01706 639355 Fax: 01706 639355 — MB ChB Makerere 1971; FRCR 1977; DMRD Lond. 1977. Cons. Radiol. Rochdale Infirm.; Clin. Director, (Clin. Area Team Lead) - Radiol., Pennine Acute Hosps. NHS Trust, Rochdale. Specialty: Radiol. Socs: Roy. Coll. Radiol. & Brit. Inst. Radiol.; BMI. Prev: Chairm. & Sen. Lect. (Diagn. Radiol.) Univ. Nairobi.; Clin. Dir. (Surg.).

RAJA, Uma Department Histopothology, St James's University Hospital, Beckett St., Leeds LS9 7TF Tel: 0113 206 4410; 51 Shelley Crescent, Oulton, Leeds LS26 8ER — MB BS Bangalore 1982 (St. John's Med. Con.) MRCPath cond. Cons. Path. (Histopah.) St. Jas. Hosp. Leeds. Specialty: Histopath. Socs: Brit. Soc. Cervical Cyno. Prev: Sen. Regist. Rotat. Leeds.

RAJAB, Hedjaz 18 Beaulieu Close, Frampton Road, Hounslow TW4 5EN — MB BS West Indies 1983; DTM RCSI 1992; FRCS 1997; MCH 1997; Cert Av Med 1998. Research Fell. Specialty: Trauma & Orthop. Surg.; Accid. & Emerg.; Occupat. Health.

RAJABALI, Shaheen 2 Manor Road, Harrow HA1 2PB Tel: 020 8861 1598; Flat 15, 2A Addington Road, Reading RG1 5PH Tel: 01734 878601 — MB BS Lond. 1995 (Univ. Coll. Lond.) BSc (Hons.) Lond. 1992. Trainee GP/SHO Reading VTS. Prev: Ho. Off. (Surg.) Thanet NHS Healthcare Trust; Ho. Off. (Med.) Mayday Healthcare NHS Trust.

RAJACK, Sacha Marie c/o Flat 2F2, 42 Spottiswoode Road, Edinburgh EH9 1DB — MB ChB Ed. 1998; MB ChB Ed 1998.

RAJADURAI, Veeravagu (retired) 40 Etonville Road, London SW17 7SL — MB BS Ceylon 1943 (Colombo) DTM & H Ceylon 1952. Asst. in Psychiat. Darenth Pk. Hosp. Dartford. Prev: Asst. Med. Off. Lond. Boro. Bexley.

RAJAGOPAL, Rajavalse Venkateshan 16 Warrington Spur, Windsor SL4 2NF Tel: 01753 864784 — MB BS Mysore 1968 (Govt. Med. Coll. Mysore) BSc Mysore 1960. Clin. Asst. (Psychiat.) St. Peters Hosp. Chertsey. Specialty: Geriat. Psychiat.

RAJAGOPAL, Ramesh Flat 11, Park House, 150 Palatine Road, Manchester M20 2QH — MB ChB Liverp. 1994.

RAJAGOPAL AROKIADASS, Sujaa Mary Hillingdon Hospital, Woodland centre, Pieldheath Road, Uxbridge UB8 3NN Tel: 01895 238282 Fax: 01895 279718 — MB BS Dr M GR University 2001. Sen. Ho. Off. (Geriat. Psychiat.) Hillingdon Hosp. Uxbridge.

RAJAGOPALAN, Bheeshma Nuffield Dept of Clinical Medicine, John Radcliffe Hospital, Oxford OX3 1UT Tel: 01865 64711 — BM BCh Oxf. 1968; DPhil Oxf. 1977, BA 1964, MA, BM BCh 1968; MRCP (UK) 1971. Clin. Sci. Med. Research Counc. & Hon. Cons. Phys. John Radcliffe Hosp. Oxf.; Reader (Med.) Univ. of Oxf.; Reader Med. 1997. Specialty: Gen. Med. Socs: Brit. Cardiac Soc. & Assn. Phys. Gt. Brit. & Irel. Prev: Med. Tutor Univ. Oxf.; Lect. (Med.) Univ. Oxf. & Hon. Sen. Regist. Oxon AHA (T); Med. Tutor Univ. Manch. & Hon. Regist. Manch. Roy. Infirm.

RAJAGOPALAN, Narayanan (retired) 3 The Limes, Water Lane, Castor, Peterborough PE5 7BH Tel: 01733 380709 — MB BS Madras 1954 (Madras Med. Coll.) BSc Madras 1948. Prev: GP P'boro.

RAJAH, Abid 41 Prospect Lane, Harpenden AL5 2PL — MB ChB Liverp. 1977; FRCA,FRARCSI. Cons. (Anaesth & Director of Intens. Care) Hemel Hempstead Hosp.

RAJAH, Moossajee Ibrahim I (retired) c/o Drive I. Barmania, 318 High Road, Leytonstone, London E11 3HS — LRCP LRCS Ed. 1940 (Roy. Colls. Ed.) LRCP LRCS Ed. LRFPS Glas. 1940.

RAJAH, Prins Arumugam Neelaranjitha 5 Cypress Close, Blackwell, Darlington DL3 8QR Tel: 01325 380300 — MB BS Ceylon 1966; MRCOG 1977; MRCS Eng. LRCP Lond. 1979; Dip. Ven. Soc. Apoth. Lond. 1982; FRCOG 1998. Cons. Genitourin. Med. Darlington Memor. Hosp. Specialty: Genitourinary Medicine.

RAJAH, Vignesh 13A Fairview Road, Chigwell IG7 6HN — MB BS Lond. 1990 (UMDS Guy's and St Thomas's) MRCP (UK) Lond.; DCH Lond. 1995. Specialist Regist. (Paediat.) All St.'s Hosp. Medway NHS Trust Kent. Specialty: Paediat. Prev: Resid. (Paediat. IC) Guy's Hosp. Lond.; SHO (Paediat.) Lewisham Hosp. Lond.

RAJAKARIAR, Ravindra Flat 4, 26 Pelham Road, London SW19 1SX — MB ChB Leic. 1995.

RAJAKARUNA, Chanaka Sandaruwan Postgraduate Deans Office, Faculty of Medicine, Robert Kilpatrick Clinical Sciences Building, Leicester Royal Infirmary, PO Box 65, Leicester LE2 7LX — MB ChB Leic. 1998; MB ChB Leic 1998.

RAJAKULASINGAM, Karalasingam Homerton University Hospital NHS Foundation Trust, Department of Respiratory Medicine/Allergy, Homerton Row, London E9 6SR Tel: 020 8510 7769 Email: raja.rajakulasingam@homerton.nhs.uk — MB BS Colombo 1982 (Univ. of Colombo) MRCP (UK) 1988; DM Soton 1996; FRCP 2001; FACP 2001. Cons. Respirat. Phyisician & Hon. Sen. Lect. Specialty: Gen. Med.; Respirat. Med. Socs: Amer. Coll.of Phys.s. & Brit. Thoracic Soc.; Bma. Prev: Sen. Regist. (Allergy, Immunol. & Thoracic Med.) Roy. Brompton Hosp. Lond.; Clin. Research Fell. & Hon. Regist. (Med.) Soton. Gen. Hosp.; Regist. (Gen. & Chest Med.) Hope Hosp. Salford.

RAJAKULENDRAN, Thambimuthu Woodfarm Health Centre, Leiden Road, Headington, Oxford OX3 8RZ Tel: 01865 762 500 — MB BS Ceylon 1973 (University of Ceylon Colombo, Sri Lanka) MRCS Eng. LRCP Lond. 1981; MRCOG 1985. GP. Specialty: Obst. & Gyn. Prev: Regist. (O & G) Univ. Hosp. of Wales Cardiff; Locum Cons. (O & G) S. Wales.

RAJAKUMAR, Rajaratnam Genitourinary Medicine Department, Derbyshire Royal Infirmary, London Road, Derby DE1 2QY Tel: 01332 347141 Fax: 01332 254872 Email: raj.rajakumar@sdah-tr.trent.nhs.uk — MB BS Sri Lanka 1972; MRCP (UK) 1983; LRCP LRCS Ed. LRCPS Glas. 1983. Cons. Genitourin. Med. Derbysh. Roy. Infirm. Specialty: Genitourinary Medicine. Special Interest: HIV Infection. Socs: BASHH.

RAJAKUMAR, Ratnasabapathy 22 Owen Gardens, Woodford Green IG8 8DJ — MB BS Sri Lanka 1974; LMSSA Lond. 1986.

RAJALINGAM, Usha Pavalalochana 16 Huntsmill, Fulbourn, Cambridge CB1 5RH — BM BS Flinders 1993.

RAJAMANOHARAN, Sasikala Watford General Hospital, Watford Sexual Health Centre, Vicarage Road, Watford WD18 9HB Tel: 01923 217319 — FRCP, MSc, DipGUM, DFFP; MB BS Colombo 1983. Cons. Genitourin. Med./HIV Watford Gen. Hosp./The Mortimer Market Centre; Thames Valley MREC Comm. Mem. Specialty: Genitourinary Medicine. Special Interest: Epidemiol.; Vulval Dis. Socs: MDU; BASHH.

RAJAMENON, Anusha 6 Hathaway Close, Bromley BR2 8RD — LRCP LRCS LRCPS Ed., Glas. 1998; LRCP Ed LRCS Ed LRCPS Glas 1998.

RAJAN, Govindan 83 Chevet Lane, Sandal, Wakefield WF2 6JE Tel: 01924 256342 — MB BS Madras 1950; BSc Madras 1944, MB BS 1950; FRCP Glas. 1981, M 1966. Cons. Paediatr. Yorks. RHA; Hon. Lect. Paediat. Univ. Leeds. Specialty: Paediat. Socs: BMA & Brit. Paediat. Assn. Prev: Sen. Regist. & Regist. Childr. Hosp. Stockton-on-Tees; Regist. (Paediat.) Inst. Paediat. Madras Med. Coll. Gen. Hosp.; India.

RAJAN, Kunnathur Thiruvenkatachari (retired) — (Christian Med. Coll. Vellore) BSc Madras 1951, MB BS 1958; DTCD Wales 1962; PhD Camb. 1970. Mem. Community Health Council,Cardiff-Welsh Assembly nomination; Providing ultrasound scanning to community. Prev: Cons., E. Glam. Gen. Hosp. Ch. Village.

RAJANATHAN, Ehamparanathan Irvine Unit, Bexhill Hospital, Holliers Hill, Bexhill-on-Sea TN40 2DZ Tel: 01424 755255 Ext: 5312; 32A Parkhurst Road, Bexhill-on-Sea TN40 1DE — MB BS Sri Lanka 1962; DPH Liverp. 1972. Clin. Med. Off. (Med. for Elderly) Bexhill Hosp. E. Sussex. Specialty: Care of the Elderly.

RAJANI, Bhavesh 7 Limetree Walk, Chorleywood, Rickmansworth WD3 4BX — MB ChB Manch. 1989. Trainee GP Edgware VTS.

RAJANI, Kanesh Keshavlal Ruh's Corner, 4 Potters Heights Close, Pinner Hill, Pinner HA5 3YW — MB ChB Manch. 1992.

RAJANI, Mukeshkumar Haridas Lister Medical Centre, Lister House, Staple Tye, Harlow CM18 7LU — MB BS Lond. 1976 (Westminster Medical School) MRCS Eng. LRCP Lond. 1976; DRCOG 1979; MRCGP 1980. Specialty: Gen. Pract.

RAJANI, Ronak 24 Malcolm Drive, Surbiton KT6 6QS — BM Soton. 1998.

RAJANI, Vakesh 7 Lime Tree Walk, Rickmansworth WD3 4BX — MB BS Lond. 1993.

RAJAP, Tuan Ilan 48 Ernest Grove, Beckenham BR3 3JF — MB BS Lond. 1994.

RAJAPAKSA, Mr Pathirannahelage Nima 20 Colts Road, Rownhams, Southampton SO16 8JX — MB BS Colombo 1980; FRCS Glas. 1990.

RAJAPAKSA, Rajapska A M Abercynon Health Centre, Abercynon, Mountain Ash CF45 4YB Tel: 01443 740447 Fax: 01443 740228.

RAJAPAKSA, Tusevnambi Jayatissa 211 Stoke Road, Slough SL2 5AX — MB BS Ceylon 1952; MRCPsych 1976. Cons. Psych. Med. St. Edwd.'s Hosp. Cheddleton. Specialty: Gen. Psychiat.

RAJAPAKSE, Indra (retired) — MB BS Ceylon 1967; Cert. Family Plann. JCC 1981.

RAJAPAKSE, Yasa Siri Bedfordshire Health, Charter House, Alma St., Luton LU1 2PL Tel: 01582 744898; 3 Farnham Way, Bedford MK41 8RE Tel: 01236 212107 — MB BS Ceylon 1963; DTPH 1971; MFCM RCP (UK) 1974; FFPHM RCP (UK) 1991. Cons. Pub. Health Med. Beds. Health Luton. Specialty: Pub. Health Med. Prev: SCMO N. Beds. HA; Med. Off. Health Anti Filariasis Campaign Colombo, Sri Lanka.

RAJAR, Ramzi Mark 1818 Great Western Road, Glasgow G13 2TN — MB ChB Dund. 1998; MB ChB Dund 1998.

RAJARATHNA SETTY, Raja Seetharamaiah (retired) Kiran, 47 Fairfield Drive, Burnley BB10 2PU Tel: 01282 425447 — (Kastruba Med. Coll.) MB BS Mysore 1966; DA Eng. 1972. Prev: Med. Asst. (Anaesth.) Burnley Gen. Hosp.

RAJARATNAM, Abharani 77 Ecton Avenue, Macclesfield SK10 1RA — MB BS Madras, India 1978.

RAJARATNAM, David Vinaya West Drive, Whalley Lane, Uplyme, Lyme Regis DT7 3UP — MRCS Eng. LRCP Lond. 1977; BSc (Hons.) Lond. 1974, MB BS 1977.

RAJARATNAM, Giridharan Department of Public Health Medicine, Bradford Health Authority, New Mill, Victoria Road, Shipley BD18 3LD Tel: 01274 366080 Fax: 01274 366060 — MB BS Lond. 1981; MSc Lond. 1986; MFCM 1989. Cons. Pub. Health Med. Bradford HA. Specialty: Pub. Health Med. Prev: Lect. (Epidemiol. & Community Med.) Univ. Wales Coll. Med.; Trainee (Community Med.) NW Thames RHA.

RAJARATNAM, Mr Koppada Department of Orthopaedics, Macclesfield District General Hospital, Victoria Road, Macclesfield SK10 3BL Tel: 01625 661316 Fax: 01625 663153; Ashramam, 77 Ecton Avenue, Macclesfield SK10 1RA — MB BS Sri Venkateswara 1975 (Kurnool Med. Coll., India) DOrth 1979; MChOrth Liverp. 1991; MS (Orth) 1 9831. Assoc. Specialist (Orthop. & Trauma) Macclesfield Dist. Gen. Hosp. Specialty: Orthop. Socs: Brit. Orthop. Assn.; BMA; World Orthop. Concern.

RAJARATNAM, Muralidharan Lister House Surgery, The Common, Hatfield AL10 0NL — MB ChB Manch. 1988. Trainee GP Burton on Trent.

RAJARATNAM, Saroja Thavapalan and Partners, 55 Little Heath Road, Bexleyheath DA7 5HL Tel: 01322 430129 Fax: 01322 440949 — MB BS Sri Lanka 1978; MB BS Sri Lanka 1978; LRCP LRCS Ed. LRCPS Glas. Edinburgh & Glasgow 1983.

RAJASANSIR, Jagatjit Gurjeet Singh The Surgery, Block Lane, Chadderton, Oldham OL9 7SG Tel: 0161 620 2321 — MB ChB Manch. 1985; BSc St. And. 1982. Trainee GP/SHO GP Oldham HA VTS.

RAJASEKARAN, Mr Jeyachandran 11 Tunnel Wood Road, Watford WD17 4SN; 43 Rainford Road, Edison NJ 08820, USA Tel: 00 1 732 767 1444 Fax: 00 1 732 767 1444 — MB BS Madurai 1974; FRCS Eng. 1981; FRCS Ed. 1981; FRCS Glas. 1981. Pres. Jersey City Med. Center New Jersey, USA. Specialty: Urol.

RAJASEKHARA, Kori Siddabasappa (Surgery), 259 Hainton Avenue, Grimsby DN32 9JX Tel: 01472 342570 Fax: 01472 250404 — MB BS Karnatak 1960; DO RCS Lond. 1970; DOMS Karnatak 1996. Hosp. Pract. (Ophth.) Grimsby. Specialty: Ophth.

RAJASINGAM, Daghni 42 Almorah Road, Hounslow TW5 9AD — MB BS Lond. 1990. Research Fell. Qu. Charlottes Hosp. Lond.

RAJASUNDARAM, S Tudor Way Surgery, 42 Tudor Way, Orpington BR5 1LH Tel: 01689 820268 Fax: 01689 839414.

RAJATHURAI, Alvappillai Doncaster Royal Infirmary, Armthorpe Road, Doncaster DN2 5NL Tel: 01302 366666; 3 Riding Close, Bessacarr, Doncaster DN4 6UZ — MB BS Ceylon 1971; MRCP (UK) 1979; MRCS Eng. LRCP Lond. 1979; FRCP Lond. 1994. Cons. Phys. (c/o the Elderly) Doncaster Roy. Infirm. Specialty: Gen. Med. Socs: Brit. Geriat. Soc.

RAJATHURAI, Thirumaran 3 Ridings Close, Doncaster DN4 6UZ — BM BS Nottm. 1998; BM BS Nottm 1998.

RAJAYOGESWARAN, Srirangini 80 Tyron Way, Sidcup DA14 6AZ Tel: 020 8300 8590 — MB BS Ceylon 1971 (Med. Coll. Peradenia) DCH RCP Lond. 1990. Clin. Med. Off. (Child Health) Greenwich HA. Socs: BMA & Nat. Assn. Family Plann. Doctors. Prev: SHO (Neonat. Paediat. & Gen. Paediat.) Gloucester Roy. Hosp.; Ho. Off. (Surg.) & Ho. Off. (Gen. Med.) Base Hosp. Gampaha, Ceylon.

RAJBEE, Faisal Tariq 38 Little Ridge Avenue, St Leonards-on-Sea, St Leonards-on-Sea TN37 7LS — MB BS Lond. 1997.

RAJBEE, Tariq Yusuf The Surgery, 38 Little Ridge Avenue, St Leonards-on-Sea TN37 7LS Tel: 01424 755355 Fax: 01424 755560 — DAB, Lond. 2000; MB BS Bihar 1965 (Darbhanga Med. Coll.) Princip. GP Hastings; Police Surg. Specialty: Gen. Med. Prev: Regist. (Surg.) JLN Med. Coll. Aligarh, India; SHO (Cas.) Staffs. Gen. Infirm. Stafford; SHO (Orthop.) Cumbld. Infirm. Carlisle.

RAJBHANDARI, Satyan Man 5 High Leys Drive, Priory Wood, Ravenshead, Nottingham NG15 9HQ; 17D Highnam Crescent Road, Sheffield S10 1BZ — MB BS Sambalpur 1989; MRCP (UK) 1993. Regist. (Gen. Med., Diabetes & Endocrinol.) Roy. Hallamsh. Hosp. Sheff. Specialty: Diabetes. Prev: Regist. (Gen. Med., Diabetes & Endocrinol.) Chesterfield Roy. Hosp. N. Derbysh.

RAJENDRA, Barathi 35 Greenfield Street, Dunkirk, Nottingham NG7 2JN — BM BS Nottm. 1995.

RAJENDRA, Shanmugarajam Flat 17, Brodie House, District General Hospital, Kings Drive, Eastbourne BN21 2YE — MB BCh BAO NUI 1988; LRCPSI 1988; MRCP (UK) 1993.

RAJENDRAM, Ranjan 41 Aelxandra Road, Hounslow TW3 4HW — MB BS Lond. 1996.

RAJENDRAM, Saddanather Doctors Mess, Tameside General Hospital, Fountain St., Ashton-under-Lyne OL6 9RW — MB BS Ceylon 1971.

RAJENDRAN, Sasha 4 Windsor Place, Dundee DD2 1BG — MB ChB Leic. 1992. SHO (O & G) Leicester Gen. Hosp. Prev: SHO (O & G) Leicester Roy. Infirm.; SHO (Neonat.) Leicester Gen. Hosp. & Leicester Roy. Infirm.

RAJENDRAN, Vijayaraghavan 9 Alford Road, High Wycombe HP12 4PT Tel: 01494 450827 — MB BS Madras 1977; MD Madras 1981; MRCP (UK) 1983.

RAJESH, Mr Pala Babu Regional Department of Thoracic Surgery, Birmingham Heartlands Hospital, Bordesley Green E., Birmingham B9 5SS Tel: 0121 424 2000 Fax: 0121 424 0562; 56 Arthur Road, Edgbaston, Birmingham B15 2UN Tel: 0121 440 1027 — MB BS Madras 1974 (Madras Med. Coll.) FRCS Ed. 1982; FRCS (Cth.) 1994; FETCS 2001. Cons. Thoracic. Surg. Birm. Heartlands Hosp. Specialty: Cardiothoracic Surg. Socs: Eur. Assn. for Cardiothoracic Surg.; Soc. Cardiothoracic Surg. GB & Irel. Prev: Hon. Sen. Regist. (Cardiothoracic Surg.) North. Gen. Hosp. Sheff.; Regist. N. Gen. Hosp. Sheff.; Regist. (Cardiothoracic Surg.) Castle Hill Hosp. Cottingham.

RAJESHWAR, Kasam The Surgery, New Road, Brownhills, Walsall WS8 6AT Tel: 01543 373214 Fax: 01543 454591 — MB BS Osmania 1965.

RAJESHWAR, Mahesh Honeywood, 3 The Fordrough, Sutton Coldfield B74 2XS — MB ChB Manch. 1997.

RAJI, Adil Mahmud 139 Harley Street, London W1G 6BG; 20 Alexandra Road, Hornsey, London N8 0PP — MB ChB Baghdad 1967. Gen. & Orthop. Surg. Lond.

RAJIV, Kumar 111 Thorpe Road, Peterborough PE3 6JQ — MRCP (UK); MB BS (Honours); MD (General Medicine); MSc (London). Assoc. Specialist in Diabetic and Cardiovasc. Med. Special Interest: Diabetic Cardiovasc. Dis.

RAJJAYABUN, Mr Paul Hosie 2A Vine Close, Clifton, Brighouse HD6 4JS Tel: 01484 719972 — MB ChB Birm. 1994; ChB Birm. 1994; FRCS Ed. 1998. 1999, Sen. SHO (Urology) City Hosp., Sunderland; 2000, Research Fell. in Urological Surg., Cancer Reseach Unit, Newc. upon Tyne; 2002, Specialist Regist. (Urology) W. Midlands Deanery. Specialty: Urol. Socs: BMA; MPS. Prev: SHO (Orthop. Trauma) Worc. Roy. Infirm.; SHO (Cardiac Surg.) Walsgrave Hosp.; SHO (Gen. Surg.) Walsgrave Hosp.

RAJKUMAR, Shivnathram The Medical Centre, 78 Oswald Road, Scunthorpe DN15 7PG Tel: 01724 843168 — MB BS Bombay 1975.

RAJLAWOT, Ganesh Pratap Flat 3, 22 Falkner Square, Liverpool L8 7NY Tel: 0151 708 8153 — MB BS Agra 1961 (Sarojini Naidu Med. Coll.) DA Agra 1963; DA Copenhagen 1972; DCH RCPSI 1981. Prev: SHO (Paediat. Med.) Leicester Gen. Hosp., Bradford Gp. Hosps. & Alder; Hey Childr. Hosp. Liverp.

RAJPURA, A I Earlsheaton Medical Centre, 252 Wakefield Road, Earlsheaton, Dewsbury WF12 8AH Tel: 01924 465511 — MRCS Eng. LRCP Lond. London; MB BS Gujarat 1972; MB BS Gujarat 1972.

RAJPURA, Anjum 79 Track Road, Batley WF17 7AB — MB ChB Birm. 1992.

RAJPURA, Arif Cheriton, 79 Track Rd, Batley WF17 7AB — MB ChB Manch. 1996.

RAJPUT, Karim Sultan 55 Portland Road, Edgbaston, Birmingham B16 9HS — MB ChB Manch. 1995. SHO (Psychiat.) All St.s Hosp. Birm. Prev: Ho. Surg. (Vasc.) Selly Oak Hosp. Birm.; Ho. Surg. (ENT) Qu. Eliz. Hosp. Birm.; Ho. Phys. Selly Oak Hosp. Birm.

RAJPUT, Mrs Kaukab Mufti Dept. of Audiological Medicine, Great Ormond Street Hospital, Great Ormond St., London WC1 3JH Tel: 0207 813 8316 Fax: 0207 833 2208; Lynfield House, Wexham St, Stoke Poges, Slough SL3 6PA Tel: 01753 663576 Fax: 01753 663576 Email: kaukab@globalnet.co.uk — MB BS Sind, Pakistan 1982; LRCP LRCS Ed. LRCPS Glas. Glas. 1987; LRCP LRCS Ed. LRCPS Glas. 1987; FRCS Glas. 1992; FRCS Glas. 1992; MSc Lond. 1995; MSc Lond. 1995. Cons. Specialty: Audiol. Med. Socs: Btritish Assoc. of Audiological Phys.; Brit. Cochlear Implant Gp.; Internat. Assoc. of Audiological Phys.

RAJPUT, Pranjivandas Bhagwandas 361 Chingford Road, Walthamstow, London E17 5AE Tel: 020 8925 4229 — MB BS Bombay 1958; DLO RCS Eng. 1967. Specialty: Otolaryngol.

RAJPUT, Rais Ahmed Dosthill and Wilnecote Street Surgery, 45 Cadogan Road, Dosthill, Tamworth B77 1PQ Tel: 01827 280800 Fax: 01827 261569; 22 Orchard Close, Dosthill, Tamworth B77 1ND — MB BS Sind 1971.

RAJPUT, Ranbir Singh 27 Daventry Road, Coventry CV3 5DJ — BM BS Nottm. 1993; BMedSci. Nottm. 1991.

RAJPUT, Satpal Springfield Medical Practice, 739-741 Stratford Road, Springfield, Birmingham B11 4DG Tel: 0121 778 4321 Fax: 0121 702 2662 — MB ChB Leic. 1984; Cert Family Plann. JCC 1987; DRCOG 1989. Prev: SHO (O & G, Gen. Med., Gen. Paediat.) Coventry HA.

RAJPUT, Vijay Kumar Springfield Medical Practice, 739-741 Stratford Road, Springfield, Birmingham B11 4DG Tel: 0121 778 4422 Fax: 0121 702 2662; 36 Inverclyde Road, Handsworth Ward, Birmingham B20 2LJ Tel: 0121 554 6741 — MB ChB Leic. 1983 (Univ. Leic.) Cert. Family Plann. JCC 1986; DRCOG 1987; Cert. JCPTGP 1988; MRCGP 1989. Med. Assessor SSAT; Mem. Disabil. Appeals Tribunal. Specialty: Gen. Pract. Prev: Clin. Asst. (Diabetes & Endocrinol.) Dudley Rd. Hosp.; Clin. Asst. (Psychiat.) All St.s Hosp.; Clin. Asst. (ENT) Heartlands Hosp.

RAJPUT, Vije Kumar Stoneydelph Medical Centre, Ellerbeck, Stoneydelph, Tamworth B77 4JA — MB ChB Manch. 1984; DObst. RCOG 1987; MRCGP 1988.

RAJSHEKHAR, Math Sangaya 19 Crooklog, Bexleyheath DA6 8DZ Tel: 020 8304 3025 — MB BS Osmania 1953 (Osmania Med. Coll. Hyderabad)

RAJU, Chintalapati Sanyasi (retired) Woodley Health Centre, Hyde Road, Woodley, Stockport SK6 1ND Tel: 0161 430 2466 Fax: 0161 406 8218 — MB BS Andhra 1967; MB BS Andhra 1967.

RAJU, Katari Singa Department of Psychiatry, Pembury Hospital, Tonbridge Road, Pembury, Tunbridge Wells TN2 4RT; 98 Headcorn Drive, Canterbury CT2 7TR — MB BS Andhra 1969; MB BS Andhra India 1969; DCH RCP Lond. 1976.

RAJU, Mr Thakur Das Yeading Court Practice, 1-2 Yeading Court, Masefield Lane, Hayes UB4 5AJ Tel: 020 8845 1515 Fax: 020 8841 1171 — LRCP LRCS Ed. 1986; MB BS Guru Nanak Dev 1977; MRCS Eng. LRCP Lond. 1986; LRCP LRCS Ed. LRCPS Glas. 1986; FRCS Ed. 1990.

RAJVANSHI, Reeta 1A Bexley Lane, Sidcup DA14 4JW — MB BS Lucknow 1966.

RAKE, Mark Oliver The Barn, Pontus Farm, Molash, Canterbury CT4 8HW Tel: 01233 740728 — MB BS Lond. 1963 (Guy's) BSc (Anat.) Lond. 1960; MRCS Eng. LRCP Lond. 1963; FRCP Lond. 1979, M 1968. Dean Kent Inst. Med. & Health Sci. Specialty: Gastroenterol. Socs: Brit. Soc. Gastroenterol. & Brit. Soc. Digestive Endoscopy.; ASME; AMEE. Prev: Cons. Phys. Kent & Canterbury Hosp.; Sen. Regist. Guy's Hosp. Lond.; Research Fell. Liver Unit King's Coll. Hosp.

RAKHIT, Anita 65 Hall Drive, London SE26 6XL — MB BS Lond. 1998; MB BS Lond 1998.

RAKHIT, Apurba Kumar 76 Market Street, Droylsden, Manchester M43 7UD Tel: 0161 370 2626; 12 Thornley Lane, Grotton, Oldham OL4 5RP Tel: 0161 624 6800 — MB BS Calcutta 1959 (Calcutta Nat. Med. Inst.) DPH Manch. 1964. Sec. Tameside LMC Ashton-under-Lyne. Specialty: Alcohol & Substance Misuse. Socs: BMA. Prev: Ho. Surg. Oldham Dist. Hosp.; Dep. MOH Saddelworth UD; Asst. Phys. Gen. Hosp. Ashton-under-Lyne.

RAKHIT, Dhrubo Jyoti — MB BS Lond. 1993; MRCP (UK) 1997. Specialist Regist. Cardiol. N. W. Thames. Specialty: Cardiol.

RAKHIT, Durgadas 4 Exmouth Place, Gourock PA19 1JE Tel: 01475 796714 — MB BS Calcutta 1967; MD Calcutta 1975; MRCOG Lond. 1984; DRCOG Lond. 1984. Assoc. Specialist (O & G) Inverclyde Roy. Hosp. Greenock. Specialty: Obst. & Gyn.

RAKHIT, Moona Kaberi 42 Copthall Lane, Gerrards Cross SL9 0DG; Kingscliffe, Bull Lane, Gerrards Cross SL9 8RF — MB BS Lond. 1989 (Charing Cross and Westminster) MRCGP 1996. Specialty: Gen. Pract.; Family Plann. & Reproduc. Health.

RAKHIT, Roby Devasish Department of Cardiology, The Rayne Institute, St Thomas's Hospital, Lambeth Palace Road, London SE1 7EH; 7 Cyprus Avenue, Finchley, London N3 1SS — MB BS Lond. 1991 (Char. Cross & Westm.) BSc (Hons.) Pharmacol. Lond. 1989; MRCP (UK) 1995. Research Regist. (Cardiol.) St. Thomas's Hosp. Lond. Specialty: Cardiol. Socs: Brit. Soc. Cardiovasc. Research; BMA; Brit. Soc. Echocardiogr. Prev: Regist. (Cardiol.) Roy. Brompton Hosp. Lond.; Regist. (Cardiol.) Hammersmith Hosp. Lond.; SHO (Neurol.) Nat. Hosp. Qu. Sq. Lond.

RAKHIT, Sreeharsha (retired) Arghya, 3 Squires Croft, Woodway Park, Coventry CV2 2RQ Tel: 024 76 612258 — MB BS Calcutta 1962 (R.G. Kar Med. Coll.) DGO Calcutta 1964; DObst RCOG 1972; DA Eng. 1974; BSc Calcutta 1956, MD (Alternative Med.) 1990; DFFP 1993; FRSH 1996.

RAKHIT, Tuhina 6 Langstrath Drive, West Bridgford, Nottingham NG2 6SD — BM BS Nottm. 1995.

RAKICKA, Helena Tameside General Hospital, Fountain Street, Ashton-under-Lyne OL6 9RW — MUDr Univ. Safarikova Czechoslovakia 1969; MUDr Univ. Safarikova, Czechoslovakia 1969; MRCP (UK) 1992; FRCP Lond. 2001. Cons. Phys. (c/o Elderly) Tameside Gen. Hosp. Ashton-under-Lyne. Specialty: Care of the Elderly. Prev: Regist. (Gen. & Geriat. Med.) Tameside Gen. Hosp. Ashton-under-Lyne.

RAKOWICZ, Anna Stefania Acorn Surgery, 136 Meeting House Lane, London SE15 2TT Tel: 020 7639 5055 Fax: 020 7732 4225; 102 Wood Vale, London SE23 3ED Tel: 020 8693 4732 — MB BS Lond. 1962 (Roy. Free) Socs: BMA. Prev: Ho. Surg. Eliz. G. Anderson Hosp. Lond.; Ho. Phys. S. Lond. Hosp. Wom. Clapham.

RAKOWICZ, Stefan Pawel Dysart House Surgery, 13 Ravensbourne Road, Bromley BR1 1HN Tel: 020 8464 0718 — MB BS Lond. 1990 (King's Coll. Sch. Med. & Dent.) BSc Lond. 1987; MRCGP 1994.

RAKOWICZ, Wojciech Piotr Dept. of Neurology, Washington University School of Medicine, Box 8228, 660 S.Euxlid Ave, St Louis MO 63110, USA Email: rakoviczw@neuro.wustl.edu; 102 Wood Vale, London SE23 3ED — MB BS Lond. 1990; BSc (Hons.) Lond. 1987, MB BS 1990; AKC Lond. 1990; MRCP (UK) 1993. Research Fell.(Neurol), Univ. of Camb. Specialty: Neurol. Socs: MDU; BMA. Prev: Regist. (Psychiat.) Maudsley Hosp. Lond.; Regist. (Med.) Poole Hosp.; SHO (Neurol.) Nat. Hosp. for Neurol. & Neurosurg. Lond.

RAKOWSKI, Jane Helene 94 Victoria Road, Formby, Liverpool L37 1LP Tel: 01704 872293 — MB ChB Liverp. 1979 (Liverpool) DCH Eng. 1981; DRCOG 1984; DPD Cardiff 1997. GP Formby; Clin. Asst. in Dermat., Roy. Liverp. Hosp. Specialty: Gen. Pract. Prev: GP Southport, Cardiff & Liverp.

RAKSHI, Jimmy Sajal 24 Westbere Road, London NW2 3SR — MB ChB Aberd. 1988.

RAKSHIT, Bhim Chandra Kings Road Surgery, 133 Kings Road, Blackburn BB2 4PY Tel: 01254 201269 Fax: 01254 200717 — MB BS Calcutta 1969.

RAKUS, Marguerita Roma Flat A, 34 Hans Road, London SW3 1RW Tel: 020 7225 2016 — MB BS Sydney 1985.

RALEVIC, Danica 45 Mawson Road, Cambridge CB1 2DZ — MB BS Lond. 1986; BA (Natural Scs.) Camb. 1981.

RALFE, Simon William Huntersmoon, School Road, Riseley, Reading RG7 1XN — MB ChB Birm. 1996; BSc 1993; ChB Birm. 1996; MBChB Birm 1996. Med. Rotat., Qu.'s Hosp. Burton-upon-Trent. Specialty: Gen. Med. Socs: Roy. Coll. Phys.s.

RALFS, Ian George William Harvey Hospital, Kennington Road, Willesborough, Ashford TN2 0LZ — MB ChB Liverp. 1970; FRCP; MRCP (UK) 1974; MSc (Immunol.) Birm. 1976; FRCP Lond. 1996. Cons. Dermat. William Harvey Hosp. Ashford. Specialty: Dermat.

RALHAN, Rekha Unsworth Medical Centre, Parr Lane, Unsworth, Bury BL9 8JR — MB ChB Dundee 1989; DRCOG 1993. Specialty: Gen. Pract.

RALL, Mathias Herbert 14 Firs Crescent, Kings Worthy, Winchester SO23 7NF — State Exam Med Freiburg 1990; State Exam Med. Freiburg 1990; DFFP 1995. Specialty: Gen. Pract.

RALLEIGH, Gita 42 Farm Avenue, Harrow HA2 7LR — MB BS Lond. 1993.

RALLI, Roger Alexander Medical Centre, HMYOI Glen Parva, Leicester LE18 4TN Tel: 0116 264 3101 Fax: 0116 264 3383 Email: roger.ralli@glenparva.hmpsha.nhs.uk — MB ChB Dundee 1976. Princip. Med. Off. Prison Dept. Home Off. Specialty: Civil Serv. Prev: Trainee GP Foyers VTS; Regist. (Psychiat.) Mapperley Hosp. Nottm.; Regist. (Anaesth.) Pinderfields Hosp. Wakefield.

RALPH, Mr David John Institute of Urology, 48 Riding House Street, London W1P 7PN Tel: 020 7486 3805 Fax: 020 7486 3810 Email: dralph@andrology.co.uk — MB BS Lond. 1984 (St Bart.) BSc Lond. 1980; FRCS Ed. 1988; FRCS Eng. 1988; FRCS (Urol.) 1994; MS Lond. 1996. Cons. (Urol.) St. Peter's Hosps. & Inst. Urol. Lond. Specialty: Urol. Special Interest: Gender dysphoria; erectile dysfunction; male Infertil. Socs: Brit. Assn. Urol. Surgs.; Internat. Soc. Impotence Research; Eur. Soc. Impotence Research.

RALPH, Debra Jane The Surgery, 22 St. Anne's Terrace, London NW8 6PH Tel: 020 7722 7389 — MB BS Lond. 1989 (St. Mary's Hosp.) DRCOG 1991; DCH RCP Lond. 1992; DFFP 1994. Specialty: Gen. Pract.

RALPH, Ian 59A Melrose Avenue, Portslade, Brighton BN41 2LT — MB BS Lond. 1990.

RALPH, Ian Fraser Longacre, 193 Moorgate Road, Rotherham S60 3BA Tel: 01709 378407 — MB ChB Aberd. 1953; DPH Ed. 1959; MFCM 1974. Dist. Med. Off. Rotherham HA. Prev: Area Med. Off. Rotherham AHA; MOH & Princip. Sch. Med. Off. Co. Boro. Rotherham; Dep. MOH Co. Boro. Stockport.

RALPH, Stanley James Derbyshire Royal Infirmary, London Road, Derby DE1 2QY — MB BS Nottm. 1982; FFA RCS Eng. 1987. Cons. Anaesth. Derbysh. Roy. Infirm. Derby. Specialty: Anaesth. Prev: Sen. Regist. (Anaesth.) Sheff.; Fell. Inten. Care Univ. Hosp. Groningen Netherlands; SHO (Anaesth.) Nott.

RALPH, Stuart John 64 East Street, Ashburton, Newton Abbot TQ13 7AX — MB BS Lond. 1998.

RALPH, Susan Gwenda Department of Genitourinary Medicine, Sunny Bank Wing, Leeds General Infirmary, Great George St., Leeds LS1 2EX Tel: 0113 292 6762 Fax: 0113 292 6387; 1 Richmondfield Garth, Barwick in Elmet, Leeds LS15 4EP — MB ChB Sheff. 1988; MRCP (UK) 1993; Dip. GU Med. Soc. Apoth. Lond. 1995; DFFP 1995. Specialist Regist. (Genitourin. Med.) Leeds Gen. Infirm. Specialty: Genitourinary Medicine.

RALPH, William Henry c/o Lynfield Mount Hospital, Heights Lane, Bradford BD9 6DP — MB BCh BAO Dub. 1994 (Univ. Dub., Trinity Coll.) Demonst. (Anat.) Roy. Coll. Surgs. Irel., Dub. Socs: BMA.

RALPHS, Alwyn Thomas Raynor Wolstanton Medical Centre, Palmerston Street, Newcastle ST5 8BN Tel: 01785 57674 — MB ChB Birm. 1987; DRCOG 1991. Trainee GP Staffs.

RALPHS, Mr David Neil Lincoln 218 Unthank Road, Norwich NR2 2AH Tel: 01603 505463 Fax: 01603 505449 Email: ralphs@norwich.com — MB BChir Camb. 1966 (Middlx.) MA Camb. 1966; FRCS Eng. 1970. p/t Cons. Surg. Norf. & Norwich Hosp.; Pres. Brit. Assn. Of Day Surg. Specialty: Gen. Surg. Special Interest: Breast and Gastrointestinal Dis. Socs: Brit. Soc. Gastroenterol. & Brit. Assn. Surg. Oncol.; Brit. Assn. Day Surg.; Brit. Assn. Surg. Oncolo. Prev: Mem. Ct. Examrs. & Regional Adviser (Surg.) RCS Eng.; Sen. Lect. & Hon. Cons. Middlx. Hosp.; Regist. (Surg.) Kettering Gen. Hosp.

RALPHS, Glenn John Gareth Abbotswood Medical Centre, Defford Road, Pershore WR10 1HZ Tel: 01386 552424 — MB ChB Birm. 1976; DRCOG 1979. Chairm. Wychavon PCG.

RALSTON, Anthony James Withington Hospital, Nell Lane, Manchester M20 2LR — MB ChB Manch. 1956; FRCP Lond. 1974, M 1961. Cons. Phys. Withington Hosp. Manch. Specialty: Gen. Med.

RALSTON, Charles Scott Birmingham Childrens Hospital NHS Trust, Steelhouse Lane, Birmingham B4 6NH Tel: 0121 333 9999 — MB BS Lond. 1980; FFA RCS Eng. 1986. Cons. Paediat. Anaesth. & Intens. Care Birm. Childr. Hosp.; Hon. Sen. Lect. Birm. Univ. Specialty: Anaesth. Socs: Assn. Anaesth.; Assn. Paediat. Anaesth. Prev: Sen. Regist. (Anaesth.) W. Midl. Area Train. Scheme.

RALSTON, Mr David Robert Dept. Of Plastic & Reconstruc. Surg., Northern General Hospital, Sheffield S5 7AV — MB ChB Manch. 1986; FRCS Eng. 1991; MD Univ. Of Sheff. 1999; FRCS 1999. Cons. Plastic & Reconstruc. Surg., North. Gen. Hosp., Sheff..; Hon. Sen. Lect., Univ. Of Sheff. Specialty: Plastic Surg. Socs: Brit. Burn Assoc.

RALSTON, Mr Gavin James 67 Dundonald Road, Kilmarnock KA1 1TQ Tel: 01563 25225 — MB ChB Ed. 1939 (Univ. Ed.) MA Ed. 1932, LLB 1935, MB ChB 1939; FRCS Ed. 1946; FRCS Glas. 1971. Prev: Cons. Surg. Kilmarnock Infirm.

RALSTON, Gavin Robert Duthie Lordswood House, 54 Lordswood Road, Harborne, Birmingham B17 9DB Tel: 0121 426 2030 Fax: 0121 428 2658 — MB ChB Birm. 1984; DA (UK) 1986; DRCOG 1990; MRCGP 1991. Hon. Sen. Lect. (Gen. Pract.) Birm. Univ.

RALSTON, Safdar James The Beeches, 142 Caldy Road, Wirral CH48 1LN — MB ChB Aberd. 1986. Specialty: Anaesth.

RALSTON, Professor Stuart Hamilton University of Edinburgh, Rheumatic Diseases Unit, Western General Hospital, Edinburgh EH4 2XU Tel: 0131 5371088 Fax: 0131 5371051 — MB ChB Glas. 1978; MRCP (UK) 1980; MD Glas. 1987; FRCPS Glas. 1991; FRCPS Ed. 1994; Fmedsci 1999. ARC Prof. of Rheum. Univ. of Edin.; Edr. Calcified Tissue Internat. 2000-. Specialty: Gen. Med.; Rheumatol. Socs: (Past. Pres. 1998-99) Bone & Tooth Soc.; (Pres. 1997-) Europ. Calcified Tissues Soc. Prev: Prof. Med. & Hon. Cons. Phys. Univ. Aberd. Med. Sch.; Wellcome Sen. Research Fell. (Clin. Sci.) Univ. Edin.

RAM, Alison Jean The Medical Centre, 12 East King Street, Helensburgh G84 7QL Tel: 01436 672277 Fax: 01436 674526; 2 Woodland Street, Helensburgh G84 8DG Tel: 01436 679 860 — MB ChB Glas. 1986; MRCGP 1990; DRCOG 1990. GP Helensburgh.

RAM, Mr Shatrughna c/o Dr S. N. Prasad, 25 Poppleton Road, Tingley, Wakefield WF3 1UX — MB BS Patna 1974; FRCSI 1985; MChOrth Liverp. 1990.

RAMA MOHANA RAO, D Sorsby Health Centre, 3 Mandeville Street, Clapton, London E5 0DH Tel: 020 8986 5613 Fax: 020 8986 8072 — MB BS Andhra, India 1974 (Guntur Medical College) BSc. Gen. Practitioner. Socs: BMA.

RAMACHANDER, Chelluri Baburao 28 Top Cross Road, Bexhill-on-Sea TN40 2RT — MB BS Madras 1965.

RAMACHANDRA, Mr Channarayapatna Ramakrishna Setty Preston Hospital, Preston Road, North Shields NE29 0LR — MB BS Mysore 1959; FRCS Eng. 1966; DLO Eng. 1973. Cons. (OtolaryngOL.) Preston Hosp. N. Shields. Specialty: Otolaryngol. Prev: Sen. Regist. (Otolaryngol.) W. Midl. RHA; Regist. (Otolaryngol.) Singleton Hosp. Swansea; Surg. Regist. Moorgate Gen. Hosp. Rotherham.

RAMACHANDRA, Rattehalli Rangappa Walsgrave Hospital, Radiology Department, Clifford Bridge Road, Coventry CV2 2DX Tel: 024 7660 2020 Fax: 024 7684 4150; 4 Broadwells Court, Westwood Heath, Coventry CV4 8JX Tel: 024 7647 1988 Email: rattehalli@hotmail.com — MB BS Mysore 1974 (Kasturba Medical College) MD Mysore 1977; DMRD UK 1981; FFR RCSI 1983. Cons. (Radiol.) Walsgrave Hosp. Coventry. Specialty: Radiol.; Gen. Med. Special Interest: Breast Cancer Screening; Lung Cancer. Socs: Roy. Coll. Radiol.; Roy. Coll. Surg. Irel. Fac. of Radiol. (Fell.); BIDA. Prev: Cons. (Radiol.) Riyadh Nat. Hosp. Riyadh; Sen. Regist. Leicester Roy. Infirm. (Teachg.) Leicester.

RAMACHANDRA, Suvendrini Department of Clinical Microscopy, 2nd Floor, New Guy's House Guy's Hospital, St Thomas St., London SE1 9RT — MB BS Sri Lanka 1981; MRCPath (Histopath.) 1991. Sen. Regist. (Histopath.) Guy's & Lewisham Hosps. Lond. Specialty: Histopath.

RAMACHANDRA, Vinodhini c/o Directorate of AnaesthesiaThe North West London Hospitals NHS Trust, Northwick Park & St Mark's Hospitals, Harrow HA1 3UJ — MB BS Colombo 1980; DA RCS Eng. 1985; FFA RCS Eng. 1986. Cons. Anaesth. Northwick Pk. & St Mark's Hosp.s,Harrow. Specialty: Anaesth. Prev: Sen. Regist. (Anaesth.) Char. Cross Hosp. Lond., Hosp Sick Childr. Gt. Ormond St. & Roy. Surrey Co. Hosp. Guildford.

RAMACHANDRA RAJU, Kalidindi Westbrook Centre, 150 Canterbury Road, Margate CT9 5DD Tel: 01843 255622 — MB BS Mysore 1973 (Kasturba Med. Coll.) Assoc. Specialist (Psychiat.) Thanet Ment. Health Unit Margate; Locum Cons. Psychiat. Specialty: Gen. Psychiat. Prev: Clin. Asst. (Psychiat.) St. Augustine's Hosp. Chartham; Regist. (Psychiat.) Cherry Knowle Hosp. Ryhope.

RAMACHANDRA RAO, Vinnakota (retired) 24 Petersham Drive, Appleton, Warrington WA4 5QF — MB BS Andhra 1972.

RAMACHANDRAM, Raja Segar Moor Green Lane Medical Centre, 339 Moor Green Lane, Moseley, Birmingham B13 8QS Tel: 0121 472 6959 — MB BCh Wales 1983; DRCOG 1987; MRCGP 1988. GP Birm. Prev: Trainee GP Cardiff VTS.

RAMACHANDRAN, Mr Kannan 22 Cumberland Drive, Royton, Oldham OL2 5AX — MB BS Madras 1980; FRCSI 1996.

RAMACHANDRAN, Kumuthini Jenner House Surgery, 159 Cove Road, Farnborough GU14 0HH Tel: 01252 548141 Fax: 01252 371516 — LRCP LRCS Ed. LRCPS Glas. 1989.

RAMACHANDRAN, Mannath Kulangara The Haven, Sandown Road, Orsett, Grays RM16 4BB — MB BS Mysore 1970.

RAMACHANDRAN, Manoj 74 Station Road, London N3 2SA — MB BS Lond. 1996.

RAMACHANDRAN, Mr Nagalingam Department of Accident & Emergency, Watford General Hospital, Vicarage Road, Watford WD18 0HB — MB BS Ceylon 1959; FRCS Ed. 1971; MRCOG 1971.

RAMACHANDRAN, Nantha Kumaran 70 Peddie Street, Top Floor Flat, Dundee DD1 5LY — MB ChB Dundee 1992.

RAMACHANDRAN, Sreenivasa (retired) 23 Bolton Road, Salford M6 7HL Tel: 0161 736 1616; 9 Victoria Road, Salford M6 Tel: 0161 789 3722 — MB BS Kerala 1964 (Med. Coll. Trivandrum) Prev: Regist. Clare Hall Hosp. S. Mimms, Hartwood Hosp. Shotts & St.

RAMACHANDRAN, Sudarshan North Staffordshire Hospital Trust, North Staffordshire Hospital, Stoke-on-Trent ST4 6QG; 70 Sir Alfreds Way, Sutton Coldfield B76 1ET — MRCS Eng. LRCP Lond. 1990. Sen. Regist., Chem. Neurol., N. Staffs. Hosp. Trust.

RAMACHANDRAN, Sunita 20 Salcombe Lodge, Lissenden Gardens, London NW5 1LZ — MB ChB Glas. 1993.

RAMACHANDRAN, Vengatasamy Queen Elizabeth Hospital, King's Lynn PE30 4ET; 6 The Dell, Bishop Auckland DL14 7HJ — MB BS Osmania 1965.

RAMACHANDRAPPA, Mr Govindappa 31 Peldon Close, Vicars Lane, Newcastle upon Tyne NE7 7PB Tel: 0191 270 2738 — MB BS Madras 1973; FRCSI 1990.

RAMADAN, Abdo Mohamed West Wales General Hospital, Carmarthen SA31 2AF; Prince Philip Hospital, Llanelli SA15 — MB BCh Alexandria, Egypt 1974.

RAMADAN, Mr Mohamed Fouad 28 Rodney Street, Liverpool L1 2TQ Tel: 0151 708 6137 Fax: 0151 932 9239; 44 Warren Road, Blundellsands, Liverpool L23 6UF Tel: 0151 931 4238 Fax: 0151 932 9239 — (Mansoura Fac. Med.) MB BCh Cairo 1968; DA Cairo 1971; DLO Eng. 1975; FRCS Ed. 1976. Cons. (ENT Surg.) Walton & Univ. Hosp. Aintree; Clin. Lect. (Otolaryng.) Univ. Liverp. Specialty: Otorhinolaryngol. Socs: Brit. Assn. Otol.; BMA; Roy. Soc. Med. Prev: Sen. Lect. (Otolaryng.) Univ. Liverp. & Mersey RHA.

RAMADAS, Ranjitharatnam Bungalow 3, Brighton General Hospital, Elm Grove, Brighton BN2 3EW — MB BS Sri Lanka 1973; LMSSA Lon. 1984.

RAMAGE, Alison Elizabeth Renfrew Health Centre, 103 Paisley Road, Renfrew PA4 8LL Tel: 0141 886 2455 Fax: 0141 855 0457; 1340 Pollokshaws Road, Glasgow G41 3RF Tel: 0141 649 2662 — MB ChB Glas. 1981; DRCOG 1984.

RAMAGE, Ian (retired) Glebe Cottage, Old Back Lane, Wiswell, Clitheroe BB7 9BS Tel: 01254 823231 — MB ChB Manch. 1954; DCH RCP Lond. 1957; FRCGP 1983, M 1965; BA Open 1995.

RAMAGE, John Keith North Hampshire Hospital, Aldermanston Rd, Basingstoke RG24 9NA — MD Lond. 1989 (Westm.) MB BS 1978; MRCP (UK) 1984; FRCP 1999. Cons. Phys. & Hepat. Gen. Med. & Gastroenterol. N. Hants. Hosp. Basingstoke Hants; Cons. Phys. Inst. of Liver Studies, Kings Coll. Hosp. Specialty: Gastroenterol. Socs: Brit. Soc. Gastroenterol.; Amer. Gastroenterol. Assn.; BASL. Prev: Sen. Regist. (Gastroenterol. & Gen. Med.) Roy. Sussex Co. Hosp. Brighton; Research Fell. (Gastroenterol.) McMaster Univ. Med. Centre, Ontario; Sen. Reg. Inst. of liver Studies, King's Coll. Hosp.

RAMAGE, Lynn 33 Dornie Place, Dundee DD2 4UD — MB ChB Aberd. 1983; MRCP (UK) 1987.

RAMAGE, Patrick Algernon James (retired) The Rowans, Fownhope, Hereford HR1 4PJ Tel: 01432 860307 Fax: 01432 860307 — MB BS Lond. 1962 (Char. Cross) Prev: GP Hereford.

RAMAGE, Philip Charles Vincent Limpsfield Road Surgery, 515 Limpsfield Road, Warlingham CR6 9LF Tel: 01883 265262 Fax: 01883 627893 — MRCS Eng. LRCP Lond. 1968 (Guy's) MRCP (UK) 1974. Dir. Interaction Systems Software; Application Cons. MFB Computers. Socs: Primary Care Spec. Gp. of Brit. Computer Soc. Prev: Specialist (Med.) Princess Mary's Hosp. Halton.

RAMAGE, Victoria Mary Wallingford Medical Practice, Reading Road, Wallingford OX10 9DU Tel: 01491 835577 — MB BS Lond. 1990, BSc (Psychol. & Basic Med. Sci.) 1987; DCH RCP Lond. 1992. Trainee GP Reading VTS. Prev: SHO (A & E) W. Middlx. Univ. Hosp. Isleworth.

RAMAKRISHNA, Gupta Mudalagiri Dasappagupta The Surgery, Bevan Close, Shotton Colliery, Durham DH6 2LQ Tel: 0191 526 1643 Fax: 0191 517 2746 — MB BS Mysore 1970. GP Durh.

RAMAKRISHNA GUPTA, Mudalagiri Dasappagupta 17 Barnard Wynd, Oakerside Park, Peterlee SR8 1LT — MB BS Mysore 1969.

Prev: SHO (Med.) Ruchill Hosp. Glas.; SHO (O & G) Robroyston Hosp. Glas.

RAMAKRISHNAN, Kattukandy Patiyeri Chipstead Valley Road Surgery, 37 Chipstead Valley Road, Coulsdon CR5 2RA Tel: 020 8660 9400; (resid.) 127 Cheam Road, Sutton SM1 2EB Tel: 020 8642 2600 — MB BS Madras 1954 (Madras Med. Coll.) Princip. GP Sutton.

RAMAKRISHNAN, Sundareswaran Weston Park Hospital, Whitham Road, Sheffield S10 2SJ Tel: 0114 226 5000 Fax: 0114 226 5512 Email: sundareswaran.ramakrishnan@sth.nhs.uk — MB BS India 1975 (Pune) MD India 1978; MPhil Bradford 1983; DMRT 1986; FRCS 1988. Cons. in Clin. Oncol. with Sheff. Teachg. Hosps. NHS Trust based at Weston Pk. Hosp., Sheff.; Vis. Cons. in Clin. Oncol., Doncaster Roy. Infirm.; Lead Clinician for Cancer Servs., Doncaster and Bassetlaw Cancer Unit. Specialty: Oncol. Socs: Brit. Oncol. Assn.; Roy. Coll. of Radiologists; Brit. Med. Assn. Prev: Sen. Regist. in Clin. Oncol., Weston Pk. Hosp., Sheff.; Regist. in Clin. Oncol., Freedom Fields Hosp., Plymouth.

RAMALINGAM, Dr Middlehouse, High St., Harby, Newark NG23 7EB — MB BS Lond. 1993.

RAMAMOORTHY, Sidha Naidu 2 Wirral View, Liverpool L19 0PU — MB BS Madras 1976; MRCS Eng. LRCP Lond. 1986.

RAMAMURTHY, Anantapur Bache 156 Roe Lane, Southport PR9 7PN — MB BS Karnatak 1964 (Kasturba Med. Coll. Mangalore) Prev: Regist. (Anaesth.) South. Gen. Hosp. Glas.

RAMAMURTHY, Laxmi 60 Ashstead Road, Brooklands, Sale M33 3PX Tel: 0161 976 3289 — MB BS Madras 1986; FRCS Ed. 1991.

RAMAN, Ashok 9 Hurst Park Road, Twyford, Reading RG10 0EZ — MB BS Lond. 1996.

RAMAN, Mr Chidambaram Medical Records Building, Barnet General Hospital, Wellhouse Lane, Barnet EN5 3DJ — MB BS Madras 1976; FRCS Ed. 1986.

RAMAN, Thirumalappa Sampangi Pallion Health Centre, Hylton Road, Sunderland SR4 7XF Tel: 0191 657 1319; 10 Thornfield Grove, Sunderland SR2 7UZ Tel: 0191 551 6257 — MB BS Bangalor 1970 (Bangalore Med. Coll.) T (GP). Princip. GP. Specialty: Gen. Pract.; Trauma & Orthop. Surg.; Gen. Psychiat. Prev: Princip. GP S.grange Med. Centre Trunk Rd. Eston Middlesbrough; Clin. Asst. (Psychiat.) St. Lukes Hosp. Middlesbrough.

RAMAN, Vivek 9 Hurst Park Road, Twyford, Reading RG10 0EZ — MB BS Lond. 1996. SHO Med. Rotat. Qu. Mary's Hosp. Sidcup, S. Lond. Specialty: Gen. Med. Prev: SHO (A & E) Univ. Hosp. Lewisham S. Lond.

RAMANA, Rajini Fulbourn Hospital, Box 357, Fulbourn, Cambridge CB1 5EF — MB BS Madras Univ. India 1984; MRCPsych Lond. 1989. Psychiat. Cambs & P'boro. Ment. Health NHS Trust Camb.

RAMANAN, Ramaratnam Basildon Hospital, Nethermayne, Basildon Tel: 01268 593983 Fax: 01268 593194 — MB BS; MRCPI; DCH. Cons. Paediat. Specialty: Paediat.

RAMANANANDAN, Avvai 17 Fraser Close, Nythe, Swindon SN3 3RP — MB BS Lond. 1996.

RAMANATHAN, Mr Chakkedath Royal Halifax Infirmary, Free School Lane, Halifax HX1 2YP Tel: 01422 357222 — MB BS Kerala 1969 (Med. Coll. Calicut) DLO Mysore 1972; DLO Eng. 1978; FRCS Glas. 1980. Assoc. Specialist (ENT) Roy. Halifax Infirm. Specialty: Otolaryngol. Socs: BMA; Semon Club.

RAMANATHAN, Jai Shankar 5 Meadowcroft, Bromley BR1 2JD — MB BS Lond. 1993; BSc (Hons) Lond. 1989. Registar (Anaesth) King Geo. Hosp. Redbridge. Specialty: Anaesth. Prev: SHO (Elderly Care) Mayday Univ. Hosp.; SHO (Med.) Norf. & Norwich Hosp.; SHO (Anaesth.) King Geo. Hosp. Redbridge.

RAMANATHAN, Manickavasagar (retired) 92 Hitchings Way, Reigate RH2 8ER Tel: 01737 244818 — MB ChB Aberd. 1961; DCP Lond 1974; DPath Eng. 1974; FRCPath 1988, M 1977.

RAMANATHAN, Mr Narayanaswami, OStJ Narayana, 23 Pincroft Wood, New Barn, Longfield DA3 7HB Tel: 01474 706473 — (Madras Med. Coll.) Dip in Med. Acupunc. (British Med. Acupunc. Society); BSc Madras 1952; MB BS Madras 1959; FRCS Ed. 1975. Indep. Med. Pract. & Hyperbaric Phys. Lond.; Med. Adviser Port of Lond. Auth. Specialty: Orthop. Socs: Fell. Roy. Soc. Med.; Eur. Undersea Biomed. Soc.; Undersea Hyperbaric Med. Soc. USA. Prev: Chief Med. Off. Nat. Dock Labour Bd. Lond.

RAMANATHAN, Ponnambalam 24 Trinty Avenue, Bush Hill Park, Enfield EN1 1HS — MB BS Sri Lanka 1973; MRCP (UK) 1983; MRCS Eng. LRCP Lond. 1984.

RAMANATHAN, Ramachandra Gary Dr Ramanathan, The Health Centre, 2-4 Bay Street, Port Glasgow PA14 5EW Tel: 01475 745321 Fax: 01475 745587 — LMSSA London 1978. GP Port Glas., Renfrewsh.; Hosp. Med. practitioner in obstetnic & gynaeological ultrasonography at the Inner chyler Roy. Hosp. IRN, Greenwich. Specialty: Acupunc.; Hypnother.

RAMANATHAN, Ravi Shankar Horley Health Centre, Kings Rd, Horley RH6 7DG; 92 Hitchings Way, Reigate RH2 8ER — MB ChB Glas. 1991; DRCOG, MRCGP.

RAMANATHAN, Satyavathi Narayana, 23 Pincroft Wood, New Barn, Longfield DA3 7HB Tel: 01474 706473 Fax: 01474 709303 Email: ramu@mcmail.com — (Madras Med. Coll.) MB BS Madras 1959; MFCH 1989; FRIPHH 1997. Specialty: Paediat. Socs: Fell. Soc. Community Med.; Fell. Roy. Soc. Med.; Brit. Paediat. Assn. & Kent Paediat. Soc. Prev: Cons. Community Paediat. Qu. Mary's Sidcup NHS Trust.

RAMANATHAN, Mr Uthaya Shankar — MB BS Lond. 1990 (Charing Cross and Westminster Medical School) BSc (Hons.) Lond. 1986, MB BS 1990; FRCOphth 1995. Cons. (Ophth.) Wolverhampton Eye Infirm.; Glacoma Fell. Birm. & Midl. Eye Centre. Specialty: Ophth. Prev: Specialist Regist. (Ophth.) Birm. & Midl. Eye Centre; SHO Rotat. (Ophth.) St. Jas. Hosp. Leeds & Bradford Roy. Infirm.; SHO (A & E) Char. Cross Hosp.

RAMANI, Pramila Consultant Pathologist, Childrens Hospital, Steelhouse Lane, Birmingham B4 6NH — MB BS Utkal 1979; PhD Lond. 1987; FRCPath 1998. Cons. Histopath. Childr.'s Hosp. Birm. Specialty: Histopath. Socs: Paediatric Pathol. Soc.; Brit. Paediatric Path. Assn. Prev: Cons. (Histopath.) Hosp. Sick Childr. Lond.; Clin. Lect. Univ. Coll. Lond.; Clin. Research Fell. ICRF.

RAMANI, Ratilal Muljibhai 10 Deer Park Way, West Wickham BR4 9QQ Tel: 020 8462 6657 — MB BS Gujarat 1970 (M.P. Shah Med. Coll. Jamnagar) DOMS Saurashtra 1972; DO Eng. 1979. Med. Pract. (Ophth.) Kent. Specialty: Ophth. Prev: Clin. Asst. (Ophth.) Centr. Middlx. Hosp. Lond.; SHO (Ophth.) St. Paul's Eye Hosp. Liverp.

RAMANNA, Marigowda (Surgery) 40 Old Hill Street, Stamford Hill, London N16 6LU Tel: 020 8802 3344; Flat 10, Caldew Court, 1 Bunns Lane, London NW7 2AW — MB BS Mysore 1970 (Mysore Med. Coll.) Dip. Pract. Dermat. Wales 1992. Specialty: Dermat. Socs: Med. Protec. Soc. Prev: SHO (Gen. Med.) Downe Hosp. Downpatrick; SHO (Infec. Dis.) Seacroft Hosp. Leeds.

RAMARAO, Mallela Venkata Ramarao, Sparkbrook Health Centre, 32 Farm Road, Birmingham B11 1LS Tel: 0121 773 2104 Fax: 0121 766 7287 — DO; MB BS Osmania 1969; DPM Lond. 1980.

RAMARAO, Paidsetty Patel and Partners, Thornley Road Surgery, Thornley Road, Wheatley Hill, Durham DH6 3NR Tel: 01429 820233 Fax: 01429 823667 — MB BS Andhra 1969. GP Durh.

RAMASAMY, Nirmalan The Surgery, 12-14 Golborne Road, London W10 5PG Tel: 020 8969 2058 Fax: 020 8964 4156 — MB ChB Birm. 1980; MB ChB. Birm. 1980; MRCP (UK) 1985; MRCGP 1988.

RAMASUBBU, Mr Krishnamurthy Flat 2, 243 Addiscombe Road, Croydon CR0 6SQ — MB BS Mysore 1972; FRCS Glas. 1980; FRCS Ed. 1980.

RAMASWAMI, Radha (retired) Kalpana, 1 Lovaine Grove, Sandal, Wakefield WF2 7NF Tel: 01924 250121 Fax: 01924 250121 — (Madras) BA Madras 1941, MB BS 1952; DCH Bombay 1955. Specialist in Community Med. (Child Health) Barnsley AHA. Prev: SCMO Barnsley AHA.

RAMASWAMI, Ravi Aravindan Medical Selection Centre, Metropolitan Police, Simpson House, Peel Centre, Aerodrome Road, London NW9 5SW Tel: 0208 358 0489 Fax: 0208 358 0407; 5 Goldsmith Way, St Albans AL3 5LH — MB BS Lond.(Royal Free Hospital) 1985 (Royal Free Hospital) MSc (Occupat. Health) Aberd. 1995; FFOM(RCP Ireland) 1997; Dip Av Med Otago 2000. Head of Medical Selection, Metropolitan Police. Specialty: Occupat. Health; Aviat. Med. Socs: Soc. Occupat. Med. & Europ. Undersea Biomed. Soc.; Underwater & Hyperbaric Med. Soc.; Aviat. Med. Soc. of Australia & New Zealand. Prev: Employm. Med. Adviser Health & Safety Exec. Scotl. E.;; Med. Off. (Undersea Med.) Inst. Naval Med.

Alverstoke;; Adjunct Ass. Prof. Dept. of Surg., Fac. of Med., Chinese Uni of Hong Kong, Shatin Hong Kong.

RAMASWAMY, Alagappan Bridge Road Surgery, 25 Bridge Road, Stockton-on-Tees TS18 3AA Tel: 01642 604117 Fax: 01642 604602 — MB BS Madras 1971; MRCGP 1981; FRCGP 2001. GP Princip. Specialty: Gen. Pract.

RAMASWAMY, Aylam Chandran 8 Hatton Road, Croydon CR0 3LX — MB BS Lond. 1982; DA (UK) 1986. SHO (ENT) Orsett Hosp. Prev: SHO (Anaesth.) Arrowe Pk. Hosp. Upton.

RAMASWAMY, Saroja (retired) 21 The Warren Drive, Wanstead, London E11 2LR Tel: 020 8989 0966 — MB BS Calcutta 1954 (Calcutta Med. Coll.) DGO 1956; FRCOG 1976, M 1959. Mem. HQ Staff MRC. Prev: Dir. Med. Train. & Research Family Plann. Assn.

RAMAYYA, Anjali 35 Aytoun Road, Pollokshiels, Glasgow G41 5HW — MB BS Osmania 1981; MRCPsych 1988.

RAMAYYA, Pradeep Department of Anaesthesia, Health Care International, Clydebank G81 4DY Tel: 0141 951 5606 Fax: 0141 951 5603; 35 Aytoun Road, Pollokshields, Glasgow G41 5HW Tel: 0141 423 6201 — MB BS Osmania 1979; FFA RCS Eng. 1984. Vice-Chairm. & Cons. Anaesth. Health Care Internat. Clydebank. Specialty: Anaesth. Socs: (Chairm.) Soc. Computing & Technol. in Anaesth. Prev: Cons. & Sen. Regist. (Anaesth.) Aberd. Roy. Infirm.; Sec. Intens. Care Computer Gp.; Regist. Prize NE Scotl. Soc. Anaesth.

RAMBIHAR, Brian Vishnu Sandy Lane Surgery, Sandy Lane, Leyland, Preston PR25 2EB Tel: 01772 909915 Fax: 01772 909911; 5 Old Oak Gardens, Walton-Le-Dale, Preston PR5 4BF Tel: 01772 627 177 Email: brian.rambihar@btinternet.com — MB BS Lond. 1986 (Char. Cross & Westm.) BSc (Hons.) Lond. 1984; MRCGP 1992; Dip. Occ. Med. 1996; ILTM 2003; Dip Med Educat Dundee 2004. GP Sandy La. Surg. Leyland & Trainer in Gen. Pract.; GP Postgrad. Tutor, Chorley & S. Ribble; Trainer in Gen. Pract.; Chair Educational Subcomittee Chorley & S. Ribble PCT; GP Appraiser; GP Appraiser Trainer; Occupational Health Phys. Preston Coll. Specialty: Gen. Pract. Socs: BMA. Prev: Trainee GP Aldergate Med. Pract. Tamworth; Trainee GP/SHO (O & G) Derby City Hosp.; SHO Rotat. (Paediat.) Dudley Rd. Hosp. Birm.

RAMCHANDANI, Mr Mahesh 39 Bankside, Westhoughton, Bolton BL5 2QP — MB ChB Manch. 1993; FRCS Ed. 1998. Specialty: Ophth.

RAMCHANDANI, Mohanlal Leigh Infirmary, The Avenue, Leigh WN7 1HS Tel: 01942 672333; The Gables, 39 Bankside, Westhoughton, Bolton BL5 2QP Tel: 01942 840126 — MB BS Karachi 1962 (Dow Med. Coll. Karachi) MRCS Eng. LRCP Lond. 1977. Assoc. Specialist (Geriat. Med.) Wigan HA. Specialty: Care of the Elderly. Socs: Fell. Roy. Soc. Med.; Brit. Geriat. Soc.; BMA.

RAMCHANDANI, Parkash The Gables 39 Bank Side, Westhoughton, Bolton BL5 2QP — MB BS Manch. 1997; MB BS Manc 1997.

RAMCHANDANI, Paul Gulab Child & Family Psychiatric Service, Sue Nicholls Centre, Manor House, Aylesbury HP20 1EG — BM Soton. 1991. Specialist Regist. Child & Family Psych. Serv. Sue Nicholls Centre Aylesbury. Specialty: Child & Adolesc. Psychiat.

RAMCHANDRA, Kanakam (retired) 44 Bakers Field, Crayford Road, London N7 0LT Tel: 020 7607 2546 — MB BS Madras 1950 (Madras Med. Coll.) DGO Madras 1952; DCH Madras 1962; DPH Newc. 1966. Prev: Prison Med. Off. HM Prison Holloway.

RAMDAHEN-GOPAL, Sangeeta Dr Deshmukh & Partners, The Medical Centre, 144-150 High Road, Willesdon Green, London NW10 2PT Tel: 020 8459 5550 Fax: 020 8451 7268 — MB BS 1991; BSc 1991 (Fatima Jinnah / Punjab Univ. Lahore, Pakistan) MRCGP 1999; DFFP 1999. Gen. Practitioner. Specialty: Gen. Pract. Socs: MRCGP; BMA.

RAMDENEE, Radhayshyam 116 Manor Drive, Upton, Wirral CH49 4PJ Tel: 0151 677 0064; 81 Leasowe Road, Wallasey, Wirral CH46 Tel: 0151 639 8271 — LRCPI & LM, LRSCI & LM 1967 (RCSI) LRCPI & LM, LRCSI & LM 1967. Socs: Wallasey Med. Soc. Prev: Regist. (Anaesth.) Qu. Mary's Hosp. Sidcup; Ho. Off. (Surg.) Vict. Hosp. Blackpool; Ho. Off. (Med.) St. Lawrence's Hosp. Dub.

RAMDEO, Anil 54 Sleapshyde Lane, Smallford, St Albans AL4 0SB — MB BCh BAO NUI 1981.

RAMELL, Michael David Barnfield Hill Surgery, 12 Barnfield Hill, Exeter EX1 1SR Tel: 01392 432761 Fax: 01392 422406 — MB BS Lond. 1983.

RAMESAR, Keith Christopher Robert Blair Pathology Department, St. John's Hospital, Livingston EH54 6PP — MB ChB Dundee 1981; MB ChB (Hons.) Dundee 1981, BMSc(Hons.) 1978; MRCPath 1987. Cons. Histopath. W. Lothian Trust. Specialty: Histopath.

RAMESH, Chandakacharla Narasimha 21 Beamsish View, Stanley DH9 0XB — MB BS Sri Venkateswara 1987.

RAMESH, Chaniyil Ayyappan St. Mary's Hospital, Whitworth Park, Manchester M13 0JU Tel: 0161 276 6200; c/o Drive S. Ramesh, Department of Paediatrics, Glan Clwyd Hospital, Bodelwyddan, Rhyl LL18 5UJ Tel: 01745 583910 — MB BS Kerala 1980; DCH RCP Glas. 1990; MRCP (UK) 1993. Regist. & Tutor (Paediat.) St. Mary's Hosp. Manch. Specialty: Paediat.

RAMESH, Cobarsanellore Belle Vue Surgery, 419 Poulton Road, Fleetwood FY7 7JY Tel: 01253 779113 Fax: 01253 770707 — MB BS Madras 1971; MB BS Madras 1971.

RAMESH, Mr Nadarajah 87 Gold Smith Avenue, London E12 6QB; 26 Lily Avenue, Colombo 6, Sri Lanka Tel: 010 941 586513 — MB BS Colombo 1986; MRCS Eng. LRCP Lond. 1991; FRCS Glas. 1992; FRCS Ed. 1993. Cons. Emerg. Phys. King Fahad Nat. Guard Hosp. Riyadh, Saudi Arabia. Specialty: Accid. & Emerg. Socs: Founder Mem. Brit. Assn. Day Case Surg.; Brit. Assn. Accid. & Emerg. Med.; Brit. Assn. Immed. Care Schemes. Prev: Sen. Regist. Fell. Emerg. Med. John Hunter Hosp. Newc. Austral.

RAMESH, Mr Subramanian West Middlesex Hospital, Twickenham Road, Isleworth TW7 6AF Email: s.ramesh@liv.ac.uk — MB BS Madras 1982; FRCS Eng. 1990; FRCS Glas. 1990. Cons. (Gen & Colorectal Surg.) W. Middlx. Univ. Hosp. Specialty: Gen. Surg. Special Interest: Colon & Rectal Cancer. Socs: BMA. Prev: Assoc. Specialist & Regist. (Surg.) Roy. Berks. Hosp. Reading; Regist. (Surg.) Basildon Hosp.; Specialist Regist. (Gen. Surg.) Liverp.

RAMESH, Venkateswaran Newcastle General Hospital, Newcastle upon Tyne NE4 6BE Tel: 0191 273 8811 — MB BS Madras 1980; DCH Eng. 1983; MRCP (UK) 1985; MRCS Eng. LRCP Lond. 1986; FRCP 1996; FRCP CH 1998. Cons. Paediat. Neurol. Newc. Gen. Hosp. Specialty: Paediat. Neurol.; Paediat. Prev: Sen. Regist. (Paediat. Neurol.) Booth Hall Childr. Hosp. Manch.; Research Fell. (Child Health) Dept. Child Health Med. Sch. Univ. Newc.; Hon. Regist. (Paediat.) Newc. Gen. Hosp.

RAMGOOLAM, Mohit Department of Psychiatry, Doncaster Royal Infirmary, Armthorpe Rd, Doncaster DN2 5LT Tel: 01302 366666 Ext: 4084 Fax: 01302 761317 — BM Soton. 1980; PhD Wales 1974, BPharm (1st cl. Hons.) 1970; MRCGP 1987; MRCPsych 1987. Cons. Old Age Psychiat. Doncaster & S. Humberside NHS Trust. Specialty: Geriat. Psychiat. Socs: Roy. Coll. of Psychiat., Mem. Prev: Cons. Old Age Psychiat. Dudley Priority Health; Cons. Old Age Psychiat. Cardiff; Sen. Regist. (Psychiat.) S. Devon.

RAMGOOLAM, Navinchandra 185 Inderwick Road, London N8 9JR — LRCPI & LM, LRSCI & LM 1975 (RCSI) LRCPI & LM, LRCSI & LM 1975. Clin. Med. Asst. Cardiac Dept. Univ. Coll. Hosp. Lond. Prev: Res. Med. Off. Civil Hosp. Port Louis, Mauritius.

RAMI REDDY, Sanampudi The Surgery, 522 Queslett Road, Great Barr, Birmingham B43 7DY Tel: 0121 360 8560 Fax: 0121 360 6833; 33 Carpenter Road, Edgbaston, Birmingham B15 2JH Tel: 0121 440 2580 — MB BS Sri Venkateswara 1972 (Kurnool Med. Coll.) Specialty: Anaesth. Prev: SHO (Anaesth.) Univ. Hosp. S. Manch.; SHO (Anaesth.) Burnley Gen. Hosp.

RAMIREZ, Professor Amanda Jane Department of Liaison Psychiatry & ICRF Psychosocial Oncology, 3rd Floor, Riddell House, St Thomas' Hospital, Lambeth Palace Road, London SE1 7EH Tel: 020 7960 5734 Fax: 020 7960 5719; 7 College Road, Dulwich Village, London SE21 7BQ Tel: 020 8693 3657 Fax: 020 8693 3657 — MB BS Lond. 1998 (Guy's) BSc (Hons. Human Genetics) Lond.; MD Lond.; MRCPsych 1987; FRCPsych 1998. Prof. (Liaison Psychiat.) Guy's & St Thos. Hosp. Trust; Dir. (Richard Dimbleby Cancer Informat. & Support Serv.) Guy's & St Thos. Cancer Centre; Dir. (Liaison Psychiat.) Guy's & St Thos. Hosp. Trust. Specialty: Gen. Psychiat.; Psychother. Socs: Exec. Comm. Liaison Psychiat. Gp. of Roy. Coll. of Psychiat.; Coun. Mem. Soc. Psychosomatic Research. Prev: Sen. Lect. & Hon. Cons. (Liaison Psychiat.) Imperial Cancer Research Fund, Clin. Oncol. Unit & Div. of Psychiat., Guy's Hosp.

RAMISHVILI, Akaki 188 Cromwell Road, London SW5 0SJ — MRCS Eng. LRCP Lond. 1949; MRCP Ed. 1961; MRCP Lond. 1961.

RAMJOHN, Mohamed Ally Ward End Medical Centre, 794A Washwood Heath Road, Ward End, Birmingham B8 2JN Tel: 0121 327 1049 Fax: 0121 327 0964; 4 Poundley Close, Castle Bromwich, Birmingham B36 9SZ — MB BCh BAO Dub. 1976 (Univ. Dub.) MA Dub. 1993, BA 1976; DRCOG 1979; DFFP 1993.

RAMKHALAWON, Meghraj 52 St Mary's Park, Louth LN11 0EF — MB BCh BAO NUI 1986; LRCPSI 1986.

RAMKISSOON, Anand Mikhail Regional Clinical Virology Laboratory, City Hospital, Edinburgh Tel: 0131 536 6334 Fax: 0131 536 6123 — MB ChB Manch. 1988; BSc (Hons.) St. And. 1983; DRCPath 1994. Regist. Reg. Clin. Urol. Laborat. Specialty: Virology. Prev: Regist. (Microbiol.) Leicester Roy. Infirm.; SHO (Path.) Roy. Preston Hosp.

RAMLI, Norlina 55 Doncaster Road, Newcastle upon Tyne NE2 1RB; 33 Grosvenor Place, Jesmond, Newcastle upon Tyne NE2 2RD Tel: 0191 2816 654 — MB BS Newc. 1997. Specialty: Ophth.

RAMNANI, Suneil Mark 8 Ambelside Drive, Walton, Wakefield WF2 6TJ Tel: 01924 258448 — MB BS Lond. 1996 (Charing Cross & Westminster Medical School) SHO (Orthop. Surg.) Castle Hill Hosp., Hull. Specialty: Trauma & Orthop. Surg. Prev: SHO, (A & E) Hull Roy. Infirm.; SHO, (A&E) Lister Hosp. Stevenage.

RAMNARINE, Vishan Dimitri Flat 11, Block 13, Good Hope Hospital, Rectory Road, Sutton Coldfield B75 7RR — MB BS West Indies 1991.

RAMON, Amos Jehoshua High Street Surgery, 69 High Street, Coningsby, Lincoln LN4 4RB Tel: 01526 344544 Fax: 01526 345540.

RAMPA, Balarami Reddy Radhika, School Lane, Trinant, Crumlin, Newport NP11 3LQ — MB BS Andhra 1964 (Guntur Med. Coll.)

RAMPERSAD, Randolph Frederick Flat 2, 211 Gipsy Road, West Norwood, London SE27 9QY — LRCPI & LM, LRSCI & LM 1958 (RCSI) LRCPI & LM, LRCSI & LM 1958. Prev: Ho. Surg. New Cross Hosp. Wolverhampton; Ho. Phys. Roy. Huddersfield Infirm.; SHO Cas. Derbysh. Roy. Infirm. Derby.

RAMPES, Hagen Barnet Enfield & Haringey Ment. Health Care NHS Trust, North West Community Mental Health Team, 7th Floor, Premier House 112 Station Road, Edgware HA8 7BJ — MB ChB Ed. 1987 (Univ. of Edin.) BSc MedSci. (Biochem.) Ed. 1985; MRCPsych 1993. Cons., Gen. Adult Psychiat. Specialty: Gen. Psychiat. Special Interest: Addictions. Prev: Cons., Gen. Adult Psychiat., W. Cannon Ment. Health NHS Trust.

RAMPHAL, Paul Shridath 57 Farm Avenue, Swanley BR8 7HZ — MB BS West Indies 1989.

RAMPHUL, Neelmanee North Tees General Hospital, Hardwick, Stockton-on-Tees TS19 8PE Tel: 01642 617617; 9 Redall Drive, Cochrane Park, Newcastle upon Tyne NE7 7LH Tel: 0199 266 9141 — MB BS Newc. 1997. SHO (Paediat.) N. Tees. Specialty: Obst. & Gyn.; Paediat. Socs: Med. Defence Union; BMA. Prev: Ho. Off. Med. S. Cleavland; Ho. Off. Surg. N. Tees.

RAMPHUL-GOKULSING, Shishana Kali 73 Mansell Road, Greenford UB6 9EJ — MB BS Lond. 1993; MRCGP.

RAMPLING, Alec Edwin, Surg. Cdr. RN (retired) Lisnamandra, Fort Road, Alverstoke, Gosport PO12 2DT Tel: 023 9258 3425 — MRCS Eng. LRCP Lond. 1957 (St. Thos.) DO Eng. 1965.

RAMPLING, Anita Margaret (retired) East Farm, Toller Whelme, Beaminster DT8 3NU Tel: 01308 862468 — MB ChB Birm. 1977; PhD Birm. 1973; MA Camb. 1979; FRCPath 1992, M 1981. Cons. Med. Microbiol. & Dir. Pub. Health Laborat. Dorchester. Prev: Cons. Med. Microbiol. Pub. Health Laborat. Camb.

RAMPLING, Constance Mary (retired) 69 Townfield Gardens, Altrincham WA14 4DT Tel: 0161 941 5809 — (Liverp.) MRCS Eng. LRCP Lond. 1937; MB ChB Liverp. 1937, CPH 1946.

RAMPLING, Kathleen 1-3 Morrowfield Avenue, Hightown, Manchester M8 9AR — MB ChB Manch. 1946.

RAMPLING, Michael John 38 Durham Road, London W5 4JP — MB ChB Dundee 1990.

RAMPLING, Professor Roy Peter Beatson Oncology Centre, Western Infirmary, Glasgow G11 6NT Tel: 0141 211 2627 Fax: 0141 211 6356 — MB BS Lond. 1979 (University College London) PhD (Phys.) Lond. 1971; MRCP (UK) 1982; FRCR 1984; FRCP Glas. 1992. Prof. of Neuro Oncol. Univ. Glas. And Hon. Cons. West. Informary; Hon. Cons. (Radiother.) West. Infirm. Glas. Specialty: Oncol.; Radiother. Socs: Fell. Roy. Coll. Phys.; Roy. Coll. Radiol. Prev: Sen. Regist. (Radiother.) Churchill Hosp. Oxf.; Regist. (Radiother.) Hammersmith Hosp. Lond.

RAMPTON, Anthony John William Harvey Hospital, Kennington Road, Willesborough, Ashford TN24 0LZ — MB BS Lond. 1980; BSc Lond. 1977, MB BS 1980; FFA RCS Eng. 1986. Cons. Anaesth. William Harvey Hosp. Ashford. Specialty: Anaesth.

RAMPTON, Professor David Stephen Royal London Hospital, Department of Gastroenterology, Whitechapel Road, London E1 1BB Tel: 020 7377 7442 Fax: 020 7377 7441 Email: d.rampton@qmul.ac.uk — BM BCh Oxf. 1973 (Oxf. & Univ. Coll. Hosp.) MA Oxf. 1970; DPhil Oxf. 1970; MRCP (UK) 1975; FRCP Lond. 1989. Cons. Gastroenterol. Roy. Lond. Hosp. & St Bart. Hosp.; Prof. of Clin. Gastroenterol., Barts & The Lond. (Queen Mary). Specialty: Gastroenterol.; Gen. Med. Special Interest: Infammatory Bowel Disease. Socs: Brit. Inflammatory Research Assn.; Brit. Soc. Gastroenterol.; Fell. Roy. Soc. Med. Prev: Cons. Phys. & Gastroenterol. Newham Gen. Hosp. & St. And. Hosp. Lond.; Lect. (Med.) Univ. Coll. Hosp. Lond.; Research Fell. (Gastroenterol.) Guy's Hosp. Lond.

RAMSAMY, Teygaraj 193 Windmill Road, London W5 4DH — MRCS Eng. LRCP Lond. 1958.

RAMSAY, Alan 18 Marchbank Gardens, Ralston, Paisley PA1 3JD Tel: 0141 810 3198 — MB ChB Aberd. 1982; FRCR 1990. Cons. Radiol. Inverclyde Roy. NHS Trust Greenock; Clin. Director; Diagnostic Serv.s. Specialty: Radiol. Socs: Scott. Radiol. Soc.

RAMSAY, Alan Drummond Histopathology Department, Great Ormond Street Hospital For Children, Great Ormond St., London WC1N 3JH Tel: 020 7829 8663 Fax: 020 7829 7875 Email: a.ramsay@ich.ucl.ac.uk — MB BS Lond. 1979; BSc (Anat.) (1st cl. Hons.) Lond. 1976; MRCPath 1985; FRCPath 1996; D.M. Soton 1997. Cons. Histopath. Gt. Ormond St. Hosp. for Childr. Specialty: Histopath. Prev: Lect. (Histopath.) Inst. Otol. & Laryngol. Lond.; Graham Schol. Dept. Histopath. Univ. Coll. Lond.; Cons. & Sen. Lect. Histopath. Soton. Gen. Hosp.

RAMSAY, Alan Livingstone 29 Church Street, Kilbarchan, Johnstone PA10 2JQ — MB ChB Glas. 1989.

RAMSAY, Andrew (retired) Ravenscraig, Frankscroft, Peebles EH45 9DX Tel: 01721 720420 Email: eahramsay@freenet.co.uk — MB ChB Ed. 1959; DObst RCOG 1966. Prev: GP Peebles.

RAMSAY, Andrew Miller (retired) Prospect House, 31 Station Road, Ossett WF5 8AY Tel: 01924 274053 — MB ChB Glas. 1929.

RAMSAY, Andrew Steven West Suffolk Hospital, Hardwick Lane, Bury St Edmunds IP33 2QZ Tel: 01284 713539 Fax: 01284 713816 Email: andrew.ramsey@wsh.nhs.uk — MB BS Lond. 1991; BSc (Hons.) Lond. 1988; FRCOphth 1993. Cons. Ophth. Surg. W. Suff. Hosps. Bury St Edmunds; Cons. Ophth. Surg. Nuffield Hosps. Bury St Edmunds. Specialty: Ophth. Special Interest: Cornea & Retinal Dis.; Laser Eye Surg.; Cataract. Socs: Fell. Roy. Coll. of Ophth.; Mem. Europ. Soc. Cataract & Refractive Surg.; Mem. UK & Irel. Soc. Cataract & Refractive Surg. Prev: Fell. (Corneal & Cataract Surg.) Moorfields Hosp. Lond.; Retinal Fell. Moorfields Hosp. Lond.

RAMSAY, Anne Elizabeth 10 Robertson Street, Dundee DD4 6EL Tel: 01382 461588 Fax: 01382 452121 Email: aeramsay@taybank.tayside.scot.nhs.uk — MB ChB Dundee 1983; MRCGP 1987; FRCGP 1998. Gen. Pract.; Advisor to the women doctors and retainers. Specialty: Family Plann. & Reproduc. Health; Acupunc. Socs: BMA; RCGP.

RAMSAY, Bruce 14 Green Walk, Berkhamsted HP4 2LW — BM Soton. 1987; MRCOG 1992. Sen. Regist. (O & G) Glos. Roy. Hosp. Specialty: Obst. & Gyn.

RAMSAY, Colin Ninian Scottish Centre for Infection & Environmental Health, Clifton House, Clifton Place, Glasgow G3 7LN Tel: 0141 300 1100 Fax: 0141 300 1170 Email: colin.ramsay@scieh.csa.scot.nhs.uk; 22 Netherbank, Edinburgh EH16 6YR Tel: 0131 672 1101 Fax: 0131 672 1101 — MB ChB Dundee 1980; DRCOG 1983; MSc Ed. 1985; MFCM 1987; FFPHM 1998. Cons. Epidemiologist (Environm. Health). Specialty: Pub. Health Med.; Epidemiol.

RAMSAY, Crichton Forbes Department of Respiratory Medicine, Norforlk and Norwich University Hospital, Norwich Coloney Lane, Norwich NR4 7UY Tel: 01603 289640 — MB ChB Ed. 1986; MRCP (UK) 1991. Cons. Phys., Respirat. and Gen. Med. Norf. and Norwich Univ. Hosp., Norwich. Specialty: Respirat. Med. Prev: Regist. (Respirat. & Gen. Med.) Edin. Teach. Hosps.; Research Regist.

(Thoracic Med.) Lond. Chest Hosp.; Specialist Regist. (Thoracic Med.) Whittingham Hosp., Roy. Lond. Hosp., St. Bart. Hosp., Lond.

RAMSAY, Deborah Ann 8 Rosebank Cottages, Edinburgh EH3 8DA — MB ChB Ed. 1993.

RAMSAY, Dorothy Hilda Elizabeth (retired) 133 Russell Road, Moseley, Birmingham B13 8RS — LRCP LRCS Ed. 1950 (Univ. Ed.) LRCP LRCS Ed. LRFPS Glas. 1950; DObst RCOG 1953; DCH Eng. 1958. Prev: Sessional Clin. Med. Off. Sandwell HA.

RAMSAY, Douglas McNab The Tors, 2 Slamannan Road, Falkirk FK1 5LG Tel: 01324 20877 — MB ChB Ed. 1965; FRCPath 1985, M 1973. Cons. Haemat. Falkirk & Stirling Roy. Infirm. Specialty: Haematology. Socs: Brit. Soc. Haematol.

RAMSAY, Duncan Winson 60 Lorne Road, Clarendon Park, Leicester LE2 1YG Tel: 0116 270 2159 — MB BS Lond. 1989 (Middlx. Hosp.) MRCP (UK) 1993; FRCR 1997. Regist. (Radiol.) Leicester Roy. Infirm. Specialty: Radiol.

RAMSAY, Esther Margaret Elizabeth (retired) 24 Lynmouth Road, Liverpool L17 6AN Tel: 0151 427 5904 — MB ChB Liverp. 1951; DPH 1956; FFCM 1981, M 1975. Prev: SCM (Med. Manpower & Postgrad. Educat.) Mersey RHA.

RAMSAY, Fiona Mary Horsham Hospital, Hurst Road, Horsham RH12 2DR; Little Duxford, 19 Langley Lane, Ifield, Crawley RH11 0NB Tel: 01293 539344 — MB BS Lond. 1977 (St. Bart.) MRCS Eng. LRCP Lond. 1977; MRCP (UK) 1982; FRCP Lond. 1995. Cons. Phys. (c/o Elderly) Surrey & Sussex Healthcare Crawley & Horsham Hosps. Specialty: Care of the Elderly. Prev: Cons. Phys. (Geriat. Med.) The Roy. Lond. Hosp.; Sen. Regist. (Geriat. Med.) St. Geo. Hosp. Lond.

RAMSAY, Helen Mary Department of Dermatology, Royal Hallamshire Hospital, Sheffield Email: helen.ramsey@sth.nhs.uk — MB ChB Birm. 1993; MRCP (UK) 1996; CCST Derm. 2002. Cons. Dermat. & Hon. Sen. Lect. Specialty: Dermat. Socs: Brit. Assn. Dermat. Dowling Club; N. Eng. Dermat. Soc. Prev: Specialist Regist. (Dermat.) N Staffs. Hosp. Centre Stoke-on-Trent.

RAMSAY, Hilary Vanessa Baddow Road Surgery, 115 Baddow Road, Chelmsford CM2 7QD; 57 Well Lane, Stock, Ingatestone CM4 9LZ Tel: 01277 841566 — MB BS Lond. 1991 (King's Coll. Sch. Med. & Dent. Lond.) BSc Lond. 1988; DRCOG 1994; MRCGP 1995. Specialty: Gen. Pract. Prev: Trainee GP/SHO Mid Essex Hosps. Chelmsford VTS; SHO (ENT) Orsett Hosp. Essex.

RAMSAY, Ian The Health Centre, 2 The Tanyard, Cumnock KA18 1BF Tel: 01290 422723 Fax: 01290 425444; 30 Oakbank Drive, Cumnock KA18 1BD Tel: 01290 420469 — MB ChB Glas. 1971 (Glasgow) Princip. GP Cumnock Ayrsh.; Med. Asst. (Geriat.) Holmhead Hosp. Ayrsh.; Exam. Med. Practit. Benefits Agency; Med.Asst. Specialty: Gen. Pract. Socs: MDDUS. Prev: SHO (Paediat.) Hawkhead Hosp. Paisley; SHO (O & G) Paisley Matern. Hosp.; Ho. Off. (Med. & Surg.) Roy. Alexandra Infirm. Paisley.

RAMSAY, Ian Douglas (cons. rooms), The Cromwell Hospital, Cromwell Road, London SW5 0TU Tel: 020 7460 5700 Fax: 020 7460 5555; (cons. Rooms), The Lister Hospital, Chelsea Bridge Road, London SW1W 8RH Tel: 020 7730 8298 Fax: 020 7259 9218; (cons. rooms), Kings Oak Hospital, Chase Farm North Side, The Ridgeway, Enfield EN2 8SD Tel: 020 8370 9505 Fax: 020 8370 9551 — (Ed.) MB ChB Ed. 1959; FRCP Ed. 1982, M 1963; MD Ed. 1964; FRCP Lond. 1979, M 1966. Cons. Endocrinol. Cromwell Hosp. Lond.; Hon. Lect. (Med.) Roy. Free Hosp. Sch. Med. Lond.; Prof. Med.& Director of Educat. (UK) St. Geo. Univ. Sch. Med. Grenada, WI. Specialty: Endocrinol. Socs: Fell. Roy. Soc. Med.; Brit. Thyroid Assn.; Ovarian Club. Prev: Cons. Endocrinol. N. Middlx. Hosp. Lond.; Lect. (Med.) King's Coll. Hosp. Med. Sch. Lond.; Research Fell. Roy. Vict. Hosp. Belf.

RAMSAY, Ian Duncan The Portland Practice, St Paul's Medical Centre, 121 Swindon Road, Cheltenham GL50 4DP Tel: 01242 707792; Westaway, Stockwell Lane, Cleeve Hill, Cheltenham GL52 3PU — MB ChB Liverp. 1975; DRCOG 1978.

RAMSAY, Ian Nairn Department of Gynaecology, Southern General Hospital, Govan Road, Glasgow G51 4TF Tel: 0141 201 1100 Fax: 0141 201 2994 — MB ChB Dundee 1981; MRCOG 1987. Cons. O & G South. Gen. Hosp. Glas. Specialty: Obst. & Gyn. Socs: Internat. Continence Soc. & Glas. Obst. Soc.; Sec./Treasuer of Internat. Continence Soc. (U.K.) Sect. Prev: Sen. Regist Rotat. (O & G) W. Scotl.; Clin. Research Assoc. Dept. O & G Univ. Newc. u Tyne; Regist. Rotat. (O & G) W. Scotl.

RAMSAY, Mr James Hamilton Hawthorn Cottage, Mildenhall, Marlborough SN8 2LR Tel: 01672 516281 — MB Camb. 1971; MA; BChir 1970; FRCS Eng. 1976. Cons. Ophth. Princess Margt. Hosp. Swindon & Ridgeway Hosp. Specialty: Ophth. Prev: Sen. Regist. Guy's Hosp. Lond. Sen. Resid. Surg. Off. Moorfields Eye; Hosp. Lond. Research Fell. Hosp. Sick Childr. Lond.

RAMSAY, James Richard 3 Green Acres, Lilley, Luton LU2 8LS — MB ChB Leeds 1997.

RAMSAY, Jane Elizabeth 14 Woodend Drive, Jordanhill, Glasgow G13 1QS — MB ChB Glas. 1991; MRCOG 1997. Specialist Regist. (O & G). Specialty: Obst. & Gyn.

RAMSAY, Jock Watson An Nead, 15 Cameron Avenue, Balloch, Inverness IV2 7JT Tel: 01463 798912 Fax: 01463 798912 Email: jock@hqhq.org — MB ChB Ed. 1984; BSc MedSci Ed. 1981; DRCOG 1989; MRCGP 1990. Professional GP Locum Highlands & Western Isles; Exec. Dir. HQHQ Ltd, Peebles, Scotl.; Assoc. Adviser in Gen. Pract., NOS Instit. of Postgrad. Educat. Raigmore Hosp., Inverness; RCGP Quality Inititives Adviser.

RAMSAY, John Henry Rolland, OBE (retired) — MB ChB Glas. 1946 (Univ. Glas.) FRFPS Glas. 1953; FRCP Glas. 1981, M 1962. Prev: Med. Dir. St. Benedicts Hospice Sunderland.

RAMSAY, John Laurence (retired) 25 Allerton Park, Leeds LS7 4ND Tel: 0113 268 4014 — MB ChB Leeds 1956; DObst RCOG 1959. Prev: Dep. Resid. Med. Off. & Ho. Phys. St. Jas. Hosp. Leeds.

RAMSAY, Jonathan Robert Spencer Willow Cottage, Baunton, Cirencester GL7 7BB — MB ChB Bristol 1978; MSc Lond. 1979; MRCP (UK) 1983; FRCR 1988. Cons. Div. Oncol. Roy. Brisbane Hosp., Austral. Specialty: Oncol. Prev: Sen. Regist. Addenbrooke's Hosp. Camb.; Fell. Harvard Med. Sch. Boston.

RAMSAY, Mr Jonathan William Alexander 15th Floor, Charing Cross Hospital, Fulham Palace Road, London W6 8RF Tel: 020 8846 7669 Fax: 020 8846 7696; Yew Trees, Southlea Road, Datchet, Slough SL3 9BY — MB BS Lond. 1977 (St. Bart.) FRCS Eng. 1982; MS Lond. 1987; FRCS (Urol.) Eng. 1988; FEBU 1992. Cons. Urol. Char. Cross Hosp., W. Middlx. Univ. Hosp. & Chelsea Westminster Hosp. Lond.; Hon. Cons. Urol. St. Lukes Hosp. for Clergy & UCH Lond.; Hon. Cons. (Urol.) King Edwd. VII Hosp. Lond.; Mem. Ct. Examrs. RCS Eng 1997; Regional adviser in Surg. (RCS 1999). Specialty: Urol. Socs: Fell. Roy. Soc. Med. (Pres. Clin. Sect. & Counc. Sect. Urol.); Brit. Assn. Urol. Surg. & Europ. Intrarenal Surg. Soc. Prev: Sen. Regist. (Urol.) St. Bart. Hosp. Lond.; Brackenbury Schol. St. Bart. Hosp.; Hon. Lect. (Lithotripsy) St. Pauls Hosp. Lond.

RAMSAY, Kirsten 59 Taymouth Road, Polmont, Falkirk FK2 0PF — MB ChB Ed. 1997.

RAMSAY, Lawrence Eccles 85 Redmires Road, Lodge Moor, Sheffield S10 4LB Tel: 0114 230 3669 — MB ChB Glas. 1967; MRCP (UK) 1970; FRCP Lond. 1983; FFPM RCP (UK) 1989. Cons. Phys. Hallamsh. Hosp. Sheff.; Reader Clin. Pharmacol. & Therap. Univ. Sheff.; Mem. Brit. Pharmacopoeia Commiss.; Mem. Comm. on Review of Med. Specialty: Gen. Med. Socs: Sec. Brit. Hypertens. Soc.; Clin. Pharmacol. Sect. Brit. Pharmacol. Soc. Prev: Lect. (Med.) Univ. Glas.

RAMSAY, Lorna Jane Information Statistics Division, Common Services Agency, Trinity Dark House, South Trinity Road, Edinburgh EH5 — MB ChB Glas. 1991 (Glasgow Uni) MB ChB (Commend.) Glas. 1991; DCH RCPS Glas. 1994; MPH Glas. 1997. Clin. Adviser to Scott. Clin. Coding Centre, ISD, Edin. Specialty: Pub. Health Med.

RAMSAY, Louise Mary 1 Erskine Avenue, Glasgow G41 5AL; The Douglas Inch Centre, 2 Woodside Terrace, Glasgow G3 7UY Tel: 0141 211 8000 Fax: 0141 211 8005 — MB ChB Glas. 1988; DRCOG 1991; MRCGP 1993; MRCPsych 1995. Sen. Regist. (Forens. Psychiat.) The Douglas Inan Centre Glas. Specialty: Forens. Psychiat. Prev: Cons. (Forens. Med.), Dougla Inch Centre.

RAMSAY, Margaret Mary Department of Obstetrics & Gynaecology, Queen's Medical Centre, Nottingham NG7 2UH Tel: 0115 924 9924 Fax: 0115 970 9776 Email: margaret.ramsay@nottingham.ac.uk; The Hayloft, Town End Court, Main Street, West Leake, Loughborough LE12 5RF Tel: 01509 852651 — (Camb.) MA Camb. 1985, BA 1981, MD 1993, MB 1984, BChir 1983; MRCP (UK) 1987; MRCOG 1989. Sen. Lect. (FetoMatern. Med.) Qu. Med. Centre Nottm. Specialty: Obst. & Gyn. Socs: Internat. Soc. Study Hypertens. in Pregn.; MacDonald Club. Prev: Vis. Asst. Prof. Physiol. Cornell Univ., USA; Train. Fell.

(FetoMatern. Med.) Nottm.; Sen. Regist. (O & G) Derby City Gen. Hosp.

RAMSAY, Mary Elizabeth Booth Public Health Laboratory Service, Communicable Disease Surveillance Centre, London NW9 5EQ — MB BS Lond. 1985. Cons. Epidemiol.

RAMSAY, Maureen Wilson The Priory Consulting Rooms, 2 Clarendon Road, Bournemouth BH4 8AH Tel: 01202 760079 — MB ChB Ed. 1979; BSc (Med. Sci.) Ed. 1976; MRCGP 1987; MRCPsych 1988. Cons. Psychiat. The Priory Hosp. Marchwood Soton. Specialty: Gen. Psychiat. Prev: Cons. Psychiat. Roy. S. Hants Hosp. Soton.

RAMSAY, Peter Denis Bewick Crescent Surgery, 27 Bewick Crescent, Newton Aycliffe DL5 5LH Tel: 01325 313289 Fax: 01325 301428 — BM BCh Oxf. 1982; DCCH RCP Ed. 1985; MRCGP 1986; DRCOG 1986. GP Newton Aycliffe.

RAMSAY, Robert Greig 15 March Road, Edinburgh EH4 3TD — MB ChB Aberd. 1985.

RAMSAY, Roger Barrington The Surgery, Scotland Street, Llanrwst LL26 0AL Tel: 01492 640411 Fax: 01492 641402; Garreg Wen, Llanddoged, Llanrwst LL26 0BJ — MB ChB Manch. 1982; DObst RCOG 1985; FRCGP 1995, M 1986.

RAMSAY, Rosalind Louisa Scutari, St Thomas' Hospital, London SE1 7EH Tel: 020 7928 9292 Fax: 020 7922 8294 — MB BS Lond. 1986; MRCPsych 1990. Cons. Psychiat. St. Thos. Hosp. Lond. Specialty: Gen. Psychiat. Prev: Sen. Regist. (Psychiat.) Maudsley & Bethlem Hosp.

RAMSAY, Rosemary The Health Centre, Redbourn, St Albans AL3 7LZ Tel: 01582 792356 — MB ChB Ed. 1986. Gen. Practitioner.

RAMSAY, Sarah Jane Top Floor Flat, Flat C, 73 Malvern Road, London NW6 5PU Tel: 020 7625 9306 — MB BS Lond. 1991; BSc Lond. (Hons.) 1988; MB BS (Hons.) Lond. 1991; FRCA 1995. Specialty: Anaesth.

RAMSAY, Scott Gordon 95 Kettil'stoun Mains, Linlithgow EH49 6SJ — MB ChB Glas. 1991 (Univ. Glas.) BSc (1st cl. Hons.) Anat. Glas. 1988; MB ChB (Commend.) Glas. 1991; MRCP (UK) 1994; MD Glas. 1999. Specialist Regist. (Geriat. Med.) & Gen. Medicene Glas. Roy. Infirm. Specialty: Care of the Elderly; Gen. Med. Socs: RCPS Glas.; Brit. Thorac. Soc.; Brit. Geriat. Soc. Prev: Career Regist. (Gen. Med.) StoneHo. Hosp. Lanarksh.; Research Fell. (Respirat. Med.) Gartnavel Gen. Hosp. Glas.; SHO Rotat. (Med.) West. Infirm. Glas.

RAMSAY, Timothy Merle 1 Bollinwood Chase, Wilmslow SK9 2DF Tel: 01625 522390 — MB ChB Dundee 1982; DA (Eng.) 1984; DRCOG 1986; FFA RCS Eng. 1988. Cons. Anaesth. Stepping Hill Hosp. Stockport. Specialty: Anaesth.

RAMSAY, Mr William Mauchline Mains, Mauchline KA5 6LL — MB ChB Ed. 1977; BSc (Hons.) Med. Sci. 1974; FRCS Ed. 1982.

RAMSAY, William Wallace (retired) 2 The Firs, Portadown, Craigavon BT63 5TA Tel: 028 3833 3597 Email: williamramsay@freewire.co.uk — MB BCh BAO 1953 (Belf.) DObst RCOG 1956; DPH 1958; FRCGP 1982, M 1965; MD Belf. 1967.

RAMSAY-BAGGS, Mr Peter Northern Ireland Regional Maxillofacial Service, The Ulster Hospital, Department Oral & Maxillofacial Surgery, Dundonald, Belfast BT16 1RF Tel: 028 90484511 Ext: 2464/028 90550418 Fax: 028 90561388 Email: peter.ramsay-baggs@ucht.n-i.nhs.uk/ramsayb@enterprise.net; Private Consulting Rooms, Holywood Dental Care, 128 High Street, Holywood BT18 Tel: 028 90423306 Fax: 028 90423313 Email: prb@maxfac.net — MB BCh BAO Belf. 1985 (Queens Univ. Belfast) BDS Lond. 1976; FFD RCSI 1986; FDS RCS Eng. 1987; FRCS Ed. 1989. Cons. Surg. (Oral & Maxillofacial Surgery) Ulster Hosp. Dundonald & Roy. Vict. Hosp. Belf.; Cons. (Oral & Maxillofacial Surg.) Daisy Hill Hosp. Newry. Specialty: Oral & Maxillofacial Surg. Special Interest: Maxillofacial Trauma; Orthognathic Surg.; Surgic. Dent. Socs: Brit. Dent. Assn.; Brit. Med. Asociation; Brit. Assn. of Oral & Maxillofacial Surgeons. Prev: Sen. Regist. Regional Oral & Maxillofacial Unit N. Irel.; Regist. (Maxillofacial) Ulster Hosp. Dundonald & Monklands Hosp. Airedrie; Regist. (Maxillofacial) Univ. Coll. Hosp. Lond.

RAMSAY SMITH, Mr Samuel Richard Department of Surgery, Victoria Hospital, Nevill Road, Lewes BN7 1PE Tel: 01273 474153 Fax: 01273 473362; 15 Arundel Street, Brighton BN2 5TG Tel: 01273 680386 — MB ChB Liverp. 1971; DCH RCP Lond. 1974; FRCS Eng. 1976; MSc Lond. 1985. Assoc. Specialist & Resid. Surg. Vict. Hosp. E. Sussex; Cons. Pub. Health E. Sussex HA. Socs: Fell. Roy. Soc. Trop. Med. & Hyg.; Assn. Med. Educat. Europ.; Assn. Surg.. E. Afr. Prev: Health of the Nation Co-ordinator Brighton; GP Hailsham E. Sussex; Safari Surg. E. Afr. Flying Doctors.

RAMSBOTHAM, Simon Edward Thornton Heath Health Centre, 61A Gillet Road, Thornton Heath CR7 8RL Tel: 020 8689 5797 Fax: 020 8665 1195; 36 Bensham Lane, Croydon CR0 2RQ Tel: 020 8689 2916 — MB BS Lond. 1973 (St. Thos.) Dip GM GP; DCH Eng. 1976; MRCGP 1980. GP Croydon. Specialty: Gen. Pract. Socs: BMA. Prev: SHO (Gen. Surg.) St. Jas. Hosp. Balham; Regist. (A & E) May Day Hosp. Thornton Health; SHO (Paediat.) Childr. Hosp. Sydenham.

RAMSBOTTOM, Norman The Wellington Hospital, Wellington Place, London NW8 9LE Tel: 020 7580 2946 Fax: 020 7637 4983; 90 Langton Way, Blackheath, London SE3 7JU Tel: 020 8858 3555 — MB BS Lond. 1964; MRCS Eng. LRCP Lond. 1964. Socs: Brit. Soc. Gastroenterol. & Physiol. Soc. Prev: Lect. (Physiol.) Guy's Hosp. Med. Sch. Lond.; Asst. Ho. Phys. & Ho. Surg. Guy's Hosp. Lond.

RAMSBOTTOM, Timothy James The Surgery, Nevells Road, Letchworth SG6 4TS Tel: 01462 675526 — BM BCh Oxf. 1993; MA Oxf. 1990; DCH RCP Lond. 1995; DFFP 1997; DRCOG 1997. GP Princip. Specialty: Gen. Pract. Socs: Christ. Med. Fellowsh. Prev: SHO (Paediat.) Roy. United Hosp. Bath; Ho. Off. (Gen. Med.) John Radcliffe Hosp. Oxf.; Ho. Off. (Gen. Surg.) Milton Keynes Gen. Hosp.

RAMSDALE, David Roland The Cardiothoracic Centre, Thomas Drive, Liverpool L14 3PE Tel: 0151 228 1616 Fax: 0151 220 8573 Email: david.ramsdale@ctc.nhs.uk — MB ChB Manch. 1975; BSc (Hons.) (Anat.) Manch. 1971; MRCP (UK) 1978; MD Manch. 1981; FRCP Lond. 1991. Cons. Cardiol. Cardiothoracic Centre Liverp. Specialty: Cardiol.

RAMSDALE, James Edward Elms Medical Centre, 31 Hoole Road, Chester CH2 3NH Tel: 01244 351000 — MB ChB Liverp. 1976.

RAMSDEN, Alexander John 15 Hazelwood Avenue, Newcastle upon Tyne NE2 3HU — MB ChB Glas. 1996.

RAMSDEN, Alistair Richard Lake House, Legh Road, Knutsford WA16 8LP; 3 Travellers Rest, Pickwick, Corsham SN13 0PP Tel: 01249 715410 — MB ChB Ed. 1997. Specialty: Gen. Surg.

RAMSDEN, Arthur Tapstone House, Hud Hey Road, Haslingden, Rossendale BB4 5JL — MB ChB Liverp. 1953. Specialty: Civil Serv. Prev: GP Haslingden; Ho. Phys. & Ho. Surg. Bury Gen. Hosp.; Med. Ref. Benefits Agency.

RAMSDEN, Clive Stuart Spring Grove House, Chapel Hill, Clayton West, Huddersfield HD8 9NH — MB ChB Manch. 1979; MRCOG 1985; MD Manch. 1989. Sen. Regist. (O & G) Leeds. Specialty: Obst. & Gyn.

RAMSDEN, Gordon Hugh Clifflands, Whitbarrow Road, Lymm WA13 9AG — MD Manch. 1991; MB ChB Manch 1979; DRCOG 1983; MRCOG 1987. Cons. O & G Chesh. Specialty: Obst. & Gyn.

RAMSDEN, Karen Lesley Department of Histopathology, Walsgrave Hospitals NHS Trust, Clifford Bridge Road, Coventry CV2 2DX — MB ChB Sheff. 1983; MRCPath 1991. Cons. Histopath. & Cytopath. Walsgrave Hosps. NHS Trust. Specialty: Histopath. Prev: Cons. in Histopath. & Cytopath. Bury Health Care NHS Trust; Sen. Regist. & Regist. (Histopath.) W. Midl. RHA; SHO (Path.) N. Manch. Gen. Hosp.

RAMSDEN, Michael John (retired) 7 Chevet Lane, Wakefield WF2 6HN Tel: 01924 255356 — (Camb. & St. Mary's) MA, MB Camb. 1959, BChir 1958; MRCS Eng. LRCP Lond. 1958; DObst RCOG 1962. Prev: Ho. Surg. & Ho. Phys. Clayton Hosp. Wakefield.

RAMSDEN, Peter Andrew Mayford House Surgery, East Road, Northallerton DL6 1NP Tel: 01609 772105 Fax: 01609 778553 — MB BS Lond. 1987; DRCOG 1991.

RAMSDEN, Mr Peter David Carr House, Great Bavington, Newcastle upon Tyne NE19 2BN — MB BS Lond. 1968; MRCS Eng. LRCP Lond. 1968; FRCS Eng. 1975. Cons. (Urol. Surg.) Freeman Hosp. Newc. Upon Tyne. Specialty: Urol.

RAMSDEN, Peter George (retired) — MB BS Lond. 1970; MRCS Eng. LRCP Lond. 1970. Appeals Serv. Med. Tribunal Mem. Prev: Gen. Practitioner.

RAMSDEN, Professor Richard Thomas Anson Medical Centre, 23 Anson Road, Manchester M14 5BZ Tel: 0161 248 2022 Fax: 0161 248 2025 Email: michael.ramsden@man.ac.uk; Brick Bank, Brick Bank Lane, Allostock, Knutsford WA16 9LY Tel: 01477

544838 — (St. And.) MB ChB St. And. 1968; FRCS Eng. 1973; FRCS (ED) (ad. Hominem) 2000. Cons. Otolaryngol. Manch. Roy. Infirm.; Hon. Prof. Otolaryngol. Univ. Manch.; Hon. Lect. Centre for Audiol., Educat. of the Deaf & Speech Path. Univ. Manch.; Edit. Bd. Jl. Laryngol. - Otol., ENT Jl. & Revue de Laryngologie Otologie & Rhinologie. Specialty: Otolaryngol. Socs: Fell. Roy. Soc. Med. (Pres, Treas. & Hon. Sec. Sect. Otol.); Corr. Mem. Die Deutsche Gesellschaft fur Hals Nasen Ohren Heilkunde; Otolaryngol. Research Soc. Prev: Sen. Regist. (Otolaryngol.) Lond. Hosp.; Sen. Regist. & Regist. Roy. Nat. Throat, Nose & Ear Hosp. Lond.; Otology and Neurotology.

RAMSDEN, Simon Steve The Pembridge Villas Surgery, 45A Pembridge Villas, London W11 3EP Tel: 020 7727 2222 Fax: 020 7792 2867; 45A Pembridge Villas, London W11 3EP Tel: 020 7727 2222 — MD Lond. 1994; MB BS 1984; MA Oxf. 1987; MRCP (UK) 1987; MRCGP 1988. Specialty: Gen. Pract. Socs: ICI Prize 1984.; Chairm. KCW Local Med. Comm. Prev: SHO (Med.) St. Mary's Hosp. Lond.; SHO (Paediat.) Univ. Coll. Hosp. Lond.

RAMSDEN, Valerie Marie Bollington Medical Centre, Wellington Road, Bollington, Macclesfield SK10 5JL Tel: 01625 572481 — MB ChB Manch. 1982; MRCP (UK) 1986; DRCOG 1988; MRCGP 1990. GP Chesh.; GPwSI Dermat. E. Chesh. Prev: Clin. Asst. in Dermat. Buxton Hosp.; Trainee GP Handforth Health Centre Chesh.; Regist. (Haemat.) Manch. Roy. Infirm.

RAMSDEN, Walter Norman (retired) 42 Repton Drive, The Westlands, Newcastle ST5 3JF Tel: 01782 617651 — MB BChir Camb. 1963 (Camb. & Lond. Hosp.) BA Camb. 1959; MRCS Eng. LRCP Lond. 1962; FFA RCS Eng. 1967. Prev: Cons. Anaesth. N. Staffs. Hosp. Trust.

RAMSDEN, William Hugh Department of Clinical Radiology, St. James's University Hospital, Beckett St., Leeds LS9 7TF Tel: 0113 243 3144 Ext: 65331 — BM Soton. 1984; FRCS Ed. 1989; FRCR 1993; T(R) (CR) 1994. Cons. Radiol. St. Jas. Univ. Hosp. Leeds. Specialty: Radiol. Prev: Sen. Regist. (Radiol.) Yorks. RHA.

RAMSEEBALUCK, Bhimduth Kempton House, Main Rd, Fleggburgh, Great Yarmouth NR29 3BA — LRCPI & LM, LRSCI & LM 1971. Specialty: Gen. Pract. Socs: BMA.

RAMSELL, Nicola Jane Annandale Surgery, 239 Mutton Lane, Potters Bar EN6 2AS Tel: 01865 374242 Fax: 01865 377826; 4 Heath Lane, Bladon, Woodstock OX20 1SB Tel: 01993 811318 — MB BS Lond. 1988 (Roy. Free Med. Sch.) DCH RCP Lond. 1991; MRCGP 1992. Prev: Trainee GP Northwick Pk. Hosp. VTS.

RAMSELL, Susan Elizabeth Grasmere House, Dugdale Hill Lane, Potters Bar EN6 2DB — MB BS Lond. 1988; DCH RCP Lond. 1990; DRCOG 1991; MRCGP 1993.

RAMSEY, Deborah Jennifer Caroline — MB BS Lond. 1996 (Char. Cross & Westm. Med. Sch. Lond.) MA Cantab. 1997; MRCP UK 1999. Research Fell. (Stroke Medicine) Kings Coll. Lond. & William Havey Hosp. Kent. Specialty: Gen. Med. Special Interest: Care of the Elderly. Prev: SHO (Med.) Lewisham Hosp,. Lond.; SHO (Haemat.) Guy's Hosp. Lond.; SHO (Med.) Guy's Hosp. Lond.

RAMSEY, Hugh Cameron Holywood Arches Health Centre, Westminster Avenue, Belfast BT4 1NS Tel: 028 9056 3354 Fax: 028 9065 3846; 14 Massey Court, Belfast BT4 3GJ — MB BCh BAO Belf. 1967; DCH RCPS Glas. 1971.

RAMSEY, James Kenneth Banbridge Medical Group Centre, Linenhall Street, Banbridge BT32 3EG — MB BCh BAO Belf. 1970.

RAMSEY, Joan Atkinson (retired) 14 Massey Court, Belfast BT4 3GJ — MB BCh BAO Belf. 1967. Med. Off. Cytopath., Belf. City Hosp.

RAMSEY, John Charles Patrick 59 Eglantine Avenue, Belfast BT9 6EW Tel: 01232 280167 — MB BCh BAO Dub. 1985; FRCR 1991. Cons. Radiol. Belf. City Hosp. Specialty: Radiol.

RAMSEY, John M 22 Shirley Avenue, Cheam, Sutton SM2 7QR Tel: 020 8642 3452 — MD Tehran 1959; MRCS Eng. LRCP Lond. 1974.

RAMSEY, Marianne Clare 53 Englands Lane, Loughton IG10 2QX — MB BS Lond. 1987.

RAMSEY, Mark William Regional Cardiac Centre, Morriston Hospital, Swansea NHS Trust, Swansea SA6 6NL Tel: 01792 704123 Fax: 01792 704140 Email: mark.ramsey@swansea-tr.wales.nhs.uk — BM BS Nottm. 1984 (Univ. of Nottingham) BMedSci 1982; MRCP (UK) 1987; DM Nottm. 1997; FRCP 2001. Cons. Cardiol. Morriston Hosp. Swansea NHS Trust; Sen. Clin. Tutor, Swansea Clin. Sch. Swansea. Specialty: Cardiol. Special Interest: Arterial Mech.; Echocardiography; Interventional Cardiol. Socs: Brit. Cardiac Soc.; Brit. Cardiovasc. Interven. Soc.; Brit. Soc. Echocardiogr. Prev: Lect. & Hon. Sen. Regist. Univ. Wales Coll. Med. & Univ. Hosp. Wales Cardiff.; Regist. (Med.) Newc. Gp. Hosps.

RAMSEY, Pamela May Allendale, 22 Shirley Avenue, Cheam, Sutton SM2 7QR Tel: 020 8642 3452 — MB BS Durh. 1966.

RAMSEY, Peter Jerry 11A Ballymoney Road, Banbridge BT32 4DS — MB ChB Aberd. 1997.

RAMSEY, Thomas Linton Knockan Road, Broughshane, Ballymena BT42 Tel: 01648 2233 — MRCS Eng. LRCP Lond. 1970. SHO (Med.) Mid-Ulster Hosp. Magherafelt. Prev: Ho. Surg., Ho. Phys. & SHO (O & G) Mid-Ulster Hosp.

RAMSHAW, Andrew Lilwall The Park Medical Group, Fawdon Park Road, Newcastle upon Tyne NE3 2PE Tel: 0191 285 1763 Fax: 0191 284 2374; Park Medical Group, Kingston Pk Avenue, Kingston Park, Newcastle upon Tyne NE3 2HB Tel: 0191 286 0022 Fax: 0191 271 2544 — MB BS Newc. 1988; MRCGP 1993; DFFP 1993; DRCOG 1993. Prev: Trainee GP Newc.

RAMSIS, Helen Elizabeth 44 Lindley Road, London E10 6QT — MRCS Eng. LRCP Lond. 1978 (Liverp.) DO RCS Eng. 1986; FRCOphth 1990. Specialty: Ophth. Socs: BMA, Fellow of RSM. Prev: Eye Bank Off. Moorfields Eye Hosp. Lond.; SHO (Ophth.) N. Middlx. Hosp. Lond. & York Dist. Hosp.; SHO (Ophth.) Myland Hosp. Colchester & Eye, Ear & Throat Hosp. Shrewsbury.

RAMSTEAD, Mr Keith Douglas 20 Gilleney Grove, Whiston, Prescot L35 7NL Tel: 0151 431 0252 Fax: 0151 431 0700 — MB ChB Manch. 1976; BSc (2nd cl. Hons.) (Anat.) Manch. 1973; FRCS Ed. 1980; FRCS Eng. 1981; FRCS (Cardiothor Surg.) Ed. 1985; T(S) 1991. Staff Grade (A & E) Rochdale Healthcare NHS Trust. Specialty: Accid. & Emerg. Prev: Sen. Regist. Cardiothoracic Surg. S.E. Thames RHA; Regist. Cardiothoracic Surg. Wythenshawe Hosp. Manch.; Ho. Surg. Profess. Unit Withington Hosp. Manch.

RAMSTER, David Guy 33 Welshwood Park Road, Colchester CO4 3HZ Tel: 01206 861191 — MB BChir Camb. 1971; MA Camb. 1972, MB BChir 1971; MRCPsych 1976. Opinion Apptd. Doctor Ment. Health Act Commiss. Specialty: Gen. Psychiat. Prev: Cons. Psychiat. NE Essex Ment. Health Servs. Colchester.; Sen. Regist. (Psychiat.) Old Manor Hosp. Salisbury; Regist. (Psychiat.) E. Anglian RHB.

RAMU, V K Crescent Surgery, 8 The Crescent, Halfway, Sheerness ME12 3BQ Tel: 01795 662941 — MB BS Kerala 1973; MB BS Kerala 1973.

RAMUS, Mr Neville Ian Taunton & Somerset Hospital, Musgrove Park, Taunton TA1 5DA Tel: 01823 342104 Fax: 01823 323691; Thomas's House, Oake, Taunton TA4 1AR Tel: 01823 461974 Fax: 01823 461974 — MB BS Lond. 1969 (St Mary's) FRCS Eng. 1973; MD Lond. 1978. Cons. Surg. Som. HA; Surg. Tutor to RCS Eng.; Chairm. SW Regional BST Comm.; Mem.Counc. Surgic. Sect. RSM; Mem.Council of ASGBI Intercollegiate Examiner, Ct. Examrs. RCS Eng. Specialty: Gen. Surg. Socs: Internat. Assn. Endocrine Surgs.; Brit. Assn. Surg. Oncol.; Brit. Soc. Gastroenterol. Prev: Sen. Regist. (Surg.) Bristol Roy. Infirm.; Research Fell. (Surg.) Univ. Texas Med. Br. Galveston, USA.

RAMWELL, John Department of Anaesthesia, Cheriton House, South Cleveland Hospital, Marton Road, Middlesbrough TS4 3BW Tel: 01642 854600; 87 Davenport Road, Yarm on Tees, Yarm TS15 9TN Tel: 01642 790372 — MB BS Newc. 1980; DA (UK) 1988. Assoc. Specialist Anaesth. S. Tees Acute Hosps. Trust. Specialty: Anaesth.

RAMZAN, Asif Yusif St Luke's Hospital, The Hutton Unit, Marton Road, Middlesbrough TS4 3AF — MB ChB Sheff. 1993; MRCPsych 1998. Cons. Forens. Psychiat. Hutton Centre, Middlesborough. Specialty: Neuropath. Prev: Specialist Regist., Forens. Psychiat. Newton Lodge Regional. Secure Unit. Wakefield.

RAMZAN, Mohammed Ascot Medical Centre, 690 Osmaston Road, Derby DE24 8GT Tel: 01332 348845 — MB ChB Manch. 1981; DRCOG 1985.

RANA, Arup Kumar 122 High Street, Hook, Goole DN14 5PJ — MB BS Calcutta 1972 (R.G. Kar Med. Coll.) Assoc. Specialist (Orthop.) Pontefract Gen. Infirm. Specialty: Orthop. Prev: SHO (A & E) Weymouth & Dist. Hosp.; SHO (Urol.) Bart. Hosp. Lond.; SHO (Med.) Elderly St. John Hosp. Goole.

RANA, Brijender Singh West Kent Health Authority, Preston Hall, Aylesford ME20 7NJ Tel: 01622 710161 Fax: 01622 719802; 9 College Drive, Tunbridge Wells TN2 3PN — MB ChB Dundee 1975; DTM & H Liverp. 1978; MRCP (UK) 1981; MFPHM RCP (UK) 1991. Cons., Pub. Health Med. Specialty: Pub. Health Med.

RANA, Bushra Shahida 67A Stour Road, Christchurch BH23 1LN — MB BS Lond. 1993.

RANA, Dur-E-Sameen 63 Woodlands Road, Ilford IG1 1JN — MB BS Lond. 1994.

RANA, Durgesh Nandini Manchester Royal Infirmary, Cytology Centre, Clinical Sciences Building 2, Oxford Road, Manchester M13 9WW — MB BS Rajasthan 1989. Cons. Cytopathologist Centr. Manch. & Manch. Univ. Hosps. Specialty: Histopath. Special Interest: Cytopathology.

RANA, Hitesh Dahyabhai 6 Barkby, Lower Earley, Reading RG6 3DY Tel: 0118 987 6548 — MB BS Bombay 1992. SHO (Paediat.) Yeovil Hosp. Som. Specialty: Orthop.

RANA, Kamlesh 23 Prestbury Road, Aston, Birmingham B6 6EP — BM BS Nottm. 1991.

RANA, Muhammad Zubair Khan 67A Stour Road, Christchurch BH23 1LN; Royal Bournemouth Hospital, Bournemouth BH7 7DW Tel: 01202 704590 Fax: 01202 704589 — (Nishter Med. Coll. Multan) BSc, MB BS Panjab (Pakistan) 1965; MRCP (UK) 1975; FRCP Ed. 1985; FRCP Lond. 1985; FRCP Glas. 1994. Cons. Phys. (Geriat. Med.) Wessex RHA. Specialty: Gen. Med. Socs: Fell. Internat. Coll. Angiol.; Brit. Soc. Digestive Endoscopy.; Brit. Soc. Geriat.s. Prev: Sen. Regist. (Geriat. Med.) Soton. Gen. Hosp.; Regist. (Med.) Liaquat. Med. Coll. Hosp. Hyderabad, Pakistan; Regist. (Geriat. Med.) Battle Hosp. Reading.

RANA, Mr Pradip Shumshere St. Peter's District General Hospital, Guildford Road, Chertsey KT16 0PZ Tel: 0193 287 2000 Fax: 01276 858290/01932 873352 Email: prana@doctors.org.uk; 31 Red Lion Road, Chobham, Woking GU24 8RG Tel: 01276 857001 Fax: 01276 858290 — (Calcutta Medical College) FRCS Ed. 1976. Cons. Surg. A & E Dept. St. Peter's Dist. Gen. Hosp. Chertsey. Specialty: Accid. & Emerg.; Gen. Surg. Socs: FFAEM (Founding Fell.).

RANA, Pratap S Geriatric Medicine (Wd. 6/7), Huddersfield Royal Infirmary, Acre Street, Huddersfield HD3 3EA Tel: 01484 342704 Fax: 01484 347152 — MD Delhi 1989; MRCP (UK) Ed. 1992; MB BS Delhi 1986 (Maulawa Azad Med. Coll.) Specialty: Gen. Med.; Gastroenterol. Socs: Brit. Geriat.s Soc.; Brit. Soc. of Gastroenterol.; Roy. Coll. of Phys.s, Lond. Prev: Specialist Regist., Geriat. Med., Soton. Gen. Hosp.

RANA, Sanjeev Kumar 42 Hartington Road, Manchester M21 8UY — MB BS Lond. 1995.

RANA, Sunita 27 Whitton Street, Wednesbury WS10 8BA — MB ChB Leic. 1995.

RANA, Tanvir Ahmad 21 McKenzie Court, Northern Birmingham Community NHS Trust, All Saints Hospital, Lodge Road, Hockley, Birmingham B18 5SD; 37 Limetree Road, Sutton Coldfield B74 3SG — MB BS Punjab 1985.

RANA, Tasneem 235 Crookesmoor Road, Sheffield S6 3FQ — MB ChB Sheff. 1994.

RANABOLDO, Mr Charles Jean Salisbury District Hospital, Salisbury SP5 8BJ Tel: 01722 425290 Email: cranaboldo@compuserve.com — BM Soton. 1984; FRCS Eng 1989; FRCS Gen 1996; MS Soton 1997. Cons. (Gen. & Vasc. Surg.) Salisbury Dist. Hosp. Specialty: Gen. Surg. Socs: Assn. Surg. GB & Irel.; Assoc. Endoscopic Surg.; Europ. Vasc. Surg. Soc. Prev: Sen. Regist. Roy. United Hosp. Bath; Regist. (Surg.) Portsmouth Hosps.; Research Fell. (Vasc.) Soton. Univ. Hosps.

RANADE, Joothica Ulhas The Surgery, 25 Chichele Road, London NW2 3AN Tel: 020 8452 4666 Fax: 020 8450 3680 — MB BS Bombay 1970.

RANAGHAN, Elizabeth Anne 55 Maryville Park, Belfast BT9 6LP — MB BCh BAO Belf. 1985.

RANASINGHE, Aaron Matthew 1 Westend Villas, Newbury Park, Ledbury HR8 1AX — MB ChB Birm. 1997.

RANASINGHE, Charles Lionel (retired) 2 Willow Lea, Oxton, Birkenhead L43 2GO — MB BS Lond. 1959.

RANASINGHE, David Nihal Essex Rivers Healthcare NHS Trust, Colchester General Hospital, Turner Road, Colchester CO4 5JL Tel: 01206 853535 — MB BS Colombo 1980 (University of Colombo, Sri Lanka) DA (UK) 1986; FFA RCS Eng. 1989; DEAA 1995. Cons. Anaesth. Essex Rivers Healthcare NHS Trust Colchester Gen. Hosp. Specialty: Anaesth. Prev: Cons. Anaesth. St. Albans & Hemel Hempstead NHS Trust; Sen. Regist. Rotat. (Anaesth.) Roy. Free Hosp. Lond.; Post-Fellowsh. Regist. Harefield Hosp. Middlx.

RANASINGHE, Don Upali Church House Surgery, 3 Church Passage, Barnet EN5 4QS Tel: 020 8449 9622; Church House Surgery, 3 Church Passage, Wood St., Barnet EN5 4QS Tel: 020 8449 9622 — MB BS Sri Lanka 1975 (Kandy, Sri Lanka) MRCOG 1989. GP Ch. Ho. Surg.

RANASINGHE, Dulmini Piyawandi 106 Poverest Road, Orpington BR5 2DQ — MB ChB Liverp. 1998; MB ChB Liverp 1998.

RANASINGHE, Hapu Arachchillage Newton 14 Clifton Avenue, Culcheth, Warrington WA3 4PD Tel: 01925 763067; Hollins Park Hospital, Hollins Lane, Winwick, Warrington WA3 Tel: 01925 664000 — (Ceylon) MB BS Ceylon 1969; DPM Lond. 1981; MRCPsych 1982. Cons. Psychiat. Hollins Pk. Hosp. Warrington; Cons. Psychiat. Winwick Hosp. Warrington. Specialty: Gen. Psychiat. Prev: Cons. Psychiat. NewCh. Hosp. Warrington; Staff Psychiat. Lakehead Psychiat. Hosp. Thunderbay, Ontario, Canada; Cons. Psychiat. Winwick Hosp. Warrington.

RANASINGHE, Harischandra 71 Montagu Avenue, Gosforth, Newcastle upon Tyne NE3 4JN — MB BS Ceylon 1955 (Colombo) FRCP Ed. 1975, M 1960; DMJ (Clin. & Path.) Soc. Apoth. Lond. 1968. Sen. Lect. (Forens. Path.) Univ. Newc.; Hon. Cons. Newc. AHA (T).

RANASINGHE, Nalini Church House Surgery, 3 Church Passage, Barnet EN5 4QS Tel: 020 8449 9622; 14 Ashurst Road, Barnet EN4 9LF — MB BS Sri Lanka 1975 (Colombo Sri Lanka) MRCP (UK) 1986. GP Ch. Hse. Surg. Barnet.

RANASINGHE, Pandikoralalage Nilamani Ianthi 35 Hollymead Close, Colchester CO4 5JU — MB BS Colombo 1980.

RANASINGHE, Renuka Sharon 15 Marshall Road, Cambridge CB1 7TY — MB BS Colombo 1990 (Roy. Free Hosp. Sch. Med.) MRCS Eng. LRCP Lond. 1990; DCH RCP Lond. 1994; DFFP 1995; DRCOG 1995; MRCGP 1995. Clin. Asst. Renal Dialysis Unit Addenbrooke's Hosp. Camb. Prev: Trainee GP/SHO Addenbrooke's Hosp. Camb. VTS; Ho. Phys. (Med.) Roy. Free Hosp. Lond.

RANASINGHE, Mr Suraj Elsham House, Cliff Gardens, Scunthorpe DN15 7BH — MB BS Colombo 1986; FRCS Ed. 1993. Staff Grade (A & E) Roy. Lancaster Infirm.

RANASINGHE, Wijesundara Appuhamillage Edmund Peiris National Blood Service, Cambridge Blood Centre, Long Road, Cambridge CB2 2PT Tel: 01223 548030 Fax: 01223 548136 Email: edmund.ranasinghe@nbs.nhs.uk; 44 Tomlyns Close, Hutton, Brentwood CM13 1PU — MB BS Ceylon 1967; FRCPath 1992, M 1980; MSc (Immunol.) Lond. 1989. Cons. Haemat. Nat. Blood Serv. Cambridge Blood Centre. Specialty: Haematology. Socs: Brit. Blood Transfus. Soc.; Brit. Med. Assn. Prev: Cons. Haemat. Nat. Blood Serv. Brentwood; Research Fell. N. Lond. Blood Transfus. Centre Edgware, Middlx.; Cons. Haemat. & Chief of Path. Abdulla Fouad Hosp. Dammam, Saudi Arabia.

RANASINHA, Kingsley Woodward Department of Medicine, Epsom General Hospital, Dorking Road, Epsom KT18 7EG Tel: 01372 735104 Fax: 01372 735261; Wedgwood, Woodcote Pk Road, Epsom KT18 7EY Tel: 01372 720240 — MD Ceylon 1970 (Colombo) MB BS Ceylon 1960; FRCP Ed. 1982, M 1966; FRCP Lond. 1981, M 1967; FCCP Ceylon 1986. Cons. Phys. Epsom Gen. Hosp., Epsom & St. Helier Health Care Trust Gen. Med. & Elderly Care. Specialty: Gen. Med.; Care of the Elderly; Neurol. Socs: Brit. Geriat. Soc. & Brit. Soc. Digestive Endoscopy; Sri Lanka Med. Assoc; Fell. of the Ceylon Coll. of Phys.s Uhniversity of Ceylon M 1980. Prev: SHO (Gen. Med.) & Regist. (Gen. Med.) Epsom Dist. Hosp.; Sen. Lect. in Med. Univ. Ceylon Peradeniya.

RANAWAT, Nitranjan Singh Colchester General Hospital, Colchester CO4 5JL Tel: 01206 853535; 9 Lexden Court, Lexden, Colchester CO3 3QP Tel: 01206 563233 — MB BS Indore 1966. Assoc. Specialist (Surg.) Colchester Gen. Hosp. & Black Notley Regional Orthop. Centre NE Thames RHA. Specialty: Orthop. Socs: Fell. BOA. Prev: Research Fell. (Orthop.) Hosp. Special Surg. New York; Regist. (Orthop.) Warwick Hosp.

RANCE, Bernard Harry Melide, Hallgate, Gedney, Spalding PE12 0AH — MB ChB Leeds 1956; MFOM RCP Lond. 1982.

Specialty: Gen. Pract.; Aviat. Med.; Occupat. Health. Socs: Aerospace Med. Assn.; Soc. Occupat. Med.; Ergonomics Soc.

RANCE, Mr Christopher Hugh City Hospital NG5 1PB Tel: 0115 9691 169 Ext: 46453 Fax: 0115 8402 679 Email: crance@ncht.trent.nhs.uk — MB BS Lond. 1971; MRCS Eng. LRCP Lond. 1971 (St Marys Hosp., Paddington) BSc, Lond. 1968; Dip.Obst., RCOG., FRACS 1978; FRCS, Eng. 2000. Cons. Paediatric Urol., City & Univ. Hosp., Nottm.; Cons. Paediatric Urol., Derby Children's Hosp., Lincoln Co. Hosp. Specialty: Paediat. Special Interest: Hypospadias; Urology. Socs: Brit. Assn. of Paediatric Surg.; Brit. Assn. of Paediatric Urol.; Europ. Soc. of Paediatric Urol. Prev: Cons. Paediatric Surg., Canberra Hosp., Australia.

RANCE, David Baskerville Liquorpond Street Surgery, 10 Liquorpond Street, Boston PE21 8UE Tel: 01205 362763 Fax: 01205 358918; 63 Linden Way, Boston PE21 9DT Tel: 01205 353649 — MRCS Eng. LRCP Lond. 1979 (St. Mary's) DCH RCP Lond. 1983; DRCOG 1984; MRCGP 1986. Prev: Clin. Asst. (Paediat.) Pilgrim Hosp. Boston Lincs.

RANCE, Jacqueline Margaret St Neots Surgery, 47 Wolseley Road, Plymouth PL2 3BJ Tel: 01752 561305 Fax: 01752 605565 — MB ChB Manch. 1976.

RAND, Mr Christopher Consultant Orthopaedic Surgeon, Princess Royal University Hospital, Farnborough Common, Orpington BR6 8ND Tel: 01689 865 698 Fax: 01689 864 451; 45 Constance Crescent, Hayes, Bromley BR2 7QH Tel: 020 8462 3184 — MB BS Lond. 1977 (Lond. Hosp.) BSc Leicester 1969; FRCS Ed. 1982; FRCS Ed. (Orth.) 1988. Cons. Orthop. Surg. Bromley Hosp. Specialty: Orthop. Prev: Cons. Orthop. Surg. Medway Hosp. Kent; Sen. Regist. Guy's & St. Thos. Hosp. Lond.; Anat. Demonst. Lond. Hosp. Med. Coll.

RAND, Julia Irene 4 Meadow Way, Hitchin SG5 2BN — MB BS Newc. 1990.

RAND, Mr Roger John Bradford Royal Infirmary, Duckworth Lane, Bradford BD9 6RJ Tel: 01274 364891 Fax: 01274 366690 Email: roger.rand@bradfordhospitals.nhs.uk; Ghyll Crest, 30 Ghyllwood Drive, Bingley BD16 1NF Tel: 01274 564190 — MB ChB Leeds 1968; DCH Eng. 1971; MD Leeds 1980; FRCOG 1986. Cons. O & G Bradford Hosps. Trust. Specialty: Obst. & Gyn. Special Interest: Colposcopy; Gyn. Oncol. Socs: BSCCP; Fell. N. Eng. Obst. & Gyn. Soc.-Pres.; RSM.

RAND, Walter (retired) Riftswood, 6 The Paddock, Walbottle Village, Newcastle upon Tyne NE15 8JG Tel: 0191 267 3238 — MB BS Durh. 1954.

RANDALL, Anthony Alexander Stephen South Oxford Health Centre, Lake Street, Oxford OX1 4RP Tel: 01865 244428 Fax: 01865 200985 — MB BS Lond. 1976 (St. Bart.) MA Oxf. 1976; Cert. Family Plann. JCC 1982; MRCGP 1982. GP Tutor (Pub. Health & Primary Care) Univ. Oxf. Prev: Trainee GP Oxf. VTS; Ho. Phys. Profess. Med. Unit Addenbrooke's Hosp. Camb.; Ho. Surg. St. Bart. Hosp. Lond.

RANDALL, Barbara Joy Dept. of Cellular Pathology, Medway Maritime Hospital, Gillingham ME7 5NY Tel: 01634 830000 — MB BChir Camb. 1979; MA Camb. 1981, BA 1976; MRCPath 1989; FRCPath 1997. Cons. Histopath. Medway HA. Specialty: Histopath. Socs: Assn. Clin. Path. & Internat. Acad. Path.; Brit. Soc. for Clin. Cytol. Prev: Sen. Regist. (Histopath.) Middlesbrough Gen. Hosp. & Roy. Vict. Infirm. Newc.; Regist. (Histopath.) Leicester Roy. Infirm. & Roy. Hants. Co. Hosp. Winchester; SHO (Path.) Brook Gen. Hosp. Lond.

RANDALL, Christine Elms Surgery, 5 Derby Street, Ormskirk L39 2BJ — MB ChB Liverp. 1985 (Liverpool) BSc (Hons.) Biochem. Liverp. 1982; MRCP (UK) 1988; MRCGP 1992. GP. Specialty: Gen. Pract. Socs: RCP; RCGP. Prev: SHO Med. Walton Hosp. Liverp.; SHO (O & G) Wellington, NZ.

RANDALL, Mr Christopher John Southampton University Hospitals Trust, St Mary's Road, Southampton SO14 0YG Tel: 02380 825079 — MB BS Lond. 1976; FRCS Eng. 1980. Cons. Otolaryngologist, Head and Neck Surg. Soton. Univ. Hosp. Specialty: Otorhinolaryngol. Prev: Sen. Regist. (ENT) St. Mary's Hosp. & Roy. Marsden Hosp. Lond.; Regist. (ENT) St. Mary's Hosp. Lond.; SHO (Surg.) Bristol Roy. Infirm.

RANDALL, Colin Frederick (retired) 7 Higher Port View, Saltash PL12 4BU — MB BS Lond. 1968 (Univ. Coll. Hosp.) MRCS Eng. LRCP Lond. 1968; DCH Eng. 1970; MRCP (UK) 1972; MRCGP 1974; FRCGP 1997, MD 2001. Hon. Lect. Plymouth Postgrad. Med. Sch. Plymouth Univ.; Course Organiser Plymouth VTS; Teach. (Gen. Pract.) Bristol Univ.; Hon. Research Fell. (Rheumatology) Plymouth NHS Trust. Prev: Princip. Trainer (Gen. Pract.) Saltash.

RANDALL, David George Stewart 16 Ravensbourne Gardens, London W13 8EW Tel: 020 8997 7227 — MB BS Lond. 1954 (Lond. Hosp.) Phys. USAF Hosp. S. Ruislip. Socs: Fell. Roy. Soc. Med. Prev: Ho. Phys. King Edwd. Memor. Hosp. Ealing; Ho. Surg. Hillingdon Hosp. Uxbridge.

RANDALL, Mr Derrick Henry (retired) 20 Stradbroke Road, Southwold IP18 6LQ Tel: 01502 723944 — MB BS Lond. 1951 (Westm.) MRCS Eng. LRCP Lond. 1943; FRCS Eng. 1948; MB BS (Univ. Medal) Lond. 1951. Prev: Cons. Surg. Roy. Hallamsh. Hosp. Sheff.

RANDALL, Elizabeth Mary The Health Centre, 68 Pipeland Road, St Andrews KY16 8JZ Tel: 01334 473441 Fax: 01334 466508; Tosh, Dunino, St Andrews KY16 8LT — MB ChB Leeds 1977; DRCOG 1979.

RANDALL, Fiona Maria Christchurch Hospital, The Macmillan Unit, Fairmile Road, Christchurch BH23 2JX Fax: 01202 705213 — MB BS Lond. 1977 (Westm. Hosp.) FRCP Lond. 1993; PHd Glasgow 2000. Cons. (Palliat. Med.) Roy. Bournemouth & ChristCh. Hosp. Trust; Sen. Clin. Teach. Soton. Med. Sch. Specialty: Palliat. Med. Special Interest: Healthcare Ethics. Socs: Association for Palliative Medicine.

RANDALL, Grahame Robert Haslemere Health Centre, Haslemere GU27 3BQ Tel: 01428 653881 Fax: 01428 645068 — MB BS Lond. 1963 (King's Coll. Hosp.) MRCS Eng. LRCP Lond. 1963; DObst RCOG 1967. Hosp. Pract. Haslemere & Dist. Hosp. Prev: Med. Off. S. Pacific Health Serv.; Ho. Surg. (Orthop. & Urol.) King's Coll. Hosp. Lond.

RANDALL, Jean Margaret The Old Vicarage, Iford, Lewes BN7 3EH — MB BS Lond. 1948 (Roy. Free) MRCS Eng., LRCP Lond. 1948. Clin. Asst. Nuclear Med. Dept. Roy. Sussex Co. Hosp. Prev: Anaesth. Regist. Edgware Gen. Hosp.; Res. Anaesth. Addenbrooke's Hosp. Camb.; Ho. Phys. Roy. Free Hosp.

RANDALL, John Charles Montague Health Centre, Oakenhurst Road, Blackburn BB2 1PP Tel: 01254 268436 Fax: 01254 268440 — MB ChB Manch. 1988; DRCOG 1991; MRCGP 1992. Company Med. Adviser Akzo Nobel Decorative Coatings Darwen, Lancs.; Mod. Adviser St. Wilfrids Sch. Blackburn. Specialty: Occupat. Health. Prev: Company Med. Adviser Sappi, Europe & Paper Mill Blackburn; Trainee GP Blackburn, Hyndburn & Ribble Valley HA VTS.

RANDALL, John Martin Peterborough District Hospital, Thorpe Road, Peterborough PE3 6; The Cedars, 82 Church St, Market Deeping, Peterborough PE6 8AL — MD Manch. 1990; MB ChB 1980; MRCOG 1987. Cons. O & G P'boro. Dist. Hosp. Specialty: Obst. & Gyn. Prev: Sen. Regist. (O & G) St. Jas. Hosp. & Gen. Infirm. Leeds; Clin. Research Fell. (O & G) Univ. Aberd.; Regist. Newc. Gen. Hosp.

RANDALL, Mr Julian Woodsetton Medical Centre, 40 Bourne Street, Woodsetton, Dudley DY3 6AF Tel: 01902 883348 Fax: 01902 878954; Acre-Rise Cottage, Upper Ludstone, Claverley, Wolverhampton WV5 7DH Tel: 01746 710634 — MB BCh Wales 1978; FRCS Eng. 1983. GP Dudley W. Midl.; Clin. Med. Off. Family Plann. Clinic Dudley. Specialty: Family Plann. & Reproduc. Health. Socs: Society of Medical Writers.

RANDALL, Keith John (retired) Red Tree House, Pine Glade, Keston Park, Orpington BR6 8NT Tel: 01689 853054 — MRCS Eng. LRCP Lond. 1943 (St. Bart.) MD (Path.) Lond. 1947, MB BS 1944; FRCPath 1964. Hon. Cons. Path. Bromley & Tunbridge Wells HAs. Prev: Sen. Regist. Path. St. Alfege's Hosp. Lond.

RANDALL, Kristen Anaesthetic Department, Worthing & Southlands Hospital, Worthing Hospital, Lyndhurst Road, Worthing BN11 2DH — MB BS Melbourne 1990.

RANDALL, Lisa Sarah, Surg. Lt. RN Retd. 6 Castlemans Lane, Hayling Island PO11 0PZ — BM Soton. 1991; DFFP 1997; DRCOG 1997; DOCGMeds. 1998; MRCGP 1998. GP Portsmouth; GP non-Princip. Specialty: Gen. Pract. Prev: Trainee GP RNH Haslar; Med. Off. HMS Osprey & HMS Endurance.

RANDALL, Marc Stewart Leeds General Infirmary, Great George St., Leeds LS1 3EX; 58 St Johns Road, Penn, High Wycombe HP10 8HU Tel: 01494 812530 — MB ChB Leeds 1998. Specialty: Gen. Surg.

RANDALL, Michaela Elizabeth Helen Falloden Way Practice, Henleage, Bristol BS9 4HT; 31 Elmlea Avenue, Stoke Bishop, Bristol BS9 3UU Tel: 0117 982 3706 — MB BS Nottm. 1982; BMedSci (Hons.) Nottm. 1980; DRCOG 1986. Flexible Careers Scheme GP Falloden Way Pract. Bristol. Prev: GP Principle Bristol Univ. Health Serv.; Asst. GP BedGr. Health Centre Aylesbury; Civil. Med. Off. Kowloon Gp. Pract. Brit. Milit. Hosp. Hong Kong.

RANDALL, Nigel Peter Crispian c/o Department of Anaesthesia, Victoria Hospital, Whinney Heys Road, Blackpool FY3 8NR — BM Soton. 1979; FFARCS Eng. 1984. Cons. Anaesth. Vict. Hosp. Blackpool. Specialty: Anaesth. Prev: Sen. Regist. (Anaesth.) N. West. RHA.

RANDALL, Peter Graham Sandown Medical Centre, Melville Street, Sandown PO36 8LD Tel: 01983 402464 Fax: 01983 405781 Email: peter.randall@gp-j84013.nhs.uk; Spring Chase, Westhill Manor, Westhill Road, Shanklin PO37 6QB Tel: 01983 863962 Fax: 01983 405781 — BM Soton. 1979; DRCOG 1981; DCH RCP Lond. 1982; MRCGP 1983; DFFP 1990; DMS Med. Soc. Apoth. Lond. 1995. GP Trainer; CHD lead for IW PCT; orthopaedic Phys. Specialty: Orthop. Prev: Exec. Bd. Mem., Isle of Wight PCT.

RANDALL, Peter John 104 Chapel Lane, Ravenshead, Nottingham NG15 9DH Tel: 01623 795606 — BM BS Nottm. 1976; PhD Nottm. 1972, BM BS 1976, BMedSci 1973; FFA RCS Eng. 1983. Cons. Anaesth. Centr. Nottm. HA. Specialty: Anaesth.

RANDALL, Mr Philip Edward North Manchester Hospital, Delauney Road, Manchester M20 4QP; 9 Ashwood, Oldham OL9 9TR — MB ChB Bristol 1973; BSc (Anat. 1st cl. Hons.) Bristol 1971; FRCS Eng. 1978; FFAEM 1993. Cons. A & E N. Manch. Gen. Hosp. Trust Med. Director. Specialty: Accid. & Emerg. Prev: Lect. Surg. (A & E) & Hon. Sen. Regist. Univ. Manch.

RANDALL, Raymond 22 Ethelbert Gardens, Ilford IG2 6UN Tel: 020 8551 3134; 2 Savoy Court, Firecrest Drive, West Heath Road, Hampstead, London NW3 7NF Tel: 020 7431 2422 Fax: 020 7431 2422 — LRCP LRCS Ed. LRFPS Glas. 1959 (RCSI & W. Lond.) DObst. RCOG 1961. Socs: BMA. Prev: Ho. Phys. W. Lond. Hosp.; Ho. Surg. New End Hosp. Hampstead; Ho. Surg. (Obst.) Whittington Hosp. Lond.

RANDALL, Reginald John (retired) 3 Georgian Close, Ringwood BH24 1SA Tel: 01425 475412 — MRCS Eng. LRCP Lond. 1946 (Westm.) Prev: GP Totton.

RANDALL, Richard Isidore (retired) Flat1, 15 Heath Drive, London NW3 7SN Tel: 020 7435 0736 — (St. Geo.) MRCS Eng. LRCP Lond. 1941. Prev: Capt. RAMC.

RANDALL, Sally Jane Guy's & St Thomas' NHS Trust, St Thomas' Hospital, Occupational Health Dept, London SE1 7EH — MB BS Lond. 1993; MRCP 1997; AFOM 2001.

RANDALL, Sarah Ella Gordon Unit, St. Mary's Hospital, Milton Road, Portsmouth PO3 6AD Tel: 023 92 866304 Fax: 023 92 866311 — MB ChB Manch. 1973; FRCOG 1993, M 1978; MD Manch. 1983; MFFP 1993. Cons. Community Gyn. Portsmouth Healthcare Trust; Chairm. Workforce Plann. Commitee. Specialty: Family Plann. & Reproduc. Health. Socs: Brit. Menopause Soc. Prev: Hon. Sec. Fac. Family Plann. & Reproductive Health Care; Vice Chairm. Fac. of Family Plann. & Reproductive Health Care.

RANDALL, Susan Carol 37 Orient Road, Salford M6 8LE Fax: 0161 789 3029 — MB ChB Bristol 1973; Cert. Family Plann. JCC 1978. GP Salford FPC.

RANDALL, Tania Mia Kristin 168 High Street, Harston, Cambridge CB2 5QD — MB ChB Leeds 1993; MRCP (UK) 1998. CCST Paediatrics 2003. SHO Psychiatry. Barrow Hospital Bristol. Specialty: Paediat.; Gen. Psychiat.

RANDALL, Vivienne Rosemary Buckland Medical Centre, 24 Gamble Road, Portsmouth PO2 7BN Tel: 023 9266 0910 Fax: 023 9267 8175 — MB ChB Sheff. 1983; MRCGP 1988. Trainer (Gen. Pract.) Portsmouth.

RANDALLS, Peter Bryce 27 Woodland Avenue, Teignmouth TQ14 8UU Tel: 01626 770848 — MB ChB Glas. 1983; BSc (1st cl. Hons.) Glas. 1978; FFA RCS 1988. Cons. Anaesth. & Intens. Care Torbay Hosp. Torquay. Specialty: Anaesth.

RANDELL, David Thomas Henry Ty Darren, 38 Nant y Felin, Efail Isaf, Pontypridd CF38 1YY — MB ChB Bristol 1960; DObst RCOG 1962. Prev: Ho. Surg. (Obst.) Southmead Hosp. Bristol; Sen. Ho. Off. Anaesth. United Bristol Hosps.; Ho. Surg. & Ho. Phys. Bristol Roy. Infirm.

RANDELL, Peter 25 Bruce Avenue, Worthing BN11 5JU Tel: 01903 242402 — MB BChir Camb. 1967; DPM Eng. 1972; MRCPsych 1974. Specialty: Psychother.; Physiother.

RANDELL, Richard Arthur (retired) Newstone House, High St., Scaldwell, Northampton NN6 9JS Tel: 01604 881595 — MB BChir Camb. 1960 (Camb. & Univ. Coll. Hosp.) MA Camb. 1986, BA 1957; DIH Soc Apoth. Lond. 1972; AFOM RCP Lond. 1978. Occupat. Health Phys. (Occupat. Health) Northampton Gen. Hosp.; Cons. Occupat. Health Phys. Various Companies. Prev: Emplym. Med. Advisor Health & Safety Exec.

RANDELL, Roy 341 Broomfield Road, Chelmsford CM1 4DX Tel: 01245 57595 — MB BChir Camb. 1946 (Camb. & Char. Cross) MRCS Eng. LRCP Lond. 1945. Prev: Dept. Demonst. Anat. Camb. Univ.; Ho. Surg. O & G Ashridge E.M.S. Hosp.

RANDERSON, Jonathan Michael Dewar and Randerson, The Health Centre, 1 Bridgeway Centre, Meadows, Nottingham NG2 2JG; Rothsay House, 1 Trevelyan Road, West Bridgford, Nottingham NG2 5GY — BM BS Nottm. 1984; BMedSci Nottm. 1982, BM BS 1984. GP Notts. Prev: Trainee GP Mansfield.

RANDEV, Barkha — MB ChB Liverp. 1998; DRCOG 2000; DFFP 2002.

RANDEV, Mrs Parveen 8 Benenden Way, Ashby-de-la-Zouch LE65 2QS — MB ChB Leeds 1989; DRCOG 1996.

RANDEV, Pawan Kumar 8 Benenden Way, Ashby-de-la-Zouch LE65 2QS — MB ChB Sheff. 1986; BMedSci (Hons.) Sheff. 1985; MRCS Eng. LRCP Lond. 1986; MRCP (UK) 1991; DRCOG 1993; DCH RCP Lond. 1994; MRCGP 1994. Specialty: Gen. Pract.

RANDFIELD, Helen Ferrars Dollar Health Centre, Park Place, Dollar FK14 7AA Tel: 01259 742120 Fax: 01259 743053; 23 Ladysneur Road, Cambuskenneth, Stirling FK9 5NN Tel: 01786 462206 Email: simon@randfield.freeserve.co.uk — MB ChB Birm. 1990 (Birmingham) DFFP 1995; DRCOG 1995; MRCGP (Distinc.) 1996. GP. Specialty: Gen. Pract. Prev: GP/Regist. DunbLa. Health Centre; Ho. Off. (Med.) Selly Oak Hosp.; Ho. off. (Surg.) Kidderminster Gen. Hosp.

RANDFIELD, Richard Simon c/o Crieff Health Centre, King St., Crieff PH7 3SA Tel: 01764 656283 — MB ChB Birm. 1990; DRCOG 1996. GP Regist. Crieff H/L Crieff. Specialty: Gen. Pract. Prev: Med. Off. Hlabisa, Kwazulu, Natal; Trainee GP/SHO Stirling Roy. Infirm.

RANDHAWA, Brijinder 21 Belbush Avenue, Sandhills, Oxford OX3 8EA — MB BS Sydney 1988.

RANDHAWA, Joginder Singh 283 Hollyhedge Road, Wythenshawe, Manchester M22 4QR Tel: 0161 428 9411 — MB BS Panjab Univ. 1967 (Medical College Amritsar, India) GP. Specialty: Gen. Med.; Acupunc.

RANDHAWA, Neil Andrew — MB ChB Birm. 1991; ChB Birm. 1991.

RANDHAWA, Rajbir Singh 119 Oswald Road, Southall UB1 1HJ — MB BS Lond. 1982.

RANDHAWA, Samarjit Singh Regional Medical Centre, RAF Wyton, Huntingdon PE17 2EA Tel: 01480 52451; 11 Warren Road, St. Ives, Huntingdon PE27 5NX — MB BS Newc. 1975 (Newcastle upon Tyne) FRCS Eng. 1980; DRCOG 1982; DFPP 1996. Civil. Med. Pract. Huntingdon. Specialty: Gen. Pract.

RANDHAWA, Veena 269 Gillott Road, Birmingham B16 0RX — MB ChB Leeds 1997.

RANDLE, Guy Hawksworth 80 Lairgate, Beverley HU17 8EU Tel: 01482 861020 — MB BS Lond. 1965 (St. Bart. & Liverp.) MRCS Eng. LRCP Lond. 1963; LMSSA Lond. 1963; DObst RCOG 1965; FRCOG 1982, M 1969. Locum Cons. O & G. Specialty: Obst. & Gyn. Socs: NINES Obst. & Gyn. Soc.; Worshipful Soc. Apoth. Lond.; N. Eng. Obst. & Gyn. Soc. & Hull Med. Soc. Prev: Cons. O & G E. Yorks. Hosps. Trust; Med. Dir. E. Yorks. Hosps. Trust.

RANDLE, Mark Chastleton Medical Group, St. Margaret's Medical Surgery, St. Margaret's Garth, Durham DH1 4DS — MB BS Lond. 1990.

RANDLE, Martin Philip The Surgery, 131 Goldsmith Avenue, Milton, Portsmouth PO4 8QZ Email: mprandle@doctors.org.uk — MB ChB Leeds 1975; RAMC(V) RRV; FRCSEd 1981; MRCOG 1981; LMCC 1984. Hosp. Practitioner, Dept. Surg., St Marys Hosp. Portsmouth.

RANDLE, Professor Sir Philip John (retired) Department of Clinical Biochemistry, Radcliffe Infirmary, Oxford OX2 6HE Tel:

01865 224001 Fax: 01865 224000; 11 Fitzherbert Close, Iffley, Oxford OX4 4EN Tel: 01865 773115 — MB BChir Camb. 1951 (Univ. Coll. Hosp.) PhD 1955, MA 1951, MD 1964, Camb.; FRCP Lond. 1972, M 1964; FRS 1983. Emerit. Prof. Clin. Biochem. Univ. Oxf.; Fell. Hertford Coll. Oxf. Prev: Prof. Biochem. Univ. Bristol.

RANDS, Catherine Elizabeth Hinchingbrooke Primary Care Trust, Primrose Lane, Huntingdon PE29 1WG Tel: 01480 415211 — MB BCh Wales 1989; MRCP (UK) 1994. Assoc. Specialist Community Paediat. Specialty: Community Child Health. Socs: Brit. Assn. Community Child Health; RCPCH. Prev: Lect. (Community Child Health) Univ. Nottm.; Regist. (Paediat.) Lincoln Co. Hosp. & Nottm. City Hosp. Trust; SHO (Community Paediat.) S. Birm. HA.

RANDS, David Allan (retired) Frenches Hill, The Frenches, Romsey SO51 6FE Tel: 01794 518727 Email: darands@aol.com — (Univ. Coll. Hosp.) MB BS Lond. 1952; MRCS Eng. LRCP Lond. 1952; MRCGP 1969. Prev: Ho. Phys. Univ. Coll. Hosp.

RANDS, Gianetta Susan Jane Camden and Islington Community Services NHS Trust, The Whittington Hospital, A8, Archway Wing, 4th Floor, Highgate Hill, London N19 5NF Tel: 020 7530 2306 Fax: 020 7530 2304 — MB BS Lond. 1981 (Royal Free Hospital London) BA Oxf. 1976; DRCOG 1983; MRCGP 1985; MRCPsych. 1988. Cons. Psychiat. Old Age Camden & Islington Community Health Servs. NHS Trust; Assoc. Clin. Tutor & Specialty Tutor in Psychiat. Camden & Islington Community Serv. NHS Trust; Hon. Sen. Lect., VCLMS; Progr. Dir. N. Thames Teachg. Hosps. Psychiat. Rotat. Specialty: Geriat. Psychiat.; Gen. Psychiat. Prev: Sen. Regist. Maudsley Hosp. Lond.

RANE, Mr Abhay Muralidhar — MB BS Poona 1983 (Poona, India) MChOrth Liverp. 1983; FRCS Glas. 1993; Dip. Urol. Lond 1995. Cons. Urol., Surrey and Sussex Healthcare. Specialty: Urol. Socs: Full Mem. BAUS.

RANE, Vasudha Ajay c/o University Department of Obstetrics & Gynaecology, Level 19, Gledhow Wing, St James' Hospital, Beckett St., Leeds LS9 7TF; 16 Eversley Court, Sherburn in Elmet, Leeds LS25 6BP — MB BS Poona 1989.

RANEEM, Iqbal Flat 4 Teynham Court, No 29 Woodside Avenue, Woodside Park, London N12 8AU — MB BS Ceylon 1967; DCH Ceylon 1978; DPM Dublin 1986. Assoc. Specialist (Ment. Handicap). Special Interest: Psychiat.

RANG, Elizabeth Harvey Merton sutton Wandsworth HA, Cranmer Road, Mitcham CR4 4TP Tel: 020 8648 3021; 1 Belvedere Drive, Wimbledon, London SW19 7BX Tel: 020 8947 7603 — MB BS Lond. 1959 (Univ. Coll. Hosp.) MB BS (Hons.) Lond. 1959; DObst RCOG 1962; MFCM 1987; FFPHM RCP (UK) 1993. Cons. Pub. Health Med. Merton & Sutton & Wandsworth Health. Specialty: Pub. Health Med. Socs: BMA (Treas. Merton & Sutton Div.); Roy. Soc. Med. Prev: Clin. Asst. Roy. Marsden Hosp. Lond.; Clin. Research Fell. St. Geo. Hosp. Lond.; Lect. Nuffield Dept. Med. Oxf.

RANGANATH, Lakshminarayan Rao Department of Chemical Pathology, Epsom District Hospital, Dorking Road, Epsom KT18 7EG Tel: 013727 26100 — MB BS Madras 1976; MSc Clin. Biochem. Surrey 1987; MRCP (UK) 1988.

RANGANATHAN, Srinivasan 301 Birmingham Road, Redditch B97 6EH — MD Mysore 1979 (Kasturba Med. Coll.) MB BS 1974. SHO (Gen. Med.) Withybush Hosp. HaverfordW..

RANGANATHAN, Sudha 110 Shaftesbury Avenue, Kenton, Harrow HA3 0RF Tel: 020 8909 2967 Fax: 020 8930 2259 Email: singasudha@hotmail.com — MB BS Madras, India 1967. Socs: BMA. Prev: GP Singapore.

RANGARAJAN, Thangaperumal Prince Charles Hospital, Merthyr Tydfil CF47 9DT — MB BS Madras 1975; MRCP (UK) 1986. Cons. (Community Paediat.) P. Chas. Hosp.

RANGASAMI, Jayanti Jairaj West Middlesex University Hospital, Paediatric Department, Twickenham Road, Isleworth TW7 6AF Tel: 020 8321 6164 Fax: 020 8321 6410 Email: jayanti.rangasami@wmuh-tr.nthames.nhs.uk; 255B Jersey Road, Isleworth TW7 4RF Tel: 020 8569 7840 Fax: 020 8569 7840 Email: jayantirangasami@hotmail.com — MB BS Sambalpur 1978 (V.S.S. Medical College, BURLA, SAMBALPUR, INDIA.) DCH 1980; MRCP (UK) 1990; MRCPCH 1997. Cons. Paediat. Middlx. Univ. Hosp. Specialty: Paediat. Socs: BMA; Brit. Soc. Paediat. Endocrinol.; MRCPCH. Prev: Lect. & Sen. Regist. (Child Health) Univ. Aberd.; Regist. Merton & Sutton HA; Hon. Sen. Regist. & Lect. (Child Health) Univ. Nottm.

RANGASWAMY, Venkataiah 23 Melbourne Road, Christchurch BH23 2HY — MB BS Mysore 1968.

RANGE, Simon Paul Department Respiratory Medicine, Glenfield Hospital, Groby Rd, Leicester LE3 9QP; 1 Tansley House Gardens, Tansley, Matlock DE4 5HQ — MB ChB Birm. 1990 (Birmingham) MRCP (UK) 1993; DM (Nottingham) 2000. Cons. Respirat. Phys., Glenfield Hosp., Leicester. Specialty: Gen. Med.; Respirat. Med. Socs: Brit. Thoracic Soc.; BMA; Amer. Coll. Chest Phys.s.

RANGECROFT, Mr Laurence Department of Paediatric Surgery, The Royal Victoria Infirmary, Queen Victoria Road, Newcastle upon Tyne NE1 4LP Tel: 0191 282 4711 Fax: 0191 227 5276; 17 The Poplars, Gosforth, Newcastle upon Tyne NE3 4AE Tel: 0191 285 0275 — (Newc. u. Tyne) MB BS Newc. 1970; FRCS Eng. 1975. Cons. Paediat. Surg. & Urol. Roy. Vict. Infirm. Newc. u. Tyne. Specialty: Paediat. Surg. Socs: Assoc. Mem. BAUS; Eur. Soc. Paediat. Urol.; Hon. Sec. And Treas.. Brit. Assn. Paediat. Surgs. Prev: Sen. Regist. (Paediat. Surg.) Alder Hey Childr. Hosp. Liverp.; Sen. Regist. (Paediat. Surg.) Hosp. Sick Childr. Dub.; Regist. (Paediat. Surg.) Roy. Childr. Hosp. Melbourne, Austral.

RANGECROFT, Margaret Ellen Haslam Regional Department of Psychotherapy, Claremont House, off Framlington Place, Newcastle upon Tyne NE1 4AA Tel: 0191 282 4542 Fax: 01912824542 Email: claremontpu@yahoo.com — (Newcastle upon Tyne) MB BS Newc. 1970; MRCPsych 1990; TQAP 1997. Cons. Psychotherapist Regional Dept. Psychother. Claremont Ho. Newc. Specialty: Psychother. Socs: MRCPsych; Brit. ConFederat. of Psychotherapists; NEAPP. Prev: GP Sefton FPC; Ho. Phys. & Ho. Surg. Roy. Vict. Infirm. Newc.; Med. Off. Univ. Newc.

RANGECROFT, Ronald George (retired) East of Eden, 62 Victoria Place, Carlisle CA1 1LR Tel: 01228 522699 — MB ChB Ed. 1959; LMCC 1961; FRCOG 1979, M 1966. Prev: Cons. Gyn. City Gen. Hosp. Carlisle.

RANGEDARA, Don Chandrasiri Epsom General Hospital, Dorking Road, Epsom KT18 7EG; 91 Holmwood Road, Cheam, Sutton SM2 7JP — MB BS Ceylon 1971 (Colombo) FRCP 1977; MRCP (UK) 1979. Sen. Regist. Dept. Geriat. & Gen. Med. Guy's Hosp. Lond.; Cons. Phys., Epsom Gen. Hosp. Specialty: Gen. Med.; Care of the Elderly.

RANGEL, Richard Lawrence Caerleon Surgery, Dover Street, Bilston WV14 6AL Tel: 01902 493426 Fax: 01902 490096; 7 Wightwick Hall Road, Wightwick, Wolverhampton WV6 8BZ Tel: 01902 765486 — MB BS Bombay 1970 (Topiwala Nat. Med. Coll.)

RANGER, Alistair Frank The Surgery, Lorne Street, Lochgilphead PA31 8LU Tel: 01546 602921 Fax: 01546 606735 Email: administrator@gp84415.ac-hb.scot.nhs.uk; Tigh an Inis, Kilmichael Glassary, Lochgilphead PA31 8QA Tel: 01546 605229 — MB ChB Dundee 1977; DRCOG 1979. Sen. Partner in Gen. Pract. Specialty: Accid. & Emerg. Prev: SHO (Gen. Med.) Co. Hosp. Oban.

RANGER, Mr Ian 15 Colney Lane, Norwich NR4 7RE Tel: 01603 54968 — MB BS Lond. 1947 (Middlx.) MS Lond. 1963, MB BS 1947; FRCS Eng. 1952. Prev: Chief Asst. Dept. Surg. Studies, Asst. Bland. Sutton Inst. Path. & Ho. Surg. Middlx. Hosp. Lond.

RANGER, Michael White Lodge, 330 Prestbury Road, Prestbury, Cheltenham GL52 3DD — MB BS Lond. 1973; AFOM RCP Lond. 1982; DAvMed RCP Lond. 1982; MRAeS Lond. 1988; QHS 2002. Specialty: Accid. & Emerg.

RANGI, Permjit Singh 21 Everton Road, Sheffield S11 8RY — MB ChB Sheff. 1995.

RANGR, Priya 2 Queen Victoria Avenue, Wembley HA0 4RW — MB BS Lond. 1996.

RANGWALA, Goolamali Dawoodbhai Mizzen Road Surgery, 5 Mizzen Road, Hull HU6 7AG Tel: 01482 854574 Fax: 01482 854576 — MB BS Ranchi 1968 (Mahatma Gandhi Memor. Med. Coll. Jamshedpur) DLO Eng. 1977.

RANGWANI, Pushpa M (Surgery) 226 Derby Road, Lenton, Nottingham NG7 1PR Tel: 0115 941 1208; 6 Rectory Gardens, Wollaton Village, Nottingham NG8 2AR Tel: 0115 928 4687 — MB BS Sind 1968 (Liaquat Med. Coll. Hyderabad) DObst RCOG 1970.

RANI, Raj 173 Hill Lane, Southampton SO15 7UA — MB ChB Leic. 1996.

RANIWALLA, Joher 27 Lydney Park, West Bridgford, Nottingham NG2 7TJ — BM Soton. 1984.

RANJADAYALAN, Kulasegaram Glen Road, Plaistow, London E13 Tel: 020 7363 8039 Email: kala.ranjan@newhamhealth.nhs.uk; 59A Lord Avenue, Clayhall, Ilford IG5 0HN — MB BS Sri Lanka 1979; MD Sri Lanka 1985; FRCP Ed. 1997, MRCP 1987; MPhil Lond. 1994; FRCP Lond. 1999. Cons. Phys. (Cardiol.) Newham Gen. Hosp.; Examr. Dent. Studs. 1995-. Specialty: Cardiol. Socs: BMA; Brit. Cardiac Soc.; Brit. Soc. Echocardiogr. Prev: Staff Phys. (Cardiol. & Chest Med.) Newham HA; Examr. MRCP (PACES) RCP (Lon) RCP (Ed).

RANJAN KUMAR, Pejaver Department of Paediatrics, Armed Forces Hospital, Tabuk, Saudi Arabia Tel: 00 966 4 4234426 Fax: 00 966 4 4222324; c/o Dr N. Subash, 46 Church St, Wootton, Ryde PO33 4PY — MB BS Bangalore 1980; MRCPI 1991. Cons. Paediat. Armed Forces Hosp. Tabuk, Saudi Arabia. Specialty: Paediat. Socs: Fell. Neonat. Soc.; Fell. Roy. Soc. Trop. Med. & Hyg. Prev: Cons. Paediat. NW Armed Forces Hosp. Tabuk, Saudi Arabia.

RANJIT, Rajalingam Dainton Cross, Marldon Road, Ipplepen, Newton Abbot TQ12 5TY — MB BS Peradeniya 1979; MRCOG 1988. Assoc. Specialist (O & G) Torbay Hosp. Torquay. Specialty: Obst. & Gyn. Prev: Regist. (O & G) Ipswich Hosp.; Regist. (O & G) Basildon Hosp. Essex; SHO (O & G) Norf. & Norwich Hosp.

RANJITHAKUMAR, Subathira Manor House Health Centre, Manor Lane, Feltham TW13 4JQ — MB BS Sri Lanka 1976; DRCOG; MRCS Eng. LRCP Lond. 1986. GP. Socs: MDU. Prev: Trainee GP Lightwater; Sen. Ho. Off. (A & E) King Geo. Hosp. Ilford; Sen. Ho. Off. (Geriat. Med.) Qu. Eliz. Hosp. Welwyn Gdn. City.

RANJITKUMAR, Sumathi 5 Heathercroft, Roxholme Gardens, Leeds LS7 4HF — MB BS Madras 1988.

RANK, Katherine Margaret 19 East Street, Salisbury SP2 7SF — MB BS Lond. 1997.

RANK, Timothy John 2 Hailey Lane, Hertford SG13 7NX — MB BS Lond. 1996.

RANKEN, Anne Muriel (retired) 22 Lower Street, Pulborough RH20 2BL — (Roy. Free) MB BS Lond. 1952; MRCS Eng. LRCP Lond. 1952. Prev: Assoc. Specialist Haemat. & Histol. Depts. St. Richards Hosp. Chichester.

RANKIN, Andrew Coats Department of Medical Cardiology, Royal Infirmary, 10 Alexandra Parade, Glasgow G31 2ER Tel: 0141 211 4833 Fax: 0141 552 4683; Glen Hall, 14 Cairns Drive, Milngavie, Glasgow G62 8AJ — MB ChB Glas. 1977; DRCOG 1979; MRCP (UK) 1980; BSc (Hons.) Glas. 1975, MD 1985; FRCP Glas. 1994. Sen. Lect. (Med. Cardiol.) Roy. Infirm. Glas. Specialty: Cardiol.

RANKIN, Angela 22 Queen Edith's Way, Cambridge CB1 7PN — MB ChB Sheff. 1972; BSc Sheff. 1969, MB ChB 1972; MRCPath 1979. Assoc. Specialist Regional Transfus. Centre Camb. Prev: Sen. Regist. (Haemat.) Hosp. Sick Childr. Lond.; Sen. Regist. Dept. Haemat. Lond. Hosp. (Whitechapel); Regist. (Haemat.) Univ. Dept. Haemat. Sheff.

RANKIN, Archibald Macpherson (retired) Hill House, Aspatria, Wigton CA7 3HG Tel: 016973 20607 — MB ChB Glas. 1950 (Glas) FRCGP 1986, M 1972. Prev: Chairm. Cumbria Family Pract. Comm.

RANKIN, David Craig Turnbull (retired) 3 Westwinds, 27 Bowleaze Coveway, Weymouth DT3 6PL Tel: 01305 834374 — (Glas.) MB ChB Glas. 1948. Prev: GP Dorchester.

RANKIN, Donald Watson (retired) 58 Bennochy Road, Kirkcaldy KY2 5RB Tel: 01592 267847 — MB ChB Ed. 1963; DObst RCOG 1966; FRCPsych 1990, M 1979; MPhil Ed. 1981. Prev: Dir. Scott. Health Advis. Serv.

RANKIN, Professor Elaine Mary Department of Cancer Medicine, University of Dundee, Ninewells Hospital and Medical School, Dundee DD1 9SY Tel: 01382 425543 Fax: 01382 632885 Email: e.m.rankin@dundee.ac.uk — FRCP Glas.; BSc (Med. Sci.) St. And. 1973; MB ChB (Hons.) Manch. 1976; MD Manch. 1984. Prof. Cancer Med. Univ. of Dundee; Hon. Cons. (Cancer Med.) Ninewells Hosp. Tayside Health Board. Specialty: Oncol. Socs: Europ. Organisation for Treatm. of Cancer, Melanoma Group & Lung Group; Brit. Assn. Cancer Research. Prev: Cons. (Med. Oncol.) Netherlands Cancer Inst., Amsterdam, The Netherlands; Sen. Lect. & Hon. Cons. Phys. Univ. Glas. & CRC Dept. Med. Oncol. Glas.; Lect. (Med. Oncol.) Guy's Hosp. Lond.

RANKIN, Elizabeth Catherine Cameron Department of Rheumatology, University Hospital Birmingham NHS Trust, Selly Oak, Birmingham B29 6JF Tel: 0121 627 1627 Fax: 0121 627 8480 — BM BCh Oxf. 1988; MA Oxf. 1986; MRCP (UK) 1991; PhD Lond. 1995. Cons. Rheum. Univ. Hosp. Birm. HHS Trust. Specialty: Rheumatol. Prev: Sen. Regist. (Rheum.) Bristol Roy. Infirm.; Research Regist. & Regist. (Med.) Middlx. Hosp. Lond.; SHO (Gen. Med.) City Gen. Hosp. Stoke on Trent.

RANKIN, Elizabeth Margaret 15 Burnside Road, Burnside, Glasgow G73 4RL — MB ChB Glas. 1974.

RANKIN, George Lloyd Sinnett (retired) Herons, Barnston, Dunmow CM6 3PP — (Camb. & Guy's) MRCS Eng. LRCP Lond. 1952; MB BChir Camb. 1953; MA Camb. 1953; FRCOG 1973, M 1960, DObst 1957. Prev: Hon. Cons. Gyn. Chelmsford Gp. Hosps.

RANKIN, James Sinnett Pershore Health Centre, Priest Lane, Pershore WR10 1RD Tel: 01386 502030 Fax: 01386 502058 Email: jamesrankin@onetel.net.uk; Butts Bank, Great Comberton, Pershore WR10 3DP Tel: 01386 710018 — MB BS Lond. 1982 (Guy's) MRCS Eng. LRCP Lond. 1982; DRCOG 1990.

RANKIN, John (retired) 38 Glasgow Road, Dennyloanhead, Bonnybridge FK4 1QG Tel: 01324 813471 — MB ChB Glas. 1952.

RANKIN, John Graham Dovercourt Health Centre, 407 Main Road, Dovercourt, Harwich CO12 4ET Tel: 01255 506451; Millbank, 119 Fronks Road, Dovercourt, Harwich CO12 4EF Tel: 01255 503835 — (St. Geo.) MB BS Lond. 1963; MRCS Eng. LRCP Lond. 1963; DObst RCOG 1966; MRCGP 1980. Med. Staff Harwich Dist. Hosp. Socs: Colchester Med. Soc.

RANKIN, John Nestor (retired) Nia-Roo, 33 Crosshill Road, Strathaven ML10 6DS Tel: 01357 521580 — LRCP LRCS Ed. LRFPS Glas. 1946 (St. Mungo's Coll. Glas.)

RANKIN, John Nestor Edgar Park Avenue Medical Centre, 9 Park Avenue, Stirling FK8 2QR Tel: 01786 473529; 1 Anne Drive, Bridge of Allan, Stirling FK9 4RE — MB ChB Glas. 1973; DFM Glas. 1990.

RANKIN, Julia Addenbrooke's Hospital, Department of Medical Genetics, Box 134, Hills Road, Cambridge CB2 2QQ; 11 Argyle Street, Cambridge CB1 3LR — MB ChB Manch. 1990 (Manchester) BSc (Hons.) Pharmacol. 1987; MRCP (UK) 1993; PhD 1998. Clin. Lect., Medial Genetics, Addgnbrooke's Hosp., Camb. Specialty: Genetics. Prev: MRC Clin. Train. Fell. (Clin. Genetics) Univ. Newc.

RANKIN, Lisa Cherry Grantham North Lodge, Minnetts Hill, Syston Park, Grantham NG32 2BU — MB ChB Glas. 1997.

RANKIN, Marion Tigh Sona, Neilston Walk, Kilsyth, Glasgow G65 9PL — MB Glas. 1977; FRCS Ed. 1981. Clin. Asst. Stobhill NHS Trust Glas. Specialty: Obst. & Gyn. Socs: Med. Wom. Internat. Assn.; Med. Wom. Federat.; Brit. Menopause Soc.

RANKIN, Nicol Elliot (retired) 22 Queen Ediths Way, Cambridge CB1 7PN — MB BS Lond. 1945 (St. Thos.) MRCS Eng. LRCP Lond. 1944; DPath Eng. 1955; FRCPath 1970, M 1963. Prev: Cons. Path. Yeovil Dist. Hosp. & Boston Hosp. Gp.

RANKIN, Paul Vincent 97 Mayogall Road, Magherafelt BT45 8PJ — MB BCh BAO Belf. 1987.

RANKIN, Philip Michael Kilsyth Medical Partnership, Kilsyth Health Centre, Burngreen Park, Glasgow G65 0HU Tel: 01236 822081 Fax: 01236 826231 — MB ChB Glas. 1977; DRCOG 1980; MRCGP 1981.

RANKIN, Rosslyn Department of Pathology, Raigmore Hospital, Inverness IV2 3UJ — MB ChB Glas. 1978. Cons. Path. Raigmore Hosp. Inverness. Specialty: Histopath.; Forens. Path. Socs: Roy. Coll. Path. Prev: Cons. Histopath. Univ. Aberd.

RANKIN, Sheila Campbell X-Ray Department, 2nd Floor Guy's Tower, Guy's Hospital, London SE1 9RT Tel: 020 7955 4258 — MB BS Lond. 1972; MRCS Eng. LRCP Lond. 1972; DCH Eng. 1974; DMRD Eng. 1977; Amer. Bd. of Radiol. 1980; FRCR 1981. Cons. Radiol. Guy's Hosp. Lond. Specialty: Radiol. Prev: Sen. Research Fell. (Computerised Tomography) St. Thos. Hosp. Lond.; Resid. (Radiol.) Tufts, New. Eng. Med. Centre Boston, USA; Regist. (Radiol.) King's Coll. Hosp. Lond.

RANKIN, Mr Simon James Adrian 9 St Ellen's, Edenderry, Belfast BT8 8JN — MB BCh BAO Belf. 1985; FRCS Ed. 1990; FCOphth 1990.

RANKIN, Susan Miriam 50 West End, Langtoft, Peterborough PE6 9LU — MB BS Lond. 1987 (Royal Free Hosp.) DRCOG 1991; MRCGP 1996.

RANKIN, Wendy Joan Wythenshawe Health Care Centre, Stancliffe Rd, Manchester M22 4PJ Tel: 0161 946 9415 Fax: 0161 946 9417 Email: wendy.rankin@mch-tr.nwest.nhs.uk; Wood Lea, 229 Mottram Road, Stalybridge SK15 2RF — MB ChB Manch. 1979; MRCP (UK) 1983; FRCP Lond. 1996. Cons. Paediat.

(Community Child Health) Manch. Health Trust; Lect. Manch. Univ. Specialty: Community Child Health. Prev: Sen. Regist. (Community Paediat.) Salford HA.

RANKIN, William Thomas (retired) 19 Gloucester Avenue, Clarkston, Glasgow G76 7LH — MB ChB Glas. 1926.

RANKINE, Anne Eleanor (retired) 17 Queensferry Road, Edinburgh EH4 3HB Tel: 0131 332 3230 — MB ChB Ed. 1949; DRCOG 1952. Prev: Ho. Phys. Tynemouth Infirm.

RANKINE, George (retired) The Barn, 106A The Causeway, Petersfield GU31 4LL Tel: 01730 267538 Fax: 01730 267538 — MB ChB St. And. 1944 (St. And. & Duke Univ.) BSc St. And. 1941; MD Duke Univ. 1944; MRCGP 1952. Prev: Maj. RAMC.

RANKINE, James Julian St James's Univ. Hospital, Beckett SL, Leeds LS9 7TF Tel: 0113 206 4807 Fax: 0113 2064 587 — MB ChB Ed. 1986; MRCP (UK) 1991; MRad(D) Aberd. 1993; FRCR 1994; MD (Manchester) 1998. Cons. (Diagn. Radiol), St Jas. Univ. Hosp., Leeds.; Hon. Clin. Sen. Lect., Univ. of Leeds. Specialty: Radiol. Socs: Mem. Brit. Soc. Skeletal Radiol.; Mem. Europ. Soc. Skeletal Radiol. Prev: Lect. (Diagn. Radiol.) Univ. Manch.; Sen. Regist. Univ. Hosps. S. Manch.; Regist. (Radiol.) Aberd. Roy. Infirm.

RANKINE, Susan Elizabeth Victoria Medical Centre, 7 Longmoore Street, London SW1V 1JH Tel: 020 7821 1531 Fax: 020 7233 5995; 12 Bloomfield Terrace, London SW1W 8PG Tel: 020 7730 4820 — MB BS Lond. 1983 (Univ. Coll. Hosp.) DFFP 1988; DRCOG 1988; MRCGP 1989; DCH RCP Lond. 1989. Specialty: Paediat.

RANMUTHU, Anoma Hemantha Charlton House Medical Centre, 581 High Road, Tottenham, London N17 6SB Tel: 020 8808 2837 Fax: 020 8801 4179; 5 The Leys, Hampstead Garden Suburb, London N2 0HE — MB BS Colombo 1979; LRCP LRCS Ed. LRCPS Glas. 1986.

RANN, Sarah Frances Great Shelford Health Centre, Ashen Green, Great Shelford, Cambridge CB2 5EY Tel: 01223 843661 Fax: 01223 844569 — MB BS Lond. 1982; DCH RCP Lond. 1985; DRCOG 1985; Cert. Family Plann. JCC 1985; DFFP 1994; MRCGP 2002. Prev: GP Cambs. Retainer Scheme; Haemophilia Centre RCH & Alfred Hosp. Melbourne, Austral.

RANNAN-ELIYA, Ronald Walter Daniel Gomes 7 Stow Gardens, Withington, Manchester M20 8HT — MRCS Eng. LRCP Lond. 1960; LMSSA Lond. 1960.

RANNAN-ELIYA, Mr Sahan Viraj Dept. of Plastic and Reconstructive Surgery, Radcliff Infirmary, Oxford; 20 Orchard Rise, Croydon CR0 7QY Tel: 020 8776 1583 — BM BCh Oxf. 1994 (PreClinical- Cambridge, Clinical- Oxford) MA Camb. 1995; FRCS (Enl) 1998. SHO Rotat. (Surg.) Oxf. Specialty: Gen. Surg.

RANNAN-ELIYA, Yi Fan Paediatric Department, Norfolk & Norwich University Hospital, Colney Lane, Norwich NR4 7UY — BM BCh Oxf. 1997 (Oxf) MA; MRCPCH; DCH. SpR (Paediat.) Norf. & Norwich Hosp. Norwich. Specialty: Paediat. Prev: SHO Paediat. N.ampton. Gen. Hosp.

RANNIE, Gordon Hugh The Surgery, The Meads, Kington HR5 3DQ Tel: 01544 230302 Fax: 01544 230824; Sharkham, Lyonshall, Kington HR5 3HT Tel: 01544 340449 — BM BCh Oxf. 1971 (Oxford) BA (Physiol.) Oxf. 1967, BM BCh 1971; PhD Ed. 1978. Specialty: Gen. Pract. Prev: Lect. & MRC Jun. Research Fell. (Path.) Univ. Manch.; MRC Research Fell. (Path.) Univ. Edin; Regist. (Path.) Dept. Med. Sch. Edin. Univ.

RANNIE, Ian (retired) Ian Rannie, Apartment G, 8 Osborne Villas, Newcastle upon Tyne NE2 1JU Tel: 0191 281 3163 — MB ChB Glas. 1938; BSc (Pure Sci.) Glas. 1935; BSc (Hons. Path. & Bact.) 1939; FRCPath 1963; FIBiol 1963. Prev: Prof. Path. Dent. Sch. Univ. Newc.

RANOLE, Anna-Lisa Gwynton Pendre Surgery, Clayton Road, Mold CH7 1SS; 3 Church Farm Cottages, Church Lane, Guilden Sutton, Chester CH3 7EW Tel: 01244 301841 — MB ChB Liverp. 1994 (Liverp) DRCOG 1997; DFFP 1997. Asst. in Gen. Pract. Specialty: Gen. Pract. Prev: GP Reg; SHO paediat.; SHO Psych.

RANOTE, A S — MB BS Punjabi U 1965; MS Punjabi U 1968.

RANOTE, S R Harpurhey Health Centre, 1 Church Lane, Harpurhey, Manchester M9 4BE Tel: 0161 205 1541 Fax: 0161 202 3700 — MB BS Panjab 1968; MB BS Panjab 1968.

RANOTE, Sandeep — MB ChB Manch. 1996; MRCPsych 2000.

RANPURA, Niksha 509 Saffron Lane, Leicester LE2 6UL — MB ChB Manch. 1994; MRCGP; DRCOG.

RANSCOMBE, Brian John The Health Centre, Skimped Hill, Bracknell RG12 1LH Tel: 01344 485333 Fax: 01344 890429; Highlands, Locks Ride, Chavey Down, Ascot SL5 8RA Tel: 01344 884833 Fax: 01344 300137 — MB BS Lond. 1960 (Westm.) MRCS Eng. LRCP Lond. 1959; DObst RCOG 1962; MRCGP 1980; Cert. Av. Med. 1986. Hosp. Pract. (Psychiat.) Churchill Ho. Hosp. Bracknell; Extern. Advis. to Ombudsman. Socs: (Ex-Pres.) Windsor Med. Soc.; Appeals Serv.s. Prev: SHO (Obst.) Lambeth Hosp.; Ho. Surg. Westm. Childr. Hosp.; Ho. Phys. Westm. Hosp.

RANSFORD, Mr Andrew Oliver 5 Fordington Road, London N6 4TD Tel: 020 8883 3317 Fax: 020 8374 3936 — MB BChir Camb. 1966 (Univ. Coll. Hosp.) BA Camb. 1966; FRCS Eng. 1970. Medics legal Pract. Specialty: Orthop. Socs: Pres. Brit. Cervical Spine Soc.; Pres. Brit. Scolosis Soc. Prev: Cons. Orthop. Surg. Roy. Nat. Orthop. Hosp. Lond.; Cons. Orthop. Surg. Univ. Coll. Hosp. Lond.; Sen. Regist. Roy. Nat. Orthop. Hosp. Lond.

RANSFORD, Jacques 40 West Bank Avenue, Mansfield NG19 7BP — MB ChB Liverp. 1998; MB ChB Liverp 1998.

RANSFORD, Rupert Alistair Joseph County Hall, Union Walk, Hereford HR1 2ER Tel: 01432 364064; Coddington, Ledbury HR8 1JH — MB BS Lond. 1988; MRCP (UK) 1992; DRCOG 1993; MRCGP 1994. Specialist Regist. (Gastroenterol.) Hereford Co. Hosp.s. Specialty: Gastroenterol.; Gen. Med. Socs: BMA; (Dinner Sec.) Herefordsh. Med. Soc.; Roy. Coll. Phys.s. Prev: Staff Phys. Co. Hosp. Hereford; GP/Regist. Hereford; Regist. (Med.) Hereford.

RANSLEY, Mr Philip Goddard 234 Gt. Portland Street, London W1W 5QT Tel: 020 7390 8323 Fax: 020 7390 8324 Email: pgr2@doctors.org.uk; 30 Orde Hall St, London WC1N 3JW Tel: 020 7831 5078 — MA, MB Camb. 1967, BChir 1966; FRCS Eng. 1971. Cons. Surg. Urol. Hosp. Sick Childr. Gt. Ormond St. Lond.; Sen. Lect. (Paediat. Urol.) Inst. Child Health Univ. Lond.; Cons. Surg. Urol. Guy's Hosp. Specialty: Urol. Socs: Fell. Roy. Soc. Med.; Assoc. Mem. BAUS; Europ. Soc. for Paediatric Urol. (Pres. 1995 - 1999) Prev: Cons. Surg. (Urol) St Peter's Hosp.s Lond.; Sen. Regist. (Surg.) Hosp. Sick Childr. Gt. Ormond St. Lond.; Sen. Regist. St. Peter's Hosps. Lond.

RANSLEY, Yvonne Florence (retired) 119 Greenway, The Wells, Epsom KT18 7HY Tel: 01372 725025 — MB BS Lond. 1960 (Roy. Free) DCH Eng. 1964; DObst RCOG 1964; MRCP (UK) 1971; FRCP Lond. 1985; FRCPCH 1990. Cons. Paediat. Epsom Health Care Trust; Hon. Sen. Lect. St. Geo. Hosp. Med. Sch. Univ. Lond. Prev: Sen. Regist. (Paediat.) Qu. Mary's Hosp. Childr. Carshalton.

RANSOM, Margaret Jane Brough (retired) Hammonds Farm, Pirton, Hitchin SG5 3QN — MB BChir Camb. 1962 (St. Thos. & Addenbrooke's Hosps.) MA Camb. 1971. Prev: Clin. Asst. (Orthop. Fract.) Lister Hosp. Stevenage.

RANSOM, Mr Paul Alan Emergency Dept, Royal Sussex County Hospital, Eastern Road, Brighton BN2 5BE Tel: 02273 696955 Email: paul.ransom@bsuh.nhs.uk; 24 Friars Walk, Lewes, Brighton BN7 2LF — MB ChB Manch. 1993; FRCS Ed.; FFAEM 1993. Cons. Roy. Sussex Co. Hosp. Brighton.

RANSOM, Ruth Mary (retired) Armingland, Church St., Stiffkey, Wells-next-the-Sea NR23 1QJ Tel: 01328 830581 — MB BCh BAO Dub. 1951; BSc Lond.; MD Dub. 1956, BA; FRCPath 1975, M 1964. Prev: Cons. (Morbid Anat.) Watford Gp. Laborat. N.W. Thames RHA.

RANSOM, Mr William Thomas McLean 13 Hampton Grove, Epsom KT17 1LA Tel: 0 7020 991144 Fax: 0 7020 991166 Email: mac@macran.demon.co.uk — MB ChB Bristol 1979 (Univ. Bristol) FRCS Eng. 1983; DRCOG 1986; MRCGP 1987; DMJ(Clin) Soc. Apoth. Lond. 1996; Barrister at Law, 1999 University West England 1996. Indep. Forens. Phys. Metrop. Police; HM Asst. Dep. Coroner St Pancras. Specialty: Forens. Path. Socs: FRSM. Prev: GP Epsom.

RANSOME, Jennifer Anne Stonefield Street Surgery, 21 Stonefield Street, Milnrow, Rochdale OL16 4JQ Tel: 01706 46234 Fax: 01706 527946 — MB ChB Manch. 1987; BSc Manch. 1984; MRCGP 1991; DRCOG 1991. Prev: Ho. Off. (Surg. & Med.) Birch Hill Hosp. Rochdale.

RANSOME, Peter John 520 Burnley Road, Todmorden OL14 8JF — MB BS Durh. 1963.

RANSOME (MRS HERON), Joselen 10 Rushmere Place, London SW19 5RP — MB BS Lond. 1949 (Roy Free) MRCS Eng. LRCP Lond. 1949; FRCS Eng. 1958. Hon. Cons. Otolaryngol. Char. Cross Hosp. Lond. Specialty: Otolaryngol. Socs: Fell. Roy. Soc. Med.; Hon.

Life Mem. (Ex-Hon. Sec.) Brit. Assn. Otolaryngol. Prev: Cons. Otolaryngol. Metrop. ENT Hosp. & Char. Cross Hosp. Lond.; Sen. Regist. (ENT) Roy. Free Hosp.; Regist. Roy. Nat. Throat, Nose & Ear Hosp. Lond.

RANSON, Malcolm Richard Department of Medical Oncology, Christie Hospital and Holt Radium Inst., Manchester; 140 Woodsmoor Lane, Woodsmoor, Stockport SK2 8TJ — MB ChB Manch. 1982; BSc (Hons.) Manch. 1979; MRCP (UK) 1985; PhD Manch. 1990. Sen. Lect. (Med. Oncol.) Christie Hosp. Manch. Specialty: Oncol. Prev: EORTC/NCI Exchange Fellowship Award; CRC Clin. Research Fell.

RANSON, Rosalind Woodside Health Centre, 3 Enmore Road, London SE25 5NT; Ash Tree Cottage, Mount Gardens, Sydenham, London SE26 4NG Tel: 020 8699 6976 — MB BS Lond. 1988; MA Med. Ethics & Law, Kings Coll. Lond.; MRCGP 1994. GP Tutor for Non Principles.

RANSON, Sarah Ann Sherries, Upper Warren Avenue, Caversham, Reading RG4 7ED — MB BS Lond. 1994.

RANU, Amandeep Singh 8 Aldington Close, Dagenham RM8 1YQ — MB ChB Manch. 1993 (Manchester) DRCOG, 1997; DFFP 1997; DCH 1998; MRCGP, 1998; Dip Occ Med 2002. Specialty: Gen. Pract.

RANU, Harpal Kaur The Surgery, 406 Lobley Hill Road, Gateshead NE11 0BS Tel: 0191 604380; 44 Gresham Road, Osterley, Isleworth Tel: 020 8570 8319 — MRCS Eng. LRCP Lond. 1975 (Med. Coll. Amritsar) MD Panjab (India) 1971, MB BS 1963; Cert. Family Plann. & IUD Family Plann. Assn 1972; DObst RCOG 1974; MRCGP 1976. Local Med. Off. Civil Serv.; Mem. Gateshead Local Med. Comm. Socs: BMA. Prev: SHO (O & G) Northwick Pk. Hosp. & Clin. Research Centre; Harrow; Ho. Off. (Surg.) Roy. E. Sussex Hosp. Hastings.

RANU, Navjot Singh 34 Gregory Avenue, Stivichall, Coventry CV3 6DL Email: navranu@hotmail.com — BM Soton. 1993; MRCGP 2001; DRCOG 2001. Police Surg., Forens. Med. Examr. Specialty: Gen. Pract. Special Interest: Forens. Med..

RAO, Abbaraju Mohan 25 Dibbins Green, Bromborough, Wirral CH63 0QF Tel: 0151 334 1580 Fax: 0151 334 1580; 25 Dibbins Green, Bromborough, Wirral CH63 0QF Tel: 0151 334 1580 Fax: 0151 334 1580 — MB BS Osmania 1979; FFA RCSI 1989. Cons. (Anaesth.) Arrowe Pk. Hosp. Wirral. Specialty: Anaesth. Socs: Obst. Anaesth. Assn.; Soc. Computing & Tech. Anaesth. Prev: Sen. Regist. (Anaesth.) Mersey RHA; Staff Grade (Anaesth.) N. Tees Gen. Hosp. Stockton-on-Tees; Regist. (Anaesth.) Hull Roy. Infirm.

RAO, Amirchetty Rajeshwar The Surgery, 112 Watnall Road, Hucknall, Nottingham NG15 7JP Tel: 0115 963 2184 Fax: 0115 955 6311.

RAO, Anupama Len Valley Practice, Tithe Yard, Church Square, Lenham, Maidstone ME17 2PJ Tel: 01622 858341 Fax: 01622 859659 — MB BS Lond. 1989 (St George's Hospital Medical School) DCH RCP Lond. 1992; MRCGP 1994. Clin. Asst. (Dermat.) Maidstone; Mem. Steering Gp. Maidstone PCG; Young Practitioners Represen. Kent Trainers Selection Comm. Prev: Trainee GP/SHO (Med.) Maidstone Hosp.

RAO, Bethapudy Ratna Sunder 13A Lime Tree Road, Norwich NR2 2NQ — MB BS Mysore 1972 (Kasturba Med. Coll. Mangalore) SHO N.-E. Health Bd. Irel. Prev: Med. Off. Leprosy Miss. Hosp. Vilianagaram, India; SHO Sligo Gen. Hosp. & Co. Surg. Hosp. Cavan.

RAO, Chandini 55 Lyntham Road, Fulwood, Preston PR2 8JD — MB BS Newc. 1993.

RAO, Mr Chirivella Screenivasa A3 Main Residences, Shotley Bridge General Hospital, Consett DH8 0NB — MB BS Sri Venkateswara 1977; FRCS Glas. 1993.

RAO, Professor Chitaldroog Ramachandra (retired) — MB BS Mysore 1958 (Mysore Med. Coll.) FRCP Ed. 1974, M 1959; DTM & H Liverp. 1959; FCCP 1975. Prev: Cons. (Cardiol. & Geriat.) Thanet Dist. Gen. Hosp. Kent.

RAO, Gita Satish Ida Darwin Hospital, Fulbourn, Cambridge CB1 5EE Tel: 01223 884000 Fax: 01223 884003; 245 Hills Road, Cambridge CB2 2RP Tel: 01223 240970 Fax: 01223 240970 — MB BS Bombay 1966. Psychiat. Ida Darwin & Fulbourn Hosps. Camb. Specialty: Ment. Health. Prev: Research Fell. (Path. & Cancer Research) Addenbrooke's Hosp. Camb.

RAO, Gutta Hanumanta Rao and Partners, 90 Darnley Road, Gravesend DA11 0SW Tel: 01474 355331 Fax: 01474 324407 — MB BS Bangalor 1967 (Bangalore) MB BS Bangalore 1967. Community Family Plann. Doctor Thameslink Healthcare Servs. NHS Trust Gravesend. Prev: Clin. Asst. (Orthop.) Dartford & Gravesham HA.; Regist. (Orthop.) Medway & Gravesend Gp. Hosps.

RAO, Hindnavis Sudhakar The Surgery, Wickford Avenue, Pitsea, Basildon SS13 3HQ Tel: 01268 583288 Fax: 01268 581586 — MB BS Osmania 1972.

RAO, Ivatury Venkata c/o Drive V. R. Mamilla, 42 Heath Road, Barming, Maidstone ME16 9LG — MB BS Andhra 1967.

RAO, Jammi Nagaraj North Birmingham Primary Care Trust, 400 Aldridge Road, Perry Barr, Birmingham B44 8PH Tel: 0121 332 1900 Fax: 0121 332 1901 Email: jammi.rao@northbirminghampct.nhs.uk — MB BS Nagpur 1975; MD Nagpur 1978; MRCP (UK) 1984; DCH RCP Lond. 1985; BA Open 1990; MFPHM 1990; FRCP 1998; FFPHM 1999. Director Pub. Health N. Birm. PCT; Chairm., W. Midlands Multi-centre Research Ethics Comm.; Hon. Sen. Clin. Lect. (Pub. Health & Epidemiol.) Univ. of Birm. Specialty: Pub. Health Med. Prev: Cons. Pub. Health Sandwell HA; Assoc. Fell. Sch. Postgrad. Med. Educat. Univ. Warwick; Sen. Regist. (Pub. Health Med.) Sandwell HA.

RAO, Mr Janardhan 12 Burnside Close, Stalybridge SK15 2TW — MB ChB Manch. 1991 (St Andrews) BSc (Hons.) St. And. 1988; FRCS Ed. 1995; FRCS (Orth & Trauma) 2001. Orthop. Specialist Regist. E. Anglia Orthop. Rotat. Specialty: Orthop. Prev: SHO (Burns & Plastic Surg.) Withington Hosp. Manch.; SHO (Orthop., A & E & Neurosurg.) Addenbrooke's Hosp. Camb.

RAO, Janneca Janarduana — MB BS Sampalpur 1972; LRCS Edin. 1982; LRCP Edin. 1982; LRCPS Glasg. 1982. Cons (Anaeth.) Univ. Hosp. of N. Tees Stockton. Specialty: Anaesth.

RAO, Kanangi Srinivasa 6 Roman Way, Sandbach CW11 3EN — MB BS Madras 1968 (Kilpauk Med. Coll.) Cons. Psychiat. Leighton Hosp. Crewe. Specialty: Geriat. Psychiat. Prev: SHO Leighton Hosp. Crewe.

RAO, Kanchikatta Prabhakar — MB BS India 1970 (Kasrurba Med. Coll., Manipal/ Mangalore) General/ Adult Psychiat. Derbysh. Ment. Health Trust. Specialty: Gen. Psychiat. Special Interest: Eating Disorders. Prev: Cons. Psychiat. in Cleeveland.

RAO, Kandukuri Rajeshwar Poole Hospital, Department of Paediatrics, Poole BH15 2JB Email: raj.rao@poole.nhs.uk — MB BS Delhi 1981 (Univ. Coll. of Med. Sci.) DCH 1982; MRCP Lond. 1991; FRCPCH Lond. 2004. Cons. Paediat., Poole Hosp. NHS Trust, Poole. Specialty: Paediat. Special Interest: Allergy; Neonatology; Respirat. Dis. Socs: BSACI; BAPM. Prev: Cons. Paediat., James Paget Healthcare Trust, Gt. Yarmouth; Sen. Regist. in Paediat., Soton. Univ. Hosps. Trust.

RAO, Karra Arjun 9 College Heights, 246-252 St John St., London EC1V 4PH — MB ChB Dundee 1987; BMSc Dund 1984, MB ChB 1987. SHO (O & G) Singleton Dist. Hosp. Sketty. Prev: Ho. Off. (Gen. Surg.) Singleton Dist. Hosp.; SHO Princess of Wales Hosp. Bridgend; Trainee GP Bridgend VTS.

RAO, Karthik Department of Anaesthetics, Bradford Royal Infirmary, Bradford BD9 6RJ Tel: 01274 366655 Email: drkart_2000@yahoo.com; Flat 5, Block A, Temple Bank Flats, Duckworth Lane, Bradford BD9 6TB — MB BS Karnatak 1998. SHO (Anaesth) Brad. Roy. Inf. Specialty: Anaesth. Special Interest: Paediatric Anaesth. Socs: MDV. Prev: Sen. Ho. Off. (Anaesth.) Airedale Gen. Hosp. NHS Trust.

RAO, Kavery Derby Royal Infirmary, Eye Clinic, London Road, Derby DE1 2QY — MB BS Mysore 1975.

RAO, Kusumeswara Chittajallu Audley Surgery, 2-4 Lincoln Close, Audley Range, Blackburn BB1 1NY Tel: 01254 671560 Fax: 01254 696679 — MB BS Andhra 1962 (Andhra Med. Coll.) DCH Andhra 1964.

RAO, M S Princes Road Surgery, 116 Princes Road, Liverpool L8 2UL Tel: 0151 727 3434.

RAO, Madduri Joadadish Bulwell Health Centre, Main St., Bulwell, Nottingham NG6 8QJ.

RAO, Madipalli Venkateswara Glen Road Medical Centre, 1-9 Glen Road, London E13 8RU Tel: 020 7476 3434 — MB BS Andhra 1972 (Andhra Med. Coll. Visakhapatnam) GP Princip. Specialty: Gen. Pract. Socs: BMA; MPS; ODA. Prev: Trainee GP Asst.; GP Princip.

RAO, Mala Langley Mill Cottage, Colne Engaine, Colchester CO6 2JL Tel: 01787 472642 — MB BS Delhi 1977; DA Eng. 1981; MSc Community Med. Lond. 1983; MFCM 1986; FFPHM RCP (UK) 1993. Dir. Pub. Health S. Essex HA. Specialty: Pub. Health Med. Prev: Cons. Pub. Health NE Essex HA Dist. Off. Cochester.

RAO, Mannige Rahul South London & Maudsley NHS Trust, Job Ward, GUY's Hospital, London SE1 9RT — MB BS Lond. 1989; BSc Lond. 1986; MRCPsych 1994; MD Lond. 1999. Cons./Sen Lect., GUY's Hosp. Lond. Specialty: Geriat. Psychiat. Socs: Brit. Neuropsychiat. Assn.; Train. Mem. Brit. Assn. Psychopharmacol.; Brit. Geriat.s Soc. Prev: Sen. Regist. (Psychiat.) Maudsley Hosp. Lond.; Regist. (Psychiat.) Fulbourn Hosp. Camb. & W. Suff. Hosp. Bury St. Edmunds; SHO (Psychiat.) Fulbourn Hosp. Camb.

RAO, Mannige Sateesh 245 Hills Road, Cambridge CB2 2RP Tel: 01223 240970 — MB BS Agra 1957 (Indore, India) Cons. Phys. Med. for Elderly/Integrated Med. Edith Cavell Hosp. Specialty: Gen. Med.; Neurol. Socs: BMA; Brit. Geriat.s Soc. Prev: Geriat. Newmarket Gen. Hosp. E. Anglian RHA; Regist. (Med.) Chesterton Hosp. Camb.

RAO, Narayan 33 Penrose Street, London SE17 3DW Tel: 020 7703 3677 — MB BS Osmania 1958 (Osmania Med. Coll. Hyderabad)

RAO, Padma 180 Hollywood Avenue, Gosforth, Newcastle upon Tyne NE3 5BU Tel: 0191 285 1390 — MB BS Lond. 1989 (St Mary's Hosp.) BSc (1st. cl. Hons.) Lond. 1986; MRCP (UK) 1993; FRCR (UK) 1996. Lect. (Paediat. Radiol.) Roy. Liverp. Childr. Hosp. Specialty: Radiol. Socs: Roy. Coll. Radiol.; Roy. Coll. Phys. Edin.; BMA. Prev: Sen. Regist. (Diagn. Radiol.) Newc. Hosps.; Regist. (Diag. Radiol.) Newc. Hosp.; SHO Rotat. (Gastroenterol. & Gen. Med.) Northwick Pk. Hosp. Harrow.

RAO, Pappu Bhogeswara Solway Health Services, 11 Roper Street, Workington CA14 3BY Tel: 01900 602997 Fax: 01900 870142 — MB BS Andhra 1971; MB BS 1971 Andhra. GP Workington, Cumbria.

RAO, Poduri Jaya 31A Willows Drive, Failsworth, Manchester M35 0PZ Tel: 0161 682 4437 — MB BS Andhra 1973. Staff Grade Roy. Oldham Hosp.

RAO, Ponnaganti Chandrasekhara 17 Staverton Leys, Rugby CV22 5RD — MB BS Sri Venkateswara 1972; DA Eng. 1979. Staff Grade (Anaesth.) Hosp. St Cross Rugby. Specialty: Anaesth. Prev: Regist. (Anaesth.) Roy. Infirm. Dumfries, Qu. Eliz. Hosp. Gateshead & Neath Gen. Hosp.

RAO, Premanand Bhaskeranand Kenley Parade Surgery, 4-6 Kenley Parade, Sheil Road, Liverpool L6 3BP Tel: 0151 263 6588 Fax: 0151 263 4723; 8 Hayles Grove, Gateacre, Liverpool L25 4SL — MB BS Karnatak 1963 (Kasturba Med. Coll. Mangalore) Specialty: Respirat. Med.

RAO, Puvvada Jagadishwara Birkdale Practice, 147 Liverpool Road, Birkdale, Southport PR8 4NT Tel: 01704 566277 Fax: 01704 563007.

RAO, Ravi Madduri 76 Comeragh Road, London W14 9HR — MB BChir Camb. 1993; MA Camb. 1993; MRCP (UK) 1995. Regist. Rheum. Unit Hammersmith Hosp. Lond. Specialty: Rehabil. Med.; Rheumatol.

RAO, Sharon Vinnakota 24 Petersham Drive, Appleton, Warrington WA4 5QF — MB ChB Dund. 1998; MB ChB Dund 1998.

RAO, Sheela 13 Padstow Drive, Bramhall, Stockport SK7 2HU — MB BS Lond. 1993.

RAO, Sridevi Kamma 13 Farnham House, Harewood Avenue, London NW1 6NT — MB BS Lond. 1996.

RAO, Sudha 15 Battersby Close, Yarm TS15 9RX Tel: 01642 879754 Fax: 01642 879754 — MB BS Madras 1974; MRCOG 1990. Specialty: Obst. & Gyn.

RAO, Mr Sudhir Gururaja Queen Mary's Hospital, Sidcup BR5 2RH; 46 Spring Shaw Road, Orpington BR5 2RH Tel: 0958 632831 Fax: 020 8300 9294 Email: sudhir.rao@virgin.net — MB BS Bombay 1985; FRCS Glas. 1989; FRCS Ed. 1989; MChOrth. Liverp. 1991; FRCS (Orth.) 1996; FRCS (Eng.) 1998. Cons. Orthopaedic Surg. Qu. Mary's Hosp. Sidcup; Cons. Orthopaedic Surg. The Blackheath Hosp., Lond. Bridge Hosp. & Chelsfield Pasrk Hosp., Kent; Cons. Orthopaedic Surg. Lond. Bridge Hosp.; Cons. Orthopaedic Surg. Chelsfield Pk. Hosp. Chelsfield, Kent. Specialty: Trauma & Orthop. Surg.; Sports Med.; Medico Legal. Socs: Fell. BOA; Brit. Assn. Surg. Knee; BMA. Prev: Cons. Orthopaedic Surg. Univ. Hosp. Lewisham; Sen. Regist. (Orthop.) N. W. Region Train. Progr.

RAO, Sumant Kogganna Damien's Mill, Datchet Road, Windsor SL4 Tel: 0175 35 52303 — MB BS Bombay 1958 (Seth G.S. Med. Coll.) MRCP Lond. 1969; MRCP Glas. 1969. Cons. Phys. Canad. Red Cross, Maidenhead, Slough & Windsor Hosps. Specialty: Gen. Med. Socs: Fell. Amer. Coll. Chest Phys.; Brit. Pharmacol. Soc. Prev: Sen. Regist. (Geriat. Med.) Centr. & Middlx. Hosps. Lond.; Hon. Sen. Regist. Hammersmith Hosp. & Roy. Postgrad. Med. Sch.; Hon. Research Asst. Dept. Cardiol. Northwick Pk. Hosp. Harrow.

RAO, Suryadevara Yadu Purna Chandra Prasada Belgrave Medical Centre, 116 Belgrave Road, Dresden, Stoke-on-Trent ST3 4LR Tel: 01782 593344 Fax: 01782 593305 Email: prasad.rao@nshawebmail.nhs.uk; Fairfield House, 169 Barlaston Old Road, Trentham, Stoke-on-Trent ST4 8HJ Tel: 01782 646099 Fax: 01782 659125 Email: prasadraos@aol.com — (Andhra Med. Coll. Visakhapatnam) MB BS Andhra 1973. Clin. Exec. Chair S. Stoke PCT; Chairman, North Staffordshire Doctor's Cooperative, Stoke on Trent. Socs: Chairm. Doctors Co-op. N. Staffs; Chairman, Association Primary Care Groups/Trusts; President North Staffordshire Division, British International Doctors Association. Prev: SHO (Gen. Surg.) Guest Hosp. Dudley; SHO (Orthop.) Gloucester Roy. Hosp. & Standish Hosp. StoneHo..

RAO, Tadepalli Lakshmi Narasimha 40-42 Atherstone Avenue, Netherton, Peterborough PE3 9TY Tel: 01733 333788 Fax: 01733 333788 — MB BS Osmania 1972; DO RCPSI 1978; MCOphth 1988. Ophth.Med. Practitioners. Specialty: Ophth. Socs: RCOphth; Brit. Contact Lens Assoc; Brit. Excimer Laser Soc. Prev: Regist. (Ophth.) Northampton Gen. Hosp.; SHO (Ophth.) P'boro. Hosp.; Laser Ophth., Optimax laser eye clinic, Manch.

RAO, Valluri Ranganadha 42 Landseer Avenue, Tingley, Wakefield WF3 1UE Tel: 0113 253 2278 — MB BS Andhra 1953; BSc Andhra 1953; DPH Liverp. 1967; Cert FPA 1968; FRSH 1970; MFCM 1974; MFPHM 1989. Socs: Fac. Community Health; BMA. Prev: SCM Wakefield & Sandwell HA; Med. Off. Environm. Health Sandwell DC.

RAO, Vasanampalli Meena Kamalakshi 59 The Broadway, Dudley DY1 4AP — MB BS Lond. 1996. Dept.of Paed.Neorology,Birm. Childr.s Hosp.k, Birm. B4 6NH. Specialty: Paediat.; Neurol.

RAO, Vibha Rohit 7 Tapley Road, Chelmsford CM1 4XY Tel: 01245 441370 — MB BS Bombay 1972 (Grant Med. Coll.) FRCS Ed. 1978. Clin. Asst. (Ophth.) Lond. Hosp.

RAO, Mr Victor Moor Green Lane Medical Centre, 339 Moor Green Lane, Moseley, Birmingham B13 8QS Tel: 0121 472 6959 — MB BS Calcutta 1952; MS Calcutta 1962, MB BS 1952; FRCS Eng. 1957. Clin. Asst. Migraine Research Clinic Birm.

RAO, Vidya Digambar 63 Brace Street Health Centre, Walsall WS1 3PS — MB BS 1974; MD (Paediat.) Osmania 1979; DCH RCP Lond. 1984; MRCP (UK) 1990; Dip (Child Stud.) Lond. 2001; MA (Child Stud.) Lond. 2002. Cons. (Paediat.) Walsall PCT. Prev: Staff Grade (Paediat.) Good Hope Hosp. Walsall; Lect. (Child Health) Univ. Of Nottm.; Clin. Med. Off. N. Birm. & Bromsgrove & Redditch HAS.

RAO, Vuppala Radha Kishan 34 Albyfield, Bromley BR1 2HZ — MB BS Osmania 1969.

RAO, Vyakaranam Padmavathi Halling Medical Centre, Ferry Road, Halling, Rochester ME2 1NP Tel: 01634 240238; 62 Rochester Road, Halling, Rochester ME2 1AH — MB BS Osmania 1965 (Gandhi Med. Coll. Hyderabad) DA Eng. 1976. Prev: Clin. Asst. (Anaesth.) Epsom Dist. Hosp.; SHO (O & G) All St.s Hosp. Chatham; Capt. IAMC.

RAO, Mr Yella Veera Venkata Satya Dr Yus Rao, Greenfields Medical Centre, 12 Terrace Street, Nottingham NG7 6ER Tel: 0115 942 3582 Fax: 0115 900 2330; 9 Pavilion Road, Nottingham NG5 8NL Tel: 0115 926 0274 — MB BS Andhra 1967; FRCS Eng. 1976. Med. Bd.ing Off. DHSS Nottm.; Med. Off. (Disabil. Med.) City Hosp. Nottm. Specialty: Disabil. Med.; Rehabil. Med. Prev: SHO (Gen. Surg.) Corbett Hosp. Stourbridge; Cas. Off. King Edwd. VII Hosp. Windsor; SHO (Orthop.) Good Hope Gen. Hosp. Sutton Coldfield.

RAO, Yerramilli Balavenkata Janardhan (John) Calnwood Court, Calnwood Road, Luton LU4 0LX Tel: 01582 704162 Fax:

01582 709164 — MB BS Andhra 1967; DPM; FRCPsych. Cons. Psychiat. Beds. & Luton NHS Trust. Specialty: Gen. Psychiat. Special Interest: Post Traumatic Stress Disorder.

RAOOF, Abdur 5 Groveside Crescent, Clifton Village, Nottingham NG11 8NT Tel: 0115 984 2959 — MRCS Eng. LRCP Lond. 1969 (Nishtar Med. Coll.) BSc, MB BS Punjab 1958; DIH Soc. Apoth. Lond. 1973; MFOM RCP Lond. 1978. Indep. Cons. Ocupational Med.. Specialty: Occupat. Health. Socs: Soc. Occupat. Med.; Brit. Occupat. Hyg. Soc. Prev: Occupat. Health Phys. Nottm. CC; Med. Off. Nat. Coal Bd. (NE Area), Roy. Ordnance Fact. Nottm. & COD Chilwell MOD.

RAOOF, Mr Hikmat Yousif 9 St Leonards Close, Welling DA16 2DN — MB ChB Mosul 1973; FRCS Glas. 1987.

RAOUF, Ali Hameed 32 Middlemore, Southfields, Northampton NN3 5DE — MB ChB Baghdad 1973; MRCP (UK) 1983.

RAPADO SANTAOLALLA, Mr Fernando 115 Smithfield Buildings, 44 Tib Street, Manchester M4 1LA Tel: 0161 839 6939 Email: frapado@talk21.com — LMS Cantabria 1990 (Santander Med. Sch.) FRCS (ENT) 1997. Specialist Regist. (ENT) Hope Hospital-Royal Manch. Children's Hosp. Specialty: Otorhinolaryngol. Special Interest: Rhinology, Undergraduate and Postgrad. Teachg. Socs: BMA; Manch. Med. Soc.; Med. Defence Union. Prev: Specialist Regist. (Otolaryngol.) NW Reg. Train. Scheme; Specialist Regist. (ENT) Blackburn Roy. Infirm. Blackburn; Demonst. (Anat.) Dept. Biomed. Sci. Univ. Sheff.

RAPEPORT, William Garth GlaxoWellcome RID, Greenford Road, Greenford UB6 Tel: 020 8966 3073 Fax: 020 8966 2757 — MB BCh Witwatersrand 1977; MRCP (UK) 1979; FFPM RCP (UK) 1995. Worldwide Dir. (Clin. Pharmacol.) Glaxo Wellcome Greenford; Vis. Prof. Dept. Pharmacol. & Therap. Univ. Liverp. Specialty: Pharmacology. Socs: Brit. Pharm. Soc. Prev: Dir. Early Clin. Research Gp. Pfizer Centr. Research Sandwich Kent; Hon. Sen. Regist. & MRC Clin. Scientist MRC Univ. Dept. Clin. Pharmacol. Radcliffe Infirm. Oxf.; Regist. Univ. Dept. Med. Gardiner Inst. West. Infirm. Glas.

RAPER, Joan Marjorie 12 ladywood Mead, Asket Hill, Leeds LS8 2LZ — MB ChB Leeds 1937.

RAPER, John Malcolm (retired) Hilltop, 13 Meadow Croft, Draughton, Skipton BD23 6EG Tel: 01756 710367 — MB ChB Leeds 1961; FFA RCS Eng. 1967. Prev: Cons. Anaesth. Airedale Gen. Hosp. E.burn.

RAPER, Joyce Agnes (retired) Owl End, 64 Stoughton Lane, Stoughton, Leicester LE2 2FH Tel: 0116 271 3331 — MB ChB Manch. 1952; DCH Eng. 1955.

RAPER, Sally Clair 80 Clough Road, Golcar, Huddersfield HD7 4JX — MB BS Newc. 1997.

RAPHAEL, Alison Mary Cherryvalley Health Centre, Kings Square, Belfast BT5 7AR; 8 Wandsworth Drive, Belfast BT4 2BJ Tel: 653874 — MB BCh BAO Belf. 1973.

RAPHAEL, Frances Jane Springfield Hospital, Glenburnie Road, Tooting, London SW17 — MB BS Lond. 1987; MRCPsych 1991; MD Llondon 1999. Cons. Psychiat. S. W. Lond. and St Geo.s, NHS Trust, Tooting Lond.. Specialty: Gen. Psychiat. Prev: Lect. (Community Psychiat.) St. Geo. Hosp. Med. Sch.; Lect. (Gen. Psychiat.) Lond.; Regist. Rotat. (Psychiat.) St. Geo. Hosp. Lond.

RAPHAEL, George Anton Jayaseelan 1 Marsden Road, Cleadon Village, Sunderland SR6 7RA Tel: 0191 537 2198 — MB BS Ceylon 1969; DA (UK) 1979; FFA RCSI 1988. Locum Cons. & Assoc. Specialist (Anaesth.) S. Tyneside Health Care Trust. Specialty: Anaesth. Prev: Staff Grade (Anaesth.) Freeman Hosp. Newc.

RAPHAEL, Maurice John 126 Harley Street, London W1N 1AH Tel: 020 7935 4072; 37 Rotherwick Road, London NW11 7DD Tel: 020 8201 9065 — MD Camb. 1971, MB 1959, BChir 1958; DObst RCOG 1960; FRCP Lond. 1978, M 1961; DMRD Eng. 1961; FFR 1964. Cons. Radiol. Middlx. Hosp. Lond. Specialty: Radiol. Socs: Fell. Roy. Soc. Med.; Brit. Inst. Radiol.

RAPHAEL, Montague, MBE 20 Bordeaux Close, Northfield Green, Sunderland SR3 2SR Tel: 0191 528 0784 — LRCP LRCS Ed. LRFPS Glas. Ed. 1950 (Roy. Colls. & Univ. Ed.) MRCGP 1958. Med. Adviser Benefits Agency Sunderland. Prev: Clin. Asst. Gen. Hosp. & Roy. Infirm. Sunderland; Ho. Surg. N. Ormesby Hosp.; Med. Off. Remploy Sunderland.

RAPHAEL, Nabil St Marks Medical Centre, 24 Wrottesley Road, Plumstead, London SE18 3EP Tel: 020 8854 6262 Fax: 020 8317 3098 — MRCS Eng. LRCP Lond. 1979; MRCOG 1983.

RAPHAEL, Olga Rachel (retired) Briar Cottage, 154 Tilt Road, Cobham KT11 3HR Tel: 01932 867370 — (Sheff.) MB ChB Sheff. 1951. Prev: Clin. Med. Off. Kingston & Esher HA.

RAPLEY, David Michael The Castle Medical Centre, 22 Bertie Road, Kenilworth CV8 1JP Tel: 01926 857331 Fax: 01926 851070; 2 Amherst Road, Kenilworth CV8 1AH Tel: 01926 512192 — MB ChB Birm. 1980 (Birmingham) MRCGP 1984; Cert. Family Plann. JCC 1984. Course Organiser Coventry & Warks.; Mem. Warks. MAAG; Hon. Sen. Clin. Lect. (Gen. Pract.) Warwick Univ. Socs: (Hon. Sec.) Midl. Fac. RCGP. Prev: GP Postgrad. Tutor S. Warks.

RAPOPORT, Jill Honnage Brook Medical Centre, Hannage Way, Wirksworth, Matlock DE4 4JG Tel: 01629 822434; 7 Yokecliffe Hill, Wirksworth, Derby DE4 4PE Tel: 01629 823515 — BM BS Nottm. 1975; BMedSci Nottm. 1973; DRCOG 1978; Cert JCC Lond. 1979; MRCGP 1979; LF HOM 1997.

RAPP, D A Simmons and Partners, Chalkhill Health Centre, Rook Close, off Chalkhill Road, Wembley HA9 9BQ Tel: 020 8901 1144 Fax: 020 8908 6945 Email: rapphussain@gp-e84033.nhs.uk — MB BS London 1977; MB BS London 1977.

RAPPAPORT, Ruth Alison (retired) 7 Howard Walk, London N2 0HB Tel: 020 8455 4813 — (Glasgow) MB ChB Glas. 1946; DPM Lond. 1950. Prev: Cons. (Child & Adoles. Psychiat.) Redbridge Child Guid.

RAPPORT, Henry Maurice, MBE (retired) Kockmaroon, 37 Brandreth Road, Penylan, Cardiff CF23 5NW Tel: 029 2046 0255 — MRCS Eng. LRCP Lond. 1937 (Cardiff) FRCGP 1975, M 1956. Clin. Asst. Marie Curie Hospice Penarth S. Glam. Prev: Ho. Surg., Ho. Phys. & Cas. Surg. Off. Cardiff Roy. Infirm.

RAPTOPOULOS, Paul — MD Thessalonika 1967 (Thessaloike) MRCPsych 1976; MFPM 1990; FFPM RCP (UK) 1996. Sen. Med. Off. Meds. Control Agency DoH Lond. Specialty: Pharmaceutical Medicine. Prev: Clin. Projects Manager, Pharmaceutical Industry; Research Sen. Regist. & Hon. Lect. St. Mary's Hosp. Med. Sch. Lond.

RARATY, Mrs Catherine Carmel Westford Lodge, Merrill's Lane, Upton, Wirral CH49 0UA Tel: 0151 605 0205 Email: c.raraty@virgin.net — MB ChB Leeds 1989; FRCS Ed. 1997. Specialty: Plastic Surg.

RARATY, Mr Michael Godwin Thomas Westford Lodge, Merrill's Lane, Upton, Wirral CH49 0UA Tel: 0151 605 0205 Email: m.raraty@virgin.net — MB BS Newc. 1989 (Newc. u tyne) FRCS Eng. 1994. Clin. Research Fell. (Dept. Surg.) Univ. of Liverp. Specialty: Gen. Surg. Prev: Regist. (Gen. Surg.) Arrowe Pk. Hosp. Wirral.

RARITY, Russell Alexander Gilbert Bain Hospital, Lerwick ZE1 0TB Tel: 01595 743007; 1 Hayfield Court, Commercial St, Lerwick ZE1 0AN Tel: 01595 692589 — MB BChir Camb. 1988; MA Camb. 1992; FRCA 1994. Cons. Anaesth., Gilbert Bain Hosp., Shetland Is.s.; Med. Serv.s Manager-Shetland Health Bd.. Specialty: Anaesth. Socs: FRSM; Mem. Intens. Care Soc.; Mem. Assn. Anaesth. GB & Irel. Prev: Sen. Regist. (Anaesth.) Roy. Berks. Hosp. Reading & Anglia & Oxf. RHA; Regist. Rotat. (Anaesth.) Oxf. RHA & Aylesbury Vale HA.

RASAIAH, Dorairetnam (retired) The Paddock, Leigh, Sherborne DT9 6HW Tel: 01935 873229 — MB ChB St. And. 1963. Prev: SHO (Fract. & Orthop.) Dundee Roy. Infirm.

RASAIAH, Selva Launceston Close Surgery, 9-10 Launceton Close, Winsford CW7 1LY Tel: 01606 861200 — MB ChB Manch. 1987. Trainee GP Sandbach.

RASAMUTHIAH, Thuraiappah Calnwood Court, Calnwood Road, Luton LU4 0LX Tel: 01582 709150 Fax: 01582 709151; 11 Hayton Close, Luton LU3 4HD Tel: 01582 596710 — MB BS Colombo 1968 (University of Ceylon, Colombo, Srilanka) Assoc. Specialist Psychiat. Dept., Beds & Luton Community NHS Trust, Luton. Specialty: Ment. Health; Gen. Psychiat.; Psychother. Socs: Affil. Mem., Roy. Coll. of Psychiat.s.

RASANAYAGAM, Stephen Romesh 36A Atherston, Warmley, Bristol BS30 8YB Tel: 0117 947 5072 — MB BS Lond. 1987.

RASARATNAM, Renuga Harperbury, Harper Lane, Shenley, Radlett WD7 9HQ Tel: 01923 427222; 7 Tithe Farm Close, South Harrow, Harrow HA2 9DP Tel: 01273 555382/020 8933 2284 Fax: 01273 556093 Email: hempling@btinternet.com/ renuga@lineone.net — MB BS Columbo 1972; BC Psych 1995; MRC Psych 1996. Specialist Regist. (Psychiat. of Learning

Disabilities) Horizon NHS Trust Shenley. Specialty: Ment. Health; Gen. Psychiat. Prev: Staff Grade Psychiat. (Acute Adult Psychiat.) Northwick Pk. Hosp. Harrow; Regist. Rotat. (Psychiat.) S. Essex Train. Scheme.

RASBURN, Barbara 27 Grayling Road, London N16 0BL; 92A Lordship Park, London N16 5UA — MB BS Lond. 1991.

RASCHID, Muhammad Salman — MB Camb. 1964; BChir 1963.

RASCHKES, Beena Jacqueline The Surgery, Main Street, Bridge of Earn, Perth PH2 9PL — MB ChB Manch. 1982; BSc (Med. Sci.) St. And. 1979; DCH RCP Lond. 1984; DRCOG 1984; DFFP 1994. Prev: Trainee GP Timperley; SHO (O & G) Wythenshawe Hosp. Manch.; SHO (Paediat.) Booth Hall Childr. Hosp. Manch.

RASDALE, Paul Dingwall Medical Group, The Health Centre, Ferry Road, Dingwall IV15 9QS Tel: 01349 863034 Fax: 01349 862022 — MB ChB Glas. 1977; MRCP (UK) 1980; FRCP Glas. 1994. Specialty: Gen. Pract.

RASH, Amar 46 Leegate Road, Stockport SK4 4AX — MB ChB Sheff. 1994 (Sheffield) MRCP (UK) 1998. SHO (Med.) Chesterfield & N. Derbysh. Roy. Hosp. Specialty: Gen. Med.

RASH, Guy James Eric Lawson Road Health Centre, Lawson Road, Norwich NR3 4LE Tel: 01603 427096 Fax: 01603 403074; 23 Hanover Road, Norwich NR2 2HD — MB BS Lond. 1990 (St Bartholomew's Med. School) MRCP (UK) 1994; MRCGP (Dist.) 1998.

RASH, Ramakant Maganlal (retired) 46 Leegate Road, Heaton Moor, Stockport SK4 4AX Tel: 0161 432 1085 — MB ChB Manch. 1962; BSc (Hons. Anat.) Manch. 1959, MB ChB 1962; FRCP Lond. 1984, M 1967. Prev: Cons. Phys. (Geriat. Med.) Wythenshawe Hosp. Manch.

RASHBASS, Barbara Joan — MB BS Univ. Coll. Lond. 1958 F 1999 (Univ. Coll. Hosp.) DCH Eng. 1961; DPH Eng. 1968; FRCP Lond. 1995. Barrister-at-Law. Socs: Medico-Legal Soc.; Roy. Soc. Med. Prev: Non-Exec. Dir. Harrow & Hillingdon Healthcare Trust; Dir. & Sec. Wolfson Foundat. & Family Charitable Trust; PMO H.Q. Staff Med. Research Counc.

RASHBASS, Jeremy Lewis Clinical and Biomedical Computing Unit, Addenbrooke's Hospital, Cambridge CB2 2SP Tel: 01223 765 355 Fax: 01223 765 505 Email: jem@cbcu.cam.ac.uk — MB BS Lond. 1987 (Univ. Coll. Lond.) BSc (Hons.) Anat. Lond 1983; PhD Camb. 1991; MRCPath 1995; FRCPath 2003. Dir. BioMed. Computing Camb. Univ. Camb.; Hon. Cons. Haemat. Histopath.; Non-Exec. Dir. NHS Informat. Auth.; Director, Centre for Applied Research in Educational Technologies, Camb. Univ. Specialty: Histopath.; Haematology. Prev: Clin. Research Fell. Cancer Research Campaign Camb.

RASHBROOK, Patricia Sybil Evenfield Centre, West Hill Road, St Leonards-on-Sea TN38 0NE — MB ChB Sheff. 1967; MSc Lond. 1972; MRCPsych 1985.

RASHED, Khalid Areef Mustafa Yeovil District Hospital, Higher Kingston, Yeovil BA21 4AT Tel: 01935 707344 Fax: 01935 384446 Email: rashk@est.nhs.uk; Al-Gazal, Queen St, Tintinhull, Yeovil BA22 8PG Tel: 01935 825253 — MB ChB Mosul 1979 (Mosul Univ.) MRCPI 1986; MRCP (UK) 1987. Cons. Gen. & Geriat. Med. E. Som. NHS Trust Yeovil. Specialty: Gen. Med. Special Interest: Care of the Elderly; Stroke. Socs: Brit Geriat. Soc. Prev: Sen. Regist. (Gen. & Geriat. Med.) SE Thames RHA; Regist. (Geriat.) Ealing Hosp. Middlx.; Research Regist. (Cardiol.) Bath.

RASHED, Mr Mohamed Daw Kettering General Hospital, Rothwell Road, Kettering NN16 8VZ Tel: 01536 492000; 3 Keating Close, Barton Sea Grave, Kettering NN15 5JA — MB BCh Tripoli 1981; FRCS Ed. 1989; FRCS (Gen.) 1998; FRCS Ed (Gen) 1998. Cons. Surg. Specialty: Gen. Surg. Socs: Mem. Assn. Cloproctol. GB & Irel.; Assoc of Surg.s of Gt. Brit. Irel..

RASHED, Nabil Fathalla Psychiatric Department, Queens Park Hospital, Blackburn BB2 3HH Tel: 01254 63555; 23 Walton Crescent, Blackburn BB2 3TQ Tel: 01254 665060 — MB ChB Alexandria 1967; DPM Eng. 1978. Specialty: Gen. Med. Socs: BMA. Prev: Med. Asst. (Psychiat.) Qu.'s Pk. Hosp. Blackburn.

RASHEED, Ali 257 Arethusa Way, Bisley, Woking GU24 9BU Tel: 01483 480097 — MB ChB Ed. 1969 (Edinburgh University) BSc Ed. 1966; DTM & H RCP Lond. 1971; T(GP) 1992; AMP (Aerospace Medicine Primary) Air Univ. Texas 1996. Out of Hours Locum Duty Dr. In S.E. Surrey Region. Specialty: Infec. Dis. Socs: Roy. Coll. Gen. Pract.; Nat. Assn. Non-Princip.; Roy. Soc. Med. Prev: GP Princip. Camberley Surrey; Med. Off. Govt. of Malaysia; U.N. Exam. Phys. RePub. of Maldives.

RASHEED, Farhat 7 Woodfield Road, Middleton, Manchester M24 1NF — MB ChB Manch. 1997.

RASHEED, Mohamed Haroon The Surgery, 77 Sandy Lane, Mansfield NG18 2LT Tel: 01623 656055 Fax: 01623 424898 — MB BS Madras 1967.

RASHEED, Mr Sohail 10 Lenten Grove, Hopwood, Heywood OL10 2LR — MB BS Punjab 1988; FRCSI 1993.

RASHEED, Sultana Amtul Ahad 18 Wessex Gardens, London NW11 9RT Tel: 020 8445 3496 — MB ChB Sheff. 1994.

RASHID, Mr Abbas Cardiothoracic Centre, Thomas Drive, Liverpool L14 3PE Tel: 0151 293 2463 Fax: 0151 293 2254 Email: a.rashid@ctc.nhs.uk — MD Tehran; FRCS Eng. Cons. Cardiac Surg. and Lead Cons. in Thoracic Surg., The Cardio-Thoracic Centre, Liverp. Specialty: Cardiol. Socs: Europan Associcaton of Cardio Thoracic Surgeons.

RASHID, Abdul Azeem Waqar 3 Ambleside Avenue, Bradford BD9 5NX — MB ChB Leeds 1995.

RASHID, Abutaleb Muhammed Fazlur Consultant Histopathologist, Darent Valley Hospital, Dartford DA2 2DA Tel: 01322 428489 Fax: 01322 428493 — MB BS Dacca 1961 (Dacca Med. Coll.) MSc (Path.) Dacca 1967; FRCPath 1990, M 1978. Cons. Histopath. Darent Valley Hosp. Specialty: Histopath. Socs: Clin. Path. Assn.; Brit. Clin. Cytol. Soc.; Roy. Soc. Med. Prev: Sen. Regist. (Histopath. & Morbid Anat.) Soton. Gen. Hosp.; Regist. in Path., Roy. Sussex Co. Hosp., Brighton.; Ex. Clin. Director of Path., Dartford & Gravesham.

RASHID, Ahmad Yusafi 90 North Hyde Road, Hayes UB3 4NF Tel: 020 8573 8560 Fax: 020 8569 0551; 11 Youlden Drive, Camberley GU15 1AL Tel: 01276 20750 — (King Edwd. Med. Coll. Lahore) BSc Punjab (Pakistan) 1955; MB BS Punjab 1962. GP Clin. Asst. (Ophth.) Hillingdon Hosp. Uxbridge. Socs: BMA. Prev: Clin. Asst. (Ophth.) Hillingdon Hosp. Uxbridge; Staff Phys. Horton Hosp. Epsom; Clin. Asst. (Ophth.) St. And. Hosp. Bow.

RASHID, Alan Hasnat 33 Hervey Close, London N3 2HG — MB BS Lond. 1994.

RASHID, Aly Countesthorpe Health Centre, Central Street, Countesthorpe, Leicester LE8 5QJ Tel: 0116 277 6336 — MB ChB Manch. 1982; DRCOG 1985; FRCGP 191991, M 1986; MD Manch. 1995. GP Leics.; Assoc. Adviser (Gen. Pract.) Univ. Leicester. Prev: Nat. Chairm. (Educat.) RCGP.

RASHID, Asrar Dept of Paediatrics, Birmingham Heartlands Hospital, Birmingham B9 5SS; 55 Leicester Road, Luton LU4 8SF — MB ChB Aberd. 1992. Specialist Regist. Paediat. Birm. Heartlands. Hosp. Specialty: Paediat.

RASHID, Attiya 90B Plaistow Lane, Bromley BR1 3JE — MB BS Lond. 1998; MB BS Lond 1998.

RASHID, Badr Ur 28 Corringham Road, Wembley HA9 9PY — MB BS Karachi 1971; DTM & H RCP Lond. 1981.

RASHID, Mr Hisham Ikram King's College Hospital, Denmark Hill, London SE5 9RS Tel: 020 7346 3339 Fax: 020 7346 4439 — MB BCh Cairo 1984; MSc Cairo 1991; FRCS Eng. 1993; MSc Lond. 1996; FRCS (Gen. Surg.) 2000. Cons. Vasc. Surg. Specialty: Gen. Surg. Socs: Assn. Surg. GB & Irel.; Fell. VSS; Fell. ESVS. Prev: SE. Thames SpR Rotat.

RASHID, Irme 23 Cottrell Road, Bristol BS5 6TH — MB BS Lond. 1993.

RASHID, Khalid 42 Fairfield Road, Scunthorpe DN15 8DQ — MB BS Bahauddin Zakariya Univ. Pakistan 1984; MB BS Bahauddin Zakariya U Pakistan 1984.

RASHID, Masoud 39 Froghall Terrace, Aberdeen AB24 3JP — MB ChB Aberd. 1997.

RASHID, Mohammed Abdur 41 Sutherland Grove, London SW18 5QP Tel: 020 8788 6047 — MB BS Karachi 1961 (Dow Med. Coll.) DTM & H Liverp. 1963.

RASHID, Mr Najam Zafar Accident & Emergency Department, Manor Hospital, Moat Road, Walsall WS2 9PS Tel: 01922 721172 Fax: 01922 611902 — MB ChB Birm. 1987 (Birmingham University) FRCS Ed. 1993; FFAEM 1997. Cons. (A & E). Specialty: Accid. & Emerg.

RASHID, Nassim Akhtar Ashgrove Surgery, Cow Lane, Knottingley WF11 9BZ — MB ChB Sheff. 1996.

RASHID, Rafaqut 9 Thorn Grove, Heaton, Bradford BD9 6LT — MB ChB Liverp. 1996.

RASHID, Raza-Ullah 4 Selwyn Road, London E3 5EA — MB BS Lond. 1996.

RASHID, Regina 10 Chelmsford Drive, Glasgow G12 0NA — MB ChB Glas. 1993.

RASHID, S Deepcar Medical Centre, 241-245 Manchester Road, Deepcar, Sheffield S36 2QZ Tel: 0114 288 2146.

RASHID, Sakina Department of Genitourinary Medicine, Sunderland Royal Hospital, Sunderland SR4 7TP Tel: 0191 569 9022 Fax: 0191 569 9244; 5 Eastfield, Peterlee SR8 4SS Tel: 0191 586 7917 — MB BS (Pakistan) 1965; DObst E. Afr. 1970; MMed Makerere 1971; FRCOG 1989. Cons. Genitourin. Med. City Hosps. Sunderland & S. Tyneside Dist. Hosp. Specialty: Genitourinary Medicine. Prev: Cons. Venereol. Sunderland & S. Tyneside AHA's & Newc. AHA (T).

RASHID, Shah Mohammad 32 Woodlands Road, Stalybridge SK15 2SQ Tel: 0161 338 3996 — MB BS Karachi 1957; DA Eng. 1964.

RASHID, Sheikh Abdur Rashid and Partners, Rycroft Primary Care Centre, Madeley Road, Havercroft, Wakefield WF4 2QG Tel: 01226 725555 Fax: 01226 700051; 6 Chevet Croft, Sandal, Wakefield WF4 2AX — MB BS Jammu & Kashmir 1969; MD Kashmir 1974; Dip. Thoracic Med. Lond 1988; DFFP 1996. Socs: Brit. Thorac. Soc.

RASHID, Sheikh Tawqeer 6 Chevet Croft, Sandal, Wakefield WF2 6QR — BChir Camb. 1996.

RASHID, Waqar — MB BS Lond. 1996; BSc Lond. 1994; MRCP (UK) 2000. Clin. Research Fell. (Neuro.) UCL Qu. Sq. Lond. Socs: Med. Protec. Soc. Prev: LAT Regist. (Neuro.) Newc. Gen. North. Deanery; SHO (Med.) City Hosp. Birm.; SHO (Med.) S. Cleveland Hosp. Middlesbrough.

RASHID, Yousef 277 Shrewsbury Road, London E7 8QU — MB BS Lond. 1992.

RASHID, Zafar Iqbal — BChir Camb. 1985 (Cambridge) BMSc (Pharmacol.) Dund 1983; DRCOG 1991; FRCA 1994. Cons., (Anaesth. & IC) Med. Stoke Mandeville Hosp. Aylesbury. Specialty: Anaesth.; Intens. Care. Socs: Assn. Anaesth.; Intens. Care Soc.; BMA. Prev: Specialist Regist. Rotat. (Anaesth.) Nuffield Dept. Anaesth. Oxf.; SHO (Anaesth.) Roy. Berks. Hosp. Reading; Trainee GP Centr. Milton Keynes Med. Centre VTS.

RASHIQ, Hunaid Noorudin 55 Broadlands Avenue, Chesham HP5 1AL — MB BChir Camb. 1992.

RASIAH, Norbert Jagadeesan 102 Queen Elizabeth Drive, London N14 6RE — MB BS Sri Lanka 1974; LRCP LRCS Ed. LRCPS Glas. 1986.

RASLAN, Mr Fateh Cons. Gyn., W. Middlx. Univ. Hosp., Twickenham Rd, Isleworth TW7 6AF Tel: 0208 565 5118 Fax: 0208 565 5428 Email: info@drraslan.com — MB BCh Cairo 1984 (Cairo Univ.) MRCOG 1992. Regist. (Obst.& Gyn.) W. Middlx. Univ. Hosp. Specialty: Obst. & Gyn.

RASMUSSEN, Jill Galloway Chisnall Psynapse, Independent Consultant in Psychiatry and Neurology, Arlington Cottage, Spook Hill, North Holmwood, Dorking RH5 4HH Tel: 01306 883272 Fax: 01306 740911 — MB ChB Manch. 1972; DRCOG 1976; MRCGP 1976; MFPM RCP (UK) 1991; Dip. Ther. 1997; FFPMRCP 1999. Indep. Cons. Dorking; Salaried GP. Specialty: Gen. Psychiat. Socs: Collegium Internat.e Neuropsycho Pharmacologicum (CINP); Eur. Coll. Neuropsychopharm.; Brit. Assn. Psychopharmacol. Prev: Sen. Positions in Lundbeck, Smithkline Beecham & Wellcome.

RASOOL, Hufrish 102 Valley Drive, Kirkella, Hull HU10 7PW — MB BS Karachi 1978; MRCPsych 1990. Cons. Child & Adolesc. Psychiat. W.-End Child, Adolesc. & Family Serv. Hull. Specialty: Child & Adolesc. Psychiat. Prev: Sen. Regist. Rotat. (Child & Adolesc. Psychiat.) St. Jas. Univ. Hosp. Leeds.

RASOOL, Mushtaq Abdul 102 Valley Drive, Kirkella, Hull HU10 7PW — MB BS Karachi 1978; DO RCPSI 1986. Med. Pract. (Ophth.) Humberside. Specialty: Ophth.

RASOOL, Shafquth The Health Centre, Queensway, Billingham TS23 2LA — MB BS Bahauddin Zakariya Univ. Pakistan 1985; MB BS Bahauddin Zakariya Pakistan 1985; MRCP (UK) 1992.

RASOOL, Tahira Parveen 81 Ferryfield, Edinburgh EH5 2PS — MB ChB Glas. 1990; DRCOG 1993; MRCGP 1994.

RASOOLY, Mr Raphael 62 Chatsworth Rd, London NW2 4DD Tel: 020 84514211 — MD Israel 1987; FRCS Glas. 1994.

RASOR, Mr Paul Andrew, Lt.-Col. RAMC Retd. Rectory Road Surgery, 7 Rectory Road, Rowhedge, Colchester CO5 7HP Tel: 01206 728585 Fax: 01206 729262; Ardgowan House, 96 Spring Lane, Fordham Heath, Colchester CO3 9TG — MB BS Lond. 1975 (Char. Cross) BSc Hull 1967; MRCS Eng. LRCP Lond. 1975; FRCS Ed. 1984. Specialty: Gen. Pract. Socs: BMA; MRCS (Ed.). Prev: Sen. Specialist (Orthop.) Qu. Eliz. Milit. Hosp. Lond.; Ho. Surg. & Ho. Phys. Char. Cross Hosp. Lond.; Regtl. Med. Off. RAMC 2/2 Gurkha Rifles.

RASOUL, Mustafa Salim Laburnum Medical Group, 14 Laburnum Terrace, Ashington NE63 0XX Tel: 01670 813376 Fax: 01670 854346 — MB BS Newc. 1973; BSc Newc. 1971.

RASSAM, Saad Munir Bashir Queen Mary's Hospital, Sidcup DA14 6LT Tel: 020 8308 3023 Fax: 020 8308 3153 Email: saad.rassam@qms-tr.sthames.nhs.uk — MB ChB Baghdad 1980; MRCP (UK) 1989; MRCPath 1991; FRCP Lond. 1997; FRCPath 1999. Cons. Haemat. & Oncol. Qu. Mary's Sidcup NHS Trust. Specialty: Haematology; Oncol. Special Interest: Adoptive Immunother. and tumour Immunol.; Lymphoma Ther.; Cancer immunotherapy. Socs: Brit. Soc. Haematol.; Amer. Soc. of Haemat.; Amer. Soc. Of Clin. Oncol. Prev: Lect. & Hon. Sen. Regist. (Haemat. & Oncol.) Hosp. for Sick Childr. Gt. Ormond St. & Univ. Coll. Hosp. Lond.; Regist. (Haemat.) Edgware Gen. Hosp.

RASSAM, Salwan Munir Bashir Eye Department, Worthing Hospital, Lyndhurst Road, Worthing BN11 2DH Tel: 01903 205111 Ext: 4039 Email: sal.rassam@wash.nhs.uk — MB BCh BAO NUI 1985; LRCPI & LM LRCSI & LM 1985; DO RCS Eng. 1990; FRCOphth 1992, M 1990; MD NUI 1994. Cons. Opthalmologist, Worthing Hosp, Worthing, W. Sussex.; Dir. of Research, Worthing Hosp. Specialty: Ophth. Special Interest: Refractive Cataract Surg.; Dis. of the Retina; Vitreoretinal Surg. Socs: Europ. Vitreoretinal Soc.; Europ. Soc. for Cataract and Refractive Surg.; Brit. and Eire Vitreoretinal Soc. Prev: Hon. Regist. Hammersmith Hosp. Lond.

RASTALL, Sarah Jane 101 Upper Gungate, Tamworth B79 8AX — MB ChB Birm. 1996; ChB Birm. 1996.

RASTOGI, Amit 17 The Moorlands, Sutton Coldfield B74 2RF — MB ChB Leic. 1994.

RASTOGI, Gulab Chand Paediatrics Department, Wycombe General Hospital, Queen Alexandra Road, High Wycombe HP11 2TT Tel: 01494 526161 Fax: 01494 425007 — MB BS Lucknow 1974 (King George Medical College, Lucknow India) DCH Lucknow 1976; MD (Paediat.) Lucknow 1978; MRCP (UK) 1987; FRCPCH 1997. Cons. Paediat. Wycombe Gen. Hosp. Specialty: Paediat.; Respirat. Med.; Oncol. Prev: Cons. Paediat. Princess Roy. Hosp. NHS Trust Telford; Staff Grade (Paediat.) Ealing Hosp. Middlx.; Regist. (Paediat.) W. Middlx. Hosp.

RASTOGI, Navin Chandra Horsefair Practice, Horse Fair, Rugeley WS15 2EL Tel: 01889 582244 Fax: 01899 582244; 24 Elm Close, Bolsover, Chesterfield S44 6EA Tel: 01246 823283 — MB BS Calcutta 1972; DA (UK) 1976. Specialty: Accid. & Emerg.

RASTOGI, Robin 127 Longwood Gardens, Clayhall, Ilford IG5 0EG — MB BS Lond. 1998; MRCGP; DRCOG; BSc.

RASTOGI, S Kensington Medical Centre, 17 Fielding Street, Liverpool L6 9AP Tel: 0151 263 3085.

RASTOGI, Sudhir Chandra St. Ann's Hospital, Haven Road, Canford Cliffs, Poole BH13 7LN Tel: 01202 708881 Fax: 01202 707628; 8 Roslin Road S., Talbot Woods, Bournemouth BH3 7EF Tel: 01202 532924 — MB BS Kanpur 1970 (G.S.V.M. Med. Coll. Kanpur) FRCPsych. 1992, M 1977; DPM Eng. 1978. Cons. Psychiat. E. Dorset HA. Specialty: Gen. Psychiat. Prev: Sen. Regist. (Psychiat.) St. Ann's Hosp. Poole; Regist. (Psychiat.) Airedale Gen. Hosp. Steeton.

RASTOGI, Tej Krishan Gillmoss Medical Centre, 48 Petherick Road, Liverpool L11 0AG Tel: 0151 546 3867 — MB BS Lucknow 1972.

RASTOMJEE, Cawas Dirk — MB BS Lond. 1996.

RASUL, Ameen — MB ChB Liverp. 1989; DRCOG 1993. Gen. Practitioner.

RASUL, Shahid Rosevale, Hilton Rd, Alloa FK10 3SG — MB ChB Dundee 1997.

RATAN, Dev Anand Leicestershire Mental Health Service, Bradgate Mental Health Unit, Leicester LE3 9EJ Tel: 0116 250 2661 — MB BS West Indies 1983; MRCPsych 1993. Cons. Psychiat. (Adult & Gen. Psychiat.). Specialty: Gen. Psychiat.

RATAN, Hari Lakshmi 34 Melrose Road, Upper Shirley, Southampton SO15 7PA — BM BS Nottm. 1998; BM BS Nottm 1998.

RATAN, Joanna Caroline — BM BS Nottm. 1998 (Notts) DRCOG; BMedSci Notts. 1996.

RATANI, Tajbano Hassanali 156 Prestonfield, Milngavie, Glasgow G62 7QA — MB BS Karachi 1962.

RATCHFORD, Mr Andrew Martin 62 Bates Lane, Helsby, Warrington WA6 9LF — MB BS Newc. 1992; FRCS Eng. 1996. Specialist Regist. (A & E) N.n. Deanery Rotat. Specialty: Accid. & Emerg. Prev: SHO (A & E) Newc. Gen. Hosp.

RATCHFORD, Joseph Anthony (retired) 24 Brock Mill Lane, Wigan WN1 2NZ — MB ChB Liverp. 1962. Prev: Ho. Off. Ormskirk & Dist. Gen. Hosp.

RATCLIFF, Arthur Jamieson Department of Anaesthetics, Perth Royal Infirmary, Perth PH1 1NX Tel: 01738 623311 Email: arthur.ratcliff@tuht.scot.nhs.uk; Easter Hill, 16 Gannochy Road, Perth PH2 7EF — MB ChB Ed. 1981 (Edinburgh) FRCA 1985. Cons. Anaesth. Perth Roy. Infirm. Specialty: Anaesth. Socs: Roy. Coll. of Anaesthetists; Assn. of Anaesthetists; Scott. Soc. of Anaesthetists. Prev: Sen. Regist. (Anaesth.) Manch. Roy. Infirm.; Clin. Fell. Roy. Vict. Hosp. Montreal; SHO (Anaesth.) Aberd. Infirm.

RATCLIFFE, Andrew Brian 4 Old Church Close, Quarndon, Derby DE22 5JF — MB ChB Leic. 1997.

RATCLIFFE, Brendan Laurence 17 Welbeck Close, Middlewich CW10 9HX — MB ChB Manch. 1980; BSc Manch. 1977, MB ChB 1980; FFA RCS Eng. 1984; MRCGP 1985. GP Knutsford. Specialty: Anaesth. Prev: Clin. Asst. (Anaesth.) Warrington Dist. Gen. Hosp.; Regist./Tutor (Anaesth.) Aberd. Hosp.; SHO (Anaesth.) Manch. Roy. Infirm.

RATCLIFFE, Charles George Old Peppard Farm House, Church Lane, Rotherfield Peppard, Henley-on-Thames RG9 5JU Tel: 01491 628698 Fax: 01491 628094 — MB ChB Sheff. 1984; MSc (Solid State Physics) Manch. 1973, BSc (Electronics) 1972.

RATCLIFFE, Christopher Alan Churchtown Medical Centre, 137 Cambridge Road, Southport PR9 7LT — MB ChB Manch. 1978.

RATCLIFFE, David Malcolm Fort House Surgery, 32 Hersham Road, Walton-on-Thames KT12 1UX Tel: 01932 253055 Fax: 01932 225910; Stretton House, 63 Winchester Road, Walton-on-Thames KT12 2RH — MB BS Lond. 1980 (Charing Cross) MRCP Lond. 1984; DRCOG 1987; MRCGP 1988; BSc 1997. Specialty: Gen. Pract. Prev: Chas. Wolfson Research Fell. City of Lond. Migraine Clinic; Regist. (Nephrol.) John Ratcliffe Hosp. Oxf.

RATCLIFFE, David Stephen Chorlton Health Centre, 1 Nicolas Road, Chorlton, Manchester M21 9NJ Tel: 0161 860 4545 Fax: 0161 860 4565; 25 Westfield Road, Chorlton, Manchester M21 0SW — MB ChB Manch. 1992 (Manchester) DCH 1994; MRCGP 1997. GP; Clin. Asst. A & E. Specialty: Accid. & Emerg.

RATCLIFFE, Francis Hubert (retired) 2 Clipston Lane, Normanton on the Wolds, Nottingham NG12 5NW — MB ChB Manch. 1960; DObst RCOG 1962. Prev: SHO Crumpsall Hosp. Manch.

RATCLIFFE, Guy Edmund, Brigadier late RAMC The Medical Council on Alocohol, 3 St Andrew's Place, London NW1 4LB Tel: 0207 487 4445 Fax: 0207 935 4479 Email: mca@medicouncilalcol.demon.co.uk — (Guy's) MB BS Lond. 1966; MRCS Eng. LRCP Lond. 1966; MRCPI 1980; MRCP (UK) 1988; MSc (Nuclear Med.) Lond. 1990; FRCP Lond. 1993. Exec. Direc. The Med. Counc. on Alcoholism.; Represen. Col. Commandant RAMC; HQ Army Med. Serv.s, Slim Rd., Camberley, Surrey GU15 4NP. Specialty: Endocrinol.; Gen. Med. Socs: BAMM; Med. Counc. on Alcohol. Prev: Commanding Off. Qu. Eliz. Milit. Hosp.; Cons. Phys. & Clin. Tutor Qu. Eliz. Milit. Hosp.; Sen. Med. Off. & Cons. Phys. BMH Dharan., Nepal.

RATCLIFFE, Helen Diane 13 Bonnytoun Avenue, Linlithgow EH49 7JR — MB ChB Aberd. 1997.

RATCLIFFE, Jane Margaret Royal Liverpool Children's NHS Trust, Alder Hey, Eaton Road, Liverpool L12 2AP Tel: 0151 228 4811 Fax: 0151 252 5771 Email: jane.ratcliffe@rlch-tr.nwest.nhs.uk — MB ChB Manch. 1977; FRCP Lond. 1995, M Glas. 1980; FRCPCH 1997. Cons. Paediat. (Intens. Care) Roy. Liverp. Childr. Hosp. Specialty: Paediat.; Intens. Care. Socs: Roy. Coll. Paediat. & Child Health; Paediat. Intens. Care Soc. Prev: Sen. Regist. (Paediat.) The Hosp. for Sick Childr. Lond.; ICU Fell. Hosp. Sick Childr. Toronto, Canada; Brit. Heart Foundat. Research Fell.

RATCLIFFE, Professor John Graham Carreg Pen-Las, Dinas, Newport SA42 0SD Tel: 01348 811568 Fax: 01348 811568 Email: jgratcliffe@aol.com — BM BCh Oxf. 1963; MSc Lond. 1968; DM Oxf. 1972; FRCPath 1985, M 1975; FRCP Glas. 1982, M 1979. Emerit. Prof. Clin. Chem. Univ. Birm. Med. Sch. Specialty: Chem. Path. Prev: Hon. Sen. Research Fell. Univ. Birm. Med. Sch.; Prof. Chem. Pathol. Univ. Manch. Med. Sch.; Cons. Clin. Biochem. & Hon. Lect. Glas. Roy. Infirm.

RATCLIFFE, Joy York House, Manchester Royal Infirmary, Oxford Road, Manchester M13 9WL Tel: 0161 276 5307 — MB ChB Manch. 1988 (Manchester) MRCPsych 1993; MSc 1996.

RATCLIFFE, Marcia Alexandra Ward 16, Aberdeen Royal Infirmary, Aberdeen AB25 1LD — MB BS Newc. 1975; MRCP (UK) 1980; MD Newc. 1993; FRCP UK 1999. Specialty: Haematology.

RATCLIFFE, Mary Jean Rhoslan Surgery, 4 Pwllycrochan Avenue, Colwyn Bay LL29 7DA — MB ChB Manch. 1983; DRCOG 1986; DCH RCP 1987.

RATCLIFFE, Mary Jennine Helen 148 Hammersmith Grove, London W6 7HE — MB BS Lond. 1994.

RATCLIFFE, Norman Arthur 7 Onslow Way, Pyrford, Woking GU22 8QX Tel: 0193 23 42832 — MB Camb. 1970 (Univ. Coll. Hosp.) BChir 1969; MRCPath 1976. Cons. Path. St. Peter's Hosp. Chertsey. Specialty: Pathology, General. Prev: Lect. Dept. Histopath. St. Geo. Hosp. Lond.

RATCLIFFE, Mr Peter John Hucks Farmhouse, Willow Road, Martley, Worcester WR6 6PS — MB BS Lond. 1981; FRCS Eng. 1986.

RATCLIFFE, Peter John Nuffield Department of Medicine, Level 7, John Radcliffe Hospital, Oxford OX3 9DU; Manor Farmhouse, 17 Church Street, Kidlington, Oxford OX5 2BA — MD Camb. 1986; MB ChB Camb. 1978; MRCP (UK) 1980; FRCP 1996; FRS 2002; FMedSci 2002. Nuffield Prof. of Med., Univ. of Oxf. Specialty: Nephrol.; Gen. Med. Special Interest: The Biol. of Hypoxia. Socs: Assn. of Physicians; Internat. Soc. of Nephrol.; Renal Assn. Prev: Wellcome Sen. Fell. (Clin. Sci.) Nuffield Dept. Med. John Radcliffe Hosp. Oxf.; Prof. Renal Med. & Hon. Cons. Phys. Inst. Molecular Med. John Radcliffe Hosp. Oxf.

RATCLIFFE, Peter Wilfred 74 Thurleigh Road, London SW12 8UD Tel: 020 8675 3128 — MB BS Sydney 1962; DMRD Eng. 1966; MSc Lond. 1980. Med. Adviser Dept. Social Security Lond. Specialty: Occupat. Health; Disabil. Med.; Radiol. Socs: Soc. Occupat. Med.; Roy. Coll. Radiol.; Assoc. Mem. Austral. Fac. Occupat. Med.

RATCLIFFE, Rosalind Margaret Hall 102 Onslow Gardens, Wallington SM6 9QG Tel: 020 8647 5997 — MB BS Lond. 1964 (St. Bart.) LMSSA Lond. 1964; DA Eng. 1966; FFA RCS Eng. 1973. Cons. Anaesth. E. Surrey Health Dist. Specialty: Anaesth. Prev: Sen. Regist. (Anaesth.) Char. Cross. Hosp. Lond.; Regist. (Anaesth.) Eastman Dent. Hosp.; Regist. (Anaesth.) St. Helier Hosp. Carshalton.

RATCLIFFE, Shirley Geraldine (retired) Medical Unit, Institute of Child Health, 30 Guilford St., London WC1N 1EH Tel: 020 7242 9789 Fax: 020 7831 1481; Elphinstone, Honeypot Lane, Edenbridge TN8 6QJ Tel: 01732 863235 Fax: 01732 860178 Email: shirley@elphin-stone.fsnet.co.uk — MB BS Lond. 1956 (Roy. Free Hosp. Sch. of Med. Lond.) MRCS Eng. LRCP Lond. 1956; DCH Eng. 1958; FRCP Ed. 1977, M 1960. Mem. Scientif. Staff & Hon. Cons. Paediat. MRC Human Genetics Unit West. Gen. Hosp. Edin.; Hon. Sen. Lect. Inst. Child Health Lond. Prev: Lect. (Child Life & Health) Univ. Edin.

RATCLIFFE, Victoria Ann 38 Hedingham Way, Mickleover, Derby DE3 0NX — BChir Camb. 1996.

RATE, Mr Anthony John Royal Oldham Hospital, Rochdale Road, Oldham OL1 2JH — MB ChB Manch. 1987; MD Manchester 1995 (Gold Medal); FRCS Eng. 1991; FRCS (Gen Surg.) 1998. Cons. Surg (Colorectal Surg.), The Roy. Odham Hosp. Specialty: Gen. Surg. Socs: Assoc of Coloproculogists, GB & Ire. Prev: Specialist Regist. Hope Hosp. Salford, The Christie Hosp.

RATH, Sucheta 5 Frankton Avenue, Haywards Heath RH16 3QX Tel: 01444 459390; Ashoak Nivans, 106 Folders Lane, Burgess Hill RH15 0DX Tel: 01444 230504 Fax: 01444 230504 — MB BS Berhampur 1972; MB BS Berhampur, India 1972. Clin. Asst. (Psychiat. & Subst. Misuse) S. Downs Health NHS Trust Brighton.

RATHAKRISHNAN, Rahul 24 Malcolm Drive, Surbiton KT6 6QS — BM Soton. 1998.

RATHBONE, Anthony Reynolds Telford & Wrekin Pct, Sommerfeld House, Sommerfeld Road, Trench Lock, Telford TF1 5RY Tel: 01952 265 191 Fax: 01952 265 197; 11 Harwin Close, Aldersley, Wolverhampton WV6 9LF Tel: 01902 562 126 — MB BS Lond. 1976 (Middlx.) BA Oxf. 1968; MRCGP 1980; DRCOG 1989. Med. Adviser (Primary Care) Shrops. HA. Prev: GP Telford.

RATHBONE, Barrie John Leicester Royal Infirmary, Infirmary Square, Leicester LE1 5WW Tel: 0116 254 1414 Fax: 0116 258 6985; Claremont House, 20 Nether Hall Lane, Leicester LE4 4DT — MB BS Lond. 1978; MRCP (UK) 1983; MD Lond. 1990; FRCP Lond. 1993. Cons. Phys. & Gastroenterol. Leicester Roy. Infirm. Specialty: Gastroenterol. Socs: Brit. Soc. Gastroenterol. Prev: Sen. Regist. Leeds.

RATHBONE, Elizabeth Ironbridge Medical Practice, Trinity Hall, Dale Road, Coalbrookdale, Telford TF8 7DT Tel: 01952 432568; 8 Station Road, Madeley, Telford TF7 5BA — MB BS Lond. 1976; MRCGP 1980.

RATHBONE, Gillian Valerie The Leicestershire Hospice, Groby Road, Leicester LE3 9QE Tel: 0116 231 3771 Fax: 0116 232 0312; Claremont House, 20 Nether Hall Lane, Birstall, Leicester LE4 4DT — MB BS Lond. 1979; MRCGP 1983; DRCOG 1984; Cert. FPA 1985. Cons. Phys. (Palliat. Med.) Leics. Hospice. Specialty: Palliat. Med. Prev: Med. Dir. Sye Ryder Hospice Staunton.

RATHBONE, Nia 39 North Street, Sandycroft, Deeside CH5 2PP — MB BCh Wales 1996.

RATHBONE, Philip Sean Long Clawson Medical Practice, The Surgery, The Sands, Melton Mowbray LE14 4PA; Ash Gables, 16 Scalford Road, Eastwell, Melton Mowbray LE14 4EJ — MB ChB Sheff. 1991; MRCGP 1996'; BMedSci Sheff. 1989.

RATHBONE, Richard George Elm Lodge Surgery, 2 Burbage Road, London SE24 9HJ Tel: 020 7274 6138 Fax: 020 7924 0710; 31 Hitherwood Drive, London SE19 1XA Tel: 020 8670 5806 — (King's Coll. Hosp.) MB BS Lond. 1961; MRCS Eng. LRCP Lond. 1961; DObst RCOG 1963; MRCGP 1975. Partially Retd. Prev: Med. Off. Baptist Miss. Soc.

RATHBORNE, Andrew Charles Springfield Surgery, Springfield Way, Brackley NN13 6JJ Tel: 01280 703431 Fax: 01280 703241 — MB BS Lond. 1993 (Roy. Free Hosp. Sch. Med.) DRCOG 1995; DCH RCP Lond. 1996; MRCGP 1997. GP Princip. Springfield Surg. Specialty: Gen. Pract.

RATHE, Mark Penketh Health Centre, Honiton Way, Penketh, Warrington WA5 2EY Tel: 01925 725644 Fax: 01925 791017; 3 Rawcliffe Close, Balmoral Park, Widnes WA8 9FZ — MB ChB Liverp. 1984; DRCOG 1987; Dip. Occ. Med. 1996. Specialty: Gen. Pract.

RATHER, Mr Ghualam Mohammed 19 Wordsworth Avenue, London E18 2HD — MB BS Jammu & Kashmir 1972; FRCS Glas. 1981; FRCS Ed. 1983.

RATHI, Ashok Kumar The Surgery, 5 Rupert Street, Biddulph, Stoke-on-Trent ST8 6EB Tel: 01782 514674 Fax: 01782 523044 — MB BS Jiwaji 1974; MB BS Jiwaji 1974.

RATHI, Rajendra Kumar Atkinson Health Centre, Market Street, Barrow-in-Furness LA14 2LR Tel: 01229 821030 Fax: 01229 827171 — MB BS Indore 1972. GP Barrow-in-Furness, Cumbria.

RATHMELL, Adrian John South Cleveland Hospital, Marton Road, Middlesbrough TS4 3BW Tel: 01642 850850 Fax: 01642 824877 — MB ChB Leeds 1981; MRCP (UK) 1984; FRCR 1989. Cons. Radiother. & Oncol. S. Cleveland Hosp. Middlesbrough. Specialty: Oncol.

RATHNAVARMA, Mr Chintalapati Venkata Rama c/o Drive L. Chandrasekaran, 6 Ashenden Road, Guildford GU2 7UU — MB BS Poona 1985; FRCS Glas. 1990.

RATHOD, Bhupendra Kumar Older Persons CMHT, Plank Lane, Leigh WN7 4QE — MB BS Jabalpur 1966 (Govt. Med. Coll.) BSc Jabalpur 1960, MB BS 1966; DPM Eng. 1972; FRCPsych 1992, M 1975. Cons. Psychiat. Leigh Infirm. Specialty: Gen. Psychiat.

RATHOD, Nehkant Hamermall (retired) Corsletts Farm, Broadbridge Heath, Horsham RH12 3LD Tel: 01403 60176 — MB BS Bombay 1948 (Grant Med. Coll.) DPM Lond. 1956; FRCP Lond. 1978, M 1963; FRCPsych 1973, M 1971. Cons. Psychiat. Cuckfield & Crawley Health Dist. Prev: Cons. to WHO.

RATHOD, Ramniklal Chimanlal 18 Quarry Park Road, Cheam, Sutton SM1 2DN — MB BS Gujarat 1970.

RATHOD, Shanaya — MB BS 1992 (Mahatma Ghandi Inst. of Med. Sci., India) MRCPsych Lond. 1998; Cert. in Health Servs. Managem., Inst. Of Health Care Managem. 2000. Specialist Regist. Psychiat., Moorgreen Hosp. Soton. Specialty: Gen. Psychiat. Socs: Roy. Coll. Psychiat.s. Prev: SpR. Psychiat., Pk.lands Hosp, Basingstoke; Lect./SpR, Roy. S. Hants Hosp., Soton.; SpR., Seymore Clinic, Swindon.

RATHOD, Sunil Lal Bramblys Grange Health Centre, Bramblys Drive, Basingstoke RG21 8UW Tel: 01256 467778 Fax: 01256 814190 — MB BS Saurashtra 1988.

RATHORE, Mr Chandra Kishore 6A Elm Park Road, London N3 1EB — MB BS Agra 1961 (S.N. Med. Coll.) MS Agra 1964, MB BS 1961; FRCS Ed. 1970; FICS 1971.

RATHORE, Jaswant Singh 2 Ploughmans Walk, Heathbrook Farm, Wall Heath, Kingswinford DY6 0DX — MB ChB Manch. 1980; DRCOG 1983; MRCGP (Distinc.) 1985.

RATHWELL, Claire Alison 13 Campion Close, Croydon CR0 5SN — MB BS Lond. 1992.

RATI, Naresh The Laurie Pike Health Centre, 95 Birchfield Road, Handsworth, Birmingham B19 1LH Tel: 0121 554 0621 Fax: 0121 554 6163 — MB ChB Manch. 1993. Specialty: Gen. Pract.

RATIB, Karim 56 Clarence Road, Kings Heath, Birmingham B13 9UH — MB ChB Birm. 1996; ChB Birm. 1996.

RATIP, Siret 34 Sutherland Avenue, London W9 2HQ — MB BS Lond. 1987.

RATLIFF, Mr Anthony Hugh Cyril (retired) 2 Clifton Park, Bristol BS8 3BS Tel: 0117 973 4500 Fax: 0117 973 0887; Esk House, 6 The Avenue, Sneyd Park, Bristol BS9 1PA Tel: 0117 968 3777 — MB ChB Manch. 1945; MB ChB (Distinc. Surg.) Manch. 1945; MRCS Eng. LRCP Lond. 1945; FRCS Eng. 1951; ChM Bristol 1968; FCPSP (Hon.) 1991. Special Lect. (Orthop. Surg.) Univ. Bristol. Prev: Cons. Orthop. Surg. Avon HA.

RATLIFF, Mr David Anthony Northampton General Hospital NHS Trust, Cliftonville, Northampton NN1 5BD Tel: 01604 634700 Fax: 01604 544312; 15 Mears Ashby Road, Earls Barton, Northampton NN6 0HQ Tel: 01604 812731 Fax: 01604 812731 — MB ChB Birm. 1977; MRCP (UK) 1980; FRCS Ed. 1982; FRCS Eng. 1982; MD Birm. 1985; FRCP 2001. Cons. Surg. (Gen. & Vasc. Surg.) Northampton Gen. Hosp. NHS Trust. Specialty: Gen. Surg. Socs: Vasc. Surg. Soc.; Assn. Surg.; Brit. Assn. Endocrine Surgs. Prev: Sen. Lect. & Hon. Cons. Surg. Leicester Roy. Infirm. & Univ. Leicester; Clin. Fell. (Vasc. Surg.) Univ. Brit. Columbia, Vancouver, Canada; Sen. Regist. (Gen. Surg.) W. Midl. RHA.

RATNAIKE, Mr Nimal Dushyantha Anthony Commonfield Road Surgery, 156 Commonfield Road, Woodchurch, Birkenhead CH49 7LP Tel: 0151 677 0016 — MB BS Lond. 1988 (St. Mary's) FRCS Eng. 1993; DFFP 1995; DRCOG 1995. Specialty: Gen. Pract. Prev: GP/Regist. Rugby VTS; SHO (O & G) Hosp. of St Cross Rugby.; SHO (Surg.) Medway Hosp. Gillingham.

RATNAKUMAR, Mr Kandiah 5 Abbotswood Gardens, Ilford IG5 0BG — MB BS Sri Lanka 1976; MRCS Eng. LRCP Lond. 1984; FRCS RCPS Glas. 1987.

RATNAKUMAR, Sarojinidevi 5 Abbotswood Gardens, Ilford IG5 0BG — MB BS Sri Lanka 1976.

RATNAM, Dharshini Sumitha John Howard Centre, 2 Crozier Terrace, Hackney, London E9 6AT Tel: 020 8919 8084 — MB BS Lond. 1992 (St Bartholomews Medical School) MRCPsych 1996. Specialist Regist. (Forens. Psychiat.), John Howard Centre. Specialty: Forens. Psychiat.

RATNARAJAH, Christine Rukma 1 Tarragon Way, Shoreham-by-Sea BN43 6JG — MB BS Sri Lanka 1974.

RATNARAJAH, Karunadevy 7 Elmer Close, Enfield EN2 7EZ Tel: 020 8364 4566 Fax: 020 8364 4566 — MB BS Peradeniya 1980; DA (UK) 1986; MRCS Eng. LRCP Lond. 1988. Clin. Asst., (A&E), Dept. (p/t); GP. Specialty: Gen. Pract.; Accid. & Emerg. Prev: SHO (O & G), Pediatrics, Psychiat.

RATNARAJAH, Mark Rauindran 55 Macmillan Way, Tooting Bec, London SW17 6AS — BM BCh Oxf. 1996.

RATNARAJAN, Nadarajan Woodlands Surgery, Woodlands Walk, Off Trafalgar Road, London SE10 9UB Tel: 020 8858 0689 Fax: 020 8293 9615 — MB BS Sri Lanka 1975; MRCS Eng LRCP Lond 1986.

RATNARAJAN, Subathira Thevy Woodlands Surgery, Woodlands Walk, Off Trafalgar Road, London SE10 9UB Tel: 020 8858 0689

Fax: 020 8293 9615 — MB BS Sri Lanka 1975; MRCS Eng LRCP Lond 1985.

RATNASABAPATHY, Lawrence 22 Elmcroft Avenue, London NW11 0RR Tel: 020 8449 5707 Fax: 020 8732 4617 — MB BS Ceylon 1966; DPM Eng. 1970; MRCPsych 1972. Cons. Psychiat. Barnet Gen. Hosp. & Napsbury Hosp. St. Albans; Hon. Cons. Lond. Hosp.; Clin. Tutor Univ. Lond.; Lead Clin. Barnet Healthcare Trust. Specialty: Gen. Psychiat.

RATNASABAPATHY, Urmila 8 Simpson Street, Crosshouse, Kilmarnock KA2 0BD — MB BCh BAO Belf. 1993.

RATNASINGAM, Latha 178 Queens Road, London SW19 8LX — MB BCh BAO NUI 1993.

RATNASINGHAM, Priyan 3 Beech Grove, Cliffsend, Ramsgate CT12 5LD — MB BS Lond. 1998; MB BS Lond 1998.

RATNATUNGA, Mr Chandana Premukh Department of Cardiothoracic Surgery, John Radcliffe Hospital, Headley Way, Oxford OX3 9DU Tel: 01865 220442 — MB BS Lond. 1980 (St Bartholomew's Hospital London) BSc Lond 1977; FRCS Ed. 1984; FRCS Eng. 1986; MS Lond. 1991; FRCS (Cth) 1994. Cons. Cardiothoracic Surg. John Radcliffe Hosp. Oxf.; Clin. Director, Cardiothoracic Surg., John Radcliffe Hosp., Oxf. Specialty: Cardiothoracic Surg. Special Interest: Aortic and Mitral valve Surgery.

RATNAVAL, Nandiran 20 Addison House, Grove End Road, London NW8 9EH — MB BS Lond. 1995.

RATNAVEL, Chenji Dakshinamurthi Flat 3, 29 New Walk, Beverley HU17 7DR — MB BS Madras 1982; LMSSA Lond. 1989.

RATNAVEL, Kathir Khanta 3 Molly Road, Jonesborough, Newry BT35 8HY — MRCS Eng. LRCP Lond. 1970 (Oxf.) DA Eng. 1973; FFA RCSI 1975; MA, MD Sri Lanka 1988. Cons. Anaesth. Our Lady's Hosp. Navan Eire. Specialty: Anaesth. Socs: Fell. Roy. Soc. Med.; Brit. Med. Acupunct. Soc.; Assn. Anaesth. Prev: Cons. Anaesth. Co. Hosp. Wexford Eire & St. Catherine's Co. Hosp. Tralee Eire; Regist. St. Bart. Hosp. Lond.

RATNAVEL, Rathini St. Philips Health Service, London School of Economics & Political Science, Sheffield St., London WC2 2AE Tel: 020 7955 7016 Fax: 020 7955 6818 — MB BS Lond. 1989 (UCL Hosps. Med. Sch.) BA Oxf. 1986; BA Oxf. 1986; DRCOG 1992; DRCOG 1992; MRCGP 1993; MRCGP 1993; DFFP 1993; DFFP 1993. Gen. Practitioner, St. Philips Med. Centre. Prev: Partner, Taylor Pract. Hornsey Rise 1994-1996; Trainee GP Edgware VTS.

RATNAVEL, Ravi Chandran Buckinghamshire Hospitals NHS Trust, Mandeville Road, Aylesbury HP21 8AL Tel: 01296 315551 Fax: 01296 315796 Email: ratnavel@talk21.com — MB BS Lond. 1988 (Oxford University UMDS (St Thomas' Campus)) BA 1985; MRCP (UK) 1991; DM Oxf. 1997; FRCP UK 2002. p/t Cons. (Dermatol.) Bucks. Hosps. NHS Trust; Hon. Cons. (Dermat.) Churchill Hosp. Oxf.; Hon. Assoc. Prof., Georgetown Univ.; Hon. Assoc. Teach., Univ. of Wales Med. Sch. Specialty: Dermat. Special Interest: Dermatopathology; Disorders of keratinization; Skin cancer. Socs: FRSM; Soc. Worshipful Apoth.; Brit. Assn. of Dermatol. Prev: Sen. Regist. St. John's Inst. of Dermat. Lond.; Hon. Sen. Regist. & MRC Train. Fell. Roy. Lond. Hosp. Med. Coll.; Regist. (Dermat.) Addenbrooke's Hosp. Camb.

RATNAVEL, Saravanamuttu (retired) 47 Grove Court, Grove End Road, London NW8 9EP — (Ceylon) MB BS Ceylon 1957; DA Eng. 1963; FFA RCS Eng. 1967. Prev: Cons. Anaesth. Rotherham & MexBoro. Gp. Hosps.

RATNAVEL, Thambipillai Upton Road Surgery, 30 Upton Road, Watford WD18 0JS Tel: 01923 226266 Fax: 01923 222324; 20 Langley Way, Watford WD17 3EQ Tel: 01923 225850 — MB BS Ceylon 1961; DIH Eng. 1970; DIH Soc. Apoth. Lond. 1970.

RATNAYAKA, Bethmage Dona Malkanthi Childrens Hospital, Uttoxeter Road, Derby DE22 3NE; 17 Foxbrook Close, Littleover, Derby DE23 3ZJ Tel: 01332 510502 — MB BS Colombo 1986; MRCP (UK) 1994; MMed Sc (Keele Univ.) 1999. Cons. Paediat. Children's Hosp. Derby. Specialty: Paediat. Socs: Roy. Coll. of Paediat.s. Prev: Specialist Regist. (Paediat.) Childr.s Hosp. Derby.

RATNAYAKE, Bernadette Chandrika Nilmini RTR Healthcare NHS Trust, Queen Marys University Hospital, Roehampton Lane, London SW15 5PN — MB BS Sri Lanka 1985; FRCA 1992.

RATNESWARAN, Mrs Dhiyaki Highfield Surgery, Jupiter Drive, Hemel Hempstead HP2 5NU; 10 Filmer Road, Leagrave, Luton LU4 9BX — MB BS Andra 1978; BA Madras 1970; DObst. RCPI 1988; Cert. Family Plann. JCC 1990. Specialty: Alcohol & Substance Misuse. Socs: Med. Protec. Soc. Prev: SHO (Psychiat.) Luton Hosp.; Trainee GP Hemel Hempstead; SHO (Paediat.) W. Herts. Hosp. Hemel Hempstead.

RATNESWAREN, Nageswary 32 Albyfield, Bickley, Bromley BR1 2HZ Tel: 020 8467 8453 — MB BS Colombo 1981; MRCS Eng. LRCP Lond. 1986; DRCOG 1988; DCH RCP Lond. 1989. SHO (Paediat. Med.) Edgware Gen. Hosp. Middlx. Prev: SHO (O & G) Edgware Gen. Hosp.; SHO (Geriat./Gen. Med.) Bedford Gen. Hosp.

RATNESWAREN, Suppiah The Surgery, 145 White Horse Hill, Chislehurst BR7 6DH Tel: 020 8857 4546 Fax: 020 8857 7778; 32 Albyfield, Bickley, Bromley BR1 2HZ Tel: 020 8295 1982 — MRCS Eng. LRCP Lond. 1978. Specialty: Gen. Pract. Socs: MRCGP; MRCP (UK). Prev: Regist. (Cardiol. & Chest Med.) Watford Gen. Hosp.; Regist. (Med., Diabetes, Endocrin., Gastroenterol. & Chest Med.) Roy. Infirm. Stirling.

RATOFF, Jonathan Charles 1 Brick Kiln Lane, Rufford, Ormskirk L40 1SY — MB BS Lond. 1994; MRCPI Dublin 1999. Clin. Research Fellow, King's Coll. Lond., 2001 -; SpR Respiratory & GM, South Thames Region, 1999 -.

RATRA, Surjan Singh Wolverhampton Health Care NHS Trust, Red Hill Street Clinic, Red Hill St., Wolverhampton WV1 1NR Tel: 01902 444325; White House, 559 Birmingham Road, Marlbrook, Bromsgrove B61 0HY Tel: 0121 445 1165 Fax: 0121 447 8363 — MB BS 1969 (S.N. Med. Coll.) BSc Agra 1963; MB BS Agra 1969; DPM Eng. 1979; Cert. Community Paediat. Warwick 1981. SCMO Wolverhampton HA; Sen. Med. Off. HMP Redditch. Specialty: Child & Adolesc. Psychiat.; Ment. Health; Community Child Health. Socs: MRCPCH; Fac. Comm. Health & Med.

RATSEY, David Hugh Kerr 2 Harley Street, London W1N 1AA Tel: 020 7589 2776 Fax: 020 7323 5743; 204 Raleigh House, Dolphin Square, London SW1V 3NP Tel: 020 7798 8800 — MB BS Lond. 1967 (St. Bart.) FFHom 1992, M 1980. Homoeop. Phys. Lond.; Cons. Homoeop. Phys. Kent & Sussex Weald NHS Trust. Specialty: Homeop. Med. Socs: BMA; Fell. Med. Soc. of Lond. Prev: Clin. Asst. Roy. Lond. Homoeop. Hosp.

RATTAN, Dapinder Singh Allum Medical Centre, Fairlop Road, Leytonstone, London E11 1BN Tel: 020 8539 2513 Fax: 020 8558 0525 — MRCS Eng. LRCP Lond. 1989.

RATTI, Bandna Moona 23 St Marks Road, Maidenhead SL6 6DG — MB ChB Liverp. 1993.

RATTI, Naveen 2 Siskin Green, Liverpool L25 4RY — MB ChB Liverp. 1990.

RATTIGAN, Siobhan Mary Ophthalmology Department, University Hospital Wales, Heath Park, Cardiff CF4 4XW; 4 Great Burnet Close, St Mellons, Cardiff CF3 0RJ — MB BCh BAO NUI 1989.

RATTNER, Gil Jonathan c/o Thorpe Health Centre, St. Williams Way, Thorpe St Andrew, Norwich NR7 0AJ Tel: 01603 701010 Fax: 01603 701942 Email: alambert@gtnet.gov.uk — MB ChB Glas. 1987; BSc (Hons.) St. And. 1983. GP Principal; Clin. Asst. in ENT Cromer Hosp. Specialty: Otorhinolaryngol. Special Interest: Diabetes; ENT.

RAU, Donald (retired) 29 Downside Crescent, London NW3 2AN Tel: 020 7794 3636 Fax: 01793 750800 — (Westm.) MB BS Lond. 1960.

RAU, Udipi Badri Narayana Trent Meadows Medical Centre, 87 Wood Street, Burton-on-Trent DE14 3AA Tel: 01283 845555 Fax: 01283 845222; Anand, Craythorne Road, Stretton, Burton-on-Trent DE13 0AZ Tel: 01283 564168 — (Madras Med. Coll.) MB BS Madras 1966; DLO Madras 1968; DLO Eng. 1973. GP Burton-on-Trent. Prev: Clin. Asst. (ENT) Dist. Hosp. Burton on Trent & Roy. Infirm. Derby.

RAUBITSCHEK, Eugene The Surgery, 103 Main Street, Addingham, Ilkley LS29 0PD Tel: 01943 830367 Fax: 01943 831287 — (Manch.) MB ChB Manch. 1965; DMRT Eng. 1969. Clin. Asst., Gastroenterol., Chemother. Specialty: Gastroenterol. Socs: Roy. Soc. Med.

RAUCHENBERG, Peter Michael The Caludon Centre, Walsgrave General Hospital, Clifford Bridge Road, Coventry CV2 2TE Tel: 024 76 602266 Fax: 024 76 538920 — MRCS Eng. LRCP Lond. 1971 (Prague & Oxf.) MRCPsych 1975. Cons. Psychiat. The Caludon Centre Coventry. Specialty: Gen. Psychiat. Prev: Cons. Psychiat. Highcroft Hosp. Birm.; Sen. Regist. (Psychiat.) Birm. AHA; Hon. Clin. Lect. (Psychiat.) Birm. Univ.

RAUDNITZ, Leslie Camill Bradley The Chestnuts, Green End Road, Boxmoor, Hemel Hempstead HP1 1 — MB BS Lond. 1970; MA Camb. 1964; MRCS Eng. LRCP Lond. 1966.

RAUF, Mr Abdul Ophthalmology Department, Queens Hospital, Belvedere Road, Burton-on-Trent DE13 0RB Tel: 01283 566333 Ext: 5260 Email: raufa@doctors.org.uk; Garden Cottage, Newton Road, Burton-on-Trent DE15 0TF — MB BS Lond. 1983 (Roy. Free Hosp. Sch. Med.) FRCS Glas. 1990; FRCOphth 1991. Cons. Ophth., Qu.'s Hosp., Burton-Upon-Trent. Specialty: Ophth. Socs: Brit. Med. assoc.; Roy. Coll. Ophth.; Roy. Soc. of Med. Prev: 1996-1999 Specialist Regist. And Fell. at Moorfields Eye Hosp., Lond.

RAUF, Abdul Healey Surgery, Whitworth Road, Rochdale OL12 0SN — MB BS Sind 1964.

RAUF, Mr Khawaja Gulraiz Lenham, Maybury Hill, Woking GU22 8AL — MB BS Punjab 1982; FRCS Eng. 1988.

RAUH, Peter Braxton Chinthurst Lodge, Wonersh, Guildford GU5 0PH Tel: 01483 458317 — MB BS Lond. 1992 (St Georges) MSc Biochem. Endocrinol. Sussex 1986; FRCS Lond. 1996. Specialist Regist. (Orthop.) S.W. Thames. Specialty: Trauma & Orthop. Surg. Socs: Soc. for the Relief of Widows and Orphans of Med. Men.

RAULT, John Peter Richard 32 Balfour Road, Bromley BR2 9SL — MB BS Lond. 1986; Cert. Family Plann. JCC 1990; MRCGP 1991.

RAUNIAR, Arun Kumar 19 Leicester Close, Ipswich IP2 9EX — MB BS Calcutta 1978.

RAUT, Rajeev 10 Allderidge Avenue, Hull HU5 4EQ — MB ChB Dundee 1989.

RAUT, Suresh Laxman 21 Colebourne Road, Birmingham B13 0EZ Tel: 0121 65746 — MB BS Bombay 1979; PhD Lond. 1971; MSc Bombay 1966, BSc (Hons.) 1963, MB BS 1979; LMSSA 1982. Specialty: Gen. Pract.

RAUT, Mr Videshnandan Vijayanand Centre for Hip Surgery, Wrightington Hospital, Hall Lane, Appley Bridge, Wigan WN6 9EP Tel: 01257 256304; Foxgloves, Wood Lane, Parbold, Wigan WN8 7TH — MB BS Bombay 1980; MS (Orthop.) Bombay 1984; DNBOrth. New Delhi 1985; MChOrth. Liverp. 1992; FRCS (Orth.) Ed. 1996. Cons. Orthop. Surg. Wrightington Hosp. & Chorley Hosp. Lancs. Specialty: Orthop. Special Interest: Arthroscopic Knee Surg.; Primary & Revision Hips & Knees. Socs: Brit. Hip Soc. Prev: Sen. Orthop. Regist. Birm. Rotat.; Sen. Surg. Fell. (Revision Surg.) Wrightington Hosp.

RAUT, Mr Vivek Vijayanand 12 Calnewood Road, Luton LU4 0ET — MB BS Bombay 1986; FRCSI 1996.

RAUTRAY, Ramesh Chandra Primrose Bank Medical Centre, Blackburn BB1 5ER Tel: 01254 672132 Fax: 01254 699189; Utkalika, Park Crescent, Blackburn BB2 6DQ Tel: 01254 672132 Fax: 01254 672132 — MB BS Utkal 1970 (S.C.B. Med. Coll. Cuttack) MD Patna 1971; Hon. Fell. Internat. Coll. Angiol. 1977; Cert. Family Plann. JCC 1981; Dip. Acupunc. Liverp. 1983; Dip. Ven. Apoth. Lond. 1985; DCH RCP Lond. 1985; Dip. Pract. Dermat. Wales 1992; DFFP 1993; DRCOG 1993. Clin. Asst. (Med.) Blackburn Roy. Infirm. Specialty: Pharmacology. Socs: Overseas Doctors Assn. (Sec. Blackburn Div.); (Chairm.) BMA; Indian Med. Assn. Prev: Regist. (Med.) Monklands Dist. Gen. Hosp. Airdrie; Regist. (Med.) Leicester Gen. Hosp.; SHO (Gen. & Geriat. Med.) Isebrook Hosp. WellingBoro.

RAUTRAY, Reena Primrose Bank Medical Centre, Blackburn BB1 5ER — MB BS Utkal 1971.

RAUZ, Saaeha Academic Unit of Ophthalmology, Division of Immunity and Infection, University of Birmingham, Birmingham & Midland Eye Centre, City Hospital, Dudley Road, Birmingham B18 7QU Email: s.rauz@bham.ac.uk — MB BS Lond. 1990 (UMDS Guy's & St. Thos. Hosps. Lond.) FRCOphth 1995; PhD 2002. Sen. Lect. (Ophthalmology) The Univ. of Birm.; Cons. (Ophth.) Birm. and Midl. Eye Centre. Specialty: Ophth. Prev: Corneal and Extern. Dis. Fell. Moorfields Eye Hosp. Lond.; Med. Research Counc. Clin. Fell. (Ophthalmology) The Univ. of Birm.; Clin. Lect. (Ophthalmology), The Univ. of Birm.

RAVAGO, Eranio 467 Kingston Road, Epsom Ewell, Epsom KT19 0DJ — MD Far East. Univ. Philippines 1970. Staff Grade (Anaesth.) Epsom Health Care & Trust. Specialty: Anaesth.

RAVAL, Jayantkumar Kantilal Walderslade Village Surgery, 62A Robin Hood Lane, Walderslade, Chatham ME5 9LD Tel: 01634 687250; 12 Fernbank Close, Chatham ME5 9NH Tel: 01634 865232 — MB BS Bombay 1972.

RAVAL, Mark Mukund The Surgery, 24 Broadwater Road, Worthing BN14 8AB Tel: 01903 231701 — BM Soton. 1986.

RAVAL, Pradyumna Bhuralal Stonecross Surgery, 25 Street End Road, Chatham ME5 0AA Tel: 01634 842334 — (M.G.M. Med. Coll.) MB BS Indore 1966; MRCS Eng. LRCP Lond. 1974. GP Princip. Socs: MPS; BMA.

RAVAL, Veena Pradyumna Blue Bell Hill Village, 82 Common Road, Chatham ME5 9RG Tel: 01634 670630 — (M.G.M. Med. Coll.) MB BS Indore 1966; DRCOG 1974; MRCS Eng. LRCP Lond. 1975; DCCH 1983; MFCH 1989. SCMO Community Child Health Dept. Kent. Specialty: Audiol. Med. Socs: Fac. Comm. Health.

RAVALIA, Abdulsatar Department of Anaesthesia, Kingston Hospital, Kingston upon Thames KT2 7QB Tel: 020 8546 7711; 69 Bodley Road, New Malden KT3 5QJ Tel: 020 8949 1268 — MB ChB Zimbabwe 1978; FFA RCS Eng. 1986. Cons. Anaesth. Kingston NHS Trust. Specialty: Anaesth. Socs: MDUn & Intens. Care Soc. Prev: Cons. Anaesth. Walsgrave Hosp. Coventry; Sen. Regist. (Anaesth.) Middlx. Hosp. Lond.; SHO (Anaesth.) Harari Zimbabwe.

RAVAT, Farhana Esmail 7 Greenhead Avenue, Little Harwood, Blackburn BB1 5PR — MB BS Lond. 1996.

RAVAT, Sangita Wigston Central Surgery, 48 Leicester Road, Wigston LE18 1DR — MB ChB Glas. 1990; MRCGP 1994.

RAVEENTHIRANATHAN, Chandraprabha 14 Thorndene, Elderslie, Johnstone PA5 9DA — MB BS Ceylon 1972; DObst RCOG 1975; LRCP LRCS Ed. LRCPS Glas. 1975. Clin. Med. Off. Forth Valley Health Bd. Prev: Clin. Med. Off. Gtr. Glas. Health Bd.; Regist. (O & G) Falkirk & Dist. Roy. Infirm.; Regist. (O & G) Rankin Memor. Hosp. Greenock.

RAVEN, Peter William Dept. of Mental Health Sciences, Royal Free & Univ. Coll. Medical School, UCL Royal Free Campus, Rowland Hill St., London NW3 2PF Tel: 0207 830 2280 — MB BS Lond. 1985 (St. Bartholomews Hospital Medical College) PhD(Endocrinology), Lond. 1983, BSc (Hons. Biochem.) 1979; MRCP (UK) 1989; MRCPsych 1992. Sen. Lect. Psychiat. Hon. Cons. Psychiat. UCL, Lond. Specialty: Gen. Psychiat. Prev: Regist. (Psychiat.) Bethlem Roy. & Maudsley Hosp. Lond.; Hon. Sen. Regist. (Psychiat.) Bethlem Roy. & Maudsley Hosp. Lond.; Lect. (Affective Disorders) Inst. Psychiat. Lond.

RAVEN, Sarah Clare Perch Hill Farm, Brightling, Robertsbridge TN32 5HP — MB BS Lond. 1992.

RAVENSCROFT, Andrew John FLat 4, Ashfield House, 8 Grove Road, Leeds LS6 2EQ — MB ChB Leeds 1988; DA (UK) 1991.

RAVENSCROFT, Jane Catherine Queens Medical Centre, Castle Boulevard, Nottingham NG7 2UH — MB ChB Leeds 1988; MRCGP; MRCP (UK) 1991. p/t Cons. Dermatol. Queens Med. Centre Nottm.; Cons. Dermatol. Kings Mill Hosp. Mansfield. Specialty: Dermat. Special Interest: Paediatric Dermat. Socs: British Association of Dermatologists; British Association of Paediatric Dermatologists. Prev: Trainee GP Leeds VTS.; Regist. (Dermat.) Leeds. Gen. Infirm. Leeds.

RAVENSCROFT, Peter James Directorate of Anaesthesia, Taunton & Somerset Hospital, Musgrove Park, Taunton TA1 5DH Tel: 01823 342 114 Fax: 01823 342 526 Email: peter.ravenscroft@tst.nhs.uk — MB BS Lond. 1974 (St Bart.) MRCS Eng. LRCP Lond. 1974; LMSSA Lond. 1974; DRCOG 1978; FRCA Eng. 1979. Cons. Anaesth. Taunton & Som. NHS Trust; Cons. Anaest. StapleGr. Anast. Gp. Specialty: Anaesth.; Intens. Care. Socs: Assn. Anaesth. Gt. Brit. & Irel.; W. Som. Med. Club Treas.; Local Negotiating Comm. Chairm. Prev: Cons. Anaesth. Som. HA; Sen. Regist. Nuffield Dept. Anaesth. Oxf. & Wycombe HAs; Regist. (Anaesth.) Centr.lasarettet Vasterás Sweden.

RAVENSCROFT, Sarah Jane Kingley Cottage, 6 Downs Road, West Stoke, Chichester PO18 9BH — MB BS Lond. 1996.

RAVETTO, Marc Peter Celestine 88 Greenside Road, Croydon CR0 3PN Tel: 020 8240 0072/020 8240 0074 Email: marc.ravetto@gp-h83631.nhs.uk — MB BS Lond. 1991; DRCOG 1994; MRCGP 1996. GP Princip.

RAVETTO, Savino 42 Graham Road, Mitcham CR4 2HA Tel: 020 8648 2432 Fax: 020 8646 8249; 57 All Saints Road, Sutton SM1 3DQ Tel: 020 8644 1974 — (Univ. Coll. Hosp.) MB BS Lond. 1957; MRCS Eng. LRCP Lond. 1957. Prev: Regist. (Med.) E. Birm.

Hosp.; Ho. Phys. St. Jas. Hosp. Balham; Ho. Surg. (O & G) Nelson Hosp. Merton.

RAVEY, Moira 29 Menlove Mansions, Menlove Gardens W., Woolton, Liverpool L18 2HY — MB ChB Liverp. 1961; DPM Eng. 1966; MRCPsych 1972. Cons. Psychitrist. Specialty: Gen. Psychiat. Socs: MHRI. Prev: Cons. Psychiat. Whiston Hosp.

RAVI, Asha New Street Health Centre, Upper New Street, Barnsley S70 1LP Tel: 01226 730000 Email: asharavi@doctors.org.uk — MB BS Nagpur 1979; MD (Gen. Med.) Nagpur Univ. 1982; MRCPI 1990; Dip. Community Child Health, Sheffield University 1992; M.Med,sc Leeds Univ. 1998. Cons.Paediat. (Community) Barnsley Communjity & Priority Serv.s (NHS) Trust, Barnsley. Specialty: Community Child Health. Socs: Roy. Coll. of Paediat. & Clin. Health (Fell.); Brit. Paediatric Neurol. Assn.; Brit. Assn. of Community Child Health. Prev: Clin. Med. Off. (Child Health) Pontefract Gen. Infirm.; Regist. & SHO (Paediat.) Barnsley Dist. Gen. Hosp.; Sen. Regist. (Community Paediat.) Leeds Community & Ment. Health Trust Leeds.

RAVI, Kambhammettu West Leeds Medical Practice, 289 Lower Wortley Place, Lower Wortley, Leeds LS12 4PZ Tel: 0113 279 9190 Fax: 0113 279 9204 — MB BS Andhra 1972. Medico Legal Servs. to Solicitors; Police Surg. Leeds & Bradford Cities. Specialty: Forens. Psychiat. Socs: Fell. Roy. Soc. Med.; Amer. Acad. Forens. Scis.; Assn. Police Surg.

RAVI, Mr Ramachandran Darent Valley Hospital, Dartford DA2 8DA Tel: 01322 428612 Fax: 01322 428779 — MB BS New Delhi 1980 (All India Inst. of Med. Sci., New Delhi, India) FEBU; MCh; MS; FRCS Glas.; FRCS Edin.; FRCS (Urol). Cons. Urol., Darent Valley Hosp., Dartford. Specialty: Urol. Socs: Brit. Assn. of Urological Surgeons; BMA.

RAVI, Mr Srinivasan Blackpool Victoria Hospital, Blackpool FY3 8BD Tel: 01253 300000; Baliyeur, The Oaks, Poulton-le-Fylde FY6 7HG — MB BS Mysore 1977; MS (Gen. Surg.) Madras 1979; FRCS Ed. 1982; FRCS (Eng.) 1996. Cons. Gen. Surg. Blackpool Vict. Hosp.; Surgic. Tutor - Roy. Coll. of Surg.s. Specialty: Gen. Surg. Socs: Assn. of Surg.s of Eng.; Assn. of ColoProctol.; Assn. of Endoscopic Surg.s. Prev: Sen. Regist. Leicester Roy. Infirm.; Regist. Lincoln Co. Hosp.; Regist. Newham & St. And. Hosp. Lond.

RAVI, Swaminathan Cope Street Surgery, 2a Cope St, Barnsley S70 4HY Tel: 01226 244476 Fax: 01226 767349 — MB BS Madras 1974; MRCP UIC; DA. GP Barnsley, S. Yorks.

RAVICHANDRAN, Mr Duraisamy Luton & Dunstable Hospital, Lewsey Road, Luton LU4 0DZ — MB BS Colombo 1986; FRCS Eng. 1991; PhD Univ. Of Soton. 1999. Specialty: Gen. Surg. Prev: Regist. (Surg.)Addenbrooke's Hosp. Camb.

RAVICHANDRAN, Mr Ganapathiraju Princess Royal Spinal Injuries Unit, Osborn Building, Northern General Hospital, Sheffield S5 7AU Tel: 0114 271 5647 Fax: 0114 271 5649 Email: ravichandran@btinternet.com — MB BS Madras 1972 (Jawaharlal Inst. Postgrad. Med. Pondicherry) BSc Annamalai 1964; FRCS Ed. 1976; T(S) 1994. Cons. Spinal Injuries Osborn Bldg., N. Gen. Hosp. Specialty: Orthop.; Rehabil. Med. Socs: Internat. Med. Soc. Paraplegia; Eur. Tissue Repair Soc.; Brit. Soc. Rehab.Med. (BSRM). Prev: Cons. Spinal Injuries Lodge Moor Hosp.; Sen. Regist. (Spinal Injuries) Stoke Mandeville Hosp. Aylesbury; Back Research Fell. Harlow Wood Orthop. Hosp. Mansfield.

RAVICHANDRAN, Subbiah Sadhashivan 6 Woodbridge Road, Newcastle ST5 4LA — MB BS Madras 1986.

RAVIKUMAR, Mr Aloor 9 Fenton Place, Monifieth, Dundee DD5 4SE Tel: 01382 534000 — MB BS Osmania 1979; FRCS Glas. 1989. Regist. (Orthop. & Trauma) Law Hosp. Lanarksh. Specialty: Orthop. Prev: SHO (Surg. & Urol.) Southlands Hosp. Sussex; SHO (Surg. & Orthop.) Worthing Hosps. Sussex; SHO (Orthop.) St. Jas. Hosp. Lond.

RAVIKUMAR, Ratukondla 50A Anmersh Grove, Stanmore HA7 1PA — MB BS Madras 1980.

RAVIKUMAR, Velupillai 67 Welbeck Road, Harrow HA2 0RU — LMSSA Lond. 1995.

RAVINDRA KUMAR, Kedia Leighton Hospital, Midcheshire Hospital NHS Trust, Middlewich Road, Crewe CW1 4QJ Tel: 01270 612419 Fax: 01270 612449 Email: ravindra.kedia@mcht.nhs.uk — MB BS GSVM Med. Coll. Kanpur India 1981; FRCP. Cons. Phys. Gen. & Respirat. Med. Leighton Hosp. Crewe; Coll. Tutor Roy. Coll. of Physicians Lond.; Mem. of BTS, ATS, ERS, Norwich Med. Soc. Specialty: Respirat. Med.; Cardiol. Special Interest: Asthma; Lung Cancer; Occupational Lung Diseases. Socs: Brit. Thoracic Soc.; Amer. Thoracic Soc.; Europ. Respirat. Soc. Prev: Regist. (Gen. & Respirat. Med.)\; N. E. Med. Rotat. Freeman Hosp. Newc.

RAVINDRA NATH, Arepalli Accident & Emergency Department, County Hospital, Louth LN11 0EU Tel: 01507 600100; 6 Blue Stone Rise, Louth LN11 9XZ Tel: 01507 609037 — MB BS Andhra 1975; MS Delhi 1980. Staff Grade A & E Co. Hosp. Louth. Specialty: Accid. & Emerg. Socs: BMA.

RAVINDRABABU, Gottipati 61 Hagley Road W., Birmingham B17 8AE — MB BS Karnatak 1972.

RAVINDRAN, Anchery Health Centre, Welbeck St., Castleford WF10 1DP Tel: 01977 552041 Fax: 01977 519342; 6 Manor Garth, Ledsham, South Milford, Leeds LS25 5LZ Tel: 01977 682876 Fax: 01977 685970 — (Madras) MB BS Madras 1953; BSc Madras 1953. Hosp. Pract. (Thoracic. Med.) Gen. Infirm. Pontefract. Specialty: Accid. & Emerg. Socs: Fell. Roy. Soc. Med.; BMA, RSM & RCGP. Prev: Regist. (Med.) Roy. Infirm. Halifax; SHO Warrington Infirm.; Ho. Phys. Gen. Hosp. Dewsbury.

RAVINDRAN, Arumugavadivelu 54 Bursland Road, Enfield EN3 7EX Tel: 020 8804 6186 — MB BS Ceylon 1971. SHO Psychiat. Unit Northwick Pk. Hosp. Harrow.

RAVINDRAN, Thambar Sabaratnam Ravindran, East Park Medical Practice, Jonesfield Crescent, Wolverhampton WV1 2LW Tel: 01902 455422 Fax: 01902 454131; Longwood, 26 Wergs Road, Tettenhall, Wolverhampton WV6 8TD Tel: 01902 579228 — MB BS Sri Lanka 1973; MRCS Eng. LRCP Lond. 1979; MRCP (UK) 1981; MRCGP 1983; DCH RCP Lond. 1990; MSc (Dermat.) Oxf. 1995; FRCP (UK) 1998. Clin. Asst. (Dermat.) Wolverhampton & Dudley. Specialty: Dermat.

RAVINE, David Medical Genetics Service for Wales, University Hospital of Wales, Heath Park, Cardiff CF14 4XW Tel: 029 2074 5008 Fax: 029 2074 7603 — MB BS Western Australia 1980 (University Western Australia) BMedSc (Hons.) 1980; FRACP 1990; MS Melbourne 1994; DRCPath 1998; MRCP 2000. Cons. Molecular Genetic Med. (Med. Genetics & Med. Biochem.ry) Univ. Hosp. Wales Cardiff. Specialty: Genetics; Paediat. Socs: Brit. Soc. Human Genetics; Amer. Soc. Human Genetics; Human Genet. Soc. of Austral.

RAVISEKAR, Mr Oduru West Suffolk General Hospital, Hardwick Lane, Bury St Edmunds IP33 2QZ — MB BS Madras 1977; FRCSI 1991. Specialty: Gen. Surg.

RAVISHANKAR, Guhendran St James Medical Centre, 189A St James Road, Croydon CR0 2BZ — MB BS Madras 1979; DMedRehab RCP Lond. 1984; LRCP LRCS Ed., LRCPS Glas. 1987.

RAVISHANKAR, Mr Ramachandran Royal Oldham Hospital, Rochdae Road, Oldham OL1 2JH Tel: 0161 624 0420 Fax: 0161 627 8497 Email: rshankar_orth@hotmail.com; 14 Spring Bank Lane, Bamford, Rochdale OL11 5SF Tel: 01706 356944 Fax: 01706 356944 — MB BS Mysore 1981 (Mysore Med. Coll., India) DOrth Madras 1983; MS (Orth) Madras 1985; MChOrth Liverp. 1994. Assoc. Specialist (Orthop.) Roy. Oldham Hosp. Specialty: Orthop. Socs: Brit. Orthop. Assn.; Internat.l Affil. Mem.; Amer. Acad. of Orthopaedic Surg.s. Prev: Sen. Regist. (Orthop.) Bradford Roy. Infirm.; Regist. (Orthop.) Russells Hall Hosp. Dudley, Corbett Hosp. Stourbridge, Alder Hey Childr. Hosp. Liverp. & Roy. Albert Edwd. Infirm. Wigan.

RAW, Anthony John Askham, RD Farnham Health Centre, East Street, Farnham GU9 7SA Tel: 01252 723122 Fax: 01252 728302; Ridgewood House, Highlands Close, Farnham GU9 8SP — MB BS Lond. 1968 (Westm.) MRCS Eng. LRCP Lond. 1968. Prev: Ho. Surg. Westm. Hosp. Lond.; Ho. Phys. Soton. Gen. Hosp.

RAW, David Stuart Sunnyside Doctors Surgery, 150 Fratton Road, Portsmouth PO1 5DH Tel: 023 9282 4725 Fax: 023 9286 1014 Email: david.raw@gp-j80209.nhs.uk; 16 St. Edwards Road, Southsea PO5 3DJ Tel: 023 92 731481 — MB BS Lond. 1973 (St. Mary's) MRCS Eng. LRCP Lond. 1973; DObst RCOG 1975; DCH Eng. 1976; FRCGP 1996; MA Portsmouth Univ. 1998. GP; Assoc. Sen. Lect. Sch. of Postgrad. Med. Portsmouth Univ. Prev: Trainee GP Bristol; SHO (Psychiat.) Barrow Hosp.; SHO (A & E) Bristol Roy. Infirm.

RAW, Jason Michael Royal Bolton Hospital, Farnworth, Bolton BL4 0JR — MB ChB Dundee 1997.

RAWAL, Bandhana Kumari Medical Department, Glaxo Wellcome UK Ltd., Stockley Park W., Uxbridge UB11 1BT — MB BS Lond. 1985; MSc (Distinc.) Lond. 1989, BSc (1st cl. Hons.) 1982; MRCPath 1992. Sen. Med. Adviser Glaxo plc Uxbridge. Specialty: Pharmaceutical Medicine. Prev: Clin. Research Fell. (Virol.) St. Geo. Hosp. Lond.

RAWAL, Jewan Lal 39 Nelmes Crescent, Hornchurch RM11 2PX Tel: 01708 621179 Fax: 01708 782308 Email: jeewarnl @hotmail.com — MB BS Delhi 1975; MRCPI; MRCPCH; MD. Cons. Pediatrician; Med. Dir. Specialty: Paediat.; Neonat. Socs: RCDH; BMA.

RAWAL, Krishna Mark, Surg. Lt.-Cdr. RN 52 Guildown Road, Guildford GU2 4EY Tel: 01483 538560 — MB BS Lond. 1990 (GUYs Hosp. Med. School) Dip RHC Aberdeen Nov 1993. Med. Off., Roy. Navy. Prev: Med. Off. RN; SHO (A & E) Poole Hosp. Trust Dorset; Med. Off. Brit. Antarctic Survey.

RAWAL, Parmjit 110 Bakers Lane, Sutton Coldfield B74 2BA — MB ChB Leeds 1997.

RAWAL, Ram Swarup (retired) 31 Riffel Road, London NW2 4PB Tel: 020 8450 7455 Mob: 07956 971907 Fax: 020 8450 1353 Email: rsrawal@yahoo.com; 31 Riffel Road, London NW2 4PB Tel: 020 8452 7455 Mob: 07956 971907 Fax: 020 8450 1353 Email: rsrawal@yahoo.com — MB BS Lucknow 1954 (King Geo. Med. Coll. Lucknow) LCPS Bombay 1951; Lucknow 1954; MD Anaesth. Panjab 1958; DA Eng. 1966; Dip. Ven. Liverp. 1971; MFHom Lond. 1972. Prev: Cons. Anaesth. N.W. Metrop. Bd. Hosp. & Wembley Hosp.

RAWAL, Miss Shashi Bala 'Bow Green', Prestbury Road, Wilmslow SK9 2LL — MB BS Delhi 1972 (Lady Hardinge Med. Coll.) DObst RCOG 1974; DA Eng. 1976; FFA RCSI 1977. Cons. Anaesth. Macclesfield Dist. Chesh. Specialty: Anaesth. Socs: BMA & Assn. Anaesth. Gt. Brit. & Irel. Prev: Cons. Anaesth. Qu. Eliz. Hosp. Barbados, W. Indies; Sen. Regist. Yorks. RHA.

RAWBONE, Roger Geoffrey Health & Safety Executive, Magdalen House, Stanley Precinct, Bootle L20 3QZ Tel: 0151 951 4555 Fax: 0151 951 3180 Email: roger.rawbone@hse.gsi.gov.uk; 38 South Parade, Bramhall, Stockport SK7 3BJ — MB BS Lond. 1969 (Char. Cross) MRCS Eng. LRCP Lond. 1969; MD Lond. 1995; MA Manc. 2001; FFOM (Hon.) 2001. Head of the Med. Unit Health & Safety Exec. Bootle. Specialty: Occupat. Health. Prev: Sen. Manager R & D/Occupat. Health Servs. Gallaher Ltd.; Research Fell. Cardiopulm. Laborats. Dept. of Med. Char Cross Hosp. Med. Sch. Lond.; Cons. Adviser to Nat. Childr. Bureau.

RAWCLIFFE, Debra Samantha Honley Surgery, Marsh Gardens, Honley, Huddersfield HD9 6AG Tel: 01484 303366 Fax: 01484 303365 — MB ChB Leeds 1987.

RAWCLIFFE, Jacqueline Anne The Health Centre, Bailey Street, Old Basford, Nottingham NG6 0HD Tel: 0115 978 1231 Fax: 0115 979 0419; 18 Villiers Road, West Bridgford, Nottingham NG2 6FR Tel: 0115 923 2560 — MB ChB Manch. 1988; DCH RCP Lond. 1991; DRCOG 1992; MRCGP 1993.

RAWCLIFFE, John Francis Xavier 10 Downs Avenue, Dartford DA1 1SU — MB BS Lond. 1983.

RAWCLIFFE, Peter Morgan Botley Medical Centre, Elms Road, Botley, Oxford OX2 9JS Tel: 01865 248719 Fax: 01865 728116 — MB Camb. 1974 (Lond. Hosp.) MA Camb. 1970, MB 1974, BChir 1973. GP Oxf. Prev: MRC Research Fell. Gastroenterol. Unit Radcliffe Infirm. Oxf.; Coeliac Trust Research Fell. & Hon. Regist. Nuffield Dept. Clin. Med. Radcliffe Infirm. Oxf.; SHO (Gastroenterol.) Hammersmith Hosp. Lond.

RAWCLIFFE, Philip John 6 Wellington Road, Ombersley, Droitwich WR9 0DZ — MB ChB Liverp. 1974.

RAWDEN, Alison Margaret Birchwood Medical Practice, Jasmin Road, Lincoln LN6 0QQ Tel: 01522 501111; Rustaley, Fen Lane, Owmby-by-Spital, Market Rasen LN8 2HP — MB ChB Leic. 1990; MRCGP 1994.

RAWDON, Catherine Mary Riverside Practice, Upper Main Street, Strabane BT82 8AS — MB BCh BAO NUI 1978; MRCGP 1984.

RAWDON SMITH, Henry Stewart Russets, 9c Irving Burgess Close, Whittlesey, Peterborough PE7 1QB Tel: 01733 206664 — (Middlx.) MB BS Lond. 1959; DObst RCOG 1964. Prev: GP Newton Abbot.

RAWEILY, Essam Aldin Awad Epsom General Hospital, Dorking Road, Epsom KT18 7EG; 19 De Burgh Gardens, Tadworth KT20 5LU Fax: 07092 261960 Email: essam.raweily@doctors.org.uk — MB BS Jordan 1987; MRCPath 1991; FRCPath 2000. Cons. Histopath./Cytopath. Epsom & St Helier NHS Trust; Cons. Path. Shirley Oaks Hosp. Croydon; Cons. Path. Ashtead Hosp. Specialty: Pathology, General. Special Interest: Cytopathology; Dermatopathology. Socs: Internat. Acad. Path.; Assn. Clin. Path.; Brit. Soc. Dermatopath. Prev: Cons. Path. Mayday Hosp. Croydon; Assoc. Prof. Jordan Univ. Sci. & Technol.

RAWES, Geoffrey Douglas Dr Geoff Rawes Surgery, The Harbour Suite, Blyth Hospital, Blyth NE24 1DX Tel: 01670 396550 Fax: 01670 396556; 1 Holywell Avenue, Whitley Bay NE26 3AH Tel: 0191 252 5728 — MB BS Newc. 1968; DObst RCOG 1970; MRCGP 1974. Specialty: Occupat. Health.

RAWES, James Charteris Lea (retired) Falcons, Little Easton, Dunmow CM6 2JH Tel: 01371 872640 — MB BChir Camb. 1954 (St. Thos.) DObst RCOG 1959; DCH Eng. 1960. Prev: GP Dunmow. Essex.

RAWES, Mr Malcolm Lindsay Department of Orthopaedic Surgery, Pinderfields General Hospital, Aberford Road, Wakefield WF1 4DG Tel: 01924 212546 Fax: 01924 212614 — MB ChB Leeds 1986 (Univ. Leeds) BSc (Hons.) Leeds 1983; FRCS Eng. 1990; MCh (Orth.) Liverp. 1995; FRCS (Orth.) 1996. Cons. Orthop. Surg. Pinderfield Gen. Hosp. Aberford Rd. Wakefield W. Yorks.; Hon. Sen. Lect., Univ. of Leeds. Specialty: Orthop.; Trauma & Orthop. Surg.; Medico Legal. Socs: Brit. Orthop. Research Soc.; Brit. Trauma Soc.; Fell. BOA. Prev: Lect. (Clin.) & Hon. Sen. Regist. Univ. Liverp.; Career Regist. Rotat. (Orthop.) Leicester & Lincoln Train. Scheme; Tutor (Surg.) Gen. Infirm. Leeds.

RAWLE, Michael Stirling Mill Bank Surgery, Water Street, Stafford ST16 2AG Tel: 01785 258348 Fax: 01785 227144; 16 White Oaks, Wildwood, Stafford ST17 4SL — MB BS Lond. 1977 (St. Mary's) MRCS Eng. LRCP Lond. 1976. Clin. Asst. Cardiol. Stafford Day.

RAWLENCE, Patrick Donnithorne (retired) The Close, Station Road, Pulham Market, Diss IP21 4TD Tel: 01379 676285 — (St. Thos.) MB BS Lond. 1940. Prev: GP Pulham Market.

RAWLES, John Michael (retired) Brunnion Minor, Lelant Downs, Hayle TR27 6NT Tel: 01736 740983 Fax: 01736 740067 Email: john.rawles@btinternet.com — MB BS Lond. 1964 (Univ. Coll. Hosp.) BSc Lond. 1960; FRCP Lond. 1982, M 1969; FRCP Ed. 1989. Prev: Hon. Sen. Lect. (Med.) Univ. Aberd.

RAWLIN, Michael Eyre Medical Centre, New St., Dinnington, Sheffield S25 2EX Tel: 01909 562207 — MB ChB Sheff. 1959; MRCGP 1990.

RAWLING, Angela Heather Dr Rawling and Partners, Springs Lane, Ilkley LS29 8TH Tel: 01943 604455 Fax: 01943 604466; Maxwell House, Maxwell Road, Ilkley LS29 8RP Tel: 01943 816588 Email: angela@rawling.force9.co.uk — MB ChB Manch. 1970; DObst RCOG 1972. Prev: Clin. Asst. (ENT Surg.) Airedale HA.

RAWLING, Keith Gordon Kintyre, Dene Road, Dalton-on-Dale, Seaham — MB BS Lond. 1976.

RAWLING, Roger Graham Springs Medical Centre, Springs Lane, Ilkley LS29 8TH Tel: 01943 604455 Fax: 01943 604466; Maxwell House, Maxwell Road, Ilkley LS29 8RP Tel: 01943 816588 Email: graham@rawling.force9.co.uk — MB ChB Manch. 1970; DObst RCOG 1973; MRCGP 1975. Specialty: Gen. Pract. Socs: Soc. Occupat. Med.

RAWLINGS, David Medical Imaging Deot, Cross house Hospital, Kilmarnock KA2 0BE Email: david.rawlings@aaaht.scot.nhs.uk; 34 Castlehill Road, Ayr KA7 2HZ — MB ChB Ed. 1982; FRCR; DMRD Aberd. 1987. Cons. Radiol. CrossHo. Hosp. Kilmarnock. Specialty: Radiol. Prev: Sen. Regist. (Radiol.) Newc. Roy. Vict. Infirm.

RAWLINGS, Elizabeth Lexden, Hartley Avenue, Mannamead, Plymouth PL3 5HR Tel: 01752 662323 — MB BCh Wales 1968; BSc Wales 1965; FFA RCS Eng. 1972. Cons. Anaesth. Plymouth Gen. Hosp. Specialty: Anaesth.

RAWLINGS, Mr Ian David Mount Gould Hospital, Plymouth PL4 — MB BS Lond. 1969; FRCS Eng. 1974. Cons. Orthop. Surg. Plymouth Health Auth. Specialty: Orthop.

RAWLINGS, Kate 14A Westfield Road, Ealing, London W13 9JR — MB ChB Leic. 1998; MRCPCH.

RAWLINGS, Keith Leonard Balmoral Surgery, 1 Victoria Road, Deal CT14 7AU Tel: 01304 373444; 19 Archery Square, Walmer,

Deal CT14 7JA — MB ChB Sheff. 1976. Clin. Asst. (Dermat.) SE Kent Hosps. Trust. Specialty: Gen. Pract. Prev: Surg. Lt.-Cdr. RN.

RAWLINGS, Pamela Jane 12 Tapton Park Mount, Ranmoor, Sheffield S10 3FH — MB ChB Sheff. 1985; DRCOG 1989; MRCGP 1990; T(GP) 1991; DOCCMed 2003. Trainee GP Sheff. VTS.

RAWLINGSON, Christopher John 43 Tavistock Road, Basildon SS15 5QF — MB BS Lond. 1994.

RAWLINS, David Charles Green Farm, Chantry, Frome BA11 3LY Tel: 01373 836252 — (Lond. Hosp.) MB BS Lond. 1959. Socs: Fell. Roy. Soc. Med. Prev: Receiv. Room Off. Lond. Hosp.; Med. Regist. Barnet Gen. Hosp.; Regist. (VD) St. Mary's Hosp. Lond.

RAWLINS, Dawn Betty Home Ground Surgery, Thames Avenue, Swindon SN2 3QQ Tel: 01793 692880; 42 The Willows, Highworth, Swindon SN6 7PH Tel: 01793 763494 — MB ChB Leeds 1982. GP Highworth, Swindon. Specialty: Gen. Pract.

RAWLINS, Sir John Stuart Pepys, KBE, OBE, MBE, Surg. Vice-Admiral (retired) Little Cross, Holne, Newton Abbot TQ13 7RS Tel: 01364 631249 Fax: 01364 631400 — (Oxf. & St. Bart.) Fell. Roy. Soc. Med. (FRSM); FRACS (Fell. Roy. Aeronautical Soc.); BM BCh Oxf. 1946; MA Oxf. 1946; FRCP Lond. 1978, M 1973; MFOM 1975; FFCM 1976. Hon. Fell. Univ. Coll. Oxf.; Hon. Research Fell. Univ. Lancaster; Hon. Doctor Technol. Robt. Gordon's Inst. of Technol. Prev: Hon. Phys. to HM the Qu.

RAWLINS, Professor Sir Michael David Woolson Unit of Clinical Pharmacology, The University of Newcastle, Medical School, Newcastle Tel: 0191 222 8041 Fax: 0191 232 3613 Email: m.d.rawlins@ncl.ac.uk — MB BS (Hons.) Lond. 1965 (St. Thos.) FRCP Lond. 1977, M 1968; BSc Lond. 1962, MD 1973; FRCP Ed. 1987; FFPM RCP (UK) 1989. Chairm. Nat. Inst. Clin. Excellence; Prof. Clin. Pharmacol. Univ. Newc.; Hon. Cons. Clin. Pharmacol. Freeman Hosp. & Roy. Vict. Infirm. Newc. Specialty: Pharmacology. Socs: Brit. Pharm. Soc.; Assn. Phys.; Chair, Nat. Inst for Clin. Excellence. Prev: Sen. Regist. (Clin. Pharmacol.) Hammersmith Hosp. Lond.; Lect. (Med.) St. Thos. Hosp. Med. Sch. Lond.; Ho. Phys. & Ho. Phys. (Neurol.) St. Thos. Hosp. Lond.

RAWLINS, Mr Richard Duddingston The Manor Hospital, Biddenham, Bedford MK40 4AW Tel: 01234 364252 Fax: 01234 325001; 13 Pemberley Avenue, Bedford MK40 2LE Tel: 01234 211882 Fax: 01234 217520 — MB BS Lond. 1968 (Middlx.) FRCS Eng. 1975; Spec. Accredit. Orthop. RCS Eng. 1981; MBA Keele 1996. Cons. Orthop. Surg. Bedford Gen. Hosp.; Mem. Jt. Cons. Comm.; Mem. Chiropodists Bd. CPSM Policy Bd. Nat. Centre for Clin. Audit; Chairm. Clin. Audit Commit. BMA; Mem. Policy. Bd. Nat. Centre for Clin. Audit; Chairm., Advisery Counc. Health Quality Serv. Specialty: Orthop.; Medico Legal. Socs: (Ex-Pres.) Brit. Orthop. Trainees Assn.; Brit. Assn. for Surg. of Knee; Brit. Hip Soc. Prev: Sen. Regist. (Orthop.) Guy's Hosp. Lond.; Lect. King's Coll. Lond.

RAWLINSON, Alicia Community Child Health Paediatrics, Royal Gwent Hospital, Newport NP20 2UB Tel: 01633 238999 Fax: 01633 656309 — MB ChB Sheff. 1976; LMCC 1980; MRCP (UK) 1982; DCH RCP Lond. 1982; MRCGP 1984; FRCPCH 1997. Cons. Community Paediat. Glan Hafren NHS Trust. Specialty: Community Child Health. Socs: Brit. Paediat. Assn.; Brit. Assn. Community Child Health. Prev: SCMO (Community Paediat.) Southmead Hosp. Bristol; Regist. Childr. Hosp. Sheff.

RAWLINSON, Andrew John Yarm Medical Centre, 1 Worsall Road, Yarm TS15 9DD Tel: 01642 786422 Fax: 01642 785617; 684 Yarm Road, Eaglescliffe, Stockton-on-Tees TS16 0DP Tel: 01642 784313 — MB ChB Bristol 1973. Prev: Trainee GP Shrewsbury VTS.

RAWLINSON, Fiona Mary Brynlea Hey, The Downs, St. Lythan's, Cardiff CF5 6SB — MB BChir Camb. 1988; DRCOG 1992; MRCGP 1993; Dip Palliat Med Wales 1995; CCST (Palliat. Med.) 2003. Course Tutor Diploma in Palliat. Med. (UWCM); Hon. Lect. Univ. Cape Town. Specialty: Palliat. Med. Prev: Sen. Regist. AllWales Palliat. Med. Higher Rotat. Train.; SR. Bridgend & Dist. NHS Trust; Staff Grade (Palliat. Care) Ybwthyn Palliat. Care Unit Pontypridd.

RAWLINSON, Graham Vaughan Lodgeside Surgery, 22 Lodgeside Avenue, Kingswood, Bristol BS15 1WW Tel: 0117 961 5666 Fax: 0117 947 6854; 328 Canford Lane, Westbury-on-Trym, Bristol BS9 3PW — MB ChB Sheff. 1976; LMCC 1980; MRCGP 1982; DRCOG 1982. Course Organiser Univ. Bristol VTS; Assoc. Regional Adviser Gloucester, Avon & Som; Examr. Roy. Coll. Gen. Pract. Socs: Cossham Med. Soc. Prev: Clin. Asst. (Orthop. Med.) Southmead Hosp. Bristol; GP Trainer Southmead Hosp. Bristol.

RAWLINSON, Howard Rowan Duncan (retired) — MRCS Eng. LRCP Lond. 1967 (Manch.) Prev: Ho. Phys. Hope Hosp. Salford.

RAWLINSON, Mr James Keith McClure Glenburn, 6 Oldfield Road, Heswall, Wirral CH60 6SE Tel: 0151 342 2232 — MB ChB Liverp. 1947; ChM Liverp. 1960, MB ChB 1947; FRCS Eng. 1951. Prev: Cons. (Urol.) Walton Hosp. Liverp.

RAWLINSON, Rev. James Nigel Accident and Emergency Department, Bristol Royal Infirmary, Marlborough St., Bristol BS2 8HW Tel: 0117 928 2713; Glen Boyd House, 38 Court View, Wick BS30 5QP — MB BChir Camb. 1980; BA Camb. 1980; FRCS Ed. 1986; FFAEM 1998; Dip. Applied Theology 1999. Cons., (A & E) Bristol Roy. Infirm.; Priest, Bath & Wells Diocese All St.s Ch. Weston Bath & Bristol Roy. Infirm.; Clin. Sub. Dean HBHT Brit. Med. Sch. Specialty: Accid. & Emerg. Prev: Hon. Sen. Regist. (Neurosurg.) Frenchay Hosp. Bristol; SHO Rotat. (Gen. Surg.) Roy. United Hosp. Bath.; Demonst. (Anat.) Emmanuel Coll. & Dept. Anat. Univ. Camb.

RAWLINSON, John Hunters Way Medical Centre, Hunters Way, Kimbolton, Huntingdon PE18 0HY Tel: 01480 860205 Fax: 01480 861590 — MRCS Eng. LRCP Lond. 1971 (Guy's) BSc Lond. 1967, MB BS 1971. Clin. Asst. (Ophth.) Hinchingbrooke Hosp. Huntington. Prev: Med. Off. Save Childr. Fund Yemen; Demonst. Anat. Aberd. Univ.; SHO (O & G) Raigmore Hosp. Inverness.

RAWLINSON, John Robert Radnor House Practice, 25 London Road, Ascot SL5 7EN Tel: 01344 874011 Fax: 01344 628868 Email: j.rawlinson@ntlworld.com — BM BCh Oxf. 1979; O.U.; MA Oxf. 1979; Cert. Family Plann. JCC 1984; Cert. Managem. 1996. GP Princip. Ascot; Educat. Lead Windsor Ascot & Maidenhead PCT; Mem. (Chairm.) LMC; Mem. (Chairm.) Regional Gen. Pract. Advis. Comm. Specialty: Gen. Pract. Socs: Roy. Soc. Med. Prev: Mem. Winder & Ascot PCG; Mem. GMSC.

RAWLINSON, Marmaduke Peter Goodwin (retired) Silver Birches, London Road, Ringles Cross, Uckfield TN22 1HF Tel: 01825 762525 — MRCS Eng. LRCP Lond. 1940 (Camb. & Westm.) MA (Hnrs.) Camb. 1941; DPH Lond. 1947. Prev: Med. Off. i/c U.K. Canad. High Commiss.

RAWLINSON, Peter Samuel Marshall Hatton Farm House, Abernethy, Perth PH2 9LN — BSc (Med. Sci.) St. And. 1979; MB ChB Manch. 1982; MRCP (UK) 1986; MRCPath 1993. Cons. Haemat. E. of Scotl. Blood Transfus. Ninewells Hosp. Dundee. Specialty: Blood Transfus. Prev: Cons. Haemat. Army Blood Supply Depot Aldershot; Sen. Regist. (Haemat. & Blood Transfus.) Yorksh. Blood Transfus. Serv.; Regist. (Haemat.) Glas. Roy. Infirm.

RAWLINSON, Sarah Meregan Basement Flat, 6 Miles Road, Bristol BS8 2JN — MB BS Lond. 1990.

RAWLINSON, William Arnold Lewin Oaklands Park, High Hatch Lane, Hurstpierpoint, Hassocks BN6 9LH Tel: 01273 832404 Email: william.rawlinson@bsuh.nhs.uk — BM BCh Oxf. 1971 (Lond. Hosp.) MA Oxf. 1973; FRCA. 1976. Cons. Anaesth. Princess Roy. Hosp. Haywards Heath; Clin. Director Brighton & Sussex Univ. Hosps. NHS Trust. Specialty: Anaesth. Socs: Brit. Assn. Med. Managers & Neuroanaesth. Soc.; Assn. Anaesth.; Anaesthetists in Management. Prev: Gen. Manager Mid-Downs E. Unit; Sen. Regist. Nuffield Dept. Anaesth. Oxf.; Ho. Surg. & Ho. Phys. Lond. Hosp.

RAWLINSON, Zoe Louise — MB BS Lond. 1998; MB BS Lond 1998.

RAWLL, Christopher Charles Gadsdon, OStJ British Airways Health Services, Speed Bird House, PO Box 10, London Airport, Hounslow TW6 2JA Tel: 020 8562 5671 Fax: 020 8562 9992; 3 Cavendish Court, Cardigan Road, Richmond TW10 6BL Tel: 020 8948 2838 — MB ChB Birm. 1953; CIH St. And. 1964; DTPH Lond 1965; FFOM RCP Lond. 1988, MFOM 1978. Cons. Occupat. Phys. Brit. Airways Health Servs.; Mem. Internat. Commiss. on Occupat. Health. Specialty: Occupat. Health. Socs: Soc. Occupat. Med. Prev: Cons. Ocupational Phys. Brit. Airways Health Serv..; Wing Cdr. RAF Med. Br..

RAWORTH, Ronald Eric (retired) 20 Lodges Grove, Bare, Morecambe LA4 6HE — MB ChB Manch. 1950 (Manchester) DObst RCOG 1963; DPH (Distinc.) Liverp. 1973; MFCM 1977. Prev: SCM Burnley DHA.

RAWSE, Helen Elizabeth Louise — MB ChB Glas. 1998.

RAWSON, Aneil Flat 8, Tall Trees, 8 Mersey Road, Manchester M20 2PE — MB ChB Sheff. 1991.

RAWSON, Anjali 46 Quarry Lane, Sheffield S11 9EB — MB BS Lond. 1990.

RAWSON, Annette Barbara, OBE (retired) 6 Cecil Close, Mount Avenue, Ealing, London W5 2RB — (St. Mary's) MB BS Lond. 1953; MRCS Eng. LRCP Lond. 1953; FRCP Lond. 1976, M 1955; MFCM 1974. Prev: Sen. Med. Off. DHSS.

RAWSON, Donald Alexander (retired) Kavalla, Mauchline KA5 5AN Tel: 01290 550268 — (Univ. Glas.) MB ChB Glas. 1943. Prev: Hon. Capt. RAMC.

RAWSON, Isabel Anne 145 Almsford Drive, Harrogate HG2 8EE — MB ChB Sheff. 1979; MRCGP 1985. Specialty: Community Child Health.

RAWSON, Lucy Elisabeth The Surgery, Tanners Meadow, Brockham, Betchworth RH3 7NJ Tel: 01737 843259 Fax: 01737 845184; Greenbanks, Old Road, Buckland, Betchworth RH3 7DU — BSc (Hons.) Lond. 1986, MB BS 1989; DRCOG 1992; MRCGP 1993; Cert. Prescribed Equiv. Exp. JCPTGP 1993; DCH RCP Lond. 1993. Prev: Trainee GP E. Surrey VTS.

RAWSON, Malcolm David 19 The Paddocks, Kirk Ella, Hull HU10 7PF Tel: 01482 655351 — MRCS Eng. LRCP Lond. 1956; MD Leeds 1976, MB ChB 1956; FRCP Lond. 1977, M 1959; DMRD Eng. 1961; FFR 1963; FRCR 1975. Cons. Neurol. The BUPA Hosp., Anlaby, Hull. Specialty: Neurol. Prev: Sen. Regist. Univ. Dept. Neurol. Manch. Roy. Infirm.; Sen. Research Fell. Yale Univ. Med. Sch. New Haven, USA; Ho. Surg. & Ho. Phys. Leeds Gen. Infirm.

RAWSTHORNE, Anne Margaret The Crofts, Wrenbury Road, Aston, Nantwich CW5 8DQ Tel: 01270 780244 — (Aberd.) MB ChB Aberd. 1965. Clin. Asst. (Psychiat.) Leighton Hosp. Crewe. Prev: SHO (Psychiat.) Ross Clinic Aberd.; Ho. Surg. (Gyn.) Aberd. Roy. Infirm.; Ho. Phys. (Gen. Med.) Roy. North. Infirm. Inverness.

RAWSTHORNE, Mr George Brian The Crofts, Wrenbury Road, Aston, Nantwich CW5 8DQ — MB ChB Aberd. 1965; FRCS Ed. 1970; FRCS Eng. 1973. Cons. Surg. Leighton Hosp. Crewe. Specialty: Gen. Surg. Prev: Sen. Regist. (Surg.) Liverp. RHB; Regist. Merseyside RHA; SHO Woodend Hosp. Aberd.

RAWSTORNE, Steven Well Lane Surgery, Well Lane, Stow on the Wold, Cheltenham GL54 1EQ Tel: 01451 830625 Fax: 01451 830693 Email: rawstorne@rcsed.ac.uk; Gloucestershire Ambulance Service NHS Trust, Tri-service Emergency Centre, Waterwells Drive, Waterwells Business Park, Quedgeley, Gloucester GL2 2BA Tel: 01452 753078 Email: steven.rawstorne@glosamb.swest.nhs.uk — MB BS Lond. 1982 (Guy's) BSc (Hons.) Biochem. Lond. 1979; DCH RCP Lond. 1984; MRCGP 1986; DRCOG 1986; FRCP 2001; FIMC RCS (Ed.) 2001. p/t GP Stow on the Wold; Med. Director Gloucestershire Ambul. Serv. NHS Trust. Prev: Trainee GP Chipping Norton Oxon.; Ho. Surg. Guy's Hosp. Lond.; Ho. Phys. Lewisham Hosp. Lond.

RAWSTRON, John Roberts, TD (retired) 5 HighStreet, Watlington OX49 5PZ Tel: 01491 613108 — MRCS Eng. LRCP Lond. 1954 (King's Coll. Hosp.) MD Lond. 1964, MB BS 1954; DPath Eng. 1960; FRCPath 1976, M 1964. Cons. Clin. Pathol. Amersham & High Wycombe Area Dept. of Path.; Maj. RAMC (TA). Prev: Sen. Lect. in Clin. Path. King's Coll. Hosp. Med. Sch.

RAY, Amar Kumar (retired) Hollybank, Rectory Lane, Heswall, Wirral CH60 4RZ Tel: 0151 342 5868 — (R.G. Kar Med. Coll.) MB BS Calcutta 1957; FFA RCS Eng. 1965. Cons. Anaesth. Mersey RHA. Prev: Sen. Regist. United Liverp. Hosps. & Liverp RHB.

RAY, Mr Amares Chandra 30 Havenwood Road, Whitley, Wigan WN1 2PA — MB BS Calcutta 1965; FRCS Eng. 1971; FRCS Ed. 1971.

RAY, Aparna 2c Sandy Lane, Hampton Wick, Kingston upon Thames KT1 4BB — MB BS Lond. 1998; MB BS Lond 1998.

RAY, Mr Ashoke Kumar 32 Monkhams Drive, Woodford Green IG8 0LE Tel: 020 8504 0179 — MB BS Calcutta 1958 (Calcutta Med. Coll.) DGO Calcutta 1960; MRCOG 1964; FRCS Canada 1968.

RAY, Mr Atanu Dept. of Surgery, Whiston Hospital, Prescot L35 5DR Tel: 0151 426 1600 — MB ChB Zambia 1983; BSc Zambia 1980; FRCS Glas. 1990. Specialty: Urol.

RAY, Bibhas Chandra Braidholm, 3 Kenmure Road, White Craigs, Glasgow G46 6TU Tel: 0141 585 3139 Email: drbibhasray@hotmail.com — MB BS Calcutta 1974; MD Calcutta 1977; DObst RCPI 1988; MRCOG 1988; MFFP 1993; FRCOG 2000. Assoc. Specialist (Obst. & Gyn.) Roy. Alexandra Hosp. & Paisley Matern. Unit. Specialty: Obst. & Gyn. Socs: Brit. Colposcopy Soc. & Brit. Ultrasound Soc. Prev: Regist. (O & G) Inverclyde Roy. Hosp. Greenock; Regist. (O & G) Jersey Gen. Hosp. CI.

RAY, Carol Kanti 14 Lower Ladyes Hills, Kenilworth CV8 2GN — MB ChB Birm. 1997.

RAY, Coralie Sunanda 6 Friars Mews, Pinwell Road, Lewes BN7 2LW Tel: 01273 480945 — MB BS Lond. 1981 (Char. Cross) BSc (Basic. Med. Sci. with Med. Sociol.) Lond.; MSc (Community Health in Developing Countries) Lond. 1983; MPH Birm. 1997. Cons. in Pub. Health, Brighton and Hove City PCT; Edit. Bd. Reproduc. Health Matters (Lond.); Edit. Bd. AIDS Action (Lond.). Specialty: Pub. Health Med. Prev: Research Fell. & Lect. (Community Med.) Univ. Zimbabwe; Med. Off. Harare City Health, Zimbabwe.

RAY, David Charles Department of Anaesthesia, Critical Care and Pain Medicine, Royal Infirmary, Little France Crescent, Edinburgh EH16 4SA Tel: 0131 242 3215 Email: david.ray@luht.scot.nhs.uk; Easterhill, 13 Galachlaw Shot, Edinburgh EH10 7JF — MB ChB Ed. 1983; FRCA 1989; MD Ed. 1992. Cons. Anaesth. & Intens. Care Roy. Infirm. Edin.; Hon. Clin. Sen. Lect., Univ. of Edin. Specialty: Anaesth.; Intens. Care. Special Interest: Anaesth. for Ophthalmological Surg.; Anaesth. for Trauma Orthop. Socs: Assn. Anaesth.; Intens. Care Soc.; Scott. Intens. Care Soc. Prev: Sen. Regist. (Anaesth.) Roy. Infirm. Edin.; Sen. Regist. (Anaesth.) Christchuch, NZ; Regist. (Anaesth.) Roy. Infirm. Edin. Train. Scheme.

RAY, David William 270 Brooklands Road, Manchester M23 9HD Tel: 0161 962 6049 Fax: 0161 275 5958 — MB ChB Manch. 1987; MRCP (UK) 1990; PhD Manch. 1994. Research Fell., Manch. Univ. Specialty: Diabetes; Gen. Med. Socs: N. W. Eudocrae Soc.; Soc. Eudocreuology. Prev: Lect. (Med.) Manch. Univ.; Vis. Fell. Cedars-Sinai Med., Center, Los Angeles, USA.

RAY, Debendra 157 Cambridge Road, Seven Kings, Ilford IG3 8LZ — MB BS Utkal 1967; MRCPsych 1974.

RAY, Debi 32 Monkhams Drive, Woodford Green IG8 0LE — MB BS Lond. 1998; MB BS Lond 1998.

RAY, Mr Dilip Kumar 3 Regpree Court, 45-47 South Park Road, Wimbledon, London SW19 8RS — MB BS Calcutta 1972 (Calcutta Nat. Medical Coll., INDIA) FRCS Ed. 1984. Specialty: Urol.

RAY, Dipak Kumar 36 Lilian Road, Blackwood NP12 1DN Tel: 01495 224267 — MB BS Calcutta 1955; MRCGP 1971.

RAY, Dipak Kumar University Hospital of Hartlepool, Holdforth Road, Hartlepool TS26 9NU — MB BS Calcutta 1990; MD Manipal, India 1995; MRCP (UK) 2000. Staff Grade Phys. Specialty: Rheumatol.

RAY, Dominic Andres Anthony Golden Jubilee National Hospital, Beardmore St., Clydebank G81 4HX — MB ChB Birm. 1982; DA (UK) 1985; FRCA 1987; MSc Birm. 1991. Dir. of Cardiac Anaesth. Health Care Internat. Glas. Specialty: Anaesth.; Intens. Care. Socs: Soc. Computing & Technol. in Anaesth.; UK Assoc. Cardiothoracic Anaesth.; Eur. Assoc. Cardiothoracic Anaesth. Prev: Sen. Regist. (Anaesth.) W. Midl. Train. Scheme; Regist. (Anaesth.) Centr. Birm.; Regist. (Anaesth.) Russells Hall Hosp. Dudley.

RAY, Elizabeth Helen 12 St Gerards Road, Solihull B91 1TZ; 7 Canons Way, Tavistock PL19 8BJ Tel: 01822 614775 — MB ChB Leic. 1995.

RAY, Gautam 13 Abbots Lane, Kenley CR8 5JB — MB BS Lond. 1989.

RAY, J N The Medical Centre, Gun Lane, Strood, Rochester ME2 4UW Tel: 01634 727888 — MB BS Patna 1973; MB BS Patna 1973.

RAY, Jacqueline Anne Adam Practice, Upton Health Centre, Blandford Road North, Poole BH16 5PW Tel: 01202 622339; Elisir, 231 Sandbanks Road, Lilliput, Poole BH14 8EY — BM Soton. 1988; DRCOG 1991; MRCGP 1992. Clin. Asst. (A & E) Poole Hosp. Trust. Specialty: Accid. & Emerg. Socs: MDU; MSS. Prev: Trainee GP Lymington Hants.; SHO (A & E) Soton. Gen. Hosp.; SHO (Med.) Lymington Hosp.

RAY, Jagadis Chandra The Surgery, 117 Fulbourne Road, Walthamstow, London E17 4HA Tel: 020 8527 6373 — MB BS Calcutta 1958.

RAY, Julian Lincoln Addenbrooke's Hospital, Department of Clinical Neurophysiology, Box 124, Cambridge CB2 2QQ Tel: 01223 217136 Fax: 01223 336941 — MB BS Lond. 1994; BSc (Physiol.) 1991; MRCP UK 1999. Specialist Regist., Clin. Neuropath., Addenbrooke's Hosp. Camb. Specialty: Clin. Neurophysiol. Prev: SHO, Med. Rotat., Norf. & Norwich Hosp.

RAY, Kamala Braidholm, 3 Kenmure Road, Glasgow Whitecraigs, Glasgow G46 6TU Tel: 0141 585 3139 — MB BS Patna 1974 (P. of Wales Med. Coll.) DCH Eng. 1980; DCH RCPSI 1980; MRCPI 1985. Regist. (Med. Paediat.) Inverclyde Roy. Hosp. Greenock; Clin. Med. Off. Lanarksh.; Assoc. Specialist (Community Child Health) Lanarksh. Specialty: Paediat. Socs: Ordinary Mem. Roy. Coll. Paediat. & Child Health; Roy. Coll. Phys. of Irel.; Fell. Soc. Pub. Health. Prev: Regist. (Med. Paediat.) Roy. Liverp. Childr. Hosp. Heswall; SHO (Med. Paediat.) Marston Green Hosp., E. Birm. Hosp. & Sydenham Childr. Hosp. Lond.

RAY, Mr Kartik Chandra Sai Medical Centre, 10 Moat Road, Walsall WS2 9PJ Fax: 01922 614088; 10 Moat Road, Walsall WS2 9PJ Tel: 01922 647353 Fax: 01922 614088 — MB BS Calcutta 1966; MD Act Medicine; Dip. Med. Acupunc; DGO 1968; MS Bihar 1969; MRCOG 1976; FICS 1978. Vis. Gyn. Colthorpe Nursing Home Birm. Specialty: Obst. & Gyn. Socs: Med. Protec. Soc.; Brit. Accupunc. Soc. Prev: Cons. Gyn. Leeds Private Hosp.

RAY, Kausik Kumar Timi Study Group, Brighams Womans Hospital, 1st Floor, 350 Longwood Avenue, Boston MA 02115 — MB ChB Birm. 1991 (Birmingham) BSc (Hons. Pharm.) Birm. 1988; MRCP (Ed.) 1994; MD harvard Medical School 2003. Spr Cardiol., N. trent. Specialty: Cardiol.; Gen. Med. Socs: BMA; Fell. Roy. Soc. Med. Prev: Ho. Phys. E. Birm. Hosp.; Ho. Surg. Good Hope Dist. Gen. Hosp. Sutton Coldfield.; Career SHO Rotat. (Med.) Dudley Rd. Hosp. Birm.

RAY, Lesley Carol Windyridge, Forge Lane, Little Aston, Sutton Coldfield B74 3BE — MB BS Lond. 1993.

RAY, Mary 5 St Margaret's Close, Shady Bower, Salisbury SP1 2RY Tel: 01722 336967 — MB BS Poona 1980; MRCP Ed. 1986.

RAY, Nandini Whipps Cross Hospital, Leytonstone, London E11 1NR Tel: 020 8539 5522 — MB BS Calcutta 1984; MCOphth 1990; FCOphth 1991.

RAY, Narendra Kumar Victoria Road Health Centre, Victoria Road, Washington NE37 2PU Tel: 0191 415 5656 Fax: 0191 417 8100; 1 Dalmahoy, Washington NE37 1SF — MB BS Utkal 1972. GP Washington Tyne & Wear. Specialty: Gen. Pract. Special Interest: Paediat.

RAY, Natasha 29 Bishop's Road, Trumpington, Cambridge CB2 2NQ — MB BS Lond. 1998; MRCGP; MB BS Lond 1998.

RAY, Nicolette Louise Flat 13, Arnhem Wharf, 2 Arnhem Place, London E14 3RU — MB BS Lond. 1996.

RAY, Paramita 28 Whitwell Acres, High Shincliffe, Durham DH1 2PX — MB ChB Dundee 1994; DRCO 1997. SHO. Specialty: Anaesth. Socs: MPS.

RAY, Pijush Kanti Department of Medicine, Warwick Hospital, Lakin Road, Warwick CV 34 5BW Tel: 01926 495321 Fax: 01926 482609 — MB BS Calcutta 1987; MD Calcutta 1992; MRCP UK 1997. Cons. Geriat. and Phys. S. Warks. Gen. Hosps. NHS Trust; Cons. Geriat. and Phys., Roy. Leamington Spa Rehabil. Hosp. Specialty: Gen. Med.; Care of the Elderly. Special Interest: Falls; Orthogeriatrics; Osteoparosis. Socs: Brit. Geriat. Soc.; Brit. Med. Assn. Prev: Specialist Regist. Gen. Med. and Geriat. Med., Univ. Hosp. Birm.; Specialist Regist. Gen. Med. and Geriat. Med., City Hosp., Dudley Rd., Birm.; Specialist Regist. Gen. Med. and Geriat. Med., Goop Hope Hosp. NHS Trust, Sutton Coldfield.

RAY, Mr Prabhat Kumar 3 Balfron Place, Aberdeen AB15 6HW Tel: 01224 314034 — MB BS Calcutta 1949; DO Eng. 1953; FRCS Ed. 1964. Cons. Ophth. Aberd. Teach. Hosps.; Sen. Clin. Lect. in Ophth. Aberd. Univ. Specialty: Ophth. Prev: Regist. Glas. Eye Infirm.; Clin. Tutor in Ophth. Aberd. Univ. & Sen. Regist. Aberd. Gen. Hosps.; Cons. Ophth. Lanarksh. Area.

RAY, Roberta Jane Department of Anaesthetics, Salisbury District Hospital, Salisbury Tel: 01722 336262; Awbridge Farm, Dunbridge Lane, Awbridge, Romsey SO51 0GQ Tel: 01794 340095 — MB ChB Leeds 1978; FFA RCSI 1984. Cons. Anaesth. Salisbury Dist. Hosp. Specialty: Anaesth.

RAY, Ronnie Aurun 12 Wildwood Gardens, Apartment F/2, Port Washington, New York NY 11050, USA; 20 Heathfielde, Lyttelton Road, London N2 0EE — MB BS Lond. 1984; BSc Lond. 1980; US Boards in Anat. Clin. Path. 1990. Attend. Pathologist St. Vincents Hosp. Richmond, USA. Specialty: Histopath. Socs: Univ. Lond. Convocation & NY Path. Soc. Prev: Attend. Pathologist Glen Core, NY, USA; Sen. Regist. Roy. Free Hosp. Lond.; Fell. Gastrointestinal & Surg. Path. New Eng. Deacones Hosp. Boston, USA.

RAY, Ruth Elaine Easterhill, Galachlaw Shot, Edinburgh EH10 7JF Tel: 0131 445 5676 — MB ChB Ed. 1982; BSc Med. Sc. Ed. 1979, MB ChB 1982; MRCGP 1986; DRCOG 1986. Staff Grade (Dermat.) Edin. Specialty: Dermat.

RAY, Sarbani 30 Colin Gardens, London NW9 6EJ — MB ChB Birm. 1993.

RAY, Simon Guy Department of Cardiology, Wythenshawe Hospital, Southmoor Road, Manchester M23 9LT Tel: 0161 291 2402 Fax: 0161 291 2389 — MB ChB Bristol 1983; MD Bristol 1993, BSc (Hons.) 1980; MRCP (UK) 1986; FACC 1996; FRCP 1999; FESC 2001. Cons. Cardiol. Regional Cardiothoracic Centre Wythenshawe Hosp. Manch. Specialty: Cardiol. Prev: Sen. Fell. (Cardiol.) Vancouver Hosp. Vancouver, Canada; Sen. Regist. (Cardiol.) Cardiothoracic Centre Liverp.; Regist. (Cardiol.) Freeman Hosp. Newc. u. Tyne.

RAY, Sisir Beaufort Gardens Surgery, 2 Beaufort Gardens, Hendon, London NW4 3QP Tel: 020 8202 2141 Fax: 020 8203 3638 Email: harleystmedicare@yahoo.co.uk — MB BS Calcutta 1961 (Medical coll. Calcutta)

RAY, Subal Chandra Walton Hospital, Chesterfield S40 3HN Tel: 01246 277271; 28 Carnoustie Avenue, Walton, Chesterfield S40 3NN Tel: 01246 204852 — MB BS Calcutta 1968; DCH Calcutta 1970; DTM & H Liverp. 1985; FCCP USA 1991. Staff Grade Phys. (Med. for Elderly) Walton Hosp. Chesterfield. Specialty: Care of the Elderly. Prev: Indep. Pract. India; SHO (Acute Med. for Elderly) Luton & Dunstable Hosp. & St. Lukes Hosp. Huddersfield; SHO (Rheum. & Rehabil. & Gen. Med.) Morriston Hosp. Wales.

RAY, Subrata Newtown Health Centre, 171 Melbourne Avenue, Newtown, Birmingham B19 2JA Tel: 0121 554 7541 Fax: 0121 515 4447; 20 Heaton Drive, Edgbaston, Birmingham B15 3LW Tel: 0121 454 0395 — MB BS Calcutta 1964 (R.G. Kar Med. Coll.) DObst RCOG 1971; MFFP 1993.

RAY, Mr Sudip Abhijit New Victoria Hospital, 184 Coombe Lane West, Kingston upon Thames KT2 7EG Tel: 020 8878 5745 Fax: 020 8878 8113 Email: sudip_a_ray@hotmail.com — MB BS Lond. 1986 (Westm.) MA Oxf. 1987; FRCS Lond. 1990; MS Lond. 1996; FRCS (Gen.) 1997. Cons. Vasc. & Gen. Surg. Kingston, Roehampton & Char. Cross Hosp. Specialty: Gen. Surg. Prev: Sen. Regist. (Surg.) St Geo. Hosp. Lond.; Sen. Regist. (Surg.) St Thos. Hosp. Lond.

RAY, Sukamal 51 Golders Gardens, London NW11 9BS Tel: 020 8458 6093 — MB BS Calcutta 1956; DA Eng. 1962; FFA RCS Eng. 1969. Specialty: Anaesth. Socs: Assn. Anaesths. Gt. Brit. Prev: Anaesth. Regist. Derbysh. Roy. Infirm., Centr. Middlx. Gp. Hosps. & Roy. Nat. Throat, Nose & Ear Hosp.

RAY-CHAUDHURI, Dominic Sunay 8 Elsee Road, Rugby CV21 3BA — MB BS Lond. 1990; MRCP (UK) 1993. Regist. (Radiol.) Roy. Hallamsh. Hosp. Sheff. Specialty: Radiol.

RAY CHAUDHURI, Kallol 42 Minet Avenue, London NW10 8AH Tel: 020 8965 8937; 8 Williams Lane, Calcutta 700009, India Tel: 50 0669 — MB BS Calcutta 1983; MRCP (UK) 1986. Lect. & Hon. Sen. Regist. (Neurol.) King's Coll. Hosp. & Maudsley Hosp. Lond. Specialty: Neurol. Socs: Clin. Autonomic Res. Soc. & Lond. Hypertens. Soc. Prev: Lect. Leicester Univ.; Research Fell. Inst. Neurol. & Nat. Hosp. Neurol. & Neurosurg. & St. Mary's Hosp. Med. Sch. Lond.; Regist. (Neurol.) Hammersmith Hosp. Lond.

RAY CHAUDHURI, Rita 96 Moorland View Road, Walton, Chesterfield S40 3DF — MB BS Mysore 1976. Sessional Med. Off. Blood Transfus. Trent Region Sheff.. Specialty: Blood Transfus.

RAY-CHAUDHURI, Simon Bibek 8 Elsee Road, Rugby CV21 3BA — MB BS Lond. 1990.

RAYANI, Ashok Patel Grove Medical Centre, 6 Uplands Terrace, Uplands, Swansea SA2 0GU Tel: 01792 643000 Fax: 01792 472800 — MB BCh Wales 1982 (Welsh Nat. Sc. Med.) MRCGP 1986. GP Walter Rd. Med. Gp.

RAYAT, Salinder Theobald Centre, 119-121 Theobald Street, Borehamwood WD6 4PU Tel: 020 8953 3355 — MB BS Lond. 1985; AKC.

RAYATT, Mr Sukhbir Singh Dept of Plastic Surgery, Sandwell Healthcare NHS Trust, West Bromwich B71 4HJ; 163 Horsenden Lane South, Perivale, Greenford UB6 7NR — MB BS Lond. 1993 (UMDS St. Thos.) BDS Lond. 1984; LDS RCS Eng. 1985; FDS RCS Eng. 1992; FRCS Eng. 1996. Specialty: Plastic Surg.

RAYBOULD, Adrian David University College Hospital of Wales, Heath Park, Cardiff CF14 4XN — MB BS Lond. 1993; BSc Lond.

1990; MRCP (UK) 1997. Specialist Regist. (Cardiol.) Univ. Hosp. of Wales Cardiff. Specialty: Cardiol.

RAYBOULD, Ronald Henry (retired) 3 Wharfedale Rise, Bradford BD9 6AU Tel: 01274 543493 — (Leeds) MB ChB Leeds 1958. Prev: GP Bradford.

RAYBOULD, Sarah Anne John Tasker House Surgery, 56 New Street, Great Dunmow, Dunmow CM6 1BH Tel: 01371 872121 Fax: 01371 873793 — BSc Wales 1978, MB BCh 1981; MRCP (UK) 1984; DRCOG 1988; DCH RCP Lond. 1988.

RAYCHAUDHURI, Mr Kaustabh (Ray) — LRCP Lond. 1989; MRCS Lond. 1989; MRCOG UK 1993. Cons. O & G Barnsley Dist. Gen. Hosp. Specialty: Obst. & Gyn. Socs: Brit. Soc. of Gyn. Endoscopy; Brit. Soc. of Fetal & Matern. Med.; Brit Soc. of Colp & Cervical Cytol.

RAYCHAUDHURI, Sujay c/o Mr J.P. Sinha, 71 Sussex Road, Watford WD24 5HR — MB BS Calcutta 1988.

RAYMAKERS, Katharine Lois Maria The Health Centre, Madeira Road, West Byfleet, Weybridge Tel: 01932 340411; Summerhill Cottage, 9 Crawley Hill, Camberley GU15 2DA — MB BS Lond. 1986; DRCOG 1989; MRCGP 1996. Specialty: Obst. & Gyn.

RAYMAKERS, Mr Roeland Leonard Wheelwrights, 5 Top Yard Farm, Great Bowden, Market Harborough LE16 7JB Tel: 01858 466605 — MB BS Lond. 1957 (Westm.) MRCS Eng. LRCP Lond. 1957; FRCS Eng. 1965. Sen. Fell. Brit. Orthop. Ass. Specialty: Orthop. Socs: BMA; Sen. Fell. Brit. Orthop. Assn. Prev: Emerit. Cons. Orthop. Surg. Leicester AHA; Clin. Head Orthop. Serv. Leic. Roy. Infirm.; Sen. Regist. Harlow Wood Orthop. Hosp.

RAYMAN, Gerrard Diabetic Centre, Ipswich Hospital, Ipswich IP4 5PD Tel: 01473 704183 Fax: 01473 704197 — MB BS Lond. 1976 (Middlesex Hosp) MRCP (UK) 1979; MD Lond. 1992; FRCP Lond 1998. Cons. Phys. (Gen. Med., Diabetes & Endocrinol.) Ipswich Hosp. Specialty: Diabetes; Endocrinol.; Gen. Med.

RAYMENT, Alan Overdale Medical Practice, 207 Victoria Avenue, Borrowash, Derby DE72 3BH Tel: 01332 280800 Fax: 01332 669256 — MB ChB Manch. 1969; DObst RCOG 1971. Socs: BMA. Prev: Ho. Off. Dept. Med. & Ho. Surg. Manch. Roy. Infirm.; SHO (Anaesth. & O & G) Nott. City Hosp.

RAYMENT, Rachel 32 Green Ridges, Oxford OX3 8PL Email: rachel.rayment@ntlworld.com — MB ChB Bristol 1991; MRCP 1994; MRCPath 1999. Research Regist. John Radcliffe Hosp. Oxf. Specialty: Haematology.

RAYMOND, Christopher John Parkfield Medical Centre, Sefton Road, New Ferry, Wirral CH62 5HS Tel: 0151 644 0055 Fax: 0151 643 1679; Redwynde, 4 North Close, Bromborough, Wirral CH62 2BU Tel: 0151 334 5206 — MB ChB Liverp. 1979; DRCOG 1982. Prev: Trainee GP/SHO Clatterbridge Hosp. Bebington VTS; Ho. Off. Roy. Liverp. Hosp.

RAYMOND, Frances Lucy Dept. Medical Genetics, Cambridge Inst. Of Medical Research, Addenbrookes Hospital, Cambridge CB2 2XY — MB BS Lond. 1989; MA Oxf. 1981, DPhil 1984; MRCP (UK) 1992; FRCP 2002.

RAYMOND, Frank Damian 230 Cambridge Road, Hitchin SG4 0JW Tel: 01462 53159 — MB BS Lond. 1988; PhD Lond. 1981, MSc 1976, BSc (Hon) 1974.

RAYMOND, George Philip Maurice 21 Brampton Grove, London NW4 4AE — MB ChB Ed. 1951; DA Eng. 1957. Prev: Regist. (Anaesth.) Poplar Hosp.; SHO (Surg. & Orthop.) Ipswich & E. Suff. Hosp.; SHO (O & G) W.wood Hosp. Beverley.

RAYMOND, Martin Paul — MB BS Lond. 1998.

RAYMOND, Mr Santhiapillai Paulpillai 11 Faircross Way, St Albans AL1 4RT — MB BS Sri Lanka 1972; FRCS Ed. 1983.

RAYMOND, Thomas Michael James Richard Low Green Farm, Lindale, Grange-over-Sands LA11 6ND — MB BS Lond. 1996.

RAYMOND-JONES, John Graham 21 Barn Close, Camberley GU15 2HW — MB BS Lond. 1963.

RAYMONT, Vanessa 139 St Josephs Vale, London SE3 0XQ — MB ChB Birm. 1993; MRCPsych 1998. Specialist Regist. Psychiat. Maudsley Hosp, Lond. Specialty: Gen. Psychiat.; Geriat. Psychiat. Prev: Regist. Rotat. & SHO Rotat. (Psychiat.) St. Geo. Hosp. Lond.; Ho. Off. Medway Hosp. Gillingham & Bromley Hosp. Kent.

RAYNAL, Anne Louise EMAS, HSE, Intercity House, Mitchell Lane, Bristol BS1 6AN Tel: 01179 886003 — MB ChB Cape Town 1979; MSc Lond. 1982; DPH RIPHH 1982; MFPHM RCP (UK) 1989; MFOM RCP Lond. 1994, AFOM 1992. Her Majesty's Insp. of Health & Safety (Med.) Wales & W.Region, Bristol. Specialty: Occupat. Health. Socs: Soc. Occupat. Med. (SW Br.). Prev: Regional Med. Advisor Brit. Gas W. Midl.; Mine Med. Off. E. Rand Proprietary Mine S. Afr.; Regist. (Community Health) Univ. Witwaterand.

RAYNE, David Saint Hildas Surgery, 50 St Hildas Street, Sherburn, Malton YO17 8PH; 5 Saint Hilda's Crescent, Sherburn, Malton YO17 8PJ Tel: 01944 710175 — MB BS Lond. 1977 (Univ. Coll. Hosp.) Hosp. Practitioner (Gastroenterol.) ScarBoro. HA. Specialty: Gen. Pract.; Gastroenterol.

RAYNER, Caroline Ann Longshoot Health Centre, Scholes, Wigan WN1 3NH Tel: 01942 242610 Fax: 01942 826612 — MB ChB Manch. 1986; DCH RCP Lond. 1991; MRCGP 1992. Trainee GP/SHO Bolton Gen. Hosp. VTS.

RAYNER, Charlotte Frances Jessica St George's Hospital, Chest Clinic, Blackshaw Road, London SW17 UQT Tel: 020 8725 1261 Fax: 020 8725 3309 Email: charlotte.rayner@stgeorges.nhs.uk — MB BS Lond. 1985 (St Thos.) MD, FRCP. Cons. Gen. & Respirat. Phys. St Geo. Hosp. Lond.; Hon. Cons., Roy. Marsden, Lond.; Cons., Parkside Hosp., Lond.; Cons., St Anthonys Hosp., Lond.; Cons., Qu. Mary's Hosp., Lond. Specialty: Respirat. Med.; Gen. Med.

RAYNER, Christopher Martin 6 White House Drive, Guildford GU1 2SU — MB BS Lond. 1972; DObst RCOG 1974; MRCGP 1976.

RAYNER, Clare Rachel North Manchester General Hospital, Delaunay's Road, Manchester M8 — MB ChB Manch. 1990; MRCGP 1994. Specialist Regist. Occupat. Health N. W. Region. Specialty: Occupat. Health.

RAYNER, Mr Colin Robert Wilfred BUPA Parkway Hospital, 1 Damson parkway, Solihull B91 2PP; 64 Wellington Road, Edgbaston, Birmingham B15 2ET Tel: 0121 244 8566 — (Middlx.) MB BS Lond. 1964; FRCS Eng. 1969; MS Lond. 1978; FRCS Ed. 1982. Cons. Plastic SurgBupa Pk.way Hosp; Clin. Dir. Burns & Plastic Surg. Birm.; BUPA S. Bank Hosp Worcester. Specialty: Plastic Surg. Prev: Cons. Plastic Surg. S. Birm. HA; Cons. Plastic Surg. Grampian HB; Clin dir.Burns & Plastic Surg. Univ.Hosp.Birm.

RAYNER, Helen Catherine Anne 291 Milkwood Road, Herne Hill, London SE24 0HE — MB BS Lond. 1986.

RAYNER, Hugh Clive Birmingham Heartlands Hospital, Bordesley Green E., Birmingham B9 5SS Tel: 0121 424 2158 Fax: 0121 424 1159 — MB BS Lond. 1981; MA Camb. 1982; MRCP (UK) 1984; MD Leic. 1990; Dip. Med. Educat. Dund 1996; FRCP 1998. Cons. Renal. Med. Birm. Heartlands Hosp.; Hon. Clin. Sen. Lect. Univ. Birm.; Med. Director (Med.Serv.s) Birm. Heartlands and Solihull NHS Trust (Teachg.). Specialty: Nephrol. Socs: Assn. for Study of Med. Educat.; Renal Assn.; Amer. Soc. Nephrol. Prev: Sen. Regist. (Nephrol. & Gen. Med.) Leeds Gen. Infirm. & St. Jas. Univ. Hosp. Leeds; Renal Fell. P. Henry's Hosp. Melbourne, Austral.; NKRF Research Fell. (Renal Med.) Leic.

RAYNER, Ian Robert Bridge House, 509 Aldridge Road, Birmingham B44 8NA Tel: 0121 685 6730 Fax: 0121 344 4645; 5 Oakwood Close, Shenstone, Lichfield WS14 0JJ Email: irayn5@msn.com — MB ChB Birm. 1983; MRCPsych 1990. Cons. Old Age Psychiat.; Birm. & Solihull Ment. Health Trust. Specialty: Geriat. Psychiat. Prev: Regist. Rotat. (Psychiat.) Birm.

RAYNER, Jane Ann The White House, Stoney Lane, Coleorton, Leicester LE67 8JJ — MB ChB Sheff. 1987; MRCGP (Distinc.) 1992; DRCOG 1992. Staff Grade Phys. (Diabetes & Med.) Derbysh. Roy. Infirm. Derby; Chief Med. Mem. Appeals Serv. Specialty: Diabetes. Prev: Med. Assessor for Indep. Tribunal Serv.

RAYNER, Jonathan Machan Hockin Ramsbury Surgery, High Street, Ramsbury, Marlborough SN8 2QT Tel: 01672 520366 Fax: 01672 520180; Yew Tree House, South St, Aldbourne, Marlborough SN8 2DW Tel: 01672 541418 Fax: 01672 541419 Email: raynerjmh@hotmail.com — MB BS Lond. 1983; DCH RCP Lond. 1988; D. Occ. Med. 2001.

RAYNER, Juliet Mary The Surgery, Elsenham, Bishop's Stortford CM22 6LA Tel: 01279 814730 Fax: 01279 647342; Blythwood Lodge, 68 Silver St, Stansted Mountfitchet, Stansted CM24 8HD Tel: 01279 812271 — MB ChB Birm. 1972; DObst RCOG 1974.

RAYNER, Kirsty Elizabeth Ballaghy, Bovingdon Green, Marlow SL7 2JQ Tel: 01628 486895 — MB ChB Birm. 1997 (Birmingham) SHO, (O & G) Wycombe Gen.Hosp. Specialty: Obst. & Gyn. Socs: BMA; MDU. Prev: SHO A&E Swindon; PRHO. Off. (Surg.) Kidderminster Gen. Hosp.; PRHO Med. Sandwell Gen.

RAYNER, Linda Dawn — MB ChB Bristol 1977; DRCOG 1980. Asst. GP, Badewell Med. Centre, Bristol. Specialty: Gen. Pract. Prev: Clin. Med. Off. (Disabelm. Serv.) Southmead Hosp. Bristol.; Clin. Asst. Psychiat. Barrow Hosp. Bristol.; Clin. Med. Off. (Family Plann.) Southmead Hosp. Bristol.

RAYNER, Lisa White House, Bardsea, Ulverston LA12 9QT — MB ChB Leeds 1993.

RAYNER, Mary Millicent (retired) The White House, 33 Meadow Hill Road, King's Norton, Birmingham B38 8DF Tel: 0121 458 6595 Fax: 0121 458 6595 — MRCS Eng. LRCP Lond. 1947; MRCGP 1973. Prev: Med. Off. Bournville Trust Almsho.

RAYNER, Nigel 1 Rose Cottages, Bissoe Road, Carnon Downs, Truro TR3 6JA — MB ChB Leic. 1990.

RAYNER, Paul Henry Walter Institute of Child Health, Clinical Research Block, Whittall St., Birmingham B4 6NH Tel: 0121 333 9999 Fax: 0121 333 8701; 219 Harborne Park Road, Harborne, Birmingham B17 0BQ Tel: 0121 426 5870 Fax: 0121 428 4414 — (Birm.) BSc (Hons.) Birm. 1957; MB ChB Birm. 1960; FRCP Lond. 1978, M 1964; FRCPCH 1997. Hon. Sen. Research Fell. & Hon. Cons. Paediat. Childr. Hosp. Birm. Specialty: Paediat. Prev: Sen. Lect. (Paediat.) Univ. Birm.

RAYNER, Philip Michael Charles The Calverton Practice, 2A St. Wilfrids Square, Calverton, Nottingham NG14 6FP Tel: 0115 965 2294 Fax: 0115 965 5898; 11 Beaumont Avenue, Southwell NG25 0BB — MB ChB Leeds 1985 (Univ. Leeds) MB ChB (Hons.) Leeds 1985; MRCP (UK) 1989; MRCGP 1995. Specialty: Paediat. Prev: Regist. Adelaide Childr. Hosp. S. Austral.

RAYNER, Philip Robert 5 Priory Close, Walton, Chesterfield S42 7HQ — MB ChB Sheff. 1975; BSc (Hons.) Lond. 1972; FFA RCS Eng. 1980; FFA RCSI 1980. Cons. Anaesth. N. Derbysh. HA. Specialty: Anaesth.

RAYNER, Robin Arthur Manor Farm Medical Centre, Mangate Street, Swaffham PE37 7QN Tel: 01760 721786 Fax: 01760 723703; Hill House, North Pickenham, Swaffham PE37 8JZ Tel: 01760 440679 — MB BS Lond. 1971 (St. Bart.) MRCS Eng. LRCP Lond. 1971; DObst RCOG 1973; Cert. JCC Lond. 1977. Specialty: Gen. Pract. Socs: BMA. Prev: Med. Off. DoH Bermuda; SHO (Paediat.) Pembury Hosp. Kent.; SHO (O & G) Freedom Fields Hosp. Plymouth.

RAYNER, Rosemary Jane Department of Paediatrics, New Cross Hospital, Wolverhampton WV10 0QP Tel: 01902 307999 Fax: 01902 643051; 100 Streetly Lane, Four Oaks, Sutton Coldfield B74 4TB Tel: 0121 353 0854 Fax: 01902 643051 — MB BS Lond. 1981 (Cambridge/London Hospital) MA Camb. 1982; DCH RCP Lond. 1983; MRCP (UK) 1984; DM Nottm. 1991; FRCPCH 1997. Cons. Paediat. Wolverhampton; Clin. Dir. Child. Servs. Roy. Wolverhampton Hosps. NHS Trust; Hon. Sen. Lect. Univ. Birm. Med. Sch. Specialty: Paediat. Socs: MDU; BMA & Brit. Paediat. Respirat. Gp.; Roy. Coll. Paeds. & Child Health - Clin. Directors Gp.. Prev: Research Fell. (Cystic Fibrosis) City Hosp. Nottm.; Sen. Regist. (Paediat.) Leeds; Regist. (Paediat.) City Hosp. Nottm.

RAYNER, Sandra Anne Immunology Department, ICSM, Hammersmith Hospital, Du Cane Road, London W12 0NN Tel: 020 8383 8174 Fax: 020 8383 2788; Flat 2, 17 Adamson Road, London NW3 3HV Tel: 020 7586 7920 — MB BChir Camb. 1988; MA Camb. 1990, BA 1986; FRCOphth 1994. Research Regist. (Immunol.) Hammersmith Hosp. Lond. Specialty: Ophth.

RAYNER, Sarah Ann Louise 45 Malvern Avenue, Fareham PO14 1QB — MB ChB Bristol 1998.

RAYNER, Shaun Price and Partners, The Surgery, Park Road, Holbeach, Spalding PE12 7EE Tel: 01406 423288 Fax: 01406 426284; White House, Bardsea, Ulverston LA12 9QT Tel: 01229 88542 — MB ChB Leeds 1985. Trainee GP Hull VTS. Prev: Ho. Off. (Med. & Surg.) Airedale Gen. Hosp. Steeton.

RAYNER, Mr Simeon Sharratt Lister House Surgery, Lister House, 53 Harrington Street, Pear Tree, Derby DE23 8PF Tel: 01332 271212 Fax: 01332 271939; 26 Stourport Drive, Chellaston, Derby DE73 1PX Tel: 01332 705440 — MB BS Lond. 1985; MA Oxf. 1986; FRCS Ed. 1989; FRCS Eng. 1989; MRCGP 1992; DRCOG 1992. Prev: Trainee GP Midway; SHO (Geriat. Med.) Derbysh. Roy. Infirm.

RAYNER, Thomas William (retired) The Cedars, Kenninghall, Norwich NR16 2ED Tel: 0195 388 8242 — MB BChir Camb. 1952; MRCGP 1968.

RAYNER, Tiina Alexandra 35 Tithebarn Street, Poulton-le-Fylde FY6 7BY — MB ChB Liverp. 1994. SHO (Med.) Blackpool Vict. NHS Trust. Specialty: Gen. Med. Prev: Ho. Off. Aintree Hosps. Trust Liverp.

RAYNES, Richard Hollings (retired) 88 Narrow Street, London E14 8BP — (St. Thos.) MB BS Lond. 1958; DPH London 1968; MFCM 1974. Prev: Med. Off. DHSS.

RAYNOR, Katherine Louise 9 Northeron, West Cross, Swansea SA3 5PJ Tel: 01792 401175 — MB BCh Wales 1997 (Cardiff) SHO Paediat., Singleton Hosp., Swansea. Specialty: Paediat.; Gen. Pract. Socs: MPS; BMA. Prev: SHO O & G - Singleton; SHO ENT - Singleton; SHO Ophth. - Singleton.

RAYNOR, Mathew Keith 31 Cranston Drive, Sale M33 2PB — MB ChB Manch. 1994. Specialist Regist., Manch. Roy. Eye Hosp. Specialty: Ophth. Prev: SHO (Ophth.) Soton. Eye Unit.

RAYNOR, Yvonne Margaret Marsh Street Surgery, 25A Marsh Street, Rothwell, Leeds LS26 0AG Tel: 0113 282 1571 Fax: 0113 282 4720 — MB ChB Leeds 1979; DRCOG 1982; Cert. Family Plann. JCC 1982.

RAYNSFORD, Andrew David Singleton Hospital, Swansea SA2 8QA — MB ChB Birm. 1986.

RAYTER, Mr Zenon Department of Surgery, Level 4, Bristol Royal Infirmary, Bristol BS2 8HW Tel: 0117 928 2883; 3 Royal York Mews, Royal York Crescent, Bristol BS8 4LF — MB BS Lond. 1977 (St. Geo.) FRCS Eng. 1981; BSc (Hons.) Lond. 1972, MS 1988. Cons. Surg. Bristol Roy. Infirm.; Hon. Sen. Lect. (Surg.) Bristol. Specialty: Gen. Surg. Socs: Brit. Assn. Surgic. Oncol.; Brit. Assn. Cancer Research; Roy. Soc. Med. (Counc. Mem. Sect. Surg.). Prev: Sen. Regist. (Surg.) & Regist. St. Geo. Hosp. Lond.; Regist. (Surg.) St. Jas. Hosp. Lond.; Research Fell. Roy. Marsden Hosp.

RAYTON, Edgar Leo The Surgery, 1 Manor House Lane, Yardley, Birmingham B26 1PE Tel: 0121 743 2273 Fax: 0121 722 2037 — MB ChB Sheff. 1960. Prev: Asst. Cas. Off. Roy. Hosp. Sheff.; Sen. Ho. Off. O & G Moorgate Gen. Hosp. Rotherham; Sen. Ho. Off. Paediat. City Gen. Hosp. Sheff.

RAZA, Asif 4 Lochview Drive, Hogganfield Park, Glasgow G33 1QF — MB ChB Glas. 1991.

RAZA, Karim MRC Centre for Immune Regulation, Division of Immunity & Infection, University of Birmingham, Birmingham B15 2TT — BM BCh Oxf. 1993; MRCP (UK) 1996. ARC Clin. Research Fell., Rheum. Univ. of Birm., Birm. Specialty: Rheumatol. Prev: Research Fell. (Rheum.) Roy. Nat. Hosp. Rheumatic Dis.; SHO Rotat. (Med.) Qu. Med. Centre Nottm.; Rhematology Specialist Regist., City Hosp., Birm.

RAZA, Kausar X Ray Department, Hillingdon Hospital, Uxbridge UB8 3NN Tel: 01895 279327 Fax: 01895 279865 Email: kausar.raza@thh.nhs.uk — MB BS Pakistan; FRCR; DMRD Lond.; FFR. p/t Cons. Radiologist, Hillingdon Hosp.; Cons. Breast Radiologist, N. Lond. Breast Screening Unit, Edgware. Specialty: Radiol. Socs: RCR Breast Group; Uk Paediatric Radiologists Gp. Prev: Specialist Regist. northwick Pk. Hosp., Harrow.

RAZA, Kazmi (retired) 58 Highfield Avenue, London NW11 9UD — MB BS Patna 1958; MS Patna 1965, MB BS 1958, DGO 1963; DRCOG 1969; FRCOG 1988, M 1970; FRCS Eng. 1989.

RAZA, Mr Masood 155 Albert Road, London N22 7AQ — MB BS Karachi 1983; FRCS Glas. 1991.

RAZA, Mohsin Primary Health Care Medical Centre, 31 Wargrave Road, Newton-le-Willows WA12 9QN Tel: 01925 220469 — MB BS Punjab 1967 (King Edwd. Med. Coll. Lahore) MB BS Punjab (Pakistan) 1967; DA Eng. 1969. Prev: Regist. (Anaesth.) Lincoln Co. Hosp., St. Geo. Hosp. Lincoln & Vict. Hosp. Kirkcaldy.

RAZA, Muhammad Naeem Dorset Renal Unit, Dorset County Hospital, Williams Avenue, Dorchester DT1 2JY Tel: 01305 251150 Fax: 01305 254756 — MB BS Punjab 1988 (Punjab Med. Coll. - Faisalabad, Pakistan) MRCP (UK) Roy. Coll. of Physicians Lond. Assoc. Specialist Renal Med. Dorset Renal Unit Dorset Co. Hosp. Specialty: Nephrol. Prev: Staff Nephrologist, Dorset Renal Unit, Dorset Co. Hosp.; SHO Med. Rotat., Dorchester; Regist. (Renal Med.) Dorset Renal Unit Dorchester.

RAZA, Mr Naeem 82 Salmon Street, London NW9 8PU — MB BS Karachi 1984; FRCS Eng. 1991.

RAZA, Syed Safdar St Nicholas Health Centre, Saunder Bank, Burnley BB11 2EN Tel: 01282 423677 Fax: 01282 832945 — MB BS Bihar 1969; MB BS Bihar 1969.

RAZA, Tanzeem Haider Acute Medicine, Royal Bournemouth Hospital, Bournemouth BH7 7DW Tel: 01202 704416 Fax: 01202 704435 Email: tanzeem.raza@rbch-tr.swest.nhs.uk — (King Edward Medical College, Lahore) MB BS Punjab, Pakistan; MCPS Karachi 1982; BSc Lahore 1985; FRCP Edin. 1996; FRCP London 1999. Cons. Phys. Gen. Med. Specialty: Gen. Med. Socs: Brit. Med. Assn.; Soc. for Acute Med.; Assn. for Study of Med. Educat. Prev: Assoc. Prof. Of Med., King Edwd. Med. Col.; Assist. Prof. of Med.; Semior Regist.

RAZA, Mr Zahid Royal Infirmary of Edinburgh, Vascular Unit, Ward 105, Old Dalkeith Road, Edinburgh EH16 4SU Tel: 0131 2423584; BUPA Murrayfield Hospital, 122 Corstorphine Road, Edinburgh EH12 6UD Tel: 0131 3340363; West Langton Farm, East Calder, Livingston EH53 0JW Tel: 01506 880159 Email: zraza@doctors.org.uk — MB ChB Dundee 1990; FRCS Ed. 1994; FRCS (Gen.) Ed. 2002; MD Dundee 2004. Cons. Vasc. Surg. & Hon. Sen. Lect. Roy. Infirm. Edin. Specialty: Gen. Surg. Special Interest: Vasc. Access, Claudication, Aortic Aneurysm Surg., Limb Salvage Surg. Prev: Specialist Regist. (Vasc. Surg.) S. E. Scot. (Ed.) HST Rotat.; Research Regist. (Vasc. Surg.) Ninewells Hosp. Dundee; SHO Rotat. (Gen. Surg.) Ninewells Hosp. & Med. Sch. Dundee.

RAZAK, Dr 26 Apple Close, Tilehurst, Reading RG31 6UR Tel: 01734 423916 Fax: 01734 423916 — MB BS Karachi 1965; DPM Eng. 1970; MRCPsych 1973; T(Psych) 1991. Hon. Cons. Trans-Cultural Psychiat. Oxf. RHA. Specialty: Gen. Psychiat. Socs: BMA. Prev: Sen. Regist. (Psychiat.) Barnet Gen. Hosp.; Sen. Regist. (Psychiat.) Napsbury Hosp.; Regist. (Psychiat.) Tooting Bec Hosp. Lond.

RAZAVI, Lawrence Michael 205 Grove End Gardens, Grove End Road, St Johns Wood, London NW8 9LT — MB BS Lond. 1960; MRCS Eng. LRCP Lond. 1960; MPH Harvard 1962. Adviser (Genetics) WHO. Specialty: Pub. Health Med. Socs: Fell. Roy. Soc. Med.; Harv. Med. Alumni Assn. Prev: Acad. (Med.) Oxf., Stanford & Harvard.

RAZIS, Platon Anthony Department of Anaesthesia, St. George's Healthcare NHS Trust, Blackshaw Road, Tooting, London SW17 0QT Tel: 020 8725 3316 Fax: 020 8767 5216 Email: raz@windward.freeserve.co.uk — MB ChB Rhodesia 1979; LRCP LRCS Ed. LRCPS Glas. 1979; FFA RCS Eng. 1985. Cons. Anaesth. St. Geo. & Atkinson Morley's Hosp. Lond. Specialty: Anaesth.; Intens. Care. Socs: Assn. Anaesth.; Neuroanaesth. Soc.; Intens. Care Soc. Prev: Sen. Regist. (Anaesth.) Univ. Coll. Hosp. Lond.; Regist. (Anaesth.) St. Geo. Hosp. Lond.; SHO (Anaesth.) Whittington & Univ. Coll. Hosps. Lond.

RAZOUQI, Bashar Mikail 5 Piper Close, Danes Court, Cardiff CF5 2RB — MB ChB Baghdad 1985.

RAZVI, Freda Miriam 15 Beresford Park, Sunderland SR2 7JU; 21 Brandling Park,, Jesmond, Newcastle upon Tyne NE2 4RR Tel: 0191 281 1133 — MB ChB Dundee 1993; MRCP UK 1997. Research Fell. (Diabetes & Endocrinol.) City Hosps. NHS Trust Birm. Specialty: Diabetes; Endocrinol.; Gen. Med. Socs: BMA; MDU; BDA. Prev: SHO Rotat. (Gen. Med.) S. Tees Acute NHS Trust Middlesbrough.

RAZVI, Syed Ahmed Hussain Walton Village Medical Centre, 172 Walton Village, Liverpool L4 6TW Tel: 0151 525 8254 Fax: 0151 525 6448 — MB BS Bangalore 1970; DTM & H Liverp. 1983. Specialty: Gen. Pract. Socs: Med. St Pauls. Prev: GP Saudi Arabia & Iran; Asst. Surg. Minto Eye Hosp., Bangalore.

RAZVI, Syed Omar (retired) 15 Beresford Park, Sunderland SR2 7JU Tel: 0191 565 3486 — MB BS Osmania 1955, DCP 1961. Prev: Haemat. S. Shields Gen. Hosp.

RAZVI, Syed Salman Queen Elizabeth Hospital, Department of Endocrinology, Gateshead NE9 6SY Tel: 0191 403 2754/0191 403 6186 — MB BS 1996; MRCP 2000. Specialist Regist. (Endocrinol.) Qu. Eliz. Hosp. Gateshead. Specialty: Endocrinol.; Diabetes.

RAZZAK, Abdul 5 Heycroft, Whitefield, Manchester M45 7HX Tel: 0161 796 7063 — MB BS Karachi 1965 (Dow Med. Coll. Karachi) BSc Karachi 1959, MB BS 1965; DA Eng. 1967; FFA RCS Eng. 1971. Cons. Anaesth. Manch. AHA (T). Specialty: Anaesth.

RAZZAK, Abdul Haji Moosa Haji Wali Muhammad Department of Psychiatry, Charing Cross Hospital, Fulham Palace Road, London W6 8RP Tel: 020 8846 1513 — MB BS Karachi 1981; MRCPsych 1988. Research Asst. (Psychiat.) Char. Cross & West. Med. Sch. Lond. Specialty: Gen. Psychiat. Prev: Regist. & Lect. Acad. Unit Horton Hosp. Epsom; Regist. Crichton Roy. Hosp. Dumfries.

RAZZAK, David (retired) Bas Séjour, Ruette des Fries, Cobo, Guernsey GY5 7PW Tel: 01481 257456 — BM BCh Oxf. 1948 (Oxf. & Lond. Hosp.) DObst RCOG 1950; MA Oxf. 1951; DA Eng. 1972. Prev: GP & Chairm. Med. Staff Comm. Princess Eliz. Hosp. Guernsey.

RAZZAK, Muna Salih Abdul Parkside Surgery, Tawney Street, Boston PE21 6PF Tel: 01205 365881 Fax: 01322 861471 Email: ikdickinson@tinyworld.co.uk; The Burrows, Hall Lane, Frampton, Boston PE20 1AB Tel: 01205 722129 — MB ChB Baghdad 1978. GP Boston Lincs.; Clin. Asst. Oncol. Specialty: Gen. Pract.

RAZZAQ, Furhan 59 Heathside Road, Withington, Manchester M20 4XH — MB ChB Manch. 1995 (Manchester) MRCP (UK) 1999; DRCOG (UK) 2001. Specialty: Gen. Med.; Respirat. Med.

RAZZAQ, Ghizala Flat 3, 19 Leamington Terrace, Edinburgh EH10 4JP — MB ChB Manch. 1990.

RAZZAQ, Isma 51 Talbot Crescent, Leeds LS8 1AL — MB ChB Leeds 1993.

RAZZAQ, Nasrin 17 Park Road, London NW4 3PT — MB ChB Manch. 1993.

RAZZAQ, Mr Quaisar Mahmood 67 Longspring, Watford WD24 6QA Tel: 01923 441274 Fax: 01923 336648 — MB ChB Aberd. 1985; FRCS Glas. 1991; FMGEMS 1992. Cons. (A & E) N. Hants. Hosp. Basingstoke. Specialty: Accid. & Emerg. Prev: Regist. (A & E) Good Hope Hosp. Birm.; Regist. (Cardiothoracic Surg.) W. Midl. RHA; SHO & Regist. (Cardiothoracic Surg.) St. Thos. Hosp. Lond.

RAZZAQ, Rubeena 17 Norford Way, Rochdale OL11 5QS Tel: 01706 32827 — MB ChB Manch. 1988; FRCR (UK) 1995, MRCP (UK) 1991. Cons. Radiol., Bolton Hosp. Bolton. Specialty: Radiol. Prev: Regist. (Diagnostic Radiol.) Manch.; SHO (Med. Oncol. & Radiotherap.) Christie Hosp. Manch.; SHO (Med.) Burnley Gen. Hosp. & Wythenshawe Hosp. Manch.

RAZZAQUE, Mira Flat 37 Penthouse, Matheson Lang House, Baylis Road, Waterloo, London SE1 7AN Tel: 020 7928 5690 — MB BS Lond. 1990 (Middlx. Hosp. Univ. Coll. Med. Sch.) MRCP 1992; FFA & Dub. 1997. Specialist Regist. Rotat. (Anaesth.) NW Thames Middlx. Hosp. & Univ. Coll. Hosp. Specialty: Anaesth. Socs: Med. Protec. Soc.; MRCAnaesth. & Dub./Lond.

RAZZAQUE, Mohammed Abdur Calderstones NHS Trust, Mitton Road, Whalley, Clitheroe BB7 9PE Tel: 01254 821312 Fax: 01254 823023; Silverley, Whitehall Terrace, Darwen BB3 2LL Tel: 01254 775808 — MB BS Rajshahi 1965; Annual Cert. of Completion of CPD, Roy. Coll. Psych.; FRCPsych Lond.; Dip. Psychol. Med. RCP Lond. RCS Eng. 1973; DFFP Lond. 1980; Cert. Psychosexual Counselling Manch. 1982. Cons. Psychiat. (Ment. Handicap) N. West. RHA & Med. Dir. Calderstone NHS Trust. Specialty: Ment. Health; Forens. Psychiat. Socs: Fell. Roy. Soc. Health. Prev: Sen. Regist. (Ment. Health & Develop. Paediat.) Regist. (Psychiat.).

RAZZELL, Philip John Town Medical Centre, 25 London Road, Sevenoaks TN13 1AR Tel: 01732 454545 — MB BS Lond. 1980 (Guy's) BSc (Hons.) Lond. 1977; MRCS Eng. LRCP Lond. 1980; DRCOG 1982; DGM RCP Lond. 1996. Hosp. Pract. (Geriat. Med.) S.W. Kent PCT, Sevenoaks Hosp. Kent; Hosp. Pract.(Ment. Health Serv.s for Older People) W. Kent Health & Social Care Trust NHS Trust, Darent Ho. Sevenoaks Hosp. Kent.

REA, Anthony James Cumberland Infirmary , Genito-Urinary Medicine, Carlisle CA2 7HY Tel: 01228 523444 — MB BS Lond. 1988 (Char. Cross & Westm. Med. Sch.) BSc (Hons.) Pharmacol. & Therap. Lond. 1984; MRCS Eng. LRCP Lond. 1988; MRCP (UK) 1993; FRCP Lond. 2002; MPH Leeds 2002. Cons Genito-Urinary Med., Cumbld. Infirm., Carlisle; Lect. in Pub. Health, Nuffield Inst., Univ. of Leeds. Specialty: Genitourinary Medicine. Special Interest: Academic Public Health. Socs: BASHH. Prev: Lect. (HIV & Genitourin. Med.) Kings Coll. Hosp.; Regist. (HIV & Genitourin. Med.) Roy. Lond. Hosp.; Ho. Off. (Med.) St. Stephens Hosp. Fulham.

REA, Daniel William 7 Serpentine Road, Selly Park, Birmingham B29 7HU; 4 Queens Gate Villas, Victoria Pk Road, London E9 7BU — MB BS Lond. 1986; BSc (Hons.) Bristol 1981; MRCP (UK) 1990.

REA, Duncan Patrick Alconbury and Brampton Surgeries, The Surgery, School Lane, Alconbury, Huntingdon PE28 4EQ Tel: 01480 890281 Fax: 01480 891787 — BM BCh Oxf. 1992; MA Camb. 1993; DRCOG 1995; MRCGP 1996. Partner GP Pract. Sch. La. Alconbury Huntingdon.

REA, George Rupert Albertville Surgery, 16 McCandless Street, Crumlin Road, Belfast BT13 1RU Tel: 028 9074 6308 Fax: 028 9074 9847; 69 Broadacres, Temple Patrick, Ballyclare BT39 0AY — (Queens University of Belfast) MB BCh BAO Belf. 1966; DObst RCOG 1970; MRCGP 1972. Specialty: Gen. Pract. Socs: Fell. Ulster Med. Soc.; BMA (Ex-Chairm. East. Div. N. Irel.).

REA, Irene Maeve — MB BCh BAO Belf. 1972; MD Belf. 1986 BSc 1969; MRCP (UK) 1979; FRCP Ed. 1991; FRCP Lond. 1993. Cons. Phys. (Geriat. Med.) Belf. City Hosp.; Sen. Lect. Qu. Univ. Belf. Specialty: Care of the Elderly. Socs: Brit. Geriat. Soc.; Brit. Soc. of Immunol.; Irish Gerontology Soc.

REA, Rt. Hon. Lord John Nicolas (retired) 11 Anson Road, London N7 0RB Tel: 020 7607 0546 Fax: 020 7687 1219 Email: reajn@parliament.uk — (Camb. & Univ. Coll. Hosp.) MB BChir Camb. 1955; DObst RCOG 1956; DCH Eng. 1957; DPH Lond. 1966; MD Camb. 1969; FRCGP 1989, M 1971. Prev: Princip. GP Lond.

REA, Margaret Alice Skeoge House, Brookeborough, Enniskillen BT94 4GN — MB BCh BAO Belf. 1993.

REA, Owen Henry The Terrace Surgery, 2 Dhu Varren Park, Portrush BT56 8EL Tel: 028 7082 4637 Fax: 028 7082 4637 — MB BCh BAO Belf. 1984.

REA, Mr Peter Anthony The Leicester Royal Infirmary, Department Of Ear Nose and Throat Surgery, Infirmary Square, Leicester LE1 5WW Tel: 0116 2585242; BUPA Hospital Leicester, Gartree Road, Oadby, Leicester LE2 2FF Tel: 0116 2653014 — BM BCh Oxf. 1991 (Camb. and Oxf.) MA Camb. 1988; FRCS Eng. 1995; FRCS (OTO) 1997. Cons. Surg. (adult and paediatric ENT Surg.). Specialty: Otorhinolaryngol. Special Interest: balance disorders and vertigo, Otol., paediatric ENT, rhinology. Socs: MPS, BMA, FRCS, BAPO, EAONO, BAO-HNS, RSM.

REA, Richard Ernest Ballymena Health Centre, Cushendall Road, Ballymena BT43 6HQ Tel: 028 2564 2181 Fax: 028 2565 8919 — MB ChB Ed. 1969; BSc Ed. 1966, MB ChB 1969; FRCGP 1991, M 1975; MICGP 1987.

REA, Rustam Denzil 69 BRoadacres, Templepatrick, Ballyclare BT39 0AY; 15 Far Rye, Wollaton, Nottingham NG8 1GJ — BM BCh Oxf. 1996. Specialist Regist. (Diabetes) Nottm. City Hosp. Specialty: Gen. Med.

REA, Shelagh Mary Ardvilla, 9 Victoria Park, Londonderry BT47 2AD Tel: 02871 348563 — MB BCh BAO Belf. 1974; MRCPsych 1978. Cons. Psychiat. (Old Age Psychiat.), Foyle Health and Social Serv.s Trust. Specialty: Geriat. Psychiat. Socs: Mem. Roy. Coll. Psychiatr.; Ulster Med. Soc.; Brit. Feriatric Soc.

REA, Vanree Alne Cross, Alne, York YO61 1SD — MB BCh BAO Belf. 1964; DA RCPSI 1968.

REA, William Edward Flat 10, Grenofen House, Grenofen, Tavistock PL19 9ES — MB BS Lond. 1996.

REACHER, Mark Henry — MD Lond. 1995 (Westm.) MB BS 1976; FRCS (Gen. Surg.) Eng. 1981; FRCS (Ophth.) Glas. 1984; MPH Johns Hopkins Univ. 1988; DPH Camb. 1994; MFPHM 1995; FFPHM 2002.

READ, Andrew Mabyn (retired) 26 Magdala Road, Cosham, Portsmouth PO6 2QG Tel: 023 9237 8185 — MRCS Eng. LRCP Lond. 1942 (St. Thos.) Prev: Asst. Phys. Chest. Clinic Portsmouth.

READ, Annette Catherine Plymouth Community Drugs Service, Plymouth Primary Care Trust, Damerel House, Damerel Cl., off Madden Road, Devonport, Plymouth PL1 4JZ Tel: 01752 56670 Fax: 01752 56670 — MB BS Lond. 1973 (London Hospital) BSc (Anat.) Lond. 1970; MRCPsych 1978; FRCPsych 1999. Cons. Psychiat. Plymouth Comm.NHS Trust. Specialty: Gen. Psychiat. Prev: Sen. Regist. (Psychiat.) Roy. United Hosp. Bath; Sen. Research Assoc. Avon Drug Research & Rehabil. Project Bristol; Sen. Regist. (Psychiat.) Glenside Hosp. Bristol.

READ, Bruce Alfred Norman 4 Llington Close, Lichfield WS13 7AL Tel: 01543 262843 Email: bamyread@aol.com — MB BS Lond. 1966 (Lond. Hosp.) MRCS Eng. LRCP Lond. 1965. Prev: Regist. (Clin. Path,) Guy's Hosp. Lond.; Regist. (Path.) Groote Scheur Hosp., Cape Town.

READ, Catherine Anne Fairways, Saltergate Lane, Bamford, Hope Valley S33 0BE — MB ChB Sheff. 1983.

READ, Mr Colin Andrew 52A Ounsdale Road, Wombourne, Wolverhampton WV5 8BH Email: drcolinread@hotmail.com — MB ChB Leic. 1992; FRCS Lond. 1996; FFAEM Lond. 2001. Cons. in A&E Med., Dudley. Specialty: Accid. & Emerg. Prev: SPR Leicester.

READ, David Edward The Wistaria Practice, Wistaria Court, 18 Avebye Riad, Lymington SO41 9PJ Tel: 01590 672212 Fax: 01590 679930 — MB BS Lond. 1975 (Char. Cross) MRCS Eng. LRCP Lond. 1975; FRCA. 1982; DRCOG 1984; MRCGP 1994. Specialty: Anaesth. Prev: Regist. (Anaesth.) Soton HA; Trainee GP Soton VTS.

READ, David Henry Princess Royal Hospital, Lewes Road, Haywards Heath RH16 4EX — MB ChB Bristol 1973; BSc (Hons.) Bristol 1970, MB ChB 1973; FFA RCS Eng. 1979. Cons. Anaesth. S.W. Thames RHA Princess Roy. Hosp. Specialty: Anaesth.

READ, David John District General Hospital, Turner Road, Colchester CO4 — BM BCh Oxf. 1971; MRCP (U.K.) 1974.

READ, Lady (Frances Edna) 173 Bickenhall Mansions, Baker St., London W1U 6BU Tel: 020 7935 3629 — MB BCh BAO Dub. 1929 (T.C. Dub.) BA, MB BCh BAO Dub. 1929; FFA RCSI 1960. Hon. Cons. Anaesth. Samarit. Hosp. Wom.; Hon. Anaesth. Chelsea Hosp. Wom. Specialty: Anaesth. Prev: Sen. Res. Anaesth. Char. Cross Hosp.; Dep. Anaesth. Roy. Nat. Orthop. Hosp.; Hon. Anaesth. All St.s' Genitourin. Hosp.

READ, Gordon Alistair 6 Kennesbourne Court, Tuffnells Way, Harpenden AL5 3HT Tel: 01582 712 684 Email: gordanaread@aol.com — (Birmingham) MB ChB Birm. 1966; DMRT Liverp. 1977; FRCR Lond. 1980. Cons. Clin. Oncologist N. Middlx. Univ. Hosp.; Hon. Cons. Clin. Oncol. & Radiat. Ther. Trent RHA; Cons. Clin. Oncol. Hosp. St. John & St. Eliz. Lond.; PPP/Columia Gp. of Hosps., The Lond. Clinic, The Cromwell Hosp. The Lond. Bridge. Specialty: Oncol.; Radiother. Socs: Fell. Roy. Coll. Radiologists; Brit. Inst. Radiol.; Roy. Soc. Med. Prev: Med. Adviser,Oncol.Internat. DC Ltd; Cons. Radiother. & Oncol. Lincs.; Sen. Regist. (Radiother.) West. Gen. Hosp. Edin.

READ, Graham Royal Preston Hospital, Sharoe Green Lane N., Fulwood, Preston PR2 9HT Tel: 01772 522089 Fax: 01772 522178 Email: graham.read@lthtr.nhs.uk — MB BChir Camb. 1972 (Cambridge) MA Camb. 1972; MRCP (UK) 1974; FRCR 1978; FRCP 2001. Cons. Clin. Oncol. Roy. Preston Hosp.; Med. Director, Lanc & S.Cumbria cancer network. Specialty: Oncol.; Radiother. Socs: Amer. Soc. Clin. Oncol.; Brit. Assn. Cancer Research; Amer. Soc. Therapeutic Radiol. & Oncol. Prev: Cons. Clin. Oncol., Christie Hosp. Manch.; Sen. Regist. (Radiother.) & Regist. (Radiother.) Christie Hosp. Manch.; Sen. Health Off. (Gastroenterol.) Manch. Roy. Infirm.

READ, Gregory Martin Fressingfield Medical Centre, New Street, Fressingfield, Eye IP21 5PJ Tel: 01379 586227 Fax: 01379 588265; Old Leaf Cottage, Earsham Road, Hedenham, Bungay NR35 2DF Tel: 01508 482581 Email: gregread@doctors.org.uk — MB ChB Manch. 1979 (Univ. Manch.) DRCOG 1984. Specialty: Gen. Pract. Special Interest: Acupunc.; Palliat. Care. Socs: BMA; BMAS. Prev: SHO (Neonat. Paediat.) Bristol Matern. Hosp.; SHO (Radiother. & Oncol.) Cheltenham Gen. Hosp.; SHO (Ophth.) Leighton Hosp.

READ, Heather Susan 8 Bryce Avenue, Edinburgh EH7 6TX — MB ChB Ed. 1991; BSc (Med. Sci.) St. And. 1987; FRCS Ed. 1995. Regist. (Orthop.) Princess Margt. Rose Hosp. Edin. Specialty: Orthop. Prev: SHO Rotat. (Surg.) SE Scotl.

READ, James Adam Poole Gatton Surgery, Sutton Scotney, Winchester SO21 3LE — MB BS Lond. 1993 (Guy's Hosp. Lond.) MA Camb. 1990; DRCOG 1995; DCH RCP Lond. 1996; MRCGP 1997; MRCGP 1997.

READ, James Michael 5 Strathavon Close, Cranleigh GU6 8PW — BM BS Nottm. 1998; BM BS Nottm 1998.

READ, Jason Matthew 12 Bramber Way, Burgess Hill RH15 8JX — MB ChB Liverp. 1996.

READ, Jennifer Mary 24 Beck Road, London E8 4RE — MB BS Lond. 1991.

READ, Joan Margaret 1 Jacklyns Close, Alresford SO24 9LL — MB BS Lond. 1957.

READ, Mr John Lewis (retired) Wroxham, 196 North Road, Hertford SG14 2PJ Tel: 01992 586820 — MB BS Lond. 1954 (Univ. Coll. Hosp.) FRCS Ed. 1966. Prev: Cons. Orthop. Surg. Princess Alexandra Hosp. Harlow, Co. Hosp. Hertford & Qu. Eliz. II Hosp. Welwyn Gdn. City.

READ, John Robert Montresor Anaesthetics Department, Aberdeen Royal Infirmary, Aberdeen AB11 6YG — MB ChB Dundee 1983; BSc Dund. 1979; FCAnaesth. 1991; DA (UK) 1991. Sen. Regist. (Anaesth.) Aberd. Roy. Infirm. Specialty: Anaesth. Prev: Regist. (Anaesth.) Roy. Infirm. Edin.

READ, John Roderick Dept of Histopathology, Hull Royal Infirmary, Anlaby Rd, Hull HU3 2JZ Tel: 01482 607711; 3 St. Matthew's Court, Minster Moorgate, Beverley HU17 8JH Tel: 01482 864051 — MB ChB Birm. 1969; BSc Birm. 1966; FRCPath 1988, M 1976. Cons. Histopath. Specialty: Histopath. Prev: Sen. Regist. (Morbid Anat.) King's Coll. Hosp. & Kingston-on-Thames; Hosp.; Regist. (Path.) Bristol Roy. Infirm.

READ, Jonathan Asher Jason Marcus 86 Stopples Lane, Hordle, Lymington SO41 0GL — MB BS Lond. 1998; MB BS Lond 1998.

READ, Juliette Helen Mary The Oak House, St Ann's Hospital, St Ann's Road, London N15 3TH Tel: 020 8442 6000 — MB ChB Liverp. 1990. SHO (Psychiat.) St Anns Hosp. Lond. Specialty: Gen. Psychiat.

READ, Katherine Gwenda 3 Arlington Villas, Bristol BS8 2ED — MB ChB Bristol 1998.

READ, Kathleen Margaret Long View, Castle Rise, Spittal, Haverfordwest SA62 5QW — MB ChB Liverp. 1971.

READ, Mr Laurence Droitwich Private Hospital, St Andrew's Road, Droitwich WR9 8DN Tel: 01905 794793 — MB BS Lond. 1971 (St. Bart.) BSc (Zool., Hons.) Lond. 1960, MB BS 1971; MRCS Eng. LRCP Lond. 1971; FRCS Eng. 1977. Cons. Orthop. & Traum. Surg. Alexandra Hosp., BromsGr. & Redditch HA. Specialty: Orthop. Socs: Brit. Orthop. Assn. & Orthop. Foot Soc. Prev: Clin. Lect. (Orthop.) & Hon. Sen. Regist. Univ. Dept. Orthop. Surg.; Hope Hosp. Salford, Lancs.; Regist. (Orthop.) Nuffield Orthop. Centre Headington.

READ, Lucien (retired) 20 Pleck Farm Avenue, Blackburn BB1 8PE Tel: 01254 53789 — MB BChir Camb. 1941 (St. Mary's) MRCS Eng. LRCP Lond. 1940. Hon. Cons. Venereol. Blackburn, Burnley, Chorley & Bury Hosp. Gps. Prev: Venereol. Co. Boro. Oldham.

READ, Malcolm Trevor Fitzwalter 7 Waterden Road, Guildford GU1 2AN Tel: 01483 566442 Fax: 01483 566442; Barbican Health, 3 White Lyon Court, The Barbican, London EC2Y 3EA Tel: 020 7588 3146 Fax: 020 7628 1831 — (Camb. & St. Thos.) FRCSP(E) Wol; MA Camb. 1966; MB Camb. 1967, BChir 1966; DObst RCOG 1969; MRCGP 1977; DMS Med. Soc. Apoth. Lond. 1994; FISM 1999. Orthop. & Sport Phys. Barbican Health Clinic & Guildford; Lect. & Examr. MSc Course Sports Med. Lond. Hosp. & Soc. Apoth. Specialty: Orthop.; Sports Med.; Rehabil. Med. Socs: Pres. UKADIS.; Roy. Soc. Med.; Brit. Inst. Musculoskeletal Med. Prev: Med. Off. English Commonw. & Brit. Olympic Teams.

READ, Maria Grazyna, MBE — MB ChB Sheff. 1972; DCH Eng. 1974. Semor Partner, DoverCt. Surg. Specialty: Respirat. Med. Prev: Research Fell. (Gastroenterol.) Roy. Hallamsh. Hosp. Sheff.; Research Fell. Univ. Texas Dallas, USA.

READ, Martyn Sinclair Department of Anaeshetics, University Hospital of Wales, Heath Park, Cardiff CF14 4XW Tel: 029 2074 3107 Fax: 029 2074 7203 — MB BS Lond. 1981; FFA RCS Eng. 1986. Cons. Anaesth. & ITU Univ. Hosp. Wales Cardiff. Specialty: Anaesth. Prev: Sen. Regist. (Anaesth.) Morriston Hosp. Swansea & Univ. Hosp. Wales Cardiff; Research Asst. (Anaesth.) Univ. Hosp. Wales Cardiff; Regist. & SHO (Anaesth.) St. Mary's Hosp. Lond.

READ, Mr Michael David Maternity Department, Gloucestershire Royal Hospital, Great Western Road, Gloucester GL1 3NN Tel: 01452 528555 Fax: 01452 395556 — MD 1981, MB ChB Manch. 1970; FRCS Ed. 1976; FRCOG 1991, M 1976; FRACOG 1981, M 1981. Cons. O & G Glos. Roy. Hosp. Specialty: Obst. & Gyn.

READ, Nathanael Peter (retired) Meadow Lea, Herne Common, Herne Bay CT6 7LB Tel: 01227 375569; The Stowe, Amberley, Arundel BN18 9NN Tel: 01798 831423 — (Middlx.) MRCS Eng. LRCP Lond. 1942; DA Eng. 1949; FFA RCS Eng. 1954. Prev: Cons. Anaesth. Canterbury & Isle of Thanet Hosp. Gps.

READ, Neil Edward Sandpiper, Turvey Mill, Turvey, Bedford MK43 8ET — MB BS Lond. 1997.

READ, Nicholas John Blackmore Health Centre, Blackmore Drive, Sidmouth EX10 8ET Tel: 01395 512601 Fax: 01395 578408 — MB BS Lond. 1984 (Middlx. Hosp. Med. Sch.) MRCGP 1988; DRCOG 1990. Specialty: Care of the Elderly. Prev: GP Melbourne, Austral.; Trainee GP Exeter VTS; SHO (O & G) Odstock Hosp. Salisbury.

READ, Professor Nicholas Wallace Centre for Human Nutrition, Northern General Hospital, Sheffield S5 7AU Tel: 0114 242 1528 Fax: 0114 261 0112 Email: n.w.read@sheffield.ac.uk; 74 Nairn Street, Crookes, Sheffield S10 1UN Tel: 0114 267 8633 Email: N.W.Read@sheffield.ac.uk — MB BChir Camb. 1971 (Camb. & Lond. Hosp.) MRCP (UK) 1972; MA Camb. 1975, MD 1981; FRCP Lond. 1985; MA Sheffield 1997. Cons. Phys. Psychoanal. Psychotherapist North. Gen. Hosp. Shefield, Comm. Helth Sheff. Trust; Hon. Cons. Gastroenterol. Trent RHA 1981; Analyt. Psychotherapist 1993. Specialty: Gastroenterol.; Psychother. Socs: Brit. Soc. Gastroenterol.; UK Counc. for Psychother.; Amer. Gastroenterol. Assoc. Prev: Dir. Sheff. Univ. Centre for Human Nutrit. 1990; Prof. Integrated Med. Univ. Sheff.1998-2001; Prof. Gastrointestinal Physiol. & Nutrit. Univ. Sheff. 1988-1990.

READ, Peter (retired) 15 Testwood Court, Clifton Gardens, Folkestone CT20 2EF Tel: 01303 210090 — MRCS Eng. LRCP Lond. 1947 (Guy's) Prev: Receiv. Room Off. Poplar Hosp.

READ, Peter Brydon (retired) Lane's End, Bowling Green Lane, Hanley Castle, Worcester WR8 0BP Tel: 01684 592776 — (Middlx.) MB BS Lond. 1954; DObst RCOG 1960; DPM Eng. 1965. Indep. Psychother. Worcs. Prev: Regist. Psychiat. Shenley Hosp.

READ, Peter Robert, CBE Marchfields, Cockpole Green, Wargrave, Reading RG10 8NL Tel: 01189 401277 Fax: 01189 404287 — (Char. Cross) MB BS Lond. 1964; DObst RCOG 1967; FFPM RCP (UK) 1989; DSc (Hon.) De Montfont 1994; FRCP Lond. 1996. Non Exec. Director Collect Gp. Plc; Non Exec Director Vernalis Plc; Non Exec. Director SCC Internat. Plc; Non Exec. Director Innogenetics; Director SEEDA (South E. Eng. Developm. Agency); Chairm. Hoechst Unlimited. Prev: SHO, Ho. Phys. & Ho. Surg. Char. Cross Hosp. Lond.; Dir. Datapharm. Pub.ats. Ltd.; Non-Exec. Dir. Hoechst Schering Agrevo UK Ltd.

READ, Mrs Priscilla Elise Smithy Hall, Cookridge Lane, Leeds LS16 7NE — BM BCh Oxf. 1971; DCH Eng. 1974.

READ, Professor Robert Charles Infectious Diseases Unit, Royal Hallamshire Hospital, Sheffield S10 2JF Tel: 0114 271 3561 Fax: 0114 275 3061 Email: r.c.read@sheffield.ac.uk — MB ChB Sheff. 1982; MD Sheff. 1992, BMedSci 1980; MRCP (UK) 1985; FRCP 1998. Cons. Phys. & Reader (Infec. Dis.) Centr. Sheff. Univ. Hosps.; Cons. Phys. & Prof. (Infectious Diseases) Sheff. Teaching Hosp. Specialty: Infec. Dis.; Gen. Med.; Trop. Med. Socs: Infect. Dis. Soc. Amer.; Brit. Infect. Soc. (Meetings Sec.); Mem. Counc. Europ. Soc. Clin. Microbiol. & Infec. Diseases. Prev: Peel Trav. Fell. San Francisco Gen. Hosp. USA; Clin. Research Fell. Nat. Heart & Lung Inst. Roy. Brompton Hosp. Lond.; Regist. & Hon. Lect. (Med.) Northwick Pk. Hosp. & Clin. Research Centre Harrow.

READ, Ruth Elizabeth Northview Farm, Beaumont, Carlisle CA5 6EF — MB ChB Sheff. 1988; MRCP (UK) 1992; CCST 1997. Consultant A&E, Cumberland Infirmary, Carlisle. Specialty: Accid. & Emerg. Prev: Sen. Regist. (A & E) South. Gen. Hosp. Glas.; Career Regist. & SHO (A & E) Glas. Roy. Infirm.; SHO (Med.) Morriston Hosp. Swansea.

READ, Simon Mihill The Old Vicarage, Spilsby Road, Horncastle LN9 6AL Tel: 01507 522477 Fax: 01507 522997; 40 Elmhirst Road, Horncastle LN9 5LU Tel: 01507 527108 Email: simon.read@virgin.net — MB ChB Leeds 1982; BSc Leeds 1979, MB ChB 1982; DRCOG 1987. Princip. GP Horncastle.

READ, Professor Stephen Geoffrey University of Huddersfield, Ramsden Building, Queensgate, Huddersfield HD1 3DH Tel: 01484 473498 Fax: 01484 472794 Email: s.read@hud.ac.uk — MB BS Lond. 1975; MRCS Eng. LRCP Lond. 1975; MRCPsych. 1981; FRCPsych 1997; MD (Leeds) 1997. Prof. of Psychiat. & Cons. in Psychiat. in Learning Disabil. Huddersfield & S. W. Yorks. Ment. Health NHS Trust. Specialty: Ment. Health. Prev: Sen. Lect. & Cons. in Psychiat. in Learning Disabil., Univ. of Leeds & Leeds Community & Ment. Health Servs. (Teachg.) Trust.

READ, Timothy Rupert Charles Department Psychiatry, Royal London Hospital, Whitechapel, London E1 1BB Tel: 020 7375 1052 — MB BS Lond. 1982 (Westm.) BSc (Hons.) Lond. 1979, MB BS 1982; MRCPsych. 1988. Cons. Psychiat.& Hon. Sec. Roy. Lond. Hosp. Trust; Clin. Director Adult Ment. Health. Specialty: Gen. Psychiat.; Psychother. Socs: Inst. Gp. Anal.; Gp. Analyt. Soc. Prev: Sen. Regist. (Psychiat.) Univ. Coll. Hosp. Lond.; Clin. Lect. (Psychiat. Middlx. Hosp. Lond.; Regist. (Psychiat.) St. Geo. Hosp. Lond.

READ, Zoe Helen 40 Lindford Chase, Lindford, Bordon GU35 0TB — MB BS Lond. 1998; MB BS Lond 1998.

READE, David William The Orrell Park Surgery, 46 Moss Lane, Orrell Park, Liverpool L9 8AL Tel: 0151 525 2736 Fax: 0151 524 1037; 6 Rose Place, Aughton, Ormskirk L39 4UJ Tel: 01695 422129 — MB ChB Liverp. 1986 (Liverpool) MRCGP 1991. Hosp. Pract. (Thoracic Med.) Aintree Chest Centre Fazakerley Hosp.

Liverp.; Treas. Continuing Educat. Support Gp.; Chairm. Liverp. MAAG. Prev: Trainee GP Maghull Liverp.; SHO (A & E) Walton Gen. Hosp. Liverp.; SHO (Anaesth.) Walton Gen. Hosp. Liverp.

READER, Andrew Graham Maxwell — MB BS Lond. 1982 (Lond. Hosp.) DRCOG 1986; MRCGP 1986; Cert. Family Plann. JCC 1987. Specialty: Gen. Pract. Prev: Trainee GP Shoreham-by-Sea W. Sussex VTS & Worthing VTS; SHO (Psychiat.) Brighton HA.

READER, Antony Maxwell (retired) 5 The Saltings, Birdham, Chichester PO20 7JA Tel: 01243 514853 — MB BS Lond. 1950 (Guy's) MRCS Eng. LRCP Lond. 1950; DObst RCOG 1955. Prev: Med. Staff Horsham Hosp.

READER, Carole Alison Stanton House, Hyde Lane, Newnham GL14 1HQ — MB BCh Wales 1984; BPharm (Hons.) Wales 1974, MB BCh 1984. GP Glos. Asst.; Sen. Clin. Med. Off. (Family Plann.).

READER, Claire Elizabeth 27 Coral Drive, Ipswich IP1 5HP — BM BS Nottm. 1997.

READER, David Cedric, Group Capt. RAF Med. Br. (retired) Kingsmede, Crondall Road, Crookham Village, Fleet GU51 5SU — (Univ. Coll. Hosp.) PhD Lond. 1975, BSc (Physiol.) 1958; MB BS Lond. 1961; MRCS Eng. LRCP Lond. 1961. Prev: Commanding Off. Aviat. Med. Train. Centre.

READER, Frances Clare Ipswich Hospital NHS Trust, Heath Road, Ipswich IP4 5PD Tel: 01473 703016 Fax: 01473 703015 — MB BS Lond. 1973 (Univ. Coll. Hosp.) FRCOG 1995, M 1982; MFFP 1993. Cons. Reproduc. Health Ipswich Hosps. NHS Trust; Cons. Reproduc. Health, Suff. W. PCT, Bury St Edmunds. Specialty: Family Plann. & Reproduc. Health; Psychosexual Med. Socs: Fac. Fam. Plann. & Reproduc. Health; RCOG; Brit. Assn. for Sexual and Relationship Ther. Prev: Edr. in Chief, Jl. of Family Plann. and Reproductive Health Care.

READER, Peter Mark Suthergrey House Surgery, 37A St. Johns Road, Watford WD17 1LS Tel: 01923 224424 Fax: 01923 243710; 24 Bisham Gardens, Highgate, London N6 6DD — MB BS Lond. 1988 (Roy. Free Hosp.) DCH RCP Lond. 1990; MRCGP 1992. Pract. Partner Watfert Herts.; Chairm. Watford & Three Rivers PCG. Prev: Trainee GP Northwick Pk. Hosp. Harrow VTS.

READING, Mr Alexander David The Alexandra Hospital, Woodrow Drive, Redditch B98 7UB Tel: 01527 503030 Fax: 01527 517432; Camelot Cottage, Ilington, Worcester WR7 4DH Email: alexreading@hotmail.com — MB ChB Glas. 1990; FRCS Eng. 1994; FRCS 2000; MD Leicester 2001. Cons. Orthop. & Truama. Specialty: Orthop. Socs: BORS; BOA (Ass). Prev: HIP Fell. Bristol; Specialist Regist. Rotat. (Orthop.) W. Scotl.; Clin. Research Fell. (Orthop.) Leicester & Rugby.

READING, Catherine Althea The Priory Surgery, 326 Wells Road, Bristol BS4 2QJ Tel: 0117 949 3988 Fax: 0117 778250 — MB BS Lond. 1975 (Middlx.) DCH Eng. 1978; DRCOG 1979; MRCP (UK) 1980. Prev: SHO (Paediat.) Roy. United & St. Martins Hosp. Bath; SHO (Obst.) Southmead Hosp. Bristol; SHO (Paediat.) Freedom Fields Hosp. Plymouth.

READING, James Henry Medical Centre, Rushden NN10 9TU Tel: 01933 314836 — MB BS Lond. 1950 (St. Bart.) MRCS Eng. LRCP Lond. 1950; DTM & H Eng. 1963; DTM & H Lond 1963. Local Treasury Med. Off.; Med. Off. Shaftesbury Soc. Homes for Disabled. Prev: Specialist in Med. RAF Hosp. Uxbridge; Ho. Phys. & Ho. Surg. St. John's Hosp. Lewisham; Ho. Surg. (Obst.) Lewisham Gen. Hosp.

READING, Jane Maralyn 11 Glover Close, Sawston, Cambridge CB2 4UP — MB BS Lond. 1978; MRCS (Eng.) 1978; LRCP Lond. 1978; Cert FPA 1981; T(GP) 1991.

READING, Jonathan Graham Ryders Farm, Manchester Rd, Kearsley, Bolton BL4 8RU — MB ChB Ed. 1997.

READING, Nicholas Graham Whipps Cross Hospital, Whipps Cross Road, London E11 1NR Tel: 020 8535 6652 Fax: 020 8535 6719; 48 Inderwick Road, London N8 9LD Tel: 020 8341 9726 — MB BChir Camb. 1979 (Middlx.) MRCP (UK) 1982; MA Camb. 1982; FRCR 1985. Cons. Radiol. Whipps Cross Hosp. Lond. Specialty: Radiol. Prev: SHO (Neurol.) Nat. Hosp. Nerv. Dis. Qu. Sq. Lond.; SHO (Med.) Whittington Hosp. Lond.; SHO (Clin. Pharmacol.) Hammersmith Hosp. Lond.

READING, Paul James 64 Gayton House, Knapp Road, Bow, London E3 4BX — MB BChir Camb. 1986.

READING, Richard Fletcher Jenny Wind Childrens Department, Norfolk and Norwich University Hospital, Colney Lane, Norwich NR4 7UY Tel: 01603 287624 Fax: 01603 287584 — MB BChir Camb.; MD; MRCP UK; FRCPCH. Cons. Paediat.; Hon. Sen. Lect., Sch. of Med., Health and Pract., Univ. of W. Anglia, Norwich. Specialty: Community Child Health. Socs: Roy. Coll. of Paediat. and Child Health; Brit. Assn. of Community Child Health.

READINGS, Stella Madeleine (retired) Aston Mill Granary, Warren Lane, Aston Crews, Ross-on-Wye HR9 7LT — MB BS Lond. 1957 (St. Geo.)

REAICH, David Renal Unit, The James Cook University Hospital, Middlesbrough TS4 3BN; 12 Cringle Moor Chase, Great Broughton, Middlesbrough TS9 7HS — MB ChB Aberd. 1986; MRCP (UK) 1989; MD Aberd. 1996; FRCP London 2000. Cons. Nephrol. James Cook Univ. Hosp. Middlesbrough. Specialty: Gen. Med.; Nephrol.

REAKES, Ruth Elisabeth May The Straw House, Roundabout Lane, Winnersh, Wokingham RG41 5AD — MB BS Lond. 1985.

REAM, Janet Elizabeth Fender Way Health Centre, Fender Way, Birkenhead CH43 9QS Tel: 0151 677 9103 Fax: 0151 604 0392 — MB ChB Liverp. 1980.

REAM, Judith Ann 25 Valley Drive, Handforth, Wilmslow SK9 3DN — MB ChB Glas. 1977; MRCGP.

REAN, Yvette Maria 36 Lytton Road, Barnet EN5 5BY — MB BS Lond. 1992.

REANEY, Elizabeth Ann 3 Linsey's Hill, Armagh BT61 9HD — MB BCh BAO Belf. 1980; DCCH RCP Ed. Specialist Registrarin Pub. Health Med. Specialty: Pub. Health Med. Socs: BACCH; BACDA.

REANEY, Susan Margaret York District Hospital, Wigginton Road, York YO31 8HE — MB ChB Liverp. 1983; DMRD Liverp. 1988; FRCR 1990. Cons. Radiologist, York Dist. Hosp. from Jan. 2002. Specialty: Radiol. Prev: Cons. Radiologist, S. Winchester Univ. Hosps. Trust 1995-2001.

REARDON, Jeffrey Allan Mayday Hospital, Thornton Heath Tel: 020 8401 3010 Fax: 020 8401 3009; 4 Selwyn Road, New Malden KT3 5AT Tel: 020 8949 3263 Fax: 020 8715 4603 — (Queensland) MB BS Queensland. 1970; MRCP (UK) 1975. Cons. Croydon HA. Specialty: Rehabil. Med.; Rheumatol. Prev: Sen. Regist. Kennedy Inst. Rheum. Lond.

REARDON, Michael Francis Department of Geriatric Medicine, Worthing and Southlands Hospital, Worthing BN11 2DH Tel: 01903 205111 — MB BCh BAO NUI 1989; MRCPI 1992. Cons. Geriat. Med. Worthing Hosp. W. Sussex. Specialty: Care of the Elderly. Socs: Brit. Geriat. Soc.; Irish Gerontol. Soc. Prev: Sen. Regist. (Geriat. Med.) St. Richards Hosp. Chichester.

REARY, Stuart Stonehaven Medical Group, Stionehaven Medical Centre, 32 Robert Street, Stonehaven AB39 2EL Tel: 01569 762945 Fax: 01569 766552; Flat 18, Cedar Court, Ashgrove Road, Aberdeen AB25 3BJ Tel: 01224 276095 Email: stureary@hotmail.com — MB ChB Aberd. 1997; BSc (Med. Sci.) 1995. Specialty: Care of the Elderly.

REASBECK, Mr Philip George Lincoln County Hospital, Greenwell Road, Lincoln LN2 5QY Tel: 01522 512512 Fax: 01522 573629; The Grove, Ramsgate Road, Louth LN11 0NH Tel: 01507 607525 Fax: 01507 607525 — MD Camb. 1985 (Guy's) MA Camb. 1975, MD 1985, MB 1975, BChir 1974; MRCP (UK) 1976; FRCS Eng. 1978; FRACS 1982. Cons. Surg. Lincoln Co. Hosp. Trent RHA. Specialty: Gen. Surg. Socs: Assn. Surg.; Assn. ColoProctol.; Assn. Upper G.I. Surg. Prev: Sen. Lect. (Surg.) Univ. Queensland & Cons. Surg. Princess Alexandra Hosp. Brisbane, Austral.; Sen. Lect. (Surg.) Univ. Otago Med. Sch. & Cons. Surg. Dunedin Hosp., NZ; Sen. Lect. (Surg.) Univ. Hong Kong & Cons. Surg. Qu. Mary Hosp., Hong Kong.

***REAVELEY, Anne Mary** 4 Parklawn Avenue, Epsom KT18 7SQ Tel: 01372 725054 — BM BS Nottm. 1998; BM BS Nottm 1998. PRHO Surg., Nottm. City Hosp. Nottm. Specialty: Gen. Surg. Socs: BMA; Med. Protec. Soc. Prev: PRHO Med, Derbysh. Roy. Infirm.

REAVES, Charles Stuart Charters Surgery, 38 Polsloe Road, Exeter EX1 2DW Tel: 01392 273805 — MRCS Eng. LRCP Lond. 1971.

REAVES, Elizabeth Chance Charters Surgery, 38 Polsloe Road, Exeter EX1 2DW Tel: 01392 273805; Deep Dene House, Deep Dene Park, Wonford Road, Exeter EX2 4PH — MB ChB St. And. 1970.

REAVEY, James Kenilworth Medical Centre, 1 Kenilworth Court, Greenfields, Glasgow G67 1BP — MB ChB Glas. 1970.

REAVLEY, Caroline Mary Three Ways, The Saltway, Astwood Bank, Redditch B96 6NE — MB BS Lond. 1987; BSc (Hons.) Lond. 1981; MRCP (UK) 1991; FRCA 1995.

REAVLEY, Paul David Alexander Barmoor Ridge, Berwick-upon-Tweed TD15 2QD — MB ChB Dund. 1998; MB ChB Dund 1998.

REAVLEY, Saffron Beryl Sea Mills Surgery, 2 Riverdeane, Bristol BS9 7HL — MB ChB Manch. 1995.

REAY, Barbara Ann 10 Meadowview Drive, Inchture, Perth PH14 9RQ — MB ChB Dundee 1980. Staff Grade (Anaesth.) Perth Roy. Infirm. Specialty: Anaesth. Prev: Regist. (Anaesth.) Ninewells Hosp. & Med. Sch. Dundee.

REAY, Sir (Hubert) Alan (John), KBE (retired) 63 Madrid Road, Barnes, London SW13 9PQ Tel: 020 8748 2482 Fax: 020 8748 2482 — MB ChB Ed. 1948 (Univ. Ed.) DTM & H 1954; FRCP Lond. 1973, M 1955; FRCP Ed. 1968, M 1955; DCH RCP Lond. 1957; FRCGP 1985; FRCPCH 1996. Pres. Friends St. Thos. Hosp.; Chairm. Lambeth ClubHo. for Ment.ly Ill People. Prev: Chairm. Lambeth Health Care NHS Trust.

REAY, John Mark Ridley The Surgery, Pickering Road, West Ayton, Scarborough YO13 9JF Tel: 01723 863100 Fax: 01723 862902 Email: john.reay@nhs.net — MB BChir Camb. 1986; DRCOG 1990; MRCGP 1990. Clin. Asst., Rheum., Scarborough Hosp. Special Interest: Musculoskeletal Med.; Rheum. Socs: Primary Care Rheum. Soc. Prev: SHO (Paediat.) York Dist. Hosp.; Trainee GP York Dist. Hosp. VTS; Ho. Surg. W. Suff. Hosp. Bury St. Edmunds.

REAY, Katherine Annette Park Parade Surgery, 69 Park Parade, Whitley Bay NE26 1DU Tel: 0191 252 3135 Fax: 0191 253 3566 — MB BS Newc. 1989; DRCOG 1993; MRCGP 1993. Specialty: Gen. Pract. Socs: Brit. Med. Acupunct. Soc. Prev: Trainee GP/SHO Northumbria VTS Newc.

REAY, Lewis Mackay Department of Public Health, Argyll & Clyde Health Board, Ross House, Paisley PA2 7BN Tel: 0141 842 7207 Fax: 0141 848 0165 Email: lewis.reay@achb.scot.nhs.uk; 3 Sinclair Lane, Helensburgh G84 9DB — (St. And.) MB ChB St. And. 1969; DObst RCOG 1975; FRCGP 1994, M 1977; MPH Glas. 1986; M 1988; FFPH 1998; FRCP Glas. 2003. Cons. Pub. Health Med. Argyll & Clyde HB; Hon. Clin. Sen. Lect. Univ. Glas. Specialty: Pub. Health Med. Prev: GP Strachur; GP Tadcaster.

REAY, Pamela Livingstone 3 Sinclair Lane, Helensburgh G84 9DB — MB ChB St. And. 1969.

REAY, Stephen 47 Crown Road, Belle Vue, Carlisle CA2 7QQ — MB ChB Liverp. 1978; MRCGP 1982.

REAY, William Anthony (retired) Caroltina Lodge, The Spinney, Kenilworth Road, Coventry CV4 7AG Tel: 024 76 418855 — MB BS Durh. 1957 (Newc.) DObst RCOG 1969; MRCGP 1977. GP Coventry. Prev: Regtl. Med. Off. 1/2Nd K.E.O. Goorkhas.

REAY-JONES, Martin Henry Havelock (retired) Dukes Mount, Lunghurst Road, Woldingham, Caterham CR3 7HE Tel: 01883 652374 — (St. Thos.) MB BS Lond. 1962. Prev: GP Caterham Valley Med. Pract. Caterham.

REAY-JONES, Mr Nicholas Havelock John 23 Talbot Street, Hitchin SG5 2QU Tel: 01462 435656 Email: nreayjones@aol.com — MB BS Lond. 1990; BSc Lond. 1989; FRSC. Eng. 1995. Specialist Regist., Gen. Surg., N. Thames, (W.). Specialty: Gen. Surg.

REBEL, David John Kent House Surgery, 36 Station Road, Longfield DA3 7QD Tel: 01474 703550 — MB BS Lond. 1973; DObst RCOG 1975. Prev: Ho. Phys. King's Coll. Hosp. Lond.; Ho. Surg. Joyce Green Hosp. Dartford; SHO (Obst.) W. Hill Hosp. Dartford.

REBELLO, Alan Joseph Anthony (retired) Silsden, Gib Lane, Houghton, Preston PR5 0RU Tel: 0125 485 4498 — MB BS Bombay 1950 (Seth G.S. Med. Coll. Bombay) Prev: Regist. Wakefield A & B Hosp. Gps.

REBELLO, Gemma Department of CYTO Pathology, Forth Park Hospital, 30 Bennochy Road, Kirkcaldy KY2 5RA Tel: 01592 643355 Ext: 2783 Fax: 01592 642376; 9 Blackford Hill View, Edinburgh EH9 3HD Tel: 0131 667 2428 — MB BS Madras 1966 (Christian Med. Coll., Vellore, Tamilnadu, S. India) FRCPath 1990, M 1978; Dip RC Path. 1996. Cons. Cytopath. & Head of Dept. of Cytopath. Fife Acute Hosps. NHS Trust. Forth Pk. Hosp. 30 Bennochy Rd. Kirkaldy KY2 5RA; Assoc. Specialist Lothian Colposcopy Clinic, Elsie Inglis Suite Roy. Infirm Edin NHS Trust. Specialty: Histopath. Socs: Brit. Soc. Colpos. & Cerv. Path. Prev: Lect. & Assoc. Specialist (Path. Cervical Cytol.) Univ. Edin.; Sen. Regist. (Path.) Roy. Infirm. Edin.; Regist. (Path) & Regist. (Neuropath.) Roy. Infirm. Edin.

REBSTEIN, Julia Water Lanes Cottage, Ville Amphrey, St Martin's, Guernsey GY4 6DT — MB BS Lond. 1997; MRCGP 2003.

RECALDIN, Stephen 137 Westley Road, Bury St Edmunds IP33 3SE Email: stephen@recaldin.f9.co.uk — BSc Lond. 1980, MB BS 1983; DCH RCP Lond. 1986; MRCGP 1988; DRCOG 1988. Civil. Med. Pract. 48 MG Hosp. RAF Lakenheath Suff. Specialty: Gen. Med.

RECK, Miss Anne Christina Royal Eye Infirmary, Dorset County Hospital, Williams Avenue, Dorchester DT1 2JY Tel: 01305 255186 Fax: 01305 255374 — Cand Med Copenhagen; FRCS; FRCOphth. Cons. Ophth. Surg., W. Dorset NHS Trust; Winterbourne Hospital, Dorchester. Specialty: Gen. Surg.; Ophth. Special Interest: Macular Degeneration; Diabetic Retinopathy; Cataract Surg. Prev: Consultant Ophthalmologist, Colchester; Fell. in Med. Retina, Moorfield Eye Hosp.; Specialist Regist. Wessex Region.

RECKLESS, Helena Marigold (retired) Pembroke House, Mullion, Helston TR12 7HN Tel: 01326 240159 — (Roy. Free) MB BS Lond. 1946; DCH Eng. 1948. Prev: Jun. Specialist in Med. Brit. Milit. Hosp. Singapore.

RECKLESS, John Phillip David Royal United Hospital, Combe Park, Bath BA1 3NG Tel: 01225 824527 Fax: 01225 824529 Email: john.reckless@ruh-bath.swest.nhs.uk; Manor Farm House, Buckland Dinham, Frome BA11 2QS Tel: 01373 461841 — MB BS Lond. 1968 (St. Bart.) MRCS Eng. LRCP Lond. 1968; MRCP (UK) 1972; MD Lond. 1977; FRCP Lond. 1985; DSc London 2002. Cons. Phys. Roy. United Hosp. Bath; Hon. Reader Dept. Med. Sci. Med. Univ. Bath; Hon. Reader (Biochem.) Univ. Bath. Specialty: Endocrinol.; Diabetes; Gen. Med. Socs: Fell. Roy. Soc. Med.; Diabetes UK; Nat. Osteop. Soc. Prev: Sen. Regist. (Med.) Hallamsh. Hosp. Sheff.; MRC Trav. Fell. Div. Metab. Dis. Univ. Calif. San Diego, USA; Hon. Sen. Regist. (Med.) & Research Fell. St. Bart. Hosp. Lond.

RECORD, Carol Stoke Mandeville Hospital, Buckinghamshire Hospitals NHS Trust, Mandeville Road, Aylesbury HP21 8AL Tel: 01296 316916; Western House, West St, Marlow SL7 2BS — MB BS Lond. 1978; BA Oxf. 1975; MRCP (UK) 1982; FRCR 1985. Cons. Radiol. Stoke Mandeville Hosp. Aylesbury. Specialty: Radiol. Special Interest: Breast Imaging & Diag. Socs: Roy. Coll. of Radiologists. Prev: Sen. Regist. (Radiol.) Northwick Pk. Hosp. Lond.

RECORD, Charles Anthony Frome Valley Medical Centre, 2 Court Road, Frampton Cotterell, Bristol BS36 2DE — MB BS Lond. 1989 (St. Thos. Hosp. Lond.) MRCP (UK) 1993; DRCOG 1995; MRCGP 1997. GP Locum. Specialty: Gen. Pract.

RECORD, Christopher Oswald 26 The Grove, Gosforth, Newcastle upon Tyne NE3 1NE Tel: 0191 284 2273 — MB BS Lond. 1966 (Lond. Hosp.) FRCP 1981, M 1968; DCC (Biochem.) Chelsea Coll. Sc. & Technol. 1968; DPhil Oxf. 1973. Cons. Phys. Roy. Vict. Infirm. Newc. Specialty: Gastroenterol. Socs: Assn. Phys.& Brit. Soc. Gastroenterol. Prev: Sen. Regist. (Med.) Lond. Hosp.; Research Fell. Nuffield Dept. Clin. Med. Univ. Oxf.; Hon. Lect. King's Coll. Hosp. Med. Sch. Lond.

RECORD, Dorothy Maud Hope Cottage, Twitchen, Craven Arms SY7 0HN Tel: 0158 87 334 — MB ChB Birm. 1945. Prev: Res. Med. Off. Little Bromwich Isolat. Hosp. Birm.

RECORD, Jane Louise 9 Cillocks Close, Hoddesdon EN11 8QT — MB ChB Leeds 1991.

RECORD, Marion Eva (retired) St. Hildas Priory, Sneaton Castle, Whitby YO21 3QN Tel: 01947 602079 — MRCS Eng. LRCP Lond. 1950 (Leeds) DA Eng. 1955; FFA RCS Eng. 1957. Prev: Med. Off. Martin Hse. Childr. Hospice.

RECORDON, John Piers (retired) 3 Vicarage Drive, Grantchester, Cambridge CB3 9NG Tel: 01223 841342 — (St. Bart) MA, MB Camb. 1961, BChir 1960.

REDD, Reginald Alfred Stanley (retired) Woodlands, South Close Green, Redhill RH1 3DU Tel: 01737 643179 — MB BS Lond. 1952 (Lond. Hosp.) Prev: Med. Off. Roy. Earlswood Hosp. Redhill.

REDDEN, Mr Jonathan Francis Doncaster Royal Infirmary, Armthorpe Road, Doncaster DN2 5LJ Tel: 01302 366666 — MB BS Lond. 1970; MRCS Eng. LRCP Lond. 1970; FRCS Eng. 1975; FRCS Ed. (Orth.) 1980. Cons. (Orthop. Surg.) Doncaster Roy. Infirm.; Vis. Prof. (Orthop. Surg.) Beijing Med. Univ.; Hon. Cons. (Orthop. Surg.) Dandong No.2 Hosp. Liaoning Peoples RePub. of China. Specialty: Orthop. Special Interest: Knee Surg.; Paediatric Orthop. Prev: Sen. Regist. (Orthop. Surg.) Edin.; Lect. (Orthop.) Surg. Wellington, NZ.

REDDIE, Ethel Mary The Landscape, 41 East Road, Bromsgrove B60 2NW Tel: 01527 872055 — MB BS Lond. 1953; MRCPsych

1978. Indep. Psychother. BromsGr. Prev: Cons. Psychiat. Kidderminster Gen. Hosp.

REDDING, Georgina Anne Catling, Rosehill, Ladock, Truro TR2 4PQ — MB BChir Camb. 1972; MB Camb. 1972, MA, BChir 1971; DCH Eng. 1974; DPM Eng. 1976; MRCPsych 1976. Cons. (Child Psychiat.) Cornw. DHA. Specialty: Child & Adolesc. Psychiat. Prev: Sen. Regist. (Child Psychiat.) Guy's Hosp. Lond.

REDDING, Helen Louise 69 Ryegate Road, Sheffield S10 5FB — MB ChB Sheff. 1995.

REDDING, Penelope Jane Lea Rig, 133 Maxwell Drive, Pollokshields, Glasgow G41 5AE Tel: 0141 427 0149 — MB BS Lond. 1974; MRCS Eng. LRCP Lond. 1974; FRCPath 1995, M 1983. Cons. and Injection Control Doctor Bacteriol. Vict. Infirm. Glas.; Hon. Clin. Lect. Univ. Glas. Specialty: Med. Microbiol. Prev: Sen. Regist. & Regist. (Microbiol. & Immunol.) West. Infirm. Glas.; Asst. Lect. (Microbiol.) St. Thos. Hosp. Lond.

REDDING, Vincent Joseph (retired) The Grange, Cossington, Leicester LE7 4UZ Tel: 01509 812810 — (St. Thos.) MD Lond. 1974, MB BS 1952. Prev: Emerit. Cons. Cardiol. Leicester HA.

REDDING, Warren 5 Holroyd Road, Putney, London SW15 6LN Tel: 020 8788 7190 — (Westm.) MRCS Eng. LRCP Lond. 1956.

REDDING, Mr Warren Howard Tennyson House, 2 High St., Thurlby, Bourne PE10 0EE — MB BS Lond. 1976; FRCS Eng. 1980.

REDDINGTON, Jacqueline Anne The Village Surgery, Elbow Lane, Liverpool L37 4AW Tel: 01704 878661 Fax: 01704 832488 — MB ChB Liverp. 1989.

REDDY, Dr Hodge Road, 56 Hodge Road, Walker Worsley, Manchester M28 3AU.

REDDY, Annaparreddy Venkata Gurava c/o Drive K. Sastrulu, 18 Hornby Lane, Calderstones, Liverpool L18 3HH Tel: 0151 722 5832 — MB BS Nagarjuna 1984.

REDDY, Ayalam Nandini Copperfield, Church St., Tempsford, Sandy SG19 2AN — MB BS Osmania 1977. Specialty: Ment. Health.

REDDY, C Narayana Deneside Medical Centre, The Avenue, Deneside, Seaham SR7 8LF Tel: 0191 513 0202 Fax: 0191 581 6764; 39 Middleton Close, Seaton, Seaham SR7 0PQ Tel: 0191 581 9515 — MB BS Bangalore 1972; MB BS 1972 Bangalore. GP Seaham, Co. Durh. Specialty: Gen. Pract.; Cardiol.; Care of the Elderly.

REDDY, Challa Prabhakar The Vale Surgery, 97 The Vale, Acton, London W3 7RG Tel: 020 8743 4086 — MB BS Osmania 1964 (Gandhi Med. Coll. Hyderabad) Socs: BMA. Prev: SHO Geriat. Mt. Pleasant Hosp. Chepstow. Regist. (Gen. Med.) Dist.; Gen. Hosp. W. Bromwich.

REDDY, Diggireddy Pratap 66 Rhydelig Avenue, Heath, Cardiff CF4 4DE Tel: 029 2061 7598 — (Osmania Med. Coll. Hyderabad) MB BS Osmania 1960. Assoc. Specialist (Trauma & Orthop.) E. Glam. Health Trust. Specialty: Accid. & Emerg.

REDDY, Eileen 76 Rosemary Hill Road, Little Aston, Sutton Coldfield B74 4HJ — LRCP LRCS LRFPS Glas. 1952 (RCS Ed.) DPH Ed. 1954. Prev: Asst. Med. Off. Midlothian & Peebles Cos.; Asst. Div. Med. Off. Lancs. CC; Ho. Surg. & Ho. Phys. Warrington Gen. Hosp.

REDDY, Gaddam Madhusudan Red House Surgery, 127 Renfrew Road, Hylton Red House, Sunderland SR5 5PS Tel: 0191 548 1269 Fax: 0191 549 8998 — MB BS Osmania 1965. GP Sunderland.

REDDY, Mr Geetla Vijender Snow Hill Medical Centre, 6 Snow Hill Road, Shelton, Stoke-on-Trent ST1 4LT Tel: 01782 219906 — MB BS Osmania 1971; DLO RCS Eng. 1984; FRCS Ed. 1985; T(GP) 1992. Specialty: Otorhinolaryngol. Prev: Trainee GP Swindon VTS; Regist. (ENT) Stoke Mandeville Hosp. Aylesbury; SHO (A & E) Milton Keynes Hosp.

REDDY, Mr Gopinath Northampton General Hospital, Cliftonville, Northampton NN1 5BD — MB BS Lond. 1992 (Guy's Hosp. Lond.) BSc (Clin. Pharmacol.) Lond. 1988; FRCOphth 1997. Cons. Ophth. Northampton Gen. Hosp. Specialty: Ophth. Prev: SHO (Ophth.) Kingston Hosp. Lond.; SHO (Ophth.) St Geo.s Hosp. Lond.; Specialist Regist. (Ophth.) Soton. Gen. Hosp.

REDDY, Mr Gudimetla Adi Narayana c/o Mr N.R. Padala, 6 Fitzgerald St., Preston PR1 5EN — MB BS Andhra 1984; FRCS Glas. 1993.

REDDY, Jason BUPA Wellness, Blackberry Clinic, Blackberry Court, Milton Keynes MK7 7PB Tel: 01908 604666 Fax: 01908 541337 Email: reddyj@bupa.com; NHS, DE PARYS H.C., 23 DE PARYS AVE, BEDFORD MK40 2TX; De Parys Health Centre, 23 de Parys Avenue, Bedford MK40 2TX Tel: 01234 350022 Email: aax19@dial.pipex.com; 25 Fountains Road, Bedford MK41 8NU Tel: 01234 351304 Fax: 01234 351304 Email: dr.jason.reddy@dial.pipex.com — MB BS Lond. 1990 (Univ. Coll. Hosp.) DCH RCP Lond. 1993; DFFP 1994; DRCOG 1996. p/t Lead Physician/Physician in Charge BUPA Wellness Blackberry Clinic Milton Keynes; NHS Salaried GP; Private GP Bedford. Specialty: Gen. Pract.; Occupat. Health. Special Interest: Primary Care; Screening; Occupat. Health. Socs: Mem. of the Fac. of pre-Hosp. c/o the Roy. Coll. of Surg.s (Edin.). Prev: Lead Physician/Physician in Charge BUPA Wellness Lond.; Sen. Ship's Doctor P & O/P.ss Cruises Ltd.; Trainee GP/SHO (Gen. Med.) Milton Keynes Gen. Hosp.

REDDY, Mr Kamireddy Marcus Flat 12, Lantern Court, 99 Worple Road, Wimbledon, London SW20 8HB Tel: 020 8286 1797 Fax: 079 3221 0837 — MB BS Lond. 1992 (St. George's Hospital Medical School London) BSc Basic Med. Scs. & Pharmacol. Lond. 1989; FRCS (Eng.) 1997. Hon. Research Fell. & Specialist Regist., (Gen. Surg.) St. Geo. Hosp. Med. Sch. Lond.& Kingston Hosp.,Kingston-Upon-Thames. Specialty: Gen. Surg. Socs: Assoc. Mem. Assn. Surg. GB & Irel.; Assoc. Mem. Brit. Assn. Surg. Oncol.

REDDY, Kamireddy Prema Elm House Surgery, 29 Beckenham Road, Beckenham BR3 4PR Tel: 020 8650 0173 Fax: 020 8663 3911; Marley Hayes, Oldfield Road, Bromley BR1 2LE — MB BS Lond. 1989 (GUYS (UNDS))

REDDY, Kaukutla Venkat Deneside Medical Centre, The Avenue, Deneside, Seaham SR7 8LF Tel: 0191 513 0202 Fax: 0191 581 6764; 11 Lodgeside Meadow, Burdon, Sunderland SR3 2PN — MB BS Osmania 1971; MB BS 1971 Osmania. GP Seaham, Co. Durh.

REDDY, Kishore Department of Radiology, Medway Hospital, Windmill Road, Gillingham ME7 5NY Tel: 01634 830000 Fax: 01634 401177; 119 Wigmore Road, Gillingham ME8 0TH — MB BS Mysore 1976; DMRD Eng. 1984; FRCR 1986. Cons. Radiol. Medway Hosp. Gillingham. Specialty: Radiol.

REDDY, Kokkanda S P Joshi and Reddy, Aston Health Centre, 175 Trinity Road, Birmingham B6 6JA Tel: 0121 327 0144 Fax: 0121 326 9784 — MB BS Osmania 1971; MB BS Osmania 1971.

REDDY, Kothur Suresh Health Centre, Cramlington NE23 6QN Tel: 01670 714581 — MB BS Osmania 1961 (Osmania Med. Coll. Hyderabad) DTCD Wales 1971.

REDDY, Mr Maddy Ashwin 13 Mill Close, Nuneaton CV11 6QD — BChir Camb. 1992 (Cambridge University) MA (Cantab) 1990; FRCOphth 1997. Specialist Regist., E. Anglican Rotat. Specialty: Ophth.

REDDY, Mr Majjiga Rajashekar House 5, The Green, Wylde Green Road, Sutton Coldfield B72 1JB — MRCS Eng. LRCP Lond. 1987; FRCS Glas. 1993. Specialty: Trauma & Orthop. Surg.

REDDY, Mamatha St Thomas' Hospital, Department of Radiology, Lambeth Wing, Lambeth Palace Rd, London SE1 7EH Tel: 0207 928 9292 — MB BS Lond. 1993; BSc (1st cl. Hons.) Lond. 1990; MRCP (Lond.) 1997; FRCR Lond. 1998. Specialist Regist. Radio. Guys & St Thos. Hosp. NHS Trust Lond. SEI. Specialty: Radiol. Prev: SHO Gen. Med. St. Geos. Hosp. Tooting, Lond.

REDDY, Nallamilli Somasekhara Research & Teaching Centre, Royal Orthopaedic Hospital, The Woodlands, Northfield, Birmingham B31 2AP — MB BS Andhra 1984.

REDDY, Paul Joseph Hill Farm Oast, Yalding Hill, Yalding, Maidstone ME18 6AN; Mid Kent Trust, Hermitage Lane, Maidstone ME16 9QQ Tel: 01622 729000 — LRCPI & LM, LRSCI & LM 1977 (Royal College Surgeons Ireland) FRCSI 1981; FRCS 1983. Cons. Urol. Specialty: Urol. Socs: BAUS; R.S.M.

REDDY, Prashanthi 41A Guilford Road, Stoneygate, Leicester LE2 2RD — MB ChB Leic. 1997.

REDDY, Mrs Ragini Majjiga Walsall Manor NHS Trust, Moat Road, Walsall WS2 9PS Tel: 01922 721172 — MB BS Osmania; MRCOG. Cons. Gynaecologist. Specialty: Obst. & Gyn. Socs: MPS.

REDDY, Ramchandra (retired) 13 Mill Close, Nuneaton CV11 6QD — MB BS Osmania 1964 (Gandhi Med. Sch. Hyderabad) Prev: GP Bedworth.

REDDY, Sathineni Venkateshwar Wickersley Health Centre, Poplar Glade, Wickersley, Rotherham S66 2JQ Tel: 01709 549610 Fax: 01709 702470 — MB ChB Leic. 1996.

REDDY, Soma Sudershan Newmains Health Centre, 18 Manse Road, Newmains, Wishaw ML2 9AX Tel: 01698 383296 Fax: 01698 387157.

REDDY, Subbalekshmi Runwell Hospital, Wickford SS11 7XX; Oakdene, Bicknacre, Chelmsford CM3 4HA — MB BS Kerala 1970 (Trivandrum Med. Coll.) DPM Eng. 1982; MRCPsych 1983. Cons. Psychiat. Mid. Essex HA; Cons. Psychiat. Southend Community Care Trust. Specialty: Gen. Psychiat. Prev: Regist. (Psychiat.) Runwell Hosp. Wickford; Regist. (Psychiat.) City Gen. Hosp. Stoke-on-Trent; SHO (Gen. Med.) Preston Hosp. N. Shields.

REDDY, Mr Thimmareddy Narayana Staffs District General Hospital, Weston Road, Stafford ST16 3SA Tel: 01785 57731 & 58251; 34 Museum Road, Bangalore, India — MB BS Mysore 1970 (Mysore Med. Coll.) BSc Mysore 1962, MB BS 1970; DLO Eng. 1973; FRCS Glas. 1981. Cons. ENT Surg. Mid Staffs. HA. Specialty: Otolaryngol. Prev: Regist. (ENT) Dartford & Gravesham HA & Barking & Havering HA; Regist. (ENT) Rochdale HA; Sen. Regist. (ENT) W. Midl. RHA.

REDDY, Vatrapu Laxmi Narayana Stantonbury Health Centre, Purbeck, Stantonbury, Milton Keynes MK14 6BL Tel: 01908 316262 — MB BS Andhra 1965 (Andhra Med. Coll.) Prev: Regist. Mapperley Hosp. Nottm.

REDDY, Veena 114 Cherry Crescent, Rossendale BB4 6DS — MB BS Lond. 1998; MB BS Lond 1998.

REDDY, Vuchuru Anila Prem 2 Horton Grove, Monkspath, Solihull B90 4UZ — MB ChB Aberd. 1984.

REDELINGHUYS, Johan 50 Clonmore Street, Southfields, London SW18 5EY — MB ChB Pretoria 1992.

REDENHAM, Antonio Jay 50 Thorpewood Avenue, Sydenham, London SE26 4BX — (St. Geo.) MRCS Eng. LRCP Lond. 1950. Prev: Ho. Off. Lambeth Hosp. Lond.

REDER, Peter Child & Family Consultation Centre, 1 Wolverton Gardens, London W6 7DY Tel: 020 8846 7806 Fax: 020 8846 7817; 20 Devereux Lane, Barnes, London SW13 8DA Tel: 020 8748 9805 — MB ChB Birm 1969; DObst RCOG 1971; DCH Eng. 1972; DPM Eng. 1974; FRCPsych 1993, M 1975. Mem. Teachg. Staff Inst. Family Ther. Lond.; Dir. Centre for Relationship Studies Lond. Specialty: Child & Adolesc. Psychiat. Prev: Cons. Child Psychiat. Newham Child Guid. Clin. Lond.; Sen. Regist. (Psychiat.) Dept. Childr. & Parents Tavistock Clinic Lond.

REDFEARN, Anabel Blyth Health Centre, Thoroton Street, Blyth NE24 1DX — MB BS Newc. 1987 (Newcastle upon Tyne) MRCP (UK) 1991. Cons. Paediat. with an interest in Community Child Health, N.umberland, Northumbria & N. Tyneside Trust, based at Blyth. Specialty: Community Child Health. Special Interest: Childr. Looked After, Adoption and Fostering. Socs: MRCPCH; MDU; CPRG. Prev: Regist. (Paediat.) North. Region; Sen. Regist. (Community Child Health) Newc. u. Tyne Flexible Train Scheme.

REDFEARN, Auberon Emergency Bed Service, Fielden House, 28 London Bridge St., London SE1 9SG Tel: 020 7407 7181 Fax: 020 7357 6705; 11 Glossop Road, Sanderstead, South Croydon CR2 0PW Tel: 020 8657 6039 — MB BChir Camb. 1976; MA Camb. 1959. SCMO Emerg. Bed. Servs. Lambeth, Southwark & Lewisham FHSA Lond. Specialty: Chem. Path. Socs: Camb. Univ. Med. Soc.; St. Bart. Hosp. Med. Coll. Alumni Assn. Prev: Regist. (Chem. Path.) St. Geo. Hosp. Lond.; Regist. (Chem. Path.) & SHO (Path.) Mayday Hosp. Croydon.

REDFEARN, Damian Paul 99 St Leonard's Road, Leicester LE2 1WT — MB ChB Leic. 1993.

REDFEARN, Edward 11 The Vale, MacKenzie Road, Birmingham B11 4EN Tel: 0121 449 3903 — MB Camb. 1955 (Camb. & Middlx.) BA Camb. 1951, MB 1955, BChir 1954; DObst RCOG 1957. Founder Mem. Lect. (Ex-Chairm.) Brit. Med. Accupunc. Soc. Prev: Ho. Phys. & Ho. Surg. Middlx. Hosp.

REDFEARN, Joseph William Thorpe London House, 90/92 High St, Brightlingsea, Colchester CO7 0EG Tel: 01206 305374 — (Univ. Camb. & Johns Hopkins Univ.) MRCS Eng. LRCP Lond. 1945; MD Johns Hopkins Univ. 1946; MB BChir Camb. 1946; DPM Lond. 1948; MA Camb. 1945, MD 1956; MD Camb. 1957MD Camb. 1957; MRCPsych 1971. Train. Analyst Soc. Analyt. Psychol. Specialty: Psychother. Prev: Psychotherap. Middlx. Hosp.; on Extern. Scientif. Staff. Med. Research Counc.; Head of Physiol. Sect. Army Operat. Research Gp.

REDFEARN, Peter Matthew The Grange Road Practice, 108 Grange Road, London SE1 3BW Tel: 020 7237 1078 Fax: 020 7771 3550 — MB BS Lond. 1988 (Univ. Lond., King's Coll. Sch. Med. & Dent.) Specialty: Gen. Pract. Socs: BMA.

REDFEARN, Simon William Birchwood Medical Centre, 15 Benson Road, Birchwood, Warrington WA3 7PJ Tel: 01925 823502 Fax: 01925 852422; 9 Pool Lane, Lymm WA13 9BJ Tel: 01925 754345 — MB ChB Liverp. 1979; MRCP (UK) 1982; DRCOG 1983; MRCGP 1986. Prev: SHO (Paediat.) Alder Hey Childr. Hosp. Liverp.; SHO (O & G) Liverp. Matern. Hosp.; SHO (Gyn.) & (Med.) Rotat. Roy. Liverp. Hosp.

REDFERN, Andrew Christopher Home Farm Cottage, Barton Road, Market Bosworth, Nuneaton CV13 0LQ — BChir Camb. 1990.

REDFERN, Mr Daniel Richard Malachy Hammersmith Hospital, Du Cane Road, London W12 0HS Tel: 020 8743 2030; 13 Canopus Way, Stanwell, Staines TW19 7TA — MB BS Lond. 1988 (St. Barts. Lond.) MA (Hons.) Oxf. 1985; FRCS Eng. 1992. Specialist Regist. (Orthop.) Hammersmith Hosp. Lond. Specialty: Orthop. Socs: BMA; BOTA. Prev: Laming Evans Fell.; Regist. (Orthop.) Hammersmith Hosp. Lond.; SHO (Orthop.) Ashford Hosp. Middlx.

REDFERN, Emma 18 Ulviet Gate, High Legh, Knutsford WA16 6TT Tel: 01925 754 4356 — MB ChB Sheff. 1997. Ho. Off. Urol. Roy. Hallamsh. Hosp. Sheff.; SHO VTS in Sheff. Rotat. GP (Med. A & E, Obstretrics, Gyn. & Paediat. Specialty: Gen. Pract.

REDFERN, Hyla Mary (retired) Swallow Barn, Andrew House, Stainton, Penrith CA11 0ES — MRCS Eng. LRCP Lond. 1950 (Sheff.) DPH Eng. 1969; MFCM 1974. Prev: SCMO Notts. AHA (T).

REDFERN, John North, TD (retired) Greenacre, Kemp Road, Swanland, North Ferriby HU14 3LZ — MB BChir Camb. 1950 (Middlx.) BA Camb. 1948, MB BChir 1950; DObst RCOG 1951. Prev: Ho. Surg. Hull Matern. Hosp.

REDFERN, Lisa 22 Noel Gate, Aughton, Ormskirk L39 5EG Tel: 01695 421606 Email: lredfernp@btopenworld.com — MB ChB Manch. 1994; BSc (Hons.) Manch. 1991; MRCP (Edin) 1998. Regist. (Paediat.) Roy. Manch. Childrens Hosp. Specialty: Paediat. Prev: Regist. (Paediat.) St Marys' Hosp. for Wom. and Childr. Manch.; Regist. (Paediat.) Roy. Vict. Infirm., Newc. on Tyne; Regist. (Paediat.) Qu. Eliz. Hosp., Gatehead, Tyne and Wear.

REDFERN, Mark Adrian Ashfield House, Forest Road, Annesley Woodhouse, Kirkby in Ashfield, Nottingham NG17 9JB Tel: 01623 752295/153 — BM BS Nottm. 1980.

REDFERN, Michael (retired) 2 Lower Faircox, Henfield BN5 9UT Tel: 01273 491 811 — MB BS Lond. 1969; MRCS Eng. LRCP Lond. 1969; MRCGP 1979; MA Soton. 1994. Prev: GP N.bourne Med. Centre Shoreham-by-Sea.

REDFERN, Nancy Royal Victoria Infirmary, Queen Victoria Road, Newcastle upon Tyne NE1 4LP Tel: 0191 273 8811 — MB BS Lond. 1979; BSc Lond. 1977; FRCA 1983. Cons. Anaesth. Roy. Vict. Infirm.; Assoc. Postgrad. Dean Newc. Specialty: Anaesth.

REDFERN, Richard Fort House Surgery, 32 Hersham Road, Walton-on-Thames KT12 1UX Tel: 01932 253055 Fax: 01932 225910; 17 Connaught Drive, Weybridge KT13 0XA — MB BS Lond. 1989 (Char. Cross & West. Med. Sch.) MRCGP 1994. Specialty: Gen. Pract.

REDFERN, Mr Robert Michael Department of Neurosurgery, Morriston Hospital, Swansea SA6 6PN Tel: 01792 703382 Fax: 01792 703455; Glyncasnod Farm, Felindre, Swansea SA5 7PU Tel: 01269 592145 — MB BS Lond. 1977 (Lond. Hosp.) FRCS Eng. 1983. Cons. Neurosurg. Directorate of Neurosci. Morriston Hosp. Swansea. Specialty: Neurosurg. Socs: BMA; Soc. Brit. Neurol. Surgs. Prev: Sen. Regist. (Neurosurg.) Brook Hosp. & Maudsley Hosp.; Regist. (Neurosurg.) Walton Hosp. Liverp.

REDFERN, Suzanne Jane 7A Monsell Dr, Leicester LE2 8PP — MB ChB Birm. 1997.

REDFERN, Mr Thomas Roberton Department of Orthopaedic Surgery, Leighton Hospital, Middlewich Road, Crewe CW1 4QJ Tel: 01270 612258 Fax: 01270 612043 Email: thomas.redfern@mcht.nhs.uk; The Grange, Wrenbury, Nantwich CW5 8HA Tel: 01270 780873 Fax: 01270 780873 — MB ChB Manch. 1976; FRCS Ed. 1981; MChOrth. Liverp. 1984. Cons. Surg. Orthop. Leighton Hosp. Specialty: Orthop. Socs: Brit. Elbow and Shoulder Soc.; Europ. Soc. for Surg. of Shoulder and Elbow. Prev: Sen. Regist. (Orthop. Surg.) Mersey RHA.

REDFERNE, Jennifer Halina The Residence, 3 Church Lane, Osgathorpe, Loughborough LE12 9SY — MB BS Lond. 1988 (St. Mary's) DRCOG 1990; DGM RCP Lond. 1992; DFFP 1993; MRCGP 1997. Specialty: Gen. Pract.

REDFORD, Anthony (retired) 11 Malvern Road, Knutsford WA16 0EH Tel: 01565 634600 — MB ChB Manch. 1961. Prev: Sen. Partner Manch. Rd. Med. Centre, Knutsford Chesh.

REDFORD, Mr David Humphrey Alexander 11 Kennedy Road, Shrewsbury SY3 7AD Tel: 01743 353541 — MB ChB Bristol 1972; FRCS Eng. 1977; FRCOG 1993, M 1978. Cons. O & G Roy. Shrewsbury Hosp. NHS Trust. Specialty: Obst. & Gyn. Prev: Sen. Regist. (O & G) Gtr. Glas. HB; Lect. (O & G) Univ. Bristol.

REDGMENT, Christopher John 112A Harley Street, London W1N 1AF Tel: 020 7224 0707 Fax: 020 7224 3102 — MB ChB Zimbabwe 1983; MRCOG 1991.

REDGRAVE, Allan Paul Public Health Department, Rotherham Health Authority, 220 Badsley Moor Lane, Rotherham S65 2QU Tel: 01709 302164 Fax: 01709 302175; 108 Carr Road, Walkley, Sheffield S6 2WZ Tel: 0114 233 6020 — MB ChB Bristol 1975; DRCOG 1979; MRCGP 1987; MFPHM RCP (UK) 1995. Cons. Pub. Health Med. Rotherham HA. Specialty: Pub. Health Med. Prev: GP Sheff.

REDGRAVE, Elizabeth Ann Casitas, Goodwood Rise, Marlow Bottom, Marlow SL7 3QE Tel: 01628 483021 Fax: 01628 474322 — MB BS Lond. 1985 (Char. Cross Hosp. Med. Sch.) BSc Lond. 1981. Orthop. Phys. Redgrave Clinic Bucks. Specialty: Sports Med. Socs: Brit. Assn. Sport & Med.; Brit. Med. Acupunct. Soc. Prev: SHO (Surg.) Char. Cross Hosp. Lond.; Chief Med. Off. GB Rowing Team; Regional Med. Off. LTA.

REDHEAD, Doris Nicol Department of Clinical Radiology, Royal Infirmary of Edinburgh, 51 Little France Crescent, Edinburgh EH16 4SA Tel: 0131 242 3772 — (Ed.) MB ChB Ed. 1966; DMRD Ed. 1975; FRCR 1978; FRCP 2003. Cons. (Radiol.) Roy. Infirm. Ed. Specialty: Radiol. Socs: BMA; Roy. Coll. Radiol.; Soc. Minimal Invasive Ther.

REDHEAD, Julian Bladen Gonne St Mary's Hospital, Praed Street, Paddington, London Tel: 020 7886 1200 Email: julian.redhead@st-marys.nhs.uk — MB BS Lond. 1991; FFAEM; MRCP. Cons. Emerg. Med., St Mary's Hosp., Lond.; Cons. Emerg. Med., Ealing Hosp., Southall. Specialty: Accid. & Emerg.; Sports Med.; Medico Legal.

REDHEAD, Keith Andrew St James House Surgery, County Court Road, King's Lynn PE30 5SY Tel: 01553 774221 Fax: 01553 692181 Email: keith.redhead@nhs.net — MB ChB Manch. 1979; DRCOG 1986; MRCGP 1987; MFFP 1993; FRCGP 2001. GP Princip. King's Lynn; GP Specialist (Epilepsy) Qu. Eliz. Hosp. King's Lynn; Course Organiser, King's Lynn Gen. Pract. Train. Scheme. Prev: Trainee GP King's Lynn VTS; Dist. Med. Insp. S. Sudan.; Instruc. Doctor (Family Plann.) King's Lynn.

REDHEAD, Robert Gonne (retired) 3 Ashfield Close, Petersham, Richmond TW10 7AF Tel: 020 8940 9336 — (St. Mary's) MB BS Lond. 1951; MRCS Eng. LRCP Lond. 1951; PhD Surrey 1974. Prev: Cons. Rehahit. Qu. Mary's Univer. Hosp. Lond.

REDINGTON, Alan Norton Tregony Road Surgery, Tregony Road, Probus, Truro TR2 4JZ; Trencreek Barn, Tregony, Truro TR2 5SY Tel: 01872 530880 — (Birm.) MB ChB Birm. 1968; DObst RCOG 1970; DCH Eng. 1972; MRCGP 1974.

REDINGTON, Professor Andrew Nicholas Great Ormond Street Hospital for Children, Great Ormond St., London WC1N 3JH Tel: 020 7405 9200 Fax: 020 7813 8263; 3 West Park Road, Kew, Richmond TW9 4DB Tel: 020 8876 3635 Email: reding@ibm.net — MB BS Lond. 1981; MRCP (UK) 1984; MD Lond. 1988; FRCP Lond. 1994. Cons. Paediat. (Cardiol.) Gt. Ormond St. Hosp. for Childr. Specialty: Paediat. Cardiol. Prev: Cons. Paediat. (Cardiol.) Roy. Brompton Hosp., Lond.; Prof. Congen. Heart Dis. Nat. Heart & Lung Inst. Imperial Coll. of Sci., Technolgoy & Med., Lond.; Sen. Regist. (Paediat. Cardiol.) Brompton Hosp. Lond.

REDINGTON, Anthony Edward Academic Department of Medicine, Castle Hill Hospital, Cottingham HU16 5JQ Tel: 01482 624067 Fax: 01482 624068 Email: a.e.redington@hull.ac.uk; 55a Gubyon Avenue, Herne Hill, London SE24 0DU Tel: 020 7737 6050 — MB BS Lond. 1984 (Oxf./King's Coll. Hosp.) BA Oxf. 1981; MRCP (UK) 1988; DM Soton. 1997; MA Oxf. 1997. Sen. Lect., Univ. of Hull; Hon. Cons. Phys., Hull & E. Riding Hosp. NHS Trust. Specialty: Respirat. Med. Socs: Amer. Thoracic Soc.; Brit. Thorac. Soc.; Brit. Soc. Allergy & Clin. Immunol. Prev: Lect. & Hon. Sen. Regist. Guy's Hosp. Lond.; Postdoctoral Research Fell. (Pathol.), McMaster Univ. Ontario, Canada.

REDLAFF, Leszek Dr Doris and Partners, The medical Centre, Vicarage Road, Derby DE3 0HA Tel: 01332 513283 Fax: 01332 518569 — MB ChB Manch. 1991; DFFP 1994; DRCOG 1994; Cert. Prescribed Equiv. Exp. JCPTGP 1995; MRCGP 1995. Prev: Trainee GP Stockport VTS.

REDMAN, Alan Geddis Oscar 52 Morris Lane, Bath BA1 7PS — MB BS Lond. 1994.

REDMAN, Mr Charles William Everett Maternity Building, North Staffs Hospital, Newcastle Road, Stoke-on-Trent ST4 6QG Tel: 01782 553460 Fax: 01782 553460; South Wing, The Old Rectory, Dalbury DE6 5BR Tel: 01283 734173 — MD Manch. 1989 (Manchester) MB ChB 1978; MRCOG 1983; FRCS Ed. 1984; FRCOG 1997. Cons. O & G N. N. Staffs Hosp. Specialty: Obst. & Gyn. Socs: Liveryman Worshipful Soc. Apoth.; Asst. Sec. Brit. Soc. Colposcopy & Cervical Path. Prev: Sen. Lect. (O & G) Sch. of Physiol. Sci.s & Postgrad. Med. Univ. Keele; Lect. Univ. Birm.; CRC Research Fell. Univ. Birm.

REDMAN, Christopher Willard George Nuffield Department of Obstetrics & Gynaecology, John Radcliffe Hospital, Oxford OX3 9DU — MB BChir Camb. 1967; FRCP Lond. 1981, M 1971; FRCOG 1993. Clin. Prof. & Cons. Obst. Med. John Radcliffe Hosp. Oxf. Specialty: Gen. Med. Prev: Lect. Dept. Regius Prof. Med. Radcliffe Infirm. Oxf.

REDMAN, David Robert Oscar Anaesthetic Department, Watford General Hospital, Vicarage Road, Watford WD18 0HB — MB BS Lond. 1976 (Middlx.) FFA RCS Eng. 1981. Cons. Anaesth. Watford Gen. Hosp. Herts. Specialty: Anaesth. Socs: Assn. Anaesth. Prev: Sen. Regist. Rotat. (Anaesth.) St. Mary's Hosp. Lond. Nat. Hosp. Nerv. Dis. Edgware Gen. Hosp. & Roy. Marsden Hosp. Lond.; Regist. (Anaesth.) Roy. Free Hosp. Lond.; SHO (Anaesth.) St. Thos. Hosp. Lond.

REDMAN, Fraces Kate — MB BCh Wales 2002; BSc Wales 2000. Ho. Off. P. Philip Hosp. Lanelli.

REDMAN, Helen Kathleen Anne Kingsfield Medical Centre, 146 Alcester Road South, Kings Heath, Birmingham B14 6AA Tel: 0121 444 2054 Fax: 0121 443 5856; 43 Chantry Road, Moseley, Birmingham B13 8DN — MB ChB Birm. 1991; DGM RCP Lond. 1994; MRCGP 1995. GP Princip. BromsGr. Prev: Clin. Asst., (GP) BromsGr.; Trainee GP Redditch VTS.

REDMAN, James Houston 1 The Gatehouse, Rochester ME15 0SG Tel: 01634 848202 Fax: 01634 847808; West Street, Hunton, Maidstone ME15 0SB — MB ChB Sheff. 1982; MRCGP 1987; AFOM RCP (UK) 1994; DMJ (Clin) 2000. GP & Occupat. Phys. Rochester. Specialty: Occupat. Health; Forens. Path.; Gen. Pract. Socs: Occupat. Med. Soc. Prev: Army Med. Off.

REDMAN, Jonathan Warwick Rosslyn Cottage, Sinderby, Thirsk YO7 4JD — MB ChB Ed. 1993. Specialty: Anaesth. Socs: Scott. Soc. Anaesth.; SE Scotl. Soc. Anaesth.

REDMAN, Leonard Rountree (retired) 52 Morris Lane, Bathford, Bath BA1 7PS Tel: 01225 858202 — MB BCh BAO Dub. 1957; DA Eng. 1960; DObst RCOG 1960; FFA RCS Eng. 1963. Cons. Anaesth. Bath Clin. Area. Prev: Jt. Sen. Regist. Anaesth. St. Thos. Hosp. & Nat. Heart Hosp. Lond.

REDMAN, Pamela Joan Ulverston Health Centre, Victoria Road, Ulverston LA12 0EW Tel: 01229 582588 — MB ChB Ed. 1984; MRCGP 1989. GP. Prev: SHO (Haemat.) Memor. Hosp. Darlington; Trainee GP Durh. & Gateshead.; Clin. Asst. (Obst. & Gyn.) Furness Hosp. Trust Barrow in Furness.

REDMAN, Richard Carlyle Burnham Market Surgery, Church Walk, Burnham Market, King's Lynn PE31 8DH Tel: 01328 737000 Fax: 01328 730104 Email: richard.redman@nhs.net — MB Camb. 1971, BChir 1970; MRCGP 1975. W. Norf. PCT Clin. Governance Jt. Lead. Prev: Treas. EMIS NUG; Mem. Core Gp. GP Working Party Read Codes (CCC Loughborough).

REDMAN, Sarah Patricia The Surgery, 1 Hammersmith Bridge Road, London W6 9DU Tel: 020 8748 5246 Fax: 020 8748 5248 — MB BS Lond. 1993 (Charing Cross & Westminster) DCH 1995; DRCOG 1998; MRCGP 1999. Specialty: Gen. Pract.

REDMAN, Susan Deborah Dingle Cottage, North Drive, Angmering, Littlehampton BN16 4JJ — MB ChB Bristol 1998. SHO, Med., MusGr. Pk. Hosp., Taunton, Som. Specialty: Gen. Med.

REDMAN, Thomas Malcolm Walker (retired) 27 Carnreagh, Hillsborough BT26 6LJ — MB BCh BAO Dub. 1948. Prev: Ho. Phys. Chase Farm Hosp. Enfield.

REDMAN, Victor Leonard (retired) Cedarwood, Smith Lane, Snitterfield, Stratford-upon-Avon CV37 0JY — (St. Bart.) MRCS Eng. LRCP Lond. 1939. Prev: Med. Off. DHSS.

REDMEN, J Ebejer (retired) Dormers, Heath Lane, Munstead, Godalming GU7 1UN Tel: 01483 415693 — MD Malta 1955; BPharm 1953; DA Eng. 1962; FFA RCS Eng. 1967. Prev: Cons. Anaesth. Guildford & Godalming Gp. Hosps.

REDMILL, Brian Sidney Department of Ophthalmology, St George's Hospital, Blackshaw Road, London SW17 0QT Tel: 020 8672 1255 Fax: 020 8725 3026; 29 Kenley Walk, North Cheam, Sutton SM3 8ES Tel: 020 8644 9288 — MB BChir Camb. 1987; FRCOphth 1991. Specialist Regist. (Ophth.) St. Geos. Hosp. Lond. Specialty: Ophth. Prev: Research Fell. Univ. Aberd.; Sen. Regist. St. John Ophth. Hosp., Jerusalem.

REDMILL, Duncan Allen 30 Princeton Road, Bangor BT20 3TA — MB BCh BAO Belf. 1994. Specialty: Gen. Surg. Prev: SHO (Surgic.) Whiteabbey Hosp. Belf.; SHO (Surgic. & A & E) Antrim Area Hosp.

REDMOND, Professor Anthony Damien, OBE 27 Byrom Street, Manchester M3 4PF Tel: 0161 832 9935 Fax: 0161 833 0643 Email: profadr@aol.com — MB ChB Manch. 1975 (Manchester) MD Manch. 1979; MRCP (UK) 1981; FRCS Ed. 1982; FRCPS Glas. 1991; FFAEM 1993; Dip IMC 1995; FIMC RCS Ed. 2002. Cons. (Trauma/Emergency Med.) Manch. Specialty: Accid. & Emerg. Special Interest: Disaster Med.; Soft Tissue Injuries; The Managem. of Maj. Trauma. Socs: Fell. Roy. Soc. Med.; N. Staff. Med. Inst.; Manch. Med. Soc. Prev: Prof. Emerg. Med. Keele Univ.; Cons. A & E Med. Univ. Hosp. S. Manch.; Sen. Regist. (A & E Med.) Hope Hosp. Manch.

REDMOND, Brian 10 Hollins Drive, Middleton, Manchester M24 5LN Tel: 0161 643 3314 — MB BCh BAO Dub. 1946 (T.C. Dub.) Mem. Frank Lord Postgrad. Centre Oldham. Specialty: Dermat. Socs: BMA. Prev: Cas. Off. Sir P. Dun's Hosp. Dub.; Ho. Surg. (Orthop. & Anaesth.) Mansfield Hosp.

REDMOND, Elizabeth Jane Countess of Chester Hospital, Liverpool Road, Chester CH2 1UL — MB ChB Liverp. 1985. Specialty: Gen. Surg.

REDMOND, John V Elm Lodge Surgery, 43 Gloucester Road North, Bristol BS7 0SN Tel: 0117 969 0909 Fax: 0117 983 9969; 22 Malmains Drive, Frenchay, Bristol BS16 1PQ Tel: 0117 956 7909 — MB BCh BAO Dub. 1975 (Univ. Coll. Dub.) DCH Dub. 1979; DRCOG 1980; MRCGP 1981. GP; Med. Bristol Rugby Club & St Mary's O.B. Rugby football Club. Specialty: Gen. Pract.; Sports Med. Socs: Frenchay Hosp. Med. Postgrad. Soc.; Cossham Med. Soc.; Brit. Assn. Sport & Med. Prev: Trainee GP Bedford VTS; SHO (Med.) Regional Hosp. Galway; SHO (Med.) St. Jas. Hosp. Dub.

REDMOND, Maureen Joan — MB ChB Liverp. 1976.

REDMOND, Michael Robert Broughshane Medical Practice, 76 Main Street, Broughshane, Ballymena BT42 4JP Tel: 028 2586 1214 Fax: 028 2586 2281 — MB ChB Dundee 1991.

REDMOND, Oonagh Aileen Beatrice (retired) Royal Belfast Hospital for Sick Children, Falls Road, Belfast BT12 6BE Tel: 01232 240503; 4 Rosevale Close, Drumbeg, Dunmurry, Belfast BT17 9LQ Tel: 02890 612024 — (TC Dub.) FRCPCH; MB BCh BAO Dub. 1959; DCH Eng. 1961; FRCPI 1981, M 1964. Cons. Paediatr. Roy. Belf. Hosp. Sick Childr. Prev: Sen. Research Fell. Dept. Paediat. Univ. Cape Town S. Afr.

REDMOND, Peter Vincent Stephen Ellergreen Medical Centre, 24 Carr Lane, Norris Green, Liverpool L11 2YA Tel: 0151 256 9800 Fax: 0151 256 5765 — MB ChB Liverp. 1981.

REDMOND, Mr Richard Maguire c/o Department of Ophthalmology, Scarborough Hospital, Scarborough YO12 6QL Tel: 01723 368111 Email: rmr@dsl.pipex.com — MB ChB Bristol 1981; MSc (Med. Sci.) Glas. 1984; FRCS (Ophth.) Lond. 1987; DO RCS Eng. 1987. Cons. Ophth. Surg. ScarBoro. Hosp. Specialty: Ophth. Prev: Sen. Regist. Moorfields Eye Hosp. Lond.; SHO Bristol Eye Hosp.; SHO (Neurosurg.) Frenchay Hosp. Bristol.

REDMOND, Robert Anthony Alexander Broughshane Medical Practice, 76 Main Street, Broughshane, Ballymena BT42 4JP Tel: 028 2586 1214 Fax: 028 2586 2281 — MB BCh BAO Belf. 1964; DObst RCOG 1966; DCH RCPSI 1975; MRCGP 1975. Socs: BMA. Prev: Ho. Off. Belf. City Hosp.; SHO (Midw.) Ards Hosp.; SHO Ulster Hosp. Sick Childr.

REDMOND, Stephen James Ellergreen Medical Centre, 24 Carr Lane, Norris Green, Liverpool L11 2YA Tel: 0151 256 9800 Fax: 0151 256 5765; 95 Queens Drive, Liverpool L15 7ND Tel: 0151 737 1719 — MB BS Lond. 1978; DCH RCP Lond. 1983.

REDMOND, Timothy Kevin 33 Score Lane, Childwall, Liverpool L16 6AN Tel: 0151 722 6312 — MB BS Lond. 1978 (Lond. Hosp.) MB BS (Hons._Distinc. Surg.) Lond. 1978; MA Camb. 1979; MRCP (UK) 1981; DCH Eng. 1981.

REDMOND, Vera Alexandra Broughshane Medical Practice, 76 Main Street, Broughshane, Ballymena BT42 4JP Tel: 028 2586 1214 Fax: 028 2586 2281 — MB BCh BAO Belf. 1965. Princip. Gen. Pract. & Community Family Plann. Dr. Socs: Mem. Fac. of Family Plann. and Reproductive Health Care. Prev: Ho. Off. Ards Hosp. Newtownards.

REDMORE, Michael John The Grange Clinic, Westfield Avenue, Malpas, Newport NP20 6EY Tel: 01633 855521 Fax: 01633 859490; 103 Ringwood Hill, Newport NP19 9EA — MB BS Nottm. 1982; DRCOG 1985; MRCGP 1986.

REDPATH, Alexander 5 Woodside, Hexham NE46 1HU — MB ChB Dundee 1975; FFA RCS Eng. 1980. Cons. Anaesth. Hexham Gen. Hosp. Specialty: Anaesth.

REDPATH, Anne Margaret Abbey House Medical Practice, Golding Close, Daventry — MB ChB Birm. 1995; BDS Lond. 1987; DRCOG 1997; DFFP 2000; MRCGP 2002. GP Partner; Clin. Asst., Maxillofacial Surg., Univ. Hosps. Coventry & Warks. NHS Trust, Coventry & Warks. Hosp., Stoney Stanton Rd, Coventry. Socs: BMA; Rugby & Dist. Med. Soc. Prev: SHO (Oral Surg.) Soton. Gen. Hosp.; Ho. Off. (Surg. & Med.) Northampton Gen. Hosp.

REDPATH, Calum Jon 29 Stevenson Road, Edinburgh EH11 2SH — MB ChB Glas. 1997.

REDPATH, Douglas (retired) Nuthatch, Low St., Burton-in-Lonsdale, Carnforth LA6 3LF — LMSSA Lond. 1949 (Guy's) MRCGP 1958.

REDPATH, James Barron Scott 11 Orion Way, Carluke ML8 5TP — MB ChB Ed. 1971; FFA RCS Eng. 1978. Specialty: Anaesth.

REDPATH, Marion 28 Hayfield Road, Kirkcaldy KY2 5DG — MB ChB Dundee 1979.

REDPATH, Sharon Carlisle House, 53 Lagland Street, Poole BH15 1QD Tel: 01202 678484 Fax: 01202 660507 — MB BS Lond. 1981; DRCOG 1983; DCH RCP Lond. 1985; MRCGP 1986.

REDPATH, Trevor Henry (retired) Manor Foram, Blockford, Yeovil BA22 7EE Tel: 01963 441374 — (Guy's) FDS RCS Eng. 1967, LDS 1958; MRCS Eng. LRCP Lond. 1964. Cons. Oral & Maxillofacial Surg. Soton. Univ. Teach. Hosp. & N. Hants. Dist. HA.

REDSHAW, Gillian Clare Temple — BM Soton. 1986. Specialty: Dermat.

REDSTONE, David 7 Charlotte Road, London SW13 9QJ — MB ChB St. And. 1955; DCH Eng. 1960. Lect. Paediat. & Hon. Lect. Chem. Path. St. Mary's Hosp. Med. Sch. Lond. Prev: RAF Med. Br.; Regist. in Clin. Path. St. Mary's Hosp. Lond.

REDVERS, Amanda 88 Gascoigne Road, New Addington, Croydon CR0 0NE — MB BS Lond. 1996.

REDWOOD, David Robert St. Anthony's Hospital, North Cheam, Sutton SM3 9DW Tel: 020 8337 6691; Oakwood Cottage, Ide Hill Road, Ide Hill, Sevenoaks TN14 6JY — MB BChir Camb. 1961; MA Camb. 1962; FRCP Lond. 1979, M 1963. Cons. Cardiol. St. Anthony's Hosp. N. Cheam. Specialty: Cardiol. Prev: Cons. Cardiol. SW Thames Regional Cardiothoracic Unit; Hon. Sen. Lect. St. Geo. Hosp. Med. Sch. Lond.; Vis. Scientist & Chief Cardiovasc. Diag. Nat. Inst. of Health Bethesda, USA.

REDWOOD, Michael David The Surgery, 25 Alms Hill, Bourn, Cambridge CB3 7SH Tel: 01954 719313 Fax: 01954 718012 — MB BS Lond. 1987 (St. Thos.) DCH RCP Lond. 1991; DRCOG 1992; MRCGP 1993; T(GP) 1993.

REDWOOD, Mr Nicholas Frederick Wakerley Dept of Surgery, The Queen Elizabeth Hospital, Gayton Road, King's Lynn PE30 4ET — MB BS Lond. 1984; FRCS Eng. 1990. Cons. Gen. & Vasc. Surg. Specialty: Gen. Surg. Prev: Sen. Regist., Northern Region Vasc. Unit, Newc.

REDWOOD, Rebekah 183 Cator Lane N., Chilwell, Nottingham NG9 4BL — BM BS Nottm. 1998; BM BS Nottm 1998.

REDWOOD, Simon Robert Cardiothoraci Centre, St Thomas's Hospital, Lambeth Palace Road, London SE1 7EH Tel: 020 7960 5638 Fax: 020 7401 3527 — MB BS Lond. 1987 (St. Geo. Hosp. Med. Sch.) MRCP (UK) 1990; MD Lond. 1996; FACC 2001. Sen. Lec./Cons Cardiol St. Thos. Hosp. Lond. Specialty: Cardiol.; Gen. Med. Prev: Interven. Fell. (Cardiol.) Washington Cardiol. Center Washington, DC, USA; Clin. Research Regist. (Cardiol.) St. Geo. Hosp. Med. Sch.; Regist. (Cardiol.) Roy. Free Hosp. Lond.

REDZISZ, Boleslaw 57 Queens Road, Leicester LE8 4EH — MD Beirut 1946.

REE, Christopher James Brooklea Health Centre, Wick Rd., Brislington, Bristol Tel: 0117 971 1211 Fax: 0117 972 3169 Email: chris.lee@dial.pipex.com — MB ChB Bristol 1983; MA Oxf. 1980; MRCGP 1987; DRCOG 1987; DCH RCP Lond. 1988.

REEBACK, Jane Susan 40 St Marys Avenue, Northwood HA6 3AZ — MB BS Lond. 1972 (Lond. Hosp.) BSc (Hons.) Lond. 1969, MB BS (Hons.) 1972; MRCP (UK) 1975. Clin. Asst. (Rheum.) Edgware Gen. Hosp. Specialty: Rehabil. Med.; Rheumatol. Socs: Brit. Soc. Rheum. Prev: Sen. Regist. (Rheum.) Lond. Hosp.; Regist. Guy's Hosp. Lond.; SHO (Med.) & Ho. Phys. Lond. Hosp.

REECE, Alastair Hugh Mackintosh Wexham Park Hospital, Slough SL2 4HL Tel: 01753 633000; 1 Hockley Lane, Stoke Poges, Slough SL2 4QF Tel: 01753 663480 — MB ChB Dundee 1975; MSc Cardiff 1999. Hosp. Pract. Chronic Pain Clinic. Specialty: Rehabil. Med.

REECE, Mr Anthony Thomas Christopher Freeman Hospital, High Heaton, Newcastle upon Tyne NE7 7DN; 117 Glenthorn Road, Jesmond, Newcastle upon Tyne NE2 3HJ — MB ChB Dundee 1983; FRCS Eng. 1988. Sen. Regist. Rotat. (Orthop.) Newc. & Sunderland N. RHA. Specialty: Orthop. Prev: Smith & Nephew Trauma Research Fell. Univ. Dept. Orthop. Glenfield Gen. Hosp. Leic.; W. Scotl. Surg. Rotat. Glas. Roy. Infirm.; Regist. (Orthop.) Leicester Roy. Infirm.

REECE, Ashley 37 Kingfisher Way, Leeds LS17 8XA — MB ChB Leeds 1995.

REECE, Dorothy Ann Moor House, Friar Terrace, Hartlepool TS24 0PF Tel: 01429 66803 — MB BS Durh. 1958. Prev: SHO Sunderland Childr. Hosp.; Ho. Phys. Roy. Vict. Infirm. Newc.; Ho. Surg. Newc. Gen. Hosp.

REECE, Elizabeth Victoria — MB BCh Wales 1992; DRCOG; DFFP; DCH; MRCGP (merit) 1999. GP VTS Bath. Specialty: Gen. Pract.

REECE, Gillian June Kenmure Medical Practice, 7 Springfield Road, Bishopbriggs, Glasgow G66 7PJ; 3 Kirklee Quadrant, Kelvinside, Glasgow G12 0TR — MB ChB Glas. 1985; DA (UK) 1989; DCH RCP Lond. 1992; DRCOG 1992; MRCGP 1992; DFFP 1997.

REECE, Mr Ian James Ravenshill, Llanishen Hill, Llanishen, Chepstow NP16 6QS Tel: 01600 860009 Fax: 01600 869039 — MB BS Lond. 1974 (St Bart.) MDCH; FFAEM; MRCS Eng. LRCP Lond. 1974; FRCS Eng. 1979. Medico-legal Pract. Specialty: Cardiothoracic Surg.; Surgery, Vascular; Accid. & Emerg. Special Interest: Cardiac; Chest; Muscular Injuries. Prev: Cons. (A & E Med.) Pr. Chas. Hosp. Merthyr Tydfil & Roy. Hosp. Haslar; Cons. (Cardiac Surg.) Glas. Roy. Infirm.; Sen. Regist. (Cardiothoracic Surg.) Glas. Roy. Infirm.

REECE, Michael Frederick (retired) Moor House, Friar Terrace, Hartlepool TS24 0PF Tel: 01429 266803 — MB BS Durh. 1958; MRCGP 1967. Hosp. Pract. (Med.) Hartlepool Gen. Hosp.; Clin. Tutor Univ. Newc. Prev: GP Hartlepool.

REECE, Mr Michael William (retired) September Cottage, Yeoland Down, Yelverton PL20 6BY Tel: 01822 852037 Email: mwreece@globalnet.co.uk — (St. Thos.) MB BS Lond. 1948; FRCS Eng. 1953. Prev: Cons. Surg. Plymouth HA.

REECE, Richard John Department of Rheumatology, Huddersfield Royal Infirmary, Acre Street, Lindley, Huddersfield HD3 3EA Tel: 01484 342990 Fax: 01484 342241 — MB BCh Wales 1987 (Univ. of Wales Coll. of Med.) FRCP 2002. Cons. and Hon. Sen. Lect. in Rheum. Specialty: Rheumatol. Special Interest: Arthroscopy; osteoarthritis; Synovitis. Socs: Brit. Soc. Rheum. Prev: Regist. (Renal & Gen. Med.) Roy. Devon & Exeter Hosp.; Regist. Roy. Devon & Exeter Hosps.; SHO (Gen. Med.) Northampton Gen. Hosp.

REECE, Mr Victor Alan Cyril, RD South Tyneside District Hospital, Accident & Emergency Department, South Shields NE34 0PL Tel: 0191 202 4049 Fax: 0191 202 4049 Email: alan.reece@sthct.nhs.uk; 72 Moorfield Gardens, Cleadon, Sunderland SR6 7TP Tel: 0191 537 4817 Email: reece.alan@virgin.net — (Newc. u. Tyne) BSc Newc. 1967; MB BS Newc. 1970; FRCS Eng. 1975; FFAEM 1993. Cons. A & E S. Tyneside Dist. Hosp. S. Shields. Specialty: Accid. & Emerg. Socs: Assoc. Mem. Brit. Hyperbaric Assn.; Brit. Assn. Accid. & Emerg. Med.; Fell. Roy. Soc. Med. Prev: Surg. Cdr. RNR; Co Surg St John Amb; Chairm. Med. Advis. Gp. Northumbria Ambul. Serv.

REECE-SMITH, Mr Howard St Anthonys, 95 Reading Road, Finchampstead, Wokingham RG40 4RD — MB BS Lond. 1973 (Lond. Hosp.) FRCS Eng. 1978; MS Lond. 1981. Cons. Surg. Reading Hosps. Specialty: Gen. Surg. Socs: ASGBI; ACPGBI. Prev: Sen. Surg. Regist. Roy. United Hosp. Bath; Hanson Trust Surg. Research Fell. John Radcliffe Hosp. Oxf.; Cons. Surg. Battle Hosp. Reading.

REED, Alice 2 The Woodlands, Slad Road, Stroud GL5 1QE — MRCS Eng. LRCP Lond. 1945 (Leeds) MRCS Eng., LRCP Lond. 1945. Prev: Leeds & Matern. Hosp. Leeds.

REED, Alison The Reaside Clinic, Birmingham Great Park., Bristol Road South, Birmingham B45 9BE Tel: 0121 678 3052 — MB BS Lond. 1983; MRCP (UK) 1987; MRCPsych 1989. Sen. Lect. in Forens. Psychiat. Uni. Of Birm., Hon. Cons. Readside Clinic, Birm.. Specialty: Forens. Psychiat. Prev: Research Worker Inst. Psychiat. & Hon. Sen. Regist. Maudsley Hosp.; Sen.Regist. Rotat. (Forens.Psychiat.) Maudsley Hosp.; Sen. Regist. (Forens. Psychiat)Readside Clinic.

REED, Andrew John Cantilupe Surgery, 49-51 St. Owen Street, Hereford HR1 2JB Tel: 01432 268031 Fax: 01432 352584 — MB BS Lond. 1961 (Westm.) DObst RCOG 1968. Socs: Past-Pres. Herts. Med. Soc. Prev: Ho. Surg. Gordon Hosp. Lond.; Surg. Lt.-Cdr. RN.

REED, Andrew Mark 143 Butchers Lane, Mereworth, Maidstone ME18 5QD — MB BS Lond. 1997.

REED, Anne Elisabeth Ryder Taunton Road Medical Centre, 12-16 Taunton Road, Bridgwater TA6 3LS Tel: 01278 720000 Fax: 01278 423691; 78 Wembdon Hill, Bridgwater TA6 7PZ — MB BS Lond. 1974 (Lond. Hosp.)

REED, Anne Mary 7 Rede Place, London W2 4TU — MB BS Lond. 1988.

REED, Anthony Birbeck Medical Group, Penrith Health Centre, Bridge Lane, Penrith CA11 8HW Tel: 01768 245200 Fax: 01768 245295; Ellangowan, Pooley Bridge, Penrith CA10 2NG Tel: 01768 486256 Fax: 01768 486256 — MB BS Newc. 1968; FRCGP 1984, M 1972; DObst RCOG 1972. Examr. RCGP. Prev: Trainee GP Newc. VTS; Ho. Phys. & Ho. Surg. Roy. Vict. Infirm. Newc.; chairm.eden valley Pcg.

REED, Anthony Bridge Cottage Surgery, 41 High Street, Welwyn AL6 9EF Tel: 01438 715044 Fax: 01438 714013; The Thatched Cottage, Walkern Road, Watton-at-Stone, Hertford SG14 3RN Tel: 01920 832118 Email: areeddoc@aol.com — MB BS Lond. 1981 (St. Mary's) DRCOG 1985. GP Welwyn. Specialty: Gen. Pract. Prev: Ship's Phys. Wind Star Miami; SHO Qu. Eliz. II Hosp. Welwyn Garden City; Trainee GP Welwyn Garden City VTS.

REED, Anthony Raddon 2 Wanstead Place, London E11 2SW — MB ChB Cape Town 1989.

REED, Antonia Lucy — MB ChB Leeds 1996; DCH Lond. 2001. Specialty: Gen. Pract.

REED, Derwyn Huw Nevill Hall And District Hospital Trust, Abergavenny NP7 7EG — MB BS Lond. 1982; MA Camb. 1982, BA 1979; MRCP (UK) 1985; FRCR 1988. Cons. Diag. Radiol. Nevill Hall Hosp. Abergavenny. Specialty: Radiol. Prev: Sen. Regist. (Diag. Radiol.) Univ. Hosp. Wales Cardiff; Regist. (Diag. Radiol.) Addenbrooke's Hosp. Camb.; SHO (Gen. Med.) Univ. Coll. Hosp. Lond.

REED, Dianna Tracy — MB ChB Aberd. 1993; DFFP, DRCOG, MRCGP. CMO Family Plann., Arbroath / Staff Grade Community Paediat.(SO/SG split), Angus. Specialty: Family Plann. & Reproduc. Health; Community Child Health. Socs: MRCGP; DRCOG. Prev: Trainee GP Dumfries VTS.; GP Trainee.

REED, Elizabeth Alice — MB ChB Ed. 1983 (Edinburgh) BSc (Med. Sci.) Ed. 1980, MB ChB 1983; MRCP)UK) 1988. Locum cons Geriat. med. Specialty: Care of the Elderly; Rheumatol.; Gen. Med.

Socs: Brit Geriat. soc. Prev: Sen Reg gen & Geriat. med, Glan clwyd hosp & Roy. Liverp. Hosp; Research Regist. (Med. for Elderly) Woodend Hosp. Aberd.; Regist. (Med.) Rotherham Dist. Gen. Hosp.

REED, Freda Susanne (retired) Castle Cottage, Chilham, Canterbury CT4 8DB Tel: 01227 730330 — MB BS Lond. 1946 (W. Lond. & Univ. Coll. Lond.) MRCS Eng. LRCP Lond. 1946; DPM Eng. 1962; FRCPsych 1979, M 1973. Hon. Cons. Psychiat. Maidstone HA.; Vis. Psychiat. H.M. Prison Canterbury. Prev: SCMO (Child & Family Psychiat.) Dover.

REED, Heather La Tourelle, Ruette de la Generotte, Castel, Guernsey GY5 7PG Tel: 01481 252511 — MB BS Lond. 1976 (St. George's Hospital Medical School) MRCOG 1989. Cons. (O & G) Princess Eliz. Hosp. Guernsey. Specialty: Obst. & Gyn. Prev: Sen. Regist. (O & G) Derriford Hosp. Plymouth.

REED, Hilary Willow Tree House, Westleigh Drive, Bromley BR1 2PN — MB BS Lond. 1956 (Guy's) MRCS Eng. LRCP Lond. 1956; DObst RCOG 1958; DCH Eng. 1958; MRCPCH 1986. Audiology (Bromley).

REED, Ian Alan Albion House Surgery, Albion Street, Brierley Hill DY5 3EE Tel: 01384 70220 Fax: 01384 78284; 269 Hagley Road, Stourbridge DY9 0RJ Email: ian_reed@bigfoot.com — MB BCh Wales 1987 (University Wales) DRCOG 1990; Cert. Family Plann. JCC 1990; T (GP) 1991; MRCGP 1994. Princip. GP. Specialty: Cardiol. Socs: BMA & Roy. Coll. GPs.

REED, Isabel Therese Delma Bushyfields Hospital, Russell Hall, Dudley DY1 2LZ; 269 Hagley Road, Stourbridge DY9 0RJ — MB BCh Wales 1987. Clin. Asst. (Psychiat.) Lucy Baldwin Hosp. Stourport-on-Severn. Specialty: Gen. Psychiat. Socs: BMA.

REED, Joanna Bell Hinchingbrooke Hospital, Hinchingbrooke, Huntingdon PE18 8NT — BM BS Nottm. 1987; BMedSci (Hons.) Nottm. 1985; FRCS Eng. 1992. Specialty: Gen. Surg. Prev: Sen. Research Assoc. (Surg.) Univ. Newc.; Specialist Regist. (Gen. Surg.) N. Region.

REED, John (retired) Trenhale, Treseders Gdn, Truro TR1 1TR Tel: 01872 278612 — (Sheff.) BSc (Hons. Physiol.) Sheff. 1936, MB ChB 1939; DPH Manch. 1948.

REED, John Langdale, CB HM Inspectorate of Prisons, Home Office, 50 Queen Anne's Gate, London SW1H 9AT Tel: 020 7273 2305 Fax: 020 7273 4087; Willow Tree House, Westleigh Drive, Bromley BR1 2PN Tel: 020 8467 1452 Fax: 020 8249 4940 — MB BChir Camb. 1956 (Guy's) FRCP Lond. 1974, M 1958; DPM Lond. 1964; FRCPsych 1974, M 1971. Prev: Med. Insp. HM Inspectorate of Prisons Lond.; Special Adviser Ment. Health & Community Care Div. DoH; Qu. Hon. Phys.

REED, John Matheson Heathfield, Collinswood Road, Farnham Common, Slough SL2 3LH Tel: 01753 5316 — MRCS Eng. LRCP Lond. 1945 (St. Thos.)

REED, John Paul Front Street Surgery, 14 Front Street, Acomb, York YO24 3BZ Tel: 01904 794141 Fax: 01904 788304 — MB BS Newc. 1991.

REED, John Richard 26c Nassington Road, London NW3 2UD — MB BS Lond. 1991; MRCP (UK) 1996. Specialty: Dermat.

REED, Laurence John 12 Trinity Church Square, London SE1 4HU; Department of Psychological Medicine, Institute of Psychiatry, De Crespigny Park, Denmark Hill, London SE5 8AF — MB BS Lond. 1994.

REED, Lesley 3 Lower Hall Road, Lascelles Hall, Huddersfield HD5 0AZ — MB ChB Leeds 1984.

REED, Linda 27 Lilburn Close, East Boldon NE36 0TZ — BM BS Nottm. 1986; DCH RCP Lond. 1990; MRCGP 1990.

REED, Professor Malcolm Walter Ronald Academic Surgical Oncology Unit, University of Sheffield, K Floor, Royal Hallamshire Hospital, Sheffield S10 2JF Tel: 0114 271 3326 Fax: 0114 271 3314 Email: m.w.reed@shef.ac.uk — MB ChB Sheff. 1981; FRCS Eng. 1986; BMedSci Sheff. 1979, MD 1990. Prof. Surg. Oncol./ Hon. Cons. Surg, Univ. of Sheff., Roy. Hallamshire Hosp. Prev: Cons. Surg. Roy. Hallamshire Hosp. Sheff.; Sen. Lect. (Surg.) Univ. Sheff.; Regist. Sheff. & Lincoln HAs.

REED, Mark Geoffrey 30 Crescent Road, Kingston upon Thames KT2 7RG — BM BCh Oxf. 1998; BM BCh Oxf 1998.

REED, Mr Michael Richard Northumbria Healthcare NHS Trust, Orthopaedics Department, North Tyneside General Hospital, Rake Lane, North Shields NE29 8NH — MB BS Newc. 1992; FRCS Ed. 1996. Cons. Orthop. Surg. Northumbria Healthcare NHS Trust. Specialty: Orthop. Socs: Brit. Orthop. Research Soc. Prev: Specialist Regist. (Orthop.) North. Deanery.

REED, Michelle 52 Commercial Road, Machen, Caerphilly CF83 8PG — MB BS Lond. 1998; MB BS Lond 1998.

REED, Natasha Jane Hunter 15 Kings Road, Cambridge CB3 9DY — MB BS Lond. 1994. Specialty: Gen. Psychiat.

REED, Nicholas Guy — BM BS Nottm. 1983; BMedSci Nottm. 1981; DRCOG 1985; MRCGP 1987. GP; Chairm. WellingBoro. PCG. Specialty: Gen. Pract.; Medico Legal; Occupat. Health. Socs: Soc. Occupat. Med.; N.ants. Medico-legal Soc. Prev: Trainee GP Croydon HA VTS; Ho. Phys. Edgware Gen. Hosp.; Ho. Surg. Mayday Hosp. Croydon.

REED, Nicholas Laurence Cobwebs, 14 Carvers Lane, Ringwood BN24 1LB — BM Soton. 1995; MRCP (UK) 1999; FRCR (LON) 2003.

REED, Nicholas Norman Stone House, West Felton, Oswestry SY11 4EH — BM BS Nottm. 1986. Specialty: Obst. & Gyn.

REED, Nicholas Simon Ephraim Western Infirmary , Beatson Oncology Centre, Dumbarton Road, Glasgow G11 6NT Tel: 0141 211 2658 Fax: 0141 211 6356 Email: nick.reed@northglasgow.scot.nhs.uk; 15 Cleveden Road, Glasgow G12 0PQ Email: nicksreed@aol.com — MB BS Lond. 1976 (Roy. Free) MRCS Eng. LRCP Lond. 1976; MRCP (UK) 1979; FRCR 1982; FRCP Glas. 1988. Cons. (Clin. Oncol.) West. Gen. Infirm. Glas.; Chairm. EORTC Gyn. Cancer Gp. Specialty: Oncol.; Radiother. Prev: Clin. Dir. Beatson Oncol. Centre Glas.; Sen. Regist. (Radiother. & Oncol.) Wessex Radiother. Centre Soton.; Regist. (Radiother. & Oncol.) Hammersmith Hosp. Lond.

REED, Pamela Jean (retired) 11 Rossett Beck, Harrogate HG2 9NT — MB ChB Leeds 1956.

REED, Paul Francis Queens Park Hospital, Haslingden Rd, Blackburn BB2 3HH Tel: 01254 293403 Fax: 01254 293856 — MB ChB Manch. 1984; MRCPsych 1989; MSc Manch. 1993. Cons. Psychiat. Lancashire Care NHS Trust. Specialty: Gen. Psychiat. Socs: Roy. Coll. Psychiat.; Brit. Med. Assoc.; Brit. Assn. Of PsychoPharmacol. Prev: Cons (Psychiat.) Roy. Bolton Hosp.; Cons. (Psychiat.) Ment. Health Serv.s of Salford NHS Trust.

REED, Paul Nicholas 19 Regency Way, Peterborough PE3 6HJ — MB BS Lond. 1977 (St. Mary's) MRCS Eng. LRCP Lond. 1977; FFA RCS Eng. 1983. Cons. Anaesth. P'boro. NHS Trust. Specialty: Anaesth. Socs: Assn. Anaesth.; Brit. Hyperbaric Assn.; (Hon. Sec.) Sheff. & E. Midl. Soc. Anaesth. Prev: Sen. Regist. (Anaesth.) Leic. HA; Sen. Specialist Anaesth. RAMC; Regtl. Med. Off. 3rd Roy. Ang./2nd RRF.

REED, Peter Austin The Lodge, Newton Road, Emberton, Olney MK46 5JJ Tel: 01234 241925 — BM BS Nottm. 1976; FFA RCS Eng. 1981. Cons. Anaesth. Milton Keynes Gen. Dist. Hosp. Specialty: Anaesth.

REED, Peter Dennis Taunton Road Medical Centre, 12-16 Taunton Road, Bridgwater TA6 3LS Tel: 01278 444400 Fax: 01278 423691 — MB BS Lond. 1974 (Lond. Hosp.) DA Eng. 1978.

REED, Peter Ivan (retired) — MB BS Lond. 1953 (King's Coll. Hosp.) MRCS Eng. LRCP Lond. 1953; LMCC 1957; CRCP Canada 1959; FRCP Lond. 1976, M 1963; FRCP Canada 1972. Prev: Cons. Phys. Hammersmith Hosp. & Heatherwood & Wexham Pk. Hosp. Trust.

REED, Phillip David Barnsley District General Hospital NHS Trust, Pogmore Road, Barnsley S75 2EP — MB ChB Sheff. 1992.

REED, Richard William Holland House, 31 Church Road, Lytham, Lytham St Annes FY8 5LL Tel: 01253 794999 Fax: 01253 795744; 12 Eden Avenue, Lytham, Lytham St Annes FY8 5PS Tel: 01253 730500 — MB ChB Manch. 1975; MRCGP 1982. Clin. Asst. (Cardiol.) Vict. Hosp. Blackpool. Prev: SHO (Obst.) & SHO (Paediat.) Vict. Hosp. Blackpool.

REED, Roderick Alan Wendover Health Centre, Aylesbury Road, Wendover, Aylesbury HP22 6LD Tel: 01296 623452 — MB BS Lond. 1983 (King's Coll. Lond.) DRCOG 1990; MRCGP 1995.

REED, Ruth Catherine Dalston Medical Group, Townhead Road, Dalston, Carlisle CA5 7PZ — MB BS Newcastle 1980; MRCGP 1984. GP Carlisle.

REED, Susan Margaret Quarry Dene, Owl Lane, Gawthorpe, Ossett WF5 9AU Tel: 01924 270749 — MB ChB Manch. 1975; BSc St. And. 1972. Med. Adviser DWP. Prev: Trainee GP Leeds VTS;

Sen. Med. Off. (Child Health) Bradford HA; Ho. Phys. & Ho. Surg. Derby City Hosp.

REED, Sylvia Elsie (retired) 57 Watford Road, St Albans AL1 2AE — MB BChir Camb. 1954; FRCPath 1978, M 1972. Prev: Mem. Scientif. Staff MRC.

REED, Timothy John Haven Health Surgery, Grange Farm Avenue, Felixstowe IP11 2FB Tel: 01394 670107 Fax: 01394 282872 — MB BS Lond. 1985; MA Camb. 1980; DRCOG 1988; DCH RCP Lond. 1989; MRCGP 1990.

REEDER, Judith Alison Dr A Willis and Partners, King Edward Road Surgery, Christchurch Medical Centre, King Edward Road, Northampton NN1 5LY Tel: 01604 633466 Fax: 01604 603227 Email: judith-sood@ntlworld.com; 45 Thorburn Road, Weston Favell, Northampton NN3 3DA Tel: 01604 401426 — MB ChB Leeds 1985; DCH RCP Lond. 1988; DRCOG 1989; MRCGP 1990. Prev: Ho. Phys. Chapel Allerton Hosp. Leeds; Ho. Surg. Wycombe Gen. Hosp.

REEDER, Martin Kingston 9 East Cottages, Shipton Road, Clifton, York YO30 5RH — MB BS Lond. 1979 (St. Bart.) BSc Lond. 1976, MB BS 1979; MRCP (UK) 1983; FFA RCS 1987. Specialty: Anaesth.

REEDER, Sally Ann 18 Kendal Green, Kendal LA9 5PN Tel: 01539 720821 — MB ChB Dundee 1986. Salaried Gen. Practitioner; Med. Director Out-of-Hours Co-op.

REEK, Christine Radiology Department, University Hospital of Leicester NHS Trust, Glenfield Hospital, Groby Road, Leicester LE3 9QP Tel: 0116 256 3093 Fax: 0116 256 3886 — MB ChB Manch. 1979; BSc (Hons.) Manch. 1976, MB ChB 1979; FRCR 1985. Cons. Radiol. (Cardiac Radiol.) Glenfield Hosp. Leics. Specialty: Radiol. Prev: Fell. (Cardiovasc. Radiol.) Green La. Hosp. Auckland, NZ; Sen. Regist. (Cardiac. Radiol.) Groby Rd. Hosp. Leics.; Sen. Regist. (Diag. Radiol.) Leics.

REEKIE, Alexander Euan Mackay (retired) Birchwood House, Sandyloan Crescent, Laurieston, Falkirk FK2 9NG Tel: 01324 623860 — MB ChB Ed. 1951. Prev: Res. Med. & Orthop. Ho. Off. Law Hosp. Carluke.

REEKIE, Elizabeth Heather (retired) Birchwood House, Sandyloan Crescent, Laurieston, Falkirk FK2 9NG Tel: 01324 623860 — MB ChB Ed. 1955. Prev: GP Falkirk.

REEKIE, Ian (retired) Mann Cottage, Moreton-in-Marsh GL56 0LA Tel: 01608 650764 Fax: 01608 650996; Wold House, Blockley, Moreton-in-Marsh GL56 9BA Tel: 01386 700546 — (Guy's) MB BS Lond. 1964; MRCS Eng. LRCP Lond. 1966; DObst RCOG 1969. Prev: Cas. Off. Guy's Hosp.

REEKIE, Robert Andrew, OBE Ash Tree House, Hyde Lane, Marlborough SN8 1JN Tel: 01672 512083 Email: andrewreekie@doctors.org.uk — MB BChir Camb. 1966 (Camb. & St. Geo.) MRCS Eng. LRCP Lond. 1966; MA Camb. 1966; DObst RCOG 1970; DCH Eng. 1976; MRCGP 1977; DTM & H Liverp. 1988; DPD Wales 1990. Socs: Fell. of the Roy. Soc. of Trop. Med. and Hyg.

REEKIE, Robert Morris ClinTrials Research Ltd., 1 Cadogan Square, Cadogan St., Glasgow G2 7HF Tel: 0141 222 5500 Fax: 0141 222 5511; Robertloan House, 32 Main St, Loans, Troon KA10 7EX — MB ChB Ed. 1982; BSc (Hons.) St. And. 1979; Dip. Pharm. Med. RCP 1988; MFPM 1990; MBA Nottm. 1995. Sen. Dir., Med. & Regulatory Clin. Trials Research Ltd Glas. Specialty: Pharmaceutical Medicine. Prev: Med. Dir. DAR Ltd.; Head Clin. Developm. & Internat. Managem. Boots Pharmaceut. Nottm.

REEKS, John Lionel Prestonpans Health Centre, Preston Road, Prestonpans EH32 9QS Tel: 01875 52606 — MB ChB Dundee 1973.

REES, Alan Martin Y Delyn, Llangan, Bridgend CF35 5DR — MB BCh Wales 1976.

REES, Alexandra Elizabeth Joy Llandough Hospital, Penylan Road, Penarth, Cardiff CF64 2XX Tel: 029 2071 5528 Fax: 029 2071 6112 Email: alexandra.rees@cardiffandvale.wales.nhs.uk — MB ChB Liverp. 1981; Dip. Obst.; MRCOG 1987; FRCOG 1997. Cons. O & G Llandough Hosp. Cardiff. Specialty: Obst. & Gyn. Socs: RCOG; BMFMS; BAPM. Prev: Sen. Regist. Morriston Hosp. Swansea & Llandough Hosp. Cardiff; Perinatal Fell. (Reproduc. Med.) Groote Schurr Hosp. Cape Town.

REES, Alice Mary 38 Church Street, Lenton, Nottingham NG7 2FF — BM BS Nottm. 1998; BM BS Nottm 1998.

REES, Allison Noreen Waterloo Road Surgery, 178 Waterloo Road, Blackpool FY4 3AD Tel: 01253 348619 Fax: 01253 404330 — MB ChB Manch. 1990 (St. And. & Manch.) BSc (Med. Sci.) Manch. 1987; DRCOG 1993; MRCGP 1994; DCH RCP Lond. 1995.

REES, Alun (retired) Combedene, Broadwell Close, Combe St Nicholas, Chard TA20 3PB — MRCS Eng. LRCP Lond. 1942 (Middlx.)

REES, Mr Alun 25 Lakeside Drive, Lakeside Est., Cyncoed, Cardiff CF23 6DF — MB BCh Wales 1963; FRCS Eng. 1970.

REES, Alun David Meddygfa Pengorof, Gorof Road, Ystradgynlais, Swansea SA9 1DS Tel: 01639 843221 Fax: 01639 843790 — MB BCh Wales 1978.

REES, Alyson Frances Park Medical Centre, Ball Haye Road, Leek ST13 6QP; Luxmore, Buxton Road, Leek ST13 6NE — MB ChB Liverp. 1982; MRCGP 1986. Specialty: Gen. Pract.

REES, Amanda Jane Severne Rotherham General Hospital, Moorgate Road, Rotherham S60 2UD Tel: 01709 824581 — MB BChir Camb. 1983; FRCS Eng. 1986; FRCS (Orth.) 1993. Cons. Orthop. Rotherham Gen. Hosp. Specialty: Orthop. Prev: Clin. Lect. (Orthop.) Sheff.

REES, Andrew Hugh The Surgery, 113 Church Lane, Stechford, Birmingham B33 9EJ Tel: 0121 783 2861 — MB ChB Birm. 1965; DObst RCOG 1968.

REES, Andrew Jackson 20 The Chanonry, Aberdeen AB24 1RQ — MB ChB Liverp. 1969; MRCP (UK) 1972; MSc Lond. 1979; FRCP Lond. 1 9832. Prof. Nephrol. Roy. Postgrad. Med. Sch. Hammersmith Hosp. Lond.; Hon. Sen. Lect. Roy. Postgrad. Med. Sch. Lond. Socs: Assn. Phys. & Internat. Soc. Nephrol. Prev: Cons. Phys. (Nephrol.) Hammersmith Hosp. Lond.

REES, Angela Lynn 23 Denby Drive, Cleethorpes DN35 9QQ — MB BS Lond. 1996.

REES, Ann Old Oaks, Nantgaredig, Carmarthen SA32 7LJ — MB BCh Wales 1965.

REES, Anne Margaret Deparment of Community Child Health, Trinity Buildings, 21 Orchard St., Swansea SA1 5AT Tel: 01792 651501 — MB BCh Wales 1978; DCH RCP Lond. 1982; MRCGP 1984. Staff Grade Community Paediat. Specialty: Community Child Health.

REES, Bethan Margaret Penylan Surgery, 74 Penylan Road, Cardiff CF23 5SY Tel: 029 2049 8181 Fax: 029 2049 1507; 1 St. Edeyrn's Close, Cyncoed, Cardiff CF23 6TH Tel: 029 2076 3153 — MB BCh Wales 1972; DObst RCOG 1974.

REES, Bethan Wyn 14 Mylne Close, Upper Mall, London W6 9TE — MB BCh Wales 1994.

REES, Betty 9B Fulwood Park, Liverpool L17 5AA — MB ChB Liverp. 1942; MD 1950. Prev: Cons. Genito-Urinary Phys., Roy. Liverp. Univ. Hosp.; Head of Univ. Dept. of G-V Med.

REES, Mr Brian Idris St. David's, The Avenue, Llandaff, Cardiff CF5 2L Tel: 029 2056 3109 — MB BChir Camb. 1970 (Camb. & St. Bart.) MA, MB Camb. 1970, BChir 1969; MRCS Eng. LRCP Lond. 1969; FRCS Eng. 1974. Cons. Surg. Univ. Hosp. Wales Cardiff.; Specialist Adviser in Gen. Surg. S. Wales; Chairm. Welsh Bd. Roy. Coll. of Surgeons of Eng.; Director Wales Inst. Minimal Acces Ther.; Lead Cancer Clinician SE Wales Network. Specialty: Gen. Surg. Special Interest: Hernia, colorectal and laparo-endoscopic Surg. Socs: Pres. Welsh Surgic. Soc. Prev: Sen. Regist. Hosp. Sick Childr. Lond.; Sen. Regist. (Surg.) Univ. Hosp. Wales Cardiff; Regist. (Rotat.) Univ. Hosp. Wales.

REES, Bryn Spencer James Melville Street Surgery, 17 Melville Street, Ryde PO33 2AF Tel: 01983 811431 Fax: 01983 817215 — MB BS Lond. 1975; MRCS Eng. LRCP Lond. 1975; MRCGP 1980.

REES, Catherine Mary Evans (retired) Pant-Y-Castell, Solva, Haverfordwest SA62 6XB Tel: 01437 721381 — MB BChir Camb. 1946 (Camb. & Manch.) MA Camb. 1950 MB BChir 1946; MRCS Eng. LRCP Lond. 1946. Prev: Clin. Med. Off. Dyfed AHA.

REES, Charles Robert Penny's Hill Practice, St Mary's Road, Ferndown BH22 9HB Tel: 01202 897200 Fax: 01202 877753; 13A Pine Vale Crescent, Redhill, Bournemouth BH10 6BG Tel: 01202 251737 — MB ChB Leeds 1968; DObst RCOG 1970; MRCGP 1976. GP Tutor E. Dorset. Specialty: Gen. Pract. Prev: SHO (Cas. & Orthop.) Poole Gen. Hosp.; SHO (Obst.) Leeds Matern. Hosp.; Ho. Surg. Leeds Gen. Infirm.

REES, Clare Miranda 17 Miles Road, Bristol BS8 2JW Tel: 0117 973 4331 Fax: 0117 973 4331 — MB ChB Bristol 1997. Anat.

Demonst., Bristol Univ. Bristol; RMO St. Mary's Hosp. Burton. Specialty: Gen. Surg. Socs: BMA. Prev: SHO (A & E) Bristol Roy. Infirm.

REES, Colin John South Tyneside Healthcare NHS Trust, Harton Lane, South Shields NE34 0PL Tel: 0191 202 4028 Email: colin.rees@sthct.nhs.uk — MB BS Newc. 1990; FRCP 2004. Cons. Gastroenterol. Specialty: Gastroenterol. Prev: Regist. (Gastroenterol. & Gen. Med.) North. Region; Research Fell. Roy. Vict. Infirm. Newc. u. Tyne.

REES, Constance Margaret Pascal John Radcliffe Hospital, Nuffield Department of Obstetrics & Gynaecology, Headington, Oxford OX3 9DU — MB BS Lond. 1975 (St George's Hosp. Lond.) BSc (1st cl. Hons.) Lond. 1972; MRCOG 1985; DPhil Oxf. 1984, MA 1988. Reader (Reproduct. Med.) John Radcliffe Hosp. Oxf. Specialty: Obst. & Gyn. Socs: (Counc.) Brit. Menopause Soc.; Endocrine Soc.; Soc. Study of Fertil. Prev: MRC Train. Fell. 1979-1983.; Edr. in Chief Jl. Brit. Menopause Soc.

REES, Corinne Alison 46 Clifton Park Road, Bristol BS8 3HN — MB ChB Bristol 1976; MA Oxf. 1977; MRCP (UK) 1979. Assoc. Specialist (Community Paediat.) & Med. Adviser to Avon AdoptionAgency, United Bristol Healthcare NHS Trust. Specialty: Community Child Health. Prev: Sen. Regist. (Paediat. with Interest in Community Child Health) SW RHA; Regist. (Paediat.) Sheff. Childr. Hosp. & Birm. Childr. Hosp.

REES, Dafydd Aled Cerdd-y-Don, Feidr Brenin, Newport SA42 0RZ — MB BCh Wales 1993.

REES, Mr David Department of Orthopaedic Surgery, Robert Jones & Agnus Hunt Orthopaedic Hospital, Oswestry Tel: 01691 404167; Springfields, Kidderton Lane, Brindley, Nantwich CW5 8JD — MB BS Lond. 1976; FRCS Ed. 1981; FRCS Eng. 1982; MChOrth Liverp. 1985. Cons. Surg. (Orthop.) Orthop. Hosp. Oswestry. Specialty: Sports Med. Prev: Cons. Surg. (Orthop.) Leighton Hosp. Crewe; Sen. Regist. (Orthop.) Roy. Liverp. Hosp.; Ho. Surg. St. Bart. Hosp. Lond.

REES, David Alun (retired) 44 College Street, Bury St Edmunds IP33 1NL — MRCS Eng. LRCP Lond. 1962 (Camb. & Guy's) MA, MB BChir Camb. 1962; FRCOG 1981, M (Gold Medal) 1968. Cons. (O & G) W. Suff. Hosp. Prev: Sen. Regist. O & G St. Mary's Hosp. Lond. & United Camb.

REES, David Alun Wordsley Green Health Centre, Wordsley Green, Wordsley, Stourbridge DY8 5PD Tel: 01384 277591 Fax: 01384 401156 — MB BCh Wales 1968.

REES, David Charles Department of Paediatric Haematology, King's College Hospital, Denmark Hill, London SE5 9RS Tel: 020 7346 3242 Fax: 020 7346 3519 Email: david.rees@kcl.ac.uk — MB BS Lond. 1987; MRCP (UK) 1990; MRCPath 1998; FRCP UK 2004. Sen. Lect. / Hon. Cons., King's Coll. Hosp., Lond.; Hon. Cons. in Paediatric Haemat., Guys and St Thomas' Hosp. Trust, Lond. Specialty: Haematology. Special Interest: Inherited Red Cell Disorders. Prev: Cons. Haematologist, Sheff. Children's Hosp. and Roy. Hallamshire Hosp., Sheff.

REES, David Garfield Panty Scallog Farm, Sennybridge, Brecon LD3 8PT Tel: 01874 636427 — MB BCh Wales 1965. SCMO Powys HA.

REES, David Geraint The Valley, Narberth SA67 8BS — MB BCh Wales 1965.

REES, David Henry Everard Bearwood House, Pembridge, Leominster HR6 9EE Tel: 01544 388613 — MB BS Lond. 1986; MRCP (UK) 1990; FRCP 2001. Cons. Rheumatologist. Specialty: Gen. Med.; Rehabil. Med. Prev: Sen. Regis. Char. Cross, Westminster & Chelsea & St Mary's Hosp. Lond.; Research Regist., Dept of Immunol. St Geo.s Hosp., Lond..; SHO in Nephetologist, Cardiol., Endocrinol. Westminster Hosp. & Char. Cross Hosp., Lond.

REES, David Rhydian The Ashgrove Surgery, Morgan Street, Pontypridd CF37 2DR Tel: 01443 404444 Fax: 01443 480917; 50 Summerfield Drive, Llantrisant, Pontyclun CF72 8QF Tel: 01443 237886 — MB BCh Wales 1984; BSc Wales 1979, MB BCh 1984.

REES, Dawn Elizabeth 24 Fleurs Avenue, Glasgow G41 5AP — MB ChB Glas. 1990.

REES, Diana Gillian Department of Anaesthesia, Whipps Cross University Hospital, Whipps Cross Road, London E11 1NR Tel: 020 8535 6614 Fax: 0208 535 6467; Parnassus, Park Hill, Loughton IG10 4ES Tel: 020 8508 8673 Fax: 020 8508 8673 — MB BS Lond. 1972 (St. Bart.) MRCS Eng. LRCP Lond. 1972; FFA RCS Eng. 1977. Cons. Anaesth. Whipps Cross Univ. Hosp. Clin. Director, Critical Care, Whipps Cross Univ. Hosp. Specialty: Anaesth. Socs: BMA; Assn. Anaesth. Prev: Sen. Regist. (Anaesth.) St. Bart. Hosp. Lond.; Regist. (Anaesth.) Hosp. Sick Childr. Lond.

REES, Edgar Lowell Cross Cottage, Rushlake Green, Heathfield TN21 9QG — MB BS Lond. 1955.

REES, Elizabeth Napier 5 Sundbury Rise, Birmingham B31 2EZ — MB ChB Birm. 1987.

REES, Ernest Gwyn (retired) 12 Mill Road, Salisbury SP2 7RZ Tel: 01722 334944 — MB BS Lond. 1948 (St Bart.) MRCS Eng. LRCP Lond. 1948; FRCP Lond. 1988, M 1950; FRCPath 1972. Prev: Cons. Haemat. Salop AHA.

REES, Esther Hughes (retired) High Ridge, Mathern, Chepstow NP16 6JD — MB BCh Wales 1950; DPH Wales 1971; MFCM 1974. JP. Prev: SCM Gwent HA.

REES, Evan Glyn (retired) Sycharth, Feidr Henffordd, Cardigan SA43 — MB BCh Wales 1948.

REES, Gareth Ambrose Dyfed, TD (retired) — MB BCh Wales 1956; FFA RCS Eng. 1963. Prev: Cons. Anaesth. Univ. Hosp. Wales Cardiff.

REES, Gareth Bowen 21 Ogmore Drive, Nottage, Porthcawl CF36 3HR — MB BChir Camb. 1977; MA, MB Camb. 1977, BChir 1976; MRCOG 1986; DM Nottm. 1989.

REES, Gareth John Glyn Bristol Haematology & Oncology Centre, Horfield Road, Bristol BS2 8ED Tel: 0117 928 2412 Fax: 0117 928 4409 Email: gareth.rees@ubht.swest.nhs.uk; 46 Clifton Park Road, Clifton, Bristol BS8 3HN Tel: 0117 973 7712 Email: garethrees@doctors.org.uk — MB BCh Cymru 1972 (Ysgol Feddygol Cymru) MRCP (UK) 1975; FRCR 1981; FRCP 1998. Cons. Clin. Oncol. Bristol Haemat. & Oncol. Centre & Roy. United Hosp. Bath. Specialty: Oncol. Socs: Founder Mem. Brit. Oncol. Assn. Prev: Clin. Director Bristol Haemat. & Oncol. Centre; Sen. Regist. (Radiotherap. & Oncol.) Weston Pk. Hosp. Sheff.; Med. Off. Montebello Mission Hosp. Natal, S. Afr.

REES, Mr Gareth Mervyn (retired) — (St. Mary's) MS Lond. 1972, MB BS (Hons.) 1960; FRCP Lond. 1983, M 1963; FRCS Eng. 1966. Prev: Emerit. Cons. Cardiothoracic Surg. St. Bart. Hosp. Lond.

REES, Geraint Ellis University College London, Institute of Cognitive Neuroscience, 17 Queen Square, London WC1N 3AR Tel: 020 7679 5496 Fax: 020 7813 1420 Email: g.rees@fil.ion.ucl.ac.uk; 20 Nella Road, London W6 9PB — BM BCh Oxf. 1991; BA Camb. 1988; MRCP (UK) 1994; PhD (UCL) 1999. Wellcome Senior Clinical Fellow, Institute of Neurology, London. Specialty: Cognitive Neurology; Functional neuroimaging. Special Interest: Cognitive Neurol.; Functional Neuroimaging. Socs: Assoc. of British Neurologists; Experimental Psychology Soc.; Vision Sci. Soc. Prev: Research Fellow (Cog. Neurol), Institute Neurol. London.

REES, Gerwyn 5 Brookes Lane, Whalley, Clitheroe BB7 9RG — MB ChB Aberd. 1996. SHO Anaesth., S. Warks. Hosp. NHS. Aug 99 - Aug 00. Specialty: Anaesth.

REES, Geryl Anne Ovoca, 460 Didsbury Road, Heaton Mersey, Stockport SK4 3BT — BM BS Nottm. 1975; BMedSci Nottm. 1973, BM BS 1975; DRCOG 1977; MRCGP 1979.

REES, Gillian Frances Margaret 48 The Drive, Northwood HA6 1HP Tel: 01923 822004 — MB ChB Liverp. 1972; DRCOG 1974. Clin. Asst. (Rheum.) Northwick Pk. & Mt. Vernon Hosps. Specialty: Rehabil. Med.; Rheumatol. Prev: Asst. GP N. Lond.

REES, Gillian Lesley 154 Ravenhurst Road, Birmingham B17 9HS — MB ChB Birm. 1986; DRCOG 1988.

REES, Gwyneth Lodwick 36 Macfarlane Road, Bearsden, Glasgow G61 2LZ — MB ChB Glas. 1990. Specialty: Child & Adolesc. Psychiat. Prev: Ho. Off. (Med.) Heathfield Hosp. Ayr; Ho. Off. (Surg.) Monklands Hosp. Airdrie.

REES, Mr Harland (retired) Kensworth Gorse, Kensworth Road, Dunstable LU6 3RF Tel: 01582 872411 — BM BCh Oxf. 1936 (Oxf. & Char. Cross) MA, MCh 1941, BA, BM BCh Oxf. 1936; FRCS Eng. 1941. Prev: Lt.-Col. RAMC, OC Surg. Div. 53 I.G.H.(C.).

REES, Harvey James Grove Road Day Hospital, 12 Grove Road, Clifton, Bristol BS6 6UJ Tel: 0117 973 0225 — MB BCh Wales 1989; MRCPsych 1995. Cons. Adult Psychiat. Specialty: Gen. Psychiat.

REES, Haydn Griffith 24 Fernhill Close, Mayals, Swansea SA3 5BX — MB BCh Wales 1967. Prev: GP Swansea.

REES, Helen Louise Flat 96 Finchley Court, Ballards Lane, London N3 1NJ — MB BS Lond. 1991.

REES, Helen Mary Church Lane Surgery, Church Lane, Boroughbridge, York YO51 9BD Tel: 01423 322309 Fax: 01423 324458; Coverpoint, Scarah Lane, Burton Leonard, Harrogate HG3 3SZ Tel: 01765 676566 — BMedSci Nottm. 1987; BM BS (Hons.) Nottm. 1989; DCH RCP Lond. 1991; MRCGP 1993. Princip. in Gen. Pract. Specialty: Gen. Pract. Prev: SHO (Cas.) Harrogate Dist. Hosp.; SHO (O & G & Geriat.) Harrogate Gen. Hosp.

REES, Helene Ceredwyn Hammersmith Hospitals NHS Trust, Dept. of Histopathology, Charing CrossHospital, Fulham Palace Road, London W6 8RF Tel: 020 8846 7150; 72 Mortlake Road, Kew, Richmond TW9 4AS — MB BS Melbourne 1972; FRCPA 1980; MRCPath 1984; LLB 1996; FRCPath 1996. Cons. Histopath. Char. Cross Hosp. Specialty: Histopath. Socs: (Vice-Pres.) Med. Soc. Lond. (Ex-Sen. & Jun. Sec.); Liveryman Soc. Apoth.; Soc. of Doctors in Law. Prev: Sen. Lect. & Hon. Cons. Histopath. St. Bart. & Homerton Hosps. Lond.; Sen. Regist. (Histopath.) Hammersmith Hosp. Lond.

REES, Hilary Margaret The Caxton Surgery, Oswald Road, Oswestry SY11 1RD Tel: 01691 654646 Fax: 01691 670994; Pentlands, 93 Oakhurst Road, Oswestry SY11 1BL — MB BChir Camb. 1975; DRCOG 1979; DCH Eng. 1981.

REES, Howard William (retired) Cedar Ridge, Gate Burton, Gainsborough DN21 5BG Tel: 0142 771207; The Graig, Langland Bay, Swansea SA3 4QG Tel: 01792 366268 — MRCS Eng. LRCP Lond. 1936 (Middlx.) MRCS Eng LRCP Lond. 1936. Prev: Ho. Phys. Middlx. Hosp. & Brompton Hosp. Sanat. Frimley.

REES, Hugh Edward Gordon London Road Medical Centre, 2 London Road, Uppingham, Oakham LE15 9TJ Tel: 01248 715250 Fax: 01572 821145; Carey's House, 4 Church Lane, Barrowden, Oakham LE15 8ED Tel: 01572 747420 — MB BS Lond. 1966 (Guy's) MRCS Eng. LRCP Lond. 1966; DObst RCOG 1968. Prev: Clin. Asst. (Orthop.) Rutland Memor. Hosp. Oakham; Ho. Surg. (Obst.) Brighton Gen. Hosp.; Ho. Surg. & Ho. Phys. (Cas. & Orthop.) Roy. Sussex Co. Hosp. Brighton.

REES, Huw Garwood UWCM Therapeutics & Toxicology Centre, Academic Centre, Llandough Hospital, Cardiff CF64 2XX Tel: 029 2071 6944 Fax: 029 2070 3454 — MB BCh Wales 1979 (Welsh Nat. Sch. Med.) Cert. Family Plann. RCOG 1982; DRCOG 1983; MRCGP 1985; MFOM RCP Lond. 1993, AFOM 1991; FFOM 1999. Sen. Res. Fell. Occupat. Med. & Toxicology, UWCM, Cardiff; Cons. Occupat. Med. Powys LHB. Specialty: Occupat. Health. Socs: BMA & Soc. Occupat. Med.; BOHS. Prev: Sen. Lect. Occupat. Med. & Toxicology, UWCM, Cardiff; Hon. Cons. Occupat. Med. Llandough Hosp. NHS Trust Cardiff; Cons. Occupat. Med., Univ. Hosp. of Wales, Cardiff.

REES, Ian Walter James Winstanley Drive Surgery, 138 Winstanley Drive, Leicester LE3 1PB Tel: 0116 285 8435 Fax: 0116 275 5416; 17 Wentworth Green, Kirby Muxloe, Leicester LE9 2EQ Tel: 0116 238 7256 — MB ChB Leic. 1982; DRCOG 1985; DCH RCP Lond. 1989. Forens. Med. Examr. Leics. Constab.; Medical Referee for Leicestershire Crematoria. Specialty: Gen. Med.; Alcohol & Substance Misuse. Socs: Brit. Assn. Sport & Med. Prev: Clin. Asst. (Rheum.) Leicester; SHO (Obst. Gyn.) Leicester Gen. Hosp.; SHO (Paediat.) Leicester Gen. Hosp.

REES, Jane Susan 9 Kensinton Drive, Willaston, Nantwich CW5 7HL Fax: 01270 664930 — MB BS Lond. 1970; DObst RCOG 1973; MRCGP 1984; MA Med. Ethics. Keele Uni 2000. Med. Adviser to Shrops. Primary Care Audit Gp..; Occupational Health - Sema Gp. Vibreation white Fincter Scheme.; Assoc. Lect. open Uni. Prev: GP Llanfyllin, Powys.

REES, Jeni Hook Surgery, Reading Road, Hook RG27 9ED — BM Soton. 1992; DRCOG 1994; MRCGP 1996. Specialty: Gen. Pract.

REES, Jennifer Ann (retired) Yaffle Lodge, Bleasby Road, Thurgarton, Nottingham NG14 7FW — MB BS Lond. 1963 (Roy. Free) MRCS Eng. LRCP Lond. 1963; DObst RCOG 1965. Prev: GP Thurgarton.

REES, Jeremy Harry National Hospital for Neurology & Neurosurgery, Institute of Neurology, London WC1N 3BG Tel: 020 7837 3611 Ext: 3021 Fax: 020 7676 2167 Email: j.rees@ion.ucl.ac.uk — MB BS Lond. 1988 (University coll. & Middx) BSc Lond. 1985; MRCP UK 1991; PhD Lond 1995. Sen. Lect., Neuro-onclogy, Inst. of Neurol., UCL.; Hon. Cons. Neurol., Nat. Hosp. For Neurol. & Neurosurg., Roy. Marsden Hosp. Middlx. Univ. Coll. Hosp. Trust. Specialty: Neurol. Special Interest: Low-grade gliomas and paraneoplastic Neurol. disorders; Neuro-oncology. Socs: Brit. Neuro-Oncol. Gp.; Mem. Assn. Brit. Neurol.; Europ. Assn Neuro-Oncol. Prev: Regist. (Neurol.) St. Thos. Hosp. Lond.; Regist. (Neurol.) Nat. Hosp. Neurol. & Neurosurg. Lond.; Regist. (Neurol.) Roy. Free Hosp. Lond.

REES, Joanna Deborah Suzanne 84 Sevington Road, London NW4 3RS Tel: 020 8202 0248 — MB BS Lond. 1994; MRCGP with merit 2001. Gen. Practitioner. Prev: Ho. Off. (Med. & Radiother.) Mt. Vernon Hosp. N.wood.; Ho. Off. (Surg. & Urol.) Luton & Dunstable Hosp.; GP Regist. - Challihill Med. Centre.

REES, John Pomeroy, Chineham Lane, Sherborne St John, Basingstoke RG24 9LR — MB BS Lond. 1980.

REES, John Alan Evan c/o Ward B7, UHW, Heath Park, Cardiff CF14 4XW Tel: 02920 743000 Fax: 02920 744581 Email: alan.rees@cardiffandvale.wales.nhs.uk — MB BCh (1st Class Honours) Wales 1978; FRCP Lond.; MD Wales; BSc., MD, FRCP; BIOCHEM, Liverpool Univ. 1973. Cons. Phys. With an interest in diabetes, Endocrinol. and Metab. Specialty: Diabetes; Endocrinol. Socs: Heart UK; Europ. Atherosclerosis Soc.; Amer. Diaretes Assn. Prev: Lect. (Med.) Univ. Wales Coll. Med. Cardiff; Research Fell. St. Bart. Hosp. Lond.; Welcome Sen. Research Fell. Clin. Med.

REES, John Andrew 9 Castle Quay, Castle Boulevart, Nottingham NG7 1FW — (St. Geo.) MB BS Lond. 1967.

REES, John Donald George Woodbridge Hill Surgery, 1 Deerbarn Road, Guildford GU2 8YB Tel: 01483 562230 Fax: 01483 452442; 10 Woodlands Road, Loughor, Swansea SA4 6PS — MB BS Lond. 1986 (St Georges Hospital) DCH RCP Lond. 1989; DRCOG 1990; MRCGP 1992; Dip Occupational Health R. C. P. Lond. 1996. Prev: Trainee GP Milton Keynes Gen. Hosp. VTS.; Ho. Off. (Med.) Frimley Pk. Hosp.; Ho. Off. (Surg.) St. James'. Hosp. Lond.

REES, John Edward Peter 11 Northmead, Narberth SA67 7DN; Rosebank, Upper Cynor Place, off Cae Siriol, Ynyshir, Porth CF39 0NW — MB BCh Wales 1981.

REES, John Eric 45 Heol Ebrandy, Pontyberem, Llanelli SA15 5DG — MRCS Eng. LRCP Lond. 1978.

REES, John Esmond (retired) Nuffield Hospital, 55 New Church Road, Hove BN3 4BG Tel: 01273 720217 Fax: 01273 220919; Silver Trees, South Bank, Hassocks BN6 8JP — (Camb. & St. Thos.) MA, MD Camb. 1973, MB 1966, BChir 1965; FRCP Lond. 1982, M 1968. Hon. Cons. Neurol. Brighton & Mid Sussex NHs Trust; Vis. Research Fell. Sussex Univ. Prev: Sen. Regist. (Neurol.) King's Coll. Hosp. Lond.

REES, John Henry Thomas (retired) Kings Park, St. Clears, Carmarthen SA33 4AX Tel: 01994 230420 — (Lond. Hosp.) MRCS Eng. LRCP Lond. 1944. Prev: Med. Off. Min. of Supply Experim. Establishm. Pendine.

REES, John Howell Norfolk Health,Norfolk Health Authority, St Andrew's House, Northside, St Andrews, Business Park, Thorpe St Andrew, Norwich NR7 0HT Tel: 01603 300600; 15 Coniston Close, South Wootton, King's Lynn PE30 3NL Tel: 01553 679304 Fax: 01553 679304 — MB ChB Manch. 1975; MRCGP 1981; MFPHM RCP (UK) 1989. Cons. Pub. Health, Norf. HA & PH Exec. Mem. W. Norf PCT. Specialty: Pub. Health Med. Prev: Sen. Med. Off. DoH HCD-PH Div. Leeds; Dir. Pub. Health W. Norf. & Wisbech HA; Sen. Regist. (Community Med.) E. Anglian RHA.

REES, John Hywel (retired) 15 Northanger Court, Grove St., Bath BA2 6PE Tel: 01225 469728; 373 Route de Valbonne, Villa 16, Biot 06410, France Tel: 00 33 0 493651694 — MB BS Lond. 1950 (St. Bart.) MRCS Eng. LRCP Lond. 1950; MRCGP 1965.

REES, John Idwal Stephen Department of Radiology, University Hospital of Wales, Heath Park, Cardiff CF14 4XW — MB BCh Wales 1984; BSc Wales 1979, MB BCh 1984; FRCR 1989. Cons. Radiol. Univ. Hosp. Wales Cardiff. Specialty: Nuclear Med.

REES, John Kempton Harold Cambridge Institute of Medical Research, Department of Haematology, University of Cambridge, Hills Road, Cambridge CB2 2XY Tel: 01223 336836 Fax: 01223 336827 Email: jkr1000@cam.ac.uk; 14 Babraham Road, Cambridge CB2 2RA — MB BCh Wales 1963 (Cardiff) MRCP UK 1970; Hon. MA Camb. 1974; FRCP 1998. Lect. (Haemat.) Univ. Camb. Specialty: Haematology. Special Interest: Haematological Malignancy. Socs: Brit. Soc. Haematol.; Eur. Haematol. Assn.; Amer. Soc. Haemat. Prev: Lect. (Haemat.) St Thos. Hosp. Lond.

REES, John Kenneth (retired) Cleveland Lodge, The Strand, Ryde PO33 1J — MRCS Eng. LRCP Lond. 1960; DA Eng. 1963. Prev: Dep. Police Surg. I. of Wight.

REES, John Llewelyn Rees, Hoe, Rostron and James, Lister House Surgery, Bollams Mead, Wiveliscombe, Taunton TA4 2PH Tel: 01984 623471 Fax: 01984 624357; Hartswell House, Wiveliscombe, Taunton TA4 2NF Tel: 01984 623343 — (St. Thos.) MB BChir Camb. 1964; DObst RCOG 1965. Specialty: Gen. Pract. Prev: Ho. Off. (Paediat.) Cardiff Roy. Infirm.; Ho. Off. (Obst.) & Ho. Surg. (ENT) St. Thos. Hosp. Lond.

REES, John Russell Litfield House, Litfield Place, Clifton Down, Bristol BS8 3LS Tel: 0117 973 1323; Friars Halt, St. Mary's Road, Leigh Woods, Bristol BS8 3PY Tel: 0117 973 5049 — (Guy's) MA, MD Camb. 1959, BA 1951; MB BChir Camb. 1951; FRCP Lond. 1973, M 1956. Emerit. Cons. Cardiol. United Bristol Healthcare NHS Trust; Chief. Med. Off. Clerical Med. Investment GP. Specialty: Cardiol. Socs: Med. Res. Soc.; Brit. Cardiac Soc. Prev: Cons. Cardiol. Bristol Roy. Hosp. & S. West. RHA; Sen. Regist. (Med.) Westm. Hosp. Lond.; Regist. (Med.) Guy's Hosp. Lond.

REES, John Sebastian Corbett House Surgery, Avondale Road, Bristol BS5 9QX Tel: 0117 955 7474 Fax: 0117 955 5402 — BM BCh Oxf. 1973 (Oxf. & St. Thos.) MRCS Eng. LRCP Lond. 1973; DObst RCOG 1975; MRCGP 1979. Prev: SHO (A & E) & SHO (O & G) Plymouth Gen. Hosp.

REES, John Wilson Fforestfach Medical Centre, 118 Ravenhill road, Fforestfach, Swansea SA5 5AA Tel: 01792 581666; 2 Somerville Court, Sketty, Swansea SA2 0RY — MB BS Lond. 1976; DCH RCP Lond. 1981; MRCGP 1983.

REES, Jonathan Edward Gooderid 8 Meadowbrook Close, Exeter EX4 2NN — MB ChB Bristol 1995.

REES, Professor Jonathan Laurence Department Dermatology, Medical School, Framlington Place, Newcastle upon Tyne NE2 4HH Tel: 0191 222 8936 Fax: 0191 222 7094; 19 Carr Field, Eland Haugh, Ponteland, Newcastle upon Tyne NE20 9XR Tel: 01661 825782 — MB BS Newc. 1982; BMedSc (1st. cl. Hons.) Newc. 1981; MB BS (Hons.) Newc 1982; MRCP (UK) 1985; FRCP 1993. Prof. & Hon. Cons. Dermat. Roy. Vict. Infirm. Newc. u. Tyne. Specialty: Dermat. Prev: MRC Clinician Scientist Univ. Newc.; Vis. Scientist Univ. Strasbourg; Regist. (Dermat.) Allgemeines Krankenhaus, Vienna.

REES, Jonathan Lloyd Fronhaul, Pentwyn Deintyr, Treharris CF46 5EA — MB BS Lond. 1992.

REES, Jonathan Richard Edward United Bristol Health Care Trust, Bristol Royal Infirmary, Upper Maudlin St., Bristol BS2 8UW Tel: 0117 923 0000; Fairways, 11 Cecil Road, Gowerton, Swansea SA4 3DF Tel: 01792 873275 — MB ChB Bristol 1997. Demonst. (Anat.) & SHO (A & E) Bristol Roy. Infirm. Prev: Ho. Surg. (Gen. Surg.) Bristol Roy. Infirm.; Ho. Phys. (Cardiol.) Roy. Devon & Exeter Hosp.

REES, Joseph Philip Mervyn 13 Second Cross Road, Twickenham TW2 5QY — MB BS Lond. 1989.

REES, Judith Elizabeth 78 Herongate Road, Wanstead, London E12 5EQ — MB BS Lond. 1974 (Lond. Hosp.) BSc Lond. 1971, MB BS 1974; DCH Eng. 1977.

REES, Julia Alison Occupational Health Department, Epsom General Hosptial, Dorking Road, Epsom KT18 7EG Tel: 01372 735377 Fax: 01372 743421; One Northweald Lane, Royal Park Gate, Kingston upon Thames KT2 5GL Tel: 020 8549 4586 — BM Soton. 1981. Clin. Asst. (Occupat. Health) Kingston Hosp. NHS Trust. Specialty: Occupat. Health. Prev: Med. Off. Lond. Boro. Ealing; Med. Off. Thos. Cook Ltd.; Clin. Asst. (Occupat. Health) W. Dorset HA.

REES, Julia Anne Department of Histopathology, North Middlesex Hospital, Sterling Way, London N18 1QX Tel: 020 8887 2275 Fax: 020 8887 2569 — MB BS Lond. 1990; BSc (Hons.) Pharmacol. Lond. 1986; MRCPath 1999. Cons. Histocytopathologist, Dept Histopath., N. Middlx Hosp. Lond.. Specialty: Histopath.

REES, Katherine Sian Plas Caer Pwsan, Clynnog Fawr, Caernarfon LL54 5PF — MB BS Lond. 1995.

REES, Lesley Great Ormond Street Hospital for Children, Renal Unit, London WC1N 3JH Tel: 020 7813 8346 Email: reesl@gosh.nhs.uk — MB ChB Manch. 1974 (Manchester) MRCP (UK) 1977; MD Manch. 1982; T(M) 1991; FRCP Lond. 1994; FRCPH 1998. Cons. Paediat. Nephrol. Gt. Ormond St. NHS Trust Lond. Specialty: Paediat. Special Interest: Paediatric Nephrol. Socs: Roy. Coll. of Physicains; Roy. Coll. Paediat. & Child Health; (Secretary) Brit. Assoc. Paediatric Nephrol. Prev: Cons. Paediat. Nephrol. Roy. Free Hosp. & Hosp. for Sick Childr. Lond.; Lect. (Paediat.) Guy's Hosp. Lond.

REES, Lesley Howard, DBE 23 Church Row, Hampstead, London NW3 6UP Tel: 020 7794 4936 — MB BS Lond. 1965 (St. Bart.) MB BS (Hons.) Lond. 1965; FRCP Lond. 1979, M 1968; MSc Lond. 1974, DSc 1989, MD 1972; FRCPath 1988, M 1976. Prof. Chem. Endocrinol. St. Bart. Hosp. Med. Coll. Lond.; Hon. Cons. St. Bart. Hosp. Lond. Specialty: Endocrinol. Socs: Fell. Roy. Soc. Med.; Soc. Endocrinol.; (Sec. Gen.) Internat. Endocrine Soc. Prev: Ho. Phys. St. Bart. Hosp. Lond. & Hammersmith Hosp. & Roy. Postgrad. Med. Sch. Lond.; Clin. Research Fell. Endocrine Unit Univ. Oregon Med. Sch. Portland, USA.

REES, Lynne Justine Brynhyfryd Surgery, Brynhyfryd, Swansea SA1 9EB Tel: 01792 655083; 12 Pennard Road, Kittle, Swansea SA3 3JS Tel: 01792 233645 Email: rees.etal@zoom.co.uk — MB BCh Wales 1991; BSc (Hons.) Cardiff 1988; DCH RCP Lond. 1994; DRCOG 1994; MRCGP 1995; Dip Pract Derm 1997. Gen. Pract. - Half Time Princip.; Clin. Asst. (A & E) Morriston Hosp. Swansea. Specialty: Gen. Pract. Prev: Trainee GP Swansea VTS.

REES, Mandy Flat 10, 118 Kingston Road, London SW19 1LY Tel: 020 8542 2020 — MB BS Lond. 1991 (St. Bartholomews) FRCA 1997. Specialist Regist. Anaesth., St Geo.s Hosp. Lond. Specialty: Anaesth.

REES, Mary Aldery Hey Childrens Hospital, Department of Community Paediatrics, Eaton Road, West Derby, Liverpool L12 2AP Tel: 0151 228 4811 Fax: 0151 252 5120 — MB BS Lond. 1967 (St. Bart.) MRCS Eng. LRCP Lond. 1967; DObst RCOG 1969; Cert. JCC Lond. 1977. Cons. Community Paediat. Alder Hey Childr. Hosp. Liverp. Specialty: Community Child Health. Socs: Inst. Psychosexual Med.; Brit. Paediat. Assn. Prev: SCMO (Family Plann., Genitourin. Med. & Community Paediat.) Hastings Dist HA.

REES, Mary Carol 21A West Heath Road, London NW3 7UU — MB Camb. 1962; BChir 1961.

REES, Mary Patricia Pen-y-Bryn, Danesfield Drive, Leominster HR6 8HW — MB BCh Wales 1965 (Cardiff) DObst RCOG 1967. Clin. Asst. (Sexual Health) Gaol St. Hereford. Prev: Clin. Med. Off. Herefordsh. HA.; Clin. Asst. Genitourin. Med. Hereford Co. Hosp.; Med. Off. Family Plann. Assn.

REES, Menna Stockton Heath Medical Centre, The Forge, London Road, Warrington WA4 6HJ Tel: 01925 604427 Fax: 01925 210501; 51 Pepper Street, Lymm WA13 0JG Tel: 0192 575 4069 — MB BCh Wales 1972; DObst RCOG 1974; MRCGP 1976. GP Warrington; Clin. Asst. (Colposcopy) Warrington Hosp. Socs: (Comm. Mem.) NW Soc. Study Sexual Med. Prev: Phys. Rochester State Hosp., USA:; SHO (O & G & Paediat.) Univ. Hosp. Wales Cardiff.

REES, Mr Myrddin North Hampshire Hospital, Aldermaston Road, Basingstoke RG24 9NA Tel: 01256 473202 Fax: 01256 313512; Old Rectory, Church Lane, Worting, Basingstoke RG23 8PX Tel: 01256 320208 Fax: 01256 350818 — MB BS Lond. 1973 (Westm.) MRCS Eng. LRCP Lond. 1973; FRCS Eng. 1977; MS Lond. 1983. Cons. Surg. N. Hants. Hosp. Specialty: Gen. Surg. Socs: Roy. Soc. Med. (Vice-Pres. Surg. Sector); RSM Pres. Surg. Sect. (Past); AUGIS Mem. of Educat. Comm. (Past). Prev: Sen. Regist. St. Geo. Hosp. Lond.; Research Fell. Ochner Med. Inst. New Orleans, USA.

REES, Olwen Vivien (retired) 52 Southlands Drive, West Cross, Swansea SA3 5RA Tel: 01792 404144 — MB BCh Wales 1945 (Cardiff) BSc Wales 1941; DPhysMed. Eng. 1961. Cons. Rheum. & Rehabil. W. Glam. AHA. Prev: Asst. Med. Off. W. Glam. AHA.

REES, Paul Ash Tree House, Church Street, Kirkham, Preston PR4 2SE Tel: 01772 686688 Fax: 01772 672054; 2 Bryning Avenue, Wrea Green, Preston PR4 2WL — MB ChB Manch. 1976.

REES, Paul Stuart Chadwick 66 Heol Maengwyn, Machynlleth, Meifod — MB BS Lond. 1996.

REES, Peter John Guy's Hospital, London SE1 9RT Tel: 020 7188 3739 Fax: 020 7188 3737 Email: john.rees@kcl.ac.uk — MB BChir Camb. 1974; FRCP Lond. 1988, M 1975; MA Camb. 1974, MD 1982. Cons. Phys. Guy's Hosp. Lond.; Sen. Lect. (Med.) UMDS Guy's Campus Lond. Specialty: Gen. Med. Special Interest: COPD; Medical Education; Sleep Apnoea.

REES, Philip Grufydd Great Ormond Street Hospital for Children, NHS Trust, Great Ormond St., London WC1N 3JH Tel: 020 7829 8839 Fax: 020 7829 8673 Email: reesp@gosh.nhs.uk — MB BCh Wales 1969; BSc Wales 1966; DRCOG 1971; MRCP (UK) 1973;

DCH RCP Lond. 1974; FRCP Lond. 1987; FRCPCH 1997. Cons. Paediat. Cardiol., Gt. Ormond St. Hosp. Childr., Lond.; Hon. Cons. Cardiol., Roy. Lond., Roy. Surrey, Lodon Co., Heatherwood, Wexham Pk., Ealling, Luton, & Northampton Gen. Hosps. Specialty: Paediat. Cardiol. Special Interest: Pacing; Transpl. Socs: Roy. Coll. of Child Health; Roy. Coll. of Phys. Prev: Sen. Regist. at Gt. Ormond St. Hosp.

REES, Philip Howell, OBE 21A West Heath Road, London NW3 7UU — MB Camb. 1962; BChir 1961; FRCP Ed. 1980; FRCP Lond. 1980.

REES, Philip John Richards and Partners, Llanfair Surgery, Llanfair Road, Llandovery SA20 0HY Tel: 01550 720648 Fax: 01550 721428; Ty-Cerian, Llandovery SA20 0YF Tel: 01550 721428 — MB BS Lond. 1982 (St. Bart.) DRCOG 1984; MRCGP 1990. Hosp. Pract. Llandovery Cottage Hosp. Prev: Trainee GP St. Albans & Llandovery VTS; SHO (Radiother.) St. Bart. Hosp. Lond.; Ho. Off. St. Bart. Hosp. Lond.

REES, Philippa Helen Buckland — MB ChB Zimbabwe 1984; LRCP LRCS Ed. LRCPS Glas. 1987; DA (UK) 1990; MRCGP 1991.

REES, Richard Gwyn Department of Rheumatology, St. Mary's Hospital, Praed St., London W2 1NY Tel: 020 7886 1046 Fax: 020 7886 6083 — MB BCh Wales 1980; MRCP (UK) 1985; FRCP 1997. Cons. Rheum. St. Mary's Hosp. NHS Trust Lond.; Hon. Clin Sen. Lect. Imperial Coll. Sch. of Med. Specialty: Rheumatol. Socs: Fell. Roy. Soc. Med.; Brit. Soc. Rheum.; Fell. Med. Soc. Lond. Prev: Sen. Regist. (Med. & Rheum.) Char. Cross Hosp. & Qu. Mary's Hosp. Roehampton; Arthritis & Rheum. Counc. Research Fell. (Rheum.) Westm. Hosp. Lond.; Resid. Med. Off. & Regist. (Med.) Westm. Hosp. Lond.

REES, Richard John, RD London Road Surgery, 31 London Road, Sittingbourne ME10 1NQ Tel: 01795 472534/425439 — MB BS Lond. 1970 (Westm.) AKC. Police Surg.; Admiralty Surg. & Agent. Prev: SHO (O & G) Soton. Gen. Hosp.; SHO (A & E) St. Stephens Hosp. Lond.; Surg. Lt.-Cdr. RNR.

REES, Mr Richard Wellesley Morgan (retired) Caer Wigau Isaf Farm, Nr. Pendoylan, Cowbridge CF71 7UJ Tel: 01446 760227 — MB ChB Birm. 1957; FRCS Ed. 1966; FRCS Eng. 1966. Cons. Urol. Dept. Urol. Univ. Hosp. of Wales, Cardiff; Hon. Clin. Teach. Univ. Wales Coll. Med. Prev: Ho. Surg. United Birm. Hosps.

REES, Robert Griffiths (retired) West Winds, 44 Great Lane, Frisby-on-the-Wreake, Melton Mowbray LE14 2PB Tel: 01664 434874 — MB BS Lond. 1942 (St. Bart.) MRCS Eng. LRCP Lond. 1942. Prev: Ho. Surg. Mt. Vernon Hosp. & Radium Inst. Northwood.

REES, Robert Simon Owen (retired) Rubbin Cottage, Treyford, Midhurst GU29 0LD Tel: 01730 825444 — (Westm.) MA, MB Camb. 1958, BChir 1957; MRCS Eng. LRCP Lond. 1957; DMRD Eng. 1962; FRCP Lond. 1975, M 1963; FFR 1965; FRCR 1975. Prev: Dir. Radiol. Roy. Brompton Lond.

REES, Robin James 31 Oakfield Road, Shrewsbury SY3 8AD — MB ChB Birm. 1993; FRCS.

REES, Roger Thomas Norfolk And Norwich University Hospital NHS Trust, Colney Lane, Norwich NR4 7UY Tel: 01603 286286 Fax: 01603 288299; 9 The St, Brooke, Norwich NR15 1JW Tel: 01508 550431 Fax: 01508 550431 — MB BS Lond. 1971 (Roy. Dent. & St. Bart.) BDS 1967; FDS RCS Eng. 1974, LDS 1968; MRCS Eng. LRCP Lond. 1971. Cons. Oral & Maxillofacial Surg. Norf. & Norwich NHS Trust & Jas. Paget NHS Trust. Specialty: Oral & Maxillofacial Surg. Socs: Fell. Brit. Assn. Oral & Maxillofacial Surg. Prev: Sen. Regist. (Oral Surg.) King's Coll. Hosp. Dent. Sch. & Qu. Vict. Hosp. E. Grinstead.

REES, Romilly Whitchurch Health Centre, Armada Road, Bristol BS14 0SU Tel: 01275 832285 Fax: 01275 540035; 63 Charlton Road, Keynsham, Bristol BS31 2JQ — MB ChB Manch. 1987; DCH RCP Lond. 1990; DRCOG 1991; MRCGP 1991; DGM RCP Lond. 1992. Socs: BMA. Prev: Staff Grade Geriat. St. David's Hosp. Brecon.

REES, Ruth Margaret Westerhope Medical Group, 377 Stamfordham Road, Westerhope, Newcastle upon Tyne NE5 2LH Tel: 0191 243 7000 Fax: 0191 243 7006 — MB BS Newc. 1993. GP Regist. Longrigg Med. Centre Gateshead. Prev: SHO (Gen. Med. & Elderly Care) N. Tees Gen. Hosp. Stockton on Tees.

***REES, Samantha Jane** Beechfield House, 30 Parrys Lane, Stoke Bishop, Bristol BS9 1AA — MB BS Lond. 1998 (St. Bartholomew's & The Royal London.) BSc (Hons) London 1995; MB BS Lond 1998. SHO, (A&E) Winchester, RHCH. Specialty: Gen. Surg. Prev: PRHO Gen. Surg. Chelmsford.; PRHO Gen. Med. Winchester, RHCH.

REES, Sheridan Giles Oliver — MB BS Lond. 1990 (St Bart.) FRCA 1996; Cert Med Educat Dundee 2002. Cons. (Full Time) Anaesth. Gloucestershire Hosps. N.H.S. Trust. Specialty: Anaesth.; Educat. Socs: Higher Educat. Acad.; Assn. of Anaesthetists of Gt. Britain & Irel.; Obst. Anaesth. Assn.

REES, Sian 16 High Street, Caerleon, Newport NP18 1AG — MB BS Lond. 1985; BA Oxf. 1982.

REES, Simon Delme Rogers DVLA, Drivers Medical Group, 2 Sandringham Park, Swansea Vale 1, Swansea SA6 8QD Email: simon.rees@dvla.gsi.gov.uk — MB BS Lond. 1989; BSc Lond. 1986. Med. Advis. to DVLA. Prev: Trainee GP Plymouth.; SHO (Med.) Derriford Hosp. Plymouth & Westm. Hosp. Lond.; Ho. Off. (Med.) Westm. Hosp. Lond.

REES, Sonja 104 Oxclose Lane, Arnold, Nottingham NG5 6FX — State Exam Med. Frankfurt 1991.

REES, Stephen Osborn Glaslyn, 7 Cilonen Road, Three Crosses, Swansea SA4 3PH — MB BCh Wales 1985.

REES, Timothy Seaborn The Redcliffe Surgery, 10 Redcliffe St., Chelsea, London SW10 9DT Tel: 020 7460 2222 Fax: 020 7460 0116 Email: tim.rees@nhs.net — MB BS Lond. 1986 (Char. Cross & Westm.) BSc Lond. 1983; DRCOG 1990; Cert. Family Plann. JCC 1991; MRCGP 1992. Course Org., Riverside VTS, Chelsea& westm. Hosp. Prev: Clin. Asst. (Genitourin. Med.) Jas. Pringle Hse. Lond.; SHO (O & G) W. Lond. & Char. Cross Hosps. Lond.; Research Regist. (MRC HIV Trials) Char. Cross Hosp. Lond.

REES, Trevor Percival Greensward Surgery, Greensward Lane, Hockley SS5 5HQ Tel: 01702 202353 Fax: 01702 204535; Greenacre, Mayes Lane, Danbury, Chelmsford CM3 4NJ Tel: 01245 222016 Fax: 01245 222016 — MB BS Lond. 1973 (Lond. Hosp.) DObst RCOG 1975; Cert. Family Plann. JCC Lond. 1976; Cert. Av Med. MoD (Air) & CAA. 1980. Sen. Med. Off. HM Prison & Youth Custody Centre Hockley; GP Tutor St. Bart. Hosp. & Lond. Hosp.; Examr. Brit. Red Cross. Specialty: Aviat. Med. Socs: Brit. Soc. Med. & Dent. Hypn. (Metrop. Br.). Prev: SHO (O & G), Ho. Phys. & Ho. Surg. Rochford Gen. Hosp.

REES, Trevor William Hawthorns Surgery, 331 Birmingham Road, Sutton Coldfield B72 1DL Tel: 0121 373 2211 Fax: 0121 382 1274; 30 Beech Hill Road, Wylde Green, Sutton Coldfield B72 1DT Tel: 0121 382 0090 — MB ChB Birm. 1979.

REES, Tudor Williams (retired) Llys Deri, Heol Henfwlch, Carmarthen SA33 6AJ — (Cardiff) MB BCh Wales 1963; DPM Eng. 1972; MRCPsych 1973. Prev: Indep. Psychiat. Servs. Carmarthen.

REES, William David Wynne Department Gastroenterology, Hope Hospital, Salford M6 8HD Tel: 0161 789 7373 Fax: 0161 787 5366 Email: wynne.rees@srht.nhs.uk — MD Wales 1978 (University of Wales School of Medicine) MB BCh 1972; MRCP (UK) 1974; FRCP Lond. 1992. Cons. Phys. & Gastroenterol. Univ. Manch. Sch. Med. Hope Hosp. Salford; Dep. Regional Adviser, Roy. Coll. of Phys.s, Lond.; Hon. Reader (Med.) Univ. Manch. Med. Sch. Specialty: Gastroenterol. Socs: Brit. Soc. of Gastroenterol. - Mem.; Amer. Gastroenterol. Assn. Mem.; Brit. Assn. of Med. Managers - Meb. Prev: Wellcome Research Fell. & Lect. (Med.) Univ. Manch.; Hon. Cons. Phys. Salford HA; Research Fell. (Gastroenterol.) Mayo Clin. Rochester, USA.

REES, William Dewi (retired) Plott Cottage, Plott Lane, Stretton-on-Dunsmore, Rugby CV23 9HL Tel: 024 7654 4363 — MB BS Lond. 1956 (St. Thos.) FRCGP 1974, M 1966; MD Lond. 1971. Prev: Med. Dir. St. Mary's Hospice Birm.

REES, William Euros Lloyd 42 Church Road, Tonteg, Pontypridd CF38 1EL Tel: 01443 202629 — MB ChB St. And. 1957; DO RCS Eng. 1960; FCOphth 1990. Surg. (Ophth.) E. Glam. Hosp. & Bridgend Gen. Hosp.; Dir. Ophth. Treatm. Centre Bridgend.

REES, William Henry Russell The Mynde House, Caerleon, Newport NP18 1AG — MB BS Lond. 1949.

REES, William Michael Thomas (retired) Ty Petroc, Little Petherick, Wadebridge PL27 7QT — MRCS Eng. LRCP Lond. 1963 (Guy's) Maj. RAMC RARO. Prev: Hon. Med. Adviser RNLI.

REES, Yvonne Afallon, New Quay SA45 9TY — MB BCh Wales 1978; DMRD Wales 1983; FRCR 1984. Cons. Radiol. Leicester Roy. Infirm. & Leicester Gen. Hosp. Specialty: Radiol.

REES-JONES, Mrs Adrienne Camois Court, Barcombe, Lewes BN8 5BH Tel: 01273 400507 Fax: 01273 401901 — MB BCh BAO

Belf. 1967; Dip. Sports Med. Scotl. 1991. Assoc. Specialist (Rheum.) Eastbourne Dist. Gen. Hosp. Specialty: Rehabil. Med.; Rheumatol. Socs: BIMM; BASM; BMA.

REES-JONES, Elizabeth Corinne Ty'r Felin Surgery, Cecil Road, Gorseinon, Swansea SA4 4BY Tel: 01792 898844 — MB BS Lond. 1975; MRCS Eng. LRCP Lond. 1974; DRCOG 1976; DCH Eng. 1977. Prev: Ho. Surg. Char. Cross Hosp. Lond.; Ho. Phys. Canad. Red Cross Memor. Hosp. Taplow.

REES-JONES, Susan Victoria West End Surgery, Moorgreen Road, West End, Southampton SO30 3PY Tel: 023 8047 2126/8039 9200 Fax: 023 8039 9201; Shirral House, Shedfield, Southampton SO32 2HY Tel: 01329 832137 — MB BS Lond. 1973 (Char. Cross Hosp. Lond.) MRCS Eng. LRCP Lond. 1973. Specialty: Obst. & Gyn. Prev: Ho. Phys. & Ho. Surg. & SHO (A & E) Basingstoke & Dist.; Hosp.

REES-JONES, Thomas Glyn, Col. late RAMC (retired) 70 Bouverie Avenue, Salisbury SP2 8DX Tel: 01722 335041 — (Guy's) MRCS Eng. LRCP Lond. 1952; DObst RCOG 1964; MRCGP 1971; DCH Eng. 1972. Prev: Sen. Med. Off. Med. Centre Army Air Corps. Middle Wallop.

REESE, Alan John Morris, TD, OStJ (retired) 9 Hopping Lane, Canonbury, London N1 2NU Tel: 020 7226 2088 — (St. Bart.) MB BS Lond. 1943; LMSSA Lond. 1943; MD Lond. 1951; FRCPath 1968, M 1963. JP.; Barrister-at-Law, Middle Temple; Lt.-Col. RAMC RARO. Prev: Sen. Lect. (Path.) Inst. Basic Med. Sc. Univ. Lond.

REESE, Christopher David 27 St Lukes Place, Cheltenham GL53 7JL — MB BCh Wales 1992 (Univ. of Wales Coll. Of Med.) MRCP (UK) 1998. Clin. Fell. Paediat. IC, Bristol Childr.s Hosp. Specialty: Paediat. Prev: Regist. (Paediat.) Cheltenham Gen. Hosp.; Regist. (Paediat.) Wom.s & Child. Hosp. Adelaide.

REEVE, Abigail Amelia 8 Oates Way, Ramsey, Huntingdon PE26 1UX — MB ChB Leic. 1997. Pre-registrat. Ho. Off. (Gen. Surg.) Pilgrim Hosp. Boston. Socs: BMA; MDU.

REEVE, Anne Catherine 97 Boundary Road, Walthamstow, London E17 8NQ — MB ChB Sheff. 1983; MRCPsych 1988. Sen. Regist. (Child & Adolesc. Psychiat.) Child & Family Consultation Serv. Waltham Forest HA. Specialty: Child & Adolesc. Psychiat. Socs: BMA; Roy. Coll. Psychiat. (E. Anglian CTC Rep.). Prev: Regist. (Psychiat.) Whipps Cross, Claybury & Chase Farm Hosps.

REEVE, Anne Patricia Mary The Surgery, 82 St Ann St., Salisbury SP1 2PT Tel: 01722 322624 — MB BS Lond. 1975; MA (Physiol. Scs.) Oxf. 1976; DCH Eng. 1982. GP. Specialty: Paediat. Prev: SHO (Paediat.) Norf. & Norwich Hosp.; SHO (O & G) W. Suff. Hosp. Bury St. Edmunds; Partner Gen. Pract. Cotswolds.

REEVE, Brian John Norton Brook Medical Centre, Cookworthy Road, Kingsbridge TQ7 1AE Tel: 01548 853551 Fax: 01548 857741 — MB BS Lond. 1976 (Lond. Hosp.) MRCGP 1980; DRCOG 1980; DCH RCP Lond. 1982.

REEVE, Howard Sydney (retired) Netherton, Leeks Hill, Melton, Woodbridge IP12 1LW Tel: 01394 382727 — (Guy's) MSc (Med.) Lond. 1982, MB BS 1952; MRCGP 1959; DIH Eng. 1980; MFOM RCP Lond. 1983, AFOM 1981. Cons. Phys. Occupat. Med. RCP. Prev: Med. Adviser (Occupat. Health) Felixstowe Dock & Railway Co.

REEVE, Hugh Anthony Brinnington Health Centre, Brinnington Road, Stockport SK5 8BS Tel: 0161 430 4002 Fax: 0161 430 7918; 28 Amherst Road, Withington, Manchester M20 4NS Tel: 0161 286 2271 — MB ChB Manchester 1981; MBCHB Manchester 1981; MRCGP (London RCGP) 1985. Princip. Gen. Pract.; Course Organiser Stockport GP VTS; Chairm. Stockport PCG Clin. Governance Comm. Specialty: Gen. Pract. Prev: Med.Advis.Stockport HA (1993-1996); Lect. GP. Univ. Manch. (1986-1993).

REEVE, Joanne Lucy 25 Bryanston Road, Liverpool L17 7AL — MB ChB Liverp. 1997; MPH 2002 Liverpool; BClinSci, (Hons) Liverp. 1994; MB ChB (Hons.) Liverp. 1997; MRCGP 2001. Specialty: Gen. Med.

REEVE, Jonathan 38 Hugh Street, London SW1V 1RP Tel: 020 7834 5166 — BM BCh Oxf. 1968; DM Oxf. 1976, BM BCh 1968; MRCP (UK) 1970; MSc Lond. (Nuclear Med.) 1972; FRCP Lond. 1983; DSc Oxf. 1984. MRC Clin. Scientif. Staff Clin. Research Centre; Hon. Cons. Phys. Northwick Pk. Hosp. Harrow. Specialty: Gen. Med.

REEVE, Marjorie 592 Wells Road, Bristol BS14 9BD Tel: 01275 832102 — MB ChB Bristol 1940.

REEVE, Norman Leonard Department of Pathology, Stepping Hill Hospital, Poplar Grove, Stockport SK2 7JE Tel: 0161 419 5605 Fax: 0161 419 5668 Email: norman.reeve@stockport-tr.nwest.nhs.uk — MB ChB Manch. 1973; BSc (Anat.) Manch. 1970; FRCPath 1992, M 1979. Cons. Histopath. Stepping Hill Hosp. Stockport. Specialty: Histopath. Special Interest: Uropathology. Socs: Manch. Med. Soc.; ACP; IAO. Prev: Lect. (Path.) Univ. Manch.; Ho. Surg. Manch. Roy. Infirm.; Ho. Phys. Withington Hosp. Manch.

REEVE, Robert George X Ray Department, Kettering & Dist. Gen Hospital, Rothwell Road, Kettering NN16 8UZ Tel: 01536 492505 Fax: 01536 492473 Email: robert.reeve@kgh.nhs.uk — MB ChB Liverp. 1979 (Liverpool) DMRD Liverp. 1984; FRCR 1986. Cons. Radiol. Kettering & Dist. Gen. Hosp. Specialty: Radiol. Prev: Sen. Regist. Mersey RHA.

REEVE, Roy Stephen Histopathology Department Hope Hospital, Eccles Old Road, Salford M6 8HD — MB BChir Camb. 1977; MA Camb. 1979; FRCPath 1992, M 1982. Cons. Histopath. Hope Hosp. Salford. Specialty: Histopath. Prev: Sen. Regist. (Histopath.) Nottm.

REEVE, Samantha 67 Acacia Grove, New Malden KT3 3BU — MB BS Lond. 1997.

REEVE, Sandra Dawn 24 Amberwood Drive, Christchurch BH23 5RU — MB BS Lond. 1993.

REEVE, William Grant Glasgow Royal Infirmary, Glasgow G4 0SF; 16 South Erskine Park, Bearsden, Glasgow G61 4NA — BM Soton. 1981; DRCOG 1983; FFARCS Eng. 1988. Cons. Anaesth. Glas. Roy. Infirm. Specialty: Anaesth.

REEVES, David Mark 25 Lon-y-Dail, Cardiff CF14 6DZ — MB ChB Bristol 1992.

REEVES, Professor David Sims 4 Parkfield Road, Pucklechurch, Bristol BS16 9PN Tel: 0117 937 3241 Fax: 0117 937 4024 Email: davidreeves2@aol.com — (Westm.) MRCS Eng. LRCP Lond. 1961; MB BS (Hons.) Lond. 1961; DA Eng. 1963; FRCPath 1982, M 1970; MD Bristol 1989. Hon. Prof, Univ. Bristol.; Hon. Emerit. Cons.N. Bristol NHS Trust; Edr.-in-chief, Jl. of Antimicrobiol chemother. Specialty: Med. Microbiol.; Med. Publishing; Medico Legal. Socs: Hon. Life Mem. Brit. Soc. Antimirobial Chemother.; Past Pres., Assn. Med. Microbiol. Prev: Med. Dir. & Cons. Microbiol. Southmead Health Servs. NHS Trust Bristol; Lect. (Bact.) St. Mary's Med. Sch. Lond.

REEVES, Diana Mary 50 Dore Avenue, North Hykeham, Lincoln LN6 8LW — MB ChB Aberd. 1965; DCH RCPS Glas. 1980.

REEVES, Edward Rupert James Rose Cottage, Tutts Clump, Bradfield, Reading RG7 6LL Tel: 01734 744520 — MB BS Lond. 1991; MA (Hons.) Oxf. 1993.

REEVES, Elizabeth Mary 32 Listley Street, Bridgnorth WV16 4AW — MB ChB Birm. 1992.

REEVES, Graham Edgar 220 Redland Road, Bristol BS6 6YR Tel: 0117 973 2800 — MRCS Eng. LRCP Lond. 1962 (Lond. Hosp.)

REEVES, Helen Louise 98 The Avenue, Stoke-on-Trent ST4 6BZ; Flat 3, 16 Tankerville Terrace, Jesmond, Newcastle upon Tyne NE2 3AH Tel: 0191 281 5125 — BM BS Nottm. 1990; BMedSci. Nottm. 1988. Specialist Regist. (Gastro enterol.) Newc.-upon-Tyne. Specialty: Gastroenterol. Prev: Wellcome Trust Clin. Research Fell.

REEVES, Iain Christopher 2F2 15 Spittal Street, Edinburgh EH3 9DY — MB ChB Ed. 1998; MB ChB Ed 1998.

REEVES, Iris Agnes (retired) 86 Holland Road, Maidstone ME14 1UT Tel: 01622 661980 — MRCS Eng. LRCP Lond. 1950 (Roy. Free) Prev: Research Clin. Epidemiol. Unit Univ. Oxf.

REEVES, James Hargrave Kirk (retired) Chapel Row Surgery, The Avenue, Bucklebury, Reading RG7 6NS Tel: 01734 713252 Fax: 01734 714161; Rose Cottage, Tutts Clump, Bradfield, Reading RG7 6LL Tel: 0118 974 4520 Email: reeves3@supanet.com — MB BS Lond. 1960 (King's Coll. Hosp.) MRCS Eng. LRCP Lond. 1960. Prev: Resid. Med. Off. Mersey Gen. Hosp. Tasmania.

REEVES, Jane Philippa Well House, Well Lane, Upper Broughton, Melton Mowbray LE14 3BL — MB BS Lond. 1984.

REEVES, Kenneth Edgar Gabriel Clanricarde House Surgery, Clanricarde Road, Tunbridge Wells TN1 1PJ Tel: 01892 546422 Fax: 01892 533987 — MB BS Lond. 1972 (King's Coll. Hosp.) DObst RCOG 1976; MRCGP 1977. G. P. Represen., W. Kent Area Health Auth.; Osteoporosis Comm. Specialty: Medico Legal.

REEVES, Malcolm Thomas Newington Road Surgery, 100 Newington Road, Ramsgate CT12 6EW Tel: 01843 595951 Fax: 01843 853387 — MB ChB Liverp. 1969.

REEVES, Mark Andrew Trescobeas Surgery, Trescobeas Road, Falmouth TR11 2UN Tel: 01326 434888 Fax: 01326 434899; Holyrood, 43 Wood Lane, Falmouth TR11 4RB — MB BS Lond. 1983; AKC 1983; BSc (Biochem.) Lond. 1980, MB BS 1983; DRCOG 1985; DCH RCP Lond. 1987; MRCGP 1988.

REEVES, Nicola Ann 154 Howard Drive, Maidstone ME16 0QB Tel: 01622 757185 — MB BS Lond. 1993 (Lond. Hosp. Med. Coll.) SHO (Paediat.) Luton & Dunstable Hosp. Luton Beds. Specialty: Accid. & Emerg. Socs: BAEM Full Mem.ship. Prev: SHO (Neurosurg.) Old Ch. Hosp. Romford Essex; SHO (A & E) Basildon Hosp. Essex; SHO (Orthop. & Trauma) Qu. Mary's Hosp. Sidcup.

REEVES, Peter (retired) Ash Tree Cottage, Chapel Lane, Caunton, Newark NG23 6AN Tel: 01636 636209 — MB ChB Sheff. 1956; Cert Contracep. & Family Plann. RCOG, RCGP &; Cert FPA 1975.

REEVES, Peter Olaf Longacre, Wyke Lane, Farndon, Newark NG24 3SP — MRCS Eng. LRCP Lond. 1955; DPM Eng. 1962; FRCPsych 1984, M 1971. Cons. (Foren. Psychiat.) Rampton Hosp. Specialty: Forens. Psychiat. Prev: Cons. Psychiat. Balderton Hosp. Newark.

REEVES, Richard George William (retired) Holyrood House, Chard TA20 2DN Tel: 0146 063333 — MB ChB Birm. 1944.

REEVES, Robert Walter Kingham The Priory Hospital Bristol, Heath House Lane, Bristol BS16 1EQ — MB BS Lond. 1959 (Roy. Lond. Hosp.) DPM Eng. 1965; FRCPsych 1987, M 1972. Cons. Forens. Psychiat. The Priory Hosp. Bristol. Specialty: Forens. Psychiat. Prev: Mem. Parole Bd.; Med. Dir. Fromeside Clinic Bristol (Regional Secure Unit); Cons. Psychiat. Broadmoor Hosp. Med. Off. HM Remand Centre, PuckleCh. & HM Prison Bristol.

REEVES, Simon David Fenton and Partners, Medical Centre, Burgage Green, Southwell NG25 0EW; 1 Lambs Meadow, Mansfield Road, Edingley, Newark NG22 8BG Tel: 01623 882611 — BM BS Nottm. 1988; BMedSci (Hons.) Nottm. 1986; MRCP (UK) 1992; MRCGP 1994.

REEVES, Susan Elizabeth Telford & Wrekin PCT, Services for Children and Young People, Longbow House, Harlescott Lane, Shrewsbury SY1 3AS Tel: 01743 450800 — MB BS Lond. 1982; MA Camb. 1983; DRCOG 1986. Specialty: Community Child Health. Prev: Clin. Med. Off. Shrops. HA.

REEVES, Susan Mary Manchester Road Medical Centre, 27-31 Manchester Road, Knutsford WA16 0LY Tel: 01565 633101 Fax: 01565 750135; 22 Comber Way, Knutsford WA16 9BT Tel: 01565 755286 — MB BS Lond. 1987 (Char. Cross & Westm.) DRCOG 1991; MRCGP 1993. Gp. Socs: BMA. Prev: Trainee GP Macclesfield; SHO (Psychiat., Paediat. & O & G) Qu. Eliz. II Hosp. Welwyn Gdn. City.

REEVES, Suzanne Jane Hey Tor Oakfield, Huddersfield Road, Stalybridge SK15 3PY — MB ChB Manch. 1992.

REEVES, Wendy Jane Tadcaster Medical Centre, Crab Garth, Tadcaster LS24 8HD Tel: 01937 530082 Fax: 01937 530192 — (Sheff. Univ.) BSc (Hons.) Sheff. 1982, MB ChB 1986; DRCOG 1988; DCH RCPS Glas. 1989; MRCGP 1990. Prev: Trainee GP Leeds VTS; Ho. Off. (Gen. Surg.) Huddersfield Roy. Infirm.; Ho. Off. (Gen. Med. & Dermat.) Rotherham Dist. Gen. Hosp.

REEVES, Professor William Gordon Court Cottage, Cricket Malherbie, Ilminster TA19 0PW Tel: 01460 53080 — MB BS Lond. 1964 (Guy's) BSc (1st cl. Hons.) Lond. 1961; MRCS Eng. LRCP Lond. 1964; FRCP Lond 1978, M 1966; FRCPath 1985. Author, Edr. & Cons. Specialty: Immunol. Prev: Prof. Immunol. & Head Dept. Microbiol. & Immunol. Coll. Med. Sultan Qaboos Univ., Oman; Edr. The Lancet; Prof. & Cons. Immunol. Univ. Hosp. Qu. Med. Centre Nottm. & Nottm. Univ. Med. Sch.

REFAAT, Rafik The Royal London Hospital, The Coborn Adolescent Service, St Clemets Site, 2a Bow Road, London E3 4LL Tel: 020 7377 7904 Fax: 020 8880 6222 — MB BCh Ain Shams 1984; MRCPsych Lond. 1995. Cons. (Psychiat., Child & Adolesc.) The Roy. Hosp. Lond. Specialty: Child & Adolesc. Psychiat.

REFAAT, Refaat Faiq Eye Dept, Pilgrim Hospital, Boston PE21 9QS — MB ChB Alexandria 1970; DO RCPSI 1986. Specialty: Ophth.

REFFITT, David Michael Lewisham Hospital, Hihg Street, Lewisham, London SE13 6LH — MB ChB Bristol 1990. Cons. Gastroenterol.

REFSON, Alicia Rebekah Garden Flat, 6 Phillimore Gardens, London W8 7QD — MB BS Lond. 1998; MB BS Lond 1998.

REFSON, Mr Jonathan Simon The Granary, Clementsbury, Brickendon Lane, Brickendon, Hertford SG13 8FG — MB BS Lond. 1988; FRCS Eng. 1992; MS Lond. 2000. Cons. Gen. & Vasc., Princess Alexandra Hosp., Essex. Specialty: Gen. Surg.

REFSUM, Mr Erling 142 Humber Road, London SE3 7LY — MB BS Lond. 1978 (Guy's) FRCS Ed. 1983.

REFSUM, Miss Sigrid Elisabet Belfast City Hospital, Lisburn Road, Belfast BT9 7AB Tel: 028 9032 9241 Fax: 028 9032 6614; 2 Malone Hill Park, Belfast BT9 6RD Tel: 028 9066 6613 Email: srefsum@aol.com — MB BCh BAO Belf. 1985 (Queen's Univ. Belf.) BSc (Hons.) Manch. 1980; FRCS Ed. 1989; MD Belf. 1997. Cons. (Gen. & Breast Surg.) Belf. City Hosp. N. Irel. Specialty: Gen. Surg. Special Interest: Breast Reconstruction. Socs: Ulster Med. Soc.; BMA; BASO.

REGAN, Alison Fiona Margaret National Blood Service, North London Centre, Colindale Avenue, London NW9 5BG Email: fiona.regan@nbs.nhs.uk — MB BS Lond. 1987 (Middlesex Hospital Medical School (82-87)) MRCP (UK) 1991; MRCPath 1998. Jt. Post Cons. Haematologist - Nat. Blood Serv. and Hammersmith Hosps. NHS Trust. Specialty: Blood Transfus.; Haematology. Prev: Research Fell. N. Lond. Blood Transfus. Centre.; Regist. (Haemat.) Soton. Gen. Hosp.; SHO Rotat. (Med.) Soton. Gen. Hosp.

REGAN, Ciaran Campbell TFR, 41A Broughton St., Edinburgh EH1 3JU — MB ChB Ed. 1996.

REGAN, Dermot Martin 54 St Mark's Road, Sale M33 6SA — MB BCh Wales 1984.

REGAN, Fiona Mary 116 Pennard Drive, Southgate, Swansea SA3 2DP — MB ChB Leic. 1994. Specialty: Paediat. Socs: BMA & Med. Sickness Soc.

REGAN, Joanna Margaret The Old Farmhouse, Pinn Lane, Exeter EX1 3RG; The Old Farmhouse, Pinn Lane, Exeter EX1 3RG Tel: 01392 464816 — MB BS Lond. 1992 (St. Geo. Hosp. Lond.) DCH RCP Lond. 1995; DRCOG 1996; DFFP 1997; MRGP 1997; DPD 2000. Clin. Asst. in Dermat. Roy. Devon & Exeter Hosp.; GP Non-Princip. Exeter; CMO Family Plann. Specialty: Dermat.; Family Plann. & Reproduc. Health. Prev: GP/Regist. Newport; SHO (Gen. Adult Psychiat.) St. Cadoc's Hosp. Caerleon Gwent; SHO (O & G) Roy. Gwent Hosp. Newport.

REGAN, Judith Louise 9 Frognal Court, Finchley Road, London NW3 5HL — MB BS Lond. 1998; MB BS Lond 1998.

REGAN, Kathryn Jane Trevose, Oakland Av, Farnham GU9 9DX — BM BCh Oxf. 1997.

REGAN, Professor Lesley Imperial College London, St Mary's Hospital, Norfolk Place, London W2 1PG Tel: 020 7886 1050 Fax: 020 7886 6054 Email: l.regan@imperial.ac.uk — MB BS Lond. 1980 (Royal Free, Lond.) MRCOG 1985; MD Lond. 1989; FRCOG 1998. Prof. & Head of Dept. O & G ICSM at St. Mary's; Hon. Cons. (Obst. & Gyn.) at St. Mary's. Specialty: Obst. & Gyn. Socs: Soc.for Gyn. Investig.; Gyn. Vis. Soc.; Expert (Reproduc. Med.) Fed. of Int. Obst. & Gyn. Prev: Sen. Lect. (O & G) St. Mary's; Sen. Regist. (O & G) Addenbrooke's Hosp. Camb.; Fell. & Dir. Med. Studies Girton Coll. Camb.

REGAN, Marian Rose Derbyshire Royal Infirmary, London Road, Derby DE1 2QY Tel: 01332 347141 Fax: 01332 254989 — MB BCh BAO NUI 1984 (University College Dublin) FRCP. Cons. Rheum. Derbysh. Roy. Infirm. Specialty: Rheumatol.

REGAN, Millicent Maire Corban 83 Cambridge Road, Gt Crosby, Liverpool L23 7TX — (Liverp.) MB ChB Liverp. 1948, DPH 1962; MFCM 1974.

REGAN, Richard John Riva, 54 North Park, Gerrards Cross SL9 8JR Tel: 01753 887057 — MB BS Sydney 1965; MRCP (UK) 1970; FRCP Lond. 1993. Cons. Phys. Gen. Med. & Geriat. Amersham Gen. Hosp. Oxf. RHA. Specialty: Gen. Med. Socs: Renal Assn. & Brit. Geriat. Soc. Prev: Sen. Regist. (Gen. Med. & Nephrol.) Hants, AHA (T); Regist. (Nephrol.) St. Jas. Univ. Hosp. Leeds.

REGE, Kanchan Pandurang Hinchingbrooke Healthcare Trust, Hinchingbrooke Park, Huntingdon PE29 6NT Tel: 01480 416155 Fax: 01480 416527 Email: kanchan.rege@hinchingbrooke.nhs.uk — MB BChir Camb. 1990; MA Cantab. 1990; MRCP (UK) 1992; MRCPath 1997; FRCPath 2005. Cons. Haematologist, Hinchingbrooke Hosp., Huntingdon; Cons. Haematologist, Papworth Hosp., Camb. Specialty: Haematology. Prev: Regist. (Haemat.) Hammersmith Hosp. Lond.; Sen. Regist. (Haemat.) St. Geo. Hosp. Lond.

REGINALD, Philip Wallace Department of Obstetrics & Gynaecology, Wexham Park Hospital, Slough Tel: 01753 34567 — MD Lond. 1989; MB BS Bangalore 1976; MRCOG 1981. Cons. O & G Wexham Pk. Hosp. Slough. Specialty: Obst. & Gyn. Prev: Lect. & Sen. Regist. (O & G) St. Mary's Hosp. Lond.

REGISTER, Paula Wendy Lyndale, Poundstock, Bude EX23 0AU — BM BS Nottm. 1998; BM BS Nottm 1998.

REGLINSKI, Frank Andrew The Surgery, Anderson Drive, Leslie, Glenrothes KY6 3LQ Tel: 01592 620222 Fax: 01592 620553 — MB ChB Dundee 1983. GP Glenrothes, Fife.

REGNARD, Claud Francis Bernard St. Oswalds Hospice, Regent Avenue, Gosforth, Newcastle upon Tyne NE3 1EE Tel: 0191 285 0063 Fax: 0191 284 8004 — MB ChB Dundee 1976; BMSc (Hons.) Dund 1973; MRCP (UK) 1996; FRCP (UK) 1998. Cons.(Palliat. Med.)St. Oswald's Hospice & Newc.Northgate & Prudhoe NHS Trust. Specialty: Palliat. Med. Socs: Assn. Palliat. Med; Assoc. Mem. Europe Assoc. Palliat. Care; Internat. Assn. Study Pain. Prev: Macmillan Fell. (Palliat. Care) Churchill Hosp. Oxf..; Hon. Clin. Lect. (Pharmacol. Scis.) Univ. of Newc.

REGUNATHAN, Ponniah The Surgery, 238 Headstone Lane, Harrow HA2 5EF Tel: 020 8428 1211 Fax: 020 8428 9434 — (Ceylon) MB BS Ceylon 1959; PhD Ed. 1971. Specialty: Immunol. Socs: BMA; Med. Protec. Soc.

REHANA, Hussain Akhter 8 Rhindmuir Grove, Baillieston, Glasgow G69 6NE — MB BS Punjab 1965.

REHLING, Graham Hugh Psychotherapy Department, 2 Cossington Road, Canterbury CT1 3HU — MB BS Lond. 1977; MRCPsych 1981; MSc Lond. 1985. Cons. Psychiat. & Psychotherapist E. Kent Community NHS Trust. Specialty: Psychother.; Gen. Psychiat. Prev: Cons. Psychiat. SE Kent HA; Sen. Regist. Camb.; Regist. Guy's Hosp. Lond.

REHMAN, Alim John 93 Harley Street, London W1G 6AD Tel: 020 7935 2079 Fax: 020 7487 2831 — MB BS Lond. 1985 (St. Mary's Hosp. Med. Sch. Lond.) D.Occ.Med. RCP Lond. 1996. Chief Med. Off. Arcadia plc Debenhams plc & Nat. Hist. Museum; Occupat. Phys. StoreHo. plc. The Arcadia plc, Hypo Bank, Vivat Holding plc Lee Cooper Jeans & Star Mining, Siberia; Chief Med. Off. Marshalls plc, Hamptons, Internat. Specialty: Occupat. Health. Socs: Fell. Roy. Soc. Med.; Soc. Occupat. Med.; Fell. Roy. Geogr. Soc. Prev: Chief Med. Off. Union Bank of Switz.; Med. Off. Boxing Bd. of Control.

REHMAN, Faiz Ur Norfolk Square Surgery, 14 Aldwick Road, Bognor Regis PO21 2LJ Tel: 01243 821404 Fax: 01243 841404; The Rubens, 105 Marshall Avenue, Bognor Regis PO21 2TN Tel: 01243 822227 — MB BS Punjab 1965 (Nishtar Med. Coll. Multan) MB BS Punjab (Pakistan) 1965. Cas. Surg. (GP) Bognor War Memor. Hosp. Socs: Fam. Plann. Doctors Assn.; (Jt. Sec.) BMA (W. Sussex Br.). Prev: Regist. (Orthop.) Nishtar Med. Coll. Hosp. Multan, Pakistan.

REHMAN, Humaira 15 Ruby Close, Slough SL1 9DZ — MB BS Lond. 1994.

REHMAN, Jahangir — MB BS Newc. 1998; MB BS Newc 1998. Specialty: Gen. Med.

REHMAN, Mohammed Javed 224 Upper Woodlands Road, Bradford BD8 9JQ — MB ChB Manch. 1994.

REHMAN, Mr Shafiq-Ur 93 South Street, Savile Town, Dewsbury WF12 9NG — MB BS Karachi 1978; FRCS Glas. 1985.

REHMAN, Shamim-ur Salford Medical Centre, 194 Langworthy Road, Salford M6 5PP Tel: 0161 736 2651 Fax: 0161 745 8955 — MB BS Karachi 1966.

REHMAN, Sheikh Abdul 2 Midfield, Langho, Blackburn BB6 8HF Tel: 01254 249994 — MB BS Punjab 1949 (King Edwd. Med. Coll. Lahore) MRCP (UK) 1973; FRCP Glas. 1990. Cons. Phys. Geriat. Med. Blackburn Health Dist. Specialty: Gen. Med. Prev: Ho. Surg. (ENT) & Med. Off. Tuberc. Outpat. Dept. Mayo Hosp. Lahore; JHMO (Chest Dis.) Ladywell Hosp. Salford.

REHMAN, Mrs Zeb 4 Hillbury Road, London SW17 8JT — MB BS Punjab 1964; MB BS Punjab (Pakistan) 1964.

REHMAN, Zia-ur Church Street Surgery, 112 Church Street, Flint CH6 5AF Tel: 01352 733194 Fax: 01352 763669 — MB BS Punjab 1962 (Nishtar Med. Coll. Multan) MB BS Punjab (Pakistan) 1962.

REHMANY, Khalid Mahmood Avian Nook, Coleshill Heath Road, Marston Green, Birmingham B37 7HU — MB BS Karachi 1959 (Dow Med. Coll.) DA Eng. 1965. Prev: Regist. Selly Oak Hosp. Birm.

REICHENBERG, Frances Pauline Newtown Hospital, Child & Family Service, Newtown Road, Worcester WR5 1JG — MB BS Lond. 1984; BSc Lond.; CCST (Child & Adolesc. Psychiat.); MRCPsych 1984. Locum Cons. (Child & Adolesc. Psychiat.). Specialty: Child & Adolesc. Psychiat.

REICHHELM, Thomas 1 Boughton Church Cottages, South St., Boughton-under-Blean, Faversham ME13 9NB — State Exam Med Freiburg 1992; DRCOG 1995. GP Regist. Canterbury VTS.

REICHL, Mr Michael Accident & Emergency Department, Poole Hospital, Longfleet Road, Poole BH15 2JB Tel: 01202 442660 Fax: 01202 448207 — MB BS Lond. 1978 (Univ. Coll. Hosp.) FRCS Ed. 1983; FRCS Ed. 1983. Cons. A & E Poole Hosp. NHS Trust & Roy. Bournemouth Hosp. Specialty: Accid. & Emerg. Prev: Sen. Regist. (A & E) Soton. Gen. Hosp.; Regist. (Accid & Emerg.) Leic. Roy. Infirm.; Regist. (Surg.) Stepping Hill Hosp. Stockport.

REID, Abigail Simpson (retired) 36 Tinto Road, Newlands, Glasgow G43 2AP Tel: 0141 637 1790 — MB ChB Glas. 1956. Prev: Assoc. Specialist Cytol. Path. Dept. Roy. Alexandra Hosp. Paisley.

REID, Ainsley Well Street Surgery, Well Street, Montgomery SY15 6PF Tel: 01686 668217 Fax: 01686 668599; RAOBH Haven, Kingsland Bridge Rd, Shrewsbury SY3 7AQ Tel: 01743 243790 — MB ChB Aberd. 1976; DRCOG 1980; MRCGP 1982; MFFP 1993. GP Princip.; Chairman Dyfed Powys Health In.; Chairm. Specialized Health Serv. Commiss. for Wales. Socs: Montgomery Med. Soc.

REID, Alan Iain Tranent Medical Practice, Loch Road, Tranent EH33 2JX — MB ChB Glas. 1975.

REID, Alan Robert, TD Occupational Health Service, The Boots Company PLC, 1 Thane Road W., Nottingham NG2 3AA Tel: 0115 959 3656 Fax: 0115 959 4867; 7 Wemyss Gardens, Wollaton Park, Nottingham NG8 1BJ Tel: 0115 970 8138 — MB ChB Aberd. 1966; DIH Soc. Apoth. Lond. 1980; FFOM RCP Lond. 1987, M 1982; FRCP Lond. 1993. Chief Med. Off. (Occupat. Health Serv.) The Boots Co. PLC; Lt.-Col. RAMC(V). Specialty: Occupat. Health. Socs: Fell. Soc. Occupat. Med. Prev: Sen. Occupat. Phys. Centr. Electricity Generating Bd. Lond. HQ; Med. Off. ICI Petrochem. Div. Middlesbrough; Ho. Off. (Surg.) Roy. Hosp. Sick Childr. & (Med.) Woodend Hosp. Aberd.

REID, Alan Stuart 4 Wheatfields, Enfield EN3 5DW — MB ChB Birm. 1997.

REID, Alastair Gilmour 2 (TFL) Lauriston Park, Edinburgh EH3 9JA Tel: 0131 229 1665; TFL, 2 Lauriston Park, Edinburgh EH3 9JA — MB ChB Ed. 1991. Prev: Ho. Off. West. Gen. Hosp. Edin.; Ho. Off. (Surg.) Orkney.

REID, Alastair Grant Parkfield Health Centre, Sefton Road, New Ferry, Wirral CH62 5HS Tel: 0151 644 6665; Plymyard Cottage, 48 Plymyard Avenue, Bromborough, Wirral CH62 6BW Tel: 0151 328 1007 — MRCS Eng. LRCP Lond. 1960 (Liverp.) DObst RCOG 1963. Chief Med. Off. Aintree Motor Cycle Club. Prev: Vis. Med. Off. Birkenhead Matern. Hosp.; Regist. (Cas.) Roy. Infirm. Liverp.; SHO (O & G) & Ho. Phys. (Paediat.) Clatterbridge Hosp.

REID, Alastair James Mayne Department of Child Health, Queen's University of Belfast, Institute of Clinical Science, Belfast BT12 6BJ — MB BCh BAO Belf. 1990. Specialty: Paediat.

REID, Alastair Norman Crawford, Wing Cdr. c/o Director General Medical Services (Royal Air Force), Headquarters Personnel and Training Command, Royal Air Force Innsworth, Gloucester GL3 1EZ Tel: 01452 712612 Ext: 5853 Email: ancreid@doctors.org.uk — MB ChB Glas. 1983; DRCOG 1986; MRCGP 1987; DAvMED 1998; MSc (Occupat. Health) Aberd. 2003; MFOM 2004. Specialty: Occupat. Health.

REID, Alexander Colinton, St. Martin's Crescent, Caerphilly CF8 — MB ChB Ed. 1946.

REID, Alexander Graham Mayfield Road Surgery, 125 Mayfield Road, Edinburgh EH9 3AJ Tel: 0131 668 1095 Fax: 0131 662 1734; 2A Church Hill, Edinburgh EH10 4BQ Tel: 0131 447 5510 — MB ChB Glas. 1966; MRCGP 1970.

REID, Alick Mitchell (retired) 108 Southbrae Drive, Glasgow G13 1TZ Tel: 0141 959 3083 — MB ChB Glas. 1949; DObst RCOG 1951; FRCA Eng. 1955. Prev: Cons. Anaesth.. Glas. Roy. Infirm.

REID, Allan William Department of Radiology, Glasgow Royal Infirmary, 16 Alexandra Parade, Glasgow G31 2ER Tel: 0141 211 4783 Fax: 0141 211 4781; 3 Sydenham Road, Glasgow G12 9NT Tel: 0141 334 9112 — MB ChB Glas. 1980; DRCOG 1982; FRCR

1986. Cons. (Radiol.) Glas. Roy. Infirm.; Clin. Dir. Imaging Directorate Glas. Roy. Infirm.; Hon. Clin. Sen. Lect. Glas. Univ.; Cons. (Radiol.) Ross Hall Hosp. Glas. Specialty: Radiol. Socs: Roy. Med. Chir. Soc. of Glas.; Scott. Radiological Soc.

REID, Allison Anna Balmore Road Surgery, 138-142 Balmore Road, Glasgow G22 6LJ Tel: 0141 531 9393 Fax: 0141 531 9389 — MB ChB Glas. 1991.

REID, Allyn Costandine Cleveland Clinic, 12 Cleveland Road, St Helier, Jersey JE1 4HD Tel: 01534 722381/734121 — MB BS Lond. 1971; DRCOG 1976. Specialty: Gen. Med.

REID, Andrew Hamilton The Cottage, Main St., Longforgan, Dundee DD2 5ET Tel: 01382 360247 — MD Dundee 1972 (St. And.) MB ChB St. And. 1965; DPM Ed. & Glas. 1968; FRCP Ed. 1980, M 1970; FRCPsych 1980, M 1972. Cons. Psychiat. Dundee Psychiat. Servs. (Tayside HB.). Specialty: Gen. Psychiat. Socs: Hon. Sen. Lect. (Psychiat.) Univ. Dundee; Fell. Roy. Soc. Med.; BMA. Prev: Lect. (Psychiat.) Univ. Dundee; Sen. Regist. (Psychiat.) Dundee Psychiat. Servs.; Ho. Surg. & Ho. Phys. Dundee Roy. Infirm.

REID, Mr Andrew Peter 68 Gillhurst Road, Harborne, Birmingham B17 8PB — MB ChB Birm. 1978; FRCS Ed. 1984. Cons. ENT Surg. Univ. Hosp. Birm. NHS Trust, Birm. Childrens Hosp. Specialty: Otolaryngol.

REID, Andrew Scott St Pancras Coroner's Court, Camley Street, London NW1 0PP Tel: 020 7387 4884 Fax: 020 7383 2485 — BM BS Nottm. 1988; BMedSci Nottm. 1986. Coroner Inner N. Lond.; Chairm. Ment. Health Review Tribunal. Specialty: Forens. Path. Socs: Fell. Roy. Soc. Med.; Medico-legal Soc.; Coroners Soc. Eng. & Wales. Prev: Asst. Dep. Coroner Nottm.; Regist. City & Univ. Hosps. Nottm.; Temp. Lect. (Human Morphol.) Univ. Nottm. Med. Sch.

REID, Angela Rosemary Community Paediatrics, Lawson Memorial Hospital, Golspie Tel: 01408 633157; The Old Manse of Creich, Bonar Bridge, Ardgay IV24 3AB Tel: 01863 766257 — MB ChB Ed. 1970; BSc, MB ChB Ed. 1970. Community Paediat. Sutherland & E. Ross-sh. Specialty: Community Child Health. Prev: GP Tain Ross Shire.

REID, Anne Grampian Health Board, Summerfield House, 2 Eday Road, Aberdeen AB15 6RE Tel: 01224 404008 Fax: 01224 404014; 22 Burns Road, Aberdeen AB15 4NS Tel: 01224 318130 Email: arjazz22@aol.com — MB ChB Aberd. 1971. Med. Off. (Communicable Dis.s) Grampian HB. Specialty: Infec. Dis. Prev: Med. Edr. Gtr. Glas. HB; Regist. (Community Med.) Grampian HB; Research Off. (Biomed., Physics & Bioeng.) Univ. Aberd.

REID, Anthony Donald Worden Medical Centre, West Paddock, Leyland, Preston PR25 1HR Tel: 01772 423555 Fax: 01772 623878 — MB ChB Manch. 1987; DRCOG 1990; MRCGP 1991. Specialty: Gen. Psychiat. Prev: Trainee GP Bury VTS.

REID, Basil Raymond 19 Burghley Avenue, New Malden KT3 4SW — MB BCh BAO Belf. 1964; DMRD Eng. 1969; FFR 1972; FRCR 1975.

REID, Mr Brian Alexander, Wing Cdr. RAF Med. Br. Retd. (retired) Department Obstetrics & Gynaecology, Claydon Wing, Stoke Mandeville Hospital NHS Trust, Aylesbury HP21 8AL Tel: 01296 315201; Four Winds, Henton, Chinnor OX39 4AE Email: bareid@btinternet.com — MB ChB Glas. 1980 (Univ. Glas.) MRCGP 1984; DCH RCP Lond. 1986; DRCOG 1987; MRCOG 1990; T(OG) 1994; MFFP 1995. Cons O&G Stoke Mandeville Hosp. NHS Trust, Aylesbury; Cons. O & G Stoke Mandeville Hosp. NHS Trust. Prev: Hon. Sen. Regist. (O & G) Glas. Roy. Infirm.

REID, Carolyn Anne Department of Plastic Surgery, Royal Victoria Infirmary, Queen Victoria Road, Newcastle upon Tyne NE1 4LP Tel: 0191 232 5131 — MB BS Newc. 1969; FRCS Ed. 1975. Cons. Plastic Surg. Roy. Vict. Infirm. Newc. u. Tyne. Specialty: Plastic Surg. Socs: Brit. Burns Assn.

REID, Catriona Mary 16 Darlington Place, Bath BA2 6BX — MB ChB Ed. 1968; DObst RCOG 1970; MFFP RCOG 1993. Manager Adult Health Servs. Bath & W. Community NHS Trust; Med. Off. Bath Univ. Specialty: Family Plann. & Reproduc. Health.

REID, Cecil David Leo Meadway, Royston Grove, Hatch End, Pinner HA5 4HF — MB BS Lond. 1966 (Univ. Coll. Hosp.) BSc Lond. 1963; DCH Eng. 1971; FRCP Lond. 1977; FRCPath 1981. Cons. Haemat. Northwick Pk. Hosp. Specialty: Haematology. Prev: Hon. Sen. Regist. (Haemat.) Northwick Pk. Hosp. Harrow.

REID, Charles Henry (retired) The Firs, Cross in Hand, Heathfield TN21 0LT Tel: 01435 862021 Fax: 01435 867522; 31 Frenches Farm Drive, Heathfield TN21 8BQ — BM BCh Oxf. 1975; BA Oxf. 1972. Prev: Regist. (Orthop.) Eastbourne Dist. Gen. Hosp.

REID, Christopher John Douglas Department of Paediatric Nephrology & Urology, 9th Floor, Guy's Hospital, St Thomas St., London SE1 9RT Tel: 020 7955 5000 Email: christopher.reid@kcl.ac.uk; 244 Barry Road, East Dulwich, London SE22 0JS — MB ChB Liverp. 1983; MRCP (UK) 1987. Cons. Paediat. Nephrol. Guy's & St. Thos. NHS Trust Lond. Specialty: Paediat. Prev: Sen. Regist. (Paediat.) Guy's & St. Thos. NHS Trust Lond.

REID, Christopher Joseph 15 Shearwater, Whitburn, Sunderland SR6 7SF — MB BS Newc. 1992.

REID, Christopher Michael Barrett Holland House, 31 Church Road, Lytham, Lytham St Annes FY8 5LL Tel: 01253 794999 Fax: 01253 795744; Eden House, 1 Eden Avenue, Lytham, Lytham St Annes FY8 5PS Tel: 01253 730705 Fax: 01253 730705 Email: michaelreid@edenhouse100.freeserve.co.uk — MB BCh BAO Dub. 1969 (Trinity Coll. Dub.) DObst RCOG 1971; MA Dub. 1992. GP Lytham Lancs.; PEC Mem. Fylde PCT; Board Mem. Fylde PCT; Mem. (Vice-Chairm.) NW Lancs. LMC; Hon. Med. Off. Lytham Lifeboat Station; Clin. Asst. (Cardiol.) Vict. Hosp. Blackpool. Specialty: Gen. Pract. Prev: SHO (Med. & Surg.) Roy. Manch. Child. Hosp. Pendlebury; Ho. Phys. & Ho. Surg. Roy. City Dub. Hosp.; Ho. Off. Glenroyd Matern. Hosp. Blackpool.

REID, Clifford Gordon A & E Medicine, North Hampshire Hospital, Basingstoke RG24 9NA — BM Soton. 1991; MRCP (UK) 1994. Specialist Regist. A&E Med. N. Hants. Hosp.

REID, Mr Clive Douglas Department of Plastic & Reconstructive Surgery, Frenchay Hospital, Bristol BS16 1LE Tel: 0117 9753993 Fax: 0117 975 3846 — MB ChB Dundee 1970; FRCS Glas. 1975. Cons. Plastic Surg. Frenchay Hosp. Specialty: Plastic Surg. Socs: Brit. Assn. Plastic Surg.; Aesthetic Plastic Surgs.; Brit. Assn. Aesthetic Plastic Surgs.

REID, Colette Mary Department of Palliative Medicine, Bristol Oncolgy Centre, Horfield Road, Bristol BS2 8ED Tel: 0117 9283507 Email: colette.reid@bristol.ac.uk; 1 Bankside Cottages, Church Lane, Owslebury, Winchester SO21 1LU — MB ChB Glas. 1989; DRCOG 1994; MRCGP 1995. Staff Grade (Palliat. Med.) Countess Mounbatten Ho. Soton.; SPR Palliant Med. Specialty: Palliat. Med.

REID, Colin Flat N Melville Court, 75 Rose St., Aberdeen AB10 1UH Tel: 01224 637556 Fax: 01224 637556 — MB ChB Aberd. 1990; DA (UK) 1992; FRCA 1994. Cons. Anaesth., Aberd. Roy. Infirm., Aberd. Specialty: Anaesth. Prev: Clin. Fell. Cardiothoracic Anaesth., Roy. Brompton Hosp. Lond.; Specialist Regist. (Anaesth. & Intens. Care) Aberd. Roy. Infirm.; Regist. (Anaesth.) Raigmore Hosp. Inverness.

REID, Colin Brown Charleston Surgery, South Campbell Street, Paisley PA2 6LR Tel: 0141 889 4373 Fax: 0141 848 0648; 103 Arkleston Road, Paisley PA1 3TY — MB ChB Glas. 1975 (Glasgow University) DRCOG 1978; MRCGP 1980. Clin. Asst. (Haemat.) Roy. Infirm. Glas.; Clin. Tutor, Univ. of Glas.

REID, Colin James Hunter Lodge, Oving, Chichester PO20 2BT Tel: 01243 532254 Fax: 01243 532254 — MB BS Lond. 1973 (St. Bart.) MRCS Eng. LRCP Lond. 1973; MRCP (UK) 1976; FRCP Lond. 1994. Cons. Phys. Cardiol. Roy. W. Sussex Hosp. Chichester. Specialty: Cardiol. Socs: Brit. Cardiac Soc. Prev: Sen. Regist. (Cardiol.) Roy. Free Hosp. Lond. & Harefield Hosp.; Regist. (Med.) St. Thos. Hosp. Lond.; Regist. Nat. Heart Hosp. Lond.

REID, Crawford Russell Greenshields 20 Back Road, Dollar FK14 7EA — MB ChB Dundee 1979.

REID, Professor Daniel, OBE (retired) 29 Arkleston Road, Paisley PA1 3TE Tel: 0141 889 4873 — MB ChB Glas. 1958 (Univ. Glas.) DPH Eng. 1967; MD (Commend.) Glas. 1969; FFPHM RCP (UK) 1978, M 1974; FRCP Glas. 1983, M 1980; FRCP Ed. 1994; FRS Ed. 1997. Prev: Dir. Scott. Centre for Infec. & Environm. Health Ruchill Hosp. Glas.

REID, David Arthur Rowan House, Whyteman's Brae, Kirkcaldy KY1 2LS Tel: 01592 643355 — MB ChB Ed. 1985; DRCOG 1990; MRCPsych 1992; Dip. Cog. Psychol. Dund 1996. Cons. Psychiat. Whyteman's Brae Hosp. Kirkcaldy. Specialty: Gen. Psychiat. Prev: Lect. & Hon. Sen. Regist. (Psychiat.) Univ. Dundee.; Regist. Rotat. Roy. Dundee Liff Hosp.; Trainee GP Fife HB VTS:.

REID, David Coutts Tayside Health Screening Clinic, 313 Strath Martine Road, Dundee DD3 8ND Tel: 01382 832600 — MB ChB

Dundee 1977; T(GP) 1991. Med. Adviser for Benefits Agency; Health Screening & Occupat. Health Clinic. Specialty: Disabil. Med. Socs: Fell. Roy. Soc. Med.; Brit. Soc. Med. & Dent. Hypn.; Brit. Med. Acupunct. Soc.

REID, David Graham 20 Parade, Berwick-upon-Tweed TD15 1DF — MB ChB St And. 1964; DPM Eng. 1969; MRCPsych 1972. Specialty: Gen. Psychiat. Prev: Hon. Sen. Lect. (Psychiat.) Univ. Aberd.; Cons. Psychiat. Craig Dunain Hosp. Inverness; Cons. Psychiat. Parkside Hosp. Macclesfield.

REID, David Hamilton Struthers Medical Institute for Research into Child Cruelty, Step Rock House, St Andrews KY16 9AT — MD St. And. 1969; MB ChB 1956; FRCP Ed. 1972, M 1963; CIH Dund 1981; FRCPCH 1997. Cons. Paediat. & Dir. MIRIC St. And. Specialty: Paediat. Socs: MRCPCH. Prev: Cons. Paediat. Mersey Regional HB; MRC Research Fell. (Child Health) Univ. Aberd.; Resid. Childr. Hosp. of Philadelphia, USA.

REID, Mr David Lauriston Lincoln 26 Foxborough Gardens, Bradley Stoke, Bristol BS32 0BT — BM Soton. 1987; FRCS Ed. 1992.

REID, Professor David Macaulay Medical School, Foresterhill, Aberdeen AB25 2ZD Tel: 01224 681818 Email: d.m.reid@abdn.ac.uk; 25 Friarsfield Road, Cults, Aberdeen AB15 9LB Tel: 01224 867874 — MD Aberd. 1985; MB ChB 1975; MRCP (UK) 1978; FRCP Ed. 1989. Prof. of Rheum. & Head of Dept. of Med. & Therap., Univ. of Aberd.; Hon. Cons. Aberd. Roy. Hosps. NHS Trust. Specialty: Rheumatol. Socs: Scientif. Advis. Comm., ARC; Chair Scientif. Advis. Gp. NOS; Brit Soc Rheum. Prev: Cons. Rheumatologist, Grampian HB; Sen. Regist. (Med. & Rheum.) Grampian HB; Lect. Med. (Rheum.) Univ. Edin.

REID, David Mark Rutherglen Primary Care Centre, 130 Stonelaw Road, Rutherglen, Glasgow G73 2PQ Tel: 0141 531 6010 Fax: 0141 613 3460; 2 Victoria Lane, Mearnskirk Road, Newton Mearns, Glasgow G77 5TP — MB ChB Glas. 1978; Dip. Forens. Med. Glas. 1992.

REID, Mr Donald Alexander Highbird, The Turnpike, Halam, Newark NG22 8AE — MB ChB Dundee 1973; FRCS Ed. 1979.

REID, Mr Donald Benjamin Vascular & Endovascular Institute, Wishaw Hospital, Wishaw ML2 7NE — MB ChB Glas. 1983; FRCS Glas. 1987; MD Glas. 1991; FRCS (Surg.) 1995. Cons., Vasc. & EndoVasc. Surg., Vasc. & EndoVasc. Inst., Wishaw Hosp. Scotl.; Hon. Sen. Clin. Lect., Univ. of Glas. Specialty: Vasc. Med. Socs: (Counc.) Roy. M-C Soc.; W Scotl. Surg. Assn.; Internat. Soc. EndoVasc. Specialists. Prev: Fell. (Cardiovasc.) Arizona Heart Inst. Phoenix, Arizona, USA; Regist. (Surg.) Univ. Dept. Surg. Roy. Infirm. Glas.; Clin. Fell. & Sen. Regist. (Surg.) Unit for Peripheral Vasc. Surg. Glas. Roy. Infirm.

REID, Mr Donald James 43 East End Lane, Ditchling, Hassocks BN6 8UP Tel: 01273 842348 Fax: 01273 842348 Email: thereids@hemscott.net — (St. Thos. Hosp. & Oxf.) BM BCh Oxf. 1954; FRCS Ed. 1960; FRCS Eng. 1960; MA Oxf. 1954, MCh 1967, DM 1967. Specialty: Gen. Surg. Socs: Fell. Assn. Surgs.; Fell. Roy. Soc. Med. Prev: Research fell. Mayo Clinic USA; Cons. Surg. Princess Roy. Hosp. Haywards Heath & Roy. Sussex Co. Hosp. Brighton; Sen. Regist. (Surg.) St. Thos. Hosp. Lond.

REID, Doreen Isobel Leslie Clinic, Anderson Drive, Leslie, Glenrothes KY6 3LG Tel: 01592 743388; Aviemore, 16 Largo Road, Lundin Links, Leven KY8 6DH Tel: 01333 320268 — MB ChB Aberd. 1966. SCMO (Community Child Health) Fife HB. Specialty: Community Child Health. Socs: Fac. Community Health; BMA; Soc. Pub. Health.

REID, Dorte Elisabeth Bjorchmar Hunter Lodge, Oving, Chichester PO20 2BT Fax: 01243 532254 — MD Odense 1983. Med. Off. (Orthop.) King Edwd. VII Hosp. Midhurst.

REID, Mr Douglas Andrew Campbell (retired) Croft House, 6 Buxton Road, Eastbourne BN20 7LA Tel: 01323 732631 — MB BS Lond. 1943 (Lond. Hosp.) MRCS Eng. LRCP Lond. 1943; FRCS Eng. 1949. Prev: Hon. Lect. Univ. Sheff.

REID, Douglas Simpson Regional Cardiothoracic Centre, Freeman Hospital, Freeman Road High Heaton, Newcastle upon Tyne NE7 7DN Tel: 0191 284 3111 Fax: 0191 213 0174 Email: d.s.reid@ncl.ac.uk; 25 Moor Road S., Gosforth, Newcastle upon Tyne NE3 1NP Tel: 0191 284 7737 Fax: 0191 285 8824 — (Glas.) FRCP Lond. 1981, M 1968; FRCP Glas. 1980, M 1968. Cons. Cardiol. Regional Cardiothoracic Unit Freeman Hosp. Newc. Specialty: Cardiol. Socs: Fell.Europ. Soc. Cardiol.; Brit. Cardiac Soc.; Scott. Cardiac Soc. Prev: Sen. Regist. (Cardiol.) Newc. Gen. Hosp.; Brit. Amer. Research Fell.; Regist. (Med.) Roy. Postgrad. Med. Sch. Hammersmith Hosp.

REID, Duncan Andrew Colinton Surgery, 296B Colinton Road, Edinburgh EH13 0LB Tel: 0131 441 4555 Fax: 0131 441 3963; 296B Colinton Road, Edinburgh EH13 0LB Tel: 0131 441 4555 — MB ChB Ed. 1987; BSc Hons. (Path.) Ed. 1985, MB ChB 1987; MRCGP 1991. Trainee GP Gtr. Glas. VTS.

REID, Elspeth Kathleen 2 Bogton Avenue, Glasgow G44 3JJ — MB ChB Glas. 1988; DA (UK) 1992. SHO (Anaesth.) Roy. United Hosp. Bath. Prev: SHO (A & E) Falkirk Roy. Infirm.; SHO (Anaesth.) Basildon Hosp. Essex; Ho. Off. (Med.) Edin. Roy. Infirm.

REID, Evan Arthur Leslie Department of Medical Genetics, Addenbrooke's NHS Trust, Addenbrooke's Hospital, Hills Road, Cambridge CB2 2QQ — MB ChB Glas. 1991; BSc (Hons.) Glas. 1988; MB ChB (Hons.) Glas. 1991; MRCP (UK) 1994. Lect. & Hon. Cons. Specialty: Genetics. Socs: Soc. Brit. Human Genetics. Prev: Wellcome Research Train. Fell. & Hon. Sen. Regist. Camb. Univ. & Addenbrooke's NHS Trust Camb.; Clin. Lect. (Med. Genetics); Career Regist. (Med. Genetics) Yorkhill NHS Trust Glas.

REID, Fergus Macdonald Hayfield, Rockcliffe, Carlisle CA6 4AA — MB ChB Glas. 1997.

REID, Fiona Margaret 68 Craigleith View, Edinburgh EH4 3JY — MB ChB Aberd. 1993.

REID, Fiona Mary Kantara, Chapel Lane, Elsham, Brigg DN20 0RN — MB ChB Manch. 1992.

REID, Frances Crowmere House, Broad Oak Crescent, Bayston Hill, Shrewsbury SY3 0NE Tel: 01743 873284 Fax: 01743 873284 Email: frankiereid@doctors.org.uk — MB ChB Birm. 1977. Clin. Asst. (Anaesth.) Roy. Shrewsbury Hosp.; Private Acupunc. Specialty: Anaesth. Socs: Accred. Mem. Brit. Med. Acupunc. Soc.

REID, Gael Susan 66 Bonhard Road, Scone, Perth PH2 6QB — MB ChB Dundee 1978.

REID, Gavin Desmond 11 Scrabo Road, Newtownards BT23 4NW — MB ChB Dund. 1998; MB ChB Dund 1998.

REID, Geoffrey Ewing, Group Capt. RAF Med. Br. Department of Community Mental Health, RAF Brize Norton, Carterton OX18 3LX Tel: 01993 897999 Fax: 01993 897555 Email: geoffreid@beeb.net — MB ChB Manch. 1974; MRCPsych 1981; T(Psych) 1991; DAvMed FOM RCP Lond. 1993; FRCPsych 1998. Cons. Adviser (Psychiat.) RAF. Specialty: Gen. Psychiat.; Aviat. Med. Special Interest: Occupational & Aviat. psychiatric issues. Socs: Fell. Roy. Soc. Med.; BMA. Prev: Head of Dept. RAF Psychiat. Centre Wroughton, Swindon; Cons. Psychiat. RAF Germany; Cons. Psychiat. (Community Psychiat.) RAF Nocton Hall.

REID, Mr Gordon Findlay Montague Medical Centre, Fifth Avenue, Goole DN14 6JD Tel: 01405 767600 Fax: 01405 726126 — MB ChB Aberd. 1968; FRCS Ed. 1972. GP Goole.

REID, Hamish Andrew Harman Penicuik Health Centre, 37 Imrie Place, Penicuik EH26 8LF Tel: 01968 672612 Fax: 01968 671543 — MB ChB Dundee 1985; DRCOG 1988; DO RCS Eng. 1990; MCOphth 1990; MRCGP 1992.

REID, Hamish La Mont BUPA Wellness, 2-6 Austin Friars, London EC2N 2HD — MB BS Lond. 1981 (Westm.) MRCGP Westm. 1988. Prev: Resid. Amer. Hosp., Paris; SHO (Gyn.) Westm. Med. Sch. Profess. Unit; Ho. Surg. Westm. Hosp. Surg. Unit.

REID, Helen Susanna 43 East End Lane, Ditchling, Hassocks BN6 8UP — MB BS Lond. 1991 (Roy. Free) MB BS (Distinc.) Pharmacol. Lond. 1991; MRCP (UK) 1994; FRCR 1997. Regist. (Radiol.) John Radcliife Hosp. Oxf. Specialty: Radiol.

REID, Hugh Aymer Stewart Department of Pathology, Enfield District Hospital, Chace Wing, The Ridgeway, Enfield EN2 8JL — MB BS Lond. 1965 (St. Mary's) DObst RCOG 1967; FRCPath 1986. Cons. Histopath. Enfield Dist. Hosp. (Chace Wing). Specialty: Histopath. Socs: Assn. Clin. Path.; Internat. Acad. Path. (Brit. Div.). Prev: Sen. Regist. (Histopath.) St. Mary's Hosp. Lond.; Lect. Bland Sutton Inst. Path. Middlx. Hosp. Lond.

REID, Hugh Conn Dunure, 553 Upper Wortley Road, Thorpe Hesley, Rotherham S61 2SZ Tel: 0114 246 7952 — MB ChB Glas. 1955; MRCGP 1965; MFHom 1984.

REID, Mr Hugh Conn (retired) 2 Machrie Drive, Newton Mearns, Glasgow G77 6LB — MB ChB Glas. 1944; FRCS Ed. 1950. Cons. Surg. Vict. Infirm. Glas. Prev: Ho. Surg. Vict. Infirm. Glas.

REID, Iain Andrew Greystones, Quarry Cottages, Off Foel Road, Dyserth, Rhyl LL18 6AR Tel: 01745 571960 Email: ian.reid@xenocide.freeserve.co.uk — MB ChB Ed. 1993. GP Regist. Specialty: Gen. Pract.

REID, Ian Cameron Templeton Farm, Newtyle, Blairgowrie PH12 8SQ — MB ChB Aberd. 1983; BMedBiol 1983. Lect. Dept. Ment. Health Aberd. Univ. Prev: Regist. Psychiat. Ross Clin. Aberd.

REID, Ian Leslie Northcote Surgery, 2 Victoria Circus, Glasgow G12 9LD Tel: 0141 339 3211 Fax: 0141 357 4480 — MB ChB Glas. 1971.

REID, Ian Nicol Department of Histopathology, York Hospital, Wiggington Road, York YO31 8HE Tel: 01904 453039 Fax: 01904 635823 Email: ian.n.reid@york.nhs.uk; Carlton Farm, Nun Monkton, York YO26 8EJ Tel: 01423 331014 — MB ChB Aberd. 1973; FRCPath 1992, M 1980. Cons. Histopath. York Dist. Hosp. Specialty: Histopath. Prev: Cons. Histopath. York & Northallerton HAs; Lect. (Forens. Med.) Path. Leeds; Lect. (Path.) Univ. Aberd.

REID, Iona Margaret Victoria Infirmary, Langside Road, Glasgow G42 9TT Tel: 0141 201 5454 Fax: 0141 201 5117 — MB BCh BAO Dub. 1985; FRCSI 1989; MD Dub. 1994. Sen. Lect./Hon. Cons. Surg. Univ. of Glas. & Vict. Infirm. Glas. Specialty: Gen. Surg. Prev: Lect. & Sen. Regist. (Gen. Surg.) N. Gen. Hosp. Sheff.

REID, Irvine Raeburn Durie (retired) 20 Bath Road, Felixstowe IP11 7JW Tel: 01394 284595 — MB BChir Camb. 1953 (Guy's)

REID, Isabel Anne Claire Skegoneill Health Centre, 195 Skegoneill Avenue, Belfast BT15 3LL Tel: 028 9077 2471 Fax: 028 9077 2449; 28 Church Avenue, Jordanstown, Newtownabbey BT37 0PJ — MB BCh BAO Belf. 1961.

REID, Jacqueline Anne Neonatal Unit, Aberdeen Maternity Hospital, Cornhill Road, Aberdeen AB25 2ZL Tel: 01224 552660 Fax: 01224 554604; 142 Osborne Place, Aberdeen AB25 2DU — MB ChB Aberd. 1973. Assoc. Specialist (Med. Paediat.) Aberd. Matern. Hosp. Specialty: Neonat.

REID, Jacqueline Anneta 56 Peveril Road, Beeston, Nottingham NG9 2HU — MB ChB Leeds 1992.

REID, James 4 Somerby Drive, Solihull B91 3YY — BM BCh Oxf. 1989; BA (Hons.) Camb. 1986; MRCP (UK) 1993; FRCP Lond. 2004. Cons., Med. & Geriat. Med., Leicester Roy. Infirm. Specialty: Care of the Elderly. Socs: Brit. Geriat. Soc.; W Midl. Inst. for Age & Ageing. Prev: Sen. Regist. (Geriat. Med.) Walsall Manor Hosp.

REID, James Edmund (retired) 4 Cranmore Park, Belfast BT9 6JG Tel: 028 9066 6238 — MB BCh BAO Belf. 1946; DA RCPSI 1949; DA Eng. 1952. Prev: Cons. Anaesth. Belf. Gp. Hosps. & Craigavon/Banbridge Unit.

REID, James Paterson (retired) Belair, St Mary Street, Kirkcudbright DG6 4AH Tel: 01557331243 — MB ChB Glas. 1950.

REID, Jane Helen Whitefriars Surgery, Whitefriars Street, Perth PH1 1PP Tel: 01738 625842 Fax: 01738 445030 — MB ChB Aberd. 1980; DRCOG 1983; DCH RCPS Glas. 1985; MRCGP 1986. p/t Gen. Practitioner Partner. Prev: Clin. Med. Off. Tayside Health Bd.

REID, Jean Perry Smellie 19 Humbie Lawns, Newton Mearns, Glasgow G77 5EA — MB ChB Glas. 1978; MRCPsych 1990. Cons. Psychiat. Gartnavel Roy. Hosp. Glas. Specialty: Gen. Psychiat.

REID, Jennifer Anne 15 Park Avenue, Crossgates, Leeds LS15 8EN — MB BS Newc. 1994.

REID, Jennifer Susan — MB ChB Birm. 1998.

REID, Jeremy Michael Southampton University Hospitals NHS Trust, Shackleton Department of Anaesthetics, Southampton General Hospital, Tremona Road, Southampton SO16 6YD Tel: 023 8077 7222; 10 Five Elms Drive, Romsey SO51 5RN Tel: 01794 522879 Email: jeremymreid@hotmail.com — BM Soton. 1992; MRCP (UK) 1995; FRCA 2001; MPhil (Med. Law) Glas. 2004. SpR in Anaesthetics, Wessex Rotation. Specialty: Anaesth.; Intens. Care. Prev: SHO (Anaesth.) Soton. Univ. Hosp. Trust; Regist. (Cardiol.) Jersey Gen. Hosp.; Regist. (Cardiol.) W. Dorset Gen. Hosps. NHS Trust.

REID, Joan Elizabeth Musgrave Park Hospital, Stockman's lane, Belfast BT9 7JB — MB BCh BAO Belf. 1992 (Queen's University, Belfast) FFARCSI 1998. p/t Cons. in Anaesth. and Pain Managem. Musgrave Pk. Hosp., Belf. Specialty: Anaesth. Special Interest: Chronic Pain. Socs: Assn. Anaesth.; Brit. Med. Assn.; The Pain Soc. Prev: Specialist Registrar in Royal Group of Hospitals Trust; Cons. in Anaesth. Craigavon Area Hosp., Craigavon.

REID, Joan Maud Magill (retired) 25 Craigarogan Road, Mallusk, Newtownabbey BT36 4RA — MB BCh BAO Belf. 1957.

REID, John Forth Valley Acute Hospitals NHS Trust, Westburn Ave, Falkirk FK1 5ST Tel: 01324 678506 Fax: 01324 678523 Email: john.reid@fvah.scot.nhs.uk; 7 Clarendon Place, Stirling FK8 2QW Email: drjohnreid@aol.com — MB ChB Ed. 1973; BSc (Hons.) Ed. 1970, MB ChB 1973; DObst RCOG 1976; MRCP (UK) 1977; FRCP Ed. 1989. Med. Dir., Forth Valley Acute Hosp.s NHS Trust. Specialty: Care of the Elderly. Prev: Sen. Regist. Vict. Geriat. Unit Glas.; Lect. (Therap. & Clin. Phamacol.) Univ. Edin.; Cons. Phys. (Geriat. Med.) Stirling Roy. Infirm.

REID, John Bon Air Consulting Rooms, St Saviour, Jersey JE2 7LJ Tel: 01534 66127 Fax: 01534 864869; Hunters Moon, Route de la Trinite, Trinity, Jersey JE3 5JP Tel: 01534 863004 — MB ChB Aberd. 1959; MD Aberd. 1967. Cons. Dermat. Bon Air Nursing Home Jersey. Specialty: Dermat. Socs: Fell. Roy. Soc. Med. (Mem. Sect. Dermat.); Fell. Internat. Soc. Dermat. Surg. Prev: Squibb Research Fell. (Dermat.) & Hon. Regist. Manch. & Salford Hosps. Skin Dis.; Regist. (Dermat.) Leeds Regional Hosp. Bd. (Bradford Roy. & St. Lukes Hosp.).

REID, John David Posterngate Surgery, Portholme Road, Selby YO8 4QH Tel: 01757 700561 Fax: 01757 213295; Briarfields, Lordship Lane, Wistow, Selby YO8 3XE Tel: 01757 268473 Email: jreid@posterngate.co.uk — MB ChB Ed. 1979 (Edin.) DRCOG 1981. Specialty: Gen. Pract.

REID, John Henderson Radiology Department, Borders General Hospital, Melrose TD6 9BS Fax: 01896 826438 — MB ChB Glas. 1979; DMRD Ed. 1983; FRCR 1984. Cons. Borders Gen. Hosp.; Asst. Med. Director, Borders Gen.Hosp. Specialty: Radiol. Socs: Roy. Coll. Radiol.; Brit. Inst. Radiol. Prev: Cons. (Radiodiagnostics) Edin. Roy. Infirm.; Sen. Regist. (Radiodiagnosics) Edin. Roy. Infirm.

REID, John Jeffrey Kiveton Park Primary Care Centre, Chapel Way, Kiveton Park, Sheffield S26 6QU Tel: 01909 770213 Fax: 01909 510108 — MB ChB Sheff. 1984; DRCOG 1989. Prev: Trainee GP Bassetlaw VTS; SHO (Dermat.) Grimsby Dist. Gen. Hosp.; SHO (Rheum. & Rehabil.) Norwich HA.

REID, John Low University Division of Cardiovascular and Medical Sciences, Gardiner Institute, Western Infirmary, Glasgow G11 6NT Tel: 0141 211 2886 Fax: 0141 339 2800 — BM BCh Oxf. 1967; MRCP (UK) 1970; BA Oxf. 1964, DM 1975; FRCP Glas. 1979; FRCP Lond. 1986; FRSE 1995; FRCP Irel. 1997; F.Med.Sci. 1998. Regius Prof. Med. & Therap. Univ. Glas.; Cons. Phys. West. Infirm. Glas. Specialty: Pharmacology. Socs: Fell. Roy Soc. Edin.; Med. Res. Soc.; Brit. Pharm. Soc. Prev: Regius. Prof. Mat. Med. Univ. Glas.; Reader (Clin. Pharmacol.) & Cons. Phys. Roy. Postgrad. Med. Sch. Hammersmith Hosp. Lond.

REID, John Matheson (retired) 44 Eaglesham Road, Clarkston, Glasgow G76 7TW Tel: 0141 644 1069 — MB ChB Glas. 1949; FRCP Ed. 1969, M 1954; MD (High Commend.) Glas. 1957. Prev: Cons. Phys. (Cardiol.) West. Infirm. Glas. & Roy. Hosp. Sick Childr. Glas.

REID, John Priestley NHS Grampian, Westholme, Queen's Road, Aberdeen AB15 6LS Tel: 01224 556563 Ext: 56563 Fax: 01224 556862 Ext: 56862 Email: john.reid@gpct.grampian.scot.nhs.uk — MB ChB Aberd. 1971; BA (OU) 1997; FRCGP 2003. Med. Prescribing Adviser Grampian Primary Care Trust. Specialty: Pharmaceutical Medicine. Prev: Region. Med. Off. Scott. Home & Health Dept., Glas.; Clin. Lect. (Gen. Pract.) Aberd.; GP Aberd.

REID, John Smith Hall Alford Medical Practice, 2 Gordon Road, Alford AB33 8AL Tel: 019755 62253 Fax: 019755 62613; West Lodge, Montgarrie Road, Alford AB33 8AE Tel: 019755 62978 — MB ChB Aberd. 1976; DRCOG 1980; MRCGP 1981. Teach. Fell. (Gen. Pract.) Univ. Aberd.

REID, Joseph McKinstry George Street Surgery, 99 George Street, Dumfries DG1 1DS Tel: 01387 253333 Fax: 01387 253301; 9 Robertson Avenue, Dumfries DG1 4EY Tel: 01387 264463 — MB ChB Glas. 1979; DRCOG 1981; MRCGP 1983; DGM RCP Lond. 1986.

REID, Joyce Allison 6 Hamilton Avenue, Glasgow G41 4JF — MB ChB Glas. 1978; DRCOG 1980; FFA RCS Eng. 1983. Sen. Regist. (Anaesth.) West. Infirm. Glas. Specialty: Anaesth. Socs: BMA & W. Scotl. Soc. Anaesth. Prev: Regist. (Anaesth.) Vict. Infirm. Glas.; Research Regist. (Anaesth.) Univ. Dept. Glas. Roy. Infirm.

REID, Judith Eileen Infertility Clinic, Farnborough Hospital, Farnborough Common, Farnborough BR6 8ND Tel: 01689 814157; 2 April Close, Green Street Green, Orpington BR6 6NA Tel: 01689 857027 — MB ChB Manch. 1981. Clin. Asst. (O & G) Orpington & Beckenham Hosp. Specialty: Obst. & Gyn. Prev: Regist. (O & G) FarnBoro. Hosp. & Whittington Hosp.

REID, Julie Ann 143 Old Ballymoney Road, Ballymena BT43 6SL Tel: 028 2541 3601 — MB BCh BAO Belf. 1997 (Queen's University, Belfast) Specialty: Gen. Surg.

REID, Karen Wright The Coach House, Sandy Lane, Guildford GU3 1HF Tel: 01483 569125 — MB BChir Camb. 1985 (Addenbrooke's Clin. Med. Sch.) MA Camb. 1986; DRCOG 1986; MRCGP 1991. Prev: GP Groombridge; SHO (ENT) Kent & Sussex Hosp. Tunbridge Wells; Trainee GP E. Grinstead.

REID, Kathleen Annie — MB ChB Glas. 1977.

REID, Kathleen May (retired) 17 Gallery Lane, Holymoorside, Chesterfield S42 7ER — MRCS Eng. LRCP Lond. 1954 (St. Bart.) Prev: Sen. Med. Off. (Family Plann.) N. Derbysh. HA.

REID, Keith 5 Blandfield Road, London SW12 8BQ — MB ChB Manch. 1990. Research Med. Off. (Applied Physiol.) Centre for Human Sci.s Dera FarnBoro. Specialty: Anat.

REID, Kingsley, SBStJ Sunfield Medical Centre, Sunfield Place, Stanningley, Leeds Tel: 0113 257 0361 Fax: 0113 236 3261; Windrush, Apperley Lane, Rawdon, Leeds LS19 7DX — MB ChB Ed. 1964; DObst RCOG 1966; MRCGP 1978. Clin. Asst. (Dermat.) Bradford Roy. Infirm.; Area Surg. St John Ambul. Specialty: Dermat. Prev: SHO (Anaesth.) St. Luke's Hosp. Bradford; Ho. Surg. Bangour Gen. Hosp. W. Lothian; Ho. Phys. W. Gen. Hosp. Edin.

REID, Kirsty Jane Dunadd, Tulloch Avenue, Dingwall IV15 9TU — MB ChB Glas. 1993.

REID, Malcolm Fraser University Hospital, Nottingham NG7 2UH — BM BS Nottm. 1980; FFA RCS Lond. 1985. Cons. Notts. HA. Specialty: Anaesth.

REID, Margaret 15 Sturdee Gardens, Jesmond, Newcastle upon Tyne NE2 3QU — MB BS Lond. 1984. Specialty: Gen. Pract.; Homeop. Med. Socs: MFHom.

REID, Margaret Jarvie Gray (retired) Craigelvan, Elmira Road, Muirhead, Chryston, Glasgow G69 9EJ Tel: 0141 779 2366 — (Glas.) LRCP LRCS Ed. LRFPS Glas. 1949. Prev: Ho. Surg. Glas. Roy. Infirm.

REID, Margaret Mary Gateacre Brow Surgery, 1 Gateacre Brow, Liverpool L25 3PA Tel: 0151 428 1851 — MB ChB Liverp. 1978; DCH Eng. 1981; MRCGP 1986.

REID, Marguerite Marion Wilson (retired) 108 Southbrae Drive, Glasgow G13 1TZ Tel: 0141 959 3083 — (Glas.) MB ChB Glas. 1963; DA Eng. 1966. Prev: Assoc. Specialist (Cytol.) Vale of Leven Hosp. Alexandria, Dunbaronsh..

REID, Marion Bernadette Department of Cellular Pathology, Stoke Mandeville Hospital, Aylesbury HP21 8AL Tel: 01296 315340; 22 Arnold Way, Thame OX9 2QA — MB ChB Manch. 1978 (St. And. & Manch.) MRCPath 1986. Cons. (Cell. Path.) Stoke Mandeville Aylesbury Hosp. Specialty: Histopath. Prev: Sen. Regist. (Histopath.) Oxf. RHA; Regist. (Histopath.) Bradford HA; SHO (Histopath.) Withenshawe Manch.

REID, Mark Andrew 56 Upper Malone Gardens, Belfast BT9 6LY Tel: 01232 612986 — MB BCh BAO Belf. 1988; MRCP (UK) 1992; FRCA 1995.

REID, Mark McClean Royal Belfast Hospital For Sick Children, Falls Road, Belfast BT12; 10 Kensington Gardens, Hillsborough BT26 6HP — MB BCh BAO Belf. 1962 (Queen's Belf.) DCH RCPS Glas. 1965; FRCP Glas. 1978, M 1967; FRCPI 1991, M 1990; FRCP Ed. 1994. Cons. Neonat. Roy. Matern. Hosp. Sick Childr. & City Hosps. Belf.; Chairm. of Staff Roy. Matern. Hosp. Belf. & Roy. Belf. Hosp. Sick Childr. Specialty: Paediat. Socs: BMA; (Ex-Pres.) Irish Perinatal Soc.; (Counc.) RCP. Prev: Cons. Paediat. Craigavon Hosp., S. Tyrone Hosp. & Roy. Belf. Hosp. Sick Childr.; Resid. Fell. Toronto Hosp. Sick Childr., Canada; Regist. Roy. Belf. Hosp. Sick Childr.

REID, Maureen 23 South Street, St Andrews KY16 9QS — MB ChB Ed. 1977 (Edinburgh) MRCGP 1982; MRCPsych 1983. GP Retainer Scheme. Prev: GP E. Lothian.; Regist. (Psychiat.) Rosslynee Hosp. Midlothian.

REID, Maurice 45 Parsons Walk, Wigan WN1 1RU — MB ChB Manch. 1974. Specialty: Sports Med.

REID, Michael Macdonald Department Haematology, Royal Victoria Infirmary, Newcastle upon Tyne NE1 4LP Tel: 0191 232 5131; 33 St. George's Terrace, Jesmond, Newcastle upon Tyne NE2 2SU — MB BS Lond. 1971 (St. Thos.) DCH RCPS Glas. 1973; FRCP Lond. 1990, M (UK) 1977; BSc (Physiol.) Lond. 1968, MD 1981; FRCPath 1996, M 1983; FRCPCH 1997, M 1996. Cons. Haemat. Roy. Vict. Infirm. Newc.; Hon. Sen. Lect. (Med. & Child Health) Univ. Newc. Specialty: Haematology. Socs: Brit. Soc. Haematol.; Brit. Paediat. Assn.; Assn. Clin. Path. Prev: Sen. Regist. (Haemat.) Roy. Vict. Infirm. Newc.; Research Fell. (Paediat. Oncol.) Sidney Farber Cancer Inst. Boston, USA; Research Assoc. (Child Health) Univ. Newc.

REID, Morag Marsaili MacColl 282 Ferry Road, Edinburgh EH5 3NP — MB ChB Bristol 1998; BSc 1995; MRCP 2001; DRCOG 2002; MRCGP 2003.

REID, Moyra Janette 22 Brines Orchard, Templecombe BA8 0JL — BM BCh Oxf. 1997.

REID, Nicholas Cunningham Green Lane Hospital, Devizes SN10 5DS Tel: 01380 731200 Fax: 01380 731308 — MB ChB Manch. 1978; BSc St. And. 1975; MRCPsych 1986; MPhil Ed. 1988. Cons. Psychiat. Avon & Wilts. Ment. Health Partnership Trust. Specialty: Gen. Psychiat. Prev: Sen. Regist. Roy. S. Hants. Hosp. Soton.; Regist. (Psychiat.) Roy. Edin. Hosp.; Area Med. Off. Kandrian W. New Brit. Papua New Guinea.

REID, Nigel Charles Ronald Wyman (retired) Reid, Broadlands Harbour, Stubb Lane, Broad Oak, Brede, Rye TN31 6BS Tel: 01424 882427 — MD Camb. 1969 (St. Thos.) MA, MB BChir 1956; FRCP Lond. 1976, M 1962. Prev: Cons. Phys. (Gastroenterol.) Hastings HA.

REID, Nigel George Bruce Horse Fair Surgery, 12 Horse Fair, Banbury OX16 0AJ Tel: 01295 259484 Fax: 01295 279293 — MB BChir Camb. 1974; MA Camb. 1974; MRCGP 1980. Specialty: Gen. Pract. Prev: Hon. Med. Advis. Yarmouth Life Boat; RMO 1 Chesh.

REID, Patrick Julian 2 Harlands Grove, Orpington BR6 7WB — MB BS Lond. 1998; MB BS Lond 1998.

REID, Paul John 6 Lamb Terrace, Arbroath DD11 4HD — MB ChB Aberd. 1996.

REID, Paul Vincent 284 Lees Road, Oldham OL4 1PA — MB ChB Manch. 1979; MRCGP 1983. Socs: Brit. Med. Acupunct. Soc.

REID, Paula Elizabeth 2/64 Edenderry Village, Belfast BT8 8LQ Tel: 01232 645523 — MB BCh BAO Belf. 1992 (Queens Univ. Belfast) Regis., Phys. Asst., Dermat. Specialty: Dermat. Prev: Lats Dermat.; SHO Dermat.

REID, Peter Cameron 1 Hawsley Road, Harpenden AL5 2BL Tel: 01582 763261 — BSc (Hons. Anat.) Manch. 1976; MB ChB Manch. 1979; MRCOG 1985; MD Manch. 1989; FRCOG 1998. Cons. Obst. Luton & Dunstable NHS Trust Hosp. Specialty: Obst. & Gyn. Prev: Sen. Regist. North. Gen. Hosp. Sheff.; Research Regist. North. Gen. Hosp. Sheff.; Regist. Watford Gen. Hosp.

REID, Peter Geddes Countess of Chester Hospital, Liverpool Road, Chester CH2 1UL Tel: 01244 366305 Fax: 01244 366455; 48 Cinder Lane, Guilden Sutton, Chester CH3 7EN — MD Ed. 1991; MB ChB 1979; MRCP (UK) 1982; FRCP UK 1997. Cons. Phys. Cardiol. Countess of Chester Hosp. NHS Trust.; Vis. Cardiol. Cardiothoracic Centre Liverp. Specialty: Cardiol.; Gen. Med. Prev: Sen. Research Regist. (Cardiol.) Roy. Vict. Infirm. Newc.; Regist. (Cardiol.) Freeman Hosp. Newc. u. Tyne; Clin. Research Off. & Hon. Regist. S. Glam HA.

REID, Peter Trevor 3 Kinedar Crescent, Belmont, Belfast BT4 3LY — MB BCh BAO Belf. 1988.

REID, Philip John The Surgery, 45A Pembridge Villas, London W11 3EP Tel: 020 7727 2222 Fax: 020 7792 2867 — MB BS Lond. 1989 (Oxford and St Mary's London) BA Oxf. 1986; MRCP (UK) 1992; DRCOG 1993; MRCGP 1995. Sec. to Trustees & Vice-Princip. Wytham Hall. Specialty: Gen. Pract. Prev: Trainee GP Lond. VTS; SHO (O & G) Hillingdon Hosp. Uxbridge; SHO Rotat. (Gen. Med.) St. Mary's Hosp. Lond.

REID, Miss Priscilla Margaret A&E Department, The Lister Hospital, Stevenage SG1 4AB Tel: 01223 217118/01438 314333 Ext: 5162 — MB BCh Wales 1976; FRCS Eng. 1982; FFAEM 1996; MA MA (ed) 2001. Cons. A & E The Lister Hosp. Specialty: Accid. & Emerg. Socs: BAEM; FRCS; Fell. FAEM. Prev: Regist. (A & E & Neurosurg.) Addenbrooke's Hosp. Camb.; Sen. Regist. (A & E) Addenbrooke's Hosp. Camb.

REID, Rachel Elizabeth Glen 144 Tile Cross Road, Tile Cross, Birmingham B33 0LU Tel: 0121 779 2711; 4 Scomerby Drive, Solihull B91 3YY — MB BChir Camb. 1990; MA Camb. 1991. GP Partner; Clin. Asst. (Psychiat.). Specialty: Gen. Pract.

REID, Richard David Bangor Health Centre, Newtownards Road, Bangor BT20 4LD Tel: 028 9146 9111; 148 Groomsport Road, Bangor BT20 5PE — MB BCh BAO Belf. 1985; DRCOG 1987; MRCGP 1989; DCH Dub. 1990. Specialty: Gen. Med.

REID, Richard Ian East Hampshire PCT, Department of Medicine for the Elderly, Queen Alexandra Hospital, Portsmouth PO6 3LY Tel: 023 92 286891 Fax: 023 92 200381 — MB ChB Glas. 1974; MRCP (UK) 1978; FRCP Glas. 1990; FRCP Lond. 1992. Cons. Phys. (Elderly Med.) Portsmouth Healthcare Trust; Med. Dir. East Hampshire PCT. Specialty: Care of the Elderly. Socs: Brit. Geriat. Soc. Prev: Sen. Regist. (Geriat. Med.) Portsmouth & SE Hants. & Soton. & SW Hants. Health Dists.; Regist. (Gen. Med.) Kilmarnock Infirm.; SHO (Med. Cardiol.) Glas. Roy. Infirm.

REID, Robert Alasdair World Health Organization, Stop TB Department, Avenue Appia 20, Geneva 27, Switzerland Tel: 00 41 22 791 4409 Fax: 00 41 22 791 4268 Email: reida@who.int — MB ChB Aberd. 1990; MRCP (UK) 1993; DTM & H Liverp. 1995; DFPHM 2001; MD Aberd. 2003. Sen. Clin. Research Off. Liverp. Sch. Trop. Med.; Med. Off. TB/HIV World Health Organisation. Specialty: Pub. Health Med. Prev: Med. Off. Hlabisa Hosp., S. Afr.; Regist. (Infec. Dis.) Fazakerley Hosp. Liverp.; SHO (Med.) Clwyd HA.

REID, Robert Pearson 19 Humbie Lawns, Newton Mearns, Glasgow G77 5EA — MB ChB Glas. 1978; BSc Glas. 1975, MB ChB 1978; MRCPath 1984.

REID, Rosemary Anne Cholderton House, Cholderton, Salisbury SP4 0DW — MB BS Lond. 1982; MRCOG 1989.

REID, Ross Paterson Glover Street Medical Centre, 133 Glover Street, Perth PH2 0JB Tel: 01738 639748 Fax: 01738 635133; 66 Bonhard Road, Scone, Perth PH2 6QB — MB ChB Dundee 1978; MRCGP 1984; FRCGP 2002.

REID, Russell Warwick Stedman 10 Warwick Road, London SW5 9UH Tel: 020 7373 0901 Fax: 020 7244 0900 — MB ChB Otago 1967; FRCPsych Lond. 1995. Cons. Psychiat. Hillingdon Hosp. PCT. Specialty: Gen. Psychiat. Special Interest: Gender Identity Disorders.

REID, Sara Elizabeth 41 Eglantine Park, Hillsborough BT26 6HL Tel: 01846 688140 Fax: 0802 364559 — MB BCh BAO Belf. 1993 (Queen's University Belfast) DCH 1997; DRCOG 1997; MRCGP (distinction) 1998; DFFP 1998. GP Locum. Socs: BMA; RCGP. Prev: GP Regist. HillsBoro. H.C. Co. Down; SHO (O & G); SHO (Paediat.).

REID, Sheilagh Vivienne 29 St. Thomas Road, Mount Merrion, Blackrock, County Dublin, Republic of Ireland; 2 Hayes Farm Court, Ticknall, Derby DE73 1JE Tel: 01332 864351 Email: mullreid@aol.com — MB BCh BAO Dub. 1992; MB BCh Dub. 1992; FRCS Lond. 1997. Research Regist. Hallamshire Hosp. Sheff. Specialty: Urol. Socs: BMA; Fell. Roy. coll. Surgs. Eng.

REID, Simon Alexander 37 Talbot Street, Cardiff CF11 9BW Tel: 029 2025 3586 — MB BS Newc. 1994; DTM & H Liverp. 1997; MRCP, Uk 1998; FRCA 2002. SpR Anaesth. Welsh Region. Specialty: Anaesth. Prev: Sen. H. Off. (Med.) Roy. Vict. Hosp. Blackpool, (Med); SHO Tamanaki Hosp. New Zealand. (Med); SHO (Anaesth.) Gwynedd Hosp. NHS Trust.

REID, Simon Charles Radbrook Green Surgery, Bank Farm Road, Shrewsbury SY3 6DU Tel: 01743 231816 Fax: 01743 344099 — MB ChB Birm. 1977 (Birmingham) MRCGP 1986. GP Princip.; Clin. Assist. - Procedural Dermatol., Roy. Shrewsbury Hosp., Shrewsbury.; Course Orginiser Shrops. VTS. Prev: Vis. Educat. Cons., Brit. Internat. Healthcare., Macedonia. 1999-2001.

REID, Simon Charles Thomas Waverly Medical Centre, Dalrymple St, Stranraer DG9 7HG Tel: 01776 706513; Larg House, Larg Road, Stranraer DG9 0JN Tel: 01776 3228 — MB BCh BAO Belf. 1985; DRCOG 1990; MRCGP 1991; LFHom RCP Lond. 1996. Prev: Trainee GP Girvan Ayrsh.; SHO (Gen. Med.) North. Health & Social Serv. Bd. GP VTS; SHO (Cas.) Belf. City Hosp.

REID, Steven Patrick John Holland House, 31 Church Road, Lytham, Lytham St Annes FY8 5LL Tel: 01253 794999 Fax: 01253 795744 — MB BCh BAO Dub. 1971 (T.C. Dub.) MA Dub. 1977, BA 1969; MB BCh BAO (Hons.) Dub. 1971; LM Rotunda 1972; FRCS Eng. 1977; MRCGP 1979. Clin. Asst. (Orthop. & Surg.) Lytham Hosp. Socs: Brit. Soc. Med. & Dent. Hypn. Prev: Tutor (Surg.) Univ. Manch.; Demonst. (Anat.) TC Dub.; Ho. Phys. & Ho. Surg. Dr. Steevens Hosp. Dub.

REID, Susan Rachel 98 Pilmuir Street, Dunfermline KY12 0ND — MB ChB Aberd. 1985.

REID, Suzanne 15 Beverley Gardens, London SW13 0LZ — MB BS Lond. 1990.

REID, Thomas Myles Sutherland Microbiology Department, Aberdeen Royal Infirmary, Aberdeen AB25 2ZN Tel: 01224 554954 Fax: 01224 550632 Email: thomas.reid@arh.grampian.scot.nhs.uk; 22 Gordondale Road, Aberdeen AB15 5LZ Tel: 01224 633665 — MB ChB Aberd. 1972; BMedBiol (Immunol.) 1969; FRCPath 1991, M 1979; MRCP Ed (UK) 1988; FRCP Ed. 1991. Head of Serv. & Cons. Microbiol. Grampian Univ. Hopitals NHS Trust; Hon. Sen. Lect. (Bact.) Univ. Aberd. Specialty: Med. Microbiol. Socs: (Hon. Sec.) Aberd. M-C Soc. 1988-2002; Pres. Aberd. M-C Soc. 2002-2003. Prev: Lect. (Bact.) Aberd. Univ.

REID, Veronica Theresa Monklands Hospital, Anaesthetic Department, Monkscourt Avenue, Airdrie ML6 0JS Tel: 01236 748748 — MB ChB Glasg. 1970 (Glasgow) FRCA 1975. Cons. (Anaesth.) Monklands Dist. Gen. Hosp. Airdrie. Specialty: Anaesth. Socs: BMA & Assn. Anaesth.; Chairm., Scott. LNC Forum; Mem. Scott. Counc. BMA. Prev: Sen. Regist. (Anaesth.) Roy. Infirm. Glas.; Regist. (Anaesth.) Stobhill Gen. Hosp. Glas.

REID, Wendy Margaret Neely The Royal Free Hosptial, Department O & G, Pond Street, London NW3 2QG Tel: 0207 830 2563 Fax: 0207 830 2261 — MB BS Lond. 1981 (Univ. Lond. Roy. Free Hosp. Sch. Med.) FRCOG 1988 (Univ. Lond. Roy. Free Hosp. Sch Med.). Cons Gynaecologist Roy. Free Hosp. Lond.; Postgrad. Dean of Med. Lond. Deanery. Specialty: Gynaecology. Special Interest: Pelvic Floor Dysfunction; Vulval Dis. Prev: Cons. Obst. & Gynaecologist Roy. Free Lond. 1994-2000.

REID, William Hayfield, Rockcliffe, Carlisle CA6 4AA Tel: 01228 74552 — MB ChB Ed. 1968; FRCOG 1988, M 1975.

REID, William 20 Johnstone Drive, Rutherglen, Glasgow G73 2PT Tel: 0141 647 1786 — MD Glas. 1990; MB ChB 1980; MRCP (UK) 1983; FRCP Glas. 1994. Cons. Phys. Med. for Elderly South. Gen. Hosp. Glas. Specialty: Care of the Elderly. Prev: Sen. Regist. (Geriat. & Gen. Med.) South. Gen. Hosp. Glas.

REID, William Alexander Pathology Department, University of Edinburgh, Edinburgh EH8 2AG Email: sandy.reid@ed.ac.uk; 8 Strathfillan Road, Edinburgh EH9 2AG — MD Glas. 1988; MB ChB Glas. 1972; MRCPath. 1980; Dip. Med. Ed. 1992. Sen. Lect. & Hon. Cons. Path. Univ. of Edin. Specialty: Pathology, General; Histopath. Socs: Path. Soc.; Roy. Coll. Path. Prev: Lect. & Hon. Cons. Path. Univ. of Leeds; Lect. Univ. Glas.

REID, Mr William Henry (retired) 6 Sutherland Avenue, Glasgow G41 4JH Tel: 0141 427 1489 — MB ChB Glas. 1955; FRCS Ed. 1959; FRFPS Glas. 1960; FRCS Eng. 1960. Vis. Prof. Bio-Engin. Strathclyde Univ. 1985; Cons. Plastic Surg. W. Scotl. Regional Plastic Surg. Serv.; Canniesburn Auxil. Hosp. Glas. Prev: Gen. Surg. Regist. Glas. Roy. Infirm.

REID-BRAIN, Hannah Euphemia (retired) c/o Mrs. C.L.D'Cruz, 37 Sarum Avenue, Melksham SN12 6BN Tel: 01225 703595 — MB BS Punjab 1929 (Lady Hardinge Med. Coll.) Prev: Orthop. Surg. Lady Harding Hosp., New Delhi.

REID MILLIGAN, David Alexander Wilson Forest Hall Medical Centre, Station Road, Forest Hall, Newcastle upon Tyne NE12 9BQ Tel: 0191 266 5823; Ovingham House, Main Road, Ovingham, Prudhoe NE42 6AG — MB ChB Dundee 1977; MRCGP 1982.

REIDY, John Quayside Medical Practice, 82-84 Strand Road, Londonderry BT48 7NN Tel: 028 7126 2790 Fax: 028 7137 3729 — LRCPI & LM, LRSCI & LM 1977; LRCPI & LM, LRCSI & LM 1977.

REIDY, John Francis Department of Radiology, Guy's Hospital, London SE1 9RT Tel: 020 7188 5565 Fax: 020 7188 5523 Email: john.reidy@gstt.nhs.uk; 19 Cumberland Street, London SW1V 4LS — (St. Geo.) MB BS Lond. 1967; MRCS Eng. LRCP Lond. 1967; MRCP (UK) 1971; DMRD Eng. 1972; FFR 1974; FRCR 1975; FRCP Lond. 1987. Cons. Radiol. Guy's Hosp. Lond.; Hon. Sen. Lect. KCL; Hon. Cons. Radiol. Gt. Ormond St. Hosp. for Childr. Specialty: Radiol. Socs: Fell. Cardiovasc. & Interven. Soc. Europe; Fell. RSM. Prev: Lect. (Radiol. Teach. & Research) St. Geo. Hosp. Med. Sch. Lond.; Sen. Regist. (Radiol.) St. Geo. Hosp. Lond.; Vis. Asst. Prof. Bowman Gray Sch. Med. N. Carolina USA.

REIDY, Mr John Joseph Department of Surgery, Inverclyde Royal Hospital, Larkfield Road, Greenock PA16 0XN Tel: 01475 656245 Fax: 01475 656139 Email: john.reidy@irh.scot.nhs.uk — MB BCh BAO NUI 1981 (Univ. Coll. Cork) FRCSI 1986; MCh NUI 1992; FRCSI (Gen.) 1995; FRCS Glas. 2002. Cons. Surg. Argyll and Clyde Hosp. NHS Trust; Hon. Clin. Sen. Lect. Univ. of Glas. Specialty: Gen. Surg.; Surgery, Vascular. Socs: Fell. Assn. Surgs.; Vasc. Surgic. Soc. GB & Irel. Prev: Sen. Regist. (Surg.) & Career Regist. W. Scotl. Higher Surg. Train. Scheme; Regist. Clin. Shock Study Gp. West. Infirm. Glas.; Surg. Fell. Train. Rotat. Regional Hosp. Wilton Cork.

REIDY, Michael Basil Courtney (retired) Blounts, Vicarage Lane, Haslemere GU27 1LQ — (T.C. Dub.) BA Dub. 1953; MB BCh BAO 1955; MB BCH BAO Trinity College Dublin 1955. Clin. Asst. (Neurol.) Roy. Surrey Co. Hosp. Guildford; Res. Med. Off. Godwin Unit Haslemere Dist. Hosp. Prev: Med. Supt. Holy Cross Hosp. Haslemere.

REIDY, Michael Jason 14 Gallows Hill, Kings Langley WD4 8PQ — MB BS Lond. 1998; MB BS Lond 1998.

REIDY, Richard Nicholas Desborough Avenue Surgery, 65 Desborough Avenue, High Wycombe HP11 2SD Tel: 01494 526006 Fax: 01494 473569; Woodbine Cottage, 81 Totteridge Lane, High Wycombe HP13 7QA Tel: 01494 527597 — MB BS Lond. 1977.

REIDY-BRADY, Nora Maria Ros Erne House, 8 Darling St., Enniskillen BT74 7EP — MB BCh BAO NUI 1948.

REIFENBERG, Naomi Ann — MB ChB Bristol 1990. Prev: SHO (Anaesth.) ScarBoro. Hosp.

REIFF, Daniel Barnett Department of Radiology, Ashford Hospital, Ashford St Peters NHS Trust, London Road, Ashford TW15 3AA Tel: 01784 884552 Fax: 01784 884041; Stoneleigh, Acrefield Road, Gerrards Cross SL9 8NA Tel: 01753 884663 — MB ChB Cape Town 1980 (Univ. Cape Town, S. Afr.) MRCP (UK) 1985; FRCR 1992; T(R) (CR) 1993. Cons. Radiol. Asford. Ashford St. Peter's NHS Trust. Specialty: Radiol. Socs: Amer. Roentgen Ray Soc.; RCR; BMA. Prev: Sen. Regist. & Regist. (Radiol.) St. Geo. Hosp. Lond.; Regist. (Med.) Hammersmith Hosp. Lond.

REILLY, Bernard Martin Aloysius Whitefriars Surgery, Whitefriars Street, Perth PH1 1PP Tel: 01738 625842 Fax: 01738 445030; 3 Tullylumb Terrace, Perth PH1 1BA Tel: 01738 643337 — MB ChB Aberd. 1986; MRCGP 1990. Prev: GP Aberd.; Trainee GP/SHO Aberd. Hosps. VTS.

REILLY, Professor Charles Stewart Department of Surgical & Anaesthetic Sciences, University of Sheffield, Royal Hallamshire Hospital, Glossop Road, Sheffield S10 2JF Tel: 0114 271 2510 Fax: 0114 271 3771 Email: c.s.reilly@sheffield.ac.uk; 242 Millhouses Lane, Sheffield S11 9JA — MB ChB Glas. 1977; FRCA 1982; MD Glas. 1989. Prof. of Anaesth. & Head of Div. of Surg. & Anaesth. Sci. Univ. Sheff.; Hon. Cons. Anaesth. Roy. Hallamsh. Hosp. Specialty: Anaesth. Prev: Sen. Lect. & Head Dept. Anaesth. Univ. Sheff.

REILLY, David Glasgow Homoeopathic Hospital, 1053 Great Western Road, Glasgow G12 0XQ Tel: 0141 211 1621 Fax: 0141 211 1631 — MB ChB Glas. 1978; MRCP Glas. 1981; MRCGP 1982; FFHom; RCP (UK) 1990, M 1983; FRCP Glas. 1993. Cons. Phys. & Dir. Acad. Depts. Glas. Homoeop. Hosp.; Hon. Sen. Lect. (Clin. Med.) Glas. Univ. Dept. Med. Specialty: Gen. Med.; Homeop. Med. Socs: Brit. Soc. Med. & Dent. Hypn.; Brit. Med. Acupunct. Soc.; Fell.- Fac. of Homeopathy. Prev: RCCM/MRC Fellowship Complementary Med. Dept. Med. Univ. Glas.; Sen. Regist. (Med.) Glas. Roy. Infirm.

REILLY, Mr David Tempest Wirral Hospital, Arrowe Park, Arrowe Park Road, Upton, Wirral CH49 5PE Tel: 0151 604 7054 Fax: 0151 604 1760; 2 Upholland, New Hey Lane, Willaston, South Wirral CH64 2UU Tel: 0151 327 4668 — MB BChir Camb. 1972 (St. Mary's Hosp. Lond.) MRCS Eng. LRCP Lond. 1971; FRCS Eng. 1977; MD Leics. 1982. Cons. Surg. Wirral Hosp. Merseyside. Specialty: Gen. Surg. Socs: Eur. Soc. Vasc. Surg.; Vasc. Surg. Soc. GB & Irel.; Assn. Surg. Prev: Cons. Surg. Watford Gen. Hosp.; Sen. Regist. (Surg.) St. Mary's Hosp. Lond.; Research Fell. (Transpl. Surg.) Univ. Leicester.

REILLY, Desmond James (retired) 1 Castleton Drive, Newton Mearns, Glasgow G77 5JU Tel: 0141 639 8286 — MB ChB Glas. 1951; DPH 1960; DIH St. And. 1966; MFCM 1974; FFPHM 1990.

REILLY, Edwin Peter Young Peoples Centre, Mount Gould Hospital, Plymouth PL4 7QD — MB BS Lond. 1976; DRCOG 1978. Staff Grade Psychiat., Young People's Centre, Mt. Gould Hosp. Specialty: Child & Adolesc. Psychiat. Prev: Princip. in Gen. Pract., Plymouth.

REILLY, Elizabeth Irene 2 Upholland, New Hey Lane, Willaston, South Wirral CH64 2UU Tel: 0151 327 4668 — MB BS Lond. 1971; DCH Eng. 1973.

REILLY, Graham David St Sampson's Medical Centre, Grandes Maisons Road, St. Sampson, Guernsey GY2 4JS; Cambrai, Le Bigard, Forest, Guernsey GY8 0HU — MB BChir Camb. 1978; MA 1978, MB BChir Camb. 1978; MRCP (UK) 1981; DRCOG 1985. Prev: Regist. (Dermat.) Roy. Hallamsh. Hosp. Sheff.

REILLY, John Tennison 79 Devonshire Road, Dore, Sheffield S17 3NU Tel: 0114 236 6043 — MD Liverp. 1986; BSc Biochem. Liverp. 1973, MB ChB 1976; MRCP (UK) 1980; MRCPath 1987; FRCP (UK) 1996; FRCPath 1997. Cons. Haemat. Roy. Hallamshire Hosp. Specialty: Haematology. Socs: BMA. Prev: Sen. Regist. (Haemat.) Roy. Liverp. Hosp.; Research Fell. (Haemat.) Roy. Liverp. Hosp.; Regist. (Haemat.) Roy. Liverp. Hosp.

REILLY, Joseph Gerard Parkside Community Mental Health Centre, Park Road N., Middlesbrough TS1 3LF Tel: 01642 230542 Fax: 01642 230542 — BM BS Nottm. 1989; BMedSci Nottm. 1987; MRCPsych 1994; Dip. Med. Sci. Newc. 1995. Cons. (Adult Psychiat.) Tees and N. E. Yorks., NHS Trust; Lead Clinician for Research and Developm. Specialty: Gen. Psychiat. Socs: Brit. Assn. Psychopharmacol. Prev: Sen. Regist. N. & Yorks. RHA; Research Regist. (Psychiat.) Roy. Vict. Infirm. Newc. u. Tyne; SHO Warlingham Pk. Hosp. Croydon.

REILLY, Margaret Mary Hartland Way Surgery, 1 Hartland Road, Shirley, Croydon CR0 8RG Tel: 020 8777 7215 Fax: 020 8777 7648; 58 Barnmead Road, Beckenham BR3 1JE Tel: 020 8777 7215 — MB BCh BAO NUI 1976; DRCOG 1979; DCH RCPSI 1980; MRCGP 1981. Socs: Croydon Medico-Legal Soc.

REILLY, Michael Patrick X-Ray Department, Altnagelvin Hospital, Londonderry BT47 6SB Tel: 01504 345171; 18 Palmerston Park, Londonderry BT47 6DJ — MB BCh BAO NUI 1982; DMRD Aberd. 1988; FRCR 1988. Cons. Radiol. Altnagelvin Area Hosp. Specialty: Radiol. Prev: Sen. Regist. (Radiol.) Univ. Hosp. S. Manch.

REILLY, Paul Alexander Joseph Frimley Park Hospital, Portsmouth Road, Camberley GU16 7UJ Tel: 01276 604348 Fax: 01276 604846 — MB ChB Aberd. 1980; MRCP (UK) 1985; FRCP Glas. 1995; FRCP Ed. 1995; FRCP Lond. 1996. Cons. Rheum. Frimley Pk. NHS Trust Hosp. Camberley. Specialty: Rheumatol. Socs: Brit. Soc. Rheum.; Windsor Med. Soc. Prev: Sen. Regist. (Rheum. & Rehabil.) E. Dorset & Salisbury HA; Research Fell. (Rheum.) Monash Med. Centre Melbourne, Austral.; Regist. (Rheum.) Roy. Nat. Hosp. Rheum Dis. Bath.

REILLY, Peter Charles Gateacre Brow Surgery, 1 Gateacre Brow, Liverpool L25 3PA Tel: 0151 428 1851; 41 Park Road, Prescot L34 3LW Tel: 0151 430 6395 — MB ChB Liverp. 1979; MRCGP 1987. GP Liverp. Prev: Ho. Off. Vict. Centr. Hosp. Wallasey; Trainee GP Whiston Hosp. VTS.

REILLY, Peter Gerard ENT Department, York District Hosptial, Wigginton Road, York YO31 8HE Tel: 01904 453900 Fax: 01904 453900 Email: pgr.york@virgin.net — MB BChir Camb. 1984 (cambridge) BSc St. And. 1981; FRCS Ed. 1989; FRCS (Orl.) 1994. Cons. ENT Surg. York Dist. Hosp.; Cons. Ent Surg. Harrogate Dist. Hosp.. Specialty: Otolaryngol. Prev: Sen. Regist. (ENT) Leicester Roy. Infirm.; Regist. (ENT) St. Bart. Hosp. Lond.; SHO (ENT) Qu. Med. Centre Nottm.

REILLY, Professor Philip Queen's University, Department of General Practice, Dunluce Health Centre, Belfast BT9 7HR Tel: 028 9020 4252 Email: p.m.reilly@qul.ac.uk; 21 Wellington Park, Belfast BT9 6DL Tel: 028 9029 2656 — (Belf.) MB BCh BAO Belf. 1968; FRCGP 1986, M 1972; MD Belf. 1985. Prof. & Head of Dept. Qu. Univ. Belf. Specialty: Gen. Pract. Socs: MICGP. Prev: UK Prescribing Fell. RCGP; Sen. Lect. (Gen. Pract.) Qu. Univ. Belf.; Lect. (Gen. Pract.) Univ. Liverp.

REILLY, Ruth Patricia Friary Surgery, Dobbin Lane, Armagh BT61 7QG Tel: 028 3752 3165 Fax: 028 3752 1514; 63 Main Street, Loughgall, Armagh BT61 8HZ — MB BCh BAO Belf. 1983; DRCOG 1986.

REILLY, Sarah Jane Cambrai, Le Bigard, Forest, Guernsey GY8 0HU — MRCS Eng. LRCP Lond. 1985. Specialty: Family Plann. & Reproduc. Health.

REILLY, Shaula Jane The Crown Medical Centre, Venture Way, Taunton TA2 8QY — MB BS Lond. 1993.

REILLY, Sheena (retired) 24 Culme Road, Mannamead, Plymouth PL3 5BJ Tel: 01752 664261 Email: she52edw@hotmail.com — MB BS (Hons.) Lond.Middx. 1976 (Middlx.) MSc (Hons.) Lond. 1979; FRCPath 1994, M 1982; Cert. Family Plann. JCC 1989. Prev: Cons. Med. Microbiol. Pub. Health Laborat. Serv. Plymouth.

REILLY, Sheila Mary 12 Papermill Road, Bromley Cross, Bolton BL7 9DF — MB ChB Leeds 1990. Regist. (Paediat.) Mater Childr. Hosp. Specialty: Paediat. Prev: SHO (Paediat.) Bolton Gen. Hosp.; Trainee GP Hull HA VTS.

REILLY, Stephen Paul Bootham Park Hospital, York YO30 7BY Tel: 01904 610777 Fax: 01904 453794 — MB BS Lond. 1976 (Royal Free) BSc (Hons.) Lond. 1973; MRCPsych 1982; MSc Manch. 1983; FRCPsych 2000. Cons. Psychiat. (Psychother.) Bootham Pk. Hosp. York.; Sen. Clin. Lect. (Psychiat. & Behavioural Sc. in Relation to Med.) Univ. of Leeds Sch Med. Specialty: Gen. Psychiat.; Psychother. Prev: Specialist Sen. Regist. (Psychother.) Manch. Roy. Infirm.; Psychiat. Heidelberg Clinic Melbourne, Austral.

REILLY, Tennison David (retired) Craigmin, Warren Road, Blundellsands, Liverpool L23 6 Tel: 0151 924 6464 — MB ChB Liverp. 1950. Prev: Ho. Surg. Liverp. Roy. Infirm.

REILLY, Terence Anthony Arthur Loxleigh, Southerndown, Vale of Glamorgan, Bridgend CF32 0RW Tel: 01656 881081 Fax: 01656 881963 — MB BCh Wales 1969; FRCGP 1985, M 1973.

REILLY, Terence Michael c/o The Retreat Hospital, 107 Heslington Road, York YO10 5BN Tel: 01904 412551 Fax: 01904 430828 — MB ChB Glas. 1971; DPM Eng. 1974; MRCPsych 1975; FRCPsych 1997. Cons. Psychiat. Retreat Hosp. York. Specialty: Gen. Psychiat. Socs: FRSM; York Med. Soc.; BMA. Prev: Sen. Regist. Maudsley Hosp. Lond.; Sen. Regist. (Psychol. Med.) St. Mary's & Middlsex Hosp. Lond.; Regist. (Pyschiatry) Middlx. Hosp. Lond.

REILLY, Timothy Gilbert Hairmyres Hospital, Eaglesham, Glasgow G75 8RG Tel: 01355 584823 Email: tim.reilly@laht.scot.nhs.uk; 1 May Terrace, Giffnock, Glasgow G46 6LD Tel: 0141 638 5769 Fax: 0141 638 5769 — MB ChB Bristol 1987; MRCP (UK) 1992; MD Bristol 1998. Cons. Phys. & Gastroenterologist Hairmyres Hosp. Specialty: Gastroenterol. Special Interest: Diagnostic and Theraputic Upper and Lower Gastrointestinal Endoscopy. Socs: Brit. Soc. of Gastroenterol. Prev: Clin. Research Fell. (Gastroenterol.) Qu. Eliz. Hosp. Birm.; Regist. Rotat. (Med.) E. Birm.; Sen. Regist. (Gastroenterol.) Glas. Roy. Infirm.

REILY, Clive Michael The Health Centre, High Street, Bedworth, Nuneaton CV12 8NQ Tel: 024 7631 5827 Fax: 024 7631 0580 — MB BChir Camb. 1985 (Cambridge University) MA Camb. 1985. Gen. Practitioner, Bedworh Health Centre; Clin. Asst. (Cardiol.) Geo. Eliot Hosp. Nuneaton. Specialty: Gen. Pract. Prev: Regist. (Cardiol. & Gen. Med.) Walsgrave Hosp. Coventry.

REIMAN, Gunnar (retired) Saffron Lane Health Centre, 612 Saffron Lane, Leicester LE2 6TD Tel: 0116 291 1212 Fax: 0116 291 0300; 531 Welford Road, Leicester LE2 6FN Tel: 0116 270 6317 — (King's Coll. Hosp.) MB BS Lond. 1960; MRCS Eng. LRCP Lond. 1960; DObst RCOG 1962. Prev: SHO & Ho. Off. (Surg.) Leicester Roy. Infirm.

REIN, Howard Irving Village Surgery, Gillett Road, Talbot Village, Poole BH12 5BF Tel: 01202 525252 Fax: 01202 533956 — MB ChB Leeds 1967; DObst RCOG 1969. Police Surg. Socs: Assn. Police Surg. Prev: Ho. Surg. (Obst.) Boscombe Hosp.

REINALD, Florian Nicolas Christian 112A West End Lane, London NW6 2LS — MB BS Lond. 1998; MB BS Lond 1998.

REINHARDT, Alistair Karl Centre For Respiratory Research, University College London, Rayne Institute, 5 University Street, London WC1E 6JJ Tel: 020 7679 6976/0207 790 6418 Fax: 020 7679 6973 Email: natwatt@fsmail.net — MB BChir Camb. 1993; MA (Hons.) Camb. 1993; MB Camb. 1993; MRCP (UK) 1995. Wellcome Trust Clin. Research Fell. Respirat. Med., Centre for Respirat. research, UCL Lond. Specialty: Respirat. Med.; Gen. Med. Prev: SpR (Gen & Respirat. Med.) Roy. Lond. Hosp., Lond; Specialist Regist. (Gen. & Respirat. Med.) OldCh. Hosp.; SHO (Gen. Med.) St. Geo. Hosp. Lond.

REINHOLD, Piers Hayward Fakenham Medical Practice, The Fakenham Medical Centre, Greenway Lane, Fakenham NR21 8ET Tel: 01328 851321 Fax: 01328 851412 Email: piersreinhold@hotmail.com; Holly Farm House, Wood Norton Road, Stibbard, Fakenham NR21 0EX Tel: 01328 829295 Fax: 01328 851412 — (Guy's) MRCS Eng. LRCP Lond. 1970; DObst RCOG 1975; MRCGP 1976. Clin. Asst. Cranmer Ho. Hosp. Unit Fakenham Norf. Prev: SHO (Cas.) & Ho. Surg. (ENT) Guy's Hosp. Lond.; Med. Off. Brit. Milit. Hosp. Berlin.

REINSTEIN, Dan Zoltan 15 Sydney House, Woodstock Road, London W4 1DP Tel: 020 8994 2890 Fax: 020 8995 0915 Email: danreinstein@compuserve.com — MB BChir Camb. 1989 (Camb. Univ./ Univ. Coll. Lond. Medical School) FRCS (C); MA Camb. 1988. Asst. Prof. of Ophth. Weill Med. Coll. Of Cosrell Univ. NY. USA; Professeur Associe Univ. de Paris France. Specialty: Ophth.

REISER, Jan Lister Hospital, Corey's Mill Lane, Stevenage SG1 4AB Tel: 01438 781010 Email: dr.reiser@lister.org.uk; 24 Chiltern Road, Hitchin SG4 9PJ Tel: 01462 452765 Email: reiserjan@hotmail.com — MB BS Lond. 1975 (Charing Cross Hospital London) MRCS Eng. LRCP Lond. 1975; DCH Eng. 1978; MRCP (UK) 1980; MD Lond. 1994; FRCPCH 1996; FRCP (L) 1996. Cons. Paediat. Lister Hosp. Stevenage. Specialty: Paediat. Special Interest: Paediatric Allergy; Paediatric Respirat. Dis. Socs: Brit. Paediat. Respirat. Soc.; Brit. Soc. Allergy & Clin. Immunol.

REISIG, Veronika Maria Theresia 44 Denholme Road, Oxenhope, Keighley BD22 9SJ — State Exam Med Marburg 1993; MD Marburg 1994; MRCP (UK) 1996; MPH 1998. Specialist Regist. (Pub. Health Med.) N. & Yorks. Region. Specialty: Pub. Health Med.

REISLER, Ronald Business Aviation Facilities, Hangar 7, Faireys Way, Manchester Airport West, Manchester M90 5NE Tel: 0161 436 0129 Fax: 0161 436 0129 Email: avmed2000@northernexec.com; 11 Wicker Lane, Hale Barns, Altrincham WA15 0HG Tel: 0161 980 2024 — MB ChB Leeds 1950. Med. Examr. Min. of Aviat. CAA Lond., Federal Aviat. USA, Austral. CAA & Canad. CAA; Sen. Aviat. Med. Examr. Federal Aviat. Auth.; Med. Off. Monarch Airlines; Med. Off. Brit. Aerospace AVRO Internat. Aerospace Woodford; Med. Off. Air 2000 Manch. & Airtours Manch.; Med. Off. Flying Colours Manch. Specialty: Aviat. Med. Prev: GP Stockport.

REISNER, Colin Queen's Hospital, Burton-on-Trent DE13 0RB Tel: 01283 566333 — MB BChir Camb. 1972 (St. Bart.) MRCP (UK) 1974; FRCP Lond. 1989. Cons. Phys. (c/o Elderly) Burton Hosp. Specialty: Care of the Elderly. Prev: Cons. Phys. (Geriat. Med.) Lond. Hosp.; Hon. Sen. Regist. (Med.) St. Bart. Hosp. Lond.; Interne des Hôp. de Paris, France.

REISS, David Dept. of Forensic Mental Health Science, Institute of Psychiatry, KCL, De Crespigny Park, Demark Hill, London SE5 8AF Tel: 020 7919 0123 Fax: 020 7919 3754 Email: d.reiss@iop.kcl.ac.uk — BChir Camb. 1988; MB Camb. 1987; MA Camb. 1987; MRCPsych 1992; MPhil Lond. 1994; Dip. Forens. Psychiat. Lond. 1996. Director Teachg. unit, dept. of Forens. Psychiat., KCL; Hon. Cons. Forens. Psychiat., Maudsley Hosp. Specialty: Forens. Psychiat. Socs: Roy. Soc. Med. Prev: Clin. Lect. (Victimoclgy & Forens. Psychiat.) Inst. Psychiat.; Sen. Regist. (Forens. Psychiat.) Bethlem Maudsley Hosp. Lond; Regist. Rotat. (Psychiat.) Roy. Free & Friern Hosp. Postgrad. Train. Scheme.

REISS, Janet Elizabeth Department of Child Life & Health, University of Edinburgh, 20 Sylvan Place, Edinburgh EH9 1UW Tel: 0131 536 4350; 53 McDonald Road, Edinburgh EH7 4LY Tel: 0131 556 7534 — MB ChB Ed. 1991 (Univ. Ed.) BSc (Hons.) Med. Sci. Pharm. Ed. 1989; MRCP (UK) 1995. Research Fell. (Child Life & Health) Univ. Edin. Specialty: Neonat. Socs: Roy. Coll. Paediat. & Child Health; BMA; RCP Edin. Prev: SHO III (Paediat.) SE Scotl.; SHO (Paediat., Neonates & Med.) Lothian HB.

REISS, Mary Catherine — MB ChB Leeds 1988; MRCOG 1998. Regist. Rotat. (O & G) N. & Yorks. RHA. Specialty: Obst. & Gyn. Prev: SHO (O & G) Bradford, St. Jas. Hosp. Leeds & York Dist. Hosp.

REISS, Stefan Horatio 31 Hull Road, Cottingham HU16 4PN — MRCS Eng. LRCP Lond. 1976.

REISS, Stephen Butts New Sheepmarket Surgery, Ryhall Road, Stamford PE9 1YA Tel: 01780 758123 Fax: 01780 758102 — BM BS Nottm. 1983; DRCOG 1986; MRCP (UK) Paediat. 1987; MRCGP 1991. Prev: Exchange Regist. Roy. Childr. Hosp. Melbourne, Australia.

REISSIS, Mr Nikolaos Watford General Hospital, Vicarage Road, Watford WD18 0HB Tel: 01923 217765 Fax: 01923 217859 Email: angela.gregg@whht.nhs.uk — Ptychio Iatrikes Thessaloniki 1981; Europ Accredit Orthop Surg 1994. p/t Cons. Orthop. Surg., W.

Herts. NHS Trust. Specialty: Trauma & Orthop. Surg. Socs: BMA; BSSH. Prev: Specialist Regist., Roy. Nat. Orthopaedic Hosp.

REISSMANN, Gerard Francis Ethel Street Surgery, 88/90 Ethel Street, Benwell, Newcastle upon Tyne NE4 8QA Tel: 0191 219 5456 Fax: 0191 226 0300 — MB BS Newc. 1985; BMedSc Newc. 1984.

REITANO, Teresa Medical Centre, 12 East King Street, Helensburgh G84 7QL Tel: 01436 673366 Fax: 01436 679715 — MB ChB Glas. 1992.

REITER, Marianne Eva Karoline 6 Bro Crannog, Llangrannog, Llandysul SA44 6RY — State Exam Med. Freiburg 1987.

***REITH, Christina Alison** Lecropt House, Bridge of Allan, Stirling FK9 4NB — MB ChB (Hons) Glas. 1998; MRCP UK; BSc (Hons) Glas 1995; MB ChB Glas 1998. SHO Med.Glasgoe.Roy.Infirm.; Drug Safety Physician, Roche Pharmaceuticals. Specialty: Gen. Med.; Alcohol & Substance Misuse. Socs: BMA; Med. Chir. Soc.

REITH, Hellen Lind (retired) 4 Kenfield Crescent, Aberdeen AB15 7UQ Tel: 01224 318530 — MB ChB Aberd. 1938; FRCOG 1971, M 1951. Prev: Cons. O & G Co. Renfrew.;.

REITH, Sheila Baillie Mackenzie Lecropt House, Lecropt, Bridge of Allan, Stirling FK9 4NB — MB BS Lond. 1962 (Univ. Coll. Hosp.) BSc (Hons.) Lond. 1959; MRCP Lond. 1965; FRCP Glas. 1983; FRCP Lond. 1990; FRCP Ed 1998. Prev. Cons. Phys. Stirling Roy. Infirm.; Hon. Sen. Lect. Univ. Glas. Specialty: Gen. Med.; Diabetes; Endocrinol. Socs: Eur. Assn. for Study Diabetes; Caledonian Endocrine Soc. Prev: Cons. Phys. St. Jas. & St. Geo. Hosp. Lond.; Hon. Sen. Lect. St. Geo. Hosp. Med. Sch. Lond.; Regist. (Med.) Univ. Coll. Hosp. Lond.

REITH, William Westburn Medical Group, Foresterhill Health Centre, Westburn Road, Aberdeen AB25 2AY Tel: 01224 559595 Fax: 01224 559597; 54 Gray Street, Aberdeen AB10 6JE Tel: 01224 326380 Fax: 01224 322098 — MB ChB Ed. 1974; BSc (Med. Sci.) Ed. 1971; FRCGP 1991, M 1978; FRCP Ed. 1994. Princip. in Gen. Pract.; Chairm., Scott. Counc. RCGP. Prev: Regional Adviser Gen. Pract. NE. Scotl.; Special Adviser (Primary Care) SCPMDE; Hon. Sec. (Counc.) RCGP.

REIVE, Alyson Ronald Southside Surgery, 17 Bernard Terrace, Edinburgh EH8 9NU Tel: 0131 662 1633/0131 667 2240 — MB ChB Ed. 1984; DCH RCPS Glas. 1987; MRCGP 1988. GP Princip. S.side surgry Edin.; Clin. Asst., Cardiol., Roy. Infirm. of Edin. Prev: GP Retainer, Grange Med. Gp., Edin.; GP Dhaka Bangladesh.

REJ, Edward Priory Fields Surgery, Nursery Road, Huntingdon PE29 3RL Tel: 01480 52361 Fax: 01480 434640 — MB BS Lond. 1989; MRCGP 1995.

REJALI, Mr Stephen Dariush 58 Craigton Drive, Newton Mearns, Glasgow G77 6TD Tel: 0141 639 5527 — MB ChB Manch. 1992 (Manchester) BSc (Hons.) Immunol Experim Oncol, 1989; FRCS CSiG (Eng.) 1996; FRCS CSiG with Otolarying (Eng.) 1998. Regist. (OtoLaryngol.) Monklanh Hosp. Airdric. Specialty: Otorhinolaryngol.; Otolaryngol. Socs: Manch. Med. Soc.; BAO - HNS; ORS. Prev: Hope Hosp. Sa ENT SHO; Manch. Roy. Infirm. Manch. ENT Gen. Surg.

REJMAN, Andrzej Stefan Miroslaw, OStJ Leicester Royal Infirmary, Department of Haematology, Infirmary Square, Leicester LE1 5WW; 15 Selwyn Road, New Malden KT3 5AU Tel: 020 8942 1767 — MB BS Lond. 1976; MRCP (UK) 1979; MD Lond. 1984; FRCPath 1996, M 1986; FRCP Lond. 1996. Cons. Haemat. Leics. Roy. Inf. Specialty: Haematology. Socs: Brit. Soc. Haematol.; Assn. Clin. Path. Prev: Sen. Med. Off. DOH & Hon. Cons. Haemat. St Thos. Hosp. Lond.; Area Surg. St John Ambul. SW Area Lond.; Lect. (Haemat.) Guy's Hosp. Med. Sch. Lond.

RELF, Christine Marjorie — MB BChir Camb. 1970 (St. Geo.) DObst RCOG 1972. Locum GP W. Cornw. Socs: BMA. Prev: Police Surg. Devon & Cornw. Constab.; Med. Off. Sanaa, Yemen Arab Rep.; Med. Off. Res al Khaimeh.

RELTON, Peter George Sparks Chadwick House, 127 York Road, Hartlepool TS26 9DN Tel: 01429 234646 Fax: 01429 861559; Parkmead, Elwick Road, Hartlepool TS26 0DW Tel: 01429 273628 Fax: 01429 273628 — MB BS Lond. 1960 (Westm.) Prev: Ho. Surg. (Obst.) N. Middlx. Hosp. Lond.; Ho. Surg. & Cas. Off. Westm. Hosp.

REMBACKEN, Bjorn Joakim 15 Wayland Close, Adel, Leeds LS16 8LT — MB ChB Leic. 1987; MRCP (UK) 1990; MD 2003. Specialty: Gastroenterol.

REMEH, Bashir Sayed 25 Pearson Road, Ipswich IP3 8NL — MB BCh Al Fateh, Libya 1991; MRCP (UK) 1990.

REMFRY, Christopher John Charles Hadwen Medical Practice, Glevum Way Surgery, Abbeydale, Gloucester GL4 4BL Tel: 01452 529933; The Coach House, Tewkesbury Road, The Leigh, Gloucester GL19 4BP — MB BChir Camb. 1989; MA Camb. 1992; DCH RCP Lond. 1992; MRCGP 1993.

REMFRY, Rita Mariaselvi Rosebank Surgery, 153B Stroud Road, Gloucester GL1 5JQ Tel: 01452 522767; Rosebank Surgery, 1538 Stroud Road, Gloucester GL1 5JQ Tel: 01452 522767 — MB ChB Glas. 1990 (Glasgow University) DRCOG 1994; MRCGP 1995. Socs: RCGP; BMA; Fac. Fam. Plann. Prev: Clin. Asst. (Diabetes).

REMINGTON, George Arthur 41 Sunnyfield, Mill Hill, London NW7 4RD — MB BS Lond. 1976 (Univ. Coll. Hosp.) OBE; O.St.J.; BSc (Pharmacol.) Lond. 1973, MB BS 1976; AFOM RCP Lond. 1984; MSc Lond 1984; MFOM RCP Lond. 1990. Chief Med. Off. Roy. Sun Alliance. Specialty: Occupat. Health. Prev: SHO (Paediat.) Northwick Pk. Hosp. Harrow; Ho. Surg. Univ. Coll. Hosp.; Ho. Phys. Barnet Gen. Hosp.

REMINGTON, Kathryn Naomi 41 Sunnyfield, Mill Hill, London NW7 4RD — MB BS Lond. 1978 (Roy. Free) BSc (Hons.) (Pharmacol.) Lond. 1973, MB BS 1978. Prev: Ho. Phys. Roy. Free Hosp. Lond.; SHO (Cas. & Orthop.) & Ho. Surg. Barnet Gen. Hosp.

REMINGTON, Shirley Ann Mary Barrfield, Prescot Road, Hale, Altrincham WA15 9PZ — MB ChB Manch. 1979; BSc (Med. Sci.) St. And. 1976; MB ChB (Hons. & Distinc.) Manch. 1979; FFA RCS Eng. 1984. Specialty: Anaesth.

RENBOURN, Edward Tobias 8 Garrick Way, Frimley Green, Camberley GU16 6LY — MRCS Eng. LRCP Lond. 1931; MD Lond. 1934, MB 1931; MRCP Lond. 1932.

RENDALL, Charles Mark Shuttleworth Giffords P.C.C., Spa Road, Melksham SN12 7EA Tel: 01225 703370 — MB BS Lond. 1966 (St. Bart.) MRCS Eng. LRCP Lond. 1966; DA Eng. 1970; DObst RCOG 1973. Prev: Surg. Lt. RN.

RENDALL, David Charles Shuttleworth (retired) 12 West Quay, Abingdon Marina, Abingdon OX14 5TL Tel: 01235 520389 — MRCS Eng. LRCP Lond. 1937 (St. Bart.) Prev: Surg. Lt.-Cdr. RNVR.

RENDALL, Jacqueline Carole 22 Circular Road, Newtownabbey BT37 0RF — MB BCh BAO Belf. 1993.

RENDALL, Joan (retired) Firle, Peaslake, Guildford GU5 9PA Tel: 01306 730630 — MB BS Lond. 1948 (Roy. Free) MRCS Eng. LRCP Lond. 1947. Prev: Ho. Phys. Vict. Hosp. Sick Childr. Hull.

RENDALL, Jonathan Richard Shuttleworth Hereford County Hospital, Union Walk, Hereford HR1 2ER Tel: 01432 364132 — MB BS Lond. 1969 (St. Bart.) MRCS Eng. LRCP Lond. 1969; MRCP (UK) 1972; FRCP Lond. 1989. Cons. Dermat. Hereford Hosps. NHS Trust. Specialty: Dermat.

RENDALL, Mr Max (retired) 4 Ladbroke Square, London W11 3LX Tel: 020 7221 4878 — MB BChir Camb. 1960 (Middlx.) MRCS Eng. LRCP Lond. 1959; BA Camb. 1960; FRCS Eng. 1964. Prev: Clin. Supt. & Cons. Surg. Guy's Hosp. Lond.

RENDEL, Susan Elizabeth Halstead The Falkland Surgery, Monks Lane, Newbury RG14 7DF Tel: 01635 40160 — MB BS Lond. 1975; BA (Hons.) Oxf. 1972; DRCOG 1977; MRCP (UK) 1978.

RENDELL, Christine Muriel (retired) 1 The Crossway, Mottingham, London SE9 4JJ Tel: 020 8857 4071 — MB ChB Bristol 1941; DA Eng. 1943; FFA RCS Eng. 1954.

RENDELL, Jean Angus (retired) 88 Abbey Meadows, Kirkhill, Morpeth NE61 2YA Tel: 01670 514922 — MB BS Durh. 1945; DObst RCOG 1948. Prev: SCMO N. Tyneside HA.

RENDER, Christina Anne (retired) 7 Speckled Wood Road, Sherborne St John, Basingstoke RG24 9SR — MB ChB Ed. 1984 (Edinb.) FRCA 1993. Sen. Regist. (Anaesth.) Wessex Region. Prev: Regist. (Anaesth.) St. Geo. Hosp. Lond.

RENDLE, Derek Ernest Estover, Brynhafod, Cardigan SA43 1NS — MB BS Lond. 1956 (St. Thos.) DA Eng. 1963; DObst. RCOG 1963.

RENE, Mr Cornelius Hinchinbrooke Hospital, Hinchinbrooke Park, Huntingdon PE29 6NT Tel: 01480 416561 — MB BS Lond. 1985 (Middlesex Hospital Medical School) FRCOphth 1992. Cons. Ophth., Hinchinbrooke Hosp., Huntingdon; Cons. Ophth., Addenbrookes Hosp. Camb. Specialty: Ophth. Socs: BMA; British Oculoplastic Surgery Society; Fellow Royal Colege Of Ophthalmologists. Prev:

Fell. Ocular Adnexal Surg., Moorfields EH, Lond.; Fell. In Ocular Adnexal Surg., Qu.s MC, Nottm.; Sen. Reg, Ophth., W Midl.s Rotat.

RENEHAN, Andrew Gerard 1 The Willows, Chorltonville, Manchester M21 8FQ — MB ChB Manch. 1995; BDentSc. Dub. 1986; FDS RCS Ed. 1989; FRCS Eng. 1997. Hon. Lect. in Surgery/Senior Research Fell.; SpR (Gen. Surg.) N. W. Deanery. Specialty: Gen. Surg. Socs: Dent. Fell. RCS Edin.; Assn. of Colopeochology of GB & Ire (Assoc. Mem); Fell. Roy. Coll. Surg Eng (Gen. Surg.). Prev: Research Fell., Christie Hosp. Manch.; SHO Rotat. (Gen. Surg.) S. Manch.; Ho. Off. (Med. & Surg.) Withington Hosp. Manch.

RENFREW, Anne Catherine 27B The Gables, Haddenham, Aylesbury HP17 8AD — MB ChB Glas. 1975; MRCOG 1981.

RENFREW, Christopher Charles Hermes Lodge, Bredons Norton, Tewkesbury GL20 7EZ — MB BS Lond. 1983 (Roy. Free) DRCOG 1986; MRCGP 1995. Managing Dir. Montpellier Health Care Ltd. Cheltenham. Specialty: Gen. Pract. Prev: Trainee GP Tewkesbury.

RENFREW, Craig William 2 Cherryvalley Gardens, Belfast BT5 6PQ — MB BCh BAO Belf. 1990; FRCA 1994.

RENFREW, Dawn Margaret Burnhead Frm., Netherburn, Larkhall ML9 3DQ — MB ChB Ed. 1989.

RENFREW, Ian 112A Agar Grove, London NW1 9TY — MB BS Lond. 1994.

RENFREW, Margaret Addie East Lodge, Barnhill, Perth PH2 7AT Tel: 01738 21097 — Mem. BMA; MB ChB Glas. 1958. Prev: Ho. Surg. Greenock Roy. Infirm.; Ho. Phys. Larkfield Hosp. Greenock; Regist. Anaesth. Roy. Halifax Infirm.

RENGAN, Mr Dhanakodi Chettiar No. 5 Sandiway, Chesterfield S40 3HG — MB BS Madras 1983; FRCS Glas. 1989.

RENKEMA, Saskia Eva Blackthorn Medical Centre, St Andrews Road, Barming, Maidstone ME16 9AL — Artsexamen Utrecht 1989; DRCOG 1994. GP FCS.

RENNER, Norren Edward Awunor (retired) 13 Dalmeny Court, Duke St., St James's, London SW1 6BL; 19 Charlton Court, Brancote Road, Prenton CH43 6XE Tel: 0151 652 3589 Fax: 0151 652 3589 — MB ChB Ed. 1949 (University of Edinburgh) DO Eng. 1956; FDS RCS Eng. 1970, L 1965.

RENNER, Suzanne Louise Shipley Hill Farmhouse, Alnwick NE66 2LX — MB BS Newc. 1997; MRCGP Lond. 2003.

RENNICK, Charles Burridge (retired) 36K Maybole Rd, Ayr KA7 4SF Tel: 01292 440291 — MB ChB Glas. 1953; DObst RCOG 1957; MRCGP 1976. Prev: GP Ayr.

RENNIE, Agnes Lees 23 Lady Jane Gate, Bothwell, Glasgow G71 8BW — MB ChB Glas. 1968; DObst RCOG 1970; DA Eng. 1971; FFA RCS Eng. 1974. Cons. Anaesth. Monklands Dist. Hosp. Specialty: Anaesth. Prev: Cons. (Anaesth.) Rutherglen Matern. Hosp. & Vict. Infirm. Glas.; Sen. Regist. (Anaesth.) Dundee Teachg. Hosps.; Regist. (Anaesth.) Vict. Infirm. Glas.

RENNIE, Alan Nisbet Thornliebank Health Centre, Glasgow G46 8HY Tel: 0141 620 2222 Fax: 0141 638 7554; Glebe Capel, Newton Mearns, Glasgow G77 6JW Tel: 0141 639 5071 — MB ChB Glas. 1965; DObst RCOG 1967; MRCGP 1977. Socs: BMA. Prev: Ho. Surg. Glas. Roy. Infirm.; Ho. Phys. Vict. Infirm. Glas.; Ho. Surg. Glas. Roy. Matern. & Wom. Hosp.

RENNIE, Mr Alexander Milne (retired) Place of Bridgefoot, Caskieben, Kinellar, Aberdeen AB21 0SY Tel: 0122 479273 — MB ChB Aberd. 1933; MB ChB (Hnrs.) Aberd. 1933; FRCS Eng. 1937; FRCS Ed. 1959. Prev: Sen. Cons. (Orthop. Surg.) Min. Health Kuwait.

RENNIE, Alison Cunningham Dr Alison Rennie, Consultant Paediatrician, Southbank Child Centre, 207 Old Rutherglen Rd, Glasgow G5 0RE Tel: 0141 201 0908 — MB ChB Dundee 1989; MRCPCH founder; MRCP (UK) 1993. Roy. Hosp. Sick Childr. Glas. Specialty: Paediat. Socs: Roy. Coll. Paediat. & Child Health.

RENNIE, Mr Alistair George Robert (retired) Altacraig, 26 Leighton Gardens, Ellon AB41 9BH Tel: 01358 720442 Fax: 01358 725236 Email: alastiarrennie@hotmail.com — MB ChB Glas. 1966; FRCS Ed. 1977; FCOphth 1989. Prev: Med. Off. Malaita Brit. Solomon Isls.

RENNIE, Andrew Robertson (retired) 20 Roman Road, Ayr KA7 3SZ — MB ChB Glas. 1941 (Univ. Glas.) BSc Glas. 1938; DPM Eng. 1969. Prev: Assoc. Specialist (Psychiat.) Ailsa Hosp. Ayr.

RENNIE, Mr Christopher Douglas Droitwich Private Hospital, St. Andrews Road, Droitwich WR9 8DN Tel: 01905 794793; Copcot House, Salwarpe, Droitwich WR9 7JB Tel: 01905 796798 Fax: 01905 796772 — MB ChB Birm. 1972; BSc (Hons.) (Anat.) Birm. 1969; FRCS Eng. 1977. Cons. Urol. Alexandra NHS Health Trust. Specialty: Urol. Prev: Sen. Regist. Qu. Eliz. Hosp. Birm. & St. Peters Hosps. Lond.; Regist. Northwick Pk. Hosp. Harrow.

RENNIE, Fay Margaret (retired) 65 Friary Park, Ballabeg, Castletown IM9 4EP — MB ChB St. And. 1952; MRCOG 1961. Prev: Cas. Off. Nobles. Hosp. Douglas Isle of Man.

RENNIE, Ian George 33 Shrublands Road, Berkhamsted HP4 3HX Tel: 0144 286 6016 — MRCS Eng. LRCP Lond. 1968; DObst RCOG 1969; DIH Eng. 1981; FFOM RCP Lond. 1992, MFOM 1984. Chief Med. Off. Kodak Ltd. Specialty: Occupat. Health. Socs: Fell. Roy. Soc. Med.; BMA. Prev: Sen. Med. Off. Lucas CAV; Med. Off. Lucas Aerospace, Lucas CAV & Lucas Elec. Companies; Trainee GP Newport Isle of Wight.

RENNIE, Professor Ian George Royal Hallamshire Hospital, Department Ophthalmology and Orthoptics, University of Sheffield, Glossop Road, Sheffield S10 2JF Tel: 0114 276 6222 Fax: 0114 276 6381; Church Lane House, Litton Mews, Buxton SK17 8QU Tel: 01298 871586 — MB ChB Sheff. 1976; FRCS Ed. 1981; FCOphth 1989. Prof. Ophth. Univ. Sheff.; Edr. Oxf. Congr..; Hon. Cons. Ophth. Roy. Hallamsh. Hosp., Sheff.; Edr. Eye. Specialty: Ophth. Socs: Mem. Counc. Coll. of Opthalmologists.

RENNIE, Ian Michael 16 Crawfordsburn Road, Bangor BT19 1BE — MB BCh BAO Belf. 1994.

RENNIE, Janet Mary 4th Floor Golden Jubilee Wing, King's College Hospital, Denmark Hill, London SE5 9RS Tel: 020 7737 4000 Ext: 4344 Fax: 020 7582 8353 Email: janet.rennie@kcl.ac.uk — (Sheffield) MB ChB Sheffield 1978; MRCP (UK) 1981; DCH RCP Lond 1982; MD Sheffield 1986; FRCPCH 1993; MA Cambridge 1994; FRCP Lond 1994. Cons. Neonat. Med. King's Coll. Hosp. Lond.; Chair CSAC, RCPCH. Specialty: Neonat.; Paediat. Socs: Brit. Med. Ultrasound Soc.; Brit. Assn. Perinatal Med.; Roy. Soc. of Med. Prev: Cons. Neonat. Med. Rosie Matern. Hosp. Camb.; Research Fell. (Neonat. Med.) Univ. Liverp.; Lect. (Paediat.) Univ. Camb.

RENNIE, Jean Ann The Kitchen, Cullen House, Cullen, Buckie AB56 4XW — MB ChB St. And. 1965; DObst RCOG 1976. Self-Employed GP Non-Princip. Specialty: Gen. Pract. Socs: BMA; Med. Wom. Federat.; Roy. Soc. Med. Prev: SHO Elsie Inglis Memor. Matern. Hosp. Edin.; Ho. Surg. (Gyn.) & Ho. Phys. Bruntsfield Hosp. Edin.

RENNIE, Jean Gibson (retired) Penchrise Peel, Hawick TD9 9UA Tel: 01450 375076 — MB ChB Glas. 1958 (Glasgow) MRCGP 1974. Prev: GP GulLa. E. Lothian.

RENNIE, Mr John Aubery Department of Surgery, King's College Hosp., London SE5 9RS Tel: 020 7346 3268 Fax: 020 7346 3438 Email: johnrennie40@hotmail.com — MRCS Eng. LRCP Lond. 1970 (St. Bart.) MS Lond. 1984, MB BS 1970; DTM & H Liverp. 1974; FRCS Eng. 1975. Sen. Lect. & Hon. Cons. Surg. King's Coll. Hosp. Lond. Specialty: Gastroenterol. Socs: Fell. Roy. Soc. Med. (Surg. & Coloproctocolectmy Sect.); Assn. Surgs.; Assoc. of Colorectal Surg. Prev: Lect. Char. Cross. Hosp. Lond.; Regist. St. Mark's Hosp. Dis. Colon & Rectum Lond. & Duncan Hosp.; Raxaul, India.

RENNIE, Louise Morag 192/3 Causewayside, Edinburgh EH9 1PN — MB ChB Ed. 1998; MB ChB Ed 1998.

RENNIE, Mary (retired) 25 St Margaret's Road, Ruislip HA4 7NX Tel: 01895 639700 — MB ChB St. And. 1938; MB ChB (Commend.) St. And. 1938, DPH 1940; DCH Eng. 1955. Prev: Asst. MOH (Matern. & Child. Welf.) Sheff.

RENNIE, Morag Lilian (retired) 1 Leemuir View, Carluke ML8 4AN Tel: 01555 771361 — MB ChB Glas. 1968; DPM Eng. 1972; FRCPsych 1996, M 1974. Cons. Psychiat. & Psychiat. of Old Age Law Hosp. Lanarksh. Prev: Cons. Psychiat. Hartwood Hosp. Shotts.

RENNIE, Peter Robertson North Bradford Primary Care Trust, New Mill, Victoria Rd, Bradford BD18 3LD Tel: 01274 366001; 23 Cleasby Road, Menston, Ilkley LS29 6JE Tel: 01943 874943 — MB ChB Ed. 1971.

RENNIE, Robert Alexander (retired) Jenner Health Centre, Turners Lane, Whittlesey, Peterborough PE7 1EJ Tel: 01733 203601 Fax: 01733 206210 — BSc (Hons. Anat.) Manch. 1965, MB ChB 1968; DCH RCPS Glas. 1970; DObst RCOG 1971.

RENNIE, Sandra Mary 28 Southey Street, Keswick CA12 4EF — MB ChB Ed. 1996.

RENNINSON, John Neal Royal Devon and Exeter Hospital, (Heavitree), Gladstone Road, Exeter EX1 2ED Tel: 01392 405052 — MB ChB Manch. 1985; DA (UK) 1990; MRCOG 1991. Cons. Roy. Devon & Exeter NHS Trust. Specialty: Obst. & Gyn.

RENNISON, Claire Marie 1 Rothley Avenue, Ashington NE63 0LG — MB ChB Dund. 1998; MB ChB Dund 1998.

RENNY, Francis Hugh Blakiston Shirley House, 186 Bridgnorth Road, Wollaston, Stourbridge DY8 3PN Tel: 0138 43 77257 — MB ChB Birm. 1969; DMRD Eng 1977; FRCR 1978. Cons. Radiol. Dudley AHA. Specialty: Radiol.

RENNY, Mr Nicholas Michael Charles Dept. Maxillofacial surgery, Aberdeen Royal Infirmary, Foresterhill, Aberdeen AB25 2ZN Tel: 01330 860859 Fax: 01224 840925; Skene House, Lyne of Skene, Skene AB32 7BQ Tel: 01330 860859 Fax: 01330 860859 — MB BS Lond. 1988 (Charing Cross and Westminster) BDS Ed. 1981; FDS RCS Eng. 1990; FRCS Ed. 1991. Head of Serv., Cons. & Hon. Sen.Lect. Oral & Maxillofacial Surg. Aberd.; Hon. Sen. Lect. Aberd. Univ. Specialty: Oral & Maxillofacial Surg. Socs: Fell. Brit. Assn. Oral & Maxillofacial Surg.; Craniofacial Soc. Prev: Sen. Regist. (Oral & Maxillofacial Surg.) North. Region.; Regist. (Oral & Maxillofacial Surg.) Lothian & Borders HB; Regist. (Gen. Surg.) Roy. Infirm. Edin.

RENOUF, Adrian Charles Dominic Chapel Platt Surgery, 1901 Fore Street, Topsham, Exeter EX3 0HE Tel: 01392 875777 Fax: 01392 875777; Court Dairy Farm, Clyst St. George, Exeter EX3 0NP Tel: 01392 874854 — MB BS Lond. 1978 (St. Bart.) MRCS Eng. LRCP Lond. 1978; DRCOG 1986. Princip. GP Clin. Asst. Cardiol. Dept. RD&E Exeter. Specialty: Gen. Med. Prev: Surg. Lt. RN. SMO D5.

RENSHAW, Anthony John Neil Werneth, 31 The Baulk, Worksop S81 0HU Tel: 01909 500990 — MRCS Eng. LRCP Lond. 1973 (Guy's) FFA RCS Eng. 1977. Cons. Anaesth. Bassetlaw Hosp. & Community Servs. NHS Trust. Specialty: Anaesth. Socs: Obst. Anaesth. Assn.; Assn. Anaesth. Prev: Cons. Anaesth. Worksop & Retford Dist.; Sen. Regist. & Regist. (Anaesth.) Roy. Infirm. Edin.; SHO (Anaesth.) Salisbury Hosp. Gp.

RENSHAW, Joanne Claire — MB ChB Birm. 1986; DRCOG 1989; DCH RCP Lond. 1990; MRCP 1991; MSc 2003. Sen. Regis. Poole Hosp. NHS Trust, Cons., Paediat., Poole Hosp. NHS Trust. Specialty: Paediat. Socs: Roy. Coll. of Paedaitricse Child Health. Prev: Sen. Regist. United Bristol Healthcare Trust; Regist. (Paediat.) Mersey RHA Liverp.

RENSHAW, Neil David Felixstowe Road Surgery, 235 Felixstowe Road, Ipswich IP3 9BN Tel: 01473 719112; 14 Glemham Drive, Rushmere, Ipswich IP4 5BH Tel: 01473 716357 — MB BS Lond. 1988; BSc Lond. 1985; DRCOG 1990; DCH RCP Lond. 1992; MRCGP 1992. Prev: Trainee GP/SHO Ipswich VTS.

RENSHAW, Piers Robin 30 Thomson Street, Aberdeen AB25 2QQ — MB ChB Aberd. 1991.

RENSHAW, Stephanie Barbara Helen Dumbarton Health Centre, Station Road, Dumbarton G82 1PW Tel: 01389 602633 Fax: 10289 602623 — MB ChB Manch. 1973; DObst RCOG 1976; Dip Palliat Med Glas. 1998. Prev: Trainee GP Helensburgh.

RENSHAW, Veronique (retired) — MD Bordeaux 1973; CPEBH 1975; CES 1977. Cons. Anaesth. Furness Gen. Hosp. Barrow-in-Furness. Prev: Cons. Anaesth. C H Lourdes France.

RENTON, Mr Charles James Crawford (retired) Mavis Holt, 35 Hampton Park Road, Hereford HR1 1TH Tel: 01432 268079 — MB ChB Glas. 1953; FRCS Ed. 1958; FRFPS Glas. 1960; FRCS Eng. 1960. Cons. Surg. Co. Hosp. Hereford. Prev: Sen. Regist. (Surg.) Roy. Hosp. Sheff. & Hon. Clin. Tutor (Surg.) Univ. Sheff.

RENTON, Mary Collette Blaise Leah Islington Square Surgery, 3 Islington Square, Liverpool L3 8DD Tel: 0151 207 0848 — BM BCh Oxf. 1975; BA Oxf. 1972, BM BCh 1975.

RENTON, Nicholas James Petersfield Hospital, Petersfield GU32 3LB Tel: 01730 263221 Fax: 01730 268218; St James' Hospital, Locksway Road, Portsmouth PO4 8LD Tel: 01705 822331 — (St Bartholomews Hospital) MRCS Eng. LRCP Lond. 1970; MB BS Lond. 1970; MRCPsych 1976; FRCPsych 1997. Cons. Psychiat. Portsmouth & S.E. Hants. HA. Specialty: Gen. Psychiat.

RENTON, Peter Heap (retired) Green Oaks, Chapel Road, Alderley Edge SK9 7DX Tel: 01625 583225 — MD Manch. 1949; BSc Manch. 1940, MD 1949, MB ChB 1943; FRCPath 1964. Dep. Dir. Regional Blood Transfus. Centre Manch.

RENTON, Sophie Caroline Northwick Park Hosptial, Watford Road, Harrow HA1 3UJ Tel: 020 8869 2617 Fax: 020 8869 2571 Email: sophie.renton@nwlh.nhs.uk; 4 Somerset Road, London W13 9PB Tel: 020 8810 1473 — MB BS Lond. 1983; FRCS Eng. 1988; MS Lond. 1994; FRCS (Gen.) 1996. Cons. Vasc. Surg. Northwick Pk. Hosp. Harrow; Clin. Director for Surg., NWLH NHS Trust. Specialty: Gen. Surg. Socs: Vasc. Surgic. Soc.; Europ. Vasc. Surgic. Soc. Prev: Sen. Regist. St. Mary's, Hammersmith & Allied Hosps.; Career Regist. SW Thames; Research Fell. (Vasc. Surg.) E.cott St. Mary's Hosp. Med. Sch. Lond.

RENTOUL, James Woods (retired) Pine Cottage, 36 Fore St., Tregony, Truro TR2 5RN Tel: 0187 253233 — MRCS Eng. LRCP Lond. 1952. Prev: RAMC.

RENTOUL, Jocelyn Roelanda 25 Lawmarnock Crescent, Bridge of Weir PA11 3AS — MB ChB Glas. 1971. Specialty: Occupat. Health. Socs: Soc. Occupat. Med. Prev: Regist. (Dermat.) West. Infirm. Glas.; SHO (Dermat.) Vict. Infirm. Glas.; SHO (Dermat.) South. Gen. Hosp. Glas.

RENVOIZE, Edward Bernard Lytham Hostpial, Warton St., Lytham St Annes FY8 5EE — MB ChB Ed. 1971; DPM Leeds 1975; MRCPsych 1976; MB Ed. 1983; MPH Leeds 1988; MFPHM RCP 1991; FRCPsych 1996; FFPHM RCP 1998. Cons. Psych. (Old Age Psych.) Lancs. Care NHS Trust. Specialty: Geriat. Psychiat. Prev: Cons. Psychiat. (Old Age Psych.) & Dir. Research & Developm., Blackpool Wyre & Fylde Comm. Health Servs. NHS Trust; Cons. in Clin. Audit, Leeds Gen. Inf.; Cons. Psych. Bootham Pk. Hosp. York.

RENWICK, Alexander Colquhoun (retired) 8 Tummel Place, Comrie, Crieff PH6 2PG — MB ChB Glas. 1968; DObst 1970. Prev: GP Dunfermline.

RENWICK, Mr Andrew Austin Rookesbury, Findhorn Road, Forres IV36 3TR Tel: 01309 674046; 111 Balshagray Avenue, Jordanhill, Glasgow G11 7EG Tel: 0141 959 6809 — MB ChB Aberd. 1991; FRCS Ed. 1995; FRCS Glas. 1995. Specialist Regist. Dept. of Gen. Surg.; Fell. Surg. RCP Surg. Glas. Coll. Counc. Specialty: Gen. Surg. Socs: Med. & Defence Union Scotl.; BMA; RCPS Glas. (Counc.lor). Prev: CrossHo. Hosp. Kilmarnock; Monklands Hosp. Airdrie; Stirling Roy. Inf.

RENWICK, Caroline Joy Casse Airthrey Park Medical Centre, Hermitage Road, Stirling University, Stirling FK9 4NJ Tel: 01786 463831 Fax: 01786 447482; 3 The Yetts, Cambusbarron, Stirling FK7 9NJ Tel: 01786 461930 — MB ChB Ed. 1969; MFFP 1992. Sen. Clin. Med. Off. (Family Plann. Servs.) Forth Valley HB.; Med. Off. (Family Plann. Servs.) HM Cornston Vale Inst. Prev: Clin. Asst. (Genitourin. Med.) Forth Valley HB; SHO (O & G) Simpson Memor. Matern. Pavil. & Roy. Infirm. Edin.; SHO (Paediat.) Northampton Gen. Hosp.

RENWICK, Colin Jeffrey Townhead Surgeries, Townhead, Settle BD24 9JA Tel: 01729 822611 Fax: 01729 892916 — MB ChB Leeds 1986; MRCGP 1990; DGM RCP Lond. 1992.

RENWICK, Deborah Susan Department of Medicine for the Elderly, St. James's Hospital, Leeds; 83 Blackmoor Court, Alwoodley, Leeds LS17 7RT — MB ChB Ed. 1987; BSc (Med. Sci.) Ed. 1985, MB ChB 1987; MRCP (UK) 1990. Sen. Regist. (Med. & Med. for Elderly) Yorks. RHA. Specialty: Gen. Med. Socs: BMA & Brit. Geriat. Soc.

RENWICK, Eilidh Catriona Drs Borthwick, Harris, Shadbolt & Renwick, 24 Quarry St, Johnstone PA5 8DZ Tel: 01505 321733; 96 Southbrae Drive, Jordanhill, Glasgow G13 1TZ Tel: 0141 959 1310 Email: c.renwick@btopenworld.com — MB ChB Glas. 1985. p/t GP Princip.; Clin. Asst. (Learning Disabilities) Merchiston Hosp. Brookfield Johnstone. Prev: GP Maybole, Ayrsh.

RENWICK, George Kerr (retired) 5 Roundwood Road, Baildon, Shipley BD17 7JZ — MRCS Eng. LRCP Lond. 1961 (W. Lond.) Prev: Sir Titus Salt's Hosp. Shipley.

RENWICK, Jill Andrae Claughton Medical Centre, 161 Park Road North, Birkenhead CH41 0DD Tel: 0151 652 1688 Fax: 0151 670 0565; 5 Howbeck Road, Oxton, Prenton CH43 6TD Tel: 0151 652 7306 — MB ChB Liverp. 1977; DRCOG 1980; Cert. (Managem. of Drug Misuse) 2002; Dip. Primary Care (Diabetic Managem.) 2003. Clin. Asst. Wirral Drug Unit St. Catherines Hosp., Wirral. Socs: BMA.

RENWICK, Mr Paul Malcolm Hull Royal Infirmary, Anlaby Road, Hull HU3 2LZ — BM BS Nottm. 1983; FRCS Ed. 1992. Specialty: Gen. Surg. Prev: Sen. Regist. (Vasc. Surg.) St Jas. Univ. Hosp. Leeds;

Career Regist. (Gen. Surg.) Scunthorpe Gen. Hosp.; Regist. (Gen. Surg.) Grimsby Dist. Gen. Hosp.

RENWICK, Sally Jane Epsom & St Helier University Hospital NHS Trust, St Helier Hospital, Wrythe Lane, Carshalton SM2 1AA — MB BS Lond. 1991 (St George's Hospital Medical School London) DA (UK) 1994; FRCA (UK) 1997. Cons. Anaesth. Epsom & St Helier NHS Trust. Specialty: Anaesth. Socs: Roy. Coll. of Anaethetists; Obstetris Anaesth.s Assoc.; Assoc. of Paediatric Anaethetists. Prev: Specialist Regist., (Anaesth./PICU), St Geo.'s Hosp.Lond; Specialist Regist., (Anaesth.), Gt. Ormond St. Hosp.; Specialist Regist., (Anaesth.) Chelsea & Westm. Hosp. Lond.

RENWICK, Sheila Jane Kerr Gilsyke House, 212A Selby Road, Halton, Leeds LS15 0LF Tel: 0113 295 2710 Fax: 0113 295 2713; 83 Parkside Road, Meanwood, Leeds LS6 4NA Tel: 0113 275 0291 — MB ChB Manch. 1985; Cert. Family Plann. JCC 1991. Clin. Asst. GUM, LGI. Specialty: Gen. Pract. Prev: Clin. Asst. (A & E) Leeds Gen. Infirm.; GP.

RENWICK, Sonia Ruth Department of Anaesthetics, Royal Free Hospital, Pond Street, London NW3 2QG — MB BChir Camb. 1988 (Cambridge) MA Camb. 1989, MB 1988, BChir 1988; MRCP (UK) 1992; FRCA 1994. Cons. (Anaesth.) Roy. Free Hosp. Lond. Specialty: Anaesth. Prev: Regist. (Anaesth.) Char. Cross Hosp. Lond.; SpR Hammersmith Hosp.; Reg. (Anaesth.) Gt. Ormond St. Hosp. Lond.

RENYARD, Mr Harold Holmwood (retired) Holmwood, 15 The Spinney, Elston, Newark NG23 5PE Tel: 01636 525204 — MB BS Lond. 1940 (King's Coll. Hosp.) MRCS Eng. LRCP Lond. 1940; FRCS Eng. 1948; MS Lond. 1952. Prev: Cons. Surg. Nottm. & Newark Hosps.

REPPER, James Alexander Elmbank Group, Foresterhill Health Centre, Westburn Road, Aberdeen AB25 2AY Tel: 01224 696949 Fax: 01224 691650; Kings Lodge, 14 Kingsgate, Aberdeen AB15 4EJ — MB ChB Aberd. 1980; FRCGP 1994, M 1984. Sen. Research Fell. (Gen. Pract.) Univ. Aberd.; Assoc. Regional Adviser N. E. Scot. Socs: M-C Soc. Aberd.; Brit. Med. Acupunct. Soc. Prev: Recertification Fell. Roy. Coll. Gen. Practs.

REQUENA DURAN, Maria del Mar Department of General Surgery, Royal Berkshire Hospital, London Road, Reading RG1 5AN Tel: 01734 875111; 16 Bradley Gardens, Ealing, London W13 8HF Tel: 020 8081 6561 — LMS La Laguna 1992. SHO Rotat. (Gen. Surg.) Roy. Berks. Hosp. & Battle NHS Trust. Specialty: Gen. Surg. Prev: SHO (Urol. & Orthop.) Roy. Berks. Hosp.

RERRIE, Mr John David (retired) 14A Green Lane, Leominster HR6 8QJ — (Univ. Coll. W. Indies) MB BS Lond. 1960; FRCS Ed. 1972; FRCOphth 1988. Prev: Cons. Ophth. Surg. P'boro. Dist. & Stamford & Rutland Hosps.

RESEK, George Emile 135 Harley Street, London W1G 6BE Tel: 020 7935 6032 Fax: 020 7935 3148 — MD Amer. Univ. Beirut 1976; MRCPsych 1980. Ex-Med. Dir. (Psychol. Med.) Cromwell Hosp. Lond. Specialty: Gen. Psychiat. Socs: Indep. Doctors Forum; RCPsych (Sect. Psychother. & Social & Community Psychiat.); Brit. Neuropsychiat. Assn. Prev: Lect. Univ. Coll. Hosp. Lond.; Sen. Regist. MRC Graylingwell Hosp. Chichester; Regist. Roy. Edin. Hosp.

RESHAMWALA, Niranjan Kantilal Doctors' Mess, Corbett Hospital, Amblecote, Stourbridge DY8 4JB Tel: 01384 456111; 18 Chawn Park Drive, Pedmore, Stourbridge DY9 0YG Tel: 01384 392960 — (Grant Med. Coll.) MB BS Bombay 1962; DA Bombay 1965; DA Eng. 1969. Clin. Asst. (Anaesth.) Corbett Hosp. Stourbridge. Specialty: Anaesth.

RESHAMWALLA, Daulat Khanum Nooredin The Surgery, 277 Fore Street, Edmonton, London N9 0PD — MB BS Osmania 1965.

RESHI, Sajjad Hussain c/o 40 Adelaide Avenue, Brockley, London SE4 1YR — MB BS Jammu & Kashmir 1973 (Med. Coll. Srinagar) MRCP (UK) 1984. Specialty: Cardiol.

RESNICK, Jeremy Victor Nottinghamshire Healthcare NHS Trust, The Wells Road Centre, The Wells Road, Nottingham NG3 3AA Tel: 0115 955 5389 Fax: 0115 952 9420 — MB ChB Stellenbosch 1981; MRCPsych 1989; DPM Dublin 1990; Dip Forens Psychother Lond 1994. Cons. Forens. Pychiatrist Nottm. Forens. Serv. Nottm. Healthcare Trust. Specialty: Forens. Psychiat. Prev: Cons. Forens. Pychiatrist Rampton Hosp.

RESOULY, Mr Adel ENT Department, Queen Alexandra Hospital, Portsmouth NHS Trust, Portsmouth PO6 3LY Tel: 023 92 286377; Southlands, Prinsted Lane, Emsworth PO10 8HS Tel: 01243 373900 — MB ChB Bristol 1966; FRCS (Orl.) Ed. 1971; FRCS Eng. 1998. Cons. Otolayngol., Head & Neck Surg. (ENT) Portsmouth NHS Trust; Hon. Civil Cons. Roy. Naval Hosp. Haslar. Specialty: Gen. Surg. Socs: BMA; Roy. Soc. Med.; Brit. Assoc. of Head & Neck Surg.s. Prev: Sen. Regist. (ENT) Soton. Univ. Hosp. & Wessex RHB; Regist. (ENT) United Bristol Hosps. & S. West. RHB; SHO Radcliffe Infirm. Oxf.

RESTALL, John, OStJ, Brigadier late RAMC Retd. Maple Lodge, Frimley Hall Drive, Camberley GU15 2BE Tel: 01276 62380 — MB BS Lond. 1958 (St. Thos.) FFA RCS Eng. 1967. Cons. Anaesth. Heatherwood & Wexham Pk. Trust. Specialty: Anaesth. Socs: BMA & Assn. Anaesth. Prev: Cons. Adviser Anaesth. & Resusc. to Army; Regist. & SHO (Anaesth.) St. Thos. Hosp. Lond.; SHO (Anaesth.) Soton. Gp. Hosps.

RESTELL, Carol Ann Burvill House Surgery, 52 Dellfield Road, Hatfield AL10 8HP Tel: 01707 269091; 16 Rodney Avenue, St Albans AL1 5SX — MB BS Lond. 1979; FRCGP 2003. Trainer (Gen. Pract.) Hatfield. Specialty: Gen. Pract.

RESTON, Peter John James X-Ray Department, Ormskirk Hospital, Ormskirk L39 2AZ Tel: 01695 656571 Fax: 01695 656571; 20A Tower Hill, Ormskirk L39 2EF — MB ChB Liverp. 1970; DMRD Liverp. 1974; FRCR 1976. Cons. (Radiol.) Ormskirk & Dist. Gen. Hosp. Specialty: Radiol.

RESTON, Samuel Craig Flat 4, 22 Crescent Road, Gosport PO12 2DH — MB ChB Glas. 1995. Specialty: Trauma & Orthop. Surg.

RESTORICK, Helen Margaret Woodthorpe, 61 Leigh Hill Road, Cobham KT11 2HY — MB BS Lond. 1994; MRCGP; BSc Lond. 1990; DRCOG 1997.

RESTRICK, Louise Jane Department of Respiratory Medicine, The Whittington Hospital, Highgate Hill, London N19 5NF Tel: 020 7288 5353/020 86721255 Ext: 1225 — MB BS Lond. 1986 (Cambridge University London Hospital Medical School) MRCP (UK) 1989; MD Lond. 1997; FRCP 2000. Cons. Phys. & Hon. Sen. Lect. Respirat & Gen. Med. Whitt. Hosp. Lond. Specialty: Respirat. Med. Prev: Research Fell. (Thoracic Med.) King's Coll. Sch. Med. & Dent. Lond.; Sen. Regist. (Thoracic & Gen. Med.) Roy. Lond. Hosp. & Lond. Chest Hosp.

RETHINASAMY, Edward Lewis 12 Ophir Gardens, Belfast BT15 5EP — MB BCh BAO Belf. 1985.

RETI, Shane Raymond Heron Hill, Lower Road, One House, Stowmarket IP14 3BX — MB ChB Auckland 1988.

RETSAS, Spyros Department of Medical Oncology, Cromwell Hospital, Cromwell Road, London SW5 0TU Email: s.retsas@ic.ac.uk — (Aristotle Univ. Thessaloniki) Ptychio Iatrikes Aristotle 1967; LMSSA Lond. 1971; MRCS Eng. LRCP Lond. 1972; MRCP (UK) 1975; MD (Thesis) Athens 1979; FRCP Lond. 1994. Cons. (Med. Oncol.) Cromwell Hosp. Cromwell Rd. Lond.; Mem. Edit Bd. Seminars in Oncol.; Mem. Edit. Bd. Melanoma Research. Specialty: Oncol. Special Interest: Malig. Melanoma; Renal cancer. Socs: Fell. Roy. Soc. Med.; Amer. Soc. Clin. Oncol.; Brit. Assn. Cancer Phys. Prev: Cons. Med. Oncol. Char. Cross & Chelsea & Westm. Hosp. Lond.; Sen. Lect. (Med. Oncol.) & Hon. Cons. Phys. Westm. Med. Sch. Lond.; Sen. Ho. Phys. (Med. Oncol.) Roy. Marsden Hosp. Sutton.

RETTIE, George Kelly Cargill (retired) 58 Napier Court, Ranelagh Gardens, London SW6 3UX Tel: 020 7736 0921 Email: george.rettie@virgin.net — MB BS Lond. 1941 (Middlx.) MRCS Eng. LRCP Lond. 1941; MD Lond. 1948. Prev: Phys. Imperial Life Assur. Company of Canada.

RETTMAN, Christopher Department of Pathology, North Tees General Hospital, Hardwick, Stockton-on-Tees TS19 8PE Tel: 01642 617617 Fax: 01642 624116 — (Warsaw, Poland) Lekarz Warsaw 1966; MD Warsaw Med. Sch. 1975; FRCPath 1997, MRCPath 1986. Cons. Histopath. N. Tees HA. Specialty: Histopath. Socs: ACP; BMA; BSCC. Prev: Dept. Path. Inst. Paediat. Warsaw, Poland; Dept. Path. Univ. of Jos; Dept. Path. Newc. Gen. Hosp.

RETZLAW, Elsa 47 Rutland Court, Denmark Hill, London SE5 8ED — MD Vienna 1937. Prev: Med. Off. Epsom Co. Hosp. & St. Augustine's Hosp. Chartham Down.

REUBEN, Adam Dov 113 Kineton Green Road, Solihull B92 7DT — MB ChB Bristol 1997.

REUBEN, Joselle Raymond 99 Regal Way, Kenton, Harrow HA3 0SG — MB ChB Cape Town 1956.

REUBEN, Mark Jonathan Westcotes Health Centre, Fosse Road South, Leicester LE3 0LP Tel: 0116 254 1800 — MB BChir Camb. 1979; BSc Pharm. Lond. 1976; DRCOG 1983.

REUBEN, Simon Francis Beverley, Brimstage Road, Heswall, Wirral CH60 1XG — MB ChB Manch. 1990.

REUBIN, Richard David Cassio Surgery, 62-68 Merton Road, Watford WD18 0WL Tel: 01923 226011 Fax: 01923 817342 — MB ChB Birm. 1973. Specialty: Gen. Pract. Prev: Dir. Med. Servs. N.ants. FHSA; Ships Surg. P & O SN Company Lond.; Ho. Off. Birm. Gen. Hosp.

REUTER, Simone 12 Gladstone Road, Chesterfield S40 4TE — State Exam Med Frankfurt 1990.

REVEL, Jean-Claude Ananda Medwyn, Moores Road, Dorking RH4 2BG Tel: 01306 882422 — MB BS Mysore 1974; DObst. RCOG 1981. Med. Off. Harrowlands Rehabil. Unit Dorking; Clin. Asst. (Diabetes) Epsom Gen. Hosp. Socs: BMA. Prev: SHO (Med.) Dorking Gen. Hosp.; SHO (Obst.) Redhill Gen. Hosp.; SHO (A & E) E. Surrey Hosp. Redhill.

REVELEY, Adrianne (retired) 17 College Gardens, London SE21 7BE Tel: 020 8693 1602 Fax: 020 8299 6625 — MB BCh Dub. 1972; MA; FRCPsych 1989, M 1978. Prev: Private Pract. Medico-Legal.

REVELEY, Colette Helen 89 Oakfield Road, Gateshead NE11 0AD — MB ChB Leic. 1997.

REVELEY, Professor Michael August Neuropsychpharmacology Unit, University Department of Psychiatry, Leicester General Hospital, Leicester LE5 4PW Tel: 0116 225 7924 Fax: 0116 225 7925 Email: rev@le.ac.uk — (Southwestern Med. Sch.) BA Univ. Texas 1966; MD Univ. Texas 1970; FRCPsych 1989, M 1978; PhD Lond. 1988. Specialty: Gen. Psychiat. Socs: Brit. Assn. for Psychopharmacol.; Eur. Coll. Neuropsychopharm.; Collegium Internat. Neuropsychopharmacol. Prev: Sen. Lect. (Psychiat.) Lond. Hosp. Med. Coll. Lond. & Hon. Cons. (Psychiat.) Lond. Hosp.; Sen. Lect. (Psychiat.) Inst. Psychiat. Lond. & Hon. Cons. (Psychiat.) Bethlem Roy. & Maudsley Hosp. Lond.

REVELL, Vice Admiral Anthony Leslie, CB, Surg. Vice-Admiral (retired) Willow Cottage, Domum Road, Winchester SO23 9NN Tel: 01962 843002 — MB ChB Birm. 1959; DA Eng. 1965; FFA RCS Eng. 1969; Hon. MD Birm. 1996. Prev: Hon. Surg. to HM The Qu. (1992-97).

REVELL, Claire Pamela Brentford Health Centre, Albany Road, Brentford TW8 0NE Tel: 020 8568 0771; 47 Montholme Road, Battersea, London SW11 6HX Tel: 020 7228 8053 — MB BS Lond. 1985; DCH RCP Lond. 1987; DRCOG 1989; MRCGP 1991. Specialty: Obst. & Gyn.

REVELL, Edmund Western Sussex Primary Care Trust, The Bramber Building, 9 College Lane, Chichester PO19 6FX Tel: 01243 770770; 10 First Avenue, Havant PO9 2QN — MB BS Lond. 1973 (Westm.) BSc Lond. 1970. Salaried GP W. Sussex. Prev: GP Havant; Regist. (Anaesth.) Glos. Roy. Hosp. Gloucester; Regist. (Anaesth.) Roy. Berks. Hosp. Reading.

REVELL, Paul Graeme Staffordshire General Hospital, Department of Haematology, Weston Road, Stafford ST16 3SA Tel: 01785 257731 Ext: 4750 Fax: 01785 230749 Email: jayne.anslow@msgh-tr.wmids.nhs.uk — MB BS Lond. 1981 (Guy's) BSc Lond. 1978; MRCP (UK) 1984; DCH RCP Lond. 1986; MRCPath 1992; MRCPCH 1996; FRCPCH 1997; FRCPath 2000; FRCP 2003. Cons. Haemat. Mid Staffs. Gen. Hosp. Specialty: Haematology. Special Interest: Lymphoma; Myeloproliferative Disorders; Patient Information. Prev: Sen. Regist. Rotat. (Haemat.) W. Midl. RHA; Lect. (Haemat.) United Med. & Dent. Schs. Lond.

REVELL, Professor Peter Allen (retired) Department of Histopathology, Royal Free and University College Medical School, Rowland Hill St., London NW3 2PF Tel: 020 7794 0500 Fax: 020 7435 3289; 17 Willowdene Court, Warley, Brentwood CM14 5ET Email: prevell@eastman.ucl.ac.uk — (Lond. Hosp.) PhD Lond. 1973, BSc 1964; MB BS Lond. 1967; FRCPath 1988, M 1975. Prof. Dept. Histopath. Roy. Free & Univ. Coll. Med. Sch. Lond. Prev: Reader Inst. Path. Lond. Hosp.

REVESZ, Thomas Institute of Neurology, UCL, Division of Neuropathology, Queen Square, London WC1N 3BG Tel: 020 7837 3611 Fax: 020 7916 9546 Email: t.revesz@ion.ucl.ac.uk; Institute of Neurology UCL , Queen Square Brain Bank, Department of Molecular Neuroscience, Queen Square, London WC1N 3BG — MD Budapest 1972 (Semmelweis Med. Sch. Budapest) MRCpath 1990; FRCpath 1998. Prof. of Neuropath.; Hon. Cons. Nat. Hosp. Neurol. & Neurosurg. Lond. Specialty: Neuropath. Special Interest: Neurodegenerative diseases. Socs: British Neuropathological Society; American Association of Neuropathologists; International Society of Neuropathology. Prev: Sen. Regist. (Neuropath.) Maida Vale Hosp. Lond.; Reader in Neuropath.; Senior Lecturer,Inst. Neurology,London.

REVILL, Hugh The Dog Mills Cottages, Bride, Ramsey IM7 4AD Tel: 01624 814221 — MB ChB Glas. 1946. Socs: I. of Man Med. Soc. Prev: Med. Dir. St. Bridget's Hospice I. of Man; Ho. Phys. Glas. Roy. Infirm.

REVILL, John Greenhill Health Centre, 482 Lupton Road, Sheffield S8 7NQ Tel: 0114 237 2961; 212 Eckington Road, Coal Aston, Dronfield S18 3AZ Tel: Dronfield 412671 — MB BChir Camb. 1963 (St. Geo.) MA, MB Camb. 1963, BChir 1962; DObst RCOG 1964. Socs: Camb. Univ. Med. Soc.; Brit. Hyperlipidaemia Assn. & Medac (UK). Prev: Res. Obst. Asst., Ho. Phys. & Cas. Off. St. Geo. Hosp. Lond.

REVILL, Susan Irene Llygad Yr Haul, Mountain West, Newport SA42 0QX — MB BCh Wales 1987; PhD Wales 1980, MA 1973, MB BCh 1987.

REVINGTON, Mr Peter John, TD Department of Maxillofacial Surgery, Frenchay Hospital, Bristol BS16 1LE Tel: 0117 975 3997 Fax: 0117 918 6650 Email: peter.revington@north-bristol.swest.nhs.uk — MB BS Lond. 1991 (Char. cross/Westminster) BDS 1976; MScD Wales 1980; FDS RCS Eng 1981; FRCS Eng 1993. Cons. Maxillofacial Surg. Frenchay Hosp. Bristol; Hon. Sen. Lect., Univ. Bristol. Specialty: Oral & Maxillofacial Surg. Special Interest: Salivary Gland Dis.; Facial Deformity; Cleft Lip & Palate. Socs: BMA; Fell. Brit. Assn. Maxillofacial Surg. Prev: Sen. Regist. (Oral Surg.) King's Coll. Hosp. Lond.; Regist. Bristol Roy. Infirm. & Frenchay Hosp.; SHO (Gen. Surg.) Kingston Hosp. Kingston-upon-Thames.

REVOLTA, Alexander David Castle Place Surgery, 9 Park Hill, Tiverton EX16 6RR Tel: 01884 252333 Fax: 01884 252152 — MB ChB Ed. 1970; BSc Ed. 1968, MB ChB 1970; DObst RCOG 1973; DCH Eng. 1977; MRCGP 1982. GP Trainer Tiverton.

REW, Mr David Anthony, TD Southampton University Hospitals NHS Trust, Breast & Endocrine Unit, Southampton SO14 0YG Tel: 023 8082 5445 Fax: 023 8082 5148 Email: dr1@soton.ac.uk; Wessex Nuffield Hospital, Chandlers Ford, Southampton SO53 2DW Tel: 023 8025 8423 — MB BChir Camb. 1981 (Camb. & King's Coll. Hosp.) MA Camb. 1982; FRCS Eng. 1985; MChir 1991. Cons. Surg. Hon. Sen. Lect. Soton. Univ. Hosps.; Jt. Edr. Europ. Jl. Surgic. Oncol.; Nat. Sec., Brit. Assn. of Surgic. Oncol. 2000-2002. Specialty: Gen. Surg. Socs: Nat. Sec. Brit. Assn. Surg. Oncol.; Roy. Soc. Med. (Sect. Coloproctol.); Internat. Soc. Anal. Cytol. Prev: Dir. Leicester Laser Cytometry Facility Glenfield Univ. Hosp.; Sen. Lect. (Surg.) & Hon. Cons. Surg. Univ. Leicester; Sen. Regist. (Gen. Surg.) Soton. Univ. Hosp.

REW, Robert John Applegate, 10 Trump's Orchard, Cullompton EX15 1TW Tel: 01884 34096 Email: rjrew@aol.com — (Guy's) MRCS Eng. LRCP Lond. 1960; DObst RCOG 1962; DMJ(Clin) Soc. Apoth Lond. 1979. Non-Princip. Gen. Practitioner, Cullompton Area. Specialty: Gen. Pract.; Medico Legal. Socs: BMA. Prev: Div. Police Surg. Eastbourne; Clin. Asst. (Obst.) & SHO (O & G) W. Norf. & King's Lynn Gen. Hosp.; Ho. Surg. St. John's Hosp. Lewisham.

REWHORN, Ian David 51 Heron's Way, Selly Oak, Birmingham B29 6TR — MB ChB Dundee 1980; MRCP (UK) 1985.

REWILAK, Anna Teresa Eisner, Goldman and Ship, Shipley Health Centre, Alexandra Road, Shipley BD18 3EG Tel: 01274 589160 — MB BS Lond. 1984.

REX, Stephen Douglas Suilven, The Orpines, Wateringbury, Maidstone ME18 5BP — MB BS Lond. 1994 (Roy. Free Hosp. Lond.) BSc (Hons.) Lond. 1993, MB BS 1994; MRCP (UK) 1997. Specialist Regist. (Cardiol.) N W Thames. Specialty: Cardiol.

REY, Mr Charles Humphrey Jules (retired) Reyscourt, Rue Du Friquet, Castel GY5 7SS Tel: 01481 257980 — MB BS Lond. 1953 (Guy's) MRCS Eng. LRCP Lond. 1939; FRCS Eng. 1952. Prev: Surg. Princess Eliz. Hosp. Guernsey.

REYBURN, Hugh William 88 Copleston Road, London SE15 4AG — MB BS Lond. 1974; MRCP (UK) 1979; MSc (Community Med.) Lond. 1981; MRCGP 1985; DTM & H RCP Lond. 1995.

REYES, Mr Richard John The Department of Surgery, Queen Mary's Hospital, Frognal Avenue DA14 6LT Fax: 020 8302 2678 Email: rick.reyes@qms.nhs.uk — MB BS Lond. 1985 (Westm. Med. Sch.) FRCS Eng. 1989; FRCS 1989; FRCS (Gen.) 2001; MS 2003. Cons. Breast & Gen. Surg.; SpR N. Thames. Specialty: Gen. Surg. Special Interest: Upper GI Surg.; Varcose Veins. Socs: Roy. Soc. Med.; Brit. Assn. Of Surgic. Oncol.; The Assn. of Surg. of Gt. Britain and Irel.

REYNARD, Amanda Jane 3 Greenmount Lane, Heaton, Bolton BL1 5JF — MB ChB Liverp. 1984.

REYNARD, Anthony Laurence (retired) 36 Church Lane, Eaton, Norwich NR4 6NY Tel: 01603 452504 — MRCS Eng. LRCP Lond. 1939 (King's Coll. & Westm.) DA Eng. 1949; FRCA Eng. 1953; Cert. Av. Med. 1972. Prev: Cons. Anaesth. United Norwich Hosps.

REYNARD, John Michael Department of Urology, 4th Floor Alexandra Wing, The Royal London Hospital, PO Box 59, London E1 1BB; Rosemary, Hardwick Road, Whitchurch on Thames, Reading RG8 7HH — MB BS Lond. 1987.

REYNARD, Kevin 9 Beech Walk, Adel, Leeds LS16 8NY — MB ChB Leeds 1987.

REYNARD, Timothy James Wilkinson Stable Cottage, Broad Lane, Newdigate, Dorking RH5 5AT — MB BS Lond. 1989.

REYNELL, Peter Carew 12 Park View Road, Bradford BD9 4PA Tel: 01274 546585 — BM BCh Oxf. 1942; FRCP Lond. 1962, M 1947; DM Oxf. 1951. Cons. Phys. Roy. Infirm. & St. Luke's Hosp. Bradford. Specialty: Gen. Med. Socs: Assn. Phys. Gt. Brit. & Brit. Cardiac Soc. Prev: Med. Tutor Radcliffe Infirm. Oxf.; Rockefeller Trav. Fell. Clin. Med.; Graded Phys. RAMC.

REYNER, Lindsay Jill Toddington Medical Centre, Luton Road, Toddington, Dunstable LU5 6DE Tel: 01525 872222 Fax: 01525 876711; 38 Park Mount, Harpenden AL5 3AR Tel: 01582 462808 — MB BS Lond. 1985 (Univ. Coll. Lond.) DRCOG 1988. GP. Specialty: Gen. Pract. Prev: GP Harpenden.

REYNISH, Emma Louise Preston Patrick Hall, Milnthorpe LA7 7NY Tel: 015395 67200 — MB BCh Wales 1992; MRCP (UK) 1995. SpR (GIM/Gastroenterology) West. Gen. Hosp. Edin. Specialty: Gastroenterol.

REYNOLDS, Mrs Anita 5 Kellett Mount, Leeds LS12 4AJ — MB BS Lond. 1989 (Middlx. & Univ. Coll. Lond.) MRCOphth 1993; FRCOphth 1995; MMedSci 1997. Specialist Regist. Rotat. (Ophth.) W. Midl. Specialty: Ophth. Socs: Roy. Soc. Med.; BMA.

REYNOLDS, Ann Lea (retired) 24 Christchurch Close, Edgbaston, Birmingham B15 3NE Tel: 0121 454 4680 — MB ChB Birm. 1949; FRCS Ed. 1957; FRCOG 1972, M 1959. Prev: Cons. O & G Dudley Rd. Hosp. Birm.

REYNOLDS, Anthony Douglas West Lodge, West Drive, Sudbrooke, Lincoln LN2 2RA — MB BCh Wales 1972; FFA RCS Eng. 1978. Cons. Anaesth. Co. Hosp. Lincoln. Specialty: Anaesth.

REYNOLDS, Carol Ann Brent Area Medical Centre, Anvil House, Brent Road, Highbridge TA9 4JD Tel: 01278 760313 Fax: 01278 760753 — BM Soton. 1983; DRCOG 1987; MRCGP 1989. Prev: Trainee GP Weston-Super-Mare VTS.

REYNOLDS, Caroline Dagmar — MB BS Newc. 1998.

REYNOLDS, Christopher Michael Norfolk & Waveny Mental Health Partnership NHS Trust, Hellesdon Hospital, Norwich NR6 5BE Tel: 01603 421421 Fax: 01603 421563 Email: chris.reynolds@nwmhp.nhs.uk; South Barn, Sea Palling Road, Ingham, Norwich NR12 0TW — MB BS Lond. 1969 (Roy. Free) MRCS Eng. LRCP Lond. 1969; DObst RCOG 1972; DPM Eng. 1973; FRCPsych 1993, M 1975. Cons. Psychiat. Hellesdon Hosp. Norwich. Specialty: Gen. Psychiat. Prev: Sen. Regist. (Psychiat.) St. Geo. Hosp. Lond. & W. Pk. Hosp. Epsom; Regist. (Psychiat.) Friern Hosp. Lond.

REYNOLDS, Clare Elizabeth Hudson Drive, Health Centre, Hudson Drive, Burntwood WS7 Tel: 01543 674477 — MB BS Lond. 1989 (St Bartholomews) DRCOG 1993; DFFP 1993; MRCGP 1994. Socs: BMA.

REYNOLDS, Colin Peter (retired) Serjeant Bendlowes Cottage, Brook St., Great Bardfield, Braintree CM7 4RQ Tel: 01371 810515 — MB BS Lond. 1961 (Lond. Hosp.) DObst RCOG 1964; DMRD Eng. 1977; FRCR 1979. Prev: Sen. Regist. Radio-diag. Dept. & Ho. Surg. Lond. Hosp.

REYNOLDS, Darren 3 Pallotine Walk, Beechwood Gardens, Rochdale OL11 4LS Tel: 01706 341707 — MB ChB Manch. 1993; MRCPsych 1998. Specialist Regist. Dual trainee in Gen. & Old Age Psychiat. Specialty: Gen. Psychiat.; Geriat. Psychiat.

REYNOLDS, Mr David Arturo (retired) — MB BS Lond. 1960 (Guy's) MRCS Eng. LRCP Lond. 1960; FRCS Eng. 1965. Prev: Emerit. Cons. Orthop. Surg. Guys St. Thomas NHS Trust, Lond.

REYNOLDS, David Farmer (retired) 5 Woodbury Close, Leigh-on-Sea SS9 4QT Tel: 01702 521313 — (Univ. Coll. Hosp.) MB BS Lond. 1945; DMRD Eng. 1950; FFR 1956; FRCR 1975. Prev: Cons. Radiol. Southend Hosp. Southend on Sea.

REYNOLDS, David John Morton The John Radcliffe, Oxford Radcliffe Trust, Headley Way, Oxford OX3 9DU Tel: 01865 220964 Fax: 01865 220972 — BM BCh Oxf. 1981 (Oxford) DPhil Oxf. 1994, BM BCh 1981; MA Camb. 1981; MRCP (UK) 1984; FRCP 1998. Cons. Clin. Pharmacol. & Gen. Phys. Oxf. Radcliffe Trust; Hon. Sen. Clin. Lect. (Clin. Pharmacol.) Univ. Oxf. Specialty: Pharmacology. Prev: Clin. Lect. (Clin. Pharmacol.) Univ. Oxf.

REYNOLDS, Dorothy Jean Newmarket Medical Practice, 153 Newmarket, Louth LW11 9EH Tel: 01507 603121 Fax: 01507 605916; 2 Crowtree Lane, Louth LN11 9LN Tel: 01507 603309 — MD Manch. 1991; MB ChB 1974; DRCOG 1977; DCH Eng. 1977.

REYNOLDS, E. Mark R. Reynold, MBE Stockett Lane Surgery, 3 Stockett Lane, Coxheath, Maidstone ME17 4PS Tel: 01622 745585 Fax: 01622 741987 Email: edward.reynolds@gp-g82024.nhs.uk — MB BS Lond. 1981 (St Thomas) BSc Lond. 1978; DRCOG 1983; MRCGP 1993; DCH 1993. GP Princip. Specialty: Gen. Pract. Socs: Chairm. Nat. Assn. of GP coOperat.s; Med. Director Assn. of Maidstone, Doctors on Call (MAIDDOC). Prev: GP Tutor.

REYNOLDS, Edward Henry King's College, Institute of Epileptology, Weston Education Centre, Denmark Hill Campus, Cutcombe Road, London SE5 6PJ Tel: 020 7848 5756 Fax: 020 7848 5530; Buckles, Yew Tree Bottom Road, Epsom Downs KT17 3NQ Tel: 01737 360867 Fax: 01737 363415 — MB BCh Wales 1959 (Cardiff) MRCS Eng. LRCP Lond. 1959; FRCP Lond. 1980, M 1963; MD Wales 1969; FRCPsych 1985. Cons. Neurol. & Hon. Sen. Lect. Guy's, King's & St Thos. Sch. Med. Lond. Specialty: Neurol. Special Interest: Epilepsy and Neuropsychiatry. Socs: (Past Pres) Brit.Chapter Internat. League Against Epilepsy;; Internat. League Against Epilepsy (Past Pres.); The Fund for Epilepsy (Past Chair). Prev: Regist. Nat. Hosp. Nerv. Dis. Lond. & MRC Neuropsychiat. Research Unit Carshalton; Vis. Asst. Prof. Neurol. Yale Univ. Med. Sch. New Haven USA; Chairm. Centre for Epilepsy Maudsley Hosp. Lond.

REYNOLDS, Professor Edward Osmund Royle, CBE (retired) Department of Paediatrics, University College London, Rayne Institute, University St., London WC1E 6JJ; 72 Barrowgate Road, London W4 4QU Tel: 020 8994 3326 Email: reynolds@dircon.co.uk — MB BS Lond. 1958 (St. Thos.) DCH Eng. 1961; BSc Lond. 1955, MD 1966; FRCP Lond. 1975, M 1966; FRCOG (ad eundem) 1983; FRS 1993; FRCPCH (Hons.) 1997; FMedSci (Founder) 1998. p/t Emerit. Prof. Neonat. Paediat. Univ. Coll. Lond.; Emerit. Cons. Paediat. Univ. Coll. Hosp. Lond. Prev: Prof. Neonat. Paediat. Univ. Coll. Lond.

REYNOLDS, Elizabeth Ruth 95 Cinderhill Lane, Scholar Green, Stoke-on-Trent ST7 3HR Tel: 01782 782872; 6 Sycamore Grove, Sandbach CW11 1PJ — MB ChB Birm. 1986; DCH RCP Lond. 1990. Specialty: Gen. Pract.

REYNOLDS, Professor Felicity Jane Morten (retired) St Thomas' Hospital, Department of Anaesthetics, London SE1 7EH Tel: 020 7188 0627 Email: felicity.reynolds@btinternet.com; 40 Cleaver Square, London SE11 4EA Tel: 020 7735 9357 — MB BS Lond. 1960 (St. Thos.) FRCA 1963; MD Lond. 1971; FRCOG (ad eundem) 1995. Prev: Prof. Obst. Anaesth. United Med. & Dent. Sch. & Hon. Cons. Anaesth. St. Thos. Hosp. Lond.

REYNOLDS, George Morton (retired) 131 Abergwili Road, Carmarthen SA31 2HG — BSc, MB BCh Wales 1948; DPH Eng. 1952; FFCM 1978, M 1974. Prev: Chief Admin. Med. Off. & Dir. Pub. Health Med. E. Dyfed HA.

REYNOLDS, Gerald Martin 115 Broomlands Road, Cumbernauld, Glasgow G67 2PT — MB ChB Dundee 1992.

REYNOLDS, Godfrey Alexander Market Cross Surgery, 7 Market Place, Mildenhall, Bury St Edmunds IP28 7EG Tel: 01638 713109 Fax: 01638 718615; Horne Lea, The St, Barton Mills, Bury St Edmunds IP28 6AA Tel: 01638 510241 — MB ChB Birm. 1983; BSc (Hons.) Physiol. Birm. 1980, MB ChB 1983; DRCOG 1988;

MRCGP 1989. Socs: BMA; RCGP. Prev: SHO Rotat. (Med.) Selly Oak Hosp. Birm.; Trainee GP/SHO E. Birm. Hosp. VTS.

REYNOLDS, Graham Collis Stephen Priory Fields Surgery, Nursery Road, Huntingdon PE29 3RL Tel: 01480 52361 Fax: 01480 434640 — MB BS Durh. 1966 (Durh. & Newc.) T(GP) 1990. Treas. Huntsdoc (GP Night Co-op); Clin. Asst. (Cas.) Hinchingbrooke Hosp. Huntingdon; Asst. Police Surg. Camb. Constab; Med. Adviser Camb. Amateur Gymnastics Assn. Prev: Chairm. Huntingdon GP Forum; Hon. Vis. Phys. Centr. Gippsland Hosp., Austral.; Clin. Asst. (Obst.) Matern. Unit Primrose La. Hosp. Huntingdon.

REYNOLDS, Gregory William 62 Gledhow wood Grove, Leeds LS8 1PA Tel: 0113 392 2185 — MB BS Lond. 1979; FRCP UK. Cons. Cardiol. Leeds Gen. Infirm. Specialty: Cardiol.

REYNOLDS, Mr Ian Stuart Russell Mouse Castle, Old Eign Hill, Hereford HR1 1TU Tel: 01432 69111 Fax: 01432 263499 — MB BChir Camb. 1969 (St. Thos.) MRCS Eng. LRCP Lond. 1968; MA Camb. 1969; FRCS Ed. 1974; FRCS Eng. 1975. Cons. Orthop. Surg. Hereford Gen. & Co. Hosps. Specialty: Orthop. Socs: Brit. Orthop. Assn. & BMA. Prev: Sen. Regist. (Orthop.) Birm. AHA (T) & Coventry & Warks. Hosp.; SHO (Orthop.) Rowley Bristow Orthop. Hosp. Pyrford.

REYNOLDS, Jeffrey Hugh 8 Forge Row, Saleyard Bridge, Gilwern, Abergavenny NP7 0HA — MRCS Eng. LRCP Lond. 1971.

REYNOLDS, Jennifer Heather Kendrick Surgery, 10 Kendrick Road, Sutton Coldfield B76 1EG Tel: 0121 351 2020 Fax: 0121 351 7987; 90 Orchard Road, Erdington, Birmingham B24 9JD — MB ChB Birm. 1978; DRCOG 1980; MRCGP 1982.

REYNOLDS, Jeremy James 3 Broomlands, Wirral CH60 6TF — MB ChB Bristol 1997.

REYNOLDS, John Beresford (retired) Alexandra Cottage, Dog Lane, Chlidrey, Wantage OX12 9UW — MRCS Eng. LRCP Lond. 1957 (Char. Cross) BA Camb. 1954.

REYNOLDS, John Clifford Lutterworth Health Centre, Gilmorton Road, Lutterworth LE17 4EB Tel: 01455 553531 — MB BS Lond. 1978; BSc (Biol.) (1st cl. Hons.) Sussex 1973. Clin. Asst. (Ophth.) Leics. Roy. Infirm.

REYNOLDS, John Cyril Citisport House, The Chackpit, College Road, Epsom KT17 4JA Tel: 01372 743166 Fax: 01372 743538; 40 Bunbury, Epsom KT17 4JP Tel: 01372 741939 — MB BS Lond. 1975 (Royal Free Hospital School of Medicine) MRCS Eng. LRCP Lond. 1975; MRCP (UK) 1985. Orthop. Phys. Breakspear Clinic Milton-under-Wychwood & 30A Wimpole St. Lond.; Cons. Rehabil. Med. to Metrop. Police; Cons. Sports Med. Princess Margt. Hosp. Windsor; Cons. Rheum. To Mid Surrey PCG. Specialty: Rheumatol.; Rehabil. Med.; Sports Med. Socs: Fell. Inst. Sports Med.; (Past Chairm). Brit. Med. Acupunc. Soc. Prev: Specialist (Rehabil. & Rheum.) RAF MRU Headley Ct. Surrey.; Med. Dir. Brit. Paralympic Assn.

REYNOLDS, John Francis (retired) 51 Princes Road, Wimbledon, London SW19 8RA Tel: 020 8542 2827; 4 Hillview, London SW20 0TA Tel: 0208 946 2779 — MRCS Eng. LRCP Lond. 1963 (St. Mary's) Prev: G.P. Trainer S.W.Thames.

REYNOLDS, John Haydn Department of Radiology, Birmingham Heartlands Hospital, Bordesley Green E., Birmingham B9 5ST Tel: 0121 766 6611 Fax: 0121 766 6919; 51 Glendon Way, Dorridge, Solihull B93 8SY Tel: 01564 775059 — MB ChB Manch. 1983; DMRD Aberd. 1989; FRCR 1991; T(R)(CR) 1992. Cons. Diag. Radiol. Birm. Heartlands & Solihull NHS Trust (Teachg.). Specialty: Radiol. Socs: Roy. Coll. Radiol.; Assn. Chest Radiologists. Prev: Sen. Regist. Rotat. (Diag. Radiol.) W. Midl. Train. Scheme; Regist. (Diag. Radiol.) Aberd. Roy. Infirm.; SHO (Gen. Med.) N. Manch. Gen. Hosp.

REYNOLDS, Mr Jonathan Richard Southern Derbyshire Acute Hospital Trust, Derbyshire Royal Infirmary, London Road, Derby DE1 2QY Tel: 01332 347141 Ext: 2038 Email: jrreynold@rcsed.ac.uk; The Tower, Hob Hill, Hazelwood, Belper DE56 4AL Tel: 01332 842898 Email: jrreynolds@rcsed.ac.uk — MB ChB Dundee 1978; FRCS Eng. 1982; FRCS Ed. 1982; DM Nottm. 1988. Cons. Colorectal Surg., Derby; Lead Clinician Derby Cancer Centre. Specialty: Gen. Surg. Special Interest: Coloproctology; paediatric Surg. Socs: Assn. Coloproctol.; Derby Med. Soc.; Amer. Soc. Colon & Rectal Surgeons. Prev: Serv. Director for Surg., South. Derbysh. Acute Hosp.s Trust; Sen. Regist. (Surg.) Nottm. & Derby; Regist. (Surg.) Derbysh. Roy. Infirm.

REYNOLDS, Joseph M Cornmarket Surgery, Newry Health Village, Monaghan Street, Newry BT35 6BW — MB BCh BAO NUI 1979; MRCGP 1984. GP Newry.

REYNOLDS, Karen Anne Child Development Centre, University Hospital of North Staffordshire, Newcastle Road, Stoke-on-Trent ST4 6QG — MB BS Lond. 1981; DRCOG 1984; MRCGP 1985; DCH RCP Lond. 1985; MRCP (UK) 1991; FRCPCH 1997. Cons. Community Paediat. N. Staffs. Hosp. Trust. Specialty: Paediat.

REYNOLDS, Karen Neilson 43 Brechin Road, Bishopsbriggs, Glasgow G64 1BH — MB ChB Glas. 1989.

REYNOLDS, Kate Margaret Dunchurch Surgery, Dunsmore Heath, Dunchurch, Rugby CV22 6AP Tel: 01788 522448 Fax: 01788 814609 — BM BS Nottm. 1994; MRCGP 1999. Gen. Practitioner Princip. Socs: Roy. Coll. of Gen. Practitioners; BMA.

REYNOLDS, Kathleen Margaret Mary (Karina) The Department of Obstetrics, Gynaecology and Reproductive Healthcare, St Mary's Hospital, Whitworth Park, Manchester M13 0JH Tel: 0161 276 6278 Fax: 0161 276 6134; Brooklands, 446 Hale Road, Hale Barns, Altrincham WA15 8XR — MB BCh BAO Dub. 1982; MRCOG 1988; FRCS Ed. 1991. Sen. Lect., Gyn. Oucology, Univ.of Manch.; Hon Cons. Gun. Oncol., St. Mary's & Clinstie Hosp. Manch. Specialty: Obst. & Gyn. Socs: Brit. Gyn. Cancer Soc.; Brit. Assoc. of Cancer Research; BMA. Prev: Fell. in Gyn. Oucology Universties of Toronto & Nu Master, Ontario, Canada. 1994-1996.

REYNOLDS, Kevin Vaughan St Mary's Surgery, 1johnson Street, St Mary's, Southampton SO14 1LT Tel: 023 8033 3778 Fax: 023 8021 1894 — BM Soton. 1988; DRCOG 1990; DGM RCP Lond. 1991; MRCGP 1992.

REYNOLDS, Linda June The Brooke Surgery, 20 Market Street, Hyde SK14 1AT Tel: 0161 368 3312 Fax: 0161 268 5670; 19 Peel Moat Road, Heaton Moor, Stockport SK4 4PL — MB ChB Manch. 1974. Specialty: Gen. Pract.

REYNOLDS, Lucy Jane — BM BS Nottm. 1989; DTM & H RCP Lond. 1992; MRCP (UK) 1994; MSc Lond. 2001. Consultant Paediatrician. Specialty: Paediat. Socs: Roy. Coll. Paediat. & Child Health; Fell. Roy. Soc. Trop. Med. & Hyg.; Child Pub. Health Interest Gp. Prev: Specialist Regist. (Paediat. IC) St. Mary's Hosp. Lond.; SpR (Community Paeds) Roy. Hamp. Co. Hosp., Winchester.; SpR (Community Paeds.) E+ N Herts.

REYNOLDS, Margaret Mary The Medical Centre, Hadlow Old School, School Lane, Hadlow, Tonbridge TN11 0ET Tel: 01732 850248; Little Spitzbrook, Collier St, Tonbridge TN12 9RB Tel: 0189273 291 — (Roy. Free) MRCS Eng. LRCP Lond. 1965; MRCGP 1987. Specialty: Gen. Pract. Prev: Clinic Med. Off. Family Plann. Servs. Kent AHA.

REYNOLDS, Mari Wyn Morden Hall Medical Centre, 256 Morden Road, London SW19 3DA Tel: 020 8540 0585 — MB BS Lond. 1985; DRCOG 1989; Dip. Pract. Dermat. Wales 1992.

REYNOLDS, Martin Francis 10 Duns Crescent, Wishaw ML2 8SF — MB ChB Glas. 1980; DRCOG 1987; MRCGP 1988; DAvMed FOM RCP Lond. 1990.

REYNOLDS, Martin Richard Finch (retired) Knights Cottage, Callas, Bishop Burton, Beverley HU17 8QL Tel: 01964 550276 — MB ChB Bristol 1966; DPH Bristol 1969; FFCM RCP (UK) 1980, M 1974; FFPHM RCP (UK) 1989; FRCP Lond. 1996. Prev: Assoc. Dir. Health Policy & Pub. Health E. Riding HA.

REYNOLDS, Mary Angela Ladycroft, 118 Marsh Lane, Mill Hill, London NW7 4PE Tel: 020 8906 1401 — MB BS Lond. 1963 (Char. Cross) FBIM 1979. Asst. Gen. Manager, Chief Underwriter & Chief Med. Off. Canada Life Assur. Co.; Chairm. Med Affairs Panel, Life Offices Assn. Socs: Fell. Roy. Soc. Med.; (Pres.) Assur. Med. Soc.; BMA. Prev: Med Adviser Amer. Embassy, Lond.; Ho. Surg. & Ho. Phys. St. Nicholas Hosp. Lond; Ho. Phys. Whittington Hosp. Lond.

REYNOLDS, Maureen Teresa Leeds Student Medical Practice, 4 Blenheim Court, Blenheim Walk, Leeds LS2 9AH Tel: 0113 295 4488 Fax: 0113 295 4499; 23 Shire Oak Road, Headingley, Leeds LS6 2DD Tel: 0113 275 4689 — MB ChB Bristol 1979; BSc (Physiol. Biochem.) Soton. 1974; DRCOG 1982; Dip. GU Med. Soc. Apoth. Lond. 1991; MRCP (UK) 1994. Gen. Practitioner, Leeds Stud. Med. Pract. Prev: Cons. Genitourin. Med. Leeds Gen. Infirm.

REYNOLDS, Michael Anthony Buxton Health Centre, Bath Road, Buxton SK17 6HH Tel: 01298 79251; 21 Lansdowne Road, Buxton SK17 6RR Tel: 01298 23376 — MB ChB Sheff. 1976 (Sheffield)

MRCP (UK) 1979; FRCP (Lond.) 1997; FRCPCH 1997. Cons. Community Paediat. N. Derbysh. HA. Specialty: Community Child Health. Socs: Fell. Roy. Coll. Paediat. & Child Health; Brit. Assn. Community Child Health; BACCH. Prev: SCMO Halton HA; Regist. (Paediat.) Liverp. HA.

REYNOLDS, Muriel Primrose (retired) The White House, The Heath, East Malling, West Malling ME19 6JL Tel: 01732 842549 — MB BS Lond. 1949. Prev: GP.

REYNOLDS, Neil George Yarm Medical Centre, 1 Worsall Road, Yarm TS15 9DD Tel: 01642 786422 Fax: 01642 785617 — MB ChB Leeds 1976; DRCOG 1979.

REYNOLDS, Nicholas John 1st Floor Flat, Kirkness House, 11 Edward St., Bathwick, Bath BA2 4DU — MB ChB Bristol 1994.

REYNOLDS, Professor Nicholas John Department Dermatology, Medical School, University of Newcastle Upon Tyne, Newcastle upon Tyne NE2 4HH Tel: 0191 222 8936 Email: n.j.reynolds@ncl.ac.uk — MB BS Lond. 1983 (Charing Cross Hospital Medical School) MRCP (UK) 1985; BSc Lond. 1980, MD 1995; FRCP 1999. Specialty: Dermat. Socs: Comm. Mem. Brit. Soc. for Investigative Dermat. 1997-2003; Chairm. Brit. Soc. for Investigative Dermat. 2000-2003. Prev: Sen. Regist. (Dermat.) Roy. Vict. Infirm. Newc.; Regist. Fell. & Lect. (Dermat.) Univ. Michigan, USA; Regist. (Dermat.) Bristol Roy. Infirm.

REYNOLDS, Nicholas John 46A Trevor Road, West Bridgford, Nottingham NG2 6FT — MB ChB Leeds 1995.

REYNOLDS, Nicholas Mark Temple House Surgery, Temple House, Temple Street, Keynsham, Bristol BS31 1EJ Tel: 0117 986 2406 Fax: 0117 986 5695 — MB BCh Wales 1987; DCH RCP Lond. 1991; MRCGP 1992; Dip. Ther. Wales 1998. Specialty: Gen. Pract.

REYNOLDS, Nigel Ninewells Hospital, Dundee DD1 9SY; The Peah House, Easter Ballindean, Inchture, Perth PH14 9QS — MB ChB Dundee 1989; MRCP Glas. 1993. Cons. Gastroenterology Ninewells Hosp. Dundee. Specialty: Gastroenterol.; Gen. Med.

REYNOLDS, Patricia Ann Department of Oral & Maxillofacial Surgery, Dental Institute, King's College Hospital, Denmark Hill, London SE5 9RW Tel: 020 7346 3474 Fax: 020 7346 3754 — MB BS Lond. 1984 (UMDS Guy's Hospital) BDS Lond. 1977; FDS RCS Eng. 1986; PhD Lond. 1996. Sen. Lect. (Oral. & Maxillofacial Surg.) King's Coll. Lond. Specialty: Oral & Maxillofacial Surg. Socs: Hon. Sec. Craniofacial Soc. GB; Brit. Assn. of Oral & Maxillofacial Surg.s; Univ. Teach.s Oral & Maxillofacial Surg. Prev: Lect. (Oral & Maxillofacial Surg.) King's Coll. Lond.; Regist. (Oral Med. & Oral Surg.) Guy's Hosp. Lond.

REYNOLDS, Patricia Marianne (retired) Eye Department, Kings College Hospital, Denmark Hill, London SE5 9RS — (King's Coll. Hosp.) MB BS Lond. 1963; MRCS Eng. LRCP Lond. 1963; DO Eng. 1965; AMQ 1968; MRCOphth 1989. Prev: Hon. Lect. & Assoc. Specialist (Ophth.) King's Coll. Hosp. Sch. of Med. & Dent. Lond.

REYNOLDS, Paul Dominic 5 Kellett Mount, Leeds LS12 4AJ — MB BS Lond. 1986; MRCP (UK) 1990. Specialist Regist. (Gastroenterol.) W. Yorks. Rotat. Specialty: Gastroenterol. Prev: Research Regist. (Gastroenterol.) Addenbrooke's Hosp. Camb.

REYNOLDS, Paul Jonathan Maidstone and Tunbridge Wells NHS Trust, Pembury Hospital, Pembury, Tunbridge Wells TN2 4QJ Tel: 01892 823535 — MB BS Lond. 1985; BSc (Hons.) Lond. 1982; FRCP Ed. 1996; FRCP Lond. 1998. Cons. Phys. (Med. for Elderly) Pembury Hosp. Tunbridge Wells. Specialty: Care of the Elderly; Gen. Med. Prev: Sen. Regist. (Gen. Med.) Soton. Univ. Hosps.; Sen. Regist. (Gen. Med.) Bournemouth & ChristCh. Hosps.; Regist. (Gen. Med.) Basingstoke Gen. Hosp.

REYNOLDS, Paul Joseph 27a Buxton Gardens, Acton, London W3 9LF — MB BS Lond. 1992.

REYNOLDS, Peter Maxwell Gore 3 Alloway Park, Ayr KA7 2AW Tel: 01292 262730 Email: peter@psreynolds.demon.co.uk — (Westm.) MB BChir Camb. 1970; MA Camb. 1971; MRCP (UK) 1973; FRCP Glas. 1983. Cons. Phys. (Gen. Med. & Rheum.) The Ayr Hosp. Specialty: Gen. Med.; Rheumatol. Socs: Brit. Soc. Rheum.; Scott. Soc. Phys.; BMA. Prev: Sen. Regist. Leicester Roy. Infirm.; Regist. Aberd. Roy. Infirm. & Centre for Rheum. Dis. Glas.

REYNOLDS, Peter Robert 44 Arundel Road, Kingston upon Thames KT1 3RZ Tel: 020 8942 7102 — MB BS Lond. 1990 (St. Barths.) MRCGP 1993; DRCOG 1993; MRCP (Paediat.) (UK) 1997. Paediat. Specialist Regist. (N. Thames). Specialty: Neonat.

REYNOLDS, Philip Alfred Phoenix Surgery, 9 Chesterton Lane, Cirencester GL7 1XG — MB BS Lond. 1984; BSc Lond. 1981; MRCGP 1989; DRCOG 1990; (Dip. Trav. Med.) Royal Free Hosp. 1999. Clin. Asst. Dermat. Cirencester Hosp. Socs: Christ. Med. Fellowsh.; BMA; ISTM. Prev: Trainee GP Dorset VTS; SHO (Psychiat., A & E, Orthop. & Dermat.) E. Dorset HA; SHO (O & G) Shoreham.

REYNOLDS, Philip Arthur Padgate Medical Centre, 12 Station Road South, Padgate, Warrington WA2 0RX Tel: 01925 815333 Fax: 01925 813650 — MB ChB Manch. 1986; DRCOG 1989; MRCGP 1990. Specialty: Gen. Med.

REYNOLDS, Rachel 9 Alexandra Road, Colwyn Bay LL29 7YB — BM BS Nottm. 1978.

REYNOLDS, Rebecca Mary MRC EE Unit, Southampton University Hospital NHS Trust, Tremona Road, Southampton SO16 6YD Tel: 023 8077 7624; The Coach House, Bicclescombe Pk Road, Ilfracombe EX34 8EU Tel: 01271 863686 — BM BCh Oxf. 1992; MA Oxf. 1989; MRCP (UK) 1995. Research Fell. (Med. Research Counc.) Soton. Univ. Hosps. Specialty: Gen. Med. Socs: Med. Defence Union; BMA. Prev: Regist. (Med.) Soton. Univ. Hosps.; SHO (Med.) Soton. Univ. Hosps.; Ho. Off. (Surg.) Oxf.

REYNOLDS, Robert Hugh (retired) White Briars, Slinfold, Horsham RH13 7RR Tel: 01403 790348 — MB BChir Camb. 1951 (Middlx.) DObst RCOG 1953; FRCGP 1982, M 1963; MA Camb. 1982. Prev: Nuffield Foundat. Trav. Fell. For GPs. 1964.

REYNOLDS, Mr Robert John 85A Pilton Street, Barnstaple EX31 1PQ Tel: 01271 372178 — MB ChB Ed. 1974; FRCS Eng. 1980. Specialty: Ophth.; Gen. Surg.; Pub. Health Med.

REYNOLDS, Mr Robert Philip The Health Centre, Queensway, Billingham TS23 2LA Tel: 01642 554967; 10 Crooks Barn Lane, Norton, Stockton-on-Tees TS20 1LW — MB ChB Sheff. 1975; FRCS Eng. 1981; MRCGP 1991.

REYNOLDS, Sally May Luther Street Primary Care Ltd, Luther Street, PO Box 7, Oxford OX1 1TD Tel: 01865 726008 Fax: 01865 204133 — MB ChB Bristol 1972; BA Camb. 1969. Med. Dir. Luther St. Med. Centre for Homeless Oxf.

REYNOLDS, Sarah Elizabeth Farrow Medical Centre, 117 Otley Road, Bradford BD3 0HX — MB ChB Leeds 1997; MRCGP.

REYNOLDS, Mrs Sarah Frances Cygnet Wing, Bedford Hospital South Wing, Kempston Road, Bedford MK42 9DJ Tel: 01234 355122 Fax: 01234 795782 Email: sarah.reynolds@bedhos.anglox.nhs.uk — MB BS Lond. 1988; MRCOG 1995. Cons. (O & G) Bedford Hosp. Bedford. Specialty: Obst. & Gyn. Prev: Research Fell. (Urogyn.) St. Geo. Hosp. Lond.; SpR. (O & G) St. Thomas W. Region.

REYNOLDS, Sheila Mary 4 Birchtree Close, Bowdon, Altrincham WA14 3PP Tel: 0161 928 7131 — MB ChB Manch. 1951.

REYNOLDS, Thomas Joseph UCLMS, Department of Psychiatry & Behavioural Sciences, 2nd Floor Woolfson Building, 48 Riding House St., London W1N 8AA Tel: 020 7323 1459 Email: t.reynolds@ucl.ac.uk; 59 Barry Road, London SE22 0HR — MB BCh BAO NUI 1988 (Univ. Coll. Galway) MMedSci NUI 1993; MRCPsych 1996. Clin. Research Fell. & Hon. Specialist Regist. (Psychiat. Elderly) UCLMS. Specialty: Geriat. Psychiat.

REYNOLDS, Timothy David Richard The Malthouse Surgery, The Charter, Abingdon OX14 3JY Tel: 01235 524001 Fax: 01235 532197 — MB ChB Bristol 1972; DObst RCOG 1974; MRCGP 1978.

REYNOLDS, Timothy Henry 417 Weedon Road, Duston, Northampton NN5 4EX — MB ChB Manch. 1969.

REYNOLDS, Professor Timothy Mark Queen's Hospital, Clinical Chemistry Department, Belvedere Road, Burton-on-Trent DE13 0RB Tel: 01283 511511 Ext: 4035 Fax: 01283 593064 Email: tim.reynolds@burtonh-tr.wmids.nhs.uk — MB ChB Leeds 1984; FACB 2001; MRCPath 1991; BSc (Hons.) Leeds 1981, MD 1994; FRCP (Path) 2000. Cons. Chem Path. Qu.s Hosp., Burton on Trent; Prof. Chem. Pathol. Wolverhampton Univ. Specialty: Chem. Path. Special Interest: Screening. Socs: Assn. Clin. Biochem.s (Reg. Vice Chairm.); Assn. Clin. Path. (Vice Chairm. Clin. Chem. SAC). Prev: Sen. Regist. (Chem. Path.) Univ. Hosp. Wales & Roy. Gwent Hosp. Newport; Regist. Rotat. (Chem. Path.) W. Midl.

REYNOLDS, Valerie Joan (retired) Serjeant Bendlowes Cottage, 5 Brook St, Great Bardfield, Braintree CM7 4RQ Tel: 01371 810515 — MB BS Lond. 1961 (Lond. Hosp.) MRCS Eng. LRCP Lond. 1961;

Dip. Ven. 1977. Cons. Genitourin. Med. Suff. Prev: Sen. Regist. (Genitourin. Med.) Addenbrooke's Hosp. Camb.

REYNOLDS, William Henry Ladycroft, 118 Marsh Lane, Mill Hill, London NW7 4PE Tel: 020 8906 1401 — MRCS Eng. LRCP Lond. 1929 (Cardiff) Socs: BMA. Prev: Treasury Med. Off. & Admiralty Surg. & Agent; Chairm. Med. Bd. DHSS; Edr. Catholic Med. Quar.

REYNOLDS, Zsuzanna Maria Brannams Medical Centre, Brannams Square, Kiln Lane, Barnstaple EX32 8GP Tel: 01271 329004 Fax: 01271 346785; 85A Pilton Street, Barnstaple EX31 1PQ Tel: 01271 372178 — MD Debrecen Hungary 1975; MFFP 1995; FFP &RHC, RCOG. 1995. SCHO, FP; GP. Specialty: Family Plann. & Reproduc. Health; Gen. Pract.; Ophth. Prev: CHO, FP.

REZAUL-KARIM, Sheikh Muhammad The Surgery, 108 Victoria Road, Pinxton, Nottingham NG16 6NH Tel: 01773 810207 — MB BS Dacca 1969.

REZK, Rezk Nicola 67 Lushington Hill, Wootton, Ryde PO33 4NR — MB BCh Cairo 1974; MRCOG 1983.

REZVANI, Katayoun 63 Rosebank, Holyport Road, London SW6 6LJ — MB BS Lond. 1993.

RFIDAH, El Hussein Ibrahim East Kent Hospital Trust, Queen Elizabeth, the Queen Mother Hospital, St Peters Road, Margate CT9 4AN Tel: 01843 225544 Fax: 01843 234589; 10 Bridleway Gardens, Broadstairs CT10 2LG Tel: 01843 600139 — MB BCh Al Fateh, Libya 1981; DCH Dub. 1986; MRCPI 1988; FRCPCH 1997. Cons. Paediatrist E. Kent Hosp. NHS Trust, QEQM Hosp., Margate. Specialty: Paediat. Socs: Roy. Coll. Paediatry and Childhealth; Internat. Paediatric Nephrol. Assn.; Brit. Assn. of Paediat. Nephrol. Prev: Cons. (long term locum) Paediat. Nephrol. Roy. Vict. Infirm. Newc.; Research Fell. & Regist. (Paediat.) Roy. Hosp. Sick Childr. Glas.; Regist. (Neonat..) Rutherglen Matern. Hosp.

RHEEM, Ju Yun 56 Rotherhithe Old Road, London SE16 2QD — MB BS Lond. 1997.

RHEIN, Helga Maria Muirhouse Medical Group, 1 Muirhouse Avenue, Edinburgh EH4 4PL Tel: 0131 332 2201; 37 Claremont Bank, Edinburgh EH7 4DR — State Exam Med Frankfurt 1978.

RHIND, Elizabeth (retired) 26 Countisbury Drive, Childwall, Liverpool L16 0JJ — (Liverp.) MB ChB Liverp. 1947. Anaesth Walton Prison Liverp. Prev: Anaesth. Deva, Mostyn & Leasowe Pk. Hosps.

RHIND, George Brown Dumfries & Galloway Royal Infirmary, Bankend Road, Dumfries DG2 7PE Tel: 01387 241348 Fax: 01387 241361 Email: g.rhind@dgri.scot.nhs.uk — MB ChB Glas. 1977; MRCP (UK) 1980; FRCP Ed. 1990. Cons. Phys. Specialty: Care of the Elderly. Special Interest: Parkinson's Dis. Socs: Brit. Geriat. Soc. Prev: Cons. Phys. Roodlands Hosp. Haddington.

RHIND, Gordon Baird 23 Rubislaw Terrace, Aberdeen AB10 1XE Tel: 01224 643665; 32 Harlaw Road, Aberdeen AB15 4YY Tel: 01224 310129 — MB ChB Aberd. 1965; MRCGP 1975. Hosp. Pract. (Orthop.) Aberd. Roy. Infirm.; Police Surg. Grampian Police.

RHIND, Mr James Ronald Dryburn, North Road, Durham DH1 5TW Tel: 0191 333 2279; 41 Valley Drive, Hartlepool TS26 0AL Tel: 01429 236589 — MB ChB Leeds 1965; FRCS Eng. 1972; Specialist Accredit (Urol.) RCS Lond. 1979. Cons. Urol. N. Durh. Acute Hosps NHS Trust. Specialty: Urol. Socs: Brit. Assn. Urol. Surgs.; BMA; EAU. Prev: Cons. Urol. Hartlepool & Peterlee Trust; Sen. Regist. (Urol.) Leeds AHA (T); Regist. Inst. Urol. Lond.

RHIND, Thomas Peter Ferrari Morden Hall Medical Centre, 256 Morden Road, London SW19 3DA Tel: 020 8540 0585 Fax: 020 8542 4480; 33 The Crescent, London SW19 8AW Tel: 020 8947 3233 — MB BS Lond. 1969 (Lond. Hosp.) MRCS Eng. LRCP Lond. 1969; DA Eng. 1971; MRCP (UK) 1973.

RHODEN, Frances Mary Rudrashetty and Partners, Mary Potter Health Centre, Gregory Boulevard, Hyson Green, Nottingham NG7 5HY — BM BS Nottm. 1985; MRCGP 1989; Cert. Family Plann. JCC 1989. Socs: BMA. Prev: Clin. Med. Off. Memor. Hse. Nottm. Community Health NHS Trust.

RHODEN, Harold Michael (retired) 16 Insole Grove E., Llandaff, Cardiff CF5 2HP Tel: 029 2056 3731 — MB BCh Wales 1955 (Welsh Nat. Sch. Med.) ECFMG Cert. USA 1967. Adjudicating Med. Pract. for Indust. Injuries & Prescribed Dis. Prev: Sen. Asst. Resid. Gtr. Baltimore Med. Center, USA.

RHODEN, Walter Ernest Barnsley District General Hospital, Gawber Road, Barnsley S75 2EP Tel: 01226 777868 Email: walter.rhoden@bhnft.nhs.uk — MB ChB Manch. 1984 (Univ. of Manch.) BSc St Andrews 1981. Cons. Phys. and Cardiol., Barsley Dist. Gen. Hosp.; Clin. Lead N. trent CHD Collaborative; Nat. Clin. Lead CHD Collaborative; Clin. Lead N. Trent Network of Cardiac Care. Specialty: Cardiol.; Gen. Med. Socs: Brit. Cardiac Soc.; Roy. Coll. of Physicians; BACR. Prev: RCP Tutor.

RHODES, Mr Alan (retired) Stanmore, 15 Stoneleigh Road, Gibbet Hill, Coventry CV4 7AB Tel: 024 76 414919 — MRCS Eng. LRCP Lond. 1959 (Birm.) BSc (Hons.) Birm. 1956, MB ChB (Hons.) 1959; FRCS Eng. 1966. Prev: Sen. Regist. (Surg.) United Birm. Hosps.

RHODES, Alison Jane Student Health Centre, De Montfort University, The Gateway, Leicester LE1 9BH Tel: 0116 257 7594 Fax: 0116 257 7614 — MB ChB Aberd. 1977; DRCOG 1979. GP De Montfort Surg. Specialty: Gen. Pract. Socs: Brit. Assn. Health Servs. in Higher Ed. Prev: GP Leicester Stud. Health Serv.

RHODES, Andrew Department of Intensive Care, St George's Hospital, Blacksmaw Road, Tooting, London SW17 0QT Tel: 020 8672 1225 — MB BS Lond. 1990; MRCP (UK) 1993; FRCA 1994. Cons., IC & Anaesth., St Geo.'s Hosp Lond. Specialty: Intens. Care. Prev: Regist. & SHO Rotat. (Anaesth.) St. Geo. Hosp. Lond.; SHO (Gen. Med.) St Heliers Hosp. Carshalton; SHO (Geriat. Med.) Soton. Gen. Hosp.

RHODES, Anita Izabela Kingston Hospital, Galsworthy Road, Kingston upon Thames KT2 7QB Tel: 020 8546 7711 — MB BS Lond. 1991 (SGHTIS) BSc (Hons.) Lond. 1988; MRCP (UK) 1995; FRCR Lond. 1999. Cons. Radiol., Kingston Hosp. Specialty: Radiol. Special Interest: Breast; Chest; Musculoskeletal. Socs: Fell. RCR. Prev: Regist. (Gen. Med.) St. Heliers' Hosp. Carshalton; SHO (Radiother.) Roy. Marsden Hosp. Surrey; SHO (Cardiol.) St Geo. Hosp. Lond.

RHODES, Benjamin 65 Beauval Road, London SE22 8UH — MB BS Lond. 1998; MB BS Lond 1998.

RHODES, Caroline Ann Forrest Medical Centre, 69 Mount Street, Coventry CV5 8DE Tel: 024 7667 2277 Fax: 024 7671 7352; Stanmore, 15 Stoneleigh Road, Coventry CV4 7AB Tel: 024 76 414919 — MB ChB Birm. 1977 (Birmingham) BSc Birm. 1974; MRCP (UK) 1979; DRCOG 1981. GP Coventry. Socs: LMC & BMA.

RHODES, Catharine Alison — MB ChB Bristol 1988; MRCOG 1996. Cons. Obst., Good Hope Hosp., Sutton Coldfield. Specialty: Obst. & Gyn.; Obstetrics. Prev: Specialist Regist. Heartlands Hosp. Birm.; Research Fell. (Obst. & Gyn.) Good Hope Hosp. Birm.

RHODES, Cecil David Patterson (retired) Tregare, Chagford, Newton Abbot TQ13 8AR Tel: 01647 433480 — MB BS Lond. 1958; MRCS Eng. LRCP Lond. 1958; DObst RCOG 1965; DCH Eng. 1966. Prev: Regist. (Path.) St. Geo. Hosp. Lond.

RHODES, David James (retired) The Spinney, Hunts Lane, Felmersham, Bedford MK43 7JQ Tel: 01234 782460 Fax: 01234 782086 Email: countyheart@aol.com — (Guy's) MB BS Lond. 1966; MRCS Eng. LRCP Lond. 1966; DObst RCOG 1968; MRCGP 1971; FRCP 2000. Indep. GP & Phys. Co. Heart & Healthcare Clinic Bedford.; Med. Off. to Human Stud.s Unit, (Colworth Research), UNILEVER Plc Laboratories. Prev: Gen. Practitioner, Harrold, Bedford.

RHODES, Edith (retired) 42 Erskine Hill, London NW11 6HD — MRCS Eng. LRCP Lond. 1941 (Camb. & Birm.) MD Camb. 1947, MB BChir 1942; DA Eng. 1944; FFA RCS Eng. 1955.

RHODES, Elizabeth Geraldine Helen Springfield, 34 Gorse Lane, West Kirby, Wirral CH48 8BH Tel: 01244 365377 — MD Lond. 1993; MB BS 1976; FRCP (UK) 1978; FRCPath 1989. Cons. Haemat. Countess of Chester Hosp. Specialty: Haematology. Prev: Sen. Regist. (Haemat.) Qu. Eliz. Hosp. Birm.; Regist. (Haemat.) Roy. Free Hosp. Lond.; SHO (Med.) Roy. North. Hosp. Lond.

RHODES, Ellen Linda (retired) 3 Pelhams Close, Esher KT10 8QB Tel: 01372 466127 — MB ChB Leeds 1944; DCH Eng. 1953; FRCP Lond. 1975, M 1960. Prev: Cons. Dermat. St. Helier Carshalton & Kingston Hosps.

RHODES, Gerald Anthony Barn Surgery, Christchurch Medical Centre, Purewell Cross Road, Christchurch BH23 3AF Tel: 01202 486456 Fax: 01202 486678; 8 Island View Avenue, Friars Cliff, Christchurch BH23 4DS Tel: 0145 52 72674 — LRCPI & LM, LRSCI & LM 1972; LRCPI & LM, LRCSI & LM 1972; DObst RCOG 1975.

RHODES, Helen Louise — MB ChB Manch. 1992 (University of Manchester) BSc (Hons.) 1990; MRCP (UK) 1995. Research Regis. Respirat. Paediat. Poole Hosp.; Specialist Regist. Respirat. Paediat.

Soton. Gen. Hosp. Specialty: Paediat. Socs: MRCPCH. Prev: Specialist Regist. (Paediat.), Poole Gen. Hosp.; Regist. (Paediat.) Roy. Childr.'s Hosp. Melbourne Australia; Specialist Regist. Paedriatric Intens. Care Soton. Gen. Hosp.

RHODES, John (retired) 30 Netherfield Avenue, Eastbourne BN23 7BS Tel: 01323 769368 — MB BS Lond. 1954 (St. Mary's) MRCS Eng. LRCP Lond. 1954; FFR 1962; FRCR 1975; DMRD ENG 1975. Prev: Cons. Radiol. Eastbourne HA.

RHODES, Professor John (retired) 25 Nantfawr Road, Cyncoed, Cardiff CF23 6JQ Tel: 029 20 762734 Fax: 029 20 762734 Email: drjohnrhodes@cardiff40.freeserve.co.uk — (Manch.) BSc Manch. 1957, MD 1965, MB ChB 1960; FRCP Lond. 1974, M 1962. Prof. (Hon.) 1987 Univ. Hosp. Wales Cardiff. Prev: Cons. Gastroenterol. Univ. Hosp. Wales Cardiff.

RHODES, John David (retired) 33 Scott Lane, Riddlesden, Keighley BD20 5BU Tel: 01535 669551 Email: r33jdr@doctors.org.uk — MB ChB Manch. 1958. Prev: GP Shipley, W. Yorks.

RHODES, Professor Jonathan Michael Department of Medicine, University of Liverpool, Liverpool L69 3GA Tel: 0151 706 4073 Fax: 0151 706 5802 Email: rhodesjm@liverpool.ac.uk — MB BChir Camb. 1974 (St. Thos.) MA 1973; MRCP (UK) 1975; MD Camb. 1982; FRCP Lond. 1989; FMedSci 1999. Prof. Gastroenterol. & Hon. Cons. Phys. Roy. Liverp. Hosp. Specialty: Gastroenterol. Socs: Assn. Phys. Soc.; Fell. Acad. Med. Sci; Brit. Soc. Gastroenterol. Prev: Sen. Regist. (Med.) Qu. Eliz. Hosp. Birm.; Hon. Lect. Med. Unit Roy. Free Hosp. Lond.; SHO Hammersmith Hosp. Lond.

RHODES, Juliet Elise 38 Ena Avenue, Nottingham NG2 4NB — BM BS Nottm. 1989; MRCGP (Distinc.) 1994.

RHODES, Katharine Emma The Surgery, 30 Beeston Fields Drive, Beeston, Nottingham NG9 3DB; 11 Mossdale Road, Sherwood, Nottingham NG5 3GX — BM BS Nottm. 1986; BMedSci Nottm. 1984; DGM RCP Lond. 1988; DRCOG 1990; MRCGP 1990. Lect. (Gen. Pract.) Nottm. Specialty: Palliat. Med. Socs: BMA. Prev: Trainee GP Nottm. VTS; SHO MacMillon Fell. Hayward Hse. Nottm.

RHODES, Kenneth Michael Princess Royal Hospital, Farnborough Common, Orpington BR6 8ND Tel: 01689 865847 — MB BS Lond. 1973 (Westm.) FRCP; MRCP (UK) 1978. Cons. Phys. Bromley NHS Trust. Specialty: Gen. Med.; Care of the Elderly. Socs: Brit. Geriat. Soc. Prev: Cons. Phsyician James Paget Hosp. Gt. Yarmouth; Sen. Regist. (Health c/o Elderly) Nottm.; Specialist Phys. Vanuatu, S. Pacific.

RHODES, Lesley Elizabeth Department of Medicine, University Clinical Departments, University of Liverpool, Liverpool L69 3SA Tel: 0151 706 4030 Fax: 0151 706 5842; 315 The Colonnades, Albert Dock, Liverpool L3 4AB — MB BS Lond. 1982 (Kings Coll. Hosp. Med. Sch. Lond.) BSc (1st cl. Hons.) Lond. 1979; AKC 1979; MRCP (UK) 1985; MD (Mechanisms of UVB-induced erythema) Liverp. 1995; FRCP 1999. Cons. Dermat. Roy. Liverp. Univ. Hosp.; Sen. Clin. Lect. (Med.) Univ. Liverp. Specialty: Dermat. Socs: Brit. Assn. Dermat. (Ex-Jun. Rep. Audit Sub. Comm.); Eur. Soc. Photobiol.; Comm. Mem. Brit. Photodermatol. Gp. Prev: Research Fell. Wellman Laborats. PhotoMed. Boston, Mass., USA; Sen. Regist. (Dermat. & Haemat.) Roy. Liverp. Hosp.

RHODES, Martin Moorlands Surgery, 139 Willow Road, Darlington DL3 9JP Tel: 01325 469168 — MB BS Newc. 1972; MRCGP 1976.

RHODES, Martin John 20 Briar Road, Nether Edge, Sheffield S7 1SA — MB ChB Sheff. 1993; MA Oxf. 1983. SHO, SCBU, Northern Gen. Hosp. Sheff. Specialty: Paediat. Prev: SHO (Paediat.) Sheff. Childr. Hosp.; SHO (A & E) Roy. Hallamsh. Hosp. Sheff.

RHODES, Martin Trevor The Medical Centre, 45 Enderley Road, Harrow Weald, Harrow HA3 5HF Tel: 020 8863 3333; 140 Woodcock Hill, Kenton, Harrow HA3 0JN — MB BS Lond. 1973; DObst RCOG 1975; FRCGP 1990, M 1977; MA Lond. 1997. Hon. Senoir Lect. Fac. of Med. Imperial Coll. Lond.; Mem. Panel of Assessors GMC; Cons. to the Kazakhstan Primary Health Care Project. Prev: GP Assoc. Northwick Pk. Hosp. Harrow; Assoc. Dean (Gen. Pract.) N. Thames; Trainee GP Northwick Pk. VTS.

RHODES, Mr Michael Department of General Surgery, Norfolk & Norwich NHS Trust, Norwich NR1 3SR Tel: 01603 286286 — BM BCh Oxf. 1984; MA Camb. 1985; FRCS Eng. 1988; MD Newc. 1991. Cons. Surg. Gastroenterol. Norf. & Norwich NHS Trust; Hon. Reacher Surg., UEA. Specialty: Cardiothoracic Surg. Socs: BSG; AESGBI; AGA.

RHODES, Michael John Wragby Surgery, Old Grammar School Way, Wragby, Market Rasen LN8 5DA; Yew Tree Cottage, Fen Road, Owmby-by-Spital, Market Rasen LN8 2HP — BM BS Nottm. 1978; BMedSci (Hons.) Nottm. 1976; DRCOG 1981; MRCGP 1982; MPH Leeds 1984.

RHODES, Nicholas Duncan 3 Clarence Grove, Horsforth, Leeds LS18 4LA — MB ChB Leeds 1996.

RHODES, Paul Charles Burnley Wood Medical Centre, 50 Parliament Street, Burnley BB11 3JX Tel: 01282 425521 Fax: 01282 832556; 3 Clover Crescent, Ightenhill, Burnley BB12 0EX Tel: 01282 454956 — MB ChB Manch. 1980.

RHODES, Paul Martin Scotstown Medical Centre, Cairnfold Road, Bridge of Don, Aberdeen AB22 8LD Tel: 01224 702149 Fax: 01224 706688 — MB ChB Aberd. 1977; MRCGP 1981.

RHODES, Peter 25 Nant Fawr Road, Cyncoed, Cardiff CF23 6JQ Tel: 029 20 762 734 Fax: 01222 762734 — MB BChir Camb. 1989; BA Camb. 1986; MA Camb. 1992; MRCP (UK) 1992; MD Camb. 1995; FRCA 1997. Specialist Regist. (Intens. Care/Anaesth.) Soton. Gen. Hosp. Soton. Specialty: Intens. Care. Prev: Resid./SHO (Intens. Care Med.) Univ. Hosp. Wales Cardiff; Brit. Heart Foundat. Research Fell. & Hon. Med. Regist. Wellcome Research Laborats. Beckenham; SHO Rotat. (Gen. Med.) Soton. Univ. Teachg. Hosps.

RHODES, Richard Jonathan Richmond Group Medical Centre, 1 Albion Street, Ashton-under-Lyne OL6 6HF Tel: 0161 339 9161 Fax: 0161 343 5131; 7 Clifton Road, Heaton Moor, Stockport SK4 4DD — MB ChB Manch. 1971 (Manchester) BSc (Hons.) (Elec. Engin.) Manch. 1964; MRCS Eng. LRCP Lond. 1971; FRCOG 1995, M 1978; MFFP 1993. GP Ashton-under-Lyne; Instruc. Doctor (Family Plann.) Tameside AHA. Specialty: Obst. & Gyn.; Family Plann. & Reproduc. Health. Socs: NW Soc. Study of Sexual Med. & Family Plann.; Chairm. W. Pennine LMC. Prev: Regist. (O & G) Tameside Gen. Hosp. Ashton-under-Lyne; Surg. Lt. RN.

RHODES, Richard Ronald Queensway Medical Centre, Doctors Surgery, Queensway, Poulton-le-Fylde FY6 7ST Tel: 01253 890219 Fax: 01253 894222; Hurstwood, 133 Carr Head Lane, Poulton-le-Fylde FY6 8EG — MB ChB Manch. 1982; DRCOG 1984; MRCGP 1986; DCH RCP Lond. 1986.

RHODES, Simon 8 Emery Close, Altrincham WA14 1NJ — MB ChB Manch. 1998; MB ChB Manch 1998.

RHODES, Simon Mitchell Edenfield Road Surgery, Cutgate Shopping Precinct, Edenfield Road, Rochdale OL11 5AQ Tel: 01706 344044 Fax: 01706 526882; 19 Passmonds Way, Rochdale OL11 5AN Tel: 01706 868810 Fax: 01706 868810 — MB ChB Manch. 1985; BSc (Hons.) Med. Sci. St. And. 1982; DRCOG 1988. GP Princip. Rochdale. Prev: Trainee GP Rochdale VTS.

RHODES, Steven Myatt and Rhodes, Hermitage Surgery, Dammas Lane, Swindon SN1 3EF Tel: 01793 522492 Fax: 01793 512520 — MB ChB Manch. 1982; DRCOG 1985; MRCGP 1986.

RHYS, Anne Student Health Centre, 1 Marine Terrace, Aberystwyth SY23 2AZ Tel: 01970 622086 Fax: 01970 621914 Email: ahr@aber.ac.uk; Plas Bronmeurig, Ystrad Meurig SY25 6AA — MB BCh Wales 1959 (Cardiff) MB BCh (Distinc. Path. & Surg.) Wales 1959; DPM Eng. 1967; MFCM RCP (UK) 1974; MRCPsych 1984. Cardiff Med. Soc. Prize 1959; Howell Rees Schol. Med. Univ. Wales; Sen. Clin. Med. Off. (Ment. Health) Ceredigion Health Dist.; Univ. Wales Psych. Specialty: Gen. Psychiat. Socs: Y Gymdeithas Feddygol. Prev: Regist. Hensol Castle Psychiat. Hosp.; SHO Dept. Psych. Med. Middlx. Hosp. Lond.; Ho. Off. United Cardiff Hosps. Llandough.

RHYS, Gwion Gwyddfor, Bow Street SY24 5BJ — MB ChB Manch. 1996.

RHYS, Rhian Department of Radiology, Royal Glamorgan Hospital, Ynysmaerdy, Llantrisant CF72 8YR Tel: 01443 443443; 12 Bloom Street, Pontcanna CF11 9QE — MB BCh Wales 1985 (Welsch National School of Medicine) FRCS Eng. 1990; FRCR 1996. Cons. Radiol., Roy. Glam. Hosp., Cardiff. Specialty: Radiol. Socs: Roy. Coll. of Radiologists; Head and Neck Sect. of Roy. Soc. of Med. Prev: Specialist Regist. (Radiol.) Univ. Hosp. Wales Cardiff.; Regist. (ENT) Univ. Hosp. Wales Cardiff; SHO (Surg.) Roy. Marsden Hosp. Lond.

RHYS, William Joseph St Ervyl-Glyndwr, CStJ Plas Bronmeurig, Ystrad Meurig SY25 6AA Tel: 01974 831650; Minffordd, Llangadog SA19 9BU Tel: 0155 03 496 — MB BS Lond. 1948 (Cardiff & Guy's) BSc Wales 1945; MRCOG 1961, DObst 1950; MA Camb. 1950; DPH Wales 1966; MFCM 1974. High Sheriff Co. Dyfed; Cons. Community Phys. Ceredigion; Med. Adviser Environm. Health

Ceredigion; Hon. Med. Adviser Welsh Nat. Water Developm. Auth. Socs: Fell. Soc. Community Med.; Nat. Assn. Community Phys. Prev: Squadron Ldr. Inst. Aviat. Med. FarnBoro.; Dist. Community Phys. Ceredigion Health Dist.; Ho. Surg. (O & G) Hammersmith Hosp. Lond.

RHYS-DAVIES, Mrs Harriet Emily, MBE (retired) Caledon Cottage, South St., Milborne Port, Sherborne DT9 5DH Tel: 01963 250355 — MB BCh BAO Belf. 1947; DCH Eng. 1950; DObst RCOG 1951.

RHYS-DAVIES, Nigel College Surgery, College Road, Cullompton EX15 1TG Tel: 01884 32373 Fax: 01884 35541; Hayes, Halberton Road, Willand, Cullompton EX15 2QF Tel: 01884 820411 — MB BChir Camb. 1967; MA, MB Camb. 1967, BChir 1966; MRCGP 1976. Specialty: Gen. Pract. Prev: Ho. Surg. & SHO Cas. Dept. Middlx. Hosp. Lond.; SHO Gyn & Obst. Chase Farm Hosp. Enfield.

RHYS-DAVIES, Simon Tudur Stickney Surgery, Main Road, Stickney, Boston PE22 8AA Tel: 01205 480237 Fax: 01205 480987; The Chestnuts, Royal Oak Lane, New Bolingbroke, Boston PE22 7LF — MB ChB Birm. 1976; DCH Eng. 1980. Trainee Gen. Pract. Lincoln Vocational Train. Scheme. Socs: BMA. Prev: SHO (Obst., Med. & Cas.) Lincs. AHA.

RHYS-DILLON, Cristyn Ceril Glyn Tg Crwn, Cwmcidy, Porthkerry Park, Barry CF62 3BY Tel: 01974 831650; 23 Cressy Road, Cardiff CF23 5BE Tel: 01222 452686 Email: rhys-dillon@easynet.co.uk — MB BChir Camb. 1992 (Camb. Sch. Med.) MA Camb. 1994; MRCP (Lond.) 1997; DSEM 2002. Cons. Rheumatologist, Roy. Glam. Hosp. 2004. Specialty: Rheumatol. Socs: Y Gymdeithas Feddygol; Brit. Soc. of Rheum. Prev: SHO (Rheum.) Roy. Lond. Hosp. Lond.; Asst. (Nephrol.) St. Luc., Brussels; SHO (Neurol.) Guy's Hosp. Lond.

RHYS EVANS, Gwilym, MC 2 Camperdown Avenue, Chester-le-Street DH3 4AB Tel: 0191 388 3173 — MB BS Lond. 1940 (St. Bart.) DLO Eng. 1947. Hon. Surg. (Otolaryngol.) Sunderland HA. Specialty: Otorhinolaryngol. Prev: Sen. Regist. (ENT) Coventry & Warw. Hosp.; Regist. Roy. Nat. Throat, Nose & Ear Hosp.; Ho. Surg. (ENT) St. Bart. Hosp. Lond.

RHYS EVANS, Mr Peter Howell The Royal Marsden Hospital, Fulham Road, London SW3 6JJ Tel: 020 7808 2209 Fax: 020 7808 2235; The Halt, Smugglers Way, The Sands, Farnham GU10 1NB Tel: 01252 782327 Fax: 01252 782327 Email: peterre@globalnet.co.uk — MB BS Lond. 1971 (St. Bart.) MRCS Eng. LRCP Lond. 1971; FRCS Eng. 1978; Dip. Carcinol. Cervicofaciale Paris 1981. Cons. Otolaryngologist, Head & Neck Surg., Roy. Marsden & King Edwd. VII Hosp., Lond.; Vis. Cons. St. Bernard's Hosp., Gibraltar; Hon. Cons. ENT RN; Vis. Pres. Yale Univ., June 1999; Leon Goldman Vis. Prof. Inst. Cape Town, S. Africa. Specialty: Otolaryngol. Socs: FRSM (Counc.); Counc. Otolaryngol. Research Soc.; Fell. Amer. Head & Neck Soc. Prev: Sen. Regist. Roy. Nat. Throat, Nose & Ear Hosp. Lond. & W. Midl.; Sen. Lect. & Cons. OtyoLaryngol. Qu. Eliz. Hosp. Univ. Birminham; Interne Etranger (OtorhinoLaryngol.) Gustave-Roussy Inst., Paris.

RIACH, Ian Charles Frazer Corronich, Boat of Garten PH24 3BU Tel: 01479 357; 16 Aignish, Point, Isle of Lewis HS2 Tel: 01851 870744 — MB ChB Ed. 1958; DMRD 1963. Cons. Radiol. West. Isles Hosp. Stornoway, I. of Lewis. Specialty: Radiol. Socs: BMA, Roy. Coll. Radiols. & Brit. Soc. Gastro-Enterol. Prev: Chief Radiol. Sultanate of Oman & Head Radiol. Roy. Hosp. Muscat; Cons. Radiol. N. Birm. Health Dist.; Sen. Regist. (Radiol.) Childr. & Dudley Rd. Hosps. Birm.

RIAD, Mr Hany Naim Renal Transplant Unit, Manchester Royal Infirmary, Oxford Road, Manchester M13 9WL Tel: 0161 276 4976 Fax: 0161 276 8020 Email: hamy.riad@cmmc.nhs.uk — MB BCh Cairo 1973; FRCS Glas. 1983. Cons. Surg. in Transplantartion and Renal Failure Surg., Manch. Roy. Infirm. Specialty: Transpl. Surg. Socs: Brit. Tranplantation Soc. Prev: Cons. Surg. in Transplantartion and Renal Failure Surg., Roy. Devon and Exeter Hosp.

RIAD, Mr Magdy Mohamed Amin ENT Department, Ninewells Hospital, Dundee DD1 9SY — MB ChB Ain Shams 1979; MSc (Otolaryngol.) 1983; FRCS Ed. 1986; MD (Otolaryngol.) 1986. Cons ENT Surg. Ninewells Hosp., Dundee; Prof. (Otolalrygol.) Ain Shams Univ. Cairo, Egypt; Sen. Lect. in Otolaryngol., Univ. of Dundee. Specialty: Otolaryngol. Socs: Collegium Otorhinolaryng. Assn.; Scott. Otolaryngol. Soc.; Brit. Assn. Otol. & Head & Neck Surg.

RIAL, Susan Carolyn The Green Practice, Waterside Health Centre, Beaulieu Road, Hythe SO45 5WX Tel: 023 8084 5955 Fax: 023 8084 1292; Bowness, 1 Forest Front, Butts Ash, Hythe, Southampton SO45 3RG Tel: 02380 844712 — MB BS Lond. 1976 (Middlx.) Prev: SHO (O & G) Soton. Gen. Hosp.; SHO (Rheum.) & Ho. Surg. Middlx. Hosp. Lond.; Ho. Phys. Watford Gen. Hosp.

RIAZ, A Breckfield Road North Surgery, 141 Breckfield Road North, Liverpool L5 4QT Tel: 0151 263 6534.

RIAZ, Amjid The Surgery, 691 Coventry Road, Small Heath, Birmingham B10 0JL Tel: 0121 773 4931 Fax: 0121 753 2210 — MB ChB Leeds 1991.

RIAZ, Muhammad 2/2, 41 Annette Street, Glasgow G42 8EH — MB BS Punjab 1973; MRCOG 1993.

RIAZ, Mr Nadeem Uddin 14 Condor Court, Guildford GU2 4BP — MB BS Punjab 1982; DO RCS Eng. 1989; FRCS Ed. 1990; FCOphth 1990.

RIAZ, Sabiha 839 Finchley Road, Golders Green, London NW11 8NA Tel: 020 8458 4321; 89-B Hali Road, Gulberg II, Lahore, Pakistan Tel: 0142 874012 — MB BS Punjab 1975; MRCPath 1987; FRCPath 1997. Specialty: Histopath.

RIAZ, Sarah Naz — MB BS Lond. 1995; BSc (Pharmacol.) Lond. 1992; MRCP 2001. Specialist Regist. St Mary's Hosp. Specialty: Dermat. Socs: MDU.

RIAZ, Yasmin 107 Bramfield Road, London SW11 6PZ — MB BS Lond. 1995.

RIBBANS, Mr William John Northampton General Hospital, Cliftonville, Northampton NN1 5BD Tel: 01604 545943 Email: wjribbans@uk-consultants.co.uk — MB BS Lond. 1980 (Roy Free) BSc (Hons.) Lond. 1977; FRCS Ed. 1985; MChOrth Liverp. 1990; FRCS Ed. (Orth.) 1990; FRCS Eng. 2001; PhD 2003. Cons. Orthop. Surg. Northampton Gen. Hosp. Specialty: Orthop. Socs: Fell. BOA; BMA; BOFSS. Prev: Cons. Orthop. Surg. Roy. Free Hosp. Lond.; Clin. Fell. (Orthop. Surg.) Harvard; Sen. Regist. (Orthop. Surg.) Middlx. Hosp.

RIBBENS, Susara Cornelia 25 Staples Road, Loughton IG10 1HP — MB ChB Pretoria 1995.

RIBCHESTER, John Martin Whitstable Health Centre, Harbour Street, Whitstable CT5 1BZ Tel: 01227 794555 Fax: 01227 794677; 12 Grove Court Farm, Colonels Lane, Boughton-under-Blean, Faversham ME13 9SH — MB BS Lond. 1975 (King's Coll. Hosp.) DCH Eng. 1979. GP Whitstable; PEC Co-Chairm. Canterbury & Coastal PCT. Socs: Beckett Med. Soc. Prev: Clin. Asst. (Surg.) Qu. Vict. Memor. Hosp.; Jun. Lect. & Demonst. (Anat.) Middlx. Hosp. Med. Sch. Lond.; SHO Rotat. (Surg.) Kent & Canterbury Hosp.

RIBEIRO, Mr Alvin Anthony Hospital of St Cross, Barby Road, Rugby CV22 5PX Tel: 01788 572831; 132/134 Pytchley Road, Rugby CV22 5NG Tel: 01788 575009 — MB BS Univ. W. Indies 1974; FRCS Ed. 1980. Staff Doctor (A & E) Hosp. of St. Cross Rugby. Specialty: Accid. & Emerg.

RIBEIRO, Anthony 4 Erica Grove, Manor Park, Marton, Middlesbrough TS7 8RY — MD Lucknow 1959 (King Geo. Med. Coll. Lucknow) MB BS 1954, DMRE 1956; DMRT Eng. 1963; DMRD Eng. 1968. Radiol. Duchess of Kent's Milit. Hosp. Catterick.

RIBEIRO, Mr Bernard Francisco (cons. rooms), The Essex Nuffield Hospital, Brentwood CM15 8EH Tel: 01277 695695 Fax: 01277 201158 Email: bernard@fribeiro.freeserve.co.uk; Merivale, Howe Green, Sandon, Chelmsford CM2 7TQ Tel: 01245 472158 Fax: 01245 473137 — MB BS Lond. 1967 (Middlx.) MRCS Eng. LRCP Lond. 1967; FRCS Eng. 1972. Cons. Surg. Basildon & Thurrock Univ. Hosps. NHS Trust; Dir. of Undergrad. Educat. (Surg.). Specialty: Gen. Surg. Socs: Fell. Roy. Soc. Med.; Fell. Assn. Surgs. (Past-Pres.); Roy. Coll. Of Surg. Engl. (Counc. Mem.). Prev: Sen. Regist. (Surg.) Middlx. & Centr. Middlx. Hosps.; Lect. (Surg.) Ghana Med. Sch. Accra.

RIBEIRO, Cedric Albert Balham Health Centre, 120 Bedford Hill, London SW12 9HS Tel: 020 8673 1720 Fax: 020 8673 1549 — MB BS Mysore 1978 (Kasturba Med. Coll. Mangalore) BSc (Hons.) Bombay 1972; LRCP LRCS Ed. LRCP Glas. 1979; DTM & H Liverp. 1980. Clin. Asst. EMI Unit Springfield Hosp. Lond. Prev: Asst. GP Lond.; SHO (A & E & O & G) Arrowe Pk. Hosp. Wirral; SHO (Paediat.) Birkenhead Childr. Hosp.

RIBEIRO, Charles Donald NPHS Microbiology, Llandough Hospital, Penarth CF64 2XX Tel: 029 2071 5152 Fax: 029 2071 5134 Email: donald.ribeiro@nphs.wales.nhs.uk — (Cardiff) MB BCh Wales 1969; Dip. Bact. Manch. 1975; FRCPath 1988, M 1976. Cons. Microbiol. Nat. Pub. Health Serv. Cardiff.; Hon. Clin. Teach.,

Univ. of Wales Coll. of Med. Specialty: Med. Microbiol. Socs: Assn. Clin. Path.Past Sect, Cambrian Br..; Cardiff Med. Soc. (Past-Pres.); Brit. Infec. Soc. (Past Sect.) Eng. Br. Brit.Soc. Study of Infec. Dis.s. Prev: Cons. Microbiol. & Ass. Dir. Cardiff Pub. Health Laborat.; Sen. Regist. (Bact.) Manch. AHA (T); Ho. Phys. Llandough Hosp. Penarth.

RIBEIRO, Maria Dulce Correia 2nd Floor, 126 Amhurst Road, London E8 2AG — MB BS Lond. 1986. SHO Rotat. (Gen. Med.) Kent & Canterbury Hosp.

RIBEIRO, Neil McLaren Northcroft Surgery, Northcroft Lane, Newbury RG14 1BU Tel: 01635 31575 Fax: 01635 551857 — BM Soton. 1981; DRCOG 1985.

RIBERA CORTADA, Inmaculada 3 The Grange, Walton-on-Thames KT12 3HN — LMS Lleida 1994.

RIBES PASTOR, Purificacion Anaesthetic Department, Stoke Mandeville Hospital, Mandeville Road, Aylesbury HP21 8AL Tel: 01296 315262 — LMS Valencia 1989 (Valencia (Spain)) LMS Valencia 1988; MSc 1989; FFARCSI 1996; FRCA 1996. Cons., (Anaesth.) Stoke Mandeville Hosp. Aylesbury. Specialty: Anaesth.; Intens. Care. Socs: BMA; AAGBI; OAA. Prev: Regist. (Anaesth.) Cardiff & Wrexham; Specialist Regist. (Anaesth.) Swansea, Morriston & Singleton Hosps.

RIBET, Lartigue Pierre (retired) Speranza, Turketel Road, Folkestone CT20 2PA Tel: 01303 242065 — MB BS Lond. 1944 (Guy's) Prev: ENT Regist. S.E. Kent Hosp. Gp.

RIBET, Philippe William Lartigue Old Court House Surgery, 27 Wood Street, Barnet EN5 4BB Tel: 020 8449 2388; 21 Camlet Way, Hadley Wood, Barnet EN4 0LH Tel: 020 8449 1120 — MB BS Lond. 1971 (Guy's) MRCS Eng. LRCP Lond. 1971.

RIBET, Roisin Patricia Old Court House Surgery, 27 Wood Street, Barnet EN5 4BB Tel: 020 8449 2388; 21 Camlet Way, Hadley Wood, Barnet EN4 0LH Tel: 020 8449 1120 — MB BS Lond. 1969 (Char. Cross) MRCS Eng. LRCP Lond. 1969; DCH Eng. 1971.

RICCIO, Massimo The Priory Hospital, Priory Lane, London SW15 5JJ Tel: 020 8392 4225 Fax: 020 8392 8995 Email: massimoriccio@.prioryhealthcare.com — State DMS Milan 1978 (Univ. Milan) MRCPsych 1987; T(Psych) 1991; FRCPsych 1997. Cons. Adult Gen. Psychiat. Priory Hosp. Lond.; Med. Dir.; Hon. Sen. Lect. Char. Cross & Westm. Med. Sch. Specialty: Gen. Psychiat. Prev: Cons. Adult Gen. Psychiat. Chelsea & Westm. Hosp. Lond.; Lect. & Hon. Sen. Regist. (Psychiat.) Char. Cross Hosp. Lond.; Regist. & SHO Rotat. (Psychiat.) Char. Cross & Westm. Hosp.

RICE, Alexandra Joan Quains, Woodlands Road W., Virginia Water GU25 4PL — MB BChir Camb. 1994 (Univ. Camb.) MA Camb. 1996, BA (Hons.) 1992. Specialist Regist. (Histopath.) N. Thames Deanery. Specialty: Histopath. Socs: Train. Mem. Path. Soc.; Train. Mem. Internat. Acid. Path.

RICE, Andrew Sven Cracroft Pain Research, Dept. Anaesthetics, Imperial College, Chelsea & Westminster Hospital Campus, 369 Fulham Road, London W2 1NY Tel: 020 87468156 Fax: 020 82375709 Email: a.rice@ic.ac.uk — MB BS Lond. 1982 (St. Mary's) FFA RCS Eng. 1987; MD (St. Thomas's) Lond. 1991. Sen. Lect. (Anaesth.) Imperial Coll. Lond.; Hon. Cons. Chronic Pain Managem., Chelsea & Westminster Hosp. Lond. Specialty: Anaesth. Socs: Pain Soc.; Physiol. Soc.; Soc. for Neurosci. Prev: Sen. Regist. (Anaesth.) Oxf.; Regist. (Anaesth.) & Research Fell. (Neurophysiol.) St. Thos. Hosp. Lond.; Hon. Cons. Pain Relief, St. Marys Hosp. Lond.

RICE, Christopher Paul 9 Meaford Road, Barlaston, Stoke-on-Trent ST12 9EE — MB ChB Birm. 1968; FFA RCS Eng. 1972. Cons. Anaesth. City Gen. Hosp. Stoke-on-Trent. Specialty: Anaesth.

RICE, Denis Fitzsimons (retired) 9 Buckingham Court, Westwood Road, Southampton SO17 1HD Tel: 023 8055 2172 — MB ChB Liverp. 1953. Prev: PMO DHSS.

RICE, Edward Alexander 76 Park View, Cloughoge, Newry BT35 8LX — MB BCh BAO Belf. 1997.

RICE, Edward Francis (retired) 15 The Marches, Kingfold, Horsham RH12 3SY — MRCS Eng. LRCP Lond. 1955 (Birm.) DObst RCOG 1959. Prev: Obst. Ho. Surg. Marston Green Matern. Hosp. Birm.

RICE, Elizabeth Daphne Beechcroft, Community Mental Health Services for Older Peopla, Hillcroft House, Rooke's Way, Thatcham RG18 3 HR Tel: 01635 292070 — MB BS Lond. 1975 (Westm.) MRCS Eng. LRCP Lond. 1975; FRCPsych 1999. Cons. Psychiat. (Old Age) Berks. Healthcare NHS Trust. Specialty: Geriat. Psychiat. Prev: Higher Specialist Train. (Gen. & Old Age Psychiat.) Nottm.

RICE, Gillian Adele Dean Lane Family Practice, 1 Dean Lane, Bedminster, Bristol BS3 1DE Fax: 0117 953 0699 — MB ChB Birm. 1980; MRCP (UK) 1983; MPhil Camb. 1984; MRCGP 1985. GP. Specialty: Gen. Pract.

RICE, Mr Graham John (retired) The Coach House, Bitham Hall, Avon Dassett, Southam CV47 2AH Tel: 01295 690255 — MB ChB Birm. 1952; FRCS Ed. 1961; FRCS Eng. 1961. Prev: Cons. ENT Surg. Coventry Gp. Hosps.

RICE, Hugh Macan Three Gables, Nimms Meadow, Great Shefford, Hungerford RG17 7BZ Tel: 01488 648530 — MB BS Lond. 1939 (Westm.) MRCS Eng. LRCP Lond. 1938; MD Lond. 1947; FRCPath 1963. Cons. Path. Emerit. Gen. Hosp. Nottm. Specialty: Pathology, General. Socs: (Ex-Vice Pres.) Assn. Clin. Path.; Path. Soc. Prev: Cons. Path. Gen. Hosp., Childr. Hosp. & Highbury Hosp. Nottm.; Maj. RAMC; Ho. Surg. Westm. Hosp. Lond.

RICE, Mr Jonathan George The Medical Specialist Group, PO Box 113, Alexandra House, Les Frieteaux, St Martins, Guernsey GY1 3EX Tel: 01481 238565 Fax: 01481 237782 — MB BS Adelaide 1988; FRCS; FRACS. Cons. Surg. Med. Specialist Gp. Guernsey; Cons. Surg. Princess Eliz. Hosp. St Martins. Specialty: Surgery, Vascular. Special Interest: Malig. Melanoma.

RICE, Karl Joseph Lyndhurst, Eureka Place, Ebbw Vale NP23 6PN Tel: 01495 353700 Fax: 01495 353737 — MB BCh BAO Belf. 1983; MRCPsych 1988. Cons. Psychiat. Ebbw Vale. Specialty: Gen. Psychiat. Prev: Sen. Regist. Rotat. (Psychiat.) S. Wales.

RICE, Katherine Mary 34 Kings Road, Walton-on-Thames KT12 2RA — MB BS Lond. 1987; BSc Lond. 1984, MB BS 1987; MRCP (UK) 1990. Specialist Regist. Rotat. (Haemat.) SW Thames. Specialty: Haematology. Prev: Regist. (Haemat.) St. Thos. Hosp. Lond., Roy. Hallamsh. & North. Gen. Hosp. Sheff.

RICE, Katherine Victoria Romaine 17 Minster Road, West Hamstead, London NW2 3SE Tel: 020 842 1039 — MB ChB Ed. 1997; BSc. Pharm (Edinb) 1995. SHO, Renal Med., Roy. Free Hosp. Lond. Specialty: Nephrol. Socs: BMA. Prev: SHO A & E; SHO Surg., Edinb. Roy. Infirm.; SHO Medium Eastern Gen Hosp. Edin.

RICE, Mary (retired) 18 Shepherds Way, Liphook GU30 7HF Tel: 01428 723618 — MB BS Lond. 1963 (Guy's) BA (Hons.) (French) Lond. 1951; MRCS Eng. LRCP Lond. 1963; DPM Eng. 1966; MRCPsych 1977. Prev: Cons. Psychiat. (Psychogeriat.) & Sen. Regist. Graylingwell Hosp. Chichester.

RICE, Michael Hugh Cracroft (retired) River Lodge Surgery, Malling Street, Lewes BN7 2RD Tel: 01273 472233 Fax: 01273 486879 — MB BChir Camb. 1961; MA Camb. 1961; DObst RCOG 1963. Prev: Med. Off. Brit. Antarctic Survey.

RICE, Neil Elliot Doctors Quarters, Chase Farm Hospital, The Ridgeway, Enfield EN2 8JL; 34 Waterman Way, Wapping, London E1W 2QN Tel: 020 7702 3785 — MB ChB Pretoria 1990; DA 1996. Specialty: Anaesth.

RICE, Paul DSH Chemical & Biological Sciences, Building 04, Porton Down, Salisbury SP4 0JQ Tel: 01980 613517 Fax: 01980 613741; 35 Cygnet Drive, Willow Mead, Amesbury, Salisbury SP4 8LQ Tel: 01980 653501 — BM Soton. 1982 (Univ. Soton.) MRCPath 1993; FRCPath 2002. Specialty: Civil Serv.; Histopath. Prev: Med. Off. Chem. Defence Estab. Porton Down; Regist. (Histopath.) & SHO Soton. Gen. Hosp.; Ho. Off. (Med.) Basingstoke Dist. Hosp.

RICE, Peter Francis Leach Heath Medical Centre, Leach Heath Lane, Rubery, Birmingham B45 9BU Tel: 0121 453 3516 Fax: 0121 457 9256; 3 Laurel Gardens, Barnt Green, Birmingham B45 8RP Tel: 0121 447 7140 Email: rice5birm@aol.com — MB ChB Birm. 1983 (University of Birmingham) DRCOG 1986; MRCGP 1987.

RICE, Peter Martin Sunnyside Royal Hospital, Montrose DD10 9JP Tel: 0167 483361 Email: peter.rice@tpct.scot.nhs.uk; Keepers Cottage, Crow Wood, Meigle, Blairgowrie PH12 8RB — MB ChB Glas. 1981; MRCPsych. 1986. Cons. Psychiat. Tayside HB; Hon. Sen. Lect. Univ. Dundee. Specialty: Alcohol & Substance Misuse. Prev: Lect. (Psychiat.) Univ. Dundee; Regist. (Psychiat.) Murray Roy. Hosp. Perth; Regist. (Psychiat.) South. Gen. Hosp. & Leverndale Hosp. Glas.

RICE, Philip Stuart Department of Virology, St Georges.Hosp., 1st Floor Jenner Wing Blackshaw Road, London SW17 0QT Tel: 020 8725 5734 Fax: 020 8725 5694 Email: p.rice@sghms.ac.uk; 34

Kings Road, Walton-on-Thames KT12 2RA Tel: 01932 888774 — MB BS Lond. 1987 (St Thomas' Hospital Medical School) BSc (Hons.) Lond. 1984, MB BS 1987; DRCPath 1994; MRCPath 1998. Cons.Virol./Hon.Sen.Lect.St Geo.s Hosp. Specialty: Virology. Socs: Soc. Gen. Microbiol.; Amer. Soc. for MicroBiol. Prev: Sen. Regist. (Virol.) St. Thos. Hosp. Lond.

RICE, Robert Harold Wynne Hill Surgery, 51 Hill Street, Lurgan, Craigavon BT66 6BW — MB BCh BAO Belf. 1970; DRCOG 1979.

RICE-EDWARDS, Mr John Martin Charing Cross Hospital, Fulham Palace Road, London W6 8RF Tel: 020 8846 1182 Fax: 020 8846 7487; Ham House Stables, Ham, Richmond TW10 7RS Tel: 020 8940 6605 — (Oxf.) MA, BM BCh Oxf. 1960; FRCS Eng. 1965. Cons. Neurosurg. Dept. Neurosci. Char. Cross Char. Cross Hosp. Hammesmith Hosp. Trust. Specialty: Neurosurg. Prev: Ho. Phys. & Ho. Surg. Radcliffe Infirm. Oxf.; Sen. Regist. Nat. Hosp. Nerv. Dis. Lond.

RICE-EDWARDS, Susan Anne 41 George Street, Berkhamsted HP4 2EG Tel: 01442 873834 — MRCS Eng. LRCP Lond. 1966 (St. Mary's) DObst RCOG 1968; DO Eng. 1975. Socs: BMA. Prev: PMO Umtata Hosp. Transkei, S. Africa; Med. Off. Jane Furse Memor. Hosp. Sekhukhuneland, S. Africa.

RICE-JONES, Matilda Claire The Surgery, 1 Glebe Road, Barnes, London SW13 0DR Tel: 020 8748 1065 Fax: 020 8741 8665 — MB BCh Wales 1991; DCH RCP Lond. 1994; DRCOG 1994; MRCGP 1996.

RICE-OXLEY, Charles Patrick Martins Oak Surgery, 36 High Street, Battle TN33 0EA Tel: 01424 772263/772060; Lower Almonry Farm House, North Trade Road, Battle TN33 0HS — BM BCh Oxf. 1973; MRCP (UK) 1977.

RICE-OXLEY, John Michael 9 Blyth Grove, Worksop S81 0JG Tel: 01909 472082 — BM BCh Oxf. 1943; MA Oxf. 1945; FRCP Lond. 1971, M 1948; DM Oxf. 1950. Emerit. Cons. Phys. Bassetlaw HA. Specialty: Gen. Med. Socs: Fell. Roy. Soc. Med.; E. Midl. Soc. Phys. Prev: Cons. Phys. Roy. Hosp. Chesterfield & Bassetlaw HA; Sen. Med. Regist. Radcliffe Infirm. Oxf.; Capt. RAMC.

RICE-OXLEY, Margaret The Royal West Sussex Trust, St Richards Hospital, Spitalfield Lane, Chichester PO19 6SE; Lower Almonry Farm House, 43 North Trade Road, Battle TN33 0HS — BM BCh Oxf. 1973; FRCP Lond. 1996. Cons. Rehabil. Med. St Richards Hosp. Chichester. Specialty: Rehabil. Med. Prev: Sen. Regist. (Rehabil. Med.) Northwick Pk.; Assoc. Specialist (Neurol.) Brighton & Worthing.

RICH, Mr Alan John Postgraduate Institute of Medicine & Dentistry, Newcastle upon Tyne NE2 4AB Tel: 0191 222 5151 Fax: 0870 168 9178 Email: a.j.rich@ncl.ac.uk; Sunderland Royal Hospital, Kayll Road, Sunderland SR4 7TP — MB BS Newc. 1968; FRCS Ed. 1974; FRCS Eng. 1974; MD Newc. 1982. Assoc Dean (Postgrad. Inst. Med. & Dent.) Univ. Newc. u. Tyne; Cons. Surg. Sunderland Roy Hosp. Specialty: Gen. Surg. Prev: Lect. (Surg.) Roy. Vict. Infirm. Newc.; Arris & Gale Lect. RCS Eng.; Dir. Postgrad Med. Educat. City Hosp. Sunderland.

RICH, Delyth Ann 72 Hereford Road, Abergavenny NP7 6AB — MB BS Lond. 1990 (St. Geos. Hosp.) Dip RCOG / RGR; BSc Lond. 1987; MRCOG 1997. Regist. (O & G) Wales; Cons. Obstetrician & Gynaecologist - Nevill Hall Hosp., Abergavenny (June 2002 -). Specialty: Obst. & Gyn. Prev: SGR Nevill Hall Hosp.; SpR Roy. Gwent Hosp.; SpR Llandough.

RICH, Elizabeth Margaret c/o National Westminster Bank plc, Kentish Town Branch, 170 Kentish Town Road, London NW5 2DG — MB ChB New Zealand 1957 (Otago) DPM Eng. 1965; FRCPsych. 1986, M 1973; T(Psych.) 1991. Prev: SCMO (Ment. Health) City & Hackney (St. Bart.) Health Dist. (T).

RICH, Graham Francis Newcastle & North Tyneside Health Authority, Benfield Road, Newcastle upon Tyne NE6 4PF Tel: 0191 219 6046 Fax: 0191 219 6084 Email: graham.rich@nant-ha.northy.nhs.uk; 9 Osborne Avenue, Newcastle upon Tyne NE2 1JQ — MB BS Lond. 1985; BSc Lond. 1982; DCH RCP Lond. 1987; DRCOG 1989; Dip. IMC RCS Ed. 1989; MRCGP 1991; MBA Insead France 1992. Dir. Commissioning & Primary Care Newc. & N. Tyneside HA. Socs: Brit. Assn. Med. Managers. Prev: Managem. Cons. Boston Consg. Gp. Inc., Mass., USA; Sen. Health Policy Analyst Jackson Hole Gp.; Sen. Med. Off. NHS Exec.

RICH, Jennifer (retired) Shay Lane Medical Centre, Shay Lane, Hale, Altrincham WA15 8NZ Tel: 0161 980 3835 Fax: 0161 903 9848; 4 Poppy Close, Brooklands, Manchester M23 9TF Tel: 0161 998 5194 — (Ed.) MB ChB Ed. 1962. Prev: Ho. Surg. & Ho. Phys. Hope Hosp. Salford.

RICH, John Albert (retired) Curlew Cottage, 8 Heather Grove, Warkworth, Morpeth NE65 0YS Tel: 01665 712991 — MRCS Eng. LRCP Lond. 1940 (Middlx.) DIH Soc. Apoth. Lond. 1975. Prev: Employm. Med. Adviser EMAS.

RICH, Kathleen Marian (retired) 18 Mulberry Lane, Cosham, Portsmouth PO6 2QU Tel: 023 9237 8295 — (St. Mary's) MB BS Lond. 1956; MRCS Eng. LRCP Lond. 1956. Prev: Gen.Med.Pract.Portsmouth.

RICH, Martin George 75 Collinson Road, Hartcliffe, Bristol BS13 9PH — BM Soton. 1979.

RICH, Paul Antony St Georges Hospital, Blackshaw Road, London SW17 0QT Tel: 020 8725 3316; 25 Cottenham Park Road, West Wimbledon, London SW20 0RX Tel: 020 8944 1778 Fax: 020 8725 3135 — (Univ. Coll. Lond.) BSc (Hons.) (Immunol. & Genetics) Lond. 1981; MB BS Lond. 1984; FRCA. 1990. Cons. Anaesth. St. Geo.s's Hosp. Lond. Specialty: Anaesth. Socs: Assn. Anaesth.; Difficult Airway Soc.; Soc. for Computing & Technol. in Anaesth. (SCATA). Prev: Sen. Regist. (Anaesth.) Middlsex Hosp. Lond.

RICH, Paula Naomi 43 Dawpool Drive, Bromborough, Wirral CH62 6DE — MB BS Lond. 1998; MB BS Lond 1998.

RICH, Philip Malcolm Top Flat, 27 Warrington Crescent, London W9 1ED — MB BS Lond. 1989; BSc (Hons.) Lond. 1986, MB BS 1989.

RICH, Mr Walter John Cecil Christopher (retired) Springfield House, Hensleigh Drive, Exeter EX2 4NZ Tel: 01392 259967 Fax: 01392 498172 — (Bristol) MB ChB Bristol 1960; DO Eng. 1964; FRCS Ed. 1967; FRCS Eng. 1967; FRCOphth 1989. Prev: Chairm. SAC Ophth.

RICHARD, Bella Lucy Day Hospital, Nevill Hall Hospital, Abergavenny NP7 7EG — MB BS Madras 1988; Dip Geriatric Med 1996, RCOP; MRCP (UK) 1993. Staff Phsician in Adult Med., Gwent Health Care, NHS Trust, Abergavenny. Specialty: Care of the Elderly. Socs: BGS.

RICHARD, Christopher John Department of Anaesthetics, Borders General Hospital, Melrose TD6 9BS Tel: 01896 826000; Mertoun School House, Clintmains, St. Boswells, Melrose TD6 0DY Tel: 01835 823470 — MB ChB Manch. 1982; BSc (Med. Sci.) St. And. 1979; DA (UK) 1986; FRCA 1992. Cons. Anaesth. Borders Gen. Hosp. NHS Trust Melrose. Specialty: Anaesth.

RICHARD, Mr Derek Randal (retired) Flexfield House, 91 The Street, Mereworth, Maidstone ME18 5LU Tel: 01622 817867 — BM BCh Oxf. 1948 (Oxf. & Middlx.) FRCS Eng. 1955; MA Oxf. 1962. Hon. Cons. Orthop. Surg. Whipps Cross Hosp. Prev: Cons. Orthop. Surg. Whipps Cross & Wanstead Hosps. Lond.

RICHARD, Helen Winifred Occupational Health Unit, Staffordshire County Council, 15 Tipping Street, Stafford ST16 2LN Tel: 01785 276282; Virginia Cottage, Brook End, Longdon, Rugeley WS15 4PD Tel: 01543 491161 — MB ChB Birm. 1972 (Birmingham Univ.) DObst RCOG 1975. Med. Adviser, Ocupational Health Unit, Staffs. Co. Counc. Specialty: Occupat. Health. Socs: ALAMA; Soc. Occupat. Med. Prev: Med. Off. Marks & Spencer Plc W. Midl.; Gen. Practitioner, Sutton Coldfield.

RICHARD, Karen West Murray Royal Hospital, Perth PH2 7BH Tel: 01738 621151; Craigard, 14 Birkhill Avenue, Wormit, Newport-on-Tay DD6 8PX Email: karen.richard@btinternet.com — MB ChB Ed. 1982; MRCPsych 1986. Cons. Forens. Psychiat. Murray Roy. Hosp. Perth; Hon. Sen. Lect. (Psychiat.) Univ. of Dundee. Specialty: Forens. Psychiat.

RICHARDS, Mr Adrian Mark Stoke Maderville Hospital, Madeville Road, Aylesbury Tel: 01296 315117 — MB BS Lond. 1988; FRCS (Plas.); MSc. Cons. (Plastic. Surg.) Stoke Manderville & Aylesbury & Northampton Gen. Hosps.; Private Pract. Cons. (Plastic Surg.) Three Shires & Northampton & Paddocks Hosps. Specialty: Plastic Surg.

RICHARDS, Mr Andrew Barnett Glenthorn, Cleeve Road, Goring on Thames, Reading RG8 9BJ Tel: 01491 872296; (cons. room), 72 Berkeley Avenue, Reading RG1 6HY Tel: 01734 584711 — MRCS Eng. LRCP Lond. 1958 (Camb. & Guy's) MB Camb. 1959, BChir 1958; DO Eng. 1964; FRCS (Ophth.) Eng. 1967. Cons. Ophth. Roy. Berks. Hosp. Reading & Townlands Hosp. Henley. Specialty: Ophth. Socs: Ophth. Soc. & Oxf. Ophth. Congr. Prev: Lect. Profess. Unit

Moorfields Eye Hosp. Lond.; Asst. Resid. in Neurol. Johns Hopkins Hosp. Baltimore, U.S.A.; Sen. Res. Moorfields Eye Hosp.

RICHARDS, Andrew Michael 64 West Cross Lane, Westcross, Swansea SA3 5LU — MB BS Lond. 1996.

RICHARDS, Andrew Philip X-Ray Department, Prince Philip Hospital, Llanelli SA14 8QF Tel: 01554 756567 Email: andrew.richards@carmarthen.wales.nhs.uk; 17 Swiss Valley, Llanelli SA14 8BS Tel: 01554 774247 — MB ChB Leeds 1986; BSc Leeds 1983; MRCP (UK) 1989; FRCR 1993. Cons. Radiol. P. Philip Hosp. Llanelli. Specialty: Radiol. Socs: BMA. Prev: Sen. Regist. (Radiol.) Yorks. RHA.

RICHARDS, Anne Elizabeth Magdalen Medical Practice, Lawson Road, Norwich NR3 4LF Tel: 01603 475555 Fax: 01603 477747 — MB ChB Leeds 1983; DRCOG 1986; DCH RCP Lond. 1989. Prev: GP Kempston; Trainee GP/SHO Bedford Gen. Hosp. VTS; SHO (Ophth.) Newc. Gen. Hosp.

RICHARDS, Anthony Arthur (retired) 140A Doddington Road, Lincoln LN6 7HB — MB ChB Sheff. 1960. Prev: GP Lincoln.

RICHARDS, Mr Anthony Brynmor The North Hampshire Hospital, Aldermaston Road, Basingstoke RG24 9NA Tel: 01256 313556 Fax: 01256 313532; The Hampshire Clinic, Basing Road, Basingstoke RG24 7AL Tel: 01256 357111 — MB BChir Camb. 1962 (Camb. & Guy's) MRCS Eng. LRCP Lond. 1961; MChir Camb. 1966, MA 1962; FRCS Eng. 1966. Cons. Urol. N. Hants. Hosp. Specialty: Urol. Socs: Fell. Assn. Surgs.; Brit. Assn. Urol. Surgs. Prev: Sen. Regist. (Surg.) Guy's Hosp. Lond.; Regist. (Surg.) Roy. Surrey Co. Hosp. Guildford; Ho. Surg. Guy's Hosp. Lond.

RICHARDS, Mr Anthony Edwin Stewart Headcorn Manor, Church Walk, Headcorn, Ashford TN27 9NP Tel: 01622 890907 — MB BS Lond. 1963 (Lond. Hosp.) MRCS Eng. LRCP Lond. 1963; FRCS Eng. 1967; FRCS Ed. 1970. Self Employed. Specialty: Otolaryngol. Socs: Fell. Roy. Soc. Med. Prev: Cons. (ENT) Char. Cross Hosp. Lond.; Sen. Regist. (ENT) St. Mary's Hosp. Lond.; Sen. Regist. & Regist. Roy. Nat. Throat, Nose & Ear Hosp. Lond.

RICHARDS, Anthony John Worthing and Southlands Hospitals NHS Trust, Worthing Hospital, Lyndhurst Road, Worthing BH11 2DH Tel: 01903 205111 Fax: 01903 285045 — MB BS Lond. 1963 (Guy's) MRCS Eng. LRCP Lond. 1963; FRCP Lond. 1986, M 1968; DPhysMed Eng. 1974. Cons. Rheum. Worthing & Southlands NHS Trust. Specialty: Rheumatol. Socs: Fell. Roy. Soc. Med.; BMA; Brit. Soc. Rheum. Prev: Sen. Regist. (Rheum. & Rehabil.) King's Coll. Hosp. Lond.; Asst. Prof. Med. McMaster Univ., Canada; Regist. (Med.) Westm. Hosp. Lond.

RICHARDS, Antony Lawrence — MB ChB Manch. 1987; MRCP (UF), 1991; FRCA 1993. Cons., Anaesth. & IC, Roy. Oldham Hosp. Specialty: Anaesth.

RICHARDS, Arthur David, Squadron Ldr. RAF Med. Br. Retd. Winch Lane Surgery, Winch Lane, Haverfordwest SA61 1RN Tel: 01437 762333 Fax: 01437 766912; Ty Newydd, Suttonfold, Sutton, Haverfordwest SA62 3LP Tel: 01437 769031 — MB BCh Wales 1983; MRCGP 1988. Prev: Sen. Med. Off., Sen. Med. Off., RAF Brawdy.

RICHARDS, Arthur Forbister Park Surgery, Windsor Street, Trecynon, Aberdare CF44 8LL Tel: 01685 872040 Fax: 01685 883696; Nant Goch, Merthyr Road, Llwydcoed, Aberdare CF44 0UT Tel: 01685 872239 — MB ChB Sheff. 1957; DObst RCOG 1961.

RICHARDS, Miss Aurelia ENT Department, Guys Hospital, St Thomas St., London SE1 9RT Tel: 020 7955 5000 Ext: 4349or 4350; 4 Chadworth Way, Claygate, Esher KT10 9DB — MB ChB Aberd. 1985 (Aberdeen University) DLO RCS Eng. 1988; FRCS Eng. 1992; Mphi l(Univ. of Sussex), 1996; FRCS (Orlhns) 1998. Sen. Regist. (ENT Surg.) SE Thames HA. Specialty: Otolaryngol. Socs: Assoc. Mem. BAOL HNS; BAPO; ORS. Prev: Sen. Regist. (ENT Surg.) Lewisham Hosp.; Regist. (ENT Surg.) Brighton HA.; SPR (Ent Surg) Hosp. for Sick Childr. Gt. Ormond St.

RICHARDS, Barbara Anne 30 Park Road, Watford WD17 4QN Tel: 01923 241551 Fax: 01923 241551 — MB BS Lond. 1956 (Univ. Coll. Hosp.) DObst RCOG 1958; MFFP 1993. SCMO (Family Plann.) W. Herts. Community Trust. Prev: Asst. Co. Med. Off. Herts. CC; Ho. Surg. (Obst.) & Ho. Phys. Univ. Coll. Hosp. Lond.

RICHARDS, Barry Wyndham (retired) 102B Effra Road, Wimbledon, London SW19 8PR — MRCS Eng. LRCP Lond. 1939; FRCPsych 1971 (Founder Fell.); DPM Lond. 1948.

RICHARDS, Basil Francis Greystones, Beach Road, Llantwit Major CF61 9RF Tel: 014465 2607 — MRCS Eng. LRCP Lond. 1946.

RICHARDS, Bruce William (retired) 15 The Glade, Endcliffe Vale Road, Sheffield S10 3FQ Tel: 0114 266 8354 — MB BS Lond. 1948 (St. Thos.) MRCS Eng. LRCP Lond. 1948; DObst RCOG 1954; MRCGP 1973; MFCM RCP 1982. Prev: Regional SCM (Health Care Plann.) Trent RHA.

RICHARDS, Catherine Amelia Lucy The Hollies, 4 St. Athans Walk, Harrogate HG2 9DU Tel: 01423 565264 — MB BCh Wales 1987 (Univ. Wales Coll. Med.) MRCP (UK) 1990; MPH Leeds 1993; MFPHM RCP (UK) 1996; MRCGP 1996. GP, Leeds. Specialty: Gen. Pract. Prev: Sen. Regist. (Pub. Health Med.) N. & Yorks. Region; Vis. Lect (Pub. Health) Nuffield Inst. for Health 1998.

RICHARDS, Mrs Catherine Anne University Hospital Lewisham, Department of Paediatrics, Lewisham High Street, London SE13 6LH — MB BChir Camb. 1989; FRCS Eng. 1993; FRCS (Paed.) Eng. 2000; M Chir Camb. 2001. Cons. (Paediat. & Neonat. Surg.) Univ. Hosp. Lewsiham Lond. Specialty: Paediat. Surg. Special Interest: Gastroenterol. Prev: Specialist Regist., (Paediat. Surg.), Lewisham; Specialist Regist., (Paediat. Surg.), St Geo.s; Specialist Regist., Roy. Lond. Hosp.

RICHARDS, Catherine Jane 16 Ashtree Road, Cosby, Leicester LE9 1UA — BM BS Nottm. 1990; BMedSci (Hons.) 1988. SHO (Histopath.) Leicester Roy. Infirm.

RICHARDS, Catherine Meredith 40 Birkenpale, Sheffield S6 3NJ Tel: 0114 234 8848 — MB BChir Camb. 1977; DRCOG 1979.

RICHARDS, Celia Ann Beech House, Post Office Lane, Lyndon, Rutland, Oakham LE15 8TZ Tel: 01572 737718 — MB BS Lond. 1971 (Westm.) MRCS Eng. LRCP Lond. 1971; DObst Auckland 1975. Med. Off. (Family Plann.) Market HarBoro.; Clin. Asst. (Ophth.) Leicester Roy. Infirm. Specialty: Ophth.; Family Plann. & Reproduc. Health. Socs: Fac. Family Plann. Prev: GP Corby; Ho. Surg. (Radiother.) Westm. Hosp. Lond.; Ho. Phys. Putney Hosp.

RICHARDS, Christopher Graham Morgan Royal Victoria Infirmary, Queen Victoria Road, Newcastle upon Tyne NE1 4LP Tel: 0191 232 5131; 25 Brandling Place S., Jesmond, Newcastle upon Tyne NE2 4RU Tel: 0191 281 2825 — MB BS Lond. 1985 (Oxford - Preclinical Lond. (BARTS) Clinical) BA Oxf. 1982; MRCP (UK) 1988. Cons. Paediat., Roy. Vic. Infirm., Newc. Specialty: Paediat. Prev: Clin. Lect. (Paediat.) & Hon. Sen. Regist. John Radcliffe Hosp. Oxf.; Tutor (Child Heath) & Hon. Regist. (Paediat.) Roy. Manch. Childr. Hosp.; SHO (Paediat.) Newc. & N. Tyneside HAs.

RICHARDS, Christopher Mordaunt 4 St Ronans Avenue, Redland, Bristol BS6 6EP Tel: 0117 909 3474 Fax: 0117 909 3474 — MB ChB Bristol 1972; MB ChB (Hons.) Bristol 1972; DCH Eng. 1974; DObst RCOG 1975; MRCGP 1976. Indep. Psychother. Bristol. Specialty: Psychother. Prev: GP Keynsham; Trainee GP Newc. VTS; Ho. Phys. & Ho. Surg. Southmead Hosp. Bristol.

RICHARDS, Clifford Brookvale Practice, Hallwood Health Centre, Hospital Way, Runcorn WA7 2UT Tel: 01928 718182 Fax: 01928 790716 — MRCS Eng. LRCP Lond. 1978; DRCOG 1982; MRCGP 1984.

RICHARDS, Clive Haskell Lister Medical Centre, Lister House, Staple Tye, Harlow CM18 7LU Tel: 01279 414882 Fax: 01279 439600 — MB BS Lond. 1970; MRCS Eng. LRCP Lond. 1970; DObst RCOG 1973. Prev: Ho. Phys. & Ho. Surg. St. Margt.s Hosp. Epping; SHO (O & G) St. And. Hosp. Billericay; Resid. in Paediat. Univ. Alberta Hosp. Edmonton, Canada.

RICHARDS, Clive Wynford 8 Park Terrace, The Park, Nottingham NG1 5DN — MB ChB Bristol 1971; DObst RCOG 1973; DA Eng. 1974; FRCGP 1985, M 1976; MSc (Health Care) Exeter 1988; MFPHM RCP (UK) 1994. Dir. Public Health, Rushcliffe Prim. Care Trust; GP Nottm. Specialty: Pub. Health Med. Prev: Cons. Pub. Health Med. Nottm. Health; GP Avon.

RICHARDS, Colin John Tychwyth, The Downs, St Nicholas, Cardiff CF5 6SB; Glamorgan House, Croescadarn Road, Pentwyn, Cardiff — MB BS Lond. 1963 (St. Bart.) FRCOG 1983, M 1970. Cons. (O & G) Mid. Glam. AHA. Specialty: Obst. & Gyn. Prev: Ho. Surg. St. Bart. Hosp. Lond.; Sen. Regist. (O & G) S. Glam. AHA; SHO (O & G) Hammersmith Hosp. Lond.

RICHARDS, Dafydd Gwilym X-Ray Department, Morriston Hospital, Swansea SA6 6NL; 19 Daphne Road, Penywern, Neath SA10 8DP — MRCS Eng. LRCP Lond. 1976 (St. Mary's) BSc (Hons.) Lond. 1973, MB BS 1976; MRCP (UK) 1980; FRCR 1984. Cons.

Radiol. Morriston Hosp. Swansea. Specialty: Radiol. Prev: Sen. Regist. (Radiol.) Univ. Hosp. Wales Cardiff.; Regist. Rotat. (Med.) Univ. Hosp. Wales Cardiff; SHO (Med.) City Hosp. Nottm.

RICHARDS, Daphne Patricia (retired) 2 Harvest Bank Road, West Wickham BR4 9DJ Tel: 020 8325 8648 — (Roy. Free) MB BS Lond. 1961; DCH Eng. 1965; DPH Eng. 1970; MFCM 1974. Prev: SCM Croydon DHA.

RICHARDS, David c/o Mr G. Richards, 2 Moor Copse Close, Reading RG6 7NA — MB BS Lond. 1984.

RICHARDS, David Allan North Devon District Hospital, Microbiology Dept, Barnstaple EX31 4JB — MB BS Lond. 1985; MRCPath 2001. Cons. Med. Microbiologist North. Devon Healthcare NHS Trust Barnstable. Specialty: Med. Microbiol.

RICHARDS, David Anthony 278 Hills Road, Cambridge CB2 2QE Tel: 01223 247086 — MRCS Eng. LRCP Lond. 1966 (King's Coll. Hosp.) MD Lond. 1977, MB BS 1966. Scientif. Admin., Dept. of Oncol., Addenbrooke's Hosp., Camb. Socs: Brit. Pharmacol. Soc. & Soc. Drug Research. Prev: Vice-Pres. Clin. Operats. Arigen Europ.; Hon. Research Fell. UCH Med. Sch. Lond.

RICHARDS, David Anthony (retired) (Main Surgery) North Cardiff Medical Centre, Excaliber Drive, Thornhill, Cardiff CF14 9BB Tel: 029 2075 0322 Fax: 029 2075 7705; 40 Mill Wood, Lisvane, Cardiff CF14 0TL Tel: 029 2075 0322 — MRCS Eng. LRCP Lond. 1959; MB Camb. 1960, BChir 1959; DObst RCOG 1962; MRCGP 1974. Prev: Clin. Asst. WhitCh. Hosp. Cardiff.

RICHARDS, David Brynmor (retired) 14 Main Road, Bryncoch, Neath SA10 7PD — MB BCh Wales 1944; MD Lond. 1951, MB BS 1945.

RICHARDS, David Edwin William McGregor Laserase, Laser Dermatological Clinic, Royal Liverpool University Hospital, Prescot St., Liverpool L7 8XP Tel: 0151 708 9994 Fax: 01244 677671; Mill Hill Cottage, Rake Lane, Eccleston, Chester CH4 9JN Tel: 01244 677445 Fax: 01244 677671 — MB BCh Wales 1984; Cert. Family Plann. JCC 1990. Clin. Dir. Laserase, Laser Dermatological Clinic Roy. Liverp. Univ. Hosp. Specialty: Dermat. Prev: GP Birkenhead.

RICHARDS, Mr David Gwilym Department of Surgery, West Cumberland Hospital, Hensingham, Whitehaven CA28 8JG Tel: 01946 693181; Ghyll Head, Low Moresby, Whitehaven CA28 6RU — MB ChB Sheff. 1970; FRCS Eng. 1974. Cons. Gen. Surg. W. Cumbld. Hosp. Specialty: Gen. Surg. Prev: Lect. Surg. Univ. Sheff. North. Gen. Hosp.

RICHARDS, Mr David Michael Royal Oldham Hospital, Rochdale Road, Oldham OL1 2JH — MB ChB Manch. 1987; FRCS Glas. 1989; FRCS Eng. 1992; MD Manch. 1996. Specialty: Gen. Surg. Socs: Manch. Med. Soc. Prev: Sen. Regist. (Gen. Surg.) Hope Hosp. Salford; Sen. Regist. Blackburn Roy. Infirm.; Sen. Regist. Manch. Roy. Infirm.

RICHARDS, David Stephen Hagley Surgery, 1 Victoria Passage, Hagley, Stourbridge DY9 0NH Tel: 01562 881700 Fax: 01562 887185; 19 Woodland Avenue, Hagley, Stourbridge DY8 2XQ MB ChB Birm. 1987. SHO Kidderminster & Dist. HA GP VTS. Prev: Ho. Off. (Gen. Med.) City Gen. Hosp. Stoke on Trent; Ho. Off. (Gen. Surg. & Urol.) Dudley Rd. Hosp. Birm.

RICHARDS, David William Lawson Department of Genitourinary Medicine, Woolman Hill, Aberdeen AB25 1 Tel: 01224 641104; Ambleside, 143 North Deeside Road, Milltimber, Milltimber AB13 0JS Tel: 01224 868855 — MB ChB Aberd. 1965; DObst RCOG 1967; MRCGP 1975. Assoc. Specialist (Genitourin. Med.) Aberd. Roy. Infirm.; Clin. Lect. (Genitourin. Med.) Univ. Aberd. Specialty: Genitourinary Medicine. Socs: BMA & Scott. Comm. for Hosp. Med. Servs. Prev: Regist. (Med.) Aberd. Gen. Hosps.; SHO (Med.) City Hosp. Aberd.; Res. Ho. Off. (Surg. & Med.) Aberd. Gen. Hosp.

RICHARDS, Dawn 39 Kingsbury Road, London NW9 7HY; 59 Woodlands Road, Irchester, Wellingborough NN29 7BU — MB BS Lond. 1983 (Guy's) BSc Lond. 1980, MB BS 1983; MRCGP 1987. GP Lond.

RICHARDS, Denis John Rushden Medical Centre, Adnitt Road, Rushden NN10 9TU Tel: 01933 412444 Fax: 01933 317666 — MB ChB Birm. 1979. Prev: Ho. Surg. (Profess. & Cardiothoracic Units) Qu. Eliz. Hosp.; Trainee GP Northampton VTS.

RICHARDS, Mr Derek James (cons. rooms), 1 Arlington Road, Eastbourne BN21 1DH Tel: 01323 734030 Fax: 01323 734030; Clare Glen, Rock's Lane, High Hurstwood, Uckfield TN22 4BN Tel: 01825 733306 Fax: 01825 733306 — MB BChir Camb. 1959 (Camb. & Guy's) MA, MB Camb. 1959, BChir 1958; MRCS Eng. LRCP Lond. 1958; FRCS Eng. 1964. Cons. Surg. Orthop. Horder Centre for Arthritis CrowBoro. Specialty: Orthop. Socs: Fell. BOA. Prev: Cons. Surg. Orthop. Dist. Gen. Hosp. Eastbourne; Sen. Regist. (Orthop.) Univ. Coll. Hosp. Lond.; Regist. (Orthop.) & Ho. Surg. Guy's Hosp. Lond.

RICHARDS, Edward Michael Department Paediatric Haematology, St. James's Hospital, Leeds — BM BCh Oxf. 1987; BA Oxf. 1984; MRCP (UK) 1990; MRCPath 1997; DM Oxf. 1998. Cons. Paediat. Haematologist St. Jas. Hosp. Leeds. Specialty: Haematology. Socs: Brit. Soc. Haematol. Prev: Sen. Regist. (Haemat.) Centr. Sheffild Univ. Hosps.; Regist. (Haemat.) Addenbrooke's Hosp. Camb.; SHO (Gen. Med.) Swansea.

RICHARDS, Emily Dorothy Jean (retired) The Mount, Rudry Road, Lisvane, Cardiff CF14 0SN Tel: 029 2075 2660 — MB ChB Ed. 1946 (Univ. Ed.) Prev: Clin. Med. Off. Mid Glam. AHA.

RICHARDS, Emma Rachel Donmall and Partners, 87 Albion Street, London SE16 7JX Tel: 020 7237 2092 Fax: 020 7231 1435 — BM BS Nottm. 1991; DGM RCP Lond. 1993; MRCP (UK) 1994; DCH RCP Lond. 1995. GP Asst./Research Assoc. Prev: SLOUTS SHO.

RICHARDS, Eurfyl Lowesmoor Medical Centre, 93 Lowesmoor, Worcester WR1 2SA Tel: 01905 723441 Fax: 01905 724987; Linacre, 7 Lansdowne Crescent, Worcester WR3 8JE Tel: 01905 25127 — (Cardiff) MB BCh Wales 1957; DCH Eng. 1962; DObst RCOG 1963. Prev: SHO (Med. & Child Health), Ho. Phys. & Ho. Surg. Llandough Hosp. Penarth.

RICHARDS, Evan Huw (retired) 8 Fleetwood Avenue, Powick, Worcester WR2 4PY — MB BChir Camb. 1960 (Camb. & Lond. Hosp.) MA, MB Camb. 1960, BChir 1959; DPM Ed. & Glas. 1965; FRCPsych 1988, M 1972. Prev: Cons. Psychiat. S. Worcs. Hosp. Gp.

RICHARDS, Evan Thomas Eric (retired) Biscovey, Trewithen Road, Penzance TR18 4LS — (St. Mary's) LMSSA Lond. 1956; MB BS Lond. 1957. Prev: Ho. Surg. & Ho. Phys. Harold Wood Hosp.

RICHARDS, Fiona Ann Hill Brow Surgery, Long Croft, Mapplewell, Barnsley S75 6FH Tel: 01226 383131 Fax: 01226 380100; Tudor Lodge, Miry Lane, Thongsbridge, Holmfirth HD9 7SW — MB ChB Sheff. 1988; DRCOG 1992; MRCGP 1993. Specialty: Family Plann. & Reproduc. Health. Socs: BMA. Prev: Trainee GP Sheff. VTS; Ho. Off. (Med. & Surg.) Rotherham Dist. Gen. Hosp.

RICHARDS, Miss Frances Helen Patricia (retired) Cedarcroft House, Broad Bush, Blunsdon, Swindon SN26 7DH — MB BS Lond. 1975 (Univ. Coll. Hosp.) DRCOG 1977; DO Eng. 1980; FRCS Eng. (Ophth.) 1982; FCOphth. 1988. Prev: Cons. Ophth. Princess Margt. Hosp. Swindon.

RICHARDS, Frances Marie (retired) 3 Thompson Avenue, Cardiff CF5 1EX Tel: 029 2056 3771 — MB BCh Wales 1948 (Cardiff) BSc 1945; DObst RCOG 1950; DCH Eng. 1951; DPH Wales 1969; FFCM 1978, M 1974. Prev: Sen. Med. Off. Welsh Office, Cardiff. Jt. Med. Off. City of Cardiff.

RICHARDS, Francis James Abel Bay View, Cadgwith, Helston TR12 7JL Tel: 01326 290524; 4 Harriers Close, Ealing, London W5 3UA Tel: 020 8579 5499 — MB BS Lond. 1996 (King's Coll.) GP VTS SHO Rotat. King Geo. Hosp. Ilford. Prev: Ho. Off. (Surg.) Bromley Hosp.; Ho. Off. (Med.) Bromley Hosp.

RICHARDS, Gareth David Huw The Surgery, 36 The Street, Capel St Mary, Ipswich IP9 2EE Tel: 01473 310203 Fax: 01473 311722; The Granary, Mill Lane, Upper Layham, Ipswich IP7 5JY Tel: 01473 824869 — MB BS Lond. 1984 (Roy. Free) Prev: Trainee GP Braintree; SHO (O & G) St. John's Hosp. Chelmsford.; SHO (Paediat. & Cas.) Colchester Gen. Hosp.

RICHARDS, Gareth Justin 72 Forest Drive, Theydon Bois, Epping CM16 7EZ — MB BS Lond. 1993.

RICHARDS, Gareth Lloyd 6 Grange Crescent, Coychurch, Bridgend CF35 5HP — MB BCh Wales 1996. Specialty: Gen. Pract.

RICHARDS, Gillian Anne Corner Place Surgery, 46A Dartmouth Road, Paignton TQ4 5AH Tel: 01803 557458 Fax: 01803 524844 Email: gillian.richards@nhs.net — MB BS Lond. 1983 (Guy's Hospital) DRCOG 1986; MRCGP 1987. Specialty: Gen. Pract.

RICHARDS, Glenn Paul Ironbridge Medical Practice, Trinity Hall, Dale Road, Telford TF8 7DT Tel: 01952 432568 Email: glenn.richards@gp-m82606.nhs.uk — MB BS Lond. 1979; DRCOG 1983.

RICHARDS, Gwen Health Centre, New Street, Beaumaris LL58 8EL Tel: 01248 810818 Fax: 01248 811589; Godreddi Bach, Llanddona, Beaumaris LL58 8UY Tel: 01248 810330 Fax: 01248 810330 — MB BCh Wales 1976; DRCOG 1980; MRCGP 1980. Specialty: Gen. Pract.

RICHARDS, Gwyneth (retired) 21 Meadway, Rustington, Littlehampton BN16 2DD — LRCP LRCS Ed. LRFPS Glas. 1949; DObst RCOG 1951; DCH Eng. 1959; MFCM 1974. Prev: Area SCM (Child Health) W. Sussex AHA.

RICHARDS, Hannah Catharine Mary 15 Forsyth Road, Newcastle upon Tyne NE2 3DB — MB BS Newc. 1998; MB BS Newc 1998.

RICHARDS, Mr Harold James (retired) 13 Green Street, Riverside, Cardiff CF11 6LN Tel: 029 20 224105 — MB BS Lond. 1938 (Univ. Coll. Hosp.) MRCS Eng. LRCP Lond. 1938; FRCS Eng. 1941; DA Eng. 1942. Cons. Orthop. Surg. Univ. Hosp. Wales & P. of Wales Orthop. Hosp. Cardiff. Prev: Res. Surg. Off. Robt. Jones & Agnes Hunt Orthop. Hosp.

RICHARDS, Hayley Weavers Croft, Field Road, Stroud GL5 2HZ — MB ChB Bristol 1986; DRCOG 1988; MRCGP 1990; MRCPsych 1993. Cons. Psychiat. Specialty: Geriat. Psychiat. Prev: Regist. (Psychiat.) SW RHA.

RICHARDS, Hilary (retired) 102 Fernedene Road, London SE24 0AA — MB BS Lond. 1955 (Univ. Coll. Hosp.) DPM Eng. 1960; MRCPsych 1973. Hon. Research Fell. Inst. Psychiat. Prev: Cons. Psychiat. Merton Child Guid. Serv. Lond.

RICHARDS, Iain McKay Portland Road Surgery, 31 Portland Road, Kilmarnock KA1 2DJ Tel: 01563 522118 Fax: 01563 573562 — MB ChB Glas. 1982; BSc (Hons.) Glas. 1979; MRCP (UK) 1985; MRCGP 1990.

RICHARDS, Ian Michael Corner Place Surgery, 46A Dartmouth Road, Paignton TQ4 5AH Tel: 01803 557458 Fax: 01803 524844 Email: ian.richards@nhs.net — MB BS Lond. 1983 (Middlesex Hospital) MRCGP 1987. Specialty: Gen. Pract.

RICHARDS, Jane Elizabeth GUM Clinic, Newcastle General Hospital, Westgate Road, Newcastle upon Tyne NE4 6BE Tel: 0191 256 3256 — MB BS Lond. 1986 (The London Hospital) MRCGP 1991; DRCOG 1991. Staff Grade Genito Urin. Med. Newc. Gen. Hosp. Specialty: Genitourinary Medicine.

RICHARDS, Janet Elizabeth Hamilton 19 Woodland Avenue, Hagley, Stourbridge DY8 2XQ — MB ChB Birm. 1989.

RICHARDS, Janice Gwendoline Milman Road Health Centre, Milman Road, Reading RG2 0AR Tel: 0118 9862285 Fax: 0118 975 5033; Thornton, 117 Cockney Hill, Reading RG30 4EY — MB BS Lond. 1974 (King's Coll. Hosp.) MRCS Eng. LRCP Lond. 1974; DObst RCOG 1976; Cert JCC Lond. 1976. Prev: Ho. Off. (Med.) Dulwich Hosp. Lond.; Ho. Surg. Brook Gen. Hosp. Woolwich; Ho. Off. (O & G) Whipps Cross Hosp. Leytonstone.

RICHARDS, Jean Margaret 62 Lauderdale Tower, Barbican, London EC2Y 8BY Tel: 07939 843231 — MB BS Lond. 1963 (Lond. Hosp.) MRCS Eng. LRCP Lond. 1963; FFCM 1982, M 1974. Indep. Pub. Health Cons. Lond.; Hon. Lect. Lond. Hosp. Med. Coll. Specialty: Pub. Health Med. Prev: Dir. Pub. Health Tower Hamlets; Specialist in Community Med. (Child Health) City & E. Lond. AHA (T); PMO Lond. Boro. Tower Hamlets.

RICHARDS, Jeffrey Brereton Cumberland House, Jordangate, Macclesfield SK10 1EG Tel: 01625 428081 Fax: 01625 503128; 77 Bishopton Drive, Henbury, Macclesfield SK11 8TS Tel: 01625 610545 — MB ChB Manch. 1977 (Manchester) BSc (Hons.) (Chem. Engineering) Leeds 1967; DCH RCPS Glas. 1980; MRCGP 1981; Dip. Palliat. Med., Wales 1998. GP Macclesfield; Hospice Pract. E. Chesh. Hospice. Prev: GP Trainer; GP Appraiser; Trainee GP Macclesfield Hosps. VTS.

RICHARDS, Joan Mary (retired) 38 Sitwell Way, Sandfields, Port Talbot SA12 6BL Tel: 01639 771065 — MB BCh Wales 1954 (Cardiff)

RICHARDS, John Desmond Morgan Parkfield Lodge, 30 Park Road, Watford WD17 4QN Tel: 01923 241551 Fax: 01923 241551 — MB BChir Camb. 1957 (Univ. Coll. Hosp.) MA Camb. Prize 1955; MRCS Eng. LRCP Lond. 1956; FRCP Ed. 1971, M 1961; FRCPath 1975, M 1963; MD (Raymond Horton-Smith prize & Sir Lionel Whitby Med) 1965; FRCP Lond. 1987. Emerit. Cons. Haemat. & Phys. Univ. Coll. Hosp. Lond. Specialty: Gen. Med.; Haematology. Prev: Sen. Regist. Univ. Coll. Hosp. Lond.; Ho. Phys. & Ho. Surg. Univ. Coll. Hosp. Lond.

RICHARDS, John Lewis The Firs, Old Lane, Peterstow, Ross-on-Wye HR9 6LB — MRCS Eng. LRCP Lond. 1948 (Middlx.) MRCPath 1971. Prev: Ho. Phys. & Cas. Off. Hounslow Hosp. & Hertford Co. Hosp.; Ho. Surg. Roy. Gwent Hosp. Newport.

RICHARDS, John Llewellyn Richards and Partners, Llanfair Surgery, Llanfair Road, Llandovery SA20 0HY Tel: 01550 720648 Fax: 01550 721428 — MB BCh Wales 1973; DRCOG 1975; DCH Eng. 1976; MRCGP 1977.

RICHARDS, Jonathan David Gwanwr-Fryn, Clydach Road, Ynysybwl, Pontypridd CF37 3LX — MB BS Lond. 1986.

RICHARDS, Professor Jonathan Philip Ty Morlais, Berry Square, Merthyr Tydfil CF48 3AL Tel: 01685 722782 Fax: 01685 722951; 20 The Grove, Merthyr Tydfil CF47 8YR Email: pagchair@dial.pipex.com — (Wales) BSc (Hons.) Anat. Wales 1976, MB BCh 1979; DRCOG 1983; MRCGP 1984. GP Merthyr Tydfil.; Ext. Prof. Prim. Care Sch. of Nurs. & Midw. Univ. Glam.; Chair/Bro Taf Prim. Care Aud. Gp. Prev: Lect. Univ. Wales Coll. Med.

RICHARDS, Josephine Anne 60 Hall Green, Malvern WR14 3QX — MB BCh Wales 1986; MRCPsych 1992.

RICHARDS, Judit Public Health Laboratory, Bowthorpe Road, Norwich NR2 3TX Tel: 01603 611816 — Medico Buenos Aires 1976; MRCPath 1988; T(Path.) 1991; FRCPath 1998. Cons. Microbiologist Norwich Pub. Health Laborat.; Hon. Lect. Sch. Biological Sci. Univ. E. Anglia; Hon. Sen. Lect. Sch. of Health Policy & Pract., Univ. E. Anglia. Specialty: Med. Microbiol. Socs: Hosp. Infec. Soc.; Assoc. Med. MicroBiol. Prev: Sen. Regist. (Microbiol.) Newc.; Regist. (Microbiol.) Leicester Roy. Infirm. & Ipswich.

RICHARDS, Julia Marjorie 72 Forest Drive, Theydon Bois, Epping CM16 7EZ — MB BS Lond. 1995.

RICHARDS, Julie Louise Valentine House, 1079 Rochdale Road, Manchester M9 8AJ Tel: 0161 740 2524 Fax: 0161 795 2531; 21 Oulder Hill Drive, Bamford, Rochdale OL11 5LB Tel: 01706 712168 — MB ChB Manch. 1987. GP Princip. Manch. Specialty: Gen. Pract. Prev: Trainee GP Falkirk Scotl. & Heywood Lancs.; SHO (Paediat.) Roy. Hosp. Sick Childr. Glas.

RICHARDS, Justin Paul DDS Medicines Research Ltd, Ninewells Hospital & Medical School, Dundee DD1 9SY — MB ChB Liverp. 1984; FRCA 1994. Med. Dir.; Hon. Cons. Anaesth. Specialty: Pharmaceutical Medicine. Socs: Assn. Anaesth.; Fell. Roy. Coll. Anaesth. Prev: Sen. Regist. (Anaesth.) NW RHA.

RICHARDS, Keith Fforestfach Medical Centre, 118 Ravenhill Road, Fforestfach, Swansea SA5 5AA Tel: 01792 581666 Fax: 01792 585332; 8 Woodlands Terrace, Caerau, Maesteg, Bridgend CF32 7LB — MB BCh Wales 1972; DObst RCOG 1975; MRCGP 1976.

RICHARDS, Kirsten Jayne Campbell 84 Hull Road, Hedon, Hull HU12 8DJ — MB ChB Sheff. 1994.

RICHARDS, Leslie Frisby (Surgery) Ravenscourt, Barry Tel: 01446 733515 & 734744; 63 The Parade, Barry CF62 6SG Tel: 01446 734973 — MRCS Eng. LRCP Lond. 1945 (St. Mary's) DObst RCOG 1947. Prev: Ho. Surg. & Ho. Surg. (O & G) Roy. Infirm. Cardiff.

RICHARDS, Lorna Alison 133 Overslade Lane, Rugby CV22 6EF — MB ChB Birm. 1995; ChB Birm. 1995.

RICHARDS, Louise Eleanor Jane Burford House, 5 St Davids Drive, Cherry Orchard, Evesham WR11 2AS — BM Soton. 1998.

RICHARDS, Louise Marie Elaine 21 Bow Lane, Finchley, London N12 0JR — MB ChB Manch. 1992; DCH RCP Lond. 1996. Regist. (Forens. Psychiat.) Roy. Free Hosp. Rotat. Specialty: Psychother. Prev: Regist. (Child & Adolesc. Psychiat.) Lond.; Regist. Rotat. (Psychiat.) Roy. Free Hosp. Lond.; Regist. (Psychiat. of Old Age) St. Anne's Hosp. Lond.

RICHARDS, Mair 96 Hunter House Road, Sheffield S11 8TW — MB ChB Bristol 1975; DCH Eng. 1979; MRCP UK 1981. Cons. Community Paediat. Community Health, Sheff. Specialty: Paediat. Socs: Brit. Paediat. Assn.; Brit. Soc. Audiol. Prev: Hon. Clin. Lect. Paediat. Univ. Sheff.; SCMO (Child Health) Sheff. HA.

RICHARDS, Margaret Anne 83 Sutton Heights, Albion Road, Sutton SM2 5TD — MB BS Lond. 1990.

RICHARDS, Margaret Cecil (retired) 5 Marston Lane, Norwich NR4 6LZ Tel: 01603 452505 Fax: 01603 452505 Email: 106313.1216@compuserve.com — MB BS Lond. 1949 (Roy. Free) Prev: Clin. Med. Off. Norf. AHA.

RICHARDS, Margaret Helen Jean (retired) 2 Heol-Y-Pavin, Llandaff, Cardiff CF5 2EG — MB BCh Wales 1950 (Cardiff) FRCGP 1975. Prev: Regist. (Med.) Min. of Pens. Hosp. Rookwood, Cardiff.

RICHARDS, Martyn James Penn Hill Surgery, St Nicholas Close, Yeovil BA20 1SB Tel: 01935 74005 Fax: 01935 421841; 52 Grove Avenue, Yeovil BA20 2BE — MB BChir Camb. 1984 (St. And.) BSc (Hons.) St. And. 1982; MA Camb. 1984; DObst RCOG 1988; DGM RCP Lond. 1988; MRCGP 1990; Dip. Pract. Dermat. Wales 1994; Cert. Av. Med. 1996. Trainer (Gen. Pract.) Yeovil. Specialty: Dermat. Socs: Brist. M-C Soc.; BMA. Prev: SHO (O & G, Cardiol. & Paediat.) Southmead Hosp. Bristol; Ho. Surg. Norf. & Norwich Hosp.

RICHARDS, Mary Elizabeth (retired) 36 Le More, Four Oaks, Sutton Coldfield B74 2XY Tel: 0121 308 6314 — (Cardiff) BSc Wales 1940; MB ChB Wales 1943; MRCOG 1949. Prev: Sen. Med. Off. (Family Plann. Serv.) Dudley, Sandwell & Walsall DHA's.

RICHARDS, Megan Branwen (retired) Norlands, Clytha Park Road, Newport NP20 4NA Tel: 01633 264535 — (Cardiff) BSc Wales 1939; MB BCh Wales 1942. JP.; Chairm. Med. Bds. Min. of Social Security. Prev: GP Rhymney, Gwent.

RICHARDS, Professor Michael Adrian St. Thomas' Hospital, Department of Palliative Medicine, London SE1 7EH Tel: 020 7188 4732 Fax: 020 7188 4720; 42 Liberia Road, Highbury, London N5 1JR Tel: 020 7226 6808 Fax: 020 7226 6808 — MB BChir Camb. 1978; MRCP (UK) 1979; MA Camb. 1987, MD 1988; FRCP Lond. 1993. Nat. Cancer Dir. Dept. of Health Lond.; Chairm. Div. of Oncol. & Palliat. Care Guy's, King's & St. Thomas' Med. Sch. Specialty: Palliat. Med.; Oncol. Prev: Prof. Palliat. Med. & Clin. Dir. (Cancer Servs.) Guy's & St. Thos. Hosp. Lond.; Reader (Med. Oncol.) & Sen. Lect. (Med. Oncol.) Guy's & St. Thos. Hosp. Lond.; ICRF Research Fell. (Med. Oncol.) St. Bart. Hosp. Lond.

RICHARDS, Michael John Albany Surgery, Albany Street, Newton Abbot TQ12 2TX Tel: 01626 334411 Fax: 01626 335663; Springbank, Croft Road, East Ogwell, Newton Abbot TQ12 6BA Tel: 01626 56261 — MB BS Lond. 1982 (Guy's) MA Camb. 1982; DRCOG 1986; MRCGP 1986. Prev: SHO (Paediat., Psychiat., O & G & Med.) Taunton Hosp. VTS.

RICHARDS, Michael John c/o Anaesthetic Department, Cheltenham General Hospital, Sandford Road, Cheltenham GL53 7AN — MB BCh Wales 1976; FFA RCS Eng. 1984. Cons. Anaesth. Cheltenham Gen. Hosp. Specialty: Anaesth. Prev: Carey Coombs Research Fell. Bristol Roy. Infirm.; Cons. Anaesth. Middlemore Hosp. NZ.

RICHARDS, Michael John 60 Hall Green, Malvern WR14 3QX Tel: 01689 863942 — BM Soton. 1993. SHO (Cardiol.) Soton. Gen. Hosp. Specialty: Cardiol. Prev: SHO (Gen. Med.) & Ho. Phys. Roy. S. Hants. Hosp.

RICHARDS, Michael Lindsay Richards and Partners, The Surgery, North Street, Langport TA10 9RH Tel: 01458 250464 Fax: 01458 253246; Croftlands, School St, Drayton, Langport TA10 0LW — MB ChB Bristol 1968; DObst RCOG 1969. Prev: Med. Off. Roy. Flying Doctor Serv. Austral.

RICHARDS, Myrtle Vivien (retired) 29A Arlington Avenue, Leamington Spa CV32 5UD Tel: 01926 422485 — MB ChB Ed. 1946; DCH Eng. 1951; DPH Lond. 1952; MFCM 1972. Specialist in Community Med. S. Warks. HA. Prev: PMO Warks. AHA.

RICHARDS, Nicholas Christopher Guyon, SBStJ Telford Occupational Health Service, Occupational Health Centre, Halesfield 13, Telford TF7 4PL Tel: 01952 581251 Fax: 01952 581251; 4 Cavendish Close, Bicton Heath, Shrewsbury SY3 5PG Email: nickrichards@doctors.org.uk — MB BS Lond. 1965 (St. Bart.) DIH Soc. Apoth. Lond. 1971; DObst RCOG 1972; MRCGP 1974; MFOM RCP Lond. 1997, A 1991. Atos Origin; Med. Adviser to Private Health Care; Med. Dir. of Telford Ocupational Health Serv. Specialty: Occupat. Health. Socs: Soc. Occupat. Med.; BMA; FOM. Prev: Surg. Lt. Cdr. HMNB Portsmouth; GP S. Wales.; CMP RAF St Athan S. Wales.

RICHARDS, Nicholas Talbot Department of Nephrology, Queen Elizabeth Hospital, Edgbaston, Birmingham B15 2TH Tel: 0121 627 2201 Fax: 0121 697 8406 — MD Lond. 1992; BSc Pharmacol. Lond. 1978, MB BS 1981; MRCP (UK) 1992; FRCP 1996. Cons. Nephrol. & Phys. Qu. Eliz. Hosp. Birm. Specialty: Nephrol.

RICHARDS, Paul London Road Surgery, 64 London Road, Wickford SS12 0AH Tel: 01268 765533 Fax: 01268 570762 Email: paul@medex.org.uk — MB ChB Manch. 1987; T(GP) 1992; MRCGP 1992; MSc Med Sci (Glas) 2001. Specialty: Gen. Pract.

RICHARDS, Paul Rees Nant Goch, Merthyr Road, Llwydcoed, Aberdare CF44 0UT — MB ChB Sheff. 1989; DAvMED; AFOM.

RICHARDS, Paula Jane University Hospital of North Staffordshire, X Ray Department, Princes Road, Heartshill, Stoke-on-Trent ST4 7LN Tel: 01782 554752 Fax: 01782 747552 Email: paulaj.richards@uhns.nhs.uk — MB BS Lond. 1987 (Guy's Hospital) BSc (Hons.) 1984 Path. & Med. Sci. Lond.; MRCP (UK) 1990; FRCR 1995. Cons. Musculoskeletal & Trauma Radilogist; Sen. Clin. Lect., Keele Univ. Staffs.. Specialty: Sports Med. Socs: Brit. Trauma Soc.; Brit. Soc. Of Skeletal Radiologists; BMA. Prev: SHO (Renal) Guy's Hosp. Lond.; SHO Rotat. (Med.) Guy's & Lewisham Hosp. Lond.; Sen. Regist. (Diag. Radiol.) St. Bart. Hosp. Lond.

RICHARDS, Mr Peter Gerald Department of Neurosurgery, The Radcliffe Infirmary, Woodstock Road, Oxford OX2 6HE Tel: 01865 228507 Fax: 01865 224898 Email: prichards@btinternet.com — MB BS Lond. 1977 (Middlx.) FRCS Ed. 1981; FRCPCH 1998; FRCS Eng 1999. Cons. Paediat. Neurosurg. Radcliffe Infirm. Oxf. Specialty: Neurosurg. Prev: Cons. Neurosurg. Char. Cross Hosp. Lond.; Cons. Paediat. Neurosurg. Chelsea & Westm. Hosp. Lond.

RICHARDS, Peter Llewellyn Wickham Surgery, Station Road, Wickham, Fareham PO17 5JL Tel: 01329 833121 Fax: 01329 832443; Speedfield House, Ingoldfield Lane, Newtown, Fareham PO17 6LF Tel: 01329 833262 — MB BS Lond. 1975; MRCS Eng. LRCP Lond. 1975; MRCP (UK) 1979; DRCOG 1980. Prev: Clin. Asst. (Rheum.) Portsmouth.

RICHARDS, Peter William St Sampson's Medical Centre, Grandes Maisons Road, St. Sampson, Guernsey GY2 4JS; L'aumone & St. Sampsons Practice, Plaisance, Candie Road, Castel, Guernsey GY5 7BX — MB ChB (Hons.) 1983; DRCOG 1986; DCH RCP Lond. 1986; MRCGP 1988. Prev: Trainee GP Winchester VTS.

RICHARDS, Mr Philip Alfred Flemish House, Chapel Lane, Dudleston Heath, Ellesmere SY12 9LZ — MB ChB Ed. 1981; FRCS Ed. 1986. Assoc. Specialist (Surg.) Wrexham Maelor Hosp. Specialty: Gen. Surg.

RICHARDS, Philip Warren 113 Dunedin Road, Birmingham B44 9DL — MB ChB Leeds 1994.

RICHARDS, Philippa Eloise Inez 4 Sylvan Drive, Coventry CV3 6AB — MB BS Lond. 1996.

RICHARDS, Rachel (retired) Amberley, Well-Meadows, Shaw, Newbury RG14 2DS — MRCS Eng. LRCP Lond. 1945 (Cardiff) FRCOG 1989, M 1957, DObst 1947. Gyn. Asst. Newbury Dist. Hosp. Prev: Res. Obst. Off. Univ. Obst. Unit, Southmead Hosp. Bristol.

RICHARDS, Richard George Newark and Sherwood PCT, 65 Northgate, Newark NG24 1HD Tel: 01636 700236; The Old Rectory, 35 High St., Brant Broughton, Lincoln LN5 0SL — MB BS Newc. 1980. Dir. Of Pub. Health Newark & Sherwood PCT Newark. Specialty: Pub. Health Med. Prev: Cons., Pub. Health Med., Nth Nott. Health Auth..

RICHARDS, Richard Michael (retired) 2 Heol y Pavin, Llandaff, Cardiff CF5 2EG Tel: 029 2056 3241 — MB BCh Wales 1949 (Cardiff) BSc, MB BCh Wales 1949; FRCGP 1976, M 1959. Prev: Ho. Surg. Obst. Dept. St. David's Hosp. Cardiff.

RICHARDS, Mr Robert Hargest Orthopaedic Department, Queen Alexandra Hospital, Cosham, Portsmouth PO6 3LY; Corkallian, 10 Cold Harbour Close, Wickham, Fareham PO17 5PT Tel: 01329 834910 — BM BCh Oxf. 1982; MA Camb. 1983; FRCS Eng. 1986. Cons. Orthop. Surg. Qu. Alexandra Hosp. Portsmouth. Specialty: Orthop. Special Interest: Trauma Surg. Socs: Fell. BOA; Brit. Soc. Childr. Orthop. Surg. Prev: Sen. Regist. (Orthop.) Soton. Gen. Hosp.; Regist. Rotat. (Orthop.) Lord Mayor Treloar Hosp. Alton.

RICHARDS, Robert William Drayton Medical Practices, The Health Centre, Cheshire St., Market Drayton TF9 3BS Tel: 01630 652158 — MB ChB Aberd. 1989; DRCOG 1993; MRCGP 1994.

RICHARDS, Rosemary Kyffin Gloucestershire Partnership NHS, Child & Adolescent Services, Cleeve House, Horton Road, Gloucester GL1 3PX Tel: 01452 891312 — BM (Hons.) Soton. 1982; BSc (Hons.) Bristol 1972 1972; PhD Nottm. 1979, MA Nottm. 1974 1979; DRCOG 1984 1984; MRCPsych 1994 1994; C. Psychol. 1997 1997. p/t Cons. Child, Adolesc. & Family Psychiat. Gloucestershire Partnership NHS. Specialty: Child & Adolesc. Psychiat. Socs: Brit. Psychol. Soc.; Asson. Child Psychol. & Psych. Prev: Sen. Regist.

(Child Psychiat.) United Bristol Hosps. Trust; Regist. & SHO (Psychiat.) Bristol & Weston HA; Sen. Regist. (Child Psychiat.) W. Midl.

RICHARDS, Sally Flat 5, 67 Pen-y-lan Road, Roath, Cardiff CF23 5HZ — MB BCh Wales 1998.

RICHARDS, Sarah Elizabeth Heathville Road Surgery, 5 Heathville Road, Gloucester GL1 3DP Tel: 01452 528299 Fax: 01452 522959 — MB ChB Sheff. 1988.

RICHARDS, Sarah Kathryn 6 Coppice View, Weavering, Maidstone ME14 5TX — MB ChB Bristol 1997.

***RICHARDS, Sarah Vivien** Ringmer Surgery, Anchor Field, Ringmer, Lewes BN8 5QN — MB BS Lond. 1998 (St.Georges.Hosp) DGM 2000; DRCOG 2001; DFFP 2001. VTS.Brighton.Gen. Specialty: Gen. Pract.

RICHARDS, Selwyn Charles Morgan Department of Rheumatology, Poole NHS Trust, Poole BH15 2JB Tel: 01202 448613 Fax: 01202 660147 Email: selwynrichards@lineone.net; 48 Pilford Heath Road, Colehill, Wimborne BU21 2NB Tel: 01202 888610 — BM BCh Oxf. 1991; MA Camb. 1991; MRCP (UK) 1994; Dip. Sports Med. (Scot.) 1997. Cons. Rheumatologist. Specialty: Rheumatol.; Sports Med.; Research. Socs: Brit. Soc. Rheum.; Brit. Pain Soc.; Chronic fatigue Network. Prev: NHS Research Train. Fell., Kings Coll. Hosp.; Specialist Regist., Rheum., S. Thames; SHO City Hosp. Nottm.

RICHARDS, Sheila Mary 133 Overslade Lane, Rugby CV22 6EF — MB BS Lond. 1993 (St George's, Lond.) DRCOG 1997; DFFP 1997; MRCGP 1998. Specialty: Community Child Health; Family Plann. & Reproduc. Health.

RICHARDS, Shirley Jane, OBE (retired) Quarryfield House, Whitestone, Exeter EX4 2JS Tel: 01392 811492 Fax: 01392 811489 Email: dr_j_richards@compuserve.com — MB BS Lond. 1957 (Univ. Coll. Hosp.) MRCS Eng. LRCP Lond. 1957; DObst RCOG 1960; DCH Eng. 1961; FRCGP 1978, M 1970. Prev: Locum, Gen. Practitioner.

RICHARDS, Simon David Thorney Medical Practice, Wisbech Road, Thorney, Peterborough PE6 0SD Tel: 01733 270219 Fax: 01733 270860; 7 The Willows, Glinton, Peterborough PE6 7NE Tel: 01733 253445 Fax: 01733 270860 — MB BChir Camb. 1983; BSc St. And. 1980; MRCGP 1988; DRCOG 1991. Prev: Trainee GP/SHO Rotat. Camb. Milit. Hosp. VTS; Regtl. Med. Off. 17/21 Lancers (GP VTS); RMO 1 King's.

RICHARDS, Stella Jane St Sampson's Medical Centre, Grandes Maisons Road, St. Sampson, Guernsey GY2 4JS Tel: 01481 45915; Plaisance, Rue De Candie, Castel, Guernsey GY5 7BX Tel: 01481 52038 — MB ChB Bristol 1983; DRCOG 1987; MRCGP 1988. GP. Specialty: Obst. & Gyn. Socs: MDU. Prev: Trainee GP Bournemouth VTS; Trainee Year, Bishops Waltham; SHO (Cas.) Weston-Super-Mare.

RICHARDS, Stephen Andrew The Health Centre, Wayside Green, Woodcote, Reading RG8 0QL Tel: 01491 680686 Fax: 01491 682264; Yew Tree Farm House, Behoes Lane, Woodcote, Reading RG8 0PP — MB BChir Camb. 1982; MA Camb. 1983; DCH RCP Lond. 1984; DRCOG 1985; MRCGP 1986; Dip. Therapeutics 1990. PEC Chair SE Oxon. PCT.

RICHARDS, Stephen Miles 98 St Martins Road, Finham, Coventry CV3 6ER — MB BS Lond. 1980 (Univ. Coll. Hosp.) BSc Lond. 1976, MB BS 1980.

RICHARDS, Stuart David 278 Hills Road, Cambridge CB2 2QE — BM BS Nottm. 1997.

RICHARDS, Sylvia Théone Mary 18 Rose Close, Hedge End, Southampton SO30 2GR Tel: 023 8055 4625 — MB ChB Liverp. 1974.

RICHARDS, Tessa Jane Louise 30 Dartmouth Row, Greenwich, London SE10 8AW — MB ChB Leeds 1973 (Leeds & Guy's) MRCP (UK) 1976; MRCGP 1982. Asst. Edr. Brit. Med. Jl. Socs: BMA.

RICHARDS, Thomas Arthur (retired) 84 St George's Avenue, Northampton NN2 6JF Tel: 01604 714044 — MB BS Lond. 1945 (King's Coll. Hosp.) MD Lond. 1949; MRCP Lond. 1949; DObst RCOG 1954.

RICHARDS, Thomas Harold (retired) Ra-Mo-Ana, 8 Cwmbach Road, Llanelli SA15 4EP Tel: 01554 750429 — MB BS Lond. 1944 (Univ. Coll. Hosp.) MRCS Eng. LRCP Lond. 1944; MRCGP 1955. Prev: Ho. Phys. Brit. Postgrad. Med. Sch. Hammersmith & E. Suff. & Ipswich Hosp.

RICHARDS, Thomas Martin (retired) Turf Run, Bunch Lane, Haslemere GU27 1AE Tel: 01428 642582 Fax: 01428 642582 Email: tom@richardst.freeserve.co.uk — (St. Thos.) MB BS Lond. 1954; DObst RCOG 1956. Prev: Ho. Surg. Salisbury Gen. Hosp.

RICHARDS, Thomas Vincent Howells 44 Dinam Street, Nantymoel, Bridgend CF32 7PU — MRCS Eng. LRCP Lond. 1939.

RICHARDS, Veronica Jane Weir Cottage, Fladbury, Pershore WR10 2QA Tel: 01386 860668 — MB ChB Birm. 1962.

RICHARDS AFFONSO, Nicola Wokingham CAM HS, Wokingham Hospital, Barkham Road, Wokingham RG41 2RE Tel: 01189 495060 — MB ChB Bristol 1991; MA Oxf. 1985; MRCPsych 1997. SPR. Rotat. (Psychiat.) Oxf. Regional Train. Scheme in Child and Adolesc. Psychiat. Specialty: Child & Adolesc. Psychiat.

RICHARDSON, Abby Jane Wellside Surgery, 45 High St., Sawtry, Huntingdon PE28 5SU — MB ChB Leic. 1992.

RICHARDSON, Adrian Law Medical Group Practice, 9 Wrottesley Road, London NW10 5UY Tel: 020 8965 8011 Fax: 020 8961 6239; 10 Crooked Usage, Church End, Finchley, London N3 3HB Tel: 020 8349 3563 — MB BS Lond. 1980 (Middlx.) MRCP (UK) 1984; DCH RCP Lond. 1987; MRCGP 1988. Prev: Clin. Research Fell. King's Coll. Hosp. Lond.; Regist. (Med.) Hillingdon Hosp. Uxbridge.

RICHARDSON, Adrian Scott Fernville Surgery, Midland Road, Hemel Hempstead HP2 5BL Tel: 01442 213919 Fax: 01442 216433 — MB ChB Ed. 1992 (Edinburgh) BMedSci Ed. 1990; MRCP (UK) 1995; MRCGP 1997. Partner. Hemel Hempstead. Specialty: Gen. Med.

RICHARDSON, Mr Alan Ernest 6 Southwood Avenue, Kingston upon Thames KT2 7HD Tel: 020 8942 6476 — MB BS Lond. 1949 (Guy's) MRCS Eng. LRCP Lond. 1949; FRCS Eng. 1955; FRCS Ed. 1955. Hon. Cons. Neurosurg. St. Geo. Hosp. Lond. & SW Thames RHA; Teach. (Surg.) St. Geo. Hosp. Med. Sch. (Univ. Lond.); Vis. Surg. Mayday Hosp. Croydon & Accid. Centre St. Peter's Hosp. Chertsey; Hon. Cons Neurosurg. Wolfson Med. Rehabil. Centre. Specialty: Neurosurg. Socs: Fell. Roy. Soc. Med.; Soc. Brit. Neurol. Surgs.; Amer. Assn. Neurol. Surgs. Prev: Research Fell. (Neurosurg.) St. Geo. Hosp. Lond.; 1st Asst. (Neurosurg.) St. Geo. Hosp. Lond. & Nat. Hosp. Nerv. Dis. QuSq.

RICHARDSON, Alfred Ian, MBE (retired) Laggan, Mullach Na Beinne, Highland, Newtonmore PH20 1DT Tel: 01528 544240 — LRCP LRCS Ed. 1947 (Roy. Colls. Ed.) LRFPS Glas. 1947. Prev: Med. Pract. Highlands & Is.s Med. Serv.

RICHARDSON, Alison Parkway Medical Centre, 2 Frenton Close, Chapel House Estate, Newcastle upon Tyne NE5 1EH Tel: 0191 267 1313 Fax: 0191 229 0630; 7 Sunnidale, Fellside Park, Whickham, Newcastle upon Tyne NE16 5TT Tel: 0191 488 4010 — MB BS Newc. 1980; DRCOG 1983; MRCGP 1984.

RICHARDSON, Andrew Grant Prudhoe Hospital, Prudhoe NE42 5NT — MB ChB Leeds 1994; MRCPsych 1999. Cons. (Psychiat.) Child & Adolesc. Learn. Dis. Prudhoe Hosp. Specialty: Gen. Psychiat. Prev: Sen. Unified SHO. (Gen. Adult Psychiat.) Newc. Gen. Hosp.; Sen. Unified SHO (Child & Adolesc. Psychiat.) Sunderland Roy. Infirm.; Sen. Unified SHO (Old Age Psychiat.) Chester-le-St. Hosp.

RICHARDSON, Andrew James Worcester & District HA, Isaac Maddox House, Shrub Hill Road, Worcester WR4 9RW — MB ChB Manch. 1985; BSc St. And. 1982; MFPHM RCP (UK) 1992. Cons. Pub. Health Med. & Dir. Commissioning Worcs. Dist. HA. Specialty: Pub. Health Med. Prev: Sen. Regist. (Pub. Health Med.) Wessex RHA & Bath Dist. HA.

RICHARDSON, Andrew Julian 35 Hilltop Way, Salisbury SP1 3QY — MB BS Lond. 1997; BSc Lond. 1994; MRCP 2000. SpR in Anaestesia, Wessex rotation.

RICHARDSON, Andrew Mark Edward McLaughlin and Partners, 27-29 Derby Road, North End, Portsmouth PO2 8HP Tel: 023 9266 3024 Fax: 023 9265 4991 — MB BS Lond. 1989; BSc Lond. 1984, MB BS 1989.

RICHARDSON, Andrew Paul Cormer Place Surgery, 46A Dartmouth Road, Paignton TQ4 5AH Tel: 01803 557458; The Gables, 31 St. Matthews Road, Chelston, Torquay TQ2 6JA Tel: 01803 606161 — MB ChB Birm. 1984; DA (UK) 1986; DCH RCP Lond. 1987; DRCOG 1988; MRCGP 1989.

RICHARDSON, Benjamin Peter The Surgery, Ewyas Harold, Hereford HR2 0EU Tel: 01981 240320 Fax: 01981 241023; Merton

Lodge, Ewyas Harold, Hereford HR2 0HU Tel: 01981 240320 Fax: 01981 241023 — MB ChB Birm. 1971; DObst RCOG 1973; MRCP (UK) 1974.

RICHARDSON, Bernard William Thomas (retired) Stable Cottage, Chequers Lane, Watford WD25 0GP Tel: 01923 672238 — LRCP LRCS Ed. LRFPS Glas. 1946. Prev: Med. Off. Beckenham Hosp. & Leavesden Hosp. Abbot's Langley.

RICHARDSON, Brian David 23 Allenbys Chase, Sutton Bridge, Spalding PE12 9SY — MB ChB Leeds 1989; MRCP 1994; CCST Gen. & Respiratory Med. 2000.

RICHARDSON, Bruce The Surgery, The Brooklands, Leek Road, Waterhouses, Stoke-on-Trent ST10 3HN — MB ChB Sheff. 1971; DObst RCOG 1973.

RICHARDSON, Caroline Annie 23 Sandringham Road, Gosforth, Newcastle upon Tyne NE3 1QB — MB BS Newc. 1992.

RICHARDSON, Catherine Margaret The Old Stores Cottage, Weston Underwood, Ashbourne DE6 4PA — MB ChB Leic. 1996.

RICHARDSON, Charles Edward 21 Park Avenue, Mumbles, Swansea SA3 4DU — MB ChB Birm. 1989; BSc (Hons.) Birm. 1986; MRCP (UK) 1992.

RICHARDSON, Clare Denise Pitsmoor Surgery, 151 Burngreave Road, Sheffield S3 9DL Tel: 0114 272 8228 — MB ChB Sheff. 1983; MRCGP 1987; DCH RCP Lond. 1987; DCCH Sheff. 1989.

RICHARDSON, David 89 Bedford Road, Sutton Coldfield B75 6BG Tel: 0121 378 3374 — MB ChB Birm. 1975 (Birmingham) BSc (Hons.) Sheff. 1962.

RICHARDSON, Mr David Maxillofacial Unit, Aintree Hospitals NHS Trust, Walton Hospital, Rice Lane, Liverpool L9 1AE Tel: 0151 529 4786 Fax: 0151 529 4358; Maxillofacial Unit, Chester Royal Infirmary, Nicholas St, Chester CH1 2AZ Tel: 01244 363056 Fax: 01244 363056 — MB BS Lond. 1987; BDS Lond. 1979; FDS RCS Eng. 1990; FRCS Eng. 1991. Cons. Oral & Maxillofacial Surg. Aintree Hosps NHS Trust Liverp. & Countess of Chester NHS Trust. Specialty: Oral & Maxillofacial Surg. Socs: Fell. Brit. Assn. Oral & Maxillofacial Surg. Prev: Sen. Regist. & Regist. Rotat. (Maxillofacial Surg.) Mersey Region.

RICHARDSON, David Andrew — MB ChB Glas. 1977. GP Princip. Catrine.; Clin. Plann. Adviser Ayrsh. & Arran Health Bd., Ayr. Prev: Trainee Gen. Pract. Ayrsh. & Arran Vocational. Surgic. Ho. Off.; Med. Ho. Off. Ballochmyle Hosp.

RICHARDSON, David Andrew Wansbeck General Hospital, Woodhorn Lane, Ashington NE63 9JJ — MB ChB Leeds 1986; MRCP (UK) 1993; MD Newc. 2002. Cons. Physician/Geriatrician Wansbeck Gen. Hosp. Ashington. Specialty: Care of the Elderly. Socs: Brit. Geriat. Soc.; BMA; Soc. of Geriat. Cardiol.

RICHARDSON, David Leslie Department Diagnostic Radiology, Royal Victoria Infirmary, Queen Victoria Road, Newcastle upon Tyne NE1 4LP Tel: 0191 232 5131 Fax: 0191 227 5223; Fell View, 8 Deepdale Close, Whickham, Newcastle upon Tyne NE16 5SN Tel: 0191 488 4010 — MB BS Newc. 1980; FRCR 1987. Cons. Radiol. Roy. Vict. Infirm. Specialty: Radiol. Prev: Cons. Radiol. Newc. Gen. & Freeman Hosps.; Sen. Regist. (Radiol.) Newc. u Tyne.

RICHARDSON, David Peter Mitchell Road Surgery, 9 Mitchell Road, Canferd Heath, Poole BH17 8UE Tel: 01202 672474 Fax: 01202 660926 — MB BS Lond. 1985.

RICHARDSON, Deborah Susan Southampton General Hospital, Dept. of Haematology, Tremona Road, Southampton SO16 6YD Tel: 02380 796164 Fax: 02380 794134 Email: deborah.richardson@suht.swest.nhs.uk — MB BChir Camb. 1989 (Univ. Camb.) MA Camb. 1991, BA (Hons.) 1987; MRCP (UK) 1993; MRC Path 1999. Cons. Haemat.S.ampton Univ. Hosp..; Hon.Sen. Lect. Univ. of Southampton Sch. Of Med. Specialty: Haematology. Socs: Brit. Soc. Haematol.; Amer. Soc .Haemat.; Eur. Haematol. Assn. Prev: Sspecialist Regist. & Hon. Lect. St Barts & Roy. Lond. Hosps.

RICHARDSON, Donald Stockingwood Farmhouse, Hillesden, Buckingham MK18 4DE — MB ChB Leeds 1989.

RICHARDSON, Donald Arthur 1 Cherry Tree Rise, Walkern, Stevenage SG2 7JL Tel: 01438 861349 — (Westm.) MB BS Lond. 1956; DObst RCOG 1958; M 1964; FRCGP 1984. Treas. Cameron Fund. Socs: BMA; RSM. Prev: GP St. Albans.

RICHARDSON, Dorothy Evelyn Margaret Carradale, Whimple, Exeter EX5 2PL — MRCS Eng. LRCP Lond. 1938 (King's Coll. Lond. & Bristol) Prev: Ho. Surg. Res. Anaesth. & Sen. Ho. Phys. Roy. Infirm. Bristol.

RICHARDSON, Elizabeth Margaret Bro Cerwyn Centre, Fishguard Road, Haverfordwest Tel: 01437 772826 Fax: 01437 772834 — MB BCh Wales 1982 (Cardiff) MRCPsych. 1989. Consultant Psychiatrist, General Adult. Specialty: Care of the Elderly.

RICHARDSON, Elspeth Mary (retired) — MB ChB Liverp. 1948. Prev: GP Liverp. VTS.

RICHARDSON, Esther Joy Laura PO Box 13787, London N14 4WD Email: gpax@supanet.com — MB BChir Camb. 1992; MRCGP. Specialty: Gen. Pract. Socs: Mem. of Roy. Coll. of Gen. Practitioners.

RICHARDSON, Ethel Anne (retired) 5 Colletts Close, Corfe Castle, Wareham BH20 5HG — (Leeds) MRCS Eng. LRCP Lond. 1954; MB ChB Leeds 1955; DCH Eng. 1959; FRCPath 1986, M 1974. Prev: Cons. Microbiol. (Pub. Health & Hosp. Microbiol. Laborat.) Poole Gen. Hosp.

RICHARDSON, Fiona Mary Millburn, 2 Milton of Straloch, Newmacher, Aberdeen AB21 0QE — MB ChB Aberd. 1988; MRCGP 1993.

RICHARDSON, Mr Francis John Accident & Emergency Department, Royal Gwent Hospital, Cardiff Road, Newport NP20 2UB Tel: 01633 234065 Fax: 01633 238966 — MB ChB Liverp. 1981; FRCS Ed. 1988; Dip IMC RCS Ed. 1989; DA (UK) 1990; FFAEM 1997; Dip Med Educ. 1999. Cons. (A & E Med.) Roy. Gwent Hosp. Newport S. Wales. Specialty: Accid. & Emerg. Socs: Brit. Assn. Accid. & Emerg. Med.; BASICS; BMA. Prev: Sen. Regist. (A & E Med.) Cardiff Roy. Infirm.; Regist. (A & E) W. Midl. RHA; Sen. Med. Off. Johannesburg Trauma Unit.

RICHARDSON, Fraser Elmbank Group, Foresterhill Health Centre, Westburn Road, Aberdeen AB25 2AY Tel: 01224 696949 Fax: 01224 691650; 13 Earlswells Road, Fairacres, Cults, Aberdeen AB15 9NY Tel: 01224 867286 Fax: 01224 691650 — MB ChB Aberd. 1968. Med. Off. Offshore Oil Indust.; Sen. Lect. (Gen. Pract.) Univ. Aberd. Specialty: Gen. Pract. Socs: Aberd. M-C Soc. Prev: Regist. (Med.) Aberd. Roy. Infirm.

RICHARDSON, Gail 12 Nelson Street, King's Lynn PE30 5DY — MB BS Lond. 1990; BSc (Hons.) Lond. 1987; MRCP (UK) 1994. Regist. Rotat. (Cardiol.) Chase Farm., Roy. Free & Lond. Chest Hosps. Specialty: Cardiol. Prev: SHO Rotat. (Med.) St. Bart. Hosp. Lond.

RICHARDSON, Giles Lindley Flat 4, Pembroke Mansions, 1-3 Oakfield Road, Clifton, Bristol BS8 2AH Tel: 01177 973 4766 Email: gilesrich@hotmail.com — MB ChB Bristol 1994. Specialty: Paediat.

RICHARDSON, Gillian — MB BCh Wales 1985; MRCGP (Distinc.) 1990; MPH Wales 1997; MFPHMI Dublin 2001. Spcialist Pub. Health and policy BroTaf Health Auth., Cardiff, Wales. Specialty: Pub. Health Med.; Epidemiol.; Gen. Pract. Socs: BMA; Christian Med. Fellowsh. Prev: SpR Pub. Health Med. BroTaf Health Auth.; SpR Pub. Health Med. Mid Glam. Health Auth.; Lect. Univ. Wales Coll. of Med.

RICHARDSON, Graham Andrew Offshore, 10 Stein Road, Southbourne, Emsworth PO10 8LD — MRCS Eng. LRCP Lond. 1958 (Univ. Coll. Hosp.) MD Lond. 1969, MB BS 1958; MRCP (U.K.) 1970. Cons. Phys. & Cons. Chest Phys. Torbay Hosp. Torquay. Specialty: Respirat. Med. Socs: Fell. Med. Soc. Lond. Prev: Sen. Rgis.Univ. Coll. Hosp. Resid. Med Off. Univ Coll Hosp. Lond.. HO,Ssurg Univ. Coll Hosp.

RICHARDSON, Gregory James Ronald Lime Trees, Child Adolescent and Family Unit, 31 Shipton Road, York YO30 5RF Tel: 01904 652908 Fax: 01904 632893 — MB ChB Liverp. 1971; MRCS Eng. LRCP Lond. 1971; DCH Eng. 1975; FRCPsych. 1991, M 1977; DPM Leeds 1977; FRCPCH 1997. Cons. Child Adolesc. & Family Psychiat. Lime Trees York; Hon. Lect. Child & Adolesc. Psychiat. Univ. Leeds.; Vis. Fell. Univ. York; Specialist Adviser to the health Advisery Serv. Specialty: Child & Adolesc. Psychiat. Socs: Fell. Roy. Coll. Psychiat.; Fell. Roy. Coll. Peadiat. & Child Health; BMA. Prev: Cons. Child & Adolesc. Psychiat. Harrogate & Northallerton HAs; Med. Off. Save the Childr. Fund Mother & Child Health Unit Torit, Sudan; Resid. (Child & Adolesc. Psychiat.) Hosp. Sick Childr. Toronto, Canada.

RICHARDSON, Hanora Bernadette Mary Thornley Street Surgery, 40 Thornley Street, Wolverhampton WV1 1JP Tel: 01902

26843 Fax: 01902 688500 — MB BCh BAO Dub. 1987; MB BCh BAO (Dub) 1987.

RICHARDSON, Hazel Joan Richardson & Ilves, 351 Danebury Avenue, London SW15 4DU Tel: 020 8876 6666 Fax: 020 8878 2629; 58 Temple Sheen Road, London SW14 7QG — BM BCh Oxf. 1968; MA Oxf. 1968; MRCGP 1981.

RICHARDSON, Helen Diane Department of Diagnostic Radiology, Kingston Hospital NHS Trust, Galsworthy Road, Kingston upon Thames KT2 7QB Tel: 0208 546 7711 — MB BS Lond. 1991 (St. Geo. Hosp. Lond.) BSc Lond. 1988; MRCP (UK) 1995; FRCR UK 2000. Cons. Radiol. Kingston Hosp. Surrey. Specialty: Radiol. Prev: Regist. (Toxicol.) Guy's Hosp. Lond.; SHO (Med.) Medway Hosp. Gillingham & King's Coll. Hosp. Lond.; Specialist Regist. (Clin. Radiol.) King's Coll. Hosp. Lond.

RICHARDSON, Ian Harold (retired) Hill Orchard, Blenheim Hill, Harwell, Didcot OX11 0DS Tel: 01235 835222 Fax: 01235 835222 — MRCS Eng. LRCP Lond. 1949 (Middlx.) Prev: Jun. Regist., Ho. Surg. & Ho. Phys. (Paediat.) St. Helier Hosp. Carshalton.

RICHARDSON, Ian Milne (retired) Rockland, 9 Grampian Avenue, Auchterarder PH3 1NY Tel: 01764 63826 — MB ChB Ed. 1944 (Univ. Ed.) MB ChB (Hons.) Ed. 1944; FRCP Ed. 1956, M 1946; DPH Glas. 1948; MD (High Commend.) Ed. 1953; PhD Aberd. 1956; FRCGP 1973, M 1968. Prev: James Mackenzie Prof. Gen. Pract. Univ. Aberd.

RICHARDSON, Ian Robert The Clinic, 4 Firs Entry, Bannockburn, Stirling FK7 0HW Tel: 01786 813435 Fax: 01786 817545 — MB ChB Glas. 1963; DObst RCOG 1966. Hosp. Pract. Bannockburn Hosp. Socs: BMA. Prev: Ho. Off. Stirling Roy. Infirm. & Ayrsh. Centr. Matern. Hosp. Irvine; Ho. Surg. S. Gen. Hosp. Glas.

RICHARDSON, James Hackwood Partnership, Essex House, Worting Road, Basingstoke RG21 8SU; The Rose, Basingstoke Road, Ramsdell, Basingstoke RG26 5RB Tel: 01256 850345 — MB BS Lond. 1974 (Guy's) MRCS Eng. LRCP Lond. 1974; DObst RCOG 1976; Cert JCC Lond. 1976; Dip Occ. Med. 1996.

RICHARDSON, Professor James Bruce Institute of Orthopaedics, Robert Jones and Agnes Hunt Orthopaedic & District Hospital NHS Trust, Oswestry SY10 7AG Tel: 01691 404386 Fax: 01691 404071 Email: james.richardson@rjah.nhs.uk — MB ChB Aberd. 1977; FRCS Ed. 1984; MD Aberd. 1989. Prof. Keele Univ. Specialty: Orthop. Socs: Brit. Orthop. Assn.; Assn. Prof.s of Orthop. Surg.; Knee Soc. Prev: Sen. Lect. & Hon. Cons. Leicester; RSO (Orthop.) Oswestry.

RICHARDSON, Jane 8 Briarwood Close, Brynoch, Neath SA10 7UH — MB BCh Wales 1983.

RICHARDSON, Jeanette Olga Concorde Cottage, Ellingstring, Ripon HG4 4PW — MB ChB Ed. 1997.

RICHARDSON, Jennifer Barbara Ladthorne Grange, Brownstow, Modbury, Ivybridge PL21 0SH — MB ChB Liverp. 1978; DA Eng. 1982.

RICHARDSON, Jeremy Peter Allan Sutton Hill Medical Practice, Maythorne Close, Sutton Hill, Telford TF7 4DH Tel: 01952 586471 Fax: 01952 588029; 3 Grange Farm View, Telford TF3 1DX — MB BS Lond. 1977; BSc Lond. 1974; MRCGP 1981. Hosp. Practitioner Psychiat. Shrops. Community & Ment. Health Servs. Trust.

RICHARDSON, Jeremy Robert Millburn, 2 Milton of Staloch, Newmachar, Aberdeen AB21 0QE — MB ChB Aberd. 1989; MRCP (UK) 1993. Specialist Regist. (A & E) Aberd. Roy. Hosps. NHS Trust. Specialty: Accid. & Emerg. Prev: Career Regist. (Clin. Pharmacol.) Aberd. Roy. Hosps. NHS Trust & Raigmore Hosp. Inverness; Clin. Research Fell. (Med. & Therap.) Aberd. Univ.; SHO (Gen. Med.) Aberd. Hosps.

RICHARDSON, Joanna Rachel Island Health, 145 East Ferry Road, London E14 3BQ Tel: 020 7363 1111 Fax: 020 7363 1112 — MB BS Lond. 1984; MRCP (UK) 1988; DRCOG 1988; DCH RCP Lond. 1988; MRCGP 1989. Princip. GP Lond. Prev: Trainee GP Roy. Free Hosp. Lond. VTS; SHO (Cardiol.) Hammersmith Hosp. Lond.; Ho. Off. Med. Unit Roy. Free Hosp. Lond.

RICHARDSON, Mr John 14 Drumoyne Close, Greenacres, E. Herrington, Sunderland SR3 3SD Tel: 0191 528 0704 — (Newc.) MB BS Durh. 1963; DO Eng. 1967; FRCS Eng. 1968; FRCOphth 1989. Cons. Ophth. Sunderland Eye Infirm. Specialty: Ophth. Socs: Fac. Ophthalmol.; N. Eng. Ophth. Soc. Prev: Sen. Regist & Regist. Eye Dept. Vict. Infirm. Newc.; SHO Oxf. Eye Hosp.

RICHARDSON, Mr John Anthony Rumwell Lodge, Rumwell, Taunton TA4 1EJ — MB ChB Bristol 1966; MRCOG 1973, DObst 1966; FRCS Ed. 1973. Cons. (O & G) MusGr. Pk. Hosp. Specialty: Obst. & Gyn. Prev: Lect. (O & G) Univ. Bristol; Regist. (O & G) S. W. RHB.

RICHARDSON, Professor John Carter, OStJ, Colonel L/RAMC Retd. 1 Franklin Place, Chichester PO19 1BL Tel: 01243 780786 Fax: 01243 773348 — MB BChir Camb. 1968 (Camb. & St. Bart.) MRCS Eng. LRCP Lond. 1967; MA Camb. 1968; FRCGP 1996, M 1974; DRCOG 1977; MSc (GP) Lond. 1990; MMedSc. (Occupat. Health) Birm. 1992; FFOM RCPI 1995. p/t GP Non Principal; Med. Adviser Roy. Brit. Legion Pilgrimage Dept.; Hon. Sen. Research Fell. Centre for Hist. of Med. Birm. Univ. Specialty: Occupat. Health; Gen. Pract. Socs: Fell. Roy. Soc. Med.; Fell. Hunt. Soc.; Fell. Med.Soc. Lond. Prev: GP Brackley; Defence Emeritus Prof. of GP,Royal Centre Defence Medicine.

RICHARDSON, John Craig (retired) 56 Porth y Felin, Holyhead LL65 1BD Tel: 01407 760206 — MB ChB Liverp. 1949; DA Eng. 1952; FFA RCS Eng. 1954. Prev: Cons. Anaesth. Liverp. Regional Cardiothoracic Surg. Centre & Mill Rd. Matern. Hosp. Liverp.

RICHARDSON, John Francis (retired) 12 Kings Hall Road, Beckenham BR3 1LU — MB BS Lond. 1963 (Lond. Hosp.) MRCP (U.K.) 1970. Prev: Ho. Surg. Lond. Hosp.

RICHARDSON, John Patrick Stuart Church Field Medical Centre, Church Field, Camelford PL32 9YT Tel: 01840 213894; The Old Farm House, Condolden, Tintagel PL34 0HJ Tel: 01840 212818 Email: condolden@aol.com — MB BS Lond. 1964; MRCS Eng. LRCP Lond. 1964.

RICHARDSON, John Pierre Ryder, VRD (retired) Westhill, Saxmundham IP17 1DT Tel: 01728 602376 — MRCS Eng. LRCP Lond. 1946 (Lond. Hosp.) Prev: Ho. Phys., Ho. Surg. Lond. Hosp.

RICHARDSON, John Sherbrooke Mount Chambers, 92 Coggeshall Road, Braintree CM7 9BY Tel: 01376 553415 Fax: 01376 552451 — MB Camb. 1969 (Camb. & St. Thos.) BChir 1968; DObst RCOG 1971; DA Eng. 1971; MRCGP 1974.

RICHARDSON, John Stuart Carradale, Whimple, Exeter EX5 2PL — (Bristol) M.B., Ch.B. Bristol 1938. Prev: Squadron Ldr. R.A.F. Med. Br.

RICHARDSON, John Warlow Holderness Road Surgery, 445 Holderness Road, Hull HU8 8JS Tel: 01482 374255 Fax: 01482 790301 — MB Camb. 1978; BChir 1977; MRCP (UK) 1979; DRCOG 1983; MRCGP 1984.

RICHARDSON, Mr John Wilberforce, OBE, Surg. Capt. RN (retired) 1 Leep Lane, Clayhall Road, Alverstoke, Gosport PO12 2BE Tel: 023 9258 1543 — MB BS Lond. 1953 (Univ. Coll. Hosp.) FRCS Eng. 1961. Prev: Dean of Naval Med.

RICHARDSON, Jonathan Department Anaesthetics, Bradford Royal Infirmary, Bradford BD9 6J Tel: 01274 364065 Fax: 01274 366548 — MB ChB Liverpool 1977; MRCP Liverpool 1982; FFARCSI Liverpool 1985; MD Liverpool 1994; FRCP 1999; FIPP 2003. Cons. Anaesth., Specialist in pain. Specialty: Anaesth. Socs: Internatioanl Spinal Injection Soc.; Pain Soc.; Pain Interven. Interest Gp.

RICHARDSON, Jonathan Charles Willerton The Surgery, Mount Avenue, Shenfield, Brentwood CM13 2NL Tel: 01277 224612 Fax: 01277 201218; 27 Coombe Rise, Shenfield, Brentwood CM15 8JJ — MB Camb. 1983; BSc (Hons.) Physiol. St. And. 1975; PhD Ed. 1979; BChir 1982. Socs: Assoc. RCGP; Fell. Amer. Soc. for Laser Med. & Surg. Prev: Regist. (Med.) Qu. Med. Centre Nottm.; SHO (O & G) Newmarket Gen. Hosp.; Ho. Phys. Addenbrookes Hosp. Camb.

RICHARDSON, Jonathan Paul 26 Ruthven Street, Glasgow G12 9BT — MB ChB Glas. 1997.

RICHARDSON, Joyce Elizabeth (retired) Cruachan, 17 Caiystane Avenue, Edinburgh EH10 6SA Tel: 0141 943 0678 — (Edinburgh) MB ChB Ed. 1957; DCH RFPS Glas. 1960; FRCP Ed. 1979, M 1967; FRCP Glas. 1983, M 1980; FRCP 1997. Cons. Med. Paediat. Lomond Healthcare NHS Trust & Roy. Hosp. Sick Childr. Glas. Prev: Sen. Regist. (Med. Paediat.) Roy. Aberd. Childr. Hosp.

RICHARDSON, Judith Anne South Manchester NHS Primary Care Trust, 1st Floor, Home 4, Withington Hsopital, Nell Lane, West Didsbury, Manchester M20 2LR Tel: 0161 6114702 Mob: 07736 713921 Fax: 0161 6113900 — MB BS Lond. 1986 (Middlesex Hosp. Medical School) MPH Leeds 1992; MRCGP 1996; MFPHM RCP (UK) 1996. p/t Dir, of Public Health, South Manchester Primary

Care Trust. Specialty: Pub. Health Med. Prev: Cons., (Pub. Health Med.) Manch. Health Auth., (p/t).

RICHARDSON, Judith Mary University Health Service, University of Edinburgh, Richard Verney Health Centre, Edinburgh EH8 9AL Tel: 0131 650 2777 Fax: 0131 662 1813; Easter Walstone, Penicuik EH26 9LS Tel: 01968 677822 — MB ChB Ed. 1990; DRCOG 1993; DCH RCPS Glas. 1993; MRCGP 1994. Specialty: Gen. Pract.

RICHARDSON, Justin Charles 36 Westfield Close, Bath BA2 2EB — MB BS Lond. 1990.

RICHARDSON, Karen Lee 9 Baslow Road, Eastbourne BN20 7UL — BMed (Hons.) NSW 1987; MRCP (UK) 1993. Clin. Research Fell. & Med. Regist. (Gen. Med., Rheum. & Haemat.) Eastbourne Gen. Hosp. Specialty: Gen. Med. Socs: Assoc. Mem. Austral. & NZ Intens. Care Soc.

RICHARDSON, Madeleine Helen 51 Cossington Road, Canterbury CT1 3HX Tel: 01227 763377 Fax: 01227 786908 — MB BS Lond. 1974; DA Eng. 1976.

RICHARDSON, Mark Lindum Medical Practice, 1 Cabourne Court, Cabourne Avenue, Lincoln LN2 2JP Tel: 01522 569033 Fax: 01522 576713; Merriott, 11 Eastfield Lane, Welton, Lincoln LN2 3NA Email: mark.scothern@lineone.net — MB ChB Liverp. 1982. Special Interest: drug misuse.

RICHARDSON, Michael Ian Hadleigh House, 20 Kirkway, Broadstone BH18 8EE Tel: 01202 692268 Fax: 01202 658954 — MB ChB Bristol 1974; MRCP (UK) 1977; DRCOG 1978.

RICHARDSON, Michael John Altrincham Medical Practice, Normans Place, Altrincham WA14 2AB Tel: 0161 928 2424; 2 Groby Road, Altrincham WA14 1RS Tel: 0161 929 6053 — MB ChB Manch. 1988; BSc (Med Sci.) St. And. 1985; DRCOG 1991; MRCGP 1992.

RICHARDSON, Michael John North Brink Practice, 7 North Brink, Wisbech PE13 1JR Tel: 01945 585121 Fax: 01945 476423 — BM BS Nottm. 1981; BMedSci Nottm. 1979, BM BS 1981; MRCGP 1987.

RICHARDSON, Michael Robert Westmount Assessment and Rehabilitation Centre, Overdale, Westmount, St Helier, Jersey JE2 3LP Tel: 01534 623060 Fax: 01534 623098 Email: M.Richardson@health.gov.je — MB ChB Ed. 1982 (Edin.) BSc (Med. Sci.) Ed; FRCP Lond. 1997, M 1986. Cons. Phys. Gen. Hosp. St. Helier, Jersey. Specialty: Gen. Med.; Care of the Elderly; Rheumatol.

RICHARDSON, Mr Nigel George Boyd Broomfield Hospital , Department of Surgery, Court Road, Broomfield, Chelmsford CM1 7ET Tel: 01245 516064 Fax: 01245 514858 Email: nigel.richardson@meht.nhs.uk; The Old School House, The Street, Little Dunmow, Dunmow CM6 3HT Tel: 01371 821303 Email: nigel.richardson@virgin.net — MB BS Lond. 1986 (St George's Hospital Medical School) FRCS Eng. 1991; MS Lond. 1996; FRCS (Gen.) 1998. Cons. (Colorectal & Gen. Surg.). Specialty: Gen. Surg. Special Interest: Colorectal Surg.; Minimal Access Surg. Socs: RSM; Assoc. of Surg.s of GB & Ire; Assoc. of ColoProctol. of GB & Ire. Prev: S. Thames (WEST), Surgic. Train. Schemes.

RICHARDSON, Paul Millmead, 61 Hall Ing Lane, Honley, Holmfirth HD9 6QW Tel: 01484 667681 — MB ChB Leeds 1984; MRCGP Edin. 1990. GP Huddersfield. Special Interest: Sports Med., Acupunc., Musculoskeletal Med. & Minor Surg. in Gen. Pract. Socs: BMA; RCGP; Brit. Med. Acupunct. Soc. Prev: GP Bradford.

RICHARDSON, Paul 45 Yew Tree Lane, West Derby, Liverpool L12 9HG — MB BS Newc. 1990; MRCP (UK) 1994.

RICHARDSON, Paul Gerard Guy 38 Fontarabia Road, Battersea, London SW11 5PF — MB BS Lond. 1986.

RICHARDSON, Paul Sebastian (retired) Department of Physiology, St. George's Hospital Medical School, London SW17 0RE; 45 Hazlewell Road, London SW15 6LS — BM BCh Oxf. 1968 (St. Geo.) DM Oxf. 1974, MA, BM BCh 1968. Reader Physiol. St. Geo. Hosp. Tooting.

RICHARDSON, Paul Stuart The Surgery, Bengal Street, Leigh WN7 1YA Tel: 01942 605506 Fax: 01942 680109 — AKC; BSc, MB BS Lond. 1979; DRCOG 1982; DCH RCP Lond. 1983; MRCGP 1983.

RICHARDSON, Peter Craig 3 Kings Mill Road, Driffield YO25 6TT — BM BS Nottm. 1983.

RICHARDSON, Peter John Cromwell Hospital, 4 Pennant Mews, London W8 5JN Tel: 020 7460 5667 Fax: 020 7244 6429 Email: pjrichardson@boltblue.com; 10 Girton House, Manor Fields, Putney Hill, London SW15 3LN Tel: 020 8788 6860 Fax: 020 7244 6429 — MB BS Lond. 1963 (King's Coll. Hosp.) FRCP Lond. 1985, M 1969; MD (Cardiol.) Lond 1984. Cons. Cardiol. & Director of Cardiol., Cromwell Hosp., Lond.; Emerit. Cons. Cardiol., Kings Coll. Hosp., Lond. Specialty: Cardiol. Special Interest: Cardiomyopathies; Coronary Artery Dis.; Hypertens. Socs: Brit. Cardiac Soc.; Europ. Soc. of Cardiol.; World heart Federat., -Counc. on cardiomyopathies. Prev: Cons. Cardiol., Kings Coll. Hosp., Lond.

RICHARDSON, Richard James 7 Emlyn Road, London W12 9TF Tel: 020 8749 4411 Fax: 020 8749 4422 Email: rjrichardson@btinternet.com — MB BS Lond. 1973 (Middlx.) FRCP London; FRCPCH; BSc Lond. 1969; MRCP (UK) 1977; DCH Eng. 1977; DTM & H Liverp. 1979. Chairm. Richardson Cons. U.K. Ltd. 7 Emlyn Rd., Lond. W12 9TF; Cons. Paediat. Gt. Ormond St. Hosp. Childr. Lond.; Hon. Cons. Paediatr., Portland Hosp. for Wom. and Childr..; Chairm. E-Health working group, Europe Health Tele. Assoc; Chairm.- Clin. Director, Health Systems Consultants Ltd. Specialty: Paediat. Special Interest: Childr. with special needs. Socs: Fell. Roy. Soc. Med.; Fell. Roy. Soc. Trop. Med.; Fell. Roy. Coll. Paediat. Prev: Sub-Dean & Sen. Lect. Centre for Internat. Child Health Inst. Child Health Lond.; Cons. Paediat. MoH Oman & Brunei.

RICHARDSON, Robert Galloway Apple Tree Cottage, French Street, Westerham TN16 1PW Tel: 01959 563942 Fax: 01959 563942 — BM BCh Oxf. 1951 (Oxf. & Middlx.) MA Oxf. 1951; LMSSA Lond. 1951. Socs: Fell. Roy. Soc. Med.; Brit. Soc. Hist. of Med. Prev: Edt. Spectrum Internat.; Edr. Abbottempo; Med. Edr. Butterworth's Med. Pub.ats.

RICHARDSON, Robert John Ormeau Road Surgery, 137 Ormeau Road, Belfast BT7 1SN — MB BCh BAO Belf. 1965; MRCGP 1971.

RICHARDSON, Mr (Robert) Simon (retired) Braeburn, Eglingham, Alnwick Tel: 01665 578448 — MB BS Lond. 1960 (St. Mary's) FRCS Eng. 1967; Specialist Accredit (Orthop.) RCS Eng. 1975. Prev: Sen. Regist. (Orthop.) St. Geo. Hosp. Lond.

RICHARDSON, Robert William Hartlepool Health Centre, Victoria Road, Hartlepool Tel: 01429 273191; 33 Parklands Way, Hartlepool TS26 0AP Tel: 01429 272593 — MB ChB Leeds 1956. Socs: BMA. Prev: Ho. Surg. (Gen. Surg.) & Ho. Phys. (Obst. & Gen. Med.) St. Jas. Hosp. Leeds; Clin. Asst. (Occupat. Health) Hartlepool HA.

RICHARDSON, Rosalind Patricia c/o Lagan Valley Hospital, Hillsborough Road, Lisburn BT28 1JP — MB BCh BAO Belf. 1988.

RICHARDSON, Rosemary The Old Farm House, Condolden, Tintagel PL34 0HJ Tel: 01840 212818 Mob: 07971 169335 Fax: 01840 212818 Email: condolden@aol.com; Treliske, Treloyhan Close, St Ives TR26 2AJ — (Bart's) MRCPCH; MB BS Lond. 1966; MRCS Eng. LRCP Lond. 1966; DCH RCP Lond. 1969; DRCOG 1969. Assoc. Specialist (Community Child Health) RCHT Treliske Truro & Plymouth Hosps. NHS Trust. Specialty: Community Child Health. Socs: Fac. Community Health; Brit. Paediat. Assn. Prev: Staff Paediat. (Community Child Health) E. Cornw.; Staff Paediat. (Community Child Health) Moorland Rd. Health Clinic St. Austell.

RICHARDSON, Sally Ann Whitley Road Health Centre, Whitley Road, Whitley Bay NE26 2ND Tel: 0191 253 1113; 4 The Crossway, Morpeth NE61 2DA Tel: 01670 510382 — MB BS Newc. 1982 (Newcastle-upon-Tyne) DCCH RCGP & FCM 1985; DRCOG 1986; MRCGP 1986.

RICHARDSON, Sharon Jane Keepers Gate, Hunstanton Road, Heacham, King's Lynn PE31 7JU Email: keepersgate@heacham.fsnet.co.uk — MB ChB Bristol 1984; DA (UK) 1988. Staff Grade (Anaesth.) Qu. Eliz. Hosp. King's Lynn. Specialty: Anaesth. Prev: Clin. Asst. (Anaesth.) Qu. Eliz. Hosp. King's Lynn.

RICHARDSON, Sian Margaret 22 Charlton-on-the-Hill, Charlton Marshall, Blandford Forum DT11 9NR — MB ChB Dundee 1984.

RICHARDSON, Stephen 53 Red Scar Lane, Newby, Scarborough YO12 5RH — MB ChB Manch. 1979; DA UK 1982; MRCGP 1984. Specialty: Anaesth.

RICHARDSON, Stephen Andrew Child Health Directorate, Westgate House, Southmead Hospital, Bristol BS10 5NB Tel: 0117 959 5355 Fax: 0117 959 5363; 12 The Orchards, Landkey, Barnstaple EX32 0QP — MB BS Lond. 1975 (St. Thos.) BSc (

Physiology) London 1972; MSc Lond. 1990, BSc 1972; DRCOG 1979; DCH RCP Lond. 1979; DTM & H Liverp. 1980; MRCGP 1983; MRCPCH 1996; DLSHTM Lond. 1997; FRCPCH 1998. Specialty: Paediat.; Community Child Health. Socs: Christ. Med. Fellowsh.; BMA; Neonat. Soc. Prev: Tutor & Lect. (Paediat.) Lilongwe Sch. for Health Sci.s & Kamuzu Centr. Hosp. Lilongwe, Malawi; Cons. Paediat. N. Devon. Distict Hosp. Barnstaple (1992-1999); Cons. Paediat.,Roy. Naval Hosp., Gibraltar (1999-2001).

RICHARDSON, Stephen Geoffrey Belfast City Hospital, Belfast BT9 7AB Tel: 01232 263834 Fax: 01232 263583 Email: geoff.richardson@bch.n-i.nhs.uk — MD Belf. 1987; MB BCh BAO 1981; MRCP (UK) 1984; FRCP Lond 1997. Cons. Cardiol. Belf. City Hosp. Specialty: Cardiol. Socs: Brit. Cardiac Soc.; Irish Cardiac Soc. Prev: Sen. Regist. (Cardiol.) Belf. City Hosp.

RICHARDSON, Stephen Guy Noel Haematology Department, Russells Hall Hospital, Dudley DY1 2HQ Tel: 01384 244158 — MB ChB Birm. 1966; MRCP (UK) 1970; M 1976; FRCPath 1988; FRCP 1990; FRCP Lond. 1991. Cons. Haemat. Dudley AHA. Specialty: Haematology. Prev: Sen. Regist. (Haemat.) Qu. Eliz. Hosp. Birm.; Regist. (Med.) N. Staffs. Roy. Infirm. Stoke-on-Trent; Sen. Regist. (Haemat.) Univ. Hosp. W. Indies Kingston, Jamaica.

RICHARDSON, Susan Mary Family Planning Clinic, Keighley Health Centre, Oakworth Road, Keighley BD21 1SA Tel: 01535 606111; 37 Main Street, Farnhill, Keighley BD20 9BJ Tel: 01535 633205 Fax: 01535 295636 — MB ChB Liverp. 1966; MFFP 1993. Cons. in Sexual & Reproductive Health, Airedale PCT, Keighley Health Centre; Research Assoc. Univ. of Exeter. Specialty: Family Plann. & Reproduc. Health. Special Interest: HRT/ Menopause Research. Socs: Fac. Fam. Plann. & Reproductive Health Care.

RICHARDSON, Suzanne Margaret The Croft, Great Wymondley, Hitchin SG4 7EU Tel: 01438 354081 Fax: 01438 357005 — MB BS Lond. 1972; MRCS Eng. LRCP Lond. 1972.

RICHARDSON, Sylvia (retired) 34 Linden Drive, Evington, Leicester LE5 6AH Tel: 0116 273 6302 — MB BS Durh. 1960 (Newc.) Med. Asst. (Anaesth.) Leicester Community Dent. Serv. Prev: Med. Asst. (Anaesth.) Harlow Wood Orthop. Hosp.

RICHARDSON, Thomas (retired) 20 Rivergrove Park, Rectory Road, Beckenham BR3 1HX Tel: 020 8650 5654 — MB BCh BAO NUI 1926 (Univ. Coll. Cork)

RICHARDSON, Thomas James 33 Kinghorn Road, Kirkcaldy KY1 1SU — MB ChB Ed. 1966; DObst RCOG 1968. Socs: BMA. Prev: Surg. Resid. City Hosp. Edin.; Med. Resid. Roodlands Hosp. Haddington; SHO Simpson Memor. Matern. Pavil. Edin.

RICHARDSON, Thomas Noel Anthony The Surgery, 10 Bolton Road, Eastbourne BN21 3JY Tel: 01323 730537 Fax: 01323 412759; 4 Ocklynge Avenue, Eastbourne BN21 2QD Tel: 01323 737092 — MB BS Lond. 1975 (Kings Coll. Hosp.)

RICHARDSON, Timothy Old Cottage Hospital Surgery, Alexandra Road, Epsom KT17 4BL Tel: 01372 724434 Fax: 01372 748171; 3 Ladbroke Road, Epsom KT18 5BG Tel: 01372 722344 — MB BS Lond. 1979; MRCGP 1983. Mem. E. Surrey LMC (Mid Surrey Represen.); Dir. Epsom Med. Serv. Ltd; Dir. Epsom Day Surg. Ltd. Specialty: Gen. Med.; Diabetes; Urol. Prev: GP Trainer SW Thames; Exec. Partner; Bd. Mem. Mid Surrey PCG.

RICHARDSON, Tina Clare Arnold Lodge, East Midlands Centre for Forensic Mental Health, Cordelia Close, Leicester LE5 0LE Tel: 0116 225 6052 — MB ChB Leic. 1991; BSc Leic. 1988. SHO (Psychiat.) Leicester Hosps. Specialty: Gen. Psychiat. Socs: BMA. Prev: SHO Rotat. (O & G) Leicester Hosps.

RICHARDSON, Tristan Ian Laurent 49 Whiteknights Road, Reading RG6 7BB — MB BS Lond. 1993 (Univ. Coll. Lond.) BSc (Hons.) Lond. 1990; MRCP (UK) 1996. SHO (Med.) Derriford Hosp. Plymouth. Specialty: Gen. Med.

RICHARDSON, Wendy Lisa Pear Tree Surgery, 28 Meadow Close, Kingsbury, Tamworth B78 2NR Tel: 01827 872755; 14 Avon, Hockley, Tamworth B77 5QA — MB Camb. 1985; MA Oxf. 1982; BChir 1984. Socs: DRCOG.

RICHARDSON, Wilfred Thomas University of Hull, 187 Cottingham Road, Hull HU5 Tel: 01482 465633 — MB BS Durh. 1949 (Newc. upon Tyne) DPH Lond. 1957; DTM & H Eng. 1956, DIH 1957; MFCM 1974; MFOM RCP Lond. 1978. Dir. Univ. Health Serv. Prev: Lt.-Col. RAMC.

RICHARDSON, William 298 Lower Eastern Green Lane, Coventry CV5 7DT — MB ChB Sheff. 1988.

RICHARDSON, William Arthur Welburn 4 Summerhill, E. Herrington, Sunderland SR3 3NH — MB BS Newc. 1986. Project Ldr. of the Pennywell Project; Clin. Lect. centre for Health Studies Durh. Univ. Socs: BMA; MDU.

RICHARDSON, William Nicholas 29 Park Road, Welton, Brough HU15 1NW Email: jojo-gunne@blueyonder.co.uk — MB ChB Dundee 1980; FFA RCSI 1985. Specialty: Anaesth.

RICHARDSON, William Robert Dept. of Homoeop. Med., Old Swan Health Centre, St Oswalds St., Liverpool L13 2BY Tel: 0151 228 6808 Fax: 0151 228 8368 — (St. Thos.) MRCS Eng. LRCP Lond. 1967; MB BS Lond. 1967; FRCS Eng. 1972; FFHom 1989, M 1985; MRCGP 1991. Cons. Homoeop. Med. Liverp. Reg. Homeop. Med. Dept. Specialty: Homeop. Med. Socs: BMA; Brit. Med. Acupunct. Soc.; Liverp. Med. Inst. Prev: GP St. Asaph N. Wales; GP Beccles, Suff.

RICHARDSON, William Wigham Independent Medical Clinic, The Old Orchard Surgery, South Street, Wilton, Salisbury SP2 0JU Tel: 01722 741314 Fax: 01722 746616; Manor Cottage, Durnford Road, Stratford Sub Castle, Salisbury SP1 3YP Tel: 01722 331239 — MB Camb. 1974 (Camb. & St. Bart.) MA Camb. 1971; BChir Camb. 1973; MRCP (UK) 1978. Indep. Med. Acupunc. Salisbury. Socs: Brit. Med. Acupunct. Soc.; Brit. Soc. Allergy, Environm. & Nutrit. Med. Prev: GP Asst. Wilton, Salisbury; GP Salisbury; Princip. Tutor & Hon. Sen. Regist. (Paediat.) Univ. Leeds & Leeds Gen. Infirm.

RICHBELL, Jane Louise 18 Craneswater Park, Southsea PO4 0NT — MB ChB Birm. 1985; DRCOG 1988; MRCGP 1989. GP Portsmouth.

RICHENBERG, Jonathan Leonard — BM BCh Oxf. 1990; MA Camb. 1989; MRCP (UK) 1993; FRCR (Lond.) 1997. Cons. (Radiol.) Royal Sussex County Hospital. Specialty: Radiol. Special Interest: Urological & Gyn. imaging. Prev: Fell., St Pauls Hosp., Vancouver BC Canada; Sen. Regist., UCLH Dept. of Radiol. Lond..; Cons. Radiologist, RSCH, Brighton. Speciality: Uroradiologist & Interven.al Radiol., Fertil. Imaging.

RICHENS, Alan (retired) Pailton Lodge, Conventry Road, Pailton, Rugby CV23 0QA — MB BS Lond. 1962; BSc (Physiol.) 1964; PhD Lond. 1968; FRCP Lond. 1979, M 1969. Prev: Prof. of Clin. Pharmacol. Inst. Neurol. Lond.

RICHENS, Mr David Department of Cardiothoracic Surgery, Nottingham City Hospital, Hucknall Road, Nottingham NG5 1PB Tel: 0115 969 1169 Email: drichens@ncht.trent.nhs.uk; 145 Musters Road, West Bridgford, Nottingham NG2 7AF Tel: 0115 981 3260 — MB BS Lond. 1981 (Kings Coll. Hosp.) FRCS Glas. 1986; FETCS 1999. Cons. Cardiac Surg. Nottm. City Hosp.; Clin. Dir. Division of Surg. Notts. City Hosp.; Intern. Prof. Adv. To Ombardsman. Specialty: Cardiothoracic Surg. Socs: Soc. Cardiothoracic Surg. GB & Irel.; Eur. Assn. Cardiothoracic Surg. Prev: Cons. Cardiac Surg. Roy. Infirm. Glas.; Sen. Regist. (Cardiothoracic Surg.) Soton. Gen. Hosp.; Sen. Regist. (Cardiopulm. Transpl.) St. Vincents Hosp., Sydney.

RICHENS, John Everard Department of Sexually Transmitted Diseases, The Mortimer Market Centre, Mortimer Market, off Capper St., London WC1E 6AU Tel: 020 7380 9660 Fax: 020 7380 9669; 11 Barton Close, Cambridge CB3 9LQ Tel: 01223 324172 — MB BS Lond. 1979; MA Camb. 1978; MRCS Eng. LRCP Lond. 1978; MRCP (UK) 1983; MSc Lond. 1983; FRCP Ed. 1990. Clin. Lect. Dept. STD's Univ. Coll. Lond. Specialty: Genitourinary Medicine. Socs: Fell. Roy. Soc. Trop. Med. & Hyg.; Med. Soc. Papua New Guinea; Med. Soc. Study VD. Prev: Clin. Lect. Lond. Sch. Hyg. & Trop. Med.; Specialist Med. Off. Goroka Base Hosp., Papua New Guinea; Regist. (Gen. Med.) Northampton Gen. Hosp.

RICHER, Lorna Audrey (retired) Morcote, 6 Hawkmoor Parke, Bovey Tracey, Newton Abbot TQ13 9NL — (King's Coll. Hosp.) MB BS Lond. 1961; MRCS Eng. LRCP Lond. 1961; DObst RCOG 1962; DA Eng. 1964; FFA RCS Eng. 1970. Prev: Cons. Anaesth. Roy. United Hosp. NHS Trust, Bath.

RICHER, Mr Reginald George (retired) Morcote, 6 Hawkmoor Parke, Bovey Tracey, Newton Abbot TQ13 9NL Tel: 01626 835422 Email: richer@morcote.fsnet.co.uk — MRCS Eng. LRCP Lond. Londres 1961 (King's Coll. Hosp.) MB BS London; DO Eng. 1968; FRCS Ed. 1970; FRCOphth 1989. Prev: Med. Off. Colombo Plan Med. Team Vientiane, Laos.

RICHES, Professor David John (retired) 8 Elsworth Place, Hills Road, Cambridge CB2 2RG Tel: 01223 512852 Email:

d.riches@ntlworld.com — MB BS Lond. 1969 (St. Thos.) BSc Lond. 1964, PhD 1969; MRCS Eng. LRCP Lond. 1969. Emerit. Prof. Anat. Qu. Mary & Westfield Coll. Lond. Prev: Prof. Anat. Chinese Univ. Hong Kong.

RICHES, Elizabeth Chatsworth Road Medical Centre, Chatsworth Road, Brampton, Chesterfield S40 3PY Tel: 01246 568065 Fax: 01246 567116; Newfield Cottage, Hemming Green, Brampton S42 7JQ — MB ChB Sheff. 1991; DFFP 1993; DRCOG 1994; MRCGP 1995. GP Princip. Chesterfield.

RICHES, Harry Ralph Claude (retired) 2 South Approach, Moor Park, Northwood HA6 2ET Tel: 01923 823330 Fax: 01923 841421 Email: harry.riches@btopenworld.com — (Guy's) MD Lond. 1956, MB BS 1948; MRCS Eng. LRCP Lond. 1948; FRCP Lond. 1974, M 1952. Hon. Cons. Phys. Harefield Hosp. Prev: Cons. Phys. Harefield, Mt. Vernon & Wembley Hosps.

RICHES, Helen Isobel Restalrig Park Medical Centre, 40 Alemoor Crescent, Edinburgh EH7 6UJ Tel: 0131 554 2141 Fax: 0131 554 5363 — MB ChB Ed. 1992.

RICHES, Marilyn Celia The Surgery, 29 Derry Downs, Orpington BR5 4DU Tel: 01689 820036 Fax: 01689 819768; Holly Cottage, Chelsfield Lane, Orpington BR6 7RP Tel: 01689 837294 — MB BS Lond. 1966 (Roy. Free) MRCS Eng. LRCP Lond. 1966.

RICHES, Susanna Marie-Therese Viewfield, Balmore, Torrance, Glasgow G64 4AE — MB ChB Ed. 1993.

RICHEY, Edmund Eric (retired) 20 Lawnakilla Park, Enniskillen BT74 7JN Tel: 028 6632 2104 — MB BCh BAO Belf. 1962; LAH Dub. 1964; FFA RCSI 1969.

***RICHEY, Helen Claire** 4 Algeo Drive, Enniskillen BT74 6JL Tel: 01365 322104 Email: clairerichey@yahoo.com — MB ChB Dund. 1998; MB ChB Dund 1998. PRHO Altnagelvin Hosp. Londonderry. Specialty: Gen. Surg. Socs: Ulster Med. Soc.

RICHEY, Ruth Elizabeth Margaret Enniskillen Health Centre, Enniskillen BT74 6AY Tel: 028 6632 2707 — MB BCh BAO Belf. 1994 (Queen's University Belfast) DCH Coll. Surgeons 1997; DRCOG RCObst&Gyn. UK 1998. Specialty: Gen. Pract.

RICHI, Mohammed Nabil Mahmoud c/o Drive J.M. Feloy, Holmwood, Staverton, Totnes TQ9 6NX — LRCP LRCS Ed. 1985; MD Aleppo 1976; LRCP LRCS Ed. LRCPS Glas. 1985; MRCPI 1986.

RICHINGS, Ceri Ian 47 Cartland Road, Stirchley, Birmingham B30 2SD — MB ChB Leic. 1989.

RICHINGS, Jane Carol Hinchliffe (retired) 65A Carlisle Mansions, Carlisle Place, London SW1P 1HZ Tel: 020 7828 1816 — MB BS Lond. 1957 (St. Bart.) DCH Eng. 1961; MRCP Lond. 1965; BA 1991.

RICHMAN, Anna Victoria The Hesketh Centre, 51-55 Albert Road, Southport PR9 0LT Tel: 01704 383172 — MB ChB Liverp. 1996. SpR (Old Age Psychiat.) Liverp. Specialty: Gen. Psychiat. Prev: SHO (Psychiat.) in Liverp.

RICHMAN, Geoffrey 138 Fordwych Road, London NW2 3PA Tel: 020 8452 7646 — BM BCh Oxf. 1956.

RICHMAN, Naomi Shirley The Medical Foundation For The Care, 96-98 Grafton Road, London NW5 3EJ Tel: 020 7813 9999; 17 Holmesdale Road, London N6 5TH Tel: 020 8348 9497 — BM BCh Oxf. 1958 (Middlx.) MSc (Epidemiol.) Columbia Univ. New York 1969; FRCPsych 1981, M 1973. Indep. Cons. Lond. Specialty: Child & Adolesc. Psychiat. Prev: Adviser (Child Ment. Health) Min. of Educat., Mozambique; Hon. Cons. Hosp. Sick Childr. Gt. Ormond St. Lond.; Reader Inst. Child Health Lond.

RICHMAN, Sharon Windmill Lodge Centre for Childrens Services, Hounslow and Spelthorne Community and Mental Health NHS Trust, Uxbridge Road, Southall UB1 3EU Tel: 020 8354 8862 Fax: 020 8354 8948; 1 Winscombe Crescent, Ealing, London W5 1AZ — MB BS Lond. 1978 (Middlx. Hosp. Med. Sch.) DCH RCP Lond. 1983; MRCP (UK) 1985. Cons. Paediat. (Community Child Health) Hounslow & Spelthome community & Ment. Health NHS Trust. Specialty: Community Child Health. Prev: Lect. (Community Paediat.) St. Mary's Hosp. Med. Sch. Lond. Univ.

RICHMOND, Catherine Ellen West Middlesex University Hospital, Department of Anaesthetics, Twickenham Road, Isleworth TW7 6AF Tel: 020 8997 1270; 48 Lynwood Road, Ealing, London W5 1JJ — MB ChB Manch. 1986; BSc (Hons.) Manch. 1984; MB ChB (Hons.) Manch. 1986; MRCP (UK) 1989; FRCA 1991. Cons. Anaesth. W. Middlx. Univ. Hosp. Isleworth. Specialty: Anaesth. Socs: MRCAnaesth.; Assn. Anaesth.; BMA. Prev: Sen. Regist. (Anaesth.) Univ. Coll. Lond. Hosps.; Regist. (Anaesth.) Gt. Ormond St. Hosp. for Sick Childr. Lond. & Middlx. Hosp. Lond.; Regist. Rotat. (Anaesth.) NW Region.

RICHMOND, Charles Steven Ashley The Old Brokes Farmhouse, Brokes, Hudswell, Richmond DL11 6DD; South Lodge, Heath Side, London NW3 1BL — MB BS Lond. 1996.

RICHMOND, David Hugh Liverpool Womens Hospital, Liverpool L8 7SS Tel: 0151 708 9988; Heatherlea, Welstone Lane, West Kirby, Wirral CH48 7HG Tel: 0151 248 7119 — MD Ed. 1988; BSc Ed. 1974, MD 1988, MB ChB 1977; MRCOG 1982; FRCOG 1995. Cons. & Med. Dir. O & G Liverp. Wom. Hosp. Specialty: Obst. & Gyn. Socs: Gyn. Club & Internat. Continency Soc. Prev: Sen. Lect. (O & G) Univ. Liverp.

RICHMOND, David John Hamilton Dept. of Anaesthetics, New Cross Hospital, Wolverhampton WV10 0QP Tel: 01902 367999; Greenways, StockwellEnd, Tettenhall, Wolverhampton WV6 9PH Tel: 01902 751448 Email: djhrichmond@lineone.net — MB BChir Camb. 1964 (Camb. & Guy's) MA Camb. 1963; MRCS Eng. LRCP Lond. 1963; DObst RCOG 1965; DA Eng. 1966; FFA RCS Eng. 1969. Cons. Anaesth. Roy. Wolverhampton Hosps. NHS Trust. Specialty: Anaesth. Socs: Fell. Birm. & Midl. Obst. & Gyn. Soc.; Obst. Anaesth. Assn. Prev: Sen. Regist. (Anaesth.) United Birm. Hosps.; Regist. (Anaesth.) St. Bart. Hosp. Lond. & St. Geo. Hosp. Lond.

RICHMOND, Eunice Edith Upton Group Practice, 32 Ford Road, Wirral CH49 0TF Tel: 0151 677 0486 Fax: 0151 604 0635; 21 Manor Road, Upton, Wirral CH49 6JE — MB ChB Manch. 1981; DRCOG 1986. GP Upton.

RICHMOND, Geoffrey Alan The Surgery, Limes Avenue, Alfreton DE55 7DW Tel: 01773 832749 Fax: 01773 832921 — (Sheff.) MB ChB Sheff. 1967; DObst RCOG 1969; MRCGP 1973. Chairm. Derby Obst. Gp. Socs: Derby Med. Soc. & Nott. M-C Soc. Prev: SHO Jessop Hosp. Wom. Sheff.; Ho. Off. (Med.) North. Gen. Hosp. Sheff.; Ho. Off. (Surg.) Roy. Hosp. Sheff.

RICHMOND, Geoffrey Oliffe Claremont Medical Practice, Exmouth Health Centre, Claremont Grove, Exmouth EX8 2JF Tel: 01395 273666 Fax: 01395 223301 Email: claremont@eclipse.co.uk; Merrion House, 1 Merrion Avenue, Exmouth EX8 2HX Tel: 01395 279164 — MB BS Lond. 1974 (Roy. Free) MRCS Eng. LRCP Lond. 1974; DRCOG 1977; MRCGP 1979. Prev: Trainee GP Exeter VTS; Ho. Phys. W. Kent Gen. Hosp. Maidstone; Ho. Surg. (Orthop.) Roy. Free Hosp. Lond.

RICHMOND, Hannah Georgina — BM BS Nottm. 1998. PRHO Surg., James Paget Hosp, Gorleston. Specialty: Gen. Surg. Prev: PRHO Med. 18/98-02/99 James Paget Hosp, Gorleston.

RICHMOND, Helen Susan 6 Balmore Drive, Caversham, Reading RG4 8NL — MB BCh Wales 1998.

RICHMOND, Hendry Gilmour (retired) Ridgeleigh, 50 Crown Drive, Inverness IV2 3QG Tel: 01463 232895 — MD Aberd. 1958; MB ChB 1948; FRCPath 1971. Prev: Cons. Path. Highland HB.

RICHMOND, Henry Auld Nisbet Towerdene, 14 Langside Drive, Glasgow G43 2EQ — MB ChB Glas. 1946 (Univ. Glas.) MFOM RCP Lond. 1982; MRCP (UK) 1983; FRCP Glas. 1985. Sen. Med. Off. Univ. Glas.; Princip. Med. Off. Scott. Mutual Assur. Soc. Socs: BMA. Prev: Res. Asst. (ENT & Phys.) West. Infirm. Glas.

RICHMOND, Iain Miller Moreton Cross Group Practice, Ashton House, Chadwick Street, Moreton, Wirral L46 7US Tel: 0151 678 0993; 21 Manor Drive, Upton, Wirral CH49 6JE — MB ChB Manch. 1980; BSc St. And. 1977; DRCOG 1986.

RICHMOND, Ian Department of Histopathology, Castle Hill Hospital, Cottingham HU16 Tel: 01482 623288 Fax: 01482 623290; Elm Cottage, 13 Mill St, Hutton, Driffield YO25 9PU Tel: 01377 270529 — MB ChB Manch. 1986; MRCPath 1994; MD Manch. 1996. Cons. Histopath. Castle Hill Hosp. Cottingham; Hon. Clin. Sen. Lect. Fac. Health Hull Univ. Sch. Med. Specialty: Histopath. Prev: Sen. Regist. Rotat. (Histopath.) N. West. RHA; Research Fell. (Path.) Freeman Hosp. Newc. u. Tyne; Regist. (Histopath.) Blackburn Roy. Infirm.

RICHMOND, James Brown 3 Bridge Street, Otley LS21 1BQ Tel: 01943 464001 Fax: 01943 850849; Creskeld Gardens, Bramhope, Leeds LS16 9EN — MB ChB Leeds 1955.

RICHMOND, Jane Rowena Queen Mother's Hospital, Yorkhill, Glasgow G3 8SJ; 35 Scotland Street, Edinburgh EH3 6PY — MB

ChB Ed. 1993; MRCOG 1998. Specialist Regist. (O & G) Qu. Mother's Hosp. Glas. Specialty: Obst. & Gyn.

RICHMOND, Jennifer Kay 24 Llantrisant Rise, Llandaff, Cardiff CF5 2PG Tel: 029 2057 8089 — (Cardiff) MB BCh Wales 1968; DCH Eng. 1970; DCH 1970; DObst RCOG 1972; FRCGP 1987, M 1976; MICGP 1987; MFCM RCP 1989; T(PHM) 1991; T(GP) 1991; FFPHM RCP (UK) 1997. Indep. Cons. Specialty: Gen. Pract. Prev: Princip. Med. Off. Welsh Off. Cardiff; Sen. Med. Off. & Med. Off. Welsh Off.; GP Barry.

RICHMOND, Professor John, CBE (retired) 15 Church Hill, Edinburgh EH10 4BG Tel: 0131 447 2760 — MB ChB Ed. 1948; FRCP Ed. 1963, M 1955; FRCPI 1990; FCP(SA) (Hon.) 1991; FRSE 1992; FRCP Lond. 1970, M 1957; MD Ed. 1963; FRCPS 1988; FFPM (Hon.) 1989; FACP (Hon.) 1989; FRACP (Hon.) 1990; FFPHM (Hon.) 1990; FRCS Ed. 1990. Prev: Emerit. Prof. Med. Univ. Sheff.

RICHMOND, John Paul 46 Devon Street, St Helens WA10 4HT — MB ChB Dund. 1998; MB ChB Dund 1998.

RICHMOND, Mr Jonathan David P.O. Box 6779, Dundee DD1 9WN Tel: 01382 223189 — MB ChB Ed. 1977; BSc (Hons.) Ed. 1974, MB ChB 1977; FRCS Ed. 1981. Govt. Servant Home Office.

RICHMOND, Marion Laurel St Patrick Surgery, 4 Laurel St Patrick, Glasgow G3 6JB Tel: 0141 332 5553 Fax: 0141 332 5557 — MB ChB Glas. 1967.

RICHMOND, Maureen Shannon 20 Kirby Park, Wirral CH48 7HJ — MB ChB Ed. 1979; BSc Ed. 1976, MB ChB 1979. SHO (Paediat.) Wirral.

RICHMOND, Moses (retired) 66 Chatsworth Road, London NW2 4DD — (Lond. Hosp.) MRCS Eng. LRCP Lond. 1933. Prev: Sen. Ho. Phys. & Cas. Off. Roy. Infirm. Oldham.

RICHMOND, Mr Paul John Murray 48 Lynwood Road, Ealing, London W5 1JJ Tel: 020 8997 1270 — MB ChB Aberd. 1986; FRCS Ed. 1991. Cons.Urol., Durh. Hosp. Durh.. Specialty: Urol. Socs: BMA; Brit. Assn. Urol. Surgs.; RCS Edin. Prev: Sen.Regist.(Urol) UCLH; Sen. Regist. (Urol.) Whipps Cross; Sen. Regist. (Urol.) Roy. Free Hosp. Lond.

RICHMOND, Mr Peter William Emergency Unit, University Hospital of Wales, Heath Park, Cardiff CF14 4XW Tel: 029 2074 8004 Fax: 029 2074 8062 Email: peter.richmond@cardiffandvale.wales.nhs.uk — MB ChB Liverp. 1977; FRCS Ed. 1981; FRCS Eng. 1982. Cons. Accid. Emerg. Med. Univ. Hosp. Of Wales. Specialty: Accid. & Emerg.

RICHMOND, Peter William (retired) 74B Thorndon Gardens, Stoneleigh, Epsom KT19 0QJ Tel: 020 8393 6906 — MB ChB NZ 1949 (Otago) MRCP Lond. 1955; DPM Eng. 1960; MRCPsych 1971. Hon. Cons. Psychiat. Riverside HA. Prev: Cons. Psychiat. & Med. Admin. Banstead Hosp.

RICHMOND, Rhianne Mary Linwood Health Centre, Ardlamont Square, Linwood, Paisley PA3 3DE Tel: 01505 321051 Fax: 01505 383302 — MB ChB Glas. 1986 (Univ. Glas.) DRCOG 1991; MRCGP 1992; DFFP 1993. GP Princ. Since 1992; Clin. Med. Off. (Family Plann. & Well Wom. Servs.) Renfrewsh. Healthcare NHS Trust; Licenced Assoc. Fac. Homoeop. Socs: BMA. Prev: Trainee GP Glas.

RICHMOND, Robert (retired) Eliock Dower House, Sanquhar DG4 6LD Tel: 01659 50254 — MB ChB Glas. 1951. Prev: Ho. Phys. Stobhill Hosp. Glas.

RICHMOND, Ruth Borders Rheumatology Service, Borders General Hospital, Melrose TD6 9BS Tel: 01896 826665 Fax: 01896 826663 — MB BS Lond. 1989; MRCP (UK) 1993. Cons. Rheumt., Borders Primary Care Trust. Specialty: Gen. Med.; Rheumatol. Socs: Collegiate Mem. Roy. Coll. Of Phys.s; Brit. Soc. Rheum.; Scott. Soc. Phys.s. Prev: Cons. Rheumatologist, Rheumatic Dis.s Unit, West. Gen. Hosp., Crewe Rd, S. Edin.,EH4 2XU; Specialist Regist. (Med & Rheum.) Edin.; SHO Rotat. (Med.) Roy. Lond. Hosp.

RICHMOND, Samuel William John Paediatrics, Northern Congenital Abnormality Survey, Maternity Service Office, Newcastle upon Tyne NE2 4AA; 28 Hedley Street, Gosforth, Newcastle upon Tyne NE3 1DL — MB BS Newc. 1972; MRCP (UK) 1983.

RICHMOND, Shirley Jean (retired) Clinical Virology Manchester Central Laboratory Services, 3rd Floor, Clinical Services Building, Manchester Royal Infirmary, Oxford Road, Manchester M13 9WL — MD Camb. 1976; MB 1960, BChir 1959. Prev: Reader (Med. Virol.) Univ. Manch.

RICHMOND, Susanna Mary 2 The Chase, Silverdale, Carnforth LA5 0UT — MB ChB Liverp. 1988; FRCA 1994. Specialty: Anaesth.

RICHMOND, Mr Thomas Randall Anderson (retired) 7 Calder Drive, Cambuslang, Glasgow G72 8NE Tel: 0141 641 1640 — (Univ. Glas.) BSc Glas. 1938; MB ChB Glas. 1941; FRFPS Glas. 1949; FRCS Glas. 1962. Prev: Regist. (Surg.) & Ho. Phys. Glas. Roy. Infirm.

RICHOLD, Jonathan Paul Garforth Medical Centre, Church Lane, Garforth, Leeds LS25 1ER Tel: 0113 286 5311 Fax: 0113 281 2679; 2 The Coach House, Manor Farm, Main Street, Aberford, Leeds LS25 3AA — MB BS Newc. 1978; DRCOG 1981; MRCGP 1982. Clin. Asst. (Endoscopy) Seacroft Hosp. Leeds; GP Trainer Leeds. Prev: Trainee GP Airedale Gen. Hosp. Steeton VTS.

RICHTER, Alex Gisela 30 Gloucester Road, Kew, Richmond TW9 3BU — MB ChB Birm. 1996; ChB Birm. 1996.

RICHTER, George 184 Nevill Avenue, Hove BN3 7NG Tel: 01273 821517 — MD Charles U Prague 1971; Dip. Trop. Dis. UPDL Prague 1978. Staff Specialist (O & G) Crawley Hosp. E. Sussex. Specialty: Obst. & Gyn. Prev: Sen. Regist. (O & G) St. Luke's Hosp. Malta.

RICKARD, Alison Jill Alton Health Centre, Anstey Road, Alton GU34 2QX Tel: 01420 84676 Fax: 01420 542975 Email: alisonrickard@thewilsonpractice.co.uk; 18 Beechlands Road, Medstead, Alton GU34 5EQ — BM BCh Oxf. 1989 (Oxford University) BA Oxf. 1986; DRCOG 1994; MRCGP 1994; Dip. Occ. Med. 1998. Specialty: Gen. Pract. Prev: SHO Spinal Unit Salisbury Dist. Hosp.; SHO (Med.) Derriford Hosp. Plymouth; Trainee GP Plymouth.

RICKARD, Anne Macleod Wellington Medical Centre, Bulford, Wellington TA21 8PW Tel: 01823 663551 Fax: 01823 660650 — MB BS Lond. 1979 (Royal London Hospital) GP; Skin Laser Specialist. Specialty: Gen. Pract.

RICKARD, Rory Frederick c/o Institute of Naval Medicine, Alverstoke, Gosport PO12 2DL — MB BCh BAO Belf. 1992; FRCS Ed. 1999.

RICKARD, Samantha Peggy Louise Reidfield Cottage, Budworth Heath, Northwich CW9 6NQ — MB ChB Sheff. 1997.

RICKARDS, Angela Frances Blomfield Practice, Nursery Lane Surgery, 150 Nursery Lane, Leeds LS17 7AQ Tel: 0113 293444 Fax: 0113 295 3440; 56 Larkfield Avenue, Rawdon, Leeds LS19 6EN — MB ChB Leeds 1990; DRCOG 1993; MRCGP 1994; DTM & H Liverp. 1994. Princip. GP.

RICKARDS, Christopher Morriston Hospital, Morriston, Swansea SA6 6NL Tel: 01792 702222 — MB ChB Manch. 1987; MB ChB (Hons.) Manch. 1987; MRCP (UK) 1990; MD Manchester 1994; BSc (Hons.) Manch. 1985, MD 1994. Cons. Neurol. Specialty: Neurol.

RICKARDS, David Department of Radiology, University College London, London W1N 8AA Tel: 020 7380 9070 Fax: 020 7486 1084; 136 Harley Street, London W1N 1AH Tel: 020 7637 8207 Fax: 020 7436 7059 — MRCS Eng. LRCP Lond. 1972; FFR (D) S. Afr. 1980; FRCR 1982. Cons. Uroradiol. Univ. Coll. Lond. Hosp. & Inst. Urol. Lond. Specialty: Urol. Socs: (Counc.) Brit. Inst. of Radiol. Prev: Regist. (Radiol.) K. Edwd. VII Hosp. Congella, Roy. S. Afr.; Lect. (Radiol.) Univ. Manch.

RICKARDS, David Francis Tingle's Farm, 15 Wood Side Lane, Grenoside, Sheffield S35 8RW — MB ChB Sheff. 1960; MRCGP 1969. Socs: Soc. Occupat. Med.

RICKARDS, Edward Hugh Galbraith 44 Franklin Road, Cotteridge, Birmingham B30 2HG Tel: 0121 627 2834 — MB ChB Birm. 1988; ChB Birm. 1988; MRCPsych 1993; MMedSci 1994. Cons. (Neuropsychiat. & Gen. Psychiat.) Qu. Eliz. Psychiat. Hosp. Birm.; Hon. Sen. Clin. Lect. (Psychiat.) Birm. Univ.; Hon. Clin. Asst. Nat. Hosp. Qu. Sq. Lond. Specialty: Gen. Psychiat. Socs: Brain Res. Assn.; Huntington's Dis. Assn.; Tourette's Syndrome Assn. Prev: Sen. Regist. (NeuroPsychiat.) Qu. Eliz. Psychiat. Hosp. Birm.; Regist. (Psychiat.) Birm. VTS; Sen. Reg. (Psychiat.) W. Midl.

RICKARDS, Francis Sylvester (retired) 15 St Oswald's Close, Oswaldkirk, Helmsley, York YO62 5YH Tel: 01439 788661 Fax: 01439 788661 — (Liverp.) MB ChB Liverp. 1941.

RICKARDS, Mabli Ann (retired) 15 Sunningdale, W. Monkseaton, Whitley Bay NE25 9YF — MB BCh Wales 1963; AFOM RCP Lond. 1983. Prev: Sen. Med. Off. (Radiol.) Brit. Coal Wath-on-Dearne S. Yorks.

RICKARDS, Manisha Gowerton Medical Centre, Mill Street, Gowerton, Swansea SA4 3ED Tel: 01792 872404 Fax: 01792 875170 — MB ChB Manch. 1986; DRCOG 1992. Specialty: Gen. Pract.

RICKARDS, Mr Michael Queen Elizabeth Hospital,Sheriff Hill, Gateshead NE9 6SX Tel: 0191 482 0000 — MB BS Newc. 1989; FRCS Ed. 1994; FFAEM 1998. Cons. (A&E) Med., Qu. Eliz. Hosp. Gateshead. Specialty: Accid. & Emerg.

RICKARDS, Nigel Peter 38 Crewe Road, Alsager, Stoke-on-Trent ST7 2ET Tel: 01270 882004; Four Winds, 6 Dunnocksfold Road, Alsager, Stoke-on-Trent ST7 2TJ — MB ChB Ed. 1980.

RICKENBACH, Carol Ann Mary High Street Surgery, 75 High Street, Minster, Ramsgate CT12 4AB Tel: 01843 821333 Fax: 01843 823146 — MB BS Lond. 1989 (Char. Cross & Westminster) DCH RCP Lond. 1993; DRCOG 1994; MRCGP 1995.

RICKENBACH, Mark Alan Park Surgery, Hursley Road, Chandlers Ford, Eastleigh SO22 5DH; West Deanery, Postgraduate Medical and Dental Education, Highcroft, winchester SO22 5DH Tel: 01962 863511 Ext. 545 Fax: 01705 866849 — MB BS Lond. 1984; BSc Lond. 1981; DCH RCP Lond. 1988; MRCP (UK) 1988; DFFP 1989; T(GP) 1992; MRCGP 1992; FRCGP 2000; PhD 2003; FRCP 2003; ILTM 2003. GP; Course Organiser for Hosp. Gen. Pract. Train. Scheme; Coordinator Wessex Research Club (WREc); Research Stud.ship NHS R&D (PHD); GP Trainer; Bd. Mem. E.leigh N. PCT; Ass. Dir. GP SHO Educat.; Ass. Dir. GP SHO Educat., Asst. Dean, flexible training. Socs: BMA; RCGP (Mem. Research & Educat. Subcomm.) (Fell.); Roy. Coll. Phys.t (Mem.). Prev: Regist. (Med.) Sir Chas. Gairdner Hosp. Perth, W. Austral.; SHO (O & G) St. Richard's Hosp. Chichester; SHO (Ophth. & Med.) St. Mary's & Qu. Alexandra Hosps. Portsmouth.

RICKERBY, Elizabeth Jane Cumberland Infirmary, Carlisle CA2 7HY; Southwaite Park, Southwaite, Carlisle CA4 0LN Tel: 0169 74 73200 Email: rickerby@dial.pipex.com — MB ChB Dundee 1978; DA 1982. p/t Clin. Asst. (Gyn.) Cumberld. Infirm. Carlisle. Specialty: Obst. & Gyn.; Nuclear Med. Prev: SHO & Regist. (Anaesth.) Cumberld. Infirm. Carlisle; SHO (O & G) City Gen. Hosp. Carlisle.

RICKERBY, John Dr A Willis and Partners, King Edward Road Surgery, Christchurch Medical Centre, Northampton NN1 5LY Tel: 01604 633466 Fax: 01604 603227; 10 Trinity Avenue, Northampton NN2 6JJ — MB BS Lond. 1981; BSc Lond. 1978; DRCOG 1983; DCH RCP Lond. 1984; FRCGP 1995, M 1988; MSc (Oxon) 2002.

RICKETS, Mark Nightingale Practice, 10 Kenninghall Road, Clapton, London E5 8BY Tel: 020 8985 8388 Fax: 020 8986 6004; 32 Sidney Road, London N22 8LU Tel: 020 8829 9042 — MB BS Lond. 1988; BSc (Physiol.) Bristol 1982; DGM RCP Lond. 1992; MRCGP 1994; DRCOG 1994. GP Princip.; Clincial Lect. St. Bartholomews & Roy. Lond. Hosp. Med. Sch.

RICKETT, Andrew Brian 37 Beechings Close, Countesthorpe, Leicester LE8 5PA — MB ChB Leic. 1985; FRCR 1992. Cons. Radiol. Leicester. Specialty: Radiol. Prev: Sen. Regist. & Regist. (Radiol.) Leicester; SHO (Cardiol. & Neonates) Centr. Birm. HA; SHO (Paediat. & Neonates) Leics. HA.

RICKETTS, Mr David Mark Princess Royal Hospital, Lewes Road, Haywards Heath RH16 4EX Tel: 01444 441881 — MB BCh Witwatersrand 1982; FRCS Eng. 1988; FRCS (Orth.) 1995. Cons. Orthop. Surg. Princess Roy. Hosp. Haywards Heath. Specialty: Orthop. Prev: Sen. Regist. Bristol Roy. Infirm.; Regist. St. Mary's & Char. Cross Hosps.

RICKETTS, Karen Jane Norven, 19 Lutterworth Close, Bracknell RG42 2NW — MB ChB Leeds 1996; MRCP (UK) 2000. SpR Palliat. Care S. W. Rotat. commencing at Plymouth. Specialty: Gen. Med. Prev: SHO Med. Rotat. Wakefield Pinderfields Hosp.

RICKETTS, Nora Elizabeth Marjorie Tayview Medical Practice, 16 Victoria Street, Newport-on-Tay DD6 8DJ Tel: 01382 543251 Fax: 01382 542052; Wellgate House, 78 West Road, Newport-on-Tay DD6 8HP Tel: 01382 542851 — MB ChB Dundee 1975; BSc St. And. 1972; DRCOG 1977. Prev: Regist. (Obst.) Ninewells Hosp. Dundee; Trainee GP Alyth VTS; SHO (Geriat.) Ashludie Hosp. Dundee.

RICKFORD, Mr Christopher Richard Keevil Pensylva, Kenwyn Close, Truro TR1 3DX Tel: 01872 272039 Fax: 01872 272039 Email: crrickford@tinyworld.co.uk — MB BChir Camb. 1967 (St. Thos.) MA, Camb. 1967; FRCS Eng. 1970. Cons. Gen. Surg. Roy. Cornw. Hosp. Trust Truro. Specialty: Gen. Surg. Socs: Fell. Roy. Soc. Med.; BMA. Prev: Sen. Regist. (Surg.) St. Thos. Hosp. Lond. & St. Helier Hosp. Carshalton; Regist. Rotat. (Surg.) St. Thos. Hosp. Lond.

RICKFORD, William Jeremy Keevil Department of Anaesthetics, Lister Hospital NHS Trust, Corey's Mill Lane, Stevenage SG1 4AB Tel: 01438 314333; Rushcroft, Green End, Weston, Hitchin SG4 7AL Tel: 01462 790323 Fax: 01462 790163 — (St. Thos.) MB BS Lond. 1973; FFA RCSI 1980; FRCA 1981. Cons. Anaesth. Lister Hosp. Stevenage. Specialty: Anaesth. Socs: Fell. Roy. Soc. Med. Prev: Vis. Asst. Prof. (Anaesth.) Univ. Maryland Hosp. Baltimore, USA; Sen. Regist. (Anaesth.) Nat. Heart Hosp. & Hosp. for Sick Childr. Gt. Ormond St. Lond., Nat. Hosp. Nerv. Dis. Lond. & St. Thos. Hosp.

RICKHUSS, Mr Peter Kenneth Ninewells Hospital, Dundee DD1 9SG Tel: 01382 660111 Fax: 01382 360688 Email: peter@balruddery.com — MB ChB Dundee 1985; FRCS Edin. 1990; FRCS Ed. Orth. 1996. Cons. (Orthop. Surg.), Ninewells Hosp., Dundee; Hon. Sen. Lect., Univ. of Dundee. Specialty: Trauma & Orthop. Surg. Socs: BMA; BOA.

RICKINSON, John Derek (retired) Yew Court, Scalby, Scarborough YO13 0NN — MB BS Durh. 1950 (Newc.) MRCGP 1963. Mem. Med. Bds. DHSS. Prev: Sec. Newc. Local Med. Comm.

RICKMAN, Angus James 66 Ridgeway Road, Timperley, Altrincham WA15 7HD — MB ChB Leic. 1994.

RICKMAN, Mark Sean 206 Hinde House Lane, Sheffield S4 8HD — MB ChB Sheff. 1994.

***RICKUS, Katherine Patricia Ann** 142 Cleveden Road, Glasgow G12 0LA Tel: 0141 339 6708 Email: katherine.rickus@doctors.org.uk — MB ChB Ed. 1998 (Edinburgh University) BSc (Med Sci) Psychology 1996; MBChB 1998; MB ChB Ed 1998.

RICKWOOD, Mr Anthony Michael Kent Royal Liverpool Childrens Hospital, Eaton Road, Liverpool L12 2AP Tel: 0151 228 4811; 51 Dudlow Lane, Liverpool L18 2EX Tel: 0151 737 1265 — BM BCh Oxf. 1965; FRCS Eng. 1972. Cons. Paediat. Urol. Roy. Liverp. Childr. Hosp. Specialty: Urol. Prev: Sen. Regist. (Surg.) Sheff. Childr. Hosp.; Cons. Spinal Injuries Unit Lodgemoor Hosp. Sheff.

RICKWOOD, Ellis Paul — MB ChB Leeds 1990; DRCOG 1993; MRCGP 1994. Specialty: Gen. Pract.

RIDDELL, Alastair James Pharmagene Laboratories Ltd, 2A Orchard Road, Royston SG8 5HD Tel: 01763 211600 Fax: 01763 211556 Email: alastair.riddell@pharmagene.com; Kia Ora, 64 Lymington Bottom, Four Marks, Alton GU34 5AH Tel: 01962 772667 Fax: 01962 773033 — MB ChB Birm. 1977 (Univ. Birm.) BSc (Hons.) (Biol. Scs.) Aston 1971; MSc (Anat.) Birm. 1973; MRCGP 1982; MFPM RCP (UK) 1992. CEO Pharmagene Laborat. Ltd. Royston. Specialty: Pharmaceutical Medicine. Socs: Fell. Roy. Soc. Med.; Soc. Nuclear Med. Prev: Managing Dir. Caremark Ltd. Harlow; SHO (Med.) Brit. Milit. Hosp. Rinteln; SHO (O & G) Roy. Berks. Hosp. Reading.

RIDDELL, Angela Mary Department of Radiology, Royal Marsden Hospital, Fulham, London — MB BS Lond. 1994 (Univ. Coll. Lond.) BSc Lond. 1991; FRCS Eng. 1998; FRCR 2001. Research Fellow. Specialty: Radiol. Prev: Regist. Radiol.

RIDDELL, Anna Felicity 44 Coity Road, London NW5 4RY — MB BS Lond. 1994. Specialty: Paediat. Socs: Med. Wom. Federat.; BMA.

RIDDELL, Christopher William Grove Surgery, Grove Lane, Thetford IP24 2HY Tel: 01842 752285 Fax: 01842 751316; 63 Arlington Way, Thetford IP24 2DZ Tel: 01842 754928 — MB BS Lond. 1976 (St. Mary's) MRCS Eng. LRCP Lond. 1976. Specialty: Gen. Pract.

RIDDELL, Claire — BM BCh Oxf. 1993 (Oxford) MA Oxf.; FRCOphth. Specialty: Ophth.

RIDDELL, David Ian, MBE, Surg. Cdr. RN Retd. Dornoch Lodge, Glen Lyon, Aberfeldy PH15 2NH — MD Dundee 1984; MB ChB 1974.

RIDDELL, David John Goyt Valley Medical Practice, Chapel Street, Whaley Bridge, High Peak SK23 7SR Tel: 01663 732911 Fax: 01663 735702; The Old Vicarage, 23 High St, Chapel-en-le-Frith, High Peak SK23 0HD Tel: 01298 812201 — MB ChB Sheff. 1981; DRCOG 1985; MRCGP 1986.

RIDDELL, Elizabeth Mary 60 Lanton Road, Newlands, Glasgow G43 2SR Tel: 0141 633 2453 — MB ChB Glas. 1958; DObst

RCOG 1960; DPath Eng. 1964; FRCPath 1979, M 1967. Prev: Cons. Haematol. Vict. Infirm. Glas.; Cons. Pathol. St. James' Hosp. Lond.; Lect. Haematol. St. Geo. Hosp. Med. Sch.

RIDDELL, Gareth 15 Oakleigh Park, Belfast BT6 8RF Tel: 02890 507 379 — MB BCh BAO 1996 (Queens Belfast) SpR Respirat. Med. Belf. City Hosp. Prev: SHO Belf. City Hosp. Belf., Northern Irel.; Resid. MO Roy. Brisbane Hosp. & Tweed Heads Hosp. Australia; Clin. Tutor St George's Med. Sch. W. Indies.

RIDDELL, John Alistair, OBE (retired) 27 Upper Glenburn Road, Bearsden, Glasgow G61 4BN — MB ChB Glas. 1953; FRCGP 1983, M 1966; FRCP Glas. 1996. Prev: Med. Sec. Glas. Local Med. Comm. 1978 - 1991.

RIDDELL, John Wilson Royal Victoria Hospital, Grosvenor Road, Belfast BT12 6BA Tel: 01232 240503 — MB BCh BAO Belf. 1994 (Qu. Univ. Belf.) SHO (Med.) Roy. Vict. Hsopital Belf. Specialty: Gen. Med. Socs: MRCP (Lond.). Prev: SHO (Med.) Erne Hosp. NI; Resid. MO, P. Cha. Hosp., Brisbane, Australia; Resid. MO, Caboolture Hosp, Queensland, Australia.

RIDDELL, Jonathan Douglas Highgate Group Practice, 44 North Hill, London N6 4QA Tel: 020 8340 6628 Fax: 020 8342 8428; 15 Park Avenue S., London N8 8LU Tel: 020 8341 1026 — MB BS Lond. 1975; MRCGP 1980. GP Trainer Whittington Hosp. Lond. VTS.

RIDDELL, Margaret Anthea (retired) The Dale, Bayswater Farm Road, Headington, Oxford OX3 8BX Tel: 01865 750981; 97 High Street, Standlake, Witney OX29 7RH Tel: 01865 300964 — (Royal Free Hospital) MRCS Eng. LRCP Lond. 1954; MB BS Lond. 1955. Prev: GP Oxf.

RIDDELL, Michael James (retired) Dornoch Lodge, Glenlyon, Aberfeldy PH15 2NH Tel: 01887 877244 — MB BS (Hons.) Lond. 1941 (St. Thos.) MRCS Eng. LRCP Lond. 1941; MRCP Lond. 1948; BSc (1st cl. Hons. Physiol.) Lond. 1938, MD 1951; FRCP Glas. 1970, M 1965.

RIDDELL, Niall Jervis Swallowfield Medical Practice, The Street, Swallowfield, Reading RG7 1QY Tel: 0118 988 3134 Fax: 0118 988 5759 — MB BChir Camb. 1977; MA Camb. 1977; MRCP (UK) 1982; DRCOG 1984; MRCGP 1984. Hosp. Pract. (Gastroenterol.) Battle Hosp. Reading. Prev: Regist. (Med.) Camb. Milit. Hosp. Aldershot; Ho. Off. (Orthop.) St. Thos. Hosp. Lond.; Ho. Phys. Soton. Gen. Hosp.

RIDDELL, Philip Leslie 23 Gillhurst Road, Harborne, Birmingham B17 8QS Tel: 0121 682 4926 Email: riddell@thefreeinternet.co.uk — MB ChB Aberd. 1973; FRCA; FFA RCS Eng. 1978. Cons. (Anaesth.) Selly Oak Hosp. Birm. Specialty: Anaesth. Prev: Sen. Regist. (Anaesth.) Midl. Anaesth. Train. Scheme; Regist. (Anaesth.) Aberd. Roy. Infirm.

RIDDELL, Rebecca Ellen Mary Esslemont Group, Foresterhill Health Centre, Westburn Road, Aberdeen AB25 2AY Tel: 01224 559666 Fax: 01224 559349; 75 Braemar Place, Aberdeen AB10 6EQ — MB ChB Aberd. 1990; MRCGP 1994. Clin. Sen. Lect. Dept. GP Aberd.

RIDDELL, William Stuart The Health Centre, The Square, Whitwell, Worksop S80 4QR Tel: 01909 720236 Fax: 01909 720236 — MB ChB Sheff. 1987; MRCGP 1993.

RIDDICK, Mr Antony Charles Paul 4 Orchard Street, Bury St Edmunds IP33 1EH — BM BS Nottm. 1992; FRCS Ed. 1996. SHO (Urol.) Nottm. City Hosp. Specialty: Urol. Prev: SHO (Gen. Surg.) Derby City Hosp. & Qu. Med. Centre Nottm.; SHO (Orthop.) Qu. Med. Centre Nottm.

RIDDICK, David George Bushman, Col. late RAMC Retd. (retired) Tudor Cottage, Church Lane, Flyford Flavell, Worcester WR7 4BZ Tel: 01386 462631 — MRCS Eng. LRCP Lond. 1948 (St. Mary's) DA Eng. 1954; DTM & H RCP Lond. 1962; MFCM 1974. Prev: Med. Off. DSS.

RIDDINGTON, David William Department Anaesthetics, Queen Elizabeth Hospital, Edgbaston, Birmingham B15 2TH Tel: 0121 472 1311 Fax: 0121 697 8359 — MB ChB Birm. 1984; DA (UK) 1986; FCAnaesth 1990. Cons. Anaesth. Univ. Hosps. Birm. NHS Trust. Specialty: Anaesth.; Intens. Care. Prev: Sen. Regist. (Anaesth.) W. Midl. RHA.; Regist. (Anaesth.) P'boro. Hosps.; Regist. (Anaesth.) Leicester Hosps.

RIDDLE, Mr Andrew Forsyth Victoria Wing, Nuffield Hospital, Shores Road, Woking GU21 4BY Tel: 01483 227800 — MB BS Newc. 1977; MRCGP 1981; FRCOG 1998. Cons. O & G Frimley Pk. Hosp. Camberley SurreyClin. director Obtetrics & Gyn..; Med. Dir. Assisted Conception Unit Woking Nuffield Hosp.; Chair, Clin. Audit, Frimley Pk. Hosp. Specialty: Obst. & Gyn. Socs: Roy. Soc. Med.; Brit. Fertil. Soc.; Eur. Soc. Human Reproduc. & Embryol. Prev: Sen. Regist. (O & G) King's Coll. Hosp. Lond.; Clin. Research Fell. (Reproduct. Endocrinol. & Infertil.) King's Coll. Hosp. Lond.

RIDDLE, Fiona Jane The Village Green Surgery, The Green, Wallsend NE28 6BB Tel: 0191 295 8500 Fax: 0191 295 8519; 48 Elsdon Road, Gosforth, Newcastle upon Tyne NE3 1HY — MB BS Newc. 1985; Cert. Family Plann. JCC 1987; MRCGP 1989. Specialty: Obst. & Gyn. Prev: Trainee GP Newc. VTS.

RIDDLE, Henry Francis Valentine (retired) Craigview, Chapelgreen, Earlsferry, Leven KY9 1AD Tel: 01333 330965 Fax: 01333 330965 Email: valentineriddle@aol.com — MB ChB Liverp. 1959; PhD Liverp. 1957, BSc (Hons. Physiol.) 1952; MRCGP 1968; MD Liverp. 1970; FFOM RCP Lond. 1988, M 1983. Prev: Dir. Fife HB Occupat. Health Serv.

RIDDLE, Ian Forsyth Department of Anaesthesia, The James Cook University Hospital, Marton Road, Middlesbrough TS4 3BW Tel: 01642 850850 Fax: 01642 824877 — MB BS Newc. 1974. Cons. Anaesth. S. Tees Acute Trust Middlesbrough. Specialty: Anaesth.

RIDDLE, Miles Andrew Rosemount, Jenny Brough Lane, Hessle HU13 0JX — MB ChB Ed. 1996.

RIDDLE, Peter Napier (retired) 4 Arnett Close, Rickmansworth WD3 4DB Tel: 01923 778010; Shearwater, Maloes, Haverfordwest SA62 3BQ Tel: 01646 636719 — MB BS Lond. 1962 (St. Bart.) BSc Lond. 1954. Prev: Cons. Applied Microscopy Laborat. Imperial Cancer Research Fund.

RIDDLE, Mr Peter Riversdale (retired) Fitz Farm, Dinton, Salisbury SP3 5DZ Tel: 01722 716255 — MB BS Lond. 1957 (St. Geo.) MRCS Eng. LRCP Lond. 1957; FRCS Eng. 1963; MS Lond. 1968. Prev: Emerit. Surg. UCL Hosp. & St. Peters Hosp. Lond.

RIDDLE, Philippa Jane Radiotherapy Department, Churchill Hospital, Oxford OX3 7XG Tel: 01865 741841 Email: pipriddle@aol.com; 6 Murrayfield Gardens, Edinburgh EH12 6DF — BChir Camb. 1991 (Char. Cross & Westm.) MA Camb. 1992; MRCP (UK) 1994; FRCR May 1999. Specialist Regist. (Clin. Oncol.) Churchill Hosp. Oxf. Specialty: Oncol.; Radiother.

RIDDLE, Robert Womack (retired) The Walled Garden, 21 Middle St., Shoreham-by-Sea BN43 5DP Tel: 01273 454262 — MB BS Durh. 1932 (Newc.) BHyg., DPH 1934. Prev: Ho. Surg. Roy. Vict. Hosp. Newc.

RIDDLE, William James Robert Herdmanflat Hospital, Haddington EH41 3BU Tel: 0131 536 8515 Fax: 0131 536 8544 — MB ChB Aberd. 1982; MRCPsych 1992; MPhil Ed. 1995. Cons. Gen. Adult Psychiat. Herdmanflat Hosp. Haddington. Specialty: Gen. Psychiat. Special Interest: Diag. and Treatm. of mood and anxiety. Socs: Brit.Assoc. fro PsychoPharmacol., Mem.. Prev: Sen. Regist. Roy. Cornw. Hosp. Aberd.; Research Fell. MRC Brain Metab. Unit Edin.; Regist. Roy. Edin. Hosp.

RIDDOCH, Andrew James Cornwall Road Surgery, 15 Cornwall Road, Dorchester DT1 1RU Tel: 01305 251128 — MB BS Lond. 1989 (St Bartholomews London) DRCOG 1994; MRCGP 1998.

RIDDOCH, Donald 5 Davenport Road, Coventry CV7 6QA Tel: 024 7667 2997; 9 Alder Lane, Balsall Common, Coventry CV7 7DZ — MB ChB Birm. 1960; FRCP Lond. 1980, M 1964. Cons. Neurol. Specialty: Neurol. Socs: BMA & Assn. Brit. Neurol. Prev: Sen. Regist. (Neurol.) United Birm. Hosps.

RIDDOCH, Margaret Elsie (retired) 33 Millfield, Kirkton, Livingston EH54 7AR Tel: 01506 493574 — MB ChB Ed. 1951 (Edinburgh University) FFA RCS Eng. 1959; MRCGP 1977. Prev: Cons. Anaesth. Bangour Gen. Hosp. & GP Howden Health Centre Livingston.

RIDDOLLS, Lucy Elizabeth (retired) Aislaby Lodge, Aislaby, Whitby YO21 1SY Tel: 01947 810419 — MB BS Lond. 1949 (Roy. Free) MRCS Eng. LRCP Lond. 1949. Prev: SCMO (Child Health) ScarBoro. HA.

RIDEHALGH, Harry (retired) 176 Bramhall Moor Lane, Hazel Grove, Stockport SK7 5BE Tel: 0161 483 2267 — (St. And.) MB ChB (Commend.) St. And. 1958. Prev: Ho. Surg. & Ho. Phys. Co. Hosp. Lincoln.

RIDEN, Donald Keith dept. Oral & Maxillofacial Surgery, Derriford Hospital, Plymouth; 25 Easterdown Close, Plymstock, Plymouth PL9 8SR Fax: 01752 494155 — BM Soton. 1988; FDS 1994; FRCS

1996; FRCS (OMFS0) 1998. Specialist. Regist. (Oral & Maxillofacial Surg.) Derriford Hosp. Plymouth. Specialty: Oral & Maxillofacial Surg.

RIDER, James Gordon (retired) Ravensthorpe, Doctors Lane, Hutton Rudby, Yarm TS15 0EQ Tel: 01642 700143 Fax: 01642 700305 Email: gordon.rider@lineone.net — MB ChB Ed. 1951 (Univ. Ed.) DObst RCOG 1953; FRCGP 1980, M 1959. Prev: Ho. Surg. Simpson Memor. Matern. Pavil. Edin.

RIDER, Mr Mark Ainsley 13 Fulwith Drive, Harrogate HG2 8HW — MB ChB Dundee 1987; FRCS Ed. 1993.

RIDGE, Alan Timothy Carlton House Surgery, 28 Tenniswood Road, Enfield EN1 3LL Tel: 020 8363 7575 Fax: 020 8366 8228 Email: tim.ridge@gp-f85027.nhs.uk; 207 Lavender Hill, Enfield EN2 8RW Email: timridge1@compuserve.com — MB BS Lond. 1972 (Lond. Hosp.) Cert FPA 1974; MRCGP 1976. Specialty: Gen. Pract. Socs: (Vice-Chairm.) Doctor-Healer Network; Brit. Holistic Med. Assn. Prev: Trainee GP Ipswich VTS; Ho. Surg. (Gen. Surg. & Orthop.) Ipswich Hosp.; Ho. Phys. Ipswich Hosp. (Heath Rd. Wing).

RIDGE, Anna Louise The Limes, Randalls Green, Chalford Hill, Stroud GL6 8EE — MB ChB Birm. 1998.

RIDGE, Mr Jeremy Andrew Francis Hopton Hall, Mirfield WF14 8EL Tel: 01924 497272 Fax: 01924 497270 — MB BS Lond. 1981; MRCS Eng. LRCP Lond. 1980; LMSSA Lond. 1980; FRCS Ed. 1986. Cons. Orthop. Surg. Dewsbury Dist. Hosp. Specialty: Orthop. Socs: Fell. BOA; BMA. Prev: Cons. Orthop. Surg. Manor Hse. Hosp.; Regist. (Orthop. Surg.) Barnet Gen. Hosp.; Regist. (Gen. Surg. & Orthop.) Mt. Vernon Hosp. Northwood.

RIDGEWELL, Mark Charles Kings Road Surgery, 2-6 Kings Road, Mumbles, Swansea SA3 4AJ Tel: 01792 360933 Fax: 01792 368930; 61 Hendrefoilan Road, Sketty, Swansea SA2 9LU — MB BS Lond. 1986 (St. Mary's Hosp. Lond.) MRCGP 1990; DRCOG 1990; Cert Family Planning JCC 1990; Dip Sports Med RCPS, Glas. 1999; MSc (Sport & Exercise Med.) Uni. Bath 2001. Specialty: Gen. Pract.; Sports Med. Socs: (Sec.) Brit. Assn. Sport & Exercise Med.; UK Assn. Of Doctors In Sport.

RIDGWAY, Mr Alan Edward Andrew Russell House, Russell Road, Manchester M16 8AR Tel: 0161 862 9568 Fax: 0161 227 9405; 23 Beeston Rd, Sale M33 5AQ Tel: 0161 973 9479 Fax: 0161 973 9479 Email: alan.e.ridgway@manchester.ac.uk — MB Cantab 1964 (Lond. Hosp.) FRCOphth; MRCS Eng. LRCP Lond. 1964; BChir Camb. 1965; DO Eng 1967; FRCS Eng 1970. Hon. Cons. Surg. Manch. Roy. Eye Hosp.; Hon. Research Fell. Dept. Of Opthalmology, Uni. Manc. Specialty: Ophth. Special Interest: Corneal Dystrophies. Socs: Fell. Roy. Soc. Med. (Ex Vice-Pres. Counc. Sect. Ophth.); (Ex-Pres.) N. of Eng. Ophth. Soc.; Delegue Britannique Soc. Francaise D'Ophtalmologie. Prev: Sen. Regist. Birm. & Midl. Eye Hosp.; Regist. (Ophth.) Cardiff Roy. Infirm.; SHO Oxf. Eye Hosp.

RIDGWAY, Brian Arthur Firth Park Surgery, 400 Firth Park Road, Sheffield S5 6HH Tel: 0114 242 6406 — MB ChB Sheff. 1960; BSc (Hons. Biochem.) Sheff. 1963, MB ChB 1960; MRCGP 1970. Prev: Research Asst. Med. Profess. Unit Roy. Hosp. Sheff.; Ho. Surg. Roy. Infirm. Sheff.; Ho. Phys. Childr. Hosp. Sheff.

RIDGWAY, Daniel Mark University of Leeds, Department of Surgery, Yorkshire Deanery, Willow Terrace Road, Leeds LS2 9JT — MB ChB Leic. 1997.

RIDGWAY, Elisabeth Jane Department of Microbiology, Royal Hallamshire Hospital, Glossop Road, Sheffield S10 2JF Tel: 0114 271 2610 Fax: 0114 278 9376 Email: elisabeth.ridgway@sth.nhs.uk — MB BS Lond. 1985 (St Barts. Hosp.) BSc (Hons.) Lond. 1982, MB BS 1985; MRCPath 1992; MD University of Liverpool 1999; FRCPath 2000. Cons. Microbiol. Roy. Hallamshire Hosp. Sheff.; Hon. Sen. Clin. Lect. Univ. of Sheff. Specialty: Med. Microbiol. Socs: Hosp. Infec. Soc.

RIDGWAY, Elizabeth Susan 8 Monmouth Close, Chiswick, London W4 5DQ Tel: 020 8742 1386; 10 Nethercote,, Newton Burgoland, Leicester LE67 2ST Tel: 01530 272205 — MB BS Lond. 1994; BSc (Hons.) Lond. 1992.

RIDGWAY, Geoffrey Lindsay Department of Health, Skipton House, London Road, London SE1 6LH Tel: 0207 972 5325 Fax: 0207 172 6169 Email: geoff.ridgway@dh.gsi.gov.uk/ gl.ridg@dial.pipex.com; 23 Richmond Road, New Barnet EN5 1SA Tel: 020 8441 1732 Fax: 020 8441 1732 — MB BS Lond. 1971 (Royal Free) MRCS Eng. LRCP Lond. 1971; FRCPath 1989, M 1977; BSc (Special Zool.) Lond. 1966, MD 1977; MRCP (UK) 1996; Hon Dip. Hic 1999; FRCP 2000. Sen. Med. Off. (P/T), Dept. Health Eng.; Hon. Sen. Lect. UCL & Lond. Sch. of Hyg. & Trop. Med. Specialty: Med. Microbiol. Special Interest: Med. Microbiol., Chlamydial Infections, Decontamination Sci. Socs: Roy. Soc. Med. (Counc. Path.); Brit. Soc. Antimicrob. Chemother.; Hosp. Infec. Soc. Prev: Cons. Microbiologist Univ. Coll. Lond. Hosps.; Hon. Cons. Microbiol. Roy. Nat. Heart & Brompton Hosp. Gp.; Sen. Regist. (MicroBiol.) Univ. Coll. Lond. Hosps.

RIDGWAY, John Charles Quinton Family Practice, 406 Quinton Road West, Quinton, Birmingham B32 1QG Tel: 0121 421 6011; Chestnut Lodge, Court Road, Upper Strensham, Worcester WR8 9LP — (St. And.) MB ChB St. And. 1968. Prev: SHO (Obst.) Northampton Gen. Hosp.; Ho. Off. Stratford Gen. Hosp.

RIDGWAY, Stephen David Flat 8, 2 Craddock Court, 30 Bodenham Road, Hereford HR1 2TS — MB BCh Wales 1994.

RIDGWAY, Timothy John 53 West Coats Road, Cambuslang, Glasgow G72 8AE — MB ChB Ed. 1989; FFARCSI 1997.

RIDING, Blodwen Eleanor Joyce (retired) Maddenii, 5 Lon Cynan, Abergele LL22 7JA Tel: 01745 824435 — MB ChB Liverp. 1950; DA Eng. 1959; DPM Eng. 1972; MRCPsych 1973. Prev: Cons. Psychiat. Fazakerley, Walton & Rainhill Hosps.

RIDING, Graham Stuart Garnett Victoria Hospital, Blackpool FY3 8NR Tel: 01253 300000; 39 South Road, Bretherton, Preston PR26 9AB — MB ChB Manch. 1991; BSc (Physiol.) Manch. 1988. SHO (Gen. Surg.) Vict. Hosp. Blackpool. Prev: SHO (A & E) Roy. Preston Hosp.; Ho. Off. (Med.) Qu. Eliz. Hosp. Blackburn; Ho. Off. (Surg.) Roy. Preston Hosp.

RIDING, John Edmund, CBE (retired) Maddenii, 5 Lon Cynan, Abergele LL22 7JA Tel: 01745 824435 — MD Liverp. 1959; MB ChB 1947; DA Eng. 1951; FFA RCS Eng. 1954; Hon. FFA RACS 1979; FRCS Eng. 1980. Prev: Cons. Anaesth. Liverp. HA.

RIDING, Katie Jane Sherwood House, Division Lane, Blackpool FY4 5DZ — MB ChB Manch. 1997.

RIDING, Sarah Margaret Easthope Road Medical Centre, Easthope Road, Church Stretton SY6 6BL Tel: 01694 722127 Fax: 01694 724604 — MB ChB Birm. 1987; MRCGP 1995.

RIDING, William Douglas Currajong, Avenue Farm Lane, Wilden, Bedford MK44 2PY Tel: 01234 771669 Fax: 01234 771669 — (Camb. & Liverp.) MA Camb. 1961, BA 1957; MB BChir Camb. 1960; MRCS Eng. LRCP Lond. 1960; FRCP Lond. 1983, M 1964. Cons. Phys. Bedford Hosp.; JP. Specialty: Gen. Med. Socs: Brit. Thorac. Soc.& BMA. Prev: Sen. Regist. (Med.) United Manch. Hosps.

RIDINGS, Philip Charles 95 Seaford Road, London W13 9HS — BM Soton. 1987.

RIDLER, Andrew Hughes Blackmore Health Centre, Blackmore Drive, Sidmouth EX10 8ET Tel: 01395 512601 Fax: 01395 578408; Rosemead, Hillside Road, Sidmouth EX10 8JF Tel: 01395 512601 — MB BChir Camb. 1973; MA Camb. 1973; DObst RCOG 1975; Cert Family Plann. RCOG RCGP & FPA 1976.

RIDLER, Brigid Mary Fitzclarence Royal Devon & Exeter Hospital (Wonford), Exeter EX2 5DW Tel: 01392 402759 Fax: 01392 402759 Email: bmfridler@hotmail.com — MB ChB Sheff. 1972; DObst RCOG 1974; Cert. Family Plann. JCC 1975. Research Assoc. (Vasc.) Vasc. Surgic. Soc. & Clin. Blood Conservation Coordinator (Staff Grade) Roy. Devon & Exeter Hosp. Socs: Devon & Exeter Med. Soc.; Antilogus Transfusion Spec. Int. Group; Brit. Blood Transf. Soc. Prev: Trainee GP Wessex VTS; A&E & Clin. Ass. Surg., Roy. Dev. & Exeter Hosp. Drs. Retainer Scheme.

RIDLER, Samantha Louise 1 Arrowfield Close, Bristol BS14 0UQ — BM BS Nottm. 1994.

RIDLER, Simon John 56 Knutsford Road, Alderly Drive SK9 7SF — MB ChB Manch. 1997.

RIDLEY, Alan Eastling 19 Hillsden Road, Whitley Bay NE25 9XF; 19 Hillsden Road, Whitley Bay NE25 9XF Tel: 0191 251 0091 — MB BS Durh. 1954; DObst RCOG 1960; MRCGP 1967. Indep. GP Whitley Bay. Prev: GP N. Shields Tyne & Wear.

RIDLEY, Alan Ridley (retired) Five Winds, 174 Pennsylvania Road, Exeter EX4 6DZ Tel: 01392 216679 — MB BS Durh. 1955; FRCP Lond. 1975, M 1959; PhD Durh. 1962; MD (Distinc.) Newc. 1964. Prev: Sen. Cons. Neurol. Lond. Hosp.

RIDLEY, Colin Charles Sheridan The Regional Child & Adolescent Unit, Park View Clinic, 60 Queensbridge Road, Moseley, Birmingham B13 8QE Tel: 0121 243 2000 Fax: 0121 243 2010; Cornerstone, Cofton Church Lane, Cofton Hacket, Birmingham B45 8BB Tel: 0121 445 2515 — MB BS Lond. 1978 (St. Geo.

Hosp. Lond.) AKC 1978; Dip. Social Learn Theory & Pract. in App Settings Leic. 1988; Dip. Psychoanal. Observat. Studies E. Lond. 1995. Assoc. Specialist Irwin Unit Pk. View Clinic Birm. Specialty: Child & Adolesc. Psychiat. Socs: Affil. Roy. Coll. Psychiat. Prev: Staff Grade Doctor Irwin Unit Pk. View Clinic Birm.

RIDLEY, David Curtis Greystoke Surgery, Kings Avenue, Morpeth NE61 15A Tel: 01670 511393 — MB ChB Sheff. 1980. Specialty: Gen. Pract.

RIDLEY, David Malcolm 52 Stangate, Royal St., London SE1 7EQ — MB ChB Aberd. 1972; MRCOG 1978.

RIDLEY, Diane Melbourne Park Medical Centre, Melbourne Road, Aspley, Nottingham NG8 5HL Tel: 0115 978 6114 Fax: 0115 924 9334 — BM BS Nottm. 1994; MRCGP 1998; DFFP Loc Lut 1999. Gen. Practitioner Nottm. Specialty: Gen. Pract.

RIDLEY, John Graham Haltwhistle Health Centre, Greencroft Avenue, Haltwhistle NE49 9AP Tel: 01434 320077 Fax: 01434 320674 — MB ChB Bristol 1975; BA Camb. 1965.

RIDLEY, Joy 27 Little Moor Hill, Smethwick B67 7BG — MB ChB Aberd. 1998; MB ChB Aberd 1998.

RIDLEY, Malcolm Gavin Grove House Surgery, 80 Pryors Lane, Rose Green, Bognor Regis PO21 4JB Tel: 01243 265222 Fax: 01243 268693 Email: ridley@solutions-inc.co.uk — MB BS Lond. 1967 (St. Thos.) DA Eng. 1969. Clin. Head in Commisioning and PEC Mem., West. Sussex PCT. Specialty: Gen. Pract. Prev: Ho. Off. St. Richard's Hosp. Chichester; Resid. (Anaesth.) St. Thos. Hosp. Lond.; Regtl. Med. Off. 21st S.A.S. Regt. (AVR).

RIDLEY, Martin Grant 35 Plainwood Close, Summersdale, Chichester PO19 4YB Tel: 01243 532164 Fax: 01242 532164 Email: martin.ridley@plainwood.demon.uk — MB BS Lond. 1978 (King's Coll. Hosp.) MRCP (UK) 1981; FRCP 1997. Cons. Rheum. with interest Gen. Med. St. Richard's Hosp. Chichester; Med. Director Roy. W. Sussex Trust. Specialty: Rheumatol.; Gen. Med. Socs: Brit. Soc. Rheum. Prev: Sen. Regist. (Rheum.) St. Thos. Hosp. Lond.; Research Fell. Rheum. Dis. Unit Guy's Hosp. Med. Sch. Lond.; Regist. (Gen. Med.) Bath Health Dist.

RIDLEY, Nancye Mary (retired) 12 Brooklands Close, Fordwich, Canterbury CT2 0BT — MRCS Eng. LRCP Lond. 1942 (Univ. Coll. & W. Lond. Hosp.) Prev: Med. Off. Nixon Memor. Hosp. Sierra Leone.

RIDLEY, Mr Nicholas Harold Lloyd Keeper's Cottage, Stapleford, Salisbury SP3 4LT Tel: 01722 790209 — (Camb. & St. Thos.) Hon. FICS; MRCS Eng. LRCP Lond. 1930; MA 1927 Camb. (Nat. Sc. Trip.) 1927, MD 1945, MA, MB BChir 1931; FRCS Eng. 1932; FRS 1986; FRCOphth. Hon. 1989; Hon. DSc City 1990. Hon. Cons. Surg. Ophth. Dept. St. Thos. Hosp.; Hon. Cons. Moorfields Eye Hosp. Specialty: Ophth. Socs: Hon. Fell. Roy. Soc. Med.; Hon. Mem. Oxf. Ophth. Congr.; Hon. Life Pres. Internat. Intraocular Implant Club. Prev: Mem. Expert Advis. Panel on Parasitic Dis. (Filariasis) WHO; Temp. Maj. RAMC; Chief Asst., &c. St. Thos. Hosp. & Moorfields Eye Hosp.

RIDLEY, Nicholas Terence Francis The Green, Stratton Audley, Bicester OX27 9BJ — MB ChB Zimbabwe 1983; LRCP LRCS Ed. LRCPS Glas. 1983; MRCP (UK) 1988; FRCR 1993.

RIDLEY, Nicola Anne Deneside, 1 Roslyn Road, Hathersage, Hope Valley S32 1BY — MB BChir Camb. 1989; DFFP.

RIDLEY, Patricia Graham Haltwhistle Health Centre, Greencroft Avenue, Haltwhistle NE49 9AP Tel: 01434 320077 Fax: 01434 320674; The Pikes, Haltwhistle NE49 9JL Tel: 01434 320346 — MB BS Newc. 1968.

RIDLEY, Paul Damien Chatswood, North Marine Road, Flamborough, Bridlington YO15 1LG — MB BS Lond. 1982.

RIDLEY, Philippa 13 Cotham Gardens, Bristol BS6 6HD — BM BS Nottm. 1994.

RIDLEY, Philippa Jane Brackendale, Parkside, Hale, Farnham GU9 0JP — MB BS Lond. 1998; MB BS Lond 1998.

RIDLEY, Mr Robert Edward Wilson (retired) The Old Vicarage, Dinnington, Newcastle upon Tyne NE13 7AA Tel: 01661 24585 — MB BS Durh. 1963; FRCOphth; LMCC 1967; DO Eng. 1973; FRCS Ed. 1977. Prev: Hon. Clin. Lect. in Ophth. Newc. Univ.

RIDLEY, Saxon Alan Norfolk and Norwich Hospital, Brunswich Road, Norwich NR1 3SR Tel: 01603 286286 — MB BS Lond. 1981; FFA RCS Eng. 1985; MD Lond. 1995. Cons. Anaesth. & Intens. Care Norf. & Norwich Hosp.; Hon. Sen. Lect. Univ. E. Anglia. Specialty: Anaesth.; Intens. Care. Socs: Hon. Sec. Intens. Care Soc. Prev: Sen. Regist. (Anaesth.) West. Infirm. Glas.; Clin. Research Fell. Clin. Shock Study in West. Infirm. Glas.; Regist. (Anaesth.) The Hosp. for Sick Childr. Gt. Ormond St. Lond.

RIDOUT, Aileen Betty (retired) 4 Mulgrave Road, Croydon CR0 1BL Tel: 020 8688 5257 — MB BS Lond. 1954 (Roy. Free) MRCS Eng. LRCP Lond. 1954; DPH Eng. 1961; FFCM 1978, M 1973. Specialist in Community Med. (Med. Staffing & Postgrad. Med. Educat.) SE Thames RHA; Barrister-at-Law Gray's Inn 1972. Prev: Dep. Med. Off. Health Lond. Boro. S.wark.

RIDOUT, Dorothy Mary (retired) 36 Parkside Road, Leeds LS6 4QG Tel: 0113 275 2311 — (Roy. Free) MB BS Lond. 1943; FRCOG 1986, M 1951; FRCS Eng. 1952.

RIDOUT, Sally Marshall Long Meadow, Gravel Pit Road, Wooton Bridge, Ryde PO33 4RB — BM Soton. 1985; DRCOG 1989; MRCGP 1990.

RIDOUT, Simon Scott Hawkmoor House, Tavistock PL19 8PA — MB BS Lond. 1976 (Middlx.) MSc (Human Appl. Physiol.) Lond. 1985; MFOM RCP Lond. 1994, AFOM 1987. Company Med. Off., Devonport Roy. Dockyard Hsp. Specialty: Occupat. Health. Prev: Employm. Med. Adviser Health & Safety Exec. Som.; RN Med. Off.; Ho. Surg. Middlx. Hosp. Lond.

RIDPATH, Joanne Homestead, 13 Hillside Walk, Brentwood CM14 4RA Tel: 01277 211802; Padstones, 7 Back Lane, Ripley, Harrogate HG3 3AE Tel: 01423 772271 — BM Soton. 1991 (Southampton) MRCP (UK) 1996. Cons. Gastroenterol./Phys. Harrogate Dist. Hosp. N. Yorks. Specialty: Gastroenterol.; Gen. Med. Prev: SpR rotation (Gastro./GenMed) Yorks. Reg. '97-'03; SHO St. Jas. Univ. Hosp. Leeds '93-'97.

RIDSDALE, Leone Lorna Dept. of Clinical Neuroscieces, Guy's, King's and St Thomas's School of Medicine, Division of Clinical Neurosciences, King's College Hospital, Denmark Hill, London SE5 9RS Tel: 020 848 5150 Fax: 020 848 5781 Email: l.ridsdale@iop.kcl.ac.uk — MD McMaster Univ. Canada 1974 (McMaster Univ., Canada) BA Kent 1969; PhD Lond. 1994, MSc 1970; FRCPC 1979; FRCGP 1994, M 1981. Reader & Hon. Cons. (Gen. Pract.& Neurol.)Guy's, Kings, & St. Thomas Sch. of Med. Lond.; Sen. Lect. in Neurol. Guy's Kings and St Thomas Sch. of Med. Specialty: Gen. Pract.; Neurol. Socs: Amer. Acad. Neurol.; Fell. Roy. Coll. Phys. Canada.; Fell. Roy. Coll. GPs. Prev: Sen. Regist., Nat. Hosp. for Neurol.; Chief Neurol. Resid. & Fell. The Montreal Neurol. Inst. Canada; Lect. Univ. Coll. & Middlx. Hosp.

RIDSDALE, Patricia Anne Tadley Medical Partnership, Holmwood Health Centre, Franklin Avenue, Tadley RG26 6ER Tel: 0118 981 166; The Natural Practice, 106 Stockbridge Road, Winchester SO22 6RL Tel: 01962 856310 Fax: 01962 852104 Email: enquiries@thenaturalpractice.com — MB ChB Birm. 1987; MRCGP 1992; DRCOG 1992; MFHom 2004. Special Interest: diving and subaqua Med.; homeopathy.

RIDSDILL SMITH, Geoffrey Patrick The Burwell Surgery, Newmarket Road, Burwell, Cambridge CB5 0AE Tel: 01638 741234 Fax: 01638 743948; The Abbey, Swaffham Bulbeck, Cambridge CB5 0NQ — MB Camb. 1977 (University of Cambridge) MA Cambridge 1966; BChir 1976; DRCOG 1978. Trainer (Gen. Pract.) Camb. VTS.

RIDSDILL SMITH, Philip Anthony Haslemere Health Centre, Church Lane, Haslemere GU27 2BQ Tel: 01483 783023 Fax: 01428 645065 — MB BS Lond. 1993; MRCGP; Dip Occ Med; DCH RCP Lond. 1995; DFFP 1998; DRCOG 1998. GP Partner. Specialty: Gen. Pract. Prev: GP Regist. St Clements Winchester, Bapdune Ho. Guildford; SHO Rotat. (Paediat.) Soton. Gen. Hosp.

RIDSDILL SMITH, Robin Michael 241 Woodlands Road, Aylesford, Aylesford ME20 7QF Tel: 01622 717324 Fax: 01622 882304 Email: robin.ridsdill.591@aol.com — (St. Bart.) MRCS Eng. LRCP Lond. 1958; MB BChir Camb. 1959; DObst RCOG 1960; FRCGP 1981, M 1968. GP Locum. Specialty: Gen. Pract. Socs: Roy. Coll. Gen. Pract. Prev: GP Thornhills Med. Gp.; Ho. Surg. (Obst.) Norf. & Norwich Hosp.; Ho. Phys. Jenny Lind Childr. Hosp. Norwich.

RIDSDILL-SMITH, William Patrick The Health Centre, Woolpit, Bury St Edmunds IP30 9QU — MB BChir Camb. 1993; MRCGP 1997.

RIDYARD, John Bolton 9 The Meadows, Rainhill, Prescot L35 0PQ — MA Camb. 1966; MD Liverp. 1978, MB ChB 1968; MRCP (UK) 1972; FRCP Lond. 1986. Cons. Phys. Whiston Hosp. Prescot; Clin. Lect. Liverp. Univ. Specialty: Gen. Med.; Respirat. Med. Socs: Liverp. Med. Inst. & Brit. Thoracic Soc. Prev: Lect. (Med.)

Ahmadu Bello Univ. Hosp. Zaria, Nigeria; Sen. Med. Regist. Broadgreen Hosp. Liverp.; Ho. Phys. & Ho. Surg. Roy. South. Hosp. Liverp.

RIEBERER, Gabriela Clair Academic Unit, Royal London Homoeopathic Hospital, Great Ormond St., London WC1N 3HR Tel: 020 7833 7223 Fax: 020 7833 7212 — State Exam Med Gottingen 1987; PhD Gottingen 1991; MFHom Lond. 1993. Specialist Homoeop. Phys. Bradford & Acad. Unit Roy. Lond. Homoeop. Hosp. Specialty: Homeop. Med. Prev: Clin. Asst. Glas. Homoeop. Hosp.

RIECK, Jonathan 7 Mount Mews, High St., Hampton on Thames, Hampton TW12 2SH Tel: 020 8979 2262 — MB BS Lond. 1983.

RIEDEL, Mr John Adolf (retired) 1 Dovedale Road, Leicester LE2 2DN Tel: 0116 270 5068 — MB ChB Ed. 1948; Med. Dipl. Amsterdam 1949; FRCS Ed. 1956; FRCOG 1973, M 1959. Cons. O & G Leicester Roy. Infirm. Prev: Resid. Simpson Matern. Pavil. Edin. Roy. Infirm.

RIEGER, Christopher Andrew Cardiff Road Surgery, 12 Cardiff Road, Luton LU1 1QG Tel: 01582 722148 Fax: 01582 485721; 56 Masefield Road, Harpenden AL5 4JR — MB BS Lond. 1975 (Lond. Hosp.) DRCOG 1979; MRCGP 1981. Vis. Med. Off. Luton Day Centre for the Homeless. Socs: BMA.

RIEU, Edward Christopher Suthergrey House Surgery, 37A St. Johns Road, Watford WD17 1LS Tel: 01923 224424 Fax: 01923 243710; Merrowdown, Burtons Lane, Chalfont St Giles HP8 4BD — MB BS Lond. 1979; DRCOG 1982; MRCP (UK) 1987.

RIFAAT, Mr Mohammed Maidstone and Tunbridge Wells NHS Trust, Eye, Ear & Mouth Unit, Hermitage Lane, Maidstone ME16 9QQ — MB BCh Ain Shams 1987; FRCS (Ophth.) Ed. 1998. Assoc. Specialist (Ophth.) Maistone & Tunbridge Wells NHS Trust. Specialty: Ophth. Special Interest: Med. Ophth.

RIFAT-GHAFFAR, Dr The Surgery, Abbey Square, Walsall WS3 2RH Tel: 01922 408416 Fax: 01922 400372; 418 Sutton Road, Walsall WS5 3BA Tel: 01922 614269 — MB BS Patna 1974 (P. of Wales Med. Coll.) GP. Specialty: Obst. & Gyn.; Family Plann. & Reproduc. Health; Dermat.

RIFKIN, Larry Maudsley Hospital, 103 Denmark Hill, London SE5 8AF Tel: 020 7740 5091 Fax: 020 7701 5092 — MB BCh Witwatersrand 1984; MRCPsych 1991. Cons. Psychiat. Maudsley Hosp.; Hon. Sen. Lect. Inst. Isyemiat. IOP. Specialty: Gen. Psychiat.

RIFKIN, Shelley 21 Woodfield Way, London N11 2NP — MB BCh Witwatesrand 1986; MB BCh Witwatersrand 1986.

RIGBY, Andrew Neil Church Street Surgery, 77 Church Street, Tewkesbury GL20 5RY Tel: 01684 292343 Fax: 01684 274305; Upper Westcroft, Westmancote, Tewkesbury GL20 7ES Tel: 01684 772412 — MB BS Lond. 1973 (Middlx.) DRCOG 1978; DGM 1996. Med. Off. Tewkesbury Hosp. Specialty: Gen. Pract. Prev: Asst. Lect. (Path.) St. Thos. Hosp. Med. Sch. Lond.; Ho. Surg. W. Norwich Hosp.; Ho. Phys. Centr. Middlx. Hosp. Lond.

RIGBY, Anthony John Brundall Medical Centre, The Dales, Brundall, Norwich NR13 5RP Tel: 01603 712255 Fax: 01603 712156; Alveston House, Yarmouth Road, Blofield, Norwich NR13 4LQ Tel: 01603 713904 — MB BS Lond. 1969; Univ. Coll. Hosp; DObst RCOG 1970. Prev: SHO (O & G) Hillingdon Hosp. Middlx.; SHO (Paediat.) & Ho. Phys. Warwick Gen. Hosp.; Ho. Off. (Surg.) Univ. Coll. Hosp. Lond.

RIGBY, Carolyn Jane North Tees General Hospital, Stockton-on-Tees TS19 8PE — MB BS Newc. 1989. SHO (Gen. Med.) N. Tees Gen. Hosp.

RIGBY, Mr Christopher Colton (retired) Newvale, 7 Clyro Place, Sutton Cum Lound, Retford DN22 8PE Tel: 01777 700469 — MB ChB Sheff. 1960; FRCS Eng. 1967. InDepend. private Pract. - Gen. and Vasc. Surg. Prev: Sen. Regist. (Surg.) Nottm. Gen. Hosp. & Roy. Hosp. Sheff.

RIGBY, Christopher Harold Lester (retired) The Elms Medical Practice, Hoo, Rochester ME3 9AE Tel: 01634 250142; Little Owls, Barn St, St. Mary Hoo, Rochester ME3 8RN Tel: 01634 270396 — MB BChir Camb. 1963 (St. Geo.) MA, MB Camb. 1963, BChir 1962; DCH Eng. 1964. Prev: Regist. (Med.) Mayday Hosp.

RIGBY, Claire Miranda 7 Salter Road, Sandbanks, Poole BH13 7RQ; The Porch Surgery, Corsham — MB BS Lond. 1991. GP Retainer. Prev: SHO (Med.) Lister Hosp. Stevenage.

RIGBY, David Jeffrey North Lochs Medical Practice, Gleann Mor, Lochs, Isle of Lewis HS2 9JP Tel: 01851 860222 Fax: 01851 860611 — MB ChB Dundee 1990. SHO (O & G) Vale of Leven Dist. Gen. Hosp. Dunbartonsh. Specialty: Obst. & Gyn.

RIGBY, Diana Queensway Surgery, 75 Queensway, Southend-on-Sea SS1 2AB; 24 Kings Road, Westcliff on Sea SS0 8LL — MB BS Lond. 1979; MRCP (UK) 1982. GP S.end.

RIGBY, George Vernon 2 The Grange, 85 High St., Iver SL0 9PN — MB BS Lond. 1971; BSc (Special, Physiol., Hons.); MRCP (UK) 1977.

RIGBY, Mr Howard Seymour Department of Pathology, Frenchay Hospital, Bristol BS16 1LE — BM BS Nottm. 1976; DM Nottm. 1986, BM BS 1976; FRCS Eng. 1980; FRCPath 1991. Cons. Histopath. Frenchay Hosp. Bristol. Specialty: Histopath.

RIGBY, John Anthony (retired) T. S. Hattersley & Son Ltd., 63 Weymouth Road, Eccles, Manchester M30 8TH Tel: 0161 789 1374 Fax: 0161 787 8632; Waterfield, Barber Green, Grange-over-Sands LA11 6HU Tel: 01539 536470 — MB ChB Birm. 1954; DObst RCOG 1960; DIH Soc. Apoth. Lond. 1976; FFOM RCP Lond. 1992, MFOM 1983. Chief. Exec. & Occupat. Phys. T.S. Hattersley & Son. Ltd. Eccles. Prev: Chief Med. Adviser VSEL plc Barrow-in-Furness.

RIGBY, John Christopher Hesketh Centre, Albert Road, Southport PR9 0LT; 9 Delamere Road, Aimsdale, Southport PR8 2RD — MB ChB Leeds 1977; DRCOG 1980; MRCPsych 1984; MMedSc Aberd. 1986; FRCPsych 1996. Cons. Psychiat. Southport; Med. Dir. Specialty: Geriat. Psychiat. Prev: Postgrad. Clin. Tutor; Specialist Scheme Organiser (Mersey Drantry); Sec. BMA.

RIGBY, John Gilbert (retired) 3 Bertram Drive, Meols, Hoylake, Wirral L47; 1 Woodland Avenue, Meols, Wirral CH47 5BA — MB ChB Liverp. 1951; DObst RCOG 1956. Prev: GP Hoylake.

RIGBY, John Martin 52 Towan Blystra Road, Newquay TR7 2RP — MB ChB Leic. 1992.

RIGBY, John Peter Vernon, TD Huntsmoor Weir, Old Mill Lane, Cowley, Uxbridge UB8 2JH Tel: 01895 234898 — (Oxf. & St. Thos.) BA (Hons. Physiol. & Nat. Sc.) Oxf. 1937; BM BCh Oxf. 1942; MA Oxf. 1942; MRCS Eng. LRCP Lond. 1942; Cert. FPA 1979. Emerit. Cons. Phys. Guy's Hosp. Lond.; Phys. (Approved Under Sect. 12 Ment. Health Act 1983). Specialty: Respirat. Med. Socs: Harveian Soc.; Brit. Thorac. Soc.; Roy. Brompton Hosp. Soc. Prev: Cons. Phys. Deptford Chest Clinic Lond.; Ho. Phys. Brompton Hosp. Dis. Chest; Cas. Phys. and Med. Reg. St Mary's Hosp. Lond.

RIGBY, Kathryn Ann 34 Church Lane, Bessacarr, Doncaster DN4 6QA — MB ChB Leeds 1994.

RIGBY, Marcus Thornburn Waterside, Haye Lane, Mappleborough Green, Studley B80 7BX Tel: 01527 852873 — MB ChB Birm. 1955.

RIGBY, Michael Charles Barn Acre, Bishops Frome, Worcester WR6 5AS — MB BS Lond. 1992; FRCS 1996. Specialty: Orthop.

RIGBY, Michael Francis Beech Lodge, Department of Psychotherapy, Carleton Clinic, Comwhinton Drive, Carlisle CA1 3SX Tel: 01228 602392 Email: mike.rigby@ncumbria.nhs.uk — MB BS Lond. 1982 (Westm.) BSc (1st cl. Hons.) Lond. 1979; DA (UK) 1986; MRCPsych 1992. Cons. (Psychotherapist) Beech Lodge Carleton Clinic Carlisle. Specialty: Psychother. Special Interest: Gp. Anal.; Personality Disorder; Staff Train. Prev: Cons. (Psychotherapist) N. Cumbria Psychother. Serv.; Sen. Regist. (Psychother.) St. Geo. Hosp. & Henderson Hosp. Lond.; Regist. (Psychiat.) Char. Cross Hosp. Lond.

RIGBY, Michael Laurence Royal Brompton Hospital, Sydney St., London SW3 6NP Tel: 020 7351 8542 Fax: 020 7351 8547 — (Leeds) MB ChB Leeds 1970; MRCP (UK) 1974; MD Leeds 1984; FRCP Lond. 1988; FRCPCH 1997. Dir. & Cons. Paediat. Cardiol. Roy. Brompton Hosp. Lond. Specialty: Paediat. Cardiol. Special Interest: Interventional Cardiac Catheterisation. Socs: Brit. Cardiac Soc.; Brit. Paediatric Cardiac Assn.; Assn. for Europ. Paediatric Cardiol. Prev: Canad. Heart Foundat. Fell. Hosp. Sick Childr. Toronto, Canada.

RIGBY, Paul Stockbridge Village Health Centre, Leachcroft, Waterpark Drive, Liverpool L28 1ST Tel: 0151 489 9924; 8 Campsey Ash, Widnes WA8 9GP — MB ChB Liverp. 1987; DRCOG 1992; MRCGP 1995.

RIGBY, Peter John Readesmoor Medical Group Practice, 29-29A West Street, Congleton CW12 1JP Tel: 01260 276161 Fax: 01260 297340; 67 Ennerdale Drive, Congleton CW12 4FJ — MB ChB Sheff. 1985; MRCGP 1989; DRCOG 1989.

RIGBY, Philip (retired) 7 Azalea Road, Wick St Lawrence, Weston Super Mare BS22 9TN Tel: 01934 521964 Email: drrigby@globalnet.co.uk — MB ChB Birm. 1946; DTM & H Liverp. 1960; DPhysMed Eng. 1970. Prev: Cons. Rehabil. Raigmore Hosp. Inverness.

RIGBY, Shirley Patricia 20 Appleby Close, Twickenham TW2 5NA Tel: 020 8898 0945 — MB BS Lond. 1988 (Charing Cross & Westm. Med. Sch.) BSc (Hons.) Lond. 1985, MB BS 1988; MRCP (UK) 1991. Specialist Regist. Northwick Pk. Hosp. Specialty: Rehabil. Med.; Rheumatol.

RIGBY-JONES, Timothy Grosvenor Medical Centre, Grosvenor Street, Crewe CW1 3HB Tel: 01270 256348 Fax: 01270 250786; Laburnum Cottage, Audlem Road, Hatherton, Nantwich CW5 7QT Tel: 01270 841251 — MB BChir Camb. 1968 (Camb. & Westm.) MA, MB Camb. 1968, BChir 1967; MRCS Eng. LRCP Lond. 1967; DObst RCOG 1969; DCH Eng. 1970. Prev: Ho. Surg. Gordon Hosp. Lond.; Ho. Off. (Obst. & Med.) Crumpsall Hosp. Manch.; SHO Booth Hall Childr. Hosp. Manch.

RIGDEN, Brian Richard Queensview Medical Centre, Thornton Road, Northampton NN2 6LS; Home Close, Moulton Lane, Boughton, Northampton NN2 8RF Tel: 01604 847964 — MB ChB Leic. 1983 (Leicester) DRCOG 1987.

RIGDEN, Jessica 1/6 Saxe Coburg Terrace, Edinburgh EH3 5BU — MB ChB Ed. 1992; MRCGP 1996. Specialty: Gen. Pract.

RIGDEN, Susan Patricia Alice Guy's Hospital , Guy's and St Thomas' NHS Foundation Trust, Department of Paediatric Nephrology, 9th Floor Guy's Tower, London SE1 9RT Tel: 020 7188 4586 Fax: 020 7188 4591 Email: sue.rigden@gstt.nhs.uk; 205 John Ruskin Street, London SE5 0PT Tel: 0207 703 4860 Email: sue.rigden@virgin.net — (Roy. Free) MB BS Lond. 1972; MRCP (UK) 1976; FRCP Lond. 1990. Cons. Paediat. Nephrol. Guy's Hosp. Lond. Specialty: Paediat.

RIGG, Alastair William Gretna Surgery, Central Avenue, Gretna DG16 5NA Tel: 01461 338317 Fax: 01461 339244 Email: drrigg@y18428.dghb.scot.nhs.uk; 3 The Meadow, Eaglesfield, Lockerbie DG11 3PH Tel: 01461 500565 Email: alrigg@hotmail.com — MB ChB Ed. 1980; BSc (Med. Sci.) Ed. 1977; DRCOG 1984; MRCGP 1985. Specialty: Gen. Pract. Socs: Christ. Med. Fellowsh.

RIGG, Christopher Donald Anaesthetics Department, Hull Royal Infirmary, Andhy Road, Kingston upon Thames; 5 St Pauls Close, Northallerton DL7 8YN Tel: 01608 770814 — MB ChB Ed. 1985; BSc (Hons.) Ed. 1983; DA (UK) 1989; DCH RCP Lond. 1990; DRCOG 1991; FRCA 1994. Cons. Anaesth. Hull Roy. Infirm.; Regist. (Anaesth.) Newc.; Specialist Regist, (Anaesth.) Newc. Specialty: Anaesth. Socs: Roy. Soc. Med. (Edin. Br.); BMA. Prev: Trainee GP Northallerton VTS.

RIGG, Emma Louise 41 The Valley, Comberton, Cambridge CB3 7DF — MB BS Lond. 1998; MB BS Lond 1998.

RIGG, John Harvey White Lodge, 28 Waterloo Road, Birkdale, Southport PR8 2NG Tel: 01704 569619 Fax: 01704 569619; White Lodge, 28 Waterloo Road, Birkdale, Southport PR8 2NG Tel: 01704 569619 Fax: 01704 569619 — (Edinburgh) MB ChB Ed. 1966; DObst RCOG 1969. Med. Off. Roy. & Ancient Golf Club St. And.; Med. Off. Birkdale Sch. for Hearing Impaired Childr.; Chairm. Southport & Formby Fundholders Assn.; Chief Med. Off. Roy. and Ancient Golf Club of St. Andrews. Specialty: Gen. Med.; Sports Med.; Medico Legal. Socs: (Ex-Pres.) S.port Med. Soc. Prev: Rotat. Intern. New Hanover Memor. Hosp. Wilmington, N. Carolina; Cas. Off. Roy. Albert Edwd. Infirm. Wigan; SHO (O & G) Roy. Infirm. Perth.

RIGG, Kathleen Jessie (retired) 14 Sherlock Close, Cambridge CB3 0HW — MB BS Lond. 1947 (Roy. Free) DCP Lond. 1956; MRCPath 1964. Prev: Cons. Haemat. Salford AHA (T).

RIGG, Mr Keith Malcolm Nottingham City Hospital NHS Trust, Hucknall Road, Nottingham NG5 1PB Tel: 0115 969 1169 Fax: 0115 962 7678 Email: krigg@ncht.trent.nhs.uk — MB BS Newc. 1981; FRCS Eng. 1986; MD Newc. 1991. City Hosp. Nottm. & Cons. Gen. Surg.. Specialty: Gen. Surg.; Transpl. Surg. Prev: 1st. Asst. & Hon. Sen. Regist. (Transpl.) Univ. Newc. u Tyne; Regist. (Surg.) N. Tees Gen. Hosp.; Clin. Research Fell. Univ. Newc.

RIGG, Kenneth Stephen The Deeping Practice, Godsey Lane, Market Deeping, Peterborough PE6 8DD — MB ChB Leic. 1982; DRCOG 1984; MRCGP 1986.

RIGG, Nancy Dunlop 3 The Meadows, Eaglesfield, Lockerbie DG11 3PH — MB ChB Ed. 1981; BSc (Med. Sci.) Ed. 1978, MB ChB 1981; (Diploma Primary Care Rheumat. Soc.) Bath 1999. Staff Grade in Haemat. & Clin. Oncol., Dumfries & Galloway Roayl Infirm., Dumfries. Specialty: Oncol.; Family Planning; Gen. Pract. Prev: Cas. Off. Cumbld. Infirm. Carlisle.; Clin. Asst. (Rheum.) Cumbld. Infirm. Carlisle; Clin. Med. Off. Family Plann., N.bank Dumfries.

RIGG, Philip Prospect Road Surgery, 174 Prospect Road, Scarborough YO12 7LB Tel: 01723 360178 — MB ChB Sheff. 1975; DRCOG 1977; FFA RCS Eng. 1980; MRCGP 1997. Specialty: Anaesth.

RIGG, Rita Charlotte The Hermitages Medical Practice, 5 Hermitage Terrace, Edinburgh EH10 4RP Tel: 0131 447 6277 Fax: 0131 447 9866; 30 Morningside Place, Edinburgh EH10 5EY — MB BCh BAO Dub. 1973 (Trinity Coll. Dub.) MRCGP 1996. Princip.; Dip. Family Med. Chinese Univ. Hong Kong 1991. Specialty: Gen. Pract. Socs: BMA & Assoc. Mem. Hong Kong Coll. Gen. Practs.; Roy. Coll. Gen. Pract. Prev: Med. Off. United States Consulate Bombay, India; Assoc. GP, Hong Kong.

RIGGS, Mary Alexandra Surgery, 2 Wellington Avenue, Aldershot GU11 1SD Tel: 01252 332210 Fax: 01252 312490; April Cottage, Portesbery Road, Camberley GU15 3TF Tel: 01276 21075 — BM BCh Oxf. 1973; DCH Eng. 1976.

RIGLER, Malcolm Stuart Withymoor Village Surgery, Turners Lane, Brierley Hill DY5 2PG Tel: 01384 573670 — MB ChB Bristol 1971; DObst RCOG 1973. Specialty: Epidemiol. Socs: Social Hist. Medico Social Soc. Prev: Regist. Community Med. S. West. RHA.

RIGNEY, Anne Theresa Roysia Surgery, Burns Road, Royston SG8 5PT Tel: 01763 243166 Fax: 01763 245315; 7 Valley Rise, Royston SG8 9EY Tel: 01763 242686 — LRCPI & LM, LRSCI & LM 1972 (RCSI) LRCPI & LM, LRCSI & LM 1972; DCH RCPSI 1975; DRCOG 1977. Prev: Ho. Off. (Paediat.) Whipps Cross Hosp. Lond.; SHO (Med.) Jervis St. Hosp. Dub.; Ho. Off. (Obst.) Mother's Hosp. Lond.

RIHAN, Mr Robert Stanley (retired) Foxgloves, Foscot, Chipping Norton OX7 6RP Tel: 01608 658280 — (Birm.) MB ChB Birm. 1951; MRCS Eng. LRCP Lond. 1951; FRCS Eng. 1959. Prev: Cons. Surg. N. Birm. Dist. Hosp. Gp.

RIISNAES, Annette May Silverdale Drive Health Centre, 6 Silverdale Drive, Thurmaston, Leicester LE4 8NN — MB ChB Bristol 1979; DRCOG 1985. Gen. Practitioner, Thurmaston, Leicester. Prev: GP Bedford.; Trainee GP Mansfield VTS.

RILEY, Adrian Patrick Queens Road Surgery, 8 Queens Road, Portsmouth PO2 7NX — MB ChB Birm. 1967; DObst RCOG 1969; DA Eng. 1972.

RILEY, Professor Alan John, OStJ Lancs. Postgrad. School of Medicine and Health University of Central Lancs., Harrington Building, Preston PR1 2HE Tel: 01772 892791 Fax: 01772 892992 Email: alanriley@doctor.org.uk; Kings Park, Cwmann, Lampeter SA 48 8HQ Tel: 01772 731500 Email: alanriley@doctors.org.uk — MB BS Lond. 1967 (Char. Cross) MRCS Eng. LRCP Lond. 1967; DObst RCOG 1969; MSc Manch. 1976; FFPM RCP (UK) 1992, M 1989. Prof. of Sexual Med., Univ. of Centr. Lancs.; Med. Edr. Sexual & Marital Ther.; Cons. Pharmaceut. Med. Specialty: Psychosexual Med. Socs: Fell. Roy. Soc. Med.; Assn. for Marital & Sexual Therapists; BMA. Prev: Edr. Brit. Jl. Sexual Med. & Jl. Sexual Health; Head New Chem. Entities Glaxo Gp. Research.

RILEY, Annette Department of Pathology, Stirling Royal Infirmary, Livilands, Stirling FK8 2AU Tel: 01786 434000 Fax: 01786 449233 — MB ChB Glas. 1985; BSc (Hons.) Glas. 1982, MB ChB 1985; FRCPath 2000; (DFMS) Glasgow 2001. Cons. (Path.) Stirling Roy. Infirm. Stirling. Specialty: Pathology, General. Socs: Assn. Clin. Path.; Internat. Acad. of Pathol.; Brit. Soc. for Clin. Cytol. Prev: Sen. Regist. (Path.) & Hon. Lect. W. Infirm. Glas.; Regist. (Path.) West. Infirm. Glas.

RILEY, Anthony John Bellevue Surgery, Bellevue Terrace, Newport NP20 2WQ Tel: 01633 256337 Fax: 01633 222856 — MB BCh Wales 1992 (Cardiff) DCH 1996; MRCGP 1999. GP Princip.

RILEY, Bernard, MBE Adult Intensive Care Unit, Queen's Medical Centre, University Hospital, Nottingham NG7 2UH Tel: 0115 924 9924 Fax: 0115 970 9910; The Corner House, 32 Browns Lane, E. Bridgford, Nottingham NG13 8PL — MB BS Lond. 1978 (St. Geo.) BSc Lond. 1975; MRCS Eng. LRCP Lond. 1978; FFA RCS Eng. 1982.

Cons. Anaesth. & Adult Intens. Care Qu. Med. Centre Univ. Hosp. NHS Trust Nottm. Specialty: Intens. Care. Prev: Cons. Anaesth. & Intens. Care Char. Cross & Westm. Hosp. Lond.; Sen. Regist. (Anaesth. & Intens. Care) Roy. Surrey Co. Hosp. Guildford.
RILEY, Christine Elizabeth Torrington Speedwell Practice, Health Centre, Torrington Park, London N12 9SS Tel: 020 8445 7261 Fax: 020 8343 9122; 2 The Grange, Grange Avenue, Totteridge, London N20 8AB Tel: 020 8445 5687 — (Univ. Coll. Hosp.) MB BS Lond. 1960; MRCS Eng. LRCP Lond. 1960. Specialty: Obst. & Gyn. Socs: Roy. Soc. Med.; Brit. Med. Acupunct. Soc. Prev: Ho. Surg. New End Hosp. Hampstead; Ho. Phys. S. Lond. Hosp.
RILEY, Christopher John (retired) 4 Riverside Close, Halton on Lune, Lancaster LA2 6NA Tel: 01524 811513 — MB ChB Manch. 1959; DObst RCOG 1961; MRCP Glas. 1966; MRCP Lond. 1967. Prev: GP Lancaster.
RILEY, Colin Christopher (retired) — (Univ. Coll. Hosp.) MB BS Lond. 1953; DObst RCOG 1954; MRCGP 1966. Prev: Ho. Surg. (Obst.) Univ. Coll. Hosp. Lond.
RILEY, Damian James 99 Harboro Road, Sale M33 6GH — MB ChB Manch. 1987.
RILEY, Mr David Orthopaedic Department, Pontefract General Infirmary, Pontefract WF8 1PL Tel: 01977 606469 Fax: 01977 606723 — MB ChB Leeds 1977; FRCS Ed. 1982; FRCS Eng. 1982. Cons. Orthop. Surg. Pontefract Gen. Infirm. Specialty: Orthop. Socs: Fell. BOA; Brit. Soc. Childr. Orthop. Surg. Prev: Regist. (Orthop.) King's Coll. Hosp. Lond.; Ho. Surg. Chapel Allerton Hosp. Leeds; Ho. Phys. Leeds Gen. Infirm.
RILEY, David John Church Street Surgery, Church Street, Spalding PE11 2PB Tel: 01775 722189 Fax: 01775 712164; 6 Amsterdam Gardens, Spalding PE11 3HY — MB ChB Liverp. 1978; DRCOG 1983. Prev: SHO (Med./Geriat., Paediat. & O & G) Whiston & St. Helen's; Hosps. Merseyside.
RILEY, Deborah Anne Grovelands Medical Centre, 701 Oxford Road, Reading RG30 1HG Tel: 0118 958 2525 Fax: 0118 950 9284 — BM BCh Oxf. 1988; MA Camb. 1989; MRCGP 1996. Prev: Trainee GP Reading VTS.
RILEY, Diana Margaret The Red House, Wendover, Aylesbury HP22 6JQ Tel: 01296 622477 Fax: 01296 624727 Email: dmriley@cwcom.net — MB BS Lond. 1953 (Univ. Coll. Hosp.) MRCS Eng. LRCP Lond. 1953; FRCPsych 1988, M 1974; DPM Eng. 1974. Indep. Cons. Chiltern Hosp. Gt. Missenden, Bucks. & Portland Hosp. Lond.; Trustee Bucks. Assn. for Ment. Health. Specialty: Gen. Psychiat. Socs: Marcé Soc.; Roy. Soc. Med.; ISPOG. Prev: Sen. Regist. (Psychiat.) St. John's Hosp. Stone; Civil Med. Pract. RAF Halton; Ho. Phys. & Ho. Surg. Univ. Coll. Hosp. Lond.
RILEY, Donald Owen (retired) 44 Moat Road, Loughborough LE11 3PN Tel: 01509 266300 Email: don@doriley.demon.co.uk — (Sheff.) MB ChB Sheff. 1959; DObst RCOG 1962; DA Eng. 1962; MRCGP 1982.
RILEY, Esther Turner (retired) 118 Whitecrest, Great Barr, Birmingham B43 6EN Tel: 0121 357 5608 — MB ChB Ed. 1941.
RILEY, Gaynor Ann Caldbergh Cottage, Caldbergh, Middleham, Leyburn DL8 4RW — MB ChB Liverp. 1990.
RILEY, Gillian A Carlton Medical Practice, 252 Girlington Road, Bradford BD8 9PB Tel: 01274 544742 Fax: 01274 483362; 10 Salisbury Avenue, Baildon, Shipley BD17 5AA — MB ChB Leeds 1973; DObst RCOG 1976; MRCGP 1977.
RILEY, Jane Maria Flat 2, Straysyde House, Cavendish Avenue, Harrogate HG2 8HX — BM BS Nottm. 1990. Trainee GP/SHO W. Cumbld. Hosp. VTS.
RILEY, Janet Priscilla Mary Rowley Medical Practice, 65 Hawes Lane, Rowley Regis B65 9AJ Tel: 0121 559 2449 Fax: 0121 559 8579; 132 Barrs Road, Cradley Heath, Cradley Heath B64 7EZ Tel: 01384 560701 — (Leeds) MB ChB Leeds 1966; DCH Eng. 1968. Hon. Med. Adviser City of Birm. Symphony Orchestra. Specialty: Paediat. Prev: Ho. Phys. (Paediat.) Selly Oak Hosp. Birm.; Ho. Phys. Med. Unit St. Mary's Hosp. Lond.; Ho. Surg. King Edwd. Memor. Hosp. Ealing.
RILEY, John Ernest The Old School Medical Practice, Horseman Lane, Copmanthorpe, York YO23 3UA; Hunters Lodge, Moor Monkton, York YO26 8JA — MB ChB Leeds 1972; DObst RCOG 1974; MRCEP 1977.
RILEY, John Lawson (retired) 4 Farnham Close, Baildon, Shipley BD17 6SF Tel: 01274 590080 — MB ChB Ed. 1954 (Ediburgh) Prev: Ho. Surg. St. Luke's Hosp. Bradford & Huddersfield Roy. Infirm.
RILEY, Kate Health Centre, Victoria Sq, Portishead, Bristol BS20 6AQ Tel: 01275 847474 Fax: 01275 817516 — BM Soton. 1981.
RILEY, Katharine Julia 8 Snab Wood Close, Little Neston, South Wirral CH64 0UP — MB ChB Manch. 1986; MRCP (UK) 1990; MRCGP 1991.
RILEY, Kevin Paul The Surgery, 4-6 High Street, kinver, Stourbridge DY7 6HG Tel: 01384 873311 Fax: 01384 877328 — MB BCh Wales 1981.
RILEY, Lindsay Michael Garden Lane Medical Centre, 19 Garden Lane, Chester CH1 4EN Tel: 01244 346677 Fax: 01244 310094 — MB ChB Manch. 1976; BSc (Med. Sci.) St. And. 1974.
RILEY, Louise 99 Harboro Road, Sale M33 6GH — MB ChB Manch. 1987.
RILEY, Marshall Seth 20 Tullyhubbert Road, Moneyrea, Newtownards BT23 6BY — MB BCh BAO Belf. 1983; MRCP (UK) 1986; BSc Belf. 1980, MD 1990. Specialty: Respirat. Med.
RILEY, Martin 55 Borfa Green, Welshpool SY21 7QF — MB BCh Wales 1971; BSc (Hons. Physiol.) Wales 1971, MB BCh (Hons.) 1974; MRCP (U.K.) 1976; DRCOG 1977.
RILEY, Neville Paul Sycamores, The Street, All Cannings, Devizes SN10 3PA — MB BS Newc. 1977.
RILEY, Pamela Margaret 5 Hoghton Close, Lancaster LA1 5UF; 2 South Barn, Burrow Rd, Lancaster LA1 0PG Tel: 01524 752355 — MB ChB Manch. 1994; DFFP 1997. LOCUM GP; SHO Dermat. Qu Vict Hosp. Morecambe. Specialty: Gen. Pract.
RILEY, Professor Patrick Anthony (retired) 2 The Grange, Grange Avenue, London N20 8AB Tel: 020 8445 5687 Fax: 020 8446 6173 — (Univ. Coll. Hosp.) MB BS Lond. 1960; FRCPath. 1985, M 1980; PhD Lond. 1965, DSc 1990. Editor, Melanoma Research, (Publ. by LWW,Lond.). Prev: Beit Memor. Research Fell. (Chem. Path.) & Sen. Lect. (Biochem. Path.)Univ. Coll. Hosp. Med. Sch. Lond.
RILEY, Paul Adrian Fraser (retired) Le Pommier, La Rue Des Bordes, St Peter Port, Guernsey GY7 9PX Tel: 01481 65505 — MB ChB Dundee 1972; DRCOG 1978; FRCP Lond. 1994. Prev: Phys. Princess Eliz. Hosp. Guernsey.
RILEY, Paul Brook Rambleside, 94 Kingsway, Scunthorpe DN15 7ER Tel: 01724 840089 — MB BS Lond. 1942 (St. Thos.) MRCS Eng. LRCP Lond. 1939. Prev: Ho. Phys. Roy. Hosp. Bristol; Regist. Bristol Matern. Hosp.; Capt. RAMC.
RILEY, Mr Peter Latham House Medical Practice, Sage Cross Street, Melton Mowbray LE13 1NX Tel: 01664 854949 Fax: 01664 501825 — MB ChB Manch. 1973; DObst RCOG 1975; MRCOG 1980; DA (SA) 1984; FRCS Glas. 1987. Hosp. Pract. (Gen. & Plastic Surg.) War Memor. Hosp., Melton Mowbray. Prev: Trainee GP Measham Med. Unit Burton on Trent; Regist. (Plastic Surg.) Harare, Zimbabwe.
RILEY, Peter Andrew 23 Woodlands Avenue, Worcester Park KT4 7AL — MB BS Lond. 1986; MD Lond. 1993; MRCPath 1993. Cons. Med. Microbiologist and Honary Sen. Lect., St George's Hosp. Lond. Prev: Lect. (Med. Microbiol.) UMDS Lond.; Asst. Lect. (Path.) UMDS Guy's & St. Thos. Hosps. Lond.; Ho. Surg. (Orthop. & Gen. Surg.) St. Thos. Hosp. Lond.
RILEY, Peter Frederick Blagbrough (retired) Strawberry Farmhouse, Up Somborne, Stockbridge SO20 6RB Tel: 01794 388078 — MRCS Eng. LRCP Lond. 1949 (Lond. Hosp.) Prev: Ho. Phys. & Ho. Surg. Lond. Hosp.
RILEY, Peter John The Hunting Clinic, 55 St Lukes Road, Maidenhead SL6 7DN Tel: 01628 622261 — (Middlx.) MB BS Lond. 1968. Med. Dir. Maidenhead Inst. Rotterdam, Holland; Med. Dir. Hunting Clinic Maidenhead.
RILEY, Peter Leslie — MB ChB Liverp. 1984; MRCP (UK) 1991; FRCR 1998. Cons. Radiol. Qu. Eliz. Hosp. Univ. Hosp. Birm. NHS Trust Metchley Pk. Rd., Edgbaston.B15 2TH. Specialty: Radiol.
RILEY, Raymond Eric 11 Tixover Park, Stamford PE9 3QN Tel: 01780 444454 — (Leeds) MB ChB Leeds 1944.
RILEY, Sara Jane Gosbury Hill Health Centre, Orchard Gardens, Chessington KT9 1AG Tel: 020 8397 7019 — MB BS Lond. 1986; DRCOG 1991. Prev: Trainee GP Brighton.
RILEY, Stephanie Elisabeth Glan-y-Mor, Manorbier, Tenby SA70 7TE — MB ChB Bristol 1988.

RILEY, Stephen George University Hospital of Wales, Institute of Nephrology, Heath Park, Cardiff CF14 4XN — MB BCh Wales 1993 (Univ. Wales Coll. Med.) MRCP UK 1996. Specialitst Regist. Inst. Nephrol. Cardiff. Specialty: Nephrol. Prev: Regist. (Renal & Med.) Wrexham Maelor Hosp.; SHO (Neurol.) Univ. Hosp. Wales Cardiff.

RILEY, Stephen Peter John Ryle Health Centre, Southchurch Drive, Clifton, Nottingham NG11 8EW Tel: 0115 921 2970 — BM BS Nottm. 1983.

RILEY, Steven Frederick Surrey Lodge Practice, 11 Anson Road, Victoria Park, Manchester M14 5BY Tel: 0161 224 2471 Fax: 0161 257 2264 — MB BS Lond. 1974 (Univ. Coll. Hosp.) MRCOG 1980; MSc Glasg. 2002.

RILEY, Stuart Anthony 24 Sefton Road, Sheffield S10 3TP — MB ChB Leeds 1979; MRCP (UK) 1983; FRCP 1996. Cons. Phys. & Gastroenterol. N. Gen. Hosp. Sheff. Specialty: Gastroenterol.

RILEY, Susan Jennifer Hurst Farm Surgery, Chapel Lane, Milford, Godalming GU8 6HU Tel: 01483 415885 Fax: 01483 42006 — MB BS Lond. 1980 (Middlx.) DRCOG 1984.

RILEY, Mr Timothy Brian Hugh (retired) Church End, Biddenham, Bedford MK40 4AW — MB BChir Camb. 1963 (Westm.) BChir 1962; MRCS Eng. LRCP Lond. 1963; FRCS Eng. 1972. Prev: Cons. Surg. (Orthop. & Trauma) Bedford Hosp. NHS Trust.

RILEY, Unell Barrington George 155 Shakespeare Road, Herne Hill, London SE24 0PY — MB BS Lond. 1986.

RILEY, Vincent Charles 3 Meadow Road, Woodhouse Eaves, Loughborough LE12 8SA — MB ChB Birm. 1970; DTM & H Liverp. 1972; Dip Ven Soc. Apoth, Lond. 1976; MRCGP 1981. Cons. Genitourin. Med. Leics. AHA (T). Specialty: Genitourinary Medicine. Prev: Med. Off. (Gen. Duties) Govt. Seychelles; Sen. Regist. (Venereol.) Nottm. Gen. Hosp.; Med. Off. (Gen. Duties) Govt. St Lucia.

RILEY, Walter Riddell, Capt. RAMC (retired) The Old Rectory, Chapel Lane, Holcombe, Bury BL8 4NB Tel: 01706 822350 — (Manch) MB ChB Manch. 1948; MRCS Eng. LRCP Lond. 1948. Prev: Ho. Phys. & Ho. Surg. Crumpsall Hosp. Manch.

RILSTONE, Francis William Borlase Barnhall Cottage, 40 High St., Stock, Ingatestone CM4 9BW Tel: 01277 840370 — (Guy's) MRCS Eng. LRCP Lond. 1939. JP. Prev: Surg. EMS S. Middlx. Fev. Hosp.; Out-pat. Off. Guy's Hosp.; ENT Ho. Surg. Kent Co. Ophth. & Aural Hosp. Maidstone.

RIMELL, Phillip John Steep Holm, Bronwydd Road, Carmarthen SA31 2A — MB BCh Wales 1971; FFA RCS Eng. 1975. Cons. (Anaesth.) W. Wales Gen. Hosp. Carmarthen. Specialty: Anaesth. Socs: Assn. Anaesth. Gt. Brit. & Irel. & Hosp. Cons. & Specialists Assn. Prev: Capt. RAMC (V); Sen. Regist. (Anaesth.) Univ. Hosp. Wales Cardiff; Clin. Fell. (Anaesth.) McGill Univ. Roy. Vict. Hosp. Montreal.

RIMINGTON, Jane Elizabeth Old Forge Surgery, Red Lion Yard, Hawkshead, Ambleside LA22 0NU Tel: 015394 360246 — MB ChB 1984 (Leeds) DRCOG 1987; MRCP 1989; (Dip. Family Medicine) Melborne 1997. p/t Assoc. GP; Med. Man. NBDC. Socs: Roy. Coll. of GPs. Prev: GP, Bradford.

RIMINGTON, John 3 Ballakeyll, Colby, Castletown IM9 4AY Tel: 01624 834937 — MB ChB Manch. 1947; MD Manch. 1968; MFCH 1991. Specialty: Respirat. Med. Socs: BMA & I. of Man Med. Soc.; Fell. Roy. Soc. Health and Hyg. Prev: Cons. Chest. Phys. & Med. Dir. Gtr. Manch. Mobile Chest X-Ray Serv. St. Thos. Hosp. Stockport; Regist. (Chest Dis.) Stockport, Macclesfield & Buxton Hosp. Gp.

RIMINGTON, Mr Peter David Department of Urology, Eastbourne District General Hospital, Kings Way, Eastbourne BN21 2UD Tel: 01323 413 700 Fax: 01323 414954 Email: peter.rimington@esht.nhs.uk — MB BCh Stellenbosch 1979; Mmed (Utol), Stellenbosch 1990; FCS, (SA)(Utol) 1991. Cons. Utology, Oncol. Minimally Invasive Surg., Eastbourne Dist. Gen. Hosp.; Hon. Cons. Urol., Epsom & St Helliets, Lond.; Hon. Cons. Urol., Chase Farm Hosp., Lond.; Hon. Cons. Urol., Guys & St Thomas Hosps., Lond. Specialty: Urol. Socs: Roy. Soc. of Med.; Brit. Soc. of Oncol.; BAUS (Brit. Assn. of Urological Surg.) Sect. of Endocrinol.

RIMMER, Alison Sheffield Occupational Health Service, Northern General Hospital, Herries Road, Sheffield S5 7AU Tel: 0114 271 4161 Fax: 0114 244 4470; 10 Belgrave Road, Ranmoor, Sheffield S10 3LN — MB BCh Wales 1978; FFOM RCP Lond. 1994, MFOM 1987; FRCP Lond. 1994. Cons. Occupat. Phys. & Dir. Occupat. Health Serv. Sheff. Occupat. Health Serv. N. Gen. Hosp. NHS Trust; Hon. Sen. Lect. (Pub. Health Med.) Univ. Sheff. Specialty: Occupat. Health. Socs: (Sec.) Assn. of NHS Occupat. Phys.; Soc. Occupat. Med. Prev: Area Med. Off. Brit. Coal Corp.

RIMMER, Anthony Francis George Dapdune House Surgery, Wharf Road, Guildford GU1 4RP Tel: 01483 573336 Fax: 01483 306602 — MB ChB Liverp. 1979; DA Eng. 1981; DRCOG 1984.

RIMMER, Anthony Joseph Bewsey Street Medical Centre, 40-42 Bewsey Street, Warrington WA2 7JE Tel: 01925 635837 Fax: 01925 630353 — MB ChB Leeds 1984; DGM RCP Lond. 1987; MRCGP 1988. Socs: BMA. Prev: Trainee GP Grimsby VTS; Ho. Off. (Gen. Med. & Cardiol.) Leeds Gen. Infirm; Ho. Off. (Gen. Surg. & Orthop.) Pinderfields Gen. Hosp. Wakefield.

RIMMER, Brenda Kathleen c/o Barclays Bank, Smithfield Branch, 89 Charterhouse St., London EC1M 6HR — MB BS Lond. 1953 (St. Bart.) DPH Eng. 1957, DA 1958.

RIMMER, Caroline Jeanie Hill House, Eversley, Hook RG27 0QA — MB ChB Liverp. 1993; MRCOG 1999. Specialty: Obst. & Gyn.

RIMMER, Caroline Susan Department of Genitourinary Medicine, Royal Infirmary, Edinburgh EH3 9YW Tel: 0131 536 1000; Woodhall Lodge, 162 Woodhall Road, Colinton, Edinburgh EH13 0PJ Tel: 0131 441 5044 — MB BS Lond. 1987; BSc Lond. 1984; Cert. Family Plann. JCC 1990. Clin. Asst. (Genitourin.) Roy. Infirm. Edin. Specialty: Genitourinary Medicine. Prev: SHO (Genitourin. Med.) Roy. Infirm. Edin.; SHO (Family Plann. & Wom. Health) Lothian HB; SHO (Communicable Dis.) St. Geo. Hosp. Lond.

RIMMER, David Bernard Department of Pathology, Bedford Hospital, Kempston Road, Bedford MK42 9DJ Tel: 01234 792162 Fax: 01234 792161 — BM BCh Oxf. 1970; MRCS Eng. LRCP Lond. 1970; FRCPath 1988, M 1976; MA Oxf. 1976. Cons. Histopath. Bedford Hosp. Specialty: Histopath. Prev: Lect. (Path.) Univ. Bristol Med. Sch.; Lect. (Histopath.) St. Bart. Hosp. Med. Coll. Lond.; SHO (Path.) Northwick Pk. Hosp. Harrow.

RIMMER, David Richard John Elliot Unit, Birch Hill Hospital, Rochdale OL12 9QB — BM BS Nottm. 1985; BMedSci (Hons.) Nottm. 1985; MRCPsych 1993. Locum Cons. (Psychiat.). Prev: Assoc. Specialist (Psychiat.) Bolton Gen. Hosp.; Assoc. Specialist (Psychiat.) Birch Hill Hosp. Rochdale.

RIMMER, Diana Mary Duckworth 75 Creffield Road, London W3 9PS Tel: 020 8992 8857 — MB BS Lond. 1965 (St. Thos.) FRCPath 1984, M 1972. Prev: Cons. Microbiol., Hillingdon Hosp., Uxbridge.

RIMMER, Elizabeth Mary Argyll and Clyde Health Board, Ross House, Hawkhead Road, Paisley PA2 7BN Tel: 0141 842 7327 Fax: 0141 848 0165; 18 Craigmillar Avenue, Milngavie, Glasgow G62 8AX Tel: 0141 956 4626 — MB ChB Liverp. 1977; MRCP (UK) 1979; MD Liverp. 1987; MRCGP 1990; FRCP Glas. 1996. Med. Prescribing Adviser Argyll & Clyde HB. Specialty: Pharmacology. Prev: Research. Fell. (Clin. Pharmacol.) Univ. Wales Coll. Med. Cardiff; Sen. Regist. (Clin. Pharmacol. & Gen. Med.) Univ. Hosp. Wales Cardiff.

RIMMER, Judith Mary Manor Practice, James Preston Health Centre, 61 Holland Road, Sutton Coldfield B72 1RL Tel: 0121 354 2032 Fax: 0121 321 1779 — MB ChB Birm. 1986; MRCGP 1990.

RIMMER, Mr Martin Gerard 3 Woodford Road, Windle, St Helens WA10 6JA — MB BS Lond. 1983 (Middlx.) BSc (Hons.) Lond. 1980, MB BS 1983; FRCS Ed. 1989; DRCOG 1995. GP Princip. Garden City Pract. Welwyn Garden City. Specialty: Gen. Pract. Prev: SHO Rotat. (Surg.) Plymouth HA; Cas. Surg. Off. Middlx. Hosp. Lond.; Ho. Surg. Middlx. Hosp. Lond.

RIMMER, Martin Joseph 45 Goodwins Road, King's Lynn PE30 5QX Tel: 01553 775022 — MB Camb. 1977; BChir 1976; MRCP (UK) 1979; FRCR 1983. Cons. (Radiol.) Qu. Eliz. Hosp. Kings Lynn. Specialty: Radiol. Prev: Sen. Regist. (Radiol.) Addenbrookes Hosp. Camb.

RIMMER, Maurus Euan Winterdyne, Flowers Hill, Pangbourne, Reading RG8 7BD Tel: 0118 984 4926 Fax: 0118 987 7067 Email: maurusrimmer@hotmail.com — MB BS Lond. 1965 (St. Bart.) MRCS Eng. LRCP Lond. 1965; DObst RCOG 1971; FRCA 1974. Cons. Anaesth. Roy. Berks. & Battle Hosps. NH Trust. Specialty: Anaesth. Socs: Assn. Anaesth.; Fellow RSM. Prev: Sen. Regist. (Anaesth.) Soton. Univ. Hosps.; Clin. Research Fell. Hosp. Sick Childr. Toronto, Canada; Regist. Rotat. (Anaesth.) Westm. Hosp. & Qu. Vict. Hosp. E. Grinstead.

RIMMER, Roger Osborne (retired) 75 Charlemont Avenue, West Bromwich B71 3BZ — (Birm.) MB ChB Birm. 1955. Prev: Ho. Phys. Ho. Surg. & O & G Ho. Surg. Hallam Hosp. W.

RIMMER, Stephen Flat 22/1, The Grassmarket, Edinburgh EH1 2HY — MB BS Sydney 1990.

RIMMER, Sylvia 12 Stanhope Road, Bowdon, Altrincham WA14 3JU — MB ChB Manch. 1967; DMRD Liverp. 1971; FRCR 1974. Cons. Radiologist, Centr. Manch. and Manch. Children's Univ. Hosps. NHS Trust. Specialty: Radiol. Prev: SHO (Med.) Mossley Hill Hosp. Liverp. RHB; SHO (Radiol.) United Liverp. Hosps.; Regist. Radiol. BRd. Green Hosp. Liverp.

RIMMER, Mr Timothy John Peterborough District Hospital, Eye Department, Thorpe Road, Peterborough PE3 6DA Tel: 01733 874018 Fax: 01733 875281; 64 High Street, St. Martins, Stamford PE9 2LA Tel: 01780 756611 Email: timothy.rimmer@talk21.com — MB ChB Liverp. 1979; FRCS Ed. 1987; FRCOphth 1989; PhD N. West. Univ. Evanston, Ill., USA 1991. Cons. Ophth. P'boro. Dist. Hosp. Specialty: Ophth. Prev: Sen. Regist. (Ophth.) Leicester Roy. Infirm.; Research Assoc. Biomed. Engineer. Dept. N.W.. Univ. Illinois, USA; Sen. Regist. St. John Ophth. Hosp. Jerusalem.

RIMMER, Trevor William East Cheshire NHS Trust, Macclesfield DGH, Victoria Rd, Macclesfield SK10 3BL Tel: 01625 663177 Fax: 01625 661378 Email: trevor.rimmer@echeshire-tr.nwest.nhs.uk — MB BCh Wales 1979 (Welsh National School Medicine) MRCP (UK) 1983; DRCOG 1986; FRCP Ed. 1998; FRCP London 2002. Macmillan Cons. In Pall. Med., E. Chesh. NHS Trust; Med. Dir. E. Chesh. Hospice. Specialty: Palliat. Med. Socs: Assn. Palliat. Med.; BMA; Roy. Soc. Med. Prev: Cons. Palliat. Med. St. Catherine's Hospice ScarBoro.; Sen. Regist (Palliat Med) Michael Sobell Hse & Mt. Vernon Hosp. Middx; GP Seven Sisters, W. Glam.

RIMMER, Yvonne Louise 14a Birckbeck Avenue, London W3 6HX — MB BS Lond. 1996.

RINALDI, Christopher Aldo Royal Devon & Exeter Hospital, Barrack Road, Exeter EX2 5DW — MB BS Lond. 1990 (King's Coll. Hosp. Med. & Dent. Sch.) MRCP (UK) 1993; MD (Lond.) 2001. Cons. Roy. Devon & Exeter Hosp. Specialty: Cardiol. Prev: Specialist Regist. (Cardiol.) Guy's & St Thos. Healthcare Trust; Research Fell. (Cardiol.) Roy. Postgrad. Med. Sch.

RINCON AZNAR, Cristobal Department of Anaesthesia, West Wales General Hospital, Carmarthen SA31 2AF — LMS Valencia 1983.

RING, Alistair Edward 50 Thorn Park, Mannamead, Plymouth PL3 4TF Tel: 01752 250765 — BM BCh Oxf. 1997 (Oxf. Clin. Sch.) MA (Hons.) Cantab. 1994. SHO, Med, Roal Postgrad. Med. Sch., Hammersmith Hosp.; Ho. Off. (Surg.) Roy. United Hosp. Bath. Specialty: Gen. Med. Prev: SHO, (Med) Roy. Brompton Hosp.; Hse. Off. (Med.) Oxf. John Radcliffe Hosp.

RING, Helen Patricia (retired) Senacre Wood Surgery, Reculver Walk, Senacre, Maidstone ME15 8SW Tel: 01622 761963; 60 Sheppey Road, Loose Court, Loose, Maidstone ME15 9SS — MB BCh BAO Dub. 1969; DObst RCOG 1971; DCH Eng. 1972. Prev: Trainee Gen. Pract. King's Lynn Vocational Train. Scheme.

RING, Howard Anton Development Psychiatry, University of Cambridge, Douglas House, 18b Trumpington Road, Cambridge CB2 2AH Tel: 01223 746121 Fax: 01223 746122 Email: har28@cam.ac.uk — MB BS Lond. 1984; MRCPsych 1989; BSc Lond. 1981, MD 1994. Psychiatry Lect. Camb. Specialty: Gen. Psychiat. Socs: Hon. Sec. Assn. Univ. Teachs. of Psychiat.; Chairm.. Roy. Coll. of Psychiat.s, s/i grp in neuropsychiatry. Prev: Sen. Regist. (Psychiat.) Maudsley Hosp. Lond.; Reader in Neuropsychiatry Barts and the Lond. Sch. of Med.; Hon. Sen. Lect. (Neuropsychiat.) Inst. Neurol. Lond.

RING, Jonathan Paul George Pewsey Surgery, High Street, Pewsey SN9 5AQ Tel: 01672 563511 Fax: 01672 563004; The Dairy House, Easton Royal, Pewsey SN9 5LZ Tel: 01672 810134 — MB ChB Bristol 1987; BSc (Hons.) Bristol 1984; DRCOG 1990; MRCGP 1991. Prev: Trainee GP N. Wilts. VTS.

RING, Kathleen Patricia The Crescent Surgery, 38 Marion Crescent, St Mary Cray, Orpington BR5 2DD Tel: 01689 818696; 1 Greenwood Close, Petts Wood, Orpington BR5 1QG Tel: 01689 601015 — MB BS Lond. 1978 (Lond. Hosp. Med. Coll.) MRCGP 1984. GP Tutor FarnBoro. Postgrad. Centre. Prev: Trainee GP Epsom Dist. Hosp. VTS.

RING, Nicholas John Department of Diagnostic Radiology, Derriford Hospital, Plymouth PL6 8DH Tel: 01752 792701 Fax: 01752 792853; 8 Venn Court, Hartley, Plymouth PL3 5NS Tel: 01752 795463 — MB BS Lond. 1970 (St. Bart.) MRCS Eng. LRCP Lond. 1970; DObst RCOG 1973; DMRD Eng. 1978; FRCR 1979. Cons. Radiol. Plymouth Hosps. NHS Trust. Specialty: Radiol. Prev: Sen. Regist. (Radiol.) Bristol Roy. Infirm.

RING, Nicholas Paul The Surgery, 58 Pembroke Road, Clifton, Bristol BS8 3DT Tel: 0117 974 1452 Fax: 0117 923 8040 — MB ChB Bristol 1982.

RING, Noreen Mary 32 Hawthorn Lane, Wilmslow SK9 5DG — MB BCh BAO NUI 1983.

RING, Mr Peter Alexander (cons. rooms), Gatwick Park Hospital, Povey Cross Road, Horley RH6 0BB Tel: 01293 785511; Eversfield, Denne Park, Horsham RH13 7AY Tel: 01403 257424 Fax: 01403 261998 — MRCS Eng. LRCP Lond. 1945 (Univ. Coll. Hosp.) MS Lond. 1956, MB BS 1945; FRCS Eng. 1948. Cons. Orthop. Surg. Gatwick Pk. Hosp. Specialty: Orthop. Socs: Fell. BOA; Fell. Roy. Soc. Med. Prev: Cons. Orthop. Surg. E. Surrey; Laming Evans Sen. Orthop. Research Fell. RCS Eng.; Regist. (Surg.) Roy. Nat. Orthop. Hosp. & Univ. Coll. Hosp.

RING, Stella Muriel (retired) 81 Salterton Road, Exmouth EX8 2EW Tel: 01395 278919 — MB BS Lond. 1946 (Univ. Coll. Hosp.) MRCS Eng. LRCP Lond. 1946; DCH Eng. 1949, DPM 1965. Prev: Assoc. Specialist in Child & Adolesc. Psychiat. Croydon Child & Family Clinic.

RING, Susan Jane Countesthorpe Health Centre, Central Street, Countesthorpe, Leicester LE8 5QJ Tel: 0116 277 6336; Straw Hall, Peatling Parva, Lutterworth LE17 5QB Tel: 0116 277 6336 — MB ChB Leic. 1984; DRCOG 1988; MRCGP 1990. GP Countesthorpe.

RINGER, Wilbur Steven 131 Woodmansterne Road, Carshalton Beeches, Carshalton SM5 4AF Tel: 020 8395 0318 — MB BCh Wales 1968; BSc (Hons. Physiol.) Wales 1965; MB BCh (Distinc. Anat., Physiol. & Pharmacol.) Wales 1968; MRNZCGP 1986. Sen. Med. Adviser Benefits Agency Med. Servs. DSS for SE Eng. Prev: GP Ystad Mynach; GP Auckland, NZ; Industr. Phys. Alex Harvey's Industries, Auckland, NZ.

RINGLAND, Raymond Alexander 7A Moneylane Road, Dundrum, Newcastle BT33 0NR Tel: 013967 51348 Email: u01rar@doctors.org.uk — MB ChB Aberd. 1997 (Univ. of Aberdeen) MB ChB Aberd. 1997(with comm.). SHO, Med., Downe Hosp., Downpatrick, Co.down. Specialty: Gen. Med. Prev: SHO Med. Oncol. Belf. City Hosp.; Jun. Ho. Off. Gen. Med. Aberd. Roy. Infirm.; Jun. Ho. Off. Gen. Surg. Aberd. Roy. Infirm.

RINGROSE, Caroline Suzanne 2 Boyce Street, Walkley, Sheffield S6 3JS — MB ChB Sheff. 1998; MB ChB Sheff 1998.

RINGROSE, David Karl 45 Somerford Way, Rotherhithe, London SE16 6QN — MB BS Lond. 1988 (UMDS Guy's Campus) DA (UK) 1990; FRCA 1993. Sen. Regist. (Anaesth.) Guy's Hosp. Lond. Specialty: Anaesth. Prev: Regist. (Anaesth.) St. Thos. Hosp. Lond.; SHO (Anaesth.) Char. Cross Hosp. Lond.; SHO (Neonat. Intens. Care) St. Geo. Hosp. Lond.

RINGROSE, Dora Winifred (retired) The Dovecote, Clay Lane, Newbridge, Yarmouth PO41 0UA — MB BChir Camb. 1950 (Camb. & Manch.) BA Camb. 1947. Prev: Regist. (Path.) United Sheff. Hosps.

RINGROSE, Timothy Richard 32 Valley View, Jesmond, Newcastle upon Tyne NE2 2JS — MB BCh Wales 1990.

RINSLER, Albert Henry (retired) 9 Kingsley Way, London N2 0EH Tel: 020 8455 8864 — (King's Coll. Hosp.) MRCS Eng. LRCP Lond. 1947; MRCGP 1965; DHMSA 1990. Prev: Ho. Phys. Pneumoconiosis Research Unit, MRC Llandough Hosp. Penarth.

RINSLER, Michael Gerald Royal College of Pathologists, 2 Carlton House Terrace, London SW1Y 5AF; 49 Wellington Court, Wellington Road, London NW8 9TB — MB BChir Camb. 1950 (Camb. & King's Coll. Hosp.) MD Camb. 1958, MA, MB BChir 1950; FRCPath 1970, M 1964. Dir. of Studies Roy. Coll. Path. Specialty: Chem. Path. Socs: Fell. Roy. Soc. Med. Prev: Cons. Chem. Pathol. Northwick Pk. Hosp.; Cons. Chem. Pathol. Chelsea & Kensington Gp. Hosps.; Research Asst. Sect. Radiobiol., Radiother. Dept. Roy. Marsden Hosp.

RINTALA, Risto Juhana Institute of Child Health, Alder Hey Children's Hospital, Eaton Road, West Derby, Liverpool L12 2AP — Lic Med Helsinki 1975; Lic Med. Helsinki 1975.

RINTOUL, Mr Andrew Johnstone, Surg. Capt. RN Retd. (retired) 9 Clayhall Road, Alverstoke, Gosport PO12 2BB Tel: 023 9258 2387 — MB ChB Glas. 1956; DO Eng. 1962; FRCS Eng. 1968; FCOphth 1989. Hon. Cons. Ophth. RNLI. Prev: Cons. & Adviser Ophth. MDG (Naval).

RINTOUL, Doreen Margaret Mary 15 Dunkeld Road, Talbot Woods, Bournemouth BH3 7EN Tel: 01202 317660 — MB BS Lond. 1961 (St. Thos.) MRCS Eng. LRCP Lond. 1961.

RINTOUL, Robert Campbell Papworth Hospital, Department of Thoracic Oncology, Papworth Everard, Cambridge CB3 8RE Tel: 01480 830541 Fax: 01480 364331 Email: robertrintoul@yahoo.co.uk — MB ChB Ed. 1992; BSc (Hons.) St. And. 1990; MRCP (UK) 1995; PhD (Cell Biol. of lung cancer) Ed. 2002. Specialty: Respirat. Med.; Gen. Med. Prev: Specialist Regist. (Respirat. Med. and Gen. Internal Med.) SE Scotl.; SHO (Med.) St. Thos. Hosp. Lond.; SHO (Med.) Hammersmith Hosp. Lond. & Roy. Infirm. Edin.

RINTOUL, Mr Robert Forbes (retired) Brambles, Chapel Lane, Abergavenny NP7 7BT Tel: 01873 853658 Fax: 01873 850718 Email: rfrintoul@rcsed.ac.uk — MB ChB Ed. 1960; FRCS Ed. 1964; FRCS Eng. 1965. Prev: Cons. Gen. Surg. Nevill Hall Hosp. Abergavenny.

RINTOUL, Russell Campbell (retired) The Cottage, Frostenden Corner, Frostenden, Beccles NR34 7JA Tel: 01502 578507 — MB BS Lond. 1957 (Kings Coll & St. Geo.) LMSSA Lond. 1955. Prev: SHO King's Coll. & St. George's Hosp. Lond.

RIORDAN-EVA, Mr Paul Department of Ophthalmology, King's College Hospital, Denmark Hill, London SE5 9RS Tel: 020 7346 1524 Fax: 020 7346 3738 Email: paul.riordan-eva@kingsch.nhs.uk — MB BChir Camb. 1982 (St Thomas' Hosp. Lond.) MA Camb. 1984; FRCS Eng. 1988; FRCOphth 1989. Cons. Ophth. King's Coll. Hosp. Lond.; Hon. Cons., Neuro-Ophth., Nat. Hosp. For Neurol. and Neurosurg., Lond.. Specialty: Ophth. Socs: FRSM; Corr. Mem. N. Amer. Neuro-Ophth. Soc.; Mem. Assn. Brit. Neurologists. Prev: Cons. Ophth. W. Kent Eye Centre FarnBoro. Hosp. Kent; Cons. Neuro-Ophth. Nat. Hosp. Neurol. & Neurosurg. & Moorfields Eye Hosp. Lond.; Sen. Regist. (Neuro-Ophth.) Nat. Hosp. Neurol. & Neurosurg. Lond.

RIORDAN, Denise Mary Child Health Directorate, Albion Road Resource Centre, Albion Road, North Shields NE29 0HG — MB BS Newc. 1987; MRCPsych 1992. Sen. Regist. (Child & Adolesc. Psychiat.) Prestwich Hosp. Manch. Specialty: Child & Adolesc. Psychiat. Prev: Regist. (Psychiat.) N. West. RHA; Regist. Rotat. (Psychiat.) North. RHA Scheme; Ho. Surg. Roy. Vict. Infirm. Newc.

RIORDAN, Frederick Andrew Ian Department of Paediatrics, Birmingham Heartlands Hospital, Bordesley Green E., Birmingham B9 5SS Tel: 0121 424 0823 Fax: 0121 424 0827 — BM Soton. 1984; MRCP (UK) 1989; DTM & H Liverp. 1995; MRCPCH 1996; MD Liverp. 1996; FRCPCH 1997. Cons. Paediat. Birm. Heartlands Hosp. Specialty: Paediat. Socs: Paediat. Research Soc.; Brit. Paediatric Allergy Immunity Infec. Gp. (Sec.). Prev: Lect. (Paediat. & Child Health) Birm. Univ.; Research Fell. Liverp. Univ.

RIORDAN, John Finbar General Office, Central Middlesex Hospital NHS Trust, Acton Lane, London NW10 7NS Tel: 020 8453 2327 Fax: 020 8453 2091 Email: john.riordan@cmh-tr.nthames.nhs.uk; 36 Woodville Gardens, Ealing, London W5 2LQ Tel: 020 8997 2319 Fax: 020 8997 2319 — (Cork) MB BCh BAO NUI 1963; FRCP Lond. 1982, M 1966. Med. Dir. Centr. Middlx. Hosp. NHS Trust; Cons. Phys. Centr. Middlx. Hosp. & Willesden Chest Clinic; Hon. Clin. Sen. Lect. (Med.) Imperial Coll. Sch. of Med.; Cons. Phys. Clementine Churchill Hosp. Harrow. Specialty: Gen. Med.; Respirat. Med. Socs: Fell. Roy. Soc. Med.; Brit. Thorac. Soc. Prev: Cons. Phys. Dudley Rd. Hosp. Birm.; Lect. (Med.) Middlx. Hosp. Med. Sch. Lond.

RIORDAN, Richard David — MB BS Lond. 1994; BSc (Hons) Lond. 1991; MRCP (UK) 1998; FRCR 2001. Specialist Regist. Radiol., Derriford Hosp., Plymouth. Specialty: Radiol. Socs: RCR Assoc.; BMA.

RIORDAN, Terence Public Health Laboratory, Royal Devon & Exeter Hospital, Church Lane, Exeter EX2 5AD Tel: 01392 402973 — MB Camb. 1976 (King's Coll. Hosp.) BChir 1975; MRCP (UK) 1978; MRCPath 1981. Cons. Microbiol. Pub. Health Laborat. Roy. Devon & Exeter Hosp. Specialty: Med. Microbiol. Prev: Cons. Microbiol. Pub. Health Laborat. Withington Hosp. Manch.

RIORDAN, Thomas Prior Swn-y-Don, 15 Rotherslade Road, Langland, Swansea SA3 4QW — MD NUI 1948 (Cork) MB BCh BAO 1936; DPM Eng. 1939; FRCPsych 1972. Prev: Cons. Psychiat. Hosp. Advis. Serv.; Med. Supt. Cefn Coed Hosp. Swansea; Specialist Psychiat. RAMC.

RIOU, Mr Peter John Derriford Hospital, Accident & Emergency Department, Derriford Road, Plymouth PL6 8DH — MB BS Lond. 1991 (Charing Cross and Westminster Hospital London) BA (Physiol. Scs) Oxf. 1988; FRCS Eng. 1996; FFAEM 2001. Specialist Regist. Derriford Hosp. Plymouth Devon. Specialty: Accid. & Emerg. Prev: Sen. Clin. Fell. (A & E) Roy. Devon & Exeter Hosp. Wonford.

RIPLEY, Colin Stephen 3 Fitzroy Terrace, Perth PH2 7HZ — MB ChB Dundee 1996. Specialty: Gen. Med.

RIPLEY, George Salvarani Bulwell Health Centre, Main Street, Bulwell, Nottingham NG6 8QJ Tel: 0115 977 1181 Fax: 0115 977 1377 — MB ChB Sheff. 1974; MRCGP 1978.

RIPLEY, James Stuart Medical Centre, Caledonian Road, Perth PH2 8HH Tel: 01738 628234 Fax: 01738 624945; 3 Fitzroy Terrace, Perth PH2 7HZ Tel: 01738 624756 — MB ChB St. And. 1968.

RIPLEY, Joan Ruth (retired) 1 Aldenham Grove, Radlett WD7 7BN Tel: 01923 854357 — MB BS Lond. 1954 (Middlx.) Cert Family Plann. JCC Lond. 1977; FRCPCH 1997. Med. Convocation Senator, Univ. Lond. Prev: Sen. Med. Off. (Child Health & Audiol.) Barnet HA.

RIPLEY, Linda Hilary 12 Farm Lane, Tonbridge TN10 3DG — MB ChB Ed. 1973; BSc (Med. Sci.) Ed. 1970, MB ChB 1973; DObst RCOG 1975. Clin. Med. Off. S.E. Thames RHA. Prev: SHO (Obst.) Firs Matern. Hosp. Nottm.; Ho. Surg. Warrington Gen. Hosp.; Ho. Phys. Leighton Hosp. Crewe.

RIPLEY, Maurice Ian eThe Five Bells, Main St., Claypole, Newark NG23 5BJ — MB ChB Sheff. 1976.

RIPLEY, Pamela 48 Overstrand Road, Cromer NR27 0AJ Tel: 01263 513148 Fax: 01263 515264 — MRCS Eng. LRCP Lond. London 1981; MRCS Eng. LRCP Lond. London 1981.

RIPMAN, Mr Hujohn Armstrong (retired) Red House, Sproughton, Ipswich IP8 3AT Tel: 01473 253325 — MB BS Lond. 1942 (Guy's) MRCS Eng. LRCP Lond. 1941; FRCOG 1961, M 1948; FRCS Eng. 1949. Prev: Cons. O & G Ipswich Hosp. Gp.

RIPPIN, Jouathan David Birmingham Heartlands Hospital., Bordesley Green E., Bondesley Green, Birmingham Tel: 0121 766 6611; Flat 1, 79 Springfield Road, Kings Heath, Birmingham B14 7DU — MB BS Lond. 1994 (Univ. of Cambridge & Charring Cross Med. School) BA Cantab 1991; MRCP 1998. Specialty: Gen. Med.

RIPPINGALE, Catherine 43 Liberty Avenue, London SW19 2QS — MB BS Lond. 1996.

RIPPON, Clare 2 Strand Road, Carlisle CA1 1NB — MB ChB Manch. 1994. SHO (O & G) The Roy. Oldham Hosp. Specialty: Obst. & Gyn. Prev: Ho. Off. (Med., Neurol. & Rheum.) N. Manch. Gen. Hosp.; Ho. Off. (Gen. Surg.) The Roy. Oldham Hosp.

RIPPON, Doreen Aldebaran, 37 Carr Hill Lane, Sleights, Whitby YO21 1RS — MB ChB Liverp. 1950.

RIPPON, Lisa Maria — MB BS Newc. 1992.

RIPPY, Elisabeth Ellen 176 Spixworth Road, Norwich NR6 7EQ — MB BS Lond. 1995.

RISDALL, Jane Elizabeth, Surg. Cdr. RN Institute of Naval Medicine, Alvestoke, Gosport PO12 2DL Fax: 023 9250 4823/023 9276 8426 — MB BS Newc. 1984 (Newcastle upon Tyne) MA Camb. 1985; DA (UK) 1989; FFA RCSI 1992. Cons. Anaesth. Roy. Navy; Hon. Cons. Soton. Gen. Hosp.; Sen. Med. Off., Hyperbaric Med., Inst. of Naval Med., Alverstoke, Gosport, Hants. Specialty: Anaesth.; Intens. Care. Prev: Sen. Regist. (Anaesth.) RN Hosp. Haslar & Addenbrooke's Hosp. Camb.; Regist. (Anaesth.) Roy. Infirm. Edin.; SHO & Regist. (Anaesth.) South. Gen. Hosp. Glas.

RISDON, Rupert Anthony Hospital for Sick Children, Department of Histopathology, Great Ormond St., London WC1N 3JH Tel: 020 7405 9200 Fax: 020 7813 1170; 4 Byfeld Gardens, London SW13 9HP Tel: 020 8748 7028 — MB BS Lond. 1962 (Char. Cross) MRCS Eng. LRCP Lond. 1962; FRCPath. 1980, M 1968; MD Lond. 1972. Emerit. Prof. Histopath. Hosp. Sick Childr. Gt. Ormond St. Prev: Reader (Morbid Anat.) Lond. Hosp. Med. Coll.; Cons. (Histopath.) Addenbrooke's Hosp. Camb.; Lect. in Histopath. Char. Cross Hosp. Med. Sch.

RISEBURY, Michael John 77 Southwood, Coulby Newham, Middlesbrough TS8 0UF — MB BS Lond. 1998; MB BS Lond 1998.

RISHI, Nand Prakash Gillingham Medical Centre, Woodlands Road, Gillingham ME7 2BU Tel: 01634 854431 — MB BS Vikram 1961 (Gandhi Med. Coll. Bhopal) DCH Eng. 1971; MRCGP 1978.

RISHKO, Alun John 39 Glenroy Street, Roath, Cardiff CF24 3JX — MB BCh Wales 1997.

RISHTON, Patricia Haslingden Health Centre, Manchester Road, Haslingden, Rossendale BB4 5SL Tel: 01706 212518 Fax: 01706 218112 — MB ChB Manch. 1979; DRCOG 1982. Specialty: Family Plann. & Reproduc. Health.

RISHWORTH, Ruth Hannah Friars Close, Goathland, York YO22 5JU — MB BS Durh. 1957.

RISHWORTH, Vivienne Cecilia The Health Centre, Brightwells, Farnham GU9 7SA Tel: 01252 712572 Fax: 01252 716336; Foxgreyden, Parkside, Farnham GU9 0JP Tel: 01252 724643 — MB BCh Wales 1980; DObst RCOG 1984.

RISK, Ahmad Mahmoud Mohamed 3 Adelaide Crescent, Hove BN3 2JD Tel: 01273 724866; 3 Adelaide Crescent, Hove BN3 2JD Tel: 01273 724866 Fax: 01273 774614 — MB BCh Univ. Ain Shams 1973 (Ain Shams) MB BCh Ain Shams 1973. Private Primary Care Phys.; Edr. Health Informatics Europe; Med. Dir. eHealth R+D Ltd. Socs: Chairm. Brit. Healthcare Internet Assn.; Mem. Bd. Dir. Internet Healthcare Coalition. Prev: GP Reigate; Med. Off. Roy. Engineers; Med. Off. Mustique Co., W.I.

RISK, Winifred Jessie Hillside, 38 Back Road, Dollar FK14 7EA Tel: 01259 742176 — (Univ. Glas.) MB ChB Glas. 1938. Prev: Ho. Surg. & Ho. Phys. Glas. Roy. Infirm.; Squadron Ldr. RAF Med. Br.; Dep. Div. Moh Bucks. CC.

RISSIK, Judith Mary St Thomas' Hospital, Neonatel Unit, 6th Floor North Wing, Lambeth Palace Road, London SE1 7EH Tel: 020 7928 9292 Fax: 020 7960 5707; Rock Robin, Underriver, Sevenoaks TN15 0SL — MB BS Lond. 1961; DCH RCP Lond. 1963d. 1960; BSc (Anat.) Lond. 1958. MB BS 1961; DObst RCOG 1962; MRCP Lond. 1966. Assoc. Specialist (Neonat.) St Thomas Hosp. Lond. Specialty: Paediat. Special Interest: Neonatology.

RISSIK, Kate Matrjorie Rock Robin, Underriver, Sevenoaks TN15 0SL — BM BCh Oxf. 1998; BM BCh Oxf 1998.

RIST, Colin Leslie Department Haematology, Worthing Hospital, Worthing BN11 2DH — BM BCh Oxf. 1971; MA,BM BCh Oxf. 1971; MRCP (UK) 1974; FRCPath 1990, M 1978; FRCP Lond. 1991. Cons. Haemat. Worthing & Southlands NHS Trust. Specialty: Haematology. Socs: Brit. Soc. Haematol. Prev: Sen. Regist. (Haematol.) Bristol Roy. Infirm.; Regist. Addenbrooke's Hosp. Camb.; SHO Radcliffe Infirm. Oxf.

RISTIC, Charles Dominic Haxby & Wigginton Health Centre, The Village, Wigginton, York YO32 2LL Tel: 01904 760125 — BM BS Nottm. 1983; MRCGP 1987.

RITCH, Genevra Mary (retired) 7 Elmwood Manor, Bothwell, Glasgow G71 8EA — MB ChB Ed. 1959; DA Eng. 1961. Assoc. Specialist (Rheum. & Rehabil.) Lanarksh. HB.

RITCHIE, Alasdair Nicolson 140 Thurston Road, Glasgow G52 2AL Tel: 0141 883 8838 — MB ChB Glas. 1986 (Glasgow) MRCGP 1992; DRCOG 1992.

RITCHIE, Mr Alastair William Scarth Urology Department, Gloucestershire Royal Hospital, Great Western Road, Gloucester GL1 3NN Tel: 01452 394902 Fax: 01452 386628; New Hall, Tibberton, Gloucester GL2 8EB Tel: 01452 790302 Fax: 01452 790763 — MB ChB Ed. 1976 (Edinburgh) FRCS Ed. 1980; BSc (Med. Sci.) Ed. 1973, MD 1985. Cons. Urol. Surg. Glos. Roy. Hosp. Specialty: Urol. Socs: Brit. Assn. Urol. Surgs.; Brit. Assn. Cancer Research. Prev: Sen. Lect. (Urol.) Univ. Edin.; Sen. Regist. (Urol.) Lothian HB; Regist. (Urol.) Liverp. HA.

RITCHIE, Alison Frances Highview Surgery, 20 Southgate Road, Potters Bar EN6 5DZ Tel: 01933 396000; 2 Grange Farm, Church Road, Hargrave, Wellingborough NN9 6BQ Tel: 01933 460850 Fax: 01933 460850 — MB BS Lond. 1985 (Univ. Coll. Hosp. Lond.) BSc Lond. 1982; DRCOG 1988; MRCGP 1989. Specialty: Gen. Pract. Prev: Regist. (A & E) Monash Univ. Med. Centre Vict., Austral.

RITCHIE, Alison Morag The Viaduct Medical Practice, Denburn Health Centre, Rosemount Viaduct, Aberdeen AB25 1QB Tel: 01224 644744 Fax: 01224 555232; Westwinds, Fowlershill, Dyce, Aberdeen AB21 7AQ — MB ChB Aberd. 1979 (Aberdeen) DRCOG 1982; MRCGP 1983; MFHom 1999. Clin. Sen. Lect. Dept. Gen. Pract. Aberd. Univ.

RITCHIE, Andrew Ferrier The Health Centre, Lawson St., Stockton-on-Tees TS18 1HX Tel: 01642 607435 — MB ChB Glas. 1940; DPH Eng. 1947. Socs: BMA & Assn. Indust. Med. Offs.

RITCHIE, Mr Andrew John Papworth Hospital NHS Trust, Papworth Everard, Cambridge CB3 8RE Fax: 01480 364740 Email: ritchie25@hotmail.com — MD Belf. 1992 (Glasgow) BSc (1st. cl. Hons.) Glas. 1979, MB ChB 1984; FRCS Ed. 1989; FRCSI 1989; PhD Belf. 1993. Cons. Cardiothoracic & Transp. Surg. Papworth NHS Trust Camb. Specialty: Cardiothoracic Surg.; Transpl. Surg. Socs: EACTA; ISHLT; Soc. & Cardiothoracic Surg.s. Prev: Cardiothoracic Surg. Sen. Regist. Freeman Hosp. Newc.; Cardiothoracic Surg. Regist. Aberd. Roy. Infirm.; Regist. (Surg.) Waveney Hosp. Ballymena.

RITCHIE, Arthur James 10 Aytoun Road, Glasgow G41 5RN — LRCP Ed. 1931; LRCP, LRCS Ed. LRFPS Glas. 1931.

RITCHIE, Brian William Drymen Road Surgery, 160 Drymen Road, Bearsden, Glasgow G61 3RD Tel: 0141 942 6644 — MB ChB Glas. 1980; MRCGP 1990.

RITCHIE, Campbell James Cook University Hospital, Marton Rd, Middlesbrough TS4 3BW Tel: 01642 850850 ext5647 — MB BChir Camb. 1978 (Camb. & King's Coll. Hosp.) MA Camb; MRCPath 1984. Cons. (Histopath./Cytopath.) James Cook Univ.. Hosp. Specialty: Histopath. Socs: Assn. Clin. Path. & Internat. Acad. Path. Prev: SHO Regist. & Sen. Regist. (Histopath.) Leicester Hosps, Qu. Med. Centre Nottm. & Kettering Gen. Hosp.; SHO (Path.) Univ. Hosp. Wales & Llandough Hosp. Penarth.

RITCHIE, Caroline Ann Margaret 568 Lanark Road W., Balerno EH14 7BN — MB ChB Aberd. 1994. SHO (Psychiat.) Falkirk & Dist. Roy. Infirm. Specialty: Gen. Psychiat. Prev: SHO Rotat. (Psychiat.) N. Glas.; SHO (Rehabil. Med.) Astley Ainslie Hosp. Edin.

RITCHIE, Catherine Marian 171 Clare Road, Waringstown, Craigavon BT66 7SE — MD Belf. 1986; MB BCh BAO 1978; MRCP (UK) 1981. Cons. Phys. Craigavon Area Hosp. Specialty: Gen. Med.; Endocrinol.; Diabetes.

RITCHIE, Catriona Milne Davidson 4 Dudley Gardens, Edinburgh EH6 4PY — MB ChB Manch. 1997.

RITCHIE, Craig William 26 Beechgrove Avenue, Aberdeen AB15 5EJ — MB ChB Aberd. 1991.

RITCHIE, David Alfred Rattray (retired) 68 Bonhard Road, Scone, Perth PH2 6QB — MB ChB Aberd. 1946; DMRD Ed. 1952. Prev: Cons. Radiol. Perth & Kinross Health Dist.

RITCHIE, David Alistair 3 Townfield Road, Wirral CH48 7EY — MB ChB Glas. 1981; FRCR Lond. 1987. Specialty: Radiol.

RITCHIE, Mr David Andrew William 1 Naseby Avenue, Broomhill, Glasgow G11 7JQ — MB ChB Aberd. 1977; FRCS Ed. 1985. Cons. A & E Med. Glas. Specialty: Accid. & Emerg.

RITCHIE, Derek Keith 43 Dura Street, Dundee DD4 6SW Tel: 01382 451100 Fax: 01382 453679 Email: dritchie@terra.finix.org.uk; 91 Camphill Road, Broughty Ferry, Dundee DD5 2NE — MB ChB Dundee 1978; MRCGP 1982; DRCOG 1983. Princip. GP Dundee. Socs: (Treas.) Dundee Med. Chub; Forfarshire Med. Assn.; Scott. Heart & Arterial Risk Preven. Gp. (SHARP).

RITCHIE, Diana Margaret 14A Kirklee Circus, Glasgow G12 0TW — MD Glas. 1988; MB ChB 1977; MRCP (UK) 1980; FRCR 1992. Cons. Clin. Oncol. Boston Oncol. Centre Glas. Specialty: Oncol.; Radiother.

RITCHIE, Elizabeth Lambie 12 Ravelston Park, Edinburgh EH4 3DX Tel: 0131 332 6560 — MB ChB Ed. 1940 (Edinburgh)

RITCHIE, Elizabeth Lorraine — MB ChB Glas. 1991 (Glasgow) DCH RCPS Glas 1994; MRCGP Glasgow 1995; FRCA 2001. Specialist Regist. Anaesthetics. Specialty: Anaesth. Prev: Sen. Health Off., Anaesth.

RITCHIE, Elizabeth Rosemary Joyce (retired) Springbank, Kilchattan Bay, Rothesay PA20 9NL Tel: 01700 831269 — MB ChB Glas. 1955; DObst RCOG 1958. Prev: GP Alexandria Dunbartonsh.

RITCHIE, Emma Catriona The Hedges Medical Centre, Pasley Road, Eyres Monsell, Leicester LE2 9BU Tel: 0116 225 1277 — MB ChB Ed. 1985; DCH RCP Lond. 1988; MRCOG 1990. Regist. (O & G) Leic. Gen. Hosp. Specialty: Obst. & Gyn. Prev: Regist. (O & G) Marston Green Hosp. Birm.

RITCHIE, Ewan Douglas Consultant in Anaesthesia, Department of Anaesthesia, Perth Royal Infirmary, Perth Tel: 01738 623311; 18 Corsie Avenue, Kinnoull Hill, Perth PH2 7BS Tel: 01738 625378 — MB ChB Aberd. 1989; FRCA 1993. Cons. (Anaesth.) Perth Roy. Infirm. Perth. Specialty: Anaesth. Prev: Clin. research fell. (Anaesth.) Toronto Hosp., Canada; Sen. Regist. (Anaesth.) Aberd. Roy. Infirm.

RITCHIE, Fiona Anne 14 Clive Road, Balsall Common, Coventry CV7 7DW — MB ChB Bristol 1978; MRCGP 1986.

RITCHIE, Fiona Hilda 49 James Street, Lossiemouth IV31 6BX — MB ChB Aberd. 1994 (Aberdeen) MRCGP 1998. Specialty: Gen. Pract.

RITCHIE, Grace Macfarlane (retired) The Anchorage, Burghead Road, Alves, Elgin IV30 8UY Tel: 01343 850274 — (Univ. Glas.) MB ChB Glas. 1945. Prev: Sen. Regist. (Path.) Glas. North. Hosp. Gp. & West. Dist. Hosp. Glas.

RITCHIE, Ian (retired) 7 Grizedale Close, Grantham NG31 8QY — MB BCh BAO Dub. 1969 (TC Dub.) BA, MB BCh BAO Dub. 1969; DObst RCOG 1971; DCH Eng. 1971; DTM & H Liverp. 1971. Locum work. Prev: Dist. Med. Off. Beaufort, Sabah.

RITCHIE, Mr Ian Kristensen Department of Orthopaedic & Trauma Surgery, Stirling Royal Infirmary, Stirling FK8 2AU Tel: 01786 434073 Fax: 01786 434432 Email: ian.ritchie@frah.scot.nhs.uk; 13 Abercromby Place, Stirling FK8 2QP Tel: 01786 474530 Fax: 01786 434432 Email: ian.ritchie4@btinternet.com — MB ChB Aberd. 1977; FRCS Ed. 1984; FRCS Ed. (Orth.) 1990. Cons. Orthop. Surg. Stirling Roy. Infirm. NHS Trust; Civil. Cons. Orthop. Surg. RN Scotl.; Clin. Sen. Lect. (Orthop.) Univ. Dundee; Director of Surgical Training. Specialty: Orthop. Socs: Fell. BOA; Assoc. Brit. Soc. for Surg. of the Hand. Prev: Sen. Regist. (Orthop.) Aberd. Roy. Infirm.; Convener of Educating Cons. Courses RCS Ed.

RITCHIE, Ian Samuel Daniel 62 Maryville Park, Belfast BT9 6LQ — MB BCh BAO Belf. 1992.

RITCHIE, Ian William William Street Surgery, 67 William Street, Herne Bay CT6 5NR Tel: 01227 740000 Fax: 01227 742729; The Six Bells, Church Lane, Chiswet, Canterbury CT3 4OX — MB ChB Aberd. 1972; DObst RCOG 1975; MRCGP 1980.

RITCHIE, Iris Margaret The Clinic, Drummore, Stranraer DG9 9QQ Tel: 01776 840205 Fax: 01776 840390 — MB BCh BAO Belf. 1984; DRCOG 1988; MRCGP 1989; DCH RCP Lond. 1990. GP Drummore. Specialty: Gen. Pract.

RITCHIE, James Morrison Garth, Strathmore Avenue, Kirriemuir — MB ChB Glas. 1919; DPH 1920. Prev: Dir. Typhoid Research Laborat. Geo.town, Brit. Guiana & Pub.; Health Laborat. (Med. Research Counc.) Birkenhead.

RITCHIE, Jane Patricia Birling Ward, Preston Hall Hospital, Maidstone ME20 7NJ Tel: 01622 255642 Fax: 01622 225658 — MB ChB Ed. 1977 (Edin.) DCH RCPS Glas. 1980; MRCP (UK) 1985; MTrop. Paediat. Liverp. 1992. Cons. Community Paediat. Maidstone and Tunbridge Wells NHS Trust. Specialty: Community Child Health. Socs: BACCH; ICHG; Fell. Roy. Coll. Paediat. & Child Health. Prev: Cons. Community Paediat. Medway Trust; Sen. Regist. (Community Paediat.) Roy. Liverp. Childr. NHS Trust; Paediat. Community Based Rehabil. Project, Jamaica.

RITCHIE, Janice 898 Govan Road, Glasgow G51 3DL — MB ChB Glas. 1995.

RITCHIE, Jean Katherine (retired) Angkor, 5 Park Avenue, Hutton, Brentwood CM13 2QL — (Oxf. & Leeds) BM BCh Oxf. 1946; DMRT 1950; MRCP Lond. 1953; FFR 1955; DM Oxf. 1972. Prev: Dir. of Research (Records) St. Marks Hosp. Lond.

RITCHIE, Jessie More Ramsay 21 Culbowie Crescent, Buchlyvie, Stirling FK8 3NH Tel: 01360 850406 — MB ChB Glas. 1950.

RITCHIE, Joan Moira St. John's Hospital, Community Child Health, Howden, Livingston EH54 6PP Tel: 01506 419666 Fax: 01506 416484 Email: joan.ritchie@wlt.scot.nhs.uk; Green Gables, 9 Riselaw Crescent, Edinburgh EH10 6HN Tel: 0131 447 3192 — MB ChB Dundee 1976; MRCGP 1982; DCH RCP Glas. 1982; DCCH RCP Ed. 1984. Assoc. Specialist. Specialty: Community Child Health. Prev: SCMO (Child Health) W. Lothian NHS Trust.

RITCHIE, John Matheson (retired) Oldways, Castle Road, Wellingborough NN8 1LL Tel: 01933 222130 — MB BS Lond. 1952 (Middlx.) FRCOG 1977, M 1964. Prev: Cons. (O & G) Kettering & Dist. Hosp. Gp.

RITCHIE, Keith Anthony Woodlands Surgery, 146 Halfway St., Sidcup DA15 8DF Tel: 020 8300 1680 Fax: 020 8309 7020 — MB BS Lond. 1980 (Guy's) BSc Hons Lond. 1977; MRCS LRCP Lond. 1980; DRCOG 1985. GP. Specialty: Gen. Pract.; Care of the Elderly; Psychosexual Med.

RITCHIE, Kenneth Brian Inverkeithing Medical Group, 5 Friary Court, Inverkeithing KY11 1NU Tel: 01383 413234 Fax: 01383 410098; Fernbank, North Queensferry, Inverkeithing KY11 1HB Tel: 01383 413508 Fax: 01383 627527 Email: drkritchie@aol.com — (Aberd.) MB ChB Aberd. 1967; DObst RCOG 1969. GP Princip.; Adviser Fife Health Bd. Socs: Brit. Soc. Med. & Dent. Hypn.; Assoc. Fac. Homeopath. Prev: Ho. Surg. & Ho. Phys. Dumfries Roy. Infirm.; Ho. Surg. O & G Falkirk & Dist. Roy. Infirm.; SHO Seafield Childr. Hosp. Ayr.

RITCHIE, Kenneth Henry, Squadron Ldr. RAF (retired) Newlands Farm, Winsor Road, Winsor, Southampton SO40 2HE Tel: 023 8081 4264 — MRCS Eng. LRCP Lond. 1949 (King's Coll. Hosp.) Prev: Ho. Phys. Diabetic Dept. King's Coll. Hosp.

RITCHIE, Professor Lewis Duthie Health Centre, Forrest Road, Peterhead AB42 2TX Tel: 01779 474841 Fax: 01779 474651; Department of General Practice and Primary Care, University of Aberdeen, Westburn Road, Aberdeen AB25 2AY Tel: 01224 681818 Fax: 01224 840683 — MB ChB Aberd. 1978; MB ChB (Commend.) Aberd. 1978; DRCOG 1980; FRCGP 1994, M 1982; FFPHM RCP (UK) 1993, M 1989; MSc Ed. (Comm. Med.) 1982, BSc (Chem.) 1978, MD 1993; FRCP Ed. 1995. Mackenzie Prof. & Head Gen. Pract. Univ. Aberd.; Hon. Cons. Pub. Health Med. Grampian HB. Specialty: Gen. Pract. Socs: Fell. Roy. Soc. Med.; Brit. Computer Soc. Prev: Cons. Pub. Health Med. Grampian HB; SHO (Gen. Med.) Aberd. Roy. Infirm.; SHO (Obst.) Aberd. Matern. Hosp.

RITCHIE, Neil Jonathan 61 Cavendish Road, Matlock DE4 3HD — MB ChB Leic. 1996.

RITCHIE, Peter Lowfield Farm, 18 Durham Road, Wolviston, Billingham TS22 5LP — MB ChB Dundee 1975; FFA RCS Eng. 1981. Cons. Anaesth. N. Tees Gen. Hosp. Stockton-on-Tees. Specialty: Anaesth.; Intens. Care.

RITCHIE, Peter Andrew Gloucestershire Hospitals NHS Trust, Department of Anaesthesia, Cheltenham General Hospital, Sandford Road, Cheltenham GL53 7AN Tel: 0845 422 4143 Fax: 0845 422 3405 Email: peter.ritchie@glos.nhs.uk — MB BS Lond. 1977 (King's Coll. Hosp.) BSc (Hons. Pharmacol.) Lond.; FRCA 1982. Cons. Anaesth. Gloucestershire Hosp. NHS Trust. Specialty: Anaesth. Special Interest: Med. Politics. Prev: Cons. Anaesth. Cheltenham NHS Trust.

RITCHIE, Rhoda Marjorie 466 Kilmarnock Road, Glasgow G43 2BS Tel: 0141 637 0701 — MB ChB Glas. 1950.

RITCHIE, Robert Tyrie (retired) — MB ChB Ed. 1944; FRCP Ed. 1966, M 1949. Prev: Cons. Phys. (Geriat.) Dundee & Angus Geriat. Serv.

RITCHIE, Robina Donaldson Skene Medical Group, Westhill Drive, Westhill AB32 6FY Tel: 01224 742213 Fax: 01224 744664; 9 Fallow Road, Westhill AB32 6PT — MB ChB Aberd. 1980. Specialty: Gen. Pract.

RITCHIE, Sara Spitalfields Practice, Tower Hamlets, 20 Old Montague Street, London E1 5PB — MB ChB Ed. 1993. GP Spitalfields Pract. Tower Hamlets Lond. Specialty: Accid. & Emerg. Prev: SHO (A & E) Hull Roy. Infirm.; SHO (Psychiat.) St. Jas. Univ. Hosp. Leeds; Ho. Off. (Surg.) West. Gen. Hosp. Edin.

RITCHIE, Sharon Anne The Surgery, John Street, Bellshill ML4 1RJ Tel: 01698 747195; East Belmont Orchard, By Overtown, Wishaw MC2 0RU — MB ChB Aberd. 1992; MRCGP 1996; DRCOG 1997. Specialty: Gen. Pract.

RITCHIE, Stuart Norman Parkview resource Centre, 152 Wellshot Road, Tollcross, Glasgow G32 7AX Tel: 0141 303 8818 — MB ChB Glas. 1988; MD; MRCPsych. Cons. In old age Psychiat. Pk.ehead Hosp. Salamanca St, Glas. G32. Specialty: Geriat. Psychiat. Prev: Career Regist. (Psychiat.) Gartnavel Roy. Hosp. Glas.

RITCHIE, Vaughn Health Centre, Blackfaulds Place, Fauldhouse, Bathgate EH47 9AS Tel: 01501 770282 Fax: 01501 772515; Bouley, Main St, Longridge, Bathgate EH47 8AE Tel: 01501 771162 — MB ChB Dundee 1981. GP FauldHo. Health Centre W. Lothian VTS.

RITCHIE, William Alan Howard Antrim Hospital, 45 Bush Road, Antrim BT41 2RL Tel: 02899 442 4263 Fax: 0289 442 4868 Email:

alan.ritchie@ah.m-l.nhs.uk — MB BCh BAO Belf. 1971; FRCOG 1990, M 1975. Cons Obst. & Gyn., Antrim Hosp. Specialty: Obst. & Gyn. Socs: Irish Perinatal Soc.; Ulster Med. Soc.; RSM. Prev: Cons Obst. & Gyn. Waveney Hosp. Ballymena.

RITCHIE, William Neil National Public Health Service, P.O. Box 13, St David's Hospital, Carmarthen SA31 3YH Tel: 01267 225225 Fax: 01267 223337 Email: william.ritchie@nphs.wales.nhs.uk; The Old Rectory, Garthbrengy, Brecon LD3 9TD Tel: 01874 624372 — MB BS Lond. 1971 (Middlx.) DPH Sydney 1977; MFCM 1987; FFPHM RCP Lond. 1994. Specialty: Pub. Health Med. Socs: Soc. of Social Med. (Memb).

RITCHIE, William Primrose 466 Kilmarnock Road, Glasgow G43 2BS Tel: 0141 637 0701 — MB ChB Glas. 1952.

RITSON, Edward Bruce Honorary Consultant, Royal Edinburgh Hospital, Morninside Park, Edinburgh EH10 5HF Fax: 0131 537 6108; 4 McLaren Road, Edinburgh EH9 2BH Tel: 0131 667 1735 — (Ed.) MB ChB Ed. 1961; DPM 1964, Dip. Psych 1964; MD Ed. 1967; Dip. Community Ment. Health Harvard 1967; FRCPsych 1980, M 1971; FRCP Ed. 1987. Clin. Dir. & Cons. Roy. Edin. Hosp.; Sen. Lect. Edin. Univ.; Chairm. DVLA Alcohol Drugs Ment. Comm.; Mem. Alcohol Educat. Research Counc. Specialty: Gen. Psychiat. Socs: Soc. Study of Addic.; Med. Counc. Alcohol.; Roy. Coll. Psychiat. (Former Fac. Chairm. Subst. Misuse). Prev: Dir. Sheff. Region Addic. Unit; Sen. Regist. Roy. Edin. Hosp.; Research Fell. Harvard Med. Sch. Boston, USA.

RITSON, Roger Harry Hailwood Medical Centre, 2 Hailwood Court, Governors Hill, Douglas IM2 7EA Tel: 01624 67544 Fax: 01624 616290; Ballafletcher, Poultry Farm Cottage, Ballafletcher Road, Braddan, Douglas IM4 4QL Tel: 01624 623219 — MB ChB Manch. 1966; MRCS Eng. LRCP Lond. 1966. Approved under Sect. 28(2) Ment. Health Act. Specialty: Pharmacology. Socs: BMA. Prev: Ho. Phys. Ho. Off. (O & G) & Regist. Psychiat. Ashton Gen.; Hosp.

RITTER, Alison Clare Jarvis and Partners, Westbrook Medical Centre, 301-302 Westbrook Centre, Warrington WA5 8UF Tel: 01925 654152 Fax: 01925 632612; 83 Stonehill Close, Appleton, Warrington WA4 5QD Tel: 01925 265899 — MB ChB Birm. 1989; DCH RCP Lond. 1992; DFFP 1993. Prev: Trainee GP Wirral HA VTS; SHO (Psychiat.) Arrowe Pk. Hosp. Liverp.

RITTER, Professor James Michael St. Thomas' Hospital, Department Clinical Pharmacology, Lambeth Palace Road, London SE1 7EH Tel: 020 7928 9292 ext 2250 Fax: 020 7401 2242 Email: james.ritter@kcl.ac.uk; 20 Vine Road, London SW13 0NE Tel: 020 8878 2381 Fax: 020 8878 9256 — BM BCh Oxf. 1974 (Oxf. Univ.) MA Oxf. 1970; DPhil (Oxf) 1970; MRCP (UK) 1976; FRCP Lond. 1994; FMedSci 2002. Prof. Clin. Pharmacol. GKT St. Thos. Hosp. Kings Coll. Lond.; Hon. Cons. Phys. Guy's & St. Thos. Hosps. Lond. Specialty: Pharmacology. Socs: Brit. Pharm. Soc.; Assn. Phys.; Med. Res. Soc. Prev: Sen. Lect. (Clin. Pharmacol.) Roy. Postgrad. Med. Sch. Lond.; Asst. Prof. Med. Case West. Reserve Univ. Cleveland Ohio, OH, USA; Asst. Chief of Serv. (Med.) Johns Hopkins Hosp. Baltimore MD, USA.

RITTEY, Christopher Donald Clement The Ryegate Childrens Centre, Tapton Crescent Road, Sheffield S10 5DD Tel: 0114 267 0237 Fax: 0114 267 8296; 45 Redmires Road, Sheffield S10 4LB Tel: 0114 230 2059 Fax: 0114 230 2671 Email: c.d.rittey@sheffield.ac.uk — MB ChB Ed. 1982; FRCP 1997; FRCPch 1997. Cons. Paediat. Neurol. Ryegate Childr. Centre Sheff. Specialty: Paediat. Neurol. Prev: Sen. Regist. & Regist. (Paediat.) Roy. Hosp. Sick Childr. Glas.; Regist. (Paediat.) Rutherglen Matern. Hosp. Glas.; SHO (Paediat.) Stobhill Gen. Hosp. & Roy. Hosp. Sick Childr. Glas.

RITTOO, Dev Bhuruth 8 Addison Close, Chorlton-on-Medlock, Manchester M13 9SB — MB ChB Manch. 1982.

RITTOO, Dylmitr Department of Cardiology, Arrowe Park Hospital, Upton CH49 5PE Tel: 0151 604 7250 Email: drittoo@yahoo.co.uk — MD Manch. 1993 (Manchester University) MB ChB 1984; MRCP (UK) 1988. Cons. Cardiologist Arrowe Pk. Hosp.; Regist. (Med.) Roy. Liverp. Hosp.; Fell. Interven.al Cardiol., Halifax, Nova Scotia; Research Fell. KCH Lond. Specialty: Cardiol. Prev: Lect. (Cardiol) Manch. Roy. Infirm.; Research Fell. (Cardiol.) West. Gen. Hosp. Edin.

RITTOO, Mr Dynesh 8 Addison Close, Chorlton on Medlock, Manchester M13 9SB — MB ChB Manch. 1991; FRCS 1995. Research Fell. Selly Oak Univ. Hosp. Birm. Specialty: Gen. Surg.; Vasc. Med. Prev: Regist. (Surg.) Bury Gen. Hosp.; Regist. (Surg.) Blackburn Roy. Infirm.

RITZEMA-CARTER, Jay Lynn Tamara The Old Post House, Crazies Hill, Reading RG10 8LU Tel: 01189 403437 — BM Soton. 1998. PRHO Med., Soton. Gen. Hosp. Specialty: Gen. Med.

RIUSECH MAS, Ines Flat 11, Warehouse 13, Kingston St., Hull HU1 2DZ — LMS U Autonoma Barcelona 1990.

RIVAS, Peter Hugh (retired) 57 Hemingford Road, Islington, London N1 1BY Tel: 020 7609 8717 — MRCS Eng. LRCP Lond. 1972 (Lond. Hosp.) MB BS Lond. 1972, BDS 1967; FDS RCS Eng. 1975. Cons. Oral Surg. & Dent. Supt. Univ. Coll. Hosp. Lond. Prev: Sen. Regist. (Oral Surg.) Mt. Vernon Hosp. Northwood.

RIVERA DE ZEA, Antonio 21 Averon Rise, Oldham OL1 4NX — LMS Malaga 1993.

RIVEROS HUCKSTADT, Maria del Pilar Flat 4, 71 Richmond Road, Worthing BN11 4AQ — LMS Seville 1988.

RIVERS, David (retired) 181 Cromwell Lane, Burton Green, Coventry CV4 8AN Tel: 024 7646 6198 — (St. Mungo's Coll. Glas.) LMSSA Lond. 1946; MRCGP 1965. Prev: Pathol. Pneumoconiosis Research Unit Llandough Hosp.

RIVERS, Jane Ann The Park Medical Practice, Maine Drive Clinic, Maine Drive, Derby DE21 6LA Tel: 01332 665522 Fax: 01332 678210 — MB ChB Leic. 1983 (Leicester) BPharm. Lond. 1974; MSc CNAA 1978; DRCOG 1986; MRCGP 1988.

RIVERS, John Somers (retired) Homeland, Balscote, Banbury OX15 6JP Tel: 01295 730672 — MB BChir Camb. 1946 (Camb. & Middlx.) MA Camb. 1947, MB BChir. 1946. Prev: GP Lincs.

RIVERS, John William Shanklin Medical Centre, 1 Carter Road, Shanklin PO37 7HR Tel: 01983 862245 Fax: 01983 862310; Apse Manor, Apse Manor Road, Shanklin PO37 7PN Tel: 01983 867677 — MB BS Lond. 1982; BSc Lond. 1979; DCH RCP Lond. 1984; DRCOG 1986; MRCGP (Distinc.) 1986. Chairm. IDOC (Isle of Wight GP Co-op.). Prev: Trainee GP Crawley VTS.

RIVERS, Malcolm Derek 16 Oatlands, Crawley RH11 8EQ — MB ChB Sheff. 1997.

RIVERS, Nigel 26 Westholme Close, Woodbridge IP12 4BE Tel: 01394 383120 — MRCS Eng. LRCP Lond. 1949 (Middlx.) LMSSA Lond. 1948; DPM Eng. 1967. Assoc. Specialist (Psychiat.) St. Audry's Hosp. Woodbridge. Specialty: Gen. Psychiat. Socs: Soc. Clin. Psychiat.; Assn. Behavioural Clinicians. Prev: JHMO (Psychiat.) Clifton Hosp. York; Regist. Mt. Vernon Hosp. Northwood & Harrow Chest Clinic; Ho. Surg. Middlx. Hosp.

RIVERS, Rodney Peter Aldridge Imperial College School of Medicine, St Mary's Campus, London W2 1PG Tel: 020 7886 6103 Fax: 020 7886 6284 Email: r.p.rivers@ic.ac.uk — MB Camb. 1966; BChir 1965; MRCP (U.K.) 1970; FRCP Lond. 1980. Reader (Paediat.) Imperial Coll. Sch. of Med. Specialty: Paediat. Socs: Neonat. Soc. & Europ. Soc. Paediat. Research.

RIVETT, Anne Williton and Watchet Surgeries, Robert Street, Williton, Taunton TA4 4QE Tel: 01984 632701 Fax: 01984 633933; Chilcombe House, 30 Trendle Lane, Bicknoller, Taunton TA4 4EG Tel: 0198 46 56243 — MB ChB Bristol 1978.

RIVETT, Geoffrey Christopher (retired) 173 Shakespeare Tower, Barbican, London EC2Y 8DR Tel: 020 7786 9617 Email: geoffrey@rivett.net — BM BCh Oxf. 1956 (Oxf. & Univ. Coll. Hosp.) MA (1st cl. Hons.) Oxf. 1957; DObst RCOG 1958; FRCGP 1987, M 1965. Prev: Sen. Princip. Med. Off. DoH.

RIVETT, James Frederick Drayton and St Faiths Medical Practice, 8 Manor Farm Close, Drayton, Norwich NR8 6EE Tel: 01603 867532 — MRCS Eng. LRCP Lond. 1977 (Guy's) BSc Lond. 1974, MB BS 1977; MRCGP 1983; AFOM RCP Lond. 1994.

RIVETT, Joan Dorothy (retired) 26 Whalley Drive, Bletchley, Milton Keynes MK3 6HP Tel: 01908 373222 — BM BCh Oxf. 1957 (Oxf. & Lond. Hosp.) MA Oxf. 1958, BM BCh 1957; FRCPath 1981, M 1969. Prev: Cons. Histopath. Stoke Mandeville Hosp. Aylesbury.

RIVETT, John Graham Martins Oak Surgery, 36 High Street, Battle TN33 0EA Tel: 01424 772263/772060 — MB BS Lond. 1985; MA Oxf. 1986; DA (UK) 1988; MRCGP 1989; DRCOG 1990; DCH RCP Lond. 1992. Prev: Dist. Med. Off. Roddickton Newfld., Canada; Resid. Med. Off. The Childr. Hosp. Sydney, Austral.; Trainee GP Lostwithiel Cornw. VTS.

RIVETT, Katharine Alison 45 Paterson Close, Stocksbridge, Sheffield S36 1JQ — MB ChB Sheff. 1997 (Sheffield) SHO, A&E, Northern Gen. Hosp., Sheff.; VTS Trainee. Specialty: Accid. &

Emerg.; Gen. Pract. Prev: GP Reg., FarLa. Surg. Sheff.; Ho. Off. InMed., Rotherham Dist. Gen.; HO, Surg., Bassetlaw, Dist., Gen.

RIVETT, Paula Maria Catslide Cottage, Caldbec Hill, Battle TN33 0JS Tel: 01424 775673 — MB BS Lond. 1987; DGM RCP Lond. 1990; DRCOG 1992. Prev: Trainee GP Taunton; Dist. Med. Off. Newfld., Canada; Resid. Med. Off. Childr. Hosp. Camperdown, Sydney, Austral.

RIVETT, Robert Stephen Williton and Watchet Surgeries, Robert Street, Williton, Taunton TA4 4QE Tel: 01984 632701 Fax: 01984 633933; Chilcombe House, 30 Trendle Lane, Bicknoller, Taunton TA4 4EG Tel: 01984 656243 — MB ChB Bristol 1978; Dip. Med. Educat. Dund; DRCOG 1981; MRCP (UK) 1981; FRCGP 1996, M 1982. GP Williton Surg. Williton Som. Prev: RCGP Internat. Developm. Adviser Lebanon.

RIVLIN, Ian 17 Dobcroft Close, Ecclesall, Sheffield S11 9LL — MB ChB Sheff. 1984. SHO (O & G) Rotherham Dist. Gen. Hosp. Socs: BMA & Med. Protec. Soc. Prev: SHO (Geriat.) Rotherham Dist. Gen. Infirm.; Ho. Off. (Gen. Med.) Rotherham Dist. Gen. Hosp.; Ho. Off. (ENT, Renal Transpl. & Gen. Surg.) Roy. Hallamsh. Hosp. Sheff.

RIVLIN, Joseph Joel (retired) Parkfield, Courtenay Road, Liverpool L25 4RL Tel: 0151 428 1203 Email: jrnw00224@blueyonder.co.uk — (Liverp.) MB ChB Liverp. 1943; MRCS Eng. LRCP Lond. 1943; MLCOM 1969; MSc Liverp. 1997. Prev: Cons. Osteop. Phys. Liverp.

RIVLIN, Rosa Sutton 9 Clarendon Court, Eastbury Avenue, Northwood HA6 3LN Tel: 01923 836713 — MRCS Eng. LRCP Lond. 1947 (Cardiff) CPH Wales 1950. Locum GP Middlx. Socs: BMA & Cardiff Med. Soc. Prev: GP Cardiff; Research Asst. (Social & Occupat. Med.) Welsh Nat. Sch. Med. Cardiff; Ho. Surg. (Radiother.) Brit. Postgrad. Med. Sch. Hammersmith.

RIVRON, Marilyn Joy 24 Station Road, Radyr, Cardiff CF15 8AA — MB BCh Wales 1979; BSc Wales 1976; MRCGP 1983. Community Paediat. Cardiff & Vale NHS Trust. Specialty: Community Child Health; Paediat. Prev: Clin. Med. Off. (Community Child Health) Lothian HB.

RIVRON, Mr Raymond Peter Royal Glamorgan Hospital, Ynysmaerdy, Llantrisant CF72 8XR Tel: 01443 443443 Fax: 01443 443248 — MB BCh Wales 1979; BSc Wales 1976; FRCS Eng. 1986; MD Wales 1995. Cons. Otolaryngol. Taff Ely Health Unit. Specialty: Otolaryngol. Prev: Sen. Regist. (Otolaryngol.) Lothian HB Edin.; Regist. (Otolaryngol.) Leeds HA; Lect. & Hon. Regist. Dept. Clin. Surg. (Otolaryng.) Univ. Edin.

RIX, Bruce David The Ongar Health Centre, Great Bansons, Bansons Lane, Ongar CM5 9EF Tel: 01277 363028 Fax: 01277 365264; Coopers, Coopers Hill, Marden Ash, Ongar CM5 9EG Tel: 01277 362912 — MB BS Lond. 1974; MRCS Eng. LRCP Lond. 1974; MRCGP 1981. Clin. Asst. (Rheum.) Broomfield Hosp. Chelmsford. Prev: SHO Broomfield Hosp. Chelmsford; Ho. Phys. Plumstead Hosp. Lond.; Ho. Surg. Guy's Hosp. Lond.

RIX, David Alan Antler Cottage, Dalton, Newcastle upon Tyne NE18 0AA — MB BS Newc. 1989.

RIX, Gerald Henner West Suffolk Hospital, Hardwick Lane, Bury St Edmunds IP33 2QZ; 8 Loch of Liff Road, Liff, Dundee DD2 5NE — MB BChir Camb. 1992 (Addenbrooke's Hosp. Camb.) BA (Hons.) Physiol. Sci. Oxf. 1989. SHO Rotat. (Gen. Surg.) W. Suff. Hosp. Bury St. Edmunds. Prev: SHO Rotat.(A & E Trauma, Orthop. & Neurosurg.) Addenbrooke's Hosp. Camb.; Ho. Off. (Gen. Med.) Ipswich Hosp.; Ho. Off. (Gen. Surg.) Addenbrooke's Hosp. Camb.

RIX, Keith John Barkclay The Grange, 92 Whitcliffe Rd, Cleckheaton BD19 3DR Tel: 01274 878604 Fax: 01274 869898 — MB ChB Aberd. 1975; MD Aberd. 1986, BMedBiol. (Hons.) 1972; FRCPsych 1992, M 1979; MPhil Ed. 1980; CBiol. 1986; MAE 1995; MEWI 1997. Cons. Forens. Psychiat. The Grange Consg. Rooms, Cleckheaton; Vis. Cons. Psychiat. HM Prison Leeds; Mem. Inst. Biol. & Inst. Health Educat. Specialty: Forens. Psychiat.; Medico Legal; Gen. Psychiat. Socs: Acad. Experts; Fell. RSM; Med. Sec. Leeds & W. Riding Medico-Legal Soc. Prev: Cons. Forens. Psych., Leeds CMH Trust; Lect. (Psychiat.) Univ. Manch.; Regist. (Psychiat.) Roy. Edin. Hosp.

RIX, Robert Daren 24 Kennet Close, Upminster RM14 1ST — MB ChB Sheff. 1989.

RIX, Stephen Mark c/o 24 Hill View, Langthorpe, Boroughbridge, York YO51 9BE — MB BS Newc. 1996.

RIX, Susan Paula 38 Parsonage Street, Dursley GL11 4AA — MB BS Lond. 1989.

RIX, Thomas Elliott 12 Abinger Way, Eaton, Norwich NR4 6NA — BChir Camb. 1995.

RIXOM, James Andrew West Hallam Medical Centre, The Dales, West Hallam, Derby DE7 6GR Tel: 0115 932 5462 — MB BCh Wales 1982; DRCOG 1986; MRCGP 1989.

RIXON, Peter Ernest (retired) Rosemary Cottage, Chillesford, Woodbridge IP12 3PU Tel: 01394 450512 — MB ChB Aberd. 1949; DPM Eng. 1956; MRCPsych 1971. Prev: Cons. Psychiat. St. Audry's Hosp. Melton & St. Geo. Hosp. Morpeth.

RIXON, Rebekah Ann Limewood Farm, Ashford Hill Road, Ashford Hill, Thatcham RG19 8BB — MB ChB Leeds 1998.

RIYAMI, Bazdawi Mohammed Said 202 Kirkintilloch Road, Bishopbriggs, Glasgow G64 2ND — MB ChB Baghdad 1971; DTM & H Liverp. 1974; DTCD Wales 1975; MRCP (UK) 1976.

RIZA, Mr Ibrahim Mohamed Department of Vascular Surgery, Manchester Royal Infirmary, Oxford Road, Manchester M13 9WL Tel: 0161 276 4525; 49 Calder Drive, Walmley, Sutton Coldfield B76 1YR Tel: 0121 313 0340 Email: viriza@btinternet.com — MB BS Mangalore 1990 (Kasturba Med. Coll. Manipal, India) FRCS Glas. 1994; FRCS Glas. 1994. Research Fell. Vasc. Surg. Manch. Roy. Infirm. Specialty: Gen. Surg. Prev: SPR (Gen. Surg.) Roy. Infirm. Edin.; Clin. Fell. Vasc. Surg.; SPR Vasc. Surg. Rlutt Liverp.

RIZK, Mr Mohib Samy Rosedale, West Ella Road, West Ella, Hull HU10 7SF — MB ChB Alexandria 1967; FRCS Ed. 1981.

RIZK, Nader Fouad St. John's Well, 109 Manor Road, Bottesford, Scunthorpe DN16 3PT Tel: 01724 840404 Fax: 01724 271437 — (Cairo) MB BCh Cairo 1968; LRCP LRCS Ed. LRCPS Glas. 1974. Prev: Trainee GP Aberd. VTS; SHO (Obst.) Mayday Hosp. Thornton Heath; SHO (Orthop.) Roy. Nat. Orthop. Hosp. Stanmore.

RIZK, Mr Samir Nessim Morcos 51 Cropwell Road, Radcliffe-on-Trent, Nottingham NG12 2FQ Tel: 0115 933 6675 Fax: 0115 933 6775 — (Cairo) MB BCh Cairo 1956; DO Eng. 1961; LMSSA Lond. 1962; FRCS Eng. 1963; FRCOpth 1989. Cons. Ophth. Surg. Pk. Hosp. Nottm.; Nottm. Nuffield Hosp. Specialty: Ophth. Prev: Ho. Phys. & Ho. Surg. Univ. Hosp. Cairo; Sen. Regist. Roy. Hosp. & Roy. Infirm. Sheff.; Regist. Nottm. Eye Hosp.

RIZKI, Sabiha 134 Albury Drive, Pinner HA5 3RG — MB BS Osmania 1965.

RIZVI, Fakhrul Hassan 3 Queen Anne Street, Stoke-on-Trent ST4 2EQ — MB BS Karachi 1975; MRCS LRCP Lond. 1980.

RIZVI, Imtiaz Hussain Consultant Radiologist, Diana, Princess of Wales Hospital, Scartho Road, Grimsby DN33 2BA Tel: 01472 276310 (Home)/01472 874111 Ext: 7724 Email: rizvi33@hotmail.com — MB BS Sind. 1964; DMRD Lond. 1972; FRCS UK 1975. Cons. Radiologist, Diana, Princess of Wales Hosp., Scartho Rd., Grimsby. Specialty: Radiol. Socs: Fell., Roy. Coll. of Radiologist, UK; Radiological Soc. of Pakistan; Ultrasound Soc. of Pakistan. Prev: Prof. and Chairm., Radiol. Dept., Aga Khan Univ. Hosp., Karachi, Pakistan, Nov. 1994 to Dec. 1999.

RIZVI, Negheth 18 Church Path, London W4 5BJ — MB BS Lond. 1996.

RIZVI, Qasim Raza 3 Poplar Road, Manchester M19 1QH Tel: 0161 286 8658 — MB ChB Dundee 1992; MRCS (I & II) Eng. 1997. Specialist Regist. (Radiol.) Liverp. Specialty: Radiol. Prev: SHO (ENT) N. Manch. Gen. Hosp.; SHO (Neurosurg.) Manch. Roy. Infirm.

RIZVI, Syed Akhlaq Hussain Consultant Physician, Watford General Hospital, Vicarage Road, Watford WD18 0HB Tel: 01923 217768 Fax: 01923 217715; 43 Marlings, Park Avenue, Chislehurst BR7 6RD Tel: 01689 608376 — MB BS Karachi 1979 (Dow Medical College, Karachi) MRCP (UK) 1991; Dip. Cardiol. Lond 1992. Cons. Phys., Watford Gen. Hosp., Watford, Herts WP1 8HB. Specialty: Care of the Elderly. Socs: BMA; Brit. Geriat. Soc.

RIZVI, Mr Syed Ishtiaq Hussain 3 Lessingham Avenue, Clayhall, Ilford IG5 0BJ — MB BS Punjab 1979 (Nishtar Med. Coll. Mutan, Univ. of The Punjab, Lahore, Pakistan) BSc Principles 1975; FRCSI 1990. Staff Grade Doctor, (A & E), King Geo. Hosp. Barley La., Good Mayes, Essex. Specialty: Accid. & Emerg.; Gen. Surg.; Urol. Socs: Roy.Soc. of Med.; BMA; Pakistan Med. & Dent. Counc. Prev: Cons Surg., Rasheed Hosp, Lahore.; Asstt. Prof., Cons. Surg., Punjab Med. Coll. Faisalabacl, Pakistan.

RIZVI, Syed Pervez Jamal 193 Homerton High Street, Hackney, London E9 6BB — MB BS Lucknow 1978.

RIZVI, Syed Shakil Ahmed Flat 2, Block 7, St. Peter's District General Hospital, Guildford Road, Ottershaw, Chertsey KT16 0PZ —

MB BS Punjab 1975; DCH RCPS Glas. 1983; MRCP (UK) 1991. Specialty: Paediat. Prev: Regist. (Paediat.) Roy. Alexandra Hosp. Paisley.; Regist. (Paediat.) Bellshill Matern. Hosp., Law Hosp. Carluke & Vale of Leven Hosp. Dunbartonsh.

RIZVI, Mr Syed Tanveer Mustafa 8 Calside Place, Dumfries DG1 4AW — MB BS Sind 1986; MB BS Sind Pakistan 1986; FRCS Glas. 1992.

RIZWAN, Muhammad Raziuddin 26 Salisbury Avenue, Swanley BR8 8DG Tel: 01322 666693 — MB BS Karachi 1976; DA (UK) 1987. SHO. Specialty: Gen. Psychiat.; Geriat. Psychiat.

RIZZA, Charles Rocco Carmine (retired) 24 Ickford Road, Tiddington, Oxford OX9 2LR Tel: 01844 339335 Email: crrizza@aol.com — (St. And.) MB ChB St. And. 1955; MD (Gold Medal) St. And. 1962; FRCP Ed. 1972, M 1964. Cons. Phys. Oxf. Haemophilia Centre Churchill Hosp.; Clin. Lect. (Haemat.) Univ. Oxf. Prev: Ho. Phys. Therap. Unit Maryfield Hosp. Dundee.

RIZZO-NAUDI, Joseph Louis Whitchurch Surgery, 49 Oving Road, Whitchurch, Aylesbury HP22 4JF Tel: 01296 641203 Fax: 01296 640021 — MRCS Eng. LRCP Lond. 1979; MRCP (UK) 1985; MRCGP 1991.

ROACH, Diana Louise 27 Grange Street, Port Talbot SA13 1EN — BM Soton. 1991.

ROACH, Emma 93 Octavia Terrace, Greenock PA16 7PY — MB ChB Aberd. 1997.

ROACH, Huw David Universtiy Hospital Of Wales, Heath Park, Cardiff CF4 4XW Tel: 029 2074 3030; 19 Clodien Avenue, Cardiff CF14 3NL Tel: 029 2052 1034 — MB BS Lond. 1994 (Univ. Coll. Lond. Med. Sch.) MRCP (UK); BSc (Hons.) Lond. 1991. Specialist Regist. (Radiol.) Univ. Hosp. Wales Cardiff. Specialty: Radiol. Prev: SHO (Med.) Plymouth Hosps.; SHO (Elderly Care) Univ. Coll. Hosps. Lond.; SHO (A & E) Southmead Hosp. Bristol.

ROACH, Richard Tremayne Springhouse, St Marys Lane, Hertford SG14 2LF — MB BS Lond. 1994.

ROACH, Sue Claire Middle Flat, 27 Spath Road, Manchester M20 2QT — MB ChB Manch. 1995.

ROADS, Peter George (retired) Pasture Cottage, Dinton, Aylesbury HP17 8UZ Tel: 01296 748504 — MRCS Eng. LRCP Lond. 1943 (St. Mary's) MD Lond.; MB BS Lond. 1948; DPH Lond. 1949; FFCM 1974; FFPHM 1989. Med. Ref. for Cremat. Prev: Regional Med. Off. SW Thames RHA.

ROAF, Mr Robert 88 Upton Park, Chester CH2 1DQ Tel: 01244 376911 Email: robertroaf@aol.com — (Oxf.) MRCS Eng. LRCP Lond. 1937; BM BCh Oxf. 1938; MA Oxf. 1938; FRCS Ed. 1939; FRCS Eng. 1942; MCh Orth. Liverp. 1946. Cons. Orthop. Surg. United Liverp. Hosp. & Robt. Jones & Agnes Hunt Orthop. Hosp. Oswestry; Hon. Acad.ian Acad. Med. Singapore; Emerit. Prof. Orthop. Surg. Univ. Liverp. Specialty: Orthop. Socs: Fell. BOA; Hon. Fell. Indian Orthop. Assn.; Hon. Fell. Singapore Orthop. Assn. Prev: Dir. of Clin. Studies & Research Robt. Jones & Agnes Hunt Orthop. Hosp. Oswestry; Vis. Orthop. Surg. Irwin Hosp., New Delhi.

ROAN, Christian Anne MacGregor 2 Regent Square, Lenzie, Glasgow G66 5AE — MB ChB Glas. 1967; DObst RCOG 1969. Prev: GP StenHo.muir.

RÖHRICHT, Frank Michael East London & The City Mental Health NHS Trust, Newham Centre for Mental Health, Glen Road, London E13 8SP Tel: 020 7540 4380 Fax: 020 7540 2971 Email: frank.rohricht@elcmht.nhs.uk — State Exam Med Berlin 1990; MB BS; MD; MRCPsych. Cons. Psychiat. & Clin. Dir. Specialty: Gen. Psychiat. Special Interest: Body Image Disorders; Body Psychother.; Psychother. in Psychosis.

ROBACK, Sharon Denise 11 Canterbury Close, Chigwell IG7 6HG — MB ChB Manch. 1989; DCH RCP Lond. 1992; DRCOG 1993; MRCGP 1994. Socs: BMA; RCGP. Prev: Retainer GP Watford.

ROBAK, Krzysztof Robert 10 Grove Court, Walton Road, East Molesey KT8 0DG — Lekarz Warsaw 1973.

ROBARDS, Martin Frank Childrens Department, Pembury Hospital, Tunbridge Wells TN2 4QJ Tel: 01892 823535 Fax: 01892 825246 — MB BS Lond. 1967 (St. Thos.) BSc (Physiol.) Lond. 1964; FRCPCH 1993. Cons. Paediat. Pembury Hosp. Kent. Specialty: Paediat. Socs: BMA; Roy. Coll. of Paediat. & Child Health. Prev: Sen. Regist. (Paediat.) Liverp. AHA (T); Regist. (Paediat.) Hosp. Sick Childr. Gt. Ormond St.; SHO (Paediat.) St. Thos. Hosp. Lond.

ROBARTS, James Herbert (retired) Cnoc Nan Caoraich, 233 Bruernish, Castlebay HS9 5UY Tel: 01871 890381 — (Ed.) MB ChB Ed. 1939. Prev: Res. Ho. Surg. & Ho. Phys. Deaconess Hosp. Edin.

ROBARTS, Philip James Barbers Orchard, Colam Lane, Little Baddow, Chelmsford CM3 4SY — MB ChB Ed. 1975; FRCOG 1994, M 1981. Cons. O & G St. John's Hosp. Chelmsford. Specialty: Obst. & Gyn.

ROBARTS, Mr William Martin 31 Sloane Avenue, London SW3 3JB Tel: 020 7589 6666 Fax: 020 7584 3871 — MB BChir Camb. 1968 (Camb. & Middlx.) MA Camb. 1968; FRCS Eng. 1973. Prev: Regist. (Surg.) Middlx. Hosp. Lond. & Cheltenham Gen. Hosp.; Ho. Phys. Centr. Middlx. Hosp.

ROBAYO CASTILLO, Luisa Victoria 35 Helena Road, London NW10 1HY Tel: 020 8452 6251 — LMS Bilbao 1985; MSc (Nutrit.) Lond. 1990.

ROBB, Agnes Kate (retired) 89 Westfield Road, Leicester LE3 6HW Tel: 0116 285 8056 — MB ChB Aberd. 1932. Prev: Med. Off. Leics. AHA (T) (Leicester).

ROBB, Alastair Keith 87 Anchorsholme Lane, Blackpool — MB ChB Liverp. 1985.

ROBB, Angela Garstang Road Surgery, 63-65 Garstang Road, Preston PR1 1LB Tel: 01772 253554 Fax: 01772 909131; Barnsfield, Eaves Green Lane, Goosnargh, Preston PR3 2FE — MB BChir Camb. 1987; GP Appraiser; MA Camb. 1988; DRCOG 1992; MRCGP (Distinc.) 1992; MFFP 1993; GP Tr. 1998; FRCGP (FBA) 1998; RCGP QPA Assessor 1999. Family Plann. Instruc. Doctor. Specialty: Gen. Psychiat. Socs: Brit. Med. Acupunct. Soc. Prev: Examr. RCGP.

ROBB, Anne Gillespie 29 Hope Street, Lanark ML11 7NE Tel: 01555 662812 — Dip. Med. Acupunc. - BMAS; MB ChB Glas. 1970; DObst RCOG 1971; MFHom 1990. Indep. Pract. (Homoeop. Acupunc.) Lanark. Specialty: Homeop. Med. Socs: Brit. Med. Acupunct. Soc. Prev: Clin. Asst. Glas. Homoeop. Hosp.

ROBB, Curtis Alexander 12 Hightor Road, Liverpool L25 6DL — MB ChB Sheff. 1997.

ROBB, Dorothy Elizabeth (retired) Flat 1, 105 Marlborough Park S., Belfast BT9 6HT Tel: 02890 381053 — (Belf.) MB BCh BAO Belf. 1950; DObst RCOG 1958.

ROBB, Elaine Masonic House Surgery, 26 High Street, Buckingham MK18 1NU Tel: 01280 816450 Fax: 01280 823885; The Old School House, Shalstone, Buckingham MK18 5LT Tel: 01280 702476 — MB BS Lond. 1980; DRCOG; MRCGP; MRCS Eng. LRCP Lond. 1980.

ROBB, Geoffrey Hugh Ashtead Hospital, Ashtead KT21 2SB Tel: 01372 276161 Fax: 01372 278704; Heath House, Headley, Epsom KT18 6NJ Tel: 01372 377227 Fax: 01372 377748 — MB ChB Bristol 1961; DObst RCOG 1963; FRCP Lond. 1982, M 1966. Cons. Phys. Epsom Gen. Hosp.; Chief Med. Off Pension & Annuity Friendly Soc.; Chief Med. Off. Friends Provident Life Off.; Chief Med. Off. UNUM Ltd; Co-Edr. Med. Selection of Life Risks 4th Edition Macmillan; Chief Med. Off. R.G.A. (UK) Ltd. Specialty: Gen. Med. Socs: Soc. Occupat. Med.; Brit. Diabetic Assn. (Med. & Scientif. Sect); Assn. Study Obesity. Prev: Sen. Regist. (Cardiol.) Groote Schuur Hosp., Cape Town; Counc.lor RCP Lond.; Presidetn Assur. Med. Soc.

ROBB, Graeme Anthony Garstang Road Surgery, 63-65 Garstang Road, Preston PR1 1LB Tel: 01772 253554 Fax: 01772 909131; Barnsfield, Eaves Green Lane, Goosnargh, Preston PR3 2FE Tel: 01772 861188 — MB BChir Camb. 1985; MA Camb. 1987, BA 1983; DRCOG 1988; MRCGP 1991. Princip. GP; Course Oganiser Preston Hosp. VTS Preston; Trainer. Socs: BMA; Roy. Coll. Gen. Pract. Prev: Trainee GP Preston VTS; SHO (Obst. & Gen.) Sharoe Green Hosp. Preston; SHO (A & E & Psychiat.) Preston.

ROBB, Henry Morgan Falkirk & District, Royal Infirmary Trust, Falkirk FK1 Tel: 01324 624000; 10 The Glebe, Linlithgow EH49 6SG — MB ChB Dundee 1982; FFA RCS Eng. 1987; MSc Glas. 1988. Cons. Anaesth. Falkirk. Specialty: Anaesth. Prev: Sen. Regist. (Anaesth.) Glas.

ROBB, Mr James Eybers Royal Hospital for Sick Children, Edinburgh EH9 1LF Tel: 0131 536 0834 Fax: 0131 536 0852; Royal Infirmary of Edinburgh, Edinburgh EH16 4SU — MB ChB Dundee 1975 (St And. & Dundee) BSc St. And. 1972; FRCS Glas. 1980; FRCS Ed. 1980; FRCP Edin. 2002; MD St. And. 2004. Cons. Orthop. Surg. Roy. Hosp. for Sick Childr. Edin. Specialty: Orthop.

ROBB, John Daniel 85 Charlotte Street, Ballymoney BT53 6AZ — MB BS Newc. 1996.

ROBB, Mr John Daniel Alexander Model Farm, Ballymoney BT53 6BX — MB BCh BAO Belf. 1957; FRCS Eng. 1961. Cons. Surg. Route Hosp. Ballymoney. Prev: Sen. Lect. in Surg. Qu. Univ. Belf. & Roy. Vict. Hosp. Belf.

ROBB, John Joseph Braemar, 52 Belfast Road, Antrim BT41 1PB Tel: 01849 3376 — MB BCh BAO Belf. 1956; LRCP LRCS Ed. LRFPS Glas. 1956; DPH Belf. 1958; FRCPI 1979, M 1967; DCH RCPSI 1972. Cons. Phys. Antrim & Ballymena Health Dist. Specialty: Gen. Med. Prev: Ho. Phys. & Ho. Surg. Londonderry Gp. Hosps.; Med. Asst. Downe Hosp. Downpatrick & Belf. City Hosp.

ROBB, Katherine Hilary 83 Front Road, Drumbo, Lisburn BT27 5JX — MB BCh BAO Belf. 1996.

ROBB, Olive Jean 3 Lomond Drive, Carnoustie DD7 6DN — MB ChB Aberd. 1978.

ROBB, Patricia Marlowe (retired) 48 Montclair Drive, Liverpool L18 0HB Tel: 0151 475 0203 — (Ed.) MB ChB Ed. 1950; FRCP Ed. 1971, M 1954; FRCPath 1974, M 1963. Prev: Cons. Haemat. Walton Hosp. Liverp.

ROBB, Mr Peter John Epsom General Hospital, Epsom KT18 7EG; Ashtead Hospital, Ashtead KT21 2SB — MB BS Lond. 1981 (Lond. Hosp.) BSc (1st cl. Hons.) Lond. 1978, MB BS 1981; FRCS Eng. 1985; FRCS Ed. 1985. Cons. ENT. Surg. Epsom Health Care. Hon. Cons. Ent Surg. The Childern's Trust, Tadworth. Specialty: Otorhinolaryngol. Socs: Fell. Roy. Soc. Med.; Brit. Assn. Paediat. Otol. Prev: Sen. Regist. (ENT) Guy's Hosp. Lond.; Research Fell. Univ. Washington, Seattle, USA; Fell. (Paediat. Laryngol.) Childr. Hosp. Sydney, Austral.

ROBB, Robert Cleghorn, OBE (retired) La Ferronerie, Sark, Guernsey GY9 0SA Tel: 01481 832128 — (Univ. Glas.) MB ChB Glas. 1946; DPhysMed. Eng. 1952; DPH Lond. 1959; DIH Eng. 1960. Prev: Med. Off. Sark.

ROBB, Stephanie Ann The Newcomen Centre, Guys Hospital, St Thomas St., London SE1 1RT Tel: 020 7955 4498 Fax: 020 7955 2819 Email: stephanie.robb@gott.sthames.nhs.uk — MB BS Newc. 1977; FRCP CH; MRCP (UK) 1979; MD Newc. 1987; FRCP Lond. 1994. Cons. Paediat. Neurol. Guy's Hosp. Lond. Specialty: Paediat. Neurol. Prev: Sen. Regist. Hosp. Sick Childr. Lond.; Regist. Hammersmith Hosp. Lond.; MRC Train. Fell. (Neurol. Sci.) Roy. Free Hosp. Sch. Med. Lond.

ROBBE, Iain James University of Wales College of Medicine, Temple of Peace, Cathays Park, Cardiff CF10 3NW Tel: 029 2040 2480 Fax: 029 2040 2504 Email: robbe@cardiff.ac.uk; Whip's Cottage, Dawn of Day, Grosmont, Abergavenny NP7 8LT Tel: 01873 821331 — MB BS Lond. 1980 (Westm.) MRCS Eng. LRCP Lond. 1980; BSc Lond. 1977, MSc (Community Med.) 1985; FFPHM RCP (UK) 1995, M 1987. Sen. Lect. (Pub. Health Med.) Univ. Wales Coll. Med. Cardiff. Specialty: Pub. Health Med. Prev: Sen. Regist. (Community Med.) Oxf. RHA; Regist. (Radiol.) Addenbrookes Hosp. Cambs.; SHO Rotat. (Paediat.) Westm. Chidr. Hosp. Lond.

ROBBIE, Douglas Stewart (retired) 17 Filmer Road, London SW6 7BU — (Aberd.) (Commendation) MB ChB Aberd. 1954; FFA RCS Eng. 1960. Prev: Cons. Anaesth. (i/c Pain Clinic) Roy. Marsden Hosp. Lond.

ROBBIE, Nicola 37 Broad Oak Road, Worsley, Manchester M28 2TL — MB ChB Manch. 1989; MRCP Paediat. (UK) 1994. GP Retainee, Manch. Specialty: Gen. Pract. Prev: Regist. (Paediat.) Trafford Gen. Hosp. Manch.

ROBBIE, Rosalene Betsy RGIT Health, RGIT Ltd., 338 King St., Aberdeen AB24 5BQ Tel: 01224 619619 Fax: 01224 619519; 69 Woodend Place, Aberdeen AB15 6AP — MB ChB Aberd. 1974; Dip. Occ. Med. RCP Lond. 1996. Occupat. Phys. RGIT Health Aberd.. Specialty: Occupat. Health. Prev: Occupat. Phys. (Occupat. Health) RGIT Ltd Aberd.

ROBBINS, Aphra Giorgina Flat 3F3 96 Marchmont Road, Edinburgh EH9 1HR — MB ChB Ed. 1998; MB ChB Ed 1998.

ROBBINS, Gerard Department of Haematology, Royal Surrey County Hospital, Egerton Road, Guildford GU2 7XX Tel: 01483 464122 Fax: 01483 464072 — MB BS Lond. 1976 (Guy's) BSc Lond. 1973; MRCP (UK) 1978; MRCPath 1984. Cons. Haemat. Roy. Surrey Co. Hosp. Guildford; Med. Director Roy. Surrey Co. Hosp. Guildford. Specialty: Haematology. Prev: Co-ordinator Bone Marrow Transp. Progr. Roy. Free Hosp. Lond.; Sen. Regist. (Haemat.) Hillingdon Hosp. & Roy. Free Hosp. Lond.

ROBBINS, Graham Mark 24 Harwood Close, Tewin, Welwyn AL6 0LF — MB BS Lond. 1987.

ROBBINS, Judy Caroline Victoria House Surgery, 33 Victoria Road, Swindon SN1 3AW Tel: 01793 536515; Garden Cottage, Broadbush, Swindon SN26 7AJ Tel: 01793 728559 — MB BS Lond. 1985; DFFP 1992; DGM RCP Lond. 1992; MRCGP 1993; DRCOG 1994. Prev: Trainee GP Twickenham; SHO (O & G) Wexham Pk. Slough; SHO (Gen. Med.) W. Middlx. Hosp.

ROBBINS, Justin Alexander Baird Church View Surgery, 30 Holland Road, Plymstock, Plymouth PL9 9BN Tel: 01752 403206 — MB BS Lond. 1966 (St. Thos.) DObst RCOG 1968; MRCP (U.K.) 1970. Prev: Med. Regist. Hither Green Hosp. Lond.; Sen. Med. Regist. Kitwe Centr. Hosp. Zambia.

ROBBINS, Matthew Charles Oliver 80 Stratford Street, Upper Stoke, Coventry CV2 4NJ — MB BS Lond. 1994. Specialty: Paediat.

ROBBINS, Nancy Estelle (retired) Heacham Lodge, Lodge Road, Heacham, King's Lynn PE31 7AZ Tel: 01485 71582 — (Roy. Free) MRCS Eng. LRCP Lond. 1938.

ROBBINS, Professor Peter Alistair The University Laboratory of Physiology, Parks Road, Oxford OX1 3PT Tel: 01865 272490 Fax: 01865 282486 Email: peter.robbins@physiol.ox.ac.uk — BM BCh Oxf. 1984 (Oxford) BA (Physiol.) Oxf. 1978; MA, DPhil Oxf. 1981; BA (Maths.) Open 1993. Prof. (Physiol.) & Fell. Qu.'s Coll. Oxf. Specialty: Clin. Physiol. Socs: BMA; Physiol. Soc.; Amer. Physiol. Soc.

ROBBINS, Sarah Anne 50 Croftdown Road, London NW5 1EN — MB BS Lond. 1989; DRCOG 1992. Trainee GP Roy. Hants. Co. Hosp. Winchester VTS. Prev: SHO (A & E) Roy. Hants. Co. Hosp. Winchester; Ho. Surg. St. Mary's Hosp. Portsmouth.

ROBBINS, Sian Eryl 1 Tithe Barn, Main St., Merton, Bicester OX25 2NF — MB BS Lond. 1987; MRCP (UK) 1990; FRCR 1995. Sen. Regist. (Radiol.) Bristol Roy. Infirm. Specialty: Radiol. Prev: Regist. (Med.) Southmead Hosp. Bristol & Princess Margt. Hosp. Swindon; SHO (Renal Med.) Southmead Hosp. Bristol.

ROBBINS-CHERRY, Anthony Martin Sturton Road Surgery, 12 Sturton Road, Saxilby, Lincoln LN1 2PG Tel: 01522 702791 Fax: 01522 704434; 43 Station Road, Thorpe-on-the-Hill, Lincoln LN1 2RR Tel: 01522 731591 — MB BS Lond. 1973 (St. Marys) BSc (Hons. 1st cl.) Lond. 1970; MRCS Eng. LRCP Lond. 1973.

ROBERSON, Frances Elizabeth Delaforce Ridgeway Practice, Plympton Health Centre, Mudgeway, Plymouth PL7 1AD Tel: 01752 345317 — MB BS Lond. 1979 (St. Bart.) DCH Glasgow; DRCOG Lond. Gen. Practitioner Chaddlewood Surg. Plympton. Prev: Trainee GP Saltash VTS.

ROBERT, Pratima Shalini 24A Tutbury Avenue, Cannonhill, Coventry CV4 7BJ Tel: 024 76 415631 — MB BS Nagpur 1965 (Nagpur Med. Coll.) DCH RCPS Glas. 1969. SCMO (Child Health) Coventry. Specialty: Community Child Health. Prev: Med. Off. Coventry AHA.

ROBERTON, Mary 24 Bertie Road, Cumnor, Oxford OX2 9PS Tel: 01865 862308 — MB BS Lond. 1963 (King's Coll. Hosp.) MRCS Eng. LRCP Lond. 1963; MRCPCH 1996. Community Paediat. & Occupat. Phys. Oxf. Specialty: Community Child Health. Socs: Fac. Community Health; BPA; ANHOPSOM.

ROBERTON, Norman Reid Clifford (retired) Sea Cottage, Lower Harrapool, Broadford, Isle of Skye IV49 9AQ Tel: 01471 822467 Fax: 01471 822095 — MB BChir Camb. 1964 (Camb. & Univ. Coll. Hosp.) MA, MB Camb. 1964, BChir 1963; FRCP Lond. 1979, M 1965. Prev: Cons. Paediat. Addenbrooke's Hosp. Camb. & Newmarket Gen. Hosp.

ROBERTS, Adam Paul 73 Dacre Park, London SE13 5BX — MB ChB Manch. 1993.

ROBERTS, Adrian 102 Cyncoed Road, Cardiff CF23 5SJ Tel: 029 2048 3005 — MB BCh BAO Belf. 1968; FRCOG 1989, M 1973. Cons. O & G Llandough Hosp. NHS Trust Penarth. Specialty: Obst. & Gyn. Prev: Lect. (O & G) Welsh Nat. Sch. Med. Cardiff.

ROBERTS, Adrian Bernard Government Buildings, Otley Road, Lawnswood, Leeds LS16 5PU — MB ChB Manch. 1973; DObst RCOG 1975; Cert. JCC Lond. 1977. Professional Support Manager, SchlumbergerSEma Med. Servs., Leeds. Specialty: Civil Serv. Prev: GP Leeds; SHO (O & G & Paediat.) Bolton Dist. Hosp.

ROBERTS, Adrian Brian Bowling Green Surgery, Bowling Green, Constantine, Falmouth TR11 5AP Tel: 01326 340666 Fax: 01326

340968 — MB ChB Bristol 1969; BSc Bristol 1965; DCH RCP Lond. 1971; MRCP (UK) 1973; DTM & H Liverp. 1978; FRCGP 1993, M 1979. Course Organiser Cornw. VTS. Prev: Cons. Phys. Gilbert & Ellice Is.s & Solomon Is.s.

ROBERTS, Alan Grove Medical Centre, 27 Grove Road, Wallasey CH45 3HE Tel: 0151 691 1112 Fax: 0151 637 0266; Grosvenor, 14 Linksview, Wallasey CH45 0NQ Tel: 0151 691 1112 Fax: 0151 637 0266 — MB ChB Liverp. 1975. Forens. Med. Examr. & Locality Facilitator Merseyside.

ROBERTS, Aled Wyn University Hospital of Wales, Ward B7, Health Park, Cardiff CF14 4XW Email: aledwynroberts@hotmail.com — MB BCh Wales 1996 (UWCM) MRCP, (Lond). Specilaist Regist. in Diabetes/Endocrinol./Internal Med., All Wales Higher Train. Progr. in Diabetes and Endocrinol. Specialty: Gen. Med.; Diabetes. Special Interest: PPAR Gamma.

ROBERTS, Alexandra Claire 14 Eewrland, Barnton, Edinburgh EH4 6DH — MB ChB Birm. 1996; ChB Birm. 1996.

ROBERTS, Alfred Edward (retired) 18 Riverview Crescent, Cardross, Dumbarton G82 5LT Tel: 01389 841007 — MB ChB Glas. 1957.

ROBERTS, Alice Mahala 8 Islivig, Wig, Isle of Lewis HS2 9HA — MB BS Newc. 1992; MRCPsych 1998. SHO (Psychiat.) & Prof. Cook St Martins Hosp. Canterbury; Specialist Regist. in old age Psychiat., Lewisham Hosp. Specialty: Geriat. Psychiat. Prev: SHO (Psychiat.) Bexley Hosp.; SHO (Psychiat.) S.W.ern UMDS Psychiat. Rotat.

ROBERTS, Alison Joan 121 Brookhouse Hill, Fulwood, Sheffield S10 3TE — MB ChB Sheff. 1996.

ROBERTS, Alison Margaret Idle Medical Centre, 440 Highfield ROAd, Idle, Bradford BD10 8RU Tel: 01274 771999 Fax: 01274 772001; 3 Beechwood Grove, Ilkley LS29 9AX Tel: 01943 600480 — MB BS Lond. 1981; MRCPsych 1985; MRCGP 1987. GP Idle Bradford.

ROBERTS, Amanda Jane Cardiff & District NHS Trust, Lansdowne Hospital, Sanatorillm, Canton, Cardiff CF1 8TE Tel: 029 2037 2451; 25 Lon-y-Fro, Pentyrch, Cardiff CF15 9TE — MB BCh Wales 1982 (Univ. Wales Sch. Med.) MRCGP 1986; DCH RCP Lond. 1996. SCMO (Audiol.) Cardiff Community Healthcare NHS Trust. Specialty: Audiol. Med. Socs: Roy. Coll. Paediat. & Child Health.

ROBERTS, Amanda Jane 36 Queen Alexandra Mansions, Judd St., London WC1H 9DQ — MB BChir Camb. 1982; MA Camb. 1983, MB BChir 1982. SHO (Gen. Med.) St. Stephens Hosp. Lond. Prev: Research Regist. (Genito-Urin. Med.) Middlx. Hosp. Lond.; SHO (Dermat.) Middlx. Hosp. Lond.; SHO (Genito-Urin. Med.) Middlx. Hosp. Lond.

ROBERTS, Mr Andrew Patrick Children's Unit, Robert Jones & Agnes Hunt Orthopaedic Hospital, Oswestry SY10 7AG Tel: 01691 404573 Fax: 01691 679471; Starlings Castle, Bron y Garth, Oswestry SY10 7NU Tel: 01691 718103 — MB ChB Birm. 1980; FRCS Eng. 1985; DM Nottm. 1991. Cons. Orthop. Surg. Robt. Jones & Agnes Hunt Orthop. Hosp. Oswestry. Specialty: Orthop. Socs: Fell. BOA; BMA; Eur. Soc. Movement Anal. in Childr. Prev: Sen. Regist. Rotat. (Orthop.) QMC Nottm.; Hon. Sen. Lect. Univ. Keele.

ROBERTS, Andrew Steven 18 Chantry Grove, Bristol BS11 0QH — MB ChB Liverp. 1994; DRCOG 1996. Vocational Trainee (Gen. Pract.) Southport Merseyside. Specialty: Gen. Pract.

ROBERTS, Angela Department of Dermatology, King Edward VII Hospital, Windsor SL4 3DP Tel: 01753 860441 Fax: 01753 636107; 111 Western Avenue, Woodley, Reading RG5 3BL — (Lond. Hosp.) MB BS Lond. 1970; DObst RCOG 1972; MRCP (UK) 1974. Cons. Dermat. King Edwd. VII Hosp. Windsor. Specialty: Dermat. Prev: Sen. Regist. (Dermat.) Char. Cross Hosp. Lond; Regist. (Dermat.) Roy. Berks. Hosp. Reading.

ROBERTS, Angela Judith Brent Child & Family Clinic, Warranty House, Dudden Hill Lane, London NW10 1DL Tel: 0208 208 7200 Fax: 0208 208 2635 — MB BS Lond. 1981 (Char. Cross) DCH RCP Lond. 1983; MRCPsych 1990. Specialty: Child & Adolesc. Psychiat. Prev: Sen. Regist. (Child & Adolesc. Psychiat.) Tavistock Clinic Lond.; Regist. Rotat. (Psychiat.) St. Mary's Hosp. Lond.; SHO & Regist. (Paediat.) Qu. Eliz. Hosp. Sick Childr. Lond.

ROBERTS, Angus Murray, RD The Sycamores, Rectory Road, Padworth Common, Reading RG7 4JD Tel: 0118 970 0021 Fax: 0118 970 0463 — (Guy's) MB BS Lond. 1965; MRCS Eng. LRCP Lond. 1965; FFOM RCP Lond. 1993; FRCP London 1999. Cons. Ocupational Phys.; Surg.Cdr. RNR. Specialty: Occupat. Health. Socs: Fell. Roy. Soc. Med.; Fell. Amer. Coll. Occupat. & Environm. Med.; Soc. Occupat. Med. Prev: Chief Med. Off. ICL; Med. Adviser Atomic Weapons Research Establishm. Aldermaston; Sen. Med. Off. Brit. Nuclear Fuels Ltd.

ROBERTS, Ann Whyteleafe Surgery, 19 Station Road, Whyteleafe CR3 0EP Tel: 01883 624181 Fax: 01883 622498; 3 Wheat Knoll, Kenley CR8 5JT Tel: 020 8645 0272 Email: drann@saqnet.co.uk — MB BS Lond. 1980 (Guy's Hospital) DRCOG 1983.

ROBERTS, Ann Gertrud Department of Psychiatry, Queen Elizabeth II Hospital, Howlands, Welwyn Garden City AL7 4HQ Fax: 01707 365169 — MB BS Lond. 1984; BA Camb. 1981; DCH RCP Lond. 1987; MRCGP 1988; DRCOG 1988; MRCPsych 1993. Cons. Gen. Adult Psychiat. QE2 Hosp. Welwyn Garden City. Special Interest: Liaison and Perinatal Psychiat.

ROBERTS, Anna Izabela 12 Clay Street, Burton-on-Trent DE15 9BB — BM BS Nottm. 1986.

ROBERTS, Anne Elizabeth Nursery Park Medical Group, Nursery Park, Ashington NE63 0HP; The Grange, Longhirst Road, Morpeth NE61 3LG — MB ChB Bristol 1980; MB ChB (Hons) Bristol 1980; MRCP (UK) 1983; DCH RCP Lond. 1983; DA Eng. 1984; DRCOG 1985. Prev: GP Retainer Morpeth.

ROBERTS, Anne Patricia 79 Kidbrooke Grove, London SE3 0LQ — MB BS Lond. 1960 (Univ. Coll. Hosp.) MRCS Eng. LRCP Lond. 1960; FRCOG 1979, M 1965. Cons. Gynaecologist, Lond. Indep. Hosp. Stepney Green; Hon. Specialist Dispensaire Francais, 6 Osnaburgh St. NW1 3DH. Specialty: Gynaecology. Prev: Cons. O & G Newham Gen. Hosp. Lond.

ROBERTS, Anthony Deans Guthrie Queens Hospital, Belvedere Road, Burton-on-Trent DE13 0RB Tel: 01283 566333 Fax: 01283 593037 Email: adgroberts@virgin.net — MB ChB Glas. 1977; MRCOG Lond. 1982; MD Glas. 1987; FRCOG Lond. 1995. Cons. O & G Qu.s Hosp. Burton upon Trent; Hon. Clin. Sen. Lect. Univ. of Birm.; RCOG Regional Adviser; Chairm. - Med. Staff Comm.- Qu.s Hosp. Specialty: Obst. & Gyn. Special Interest: Colposcopy; Gynae Oncol. Socs: Brit. Med. Assn. Prev: Sen. Regist. (O & G) Leicester Roy. Infirm.; Regist. (O & G) Qu. Mothers & Stobhill Hosps. Glas.; Clin. Teach. Univ. Leic. & Examr. Leics. Univ. Med. Sch.

ROBERTS, Anthony Herber 74 Harley Street, London W1G 7HQ Tel: 020 7580 0731 — MB BS Lond. 1959 (St. Thos.) MRCS Eng. LRCP Lond. 1959; DPM Eng. 1962; FRCP Lond. 1977, M 1964; PhD Lond. 1979, MD 1969. Cons. Neurol. Lond. Specialty: Neurol. Prev: Cons. Neurol. SE Thames Regional Neurol. Centre; Sen. Regist. (Neurol.) Lond. Hosp.; Regist. (Med.) St. Thos. Hosp. Lond.

ROBERTS, Mr Anthony Howard Norman Department of Plastic Surgery, Stoke Mandeville Hospital, Aylesbury HP21 8AL Tel: 01296 315116; The Old House, Whitchurch, Aylesbury HP22 4JX Tel: 01296 641232 Fax: 01296 641820 — BM BCh Oxf. 1972 (Cambridge/Oxford) BSc Leeds 1961; MA Camb. 1972, BA 1969; MA Oxf. 1971; FRCS Eng. 1976. Cons. Plastic & Hand Surg. Stoke Mandeville Hosp. Aylesbury; Dir. Research Stoke Mandeville Burns & Reconstruc. Surg. Research Trust; Civil.. Cons. Advis. Plastic Surg. RAF; Hon. Sen. Lect. Dept. Surg. UCL; Vis. Prof. Dept. Surg. Chinese Univ., Hong Kong. Specialty: Plastic Surg. Socs: Brit. Soc. Surg. of Hand & Mem .Brit. Assn. Plastic Surgs.; Brit. Burn Assn. (Exec. Cttee); Chairm. Burn Preven. (Cttee). Prev: Sen. Regist. (Plastic Surg.) St. Luke's Hosp. Bradford & St. Jas. Hosp. Leeds; Research Fell. (Microsurg.) St. Vincent's Hosp. Melbourne, Austral.; Cons. Plastic & Hand Surg. Stoke Mandeville Hosp. Aylesbury.

ROBERTS, Anthony John (retired) The Old Vicarage, Berry Pomeroy, Totnes TQ9 9LH; Hilden Hall, Hammersley Lane, Penn, High Wycombe HP10 8HE — MB BS Lond. 1968; DObst RCOG 1970.

ROBERTS, Anthony Philip Wyke Regis Health Centre, Portland Road, Wyke Regis, Weymouth DT4 9BE Tel: 01305 782226 Fax: 01305 760549; 2 Russell Avenue, Weymouth DT4 9RA — MB ChB Bristol 1979; DRCOG 1982. Prev: Med. Superinten. Methodist Hosp. Semonkong Lesotho Africa.

ROBERTS, Anthony Waldron Moore Street Health Centre, 77 Moore Street, Bootle L20 4SE Tel: 0151 944 1066 Fax: 0151 933 4715 — MB ChB Dundee 1978.

ROBERTS, Antony Paul 3 East Street, Wardle, Rochdale OL16 2EG — MB ChB Leeds 1984. Trainee GP Stepping Hill Hosp. Stockport VTS.

ROBERTS, Archibald Peter (retired) 19 The Shimmings, Boxgrove Road, Guildford GU1 2NG — MB BS Lond. 1946 (St. Thos.) FRCPCH; MRCS Eng. LRCP Lond. 1945; DCH Eng. 1946; FRCP Lond. 1975, M 1952. Prev: Cons. Paediat. Bradford & Airedale Hosp. Gps.

ROBERTS, Arthur Bodowen Surgery, Halkyn Road, Holywell CH8 7GA Tel: 01352 710529 Fax: 01352 710784 — MB ChB Liverp. 1969. Prev: SHO (Orthop.) Birkenhead Gen. Hosp.; Ho. Phys. & Ho. Surg. St. Catherine's Hosp. Birkenhead.

ROBERTS, Arthur Westwood (retired) The Surgery, 1 Ratcliffe Road, Atherstone CV9 1EY Tel: 01827 713664 Fax: 01827 713666; 2 Witherley Road, Atherstone CV9 1LY Tel: 01827 712119 — MB BS Lond. 1950 (King's Coll. Hosp.) MRCS Eng. LRCP Lond. 1950. Prev: Cas. Off. & Ho. Surg. King's Coll. Hosp.

ROBERTS, Austin Parry Department of Mental Health, Friarage Hospital, Northallerton DL6 1JG Tel: 01609 763438 Fax: 01609 778066 — MB BChir Camb. 1987; MA Camb. 1987; MRCPsych 1992. Cons. Psychiat. for Older People Friarage Hosp. Northallerton. Specialty: Geriat. Psychiat. Socs: Roy. Coll. Psychiatr.; BMA. Prev: Sen. Regist. (Psychiat.) Univ. Coll. Hosp. & Middlx. Hosp Lond.; SHO & Regist. Rotat. (Psychiat.) N. Yorks. Train. Scheme; Ho. Off. (Gen. Surg. & Urol.) Newmarket Gen. Hosp.

ROBERTS, Barbara Cecily The Lodge, 8 Drysgol Road, Radyr, Cardiff CF15 8BT Tel: 029 2084 2469 — (Cardiff) BSc Wales 1938, MB BCh 1941; DA Eng. 1945; FFA RCS Eng. 1953. Cons. Anaesth. Univ. Hosp. Wales (Cardiff) Gp. Hosps. Specialty: Anaesth. Socs: Assn. Anaesths.; Cardiff Med. Soc.; Fell. Roy. Soc. Med. Prev: Sen. Res. Anaesth. Co. Hosp. FarnBoro., Lond. Hosp. & Roy. Infirm.; Cardiff.

ROBERTS, Barbara Kathleen 2 Lesley Avenue, Canterbury CT1 3LF Tel: 01227 51072 — MB ChB Liverp. 1944; MRCS Eng. LRCP Lond. 1944.

ROBERTS, Beatrice Jane Number 18 Surgery, 18 Upper Oldfield Park, Bath BA23JZ Tel: 01225 427403; 15 Upper Oldfield Park, Bath BA2 3JX — MB BS Lond. 1987; DRCOG 1991; MRCGP 1992. p/t Returner GP. Specialty: Gen. Pract. Socs: BMA. Prev: GP Gable House Surgery, Malmesbury.

ROBERTS, Bernard Lyall 88 Corringham Road, London NW11 7EB — MB ChB Manch. 1973; FRCPsych 19896, M 1979. Cons. Psychotherapist Brent Kensington Chelsea & Westminster Ment. NHS; Cons. Psychotherapist St Geo.s & SW Thames Ment. Health NHS Trust. Specialty: Psychother. Socs: Brit. Psychoanal. Soc. Prev: Sen. Regist. (Psychother.) Tavistock Clinic Lond. & Cassel Hosp. Richmond; Regist. (Psychiat.) Lond. Hosp.; Cons. Psychother. & Med. Dir. Kingston & Kingston & Dist. Community NHS Trust.

ROBERTS, Bethan Non 226 Caerphilly Road, Cardiff CF14 4NR — MB BCh Wales 1991.

ROBERTS, Bryn Merllyn, Henllan, Denbigh LL16 5DF — MB BCh Wales 1987.

ROBERTS, Mr Carl Jessamine House, Hamsterley, Bishop Auckland DL13 3QF — MB BS Newc. 1970; FRCS Eng. 1975. Cons. Urol. Bishop Auckland Gen. Hosp. & Univ. Hosp. Of N. Durh.. Durh. Specialty: Urol. Socs: BMA; Brit. Assn. Urol. Surgs. Prev: Sen. Regist. (Gen. Surg. & Urol.) Newc. Hosps.; Regist. (Gen. Surg.) Norwich Hosps.; Research Fell. Univ. Calif. San Francisco, USA.

ROBERTS, Caroline Anne Thorkhill Road Surgery, 115A Thorkhill Road, Thames Ditton KT7 0UW Tel: 020 8398 3141 Fax: 020 8398 7836 — MB BS Lond. 1977 (St. Mary's) DCH Eng. 1980; MRCGP 1982; DGM RCP Lond. 1986.

ROBERTS, Caroline Evelyn Ann St Peter's Medical Centre, 30-36 Oxford Street, Brighton BN1 4LA Tel: 01273 606006 Fax: 01273 623896; 18 Tongdean Avenue, Hove BN3 6TL — MB BS Lond. 1968; MRCS Eng. LRCP Lond. 1968; MFFP 1993. Tutor Family Plann. JCC. Prev: SHO (Paediat.) W. Middlx. Hosp. Isleworth; SHO (Gyn.) St. Olave's Hosp. Lond.; SHO (Obst.) Roy. Sussex Co. Hosp. Brighton.

ROBERTS, Miss Catharine Helen Homerton Hospital, Homerton Road, London E9 6SR Tel: 020 8510 7595 Fax: 020 8510 7787 Email: cathy.roberts@homerton.nhs.uk — MB BS Lond. 1990 (University of London) MRCOG 1995. Cons. Obst. and Gynaecologist, Homerton Hosp., Lond. Specialty: Obst. & Gyn.

ROBERTS, Catherine Elizabeth Patricia (retired) Clinton House, 31 Trefusis Road, Flushing, Falmouth TR11 5TZ — MB ChB Glas. 1943. Prev: Clin. Med. Off. Kent HA.

ROBERTS, Catherine Jane Riversdale Surgery, 51 Woodcroft Road, Wylam NE41 8DH Tel: 01661 852208 Fax: 01661 853779; 6 Village W., Ryton Old Village, Ryton NE40 3QD — BM BS Nottm. 1985; BMedSci Nottm. 1983; DRCOG 1988; MRCGP 1989. Specialty: Gen. Pract.

ROBERTS, Catherine Louise Dept. of Radiology, Huddersfield Royal Infirmary, Acre Street, Lindley, Huddersfield HD3 3EA — MB BS Newc. (Honours) 1990 (Newc. u. Tyne) MRCP (UK) 1993; FRCR 1996. Cons. Radiol., Radiol. Dept. Huddersfield Roy. Infirm. Specialty: Radiol. Prev: Specialist Regist. (Radiol.) Leeds & Bradford Scheme; SHO Rotat. (Med.) Newc. HA.

ROBERTS, Mr Ceri Department of Otorhinolaryngology, Princess of Wales Hospital, Coity Road, Bridgend CF31 1RQ — MB BS Lond. 1978; FRCS Ed. 1985. Specialty: Otorhinolaryngol.

ROBERTS, Charles Andrew — MB ChB Manch. 1988; BSc (Hons.) (Physiol.) Wales 1977; MSc (Physiol.) Aberd. 1979; DCH RCP Lond. 1990; DRCOG 1992; MRCGP 1992. Prev: Clin. Asst. (Dermat.) Leighton Hosp. Crewe.

ROBERTS, Charles Christopher Nicholson Sarum House Surgery, 3 St. Ethelbert Street, Hereford HR1 2NS Tel: 01432 265422 Fax: 01432 358440 — MB BChir Camb. 1966 (Middlx.) MA, MB Camb. 1966, BChir 1965; DObst RCOG 1968. Socs: BMA. Prev: Res. Med. Off. King Edwd. VII Memor. Hosp. Bermuda; Ho. Surg. (Obst.) Whittington Hosp. Lond.; Ho. Surg. Middlx. Hosp. Lond.

ROBERTS, Christine 27A Shirley Drive, Hove BN3 6NQ — MB ChB Birm. 1985; ChB Birm. 1985. GP Hove Retainer Scheme.

ROBERTS, Christopher David Palace Road Surgery, 3 Palace Road, London SW2 3DY Tel: 020 8674 2083 Fax: 020 8674 6040 — MB BS Lond. 1971; DObst RCOG 1973. Socs: BMA. Prev: SHO (O & G & Cas.) Whipps Cross Hosp. Lond.; SHO (Paediat.) Paddington Green Childr. Hosp. Lond.

ROBERTS, Christopher James Department of Anaesthesia, Gloucester Royal Hospital, Gloucester GL1 3NN Tel: 01452 528555 Fax: 01452 394249 — BM BCh Oxf. 1980; BA Camb. 1977; FFA RCS Eng. 1988. Cons. Anaesth. & Intens. Care Glos. Roy. Hosp. Specialty: Anaesth. Socs: Intens. Care Soc.; Assn. Anaesth. of GB & Irel.; BMA. Prev: Sen. Regist. Nuffield Dept. Anaesth. Oxf.; Regist. (Anaesth.) Bristol & Weston Hosps.; Anaesth. Project Orbis Inc. New York, USA.

ROBERTS, Christopher Mark — MB BS Lond. 1991; MRCPsych 1995.

ROBERTS, Professor Christopher Michael Whipps Cross University Hospital, Chest Clinic, London E11 1NR Tel: 020 8535 6782 Fax: 020 8535 6709; St Bartholomew's Hospital, Queen Mary Westfield Bart's & The London Medical College, Robin Brooke Centre, West Smithfield, London EC1A — MB ChB Liverp. 1980; MRCP (UK) 1983; MD Liverp. 1992; FRCP Lond. 1996; MA (Med. Educat. (Distinction)) APU 2004. Cons. Phys. Thoracic Med. Whipps Cross Univ. Hosp. Lond.; Prof. of Med. Educat. for Clin. Pract.; Dir. Med. Educat. Forest Healthcare Trust; Assoc. Director Clin. Effectiveness Unit, Roy. Coll. of Physicans of Lond.. Specialty: Respirat. Med. Special Interest: COPD; Med. Educat. Socs: Brit. Thorac. Soc.; Mem. Audit Sub Comm.; Inst. Learning & Teachg. Higher Educat. Prev: Sen. Regist. (Thoracic Med.) Univ. Coll. & Lond. Chest Hosps.; Sen. Regist. St Vincents Hosp. Sydney; Hon. Sen. Lect. St. Bart Hosp. Med. Coll.

ROBERTS, Christopher Michael The Surgery, Gaywood House, North St, Bedminster, Bristol BS3 3AZ Tel: 0117 966 1412 Fax: 0117 953 1250; Battens House, Jacklands Bridge, Tickenham, Clevedon BS21 6SG — MRCS Eng. LRCP Lond. 1973; LMSSA Lond. 1973. Prev: Trainee GP Bristol VTS; Regist. (Anaesth.) Bristol Roy. Infirm.; Chief Med. Off. Anguilla, W. Indies.

ROBERTS, Christopher Paul 14 Wimbish Road, Papworth Everard, Cambridge CB3 8XJ — MB BS Lond. 1992 (UMDS) FRCS Eng. 1996. Specialty: Orthop.

ROBERTS, Clare Judith Southampton Eye Unit, Southampton General Hospital, Tremona Road, Southampton SO16 6YD; Flat 12 Pavilion Court, 74 Northlands Road, Southampton SO15 2NN — BM BCh Oxf. 1991; MA Camb. 1992; FRCOphth 1995. Regist. Soton. Eye Unit Soton. Gen. Hosp. Specialty: Ophth.

ROBERTS, Clive John Charlton Centre for medical Education, 39 - 41 St Michael's Hill, Bristol BS2 8DZ Tel: 0117 954 6513 Fax: 0117 954 6514 Email: c.j.c.roberts@bristol.ac.uk; Clapton Wick

Farm, Clevedon Lane, Clevedon BS21 7AG Tel: 01275 852403 — MD Bristol 1979 (King's Coll. Hosp.) MB BS Lond 1969; MRCS Eng. LRCP Lond 1969; MRCP UK 1973; FRCP Lond 1987; ILTM (Inst. Of Learning & Teaching) 2001. Sen. Lect. (Clin. Pharmacol.)/Clin. Dean Bristol Univ.; Hon. Cons. Phys. Bristol Roy. Infirm. Specialty: Pharmacology; Gen. Med. Socs: Brit. Pharm. Soc.; Assn. For Med. Educat. In Europe. Prev: Regional Adviser (SW) Roy. Coll. Phys.; Asst. Lect. (Clin. Pharmacol.) Lond. Hosp. Med. Coll.; Regist. (Med.) Plymouth Gen. Hosp.

ROBERTS, Clive Julian Thornbury Health Centre, Eastland Road, Thornbury, Bristol BS35 1DP Tel: 01454 412599 Fax: 01454 41911 — MB ChB Bristol 1985; BSc (Hons.) Bristol 1982, MB ChB (Hons.) 1985; DRCOG 1987; MRCGP 1989. Prev: Trainee GP Bristol VTS; SHO (Obst.) Bristol Matern. Hosp.; SHO (Psychiat. & Geriat.) Ham Green Hosp. Bristol.

ROBERTS, Professor Colin Microbiol. Dept., Level 6, The John Radcliffe Hospital, Oxford OX3 9DU Tel: 01865 220886 Fax: 01865 220890 Email: colin.roberts@orh.nhs.uk — MB ChB Liverp. 1963; FFPHM; BSc Liverp. 1960, MD 1968; Dip. Bact. Manch. 1972; FRCPath 1986, M 1973; FRCP (UK) 1999. M RCP 1996; FRCPCH (Hon.) 1996; FFpath (I) 2000. Locum Cons. John Radcliffe Hosp, Oxf.; Vis. Prof. Univ. Strathclyde; Vis. Prof. Lond. Sch. of Trop. Med. and Hyg.. Specialty: Med. Microbiol. Socs: (Pres.) Assn. Med. Microbiol. Prev: Med. & Scientif. Postgrad.Deran Pub. Health Lab Serv. Lond; Dep. Dir. PHLS; Cons. Med. Microbiol. & Sen. Microbiol. Pub. Health Laborat. Liverp.

ROBERTS, Professor Colin John (retired) Department Epidemiology & Public Health, University of Wales, College of Medicine, Heath Park, Cardiff CF14 4XN Tel: 029 2075 0435 Fax: 029 2074 2898; Exmoor, 10 Llangorse Road, Cyncoed, Cardiff CF23 6PF Tel: 029 2075 4748 Fax: 029 2076 1076 — MRCS Eng. LRCP Lond. 1958 (Birm.) MD Birm. 1966, MB ChB 1958; DObst RCOG 1960; DPH Wales 1964; PhD Wales 1970; FFPHM 1977, M 1974; FRCR 1984. Prof. Epidemiol. & Pub. Health Univ. Wales Coll. Med. Cardiff; Hon. Cons. Pub. Health Med. S. Glam. HA (T). Prev: Sen. Lect. Univ. Wales Coll. Med. Cardiff.

ROBERTS, Dafydd Llewelyn Lloyd Singleton Hospital, Department of Dermatology, Sketty, Swansea SA2 8QA Tel: 01792 285324 Email: dafydd.roberts@swansea-tr.wales.nhs.uk — MB BS Lond. 1972 (Lond. Hosp.) MRCP (UK) 1975; FRCP Lond. 1994. Cons. Dermatol. Swansea NHS Trust. Specialty: Dermat. Special Interest: Malig. Melanoma; Pigmented Lesions; Skin Cancer. Socs: Fell. RSM; Fell. Amer. Acad. Dermat.; Brit. Assn. Dermat. Prev: Sen. Regist. (Dermat.) N. Staffs. Hosp. Centre Stoke-on-Trent; Regist. (Dermat. & Gen. Med.) Univ. Hosp. Wales, Cardiff; Med. Off. King Edwd. VII Memor. Hosp. Bermuda.

ROBERTS, David Arthur Thomas Gwyninydd, Gorrig Road, Llandysul SA44 4LF — MB ChB Birm. 1973.

ROBERTS, David Edward X-Ray Department, Morriston Hospital, Swansea SA6 6NL Tel: 01792 703636 — MB BCh Wales 1986; DMRD Liverp. 1991; FRCR 1993. Cons. Radiol. Morriston Hosp. Swansea. Specialty: Radiol.

ROBERTS, David Frost St Mark's Dee View Surgery, Church Street, Connah's Quay, Deeside CH5 4AD Tel: 01244 812003 Fax: 01244 822609 — MB BCh Wales 1977.

ROBERTS, David Gareth Vaughan Wendover, 170 Downend Road, Bristol BS16 5EB — MB BS Lond. 1976; MRCP (UK) 1981. Cons. Paediat. Community Child Health Frenchay Health Care Trust Bristol. Specialty: Paediat. Prev: SCMO Frenchay HA; Lect. (Child Health) Univ. Bristol; Regist. Birm. Childr. Hosp.

ROBERTS, David Geoffrey St Thomas Road Surgery, St. Thomas Road, Featherstone, Pontefract WF7 5HE Tel: 01977 792212 Fax: 01977 600278 — MB ChB Sheff. 1982.

ROBERTS, David Griffith Ty Isa, Corwen LL21 9EF Tel: 01490 2412 — MRCS Eng. LRCP Lond. 1943.

ROBERTS, David Hesketh Victoria Hospital, Whinney Heys Rd, Blackpool FY3 8NR Tel: 01253 303611 Fax: 01253 306941 — MB BCh Wales 1978; MRCP (UK) 1981; MD Liverp. 1991; FESC 1999; FRCP 1999; FACC 1999. Cons. Cardiol., Blackpool. Specialty: Cardiol. Socs: Brit. Hypertens. Soc. & Brit. Pacing & Electrophysiol. Gp.; Mem. of Brit. Cardiac Soc.; Fell. of Amer. Coll. of Cardiol. Prev: Sen. Regist. (Cardiol.) Qu. Eliz. Hosp. Birm.; Regist. (Cardiol.) Regional Cardiac Unit Broadgreen Hosp. Liverp.; Lect. (Clin. Pharmacol. & Therap.) Univ. Liverp.

ROBERTS, David Hywel Griffith Great Staughton Surgery, 57 The Highway, Great Staughton, Huntingdon PE19 5DA Tel: 01480 860770 Fax: 01480 861514 — MB ChB Manch. 1982; BSc St. And. 1979; DRCOG 1985; MRCGP 1986. GP; Mem. Caring Professions Concern; Princip. Police Surg. Cambridgeshire. Specialty: Gen. Pract. Socs: BMA. Prev: Princip. GP Altrincham Chesh.; Trainee GP Univ. Manch. Dept. Gen. Pract. VTS; Trainee GP Tameside Gen. Hosp. VTS.

ROBERTS, David John Molecular Parasitology Group, Institute of Molecular Medicine, John Radcliffe Hospital, Headington, Oxford OX3 9DU Tel: 01865 222302 Fax: 01865 222444; 3 Fulwell, Chipping Norton OX7 4EN Tel: 01608 677125 — MB ChB Liverp. 1983; DPhil Liverp. 1994, MB ChB 1983; MRCP (UK) 1986; DTM & H Liverp. 1989. Hon. Sen. Regist. (Haemat.) John Radcliffe Hosp. Oxf.; Wellcome Fellowship Inst. of Molecular Med. John Radcliffe Hosp. Oxf. Specialty: Trop. Med. Prev: Regist. (Haemat.) Roy. Liverp. Hosp.; Ho. Off. (Profess. Med. & Surg. Units) Roy. Liverp. Hosp.; SHO (Gen. Med.) Walton & Fazakerley Hosps.

ROBERTS, David Lloyd Oak Hill Health Centre, Oak Hill Road, Surbiton KT6 6EN Tel: 020 8399 6622 Fax: 020 8390 4470; 18 The Ridge, Surbiton KT5 8HX — MB ChB Manch. 1961; DObst RCOG 1967. Clin. Asst. Endoscopy Unit Kingston Hosp. Surrey. Prev: Clin. Asst. (Surg.) Surbiton Gen. Hosp.; SHO (Neurosurg. & Plastic Surg.) Frenchay Hosp. Bristol; Ho. Surg. (Orthop.) Manch. Roy. Infirm.

ROBERTS, Mr David Michael Stepping Stones, 9 Over Lane, Almondsbury, Bristol BS32 4BL — MB BS Lond. 1963 (King's Coll. Lond. & Liverp.) MRCS Eng. LRCP Lond. 1963; DObst RCOG 1965; FRCS Eng. 1970; DIH Eng. 1982; MFOM RCP Lond. 1983, A 1982. Sen. Med. Off. Rolls-Royce Plc. Socs: Soc. Occupat. Med. & Brit. Occupat. Hyg. Soc. Prev: Sen. Med. Adviser Standard Telephones & Cables Plc.; Dep. Med. Dir. Harlow Indust. Health Serv.

ROBERTS, David Michael, Maj.-Gen. late RAMC Retd. (retired) — MB BS Lond. 1954 (Roy. Free) FRCP Ed. 1975, M 1965; MD Lond. 1971; FRCP Lond. 1985, M 1978. Prev: Dir. of Army Med. & Cons. Phys. to Army.

ROBERTS, David Michael Rosebank Surgery, 153B Stroud Road, Gloucester GL1 5JQ Tel: 01452 543000 Fax: 01452 387807 Email: mike.roberts@gp-l84050.nhs.uk; 90 Hucclecote Road, Hucclecote, Gloucester GL3 3RU Tel: 01452 547566 — MB ChB Bristol 1982; Family planning diploma 1988; DRCOG 1988; T(GP) 1991. Gen. practitioner, Rosebank health; Chair Glos. + S. Tewkesbury PCG. Prev: SHO (Med. & Anaesth.) Glos. Roy. Hosp.

ROBERTS, David Michael (retired) 27 Huntsmans Corner, Wrexham LL12 7UE Tel: 01978 364307 — MB ChB Birm. 1963; DObst RCOG 1965; FFOM RCP Lond. 1994, MFOM 1986, AFOM 1984. Prev: Ho. Surg., Ho. Phys. & Ho. Surg. (O & G) Manor Hosp. Walsall.

ROBERTS, Mr David Newton 55 Harley Street, London W1G 8QR Tel: 020 7580 1481 Fax: 020 7631 0807 Email: dr@easynet.co.uk — MB BS Lond. 1987 (St. Thomas') BSc (Anat.) Lond. 1984, MB BS 1987; FRCS (Gen. Surg.) Lond. 1992; FRCS (Otol.) Lond. 1993; FRCS (Orl) 1996. Cons., Otorhubinolaryng., GUYs & St Thomas NHS Trust; Hon.Cons. King Edwd. V11's (Sister Agnes). Specialty: Otorhinolaryngol. Socs: Europ. Acad. of Facial Plastic Surg.. (Bd. Mem.); Europ. Rhinological Soc. (Mem.). Prev: Research Fell. Roy. Postgrad. Med. Sch. Hammersmith Hosp. Lond.; Fell. (Facial Plastic Surg.) The Europ. Acad. of Facial Plastic Surg.; Sen. Regist. (Otorhinolaryngol.) Roy. Nat. Throat, Nose & Ear Hosp. Lond.

ROBERTS, David Powys Wynn 8 Trefonwys, Bangor LL57 2HU — MB ChB Birm. 1952; MRCS Eng. LRCP Lond. 1953; DObst RCOG 1955; DPH Liverp. 1957; MFCM 1974. Specialist in Community Med. Gwynedd AHA. Socs: BMA. Prev: MOH West. Flints. CC; Dep. MOH Blackpool; Asst. MOH Chester.

ROBERTS, David Robert Ainsley 126 Crossbrook Street, Cheshunt, Waltham Cross EN8 8JH; 55 Trinity Street, Enfield EN2 6NT — MB BS Lond. 1992.

ROBERTS, David Ronald Digby Freeman Hospital, High Heaton, Newcastle upon Tyne NE7 7DN Tel: 0191 223 1304 Fax: 0191 223 1337 — MB ChB Manch. 1981 (Manchester) BSc (Hons.) Physiol. Manch. 1978, MB ChB 1981; FRCA 1988. Cons. Anaesth. Freeman Hosp. Specialty: Anaesth. Prev: Sen. Regist. Newc.; Regist. & SHO (Anaesth.) RN; Med. Off. Roy. Marines.

ROBERTS, Mr David St Clair (retired) Beechfield, 25 Bolnore Road, Haywards Heath RH16 4AB Tel: 01444 413507 — BM BCh Oxf. 1945; MA, BM BCh Oxf. 1945; FRCS Eng. (Ophth.) 1956; FCOphth 1989. Mem. Oxf. Ophth. Congr. Prev: Mem. Ct. of Examrs. RCS Eng.

ROBERTS, David Thomas 282 Ladybrook Lane, Mansfield NG19 6QL — MB BS Lond. 1980; MRCPsych 1988.

ROBERTS, David Trevor Southern General Hospital, 1345 Govan Rd, Glasgow G51 4TF Tel: 0141 201 1567 Fax: 0141 201 2990; 17c Mains Avenue, Glasgow G46 6QY Tel: 0141 638 8258 — MB ChB Glas. 1970; MRCP (UK) 1973; FRCP Glas. 1984. Cons. Dermat. South. Gen. Hosp. & Vict. Infirm. Glas.; Hon. Sen. Lect. Univ. Glas. Specialty: Dermat. Prev: Cons. Dermat. West. Infirm. & Roy. Hosp. Sick Childr. Glas.; Sen. Regist. (Dermat.) Roy. Infirm. Glas.; Regist. (Dermat.) West. Infirm. Glas.

ROBERTS, Derrick (retired) 340 Upper Richmond Road, Putney, London SW15 6TL Tel: 020 8788 0686 — MB BS Lond. 1954 (St. Geo.) MRCS Eng. LRCP Lond. 1954. Prev: Ho. Surg. Vict. Hosp. Childr. Lond.

ROBERTS, Devender 12 Elmsdale Road, Liverpool L18 1LX — MB ChB Liverp. 1989; MRCOG 1995. Lect., Univ. Dept. of (O & G), Univ. of Liverp., Liverp. Wom.'s Hosp. Specialty: Obst. & Gyn. Prev: Specialist Regist., Mersey Rotat.; SHO Countess of Chester Hosp.

ROBERTS, Dewi Wyn (retired) Derwen Deg, Hwfa Road, Bangor LL57 2BN — MB BChir Camb. 1965 (Westm.) MRCS Eng. LRCP Lond. 1964; MA Camb. 1965. Prev: GP Daventry.

ROBERTS, Diana Mary Bron Heulog, Four Mile Bridge, Holyhead LL65 2HX — MB BS Newc. 1972; MRCGP.

ROBERTS, Dilys Yvonne 7 Fieldside, Hawarden, Deeside CH5 3JB — MB BCh Wales 1977.

ROBERTS, Donald James (retired) Wild Acre, 15 Ashley Drive N., Ashley Heath, Ringwood BH24 2JL Tel: 01425 471624 — (Camb. & Guy's) MRCS Eng. LRCP Lond. 1954; MB BChir Camb. 1956; MA Camb. 1956; DPH Leeds 1959; FFCM 1980, M 1972; FFPHM 1989. Prev: DMO St. Helens & Knowsley HA.

ROBERTS, Doreen Jean Central Manchester Primary Care Trust, Mauldeth House, Mauldeth Road South, Manchester M21 7RL; 3 Linden Road, Manchester M20 2QJ Tel: 0161 445 4308 — MB ChB Manch. 1964; MSc (Clin. Audiol.) Manch. 1987, BSc (Hons. Anat.) 1961. Cons. Audiological Phys. Centr. Manch. PCT. Socs: Fell. Manch. Med. Soc. Prev: SCMO (Audiol. Med.) S. Mancunian Community Health NHS Trust; SHO (Geriat.) Barnes Hosp. Manch.; Family Plann. Assn. Clinic Doctor.

ROBERTS, Dorothy Margaret Haver, OStJ (retired) Field Barn Farm, Hampton Poyle, Kidlington OX5 2PY Tel: 01865 374773 — MB BS Durh. 1955; MRCS Eng. LRCP Lond. 1955; DPH Bristol 1968; MFCM 1974. Prev: PMO Oxf. Health Auth.

ROBERTS, Dubravka Stefica 19 Woodhall Lane, Balsham, Cambridge CB1 6DT — MB ChB Birm. 1980; MRCP (UK) 1985. Specialty: Paediat. Prev: Sen. Regist. (Paediat.) Addenbrooke's Hosp. Camb.

ROBERTS, Edward Morgan Fairfield Medical Centre, Julian Terrace, Port Talbot SA12 6UQ Tel: 01639 890916; 7 Tenacre Wood, Margam, Port Talbot SA13 2SU Tel: 01639 897706 — (Welsh National School of Medicine) MB BCh Wales 1970; MRCGP 1977; FRCGP 1996. Chairm. Neath Port Talbot LHB; Trust Practitioner (Geriat.) Bromorgannwg NHS Trust. Specialty: Gen. Pract.; Care of the Elderly. Socs: BMA (Ex-Chairm. W. Glam. Div.). Prev: CME Tutor Neath Postgrad. Centre; Course Organiser Neath Postgrad.; Chairm. & Sec. W. Glam. LMC (Ex. Mem. W. Glam. FPC).

ROBERTS, Edwin George Gerald (retired) Marford Gate, Marford, Wrexham LL12 8SF Tel: 01978 852217 — MRCS Eng. LRCP Lond. 1945 (Cardiff) BSc (Distinc. Anat.) 1941, MB BCh Wales 1944; FRCP Lond. 1971, M 1947; DCH Eng. 1949; FRCPCH 1997. Cons. Paediat. Clwyd & Powys AHAs, Wrexham; Hon. Cons. Paediat. Robt. Jones & Agnes Hunt Orthop. Hosp. Oswestry. Prev: Regist. (Paediat.) Roy. Infirm. Cardiff.

ROBERTS, Eiry Wyn Lilly Research Centre Ltd., Erlwood Manor, Windlesham GU20 6PH — MB BS Lond. 1987 (St. Bart. Med. Coll.) BSc (Pharmacol.) Lond. 1983; MRCP (UK) 1990; Dip. Pharm. Med. RCP (UK) 1994. Dir. Clin. Pharmacol. (Europe) Lilly Research Centre Ltd. Surrey. Specialty: Pharmacology. Socs: Roy. Soc. Med.

ROBERTS, Elaine Quarry Farm, Sandy Lane N., Irbymill Hill, Irby, Wirral L61 4XW — MB ChB Liverp. 1986. Clin. Med. Off. (Paediat.) Liverp. HA.

ROBERTS, Elisabeth Damaris (retired) 31 Park Gates Drive, Cheadle Hulme, Cheadle SK8 7DD Tel: 0161 485 4975 Email: damaris_roberts@hotmail.com — (Manch.) MB ChB Manch. 1956; DA Eng. 1959. Prev: Clin. Med. Off. S. Manch. HA.

ROBERTS, Elizabeth Jane Queen Marys Sidcup NHS Trust, Sidcup DA14 6LT Tel: 020 8302 2678 Fax: 020 8308 3052 Email: elizabeth.roberts@gns.nhs.uk — BM Soton. 1978 (Univ. Soton.) FFA RCS Eng. 1985. Cons. Anaesth. Qu. Mary's Hosp. Sidcup. Specialty: Anaesth. Socs: Obsteric Anaesthetics Assn.; H.C.S.A; B.M.A. Prev: Sen. Regist. Rotat. (Anaesth) Soton. Gen. Hosp. & Roy. Hants. Co. Hosp. Winchester.

ROBERTS, Elizabeth June Dunchurch Surgery, Dunsmore Heath, Dunchurch, Rugby CV22 6AP Tel: 01788 522448 Fax: 01788 814609 — BM Soton. 1987; MRCGP 1991 (Southampton)

ROBERTS, Elizabeth Merryl Plains View Surgery, 57 Plains Rd, Mapperley, Nottingham NG3 5LB Tel: 0115 962 1717; 8 Highcroft, Woodthorpe, Nottingham NG3 5LP Tel: 0115 967 0613 — MB ChB Manch. 1989; BSc St. And. 1986; MRCGP 1996. GP Retainer, Plains View Surg. Nottm.; Salaried GP, Plains View Surgery. Socs: Roy. Coll. of Gen. Practitioners. Prev: Trainee GP Stockport; SHO (O & G) Hope Hosp. Manch.; GP Retainer.

ROBERTS, Elizabeth St Clair (retired) Beechfield, 25 Bolnore Road, Haywards Heath RH16 4AB Tel: 01444 413507 — BM BCh Oxf. 1945; MA, BM BCh Oxon. 1945; DCH Eng. 1948. Prev: Clin. Asst. (Dermat.) Brighton & Cuckfield & Crawley Health Dists.

ROBERTS, Elved Bryn — MB ChB Liverp. 1993; MRCP (UK) 1997. Specialist Regist. (Cardiol.) Mersey Region. Specialty: Cardiol. Socs: BMA.

ROBERTS, Elwyn Bron Derw, Garth Road, Bangor LL57 2RS Tel: 01248 370900; Cil-y-Bont, Treborth Road, Bangor LL57 2RJ Tel: 01248 353312 — MB BCh Wales 1959 (Cardiff) DPH 1962; DObst RCOG 1964. Socs: BMA. Prev: Ho. Surg. ENT & Ophth. Depts. Cardiff Roy. Infirm.; SHO (Paediat.) & Ho. Surg. (Obst.) St. David's Hosp. Bangor.

ROBERTS, Eric Lloyd (retired) Lower Hisley, Lustleigh, Newton Abbot TQ13 9SH Tel: 0164 77 389 — MB ChB Liverp. 1923. Prev: Ho. Surg. Roy. Liverp. Childr. Hosp. & Special Depts. Liverp. Roy.

ROBERTS, Eric Lloyd Kyle Firth, Lon-y-Bryn, Treardour Bay, Anglesey LL65 2BQ Tel: 01407 860619; Euron, 1 Garth Drive, Gaerwen LL60 6DH Tel: 01248 421683 — MB ChB Liverp. 1962. Prev: SHO Radiol. Liverp. Roy. Infirm. Ho. Phys. Wiston Hosp. Prescot; Ho. Surg. Ormskirk & Dist. Gen. Hosp.

ROBERTS, Ernest Forbes (retired) 90 Park Road, London W4 3HL Tel: 020 8995 2583 — LMSSA Lond. 1944 (Camb. & St. Geo.) MA Camb. 1943; MRCGP 1953. Prev: GP Lond.

ROBERTS, Ernest Theodore (retired) The Torrs, 101 Havant Road, East Cosham, Portsmouth PO6 2JE Tel: 023 9237 9726 — MB BChir Camb. 1947 (Camb. & St. Thos.) BA Camb. 1944, MA 1949, MB BChir 1947. Prev: Cas. Off. & Ho. Phys. St. Thos. Hosp.

ROBERTS, Fiona 17 Kirklee Circus, Glasgow G12 0TW Email: froberts@cableinet.co.uk; f.roberts@spr.co.uk — MB ChB Glas. 1991 (Glasgow) BSc Glas. 1989, MB ChB 1991; Dip RCPath 1995; MRCPath Glas. 1998; MD 1998. Cons. Dept. Path. Vict. Infirm. Glas. Specialty: Histopath.

ROBERTS, Fiona Cookridge Hospital, Leeds LS16 6QB Tel: 0113 392 4428 — MB BS Lond. 1981; MA (Hons.) Camb. 1981; MRCP (UK) 1985; FRCR 1990; MD Lond. 1994. Cons. Clin. Oncol. Cookridge Hosp. Leeds. Specialty: Oncol.; Radiother.

ROBERTS, Fiona Edith Vivian (retired) Whitchurch Surgery, 49 Oving Road, Whitchurch, Aylesbury HP22 4JF Tel: 01296 641203 Fax: 01296 640021; The Old House, Whitchurch, Aylesbury HP22 4JX Tel: 01296 641232 Fax: 01296 641820 — MB BS Lond. 1968 (St. Bart.) MRCS Eng. LRCP Lond. 1968; DObst RCOG 1971; DCH RCP Lond. 1973; MRCGP 1975.

ROBERTS, Fleur Elizabeth 157 Quinton Road, Harborne, Birmingham B17 0PY — MB ChB Birm. 1997; ChB Birm. 1997.

ROBERTS, Francis Paul Washford House, Claybrook Drive, Redditch B98 0DU Tel: 01527 517747 Fax: 01527 525934 — MB ChB Birm. 1967 (Birmingham) MRCS Eng. LRCP Lond. 1967; DIH Eng. 1979; FFOM RCP Lond. 1993, MFOM 1984. Director, Med. Serv.s, Marsh Heath Ltd (UK). Specialty: Occupat. Health. Socs: Soc.

Occupat. Med.; Fell., Roy. Soc. of Med. Prev: Sen. Employm. Med. Adviser to the Health & Safety Exec. W. Midl.; Company Med. Adviser Lucas Elec. Ltd. Birm.; Health Progr. Manager & Sen. Med. Adviser Lucas Varity plc Solihull.

ROBERTS, Frederick David (retired) 5 Manor Farm Close, Gate Lane, Broughton, Kettering NN14 1SL Tel: 01536 791515 Email: davidroberts@doctors.org.uk — (Leeds) MRCS Eng. LRCP Lond. 1967; DObst RCOG 1972. p/t Indep. Dispensing Cons.; Edr. Non-Princip., Locum GP. Prev: SHO (Paediat.) Herts. & Essex Gen. Hosp. Bishop's Stortford.

ROBERTS, Frederick John (retired) Hilltop, 2 West Road, Prenton, Prenton CH43 9RP Tel: 0151 677 4087 Email: fj.roberts@ntlworld.com — MD Bristol 1974 (K.C.H.) MB BS Lond. 1956; MRCS Eng. LRCP Lond. 1956; DPM Durham. 1960; FRCP Ed. 1982, M 1961; FRACP 1978; FRANZCP 1979; FRCPsych. 1979. Prev: Prof. Psychol. Med. Univ. of Otago, NZ.

ROBERTS, Frederick Leighton 18 Penleonard Close, Exeter EX2 4NY Tel: 01392 420077 — MB ChB Bristol 1978; FFA RCS Eng. 1982. Cons. Anaesth. Roy. Devon & Exeter Hosp. Specialty: Anaesth. Prev: Sen. Regist. (Anaesth.) Bristol; Regist. (Anaesth.) Cardiff; Vis. Asst. Prof. Anaesth. Madison Wisconsin.

ROBERTS, Gareth Endaf Wyn Bryn Dedwydd, 8 Trefonwys, Bangor LL57 2HU Tel: 01248 352297 — MB ChB Liverp. 1994; BSc (Hons.) Physiol. Liverp. 1991, MB ChB 1994. Ho. Off. (Med. & Surg.) Aintree Trust Hosps. Liverp. Socs: Y Gymdeithias Feddygol.

ROBERTS, Gareth Rhys The Surgery, Market Square, Masham, Ripon HG4 4DZ — MB ChB (Hons.) Manch. 1994; BSc (Hons.) Manch. 1991. Specialty: Gen. Pract. Socs: Roy. Coll. GP's.

ROBERTS, Geoffrey Cyril Stuart 4 Newhaven Road, New Brighton, Wallasey CH45 1HS — MB ChB Liverp. 1952. Prev: Orthop. Ho. Surg. & Cas. Off. David Lewis North. Hosp.

ROBERTS, Geoffrey David Upper Gordon Road Surgery, 37 Upper Gordon Road, Camberley GU15 2HJ Tel: 01276 26424 Fax: 01276 63486; 2 Kingsley Avenue, Camberley GU15 2LZ Tel: 01276 27770 — MB ChB Manch. 1973 (Manchester University) FRCGP 1992, M 1978; MRCP (UK) 1980; DCH Eng. 1980. Primary Care Lead, Nat. Body Progr. (Modernisation Agency); Sen. Tutor & Hon. Sen. Lect. (Gen. Pract.) St. Geo. Hosp. Med. Sch. Lond.; Educat. Adviser W. Surrey HA. Specialty: Gen. Pract. Socs: Fell.RCGP; Centre for Advancem. of Interprofessional Educat.; Commiss. on Primary Care. Prev: Cons. Primary Care MSW HA; Chairm. Anticipatory Care Teams; Educat.l Adviser RCGP.

ROBERTS, Geoffrey James 24 Springmeadow, Charlesworth, Glossop SK13 5HP Tel: 01457 867027 Fax: 01457 858048 — MB ChB Manch. 1972. Med. Dir. 5 Boroughs Partnership NHS Trust; Chief Examr. Health Inst. Risk Managem.; Mem. Ment. Health ACT Commision. Socs: Manch. Med. Soc. Prev: Head Risk Managem. Med. Defence Union; Med. Dir. & Dir. Ment. Health Servs. Worthing Priority Care NHS Trust.

ROBERTS, Geoffrey Stafford (retired) 14 Stevens Road, Heswall, Wirral CH60 1XS — MB ChB Liverp. 1953; MRCS Eng. LRCP Lond. 1953; FRCGP 1980, M 1965. Prev: Mem. Disabil. Appeal Tribunals Indep. Tribunal Serv.

ROBERTS, Geraint (retired) 2 Penybanc, Tanerdy, Carmarthen SA31 2HA Tel: 01267 234099 — MB BCh Wales 1964 (Cardiff) FRCOG 1982, M 1969. Cons. O & G W. Wales Gen. Hosp.; Hon. Clin. Teach. Univ. Wales Coll. Med. & Univ. Lond. Prev: Sen. Regist. (O & G) Welsh Hosp. Bd. & Univ. Hosp. Wales Gp. Hosps.

ROBERTS, Geraint Llion Wyn 8 Trefonwys, Bangor LL57 2HU — MB ChB Liverp. 1997 (Liverpool)

ROBERTS, Gerard William Madeira Road Surgery, 1A Madeira Road, Parkstone, Poole BH14 9ET Tel: 01202 741345; 14 Eaton Road, Branksome Park, Poole BH13 6DG Tel: 01202 757613 Fax: 01202 757613 Email: gerry.roberts@dial.pipex.com — MB ChB Bristol 1980; MBA Bournemouth; DCH; MRCGP; FFARCS. GP Princip.; Lect. in Gen. Med. Diag. AngloEurop. Chirpractic Coll.; Dir. Poole Hyperbaric Centre Ltd. Specialty: Gen. Pract. Socs: BMA; Undersea & Hyperbaric Med. Soc.

ROBERTS, Gillian Catherine 7 Hawick Avenue, Paisley PA2 9LD — MB ChB Glas. 1998; MB ChB Glas 1998.

ROBERTS, Gillian Margaret (retired) Bryn Arlais, Llanaelhaearn, Caernarfon LL54 5AG — BM BCh Oxf. 1960 (Oxf. & Univ. Coll. Hosp.) MA, BM BCh Oxf. 1960; MRCOG 1967. Prev: Regist. (O & G) King's Coll. Hosp. Gp. Hosps.

ROBERTS, Glenn Anthony North Devon District Hospital, Raleigh Park, Barnstaple EX31 4JB Tel: 01271 22577 — MB ChB Bristol 1979. Cons. Psychiat. N. Devon. Specialty: Gen. Psychiat. Prev: Sen. Regist. (Adult Psychiat.) Wessex RHA.

ROBERTS, Glyn Hywel Plas Meddyg Surgery, Station Road, Ruthin LL15 1BP Tel: 01824 702255 Fax: 01824 707221; Plas Meddyg, Station Road, Ruthin LL15 1BP Tel: 01824 702255 — MB BS Lond. 1981 (St. Bart.) BSc (Hons.) (Biochem.) Lond. 1978; MRCS Eng. LRCP Lond. 1981; Cert. Family Plann. JCC 1986; DRCOG 1986; DFFP 1994. Hon. Med. Advis. Welsh Wom's Hockey Assn. Specialty: Orthop. Prev: SHO (Orthop.) Roy. Nat. Orthop. Hosp. Lond.

ROBERTS, Graham Alexander 10 Garw-Wood Drive, Croesyceiliog, Cwmbran NP44 2QJ — MB BS Lond. 1991.

ROBERTS, Graham Colin — BM BCh Oxf. 1993; MRCP (UK); MRCPCH; MA Oxf. 1996; MSc London 2001; DM Oxf 2003. Specialist Regist. (Paediat.) N. Thames. Specialty: Paediat. Prev: Regist. (Paediat.) St. Mary's Hosp. Lond.; SHO Rotat. St. Jas. Univ. Hosp. Leeds; Ho. Off. (Paediat. Surg.) Roy. Hosp. Sick Childr. Glas.

ROBERTS, Graham Ivor (retired) 18 Chantry Grove, Lawrence Weston, Bristol BS11 0QH Tel: 0117 982 7710 — LRCP and SI 1954 (RCSI) LRCPI & LM, LRCSI & LM 1954. Prev: Saiburi, Christian Hosp., Thailand.

ROBERTS, Gregory Anthony Manor Road Surgery, 31 Manor Road, Folkestone CT20 2SE Tel: 01303 851122 — MB BChir Camb. 1991 (Cambridge) Specialty: Gen. Pract.

ROBERTS, Mr Griffith Ithel (retired) Rutherglen, 17 Wexham St., Beaumaris LL58 8HW Tel: 01248 810707 — MB ChB Liverp. 1938; FRCS Ed. 1943; MChOrth. Liverp. 1947. Prev: Ships Surg. Roy. Fleet Auxil.

ROBERTS, Gwyn Haydn Berllys, Penaber, Criccieth LL52 0ES — MB BCh Wales 1993.

ROBERTS, Mr Gwyn Richard Ellis (retired) Beech Farm House, Sedlescombe, Battle TN33 0QS Tel: 01424 870 267 — MRCS Eng. LRCP Lond. 1955 (Lond. Hosp.) MS Lond. 1973, MB BS 1955; FRCS Eng. 1960; FRCS Ed. 1960. Prev: Cons. Surg. Roy. E. Sussex & St. Helen's Hosps. Hastings & Bexhill Hosp.

ROBERTS, Gwyneth Margaret (retired) 65 Beacon Way, Rickmansworth WD3 7PB Tel: 01923 897500 — MB ChB Manch. 1954. Prev: Ho. Phys. Crumpsall Hosp. Manch.

ROBERTS, Gwynfor Health Centre, Llanfairpwllgwyngyll LL61 5YZ Tel: 01248 714388 Fax: 01248 715826; Carreg Lwyd, Ffordd Pentraeth, Menai Bridge LL59 5HU Tel: 01248 712448 — MB BCh Wales 1969; BSc Wales 1966.

ROBERTS, Gwynneth Ann 48 Redwood Road, Kinver, Stourbridge DY7 6JR Tel: 01384 877351; Midlands Occupational Health Service, 83 Birmingham Road, West Bromwich B70 6PX Tel: 0121 601 4041 — MB BCh Wales 1981 (Welsh National School of Medicine) BSc (1st cl. Hons.) Wales 1978; MRCP (UK) 1985; MFOM RCP Lond. 1995, AFOM 1990. Med. Off. Midl. Occupat. Health Serv. W. Bromwich. Specialty: Occupat. Health. Socs: Soc. Occupat. Med. (Treas. W. Midl.s Gp. 1998).

ROBERTS, Harold Edward Saltaire Medical Centre, Richmond Road, Shipley BD18 4RX Tel: 01274 593101 Fax: 01274 772588 — MB ChB Leeds 1968. Socs: Bradford M-C Soc.

ROBERTS, Harold Ellison (retired) 20 Clifford Road, Sheffield S11 9AQ Tel: 0114 255 1473 — BM BCh Oxf. 1957 (Oxf. & Lond. Hosp.) MRCS Eng. LRCP Lond. 1949. Med. Off. Sheff. Regional Blood Transfus. Centre.

ROBERTS, Helen Clare Elderly Care Unit, Level G, West Wing, Southampton General Hospital, Tremona Road, Shirley, Southampton SO16 6YD Tel: 023 8079 4354 Fax: 023 8079 6965 — MB ChB Birm. 1984; BSc (Hons.) Birm. 1981; MRCP (UK) 1989; FRCP (UK) 1999. Sen. Lect. and Hon. Cons. (Elderly Care) Soton. Gen. Hosp. Specialty: Care of the Elderly. Socs: BMA; Brit. Geriat. Soc. Prev: Sen. Regist. (Geriat. Med.) Qu. Alexandra Hosp. Portsmouth & Soton. Gen. Hosp.; Regist. (Gen. Med.) Gen. Hosp. St. Helier Jersey & Roy. S. Hants. Hosp. Soton.

ROBERTS, Helen Judith Margaret Farnham Health Centre, Brightwells, Farnham GU9 7SA Tel: 01252 723122; 37 Weydon Hill Road, Farnham GU9 8NX Tel: 01252 733630 Fax: 01252 733630 — MB BS Lond. 1988 (Univ. Coll. Hosp. Med. Sch.) SCMO Jarvis Breast Screening Centre Guildford. Prev: Trainee GP Yeovil Dist. Hosp.

ROBERTS, Helen Louise 26 Oldacres, Maidenhead SL6 1XJ — MB ChB Sheff. 1996.

ROBERTS, Helen May Dinas Point, Y Felinheli LL56 4RX — MB BCh Wales 1973; CCST 1998.

ROBERTS, Mr Henry (retired) — MD Liverp. 1951; MB ChB 1945; FRCOG 1961, M 1951; FRCS Ed. 1956. Cons. O & G United Birm. Hosps. Prev: Regist. (Obst.) & Tutor, Mill Rd. Matern. Hosp. Liverp.

ROBERTS, Henry Lomax, Col. late RAMC (retired) 11 Pendleton Close, Redhill RH1 6QY Tel: 01737 760669 — MB ChB Leeds 1954; DTM & H Eng. 1964. Prev: Dir. Med. Servs. Sultans' Armed Forces Oman.

ROBERTS, Honor Susan Anne Department of Microbiology, Farnborough Hospital, Farnborough Common, Orpington BR6 8ND Tel: 01689 814110 Fax: 01689 814031 — MRCS Eng. LRCP Lond. 1979; MSc (Microbiol.) Lond. 1987, BSc (Hons. Path.) 1976, MB BS 1979; FRCPath 1986. Cons. Microbiol. Bromley Hosp.s NHS Trust. Specialty: Med. Microbiol. Prev: Sen. Regist. (Microbiol.) Guy's Hosp. Lond. & Pub. Health Laborat. Serv. Ashford Kent.

ROBERTS, Howard Frederick 73, Onslow Gardens, London N10 3JY Tel: 020 8883 7473 Fax: 020 8883 7473 — (Lond. Hosp.) MPhil Lond. 1973, MB BS 1963; MRCP Lond. 1969; MRCPsych 1974. Cons. Child & Adolesc. Psychiat. S. Lond. and Maudsley NHS Trust. Specialty: Child & Adolesc. Psychiat. Socs: Assoc. Mem. Brit. Psychoanalyt. Soc. Prev: Regist. & Hon. Sen. Regist. Maudsley Hosp. Lond.; Research Worker Inst. Psychiat. Lond.

ROBERTS, Hugh Richard Sydney 18 Gosset Street, St Albans, Christchurch, New Zealand; 19 St. Thomas Road, London N4 2QH — MB BS Lond. 1987 (Char. Cross & Westm.) MRCP (UK) 1990; FRCR 1994; MD Lond. 1996. Cons. Radiol. & Hon. Sen. Lect. ChristCh. Pub. Hosp. NZ. Specialty: Radiol. Prev: Sen. Regist. (Radiol.) Univ. Coll. Lond. Hosps.; Clin. Lect. (Surg.) Univ. Coll. Lond.; Regist. (Med.) Jersey Gen. Hosp.

ROBERTS, Mr Humphrey Richard Medwyn (retired) 64 Chartfield Avenue, London SW15 6HQ Tel: 020 8789 1758 — BChir Camb. 1957 (Camb. & Westm.) FRCS Eng. 1961, LRCP Lond. 1957; MB Camb. 1958; MA Camb. 1958; FRCOG 1978, M 1965. Prev: Cons. O & G Westm. Hosp. Lond.

ROBERTS, Huw Gruffydd Tenby Surgery, The Norton, Tenby SA70 8AB Tel: 01834 844161 Fax: 01834 844227; Ger-y-Rhyd, St. Florence, Tenby SA70 8LJ — MB BS Lond. 1973; BSc Lond. 1973, MB BS 1973.

ROBERTS, Huw Lewis Liverpool House, Waunfawr, Caernarfon LL55 4YY Tel: 01286 650223 Fax: 01286 650714; Y Culfor, Bangor Road, Caernarfon LL55 1LN Tel: 01286 671067 — MB ChB (Hons) Liverp. 1971; MRCS Eng. LRCP Lond. 1971; MRCP (UK) 1974. Socs: Gymdeithas Feddygol; BMA. Prev: Resid. & Fell. (Med.) Johns Hopkins Hosp. Baltimore, USA; Regist. David Lewis North. Hosp. Liverp.; Ho. Off. Liverp. Roy. Infirm.

ROBERTS, Ian Queens Hospital, Burton Hospitals NHS Trust, Belvedere Road, Burton-on-Trent DE13 0RB; 51 Main Street, Rosliston, Swadlincote DE12 8JW — MB ChB Leic. 1986 (Leicester) DA (UK) 1988; FRCA 1995; M.Med Sci. (Distinction) 1998. Cons. Anaesth. Specialty: Anaesth.; Intens. Care. Prev: Regist. (Anaesth.) N. Staffs. Hosps.

ROBERTS, Ian Station Road Health Centre, Station Road, Haydock, St Helens NA11 0JN Tel: 01744 22272; 6 Elmsfield Park, Aughton Green, Ormskirk L39 6TJ — MB ChB Liverp. 1973; DCH Eng. 1976; Dip. Pract. Dermat. Wales 1990. GP St. Helens Merseyside. Socs: Fac. Community Health.

ROBERTS, Ian Cobtree Medical Practice, Southways, Sutton Valence, Maidstone ME17 3HG Tel: 01622 843800 Fax: 01622 844184; Gladstones, The Quarries, Boughton Monchelsea, Maidstone ME17 4NJ — MB BS Lond. 1971; MRCS Eng. LRCP Lond. 1971; MRCP (UK) 1975; DRCOG 1976.

ROBERTS, Ian Ellis Meddygfa, Canolfan, Iechyd, Bala LL23 7BA Tel: 01678 520308 — MB ChB Liverp. 1958. Socs: BMA. Prev: Ho. Phys., Ho. Surg. & Ho. Surg. (Obst.) Sefton Gen. Hosp.; Res. Med. Off. Colwyn Bay & W. Denbighsh. Hosp.

ROBERTS, Ian Forrest Chesterfield and North Derbyshire Royal Hospital, Calow, Chesterfield S44 5BL Tel: 01246 277271 Fax: 01246 552620; Cornerstone Cottage, 209 Walton Back Lane, Walton, Chesterfield S42 7LP Tel: 01246 569789 Email: ian@wbl209.fsnet.co.uk — (Guy's) MB BS Lond. 1966; MRCS Eng. LRCP Lond. 1966; MRCP (UK) 1969; FRCP Lond. 1991; FRCPCH 1997. Cons. Paediat. Chesterfield & N. Derbysh. Roy. Hosp. Specialty: Paediat.; Diabetes; Rheumatol. Special Interest: Diabetes; Rheumatology. Socs: Hon. Sec. Chesterfield Med. Soc.; E. Mids. Med. Soc; Trent Regional Paediat. Soc. Prev: Sen. Regist. St. Geo. Hosp. Lond.; SHO Hammersmith Hosp. Lond.; Ho. Phys. Evelina Childr. Hosp. S.wark.

ROBERTS, Professor Ian Gray Child Health Monitoring Unit, Department of Edipemiology & Biostatistics, Institute of Child Health, 30 Guildford St., London WC1N 1EH — MB BCh Wales 1985. Specialty: Epidemiol.

ROBERTS, Ian Simon David Dept. of Cellular Pathology, John Radcliffe Hospital, Headington, Oxford OX3 9DU Tel: 01865 222889 Fax: 01865 220519 Email: ian.roberts@orh.nhs.uk — MB ChB Manch. 1985; MRCPath 1993. Cons. Pathologist Oxf. Radcliffe Hosp.; Hon. Sen. Lect. The Univ. of Oxf. Specialty: Histopath. Prev: Lect. (Path.) Univ. Manch.; Sen. Regist. (Histopath.) NW Region; Regist. (Histopath.) Merseyside Region.

ROBERTS, Ifor John Wynn 3A New Street, Pwllheli LL53 5HT — MB ChB Ed. 1966.

ROBERTS, Iorwerth, MM (retired) 209 Pitshanger Lane, Ealing, London W5 1RQ — MB BS Lond. 1956 (St. Bart) MRCS Eng. LRCP Lond. 1956; DObst RCOG 1958.

ROBERTS, Professor Irene Anne Graham Department of Haematology, Imperial College Hammersmith Campus, Du Lane Road, London W12 0NN Tel: 0208 383 4017 Fax: 0208 742 9335 — MB ChB Glas. 1978; DRCOG 1980; MRCP (UK) 1981; MRCPath 1987; MD (Hons.) Glas. 1988; T(Path) 1991; T(M) 1991; FRCP Glas. 1992; FRCP Lond. 1994. Prof. of Paediatric Haemat., Imperial Coll. Sch. of Med., Hammersmith Campus; Hon. Cons. Paediat. Haemat. Hammersmith Hosp. Lond.; Hon. Cons. Paediat. Haemat. St. Mary's Hosp., Paddington, Lond. Specialty: Haematology. Prev: Sen. Lect. (Haemat.) Roy. Postgrad. Med. Sch. Univ. Lond.

ROBERTS, Irene Elizabeth Maesyrhedydd, Pencefn Road, Dolgellau LL40 2ET — MB BCh Wales 1964 (Cardiff) Clin. Med. Off. N. W. Wales NHS Trust. Prev: Ho. Phys., Ho. Surg. & SHO Paediat. Maelor Gen. Hosp.

ROBERTS, Mr Iwan Francis 45 Stroud Road, Wimbledon Park, London SW19 8DQ — MB BS Lond. 1987; BA Oxf. 1984; FRCS Eng. 1991. Regist. (Radiol.) St. Geo. Hosp. Lond. Specialty: Radiol. Prev: Regist. (Paediat. Surg.) St. Geo. Hosp. Lond.; Demonst., SHO (Anat.) & Phys. (Accid. & Emerg.) St. Mary's Hosp. & Med. Sch. Lond.; SHO (Gen. Surg.) Bristol & Weston HA.

ROBERTS, Jack (retired) 28 Altar Drive, Bradford BD9 5QD Tel: 01274 226992 Email: jack.roberts@virgin.net — (Oxf.) MA Oxf. 1947, BM BCh 1944. Prev: Res. Anaesth. Roy. Berks. Hosp. Reading.

ROBERTS, Jacqueline Mary Putneymead Medical Centre, 350 Upper Richmond Road, London SW15 6TL Tel: 020 8788 0686 — MB BS Lond. 1984. GP Princip. Specialty: Rehabil. Med.; Rheumatol. Prev: Trainee GP Richmond Twickenham & Roehampton HA VTS; Ho. Phys. (Gen. Med. & Radiother.) Essex Co. Hosp. Colchester; Ho. Surg. (Gen. Surg. & Orthop.) & SHO (A & E) Qu. Mary's Hosp. Roehampton.

ROBERTS, James (retired) 459 Altrincham Road, Wythenshawe, Manchester M23 1AA Tel: 0161 998 3326 — MB ChB Manch. 1957; DObst RCOG 1959; FRCGP 1975, M 1965. Prev: Regional Adviser (Gen. Pract.) Univ. Dept. Postgrad. Med. Studies Manch. Univ.

ROBERTS, James Hugh St Mary's Surgery, Windermere LA23 1BA — MB ChB Leeds 1989. SHO (Orthop.) Norf. & Norwich Hosp. Prev: SHO (A & E) & Demonst. (Anat.) Leics. Roy. Infirm.; Ho. Off. Leeds Gen. Infirm. & St. Jas. Hosp. Leeds.

ROBERTS, James Hugh Medwyn — MB BS Lond. 1993 (St Mary's Hosp. Med. School.) BSc (Hons. Human Biol.) UCL 1990; FRCA 2002. Specialist Regist. (Anaesth.) N. Centr. Lond. Rotat. Specialty: Anaesth. Socs: Roy. Soc. of Med. Prev: SHO (Anaesth.), Northwick Pk. Hosp. Lond.

ROBERTS, James John Kennedy HM Prison & Institution, Cornton Vale, Stirling FK9 5NU Tel: 01786 832591 Fax: 01786 834467; 12 Winton Circus, Saltcoats KA21 5DA Tel: 01294 461798 — MB ChB Ed. 1976; BSc Ed. 1973; MRCGP 1980. Med. Off. HM Prison & Inst. Cornton Vale Stirling. Specialty: Alcohol & Substance Misuse. Prev: Clin. Asst. (Med.) West. Gen. Hosp. Edin.; GP MuirHo.

ROBERTS, James Kennedy Walnut Tree Cottage, Waterley Bottom, North Nibley, Dursley GL11 6EG Tel: 01453 543186 — MB BS Lond. 1968 (St. Thos.) MRCS Eng. LRCP Lond. 1968; DObst RCOG 1973.

ROBERTS, James Michael Beech House Surgery, Beech House, 69 Vale Street, Denbigh LL16 3AY Tel: 01745 812863 Fax: 01745 816574; Llys Hedydd, Llansannan Road, Henllan, Denbigh LL16 5DE — MB BCh Wales 1985; DRCOG 1990. Specialty: Endocrinol.

ROBERTS, James Trevor Newcastle General Hospital, Northern Centre for Cancer Treatment, Westgate Road, Newcastle upon Tyne NE4 6BE Tel: 0191 256 3543 Fax: 0191 256 3670; 31 Eskdale Terrace, Jesmond, Newcastle upon Tyne NE2 4DN Tel: 0191 281 1872 — MB BS Lond. 1973 (Westm.) MRCP (UK) 1976; FRCR 1978; FRCP Lond. 1993. Cons. Clin. Oncol. N. Centre for Cancer Treatm. Specialty: Oncol. Socs: Fell. Roy. Soc. Med.; Brit. Inst. Radiol.; Estro Europ. Soc. of Therapeutic Radiol. and Oncol. Prev: Cons. Radiother. & Oncol. Newc. HA; Lect. (Clin. Oncol.) Univ. Camb.; Sen. Regist. (Radiother. & Oncol.) Addenbrooke's Hosp. Camb.

ROBERTS, Jane Elisabeth Camden & Islington Community Health Services NHS Trust, Child & Family Psychiatry, Whittington Hospital, London N19 5NF Tel: 020 7530 2444 Fax: 020 7530 2479 — MB ChB Bristol 1980; MRCP (UK) 1983; MRCPsych 1986; MSc Brunel 1991. Cons. Child & Adolesc. Psychiat. Camden & Islington Community Health Servs. NHS Trust Lond. Specialty: Child & Adolesc. Psychiat. Prev: Sen. Regist. (Child Psychiat.) Tavistock Clin. Lond.; Regist. (Psychiat.) Maudsley Hosp. Lond.; SHO (Paediat.) Qu. Eliz. Hosp. Childr. Lond.

ROBERTS, Jane Elizabeth 14 Kiltongue Cottages, Monklands Hospital, Airdrie ML6 0JS Tel: 01236 713053; 17c Mains Avenue, Giffnock, Glasgow G46 6QY Tel: 0141 638 8258 — (Aberd.) MB ChB Aberd. 1969; DObst 1971; FRCOG 1990, M 1975; FRCP Glas. 1994 M 1992; CFM 1995. Cons. Genitourin. Med. Lanarksh. Specialty: Genitourinary Medicine. Prev: Regist. (O & G) Qu. Mother's Hosp. Glas. & West. Infirm. Glas.; Cons. Genitourin. Med. Greater Glas. HB.

ROBERTS, Jane Hazel Alma Street Medical Centre, Alma St., Stockton-on-Tees, Middlesbrough TS1 2AP Tel: 01642 670248; 69 Barker Road, Linthorpe, Middlesbrough TS5 5EW Tel: 01642 607248 — MB ChB Sheff. 1988; BMedSci Sheff. 1986; MRCGP 1997. Lect. Primary Health Care, Univ. Of Durh. Specialty: Gen. Pract.

ROBERTS, Jane Mary Truan Bach, Cerrigceinwen, Bodorgan LL62 5DH — MB ChB Sheff. 1994.

ROBERTS, Janet Catherine (retired) Marnie, Roseacre Road, Roseacre, Preston PR4 3UE — MB ChB Liverp. 1971; DA Eng. 1973; FFA RCS Eng. 1975. Prev: Cons. Anaesth. Blackpool Vict. Hosp.

ROBERTS, Janet Eleanor 1 Risca Road, Rogerstone, Newport NP10 9FZ — MB BCh Wales 1973; BSc Hull 1968.

ROBERTS, Mr Jason Lloyd Barclay 10 Lochard Cottages, Kinlochard, Aberfoyle, Stirling FK8 3TL — MB ChB Leic. 1994 (University of Leicester) FRCS Pt. A Ed. 1998; FRCS Pt. B Glas. 1998. SpR Orthop. & Trauma Surg. W. of Scotl. Rotat. Specialty: Gen. Surg. Prev: SHO (Orthop.) Western Infirm. Glas.; SHO (Gen./Vasc. Surg.) Gartnavel & West. Infirm. Glas.; SHO (Orthop.) Qu. Med. Centre Nottm.

ROBERTS, Jeffrey Paul Hazel Cottage, 42 Stubbs Wood, Chesham HP5 3RL Tel: 01494 724466 Fax: 01494 724466 — BM BCh Oxf. 1969; DPM Eng. 1973; FRCPsych 1992, M 1973; MA Oxf. 1975. Vis. Cons. Grovelands Priory Hosp. Lond.; Non-Exec. Dir. Grendon & Springhill Prisons, Grendon Underwood nr. Aylesbury; Mem. Inst. Gp. Anal.; Mem. Managem. Gp. Analytic Pract. Specialty: Psychother. Socs: Fell. Roy. Soc. Med.; Gp. Analyt. Soc. Prev: Cons. Psychother. The Roy. Lond. Hosp. & St. Clements Hosp. Lond.; Hon. Cons. Psychother. Guy's Hosp. Lond.; Cons. Psychother. Ingrebourne Centre St. Geo. Hosp. HornCh.

ROBERTS, Jeremy Christopher Radnor Street Surgery, 3 Radnor Street, Glasgow G3 7UA Tel: 0141 334 6111 — MB ChB Glas. 1977; MRCPsych 1981; DRCOG 1984.

ROBERTS, Jeremy Mark — MB BS Lond. 1983 (Roy. Free) MRCPsych 1990. Cons. Psychiat. (Gen. Psychiat.) Wonford Ho. Hosp. Exeter. Specialty: Gen. Psychiat. Prev: Trainee Psychiat. Exeter HA Scheme; Trainee GP Coventry VTS; Sen. Regist. Rotat. (Psychiat.) Bristol.

ROBERTS, Mr Jeremy Openshaw City General Hospital, Newcastle Road, Stoke-on-Trent ST4 6QG Tel: 01782 715444; North Staffordshire Nuffield Hospital, Clayton Road, Newcastle ST5 4DB Tel: 01782 625431 — MB BS Lond. 1977; MA Camb. 1978; FRCS Eng. 1983; MS Lond. 1991. Cons. Plastic Surg. City Gen. Hosp. Stoke-on-Trent. Specialty: Plastic Surg. Prev: Sen. Regist. (Plastic Surg.) Canniesburn Hosp. Glas.; Regist. (Plastic Surg.) Stoke Mandeville Hosp. Aylesbury; Lect. (Surg.) Char. Cross & Westm. Med. Sch.

ROBERTS, Joanne Linda Amwell Street Surgery, 19 Amwell Street, Hoddesdon EN11 8TS Tel: 01992 464147 Fax: 01992 708698 — MB BS Lond. 1987.

ROBERTS, John (retired) 1 Keyes Avenue, Roath Park, Cardiff CF23 5QQ Tel: 029 2075 1466 — MB BCh Wales 1952. Prev: GP Cardiff.

ROBERTS, John 89 Northfield Broadway, Edinburgh EH8 7RX Tel: 0131 657 5444 Fax: 0131 669 8116 — MB ChB Ed. 1958. Socs: BMA. Prev: Ho. Phys. Cumbld. Infirm. Carlisle; Ho. Surg. Falkirk Roy. Infirm.; Ho. Off. (Obst.) City Matern. Hosp. Carlisle.

ROBERTS, John Alan Medical Unit, Royal Hampshire County Hospital, Winchester SO22 5DG Tel: 01962 824775 Fax: 01962 825227; Sainfoin, Winchester Hill, Romsey SO51 7NL Email: alan@roberty@virgin.net — MB ChB Glas. 1978; MRCP (UK) 1982; BSc (Hons.) (Microbiol.) Glas. 1973, MD 1988; FRCP Lond. 1996. Cons. Gen. & Thoracic Med. Roy. Hants. Co. Hosp. Specialty: Respirat. Med. Socs: Brit. Thorac. Soc. Prev: Sen. Regist. (Internal & Respirat. Med.) Soton. Gen. Hosp.; Regist. (Respirat. Med.) West. Infirm. & Kt.swood Hosp. Glas.; Hon. Research Fell. Strathclyde Univ. Glas.

ROBERTS, Mr John Andrew Diana, Princess of Wales Hospital, Scartho Road, Grimsby DN33 2BA Tel: 01472 74111; Stone House, Stainton le Vale, Market Rasen LN8 6HP Tel: 01472 398605 — MB ChB Bristol 1976; FRCS Glas. 1981. Cons. Surg. Orthop. & Trauma Grimsby Dist. Gen. Hosp. Specialty: Orthop. Socs: BMA; BOA. Prev: Sen. Regist. (Orthop.) West. Infirm. Glas.

ROBERTS, Mr John Bernard Michael (retired) Dormers, Woodlands Road, Portishead, Bristol BS20 7HE Tel: 01275 843254 — (Leeds) ChM Leeds 1963, MB ChB 1952; FRCS Eng. 1957; FRCGP 1990. Med. Postgrad. Dean Univ. Bristol. Prev: Cons. Urol. Surg. Bristol Roy. Infirm.

ROBERTS, John Brian Priory Medical Group, 19 Albion Road, North Shields NE29 0HT Tel: 0191 257 0223 — MB BS Newc. 1978.

ROBERTS, John Clive (retired) Long Acre, Riverside Road, Dittisham, Dartmouth TQ6 0HS Tel: 01803 722273 — MB BS Lond. 1959 (St. Mary's) LMSSA Lond. 1959; FFA RCS Eng. 1965. Cons. Anaesth. St. Mary's Hosp. Lond. Prev: Sen. Regist. (Anaesth.) & Ho. Surg. Surgic. Unit St. Mary's Hosp. Lond.

ROBERTS, John David Victoria Road Health Centre, Victoria Road, Rhymney NP22 5NU Tel: 01685 840627 Fax: 01685 843100 — MB ChB Liverp. 1977; MRCS Eng. LRCP Lond. 1977.

ROBERTS, John Gareth BarlowHolsy Srgery, 22 Haniton Terrace, Milfund Daien, Pembroke SA73 35L Tel: 01646 690674 — MB BS Lond. 1982. Specialty: Paediat. Dent.

ROBERTS, Mr John Gethin Glan-y-Menai, Glyn Garth, Menai Bridge LL59 5NS — BM BCh Oxf. 1967 (Oxf. & Lond. Hosp.) MA; FRCS Eng. 1972. Cons. Urol. Llanelli Dynefur Trust Llanelli. Specialty: Urol. Prev: Sen. Regist. (Urol.) Univ. Hosp. Wales Cardiff; Sen. Regist. (Gen. Surg.) S. Glam. (T) & Clwyd HAs.; Cancer Research Campaign Research Fell. Univ. Hosp. Wales.

ROBERTS, John Guymer The Surgery, Caerffynon, Dolgellau LL40 1LY; Maesyrhedydd, Pencefn Road, Dolgellau LL40 2ET Tel: 01341 422775 — MB BCh Wales 1964; DObst RCOG 1966; MRCGP 1969; FRCGP 1990. Clin. Asst. (Geriat.) Dolgellau & Barmouth Dist. Hosp.; Police Surg. Dolgellau & Dist.; Chairm. Meirionnydd Med. Soc.; Chairm. N. Wales Fac. RCGP; Sec. Gwynedd LMC. Socs: BMA. Prev: Ho. Phys., Ho. Surg. & SHO (O & G) Maelor Gen. Hosp. Wrexham.

ROBERTS, John Huw (retired) 42 Dunniwood Avenue, Bessacarr, Doncaster DN4 7JT — Cons. Radiol. Doncaster Roy. Infirm; MB ChB Liverp. 1953; DMRD Eng. 1960.

ROBERTS, John Iolo 10 Shawhill Crescent, Newton Mearns, Glasgow G77 5BY — MB ChB Dundee 1979; FRCR 1986. Cons. (Radiol.) Law Hosp. Carluke. Specialty: Radiol. Prev: Sen. Regist. (Radiol.) West. Infirm. Glas.; Regist. (Radiol.) West. Infirm. Glas.; SHO (Gen. Med.) Law Hosp. Carluke.

ROBERTS, John Kenneth 93 Chapel Street, Billericay CM12 9LR Tel: 22940 — MB BS Lond. 1952 (Middlx. Hosp.) DObst RCOG 1960. Local Civil Serv. Med. Off.; Med. Off. East. Elect. Bd. Prev: Ho. Phys. Brighton Gen. Hosp.; Ho. Surg. P. of Wales Gen. Hosp. Lond.; Obst. Sen. Ho. Off. Morriston Hosp.

ROBERTS, John Kenneth (Surgery) Victoria Surgery, Holyhead LL65 1UB Tel: 01407 762713 Fax: 01407 765052; Cae Paradwys, 16 The Rise, Trearddur Bay, Holyhead LL65 2UY Tel: 01407 860529 — MB ChB Manch. 1959. Socs: BMA. Prev: Clin. Asst. (Orthop.) Gwynedd Hosp. Bangor; SHO (Orthop.) Caerns. & Anglesey Gen. Hosp. Bangor; Ho. Surg. Univ. Dept. Orthop. Manch. Roy. Infirm.

ROBERTS, John McKinlay Norcliffe Morris Dean, Henley-by-Fosbury, Marlborough SN8 3RJ Tel: 01264 731250 — (St. Thos.) MB BS Lond. 1951. Prev: Regist. (Med.) St. Mary's Hosp. Portsmouth; Demonst. (Clin. Path.) & Ho. Phys. St. Thos. Hosp.

ROBERTS, John Michael Queen Street House, Queen St., Twyford, Winchester SO21 1QG Tel: 01962 712165 — MRCS Eng. LRCP Lond. 1945 (Camb. & St. Bart.) BA Camb. 1941, MB BChir 1949. Socs: BMA. Prev: Regist. (Surg.) St. Bart. Hosp.; Asst. Lect. (Anat.) Char. Cross Hosp. Med. Sch.; Surg. Falkland Is.s Dependency Survey.

ROBERTS, John Rees, VRD Iona, St. Margarets Road, Hoylake, Wirral CH47 1HX Tel: 0151 632 4636 — MD Liverp. 1958; MB ChB 1948; FRCP Lond. 1972, M 1953. Emerit. Cons. Paediat. Roy. Liverp. Childr. Hosp.; Emerit. Cons. Paediat. Neurol. Liverp. RHB. Specialty: Neurol. Socs: Brit. Paediat. Neurol. Assn.; Assn. Brit. Neurols. Prev: Hon. Phys. to HM The Qu.; Surg. Capt. RNR; Fullbright Schol. 1955-56.

ROBERTS, John Richard Lloyd 9a Wilbraham Place, London SW1X 9A Tel: 020 7730 7928 Fax: 020 7823 5606; 17 Perrymead Street, London SW6 3SW Tel: 020 7736 7220 Fax: 020 7731 2732 — MB BChir Camb. 1960 (Westm.) MA, MB Camb. 1960, BChir 1959; MRCS Eng. LRCP Lond. 1959. GP Lond.; Med. Off. Hellenic Coll.; Sen. Examr. Scott. Widows Fund. Prev: Med. Off. Staff Occupat. Health Unit Chelsea & Westm. Hosp.; Ho. Phys. Westm. Hosp. Lond.; Ho. Surg. Addenbrooke's Hosp. Camb.

ROBERTS, John Taylor 15 Wootton Way, Newnham, Cambridge CB3 9LX Tel: 01223 63539 — MB BS Lond. 1956 (St. Mary's) DPH Lond. 1960; MFCM 1974.

ROBERTS, John Wyn Anaesthetic Dept, Royal Bolton Hospital, Minerva Road, Farnworth, Bolton BL4 0JR Tel: 01204 390762; 18 Dimple Park, Egerton, Bolton BL7 9QE — MB BCh Wales 1987 (Univ. Wales Coll. Med.) DRCOG 1992; DA (UK) 1993; FRCA 1996. Cons., (Anaesth.), Bolton Roy. Infirmiry, Bolton, Lancs. Specialty: Anaesth. Socs: Obst. Anaesth. Assocn. & Difficult Airway Soc. Prev: Trainee GP Mold.

ROBERTS, John Wynne The Bousfield Surgery, Westminster Road, Liverpool L4 4PP Tel: 0151 207 0813 — MRCS Eng. LRCP Lond. 1979 (Liverp.) DRCOG 1982.

ROBERTS, Jon Hilton Windmill Health Centre, Mill Green, Leeds LS14 5JS Tel: 0113 273 3733 Fax: 0113 232 3202; 6 Moor Allerton Drive, Leeds LS17 6RZ — MB ChB Manch. 1984; DRCOG 1987.

ROBERTS, Jonathan David Vaughan Mayfield Medical Centre, 37 Totnes Road, Paignton TQ4 5LA Tel: 01803 558257 Fax: 01803 663353; Orchard Lodge, Old Road, Harbertonford, Totnes TQ9 7TA Tel: 01803 732879 — MB BS Lond. 1985; DCH RCP Lond. 1990; MRCGP 1991. GP Princip.; Hon. Lect. Plymouth Postgrad. Med. Sch. Socs: Primary Care Gastroenterol. Soc. Prev: SHO (Paediat.) Plymouth HA; SHO (Geriat.) W. Dorset HA; SHO (A & E) Torbay HA.

ROBERTS, Mr Jonathan Verrier 23 Barnsbury Square, London N1 1JP — MB BCh Wales 1978; FRCS Eng. 1984. Clin. Research Fell. Dept. Surg. King's Coll. Hosp. Lond. Prev: Regist. (Gen. Surg.) Lond. Hosp. Whitechapel; Regist. (Gen. Surg.) Orsett Hosp. Grays; SHO (Gen. Surg.) Battle Hosp. Reading.

ROBERTS, Judith Alison Dr H M Freeman and Partners, 12 Durham Road, Raynes Park, London SW20 0TW Tel: 020 8946 0069 Fax: 020 8944 2927; 23 Bernard Gardens, Wimbledon, London SW19 7BE — BM BS Nottm. 1984; BMedSci Nottm. 1982; MRCGP 1989; DRCOG 1989. Clin. Asst. Morris Markowe Unit Springfield Hosp. Lond.

ROBERTS, Judith Mary 122 Fernbrook Road, Wither Green, London SE13 5NH — MB ChB Birm. 1994; ChB Birm. 1994; DRCOG 1998. Specialty: Gen. Pract.

ROBERTS, Julia Elvin Doncaster Royal Infirmary, Armthorpe Road, Doncaster DN2 5LT — MB ChB Leeds 1979; MRCPsych. 1984; T(Psych) 1991. Cons. Psychiat. Doncaster Healthcare NHS Trust. Specialty: Gen. Psychiat. Prev: Sen. Regist. (Psychiat.) Trent RHA.

ROBERTS, Julian Crown House Surgery, Chapelgate, Retford DN22 6NX Tel: 01777 703672 Fax: 01777 710534 — MB ChB Liverp. 1982. Specialty: Gen. Pract. Special Interest: Leg elongation in the gullible adult.

ROBERTS, Julian Foley Ridge Medical Practice, 3 Paternoster Lane, Bradford BD7 3EE Tel: 01274 322822 Fax: 01274 322833 — MB BS Lond. 1980; MRCGP 1985; MPH Leeds 1990; MFPHM 1991. Salaried GP, Ridge Med. Pract., Bradford. Specialty: Pub. Health Med. Prev: Cons. Pub. Health Med. Bradford HA.

ROBERTS, Julian Mervyn, OBE (retired) Linden Lea, Moor Lane, Menston, Ilkley LS29 6AP Tel: 01943 872574 — MD Ed. MBchb 1947 1958 (Univ. Ed.) MD (Commend.) Ed. 1958, MB ChB 1947; DPM Leeds 1951; FRCPsych 1971. Prev: Cons. Psychiat. St. Jas. Hosp. Leeds.

ROBERTS, Mr Julian Paul 81 Clarendon Road, Fulwood, Sheffield S10 3TQ Tel: 0114 263 0737 — BM Soton. 1980; FRCS Eng. 1986; FRCS Ed. 1986; MS Soton. 1992; FRCS (Paediat.) 1994. Cons. Paediat. Surg. Sheff. Childr. Hosp. Specialty: Paediat. Surg. Prev: Regist. (Paediat. Surg.) Roy. Childr. Hosp., Melbourne; Sen. Regist. (Paediat. Surg.) Soton. Gen. Hosp.

ROBERTS, Julie Cheyne Walk Clinic, 3 Cheyne Walk, Northampton NN1 5PT Tel: 01604 231438 Fax: 01604 603823 Email: pam.tates.@nchc-tr.anglox.nhs.uk — MB BCh Wales 1972 (University of Wales) MRCPsych 1984; MBA 1998; FRCPsych 1999. Cons. Psychother. Cheyne Walk Clinic Northampton. Specialty: Psychother. Socs: Fell.Roy. Soc. of Med.; Mem. Inst. Gp. Anal.; Mem. Gp. Analytic Soc. Prev: Sen. Regist. (Psychother.) Cheyne Walk Clinic Northampton; Regist. (Psychiat.) St. Crispin Hosp. Northampton; SHO (Psychiat.) Univ. Hosp. Wales Cardiff.

ROBERTS, Juliet Catherine Udal 8 Michael Close, Maidenhead SL6 4PD — BM (Hons.) Soton. 1992; MRCP (UK) 1995; Dip Pharm Med 2000; MFPM 2002. Senior Med. Advisor Cardiovasc. Dept. Boehringer-Ingelheim Ltd. Bracknell. Specialty: Pharmaceutical Medicine. Prev: Regist. (Gen. Med.) John Radcliffe Hosp. Oxf.; SHO (Gen. Med.) Roy. Hants. Co. Hosp. Winchester; SHO (Radiother.) Roy. S. Hants. Hosp.

ROBERTS, Juliet Margaret 51 Lansdowne Road, Tonbridge TN9 1JD — MB ChB Leeds 1986.

ROBERTS, June Margaret (retired) 2 Manor Close, Bramhope, Leeds LS16 9HQ — MB ChB Leeds 1955; DA Eng. 1960; FFA RCS Eng. 1964.

ROBERTS, Justin 14 Moorside Lane, Parkside, Neston, South Wirral CH64 6QP — MB ChB Manch. 1995.

ROBERTS, Kathleen Elizabeth Victoria Health Centre, 5 Suffrage Street, Smethwick, Warley B66 3PZ — MB ChB Birm. 1971; DObst RCOG 1973; MRCGP 1976.

ROBERTS, Mr Keith Danford (retired) 75 Reddings Road, Moseley, Birmingham B13 8LP Tel: 0121 449 1959 — MB ChB (2nd cl. Hons.) Birm. 1945; MRCS Eng. LRCP Lond. 1946; FRCS Eng. 1950; ChM Birm. 1958. Hon. Cons. Cardiothoracic Surg. Centr. Birm. HA; Hon. Cons. Thoracic Surg. W. Midl. HA. Prev: Asst. Lect. (Anat.) Univ. Birm.

ROBERTS, Keith Michael 33 George V Avenue, Worthing BN11 5SE — MB BS Lond. 1981.

ROBERTS, Kenneth Norman Rose Cottage, Barracks Lane, Ravensmoor, Nantwich CW5 8PR — MB BS Newc. 1973; DRCOG 1981.

ROBERTS, Kim Elizabeth St Clements Partnership, Tanner Street, Winchester SO23 8AD Tel: 01962 852211 Fax: 01962 856010; Derwent House, Stoke Charity Road, Kingsworthy, Winchester SO21 2RP — BM Soton. 1983; DGM RCP Lond. 1985; DCH RCP Lond. 1985; DRCOG 1986.

ROBERTS, Laura Gwendoline Ruth Maes Cadarn, Llanelidan, Ruthin LL15 2RD Tel: 01824 710218; Flat 1, 34 Cleveland Way, Whitechapel Way, London E1 4UF — MB BS Lond. 1996 (The

Royal London Hosp. Med. Coll.) Clin. Research Fell. Inst. of Reproductive & Developm. Med. Imperial Coll. Specialty: Obst. & Gyn. Prev: SHO. O & G Greenwich DGH. Greenwich Lond.; SHO O & G. Kings Coll. Hosp. Camberwell; Ho. Off. Surg. Roy. Lond. Hosp. Whitechapel.

ROBERTS, Lawrence John Scunthorpe General Hospital, Cliff Gardens, Scunthorpe DN15 7BH Tel: 01742 290020; Leek House, Leek Hill, Winterton, Scunthorpe DN15 9SR Tel: 01724 734384 Fax: 01724 734646 — MB BS Lond. 1981; MRCGP 1986; MRCOG 1990. Cons. O & G Scunthorpe & Goole Hosps. Trust. Specialty: Obst. & Gyn. Prev: Sen. Cons. O & G BMH Rinteln.

ROBERTS, Lesley Susan Agnes Ridge End, The Drive, Wimbledon, London SW20 8TG — MB BS Lond. 1993 (GUYS) Specialist Regist. (O & G).

ROBERTS, Linda Caroline York House Medical Centre, Heathside Road, Woking GU22 7XL Tel: 01483 761100 Fax: 01483 751185; Meadow Croft, 25 Wexfenne Gardens, Woking GU22 8TX — MB BS Lond. 1985; DRCOG 1988.

ROBERTS, Lindsay Ann Cheltenham Road Surgery, 16 Cheltenham Road, Gloucester GL2 0LS Tel: 01452 522575 Fax: 01452 304321; 9 Red Admiral Drive, Abbeymead, Gloucester GL4 5EA — MB ChB Leeds 1980; DRCOG 1983; MRCGP 1984; DA (UK) 1987. Prev: SHO (Anaesth.) ScarBoro. Hosp.

ROBERTS, Lisa Helen 6 Dunmoor Grove, Ingleby Barwick, Stockton-on-Tees TS17 0QW — MB ChB Birm. 1993.

ROBERTS, Lisa Maxine Barclays Bank Plc, 83 Wandsworth High Street, London SW18 2PR — MB BS Lond. 1991 (St Georges) DRCOG 1995; MRCGP 1997. VTS S. Lond. Specialty: Gen. Pract. Prev: GP Regist. Bournemouth.

ROBERTS, Llinos Rhianedd Llys y Coed, Meirion La, Bangor LL57 2BU Email: llin3@hotmail.com — MB BCh Wales 1997.

ROBERTS, Lorna Jane 5 Comfrey Close, Romsey SO51 7RE — BChir Camb. 1991. Specialist Regist. (Anaesth.) Salsbury Dist. Hosp. Specialty: Anaesth.

ROBERTS, Miss Louise Anne Kent & Sussex Hospital, Mount Ephraim, Tunbridge Wells TN4 8AT Tel: 01892 526111 — MB BS Lond. 1983; FFAEM; FRCS (A&E) Ed. 1991. Cons., A & E. Specialty: Accid. & Emerg.

ROBERTS, Lucy Lizette 2 Cavendish Dr, Edgware HA8 7NR — MB ChB Ed. 1997.

ROBERTS, Lynn 35 Selby Lane, Keyworth, Nottingham NG12 5AQ Tel: 0115 937 2406 — MB ChB Dundee 1978; DA Eng. 1983. Prev: Regist. (Anaesth.) Airedale Gen. Hosp.

ROBERTS, Maiben Brian Ronayne 6 Ismay Wharf, Maryport CA15 8AX Tel: 01900 812166 — MB BCh BAO Dub. 1961 (TC Dub.) DCH RCP Lond. 1966; FRCPI 1983, M 1968; FRCPCH 1998. Locum Cons. Paediat. Specialty: Paediat. Socs: HCSA. Prev: Cons. Paediat. W. Cumbria Health Dist.; Sen. Regist. Paediat. Dept. Radcliffe Infirm. Oxf.; Paediat. Specialist Sarawak, Malaysia.

ROBERTS, Margaret Ann Mansionhouse Unit, Victoria Infirmary, South Glasgow University Hospitals NHS Trust, Mansionhouse Road, Glasgow G41 3DX Tel: 0141 201 6129 Fax: 0141 201 6159 — MD Birm. 1988 (Birmingham University) MRCP (UK) 1976; FRCP Glas. 1986; FRCP Ed. 1994; FRCP Lond. 1998. Cons. Phys. Geriat. Med. Vict. Infirm. Glas. Specialty: Care of the Elderly. Socs: Brit. Geriat. Soc. Prev: Sen. Regist. (Geriat. Med.) Stobhill Hosp. Glas.; Regist. (Med.) South. Gen. Hosp. Glas.; Regist. (Geriat. Med.) South. Gen. Hosp. Glas.

ROBERTS, Margaret Delyth Woodland Avenue Practice, 30 Woodland Avenue, Luton LU3 1RW Tel: 01582 572239 Fax: 01582 494227; 14 The Avenue, Flitwick, Bedford MK45 1BP Tel: 01525 712381 — MB ChB Liverp. 1972; Cert Contracep. & Family Plann. RCOG & RCGP & Family Plann. Assn. 1975; MRCGP 1978. Bd. Mem. Luton PCG. Prev: SHO (Dermat.) Newsham Gen. Hosp. Liverp.; SHO (Psychiat.) Sefton Gen. Hosp. Liverp.

ROBERTS, Margaret Jane Chirk Surgery, Chirk, Wrexham LL14 5BS — BM BCh Oxf. 1987; MA Camb. 1988; MRCP (UK) 1991; DRCOG 1992; MRCGP 1994. Gen. Practitioner, Chirk; Clin. Asst., Wrexham Rheum.

ROBERTS, Marguerite Morrell (retired) 2 Birch Cottage, Werneth Low, Hyde SK14 3AD — MB ChB Manch. 1963; MRCP (UK) 1971; FRCP Lond. 1985. Salford Roy. Hosp.s NHS Trust, N. Manch. Healthcare, W. Pennine Health Auth.

ROBERTS, Marian Elizabeth The Doctors Centre, 41 Broomwood Road, Orpington BR5 2JP Tel: 01689 832454 Fax: 01689 826165; 13 Meadow Way, Farnborough Park, Orpington BR6 8LN Tel: 01689 55730 — MRCS Eng. LRCP Lond. 1967 (St. Bart.) MB BS (Hnrs. Path., Obst. & Gyn.) Lond. 1967; DObst RCOG 1969; MRCGP 1981. Prev: Ho. Surg. P. of Wales Hosp. Tottenham; Ho. Off. (Med.) St. Bart. Hosp. Lond.; SHO (Obst.) Brit. Hosp. Mothers & Babies Woolwich.

ROBERTS, Marion Jean 12 Athol Road, Bramhall, Stockport SK7 1BS — MB ChB Manch. 1994.

ROBERTS, Mark Women's Services, Royal Victoria Infirmary, Newcastle upon Tyne Tel: 0191 282 5861 Email: mark.roberts@nuth.northy.nhs.uk — MB ChB Liverp. 1986; MRCOG 1991; MD Newc. 1997. Cons. (Gynae. Surg.) Roy. Vict. Infirm. Newc. Specialty: Obst. & Gyn. Prev: Research Regist. (O & G) Univ. Newc. u. Tyne.; Research Regist. Princess Mary Matern. Hosp. Newc.

ROBERTS, Mark Andrew — MB ChB Liverp. 1982; MRCP Ed. 1985; MRCPsych 1991. Cons. Forens. Psychiat. Specialty: Forens. Psychiat.

ROBERTS, Mark Eldon Department of Neurology, House 4, Withington Hospital, Nell Lane, West Didsbury, Manchester M20 2LR — MB ChB Liverp. 1989 (Liverpool) BSc (Hons.) Physiol. Liverp. 1986; MRCP (UK) 1992; MD Liverp. 1999. (Neurol.) Cons. Hope Hosp., Manch. Specialty: Neurol. Socs: Assoc. Mem. Assn. Brit. Neurol. Prev: Clin. Research Regist. Inst. Molecular Med. (Dept. Neurosci.) Oxf.; SHO (Neurol.) Nat. Hosp. for Neurol. Lond.; SHO Rotat. (Med.) N. Manch. Gen. Hosp.

ROBERTS, Mark Howard Wakley c/o New Road Rehabilitation Unit, Cumberland Infirmary, Carlisle CA2 7HY Tel: 01228 523444 — MB ChB Leeds 1980; FRCP; BA Oxf. 1973; MRCP (UK) 1983; DM Soton. 1991. Cons. (Rehabil. Med.) N. Cumbria. Specialty: Rehabil. Med.; Rheumatol.

ROBERTS, Mark Theodore Milward Adenbrooke's Hospital, D10 Ward, Box 25, Infectious Diseases Unit, Cambridge CB2 2QQ Tel: 01223 245151 Fax: 01223 586874 — MB BS Lond. 1994; MA Camb. 1995; MRCP (UK) 1998; DTM & H Liverpool 1999. Specialty: Gen. Med.; Infec. Dis. Prev: Med. Regist. John Radcliffe Hosp. Oxf.; SHO (Med.) St. Richard's Hosp. Chichester.

ROBERTS, Martin David Victoria Street Surgery, 1 Victoria Street, Norwich NR1 3XQ Tel: 01603 620872 — MB BS Lond. 1980; DA Eng. 1984; DRCOG 1985; MRCGP 1986.

ROBERTS, Mary Annette Abbey Surgery, 28 Plymouth Road, Tavistock PL19 8BU Tel: 01822 612247 Fax: 01822 618771 — MB BCh Wales 1980; DCH RCPS Glas. 1986.

ROBERTS, Mary Elisabeth The Writtle Surgery, 16A Lordship Road, Writtle, Chelmsford CM1 3EH Tel: 01245 421205 Fax: 01245 422094; 4 Great Godfreys, Writtle, Chelmsford CM1 3PQ — MB ChB Leeds 1968.

ROBERTS, Mary Louise 3 Elm Road, Prenton, Birkenhead CH42 9NY Tel: 0151 608 1220 — MB ChB Manch. 1975; BSc (Hons.) Med. Biochem. Manch. 1972; RMN (Hon.) 1975; BD BS (Research) 1977. Psychoanalyst. Socs: BMA; Anthroposop. Med. Assn.; Brit. Soc. Rehab. Med. Prev: Phys. NATO Forces.

ROBERTS, Megan Charlotte Richmond Royal Hamlet, Kewfoot Road, Richmond TW9 2TE Tel: 020 8355 1967 — MB BS Lond. 1986; MRCPsych 1991. Cons. Gen. Adult Psychait. Qu. Mary's Univ. Hosp Roehampton. Specialty: Gen. Psychiat. Prev: Regist. (Psychiat.) St. Mary's Hosp. Lond.

ROBERTS, Merryl Wynne (retired) 16 Ethelbert Road, Canterbury CT1 3NE Tel: 01227 760294 Fax: 01227 781377 — MB ChB St. And. 1964. SCMO Canterbury & Thanet Health Dist. Prev: Asst. Med. Off. Med. Centre Univ. Kent Canterbury.

ROBERTS, Michael 67 Tenby Road, Moseley, Birmingham B13 9LY — MB ChB Birm. 1987; BSc Birm. 1984, MB ChB 1987; MRCGP 1992.

ROBERTS, Michael Andrew Mor A Mon, Meirion Lane, Bangor LL57 2BU — MB ChB Bristol 1998.

ROBERTS, Michael Bradfield (retired) Westover, Lansdown Road, Bath BA1 5RB — MB ChB Bristol 1967; DMRD Eng. 1971; FFR 1973; FRCR 1975. Cons. Radiol. Bath Health Dist. Prev: Sen. Regist. (Radiodiag.) United Bristol Hosps.

ROBERTS, Michael George (retired) 13 Linnet Hill, Rochdale OL11 4DA Tel: 01706 49899 — MB ChB Manch. 1957; BSc

(Hons.) Manch. 1954, MB ChB 1957; FFA RCS Eng. 1964. Cons. Anaesth. Rochdale & Dist. Hosp. Gp. Fell. Manch. Med. Soc. Prev: Regist. Anaesth. Manch. Roy. Infirm. & Pk. Hosp. Davyhulme.

ROBERTS, Mr Michael John 112 Harnham Road, Salisbury SP2 8JW — MB BS Lond. 1985; FRCS Eng. 1990.

ROBERTS, Michael John Desmond Regional Medical Cardiology Centre, Royal Victoria Hospital, Belfast BT12 6BA; 9 Trossachs Park, Belfast BT10 0AX Tel: 02890 612561 — MB ChB Ed. 1984 (Edinburgh University) FRCP Lond.; FRCPI; MRCP (UK) 1987; MD Belf. 1992. Cons. Cardiol. Roy. Vict. Hosp. Belf. Specialty: Cardiol.

ROBERTS, Miranda Jane Lister Medical Centre, Lister House, Staple Tye, Harlow CM18 7LU Tel: 01279 414882 Fax: 01279 439600; 23 Foxley Drive, Bishop's Stortford CM23 2EB Tel: 01279 755732 — MB BS Lond. 1985. GP Lister Med. Centre Harlow. Prev: Trainee GP Harlow.

ROBERTS, Monica Annette (retired) Faraway, Hill Top, Beaulieu, Brockenhurst SO42 7YT — MB BCh BAO Dub. 1947 (T.C. Dub.) Prev: Res. Med. Off. Odstock Hosp. Salisbury.

ROBERTS, Morian 3 Gilfach Road, Rhydding, Neath SA10 8EH — MB BS Lond. 1974.

ROBERTS, Neil Springbank Barn, Gossefoot Lane, Nabs Head, Samlesbury, Preston PR5 0UQ — MB ChB Dundee 1996.

ROBERTS, Neil Stockwell Lodge Medical Centre, Rosedale Way, Cheshunt, Waltham Cross EN7 6HL Tel: 01992 624408 Fax: 01992 626206.

ROBERTS, Nest Enerys Morris Chelsea & Westminster Hospital, 369 Fulham Road, London SW10 9NH Tel: 020 8237 5293 Fax: 020 8746 8578; Great Ormond Street Hospital, London WC1N 3JH Tel: 020 7405 9200 — MB BS Lond. 1983; MRCP (UK) 1987; BSc Lond. 1980, MD 1993; FRCP UK 2000. p/t Cons. Dermat. Chelsea & Westm. Hosp.; Hon. Cons. Paediat. Dermat. Gt. Ormond St. Hosp. for Childr. Lond.; Hon. Lect. (Pharmacol.) Kings Coll. Lond. Specialty: Dermat. Special Interest: Paediatric Dermatology. Socs: Roy. Soc. Med.; Brit. Assn. Dermat.; Brit. Soc. Allergy & Clin. Immunol. Prev: Cons. Dermat. Qu. Mary's Univ. Hosp. Roehampton; Sen. Regist. (Dermat.) Chelsea & Westm. Hosp. Lond.; Regist. (Dermat.) Westm. Hosp. Lond.

ROBERTS, Nesta Gwendolyn (retired) Gorwel, Llanarth SA47 0NN Tel: 01545 580204 — MRCS Eng. LRCP Lond. 1946.

ROBERTS, Nicholas Adrian Department of Medicine for the Elderly, Queens Park Hospital, Blackburn BB2 3HH Tel: 01254 293865 Fax: 01254 293864 — MB ChB Manch. 1981 (Manchester) MRCP (UK) 1985; FRCP 1996. Cons. Phys. Med. for Elderly Qu.s Pk. Hosp. Blackburn. Specialty: Care of the Elderly. Socs: Brit. Geriat. Soc.; Brit. Soc. Research on Ageing; Brit. Stroke Research Gp.

ROBERTS, Nicholas Ian Swallow Barn, Denbury Green, Denbury, Newton Abbot TQ12 6DQ — MB ChB Bristol 1986; DA 1988.

ROBERTS, Nicola Jane Forest End Surgery, Forest End, Waterlooville PO7 7AH — MB BS Lond. 1977 (Univ. Coll. Hosp.) MRCGP; FP Cert.; MRCP; BSc; DRCOG. GP; Course Organiser, Portsmouth Vocational Train. Scheme; GP Trainer. Specialty: Gen. Med.; Educat.

ROBERTS, Nigel George 2 Little Aston Hall, Streetly, Sutton Coldfield B74 3BH Tel: 0121 353 0608 Fax: 0121 352 1929; Bora-Bora, Paynes Bay, St James, Barbados, West Indies Tel: 00 1 246 432 7345 Fax: 00 1 432 2824 8125 — MRCS Eng. LRCP Lond. 1966; MB BS Lond. 1966. Fleet Med. Cons. Cunard Lines Ltd. Prev: PMO RMS Qu. Eliz. 2 Cunard Lines Ltd.

ROBERTS, Norman Glynne (retired) The Chalet, Marine Drive, Llandudno LL30 2QZ Tel: 01492 77250 — MB ChB Liverp. 1956; DObst RCOG 1958.

ROBERTS, Olumuyiwa Adebola 30C Rhyl Street, London NW5 3HA; 14 Damers Court, Damers Road, Dorchester DT1 2JR Tel: 01305 254595 — MB BS Ibadan 1978; MRCOG 1993. Regist. W. Dorset Gen. Hosp. Socs: BMA & Nigerian Med. Soc.

ROBERTS, Pamela Dorothy (retired) Hilltop, 2 West Road, Prenton, Prenton CH43 9RP Tel: 0151 677 4087 Email: fj.roberts@ntlworld.com — MB BS Lond. 1956; MRCS Eng. LRCP Lond. 1956; DPM Eng. 1966; MRANZCP 1977. Prev: Cons. Child & Adolesc. Psychiat. Merseyside RHA.

ROBERTS, Pamela Fay Caterham Valley Medical Practice, Eothen House, Eothen Close, Caterham CR3 6JU Tel: 01883 347811 Fax: 01883 342929; 76 Tupwood Lane, Caterham CR3 6DP Tel: 01883 347805 — MB BS Lond. 1978 (Char. Cross) DRCOG 1981; MRCGP 1982.

ROBERTS, Pamela Joan (retired) The Cottage, Woodfield Lane, Woodfield Avenue, London SW16 1LF Tel: 020 8769 7901 — MB BS Ceylon 1951. Prev: Clin. Med. Off. Merton & Sutton DHA.

ROBERTS, Patrick James 12 Larkhill Lane, Formby, Liverpool L37 1LX — MB BS Lond. 1991.

ROBERTS, Patrick John Torbay Hospital, Department of Haematology, Lawes Bridge, Torquay TQ2 7AA — BM Soton. 1993; MRCP (UK) 1997; MRCPath 2003. Cons. Haemat. Specialty: Haematology. Prev: Specialist Regist. (Haemat.) Leicester Roy. Infirm. Leicester.

ROBERTS, Mr Paul Elmwood House, Elm Road, Tutshill, Chepstow NP16 7BX Tel: 01291 629490 Fax: 01291 629490 — MB BS Lond. 1981 (St Mary's) MB BS (Hons.) Lond. 1981; MA Oxf. 1983; FRCS Lond. 1986. Cons. Orthop. Surg. Roy. Gwent Hosp. Newport. Specialty: Orthop. Socs: Brit. Orthop. Research Soc.; Brit. Orthop. Assn.; Brit. Hip Soc.

ROBERTS, Paul Douglas Iona, 13 Green East Road, Jordans, Beaconsfield HP9 2SU — MD Leeds 1958; MB ChB 1948; DPath. Eng. 1954. Socs: Brit. Soc. Haemat. Prev: Cons. Haematol. W. Middlx. Hosp. Isleworth; Hon. Sen. Lect. Univ. Lond.; Sen. Regist. Lond. Hosp.

ROBERTS, Paul Richard Wessex & Cardiothoracic Centre, Southampton General Hospital, Tremona Road, Southampton SO16 6YD — MB ChB Leeds 1990; MRCP (UK) 1993.

ROBERTS, Paula Bowling Green Surgery, Bowling Green, Constantine, Falmouth TR11 5AP Tel: 01326 340666 Fax: 01326 340968 — MB ChB Bristol 1970; DRCOG 1973; Cert. Family Plann. JCC 1975; MRCGP 1986. Trainer (Gen. Pract.) Cornw. VTS. Prev: Family Plann. Off. Gilbert & Ellice Is.

ROBERTS, Paula-Jayne Seven Brooks Medical Centre, Church St., Atherton, Manchester M46 9DE Tel: 01942 873533 Fax: 01942 873859; 2 The Rookery, Newton-le-Willows WA12 9PW Tel: 01925 290181 — MB ChB Manch. 1986; BSc (Hons.) Physiol. Manch. 1983; DRCOG 1988; DCH RCPS Glas. 1989; MRCGP 1990; DCCH RCP Ed. 1992; DFFP 1995. GP Manch.; Hon. Research Fell. Nat. Primary Care Research & Developm. Centre Manch. Univ. Socs: Brit. Menopause Soc.; Brit. Med. Acupunct. Soc.; Internat. Menopause Soc. Prev: Clin. Med. Off. (Paediat.) Warrington Trust; Clin. Med. Off. (Family Plann.) Wigan Trust.; Clin. Med. Off. Ashton in Makerfield Wigan.

ROBERTS, Pauline 17 Parkanuar Avenue, Thorpe Bay, Southend-on-Sea SS1 3HX — MB BS Lond. 1976; MRCPsych. 1982.

ROBERTS, Peter John Cookham Medical Centre, Lower Road, Cookham, Maidenhead SL6 9HX — MB BS Lond. 1996 (St Marys Hospital Imperial College) BSc Lond. 1993; DCH Lond. 2001. GP. Specialty: Gen. Pract. Prev: SHO Rotat. (Anaesth.) Hillingdon Hosp./Mt. Vernon Hosp.; Chelsea & Westminster (A & E) St Marys Hosp. Med. & Surgic. Ho. Jobs.

ROBERTS, Mr Peter Neil Oak House, Eastwood Business Village, Coventry CV3 2UB Tel: 02476 561900; 64 Purnells Way, Knowle, Solihull B93 9EE Tel: 01564 772841 — (Birmingham) MB ChB Birm. 1969; FRCS Eng. 1975. Cons. Gen. & Vasc. Surg. Walsgrave Hosp. Coventry. Specialty: Gen. Surg.

ROBERTS, Peter Richard Gerald 6 Seaburn Drive, Houghton-le-Spring DH4 5DW; 27 Maindy Road, Cathays, Cardiff CF24 4HL Tel: 01222 232414 — MB ChB Ed. 1993. Specialist Regist. (Anaesth.) Univ. Hosp. of Wales Cardiff. Specialty: Anaesth.; Intens. Care.

ROBERTS, Philip Franklin Norfolk & Norwich University Hospital, Department of Histopathology, Colney Lane, Norwich NR4 7UY Tel: 01603 286019 Fax: 01603 286017 — MB BS Lond. 1966 (St Bart.) MRCS Eng. LRCP Lond. 1966; MRCP Lond. 1969; FRCPath 1984, M 1972; FRCP Lond. 1998. Cons. Histopath. Norf. & Norwich Hosp.; Mem. (Ct.) Univ. E. Anglia; Examr. Histopath. Roy. Coll. Paths.; Mem. Ct. Examrs. RCS Eng. Specialty: Histopath. Socs: BMA. Prev: East. Region Vice-Chair, Adv. Comm on Distinc. Awards; Dir. (Path.) Norf. & Norwich Hosp.; Regional Represen. Roy. Coll. Paths.

ROBERTS, Mr Philip Hugh Martindale, Bridgwater Road, Sidcot, Winscombe BS25 1NN Tel: 01934 844135 Fax: 01934 843075 — MB ChB Manch. 1958; FRCS Eng. 1964; FRCS Ed. 1964. Hon. Cons. Orthop. Surg. Weston Area Health Trust; Hon. Clin. Teach. Univ. Bristol. Specialty: Orthop. Socs: Fell. Bristol M-C Soc.; (Pres.)

Bristol Medico-Legal Soc. Prev: Sen. Regist. (Orthop.) Manch. Roy. Infirm.; Regist. (Orthop.) Robt. Jones & Agnes Hunt Orthop. Hosp. Oswestry; Resid. Surg. Off. Preston Roy. Infirm.

ROBERTS, Philip John 8 Fairview, Erith DA8 2PR — MB BS Lond. 1989.

ROBERTS, Mr Philip John Marsdens, 7 Brook Road, Whitchurch SY13 1QF Tel: 01948 664799 Fax: 01948 664799 — MB BS Lond. 1992 (St. Mary's Med. Sch.) BSc (Hons.) Lond. 1990; FRCS Eng. 1996; FRCS (Tr and Orth) 2002. Specialist Regist., Orthop. & Trauma, N. Staffs. Roy. Infirm., Stoke-on-Trent. Specialty: Trauma & Orthop. Surg. Socs: BOA; Brit. Orthopaedic Research Soc. Prev: McCowan Schol., St. Mary's Med. Sch., 1986, 1987 and 1988; Laming Evans research fell., Roy. Coll. Of Surgs.

ROBERTS, R Elizabeth (retired) 1 Waverley Lodge, The Knowes, Kelso TD5 7BB Tel: 01573 228153 — MB BS Lond. 1964; MRCS Eng. LRCP Lond. 1964; FFCM 1989, M 1983. Prev: Dir. Breast Test Wales.

ROBERTS, Rachel Fiona 10 Curlew Lane, Stockton-on-Tees TS20 1NA — MB ChB Leic. 1995.

ROBERTS, Rachel Penelope Ludmilla Forest Practice, 26 Pyrles Lane, Loughton IG10 2NH Tel: 020 8508 4580 Fax: 020 8508 4383 — MB BS (Hons.) Lond. 1986; MRCP (UK) 1989; DCH RCP Lond. 1990; MRCGP 1993; DFFP 1995. One session course organiser post Ilford Scheme. Prev: SHO (O & G) Homerton Hosp. Lond.; SHO (Paediat.) St. Mary's Hosp. Lond.; SHO (A & E & Med.) Char. Cross Hosp.

ROBERTS, Raine Emily Ireland, MBE 459 Altrincham Road, Wythenshawe, Manchester M23 1AA Tel: 0161 998 3326 Fax: 0161 998 3326 — MB ChB Manch. 1955; DCH Eng. 1958; FRCGP 1982, M 1968; DMJ (Clin.) Soc. Apoth. Lond. 1979. Clin. Dir. St. Mary's Centre (Sexual Assault Referral Centre) St. Mary's Hosp. Manch.; Forens. Phys. Gtr. Manch. Police. Socs: Fell. Manch. Med. Soc.; Roy. Soc. Med. (Ex-Pres. Sec. Clin. Forens. Med.). Prev: Regist. (Gen. Med.) Blackburn Roy. Infirm.; Ho. Phys. & Ho. Surg. (Neurosurg.) Manch. Roy. Infirm.; Ho. Phys. (Paediat.) Pendlebury Childr. Hosp.

ROBERTS, Ralph Neville Frank Rothschild House Surgery, Chapel Street, Tring HP23 6PU Tel: 01442 822468 Fax: 01442 825889; Dormers, Buckland Village, Aylesbury HP22 5HY Tel: 01296 630256 Fax: 01296 630256 — MB BS Lond. 1974 (Roy. Free) Specialty: Gen. Pract. Socs: Roy. Soc. Med.

ROBERTS, Ralph Nigel Duchess of Gloucester Maternity Unit, Ulster Hospital, Dundonald, Belfast BT16 1RH Tel: 02890 484511 Fax: 02890 561402 — MB BCh BAO Belf. 1983; BSc Belf. 1980; MRCP (UK) 1986; MRCOG 1989; MFFP 1993; MD Belf. 1996; FRCP Ed. 2000. Cons. (O & G) Ulster Hosp. Dundonald. Specialty: Obst. & Gyn. Socs: Brit. Med. Assn.; Ulster Obst. & Gyn. Soc.; Brit. Fertil. Soc. Prev: Sen. Regist. (O & G) Qu. Mother's Hosp. Glas.; Lect. (O & G) Univ. Edin.; Research Regist. (O & G) Roy. Matern. Hosp. Belf.

ROBERTS, Rebecca Jane 8 Woodthorn Close, Daresbury, Warrington WA4 6NQ — MB ChB Manch. 1995.

ROBERTS, Rhian Carrington 19 Green Park, Wrexham LL13 7YE Email: rhianroberts@hotmail.com — MB BCh Wales 1996.

ROBERTS, Richard Alun 21 St Georges Road, Formby, Liverpool L37 3HH — MB BCh Wales 1993.

ROBERTS, Richard Charles Ninewells Hospital and Medical School, Department of Neurology, Dundee DD1 9SY Tel: 01382 425720 Fax: 01382 425739 Email: r.c.roberts@dundee.ac.uk; 67 Camphill Road, Broughty Ferry, Dundee DD5 2LY Tel: 01382 477438 — BM BCh Oxf. 1976 (Oxford) MA, DPhil Oxf. 1974; MRCP (UK) 1979; FRCP Ed. 1994. Reader in Med., Univ. Dundee; Hon. Cons. Neurologist, NHS Tayside. Specialty: Neurol. Prev: Clin. Lect. Inst. Neurol. Qu. Sq. Lond.

ROBERTS, Richard Clive 7 Woodville Road W., Cinderford GL14 2AT — MB BS Lond. 1998; MB BS Lond 1998.

ROBERTS, Richard John Bryn Clwyd, Brookhouse, Denbigh LL16 4RF — MB BS Lond. 1986; BSc Lond. 1983; DCH RCP Lond. 1989; MPH Wales 1992; MFPHM Lond. 1995. Cons. Communicable Dis. Control N. Wales HA. Specialty: Pub. Health Med. Prev: Sen. Regist. (Pub. Health Med.) Health Prom. Auth. Wales & PHLS CDSC (Welsh Unit).

ROBERTS, Richard Norman 22 Meadow Road, Finchfield, Wolverhampton WV3 8EZ — MB ChB Birm. 1996; ChB Birm. 1996.

ROBERTS, Richard Ralton (retired) 30 Whalley Drive, Bletchley, Milton Keynes MK3 6HS Tel: 01908 373320 — MB BS Lond. 1958 (Univ. Coll. Hosp.) BSc (Anat.) Lond. 1955; MRCS Eng. LRCP Lond. 1958; DCH Eng. 1961. Prev: Ho. Phys. & Ho. Surg. Cheltenham Gen. Hosp.

ROBERTS, Robert Sion Cynfab Taleithin, Penglais Road, Aberystwyth SY23 2EU — MB BCh Wales 1989.

ROBERTS, Robin Hugh Queen Mary's Hospital, Roehampton, London SW15 5PW Tel: 0208 355 2677 Fax: 0208 355 2258; Ridge End, The Drive, Wimbledon, London SW20 8TG Email: RobinHRoberts@aol.com — MB BS Lond. 1982 (Westm.) MRCP (UK) 1985. Cons. Cardiol. Qu. Marys, Roehampton Kingston Hosp.; The Roy. Brompton Hosp.; Cons. Cardiol. Qu. Mary's Hosp.; Cons. Cardiol. Roy. Brompton Hosp., Lond. Specialty: Cardiol. Special Interest: Coronary Angiography; Heart Failure; Hypertemsion.

ROBERTS, Roma Elizabeth Willow Green Surgery, Station Road, East Preston, Littlehampton BN16 3AH Tel: 01903 758152 Fax: 01903 859986; Poundville, Roundstone Lane, Angmering, Littlehampton BN16 4AP — MB BS Lond. 1984 (St. Geo.) DRCOG 1989; Cert. Family Plann. JCC 1989. Specialty: Obst. & Gyn. Prev: Trainee GP Bordon & Liss; SHO (O & G & Paediat.) Portsmouth.

ROBERTS, Ruth Diane Department of Care of the Elderly, Weston General Hospital, Grange Road, Uphill, Weston Super Mare BS23 4TQ Tel: 01934 636363 Fax: 01934 619275; Long Meadow, 52 Church Lane, Backwell, Bristol BS48 3PQ Tel: 01275 463100 — MB BS Lond. 1969 (St. Geo.) DCH Eng. 1971. Staff Grade Doctor (c/o the Elderly) Weston Gen. Hosp. Weston-Super-Mare. Specialty: Care of the Elderly. Socs: Brit. Geriat. Soc. Prev: Clin. Asst. (Geriat. Med.) Frenchay Hosp. Bristol; Regist. (Paediat.) Qu. Charlotte's Hosp. Lond.; Regist. (Geriat. Med.) Plymouth Gen. Hosp.

ROBERTS, Ruth Esther Pennant Rosetree Cottage, High St., Elswick, Preston PR4 3ZB — MB ChB Leeds 1990; MRCP (UK) 1994. SHO (Paediat.) St. Mary's Hosp. Manch. Specialty: Paediat. Prev: SHO (Paediat.) Salford Community Health, Booth Hall Childr. Hosp. & Leeds Gen. Infirm.

ROBERTS, Sally Ann 16 Pisgah Street, Kenfig Hill, Bridgend CF33 6BY — MB ChB Bristol 1986.

ROBERTS, Sally Ann Hawthorn Cottage, Unthank, Dalston, Carlisle CA5 7BA — MB BS Newc. 1992.

ROBERTS, Sally Kathryn 52 Church Lane, Backwell, Bristol BS48 3PQ — MB BS Lond. 1998; MB BS Lond 1998.

ROBERTS, Sam Craig 30 North Deeside Road, Bieldside, Aberdeen AB15 9AB — MB ChB Aberd. 1998; MB ChB Aberd 1998.

ROBERTS, Selwyn Pennant Wythenshawe Hospital, Southmoor Road, Manchester M23 9LT; 69 Kingston Road, Manchester M20 2SB — BM BCh Oxf. 1982; MA Camb. 1982; DA (UK) 1984; FRCA. 1986. Cons. Anaesth. Univ. Hosp. Manch.; Hon. Lect. (Anaesth.) Univ. Manch. Specialty: Anaesth.

ROBERTS, Sheila Elizabeth 25 Bartle Gill Drive, Baildon, Shipley BD17 6UE — MB ChB Sheff. 1977. GP Bradford. Prev: Clin. Med. Off. (Community Child Health & Family Plann.) Yorks.

ROBERTS, Sheila Mary (retired) Derwen Deg, Hwfa Road, Bangor LL57 2BN — MB BS Lond. 1964. Prev: GP Daventry.

ROBERTS, Sheila Rosemary 74 Windermere Crescent, Looseleigh, Plymouth PL6 5HX Tel: 01752 774774 — MRCS Eng. LRCP Lond. 1976; DLO RCS Eng. 1988. Staff Grade (Ear Nose & Throat) Derriford Hosp. Plymouth. Specialty: Otorhinolaryngol. Prev: Clin. Asst. (ENT) Derriford Hosp. Plymouth.

ROBERTS, Sian Fiona, Flight Lt. RAF Med. Br. 2 Mount Cottages, Adbaston, Knighton, Stafford ST20 0QQ — MB BS Lond. 1992; MB BS (Hons.) Lond. 1992; DCH RCP Lond. 1995. Trainee GP RAF Halton Aylesbury. Prev: SHO (Paediat.) St. Geo. Hosp. Lond.; Ho. Off. (Med.) St. Bart. Hosp. Lond.; Ho. Off. (Surg.) N. Middlx. Hosp.

ROBERTS, Mr Simon Nicholas John Robert Jones & Agnes Hunt Hospital, Oswestry SY10 7AG Tel: 01691 404167 — BM BCh Oxf. 1987 (Camb. & Oxf.) MA Camb. 1988; FRCS Eng. 1992; FRCS (Orth) 1996. Cons. Orthop. & Sports Injury Surg.; Cons. Othopaedic Surg., Wrexham Maelor Hosp., Croesnewydd Rd., Wrexham CLWTD. Specialty: Sports Med.; Trauma & Orthop. Surg.; Orthop. Special Interest: Sports Injury Surg.; Knee; Shoulder. Socs: Fell. BOA; BASEM; ISAKOS.

ROBERTS, Sophie Amanda 20 Longfield Terrace, York YO30 7DJ — MB BS Newc. 1992. Regist. (Psychiat.) Bootham Pk. Hosp. York. Specialty: Gen. Psychiat.

ROBERTS, Stanley Desmond, OBE 7 Viewfort Park, Upper Malone, Dunmurry, Belfast BT17 9JY Tel: 02896 627006 Fax: 02896627006 — MB BCh BAO Belf. 1956 (Qu. Univ. Belf.) MD Belf. 1960; FRCPI 1975, M 1963; FRCP Lond. 1975, M 1963; FRCP Ed. 1996; FRCP 1997. Hon. Cons. Phys. & Rheum. Roy. Vict. Hosp. & Musgrave Pk. Hosp. Belf. Specialty: Rheumatol. Socs: Brit. Soc. Rheum.; Assn. Phys. Prev: Pres. Roy. Coll. Phys. Irel.; ARC Research Fell. At MRC Rheum. Research Unit Taplow.

ROBERTS, Stephen Arthur Paediatric Department, Wythenshawe Hospital, Southmoor Road, Manchester M23 9LT — MB ChB 1970; FRCPCH; MD Edinburgh 1982; FRCP London 1990. Cons. Paediat. Univ. Hosp. S. Manch. Specialty: Paediat. Socs: Brit. Paediat. Assn.; Brit. Soc. Allergy & Clin. Immunol.

ROBERTS, Stephen John Deben Road Surgery, 2 Deben Road, Ipswich IP1 5EN Tel: 01473 741152 Fax: 01473 743237; 2 Deben Road, Ipswich IP1 5EN — MB ChB Aberd. 1983; MRCGP 1987.

ROBERTS, Stephen Jones Llawenydd, Gwaenysgor, Rhyl LL18 6EW Tel: 01745 888588 — MB BCh Wales 1985. GP. Specialty: Community Child Health.

ROBERTS, Stephen Louis Sunnyside, 19 London Road, Woore, Crewe CW3 9SF — MB BS Lond. 1978; Dip. Bact. Manch. 1984; AFOM RCP Lond. 1990. Specialty: Occupat. Health.

ROBERTS, Stephen Owen Bellamy (retired) 14 Fendon Road, Cambridge CB1 7RT — MB BChir Camb. 1961 (Guy's) MA, MB Camb. 1961, BChir 1960; MRCS Eng. LRCP Lond. 1960; FRCP Lond. 1979, M 1964. Formerly Cons. Dermat. Addenbrookes Hosp. Camb.

ROBERTS, Steven John 1 Prospect Row, Burley-in-Wharfdale, Ilkley LS29 7AT — MB ChB Leeds 1992.

ROBERTS, Stuart Morgan Strawberry Place Surgery, 5 Strawberry Place, Morriston, Swansea SA6 7AQ Tel: 01792 522526 Fax: 01792 527530; Mayfield, 547 Clydach Road, Ynystawe, Swansea SA6 5AA Tel: 01792 845946 — MB ChB Liverp. 1970; DObst RCOG 1973; MRCGP 1975.

ROBERTS, Susan 21 Gronant .Road, Prestatyn LL19 9DT — MB ChB Leic. 1987. Specialty: Community Child Health.

ROBERTS, Susan Ann Margaret Microbiology Laboratory, Universtiy Hospital of Hartlepool, Holdforth Rd, Hartlepool TS24 9AH Tel: 01429 266654 Ext: 2420 — MRCS Eng. LRCP Lond. 1976 (Sheff.) Dip. Bact. Manch. 1981; MRCPath 1983. Cons. Med. Microbiol. N. Tees & Hartlepool NHS Trust. Specialty: Med. Microbiol. Socs: Fell. Roy. Coll. Path.

ROBERTS, Susan Elizabeth Kim East Quay Medical Centre, East Quay, Bridgwater TA6 5YB Tel: 01278 444666 Fax: 01278 445448 — MB ChB Bristol 1984; DRCOG 1988; MRCGP 1993. Prev: SHO (Gen. Med.) Weston Gen. Hosp. Weston-Super-Mare; SHO (ENT) Bath Roy. United Hosp.; SHO (A & E) Frenchay Hosp. Bristol.

ROBERTS, Susan Holt Northumbria Health Care Trust, Diabetes Resource Centre, North Tynside District General Hospital, Rake Lane, North Shields NE29 8NH Tel: 0191 293 2708 Fax: 0191 293 2734; 25 Linden Road, Newcastle upon Tyne NE3 4EY Tel: 0191 285 5004 Fax: 0191 285 5004 — MB BS Lond. 1969 (Middlx.) BSc (Physiol.) Lond. 1966; FRCP Lond. 1986, M 1972; MSc (Clin. Biochem.) Newc. 1975. Cons. Phys. (Med. & Diabetes) N. Tyneside HA. Specialty: Diabetes. Socs: Brit. Diabetic Assn.; Educat. Advis. Comm. Prev: Regist. (Gastroenterol.) Roy. Vict. Infirm. Newc.; Lect. (Med.) Memor. Univ. of Newfld. St. John's, Canada; Sen. Regist. (Research) Dept. Med. Newc. Gen. Hosp.

ROBERTS, Suzanne Hannah Kaleidescope Project, 40-46 Cromwell Road, Kingston upon Thames KT2 6RE — MB ChB Sheff. 1974; DRCOG 1976; DTM & H Liverp. 1991. Ministerial Stud. S. Wales Baptist Coll. Cardiff. Specialty: Pub. Health Med. Prev: ACRIS Community Health Progr., Mozambique; Clinician i/c BBS Ruhea Clinic Community Health Progr., Bangladesh; Clin. Med. Off. Greenwich HA.

ROBERTS, Sylvia Ann Ashley Centre Surgery, Ashley Square, Epsom KT18 5DD Tel: 01372 723668 Fax: 01372 726796 — MB ChB Leeds 1974; DRCOG 1976; DCH Eng. 1977; MRCGP 1978.

ROBERTS, Teresa Agnes Gunn, Roberts, Fourie and Cooper, Witton Medical Centre, 29-31 Preston Old Road, Blackburn BB2 2SU Tel: 01254 262123 Fax: 01254 695759; The Old Barn, Bowfields Lane, Balderstone, Blackburn BB2 7LW — MB ChB Manch. 1983. Princip. in Gen. Pract., Blackburn. Specialty: Diabetes. Prev: Community Med. Off. Burnley, Pendle & Rossendale HA.

ROBERTS, Teresa Catherine 78 Wymondley Road, Hitchin SG4 9PT — BM BS Nottm. 1984; DRCOG 1989. Specialty: Gen. Pract.

ROBERTS, Thomas Gwyn Beechley Medical Centre, 73 Ruabon Road, Wrexham LL13 7PU Tel: 01978 361279 Fax: 01978 350915; T'Yr Gloch Farm, Talwyn, Coedpoeth, Wrexham LL11 3BY — MB ChB Liverp. 1976; MRCP (UK) 1978; MRCGP 1983; DCH RCP Lond. 1983.

ROBERTS, Timothy Edward Flat 1, 39 Hanover Square, Leeds L53 1BQ Email: teroberts85@hotmail .com — MB ChB Leeds 1997. Gen. Practitioner.

ROBERTS, Timothy Lloyd North Devon District Hospital, Raleigh Park, Barnstaple EX31 4JB Tel: 01271 322418 Fax: 01271 322709; Herders, Kings Heanton, Barnstaple EX31 4ED Tel: 01271 346418 — MB BS Lond. 1982 (Middlx.) BSc Physiol. (Hons.) Lond. 1979, MB BS 1982; MRCP (UK) 1985; MD Lond. 1995; FRCP London 2000. Cons. Cardiol. and Phys. N. Devon Dist. Hosp. Specialty: Cardiol.; Gen. Med. Socs: Brit. Cardiac Soc. Prev: Regist. (Cardiol.) Soton. Gen. Hosp.; Lect. (Preven. Cardiol.) Univ. Soton.; Clin. Research Phys. Wellcome Foundat.

ROBERTS, Trevor John Hyde Bungeons Farm Cottage, Barking, Ipswich IP6 8HN — MB BS Lond. 1962; DObst RCOG 1965; MRCS Eng. LRCP Lond. 1965. Med. Off. Nat. Blood Serv. Camb. Specialty: Blood Transfus.

ROBERTS, Professor Trudie Elizabeth Medical Education Unit, Level 7 Worsley Building, University or Leeds Medical School, Leeds LS2 9JT Tel: 0113 343 1657 Fax: 0113 343 4910 Email: t.e.roberts@leeds.ac.uk — MB ChB Manch. 1979; PhD Manch. 1987, BSc (Hons.) (Anat.) 1976, MB ChB 1979; MRCP (UK) 1982; FRCP 1999. Prof. of Med. Educat. and Director of the Med. Educat. Unit; Hon. Cons. Leeds Acute Trust. Specialty: Gen. Med.

ROBERTS, Vivienne Margaret Twyford Surgery, Loddon Hall Road, Twyford, Reading RG10 9JA Tel: 0118 934 0112 Fax: 0118 934 1048 — MB BS Newc. 1979; DCH RCP Lond. 1983; MRCGP 1988.

ROBERTS, William (retired) 19 West Road, Irvine KA12 8RE — (Anderson Coll. Glas.) LRCP LRCS Ed. LRFPS Glas. 1945; FRFPS Glas. 1951; FRCP Glas. 1973, M 1962. Prev: Cons. Phys. (with Responsibil. For Infec. Dis.) Ayrsh. Centr. Hosp. Irvine.

ROBERTS, William James Cynfab (retired) Taleithin, Penglais Road, Aberystwyth SY23 2EU Tel: 01970 623321 — MB BChir Camb. 1964 (Camb. & St Mary's) MA Camb. 1963; DObst RCOG 1966; FRCGP 1988, M 1977. Prev: Treasury Med. Off.

ROBERTS, William Owen Bryn Awel, Gyrngoch, Clynnogfawr, Caernarfon LL54 5PG — MB ChB Liverp. 1966; DObst RCOG 1970; FFA RCSI 1973; FFA RCS Eng. 1974. Cons. Anaesth. Caerns. & Anglesey & St. David's Hosps. Bangor, Eryri; Hosp. Caernarfon & Caernarfon Eye & Cott. Hosp. Specialty: Anaesth. Prev: Med. Off. Zambian Flying Doctor Serv.

ROBERTS, William Thomas — MB ChB Liverp. 1975; Cert. Family Plann. JCC 1980; Dip. ALS RCS Eng. 1996; Dip. ATLS RCS Eng. 1996. GP with Halton PCT. Specialty: Accid. & Emerg. Prev: SHO (Cas. & Gen. Surg.) Walton & Fazakerley Hosp. Liverp.; Lect. (Anat.) Univ. Manch.; Ho. Off. St. Helens Hosp.

ROBERTS-HAREWOOD, Marilyn-Rae Diane — MB BS Lond. 1989 (St. Geos.) MRCP (UK) 1993. SpR (Haemat.). Specialty: Haematology. Prev: Clin. Research Fell. (Haemat.).

ROBERTS-HARRY, Nest Gwenllian (retired) 20 Cimla Road, Neath SA11 3PP Tel: 01639 4601 — (Cardiff) BSc, MB BCh Wales, 1941; DCH Eng. 1947. Prev: Ho. Phys. Llandough Hosp. Penarth.

ROBERTS-HARRY, Mr Thomas John West Wales General Hospital, Department of Ophthalmology, Carmarthen SA31 2AF — MB BS Lond. 1979; MRCS Eng. LRCP Lond. 1978; FRCS Ed. 1986; FRCOphth 1994. Cons. (Ophth.) W. Wales Gen. Hosp. Specialty: Ophth. Prev: Sen. Regist. Rotat. (Ophth.) Univ. Coll., Roy. Free, St Bart. & Moorfields Eye Hosp. Lond.

ROBERTS-PUW, Elin Hanna Conwy & Denbighshire Health Trust, Health Premises, Argyll Road, Llandudno LL30 1DF Tel: 01492 862000 — MB BCh Wales 1982. SCMO Aberconwy. Specialty: Community Child Health. Socs: BMA; Welsh Med. Soc.; BACCH.

ROBERTS-SHEPHARD, Alison 2 Albury Avenue, Sutton SM2 7JT — MB BS Lond. 1977; DRCOG 1979; DCH Eng. 1980; MRCGP 2001.

ROBERTS-THOMSON, Mr James Harold 38 Caves Lane, Bedford MK40 3DP — MB BS Tasmania 1977; BMedSc Tasmania 1980, MB BS 1977; FRCS Glas. 1986.

ROBERTSHAW, Barbara Ann Earls House Hospital, Durham DH1 5RE Tel: 0191 333 6296 Fax: 0191 333 6528 — (Galway) MB BCh BAO NUI 1967; DPM Dub. 1972; FRCPsych 1996, M 1974. Assoc. Med. Dir.Learning Disabil.Co. Durh. & Darlington Priority Serv. NHS Trust; Assessor for Advis. Appts. Comms. (Cons. & Hon. Cons.) Roy. Coll. Psychiat. Specialty: Gen. Psychiat. Prev: Regist. St. Patrick's Hosp. Dub. & Earls Ho. Hosp. Durh.; SHO Stewart's Hosp. Palmerstown.

ROBERTSHAW, Carolyn Jane Thames Valley Hospice, Hatch Lane, Windsor SL4 3RW Tel: 01753 842121 Fax: 01753 832886; Willowtree House, 50 Alma Road, Windsor SL4 3HA Tel: 01753 832685 — MB ChB Manch. 1985; Dip Palliat Med Cardiff; Dip Med Ac; BSc St. And. 1982; DCH RCP Lond. 1987; MRCGP 1989; DRCOG 1989. Med. Dir. Thames Valley Hospice Windsor. Specialty: Gen. Pract. Special Interest: Acupunc.; Palliat. Med. Socs: Brit. Med. Acupunct. Soc.; BMA. Prev: GP Windsor; Trainee GP Milnthorpe & Bracknell; SHO (Paediat.) Roy. Lancaster Infirm.

ROBERTSHAW, Denise Elizabeth (retired) Flat 2 Springhead Court, 444 Haworth Road, Allerton, Bradford BD15 9LL Tel: 01274 544511 — MB ChB Ed. 1958; DPH Leeds 1965; DCH Eng. 1966; MFCM 1974. Prev: Cons. Pub. Health Med. Leeds Health Dist.

ROBERTSHAW, Heidi Jane 16 Barmouth Road, London SW18 2DN; Anaesthetic Department, St Mary's Hospital, Praed St., London W2 1NY — (St. Bartholomew's Hospital) MB BS Lond. 1993; FRCA 1998. Anaesth. Regist. St Marys Hosp. Lond. Specialty: Anaesth.

ROBERTSHAW, John Keith 150 Longmoor Lane, Breaston, Derby DE72 3BE — MB ChB Bristol 1981.

ROBERTSHAW, Katharine Anna Derbyshire Children's Hopital, Uttoxeter Road, Derby DE22 3NE Tel: 01132 340131 — MB ChB Leeds 1993; MCRP (Edin.) (Paeds) 1996. SpR in Community Paediat., Derbysh. Childr.'s Hosp. Derby. Specialty: Paediat. Socs: MRCPCH.

ROBERTSHAW, Mary Freda Ribbleton Medical Surgery, 243 Ribbleton Ave, Ribbleton, Preston PR2 6RD — MB ChB Manch. 1974.

ROBERTSHAW, Nancy Miriam Elsie (retired) Beech Bank, Beetham, Milnthorpe LA7 7AL Tel: 015395 62651 — MB ChB St. And. 1945; BSc St. And. 1942; DObst RCOG 1948; DCH Eng. 1953; DPM Eng. 1967. Prev: Assoc. Specialist (Psychiat.) Leighton Hosp. Crewe.

ROBERTSHAW, Richard Three Hollies, Brilly Green, Whitney-on-Wye, Hereford HR3 6HZ — MB BS Lond. 1962 (King's Coll. Hosp.) MRCS Eng. LRCP Lond. 1961; DA Eng. 1963; FFA RCS Eng. 1966. p/t Cons. (Palliat. Care & Pain Managem.) Qu. Eliz. Hosp. King's Lynn. Specialty: Anaesth. Prev: Cons. (Anaesth. & Chronic Pain Managem.) Peterboro. Dist. Hosp.; Staff Anaesth. Trail-Tadenal Hosp. Canada; Clin. Research Fell. (Anaesth.) Hosp. Sick Childr. Toronto.

ROBERTSHAW, William Edward Guy West House Farm, Bishop Middleham, Ferryhill DL17 9DY — MB BS Newc. 1986; MRCPsych. 1991. Trainee GP Cleveland VTS. Prev: Regist. (Psychiat.) Airedale Gen. Hosp. Keighley.

ROBERTSON, Adam Alan (retired) 2 Rothsay Place, Edinburgh EH3 7SL Tel: 0131 226 4961 — MB ChB Ed. 1951; MRCGP 1963. Prev: MuirHo. Med. Gp.

ROBERTSON, Agnes Helen Angela Riverbank Practice, Janet St., Thurso KW14 7AR Tel: 01847 892027; Bruan Lodge, Mid Clyth, Lybster KW3 6BA Tel: 01593 721296 — MB ChB Ed. 1974; BSc Ed. 1971; DFFP 1997. Princip. (p/t), Riverbank Pract., Thurso, Caithness. Socs: BMA; MDDUS. Prev: Assoc. GP Lybster & Dunbeath Pract.s.

ROBERTSON, Aileen Patricia Albany House Medical Centre, 3 Queen Street, Wellingborough NN8 4RW Tel: 01933 222309 Fax: 01993 229236 — MB ChB Dundee 1985; DCH RCP Lond. 1989; DRCOG 1989.

ROBERTSON, Alasdair Neil 1 Kylepark Crescent, Uddingston, Glasgow G71 7DQ — MB ChB Glas. 1995.

ROBERTSON, Alastair Scott University Hospital Birmingham, Occupational Health Department, Woodlands Nurses Home, Selly Oak Hospital, Birmingham B29 6JF Tel: 0121 627 8286 Fax: 0121 627 8312; 9 St Bernards Road, Olton, Solihull B92 7AU Tel: 0121 707 5639 — MB ChB Aberd. 1978; MRCP (UK) 1981; MFOM RCP 1992, AFOM 1989; FFOM 1997; FRCP 1998. Cons. Occupat. Health Univ. Hosp. Birm. NHS Trust; Cons. Occupat. Respirat. Dis. Birm. Chest Clinic; Hon. Sen. Lect. Univ. Birm. Specialty: Occupat. Health. Socs: Brit. Thorac. Soc. & Soc. Occupat. Med.; Assn. Nat. Health Servs. Occupat. Phys. Prev: Lect. (Occupat. Health) Univ. Birm.; Regist. (Respirat. Dis.) Kings Cross Hosp. Dundee; Ho. Surg. & Ho. Phys. Roy. Infirm. Aberd.

ROBERTSON, Alastair Wilson (retired) Haworth, Lundin Links, Lower Largo, Leven KY8 6AH Tel: 01333 320335 — (St. And.) MB ChB (Commend.) St. And. 1949; DIH Soc. Apoth. Lond. 1976; CIH Dund 1976; MFOM RCP Lond. 1984. Prev: Occupat. Phys. St. And. Univ. Fife.

ROBERTSON, Alexander Delamere, West End Lane, Warton, Preston PR4 1TA — LRCP LRCS Ed. 1939; LRCP LRCS Ed. LRFPS Glas. 1939.

ROBERTSON, Mr Alexander Alan 22 Dumyat Drive, Falkirk FK1 5PD Tel: 01324 24430 — MB ChB Glas. 1949; FRCS Ed. 1957. Cons. Orthop. Surg. Stirlingsh. Area, Falkirk & Dist., & Stirling Roy. Infirms. Specialty: Orthop. Prev: Cons. Orthop. Surg. Norf. & Norwich & Gt. Yarmouth Hosps.; Sen. Regist. Orthop. Dundee Roy. Infirm. & Bridge of Earn Hosp.; Orthop. Regist. West. Infirm. Glas.

ROBERTSON, Alick John Cuminestown, 8 Long Hey Road, Caldy, Wirral CH48 1LZ Tel: 0151 625 7248 Fax: 0151 625 0807 Email: drajrcaldy@onetel.net.uk — MB ChB Liverp. 1942; FRCP Lond. 1964, M 1949; MD Liverp. 1951; MFOM RCP Lond. 1983. Cons. WHO (Afghanistan); Mem. Inst. & Emerit. Cons. Phys. King Edwd. VII Hosp. Midhurst; Examr. Milroy Lect. & Fitzpatrick Lect. RCP Lond.; Emerit. Cons. Phys. & Phys. Heart Dept. Roy. Liverp. Univ. Hosp. Specialty: Gen. Med.; Respirat. Med.; Occupat. Health. Socs: Thoracic Soc.; Assn. Phys.; Internat. Soc. Internal Med. Prev: Edr. Thorax; Samuel Memor. Schol. 1951.

ROBERTSON, Alistair Charles The Health Centre, 11 Hull Road, Hessle HU13 9LU Tel: 01482 634331 — MB ChB Aberd. 1968. Prev: Ho. Phys. City Hosp. Aberd.; Ho. Surg. Dumfries & Galloway Roy. Infirm.

ROBERTSON, Alistair John Pathology Department, Ninewells Hospital & Medical School, Dundee DD1 9SY Tel: 01382 660111 Fax: 01382 640966; Glendale, Kilspindie, Errol, Perth PH2 7RX — MB ChB Aberd. 1975; BMedBiol (Hons.) 1972; FRCPath 1993. Clin. Gp. Director, Clin. support Serv.s, Tayside Teachg. Hosp.s NHS Trust.; Cons. & Hon. Sen. Lect. (Path.) Dundee Tech. Hosp. NHS Trust. Specialty: Pathology, General. Socs: Internat. Acad. Path. & Assn. Clin. Pathols. Prev: Lect. & Hon. Sen. Regist. (Path.) Univ. Dundee at Ninewells Hosp.; Cons. in Admin. Charge Lab. Servs. Perth & Kinross Dist.

ROBERTSON, Alistair Stuart Manor House Surgery, Providence Place, Bridlington YO15 2QW; 11 Second Avenue, Bridlington YO15 2LL — MB ChB Leeds 1985; BSc (Hons.) (Physiol.) Leeds 1982, MB ChB 1985; MRCGP 1989; DRCOG 1989. GP N. Humberside.

ROBERTSON, Amanda May 7 Hatfield Close, Maidenhead SL6 4RJ — MB BS Lond. 1990.

ROBERTSON, Andrea c/o 52 High Ridge, Hythe CT21 5TF — MB ChB Leic. 1992.

ROBERTSON, Andrew The Medical Centre, Station Avenue, Bridlington YO16 4LZ Tel: 01262 670686 Fax: 01262 401685; Westerlands, 95 Martongate, Bridlington YO16 6YE Tel: 01262 672128 — MB ChB Glas. 1954; DObst RCOG 1956.

ROBERTSON, Andrew George Colin Fyrish, Fordyce Terrace, New Deer, Turriff AB53 6WE Tel: 01771 644675 Fax: 01771 653294 Email: andrewrobertson@btinternet.com — MB ChB Aberd. 1974; DObst RCOG 1976; MRCGP 1978; FRCGP 2003.

ROBERTSON, Andrew Gerard 44 Lubnaig Road, Newlands, Glasgow G43 2RX — MB ChB Glas. 1975; PhD Glas. 1970, BSc (Hons.) 1967, MB ChB 1975; FRCR 1980; FRCP Glas. 1988, M 1986. Cons. Radiol. & Oncol. Beatson Oncol. Centre Glas.; Assoc. Treas. Head & Neck Oncol. Gt. Brit. Specialty: Oncol.; Radiother. Prev: Cons. (Radiol. & Oncol.) Glas. Inst. Radiotherap.; Sen. Regist. (Radiother. Oncol.) Christie Hosp. & Holt Inst. Manch.

ROBERTSON, Andrew Graeme Cross Deep Surgery, 4 Cross Deep, Twickenham TW1 4QP Tel: 020 8892 8124 Fax: 020 8744 9801; 86 Fairfax Road, Teddington TW11 9BX Tel: 020 8943 2124 — MB ChB Aberd. 1979 (Aberdeen Univ.) DRCOG 1981; Dip (Anaesth.) 1983; MRCGP 1985; Dip Sports Med. 1990; MLCOM 1991. GP; Sports Phys.; Med. Off. Rugby Football Union, Twickenham. Specialty: Sports Med. Socs: Lond. Coll. Osteop. Med.; Brit. Assoc of Sports Med.

ROBERTSON, Andrew James The Surgery, East Grinstead Road, Lingfield RH7 6ER Tel: 01342 833456 Fax: 01342 836347; Beechlands, Dormans Park, East Grinstead RH19 2NG Tel: 01342 870733 — MB Camb. 1966 (St. Bart.) BChir 1965; DA Eng. 1969. Prev: Ho. Surg. St. Bart. Hosp. Lond.; Regist. in Anaesth. Qu. Vict. Hosp. E. Grinstead.

ROBERTSON, Andrew Macpherson (retired) 6 Green Tree Gardens, Romiley, Stockport SK6 3JL; 6 Green Tree Gardens, Romiley, Stockport SK6 3JL Email: amrobertson@ntlworld.com/ jay_spurgate@hotmail.com — MB ChB Manch. 1976; DRCOG 1978; MRCGP 1982. Prev: Ho. Off. Manch. Roy. Infirm.

ROBERTSON, Andrew Stephen 95 Martongate, Bridlington YO16 6YE — MB BS Newc. 1983.

ROBERTSON, Angela Meadowbank Health Centre, 3 Salmon Inn Road, Polmont, Falkirk FK2 0XF Tel: 01324 715540 Fax: 01324 716723 — MB ChB Dundee 1987; MRCGP 1992. Specialty: Family Plann. & Reproduc. Health.

ROBERTSON, Mr Angus — MB ChB Ed. 1996 (St. Andrews & Edin.) BSc (Med. Sci.) St. And. 1993; MRCD Ed. 1999. SpR Orthopaedocs, Yorks. Specialty: Orthop. Socs: BMA; MDDVS (Med. & Dent. Defence Vision of scalled); BOA (Brit. Orthopadic Assn.). Prev: SHO (Accid. and Emerg.) Edin. Roy. Infirm.; Pre-Regist. H.O. (Gen. Surg.) Edin. Roy. Infirm.; Pre-Regist. H.O. (Gen. Med.) Edin. Roy. Infirm.

ROBERTSON, Anne The Health Centre, 201 Main Street, Barrhead, Glasgow G78 1SA Tel: 0141 880 6161 Fax: 0141 881 7063 — MB BS Newc. 1975; DCH RCPS Glas. 1977; DRCOG 1979; MRCGP 1980.

ROBERTSON, Anne Elizabeth (retired) 12 Milton Drive, Edinburgh EH15 2JX Tel: 0131 669 5434 — MB ChB Ed. 1939. Prev: Clin. Asst. E. & SE Scotl. Blood Transfus. Serv.

ROBERTSON, Anne Johnston 4 Ruthven Water, Aberuthven, Auchterarder PH3 1JD Tel: 01764 663570 — MB ChB Ed. 1952; DObst RCOG 1955; DPH 1959.

ROBERTSON, Annie Kirk 58 Catherine Drive, Galston KA4 8BS — MB ChB Glas. 1995.

ROBERTSON, Barbara Catto Lister House Surgery, 35 The Parade, St Helier JE2 3QQ Tel: 01534 36336 Fax: 01534 35304; 9 Le Jardin De La Chapelle, St. Aubin, St Brelade, Jersey JE3 8JL — MB ChB Aberd. 1980; DRCOG 1983; DCCH RCP Ed. 1986.

ROBERTSON, Bodil Ronnfeldt Anaesthetic Department, Kent & Canterbury Hospital, Ethelbert Road, Canterbury CT1 3NG; 36 Long Oaks Court, Sketty, Swansea SA2 0QH — MB ChB Aberd. 1989.

ROBERTSON, Brian, OStJ, TD North Lane Practice, 38 North Lane, Aldershot GU12 4QQ Tel: 01252 344434; 248 A Shawfield Road, Ash, Aldershot GU12 5DJ Tel: 01252 350294 — MRCS Eng. LRCP Lond. 1972 (Roy. Free) Col.-L/RAMC (V); Mem. Editr. Bd. Pre-Hosp. Immediate Care. Specialty: Gen. Pract. Socs: BMA; BASICS; IEM. Prev: Ho. Surg. New End Hosp. Hampstead; Ho. Phys. St. And. Hosp. Bow.

ROBERTSON, Brian John Dinnington Group Practice, Medical Centre, New Street, Dinnington, Sheffield S25 2EZ — MB ChB Dundee 1979; DRCOG 1982; MRCGP 1983. Prev: Trainee GP Doncaster VTS.; Ho. Off. (Orthop.) Vict. Hosp. Kirkcaldy; Ho. Off. (Med.) Ninewells Hosp. Dundee.

ROBERTSON, Carol Royal Cornhill Hospital, Cornhill Road, Aberdeen AB25 2ZH Tel: 01224 663131; Melrose, Station Road, Ellon AB41 9AR Tel: 01358 720577 — MB ChB Aberd. 1984 (Aberdeen) DRCOG 1987; MRCGP 1988; MRCPsych 1991; M Med Sci Aber. Uni, 1995. Cons. Grampian HB. Specialty: Gen. Psychiat. Prev: Trainee Psychiat. Aberd.

ROBERTSON, Caroline Lois Thorneloe Lodge Surgery, 29 Barbourne Road, Worcester WR1 1RU Tel: 01905 22445 — MB BS Lond. 1980 (Guy's) DRCOG 1983; MRCGP 1985.

ROBERTSON, Caroline Younger Battersby Moleigh House, Oban PA34 5JD — LRCP LRCS Ed. 1946 (Anderson & St. Mungo's Colls. Glas.) LRCP LRCS Ed. LRFPS Glas. 1946.

ROBERTSON, Carolyn Margaret McCallum 43 Hope Park Gardens, Bathgate EH48 2QT — MB ChB Ed. 1989; MRCGP 1994.

ROBERTSON, Catherine Jackson Allan (retired) Montpelier, 32 Barrhead Road, Newton Mearns, Glasgow G77 6BD Tel: 0141 639 1125 — (Anderson Coll. Glas.) LRCP LRCS Ed. LRFPS Glas. 1948. Prev: Med. Off. Child Health Ayrsh. & Arran HB.

ROBERTSON, Catriona Mary 6 Rockford Lodge, Knutsford WA16 8AH — MB ChB Dundee 1981. Specialty: Gen. Pract.

ROBERTSON, Mr Charles Stuart Worcestershire Park Hospital, Charles Hastings Way, Worcester WR5 1DD Tel: 01905 760577 Fax: 01905 760786; Hill Farm Barn, Broadwas-on-Teme, Worcester WR6 5NH Tel: 01886 821977 Fax: 01886 821977 — MB BS Lond. 1980 (Guy's) FRCS Eng. 1984; DM Nottm. 1989. Cons. Gen. & Gastrointestinal Surg. Worcester Roy. Infirm. Specialty: Gen. Surg. Socs: Assn. Surg.; Assn. Upper G.I. Surg.; Assn. Endoscopic Surgs. Prev: Sen. Regist. Newc.; Lect. Chinese Univ. of Hong Kong; Regist. Nottm.

ROBERTSON, Clare Margaret Churchill Hospital, The Ounsted Clinic, Headington, Oxford OX3 7LJ Tel: 01865 225617 Fax: 01865 225618 — MB ChB Bristol 1983; FRCPCH; MRCP (UK) 1986. Cons. Paediat. (Community Child Health) Oxf. Specialty: Paediat. Prev: Sen. Regist. (Community Paediat.) & Regist. (Paediat.) Oxf.

ROBERTSON, Clifton (retired) Castle Mound, Cressage, Shrewsbury SY5 6AD Tel: 01952 510502 — MB BS Durh. 1950 (Newc.) Prev: Ho. Phys. Childr. Dept. & Regist. (Paediat.) Roy. Vict. Infirm. Newc.

ROBERTSON, Mr Colin (retired) 3 Broomhall Avenue, Wakefield WF1 2BB Tel: 01924 373373 — MB ChB Birm. 1951; FRCS Ed. 1962; FRCS Eng. 1963. Prev: Orthop. Surg. Pinderfields Hosp. & Wakefield Gp. Hosps.

ROBERTSON, Colin Crawford (retired) 2A Green Hill Road, Leeds LS12 3QA Tel: 0113 263 8782 — MB ChB Leeds 1960; MRCS Eng. LRCP Lond. 1961. Prev: GP Leeds.

ROBERTSON, David Alasdair (retired) 54 Bay Street, Fairlie, Largs KA29 0AL Email: darmog@cwcom.net — MB ChB Aberd. 1959; FRCP Canada 1974. Prev: Cons. Psychiat. Ailsa Hosp. Ayr.

ROBERTSON, David Alexander Carmondean Medical Group, Carmondean Health Centre, Livingston EH54 8PY Tel: 01506 430031 Fax: 01506 432775 — MB ChB Ed. 1982.

ROBERTSON, Mr David Edward Assisted Conception Unit, Esperance House, Hartington Place, Eastbourne BN21 3BG Tel: 01323 410717 Fax: 01323 410626; 28 Summerdown Road, Eastbourne BN20 8DR Tel: 01323 726151 Email: der@dial.pipex.com — MB ChB Glas. 1977 (University of Glasgow) MRCOG 1982; FRCOG 1998. Med. Dir. Assisted Conception Unit Esperance Private Hosp.; Hon. Cons. (Obst. & Gyn.) Eastbourne DGH. Specialty: Obst. & Gyn. Socs: Brit. Fertil. Soc.; Amer. Fertil. Soc.; ESHRE. Prev: Cons. O & G Awali Hosp.; Regist. (O & G) Leic. Roy. Infirm.; Hall Fell. Midw. Univ. Glas.

ROBERTSON, David Eric The Old Shippon, Bradley Hall, Bradley, Frodsham, Warrington WA6 7EP Tel: 01928 733250 Fax: 0151 424 0299 — MB ChB Liverp. 1968; FRCGP 1985, M 1973; MSc (Community Med.) Manch. 1983; MFFP 1993. Cons. Pub. Health Med. Chesh. HA; Hon. Lect. (Gen. Pract.) Liverp. Univ. Specialty: Pub. Health Med.; Family Plann. & Reproduc. Health. Socs: Fell. Fac. Community Health.

ROBERTSON, David Iain Stewart 17-19 Raise Street, Saltcoats KA21 5LX Tel: 01294 605141; 4 North Crescent, Ardrossan KA22 0LY Tel: 01294 62517 — MB ChB Glas. 1955; MRCGP 1968.

ROBERTSON, David James Drumchapel Health Centre, 80-90 Kinfauns Drive, Glasgow G15 7TS Tel: 0141 211 6110 Fax: 0141 211 6117; 10 Heathfield Drive, Milngavie, Glasgow G12 0PZ — MB ChB Glas. 1978. GP Glas.

ROBERTSON, David Neil Queen Elizabeth Psychiatric Hospital, Mindelsohn Way, Vincent Drive, Edgbaston, Birmingham B15 2QZ — MB ChB Birm. 1984; MRCPsych 1992. Prev: Sen. Regist. Gen. Psychiatry) Qu. Eliz. Psychiat. Hosp. Birm.

ROBERTSON, Denis Wilson (retired) 29 Cottage Gardens, Northampton NN3 9YW Tel: 01604 413206 — MRCS Eng. LRCP

Lond. 1950 (St. Mary's) MRCGP 1967; Cert. Av Med. MoD (Air) & CAA 1973. Hon. JP; Med. Examr. Civil Aviat. Auth.

ROBERTSON, Denise Elexia Herne Hill Group Practice, 74 Herne Hill, London SE24 9QP Tel: 020 7274 3314 Fax: 020 7738 6025 — MB BS Lond. 1987.

ROBERTSON, Derek Dalkeith Medical Practice, 24 St Andrew Street, Dalkeith EH22 1AP Tel: 0131 663 2461 Fax: 0131 561 5555; Ellangowan, 6 Lothian Bank, Dalkeith EH22 3AN Tel: 0131 660 5004 — MB ChB Ed. 1977; DRCOG 1980; MRCGP 1981.

ROBERTSON, Diana Christine Foote — MB ChB Ed. 1980.

ROBERTSON, Donald Henry Mouat (retired) Calderstones, 33 Snowdon Place, Stirling FK8 2JP Tel: 01786 475634 — MB ChB Ed. 1961; FFA RCS Eng. 1966. Prev: Regist. & Sen. Regist. Roy. Infirm. Edin.

ROBERTSON, Donald Macpherson (retired) 7 Chadkirk Road, Romley, Stockport SK6 3JY — MB ChB Ed. 1938. Prev: Apptd. Fact. Doctor.

ROBERTSON, Dorothy Elizabeth (retired) 11 Woodburn Avenue, Aberdeen AB15 8JQ Tel: 01224 317606 — MB ChB Aberd. 1947. Prev: GP Aberd.

ROBERTSON, Dorothy Ruth Caddick 10 Chapel Path, Colerne, Chippenham SN14 8DL Tel: 01225 742767 — MB ChB Glas. 1976; DCH RCP Lond. 1978; MRCP (UK) 1979; DM Soton. 1994; FRCP Lond. 1997. Cons. Geriat. Med. St. Martins Hosp. Bath. Specialty: Care of the Elderly. Socs: Brit. Geriat. Soc. (Comm. Mem. s/i Gp. Pk.inson's Dis.). Prev: Regist. (Med.) Gen. Hosp. Birm.; Lect. (Geriat. Med.) Soton.; SHO (Med.) Chapel Allerton Hosp. Leeds.

ROBERTSON, Douglas Allan 27 Drummond Crescent, Inverness IV2 4QR — MB ChB Glas. 1971; MRCPath 1978. Cons. Biochem. Raigmore Hosp. Inverness. Specialty: Biochem. Prev: Sen. Regist. Clin. Biochem. Roy. Infirm. Glas.; Jun. Ho. Off. South. Gen. Hosp. Glas.; Jun. Ho. Off. West. Infirm. Glas.

ROBERTSON, Douglas Andrew Sandwell General Hospital, Lyndon, West Bromwich B71 4HJ Tel: 0121 553 1831 Fax: 0121 607 3300; Littlefield House, Market Lane, Wall, Lichfield WS14 0AU Tel: 01543 483225 Email: douglas.a.robertson@ntlworld.com — BM BCh Oxf. 1981; MA Camb. 1982, BA 1978; MRCP (UK) 1984; DM Oxf. 1991; MBA 1999; FRCP FRCP (London) 2000 2000. Cons. Phys. (Diabetes & Endocrinol.) Sandwell Gen. Hosp. W. Bromwich. Specialty: Diabetes; Endocrinol.; Gen. Pract. Socs: Diabetes UK; Soc. Endocrinol. Prev: Sen. Regist. (Diabetes) Newc.; Regist. (Renal) City Hosp. Nottm.; Research Fell. (Diabetes) Gen. Hosp. Birm.

ROBERTSON, Douglas Kerr Pennan Place Surgery, 20 Pennan Place, Glasgow G14 0EA Tel: 0141 959 1704 Fax: 0141 958 1100 — MB ChB Glas. 1977; DRCOG 1983; MRCGP 1987.

ROBERTSON, Duncan Alexander Findlay Royal United Hospital, Combe Park, Bath BA1 3NG Tel: 01225 824547 — MB ChB Leeds 1977; MD Leeds 1983, BSc (Hons.) Biochem. 1974, MB ChB 1977; MRCP (UK) 1979; FRCP Lond. 1994. Cons. Phys. & Gastroenterol. Roy. United Hosp. Bath; Hon. Sen. Lect. Univ. Bath. Specialty: Gastroenterol. Prev: Lect. (Med.) Dept. Med. II Soton Univ.; Regist. (Med.) Selly Oak Hosp. Birm.; Research Fell. (Med.) St. Jas. Univ. Hosp. Leeds.

ROBERTSON, Duncan Alexander Ramsay (retired) — MB ChB Ed. 1958. Prev: Cons. Radiol. South. Gen. Hosp. Glas.

ROBERTSON, Duncan Alexander Struan (retired) Victoria Mews, 28 Victoria St, St Annes, Alderney GY9 3TA Tel: 01481 823195 — MB ChB Bristol 1957; DObst RCOG 1959; DPM Eng. 1962.

ROBERTSON, Duncan George, Lt.-Col. RAMC OC Cattrick RRU, Teesdale Road, Catterick Garrison DL9 4ER Tel: 01748 873754; Meadow View, Moor Road, Melsonby DL10 5PF Tel: 01748 872598 — MB ChB Ed. 1985 (Edinburgh University) DCH RCP Lond. 1989; MRCGP 1991; Dip. Sport Med. Bath 2001. Prev: Trainee GP/SHO (Paediat.) Catterick; GP ChristCh., NZ.

ROBERTSON, Edwin William Alexandria Medical Centre, 46-62 Bank Street, Alexandria G83 0LS Tel: 01389 752650 Fax: 01389 752361; 29 Suffolk Street, Helensburgh G84 9QZ — MB ChB Glas. 1982.

ROBERTSON, Eileen Old Farm House, Shipley, Alnwick NE66 2LP Tel: 01665 579222 — (Newc.) M.B., B.S. Durh. 1948.

ROBERTSON, Elizabeth Ann 28 Hillview Drive, Cults, Aberdeen AB15 9SA — MB ChB Birm. 1975; FFA RCS Eng. 1979. Cons. Anaesth. Aberd. Roy. Hosps. NHS Trust. Specialty: Anaesth. Prev: Cons. Anaesth. Hairmyres Hosp. E. Kilbride.

ROBERTSON, Elizabeth Ann Burdwood Surgery, Station Road, Thatcham RG19 4 Tel: 01635 868006; Heathlands, Upper Woolhampton, Reading RG7 5UA Tel: 01189 714036 — MB ChB Birm. 1979; DRCOG 1981. GP Non-Princip. Specialty: Gen. Pract.; Haematology. Socs: MOSA; NANP. Prev: Clin. Med. Offcer (Community Child Health) W. Berks.; Clin. Asst. (Haemat.) Roy. Berks. Hosp.

ROBERTSON, Elizabeth Hutchings Lee (retired) Barra, Knockfarrie Road, Pitlochry PH16 5DN Tel: 01796 474347 — MB ChB St. And. 1952. Prev: SCMO (Community Health) W. Essex HA.

ROBERTSON, Elizabeth Margaret 95 King's Gate, Aberdeen AB15 4EN — MB ChB Aberd. 1975; DMRD Aberd. 1979; FRCR 1981. Dep. Med. Dir., Grampian Univ. Hosp. Trust; Clin. Sen. Lect. (Radiol.) Univ. Aberd.; Cons. (Radiol.) Aberd. Roy. Infirm. Grampian Univ. Hosps. Trust. Specialty: Radiol. Socs: President of Scottish Radiological Society. Prev: Clin. Director of Radiol., Aberd. Roy. Hosp.'s Trust; Sen. Regist. (Diagn. Radiol.) Qu. Mary's Hosp. Roehampton & Westm. Hosp. Lond.; Regist. (Diagn. Radiol.) Aberd. Roy. Infirm.

ROBERTSON, Elspeth Gatelawbridge House, Gatelawbridge, Thornhill DG3 5EA — MB BS Newc. 1977.

ROBERTSON, Euan Thomas Smith Flat 14, Queenscroft, Eccles, Manchester M30 9QQ — MB ChB Manch. 1997.

ROBERTSON, Fergus James Flat 12, 50 Roman Road, London E2 0LT — MB BS Lond. 1996.

ROBERTSON, Frank (retired) Crantock, 31 Durham Road, Bishop Auckland DL14 7HU Tel: 01388 602967 — MB BS Durh. 1938; MD Durh. 1940; FRCP Lond. 1968, M 1946. Hon. Cons. Phys. N. RHA. Prev: Cons. Phys. S.W. Durh. Hosp. Gp.

ROBERTSON, Garth Dundas Shatterwell House, North St., Wincanton BA9 9AZ Tel: 01963 33155 Fax: 01963 34964; London College of Osteopathic Medicine, 10 Boston Place, London NW1 6QH Tel: 020 7262 5250 — MB BCh BAO Dub. 1970; MRCP (UK) 1975; MLCOM 1988; DMS Med. Soc. Apoth. Lond. 1991. Registered Osteopath (General Osteop. Council) 1988. Specialty: Rehabil. Med.; Rheumatol.

ROBERTSON, Mr Gavin Scott Miller Department of Surgery, Leicester Royal Infirmary, Leicester LE1 5WW Tel: 0116 258 5997; Elms Farmhouse, Main Street, Peckleton, Leicester LE9 5RE — MB ChB Leic. 1984; FRCS Eng. 1988; FRCS Ed. 1988; MD Leic. 1993; FRCS (Gen) 1997. Cons., Gen. Surg., Leicester Roy. Infirm., Leicester; Train. Progr. Director in Gen. Surg. (S. Trent). Specialty: Gen. Surg. Socs: Brit. Soc. Gastroenterol.; Assn. of Surgeons of Gt. Britain and Irel.; Assn. of Endroscopic Surgeons of Gt. Britain and Irel. Prev: Hon. Sen. Regist. & Clin. Lect. (Surg.) Univ. Leic.; Sen. Regist. (Surg.) Qu. Eliz. Hosp. Adelaide Australia; Clin. Lect. & Hon. Regist. (Surg.) Univ. Leicester.

ROBERTSON, George Duncan (retired) 76 Hillpark Avenue, Edinburgh EH4 7AL Tel: 0131 336 1911 — (Ed.) MB ChB Ed. 1963; DObst RCOG 1967; DIH 1982; AFOM RCP Lond. 1982. Prev: GP Leith Occupat. Health Adviser, Med. Adviser Benefits Agency.

ROBERTSON, George Slessor (retired) Hazlewood, 12 Queen's Den, Woodend, Aberdeen AB15 8BW Tel: 01224 311903 Email: home@gsrobertson.plus.com — MB ChB Aberd. 1958; FRCA 1964; MD Aberd. 1973. Cons. Anaesth. Aberd. Roy. Infirm.

ROBERTSON, George Stuart (retired) 19 Shepherd Road, St. Annes, Lytham St Annes FY8 3JB — LRCP LRCS Ed. 1931 (Toronto) MD Toronto 1937, MB 1927; LRCP LRCS Ed. LRFPS Glas. 1931. Prev: Dep. Princip. Sch. Med. Off. Liverp.

ROBERTSON, Gordon Allan Chestertons, Burnt Hill, Yattendon, Thatcham RG18 0XD Tel: 01635 201311 — MB BS Lond. 1976 (Roy Free) MRCS Eng. LRCP Lond. 1976; DRCOG 1980; DCH Eng. 1980; MRCGP 1981. Hosp. Pract. (Neurol.) Roy. Berks. Hosp. Reading. Specialty: Gen. Pract. Prev: SHO (Med.) Nottm. Gen. Hosp.; Ho. Phys. Roy. Free Hosp. Lond.

ROBERTSON, Gordon James (retired) 20 Broadwood Park, Alloway, Ayr KA7 4XE Tel: 01292 441882 — MB ChB St. And. 1958. Prev: Ho. Phys. Heathfield Gen. Hosp. Ayr.

ROBERTSON, Graham Andrew 1 Kylepack Crescent, Uddington, Glasgow G71 7DQ — MB ChB Glas. 1995.

ROBERTSON, Grant 35 Lutton Place, Edinburgh EH8 9PF — MB ChB ED. 1994.

ROBERTSON, Heidi Joanne 37 Medina Avenue, Hinchley Wood, Esher — MB BS Lond. 1994; DRCOG; DFFP; MA Camb. 1995. Specialty: Gen. Pract.

ROBERTSON, Helen Margaret 30 Kessington Drive, Bearsden, Glasgow G61 2HG — MB ChB Glas. 1980.

ROBERTSON, Henry Keith Ceol - Mara, Tighnabruaich PA21 2BE Tel: 01700 811172 — MB ChB Ed. 1954; DTM & H 1961; DObst RCOG 1965. Specialty: Gen. Pract. Socs: BMA; RCGP (Assoc.). Prev: GP (Prinicp.) Hertford; GP (Princip.) Inverness; Med. Off. Keith Falconer Hosp. Aden.

ROBERTSON, Hugh Alexander McNeil (retired) 17A Sussex Heights, St. Margaret's Place, Brighton BN1 2FR — MD Manch. 1925 (Man.) BA Manch. 1921; LMCC 1925; MCPS Alta. 1926. Prev: Chest Cons. Dept. Nat. Health & Welf. Canad. Lond.

ROBERTSON, Iain Gregory, VRD, TD, OBE, QHP Royal Preston Hospital , Lancashire Teaching Hospitals NHS Trust, Sharoe Green Lane, Fulwood PR2 8DU Tel: 01772 522 042 Email: iain.robertson@lthtr.nhs.uk — MB ChB Manch. 1976; BSc (Hons.) Aston 1968; MPS 1969; FRCOG 1994, M 1981; MD Manch. 1984. Med. Director & Cons. Gyn. & Obst.; Dep. Lt.; Cons. Adviser in Obst. & Gyn., Army Med. Directorate, Min. of Defence. Specialty: Obst. & Gyn. Socs: BMA & N. Eng. Obst. & Gyn. Soc.; BSCCP; TENS Gyn. Soc. Prev: Territorial Army Adviser (Brigadier), Army Med. Directorate, Min. of Defence.

ROBERTSON, Mr Iain James Alexander Department Neurosurgery, Queens Medical Centre, Nottingham NG7 2UH Tel: 0115 924 9924 Ext: 42254 Email: iain.robertson@mail.qmcuh-tr.trent.nhs.uk; The Hollies, Black Lane, Chopwell Butlet, Nottingham NG12 3AD Tel: 0115 933 3672 — MB ChB Ed. 1981; FRCS Ed. 1986. Cons. Neurosurg., Queens Med. Centre, Nottm.; Cons. Neurosurg., Leicester Roy. Infirm. Specialty: Neurosurg. Special Interest: Pituitary; Skull Base. Socs: Soc. of Brit. Neurosurgeons; Europ. Skull Base. Prev: Sen. Regist. (Neurosurg.) Brook Hosp. SE Thames RHA. Cons. Neurosurg., Qu.s Med. Centre. Notts.; Regist., West. Gen. / Roy. Infirm. Edin.

ROBERTSON, Iain Kilpatrick 8 Mountbatten Way, Lutterworth LE17 4YD — MB BCh Wales 1979; BSc Wales 1976, MB BCh 1979; FFA RCS Eng. 1984. Regist. (Community Med.) Oxf. RHA. Specialty: Anaesth.

ROBERTSON, Iain Robert St James University Hospital, Beckett St., Leeds LS9 7TF — MB ChB Glas. 1984; MRCP (UK) 1988; FRCR 1991. Cons. Radiol. Dept. Diagn. Imaging St. Jas. Univ. Hosp. Leeds. Specialty: Radiol.

ROBERTSON, Iain William, RD Craigallian Avenue Surgery, 11 Craigallian Avenue, Cambuslang, Glasgow G72 8RW Tel: 0141 641 3129; 15 Burnside Road, Burnside, Glasgow G73 4RL Tel: 0141 634 4848 Email: iain.robertson3@ntlworld.com — MB ChB Glas. 1974. Specialty: Gen. Pract. Prev: Regist. (Anaesth.) Vict. Infirm. Glas.

ROBERTSON, Ian Station View Medical Centre, 29A Escomb Road, Bishop Auckland DL14 6AB Tel: 01388 663539 Fax: 01388 601847; 9 Langley Grove, Bishop Auckland DL14 6UJ — MB BS Newc. 1978; MRCGP 1982.

ROBERTSON, Ian Douglas Cityside Community Mental Health Team, 22 Crawford Square, Londonderry BT48 7HT Tel: 01504 372230 Fax: 01504 267487; 106 Seacoast Road, Limavady BT49 9EG Tel: 015047 63453 — MB ChB Aberd. 1977; MRCPsych 1985. Cons. Psychiat. Cityside Community Ment. Health Team Londonderry. Specialty: Gen. Psychiat. Prev: Sen. Regist. (Psychiat.) Tralee Gen. Hosp.; Sen. Regist. Cork Regional Hosp.; Regist. St. Anne's Hosp. Poole Dorset.

ROBERTSON, Ian James 36 Archfield Road, Cotham, Bristol BS6 6BE — MB ChB Birm. 1979; LLB (Hons.) Soton. 1971; DRCOG 1982; MRCGP 1983. Specialty: Rehabil. Med.; Rheumatol.

ROBERTSON, Ian Peter Cameron (retired) Greenbraes, 3 Westpark Gate, Saline, Dunfermline KY12 9US Tel: 01383 852000 Fax: 01383 852000 — MB ChB Glas. 1950; DLO Eng. 1958. Prev: GP Dunfermline.

ROBERTSON, James 19 Mast Lane, North Shields NE30 3DF — MB ChB Leeds 1995.

ROBERTSON, James Alexander 25 Thornhill Road, Steeton, Keighley BD20 6TN — MB ChB Leeds 1976; FFA RCS Eng. 1982. Cons. Anaesth. Airedale Gen. Hosp. Specialty: Anaesth. Prev: Sen. Regist. (Anaesth.) S.W. Region & RN Hosp. Plymouth; Hon. Regist. (Anaesth.) Soton. Gen. Hosp.

ROBERTSON, James Alexander (retired) Church Cottage, Stoke Street, Milborough, Ludlow SY8 2EJ — MB BChir Camb. 1966 (Middlx.) BA Camb. 1963, MB BChir 1966; DPM Eng. 1971; FRCPsych 1992, M 1973. Mem. Ment. Health Review Tribunal. Prev: Cons. Psychiat. Kidderminster Health Dist.

ROBERTSON, Mr James Anthony (retired) BUPA Chalybeate Hospital, Chalybeate Close, Tremona Road, Southampton SO16 6UY Tel: 023 8077 5544 Fax: 023 8070 1160; Shootash Farm, Romsey SO51 6FB — MB BS Lond. 1964 (King's Coll. Hosp.) MRCS Eng. LRCP Lond. 1964; FRCS Eng. 1969. Prev: Cons. Orthop. Surg. Soton. Univ. Hosp.

ROBERTSON, James Campbell Departments of Rheumatology and Rehabilitation, Salisbury District Hospital, Salisbury SP2 8BJ Tel: 01722 336262 Ext: 4218 Fax: 01722 337912 — MB BS Lond. 1965 (Guy's) MRCS Eng. LRCP Lond. 1965; DCH Eng. 1967; MRCP (UK) 1971; FRCP Lond. 1986. Cons. Rheum. & Rehabil. Salisbury & Soton. HAs; Life Mem. Fac. of Med., Soton. Univ. Specialty: Rehabil. Med.; Rheumatol. Socs: Brit. Soc. Rheum.; Backpain Assoc; Brit. Soc. for Rheumatism. Prev: Dir. Wessex Regional Rehabil. Unit; Cons. in Rheum. and Rehabil., Soton. Health Dist.

ROBERTSON, James Douglas Bennochy Medical Centre, 65 Bennochy Road, Kirkcaldy KY2 5RB Tel: 01592 263332 Fax: 01592 207599 — MB ChB Ed. 1974 (Edinburgh) BSc (Med. Sci.) Ed. 1971. GP Princip. Specialty: Gen. Pract. Prev: SHO (Cardiol.) West. Gen. Hosp. Edin.; SHO (Renal & Gen. Med.) Ninewells Hosp. Dundee; Ho. Surg. Roy. Infirm. Edin.

ROBERTSON, James Douglas Alexander The Cambridge Medical Group, 10A Cambridge Road, Linthorpe, Middlesbrough TS5 5NN Tel: 01642 851177 Fax: 01642 851176 — MB ChB Aberd. 1980; BMedBiol Aberd. 1978; DRCOG 1982; DCH RCPS Glas. 1983; MRCGP 1984; MSOM 1999. Clin. Asst. (Rheum.) Middlesbrough. Prev: GP Shenton Med. Gp. Singapore; Trainee GP Highland HB VTS.

ROBERTSON, James Duncan Friary Surgery, Victoria Road, Richmond DL10 4DW Tel: 01748 822306 Fax: 01748 850356 — MRCS Eng. LRCP Lond. 1966 (Char. Cross) DObst RCOG 1968. Prev: SHO (Obst.) Greenbank Matern. Hosp. Darlington; Cas. Off. & Ho. Phys. Mt. Vernon Hosp. Northwood; Ho. Surg. Wembley Hosp.

ROBERTSON, James Gordon Fergus St Nicholas Health Centre, Saunder Bank, Burnley BB11 2EN Tel: 01282 831249 Fax: 01282 425269; Utherstone, 264 Gisbyrn Road, Blacko, Nelson BB9 6LP Tel: 01282 619908 — MB ChB Dundee 1982.

ROBERTSON, James Hanson McPherson (retired) 12 The Avenue, Healing, Grimsby DN41 7NG Tel: 01472 882599 — MB ChB Manch. 1955; DPH Leeds 1963. Prev: GP The Surg. Immingham.

ROBERTSON, Professor James Ian Summers Elmbank, Manse Road, Bowling, Glasgow G60 5AA Tel: 01389 873121 Fax: 01389 890291 — (St. Mary's) FRS Ed.; FRCP Lond. 1970, M 1954, C.Biol; FI Biol; FAHA; BSc Lond. (1st cl. Hons.) 1949; MB BS (Hons. Path. & Med.) Lond. 1952; FRCP Glas. 1984; MD (Hons. Causa) Brussels 1986. Sen. Cons. (Cardiovasc. Med.) Janssen Research Foundat. Worldwide; Sen. Scientif. Adviser Janssen Internat. Research Counc. Specialty: Cardiol. Socs: Scientif. Staff, MRC Blood Pressure Unit, and Hon. Cons. Phys., West. Infirm., Glas.; Chairm., Scientif. Counc. on Hypertens., Int. Soc. And Fed. Cardiol. Prev: Vis. Prof. Med. P. of Wales Hosp. Hong Kong; Pres. Brit. Hypertens. Soc.; Pres. Internat. Soc. Hypertens.

ROBERTSON, James Lake SCBU, Arrowe Park Hospital, Upton, Liverpool — MB ChB Leeds 1989; MRCP (Paed.) 1996. Assoc. Specialist Paediat. Arrowe Pk. Hosp. Upton, Wirral. Specialty: Neonat. Special Interest: Drug Abuse in Pregnancy. Prev: Staff Grade Paediat. Arrowe Pk. Hosp. Upton, Wirral.

ROBERTSON, James Loudon West Calder Medical Practice, Dickson Street, West Calder EH55 8HB Email: james.robertson@wlt.scot.nhs.uk; Harwood House, 14 Hartwood Road, West Calder EH55 8DG Tel: 01506 873337 — MB ChB Glas. 1989; BSc (Hons) Glas. 1986; DRCOG 1993; MRCGP 1994; T(GP) 1994. Specialty: Gen. Pract. Prev: SHO (Dermat.) Ninewells Hosp. Dundee.

ROBERTSON, James Mowat Department of Oral and Maxillo-Facial Surgery, Peterborough District Hospital, Thorpe Road,

Peterborough PE3 6DA Tel: 01733 874319 Fax: 01733 875697 — MB ChB Sheff. 1972; BDS 1968; FDS RCS Eng. 1975. Cons. Oral & Maxillofacial Surg. P'boro Hosps. NHS Trust; Hon. Clin. Teach. (Oral & Maxillofacial Surg.) Univ. Sheff. Specialty: Oral & Maxillofacial Surg. Socs: Fell. BAOMFS; BMA; BDA. Prev: Sen. Regist. (Oral Surg.) Guy's Hosp. Lond. & Qu. Vict. Hosp. E. Grinstead.

ROBERTSON, James Roy Muirhouse Medical Group, 1 Muirhouse Avenue, Edinburgh EH4 4PL Tel: 0131 332 2201; 18 Henderland Road, Murrayfield, Edinburgh EH12 6BB Tel: 0131 337 4707 — MB ChB Ed. 1975 (Edinburgh) FRCGP 1988, M 1980. Lect. Univ. Edin. Prev: Regist. (Med.) Vict. Hosp. Kirkcaldy; SHO North. Gen. Hosp. Edin.; Ho. Off. Chalmers Hosp.

ROBERTSON, James Stewart, OBE (retired) Colwell, Brigg Road, Barton-upon-Humber DN18 5DH Tel: 01652 635632 Email: 113031.2524@compuserve.com — MB ChB Leeds 1949; MRCS Eng. LRCP Lond. 1949; DPH Lond. 1956; DIH Eng. 1957; MFCM 1974; FFPHM 1989. Prev: DMO Scunthorpe HA.

ROBERTSON, James Thomas Weir (retired) 6 Victoria Avenue, Woodhall Spa LN10 6TY Tel: 01526 352363 — MB ChB Glas. 1945 (Glas. & Mich.) MD (Distinc.) Mich. 1973; MRCGP 1974; DPhysMed Eng. 1975. Prev: Rockefeller Med. Stud. Univ. Mich. 1942-44.

ROBERTSON, Jane Diana 11 Ashfield Road, Cheadle, Manchester M13 0YP — MB BS Lond. 1990; BA (Hons.) Oxf. 1987; MRCP (UK) 1993.

ROBERTSON, Jane Kennedy 3 Balmore Court, Kilmacolm PA13 4LX — MB ChB Glas. 1972. Staff Grade Med. Off. Glas. & W. of Scotl. Blood Transfus. Serv. Specialty: Blood Transfus.

ROBERTSON, Jane Margaret Hillingdon Health Centre, 4 Freezeland Way, Hillingdon, Uxbridge UB10 9QF — MB BS Lond. 1996; DRCOG; MRCGP; DFFP; Dip Child Health, RCPaed & Child Health., 1999. Specialty: Gen. Pract. Prev: SHO Psychiat. (GPUTS) Hillingdon Hosp., Hillingdon, Middlx.

ROBERTSON, Janet Anne Church Place Surgery, 6 Church Place, Moffat DG10 9ES Tel: 01683 220197 — MB ChB Glas. 1985; DObst. Otago 1988; MRCGP 1990.

ROBERTSON, Janette 55 Partickhill Road, Glasgow G11 5AB — MB ChB Glas. 1993; BSc St And. 1976; PhD Sheff. 1985; MPH Glas. 1987. Sen. Partner, Kelso St. Surg.; Hon. Sen. Lect., Glas. Univ. Specialty: Gen. Pract.

ROBERTSON, Jean Lesley 15 Barclay Park, Aboyne AB34 5JF Tel: 0133 98 86679 — MB ChB Aberd. 1968.

ROBERTSON, Jeffrey Hampton (retired) 93 Shandon Park, Belfast BT5 6NY — MB BCh BAO Belf. 1954 (Qu. Univ. Belf.) MD Belf. 1958; FRCP Ed. 1981, M 1962; FRCPath 1977, M 1964. Prev: Clin. Path. Belf. City Hosp.

ROBERTSON, Jennie The Chase, Spurgrove, Frieth, Henley-on-Thames RG9 6PA Tel: 01494 881555 — MB BS Lond. 1959 (Roy. Free) MRCS Eng. LRCP Lond. 1959. Assoc. Specialist (Geriat.) St. Marks Hosp. Maidenhead. Prev: Med. Asst. (Geriat.) St. John's Hosp. Lond.; Regist. (Geriat.) St. John's Hosp. Battersea; SHO Geriat. S. West. Hosp. Lond.

ROBERTSON, Jennifer Forsyth South Queensferry Group Practice, The Health Centre, Rosebery Avenue, South Queensferry EH30 9HA Tel: 0131 331 1396 Fax: 0131 331 5783; 76 Hillpark Avenue, Edinburgh EH4 7AL Tel: 0131 336 1911 — MB ChB Ed. 1963. Prev: Med. Off. Brook Advis, Centre Edin.; Ho. Phys. & Ho. Surg. Princess Margt. Hosp. Nassau.

ROBERTSON, Joan Arden (retired) Haworth, 33 Leven Road, Lundin Links, Lower Largo, Leven KY8 6AH Tel: 01333 320335 — (Bristol) MB ChB Bristol 1949. Prev: Chairm. Scott. Family Plann. Med. Soc.

ROBERTSON, John Albert (retired) 26 Elsdon Close, Peterlee SR8 1NE Tel: 0191 586 0243 — MB BS Durh. 1938 (Newc.) Prev: Ho. Phys. & Ho. Surg. Tynemouth Jubilee Infirm.

ROBERTSON, John Forsyth Russell 114 Carfin Road, Newarthill, Motherwell ML1 5JX — MB ChB Glas. 1980.

ROBERTSON, John Gareth Jakaranda, Mosstowie, Elgin IV30 8TX — MB ChB Aberd. 1998; MB ChB Aberd 1998.

ROBERTSON, John Gordon The Health Centre, High Street, Dodworth, Barnsley S75 3RF Tel: 01226 203881 — MB ChB Aberd. 1959.

ROBERTSON, John Leslie (retired) 99 St Andrews Drive, Glasgow G41 4DH — MB ChB Glas. 1946.

ROBERTSON, John Lindsay (retired) South Acre, Galston KA4 8NB Tel: 01563 820353 — MB ChB Glas. 1951; DObst RCOG 1953. Prev: Res. Ho. Phys. Glas. Roy. Infirm. & Stobhill Hosp. Glas.

ROBERTSON, Mr John Moore 9 West Werberside, Edinburgh EH4 1SZ — MB ChB Glas. 1948; FRCS Ed. 1954. Cons. Neurosurg. S. Tees Health Dist. Specialty: Neurosurg. Prev: Sen. Regist. Glas. & W. Scotl. Neurosurg. Unit Killearn Hosp. Glas.; Surg. Regist. Stobhill Hosp. Glas.

ROBERTSON, John Murison Associated Health Specialists, Templeton Business Centre, Templeton St., Glasgow G40 1DA Tel: 0141 554 1566 Fax: 0141 554 1995 — (Guy's) MRCS Eng. LRCP Lond. 1961; MB BS Lond. 1961; AFOM RCP Lond. 1982; CIH Dund 1983. Dir. Assoc. Health Specialists Ltd. Glas. Specialty: Occupat. Health. Socs: Soc. Occupat. Med. Prev: Regional Occupat. Phys. Brit. Ship Builders (TES); Med. Off. Standard Telephones & Cables plc.

ROBERTSON, John Richard (retired) 74 Clarendon Drive, Putney, London SW15 1AH Tel: 020 8789 2661 Email: jrr_74@yahoo.com — MB ChB Ed. 1964; BSc (Hons.) Ed. 1962; DPM Eng. 1970; FRCPsych. 1989, M 1972. Prev: Cons. (Psychiat.) W. Lond. Healthcare Trust.

ROBERTSON, John Thomson (retired) 4 Ailsa Craigview, Grangemuir Court, Prestwick KA9 1GA — MB ChB Glas. 1954.

ROBERTSON, John Watt (retired) East Wing, Kincurdie House, Rosemarkie, Fortrose IV10 8SJ Tel: 01381 621388 Fax: 01381 620325 — (Aberd.) MB ChB Aberd. 1959; DObst RCOG 1962; FRCGP 1990, M 1968. Prev: Med. Prescribing Adviser West. Is. HB.

ROBERTSON, Josefina de Unamuno Viewfield Medical Centre, 3 Viewfield Place, Stirling FK8 1NJ Tel: 01786 472028 Fax: 01786 463388 — LMS Salamanca 1979; LMS 1979 Salamanca; LRCP Edin LRCS Edin LRCPS Glasg 1983. GP Stirling; Clin. Med. Off., Psychiat.; Regist. Acupunc. & Hypnotherapist. Specialty: Dermat.; Gen. Psychiat.; Family Plann. & Reproduc. Health. Socs: BMA.

ROBERTSON, Joyce Buchan Peterhead Group Practice, The Health Centre, Peterhead AB42 2XA Tel: 01774 474841 Fax: 01774 474848; Clifton House, Cruden Bay, Peterhead AB42 0HP Tel: 01779 812748 — MB ChB Aberd. 1982 (Aberdeen) DRCOG 1985; MRCGP 1986; FRCGP 2003. GP Trainer. Socs: (Ex-Chairm.) Educat. Sect. NE Scotl. Fac. RCGP. Prev: Trainee GP Aberd. VTS.

ROBERTSON, Katherine May, OBE (retired) Bragleenmore, Kilninver, Oban PA34 4UU — MB ChB Glas. 1945. Prev: Med. Tutor Lilongwe Sch. of Health Sci.s Malawi.

ROBERTSON, Katrina Jeanette PO Box 90, Ipswich IP6 9EQ — MB BS Lond. 1993.

ROBERTSON, Kenneth 19 Gardner Road, Aberdeen AB12 5TB — MB ChB Aberd. 1983; FFA RCS Eng. 1988. SHO (Anaesth.) Vict. Infirm. Glas. Prev: Ho. Phys. South. Gen. Hosp. Glas.; Ho. Surg. Vict. Infirm. Glas.

ROBERTSON, Mr Kenneth (retired) 1/10 Pentland Drive, Fairmilehead, Edinburgh EH10 6PU Tel: 0131 467 1919 — MB ChB Ed. 1946; FRCS Ed. 1951. Prev: Cons. Gen. Surg. South. Isles.

ROBERTSON, Kenneth James Royal Hopital for Sick Children, Yorkhill, Glasgow G3 8SJ Tel: 0141 201 0000 Fax: 0141 201 0671 Email: k.j.robertson@clinmed.gla.ac.uk; 16 Craigenlay Avenue, Blanefield, Glasgow G63 9DR Tel: 01360 771022 — MB ChB Aberd. 1982; FRCPCH 1997; FRCP Ed. 1998. Cons. Paediat. Yorkhill NHS Trust Glas.; Hon. Sen. Clin. Lect. Glas. Specialty: Paediat.; Diabetes. Socs: Brit. Diabetic Assn.; Advisery Counc. Internat. Soc. Paediatry & Adolesc. Diabetes. Prev: Lecture & Hon. Sen. Regist. (Child Health) Ninewells Hosp. Univ. Dundee; MRC Clin. Research Fell. (Child Health & Biochem.y Med.) Ninewells Hosp. Dundee; Registar (Paediatry) Ninewells Hosp. Dundee.

ROBERTSON, Mr Kevin William Stobhill Hospital, 130 Balomock Road, Glasgow G21 3UT — MB ChB Glas. 1988; FRCS Glas. 1992. Specialty: Gen. Surg. Socs: Roy. Coll. Phys. & Surgs. Glas. (Counc. Jun. QUA Surg.).

ROBERTSON, Laura Margaret 212 Osborne Road, Jesmond, Newcastle upon Tyne NE2 3LD — MB BS Lond. 1983; DRCOG 1985; MRCGP 1987.

ROBERTSON, Lawrence (retired) 1 Sunnyside Close, Freckleton, Preston PR4 1YJ Tel: 01772 632202 — BM BCh Oxf. 1950; MA Oxf. 1951; Dip. Bact. Lond 1953; FRCPath 1970, M 1964. Prev: Dir., Pub. Health Laborat. Preston.

ROBERTSON, Lesley Jane Aylesbury Vale Community Healthcare, Tindal Centre, Bierton Road, Aylesbury HP20 1HU — MB ChB

Aberd. 1982; MRCPsych 1988. Cons. Psychiat. Tindal Centre Aylesbury. Specialty: Gen. Psychiat.

ROBERTSON, Linda Marjorie Psychiatric Unit, Hairmyres Hospital, East Kilbride, Glasgow Tel: 0141572532; 11 Arran Gardens, Carluke ML8 4HS Tel: 01555 750582 — MB ChB Glas. 1979; DCH RCPS Glas. 1982; MRCGP 1985. Specialty: Gen. Psychiat.

ROBERTSON, Lindsay Patience 9 Queens Gate, Hillbridge, Plymouth PL1 5NQ Tel: 01752 569563 — BSc Immunology 1991 Glas. Univ.; MB ChB Glas. 1994; MRCP UK Glas. 1997; MSc Plymouth 2002. Cons. Rheumatologist, Bristol Roy. Infirm. Specialty: Rheumatol. Special Interest: Adolescent Rheumatology; Transitional Care. Socs: Brit. Soc. Rheum.; BMA. Prev: Hon. Specialist Regist., Princess Diana Hosp. for Childr., Birm.; Specialist Regist. Rheum., Derrifaord Hosp. Plymouth; Specialist Regist. Rheum., Roy. Cornw. Hosp. Truro.

ROBERTSON, Lynne Margaret 55 Osnaburgh Court, Dairsie, Cupar KY15 4SU — MB ChB Ed. 1991 (Edinburgh) MRCGP 1997; DCCH 1998. Specialist Regist. Pub. Health, Fife Health Bd., Cupar, Fife. Specialty: Pub. Health Med. Socs: BMA; RCGP. Prev: SHO Rehabil. Med., Astley Ainslie, Edinb.; Community Regist. (Paediat.) Sighthill Health Centre Edin.; GP Regist. W. End Med. Pract. Edin.

ROBERTSON, Margaret House 3, Bridlington General Hospital, Bridlington YO16 5QP; 11 Second Avenue, Bridlington YO15 2LL — MB ChB Leeds 1984; MRCGP 1988. GP N. Humberside.

ROBERTSON, Margaret Alison East Donnington Street Clinic, East Donnington Street, Darvel KA17 0JR Tel: 01560 320205 Fax: 01560 321643; 31 Milagarholm Avenue, Irvine KA12 0EL Tel: 01294 278341 — MB ChB Glas. 1988 (Univ. Glas.) DRCOG 1993. GP Darvel & Newmilns. Specialty: Gen. Pract. Socs: BMA. Prev: GP Castlemilk Health Centre Glas.; SHO (Psychiat.) St. John's Livingston; SHO (O & G) St. John's Livingston.

ROBERTSON, Margaret Elizabeth Castle Street Surgery, 67 Castle Street, Salisbury SP1 3SP Tel: 01722 322726 Fax: 01722 410315 — (Birm.) MB ChB Birm. 1967; DObst RCOG 1969. Socs: BMA. Prev: Sch. Med. Off. Wilts. AHA; SHO (Gen. Med.) Good Hope Hosp. Sutton Coldfield; Ho. Surg. Gen. Hosp. Birm.

ROBERTSON, Margaret Foster 139 Hough Green, Chester CH4 8JR — MB ChB Cape Town 1958; DPM Eng. 1966; MRCPsych 1972. Cons. Psychotherap. N. Wales. Hosp. Denbigh. Specialty: Gen. Psychiat. Socs: Fell. Roy. Coll. Psychiat. Prev: Sen. Regist. (Psychol. Med.) King's Coll. Hosp. Lond.; Regist. (Med.) Groote Schuur Hosp. Cape Town, S. Afr.; SHO (Psychiat.) Middlx. Hosp. Lond.

ROBERTSON, Margaret Jean Stark 19 Wimpole Street, London W1M ADH Tel: 020 7935 8488 Fax: 020 7636 5758; 22 Almeida Street, Islington, London N1 1TB Tel: 020 7226 2730 — (Glas.) MB ChB Glas. 1964; MRCP (UK) 1969; FFA RCS Eng. 1975; FRCP Glas. 1983. Cons. Anaesth. Newham Gen. Hosp. Lond.; Cons. Anaesth. Whittington Hosp. Lond. Specialty: Anaesth. Prev: Cons. (Anaesth.) Whittington Hosp. Lond.; Sen. Regist. Univ. Coll. Hosp. Lond.

ROBERTSON, Margaret Joy Crerar Braids Medical Practice, 6 Camus Avenue, Edinburgh EH10 6QT Tel: 0131 445 5999; Braids Medical Practice, 6 Camus Avenue, Edinburgh EH10 6QT Tel: 0131 445 5999 — MB ChB Ed. 1978; BSc Ed. 1975, MB ChB 1978; MRCGP 1982.

ROBERTSON, Margaret Mary Dorothy 44 Lubnaig Road, Newlands, Glasgow G43 2RX — MB ChB Glas. 1971; BSc Glas. 1966, MB ChB 1971; MFCM 1989. Med. Off. Gtr. Glas. Health Bd. Specialty: Community Child Health. Socs: BMA; Soc. of Pub. Health. Prev: Ho. Off. Ayr Co. Hosp. & Heathfield Gen. Hosp. Ayr.

ROBERTSON, Mary Croft (retired) Colwell, 9 Brigg Road, Barton-upon-Humber DN18 5DH Tel: 01652 635632 — MB ChB Leeds 1949. Prev: SCMO Scunthorpe Health Dist.

ROBERTSON, Professor Mary May Department of Psychiatry & Behavioural Sciences, UCLMS, Wolfson Building, 48 Riding House St., London W1N 8AA Tel: 020 7679 9471 Fax: 020 7679 9426 Email: rejummr@ucl.ac.uk; Department Neuropsychiatry Box 77, The National Hospital for Neurology & Neurosurgery, Queen Square, London WC1N 3BG Tel: 020 7837 3611 Ext: 3947 Fax: 020 7278 8772 Email: profmmr@a.o.l.com — MB ChB Cape Town 1971; FRCPsych 1991, M 1979; DPM Eng. 1979; MD Cape Town 1983. Prof. (Neuropsychiat.) Univ. Coll. Lond. Med. Sch.; Cons. Neuropsychiat. Nat. Hosp. Qu. Sq. Lond.; Hon. Med. Adviser UK & Irish Tourette Syndrome Assns.; Hon. Med. Adviser Tourette Syndrome Foundat. Canada; Hon. Med. Adviser, German Tourette Syndrome Assoc. Specialty: Gen. Psychiat. Socs: Brit. Neuropsychiat. Assn.; Exec. Comm. Internat. Neuropsychiatric Assn. Prev: Reader Univ. Coll. Lond. Med. Sch.; Sen. Lect. Univ. Coll. Lond. Med. Sch.; Sen. Regist. Rotat. Maudsley Hosp. Lond.

ROBERTSON, Matthew Henderson (retired) Barra, Knockfarrie Road, Pitlochry PH16 5DN Tel: 01796 474347 — MB ChB St. And. 1951; FRCPath 1974, M 1963. Prev: Cons. Microbiol. W. Essex Health Dist.

ROBERTSON, Mhairi Iona 7 Cameron Street, Dunfermline KY12 8DP — MB ChB Aberd. 1997.

ROBERTSON, Mr Michael Alexander Hynd Fiunary, Morvern, Oban PA34 5JQ — MB ChB Ed. 1960 (Edin.) MRCP (UK) 1965; FRCS Ed. 1993.

ROBERTSON, Moira Royal Alexandra Hospital, Corsebar Road, Paisley PA2 9PN Tel: 0141 887 9111 Ext: 4225 Fax: 0141 580 4112; 31 Newark Drive, Glasgow G41 4QA — MB ChB Glas. 1977; FRCPath; FRCP 1950; MRCP 1980; FRCP 1980. Cons. Haemat. Roy. Alexandra Hosp. Paisley. Specialty: Haematology.

ROBERTSON, Moira Carole (retired) 129 Marlborough Road, Swindon SN3 1NJ — BM BCh Oxf. 1958; FRIPHH; MA Oxf. 1959; DObst RCOG 1960; DPH Leeds 1963; DCH Eng. 1972; MFFP 1993; Dip Occ Med 1998.

ROBERTSON, Morag Wyllie (retired) 26 Heol Tyn y Cae, Rhiwbina, Cardiff CF14 6DJ Tel: 029 2061 3439 — (Glas.) MB ChB Glas. 1951. Clin. Med. Off. S. Glam. AHA. Prev: Jun. Hosp. Med. Off. Roy. Hosp. Sick Childr. Glas.

ROBERTSON, Nan Agnew 19 Glenwood Road, Kirkintilloch, Glasgow G66 4DY — MB ChB Glas. 1973.

ROBERTSON, Neil James 159 Prospect Road, Totley Rise, Sheffield S17 4HX — BM BS Nottm. 1984; MRCPath; BMedSci (Hons) Nottm. 1982, BM BS 1984.

ROBERTSON, Neil Malcolm Woodlands Med. Pract., Blue bell Wood Way, Sutton-in-Ashfield NG17 1JW Tel: 01623 514003 Fax: 01623 554514; 19 The Heyes, Ravenshead, Nottingham NG15 9AU Tel: 01623 795485 — MB BS Lond. 1977 (St. Geo. Hosp. Med. Sch.) DRCOG 1980; FRCGP 1996, M 1983. Trainer (Gen. Pract.) Mansfield VTS; Coorse Organiser Mansfield Uts. Socs: N. Notts. LMC. Prev: Mem. Centr. Notts. HA; Course Organiser Centr. Notts. VTS; Mem. Vale of Trent Fac. Bd. Rcgp.

ROBERTSON, Nicholas Craig 17 Wetherby Road, York YO26 5BS — MB BCh Wales 1993.

ROBERTSON, Nicola Jayne Dept of Paediatrics, Imperial College School of Medicine, Hammersmith Hospital Du Cane Road, London W12 0HS Tel: 020 8743 2030 Fax: 020 8740 8281 Email: n.robertson@ic.ac.uk; 10 Silver Crescent, Chiswick, London W4 5SE — MB ChB Ed. 1988 (Edin) MRCP (UK) 1995. Cons. Neonat.. Hammersmith Hosp. Specialty: Neonat.; Paediat. Socs: Brit. Med. Assn.; Brit. Assn. Perinatal Med.; Neonat..Soc. Prev: Regist. (Neonat.) Monash Med. Centre Vict., Austral.; Regist. (Paediat.) Kent & Canterbury Hosp.; SHO (Host Defence) Gt. Ormond St. Hosp.

ROBERTSON, Patrick Dugan, OBE (retired) Avila, Rockhill, Wick KW1 5TP Tel: 01955 602728 — (Aberd.) MB ChB Aberd. 1954; FRCP Ed. 1978, M 1962. Prev: Cons. Phys. Caithness Hosp. Gp.

ROBERTSON, Patrick Michael Marcham Health Centre, Marcham Road, Abingdon OX14 1BT Tel: 01235 522602; 12 Conduit Road, Abingdon OX14 1DB — MB BS Newc. 1983 (Newc. u. Tyne) BMedSc Newc. 1980; MRCP (UK) 1986; Cert. Family Plann. JCC 1989; DRCOG 1989; MRCGP 1996.

ROBERTSON, Paul 45 Oakdene Court, Culloden, Inverness IV2 7XL — MB ChB Ed. 1998; MB ChB Ed 1998.

ROBERTSON, Paula Anne Sisters Home, City Hospital, Dudley Road, Birmingham B18 7QH — MB BS W. Indies 1995.

ROBERTSON, Paula Jane 12 Swanston Avenue, Edinburgh EH10 7BU — MB ChB Dundee 1995.

ROBERTSON, Pauline Elizabeth Herdman Flat Hospital, Dunpender, Haddington EH41 3BU — MB ChB Ed. 1974; DObst RCOG 1976; MRCPsych 1985; MPhil Ed. 1988; Dip. Forens. Med. Glas 1994; FRCPsych 2003. Cons. Psychiat. Learning Disabilites Lothian PCT NHS Trust Edinburgh/ Haddington; Train. Progr. Director S.E. Scotl. Higher Train. Scheme; Psychiat. of Learning Disabilities Edin. Specialty: Gen. Psychiat. Special Interest: Epilepsy. Prev: Cons. Psychiat. (Ment. Handicap) Roy. Scott. Nat. Hosp.

Larbert; Sen. Regist. Prudhoe & N.gate Hosps. N.d.; Regist. (Psychiat.) Roy. Edin. Hosp.

ROBERTSON, Peter Dedridge Health Centre, Nigel Rise, Livingston EH54 6QQ Tel: 01506 414586 Fax: 01506 461806 — MB ChB Ed. 1984; BSc (Hons.) Ed. 1981; DRCOG 1988; Cert. Family Plann. JCC 1989; MRCGP 1989. Prev: Ho. Off. Respirat. Unit City Hosp.; SHO (Cas.) Falkirk Roy. Hosp.; SHO (O & G) Bangour Gen. Hosp.

ROBERTSON, Peter Cowe (retired) Lanercost, Cliftonville Road, Northampton NN1 5BX Tel: 01604 66434 & 34700 Email: pcrob@lanercostpcr.freeserve.co.uk — MD Dundee 1969 (St. And.) MB ChB (Hnrs.) St. And. 1956; FRCP Ed. 1973, M 1961; FRCP Lond. 1977, M 1965. Prev: Cons. Gen. Phys. Northampton Gen. Hosp.

ROBERTSON, Peter Gordon Cochrane (retired) The Surgeries, Lombard Street, Newark NG24 1XG Tel: 01636 702363 Fax: 01636 613037; Mile Tree Lodge, 114 Hawton Road, Newark NG24 4QF Tel: 01636 705505 — MB ChB St. And. 1958.

ROBERTSON, Peter Macgregor The Burdwood Surgery, Wheelers Green Way, Thatcham, Newbury RG19 4YF Tel: 01635 68006 Fax: 01635 867484 Email: peter.robertson@gp-k81102.nhs.uk; Heathlands, Upper Woolhampton, Reading RG7 5UA — MB ChB Birm. 1978; MRCGP 1984; MRCGP 1984.

ROBERTSON, Philip Royal Hospital for Sick Children, 9 Sciennes Road, Edinburgh EH9 1LQ Tel: 0131 667 1991; 15 East Terrace, South Queensferry EH30 9HS — MB ChB Dundee 1984; BDS 1978; MRCP (UK) 1993. Staff Phys. (Paediat. A & E) Roy. Hosp. for Sick Childr. Edin. Specialty: Paediat. Prev: Regist. & SHO (Paediat.) Roy. Hosp. Sick Childr. Edin.; SHO (Paediat.) Ninewells Hosp. Dundee.

ROBERTSON, Philip Warner (retired) 9 Heaton Drive, Edgbaston, Birmingham B15 3LW Tel: 0121 454 3793 — MD Liverp. 1950; MB ChB 1945; FRCP Lond. 1966, M 1949; DMRD Eng. 1968. Prev: Direct. Radiol. Serv. E. Birm. Hosp.

ROBERTSON, Richard The Health Centre, Whyteman's Brae, Kirkcaldy KY1 2NA Tel: 01592 642178 Fax: 01592 644782; 44 Boglily Road, Kirkcaldy KY2 5NF Tel: 01592 204622 — MB ChB Ed. 1967; DObst RCOG 1971; DCH Eng. 1972; MRCGP 1979.

ROBERTSON, Richard John Student Health Service, 25 Belgrave Road, Bristol BS8 2AA Tel: 0117 973 7716 Fax: 0117 970 6804 — MB ChB Ed. 1970; DObst RCOG 1972; DCH RCPS Glas. 1972; MRCGP 1975. Prev: GP Annan Dumfriessh.

ROBERTSON, Rita Mary Prisca 24 Chessington Close, Appleton, Warrington WA4 5HG — MB ChB Birm. 1982; MFPHM RCP (UK) 1992. Director of Pub. Health Warrington Primary Care Trust. Specialty: Pub. Health Med.

ROBERTSON, Robert Chapman Gibson North Glen Medical Practice, 1 Huntsmans Court, Glenrothes KY7 6SX Tel: 01592 620062 Fax: 01592 620465; Wellwood, Kettle Road, Ladybank, Cupar KY15 7PA — MB ChB Ed. 1982; DRCOG 1986.

ROBERTSON, Robert Hennedy Aultbea and Gairloch Medical Practice, The Health Centre, Auchtercairn, Gairloch IV21 2BH Tel: 01445 712229 — (St. And. & Dundee) MB ChB St. And. 1971. Socs: Assoc. Mem. RCGP; BASICS. Prev: GP Dalkeith; Med. Adviser Ethicon Ltd.

ROBERTSON, Robert John (retired) Fjaere, Brae, Shetland ZE2 9QJ Tel: 01806 522663 — MB ChB Aberd. 1958; CIH Dund 1973.

ROBERTSON, Robert St Clair Department of Diagnostic Radiology, Royal Berkshire Hospital, London Road, Reading RG1 5AN Tel: 0118 987 8035; Peacehaven, The Street, Tidmarsh, Reading RG8 8ER Tel: 0118 984 3163 — MB BS Lond. 1975 (St. Bart.) BSc Lond. 1972; MRCP (UK) 1981; DMRD 1982; FRCR 1984. Cons. Radiol. Roy. Berks. & Battle NHS Trust. Specialty: Radiol. Prev: Sen. Regist. (Radiol.) St. Bart. Hosp & Gt. Ormond St. Hosp. for Sick Childr. Lond.

ROBERTSON, Robin Andrew University of Glasgow, Department of General Practice & Primary Care, Glasgow G12 8QQ; The Lindens, 4 Balmuildy Road, Bishopbriggs, Glasgow G64 3BS — MB ChB Glas. 1964; MRCGP 1966; DObst RCOG 1966; FRCGP 1997. Sen. Clin. Tutor (Gen. Pract. & Primary Care) Univ. Glas. Prev: SHO (Matern.) Ayrsh. Centr. Hosp. Irvine.

ROBERTSON, Roderick John Hally 1A Whinbrook Gardens, Moortown, Leeds LS17 6AE — MB ChB Ed. 1975; MRCP (UK) 1979; FRCR 1986. Cons. Radiol. Killingbeck Cardiothoracic Hosp. & St. Jas. Univ. Hosp. Leeds. Specialty: Radiol.

ROBERTSON, Rosemary (retired) 33 Crofton Close, Southampton SO17 1XB Tel: 02380556482 — MB ChB Ed. 1955. Prev: SCMO (Child Health) Soton. Community Health Trust.

ROBERTSON, Sarah Jex Dept. Psychotherapy, Harewood House, Glenburnie Road, London SW17 7RD — MB BS Lond. 1976 (St. Bart.) BSc (Psych.) Lond. 1973; MRCPsych 1983. Cons. Psychother. S. W. Lond. & St. Geo.s Ment. Health NHS Trust, Lond.. Specialty: Psychother. Socs: ASSOC. Mem. Brit. Psycoanalytic Soc..; Mem. Assn. Psychoanalytic Psychother. in the NHS; Mem. Roy. Coll. Psychiatr. Prev: Sen. Regist. (Psychother.) Maudsley Hosp. Lond.; Research Worker Inst. Psychiat. Lond.; Regist. Maudsley Hosp. Lond.

ROBERTSON, Sheila Jean Barclay Crewkerne, Clovenfords, Galashiels TD1 3ND Tel: 01896 850280 — MB ChB Ed. 1955; DA Eng. 1958; FFA RCS Eng. 1964. Specialty: Anaesth. Socs: BMA. Prev: Cons. Anaesth. Borders Gen. Hosp. Melrose; Cons. Anaesth. Peel Hosp. Galashiels; Regist (Anaesth.) Bangour Gen. Hosp. & S. Som. Clin. Area.

ROBERTSON, Simon Bramwell Fyvie Oldmeldrum Medical Group, Fyvie Health Centre, 27 Parnassus Gardens, Fyvie, Turriff AB53 8QD Tel: 01651 891205 Fax: 01651 891834; Struan, School Road, Fyvie, Turriff AB53 8QE Tel: 01651 891509 — MB ChB Aberd. 1977; MRCP (UK) 1980; DRCOG 1982; Cert. Family Plann. JCC 1982; MRCGP 1983; FRCGP 2003. Princip. in Gen. Pract.; Clin. Asst. A & E Dept., Foresthill; Dep. Trainer, Grampian VTS; Chairman of Gen. Aberdeenshire Local Health Care Co-operative. Specialty: Gen. Pract. Socs: (Ex Chairm., Sec. & Treas.) Ythan Med. Soc.; Garioch Med. Assn. Prev: Trainer Grampian VTS; Regist. (Med.) Aberd. Roy. Infirm.; Research Fell. (Med.) Aberd. Univ.

ROBERTSON, Simon James 1 Hollytree Close, Gerrards Cross SL9 0JL Tel: 01753 87474; Flat 3, 4 Cavendish Place, Bath BA1 2UB Tel: 01225 332862 — BM Soton. 1994 (Southampton) SHO (Paediat.) Gloucestershire Roy. Hosp. Gloucester. Specialty: Paediat. Prev: SHO (Paediat.) Derriford Hosp. Plymouth.

ROBERTSON, Sonia Margaret Highgate Group Practice, 44 North Hill, London N6 4QA Tel: 020 8340 6628 Fax: 020 8342 8428 — MB ChB Leeds 1972.

ROBERTSON, Stephen Charles The Cameleon Centre, 34 The Avenue, Watford WD17 4AH Tel: 01923 242565 Fax: 01923 218271; 28 Park Street, Windsor SL4 1LB — MB BChir Camb. 1977; MA (Hons.) Camb. 1977.

ROBERTSON, Steven Howard, Capt. RAMC Squirrel Preys, Caldy Road, Wirral CH48 1LN — MB ChB Glas. 1986; MRCGP 1990; MRCPsych 1992.

ROBERTSON, Struan (retired) 5 Kensington Close, Rocks Road, Halifax HX3 0HX — MB ChB Ed. 1932; DOMS Eng. 1950.

ROBERTSON, Struan John Tannahill (retired) Torranroy, Evelix Road, Dornoch IV25 3HR Tel: 01862 810274 — (Univ. Glas.) MB ChB Glas. 1945; MRCGP 1968. Prev: GP Glas. Inaugural Chairm. Woodside Health Centre Glas.

ROBERTSON, Stuart Forrest (retired) 25 Hazlehead Place, Aberdeen AB15 8HD — MB ChB Aberd. 1964. Prev: SCMO (Community Health) Grampian HB.

ROBERTSON, Stuart Hamish Addington Road Surgery, 33 Addington Road, West Wickham BR4 9BW Tel: 020 8462 5771 Fax: 020 8462 8526; 3 Addington Road, West Wickham BR4 9BW Tel: 020 8462 5297 — MB BS Lond. 1976 (Roy. Free Hosp.) GP & Trainer W. Wickham; Med. Off.; Lect. & Examr. Brit. Red Cross; Chairm. EMDOC Ltd. Specialty: Psychother. Prev: Trainee GP Cirencester VTS; Ho. Surg. Edgware Gen. Hosp.; Ho. Phys. Lister Hosp. Stevenage.

ROBERTSON, Stuart Mitchell Queen Elizabeth Hospital, Stadium Road, Woolwich SE18 4QH Tel: 0208 836 5595 Email: stuart.robertson@nhs.net — MB BS Lond. 1980; FCA RCSI 1988. Cons. Anaesth.Qu. Eliz. Hosp., Woolwich, Lond. Specialty: Anaesth. Prev: Sen. Regist. Rotat. (Anaesth.) NE Thames RHA.

ROBERTSON, Stuart William 25 Hayfield Avenue, Cardiff CF5 1AL — MB ChB Ed. 1992. Specialty: Nephrol.

ROBERTSON, Susan Elizabeth The Renal Unit, Dumfries Royal Infirmary, Bankend Road, Dumfries DG1 4AP Tel: 01387 241604; Gillfoot Farm, New Abbey, Dumfries DG2 8HD Tel: 01387 850225 — MB ChB Aberd. 1986; DRCOG 1991. Staff Grade (Renal) Dumfries Roy. Infirm. Specialty: Nephrol. Prev: Trainee GP/SHO Dumfries & Galloway VTS; Ho. Off. (Med.) Dumfries Roy. Infirm.

ROBERTSON, Tanya Collette North Western Deanery, Royal Albert and Edward Infirmary, Wigan; 40 Spires Gardens, Golborne Road, Winwick, Warrington WA2 8WB Tel: 01925 637786 — MB BS Lond. 1996 (St. Georges London) MRCPCH. SpR (Paediat.) N. West. Region. Specialty: Paediat. Prev: SHO (Paediat.) United Leeds Teachg. Hosp. Leeds.

ROBERTSON, Mr Timothy Damian Warwick Hospital, Lakin Road, Warwick CV34 5BW Tel: 01926 495321 — MB ChB Birm. 1986; FRCS Ed. 1994. Cons. Orthopaedic Surg., Warwick Hosp., Warwick. Specialty: Orthop.

ROBERTSON, Professor William Bruce 3 Cambisgate, 109 Church Road, Wimbledon, London SW19 5AL Tel: 020 8947 6731 — MB ChB St. And. 1947; BSc St. And. 1944, MD 1959; FRCPath 1969, M 1963. Emerit. Prof. Histopath. (Univ. Lond.) St. Geo. Hosp. Med. Sch. Lond.; Hon. Cons. Path. St. Geo. Hosp. Specialty: Histopath. Prev: Dir. Studies Roy. Coll. Path.; Vis. Prof. Univ. Leuven, Belgium; Sen. Lect. (Morbid Anat.) Univ. W. Indies, Jamaica.

ROBERTSON, William Graham (retired) 9 Station Road, Biggleswade SG18 8AL Tel: 01767 312124 — MB ChB Ed. 1941.

ROBERTSON, William Shedden Muir The Surgery, 31 Portland Road, Kilmarnock KA1 2DJ Tel: 01563 22118; 29 Glasgow Road, Kilmarnock KA3 1TJ Tel: 01563 24869 — MB ChB Glas. 1959.

ROBERTSON-RINTOUL, James (retired) Pictavia, 11 Bonfield Road, Strathkinness, St Andrews KY16 9RR Tel: 01334 850653 — MB ChB St. And. 1951; BSc St. And. 1944; MD St. And. 1960. Prev: Reader (Clin. Anat.) Univ. St. And.

ROBERTSON-RITCHIE, Hugh The New Surgery, 128 Canterbury Road, Folkestone CT19 5SR Tel: 01303 243516 Fax: 01303 244633 Email: hughrr@doctors.org.uk — MB BS Lond. 1972 (Guy's) MRCS Eng. LRCP Lond. 1972; Cert. Family Plann. JCC 1980; MRCGP 1980; MPhil Camb. 1996; DPMSA 2000. GP Trainer. Prev: SHO (Chest Dis.) Univ. Coll. Hosp. Lond.; SHO (Radiother.) St. William's Hosp. Rochester; Ho. Surg. Greenwich Dist. Hosp. Lond.

ROBERTSON-STEEL, Iain Rhoderick Stewart West Midlands Ambulance Service, Falcon Hse, 6 The Memories, Dudley DY2 8PN Tel: 01384 215555 Fax: 01384 215559; Ivy Lodge, 17 Priorslee Village, Telford TF2 9NW — MB ChB Birm. 1979; DRCOG 1986; MRCGP 1987; Dip. IMC RCS Ed. 1991; DFFP 1994. Med. Dir., W,Midl.s Ambul. Serv., Med. Dir. NHS Dir. Birm. Black Country & Solihull; Hon. Sen. Clin. Lect. (Primary Care) Univ. Wolverhampton; Hon. Research Fell. Sch. Heath & Social Serv. Univ. of Coventry. Specialty: Accid. & Emerg. Socs: BASICS; Assoc. Fell. Fac. Accid. & Emerg. Med.; Fac. Pre Hosp. Care. Prev: RAF Med. Servs.; GP Leatherhead Surrey; Police Surg. Surrey Police.

ROBIN, Mr Ian Gibson (retired) Merchiston, 4 Lodge Gardens, Oakham LE15 6EP — MB BChir Camb. 1933 (Camb. & Guy's) MRCS Eng. LRCP Lond. 1933; MA Camb. 1933; FRCS Eng. 1935. Prev: ENT Surg. The Princess Louise (Kensington) Hosp. for Childr., Paddington Green Childr. Hosp., Roy. Chest Hosp. & Well Ho. Hosp. Lond.

ROBIN, John Gilbert The Medical Centre, 12 East King Street, Helensburgh G84 7QL Tel: 01436 672277 Fax: 01436 674526; 5 Queen's Point, Shandon, Helensburgh G84 8QZ Fax: 01436 74526 — MB ChB Glas. 1970; DObst RCOG 1973; MRCGP 1974.

ROBIN, Jonathan Mark Centre for Clinical Pharmacology, The Cruciform Project, Rayne Institute, University College London, London WC1; 25 Oak Tree Close, Virginia Water GU25 4JF — MB BS Lond. 1994 (UMDS Guy's & St. Thos.) MB BS (Hons.) Lond. 1994; MRCP (UK) 1997. Lect. (Clin. Pharmacol. & Intens. Care Med.) Univ. Coll. Lond. Specialty: Pharmacology. Prev: SHO, Roy. Brompton & Hammersm. Hosp. Lond.; HO. Phys. Guy's Hosp. Lond.

ROBIN, Nicole Marie 14 Alexandra Road, West Kirby, Wirral CH48 0RT Tel: 0151 625 3437 — MB ChB Birm. 1990; MB ChB (Hons.) Birm. 1990; MRCP (UK) 1993; DA (UK) 1994; FRCA 1996. Regist. (Anaesth.) Mersey RHA. Specialty: Anaesth.

ROBINS, Amanda Elizabetta Walnut Yard, Church St., Buckingham MK18 1BY — BM Soton. 1996. SHO (Med.) Greenwich Hosp. Lond. Specialty: Gastroenterol.; Respirat. Med. Socs: Anglo-French Med. Soc. Prev: SHO (A & E) Univ. Coll. Hosp. Lond.

ROBINS, Andrew William Department of Paediatrics, Whittington Hospital, Highgate Hill, London N19 5NF Tel: 020 7288 5188 Fax: 020 72885215 Email: andrew.robins@whittington.nhs.uk; 23 Tavistock Terrace, London N19 4BZ — MB BS Lond. 1986 (Roy. Free Hosp. Lond.) MRCPI 1990; DCH RCP Lond. 1990; MRCP (UK) 1991; MSc (Clin. Paediat.) Lond. 1996; FRCPCH 1997. Cons. Paediat. Whittington Hosp. Lond. Specialty: Paediat. Socs: Fell. Roy. Coll. Paediat. & Child Health; InterNat. Child Health Gp.; BMA. Prev: Sen. Regist. (Paediat.) N. Middlx. Hosp.; Regist. (Paediat.) Whipps Cross Hosp. Lond.; Regist. (Neonat.) Univ. Coll. Hosp. Lond.

ROBINS, David Peter Cross Keys House, South Hinkley, Oxford — BM BCh Oxf. 1969.

ROBINS, David Stuart (retired) 26 Bretby Lane, Bretby, Burton-on-Trent DE15 0QN Tel: 01283 548628 Fax: 01238 548628 Email: dave@the-robins.freeserve.co.uk — (Manch.) MB ChB Manch. 1969; DObst RCOG 1971. Prev: Ho. Surg. & Ho. Phys. Manch. Roy. Infirm.

ROBINS, David William Anaesthetic Department, North Hampshire Hospital, Basingstoke RG24 9NA Tel: 01256 313461 Fax: 01256 354224 — MB BS Lond. 1971 (Lond. Hosp.) MRCS Eng. LRCP Lond. 1971; DObst RCOG 1973; FRCA 1978. Cons. Anaesth. (Day Surg.) N. Hants. Hosp. Trust Basingstoke. Specialty: Anaesth. Socs: Eur. Soc. Anaesth.; Brit. Assn. Day Surg. Prev: Dir. ITU; Clin. Dir. (Anaesth.); Sen. Regist. (Anaesth.) Bristol Roy. Infirm., Frenchay Hosp. Bristol & Treliske Hosp. Truro.

ROBINS, Gwyn 2 Elm Grove, Gilwern, Abergavenny NP7 0BE — MRCS Eng. LRCP Lond. 1946.

ROBINS, James Brent Department of Obstetrics & Gynaecology, Inverclyde Royal Hospital, Larkfield Road, Greenock PA16 0XN Tel: 01475 633777 Fax: 01475 656188 Email: james.robins@irh.scot.nhs.uk; St. Colms, Duchal Road, Kilmacolm PA13 4AY Tel: 01505 872938 Email: robinsjim@aol.com — MB ChB Ed. 1984; MRCOG 1990; (Advanced Obst. Ultrasound Diploma) RCR/RCOG 1994; MPhil Glasgow 2002. Cons. O & G Inverclyde Roy. NHS Trust; Hon. Clinical Senior Lecturer (mem. MREC Scotland). Specialty: Obst. & Gyn. Special Interest: Med. Ethics and Law; Pre-natal screening. Socs: Brit. Med. Ultrasound Soc.; Brit. Matern. & Fetal Med. Soc.; Glas. Obst. and Gyn. Soc. Prev: Sen. Regist. (O & G) Leeds Gen. Infirm.; Regist. (O & G) Glas. Matern. Hosp.; Neonat. Research Fell. Univ. Edin. Simpson Memor. Matern. Pavil. Edin.

ROBINS, Kay — MB BS Newc. 1994.

ROBINS, Nathalie Marie Raunsley Building, Dept. Psychiatry, Manchester Royal Infirmary, Oxford Road, Manchester M13 9WL Tel: 0161 276 5365 Fax: 0161 276 5444 — MB ChB Manch. 1992; MRCPsych 1996; MSc 1999. Sen. Regist. (Psychiat.) Manch. Roy. Infirm. Specialty: Gen. Psychiat.

ROBINS, Mr Robert Henry Cradock (retired) 3 Lemon Villas, Truro TR1 2NX Tel: 01872 273689 Fax: 01872 273689; Oak Tree House, Perran-Ar-Worthal, Truro TR3 7QL Tel: 01872 863356 — (St. Bart.) MA Camb. 1949, BA (2nd cl. Nat. Sc. Trip. Pts. I & II) 1944; MB BChir Camb. 1947; FRCS Eng. 1950. Prev: Orthop. Surg. Roy. Cornw. Hosp. Truro & Cornw. & I. of Scilly DHA.

ROBINS, Sally Jane The Stubbington Medical Practice, Park Lane, Stubbington, Fareham PO14 2JP — MB BS Lond. 1992 (St Thomas) BSc (Biochem.) Lond. 1989; DRCOG 1995; DFFP 1996. GP. Specialty: Gen. Pract. Prev: GP Regist. Portsmouth; SHO c/o Elderly, Qu. Alexandra Hosp. Portsmouth.; SHO Psychiat. St Jane's Portsmouth.

ROBINS, Sandra Betty Suttons, Brownbread Street, Ashburnham, Battle TN33 9NX Tel: 01424 892410 — MB BS Lond. 1988; BSc Lond. 1985; DCH RCP Lond. 1991; DRCOG 1993. GP E. Sussex Retainer Scheme. Prev: Trainee GP Tunbridge Wells VTS.

ROBINSKA, Ewa Maria Eastfields Road Surgery, 1 Eastfields Road, Acton, London W3 0AA Tel: 020 8992 4331 — MB BS Lond. 1978 (Roy. Free) DCH RCP Lond. 1982; DRCOG 1983; MRCGP 1984. GP Acton. Prev: Ho. Surg. & Ho. Phys. Edgware Gen. Hosp.; Trainee GP Ealing VTS.; GP Greenford.

ROBINSON, Adam Corin James Diabetes Centre, Chorley Street, Bolton BL1 4AL Tel: 01204 522814 Email: acjrobninson@yahoo.com; Highfield Hospital, Manchester Road, Rochdale OL11 4LZ Tel: 01706 655121 — MB BS Lond. 1987 (King's Coll.) FRCP (UK) 1991. Cons. Diabetes & Endocrinol. Specialty: Endocrinol.; Diabetes; Gen. Med. Special Interest: Hypertens. Obesity Impotence CVrisk. Prev: Registar/Research Fell. St Mary's Paddington; Cons. QE Gateshead & Roy. Oldham Hosp.; SHO (Renal Transpl.) Roy. Free Hosp. Lond.

ROBINSON, Alan Andrew The Briars, Nethergate St., Harpley, King's Lynn PE31 6TN Tel: 01485 520644; 29 Woodcock Road, Norwich NR3 3UA Tel: 01603 425989 Fax: 01603 488315 — MB ChB Liverp. 1978; MRCP (UK) 1981; MRCGP 1986.

ROBINSON, Alexandra Jane Smallwood House, Church Green W., Redditch B97 4BD; 44 Leslie Road, Edgbaston, Birmingham B16 9DX — MB ChB Bristol 1982; MRCGP 1985; DCH RCP Lond. 1985; DRCOG 1986. Clin. Asst. (Psychiat. of Old Age & Geriat.) Redditch & Worcs. HA. Specialty: Care of the Elderly.

ROBINSON, Alexandra Louise Department of Anaesthetics, Birmingham Childrens Hospital, Ladywood Middleway, Birmingham B16 8ET; 5 St. Helier Close, Wokingham RG41 2HA — MB BS Lond. 1988; FRCA 1993. Sen. Regist. Birm. Sch. Specialty: Anaesth. Prev: Regist. Rotat. (Anaesth.) Oxf.; Regist. Rotat. (Anaesth.) Milton Keynes Gen. Hosp.; Clin. Fell. Birm. Childr. Hosp.

ROBINSON, Alfred (retired) Oakhurst, 146 Barnham Road, Barnham, Bognor Regis PO22 0EH Tel: 01243 553259 — (Guy's) MA Camb. 1968, BA 1951; MB BChir Camb. 1954; FRCP Lond. 1974, M 1961; DCH Eng. 1961. Prev: Cons. Paediat. Chichester & Worthing Trust.

ROBINSON, Alfred Alexander Thomas House Surgery, 12 East Bridge Road, Dymchurch, Romney Marsh TN29 0PF Tel: 01303 873156 Fax: 01303 874885; Moonfield, Cambers Green, Pluckley, Ashford TN27 0HR Tel: 01233 840254 — MB BS Lond. 1965 (King's Coll. Hosp.) MRCS Eng. LRCP Lond. 1965; DCH Eng. 1969; DObst RCOG 1970. GP Dymchurch. Socs: BMA.

ROBINSON, Alison Frances Central Clinic, East Lodge Court, High Street, Colchester CO1 1UJ; Priory House, 166 Rushmere Road, Ipswich IP4 3LP — MB BS Lond. 1978 (Char. Cross) MA Oxf. 1974; MRCP (UK) 1981; DCH 1981; FRCPCH 1994. Cons. Paediat. Essex Rivers Healthcare Trust; Med. Adviser to Fostering Serv. Essex Co. Counc. Specialty: Paediat.; Disabil. Med.; Child & Adolesc. Psychiat. Socs: Brit. Assn. of Adoption & Fostering; Brit. Assn. of Community Child Health; Assn. of Child Psychol. & Psychiat. Prev: Sen. Regist. (Child Health) Ipswich; SCMO (Child Health) Ipswich.

ROBINSON, Amanda Susan Ann Butt Lane Surgery, 58 Butt Lane, Leeds LS12 5AZ Tel: 0113 263 7635 Fax: 0113 279 1781; 13 Arncliffe Road, Leeds LS16 5AP Tel: 0113 274 6424 Fax: 0113 274 6424 — MB Oxf. 1976; ChB Birm. 1979; MA Oxf. 1980; DRCOG 1981; MRCGP 1983; MBA 1989. Dist. Fac. Tutor Roy. Coll. Gen. Pract.; GP Adviser Med. Serv. Commissioning Team Leeds HA; Chairm. Leeds W. PCG. Specialty: Gen. Pract. Socs: Inst. Psychosexual Med. Prev: GP Gt. Shelford Camb.

ROBINSON, Andrew Garforth Medical Centre, Church Lane, Garforth, Leeds LS25 1HB Tel: 0113 286 5311 Fax: 0113 281 2679 — MB BS Lond. 1984 (St. George's Lond.) DA (UK) l987; DRCOG 1992. GP Princip.; Clin. Asst. Anaesth. Specialty: Anaesth. Prev: Trainee GP Kingston upon Hull.

ROBINSON, Andrew David Thiele Fulton Clinic, Royal Cornhill Hospital, Aberdeen AB25 2ZW Tel: 01224 557525 — MB ChB Dundee 1978 (Dundee Univ.) MRCPsych 1985. Cons. Psychiat.

ROBINSON, Mr Andrew Hugh Neil Box 37, Addenbrooke's Hospital, Hills Road, Cambridge CB3 2QQ Tel: 01223 216426 Fax: 01223 217307; 170 Gwydir Street, Cambridge CB1 2LW — MB BS Lond. 1988; BSc Lond. 1985; FRCS Lond. 1992; FRCS (Orth.) 1996. Cons. (Trauma & Orthop.) Addenbrooke's Hosp. Camb. Specialty: Trauma & Orthop. Surg. Socs: BOA; Brit. Ohthopaedic Surg. Soc.; RSM. Prev: SHO (Surg) St. Barts Hosp. Lond.; Higher Surg. Trainee (Orthop.) E. Anglia.

ROBINSON, Andrew John Albany Surgery, Albany Street, Newton Abbot TQ12 2TX Tel: 01626 334411 Fax: 01626 335663 — MB ChB Bristol 1988; BSc (Hons.) Bristol 1985; MRCP (UK) 1991; MRCGP 1993.

ROBINSON, Angela Joyce University College Hospital, Department of Genitourinary Medicine, Mortimer Market Centre, off Capper Street, London WC1E 6AU Tel: 020 7530 5033 Fax: 020 7530 5044 Email: arobinson@gum.ucl.ac.uk; 36 Palace Road, Crouch End, London N8 8QJ — MB BS Newc. 1980; MRCP (UK) 1983; FRCP (UK) 1996. Cons. Genitourin. Med. Mortimer Market Centre Lond.; Hon. Sen. Lect. UCL. Specialty: Genitourinary Medicine. Socs: Pres. of Brit. Assn. for Sexual Health & HIV, Jt. Specialty Comm. of Genitourin. Med. Prev: Sen. Regist. (Genitourin. Med.) Roy. Hallamshire Hosp. Sheff.; Regist. (Haemat.) Univ. Hosp. Wales Cardiff.

ROBINSON, Angus John Radiotherapy Department, Churchill Hospital, Old Road, Headington, Oxford OX3 7LJ Tel: 01865 741841; 68 James Street, Oxford OX4 1EX Tel: 01865 243966 — BM BS Nottm. 1992; FRCR Part 1; BMedSci Nottm. 1990; MRCP 1996. Regist. Clin. Oncol. Oxf. Radcliffe Hosps. Specialty: Oncol.; Radiother. Prev: SHO (Oncol. & Cardiol.) St. Bart. Hosp. Lond.; SHO (Gen. & Respirat. Med.) Ealing.

ROBINSON, Ann Benedict 8 Kimblesworth Grange, Potterhouse Lane, Chester-le-Street DH2 3QS Tel: 0191 371 9141 — MB BS Lond. 1991 (King's Coll. Lond.) BSc Lond. 1988; MRCP (UK) 1995; DFFP 1996. GP Regist. Lond.

ROBINSON, Ann Chany The Mountfield Surgery, 55 Mountfield Road, Finchley, London N3 3NR Tel: 020 8346 4271 Fax: 020 8371 0187 — MB BS Lond. 1984 (Middlx. Hosp.) DRCOG 1986; DCH RCP Lond. 1987; MRCGP 1988. Specialty: Gen. Pract.

ROBINSON, Ann Judith — MB ChB Ed. 1969; BSc (Hons., Physiol.) Ed. 1966. Specialty: Gen. Psychiat. Socs: MRCPsych. Prev: Med. Research Fell. Dept. Psychiat. Nottm. Univ.; Staff Grade Community Psychait. Milton Kynes pt/t.; GP Gateshead.

ROBINSON, Ann Louise Windmill Medical Practice, 65 Shoot Up Hill, London NW2 3PS Tel: 020 8452 7646 Fax: 020 8450 2319 — MB BS Lond. 1986; DRCOG 1990; DCH RCP Lond. 1992; MRCGP 1993.

ROBINSON, Anne Caroline Radcliff Department of Radiotherapy, Southend Hospital, Prittlewell Chase, Westcliff on Sea SS0 0RY; 1 Fairview Lodge, Underwood Square, Leigh-on-Sea SS9 3QH — MB BCh BAO Dub. 1974 (TC Dub.) MRCPI 1976; DCH NUI 1977; FFR RCSI 1985; FRCR 1988; MA 1992; FRCPI 1997. Cons. Southend Hosp. Westcliff on Sea. Specialty: Oncol.; Radiother. Socs: Fell. Roy. Acad. Med. Irel.; Brit. Oncol. Assn. Prev: Sen. Regist. Christie Hosp. & Holt Radium Inst. Manch.; Radiother. St. Lukes Hosp. Dub.; Hon. Sen. Regist. Cookridge Hosp. Leeds.

ROBINSON, Anne Elizabeth (retired) 18 Hammondswick, Harpenden AL5 2NR Tel: 0158 27 13888 — (Univ. Coll. Hosp.) MB BS Lond. 1954; DObst RCOG 1955. Prev: Clin. Asst. Soho Hosp. for Wom. Lond.

ROBINSON, Anne Elizabeth 76 Birchdale Road, Appleton, Warrington WA4 5AW Tel: 01925 267045 — MB ChB Liverp. 1983; FRCS Ed. 1988; FRCS Eng. 1988; MRCGP 1990. Cons. A & E Warrington Hosp. NHS Trust. Specialty: Accid. & Emerg. Prev: Sen. Regist. (A & E) Warrington Hosp. NHS Trust; Regist. (A & E) Whittington Hosp. Lond.; Trainee GP Edgware VTS.

ROBINSON, Anne Penelope Alport Castles Farm, Alport Dale, Bamford, Hope Valley S33 0AB — MB ChB Birm. 1975; MRCP (UK) 1977.

ROBINSON, Mr Anthony Colin The Clementine Churchill Hospital, Sudbury Hill, Harrow HA1 3RX Tel: 0208 872 3899 Fax: 0208 872 3908 — MB BS Lond. 1979 (Middlx.) FRCS Eng. 1985. Cons. Otolaryngol. W. Middlx. Univ. Hosp. Isleworth. Specialty: Otolaryngol. Socs: Fell. Roy. Soc. Med.; Brit. Med. Assoc; Young Cons. Otolaryingologists Head & Neck Surg. Prev: Sen. Regist. (ENT) Roy. Free Hosp. Lond. & Roy. Surrey Co. Hosp. Guildford; Regist. (ENT) Roy, Free Hosp. Lond.; SHO (ENT) Roy. Nat. Throat, Nose & Ear Hosp. Lond.

ROBINSON, Anthony John The Great Bridge Partnerships for Health, Sai Surgery, 10 Slater Street, Great Bridge, Tipton DY4 7EY Tel: 0121 557 0122 Email: anthony.robinson@nhs.net; Meadowcroft, Stream Road, Kingswinford DY6 9NX Tel: 01384 401332 Fax: 01384 401332 Email: tony.robinson@tesco.net — MB ChB Birm. 1983; BSc (Hons.) Nottm. 1978; MRCGP 1987; DRCOG 1987; MFFP 1994; FRCGP 1997. Princip. Gen. Pract.; Trainer (Gen. Pract.) Sandwell; Assoc. Adviser Gen. Pract; Mem. Roy. Coll. GPs Exam. Bd. Specialty: Family Plann. & Reproduc. Health. Socs: Primary Care Assn. for Gastroenterol.; GP Airways Gp.; Roy. Soc. Med. Prev: Trainee GP Sandwell Dist. Gen. Hosp. W. Bromwich; Ho. Surg. Roy. Shrewsbury Hosp.; Ho. Phys. Sandwell Dist. Gen. Hosp.

ROBINSON, Anthony Michael Halton Leys, Iford Hill, Westwood, Bradford-on-Avon BA15 2BG Tel: 01225 867644 — MB BCh Wales 1985 (Welsh Nat. Sch. Med.) BSc Wales 1980; MRCP (UK) 1989; DM Nottm. 1996; FRCP (Lond.) 2001. Cons. Phys. (Diabetes & Endocrinol.) Roy. United Hosp. Bath. Specialty: Diabetes; Gen. Med.; Endocrinol. Socs: Sec. of Wessex Endocrine and Diabetes Assn. Prev: Sen. Regist. (Diabetes & Endocrinol.) Sheff. Hosps.; Regist. (Med.)

Roy. Hallamsh. Hosp. Sheff.; Research Fell. (Diabetic Med.) Qu. Med. Centre Nottm.

ROBINSON, Arthur Thomas (retired) Haddef, Tudweiliog, Pwllheli LL53 8NB — MB BS Lond. 1954 (King's Coll. Hosp.) MRCGP 1966. Prev: Ho. Surg. Orthop. & Urol. Depts. King's Coll. Hosp.

ROBINSON, Arthur William (retired) 30 Brueton Avenue, Solihull B91 3EN Tel: 0121 246 0581 — (Camb. & Univ. Coll. Hosp.) MA Camb. 1953, MD 1956; FRCR 1983. Prev: Cons. Radiol. Coventry Hosps.

ROBINSON, Ashley James Department of Diagnostic Radiology, University of Manchester Medical School, Stopford Building, Oxford Road, Manchester M13 9PT Tel: 0161 275 5114 Fax: 0161 275 5594 — MB ChB Leeds 1994; BSc (Hons.) Leeds 1991; Dip. ATLS RCS Eng. 1995; FRCR 1997. Specialist Regist. (Diagn. Radiol.) Manch. Roy Infirm. Specialty: Radiol. Prev: SHO (Gen. Med.) Sescroft Hosp. Leeds; SHO (A & E) Roy. Halifax Infirm.; Ho. Off. (Surg.) St. Jas. Hosp. Leeds.

ROBINSON, Barry George 12 Regent Road, Lowestoft NR32 1PA Tel: 01502 65252 — MB BS Lond. 1981; DRCOG 1984.

ROBINSON, Barry John Lyme Practice, Uplyme Road, Lyme Regis DT7 3LS Tel: 01297 445777 Fax: 01297 444917; Valley Farm, Rocombe, Uplyme, Lyme Regis DT7 3RR Tel: 01297 445868 Email: barry.robinson@gp-j81088.nhs.uk — BM Soton. 1983; MRCGP 1988; DRCOG 1988. Socs: Internat. Comm. Wound Managem.; Eur. Wound Managem. Assn.; Wound Care Soc. Prev: Unit Gen. Manager Lyme Community Care Unit.

ROBINSON, Basil (retired) Hasty Bank, 9 Foxglove Road, Almondbury, Huddersfield HD5 8LW Tel: 01484 532517 — MRCS Eng. LRCP Lond. 1939 (Cardiff) MRCGP 1953. Prev: Surg. Lt.-Cdr. RNVR.

ROBINSON, Benjamin Guy 186 Cathays Ter, Cardiff CF24 4HZ — MB BCh Wales 1997.

ROBINSON, Beverley Louise Department of Radiology, Royal United Hospital, Combe Park, Bath BA1 3NG Tel: 01225 825728 Fax: 01225 825515 Email: louise.robinson@ruh-bath.swest.nhs.uk; Broughton Gifford Manor, Broughton Gifford, Melksham SN12 8PP Tel: 01225 782259 Fax: 01225 783383 Email: louise.robinson@ruh-bath.swest.nhs.uk — MB BS Lond. 1981 (King's Coll Hosp. Lond.) FRCR 1988; T(R) (CR) 1993. Cons. Radiol. Roy. United Hosp. Bath. Specialty: Radiol. Prev: Cons. Radiol. St. Helier Hosp. Carshalton; Clin. Lect. MRI Dept. Guy's Hosp. Lond.; Sen. Regist. & Regist. (Radiol.) Guy's Hosp. Lond.

ROBINSON, Brian Barrow Hospital, Barrow Gurney, Bristol BS48 3SG Tel: 0117 9286644 Fax: 0117 9246650 — MB BCh Wales 1979; MRCPsych 1984. Specialty: Gen. Psychiat.

ROBINSON, Brian Fyffe The Manor House, Curry Mallet, Taunton TA3 6SU Tel: 01823 480161 Email: brianrobinson@mcmail.com — (St. Geo.) MD Lond. 1966, MB BS 1951; FRCP Lond. 1971, M 1953. Emerit. Prof. Cardiovasc. Med. Univ. of Lond. Prev: Prof. Cardiovasc. Med. St. Geo. Hosp. Med. Sch. Lond.; Reader in Cardiovasc. Med. St. Geo. Hosp. Med. Sch. Lond.; Nuffield Med. Fell. Cardiol. Br. Nat. Insts. Health Bethesda, MD.

ROBINSON, Brian Hertzel Ashchurch Surgery, 134 Askew Road, Shepherd Bush, London W12 9BP Tel: 020 8743 2920 Fax: 020 8743 1545; 20 Delamere Road, London W5 3JR Tel: 020 8567 6558 — MB BCh BAO Belf. 1959; DObst RCOG 1962. Socs: BMA. Prev: SHO Waveney Hosp. Ballymena; Ho. Phys. Belf. City Hosp. & Roy. Belf. Hosp. Sick Childr.; Ho. Surg. Musgrave Pk. Hosp. Belf.

ROBINSON, Brian Hugh Bartlett, TD Birmingham Nuffield Hospital, 22 Somerset Road, Edgbaston, Birmingham B15 2QQ Tel: 0121 456 2000 Fax: 0121 454 5293; Five Oaks, 55 Meriden Road, Hampton-in-Arden, Solihull B92 0BS Tel: 01675 442300 Fax: 01675 442300 Email: 101523.1574@compuserve.com — (Camb. & Guy's) MB BChir Camb. 1954; MA Camb. 1954; MRCS Eng. LRCP Lond. 1954; FRCP Lond. 1974, M 1959. Cons. Nephrol. Birm. Nuffield Hosp.; Hon. Cons. Phys. Birm. Heartlands Hosp. NHS Trust (Teachg.). Specialty: Nephrol. Socs: Renal Assn.; Eur. Renal Assn. Prev: Cons. Phys. & Clin. Dir. (Renal Servs.) Birm. Heartlands Hosp. NHS Trust (Teachg.); Hon. Sen. Clin. Lect. Univ. Birm.; Sen. Regist. Med. Unit Univ. Coll. Hosp.

ROBINSON, Brian Stuart Havant Health Centre Suite A, PO Box 41, Civic Centre Road, Havant PO9 2AJ Tel: 023 9248 2148 Fax: 023 9249 2524 — MB BS Lond. 1970; MRCS Eng. LRCP Lond. 1970.

ROBINSON, Brian Wilfred 137 Westbrooke Avenue, Hartlepool TS25 5HZ — MB BS Newc. 1979.

ROBINSON, Bronwen Eileen (retired) Padeswood Lodge, Padeswood, Mold CH7 4JF Tel: 01244 546420 Email: bron_robinson@lineone.net — BMedSc Otago, NZ 1952 (Otago) MB ChB NZ 1955; FRCP Lond. 1991; FRCPCH 1996. Prev: Cons. Community Paediat. Countess of Chester NHS Hosp. Trust.

ROBINSON, Bryan Laurence (retired) 16 Orkney Ct, Taplow, Maidenhead SL6 0JB Tel: 01628 669333 Fax: 01628 669333 — MB BS Lond. 1963 (Guy's) MRCS Eng. LRCP Lond. 1963; DObst RCOG 1966; MRCGP 1968. Examr. Benefits Agency Med. Serv. Prev: Med. Adviser Benefits Agency Med. Serv. DSS.

ROBINSON, Carmel Jessica Sarah 62 Downhills Road, Liverpool L23 8SP — MB BS Lond. 1992.

ROBINSON, Caroline Anne 52 The Drive, Ickenham, Uxbridge UB10 8AG — MB BS Lond. 1996.

ROBINSON, Catherine Rose Oak Street Medical Practice, 1 Oak Street, Norwich NR3 3DL Tel: 01603 613431 Fax: 01603 767209; 133 Christchurch Road, Norwich NR2 3PG — MB BS Lond. 1981; BA Oxf. 1978; DRCOG 1985; DCH RCP Lond. 1987; DTM & H 1989. Prev: Trainee GP Norwich VTS; Gen.iste Urgences Amer. Hosp., Paris.

ROBINSON, Charles Adrian 39 Honister Avenue, Newcastle upon Tyne NE2 3PA — MB BS Newc. 1988.

ROBINSON, Charles Graham Francis Department of Diagnostic Imaging, Mobay Hope Medical Centre, P.O.Box 2520, Half Moon P.O., Rose Hall, Montego Bay, Jamaica; Y Bodau O'R Cathod, Llanfallteg, Whitland SA34 0UJ — MRCS Eng. LRCP Lond. 1972 (Lond. Hosp.) DMRD Eng. 1979. Specialty: Radiol. Socs: Roy. Coll. Radiol.; Brit. Inst. Radiol.; BMA. Prev: Cons. Radiol. Withybush Gen. Hosp. HaverfordW.

ROBINSON, Charles Patrick c/o X-Ray Department, Cheltenham General Hospital, Sandford Road, Cheltenham GL53 7AN — MB BCh BAO Dub. 1971; BA Dub. 1969; MB BCh Dub. 1971; FRCR 1978. Cons. Radiol. Cheltenham Gen. Hosp. Specialty: Radiol. Prev: Cons. Radiol. Dorset Co. Hosp. Dorchester; State Specialist Radiol. Gen. Hosp. Bandar Seri Begawan Brunei; Sen. Regist. & Regist. (Radiol.) Brist. Roy. Infirm.

ROBINSON, Charles Richard The Crofters, Pool Bank Farm, Tarvin, Chester CH3 8JX Email: charles.robinson@hunterlink.net.au — MB BS Tasmania 1981; BDS Bristol 1974; DObst. Austral. 1986.

ROBINSON, Christina Jane 18 Ramsey Road, Sheffield S10 1LR — MB ChB Sheff. 1995.

ROBINSON, Christine Anne The Lodge, 4 George St. W., Luton LU1 2BJ Tel: 01582 511003 Fax: 01582 511001 — MB BChir Camb. 1983 (Camb./St. Thos.) MA Camb. 1983; MRCOG 1990; MFFP 1994; FRCOG 2003. Cons. Family Plann. & Reproduct. Health Care. Luton PCT.

ROBINSON, Christopher High Street Surgery, 1st Floor, 99 High Street, Fort William PH33 6DG Tel: 01397 703773 Fax: 01397 701068; Arkaig Cottage, Achintore Road, Fort William PH33 6RN Tel: 01397 702886 Email: cr@lochaber.almac.co.uk — MB BS Lond. 1971 (Roy. Free) DA Eng. 1973; DObst RCOG 1974. Prev: SHO (Anaesth.) Edgware Gen. Hosp.; SHO (Obst.) Vale of Leven Hosp. Alexandria; SHO (Paediat.) Law Hosp. Carluke.

ROBINSON, Christopher David The Paddock Surgery, Chapel Lane, Thornhill, Dewsbury WF12 0DH Tel: 01924 465343 Fax: 01924 455781 — MB ChB Sheff. 1982. Prev: Trainee GP Mansfield VTS; SHO (A & E) Rotherham Dist. Gen. Hosp.

ROBINSON, Christopher Gurth Goland The Medical Centre, 45 Enderley Road, Harrow Weald, Harrow HA3 5HF Tel: 020 8863 3333; 14 Evelyn Drive, Pinner HA5 4RX Tel: 020 8428 4186 — MB ChB Dundee 1977 (Dundee University) DRCOG 1979; MRCGP 1982. GP Trainer Northwick Pk. VTS. Prev: Trainee GP Harrow VTS; Ho. Surg. Canad. Red Cross Memor. Hosp. Taplow; Ho. Phys. Wexham Pk. Hosp. Slough.

ROBINSON, Christopher John Canton Health Centre, Wessex Street, Cardiff CF5 1XU Tel: 029 2039 5115 Fax: 029 2039 4846 — MB BCh Wales 1978; BA Oxf. 1975; MRCGP 1984.

ROBINSON, Christopher Michael TLF, 11 Marchmont Road, Edinburgh EH9 1EL — BM BS Nottm. 1985.

ROBINSON, Clive Flat 10, The Beeches, Simmons Way, Whetstone, London N20 — MB BS Lond. 1978; BSc. Lond. 1975, MB BS Lond. 1978.

ROBINSON, Colan Denis Belmont Surgery, 12 Belmont Road, St Austell PL25 4UJ Tel: 01726 291266 Fax: 01726 291266 — MB ChB Manch. 1983; DA (UK) 1985; DObst NZ 1987; Dip Obst Otago 1989; DCH S. Afr. 1991; MRCGP 1993; FRCGP Lond. 1999. Prev: Trainee GP Barnstaple; Princip. Med. Off. Kwazulu DoH, S. Afr.; SHO (Anaesth.) Southmead Hosp. Bristol.

ROBINSON, Damian Paul Akenside Unit, Newcastle General Hospital, Newcastle upon Tyne NE4 6BE Tel: 0191 273 6666 Fax: 0191 272 2340; 1 Sutton Close, Milton, Cambridge CB4 6DU — MB BChir Camb. 1986 (Cambridge) MA Camb. 1986; MRCPsych 1989; MFPHM RCP (UK) 1995. Cons. Psychiat. Newc. City Health Trust. Specialty: Geriat. Psychiat.; Gen. Psychiat. Prev: Sen. Regist. (Pub. Health Med.) E. Anglian RHA; Sen. Regist. Psychiat. E. Anglia.

ROBINSON, David Alan The Cross Farm, Llansoy, Usk NP15 1DE — MB BCh Wales 1979; BSc (1st cl. Hons. Chem.) Bristol 1973; MRCP (UK) 1983; FRCR 1985. Cons. Radiol. Nevill Hall Hosp., Abergavenny, Gwent. Specialty: Radiol. Socs: (Counc.) Brit. Inst. Radiol. Prev: Sen. Regist. Univ. Hosp. Wales, Cardiff; Post-Grad. Research Fell. RPMS Hammersmith Hosp. Lond.

ROBINSON, David Anthony Department of Anaesthetics, Warwick Hospital, Lakin Road, Warwick CV34 5BW Tel: 01926 495321; Thornwood, New Road, Norton Lindsey, Warwick CV35 8JB Tel: 0192 684 3386 — MB BS Lond. 1977; FFA RCS Eng. 1985. Cons. Anaesth. Warwick Hosp. Specialty: Anaesth. Socs: Obst. Anaesth. Assn. Prev: Sen. Regist. Nuffield Dept. Anaesth. Oxf.; Sen. Regist. (Anaesth.) Princess Margt. Hosp. Swindon; Vis. Asst. Prof. Anesthesiol. Univ. Texas Health Sci. Center Texas, USA.

ROBINSON, David Bird Westlakes Research Institute, International Research & Graduate Centre, Westlakes Science & Technology Park, Moor Row, Wigton CA24 3JY Tel: 01946 514000; Jenkin, Loweswater, Cockermouth CA13 0RU Tel: 079 4044 9094 Fax: 0870 056 0319 Email: david@loweswater.net — MB BS Lond. 1979. Head of Healthcare Informatics. Specialty: Research. Special Interest: Clin. terminology; Med. informatics. Prev: Med. Off. Tristan Da Cunha 1984-85.

ROBINSON, David Charles 8 High View, Ponteland, Newcastle upon Tyne NE20 9ET — MB BS Newc. 1998; MB BS Newc 1998.

ROBINSON, David Cloberry (retired) Yatton Family Practice, 155 Mendip Road, Yatton, Bristol BS49 4ER Tel: 01934 832277 Fax: 01934 876085 Email: david@drobinson36.fsnet.co.uk; Oakfield, Meeting House Lane, Claverham, Bristol BS49 4PB Tel: 01934 833002 — MB BS Lond. 1962 (Middlx.) DObst RCOG 1964. Prev: Ho. Surg. Orpington Hosp.

ROBINSON, Mr David Derek Worcestershire Royal Hospital, Charles Hastings Way, Worcester WR5 1DD Tel: 01905 763333 Fax: 01905 760166; BUPA South Bank, 139 Bath Road, Worcester WR5 3YB Tel: 01905 350003 Fax: 01905 350856 — MB BS Lond. 1983; MA Camb. 1984; FRCS Ed. 1988; FRCS (Orth.) 1995. Cons. Trauma & Orthop. Worcester Roy. Infirm. Specialty: Orthop. Prev: Sen. Regist. Robt. Jones & Agnes Hunt Hosp. Oswestry.

ROBINSON, David John Culmer 88 Christchurch Avenue, London NW6 7PE — MB BS Lond. 1971 (St. Bart.) MRCS Eng. LRCP Lond. 1971; DA Eng. 1975; FFA RCS Eng. 1978. Cons. Anaesth. St. Mary's Hosp. Lond. Specialty: Anaesth. Prev: Anaesth. RN; Ho. Phys. Hackney Hosp.; Ho. Surg. Hillingdon Hosp.

ROBINSON, David Joseph Old School Surgery, School Street, Pontyclun CF72 9AA Tel: 01443 222567 Fax: 01443 229205 — MB BCh Wales 1974; BSc Wales, MB BCh 1974; DRCOG 1977; MRCGP 1979; Dip Occ Med (RCP) 1999. Hon. Lect. UWCM. Prev: SHO (Paediat.) & (Gen. Med.) E. Glam. Gen. Hosp.

ROBINSON, David Leonard Department of Paediatrics, King George Hospital, Barley Lane, Goodmayes, Ilford IG3 8YB Tel: 020 8970 8063 Fax: 020 8970 8063 Email: david.robinson@rbhc-tr.nthames.nhs.uk; 2 Christchurch Road, Crouch End, London N8 9QL Tel: 020 341 3300 Fax: 020 341 3300 — MB BS Lond. 1976; MRCS Eng. LRCP Lond. 1976; DCH RCP Lond. 1978; MRCP (UK) 1981; MSc (Pol./Admin.) Univ. Lond. 1988. Cons. Paediat. King Geo. Hosp. Ilford. Specialty: Paediat. Prev: Lect. & Hon. Sen. Regist. The Lond. Hosp. Whitechapel; Clin. Fell. Neonatol. Hosp. for Sick Childr. Toronto.

ROBINSON, David Nicoll — MB ChB Glas. 1985; FRCA 1992; BSc Open 1996. Cons. Paediat. Anaesth., Roy. Hosp. For sick chilkdren Yorkhill NHS Trust Glas. Specialty: Anaesth. Prev: Regist. (Anaesth.) St. Geo. Hosp. Lond.; Cons. Paediatric Anaesth., Roy. Manch. Childr.s Hosp.

ROBINSON, David Timm Rose Cottage, Witton, North Walsham NR28 9UD — MB ChB Manch. 1956.

ROBINSON, Mr David William 25 Oaklands, Miskin, Pontyclun CF72 8RW — MB BS Lond. 1981; BSc (Hons) Anat. Univ. Lond. 1978; FRCS Glas. 1989; FRCS (orth) 2000.

ROBINSON, David William 143 Scalby Road, Scarborough YO12 6TB Tel: 01723 372365 — BM BCh Oxf. 1964 (Oxf. & St. Mary's) BSc, BA Oxf. 1963, MA, BM BCh 1964; MSc Leeds 1969; FRCOG 1990, M 1970. Cons. O & G ScarBoro. Health Dist. Specialty: Obst. & Gyn. Socs: N. Engl. Obst. & Gyn. Soc. Prev: Sen. Regist. (O & G) Yorks. RHA; Regist. (O & G) Radcliffe Infirm. Oxf.; Ho. Surg. & Ho. Surg. Obst. St. Mary's Hosp. Lond.

ROBINSON, David William (retired) 2 Brettles Cottages, Beacon Lane, Shalterford, Bewdley DY12 1TJ — MB ChB Birm. 1954; BSc (Hons.) Birm. 1951, MB ChB 1954. Prev: Ho. Phys. & Ho. Surg. Gen. Hosp. Birm.

ROBINSON, Derek Axland-Harwood, 15 Claremont Hill, Shrewsbury SY1 1RD Tel: 01743 243414; 10 Kerris Close, St Michaels Wood, Liverpool L17 5BY Tel: 0151 727 4883 — (Manch.) MD Manch. 1961, MB ChB 1952; DPH Lond. 1959; DCH Eng. 1959; Dip. Amer. Bd. Preven. Med. 1969; FFCM 1980, M 1976. Indep. Internat. Epidemiologist & Med. Edr. Shrewsbury. Specialty: Epidemiol.; Trop. Med.; Infec. Dis. Socs: Fell. Mass. Med. Soc. Prev: Dir. Pub. Health Shrops. HA; Sen. Clin. Lect. Liverp. Sch. Trop. Med.; Instruc. & Research Assoc. Harvard Sch. Pub. Health Boston, USA.

ROBINSON, Mr Derek Edward 2 Alma House, 25 Alma Road, Clifton, Bristol BS8 2BZ Tel: 0117 923 9041 — MB ChB Manch. 1990 (Manchester) FRCS (Ed); FRCS (Eng); BSc (Hons.) Physiol. Manch. 1990, MB ChB (Hons.) 1993. Specialist Regist. Orthop., Bristol. Specialty: Orthop.

ROBINSON, Derek Keith Queens Park Surgery, 146 Drove Road, Swindon SN1 3AS — MB BS Newc. 1989; DRCOG 1992; MRCGP 1994.

ROBINSON, Derek Shillito (retired) Walnut Tree Cottage, Evenlode, Moreton-in-Marsh GL56 0NP — MB BS Lond. 1952 (Guy's) MRCS Eng. LRCP Lond. 1952. Prev: Ho. Surg., Ho. Phys. & Cas. Off. Cheltenham Gen. Hosp.

ROBINSON, Diane Elizabeth 26 Harwood Court, Trimdon Grange, Trimdon Station TS29 6HU — MB BS Newc. 1996. Paediat. Specialty: Gen. Pract. Prev: O & G; Psychiat.; GP.

ROBINSON, Diane Patricia Mourneside Medical Centre, 1A Ballycolman Avenue, Strabane BT82 9AF Tel: 028 7138 3737 Fax: 028 7138 3979; 12 Edgewater, New Buildings, Londonderry BT47 2TE — MB BCh BAO Belf. 1983; DRCOG 1986; MRCGP 1987.

ROBINSON, Douglas Keith (retired) 78 Grafton Way, London W1T 6JF — MB BChir Camb. 1954 (Lond. Hosp.) MA, MB Camb. 1954, BChir 1953; DCH Eng. 1957. Prev: Assoc. Specialist Jas. Pringle Ho. Middlx. Hosp. Lond.

***ROBINSON, Elizabeth** Church End, Church Lane, Wylye, Warminster BA12 0QZ — MB BS Lond. 2002. Ho. Off. (Surg.) Chelsea & Westm. Hosp. Lond.

ROBINSON, Elizabeth Angela Eleanor National Blood Authority, Oak House, Reeds Crescent, Watford WD24 4QN Tel: 01923 486820 Fax: 01923 486801; Low Brandon Farm, Brandon Crescent, Shadwell, Leeds LS17 9JH — (St. Mary's) MB BS Lond. 1967; MRCS Eng. LRCP Lond. 1967; FRCPath 1986, M 1973. Med. Dir. Specialty: Haematology; Blood Transfus. Socs: Founder Mem. Brit. Blood Transfus. Soc.; UK Director Europ. Soc. Haemapheresis. - Founder Mem.; Mem. of ISBT. Prev: Chief Exec. Yorks Regional Transfus. Centre Leeds.; Hon. Sen. Clin. Lect. Dept. Med. Leeds Gen. Infirm. & St. Jas. Univ. Hosp.

ROBINSON, Elizabeth Anne (retired) Tanners Pool, Alkerton, Banbury OX15 6NL — (St. Geo.) LMSSA Lond. 1957. Assoc. Specialist Horton Gen. Hosp. Banbury. Prev: Assoc.Specialist Horton Gen.Hosp.Banbury.

ROBINSON, Elizabeth Mary O'Keefe (retired) 14 Queens Park Rise, Brighton BN2 9ZF Tel: 01273 609971 Fax: 01273 609971 — MB BS Lond. 1964 (St. Mary's) DObst RCOG 1966. Prev: Sen. GP E. Grinstead.

ROBINSON, Emiko Terasaki Wolfson College, Linton Road, Oxford OX2 6UD — LRCP LRCS Ed. LRCPS Glas. 1995.

ROBINSON, Emma Kate East Sussex Brighton and Hove Health Authority, 36-38 Friars Walk, Lewes BN7 2PB Tel: 01273 485300 Fax: 01273 403600 — MB BS Lond. 1991 (Guy's (United Medical and Dental Schools)) MSc Lond. 1998. Sen. Resist. (Pub. Health Med.) E. Sussex Brighton & Hove HA. Specialty: Pub. Health Med. Socs: BMA; Train. Mem. Fac. Pub. Health Med.; Soc. Social Med.

ROBINSON, Ernest Thomson, OBE, TD (retired) 132 Prestonfield, Milngavie, Glasgow G62 7QA Tel: 0141 563 7409 — MB ChB Glas. 1959; DObst RCOG 1962; FRCGP 1977, M 1963. Chairm. (Counc.) St. And. Ambul. Assn. Prev: Maj. RAMC (TA) Regtl. Med. Off. 154 Regt. RCT (TA).

ROBINSON, Finlay McLean The Surgery, 4 Stoke Road, Bishops Cleeve, Cheltenham GL52 8RP Tel: 01242 672007 — MB ChB Dundee 1975; BSc (Med. Sci.) St. And. 1972; DRCOG 1977; DCH Eng. 1978; MRCGP 1982.

ROBINSON, Fiona Margaret 64 Eversden Road, Harlton, Cambridge CB3 7ET — MB ChB Glas. 1983; MRCOG 1990. Regist. (O & G) W. Scotl. Rotat. Scheme. Specialty: Obst. & Gyn.

ROBINSON, Fiona Osborne The Dell, 17 Lawrie Park Crescent, London SE26 6HH Fax: 020 7346 3738 — MB BCh BAO Belf. 1986; MRCP (UK) 1989; DO RCPSI 1991; FRCOphth 1992. Cons. (Ophth.) Kings Coll. Hosp. Lond. Specialty: Ophth. Prev: Fell. with Dr Serge Morax, Foundat. Rothschild, Paris; Fell. with Dr Alan McNab Melbourne, Australia; Fell. with Mr Richard Collin. Lond.

ROBINSON, Florence Lydia 6 Dillon Heights, Armagh BT61 9HF — MB BCh BAO Belf. 1959.

ROBINSON, Frances Eileen Occupational Health Centre, Purdysborn Hospital, Saintfield Road, Belfast BT8 8BH Tel: 01232 401333; 15 Newforge Lane, Belfast BT9 5NT — MB BCh BAO Belf. 1963 (Qu. Univ. Belf.) DCH RCPS Glas. 1965; DObst RCOG 1968; MRCGP 1972. Socs: BMA. Prev: Med. Off. Qu. Eliz. Hosp. Bridgetown Barbados, Cheltenham Gen.; esbyt. Mission Hosp. Chogoria, Kenya.

ROBINSON, Frances Lenore Josephine (retired) 13 Rosemary Park, Malone Road, Belfast BT9 Tel: 028 9066 8806 — MB BCh BAO Belf. 1947; DCH Eng. 1952; MD Belf. 1952. Prev: Cons. Phys. North. Irel. Fever Hosp.

ROBINSON, Frances Patricia 8 Georgian Villas, Omagh BT79 0AT — MD Belf. 1987; MB BCh BAO Belf. 1977; FFA RCSI 1981; Dip. Pall. Med 1997. Cons. Anaesth. with s/i in Pain Relief and Palliat. Med., Sperrin Lakeland Health & Social Care Trust. Specialty: Anaesth.; Palliat. Med. Prev: Cons. Anaesth. Tyrone Co. Hosp. Omagh.

ROBINSON, Gareth Mark 7 Buckhurst Road, Frimley Green, Camberley GU16 6LH Tel: 01252 836610 — MB BS Lond. 1993. Trainee GP Frimley Pk. Hosp. VTS.

ROBINSON, Garrett Joseph (retired) 2 Thornfield Grove, Sunderland SR2 7UZ Tel: 0191 567 4144 — (Univ. Coll. Dub.) MB BCh BAO NUI 1951.

ROBINSON, Geoffrey Brian c/o Lloyds TSB Bank plc, Lloyds Court, 28 Secklow Gate, Milton Keynes MK9 3EH; 5 Shouler Close, Shenley Church End, Milton Keynes MK5 6DZ Tel: 01908 505289 Fax: 0870 056 6397 — MB BCh BAO Dub. 1961; MA Dub. 1962; DPM Eng. 1967; DClinHyp (Distinc.) Univ. Lond. 1994. Specialty: Gen. Psychiat. Socs: Brit. Soc. Experim. & Clin. Hypn.

ROBINSON, Geoffrey John Lake Road Health Centre, Nutfield Place, Portsmouth PO1 4JT Tel: 023 9282 1201 Fax: 023 9287 5658; 19 Montgomery Road, Havant PO9 2RH Tel: 023 92 471212 Email: geoff.robinson@btinternet.com — BM (Distinc. Clin. Med.) Soton. 1979; DCH Eng. 1981; DRCOG 1981; MRCGP (Distinc.) 1983; DFFP 1996. GP Trainer Portsmouth; Non-Exec. Dir. Portsmouth HA.

ROBINSON, Gillian Ada 27 Frondeg, Llandegfan, Menai Bridge LL59 5TN — BM Soton. 1978; DO RCS Eng. 1983; FRCS Ed. 1985.

ROBINSON, Gillian Elizabeth Flat 7, The Nightingales, 23 Nightingale Lane, London SW12 8TN — MB BS Lond. 1980.

ROBINSON, Gillian Mary 22 The Mall, London N14 6LN — MB BS Lond. 1990.

ROBINSON, Gordon 69 Swanland Road, Hessle HU13 0NN Tel: 01482 648721 — MB ChB Leeds 1954. Socs: BMA. Prev: Surg. Lt. RNVR; Resid. Obst. Off. Staincliffe Gen. Hosp. Dewsbury; Cas. Off. Roy. Infirm. Bradford.

ROBINSON, Graham Robert Edward Oakhurst, 146 Barnham Road, Barnham, Bognor Regis PO22 0EH Tel: 01243 553259 — MB BS Lond. 1996; MRCP Part 1 1999. SHO (p/t) (Med.) Worthing Hosp. W. Sussex; Specialist Regist., Radiol., St. Geo. Hosp. Lond. Specialty: Radiol. Socs: Roy. Soc. Med. Prev: Ho. Phys. Worthing Hosp.; Ho. Surg. Roy. Sussex Co. Hosp. Brighton; SHO,(Geriat., St Geo.'s Hosp.).

ROBINSON, Grant Trafford Michael Nevill Hall Hospital, Department of Pathology, Brecon Road, Abergavenny NP7 6AL Tel: 01873 732253 Email: grant.robinson2@gwent.wales.nhs.uk — MB BS Lond. 1986; BSc (Hons.) Lond. 1983, MB BS 1986; MRCP (UK) 1989; MRCPath 1997; FRCP 2003. Cons. Haematologist & Path. Chief of Staff Gwent Healthcare NHS Trust; Hon. Cons. Haematologist Univ. Hosp. Of Wales Cardiff. Specialty: Haematology. Special Interest: Myeloproliferative Dis. Socs: Roy. Coll. of Pathologists; Roy. Coll. of Physicians; Brit. Soc. For Haemat. Prev: Regist. (Haemat.) St. Geo. Hosp. Lond.

ROBINSON, Gwyneth Jean 592A Dorchester Road, Broad Wey, Weymouth DT3 5LL Tel: 0130 581 4833 — MB ChB Glas. 1955.

ROBINSON, Hazel Alice 29 High Street, Toller Porcorum, Dorchester DT2 0DN Tel: 01300 320961 — MB ChB Bristol 1994 (Univ. Bristol) SHO (O & G) Poole Gen. Hosp. Specialty: Obst. & Gyn. Prev: SHO (c/o Elderly & A & E) Poole Gen. Hosp.; Ho. Surg. (Urol.) Derriford Hosp. Plymouth; Ho. Off. (Med.) Torbay Hosp.

ROBINSON, Heather Elizabeth — MB BS Newc. 1998.

ROBINSON, Heather Yvonne 22 Bonython Road, Newquay TR7 3AN — MB ChB Aberd. 1989. Regist. (Psychiat.) Torbay Hosp. Specialty: Gen. Psychiat. Socs: BMA & Roy. Coll. Psychiat. Prev: SHO (Psychiat.) Torbay Hosp.; Ho. Off. (Med.) W. Cornw. Hosp.

ROBINSON, Helen Judith Department of Community Paediatrics, St. John's Hospital at Howden, Howden Road W., Livingston EH54 6PP Tel: 01506 419666; 167 Craiglea Drive, Edinburgh EH10 5PT Tel: 0131 447 1884 — MB BS Lond. 1974 (Roy. Free) MRCS Eng. LRCP Lond. 1974; DCH RCPS Glas. 1977; MRCGP 1980. Staff Grade Paediat. (Community Child Health) St. Johns. Hosp. Howden. Socs: BMA; SACCH; Wom. Med. Federat. Prev: GP Edin. & Livingston; SHO (O & G) Bangour Gen. Hosp. Broxburn.

ROBINSON, Hillary Ina (retired) The Old Rectory, Edmundbyers, Consett DH8 9NQ Tel: 01207 255634 — MRCS Eng. LRCP Lond. 1965 (King's Coll. Hosp.) FRCS Eng. 1974. Hon. Lect. Univ. Zambia Med. Sch.; Chairm. WOC (UK). Prev: Cons.Orthop. Surg. Shotley Bridge Gen. Hosp. Cons.

ROBINSON, Holly 10 Toberdowney Valley, Ballynure, Ballyclare BT39 9TS — MB BCh BAO Belf. 1996.

ROBINSON, Hugh Malcolm (retired) 14 Meads Road, Seaford BN25 1SY Tel: 01323 893157 — MRCS Eng. LRCP Lond. 1943 (Middlx.) Prev: Flight Lt. RAF Med. Br.

ROBINSON, Ian Clive Broom Leys Surgery, Broom Leys Road, Coalville LE67 4DE Tel: 01530 832095; Bay Tree House, 134 The Moor, Coleorton, Coalville LE67 8GF Tel: 01530 835170 Fax: 01530 835170 — MB BS Lond. 1978 (Univ. Coll. Hosp.) BSc Lond. 1975; DRCOG 1982; Cert. Family Plann. JCC 1982. Clin. Asst. (Clin. Genetics) Leicester Roy. Infirm.; PCG Bd. Mem. NW Leics. PCG (Finance Commissioning Lead). Specialty: Genetics. Prev: Trainee GP Leics. VTS; Ho. Phys. Roy. United Hosp. Bath; Ho. Surg. Frimley Pk. Hosp. Frimley.

ROBINSON, Ian Hardy, VRD (retired) Sherwood, 26 Fitzroy Road, Fleet, Aldershot GU51 4JJ Tel: 01252 613897 — (St. Mary's) MB BChir Camb. 1951; DObst RCOG 1956; DA Eng. 1969; FFA RCS Eng. 1971. Prev: Cons. Anaesth. Frimley Pk. Hosp.

ROBINSON, Ian Henry Warnock 59 Ballymena Road, Ballymoney BT53 7EZ — MB ChB Ed. 1998; MB ChB Ed 1998.

ROBINSON, Ian Stuart Occupational Health Unit, Force Headquarters, Northumbria Police, Ponteland, Newcastle upon Tyne NE20 0BL Tel: 01661 868865 Fax: 01661 868818; The Old Dairy, Rothley Mill, Hartburn, Morpeth NE61 4ED Tel: 01670 774298 — MB ChB Sheff. 1972; DObst RCOG 1974; AFOM 1999; D Occ med 1999. Sen. Occupat. Health Phys. Northumbria Police Force Ponteland; Princip. Med. Dir. Police Nat. Diving Sch.; Hon. Cons. S. Tyneside Dist. Gen. Hosp. Specialty: Occupat. Health. Socs: Brit. Med. Acupunct. Soc.; Assn. Local Auth. Med. Advisers; Soc. Occupat. Med. Prev: GP Sheff.; Med. Dir. Cavendish Centre.

ROBINSON, Innes (retired) Cappelle, Wereton Road, Audley, Stoke-on-Trent ST7 8EN Tel: 01782 720589 — MB ChB Birm. 1949. Prev: Ho. Phys. N. Staffs. Roy. Infirm. Stoke-on-Trent.

ROBINSON, Ira Ellen 12 Stevenage Road, London SW6 6ES — MB BS Lond. 1991.

ROBINSON, Ivan Alexandre Department of Histopathology, Derbyshire Royal Infirmary, Derby Tel: 01332 347141; 44 St. Bernard's Road, Solihull B92 8NY Tel: 0121 743 7325 Email: dr.robinson@btinternet.com — MB BCh BAO NUI 1985; LRCPSI 1985; MRCPI 1988; MRCPath 1993. Cons. Histopath. Derbysh. Roy. Infirm. Specialty: Histopath. Socs: Path. Soc.; Assn. Clin. Paths.; Brit. Soc. for Oral and Maxillofacial Path. Prev: Sen. Regist. (Histopath. & Cytopath.) St. Geo. Hosp. Lond. & Roy. Surrey Co. Hosp. Guildford.

ROBINSON, Ivor Frantisek St Johns Way Medical Centre, 96 St. Johns Way, London N19 3RN Tel: 020 7272 1585 Fax: 020 7561 1237; 1 The Chine, London N10 3PX Tel: 020 8883 8165 Email: ivorrobinson@hotmail.com — MB ChB Birm. 1970; DObst RCOG 1972; Cert FPA 1972. Med. Off. Highgate Sch. Lond.; Chairm. CAMIDOC Lond. Specialty: Gen. Pract. Socs: Med. Assn. Victims of Torture; BMA. Prev: Hon. Clin. Asst. Whittington Hosp.; Occupat. Health Med. Adviser Performing Righ Soc. Lond. & Whittington Hosp. Lond.; Staff Health Off. St. Mary's Hosp. Lond.

ROBINSON, James (retired) 11 Goose Cote Hill, Egerton, Bolton BL7 9UQ Tel: 01204 307294 — (Manch.) MB ChB Manch. 1950; MRCGP 1958. Prev: GP. Bolton.

ROBINSON, James 7 Squirrel Walk, Acresford Road, Overseal, Swadlincote DE12 6NL — MB ChB Ed. 1967.

ROBINSON, James Andrew 116 Lancaster Road, Salford M6 8AW — BM BCh Oxf. 1989.

ROBINSON, James Edward 7 Dawlish Avenue, Chadderton, Oldham OL9 0RF — MB ChB Manch. 1996.

ROBINSON, Jana Ordsall Health Centre, Regent Park Surgery, Belfort Drive, Salford M5 3PP Tel: 0161 872 2021 Fax: 0161 877 3592; 3A Bowgreen Road, Bowdon, Altrincham WA14 3LX — MRCS Eng. LRCP Lond. 1971 (Lond. Hosp.) Prev: Regist. (Paediat.) Whipps Cross Hosp. Lond.; SHO Qu. Eliz. Hosp. for Childr. Lond.; SHO Lond. Hosp.

ROBINSON, Jane Elizabeth Rebecca 27 Bainbrigge Road, Leeds LS6 3AD Tel: 0113 2740 666 — MB ChB Leeds 1995. SHO Psychiat. High Royds Hosp. Meston, Nr. Ire. Specialty: Gen. Psychiat. Socs: MPS; MMS; BMA. Prev: SHO (Psychiat.), St. James Hosp, Leeds; SHO (Oncol.) Cookridge Hosp, Leeds; SHO (A&E) Ponte Fralt, Gen. Infirm., Ponte Fralt.

ROBINSON, Jane Freya Dr Dickson & Partners, 7/8 Park St., Ripon HG4 2AX — MB ChB Leeds 1982; DRCOG 1985; MRCGP 1986; DCH RCP Lond. 1986. Retainee GP, Ripon. Specialty: Community Child Health. Prev: Clin. Med. Off. Hull HA; GP Princip., Montague Med. Centre, Goole.

ROBINSON, Janet Frances Cheslyn Cornergates, Repton, Derby DE65 6GG — MB BChir Camb. 1949 (Camb. & Roy. Free) MA, MB BChir Camb. 1949.

ROBINSON, Jean Grace Department of Child & Family Psychiatry, Royal Aberdeen Childrens Hospital, Aberdeen AB25 2ZG Tel: 01224 552706 Email: jean.robinson@arh.grampian.scot.nhs.uk; South Leylodge Farmhouse, Leylodge, Kintore, Inverurie AB51 0XY — (Aberdeen) MB ChB Aberd. 1977; MRCPsych 1982. Cons. Child & Adolesc. Psychiat. Roy. Aberd. Childr.'s Hosp. Specialty: Child & Adolesc. Psychiat.

ROBINSON, Jill Alexandra Tryst Medical Centre, 431 King St., Stenhousemuir, Larbert FK5 4HT Tel: 01324 551555; 9 Greenhorn's Well, Well Avenue, Falkirk FK1 5HL Tel: 01324 36092 — MB ChB Ed. 1986; DRCOG 1988; MRCGP 1990. Long term Locum GP StenHo.muir; Clin. Asst. Roy. Scott. Nat. Hosp. For Ment. Handicap. Prev: Partner GP Pract. Stirling; Trainee GP Tryst Med. Centre Larbert; Trainee GP/SHO (Psychiat.) Bellsdyke Hosp. Larbert VTS.

ROBINSON, Joan Florence Haringey Health Care Trust, St. Ann's Hospital, St Ann's Road, London N15; New River Health Authority, Public Health Department, Alexander Place, Lower Park Road, London N11 — MB BS Lond. 1959; DCH Eng. 1962; DPH Eng. 1963; MFPHM 1972. Sen. Med. Off. Haringey Health Care Trust & New River HA. Specialty: Pub. Health Med. Socs: Assoc. Mem. BPA; Harv. Soc. Prev: Sen. Med. Off. Lond. Boro. Haringey.

ROBINSON, Joanna Patricia Jane Barnes Close Surgery, Barnes Close, Sturminster Newton DT10 1BN Tel: 01258 474500 Fax: 01258 471547 Email: joanna.robinson@gp-J81620.nhs.uk — MB BS Lond. 1983 (Char. Cross) Cert. Family Plann. JCC 1986; DRCOG 1986; DCH RCP Lond. 1987; MRCGP 1987; DFFP 1993. GP Sturminster Newton Barnes Cl. Surg. Prev: Trainee GP Eastbourne VTS; SHO (Gen. Med.) St. Mary's Hosp. Eastbourne; SHO (O & G, Paediat. & A & E) Eastbourne Dist. Gen. Hosp.

ROBINSON, John Charles Newbury Street Practice, Wantage Health Centre, Mably Way, Wantage OX12 9BN Tel: 01235 763451 Email: john.robinson@nhs.net — MB ChB Bristol 1977; DA Eng. 1979; DRCOG 1980; MRCGP 1982. Specialty: Gen. Pract. Prev: GP; Med. Cons. to AAH Meditel; SHO (Anaesth.) Roy. United Hosp. Bath.

ROBINSON, John Easton (retired) Padeswood Lodge, Padeswood, Mold CH7 4JF Tel: 01244 546420 — MB BChir 1957 (Guy's) MA Camb. 1958; DA Eng. 1961; FFA RCS Eng. 1964. Prev: Cons. Anaesth.Chester Dist. Hosp.

ROBINSON, John Franklin (retired) 7 Farrant House, Winstanley Estate, Winstanley Road, London SW11 2ES Tel: 020 8741 0238; 41 Castelnau Mansions, Barnes Castelnau, London SW13 9QU — MB BCh Witwatersrand 1943. Med. Advis. Hamblin Film & Video (Med. & Scientif.); Script Writer & Edr. Adviser Med. Computer Animation Magic Touch Videographics Lond. Prev: Med. Dir. Med. Ltd. (Med. & Sci. Films) Lincoln.

ROBINSON, John Graham Meadowcroft Surgery, Jackson Road, Aylesbury HP19 9EX Tel: 01296 425775 Fax: 01296 330324 — MB BS Lond. 1977 (Royal London Hospital) BSc Lond. 1970; DRCOG 1980; MRCGP 1981. Specialty: Gen. Pract.

ROBINSON, John Richard (retired) 480 Banbury Road, Oxford OX2 8EN Tel: 01865 57128 — (St. Thos.) MB BS Lond. 1954; DPM Eng. 1964; FRCPsych. 1982, M 1972. Hon. Cons. Psychiat.. Oxf. Ment. Health care NHS Trust. Prev: Nuffield Research Fell. Psychiat. Littlemore Hosp. Oxf.

ROBINSON, John Stanley 49 Mavis Drive, Wirral CH49 0UN — MB ChB Liverp. 1981.

ROBINSON, Professor John Stanley 43 Goodby Road, Moseley, Birmingham B13 8RH Tel: 0121 449 8370 Fax: 0121 449 2828 — MB ChB Liverp. 1953; DA Eng. 1957; FFA RCS Eng. 1958; MD Liverp. 1960. Emerit. Prof. Univ. Birm.; Hon. Cons. Anaesth. W. Midl. RHA; Non.-Exec. Dir. W. Midl. Ambul. Serv. Trust. Specialty: Anaesth. Socs: Assn. Anaesth. Prev: Prof. Anaesth. Univ. Birm.; Cons. Anaesth. Liverp. RHB; Demonst. (Anaesth.) Univ. Liverp.

ROBINSON, Jonathan Mark 2 Shangarry Park, Belfast BT14 8JD — MB BCh BAO Belf. 1988; MRCP (UK) 1991.

ROBINSON, Miss Joy 3 Greenhead Park, Bamford, Hope Valley S33 0AS — MB ChB Sheff. 1992; FRCS Lond. 1997. Surg. Research Assoc. Univ. of Sheff. Specialty: Gen. Surg. Socs: BMA; MDU.

ROBINSON, Joyce Mawgan (retired) South Lodge, Great Bardfield, Braintree CM7 4SD Tel: 01371 810511 Fax: 01371 811428 Email: joyce.antcliffe@btinternet — (King's Coll. Hosp.) MB BS Lond. 1961; MRCS Eng. LRCP Lond. 1961. Prev: Ho. Surg. & Ho. Phys. Dulwich Hosp.

ROBINSON, Karen Anne Medical Centre, Easthope Road, Church Stretton SY6 6BL Tel: 01694 722127; Lymehurst, Longhills Road, Church Stretton SY6 6DS — MB ChB Bristol 1979; DRCOG 1982; MRCGP 1984. GP Trainer. Specialty: Gen. Pract.

ROBINSON, Karen Anne 36 South Esk Road, London E7 8EY — MB BS Lond. 1996.

ROBINSON, Karen Elizabeth 176 Main Street, High Blantyre, Blantyre, Glasgow G72 0ER — MB ChB Glas. 1991. Specialty: Anaesth.

ROBINSON, Katharine Jane 101 Wood Vale, London N10 3DL — MB BS Lond. 1996.

ROBINSON, Katharine Natasha General Hospital, Cliftonville, Northampton NN1 5BD Tel: 01604 634700 Email: natasha.robinson@ngh.nhs.uk — MB BS Lond. 1978 (St. Thos.) BA Oxf. 1975; MRCP (UK) 1980; FRCA Eng. 1983. Cons. Anaesth. Northampton Gen. Hosp. Specialty: Anaesth. Prev: Cons. Anaesth. Brook Hosp. Lond.; Sen. Regist. (Anaesth.) Brompton Hosp. Nat. Hosp. for Neurol. Lond. & Roy. Free Hosp.; Regist. Nuffield Dept. Anaesth. Oxf.

ROBINSON, Katherine Anne 110 North Parade, Ormeau Road, Belfast BT7 — MB BCh BAO Belf. 1990.

ROBINSON, Kathryn Margaret Liverpool House Surgery, 69 Risedale Road, Barrow-in-Furness LA13 9QY Tel: 01229 832232

Fax: 01229 432156 — MB ChB Dundee 1989; MRCGP 1994. Socs: Brit. Assn. Med. Acupunct.s.

ROBINSON, Keith Douglas (retired) Stoneleigh, 55 Ashwell Road, Heaton, Bradford BD9 4AX Tel: 01274 828994 — MB ChB Ed. 1958; DObst RCOG 1960; MRCGP 1969. Prev: Med. Adviser Allied Colloids plc. Bradford.

ROBINSON, Kenneth Francis (retired) Cornergates, The Pastures, Repton, Derby DE65 6GG Tel: 01283 702183 — MRCS Eng. LRCP Lond. 1950 (Guy's & Camb.) MA, MB BChir Camb. 1950; DObst RCOG 1954. Prev: GP Derbys.

ROBINSON, Kenneth Roger Health Centre, Newgate Street, Worksop S80 1HP Tel: 01909 500266 Fax: 01909 478014; Woodhurst, Sparken Hill, Worksop S80 1AX — MI NUI 1983; DRCOG 1985.

ROBINSON, Kerry Abigail 63 Queens Crescent, Chalk Farm, London NW5 4ES — MB BS Lond. 1997; MRCPCH 2002.

ROBINSON, Mr Kingsley Peter 75 Robin Hood Lane, Kingston Vale, London SW15 3QR — MRCS Eng. LRCP Lond. 1955 (Westm.) MS Lond. 1964, MB BS 1955; FRCS Ed. 1959; FRCS Eng. 1959. Project Advis. (Osseointegration) Rehabil. Centre Roehampton; Vis. Prof. (Biomedical Engin. Gp.) Univ. Surrey. Specialty: Gen. Surg. Socs: Fell. Roy. Soc. Med.; Vasc. Surg. Soc. Gt. Brit. & Irel. Prev: Sen. Lect. (Surg.) Westm. Hosp. Lond.; Cons. Surg. Westm. Hosp. Lond. & Qu. Mary's Hosp. Roehampton.

ROBINSON, Mr Lee Quenby 88 Barnston Road, Wirral CH60 1UB Tel: 0151 342 2390 — MB ChB Liverp. 1978; FRCS Eng. 1984; ChM Liverp. 1990; FRCS (Urol) 1992. Cons. Urol N. Chesh. Hosps. Specialty: Urol. Prev: Cons. Urol. Warrington Hosp. NHS Trust.

ROBINSON, Lili Ostberg Radiology Department, Leicester Royal Infirmary, Infirmary Square, Leicester LE1 5WW Tel: 0116 254 1414; 8 Outwoods Road, Loughborough LE11 3LY — MB ChB Leeds 1975; DA Eng. 1977; FRCR 1982. Cons. Radiol. Leicester Roy. Infirm. NHS Trust. Specialty: Radiol. Prev: Cons. Radiol. Qu. Mary's Hosp. Sidcup; Sen. Regist. & Regist. (Radiol.) St. Geo. Hosp. Lond.

ROBINSON, Linda Joy 275 Moor Road, Chorley PR7 2NN — MB ChB Leeds 1994.

ROBINSON, Louise Ann Saville Medical Group, 7 Saville Place, Newcastle upon Tyne NE1 8DQ Tel: 0191 232 4274 Fax: 0191 233 1050; 8 Westfield Avenue, Gosforth, Newcastle upon Tyne NE3 4YH Tel: 0191 285 4793 — MB BS Newc. 1985; DCH Lond. 1988; MRCGP 1989. Sen. Lect. (Primary Health Care) Univ. Newc. Prev: GP Sunderland.

ROBINSON, Louise Helen — MB BS Lond. 1985; FCAnaesth 1990. Staff Grade Doctor (Anaesth.) Torbay HA. Specialty: Anaesth. Prev: SHO (A & E) Poole Gen. Hosp.; SHO (Geriat.) Mt. Gould Hosp. Plymouth; Ho. Surg. Roy. Vict. Hosp. Boscombe.

ROBINSON, Madeleine Christina (retired) Rose Cottage, Sunbank Lane, Ringway, Altrincham WA15 0PZ Tel: 0161 980 3087 — MB ChB Ed. 1974; DRCOG 1981.

ROBINSON, Magda 12 Hayfield Road, Oxford OX2 6TT — BM (Hons.) Soton. 1993; DFFP 1994. Sessional Med. Off. (Family Plann.) Brook Advis. Serv. Lond. Specialty: Family Plann. & Reproduc. Health.

ROBINSON, Margaret Osborne Practice Surgery, 25 Osborne Road, Southsea PO5 3ND Tel: 023 9282 1371; 11 Great Southsea Street, Southsea PO5 3BY Fax: 01705 738587 — BM Soton. 1982 (Southampton) MRCGP 1988. SHO (Med. Rotat.) Qu. Alexandra's Hosp. Portsmouth. Specialty: Gen. Pract. Socs: Soc. Med.; Med. & Dent. Hypn. Soc. Metrop. Br.; Med. & Scientif. Network Gp.

ROBINSON, Margaret Denise 210 Whitchurch Road, Cardiff CF14 3NB Tel: 029 2062 1282; 9 Cefn Coed Gardens, Cyncoed, Cardiff CF23 6AX — MB BCh Wales 1979; BSc (Hons.) (Physiol.) Wales 1974, MB BCh 1979; DRCOG 1982.

ROBINSON, Margaret Mary (retired) Swn-y-Fenai, Bryn Ffynon Road, Port Dinorwic LL56 4SJ Tel: 01248 670389 — (Dundee) MB ChB St. And. 1939; BA (Hons.) Wales 1969. Clin. Med. Off. Gwynedd HA. Prev: Clin. Asst. (Geriat. Med.) Gwynedd AHA.

ROBINSON, Margaret Reynolds (retired) 4 Higham Lane, Tonbridge TN10 4JA — MB BS Lond. 1955 (St. Bart.) DObst RCOG 1956; DA Eng. 1961. Prev: Regist. (Anaesth.) & Sen. Ho. Off. (Anaesth. & O & G) St.

ROBINSON, Margaret Valerie Crosby House Surgery, 91 Stoke Poges Lane, Slough SL1 3NY Tel: 01753 520680 Fax: 01753 552780; 8 Ketcher Green, Binfield, Bracknell RG42 5TA — MB ChB Liverp. 1977; DRCOG 1979; MRCPsych 1982. Prev: Regist. (Psychiat.) Liverp. HA (T); Clin. Med. Off. (Psychiat.) Sefton HA.

ROBINSON, Mark Jeremy Charles 96 Poole Crescent, Birmingham B17 0PB — MB ChB Birm. 1996; ChB Birm. 1996.

ROBINSON, Marlene Jane (retired) Lime Cottage, Downside Bridge Road, Cobham KT11 3EJ Tel: 01932 862984 Fax: 01932 865328 — MB BS Lond. 1957 (St. Geo.) MRCS Eng. LRCP Lond. 1957. Prev: Clin. Asst. Dept. Ultrasound St. Luke's Hosp. Guildford.

ROBINSON, Martin Hurst Clinical Oncology, Weston Park Hospital, Whitham Road, Sheffield S10 2SJ Tel: 0114 226 5000 Fax: 0114 226 5511 Email: m.h.robinson@sheffield.ac.uk; Riplingham, Sheffield Road, Hathersage, Hope Valley S32 1DA — MB BChir Camb. 1978; MRCP (UK) 1980; MA Camb. 1983; FRCR 1986; MD Camb. 1993; FRCP 1997. Sen. lect. (Clin. Oncol.) Weston Pk. Hosp. Sheff. Specialty: Oncol.; Radiother. Socs: BOA (Hon. Sec.). Prev: Sen. Regist. (Radiother.) Roy. Marsden Hosp. Lond.; Regist. (Radiother.) Churchill Hosp. Oxf.

ROBINSON, Martyn Gerald Woodland Road Surgery, 20 Woodland Road, St Austell PL25 4QY Tel: 01726 63311; The Oak, Porthpean Road, St Austell PL25 5DG Tel: 01726 65774 — MB BS Lond. 1981; DRCOG 1981.

ROBINSON, Maryanne 10 McPherson Drive, Gourock PA19 1LJ — MB ChB Glas. 1984; DRCOG 1986.

ROBINSON, Mr Maurice Patrick 35 Rope Lane, Wells Green, Crewe CW2 6RB Tel: 01270 67237 — MB BS Lond. 1952 (Middlx.) FRCS Eng. 1958. Specialty: Orthop. Socs: Brit. Orthop. Assn. Prev: Cons. Surg. Orthop. Robt. Jones & Agnes Hunt Orthop. Hosp. & Leighton Hosp. Crewe; Sen. Regist. Middlx. Hosp. Lond.

ROBINSON, Maurice William (retired) 91 Heathermount Drive, Crowthorne RG45 6HJ Tel: 01344 774862 Fax: 01344 774862 Email: mauricewr@bigfoot.com — MB ChB Sheff. 1960 (Sheffield) DObst RCOG 1962; MRCGP 1971. Prev: GP Bracknell.

ROBINSON, Melvyn 6A Twitch Hill, Horbury, Wakefield WF4 6NA — MB ChB Liverp. 1979.

ROBINSON, Mr Melvyn Roland Griffiths (retired) The General Infirmary, Friarwood Lane, Pontefract WF8 1PL Tel: 01977 606716; 25 Went Hill Close, Ackworth, Pontefract WF7 7LP Tel: 01977 702196 — MB BS Lond. 1957 (Char. Cross) MRCS Eng. LRCP Lond. 1957; DObst RCOG 1959; FRCS Ed. 1967; FRCS Eng. 1968. Hon. Cons. Urol., Pontefract NHS Trust. Prev: Sen. Regist. & Research Fell. Inst. Urol. Lond.

ROBINSON, Michael 6 Sycamore Grove, Sandbach CW11 1PJ — MB ChB Liverp. 1986. Specialty: Gen. Pract.

ROBINSON, Michael Barney Nuffield Institute University of Leeds, 75-79 Clarendon Road, Leeds LS2 9PL Tel: 0113 245 9034 — MB BS Lond. 1982; MA Camb. 1979; MRCP (UK) 1985; MRCGP 1986; DCH RCP Lond. 1987; DRCOG 1989; MSc Lond. 1990; MFPHM RCP (UK) 1991. Sen. Lect. (Pub. Health) & Hon. Cons. Pub. Health Med. Leeds HA. Specialty: Gen. Med. Prev: Lect. (Pub. Health Med.) Lond. Sch. Hyg. & Trop. Med.

ROBINSON, Michael David In Practice Systems Ltd., The Bread Factory, 1 Broughton Street, London SW8 3QJ Tel: 020 7501 7000 Fax: 020 7501 7100 Email: mike.robinson@inps.co.uk; 33 Upfield, Horley RH6 7JY Tel: 01293 783146 Email: mike.upfielddoc@btinternet.com — MB BS Lond. 1975 (St. Mary's) MRCS Eng. LRCP Lond. 1975. Med. Dir. In Pract. Systems Ltd. Specialty: Gen. Pract. Special Interest: Med. Informatics. Prev: Med. Dir. VAMP Health Lond.; GP Surrey.

ROBINSON, Michael Edward Family Practice, 75 Cardiff Road, Dinas Powys CF64 4JT Tel: 029 2051 5455 Fax: 029 2051 5177; 22 Millbrook Heights, Dingwall, Penarth CF64 4JJ Tel: 01222 512535 — MB BCh Wales 1970. Chairm. Vale LHG. Prev: Research Regist. MRC Pneumoconiosis Unit Dept. Child Health, Llandough Hosp. Penarth.

ROBINSON, Mr Michael Harold Edward University Hospital, Queens Medical Centre, Nottingham NG5 2UH Tel: 0115 924 9924; Crodock Cottage, 74 Brook St, Wynsehold, Loughborough LE12 6TH — BM BCh Oxf. 1983; MA Camb. 1984; FRCS Eng. 1988; DM Nottm. 1996. Cons. Gen. Surg. Qu.. Med. Centre Nottm. Specialty: Gen. Surg. Socs: Assoc. of ColoProctol.; Brit.Med.Assoc. Prev: Lect. & Regist. Qu. Med. Centre Nottm.; Regist. Roy. Hosp. Gloucester; Cons. Gen. Surg. City Hosp. NHS Trust, Notts.

ROBINSON, Mr Michael John 33c Thornhill Crescent, Islington, London N1; Greenburn Croft, Balfron Station, Glasgow G63 0QY — MB BS Lond. 1981; BA Camb. 1978; FRCS Ed. 1986. Regist. Inst. Neurol. Sci. South. Gen. Hosp. Glas. Specialty: Neurol.

ROBINSON, Michael Jonathan Hope Hospital, Newborn Department, Salford M6 8HD Tel: 0161 787 5273 Fax: 0161 787 5786 — BM BCh Oxf. 1968 (Univ. Coll. Hosp.) MA, BM BCh Oxf. 1968; MRCP (UK) 1972; FRCP 1986; FRCP CH 1998. Cons. Paediat. Hope Hosp. Salford & Roy. Manch. Childr. Hosp. Specialty: Paediat. Socs: Neonat. Soc.; BAPM. Prev: Sen. Regist. St. Thos. Hosp. Lond.; Vis. Lect. Hadassah Univ. Jerusalem; Regist. Hosp. Sick Childr. Gt. Ormond St. Lond.

ROBINSON, Michael Kefford 17 Herbrand Walk, Bexhill-on-Sea TN39 4TX — MB ChB Ed. 1952.

ROBINSON, Michael Lansdale University Department of Psychiatry, Royal Liverpool Hospital, Prescot St., Liverpool L7 8XP — MD Belf. 1984; MB BCh BAO Belf. 1970; MRCP (U.K.) 1972; MRCPsych 1976; MPsychMed Liverp. 1980. Sen. Lect. (Psychiat.) Univ. Liverp. Prev: Lect. Psychiat. Univ. Liverp.; Research Worker Inst. Psychiat. Lond.; Regist. (Psychiat.) Maudsley Hosp. Lond.

ROBINSON, Michael Sandwith Tamerton, Plum Orchard, Nether Compton, Sherborne DT9 4QA — MB BS Lond. 1985; MRCGP 1993.

ROBINSON, Neil Alexander Sinclair c/o Emerg. Dept., Soton. Gen. Hosp., Tremona Road, Southampton SO16 6YD Tel: 02380 794127 Email: poppabear@hotmail.com — MB BS Lond. 1991 (Lond. Hosp. Med. Coll.) MRCP (UK) 1995; DA (UK) 1996; FFAEM 1999. Cons. in Emerg. Med., Soton. Gen. Hosp. Specialty: Accid. & Emerg. Prev: Specialist Regist. (A & E Med.) Wessex.

ROBINSON, Neville Anthony Ynysangharad Surgery, 70 Ynysangharad Road, Pontypridd CF37 4DA Tel: 01443 480521 Fax: 01443 400260 — (Charing Cross) MB, BS London 1959; DObst RCOG 1961; LMCC Medical Council Canada 1972. GP. Specialty: Gen. Pract. Socs: BMA. Prev: Chief of Staff, Dartmouth Gen. Hosp., Dartmouth, Nova Scotia, Canada.

ROBINSON, Nicholas David Penrose The Jersey Practice, Heston Health Centre, Cranford Lane, Hounslow TW5 9ER Tel: 020 8321 3434 Fax: 020 8321 3440 — BM BCh Oxf. 1979; MA Oxf. 1979, BA 1976; MRCGP 1985. Research Fell. (Primary Care) Char. Cross & Westm. Med. Sch. Socs: Hon. Sec. Brit. Computer Soc. Health Informat. Specialist Gp.; Assoc. Mem. Brit. Computer Soc.

ROBINSON, Nicholas Mark Kuenzlen 129 Fentiman Road, London SW8 1JZ Tel: 020 7735 8641 — MB BChir Camb. 1987 (Cambridge University) MA, MB BChir Camb. 1987; MRCP (UK) 1990; MD 1996. Sen. Regist. Lond. Chest Hosp. Specialty: Cardiol. Prev: Regist. (Cardiol.) King's Coll. Hosp. Lond.; Regist. (Cardiol.) Roy. Sussex Co. Hosp. Brighton; SHO (Neurol.) Nat. Hosp. Nerv. Dis. Lond.

ROBINSON, Nigel Norton Medical Centre, Billingham Road, Norton, Stockton-on-Tees TS20 2UZ Tel: 01642 360111 Fax: 01642 558672 — MB ChB Liverp. 1984; MB ChB Liverp. l984; DGM RCP Lond. 1987; MRCGP 1988; DRCOG 1988; Dip. Pract. Dermat. Wales 1992. Prev: GP Ayrsh.; Trainee GP E. Cumbria VTS; Med. Off. RAF.

ROBINSON, Oliver Patrick Waring, RD (retired) Lime Cottage, Downside Bridge Road, Cobham KT11 3EJ Tel: 01932 862984 Fax: 01932 865328 — MB BS Lond. 1953 (St. Geo.) DTM & H Eng. 1962; Dip. Pharm. Med. RCP (UK) 1976; FFPM RCP (UK) 1989. Surg. Lt.-Cdr. RNR. Prev: Med. Dir. Smithkline Beecham Pharm.

ROBINSON, Patrick Savile William Harvey Hospital, Kennington Road, Willesborough, Ashford TN24 0LZ; Mount Charles House, 5 Mount Charles Walk, Union Road Bridge, Canterbury CT4 5JS — MB BChir Camb. 1971 (St Thos.) MA Camb. 1973; MRCP (U.K.) 1974; MSc (Nuclear Med.) Lond. 1979; FRCP (UK) 1990; FRACP 1993. Cons. (Nuclear Med.) East Kent Hospitals NHS Trust. Specialty: Nuclear Med. Socs: Hon. Sec. Brit. Nuclear Med. Soc.; Soc. of Nuclear Med.; Austral. & New Zealand Soc. of Nuclear Med. Prev: Cons. (Nuclear Med.) Brighton Healthcare NHS Trust; Cons. (Nuclear Med.) Roy. Perth Hosp. WA Australia.

ROBINSON, Paul Hackness Road Surgery, 19 Hackness Road, Scarborough YO12 5SD Tel: 01723 506706 — MB ChB Sheff. 1975; FFA RCS Eng. 1980; DRCOG 1982; Cert. Family Plann. JCC 1982. Hosp. Pract. (Anaesth.) ScarBoro. Hosp. Specialty: Anaesth. Prev: Regist. (Anaesth.) ScarBoro. Hosp.; Regist. (Anaesth.) Wellington Hosp. & Dunedin Hosp., NZ; SHO (Paediat.) Bradford Childr. Hosp.

ROBINSON, Paul Derek Guy's Hospital, Department of Oral & Maxillofacial Surgery, 23rd Floor Guy's Tower, London SE1 9RT Tel: 020 7955 4419 Fax: 020 7955 4165 Email: paul.robinson@kcl.ac.uk; 2 Orchard Gate, Esher KT10 8HY — MB BS Lond. 1981; BDS Lond. 1971; FDS RCS Eng. 1976; PhD Lond. 1992. Sen. Lect. & Cons. Oral and Maxillofacial Surg. GKT Dent. Inst. Lond. Specialty: Oral & Maxillofacial Surg. Special Interest: Bone Subsitute Materials; Dentofacial Deformity. Socs: BAOMS; BDA.

ROBINSON, Paul Frank The Croft & Tinshill Medical Practice, 8 Tinshill Lane, Leeds LS16 7AP Tel: 0113 267 3462 Fax: 0113 230 0402 — MB ChB Leeds 1988; DRCOG 1994; MRCGP 1995. Specialty: Diabetes. Prev: Trainee GP Bradford VTS.

ROBINSON, Paul Hyman Royal Free Hospital, Eating Disorders Service, Department of Psychiatry, Pond Street, London NW3 2QG Tel: 020 7830 2295 Fax: 020 7830 2876 Email: paul.robinson@royalfree.nhs.uk — MB BS Lond. 1974 (Univ. Coll. Hosp.) MRCP (UK) 1977; MD Lond. 1993; BSc Lond. 1971, MD 1994; FRCPsych 1982, M 1995. Cons.(Psychiat.) Roy. Free Hosp. Lond.; Hon. Sen. Lect. Roy. Free & Univ. Coll. Med. Sch. Specialty: Gen. Psychiat. Special Interest: Psychiat., Eating Disorders. Prev: Sen. Lect. (Psychol. Med.) Kings Coll. Hosp. Sch. Med. Lond.; Wellcome Lect. (Ment. Health) Inst. Psychiat. Lond.; Cons. (Psychiat.) Gordon Hosp. Lond.

ROBINSON, Paul Jeremy Merck, Sharp & Dohme Ltd., Hertford Road, Hoddesdon EN11 9BU Tel: 01992 467272 Fax: 01992 451066 Email: paul_robinson@merck.com — MB BS Lond. 1984 (Lond. Hosp.) FFPM 2005; MFPM 1994; Dip. Pharm. Med. 1994. Director of Clin. Research, MSD (UK), Hoddesdon.; Hon. Clin. Asst. (Cardiol.) Chase Farm Hosp. Enfield. Specialty: Pharmaceutical Medicine; Cardiol. Socs: Brit. Cardiac Soc.; Brit. Hypertens. Soc. Prev: Assoc. Dir. (Clin. Research) Chiltern Internat. Ltd. Stoke Poges; Research Phys. Romford Cardiovasc. Research; SHO Rotat. (Med.) Newham Gen. Hosp. Lond.

ROBINSON, Paul John The Surgery, Station Road, Snainton, Scarborough YO13 9AP Tel: 01723 859302 Fax: 01723 859036 Email: paul01@btconnect.com; Wayside, Pickering Road, Snainton, Scarborough YO13 9AF — MB BS Lond. 1978 (London Hospital) MA Camb. 1980; DRCOG 1983; MRCGP 1983; MMEd Dundee 1998. GP ScarBoro. Prev: Course Organiser ScarBoro. VTS; Trainee GP York VTS; Ho. Off. Lond. Hosp.

ROBINSON, Peter Charles Farnham Centre For Health, Hale Road, Farnham GU9 9QS Tel: 01252 723122 Fax: 01252 728302; The Limes, 57 The St, Tongham, Farnham GU10 1DD Tel: 01252 651415 Email: pcrcabel@ntlworld.com — MB BS Lond. 1981 (St. Geo.) DRCOG 1984. Hosp. Practitioner (Genitourin. Med.) Farnham Rd. Hosp. Guildford.; GP. Acorn Community Drug & Alcohol Team Guildford. Specialty: Genitourinary Medicine. Prev: SHO (Paediat.) Roy. Surrey Co. Hosp. Guildford; SHO (O & G) Frimley Pk. Hosp.; Ho. Phys. St. Geo. Hosp. Lond.

ROBINSON, Peter Hugh 16 Courthill, Bearsden, Glasgow G61 3SN — MB BCh BAO Belf. 1981; BSc Belf. 1978, MB BCh BAO 1981; MRCP (UK) 1984.

ROBINSON, Peter John (retired) 2 Riponway, Carlton Miniott, Thirsk YO7 4LR Tel: 01845 522019 — MB ChB Leeds 1957; DTM & H Eng. 1968; MRCGP 1974.

ROBINSON, Peter John (retired) Cliff House, Chyandour, Penzance TR18 3LQ — MB BCh BAO Dub. 1958.

ROBINSON, Peter Kenneth (retired) 14 St James Villas, Winchester SO23 9SN Email: peterk.robinson@virgin.net — MB BChir Camb. 1945 (Camb. & St. Bart.) MRCS Eng. LRCP Lond. 1944; FRCP Lond. 1965, M 1945; MA Camb. 1946, MD 1956. Prev: Cons. Neurol. Hants. AHA (T).

ROBINSON, Peter William Longton Health Centre, Liverpool Road, Longton, Preston PR4 5HA Tel: 01772 615429 Fax: 01772 611094; The Sandpipers, Marsh Lane, Longton, Preston PR4 5LA — MB ChB Manch. 1974 (Manchester) DRCOG 1977; MRCGP 1986; MICGP 1987. Trainer (Gen. Pract.) Preston. Specialty: Gen. Pract.

ROBINSON, Philip Chenellor Wing X-Ray, St James University Hospital, Leeds LS7 7TF Tel: 0113 206 4807 — MB BCh BAO Belf. 1991 (Queen's Belfast) MB (Hons) BCh BAO Belf. 1991; MRCP (UK)

1994; FRCR (UK) 1998. Cons. Muscul. Radiologist, Leeds Teachg. Hosps. Specialty: Radiol. Special Interest: Musculoshelltal including Sarcoma, Sports and Ankle Imaging. Socs: Sen. RCR.

ROBINSON, Mr Philip James Southmead Hospital, ENT Department, Westbury-on-Trym, Bristol BS10 5NB Tel: 0117 959 5161 Fax: 0117 959 5850 — MB ChB Bristol 1981; FRCS (Gen. Surg.) Eng. 1986; FRCS (Orl.) Eng. 1988. Cons. Adult & Paediatric Otolaryngolist, N. Bristol NHS Trust, Bristol; Speciality Director for Otolaryngol. head and neck Surg., N. Bristol Trust. Specialty: Otolaryngol. Socs: Brit. Assn. Otolaryngol., head and neck Surg.; British Cochlear Implant Group; Brit. Assn. fo Paediatric Otolaryngol. Prev: Vice Pres., Sect. of Otol., Roy. Soc. Of Med., 1996-98.

ROBINSON, Philip Joseph Andrew 371 Shadwell Lane, Leeds LS17 8AH Tel: 0113 266 0471 — MB BS Lond. 1966 (St. Mary's) MRCP Lond. 1969; DMRD Eng. 1973; FRCR 1975; FRCP Lond. 1989. Cons. Radiol. Leeds AHA (T). Specialty: Radiol.

ROBINSON, Philip Lawrence (retired) 38 Macdona Drive, West Kirby, Wirral CH48 3JD Tel: 0151 625 6843 — MB ChB Liverp. 1942; FRCP Lond. 1972, M 1948; MD Liverp. 1949. Prev: Cons. Phys. Clatterbridge Gen. Hosp. Bebington.

ROBINSON, Philip Norman Gordon Street Surgery, 72 Gordon Street, Burton-on-Trent DE14 2JA Tel: 01283 563175 Fax: 01283 500638; 133 Field Lane, Burton-on-Trent DE13 0NJ — MB ChB Birm. 1981; DRCOG 1985.

ROBINSON, Philip William Henry (retired) 203 Haven Road, Haverfordwest SA61 1DQ Tel: 01437 768672 — (Birm.) MB ChB Birm. 1947; MRCS Eng. LRCP Lond. 1947; DA Eng. 1952; FFA RCS Eng. 1956. Prev: Cons. Anaesth. Withybush Gen Hosp. HaverfordW.

ROBINSON, Quentin Lawrence Alleyne Holly Green, 9 Moorfield Road, Ben Rhydding, Ilkley LS29 8BL Email: bnq@tesco.net — MB ChB Ed. 1965; FFA RCS Eng. 1970. Cons. Anaesth. Wharfedale Gen. Hosp.; Cons. Anaesth. The Gen. Infirm. Leeds. Specialty: Anaesth. Socs: Intractable Pain Soc. Prev: Cons. Anaesth. Ahmadu Bello Hosp. Kaduna, Nigeria; Sen. Regist. Leeds Gen. Infirm.; Regist. (Anaesth.) Roy. Infirm. Edin.

ROBINSON, Rachael Marie The Surgery, 21 Stockwell Road, Knaresborough HG5 0JY Tel: 01423 867433/01423 869633 Email: rachael@coughsandsneezes.com — MB ChB Leeds 1990; DRCOG 1994; MRCGP 1997. GP Partner; GP Trainer, Dates GPEC. Specialty: Gen. Pract. Prev: SHO (Paediat.) LG1; SHO (Palliat. Med.) St Gemmas.

ROBINSON, Mr Ralph Eldon (retired) Thaxted Lodge, 12 Babraham Road, Cambridge CB2 2RA Tel: 01223 248629 Fax: 01223 248629 — (St. Mary's) MB BS (Hons. Surg., Obst. & Gyn.) Lond. 1960; MRCS Eng. LRCP Lond. (Begley Prize in Surg.) 1960; FRCS Eng. 1964; FRCOG 1980, M 1968. Assoc. Lect. Univ. Camb. Prev: Cons. O & G Addenbrooke's Hosp. Camb. & NW Thames RHA.

ROBINSON, Ralph Henry (retired) 4 Grove Park, Bishop's Stortford CM23 2BX Tel: 01279 654612 — (Guy's) MB BS Lond. 1956; MRCS Eng. LRCP Lond. 1956; DA Eng. 1958; DTM & H Eng. 1962; FFA RCS Eng. 1963. Cons. Anaesth. Prev: Cons. (Anaesth.) E. Herts. NHS Trust.

ROBINSON, Richard Conrad Oliver and Partners, The Guildhall Surgery, Lower Baxter Street, Bury St Edmunds IP33 1ET Tel: 01284 701601 Fax: 01284 702943 — MB ChB Auckland 1975 (Auckland, New Zealand) DCH Eng. 1978; DRCOG 1979; MRCGP 1980. Specialty: Gen. Pract.

ROBINSON, Richard Edward Menaus 14 Queens Park Rise, Brighton BN2 9ZF — MB BCh Wales 1995.

ROBINSON, Richard John University Hospitals of Leicester NHS Trust, Glenfield Hospital, Groby Road, Leicester LE3 9QP Tel: 0116 287 1471 Fax: 0116 256 3422; 35 Station Road, Quorn, Loughborough LE12 8BP Email: rjrob@globalnet.co.uk — MB BS Lond. 1989 (St Mary's Hospital) BSc Lond. 1988; MRCP (UK) 1992; MD Leicester 1999. Cons. Gastroenterol./ Med., Glenfield Hosp., Leicester. Specialty: Gastroenterol. Special Interest: Inflammatory Bowel Disease; Osteoporosis; Therapeutic Endoscopy. Socs: Brit. Soc. Gastroenterol.; BMA. Prev: Specialist Regist. (Gastroenterol.) Leicester Roy. Infirm.; Research Fell. Leicester Gen. Hosp.; SHO Rotat. (Med.) Bristol Roy. Infirm.

ROBINSON, Richard John Nivana, Pinfold Lane, Fishlake, Doncaster DN7 5LA — MB ChB Manch. 1997.

ROBINSON, Richard Karl 24 Tweskard Park, Belfast BT4 2JZ — MB BCh BAO Belf. 1981.

ROBINSON, Professor Richard Oakley Newcomen Centre, Guys Hospital, London SE1 9RT Tel: 020 7955 4671 Fax: 020 7955 4950; 166 Burbage Road, Dulwich, London SE21 7AG Tel: 020 7733 9127 — (Camb. & Guy's) MB Camb. 1967, BChir 1966; FRCP Lond. 1983, M 1969. Prof. Paediat. Neurol. Guy's Hosp. Lond. Specialty: Paediat. Neurol. Socs: Brit. Paediatric Neurol. Assoc. Past Pres. Prev: Instruc. (Neurol.) Kentucky Univ. Med. Centre; Lect. (Paediat.) Oxf. Univ.; Nuffield Research Fell. Nuffield Inst. Med. Research, Oxf.

ROBINSON, Robert Anthony 7 Wilmer Crescent, Kingston upon Thames KT2 5LU — MB BS Lond. 1994.

ROBINSON, Robert Bruce (retired) 19 St Luke's Court, Hyde Lane, Marlborough SN8 1YU Tel: 01672 515749 — MB BS Lond. 1952 (Middlx.) MSc (Social Med.) Lond. 1971, MB BS 1952; FFCM RCP (UK) 1982, M 1974. JP. Prev: SCM Hants. AHA (T).

ROBINSON, Robert Timothy Charles Edward 27 Ashdell Road, Broomhill, Sheffield S10 3DA — MB ChB Liverp. 1992; MRCP (UK) 1996. Specialty: Diabetes; Endocrinol.; Gen. Med. Socs: BMA; Diabetics UK; EASD. Prev: Clin. Research Fell. (Diabetes & Endocrinol.) North. Gen. Hosp. Sheff.

ROBINSON, Ronald Arthur (retired) 14 Ramsay Garden, Edinburgh EH1 2NA Tel: 0131 225 3125 — (Queens University Belfast) MB BCh BAO Belf. 1949; DPM RCPSI 1953; FRCPsych 1973, M 1971; FRCP Ed. 1979, M 1973. Vice-Chairm. Fac. Psychiat. Of Old Age Roy. Coll. Psychiat. Prev: Sen. Lect. (Psychiat.) Univ. Edin.

ROBINSON, Rosemary Elizabeth Unversity Hospitals of Coventry & Warwickshire NHS Trust, Stoney Stanton Road, Coventry CV1 4FH Tel: 024 7622 4055 — MB BCh BAO NUI 1985 (Royal College of Surgeons in Ireland) LRCPSI 1985; BSc Dub. 1987; DO RCSI 1988; FRCSI 1990; FRCOphth 1990. Cons. (Ophth.) Univ. Hosps. Coventry & Warks. NHS Trust; Oak House, Eastwood Business Village, Eastwood Business Village, Binley Business Park, Coventry CU3 2UB, Tel: 02476561900, Fax: 02476561901. Specialty: Ophth. Prev: Sen. Regist. (Ophth.) Birm. & Midl. Eye Hosp.

ROBINSON, Ruth Christine 4 Alma Farm Road, Toddington, Dunstable LU5 6BG; 60 Wheatfield Road, Luton LU4 0SY — MB BS Lond. 1977.

ROBINSON, Ruth Elizabeth Fairthwaite Park, Cowan Bridge, Carnforth LA6 2HX Tel: 015242 72777 — MB ChB Leeds 1951. Prev: Clin. Med. Off. (Family Plann.) Airedale Med. Auth.

ROBINSON, Samuel Myles — BM BS Nottm. 1998; BMedSci. Specialty: Gen. Pract.

ROBINSON, Sandra Janice Greenwich & Bexley, Cottage Hospice, 185 Bostall Hill, Abbey Wood, London SE2 0QX Fax: 020 8312 2244; 16 Water Meadows, Fordwich, Canterbury CT2 0BF Tel: 01227 711353 — MB BS Lond. 1974 (St. Bart.) MRCS Eng. LRCP Lond. 1974; MSc. Hist. of Sci. and Med. Univ. of Lond. 1996. Med. Off. (Palliat. Care), Greenwich & Bexley Cottage Hospice Lond. Specialty: Palliat. Med. Socs: Assoc. of Palliat. Med. Prev: Clin. Asst. (Palliat. Care) Wisdom Hospice Rochester, Kent; Med. Off. Ellenor Foundat. Dartford Kent; Clin. Asst. (Ophth.) Greenwich Dist. Hosp. Lond.

ROBINSON, Sarah Julie 6 Sorrel Drive, Whiteley, Fareham PO15 7JL — BM Soton. 1996 (Southhampton) Specialty: Accid. & Emerg. Prev: SHO Orthop.; SHO Acute Gen. Med.; SHO A&E.

ROBINSON, Simon David Westgate Surgery, Westgate, Otley LS21 3HD Tel: 01943 465406 Fax: 01943 468363; The Old Vicarage, Stripe Lane, Hartwith, Harrogate HG3 3EZ — MB ChB Leeds 1982 (Leeds University) DRCOG 1985; DCH RCP Lond. 1986; MRCGP 1986. Gen. Practitioner, Westgate Surg., W.gate, Otley, Leeds LS21 3HD.

ROBINSON, Simon Haydn 35 Watery Road, Wrexham LL13 7NP — MB ChB Liverp. 1992.

ROBINSON, Simon Lee 8 Clarks Lane, Newark NG24 2EF — BM BS Nottm. 1996.

ROBINSON, Simon Paul 33 Princess Street, Oxford OX4 1DD — MB BS Lond. 1992.

ROBINSON, Simon Timothy Clarendon House, Croft Road, Ipplepen, Newton Abbot TQ12 5SS — MB BS Lond. 1997.

ROBINSON, Sophia Louise Greystones, Church St., Bloxham, Banbury OX15 4ET — MB BS Lond. 1989; MSc Lond. 1982, BSc

(Hons.) 1980, MB BS 1989. Trainee GP Banbury VTS. Prev: SHO (A & E Dermat. & O & G) Banbury VTS.

ROBINSON, Stephen Unit of Metabolic Medicine, Imperial College School of Medicine, St. Mary's Hospital, London W2 1PG Tel: 020 7886 1253 Fax: 020 7886 1790 Email: stephen.robinson@ic.ac.uk — MB BChir Camb. 1982 (Camb. & Westm.) MRCP (UK) 1987; MA Camb. 1985, MD 1997; FRCP 1999. Cons. Hon. Sen. Lect. (Gen. Med. Diabetes & Endocrinol.) St. Mary's Hosp. Lond. Specialty: Gen. Med.; Diabetes; Endocrinol. Prev: Sen. Lect., Lect. & MRC train. fell. St. Mary's Hosp. Lond.

ROBINSON, Stephen James 80 Cartington Terrace, Heaton, Newcastle upon Tyne NE6 5SH — MB BS Newc. With Merit 1998 (Newcastle) BSc Sackville NB Canada, 1989; MB BS Newc 1998. SHO Gen. Paediat., Qu.s Eliz. Hosp. Gateshead. Specialty: Paediat. Prev: HO, Med. Wansbeck Gen. Hosp. Ashington; HO, Gen. Surg., N. Tyneside Gen. Hosp. N. Shields.; SHO A&E Sunderland Roy. Hosp., Sunderland.

ROBINSON, Stephen John, Surg. Lt.-Cdr. RN Retd. Ridgeway Practice, Plympton Health Centre, Mudgeway, Plymouth PL7 1AD Tel: 01752 346634 Fax: 01752 341444; Follaton, 5 Bainbridge Avenue, Hartley, Plymouth PL3 5QY Tel: 01752 774187 Email: dr.robinson@bigfoot.com — MB BS Lond. 1986 (St Thomas' Hospital Medical School) DRCOG 1993; DFFP 1994; MRCGP 1994. GP Princip.; Police Surg. Devon & Cornw. Constab. Prev: SHO (O & G) Freedom Fields Plymouth; SHO (A & E) Derriford Hosp. Plymouth; SHO (Surg., Med. & A & E) Roy. Naval Hosp. Plymouth.

ROBINSON, Stephen Mark — MB BS Lond. 1986; DA (UK) 1989; MRCP (UK) 1991; FRCA 1992. Cons. Anaesth. & Intens. Care Southmead Hosp. Bristol. Specialty: Anaesth. Prev: Sen. Regist. Rotat. (Anaesth.) Bristol; Regist. Rotat. (Anaesth.) Avon HA; SHO (Med.) Gloucester Roy. Hosp.

ROBINSON, Stephen Paul 36 Pullens Buildings, Penton Place, London SE17 3SH — MB BS Lond. 1992 (Roy. Free Hosp.) MRCP (UK) 1995. Clin. Research Fell. & Hon. Regist. (Haemat.) Antigen Presentation Research Gp. Imperial Coll. Sch. Med. Northwick Pk. Lond. Specialty: Haematology. Prev: SHO (Med.) Northwick Pk. Hosp. Lond.

ROBINSON, Stephen Philip Rose Cottage, Sunbank Lane, Ringway, Altrincham WA15 0PZ Tel: 0161 980 1498 Fax: 0161 980 1498 Email: steverobinsonfagin@compuserve.com — MB ChB Manch. 1971; DMJ Soc. Apoth. Lond. 1984; MMJ Soc. Apoth. 1997. Fell. Inst. Med. & Bioethics Univs. Liverpo. & Manch.; Hon. Lect. (Clin. Forens. Med.) Univ. Manch.; Sen. Police Surg. Gtr. Manch. Police; Co-ordinator Forens. Acad. Gp. North.; Mem. Edit. Comm. Jl. Clin. Forens. Med. (Bk. Review Edn.).

ROBINSON, Steven John 12 The Circle, Birmingham B17 9EE — MB ChB Birm. 1995; ChB Birm. 1995.

ROBINSON, Stuart John 8 Princess Drive, Bollington, Macclesfield SK10 5ER — MB ChB Manch. 1992.

ROBINSON, Susan Institute of Psychiatry, De Crespigny Park, Denmark Hill, London SE5 8AF Tel: 020 7703 5411 — MB ChB Aberd. 1985; MRCPath 1993. Cons. Neuropath., Dept. of Neuropath. The Inst. of Psychiat. Lond. Specialty: Neuropath. Prev: Lect. (Neuropath.) St Barth. & The Roy. Lond. Sch. of Med. & Dent.; Lect. (Path.) Univ. Aberd.; SHO (Path.) Centr. Birm. HA.

ROBINSON, Susan Caroline Lavender Hill Group Practice, 19 Pountney Road, Battersea, London SW11 5TU Tel: 020 7228 4042 Fax: 020 7738 9346 — MB BChir Camb. 1984; MA Camb. 1984.

ROBINSON, Susan Elizabeth Wanstead Place Surgery, 45 Wanstead Place, Wanstead High Street, London E11 2SW Tel: 020 8989 2019 Fax: 020 8532 9124; 28 The Avenue, Wanstead, London E11 2EF — MB BS Lond. 1972 (Roy. Free) MRCS Eng. LRCP Lond. 1972; DObst RCOG 1974; MRCGP 1976; Certificate in Health Management (Keele) 1997. Sen. Partner in Gen. Pract. Prev: Trainee GP Ilford VTS.

ROBINSON, Susan Jane Regents Park Surgery, Park Street, Shirley, Southampton SO16 4RJ Tel: 023 8078 3618 Fax: 023 8070 3103; 5 Amberley Court, Ashurst Bridge, Southampton SO40 7JX — BM Soton. 1982; Cert. Family Plann. JCC 1985; DRCOG 1985; MRCGP 1987. Specialty: Gen. Pract. Prev: Trainee GP Soton. Gen. Hosp.

ROBINSON, Susan Miriam Emergency Department, Addenbrookes NHS Trust, Hills Road, Cambridge CB2 2QQ Tel: 01223 217031 Fax: 01223 217057 — MB BS Lond. 1985 (Westm. Med. Sch.) MRCP (UK) 1988; FRCS Ed. 1993; FFAEM 1995; FRCP 1999. Cons. Emerg. Med. Addenbrooke's Hosp. Camb. Specialty: Accid. & Emerg. Prev: Sen. Regist. (Emerg. Med.) E. Anglia; Regist. (Emerg. Med.) St. Mary's Hosp. Lond.

ROBINSON, Terence John The Barn, Combe Cross, Christow, Exeter EX6 7NR — MB ChB Ed. 1968; MRCPsych 1974. Cons. (Child Psychiat.) Roy. Devon & Exeter Hosp. Exeter. Specialty: Child & Adolesc. Psychiat.

ROBINSON, Thomas Anthony Sully Surgery, 25 South Road, Sully, Penarth CF64 2TG Tel: 029 2053 0255 Fax: 029 2053 0689; Sunnybank, Swaybridge Road, Sully, Penarth CF64 5UN — MB BCh Wales 1981; MRCP (UK) 1985; DRCOG 1986; MRCGP 1987. GP Sully.; Clin. Asst. Impotence Clinic Llandulch Hosp.

ROBINSON, Thomas John Bracken Hill, 101 Lisnaree Road, Banbridge BT32 4JU — MD Belf. 1967; MB BCh BAO 1961; FRCP Lond. 1980, M 1968. Cons. Phys. Craigavon Area Hosp. & Banbridge Hosp. Specialty: Gen. Med. Socs: Brit. Soc. Gastroenterol. & Irish Soc. Gastroenterol. Prev: Ho. Off. & Regist. Roy. Vict. Hosp. Belf.

ROBINSON, Timothy Dudley 7 Beulah Hill, Upper Norwood, London SE19 3LQ — MB BS Lond. 1991; Sub-specialty Accreditation in Urogynaecology 2004; CCST (Obst. & Gyn.) 2004. Locum Cons. (Obstetrician & Gynaecologist) Kings Coll. Hosp. Lond. Specialty: Obst. & Gyn.

ROBINSON, Timothy William Barton House Surgery, Barton House, Beaminster DT8 3EQ Fax: 01308 863785 — MB BS Lond. 1984; DRCOG 1987; Cert. Family Plann. JCC 1987; MRCGP 1988; LF Hom 1996; MFHom 2000. Gen. Practitioner; Homeopathic Phys.; Fac. of Homeopathy Lond. Mem. Comm., Represen.; Convenor Som. / Dorset Homeopathy Forum; Lect. Homeopathic Med., Briston Homeopathic Hosp. Specialty: Homeop. Med. Prev: Ho. Surg. Middlx. Hosp. Lond.; SHO Salisbury Hosps. VTS; Ho. Phys. Cheltenham Gen. Hosp.

ROBINSON, Tony Reynolds (retired) 5 Valley Forge Close, Tonbridge TN10 4EU Tel: 01732 360618 Fax: 01732 360618 — (Middlx.) MB BS Lond. 1957; DObst RCOG 1961. Prev: GP Tonbridge.

ROBINSON, Trevor Walter Ernest 99 Harley Street, London W1G 6AQ Tel: 020 7637 7325 Fax: 020 7637 5383; 1 Cholmeley Crescent, Highgate, London N6 5EZ Tel: 020 8348 9856 — (St. Bart.) MB Camb. 1959, BChir 1958; MRCS Eng. LRCP Lond. 1959; FRCP Lond. 1975, M 1963. Emerit. Cons. Dermat. Univ. Coll. Lond. Hosps. Specialty: Dermat. Socs: Fell. Roy. Soc. Med.; Fell. (Ex-Pres.) St. John's Hosp. Dermat. Soc. Prev: Sen. Regist. & Regist. St. Bart. Hosp. Lond.; SHO St. John's Hosp. Dis. Skin Lond.

ROBINSON, Victor Philip Iver House, 78 High St., Iver SL0 9NG Tel: 01753 652020 Fax: 01753 655459 — MB BS Lond. 1968 (St. Mary's) MRCOG 1975; FRCOG 1992. Cons. O & G Hillingdon, Mt. Vernon, Northwood & Pinner & Dist. Cottage Hosps.; Authorised Med. Examr. for the Civil Aviat. Auth. (AME). Specialty: Obst. & Gyn.; Aviat. Med. Socs: Fell. R.S.M.; B.S.P.O.G.A; Windsor Med. Sailing Soc. Prev: Sen. Regist. (Obst.) St. Geo. Hosp. Lond.; Regist. (Obst.) St. Mary's Hosp. Lond.; Resid. Med. Off. Qu. Charlotte's Matern Hosp. Lond.

ROBINSON, Waring Castlegate Surgery, Castle Street, Hertford SG14 1HH Tel: 01992 589928 — MB BS Lond. 1963 (St. Geo.)

ROBINSON, Wendy Janet Elspeth 5 Bluefield Close, Carrickfergus BT38 7XQ — MB ChB Ed. 1991; BSc (Hons.) Ed. 1989, MB ChB 1991.

ROBINSON, William Henry The Vesey Practice, James Preston Health Centre, 61 Holland Road, Sutton Coldfield B72 1RL Tel: 0121 355 5150 Fax: 0121 321 2498; 106 Tamworth Road, Sutton Coldfield B75 6DH Tel: 0121 378 0018 Fax: 0121 241 3574 — BM BCh Oxf. 1972 (Westm.) MA Oxf. 1972; MRCGP 1980; DRCOG 1981. Sen. Partner in the Vesey Pract.; Regional Med. Adviser Simply Health. Specialty: Gen. Pract. Socs: BMA. Prev: Maj. RAMC.

ROBINSON, William Michael, Col. late RAMC (retired) 4 Searle Road, Farnham GU9 8LJ — MB BCh BAO Dub. 1958; DTM & H Eng. 1960; FRCP Ed. 1976, M 1963. Asst. Surg. Roy. Hosp. Chelsea. Prev: Asst. Surg. Roy. Hosp. Chelsea.

ROBINSON-WHITE, Catherine Mary 41 Fairview Street, Cheltenham GL52 2JF — MB BS Lond. 1989.

ROBISON, Christine Royal Infirmary of Edinburgh, Anaesthetics Department, 51 Little France Crescent, Old Dalkeith Road,

Edinburgh EH3 9YW Tel: 0131 242 3224 — MB ChB Ed. 1978; BSc (Med. Sci.) Ed. 1976; FFA RCS Eng. 1984. Assoc. Specialist Lothian Univ. Hosp. Trust. Specialty: Anaesth. Socs: BMA; Ed. & E. Scot. Soc. Anaesth. Prev: Staff Anaesth. E. Gen. Hosp. Edin.; Staff Anaesth. St. John's Hosp. Livingston; Regist. (Anaesth.) Roy. Infirm. Edin.

ROBISON, Janet Margaret 83 Mountalto Avenue, Motherwell ML1 4AZ — MB ChB Glas. 1995.

ROBLES, Alfonso 1 Westfield Road, London NW7 3BJ — Medico Salvador Argentina 1974.

ROBLESS, Peter Ashley Flat 2/R, 22 Polwarth Street, Hyndland, Glasgow G12 9TY — MB ChB Aberd. 1992.

ROBLIN, David Pfizer Global Research & Development, Sandwich CT13 9NJ Tel: 01304 646210 — MB BS Lond. 1991; BSc Lond. 1988; MRCP (UK) 1994. Vice Pres. & Head of Clin. R&D, Pfizer Global Research & Developm., Sandwich; Sen. Lect. Brighton & Sussex Med. Sch. Specialty: Pharmaceutical Medicine; Infec. Dis. Socs: Roy. Soc. Pharmaceutical Med. Prev: Candidate Team Ldr., Pfizer Centr. Research; Head of Anti-Infectives, Pharma Europe, Bayer; SHO Rotat. (Med.) St. Geo. Hosp. Lond.

ROBLIN, Mr David Graham University Hospital of Wales, Heath Park, Cardiff — MB BCh Wales 1989; FRCS Ed. 1995; FRCS ORL-HNS 2001; MPhil 2002. Specialty: Otorhinolaryngol.

ROBLIN, (Karen) Jane Manor Surgery, Osler Road, Headington, Oxford OX3 9BP Tel: 01865 762535; 48 Sandfield Road, Headington, Oxford OX3 7RJ Tel: 01865 761216 — MB BS Lond. 1981; DCH RCP Lond. 1983; MRCGP 1990. GP Oxf.; Clin. Asst. (Infertil.) John Radcliffe Hosp. Oxf.; Assoc. Course Organiser Oxf. VTS. Prev: Trainee GP Oxf.; SHO (Paediat.) Kingston Hosp.; SHO (Cardiol.) Middlx. Hosp.

ROBLIN, Menna Wyn 19 Pencisely Avenue, Cardiff CF5 1DZ — MB BCh Wales 1989; DRCOG 1992; MRCGP 1993; DCH RCP Lond. 1993. Staff Grade (Community Paediat.) M. Glam. Specialty: Community Child Health.

ROBLIN, Paul 3 Coombe Neville,, Warren Road, Kingston upon Thames KT2 7HW Tel: 020 8949 4344 — MB BS Lond. 1990 (St. George's Hosp. Medical School Lond.) MSc - Sept 1998, Univ Coll of Lond.; FRCS Eng 1995. Specialist Regist. in Plastic Pan - Thames Rotat. Surg. Specialty: Plastic Surg. Prev: Specialist Reg. In Plastic Surg., Qu. Vict. Hosp, E. Grinstead, W. Sussex.

ROBLIN, Paul Howard Summertown Group Practice, 160 Banbury Road, Oxford OX2 7BS Tel: 01865 515552 Fax: 01865 311237; 48 Sandfield Road, Oxford OX3 7RJ Tel: 01865 761216 Fax: 01865 767924 — MB Camb. 1978; MB Camb., BChir 1978; MRCP (UK) 1980; DCH RCP Lond. 1983; MRCGP 1983. Specialty: Gen. Pract. Socs: Sec. Oxon. LMC; Bd. Mem. Oxf. PCG. Prev: SHO Obst. St. Mary's Hosp. Lond.; SHO Paediat. Kingston Hosp. Surrey; SHO Gen. Med. Centr. Middlx. Hosp. Lond.

ROBLIN, Sallyanne The Surgery, 43 London Road, High Wycombe HP12 4DG Tel: 01494 527036 — MB BS Lond. 1990; DRCOG 1993; MRCGP 1994; DFFP 1994. GP Asst. High Wycombe. Specialty: Gen. Pract. Prev: Asst. GP Caterham; Trainee GP E. Surrey Hosp. VTS.

ROBLING, Siri-Ann West Suffolk Hospital, Suffolk Mental Health Partnership NHS Trust, Hardwicke Lane, Bury St Edmunds IP33 2QZ Tel: 01284 713182 Fax: 01284 713694 Email: siri.robling@smhp.nhs.uk — MB BChir Camb. 1989 (St Catharines College University of Cambridge Addenbrooks Clinical Medical School, Cambridge) MRCPsych 1994. Cons. (Gen. Adult) Psychiat. W. Suff. Hosp. Bury, St, Edmunds Suff.. Specialty: Gen. Psychiat. Prev: Sen. Regist. Rotat. (Psychiat.) Addenbrookes, Hosp. Camb.; Regist. (Psychiat.) Fulbourn Hosp. Camb.

ROBLINGS, George Lindsey John (retired) Glynhir, Llanmartin Road, Langstone, Newport NP18 2JX Tel: 01633 412162 — MB BCh Wales 1959 (Cardiff) Prev: GP Newport, Gwent.

ROBSON, Alan Beech Tree Surgery, 68 Doncaster Road, Selby YO8 9AJ Tel: 01757 703933 Fax: 01757 213473; 66 Leeds Road, Selby YO8 4JQ Tel: 01757 702228 — MB ChB St. And. 1966; DObst RCOG 1968. Prev: Med. Off. Kerugoya Hosp., Kenya; SHO (Paediat.) Seafield Childr. Hosp. Ayr.; SHO (Obst.) Ayrsh. Centr. Hosp. Irvine.

ROBSON, Alastair Malcolm The Surgery, Stowe Drive, Southam, Leamington Spa CV47 1NY Tel: 01926 812577 Fax: 01926 817447 — MB BCh BAO Dub. 1971; MA Dub. 1972; DObst RCPI 1983; MICGP 1988. GP Warwicksh.

ROBSON, Lady Alice Eleanor Flat II, The Coach House, 3 Victoria Road, Preston PR2 8ND Tel: 01772 713447 — (Ed.) MB ChB Ed. 1944.

ROBSON, Mr Andrew Kenneth Department of Otolaryngology, Cumberland Infirmary, Carlisle CA2 7HT Tel: 01228 814207 Fax: 01228 814276; Holm Hill House, Hawksdale, Dalston, Carlisle CA5 7BX — MB BS Lond. 1984 (Middlx.) FRCS Eng. (Gen.) 1988; FRCS Eng. (Otol.) 1990; FRCS (Orl.) 1993. Cons. Otolaryngol. Carlisle Hosps. NHS Trust. Specialty: Otolaryngol. Prev: Sen. Regist. (Otolaryngol.) Newc. & Sunderland; Tutor Specialist (Otolaryngol.) Dunedin Pub. Hosp., NZ; Regist. (Otolaryngol.) Radcliffe Infirm. Oxf.

ROBSON, Angus Osborn (retired) The Grange, Horsenden, Princes Risborough HP27 9NE Tel: 01844 343015 — (Middlx.) MB BS Lond. 1951; FRCP Lond. 1973, M 1957; MD Lond. 1966. Prev: Sen. Regist. Roy. Vict. Infirm. Newc.

ROBSON, Barbara Edith Claire 118 Wimbledon Hill Road, London SW19 7QU Tel: 020 8946 9690 — MB BS Lond. 1952.

ROBSON, Brenda Jean (retired) 7 King John's Court, Darras Hall, Ponteland, Newcastle upon Tyne NE20 9AR Tel: 01661 823316 — MB BS Durh. 1955. Asst. Orthop. Surg. Freeman Hosp. Newc. u. Tyne. Prev: Asst. Orthop. Surg. W.J. Sanderson Orthop. Hosp. Gosforth.

ROBSON, Brian John Incle Street Surgery, 8 Incle Street, Paisley PA1 1HR Tel: 0141 889 8809 Fax: 0141 849 1474; 331 Mearns Road, Newton Mearns, Glasgow G77 5LT — MB ChB Glas. 1988; DRCOG 1991; MRCGP 1992.

ROBSON, Catherine Helen 480 Bristol Road, Selly Oak, Birmingham B29 6BD Tel: 0121 472 0129 — MB ChB Birm. 1987; MRCGP (UK) 1992.

ROBSON, Christopher Edward Cirencester Memorial centre, Sheep Street, Cirencester GL7 1RQ — MB ChB Leeds 1985; BSc Psychol. Leeds 1982, MB ChB 1985; MRCPsych 1990. Specialty: Gen. Psychiat. Prev: Sen. Regist. (Rehabil. Psychiat.) Coney Hill Hosp. Gloucester.; Sen. Regist. (Gen. Psychiat.) Southmead Gen. Hosp. Bristol & Barrow Hosp. Bristol.

ROBSON, Christopher James Lochee Health Centre, 1 Marshall Street, Lochee, Dundee DD2 3BR Tel: 01382 611283 Fax: 01382 624480; Briarbank, 7 Albert St, Monifieth, Dundee DD5 4JS Tel: 01382 532808 — MB ChB Ed. 1981; MRCGP 1985; DRCOG 1986.

ROBSON, Clare Winifred Marine Avenue Medical Centre, 64 Marine Avenue, Whitley Bay NE26 1NQ Tel: 0191 252 5317 — (Westm.) MB BS Lond. 1973; DObst RCOG 1975; MRCP (UK) 1976.

ROBSON, David Allan Haematology Department, Royal Gwent Hospital, Newport Tel: 01633 252244 — MB ChB Ed. 1980; MRCP (UK) 1985. Staff Grade (Haemat.) Roy. Gwent Hosp. Specialty: Haematology. Prev: Regist. (Haemat.) Univ. Hosp. Wales Cardiff; Regist. (Geriat.) Roy. Lancaster Infirm.; Regist. (Gen. Med.) Wythenshawe Hosp. Manch.

ROBSON, David John Queen Elizabeth Hospital, Stadium Road, Woolwich, London SE18 4QH — MB BS Lond. 1968 (Middlx.) MRCP (U.K.) 1972; FRCP Lond. 1986. Specialty: Cardiol.; Intens. Care. Socs: Brit. Cardiac Soc. Prev: Cons. Phys. Greenwich Dist. Hosp. Lond.

ROBSON, David John Biddlestone Health Group, 1 Biddlestone Road, Heaton, Newcastle upon Tyne NE6 5SL Tel: 0191 265 5755 Fax: 0192 275 5550 Email: david.robson@gp-A86010.nhs.uk — MB BS Newc. 1984; BMedSc (Hons.) Newc. 1986; MRCGP 1989. GP Princ. Heaton. Prev: Trainee GP N.d. VTS.

ROBSON, Deborah 6 Postcliffe House, Peterculter, Aberdeen AB14 0UY — MB ChB Liverp. 1996. SHO Infec. Dis.s/ Gen. Med., Aberd. Roy. Infirm., Aberd. Specialty: Gen. Med.

ROBSON, Derek Clark, Col. late RAMC (retired) 85 Queens Road, Alton GU34 1JA Tel: 01420 88984 — MB ChB Leeds 1957; BSc (Hons.) Manch. 1952; MPhil Leeds 1987, MD 1967. Prev: Dir. Army Path.

ROBSON, Derek Keith Department of Pathology, Queens Medical Centre, Clifton Boulevard, Nottingham NG7 2 Tel: 0115 942 1421; 5 Paget Crescent, Ruddington, Nottingham NG11 6FD — MB BS Lond. 1980; MRCPath 1989. Cons. Neuropath. Qu. Med. Centre Nottm. Specialty: Neuropath.

ROBSON, Donald John Longford House Surgery, Longford Road, Holyhead LL65 1TR Tel: 01407 762341 Fax: 01407 761554; 7 The

Rise, Trearddur Bay, Holyhead LL65 2UY — MB BS Newc. 1980; DRCOG 1983; MRCGP 1984. Specialty: Gen. Pract. Prev: Trainee GP Northumbria VTS; Mem. Ment. Health Task Force RCGP.

ROBSON, Duncan James Silver Lane Surgery, 1 Suffolk Court, Yeadon, Leeds LS19 7JN Tel: 0113 250 4953 Fax: 0113 250 9804; Woodlands, 9 Creskeld Garth, Bramhope, Leeds LS16 9EW — MB ChB Leeds 1978. Sen. Med. Adviser Yorks. Water Plc Bradford. Specialty: Cardiol.; Occupat. Health.

ROBSON, Elizabeth St Andrews Medical Centre, Pinewood Gardens, Southborough, Tunbridge Wells TN4 0LZ Tel: 01892 515455; 65 Southview Road, Tunbridge Wells TN4 9BU Tel: 01892 531655 Fax: 01892 531655 — MB BS Lond. 1977; AKC; DRCOG 1981; MRCGP 1982. Prev: Trainee GP Brighton VTS; Ho. Surg. Dulwich Hosp. Lond.; Ho. Phys. Gravesend & N. Kent Hosp. Gravesend.

ROBSON, Elizabeth Jane 57 Tabors Avenue, Great Baddow, Chelmsford CM2 7EJ — BM Soton. 1983.

ROBSON, Eva Gwendoline (retired) 7 Waterside, Staindrop Road, Darlington DL3 9AF Tel: 01325 488202 — MB BS Durh. 1946; DObst RCOG 1948. Prev: GP Hurworth-on-Tees.

ROBSON, Fiona Susan 58 Hollies Way, Bushby, Leicester LE7 9RJ — MB ChB Leeds 1977.

ROBSON, Georgina Mary Willett East Oxford Health Centre, Manzil Way, Cowley Road, Cowley, Oxford OX4 1XD Tel: 01865 242109; St. Marys Cottage, Church St, Beckley, Oxford OX3 9UT Tel: 01865 351637 — MB BS Lond. 1968 (Middlx.) DObst RCOG 1970.

ROBSON, Guy Ernest William 165 Bury New Road, Prestwich, Manchester M25 9PJ — MB ChB Leeds 1970; BSc (Hons.) Leeds 1967; FFA RCS Eng. 1976. Cons. N. Manch. Healthcare Trust. Specialty: Anaesth. Prev: Sen. Regist. Manch. Roy. Infirm.; Regist. Leeds Gen. Infirm.; SHO & Ho. Off. Leeds Gen. Infirm.

ROBSON, Jacqueline (retired) The Old Vicarage, 62 Williams Park, Benton, Newcastle upon Tyne NE12 8BL Tel: 0191 215 9898 — MB BS Durh. 1947 (Univ. Durh.) Prev: Anaesth. Regist., Ho. Phys. & Ho. Surg. Roy. Vict. Infirm. Newc. upon.

ROBSON, Professor Sir (James) Gordon, CBE (retired) Brendon, Lyndale, London NW2 2NY Tel: 020 7435 3762 Fax: 020 7435 3762 — MB ChB (Commend.) Glas. 1944; Hon. DSc Glas. 1990; Hon. FRCPS Glas. 1993; DA Eng. 1948; FFA RCS Eng. 1953; Hon. FFA RACS 1968; FRCS Eng. 1977; Hon. FDS RCS 1979; Hon. FFA RCSI 1980; DSc McGill 1984; Hon. FRCPC 1988. Prev: Dean Fac. Anaesth. RCS Eng.

ROBSON, James Peter West Gate Health Centre, Charleston Drive, Dundee DD2 4AD Tel: 01382 668189 Fax: 01382 665943; 8 Piperdam Drive, Fowlis, Dundee DD2 5LY — MB ChB Dundee 1988; MRCGP 1995; Dip SEM GB & I 2000.

ROBSON, James Scott (retired) 1 Grant Avenue, Colinton, Edinburgh EH13 0DS Tel: 0131 441 3508 — (Univs. Ed. & N.Y.) MB ChB (Hons.) Ed. 1945; MD Ed. 1946; FRCP Ed. 1960, M 1948; FRCP Lond. 1978, M 1978. Prev: Prof. Med. (Emerit.) Univ. Edin.

ROBSON, Mrs Jane Mary 96 Chesterton Road, Cambridge CB4 1ER Tel: 01223 365555 Fax: 01223 356848; Herrings House, Wilbraham Road, Fulbourn, Cambridge CB1 5EU Tel: 01223 880277 — (St. Thos.) MB BChir Camb. 1961; MA Camb. 1961; DObst RCOG 1962. GP; Hosp. Pract. (Geriat.). Specialty: Gen. Pract. Socs: Accred. Mem. Brit. Med. Acupunc. Soc.

ROBSON, Jannette Thwaite Street Surgery, The Chestnuts, 45 Thwaite Street, Cottingham HU16 4QX Tel: 01482 847250 Fax: 01482 848173 — MB ChB Leic. 1987; DRCOG 1990; MRCGP 1991. Prev: Trainee GP Walston, Coventry.

ROBSON, Jean, MBE (retired) New Barn Cottage, Alston Lane, Longridge, Preston PR3 3BN Tel: 01772 785395 — MB ChB Manch. 1948; DCH Eng. 1951. Prev: SCMO (Audiol.) Preston HA.

ROBSON, Jean Elizabeth Charlotte Street Surgery, 1 Charlotte Street, Dumfries DG1 2AQ Tel: 01387 267626 Fax: 01387 266824 — MB BS Lond. 1980; MRCGP 1985; DRCOG 1987; Dip. Sports Med. (Lond.) 1988; Dip Adv. Therap. 2000. Socs: Roy. Coll. Gen. Pract. & Brit. Assn. Sports Med.

ROBSON, Jennifer Jane 6 Rosevale, Hoddesdon EN11 8NR — MB BS Western Australia 1988.

ROBSON, Jo-Anna 23 Broadway, Shifnal TF11 8BB — MB ChB Glas. 1996.

ROBSON, John Dickson Hilton, New Ridley, Stocksfield NE43 7RQ — MB ChB Dundee 1980. Prev: Ho. Off. (Gen. Surg.) Arbroath; Ho. Off. (Gen. Med.) Northampton Gen. Hosp.

ROBSON, John Laidlaw Yew Tree Medical Centre, 100 Yew Tree Lane, Solihull B91 2RA Tel: 0121 705 8787 Fax: 0121 709 0240 — MB BS Newc. 1969; DObst RCOG 1972. Prev: Med.Off.jaguar Cars; med.Off.Land rover; Med.Off.Birm City FC.

ROBSON, John Peter Chrisp Street Health Centre, 100 Chrisp Street, London E14 6PG Tel: 020 7515 4860 Fax: 020 7515 3055 — MB BS Lond. 1974; MSc Lond. 1984, MB BS 1974; DRCOG 1977; DCH Eng. 1978; MRCGP 1978.

ROBSON, John Ryder (retired) The White Cottage, Newick, Lewes BN8 4SA Tel: 01825 722510 — MB BS Lond. 1960 (St. Bart.) MRCS Eng. LRCP Lond. 1960; DObst RCOG 1963. Examg. Med. Practitioner, Dept. of Work and Pens.

ROBSON, Julia Claire 115 Sherburn Way, Gateshead NE10 8TZ — MB BCh Wales 1983; DRCOG 1986; MRCGP 1987. Prev: Trainee GP E. Dist. Glas. VTS.

ROBSON, Keith Henry Bingley Health Centre, Myrtle Place, Bingley BD16 2TL Tel: 01274 362760 Fax: 01274 772345 — MB ChB Leeds 1979; DA Eng. 1982; Cert. Family Plann. JCC 1984. Prev: Trainee GP/SHO Bradford VTS; SHO (Anaesth.) Bradford Gp. Hosp.; Ho. Off. (Med.) York Dist. Hosp.

ROBSON, Mark Charlton (retired) Maple House, 28 The Green, Hurworth-on-Tees, Darlington DL2 2AA — MB BS Durh. 1947 (Newc. upon Tyne) Prev: GP Hurworth-on-Tees.

ROBSON, Mr Martin John (retired) 6 Brook Way, Christchurch BH23 4HA Tel: 01425 272522 Email: martin@robson2.fsnet.co.uk; 77 Rundle Road, Sheffield S7 1NW Tel: 0114 258 8660 — MB BS Lond. 1966 (Char. Cross) LMCC Licentiate Medical College of Canada; MRCS Eng. LRCP Lond. 1966; FRCS Eng. 1971. Cons. Orthop. Surg. (retired) Rotherham Dist. Gen. Hosp. Prev: Sen. Regist. (Orthop.) Sheff. AHA (T).

ROBSON, Matthew Town End, Far Sawrey, Ambleside LA22 0LH Tel: 015394 47427; 19 Fernbank Road, Redland, Bristol BS6 6QA Tel: 0117 944 6912 — MB ChB Bristol 1993; MRCP (UK) 1996. Clin. Fell. (Bone Marrow Transpl.) Roy. Hosp. Sick Childr. Bristol. Prev: SHO (Paediat.) Southmead Hosp. & Bristol Roy. Hosp. Sick Childr.; SHO (Neonat. Med.) St. Michael's Hosp. Bristol.

ROBSON, Melanie Jayne Level 4, Women's Centre, John Radcliffe Hospital, Headley Way, Headington, Oxford OX3 9DZ; 64 Margaret Road, Headington, Oxford OX3 8NQ Tel: 01865 760989 Email: melanie.robson@orh.nhs.uk — MB BS Lond. 1984; MRCOG 1990. Cons. Feto-Matern. Med. Wom. Centre John Radcliffe Hosp. Oxf. Specialty: Obst. & Gyn. Socs: BMUS; Brit. Matern. & Fetal Med. Soc.; Blair Bell Res. Soc. Prev: Research Fell. (Obst.) St. Geo. Hosp. Med. Sch. Lond.; Sen. Regist. Roy. United Hosp. Bath & St. Michael's Hosp. Bristol.

ROBSON, Michael Gregory Guy's Hospital, London SE1 9RT — MB BS Lond. 1992; MRCP 1995; PhD 2000.

ROBSON, Michael James Allan 25 Avondale Place, Edinburgh EH3 5HX — MB ChB Ed. 1988.

ROBSON, Michael John Pilladilly House, 17 Pilladilly, Slotforth, Lancaster LA1 4PX — MB ChB Ed. 1990; MRCPsych Roy. Coll. of Psychiat. 1999. Specialists Regist. (Gen. Adult Psychiat.) Roy. Preston Hosp. Specialty: Gen. Psychiat. Socs: Life Mem. Roy. Med. Soc. Edin. Prev: Specialist Regist., Gen Adult Psycian, Ridge Way, Lancaster.

ROBSON, Michael Stanley (retired) 4 Cefn Gethinog, Talybont-on-Usk, Brecon LD3 7YN Tel: 01874 676345 Fax: 01874 676292 Email: MrMichaelSRobson@aol.com — MB Camb. 1955; BChir 1954; DTM & H Lond. 1961.

ROBSON, Mr Michael Stephen Department of Obstetrics & Gynaecology, Wycombe General Hospital, Queen Alexanda Road, High Wycombe HP11 2TT — MB BS Lond. 1982; FRCS Eng. 1987; MRCOG 1990. Cons. O & G Wycombe Gen. Hosp. Specialty: Obst. & Gyn. Prev: Asst. Master Nat. Matern. Hosp. Dub.

ROBSON, Nicola Kay Poole Hospital, Long Fleet Road, Poole BH15 2JB — MB BChir Camb. 1985 (Cambridge University) BSc Hull 1981; BA Camb. 1983, MB BChir 1985; MA Camb. 1988; DMRD Lond. 1990; FRCR 1992; T(R) (CR) 1993. Cons. Radiol. Poole Hosp. NHS Trust. Specialty: Radiol. Socs: Assoc. Mem. Roy. Soc. Med.; BMA; BNMS. Prev: Sen. Regist. (Radiol.) Soton. Gen.

Hosp.; Regist. (Radiol.) Soton. Gen. Hosp.; SHO Rotat. (Med.) Addenbrooke's Hosp. Camb.

ROBSON, Nigel James The Surgery, 10-12 Jubilee Road, Eston, Middlesbrough TS6 9ER Tel: 01642 455524 Fax: 01642 464678 — MB ChB Leeds 1965; DObst RCOG 1967; DA Eng. 1969. Med. Dir. Cleveland Deputising Servs. Ltd.

ROBSON, Nigel Jonathan 12 Charlotte Road, Edgbaston, Birmingham B15 2NG — MB Camb. 1980; BChir 1979; FFA RCS Eng. 1983. Cons. Paediat. Anaesth. Childr. Hosp. Birm. Specialty: Anaesth.

ROBSON, Noel Leslie Kent (retired) 33 Worsley Crescent, Marton, Middlesbrough TS7 8LU Tel: 01642 315384 — MB BS Durh. 1956; DMRT Eng. 1964. Cons. Radiother. & Oncol. Regional Radiother. Serv. Newc. Hosp. & S. Cleveland Dist. Gen. Hosp. Middlesbrough; Assoc. Clin. Lect. (Radiother.) Univ. Newc. Prev: Sen. Regist. (Radiother.) Roy. Infirm. & West. Gen. Hosp. Edin.

ROBSON, Peter 1 Buttermere Avenue, Whickham, Newcastle upon Tyne NE16 4EX Tel: 0191 488 7519 — MB Camb. 1975; BA Camb. 1971, MB 1975, BChir 1974; MRCP (UK) 1977; FRCP Lond. 1989. Cons. Phys. Responsibil. c/o Elderly N. Durh. Acute Hosps. NHS Trust. Specialty: Gen. Med.

ROBSON, Peter (retired) 270 Wickham Chase, West Wickham BR4 0BS Tel: 020 8402 9517 Email: peter@drrobson.fsnet.co.uk — MB BS Lond. 1959 (King's Coll. Hosp.) MRCS Eng. LRCP Lond. 1959; DCH Eng. 1961; FRCP Ed. 1977, M 1968. Cons. Paediat. King's Coll. Hosp. Lond., Bethlem Roy. & Maudsley Hosps.; Sen. Lect. (Neuro-Developm. Paediat.) KCH Med. Sch. Lond. Prev: Cons. Paediat. Guy's Hosp. Lond.

ROBSON, Peter Anthony (retired) 17 Thornlea, Hepscott, Morpeth NE61 6NY Tel: 01670 516867 — MB BS Durh. 1956 (Newc.) Prev: Ho. Phys. (Child Health) Roy. Vict. Infirm. Newc. u. Tyne.

ROBSON, Peter Grant Ravens Craig, Main St., Kinnesswood, Kinross KY13 9HW — MB ChB Dundee 1980; DRCOG 1984; MRCGP 1984. GP Kinnesswood.

ROBSON, Mr Peter Napier (retired) The Old Vicarage, 62 Williams Park, Newcastle upon Tyne NE12 8BL — MB BS Durh. 1946; MRCS Eng. LRCP Lond. 1946; FRCS Eng. 1949. Hon. Cons. Orthop. Surg. Newc. HA.

ROBSON, Peter William 38 Keathbank Avenue, Irby, Wirral L62 4XD — MB ChB Liverp. 1989. SHO (A & E) Countess of Chester Hosp.

ROBSON, Philip John Oxford University Department of Psychiatry, The Warneford Hospital, Oxford OX3 7JX Tel: 01865 784869 — MB BS Lond. 1970; MRCP (UK) 1978; MRCPsych 1985; FRCPsych 2000. Director, Cannabinoid Research Inst.; Sen. Research Fell., Oxf. Univ. Dept. of Psychiat. Specialty: Alcohol & Substance Misuse; Medicinal cannabis research. Prev: Region Cons. & Cons. Psychiat. Subst. Misuse Oxf.; Sen. Clin. Lect. Univ. Oxf.; Clin. Lect. (Psychiat.) Univ. Oxf.

ROBSON, Piers Cowen (retired) Snuff Mill Cottage, Mitford, Morpeth NE61 3PY — MB ChB St. And. 1958; DPM Eng. 1964; MRCPsych 1971. Prev: Cons. Psychiat. St. Geo. Hosp. Morpeth & Cherry Knowle Hosp. Ryhope.

ROBSON, Richard Austin Department of Clinical Pharmacology, Roche Products, PO Box 8, Welwyn Garden City AL7 3AV — MB ChB Otago 1977.

ROBSON, Rita Ann Twickenfield, Shotley Bridge, Consett DH8 0NJ — MB ChB Manch. 1979; BSc Manch. Univ. 1976; FRCR 1985. Cons. Radiol. N. Tyneside Gen. Hosp. Northumbria Health Care NHS Trust. Specialty: Radiol. Prev: Cons. Radiol. N. Durh. Acute Hosps. NHS Trust; Sen. Regist. & Regist. (Radiol.) Roy. Vict. Infirm. Newc.

ROBSON, Robert Howard Cumberland Infirmary, Newtown Road, Carlisle CA2 7HY Tel: 01228 814032 Fax: 01228 814032 Email: howard.robson@ncumbria_acute.nhs.uk — MB BChir Camb. 1970 (Camb. & Middlx. Hosp.) MA Camb. 1970; FRCP Lond. 1988, M 1972; FRCP Ed. 1983. Cons. Phys. Cumbld. Infirm. Carlisle. Specialty: Gen. Med. Socs: Brit. Pharm. Soc.; Brit. Cardiac Soc.; Med. Res. Soc. Prev: Sen. Regist. (Clin. Pharmacol. & Therap.) Roy. Infirm. Edin.; Research Fell. Centr. Middlx. Hosp. Lond.; Regist. (Neurol.) Walton Hosp. Liverp.

ROBSON, Sarah Chainsbridge Medical Partnership, Chainbridge House, The Precinct, Blaydon-on-Tyne NE21 5BT Tel: 0191 414 2856 Fax: 0191 499 0449; Boundary House, Roseworth Terrace, Gosforth, Newcastle upon Tyne NE3 1LU Tel: 0191 213 1132 — MB BS Lond. 1985 (St Bartholomew's Hospital Medical School) DRCOG 1990; DCH RCP Lond. 1990. Specialty: Gen. Med. Prev: Trainee GP Ashford; Trainee GP W. Middlx. Univ. Hosp. VTS.

ROBSON, Professor Stephen Courtenay Department of Obstetrics & Gynaecology, University Newcastle upon Tyne, Royal Victoria Infirmary, Newcastle upon Tyne NE1 4LP Tel: 0191 232 5131 Fax: 0191 222 5066 Email: s.c.robson@ncl.ac.uk — MB BS Newc. 1982; MRCOG 1987; MD Newc. 1992. Prof. Fetal Med. Univ. Newc. u. Tyne & Roy. Vict. Infirm. Specialty: Obst. & Gyn. Prev: Sen. Lect. (Obst.) & Regist. (O & G) Roy. Vict. Infirm. Newc.; RCOG Train. Fell. (Fetal Med.) Univ. Coll. Hosp. Lond.

ROBSON, Susan Andrée University of Manchester Health and Safety Services, Waterloo Place, 182/184 Oxford Road, Manchester M13 9DG Tel: 0161 275 697011 Fax: 0161 275 6989 Email: susan.a.robson@man.ac.uk; Hollows Farm, Stamford Lane, Christleton, Chester CH3 7QD Tel: 01244 335368 — (University of Newcastle-upon-Tyne) MB BS Newc. 1968; FFOM RCP Lond. 1992, MFOM 1985; MFFP 1995; FRCP Lond. 1998. Dir. Health & Safety Servs., Univ. of Manch.; Clin. Med. Off.; family Plann.; primary care trust Chester; Hon Lect. Centre for Occup. Health Univ. Manch. Specialty: Occupat. Health; Family Plann. & Reproduc. Health. Socs: Ex Chairm. Assn. of Authorities Med. Advisers; Curr. Chairm. BMA occup. Health Comm.; Curr. Mem. bma Counc. Prev: Ho. Phys. W. Suff. Gen. Hosp.; Ho. Surg. Chester Roy. Infirm.; Country Med. health and safety, admin Ocupational health.

ROBSON, Timothy William Cassio Surgery, 62-68 Merton Road, Watford WD18 0WL Tel: 01923 226011 Fax: 01923 817342; 96 Church Road, Watford WD17 4PU Tel: 01923 225798 — MB BS Lond. 1975 (Lond. Hosp.) BSc Lond. 1972, MB BS 1975. Specialty: Alcohol & Substance Misuse. Prev: SHO (Trop. Med.) Hosp. Trop. Dis. Lond.; SHO (Med. Oncol.) Roy. Marsden Hosp. Sutton; SHO (Gen. Med. & Rheum.) Northwick Pk. Hosp.

ROBSON, Victoria-Anne Royal Victoria Infirmary, Queen Victoria Road, Newcastle upon Tyne NE1 4LP — MB BS Lond. 1991 (St. George's Hospital, University of London) BSc (Hons.) Lond. 1988; MRCP (UK) 1995; FRCA 1997; EDIC 2001. Cons. Anaesth. ITG Roy. Vict. Infirm. Newc. Specialty: Anaesth.; Intens. Care. Socs: Roy. Coll. Of Anaesth.; Assn. of Anaesth.; Intens. Care Soc. Prev: Specialist Regist. (Anaesth.) St. Marys Hosp.; SPR (Anaesth.) Hammersmith Hosp.; SPR (ITG) Newc.

ROBSON, Winifred Joan Royal Liverpool Children's NHS Trust, AlderHey, Liverpool LI2 2AP Tel: 0151 228 4811 — MB ChB Liverp. 1967; FRCS Eng. 1972; FFAEM 1994; FRCPCH 1997. Cons. Paediat.. Roy. Liverp. Childr. Hosp. Alder Hey.; Liverp. Univ.; Teachg. Asst. Specialty: Accid. & Emerg.; Paediat. Socs: BMA; Brit. Assn. Accid. & Emerg. Med.; Bd. Fac. A&E Med. Prev: Sen. Research Asst. Dept. Child Health Alder Hey Childr. Hosp.; Liverp.; Regist. (Paediat. Surg. & Urol.) Alder Hey Childr. Hosp. Liverp.

ROBY JONES, Christopher (retired) 1 Chichester Close, Instow, Bideford EX39 4JT Tel: 01271 860560 — MB ChB Liverp. 1958; FRCP Lond. 1980, M 1965. Cons. Phys. in Geriat. N. Devon Hosp. Gp. Prev: Sen. Regist. (Geriat.) Char. Cross Hosp. Gp.

ROBYNS-OWEN, David Treflan Surgery, Treflan, Lower Cardiff Road, Pwllheli LL53 5NF Tel: 01758 701457 Fax: 01758 701209; Treflan, Penlan St, Pwllheli LL53 5D Tel: 01758 612457 — MB ChB Liverp. 1979; DRCOG 1983.

ROCH-BERRY, Colin Sydney Bertram Oakfield, Badgeworth Lane, Badgeworth, Cheltenham GL51 4UQ Tel: 01242 862703 Fax: 01242 862703 Email: colin@roch-berry.net/roch-berry@doctors.net.uk — (St. Bart.) LLM 1991 Cardiff; MRCS Eng. LRCP Lond. 1968; MB BS Lond. 1969; FRCR 1975. Caldicott Guardian Gloucestershire Hosp. NHS Foundat. Trust; Fell. (Governor) Gloucestershire Univ.; Medico-legal work as Expert Witness. Specialty: Oncol. Special Interest: Medico-legal work as Expert Witness. Socs: Medico-Leg. Soc.; BMA; Roy. Soc. Med. Prev: Cons. Clin. Oncol. Glos.Oncol.Centre Cheltenham; Sen. Regist. (Radiother.) Christie Hosp. & Holt Radium Inst. Manch.

ROCHA JANEIRO, Maria Magdelena 5 Laurel Bank, The Highlands, Whitehaven CA28 6SW Tel: 01946 694324 — LMS Barcelona 1984. VTS (GP) Cumbria VTS for Gen. Pract. in W. Cumbria; GP Regist. Whitehaven. Specialty: Gen. Pract. Socs: BMA; Med. Protec. Soc. Prev: SHO (O & G) Bishop Auckland Gen. Hosp.

ROCHE, Caroline Jane Heath The Surgery, 2-4 Steerforth Street, Earlsfield, London SW18 4HL; 92 Arthur Road, London SW19 7DT Tel: 020 8947 4916 — MB BS Lond. 1955 (Univ. Coll. Hosp.) Prev: SHO (Path.) Lewisham Hosp.; Ho. Surg. Roy. Hosp. Richmond; Ho. Phys. St. Mary Abbots Hosp. Kensington.

ROCHE, David Belmont Surgery, St James Square, Wadhurst TN5 6BJ Tel: 01892 782121 Fax: 01892 783989; 3 Eastfield Cottages, Tidebrook, Wadhurst TN5 6PF Tel: 01892 783310 — MB BS Lond. 1981; BSc Lond. 1977; DRCOG 1982; MRCGP 1986. Prev: Trainee GP Tunbridge Wells VTS.

ROCHE, David Walter (retired) 92 Arthur Road, Wimbledon, London SW19 7DT Tel: 020 8947 4916 — MB BS Lond. 1956 (St. Bart.) Prev: GP Lond.

ROCHE, Denis Arthur (retired) 44 Corbett Avenue, Droitwich WR9 7BE Tel: 01905 773956 Email: denis.roche@btopenworld.com — MB BS Lond. 1951 (Middlx.) DObst RCOG 1955; DTCD Wales 1966; DTM & H Liverp. 1976; DIH Dund 1980; AFOM RCP Lond. 1982. Prev: Internat. Med. Adviser Interserve Cyprus.

ROCHE, Donal Francis Ellis The Meadows Surgery, Temple Grove, Gatehouse Lane, Burgess Hill RH15 9XN Tel: 01444 242860 Fax: 01444 870496 — MB BCh BAO NUI 1979 (University College Dublin) MRCGP 1984; DRCOG 1986; MFHom 1989. Specialty: Gen. Med.; Homeop. Med.

ROCHE, John Desmond (retired) Eden Brook, Ivy Mill Lane, Godstone RH9 8NE Tel: 01883 742251 — MRCS Eng. LRCP Lond. 1951 (Middlx.) Prev: Gen. Pract.

ROCHE, Justin Southampton General Hospital, Tremona Road, Shirley, Southampton SO16 6YD Tel: 023 8077 7222; 23 Acorn Grove, Chandlers Ford, Eastleigh SO53 4LA — MB ChB Leeds 1996. SHO Rotat. (Paediat.) Soton. Gen. Hosp. Specialty: Paediat. Prev: SHO (Paediat.) St Mary's IOW; PRHO (Paediat. & Gen. Surg.) Leeds Gen. Infirm.; PRHO (Padeiatrics) St Jas. Leeds.

ROCHE, Mary Teresa West Norwich Hospital, Bowthorpe Road, Norwich NR2 3TU — MB BCh BAO NUI 1980; MRCP (UK) 1988. Staff Doctor (Med. for Elderly) W. Norwich Hosp. Specialty: Care of the Elderly. Prev: Regist. (Gen. & Geriat. Med.) Roy. Devon & Exeter Hosp.; Regist. (Gen. Med.) Walsgrave Hosp. Coventry.

ROCHE, Monica Emmet Renal Unit, Manchester Royal Infirmary, Oxford Road, Manchester M13 9WL; 37 The Fairway, Fixby, Huddersfield HD2 2HU Tel: 01484 420918 — MB ChB Manch. 1973. Prev: Clin. Asst. Renal Unit Manch. Roy. Infirm.; Med. Pract.(Family Plann.) Rochdale; SHO (Anaesth.) & SHO (O & G) Wythenshawe Hosp. Manch.

ROCHE, Nicola Anne Royal Free Hospital, Breast Unit, Pond Street, London NW3 2QG — MB BCh BAO Dub. 1989; FRCS Ed. 1993; MCh 1999; FRCS (Gen. Surg.) 2000. Cons. Breast & Gen. Surg. Roy. Free Hosp. Lond. Specialty: Gen. Surg.

ROCHE, Ruth Elizabeth The White Rose Surgery, Exchange Street, South Elmsall, Pontefract WF9 2RD Tel: 01977 642412 Fax: 01977 641290; The Copse, Bannister Lane, Skelbrooke, Doncaster DN6 8LU Tel: 01302 723068 Fax: 01302 728330 — MB BS Lond. 1987 (St. Thos. Hosp. Lond.) DRCOG 1990; DCH RCP Lond. 1990. Clin. Asst. P. of Wales Hospice Pontefract.

ROCHE, Shane William St Marys Hospital, Praed Street, London W2 1NY Tel: 020 7886 1077; 9 Meadow View, West Street, Harrow on the Hill, Harrow HA1 3DN Tel: 020 8426 9829 — MB BCh BAO NUI 1980; LRCPI & LM, LRCSI & LM BAO 1980; MRCP (UK) 1984; FRCP 1997. Cons. Med. for Elderly St. Mary's & St. Chas. Hosp. Lond. Specialty: Care of the Elderly. Prev: Sen. Regist. (Geriat.) St. Mary's Hosp. Lond.; Regist. (Neurol.) Char. Cross Hosp. Lond.

ROCHE, Professor William Robert Patrick Department of Pathology, University of Southampton, Southampton General Hospital, Southampton SO16 6YD Tel: 023 8079 6671 Fax: 023 8079 6603 Email: wrr@soton.ac.uk — MD NUI 1986; MSc (Path.) NUI 1981, BSc (Path.) 1980, MD 1986, MB BCh BAO 1978; FRCPath 1997, MRCPath 1988; FFPath RCPI 1990. Prof. (Pathol.) Univ. Soton.; Hon. Cons. (Path.) Soton. Univ. Hosps. NHS Trust. Specialty: Histopath. Prev: Sen. Lect. Path Univ. Soton; Vis. Investig. Kolling Inst. Med. Research, Roy. N. Shore Hosp. Sydney; Asst. (Path.) Univ. Coll. Dub.

ROCHESTER, Mr John Robert 59 Barholm Road, Sheffield S10 5RR — BM Soton. 1986; FRCS Eng. 1992; MD Sheff. 1995; FRCS (Gen) 1997.

ROCHETEAU, Marc Steven Department of Anaesthetics, The Calderdale Royal Hospital, Salterhebble, Halifax HX3 0PW — MB ChB Leic. 1987.

ROCHFORD, Frances Mary Margaret 12 Newland Park, Cottingham Road, Hull HU5 2DW — MB BS Lond. 1974 (Guy's)

ROCHFORD, John James The Surgery, Templars Way, Sharnbrook, Bedford MK44 1PZ Tel: 01234 781392 Fax: 01234 781468; Jubilee House, Odell Road, Sharnbrook, Bedford MK44 1JL Tel: 01234 782473 — MB BChir Camb. 1980 (Barts.) DRCOG 1983; MRCGP 1985. Gen. Practitioner, Bedfordshire.

ROCHFORT, Andree Mary Catherine Woodlands Surgery, 1 Greenfarm Road, Ely, Cardiff CF5 4RG Tel: 029 2059 1444 — MB BCh BAO Dub. 1987; BA, MB BCh BAO Dub. 1987; MRCGP 1991. Prev: Trainee GP S. Glam. VTS; Ho. Off. (Med. Surg.) St. Jas. Hosp. Dub.

ROCHOW, Stuart Blair Victoria Hospital, Hayfield Road, Kirkcaldy KY9 1LF Tel: 01592 643355 Email: stuart.rochow@faht.scot.nhs.uk — MB ChB Ed. 1985; MRCP (UK) 1990. Cons. Phys. Vict. Hosp. Kirkcaldy; Hon. Lect., Edin. Univ. Specialty: Gen. Med. Special Interest: Parkinsons Dis.; Stroke; Syncope. Socs: Brit. Geriat. Soc.; Brit. Soc. of Echocardiography. Prev: Sen. Regist. (Gen. & Geriat. Med.) Roy. Cornw. Hosp. Truro; Regist. (Geriat.) City Hosp. Edin.

ROCK, Clare Louise Theale Medical Centre, Englefield Road, Theale, Reading RG7 5AS; Englefield Road, Theale, Reading RG7 5AS — MB ChB Birm. 1992 (Birmingham) MRCGP 1997; DFFP 1997.

ROCK, Iain William 2 Hay Park, Birmingham B5 7LT — MB ChB Birm. 1991; ChB Birm. 1991.

ROCKALL, Andrea Grace The Middlesex Hospital, Martimer St., London W1T 3AA; 9 Jackson's Lane, Highgate, London N6 5SR — MB BS Lond. 1990 (King's Coll. Hosp. Med. Sch.) BSc (1st cl. Hons.) Lond. 1987; MRCP (UK) 1993; FRCR 1997. Sen. Regist. (Radiol.) Middlx. Hosp. Lond. Specialty: Radiol. Prev: Regist. (Radiol.) St. Mary's Hosp.

ROCKALL, Linda Jane Chestnut House, St. Georges Road, Worthing BN11 2DR Tel: 01903 239861 — MB BS Lond. 1971; MRCS Eng. LRCP Lond. 1971; DMRD Eng. 1975; FRCR 1977. Cons. Radiol. Worthing & Southlands NHS Trust. Specialty: Radiol.

ROCKALL, Mr Timothy Alexander 9 Jackson's Lane, Highgate, London N6 5SR — MB BS Lond. 1988 (GUYs Hosp.) FRCS Eng. 1992; MD Lond 1998; FRCS (Gen. Surg.) 1999. Higher Surgic. Trainee St. Mary's Hosp. Lond.

ROCKE, Mr Laurence Gilmore Department Accident & Emergency, Royal Victoria Hospital, Belfast BT12 6BA Tel: 01232 240503; 83 Gransha Road, Dundonald, Belfast BT16 1XQ Tel: 01232 481621 — MB BCh BAO Belf. 1971; FRCS Ed. 1975. Cons. A & E Med. Roy. Vict. Hosp. Belf. Specialty: Accid. & Emerg. Socs: Cas. Brit. Assn. Accid. & Emerg. Med. Prev: Cons. A & E Med. Mater Infirmorum Hosp. Belf.; Sen. Regist. (A & E) Roy. Vict. Hosp. Belf.

ROCKER, Michael Daniel 35 Grantham Road, London W4 2RT — MB BS Lond. 1994; BDS Lond. 1986.

ROCKER, Philip Benjamin County Hospital, North Road, Durham DH1 4ST Tel: 0191 333 3441; 31 Stobbart Terrace, Fishburn, Stockton-on-Tees TS21 4AF — MB BS Lond. 1981; MRCPsych 1988. Locum Cons. (Psychiat.) Co. Hosp. Durh. Specialty: Gen. Psychiat. Prev: Staff Grade (Psychiat.) Co. Hosp. Durh.; Staff Grade (Psychiat.) Highfield Day Hosp. Chester-le-St.; Regist. (Psychiat.) Winterton Hosp. SW Durh.

ROCKETT, Helena Elizabeth St John St Health Centre, Mansfield NG18 1RH — MB ChB Sheff. 1979; MFFP 1994; DCCH 1995. Sen. Clin. Med. Off. St John St Clinic Mansfield. Specialty: Family Planning.

ROCKETT, James William Westgate Practice, Greenhill Health Centre, Church Street, Lichfield WS13 6JL Tel: 01543 414311 Fax: 01543 256364 — MB ChB Birm. 1991.

ROCKETT, Mark Peter 33 Sellwood Road, Abingdon OX14 1PE — MB ChB Bristol 1993.

ROCKLEY, Peter Anderson The Gold Street Surgery, Gold St., Saffron Walden CB10 1EJ Tel: 01799 525325 Fax: 01799 524042 — MB ChB St. And. 1966.

ROCKLEY, Mr Timothy Joseph The Croft House, Station Road, Rolleston-on-Dove, Burton-on-Trent DE13 9AA — MB BCh Wales 1978; FRCS Eng. 1983; T(S) 1991; MD University of Wales 1999.

Cons. ENT Surg. Burton, Lichfield & Tamworth Hosp. Specialty: Otorhinolaryngol. Prev: Sen. Regist. W. Midl. Higher Surgic. Train. Progr. in Otolaryngol.; Research Fell. Univ. Toronto, Canada.

ROCKWELL, Susan Rosemary Portslade Health Centre, Church Road, Portslade, Brighton BN41 1LX Tel: 01273 422525/418445 Fax: 01273 413510 — MB BS Lond. 1987 (Char. Cross & Westm.) DRCOG 1991; DCH RCP Lond. 1991; LFHom (Med) 2001. PEC Mem. Brighton & Hove PCT.

ROCYN-JONES, James Rowland (retired) South Lawn, 18 Hermosa Road, Teignmouth TQ14 9JZ Tel: 01626 772031 — LMSSA Lond. 1937.

ROCYN-JONES, John (retired) Melville House, Ruardean, Gloucester GL17 9US — MB BS Durh. 1964 (Newc.) DObst RCOG 1966. Prev: Ho. Phys. Paediat. St. Woolos Hosp. Newport.

RODAN, Konrad S (retired) Squirrels, Kithurst Park, Storrington, Pulborough RH20 4JH Tel: 01798 742971 — MD Prague 1938; FRCPath 1963. Prev: Dir. Path. Worthing, Southlands & Dist. Hosps.

RODD, Caroline Dawn Highfield, Alexandra Road, Crediton EX17 2DZ — MB BCh Wales 1990 (Univ. Wales Coll. Med.) DCH 1993; FRCS Eng. 1996. Lect. Vasc. Surg. Char. Cross Hosp. Lond.; Specialist Regist. N. W. Thames Rot. Specialty: Gen. Surg. Socs: Affil. Assn. Surgs. GB & Irel.; Affil. Vasc. Surg. Soc.; Assoc. of Surg.s in Train.

RODDA, Louise Claire Mullion Cottage, Church Road, Chrishall, Royston SG8 8QT — MB BS Newc. 1997.

RODDAM, Philip Adrian Kirkside Elton, Stockton-on-Tees TS21 1AG — MB ChB Ed. 1987.

RODDEN, Nigel David 350 Castlereagh Road, Belfast BT5 6AE — MB BCh BAO Belf. 1995.

RODDICK, Jonathan Neil Woodseats Medical Centre, 4 Cobnar Road, Woodseats, Sheffield S8 8QB Tel: 0114 274 0202 Fax: 0114 274 6835; 19 Hoober Road, Ecclesall, Sheffield S11 9SF Tel: 0114 235 1766 Fax: 0114 235 1766 — MB ChB Sheff. 1986; MRCGP 1990; Dip Occupat Med 1998. GP Princip. Woodseats Med. Centre; Chairm. S.W. Sheff. PCG. Specialty: Gen. Pract. Prev: Occupat. Health Adviser S. Yorks. Police.

RODDIE, Alastair Ewan 81 Harpers Lane, Bolton BL1 6HU — MB ChB Leeds 1996.

RODDIE, Alison Mary Sherwood Department Medical Genetics, Churchill Hospital, Headington, Oxford OX3 7JL; Alscot Cottage, Alscot Lane, Alscot, Princes Risborough HP27 9RU Tel: 01844 343382 — MB BS Lond. 1981 (St. Bart.) MRCP (UK) 1985. Specialty: Genetics. Socs: Fell. Roy. Soc. Med.; BMA. Prev: Sen. Regist. (Clin. Genetics) Churchill Hosp. Oxf.; Clin. Research Phys. Lilly Research Centre Ltd. Windlesham; Regist. (Haemat.) King's Coll. Hosp. Lond.

RODDIE, Katherine Anne Willowfield Surgery, 50 Castlereagh Road, Belfast BT5 5FP Tel: 028 9045 7862 Fax: 028 9045 9785 — MB BCh BAO Belf. 1973; MRCGP 1978.

RODDIE, Mary Elizabeth Department Diagnostic Radiology, Charing Cross Hospital, Fulham Palace Road, London W6 8RF Tel: 020 8383 0147 Fax: 020 8846 1861 Email: mroddie@hhnt.nhs.uk; 11 Briar Walk, London SW15 6UD — BM BS Nottm. 1983 (Univ. Nottm.) BMedSci Nottm. 1981; MRCP (UK) 1986; FRCR 1989. Cons. Radiol. Char. Cross Hosp. Specialty: Radiol. Prev: Cons. Radiol. Kingston Hosp. NHS Trust; Cons., Sen. Regist. & Regist. (Radiol.) Hammersmith Hosp. Lond.

RODDIE, Patrick Huw Department of Haematology, Western General Hospital, Crewe Road, Edinburgh EH4 2XU Tel: 0131 537 1182 Email: huw.roddie@luht.scot.nhs.uk — MB ChB Ed. 1989; MRCPath 1997; PhD 2001; FRCPE 2003. Cons. Haem., Dept. Of Haemat., WGH, Edin. Specialty: Haematology. Socs: Brit. Soc. Haemat. Prev: Cons. (Locum) Haem., Dept. of Haemat., WGH, Edin.; Clin. Research Fell. John Hughes Bennett Laborat. Western Gen. Hosp. Edin.; Sen. Regist. (Haematolgy) Western Gen. Hosp. Edin.

RODDY, Edward 18 Hartlands Road, Eccleshall, Stafford ST21 6DW Tel: 01785 850168 — BM BS Nottm. 1997. SHO (Gen. Med.) Nottm. City Hosp. Specialty: Gen. Med. Prev: Primary Ho. Off. (Gen. Med.) Nottm. City Hosp.

RODDY, Richard James 61 Clewer Park, Windsor SL4 5HD — MB BS Lond. 1996.

RODECK, Professor Charles Henry University College London, Department of Obstetrics & Gynaecology, 86-96 Chenies Mews, London WC1E 6HX Tel: 020 7679 6060 Fax: 020 7383 7429 Email: c.rodeck@ucl.ac.uk — MB BS Lond. 1969 (Univ. Coll. Lond. & Univ. Coll. Hosp. Med. Sch.) FRCOG 1986, M 1975; BSc (Anat.) Lond. 1966, DSc (Med.) 1990; FRCPath 1994; FMedSci 1998. Prof. O & G Univ. Coll. Lond. Med. Sch. Specialty: Obst. & Gyn. Socs: (Ex-Pres.) Internat. Fetal Med. & Surg. Soc.; Hon. Mem. Brit. Assn. Perinatal Med.; Pres. Internat. Soc. for Prenatal Diag. Prev: Prof. O & G Qu. Charlotte's & Chelsea Hosp. Lond.; Dir. Harris Birthright Research Centre for Fetal Med. & Sen. Lect. & Cons. O & G King's Coll. Sch. Med. & Dent.; Resid. Off. Chelsea Hosp. for Wom. & Qu. Charlotte's Hosp. Lond.

RODEN, Ann Tyndall 27 Lankers Drive, Harrow HA2 7PA Tel: 020 8866 5944; 31 Downs Avenue, Pinner HA5 5AQ Tel: 020 8866 1148 — MB BS Lond. 1959 (St. Bart.) MRCS Eng. LRCP Lond. 1959. Craniosrect Therp. & Ayuruedic Lifestyle Adviser & Lect.; Cranio Sacral Therapist 1992; Fell. Fac. Community Health. Specialty: Paediat. Special Interest: Lifestyle Nutritian. Socs: Fell. Roy. Soc. Med.; BMA. Prev: SCMO Brent & Harrow HA; SCMO Harrow HA; Clin. Med. Off. Brent & Harrow AHA.

RODEN, Clare Eileen The Clarendon Surgery, 213 Burrage Road, London SE18 7JZ Tel: 020 8854 0356 Fax: 020 8855 5484 — MB BCh Wales 1963.

RODEN, David 97 Tapton Hill Road, Sheffield S10 5GB — MB ChB Sheff. 1995.

RODEN, Marian SmithKline Beecham, The Frythe, Welwyn AL6 9AR Tel: 01438 782513 Fax: 01438 782992; La Chebassiere, 79190 Lorigne, France Tel: 00 33 5 49271452 Fax: 00 33 5 49072643 — MB BS Lond. 1976 (Roy. Free) MA Oxf. 1974; MRCS Eng. LRCP Lond. 1976; AFOM RCP Lond. 1982. Occupat. Med. Dir. SmithKline Beecham Herts. Specialty: Occupat. Health. Prev: Med. Off. Nat. West. Bank plc.; SHO (Anaesth.) Addenbrooke's Hosp. Camb.; Ho. Phys. & Ho. Surg. Roy. Free Hosp. Lond.

RODEN, Rosalind Katrina Woodlands View, Street Lane, Leeds LS8 1DF — BM BCh Oxf. 1982; FRCS Ed. 1990. Specialty: Accid. & Emerg.

RODERIC-EVANS, Jane Elizabeth The Montpelier Surgery, 2 Victoria Road, Brighton BN1 3FS Tel: 01273 328950 Fax: 01273 729767; 29 Florence Road, Brighton BN1 6DL Tel: 01273 270565 — MB BS Lond. 1978 (Lond. Hosp. Med. Coll.) DRCOG 1982; DCH RCP Lond. 1983. Specialty: Psychother. Socs: Membership Soc. Analyt. Psychol.

RODERICK, Anthony Howard (retired) Winter Haven, Bovingdon Green, Marlow SL7 2JQ Tel: 01628 474262 — MB BS Lond. 1969 (St. Bart.) MRCS Eng. LRCP Lond. 1969; DObst RCOG 1972; DA Eng. 1976. Prev: Marlow GP.

RODERICK, Eleri Mai The Surgery, Caldbeck, Wigton CA7 8DS Tel: 01697 478254 Fax: 01697 478661 — MB BCh Wales 1979; FRCGP 1994, M 1983; DRCOG 1985. Princip. in Gen. Pract.; Chairm. Cumbia Pract. Research Gp.

RODERICK, John Morgan, MC (retired) Ridge Hanger, Rake, Liss GU33 7NN Tel: 01730 893177 — MRCS Eng. LRCP Lond. 1951 (St. Mary's)

RODERICK, Paul Julian c/o Health Care Research Unit, B Floor, South Academic Block, Southampton General Hospital, Southampton SO16 6YD Tel: 02380 796532 Fax: 02380 796529 — MB BS Lond. 1982; FRCP; FFPHM; MA Camb. 1979; MRCP (UK) 1985; MSc Lond. 1989; MFPHM RCP Lond. 1990. Sen. Lect. (Pub. Health Med.) Soton. Univ. Specialty: Pub. Health Med. Special Interest: Kidney Disease; Liver Disease; Screening. Socs: Renal Assn.; Amer. Soc. of Nephrol. Prev: Sen. Regist. & Cons. Pub. Health. Med. NW Thames RHA; Regist. (Haemat.) Roy. Free Hosp.

RODGE, Sally Louise Drayton Medical Practices, The Health Centre, Cheshire Street, Market Drayton TF9 3BS Tel: 01630 658208; Ashfields, Cuddington, Malpas SY14 7EL Tel: 01948 860334 Fax: 01948 860334 — MB BS Lond. 1986 (Middlx. Hosp. Lond. Univ.) p/t GP. Specialty: Gen. Pract.

RODGER, Alan Buchanan c/o Accident and Emergency Department, Dr Grays Hospital, Elgin IV30 1SN — MB ChB Aberd. 1985. Staff Surg. (A & E) Dr Gray's Hosp. Elgin. Specialty: Accid. & Emerg. Prev: Med. Adviser Shell Expro (UK) Ltd. Aberd.

RODGER, Anthony, CStJ Birchwood Surgery, 232-240 Nevells Road, Letchworth SG6 4UB Tel: 01462 683456 — MB BS Lond. 1951 (St. Geo.) MRCS Eng. LRCP Lond. 1951. Co. Surg. St. John Ambul. Brig.; Med. Off. Letchworth Hosp. Socs: BMA. Prev: Ho. Phys. St. Geo. Hosp.; O & G Ho. Surg. Roy. Vict. Hosp. Folkestone.

RODGER, Christopher James 3 Gardenside Street, Uddingston, Glasgow G71 7BY — MB ChB Glas. 1997.

RODGER, Elaine Margaret Elizabeth 34 Regent Road, Gosforth, Newcastle upon Tyne NE3 1ED Tel: 0191 213 0688 — MB ChB Ed. 1993; FRCA 2000. Cons. Anaesth., Sunderland Roy. Hosp., Tyne & Wear. Specialty: Anaesth. Socs: Assn. Anaesth.; Obst. Anaesth. Assn.

RODGER, George Neil (retired) Kirkbank, 28 Devon Road, Dollar FK14 7EY Tel: 01259 742868 — MB ChB Glas. 1972; DObst RCOG 1974. Prev: GP.

RODGER, James 120 Blythswood Street, Glasgow G2 4EH Tel: 0141 221 5858 Fax: 0141 228 1208; 3 Gardenside Street, Uddingston, Glasgow G71 7BY Tel: 01698 813763 Fax: 01698 811776 Email: jimrodger@btinternet.com — MB ChB Glas. 1972; BSc (Hons.) Glas. 1970; FRCGP 1988, M 1979; DMJ Soc. Apoth. Lond. 1982; BA Open 1987; FRCP (Ed.) 1997. Med. Adviser MDDUS; Police Surg. Glas. Socs: Assn. Police Surg.& Brit. Acad. Forens. Sc. Prev: Princip. GP & Assoc. Adviser Hamilton.

RODGER, Jean Christine 12A Kirklee Road, Glasgow G12 0ST — MD Glas. 1975; MB ChB 1961; FRCP Glas. 1978, M 1965; FRCP Ed. 1982, M 1965; FRCP Lond. 1982, M 1966. Cons. Phys. Monklands Hosp. Airdrie. Specialty: Gen. Med. Socs: Brit. Cardiac Soc.

RODGER, Kirsteen Anne 126 Main Street, Symington, Biggar ML12 6LJ — MB ChB Glas. 1993.

RODGER, Mary Wallace Glasgow Royal Infirmary, Castle Street, Glasgow G4 0SF; 4 Dargarvel Avenue, Dumbreck, Glasgow G41 5LD Tel: 0141 419 0446 Email: mary.rodger7@virgin.net — MB ChB Ed. 1983; DRCOG 1986; MRCOG 1991; MD Edinburgh 2000. Cons. (O & G) Glas. Roy. Infirm. & Glas. Matern. Hosp. Specialty: Obst. & Gyn. Prev: Regist. (O & G) Rottenrow Hosp. Glas.; Sen.Reg.O & G GRI GRMH.

RODGER, Robert Arthur Ri Cruin, 26 Strathmore Avenue, Dunblane FK15 9HX — MB ChB Dundee 1976.

RODGER, Robert Stuart Campbell 45 Manse Road, Bearsden, Glasgow G61 3PN — MB ChB Aberd. 1977; MRCP (UK) 1980; FRCP Glas. 1990; FRCP Ed. 1991. Cons. Nephrol. West. Infirm. Glas. Specialty: Nephrol.

RODGER, Sheena Nancy Gordon 44 Leven Road, Lundin Links, Leven KY8 6AH — MB ChB Dundee 1977.

RODGER, Susan Jane Nicolson Royal Aberdeen Children's Hospital, Department of Community Child Health, Westburn Road, Aberdeen AB25 2ZG Tel: 01224 551704 Fax: 01224 551750; 43 Woodburn Gardens, Aberdeen AB15 8JT — MB ChB Aberd. 1978. Assoc. Specialist (Child Health) NHS Grampian. Specialty: Community Child Health.

RODGERS, Alan 11 Keyes Gardens, Jesmond, Newcastle upon Tyne NE2 3RA — MB BS Newc. 1980; MRCP (UK) 1983. Cons. Phys. i/c Elderly Durh. HA. Specialty: Gen. Med. Socs: Brit. Geriat. Soc. Prev: Sen. Regist. (Gen./Geriat. Med.) Newc. HA; 1st Asst. Clin. Pharmacol. Univ. Newc.

RODGERS, Alan Douglas Department of Histopathology, North Tyneside General Hospital, Rake Lane, North Shields NE29 8NH — MB BChir Camb. 1980; BA Oxf. 1971; PhD Lond. 1976; BSc St. And. 1978; MRCPath 1988. Cons. Histopath. N. Tyneside Gen. Hosp. Specialty: Histopath.

RODGERS, Alison Anne 33 Gortnaskea Road, Stewartstown, Dungannon BT71 5NY Tel: 018687 38751 — MB BCh BAO NUI 1984 (UCD) DCH 1989; DObst RCPI 1990; MRCGP 1994. Sen. Med. Off. Tansen United Mission Hosp. (Box 126 Kathmandu) Nepal. Specialty: Gen. Pract.

RODGERS, Alison Joan Cumming Stockbridge Health Centre, 1 India Place, Edinburgh EH3 6EH — MB ChB Ed. 1973; MRCGP 1982.

RODGERS, Brian The Barn, Sodom, Bodfari, Denbigh LL16 4DU Tel: 01352 720036 — MRCS Eng. LRCP Lond. 1980 (Guy's) BSc, MB BS Lond. 1979; MRCPath 1988; FRCPath 1998; DMJ (Path) 2000. Cons. Histopath. Glan Clwyd Hosp.; Cons. Forens. Pathologist. Specialty: Pathology, General. Prev: Sen. Regist. (Histopath.) Arrowe Pk. Hosp. Upton.

RODGERS, Catherine Anne Lydia Clinic, Department of Genito-Urinary Medicine, St Thomas's Hospital, Lambeth Palace Road, London SE1 7EH Tel: 020 7928 9292 — MB ChB Liverp. 1989; BSc (Med. Cell Biol.) Liverp. 1985; Dip. GU Med. Liverp. 1993; FRCP (UK) 1993. Cons. in Genitourin. Med. & HIV Med. St. Thomas' Hosp. Lond. Specialty: Genitourinary Medicine. Prev: Sen. Regist. (HIV & Genitourin. Med.) St. Mary's Hosp. NHS Trust Lond.

RODGERS, Colin Principal's Residence, Stranmillis College, Stranmillis Road, Belfast BT9 5DY — MB BCh BAO Belf. 1983.

RODGERS, Colin James 6 Woodlands Mews, Knockmore Road, Lisburn BT28 2XS — MB BCh BAO Belf. 1991; DGM RCPS Glas. 1994; DCH RCPI 1995; DRCOG 1995; MRCGP 1996. Specialty: Gen. Pract.

RODGERS, David Andrew 18 Kalendra Court, Dungannon BT71 6EB — MB BCh BAO Belf. 1988; DRCOG 1991; MRCGP 1992; DCH 1993. Locum GP.

RODGERS, David Jon Old Grammar School, Ramsey Road, St. Ives, Huntingdon PE27 5BZ Tel: 01480 466466 — MB ChB Leeds 1969; MRCP (UK) 1974. Prev: Regist. (Gen. Med.) Sheff. Roy. Infirm.; Ho. Phys. & Ho. Surg. Gen. Infirm. Leeds; Research Asst. Dept. Surg. Guy's Hosp. Lond.

RODGERS, David Marcus Farnham Road Surgery, 301 Farnham Road, Slough SL2 1HD Tel: 01753 520917 Fax: 01753 550680; Woodpeckers, 6 Egypt Wood Cottages, Farnham Common, Slough SL2 3LE Tel: 01753 643563 — MB BS Lond. 1978; DRCOG 1982; MRCGP 1989. Specialty: Gen. Psychiat.

RODGERS, Elaine Margaret Suilven, Bridge End Lane, Prestbury, Macclesfield SK10 4DJ; Suilven, Bridge End Lane, Prestbury, Macclesfield SK10 4DJ — MB ChB Ed. 1984; BSc (Hons.) Aberd. 1976; FFA RCSI 1989; FCAnaesth 1990. Regist. (Anaesth.) Westm. Hosp. Lond.; Med. Adviser ICI Pharmaceut. Chesh. Specialty: Anaesth.

RODGERS, Fiona Marie Willowbrook Health Centre, Cottingham Road, Corby NN17 3HZ — MB ChB Leic. 1982; BSc 1977.

RODGERS, Frances Russell 40 Valleyview, Clovenfords, Galashiels TD1 3NG Tel: 01896 850643 — MB ChB Glas. 1969. Assoc. Specialist Psych. Lynebank Hosp. Fife; Clin. Asst. Psychiat. Dykebar Hosp. Paisley. Socs: BMA; L.D. Sect. Roy. Coll. Psychiat. Prev: Assoc. Specialist Psych. Borders Network Team Dingleton Hosp. Melrose; Clin. Asst. Psychiat. Dykebar Hosp. Paisley.; Assoc. Specialist Psych. Dykebar Hosp. Paisley.

RODGERS, Helen Department of Medicine (Geriatrics), The Medical School, University of Newcastle upon Tyne, Framlington Place, Newcastle upon Tyne NE2 4HH Tel: 0191 222 8025 Fax: 0191 222 6043 Email: helen.rodgers@newcastle.ac.uk; 5 Camp Terrace, North Shields NE29 0NE — MB ChB Leeds 1983; MB ChB Leeds. 1983; MRCP (UK) 1986; FRCP 1998. Sen. Lect. (Stroke Med. & Servs.) Univ. Newc. u. Tyne; Hon. Cons. Neurol. Roy. Vict. Infirm. Newc.; Hon. Cons. Phys. N. Tyneside Gen. Hosp. Specialty: Care of the Elderly; Neurol.; Gen. Med.

RODGERS, Helen Clare Respiratory Unit, Anne Fergusson Building, Western General Hospital, Crewe Road South, Edinburgh EN4 2XU Tel: 0131 5373 1783; Ardmeanach, 19 Orchard Road South, Edinburgh EN4 3NE Email: helen.rodgers@boltblue.com — MB ChB Leeds 1990; MRCP (UK) 1994; DM Nottm. 2002. Specialist Regist. Respirat. Med.; Cons. Respirat. Phys. Specialty: Respirat. Med. Prev: Research Fell. (Cystic Fibrosis) City Hosp. Nottm.; Research Fell. Cystic Fibrosis Respirat. Unit West. Gen. Hosp. Edin.; SHO (Neurol.) Qu. Med. Centre Nottm.

RODGERS, Henry Jack 12 Corstorphine House Avenue, Edinburgh EH12 7AD — MB ChB Ed. 1973.

RODGERS, Ian David Sefton Park Medical Centre, Smithdown Road, Liverpool L15 2LQ Tel: 0151 734 5666 Fax: 0151 734 1321; 42 Sunny Bank Road, Liverpool L16 7PW Tel: 0151 722 7357 Fax: 0151 734 1321 — MB ChB Liverp. 1962; DObst RCOG 1964. Prev: Clin. Asst. (Med.) Mossley Hill Hosp. Liverp.; Clin. Asst. (Surg.) Liverp. Homoeop. Hosp.; Cas. Off. Roy. Liverp. Childr. Hosp.

RODGERS, James Borders General Hospital NHS Trust, Melrose TD6 9BS Tel: 01896 754333 Fax: 01896 823476 Email: james.rodgers@borders.scot.nhs.uk; 40 Valley View, Clovenfords, Galashiels TD1 3NG Tel: 01896 850643 — MB ChB Glas. 1969; FRCS Glas. 1974; FRCP Glas. 2001. Cons. Palliat. Med. Borders Gen. Hosp. NHS Trust. Specialty: Palliat. Med. Prev: Med. Dir. P. & Princess of Wales Hospice Glas.

RODGERS, John Somerset (retired) Redhill Farmhouse, Chapel Lane, Barrowden, Oakham LE15 8EB Tel: 01572 747456 — (Camb. & Sheff.) MA, MB Camb. 1964, BChir 1963; MB ChB Sheff. 1963; DObst RCOG 1965; DPH Bristol 1967; FFCM 1981, M 1974; MA

Oxf. 1975. Cons. Pub. Health Med. N.ants. HA. Prev: SCM (Social Servs.) Oxon. AHA (T).

RODGERS, Lisbeth Jane The Surgery, Fox Lane, Barnburgh, Doncaster DN5 7ET Tel: 01709 892059 Fax: 01709 888744; 2 The Cottages, Green Lane, Skellow, Doncaster DN6 8JY — MB ChB Sheff. 1976 (Sheffield) DA Eng. 1981; MSc General Practice 1998. Specialty: Gen. Pract.

RODGERS, Lorna Mary — MB BCh BAO Belf. 1983; BSc (Hons.) Biochem. Belf. 1980; MRCP (UK) 1986; MRCGP 1990; FFOM RCP(UK) 2002. Cons. Occupat. Health Belf. City Hosp. Trust. Specialty: Occupat. Health. Socs: Assn. NHS Occupat. Phys.; BMA & Soc. Occupat. Med. Prev: Sen. Regist. (Occupat. Health) South. Health & Soc. Servs. Bd. N. Irel.

RODGERS, Martin Donative, Queen St., Oadby, Leicester LE2 4NJ — MB ChB Leic. 1983.

RODGERS, Martin Eric The Willows Surgery, Lords Avenue, Salford M5 5JR Tel: 0161 736 2356 Fax: 0161 737 2265; 32 Chatsworth Road, Eccles, Manchester M30 9DY Tel: 0161 789 7661 — MB ChB Ed. 1967.

RODGERS, Mette Ewing 2 Netherford Road, London SW4 6AE — MB BS Lond. 1987; MRCOG 1993.

RODGERS, Pamela Wrightington Wigan & Leigh Trust, Wigan Lane, Wigan WN1 2NN Tel: 01942 244000; 2 Maldon Road, Ashfield Park, Standish, Wigan WN6 0EX Tel: 01257 421288 — MB ChB Manch. 1979 (Manchester) FRCR 1985. Cons. Radiol. Wigan HA. Specialty: Radiol.; Nuclear Med. Socs: Roy. Coll. Radiol.; Manch. Med. Soc.

RODGERS, Peter John Abbey Surgery, 28 Plymouth Road, Tavistock PL19 8BU Tel: 01822 612247 Fax: 01822 618771 — MB BS Lond. 1986; MRCP (UK) 1991; DRCOG 1992; MRCGP 1996.

RODGERS, Peter Matthew 57 Guilford Road, Leicester LE2 2RD — MB BS Lond. 1981; MRCP (UK) 1986. Regist. (Radiol.) Univ. Hosp. Nottm. Specialty: Radiol. Prev: SHO/Regist. Rotat. Brighton Hosps.; Cas. Off. Guy's Hosp. Lond.; SHO (Med.) Morriston Hosp. Swansea.

RODGERS, Philip Frederic Ewing Church Street Surgery, Church Street, Spalding PE11 2PB Tel: 01775 722189 Fax: 01775 712164; 22 The Terrace, London Road, Spalding PE11 2TA — MB BCh BAO Dub. 1974; DRCOG 1978. Prev: Trainee Gen. Pract. Banbury Vocational Train. Scheme.

RODGERS, Mr Richard Thomas Boycott 63 Meadow Brook Road, Northfield, Birmingham B31 1ND Tel: 0121 476 0789 Fax: 0121 604 9315 Email: rodgers@charis.co.uk — MB BS Lond. 1970 (St. Bart.) MRCS Eng. LRCP Lond. 1970; FRCS Eng. 1981. Clin. Asst. Orthop. Birm. Childrs. Hosp. Specialty: Orthop. Prev: SHO (Gen. Surg.) Derbysh. Roy. Infirm. Derby; Regist. (Orthop.) Gwynedd; Regist. (Orthop.) Roy. Orthop. Hosp. Birm.

RODGERS, Robert Colin Whitegate, Broadwath, Heads Nook, Brampton CA8 9BA — MB BCh BAO Belf. 1979; MB BCh Belf. 1979; FFA RCSI 1986. Cons. N. Cumbria Acute Hosps. NHS Trust. Specialty: Anaesth. Prev: Hon. Lect. Clin. Anaesth. Aberd. Univ.; Regist. (Anaesth.) Aberd. Hosps.

RODGERS, Stephen Arthur Clifton Street Surgery, 15-17 Clifton Street, Belfast BT13 1AD Tel: 028 9032 2330 Fax: 028 9043 9812 — MB BCh BAO Belf. 1984; DRCOG 1988; MRCGP 1991.

RODGETT, Andrew Francis Mitcheldean Surgery, Brook Street, Mitcheldean GL17 0AU Tel: 01594 542270 Fax: 01594 544897 — MB ChB Liverp. 1977; DRCOG 1981. Bd. Mem. Forest of Dean PCG.

RODGMAN, Mary Elizabeth UBHT Community Child Health Services, 4th Floor, King Square House, King Square, Bristol BS2 8EF Tel: 0117 900 2350 Fax: 0117 900 2370 Email: mary.rodgman@ubht.swest.nhs.uk — (Roy. Free) MB BS Lond. 1970; DObst RCOG 1972; DCH Eng. 1972; MRCP (UK) 1975; MFFP 1993; FRCPCH 1997. p/t Cons. Paediat. (Community Child Health) United Bristol Healthcare NHS Trust; Hon. Sen. Clin. Lect. (Child Health) Univ. Bristol. Specialty: Community Child Health. Socs: Brit. Assn. Community Child Health; Assn. Research in Infant & Child Developm.; Brit. Assn. Study & Preven. Child Abuse & Neglect. Prev: SCMO (Child Health) United Bristol Healthcare NHS Trust.

RODIE, Vanessa Angela Queen Mothers Hospital, Glasgow — MB ChB Glas. 1997; MRCOG.

RODIN, David Andrew St. Helier Hospital, Wrythe Lane, Carshalton SM5 1AA Tel: 020 8296 2114/020 8296 2580 Fax: 020 8644 4377 Email: andrew.rodin@epsom-sthelier.nhs.uk; Maplehurst, 5 High View, Cheam, Sutton SM2 7DZ — MB BS Lond. 1981 (Univ. Coll. Hosp.) MRCP (UK) 1986; BSc (Hons.) (Biochem.) Lond. 1978, MD 1991; FRCP 2000. Cons. Phys. & Endocrinol. Epsom & St. Helier NHS Trust, Carshalton, Surrey; Hon. Sen. Lect. (Endocrinol.) St. Geo. Hosp. Med. Sch. Lond.; Sub-Dean (MBBS Cycle 2), St. Geo.'s Hosp. Med. Sch., Lond..; Chairm., Diabetes & Endocrinol. Speciality Train. Comm. & Regional Speciality Adviser for Diabets & Endocrin. S. Thames W. Specialty: Endocrinol.; Diabetes; Gen. Med. Socs: Soc. for Endocrinol.; Med. & Scientif. Sect. Diabetes UK; Sutton & Dist. Med. Soc. Prev: Clin. Lect. & Hon. Sen. Regist. (Endocrinol.) St. Geo. Hosp. Med. Sch. Lond.; Mem. Clin. Sci. Staff & Hon. Sen. Regist. (Endocrinol.) MRC Clin. Research Centre & Northwick Pk. Hosp. Harrow; Regist. (Gen. Med.) Hillingdon Hosp.

RODIN, Ian — BM Soton. 1989; MRCPsych 1994. Cons. Psychiat. Portsmouth Healthcare NHS Trust; Hon. Sen. Lect., Sch. of Postgrad. Med. Univ. of Portsmouth. Specialty: Gen. Psychiat.

RODIN, Marion Josephine Seyan, Saffar and Rodin, The Health Centre, Robin Hood Lane, Sutton SM1 2RJ Tel: 020 8642 3848 Fax: 020 8286 2010; Maplehurst, 5 High View, Cheam, Sutton SM2 7DZ Fax: 020 8286 1010 — MB BS Lond. 1982 (Univ. Coll. Hosp.) MRCGP 1986. Princip. GP Health Centre, Robin Hood La., Sutton, Surrey. Specialty: Gen. Pract. Prev: GP Fairbrook Med. Centre Borehamwood.

RODIN, Philip (retired) 115 Blackheath Park, London SE3 0HA Tel: 020 8852 8814 — MB BS Lond. 1954 (Lond. Hosp.) FRCP Lond. 1977, M 1965. Prev: Cons. Venereol. Lond. Hosp.

RODITI, Eric 22 Knoll Court, Farquhar Road, London SE19 1SP Tel: 020 8670 1225 — MB ChB Manch. 1954.

RODITI, Giles Hannibal Dept of Radiology, Glasgow Royal Infirmary, 16 Alexandra Parade, Glasgow G31 2ER Tel: 0141 211 4619 Fax: 0141 211 4781 — MB ChB Aberd. 1985; DMRD Aberd. 1991; FRCR 1992; FRCP Edin 1999. Hon. Sen. Lect. Uni. Glasg. Specialty: Radiol. Socs: BIR; Fell. RCR; Fell. RCRP of Edin. Prev: Sen. Regist. (Radiol.) Aberd. Roy. Infirm.; Lect. (Hon.) Univ. Aberd.

RODMAN, Rebecca 130 Birkworth Court, Offerton, Stockport SK2 5LS — MB ChB Sheff. 1998; MB ChB Sheff 1998.

RODRICK, Caroline Jane Karis Medical Centre, Waterworks Road, Edgbaston, Birmingham B16 9AL Tel: 0121 454 0661 Fax: 0121 454 9104; 27 Cartland Road, Kings Heath, Birmingham B14 7NS Tel: 0121 444 5595 — MB ChB Birm. 1991; ChB Birm. 1991; DTM & H Liverp. 1993; DRCOG 1996; DCH 1998. GP Regist. Birm. Specialty: Gen. Pract. Prev: SHO (Paediat.) Heartlands Hosp. Birm.; SHO (O & G) Solihull; SHO (Infec. Dis.) E. Birm. HA.

RODRICK, Ian Walker Windrush Surgery, 21 West Bar Street, Banbury OX16 9SA Tel: 01295 251491 — MB ChB Ed. 1966; DObst RCOG 1972.

RODRIGUES, Anthony James Stonehurst, 46 Garretts Green Lane, Birmingham B26 2HP Tel: 0121 743 3144 — MB BS Bombay 1937 (Grant Med. Coll. Bombay) Socs: BMA. Prev: Med. Off. Saudi Arabia Mining Syndicate & Lever Bros. (India) Ltd.; Bombay.

RODRIGUES, Camilla 31 St Andrews, Grantham NG31 9PE — MB BS Nagpur 1971; MRCOG 1987; FRCOG 2000.

RODRIGUES, Christopher Arthur Kingston Hospital, Galsworthy Road, Kingston upon Thames KT2 7QB — MB BS Poona 1978 (Armed Forces Poona India) MD (Med.) Chandigarh 1980; MRCP (UK) 1982; PhD Lond. 1991; FRCP 1998. Cons. Phys. Kingston Hosp. Surrey. Prev: Research Regist. St. Mark's Hosp. Lond.; Regist. (Med.) St. Mark's Hosp. Lond.; Sen. Regist. Guy's Hosp. Lond.

RODRIGUES, Erwin Alexander Aintree Cardiac Centre, University Hospital Aintree, Longmoor Lane, Liverpool L9 7AL Tel: 0151 529 2721 Fax: 0151 529 2724 — MB ChB Ed. 1977; MRCP (UK) 1979; FICA 1988; FRCP Ed. 1992; FESC 1993; FACC 1993; FRCP Lond. 1994. Cons. Cardiol. & Clin. Dir. Aintree Cardiac Centre & Univ. Hosp. Aintree; Clin. Lect. (Med.) Univ. Liverp.; Cons. Cardiol. BUPA Murrayfield Hosp. Wirral & Abbey Sefton Hosp. Liverp. Specialty: Cardiol. Socs: Fell. AM Coll. Cardiol.; Fell. Europ. Soc. Cardiol.; Brit. Cardiac. Soc. Prev: Sen. Regist. (Gen. Med. & Cardiol.) Broadgreen Hosp. Liverp.; Research Fell. (Cardiol.) Northwick Pk. Hosp. Lond.; Regist. (Cardiol. & Gen. Med.) Roy. Infirm. Edin.

RODRIGUES, Jennifer 15 Sunnygate Road, Grassendales, Liverpool L19 9BS — MB ChB Liverp. 1992. Specialty: Anaesth.

RODRIGUES, Kevin Francis Abbey Medical Centre, 63 Central Avenue, Beeston, Nottingham NG9 2QP Tel: 0115 925 0862 Fax: 0115 922 0522.

RODRIGUES, Mervyn John Paul 30B Northbrook Road, Ilford IG1 3BS — MB ChB Manch. 1987.

RODRIGUES, Norman Felix Bonifacio London Road Surgery, 501 London Road, Thornton Heath CR7 6AR Tel: 020 8662 8640 Fax: 020 8665 5011 — MB ChB Dundee 1987; DTM & H Lond. 1993. GP. Specialty: Gen. Pract.

RODRIGUES, Rene Joseph Charles The Health Centre, 1 Dunluce Avenue, Belfast BT9 7HR Tel: 01232 204247; 33 Broughton Gardens, Belfast BT6 0BB — MB BCh BAO Belf. 1972; DCH Dub. 1974.

RODRIGUEZ, John Martin 41 Bowlingfield, Ingol, Preston PR2 7DE Tel: 01772 734511 Fax: 01572 770538 — MB BS Lond. 1979 (St. Thos.) BA (Physiol. Sci.) Oxf. 1976; MRCP (UK) 1982; FRCR 1986; T(R) (CO) 1991. Managing Dir. Socs: Collegiate Mem. RCP; Fell. Roy. Soc. Med.; BMA. Prev: Dir. & Chief (Oncol.) Suleiman Fakeeh Hosp. Jeddah, Kingdom of Saudi Arabia; Dir. (Oncol.) Al-Hada Armed Forces Hosp. Al-Taif Kingdom Saudi Arabia; Sen. Regist. SE Lond. Cancer Centre & Roy. Sussex Co. Hosp.

RODRIGUEZ ARNAO, Javier Department of Endocrinology, St. Bartholomews Hospital, West SMmithfield, London EC1A 7BE; 80 East Dulwich Road, London SE22 9AT — LMS U Complutense Madrid 1987.

RODRIGUEZ CASTELLO, Cesar Sunnyside Royal Hospital, Hillside, Montrose DD10 9JP Tel: 01674 832261 Email: cesar.rodriguez@tpct.scot.nhs.uk; Renmure, Arbroath DD11 4RZ — LMS Valencia 1991; MRCPsych 1997. Cons. Old Age Psychiat. Tayside, Primary Care Trust, Sunnyside Roy. Hosp. Montrose. Specialty: Geriat. Psychiat.

RODRIGUEZ DE LA SIERRA, Luis 15 Highwood House, 148 New Cavendish St., London W1W 6YH Tel: 020 7580 5460 Fax: 020 7637 0070 — LMS Barcelona 1969; DNPsych Barcelona 1974; MRCPsych 2001. Socs: Brit. Psychoanal. Soc.

RODRIGUEZ GARCIA, Francisco Javier Dryburn Hospital, North Road, Durham DH1 5TW Tel: 0191 333 2333 — LMS Granada 1989.

RODRIGUEZ SANTOS, Javier Department of Obstetrics & Gynaecology, Crosshouse Hospital, Kilmarnock Road, Kilmarnock KA2 0BE — LMS Navarre 1990.

RODWAY, Alexander Dominic Flat 4, 101 Finsbury Pavement, London EC2A 1RS — MB BS Lond. 1998; MB BS Lond 1998.

RODWAY, Anne Elizabeth Pauline Chantry House Surgery, High Street, Sevenoaks TN13 1HZ Tel: 01732 457996 — MB BS Lond. 1968 (St. Mary's) MRCS Eng. LRCP Lond. 1968; DObst RCOG 1970. Socs: Fell. Med. Soc. Lond. Prev: Ho. Off. (Obst.) & Ho. Surg. & Ho. Phys. St. Mary's Hosp. Lond.

RODWELL, Nicola Anne Oakfield, Hither Chantlers, Tunbridge Wells TN3 0BJ — MB ChB Birm. 1992. Specialty: Gen. Pract.

ROE, Mr Alan Martin Department of Surgery, Southmead Hospital, Bristol BS10 5NB Tel: 0117 950 5050 Fax: 0117 959 5168; 21 West Dene, Stoke Bishop, Bristol BS9 2BQ — MB ChB Dundee 1977; FRCS Eng. 1982; FRCS Ed. 1982; ChM Bristol 1988. Cons. Gen. Surg. Southmead Hosp. Bristol. Specialty: Gen. Surg. Socs: Surg. Research Soc. & Brit. Soc. Gastroenterol.; Assn. Coloproctol. Prev: Sen. Regist. (Gen. Surg.) St Mark's Hosp. Lond.; Sen. Regist. (Gen. Surg.) Southmead Hosp. Bristol & Derriford Hosp. Plymouth.

ROE, Catherine Margaret Abraham and Partners, 21-23 Morden Hill, Lewisham, London SE13 7NN Tel: 020 8469 2880 Fax: 020 8692 9399; 27 Newstead Road, Lee, London SE12 0SY Email: lesfrancoisalee@aol.com — MB BS Lond. 1985 (The Royal London Hospital) DCH RCP Lond 1988; MRCGP 1990. Specialty: Gen. Pract. Prev: SHO (O & G) Lond. Hosp. Whitechapel; SHO (Paediat.) Newham Gen. Hosp.; SHO (Med.) Basildon Hosp.

ROE, Mr David Alan 61 Station Road, Gateacre, Liverpool L25 3PY — MB ChB Liverp. 1990; MB ChB (Hons.) Liverp. 1990; FRCS Eng. 1994; FRCS Ed. 1994. SHO (Gen. Surg.) Wythenshawe Hosp. Manch. Prev: SHO Rotat. (Surg.) S. Manch.

ROE, Francis John Caldwell (retired) 11B Raymond Road, Wimbledon, London SW19 4AD Tel: 020 8946 4518 Fax: 020 8947 9171 — (Oxf. & Lond. Hosp.) BM BCh Oxf. 1948; MA Oxf. 1950, BA 1946, DM 1957; DSc Lond. 1965; FRCPath 1967. Fell. (Vice-Pres.) Marie Curie Cancer Care. Prev: Reader (Experim. Path.) Inst. Cancer Research Roy. Cancer Hosp. Lond.

ROE, Joanna The Health Centre, Creebridge, Newton Stewart DG8 6NR — MB BS Lond. 1989.

ROE, Michael Felix Edward 10 Lodge Drive, Hatfield AL9 5HN — BM BCh Oxf. 1990; MA Camb. 1991; MRCP (Paediat.) Lond. 1995. Clin. Research Fell. Dept. of Paediat. Univ. Camb. Specialty: Paediat. Prev: SHO (Paediat.) Guy's Hosp. Lond.; SHO (Obst.) Univ. Coll. Hosp. Lond.; SHO (A & E & ITU) Roy. Free Hosp. Lond.

ROE, Paul Gerald Department of Anaesthetics, Addenbrooke's Hospital, Hills Road, Cambridge CB2 2QQ Tel: 01223 217434 — MB BS Lond. 1982 (Westm.) BSc Lond. 1979; FFA RCS Eng. 1988. Cons. Anaesth. Addenbrooke's Hosp. Camb. Specialty: Anaesth. Socs: Assn. Anaesth. Prev: Vis. Asst. Prof. Dallas (1991-92); Sen. Regist. (Anaesth.) Yorks. RHA; Regist. (Anaesth.) St. Geo. Hosp. Lond.

ROE, Peter Frank (retired) Kirkmead, Staplegrove, Taunton TA2 6AP Tel: 01823 284568 — MB ChB Ed. 1955; MA Camb. 1957; FRCP Glas. 1981, M 1962; MD Ed. 1969. Prev: Cons. Geriat. Som. HA.

ROE, Robert Bradley (retired) 9 Greens Lane, Wroughton, Swindon SN4 0RJ — (Oxf. & St. Geo.) LMSSA Lond. 1952; BM BCh Oxf. 1953; MA Oxf. 1953; DObst RCOG 1955; FFA RCS Eng. 1959. Prev: Cons. Anaesth. Princess Margt. Hosp. Swindon.

ROE, Sally Elizabeth The Whitecot, Park Avenue, Farnborough, Orpington BR6 8LL — BM BCh Oxf. 1978; MRCP (UK) 1980; FRCP Lond. 1994. Cons. Geriat. Qu. Mary's Hosp. Sidcup. Specialty: Care of the Elderly.

ROE, Simon David Nottngham Renal Unit, Nottingham City Hospital, Hucknall Road, Nottingham NG5 1PB Tel: 0115 969 1169 Fax: 0115 962 7678 Email: sroe2@ncht.trent.nhs.uk — MB ChB Manch. 1991 (Univ. Manch.) MRCP (UK) 1994. Cons. Nephrologist, Nottm. City Hosp. NHS Trust; Cons. Nephrologist, Sherwood Forest Hosps. NHS Trust, Mansfield. Specialty: Nephrol.; Gen. Med. Special Interest: Renal Bone Dis. Socs: Renal Assn. Prev: Regist. (Gen. Med. & Nephrol.) Derby City Gen. Hosp.; SHO (Gen. Med.) Trafford Dist. Gen. Hosp. & Roy. Preston Hosp.; Ho. Off. (Gen. Med.) Roy. Preston Hosp.

ROE, Yvonneke Olivia Walton The Nunhead Surgery, 58 Nunhead Grove, London SE15 3LY Tel: 020 7639 2715 Fax: 020 7635 6942; 26 Rollscourt Avenue, Herne Hill, London SE24 0EA — MB BChir Camb. 1982 (St. Thos.) MA Camb. 1983; DCH RCP Lond. 1985; DRCOG 1986; MRCGP 1989. Socs: BMA; BHMA; (Counc.) SMN. Prev: SHO (Gyn.) W. Middlx. Hosp. Lond.; Ho. Phys. St. Thos. Hosp. Lond.; Ho. Surg. Qu. Mary's Hosp. Sidcup.

ROEBUCK, Eric James (retired) Earleydene, 45 Private Road, Sherwood, Nottingham NG5 4DD Tel: 0115 960 9547 — MB BS Lond. 1954 (Charing Cross Hospital) DMRD Eng. 1960; FFR 1963; FRCR 1975. Cons. Radiol. Nottm. Univ. Hosps.; Regist. Roy. Coll. Radiol.

ROEBUCK, Harold Cornerways, Woolfall Heath Avenue, Huyton, Liverpool L36 — MRCS Eng. LRCP Lond. 1941 (Leeds) Prev: Ho. Surg. Gen. Infirm. Pontefract.

ROEBUCK, Paul David Sheringham Medical Practice, Health Centre, Cromer Road, Sheringham NR26 8RT Tel: 01263 822066 Fax: 01263 823890 — MB ChB Glas. 1986; DRCOG 1989; MRCGP 1995. Specialty: Gen. Pract.

ROEDLING, Ann Sherie 30B Prince of Wales Road, London NW5 3LG — MB BS Lond. 1998; MB BS Lond 1998.

ROEHR, Stephan Patrick c/o Dr P. Waugh, Coultershaw Farm House, Station Road, Petworth GU28 0JE — State Exam Med Bochum 1992.

ROEMMELE, Barbara Jane The Clinic, Buchanan Street, Balfrom, Glasgow G63 0TS Tel: 01360 440515 — MB ChB Glas. 1985; MRCGP 1990.

ROEMMELE, Mr Peter Michael (retired) Ballinahery, Limavady BT49 0PD Tel: 0150 47 62534 — MB ChB Ed. 1943; FRCS Ed. 1948. Prev: Cons. Staff Roe Valley Hosp. & NW Gp. Altnagelvin.

ROET, Brian Charles 2 The Mews, 6 Putney Common, London SW15 1HL Tel: 020 8780 2284 Fax: 020 8780 2347 — MB BS Melbourne 1962. Specialty: Psychother. Socs: Brit. Med. & Dent. Hypn. Soc.

ROEVES, Alastair John The Randolph Surgery, 235A Elgin Avenue, London W9 1NH — MB BS Lond. 1991.

ROFAIL, Mr Stephen Dimitri 18 Ticehurst Close, Worth, Crawley RH10 7GN — MRCS Eng. LRCP Lond. 1973; MB BS Khartoum 1972; T(GP) 1991; FRCSI 1991. Specialty: Gen. Med.

ROFFE, Terence Henry Halcyon, Station Lane, Farnsfield, Newark NG22 8LB Tel: 01623 882898 — (Lond. Hosp.) MB BS (Hons.) Lond. 1950. GP Farnsfield. Socs: Fell. Roy. Coll. Gen. Pract. Prev: Demonst. (Anat.) Lond. Hosp. Med. Coll.; SHO (Surgic.) ScarBoro. Hosp.; Ho. Surg. (Orthop.) Lond. Hosp.

ROFFEY, Marc 18 Daisy Bank, Lancaster LA1 3JW — MB ChB Cape Town 1987.

ROG, David Josef 2 Chester Close, Bletchley, Milton Keynes MK3 5JY — BM BS Nottm. 1996.

ROGAHN, Detlev Countess of Chester Hospital, Liverpool Road, Chester CH2 1UL Tel: 01244 365061 — State Exam Med Berlin 1988; MRCP Edin. 1995; FRCPCH Lond. 1997; M 1997. Cons. Paediat. Specialty: Paediat. Special Interest: Neonatology.

ROGAN, Edward (retired) 3 Beechfield Avenue, Blackpool FY3 9JE Tel: 01253 315763 — LRCPI & LM, LRCSI & LM 1952; DPH Bristol 1956.

ROGAN, Jacqueline Therese 45d Deramore Park, Belfast BT9 5JX — MB BCh BAO Belf. 1987; MRCGP.

ROGAN, Patricia Mary (retired) 3 Beechfield Avenue, Blackpool FY3 9JE Tel: 01253 315763 — MB BCh BAO NUI 1952; DPM Eng. 1976.

ROGAWSKI, Mr Karol, Marian Consultant Urologist, Royal Halifax Infirmary, Free School Lane, Halifax HX1 2YP Tel: 01422 357222 Fax: 01422 321087 — Lekarz Stettin, Poland 1980; FCS (S Afr) Urology 1990; FRCS (Urol) 1995; FRCS Ed 1996. Cons. Urol. Calderdale Healthcare NHS Trust Roy. Halifax Infirm. Specialty: Urol. Socs: Brit. Assn. Urol. Surgs.; Brit. Soc. Endocrinol.; BMA BMA. Prev: Cons. Urol. Dept. Urol. Johannesburg Hosp.

ROGER, Mark Douglas 65 West End, Redruth TR15 2SQ Tel: 01209 210333 — MB ChB (Hons.) Manch. 1996; MRCP (UK); BSc (Med. Sci.) St And. 1993. SpR (Radiology) Edin. Specialty: Gen. Med. Socs: BMA; Med. Sickness Soc.; MDU. Prev: SHO (Med.) Blackburn Roy. Infirm.

ROGERS, Adrian John Western Avenue Medical Centre, Gordon Road, Blacon, Chester CH1 5PA Tel: 01244 390755 Fax: 01244 383955 — MB ChB Manch. 1985.

ROGERS, Adrian Rudd Cranmere House, Trews Weir Reach, St Leonards, Exeter EX2 4EG Tel: 01392 258562 Fax: 01392 251917 Email: a@dradrianrogers.co.uk — MB BS Lond. 1972 (Guy's) MRCS Eng. LRCP Lond. 1972; DObst RCOG 1976; MRCGP 1978. Socs: Acad. of Experts, Exeter Med. Lega Soc.

ROGERS, Alan Llynfi Surgery, Llynfi Road, Maesteg CF34 9DT Tel: 01656 732115 Fax: 01656 864451; 28 Ystad Celyn, Maesteg CF34 9LT Tel: 01656 734610 — MB BCh Wales 1970; DObst RCOG 1972; MRCGP 1986. Course Organiser Bridgend VTS.

ROGERS, Alan David The Surgery, 1 Forest Hill Road, London SE22 0SQ Tel: 020 8693 2264 Fax: 020 8299 0200 Email: alan.rogers@gp-g85001.nhs.uk — MB BS Lond. 1960 (King's Coll. Hosp.) MRCS Eng. LRCP Lond. 1960; DObst RCOG 1962. Local Treasury Med. Off.; Chairm. S. Southwark PrimaryCare Gp.

ROGERS, Alison Mary Carlisle House, 53 Lagland Street, Poole BH15 1QD Tel: 01202 678484 Fax: 01202 660507 — MB ChB Liverp. 1987. Prev: GP Wirral Merseyside.

ROGERS, Andrew John Pendeen Surgery, Kent Avenue, Ross-on-Wye HR9 5AL Tel: 01989 763535 Fax: 01989 768288 — BM BCh Oxf. 1974; MA Camb. 1974; DRCOG 1977; MRCGP 1978. Socs: BMA. Prev: Trainee GP Hereford VTS; Ho. Off. Radcliffe Infirm. Oxf.; Ho. Surg. Hereford Co. Hosp.

ROGERS, Anne Katherine Jean Elm Surgery, Leypark Walk, Estover, Plymouth PL6 8UE Tel: 01752 776772 Fax: 01752 785108 — MB ChB Manch. 1975; DCH Eng. 1977; DRCOG 1978; MRCGP 1979.

ROGERS, Mr Anthony Crawford Nugent (retired) 5 Abercromby Place, Stirling FK8 2QP Tel: 01786 473948 Email: trogersstg@aol.com — MB ChB Glas. 1963 (Glasgow) FRCS Eng. 1969; FRCS Glas. 1969. Private Pract.; 2 Session/week, Lead Clinician Cancer Servs. Redesign Unit. Prev: Regist. (Urol.) Gen. Hosp. Newc.

ROGERS, Benedict Aristotle 38 Woodham Waye, Woking GU21 5SJ — MB BS Lond. 1997 (St. Georges) BA Oxf 1994, (Christ Church). GP Regis. Redhill; BASIC's doc. (Redhill.). Specialty: Gen. Pract. Prev: A & E SHO E. Surrey; PRHO St. Geo.s Hosp. Tooting; PRHO Frinley Pk.

ROGERS, Benedict James 4 Lisle Court Cottages, Lymington SO41 5SH — MB BS Lond. 1994.

ROGERS, Bernadette Harewood Crescent Surgery, Harewood Crescent, Littledown, Bournemouth BH7 7BU Tel: 01202 309500 — MRCS Eng. LRCP Lond. 1988; DRCOG 1994; DFFP 1994. GP Princip.; Clin. Asst. Dept. GU Med., Roy. Bournemouth Hosp., Bournemouth.

ROGERS, Brian Maclean (retired) The Swan Surgery, Swan St., Petersfield GU32 3AB — MRCS Eng. LRCP Lond. 1966; BSc (Zool. & Marine Zool., Hons.) Wales 1971; DObst RCOG 1971. Prev: SHO (O & G) Groote Schuur Hosp. Cape Town, S. Afr.

ROGERS, Caroline Blair 5 Richford St, London W6 7HJ Tel: 020 8749 7883 — MB BS Lond. 1993 (St. Bartholomew's) MA Camb.; DFFP 1995; DRCOG 1996; DGM 1997. GP Regist. N. End Med. Centre Lond. Specialty: Gen. Pract.

ROGERS, Cerilan National Public Health Service for Wales, Unit 1, Charnwood Court, Nantgarw, Cardiff CF15 7QZ; Glan Nant, 70 Cemetery Road, Porth CF39 0BL Tel: 01443 681050 — MB BChir Camb. 1981; MA Camb. 1982, BA 1978; DRCOG 1984; MRCGP 1989; MFPHM RCP (UK) 1995; FFPH RCP(UK) 2001. Director Nat. Pub. Health Serv. Wales. Specialty: Pub. Health Med. Prev: Dir. Breast Test Wales; Dir. Cervical Screening Wales; Cons. (Pub. Health) N. Wales Health Auth.

ROGERS, Christina 25A Arlington Park Mansions, Sutton Lane N., London W4 4HE — MB BS Lond. 1990.

ROGERS, Christina Margaret Anaesthetics Department, Hope Hospital, Stott Lane, Salford M6 8HD Tel: 0161 787 5107/8 Fax: 0161 787 4677 Email: christina.rogers@srht.nhs.uk — MB ChB Otago 1980; FFA RCSI 1989. Cons. Anaesth. (Obst. Anaesth. & Analgesia) Hope Hosp. Salford. Specialty: Anaesth. Socs: Assn. Anaesth. GB & Irel.; Obst. Anaesth. Assn.; Manch. Med. Soc. Div. Anaesth.

ROGERS, Christopher Evan 35 Carnation Drive, Winkfield Row, Bracknell RG42 7NT — BM BCh Oxf. 1983; T(R) (CR) 1992.

ROGERS, Clare Elizabeth 35 (IF3) Lutton Place, Edinburgh EH8 9PF — MB ChB Ed. 1994.

ROGERS, Mr Colin Anthony Queen's Hospital, Belvedere Road, Burton-on-Trent DE13 0RB Tel: 01283 566333 Email: colindodgy@aol.com — MB ChB 1981 (Godffrey Huggins Sch. of Med.) FRCS Edin 1989; MSc 1995. Cons. Breast and Vasc. Surg., Queen's Hosp., Burton on Trent. Specialty: Gen. Surg.; Surgery, Vascular. Socs: VSS; Roy. Soc. of Med.; BASO.

ROGERS, Daniel George Charles Burden Centre, Frenchay Hospital, Stapleton, Bristol BS16 1JB Tel: 0117 970 1212 Fax: 0117 965 4141; Cherry House, Frampton End Road, Frampton Cotterell, Bristol BS36 2LA Tel: 01454 773166 — MB BChir Camb. 1973 (Middlx.) MA Camb. 1974; MRCP (UK) 1976; MRCPsych 1982; MD 1998. Cons. Neuropsychiat. Burden Centre, Frenchay Hosp., Bristol. Specialty: Neurol.; Gen. Psychiat. Socs: Brit. Neuropsychiat. Assn. Prev: Raymond Way Lect. Neuropsychiat. Inst. Neurol. Lond.; Regist. (Psychiat.) Roy. Free & Friern Hosps. Lond.; SHO (Neurol.) Radcliffe Infirm. Oxf. & Maudsley Hosp. Lond.

ROGERS, David Alan 71 Madeley Road, London W5 2LT Tel: 020 8991 9365 — MB BS Lond. 1963 (Univ. Coll. Hosp.) MRCOG 1972, DObst 1965. Specialty: Family Plann. & Reproduc. Health. Prev: Regist. (O & G) Princess Margt. Hosp. Nassau, Bahamas.

ROGERS, David Andrew Great Bansons, Bansons Lane, Ongar CM5 9AR Tel: 01277 363028; 66 Glovers Field, Kelvedon Hatch, Brentwood CM15 0BD — MB BS Lond. 1987; BSc Lond. 1984, MB BS 1987; DCH RCP Lond. 1990. Prev: SHO (Gen. Med. & Geriat.) Thanet Dist. Gen. Hosp.; Trainee GP Thanet VTS.

ROGERS, David Charles The Surgery, 134 Baffins Road, Portsmouth PO3 6BH Tel: 023 9282 7132 Fax: 023 9282 7025; 134 Baffins Road, Portsmouth PO3 6BH — BM BS Nottm. 1981; BMedSci. Nottm. 1979, BM BS 1981; MRCGP 1985.

ROGERS, David John Flatt Walks Health Centre, 3 Castle Meadows, Catherine Street, Whitehaven CA28 7QE Tel: 01946 692173 Fax: 01946 590406 — MB ChB Leeds 1985; DA (UK) 1988; MRCGP 1990.

ROGERS, David John Orchard Surgery, Christchurch Medical Centre, Purewell Cross Road, Christchurch BH23 3AF Tel: 01202

481902 Fax: 01202 486887 — MB BCh Wales 1975; DRCOG 1979; MRCGP 1981.

ROGERS, David John de Sola 147 Beaufort Park, London NW11 6DA Tel: 020 8458 3177 — MB ChB Birm. 1970; FFA RCS Eng. 1980. Cons. Anaesth. IVF Unit Humana Hosp. Lond. Specialty: Anaesth. Prev: Sen. Regist. (Anaesth.) St. Mary's Hosp. Lond. & Research Dept.; Anaesth. RCS Lond.; Med. Off. St. Helena, S. Atlantic.

ROGERS, David Joseph Harry (retired) 40 Sherrardspark Road, Welwyn Garden City AL8 7LB Tel: 01707 324494 — MB BS Lond. 1947 (St. Bart.) MRCS Eng. LRCP Lond. 1947; DObst RCOG 1952; MRCGP 1960; AFOM RCP Lond. 1981. Prev: Resid. Anaesth. St. Bart. Hosp. Lond.

ROGERS, Deborah Ann Lizbeth Trelawny, 78 Riddlesdown Road, Purley CR8 1DB — MB BS Lond. 1993.

ROGERS, Deborah Jayne The Forensic Medicine Unit, St George's Hospital, Hunter Wing, Cranmer Terrace, London SW17 0RE — MB BS Lond. 1983.

ROGERS, Dorian Wynne Bryncelyn, High St., Pontardawe, Swansea SA8 4JN Tel: 01792 862776 — MB BCh Wales 1981; FFA RCS Eng. 1987. Cons. Anaesth. Morriston Hosp. NHS Trust Swansea. Specialty: Anaesth. Prev: Sen. Regist. (Anaesth.) St. Geo. Hosp. Lond. & Kingston Hosp.; Regist. & Research Regist. Univ. Hosp. of Wales Cardiff; Regist. Guy's, Brighton & E. Grinstead Hosps.

ROGERS, Duncan Paul Evans — MB BS Lond. 1989 (St Mary's) DRCOG 1994; MRCGP 1995.

ROGERS, Euphemia (retired) Funchal, 1 Preston Place, Gourock PA19 1LF Tel: 01475 631240 — MB ChB Glas. 1954; BSc Glas. 1945, MB ChB 1954; DA Eng. 1959. SHMO Argyll & Clyde Health Bd.; Mem. SHMO Working Party Lond. Prev: Anaesth. Inverclyde Roy. & Dist. Hosps.

ROGERS, Frances Anne Louise Shepperton Health Centre, Shepperton Court Drive, Laleham Road, Shepperton TW17 8EJ — MB BS Lond. 1983; MRCGP 1987; DRCOG 1987; (Fac. Of Homeopathy) LFHom 1999; MFHom 2002. Specialty: Homeop. Med.

ROGERS, Gary 10 Oxford Road, Dorchester-on-Thames, Wallingford OX10 7LX — MB BS Lond. 1985.

ROGERS, Gregory James Cornwall Gardens Surgery, 77 Cornwall Gardens, Cliftonville, Margate CT9 2JF Tel: 01843 291833 Fax: 01843 293126 — MB ChB Manch. 1983; MRCGP 1987; DRCOG 1987. Specialty: Gen. Pract. Socs: Christian Med. Fellowsh.; BMA.

ROGERS, Gwyneth Yvette West Bar Surgery, 1 West Bar, Banbury OX16 9SF Tel: 01295 256261 — (St. Georges) MRCGP; MB BS Lond. 1993; DCH 1996; DRCOG 1997; DFFP 1998. GP Princip.; Clin. Med. Off. (Family Plann.). Specialty: Gen. Pract. Prev: Trainee GP Horton Gen. Hosp. Oxf. VTS.

ROGERS, Helen Jane 37 Grange Avenue, Bangor BT20 3QF — MB ChB Sheff. 1987.

ROGERS, Mr Hugh Stephen West Middlesex University Hospital Trust, Twickenham Road, Isleworth TW7 6AF Tel: 020 8321 5440 Fax: 020 8565 5440 Email: hugh.rogers@npat.nhs.uk; 179 Waldegrave Road, Teddington TW11 8LU Tel: 020 8977 6110 Fax: 020 8977 0956 — MB BChir Camb. 1975; BA Camb. 1971; FRCS Eng. 1978. Cons. Urol. & Gen. Surg. W. Middlx. Hosp. Isleworth; Clin. Head, NHS Modernisation Agency (IPH); Hon. Cons. Urol. Hammersmith Hosps. Trust. Specialty: Urol.; Gen. Surg. Socs: Brit. Assn. Urol. Surgs.; Assn. Surg.; Founder Mem. Brit. Endurol. Assn. Prev: Clin. Dir. (Elective Servs.) W. Middlx. Hosp.; Sen. Regist. (Gen. Surg.) Roy. Free Hosp. Lond.; Sen. Regist. (Urol.) Roy. Lond. Hosp.

ROGERS, Mr Ian (retired) South Tynemeade Hospital, Harton Lane, South Shields; 46 Whitburn Road, Cleadon Village, Sunderland SR6 7QS — (Glas.) MB ChB Glas. 1967; FRCS Ed. 1972; MRCP (UK) 1973; FRCP Glas. 1985. Surgic. Dir. Gen. Surg. S. Shields Hosp.; Hon. Lect. (Surg.) Newc. Univ. Prev: Sen. Regist. Glas. Roy. Infirm.

ROGERS, James Brian (retired) Porters Hill Farm, Ladywood, Droitwich WR9 0AN Tel: 01905 452397 — (Liverp.) MB ChB Liverp. 1951; MRCS Eng. LRCP Lond. 1951. Prev: Clin. Asst. Newtown Hosp. Worcester.

ROGERS, James Edwin Guy Dept of Anaesthesia, Frenchay Hospital, Bristol BS16 1LE; Ayr Cottage, 13 Sutherland Place, Bristol BS8 2TZ — MB BS Lond. 1985; MRCP (UK) 1988; FRCA 1993. Cons. Anesthetist, N. Bristol NHS Trust.; Sen. Clin. Lect. Uni. Bristol. Specialty: Anaesth.

ROGERS, Janet — MB BCh BAO Belf. 1990; DRCOG 1993; DCH RCPI 1994; MRCGP 1995.

ROGERS, Jeremy Edward Medical Informatics Group, Computer Science Department, University of Manchester, Oxford Road, Manchester M13 9PL Tel: 0161 275 6145 Fax: 0161 275 6932 Email: jeremy@cs.man.ac.uk; 44 Mill Brow, Marple Bridge, Stockport SK6 5LW — MB ChB Manch. 1989; DRCOG 1993; DFFP 1993; MRCGP 1994. Clin. Research Fell. (Med. Informatics Gp.) Univ. Manch. Socs: Brit. Med. Informat. Soc. Prev: Trainee GP Sett Valley Med. Centre; SHO (Psychiat.) Stepping Hill Hosp.

ROGERS, Joanne Mary 17 Meadowside, Adlington, Macclesfield SK10 4PE — MB ChB Manch. 1990.

ROGERS, Mr John 32 Nottingham Place, London W1U 5NR Tel: 020 7486 1515 Fax: 020 7935 4984 Email: jrogers@gordcentre.org; 32 Nottingham Place, London W1U 5NR Tel: 020 7935 4645 Fax: 020 7935 4984 — MB BS Lond. 1979 (King's Coll. Hosp.) FRCS Eng. 1985; MD Lond. 1991. Consultant Surgeon; Hon. Cons. Surg. St. Helen's & Knowsley NHS Trust; Hon. Cons. Surg. St. Mary's NHS Trust & NW Lond.; Hosps. NHS Trust, ACAD-PCP Project. Specialty: Gen. Surg.; Gastroenterol. Special Interest: Laparoscopic Lap-band Anti-obesity Surg.. Prev: Cons. Surg. Acad. Surg. Unit Roy. Lond. Hosp.; Lect. & Sen. Regist. Acad. Surg. Unit Roy. Lond. Hosp.; MRC Research Fell. (Gastroenterol.) Centr. Middlx. Hosp. Lond.

ROGERS, John Howell The Surgery, Victoria Gardens, Neath SA11 1HW; 88 Cimla Road, Neath SA11 3UD — MB BS Lond. 1964 (Middlx.) Prev: Squadron Ldr. RAF Med. Br., Sen. Med. Off. RAF Innsworth; Unit Med. Off. RAF Akrotiri, Cyprus; Ho. Surg. Middlx. Hosp. Lond.

ROGERS, Mr John Humphreys 41 Druidsville Road, Liverpool L18 3EL — BM BCh Oxf. 1965 (Oxf. & St. Thos.) MRCS Eng. LRCP Lond. 1964; BA Oxf. 1958, MA, BM BCh 1965; DLO Eng. 1969; FRCS Ed. 1970; FRCS Eng. 1971. Cons. Surg. (ENT) Liverp. AHA (T); Aurist & Laryng. RNCM. Specialty: Otolaryngol. Socs: Liverp. Med. Inst. Prev: Lect. ENT Univ. Liverp.; SHO (ENT) Bristol Roy. Hosp.; Research Fell. in Laryng. Univ. Toronto, Canada.

ROGERS, John Michael 42 Haunch Lane, Birmingham B13 0PX — MB BS Lond. 1994.

ROGERS, John Neville The Central Hospital, Hatton, Warwick CV35 7EE Tel: 01926 491861 — MB ChB Leeds 1959; DPM Eng. 1968; MRCPsych 1972. Cons. Centr. Hosp. Warwick. Prev: Sen. Regist. Graylingwell Hosp. Chichester; Regist. Shenley Hosp. St. Albans.

ROGERS, Jonathan Charles Southmead Health Centre, Ullswater Road, Bristol BS10 6DF Tel: 0117 950 7100 Fax: 0117 959 1110; 20 Windsor Road, St Andrews, Bristol BS6 5BP Tel: 0117 924 7380 Fax: 0117 944 5498 — MB ChB Bristol 1978; DRCOG 1981; MRCGP 1983. GP; Chairm. GP Specialty Working Gp. Clin. Terms; Vice Chairm. Avon Local Med. Comm.; Med. Adviser AAH Meditel. Prev: Sec. Avon Local Med. Comm.

ROGERS, Jonathan David Chawton House, St. Thomas St., Lymington SO41 9ND Tel: 01590 673063 — BChir Camb. 1965; MB 1966.

ROGERS, Jonathan Huw Price 34 Cherry Tree Road, The Bryn, Pontllanfraith, Blackwood NP12 2PY — MB BS Lond. 1993.

ROGERS, Julian Mark Courtenay Esplanade Surgery, 19 Esplanade, Ryde PO33 2EH Tel: 01983 813600 Fax: 01983 813609 — MB BS Lond. 1979; DA Eng. 1982; DRCOG 1984; MRCGP 1985; D.OCC.Med 2000.

ROGERS, Kathleen Anne (retired) 21 Broomieknowe Park, Bonnyrigg EH19 2JB Tel: 0131 660 1295 — MB ChB Glas. 1975. Prev: Occupat. Health Phys. Roy. Vict. Hosp. Edin.

ROGERS, Keith Bernard (retired) 12 Church Mount, London N2 0RP Tel: 020 8458 1956 — MD Lond. 1948 (St. Mary's) MRCS Eng., LRCP Lond. 1934; MB BS 1935; FRCPath 1963. Prev: Maj. RAMC, Path. Specialist.

ROGERS, Keith Llewellyn (retired) Farthings, The Rise, Tadworth KT20 5QT Tel: 01737 361312 — MB BS Lond. 1954 (Middlx.) MRCPath 1964. Prev: Dir. S. Lond. Blood Transfus. Centre Tooting.

ROGERS, Keith Main Pain Management Clinic, Gartnavel General Hospital, Glasgow G11 0YN Tel: 0141 334 8122; 7 Dargarvel Avenue, Dumbreck, Glasgow G41 5LD Tel: 0141 427 0853 —

(Glasgow University) BSc (1st cl. Hons. Pharmacol.) Glas. 1964, MB ChB 1972; DObst RCOG 1975; FFA RCS Eng. 1977. Cons. Anaesth. West. Infirm. Glas.; Hon. Clin. Sen. Lect. Univ. Glas. Specialty: Anaesth. Socs: Assn. Anaesth., Pain Soc. & Anaesth. Res. Soc. Prev: Sandoz Res. Fell. Dept. Mat. Med. Glas. Univ.; Regist. (Anaesth.) Glas. Roy. Infirm.; Sen. Regist. (Anaesth.) Glas. West. Infirm.

ROGERS, Professor Kenneth Plymouth Postgraduate Medical School, Derriford Hospital Level 7, Plymouth PL6 8DH Tel: 01752 782711 Fax: 01752 763531 — MB ChB Bristol 1969; MSc Birm. 1973; FRCS Eng. 1977; MD Sheff. 1989. Dean & Hon. Cons. Surg. Postgrad. Med. Sch. Derriford Hosp. Plymouth. Specialty: Gen. Surg. Socs: Brit. Assn. Surg. Oncol. & Assn. Surg. GB & Irel.; Surg. Research Soc. Prev: Prof. Surg. Univ. Sheff.; Lect. (Surg.) Welsh Nat. Sch. Med.; Regist. (Surg.) Worcester Roy. Infirm.

ROGERS, Lesley Anne Northwick Surgery, 36 Northwick Park Road, Harrow HA1 2NU Tel: 020 8427 1661; 29 Fisher Road, Harrow Weald, Harrow HA3 7JX Tel: 020 8424 0979 — MB ChB Ed. 1985; DRCOG 1987; MRCGP 1990. Med. Examr. Benefits Agency Med. Servs. Lond.; Asst. GP Harrow Retainer Scheme. Specialty: Civil Serv. Prev: Princip. GP Overdale Med. Pract. Derbysh.

ROGERS, Madeline Jane Asplands Medical Centre, Wood St., Woburn Sands, Milton Keynes MK17 8QP Tel: 01908 582069; 32 Station Road, Woburn Sands, Milton Keynes MK17 8RW Tel: 01908 583670 — MB ChB Sheff. 1977; DRCOG 1980.

ROGERS, Mark Alan 15 Mereway, Swanland, North Ferriby HU14 3QB — MB ChB Dundee 1995.

ROGERS, Mr Mark John Mid Yorkshire Hospitals NHS Trust, Pinderfields Hospital, Aberford Road, Wakefield WF1 4EE Tel: 01924 232272 Fax: 01924 213704; 38 Annandale Road, Kirk Ella, Hull HU10 7UU — MB ChB Leeds 1985; BSc Leeds 1982; FRCS Eng. 1991; FRCS Gen. 1996. Cons. (Gen. & Colorectal Surg.) Mid Yorksh. Hosps. NHS Trust. Specialty: Gen. Surg. Socs: BMA; Assn. Surg. GB & Irel.; Assn. Coloproctol. GB & Irel.

ROGERS, Mark John — MB ChB Bristol 1998.

ROGERS, Mark Simon Sutherland The Crookes Practice, 203 School Road, Sheffield S10 1GN Tel: 0114 266 0677 Fax: 0114 266 4526 — MB ChB Leeds 1993.

ROGERS, Mark Thomas Institute of Medical Genetics, University Hospitals of Wales, Heath Park, Cardiff CF14 4XN Tel: 029 2074 4022 Fax: 029 2074 7603 Email: rogersmt@cardiff.ac.uk; 4 Mitre Place, Llandaff, Cardiff CF5 2EQ Tel: 029 2056 1324 — MB BS Lond. 1984 (St. Thos.) DRCOG 1989; DCH RCP Lond. 1989; MRCGP 1990; MRCP (UK) 1995. Specialist Regist. (Clin. Genetics) Univ. Hosp. of Wales Cardiff. Specialty: Genetics. Socs: BMA; Brit. Soc. Human Genetics; Clin. Genetics Soc. Prev: Muscular Dystrophy Gp. Clin. Research Fell. (Research Regist. Med. Genetics) Univ. Wales Coll. Med. Cardiff; GP Oxf.; Trainee GP Aberystwyth VTS.

ROGERS, Martin Christopher Elm Cottage, Etchingwood, Buxted, Uckfield TN22 4PT — MB BS Lond. 1997; DRCOG 2000. GP Principal, Heathfield, E.Sussex. Specialty: Gen. Pract. Prev: GP Trainee, Hastings &Rother NHSTrust.

ROGERS, Martyn John Church Street Partnership, 30A Church Street, Bishop's Stortford CM23 2LY Tel: 01279 657636 Fax: 01279 505464; 54 Penningtons, Bishop's Stortford CM23 4LF Tel: 01279 657636 — MB BS Lond. 1982 (St Bartholomews Hospital London) MSc Lond. 1985; DRCOG 1987; MRCGP 1988; Dip Med Acupunc 1998; DFFP 1998.

ROGERS, Michael (retired) 42 Manor Road, Folksworth, Peterborough PE7 3SU Tel: 01733 241451 — MB ChB Dundee 1971; DObst RCOG 1974. Prev: Retd. Gen. Practitioner, Yaxley Gp. Pract., Yaxley, PeterBoro..

ROGERS, Michael Anthony Llynfi Surgery, Llynfi Road, Maesteg CF34 9DT Tel: 01656 732115 Fax: 01656 864451; 3 Nicholls Road, Coytrahen, Bridgend CF32 0EP — MB BCh Wales 1979; MRCGP 1983.

ROGERS, Michael Geoffrey Howden Department of Community Child Health, Alder Hey Children's Hospital, Eaton Road, Liverpool L12 2AP Tel: 0151 228 4811 Fax: 0151 252 5120; 3 Dene Cottages, Great Budworth, Northwich CW9 6HB Tel: 01606 891966 — MB BChir Camb. 1964 (Westm.) MA, MB Camb. 1964, BChir 1963; DCH Eng. 1965; DPH Lond. 1967. Sen. Lect. (Community Child Health) Univ. Liverp.; Hon. Cons. Community Paediat. Liverp. HA. Specialty: Community Child Health. Socs: Brit. Paediat. Assn. & Brit. Assn. Comm. Child Health.; Fell. Roy. Coll. of Paediat. and Child Health. Prev: Cons. Community Paediat. Macclesfield HA.

ROGERS, Michael Harvey High House, Ballinger Road, South Heath, Great Missenden HP16 9QJ — MB ChB Birm. 1953; DObst RCOG 1964; MFCM 1974; AFOM RCP Lond. 1979. Prev: Princip. Med. Off. Jt. H.Q. RAF Germany; CO RAF Hosp. Wegberg; Sen. Ho. Phys. & Obst. Ho. Surg. Manor Hosp. Walsall.

ROGERS, Moira Elizabeth Biel Mill Lodge, Dunbar EH42 1SY — MB ChB Dundee 1983. Clin. Asst. (Ophth.) St John's Hosp. Livingston W. Lothian.

ROGERS, Neil Kingsley 24 Fulney Road, Sheffield S11 7EW Tel: 0114 230 2093 — BM BCh Oxf. 1989; BSc York 1981; DPhil Oxf. 1984, BM BCh 1989; FRCOphth 1994. Cons. Ophth., Tashkent Med. Paediat. Inst., Tashkent, Uzbekistan. Specialty: Ophth. Prev: Sen. Regist. (Ophth.) Roy. Hallamsh. Hosp. Sheff.

ROGERS, Mr Norman Charles, Maj.-Gen. late RAMC Retd. (retired) 110 Mill Street, Kidlington OX5 2EF — MB BS Lond. 1939 (St. Bart.) MRCS Eng. LRCP Lond. 1939; FRCS Eng. 1949. Prev: Hon. Surg. to HM the Qu.

ROGERS, Pamela Marion 110 Mill Street, Kidlington OX5 2EF — MB ChB Birm. 1953; AFOM RCP Lond. 1982. Cons. Occupational Health Phys., Oxon. Ment. Healthcare NHS Trust; Gp. Med. Adviser Tate & Lyle plc. Socs: BMA & Soc. Occupat. Med. Prev: Occupat. Health Phys. Guy's & St. Thos. NHS Trust; Med. Off. Nurses Health Serv. & Occupat. Health Serv. Guy's Hosp. Lond.

ROGERS, Paul Bryan Berkshire Cancer Centre, Royal Berkshire Hospital, London Road, Reading RG1 5AN Tel: 0118 987 5111; 70 Westwood Drive, Little Chalfont, Amersham HP6 6RW — MB BS Lond. 1989; MRCP (UK) 1993; FRCR 1996. Cons., Clin. Oncol., Berks. Cancer centre, Roy. Berks. Hosp. Reading; Sen. Specialist Regist., Clin. Oncol., St. Batholomews Hosp.& Mt. Vernon; Vis. Worker: MRC Cell Mutation Unit, Brighton, Sussex. Specialty: Oncol.; Radiother. Socs: Amer. Soc. Clin. Oncol.; Eur. Soc. Therap. Radiol. & Oncol.; Brit. Oncol. Assn. Prev: Regist. Rotat. (Radiother. & Oncol.) Roy. Free Hosp., Middlx. Hosp. & Mt. Vernon Hosp.; SHO Rotat. (Med.) Stoke Mandeville Hosp. Aylesbury; SHO Rotat. (Radiother. & Oncol.) Mt. Vernon Hosp. & Char. Cross Hosp. Lond.

ROGERS, Paul Haydon (retired) 3A Watery Lane, Nether Heyford, Northampton NN7 3LN Tel: 01327 340126 — MB BChir Camb. 1943 (Camb. & Lond. Hosp.) FRCP Lond. 1973, M 1948; DPM Eng. 1955; FRCPsych 1974, M 1971. Prev: Cons. Psychiat. & Med. Dir. St. Crispin Hosp. Northampton.

ROGERS, Paul Nicholas 35 Spenbeck Drive, Allestree, Derby DE22 2UH — MB ChB Dundee 1994.

ROGERS, Mr Paul Noel Gartnavel General Hospital, Great Western Road, Glasgow G12 0YN — MB ChB Glas. 1977; FRCS Glas. 1981; MD Glas. 1988; MBA Open 1995. Cons. Gen. Surg. Gartnavel Gen. Hosp. Glas.; Hon. Clin. Sen. Lect. Univ. Glas. Specialty: Gen. Surg.

ROGERS, Paul Thomas College Health Centre, Geography Building, Queen Mary University of London, London E1 4NS Tel: 020 6622 4450; 16 Eltringham Street, Wandsworth, London SW18 1TE — MB BS Lond. 1984; BSc Lond. 1981; DRCOG 1988; Cert. Family Plann. JCC 1988. GP Non-Princ. Tower Hamlets. Specialty: Gen. Pract. Prev: GP Lond.

ROGERS, Paula Jane 9 Pickersleigh Road, Malvern WR14 2RP — MB ChB Liverp. 1992.

ROGERS, Peter Derek St Mary's Hospital, Department of Pain Medicine, Milton, Portsmouth PO3 6AD Tel: 023 9228 6000 Fax: 023 9286 6388 Email: peter.rogers@porthosp.nhs.uk — MB BS Lond. 1974 (Westm.) LRCP; FRCA; DA Eng. 1977. Cons. Anaesth. & Pain Managem., Portsmouth; Clin. Director Dept. of Pain Med.; Chairm. Wessex Pain Gp.; Cons. (anaesth.) Qu. Alexandra Hosp. Portsmouth. Specialty: Anaesth. Special Interest: Back & Neck Pain; Neuropathic Pain; Shoulder Pain. Socs: Internat. Assn. Study of Pain; Brit. Pain Soc.; Internat. Neuromodulation Soc.

ROGERS, Philip Peter 32 The Old Mill, Hillsborough BT26 6RA — MB BCh BAO Belf. 1996.

ROGERS, Rebecca 40 Manor Farm Close, Lympne, Hythe CT21 4EG Email: becca_rogers@yahoo.com — MB ChB Birm. 2001. GP trainee.

ROGERS, Richard Department of Anaesthetics, John Radcliffe Hospital, Headley Way, Oxford OX3 9DU Tel: 01865 741166; The Cottage, The Green, Cassington, Witney OX29 4DW Tel: 01865

881322 — MB BS Lond. 1987; BA Oxf. 1981; FRCA. 1992. Cons. Paediat. Anaesth. John Radcliffe Hosp. Oxf. Specialty: Anaesth. Prev: Sen. Regist. (Anaesth.) Gt. Ormond St. Hosp. for Childr. & St. Geos. Hosp. & St. Peter's Chertsey, St. Geo. Hosp. Lond. & Hosp. for Childr. Gt. Ormond St. Lond.; Regist. Rotat. (Anaesth.) Guildford, St. Heliers Hosp. Carshalton & St. Geo. Hosp. Lond.; SHO Rotat. (Anaesth.) Lewisham & Guy's Hosps. Lond.

ROGERS, Richard Thomas Neave Abbey Medical Centre, 63 Central Avenue, Beeston, Nottingham NG9 2QP Tel: 0115 925 0862 Fax: 0115 922 0522 — MB ChB Leic. 1983.

ROGERS, Robert Samuel Boulderson (retired) 1 Royal Crescent, Cheltenham GL50 3DB Tel: 01242 521070; Treetops, Prestbury, Cheltenham GL52 3BB — MB BS Lond. 1952; DObst RCOG 1955.

ROGERS, Sally Joy Katharine House Hospice, East End, Adderbury, Banbury OX17 3N Tel: 01295 811866; The Retreat, Chapel Lane, Stoke Bruerne, Towcester NN12 7SQ — MB BS Lond. 1980; MRCGP 1986; DRCOG 1988; Dip. Palliat. Med. 1998. Assoc. Specialist (Palliat. Med.) Katharine Ho. Hospice Banbury. Specialty: Palliat. Med.

ROGERS, Sinead Mary Harlestone Road Surgery, 117 Harlestone Road, Northampton NN5 7AQ Tel: 01604 751832 Fax: 01604 586065; 20 Church Street, Weedon, Northampton NN7 4PL Tel: 01327 340521 — MB BS Lond. 1992 (UMDS (GUYS)) DRCOG 1995; MRCGP 1996; DFFP 1996. Princip. GP, Dr Gill & Partners, N.hampton. Specialty: Gen. Pract.

ROGERS, Stephen 21 The Walk, Hengoed CF82 7AH — MB BCh Wales 1982.

ROGERS, Stephen Andrew Moordown Medical Centre, 2A Redhill Crescent, Bournemouth BH9 2XF Tel: 01202 516139 Fax: 01202 548525 — MB ChB Birm. 1977; DRCOG 1981; MRCGP 1984.

ROGERS, Stephen James 29 Kendalls Close, High Wycombe HP13 7NN — MB BS Tasmania 1987.

ROGERS, Stephen Young Fife Area Laboratory, Hayfield Road, Kirkcaldy KY2 5AG Tel: 01592 643355 Fax: 01592 647037 Email: stephen.rogers@faht.scot.nhs.uk; 2 Telny Place, Aberdour, Burntisland KY3 0TG — MB BS Newc. 1983; BA Camb. 1980; MRCP (UK) 1986; MRCPath 1992; FRCP Ed. 1996. Cons. Haemat. Vict. Hosp. Kirkcaldy; Hon. Sen. Lect. Edin. Univ.; Hon. Sen. Lect. St Andrews Univ. Specialty: Haematology. Prev: Lect. (Haemat.) Univ. Nottm.

ROGERS, Susan Diana 42 Manor Road, Folksworth, Peterborough PE7 3SU Tel: 01733 241451 Email: mikeandsue@folksworth42.fsnet.co.uk — MB ChB Dundee 1972 (Univ. Dundee) Prev: Clin. Asst. Wansford.

ROGERS, Susan Pamela 119 Markwell Road, Parsloe Road, Harlow CM19 5QU — MB BS Lond. 1990.

ROGERS, Suzanne Department of Pathology, Doncaster Royal Infirmary, Armthorpe Road, Doncaster DN2 5LT Tel: 01302 366666 Fax: 01302 553264 — MB ChB Bristol 1987; BSc Cellular Path. Bristol 1984; MRCPath 1994. Cons. Histopath. Doncaster Roy. Infirm. Specialty: Histopath. Prev: Lect. (Path.) Sheff. Univ.

ROGERS, Professor Thomas Richard Frazer Department of Infectious Diseases & Microbiology, Imperial College School of Medicine, Hammersmith Campus, Ducane Road, London W12 0NN Tel: 0208 383 3224 Fax: 0208 383 3394 — LRCPI & LM, LRSCI & LM 1972; LRCPI & LM, LRCSI & LM 1972; FRCPath 1990, M 1978; MSc Lond. 1979; FRCPI 1987, M 1985; MA (Med. Law & Ethics) 1994. Prof. Univ. Lond.; Hon. Cons. Hammersmith Hosps. Trust. Specialty: Pathology, General; Med. Microbiol. Socs: Assn. Clin. Path.; Fell. Roy. Soc. Med.; Hosp. Infec. Soc. (Chairm. 97-98). Prev: Sen. Lect. (Med. Microbiol.) Char. Cross & Westm. Med. Sch. Lond.

ROGERS, Timothy Alexander Manor Surgery, Forth Noweth, Chapel Street, Redruth TR15 1BY Tel: 01209 313313 Fax: 01209 313813 — MB BS Lond. 1975 (Westm.) MRCS Eng. LRCP Lond. 1975; DRCOG 1978; FRCGP 1993, M 1980; PGcert Ed. 2001.

ROGERS, Timothy David Herdmanflat, Aberlady Road, Haddington EH41 3BU Tel: 0131 536 8300 — MB ChB Aberd. 1983; MRCPsych 1988; MPhil Ed. 1990. Cons. Gen. Psychiat. Herdmanflat Hosp. Haddington & Roy. Infirm. Edin. Specialty: Gen. Psychiat. Prev: Sen. Regist. & Regist. (Psychiat.) Roy. Edin. Hosp.

ROGERS, Trevor Keith Chest Clinic, Doncaster Royal Infirmary, Armthorpe Road, Doncaster DN2 5LT Fax: 01302 553192 — MB ChB Bristol 1985; BSc Bristol 1982; MD Sheff. 1995; FRCP (UK) 1998. Cons. Phys. (Gen. & Chest Med.) Doncaster Roy. Infirm.; Hon. Cons. Sen. Lect., (Div. of Genomic Med., Univ. Sheff.). Specialty: Respirat. Med. Special Interest: Occupational Lung Dis. Socs: Brit. Thorac. Soc.; Amer. Thoracic Soc.; RCP London. Prev: Clinical Lect. (Med.) Univ. Sheff.; Medical Registrar, Royal Hall. Hosp., Sheffield; Med. Regist., Bristol Roy. Infirm.

ROGERS, Valerie Jean Bodymoor Heath Farm, Dog Lane, Bodymoor Heath, Sutton Coldfield B76 9JD — MB BS Lond. 1997.

ROGERS, Vincent Joseph — MB ChB Glas. 1982. Socs: Roy. Soc. Med.

ROGERS, Walter James Blachford (retired) Achmaha, Rockcliffe, Dalbeattie DG5 — MB BChir Camb. 1947; MRCS Eng. LRCP Lond. 1941; MRCP Lond. 1948; DPM Lond. 1952; FRCPsych 1971. Prev: Cons. (Child Psychiat.) Dept. Child Psychiat. Crichton Roy. Hosp.

ROGERS, Watson (retired) Little Acre, Priestlands, Sherborne DT9 4HW — MB BChir Camb. 1943 (Camb. & St. Thos.) MRCS Eng. LRCP Lond. 1942; MRCGP 1953; DA Eng. 1957. Prev: Med. Asst. Anaesth. Yeatman Hosp. Sherborne.

ROGERS, William Andrew 27 Alexandra Road, Heaton Moor, Stockport SK4 2QE — MB ChB Manch. 1989. Trainee GP/SHO (Psychiat.) Blackburn Roy. Infirm. VTS. Prev: Ho. Phys. Qu. Pk. Hosp. Blackburn; Ho. Surg. Preston Roy. Hosp.

ROGERS, William Francis (retired) 18 Tavistock Crescent, Westlands, Newcastle Under Lyme, Newcastle ST5 3NW Tel: 01782 615160 — MB BCh BAO Dub. 1940 (TC Dub.) MA Dub. 1995, BA 1938, MD 1942; Cert. VD Dr. Stevens' Hosp. Dub. 1948. Vol. Chairm. Vis. Standards/Quality Assur. Comm. Douglas MacMillan Homs Stoke on Trent. Prev: Sen. Cons. Geriat. N. Staffs. Health Dist.

ROGERS, William John Felpham and Middleton Health Centre, 109 Flansham Park, Felpham, Bognor Regis PO22 6DH Tel: 01243 582384 Fax: 01243 584933 — MB BS Lond. 1980 (St. Bart.) MRCS Eng., LRCP Lond. 1980; MRCGP 1984; DRCOG 1984. Prev: Trainee GP Mid-Sussex VTS; Ho. Surg. Roy. E. Sussex Hosp. Hastings; Ho. Phys. Frimley Pk. Hosp.

ROGERS, Zoe Jane Cockoo Lane Practice, 14 Cuckoo Lane, Hanwell, London W7 3EY — BM BCh Oxf. 1992. GP Princip. Cuckoo La. Pract. Hanwell.

ROGERSON, Charlotte Ann 19 Fry's Lane, Yateley, Yateley GU46 7TJ — BM BS Nottm. 1997.

ROGERSON, David 7 Church Road, Eggington, Derby DE65 6HP Tel: 01283 734384 Fax: 01283 734384 — MB ChB Manch. 1975 (Manchester) FFA RCSI 1978; DA Eng. 1978; MMedSci 1997. Cons. Anaesth. Derbysh. Roy. Infirm. Specialty: Anaesth.; Hypnother. Socs: Assn. Anaesth. Gt. Brit. & Irel.; Soc. Med. & Dent. Hypn.; Brit. Med. Acupunc. Soc.

ROGERSON, Grace Gilmour The Health Centre, Kilbowie Road, Clydebank G81 2TQ Tel: 0141 531 6400 Fax: 0141 531 6433; 37 Braehead Avenue, Milngavie, Glasgow G62 6DH — MB ChB Glas. 1967.

ROGERSON, Ian Michael West Chester Hospital, Liverpool Road, Chester CH2 1BQ — MB ChB Liverp. 1991. Cons. Liason Psychiat.Countess of Chester/Arrow Pk. Hosp. Specialty: Gen. Psychiat.

ROGERSON, James William 60 Hawcoat Lane, Barrow-in-Furness LA14 4HQ Tel: 01229 20542 — MRCS Eng. LRCP Lond. 1940 (Liverp.) Socs: Assoc. MRCGP; BMA. Prev: Ho. Surg. David Lewis North. Hosp. Liverp.; Asst. Phys. N. Lonsdale Hosp. Barrow; RAMC.

ROGERSON, Joseph Thomas Gerard (retired) 11 Northampton Close, Ely CB6 3QT — MB ChB Liverp. 1962; DA Eng. 1964; FFA RCS Eng. 1970. Prev: Med. Dir. St. John Ambul. Nat. HQ Lond.

ROGERSON, Lynne Joanne 74 Stones Drive, Old Stones Park, Sowerby Bridge HX6 4NY Tel: 01422 824150; 3 The Grove, Boston Spa, Wetherby LS23 6AR Tel: 01937 844029 — MB ChB Manch. 1990; MRCOG 1996. Specialist Regist. (Obstet. & Gyn.) Leeds Gen. Infirm. Specialty: Obst. & Gyn. Socs: MRCOG; BMA; BSGE.

ROGERSON, Mari Ellen 160 East Dulwich Grove, London SE22 8TB Tel: 020 8299 0499; The White House, Wycombe Road, Studley Green, High Wycombe HP14 3UY — MB BS Lond. 1986; DRCOG 1990.

ROGERSON, Mark Edward Histopathology Department, Central Pathology Laboratory, North Staffordshire Hospital, Stoke-on-Trent ST4 7PA Tel: 01782 554988; 59 Hodge Lane, Hartford, Northwich CW8 3AG Tel: 01606 74669 — MB BS Lond. 1975 (Middlx. Hosp.)

BSc Lond. 1972, MB BS 1975; MRCPath 1994. Cons. Histopath. N. Staff. Hosp. Specialty: Histopath.

ROGERSON, Mary Elizabeth Southampton General Hospital, Southampton SO16 0YD Tel: 023 8077 7222 Email: mary.rogerson@suht.swest.nhs.uk — MB BS Lond. 1981; BSc Lond. 1978, MB BS 1981; MRCP (UK) 1984; FRCP 1999. Cons. Phys. Renal Med. Soton. Univ. Hosps. Trust. Specialty: Nephrol. Prev: Clin. Lect. (Nephrol.) Inst. Urol. Lond.; Regist. Rotat. (Med.) Wessex RHA.; Sen. Regist. (Nephrol.) Wessex RHA.

ROGERSON, Mrs Myra Sylvia (retired) 31 Churchburn Drive, Loansdene, Morpeth NE61 2BZ Tel: 01670 513923 — MB ChB Ed. 1951. Prev: Assoc. Specialist St. Geo. Hosp. Morpeth.

ROGERSON, Rowland 52 Beverley Road, Kirkella, Hull HU10 7QB Tel: 01482 653277 — LMSSA Lond. 1959 (Leeds) MRCGP 1966. Med. Examr. & Adviser Offshore Oil Industries. Specialty: Occupat. Health. Socs: Hull Med. Soc.; Soc. Occupat. Health. Prev: SHO (Anaesth. & Med.) Friarage Hosp. Northallerton; Ho. Off. (Obst.) Greenbank Matern. Hosp. Darlington.

ROGERSON, Ruth Elizabeth 14 Gresley Close, Welwyn Garden City AL8 7QB Tel: 01707 339543 — MB ChB Ed. 1986; MRCGP 1990. Asst. GP Herts. Retainer Scheme. Prev: Trainee GP Qu. Eliz. II Hosp. Welwyn Gdn. City.

ROGERSON, Simon Hugh Norwood Medical Centre, 99 Abbey Road, Barrow-in-Furness LA14 5ES Tel: 01229 822024 Fax: 01229 823949; 30 Hawcoat Lane, Barrow-in-Furness LA14 4HF Tel: 01229 825561 — MB ChB Liverp. 1974. Specialty: Gen. Med. Socs: Brit. Med. Acupunct. Soc. & Med. Research Counc.; Gen. Pract. Research Framework.

ROGGER-AMIES, Andrew Melvin Acorns, Orvis Lane, East Bergholt, Colchester CO7 6TT Email: andy4sue@bigpond.net.au — MB BS Lond. 1990.

ROGOL, Benjamin Wellington Hospital, London NW8 9LE Tel: 020 7586 5959 Fax: 020 7483 0297; 14 Bracknell Gate, Frognal Lane, London NW3 7EA Tel: 020 7435 4168 — (T.C. Dub.) MA Dub 1993, BA 1934, MB BCh BAO 1936; LM Rotunda 1938. Specialty: Gen. Med. Socs: Fell. Roy. Soc. Med. & Med. Soc. Lond.; Brit. Soc. Rheum. Prev: Clin. Asst. (Dermat.) Univ. Coll. Hosp.; SHMO (Rheum.) Hackney & German Hosps.; Resid. Med. Off. Princess Louise Kens. Hosp. Childr.

ROGOL, Solomon, Capt. RAMC Retd. (retired) Flat 5, 99 Hendon Lane, London N3 3SH Tel: 020 8346 2875 — (Dub.) LRCPI & LM, LRCSI & LM 1943. Prev: Ho. Surg. Roy. Berks. Hosp. Reading & Roy. W. Hants. Hosp.

ROGOWSKI, Piotr 185 Hamstead Road, Birmingham B20 2RL Tel: 0121 554 1567 — (Wilno) Med. Dipl. Kovno 1941.

ROGSTAD, Karen Elizabeth Royal Hallamshire Hospital, Department of Genitourinary Medicine, Glossop Road, Sheffield S10 2JF Tel: 0114 270 0928 Fax: 0114 275 9081 — MB BS (Hons.) Newc. 1982; FRCP; MRCP (UK) 1985; MRCGP 1987. Cons. Genitourin. Med. Roy. Hallamsh. Hosp. Specialty: Genitourinary Medicine. Socs: MSSVD; Educat. Sub-Comm. BASHM; Chairman Adolescent Special Interest Grp. Prev: Sen. Regist. (Genitourin. Med.) City Hosp. Nottm.; Regist. (Gen. Med.) Roy. Vict. Infirm. Newc.; Workforce Officer for GUM.

ROHAN, Claire Frances Cedar House, St. Michael's Hospital, Enfield; 280 The Ridgeway, Enfield EN2 8AP — MB BCh BAO NUI 1985; MRCP (UK) 1990. Cons. Paediat. Chase Farm Hosp. Enfield. Specialty: Paediat. Socs: Roy. Coll. Paediat. & Child Health. Prev: SCMO St. Bart. NHS Trust.

ROHAN, John Stephen Lawrence House, 107 Philip Lane, Tottenham, London N15 4JR Tel: 020 8801 6640; 280 The Ridgeway, Enfield EN2 8AP — MB BCh BAO NUI 1984; DCH Dub 1986; DObst RCPI 1987; MRCGP 1988; MICGP 1988; FRCGP 2001. GP Trainer Lond.; Clin. Asst. (Ment. Handicap) Chase Farm Hosp. Enfield.; Course Organiser (Gen. Pract.) Enfield & Haringey VTS. Specialty: Gen. Med.

ROHATGI, Krishna Kumar (retired) 6 Camstradden Drive W., Bearsden, Glasgow G61 4AJ — MB BS Bihar 1961 (Darbhanga Med. Coll.) DPM Eng. 1973. Cons. Psychiat. Lanarksh. Health Bd. Prev: Sen. Regist. (Foren. Psychiat.) Gtr. Glas. Health Bd.

ROHATGI, Mahindra Kumar Sita Medical Centre, High Street, Goldenhill, Stoke-on-Trent ST6 5QJ Tel: 01782 772242 Fax: 01782 776711; 2 Sandbach Road, Church Lawton, Stoke-on-Trent ST7 3BE Tel: 01270 877910 — MB BS Jiwaji 1967; DA Eng. 1971. Specialty: Family Plann. & Reproduc. Health; Gen. Pract. Socs: Med. Protec. Soc.

ROHATGI, Shakuntla Sita Medical Centre, High Street, Goldenhill, Stoke-on-Trent ST6 5QJ Tel: 01782 772242 Fax: 01782 776711; 2 Sandbach Road, Church Lawton, Stoke-on-Trent ST7 3BE Tel: 01270 877910 — MB BS Delhi 1965 (Lady Harding Med. Coll.) MRCOG 1974. Specialty: Family Plann. & Reproduc. Health.

ROHATGI, Subir 5 Greenhill Road, Whitnash, Leamington Spa CV31 2HG — MB BS Lond. 1990.

ROHATINER, Anna Zofia Stefania 62 South Croxted Road, London SE21 8BD Email: ama.rohatiner@cancer.org.uk — MB BS LRCP (Lond.) 1974 (Guy's) MRCP (UK) 1977; MD Lond. 1984; FRCP 1999. Prof. (Haemato-Oncology & Cons. Physician) St Bartholomews Hosp. Lond.; Director, Internat. Network for Cancer Treatm. & Research. Specialty: Gen. Med.

ROHDE, Peter David (retired) 53 Harley Street, London W1G 8QP Tel: 020 7636 5901 — MB Camb. 1958 (Camb. & St. Thos.) BA Camb. 1954, MB 1958, BChir 1957; DPM Eng. 1961; MRCP Lond. 1968; FRCP Ed. 1983, M 1968; FRCPsych 1983, M 1971. Prev: Hon. Emerit. Cons. Riverside HA. Lond.

ROHDE, Simon Peter Dr H M Freeman and Partners, 12 Durham Road, Raynes Park, London SW20 0TW Tel: 020 8946 0069 Fax: 020 8944 2927 — MB BS Lond. 1987; BSc (Psychol. Med. Sci.) Lond. 1984. SHO (Obst.) W. Lond. Hosp.

ROHLFING, Robert Frederick Eaglestone Health Centre, Standing Way, Eaglestone, Milton Keynes MK6 5AZ Tel: 01908 679111 Fax: 01908 230601 — MB BS Lond. 1991. Specialty: Gen. Pract.

ROHMAN, Stephen Owen King's Surgery, Water St., Port Talbot SA12 6LF Tel: 01639 890983 Fax: 01639 870146 Email: steve.rohman@gr-w98014.wales.nhs.uk; 1 Dynevor Avenue, Neath SA10 7AG Tel: 01639 797361 Email: stephen.rohman@ntlwalls.com/steve@rohman.freeserve.co.uk — MB BS Lond. 1986 (St. Bart.) DRCOG 1989; MRCGP 1991. Clin. Asst. (Care Elderly) Cymla Hosp. Neath. Prev: Trainee GP Fairfield Med. Centre Port Talbot; SHO (Gen. Med., Geriat., O & G, Paediat. & A & E) Neath Gen. Hosp.; SHO (A & E) Roy. Gwent Hosp. Newport.

ROITH, Eva 183 Harrow Road, Wollaton Park, Nottingham NG8 1FL — MA Dub. 1958, MB BCh BAO 1949; DPH NUI 1953; DPM Eng. 1962. Prev: Sen. Med. Off. (Ment. Health) Notts. HA; Med. Off. St. Lawrence's Hosp. Caterham; SHO Kettlewell Hosp. Swanley.

ROKAN AL-MALLAK, Mr Hamid Southend Hospital, Prittlewell Chase, Westcliff on Sea SS0 0RY — MB ChB Baghdad 1973; FRCSI 1990; Dip Sports Med 1994; FFAEM 1996. Cons. A & E Med. Southend Hosp. Westcliff on Sea; Southend Hosps. NHS Tusts West-Cliff-On-Sea Essex. Specialty: Accid. & Emerg. Special Interest: Sports & Sports Related Injuries. Socs: BAEM.

ROLAN, Paul Edward Medeval Ltd., Skelton House, Manchester Science Park, Lloyd Street N., Manchester M15 6SH Tel: 0161 226 6525 Fax: 0161 226 8936 Email: p.rolan@medeval.com — MB BS Adelaide 1979; DCPSA 1985; FRACP 1985; MD Adelaide 1995; FFPM RCP (UK) 1997, MF 1996. Med. Dir. Medeval Manch.; Hon. Cons. Phys. (Neurol.) Manch. Roy. Infirm.; Dir. Neuraxis Manch. Specialty: Pharmacology. Socs: Assn. Human Pharmacol. Pharmaceut. Industry; Pharmacol. Soc.; Int. Headache Soc. Prev: Head of Clin. Pharmacokinetics Wellcome Research Laborat. UK; Dir. Med. Cairns Base Hosp. Queensland, Austral.

ROLAND, Jess 3 The Springs, Park Road, Bowdon, Altrincham WA14 3JH Tel: 0161 927 7554 — MB ChB Manch. 1945. Prev: Asst. Med. Off. Booth Hall Childr. Hosp. Manch.

ROLAND, Jill 12 Huxley Drive, Bramhall, Stockport SK7 2PH Tel: 0161 439 6973 — MRCS Eng. LRCP Lond. 1961; MSc Manch. 1981; MFCM RCP (UK) 1982; FFPHM RCP (UK) 1996. Specialty: Pub. Health Med.

ROLAND, Jonathan Michael Edith Cavell Hospital, Bretton Gate, Peterborough PE3 9GZ Tel: 01733 874217 Fax: 01733 875159 Email: jonathan.roland@pbh-tr.nhs.uk — MB BS Lond. 1972; BSc Lond. 1969, MB BS 1972; MRCP (UK) 1975; DM Nottm. 1984; FRCP Lond. 1994. Cons. Phys. PeterBoro. Hosp. NHS Trust. Specialty: Diabetes; Endocrinol.; Gen. Med. Prev: Sen. Regist. (Med.) Bristol Roy. Infirm.

ROLAND, Professor Martin Oliver, CBE National Primary Care Research & Development Centre, Williamson Building, University of

Manchester, Oxford Road, Manchester M13 9PL Tel: 0161 275 7659 Fax: 0161 275 7600 Email: m.roland@man.ac.uk; 15 Portland Road, Altrincham WA14 2PA Tel: 0161 928 1748 Fax: 0161 926 8436 — BM BCh Oxf. 1975; DRCOG 1977; MRCP (UK) 1978; FRCGP 1994, M 1979; MFPHM 1988; MA Oxf. 1976, DM 1989; F.Med Sci, 2000; FRCP, 2001. Prof. Gen. Pract. Univ. Manch.; Director Nat. Primary Care Research & Developm. Centre Univ Manch. Specialty: Gen. Pract. Prev: Dir. of Studies Gen. Pract., Camb. Univ. Sch. Clin. Med.; Lect. (Gen. Pract.) St. Thos. Hosp. Med. Sch. Lond.; Trainee GP Camb. VTS.

ROLAND, Mr Nicholas John Department of Otorhinolaryngology, Aintree NHS Trust, Liverpool Tel: 0151 529 5259 — MB ChB Liverp. 1987; FRCS Eng. 1992; MD Liverp, 1997. Cons. (Otolaryngol & Head & Neck Surg.) Aintree NHS Trust, Liverp.; Hon. Lect. (Otolaryngol. & Head & Neck Surg.) Liverp. Univ. Specialty: Otorhinolaryngol. Socs: BMA; Brit. Assn. Otol. & Head & Neck Surg.; Brit. Assn. Cancer Res. Prev: Lect. & Sen. Regist. (Otolaryngol. & Head & Neck Surg.) Roy. Liverp. Univ. Hosp.

ROLAND, Mr Peter Ernest (retired) 34 Regency House, Newbold Terrace, Leamington Spa CV32 4HD Tel: 01926 470980 — (Middlx.) MRCS Eng. LRCP Lond. 1939; MB BS Lond. 1940; DLO Eng. 1942; FRCS Ed. 1948. Prev: Cons. Surg. (ENT) Hosp. St. Cross Rugby & Coventry AHA.

ROLANT-THOMAS, Catherine Mabel (retired) Bron Menai, Cadnant Road, Menai Bridge LL59 5NG Tel: 01248 712526 — MRCS Eng. LRCP Lond. 1922 (Lond. Sch. Med. Wom., St. Mary's, Ed. & Roy. Dent. Hosp.) LDS Eng. 1924. Prev: Clin. Asst. Dent. Dept. Gt. Ormond St. Hosp. Sick Childr.

ROLES, Wendy Princess Margaret Hospital, Windsor SL4 3SJ Tel: 01753 743434; 5 The Dell, Bishopsgate Rd, Englefield Green, Egham TW20 0XY Tel: 01784 437645 Fax: 01276 431576 — MB BS Lond. 1960 (Barts) RCOG; MRCS Eng. LRCP Lond. 1960; MFFP 1993. Cons. Psychosexual Med. Princess Margt. Hosp. Windsor. Specialty: Psychosexual Med. Socs: Windsor Med. Soc. Prev: Med. Director Slough Family Plann. Clinc; Clin. Asst. Colposcopy Heatherwood Hosp. Ascot.

ROLFE, Alun Bowen The Hall, Merthyr Road, Llanfoist, Abergavenny NP7 9LR Tel: 01783 2148 — MB ChB Birm. 1954; MRCS Eng. LRCP Lond. 1954; DPM Eng. 1962; FRCPsych. 1987, M 1972. Cons. Psychiat. Llanarth Ct. Hosp. Raglan, Gwent; JP. Specialty: Gen. Psychiat. Prev: Cons. Psychiat. Pen-y-Fal Hosp. Abergavenny; Chairm. Gwent Div. Psychiat.; Mem. Ment. Health Act Commiss.

ROLFE, Diana (retired) 6 Chapman Square, Harrogate HG1 2SL Tel: 01423 567663 — MB BS Lond. 1966 (Middlx.) MRCP Lond. 1969. Prev: SHO (Rheum.) Middlx. Hosp. Lond.

ROLFE, Helena Clare Ilkley Health Centre, Springs Lane, Ilkley LS29 8TQ Tel: 01943 430005; 23 Hillside, Follifoot, Harrogate HG3 1EF Tel: 01423 879932 — MB ChB Leeds 1992; MRCGP 1996. GP Princip. Specialty: Gen. Pract. Prev: SHO (Paediat.) Dewsbury Dist. Hosp.; Trainee GP Leeds.

ROLFE, Lindsey Margaret Hammersmith Medicines Research, Central Middlesex Hospital, Acton Lane, London NW10 7NS — MB ChB Ed. 1992; MRCP (UK) 1995.

ROLFE, Michael Garland Carmel, Beech Avenue, Pennsylvania, Exeter EX4 6HE — MB BChir Camb. 1947 (Lond. Hosp.) DObst RCOG 1950; DA Eng. 1955; FFA RCS Eng. 1956. Specialty: Anaesth. Socs: Fell. Roy. Soc. Med.; Assn. Anaesths. Prev: Cons. Anaesth. Lond. Hosp. & King Geo. Hosp. Ilford; Regist. Anaesth. Roy. Nat. Throat, Nose & Ear Hosp.; Sen. Regist. Anaesth. Lond. Hosp.

ROLFE, Muriel Elisabeth (retired) The Old House, 24 High St, Bridge, Canterbury CT4 5JY Tel: 01227 832694 — MB BS Lond. 1957 (Roy. Free) MRCS Eng. LRCP Lond 1957; DO Eng 1961. Prev: Assoc. Specialist Moorfields Eye Hosp. Lond.

ROLFE, Mrs Sally Anne Portland House, 348 Vale Road, Ash Vale, Aldershot GU12 5LW — MB BS Lond. 1961 (Char. Cross)

ROLFE, Sian Eluned The Hall, Llanfoist, Abergavenny NP7 9LR — MB ChB Manch. 1985.

ROLL, Matthew Jeremy Simon 113 Overdale Road, Romiley, Stockport SK6 3EN — MB ChB Manch. 1988.

ROLLAND, Charles Frederick (retired) Knocker House, Caldbeck, Wigton CA7 8EG — MD Ed. 1953 (Camb. & Ed.) BA (Nat. Sc. Trip. Pt. I, cl. I) Camb. 1941; MB ChB 1944; FRCP Ed. 1956, M 1948; MD (High Commend.) Ed. 1953. Prev: Phys. Cumbld. Infirm. Carlisle.

ROLLAND, Douglas McIntyre Teviot Medical Practice, Teviot Road, Hawick TD9 9DT Tel: 01450 370999 Fax: 01450 371025; Westwood, Sunnyhill Road, Hawick TD9 7HT Tel: 01450 373633 — MB ChB Aberd. 1989; DCH RCPS Glas. 1991; MRCGP 1993; Cert Prescribed Equiv. Exp. JCPTGP 1993. GP Princip. Hawick. Prev: Trainee GP Borders HB VTS; Ho. Off. (Surg.) Glas. Roy. Infirm.; Ho. Off. (Med.) Woodend Hosp. Aberd.

ROLLAND, Morag Bruce Teviot Medical Practice, Hawick Health Centre, Teviot Road, Hawick TD9 9DT Tel: 01450 370999 Fax: 01450 371025; Westwood, Sunnyhill, Hawick TD9 7HT Tel: 01450 373633 — MB ChB Aberd. 1988 (Aberdeen) DCH RCPS Glas. 1990; Cert. Prescribed Equiv. Exp. JCPTGP 1992; MRCGP 1993. GP (Retainer). Prev: Trainee GP Highland HB VTS; SHO (Orthop. & Cas.) Borders HB; Resid. Med. Raigmore Hosp. Inverness.

ROLLAND, Philip Andrew 7 Bradgate Drive, Sutton Coldfield B74 4XG — BM BS Nottm. 1998; BM BS Nottm 1998.

ROLLAND, Philip Stewart Clerklands Surgery, No. 2 Vicarage Lane, Horley RH6 8AP Tel: 01293 783802; 1 Ross Close, Tilgate, Crawley RH10 5DT Tel: 01293 25204 — MB BS Lond. 1954 (Univ. Coll. Hosp.) DObst RCOG 1958. Hosp. Pract. (Gyn.) Crawley Hosp. Specialty: Obst. & Gyn. Socs: BMA. Prev: Ho. Phys. W. Kent Gen. Hosp. Maidstone; Sen. Ho. Off. Paediat. & Obst. Depts. St. Luke's Hosp. Guildford.

ROLLASON, Stuart Bernard 57 Disraeli Road, London W5 5HS — MB ChB Birm. 1985.

ROLLASON, Terence Paul — MB ChB Birm. 1976; BSc (Hons.) Birm. 1973; FRCPath 1994, M 1983. Cons. Path.; Clin. Tutor in Path., Univ. of Birm. Specialty: Histopath. Prev: Sen. Lect. (Path.) Univ. Birm.; Cons. Histopath. & Cytopath. Maelor Gen. Hosp. Wrexham; Lect. (Path.) Univ. Birm.

ROLLES, Christopher John Bassett Wood House, Bassett Wood Drive, Bassett, Southampton SO16 3PT — MB ChB Birm. 1965; MRCP (UK) 1970; FRCP Lond. 1984.

ROLLES, Mr Keith Royal Free Hospital, Department of Surgery, London NW3 2QG Tel: 0208 830 2198 Fax: 0208 830 2198 Email: keith.rolles@royalfree.nhs.uk — MB BS Lond. 1972 (Lond. Hosp.) FRCS Eng. 1976; MA Camb. 1983; BSc Lond. 1969, MS 1985. Cons. Surg. Roy. Free Hosp. Lond. Specialty: Transpl. Surg.; Gen. Surg. Socs: Transpl. Soc. & Europ. Soc. Organ Transpl.; BMA. Prev: Lect. (Surg.) & Hon. Cons. Surg. Addenbrooke's Hosp. Camb.

ROLLES, Toni Frances Bassett Wood House, Bassett Wood Drive, Bassett, Southampton SO16 3PT — MB ChB Birm. 1965; DCH Eng. 1969; MRCGP 1984.

ROLLI, Marie-Josee — MB ChB Manch. 1985.

ROLLIN, Anna-Maria Department of Anaesthetics, Epsom General Hospital, Dorking Road, Epsom KT18 7EG Tel: 01372 735270 Fax: 01372 735497; 101 College Road, Epsom KT17 4HY Tel: 01372 724772 Fax: 01372 749758 — MB BS Lond. 1970 (Guy's) FRCA Eng.; MRCS Eng. LRCP Lond. 1970; DA Eng. 1972; FFA RCS Eng. 1975. Cons. Anaesth. Epsom Gen. Hosp,Epsom St Helier Univ. NHS Trust; Hon. Cons. Anaesth. The Childrens Trust, Tadworth; Assessor in Anaesthetics, GMC, Lead; Mem. of Counc., Roy. Coll. of Anaesth.s. Specialty: Anaesth. Socs: BMA; (Ex Vice-Pres.) Assn. Anaesth. (GBI); Fell. Roy. Soc. Med. (President Elect, Sect. Anaesth.). Prev: Sen. Regist. & Regist. Guy's Hosp. Lond.; Regist. Qu. Vict. Hosp. E. Grinstead.

ROLLIN, Henry Rapoport 101 College Road, Epsom KT17 4HY Tel: 01372 724772 — MB ChB Leeds 1935; DPM Eng. 1939; MD Leeds 1947; FRCPsych 1971; FRCP Lond. 1993, M 1976; FRCPsych (Hon.) 1989. Emerit. Cons. Psychiat. Horton Hosp. Epsom. Specialty: Gen. Psychiat. Socs: Fell. Roy. Soc. Med. (Pres. Sec. Hist. of Med.). Prev: Hon. Cons. Psychiat. Qu. Eliz. Foundat. for Disabled Leatherhead; Cons. Psychiat. Horton Hosp. Epsom; Wing Cdr. (Neuro-Psychiat. Specialist) RAFVR.

ROLLINS, John William, Group Capt. RAF Med. Br. Retd. c/o National Westminster Bank, 68 Palmerston Road, Southsea PO5 3PT — MB BS Lond. 1959 (Guy's) MRCS Eng. LRCP Lond. 1959; DPM Eng. 1970; FRCPsych 1985, M 1972. Civil. Cons. Psychiat. RN Hosp. Haslar. Specialty: Gen. Psychiat.

ROLLINS, Mark David 8 Gortycavan Road, Coleraine BT51 4LT Tel: 01265 43405 Fax: 01265 50000 — MB BCh BAO Belf. 1981; DCH Dub. 1985; MRCPI (Paediat.) 1987; MD Qu. Univ. Belf. 1993.

Cons. Paediat. Coleraine Hosp. NHSSB. Specialty: Paediat. Socs: Brit. Paediat. Assn. & Irish Paediat. Assn. Prev: Sen. Regist. St. Mary's Hosp. Lond.

ROLLO, Alan Geoffrey Townhead Health Centre, 16 Alexandra Parade, Glasgow G31 2ES Tel: 0141 531 8940 Fax: 0141 531 8935; 24 Banavie Road, Dowanhill, Glasgow G11 5AN — MB ChB Glas. 1981; DRCOG 1984; MRCGP 1986.

ROLLS, Anita Seaton Hospital, Valley View Road, Seaton EX12 2DU Tel: 01297 23901; Lattenbells, Stepps Lane, Axmouth, Seaton EX12 4AR — MB BS Lond. 1963 (Guy's) MRCS Eng. LRCP Lond. 1963. Clin. Asst. (Psychogeriat.) Seaton Hosp. Specialty: Geriat. Psychiat. Prev: GP Seaton; Clin. Asst. (Psychogeriat.) Axminster Day Hosp.

ROLLS, Nigel Paul Acle Medical Centre, Bridewell Lane, Acle, Norwich NR13 3RA Tel: 01493 750888 Fax: 01493 751652; The Old Rectory, North Burlingham, Norwich NR13 4TA Tel: 01603 712221 — MB BCh Wales 1975; MRCGP 1980. Specialty: Gen. Pract.

ROLLS, Roger Lewis The Surgery, 35 Great Pulteney Street, Bath BA2 4BY Tel: 01225 464187 Fax: 01225 485305 — MB BChir Camb. 1970 (St. Bart.) MB Camb. 1970, BChir 1969; DObst RCOG 1973; MRCGP 1990. Socs: Fell. Roy. Soc. Med.; Brit. Inst. Manip. Med. Prev: Resid. (Path.) Radcliffe Infirm. Oxf.; SHO Hosp. Sick Childr. Bristol; Ho. Phys. St. Bart. Hosp. Lond.

ROLPH, Martin James William The St Lawrence Surgery, 79 St. Lanewrence Avenue, Worthing BN14 7JL Tel: 01903 237346; 12 Offington Drive, Worthing BN14 9PN — MB BS Lond. 1990; MRCGP 1994. Specialty: Palliat. Med.

ROLSTON, Eleanor Thomasine Larksfield Integrated Therapy, 21 Elizabeth Road, Walsall WS5 3PF Tel: 01922 642831 Email: rolston@gpanet.co.uk — MB BS Lond. 1952 (Univ. Coll. Hosp.) FRCPI 1986, M 1955; DPM Eng. 1962; MRCPsych 1971. Private Cons. Psychiat. and Psychotherapist; Vis. Cons. Psychiat., Woodbourne Hosp. Birm. Specialty: Gen. Psychiat.; Psychother. Socs: Mem. Wolverhampton Med. Inst..; Mem. Of the Inst. of Transactional Anal. Prev: Sen. Regist. (Psychiat.) St. Matthew's Hosp. Burntwood.; Postgrad. Clin. Tutor/Cons. Psychiat., New Cross Hosp., Wolverhampton; Cons. Psychiat., Weston Villa Addic. Unit, St Geo.s Hosp. Stafford.

ROMACHNEY, Peter 6 Herschell Street, Mill Hill, Blackburn BB2 4DQ — MB ChB Manch. 1991.

ROMAN, Fiona — MB ChB Sheff. 1987.

ROMAN, Mark Victor York Medical Group, 199 Acomb Road, Acomb, York YO24 4HD Tel: 01904 342999 — MB BS Lond. 1982 (Westm.) DRCOG 1985; MRCGP 1986. GP York.

ROMAN, Mr Raed Mikhail Singleton Hospital, Sketty, Swansea SA2 8QA — MB BCh Cairo 1975; FRCS Glas. 1983.

ROMAN, Mr Victor (retired) 46 St Helen's Lane, Leeds LS16 8BS Tel: 0113 267 7744 — MD Innsbruck 1946; FRCS Ed. 1959. Prev: Sen. Med. Off. DHSS.

ROMANES, Professor George John, CBE (retired) Camus na Feannag, Kishorn, Strathcarron IV54 8XA Tel: 01520 733273 — (Camb. & Ed.) FRS Ed.; BA Camb. 1938, PhD 1941; MB ChB Ed. 1944; FRCS Ed. 1959; Hon. DSc Glas. 1982. Prev: Prof. Anat. & Dean Fac. Med. Univ. Edin.

ROMANES, Mr Giles John, KStJ 20 Dukes Avenue, Dorchester DT1 1EN Tel: 01305 263774; Portesham House, Portesham, Weymouth DT3 4HE Tel: 01305 871300 — (Camb. & St. Mary's) MRCS Eng. LRCP Lond. 1945; MA Camb. 1949; DOMS Eng. 1950; FRCS Eng. 1975; FRCOpth 1993. Specialty: Ophth. Socs: Fell. Roy. Soc. Med.; Ophth. Soc. UK. Prev: Cons. Ophth. Surg. W. Dorset; Regist. (Plastic & Jaw) Rooksdown Hse. Basingstoke; 1st Asst. Corneo-plastic Unit & Regional Eye Bank, Qu. Vict. Hosp. E. Grinstead.

ROMANIUK, Christopher Stanley MRI Department, Clatterbridge Centre for Oncology, Bebington, Wirral CH63 4JY Tel: 0151 334 4000 Fax: 0151 604 7497 — MB ChB Manch. 1983; MRCP (UK) 1986; FRCR 1989; T(R)(CR) 1992. Cons. Radiol. (Magnetic Resonance Imaging) Clatterbridge Centre Oncol. The Wirral. Specialty: Radiol. Socs: Brit. Inst. Radiol.; Assoc. Mem. Internat. Cancer Imaging Soc. Prev: Sen. Regist. (Diag. Radiol.) St. Jas. Hosp. Leeds & Leeds Gen. Infirm.

ROMANIUK, Deirdre Annamaria Riverside Surgery, 525 New Chester Road, Rockferry, Birkenhead CH42 2AG Tel: 0151 645 3464 Fax: 0151 643 1676 — MB ChB Manch. 1983; MRCGP 1988; DRCOG 1989. Princip. in Gen. Pract. Prev: Trainee GP Leeds VTS; SHO (Obst.) Leeds Gen. Infirm.; SHO (Geriat. Med.) Manch. Roy. Infirm.

ROMANO, Paolo 56 St Kilda Road, London W13 9DE — State Exam Bologna 1993.

ROMANOS BETRAN, Maria Teresa Flat 2, 55 Shepherds Hill, London N6 5QP — LMS Saragossa 1995.

ROMANOWSKI, Charles Anthony Jozef Department of Radiology, Royal Hallamshire Hospital, Glossop Road, Sheffield S10 2JF Tel: 0114 271 2957 Fax: 0114 271 2606; Canterbury House, 50 Canterbury Avenue, Fulwood, Sheffield S10 3RU Tel: 0114 230 1230 Email: charles.romanowski@virgin.net — MB ChB Manch. 1986; BSc (Hons.) Anat. Manch. 1983; MRCP (UK) 1989; FRCR 1992. Cons. Neuroradiol. Roy. Hallamsh. Hosp. Sheff. Specialty: Radiol. Socs: Brit. Soc. Neuroradiol.; Eur. Soc. Neuroradiol. Prev: Sen. Regist. (Neuroradiol.) Manch. Roy. Infirm.

ROMAYA, Basil Francis North Lane Practice, 38 North Lane, Aldershot GU12 4QQ Tel: 01252 344434 — LMSSA London 1979; LMSSA London 1979.

ROMER, Charles The Tything Surgery, 1 The Tything, Worcester WR1 1HD Tel: 01905 26086; Manor House, Kempsey, Worcester WR5 3JZ Tel: 01905 820206 — MB BS Lond. 1947 (King's Coll. Hosp.) MRCS Eng. LRCP Lond. 1943. Prev: Surg. Lt. RNVR; Regist. (Med.) Worcester Roy. Infirm.; Phys. i/c Dept. Venereol. Worcester Roy. Infirm.

ROMER, Heike Carolyn Royal Liverpool University Hospital, Anaesthetic Office, 12th Floor, Prescott Street, Liverpool L7 8XP Tel: 0151 706 3190 Fax: 0151 706 5646 — MB BS Newc. 1987 (Newcastle upon Tyne) DA (UK) 1991; FRCA 1993. Cons. In Anaesth. and Pain Managem., Roy. Liverp. Uni.Hosp. Liverp.; Cons. In Anaesth. and Pain Managem. with admitting rights to the Lourdes Hosp. Liverp. and Murrayfield Hosp. Wirral. Specialty: Anaesth.; Medico Legal.

ROMER, Joseph Max (retired) Thornwood, 201 Victoria Road W., Thornton-Cleveleys FY5 3QE Tel: 01253 853095 — MB ChB Liverp. 1958; DObst RCOG 1964. Prev: Clin. Asst. (Psychiat.) Psychiat. Day Hosp. Blackpool.

ROMILLY, Crystal Sophia Institute of Psychiatry, Crespigny Park, Denmark Hill, London SE5 8AF Tel: 020 7848 0123 Fax: 020 7848 3754 — (Guy's Hosp. Lond.) CCST Forens Psych. 1998 (Roy Coll of Psych.); BSc (Econ.) Lond. 1978; MB BS Lond. 1987; MRCPsych 1993. Clin. Research Worker. Specialty: Forens. Psychiat. Socs: Roy. Coll. Psychiat. Prev: Sen. Regist. Maudsley Hosp. Lond.; Sen. Reg. in Forens. Psych., Bracton RSU; Sen. Reg. in Forens. Psych., Broadmoor.

ROMILLY, Sarah Ann Cassington, Fernleigh Road, Mannamead, Plymouth PL3 5AN — MB BS Lond. 1990.

ROMOTOWSKI, Louise Isobel Drumhar Health Centre, North Methven St., Perth PH1 5PD Tel: 01738 564260 Fax: 01738 564293; 3 James Place, Stanley, Perth PH1 4PD Tel: 01738 827124 — MB ChB Glas. 1974; Cert. Family Plann. JCC 1979. Staff Grade Paediat. Tayside Univ. Hosp. NHS Trust. Specialty: Community Child Health. Socs: BMA; Scott. Assn. Community Child Health; Brit. Med. Acupunct. Soc. Prev: Clin. Med. Off. (Community Child Health) Perth & Kinross Health Care; Clin. Med. Off. S. Beds. HA.

RON, Professor Maria Antonia National Hospital for Neurology & Neurosurgery, Queen Square, London WC1N 3BG Tel: 0207 676 2050 Fax: 0207 676 2051 — LMS Madrid 1966 (Madrid Med. Sch.) MRCPsych 1973; PhD Lond. 1981, MPhil 1974. Prof. of Neuropsychiatry, Inst. of Neurol., Nat. Hosp. for Neurol., UCL, Lond. Specialty: Gen. Psychiat. Socs: Royal College of Psychiat.; Royal College of Physicians; Brit. Neuropsychiatric Assn.

RONA, Roberto Jorge Department of Public Health Sciences, Division of Asthma, allergy & Lung Biology, Guy's, King's & St Thomas' School of Medicine, 6th Floor, Capital House, 42 Weston Street, London SE1 3QD Tel: 020 7848 6618 Email: roberto.rona@kcl.ac.uk — Medico Cirujano Chile; PhD Lond. 1976; MFPHM 1985; FFPHM 1990. Prof. of Pub. Health Kings Coll. Lond. Specialty: Pub. Health Med. Socs: Fac. of Pub. Health; Soc. of Social Med.; Soc. for the Study of Human Biol.

RONALD, Andrew Lindsay Department of Anaesthesia, Aberdeen Royal Infirmary, Forresterhill, Aberdeen AB25 2ZN Tel: 01224 681818 Fax: 01224 404469; 4 Ashdale Drive, Westhill AB32 6LP

Tel: 01224 743526 — MB ChB Ed. 1983; FRCA 1989. Cons. Anaesth. Aberd. Roy. Hosps. NHS Trust; Clin. Sen. Lect. (Anaesth.) Univ. Aberd. Specialty: Anaesth. Socs: Assn. Anaesth.; Hist. Anaesth. Soc. & BMA. Prev: Sen. Regist. (Anaesth.) Grampian HB; Regist. (Anaesth.) Lancaster Roy. Infirm. & Assoc. Hosps.; SHO (Anaesth.) Kidderminster Gen. Hosp.

RONALDS, Clare Mary Ladybarn Group Practice, 177 Mauldeth Road, Fallowfield, Manchester M14 6SG Tel: 0161 224 2873 Fax: 0161 225 3276 — BM BS Nottm. 1976 (Nottingham) BMedSci Nottm. 1974; MRCGP 1981. GP & Trainer Manch.; Tutor (Gen. Pract.) Univ. Manch. Specialty: Gen. Pract.

RONALDSON, Philip Noel (retired) 36 Judges Walk, Norwich NR4 7QF Tel: 01603 452097 — (Queens University Belfast) MB BCh BAO Belf. 1947. Prev: Med. Off. DHSS Norwich Bd.ing Centre 1980-1993.

RONAY, Susan Amanda Sonning Common Health Centre, Wood Lane, Sonning Common, Reading RG4 9SW Tel: 0118 972 2188 Fax: 0118 972 4633; 28 St. Barnabas Road, Emmer Green, Reading RG4 8RA — MB ChB Manch. 1985; DCH RCP Lond. 1987; DRCOG 1988; MRCGP 1989. Course Organiser Reading VTS.

RONAYNE, Karen Linda 4 Berber Close, Whiteley, Fareham PO15 7HF Tel: 01489 880913 — BM BS Nottm. 1994; DRCOG 1997. Trainee GP Portsmouth. Specialty: Gen. Pract. Prev: SHO (ENT & A & E) Qu. Alexandra Hosp. Portsmouth; Ho. Off. (Med.) MusGr. Pk. Hosp. Taunton; Ho. Off. (Surg.) Princess Margt. Hosp. Swindon.

RONCHETTI, Martin Gerard Pensilva Health Centre, School Road, Pensilva, Liskeard PL14 5RP Tel: 01579 362249 Fax: 01579 363323; Upton Farm House, Upton Cross, Liskeard PL14 5AZ Tel: 01579 362689 — MB ChB Bristol 1984; DCH RCP Lond. 1987; MRCGP 1988; DFFP 1995. Prev: SHO (O & G, Paediat. & Cas.) Roy. Cornw. Hosp. Truro.

RONDEL, Professor Richard Kavanagh 2 King George Square, Park Hill, Richmond TW10 6LG Tel: 020 8940 7852 Fax: 020 8940 7852 — MB BS Lond. 1956 (St. Geo.) DObst RCOG 1963; Dip. Pharm. Med. RCP (UK) 1976; FRCP Lond. 1992. Visiting Professor, Post Graduate Medical School. Specialty: Pharmaceutical Medicine. Socs: (Ex-Pres.) Internat. Federat. Pharmaceutical Phys.s; (Ex-Chairm.) & Hon. Life Mem.Brit. Assoc. Pharmaceutical Phys.s. Prev: Prof. Clin. Practitioner Univ. Surrey; Med. Dir. Human PsychPharmacol. Research Unit Univ. Surrey; Regist. Fac. Pharmology Med.

RONDER, Julia Therese Ticehurst House Hospital, Ticehurst, Wadhurst TN5 7HU Tel: 01580 200391 — MB BS Lond. 1986 (Univ. Coll. & Middlx.) BSc Lond. 1983; MRCPsych 1990; MD Lond. 2003. Cons. Psychiat. Young Person's Unit, Priory Ticehurst Ho. Hosp.; Hon. Lect. Guy's Hosp. Lond. Specialty: Child & Adolesc. Psychiat. Socs: Roy. Coll. Psychiats.; Assn. Child Psychol. Psychiat. Prev: Sen. Regist. Guys & St. Thos. Hosps. Lond.

RONEY, David Brian 4 Leech Street, Hyde SK14 2PF — MB ChB Manch. 1987.

RONEY, Sheila Margaret 15 Parfrey Street, London W6 9EW — MB BS Lond. 1993.

RONGHE, Milind Dattatraya Royal Hospital for Sick Children, Yorkhill NHS Trust, Dalnair Street, Glasgow G3 8SJ Tel: 0141 201 0392 Fax: 0141 201 0857 Email: milind.ronghe@yorkhill.scot.nhs.uk — MB BS Bombay 1992. Cons. (Paediat. Oncol.) Roy. Hosp. for Sick Childr. Glas.

RONN, Howard Humphrey (retired) Parsonage Farm, Edington, Westbury BA13 4QF — MB BS Lond. 1949; MB BS (Hnrs.) Lond. 1949; MRCP Lond. 1952. Prev: Surg. Lt.-Cdr. RNR.

RONSON, John Gareth The Lennard Surgery, 1-3 Lewis Road, Bishopsworth, Bristol BS13 7JD Tel: 0117 964 0900 Fax: 0117 987 3227 — MB ChB Manch. 1982 (Manchester) MRCP (UK) 1985; DRCOG 1987; MRCGP 1989.

RONSON, Julia Anne Manchester Road Surgery, 57 Manchester Road, Southport PR9 9BN Tel: 01704 532314 Fax: 01704 539740 — MB ChB Sheff. 1992.

ROOBAN, R A Carterhatch Lane Surgery, 99 Carterhatch Lane, Enfield EN1 4LA Tel: 020 8804 5312 Fax: 020 8804 5095 — MB BS Kerala 1976; MB BS Kerala 1976.

ROOBOTTOM, Carl Ashley Radiology Department, Plymouth PL6 8DH Tel: 01752 777111; Brook House, Sampford Spiney, Yelverton PL20 7QT — MB ChB Birm. 1987; BSc (1st cl. Hons.) Birm. 1986; MB ChB (Hons.) Birm. 1987; MRCP (UK) 1990; FRCR 1993. Cons. Radiol. Derriford Hosp. Plymouth. Specialty: Radiol. Socs: Brit. Soc. Interven. Radiol.; Roy. Coll. Radiol. Prev: Merck Fell. & Lect. (Radiol.) Bristol Roy. Infirm.; Regist. (Diag. Radiol.) Plymouth.; SHO (Med.) Selly Oak Birm.

ROOD, Professor Jan Philip Department of Oral & Maxillofacial Surgery, King's Dental Institute, King's College Hospital, Denmark Hill, London SE5 9RW Tel: 020 7346 3278 Fax: 020 7346 3642 — MB BS Newc. 1973; BDS Durham. 1966; FDS RCS Eng. 1972; MDS 1976; MSc Manch. 1985; FRCS Ed. 1985. Prof. Oral & Maxillofacial Surg. King's Dent. Inst. Lond. Specialty: Oral & Maxillofacial Surg. Socs: Brit. Assn. Oral Surgs. & Brit. Dent. Assn. & Brit. Assn. Day Surg. Prev: Lect. (Oral Surg.) Univ. Lond.; Sen. Lect. & Hon. Cons. Oral & Maxillofacial Surg. King's Coll. Hosp. Lond.; Prof. Oral & Maxillofacial Surg. Manch.

ROODYN, Leonard, LVO 7 Wimpole Street, London W1G 9SN Tel: 020 7323 1555 — MD Lond. 1960 (Middlx.) MB BS 1946. Cons. i/c Vaccination Serv. Hosp. Trop. Dis. Lond. Specialty: Infec. Dis. Prev: Supernum. Asst. Bland-Sutton Inst. Path. Middlx. Hosp.

ROOHANNA, Rafat 46 Overstone Road, Hammersmith, London W6 0AB Tel: 020 8748 7861 — MD Pahlavi 1966 (Pahlavi Univ.) DPM Ireland 1973; MRCPsych 1973; DPM Eng. 1973.

ROOHI, Shanila 26 Dawn Close, Ness, South Wirral CH64 4DS — MB ChB Glas. 1989.

ROOK, Christopher Demarquay 16 South Street, Oxford OX2 0BE — MB BS Lond. 1996.

ROOK, Professor Graham Arthur William Department of Bacteriology, Windeyer Building, 46 Cleveland St., London W1T 4JF Fax: 020 7636 8175 Email: g.rook@ucl.ac.uk — MB BChir Camb. 1971; MD Camb. 1978. Prof. Med. Microbiol. & Hon. Cons. Microbiol. UCL Med. Sch. Lond. Specialty: Immunol.

ROOKE, Alfred William Michael (retired) Orford House, Woodcote Grove, Meadow Hill, Coulsdon CR5 2XN Tel: 020 8660 4221 — MB BS Lond. 1930 (Univ. Coll. Hosp.) Prev: Regional Med. Off. DHSS.

ROOKE, David Kenneth Taunton Road Medical Centre, 12-16 Taunton Road, Bridgwater TA6 3LS Tel: 01278 444400 Fax: 01278 423691 — MB ChB Manch. 1977; MRCGP 1981.

ROOKE, Henry William Patrick 4 East Court, Cosham, Portsmouth PO6 2NX Tel: 023 92 373244 — (T.C. Dub.) BA Dub. 1953, MB BCh BAO 1955; DMRD Eng. 1960; FFR 1963; FRCR 1975. Specialty: Radiol. Prev: Cons. Radiol. Portsmouth Gp. Hosps.; Sen. Regist. (Radiol.) United Birm. Hosps.; Regist. Portsmouth Hosp. Gp.

ROOKE, Kenneth Christopher (retired) 22 Longlands, Worthing BN14 9NN Tel: 01903 236086 — MRCS Eng. LRCP Lond. 1962 (Guy's) Cert. Family Plann. JCC 1967; DFFP 1993. Indep. GP W. Sussex. Prev: GP Worthing.

ROOKER, Mr Guy David Cheltenham General Hospital, Sandford Road, Cheltenham GL53 7AN — MB BS Lond. 1971; MRCS Eng. LRCP Lond. 1971; FRCS Eng. 1975; FRCS Ed. (Orth.) 1981. Cons. Orthop. Surg. Cheltenham Gen. Hosp. Specialty: Orthop. Prev: Sen. Regist. (Orthop.) Radcliffe Infirm. & Nuffield Orthop. Centre; Oxf.; Regist. (Gen. Surg.) Cheltenham Gen. Hosp.

ROOKLEDGE, Marina Margaret Danetre Medical Practice, The Health Centre, London Road, Daventry NN11 4EJ Tel: 01327 703333 — MB BS Lond. 1990 (St. Thomas's Hospital Medical School London) DRCOG 1993; MRCGP 1995; DFFP 1995.

ROOKLEDGE, Mark Andrew 2 West Avenue, Pinner HA5 5BY — MB BS Lond. 1990.

ROOM, Geraldine Rainier Walden Cromwell Hospital, Cromwell Road, London SW5 0TU Tel: 020 7460 2000 Fax: 020 7460 5700 Email: grwroom@medix-uk.com; 151 Castelnau, Barnes, London SW13 9EW — MB BS Sydney 1973; FRACP Australia 1979. p/t Cons. Rheumatologist Private Practice. Specialty: Rheumatol. Socs: B.S. Rheumatology; B.S. Immunology; Austral. Rheum. Assoc. Prev: Cons. Rheumatologist, Ealing Hosp; Hon. Senior Lectuere, Imperial College; Cons. Physician/Rheumatologist, Bromley Dist.

ROOME, Jane Katherine Kingswood Surgery, Kingswood Road, Tunbridge Wells TN2 4UH Tel: 01892 511833 Email: janeroome@btinternet.com — MB BS Lond. 1992 (St Georges) DRCOG 1994; DFFP 1996; MRCGP 1996. p/t GP Asst. Specialty: Gen. Pract. Socs: Course organiser Tunbridge Wells Non Princip. Gp. Prev: GP Regist. - Rustham Tunbridge Wells; SHO Paediat. Pembury Hosp.; c/o the Elderly Pembury Hosp.

ROOME, Paul Christian The Kingswood Surgery, Kingswood Road, Tunbridge Wells TN2 4UJ Tel: 01892 511833 Fax: 01892 517597; 96 Culverden Down, Tunbridge Wells TN4 9TA — MB BS Lond. 1993 (St George's Hospital Medical School, Tooting, London) BSc (Hons.) Lond. 1990; DRCOG 1995; DFFP 1996; MRCGP 1997. Gen. Practitioner, Kingswood Surg., Tunbridge Wells, Kent; Clin. Asst. Neurol. Dept., Kent & Sussex Hosp., Tunbridge Wells.

ROOMI, Mr Riad 591 Fulham Road, London SW6 5UA Tel: 020 7385 3922 Fax: 020 7381 8180 — MB ChB Baghdad 1977 (Univ. Baghdad Coll. Med.) FICS 1988; Board Certified (Diploma), Amer Board of Hair Restoration Surg 1998. Cons. Cosmetic Surg. Lond.; Cons. Hair Restoration Surg. Specialty: Plastic Surg. Socs: Brit. Assn. Hair Restorat. Surgs.; Amer. Soc. Hair Restorat. Surg.; Amer. Acad. Cosmetic Surg. Prev: Regist. (A & E) St. Stephens Hosp. Lond.

ROOMS, Margaret (retired) 66 Blakes Lane, New Malden KT3 6NX Tel: 020 8942 3542 — (King's Coll. Hosp.) MB BS Lond. 1951; MRCS Eng. LRCP Lond. 1951; DA Eng. 1953; FFA RCS Eng. 1954. Prev: Cons. Anaesth. Qu. Mary's Hosp. Carshalton Surrey.

ROOMS, Mark Andrew, Maj. RAMC 2 (Trg) Regt AAC, Middle Wallop, Stockbridge SO20 8DY Tel: 01449 728276; 14 Roman Road, Wattisham, Ipswich IP7 7RW — BM Soton. 1988. Aircrew Train. Prev: GP Wattisham Nr. Ipswich; GP Ballykinler.

ROONEY, Barbara Ann 1 Appstree Cottages, Ockham Lane, Ockham, Woking GU23 6NR — MB BS Lond. 1982; MRCPsych 1987. Sen. Regist. (Psychiat.) St. Geo. Hosp. Atkinson Morley Hosps. Lond. Specialty: Gen. Psychiat. Prev: Sen. Regist. (Psychiat.) Qu. Mary's Univ. Hosp. Roehampton; Sen. Regist. (Psychiat.) St. Bernard's Wing Ealing Hosp., Gordon Hosp. & Qu. Mary's Univ. Hosp. Lond.

ROONEY, Christine Mary The Whitfield Practice, Hunslet Health Centre, 24 Church Street, Leeds LS10 2PE Tel: 0113 270 5194 Fax: 0113 270 2795 — MB BS Lond. 1982.

ROONEY, Clair Marie 2 Ryedale, Belmont, Durham DH1 2AL Tel: 0191 3709114 — MB BCh BAO NUI 1989 (University Coll. Dublin) DCH RCP Lond. 1991; Cert. Family Plann. JCC 1992; MRCGP 1992; DTM & H Liverp. 1993. Prev: Trainee GP Hull; Locum GP Leeds.

ROONEY, Dennis 20 Northumberland Avenue, Gosforth, Newcastle upon Tyne NE3 4XE; The Croft, Galloping Green Road, Wrekenton, Gateshead NE9 6DT — MB BS Newc. 1981; DCCH RCP Ed. 1984; MRCGP 1985; DRCOG 1985.

ROONEY, Desmond Patrick Diabetes Centre, Victoria Infirmary, Langside Rd, Glasgow G42 9TY; 2/1, 28 Bellwood ST,, Glasgow G41 3ES — MD Belf. 1991 (Queen's Univ. Belfast) MB BCh BAO 1984; MRCP (UK) 1987. Cons. Phys. Diabetes & Endocrinol. Vict. Infirm. Glas. Specialty: Diabetes; Endocrinol. Prev: Sen. Regist. Belf.; Post Doctoral Assoc. Univ. of Minnesota Minneapolis, USA.

ROONEY, Francis Joseph 22 Falkland Rise, Moortown, Leeds LS17 6JQ Tel: 0113 268 4470 Fax: 0113 268 4470 — MB ChB Leeds 1980 (Univ. Leeds) DRCOG 1983; Cert. Family Plann. JCC 1985. Specialty: Gen. Pract.; Family Plann. & Reproduc. Health; Obst. & Gyn. Prev: BAMS; GP Princip. Leeds; GP Regist. Cornw.

ROONEY, Guy Jonathan Sexual Health Dept., Great Western Hospital, Marlborough Road, Swindon SN3 6BB Tel: 01793 604038 — MB BS Lond. 1989; BSc Lond. 1986; MRCP (UK) 1993; Dip. GU Med. Soc. Apoth. Lond. 1995; DFFP 1997; Dip Sytemative Reviews Lond. 1999; FRCP 2003. Cons. (Genitourin. Med.) Gt. West. Hosp. Swindon; Cons. (Genitourin. Med), Harrison Dept, Radcliffe Infirm. Specialty: Genitourinary Medicine; HIV Med. Socs: MSSVD; BMA; AGUM. Prev: Cons., (Genitourin. - Med) Princess Margt. Hosp. Swindon, Wilts.

ROONEY, Mary Magdalen Elizabeth 174 Ferry Road, Edinburgh EH6 4NS Tel: 0131 554 8166 — MD Belf. 1988; MB BCh BAO Belf. 1980; MRCP (UK) 1983; DCH Dub. 1985. Lect. Rheum. Univ. Edin. (Rheum. Dis. Unit), N. Gen. Hosp. Edin. Prev: Research Fell. (Rheum.) St. Vincents & St. Jas. Hosps. Dub.; Regist. (Med.) Altnagelvin Hosp. Londonderry; SHO (Rheum.) Roy. Vict. Hosp. Belf.

ROONEY, Matthew Jonathan Department of Anaesthetics, Birmingham Heartlands Hospital, Bordesley Green E., Birmingham B9 5SS Tel: 0121 424 3488 Fax: 0121 424 1441 — MB BS Newc. 1986 (Newcastle-upon-Tyne) FRCA 1991. Cons. (Anaesth.) Birm. Heartland & Solihull NHS Trust; Cons. Anaesth. Birm. Heartlands & Solihull NHS Trust Birm. Specialty: Anaesth. Socs: Assn. Anaesth. & Soc. Computing & Technol. in Anaesth.; Brit. Ophth. Anaesth. Soc. Prev: Sen. Regist. Anaesth. City Hosp. Birm.; Sen. Regist. Qu. Eliz. Hosp. Birm.; Research Fell. Univ. Dept. of Anaesth. Nottm.

ROONEY, Michael Joseph Bramhall Park Medical Centre, 235 Bramhall Lane South, Bramhall, Stockport SK7 3EP Tel: 0161 440 7669 Fax: 0161 440 7671 — MB ChB Manch. 1983; MRCGP 1987; DGM RCP Lond. 1987. Prev: Trainee GP Hillingdon Hosp.

ROONEY, Nicholas Department of Cellular Pathology, Royal United Hospital, Bath BA1 3NG Tel: 01225 824705 Fax: 01225 461044 — MB ChB Bristol 1979; MRCPath 1986; MD Sheff. 1986; T(Path) 1991. Cons. Histopath. Roy. United Hosp. Bath. Specialty: Histopath. Socs: Brit. Lymphoma Path. Gp.; Sec. Brit. Lymphoma Path GP-Internat. Acad. Path. (Brit. Div.). Prev: Cons. Sen. Lect. Univ. Bristol; Lect. (Path.) Sheff. Univ. Med. Sch.; SHO (Clin. Path.) Roy. Hallamsh. Hosp. Sheff.

ROONEY, Paul Joseph Bacteriology Laboratory, Belfast City Hospital, Belfast BT9 7AB Tel: 02890 263661 Fax: 02890 263991 — MB BCh BAO Belf. 1982; BSc Belf. 1979; MB BCh Belf. 1982; MRCPath 1990; DTM & H RCP Lond. 1990. Cons. Med. Microbiol. Belf. City Hosp. Belf. Specialty: Med. Microbiol.

ROONEY, Mr Paul Stephen Royal Liverpool University Hospital, Prescot Street, Liverpool L7 8XP Tel: 0161 706 3426 Fax: 0161 706 5828; Loreto, Osbert Road, Blundellsands, Liverpool L23 6UP Tel: 0151 931 1085 — MB ChB Sheff. 1984; FRCS Ed. 1988; DM Nottm. 1994. Cons. Colorectal Surg. Roy. Liverp. Hosp. Specialty: Gen. Surg. Socs: Brit. Assn. Surgic. Oncol.; BSG; Assn. Coloproct. GB & Irel. Prev: Lect. (Gen. Surg.) Nottm.; Lect. (Surg.) 1996-1998.

ROONEY, Richard Geoffrey (retired) 45 Knowsley Road W., Blackburn BB1 9PW Tel: 01254 249008 — MB ChB Manch. 1946 (Manchester) DCH Eng. 1950.

ROONEY, Stephen James The Fields, Kingsland, Shrewsbury SY3 7AF — BM BS Nottm. 1986.

ROONEY, Veena (retired) Boundary House, Coombe Road, Salisbury SP2 8BT Tel: 01722 334282 Email: rooneybv@aol.com — (Rangoon) MB BS Rangoon 1956. SCMO Salisbury HA.

ROOPE, Richard Marcus The Whiteley Surgery, Yew Tree Drive, Whiteley, Fareham PO15 7LB Tel: 01489 881982 Fax: 01489 881980; Silverbeck, Lake Road, Curdridge, Southampton SO32 2HH Tel: 01489 795199 — MB BS Lond. 1987 (Camb. & Roy. Lond. Hosp.) BA (Psychol.) Camb. 1984, MA 1988; DGM RCP Lond. 1989; DCH RCP Lond. 1990; MRCGP 1991; DFFP 1993; Dip Occ Med RCP Lond. 1998. Med. Dir. Occupational Health Consultancy Ltd. Specialty: Rheumatol.; Occupat. Health. Socs: Christ. Med. Fellowsh. (Wessex Regional Sec.).; Soc. Occ. Med. Prev: GP Princip. Soton. & Clin. Asst. (Rheum.) Soton. Gen. Hosp.; Ho. Off. (Surg.) Epsom Dist. Hosp. Surrey.; Ho. Off. (Med. & Geriat.) Qu. Mary's Hosp. Sidcup, Kent.

ROOTH, Francis Graham (retired) 6 Church Avenue, Bristol BS9 1LD — MRCS Eng. LRCP Lond. 1964 (Middlx.) BA Camb. 1958; MPhil Lond. 1970, MD 1973, MB BS 1964; MRCPsych 1971. Cons. Psychiat. Bristol Health Dist. (T). Prev: Sen. Regist. Bethlem Roy. & Maudsley Hosps.

ROOTH, Jane Alexandra 6 Church Avenue, Stoke Bishop, Bristol BS9 1LD — MB BS Lond. 1964 (Middlx.) MRCS Eng. LRCP Lond. 1964.

ROOTS, Lila Mabel (retired) 52, Barfield Crescent, Leeds LS7 8RU Tel: 0113 268 1953 — (Leeds) MB ChB 1961; DPH Liverp. 1965; MCPS Ontario 1971; LMCC 1971; MFCM 1979; BA Leeds 1993. Prev: Dep. MOH Metro Windsor, Ont. Canada.

ROOTS, Peter James 6 Linsey Close, Hemel Hempstead HP3 8DA — BM Soton. 1996. SHO (Psychiat.) Qu. Eliz. Psychiat. Hosp. Specialty: Gen. Psychiat. Prev: Ho. Off. (Med.) Redditch Alexandra Hosp.; Ho. Off. (Surg.) Russells Hall Hosp. Dudley.

ROPE, Tamsin Caroline Maxcroft House, Hilperton Marsh, Trowbridge BA14 7PS — MB ChB Birm. 1996; ChB Birm. 1996. SHO (A & E) Glos. Roy. NHS Hosp. Specialty: Gen. Med.

ROPEL, Christine Anne 36 High Oaks Road, Welwyn Garden City AL8 7BH Tel: 01707 377414 — MB BS Lond. 1979; DMRD Eng. 1983; FRCR 1988. Cons. Diag. Radiol. Qu. Eliz. Hosp. Welwyn Gdn. City. Specialty: Radiol. Prev: Sen. Regist. (Diag. Radiol.) Char. Cross Hosp. Lond.

ROPER, Alan Frederick (retired) Bulcote Lodge, Bulcote, Nottingham NG14 5GU — MRCS Eng. LRCP Lond. 1951; FFA RCS Eng. 1958. Prev: Anaesth. S. Warw. Hosp. Gp.

ROPER, Barry Windsor Diagnostic X-Ray Department, Neath General Hospital, Neath SA11 2LQ — MB ChB Birm. 1957; MB ChB (Hons. Obst.) Birm. 1957; MRCP Lond. 1964; DMRD Eng. 1966; FFR 1969. Cons. Radiol. W. Glam. AHA. Specialty: Radiol. Socs: Brit. Med. Ultrasound Soc.; S. Wales Ultrasound Gp. Prev: Med. Regist. Dudley Rd. Hosp. Birm.; Clin. Tutor (Radiol.) Univ. Birm.; Sen. Regist. Radiol. United Birm. Hosps.

ROPER, Daniel James Springhead Medical Centre, 376 Willerby Road, Hull HU5 5JT; 376 Willerby Road, Hull HU5 5JT Tel: 01482 52263 — MB ChB Ed. 1982; MRCGP 1986. GP Hull.

ROPER, David John St Johns Medical Centre, 62 London Road, Grantham NG31 6HR Tel: 01476 590055 Fax: 01476 400042; Ashfield House, Casthorpe Road, Barrowby, Grantham NG32 1DP — MB BS Lond. 1974 (Westm.) MRCS Eng. LRCP Lond. 1974; DCH Eng. 1978; MRCGP 1979. GP Trainer Grantham. Prev: Trainee GP Cirencester VTS; Ho. Off. (Orhop. Surg.) Qu. Mary's Hosp. Roehampton; Ho. Phys. (Gen. Med.) City Hosp. Nottm.

ROPER, Emma Cathryn Sheffield Children's Hospital, Clinical Genetics Department, Western Bank, Sheffield S11 7GL Tel: 0114 271 7025 — MB ChB Leic. 1996; MRCPCH 1999. Specialist Regist. Sheff. Childr. Hosp. Specialty: Genetics. Prev: Sen. SHO (Paediat.) Kettering Gen. Hosp.; SHO (Neonatol.) Leics. Roy. Infirm.; SHO (Paediat.) Leics. Roy. Infirm.

ROPER, Gordon Paul 6 Wingate Close, Trumpington, Cambridge CB2 2HW Tel: 01223 514752 Fax: 01223 515713 — MB BCh BAO NUI 1984 (Roy Coll. Surgs. In Irel.) BSc New Brunswick 1981; LRCPI & LM, LRCSI & LM 1984. GP Clin. Asst. Addenbrooke's Hosp. Camb. Specialty: Gen. Pract. Prev: GP Regist. Buffisham Surg. Camb.; Med. Resid. Fac. Med. Memor. Univ. Newfld..; Ho. Off. Glas. Roy. Infirm. & Roy. Orthop. Hosp. Birm.

ROPER, Helen Margaret (retired) 90 Bourverie Avenue, Salisbury SP2 8DK — MB BS Lond. 1967 (Roy. Free) MRCS Eng. LRCP Lond. 1967. Prev: Clin. Med. Off. Salisbury DHA.

ROPER, Helen Patricia Department Paediatrics, Birmingham Heartlands Hospital, Bordesley Green E., Birmingham B9 5SS Tel: 0121 766 6611 Fax: 0121 773 6458 — MD Manch. 1989; MB ChB (Hons.) Manch. 1980; DCH RCP Lond. 1982; MRCP (UK) 1983; FRCP Lond. 1996. Cons. Paediat. Birm. Heartlands Hosp. Specialty: Paediat. Prev: Tutor (Child Health) Manch. Univ.

ROPER, Ian William Millward King Street Surgery, 22A King Street, Hereford HR4 9DA Tel: 01432 272181 Fax: 01432 344725 — MB ChB Leic. 1990; DRCOG 1992; Dip Thor. 1998.

ROPER, Janice Homerton Hospital, Homerton Road, London E9 6SR Tel: 020 8510 7952 Fax: 020 8510 7448; 220 Richmond Road, Hackney, London E8 3QN Tel: 020 7254 4078 Fax: 020 7254 4078 — BM BS Nottm. 1980 (Nottingham) BMedSci Nottm. 1978, BM BS 1980; MRCP (UK) 1984. Cons. (Neonat. Paediat.) Homerton Hosp. Specialty: Neonat. Socs: FRCPCH; BAPM. Prev: Cons. & Sen. Lect. (Neonat. Paediat.) Homerton Hosp. Lond.; Sen. Lect. Med. Coll. St. Bart. Hosp. Lond.; Sen. Regist. (Paediat.) Parkside HA.

ROPER, John (retired) 2 Levignen Close, Church Crookham, Fleet GU52 0TW Tel: 01252 622234 — (Westm.) MB BS Lond. 1948; MRCS Eng. LRCP Lond. 1948; FRCOG 1968, M 1954. Prev: Cons. O & G W. Surrey & NE Hants. Health Dist.

ROPER, John Patrick 7 Ashburton Avenue, Birkenhead CH43 8TJ — MB BChir Camb. 1994.

ROPER, Mr John Paul The Cottage, Old Road, Thornton in Craven, Skipton BD23 3TB Tel: 01282 843962 — MB BCh BAO Dub. 1970; FRCSI 1982; FCOphth 1988. Cons. Ophth. Burnley Gen. Hosp. Specialty: Ophth. Prev: Sen. Regist. Wolverhampton Eye Infirm.; Regist./SHO Hallamsh. Hosp. Sheff.

ROPER, Joseph Neville (retired) 40 Ranmoor Cliffe Road, Sheffield S10 3HB Tel: 0114 230 7208 — MB ChB Sheff. 1951; MRCS Eng. LRCP Lond. 1951; DObst RCOG 1955. Prev: GP Derby.

ROPER, Michael (retired) La Corderie, 3 La Vallee, Alderney GY9 3XA — MRCS Eng. LRCP Lond. 1946 (St. Mary's)

ROPER, Nicholas Alan 47 Douglas Villas, Durham DH1 1JL — BM BS Nottm. 1992; BMedSci (Hons.) Nottm. 1990; MRCP (UK) 1995. Regist. (Diabetes & Endocrinol.) Northern Deanery. Specialty: Diabetes; Endocrinol.; Gen. Med.

ROPER, Nigel David King The Surgery, Vicarage Lane, Walton on the Naze CO14 8PA Tel: 01255 674373 Fax: 01255 851005 — BM Soton. 1983.

ROPER, Paul Howard The Surgery, 2 Great Wood Road, Small Heath, Birmingham B10 9QE Tel: 0121 766 8828 Fax: 0121 773 0091 — MB ChB Manch. 1980; DCH RCP Lond. 1983; MRCGP 1985.

ROPER, Paul Winnard Roper and Partners, Syston Health Centre, Melton Road, Leicester LE7 2EQ Tel: 0116 260 9111 Fax: 0116 260 9055 — BM BCh Oxf. 1978; BA Camb. 1975; MRCGP 1986.

ROPER, Phyllis Barbara (retired) Bulcote Lodge, Burton Joyce, Nottingham NG14 5GU Tel: 0115 931 2160 — MB ChB Sheff. 1951. Prev: SCMO (Community Health) Notts. HA.

ROPER, Robin Mark Blackwater Medical Centre, Princes Road, Maldon CM9 7DS Tel: 01621 854204 Fax: 01621 850246; 1 Bergen Court, Maldon CM9 6UH — MB BS Lond. 1982; DA (UK) 1986; MRCGP 1991. Specialty: Care of the Elderly.

ROPER-HALL, Mr Michael John (cons. rooms), 38 Harborne Road, Edgbaston, Birmingham B15 3HE Tel: 0121 454 2721; 51 Church Road, Edgbaston, Birmingham B15 3SJ Tel: 0121 454 2310 Fax: 0121 454 0090 — MRCS Eng. LRCP Lond. 1945 (Birm.) MB ChB Birm. 1945; DOMS Eng. 1946; FRCS Eng. 1948; ChM Birm. 1952; FRCOphth 1988; Hon. FRCOphth 1990. Hon. Cons. Surg. Birm. & Midl. Eye Hosp.; Hon. Cons. Ophth. Qu. Eliz. Hosp. Birm. Specialty: Ophth. Socs: Fell. Roy. Soc. Med. (Ex-Pres. Sect. Ophth.). Prev: Ex-Pres. Fac. Ophths. & Ophth. Soc. UK; Mem. Bd. Governors Moorfields Eye Hosp. Special HA; Mem. Counc. & Mem. Ct. Examrs. RCS Eng. (Chairm. Specialist Advis. Comm. (Ophth.) Jt. Comm. on Higher Surg. Train.).

ROPNER, Janet Elizabeth Haematology Department, Gloucestershire Royal NHS Trust, Great Western Road, Gloucester GL1 3NN Tel: 01452 395252; Rossett, Balcarras Road, Charlton Kings, Cheltenham GL53 8QG — MB BS Lond. 1971 (Univ. Coll. Hosp.) BSc (Special) Lond. 1968; MRCP (UK) 1974; FRCPath 1994, M 1982; FRCP Lond. 1994. Cons. Haemat. Glos. Roy. Hosp. Specialty: Haematology. Prev: Sen. Regist. (Haemat.) Oxf. AHA (T); SHO (Med.) Hammersmith Hosp. Lond.; Ho. Phys. Univ. Coll. Hosp. Lond.

ROPNER, Richard John Ronald Rossett, Balcarras Road, Charlton Kings, Cheltenham GL53 8QG — MB ChB Ed. 1965; DObst RCOG 1970; DPM Eng. 1972; MRCPsych 1973. Cons. (Adult Ment. Illness & Alcoholism) Charlton La. Centre, Cheltnam. Specialty: Ment. Health. Socs: Fell. Roy. Soc. Trop. Med. & Hyg. Prev: Sen. Regist. Warneford Hosp. Oxf.; Rotating Intern Pottsville Hosp., U.S.A.; Med. Off. United Africa Co. (Nigeria) Ltd. Lagos.

ROPNER, Vivien Anne (retired) Tethermill House, 2A Millfield Road, Whickham, Newcastle upon Tyne NE16 4QA Tel: 0161 488 7908 — MB BS Durh. 1955 (Newc.) Prev: Ho. Phys., Ho. Surg. & Res. Med. Off. Roy. Vict. Infirm. Newc.

ROPPER, David Noel (retired) Pennygown House, Campbeltown PA28 6PH Tel: 01586 551050 — BSc (Hons. Physiol.) Glas. 1958; MB ChB Glas. 1961; FRCP Glas. 1981, M 1965; LMCC 1970. Prev: Cons. Geriat. Roy. Alexandra Infirm. Paisley.

ROQUES, Antoine William Wanklyn Dept. Of Haematology, Worthing Hospital, Worthing BN11 2DN Tel: 01903 205111 Fax: 01903 285072; 47 Hillside Avenue, Worthing BN14 9QS Tel: 01903 237229 — MB BS Lond. 1973 (St. Thos.) FRCP Lond. 1991, M 1976; FRCPath 1991, M 1979. Cons. Haemat. Worthing & Southlands Hosps.; Regional Adviser (Path.) S. Thames (W.). Specialty: Haematology. Socs: Brit. Soc. Haematol. Prev: Lect. (Haemat.) & Asst. Lect. (Path.) St. Thos. Hosp. Med. Sch. Lond.; Ho. Phys. St. Thos. Hosp. Lond.

ROQUES, Clare Joanna 47 Hillside Avenue, Worthing BN14 9QS — BChir Camb. 1996.

ROQUES, Thomas William 45 Rochester Road, London NW1 9JJ — BM BCh Oxf. 1994.

RORIE, David Archer Terra Nova House Medical Practice, 43 Dura Street, Dundee DD4 6SW Tel: 01382 451100 Fax: 01382 453679 — MB ChB Aberd. 1973.

RORKE, Steuart Flat C, 20A Molyneux Park Road, Tunbridge Wells TN4 8DT — MB ChB Stellenbosch 1996.

RORRISON, Hugh Webster 342A Perth Road, Dundee DD2 1EQ — MB ChB Dund. 1998; MB ChB Dund 1998; FRCA 2004.

ROSALIE, Ralph Marlborough Medical Practice, The Surgery, George Lane, Marlborough SN8 4BY Tel: 01672 512187 Fax: 01672 516809 — MB ChB Leeds 1989; DRWG; MB ChB Leeds. 1989; MRCGP 1994. SHO (A & E) Pontefract Gen. Hosp. Prev: Ho.

Off. (Surg.) Harrogate Dist. Hosp.; SHO VTS Scheme (Milton Keynes Hosp.).

ROSALKI, Sidney Bertram 10 Wimpole Mews, London W1G 8PE Tel: 020 7486 7517 Fax: 020 7486 7517 — MB BS Lond. 1953 (St. Mary's) MRCS Eng. LRCP Lond. 1953; FRCP Lond. 1981, M 1958; DSc (Med.) Lond. 1986, MD 1962; FRCPath 1975, M 1963; MCB Jt. Exam. Bd. (Hon.) 1996. Med. Dir. & Cons. Chem. Path. Omnilabs, UK; Hon. Cons. Chem. Path. Roy. Free Hosp. Lond. Specialty: Chem. Path. Socs: Fell. Roy. Soc. Med. (Ex. Pres. Sect. Path.); Internat. Soc. Clin. Enzyme; Amer. Assn. for Clin. Chem. Prev: Cons. Chem. Path. Roy. Free Hosp. Lond.; Cons. Path. St. Mary's Hosp. & Paddington Childr. Hosp. Lond.; Flight Lt. RAF Med. Br.

ROSANWO, Mr Emmanuel Olufemi 17 Stiles Road, Liverpool L33 4EA Tel: 0151 546 8900 Fax: 0151 546 8900 — MB BS Ibadan 1975; FRCS Ed. 1981. Specialty: Accid. & Emerg.

ROSANWO, Mofolusho Omobola Monisola (retired) 17 Stiles Road, Liverpool L33 4EA — MB BS Ibadan 1974; MB BS Ibadan Nigeria 1974; FFA RCSI 1983. Prev: Locum Cons. Anaesth.and Locum Assoc. Anaesth.Aintree Hosps. Fazakerley Liverp.

ROSARIO, Amanda Jane Foxhill Medical Centre, 363 Halifax Road, Sheffield S6 1AF Tel: 0114 232 2055 Fax: 0114 285 5963; 21 Ryegate Crescent, Sheffield S10 5FD — MB ChB Sheff. 1988; MRCGP 1996.

ROSBOTHAM, Jane Louise Epsom Hospital, Dorking Road, Epsom KT18 Tel: 01372 735735 Ext: 6547; 2 Spenser Avenue, Weybridge KT13 0ST — MB BS Lond. 1988 (Guy's Hospital) MRCP (UK) 1991. p/t Cons. Dermatol., Epsom Hosps. Specialty: Dermat. Special Interest: Mole Checks; Psoriasis; Skin cancer. Socs: BMA; RSM; BAD. Prev: Sen. Regist., St Georges Hosp.; Regist., St Johns Inst. of Dermat.

ROSBOTHAM-WILLIAMS, Gary Martin Holme Green, Lathom Road, Ormskirk L39 0EA — MB ChB Liverp. 1991.

ROSBOTTOM, Jane Margaret St Georges Surgery, 46A Preston New Road, Blackburn BB2 6AH Tel: 01254 53791 Fax: 01254 697221 — MB ChB Manch. 1986; MRCGP 1990; DRCOG 1990.

ROSBOTTOM, Robert Coldside Medical Practice, 129 Strathmartine Road, Dundee DD3 8DB Tel: 01382 826724 Fax: 01382 884129 — MB ChB Ed. 1974.

ROSCOE, Alan Harwood, MBE (retired) 80 Fildyke Road, Meppershall, Shefford SG17 5LU Tel: 01462 816153 — MB ChB Manch. 1954 (Manch.) DObst RCOG 1955; MRCGP 1965; DAvMed Eng. 1971; MFOM RCP Lond. 1981; MD Manch. 1983. Cons. Med. Adviser Britannia Airways Luton. Prev: Adjunct. Prof. Embry-Riddle Aeronautical Univ. Florida, USA.

ROSCOE, Bruce Luckholds Farm, Alfrick, Worcester WR6 5HW Tel: 01886 32980 — MB ChB Birm. 1964; FFA RCS Eng. 1969. Cons. (Anaesth.) Hereford & Worcester AHA. Specialty: Anaesth.

ROSCOE, Elizabeth Joy Haresfield House Surgery, 6-10 Bath Road, Worcester WR5 3EJ Tel: 01905 763161 Fax: 01905 767016; The Tynings, Church Lane, Flyford Flavell, Worcester WR7 4BZ Tel: 0138 682470 — (Birm.) MB ChB Birm. 1964. Prev: Ho. Phys. & Ho. Surg. Ronkswood Hosp. Worcester.

ROSCOE, Peter (cons. room), 11 Imperial Square, Cheltenham GL50 1QU Tel: 01242 522646 — MB ChB Ed. 1967; BSc (Hons.) Ed. 1965; MRCP (UK) 1970; FRCP Ed. 1981. Cons. Phys. Cheltenham Gen. Hosp.; Med. Dir. E. Glos. NHS Trust. Specialty: Gen. Med. Prev: Sen. Regist. (Gen. Med. & Respirat. Dis.) & Regist. (Respirat. Dis.) City Hosp. Edin.; Regist. (Gen. Med. & Clin. Toxicol.) Roy. Infirm. Edin.

ROSCOE, Sally Anne The Tynings, Church Lane, Flyford, Flavell, Worcester WR7 4BZ — MB ChB Birm. 1993.

ROSCOE, Trefor John Beighton Health Centre, Queens Road, Beighton, Sheffield S20 1BJ Tel: 0114 269 5061 — MB ChB Sheff. 1982. Lect. (GP) Univ. Sheff.; GP CME Tutor Informatics N. Trent. Specialty: Gen. Pract. Socs: Brit. Healthcare Internet Assn. Research Coordinator; GP Writers Assn.; Soc. Internet in Med. Prev: Trainee GP Worksop VTS.

ROSCROW, Suzanne Elizabeth St. Johns Hosp, Howden, Livingston EH54 6PP Tel: 01506 419666 — MB ChB Aberd. 1986; MRCPsych 1991; MPhil Ed. 1994. Cons. (Psychiat), St Johns Hosp., Livingston. Specialty: Geriat. Psychiat. Prev: Sen. Regist. (Psychiat.) Roy. Edin. Hosp.

ROSE, Adrian Paul 1 Edwen Close, Childwall, Liverpool L16 5HF — MB ChB Liverp. 1996; BDS Wales 1983; FDS Glas. 1989. SHO (Gen. Surg., Orthop., A & E, Paediat.) Basic Surgic. Regional Rotat. Whiston Dist. Gen. Hosp. Merseyside; Specialist (Oral Surg.) S. Yorks. Specialty: Orthop. Socs: Assoc. Mem. Brit. Assn. Oral & Maxillofacial Surg. Prev: Ho. Off. (Surg. & Med.) Roy. Liverp. Univ. Hosp.; Regist. (Maxillofacial Surg.) Roy. Liverp. Univ. Hosp.

ROSE, Amanda Fiona Flat 8, Albion Terrace, London Road, Reading RG1 5BG — MB BS Lond. 1982; DCH RCP Lond. 1985; MRCP Lond. 1986. Regist. (Paediat.) Roy. Berks. Hosp., Reading; Regist. (Paediat.) John Radcliffe Hosp Oxf. Specialty: Paediat. Prev: SHO (Paediat.) Gt. Ormond St. Hosp.; SHO (Paediat.) Qu. Eliz. Hosp. for Childr. Lond.; SHO (Neonat. Paediat.) Qu. Charlottes Matern. Hosp. Lond.

ROSE, Andrew John The Surgery, 5 Sloane Avenue, London SW3 3JD Tel: 020 7581 3187 Fax: 020 7225 0034 Email: chelsea.medical@nhs.net; 4 Markham Square, London SW3 4UY — MB ChB Birm. 1971; BSc (Hons.) (Physiol.) Birm. 1968; DObst RCOG 1975; Cert. Family Plann. JCC 1975; MRCGP 1976; Dip. Pharm. Med. RCP 1980; MFPM 1989. GP Princip.; Wates Gp., Macmillan Cancer Relief; Non-Exec. Chairm. J.H. Lavender & Company Ltd. W. Bromwich; Med. Off. Nat.Britannia Ltd. Specialty: Gen. Pract. Socs: Chelsea Clin. Soc.; Small Pract.s Assn.; Brit. Assn. Pharmaceut. Phys. Prev: Med. Adviser Beecham Pharmaceuts.; Examr. Dip. Nursing Univ. Lond.; Trainee GP St. Thos. Hosp. VTS & Bristol VTS.

ROSE, Andrew John Rose, Tinker and Healy, The Surgery, Bowholm, Canonbie DG14 0UX Tel: 01387 371313 Fax: 01387 371244; Chestnut Cottage, Blackford, Carlisle CA6 4EG Tel: 01228 74094 — MB ChB Manch. 1987 (Manch. Med. Sch.) DCOG 1992; MRCGP 1993. GP Canonbie Med. Pract. Specialty: Gen. Pract. Prev: VTS Carlisle.

ROSE, Barry Stuart 626 London Road, Davenham, Northwich CW9 8LG Tel: 01606 42662 — (Manch.) MRCS Eng. LRCP Lond. 1959; DObst RCOG 1963; FFHom 1982, M 1980. Specialty: Homeop. Med. Prev: Dean Fac. of Homoeop.; Pres. Fac. of Homoeop. Roy. Lond. Homoeop. Hosp. Lond.

ROSE, Caroline Jane Theatre Royal Surgery, Theatre St., Dereham NR19 2EN; Lyng House, Rectory Road, Lyng, Norwich NR9 5RA — MB ChB Bristol 1982; DRCOG 1984; MRCGP 1986. Specialty: Rheumatol.

ROSE, Catherine Elizabeth 19 Redleaf Close, Tunbridge Wells TN2 3UD — MB BS Newc. 1993 (Newcastle upon Tyne) Dip Child Health 1996; Dip of Family Plann. 2000. GP Princip. Specialty: Gen. Pract. Prev: SHO (A & E) Morriston Hosp. Swansea; SHO (Gen. Med.) Shotley Bridge Dist. Gen. Hosp. Consett; SHO (Clin. Geratol. & Rehabil.) Radcliffe Infirm. Oxf.

ROSE, Charles David Lauchlan 42 Bartholomew Villas, London NW5 2LL — MB BS Lond. 1986.

ROSE, Christopher Francis Linden Medical Group, Linden Medical Centre, Linden Avenue, Kettering NN15 7NX Tel: 01536 512104 Fax: 01536 415930; Werburgh House, 46 Cranford Road, Barton Seagrave, Kettering NN15 5JH Tel: 01536 726051 Email: chris.rose@virgin.net — MB BS Lond. 1977 (King's Coll. Lond. & St. Geo.) BSc (Hons.) Lond. 1974; DRCOG 1982; MRCGP 1984. LMC Med. Sec. 1998-; Clin. Teach. Univ. Leicester Med. Sch. 1997-. Specialty: Gen. Pract. Prev: Trainee GP Bristol VTS; SHO (Med.) Plymouth Health Dist.; Ho. Off. St. Geo. Hosp. Lond.

ROSE, Claire Michelle 2 St Anthonys Close, Ottery St Mary EX11 1EN — BM Soton. 1997.

ROSE, Daniel Murray Austhorpe View Surgery, 5 Austhorpe View, Leeds LS15 8NN Tel: 0113 260 2262 Fax: 0113 232 8090; 24 Sandhill Oval, Alwoodley, Leeds LS17 8EA Tel: 0113 268 8155 — MB BS Lond. 1974 (King's Coll. Hosp.) MRCGP 1978; Cert FPA. 1980. Clin. Asst. (A & E) St. Jas. Hosp. Leeds.; Mem. Leeds LMC. Prev: Trainee GP Leeds VTS; SHO (Obst.) St. Mary's Hosp. Leeds; SHO (Paediat.) Roy. Infirm. Huddersfield.

ROSE, David Hill Brow Surgery, Long Croft, Staincross, Barnsley S75 6FH Tel: 01226 383131 Fax: 01226 380100; 339A Darton Lane, Mapplewell, Barnsley S75 6AW Tel: 01226 387756 Email: david.rose@wdconfed.nhs.uk — MB ChB Sheff. 1981; MA Camb. 1982; DRCOG 1985; MRCGP 1985. GP; Assoc. Postgrad. Dean, S. Yorks and S. Humba. Prev: Course Organiser Barnsley VTS.

ROSE, Mr David Harold Mount Pleasant Farm, 105 Moss Lane, Bramhall, Stockport SK7 1EG Tel: 0161 439 7459 Email: d.h.rose@talk21.com — MB ChB Manch. 1962; DLO Eng. 1970; FRCS Ed. 1972. Coordinator of universal Neonat. hearing screening Progr. Stockport NHS Trust- (Part Time Cons.). Specialty: Audiol. Med. Socs: Mem. Brit. Soc. Audiol Full Mem.; Full Mem. Manch. Med. Soc. Prev: Sen. Regist. (ENT) Sheff. AHA (T); Regist. (ENT) United Sheff. Hosps.; Regist. (ENT) Stockport & Buxton Gp. Hosps.

ROSE, David John Anthony Whitecroft, Sandy Lane, Pleasington, Blackburn BB2 6RE — MB ChB Liverp. 1977; FFA RCS Eng. 1982. Cons. Anaesth. Blackburn Hosps. Specialty: Anaesth.

ROSE, David Simon Charles Department of Histopathology, Royal United Hospital of Bath, Combe Park, Weston, Bath BA1 3NG Tel: 01225 824716; 40 Combe Park, Bath BA1 3NR Tel: 01225 824963 — MB BS Lond. 1987; BSc (Hons.) Lond. 1984; DRCPath 1992; MRCPath 1995. Cons. Histopath. Roy. United Hosp. Bath. Specialty: Histopath. Prev: Sen. Regist. (Histopath.) Univ. Coll. Ldon. Med. Sch.

ROSE, Donald Hugh Department of Radiology, Nottingham City hospital NHS Trust, Hucknall Road, Nottingham NG5 1PB Tel: 0115 969 1169 Ext: 45801 Fax: 0115 962 7776 Email: drose@nchit.trent.nhs.uk; 1 Pinfold Cl, Woodborough, Nottingham NG14 6DP Tel: 0115 965 2866 Email: donrose@doctors.org.uk — (Univ. Coll. Hosp.) MRCS Eng. LRCP Lond. 1967; MB BS Lond. 1967; DMRD Eng. 1972; FFR 1974; FRCR 1975. Cons. Radiol. City Hosp. Nottm. City Hosp. Specialty: Radiol. Prev: Research Fell. Roy. Marsden Hosp. Lond.; Radiol. Sen. Regist. Guy's Hosp. Lond.

ROSE, Edward Leslie Halton General Hospital, Hospital Way, Runcorn WA7 2DA Tel: 01928 713714 Fax: 01928 753119; Bank House Farm, 287 Chester Road, Helsby, Frodsham WA6 0PT Tel: 01928 722334 — MB BS Lond. 1982 (Guy's) BA Oxf. 1979, DM 1992; FRCP Ed. 1996; FRCP 1997. Cons. Phys. (Cardiol.) North Cheshire Hospitals NHS Trust. Specialty: Cardiol. Socs: Brit. Cardiac Soc.; Brit. Soc. Echocardiogr. Prev: Regist. (Gen. Med. & Cardiol.) Aberd. Roy. Infirm.; Research Regist. (Cardiol.) Northwick Pk. Hosp. Harrow; Regist. Rotat. (Med.) Univ. Hosp. Wales Cardiff.

ROSE, Elizabeth, MBE (retired) Ernsheenie, Dalbeattie DG5 4QW — MD Ed. 1972; MB ChB 1950; FRCGP 1977, M 1965.

ROSE, Elizabeth Margaret (retired) 8 Malta Terrace, Edinburgh EH4 1HR Tel: 0131 332 5823/01786 832389 — (Edinburgh) MB ChB Ed. 1938; FRCOG 1966, M 1947. Prev: Cons. O & G Stirling Roy. Infirm. & Assoc. Hosps.

ROSE, Eric David Milton Keynes Village Practice, Griffith Gate, Middleton, Milton Keynes MK10 9BQ Tel: 01908 393979 Fax: 01908 393774 Email: 100576.2422@compuserve.com; 3 Sandpiper, Aylesbury HP19 0FP Tel: 01296 486735 Fax: 01296 331104 Email: ericdrose@compuserve.com — (St. Mary's) MRCS Eng. LRCP Lond. 1968; MB BS Lond. 1969; DObst RCOG 1971; MRCGP 1980; Cert. Family Plann. JCC 1984. GP Princip. Specialty: Gen. Pract. Socs: GP Writers Assn. Prev: Sec. Berks. & Bucks. Local Med. Comm.; GP Aylesbury; SHO (Obst.) Roy. Berks. Hosp. Reading.

ROSE, Francis George ICI, 20 Manchester Square, London W6 3AN Tel: 020 7009 5403 Fax: 020 7009 5735 Email: frank_rose@ici.com — MB ChB Liverp. 1974; DCH Eng. 1978; MRCGP 1982; FFOM RCP Lond. 1990. Gp. Vice Pres. SSHE, ICI Lond.; Bd. Mem. MEDICHEM; Bd. Mem. Internat. Commiss. Occupat. Health; Hon. Sen. Clin. Lect. Inst. Occupat. Health Univ. Birm. Specialty: Occupat. Health. Socs: MEDICHEM; Soc. Occupat. Med.; ACOEM. Prev: Chief Med. Off. ICI plc; Med. Off. HM Forces (Army); Ho. Off. Roy. Infirm. Liverp.

ROSE, Frank Clifford The London Neurological Centre, Alliance Medical, 10-11 Bulstrode Place, Marylebone Lane, London W1G 2HX Tel: 020 7935 3546 Fax: 020 7935 7215 — MB BS Lond. 1949 (King's Coll. Lond. & Westm.) MRCS Eng. LRCP Lond. 1949; DCH Eng. 1951; FRCP Lond. 1971, M 1954. Cons. Neurol. ; Founding Edr. Jl. Hist. Neurosci. Specialty: Neurol. Socs: Fell. Roy. Soc. Med. Lond. (Ex-Pres. Neurol. Sect.); Hon. Life Mem. Internat. Headache Soc.; Sec. / Treas. Gen. World Federat. of Neurol. Prev: Neurol. Regional Neurosci. Centre Char. Cross Hosp. Lond.; Dir. Acad. Unit Neurosci. Char. Cross & Westm. Med. Sch. Lond.; Cons. Neurol. Med. Ophth. Unit St. Thos. Hosp.

ROSE, Mr Geoffrey Edward 73 Harley Street, London W1G 8QJ Tel: 020 7935 5385 Fax: 020 7935 5385; Moorfields Eye Hospital, City Road, London EC1V 2PD Tel: 020 7566 2604 Fax: 020 7566 2608 Email: geoff.rose@moorfields.nhs.uk — MB BS Lond. 1979 (Kings College Hospital) BSc (Hons.) Lond. (Pharmacol.) 1976; MRCP (UK) 1982; FRCS Eng. 1985; FCOphth 1988; MS Lond. 1990; FRCOphth 1992. Cons. Ophth. Surg. Moorfields Eye Hosp. Lond.; Hon. Cons. Ophth. Surg. Hosp. Childr. Gt. Ormond St. Lond. & Roy. Vict. Hosp. Belf. Specialty: Ophth. Prev: Lect. Inst. Ophth. Lond.; Sen. Regist. & Regist. (Ophth.) Moorfields Eye Hosp. Lond.

ROSE, Gillian Karen 61 Bradford Road, Manchester M40 7EY — MB ChB Leic. 1991.

ROSE, Gillian Linda Queen Charlotte's & Chelsea Hospital, Du Cane Road, London W12 0XS Tel: 020 8383 1111 Fax: 020 8383 5250; Lisa Sainsbury,, Hammersmith Hospital, Du Cane Road, London W12 0XS — MRCS Eng. LRCP Lond. 1978 (Royal Free Hospital) MB BS 1978; MRCOG 1984; MD 1990. Cons. Gyneacologist, Qu. Charlotte's & Chelsea Hosp. Lond. Specialty: Gynaecology; Paediat. Socs: Med. Soc. Lond.; Brit. Fertil. Soc.; Brit. Soc. Paediat. & Gynae. Prev: Sen. Lect. & Hon. Cons. Qu. Charlotte's & Chelsea Hosp. Lond.; Sen. Regist. Qu. Charlotte's & Chelsea Hosps. Lond.; Research Regist. Chelsea Hosp. for Wom. Lond.

ROSE, Gillian Sarah 5 Collingham Gardens, London SW5 0HW Tel: 020 8846 6644 — MB BS Lond. 1986 (University of London) BSc (Hons.) Lond. 1983; MRCPsych 1990. Child Psychiat. InPat. Unit. Eng. Specialty: Child & Adolesc. Psychiat. Prev: Clin. Lect. & Hon. Sen. Regist. (Child & Adolesc. Psychiat.) St. Mary's Hosp. Med. Sch. Lond.; SHO (Adult Psychiat.) Fulbourn Hosp. Lond. & Barnet Gen. Hosp.; Child & Adolesc. Psychiatr. N.Herts.NHS Trust.

ROSE, Graeme Dick Orchard Medical Centre, 41 Ladywell Road, Motherwell ML1 3JX Tel: 01698 242700 Fax: 01698 242720 — MB ChB Aberd. 1971.

ROSE, Harry Kaye (retired) 9 The French Apartments, Purley CR8 2PH Tel: 020 8763 8044 — (Anderson Coll. Glas.) LRCP LRCS Ed. LRFPS Glas. 1946; DPH Glas. 1952; DPM Eng. 1955; FRCPsych 1981, M 1971. Prev: Cons. Psychiat. HM Prison Maidstone.

ROSE, Heather Mary Croft Medical Centre, 2 Glen Rd, Oadby, Leicester LE2 4PE — MB ChB Bristol 1983; DRCOG 1985; MRCGP 1987; DCH RCP Lond. 1987. GP Leicester. Prev: GP Reading; Trainee GP Bath VTS; Ho. Phys. & Ho. Surg. Frenchay Hosp. Bristol.

ROSE, Helen Frances (retired) 33 de Freville Avenue, Cambridge CB4 1HW Tel: 01223 312234 — MB BChir Camb. 1973 (Camb. & St Thos.) Clin. Med. Off. Camb. HA. Prev: Clin. Med. Off. (Child Psychiat.) Oxf. RHA.

ROSE, Henry Myer (retired) 40 Spinney Crescent, Blundellsands, Liverpool L23 8TZ Tel: 0151 924 4702 — MRCS Eng. LRCP Lond. 1942 (Univ. Coll. Hosp.) DO Eng. 1961. Prev: Ophth. Sefton & Liverp. HA (T).

ROSE, Howard James Chilcompton Surgery, Wells Road, Chilcompton, Bath BA3 4EU Tel: 01761 232231 — MB BS Lond. 1967 (St. Geo.) DObst RCOG 1969; DPM Eng. 1970. Med. Off. Downside Sch. Prev: Regist. N. Staffs. Matern. Hosp. Stoke on Trent; Regist. (Psychiat.) St. Geo. Hosp. Med. Sch.; Ho. Off. Cirencester Memor. Hosp.

ROSE, Jack Harvey (retired) 182 Clarence Gate Gardens, Glentworth St., London NW1 6AR Tel: 020 7262 9482 — MB ChB Glas. 1938.

ROSE, Jacqueline Ann The Surgery, 2 Mark Street, Rochdale OL12 9BE Tel: 01706 43183 Fax: 01706 526640 — MB ChB Manch. 1984.

ROSE, James (retired) 69 Muirfield Crescent, Dundee DD3 8QA Tel: 01382 826706 — MB ChB Aberd. 1949; FRCGP 1977, M 1971. Med. Ref. Scott. Home & Health Dept. Prev: Ho. Phys. City Hosp. Aberd.

ROSE, James Dudfield Richardson Burnock Lodge, 13 Racecourse Road, Ayr KA7 2DQ Tel: 01292 263531 — MB BChir Camb. 1973 (Camb. & Newc. u. Tyne) MRCP (UK) 1975; MA Camb. 1973, MD 1986; FRCP Glas. 1990. Cons. Phys. Ayr Hosp. Specialty: Gastroenterol. Socs: Brit. Soc. Gastroenterol.; Scot. Soc. Gastroenterol. Prev: Sen. Regist. (Gen. Med.) Llandough Hosp. & Univ. Hosp. Wales Cardiff; Regist. Addenbrooke's Hosp. Camb.; Ho. Off. Newc. u. Tyne Gen. Hosp.

ROSE, James William Peter St Clements Partnership, Tanner Street, Winchester SO23 8AD Tel: 01962 852211 Fax: 01962 856010 — MB BS Lond. 1986; BSc Lond. 1981; MRCGP 1994.

ROSE, Jane Deborah Grove Road Surgery, 25 Grove Road, Borehamwood WD6 5DX — MB ChB Manch. 1988 (Univ. Manch.) MRCGP 1993. Princip. GP Borehamwood Herts. Specialty: Gen. Pract. Prev: Trainee GP Borehamwood.

ROSE, Joanna Helen 50 St Laurence Road, Birmingham B31 2AX — MB BS Lond. 1988; DRCOG 1992; MRCGP 1993; DFFP 1994. Clin. Asst. (Genitourin. Med.) & Doctor (Family Plann.) Birm. Specialty: Family Plann. & Reproduc. Health. Prev: Trainee GP Taunton & Som. Hosp.

ROSE, Jocelyn Margaret (retired) 5 Hilary Close, Wollaton, Nottingham NG8 2SP Tel: 0115 928 4242 — MB ChB Sheff. 1961. Prev: Staff Grade (Anaesth.) Nottm. HA.

ROSE, John David Gardiner Department of Radiology, Freeman Hospital, Freeman Road, High Heaton, Newcastle upon Tyne NE7 7DN Tel: 0191 284 3111; Allendale House, Allendale Road, Hexham NE46 2DE — MB BS Lond. 1975 (Roy. Free Hosp. Lond.) FRCP Lond. 1997, M 1978; DMRD 1981; FRCR 1983. Cons. Radiol. Freeman Hosp. Newc. Specialty: Radiol. Socs: Brit. Soc. Interven. Radiol.; Brit. Inst. Radiol. & Cardiovasc. & Intervent. Radiol. Soc. Europe. Prev: Cons. Radiol. Hillingdon Hosp. Uxbridge; Regist./Sen. Regist. (Radiol.) Newc. Teach. Hosps.

ROSE, John Stuart Badgerswood Surgery, Mill Lane, Headley, Bordon GU35 8LH Tel: 01428 713511 Fax: 01428 713812; Brantfell House, New Road, Whitehill, Bordon GU35 9AX Tel: 01420 487374 — MB BS Lond. 1982 (King's Coll. Hosp.) BSc (1st cl. Hons.) Lond. 1979, MB BS 1982; DRCOG 1985; DCH RCP Lond. 1986; MRCGP 1986.

ROSE, Justine Ann 5 Badingham Drive, Fetcham, Leatherhead KT22 9ES — (C&WMS) BSc Lond. 1989, MB BS 1992; DRCOG Lond. 1996; MRCGP Lond. 1997. Asst. Gen. Pract. Fairlands Surg. Guildford. Specialty: Gen. Pract. Socs: DRCGP; MRCGP.

ROSE, Karen Ingrid 4 Belmont Crescent, Glasgow G12 8EU — MB ChB Glas. 1989; BSc (Hons.) St. And. 1983; MRCP (UK) 1992. SHO (Gen. Med.) Roy. Alexandra Hosp. Paisley. Socs: Jun. Doctors Comm. Prev: SHO Rotat. (Gen. Med.) Glas. Roy. Infirm.; Research Asst. & Ho. Off. (Med.) West. Infirm. Glas.; Ho. Off. (Surg.) Roy. Alexandra Hosp. Paisley.

ROSE, Kathleen Fionuala Allendale House, Allendale Road, Hexham NE46 2DE — MB BS Lond. 1975.

ROSE, Mr Keith Graham Surgicare, Parkway House, Palatine Road, Manchester M22 4DB Tel: 0161 945 8688 Fax: 0161 945 8689; The Nook, 1 Essex Avenue, Didsbury, Manchester M20 6AN Tel: 0161 445 5274 — MB BS Lond. 1978 (St. Thos.) MRCS Eng. LRCP Lond. 1978; FRCS Eng. 1984. Surg. Surgicare Manch. Specialty: Gen. Surg. Prev: Surg. to ICRC; Regist. St. Helier Hosp. Carshalton; SHO & Ho. Surg. St Thos. Hosp. Lond.

ROSE, Leslie (retired) 41 Burton Road, Burton-on-Trent DE14 3DL Tel: 01283 562358 — MB ChB Glas. 1949; DObst RCOG 1953. Prev: Obst. Ho. Surg. Glas. Roy. Matern. Hosp.

ROSE, Lionel Clifford (retired) Timbertop, Tye Green Village, Harlow CM18 6QY Tel: 01279 423844 — MB ChB St. And. 1958; DObst. RCOG 1960.

ROSE, Margaret Anne 2 Westview, Elm Grove, Salisbury SP1 1NE — MB BS Lond. 1983.

ROSE, Mr Martyn John Thatch, Chapel Lane, Old, Northampton NN6 9RD Tel: 01604 781333 — MB ChB Liverp. 1967; FRCS Eng. 1972. Cons. Rehabil. Med. St. And. Hosp. N.ampton. Specialty: Rheumatol.; Rehabil. Med. Prev: Sen. Regist. (Neurosurg.) Walton Hosp. Liverp.; Regist. (Neurosurg.) Inst. Neurol. Scs. Glas.; Demonst. (Anat.) Univ. Liverp.

ROSE, Mary Department of Anaesthesia, Royal Hospital for Sick Children, Sciennes Road, Edinburgh EH9 1LF Tel: 0131 536 0226 — MB BS Lond. 1985 (Royal Free) DA (UK) 1992; FRCA 1993. Cons. (Anaesth.) Roy. Hosp. for Sick Childr. Edin. Specialty: Anaesth. Socs: Assn. Anaesth.; Pain Soc.; Edin. and E. of Scotl. Soc. of Anaesth.s. Prev: Regist. (Anaesth.) ChristCh. Hosp. NZ; Regist. (Anaesth.) Derriford Hosp. Plymouth.

ROSE, Mary Walker (retired) 45 Stumperlowe Park Road, Sheffield S10 3QP Tel: 0114 230 5671 — MB ChB Sheff. 1953. Prev: Clin. Med. Off. Sheff. AHA.

ROSE, Megan Sandwell Hospital, Lyndon, West Bromwich B71 4HJ — MB ChB Birm. 1998; ChB Birm. 1998.

ROSE, Mr Michael Barritt Morriston Hospital (Department of Urology), Morriston, Swansea SA6 6NL Tel: 01792 703379; 16 Kilfield Road, Bishopston, Swansea SA3 3DL Tel: 01792 232808 — MB Camb. 1966 (St. Thos.) MA; MChir Camb. 1977, MB 1966, BChir 1965; DObst RCOG 1968; FRCS Eng. 1970. Cons. Surg. (Urol.) Swansea Health Dist. Specialty: Urol. Socs: Brit. Assn. Urol. Surgs. Prev: Sen. Regist. (Urol.) Leeds Hosp. Gp.; Regist. (Surg.) St. Thos. Hosp. Lond.; SHO (Surg.) Bath Hosp. Gp.

ROSE, Michael Norman The Limes Surgery, 172 High Street, Lye, Stourbridge DY9 8LL Tel: 01384 422234 — MB ChB Birm. 1966.

ROSE, Michael Richard King's College Hospital, Department of Neurology, Denmark Hill, London SE5 9RS Tel: 020 7346 5355 Fax: 020 7346 5329 — MB BS Lond. 1980 (Middlx.) BSc 1977; MRCP 1983; MD 1993; FRCP 1999. Cons. & Hon. Sen. Lect. (Neurol.); Cons. Neurol. Qu. Eliz. Hosp. Woolwich; Hon. Sen. Lect. (Neurol.) GKT Med. Sch. Lond.; Edr. Neuromuscular Dis. Cochrane Collaborative Review Gp. Lond.; Clin. Trials Mediator Europ. Neuromuscular Centre Baarn, Holland. Specialty: Neurol. Special Interest: Neuromuscular Dis.

ROSE, Mrs Muriel (retired) 36 Seckford Street, Woodbridge IP12 4LY — MRCS Eng. LRCP Lond. 1933 (Univ. Coll. Hosp.) BSc Lond. 1930, MD 1947, MB BS 1935; FRCOG 1962.

ROSE, Naomi Jacqueline 123 Wigton Lane, Alwoodley, Leeds LS17 8SH — MB ChB Leeds 1963.

ROSE, Nicholas David Bridgeman Littlemore Hospital, Littlemore, Oxford OX4 4XN — MB ChB Leeds 1971; FRCPsych 1992, M 1977. Cons. Psychiat. Littlemore Hosp. Oxf.; Oxf. Regional Tutor for Vis. Regist.; Oxf. Regional MRCPsych Course Organiser. Specialty: Gen. Psychiat. Prev: Cons. Community Psychiat. & Psychother. High Wycombe; Assoc. Prof. (Psychiat.) Univ. Sains, Malaysia; Lect. (Psychiat.) Univ. Oxf.

ROSE, Nigel Maxwell The Hacketts, Fromes Hill, Hereford — BM BCh Oxf. 1971; FFA RCS Eng. 1976. Specialty: Anaesth.

ROSE, Peter Garden House, Old colwall, Malvern WR13 6HF — MB ChB Sheff. 1969.

ROSE, Peter Edgar Hurstwood Park Neurological Centre, Haywards Heath RH16 4EX Tel: 01444 441881 Fax: 01444 417995 — MB BS Lond. 1973; BSc (Hons.) Lond. 1970, MB BS 1973; FRCPath 1992, M 1980. Cons. Neuropath. Hurstwood Pk. Neurol. Centre Haywards Heath; Hon. Lect. (Morbid Anat.) KCH Med. Sch. Lond. Specialty: Neuropath. Prev: Clin. Lect. (Neuropath.) Inst. Psychiat. Lond.

ROSE, Peter Edwin Warwick Hospital, Lakin Road, Warwick CV34 5BJ Tel: 01926 482600 Fax: 01926 493567; Ryderdale, Manor Lane, Pinley, Claverdon, Warwick CV35 8NH — MB ChB Dundee 1976; MRCP (UK) 1979; FRCPath 1995, M 1984; FRCP Ed. 1994. Cons. Haemat. S. Warks. HA. Specialty: Haematology.

ROSE, Peter Gerard 33 Lindisfarne Close, Jesmond, Newcastle upon Tyne NE2 2HT — MB ChB Ed. 1963; DMRD Eng. 1971; FFR 1973. Cons. Radiol. N. RHA & Newc. AHA (T); Hon. Clin. Lect. Univ. Newc. Specialty: Radiol. Socs: Brit. Med. Ultrasound Soc.; Brit. Inst. Radiol. Prev: Sen. Regist. (Radiol.) & Regist. (Radiol.) Roy. Vict. Infirm. Newc.; SHO (Med.) & Regist. (Med.) Vict. Hosp. Blackpool.

ROSE, Peter Selborne (retired) The Surgery, 59 Mansfield Road, Blidworth, Mansfield NG21 0RB Tel: 01623 795461 Fax: 01623 490514; 118 Main Road, Ravenshead, Nottingham NG15 9GW Tel: 01623 793467 — MB ChB Ed. 1966. Prev: Ho. Off. O & G Bangour Gen. Hosp. Broxburn.

ROSE, Peter William Mill Stream Surgery, Mill Stream, Benson, Wallingford OX10 6RL Tel: 01491 838286 — MB BChir Camb. 1978; MB Camb. 1978, MA, BChir 1977; DCH Eng. 1979; DRCOG 1980; FRCGP 1994, M 1981. Research Fell. ICRF GPRG Dept. Pub. Health & Primary Care Inst. Health Sci.s Oxf. Prev: Trainee GP Banbury VTS.

ROSE, Philip Alfred 30 Winscombe Way, Stanmore HA7 3AU — MB BS Lond. 1985.

ROSE, Philip Francis Doune Health Centre, Castlehill, Doune FK16 6DR Tel: 01786 841213; 9 Elm Court, Doune FK16 6JG — MB ChB Dundee 1984; MB ChB Dundee. 1984; MRCGP 1988. Specialty: Occupat. Health.

ROSE, Senga 59 Harefields, Oxford OX2 8HG Tel: 01865 56992 — MB ChB Glas. 1961. Prev: Sen. Med. Off. Coll. Health Serv. Camden & Islington AHA (T).

ROSE, Shamim Akhtar 1 Ewden Close, Abbeyfields, Childwall, Liverpool L16 5HF Tel: 0151 738 0209; Forensic Medical Services, HM Prison Altcourse, Fazakerely, Liverpool L9 7LH Tel: 0151 522

2066 Fax: 0151 522 2153 — MB ChB Liverp. 1990; DFFP 1997. Prison Med. Off. HM Prison Altcourse Liverp. Specialty: Civil Serv.; Gen. Pract.

ROSE, Mr Sidney Samuel (retired) 135 Palatine Road, West Didsbury, Manchester M20 3YA Tel: 0161 445 0128; The Homestead, Whitehall Road, Sale M33 3WJ Tel: 0161 973 4533 — MB ChB University Manch. (Hons.) 1941; FRCS Eng. 1948. Prev: Pres. Manch. Surg.

ROSE, Stephen John Department of Paediatrics, Birmingham Heartlands Hospital, Bordsley Green E., Birmingham B9 5SS Tel: 0121 424 1687 Ext: 5069 Fax: 0121 773 6458; 92 Dovehouse Lane, Solihull B91 2EG Tel: 0121 707 2311 Fax: 0121 682 8397 Email: sbrose98@aol.com — MA Camb. 1976, M BChir 1975; MRCP (UK) 1979; FRCP Lond. 1994; FRCPCH Lond. 1997. Cons. Paediat. & Hon. Sen. Lect. Univ. Birm. Heartlands Hosp. Birm. Specialty: Paediat.; Neonat. Socs: Brit. Soc. for Paediatric; Diabetes UK; Brit. Med. Assn. Prev: Lect. in Child Health, Univ. of Aberd.

ROSE, Susan Elizabeth Crawley Hospital, Child Development Centre, West Green Drive, Crawley RH11 7DH Tel: 01293 600351 Fax: 01293 600353 — MB ChB Aberd. 1980; DRCOG 1983; MRCGP 1985; DCH RCP Lond. 1986. Assoc. Specialist Surrey & Sussex Healthcare. Specialty: Community Child Health; Audiol. Med. Prev: SCMO Surrey & Sussex Healthcare; SCMO Mid Sussex NHS Trust; Sen. Clin. Med. Off. Tower Hamlets HA.

ROSE, Susan Louise Holmlea, Church Hill, Wilmington, Dartford DA2 7EH — MB BS Lond. 1989; MRCP (UK) 1994.

ROSE, Teresa Spa Surgery, 205 High Street, Boston Spa, Wetherby LS23 6PY Tel: 01937 842842 Fax: 01937 841095 — MB BS Lond. 1966 (Middlx.) MRCS Eng. LRCP Lond. 1966; MMedSc Leeds 1985. Prev: Departm. Med. Off. W. Riding CC Yorks; Ho. Surg. Profess. Surg. Unit Leeds Gen. Infirm.; Ho. Phys. Profess. Med. Unit Middlx. Hosp.

ROSE, William James McQueen 4 Ladycross Cottages, Hollow Lane, Dormansland, Lingfield RH7 6PB — MB BS Lond. 1993.

ROSEBLADE, Christopher Kenneth Wrexham Maelor Hospital, Croesnewydd Road, Wrexham LL13 7TD Tel: 01978 291100 — MB ChB Manch. 1984; BSc St. And. 1981; MA Oxf. 1983; MRCOG 1990. Cons. O & G Wrexham Maelor Hosp. Specialty: Obst. & Gyn. Socs: Fell. Roy. Soc. Med.; Internat. Continence Soc. Prev: Sen. Regist. (O & G) Withington Hosp. N. West. RHA; Regist. Rotat. Kings Coll. Hosp. & Brighton; Research Regist. (O & G) Hammersmith Hosp.

ROSEDALE, James Oriel Bernard The Marlborough Surgery, George Lane, Marlborough SN8 4BY Tel: 01672 512187; Thornsend, Kingsbury St, Marlborough SN8 1HZ — MB BS Lond. 1964 (St. Thos.) DCH Eng. 1966; DTM & H Liverp. 1966; DObst RCOG 1974. Med. Off. Savernake Hosp. MarlBoro. & MarlBoro. Coll. Prev: Med. Off. Brit. Everest Expedit. 1972; Ldr., Brit. Nepal Med. Trust, Nepal; Regist. (Paediat.) Univ. Coll. Hosp. Ibadan, Nigeria.

ROSEDALE, Neville (retired) 46 Hatherley Court, Hatherley Grove, Westbourne Grove, London W2 5RE Tel: 020 7727 9639 Email: nrosedale@hotmail.com; 23 Peveril Heights, Sentry Road, Swanage BH19 2AZ Tel: 01929 423649 Email: neville.rosedale1@btopenworld.com — (St. Bart.) MRCS Eng. LRCP Lond. 1945; FRCP Ed. 1974, M 1959. Prev: Cons. Venereol. W. Middlx. Hosp. Isleworth & Hillingdon Hosp. Uxbridge.

ROSEFIELD, Andrea Ruth 3 Mountview, Barnet Way, Mill Hill, London NW7 3HT Tel: 020 8959 4793 — MB BS Lond. 1964; MRCS Eng. LRCP Lond. 1965. Clin. Asst. (Genitourin. Med.) Mortimer Market Centre UCL Hosp.; Clin. Asst. (Genitourin. Med.) Ambrose King Centre Roy. Lond. Hosp. Specialty: Genitourinary Medicine; Occupat. Health. Socs: Soc. Occupat. Med.; Soc. Study VD.

ROSEHILL, Sydney Parkdale, 1 Edward VII Avenue, Newport NP20 4TL Tel: 01633 63467 — MB BCh BAO NUI 1939 (Cork) MRCGP 1956. Vis. Anaesth. & Med. Asst. Dermat. Dept. Roy. Gwent Hosp. Newport; Vis. Anaesth. St. Woolos Hosp. Newport; Med. Off. Alit-yr-Yn Isolat. Hosp. Socs: BMA & Soc. Anaesths. S. Wales. Prev: Res. Med. Off. St. Luke's Hosp. Huddersfield; Squardron Ldr. RAF Med. Br. 1941-45; Ho. Phys. Roy. Gwent Hosp. Newport.

ROSELL, Philip Anthony Edward Yew Tree Farmhouse, 152 Botley Road, Swanwick, Southampton SO31 1BU — MB BS Lond. 1991; BSc Lond. 1988.

ROSELLO, Natalia Susana 10 Doves Yard, Culford Road, London N1 0HQ — MB BS Lond. 1996.

ROSEMEN, Joan Jemima St Giles Surgery, 40 St. Giles Road, London SE5 7RF Tel: 020 7252 5936; 450 Westhorne Avenue, Eltham, London SE9 5LT — MB BS Newc. 1978; DCH RCP Lond. 1982; MRCGP 1984.

ROSEN, Bernard Keith Keats House, 24-26 St Thomas Street, London SE1 9RS — MB ChB Sheff. 1968; FRCPsych 1988, M 1973; MRCPsych 1973. Specialty: Gen. Psychiat. Prev: Sen. Lect. & Hon. Cons. (Psychiat.) Guy's Hosp. Lond.; Lect. & Hon. Sen. Regist. (Psychiat.) Guy's Hosp. Lond.; Vis. Lect. (Psychiat.) Memor. Univ. Newfld.

ROSEN, Calmen 26 Wolfreton Garth, Kirk Ella, Hull HU10 7AD — MRCS Eng. LRCP Lond. 1946. Socs: MRCGP.

ROSEN, Edwin David (retired) 47 Canonbury Park N., London N1 2J4 Tel: 020 7226 9823 Fax: 020 7226 9823 — MB BS Lond. 1957 (Oxf.) MRCS Eng., LRCP Lond. 1956. Mem. Med Ethic Comm. Moorfields Eye Hosp.Lond. Prev: Obst. Ho. Off. & Med. Off. Radiother. Unit Churchill Hosp. Oxf.

ROSEN, Mr Emanuel Saul (retired) 10 St John Street, Manchester M3 4DY Tel: 0161 832 8778 Fax: 0161 832 1486 Email: erosen564@aol.com — MB ChB Manch. 1961; FRCS Ed. 1967; BSc (Hons.) Manch. 1957, MD 1969; FRCOphth 1988. Cons. (Opthal.) Rosen Eye Surg. Centre, Manch.; Vis. Prof. Vision Sc. Univ. Manch.; Co-Edr. Jl. Cataract & Refractive Surg.; Hon. Cons. Ophth. Manch. Roy. Eye Hosp.

ROSEN, Jan-Paul David 49 Cholmeley Crescent, London N6 5EX — MB BS Lond. 1989; MFPM.

ROSEN, Maria Rosaline South Essex Partnership NHS Trust, Mental Health Unit, Basildon Hospital, Basildon SS16 5NL Tel: 01268 533911 — MB ChB Glas. 1965; DPM Ed. & Glas. 1970; MRCPsych 1973. Cons. Psychiat./Eating Disorders Lead Basildon Hosp. Essex. Specialty: Gen. Psychiat. Socs: BMA.

ROSEN, Maurice Howard (retired) Health E1, Homeless Medical Centre, 9-11 Brick Lane, London E1 6PU Tel: 020 7247 0090 Fax: 020 7376 0802 — (St. Mary's) MRCS Eng. LRCP Lond. 1964; DA Eng. 1966; MSc Lond. 1995; MA Lond. 1997.

ROSEN, Professor Michael, CBE 45 Hollybush Road, Cardiff CF23 6TZ Tel: 029 2075 3893 Email: rosen@mrosen.plus.com — (St. Andrews) MB ChB St. And. 1949; FFA RCS Eng. 1957; FRCOG 1989; FFA RCSI (Hons.) 1990; FRCS Eng. 1992. Chairm., World Federat. of Socs. of Anaesthesiol. Foundat. Specialty: Anaesth. Socs: Roy. Soc. Med.; Amer. Soc. Anaesthesiologists. Prev: Hon. Prof. Anaesth. Univ. Wales Coll. Med.; Pres. Roy. Coll. of Anaesths. 1988-91; Pres. Assn. of Anaesth. Gt. Britain & Irel. 1986-88.

ROSEN, Michael Philip (cons. rooms) 37 Rodney Street, Liverpool L1 9EN Tel: 0151 709 1864 Fax: 0151 428 5399; 121 Church Road, Woolton, Liverpool L25 6HT — LRCPI & LM, LRSCI & LM 1970 (RCSI) LRCPI & LM, LRCSI & LM 1970. Prev: SHO (O & G) St. Mary's Hosp. Manch. & Whiston Hosp. Prescot.

ROSEN, Mr Paul Henry Oxford Eye Hospital, Radcliffe Infirmary, Woodstock Road, Oxford OX2 Tel: 01865 224739 — MB ChB Manch. 1980; BSc (Hons.) Physiol. Manch. 1977; FRCS Glas. 1985. Cons. Ophth. Surg. Oxf. Eye Hosp. Specialty: Ophth. Socs: UK & Irel. Soc. of Cataract & Refractive Surg.; Europ. Soc. of Catarct Surg.; Amercian Acad. of Opthalmology. Prev: Lect., Fell. & Sen. Regist. Moorfields Eye Hosp. Inst. Ophth. Lond.

ROSEN, Rebecca Celia The Kings Fund, 11-13 Cavendish Square, London W1G 0AN Tel: 020 7307 2443; 32 Coleraine Road, Blackheath, London SE3 7PQ Tel: 020 8305 1694 — MB ChB Bristol 1988; DCH RCP Lond. 1991; MSc Lond. 1992; MFPHM RCP (UK) 1995; MD Bristol 1998; MFFP (RCOG0 1998. Fell. in Primary Care, The Kings Fund, Lond.; Hon. Lect. (Health Servs. Research) Lond. Sch. Hyg. & Trop. Med. Specialty: Gen. Pract.

ROSEN, Stuart David Ealing Hospital , Department of Cardiology, Uxbridge Road, Southall UB1 3HW Tel: 020 8967 5359 Fax: 020 8967 5007; Royal Brompton Hospital , Department of Clinical Cardiology, Sydney Street, London SW3 6NP Tel: 020 7351 8164 — MB BS Lond. 1985 (Cambridge University & Charing Cross & Westminster Med. Sch.) MA Camb. 1986, BA 1982; MRCP (UK) 1990; MD Lond. 1996; FRCP 2001. Sen. Lect & Hon. Cons.

Cardiol., Imperial Coll. & Royal, Hammersmith & Royal Brompton Hospitals; Director of Research & Development Ealing Hospital NHS Trust; Clinical Director of Medicines. Specialty: Cardiol. Socs: Fell. Amer. Coll. Cardiol. & Europ. Soc. Cardiol.; Brit. Cardiac Soc.; BMA. Prev: Regist. (Cardiol. & Med.) & Research SHO (Cardiol.) Char. Cross Hosp. Lond.; Clin. Scientist, MRC Clin. Scis. Centre, Hon. Lect. & Sen. Regist. (Cardiol.) RPMS, Hammersmith & St. Mary's Hosp. Lond.

ROSENBAUM, Naomi Louise 31 Mount Pleasant, Barnet EN4 9ES — MB BS Lond. 1991; DRCOG 1994; DFFP 1995. Socs: Assoc. Mem. RCGP. Prev: Trainee GP Edgware VTS.

ROSENBAUM, Mr Tomas Pedro Department of Urology, Ealing Hospital, Uxbridge Road, Southall UB1 3HW Tel: 020 8967 5778 Fax: 020 8813 8607 Email: tom.rosenbaum@eht.org.uk — Medico Buenos Aires 1973 (Univ. of Buenos Aires) MRCS Eng. LRCP Lond. 1979; FRCS Ed. 1982; FRCS (Urol.) 1994; FEBU 1996. Cons. Urol. Ealing Hosp. Southall Middlx. Specialty: Urol.; Oncol. Socs: Fell. Roy. Soc. Med.; Internat. Continence Soc.; Brit. Assn. Urol. Surg. Prev: Lect. (Urol.) Inst. Urol. Lond.; Sen. Regist. (Urol.) St. Helier Hosp. Carshalton; Sen. Regist. (Urol.) Roy. Marsden Hosp.

ROSENBERG, Aaron (retired) — LRCPI & LM, LRSCI & LM 1959; LRCPI & LM, LRCSI & LM 1959. Prev: Assoc. Specialist (Psychiat.) Prestwich Hosp. Manch.

ROSENBERG, Mr Bernard Cecil, TD Birkdale Clinic, Parkfield Road, Rotherham S65 2AJ Tel: 01709 828928 Fax: 01709 828372; Montrose, 31 Stumperlowe Crescent Road, Sheffield S10 3PQ Tel: 0114 230 8433 — MB BCh BAO Dub. 1962; MA Dub. 1992, BA 1960; DObst RCOG 1964; FRCOG 1983, M 1970. Cons. O & G Rotherham Dist. Gen. Hosp. Specialty: Obst. & Gyn. Socs: BMA; Fell. N. Eng. Obst & Gyn. Soc.; Lond. Obst & Gyn. Soc. Prev: Sen. Regist. Hammersmith Hosp. Lond.; Regist. St. Mary's Hosp. W9 & Samarit. Hosp. Lond.; Ho. Surg. & Ho. Phys. Meath Hosp. Dub.

ROSENBERG, Bethel Greyland Medical Centre, 468 Bury Old Road, Prestwich, Manchester M25 1NL Tel: 0161 819 1111 — MB BCh BAO Dub. 1962 (T.C. Dub.) BA Dub. 1961. Area Med. Off. Brit. Boxing Bd. of Control.; Occupational Health Phys. Manch. Medico Legal Assessm. Specialty: Medico Legal; Occupat. Health. Prev: SHO (Med.) Bolton Dist. Gen. Hosp.; Ho. Surg. Matern. Hosp. Hull; Ho. Phys. & Cas. Off. Meath Hosp. Dub.

ROSENBERG, David 27 Hillside Gardens, Edgware HA8 8HA — MB ChB Manch. 1993.

ROSENBERG, Mr David Averell 35 Hyndewood, Dacres Road, Forest Hill, London SE23 2NX — MB BS Lond. 1970 (Guy's) MRCS Eng. LRCP Lond. 1970; MRCOG 1977; FRCS Ed. 1979. Cons. (O & G) St. Albans City Hosp. & W. Herts. Hosp. Hemel. Specialty: Obst. & Gyn. Prev: Sen. Regist. (O & G) St. Geo.'s Hosp. Lond.; Regist. King's Coll. Hosp. Lond.

ROSENBERG, Fraser Guy The Old School House, Main Road, Scalby, Gilberdyke, Brough HU15 2UU — MB ChB Manch. 1998; MB ChB Manch 1998.

ROSENBERG, Mr Ivor Lawrence 1 Egglescliffe Court, Egglescliffe Village, Stockton-on-Tees TS16 9BU Tel: 01642 781577/ 624595 Fax: 07092 290141 Email: il.rosenberg@ntlworld.com — MB BChir Camb. 1966 (Camb. & Leeds) MA Camb. 1966; FRCS Eng. 1971; FRCS Ed. 1971; MChir Camb. 1979. Cons. Surg. Univ. Hosp. N. Tees Stockton on Tees. Specialty: Gen. Surg. Socs: Fell. Assn. Surgs.; BASO; Assn. ColoProctol. GB & Irel. Prev: Lect. (Surg.) Leeds Univ. & Hon. Sen. Regist. St Jas. Hosp. Leeds; Regist. (Surg.) Scarboro. Hosp.; SHO Hammersmith Hosp. Lond.

ROSENBERG, Jeffrey Nathan The Garden Hospital, 46-50 Sunny Gdns. Road, London NW4 1RP Tel: 020 8457 4500 Fax: 020 8457 4567 — (Guy's) MRCS Eng. LRCP Lond. 1970; MB BS Lond. 1970; MRCP (UK) 1973; FRCP Lond. 1991. Hon.Cons Rheum Roy. Nat. Orthopaedic Hosp. Specialty: Rheumatol. Socs: Fell. Med. Soc. Lond.; Fell. Zool. Soc. Lond.; Fell. Hunt. Soc. Prev: Sen. Regist. (Rheum.) Lond. Hosp.; Regist. MRC Rheum. Unit Taplow; Regist. (Med.) Guy's Hosp. Lond.

ROSENBERG, Katharine 14 Shire Oak Road, Headingley, Leeds LS6 2DL — MB ChB Leeds 1993.

ROSENBERG, Michael Alexander John South Downs Health NHS Trust, Brighton General Hospital, Elm Grove, Brighton BN2 3EW Tel: 01273 696011 Email: michael.rosenberg@southdowns.nhs.uk — MB BS Lond. 1972 (Guy's Hospital) MRCS Eng. LRCP Lond. 1972; FRCPsych 2001. p/t Cons. Psychiat. S. Downs Health NHS Trust Brighton.; Chief. Exec. Specialty: Gen. Psychiat.; Intens. Care. Prev: Cons. Psychiat. S. Downs Health NHS Trust Brighton.; Sen. Regist. (Psychiat.) St. Geo. Hosp. Lond.; Regist. (Psychiat.) St. Geo. Hosp. Lond.

ROSENBERG, Raymond Henry (retired) 59 Shearwater, New Barn, Longfield DA3 7NL Tel: 0147 47 04916 — MB ChB Cape Town 1953. Prev: Cons. Psychiat. (Ment. Handicap.) Darenth Pk. Hosp. Dartford.

ROSENBERG, Roger Martin 21 Pink Lane, Burnham, Slough SL1 8JP Tel: 01628 603278 Email: roger@rosenberg87.freeserve.co.uk — MB BCh Witwatersrand 1966; MB BCh Witwatersrand 1966; BSc (Hons.) Witwatersrand 1983. Head Clin. Strategy Glaxo Wellcome. Specialty: Pharmaceutical Medicine. Socs: FFPM. Prev: Exec. Dir. Clin. Raesearch Marion Merkell Dow Winnersh.; Dir. Strategic Drug Developm. Clintrials Research Ltd.

ROSENBERG, Ronald Basil Collegiate Medical Centre, Brideoak St., Manchester M8 0AT Tel: 0161 205 4364; Flat 2, Radnor House, 25 Upper Park Road, Braughton Pk., Salford M7 4JB Tel: 0161 740 3079 — MB ChB Manch. 1953. Hosp. Pract. Dept. Endocrinol. N. Hosp. Manch. Socs: Fell. Manch. Med. Soc.

ROSENBERG, Susan Elaine 35 Upper Park Road, Salford M7 4JB — MB ChB Manch. 1981. SHO (Neonat. Med.) St. Mary's Hosp. Manch. Prev: SHO (O & G) Univ. Hosp. S. Manch. & Withington Hosp. Manch.; SHO (Paediat.) Booth Hall Childr. Hosp. Manch.; Ho. Off. (Surg.) N. Manch. Gen. Hosp.

ROSENBERG, William Malcolm Charles Mail Point 811 Level A South Block, Southampton General Hospital, Tremona Road, Southampton SO16 6YD Tel: 02380 796883 — MB BS Lond. 1983 (Guy's) MA Camb. 1984; MRCP (UK) 1987; DPhil Oxf. 1992, MA 1992. Reader in Med. (hepatology) Univ. of Soton.; Director Wellcome trust Clin. Research Facility Soton. Univ. Hosps. Trust. Specialty: Pathology, General. Socs: Assn. of Physicians. Prev: Clin. Tutor (Med.) Univ. Oxf.

ROSENBLOOM, Lewis 83 Waterloo Warehouse, Waterloo Road, Liverpool L3 0BQ — MB ChB Liverp. 1961; FRCP Lond. 1978, M 1965; DCH Eng. 1966; FRCRCH 1997. Hon.Cons. Paediat. Neurol. Roy. Liverp. Childr. NHS Trust. Specialty: Paediat. Neurol. Prev: Research Fell. Inst. Child Health Univ. Lond.; Regist. (Paediat.) Guy's Hosp. Lond.

ROSENFELD, Kevin Mark — MB ChB Cape Town 1989. Specialty: Radiol.

ROSENFELD, Sabine (retired) 360 Brockley Road, Crofton Park, London SE4 2BY — MD Vienna 1930. Prev: Obst. Regist. Greenbank Matern. Hosp. Darlington.

ROSENFELDER, Alan Frederick Brondesbury Medical Centre, 279 Kilburn High Road, Kilburn, London NW6 7JQ Tel: 020 7624 9853 Fax: 020 7372 3660 — BSc (Hons.) Lond. 1978; MB BS Lond. 1981; DRCOG 1983; DCH RCP Lond. 1984; MRCGP 1985. Socs: Primary Care Genetics Soc.

ROSENFELDER, Eileen — MB BS Lond. 1985; BSc Hist. of Med. Lond. 1982; DRCOG 1988; DCH RCP Lond. 1988; MRCGP 1989. Specialty: Gen. Pract.

ROSENGREN, Helena 16 Rokeby Avenue, Bristol BS6 6EL — MB ChB Sheff. 1989.

ROSENTHAL, Adam Nicholas 12 Crouch Hall Road, London N8 8HU — MB BS Lond. 1992 (St. Mary's Hosp. Med. Sch. Lond.) BSc (Hons.) Physiol. Lond. 1990; DFFP 1997; MRCOG 2003. Gyna. Oncol. Research Fell. St. Barth. Hosp. Lond.; SpR Obst & Gyn Lister Hosp., Stevenage. Specialty: Obst. & Gyn. Prev: Spr Obst & Gyn St Mary's Hosp. Lond.; Spr Obst & Gyn Chelsea & Westm. Hosp. Lond.

ROSENTHAL, Diane The Surgery, 153 Park Road, London N8 8JJ Tel: 020 8340 7940 Fax: 020 8348 1530; 26 Gladwell Road, London N8 9AA — MB ChB Dundee 1977; DRCOG 1980; MRCGP 1982. Prev: Doctor/Counsellor Lond. Youth Advisory Centre; Whittington Hosp. VTS Lond. 1978-81.

ROSENTHAL, Ferdinand David 17 Knighton Grange Road, Leicester LE2 2LF Tel: 0116 270 7797 Fax: 0116 270 8737 Email: david.rosenthal@virgin.net — (King's Coll. Hosp.) MB BS Lond. 1945; FRCP Lond. 1970, M 1948; MD Lond. 1952; LLB Leic. 1991. Emerit. Cons. Phys. Leicester Roy. Infirm., Leicester Gen. Hosp. & Hinckley Hosp. Specialty: Endocrinol.; Gastroenterol. Socs: Soc. Endocrinol.; Med. Res. Soc.; Brit. Thyroid Assn. Prev: Sen. Regist.

(Med.) Leicester Roy. Infirm.; Sen. Regist. (Med.) Roy. Infirm. Sheff.; Ho. Phys. King's Coll. Hosp.

ROSENTHAL, Jane Miranda 52 Holland Park Avenue, London W11 3QY — MB BS Lond. 1992.

ROSENTHAL, Jerrold Malcolm 263 Townsend Lane, Liverpool L13 9DG Tel: 0151 226 1358; 49 Rockburn Avenue, Liverpool L25 4TN — LRCPI & LM, LRSCI & LM 1957; LRCPI & LM, LRCSI & LM 1957.

ROSENTHAL, Jonathan Joseph Park Road Surgery, 153 Park Road, London N8 8JJ Tel: 020 8340 7940 Fax: 020 8348 1530; 57 Barrington Road, Crouch End, London N8 8QT Tel: 020 8342 9893 Fax: 020 8348 5426 — MB BCh Wales 1986 (Univ. of Wales Coll. of Med., Cardiff) BSc (Hons.) Psychol. Wales 1981; DRCOG 1989; FRCGP 1997, M 1990; DFFP 1994; MSc (Gen. Pract.) Lond. 1994. Sen. Lect. (Gen. Pract.) Roy. Free & Univ. Coll. Med. Sch. Lond. - Princip. in Gen. Pract., Drs Greenbury; Course Organiser Roy. Free Hosp. VTS. Specialty: Gen. Pract. Prev: Lect. (Gen. Pract.) Roy. Free Hosp. Sch. Med. Lond.; Ho Med. Singleton Hosp. Swansea; Trainee GP/SHO Guy's Hosp. Lond. VTS.

ROSENTHAL, Keri Louise 2 The Linleys,, Weston, Bath BA1 2XE Tel: 01225484539 — MB BS Lond. 1994 (St Mary's Hospital) BSc Kings Coll. Lond. 1993; MRCGP 1998; DFFP 1998. Asst. GP -. Specialty: Gen. Pract.

ROSENTHAL, Mark Department of Paediatric Respiratory Medicine, Royal Brompton Hospital, Sydney St., London SW3 6NP Tel: 020 7351 8754 Fax: 020 7351 8763 Email: mark.rosenthal@virgin.net; 33 Methuen Park, London N10 2JR Tel: 020 8444 4123 — MB ChB Manch. 1981 (Manchester) MB ChB (Hons.) (Distinc. Paediat. Surg. Pathol.) Manch. 1981; MRCP (UK) 1984; Spec. Accredit. Paediat. JCHMT 1990; BSc (1st cl. Hons.) Pharmacol. Manch. 1978, MD 1994; FRCPH 1997; FRCP 1999. Cons. Paediat. Respirat. Phys. Roy. Brompton Hosp. Lond. & Qu. Mary's Childr. Hosp. St Helier; Vis. Prof. (Paediat.) Univ. Odessa Ukraine. Specialty: Paediat.; Respirat. Med.; Allergy. Socs: Brit. Paediat. Assn.; Brit. Thorac. Soc.; Eur. Respirat. Soc. Prev: Sen. Regist. (Paediat.) Univ. Coll. Hosp.

ROSENVINGE, Henry Paul Thornhill Unit, Moorgreen Hospital, West End, Southampton SO30 3JB Tel: 023 8047 5242 Fax: 023 8046 5014 — MB BS Lond. 1972 (King's Coll. Hosp.) FRCPsych 1991,M 1976. Cons. (Psychogeriat.) Moorgreen Hosp. Soton. Specialty: Geriat. Psychiat. Prev: Sen. Regist. (Psychiat.) Newc. Gen. Hosp.; Intern Memor. Univ. Hosps. St. John's, Newfld.; Regist. (Psychiat.) Knowle Hosp. Fareham.

ROSEVEAR, Catherine Linden Hall Surgery, Newport TF10 7HU Tel: 01952 820400 Fax: 01952 825149 — MB ChB Birm. 1981; DRCOG 1985.

ROSEVEARE, Christopher David Southern University Hospital NHS Trust, Tremona Road, Southampton SO16 6YD — BM Soton. 1991; FRCP Edin.; MRCP (UK) 1994. Consulltant Phys., Soton. Gen. Hosp. Specialty: Gen. Med.; Gastroenterol. Special Interest: Acute Med.; Gastroenterol. Socs: Treas., Soc. for Acute Med. UK. Prev: Specialist Regist. (Gen. Med. & Gastroenterol.) Qu. Alexandra Hosp., Portsmouth; Regist. (Gen. Med. & Gastroenterol.) Roy. Hants. Co. Hosp. Winchester; Regist. (Gastoenterol.) Roy. Bournemouth Hosp.

ROSEVEARE, Helen Margaret (retired) 12 Old Quay Court, Holywood BT18 0HT Tel: 028 9042 3514 — MB BChir Camb. 1951 (Camb. & W. Lond.) DTM & H Antwerp 1952. Prev: Med. Dir. Nebobongo Hosp., Zaire & Nyankunde Train. Sch. for Med.

ROSEVEARE, Martin Peter Paxton Green Health Centre, 1 Alleyn Park, London SE21 8AU Tel: 020 8670 6878 Fax: 020 8766 7057; 62 Burbage Road, London SE24 9HE — MB Camb. 1966 (Univ. Coll. Hosp.) BChir 1965; MRCOG 1970, DObst 1967; FRCOG 1991. Prev: Regist. (O & G) King Edwd. Memor. Hosp. Ealing; SHO Centr. Middlx. Hosp. Lond.; Ho. Off. Univ. Coll. Hosp. Lond.

ROSEWALL, Heidede Luise The Medical Centre, Lower Road, Cookham Rise, Maidenhead SL6 9HX Tel: 01628 524646 Fax: 01628 810201; Springfield, Hearns Lane, Gallowstree Common, Reading RG4 9DE Tel: 0118 972 1262 — MD Vienna 1966; MRCS Eng. LRCP Lond. 1972. Socs: Assoc. Homoep. Soc.

ROSEWARNE, Helen Catherine Little Orchard, The Common, Abberley, Worcester WR6 6AY — MB BS Lond. 1993.

ROSEWARNE, Melvyn Douglas 6 Beech Avenue, Worcester WR3 8PZ — MB ChB Leeds 1963; DMRD Eng. 1970; FFR 1972; FRCR 1975. Cons. Radiol. Worcester Roy. Infirm. NHS Trust. Specialty: Radiol. Prev: Sen. Regist. United Sheff. Hosps.; Instr. (Radiol.) Univ. Washington, USA.

ROSIE, Henrietta Anne c/o Drive M. B. O'Neill, 25 Durham Road, Edinburgh EH15 1NY — MB ChB Sheff. 1975.

ROSIER, Nicholas Charles Ian Clarkson Surgery, De-Havilland Road, Wisbech PE13 3AN Tel: 01945 583133 Fax: 01945 464465 — MB BS Lond. 1978 (Middlx.) DRCOG 1983. Prev: Maj. RAMC; Med. Off. Shape Belgium; Regtl. Med. Off. Qu.'s Own Hussars.

ROSIN, Louis Joseph, MBE (retired) The Coach House, Cypress Close, Blackwell, Darlington DL3 8QR Tel: 01325 467393 Fax: 01325 243413 — MB BS Durh. 1940 (Newc.) MB BS (Hons.) Durh. 1940; MRCGP 1953. Med. Ref. Darlington Crematorium. Prev: RAMC.

ROSIN, Mr Michael David Department of Cardiothoracic Surgery, 3rd Floor, Walsgrave Hospital, Clifford Bridge Road, Walsgrave, Coventry CV2 2DX Tel: 02476 538935; 4 The Moat, Coventry Road, Berkswell, Coventry CV7 7AZ — MB ChB Sheff. 1973; FRCS Ed. 1979. Cons. Cardiothoracic Surg. Walsgrave Hosp. Coventry. Specialty: Cardiothoracic Surg. Special Interest: Post Operat. Critical Care. Socs: RSM.

ROSIN, Richard Allan c/o 15 Elm Grove, London N8 9AH — BM Soton. 1988. Specialty: Gen. Pract. Prev: Regist. (Gen. Pract.) Saffron Walden; Chief Resid. (Psychiat.) Albert Einstein Coll. Med. Bronx, NY, USA.

ROSIN, Mr Richard David St Mary's Hospital, General Surgical Unit, Praed Street, London W2 1NY Tel: 020 7886 1242 Fax: 020 7886 1571 Email: rdrosin@uk-consultants.co.uk — MB BS Lond. 1966 (Westm.) MRCS Eng. LRCP Lond. 1966; FRCS Ed. 1971; FRCS Eng. 1972; MS Lond. 1977; DOHM 2003. Sen. Cons. Surg. in Gen. Surg., Surgic. Onclogy & Minimal Access Surg. St Mary's Hosp. Imp. Coll. Sch. Med. Lond.; Mem. of Counc. RCS 1994-, Vice Pres. 2004; NW Thames RHA Surgic. Adviser to RCS Ed.; Examr. RCS Ed. & FRCS Intercollegiate; Mem. of Counc. RSM 2002-; Mem. of Counc. RCS 1994-. Specialty: Gen. Surg. Socs: Fell. Assn. Surg. GB & Irel.; Fell. Internat. Coll. Surg.; Fell. Assn. Laparoscopic Surg. GB & Irel. Prev: Sen. Regist. (Surg.) Westm. Hosp. Lond.; Regist. (Surg.) St. Helier Hosp. Carshalton; Ho. Phys. Profess. Med. Unit & Ho. Surg. Profess. Surg. Unit Westm. Hosp. Lond.

ROSKELL, Derek Edward John Radcliffe Hospital, Headington, Oxford OX3 9DU — BM BCh Oxf. 1991; BA Oxf. 1988; BA Camb. 1988; MA Camb. 1992; DRCPath 1996. Cons. John Radcliffe Hosp. Oxf.; Hon. Sen. Regist. Oxf. Radcliffe NHS Trust. Specialty: Histopath. Prev: Clin. Tutor (Path.) Nuffield Dept. Path. Univ. Oxf.

ROSKELL, Helen Grace Westfield Farm, Shepherds Close, Weston-on-the-Green, Bicester OX25 3RF — BM BCh Oxf. 1998.

ROSKILLY, John Noel (retired) North View, Hawkins Lane, Rainow, Macclesfield SK10 5TL Tel: 01625 501014 — MB ChB Manch. 1958; DObst RCOG 1960; MRCGP 1968.

ROSLING, Lesley Elizabeth Annette 95 Queens Road, Richmond TW10 6HF; 8 Gilmour Circle, Constantia, Capetown 7800, South Africa — MB BS Lond. 1984; DCH RCP Lond. 1989; MRCGP 1996. SACLA health project. Specialty: Gen. Pract. Prev: GP reg.Richmond; Reg.med.King Edwd. VII Hosp.

ROSOVSKE, Bernard Merton (retired) 14 Goldfields Avenue, Greetland, Halifax HX4 8LE — LRCPI & LM, LRSCI & LM 1955; LRCPI & LM, LRCSI & LM 1955. Prev: GP Halifax.

ROSS, Adrian Piers 2 St Austell Road, Blackheath, London SE13 7EQ — MB BS Lond. 1974; DCH Eng. 1977; MRCP (UK) 1980.

ROSS, Mr Alasdair Hugh McLean Broomfield Hospital, Department of Surgery, Chelmsford CM1 7ET Tel: 01245 514094 Fax: 01245 514859 Email: hross30849@aol.com — MB ChB Ed. 1973 (Edinburgh) FRCS Ed. 1978; ChM Ed. 1985; FRCS 1999. Cons. Surg. Mid Essex Hosps. Trust. Specialty: Gen. Surg. Special Interest: Colorectal Surg.; Endocrine Surg. Socs: Assn. Coloproctol.; Brit. Assn. of Endocrine Surgs.; Roy. Soc. Med. Prev: Sen. Regist. (Surg.) St. Mark's Hosp. Lond.; Ho. Surg. & Regist. Rotat. (Surg.) Roy. Infirm. Edin.; Fell. (Surg.) Univ. Calif. Los Angeles, USA.

ROSS, Alexander 12 The Avenue, Charlton Kings, Cheltenham GL53 9BJ — MB BS Newc. 1993.

ROSS, Alice (retired) 10 West Forth Street, Cellardyke, Anstruther KY10 3HL — MB ChB Ed. 1923. Prev: Asst. MOH Hull & Huddersfield.

ROSS, Alison Wrexham Maelor Hospital, Croes Newydd Road, Wrexham LL13 7TD Tel: 01978 291100; Ochr Farm, Porch Lane, Caergwrle, Wrexham LL12 9HG Tel: 01978 760595 — MRCS Eng. LRCP Lond. 1965 (Royal Free Hospital London) MD Lond. 1972, MB BS (Hons.) 1965; FRCP Lond. 1984, M 1967. Cons. Phys. Wrexham Maelor Hosp. Specialty: Gen. Med.; Gastroenterol.

ROSS, Alison Mary Department of Medical Genetics, Argyll House, Fosterhill, Aberdeen — MB ChB Aberd. 1995; BSc Med. Sci. Aberdeen 1994.

ROSS, Alison Myron Grampain University Hospitals Trust, Department of Anaesthesia, Foresterhill, Aberdeen AB25 2ZN Tel: 01224 681818; South Burnside, Kinella, Aberdeen AB21 0TG Tel: 01224 790255 — MB ChB Aberd. 1981. Specialty: Anaesth. Prev: Regist. (Anaesth.) Aberd. Roy. Infirm.

ROSS, Mr Alistair Charles The Bath Clinic, Claverton Down Road, Bath BA2 7BR Tel: 01225 835555; Westcombe House, Combe Hay, Bath BA2 7EG Tel: 01225 836058 — MB BS Lond. 1976 (Char. Cross) MRCS Eng. LRCP Lond. 1976; FRCS Eng. 1980. Cons. Orthop. Surg. Roy. United Hosp. Bath & Roy. Nat. Hosp. Rheum. Dis. Bath; Dir., Bath & Wessex Orthop. Research Unit; Hon. Sen. Lect. Sch. Postgrad. Med. Univ. Bath. Specialty: Trauma & Orthop. Surg. Socs: Fell. Brit. Orthopaedic Assn.; Mem. Speciality Advisery Bd. in Orthop. Roy. Coll. Surg. Edin.; Past. Pres. Rheumatoid Arthritis Surgic. Soc. Prev: Sen. Regist. (Orthop.) St. Mary's Hosp. Paddington; Regist. (Surg.) Lond. Hosp.; Brit. Orthop. Assn. Europ. Trav. Schol. 1987.

ROSS, Alistair Kenneth, MBE (retired) 30 Leys Drive, Newcastle ST5 3JG Tel: 01782 614945 Email: akross@tinyworld.co.uk — MB ChB Glas. 1949; FRCGP 1974, M 1963. Prev: Med. Ref. Benefits Agency Med. Serv. DSS.

ROSS, Allan (retired) 5 Maywood Close, Beckenham Place Park, Beckenham BR3 5BW Tel: 020 8650 1647 — (Guy's) BDS Lond. 1941; LDS RCS Eng. 1941; LMSSA Lond. 1951; MRCS Eng. LRCP Lond. 1951. Prev: Lt.-Col. RAMC (TA).

ROSS, Allison Mabel Cherryvalley Health Centre, Kings Square, Belfast BT5 7BP Tel: 028 9040 1744 Fax: 028 9040 2069; 27 Fort Road, Ballylesson, Belfast BT8 8LX — MB BCh BAO Belf. 1981; DRCOG 1985; DCH RCSI 1985; MRCGP 1986. Socs: BMA & Med. Wom. Federat.

ROSS, Amanda Joy The Lennard Surgery, 1-3 Lewis Road, Bishopsworth, Bristol BS13 7JD Tel: 0117 964 0900 Fax: 0117 987 3227 — MB ChB Bristol 1992 (Bristol University) DFFP 1995; DRCOG 1995; MRCGP 1996. GP Princip. The Lennard Surg. Bristol. Specialty: Gen. Pract. Prev: GP/Regist. Frenchay Hosp. Bristol VTS.

ROSS, Andrew Mackenzie (retired) Cherry Tree Cottage, Nether Compton, Sherborne DT9 4QG Tel: 01935 812766 — MD Ed. 1937 (Univ. Ed. & Vienna) MB ChB 1924; DLO Eng. 1928. Prev: Otorhinolaryngol. Bournemouth & E. Dorset Hosp. Gp.

ROSS, Andrew Munro Northfield Health Centre, 15 St. Heliers Road, Northfield, Birmingham B31 1QT Tel: 0121 478 1850 Fax: 0121 476 0931 — (Nottm.) BMedSci. Nottm. 1979, BM BS 1981; DCH RCP Lond. 1983; DRCOG 1984; MRCGP 1985; M Med Sci. 1996; FRCGP 1999. Partner GP; Research Fell. RCGP. Specialty: Epidemiol. Prev: Trainee GP Rugby VTS.

ROSS, Angus Malcolm Rokeby Villa, The Lendings, Barnard Castle DL12 9AB — MB BS Newc. 1994.

ROSS, Anne Elizabeth West Berkshire Occupational Health, 21 Craven Road, Reading RG1 5LE Tel: 01734 877634 Fax: 01734 878778; Balnagowan, Berrick Salome, Wallingford OX10 6JQ Tel: 01865 890047 — MB ChB Manch. 1965; DObst RCOG 1967; FRCP Lond. 1996, M 1971; MSc (Occupat. Med.) Lond. 1985; FFOM RCP Lond. 1994, MFOM 1989, AFOM 1985. Cons. Occupat. Health Phys. & Specialist (Gen. & Thoracic Med.) Roy. Berks. & Battle NHS Trust. Specialty: Occupat. Health. Socs: Soc. Occupat. Med.; Brit. Thorac. Soc. Prev: Sen. Regist. (Gen. & Thoracic Med.) Battle Hosp. Reading; Regist. (Chest Dis. & Cardiol.) Baguley Hosp. Manch.; Regist. (Gen. Med.) Pk. Hosp. Davyhulme.

ROSS, Ardyn Mirande Tufnell Park Road Surgery, 244 Tufnell Park Roa, London N19 5EW Tel: 020 7272 9105 Fax: 020 7272 8996 — MB BS Lond. 1992 (Univ. Coll. Lond.) BSc (Hons.) Lond. 1989; DCH RCP Lond. 1994; DRCOG 1995. Specialty: Gen. Pract. Prev: Trainee GP Univ. Coll. Hosp. Lond. VTS.

ROSS, Arthur 3 Russell House, Eamont St., St John's Wood, London NW8 7DD Tel: 020 7722 6746 Fax: 020 7722 6746 — MB BCh BAO Dub. 1950. Prev: Mem. Lambeth, Lewisham & Southwark LMC; Clin. Asst. (ENT) St. Bart. Hosp. Lond.; Cas. Off. Hampstead Gen. Hosp.

ROSS, Audrey (retired) 4 The Redlands, Laundry Lane, Shrewsbury SY2 6ER Tel: 01743 356651 — MB ChB Manch. 1952.

ROSS, Mr Barry Alan, TD (retired) 8 The Crescent, Chapel Field, Norwich NR2 1SA Tel: 01603 623571 Fax: 01603 767851 Email: bross52593@aol.com — (Guy's) MB BS Lond. 1958; MRCS Eng. LRCP Lond. 1958; FRCS Eng. 1963. Cons. Thoracic Surg. E. Anglian RHA; Lt. Col. Cons. Surg. 257 Gen. Hosp. RAMC (V). Prev: Sen. Regist. (Thoracic Surg.) Guy's Hosp. Lond.

ROSS, Ben The Meadows Surgery, Temple Grove, Gatehouse Lane, Sussex Way, Burgess Hill RH15 9XH — MB BCh Belf. 1952. GP Burgess Hill, W. Sussex.

ROSS, Mr Brian David Glebe Cottage, Bell Lane, Cassington, Oxford OX29 4DS Tel: 01865 880629; 1291 Meadowbrook Road, Altadena CA 91001, USA Tel: 818 794 2004 — MB BS Lond. 1961; DPhil Oxf. 1966; FRCS Lond. 1973; FRCPath 1989, M 1976. Dir. Magnetic Resonance Spectroscopy Unit Huntington Med. Research Inst. Pasadena Calif., USA; Vis. Assoc. Calif. Inst. Technol.. Prev: Hon. Cons. Clin. Spectroscopy (N.M.R.) Roy. Postgrad. Med. Sch. Lond.; Cons. Chem. Path. Radcliffe Infirm. Oxf.; Univ. Lect. Metab. Med. Nuffield Dept. Med. Oxf.

ROSS, Bryan (retired) 6 Dickinson Way, North Muskham, Newark NG23 6FF — (Sheff.) MD (Commend.) Sheff. 1964, MB ChB (Hnrs.) 1959; DMRD Eng. 1969; FFR 1971; FRCR 1975. Prev: Cons. in Radiol. Centr. Sheff. Univ. Hosps. (NHS Trust).

ROSS, Callum Chalmers Yarra, Ettrickbridge, Selkirk TD7 5JN — MB ChB Aberd. 1997; MRCPsych.

ROSS, Calum Neil 44 Colney Lane, Norwich NR4 7RF — MB ChB Sheff. 1983; MRCP (UK) 1986; PhD 1996. Specialty: Nephrol.

ROSS, Caroline P\ediatric Neurology, Leicester Royal Infirmary, Leicester LE1 5WW Tel: 0116 254 1414 — MB ChB Manch. 1988; BSc (Med. Sci.) St. And. 1985; MRCP (UK) 1995; MSc (Paediatrics) University of Birmingham 1998. Cons. Paediatric NeUrol., Leicester Univ. Hosps. Trust, Leicester. Specialty: Paediat. Neurol. Socs: Brit. Paediatric Neurol. Assn.; Europ. Paediatric Neurol. Soc.; Roy. Coll. of Paediat. and Child Health. Prev: Trainee GP/SHO & Clin. Med. Off. Tameside Gen. Hosp.; SHO (Paediat.) Roy. Preston Hosp.; Regist. (Paediat.) Walsgrave Hosp. Coventry.

ROSS, Cathmar MacIver 10 Achany Road, Dingwall IV15 9JB — MB ChB Aberd. 1986. SHO (Anaesth.) Law Hosp. Carluke.

ROSS, Catriona Stirling Kirkwood St Andrew's Hospice, Henderson Street, Airdrie ML6 6DJ Tel: 01236 766951; 58 Hayford Mills, Cambusbarron, Stirling FK7 9PN Tel: 01784 451488 Email: cskross@hotmail.com — MB ChB Aberd. 1992; BMedBiol Aberd. 1989; MRCP (UK) 1995. Macmillan Consultant in Palliative Med. Specialty: Palliat. Med. Prev: Specialist Regist. Palliat. Med. N. Thames Rotat.; Spec. Reg. Palliat Med., S.E. Scotland, Rotation.

ROSS, Charles Duffin Bank House, Salter St., Stafford ST16 2JU Tel: 01785 4348 — MD Belf. 1948; MB BCh BAO 1939. Socs: BMA. Prev: Squadron Ldr. RAFVR Med. Br.; Res. Med. Off. Belf. City Hosp.; Res. Obstetr. Jubilee Matern. Hosp.

ROSS, Christine Elsie Central Manchester PCT, Wythenshawe Health Care Centre, 1 Stancliffe Road, Sharston, Manchester M22 4PJ; 196 Palatine Road, Didsbury, Manchester M20 2WG — MB ChB St. And. 1971. Staff Grade (Paediat.) Centr. Manch. PCT. Specialty: Community Child Health. Prev: Staff Grade (Paediat.), Mancunial Community NHS Trust.

ROSS, Colin Malcolm Douglas (retired) 17 Litchdon St, Barnstaple EX32 8ND — MB ChB Ed. 1955; FRCPath 1978.

ROSS, Constance Anne Cameron (retired) 21 Strathmore Court, 20 Abbey Drive, Glasgow G14 9JX Tel: 0141 959 4919 — MB ChB Glas. 1942; MD Glas. 1946; FRCPath 1976, M 1964. Prev: Cons. Virol. Regional Virus Laborat. Ruchill Hosp. Glas.

ROSS, David 32 Montacute Road, Lewes BN7 1EN — BM BCh Oxf. 1990.

ROSS, David Andrew, Lt.-Col. RAMC Chief Medical, UKSC (G), Rheindahlen BFPO 140, Germany Tel: 0049 2161 472 2926 Fax: 0049 2161 472 4601; 37A The Mall, Faversham ME13 8JN Email: doctulse@compuserve.com — MB BS Lond. 1985 (St Bartholomews Hosp.) MSc (Community Paediat.) Lond 1996; DCCH Ed. 1996; DFPHM 1998; DFFP 2000; MFPHM 2001. Chief Med., UKSC(G). Specialty: Pub. Health Med. Socs: BMA; Fell. Roy. Soc. Med.; Assoc.

Mem. Roy. Coll. Paediat., Child Health. Prev: Regist. (Community Paediat.) Brit. Milit. Hosp. Rinteln; SHO (Paediat.) Princess Margt. Hosp. Swindon; SHO (Gen. Med.) Brit. Milit. Hosp. Munster & Iserlohn.

ROSS, David Anthony Department of Epidemiology & Population Sciences, London School of Hygiene & Tropical Medicine, Keppel St., London WC1E 7HT Tel: 020 7927 2003 Fax: 020 7637 1173 — BM BCh Oxf. 1980; MSc Oxf. 1980, MA 1980, BA 1976. Sen. Lect. (Epidemiol.) Lond. Sch. Hyg. & Trop. Med. Specialty: Epidemiol. Socs: Internat. Epidemiol. Assn.; Roy. Soc. Trop. Med. & Hyg. Prev: Lect. (Epidemiol.) Lond. Sch. Hyg. & Trop. Med.; Research Fell. (Epidemiol.) Eval. & Plann. Centre for Health Care Lond. Sch. Hyg. & Trop. Med.; MRC Research Project Grantholder Trop. Med. Oxf. Univ.

ROSS, David George 13A Linden Road, Gosforth, Newcastle upon Tyne NE3 4EY — MB ChB Manch. 1997.

ROSS, Mr David John Consultant Orthopaedic Surgeon, Stirling Royal Infirmary, Stirling FK8 2AU — MB ChB Glas. 1973; FRCS Ed. 1979. Cons. Orthop. Surg. Stirling Roy. Infirm. Specialty: Orthop. Socs: Brit. Orthop. Assn.; Brit. Soc. Surg. Hand.

ROSS, David John St Richard's Hospital, Spitalfield Lane, Chichester PO19 4SE Tel: 01243 831728 Fax: 01243 831613 Email: david@boross.fsnet.co.uk — MB BS Lond. 1985; MRCP (UK) 1990; MSc (Epidemiology) Lond. 1994; MA (Cantab.) 1999. Cons. Phys. Chest Med. St. Richards Hosp., Chichester. Specialty: Respirat. Med.; Epidemiol.; Gen. Med.

ROSS, David Sloan (retired) Woodlands, 26 Kings Crescent, Elderslie, Johnstone PA5 9AA Tel: 01505 322832 — MB ChB Glas. 1956 (University of Glasgow) DPH Manch. 1960; DIH Eng. 1961; MFOM RCPI 1977; MFOM RCP Lond. 1978; MFCM RCP (UK) 1979; MFPHM RCP (UK) 1989; T(PHM) 1989; T(OM) 1989. Prev: Cons. Pub. Health Med. Argyll & Clyde HB.

ROSS, Donald (retired) 5 Riding Close, Hatchelwood Park, Bessacarr, Doncaster DN4 6UZ Tel: 01302 535247 — MB ChB Glas. 1951.

ROSS, Donald (retired) Overcombe, Lewis Lane, Chalfont St Peter, Gerrards Cross SL9 9TS Tel: 0128 13 83091 — LRCP LRCS Ed. 1927 (Univ. & Anderson Coll. Glas.) LRCP LRCS Ed. LRFPS Glas. 1927. Prev: Med. Off. Hoover Ltd. Perivale.

ROSS, Donald Ewen, Wing Cdr. Health Services Directorate, HQ Personnel and Training Command, RAF Innsworth, Gloucester GL3 1EZ Tel: 01452 712612 Ext: 5812 Email: flugharzt@luftschloss.freeserve.co.uk; Flat 4, 28 Larusdown Cresent, Cheltenham GL50 2LF Email: flugarzt@luftschloss.freeserve.co.uk — MB ChB Aberd. 1986; DCH RCPS Glas. 1990. Command Flight Med. Official Roy. Air Force. Specialty: Aviat. Med. Socs: Mem. of Aerospace Med. Assn. Prev: SMO RAF Lossiemouth; SMO RAF Sek Hong; SMO RAF Locking.

ROSS, Donald George North Burnside Croft, Clinterty, Kinellar, Aberdeen AB21 0TG — MB ChB Aberd. 1967; FFA RCS Eng. 1973. Cons. Anaesth. Grampian Health Bd. Specialty: Anaesth.

ROSS, Mr Donald Nixon 25 Upper Wimpole Street, London W1G 6NF Tel: 020 7935 8805 Fax: 020 7935 9190; 35 Cumberland Terrace, Regents Park, London NW1 4HP Tel: 020 7935 0756 — MB ChB Cape Town 1946; Hon. DSc Cape Town 1982, BSc, MB ChB 1946; FRCS Eng. 1949; FACC 1973; FACS 1976; Hon. FRCSI 1984; Hon. FRCS Thailand 1987; Hon. FACS 1993. Cons. Emerit. Card. Surg. Middlx. Hosp. Lond.; Cons. Emerit. Thoracic Surg. Guy's Hosp. Lond. Specialty: Cardiothoracic Surg. Socs: (Ex-Pres.) Soc. Thoracic Surgs. & Soc. & Assocs. Thoracic Surgs.; Hon Mem. RSM. Prev: Sen. Surg. Nat. Heart Hosp. Lond.; Dir. Dept. Surg. Inst. Cardiol. Lond.; Cardiovasc. Research Fell. & Sen. Regist. Thoracic Surg. Guy's Hosp. Lond.

ROSS, Donovan Library House Surgery, Avondale Road, Chorley PR7 2AD Tel: 01257 262081 Fax: 01257 232114; Rose Hill, Leyland Lane, Ulnes Walton, Leyland, Preston PR26 8LB Tel: 01257 450182 Email: donovan@gøvho.demon.co.uk — MB ChB Liverp. 1972; DRCOG 1977; MRCGP 1979. Specialty: Gen. Pract. Socs: Brit. Med. Acupunct. Soc. Prev: Med. Off. RAF.

ROSS, Mr Edward Raymond Smith Hope Hospital, Eccles Old Road, Salford M6 8HD — MB ChB St. And. 1971; FRCS Ed. 1976; FRACS 1983. Cons. Orthop. Surg. Hope Hosp. Manch.; Hon. Asst. Lect. Univ. Manch. Specialty: Orthop. Prev: Flight Lt. RAF Med. Br.; Sen. Regist. (Orthop.) Robt. Jones & Agnes Hunt Orthop. Hosp. OsW.ry.

ROSS, Elizabeth Jane Walker 'Eredine', Todlaw Road, Duns TD11 3EW — MB ChB Glas. 1970.

ROSS, Emma Caroline 24 Thornfield Road, London W12 8JG — MB BS Lond. 1992 (Char. Cross & Westm.) BSc (Hons.) Psychol. 1989; MRCP (UK) 1996. SHO (Neurol. & Neurosurg.) Gt. Ormond St. Hosp. Lond. Specialty: Paediat.

ROSS, Eric Buchanan (retired) The Pightle, 6 Thornlea, Hepscott, Morpeth NE61 6NY Tel: 01670 57558 — MB ChB Ed. 1943 (Univ. Ed.) MRCGP 1973. Prev: Ho. Surg. Perth Roy. Infirm.

ROSS, Eric John (retired) 47 Campden Street, London W8 7ET Tel: 020 7229 2122 Email: janericross@waitrose.com — (Univ. Coll. Hosp.) MB BS Lond. 1951; MRCS Eng. LRCP Lond. 1951; FRCP Lond. 1966, M 1955; BSc, PhD Lond., MD 1958. Prev: Emerit. Prof. Endocrinol. & Hon. Research Fell. Univ. Coll. Med. Sch. Lond.

ROSS, Ernest, AE 34 Elmfield Road, Gosforth, Newcastle upon Tyne NE3 4BA Tel: 0191 285 4107 — MB BS Durh. 1958. Med. Mem. Indep. Tribunal Serv. Prev: SHO Princess Margt. Rose Orthop. Hosp. Edin.; Regist. (Orthop.) Leicester Roy. Infirm.; Ho. Surg. (Orthop.) Roy. Vict. Infirm. Newc.

ROSS, Esther Stuart (retired) 15 Mount Avenue, Bare, Morecambe LA4 6DJ — MB ChB Glas. 1963; DPM Ed. & Glas. 1967; FRCPsych 1993, M 1973.

ROSS, Professor Euan MacDonald Child Studies, School of Law, King's College London, Strand, London WC2R 2LS Tel: 020 7848 2377 Fax: 020 7848 2910; Linklater House, Mount Park Road, Harrow HA1 3JZ Tel: 020 8864 4746 Fax: 020 8864 4746 — MB ChB Bristol 1962; DCH RCPS Glas. 1965; MRCP (UK) 1971; MD Bristol 1975; FRCP Lond. 1980; Hon. FFPHM RCP (UK) 1997; FRCPCH 1997. Specialty: Community Child Health. Socs: Brit. Paediat. Neurol. Assn.; Brit. Assn. Community Child Health; Brit. Neuro Psych. Assn. Prev: Cons. Comm. Health. S. Lond. NHS; Cons. KCH Lond.; Prof. Community Paediat. & Hon. Cons. Community Paediat. King's Coll. Univ. Lond.

ROSS, Ewen Thomas 17 North Square, Aberdeen AB11 5DX — MB ChB Ed. 1992.

ROSS, Felicity Anne Craig End, Kincraig Drive, Sevenoaks TN13 3BB; Flat 3, 1 Salisbury Road, Hove BN3 3AB — MB BS Lond. 1992; DRCOG 1996; MRCGP 1997. Specialty: Gen. Pract.

ROSS, Fiona Kathlyn 14 Upper Stoneborough Lane, Budleigh Salterton EX9 6SX — MB ChB Birm. 1985; DRCOG 1988; MRCGP 1994.

ROSS, Frances Mary Harrold Medical Practice, Peach's Close, Harrold, Bedford MK43 7DX Tel: 01234 720225 Fax: 01234 720603; 17 Brook Lane, Harrold, Bedford MK43 7BW — MB ChB Ed. 1982; DRCOG 1985; MRCGP 1988.

ROSS, Frances Mary Hunter 6 Saxe-Coburg Place, Edinburgh EH3 5BR — MRCS Eng. LRCP Lond. 1975.

ROSS, Geoffrey George 58 St Benets Road, Prittlewell, Southend-on-Sea SS2 6LF — BM Soton. 1986; BA Sheff. 1980; MRCGP 1991. Pharmaceut. Phys. Horsham. Specialty: Pharmaceutical Medicine; Gen. Pract.

ROSS, Geoffrey McEwen John O'Connell Street Medical Practice, 6 O'Connell Street, Hawick TD9 9HU Tel: 01450 372276 Fax: 01450 371564; Ravenswood, 3 West Stewart Place, Hawick TD9 8BH — MB ChB Aberd. 1976; DRCOG 1979; MRCGP 1980.

ROSS, George (retired) Ingfield House, 57 Northgate, Almondbury, Huddersfield HD5 8RY Tel: 01484 21391 — MB BCh BAO Belf. 1940 (Qu. Univ. Belf.) Prev: Mem. (Ex-Pres.) W. Riding Irish Med. Soc. Mem. BMA (Chairm. Huddersfield Div.).

ROSS, George Allen Wood Selworthy, 65 Roebuck Lane, Buckhurst Hill IG9 5QX — MB BChir Camb. 1968; MA, MB BChir Camb. 1968; DObst RCOG 1970.

ROSS, George Innes MacDonald (retired) 25 York Road, Weybridge KT13 9DY Tel: 01932 844428 — MB ChB Aberd. 1942; DCP Lond 1948; FRCPath 1966, M 1963. Prev: Cons. Path. Ashford Hosp. Middlx.

ROSS, Gillian Margaret 30 Wingrave Road, London W6 9HF — BM Soton. 1979; MRCP (UK) 1992.

ROSS, Gordon Buchan (retired) 4 The Redlands, Laundry Lane, Shrewsbury SY2 6ER Tel: 01743 356651 — MB ChB Manch. 1951.

ROSS, Greta Primary Care Services, South Block, Louth County Hospital, Louth LN11 0EU Tel: 01507 600100; 54 St Mary's Lane,

Louth LN11 0DT Tel: 01507 605232 Fax: 01507 602544 Email: drgretaross@aol.com — MB BS Sydney 1965; DCH RCP Glas. 1972; MRCGP Lond. 1977. SCMO (Sexual Health & Family Plann. Train.). Specialty: Family Plann. & Reproduc. Health.

ROSS, Mr Harvey Burton, RD (retired) Springvale, Brewery Common, Mortimer, Reading RG7 3JE Tel: 01189 332374 — MB BS Lond. 1952 (St. Bart.) MS Lond. 1966, MB BS 1952; FRCS Eng. 1957. Prev: Surg. Roy. Berks. Hosp. Reading.

ROSS, Hector John Taylor (retired) 47 Park Road, West Hagley, Stourbridge DY9 0QQ Tel: 01562 882039 — LRCP LRCS Ed. LRFPS Glas. 1935 (Anderson & St. Mungo's Colls. Glas.) FRCP Ed. 1968, M 1947. Prev: Cons. Phys. E. Birm. Hosp.

ROSS, Helen Grant (retired) 1 Springfields, Hillside, Follifoot, Harrogate HG3 1EF Tel: 01423 870465 — MB ChB St. And. 1954; DTM & H Liverp. 1966; Dip Bact . Lond. 1969; FRCPath 1984, M 1972; T(Path) 1991. Prev: Cons. Bact. Pub. Health Laborat. Seacroft Hosp. Leeds.

ROSS, Iain Sutherland Clinical Biochemistry Department, Aberdeen Royal Infirmary, Aberdeen AB25 2ZD Tel: 01224 681818 Fax: 01224 694378 — MB ChB Aberd. 1964; PhD Aberd. 1970, MB ChB 1964. Cons. i/c Dept. Clin. Biochem. Grampian HB; Clin. Sen. Lect. & Head (Clin. Biochem.) Univ. Aberd.; Dir. of Laborat. Med. Aberd. Roy. Hosps. Trust. Specialty: Biochem. Socs: Roy. Soc. Med. (Lond. Br.). Prev: Ho. Off. Woodend Gen. Hosp. Aberd. & Aberd. City Hosp.

ROSS, Ian (retired) 12 Anderson Drive, Aberdeen AB15 4TY Tel: 01224 314716 — MB ChB Aberd. 1955; MRCGP 1976. Prev: GP Aberd.

ROSS, Ian Hugh Barnard Castle Surgery, Victoria Road, Barnard Castle DL12 8HT Tel: 01833 690707 — MRCS Eng. LRCP Lond. 1968 (Roy. Free) BDS Durham. 1963; MRCS Eng. LRCP Lond. 1968 FDS RCS Eng. 1968; DObst RCOG 1971; MRCGP 1994. Socs: BMA. Prev: Regist. (Oral Surg.) Eastman Dent. Hosp. Lond.; SHO (O & G) Darlington Memor. Hosp.; Ho. Phys. Friarage Hosp. Northallerton.

ROSS, Ian Nicholas The Newpark Hospital, Boundary Road, Newark NG24 4DE Tel: 01636 685675 Email: ian.ross@sfh-tr.nhs.uk — MB BS Lond. 1972 (Roy. Free Hosp. Lond.) MRCS Eng. LRCP Lond. 1972; MRCP (UK) 1974; PhD Birm. 1980, MSc 1977; FRCP Lond. 1992. Cons. Gastroenterol., Sherwood Forest Hospitals NHS Trust. Specialty: Gastroenterol.; Gen. Med. Socs: Brit. Soc. Gastroenterol.; Brit. Med. Assn.

ROSS, Ian Ronald Francis Rose Garden Medical Centre, 4 Mill Lane, Edinburgh EH6 6TL Tel: 0131 554 1274 Fax: 0131 555 2159; 52 Hopetoun Terrace, Gullane EH3 2DD — MB ChB Ed. 1970. Med. Off. Gen. Counc. Brit. Shipping, Leith. Prev: Med. Adviser Craig & Rose Paint Co.

ROSS, Irene Rayner Portland House Surgery, 75 Mornington Road, Greenford UB6 9HN Tel: 020 8578 1730 — MB ChB Leeds 1963. Trainer (Gen. Pract.) Greenford Middlx. Specialty: Paediat. Socs: BMA. Prev: Med. Off. Lond. Boro. Ealing; SHO Claybury Hosp. Woodford Green; SHO Roy. Childr. Hosp. Melbourne.

ROSS, Jacqueline Axford 11 Petts Wood Road, Orpington BR5 1JT — MB BS Lond. 1992.

ROSS, James Douglas The Health Centre, Victoria Road, Leven KY8 4ET Tel: 01333 432577 Fax: 01333 422249 — MB ChB Aberd. 1977; DRCOG 1980; MRCGP 1982.

ROSS, James Roy Young 10 Weston Way, Weston Favell, Northampton NN3 3BL — MB BS Lond. 1972 (St. Geo.) BSc Lond. 1969, MB BS 1972; MRCP (U.K.) 1975; MRCPath 1980. Cons. Haemat. Northampton Gen. Hosp. Specialty: Haematology. Prev: Sen. Regist. (Haemat.) Childr. Hosp. Birm. SHO (Med.) N. Staffs.; Health Dist.; Ho. Phys. & Ho. Surg. Roy. S. Hants. Hosp. Soton.

ROSS, James William Buchan, Surg. Lt. RN St Budeaux Health Centre, Stirling Road, St Budeaux, Plymouth PL5 1PL Tel: 01752 361010 Fax: 01752 350675 — MB ChB Aberd. 1988; DFFP. GP Principle St Budeaux Health Centre. Prev: Trainee GP/SHO Roy. Navy Med. Off.

ROSS, Jean Mary Linklater House, Mount Pk Road, Harrow on the Hill, Harrow HA1 3JZ Tel: 020 8864 4746 Fax: 020 8864 4746 — MB ChB St. And. 1963; DObst RCOG 1965; MSc Occupat. Med. Lond. 1983; MFOM RCP 1990; FFOM 1997. Cons. (Occupat. Med.) N. W. Lond. Hosp. NHS Trust; Cons. (Occupat. Med.) Univ. of W.minster & Harrow & Hillingdon Healthcatre NHS Trust. Specialty: Occupat. Health. Special Interest: Infec.; Ment. Health. Socs: Soc. Occupat. Med.; Assn. Local Auth. Med. Advisers; Assn. NHS Occupat. Health Phys. Prev: Phys. (Occupat. Health) Unilever Lond.; Mem. Scientif. Staff (Perinatal Med.) & Clin. Asst. Clin. Research Centre Northwick Pk. Hosp.; Med. Off. Community Health Depts. Dundee & Bristol.

ROSS, Jean Ruth Williamina (retired) 17 St Joseph's Vale, Blackheath, London SE3 0XF Tel: 020 8463 0725 — (Univ. Ed.) BSc Ed. 1946, MB ChB 1947. Prev: Sen. Lect. (Anat.) Char. Cross Hosp. Med. Sch. Lond..

ROSS, Jerard 22 Culloden Road, Balloch, Inverness IV2 7HQ — MB ChB Aberd. 1994. Specialty: Paediat.; Intens. Care; Respirat. Med.

ROSS, Joan Ramsay 31 Birkhill Road, Stirling FK7 9LA — MB ChB Glas. 1973; Dip. Forens. Med. Glas 1996.

ROSS, John Alexander Strachan Department Environmental & Occupational Medicine, University of Aberdeen, Ashgrove Road W., Aberdeen AB25 2ZD Tel: 01224 681818 Fax: 01224 662990 — MB ChB Aberd. 1973; FFA RCS Eng. 1979; PhD Lond. 1986. Hon. Cons. Anaesth. Aberd. Roy. Hosp. Trust; Sen. Lect. Environment & Occupat. Med. Univ. Aberd. Specialty: Anaesth. Socs: Soc. Occupat. Med. & Assn. Anaesth. Prev: Sen. Regist. (Anaesth.) Middlx. Hosp. Lond.; Scientif. Off. MRC Div. Anaesth.; Regist. (Anaesth.) Aberd. Roy. Infirm.

ROSS, John Donald, Surg. Capt. RN Retd. The Barn, Woodscott Barton, Ilfracombe EX34 9RW Tel: 01271 864295 Fax: 01271 864295 — MRCS Eng. LRCP Lond. 1952 (St. Mary's) DPath Eng. 1965. Cons. Med. Adviser (Water Quality & Pub. Health) Thames Water Utilities. Specialty: Pub. Health Med. Socs: Fell. Roy. Soc. Med. Prev: Med. Adviser Thames Water Auth.; Dir. Health & Research (Naval).

ROSS, John Frederick Gunn 6 Saxe-Coburg Place, Edinburgh EH3 5BR Tel: 0131 332 7068 — MB ChB Aberd. 1972; DObst RCOG 1974; MRCGP 1984.

ROSS, John Hugh, MC (retired) Barkstone, 24 Overbury Road, Hereford HR1 1JE Tel: 01432 272717 — (Lond. Hosp.) MD Camb. 1959, MB BChir 1950; DObst RCOG 1952; FRCP Lond. 1970, M 1953. Prev: Cons. Phys. Heref. Hosp. Gp.

ROSS, Mr John Macaulay Hamilton (retired) C/2 Craufurdland, Braepark Road, Barnton, Edinburgh EH4 6DL Tel: 0131 339 8647 — MB ChB Ed. 1937; FRCS Ed. 1941. Prev: Cons. Surg. (Urol.) Roy. Infirm. Sunderland.

ROSS, John Macdonald, MBE (retired) Clovelly, 487 Lanark Road, Juniper Green, Edinburgh EH14 5DQ — MB ChB Ed. 1937 (Univ. Ed.) MRCGP 1976. Prev: Ho. Surg. Edin. Roy. Infirm.

ROSS, John Scott Carolside Medical Centre, 1 Carolside Gardens, Clarkston, Glasgow G76 7BX Tel: 0141 644 3511 Fax: 0141 644 5525; 9 Glebe Road, Newton Mearns, Glasgow G77 6DU — MB ChB Glas. 1980; DRCOG 1983. Hon. Clin. Sen. Lect. in Gen. Pract. Specialty: Dermat.; Pharmaceutical Medicine. Prev: Clin. Asst. Dermat.

ROSS, Jonathan Denys Crawford Whittall Street Clinic, Whittall St., Birmingham B4 6DH Tel: 0121 237 5721 Fax: 0121 237 5729 — MB ChB Aberd. 1986; MRCP (UK) 1989; MD Aberdeen 1995; FRCP (Edin.) 1998; FRCP (Lond.) 2000. Cons. (GU Med.) Birm. specialist, community NHS Trust.; Sen. Lect. Birm. Univ. 1997- Cons. Phys., Univ. Hosp. trust, Birm.. Specialty: Genitourinary Medicine; HIV Med.

ROSS, Jonathan James 6 Crossland Road, Hathersage, Hope Valley S32 1AN — MB ChB Ed. 1988; FRCA 1995. Clin. Research Assoc. (Surgic. & Anaesth. Scis.) Univ. Sheff. Specialty: Anaesth.

ROSS, Mr Jonathan James Tennent Institute of Ophthalmology, Gartnavel General Hospital, Great Western Road, Glasgow G12 0NY — MB ChB Glas. 1998; MRCS Ed. 2002; MRCOphth 2002. Specialist Regist., Ophth., Tennent Inst., Glas. Specialty: Ophth. Special Interest: Ocular Oncol.; Cornea; Oculoplastics. Prev: Specialist Regist., Ophth., Cardiff Eye Unit; Specialist Regist. Ophth., Manch. Roy. Eye Hosp.; Fell., Ophth., St Pauls Eye Unit, Liverp.

ROSS, Mr Jonathan Knox Occupational Health Department, BG Group plc, 100 Thames Valley Park Drive, Reading RG6 1PT Tel: 0118 929 3144 Fax: 0118 929 3140 Email: jonathan.ross@bg-group.com; 23 Kingsley Avenue, London W13 0EQ Tel: 020 8997 6583 — MB BS Lond. 1979 (Univ. Coll. Hosp.) BSc (Hons.) Lond. 1976; FRCS Eng. 1984; AFOM RCP Lond. 1995; MFOM RCP Lond. 1996. Chief Med. Advis. BG Gp. Specialty: Occupat. Health. Socs:

Roy. Soc. Med.; BMA. Prev: Med. Off. Brit. Antarctic Survey; Regist. (Orthop. Surg.) Hammersmith Hosp. Lond.; Regist. (Gen. Surg.) Mt. Vernon Hosp.

ROSS, Josiah (retired) 32 Montacute Road, Lewes BN7 1EN Tel: 01273 473419 Email: joeross@onetel.com — MB BCh BAO Belf. 1958 (Qu. Univ. Belf.) BSc Belf. 1955; DPM Lond. 1964; MRCPsych 1971. Prev: Cons. Child & Adolesc. Psychiat. Mid-Downs & Brighton Health Dist.

ROSS, Joy Ruth Royal Marsden Hospital, Department of Palliative Medicine, London SW3 6JJ; 59 Ann Moss Way, London SE16 2TJ — MB BS Lond. 1995. Research Fell. Roy. Marsden Hosp. Lond.

ROSS, Judith B Banff Health Centre, Clunie St., Banff AB45 1HY Tel: 01261 812027; Blackpots Farm House, Whitehills, Banff AB45 2NS Tel: 01261 861215 — MB ChB Aberd. 1982; Dip. Sports Med. 1977. GP Banff Health Centre. Specialty: Sports Med. Prev: SHO (O & G) Cresswell Matern. Hosp. Dumfries; Trainee GP Lockmaben VTS; SHO (Med.) Palmerston Pk. Hosp., NZ.

ROSS, Juliette Wembley Park Medical Centre, 21 Wembley Park Drive, Wembley HA9 8HD Tel: 020 8902 4411 Fax: 020 8795 2987; 15 Leavesden Road, Stanmore HA7 3RQ Tel: 020 8954 1851 Fax: 020 8357 0835 Email: juliette.ross@dircon.co.uk — MB BS Lond. 1981 (Middlx.) Dip.Med.ACU 2000 BMAs; MRCGP 1986. GP Tutor, Roy. Free Hosp. Med. Sch. Specialty: Gen. Pract.; Acupunc. Prev: GP Trainer (Gen. Pract.) Centr. Middlx. Scheme.

ROSS, Keith Raymond (retired) 21/182485 Windsor Gardens, Codsall, Wolverhampton WV8 2EX Tel: 01902 842432 — MB ChB Manch. 1968; FRCPCH; FRCP (UK) 1972. Prev: Cons. Paediat. Wolverhampton.

ROSS, Kenneth Grant McLagan Adolescent Forensic Service, Preswich Hospital, Bury New Road, Prestwich, Manchester M25 3BL Tel: 0161 772 3811 Fax: 0161 772 3693; 1 A Arundale Avenue, Whalley Range, Manchester M16 8LS Tel: 0161 881 6566 Email: kenny.ross@tesco.net — MB ChB Dundee 1985; MRCPsych 1994. Cons. Adolesc. Forens. Psychiat., Adolesc. Forens. Serv., Prestwich Hopsital, Manch.. Specialty: Child & Adolesc. Psychiat. Prev: Career Regist. Rotat. (Psychiat.) S. Glas.; Sen. Regist. Child Adolesc. Psychiat. Rotat. Manch.

ROSS, Mr Kenneth Raeburn Shepherds Hey, 7 Old Camp Road, Eastbourne BN20 8DH Tel: 01323 641221 — MB BS Lond. 1973 (St. Bart.) MRCS Eng. LRCP Lond. 1973; FRCS Eng. 1979. Cons. Orthop. Surg. Eastbourne Dist. Gen. Hosp. Specialty: Orthop.; Trauma & Orthop. Surg. Socs: BMA & Hunt. Soc.; Anglo-Amer. Med. Soc.(Vice-Pres.); Brit. Orthopaedic Assn. Prev: Sen. Regist. Rotat. (Orthop.) St. Bart. Hosp. Lond.; Regist. (Surg.) Mt. Vernon Hosp. Northwood; Ho. Surg. St. Bart. Hosp. Lond.

ROSS, Kevin 60 Crediton Drive, Platt Bridge, Wigan WN2 5HU — BM BS Nottm. 1997.

ROSS, Lesley Anne Royal Hospital for Sick Children, 9 Sciennes Road, Edinburgh EH9 1LF Tel: 0131 536 0000 Email: lesley.ross@luht.scot.nhs.uk — MB ChB Ed. 1985; MRCGP 1989; DRCOG 1989; DCH RCP Lond. 1991; MRCP Paediat. (UK) 1993. Cons. Paediat. Specialty: Paediat. Prev: Specialist Regist. (Paediat.) Roy. Hosp. Sick Childr. Edin.; Clin. Research Fell. (Child Life & Health) Univ. Edin.; Regist. (Paediat.) St Jas. Univ. Hosp. Leeds. & York. Dist. Hosp.

ROSS, Mr Leslie David Womens Health, St Helier Hospital, Wryth Lane, Carshalton SM5 1AA Tel: 020 8644 4343; 61 The Ridgeway, Sutton SM2 5JX Tel: 0208 643 3349 — MB BS Lond. 1974 (Guy's) MRCS Eng. LRCP Lond. 1974; FRCOG 1997, MRCOG 1980, DObst 1975; FRCS Ed. 1980. Cons. O & G St. Helier Hosp. Carshalton; Hon. Sen. Lect. Univ. Lond. Specialty: Obst. & Gyn. Socs: Fell. Roy. Soc. Med.; Soc. for the Study of Fertil. Prev: Sen. Regist. Jessop Hosp. for Wom. Sheff.; Regist. (O & G) Addenbrooke's Hosp. Camb.; Resid. Surg. Off. Hosp. Wom. Lond.

ROSS, Linda Margaret 101 Earlbank Av., Scotstoun, Glasgow G14 9DY — MB ChB Glas. 1990; MRCP (UK) 1994. Specialist Regist. (Med. Paediat.) Yorkhill NHS Trust Glas. Specialty: Paediat. Socs: BMA & RCPCH; RCPS Glas.; Scott. Paedia. Soc. Prev: SHO (Geriat. Med.) Lightburn Hosp. Glas.; SHO (A & E Med.) Glas. Roy. Infirm.; Ho. Off. (Gen. Med.) Glas. Roy. Infirm.

ROSS, Lindsey Elizabeth Dingwall Medical Group, The Health Centre, Percy Road, Dingwall IV15 9QS Tel: 01349 863033 Fax: 01349 862022; An Crasg, West Drummuie, Golspie KW10 6TA Tel: 01408 633978 Fax: 01408 634189 Email: lindsey@rossdrummuie.com — MB ChB Aberd. 1985 (Aberdeen) BSc (Hons.) Developm. Biol. Aberd. 1980, MB ChB 1985; Cert. Family Plann. JCC 1987; MRCGP 1990. GP at Ross Memorial, Dingwall; Practice Accreditation Assessor. RCGP, Scotland; JP, Sutherland; Chair, Cross Rd., E. Sutherland, Care Attendant Scheme. Specialty: Care of the Elderly; Accid. & Emerg. Socs: Highland Med. Soc.; BMA; BASICS. Prev: Hospital Pract., GP Unit Lakon Memor. Hosp. Golspie; Clinical Assistant, Golspie.

ROSS, Louis (retired) 24 Bentinck Close, Prince Albert Road, London NW8 7RY Tel: 020 7586 2992 — (Univ. Coll. Hosp.) MRCS Eng. LRCP Lond. 1939; MB BS Lond. 1941; MRCGP 1953. Prev: Clin. Asst. (Cardiol.) Middlx. Hosp. Lond.

ROSS, Mairie Annabella Rutland Place Surgery, 21 Rutland Place, Glasgow G51 1TA Tel: 0141 427 3121 Fax: 0141 427 7600 — MB ChB Ed. 1978. Specialty: Gen. Psychiat. Prev: Regist. (Psychiat.) Inverclyde Roy. Hosp. Greenock.

ROSS, Margaret Haigh (retired) (Surgery) 59 Northgate, Almondbury, Huddersfield HD5 8RX Tel: 01484 421391; Ingfield House, 57 Northgate, Almondbury, Huddersfield HD5 8RX Tel: 01484 513381 — MRCS Eng. LRCP Lond. 1964 (Sheff.) BSc Lond. 1958. Med. Off. Huddersfield Cervical Cytol. Clinic & Family Plann. Clinics; Med. Off. BrigHo. Family Plann. Comm. Prev: Staff Med. Off. Storthes Hall Ment. Hosp. Kirkburton.

ROSS, Margaret Shirley (retired) 34 Elmfield Road, Gosforth, Newcastle upon Tyne NE3 4BA Tel: 0191 285 4107 — (Durh.) MB BS Durh. 1958; DA Eng. 1984. Prev: Assoc. Specialist (Anaesth.) Sunderland Hosps.

ROSS, Margot Pamela 3 The Coombe, Dartmouth TQ6 9PG — State Exam Med. Berlin 1991.

ROSS, Martin Graham Silloth Group Medical Practice, Lanewn Terrace, Silloth, Carlisle CA7 4AH Tel: 016973 31309 Fax: 016973 32834 — MB ChB Birm. 1972.

ROSS, Melvin (retired) 9 Tillingbourne Gardens, Finchley, London N3 3JJ Tel: 020 8346 3556 — MB BS Lond. 1950 (Univ. Coll. Hosp.) MRCS Eng. LRCP Lond. 1949; FRCGP 1975, M 1960. Prev: Sen. Lect. Dept. Primary Health Care Univ. Coll. & Middlx. Sch. Med. Lond.

ROSS, Mervyn Thomas Anaesthetic Department, Level B, King's Hill Hospital, Mansfield Road, Sutton-in-Ashfield NG17 4JL; 9 Southgreen Hill, Mansfield NG18 4PU — MB ChB Ed. 1971; FFA RCS Eng. 1977. Cons. Anaesth. Centr. Notts. Health Auth. Specialty: Anaesth. Prev: Sen. Regist. (Anaesth.) Shackleton Dept. Anaesth. Soton. Gen.; Hosp.

ROSS, Michael Bilton Medical Centre, 120 Lily Road, Bradford BD8 8JT Tel: 01274 490409 Fax: 01274 499112; 2 Yate Lane, Oxenhope, Keighley BD22 9HL Tel: 01535 646763 Fax: 01535 645405 — MB BS Lond. 1975 (Univ. Coll. Hosp.) BSc (Anat.) Lond. 1972; Cert JCC Lond. 1978; DRCOG 1978; MRCP (UK) 1979; MSc Comm. Med. 1980; MRCGP 1981; DTM & H Liverp. 1984. Instruc. Doctor JCC.

ROSS, Michael Taylor General Practice Section, Division of Community Health Sciences, The University of Edinburgh, 20 West Richmond Street, Edinburgh EH8 9DX Email: m.ross@doctors.org.uk — MB ChB Ed. 1998; DRCOG; Bsc hons; MB ChB Ed. 1998; MB ChB Ed 1998; MRCGP 2003.

ROSS, Nicholas Elizlea, High St., Errol, Perth PH2 7QJ — MB ChB Dundee 1990.

ROSS, Oliver Charles Flat 1, Moray House, 4 Morden Road, London SE3 0AA; 44 Lings Coppiu, West Dalwich, London SE21 8SX — MB ChB Birm. 1989; FRCA 1994. Specialist Regist., Anaesth. St Geo.'s Hosp. Specialty: Anaesth. Socs: Assoc. of Anaesth.; Paediat. Intens. Care Soc.

ROSS, Oswald (retired) Flat 6, Fairmead Court, 1441 High Road, Whetstone, London N20 9PF Tel: 020 8343 8575 — MB BCh BAO Belf. 1946 (Qu. Univ. Belf.) DObst RCOG 1949; MRCGP 1960.

ROSS, Pamela Mary Dunn 10 Abbey Place, Airdrie ML6 9QT — MB ChB Glas. 1998; MB ChB Glas 1998.

ROSS, Pamela Susan 16 Ashdale Park, Wokingham RG40 3QS Tel: 01344 775667 — MB BChir Camb. 1982 (Middlesex) MA Camb. 1982; MRCGP 1986. GP Princip. at Heathhill Surg., Crowthorne. Specialty: Gen. Pract. Socs: MRCGP. Prev: GP Princip. at Skimped Hill Health Centre Bracknell Berks.

ROSS, Paul Alistair 16 Miles Avenue, Sandford, Wareham BH20 7AT — BM BS Nottm. 1994. Specialty: Gen. Pract.

ROSS, Paul Jonathan 99 Rivermead Court, Ranelagh Gardens, London SW6 3SB — MB BS Lond. 1990; BSc (Hons.) Lond. 1987; MRCP (UK) 1995. Research Fell. & Hon. Regist. (Med. Oncol.) Roy. Marsden NHS Trust Surrey. Prev: Regist. (Gastroenterol. & Gen. Med.) Jersey Gen. Hosp.; SHO (Med. Oncol.) Roy. Marsden NHS Trust Surrey.

ROSS, Peter John 15 Wardie Road, Edinburgh EH5 3QE — MD Wales 1979; MB ChB 1971; MRCP (UK) 1973. Managing Dir. Private Nursing Homes of Edin. Ltd. Socs: Assoc. Fell. Amer. Coll. Cardiol. Prev: Lect. & Hon. Sen. Regist. (Clin. Cardiol.) Univ. Hosp. Wales Cardiff; Cons. Cardiol. Riyadh Armed Forces Hosp. Saudi Arabia; Exchange; Fellowship Cardiovasc. Lab. Loma Linda Univ. Med. Center Calif. USA.

ROSS, Philip Wesley, TD The Old Yard, 38 High Street, Pittenweem, Anstruther KY10 2PL Tel: 0131 661 5415 — (Aberd.) MD (Commend.) Aberd. 1970; FRCPath 1988, M 1983; MRCP Ed. 1985; FIBiol 1988; FRCP Ed. 1989; FRCSed 2000. Reader (Med. Microbiol.) Bact. Univ. Edin.; Hon. Fell., Univ. of Edin.; Vis. Prof., Coll.s of Med. and Med. Sch.s in Africa and India; Hon. Cons. Roy. Infirm. Edin.; FLS; Lt.-Col. RAMC (V) Graded Cons. Path. RARO. Specialty: Med. Microbiol. Socs: Brit. Soc. Study of Infec.; Pres. Scott. Microbiol. Assn.; U.K Counc. of Inst. of Biol. Prev: Sen. Lect. (Bact.) Univ. Edin.; Lect. (Bact.) Univ. Edin. & Univ. Aberd.; Ho. Phys. & Ho. Surg. Woodend Hosp. Aberd.

ROSS, Rachael Joan Lee-on-the-Solent Health Centre, Manor Way, Lee-on-the-Solent PO13 Tel: 02392 550220; 65 The Keep, Fareham PO16 9PW Email: rachael.ross@virgin.net — MB BS Newc. 1987 (Newc. u. Tyne) DRCOG 1990; DCH RCP Lond. 1990; MRCGP 1991. GP Retainee; Clin. Asst. (Elderly Med.) Gosport War Memor. Hosp. Socs: Soc. Occupat. Med. Prev: Trainee GP Furness Gen. Hosp.

ROSS, Richard Anthony St Andrews Surgery, The Old Central School, Southover Road, Lewes BN7 1US Tel: 01273 476216 Fax: 01273 487587; Kingston Lodge, The St, Kingston, Lewes BN7 3PB Tel: 01273 476216 — MB BS Lond. 1974 (King's Coll. Hosp.) FFA RCS Eng. 1979. Hosp. Pract. Vict. Hosp. Lewes. Specialty: Anaesth.

ROSS, Professor Richard John Martin Northern General Hospital, Department of Medicine, Herries Road, Sheffield S5 7AU Tel: 0114 271 4884 Fax: 0114 256 0458 Email: r.j.ross@sheffield.ac.uk — MB BS Lond. 1979; MRCP Lond. 1982; MD Lond. 1988; FRCP Lond. 1995. Prof. & Hon. Cons. Phys. (Endocrinol.) Northern Gen. Hosp. Sheff. Specialty: Endocrinol. Prev: Sen. Lect. & Hon. Cons. Phys. (Endocrinol.) & Research Fell. St. Bart. Hosp. Lond.; Sen. Regist. (Med.) King's Coll. Hosp. Lond.

ROSS, Mr Robert Alasdair Medical Centre, Commando Trainging Centre Royal Marines, Lympstone EX8 5AX Tel: 01392 414120 Fax: 01392 414155 — MB BS Lond. 1985 (King's Coll. Hosp. Lond.) FRCS Eng. 1994; DFFP 1995.

ROSS, Robert Jeremy Pudsey Health Centre, 18 Mulberry Street, Pudsey LS28 7XP Tel: 0113 257 6711 Fax: 0113 236 3928 — MB ChB Dundee 1974.

ROSS, Robert William David 5 Chesham Terrace, Belfast BT6 8GY — MB BCh BAO NUI 1983.

ROSS, Robin Trevor Andrew (retired) Fir Trees, Lower Oakfield, Pitlochry PH16 5DS Tel: 01796 472419 — MB ChB Ed. 1959; DObst RCOG 1968. Prev: GP Pitlochry.

ROSS, Roderick Sutherland 6 Springvalley Terrace, Edinburgh EH10 4PY — MB ChB Ed. 1944. Med. Off. (Outpats.) King Faisal Milit. Hosp. Khamis, Saudi Arabia; Mem. Med. Counc. for Alcoholism & Internat. Traffic & Accid. Med. Assn.

ROSS, Mr Ronald MacFarlane (retired) Medical Director, Golden Jubilee National Hospital, National Waiting Times Centre, Special Health Board, Beardmore Street, Clydebank G81 4HX Tel: 0141 951 5665 Fax: 0141 951 5006 Email: ronald.ross@hci.co.uk; 9 Duart Drive, Newton Mearns, Glasgow G77 5DS Tel: 0141 639 4855 — MB ChB Glas. 1959; FRCS Ed. 1965; FRCS Glas. 1984. Med. Dir. Breast Surg. HCI Internat. Med. Centre Glas.. Prev: Cons. Surg. Roy. Alexandra Hosp. Paisley & Hon. Surg. Princess Louise Scott Hosp. Erskine.

ROSS, Ronald William David Saintfield Health Centre, Fairview, Saintfield, Ballynahinch BT24 7AD; 32 Kirkwood Park, Ballynahinch Road, Saintfield, Ballynahinch BT24 7DP — MB BCh BAO Belf. 1983; DRCOG 1985; MRCGP 1987. Prev: Med. Off. & SHO (Med. & Cardiol.) Ulster Hosp. Dundonald; SHO (Obst.) Ulster Hosp. Dundonald; Ho. Off. Ulster Hosp. Dundonald.

ROSS, Ruth Allyson — MB BS Lond. 1986 (King's) BSc Lond. 1983; MRCPI Irel. 1998. Specialty: Care of the Elderly.

ROSS, Sean David Greencroft Medical Centre (North), Greencroft Wynd, Annan DG12 6BG — MB BCh BAO Belf. 1986 (Qu. Univ. Belf.)

ROSS, Sheena Margaret Ayrfield, 131 Huntingdon Road, Thrapston, Kettering NN14 4NG Tel: 01832 733066 — MB ChB Ed. 1972; BSc Ed. 1969, MB ChB 1972; DRCOG 1976; FFA RCS Eng. 1979. Cons. Anaesth. Hinchingbrooke Hosp. Huntingdon. Specialty: Anaesth.

ROSS, Sheila Kerr (retired) 87a Glencairn Drive, Pollokshields, Glasgow G41 4LL Tel: 0141 424 3737 Fax: 0141 424 3747 Email: sheilak.ross@virgin.net — MB ChB Glas. 1966 (Univ. Glas.) FRCP Glas. 1981 M 1969; FRCGP 1993, M 1987. Prev: Med. Prescribing Adviser Ayrsh. & Arran HB.

ROSS, Sheila Maclean 3 Grappenhall Road, Stockton Heath, Warrington WA4 2AJ Tel: 01925 61263 — MB ChB St. And. 1946; DCH 1949. Socs: BMA. Prev: Obst. Ho. Surg. Roy. Infirm. Perth.; Jun. Med. Regist. Booth Hall Childr. Hosp. Manch.; Ho. Phys. Cumbld. Infirm. Carlisle.

ROSS, Stephen David John Exmouth Health Centre, Claremont Grove, Exmouth EX8 2JF Tel: 01395 273001 Fax: 01395 273771 — MB ChB Birm. 1985; MRCGP 1991. Specialty: Gen. Pract.

ROSS, Wendy Elizabeth St Anthony's Medical Group, Thomas Gaughan House, Pottery Bank, Newcastle upon Tyne NE6 3SW Tel: 0191 265 5689 — MB ChB Ed. 1986; BSc (Hons.) Med. Sci. Ed. 1984; DRCOG 1989; MRCGP 1991; Dip. Ther. Newc. 1994. GP Locality Represen. Specialty: Gen. Pract.

ROSS, William Alexander Fairfield Medical Practice, 22A Abban Street, Inverness IV3 8HH Tel: 01463 713939 Fax: 01463 716256 — MB ChB Aberd. 1980; MRCGP 1985. GP Inverness.

ROSS, Mr William Mackie, CBE (retired) 62 Archery Rise, Durham DH1 4LA Tel: 0191 386 9256 — (Durh.) MB BS Durh. 1945; DMRT Eng. 1948; MD Durh. 1953; FRCS Eng. 1956; FFR 1961; FRCR 1975; FRCS Ed. 1994. Prev: DL.

ROSS, Zoe Eleanor 10 Broadwell Close, Abbeymead, Gloucester GL4 4XX Tel: 01452 372882 — MB ChB Birm. 1997. GP Rotat. (VTS) Roy. Shrewsbury Hosp. Specialty: Obst. & Gyn. Prev: Hse. Off. (Med.) Roy. Shrewsbury Hosp.; Hse. Off. (Surg.) Sandwell DGH.

ROSS ERRO, Anne-Louise c/o Erro-Dann, 12 Lillian Road, London SW13 9JG — Lakarexamen Stockholm 1988.

ROSS-MARRS, Roderick Peter Rectory Road Surgery, 7 Rectory Road, Rowhedge, Colchester CO5 7HP Tel: 01206 728585 Fax: 01206 729262; Rowhedge Surgery, 7 Rectory Road, Rowhedge, Colchester CO5 7HP Tel: 01206 728585 — MB BS Lond. 1986 (Westminster) BSc (Hons.) Lond. 1981, MB BS 1986. Specialty: Gen. Pract. Prev: Partner with Drs Sarda, 1991 Patel, Getha Meadow La. Sudbury Suff.

ROSS-MAWER, Jeremy Hugh Ronald 7 South Street, Fowey PL23 1AR — MRCS Eng. LRCP Lond. 1969 (King's Coll. Hosp.) Specialty: Accid. & Emerg. Prev: GP Wilts. & Warlingham Surrey.

ROSS RUSSELL, Fiona Mary Addison House, Milston, Salisbury SP4 8HT — MB BS Lond. 1982; DCH RCP Lond. 1985; DRCOG 1986; MRCGP 1997.

ROSS RUSSELL, Ian (retired) Lernham, Barrells Down Road, Bishop's Stortford CM23 2SW Tel: 01279 651485 — MB Camb. 1955 (Camb. & St. Thos.) BChir 1954; DObst RCOG 1959. Prev: Area Surg. St. John Ambul. Brig.

ROSS RUSSELL, Ralph William (retired) 23 Regent Terrace, Edinburgh EH7 5BS — (St. Thos.) MA, MD Camb. 1958, MB BChir 1952; FRCP Lond. 1967, M 1958; DM Oxf. 1962; FRCP Ed. 1977, M 1966. Phys. (Neurol.) Guy's & St. Thos. Trust Lond. Prev: Lect. (Med.) Univ. Oxf.

ROSS RUSSELL, Robert Ian Department of Paediatrics, Addenbrooke's Hospital, Hills Road, Cambridge CB2 2QQ Tel: 01223 586795 Fax: 01223 586784; Old Tiled House, Red Cross Lane, Cambridge CB2 2QU — MB BChir Camb. 1982; BA Camb. 1979; MA Camb. 1984; MRCP (UK) 1986; MD Camb. 1995; FRCP (UK) 1997; FRCPCH 1997; ILTHE 2002. Cons. Paediat. Addenbrooke's Hosp. Camb. Specialty: Paediat.; Intens. Care; Respirat. Med. Prev: Sen. Lect. (Paediat.) King's Coll. Hosp. Lond.; Sen. Regist. (Paediat.) Hosp. Sick Childr. Gt. Ormond St. Lond.

ROSSA, Kanwaljit Kaur — MB ChB Glas. 1981 (Univ. Glas.) BSc Zambia 1977; DCH RCP Lond. 1985. Prev: Clin. Med. Off. (Community Paediat.) Sunderland HA.

ROSSALL, Adrian Michael Danebridge Medical Centre, 29 London Road, Northwich CW9 5HR Tel: 01606 45786 Fax: 01606 331977; Southdown, Sutton Field, Whitegate, Northwich CW8 2BD Tel: 01606 882278 Email: rossall@arossall.freeserve.co.uk — MRCS Eng. LRCP Lond. 1978 (Manch.) DRCOG 1985. Specialty: Gen. Pract. Prev: Hosp. Pract. (Anaesth.) Leighton Hosp. Crewe.

ROSSALL, Christopher John Deepdale Road Healthcare Centre, Deepdale Road, Preston PR1 5AF Tel: 01772 655533 Fax: 01772 653414; Brookfield Farm, Tabley Lane, Higher Bartle, Preston PR4 0LH Fax: 01772 722221 Email: haighton@aol.com — MB ChB Liverp. 1974 (Liverpool) Prev: Research Regist. Univ. Hosp. S. Manch.; SHO (Obst. & Paediat.) Tameside Gen. Hosp.; Ho. Phys. & Ho. Surg. Roy. Lancaster Infirm.

ROSSDALE, Douglas (retired) 16 Marston Close, Fairfax Road, London NW6 4EU Tel: 020 7624 0328 Fax: 020 7723 6114; 16 Marston Close, London NW6 4EU — MB BS Lond. 1948 (St. Bart.) DObst RCOG 1950. Adviser (Hyperbaric Med.) Esso Petroleum Co. Ltd. Prev: Surg. Regist. Luton & Dunstable Hosp.

ROSSDALE, Martin Roger Department of Anatomy & Developmental Biology, University College, Gower St., London WC1E 6BT; Department of Anatomy & Embryology, University College, Gower St, London WC1E 6BT — BM BCh Oxf. 1965; DM Oxf. 1978, BM BCh 1965. Sen. Lect. (Haemat.) Univ. Coll. Lond. Specialty: Haematology.

ROSSDALE, Michael George Philip The Surgery, 111 Pembroke Road, Clifton, Bristol BS8 3EU Tel: 0117 973 3790; 12 Park Grove, Henleaze, Bristol BS6 7XD — MB BChir Camb. 1980 (Univ. Coll. Hosp.) MA Camb. 1980; DCH RCP Lond. 1983; DRCOG 1984; MRCGP 1986. Hosp. Pract. (Chest Med.) Southmead Hosp. Bristol. Prev: SHO (Paediat.) Southmead Hosp. Bristol; SHO (Gen. Med.) Cheltenham Gen. Hosp.

ROSSDALE-SMITH, Georgina Jane Poplars, Chinthurst Lane, Shalford, Guildford GU4 8JS — MB BS Lond. 1975; MRCS Eng. LRCP Lond. 1974.

ROSSER, Anne Kathryn Dorothy e4 Lentran Farm Cottages, Lentran, Inverness IV3 8RL — MB ChB Manch. 1981.

ROSSER, Betsan 13 Brynygors, Morriston, Swansea SA6 6DQ — MB BCh BAO NUI 1983; LRCPI & LM, LRCSI & LM 1983; MRCPsych 1991.

ROSSER, Miss Catherine Gwyndy, Upper Garth Road, Bangor LL57 2SS — MB BCh Wales 1988.

ROSSER, Catherine Anne 15 The Walk, Hengoed CF82 7AH — BM Soton. 1994.

ROSSER, Clive Anthony Khan and Partners, Medical Centre, Church Road, Neath SA10 9DT Tel: 01639 700203 Fax: 01639 700010 — MB BS Lond. 1981.

ROSSER, David William Albert (retired) 2 Priory Avenue, Caversham, Reading RG4 7SE Tel: 01734 472431 Fax: 01734 463340 — MB BCh BAO Dub. 1959 (T.C. Dub.) BA Dub. 1959. Prev: Ho. Off. Lagan Valley Hosp. Lisburn & Roy. Berks. Hosp. Reading.

ROSSER, Edmund Mervyn (retired) 18 Eastlands Crescent, Dulwich Village, London SE21 7EG Tel: 020 8693 4883 — (St. Bart.) MB BS Lond. 1952; MRCS Eng. LRCP Lond. 1952; MRCGP 1962. Prev: Clin. Tutor (Gen. Pract.) Acad. Dept. Gen. Pract. Primary Med. Care Med. Coll. St. Bart. Hosp. Lond.

ROSSER, Elisabeth Mary Department of Clinical Genetics, Institute of Child Health, 30 Guilford St., London WC1N 1EH Tel: 020 7905 2607 Fax: 020 7813 8141 — MB BS Lond. 1986; BSc (Genetics) Lond. 1983, MB BS 1986; MRCP (UK) 1993; FRCP 2001. Cons. (Clin. Genetics) Inst. Child Health & Gt. Ormond St. Hosp. Childr. Specialty: Genetics.

ROSSER, Jeffrey Graham Rosser and Partners, Crewkerne Health Centre, Middle Path, Crewkerne TA18 8BX Tel: 01460 72435 Fax: 01460 77957 — MB ChB Birm. 1957; DO RCS 1989; MCOphth 1990.

ROSSER, Maria Alda 19 Parmin Way, Taunton TA1 2JU — MB ChB Sheff. 1982.

ROSSER, Michael John, Wing Cdr. RAF Med. Br. Retd. Lister House Surgery, 35 The Parade, St Helier JE2 3QQ Tel: 01534 736336 Fax: 01534 735304 — MB BS Lond. 1974; DAvMed 1983. Specialty: Aviat. Med. Prev: Sen. Med. Off. HQAFCENT.

ROSSER, Peggy Mildred (retired) Dorset House, Blackfriars Avenue, Droitwich WR9 8DR Tel: 01905 76471 — (Lond. Sch. Med. Wom.) MB BS Lond. 1939. Prev: Ho. Phys. Postgrad. Med. Sch.

ROSSER, Rosemary Lovann Bulwell Health Centre, Main Street, Bulwell, Nottingham NG6 8QJ Tel: 0115 927 9119 Fax: 0115 977 1236 — MB ChB Liverp. 1981; MRCS Eng. LRCP Lond. 1981; MRCGP 1988. Prev: GP Sheff.; Trainee GP Romford VTS; SHO (A & E) OldCh. Hosp.

ROSSER, Sally Anne Giffords Primary Care Centre, Spa Road, Melksham SN12 7EA Tel: 01225 703370; Hill Farm House, Seend, Melksham SN12 6RU — MB BS Lond. 1982; DCH RCP Lond. 1986; DRCOG 1987; MRCGP 1988.

ROSSER, Vaughan Charles Edgar Heavitree Health Centre, South Lawn Terrace, Exeter EX1 2RX Tel: 01392 431355 Fax: 01392 498305; Greenwood House, Ebford Lane, Ebford, Exeter EX3 0QX — MB ChB Manch. 1975; MRCGP 1980.

ROSSI, Charlotte Anne Melissa The Surgery, Welbeck Street, Creswell, Worksop S80 4HA Tel: 01909 721206; Fuchsia Cottage, 54 Bakestone Moor, Whitwell, Worksop S80 4QD — MB BS Newc. 1991; DFFP 1996; DRCOG 1998. GP Princip.; Clin. Asst. Gum. Specialty: Gen. Pract. Prev: Trainee GP Bassetlaw VTS; Trainee GP N.d. VTS.

ROSSI, Mr Leo Francis Anthony Spindleberry, Brickworth Down, Whiteparish, Salisbury SP5 2QD — MB BS Lond. 1966 (Westm.) FRCS Eng. 1971. Cons. Plastic Surg. Odstock Hosp. Salisbury. Specialty: Plastic Surg. Prev: Sen. Regist. Burns & Plastic Unit Qu. Mary's Hosp. Roehampton; Sen . Regist. Head & Neck Unit Roy. Marsden Hosp. Lond.; Dir.Wessex Regional Burns Unit.

ROSSI, Maria Kathleen Summerfield House, 2 Eday Rd, Aberdeen AB15 6RE — Dip. Fac. Public Health 2001 (Univ. La Sapienza di Roma) Laurea Medicina & Chirurgia 1989; DTM & H RCP Lond. 1995; MSc (Public Health & Health Services Research) Aberd. 2001. Specialist Regist. Pub. Health, Grampian NHS Bd., Aberd.; Hon. Lect., Pub. Health Med., Univ. of Aberd. Specialty: Pub. Health Med. Prev: Field Med. Co-Ord. MSF-B Wajir, Kenya; Field Med. Co-Ordinator MSF-B Dadaab Kenya; SHO (Gen. Med.) Aberd. Roy. Infirm.

ROSSI, Michela Whittington Hospital, Highgate Hill, London N19 5NF Tel: 020 7288 5219 Fax: 020 7288 5052 Email: michela.rossi@whittington.nhs.uk — MB BS Newc. 1990 (Newc. Upon Tyne) MRCP (UK) 1994; PhD Lond. 2001. Cons. In Endocrinol., Diabetes & Gen. Med., Whittington Hosp.Lond.; Hon. Sen. Lect., Univ. Coll. Lond. Specialty: Endocrinol.; Diabetes. Socs: Diabetes UK; Soc. of Endocrinol.; Brit. Med. Assn. Prev: Lect. in Endocrinol., Diabetes Hammersmith Hosp., Lond.

ROSSI, Steven Health Centre, Newgate Street, Worksop S80 1HP Tel: 01909 500266 Fax: 01909 478014; Fuchsia Cottage, 54 Bakestone Moor, Whitwell, Worksop S80 4QD Tel: 01909 720682 — (Newcastle upon Tyne) MB BS Newc. 1989; DRCOG 1992; MRCGP 1996. Princip. GP The Health Centre, Worksop. Specialty: Gen. Pract. Socs: RCGP; BMA. Prev: Assoc. GP Lintonville Med. Gp. Ashington; GP Regist. Cestria Health Centre Chester-le-St.; GP Regist. Seaton Hirst Med. Gp. Ashington.

ROSSI, Susan Isobel Maxwell — MB ChB Leeds 1998. HO. St.James Univ. Hosp. Specialty: Accid. & Emerg.; Gen. Pract. Prev: HO, Med., Leeds Gen. Infirm.

ROSSINI, Jane North Western RHA, Piccadilly S., Manchester; Rivendell, 56C Manchester Road, Greenfield, Oldham OL3 7HJ Tel: 01457 870470 — MB ChB Manch. 1986. Regist. (Pub. Health Med.) N. West. RHA.

ROSSITER, Anne Exeter Occupational Health Service, 79 Heavitree Road, Exeter EX1 2HZ Tel: 01392 405037 Fax: 01392 405063 Email: anne.rossiter@rdehc-tr.swest.nhs.uk; Newcombes, Newton St Cyres, Exeter EX5 5AW Tel: 01392 851235 Fax: 01392 851234 — MB BS Lond. 1978 (St Thos.) DA Eng. 1981; DRCOG 1982; MFOM Lond. 1997; FFOM Lond. 2005. p/t Cons. (Occupat. Med.) Roy. Devon & Exeter Trust Exeter. Specialty: Occupat. Health.

ROSSITER, Brian Derek Whipps Cross Hospital, London E11 — MB BS Lond. 1974; FRCP Lond. 1994. Cons. Phys. Med. for Elderly Whipps Cross Hosp. Lond. Specialty: Care of the Elderly.

ROSSITER, John Michael Alvaston Medical Centre, 14 Boulton Lane, Alvaston, Derby DE24 0GE — (Univ. Coll. Dub.) MB BCh BAO NUI 1968.

ROSSITER, Mary Anne (retired) — (Guy's) MA Camb. 1963, MB BChir 1962; MRCS Eng. LRCP Lond. 1962; DObst RCOG 1964; DCH Eng. 1966; FRCP Lond. 1985, M 1967; FRCPCH 1997. Prev: Cons. Paediat. N. Middlx. Univ. Hosp. NHS Trust.

ROSSITER, Michael Adam The Castle Practice, Health Centre, Central Street, Ludgershall, Andover SP11 9RA Tel: 01264 790356 Fax: 01264 791256; Quercus Cottage, 67 Cadley Road, Collingbourne Ducis, Marlborough SN8 3EB Tel: 01264 850107 — MB BS Lond. 1991 (Roy. Free Hosp.) DRCOG 1994; DFFP 1995; MRCGP 1996. GP Princip. Specialty: Gen. Pract.; Sports Med. Prev: Trainee GP Newquay & Cornw. VTS; Ho. Phys. & Ho. Surg. Roy. Cornw. Hosp. Treliske.

ROSSITER, Mr Nigel Daniel Orthopaedic Dept, Derriford Hospital, Plymouth PL6 8DH Tel: 01752 777111 — MB BS Lond. 1988 (London Hospital Medical College) FRCS Ed. 1993; FRCS Tr & orth 1999. Cons. T & O Derriford Hosp., Plymouth. Specialty: Orthop.; Trauma & Orthop. Surg. Socs: Brit. Orthopaedic Assn., Fell.; Brit. Trauma Soc.; Combined Serv.s Orthopaedic Soc. Prev: Trauma Fell. Texas, USA (Dallas & San Antonio); Lect. (Milit. Surg.) RAMC; Specialist Regist. (Orthop.) Oxf.

ROSSITER, Stephen Kim Wellwaters, New Street Lane, Eype, Bridport DT6 6AD — MB BCh Wales 1980; MRCPsych 1990; Dip. Addic. Behaviour (St. Georges Lond.) 1997.

ROSSON, Amanda Kate Fairfield, Wall Hill Lane, Congleton CW12 4TD — MB BS Lond. 1990; DRCOG 1993.

ROSSON, Mr John William The Royal Surrey County Hospital, Orthopaedic Department, Egerton Road, Guildford GU2 7XX — BM Soton. 1979; FRCS Ed. 1983; FRCS Eng. 1985; MS 1990. Specialty: Orthop.

ROSSOR, Eve Beatrix Mary Sheridan Centre, 5 Dugard Way, off Renfrew Road, London SE11 4TH Tel: 020 7414 1455 Fax: 020 7414 1372 Email: eve.rossor@chsltr.sthames.nhs.uk; 145 Woodwarde Road, London SE22 8UR Tel: 020 8693 0682 — MB BChir Camb. 1975; MA Camb. 1974; MRCP (UK) 1978; FRCP Lond. 1995; FRCPCH 1998. Dir. Child Health Directorate Community Health S. Lond. NHS Trust; Cons. Paediat. Dir. Learning Assessm. Clinic. Specialty: Community Child Health. Prev: Med. Dir. & Clin. Dir. Community Child Health W. Lambeth Community Care Trust; SCMO W. Lambeth HA; Regist. (Paediat.) Addenbrooke's Hosp. Camb.

ROSSOR, Professor Martin Neil The National Hospital for Neurology & Neurosurgery, Box 16, Queen Square, London WC1N 3BG Tel: 020 7829 8773 Fax: 020 7676 2066 — MB BChir Camb. 1975; MRCP (UK) 1976; MA Camb. 1975, MD 1986; FRCP Lond. 1990; FMedSci 2002. Prof. of Clin. Neurol. Inst. of Neurol., Uni. Coll. & Imperial Coll. Lond..; Hon.Cons. Nat. Hosp. for Neurol. and Neurosurg. and St Mary's Hosp., Lond..; Prof. of Clin. Neurol. (Personal Chair.) Imperial Coll. Lond. Specialty: Neurol.

ROSSOUW, Daniel John 72 Margaret Road, Barnet EN4 9NX — MB BCh Witwatersrand 1982.

ROSSWICK, Mr Robert Paul 5,Staffordshire House, 50 Broughton Park, London N3 3EG Tel: 020 8343 2878 Fax: 020 8343 2878 Email: rpr@dial.pipex.com — (Lond. Hosp.) MB BS Lond. 1955; DObst RCOG 1957; FRCS Eng. 1961; MS Univ. Illinois 1963. Emerit. Surg. St. Geo. Hosp. Lond. & Hon. Sen. Lect. (Surg.) St. Geo. Hosp. Med. Sch. Lond. Specialty: Gastroenterol.; Endocrinol.; Medico Legal. Socs: Fell. Roy. Soc. Med.; Fell. (Treas.) Med. Soc. Lond. Formerly Pres. Prev: Surg. Roy. Masonic Hosp. Lond.; Sen. Regist. & 1st Asst. (Surg.) St. Geo. Hosp. Lond.; Robt.son Exchange Fell. (Surg.) Presbyt.-St. Luke's Hosp. Chicago, USA.

ROSTED, Palle Weston Park Hospital, Whitham Road, Sheffield S10 2SJ Tel: 0114 226 5000 Fax: 0114 226 5555; 200 Abbey Lane, Sheffield S8 0BU Tel: 0114 236 0077 Fax: 0114 262 0491 Email: prosted@aol.com — MD Copenhagen 1973. Indep. Med. Acupunc. Sheff.; Cons. Med. Acupunc. Weston Pk. Hosp.; Clin. Lect. Univ. Sheff.; GMC Registered Specialist in Acupunc. Specialty: Gen. Med.; Acupunc. Socs: (Ex-Treas.) Brit. Med. Assn. Acupunc.; (Ex Vice-Chairm.) Danish Soc. Acupunc.; Treas. IACMART.

ROSTEN, Margaret Helen (retired) 160 Twickenham Road, Hanworth, Feltham TW13 6HD Tel: 020 8979 6222 — (Guy's) MB BS Lond. 1954; DCH Eng. 1957; DObst RCOG 1961.

ROSTOM, Assem Youssef The Royal Marsden Hospital, Downs road, Sutton SM2 5PT Tel: 020 8661 3169 Fax: 020 8661 3470 Email: assem.rostom@rmh.nthames.nhs.uk — MB ChB Alexandria 1967; DMRT Alexandria 1970; FRCR 1976. Cons. Clin. Oncologist Roy. Marsden Hosp. Lond.; Hon. Cons. Clin. Oncologist, St Georges Hosp., Tooting. Specialty: Oncol. Special Interest: Breast, Lung and Skin Cancer. Socs: BMA; Roy. Coll. of Radiologists. Prev: Cons. (Radiother. & Oncol.) Regional Radiother. Centre St. Luke's Hosp. Guildford.

ROSTRON, Mr Chad Kenneth St George's Hospital, Moorfields Eye Department, Blackshaw Road, London SW17 0QT Tel: 020 8725 2325 Fax: 020 8725 3026 Email: rostron@sghms.ac.uk; 10 Harley Street, London W1G 9PF Tel: 020 7483 4921 Fax: 020 7467 8312 Email: rostron@sghms.ac.uk — (Newcastle Upon Tyne) MB BS Newc. 1975; DO Eng. 1979; FRCS Eng. 1982; FRCOphth 1989. Cons. Ophth.Moorfileds Eye Dept at St. Geo. Hosp. Lond.; Hon. Sen. Lect. Univ. Lond.; Director Keratec Eye Bank, Lond. Specialty: Ophth. Special Interest: Specialist in Corneal lamellar Surgic. Techniques. Socs: Internat. Refractive Surgic. Soc.; Brit. Soc. for Refractive Surg.; United Kingdom Intraocular Implant Soc. Prev: Sen. Regist. (Ophth.) Leicester Roy. Infirm.

ROSTRON, Elizabeth Anne Church Street Practice, 8 Church Street, Southport PR9 0QT Tel: 01704 533666 Fax: 01704 539239 — MB ChB Manch. 1971.

ROSTRON, Mr Kenneth William Briggs (retired) Pentrig, Vicarage Lane, Lelant, St Ives TR26 3EA Tel: 01736 752107 — MB BChir Camb. 1937 (Camb. & Manch.) MA, MB BChir Camb. 1937; DOMS Eng. 1947; FRCS Eng. 1950.

ROSTRON, Michael Gordon Roston, James, Devine, Trepess & Burford, Lister House Surgery, Bollams Mead, Wiveliscombe, Taunton TA4 2PH Tel: 01984 623471 Fax: 01984 624357 Email: mike.roston@wiveliscombesurgery.nhs.uk; Church Hill Cottage, Halse, Taunton TA4 3AB Tel: 01823 432815 Fax: 01823 433730 — MB BS Lond. 1980 (Lond. Hosp.) DRCOG 1982; MRCGP 1984. Trainer GP Taunton.

ROSTRON, Mr Peter Kenneth Makin 25 Rodney Street, Liverpool L1 9EH Tel: 0151 709 2393 Fax: 0151 707 2456; Wensleydale Farm, Gaw Hill Lane, Aughton, Ormskirk L39 7HA Tel: 01695 422848 — MB ChB Liverp. 1967; FRCS Ed. 1973; MChOrth 1975. Specialty: Orthop. Prev: Cons. Orthop. Surg. Whiston & St. Helens Hosps.; Sen. Regist. (Orthop.) Wrightington Hosp. Appley Bridge; Demonst. (Anat.) Univ. Liverp.

ROTBLAT, Frances 50 Muswell Avenue, London N10 2EL — MB BS Lond. 1970; BSc (Hons.) Lond. 1967, MB BS 1970; FRCPath 1990, M 1978. Sen. Med. Off. Med. Control Agency DoH. Prev: Research Fell. Haemophilia Centre Roy. Free Hosp. Lond.

ROTCHFORD, Alan Paul 2 Barley Way, Rothley, Leicester LE7 7RL — BChir Camb. 1990.

ROTH, Cathy Ellen St. Thomas' Hospital, London SE1 7EH — MB BChir Camb. 1989.

ROTH, Daphne Mary Liddon (retired) 84 North End House, Fitzjames Avenue, London W14 0RX Tel: 020 7603 2384 — MB BS Lond. 1948 (Lond. Sch. Med. Wom.) MRCS Eng. LRCP Lond. 1948; DCH Eng. 1951; DObst RCOG 1952. Prev: Clin. Med. Off. (Community Health) Riverside & Wandsworth HA's.

ROTH, John Andrew (retired) 3 Clevedon Drive, Earley, Reading RG6 5XF Tel: 0118 986 7482 — (Oxf.) MB BS Lond. 1962; DO Eng. 1969. Prev: Regist. & SHO Oxf. Eye Hosp.

ROTH, Lucy Juliet 68 High Street, Great Broughton, Middlesbrough TS9 7EG — MB BS Newc. 1992.

ROTH, Sir Martin Level 9, Addenbrooke's Hospital, University of Cambridge, Hills Road, Cambridge CB2 2QQ Tel: 01223 242106 Fax: 01223 412193; Trinity College, Cambridge CB2 1TQ Tel: 01223 242106 Fax: 01223 412193 — MB BS Lond. 1943 (St. Mary's) MRCS Eng. LRCP Lond. 1941; MA Camb. 1943; FRCP Lond. 1958, M 1944; MD Lond. 1946; DPM RCPSI 1949; FRCPsych 1971; Hon. ScD Dub. 1972; Hon. FRCPS Glas. 1973; Hon. DSc Indiana 1993. Emerit. Prof. of Psychiat. Univ. Camb.; Mem. Bd. Governors St. And. Hosp. Northampton; Fell. Trinity Coll. Camb.; Hon. Fell. Inst. of Advanced Studies Indiana 1991; Hon. Fell. Coll. Med. & Surg. S. Afr.; Founder Pres. & Hon. Fell. Roy. Coll. Psychiat.; Hon. Fell. Austral. & NZ Roy. Coll. Psychiat. Specialty: Gen. Psychiat. Socs: Fell. of the Acad. of Med. Sci. Prev: Scientif. Mem. MRC Counc. & Clin. Research Bd.; Pres. Counc. & Chairm. Ct. of Electors

Appeals Comm. RCPsych. & Jt. Comm. Higher Psychiat. Train.; Vice-Pres. & Counc. Med. Defence Union.

ROTH, Michael Gilbert 3 Florence Villas, Milton Road, London SE24 0NN Tel: 020 7737 5576 Email: mike@mikeroth.force9.co.uk — (Westminster Medical School) BSc Lond. 1965, MB BS 1968.

ROTH, Simon Christhold Barnet and Chase Farm Hospitals NHS Trust, Barnet General Hospital, Wellhouse Lane, Barnet EN5 3DJ — MB BS Lond. 1982; MRCP (UK) 1986; FRCP 1997; FRCPCH 1997. Cons. Barnet Gen. Hosp.; Sen. Lect. Univ. Coll. Lond. Specialty: Paediat. Prev: Clin. Lect. (Paediat.) Univ. Coll. Hosp. Lond.; Research Regist. (Paediat.) Univ. Coll. Hosp. Lond.; Regist. (Paediat.) Whittington Hosp. Lond.

ROTHBURN, Michael Mark University Hospital Aintree, Clinical Microbiology & Health Protection Agency Collaborating Laboratory, Longmoor Lane, Liverpool L9 7AL Tel: 0151 529 4900 Fax: 0151 529 4918 — MB ChB Leeds 1979; BSc (Hons.) (Biochem. Med.) Leeds 1976, MB ChB 1979; Dip. Bact. Manch. 1984; FRCPath 1996. Cons. Med. Microbiol. Univ. Hosp. Aintree, Liverp.; Hon. Clin. Lect. Sch. of Clin. Sci. Univ. Liverp.; Med. Off. (Control of Infect.) Aintree Hosps.; Med. Off. (Control of Infect.) Walton Centre Neurol. & Neurosurg. Specialty: Med. Microbiol. Prev: Clin. Lect. Dept. Trop. Med. & Infec. Dis. Univ. Liverp.

ROTHER, Penelope Bonnyrigg Health Centre, High Street, Bonnyrigg EH19 2DA Tel: 0131 663 7272 Fax: 0131 660 5636; 21 Station Road, Loanhead EH20 9NJ Tel: 0131 440 1019 — MB ChB Ed. 1981; DRCOG 1983; MRCGP 1985.

ROTHERA, Mr Michael Patrick 20 Harrop Road, Hale, Altrincham WA15 9BZ — MB BS Lond. 1977; FRCS Eng. 1983.

ROTHERAY, Andrew David Trevaylor Road Health Centre, Trevaylor Road, Falmouth TR11 2LH Tel: 01326 317317; CHY Cara, 37 Penhale Road, Falmouth TR11 5UZ — MB ChB Liverp. 1973; BSc (Hons. Biochem.) Liverp. 1970, MB ChB 1973.

ROTHERAY, Christine Florence Royal Cornwall Hospital Trust, Treliske, Truro TR1 2XN Tel: 01872 272 4242; Eschol, 6 Mitchell Hill Terrace, Truro TR1 1HY — MB ChB Liverp. 1973 (Liverpool) D.Occ.Med. RCP Lond. 1995; AFOM RCP Lond. 1997. SHO (Gen. Med.) Roy. Cornw. Hosp. Treliske Truro. Specialty: Gen. Med. Prev: Med. Adviser (Occupat. Health) Cornw. CC; Med. Off. Assessor DSS; Clin. Asst. (Geriat.) Barncoose Hosp. Redruth.

ROTHERHAM, Joann 91 Eastfield Road, Keyingham, Hull HU12 9TP — MB BS Newc. 1994.

ROTHERHAM, Melanie Jane Farndon Green Medical Centre, 1 Farndon Green, Wollaton Park, Nottingham NG8 1DU Tel: 0115 928 8666 Fax: 0115 928 8343 — MB ChB Leeds 1988; MB ChB Leeds. 1988. GP Nottm. Prev: Trainee GP/SHO Nottm. VTS; Ho. Off. (Med.) Pinderfields Hosp. Wakefield; Ho. Off. (Surg.) Sea Croft Hosp. Leeds.

ROTHERHAM, Neil Eric 2 Waterside Close, Gamston, Nottingham NG2 6QA — MB ChB Sheff. 1986; MRCP (Pt.I) 1988; Dip. Pharm. Med. 1992; MFPM 1993. Managing Dir. Clinphone Ltd. Prev: Research Phys. Boots Pharmaceutics; SHO (Chest Med./Cardiol.) Wythenshawe Hosp. Manch.

ROTHERY, Anne Moira — MB ChB Manch. 1979; BSc St. And. 1976; DRCOG 1983; MRCGP 1984.

ROTHERY, David James Parkview Clinic, 60 Queens Bridge Road, Moseley, Birmingham B13 8QD Tel: 0121 243 2000 Fax: 0121 243 2010 Email: david.rothery@bch.nhs.uk — MB ChB Leeds 1977; FRCPsych 1995, M 1982. Cons. Psychiat. Regional Adolesc. Unit. Birm.; Sen. Clin. Lect. Univ. Birm. Specialty: Child & Adolesc. Psychiat. Prev: Sen. Regist. (Child & Adolesc. Psychiat.) W. Midl. Regional TS.

ROTHERY, Stephen Philip Stonefield Street Surgery, 21 Stonefield Street, Milnrow, Rochdale OL16 4JQ Tel: 01706 646234 Fax: 01706 527946 Email: stephen.rothery@nhs.net — MB ChB Manch. 1979; DRCOG 1982; MRCGP 1983; DCCH RCGP 1984; Cert. Family Plann. JCC 1984; CHD Diploma 2003.

ROTHMAN, Doreen, OBE (retired) 46 Alleyn Road, Dulwich, London SE21 8AL Tel: 020 8670 5297 Fax: 020 8670 5297 Email: drothman@talk21.com — (Charing Cross Hospital Medical School) BSc Lond. 1950, MB BS 1955; MRCS Eng. LRCP Lond. 1955; FRCOG 1975, M 1960, DObst 1957. Prev: Sen. Med. Off. Dept. Health & Social Security Lond.

ROTHMAN, Professor Martin Terry London Chest Hospital, Bonner Road, London E2 9JX Tel: 020 8983 2216 Fax: 020 8983 2381 Email: martin.rothman@bartsandthelondon.nhs.uk — MB ChB Manch. 1972; MRCP (UK) 1976; FRCP Lond. 1991. Cons. Cardiol. Barts and The Lond. NHS Trust, Lond.; Director of Cardiac Research and Developm., Barts and The Lond. NHS Trust; Hon. Prof. of Internat. Cardiol., Qu. Mary Univ. of Lond.; Co-Director, Cardiac Dept., Vasc. and Inflamatory Research, William Harvey Research Inst., Lond. Specialty: Cardiol. Socs: Brit. Cardiac Soc.; Brit. Cardiovasc. Interven. Soc.; Roy. Coll. of Physicians.

ROTHMAN, William Thurlow (retired) Little Wood, Woodlands Rise, Sevenoaks TN15 0HZ Tel: 01732 761445 Fax: 01732 761445 — (Cape Town) MB ChB Cape Town 1948; DMRD Eng. 1956; FFR 1961; FRCR 1975. Prev: Cons. Radiol. Tunbridge Wells & Bromley HAs.

ROTHNIE, Douglas William (retired) 38 Hartington Street, Barrow-in-Furness LA14 5SW Tel: 01229 20554; 52 Dane Avenue, Barrow-in-Furness LA14 4JY Tel: 01229 820554 — MB ChB Aberd. 1957.

ROTHNIE, James Robert (retired) Glenwood Health Centre, Napier Road, Glenrothes KY6 1HL Tel: 01592 611000 — MB ChB Glas. 1960; DA Eng. 1962; DObst RCOG 1963. Prev: Res. Med. Off. O & G Robroyston Hosp. Glas.

ROTHNIE, Mr Neil David Department Surgery, Southend Hospital NHS Trust, Prittlewell Chase, Westcliff on Sea SS0 0RY Tel: 01702 540461 Ext: 2680 — MB BS Lond. 1981 (St Bartholomews) FRCS Eng. 1986; MS Univ. of Lond. 1991. Cons. Surg. Southend Health Care Trust. Specialty: Gen. Surg. Special Interest: Breast Disease; Surgical Oncology. Prev: Sen. Regist. (Surg.) St. Bart. Hosp. Lond.

ROTHNIE, Mr Norman George (retired) 1 Ingleside Court, Upper West Terrace, Budleigh Salterton EX9 6NZ Tel: 01395 443986 — MB BS Lond. 1950 (St. Bart.) MS Lond. 1960, MB BS 1950; FRCS Eng. 1956. Prev: Sen. Surg. Regist. & Ho. Surg. Surgic. Profess. & Thoracic Units St.

ROTHNIE, Rosalind Jane Diana High Street, Great Wakering, Southend-on-Sea SS3 0EF Tel: 01702 577850 — MB BS Lond. 1981 (St. Bart.) BSc (Hons. Pharmacol.) Lond. 1978; DRCOG 1983; Cert. Family Plann. JCC 1983; DFFP 1993. Gen. Practitioner; Examr. Med. Off. DHSS; Family Plann. Off. Southend HA; Adj. Med. Off. DHSS. Specialty: Family Plann. & Reproduc. Health; Gen. Pract.; Civil Serv. Socs: Brit. Med. Assn. Prev: GP Cheshunt; SHO (O & G) St. Bart. Hosp. Lond.; SHO (A & E & Geriat. & Med.) Whipps Cross Hosp. Lond.

ROTHWELL, Anne Catherine Llandaff North Medical Centre, 99 Station Road, Llandaff North, Cardiff CF14 2FD Tel: 029 2034 2113 Fax: 029 2034 2686 — MB BCh Wales 1983.

ROTHWELL, Bryan Peter Oldbury Health Centre, Albert Street, Oldbury B69 4DE Tel: 0121 552 6747; 4 Millbrook Way, Lakeside, Brierley Hill DY5 3YY Tel: 01384 77307 — BM BCh Oxf. 1984; MA, BM BCh Oxf. 1984; DRCOG 1987; MRCGP 1988. Clin. Asst. (Neonat.) Wordsley Hosp. Stourbridge. Prev: SHO (Paediat./Obst./Med.) Burnley Gen. Hosp.

ROTHWELL, Kay The Old School Surgery, Hinckley Road, Stoney Stanton, Leicester LE9 4LJ Tel: 01455 271445 Fax: 01445 274526; 82 Underwood Drive, Stoney Stanton, Leicester LE9 4TD Tel: 01455 273181 — BM BS Nottm. 1985; BMedSci Nottm. 1983; DRCOG 1988; MRCGP 1989. GP Partner. Prev: Trainee GP/SHO Nottm. VTS; Ho. Off. (Therap.) Qu. Med. Centre Nottm.; Ho. Off. (Surg.) Derby Roy. Infirm.

ROTHWELL, Michael Peter Dept. of Anaesth., Macclesfield Hospital, Victoria Road, Macclesfield SK10 3BL Tel: 01625 661307 — MB BS Lond. 1990 (St. Marys London) FRCA 1996. Cons. Anaesth. Specialty: Anaesth.

ROTHWELL, Nicola Louise 38 Kinloch Drive, Heaton, Bolton BL1 4LZ Tel: 01204 495936; 38 Kinloch Drive, Heaton, Bolton BL1 4LZ Tel: 01204 495036 — MB ChB Birm. 1998. Surgic. HO, Qu.s Hosp., Burton-upon-Trent. Specialty: Gen. Surg.

ROTHWELL, Mr Peter James Neil Department of Urology, Blackpool Victoria Hospital NHS Trust, Whinney Heys Road, Blackpool FY3 8NR Tel: 01253 306996; 22 The Belfry, Lytham St Annes FY8 4NW Tel: 01253 731633 — MB ChB Manch. 1979; FRCS Ed. 1984; BSc Manch. 1976, MD 1991; FRCS (Urol.) 1994. Cons. Urol. Blackpool Vict. NHS Trust. Specialty: Urol. Prev: Sen. Regist. Rotat. (Urol.) NW Region.

ROTHWELL, Peter Malcolm Department of Clinical Neurosciences, Western General Hospital, Crewe Road, Edinburgh

EH4 2XU Tel: 0131 537 2129; 12 Clackmae Road, Liberton, Edinburgh EH16 6NZ Tel: 0131 658 1591 — MB ChB Ed. 1987; MRCP (UK) 1990; MD Ed. 1995. Clin. Research Fell. (Neurol.) West. Gen. Hosp. Edin. Specialty: Neurol. Prev: Regist. (Neurol.) West. Gen. Hosp. Edin.; Regist. (Med.) Falkirk & Dist. Roy. Infirm.; SHO (Med.) Cleveland Hosps.

ROTHWELL, Mr Richard Ian Cookridge Hospital, Leeds LS16 6QB Tel: 0113 267 3411 — MB BS Lond. 1966 (Middlx.) MRCS Eng. LRCP Lond. 1966; DObst RCOG 1968; FRCS Eng. 1974; FRCR 1983. Cons. Radiother. & Oncol. Cookridge Hosp. Leeds. Specialty: Oncol. Socs: BMA; Europ. Soc. Therapeutic Radiol. & Oncol.; Brit. Inst. of Radiol. Prev: Lect. (Radiother. & Oncol.) Cookridge Hosp. Univ. Leeds.; Surg. Govt. of Sabah, Malaysia; Ho. Phys. Middlx. Hosp. Lond.

ROTHWELL, Simon James St. Francis Hospital, Private Bag 11, Katete, Zambia; Thistlegrove, La Grande Route De St Laurent, St Lawrence, Jersey JE3 1FB Tel: 01534 861722 — MB BS Lond. 1990.

ROTHWELL, Susan Elizabeth 3 Chesterford House, Southacre Park, Southacre Drive, Cambridge CB2 2TZ; Barnston Oak House, Parsonage Lane, Barnston, Dunmow CM6 3PA — MB BChir Camb. 1993; BSc (1st cl. Hons.) Bradford 1983; FBCO 1988, M 1984; Dip. Opt. Gen. Optical Counc. Worsh Co Spectacle Makers, Freedom City Lond. 1984; MSc Neurosensory Physiol. Camb. 1988. SHO, (Ophth.) Roy. Bershire Hosp. Reading.; Princip. Optometrist Boots Optical Servs. Camb. Specialty: Ophth. Prev: SHO (Ophth.) King Edwd. VII Hosp., P. Chas. Eye Unit, Windsor; Ho. Off. (Gen. Surg. & Transpl.) Addenbrooke's Hosp. Camb.; Ho. Phys. (Gen. Med.) W. Suff. Hosp. Bury st Edmunds.

ROTHWELL HUGHES, Mary Elizabeth Medical Centre, Hay-on-Wye, Hereford HR3 5QX Tel: 01497 820333 — MB ChB Bristol 1987; DCH RCP Lond. 1989; DRCOG 1991; MRCGP 1992. Prev: SHO (Paediat.) S. Warks. HA.

ROTHWELL-JACKSON, Mr Richard Loxton (retired) The Conifers, Common Road, Kensworth, Dunstable LU6 2PW — MB BChir Camb. 1956 (St. Bart.) MChir Camb. 1966, MA 1956; FRCS Eng. 1960. Prev: Cons. Gen. Surg. Luton & Dunstable Hosp.

ROTMAN, Charles Morris Henry, OStJ 213 Hempstead Road, Watford WD17 3HH Tel: 01923 232010 — MRCS Eng. LRCP Lond. 1940 (King's Coll. & Char. Cross) FRIPHH; Cert. (L.S.) Royl Humane Soc.; MD Lond. 1947, MB BS 1940, DPH 1947; DCH Eng. 1949; MRCGP 1953; DMJ Soc. Apoth. Lond. 1969; MFCM 1974; AFOM RCP Lond. 1982. Mem. Middle Temple. Socs: Nutrit. Soc. & Soc. of Chem. Indust. Prev: Ho. Surg. Char. Cross Hosp.; Phys. Supt. Willesden Fev. Hosp.; Surg. Lt. RNVR 1941-46.

ROTONDETTO, Salvatore 4 Clumber Avenue, Clayton, Newcastle ST5 3AX — State Exam Naples 1991.

ROTTENBERG, Giles Tobias 11 Bromfield Street, London N1 0QA — MB BS Lond. 1988; MRCP (UK) 1991; FRCR 1994. Cons. Radiol. Guy's & St. Thom. Trust Lond. Specialty: Radiol. Prev: Sen. Regist. Middlx. Hosp. Lond.

ROTZ, Bernhard 38 Aberdare Close, Chichester PO19 6UG — State Exam Med Berlin 1991.

ROUALLE, Mr Henri Louis Marcel (retired) 89 Marsh Lane, London NW7 4LE Tel: 020 8959 6042 — MRCS Eng. LRCP Lond. 1937 (St. Bart.) MD Lond. 1940, MB BS 1937; FRCS Eng. 1940. Prev: Vis. Surg. H.M. Prison Wormwood Scrubs.

ROUD MAYNE, Catherine Charlotte Anne 10 Hunts Close, Luton LU1 5JL — MB BChir Camb. 1990.

ROUGH, Sandy Aitken 8 Grey Street, Killin FK21 8SW Tel: 01567 820704 — MB ChB Glas. 1993; DRCOG 1995; MRCGP 1998. Specialty: Gen. Pract.

ROUGHEAD, Peter (retired) 12 Anne Drive, Stenhousemuir, Larbert FK5 4JE Tel: 01324 554246 — MB ChB Glas. 1949; DPH 1954, DPM Eng. 1957; DPM Durham. 1958; FRCPsych 1992, M 1971. Prev: Cons. Psychiat. Bellsdyke Hosp. Larbert.

ROUGHNEEN, Patrick Thomas Martin The Hospital for Sick Children, Great Ormond St., London WC1N 3JH — MB ChB Leic. 1982.

ROUGHTON, Helen Clare Oakenhall Medical Practice, Bolsover Street, Hucknall, Nottingham NG15 7UA Tel: 0115 963 3511 Fax: 0115 968 0947 — BM BS Nottm. 1991.

ROUGHTON, Susanna Alice, Maj. RAMC Killead Health Centre, Killead Road, Aldergrove, Crumlin BT29 4EN — MB BS Lond. 1989 (GUY's) MRCGP Oct 1995; DFFP 1996; DSOM May 1997; Dip Imm C RCS Ed 1999. Specialty: Gen. Pract.

ROUHOLAMIN, Mr Ebrahim Worcester Royal Infirmary, Charles Hastings Way, Worcester WR5 1DD; Hallow Bank, Hallow Road, Worcester WR2 6DD Tel: 01905 423250 — MD Tehran 1969; FRCS Glas. 1984. Cons. Orthop. Surg. Worcs. & Dist. HA. Specialty: Trauma & Orthop. Surg. Special Interest: Knee Surgery. Socs: BMA; BOA.

ROULSON, Catherine Jane University Hospital, Anaesthetic Department, Lewisham High Street, London SE13 6LH Tel: 020 8333 3000 — MB ChB Manch. 1984 (Manchester University) FRCA. Cons. Anaesth. Lewisham Hosp. Specialty: Anaesth.

ROULSON, Jo-An Saville Coach House, Savile Road, Halifax HX1 2BA — MB ChB Dund. 1998; MB ChB Dund 1998.

ROULSTON, Miss Lizanne 52 Baycliff Road, West Derby, Liverpool L12 6QU Tel: 0151 228 4702 — MB ChB Liverp. 1996. SHO (Gastroenterol.) Fazakerley Hosp. Liverp. Specialty: Gastroenterol. Prev: Ho. Off. (Med. & Surg.) Fazakerley Hosp. Liverp.

ROULSTON, Rose Gwynne (retired) The Coach House, 37 Beechwood Avenue, Mirfield WF14 9LG Tel: 01924 493622 — (Dundee) MB ChB St. And. 1948. Prev: Assoc. Specialist Anaesth. Yorks. RHA.

ROUNCEFIELD, Mrs Angela Mary Bodmin Hospital, Boundary Rd, Bodmin PL31 2QT Tel: 01208 251300 Fax: 01208 251455; Broadwater, Restronguet Point, Feock, Truro TR3 7QD Tel: 01872 862751 Fax: 01872 862751 — MB ChB Liverp. 1962; DPM Eng. 1965; FRCPsych. 1984, M 1971. Cons. Psychiat. Bodmin Hosp. Bodmin; Medicla Adviser Cornw. Alcohol and Drug Agency, Truro. Specialty: Gen. Psychiat. Socs: BMA (Chairm.) Cornw. Br.; Cornw. Clin. Soc. (Past Pres.). Prev: Cons. Psychiat. N. Wales Hosp. Denbigh, & Maelor Hosp. Wrexham; Research Fell. & Hon. Sen. Regist. N. Wales Hosp. Denbigh; Regist. (Psychiat.) Sefton Gen. Hosp. Liverp.

ROUND, Alison Pamela East Devon PCT, Cecil Boyall House, Southernhay East, Exeter EX1 1PQ Tel: 01392 207457 Fax: 01392 207506 — MB ChB Bristol 1982; BSc Med. Microbiol.; MRCP (UK) 1985; MRCGP 1991. Director of Public Health, East Devon PCT. Specialty: Pub. Health Med.

ROUND, Caroline Elizabeth 121 Girton Road, Cambridge CB3 0LS — MB BS Lond. 1983.

ROUND, Jonathan Edward Collier 11 Hansler Road, London SE22 9DJ — MB BS Lond. 1990.

ROUND, Keith William Tregony Road Surgery, Tregony Road, Probus, Truro TR2 4JZ — MB ChB Ed. 1973; DObst RCOG 1976; MRCGP 1977.

ROUND, Leslie Aylesbury Partnership, Aylesbury Medical Centre, Taplow House, Thurlow Street, London SE17 2XE Tel: 020 7703 2205 — MB BS Lond. 1974; DRCOG 1977.

ROUND, Patrick Michael Glaxo Wellcome R&D, Stockley Park, Uxbridge UB11 1BT Tel: 020 8990 8214 Fax: 020 8990 8245 Email: pr43229@glaxowellcome.co.uk; 37 Brands Hill Avenue, High Wycombe HP13 5PY Tel: 01494 451205 — MB BS Lond. 1982 (Charin g Cross Hosp. Med. Sch.) FCAnaesth. 1990; AFPM/Dip Pharm Med 1995. Clin. Developm. Director, Pain & Endocrinol.,Glaxowellcome. Specialty: Pharmaceutical Medicine. Prev: Clin. Research Phys., Novo Nordisk Copenhagen.

ROUND, Percy Holcroft (retired) 40 Alfreton Road, South Normanton, Alfreton DE55 2AS Tel: 01773 811421 — MB ChB Birm. 1951. Prev: Ho. Surg. (Obst.) & Ho. Phys. Qu. Eliz. Hosp. Birm.

ROURKE, Anne 9 Woodcote Valley Road, Purley CR8 3AL — MB ChB Dundee 1973; BMSc Dund 1970; MRCPsych 1978. Assoc. Specialist Springfield Hosp. Lond. Specialty: Gen. Psychiat. Prev: Clin. Asst. Springfield Hosp. Lond.; Clin. Asst., Regist. & SHO Barrow Hosp. Barrow Gurney.

ROURKE, Anthony — MB ChB Glas. 1958. Princip. Med. Off. Scott. Prison Serv. Prev: Sen. Med. Off. H.M. Prison Serv.

***ROURKE, Duncan Matthew Carlton** 38 Darnford Lane, Lichfield WS14 9RN — MB BS Lond. 1998 (Barts & Lond.) MA Hons. (Gantab.); MB BS Lond 1998. PRHO. Specialty: Gen. Med.

ROUS, Elizabeth Mary 210 Prestbury Road, Macclesfield SK10 3HL — MB ChB Leic. 1982; DCH RCP Lond. 1985; DRCOG 1985; MRCGP 1986; MFPHM 1990; MSc Manch. 2000. Prev: Cons.

Pub. Health Med. Manch. HA.; Cons. Pub. Health. Med. Stockport H.A.; Cons. Pub. Health Med. N. West. RHA.

ROUSE, Amanda Kate — MB BS Lond. 1991; MRCP; BSc; DTM & H; MRCGP; MSc.

ROUSE, Andrew Michael Dept of Public Health and Epidemiology, University of Birmingham, Birmingham B15 2TT; Pengarn Fach, Cippin, St Dogmaels, Cardigan SA43 3LT — MB BS Lond. 1975; MRCS Eng. LRCP Lond. 1975. Sen. Lect. Pub. Health Med., Uni. Birm.

ROUSE, Brian Richard Shephall Way Surgery, 29 Shephall Way, Stevenage SG2 9QN Tel: 01438 312097 — MB BS Newc. 1978.

ROUSE, David Andrew The London Medicolegal Centre, P.O. Box 70, Billingshurst RH14 0YH Tel: 07973 548574 Fax: 01403 753524 Email: d.a.rouse@talk21.com — MB BChir Camb. 1985; MA Camb. 1985; DMJ(Path) Soc. Apoth. Lond. 1990; MRCPath 1991; FRCPath 2000. Cons. Forens. Med. & Path. Lond. Medico-Legal Centre. Specialty: Forens. Path. Socs: Brit. Acad. Forens. Scs.; Brit. Assn. in Forens. Med.; Forens. Sci. Soc. Prev: Lect. (Forens. Med.) Lond. Hosp. Med. Coll.; SHO (Histopath.) St. Bart. Hosp. Lond.; Ho. Off. Guy's Hosp. Lond.

ROUSE, Eileen Hilda (retired) Oaklee, Pound Lane, Burley, Ringwood BH24 4EE — MB BCh Witwatersrand 1953.

ROUSE, Gillian Margaret 3 The Cherry Orchard, Staverton, Cheltenham GL51 0TR Tel: 01242 680532 — MB ChB Birm. 1969; MFFP 1993. SCMO (Family Plann.) E. Glos. NHS Trust & Clin. Asst. (Haemat.) Glos. Roy. Hosp. & Cheltenham Hosp.

ROUSE, Jane Margaret The Princess Royal Hospital, Haywards Heath RH16 4EX Tel: 01444 441881; Little Orchard, Ansty, Haywards Heath RH17 5AG — MB BS Lond. 1971 (St. Mary's) FFA RCS Eng. 1976. Cons. Anaesth. Princess Roy. Hosp. Hayward Heath W.Sussex; Cons. Anaesth. Hurstwood Pk. Neurol. Unit Haywards Heath; Clin. Tutor Mid Sussex NHS Trust 1997-. Specialty: Anaesth. Socs: Roy. Coll. Anaesth.; Assoc of Anaesth. G.B. & Irel.; Neuro anaesth. Soc. Prev: Chairm. Anaesth. Div. Mid Sussex NHS Trust; Coll. Tutor (Anaesth.) RCS; Sen. Regist. (Anaesth.) St. Mary's Hosp. Lond.

ROUSE, Mary Emily 45 Regent Park Square, Glasgow G41 2AF — MB ChB Glas. 1996 (Glasgow) BSc (Hons.) Glas. 1988; PhD Glas. 1992; MB ChB (Hons.) Glas. 1996. GP Locum. Specialty: Gen. Med. Prev: SHO (Med.).

ROUSE, Michael Edward Dr M E Rouse and Partners, 24 St John's Avenue, Churchdown, Gloucester GL3 2DB Tel: 01452 713036 Fax: 01452 714726; 3 The Cherry Orchard, Staverton, Cheltenham GL51 0TR Tel: 01452 680532 — MB ChB Birm. 1968. Socs: BMA. Prev: Ho. Surg. Profess. Unit Qu. Eliz. Hosp. Birm.; Ho. Phys. & Ho. Off. (O & G) Dudley Rd. Hosp. Birm.

ROUSE, Robert Turnbull Rysseldene, 98 Conway Road, Colwyn Bay LL29 7LE Tel: 01492 532807 — MB ChB Ed. 1961.

ROUSHDI, Mr Hossam Roushdi Ibrahim Mohamed Ashford and St Peter's Hospital NHS Trust, London Road, Ashford TW15 3AA Tel: 01753 743317 Fax: 01753 743317 Email: roushdi@aol.com; Princess Margaret Hospital, Windsor, Windsor SL4 3SJ Tel: 01753 743317 Email: Roushdi@aol.com — MB ChB Alexandria 1975; MS Alexandria 1979; FRCS Glas. 1985. Cons. Orthop. Surg.(Knee Surgeon), Ashford & St. Peter's Hosp. Specialty: Orthop. Special Interest: Knee Surg. Ligament and Jt. Replacement. Socs: BOA; BASK; ILARUS.

ROUSHDY-GEMIE, May Dyke Road Surgery, 361 Dyke Road, Glasgow G13 4SQ Tel: 0141 959 2118 Fax: 0141 959 9851; 41 Rowallan Gardens, Glasgow G11 7LH Tel: 0141 334 1296 — MB ChB Glas. 1984; DRCOG 1986; MRCGP 1988. GP Glas. Retainer Scheme.

ROUSSAK, Mr Jeremy Brian St John's Buildings, 24A-28 St John St, Manchester M3 4DJ Tel: 0161 214 1500 Fax: 0161 835 3929 Email: jbr@mac.com — MB BChir Camb. 1984; MA, MB Camb. 1984, BA 1980, BChir 1983; FRCS Ed. 1988; Dip. Law 1995. Specialty: Cardiothoracic Surg. Prev: Regist. (Cardiothoracic Surg.) Roy. Brompton Nat. Heart & Lung Hosp. Lond.; Regist. (Cardiothoracic Surg.) Hammersmith Hosp. Lond.; SHO (Cardiothoracic Surg.) Hammersmith Hosp.

ROUSSAK, Neville Jack (retired) 48 Spath Road, Manchester M20 2GT Tel: 0161 445 9292 Email: roussak@btinternet.com — MB ChB Manch. 1945; BSc Manch. 1942; FRCP Lond. 1975, M 1948. Prev: Cons. Phys. Withington Hosp. Manch.

ROUSSEAU, Marek Jan 3 Canonbury, Shrewsbury SY3 7AG — MB BS Lond. 1988; BSc BPharm. (Hons.) Aberd. 1982.

ROUSSEAU, Neil Charles Brocklebank Health Centre, 249 Garratt Lane, London SW18 4UE Tel: 020 8870 1341/871 4448; 249 Garratt Lane, London SW18 4DU Tel: 020 8870 1341 — MB BS Lond. 1983; MIMC; BSc (Hons.) Lond. 1980. Demonst. (Anat.) & SHO (Cas.) Univ. Coll. Hosp. Lond. Socs: Gold Star Mem. Inner Magic Circle. Prev: SHO (Geriat., Med. & Paediat.) Roy. Free Hosp. Lond.; Ho. Off. (Surg. & A & E) Univ. Coll. Hosp. Lond.; Ho. Off. (Med.) Hillingdon Hosp.

ROUSSOUNIS, Socrates Hercules 1 Nichols Way, Wetherby LS22 6AD Tel: 01937 584178 — MB BS Lond. 1964 (St. Geo.) MRCS Eng. LRCP Lond. 1962; DObst RCOG 1966; DCH Eng. 1968; MRCP (UK) 1972; FRCP Lond. 1989. Cons. Paediat. & Dir. Regional Child Developm. Centre St. Jas. Univ. Hosp. Leeds; Hon. Sen. Lect. (Clin. Paediat.) Univ. Leeds. Specialty: Paediat. Prev: Sen. Regist. (Paediat.) Char. Cross Hosp. Lond.; Research Fell. & Ho. Phys. (Neurol.) Hosp. Sick Childr. Gt. Ormond St.Lond.

ROUT, David John Willows Medical Centre, Osbourne Drive, Queensbury, Bradford BD13 2GD Tel: 01274 882008 Fax: 01274 818447; Catherine House Farm, Catherine House Lane, Luddenden Dean, Halifax HX2 6XB Tel: 01422 882342 — MB ChB Leeds 1981; MRCGP 1987.

ROUT, Jonathan Philip Priory Avenue Surgery, 2 Priory Avenue, Caversham, Reading RG4 7SE Tel: 0118 947 2431 Fax: 0118 946 3340 — MB BS Lond. 1977 (St. Thos.) MRCGP 1982; DRCOG 1982. Prev: SHO (O & G) Roy. Berks. Hosp. Reading; SHO (Paediat.) & Ho. Phys. Battle Hosp. Reading.

ROUTH, Curtis Dudley (retired) Tintern Lodge, 86 Lion Road, Bexleyheath DA6 8PQ Tel: 020 8303 3229 — MRCS Eng. LRCP Lond. 1944 (St. Bart.) MB BS 1944; MD Lond. 1951; FRCP Lond. 1972, M 1951. Prev: Cons. Venereol. Dartford & Gravesham, Medway & Maidstone Health.

ROUTH, Guy Stephen Cheltenham General Hospital, Cheltenham GL53 7AN Tel: 01242 222222 Fax: 01242 273405 — MB BS Lond. 1974 (St. Bart.) MRCS Eng. LRCP Lond. 1973; FFA RCS Eng. 1978. Cons. Anaesth. Cheltenham Gen. Hosp. & Glos. Roy. Hosp. Gloucester. Specialty: Anaesth.; Intens. Care. Prev: Med. Dir. E. Glos. NHS Trust; Sen. Regist. (Anaesth.) Glas. Roy. Infirm.; Research Regist. (Intens. Care) West. Infirm. Glas.

ROUTH, John Eric (retired) Leyland Park, Tubwell Lane, Crowborough TN6 3RH Tel: 01892 663866 — MRCS Eng. LRCP Lond. 1950 (St. Mary's) DPH Lond. 1961; MFCM 1974. Prev: Wing Cdr. RAF Med. Br.

ROUTLEDGE, Deborah Jane 21 Coniston Av, West Jesmond, Newcastle upon Tyne NE2 3EY — MB BS Newc. 1997.

ROUTLEDGE, Helen Clare 167 College Road, Collegetown, Sandhurst GU47 0RG; 201 Sherbourne Lofts, Grosvenor Street W., Birmingham B16 8HW Tel: 0121 246 6911 Email: rutters@dial.pipex.com — MB ChB Birm. 1996 (Birmingham) BSc (Hons.) Biochem. Birm. 1994. SHO (Med.) Birm. Heartlands & Solihull NHS Trust (Teachg.). Specialty: Gen. Med.

ROUTLEDGE, Nicholas Graham High Beech Villa, Beech Road, Newport PO30 2AH — MB BS Lond. 1993.

ROUTLEDGE, Professor Philip Alexander Department of Pharmacology, Therapeutics and Toxicology, University of Wales College of Medeicine, Heath Park, Cardiff CF14 4XN Tel: 029 2074 2051 Fax: 0292074 8316 Email: 106174.22@compuserve.com — MD Newc. 1978, MB BS 1972; FRCP (UK) 1986, M 1975; FRCP Edin. 2002. Prof. Clin. Pharmacol. Univ. Wales Coll. Med. Cardiff; Dir. Therap. & Toxicol. Centre; Dir. CSM Wales; Hon. Cons. Phys. S. Glam. HA; Cons. Toxicol. Welsh Off. Specialty: Pharmacology; Gen. Med. Socs: Assn. of Phys.s of GB/NI; Brit. Pharmacol. Soc.; Brit. Toxicological Soc. Prev: Lect. (Clin. Pharmacol.) Univ. Newc.; Asst. Prof. Med. (Med. Research) Duke Univ. Durh., N. Carolina, USA; Merck, Sharpe & Dohme Internat. Fell. (Clin. Pharmacol.) Duke Univ.

ROUTLEDGE, Raymond, OStJ (retired) 9 Gowan Lea, 15 Woodford Road, Snaresbrook, London E18 2ER Tel: 020 8989 7451 — MB BChir Camb. 1953 (Char. Cross) MA Camb. 1953; MRCS Eng. LRCP Lond. 1953; DIH Eng. 1959; MFOM RCP Lond. 1978. Prev: Sen. Regional Med. Off. Brit. Telecom. Lond.

ROUTLEDGE, Raymond Crawford Hope Hospital, Eccles Old Road, Salford M6 8HD — MB ChB Manch. 1966; MRCPath 1975. Cons. Haemat. Salford AHA (T). Specialty: Haematology.

ROUTLEDGE, Richard York Bridge Surgery, 5 James Street, Morecambe LA4 5TE Tel: 01524 824149 — MB ChB Manch. 1968; MRCGP 1974.

ROUTLEDGE, Thomas Adam The Court, Chapel Lane, Winford, Bristol BS8 3DN — BM BCh Oxf. 1997.

ROUX, Bryant Raphael Flat 2, 65A Chalk Farm Road, London NW1 8AN — MB ChB Cape Town 1990.

ROUX, Hermanus Johannes 8 Harefield Close, Enfield EN2 8NQ — MB ChB Stellenbosch 1988.

ROVIRA, Peter Alan Kirkham Medical Practice, St Albans Road, Torquay TQ1 3SL Tel: 01803 323541; Red Roofs, Teignmouth Road, Maidencombe, Torquay TQ1 4TP — MB ChB Liverp. 1970.

ROW, Kandukar Prabakar 1 Coburg Gardens, Clayhall, Ilford IG5 0PP Tel: 020 8551 3478 — MB BS Madras 1941; DPH Ed. 1948; DCH Eng. 1950. Specialty: Community Child Health.

ROWAN, Ian George Ormeau Park Surgery, 281 Ormeau Road, Belfast BT7 3GG Tel: 028 9064 2914 Fax: 028 9064 3993; 281 Ormeau Road, Belfast BT7 3GG — MB BCh BAO Belf. 1980; DCH RCPSI 1982; DRCOG 1983; MRCGP 1984. GP Belf. Socs: Ulster Med. Soc.; BMA. Prev: SHO Roy. Belf. Hosp. Sick Childr. & Roy. Matern. Hosp. Belf.; Ho. Off. Roy. Vict. Hosp. Belf.

ROWAN, John 27 Surrenden Road, Brighton BN1 6PA — MB ChB Leeds 1976; DRCOG 1981; MRCGP 1981.

ROWAN, Maurice Glenn Dunluce Avenue Surgery, 1-3 Dunluce Avenue, Belfast BT9 7AW Tel: 028 9024 0884; 17 Magherlave Road, Lisburn BT28 3BW Tel: 01846 675100 Fax: 01846 628168 — (Belf.) MB BCh BAO Belf. 1968; DCH RCPSI 1970; DObst RCOG 1975. Prev: Ho. Off. Roy. Vict. Hosp. Belf.; Regist. & SHO. Roy. Belf. Hosp. Sick Childr.

ROWAN, Peter Arthur Church Hill Surgery, Station Road, Pulham Market, Diss IP21 4TX Tel: 01379 674116 Fax: 01379 608014 — MRCS Eng. LRCP Lond. 1974 (Camb. & Lond. Hosp.) LMSSA Lond. 1974; BSc (Hons) Lond. 1971, MB BS 1974; MRCP (UK) 1978; FRCP 2000. Prev: Ships Surg. RRS Discovery.

ROWAN, Peter Rowley The Priory Hospital, Priory Lane, London SW15 5JQ; 16 Dewhurst Road, London W14 0ET — MB BS Lond. 1972; MRCPsych 1977.

ROWAN, Robert Anthony (retired) Saracens Cottage, Pluckley, Ashford TN27 0SA Tel: 01233 840253 Email: tonyrow1@aol.com — MB BChir Camb. 1949 (Camb. & St. Thos.) DObst RCOG 1954; MRCGP 1971. Prev: Ho. Surg. St. Thos. Hosp. Hydestile & Roy. Portsmouth Hosp.

ROWAN, Robert Martin (retired) 13 Buchanan Street, Milngavie, Glasgow G62 8AW Tel: 0141 956 4573 — MB ChB Ed. 1959; FRCP Glas. 1979, M 1966; FRCP Edin. 1986; FRCPath 1996.

ROWAN-ROBINSON, Martin Neil Macklin Street Surgery, 90 Macklin Street, Derby DE1 1JX Tel: 01332 340381 Fax: 01332 345387; 90 Blagreaves Lane, Littleover, Derby DE23 7FP — MB ChB Bristol 1978; FRCGP 1996, M 1981; DRCOG 1982. Trainer Derby VTS. Prev: Trainee GP Chesterfield VTS; Ho. Off. (Surg.) Bristol Gen. Hosp. & Vict. Hosp. Blackpool.

ROWBOTHAM, Mr Carl 83 Mansfield Road, Aston, Sheffield S26 4UE Tel: 0114 287 2527 — BM BCh Oxf. 1993; MA (Hons.) Camb. 1994. Specialty: Urol.

ROWBOTHAM, Christopher Jeremy Frederick Falconhill, 19 St Bernards Road, Solihull B92 7AU Tel: 0121 707 6427 — MB BS Durh. 1962; MRCOG 1969. Cons. O & G Solihull & E. Birm. Health Dists. Specialty: Obst. & Gyn. Socs: BMA. Prev: Sen. Regist. O & G Birm. RHB; Regist. O & G United Birm. Hosps.; Regist. (O & G) Newc. Gen. Hosp.

ROWBOTHAM, Professor David John Department of Anaesthesia and Pain Management, Leicester Royal Infirmary, Leicester LE1 5WW Tel: 0116 258 5291 Email: djr8@le.ac.uk — MB ChB Sheff. 1978 (Sheffield) MRCP (UK) 1983; FRCSI 1985; FRCA 1986; MD Sheff. 1991. Prof. Pain Managem. & Anaesth. Leicester Roy. Infirm. Specialty: Anaesth. Socs: Eur. Soc. Anaesth. (Chairm. Pharmacol. Sub. Comm.); Coun. Mem. Pain Soc.; Anaesth. Res. Soc.

ROWBOTHAM, Hugo Dalyson 147 Harley Street, London W1G 6BL Tel: 020 7935 4444 Fax: 020 7486 9636; 11 Cromwell Crescent, London SW5 9QW Tel: 020 7603 6967 — MB BS Durh. 1965. GP Lond. Socs: BMA & Soc. Occupat. Med.

ROWBURY, Cynthia Anne Temple Fortune Health Centre, 23 Temple Fortune Lane, London NW11 7TE Tel: 020 8458 4431 — MRCS Eng. LRCP Lond. 1972; MRCP (UK) 1978.

ROWBURY, James Lionel Hide Hollow, Brookvale Orchard, Higher Ringmore Road, Shaldon, Teignmouth TQ14 0HH — MB BS Lond. 1998; MB BS Lond 1998.

ROWDEN, Jennifer Daphne Thornhill Unit, Moorgreen Hospital, West End, Southampton SO30 3JB Tel: 02380 475241/2 — BM Soton. 1980; DRCOG 1982; MRCGP 1984. Assoc. Specialist, Old Age Psychiat., W. Hants. NHS Trust, Soton.

ROWDEN, Kenneth White Singleton Medical Centre, Singleton, Ashford Tel: 01233 646036; The White House, Sheldwich Lees, Faversham ME13 0NG Fax: 01795 533200 — MB BS Lond. 1957 (Lond. Hosp.) MRCS Eng. LRCP Lond. 1957; DObst RCOG 1960; DCH Eng. 1961. Prev: Clin. Asst. (Child Psychiat.) Canterbury & Thanet Health Dist.; SHO (Paediat.) OldCh. Hosp. Romford; Ho. Surg. (Obst.) Forest Gate Hosp. Lond.

ROWE, Alan Frank 6 Gortgrannagh Drive, Wheatsheaf Heights, Coleraine BT51 3NQ Tel: 01265 54244 — MB BCh BAO Dub. 1974 (TC Dub.) BA; DRCOG 1977; MRCGP 1978. Prev: SHO (O & G) Route Hosp. Ballymoney; SHO (Psychiat.) & SHO (Med.) Whiteabbey Hosp. Newtownabbey.

ROWE, Alan Inness (retired) Garmoe, Camelford PL32 9TS Tel: 01840 212689 — (Univ. Durh. King's Coll. Med. Sch.) MB BS Durh. 1947. Prev: Ho. Surg. N. Eng. Thoracic Surg. Centre Shotley Bridge.

ROWE, Alan John, OBE (retired) Haughley Grange, Stowmarket IP14 3QT Tel: 01449 673008 Fax: 01229 774935 Email: arowe@bma.org.uk; The Grange Haughley, Stowmarket IP14 3QT Tel: 01449 673008 Fax: 01449 774935 — LMSSA Lond. 1950 (King's Coll. Lond. & Char. Cross) FRCGP 1982, M 1968. Cons. WHO; Cons. WHO. Prev: Hosp. Pract. (Rheum. & Rehabil.) Addenbrooke's Hosp. Camb.

ROWE, Alexander John Scarth Tan-yr-Allt, Bont Ystrad, Denbigh LL16 3HE — MB BS Lond. 1994.

ROWE, Angela Okehampton Medical Centre, Okehampton EX20 1AY Tel: 01837 52233 — MB BS Lond. 1987 (St. Thomas' Hospital Medical School) DCH Otago 1991; MRCGP 1994; DRCOG 1995; DFFP 1995. Asst. GP.

ROWE, Antonia Jane Trescobeas Surgery, Falmouth TR11 2UN Tel: 01326 434888 — MB ChB Bristol 1991. Retained Doctor, GP. Specialty: Gen. Pract.

ROWE, Bernard, OBE, TD, Brigadier late RAMC Retd. Central Public Health Laboratory, Colindale Avenue, London NW9 5HT Tel: 020 8200 4400 Fax: 020 8905 9992; 14 Barns Dene, Harpenden AL5 2HQ Tel: 01582 715835 — (Camb. & Univ. Coll. Hosp. Lond.) BA Camb. 1957, MA 1961; MB BChir Camb. 1961; DTM & H Eng. 1964; FRCPath 1982, M 1978. Cons. Med. Microbiol. & Dir. Div. Gastro-Intestinal Infects. Centr. Pub. Health Laborat. Colindale; Cons. Path. Defence Med. Servs.; Dir. WHO Internat. Collaborating Centre for Phage Typing & Drug Resistance of Enterobacteria. Specialty: Med. Microbiol.; Trop. Med.; Pub. Health Med. Prev: Hon. Surg. to HM The Qu.; TA Adviser to Dir. Gen. Army Med. Servs.; Maj. RAMC, Off. i/c Enteric Ref. Laborat. David Bruce Laborats.

ROWE, Brian Ramsey Northgate Medical Centre, 10 Upper Northgate Street, Chester CH1 4EE Tel: 01244 379906 Fax: 01244 379703; 6 Glan Aber Park, Hough Green, Chester CH4 8LF Tel: 01244 674448 — MB BS Newc. 1976 (Newc. u. Tyne) DRCOG 1979; MRCGP 1980. Gen. Practitioner; Clin. Asst., Chester Drugs Serv. Specialty: Gen. Pract. Socs: Bd. of Dirs. Save The Family Charity. Prev: Dist. Med. Off. Nkhata Bay, Malawi.

ROWE, Carla Jane 22 Post House Lane, Great Bookham, Leatherhead KT23 3EA — MB ChB Birm. 1993 (Birmingham) DRCOG 1997. GP Regist. Portseath Surg. Truro Cornw. Specialty: Gen. Pract. Prev: SHO (Ent.) Warwick; SHO (O & G) Banbury; SHO (Paediat.) Warwick.

ROWE, Cecil Eleanor Specialist Psychotherapy Services, Southfield House, 40 Clarendon Road, Leeds LS2 7PJ Tel: 0113 295 5430 — MB BChir Camb. 1972 (Univ. Camb. & St. Thos. Hosp. Lond.) MRCP (UK) 1974; FRCPsych 1996, M 1983; Dip. Psychother. Leeds 1983. Cons. Psychotherapist Leeds Community & Ment. Health Servs. NHS Teachg. Trust; Hon. Sen. Lect. Univ. Leeds. Specialty: Psychother. Prev: Cons. Psychother. St. Jas. Univ. Hosp. Leeds; Sen.

Regist. (Psychother.) Leeds East. HA; Regist. (Psychiat.) Newc. & York HAs.

ROWE, David Jeremy 21 Manorgate Road, Kingston upon Thames KT2 7AW — MB BS Lond. 1998; MB BS Lond 1998.

ROWE, Eleanor 20 Rowantree Rd, Milber, Newton Abbot TQ12 4LL — MB BS Lond. 1994; MRCGP.

ROWE, Fiona Jane Howard House Surgery, 31 Orwell Road, Felixstowe IP11 7DD Tel: 01394 282706 Fax: 01394 278955 — MB BS Lond. 1986 (Charing Cross, Univ. Lond.) BSc (Hons.) Leeds 1981; DRCOG 1989; MRCGP 1990.

ROWE, Gillian Mary X-Ray Department, County Hospital, Hereford HR1 2ER Tel: 01432 355444 Email: gillian.rowe@hhtr.nhs.uk; Causeway Cottage, Ravens Causeway, Wormsley, Hereford HR4 8LZ Tel: 01432 830363 — MB BS Lond. 1974 (Univ. Coll. Hosp. Med. Sch. Lond.) BSc (Biochem.) Lond. 1971; MRCPI 1983; DMRD Eng. 1983; FRCR 1984. Cons. Radiol. Herefordsh. HA. Specialty: Radiol. Special Interest: Cross Sectional Imaging; Mammography.

ROWE, Ian Francis Worcester Centre for Rheumatic Diseases, Highfield Unit, Worcestershire Royal Hospital, Worcester WR5 1DD Tel: 01905 760 460 Fax: 01905 760 460 — MB BChir Camb. 1977; MD Camb. 1985, MA 1976; MRCP (UK) 1979; FRCP Lond. 1995. Cons. Rheum. Worcester Acute Hosps. NHS,Trust, Worcester Roy. Hosp. Specialty: Rheumatol. Socs: Mem. Brit. Soc. Rheumatol. Prev: Sen. Regist. (Rheum. & Gen. Med.) Char. Cross & Westm. Hosps. Lond.; MRC Train. Fell. Immunol. Med. Unit & Hon. Sen. Regist. (Med.) Hammersmith Hosp. Lond.; Regist. (Med.) St. Thos. Hosp. Lond.

ROWE, James Benedict — BM BCh Oxf. 1994; BA Cantab. 1991; PhD Lond. UCL 2001.

ROWE, Jeremy Moseley Hall Hospital, Birmingham B13 8JL Tel: 0121 442 4321 Email: jed.rowe@southbirminghampct.nhs.uk; Mayfield, 18 Fiery Hill Road, Barnt Green, Birmingham B45 8LG Tel: 0121 445 1555 — MB ChB Birm. 1977; MRCP (UK) 1983; FRCP Lond. 1994. Cons. Geriat. Moseley Hall Hosp. Birm.; Cons. Geriat. Selly Oak Hosp., Birm. Specialty: Care of the Elderly. Special Interest: Elder Abuse; Falls; Tissue Viability. Socs: Brit. Geriat. Soc.; Soc. for Research in Rehabil.; Tissue Viability Soc. Prev: Cons. Geriat. Broadgreen Hosp. Liverp.; Lect. (Geriat. Med.) Univ. Birm. & Selly Oak Hosp.

ROWE, Mr Jeremy Geraint Rock Mill, Par PL24 2SS — BM BCh Oxf. 1988; MA Oxf. 1988, BM BCh 1988; FRCS Eng. 1992. Clin. Fell. MRC Clin. & Biochem. Magnetic Resonance Unit John Radcliffe Hosp. Oxf. Specialty: Neurosurg. Prev: SHO (Gen. Surg. & ENT) Norwich HA; SHO (Orthop. & Neurosurg.) Oxf.

ROWE, Julie Ann Adbury Springs, Adbury, Newbury RG20 4EX — MB BS Lond. 1982.

ROWE, Karen Ann Gratton Surgery, Sutton Scotney, Winchester SO21 3LE Tel: 01962 760394 — BM Soton. 1990; BSc Lond. 1980; DPhil Oxf. 1986; MRCGP 1995. GP Asst. Gratton Surg. Winchester; Retainee Gratton Surg. Winchester. Specialty: Gen. Pract. Prev: Trainee GP Hants.; Sen. Health Off. (O & G & Paediat.) Basingstoke Dist. Gen. Hosp.

ROWE, Michael John The Limes Medical Centre, 65 Leicester Road, Narborough, Leicester LE19 2DU Tel: 0116 284 1347 — MB ChB Leic. 1981. GP. Specialty: Gen. Pract.

ROWE, Michael Peter Alexandra Villa, 19 Marine Parade, Sheerness ME12 2PQ Tel: 01795 585058 Fax: 01795 585158 — MB BCh Wales 1970 (Welsh Nat. Sch. Med.) DAvMed Eng. 1977.

ROWE, Mr Mohan (retired) Phayrelands, Cummingston, Burghead, Elgin IV30 5XZ Tel: 01343 830617 — MB BS Madras 1946; FRCS Ed. 1959. Cons. Orthop. Surg. SW Durh. Hosp. Gp. Prev: Sen. Regist. (Orthop. & Traum. Surg.) Morriston Hosp. Swansea.

ROWE, Mr Paul Harold Capstan House, Western Road, Pevensey bay, Eastbourne BN24 6HG — MB BChir Camb. 1977 (Guy's) MA, MB Camb. 1977, MChir 1989, B 1976; FRCS Eng. 1981. Cons. Surg. (Gen. Surg.) Eastbourne DGH. Specialty: Gen. Surg. Socs: Fell. Med. Soc. Lond. & Roy. Soc. Med. Prev: Regist. Rotat (Sen. Surg.) Guy's Hosp. Lond.

ROWE, Paul Robert 27 Rosevalley, Threemilestone, Truro TR3 6BH — MB BCh Wales 1998.

ROWE, Penelope Claire (retired) Little Court, Matfield, Tonbridge TN12 7JX Tel: 0189 272 2153 — MB BS Lond. 1951 (Roy. Free) MRCS Eng. LRCP Lond. 1951; DObst RCOG 1953; MFFP 1993. Prev: Sen. Clin. Off. (Family Plann.) Tunbridge Wells HA.

ROWE, Peter Andrew Derriford Hospital Renal Services Directorate, Level 03, Plymouth PL6 8DH Tel: 01752 792258 Fax: 01752 774651 Email: peter.rowe@phnt.swest.nhs.uk — MB ChB Bristol 1979 (Bristol University) MRCP (UK) 1983; MD Bristol 1990; FRCP Glas. 1998; FRCP Lond 2001. Cons. Renal Phys. Derriford Hosp. Plymouth; Hon. Sen. Clin. Lect. Peninsula Med. Sch., Plymouth. Specialty: Nephrol. Special Interest: Hypertens.; Transpl. Med. Socs: Renal Assn.; Brit. Transpl. Soc.; Amer. Soc. Nephrol. Prev: Hon. Sen. Clin. Research Fell. Peninsula Med. Sch. Plymouth.

ROWE, Peter Brian Tudor Cottage, Springhill, Boldre, Lymington SO41 8NG Tel: 01590 674943; Tudor Cottage, Springhill, Boldre, Lymington SO41 8NG Tel: 01590 674943 — MB ChB Leeds 1950; FRCGP 1982, M 1965.

ROWE, Peter George Greensand Surgery, 57 Oliver Street, Ampthill, Bedford MK45 2SB Tel: 01525 631390 Fax: 01525 631393; 87 Station Road, Ampthill, Bedford MK45 2RE — MB BS Lond. 1985; DRCOG 1989; MRCGP 1994.

ROWE, Peter William c/o Children's Department, Newcastle General Hospital, Westgate Road, Newcastle upon Tyne NE4 6BE — MB BS Monash 1981.

ROWE, Rachel Elizabeth 22 Swann Lane, Cheadle SK8 7HR — BM BS Nottm. 1987; MRCP UK 1990; DM Nottm. 1995. Specialty: Diabetes; Endocrinol.; Gen. Med.

ROWE, Renarta Louise 20 Mallow Way, Rugby CV23 0UE — MB ChB Leeds 1995.

ROWE, Richard Clive Gentry Pathology Laboratory, Ipswich Hospital, Ipswich IP4 5PD Tel: 01473 712233 Ext: 5735 — MB BS Lond. 1967 (Guy's) FDS RCS Eng. 1966; MRCS Eng. LRCP Lond. 1967; FRCPath 1985, M 1973; MRCPath Lond. 1973. Cons. Pathologist in Histopath. and Cytopathology at Ipswich Hosp. NHS Trust, Ipswich, Suff. Specialty: Histopath.

ROWE, Robert Gerald (retired) Ratley Grange, Awbridge, Romsey SO51 0HN Tel: 01794 340018 — (Lond. Hosp.) MB BS Lond. 1953; MRCS Eng. LRCP Lond. 1956; FFPHM RCP (UK) 1979, M 1974. Psychother. Med. Counsellor. Prev: Psychother. Med. Counsellor.

ROWE, Sarah Catherine Hawkstone View, Longford, Market Drayton TF9 3PW — MB ChB Dundee 1984; DA (UK) 1987. GP Assistant, Wrenbury. Prev: GP Retainer Scheme Market Drayton.

ROWE, Siobhan Cringleford Surgery, Cantley Lane, Cringleford, Norwich NR4 6TA Tel: 01603 54678 Fax: 01603 58287; Keswick Cottage, Low Road, Keswick, Norwich NR4 6TZ Tel: 01603 456743 Email: siobhan@keswickcottage.com — MB BS Lond. 1988; DRCOG 1990; DCH RCP Lond. 1991; DFFP 1992; MRCGP 1993. Prev: Trainee GP/SHO Norf. & Norwich Hosp. VTS; SHO (O & G) St. Thos. Hosp. Lond.

ROWE, Steven David Mental Health Unit, Royal Bolton Hospital, Minerva Road, Farnworth, Bolton BL4 0JR Tel: 01204 390031 — MB ChB Manch. 1983; BSc Manch. 1980; T(Psychiat.) 1991. Cons. Psychiat. (Ment. Handicap)Roy. Bolton Hosp. NHS Trust. Specialty: Ment. Health. Socs: Manch. Med. Soc.; Europ. Assn. for Ment. Health and Ment. Retardation. Prev: Cons. Psychiat. (Ment.Handicap) Olive Mt. Hosp. Liverp..; Sen. Regist. (Psychiat. Ment. Handicap.) N. West. RHA; Regist. (Psychiat.) N. Manch. HA.

ROWE, Susan Margaret Llandaff North Medical Centre, 99 Station Road, Llandaff North, Cardiff CF14 2FD Tel: 01443 406813; Plot 8 Tiy-y-Coed, Nant Celwyn, Efail Isaf, Pontypridd CF38 — MB BCh Wales 1977. GP Pontypridd.

ROWE, Tracey Louise Vine Medical Centre, 69 Pemberton Road, East Molesey KT8 9LJ — MB BS Lond. 1987; DCH RCP Lond. 1990; DRCOG Lond. 1991; MRCGP 1993.

ROWE, Valerie Bewick Dartford & Darent Valley Hospital, Lions Hospice, Gravesend & Ellenor Foundation, Dartford DA2 8DA; 39 South Croxted Road, West Dulwich, London SE21 8AZ — MB BChir Camb. 1976; MA, MB Camb. 1976, BChir 1975; MRCGP 1981; Dip. Palliat. Med. Wales 1992. Cons. Lions Hospice Dartford & Darent Valley Hosp. Specialty: Palliat. Med. Prev: SHO St. Joseph's Hospice Lond.; Regist. St. Christopher's Hospice Lond.; Med. Off. Trinity Hospice Lond.

ROWE, Victor Laurie Station View Health Centre, Southfield Road, Hinckley LE10 1UA Tel: 01455 635362 — MB ChB Ed. 1977; BSc (Med. Sci.) (Hons.) Ed. 1974; DCH Eng. 1980; DRCOG 1982; MRCGP 1984. Specialty: Paediat.

ROWE, William Lawrence Department of Anaesthesia, Norfolk & Norwich Hospital, Brunswick Road, Norwich; Keswick Cottage, Low Road, Keswick, Norwich NR4 6TX Tel: 01603 456743 Fax: 01603 287886 — MB ChB Leeds 1981; DRCOG 1984; FFA RCS Eng. 1987. Cons. Anaesth. Norf. & Norwich Hosp. Specialty: Anaesth. Prev: Sen. Regist. Rotat. (Anaesth.) E. Anglia RHA; Regist. (Anaesth.) Leic. Roy. Infirm.; Regist. (Anaesth.) Dunedin, NZ.

ROWE-JONES, Mr David Colin Poole General Hospital, Longfleet Road, Poole BH15 2 Tel: 01202 675100; 6 Haig Avenue, Canford Cliffs, Poole BH13 7AJ Tel: 01202 709489 Fax: 01202 709489 — MRCS Eng. LRCP Lond. 1959 (Westm.) MS Lond. 1969, MB BS 1959; FRCS Eng. 1964. Cons. Surg. Poole Gen., & Swanage Hosps.; Hunt. Prof. RCS Eng. Specialty: Gen. Surg. Prev: Sen. Regist. (Surg.) Westm. Hosp. Lond.; Regist. (Surg.) Roy. Marsden Hosp. Lond. & Gordon Hosp. Lond.

ROWE-JONES, Mr Julian Mark Royal Surrey County Hospital, Egerton Road, Guildford GU2 7XX Tel: 01483 406637 Fax: 01483 464113; Guildford Nuffield Hospital, Stirling Road, Guildford GU2 7RF Tel: 01483 555827 Fax: 01483 555829 Email: info@noses.org.uk — MB BS Lond. 1986 (St. Thos. Hosp.) FRCS Eng. 1992; FRCS (Orl.) 1996. Cons. (Rhinol. & ENT Surg.) Roy. Surrey Co. Hosp. Guildford; Vice-President Sect. of Laryngol. and Rhinology, Roy. Soc. of Med.; Chairm., Fellowsh. Comm. of Europ. Acad. of Facial Plastic Surg. Specialty: Otorhinolaryngol. Special Interest: Endoscopic Sinus Surg.; Rhinoplasty; Nasal Deformity. Socs: Fell. Europ. Acad. Facial Plastic Surg.; Brit. Rhinological Soc.; Brit. Assn. Otorhinolaryngol. Prev: Sen. Regist. (Otorhinolaryngol.) Char. Cross Hosp. Lond.; Lect. (Rhinol.) Char. Cross & Roy. Brompton Hosp. Lond.; Regist. (ENT Surg.) St. Geo. Hosp. Lond. & Roy. Surrey Co. Hosp. Guildford.

ROWELL, Andrew Martin The Surgery, 13 Camberwell Green, London SE5 7AF Tel: 020 7703 3788 — MB BS Lond. 1978 (St. Thos.) BA Oxf. 1975; DRCOG 1981; MRCGP 1982. Forens. Med. Examr. (Metrop. Police). Prev: Ho. Surg. Qu. Mary's Hosp. Sidcup; Ho. Phys. William Harvey Hosp. Ashford; Trainee GP St. Thos. Hosp. Lond. VTS.

ROWELL, Elizabeth Rachel Martin 15 Radlyn Oval, 20 Park Avenue, Harrogate HG2 9BG Tel: 01423 566478 — MB BS Durh. 1952. Prev: Clin. Asst. (Dermat.) Gen. Infirm. Leeds & St. Jas. Hosp. Leeds; Hon. Tutor (Dermat.) Univ. Leeds; Asst. Med. Off. Dept. Stud. Health Univ. Leeds.

ROWELL, Geoffrey Humphery Robin Doctors Surgery, Pembroke Road, Framlingham, Woodbridge IP13 9HA Tel: 01728 723627 Fax: 01728 621064; Oakhill, Earl Soham, Woodbridge IP13 7SL Tel: 01728 685393 — MB Camb. 1965 (King's Coll. Hosp.) BChir 1964; DCH Eng. 1969. GP Woodbridge.

ROWELL, Professor Neville Robinson Nuffield Hospital, Outwood Lane, Horsforth, Leeds LS18 4HP Tel: 0113 258 8756 Fax: 0113 258 3108; 15 Radlyn Oval, 20 Pk Avenue, Harrogate HG2 9BG Tel: 01423 566478 Fax: 01423 709677 Email: nrowell@onetel.net.uk — (Durh.) MB BS Durh. 1949; DCH Eng. 1952; FRCP Lond. 1968, M 1957; MD Newc. 1966. Emerit. Prof. Dermat. Univ. Leeds. Specialty: Dermat. Socs: Med. Appeal Tribunal; (Ex-Pres.) Brit. Assn. Dermat. & N. Eng. Dermat. Soc. Prev: Sen. Cons. Phys. (Dermat.) Gen. Infirm. Leeds & St. Jas. Univ. Hosp. Leeds; Cons. Adviser (Dermat.) DHSS; Tutor (Dermat.) & Sen. Regist. Univ. & Gen. Infirm. Leeds.

ROWELL, Nicholas Phillip Department of Clinical Oncology, Oxford Radcliffe Hospital (Churchill Site), Oxford OX3 7LJ Tel: 01865 225681 Fax: 01865 225660 — MB BChir Camb. 1980 (King's Coll. Hosp.) MRCP (UK) 1982; FRCR 1987; MA Camb. 1980, MD 1990; FRCP Lond. 1996. Cons. & Hon. Sen. Clin. Lect. (Clin. Oncol.) Churchill Hosp. Oxf. Specialty: Oncol.; Radiother. Prev: Sen. Regist. (Radiother.) Mt. Vernon Hosp. Northwood; Clin. Research Fell. Roy. Marsden Hosp. Sutton; Regist. (Radiother.) St. Bart's. Hosp. Lond.

ROWELL, Nigel Timothy The Health Centre, PO Box 101(a), The Health Centre, 20 Cleveland Square, Middlesbrough TS1 2NX Tel: 01642 242192 Fax: 01642 231809; 34 Station Road, Stokesley, Middlesbrough TS9 5AJ Tel: 01642 711929 Fax: 01642 711929 — MB ChB Manch. 1983; BSc (Hons.) St. And. 1980; MRCGP 1987. GP Middlesbrough; Clin. Asst. (Cardiol.) S. Tees HA.; Undergrad Teach. Univ. Newc. upon Tyne. Specialty: Gen. Med. Prev: Trainee GP Cleveland VTS; SHO (Gen. Med.) S. Tees HA.

ROWELL, Patrick John Walter, TD (retired) 3 Poplar Street, Southport PR8 6DT Tel: 01704 543236 — MB ChB Liverp. 1953. Prev: Orthop. Surg. Mersey RHA.

ROWELL, Susan Roberta 6 Bracken Lane, Retford DN22 7EU — MB ChB Aberd. 1995.

ROWEN, David 5 Taw Drive, Chandlers Ford, Eastleigh SO53 4SL — MB ChB Leic. 1983.

ROWLAND, Alan Charles Medical Centre, RASU BFPO 40 — MB BS Lond. 1979 (St. Bart.) SHO (Med.) W. Suff. Hosp. Bury St. Edmunds. Prev: SHO (Anaesth.) Qu. Mary's Hosp. Sidcup; Ho. Off. (Surg.) Poole Gen. Hosp.; Ho. Phys. Rochford Gen. Hosp.

ROWLAND, Andrew George 6 Banks Cottages, Heathgreen Road, Studland, Swanage BH19 3BX — MB ChB Sheff. 1988.

ROWLAND, Andrew Graeme The Pennine Acute Hospitals NHS Trust, Paediatric Secretaries, Fairfield General Hospital, Rochdale Old Road, Bury BL9 7TD Tel: 0161 764 6081 Email: andrew.rowland@doctors.org.uk; 7 Princeton Close, College Gardens, Pendleton, Salford M6 8QL — BM BS (Hons.) Nottm. 2000; BMedSci (Hons.) Nottm. 1998; MRCPCH Lond. 2004. Specialist Regist. (Paediatrics). Specialty: Paediat. Special Interest: Paediatric Accid. & Emerg. Med. Socs: Roy. Coll. of Paediat. & Child Health.

ROWLAND, Anthony John (retired) Willowmead, Kersbrook, Budleigh Salterton EX9 7AB Tel: 01395 444057 — MB ChB Bristol 1952; DObst RCOG 1957; DPH Bristol 1961; FFCM 1977, M 1974. Prev: Cons. Communicable Dis. Control Cornw. & I. of Scilly HA.

ROWLAND, Barbara Jill, Surg. Lt. RN Retd. c/o 77 Lawsons Road, Thornton-Cleveleys FY5 4DB — MB ChB Dundee 1989; LMSSA Lond. 1982.

ROWLAND, Christopher Giles Kenton Lodge, Kenton, Exeter EX6 8JE Tel: 01626 890171 — MB BS Lond. 1971; BSc (Biochem., Hons.) Wales 1966; MRCS Eng. LRCP Lond. 1971; DMRD Eng. 1975; DMRT Eng. 1977; FRCR 1981. Cons. Radiother. & Oncol. Roy. Devon & Exeter Hosp. Exeter; Sen. Lect. (Radiother & Oncol.) Univ. of Exeter; Dir. FORCE Cancer Research Centre Exeter. Specialty: Oncol.; Radiother. Prev: Sen. Regist. (Radiother. & Oncol.) Bristol Health Dist. (T).; Sen. Regist. (Radiother. & Oncol.) Mersey Regional Centre Radiother. & Oncol. Clatterbridge Hosp. Bebington.

ROWLAND, Christopher James, OBE, OStJ (retired) 1 Woodlands Road, Surbiton KT6 6PR Tel: 020 8255 0713 — (Guy's) MB BS Lond. 1959; MRCS Eng. LRCP Lond. 1959; DObst RCOG 1961. Prev: Gen. Practitioner.

ROWLAND, Edward Department of Cardiological Sciences, St. George's Hospital Medical School, Cranmer Terrace, London SW17 0RE Tel: 020 8725 2922 Fax: 020 8767 7141 Email: erowland@sghms.ac.uk; 47 Wimpole Street, London W1M 7DG Tel: 020 7573 8899 Fax: 020 7573 8898 — MB BS Lond. 1974 (St. Bart. Hosp. Lond.) MRCS Eng. LRCP Lond. 1974; FESC 1988; FACC 1990; MD Lond. 1990; FRCP 1998. Cons. & Hon. Sen. Lect. (Cardiol.) St. Geo. Hosp. Med. Sch. Lond.; Cons. Cardiol. Papworth Hosp.; Hon. Cons. Cardiol. Hosp. Childr. Gt. Ormond St. Lond. Specialty: Cardiol. Socs: Brit. Cardiac Soc., Mem.; Brit. pacing and Electrophysiol. Gp., Counc. Mem. Prev: Lect. Nat. Heart & Lung Inst.; Brit. Heart Foundat. Fell. Roy. Postgrad. Med. Sch.

ROWLAND, Gareth David 11 Moor Grange View, West Park, Leeds LS16 5BN — MB BS Lond. 1998; MB BS Lond 1998.

ROWLAND, George Frederick Uffdown, St Mary's Road, Bowdon, Altrincham WA14 2PJ — MB ChB Ed. 1976; BSc (Hons.) Ed. 1974, MB ChB 1976; DCH Eng. 1978; FRCOG 1997. Cons. O & G Univ. Hosp. Aintree Liverp. Specialty: Obst. & Gyn. Prev: Cons. O & G Billinge Hosp. Wigan; Sen. Regist. (O & G) St. Mary's Hosp. Manch.; Specialist Bourn Hall Clinic Cambs.

ROWLAND, Gillian Pamela Child Health Department, East Yorkshire Community Health Care Trust, Temperton House, Beverley Westwood Hospital, Beverley HU17 8BU; 48 Nordham, North Cave, Brough HU15 2LT — MB ChB Manch. 1984; BSc (Med. Sci.) St. And. 1981. Specialty: Community Child Health.

ROWLAND, John Francis (retired) Rose Cottage, Heol-y-Mynydd, Southerndown, Bridgend CF32 0SN — MB ChB Bristol 1951; DPH Eng. 1960. Prev: Sen. Med. Off. (Clin.) Bridgend (Ogwr) Health Dist.

ROWLAND, Kenneth Park Road Health Centre, Park Road, Tarporley CW6 0BE Tel: 01829 732401 Fax: 01829 732404 — MB ChB Liverp. 1967. Course Organiser & Med. Adviser Chesh.

ROWLAND, Lindsey Jane Tors, Fairies Lane, Perth PH1 1NN — BChir Camb. 1995.

ROWLAND, Margaret 2 Camdale View, Ridgeway, Sheffield S12 3XQ — MB ChB Sheff. 1978.

ROWLAND, Michael Garth Murray The Conifers, 16 Hayter Close, West Wratting, Cambridge CB1 5LY Tel: 01223 290788 Fax: 01223 290415 Email: rowland550@aol.com — MB BS Durh. 1964; DCH RCP Lond. 1968; MRCP (UK) 1971; DTM & H RCP Lond. 1973; FRCP Lond. 1983; MFCM RCP (UK) 1987; FFPHM RCP (UK) 1991; FRCPCH (UK) 1997. Progr. Co-ordinator Europ. Progr. Interven. Epidemiol. Train. Paris. Specialty: Pub. Health Med.; Epidemiol. Socs: Life Fell Roy. Soc. Trop. Med. & Hyg.; Soc. Social Med. Prev: Cons. Epidemiol. AORHA & PHLS Communicable Dis. Surveillance Centre; Assoc. Dir. & Head Community Med. Div. Internat. Centre for Diarrh.l Dis. Research Bangladesh; Sen. Sci. MRC Laborat. Fajara, The Gambia.

ROWLAND, Philip Geoffrey Peverell Park Surgery, 162 Outland Road, Peverell, Plymouth PL2 3PX — MB ChB Birm. 1992; MRCGP 1997.

ROWLAND, Raymond Marc Jenner Health Centre, 201 Stanstead Road, London SE23 1HU Tel: 020 8690 2231; 34 Garlies Road, Forest Hill, London SE23 2RT — MB BS Lond. 1974 (Guy's) MRCS Eng. LRCP Lond. 1974; DRCOG 1976; MRCGP 1979.

ROWLAND, Richard George 4 Delaware Road, Lewes BN7 1LD Tel: 01273 474781 — BM BCh Oxf. 1968; DObst RCOG 1970; DA Eng. 1971; Dip. Trop. Med. Antwerp 1973; MRCGP 1984. Princip. GP, Lewes; HIV/AIDS Awareness Advisor, Rwanda. Prev: Med. Dir. Hôpital de Gahini, Rwanda.

ROWLAND, Robert George 4 Sunnydown Road, Olivers Battery, Winchester SO22 4LD — MB ChB Manch. 1987. Regist. Rotat. (Anaesth.) NW RHA. Specialty: Anaesth. Prev: SHO (Obst. & Gyn.) Roy. Preston Hosp.; SHO (Obst. & Gyn.) Chorley & Dist. Hosp.

ROWLAND, Roy MacDonald (retired) 5 Richmond Avenue, Wolverhampton WV3 9JB Tel: 01902 28748 — MB ChB Aberd. 1954. Prev: Surg. Lt. RNR.

ROWLAND, Stephen James Owlthorpe Medical Centre, Moorthorpe bank, Sheffield S20 6PD Tel: 0114 247 7852 Fax: 0114 248 3691; 2 Camdale View, Ridgeway, Sheffield S12 3XQ Tel: 0114 248 5209 — MB ChB Sheff. 1978.

ROWLAND HILL, Christopher Andrew Centre for Magnetic Resonance Investigations, Hull Royal Infirmary, Anlaby Road, Hull HU3 2JZ Email: chris.rowland-hill@hey.nhs.uk; The Nest, 56 George St, Cottingham HU16 5QP Tel: 01482 849173 Fax: 01482 849173 — MB BS Lond. 1982 (Oxford University & St. Thomas' Hospital) BA Oxf. 1979; MRCP (UK) 1985; FRCR 1990. Cons. Neuroradiol. Hull Roy. Infirm. Specialty: Radiol. Socs: BSNR; UKNG. Prev: Sen. Regist. (Radiol.) Nat. Hosp. Neurol. & Neurosurg. Lond.; Regist. (Radiol.) St. Thos. Hosp. Lond.; Regist. (Med.) Whittington Hosp. Lond.

ROWLAND-JONES, Sarah Louise Molecular Immunology Group, Institute of Molecular Medicine, John Radcliffe Hospital, Oxford OX3 9DS Tel: 01865 222316 Fax: 01865 222502; 53 Jack Straw's Lane, Headington, Oxford OX3 7DW Tel: 01865 765608 Fax: 01865 433903 — BM BCh Oxf. 1983; MA Camb. 1984; MRCP (UK) 1986; DM Oxf. 1995. MRC Sen. Clin. Fell. Nuffield Dept. Med. Inst. Molecular Med. Oxf.; Hon. Cons. Infec. Dis. John Radcliffe Hosp. Oxf. Specialty: Infec. Dis. Prev: Clin. Lect. (Molecular Immunol.) Dept. Med. Inst. Molecular Med. Oxf. & MRC Clincian Scientist Fell.; MRC Train. Fell. (Molecular Immunol.) Inst. Molecular Med. Oxf.; Regist. (Infec. Dis.) Churchill Hosp. Oxf.

ROWLAND PAYNE, Christopher Melville Edwin The London Clinic, 149 Harley Street, London W1G 6DE Tel: 020 7224 1228 Fax: 020 7487 5479 Email: crp@thelondonclinic.co.uk — (St. Bart.) MB BS 1977; MRCP (UK) 1980. Cons. Dermat. The Lond. Clin.; Hon. Cons. Dermat. Roy. Marsden Hosp. Lond.; Edr. Jl. of Cosmetic Dermat.; Cons. Dermat. St Saviour's Hosp. Hythe; Vis. Prof. Dermat. Sch. Med. Sci. Kumasi, Ghana; Prof. Clin. Dermat. Ross. Univ. Sch. Med. New York City. Specialty: Dermat. Special Interest: Medical, Surgical, Laser & Cosmetic Dermatology; Skin Malignancies. Socs: Mem Brit. Assn. Dermatol.; Mem. Hon. Soc. Francaise de Dermatol. & Syphiligraphie; Sec-Gen. (past Presid.) Europ. Soc. Cosmetic & Aesthetic Dermatol. Prev: Clin. Lect. & Hon. Sen. Regist. (Dermat.) Westm. Hosp. & Char. Cross & Westm. Med. Sch. Lond.; Regist. (Dermat.) St. Thos. Hosp. Lond.; Vis. Prof. Univ. Texas 1986.

ROWLANDS, Alan John Dept. of Paediatrics, Victoria Hospital, Blackpool FY3 8NR — MB ChB Manch. 1983; MRCP; BSc (Hons.) Med. Biochem. Manch. 1981; DGM RCP Lond. 1985; DCH RCP Lond. 1987. Prev: Hon. Sec. Tameside LMC.

ROWLANDS, Albert David (retired) Rosemullion, Turkdean, Northleach, Cheltenham GL54 3NT Tel: 01451 860683 — MB BS Lond. 1953 (Lond. Hosp.) MRCS Eng. LRCP Lond. 1952; DObst RCOG 1955; MRCGP 1963. Prev: Ho. Surg. (Neurosurg.) Lond. Hosp.

ROWLANDS, Aled Montgomery House Surgery, Piggy Lane, Bicester OX26 6HT Tel: 01869 249222 Fax: 01869 322433; The Plough House, Wendlebury, Bicester OX25 2PS Tel: 01869 321113 Fax: 01869 240694 Email: rowlands@melwood.fsnet.co.uk — MB ChB Birm. 1973 (Birmingham) DObst RCOG 1975; MRCGP 1978. Gen. Practitioner; Clin. Asst. (ENT) Banbury Hosp. Specialty: Gen. Pract.; Otolaryngol. Prev: Regist. (Med.) Whakatane Pub. Hosp. NZ; SHO (Surg.) Birm. Matern. Hosp.; Ho. Surg. Birm. Accid. Hosp.

ROWLANDS, Alison Gail Hope Lodge, 11 Poplar Road, Oxton, Birkenhead CH43 5TB Tel: 0151 652 2834 Email: cons.com@msn — MB BS Lond. 1992 (Charing Cross & Westminster London) BSc (Hons.) Lond. 1989; FRCOphth. 1997. Specialist Regist. St Paul's Eye Unit Roy. Liverp. Univ. Hosp. Specialty: Ophth. Prev: SHO (Ophth.) Birm. & Midl. Eye Centre, Kings Mill Hosp. & Kidderminster NHS Trust Hosp.

ROWLANDS, Andrew Buchan Cornhill Road, Aberdeen AB25 2ZN — MB ChB Ed. 1990; MSc Remot Health Care Robert Gordon University 1997; FRCS (A&E) Ed. 1998. Specialist Regist. A & E Med. Specialty: Accid. & Emerg. Prev: SHO A & E Med.; GP Regist.

ROWLANDS, Angela Mary Stratton Medical Centre, Hospital Road, Stratton, Bude EX23 9BP Tel: 01288 352133; Leemoor, 4 Tamor Terrace, Tavistock Road, Launceston PL15 9EU Tel: 01566 773451 Fax: 01566 777495 — MB BS Lond. 1980 (Lond. Hosp.) BSc (Hons.) Lond. 1975, MB BS 1980. Clin. Asst. in Occupat. Health, Cornw. Healthcare Trust. Prev: GP Swindon.

ROWLANDS, Ann Eleri Church Crescent Surgery, 50 Church Crescent, Finchley, London N3 1BJ Tel: 020 8346 1323 Fax: 020 8343 4026; 8 Etheldene Avenue, Muswell Hill, London N10 3QH Tel: 020 8883 4434 — MB BS Lond. 1970 (Roy. Free) MRCS Eng. LRCP Lond. 1970; DObst RCOG 1972. Prev: Ho. Surg. (Obst.) Whittington Hosp. Lond.; Ho. Phys. Eliz. G. Anderson Hosp. Lond.; Ho. Surg. Roy. Free Hosp. Lond.

ROWLANDS, Anne Kathleen (retired) 2 Brackenwood Drive, Bruntwood, Cheadle SK8 1JX Tel: 0161 491 3434 — MB ChB Manch. 1960. Prev: Clin. Med. Off. Manch. Centr. Hosp. Community Care Trust.

ROWLANDS, Professor Brian James University of Nottingham, Section of Surgery, Queen's Medical Centre, Nottingham NG7 2UH Tel: 0115 970 9245 Fax: 0115 970 9428 Email: bjr.surgery@nottingham.ac.uk — MB BS Lond. 1968 (Guy's) FRCS Eng. 1973; MD Sheff. 1978; FACS 1983; FRCSI 1988; FRCPS Glas. 1995; FRCS Ed 1995. Prof. Surg. Nottm. Univ. & Cons. Surg. Qu.'s Med. Centre and Div. GI Surg. Sci. Notts Univ Head of Sect. of Surg.; Director of Gen. Surg., Univ. Hosp. Trust, Queen's Med. Centre, Nottm. Specialty: Gen. Surg. Socs: Soc. of Acad. and Research Surg. (SARS) Pres. 2003; Chairm. RCS (Eng.) c/o the Critically Ill Pat. Working Party 1944-present; Chairm. Scientif. Comm., Ass. Surg. GB & Irel. 1997-2001. Prev: Prof. & Head of Dept. of Surg. Qu.'s Univ. of Belf.; Lect. North. Gen. Hosp. & Roy. Infirm. Sheff.; Assoc. Prof. Surg. Univ. Texas, Houston, USA.

ROWLANDS, Christopher John Anaesthetic Department, Bradford Royal Infirmary, Duckworth Lane, Bradford BD9 6RJ Tel: 01274 542200 — MB ChB Leeds 1987; DA (UK) 1993. Staff Grade Anaesth. Bradford Hosps. NHS Trust. Specialty: Anaesth.

ROWLANDS, Christopher Merlin, MBE Rowallan, 26 Uddingston Road, Bothwell, Glasgow G71 8PN Tel: 07970 309880 — MB BS Lond. 1980 (Guy's) MRCS Eng. LRCP Lond. 1979; DRCOG 1983; Dip. IMC RCS Ed. 1990; T(GP) 1991. GP Bothewell, Lanarksh.; Mem. BASICS. Specialty: Gen. Pract.; Accid. & Emerg.; Aviat. Med. Socs: MICGP; Fac. Pre Hosp. Care RCSurg. (Edin.). Prev: Emerg. Room Phys., Glagow Roy. Infirm. A & E Dept.; GP Sumburgh Shetland; Resid. Med. Off. Qu. Charlotte's Matern. Hosp. Lond.

ROWLANDS, David Bartlett Peterborough District Hospital, Thorpe Road, Peterborough PE3 6DA Tel: 01733 874000 Fax: 01733 874115; Ashfield House, Splash Lane, Castor, Peterborough PE5 7BD — MB BS 1974 (St. Bart.) MRCP (UK) 1980; MD Lond. 1987; FRCP 1995. Cons. Cardiologist, Peterborough Hospitals NHS Trust; Vis. Cardiol. Papworth Hosp. Papworth Everard Camb.; Chief Med. Adviser Pearl Assur. Company; Cons. Cardiologist, ERT (UK). Specialty: Cardiol. Socs: Brit. Cardiac Soc.; Brit. Hypertension Soc. Prev: Sen. Regist. (Med.) Mersey RHA.; Clin. Research Fell. Univ. Birm.; Hon. Regist. (Cardiol.) E. Birm. Hosp.

ROWLANDS, David Charles Department of Histopathology, New Cross Hospital, Wolverhampton WV10 0QP — BM Soton. 1982; MRCPath 1992. Cons. (Histopath.) New Cross Hosp. Wolverhampton. Specialty: Histopath. Prev: Cons. (Path.) Univ. Hosp. Birm.; Lect. (Path.) Med. Sch. Univ. Birm.; Regist. (Histopath.) Hosp. Wales Cardiff.

ROWLANDS, David Edward (retired) Plas Newydd, Penmaenmawr LL34 6RH Tel: 01492 622306 Fax: 01492 622306 — MRCS Eng. LRCP Lond. 1945 (Middlx.) DA Eng. 1951; FFA RCS Eng. 1954. Prev: Anaesth. Llandudno Gen. Hosp.

ROWLANDS, David Francis, CStJ (retired) 19 Barnlake Point, Burton, Milford Haven SA73 1PF — MB BS Lond. 1958 (St. Bart.) DObst RCOG 1960; DPH Wales 1966; MFCM 1974; MFPHM 1989. Prev: Cons. Primary Care Phys. Armed Forces Hosp. Riyadh, Saudi Arabia.

ROWLANDS, Mr David John Wirral Hospital, Arrowe Park, Upton, Wirral CH49 5PE Tel: 0151 678 5111 — MB ChB Birm. 1985; MRCOG 1990. Cons. O & G Wirral Hosp.; Hon. Clin. Lect. (Obst. & Gyn.) Univ. Liverp. Specialty: Obst. & Gyn.

ROWLANDS, Debra 44 Willowmead Drive, Prestbury, Macclesfield SK10 4DD — MB BS Newc. 1997.

ROWLANDS, Derek John The Beeches Consulting Centre, Mill Lane, Cheadle SK8 2PY Tel: 0161 491 2959 Fax: 0161 428 1589 Email: djr@djr12ecg.demon.co.uk — (Manch.) FACA; FESC; MB ChB (Hons.) Manch. 1961; FRCP Lond. 1976, M 1964; BSc (1st cl. Hons.) Manch. 1958, MD 1984; FACC 1985. p/t Hon. Cons. Cardiol. Manch. Roy. Infirm. Specialty: Cardiol. Socs: Fell. Amer. Coll. Cardiol. 1985; Brit. Cardiac Interven. Soc.; Fell.Amer.Coll Angiology 2000. Prev: MRC Trav. Fell. Mayo Clinic Rochester, Minn.; SHO (Med.) Hammersmith Hosp.; Cons. Lect. (Cardiol.) Univ. Manch.

ROWLANDS, Dorothy Ann 134 Abbeyfield Road, Sheffield S4 7AY — MB ChB Sheff. 1985.

ROWLANDS, Dorothy Mair Seymour House, Shoreham Lane, St Michael's, Tenterden TN30 6EH Tel: 01580 762967 — (Cardiff) MB BCh Wales 1966; DCH Eng. 1968. SCMO S. Kent Community NHS Trust. Specialty: Community Child Health. Prev: SHO Roy. Liverp. Childr. Hosp.; SHO Mossley Hill Hosp. Liverp.

ROWLANDS, Elwyn (retired) Flat 1, 57 Water St., Rhyl LL18 1SR — MB ChB Liverp. 1924.

ROWLANDS, Emma Celeste Dept. Medicine, 4th Floor North Block, St Thomas Hospital, Lambeth Palace Road, London SE1 7EH Tel: 020 7928 9292; 3 Lancaster Road, Uxbridge UB8 1AW Email: e.rowlands@virgin.net — MB ChB Sheff. 1992 (Sheffield) FRCOphth 1998. Research Fell., Oprthalmology, St Thomas, Lond. Specialty: Ophth.

ROWLANDS, Frances Mary 37 Redwood, Westhoughton, Bolton BL5 2RU — MB ChB Leic. 1987.

ROWLANDS, Gillian Clare 3 Kippen Drive, Clarkston, Glasgow G76 8JG Tel: 0141 644 2725 — MB ChB Aberd. 1994. GP Asst. Position ChristCh., New Zealand; GP Locum. Specialty: Gen. Pract. Socs: MRCGP. Prev: Trainee GP Kemnay Surg. Kemnay; Trainee GP Gt. West. Rd. Med. Gp., 327 Gt. W. Rd., Aberd.; SHO (A & E) Aberd. Roy. Infirm.

ROWLANDS, Gillian Patricia Acorn Practice Group, St Johns Health Centre, Oak Lane, Twickenham TW1 3PH Tel: 020 8891 0073 Fax: 020 8744 0060 — MB BS Lond. 1984; MRCP (UK) 1987; DRCOG 1989; MRCGP 1990.

ROWLANDS, Gwyn (retired) 1A Boxwell Road, Berkhamsted HP4 3ET Tel: 01442 863666 — MRCS Eng. LRCP Lond. 1951 (Lond. Hosp.) DA Eng. 1955; DObst RCOG 1959; FFPM 1989. Prev: Med. Adviser Wellcome Foundat. Ltd. Lond.

ROWLANDS, Helen Elizabeth — MB BS Lond. 1997; MRCPCH UK 2002. PICU SpR Birm. Childrens Hosp. Specialty: Paediat.

ROWLANDS, Henry Walter David Scranton House, Pantyffynnon, Ammanford SA18 3HN — MB BS Lond. 1983; MRCOG 1988; MRCGP 1989.

ROWLANDS, Idris Gwynn Lluest, Llangathen, Carmarthen SA32 8QD Tel: 015584 105 — MB BS Lond. 1969; MRCOG 1974; MRCGP 1980. GP Llandeilo, Dyfed. Prev: Regist. (Obst.) Univ. Hosp. Wales Cardiff; SHO (Endocrine), (Gyn.) & (Obst.) Jessop Hosp. Wom. Sheff.

ROWLANDS, Jennifer Louise 531 Blenheim Road, Kingswinford DY6 8SH — MB BS Lond. 1997.

ROWLANDS, John Kendrew Westway Medical Centre, Westway, Maghull, Liverpool L31 0DJ Tel: 0151 526 1121 Fax: 0151 531 2631 — MB BS Durh. 1963 (Newc.) MRCGP 1971. Hosp. Practitioner. Ashworth Hosp. Maghull. Prev: Demonst. (Path.) & SHO (Dermat.) Univ. Newc.; Lect. (Gen. Pract.) Guy's Hosp. Lond.

ROWLANDS, Mark Pendre Surgery, Coleshill Street, Holywell CH8 7RS Tel: 01352 712029 Fax: 01352 712751; Groes Faen, Babell, Holywell CH8 8QB — MB ChB Manch. 1980; DRCOG 1982; MRCGP 1984; DCH RCP Lond. 1984. Prev: Trainee GP Clwyd VTS; Clin. Med. Off. (Child Health) Clwyd HA.

ROWLANDS, Martin 6 Broadoak Road, Bramhall, Stockport SK7 3BW — MB BS Lond. 1980; MRCP (UK) 1984; MRCPath. 1989. Sen. Regist. (Haemat.) N. West. RHA. Specialty: Haematology. Prev: Regist. (Haemat.) Leic. Roy. Infirm.; SHO (Path.) Withington Hosp. Manch.

ROWLANDS, Martin 4 Hunts Lane, Stockton Heath, Warrington WA4 2DT — MB ChB Sheff. 1998; MB ChB Sheff 1998.

ROWLANDS, Mary Helena 10 Silverdale Close, Huyton, Liverpool L36 5YJ — MB ChB Dundee 1977; Cert JCC Lond. 1979; MRCPsych 1984. Med. Off. Home Off. Bristol. Socs: Guild Catholic Doctors.

ROWLANDS, Michael Philip William (retired) Lynwood, Graig Isaf, Mountain Ash CF45 3RD Tel: 01443 474287 — MB BCh Wales 1961 (Welsh Nat. Sch. of Med.) Prev: Dir. of Social Servs. Merthyr Tydfil Co. Boro.

ROWLANDS, Michael William Denton Sturt Priory Hospital, Walton-on-the-Hill, Tadworth KT20 7RQ Tel: 01737 814488 Fax: 01737 813926; 13 White Beam Way, Tadworth KT20 5DL Tel: 01737 812211 Fax: 01737 819747 Email: trudymoon@compuserve.com — MB ChB Birm. 1979; MRCPsych 1984. Staff Cons. Sturt Priory Hosp. Tadworth. Specialty: Gen. Psychiat. Prev: Cons. Psychiat. E. Surrey; Lect. (Psychol. Med.) St. Bart. Hosp. Lond.; Regist. Rotat. (Psychiat.) St. Geo. Hosp. & Centr. Birm. HA.

ROWLANDS, Molly Patricia (retired) The Gate House, Alderley, Wotton-under-Edge GL12 7QT Tel: 01453 844804 — (St. Mary's) MB BS Lond. 1968. Prev: GP Sen. Partner Cipping Surg.

ROWLANDS, Patricia Rochdale Healthcare NHS Trust, Rochdale Infirmary, Whitehall St., Rochdale OL12 0NB Tel: 01706 377777 Fax: 01706 755347; Calliard's House, Smithybridge Road, Littleborough OL15 8QF — MB ChB Leic. 1982. Assoc. Specialist (A & E Med.); Dep. Police Surg. Gtr. Manch. Police; Prison Med. Off. HMP Buckley Hall Rochdale. Specialty: Accid. & Emerg.; Gen. Pract. Prev: GP Bolton; SHO (A & E) Rochdale Infirm., SHO (Psychiat.) Oldham Roy. Infirm.

ROWLANDS, Peter Christopher Radiology Department, Royal Liverpool Hospital, Prescot St., Liverpool L7 8XP Tel: 0151 706 2733 Fax: 0151 706 5799 — BM BS Nottm. 1981; MRCP (UK) 1985; FRCR 1989. Cons. Radiol. Roy. Liverp. Hosp. Specialty: Radiol. Prev: Sen. Regist. (Radiol.) St. Mary's Hosp. Lond.; Regist. (Med.) Hackney Hosp. Lond.; SHO (Med.) Middlesbrough Hosp. Gp.

ROWLANDS, Peter Julian Cwmbran Village Surgery, Victoria Street, Cwmbran NP44 3JS Tel: 01633 871177 Fax: 01633 860234; Hill View, Michaelston-y-Fedw, Cardiff CF3 6XS — MB BCh Wales 1984; MRCGP 1989.

ROWLANDS, Philip (retired) Knowsley, Heights Lane, Rochdale OL12 0PZ Tel: 01706 644050 — (Cardiff) MB BCh Wales 1954; BSc Wales 1954; DCH Eng. 1965; MRCP Ed. 1968. Prev: GP Rochdale.

ROWLANDS, Richard Gareth 48 Sandtoft Road, Charlton, London SE7 7LR — MB ChB Manch. 1995; MRCS 1999; DLO 2002. Specialist Registrar Otolaryngology, North Thames.

ROWLANDS, Robert Paul 42 St Mary's Gate, Chesterfield S44 1bl — MB BS Newc. 1987 (Newcastle University) MRCPsych 1991.

Cons., Gen.Adult Psychiat., CHCS Chesterfield, Derbysh.. Specialty: Gen. Psychiat.

ROWLANDS, Roger John (retired) The Gate House, Alderley, Wotton-under-Edge GL12 7QT Tel: 01453 844804 — (St. Mary's) MB BS Lond. 1968; MRCS Eng. LRCP Lond. 1968; DObst RCOG 1971; MBAcA 1995; LLB (Hons.) Bristol 1995; DMed Acupunc. 1997. Prev: GP Wotton-under-Edge.

ROWLANDS, Samuel Crosfield Austy Manor, Wootton Wawen, Solihull B95 6BX Tel: 01564 793225 Fax: 01564 794935; 3 Dennis Green, Gamlingay, Sandy SG19 3LQ Tel: 01767 651897 — MB BS Lond. 1974 (Lond. Hosp.) DRCOG 1976; DCH Eng. 1978; MRCGP 1980; MFFP 1993; MD Lond. 1999. Clin. Dir. Brit. Pregnancy Advis. Serv. Specialty: Family Plann. & Reproduc. Health. Socs: Roy. Soc. Med. (Pres. Sexual Health & Reproduc. Med. Sect.). Prev: Med. Dir. EPIC Lond.; Research Asst. Margt. Pyke Centre Lond.; Trainee GP Redhill VTS.

ROWLANDS, Stephen Charles Bradford Road Medical Centre, 60 Bradford Road, Trowbridge BA14 9AR Tel: 01225 754255 Fax: 01225 774391 — MRCS Eng. LRCP Lond. 1977.

ROWLANDS, Stephen Gerent Brynmeddyg Surgery, Llanybydder SA40 9RN Tel: 01570 480244 Fax: 01570 481174 Email: stephen.rowlands@gp-w92045.wales.nhs.uk — BM BCh Oxf. 1974 (Oxford) MRCGP 1978; DRCOG 1978. GP Princip. Llanbydder; Clin. Asst. (Dermat.) W. Wales Hosp. Carmarthan. Specialty: Gen. Pract.; Dermat.

ROWLANDS, Thomas Kinya 36 Manadon Drive, Plymouth PL5 3DJ — MB ChB Manch. 1997.

ROWLANDSON, George Forrester, Bowman and Rowlandson, Berry Lane Medical Centre, Berry Lane, Preston PR3 3JJ Tel: 01772 783021 Fax: 01772 785809; Lower Cockhill Farm, Hothersll Lane, Longridge, Preston PR3 2XB — BM BS Nottm. 1984; BMedSci Nottm. 1982; DCH RCP Lond. 1987; MRCGP 1988; DRCOG 1988; Cert. Family Plann. JCC 1988.

ROWLATT, Basil (retired) The Old Vicarage, Healey, Masham, Ripon HG4 — MB BS Lond. 1941 (Guy's) MRCS Eng. LRCP Lond. 1941. Prev: Ho. Phys. Guy's Hosp.

ROWLATT, Charles (retired) 10 Hampstead Hill Gardens, London NW3 2PL Tel: 020 7435 1285 — (St. Thos.) MA, BM BCh Oxf. 1960; PhD Lond. 1971. Prev: Staff Scientist Imperial Cancer Research Fund Lond.

ROWLATT, Richard John (retired) 2 Greenbank, Ulverston LA12 7HA Tel: 01229 582536 Email: glowlamps@aol.com — (St. Thos.) MB BS Lond. 1966; MRCP (UK) 1970; DCH Eng. 1970; FRCP Lond. 1990; FRCPCH 1996. Prev: Cons. Paediat. S. Cumbria HA Barrow in Furness.

ROWLES, Mr John Marshall Derby Royal Infirmary NHS Trust, London Road, Derby DE1 2QY Tel: 01332 347141; East Midlands Nuffield Hospital, Rykneld Road, Littleover, Derby DE23 7SN Tel: 01332 517891 — BM BS Nottm. 1984; DM Nottm. 1993, BMedSci. 1982; FRCS Eng. 1988; FRCS (Orth.) 1995. Cons. Orthop. & Trauma Surg. Derbysh. Roy. Infirm. NHS Trust. Specialty: Orthop. Prev: Clin. Research Fell. Nottm., Leicester, Derby & Belf. Study Gp.

ROWLES, Nicola Horkstow Hall, Horkstow, Barton-upon-Humber DN18 6BE — MB BS Lond. 1987. Socs: BMA.

ROWLES, Susannah Victoria 11 Tivoli Road, Cheltenham GL50 2TD Tel: 0161 225 9689 — MB BS Lond. 1991 (Char. Cross & Westm.) MRCP. Specialist Regist.(Endocrinology) Manch. Specialty: Diabetes; Endocrinol.; Gen. Med.

ROWLEY, Christine 16 Tyndall House, Southmead Hospital, Southmead Road, Westbury-on-Trym, Bristol BS10 5NB; 90 Howard Road, Westbury Park, Bristol BS6 7UY — BM Soton. 1993.

ROWLEY, Professor David Ian Department of Orthopaedic & Trauma Surgery, University of Dundee, Ninewells Hospital, Dundee DD1 9SY Tel: 01382 425746 Fax: 01382 496200; Marclann Cottage, Kellie Castle, Arbroath DD11 2PB Tel: 01241 876466 Fax: 01241 431894 — MB ChB Aberd. 1976; BMedBiol Aberd. 1973; FRCS Ed. 1980; MD Sheff. 1986; FRCS Glas. 1992; FRCS England 1998. Prof. Orthop. & Trauma Surg. Univ. Dundee; Clin. Director Taysdide Univ. Hosps. Trust. Specialty: Orthop. Socs: Roy. Coll. Surg. Prev: Sen. Lect. (Orthop.) Univ. Manch.; Lect. (Orthop. Surg.) Univ. Sheff.; Sen. Lect. (Orthop. Mech.) Univ. Salford.

ROWLEY, Dorothy Elizabeth Margaret (retired) Greystead, South Road, Ashley Heath, Hale, Altrincham WA14 3HT — MB ChB Liverp. 1946; DObst RCOG 1948. Prev: SCMO Manch. AHA (T).

ROWLEY, Eric 37 Princess Way, Fleetwood FY7 8AE — MB ChB Manch. 1955. Prev: Regist. (Med.) & SHO (Neurosurg.) Preston Roy. Infirm.; Flight Lt. RAF Med. Br.

ROWLEY, Hungerford Aboyne Thomas The Limes Medical Centre, 65 Leicester Road, Narborough, Leicester LE19 2DU Tel: 0116 284 1347 Fax: 0116 275 2447; 31 Springfield Road, Leicester LE2 3BB Tel: 0116 270 5149 — MB ChB Leic. 1986; DRCOG 1990; MRCGP 1995. Specialty: Gen. Med.

ROWLEY, Jean (retired) — MB ChB Manch. 1956; DCH Eng. 1959. Prev: Med. Adviser Benefits Agency DSS.

ROWLEY, John Martin King's Mill Hospital, Mansfield Road, Sutton-in-Ashfield NG17 4JL Tel: 01623 622515 Email: john.rowley@sth-tr.nhs.uk — MB Camb. 1976; MA Camb. 1979, BA 1972, BChir 1975; MRCP (UK) 1977. Cons. Phys./Cardiol. Kings Mill Centre, Mansfield. Specialty: Cardiol. Socs: Brit. Cardiac Soc. Prev: Cons. Phys./Cardiol. Mansfield Hosps.; Lect. Dept. Med. Univ. Nottm.

ROWLEY, Kathryn Helen Mary Department of Oncology, Singleton Hospital, Sketty, Swansea SA2 8QA Tel: 01792 285455 Fax: 01792 285455 — MB BCh Wales 1985 (University of Wales College of Medicine) BSc (Med. Biochem.) Wales 1982; MRCP (UK) 1988; FRCR (Clin. Oncol.) 1994. Cons., Clincal Oncol., Swansea NHS Trust. Specialty: Oncol.; Radiother. Socs: Brit. Oncol. Assoc.; BMA-Brit. Med. Assoc.; Roy. Soc. Med. Prev: Research Fell. (Oncol.) Cancer Research Wales; Hon. Sen. Regist. Velindre Hosp. Cardiff; Regist. & SHO (Clin. Oncol.) Velindre Hosp. Cardiff.

ROWLEY, Lester John (retired) Heronswood, The Drive, Wonersh, Guildford GU5 0QW — MB BChir Camb. 1944 (Westminster)

ROWLEY, Megan Ruth Haematology Department, Kingston Hospital, Galsworthy Road, Kingston upon Thames KT2 7QB Tel: 020 8934 2706 Fax: 020 8934 3245 — MB BS Lond. 1982 (Guy's Hosp. Med. Sch.) MRCP (UK) 1985; MRCPath 1990; FRCP 1997; FRCPath 1998. Cons. Haematologist Qu. Mary's Univ. Hosp. Lond. & Kingston Hosp.; Cons. Haemat. Kingston Hosp.; Hon. Cons. Haemat. St Geo. Hosp. Specialty: Haematology. Socs: Brit. Soc. Haemat.; Assn. Clin. Path; Brit. Blood Transfus. Soc. Prev: Sen. Regist. (Haemat.) St. Geo. Hosp. Lond.; SHO Roy. Marsden Hosp. Sutton, William Harvey Hosp. Ashford & Guy's Hosp. Lond.

ROWLEY, Norman Clive (retired) The Stone House, College Road, Denstone, Uttoxeter ST14 5HR Tel: 01889 591468 — MB BChir Camb. 1971 (Camb. & Roy. Lond. Hosp.) MB Camb. 1971, Bchir,camb, 1970; MA Camb. 1971. Prev: Sen. Partner; Drs Rowley, Elsdon & Rees, Staffs.

ROWLEY, Peter David The Surgery, 18 Thurloe Street, London SW7 2SU Tel: 020 7225 2424 Fax: 020 7225 1874; 148 Felsham Road, London SW15 1DP Email: peterrowley@compuserve.com — MB BS Lond. 1979; DRCOG 1988; Dip. Pract. Dermat. Wales 1990. GP Lond. Prev: SHO (O & G) Louise Margt. Hosp. Aldershot; Ho. Phys. PeterBoro. Dist. Hosp.; Maj. RAMC.

ROWLEY JONES, David SmithKline Beecham, SB House, Great West Road, Brentford TW8 9 Tel: 020 8560 5151 — MB BChir Camb. 1972; MA, MB Camb. 1972, BChir 1971; MRCP (UK) 1977; MFPM 1990. Dir. Worldwide Med. Affairs SmithKline Beecham Brentford. Specialty: Pharmaceutical Medicine. Prev: SHO (Gen. Med.) Univ. Hosp. Wales Cardiff; Ho. Phys. (Gen. Med.) Nevill Hall Hosp. Abergavenny; Ho. Surg. (Orthop. & Traum.) Guy's Hosp. Lond.

ROWLING, Andrew James 102 Silvester Road, Waterlooville PO8 8TS — MB BCh Wales 1995.

ROWLING, Dorothy Estyn Hillcrest, Blebo Craigs, Cupar KY15 5UQ Tel: 0133 485646 — MB ChB Leeds 1938; FRCS Ed. 1949.

ROWLING, Mr John Thompson 14 Rutland Park, Sheffield S10 2PB Tel: 0114 266 4982 — MB BChir Camb. 1946 (Camb. & Leeds) MRCS Eng. LRCP Lond. 1945; FRCS Eng. 1952; MChir MA 1959; BA (Nat. Sc. Trip. Cl. II) Camb. 1942, MD 1961. Hon. Cons. Surg. Roy. Hallamsh. Hosp. Sheff. Specialty: Gen. Surg.

ROWNEY, David Antony 23 Gardners Crescent, Edinburgh EH3 8DE Tel: 0131 622 4621 — MB ChB Ed. 1990; FRCA 1996. Specialist Regist. (Anaesth.) Edin. Specialty: Anaesth.

ROWNEY, James — MB BCh BAO Belf. 1988 (Belfast) DRCOG 1991; MRCGP 1993.

ROWNEY, William Robert Finaghy Health Centre, 13-25 Finaghy Road South, Belfast BT10 0BX Tel: 028 9062 8211; Dunluce Health

Centre, Belfast BT9 7HR Tel: 01232 204245 Fax: 01232 312306 — MB BCh BAO Belf. 1961 (Qu. Univ. Belf.) DObst RCOG 1963; FRCGP 1988, M 1968; Cert. Family Plann. JCC 1976.

ROWNTREE, Barbara Mary (retired) Riverdale Cottage, West St, Soberton, Southampton SO32 3PL Tel: 01489 877373 — MRCS Eng. LRCP Lond. 1940. Prev: Med. Off. Stud. Health Serv. Univ. Soton.

ROWNTREE, Brenda Maureen (retired) Comp Corner Cottage, Borough Green, Sevenoaks TN15 8QT Tel: 01732 884151 — MB BS Durh. 1947; DObst RCOG 1949; DFFP 1993. Prev: Clin. Med. Off. Family Plann. Serv. Maidstone, Medway & Gravesham HAs.

ROWNTREE, Catherine 75 Lee Road, Blackheath, London SE3 9EN Tel: 020 8852 5622 Fax: 020 8318 2576 — MB Camb. 1972; BChir 1971; DMRD Eng. 1975; FRCR 1977. Cons. Radiol. Newham Gen. Hosp. Specialty: Radiol. Prev: Sen. Regist. Univ. Coll. Hosp. Lond. & Hosp. Sick Childr. Gt. Ormond St. Lond.; Regist. St. Bart. Hosp. Lond.

ROWNTREE, Mr Mark 75 Lee Road, Blackheath, London SE3 9EN — MB BS Lond. 1971; MB Camb. 1972, BChir 1971; FRCS Eng. 1976; FRCS Ed. 1976. Cons. Orthop. Surg. Qu. Mary's Hosp. Sidcup. Specialty: Orthop. Prev: Sen. Regist. St. Bart. Hosp. Lond.; Sen. Regist. Hosp. Sick Childr. Lond.; Sen. Regist. Roy. Nat. Orthop. Hosp. Lond.

ROWNTREE, Mr Tom (retired) Riverdale Cottage, West St, Soberton, Southampton SO32 3PL Tel: 01489 877373 — MB BChir Camb. 1941 (Rome, Camb. & St. Bart.) MRCS Eng. LRCP Lond. 1940; MS Lond. 1950, MB BS 1941; FRCS Eng. 1942; BA (Hons.) Camb. 1937, MChir 1958. Prev: Cons. Surg. Soton. & SW Hants. Health Dist. (T).

ROWSE, Mr Alistair David Russells Hall Hospital, Dudley DY1 2HQ Tel: 01384 244201 Fax: 01384 244202; 18 Phoenix Green, Edgbaston, Birmingham B15 3NR Tel: 0121 684 5945 — MB ChB Birm. 1969; MSc Birm. 1974, BSc 1966; FRCS Eng. 1976. Cons. Urol. Russells Hall Hosp. W. Midl. Specialty: Urol.

ROWSE, Elizabeth Anne (retired) Sunnyhill, Forster Road, Salcombe TQ8 9EB — MB BS Durh. 1964; MRCP (UK) 1976. Prev: Sen. Med. Adviser DVLA Swansea.

ROWSE, Nicholas James 5 Shakesspear Road, Walthamstow, London E17 6AS — MB BS Lond. 1979; DRCOG 1981.

ROWSELL, Mr Anthony Richard Department of Plastic Surgery, Guy's Hospital, St Thomas St., London SE1 9RT; 41 Leckford Road, Oxford OX2 6HY — MB BS Lond. 1968; FRCS Eng. 1975; FRACS (Plast Surg.) 1980; DPhil Oxf. 1988. Cons. Plastic Surg. Guy's Hosp. Lond. Specialty: Plastic Surg. Prev: Sen. Regist. (Plastic Surg.) Radcliffe Infirm. Oxf.; Cons. Plastic Surg. P. Henry's Hosp. Melbourne, Australia.

ROWSELL, Rhiannon Bracher AstraZeneca UK Ltd, Horizon Place, 600 Capability Green, Luton LU1 3LU Tel: 01582 836 000 — MB BCh Wales 1979; MRCP (UK) 1983; Dip Pharm. Med. RCP (UK) 1986; FFPM RCP (UK) 1994, M 1989. Med. & Regulatory Affairs Dir. AstraZeneca. Specialty: Pharmaceutical Medicine. Socs: FFPM. Prev: Med. Dir. Amersham Internat. plc; Dir. Clin. Investig. SmithKline Beecham Pharmaceut. Harlow, Essex; Regist. (Dermat.) Univ. Hosp. Wales.

ROWSON, Mr John Edmund Maxillofacial Unit, Queens Medical Centre, Derby Road, Nottingham NG7 2UH Tel: 0115 924 9924 Ext: 48916 Email: john.rowson@mail.qmcuh-tr.trent.nhs.uk — BM BS Nottm. 1986 (Nottm. Univ.) BDS Liverp. 1978; BMedSci Nottm. 1984; FDS RCS Eng. 1990; FRCS Ed. 1991. Cons. Maxillofacial Surg., Qu. Med. Centre, Nottm.; Asst. Med. Director, Surgic. Divisio, Qu. Med. Centre, Nottm.; Cons. Cleft Surg., Regional Cleft Lip & Palate Centre, Nottm. Specialty: Oral & Maxillofacial Surg. Special Interest: Cleft lip & Palate; Facial Deformity; Trauma Surg. of the face. Socs: Brit. Assn. Oral & Maxillofacial Surg.s; Europ. Assn. of Crniomaxillo Facial Surg.; BMA.

ROWSON, Mr Neil James 33 Edna Street, London SW11 3DP — MB ChB Leeds 1982; DO RCS Eng. 1988; FCOphth 1989; FRCS Glas. 1989; FRCOphth 1993. Sen. Regist. (Ophth.) Wolverhampton, Birm. & Stoke-on-Trent Hosps. Specialty: Ophth. Prev: Resid. Surg. Off. Moorfields Eye Hosp. Lond.

ROWTON-LEE, Martyn Addington Bournemouth Tel: 01202 769210 — MA, BM BCh Oxf. 1960 (Univ. Coll. Hosp.) DPM Eng. 1970; FRCPsych 1986, M 1973. Specialty: Gen. Psychiat. Prev: Cas. Surg. Off. Univ. Coll. Hosp. Lond.; Squadron Med. Off. 29th Escort Squadron; Med. Off. RN Sch. Instruc. Diving, H.M.S. Vernon, Portsmouth.

ROXBURGH, Andrew Cathcart Amherst Medical Practice, 21 St Botolphs Road, Sevenoaks TN13 3AQ Tel: 01732 459255 Fax: 01732 450751; Littlecroft, Woodland Rise, Sevenoaks TN15 0HY Tel: 01732 761159 — MB BS Lond. 1984; MA Camb. 1985. Clin. Asst. (Neuro-Rehabil.). Prev: Regist. (Med.) St. Chas. Hosp. Lond.; SHO (Renal Med.) St. Thos. Hosp. Lond.; SHO (Clin. Oncol.) Hammersmith Hosp. Lond.

ROXBURGH, Annie May (retired) c/o Barclays Bank, 1 Brompton Road, London SW1 — MB ChB Ed. 1920; DPH Ed. 1921.

ROXBURGH, Christine Macleod Campbell Mauve Practice, Drumhar Health Centre, North Methven Street, Perth PH1 5PD Tel: 01738 622421 Fax: 01738 444077 — MB ChB Glas. 1974; DObst RCOG 1976.

ROXBURGH, David Alexander The Snypes, Greenloaning, Dunblane FK15 0LZ Tel: 01786 880378 — MB ChB Ed. 1964; DMRD Eng. 1970; FRCR 1977. Cons. Radiol. Falkirk & Dist. Roy. Infirm. NHS Trust. Specialty: Radiol. Prev: Cons. Radiol. RAF.

ROXBURGH, Ian Oliphant (retired) Coverpoint, Goldsithney, Penzance TR20 9LB Tel: 01736 710635 — (Glas.) MB ChB Glas. 1952. Prev: SHO O & G Princess Beatrice Hosp. Lond.

ROXBURGH, Mr James Cathcart Department of Cardiothoracic Surgery, St Thomas Hospital, Lambeth Palace Road, London SE1 7EH Tel: 020 7928 9292 Fax: 020 7922 8005 Email: james.roxburgh@gstt.sthames.nhs.uk — (Middlesex Hospital, University of London) MB BS Lond. 1981; FRCS Eng. 1985; MS Lond. 1990; FRCS (Cth) 1992. Cons. (Cardiothoracic Surg.) St. Thos. Hosp. Lond. Specialty: Cardiothoracic Surg. Socs: Fell. Roy. Soc. Med. (Counc. Mem. of Cardiothoracic Sect.); Soc. Cardiothoracic Surg. GB & Irel. (Exec. Mem.); Surgic. Subspeciality Comm. Centr. Cons.s, BMA. Prev: Regist. (Cardiothoracic Surg.) Harefield & St. Thos. Hosp. Lond.; Sen. Regist. (Cardiothoracic Surg.) Guys & St. Thos. Hosp. Lond.; Research Fell. Middlx. Hosp. Lond.

ROXBURGH, Richard Hugh Stephen Richards 25 Birch Polygon, Rusholme, Manchester M14 5HX — MB ChB Otago 1989.

ROXBURGH, Mr Robert Alexander (retired) 6 The Court, Dunsford, Exeter EX6 7DD Tel: 01674 252251 — MB BChir Camb. 1953 (Camb. & St. Bart.) BA (Hons.) Camb. 1950; FRCS Ed. 1960; FRCS Eng. 1960; MChir Camb. 1965; MA Camb. 1965. Prev: Hon. Cons. Surg. Broomfield Hosp. Chelmsford.

ROXBURGH, Ronald Cathcart (retired) Wiggenhall House, Wiggenhall St Mary, King's Lynn PE34 3EH Tel: 01553 617333 — MB BChir Camb. 1947 (Camb. & St. Bart.) FRCP CH; MRCS Eng. LRCP Lond. 1944; DCH Eng. 1949; FRCP Lond. 1972, M 1950; MA Camb. 1961, BA (Hons.) 1942, MD 1954. Prev: Cons. Paediat. King's Lynn Dist. Gen. Hosp. & N. Cambs. Hosp. Wisbech.

ROXBURGH, Mr Stuart Thomas Dalrymple 4 Craigie Knowes Avenue, Perth PH2 0DL Tel: 01738 643347 Email: stuart.roxburgh@virgin.net — MB ChB Glas. 1974 (Glagow) FRCS Ed. 1979; FRCOphth 1989. Cons. Ophth. Tayside HB; Hon. Sen. Lect. in Ophth. Dundee Univ. Specialty: Ophth.

ROXBY, Elaine Marjory Arran Surgery, 40 Admiral Street, Glasgow G41 1HU Tel: 0141 429 2626 Fax: 0141 429 2331 — MB ChB Glas. 1971.

ROXBY, Morven (retired) Bollin Chase, Willowmead Drive, Prestbury, Macclesfield SK10 4BU Tel: 01625 829432 — MB ChB Ed. 1965; DPH Glas. 1971; MFCM 1974; FFCM 1988; FFPHM 1989. Cons. Pub. Health Med. W. Pennine HA. Prev: Dir. & Cons. Pub. Health Tameside & Glossop HA.

ROY, Alistair Ian Department of Anaesthesia, Sunderland Royal Hospital, Kayll Road, Sunderland SR4 7TP Tel: 0191 565 6256; 15 Elsdon Road, Gosforth, Newcastle upon Tyne NE3 1HY Tel: 0191 213 2877 — MB ChB Dundee 1991; BSc (Hons.) Med. Microbiol. Dund 1986. Cons. Anaesth. & Intens. Care, Sunderland Roy. Hosp. Specialty: Intens. Care; Anaesth. Prev: SHO (Anaesth.) S. Cleveland Acute Hosps. NHS Trust Middlesbrough.; Specialist Regist. (Anaesth.)Roy. Vict. Infirm., Newc. upon Tyne.

ROY, Arun Bewbush Medical Centre, Bewbush Place, Bewbush, Crawley RH11 8XT Tel: 01293 519420 — MB BS Calcutta 1961. GP Crawley, W. Sussex.

ROY, Ashok Brian Oliver Centre, Brooklands, Coleshill Road Marston Green, Birmingham B37 7HL Tel: 0121 329 4927 Fax: 0121 779 4695 Email: ashok.roy@nw-pct.nhs.uk — MB BS Madras

1978 (Cristian Medical College, Vellore, India) DPM Madras 1981; MRCPsych 1985; MA Wales 1992; FRCPsych 1998. Cons.(Psychiat.) N. Warks. PCT & S. Birm. PCT; Med. Dir. N. Warks. PCT; Sen. Clin. Lect. (Psychiat.) Birm. Univ. Specialty: Ment. Health. Prev: Sen. Regist. (Ment. Handicap) W. Midl. RHA; Regist. (Psychiat.) S. Derbysh. HA.

ROY, Asoke Haematology Department, Basingstoke District Hospital, Aldermaston Road, Basingstoke RG24 9NA Tel: 01256 473202 — MB BS Calcutta 1976; MD Chandigarh 1978. Specialty: Haematology.

ROY, Barbara Fulton Elm Hayes Surgery, High Street, Paulton, Bristol BS39 7QJ Tel: 01761 413155 Fax: 01761 410573; 1 Sleight View, Bloomfield Road, Timsbury, Bath BA2 0LL — MB ChB Dundee 1980; DRCOG 1982; MRCGP 1984. Specialty: Disabil. Med.; Homeop. Med.

ROY, Bijon Kumar St. Margaret's Hospital, Epping CM16 6TN Tel: 01378 561666; Laurels, Kendal Avenue, Epping CM16 4PL — MB BS Calcutta 1957 (Calcutta Nat. Med. Coll.) DCH Eng. 1965; FRCPI 1979, M 1976; Fell. Internat. Coll. Angiol. 1978. Cons. Phys. For the Elderly St. Margt. Hosp. Epping. Specialty: Care of the Elderly. Socs: BMA. Prev: Sen. Regist. S. West. RHA; Regist. (Med. & Paediat.) I. of Man Health Auth.; Regist. (Med.) Liverp. RHB.

ROY, Birajananda 6 Seathwaite Close, Liverpool L23 6WD — MB BS Dibrugarh 1971.

ROY, Chandra Has The Bridge Street Centre, Foundry Bridge, Abertillery NP13 1BQ Tel: 01495 322635 Fax: 01495 322621 — MB BS Patna 1974; MS Patna 1979. Specialty: Gen. Pract.

***ROY, Chandrima** 7 Moorcroft Road, Fulwood, Sheffield S10 4GS Tel: 0114 230 9188 — MB ChB Leeds 1998; BSc. Hon Pathological Sciences 1995. PRHO Gen. Med. Halifax Gen. Hosp. Halifax. Specialty: Gen. Med. Prev: PRHO Gen. Surg. Airedale Gen. Hosp. Keighley.

ROY, Christopher William — MB ChB Glas. 1975; DRCOG 1977; MRCP (UK) 1980. Cons. Rehabil. Med. S. Glas. Uni. Hosp. NHS Trust; Hon.Clin.Sen.Lect. Uni Glasg. Specialty: Rehabil. Med. Socs: Brit. Soc. Rehabil. Med.; Soc. Research. Rehabil.; Scott. Seating & Wheelchair Gp.. Prev: Sen. Lect. (Rehabil. Med.) Wellington Sch. Med. Univ. Otago, NZ.; Hon. Sen. Research Fell. Univ.Glasg.

ROY, David Charles Kirkhall Surgery, 4 Alexandra Avenue, Prestwick KA9 1AW Tel: 01292 476626 Fax: 01292 678022; 17 Duart Avenue, Prestwick KA9 1NA — MB ChB Glas. 1977; MRCGP 1981.

ROY, David Henry South London and Maudsley NHS Trust, 9th Floor, Tower Building, 11 York Road, London SE1 7NX Tel: 020 7919 2415 Email: david.roy@slam.nhs.uk.

ROY, Diane Helen 6 Sween Avenue, Braehead, Cathcart, Glasgow G44 3PD — MB ChB Dundee 1987.

ROY, Dinah Venetia The Surgery, Oxford Road, Spennymoor DL16 6BQ Tel: 01388 815081 Fax: 01388 815100 — MB BChir Camb. 1984; MA Camb. 1986, BA 1981; DA (UK) 1985; MRCGP 1989; DRCOG 1989; FRCGP 1997. GP Spennymoor, Co Durh.; Chairm. Professional Executive Committee, Sedgefeild PCT. Specialty: Gen. Pract. Socs: BMA; Roy. Coll. GPs; Hon. Treasurer N. of Eng. Fac. RCGP. Prev: GP Coxhoe, Co. Durh.; Trainee GP Dunstable VTS.

ROY, Dipak — MB BS Calcutta 1966 (NRS Medical College, Calcutta, India) Gen. Practitioner.

ROY, Dipak Kumar 4 Woodside Road, Walsall WS5 3LS — MB BS Lond. 1992.

ROY, Elizabeth Helen 363 Jamaica Street, London E1 3HU — MB BS Lond. 1998; MB BS Lond 1998.

ROY, Gwynneth Aileen 17 Copse Close, Oadby, Leicester LE2 4FD Tel: 0116 271 6429 — MB ChB Sheff. 1961; MB ChB (Hons.) Sheff. 1961; DObst RCOG 1963; DPH Bristol 1964. Specialty: Community Child Health. Prev: SCMO Leics. HA; Asst. MOH Doncaster & Lond. Boro. Barnet.

ROY, Hermione — MB ChB Leic. 1993.

ROY, Hiren 912 Walsall Road, Birmingham B42 1TG Tel: 0121 357 1250; 117A Harley Street, London W1 — MRCS Eng. LRCP Lond. 1942 (Guy's) MSc 1935, BSc 1933. Socs: BMA & Brit. Tuberc. Assn. Prev: Sen. Med. Off. & 1st Asst. to Med. Dir., Preston Hall, Maidstone; Ho. Phys. St. John's Hosp. Lewisham; Asst. Med. Off. St. Giles' Hosp. Camberwell.

ROY, Hiresh Lal High Street Surgery, 1st Floor, 97-101 High Street, Fort William PH33 6DG Tel: 01397 703773 Fax: 01397 701068; 20 Zetland Avenue, Upper Achintore, Fort William PH33 6LL Tel: 01397 705188 — MB BS Dibrugarh 1967 (Assam Med. Coll.) MS (Gen. Surg.) Calcutta 1971; Cert. Family Plann. JCC 1982; MFHom 1983. GP Princip. Specialty: Homeop. Med.; Gen. Surg.; Family Plann. & Reproduc. Health. Socs: Fac. Homoeop. Prev: Regist. (Gen. Surg.) Dunoon Gen. Hosp. W. Kent Gen. hosp; Hosp. Pract. (Gen. Surg.) Belford Hosp. Fort William; SHO (O & G) Inverclyde Roy. Infirm. Greenock.

ROY, Ian Gordon Briarswood, West Looe Hill, Looe PL13 2HW — MB BS Lond. 1985.

ROY, Ian Leslie (retired) 16 Howard Place, Carlisle CA1 1HR Tel: 01228 526385 — (Aberd.) MB ChB Aberd. 1942. Prev: Res. Ho. Surg. Rosedene Matern. Hosp. Inverness.

ROY, Jataveda Greenock Health Centre, 20 Duncan St., Greenock PA15 4LY; 10 Cowal View, Gourock PA19 1EX — MB BS Calcutta 1974. Clin. Med. Off. (Community & Sch. Health) Greenock Health Centre. Specialty: Community Child Health.

ROY, Julie Paterson 49 Machanhill, Larkhall ML9 2HZ — MB ChB Glas. 1995.

ROY, Koushik Kumar South Street Surgery, 261 South Street, Romford RM1 2BE Tel: 01708 769780 Fax: 01708 722459 — MB BS Calcutta 1959; MB BS Calcutta 1959.

ROY, Leena Parklands Hospital, Aldermaston Road, Basingstoke RG24 9RH Tel: 01256 817718 — MB BS Lond. 1982; MRCPsych 1986. Cons. Psychiat. Pk.lands Hosp. Basingstoke. Specialty: Gen. Psychiat.

ROY, Louise Kathryn Mackay Castlehill Health Centre, Castlehill, Forres IV36 1QF Tel: 01309 672233; Gairland, 8 Hay Place, Elgin IV30 1LZ — MB ChB Aberd. 1976; DRCOG 1979.

ROY, Lucy Caroline 5 Witham Close, Barley Meadows, Taunton TA1 2RR — MB ChB Bristol 1982.

ROY, Manatosh Eaglestone Health Centre, Standing Way, Eaglestone, Milton Keynes MK6 5AZ Tel: 01908 679111 Fax: 01908 230601 — Vrach Minsk Med. Inst. USSR 1980; Vrach Minsk Med Inst USSR 1980.

ROY, Manmatha Kumar Hartlepool General Hospital, Department of Anaesthesia, Holdforth Road, Hartlepool TS24 9AH Tel: 01429 266654/01429 522192/01429 522965 Fax: 01429 522194 Email: m.roy@nth.nhs.uk/mkroy01@hotmail.com; 18 The Spinney, West Park, Hartlepool TS26 0AW Tel: 01429 274180 Fax: 01429 274180 Email: mkroy01@hotmail.com — MB BS Dacca 1967 (Sir Salimullah Med. Coll.) Cons. Anaesth. (N.tees of Hartlepool. NHS Trust. Cons. Anaesth.-N. Tees and Hartlepool NHS Trust. Specialty: Anaesth. Socs: N. E. Soc. of Anaesth.; Pain Soc.; Assn. of Anaesth. of G.Band Irel. Prev: Assoc. Specialist (Anaesth.) N. RHA; Med. Asst. (Anaesth.) North. RHA.

ROY, Mausumi 20 Zetland Avenue, Upper Achintore, Fort William PH33 6LL — MB ChB Aberd. 1998; MB ChB Aberd 1998.

ROY, Meera Greenfields, Monyhull Hall Rd, Kings Norton, Birmingham B30 3QQ Tel: 0121 255 8014; 85 Monmouth Drive, Sutton Coldfield B73 6JH — MB BS Madras 1980 (Christian Medical College Vellove India) DPM Madras 1983; MRCPsych 1986; MMedSci Birm. 1991; FRCPsych 1998. Cons. Psychiat. (Learning Disabilities)Birm. Specialist Community Trust. Specialty: Ment. Health. Prev: Sen. Regist. (Ment. Handicap) W. Midl. RHA; Regist. (Psychiat.) Nottm. HA; Regist. (Psychiat.) S. Derbysh. HA.

ROY, Meghnath The Surgery, 35 Maplestead Road, Dagenham RM9 4XH Tel: 020 8595 0017 Fax: 020 8595 7741; 137 Ashburton Avenue, Ilford IG3 9EW Tel: 020 8599 4343 Fax: 020 8595 7741 — MB BS Banaras Hindu 1967; DA (UK) 1975. Specialty: Anaesth.

ROY, Munna Sudipto Kumar 40 Cecil Street, Glasgow G12 8RJ — MB ChB Glas. 1992.

ROY, Prabhat Kumar (cons. rooms), Treetops, Upper Layham, Hadleigh, Ipswich IP7 5JZ Tel: 01473 822253 — MB Calcutta 1949; DTM 1949; DPM Eng. 1954; FRCP Ed. 1975, M 1958; FRCPsych 1977, M 1972. Prev: Cons. Psychiat. Severalls Hosp. Colchester; Assoc. Prof. Psychiat. NRS Med. Coll., Calcutta.

ROY, Premananda 863 Finchley Road, London NW11 8LX — MB BS Calcutta 1950; DTM & H Eng. 1959.

ROY, Pulin Behari 6 Maesceiro, Bow Street SY24 5BG Tel: 01970 828708 — MB BS Dacca 1961; DO Eng. 1973. Prev: SHO (Ophth.)

W. Wales Gen. Hosp. Carmarthen; Regist. (Ophth.) St. Woolos Hosp. Newport.

ROY, Ramesh (retired) Radford Health Centre, Ilkeston Road, Nottingham NG7 3GW Tel: 0115 979 1313 Fax: 0115 979 1470.

ROY, Mr Raymond Robert The Oaks, 2 Sarsen Close, Halesworth IP19 8JP — MB ChB Bristol 1961; FRCS Ed. 1968; FRCS Eng. 1969; Specialist Accredit (Urol.) RCS Eng. 1974. Specialty: Urol.; Disabil. Med. Socs: Brit. Assn. Urol. Surgs. Prev: Sen. Regist. (Urol.) Manch. AHA (T); Regist. Dept. Urol. Hammersmith Hosp. & Tutor in Surg. Roy. Postgrad.; Med. Sch. Lond.

ROY, Mr Ronen 1 Rosemary Avenue, Lower Earley, Reading RG6 5YQ Tel: 01734 868557 — MB BS Calcutta 1985; FRCS Glas. 1989.

ROY, Ruby 21 Crowden Walk, Barnsley S75 2LU — MB ChB Manch. 1998; MB ChB Manch 1998.

ROY, Sabita 17 Seldon Close, Westcliff on Sea SS0 0AD Tel: 01702 334139; St Clements Hospital, 2A Bow Road, London E3 — MB BS Ravishanker 1971; MB BS Ravishankar 1971. Staff Grade (Psychiat.) St Clements Hosp. Lond. Specialty: Gen. Psychiat.

ROY, Sarah Priya 5 Parkwood Crescent, Sherwood Vale, Nottingham NG5 4EA — MB BS Lond. 1996.

ROY, Shambu Nath 1 Barbondale Grove, Knaresborough HG5 0DX Tel: 01423 864103 — MB BS Ranchi 1966 (Rajendra Med. Coll. Bihar) Staff Grade Phys. (Geriat. Med.) Harrogate Gen. Hosp. Specialty: Care of the Elderly. Prev: Regist. (Geriat. Med.) Harrogate Gen. Hosp.

ROY, Somnath (retired) 99 Pelham Avenue, Grimsby DN33 3NG Tel: 01472 878807 — (R.G. Kar Med. Coll.) MB BS Calcutta 1963; MRCP (UK) 1972; FRCP Lond. 1993. Prev: Cons. Phys. (Geriat.) Trent RHA.

ROY, Sonia Lara East Ardsley Health Centre, Bradford Road, East Ardsley, Wakefield WF3 2DN — MB ChB Sheff. 1992; MRCPsych 1997.

ROY, Subhas Chandra South Tynside District Hospital, Bede Wing, Harton Lane, South Shields NE34 0PL Tel: 0191 454 8888 — MB BS Dhaka 1964.

ROY, Sucheta The Surgery, 172 Pitfield Street, London N1 6JP — MB BS Calcutta 1967.

ROY, Sudhan Rani 3 Elmbourne Drive, Belvedere DA17 6JE — MB BS Lond. 1991.

ROY, Sunil Kanti c/o Drive R. Talukder, 3 Partridge Close, Swanlow Park, Winsford CW7 1PY — MB BS Dacca 1970; MRCS Eng. LRCP Lond. 1983; MRCP (UK) 1984.

ROY, Supriyo (retired) 17 Copse Close, Oadby, Leicester LE2 4FD — MB ChB Sheff. 1961; DCH Eng. 1963; FRCP Lond. 1984, M 1969. Emerit. Cons. Leicester UHL Trust. Prev: Cons. in Rheum. Leicester Area Hosps.

ROY, Syama Prosad 14 Read Head Road, South Shields NE34 6HT Tel: 0191 552498 & profess. 561161 — MB BS Calcutta 1962 (R.G. Kar Med. Coll.) DA Calcutta 1967; DA Eng. 1971. Assoc. Specialist (Anaesth.) S. Tyneside HA. Prev: Regist. (Anaesth.) Canad. Red Cross Memor. Hosp. Taplow; Regist. (Anaesth.) Ilford & Dist. Gp. Hosps. & Nuneaton Gp. Hosps.

ROY, Tapan Kumar The Surgery, High Street, Talke Pits, Stoke-on-Trent ST7 1QH Tel: 01782 782440 Fax: 01782 763884 — MB BS Calcutta 1956; MB BS Calcutta 1956.

ROY, William (retired) 9 Dunchattan Grove, Troon KA10 7AT Tel: 01292 317303 — MB ChB Glas. 1946 (Univ. Glas.) FRFPS Glas. 1949; FRCP Glas. 1980, M 1962; FRCGP 1974, M 1967. Prev: Regist. (Med.) Ballochmyle Hosp.

ROY, William Noel Thompson (retired) Caius House, Wooler NE71 6EE Tel: 01668 281559 — MB BS Lond. 1959 (King's Coll. Hosp.) MRCS Eng. LRCP Lond. 1959; DObst RCOG 1960. Prev: SHO (Paediat.) Preston Hosp.

ROY, William Stuart 124 Kings Road, Cardiff CF11 9DG — MB ChB Bristol 1992; MPhil Camb. 1994. SHO (Gen. Surg.) Gwynedd. Specialty: Gen. Surg.

ROY CHOUDHURY, Manik 14 Hermitage Road, Edgbaston, Birmingham B15 3UR — MB BS Calcutta 1961; FRCOG 1985, M 1969.

ROYAL, David Mark St John Manor House Surgery, Braidwood Road, Normanby, Middlesbrough TS6 0HA Tel: 01642 453338 Fax: 01642 468915; The Orchard, 648 Yarn Road, Eaglescliffe, Stockton-on-Tees TS16 0DH — MB BS Newc. 1988; DFFP 1993; DCH RCP Lond. 1993; T(GP) 1993; MRCGP 1994. Prev: Trainee GP/SHO (O & G) Darlington Memor. Hosp. Cleveland VTS.

ROYAL, Valerie Moira 526 Yarm Road, Eaglescliffe, Stockton-on-Tees TS16 0BH Tel: 01642 790204 — MB ChB Leeds 1987.

ROYAN, Caroline Nicole BUPA Wellness, 2-6 Austin Friars, London EC2N 2HD Tel: 0207 562 7371; 31 Ordnance Hill, London NW8 6PS Email: nicole@royanryan.fsnet.co.uk — MRCS Eng. LRCP Lond. 1984 (Char. Cross) MRCGP 1989; DRCOG 1990; T(GP) 1991; T(OM) 1996; MFOM RCP Lond. 1996. p/t Cons. (Occupat. Phys.) BUPA Wellness. Specialty: Occupat. Health. Socs: Soc. Occup. Med - Counc. Mem. Prev: Med. Adviser Lond. Transport Occupat. Health.

ROYCE, Samuel Lester, Capt. RAMC Retd. (retired) 1 Dovehouse Close, Whitefield, Manchester M45 7PE Tel: 0161 766 7002 — MB ChB Manch. 1947. Prev: Hosp. Clin. Practitioner (Geriatrics) Crumpsall (NMGH) Hosp.

ROYCE, Susan Margaret Top Farm, Barking Tye, Ipswich IP6 8JD Tel: 01473 658583 — MB BS Lond. 1967; MFFP 1993. Assoc. Specialist (Reproduc. & Sexual Health) Ipswich Hosp. Trust. Specialty: Family Plann. & Reproduc. Health.

ROYCROFT, Roger John Roycroft, Madden and Thomas, Chelford Surgery, Elmstead Road, Chelford, Macclesfield SK11 9BS Tel: 01625 861316 Fax: 01625 860075; Roadside House, Chelford, Macclesfield SK11 9AT Tel: 01625 861509 — MB ChB Manch. 1958; MSc Manch. 1991. Prev: Regist. Duchess of York Hosp. For Babies Manch.; SHO (O & G) Copthorne Hosp. Shrewsbury; Ho. Surg. Manch. Roy. Infirm.

ROYDE, Chaim Alexander, Maj. (retired) 10 Devonshire Court, New Hall Road, Salford M7 4JT — (Westm.) MD Lond. 1947, MB BS 1940; MRCS Eng. LRCP Lond. 1940; DPH Eng. 1947; FFCM 1979, M 1974. Prev: Area Med. Off. Bury AHA.

ROYDS-JONES, Jonathan Aidan Bridge Medical Centre, Wassand Close, Three Bridges Road, Crawley RH10 1LL Tel: 01293 526025 — MB BS Lond. 1973.

ROYLANCE, John 45 Corvedale Road, Birmingham B29 4LA — MB ChB Birm. 1968; FFA RCS Eng. 1975. Specialty: Anaesth.

ROYLANCE, Margaret Helen 79 Tennyson Avenue, Dukinfield SK16 5DR — MB ChB Leeds 1992.

ROYLANCE, Michael Kingsley Millbrook Gardens Surgery, Millbrook Gardens, Castle Cary BA7 7EE Tel: 01963 350210 Fax: 01963 350366; Joss Cottage, Church Road, Sparkford, Yeovil BA22 7JZ Tel: 01963 440577 — (Leeds) MB ChB Leeds 1969.

ROYLANCE, Pauline Deidre Tattenhall Medical Practice, Mercury House, High Street, Chester CH3 9PX Tel: 01829 770606 Fax: 01829 770144; Yew Tree Farm, Beeston Moss, Beeston, Tarporley CW6 9SU — MB ChB Manch. 1973; MSc (Primary Med. Care) Keele 1995. Specialty: Gen. Pract.

ROYLANCE, Rebecca Ruth 51 Brompton Park Crescent, Fulham, London SW6 1SW — MB BS Lond. 1991; BSc (Hons.) Lond. 1988; MRCP (UK) 1994; PhD 2000. Specialty: Oncol.

ROYLE, Mr Clive Alexander Joseph Peel Yeovil District Hospital, Yeovil BA21 4AT; Langley, Henley Road, Misterton, Crewkerne TA18 8LS Tel: 901460 78580 Email: c-royle@compuserve.com — MB BS Lond. 1980 (St Marys Hosp. Lond.) FRCS Eng. 1987; MS Soton. 1995. Cons. Gen. & Colorectal Surg. Yeovil Dist. Hosp. Specialty: Gen. Surg. Prev: Cons. Gen. Surg. Frimley Pk. Hosp. Milit. Unit; Cons. Camb. Milit. Hosp.; Sen. Regist. Soton. Prof. Unit.

ROYLE, David Andrew Birchwood Medical Centre, 15 Benson Road, Birchwood, Warrington WA3 7PJ Tel: 01925 823502 Fax: 01925 852422; Summerville House, Summrville Gardens, Grappenhall, Warrington WA4 2EG Tel: 01925 602067 — MB ChB Liverp. 1983; DRCOG 1986; Cert. Family Plann. JCC 1987; MRCGP 1988. Socs: N. Chesh. LMC; Bd. Mem. NES PCG. Prev: Trainee GP N. Staffs. VTS; SHO (Cardiothoracic Med.) & Ho. Off. Broadgreen Hosp. Liverp.

ROYLE, Deborah Jane 16 Hawthorne Rise, Answorth, Nottingham NG16 2RG — MB ChB Leeds 1992.

ROYLE, Deborah Tracy Sett Valley Medical Centre, Hyde Bank Road, New Mills, Stockport SK22 4BP Tel: 01663 743483 — MB ChB Manch. 1982; BSc (Med. Sci.) St. And. 1979; DRCOG 1985. Prev: SHO (O & G) St. Marys Hosp. Manch.; SHO (Cas.) Stockport HA; SHO (Med.) Stepping Hill Hosp. Stockport.

ROYLE, Francis Clifford William (retired) Shearwater, Salterns Lane, Old Bursledon, Southampton SO31 8DH Tel: 023 403575 Fax:

023 8040 3575 — MRCS Eng. LRCP Lond. 1946 (Camb. & St. Bart.) MA Camb. 1948. Prev: GP Soton.

ROYLE, Mr Gavin Timothy Department of Surgery, Royal South Hants Hospital, off St. Marys Road, Southampton SO14 0YG Tel: 023 80 825717 Fax: 023 80 825148 Email: royle.gavin@suht.swst.nhs.uk; Shawlands House, Shawlands Farm, Bunstead Lane, Hursley, Winchester SO21 2LQ Tel: 01962 775324 Fax: 01962 775324 — MB BS Lond. 1970 (Char. Cross.) MRCS Eng. LRCP Lond. 1970; FRCS Eng. 1974; MS Lond. 1979. Cons. Gen. Surg. Soton. Univ. Hosps.; Hon. Sen. Lect. Univ. Soton. Specialty: Gen. Surg. Socs: Surgic. Research Soc.; Assn. Surg.; Brit. Breast Gp. Prev: Sen. Lect. (Surg.) Soton Univ.; Lect. (Surg.) Mass. Gen. Hosp. Boston, USA; Clin. Lect. (Surg.) Nuffield Dept. Surg. Oxf.

ROYLE, Hannah Mary Summerside Medical Centre, 29B Summerside Place, Edinburgh EH6 4NY Tel: 0131 554 3533 Fax: 0131 554 9722; 6 James Street, Edinburgh EH15 2DS — MB ChB Ed. 1966.

ROYLE, Janice Brampton Medical Practice, 4 Market Place, Brampton CA8 1NL Tel: 01697 772551 Fax: 01697 741944 — MB ChB Manch. 1984; BSc St. And. 1981; DCH RCP Lond. 1988; DRCOG 1988; MRCGP 1989.

ROYLE, John Dinnis Great Harwood Health Centre, Water Street, Great Harwood, Blackburn BB6 7QR Email: johndroyle@tiscali.co.uk — MRCS Eng. LRCP Lond. 1972; LMSSA Lond. 1971. Princip. Med. Practitioner. Specialty: Acupunc. Socs: B.M.A.S. Prev: Regist. Psychiat. Lamont Clinic.

ROYLE, Justine Sarah 4 Ennerdale Drive, Sale M33 5NE — MB ChB Manch. 1994.

ROYLE, Martin John 6 Lyndon Drive, Liverpool L18 6HP — MB ChB Liverp. 1994.

ROYLE, Mr Michael Gordon The Hove Nuffield Hospital, 55 New Church Road, Hove BN3 4BG Tel: 01273 720217 Fax: 01273 220919 — MB BS Lond. 1960 (St. Mary's) FRCS Eng. 1965; FACS 1972. Specialty: Urol. Prev: Cons. Urol. Brighton Health Trust; Resid. (Urol.) Univ. Calif. Los. Angeles, USA; Hon. Sen. Lect. Inst. Urol. Univ. Lond.

ROYLE, Peter, Wing Cdr. RAF Med. Br. Retd. Anaesthetic Department, North Tees Hospital, Hardwick, Stockton-on-Tees TS19 8PE — MB BS Lond. Guy's 1976; FFA RCS Eng. 1983; MBA (Open Univ) 1999. Cons. Anaesth. N. Tees Hosp. Stockton-on-Tees.; Med. Director, North Tees & Hartlepool NHS Trust. Specialty: Anaesth. Prev: Cons. Anaesth. RAF Hosp. Wroughton; SHO (Anaesth.) Frimley Pk. Hosp.

ROYLE, Robert Arthur Weaverham Surgery, Northwich Road, Weaverham, Northwich CW8 3EU Tel: 01606 853106 Fax: 01606 854980 — MB ChB Sheff. 1975; MRCGP 1979.

ROYLE, Mr Stephen Gordon Stepping Hill Hospital, Poplar Grove, Hazel Grove, Stockport SK2 7JE Tel: 0161 483-1010 Ext: 4185 Fax: 0161 483-5882 Email: stephen.royle@stockport-tr.nwest.nhs.uk; Ryley Mount, 432, Buxton Road, Hazel Grove, Stockport SK2 7JQ Tel: 0161 483-9333 Fax: 0161 419-9913; Herries Cottage, Aspenshaw, Birch Vale, High Peak SK22 1AU Tel: 01663 747593 Email: steveroyle@clara.co.uk — (Manchester) MB ChB Manch. 1982; FRCS Ed. 1986; MD Manch. 1993; FRCS (Orth.) 1994. Cons. Surg. (Trauma & Orthop.) Stepping Hill Hosp. Specialty: Orthop.; Trauma & Orthop. Surg. Special Interest: Hand & Elbow Surg.; Trauma Surg. Socs: BMA, RCSEd, BOA, BSSH, RASS. Prev: Cons. Surg. (Orthop. Surg.) Trafford Gen. Hosp. Manch.; Sen. Regist. Rotat. (Orthop.) N. Manch.; Regist. (Orthop.) Salford & Wythenshawe Hosp. Manch.

ROYSAM, Chandrikha Sashidhar Samsara, 86 Kenton Road, Gosforth, Newcastle upon Tyne NE3 4NP — MB BS Bangalore 1983; MD (Am. Boards); DA (UK) Lond. 1987; FFA RCS Dub. 1989; FCAnaesth 1990. Cons. Anaesth. Freeman Hosp. Newc. Specialty: Anaesth. Prev: Resid. Harvard Univ. Boston, USA.

ROYSAM, Mr Gorur Shashidhar South Tyneside Hospital, Harton Lane, South Shields NE34 0PL Tel: 0191 202 4025 — MB BS Bangalore 1981; MRCS Eng. LRCP Lond. 1988; FCPS Glas. 1988; FRCS Ed. 1988; FRCS Glas. 1988; MChOrth Liverp. 1991; FRCS (Orth.) 1993. Sen. Regist. (Orthop. Surg.) St. Geo. Hosp.; Spine Fell. Robt. Jones Agnes Hunt Orthop. Hosp. OsW.ry. Specialty: Orthop. Prev: Regist. & Sen. Regist. St. Geo. Hosp. Lond.

ROYSTON, Ashley Melvyn The Stennack Surgery, The Old Stennack School, St Ives TR26 1RU Tel: 01736 793333 Fax: 01736 793746; Lamerton Manor, Idless, Truro TR4 9QT Tel: 01872 273890 — MB BS Lond. 1972 (Guy's) MRCS Eng. LRCP Lond. 1972; MRCP (U.K.) 1976. GP St. Ives.

ROYSTON, Mr Christopher Mackie Sheridan 43 Newlands Park, Hull HU5 Tel: 01482 42314 — MB BS Lond. 1965; MRCS Eng. LRCP Lond. 1965; FRCS Eng. 1970. Cons. (Gen. Surg.) Hull Roy. Infirm. Specialty: Gen. Surg. Prev: Sen. Regist. (Surg.) Hammersmith Hosp. Lond.; Sen. Regist. (Surg.) Northampton Gen. Hosp.; Research Assoc. Middlx. Hosp. Lond.

ROYSTON, Ian McLean Everest House Surgery, Everest Way, Hemel Hempstead HP2 4HY Tel: 01442 240422 Fax: 01442 235045 — MB BS Lond. 1974; BSc (Hons.) Liverp. 1969; MRCS Eng. LRCP Lond. 1974. GP Hemel Hempstead.

ROYSTON, Nancy (retired) Holmwood, 46 Crescent Road, Hemel Hempstead HP2 4AH Tel: 01442 65590 — MB ChB Ed. 1969; BSc (Hons.) Ed. 1967, MB ChB 1969; FFA RCS Eng. 1974. Prev: Cons. Anaesth. St. Vincents' Orthop. Hosp. E.cote.

ROYSTON, Robin Gray Psychotherapy Department, 2 Cossington Road, Canterbury CT1 3HU; The Red House, Stonewall Pk Road, Langton Green, Tunbridge Wells TN3 0HD Tel: 01892 863858 — MRCS Eng. LRCP Lond. 1974; MRCPsych 1986. Cons. Psychother. Canterbury & Thanet Trust.; Clin. Dir., Acute Psychiatric Unit, Ticehurst Ho. Hosp., E. Sussex; Hon. Research Fell. Univ. Kent. Specialty: Gen. Psychiat.; Psychother.

ROYSTON, Virginia Helen Southmead Health Centre, Ullswater Road, Bristol BS10 6DF — MB ChB Bristol 1979; BSc (Hons.) Bristol 1976; DRCOG 1982; MRCGP 1983; Cert. Family Plann. JCC 1984; DFFP 1995. GP, Southmead HC., Bristol. Prev: SCMO Avon Pregn. Advis. Serv.; GP Bristol; Ho. Off. (Med.) Univ. Bristol.

ROYTHORNE, Christopher The British Petroleum Company plc, Britannic House, 1 Finsbury Circus, London EC2M 7BA Tel: 020 7496 4126 Fax: 020 7496 4544; 1 Pine Close, North Road, Berkhamsted HP4 3BZ Tel: 01442 875496 — MB BS Newc. 1969; DIH Soc. Apoth. Lond. 1977; CIH Dund 1977; FFOM RCP Lond. 1988, MFOM 1982. Vice Pres. Health B.P. plc. Specialty: Occupat. Health. Prev: Sen. Med. Adviser BP Oil UK; Internat. Health Coordinator BHPP Lond.; Med. Dir. Conoco (UK) Ltd. Lond.

ROYTHORNE, Judith Patricia Milton House Surgery, Doctors Commons Road, Berkhamsted HP4 3BY Tel: 01442 874784 Fax: 01442 877694; 1 Pine Close, North Road, Berkhamsted HP4 3BZ Tel: 01442 875496 — MB ChB Manch. 1969.

ROZARIO, Elizabeth Liza 49B Sutton Road, Walsall WS1 2PQ — MB BS Lond. 1993.

ROZARIO, John Alfred Christopher 25 Enys Quay, Truro TR1 2HH Tel: 01872 222973 — MB BS Lond. 1953 (Guy's) MRCS Eng. LRCP Lond. 1953. Prev: Med. Supt. Gen. Hosp. Ndola, Zambia; Paediat. Ho. Phys. Freedom Fields Hosp. Plymouth; Obst. Ho. Surg. Roy Bucks. Hosp. Aylesbury.

ROZEWICZ, Deborah Phyllis Simpson House Medical Centre, 255 Eastcote Lane, South Harrow, Harrow HA2 8RS Tel: 020 8864 3466 Fax: 020 8864 1002 — MB BS Lond. 1988 (St. Geo. Hosp.) DRCOG 1991; MRCGP 1994. Simpons Ho. Med. Centre Harrow. Specialty: Gen. Pract. Prev: Trainee GP Mayday Univ. Hosp. VTS; Ho. Off. (Surg.) St. Geo. Hosp. Lond.

ROZEWICZ, Ella Chandos Crescent, 82 Chandos Crescent, Edgware HA8 6HL Tel: 020 8952 7662; 13 Sunningdale Close, Gordon Avenue, Stanmore HA7 3QL Tel: 020 8954 2848 — LMSSA Lond. 1978; MB Silesia 1963.

ROZEWICZ, Leon Michal Wimbledon CMHT, Nelson Hospital, Kingston Road, London SW20 8DB Tel: 020 8544 9799 Fax: 020 8544 9033 — MB BS Lond. 1984; MRCP (UK) 1989; MRCGP 1990; T(GP) 1991; MRCPsych 1993. Cons. Psychiat. S. W. Lond., St. Geo.'s NHS Ment. Health Trust; Hon. Sen. Lect. in Psychiat., St. Geo.'s Hosp. Med. Sch. Specialty: Gen. Psychiat. Prev: Cons. Psychiat. Centr. Middlx. Hosp. Lond.; Lect. & Hon. Sen. Regist. (Psychiat.) St. Geo. Hosp. Med. Sch. Lond.; Hon. Sen. Regist. & Research Fell. Inst. Neurol. Lond.

ROZKOVEC, Adrian Royal Bournemouth Hospital, Castle Lane E., Bournemouth BH7 7DW Tel: 01202 704596 — MB BS Lond. 1974 (Univ. Coll. Lond. & Westm.) MRCP (UK) 1977; BSc Lond. 1971, MD 1987; FRCP Lond. 1995; FESC 2001. Cons. Phys. & Cardiol. Roy. Bournemouth Hosp. Specialty: Cardiol. Socs: Fell.of the Roy. Soc. Med.; Brit. Cardiac Soc.; Brit. Pacing & Electrophysiol. Gp. Prev: Sen. Regist. (Gen. Med. & Cardiol.) Plymouth & Bristol Roy.

Infirm.; Regist. (Cardiol.) Hammersmith Hosp. Lond.; Resid. Med. Off. Nat. Heart Hosp. Lond.

ROZNER, Lorna Margaret (retired) 33 Princess Mary Court, Newcastle upon Tyne NE2 3BG Tel: 0191 281 0770 — MB BS Durh. 1947; DPH Durh. 1951. Prev: Cons. Psychiat. S. Tyneside AHA.

ROZYCKI, Andrzej Antoni 12 Tewkesbury Drive, Prestwich, Manchester M25 0HG Tel: 0161 798 7890 — Lekarz Gdansk 1957. Assoc. Specialist Prestwich Hosp. Specialty: Pub. Health Med. Socs: Ex-Pres. of Warsaw Br. Polish Psychiat. Assn.; Ex-Vice-Pres. Soc. Psychiat. Assn. Poland. Prev: Med. Direct. Drewnica Psychiat. Hosp., Warsaw.

RUAUX, Caroline Denise New Hayesbank Surgery, Cemetery Lane, Kennington, Ashford TN24 9JZ Tel: 01233 624642 Fax: 01233 637304; 7 St. Nicholas Mansions, Trinity Crescent, Tooting, London SW17 7AF — MB BS Lond. 1989; DRCOG 1991; MRCGP 1994. Prev: SHO (Geriat. Med.) Epsom Gen. Hosp.; SHO (A & E) Kingston Hosp. Lond.; SHO (O & G) St. Helier Hosp. Carshalton.

RUB, Abdul 248 Earls Court Road, London SW5 9AD Tel: 020 7373 9797; (Surgery) 26 Fourth Avenue, London W10 Tel: 020 8960 5252 — MB BS Calcutta 1954.

RUB, Hasib-ur Chislehurst Medical Practice, 42 High Street, Chislehurst BR7 5AQ Tel: 020 8467 5551 Fax: 020 8468 7658; 20 Heath Park Drive, Bromley BR1 2WQ — BM Soton. 1984; DCH RCP Lond. 1988; MRCGP 1991. Mem. LMC. Specialty: Gen. Pract. Prev: SHO (O & G) Pembury Hosp.; SHO (Paediat.) Freedon Fields Hosp. Plymouth; SHO (Med.) Lister Hosp. Stevenage.

RUB, Rebecca — MB BS Lond. 1994 (St. Geo. Hosp. Lond.) BSc (Physiol. with Basic Med. Sci.) Lond. 1991; MB BS (Hons Med.) Lond. 1994. SpR Paediat. South Thames. Specialty: Paediat. Prev: SHO (Paediat.) Roy. Surrey Co. Hosp.

RUBAN, Ernest Peter 1 Freswick Court, Hinckley LE10 0RW — BM BS Nottm. 1989; BMedSci 1987; MRCPath 1995. Specialty: Histopath.

RUBEN, Lewis Alan (retired) 4 Little Bornes, Dulwich, London SE21 8SE Tel: 020 8670 0430 — MB BCh BAO Dub. 1957; MA Dub. 1960; DObst RCOG 1962; FRCGP 1979, M 1966. Non-Exec. Dir., Southwark Primary Care Trust; GP Mem. S. E. MREC; Mem. of Counc. Assn. of Research Ethics. Prev: Dean Postgrad. Gen. Pract. Educat. S. Thomas (E.).

RUBEN, Mr Montague (retired) 20 Seven Stones Drive, Broadstairs CT10 1TW — (Guy's) MRCS Eng. LRCP Lond. 1945; DOMS Eng. 1949; FRCS Eng. 1960; LMS Barcelona 1986; FRCOphth 1989. Prev: Cons. Ophth. & Dir. Dept. Contact Lens & Prosth.s Moorfields Eye Hosp. (City Rd. Br.) Lond. & Dist. Prof. Col. Univ. Houston Texas.

RUBEN, Pamela Elaine Stockwell Group Practice, 107 Stockwell Road, Brixton, London SW9 9TJ Tel: 020 7274 3225 Fax: 020 7738 5005; 4 Little Bornes, Dulwich, London SE21 8SE Tel: 020 8670 0430 — MB BS Lond. 1963 (St. Geo.) MRCS Eng. LRCP Lond. 1963.

RUBEN, Mr Simon Timothy Holly House, High Road, Buckhurst Hill IG9 5HZ Tel: 020 8505 3311 Email: streye1@aol.com — MB BS Lond. 1985 (St. Bart. Hosp. Lond.) DO 1989; FRCS Glas. 1989; FCOphth 1990; MD Lond. 1996; BSc Lond. 1982, MD 1996. Cons. Ophth. Surg. Whipps Cross Hosp. & Harold Wood Hosp. Specialty: Ophth. Prev: Sen. Regist. Birm. Eye Hosp.; Regist. West. Ophth. Hosp.; Fell. (Glaucoma) Moorfields Eye Hosp. Lond.

RUBEN, Susan Mary — MB ChB Ed. 1978; MRCPsych 1983; FRCPsych 1992. Cons. Psychiat. Drugs & Alcohol Directorate. Specialty: Substance Misuse.

RUBENS, David Harold (retired) 25 Homecross House, Fishers Lane, Chiswick, London W4 1YA Tel: 020 8747 4962 — MB BS Lond. 1954 (Lond. Hosp.) MRCS Eng. LRCP Lond. 1954. Clin. Asst. Centr. Middlx. Hosp. Lond.; Med. Ref. Pruden. & Scott. Life Assur. Cos. Prev: Surg. Merchant Navy.

RUBENS, Michael Bernard Flat 6, Harmont House, 20 Harley St., London W1G 9PH Tel: 020 7580 1442 Fax: 020 7580 0494 — MB BS Lond. 1971; MRCS Eng. LRCP Lond. 1971; DMRD Eng. 1975; FRCR 1976. Cons. Radiol. Roy. Brompton Hosp. Lond.; Hon. Sen. Lect. Heart & Lung Inst. Univ. Lond. Specialty: Radiol. Prev: Asst. Prof. (Diagn. Radiol.) Univ. Florida, USA; Fell. (Cardiac Radiol.) Univ. Alabama, USA:; Asst. Prof. Diagn. Radiol. Univ. Miami, USA.

RUBENS, Professor Robert David 5 Currie Hill Close, Arthur Road, Wimbledon, London SW19 7DX Tel: 020 8946 0422 Email: rdrubens@doctors.org.uk — (St. Geo.) MRCS Eng. LRCP Lond. 1967; MB BS Lond. 1967; MRCP (UK) 1969; BSc Lond. 1964, MD 1974; FRCP Lond. 1984. Chief Med. Off. Swiss Re Life & Health; Chief Med. Off. Legal & Gen. Assur. Soc. Ltd. Specialty: Oncol. Socs: BMA; Amer. Soc. of Clin. Oncol.; Assur. Med. society (Pres.-elect for 2003-5). Prev: Prof. Clin. Oncol. Guy's, Kings Coll. & St Thomas's Sch. of Med. & Dent. of King's Coll. Lond. 1985-2003; Dir. Imperial Cancer Research Fund Clin. Oncol. Unit Guy's Hosp. Lond.; Regist. St. Geo. Hosp. Lond.

RUBENSTEIN, David Addenbrooke's Hospital, Cambridge CB2 2QQ Tel: 01223 216243 Fax: 01223 216056 — (Middlx.) MB BS LOnd. 1962; MRCS Eng. LRCP Lond. 1962; FRCP Lond. 1979, M 1965; MD Lond. 1971. Phys. Addenbrooke's Hosp. Camb. Specialty: Gen. Med.

RUBENSTEIN, Ian David Eagle House Surgery, 291 High Street, Ponders End, Enfield EN3 4DN Tel: 020 8351 1000 Fax: 020 8351 1007 — BM BS Nottm. 1978; BMedSci (Hons.) Nottm. 1976, BM BS 1978; DRCOG 1982; MRCGP 1983. Socs: Brit. Soc. Med. & Dent. Hypn.. Prev: Stud. Health Off. Lond. Sch. Economics.; Clin. Asst. Pain Managem. Course Whittington Hosp. Lond.

RUBENSTEIN, Punam Department of Reproductive Healthcare, Enfield Community Care Trust, Wenlock House, 1 Eaton Road, Enfield EN1 1NJ; 1 Heather Drive, Enfield EN2 8LQ — BM BS Nottm. 1978; BMedSci (Hons.) Nottm. 1976; DRCOG 1980; MFFP 1993. SCMO (Reproduc. Healthcare) Enfield Community Care Trust. Specialty: Family Plann. & Reproduc. Health. Prev: Doctor (Family Plann.& Child Health) Enfield HA.

RUBERY, Eileen Doris, CB, QHP Lecturer in Public Policy, Judge Institute of Management, University of Cambridge, Trumpington St., Cambridge CB2 1AG Tel: 01223 765879 Fax: 01223 766330 Email: e.rubery@jims.cam.ac.uk — MB ChB Sheff. 1966; FRIPHH; MB ChB (Hons.) Sheff. 1966; PhD (Biochem.) Camb. 1972; DMRT Eng. 1975; FRCR 1976; MRCPath 1989; FFPHM RCP (UK) 1994; FRCPath 1999. p/t Pub. Health Policy, Professional Career Developm., Research on Uncertainty and Decision Making; Sen. Research Fell. Girton Coll. Camb. Specialty: Pub. Health Med.; Biochem. Special Interest: Career Developm.; Pub. Policy and Decision making. Prev: Hon. Cons. Radiother. & Oncol. & Wellcome Sen. Research Fell. Addenbrooke's Hosp. Camb.; Under-Sec., Dept. of Health; Dir. Med. Studies & Sen. Research Fell. Girton Coll. Camb.

RUBIN, Alan Department of Cytology, Watford General Hospital, Vicarage Road, Watford WD18 0HB Tel: 01923 244366 Fax: 01923 217448; 69 Green Lane, Edgware HA8 7PZ Tel: 020 8958 8918 — MB BS Lond. 1983 (Roy. Free) BSc (Hons.) Lond. 1980, MB BS 1983; MRCPath 1990; FRCPath 1998. Cons. Path. Histopath. & Cytol. Mt. Vernon & Watford NHS Trust. Specialty: Histopath. Prev: Sen. Regist. (Histopath.) Univ. Coll., Middlx. & Whittington Hosps. Lond.; Regist. (Histopath.) Hammersmith Hosp. Lond.; SHO (Path.) Chase Farm Hosp. Enfield.

RUBIN, Anthony Paul 126 Harley Street, London W1G 7JS Tel: 020 7935 9409 Fax: 020 7224 3490 Email: admin@groupanaestheticservices.com — MRCS Eng. LRCP Lond. 1961 (Lond. Hosp.) MB Camb. 1962, BChir 1961; DA Eng. 1963; FFA RCS Eng. 1966. Cons. Anaesth. Nat. Orthop. Hosp. Lond. Specialty: Anaesth. Socs: Fell. Roy. Soc. Med.; Assn. Anaesths. Prev: Anaesth. Sen. Regist. Char. Cross Hosp. Lond.; Anaesth. Regist. St. Margt.'s Hosp. Epping; Jun. Anaesth. Regist. Lond. Hosp.

RUBIN, Caroline Moira Elizabeth Department of Radiology, Southampton General Hospital, Tremona Road, Southampton SO16 6UY Tel: 02380 794028 Fax: 02380 825135 Email: caroline.rubin@suht.swest.nhs.uk — MB BS Lond. 1979 (Westm.) MRCP (UK) 1982; FRCR 1986. Cons. Radiologist with a special interest in breast imaging, Soton. Univ. Hosps. NHS Trust, Soton. Specialty: Radiol. Socs: MRCP; FRCR; BMUS.

RUBIN, Gary X Ray Department, Royal Sussex County Hospital, Eastern Road, Brighton BN2 5SE; 14 Hove Park Way, Hove BN3 6PT — MB BS Lond. 1979 (St. Geo.) BSc (Hons.) Lond. 1976, MB BS 1979; FRCR 1984. Cons. (Radiol.) Roy. Sussex Co. Hosp. Brighton. Specialty: Radiol. Prev: Sen. Regist. (Radiol.) Roy. Free Hosp. Lond.; Regist. (Radiol.) Westm. Hosp. Lond.; SHO (Med.) Chase Farm Hosp. Enfield.

RUBIN, Professor Gregory Paul University of Sunderland, Centre for Primary and Community Care, Benedict Building, Sunderland SR2 7BW Tel: 0191 515 3831 Fax: 0191 515 Ext: 2741 Email: greg.rubin@sunderland.ac.uk; West Gate, Worsall Hall, Low Worsall, Yarm TS15 9PJ — MB ChB Sheff. 1974; MRCGP 1983; FRCGP 1997. Professor (Primary Care) University of Sunderland; Director, North. Primary Care Research Network (NoReN); GP Springwell Med. Gp. Specialty: Gen. Pract. Special Interest: Gastroenterol. Prev: Sen. Lect. (Primary Health Care) Univ. Teeside; NoReN Research Fell. (Primary Health Care) Newc.Univ.; Hon. Sen. Research Assoc. Dept. Primary Care Newc. Univ.

RUBIN, Mr John Rubin Royal National Throat, Nose & Ear Hospital, 330 Grays Inn Road, London WC1X 8DA Tel: 020 7915 1313 Fax: 020 7815 1388 — MD New York. Cons. ENT Surg.; Clin. Head of Serv.; Hon. Cons., Barths Hosp.; Hon. Sen. Lect., Univ. Coll., Lond. Socs: American College Surgeon; Fell. Roy. Coll. Surgeons (Eng.); BMA. Prev: Cons. ENT Surg., Lewisham Hosp.

RUBIN, Joseph (retired) 5 Whitehorn Drive, Brighton BN1 5LH Tel: 01273 557117 — LRCP LRCS Ed. 1945; LRCP LRCS Ed. LRFPS Glas. 1945; DMRD Eng. 1949. Prev: Cons. Radiol. Brighton Health Dist.

RUBIN, Professor Peter Charles Division of Therapeutics, Queen's Medical Centre, Nottingham NG7 2UH Tel: 0115 970 9905 Fax: 0115 875 4596 Email: peter.rubin@nottingham.ac.uk — BM BCh Oxf. 1974 (Camb. & Oxf.) BA Camb. 1971; MRCP (UK) 1976; DM Oxf. 1980; FRCP Lond. 1989. Prof. Therap. Univ. Nottm. Specialty: Pharmacology. Prev: Amer. Heart Assn. Research Fell. Stanford Med. Center, USA; Wellcome Trust Sen. Fell. (Mat. Med.) Univ. Glas.; Dean of Fac. of Med. & Health Sci. Univ. of Notts.

RUBIN, Philip 59 Orchard Drive, Giffnock, Glasgow G46 7AG — MB ChB Glas. 1991.

RUBIN, Susan Penelope-Ann Dept. Of Paediatrics, Queen Elizabeth Hospital, King's Lynn PE30 4ET Tel: 01553 613613 Fax: 01553 613468; Staines House, Sporle Road, Swaffham PE37 7HL — MB BS Lond. 1976 (Westm.) MRCS Eng. LRCP Lond. 1976; DCH Eng. 1979; MRCP (Paed.) 1980; FRCP Lond. 1995; FRCPCH 1997. Cons. Paediat. Qu. Eliz. Hosp. King's Lynn Norf. Specialty: Paediat. Special Interest: neonatology; Paediatric Dermatology. Socs: Roy. Coll. of Paediatricians and Child Health; Roy. Coll. of Physicians; Brit. Assn. of Perinatal Med. Prev: Fell. (Perinatol.) Hosp. Sick Childr. Toronto.

RUBINSZTEIN, David Chaim Dept. of Med. Genetics, Cambridge Institute for Medical Research, Addenbrookes Hospital, Hills Road, Cambridge CB2 2XY Tel: 01223 762608 Fax: 01223 331206 Email: dcr1000@hermes.cam.ac.uk — MB ChB Cape Town 1986; BSc (Hons. Med.) 1988; PhD 1993; MRCPath 1997; FMedSci 2004; FRCPath 2005. Reader, Molecular Neurogenetics/ Wellcome Trust Sen. Clin. Fell.; Hon. Cons., Molecular Genetics & Cytogenetics. Specialty: Genetics. Socs: Clin. Genetics Soc.; Amer. Soc. of Human Genetics; World Federat. of Neurol. Prev: Glaxo Wellcome Research Fell.; Sen. Regist., Genetic Path.

RUBINSZTEIN, Judy Sasha Department of Psychiatry, Addenbrooke's Hospital, Box 189, Cambridge CB2 2QQ Tel: 01223 336945 Email: jsr25@cam.ac.uk — MB ChB Cape Town 1991; MRCPsych. Hon. Specialist Regist.; Research Fell. Specialty: Gen. Psychiat. Prev: Specialist Regist.

RUBIO LAINEZ, Carlos Ricardo Flat 1B, 33 Belsize Park Gardens, London NW3 4JJ — LMS Cadiz 1988; MD U Autonoma Madrid 1991.

RUBIO RODRIGUEZ, Maria Del Carmen Department of Medicine, Royal Marsden Hospital, Sutton SM2 5PT — LMS Salamanca 1990.

RUBNER, Janet Vivian Bedford House Medical Centre, Glebe Street, Ashton-under-Lyne OL6 6HD Tel: 0161 330 9880 Fax: 0161 330 9393 — MB ChB Manch. 1982 (Manchester) DRCOG 1985. Specialty: Gen. Med.; Obst. & Gyn.; Paediat.

RUBRA, Timothy David Crouch End Health Centre, 45 Middle Lane, Crouch End, London N8 8PH — (Westm.) MRCS Eng. LRCP Lond. 1962; MB BS Lond. 1962; DObst RCOG 1964.

RUBY, Aisha Ejaz Medical Centre, 276 Dudley Road, Winson Green, Birmingham B18 4HL Tel: 0121 455 6170 — MB BS Patna 1973.

RUCINSKI, Jacek Medway Maritime Hospital, Department of Psychiatry, A Block, Windmill Road, Gillingham ME7 5NY Tel: 01634 833718 Fax: 01634 830082 — DM Lekarz, Gdansk 1973 (Gdansk Med. Acad.) MRCPsych 1978; DPM Eng. 1978. Cons. Psychiat.West Kent NHS and Social Care Trust; Lead Clinician, Thames Gateway NHS Trust; Second Opinion Apptd. Doctor - Ment. Health Act Commiss.; Recognised Teach. in Psychiat., Univ. of Lond.; Independent medico-legal expert; Author: revew articles in Neurology, psychiatry and Med.; book chapters on psychiatric disorders in med. Profession, self-neglect in old age. Specialty: Geriat. Psychiat.; Gen. Psychiat. Socs: MRC Psych; BMA; PMA. Prev: Sen. Regist. (Psychiat.) St. Thos. Hosp. Lond.; Regist. (Psychiat.) Guy's Hosp. Lond. & Bexley Hosp.

RUCK, Colin Stuart Kenneth, RD (retired) Sheep Plain House, Sheep Plain, Crowborough TN6 3ST Tel: 01892 653896 — (Oxf. & St. Mary's) BM BCh Oxf. 1955; BA Oxf. 1952, MA 1955; DObst RCOG 1959. Med. Off. BAMS; Med. Off. The Appeals Serv. Prev: GP CrowBoro.

RUCK, Michael John Yarnton Carteknowle and Dore Medical Practice, 1 Carterknowle Road, Sheffield S7 2DW Tel: 0114 255 1218 Fax: 0114 258 4418; 115 Osborne Road, Sheffield S11 9BB Tel: 0114 281 5546 — MB ChB Bristol 1967; MRCGP 1986. Prev: SHO (Surg. & Urol.) Sheff. Roy. Hosp.; Ho. Phys. & Ho. Surg. Roy. United Hosp. Bath; Demonst. (Anat.) Univ. Sheff.

RUCK, Sarah Elizabeth 115 Osborne Road, Brincliffe, Sheffield S11 9BB — BM BS Nottm. 1996.

RUCKERT, Linden Alexandra Louise City University, Health Centre, 20 Sebastian Street, London EC1V 0JA Tel: 020 7253 4454 Fax: 020 7477 8867 — MB BS Lond. 1985 (Univ. Lond. & Middlx. Hosp. Med. Sch.) DRCOG 1988; DFFP 1995. Gen. Practitioner. Specialty: Family Plann. & Reproduc. Health. Prev: Trainee GP Taunton VTS; Psychiat. Rotat. Glenside Hosp. Bristol.

RUCKLEY, Professor Charles Vaughan, CBE (retired) 1 Mayfield Terrace, Edinburgh EH9 1RU — (Ed.) MB ChB Ed. 1959; FRCS Ed. 1963; ChM Ed. 1970; FRCP Ed. 1993. Emerit. Prof. Vasc. Surg. Univ. Edin.; Med. Adviser, Clin. Standards Bd. for Scotl. Prev: Cons. Surg. Roy. Infirm. Edin.

RUCKLEY, Mr Robert William Darlington Memorial Hospital, Hollyhurst Road, Darlington DL3 6HX Tel: 01325 380100 Fax: 01325 743798 — MB ChB Dundee 1975 (Dundee Univ.) FRCS Eng. 1980. Cons. ENT Surg. Darlington Memor. Hosp., Bishop Auckland Gen. Hosp. & Friarage Hosp. N. Yorks.; Lionel Colledge Memor. Fell. Otolaryngol. RCS Eng. 1984-5; Exam. RCS Eng. Specialty: Otorhinolaryngol. Prev: Sen. Regist. & Hon. Lect. (ENT. Surg.) Ninewells Hosp. Dundee.; Regist. (Surg.) Ninewells Hosp. Dundee; SHO (Neurosurg. & Orthop. Surg.) & Regist. (Urol.) Dundee Roy. Infirm.

RUCKLEY, Valerie Anne (retired) 1 Mayfield Terrace, Edinburgh EH9 1RU Tel: 0131 667 8678 Fax: 0131 667 8678 — BSc Ed. 1959; MB ChB Ed. 1962; FRCP Ed. 1996. Prev: Sen. Med. Off. Chief Scientist Off. Scott. Home & Health Dept.

RUCKLIDGE, Matthew William Miles 26B Lydford Road, Maida Vale, London W9 3LU — MB BS Lond. 1994; BSc Lond. 1991. Specialist Regist. Imperial Sch. of Anaesth. Rotat. Specialty: Anaesth.

RUCKLIDGE, Miles Aspinall (retired) Old Hall Farm, Littledale Road, Brookhouse, Lancaster LA2 9PH Tel: 01524 770450 Fax: 01524 771679 — (Oxf. & Middlx.) BM BCh Oxf. 1959; MA Oxf. 1959; FFA RCS Eng. 1966. Prev: Cons. Anaesth. Roy. Lancaster Infirm.

RUDD, Ann Gloria 7 Borrowell Terrace, Kenilworth CV8 1ER — MB BCh BAO Dub. 1959 (T.C. Dub.) DObst RCOG 1962. Med. Asst. (A & E) Warwick Hosp. Socs: BMA.

RUDD, Anthony George Guy's & St Thomas' NHS Foundation Trust, Lambeth Palace Road, London SE1 7EH Tel: 020 7188 2515 Fax: 020 7928 2339 Email: anthony.rudd@kcl.ac.uk; 33 Newstead Way, Wimbledon, London SW19 5HR Tel: 020 8946 9713 Fax: 020 8286 1482 — MB BChir Camb. 1979; FRCP Lond. 1994. Cons. Phys. I/C Elderly, Guy's & St Thomas's Hosp. Lond. & Cons. Stroke Phys.; Clin. Effectiveness & Eval. Unit Roy. Coll. of Phys., Lond.; Assoc. Director. Specialty: Care of the Elderly. Prev: Lect. (Geriat. Med.) St. Geo. Hosp. Lond.

RUDD, Brigitte Caroline Hatch End Medical Centre, 577 Uxbridge Road, Hatch End, Pinner HA5 4RD Tel: 020 8428 0272 Fax: 020 8421 4109 — MB BS Lond. 1977 (St. Bart.) GP Hatch End. Prev: Ho. Surg. St. Bart. Hosp. Lond.

RUDD, Cyril 43 Coast Road, Redcar TS10 3NN Tel: 01642 484427 — LRCP LRCS Ed. 1939; LRCP LRCS Ed. LRFPS Glas. 1939.

RUDD, Gillian Nicola Osborne Building, Leicester Royal Infirmary, Leicester LE1 5WW Tel: 0116 258 7512 Fax: 0116 258 7512; High Holme, 43 High St, Hallaton, Market Harborough LE16 8UD Tel: 01858 555714 — MB ChB Birm. 1980; MRCP (UK) 1984; FRCP 2000. Cons. Phys. (Palliat. Med.) Leics. Roy. Infirm.; Cons. Leics. Hospice. Specialty: Palliat. Med.

RUDD, James Harvey Fitzgerald ACCI, Level 6 Box 110, Addenbrooke's Hospital, Hills Road, Cambridge CB2 2QQ Tel: 01223 331504 — MB ChB (Hons.) Birm. 1993; MRCP (UK) 1996; PhD Cantab. 2002. Specialist Regist., Addenbrookes Hosp., Papworth Hosp., Camb. Specialty: Cardiol. Prev: BHF Research Fell., Addenbrookes Hosp., Camb.; Assoc Lect (Med) Flinders Univ. Adelaide, Australia.; SHO (Med), Qu. Eliz., Selly Oak Hosp. Birm.

RUDD, Keith Kitson (retired) c/o 28 Greame Road, Bridlington YO16 6TQ — MB ChB Leeds 1953. Prev: Ho. Surg. Leeds Gen. Infirm.

RUDD, Margaret Elizabeth — MB ChB Glas. 1975. Staff Grade (Dermat.) Roy. Infirm. Edin. & St Johns Livingston; GP Eyre Med. Pract. Edin. Specialty: Dermat. Socs: BMA; Scott. Dermatol. Soc. Prev: GP Edin.; Med. Cytol. & Lect. (Cytopath.) Univ. Edin.

RUDD, Margaret Isobel (retired) 5 Northcroft, Winslow, Buckingham MK18 3JR Tel: 01296 713399 — MB ChB Birm. 1942. Prev: Clin. Asst. Dept. Venereol. Stoke Mandeville Hosp. Aylesbury.

RUDD, Peter Thomas Childrens Centre, Royal United Hospital, Bath BA1 3NG Tel: 01225 824393 Fax: 01225 824212; Moregrove, Perrymead, Bath BA2 5AZ Tel: 01222 833292 Fax: 01222 833292 — MB BChir Camb. 1975; DCH Eng. 1978; MRCP (UK) 1979; MA Camb. 1976, MD 1984; FRCPCh Lond. 1993. Cons. Paediat. Roy. United Hosp. Bath. Specialty: Paediat. Prev: Wellcome Fell. Univ. Alabama Birm.; Sen. Regist. (Paediat.) Norf. & Norwich Hosp.

RUDD, Robin Michael St Bartholomew's Hospital, West Smithfield, London EC1A 7BE Tel: 020 7601 7900 Fax: 020 7601 7577 Email: r.m.rudd@qmul.ac.uk; 54 New Cavendish Street, London W1G 8TQ Tel: 020 7486 3247 Fax: 020 7486 3248 Email: dr@robinrudd.com — MB BChir Camb. 1977 (Cambridge & St Georges) MRCP (UK) 1978; MA Camb. 1977, MD 1983; FRCP Lond. 1992. Cons. Phys. Lond. Chest Hosp. & St. Bart. Hosp. Specialty: Respirat. Med.; Oncol. Special Interest: Asbestos related diseases; Lung cancer; Mesothelioma. Socs: Brit. Thoracic Soc.; Amer. Thoracic Soc.; Europ. Respirat. Soc. Prev: Sen. Regist. (Med.) Lond. Chest Hosp. & St. Thos. Hosp. Lond.; Regist. (Med.) St. Geo. Hosp. Lond.

RUDD, Susan Elizabeth 27 Smedley Street, Matlock DE4 3FQ — MB ChB Leic. 1987.

RUDDELL, Kathryn Brenda Louise Winscombe Surgery, Hillyfields Way, Winscombe BS25 1AF Tel: 01934 842211 — MB BS Lond. 1983; BSc (Anat.) Lond. 1980, MB BS 1983; DRCOG 1985; MRCGP 1987.

RUDDELL, Mark Colin Nottingham Healthcare NHS Trust, Duncan MacMillan House, Porchester Road, Nottingham NG3 6AA Tel: 0115 969 1300 — BM BS Nottm. 1995; BMedSci (Hons.) Nottm. 1992. SHO (Psychiat.) Nottm. Healthcare NHS Trust. Specialty: Gen. Psychiat. Socs: BMA; MPS; Roy. Coll. Psychiat. (Inceptor).

RUDDELL, Michael Andrew Lisburn Health Centre, Linenhall Street, Lisburn BT28 1LU Tel: 028 9260 3090 Fax: 028 9250 1310; 101 Osbourne Park, Belfast BT9 6JQ — MB BCh BAO Belf. 1985 (Queen's University, Belfast) DRCOG 1989; DCH Dub. 1989; MRCGP 1990.

RUDDELL, Nigel John Dromara Surgery, Begney Hill Road, Dromore BT25 2AT Tel: 01238 532217 Fax: 01238 533301 Email: njruddell@dromarasurgery.freeserve.co.uk — MB BCh BAO Belf. 1992 (Queens Univ. Belf.) DCH RCPSI 1995; DRCOG 1996; MRCGP 1996. Princip., GP. Specialty: Accid. & Emerg. Socs: Fac. Edr., N. Ire., Fac. of Roy. Coll. Of GPs.; Brit. Assn. for Immed. Care.

RUDDELL, William Samuel John 9 Clarendon Place, Stirling FK8 2QW — MD Birm. 1979; MB ChB 1968; MRCP (UK) 1973; FRCP Ed. 1986. Cons. Phys. & Gastroenterol. Falkirk & Dist. Roy. Infirm.; Hon. Sen. Lect. (Med.) Univ. Edin. Specialty: Gastroenterol.

RUDDLE, Adrian Charles East Hants Primary Care Trust, Specialist Palliative Care Services, The Rowans, Purbrook Heath Road, Purbrook, Waterlooville PO7 5RU Tel: 023 92250001 Ext: 320 Fax: 023 92255775 — MB BS Lond. 1971 (St. Bart.) MRCS Eng. LRCP Lond. 1970; DObst RCOG 1972; MRCGP 1975; DA Eng. 1977. Cons. in Palliat. Med. Specialty: Palliat. Med. Socs: Assn. for Palliat. Med. of Gt. Britain and Irel. Prev: Chief Executive/Medical Director, St. Barnabas Hospice, Worthing; Hon. Cons. Palliat. Med. Worthing & Southlands Hosps. Trust; Sen. Regist. St. Gemma's Hospice Leeds.

RUDDLE, Jane Elizabeth 3 West Avenue, Benton, Newcastle upon Tyne NE12 9PA — MB BS Lond. 1977; MA Camb. 1978. Specialty: Nuclear Med.

RUDDLESDIN, Mr Christopher Barnsley DGH, Gawber Road, Barnsley S75 2EP Tel: 01226 777701 Fax: 01226 283020 Email: chris.ruddlesdin@bdgh-tr.trent.nhs.uk; Grove House, 5 Beech Grove, Barnsley S70 6NG Tel: 01226 283020 Email: ruddlesdin@doctors.org.uk — MB BS Lond. 1974 (Lond. Hosp.) FRCS Eng. 1979. Med. Dir., Barnsley DGH NHS Trust; Cons. Orthopaed. Surg. Barnsley DGH. Specialty: Orthop. Socs: BMA.; Mem. Brit. Assn. Med. Managers. Prev: Sen. Regist. (Orthop.) Roy. Free Hosp. & Windsor Gp. Hosp.; Regist. (Orthop.) Adelaide Childr. Hosp.; Regist. (Surg.) Lond. Hosp.

RUDDOCK, Caroline Jane The Limes Medical Centre, 65 Leicester Road, Narborough, Leicester LE19 2DU Tel: 0116 284 1347 Fax: 0116 275 2447; 23 North Avenue, Leicester LE2 1TL Tel: 0116 270 5393 — MB ChB Leic. 1989; DRCOG 1992; MRCGP 1993.

RUDDOCK, Fiona Sue Deddington Health Centre, Earls Lane, Deddington, Banbury OX15 0TQ Tel: 01869 338611 Fax: 01869 37009; 1 The Pitts, Sandford St. Martin, Oxford OX7 7AH Tel: 0160 8683 423 — MB ChB Birm. 1983; BSc (Hons.) Birm. 1980, MB ChB (Hons.) 1983; MRCP (UK) 1986; DRCOG 1989. Prev: GP Moreton-in-Marsh.; Regist. (Gen. Med.) Leicester Roy. Infirm.

RUDDOCK, John Michael Oak Villa, St. Neots Road, Coton, Cambridge CB3 7PH Tel: 01954 210760; 26 Chatworth Avenue, Cambridge CB4 3LT — MB Camb. 1971, BChir 1970; FFA RCS Eng. 1980. Cons. Anaesth. Roy. Nat. Throat Nose & Ear Hosp. Lond. WC1X 8DA. Specialty: Anaesth.

RUDDY, James Patrick 15 Queens Avenue, Meols, Wirral CH47 0LR — MB ChB Ed. 1991.

RUDDY, Michael Charles Peter 336 Landsee Road, Ipswich IP3 0EL — MB ChB Sheff. 1990.

RUDENSKI, Aram Clinical Biochemistry, Hope Hospital, Salford M6 8HD Tel: 0161 206 1490 — BM BCh Oxf. 1982; MA Camb. 1983; DPhil Oxf. 1988; MRCPath 1994. Specialty: Biochem.

RUDGE, Mr Christopher John Medical Director, UK Transplant, Fox Den Road, Bristol BS34 8RR Tel: 01179 757488 Email: chris.rudge@uktransplant.nhs.uk; Pennis Farm, Fawkham, Longfield DA3 8LZ Tel: 01474 707522 — MB BS Lond. 1972 (Guy's) BSc (Hons.) Lond. 1969; MRCS Eng. LRCP Lond. 1972; FRCS Eng. 1976. Med. Director, UK Transpl., Bristol. Specialty: Transpl. Surg. Prev: Cons. Transpl. Surg. Guy's Hosp. Lond. & St. Peter's Hosp. Lond.; Cons. Transpl. Surg. Roy. Hosps. Trust Lond.

RUDGE, James William Bridge House Medical Centre, Scholars Lane, Stratford-upon-Avon CV37 6HE Tel: 01789 292201 Fax: 01789 262087 — BM BS Nottm. 1988; BM BS (Hons.) Nottm. 1988, BMedSci (Hons.) 1986; DRCOG 1991; MRCGP 1992. Prev: Trainee GP Lincoln VTS.

RUDGE, Peter c/o National Hospital, Queen Square, London WC1N 3BG Tel: 020 7837 3611 — MB BS Lond. 1966 (St. Bart.) BSc Lond. 1963; FRCP Lond. 1981, M 1969. Cons. Neurol. Nat. Hosp. For Neurol. & Neurosurg. Qu. Sq. Lond.; Cons. Neurol. Northwick Pk. Hosp. Harrow; Hon. Cons. Neuro-optology Unit & Psychol. Dept. Nat. Hosp.; RCP Regional Adviser NE Thames; Regional Speciality Adviser N. Thames. Specialty: Neurol. Prev: Clin. Tutor Nat. Hosp. Lond.; Hon. Cons. Neurol. MRC Human Movement & balance unit Nat. Hosp. Lond.; Ho. Phys. Nat. Hosp. Nerv. Dis. Nerv. Dis. Qu. Sq.

RUDGE, Peter 44 Daniel Street, Cardiff CF24 4NY — MB BCh Wales 1993.

RUDGE, Peter John Pennine Drive Surgery, 6-8 Pennine Drive, London NW2 1PA Tel: 020 8455 9977; 133 Cricklewood Lane, London NW2 1HS Tel: 020 8452 8840 Email: peter.rudge@netalia.com — MB BS Lond. 1972 (Roy. Free Hosp. Sch. Med.) BSc Lond. 1969. Gen. Practitioner; Clin. Asst. in Dermat. The Roy. Free Hosp. Socs: Hampstead Med. Soc.; Fell. RSM.

RUDGE, Shauna Deirdre Elaine Charing Cross Hospital, Fulham Palace Road, London W6 8RF Tel: 020 8846 1234; 73A Lynton Avenue, London W13 0EA — MB BS Lond. 1986; MRCPsych 1991.

Sen. Regist. (Psychiat.) Char. Cross Hosp. Lond. Specialty: Gen. Psychiat.

RUDGE, Stuart David Castle Gardens Medical Centre, 78 East Hill, Colchester CO1 2QS Tel: 01206 866626 — MB BS Lond. 1981 (St. Bart.) DRCOG 1985; DGM RCP Lond. 1986. GP Colchester; Club Doctor Colchester United Football Club. Specialty: Alcohol & Substance Misuse. Prev: Trainee GP Colchester VTS; Ho. Surg. & Ho. Phys. Essex Co. Hosp. Colchester.

RUDGLEY, Richard John Fairholme, The Ridge, Cold Ash, Thatcham RG18 9HZ — MB BS Lond. 1986; MRCGP 1991; MRCGP 1991; DRCOG 1992.

RUDHAM, Samuel James 19 Normanby Road, Nottingham NG8 2TA — BM Soton. 1993.

RUDIN, Claudius Department of Haematology, Royal Devon and Exeter Hospital, Wonford, Exeter EX2 5DW — Diplome Federal Switzerland 1985; MRCP (UK) 1991; MRCPath 2001; MD 2001.

RUDIN, Joseph Albert Lingholm, 5 Haslemere Road, Long Eaton, Nottingham NG10 4AG Tel: 0115 973 4727 Fax: 0115 946 0197 — MB ChB Manch. 1957 (Manchester) Prev: Ho. Phys. Manch. Roy. Infirm.; Ho. Off. (Obst.) St. Mary's Hosp. Manch.; Ho. Surg. Ancoats Hosp.

RUDLAND, Edward Neville (retired) Green Westerland, Marldon, Paignton TQ3 1RR Tel: 01803 663660 Fax: 01803 663666 — (royal London Hosp) MRCS Eng. LRCP Lond. 1952; MRCGP 1969. Prev: Clin. Asst. Roy. Eye Infirm. Plymouth.

RUDLAND, Simon Victor, Surg. Lt.-Cdr. RN Retd. Stowhealth, Violet Hill House, Violet Hill Road, Stowmarket IP14 1NL Tel: 01449 776000 Fax: 01449 776005; 15 Ipswhich Road, Woodbridge IP12 4BS Tel: 01394 388821 — BM BS Nottm. 1986; BMedSci Nottm. 1984; DA (UK) 1990; DRCOG 1993; MRCGP 1994. GP Princip.; GP Professional Developm. Mentor, E. Suff. Specialty: Accid. & Emerg. Prev: Regist. (Emerg. Med.) Fremantle Hosp., West. Austral.; Med. Off. SST North. Iraq, Gulf War; Med. Off. HMS Challenger.

RUDLING, Joanne Louise 90 Lascelles Drive, Cardiff CF23 8NQ — MB BCh Wales 1994. SHO (Gen. Med.) Princess of Wales Hosp. Bridgend. Specialty: Gen. Med. Prev: SHO (A & E & Psychiat.) Princess of Wales Hosp. Bridgend; GP/Regist. Porthcawl.

RUDMAN, David John (retired) 167 Percy Road, Whitton, Twickenham TW2 6JE — MB BS Lond. 1950 (Guy's) MRCS Eng. LRCP Lond. 1945.

RUDMAN, Julie Davina Catherine Street Surgery, 3 Catherine Street, Whitehaven CA28 7PD Tel: 01946 693094 — MB ChB Leeds 1978; MB ChB 1978 Leeds. GP Whitehaven, Cumbria.

RUDMAN, Robert Jeffrey Doctors Surgery, Hinnings Road, Distington, Workington CA14 5UR Tel: 01946 830207 — MB ChB Leeds 1978. GP Workington, Cumbria.

RUDMAN, Timothy John The Health Centre, Hermitage Road, St John's, Woking GU21 8TD Tel: 01483 723451 Fax: 01483 751879; Comeragh House, Comeragh Close., Hook Heath, Woking GU22 0LZ Tel: 01483 715621 Fax: 01483 776660 — (Roy. Free) MB BS Lond. 1967; MRCS Eng. LRCP Lond. 1967; DObst RCOG 1970; DFFP 1994. Med. Ref. Home Off. Socs: Woking Med. Soc. Prev: Ho. Off. (Med. & Neurol.) Roy. Free Hosp. Lond.; Ho. Off. (Surg. & Orthop.) N. Middlx. Hosp. Lond.; Ho. Off. (Paediat.) Whipps Cross Hosp. Lond.

RUDNICK, Leanne Rose St Paul's Medical Centre, Dickson Road, Blackpool FY1 2HH Tel: 01253 623896 Fax: 01253 752818 — MB ChB Manch. 1990.

RUDNICK, Steven Phillip St George's Medical Centre, Field Road, New Brighton, Wallasey CH45 5LN Tel: 0151 630 2080 Fax: 0151 637 0370 — MB ChB Liverp. 1986. Specialty: Gen. Pract. Prev: SHO/Trainee GP Wirral HA VTS; Ho. Off. (Med. & Surg.) Arrowe Pk. Hosp. Wirral.

RUDOLF, Mary Catherine Joy Department of Community Child Health, Belmont House, Leeds General Infirmary, Leeds LS2 9NP Tel: 0113 292 6352 Fax: 0113 292 6219; 1 Crescent Gardens, Leeds LS17 8DR Tel: 0113 268 6442 — MB BS Lond. 1975 (Univ. Coll. Hosp.) BSc (Human Genetics) Lond. 1972; DCH RCP Lond. 1985; FRCPCH 1997. Cons. Community Child Health Leeds Community & Ment. Health Trust & Hon. Sen. Lect. Univ. Leeds. Specialty: Community Child Health; Paediat. Prev: Fell. (Pediat. Endocrinol.) Yale Univ, USA; Research Fell. (Ambul. Pediat.) Brown Univ., USA; Paediat. Kupat Holim Child Developm. Centre, Haifa, Israel.

RUDOLF, Michael Ealing Hospital, Uxbridge Road, Southall UB1 3HW Tel: 020 8967 5687 Fax: 020 8967 5660 Email: michael.rudolf@eht.nhs.uk — MB BChir Camb. 1970 (Middlx.) MA Camb. 1970; MRCP (UK) 1973; FRCP Lond. 1989. Cons. Phys. Ealing Hosp. Southall; Hon. Sen. Lect. (Med.) Imperial Coll. Sch. of Med. Specialty: Respirat. Med. Socs: Fell. Roy. Soc. Med. (Ex-Pres. Sect. Measurem. in Med.); (Pres.) Internat. Asthma Counc.; Brit. Thorac. Soc. (Ex chair, Standards of care Comm.). Prev: Sen. Regist. Hammersmith Hosp. Lond.; Sir Jules Thorn Research Fell. Middlx. Hosp. Med. Sch. Lond.; Regist. Prof. Med. Unit Middlx. Hosp. Lond.

RUDOLF, Noel de Montjoie 130 Harley Street, London W1G 7JU Tel: 020 7935 1825 Fax: 020 7224 7220 — BM BCh Oxf. 1959 (Oxf. & King's Coll. Hosp.) BA Oxf. 1954; MA Oxf. 1958. Cons. (Clin. Neurophysiol.) Privat. Pract. Lond. Specialty: Clin. Neurophysiol. Socs: Founder Mem. Assn. Brit. Clin. Neurophysiol.; Brit. Soc. Clin. Neurophysiol.; Fell. R.S.M. Prev: Cons. Clin. Neurophysiol. Char. Cross Hosp. & Cheyne Centre Lond.; Hon. Sen. Lect. Char. Cross & Westm. Med. Sch. Lond.; Hon. Cons. Clin. Neurophysiologist Chelsea & Westminster Hosp Lond.

RUDOLPH, Jonathan Kevin Pinn Medical Centre, 8 Eastcote Road, Pinner HA5 1HF Tel: 020 8866 5766 Fax: 020 8429 0251; 15 Brockley Close, Stanmore HA7 4QL Tel: 020 8958 2455 Fax: 020 8954 5966 — MB BCh Witwatersrand 1988; MRCGP 1994; DRCOG 1994. Specialty: Gen. Pract.

RUDOLPH, Julia The Red House, 7 High St., Barton, Cambridge CB3 7BG — MB BS Lond. 1998 (St Mary's) Jun. Ho. Off. A&E Hervey Bay.Hosp.Qu.sland AU. Specialty: Accid. & Emerg.

RUDOLPHIJ, Adelhart Jan Department ENT, St. Helier Hospital, Wrythe Lane, Carshalton SM5 1AA Tel: 020 8644 4343 Fax: 020 8296 3652; 101 Carshalton Park Road, Carshalton SM5 3SJ Tel: 020 8647 7463 — MRCS Eng. LRCP Lond. 1978; St. Mary's. Clin. Asst. (ENT) St. Helier Hosp. Carshalton. Specialty: Otolaryngol. Prev: Trainee GP Ashtead; SHO (ENT & O & G) St. Helier Hosp. Carshalton; Resid. Emerg. Med. Bermuda.

RUDOLPHY, Steven Michael c/o Coniston, 5 Wyvern Road, Purley CR8 2NQ — MB BS Lond. 1985; MRCGP 1990.

RUDRA, Hiren D (retired) 1 Oak Drive, Sawbridgeworth CM21 0AH Tel: 01279 723573 — MB BS Calcutta 1956, DGO 1958; MRCOG 1967. Dir. Harlow Occupat. Health Serv. Ltd. Prev: Regist. (O & G) Essex Gen. Hosp. Colchester & Camb. Matern. Hosp.

RUDRA, Thilaka Prakash Colchester General Hospital, Gainsborough Wing, Turner Road, Colchester CO4 5JL Tel: 01206 742535 Fax: 01206 742545 — MB BS Sri Lanka 1975; FRCP. Cons. Phys. Geriat. Med. Colchester Gen. Hosp. Specialty: Care of the Elderly.

RUDRALINGAM, Meenakshi Musgrave and Clark House, The Royal Groups of Hospitals and, Social Services Trust, Grosvenor Rd, Belfast BT12 6BA — MB BCh BAO Belf. 1997.

RUDRALINGAM, Velauthan 4A Windsor Close, Belfast BT9 6FG — MB ChB BAO Belf. 1995; MB BCh BAO Belf. 1995.

RUDRAMOORTHY, Thuraiayah 32 Hunter's Oak, Hemel Hempstead HP2 7SW Tel: 01442 232037; 32 Hunter's Oak, Hemel Hempstead HP2 7SW Tel: 01442 232037 — MB BS Ceylon 1971. Asst. GP. Specialty: Gen. Med.; Geriat. Psychiat.; Care of the Elderly. Socs: BMA. Prev: Assessor Benefit Agency.

RUDRAN, Viji Peace Children's Centre, Peace Prospect, Watford WD17 3EW — MB BS Sri Lanka 1978; DCH Eng. 1983; LRCP LRCS Ed. LRCPS Glas. 1984; MRCP (UK) 1987; FRCPCH UK 1997. Specialty: Paediat.

RUDRAPPA, Chithriki William Way Doctors Surgery, William Way, Wainfleet All Saints, Skegness PE24 4DE Tel: 01754 880212 Fax: 01754 880788 — MB BS Mysore 1968.

RUDRASHETTY, Sarojani Rudrashetty and Partners, Mary Potter Health Centre, Gregory Boulevard, Hyson Green, Nottingham NG7 5HY.

RUDWICK, Ann Louise (retired) Mellstock, 9B Westwood Road, Ryde PO33 3BJ; Mellstock, 9B Westwood Rd, Ryde PO33 3BJ Tel: 01983 568762 — (Roy. Free) BSc Durham. 1951; MB BS Lond. 1956; DCH Eng. 1959. Prev: SCMO (Child Health) Richmond, Twickenham & Roehampton HA.

RUDZINSKI, Barbara Mary 16 Broomhill Road, London SW18 4JF — MB BS Lond. 1981.

RUEL, Ann Hilary (retired) 14 Church Street, Histon, Cambridge CB4 9EP Tel: 01223 563619 — MB BS Lond. 1953 (Roy. Free) MRCS Eng. LRCP Lond. 1953; DCH Eng. 1956. Volun. Phys. Med. Foundat. for the c/o the Victims of Torture. Prev: Clin. Asst. (Child & Family Psychiat.) Camb.

RUELL, Jacqueline Ann Holcombe Water, Wiveliscombe, Taunton TA4 2SL — MB ChB Liverp. 1998; MB ChB Liverp 1998.

RUELL, Sheila Diane Fairfield Surgery, Station Road, Flookburgh, Grange-over-Sands LA11 7JY — MB ChB Liverp. 1984; DRCOG 1987; MRCGP 1988.

RUFF, Stephen James 22 Willow Way, Ponteland, Newcastle upon Tyne NE20 9RF — MB ChB Liverp. 1974; FFA RCSI 1978. Specialty: Anaesth.

RUFFE, Sarah Helen 19 Moorhead Terrace, Shipley BD18 4LB.

RUFFELL, Elizabeth Anne Eastbourne District General Hospital, Kings Drive, Eastbourne BN21 2UD — MB BS Lond. 1973 (St. Georges Hospital Medical School London) MRCP (UK) 1976; FRCR 1981; FRCP 2000. Cons. Radiol. Eastbourne Dist. Hosps. Specialty: Radiol.

RUFFETT, Douglas Ian Appleton House, Lanchester Road, Durham DH1 5XZ Tel: 0191 333 3232 Fax: 0191 333 3233; 64 Hall Drive, Acklam, Middlesbrough TS5 7EX Tel: 01642 819821 — MB BS Newc. 1971; FRCGP 1986, M 1975; MSc (Pub. Health Med.) Newc. 1995. Head of Primary Care Support Unit Co. Durh. & Tees Valley SHA. Prev: GP Middlesbrough; Regional Med. Off. DoH; Primary Care Med. Adviser Tees HA.

RUFFLE, Simon Patrick Twyford Surgery, Loddon Hall Road, Twyford, Reading RG10 9JA Tel: 0118 934 6680 Fax: 0118 934 6690 — MB BS Lond. 1992; MRCGP.

RUFFORD, Barnaby David High Trees, Lower St., Great Bealings, Woodbridge IP13 6NL — MB BS Lond. 1993.

RUFFORD, Christopher William 28 Brook Street, Woodbridge IP12 1BE Email: c.rufford@qmul.ac.uk — MB BS Lond. 1978; DRCOG 1981; DCH RCP Lond. 1983; MRCGP 1986; Dip Sports & Exercise Med. 1990. Sen. Lect. (Sports & Exercise Med.) Barts & The Lond. Hosp. Lond. Specialty: Sports Med. Special Interest: Med. Educat.; Sports Med. Prev: Trainee GP Wimbourne.

RUFFORD, Hermione Jane 46 Upcerne Road, London SW10 0SQ — MB BS Lond. 1993 (King's College School of Medicine & Dentistry London) Specialist Regist. Kent & Canterbury Hosp.; Spec. Regist. Kings Coll. Hosp. Lond.; Research Fellow Kings Coll. Hosp. Lond.; Spec. Regist. Univ. Hosp., Lewisham. Specialty: Obst. & Gyn. Prev: SHO (O & G) King's Coll. Hosp. Lond.; SHO (O & G) Roy. Sussex Co. Hosp. Brighton; SHO (A & E) King's Coll. Hosp. Lond.

RUGG, Anthony John Harrogate District Hospital, Lancaster Park Road, Harrogate HG2 7SX Tel: 01423 885959 Fax: 01423 593397; 6 St. John Street, York YO31 7QT Tel: 01904 630507 — MB ChB Birm. 1971; DCH Eng. 1973; DPM Leeds 1975; FRCPsych 1995, M 1976. Cons. Psychiat. Harrogate HA. Specialty: Gen. Psychiat. Prev: Sen. Regist. (Psychiat.) Lond. Hosp.; Regist. Naburn & Bootham Pk. Hosps.; SHO (Paediat.) Co. & Fulford Hosps. York.

RUGG, Sarah Ann Matilda The Surgery, 15 Brook Green, London W6 7BL — MB BCh Wales 1995 (Univ. Wales Coll. Med.) DFFP 1998; DCH 1999. Specialty: Gen. Pract. Prev: GP Sen. Regist., Lond.; GP Regist., Fulham, Lond.; SHO Gynaecologist/Obs., Lond.

RUGG-EASEY, Margaret Lilian (retired) 4 Wentworth Drive, Tividale, Oldbury B69 1QD Tel: 01384 850351 — MB BS Lond. 1940 (Roy. Free) MRCP Lond. 1947. Prev: Capt. RAMC.

RUGGIER, Romanie Dept of Anaesthesia, St George's Healthcare NHS Trust, London SW17 0QT Tel: 020 8725 3316 Email: ruggier@virgin.net; 5 Old Palace Lane, Richmond TW9 1PG Tel: 020 8940 4426 Fax: 020 8940 4426 — MB BS Lond. 1987 (Royal Free Hospital School of Medicine) BSc Lond. 1984; Royal College of Anaesthetists 1993. Cons. Anaesth. with s/i in Neuroanaesth. & Neurocritical Care. Specialty: Anaesth.

RUGGINS, Nigel Raymond Derbyshire Children's Hospital, Uttoxeter Road, Derby DE22 3NE Tel: 01332 340131 Fax: 01332 200857 Email: nigel.Ruggins@sdah-tr.trent.nhs.uk; 48 Hazelwood Road, Duffield, Belper DE56 4AA Tel: 01332 842347 Email: nigel.ruggins@sdah-tr.trent.nhs.uk — MB BS Lond. 1979 (Univ. Coll. Hosp.) FRCPCH; BSc (Hons.) (Human Genetics) Lond. 1979; MRCP (UK) 1986. Cons. Paediat., Derbysh. Childr. Hosp.; Serv. Director, Childrens Servs., SDAHT. Specialty: Paediat. Special Interest: Paediatric Respirat. Med. Socs: BMA; Perinatal Soc.; FRCPCH. Prev: Sen. Regist. (Paediat.) Nottm.; Research Fell., Childr. Respirat. Unit, Univ. Hosp. Nottm.

RUGGLES, Ruth Marie Brentford Health Centre, Albany Road, Brentford TW8 8DS — BM BCh Oxf. 1985; DCH RCP Lond. 1989; Cert. Family Plann. JCC 1989; DRCOG 1990; MRCGP 1991.

RUGHANI, Amar Nath Burncross Surgery, 1 Bevan Way, Chapeltown, Sheffield S35 1RN Tel: 0114 246 6052 Fax: 0114 245 0276; 519 Fulwood Road, Sheffield S10 3QB — MB BS Lond. 1982 (Roy. Lond. Hosp.) BSc Lond. 1979; DRCOG 1986; MRCGP (Distinc.) 1986; DCH RCP Lond. 1987; FRCGP 1999. Examr. RCGP; Assoc. Course Organiser Sheff. VTS; Assoc. Postgrad. Dean, S. Yorks. and Humber Deanery. Socs: Roy. Coll. of Gen. Practitioners, Treas. Sheff. Fac. & Treas. Prev: GP Tutor Continuing Professional Developm., Univ. of Sheff.

RUGHANI, Vijaykumar Gokaldas Ardgowan, Wakefield Road, Ackworth, Pontefract WF7 7DN Tel: 01977 619902 Mob: 07905 405471 — MB BS Durh. 1957.

RUGMAN, Francis Paul — MB ChB Liverp. 1977 (Univ. of Liverp.) MRCP (UK) 1983; FRCP Lond. 1996; FRCPath 1997; MSc (Distinc.) O.U. 2002; MSc open Univ. 2002. Cons. Haemat. Lancs. Teachg. Hosps. NHS Trust Preston Lancs.; Assoc. Lect. (Med. : Infec. Dis.) Open Univ. Specialty: Haematology. Special Interest: Gen. Haemat.; Haemostasis & Thrombosis. Socs: European Haematology Association; British Society of Haemostasis & Thrombosis; Chronic Lymphocytic Leukaemia Forum. Prev: Sen. Regist. (Haemat.) Roy. Liverp. Hosp.; Research Fell. (N. W. Cancer Fund) Univ. Liverp.; Regist. (Gen. Med.) Wirral Hosps.

RUHI, Shamim Osmani East Ham Memorial Hospital, Shrewsbury Road, Forest Gate, London E7 8QR Tel: 020 8586 5012 — MB BS Punjab 1977; DTCD Punjab 1979; DPMSA Punjab 1981; DHMSA Punjab 1983; MRCPsych 1985. Cons. Psychiat. Newham HA.; Unit Train. Dir. Specialty: Gen. Psychiat. Prev: Sen. Regist. (Psychiat.) St. Bart. Hosp. Lond.

RUHUL AMIN, Mir Abul Kalam Mohammed 18 Ferme Park Road, London N4 4ED Tel: 020 8340 6050 — MB BS Dacca 1956 (Dacca Med. Coll.) LMSSA Lond. 1968.

RUIGROK, Mr André St James's University Hospital, Beckett Street, Leeds LS9 7TF Tel: 0113 243 3144 Ext: 66317 Email: Andre.Ruigrok@virgin.net — Artsexamen Nijmegen 1982; FCOphth. Community Ophth. Specialty: Ophth. Special Interest: Glaucoma.

RUIZ, George Antonio 68 Endrick Gardens, Balfron, Glasgow G63 0RD — MB ChB Glas. 1996.

RUIZ, Kenneth 11 Crimicar Drive, Sheffield S10 4EF — MB ChB Sheff. 1984; BMedSci Sheff. 1982, MB ChB 1984; FRCA 1989.

RUIZ, Maria-Carmen 38 Letterfearn Drive, Glasgow G23 5JL — MB ChB Glas. 1998; MB ChB Glas 1998.

RUIZ, Ramon Gregory Gary 69 Frankfurt Road, London SE24 9NX — MB BS Lond. 1982 (King's Coll. Hosp.) BSc (Physiol.) Lond. 1979; MRCP (UK) 1986. Cons. Paediat. King's Coll. Hosp. Lond. Specialty: Paediat. Prev: Sen. Regist. (Paediat.) Dudley Rd. Hosp. Birm.; Research Regist. (Paediat.) King's Coll. Sch. Med. & Dent. Univ. Lond.

RUIZ DE ARCAUTE, Javier 21 Rozel Square, Manchester M3 4FQ — LMS Basque Provinces 1996.

RUIZ FITO, Jose Rafael ENT Department, Barnsley District General Hospital, Gawber Road,, Barnsley S75 2PW; Park View House, Barnsley Road,, Cudworth, Barnsley S72 8SY Tel: 01226 718767 — LMS Seville 1990. SHO (ENT) (Barnsley Dist. Gen. Hosp.). Specialty: Otorhinolaryngol. Prev: SHO (ENT - Barnsley Dist. Gen. Hosp.); SHO (ENT - Roy. Gwent Hosp., Newport); SHO (ENT - Singleton, Hosp., Swansea).

RUIZ GONZALEZ, Maria Chorley & South Ribble Hospital, Oakfield Unit, Preston Road, Chorley PR7 1PP Tel: 01257 245890 Fax: 01257 245281 — LMS Navarra 1992. Cons. (Psychiat.) Chorley & S. Ribble Hosp. Specialty: Gen. Psychiat. Special Interest: Mood Disorders; Psychother.

RUIZ HERRERO, Angel Luis 242 Malone Road, Belfast BT9 5LR Tel: 01232 682916; c/o Estudios No 2, Madrid 28012, Spain Tel: 00 34 1 3669401 — LMS Madrid 1989; FRCSI 1994. Career Specialist Regist. Belf. City Hosp.; Specialist Regist. (Orthop.) Rotat. Altnagelvin Hosp., Londonderry, N. Irel. Specialty: Orthop. Prev: Career Regist. Rotat. Ulster Hosp., Roy. Vict. Hosp. & Musgrave Pk. Hosp. Belf.; SHO (Surg.) Crawley Hosp. W. Sussex; SHO (Surg. & Orthop.) Princess Roy. Hosp. Haywards Heath.

RUIZ MARTIN, Marcelino Block 14, Flat 7, Good Hope Hospital, Rectory Road, Sutton Coldfield B75 7RR — LMS Granada 1992.

RUKMANI, Krishna Sastrigal The Surgery, 145 Portland Road, Hove BN3 5QJ Tel: 01273 734888 Fax: 01273 203232; 97 The Promenade, Peacehaven BN10 8LH — MB BS Calcutta 1975. Specialty: Family Plann. & Reproduc. Health.

RUKUNAYAKE, Gunasili Nimal Chandrasena 20 Claremont Gardens, Clevedon BS21 5BG — MB BS Ceylon 1968.

RULE, Mrs Elizabeth Margaret Pensby Road Surgery, 349 Pensby Road, Pensby, Wirral CH61 9NL Tel: 0151 648 1193 Fax: 0151 648 2934; 8 Brancote Road, Oxton, Birkenhead CH43 6TJ — MB ChB Liverp. 1972; BSc (Hons.) (Microbiol.) Liverp. 1972; MB ChB Liverp. 1974; DCH Eng. 1977; DRCOG 1977.

RULE, Joan Tonna Hospital, Tonna, Neath SA11 3LX Tel: 01639 635404 — MB BCh Wales 1973; FRCPsych.

RULE, Michael Jeremy Peartree Lane Surgery, 110 Peartree Lane, Welwyn Garden City AL7 3XW Tel: 01707 329292; 62 Peartree Lane, Welwyn Garden City AL7 3UH — MB BS Lond. 1981 (St. Bart.) BSc (Hons.) Lond. 1978, MB BS 1981.

RULE, Simon Alexander Joseph Derriford Road, Plymouth PL6 8DH; Stowe Hill House, Netherstowe, Lichfield WS13 6TJ — BM BS Nottm. 1987; MPhil Nottm. 1986, BMedSci 1984; MRCP 1990, FRCPA 1995. Cons. (Haematology) Derriford Hosp. Devon. Prev: SHO (Med. Rotat.) Taunton & Som. Hosp.

RULEWSKI, Nigel John 37 Saxonwood Road, Cheswick Green, Shirley, Solihull B90 4JR — MB BS Lond. 1977 (St. Bart.) DRCOG 1981; DCH RCP Lond. 1982. Vice-Pres. Med. Affairs Astra, USA.

RUMBALL, Bernard John Southview Surgery, Guildford Road, Woking GU22 7RR Tel: 01483 763186 Fax: 01483 821526 — MB BCh Wales 1982.

RUMBALL, Claire Louise Ash House, St Martin's Hospital, Midford Road, Bath BA2 5RP Tel: 01225 840132 — MB BS Newc. 1991 (Newcastle upon Tyne) MRCGP 1996; DFFP 1996. Clin. Med. Off. (Family Plann.) Bath & Wilts. Specialty: Family Plann. & Reproduc. Health; Gen. Pract.; Genitourinary Medicine.

RUMBALL, Daphne The Bure Centre, 7 Unthank Road, Norwich NR2 2PA Tel: 01603 671900 Fax: 01603 671920 — MB ChB Liverp. 1975 (Liverpool University) DRCOG 1979; MRCPsych 1981; FRCPsych 1997. Cons. Psychiat. (Addiction Psychiatry) Norf.and Waveney Ment. Health Partnership NHS Trust; Acad. Adviser, Sch. of Med., Univ. of E. Anglia. Specialty: Gen. Psychiat. Prev: Cons. Psychiat. Gt. Yarmouth & Waveney Health Dist.

RUMBLE, Mr John Anthony 45 Imperial Avenue, Westcliff on Sea SS0 8NQ Tel: 01702 337598; Finches, Church End, Paglesham, Rochford SS4 2DP Tel: 01702 258584 Fax: As Phone — (Sheffield University) MB ChB Sheff. 1955; DObst RCOG 1958; DO Eng. 1963; FRCS Eng. 1967; FCOphth 1989. Cons. Ophth. Southend Health Dist. Specialty: Ophth. Prev: Sen. Regist. (Ophth.) United Birm. Hosps.; Res. Surg. Off. Birm. & Midl. Eye Hosp.

RUMBLE, Mark Leonard Ley Surgery, Nathaniel Fish Row, 43 King Street, Great Yarmouth NR30 2PN Tel: 01493 330338 — MB ChB Dundee 1971; MA UEA 1996.

RUMBLE, Peter Bertram Castle Place Surgery, 9 Park Hill, Tiverton EX16 6RR Tel: 01884 252333 Fax: 01884 252152; Withleigh Goodman, Withleigh, Tiverton EX16 8JG — MB ChB Bristol 1978; Family Plann. Cert 1981; DRCOG 1981; MRCGP 1982. GP Tiverton Devon. Prev: GP Trainee Backwell.

RUMBOLD, Christopher Alexander Wool Surgery, Folly Lane, Wool, Wareham BH20 6DS Tel: 01929 462376; Kingsmead, Chalkpit Lane, Wool, Wareham BH20 6DW — MB BCh Wales 1974.

RUMBOLD, John Mark Michael 10 Newland Road, Bordesley Green, Birmingham B9 5PS — MB ChB Dundee 1994.

RUMFELD, Werner Robert The Cedars Surgery, 26 Swanley Centre, Swanley BR8 7AH Tel: 01322 663111/663237 Fax: 01322 614867 — State Exam Med Berlin 1976 (Freie Univ. Berlin) MD Berlin 1978; MRCGP 1990. Arzt für Innere Medizin und Rheumatologie, NR W.falen 1985. Specialty: Gastroenterol.; Rheumatol. Socs: Roy. Coll. Gen. Pract.; Med. Defence Union. Prev: Regist. (Rheum.) Univ. Hosp. Wales Cardiff; Regist. (Med.) Princess Margt. Hosp. Swindon.

RUMIAN, Adam Piotr Crossley House, Sutton Lane, London W4 4HF — MB BS Lond. 1998; MB BS Lond 1998.

RUMIAN, Ryszard (retired) Crossley House Surgery, Sutton Lane, London W4 4HF Tel: 020 8994 0342 Fax: 020 8994 6927 — LRCPI & LM, LRSCI & LM 1954 (RCSI) LRCPI & LM, LRCSI & LM 1954; DObst RCOG 1959. Clin. Asst. (Orthop.) W. Middlx. Hosp. Isleworth. Prev: Regist. (Orthop., Plastic Surg. & Cas.) W. Middlx. Hosp. Isleworth.

RUMLEY, Joseph James 37 Crofthead Street, Uddingston, Glasgow G71 7JQ — MB ChB Glas. 1998; MB ChB Glas 1998.

RUMLEY, Sally Jane Abberley cottage, Dowles Road, Bewdley DY12 2EJ — MB ChB Birm. 1990. Specialty: Gen. Pract.

RUMLEY, Simon Lawrence Paul York House Medical Centre, Stourport-on-Severn DY13 9EH Tel: 01299 827171 — MB ChB Leeds 1989; DCH RCP Lond. 1994; MRCGP 1996. GP Princip. Specialty: Otorhinolaryngol.

RUMMENS, Ian Frank Cae Glas Doctors Surgery, 34 Church Street, Oswestry SY11 2SP Tel: 01691 652929 Fax: 01691 670175 Email: ian.rummens@nhs.net; Cae Cerrig, Sweeney Mountain, Oswestry SY10 9EZ — MB ChB Birm. 1978; DRCOG 1982. Med. Off., Derwen Coll., Oswestsy SY11 3JA (1985-). Socs: Hon. Sec. Shrops. Local Med. Comm. (1986-).

RUMMENS, Laura Jane Selly Park Surgery, 2 Reaview Drive, Pershore Road, Birmingham B29 7NT Tel: 0121 472 0187 Fax: 0121 472 0187 — MB ChB Birm. 1990; DRCOG 1993; DCH RCP Lond. 1994; MRCGP 1996. Specialty: Gen. Pract.

RUMMENS, Simon David University Health Centre, Elms Road, Off Pritchatts Road, Birmingham B15 2SE Tel: 0121 414 5111 Fax: 0121 414 5108; 92 Woolacombe Lodge Road, Selly Oak, Birmingham B29 6PY Tel: 0121 414 5111 — MB ChB Birm. 1989; DRCOG 1993; MRCGP 1994.

RUMSEY, Jennifer Margaret Anne Greenbank Surgery, 1025 Stratford Road, Hall Green, Birmingham B28 8BG Tel: 0121 777 1490 Fax: 0121 778 6239; 39 Kineton Green Road, Olton, Solihull B92 7DX Tel: 0121 706 0165 — (Camb. & St. Geo.) MA, MB Camb. 1972, BChir 1971; Cert FPA 1974; DObst RCOG 1975. Prev: SHO (Ophth.) Bromley Hosp.; Ho. Off. (O & G) Lambeth Hosp.; Ho. Off. (Ophth. & ENT) St. Geo. Hosp. Lond.

RUMSEY, Sarah 5 Tylers, Sewards End, Saffron Walden CB10 2LN — MB BS Lond. 1955; DRCOG 1957; DCH RCP Lond. 1959; MLCOM 1982; MRO 1992. Med. Osteop. Essex.

RUNACRES, Anthony Selwyn Robert Blandford House Surgery, 7 London Road, Braintree CM7 2LD Tel: 01376 347100 Fax: 01376 349934 — MB Camb. 1972 (St. Bart.) BChir 1971; DObst RCOG 1975. Clin. Assist Dermat. Broomfield Hosp. Essex. Prev: Trainee Gen. Pract. Norwich Vocational Train. Scheme.

RUNAGALL, Simon Edward Loughton Mental Health Centre, 8-10 High Beech Road, Loughton IG10 4BL Tel: 020 8271 4000 Fax: 020 8271 4006 Email: simon.runagall@nemhpt.nhs.uk — MB ChB Dundee 1989; DCH RCPS Glas. 1991. Staff Grade Community Ment. Health Centre Loughton. Specialty: Gen. Psychiat. Prev: SHO (Psychiat.) Colchester; SHO (Paediat.) Harlow.

RUNCHMAN, Mr Phillip Charles, Surg. Cdr. RN — BM BCh Oxf. 1974; FRCS Eng. 1981. Cons. Gen. Surg. Specialty: Gen. Surg.

RUNCIE, Colin John Department of Anaesthetics, Western Infirmary, Glasgow G11 6NT Tel: 0141 211 2069; 18 Whittngehame Drive, Glasgow G12 0XX — MB ChB Glas. 1982; MRCP (UK) 1985; FRCA 1988; FRCP Glas. 1995. Cons. Anaesth. West. Infirm. Glas. Specialty: Anaesth.

RUNCIE, Ian James Denmans, 4 The Glebe, Lindfield, Haywards Heath RH16 2JS Tel: 01444 450639 Fax: 01444 414816 — MB BCh Wales 1975; FRCR 1982; T(R) (CR) 1991. Cons. Radiol. Princess Roy. Hosp. Haywards Heath. Specialty: Radiol.

RUNCIE, James 14 Provost Ferguson Drive, Tain IV19 1RE — MB ChB Ed. 1937; MF Hom. 1946.

RUNCIMAN, David Martin Inglis 3 Lucerne Road, Oxford OX2 7QB Tel: 01865 516696 Fax: 01865 516696 — MB BS Lond. 1988; MRCPI 1994; MRCPCH 1996. Specialist Regist. (Paediat. Cardiol.) Oxf.

RUNDELL, Timothy Roy 13 Robin Close, Stanstead Abbotts, Ware SG12 8TX — MB BS Lond. 1986; DCH RCP Lond. 1990.

RUNDLE, Catriona McHarg Tayside University Hospitals Trust, Ninewells Hospital, Dundee — MB ChB Dundee 2002. Sen. Ho. Off. in Obst. and Gyn.

RUNDLE, John Alan Little Pastures, 6 Church Road, Brackley NN13 7BU Tel: 01280 705102 Fax: 01280 705102 — (Lond.

Hosp.) MRCS Eng. LRCP Lond. 1951; FRFPS Glas. 1954; MRCP Ed. 1955; MRCP Lond. 1955; MRCP Glas. 1962; FRCP Ed. 1995. Cons. Neurol. Essex Nuffield Hosp. Brentwood., Ashcroft Clinic, Deddington, Oxon. & Hartswood Hosp. Brentwood; Vis. Phys. NHS Hosp. Essex; Phys. to Med. Foundat. Lond.; Cons. Neur. Lond. Neurol. Centre. Specialty: Neurol. Socs: BMA; Liveryman Soc. Apoth. Lond. Prev: Sen. Regist. Maida Vale Hosp.; Regist. (Med.) Hackney Hosp. & Roy. Lond. Hosp.; Ho. Phys. Nat. Hosp. Nerv. Dis. Lond.

RUNDLE, Mr John Samuel Harris 2 Dover Road, Branksome Park, Poole BH13 6DZ — MB ChB Ed. 1973; FRCS Ed. 1977. Cons. Urol. Roy. Bournemouth Hosp. Specialty: Urol.

RUNDLE, Paul Anthony Department of Opthalmology, Royal Hallamshire Hospital, Glossop Road, Sheffield S10 2JF Tel: 0114 2713619 Email: paul.rundle@sth.nhs.uk — MB BS Newc. 1988; FRCOphth Lond. 1995. Cons. Ophth., Roy. Hallamshire Hosp., Sheff.; Cons. Ophth., Claremont Hosp., Sandygate Rd., Sheff. Specialty: Ophth.; Oncol. Prev: Regist. Ophth., RVH, Belf.

RUNDLE, Philippa Kate 8 Firs Avenue, East Sheen, London SW14 7NZ — (St. Mary's) MB Camb. 1969, BChir 1968; DObst RCOG 1970; DCH Eng. 1971. Assoc. Specialist (Paediat.) St. Mary's Hosp. Lond.; Sen. Clin. Med. Off. Kingston AHA; Forens. Med. Examr. Metrop. Police. Specialty: Paediat. Prev: SCMO Kensington, Chelsea & Westm. AHA.

RUNDLE, Susan Kathleen 39 Sunnybank, Epsom KT18 7DY — BM Soton. 1995 (Southampton University Medical School) BSc Soton. 1994; MRCP 1998. SHO (Neurol.) Qu. Eliz. Hosp. Specialty: Otorhinolaryngol. Socs: BMA. Prev: SHO (Oncol.) Qu. Eliz. Hosp. Birm.; SHO (Endocrinol.) SOH Birm.; SHO (Elderly Care) SOH Birm.

RUNNETT, Craig — MB ChB Leeds 1993.

RUOSS, Mr Christopher Fredrick Combe Hill, 36 The Heights, Worthing BN14 0AJ Tel: 01903 261737 Fax: 01903 261737 — MB BS Lond. 1963 (St. Bart.) MRCS Eng. LRCP Lond. 1963; FRCS Eng. 1967; FRCOG 1982, M 1969. Cons. O & G Worthing & Southlands Hosps. Specialty: Obst. & Gyn. Socs: Blair Bell Res. Soc. Prev: Cons. Matern. & Child Health WHO Europ. Off. Copehagen, Denmark; Sen. Regist. (O & G) St. Bart. Hosp. Lond.; Resid. Med. Off. Qu. Charlotte's Matern. Hosp. Lond.

RUPAL, Anita 26 Downshall Avenue, Ilford IG3 8NB — MB ChB Aberd. 1988; DRCOG 1993.

RUPARELIA, Mr Bhanuprasad Anandji Worcestershire Royal Hospital, Charles Hastings Way, Worcester WR5 1DD Tel: 01905 760608 Fax: 01905 760787 Email: bhanu.ruparelia@nhs.net; Holly Lodge, Bosbury Road, Cradley, Malvern WR13 5LT Email: bhanu@baruparelia.freeserve.co.uk — MB BS Lond. 1976 (Guy's) BSc (Biochem.) Lond. 1973; MRCS Eng. LRCP Lond. 1976; FRCOG 1995, M 1982; FRCS Ed. 1982. Cons. O & G Worcester Roy. Hosp.; Lead Clinician, Worcester Osteoporosis Unit. Specialty: Obst. & Gyn. Special Interest: Gyn. Oncol.; Menopause; Osteoporosis. Socs: Mem. - Brit. Menopause Soc.; Mem. Brit. Soc. Colposcopy & Cytol. Pathol.; Mem. Nat. Osteoporosis Soc. Prev: Sen. Regist. Rotat. (O & G) W. Midl. RHA; Clin. Lect. & Regist. (O & G) Guy's Hosp. Lond.; Regist. (Surg.) Beckenham Gen. Hosp.

RUPARELIA, Vibha Kishor Queen Charlotte's Hospital, Goldhawk Road, London W6 Tel: 020 8748 4666; Cintamani Caravan, Wall Hall Cottages, Aldenham, Watford WD25 8AS — MB BS Lond. 1992. Research Fell. (Gyn. Oncol.) St. Thos. Hosp. Lond.; Mem. Trainees Register of RCOG. Specialty: Obst. & Gyn. Prev: SHO (O & G) St. Thos. Hosp. Lond.; SHO (O & G) Whittington Hosp. Lond.

RUPARELIA, Vrajlal Kalyanji — MB BS Rajasthan 1970 (Bikaner Medical College)

RUPASINGHE, Edmund Priyankara 13 Linden Road, Bedford MK40 2DQ Tel: 01234 273272 — MB BS Ceylon 1973; MRCS Eng. LRCP Lond. 1985. GP Bedford. Socs: BMA.

RUSBY, Jennifer Elizabeth 69 Gloucester Road, Hampton TW12 2UQ Email: rusby@hotmail.com — BM BCh Oxf. 1998. Pre Registration Ho. Off. Med., John Radcliffe Hosp., Oxf. Specialty: Accid. & Emerg. Prev: Pre-Regist. Ho. Off. Surg. Univ. Hosp. Selly Oak, Birm.

RUSCILLO, Giuseppe Antonio 38 King Street, Lancaster LA1 1RE Tel: 01524 32294 — MB ChB Sheff. 1992 (Sheffield) MRCGP 1997. GP Princip.

RUSCOE, Michael Nicholas John Manor Surgery, Forth Noweth, Chapel Street, Redruth TR15 1BY Tel: 01209 313313 Fax: 01209 313813; 12 Trewirgie Road, Redruth TR15 2SX Tel: 01209 315038 Email: mruscoe@cix.compulink.co.uk — MB ChB Leeds 1971; MB ChB (Hons.) Leeds 1971; FRCGP 1993, M 1982; MSc 1999. Assoc. Regional Adviser (Gen. Pract.) Bristol Univ. Prev: SHO (Obst.) Leeds Matern. Hosp.; Ho. Phys. St. Jas. Hosp. Leeds; Ho. Surg. Leeds Gen. Infirm.

RUSE, Gareth Antony Cheam Family Practice, The Knoll, Parkside, Cheam, Sutton SM3 8BS Tel: 020 8770 2014 Fax: 020 8770 1864 — MB BS Lond. 1985.

RUSH, Elaine Margaret Department of Anaesthesia, The Ipswich Hospital, Heath Road, Ipswich IP4 5PD Tel: 01473 712233 Fax: 01473 702006 Email: elaine.rush@ipsh-tr.anglox.nhs.uk; 18 York Road, Martlesham Heath, Ipswich IP5 3TL Email: elaine.rush@btinternet.com — MB ChB Liverp. 1976 (Liverpool) FRCA Eng. 1981; MRCP UK 1983. Cons. Anaesth. Ipswich Hosp. Specialty: Anaesth. Socs: Assn. of Anaesthetists; Intens. Care Soc.; Brit. Med. Assn.

RUSH, Jennifer Mary 26 Crossway, Petts Wood, Orpington BR5 1PE; 65-97 Lowfield Street, Dartford DA1 1HP Tel: 01322 224550 — MB BS Lond. 1984 (Royal Free Hospital London) BSc Lond. 1981, MB BS 1984; MRCP (UK) 1987; MRCGP 1990; Cert. Family Plann. JCC 1990; DRCOG 1995. GP Tutor Dartford. Specialty: Gen. Pract.

RUSH, Mark 2 Sunnyside, Washford, Watchet TA23 0LB — MB BS Lond. 1998; MB BS Lond 1998.

RUSHAMBUZA, Francis Gratian National Blood Service, Mersey and North Wales Blood Centre, West Derby St., Liverpool L7 8TW Tel: 0151 551 8862 Fax: 0151 551 8895; 2 Beech Lawn, Grassendale, Liverpool L19 0LH Tel: 0151 427 2428 — MB ChB St. And. 1968 (St. Andrews) MSc (Clin. Pharmacol.) Manch. 1974; DTM & H (Liverp.) 1996; MRCP (U.K.) 1975; FRCP Lond. 1997; DGUM & Ven (Liverp.) 1998. Cons. (Haemat.) Nat. Blood Transfus. Serv. Regional Blood Transfus. Centre Liverp. Specialty: Blood Transfus. Socs: Fell. Roy. Soc. Trop. Med. & Hyg.; Brit. Blood Transfus. Soc.; Brit. Soc. Haematol. Prev: Sen. Regist. (Haemat.) Mersey RHA.

RUSHAMBUZA, Roger Pascal Mugisha 2 Beech Lawn, Grassendale, Liverpool L19 0LH Email: roger_rushambuza@hotmail.com — MB BS Newc. 1998; MRCS Ed. 2002. SHO (A & E) N. Staffs. Hosp. Stoke-on-Trent, 1999-Feb 2000.; SHO Orthopaedics Bradford Royal Infirmary 2002-3. Specialty: Gen. Surg. Prev: SHO (Gen. Surg) Dewsbury & District Hosp. 2002; SHO (ENT) Bradford Royal Inf. 2001-2002; SHO (Ortho) St James Univ. Hosp. 2001.

RUSHBROOK, Laurence Alfred William Layer Road Surgery, Layer Road, Colchester CO2 9LA Tel: 01206 546494 Fax: 01206 369912 — MB ChB Sheff. 1974.

RUSHBROOK, Simon Matthew 5 The Ridings, Chelmsford CM2 9RR — MB BS Lond. 1997.

RUSHDY, Amal Abbas Abdel Rahman 282 Overdown Road, Reading RG31 6PP — MB BS Lond. 1985 (Guy's Hospital medical school, Univ of London) MSc (Pub. Health Med.) Lond. 1993, MB BS 1985; MRCP (UK) 1989; DTM & H Liverp. 1991; MSc (Pub. Health Med.) Lond. 1993; MFPHM 1997. Clin. Sen. Lect.,Epidemiol. & Pub. Health Univ. of Wales Coll. of Med Cardiff; Sen. Med. Off., Dept. of Health, Lond. Specialty: Pub. Health Med. Prev: Sen Reg, Pub. health Med., PHLS communicable Dis. surveillance centre Lond.; Detached Nat. Expert, DG Health & Consumer Protec., Europ. Commiss. Luxemberg; Cons epidemiologist PHLS CDSC Lond. Sen. Med. Off., Dept of health, Lond.

RUSHEN, Daniel Jon 6 Links View Avenue, Poole BH14 9QT — BM Soton. 1993.

RUSHEN, Julie Elizabeth Russell Place Farm, Wood St., Guildford GU3 3EZ; 34 Coleshill Road, Teddington TW11 0LJ — MB BS Lond. 1988; BSc (Hons.) Lond. 1987; DCH RCP Lond. 1991; DRCOG 1992; Cert. Family Plann. JCC 1992; MFFP 1993.

RUSHFORD, Carole Ann Vine Surgery, Hindhayes Lane, Street BA16 0ET Tel: 01458 841122 Fax: 01458 840044 — MB ChB Sheff. 1968; Cert. Family Plann. JCC 1984. Instruct. Doctor Family Plann. Jt. Comm. Contracept.

RUSHFORTH, Mr Graham Frederick Weaveland, Homington Road, Coombe Bissett, Salisbury SP5 4LY — MB BS Lond. 1966 (Guy's) MRCS Eng. LRCP Lond. 1966; DObst RCOG 1969; FRCS Eng. 1971. Cons. Orthop. Surg. Salisbury Health Dist. Specialty: Orthop. Prev: Sen. Orthop. Regist. St. Geo. Hosp. & S.W. Thames;

Orthop. Regist. Roy. Surrey Co. Hosp. Guildford; Surg. Regist. Northampton Gen. Hosp.

RUSHFORTH, Jean Alison — MB BCh Wales 1985; MRCP (UK) 1989. Cons. Paediat. Glos. Roy. Hosp. Specialty: Paediat. Prev: Lect. (Child Health) Univ. Wales Coll. Med. Cardiff; Regist. & SHO (Paediat.) Leeds Gen. Infirm.

RUSHMAN, Geoffrey Boswall (retired) 26 Tyrone Road, Thorpe Bay, Southend-on-Sea SS1 3HF Tel: 01702 586379 Fax: 01702 586379 — (St. Bart.) MB BS Lond. 1962; MRCS Eng. LRCP Lond. 1962; FFA RCS Eng. 1970. Cons. Anaesth. Southend Hosp., Rochford Hosp. & Runwell Hosp.; FRCA Examr. Roy. Coll. Anaesth. Prev: Sen. Regist. (Anaesth.) St. Bart. Hosp. Lond. & Northampton Gen. Hosp.

RUSHMAN, Nicholas Richard 47 Hillway, London N6 6AH — MB BS Lond. 1992.

RUSHMER, Robert Jeremy Department of Anaesthetics, Wansbeck General Hospital, Woodhorn Lane, Ashington NE63 9JJ Email: jeremy.rushmer@northumbria-healthcare.nhs.uk — MB BS Lond. 1987; BSc Lond. 1984; MRCP (UK) 1992. Clin. Director (Anaesth.) Wansbeck Gen. Hosp. Specialty: Anaesth. Prev: SHO (Anaesth.) Roy. Infirm. Edin.

RUSHTON, Andrew Michael 7 Sovereign Close, Rudheath, Northwich CW9 7XN — MB ChB Manch. 1994; FRCA; BSc St Andrews 1991. Specialty: Anaesth.

RUSHTON, Arthur Four Gables, 14 Overhill Road, Wilmslow Park, Wilmslow SK9 2BE Tel: 01625 523628 Fax: 01625 523916 Email: arthur.rushton@protherics.com — MB ChB Manch. 1969; MRCP (UK) 1972; Dip. Managem. Studies CNAA 1977; FFPM 1989. Chief. Operat. Off. Protherics plc Chesh. Specialty: Pharmaceutical Medicine. Prev: Med. Dir. Clin. Research Foundat. (UK) Ltd.; Manager (Med. Plann.) ICI Pharmaceuts.; Regist. (Med.) Aberd. Roy. Infirm.

RUSHTON, Arthur Wilsden Medical Practice, Townfield, Wilsden, Bradford BD15 0HT Tel: 01535 273227; Penhallow, Keighley Road, Denholme, Bradford BD13 4LT Tel: 01274 833508 — MB ChB Manch. 1955. Prev: Regist. (Gen. Med.) Bradford Roy. Infirm.; SHO (Med.) & Ho. Off. (O & G) St. Luke's Hosp. Bradford.

RUSHTON, Barbara Elizabeth Anne Newtown Surgery, Station Road, Liphook GU30 7DR Tel: 01428 724768 Fax: 01428 724162 Email: barbara.rushton@gp_j82164.nhs.uk; Borreraig, 3 Hollycombe Close, Liphook GU30 7HR Tel: 01428 722173 Email: barbara@therushtons.me.uk — BM BCh Oxf. 1978; BA Oxf. 1975; DRCOG 1980; MRCGP 1982; DFFP 1995. Specialty: Gen. Pract. Prev: Assoc. Specialist (Paediat.) Paddington Green Childr. Hosp. Lond.; GP Hammersmith; Trainee GP Hammersmith Hosp. VTS.

RUSHTON, Claire Ellen Roman Road Health Centre, Fishmoor Drive, Blackburn BB2 3UY Tel: 01254 664832 — BM Soton. 1978; DRCOG 1980; DCH Eng. 1981; MRCGP 1982. Socs: Chairm. of E. Lancs Small Pract.s Assn.

RUSHTON, David Ian (retired) Department of Pathology, Birmingham Womens Hospital, Edgbaston, Birmingham B15 2TG Tel: 01367 810253 Fax: 01367 810253 — MB ChB Manch. 1960; FRCPath 1980, M 1968; FRCPCH 1997. Sen. Lect. (Path.) Univ. Birm. & Birm. Wom.s Hosp.; Hon. Cons. Path. Birm. Wom. Hosp.; Vis. Prof. Path. Univ. Manitoba. Prev: Lect. (Path.) Univ. Birm.

RUSHTON, Professor David Nigel Frank Cooksey Rehab Unit, King's Healthcare, Mapother House de Crespigny Park, Denmark Hill, London SE5 8AZ Tel: 020 7346 5324 Fax: 020 7346 5346; Holly Place, 20 High St, Shoreham, Sevenoaks TN14 7TD Fax: 01959 522985 Email: david@rushtons.demon.co.uk — MB BChir Camb. 1970; MRCP (UK) 1974; MD Camb. 1978; FRCP Lond. 1989. Cons. (Rehabil.) King's Healthcare Trust. Specialty: Rehabil. Med. Socs: Physiol. Soc.; Assn. Brit. Neurols.; Brit. Soc. Rehabil. Med. Prev: Prof. Rehabil. Lond. Hosp. Med. Coll.; Reader (Neurol. & Physiol.) Inst. Psychiat. Lond.; Hon. Cons. Neurol. King's Coll. Hosp. Lond.

RUSHTON, George John 43 Hainault Road, Chigwell IG7 5DQ Tel: 020 8500 2641 — MRCS Eng. LRCP Lond. 1963 (Oxf. & St. Bart.) MA Oxf. 1960, BM BCh 1963. Prev: Ho. Phys. & Ho. Surg. Radcliffe Infirm. Oxf.

RUSHTON, Joanne Marie Cedars Surgery, 8 Cookham Road, Maidenhead SL6 8AJ Tel: 01628 620458 Fax: 01628 633270 — MB ChB Manch. 1989; DRCOG 1993; MRCGP 1994. Prev: Trainee GP Reading VTS; Ho. Off. (Surg.) N. Manch. Gen. Hosp.; Ho. Off. (Orthop. & Cas.) Princess Margt. Hosp. Swindon.

RUSHTON, Kenneth Lindsay Surrey Hampshire Borders NHS Trust, 49 Farnham Road, Guildford GU1 — MB BCh Wales 1977. Cons. in Alcohol & Subst. Misuse. Specialty: Alcohol & Substance Misuse.

RUSHTON, Michael John West Malling Group Practice, 116 High Street, Milverton, West Malling ME19 6LX Tel: 01732 870212 Fax: 01732 842437; 2 Warden Mill Close, Wateringbury, Maidstone ME18 5DJ Tel: 01622 812878 Email: mike@mrushton.demon.co.uk — MB BS Lond. 1975 (St. Thos.) BSc (Physiol.) (Hons.) Lond. 1972, MB BS 1975; DRCOG 1981. Prev: SHO (Gen. Med.) Salisbury Gen. Hosp.; SHO (Radiother. & Oncol.) Roy. Marsden Hosp. Lond.; SHO (Neurol.) St. Thos. Hosp. Lond.

RUSHTON, Mr Neil Orthopaedic Research Unit, Box 180, Addenbrooke's Hospital, Hills Road, Cambridge CB2 2QQ Tel: 01223 217551; 37 Bentley Road, Cambridge CB2 2AW — MB BS Lond. 1970 (Middlx.) MRCS Eng. LRCP Lond. 1970; FRCS Eng. 1975; MA Camb. 1979, MD 1984. Dir. of Orthop. Research Unit Camb.; Hon. Cons. Addenbrooke's Hosp. Camb.; Reader in Orthop. Surg., Univ. of Camb. Specialty: Orthop. Socs: Fell. Magadalene Coll. Camb.; Fell. BOA & Roy. Soc. Med.; Vice-Pres. Europ. Orthop. Research Soc.

RUSHTON, Neil Patrick College Surgery, College Road, Cullompton EX15 1TG Tel: 01884 32373 Fax: 01884 35541; Lower Moorhayes, Cullompton EX15 1QN Tel: 01884 33204 — MB BS Lond. 1976 (St. Geo.) MRCGP 1981. Specialty: Child & Adolesc. Psychiat. Prev: SHO (O & G) St. Geo. Hosp. Lond.; SHO (Cas.) St. Geo. Hosp.; SHO (Paediat.) Mayday Hosp. Thornton Heath.

RUSHTON, Philip John 2 The Orchard, Wolverhampton WV6 9PF — BM Soton. 1997.

RUSHTON, Prudence Felicity Old Rectory Cottage, Burway Road, Church Stretton SY6 6DP — MB BS Newc. 1978; DCH RCPS Glas. 1987. Sessional Med. Off. Wolverhampton Family Plann.; Sessional Med. Off. Shrops. Family Plann. Specialty: Family Plann. & Reproduc. Health.

RUSHTON, Rebecca Jane Emley Cottage, 8 Wood St., Skelmanthorpe, Huddersfield HD8 9BN — MB ChB Leeds 1991. Trainee GP Huddersfield VTS. Prev: Ho. Off. (Med. & Surg.) Huddersfield Roy. Infirm.

RUSHTON, Richard James (retired) Redesdale, Papworth-st-Agnes, Cambridge CB3 8QU — MB BChir Camb. 1957 (Camb. & Lond. Hosp.) MRCS Eng. LRCP Lond. 1956; MA Camb. 1957; DObst RCOG 1963; DA Eng. 1964. Prev: GP Huntingdon.

RUSHTON, Sally Catherine Doctors Surgery, Mount Chambers, 92 Coggeshall Road, Braintree CM7 9BY — MB BS Lond. 1991; BSc Lond. 1988; DRCOG 1994; MRCGP 1995. Prev: Job Sharing Princip. GP Braintree; GP Asst. Caterham.

RUSHTON, Sheila Margaret 37 Bentley Road, Cambridge CB2 2AW — MB BS Lond. 1970 (Middlx.) MRCS Eng. LRCP Lond. 1970; DA Eng. 1973.

RUSHTON, Susan Clare 4 Seagrave Close, Sonning, Reading RG4 6BB — MB ChB Liverp. 1977; DA UK 1989.

RUSHTON, Susan Rosemary Louise Woodvale, Clifford St., Chudleigh, Newton Abbot TQ13 0LH — MB BS Lond. 1976.

RUSHWORTH, Elizabeth Ann (retired) Ridings End, Headington, Oxford OX3 8TB Tel: 01865 762302 — MB BS Lond. 1948 (Univ. Coll. Hosp.) MRCS Eng. LRCP Lond. 1948; DCH Eng. 1953; MRCP Lond. 1955. Prev: Cons. Rehabil. Rivermead Rehabil. Centre Oxf.

RUSHWORTH, Miss Frances Helen Singleton Hospital, Sketty, Swansea SA1 8QA Tel: 01792 205666; 29 Bowham Avenue, Bridgend CF31 3PA Tel: 01656 653808 Email: francesthomas@waitrose.com — MB BS Lond. 1989 (St. Mary's Hosp. Lond.) DFFP 1996; MRCOG 1998. p/t Specialist Regist. Rotat., S. Wales. Specialty: Obst. & Gyn. Prev: Specialist Regist. (O & G) St Mary's Hosp. Lond.; Specialist Regist. (O & G) W. Middlx. Univ. Hosp.; SHO (O & G) St. Mary's Hosp. & Samarit. Hosp. Lond.

RUSIUS, Christopher William 74 Highfield Avenue, Burnley BB10 2PS — MB ChB Aberd. 1983; MRCPsych 1989. Cons. Community Health Sheff. Specialty: Geriat. Psychiat. Prev: Sen. Regist. & Regist. Middlewood Hosp. Sheff.; SHO Severalls Hosp. Colchester.

RUSIUS, John (retired) 74 Highfield Avenue, Burnley BB10 2PS — LRCP LRCS Ed. 1946; LRCP LRCS Ed. LRFPS Glas. 1946; DCP Lond

1955; FRCPath 1972. Prev: Cons. Pathol. Path. Laborat. Gen. Hosp. Burnley.

RUSK, Maeve (retired) 18 Morven Road, Inverness IV2 4BU Tel: 01463 232643 — MB ChB Glas. 1942; DOMS Eng. 1947. Prev: Cons. Ophth. Roy. North. Infirm. Inverness.

RUSK, Rosemary Anne 15 Harberton Park, Belfast BT9 6TW — MB BCh BAO Belf. 1987 (Queen's University Belfast) BSc (Hons.) Belf. 1984; MRCP (UK) 1991; MD 1997. Specialty: Cardiol.

RUSNAK, Alexandra Sophie Hannah 85 Teignmouth Road, London NW2 4EA — MB BS Lond. 1997.

RUSSELL, Alan John 5 St Marys Place, Bury BL9 0DZ Tel: 0161 764 7484; Dakins, Walker Fold, Bolton BL1 7PU Tel: 01204 842756 — MB ChB Birm. 1971; FRCOG 1990, M 1977. Cons. O & G Bury Health Care NHS Trust. Specialty: Obst. & Gyn. Prev: Sen. Regist. (O & G) St. Marys Hosp. Manch.; Clin. Tutor (O & G) Univ. Manch. Wythenshawe Hosp. Manch.; Regist. (Obst & Gyn.) Birm. Matern. Hosp. & Birm. & Midl. Hosp. Wom.

RUSSELL, Alan Lawrence 5 Woodborough Road, London SW15 6PX — MB BS Lond. 1963; MRCS Eng. LRCP Lond. 1963; MRCP Lond. 1966; LMCC 1970. Dir. Brampton Pain Clinic Brampton, Ont.

RUSSELL, Alan S (retired) PO Box 15, Newton-le-Willows WA12 9BF Tel: 01942 720519; Puerta 172, Calle Corbeta 10, Calpe 03710, Spain Tel: 00 3496 574 8392 — MB ChB Liverp. 1964.

RUSSELL, Alec John The Beeches, Walsham-le-Willows, Bury St Edmunds IP31 3AD Tel: 0135 98 259227 — MB BChir Camb. 1947 (St. Thos.)

RUSSELL, Alfred McCarrison 4 Friars Orchard, Salisbury SP1 2SY — MA Dub. 1986, MB BCh BAO 1942 (Dub.) MRCGP 1953. Prev: Ho. Surg. Accid. Serv. Radcliffe Infirm. Oxf.; Squadron Ldr. RAF Med. Br.

RUSSELL, Aline Joan Clayton Southern General Hospital NHS Trust, Department of Clinical Neurophysiology, Institute of Neurological Sciences, 1345 Govan Road, Glasgow G51 4TF Tel: 0141 201 2462 — MB BS Lond. 1975 (Middlx.) BSc Lond. 1972; MRCP (UK) 1979; FRCP Edin. 2003. Cons. (Clin. Neurophysiol.) South. Gen. Hosp. Specialty: Clin. Neurophysiol. Prev: Sen Regist. (Clin. Neurophysiol.) South. Gen. Hosp. NHS Trust Glas.; Clin. Asst. (EEG & Epilepsy) Falkirk Dist. Roy. Infirm.; Regist. & SHO (Paediat.) Ninewells Hosp. Dundee.

RUSSELL, Andrew Giles 37 Thirlmere Road, London N10 2DL — MB BS Lond. 1989.

RUSSELL, Andrew Gordon Blue Wing Medical Practice, Wallacetown Medical Centre, 3 Lyon Street, Dundee DD4 6RB Tel: 01382 458333 Fax: 01382 461833 — MB ChB Dundee 1986.

RUSSELL, Andrew Ian 28 All Saints Avenue, Margate CT9 5QW — MB BS Lond. 1994.

RUSSELL, Andrew McNeill 56 Spruce Avenue, Johnstone PA5 9RG — MB ChB Glas. 1998; MB ChB Glas 1998.

RUSSELL, Andrew Oldrey (retired) Sandfield Farm, Hever, Edenbridge TN8 7ES Tel: 01732 863301 — (Camb. & St. Thos.) MB BChir Camb. 1955; DObst RCOG 1955; MA Camb. 1957; DA Eng. 1959; MRCGP 1964. Prev: GP Edenbridge.

RUSSELL, Anthony James Barter Headlands Surgery, 20 Headlands, Kettering NN15 7HP Tel: 01536 518886 Fax: 01536 415385; Measures House, Grafton Underwood, Kettering NN14 3AA — MB ChB Leic. 1984; BA (Open) 1996, BSc Lond. 1978. Prev: Ho. Phys. Kettering Gen. Hosp.; Ho. Surg. Geo. Eliot Hosp. Nuneaton.

RUSSELL, Audrey Serena Melbourne Park Medical Centre, Melbourne Road, Aspley, Nottingham NG8 5HL Tel: 0115 978 6114 Fax: 0115 924 9334 — MB ChB Dundee 1983; MRCGP 1987. Specialty: Gen. Pract. Prev: Trainee GP Doncaster VTS.

RUSSELL, Barry Neil Drayton Surgery, 280 Havant Road, Drayton, Portsmouth PO6 1PA Tel: 023 9237 0422 Fax: 023 9261 8383 — MB BS Lond. 1972; DObst RCOG 1974; D Med 1999.

RUSSELL, Bernard Stephen Hawkley Brook Surgery, Highfield Grange Avenue, Wigan WN3 6SU Tel: 01942 234740 Fax: 01942 820037 — MB ChB Manch. 1981; MRCGP 1985. Princip. GP Wigan.

RUSSELL, Brian Thomas Feidrfair Health Centre, Feidrfair, Cardigan SA43 1EB Tel: 01239 612021 Fax: 01239 613373; Oakleaves, Mwtshwr, St. Dogmaels, Cardigan SA43 3HZ — MB BCh BAO Dub. 1982; DCH RCP Lond. 1985. Gen. Practioner, Cardigan Health Centre. Prev: Trainee GP Cardigan Health Centre; SHO (A & E, Med., Paediat. & O & G) Withybush Gen. Hosp. HaverfordW.

RUSSELL, Brigid Ita (retired) 36 Lancaster Road, Wimbledon, London SW19 5DD — MB ChB St. And. 1958; MA Lond. 1996. Prev: Research Assoc. Yale Univ. Med. Sch., USA.

RUSSELL, Catherine Jane Corner Cottage, Heath Lane, Crondall, Farnham GU10 5AW Tel: 01252 851190 — MB BS Lond. 1987; DCH RCP Lond. 1991; MRCGP 1992; DRCOG 1994. Specialty: Community Child Health.

RUSSELL, Cecilia Valentine (retired) Newlands, Tranwell Woods, Morpeth NE61 6AG Tel: 01670 515666 — MB ChB Aberd. 1942; DCH Eng. 1943; MD Aberd. 1946. Prev: Ho. Surg. Roy. Aberd. Childr. Hosp.

RUSSELL, Christina Joan Doctors Surgery, Half Moon Lane, Wigton CA7 9NQ Tel: 016973 42254 Fax: 016973 45464 — MB ChB Aberd. 1981.

RUSSELL, Christine Marian Lisburn Health Centre, Linenhall Street, Lisburn BT28 1LU Tel: 028 9260 3111 Fax: 028 9266 1335; 4 Harmony Hill, Lisburn BT27 4EP Tel: 028 9267 0706 — MB BCh BAO Belf. 1974 (Queen's University Belfast) DRCOG 1977; MRCGP 1980. GP Princip. Socs: Brit. Med. Assn.; Roy. Coll. of G.P's.

RUSSELL, Christopher Ian Fraser Oakspring Clinic, 17 Melbourne Terrace, Clevedon BS21 6HQ Tel: 01275 874832; Symondsdown House, Woodbury Lane, Axminster EX13 5TL — MB BS Lond. 1976; LRCP Lond. 1976; MRCS Eng. 1976; MRCP (UK) 1978; DRCOG 1983; MRCGP 1984; Dip Occ Med 2002. Prev: SHO Rotat. (Med.) Whittington Hosp. Lond.; SHO (Infec. Dis.) Coppetts Wood Hosp. Lond.; Med. Off. Swaziland Irrigation Scheme, Swaziland.

RUSSELL, Claire 53 Victoria Road, Netley Abbey, Southampton SO31 5DQ — MB BS Lond. 1986; Dip. IMC RCS Ed. 1995. Staff Grade (A & E) Soton. Gen. Hosp. Univ. NHS Trust. Specialty: Accid. & Emerg. Prev: Staff Grade (A & E) St. Mary's Hosp. Isle of Wight; Doctor & Crew Mem. 'Maiden', Whitbread Round World Yatch Race 1989/90.

RUSSELL, Claire Holly 35 Bridgend Road, Ballycarry, Carrickfergus BT38 9JZ — MB ChB Ed. 1994.

RUSSELL, Clive John McLean Tyrone County Hospital, Hospital Road, Omagh BT79 0AP Tel: 01662 245211; Lisboy House, 28 Dryarch Road, Omagh BT79 0SQ — MB BCh BAO Dub. 1972 (Tinity Dub.) MRCP (UK) 1976; FRCP Ed. 1988. Cons. Phys. Tyrone Co. Hosp. Specialty: Gen. Med. Socs: Fell. Ulster Med. Soc.; Ulster Soc. Internat. Med.; Irish Cardiac Soc. Prev: Sen. Tutor (Therap. & Pharmacol.) & Sen. Regist. Qu. Univ. Belf.

RUSSELL, Mr Colin Frederick James, Deputy Lt. Royal Victoria Hospital, Grosvenor Rd, Belfast BT12 6BA Tel: 02890 894904; 8 Deramore Dr, Malone rd, Belfast BT9 5JQ Tel: 02890 660748 Fax: 02090 660748 — MB BCh BAO Belf. 1971; BDS Belf. 1966; FRCS Ed. 1976; FRCSI 1995. Cons. Gen. & Endocrine Surg. Roy. Vict. Hosp. Belf.; Lect. Surg. Dent. Stud.s Qu.'s Univ. Belf.; Chairm. Intercollegiate Bd. in Gen. Surg. Specialty: Gen. Surg. Socs: Coun. Mem. Assoc. Surg.s Gt. Britain & Irel.; Pres. Brit. Assn. Endocrine Surg.; Exec. Counc. Intnl. Assn. Endocrine Surg.s.

RUSSELL, Colin Robert Union Street Surgery, 75 Union Street, Larkhall ML9 1DZ Tel: 01698 882105 Fax: 01698 886332 Email: colin.russell@larkhall.larpct.scot.nhs.uk; 56 Hamilton Street, Larkhall ML9 2AU Tel: 01698 886160 Email: colinrussell@blueyonder.co.uk — MB ChB Dundee 1982; DRCOG 1986.

RUSSELL, David Orchard Court Surgery, Orchard Court, Orchard Road, Darlington DL3 6HS Tel: 01325 465285 Fax: 01325 284034 — MB BS Newc. 1980; MRCGP 1988. Hon. Med. Off. Hartlepool United F.C.

RUSSELL, David Anthony Gordon House Surgery, 78 Mattock Lane, Ealing, London W13 9NZ Tel: 020 8997 9564 Fax: 020 8840 0533 — MB BS Lond. 1969 (Westm.)

RUSSELL, David Davis Gourock Health Centre, 181 Shore Street, Gourock PA19 1AQ Tel: 01475 634617; Felridge, 3 Divert Road, Gourock PA19 1DR Tel: 01475 632939 — MB ChB Glas. 1965; DObst RCOG 1967.

RUSSELL, David James Mount Pleasant Health Centre, Mount Pleasant Road, Exeter EX4 7BW Tel: 01392 55722 — MB BCh BAO Dub. 1980; MRCP (UK) 1985; MRCGP 1986; FRCGP 1999. GP

Trainer, Lead Research GP Mt. Pleasant Health Centre Research Gen. Pract.

RUSSELL, Derrick Ian Department of Oral and Maxillofacial Surgery, Victoria Infirmary, Langside, Glasgow G42 9TY Tel: 0141 201 5415; Cairnmount, Gryffe Road, Kilmacolm PA13 4AZ Tel: 01505 872393 — MB BS Lond. 1973; FDS RCS Eng. 1977, L 1967; BDS Lond. 1968; MRCS Eng. LRCP Lond. 1973; FFD RCSI 1976; FDS RCPS Glas. 1989. Cons. Oral & Maxillofacial Surg. Glas. Dent. Hosp., West. Infirm., South. Gen. Hosp. & Vict. Infirm. Glas.; Cons. Oral Surg. & Hon. Sen. Clin. Lect. Glas. Dent. Hosp. & Sch. Specialty: Oral & Maxillofacial Surg. Socs: Fell. - Brit. Assn. of Oral and Miaxillo Facial Surg.s; BMA. Prev: Sen. Regist. (Oral Surg.) Roy. Dent. Hosp. Lond. & St. Geo. Hosp. Lond.; Sen. Regist. (Oral Surg.) Guildford & Haslemere Hosps.; Sen. Regist. (Oral Surg.) St. Thos. Hosp. Lond.

RUSSELL, Mrs Diana Winifred West Gate Health Centre, Charleston Drive, Dundee DD2 4AD Tel: 01382 632771 Fax: 01382 633839; 6 Elliot Road, Dundee DD2 1TB — MB ChB Manch. 1984; BSc St. And. 1981; DRCOG 1987; MRCGP 1989; MFFP 1994. Specialty: Gen. Pract. Prev: Trainee GP Dundee VTS; Ho. Off. (Surg.) Stirling Roy. Infirm.; Ho. Off. (Med.) Falkirk Dist. Roy. Infirm.

RUSSELL, Mrs Dorothy Hazel (retired) 4 Friars Orchard, St. Ann Place, Salisbury SP1 2SY — MB BCh BAO Dub. 1941 (TC Dub.) BA, MB BCh BAO Dub. 1941. Prev: Ho. Surg. Adelaide Hosp. Dub.

RUSSELL, Douglas — MB ChB Glas. 1983; DA (UK) 1989; FRCA 1990. Cons. Anaesth. South. Gen. Hosp. Glas. Specialty: Anaesth. Socs: Hon. Sec, UK Soc. for Intravenous Anaesth. Prev: Research Fell. (Anaesth.) Univ. Glas.

RUSSELL, Douglas Robert Tower Hamlets PCT, Mile End Hospital, Bancroft Road, London E1 4DG Tel: 0208 709 5002 Mob: 07713 259271 Fax: 0208 709 5000 — MB BS Lond. 1975 (St. Bart.) BSc Lond. 1972, MB BS 1975; DRCOG 1980; MRCGP 1990. Head of GP Develop. Dyfed Powys HA; Med. Director, GP, Tower Hamlets PCT. Prev: GP Carmarthen.

RUSSELL, Elizabeth Caroline The Hildenborough Medical Group, Tonbridge Road, Hildenborough, Tonbridge TN11 9HL Tel: 01732 838777 Fax: 01732 838297 — MB BS Lond. 1983 (Guy's) MRCGP 1989; MRCPsych 1989. Specialty: Gen. Psychiat.

RUSSELL, Elizabeth Clare 55 Woodstock Road, Redland, Bristol BS6 7EW — MB ChB Birm. 1995.

RUSSELL, Professor Elizabeth Mary, CBE (retired) Kilburn, Inchgarth Road, Pitfodels, Aberdeen AB15 9NX Tel: 01224 861216 Fax: 01224 861216 Email: e.m.russell@abdn.ac.uk — MB ChB Glas. 1958; DObst RCOG 1960; FRSE 1997; MD (Commend.) Glas. 1966; Dip. Soc. Med. Ed. 1967; FFCM 1979, M 1974; MRCP (UK) 1986; FRCP Glas. 1988; FRCP Ed. 1993; MRCGP UK 2000. Prev: Chair Scottish Privacy Advosory Committee.

RUSSELL, Elspeth Margaret (retired) Downderry, 96 Carrwood, Hale Barns, Altrincham WA15 0ES Tel: 0161 980 3399 — (Edinburgh) MB ChB Ed. 1956; DCH Eng. 1959. Prev: Gen. Practitioner.

RUSSELL, Emma 71 Hookstone Drive, Harrogate HG2 8PH — MB ChB Sheff. 1998; MB ChB Sheff 1998.

RUSSELL, Erica Barbara Anne Weir 10 Greenhill Park, Edinburgh EH10 4DW Tel: 0131 447 6379 — MB ChB Aberd. 1962; DObst RCOG 1964; DSM Ed. 1969; MFCM 1974. Sen. Research Fell. Dept. Community Med. Univ. Edin. Prev: Ho. Phys. Aberd. Roy. Infirm.; Ho. Surg. Roy. Aberd. Hosp. Sick Childr.; Research Lect. Dept. Social Med. Univ. Edin.

RUSSELL, Evelyn Wythenshawe Hospital, Laureate House, Southmoor Road, Wythenshawe, Manchester M23 9LT Tel: 0161 291 6940 Fax: 0161 291 6940 — MB ChB Manch. 1989; BSc (1st. cl. Hons.) Leeds 1972; PhD Leeds 1975; MRCPsych 1994; MD Manch. 1996. Cons. (Old Age Psychiat.) Manch. Mental Health & Social Care Trust. Specialty: Geriat. Psychiat. Special Interest: Durg treatments in dementia; Psychother. for older people.

RUSSELL, Fiona Elizabeth 11 Cullen Drive, Glenrothes KY6 2JH Tel: 01592 754908 — MB ChB Dundee 1991 (Dundee University) Specialist Regist. (anaesth) Glas. Specialty: Anaesth. Prev: SHO (Anaesth.) Glas.

RUSSELL, Fiona Marion 38 Station Road, Bearsden, Glasgow G61 4AL — MB ChB Glas. 1989; FRCS Glas. 1993; FRCS Ed. 1993.

RUSSELL, Francis Ellis (retired) 9 St Bride's Road, Glasgow G43 2DU Tel: 0141 632 0081 — MB ChB Glas. 1955; DPath Eng. 1963; FRCPath 1977, M 1965. Prev: Cons. Bacteriol. Roy. Alexandra Hosp. Paisley.

RUSSELL, Frank Richard 37 Coniscliffe Road, Hartlepool TS26 0BU Tel: 01429 274568 — (Guy's) MRCS Eng. LRCP Lond. 1941; DA Eng. 1947; FFA RCS Eng. 1954. Hon. Cons. Anaesth. Hartlepool Health Dist. Specialty: Anaesth. Prev: Sen. Cons. Anaesth. Hartlepool Gp. Hosps.; Sen. Regist. Dept. Anaesth. W. Middlx. Hosp. Isleworth; Capt. RAMC.

RUSSELL, Gavin Ian Department of Nephrology, Royal Infirmary, Princes Road, Hartshill, Stoke-on-Trent ST4 7LN Tel: 01782 554167 — MD Leic. 1982; MB ChB Birm. 1973; MRCP (UK) 1978; FRCP Lond. 1994. Cons. (Renal) Phys. Specialty: Nephrol. Socs: Internat. Soc. Hypertens. & Renal Assn.; Brit. Hypertens. Soc.

RUSSELL, Professor George Department of Child Health, University of Aberdeen, Cornhill Road, Aberdeen AB25 2ZD Tel: 01224 552471 Fax: 01224 840707 Email: libra@ifb.co.uk; 12 Pinewood Avenue, Aberdeen AB15 8NB Tel: 01224 314224 Fax: 01224 314224 Email: libra@ifb.co.uk — (Aberd.) MB ChB Aberd. 1959; FRCP Lond. 1977, M 1964; FRCP Ed. 1993; FRCPCH 1996. Emeritus Professor, Child Health Univ. Aberd.; Hon. Cons. Paediat. Roy. Aberd. Childr. Hosp. Specialty: Paediat. Special Interest: Asthma; Condits. related to migraine; Cystic fibrosis. Socs: Amer. Thoracic Soc.; Eur. Respirat. Soc.; Internation Headache Soc. (Mem., Peadiatric sub-committee). Prev: Cons. Paediat. Roy. Aberd. Childr. Hosp.; Fell. (Pediat.) Univ. Colorado Med. Center Denver, USA; Prof. Paediat. Univ. Riyad, Saudi Arabia.

RUSSELL, Professor Gerald Francis Morris Hayes Grove Priory Hospital, Prestons Road, Hayes, Bromley BR2 7AS Tel: 020 8462 7722 Fax: 020 8462 5028; 3 Aberdare Close, West Wickham BR4 9LP — MD Ed. 1957; MB ChB (Hons.) Ed. 1950; FRCP Ed. 1967, M 1954; FRCP Lond. 1969, M 1955; DPM Eng. 1958; FRCPsych 1971. Dir. Eating Disorders Unit Hayes Gr. Priory Hosp. Hayes, Kent; Emerit. Prof. Psychiat. Univ. Lond.; Emerit. Cons. Phys. Bethlem Roy. & Maudsley Hosp. Lond. Specialty: Gen. Psychiat. Prev: Dean Inst. Psychiat. Univ. Lond.; Prof. Psychiat. Inst. Psychiat. Univ. Lond.; Prof. Psychiat. Roy. Free Hosp. Sch. Med. Lond.

RUSSELL, Glenn Nicholas The Cardiothoracic Centre-Liverpool, Thomas Drive, Liverpool L14 3PE Tel: 0151 228 1616 Fax: 0151 220 8573 — MB ChB Aberd. 1980; FRCA 1984. Cons. Anaesth. Cardiothoracic Centre Liverp.; Lect. (Anaesth.) Univ. Liverp. Specialty: Anaesth. Prev: Lect. (Anaesth.) Ottawa Heart Inst., Canada.

RUSSELL, Graham Alfred The Health Centre, The Park, Gloucester GL1 1XR Tel: 01452 527217 Fax: 01452 387926; 94B Stroud Road, Gloucester GL1 5AJ — MB ChB Bristol 1957; DCH Eng. 1960; DObst RCOG 1964.

RUSSELL, Graham Anthony Dept. of Histopathology, Pembury Hospital, Tunbridge Wells TN4 4QJ Tel: 01892 823535 — MB BS Lond. 1982 (Guy's) BSc (1st cl. Hons.) Lond. 1979; MRCPath 1989. Cons. Histopath.Pembury Hosp. Tunbridge Wells. Specialty: Histopath. Prev: Sen. Regist. (Histopath.) Rotat. Bristol HA; Regist. (Path.) Addenbrookes Hosp. Camb.; Ho. Surg. Guy's Hosp. Lond.

RUSSELL, Graham Thomas Bellevue Medical Centre, 26 Huntingdon Place, Edinburgh EH7 4AT Tel: 0131 556 2642 Fax: 0131 557 4430 — MB ChB Ed. 1985; DRCOG 1989; DCCH RCGP 1990; MRCGP 1990; Dip. IMC RCS Ed. 1995. Clin. Asst. (A & E) Roy. Infirm. Edin. Specialty: Gen. Pract.

RUSSELL, Grant Kingsley 7 Glanwern Avenue, Newport NP19 9BU — MB BS Lond. 1980.

RUSSELL, Guy St John Wychall Lane Surgery, 11 Wychall Lane, Kings Norton, Birmingham B38 8TE Tel: 0121 628 2345 Fax: 0121 628 8282; 16 Cotton Lane, Mosley, Birmingham B13 9SA Tel: 0121 449 1781 — MB ChB Birm. 1988; MRCGP.

RUSSELL, Harold George — MB BCh BAO Belf. 1969; DObst RCOG 1971. GP Ballycastle; Med. Off. Dalriada Hosp. Ballycastle. Prev: Capt. RAMC, Regt.. Med. Off. 1st Bn. Glos. Regt.

RUSSELL, Harriet Clare Gloucestershire Breast Screening, Linton House, Thirlestaire Road, Cheltenham GL53 7AS Tel: 01242 251081; Yew Tree House, Great Comberton, Pershore WR10 3DP Tel: 01386 710885 — MB BS Lond. 1982. Breast hys., Gloucestershire Breast Screening, Cheltenham, (p/t).

RUSSELL, Hilary Jane Department of Psychotherapy, 4 Shide Road, Newport PO30 1YQ Tel: 01983 521511; 5 Northcourt Close, Shorwell, Newport PO30 3LD — MB BS Newc. 1980. Clin. Asst. (Psychother.) Newport I. of Wight. Specialty: Psychother. Prev: Regist. (Child & Adolesc. Psychiat.) I. of Wight; Regist. (Psychiat. Rotat.) Nottm. HA.

RUSSELL, Hugh Bernard Langford (retired) 10 Greenhill Park, Edinburgh EH10 4DW Tel: 0131 447 6379 — MRCS Eng. LRCP Lond. 1941 (St. Thos.) DTM & H Liverp. 1946; DPH Lond. 1951; FFCM 1982, M 1974. Prev: Sen. Lect. Dept. Community Med. Univ. Edin.

RUSSELL, Iain Cairns Crown Avenue Surgery, 12 Crown Avenue, Inverness IV2 3NF Tel: 01463 710777 Fax: 01463 714511 — MB ChB Aberd. 1983; MRCGP 1987; DRCOG 1989. GP Crown Med. Pract.; Prison Med. Off. HM Prison Inverness. Prev: SHO & Regist. (Gen. Med.) Roy. Infirm. Hosp. Sunderland; Trainee GP N. Edin.; GP N. Edin.

RUSSELL, Iain James Brodie (retired) Highway Farm, Churton, Chester CH3 6LB Tel: 01829 270960 — MB ChB Ed. 1948 (Univ. Ed.) Prev: Capt. RAMC.

RUSSELL, Ian Alexander Elms Medical Centre, 31 Hoole Road, Chester CH2 3NH Tel: 01244 351000; Whitethorne, Long Lane, Saughall, Chester CH1 6DN Tel: 01244 880364 — MB ChB Liverp. 1970 (Lond.) DObst RCOG 1973. Hon. Treas. S. Chesh. LMC; GP Mem. Countess of Chester Hosp. Managem. Bd. Prev: SHO (Paediat. & O & G) Clatterbridge Hosp. Bebington; Asst. Surg. P & O SN Co.

RUSSELL, Ian Archibald (retired) Northfield Road Surgery, Northfield Road, Blaby, Leicester LE8 4GU Tel: 0116 277 1705; 15 Chapel Lane, Cosby, Leicester LE9 1RG Tel: 0116 286 4850 — MB BChir Camb. 1971; MA Camb. 1970; DObst RCOG 1973; MRCGP 1976; T(GP) 1991. Clin. Teach. (Gen. Pract.) Fac. Med. Leicester Univ. Prev: Ho. Surg., Ho. Phys. & Ho. Off. (O & G) Warneford Hosp. Leamington Spa.

RUSSELL, Ian Digby 22 Beechwood Court, Monyhull Hall Road, Birmingham B30 3QL — MB ChB Birm. 1991; ChB Birm. 1991.

RUSSELL, Mr Ian Dougal 4 Rural Way, Ty Coch, Swansea SA2 9NA Tel: 01792 299739 — MB BCh Wales 1988. Specialist Regist. (Trauma & Orthop.) Train. Scheme. Specialty: Trauma & Orthop. Surg.

RUSSELL, Ian Farquhar Department of Anaesthetics, Hull Royal Infirmary, Anlaby Road, Hull HU3 2JZ Tel: 01482 674542 Fax: 01482 674371; 3 The Paddock, North Ferriby HU14 3JU Tel: 01482 633267 — MB ChB Aberd. 1973; BMedBiol. (Hons.) Aberdeen 1970; FFA RCS Eng. 1977. Cons. Anaesth. Hull Matern. Hosp. Castlehill Hosp. Hull Roy. Infirm. Specialty: Anaesth. Prev: Sen. Regist. Aberd. Roy. Infirm.; Regist. Aberd. Roy. Infirm.; Sen. Res. Med. Off. Perth Med. Centre, Australia.

RUSSELL, Ian Ronald (retired) Lapley Cottage, Lothians Road, Tettenhall, Wolverhampton WV6 9PN — MB BS Lond. 1960 (St. Geo.) Prev: Med. Regist. King's Coll. Hosp. Lond. & S.E. Metrop. RHB.

RUSSELL, Ian Speirs Easington and Peterlee Medical Group, William Brown Centre, Manor Way, Peterlee SR8 5TW — MB ChB Glas. 1985. Specialty: Accid. & Emerg.

RUSSELL, James Conn 27 Ravensdene Park, Belfast BT6 0DA — MB BCh BAO Belf. 1995.

RUSSELL, James Douglas (retired) 14 Shiel Hill, Alloway, Ayr KA7 4SY — MB ChB Glas. 1957; DMRD Eng. 1971.

RUSSELL, James Gordon (retired) Kalmia, Azalea Close, Thakeham Copse, Storrington, Pulborough RH20 3PD Tel: 01903 745030 — MB ChB Aberd. 1966; DObst RCOG 1968; MRCGP 1972; Dip. Pharm. Med. RCP (UK) 1977; FFPM RCP (UK) 1990. Cons. Pharmaceut. Med. Prev: Head Med. Affairs CIBA Pharmaceut. Horsham.

RUSSELL, Professor James Knox Newlands, Tranwell Woods, Morpeth NE61 6AG Tel: 01670 515666 — MB ChB Aberd. 1942; FRCOG 1958, M 1949; MD Aberd. 1954. Emerit. Prof. Univ. Newc.; Hon. Cons. Obst. & Gyn. United Newc. Hosps. Specialty: Obst. & Gyn. Prev: Prof. (O & G) & Dean Postgrad. Med. Univ. Newc.; Cons. O & G United Newc. Hosps.; Cons. Human Reproduc. WHO.

RUSSELL, James Lockhart — MB BCh BAO Belf. 1950 (Queens University Belfast) MS (MSc) (Med. & Physiol.) Minnesota 1960; FRCP Lond. 1976. Cons. Phys. Belf. City Hosp. Specialty: Gen. Med.

RUSSELL, James Rowland Hawthorn Walop, 3 Princes Court, Coedbury, Shrewsbury SY5 9BF Tel: 01743 884593 — MB BChir Camb. 1965 (Middlx.) MA Camb. 1965; DObst RCOG 1968. Med. Off., Nuffield Hosp., Shrewsbury. Specialty: Gen. Pract. Prev: GP Sittingbourne; Ho. Surg. Thoracic Surgic. Unit Middlx. Hosp. Lond.; Sen. Med. Off. Beira Patrol.

RUSSELL, Jeremy Johnston 16 Sandringham Road, Dersingham, King's Lynn PE31 6LL Tel: 01485 543118 — MB BS Lond. 1985; DRCOG 1989; MRCGP 1989; Cert. Family Plann. JCC 1989. GP Heacham. Prev: Trainee GP King's Lynn VTS; SHO (Ophth. & ENT) Qu. Eliz. Hosp. King's Lynn.

RUSSELL, Jeremy Paul Anthony 5 Paultons Square, London SW3 5AS Tel: 020 7352 5172/020 7352 6464 Fax: 020 7352 1617 Email: thepractice@drjeremyrussell.com — MB BChir Camb. 1970 (St. Geo.) MA, BChir 1969. Med. Adviser Dupont UK Ltd.; Med. Adviser Abbey Nat. plc. Specialty: Gen. Pract.; Paediat.; Physiother. Socs: Liveryman, Worshipful Soc. Of Apoth.; Chelsea Clin. Soc. Prev: Sen. Ho. Phys. Kent & Canterbury Hosp. Canterbury; Paediat. Ho. Phys. St. Geo. Hosp. Lond.; Ho. Surg. Essex Co. Hosp. Colchester.

RUSSELL, Joan (retired) 25 Roe Lane, Southport PR9 9EB Tel: 01704 31015 — MB ChB Liverp. 1950.

RUSSELL, Joanne Rachel 40 Warren Avenue, Cheadle SK8 1ND — MB ChB Manch. 1995.

RUSSELL, Johanna Alice Withymoor Surgery, Turners Lane, Brierley Hill DY5 2PG — MB BS Lond. 1989; MFFP 1992; DCH RCP Lond. 1992; MRCGP 1993.

RUSSELL, John Arrowe Park Hospital, Upton, Wirral CH49 5PE Tel: 0151 678 5111 — MB ChB Liverp. 1975; MA Camb. 1975; MRCP (UK) 1981. Cons. Phys. Geriat. Med. Arrowe Pk. Hosp. Specialty: Care of the Elderly.

RUSSELL, John Albert Rosehill, 4 Vogrie Road, Gorebridge EH23 4HQ — MB ChB Ed. 1967; PhD Ed. 1974, BSc (Hons.) 1964, MB ChB 1967. Sen. Lect. Dept. Physiol. Med. Sch. Univ. Edin.

RUSSELL, John Alexander 254 Avenue Road Extension, Leicester LE2 3EL — MB BCh BAO Belf. 1990; MB BCh Belf. 1990.

RUSSELL, John Anderson Oliver (retired) Norah Fry Research Centre, 3 Priory Road, Bristol BS8 1TX Tel: 0117 923 8137 Fax: 0117 946 6553 Email: o.russell@bris.ac.uk; 8 Napier Road, Bristol BS6 6RT Tel: 0117 973 6759 — (Middlx.) BM BCh Oxf. 1963; MA Oxf. 1963; DPM Eng. 1968; FRCPsych 1985, M 1972. p/t Hon. Research Fell. Univ. Bristol. Prev: Reader (Ment. Health) Univ. Bristol.

RUSSELL, John Cameron The Health Centre, Holmes Road, Broxburn EH52 5JZ — MB ChB Glasgow 1980. GP Broxburn, W. Lothian.

RUSSELL, John Gerarde, Squadron Ldr. RAF Med. Br. Retd. Regional Medical Centre, Royal Air Force Lyneham, Chippenham SN15 4PZ Tel: 01249 596382 Fax: 01249 896872 — MB BS Lond. 1982; MRCGP 1986; DRCOG 1988. Civil. Med. Pract. RAF Lyneham.; GP Trainer. Specialty: Sports Med. Prev: GP Princip. Swindon; RAF Med. Off.

RUSSELL, John Graham Buchanan (retired) 96 Carrwood, Hale Barns, Altrincham WA15 0ES Tel: 0161 980 3399 — (Manchester) MB ChB Manch. 1953; DCH Eng. 1956; DObst RCOG 1958; DMRD Ed. 1961; FFR 1964; FRCR 1975. Prev: Mem. Comm. 3 Internat. Commiss. Radiol. Protec.

RUSSELL, Mr John Lambert Department of Oral Surgery, The Leeds Teaching Hospitals NHS Trust, Clarendon Way, Leeds LS2 9LU Tel: 0113 233 6219 — MB ChB Ed. 1983 (Edinburgh) BDS Ed. 1976; FDS RCS Ed. 1980; FRCS (Max. Fac.) Ed. 1989. Cons. Oral & Maxillofacial Surg. Leeds Teachg. Hosps. NHS Trust; Head of Dept.; Lead Clinician. Specialty: Oral & Maxillofacial Surg. Prev: Sen. Regist. (Oral Surg.) Leeds Dent. Hosp.

RUSSELL, John Martin Western Infirmary, Beatson Oncology Centre, Dumbarton Road, Glasgow G11 6NT Tel: 0141 211 6319 Fax: 0141 211 6356 Email: martin.russell@northglasgow.scot.nhs.uk; 19 Glen Clunie, St Leonards, East Kilbride, Glasgow G74 2JR Tel: 01355 241401 Fax: 01355 902933 Email: jmartin@russelldyce.freeserve.co.uk — MB ChB Glas. 1975; BSc (Hons. Path.) Glas. 1973; MRCP (UK) 1977; FRCR 1984; FRCP Glas. 1990. Cons. Clin. Oncol. Beatson Oncol. Centre Glas.; Hon. Clin. Sen. Lect. (Radiat. Oncol.) Univ. Glas. Specialty: Oncol. Socs: Scott. Radiol. Soc.; Brit. Prostate Gp.; Assoc. Mem. BAUS. Prev: Sen. Regist. (Radiother.) Christie Hosp. & Holt

Radium Inst. Manch.; Regist. (Radiother. & Oncol.) West. Infirm. Glas.; Regist. (Med. Oncol.) Gartnaval Gen. Hosp. Glas.

RUSSELL, Joseph George (retired) 141 Argyle Street, Heywood OL10 3SD Tel: 01706 66135 — MB BS Lond. 1957 (St. Mary's) DObst RCOG 1960; MRCGP 1965. Prev: Ho. Surg. (O & G) St. Alfege's Hosp. Greenwich.

RUSSELL, Judith Elizabeth Lisboy House, 28 Dryarch Road, Beragh, Omagh BT79 0SQ — MB BCh BAO Dub. 1974.

RUSSELL, Judith Frances Anquetil (retired) 57 Falcon Avenue, Edinburgh EH10 4AN — MB BS Lond. 1965 (Univ. Coll. Hosp.) MRCS Eng. LRCP Lond. 1965; DPM Eng. 1976; MRCPsych 1977. Prev: Indep. Cons. Psychother. Edin.

RUSSELL, Karen 79 London Road, Shrewsbury SY2 6PQ — MB ChB Manch. 1984. Community Med. Off., Sexual Health, (p/t). Specialty: Family Plann. & Reproduc. Health.

RUSSELL, Karen Anna 27 Murrayfield Gardens, Edinburgh EH12 6DG — MB ChB Bristol 1997.

RUSSELL, Keith John The Health Centre, Loch Road, Tranent EH33 2JX Tel: 01875 610697; Achray, 20 Dovecot Road, Edinburgh EH12 7LE — MB ChB Ed. 1981; DRCOG 1984; MRCGP 1985; DGM RCP Lond. 1986. GP Tranent; GP Audit Facililtor Lothian Health. Specialty: Gen. Pract. Prev: Trainee GP N. Lothian VTS; Regist. E. Lothian Geriat. Serv.

RUSSELL, Kenneth A Viewpark Health Centre, Burnhead Street, Uddingston, Glasgow G71 5SU Tel: 01698 813753 Fax: 01698 812062 — MB ChB St Andrews 1970; MB ChB St Andrews 1970.

RUSSELL, Lai Fun Mary 20 Dovecot Road, Edinburgh EH12 7LE — MB ChB Ed. 1984 (Edinburgh) MRCGP 1988; DTM & H Liverp. 1990. GP Non Princip. Prev: Trainee GP Dunfermline VTS; SHO (Infec. Dis.) Cameron Hosp. Fife; SHO (Cas.) Dunfermline & W. Fife Hosp.

RUSSELL, Leonie Kay West Suffolk Hospital, Hardwick Lane, Bury St Edmunds IP33 2QZ; c/o Mr & Mrs M. Hardy, 15 Water Lane, Flitwick, Bedford MK45 1LG — MB ChB Otago 1991.

RUSSELL, Leslie Helen Ferguson Braidcraft Medical Centre, 200 Braidcraft Road, Glasgow G53 5QD Tel: 0141 882 3396 Fax: 0141 883 3224 — MB ChB Cape Town 1981; MRCGP 1988.

RUSSELL, Lucinda Elizabeth Lingwell Croft Surgery, Ring Road, Middleton, Leeds LS10 3LT Tel: 0113 270 4848 Fax: 0113 272 0030; 26 Rose Croft, East Keswick, Leeds LS17 9HR — MB ChB Leeds 1991. GP Leeds.

RUSSELL, Manson McCausland (retired) 42 Stanton Lane, Stanton on the Wolds, Nottingham NG12 5BJ — MB BS Lond. 1946 (Middlx.) Prev: Ho. Phys. & Cas. Med. Off., & Asst. Pathol. Bland-Sutton Inst.

RUSSELL, Margaret Cleland 47 Greystone Avenue, Burnside, Rutherglen, Glasgow G73 3SN Tel: 0141 647 1355 — MB ChB Glas. 1953; DObst RCOG 1955; MRCGP 1963.

RUSSELL, Margaret Winifred (retired) Green Gables, 16 Finlaystown Road, Portglenone, Ballymena BT44 8EA Tel: 028 2582 1078 — (Qu. Univ. Belf.) MB BCh BAO. Belf. 1946. Prev: GP Portglenone Health Centre.

RUSSELL, Mark Andrew Goodwin The Flat, Ronksley Hall, Hollow Meadows, Sheffield S6 6GH; Lower Tremenheere Farm, Ludgvan, Penzance TR20 8XG Tel: 01736 331107 — MB BS Lond. 1986; BA Oxf. 1982. Specialty: Gen. Pract.

RUSSELL, Mark Humphreys 43 Princess Marys Road, Crouch Oak Green, Addlestone, Weybridge — MB BS Lond. 1972 (King's Coll. Hosp.) FFA RCS Eng. 1978. Cons. Anaesth. St. Peters Hosp. Chertsey. Specialty: Anaesth. Prev: Sen. Regist. (Anaesth.) Westm. & Soton. Hosps.; Regist. (Anaesth.) Soton. Gen. Hosp.; SHO (Nephrol.) Southmead Hosp. Bristol.

RUSSELL, Maureen Currie Felridge, 3 Divert Road, Gourock PA19 1DR Tel: 01475 32939 — MB ChB Glas. 1964. Staff Grade (O. & G. Ultrasound) Rankin Matern. Unit Inverclyde Hosp. Greenock. Specialty: Obst. & Gyn. Prev: Clin. Asst. (O & G Ultrasound) Rankin Matern. Hosp. Greenock.; Ho. Off. Med. South. Gen. Hosp. Glas.; SHO Paediat. Hawkhead Hosp. Paisley.

RUSSELL, Maurice Frederick Holywood Arches Health Centre, Westminster Avenue, Belfast BT4 1NS Tel: 01232 471188; 60 Hampton Park, Belfast BT7 3JP Tel: 01232 647942 — MD Belf. 1968; MB BCh BAO 1954; DObst RCOG 1957; FRCGP 1980, M 1966. Staff Med. Off. Ulster Hosp. Dundonald. Prev: SHO Roy. Vict. Hosp. Belf.; Ho. Off. Waveney Hosp. Ballymena & Roy. Matern. Hosp. Belf.

RUSSELL, Maurice Hugh (retired) 64 Colney Lane, Cringleford, Norwich NR4 7RF Tel: 01603 502133 — MB BChir Camb. 1948 (Westm.) MRCS Eng. LRCP Lond. 1943; DCH Eng. 1949; DObst RCOG 1950. Prev: Ho. Surg. Westm. Hosp.

RUSSELL, Professor Michael Anthony Hamilton Maudsley Hospital, Denmark Hill, London SE5 8AF Tel: 020 7703 5411 Fax: 020 7703 6197; 14 Court Lane Gardens, London SE21 7DZ Tel: 020 8693 3606 — (Oxf. & Guy's) BM BCh Oxf. 1957; MA Oxf. 1957; FCP(SA) 1963; FRCP Lond. 1982, M 1964; DPM Lond. 1968; FRCPsych 1980, M 1971. Emerit. Prof. Addic. Inst. Psychiat. Univ. Lond.; Hon. Cons. Psychiat. Maudsley Hosp. Lond.; Hon. Cons. ICRF Health Behaviour Unit, UCL. Specialty: Gen. Psychiat. Prev: Hon. Dir. ICRF Health Behaviour Unit Univ. Coll. Lond.; Mem. Med. Research Counc. Extern. Scientif. Staff.; Ho. Phys. Guy's Hosp. Lond.

RUSSELL, Moira Margaret Alice 213 Woodlands Road, Woodlands, Southampton SO40 7GJ — BM Soton. 1986.

RUSSELL, Neil John Knypersley Villas, 115 Tunstall Road, Biddulph, Stoke-on-Trent ST8 6LB Tel: 01782 523353 — MB ChB Liverp. 1982. Specialty: Gen. Pract.

RUSSELL, Nichola Antonia Danebridge Medical Centre, 29 London Road, Northwich CW9 5HR Tel: 01606 338100 Fax: 01606 331977 — MB ChB Leic. 1987; DRCOG 1991; MRCGP 1992. Prev: Trainee GP Macclesfield; SHO (Gen. Med.) Profess. Unit Univ. Hosp. S. Manch.; SHO (Gen. Med., Obst. & Gyn. & Accid. & Emerg.) Macclesfield Dist. Gen. Hosp.

RUSSELL, Nicholas John West Cumberland Hospital, Whitehaven CA28 8JG; Moor End, Irton, Holmrook CA19 1YQ — MB BChir Camb. 1978; MRCP (UK) 1980; FRCP Lond. 1996. Cons. Phys. (Geriat. Med.) W. Cumbld. Hosp. Specialty: Care of the Elderly.

RUSSELL, Nigel Charles Radbrook Green Surgery, Bank Farm Road, Shrewsbury SY3 6DU Tel: 01743 231816 Fax: 01743 344099 — MB ChB Manch. 1984.

RUSSELL, Nigel Hudson 76 Brookside Road, London NW11 9NG Tel: 020 8458 5664 — MD Liverp. 1980; MB ChB 1973; MRCP (UK) 1976. Leukaemia Research Fund Research Fell. & Hon. Lect. (Haemat.) Roy. Free Hosp. Lond. Prev: SHO (Gen. Med.) Sefton Gen. Hosp. Liverp.; Research Fell. (Haemat.) Liverp. Univ.; Leukaemia Research Fund Trav. Fell.

RUSSELL, Norman Lawn (retired) The Priory, Patermoster Row, Ottery St Mary EX11 Tel: 0140 481 2939 — MRCS Eng. LRCP Lond. 1925 (St. Geo.) MA Camb. 1922. Prev: Ho. Surg. Hosp. SS. John & Eliz. Lond.

RUSSELL, Patricia Mary 5 Quayside Close, Worsley, Manchester M28 1YB Tel: 0161 702 8963 — MB ChB Manch. 1981; DRCOG 1984; MRCGP 1985; MFHom 2001. GP. Specialty: Gen. Pract.; Homeop. Med.; Psychosexual Med. Prev: Community Med. Off. N. Manch. HA.

RUSSELL, Patrick Stanley Bruce (retired) 9 Green Lane, Croxley Green, Rickmansworth WD3 3HR Tel: 01923 772016 — MB BS Lond. 1951 (Guy's) MRCS Eng. LRCP Lond. 1950; DObst RCOG 1954. Prev: Med. Adviser Peace Hosp. Watford.

RUSSELL, Richard Edward Kynnersley Department of Thoracic Medicine, Guy's Hospital, London Bridge, London SE1 9RT Tel: 020 7955 5000; 14 Torrington Court, Crystal Palace Pk Road, London SE1 9RT Tel: 020 7955 5000 — MB BS Lond. 1992 (Guy's Hosp. Lond.) BSc Lond. 1989; MRCP (UK) 1995. Regist. (Chest Med.) Guy's Hosp. Lond. Specialty: Respirat. Med. Prev: Regist. Greenwich Dist. Hosp.; SHO Rotat. (Med.) St. Geo. Hosp. Lond.

RUSSELL, Richard Jonathan 27 Jerviston Street, Motherwell ML1 4BL — MB ChB Manch. 1997.

RUSSELL, Robert Gordon (retired) Mill Cottage, Elmley Lovett, Droitwich WR9 0PS Tel: 0129 923412 — MB ChB Birm. 1951. Prev: GP Kidderminster.

RUSSELL, Robert Graham Goodwin Department Human Metabolism & Clinical Biochemistry, Sheffield University Medical School, Beech Hill Road, Sheffield S10 2RX Tel: 0114 276 6222 Fax: 0742 726938; Ronksley Hall Farm, Hollows Meadows, Sheffield S6 6GH Tel: 0114 308437 — MB Camb. 1971; PhD Leeds 1967; BA Camb. 1962, MB 1971, BChir 1970; MRCP FRCP (UK) 1981, M 1974; FRCPath 1986, M 1974; DM Oxf. 1975. Prof. & Hon. Cons. Dept. Human Metab. & Clin. Biochem. Univ. Sheff. Med. Sch. Specialty: Biochem. Socs: Brit. Soc. Rheumat. & Endocrine Soc. Prev:

Med. Research Fell. St. Peter's Coll. Oxf.; Asst. Prof. Med. Harvard Med. Sch., U.S.A.; Sen. Lect. Univ. Bern.

RUSSELL, Robert McCulloch Ainsdale Medical Centre, 66-68 Station Road, Ainsdale, Southport PR8 3HW Tel: 01704 574137 Fax: 01704 573875 — MB ChB Ed. 1977; DRCOG 1979; MRCGP 1982.

RUSSELL, Professor Robin Irvine Department of Gastroenterology, Royal Infirmary, Glasgow G31 2ER Tel: 0141 942 6613 Fax: 0141 943 2410 Email: rirla@aol.com; 28 Ralston Road, Bearsden, Glasgow G61 3BA Tel: 0141 942 6613 Fax: 0141 943 2410 — (Glas.) MB ChB Glas. 1960; FRCP Glas. 1972, M 1965; FRCP Ed. 1976, M 1965; PhD Glas. 1976, MD 1972. Vis. Prof. Univ. Mississippi, USA, Univ. Singapore, Toronto & Univ. Glas.; NIH Washington DC USA. Specialty: Gastroenterol. Socs: Assn. Phys.; Brit. Soc. Gastroenterol.; Amer. Gastroenterol. Assn. Prev: Cons. i/c Gastroenterol. Roy. Infirm. Glas.; Lect. (Med.) Gardiner Inst. West. Infirm. Glas.; Mem. Med. & Scientif. Staff MRC Gastroenterol. Unit Lond.

RUSSELL, Robin Maxwell 31 Five Mile Drive, Oxford OX2 8HT — MB BS Lond. 1985; FRCA. 1990; MD Lond. 1997. Cons. Anaesth. Nuffield Dept. Anaesth. John Radcliffe Hosp. Oxf. Specialty: Anaesth.

RUSSELL, Mr Roland Curtis 7 West Farm Court, 12 Gatcombe Way, Barnet EN4 9TT Tel: 020 8440 0130 — MB BS Lond. 1994 (Royal Hosp. Of Lond., Whitechapel) FRCS (Eng.) 1999; FRCS Lond. 1999. SpR Orthop. N. W. Thames Rotat. Specialty: Orthop. Prev: SHO (Orthop.) Southend Dist. Hosp.

RUSSELL, Mr Ronald Christopher Gordon 40 Devonshire Place Mews, London W1G 6DD Tel: 020 7486 7602 Fax: 020 7380 9162 — (Middlx.) MB BS Lond. 1963; FRCS Eng. 1966; MS Lond. 1979. Cons. Surg. Middlx. Hosp. & King Edwd. VII Hosp. for Offs. Lond.; Pres., Assoc. of Surg.s Gt. Britain & Irel.; Chairm., Jt. Comm. On Intercollegiate Exam.s (Surg.); Chairm. Brit. Jl. Surg. Soc.; Mem. of Counc., Roy. Coll. of Surg.s. Specialty: Gen. Surg. Socs: (Counc.) Med. Defence Union. Prev: Sen. Regist. (Surg.) Centr. Middlx. Hosp. Lond.; Asst. Dir. Surg. Unit St. Mary's Hosp. Med. Sch. Lond.

RUSSELL, Sally Ann 24 Marine Road, Walmer, Deal CT14 7DN Tel: 01304 373341 Fax: 01304 372864 — MB ChB Birm. 1994. Gen. Practitioner. Specialty: Gen. Pract.

RUSSELL, Sarah Ann St. Mary's Hospital, Clinical Radiology, Hathersage Road, Manchester M13 0JH Tel: 0161 276 6136 Fax: 0161 276 8612 — MB ChB Manch. 1980; FRCR 1986. Cons. Radiol. Centr. Manch. and Manch. Childr.'s Univ. Trust; Hon. Lect. Univ. Manch.; Hon.Lect. Univ. Salford. Specialty: Radiol. Prev: Asst. Prof. Ultrasound Univ. Calif., San Francisco, USA.

RUSSELL, Scott Howard Consultant Anaesthetist, Queen Elizabeth Hospital, Edgbaston, Birmingham; 51 Bittel Road, Barnt Green, Birmingham B45 8LX — MB BS Lond. 1985; FRCA 1990. Cons. Anaesth. Qu. Eliz. Hosp. Birm. Specialty: Anaesth.

RUSSELL, Sharon Lesley Cadzow Health Centre, 187 Low Waters Road, Hamilton ML3 7QQ Tel: 01698 327028 Fax: 01698 327344 — MB ChB Glas. 1989; DRCOG 1992; MRCGP 1993; DFFP 1994.

RUSSELL, Sheena Cochrane Department of Dermatology, Queen Margaret Hospital, Whitefield Road, Dunfermline KY12 0SN — MB ChB Glas. 1985; MRCP (UK) 1989. Cons. Dermatol., Fife Acute Hosps. Trust. Specialty: Dermat. Socs: Brit. Assn. of Dermatol.s; Scott. Dermat. Soc.; Brit. Med. Assn.

RUSSELL, Sheenah Jean McKinnon (retired) Machrie, 46 Rotchell Park, Dumfries DG2 7RJ Tel: 01387 254426; Balerno, 19 John St, Largs KA30 8HY Tel: 01475 673151 — MB ChB Glas. 1943 (Univ. Glas.) MD (Commend.) Glas. 1947; DCH Eng. 1947; FRCP Ed. 1971, M 1952; DPH Glas. 1953. Prev: Cons. Paediat. Dumfries & Galloway Roy. Infirm., Cresswell Matern. & Parkhead Hosps.

RUSSELL, Stanley Samuel 5 Laybrook Lodge, 63 Snaresbrook Road, Wanstead, London E11 1SR Tel: 020 8989 5885 — MB ChB Liverp. 1954; CPH Eng. 1956.

RUSSELL, Stella Caroline Joanna Ashwell Surgery, Gardiners Lane, Ashwell, Baldock SG7 5PY Tel: 01462 742230 Fax: 01462 742764; Lordship Farm, High St, Melbourn, Royston SG8 6EB Tel: 01763 262479 — MB BS Lond. 1975; MRCS Eng. LRCP Lond. 1975; DRCOG 1978; DCH Eng. 1978; MRCGP 1979.

RUSSELL, Stephen George The Gables Medical Centre, 45 Waveney Road, Ballymena BT43 5BA Tel: 028 2565 3237 Fax: 028 2564 0754; 151 Old Cullbackey Road, Cullbackey, Ballymena BT43 5PD — MB BCh BAO Belf. 1985; DRCOG 1987; DCH RCPSI 1988; MRCGP 1989; DMH Belf. 1990. GP Ballymena. Prev: SHO (Psychiat.) Holywell Hosp. Antrim; Trainee GP Broughshane VTS; SHO Waveney Hosp. Ballymena VTS.

RUSSELL, Stephen James Department of Haematology, Addenbrooke's Hospital, Cambridge CB2 2HQ Tel: 01223 402030 Fax: 01223 402140; 2701 Salem Road South W., Rochester, Minnesota 55902, USA — MB ChB Ed. 1982; MRCP (UK) 1985; PhD Lond. 1990; MRCPath 1992; Spec. Accredit. Haemat. JCHMT 1993. MRC Sen. Fell. (Clin.) & Hon. Cons. Haemat. Univ. Camb. Specialty: Haematology. Prev: Clin. Research Fell. (Cell. & Molecular Biol.) Chester Beatty Research Inst. Lond.; Regist. (Haemat.) Univ. Coll. Hosp. Lond.; SHO (Gen. Med.) N. Tees Gen. Hosp. Stockton-on-Tees.

RUSSELL, Stephen McCausland High Street, 16 High Street, Great Baddow, Chelmsford CM2 7HQ Tel: 01245 473251 Fax: 01245 478394 — MB BS Lond. 1977.

RUSSELL, Stewart 1B1 Templeton Business Centre, Templeton St., Glasgow G40 1DA Tel: 0141 554 1566 Fax: 0141 554 1995; 185 Nithsdale Road, Pollokshields, Glasgow G41 5QR — MB ChB Dundee 1978; MRCGP 1982; D.Occ.Med. RCP Lond. 1995. Occupat. Phys. Assoc. Health Servs. Glas. Specialty: Occupat. Health. Prev: GP Trainer Glas.; Regional Med. Advisor Manor Hse. Hosp.; Med. Off. Strathclyde Buses Glas.

RUSSELL, Susan Catriona Sandra Dept. of Anaesth., Victoria Hospital, Hayfield Road, Kirkcaldy KY2 5AH — MB ChB Ed. 1987; FFA RCSI 1993; FRCA 1993. Cons. Anesthetist, Vic. Hosp. Kirkcaldy. Specialty: Anaesth.

RUSSELL, Susan Gillian Dr McElhone and Partners, Townhead Surgery, 6-8 High St., Irvine KA12 0AY Tel: 01294 273131 Fax: 01294 312832; 22 Broadwood Park, Alloway, Ayr KA7 4UR Tel: 01292 45285 — MB ChB Glas. 1979; DRCOG 1985; MRCGP 1987.

RUSSELL, Susan Ruth 140 Cranbrook Road, Bristol BS6 7DD — MB ChB Cape Town 1979; DCH RCP Lond. 1 9092.

RUSSELL, Susanne Alcorn Maryhill Health Centre, 41 Shawpark Street, Glasgow G20 9DR Tel: 0141 531 8897 Fax: 0141 531 8863; 32 Bailie Drive, Bearsden, Glasgow G61 3AH — MB ChB Glas. 1985 (Glasgow) MRCGP 1989; Dip. Forens. Med. Glas. 1989.

RUSSELL, Sylvia Ellen (retired) Burcot Grange, Greenhill, Burcot, Bromsgrove B60 1BJ Tel: 0121 445 2534 — MB ChB ChB Birm. 1946 (Birm.) JP. Prev: Assoc. Specialist (Geriat. Med.) Selly Oak Hosp. Birm.

RUSSELL, Thea Jayne 60 Old Castle Road, Glasgow G44 5TE Tel: 0141 637 6309 — MB ChB Glas. 1953; BDS Glas. 1958.

RUSSELL, Mr Thomas Department of Clinical Neurosciences, Lothian University Hospitals NHS Trust, Edinburgh EH4 2XU Tel: 0131 537 2110 Fax: 0131 537 1134 Email: tr@skull.dcn.ed.ac.uk; 15 White Dales, Edinburgh EH10 7JQ Tel: 0131 445 5920 Fax: 0131 445 5920 — MB ChB Glas. 1975 (Glasgow) BSc (Hons.) Glas. 1973; FRCS Ed. 1979; FRCS Glas. 1979; PhD Wales 1998. Cons. Neurosurg. West. Gen. Hosp. NHS Trust. Specialty: Neurosurg. Prev: Sen. Regist. (Neurosurg.) Bristol & Weston HA; Lect. & Regist. (Neurosurg.) Univ. Glas.; MRC Regist. (Neurosurg.) Inst. Neurol. Sc. Glas.

RUSSELL, Mr Thomas Simpson (retired) 60 Old Castle Road, Cathcart, Glasgow G44 5TE Tel: 0141 637 6309 — MB ChB Glas. 1949 (Glasgow) DLO Eng. 1957; FRCS Ed. 1959. Prev: Cons. ENT Surg. Vict. Infirm. & South. Gen. Hosp. Glas.

RUSSELL, Thomas Victor Nivison Willow Lodge, Auchendon Est., Holly Bush, Ayr KA6 7EB — MB ChB Glas. 1966; MRCOG 1972. Cons. Obst. & Gyn. Ayrsh. Specialty: Obst. & Gyn.

RUSSELL, Tina The New Surgery, Lindo Lodge, Lindo Close, Chesham HP5 2JN; Highfield, Bellingdon, Chesham HP5 2XN — BM BS Nottm. 1988; DRCOG 1991; MRCGP 1992. SHO (Paediat.) Cheltenham Gen. Hosp.

RUSSELL, William (retired) 36 Lancaster Road, Wimbledon, London SW19 5DD Tel: 020 8946 4265 — MB ChB St. And. 1957; Dip. Amer. Bd. Pediat. 1969; MRCGP 1983. Prev: Sen. Attend. Pediatr. Meriden-Wallingford Hosp., USA.

RUSSELL, William Carnduff Adult Intensive Care Unit, Leicester Royal Infirmary, Leicester LE1 5WW; 24 Main Street, Rotherby, Melton Mowbray LE14 2LP — MB BS Melbourne 1982; FANZCA

1994. Cons. Anaesth. & Intens. Care Leicester Roy. Infirm. Specialty: Intens. Care; Anaesth.

RUSSELL, William Francis (retired) Offerton Health Centre, 10 Offerton Lane, Offerton, Stockport SK2 5AR Tel: 0161 480 0326 — MB ChB Birm. 1977; FFA RCS 1983. Prev: Gen.Prac. Offerton Health Centre Stockport SK2 5AR (Retd. March 98).

RUSSELL, William Gordon (retired) 34 Norwood Terrace, Newport-on-Tay DD6 8DW Tel: 01382 542280 — MB ChB Ed. 1959; DObst RCOG 1962; MRCGP 1978. Prev: GP Fife.

RUSSELL, William Ian (retired) 112 Hamilton Avenue, Pollokshields, Glasgow G41 4EX Tel: 0141 427 1383 — MB ChB Glas. 1947; DObst RCOG 1949. Prev: Ho. Surg. PeterBoro. Memor. Hosp.

RUSSELL-EGGITT, Isabelle Mary Department of Ophthalmology, Great Ormond Street Hospital for Children NHS Trust, Great Ormond St., London WC1N 3JH Tel: 020 7813 8524 Fax: 020 7829 8647; Consulting Rooms, 234 Great Portland St, London W1W 5QT — MB BChir Camb. 1979; DO RCS Eng. 1983; MA Camb. 1984; FRCS (Ophth.) Eng. 1984. Cons. Paediat. Ophth. Hosp. Sick Childr. Gt. Ormond St. Lond.; Hon. Sen. Lect. Inst. Child Health Lond. Specialty: Ophth. Socs: FRCOphth. Prev: Lect. (Clin. Ophth.) Jt. Inst. Child Health & Ophth. Univ. Lond.; Resid. Surgic. Off. Moorfields Eye Hosp. Lond.; Regist. Leicester Roy. Infirm.

RUSSELL-JONES, David Lowell Burningfold Court, Dunsford, Godalming GU8 4NZ — MB BS Lond. 1985 (St. Thos. Hosp.) MD Lond. 1994. Sen. Lect. & Cons. Phys. UMDS Guy's & St. Thos. Hosp. Lond. Specialty: Gen. Med. Prev: Sen. Regist. Portsmouth & UMDS; SHO Hammersmith, Qu. Sq. & Roy. Brompton Hosps.

RUSSELL-JONES, Robin David Skin Tumour Unit, St. John's Institute of Dermatology, St Thomas Hospital, London SE1 7EH Tel: 0207 928 9292 Ext: 1333 Fax: 0207 922 8138 — MB BChir Camb. 1972 (Cambridge University) MA Camb. 1973; MRCP 1974; FRCP Lond. 1991; FRCPath 2002. p/t Dir. Skin Tumour Unit St. John's Inst. Dermat. St. Thomas' Hosp. Lond.; Hon. Sen. Lect. (Med.) Roy. Postgrad. Med. Sch. Lond.; Cons. Dermat. Ealing Hosp. Lond. Specialty: Dermat. Socs: Chair UK Skin Lymphoma Gp.; (Ex-Pres.) Dowling Club; Pres. St John's Hosp. Dermatol. Soc. (Ex-Sec.). Prev: Sen. Regist. & Tutor (Dermat. & Path.) St. John's Hosp. for Dis. of the Skin Lond.; Sen. Regist. (Dermat.) Char. Cross & Centr. Hosp. Lond.; Regist. (Dermat.) Guy's Hosp. Lond.

RUSSELL-SMITH, Edward Denham Craigshill Health Centre, Livingston EH54 5DY Tel: 01501 51931 — MB ChB Ed. 1987; DFFP; DCCH RCP Ed. 1990; DRCOG 1990; MRCGP 1992. SHO (Psychiat.) Lothian HB. Prev: Trainee GP Lothian HB; Regist. (Paediat.) Lothian HB.

RUSSELL-SMITH, Roy Barnes Thatch, Romsey Road, Awbridge, Romsey SO51 0HG Tel: 01794 40403 — MRCS Eng. LRCP Lond. 1940 (Camb. & St. Bart.) MA Camb. Prev: Capt. RAMC; Asst. Med. Off. Gr. Pk. Hosp.; Ho. Phys. St. Bart. Hosp.

RUSSELL-TAYLOR, Michelle Ann 213 Beechwood Road, Luton LU4 9RZ; 27 Columba Drive, Leighton Buzzard LU7 3YN Tel: 01525 756716 — MB BS Lond. 1991; DCH RCP Lond. 1995; MRCPI 1996. Regist. (Paediat.) Milton Keynes. Specialty: Paediat. Prev: Regist. (Paediat.) John Radcliffe Hosp.; Regist. (Paediat.) Northampton Gen.; Regist. (Paediat.) Wycombe Gen. Hosp.

RUSSELL-WEISZ, David Jonathan 10 Elizabeth Avenue, St Brelade, Jersey JE3 8GR; PO Box 63, Port Hedland WA 6721, Australia — MB ChB Dundee 1987; MRCGP 1991; DRCOG 1991; Dip IMC RCS Ed. 1992; DFFP 1992. Sen. Med. Off. E. Pilbare Health Serv. West. Austral.; Chief Med. Off. Roy. Flying Doctor Serv. Broken Hill, NSW, Austral. Specialty: Accid. & Emerg. Prev: Med. Off. Roy. Flying Doctor Serv. Broken Hill, NSW, Austral.; Med. Off. Europassistance Croydon; Trainee GP/SHO (Anaesth.) Mayday Hosp. Croydon.

RUSSELL-WELLS, Sydney John Edward (retired) Riverside, The Shoals, Irstead, Norwich NR12 8XS Tel: 01692 630301 — (St. Thos.) MB BChir Camb. 1961; DObst RCOG 1963; MA Camb. 1973; MRCGP 1974.

RUSSO, Pamela 37 Lyndon Avenue, Great Harwood, Blackburn BB6 7TP Tel: 01254 884869 — MB ChB Manch. 1966. Staff Grade Community Doctor Blackburn, Hyndburn & Ribble Valley HA. Prev: SHO (Paediat.) & Ho. Phys. Preston Roy. Infirm.

RUSSON, Lynne Julie Bradford Hospitals Trust, Bradford Email: lynne.russon@virgin.net; Holly Dene, 20 Park Crescent, Roundhay, Leeds LS8 1DH — MB ChB Leeds 1987; MRCP (UK) 1992; MA Keele 1998. p/t Con. (Palliat. Med.) Bradford Roy. Infirm. Bradford. Specialty: Palliat. Med.

RUSSON, Michael John Primrose Lane Health Centre, Primrose Lane, Wolverhampton WV10 8RN Tel: 01902 731583 Fax: 01902 305789; 32 Newbridge Crescent, Wolverhampton WV6 0LH Tel: 01902 751381 — MB BS Lond. 1981; BSc Biochem. Lond. 1977, MB BS 1981.

RUST, Jack Harold Laura Mitchell Centre, Halifax Tel: 01422 50011 — MB ChB Leeds 1947; MRCGP 1954.

RUST, Nigel Edward Frimley Green Medical Centre, Beech Road, Frimley Green, Camberley GU16 6QQ — MB BS Lond. 1955 (St. Mary's) MRCS Eng. LRCP Lond. 1955; DObst RCOG 1958. Prev: Ho. Phys. St. Mary's Hosp.; Ho. Surg. King Edwd. VIi Hosp. Windsor & St. Stephen's Hosp. Lond.

RUST, Philippa Ann 7 Salisbury Place, Langton Road, London SW9 6UW — MB BS Lond. 1996 (Guy's & St. Thomas's Hospitals) Specialty: Gen. Surg.

RUSTIN, Gordon John Sampson Mount Vernon Hospital, Cancer Treatment Centre, Northwood HA6 2RN Tel: 01923 844389 Fax: 01923 844840 Email: gordon.rustin@whht.nhs.uk — MB BS Lond. 1971 (Middlx.) MRCP (UK) 1974; MSc Lond. 1979, MD 1980; FRCP Lond. 1992. Dir. (Med. Oncol.) Mt. Vernon Hosp. Northwood; Cons. Med. Oncol. Hillingdon Hosp. Specialty: Oncol. Socs: Counc.Onocolgy Sect.RSM, ACP, ASCO; ESMO. Prev: Sen. Lect. (Med. Oncol.) & Hon. Cons. Phys. Char. Cross Hosp. Lond.; Sen. Regist. (Med. Oncol.) Char. Cross Hosp. Lond.; Research Fell. Roy. Postgrad. Med. Sch. Lond.

RUSTIN, Joanna Katie 33 Fordington Road, London N6 4TD Tel: 020 8883 4191 Fax: 020 883 4191; Cherry Tree Surgery, 26 Southern Road, London N2 9JG Tel: 020 8444 7478 Fax: 020 8444 7628 — MB BS Lond. 1979 (Middlx.) MRCGP 1983. p/t GP Partner. Specialty: Pub. Health Med. Prev: Asst. Phys. City Univ. Stud. Health Serv. Lond.; GP Lond.

RUSTIN, Malcolm Howard Albert 53 Wimpole Street, London W1G 8YH Tel: 020 7935 9266 Fax: 020 7935 3060; 33 Fordington Road, Highgate, London N6 4TD Tel: 020 8883 4191 — MB BS Lond. 1976 (Middlx.) MRCP (UK) 1980; BSc Lond. 1973, MD 1988; FRCP Lond. 1995. Cons. Dermat. Roy. Free Hosp. Lond.; Cons. Dermat. King Edwd. VII Hosp. Lond. Specialty: Dermat. Special Interest: Atopic Eczema; Skin Lasers. Socs: Fell. Amer. Acad. Dermat.; Fell. Roy. Soc. of Med.; Fell. Brit. Assn. of Dermatols. Prev: Sen. Regist. (Dermat.) Univ. Coll. Hosp. & Middlx. Hosp. Lond.; Muir Hambro Research Fell.ship Roy. Coll. Phys.; Regist. (Dermat.) St. Bart. Hosp. Lond.

RUSTOM, Jane Willow 61 New Street, Salisbury SP1 2PH Tel: 01722 334402; Jasmine Cottage, Church St, Bowerchalke, Salisbury SP5 5BH Tel: 01722 781077 — MB BS Lond. 1983; DRCOG 1987.

RUSTOM, Rana 37 Roedean Crescent, Brighton BN2 5RG Tel: 01273 602015 — MB ChB Liverp. 1980; MRCS Eng. LRCP Lond. 1980; MRCPath 1990.

RUSTON, John Joseph Smirke 6 Aldenham Grove, Radlett WD7 7BN — MB BS Lond. 1978; FFA RCS Eng. 1983. Sen. Regist. (Anaesth.) Harefield Hosp. Middlx. Specialty: Anaesth. Socs: BMA & Assn. Anaesth. Gt. Brit. & Irel. Prev: Regist. (Anaesth.) Ealing Hosp. Southall Roy. Nat. Throat, Nose & Ear Hosp. & St. Mary's Hosp. Lond. W2; Sen. Regist. (Anaesth.) Roy. Free Hosp. Lond.; Sen. Regist. (Anaesth.) Eastman Dent. Hosp. Lond.

RUSTON, Miranda Ann Bond's Cay, 6 Aldenham Grove, Radlett WD7 7BN Tel: 01923 850484 Fax: 01923 850486 Email: sam@jruston.u-net.com — MB BS Lond. 1980.

RUSTON, Robert The Surgery, 32 Clifton, York YO30 6AE Tel: 01904 653834 Fax: 01904 651442 — MB ChB Leeds 1978; MRCP (UK) 1982; MRCGP 1983; MA Leeds 1999. Mem. York Local Research Ethics Comm.; Sen. Clin. Tutor, Hull-York Med. Sch., Univ. of York. Socs: York; Leeds. Prev: Regist. (Paediat.) York Dist. Hosp.; Tutur, Med. Ethics, Univ. of Leeds.

RUT, Andrew Richard GlaxoSmithKline, Greenford Road, Greenford UB6 0HE Tel: 020 84223434 Fax: 020 84234401 Email: andrew.r.rut@gsk.com — MB BS Lond. 1985; BSc (Hons.) Lond. 1982, MB BS 1985; MRCP (UK) 1989; MD Lond. 1995. Vice Pres. Global Clin. Saftey & Pharmacovigilance - Greenford. Specialty: Genetics. Prev: Lect. & Sen. Regist. (Med.) Univ. Coll. Lond.

RUTA, Daniel Adolf Department of Epidemiology & Public Health, Ninewells Hospital & Medical School, Dundee DD1 9SY — MB BS Lond. 1985. Specialty: Epidemiol.

RUTENBERG, Sidney Mortimer Felling Health Centre, Stephenson Terrace, Felling, Gateshead NE10 9QG Tel: 0191 469 2311 Fax: 0191 438 4661; 15 Grasmere Street, Gateshead NE8 1TR Tel: 0191 477 1980 — MB BCh Witwatersrand 1970.

RUTH, Martin Joseph, Squadron Ldr. RAF Med. Br. Department of Anaesthesia, Royal Infirmary of Edinburgh, Edinburgh EH3 Tel: 0131 536 1000 — MB ChB Glas. 1990 (Univ. Glas.) DA (UK) 1995. Regist. (Anaesth.) Roy. Infirm. of Edin. Specialty: Anaesth. Prev: Regist. (Anaesth.) Roy. Infirm. Edin.; Regist. (Anaesth.) MDHU PeterBoro. Dist. Hosp.

RUTH, Pauline Mary Maindiff Court Hospital, Abergavenny NP7 8NF Tel: 01973 735508 Fax: 01633 436846 — MB BS Lond. 1981; BSc (1st cl. Hons.) Lond. 1978; MRCPsych 1987. Cons. Old Age Psychiat. Mon.; Chief of Staff Ment. Health & Learning Disabilities Gwent Healthcare NHS Trust. Specialty: Geriat. Psychiat. Prev: Head Clin. Director, Ment. Health Serv.s, Gwent Healthcare NHS Trust; Sen. Regist. Secondm. Roy. Pk. Hosp. Melbourne, Australia; Sen. Regist. Rotat. (Psychiat.) Maudsley Hosp. Lond.

RUTHERFORD, Anne Blyth and Partners, Greenock Health Centre, 20 Duncan Street, Greenock PA15 4LY Fax: 01475 725380/020 8535 6952 — MB ChB Glas. 1977; MRCGP 1981. Socs: MRCGP; BMA.

RUTHERFORD, Anne Noel New Milton Health Centre, Spencer Road, New Milton BH25 6EN Tel: 01425 621188; Squirrels Hide, The Close, Sway, Lymington SO41 6ED Tel: 01590 682906 — BM Soton. 1982. Prev: Trainee GP S.bourne VTS; Trainee GP St. Peters Hosp. Chertsey VTS.

RUTHERFORD, Anthony John Leeds General Infirmary, Clarendon Wing, Belmont Grove, Leeds LS2 9NS Tel: 0113 292 3879; Ashfield Lodge, 38 Main St, Thorner, Leeds LS14 3DX Tel: 0113 289 2345 Fax: 0113 289 2345 — MB BS Lond. 1980; MRCOG 1985; FRCOG 1998. Cons. O & G Leeds Gen. Infirm.; Director, Assisted Conception Unit; Hon. Sen. Lect, O & G. Specialty: Obst. & Gyn.

RUTHERFORD, Daniel Croftwell, Prior Muir, St Andrews KY16 8LP Tel: 01334 474209 Fax: 01334 474209 Email: dan.rutherford@virgin.net; Croftwell, Prior Muir, St Andrews KY16 8LP Email: dan.rutherford@virgin.net — MB ChB Ed. 1979 (Edinburgh) BSc Ed. 1976, MB ChB 1979; MRCP (UK) 1983; MRCGP 1985; FRCP (Edin.) 1999. p/t Med. Director www.netdoctor.co.uk Ltd.; Private GP; GP Locum. Specialty: Med. Publishing; Medico Legal. Prev: Regist. Dundee Teach. Hosps.; Regist. Gastrointestinal Unit West. Gen. Hosp. Edin.; Ho. Off. Roy. Infirm. Edin.

RUTHERFORD, Helen Jane 7 Langley Way, Hemingford Grey, Huntingdon PE28 9DB — MB BS Lond. 1992.

RUTHERFORD, James Renton Drumart Square Surgery, 1B Drumart Square, Belvoir Estate, Belfast BT8 7EY — MB BCh BAO Belf. 1982; MB BCh Belf. 1982.

RUTHERFORD, Jane Marion 20 Bradshaw Drive, Holbrook, Belper DE56 0SZ — MB ChB Ed. 1989; MRCOG 1994. Research Fell. (Obst. Med.) Qu. Med. Centre Nottm. Specialty: Obst. & Gyn. Prev: SHO (O & G) Roy. Infirm. Edin.

RUTHERFORD, Janet Angel Hill Surgery, 1 Angel Hill, Bury St Edmunds IP33 1LU Tel: 01284 753008 Fax: 01284 724744 — MB BS Lond. 1985 (St. Barth.) DRCOG 1988; MRCGP 1989; FRCGP 2002. GP.

RUTHERFORD, Jean Aitken Steel (retired) 38 Gladstone Place, Aberdeen AB10 6XA Tel: 01224 322657 — MB ChB Glas. 1948 (Univ. Glas.)

RUTHERFORD, Joan The Ridgewood Centre, Old Bisley Road, Frimley, Camberley GU16 9QE Tel: 01276 692919 Fax: 01276 605366 — MB BS Lond. 1983; MPhil Lond. 1992, BSc 1980; MRCPsych. 1987. Cons. Adult Psychiat. Ridgewood Centre Camberley. Specialty: Gen. Psychiat.

RUTHERFORD, John David Ridgefield House, 14 John Dalton St, Manchester M2 6JR Tel: 0161 872 4868 — MB ChB Sheff. 1972; BSc (Hons.) Sheff. 1969; MRCP (UK) 1981; MRCPath 1987; DMJ(Path) Soc. Apoth. Lond. 1992; FRCPath 1997; FRCP Ed. 1998. Home Off. Path.; Indep. Cons. Forens. Path. Gtr. Manch.; Hon. Lect. (Path.) Manch. Univ. Med. Sch. Specialty: Forens. Path.; Histopath. Socs: Brit. Assn. of Forens. Med.; Brit. Assn. for Forens. Odontology; Manch. & Dist. Medico-Legal Soc.

RUTHERFORD, John Hilton Donaghadee Health Centre, 3 Killaughey Road, Donaghadee BT21 0BU — MB BCh BAO Belf. 1977; DRCOG 1979; MRCGP 1981.

RUTHERFORD, John Stanley Anaesthetic Department, Dumfries & Galloway Royal Infirmary, Bankend Road, Dumfries DG1 4AP Tel: 01387 246246 Fax: 01387 241639; Greystone, 53 Moffat Road, Dumfries DG1 1NN — MB ChB Aberd. 1985; FRCA 1990. Specialty: Anaesth.

RUTHERFORD, Margaret Cooper (retired) 144 South Anderson Drive, Aberdeen AB10 7PU Tel: 01224 315808 — MB ChB Aberd. 1942.

RUTHERFORD, Margaret Elizabeth (retired) 109 Glenburn Road, Belfast BT17 9AR Tel: 01232 629004 — MB BCh BAO Dub. 1944; BA Dub. 1944. Prev: Med. Asst. (Geriat.) Leics. AHA (T).

RUTHERFORD, Mary Ann Department of Paediatrics, Hammersmith Hospital, Du Cane Road, London W12 0NN — MB ChB Bristol 1984; MRCP (Paediat.) (UK) 1987. Research Regist. (Paediat.) Hammersmith Hosp. Lond. Specialty: Paediat. Prev: SHO Qu. Eliz. Hosp. Lond.

RUTHERFORD, Peter Anthony University of Wales College of Medicine, Wrexham Maelor Hospital, Wrexham LL13 7TD Tel: 01978 727122 Fax: 01978 727124 Email: peter.rutherford@new-tr.wales.nhs.uk — MB BS Newc. 1986 (Newc. u. Tyne) BMedSc (Hons.) Newc. 1983; MB BS (Hons.) Newc. 1986; PhD Newc. 1994; FRCP Ed 1999; FRCP 2001. Med. Director NE Wales NHS Trust; Sen. Lect. (Nephrol.) & Hon. Cons. Phys. Univ. Wales Coll. of Med. Specialty: Nephrol. Socs: Renal Assn; Am. Soc. Nephrol; EOTA-ERA. Prev: Lect. (Med. & Nephrol.) Univ. Newc.; MRC Trav. Fell. Yale Univ. Sch. Med., USA; MRC Train. Fell. Univ. Newc. u. Tyne.

RUTHERFORD, Robert Andrew (retired) 6 Transy Place, Dunfermline KY12 7QN Tel: 01383 723907 — MB ChB Ed. 1938. Prev: Res. Ho. Surg. Dunfermline & W. Fife Hosp.

RUTHERFORD, Robert Gordon Fulwell Medical Centre, Ebdon Lane, off Dene Lane, Sunderland SR6 8DZ Tel: 0191 548 3635; 2 Rosedale Avenue, South Bents, Sunderland SR6 8BD — MB BS Newc. 1979; MRCGP 1983.

RUTHERFORD, Susan Jane Queen Street Surgery, 13A Queen Street, Deal CT14 6ET Tel: 01304 363181 Fax: 01304 381996 — MB BS Lond. 1986 (UMDS Guy's Hosp. Lond.) BA Oxf. 1983; DRCOG 1990. Socs: Christian Med. Fellowsh. Prev: Ho. Phys. Yeovil Dist. Hosp. Som.

RUTHERFORD, Sylvia 80 Mill Rise, Swanland, North Ferriby HU14 3PW — MB ChB Dundee 1980; DRCOG 1984. Specialty: Ophth.

RUTHERFORD, Mr William Harford, OBE (retired) 113 Glenburn Road, Dunmurry, Belfast BT17 9AR Tel: 0289 062 1622 Email: william.rutherford@ukgateway.net — (T.C. Dub.) FIFEM(Fellow of intntl.Fed.of Emerg.Med.); MB BCh BAO Dub. 1944; FRCS Ed. 1951; FRCS Eng. 1985. Prev: Preven. of Injury Adviser DHSS N. Irel.

RUTHERFURD, Harry Napier (retired) Oakley, St Mary St, Kirkcudbright DG6 4AH Tel: 01557 330266 — MB ChB Ed. 1960; DObst RCOG 1964. Estab. Med. Off. Armament Wing RARDE Kirkcudbright. Prev: Surg. Roy. Fleet Auxil. Serv.

RUTHERFURD, Jacqueline Anne Ferguson Oakley, St Mary St., Kirkcudbright DG6 4AH Tel: 01557 330266 — MB ChB Ed. 1956.

RUTHERFURD, Stewart Ferguson Armstrong and Partners, Morrab Surgery, 2 Morrab Road, Penzance TR18 4EL Tel: 01736 363866 Fax: 01736 367809; Trenow Villa, Trenow, Long Rock, Penzance TR20 8YQ Tel: 01736 710198 — MB ChB Ed. 1988 (Univ. Edin.) DGM RCP Lond. 1991; MRCGP 1995. Specialty: Gen. Pract.

RUTHVEN, Elaine 31 Portree Avenue, Broughty Ferry, Dundee DD5 3EG — MB ChB Glas. 1995. SHO (c/o Elderly) Ashludie Hosp. Dundee. Prev: SHO (Med.) Stirling Roy. Infirm.; SHO (Surg.) Dumfries & Galloway Roy. Infirm.

RUTHVEN, Ian Scott (retired) Westholme, 10 Victoria Drive, Troon KA10 6EN Tel: 01292 313006 — MB ChB Glas. 1961; DObst RCOG 1963; FRCP Glas. 1977, M 1968; FRCP Ed. 1983, M 1968; FRCPCH 1997. Cons. Paediat. Ayrsh. & Arran HB; Clin. Director (Paediat.) Ayrsh. & Arran Acute Hosp.s NHS Trust. Prev: Postgrad. Tutor S. Ayrsh. Hosps.

RUTHVEN, Jennifer Louise 31 Portree Avenue, Broughty Ferry, Dundee DD5 3EG — MB BS Manch. 1998; MB BS Manch 1998.

RUTHVEN-STUART, Ian Alexander (retired) Verney Cottage, East St., Hambledon, Waterlooville PO7 4RX Tel: 02392 632596 Fax: 02392 632596 — MB ChB Ed. 1950; DObst RCOG 1960. Hosp. Pract. Qu. Alexandra Hosp. Cosham. Prev: Regist. (Orthop.) Roy. Infirm. Edin.

RUTLAND, Andrew Frank Knowles Lilliput Surgery, Elms Avenue, Lindisfarne, Poole BH14 8EE Tel: 01202 741310 Fax: 01202 739122; 17 Brunstead Road, Branksome, Poole BH12 1EJ Tel: 01202 268958 — MB BS Lond. 1988 (Char. Cross & Westm.) MA Oxf. BA Oxf. 1985; MRCGP Lond. 1993.

RUTLAND, Eileen (retired) 111 Rotunda Road, Eastbourne BN23 6LQ Tel: 01323 737181 — (Lond. Sch. Med. Wom.) MRCS Eng. LRCP Lond. 1940.

RUTLAND, Robert Frederick Knowles 31 Beckford, Washington NE38 8TP — MB BS Lond. 1987.

RUTLEDGE, David George Alexander Inverurie Medical Group, Health Centre, 1 Constitution Street, Inverurie AB51 4SU Tel: 01467 621345 Fax: 01467 625374; 17 Wellpark, Daviot, Inverurie AB51 0NF Tel: 01467 671687 — MB BCh BAO Belf. 1987; DRCOG 1991; DCH RCP Glas. 1991; MRCGP 1992.

RUTLEDGE, Esther Mary The Valley Medical Centre, 20 Cooneen Road, Fivemiletown BT75 0ND Tel: 028 8952 1326; The Glebe, Clogher BT76 0UW Tel: 0166 25 48346 — MB BCh BAO Belf. 1960. GP Clogher. Prev: Sen. Ho. Phys. Belf. City Hosp. & Musgrave Pk. Hosp. Belf.; Sen. Ho. Surg. Tyrone Co. Hosp. Omagh.

RUTLEDGE, Gillian Jane 10 Huby Park, Huby, Leeds LS17 0EE — MB ChB Ed. 1987; DRCOG Ed. 1989; MRCGP 1991. Prev: SHO (A & E) West. Gen. Hosp. Edin; SHO (O & G) West. Gen. Hosp. Edin.

RUTLEDGE, Malcolm Robert 6 Winters Lane, Omagh BT79 0DY — MB BCh BAO Belf. 1991.

RUTLEDGE, Mary Lynda Campbell Department of Anaesthesia, Western General Hospital, Crewe Road, Edinburgh EH4 2XU Tel: 0131 537 1000 Fax: 0131 537 1025; Cedar Lodge, 74 Trinity Road, Edinburgh EH5 3JT Tel: 0131 552 4774 — MB ChB Aberd. 1974; FFA RCS Eng. 1979. Cons. Anaesth. West. Gen. Hosp. Edin. Specialty: Anaesth. Prev: Sen. Regist. & Regist. (Anaesth.) Lothian HB.

RUTLEDGE, Philip Clinikcal Pharmacology Unit, Western General Hospital, Edinburgh EH4 2XU Tel: 0131 537 1737 Fax: 0131 536 1737; 74 Trinity Road, Edinburgh EH5 3JT Tel: 0131 552 4774 — MB ChB Aberd. 1974; DRCOG 1978; FRCGP 1999. Director of Med.s Managem.. CPU. WGH. Specialty: Pharmaceutical Medicine. Prev: Med. Prescribing Adviser, Lothian Primary Trust.

RUTT, Graham Alan Doctor's Surgery, 42 Heaton Road, Heaton, Newcastle upon Tyne NE6 1SE Tel: 0191 265 5911 Fax: 0191 265 6974; 5 Parkhead Road, High heaton, Newcastle upon Tyne NE7 7DH — MB BS Newc. 1978 (Newcastle upon Tyne) MRCGP 1982; MA Dunelm 1998; FRCGP 2000. Course Organiser Northumbria VTS. Specialty: Gen. Pract.

RUTTER, Dag Allenson 2 Herbert Villas, Pelham Road, London SW19 1NW — MB BS Lond. 1991; MRCP 1996 Lond.

RUTTER, David Vivian Mimosa, 4 Windfield Drive, Winchester Hill, Romsey SO51 7RL — MB ChB Bristol 1972; DObst RCOG 1975; FFA RCS Eng. 1977. Cons. Anaesth. Soton. Univ. Trust Hosp.; Hon. Clin. Teach. Univ. Fac. Med. Soton. Specialty: Anaesth. Prev: Sen. Regist. (Anaesth.) Hammersmith Postgrad. Med. Sch. Lond.; Regist. (Anaesth.) Vásterás Hosp., Sweden; Regist. (Anaesth.) Bristol Roy. Infirm.

RUTTER, Diana Patricia Infirmary Square, Leicester LE1 5WW — MB BS Lond. 1972; MRCP (UK) 1975; FRCP Canada 1979; FRCP Lond. 1994. Cons. Paediat. Leicester Roy. Infirm., Leicester, LF1 5WW. Specialty: Paediat. Prev: Sen. Regist. Roy. Free Hosp. Lond.; Cons. Paediat. Pontefract Gen. Infirm. W.Yorks.

RUTTER, Eleanor Lucy 129 Furnis Avenue, Dore, Sheffield S17 3QN Tel: 0114 236 4308 — MB ChB Manch. 1994; MRCP. SpR Pub. Health Med. N. East. Derbysh. Specialty: Respirat. Med. Prev: SHO (Gen. Med.) Derbysh. Roy. Infirm.; Regist. (Cardiol.) Liverp. Dist. Gen. Sydney; Ho. Off. (Gen. Med.) Macclesfield Dist. Gen. Hosp.

RUTTER, Francis Clarence (retired) 446 Unthank Road, Norwich NR4 7QJ Tel: 01603 451047 Email: francis@fcrutter.me.uk — (Middlx.) MB BChir Camb. 1951; DObst RCOG 1953.

RUTTER, Mr Francis John (retired) 33 Oakfield Avenue, Wrenbury, Nantwich CW5 8ER — MB ChB Birm. 1933; DOMS 1938; FRCS Ed. 1939. Prev: Cons. W. of Eng. Eye Infirm. Exeter.

RUTTER, Harald Roderick Oxfordshire Health Authority, Old Road, Headington, Oxford OX3 7LG Tel: 01865 741174 — MB BChir Camb. 1992; MA Camb. 1992. Specialist Regist. Pub. Health Med. Oxf.shire Health Auth. Oxf. Specialty: Pub. Health Med.

RUTTER, Helen Elizabeth — MB ChB Birm. 1998.

RUTTER, Ian Paul Westcliffe Medical Centre, Westcliffe Road, Shipley BD18 3EE Tel: 01274 580787 Fax: 01274 532210; Green Bank, Otley Road, Eldwick, Bingley BD16 3DA — MB ChB Leeds 1976; MRCGP 1980. GP Co-ordinator N. Bradford Health Gain Organisation. Prev: GP Course Organiser Bradford VTS.

RUTTER, John Anthony St Thomas Health Centre, Cowick Street, St. Thomas, Exeter EX4 1HJ Tel: 01392 676677 Fax: 01392 676677; Blackdown Cottage, Heath Cross, Whitestone, Exeter EX4 2HL Tel: 01647 61305 — MB BS Lond. 1974; MRCS Eng. LRCP Lond. 1974; DRCOG 1978. GP; Clin. Ass. Exeter & Dist. Hospice. Specialty: Pub. Health Med. Prev: Med. Adviser Hospiscare Exeter.

RUTTER, Josephine (retired) 26 Kerr Crescent, Sedgefield, Stockton-on-Tees TS21 2EG Tel: 01740620472 — (Durh.) MB BS Durh. 1948; DPM Eng. 1954; DPM. Durham 1955; FRCPsych 1986, M 1971. Prev: Cons. Psychiat. Winterton Hosp. Sedgefield & SW Durh. Gp. Hosps.

RUTTER, Judith Mary 12 St Davids Crescent, Aspull, Wigan WN2 1SN — MB ChB Leeds 1991.

RUTTER, Julie Marguerite — MB ChB Leeds 1986 (Univ. Leeds) DA (UK) 1989; FRCA. 1992. Cons. Anaesthetist sherwood Forest NHS Trust. Specialty: Anaesth. Prev: Sen. Regist. Freemantle Hosp. West. Austral.; Regist. Rotat. St. Jas. Leeds & Pontefract; SHO (Paediat.) Boston.

RUTTER, Mr Kiko Roderick Peter (retired) 23 Echo Barn Lane, Farnham GU10 4NQ — MB BChir Camb. 1967 (Camb. & St. Thos.) FRCS Eng. 1971. Cons. Surg. Frimley Pk. Hosp. Prev: Lect. (Surg.) Surg. Unit St. Geo. Hosp. Lond.

RUTTER, Louise Elizabeth 27 French Laurence Way, Chalgrove, Oxford OX44 7YF — BM BCh Oxf. 1986; DRCOG 1988; DCH RCP Lond. 1988; MRCGP 1990. PMS GP, Bury Knowle Health Centre, Oxf. Prev: Retainer GP Chalfont St Peter; SHO (Palliat. Care) Arthur Rank Hse. Camb.; SHO (Geriat.) Newmarket Gen. Hosp.

RUTTER, Martin Kenneth Department of Medicine, Countess of Chester Hospital, Liverpool Road, Chester CH2 1UL — MB ChB Ed. 1985; MRCP (UK) 1991; MRCPI 1991; DGM RCP Lond. 1991. Specialty: Gen. Med.

RUTTER, Matthew David Wolfson Unit for Endoscopy, St Mark's Hospital, Watford Road, Harrow HA1 3UJ Tel: 020 8235 4025 Fax: 020 8423 3588 — MB BS Newc. 1993; MRCP (UK) 1996. Specialist Regist. (Gastroenterol. & Gen. Med.) N. Deanery; Research Fell. Gatroenterol. & Endosc. St Mark's Hosp. Specialty: Gastroenterol.

RUTTER, Michael John X-Ray Department, North Devon District Hospital, Raleigh Park, Barnstaple EX31 4JB — MB BS Lond. 1962; DMRD Eng. 1966; FFR 1969. Cons. Radiol. N. Devon Health Dist. Specialty: Radiol.

RUTTER, Professor Sir Michael Llewellyn, CBE Social Genetic & Development Psychiatry Research Centre, PO80 Institute of Psychiatry, De Crespigny Park, Denmark Hill, London SE5 8AF Tel: 020 7848 0882 Fax: 020 7848 0881; 190 Court Lane, Dulwich, London SE21 7ED — MRCS Eng. LRCP Lond. 1955; MD (Hons.) Birm. 1963, MB ChB (Distinc. Pharmacol. & Therap.) 1955; FRCP Lond. 1972, M 1958; DPM (Distinc.) Lond. 1961; FRCPsych 1971; FRS 1987. Prof. Develop. Psychopathol. Inst. Psychiat. Univ. Lond.; Hon. Cons. Phys. Maudsley Hosp. Lond. Specialty: Child & Adolesc. Psychiat. Socs: Hon. Fell. Brit. Psychol. Soc.; (Ex-Chairm.) Assn. Child Psychol. & Psychiat.; Hon. Fell. Roy. Soc. Med. Prev: Ho. Phys. & Ho. Surg. Qu. Eliz. Hosp. Birm.; Nuffield Med. Trav. Fell. Dept. Paediat. Albert Einstein Coll. Med. New York.

RUTTER, Professor Nicholas 9 Chestnut Grove, Radcliffe-on-Trent, Nottingham NG12 1AH Email: nick.rutter@nottingham.ac.uk — MD Camb. 1980; MB 1971, BChir 1970; FRCP Lond. 1987, M 1972. Prof. Paediat. Med. & Hon. Cons. Paediat. Nottm. Univ. Prev: SHO Qu. Charlottes Matern. Hosp. Lond.; SHO Hosp. Sick Childr. Gt. Ormond St. Lond.; Ho. Phys. St. Thos. Hosp. Lond.

RUTTER, Mr Peter Charles Old Farmhouse, The Pound, Cookham, Maidenhead SL6 9SA — MB BS Lond. 1975; MRCS Eng. LRCP Lond. 1975; FRCS Eng. 1980; MS Lond. 1987. Cons. Surg. Wexham Pk. Hosp. Slough. Specialty: Gen. Surg.; Vasc. Med. Prev: Sen. Regist. (Vasc.) St. Mary's Hosp. Lond.

RUTTER, Philippa 21C Fernhead Road, London W9 3EU — MB BS Lond. 1998; MB BS Lond 1998.

RUTTER, Rowena Ann Canterbury Road Surgery, 186 Canterbury Road, Davyhulme, Manchester M41 0GR Tel: 0161 748 5559 Fax: 0161 747 1997; 20 Belgrave Avenue, Flixton, Urmston, Manchester M41 8SR Tel: 0161 747 9458 — MB ChB Manch. 1971; DObst RCOG 1973. GP Partner.

RUTTER, Stephen Michael Queens Medical Centre, Nottingham NG7 2UH; 190 Court Lane, London SE21 7ED — MB ChB Bristol 1989; BSc (Hons.) Psychol. Bristol 1986; MRCP (UK) 1994. Specialist Regist. Geriats. (TRENT). Specialty: Care of the Elderly. Socs: Brithish Geriat.s Soc.; Brit. Diabetic Assoc. Prev: SHO (Med.) Kings Mill Hosp. Notts.

RUTTER, Mr Timothy Morton 2 Portobello Mews, London W11 3DQ Tel: 020 7727 6686 Email: timothymrutter@aol.com — MB ChB Ed. 1966; BSc Ed. 1963, MB ChB 1966; FRCS Ed. 1970; MRCOG 1973.

RUTTLEY, Marie-Elisabeth 11 Kirkstall Road, London SW2 4HD — MB BS Lond. 1973 (Char. Cross) MRCS Eng. LRCP Lond. 1973. Prev: Regist. (Anaesth.) Guy's Hosp. Lond.

RUTTLEY, Michael Samuel Taylor Department of Radiology, University Hospital of Wales, Cardiff CF4 4XW Tel: 029 2074 3955 Fax: 029 2074 3029; Ty'r Bont, 3 The Paddock, Cowbridge CF71 7EJ Tel: 01446 772598 — (St. Geo.) MB BS Lond. 1964; MRCS Eng. LRCP Lond. 1964; FRCP Lond. 1984, M 1967; DMRD Lond. 1969; FFR 1970. Cons. Radiol. Univ. Hosp. of Wales, Cardiff.; Clin. Dir. Radiol., Univ. Hosp. of Wales, Cardiff. Specialty: Radiol. Prev: Ho. Phys. St. Geo. Hosp. Lond.; Clin. Fell. in Radiol. Harvard Med. Sch. Boston, U.S.A.

RUTTY, Professor Guy Nathan Division of Forensic Pathology University of Leicester, Robert Kilpatrick Building Leicester Royal Enfirmary, P.O/ Box 65, Leicester LE3 7ES — MB BS Lond. 1987 (Roy. Free Sch. Med. Lond.) MRCPath 1993; Dip RCPath (Forens.) 1996; FRCPath 2002. Prof. Forens. Path.) Univ. Leicester; Cons. Path. to Home Office. Specialty: Forens. Path. Socs: Forens. Sci.. Soc.; Counc. Mem. Assn. Clin. Pathol. Prev: Sen. Lect. (Forens. Path.) Univ. Sheff.; Sen. Regist. (Histopath.) Leicester Roy. Infirm.; Regist. (Histopath.) Mt. Vernon Hosp. Northwood.

RUXTON, Andrew McCall (retired) Meadhurst, James St., Armadale, Bathgate EH48 3JG Tel: 01506 30205 — MB ChB Ed. 1948. Prev: Capt. RAMC, TA.

RUZICKA, James Mark Vincent 15 Muir Avenue, Tollerton, Nottingham NG12 4EZ — MB BS Lond. 1994; BA (Hons.) Camb. 1991. SHO (Anaesth. & IC) St. Geo.'s Hosp., Tooting. Specialty: Anaesth.; Intens. Care.

RYALL, Christopher John 3 Cavendish Road, Birkenhead CH41 8AX — MB BS Newc. 1980; BA Camb. 1974; FRCR 1986. Cons. Radiol. Broadgreen NHS Trust Liverp. Specialty: Radiol. Prev: Sen. Regist. (Diag. Radiol.) North. RHA.

RYALL, David Michael 1 Eden Park Road, Hutton Rudby, Yarm TS15 0HS — MB ChB Aberd. 1983. Cons. S. Cleveland Hosp.. Specialty: Anaesth.

RYALL, Mr Robert James (retired) Scrivelsby, Heathbourne Road, Bushey Heath, Watford WD23 1PD Tel: 020 8950 1511 Fax: 020 8950 1511 Email: bob.ryall@btinternet.com — MB BCh BAO NUI 1951; FRCS Eng. 1958; MCh NUI 1960. Fell. Roy. Soc. Med. Prev: Cons. Surg. Edgware Gen. Hosp.

RYALL, Roger Duncan Hall (retired) Hampton House, Headbourne Worthy, Winchester SO23 7JH Tel: 01962 883270 Fax: 01962 886199 — (Middlx.) MB BS Lond. 1962; MRCS Eng. LRCP Lond. 1962; DMRT Eng. 1967; FFR 1971; FRCR 1975. Clin. Tutor Univ. Soton.; Regist. (Clin. Oncol.) & Mem. Counc. Roy. Coll. Radiol. Prev: Clin. Dir. & Cons. Radiother. & Oncol. Wessex Radiother. Centre.

RYALL, Rosemary Elizabeth (retired) Hampton House, Headbourne Worthy, Winchester SO23 7JH Tel: 01962 883270 Fax: 01962 886199 — MB BS Lond. 1963; MRCS Eng. LRCP Lond. 1963. Med. Off. Wom. Screening Clinics Basingstoke, Winchester & Soton.

RYALLS, Michael Robin Royal Surrey County Hospital, Egerton Road, Guildford GU2 7XX Tel: 01483 571122 Fax: 01483 450742; Heath View, 62 Chapel Road, Tadworth KT20 5SE Tel: 01737 213289 Fax: 01737 270521 Email: drmryalls@cwcom.net — MB BCh Wales 1981 (Welsh National School Medicine) MRCP (UK) 1986. Cons. Paediat. Roy. Surrey Co. Hosp.; Hon. Cons. St. Geo. Hosp. Lond. & Roy. Marsden Hosp. Sutton. Specialty: Paediat.; Endocrinol. Socs: Fell. Roy. Coll. Paediat. & Child Health. Prev: Sen. Regist. (Paediat.) Roy. Lond. Hosp. & Hosp. Sick. Childr. Gt. Ormond St. Lond.; Hon. Regist. (Paediat.) Roy. Childr. Hosp. Melbourne, Austral.; Clin. Research Fell. Roy. Marsden Hosp. Sutton.

RYAN, Alan James The Grange Surgery, 41 York Road, Southport PR8 2AD Tel: 01704 560506 Fax: 01704 563108; 18 Allerton Road, Southport PR9 9NJ — MB ChB Liverp. 1988. Prev: Trainee GP Blackpool Vict. Hosp. VTS.

RYAN, Andrew Royal Hospitals NHS Trust, Whitechapel, London E1 1AD Tel: 020 7377 7000; 43 Liddington Road, Stratford, London E15 3PL Tel: 0958 606667 — MB BS Lond. 1996 (Lond. Hosp. Med. Coll.) BSc (Hons.) 1991. Trainee GP E. Lond. VTS. Specialty: Gen. Pract.

RYAN, Anne Marie 6 Grasmere Gardens, Belfast BT15 5EG — MB BCh BAO Belf. 1997.

RYAN, Anthony George Portishead Health Centre, Victoria Square, Portishead, Bristol BS20 6AQ Tel: 01275 847474 Fax: 01275 817516 — MB ChB Bristol 1988; DGM RCP Lond. 1992; MRCGP 1994.

RYAN, Anthony Gerard Majella Joseph c/o Department of Radiology, University Hospital of Wales & Cardiff, Heath Park, Cardiff CF4 4XW — MB BCh BAO NUI 1990 (National Univ. of Ire., Galway) MSc, DIC. Imperial Coll. Of Sci., Tech, & Med. Lond. 98; FRCSI 1995. Specialist Regist. in Clin. Radiol. Specialty: Radiol.

RYAN, Audrey Mary Longthatch, Rodmell, Lewes BN7 3HQ — MB BS Lond. 1994.

RYAN, Bernard Edmund (retired) 10 Henley Close, Rawdon, Leeds LS19 6QB — MB ChB Liverp. 1968; T(GP) 1991; DTM & H Liverp. 1996. Prev: Med. Off. Univ. Stud. Health Serv. Leeds.

RYAN, Mr Brendan Patrick Trust Headquarters, Wythenshawe Hospital, Southmoor Road, Wythenshawe, Manchester M23 9LT Tel: 0161 291 5422 Fax: 0161 291 2037 Email: brendan.ryan@smuht.nwest.nhs.uk; 10 Granville Road, Timperley, Altrincham WA15 7BE — MB BCh BAO NUI 1981 (Univ. Coll. Cork) FRCSI 1985. Med. Dir. - S. Manch. Univ. Hosp.s NHS Trust.; Cons. (A&E) Wythenshawe Hosp.. Manch.. Specialty: Accid. & Emerg. Socs: Founding Fell. Fac. A & E Med.; BASICS; Fac. of preHosp. Care (Ed). Prev: Div.al Director of Med.; Clin. Director A/E.

RYAN, Carolyn Mary Spring Gables Surgery, Clint Bank, Birstwith, Harrogate HG3 3DW — MB BCh Wales 1982; DCH RCP 1987; DRCOG 1988.

RYAN, Catherine Jane 19 Wentworth Avenue, Sheffield S11 9QX — MB ChB Leeds 1995. GP Regist. Chesterfield. Specialty: Gen. Pract.

RYAN, Christopher John Melbourne Park Medical Centre, Melbourne Road, Aspley, Nottingham NG8 5HL Tel: 0115 978 6114 Fax: 0115 924 9334; The Anchorage, Spencer Drive, Nuthall, Nottingham NG16 1DX Tel: 0115 938 4167 — (Birm.) MRCS Eng. LRCP Lond. 1969; MB ChB Birm. 1969; DObst RCOG 1972; MRCGP 1977. Princip. GP; Examg. Med. Practitioner, Nestor Disabil. Anal.; Police Surg. Notts. Constab. Socs: BMA & Assur. Med. Soc.; Fell. Roy. Soc. of Med. Prev: Trainer (Gen. Pract.) Nottm. VTS; Ho. Surg. Surgic. Profess Unit Qu. Eliz. Hosp. Birm.; SHO O & G City Hosp. Nottm.

RYAN, Claire Elizabeth 10 St Andrew's Close, Workstead, North Walsham NR28 9SG — MB ChB Glas. 1995.

RYAN, Damian Jonathan 17 Abbotswood Road, St. Francis Place, East Dulwich, London SE22 8DJ — MB BS Lond. 1992 (UMDS (Guy's)) SHO (Neurosurg.) Atkinson Morley's Hosp. Lond. Specialty: Orthop. Prev: SHO (Orthop. & Trauma) Kingston Hosp. Surrey & Soton. Gen. Hosp.; SHO (ENT) Lewisham Hosp.

RYAN, David Alan Department of Anaesthetics, The Ayr Hospital, Dalmellington Road, Ayr KA6 6DX Tel: 01292 610555 Email: david.ryan@aaaht.scot.nhs.uk — MB BS Lond. 1976; BSc (Hons.) Lond. 1973; DA Eng. 1979; FRCA Eng. 1983. Cons. (Anaesth.) The Ayr Hosp.; Director Heartstart, Ayrsh. and Arran. Specialty: Anaesth.;

Intens. Care. Prev: Cons. (Anaesth.) Bronglais Hosp. Aberystwyth; Cons. (Anaesth.) Nevill Hall Hosp. Abergavenny; Sen. Regist. S. Glam. HA.

RYAN, David Hugh Community Mental Health Centre, Manor Road, Beverley HU17 7BZ Tel: 01482 887664 Fax: 01482 880026; Park Lodge, York Road, Beverley HU17 8DP — MB ChB Bristol 1976 (Bristol Medical School) MRCPsych. 1985; MSc Bristol 1988; MD Bristol 1995. Cons. Psychiat.Hull and E. Riding, Community NHS Trust; Project Manager:Investors in Ment. Health. Specialty: Gen. Psychiat.; Geriat. Psychiat. Prev: Sen. Regist. (Psychiat.) Roy. Edin. Hosp.; Regist. (Psychiat.) Exeter.; GP Devon.

RYAN, David Peter Michael Grassendale Medical Practice, 23 Darby Road, Liverpool L19 9BP Tel: 0151 427 1214 Fax: 0151 427 0611; 8 Burrell Road, Prenton, Birkenhead CH42 8NH — MB BCh BAO NUI 1979; MRCGP 1986.

RYAN, David William Freeman Hospital, High Heaton, Newcastle upon Tyne NE7 7DN Tel: 0191 233 6161 Fax: 0191 213 1968 Email: David.Ryan@nuth.northy.nhs.uk; 63 The Grove, Gosforth, Newcastle upon Tyne NE3 1NJ Tel: 0191 285 7430 Fax: 0191 285 7430 Email: dwryn@aol.com — MB ChB Sheff. 1970; FRCA 1974. Cons. Clin. Physiol. Freeman Hosp. Trust; Meritus, Edr. c/o Critically Ill. Specialty: Intens. Care; Anaesth. Prev: Cons. & Sen. Regist. (Anaesth.) Newc. AHA (T).

RYAN, Denis 117 High Street, Clay Cross, Chesterfield S45 9DZ — MB ChB Sheff. 1954; MA (Distinc.) Sheff. 1996. Specialty: Paediat. Neurol.

RYAN, Dermot Patrick Woodbrook Medical Centre, 28 Bridge Street, Loughborough LE11 1NH Tel: 01509 239166 Fax: 01509 238747 — MB BCh BAO NUI 1977 (University College Dublin) DCH NUI 1979; DObst RCPI 1980; MRCGP 1981; MICGP 1985; DFFP 1993. GP Princip.; Clin. Tutor Leics. Univ. Med. Sch.; Civil Serv. Med. Off. LoughBoro. & Dist.; Clin. Asst. Gastroenterol. LoughBoro. Gen. Hosp. Specialty: Respirat. Med. Prev: Lect. (Clin. Med.) Univ. Leicester; Trainee GP Dub. Regional VTS.

RYAN, Elizabeth The Old Stores, Wellshead Lane, Harwell, Didcot OX11 0HD Tel: 01235 832847 — MB ChB Sheff. 1977. SCMO (Family Plann.); Privat. Relationsh. & Psychosexual Therapist. Specialty: Pub. Health Med. Socs: Accred. Mem. BASRT. Prev: Ho. Off. (Med., Dermat. & Orthop.) Sheff. AHA.

RYAN, Eugene Paul Mary The Surgery, 291 Ashby Road, Scunthorpe DN16 2AB Tel: 01724 864426/7/8 Fax: 01724 282570; Glencrest, Ermine St, Scawby, Brigg DN20 9NB Tel: 01652 57768 — MB BCh BAO Dub. 1983; DCH RCPSI 1986. Trainee GP Barton VTS. Prev: SHO (Geriat.) Castle Hill Hosp. Hull; SHO (Paediat.) Scunthorpe Gen. Hosp.; SHO (Surg.) Craigavon Gen. Hosp.

RYAN, Frances Mary 22 Sussex Way, Barnet EN4 0BJ — MB BS Lond. 1991.

RYAN, Francis Patrick Woodbine Cottage, 2 Vicarage Lane, Dore, Sheffield S17 3GX — MB ChB Sheff. 1970; MB ChB (Hons.) Sheff. 1970; MRCP (UK) 1973; FRCP Lond. 1987. Cons. Adviser, Sheff. HA. Specialty: Gastroenterol.; Gen. Med. Prev: Cons., Gastroenterol., N. Gen. Hosp., Sheff..

RYAN, George Low Hill Medical Centre, First Avenue, Low Hill, Wolverhampton WV10 9SX Tel: 01902 728861 — MB ChB Liverp. 1961; DObst RCOG 1964; MA Liverp. 1991.

RYAN, Hubert Sidney Sims The Lime Kiln, Llanvanches, Newport NP26 3AY — MB BS Lond. 1953 (St. Bart.)

RYAN, Hugh Trevor 8 Haden Road, Cradley Heath, Warley B64 6ER Tel: 01384 66479 — MD Dub. 1937; MA Dub. 1937, MD 1937, MB BCh BAO 1934. Prev: Ho. Surg. Waterloo Hosp. Liverp. & Guest Hosp. Dudley.

RYAN, James David Varley 63 The Grove, Gosforth, Newcastle upon Tyne NE3 1NJ Tel: 0191 285 7430 Fax: 0191 285 7430 — MB ChB Leic. 1997. Specialty: Gen. Med.

RYAN, Professor James Michael Department of Conflict Recovery, University College London Hospitals, 4 Taviton Street, London WC1H 0BT Tel: 020 7679 4517/020 7679 4518 Fax: 020 7813 2844 Email: james.ryan@ucl.ac.uk; 111 Alexandra Road, Farnborough GU14 6RR Tel: 01252 673565 — (Univ. Coll. Dub.) MB BCh BAO NUI 1970; FRCS Eng. 1978; MCh NUI 1990; DMCC Soc. Apoth Lond. 1994; FFAEM (Hon) Fac. Of A&M 2000. Leonard Chesh. Prof. of Conflict Recovery Univ. Coll. Lond. Hosps.; Sen. Lect. Trauma Care. Specialty: Accid. & Emerg. Socs: Fell. Milit. Surgic. Soc.; Fell. Assn. Surgs.; Assn. Milit. Surg. of the US (AMSUS). Prev: Prof. Milit. Surg. RAMC & Roy. Coll. Surg. Eng.; Cons. Surg. Brit. Milit. Hosps. Hong Kong & Dharan (Nepal); Lect. (Surg.) & Hon. Sen. Regist. Prof. Surg. Unit St. Bart. Hosp. Lond.

RYAN, Jane Alison 26 Ferndale, Waterlooville PO7 7PA — MB BS Lond. 1983; DCH RCP Lond. 1987.

RYAN, Jeremy Martin Little Holmside Hall, Burnhope, Durham DH7 0DS — MB ChB Liverp. 1985; BDS Lond. 1978; FDS RCS Eng. 1988; FRCS Ed. 1989. Cons. Oral & Maxillofacial Surg. Sunderland Roy. Hosp. & Shotley Bridge Hosp. Co. Durh. Specialty: Oral & Maxillofacial Surg.

RYAN, Joan Mary 109 Grove Hill, London E18 2HY — MB BS Lond. 1983; DCH RCP Lond. 1990; DRCOG Lond. 1990; MRCGP 1991.

RYAN, Johanna Patricia Anaesthetic Department, Bolton Hospitals NHS Trust, Minerva Road, Farmworth, Bolton BL4 0JR Tel: 01204 390762 Fax: 01204 390763; 111 Moss Lane, Ashton-on-Mersey, Sale M33 5BU — MB BCh BAO NUI 1979; FFA RCSI 1984; FFA RCS Eng. 1985; DCH RCPSI 1987. Cons. Anaesth. Bolton Hosp. Specialty: Anaesth.

RYAN, John Brendan Ash Lodge Medical Centre, 73 Old Road, Chesterfield S40 2RA Tel: 01246 203138 Fax: 01246 231824; 22 The Crescent, Holy Moorside, Chesterfield S42 7EE Tel: 01246 569736 — MB ChB Sheff. 1986. Prev: GP Sheff.

RYAN, John Francis Alverton Surgery, 7 Alverton Terrace, Penzance TR18 4JH Tel: 01736 363741 Fax: 01736 330776 — BM Soton. 1982; MRCGP 1987; DRCOG 1988. GP Penzance.

RYAN, Katherine Elizabeth Rose Haematology Department, Manchester Royal Infirmary, Oxford Road, Manchester M13 9WL Tel: 0161 276 6722 Fax: 0161 276 4814 Email: kate.ryan@cmmc.nhs.uk; 38 Belfield Road, Manchester M20 6BH — MB BS Lond. 1981 (St Georges Hosp., Lond.) MRCP (UK) 1986; MRCPath 1993; MD Lond. 1995; FRC Path 2000; FRCP 2003. Cons. (Haemat.) Manch. Roy. Infirm. Specialty: Haematology. Special Interest: Haemoglobinopathy; Lymphoma.

RYAN, Margaret Mary (retired) 55 Gleneagles Road, Urmston, Manchester M41 8SB Tel: 0161 748 8389 — MB ChB Manch. 1961; FFA RCS Eng. 1969. Prev: Cons. Anaesth. Manch. Roy. Infirm.

RYAN, Mark Francis 90 Thingwall Road, Wavertree, Liverpool L15 7LA — BM BS Nottm. 1996.

RYAN, Martin Joseph Roche (retired) Withy House, Bamber Bridge, Preston PR5 6JD Tel: 01772 628357 — MB ChB Liverp. 1942. Prev: Capt. RAMC.

RYAN, Mervyn Maurice Benjamin Longton Hall Surgery, 186 Longton Hall Road, Blurton, Stoke-on-Trent ST3 2EJ Tel: 01782 342532 — BM Soton. 1981 (Southampton) BA (Engin. Sci. & Econ.) Oxf. 1969; DRCOG 1985. GP Stoke on Trent.

RYAN, Michael Francis Department of Biochemical Medicine, Ninewells Hospital, PO Box 120, Dundee DD1 9SY — MB ChB Ed. 1987.

RYAN, Michael Francis Baronscourt Surgery, 89 Northfield Broadway, Edinburgh EH8 7RX Tel: 01661 832209 Fax: 01661 836338 — MB ChB Edinburgh 1987; MB ChB Edin. 1987. GP Prudhoe, N.d.

RYAN, Michael Patrick, MBE 26 Cluny Gardens, Edinburgh EH10 6BJ Tel: 0131 447 2347 — BM BCh Oxf. 1968 (Oxf. & St. Mary's) BSc (1st. cl. Hons.) Lond. 1959; DObst RCOG 1970; FRCGP 1987, M 1974; Dip. Community. Med. Ed. 1976; MFCM 1980. Med. Dir. Primary Care System Health Systms Div. Edin. Specialty: Pub. Health Med. Prev: Ho. Off. Cowley Rd. Hosp.; Ho. Off. Radcliffe Infirm. Oxf.; Ho. Off. Churchill Hosp. Oxf.

RYAN, Miranda Jane Residency Block, Greenwich Health Authority, Greenwich District Hospital, Vanbrugh Hill, London SE10 9HE — MB BS Lond. 1997.

RYAN, Natalie Clare 9 Town Lane, Sheet, Petersfield GU32 2AF — MB ChB Birm. 1996.

RYAN, Noel Patrick The Health Centre, 7 St Andrew's Gate, Woking GU22 7LJ Tel: 01483 857835; Glenholme, Wych Hill Lane, Woking GU22 0AH Tel: 014862 63507 — MB BCh BAO NUI 1976. Medical Homeopath. Specialty: Homeop. Med.

RYAN, Noreen Marie Ann 50 Sherrick Green Road, London NW10 1LD — MB BS Lond. 1996.

RYAN, Padraic John Joseph Glaxosmithkline, GSK House, 980 Great West Road, Brentford TW8 9ES Tel: 0208 0475351 Fax:

0208 0476960 Email: padraic.j.ryan@GSK.com — MB BCh BAO Dub. 1983 (Univ. Dub. Trinity Coll) DCH RCPSI 1986; MRCGP 1988; T(GP) 1991; MA Dub. 1992; MFOM RCP Lond. 1995; T(OM) 1995; FFOM 2000. Director Glaxosmithkline Employee health Managem. Specialty: Occupat. Health. Prev: Health & Safety Adviser Kraft Gen. Foods Ltd. Banbury.

RYAN, Patrick Benedict Forest End Surgery, Forest End, Waterlooville PO7 7AH; 26 Ferndale, Waterlooville PO7 7PA — MB BS Lond. 1983; MRCGP (Distinc.) 1987; DCH RCP Lond. 1987; DRCOG 1987.

RYAN, Paul Francis Glenmill Medical Centre, 1191 Royston Road, Glasgow G33 1EY Tel: 0141 770 4052 Fax: 0141 770 4255 — MB ChB Glas. 1979; DRCOG 1981; DCH Glas. 1981; MRCGP 1983; FRCP Glas. 1999. Clin. Asst. (Geriat. Med.) Glas.; Chairm., Dennistown L.H.C.C.

RYAN, Paul John Medway Maritime Hospital Trust, Windmill Road, Gillingham ME7 5NY Tel: 01634 833889 Fax: 01634 846661 — MB BChir Camb. 1982 (Cambridge and Guy's) MB BChir Camb. 1981; MA Camb. 1982; MRCP (UK) 1986; MSc Lond. Univ. 1991; MD Camb. 1998; FRCP 1999. Cons. Nuclear Med. Medway Hosp. Trust Gillingham.; Hon. Sen. Lect. (Nuclear Med.) Guy's Hosp.; Hon. Cons. (Nuclear Med.) Maidstone Mid. Kent Oncol. Centre. Specialty: Nuclear Med. Socs: Amer. Soc. Bone & Mineral Research; Brit. Nuclear Med. Soc.; Eur. Assn. of Nuclear Med. Prev: Sen. Regist. (Nuclear Med.) Guy's Hosp. Lond.; Lect. (Nuclear Med. & Rheum.) Guy's Hosp. Lond.

RYAN, Peter Donald 2 Upper Wimpole Street, London W1G 6LD Tel: 020 7935 9711 — MB BS Adelaide 1967; DA Eng. 1976.

RYAN, Mr Peter George, TD Sandwell & West Birmingham Hospitals NHS Trust, City Hospital, Dudley Road, Birmingham B18 7OH Tel: 0121 507 4396 Fax: 0121 507 5637 Email: peter.ryan@subh.nhs.uk; City Hospital, Dudley Road, Birmingham B90 1N2 Tel: 0121 507 4636/4396 Email: peter.ryan@swbh.nhs.uk — BM Soton. 1978; FRCS Ed. 1984; FRCS 1998. Cons. Urol. City Hosp. Sandwell & W.Birm. NHS Trust; Med. Director Sandwell & W.Birm. NHS Trust; Hon. Sen. Lect. (Surg.) Univ. Birm. Specialty: Urol. Special Interest: Radical Prostolectomy. Socs: Fell. Roy. Soc. Med.; BMA; Brit. Prostate Gp. Prev: Sen. Regist. Rotat. (Urol.) Qu. Eliz. Hosp. Birm.; Clin. Research Regist. (Urol.) St. Woolos Hosp. Newport, Gwent.

RYAN, Petrina Francis Maria O'Tierney, Murphy and Ryan, Health Centre, Summerhill, Warrenpoint, Newry BT34 3JD Tel: 028 4175 4100 Fax: 028 4175 4050; 92 Shore Road, Rostrevor, Newry BT34 3AB Tel: 02841 738661 — MB BCh BAO NUI 1987 (Royal College of Surgeons in Ireland) LRCPSI 1987; DRCOG 1991; DMH Belf. 1992; MRCGP 1992. Prev: Trainee GP Warrenpoint; SHO (O & G, Paediat., Med. Cas. & Surg.) Daisy Hill Hosp.; SHO (Psychiat.) Craigavon Area Hosp.

RYAN, Philip John Department of Respiratory Medicine, Hereford County Hospital, Hereford HR1 2ER Tel: 01432 364096 Fax: 01432 364137 Email: philipryan@btinternet.com — MB ChB Birm. 1987; MRCP (UK) 1990; MD 2000; FRCP 2001. Cons. (Thoracic Med.) Hereford Hosp. Specialty: Respirat. Med.; Gen. Med. Socs: BMA; Brit.Thoracic Soc.; Brit. Soc. Of Allergy & Clin. Immunol. Prev: Regist. (Chest Med.) Birm. Heartlands Hosp.; Regist. (Chest & Gen. Med.) Birm. Gen. Hosp.; SHO (Chest Med.) Warwick Hosp.

RYAN, Philip Michael Barnard Castle Surgery, Victoria Road, Barnard Castle DL12 8HT Tel: 01833 690707 — MB BS Lond. 1979; AFOM RCP Lond. 1991. Specialty: Occupat. Health. Prev: Trainee GP Northallerton VTS; SHO (Infect. Dis.) St. Ann's Hosp. Lond.

RYAN, Robert Alphonsus Highlands, Greenway, Somers Road, Lyme Regis DT7 3EY Tel: 01297 443745 — (Camb. & St. Thos.) MRCS Eng. LRCP Lond. 1947; MB BChir Camb. 1948; DPH RCPS Eng. 1958; MRCGP 1971; LMCC 1977. GP Ripley; Med. Off. Ripley & Dist. Hosp. Socs: Derby Med. Soc. 1960-93; Derby Med. Soc. Prev: Cas. Off. & Ho. Surg. St. Thos. Hosp.

RYAN, Robert John 12 Dows Road, Belfast BT8 8LB — MB BCh Belf. 1998; MB BCh Belf 1998.

RYAN, Robert Patton 18 St Alban Road, Bedford MK40 2NG Tel: 01234 64285 — MB BS Durh. 1953 (Newc.) DPH Bristol 1959; FFCM 1980, M 1974. DMO N. Bedfordsh. Health Auth.

RYAN, Miss Rowena Marion Northwick Park Hospital, Watford Road, Harrow HA1 3UJ Tel: 020 8869 2679 — MB BCh BAO Dub. 1982; FRCS (Gen. Surg.) Glas. 1986; FRCS (Orl.) Eng. 1989. Cons. in ENT Northwick Pk. Hillingdon. Middlx. Hosp. Specialty: Otolaryngol. Prev: Sen. Regist. Roy. Nat. Throat, Nose & Ear Hosp.

RYAN, Sean Michael 27 Cotman Close, Westleigh Avenue, London SW15 6RG — MB BS Lond. 1991.

RYAN, Sean Seosap 3 Lindstrand Gardens, Limavady BT49 0TD — MB BCh BAO Belf. 1991; Diplomate Amer. Bd. Internal Med. Chicago 2001.

RYAN, Sheila Margaret The Roseberry Centre, St. Lukes Hospital, Middlesbrough TS1 3AF Tel: 01642 854958; 33 The Front, Middleton-One-Row, Darlington DL2 1AS Tel: 01325 332456 — MB ChB Sheff. 1968 (Newc.) MRCPsych 1981. Cons. Child & Adolesc. Psychiat. St. Lukes Hosp. Middlesbrough. Specialty: Child & Adolesc. Psychiat.

RYAN, Sheila Ruth (retired) 49 Abbot's Grove, Chester CH2 1AV Tel: 01244 381071 — MB ChB Liverp. 1950; DObst RCOG 1952; DA Eng. 1954; FFA RCS Eng. 1958. Prev: SCMO Barnet HA.

RYAN, Steven William 20 Kirby Park, Wirral CH48 2HA; 19 Woodhall Close, Pudsey LS28 7TX — MD Leeds 1990, MB ChB 1981; MRCP (UK) 1984; DCH RCP Lond. 1985. Sen. Lect. (Child Health) Univ. Liverp. Prev: Tutor & Hon. Sen. Regist. (Paediat. & Child Health) Leeds Gen. Infirm.

RYAN, Terence David Richard Kinross, 8 Well Lane, Heswall, Wirral CH60 8NE — MB ChB Aberd. 1972; DObst RCOG 1974; DCH Eng. 1975; FFA RCSI 1980; FFA RCS Eng. 1981. Cons. Anaesth. Roy. Liverp. Hosp. & Liverp. Matern. Hosp. Specialty: Anaesth.

RYAN, Professor Terence John, KStJ Hill House, Abberbury Avenue, Iffley, Oxford OX4 4EU Tel: 01865 777041 — BM BCh Oxf. 1957; FRCP Lond. 1974, M 1965; DM Oxf. 1977, MA 1965. Emerit. Prof. Oxon DHA (T); Emerit. Prof. Oxf. Brooks Univ. Specialty: Dermat. Socs: Hon. Pres. Internat. Soc. Dermat.; Pres. Internat. Foundat. Dermat. Prev: Clin. Prof. Dermat. Oxf. Univ.; Hons. Cons. Dermat. Roy. Postgrad. Med. Sch. Hammersmith Hosp.; Sen. Lect. Inst. Dermat. Lond.

RYAN, Thomas Declan Salop Road Medical Centre, Salop Road, Welshpool SY21 7ER Tel: 01938 553118 Fax: 01938 553071; Springwater, Shadeoak, Guilsfield, Welshpool SY21 9BT Tel: 01938 2442 — MB BS Lond. 1977; MRCS Eng. LRCP Lond. 1977; DCH RCP Lond. 1983; DRCOG 1984. Prev: Trainee GP Betws-y-Coed; SHO Birm. Matern. Hosp.; SHO Glos. Roy. Hosp.

RYAN, Thomas George Frazer 29A Cultra Avenue, Holywood BT18 0AZ — MB BCh BAO Belf. 1981.

RYAN, Ursula (retired) Saunton, Broseley Avenue, Culcheth, Warrington WA3 Tel: 0192 576213 — MB BCh BAO NUI 1955.

RYAN, Mr William Gerard Department of Orthopaedic Surgery, F Block, Royal Bolton Hospital, Minerva Road, Farnworth, Bolton BL4 0JR Tel: 01204 390343; 1 Lyme Grove, Altrincham WA14 2AD Tel: 0161 928 6009 — MB ChB Manch. 1986; FRCS Eng. 1990; FRCS (Orth) 1996. Cons. (Orthop. Surg.) Roy. Bolton Hosp. Specialty: Trauma & Orthop. Surg. Prev: Lect. (Orthop. Surg.) Univ. Manch.; Regist. (Orthop. Surg.) Manch.; Sir Harry Platt Fell. Univ. Manch.

RYAN, William James Acre Day Hospital, Homefield Road, Worthing BN11 2HS — LRCPI & LM, LRSCI & LM 1973; LRCPI & LM, LRCSI & LM 1973; MRCPsych 1979.

RYANNA, Kimuli Barbara Wasonga 12 Vanguard Close, London E16 1PN — MB BS Lond. 1998; MB BS Lond 1998.

RYANS, Robert Ian Castle Practice, Carrickfergus Health Centre, Taylors Avenue, Carrickfergus BT38 7HT Tel: 028 9331 5805 Fax: 028 9331 5947 — MB BCh BAO Belf. 1986 (Qu. Univ. Belf.) DRCOG 1988; DMH Belf. 1990; DCH RCPSI 1990; MRCGP 1991; DFFP 1993; MSOM 1998; MD Univ. of Ulster 2004. p/t Gen. Pract., Castle Pract., Carrickfergus; Hosp. Pract. (Rheum.) Ulster Hosp. Dundonald; Musculoskeletal Prive Pract., Dundonald Physiother. & Sports Injury Clinic, Camber Rd., Dundonald. Specialty: Rheumatol.; Gen. Pract. Special Interest: Musculoskeletal Med. Prev: Trainee GP W. Lothian VTS; SHO (Gen. Med.) Ulster Hosp. Dundonald; SHO (O & G) Waveney Hosp. Ballymena.

RYATT, Kamaljit Singh Walsall Hospitals NHS Trust, Moat Road, Walsall WS2 9PS Tel: 01922 721172 Ext: 6336 Fax: 01922 656226 Email: kama;jit.ryatt@wht.walsallh-tr.wmids.nhs.uk — MD Manch. 1984 (Manchester) FRCP Lond.; MB ChB Manch. 1973; MRCP (UK) 1977. Cons. (Dermat.) Manor Hosp. Walsall & The Skin Hosp. Birm.;

Hon. Sen. Lect. Univ. Birm. Specialty: Dermat. Special Interest: Dermatopharmacology; Photobiology. Socs: Brit. Assn. of Dermatologists; Fell., Amer. Acad. of Dermat. Prev: Lect. & Hon. Sen. Regist. (Dermat.) Gen. Infirm. Leeds; Sen. Regist. (Gen. & Geriat. Med.) Hope Hosp. Salford, Withington; Hosp. Manch. & N. Manch. Gen. Hosp.

RYATT, Lisel Karen The Broadway Surgery, 3 Broadway Gardens, Monkhams Avenue, Woodford Green IG8 0HF — MB BS Lond. 1994 (Lond. Hosp. Med. Coll.) BSc Lond. 1992; DGM 1996; DRCOG 1997; DFFP 1997; MRCGP (Merit) 1998. GP Non-Princip. Specialty: Gen. Pract.

RYBA, Penelope Catherine Jane Dysart Surgery, 13 Ravensbourne Road, Bromley BR1 1HN Tel: 020 464 4138 — BM BCh Oxf. 1987; DRCOG 1990; MRCGP 1991. GP Princip. Prev: Trainee GP Oxf. VTS.

RYBINSKI, Eugene Augustyn Burncross Surgery, 1 Bevan Way, Chapeltown, Sheffield S35 1RN Tel: 0114 246 6052 Fax: 0114 245 0276 — MB ChB Sheff. 1980; MRCS Eng. LRCP Lond. 1980; MRCGP 1986.

RYBINSKI, Paul 1 Carsick Hill Way, Sheffield S10 3LY — MB BS Lond. 1998; MB BS Lond 1998.

RYCROFT, Henry David Offshore Medical Services Ltd, The Lodge, Roddinglaw Business Park, Roddinglaw Road, Edinburgh EH12 9DB Tel: 0131 333 2525 Fax: 0131 333 0929 — MB BS Lond. 1973 (St. Geo.) BSc (Physiol., Hons.) St. And. 1968; MRCS Eng. LRCP Lond. 1973; DObst RCOG 1976; T(GP) 1991. Offshore Med. Servs. Ltd, Edin.; Med. Examr.uk.Offshore.Oil.Assn; Med. Examr. Marine Safety Agency (MSA); Med. Examr. Nonwegian Maritime Directorate; Med. Examr. Dutch Min. of Mines (offshore Div.); Offshore & Diving Doctor Norwegian Directorate of Health; Health & Safety Exec. Approved Diving Doctor; HSE Approved Blood Lead Doctor; WHO Approved Yellow Fever Doctor & Immunisation Centre. Prev: Med. Adviser (Cydesdale Bank plc.) Med. Adviser Santa Fe construction Leith; Med. Adviser Rigblast Aberd.

RYCROFT, John Alfred (retired) Rushes House, Charlton, Malmesbury SN16 9EA Tel: 01666 823607 — MB BS Lond. 1951 (Guy's) DMRT Eng. 1964. Prev: Asst. Radiotherap. N. Staffs. Regional Radiother. Centre.

RYCROFT, Nicole Elizabeth Child Health Centre, Hospital Road, Bury St Edmunds IP33 3ND Tel: 01284 775075 Fax: 01284 750280 Email: n.rycroft@doctors.net.uk — MB BS Lond. 1972 (Westm.) MRCS Eng. LRCP Lond. 1972; DCH Eng. 1975. Lead Cons. Paediat. Dept. of Community Paediat.; Forens. Med. Examr. Suff. Constab. Specialty: Community Child Health; Paediat. Socs: RCPCH; Brit. Assn. Community Child Health. Prev: SCMO (Community Health) Unit W. Suff. HA; Med. Off. Community Child Health Serv. Edin.; Med. Dir. & Cons. Paediat. Community Child Health Mid Anglia Community Trust.

RYCROFT, Richard John Graham St. John's Institute of Dermatology, St. Thomas's Hospital, London SE1 7EH Tel: 020 7922 8076 Fax: 020 7620 0890; 197 Sycamore Road, Farnborough GU14 6RQ Tel: 01252 543695 — MB BChir Camb. 1971 (Guy's) DIH Eng. 1976; FFOM RCP Lond. 1991, MFOM 1982; MA Camb. 1971, MD 1982; FRCP Lond. 1987. Cons. Dermatol. St. John's Inst. Dermat. St. Thomas Hosp. Lond.; Sen. Med. Adviser (Dermat.) Health & Safety Exec. Lond. Specialty: Dermat. Socs: Fell. Roy. Soc. of Med. Lond.; Fell. of St John's Hosp. Dermatological Soc. (Past-Pres); Brit. Assn. Dermatols. Prev: Sen. Regist. (Dermat.) St. John's Hosp. Dis. Skin. Lond.; Regist. (Dermat.) Guy's Hosp. Lond.; SHO (Med.) Hammersmith Hosp. Lond.

RYDER, Christine 16 Graham Park Road, Gosforth, Newcastle upon Tyne NE3 4BH — MB ChB Ed. 1958. Socs: N. Eng. Soc. Anaesth.

RYDER, Clive Alexander John 40 Harrow Road, Selly Oak, Birmingham B29 7DN — MB ChB Birm. 1984. SHO (Med. Rotat.) Russell's Hall Hosp. Dudley.

RYDER, Geoffrey Horace (retired) 3 Jagos Slip, Packet Quays, Falmouth TR11 2UA Tel: 01326 317239 — MB BS Lond. 1955 (Char. Cross) DA Eng. 1957; FFA RCS Eng. 1965. Prev: Cons. Anaesth. Walsgrave Hosp. Coventry.

RYDER, Ian George 47 Langfield Road, Knowle, Solihull B93 9PS — MB ChB Bristol 1984; FRCA 1989. Sen. Regist. (Anaesth.) S. West. RHA. Specialty: Anaesth. Prev: Vis. Asst. Prof. Univ. Maryland, USA; Regist. (Anaesth.) Wessex Regional Train. Scheme.

RYDER, Jeffrey Eric Northdown Surgery, St Anthony's Way, Cliftonville, Margate CT9 2TR Tel: 01843 296413 Fax: 01843 231231 Email: jeffrey.ryder@gp-g82066.ns.uk; 48 Devonshire Gardens, Cliftonville, Margate CT9 3AD Tel: 01843 228339 — MB BS Lond. 1971 (Roy. Free) MRCS Eng. LRCP Lond. 1971; DObst RCOG 1973. Prev: Ho. Off. (Med.) Coppetts Wood Hosp. Lond.; Med. Off. (Surg.) St. Albans City Gen. Hosp.

RYDER, Jessica Clare Bellegrove Surgery, 174 Bellegrove Road, Welling DA16 3 EW Tel: 020 8856 9648 — MB ChB Manch. 1996; BSc St. Andrews University 1994; DFFP Lond. 2000; DRCOG Lond. 2000. Salaried Gen. Practitioner BelleGr. Surg., Welling. Specialty: Gen. Pract. Prev: GP Regist. Ct. Yard Surg., Etham; Paediatric SHO, Qu. Mary's Hosp. Sidcup.

RYDER, John James Dynamic Psychotherapy Service, Humberstone Grange Clinic, Thurmaston Lane, Leicester LE5 0TA Tel: 0116 225 6430 Fax: 0116 225 6432 — MB ChB Birm. 1974; MRCPsych 1979; S. Trent Train. In Dynamic Psychother. 2001. Cons. Psychotherapist,Dynamic Psychother. Serv. Leic. Specialty: Psychother. Prev: Cons. Psychiat. & Psychother. Heronbrook Hse. (Therap. Community for Clergy & Religious) W. Midl.

RYDER, Joseph Bryan (retired) 4 Lansdowne Court, Causey Hill, Hexham NE46 2LP Tel: 01434 603220 — MB BCh BAO Dub. 1948; MB BCh BAO (Hons.) Dub. 1944; FRCPI 1969, M 1946; MD Dub. 1948; FRCP Lond. 1972, M 1951; Cert. Internat. Med. RCPS Canada 1955. Prev: Chest Phys. Mt.ain Sanat. Hamilton, Ont.

RYDER, Kathryn Olivia PO Box 6779, Dundee DD1 9WN — MB BS Lond. 1985 (Middlesex London) BSc Lond. 1982; MRCP (UK) 1988; DPhil Oxf. 1992. Civil Servant. Specialty: Cardiol. Prev: Research Fell. John Radcliffe Hosp. Oxf.; MRC Train. Fell. (Cardiovasc. Med.) John Radcliffe Hosp. Oxf.; SHO (Med.) Northwick Pk. Hosp. Harrow.

RYDER, Patrick Gerard Matthew Ryder Clinic, 20 Dingle Road, Upholland, Skelmersdale WN8 0EN Tel: 01695 624331 — MB BCh BAO NUI 1982. SHO (A & E) Warrington Dist. Gen. Hosp., Gen. Practitioner, Upholland, Lancs.; Hosp. Practitioner Gastroenterol., Wrightington, Wigan, Leigh Hosp. Trust. Specialty: Gen. Pract. Socs: PCGS Primary Care; Gastroenterol. Dept. Prev: Mem. Professional Fees Comittee, BMA 2001-2002.

RYDER, Robert Charles 16 Llantrisant Road, Llandaff, Cardiff CF5 2PX — MB BCh Wales 1959; FRCPath 1983, M 1966. Cons. Path. Mid Glam. AHA. Specialty: Histopath.

RYDER, Robert Elford John Department of Diabetes, Endocrinology & Lipid Metabolism, City Hospital, Dudley Road, Birmingham B18 7QH Tel: 0121 554 3801 Fax: 0121 507 4988 Email: bob.ryder@swbh.nhs.uk — MB BCh Wales 1977; MRCP (UK) 1981; MD Wales 1988; T(M) 1991; FRCP Lond. 1996. Cons. Phys. Diabetes & Endocrinol. City Hosp. Birm.; Clin. (IT Lead) City Hosp. Birm. & Diabetes Lead City Hosp. Birm. Specialty: Diabetes; Endocrinol.; Gen. Med. Special Interest: Clin. IT; Diabetic Retinopathy Screening. Socs: Assn. of Brit. Clin. Diabetologists (Com. & IT Off.). Prev: Sen. Regist. (Med.) Roy. Hallamshire Hosp. Sheff.; Research Fell. Diabetic Unit Univ. Wales Coll. Med. Cardiff; Regist. (Med.) Univ. Hosp. Wales Cardiff.

RYDER, Sally-Ann 198 Dover Road, Walmer, Deal CT14 7NB — MB BS Lond. 1993.

RYDER, Stephen David Department of Medicine, 4th Floor, South Block, Queens Medical Centre, Nottingham NG7 2UH Tel: 0115 970 9155 Fax: 0115 970 9012; 31A Fernhead Road, London W9 3EX Tel: 020 8960 2975 — BM BS Nottm. 1985; MRCP (UK) 1988; DM Nottm. 1993. Cons. Hepatol. Qu. Med. Centre Nottm. Specialty: Gastroenterol. Prev: Sen. Regist. (Liver Studies) Kings Coll. Hosp. Lond.

RYDER, Timothy Simon The Surgery, 1 Kew Gardens Road, Richmond TW9 3HL Tel: 020 8940 1048 Fax: 020 8332 7644 — MB BS Lond. 1989; DRCOG 1993; MRCGP 1993.

RYDER, William (retired) Department of Anaesthesia, Royal Victoria Infirmary, Newcastle upon Tyne NE1 4LP Tel: 0191 232 5131; Bessiemont, l6 Graham Pk Road, Gosforth, Newcastle upon Tyne NE3 4BH — MB ChB Ed. 1958; DA Eng. 1963; FFA RCS Eng. 1965. Cons. Anaesth. Roy. Vict. Infirm. Newc.

RYDING, Frank Noel, OBE Pine Lodge, Dinmore Road, Bodenham, Hereford HR1 3JR — MB BS Lond. 1972 (Univ. Coll. Hosp.) Med. Off. Internat. Comm. Red Cross. Specialty: Anaesth.

Prev: Regist. (Anaesth.) Hereford HA; Med. Off. Brit. Antarctic Survey; Regist. (Anaesth.) RiksHosp.et, Oslo, Norway.

RYDON, Arthur Harold Bruce 3 Roeheath, North Chailey, Lewes BN8 4HR — (Westm.) MRCS Eng. LRCP Lond. 1945; DTM & H Eng. 1956, DPH 1957. Specialty: Pub. Health Med.; Trop. Med. Socs: Roy. Soc. Health. Prev: RAMC; Dep. MOH Mombasa, Kenya.

RYE, Adam David 43 Waterloo Gardens, Cardiff CF23 5AB Tel: 029 2074 2373 — MB ChB Bristol 1992; MRCP (UK) 1995; Dip RCPath (Royal Coll. Of Path.) 1999. Specialist Regist., Haemot., Univ. Hosp. Wales, Cardiff. Specialty: Haematology.

RYE, Gillian Patricia Osborne Avenue Surgery, 5 Osborne Avenue, Jesmond, Newcastle upon Tyne NE2 1PQ Tel: 0191 281 0041 — MB BS Newc. 1982; MRCGP 1986; DCCH Manch. 1987.

RYE, Kara Anne 21 Mill Farm Close, Dunchurch, Rugby CV22 6QL — MB ChB Leic. 1996.

RYE, Stephen St. Chad's Surgery, Midsomer Norton, Bath BA3 2UH Tel: 01761 413334 Fax: 01761 411176; Asquith House, Gurney Slade, Bath BA3 4TD Tel: 01749 840461 — (Middlx.) MRCS Eng. LRCP Lond. 1969; MB BS Lond. 1969; DObst RCOG 1971; DCH Eng. 1972; Dip. Palliat. Med. Wales 1993. Prev: SHO (Accid. & Orthop.) Kettering Hosp. Gp.; Regist. (Paediat.) Kettering Gp. Hosps.

RYECART, Christine Noel Regal Chambers, 50 Bancroft, Hitchin SG5 1LL Tel: 01462 453232 — MB BChir Camb. 1981; MA Camb. 1983; DRCOG 1987. Princip. GP Hitchin. Specialty: Gen. Pract. Prev: SHO (O & G & A & E) Lister Hosp. Stevenage; SHO (Geriat.) Hitchin Hosp.

RYLAH, Lindsey Thomas Alan Basildon Hospital, Nether Mayne, Basildon SS16 5NL Tel: 01268 533911 Fax: 01277 636459 Email: lindsey@rylah.fsnet.co.uk; 6 Penwood Close, Billericay CM11 1DY Tel: 01277 631098 — MB BS Lond. 1977 (Westm.) MRCS Eng. LRCP Lond. 1977; MRCS Eng. LRCP Lond. 1977; FFA RCS Eng. 1982; FFA RCS Eng. 1982; MBA 1996; MBA 1996; MSc 2000. Cons. Anaesth. Basildon & Thurrock Trust; Hon. Lect. St. Bart. Med. Sch. Lond.; Hon. Lect. Roy. Lond. Med. Sch. Specialty: Anaesth. Socs: Expert Panellist Comm. Safety of Med., 1999 -. Prev: Dir. Critical Care Regional Burns Unit St. And. Hosp. Billericay; Sen. Regist. (Anaesth.) Yorks. RHA; Regist. (Anaesth.) Westm. Hosp. Lond.

RYLANCE, George William School of Clinical Medical Sciences (Child Health), University of Newcastle upon Tyne, Queen Victoria Road, Newcastle upon Tyne NE1 4LP Tel: 0191 202 3033/0191 233 6161 Fax: 0191 202 3022 Email: george.rylance@ncl.ac.uk; Greystones, 24 Painshawfield Road, Stocksfield NE43 7DZ Tel: 01661 843241 — MB ChB Glas. 1970; DObst RCOG 1972; MRCP (UK) 1974; FRCPCH 1999. Cons. Paediat. & Paediat. Clin. Pharmacol. The Childr. Hosp. Birmingham; Vis. Prof. McGill Univ. Montreal; Cons. Paediat. Royal Victoria Infirmary, Newcastle upon Tyne. Specialty: Pharmacology. Prev: Lect. (Child Health) Univ. Dundee & Ninewells Hosp. Dundee; Regist. (Paediat.) Univ. Hosp. of Wales, Cardiff; SHO (Paediat.) St. Mary's Hosp. Lond.

RYLANCE, Paul Brian Renal Unit, New Cross Hospital, Wolverhampton WV10 0QP Tel: 01902 307999 Fax: 01902 643025 Email: dr.rylance@rwh-tr.nhs.uk — MB BS Lond. 1977 (St. Geo.) BSc (1st cl. Hons.) Lond. 1977; MRCP (UK) 1980; FRCP Lond. 1994. Cons. Phys. & Nephrol. New Cross Hosp. Wolverhampton; Sen. Clin. Lect. (Med.) Univ. Keele; Hon. Sen. Lect. (Nephrol.) Inst. Urol. Lond. & Univ. Wolverhampton; Chairm. Midl. Lipid Gp. Specialty: Nephrol.; Gen. Med. Socs: Renal Assoc.; Amer. Soc. Of Nephrol.; Euro. Renal Assoc. Prev: Lect. & Hon. Sen. Regist. (Nephrol.) St. Peter's Hosps., Inst. Urol. & Univ. Coll. Hosp. Lond.; Research Fell. (Nephrol.) Kings Coll. Hosp. Med. Sch.; Regist. Rotat. (Med.) St. Geo. Hosp. Lond.

RYLANCE, Wendy Sheila Duncan Street, Wolverhampton WV2 3AN Tel: 01902 459076 Fax: 01902 455309; Roughton Farm House, Roughton, Worfield, Bridgnorth WV15 5HE Tel: 01746 716399 — MB BS Lond. 1978 (St. Geo.) DCH Eng. 1980; MRCGP 1982; DRCOG 1989. GP; Hon. Lect., Univ. of Birm. Sch. of Med. Specialty: Gen. Pract. Socs: RCOGP. Prev: Jt. Chair Wolverhampton Commissioning Forum; GP Clin. Asst. (Gastroenterol.) New Cross Hosp. Wolverhampton; Clin. Asst. (Diabetes) Roy. Hosp. Wolverhampton.

RYLAND, David Andrew Rose Street, Todmorden OL14 5AT — MB BS Lond. 1967 (Guy's) MRCS Eng. LRCP Lond. 1967; MRCP (UK) 1970; MRCGP 1977. GP Tutor (Clin. Med. Educat.) Postgrad. Centre Halifax Gen. Hosp. Prev: Lect. (Epidemiol. in Gen. Pract.) Cardiothoracic Inst. Lond.; Dep. Resid. Med. Off. Brompton Hosp. Lond.; Ho. Phys. Guy's Hosp. Lond.

RYLAND, Jonathan Michael 7 Sydenham Terrace, Covington Road, Westbourne, Emsworth PO10 8SZ — MB BS Lond. 1986; BSc Lond. 1983, MB BS 1986. SHO (O & G) Lond. GP VTS.

RYLAND, Olga Blethyn (retired) St. Govans, Frances Road, Saundersfoot SA69 9AH Tel: 01834 813301 — (Roy. Free) MB BS Lond. 1942; MRCS Eng. LRCP Lond. 1942.

RYLANDS, Alison Jane 16 Coronation Drive, Crosby, Liverpool L23 3BN Tel: 0151 931 5918 — (Char. Cross & Westm.) BSc (Hons.) Manch. 1978; MB BS Lond. 1986; MA Camb. 1987; MPH Liverp. 1991; MFPHM RCP (UK) 1996. Cons. (Pub. Health Med.) Wirral Hosp. Trust. Specialty: Pub. Health Med. Prev: Regist. (Pub. Health Med.) Mersey RHA; SHO (Med.) Roy. Liverp. & Westm. Hosps.; Ho. Off. Westm. Hosp.

RYLE, Anthony Guy's Hospital, Munro Centre, London SE1 9RT Tel: 020 7378 3210; Westerlands Lodge, Graffham Road, Petworth GU28 0QF Email: rylecat@aol.com — BM BCh Oxf. 1949 (Oxf. & Univ. Coll. Hosp.) DObst RCOG 1952; DM Oxf. 1960; FRCPsych 1980, M 1973. Sen. Research Fell. Kings coll & Hon. Cons. Psychother. Div. Psychiat. Guy's Hosp. Lond. Specialty: Psychother. Socs: Roy. Soc. of Med.; Pres., Assn. of Cognitive Analytic Ther. Prev: Cons. Psychother. St. Thos. Hosp. Lond.; Ho. Surg. (Obst.) & Ho. Phys. Univ. Coll. Hosp.; Ho. Surg. Colindale Sanat.

RYLE, Cym Anthony Havant Health Centre Suite C, PO Box 44, Havant PO9 2AT Tel: 023 9247 4351 Fax: 023 9249 2524 — BM Soton. 1977; DRCOG 1979; DCH Eng. 1980; MRCGP 1981. GP Princip.; Bd. Mem. & Clin. Governance Lead E. Hants PCG.

RYLE, Derek Marsden 1 Holmesdale Road, Teddington TW11 9LJ Tel: 020 8977 2220 — (Middlx.) MB BS Lond. 1949; AFOM RCP Lond. 1980. Prev: Ho. Off. Mt. Vernon Hosp. & Radium Inst. N.wood, Char. Cross Hosp.; Unit, Northwood & Kingsbury Matern. Hosp. Lond.

RYLE, Frederick Robert (retired) Whitmoor, Chalk Pit Lane, Monxton, Andover SP11 8AR Tel: 01264 710388 — MB BChir Camb. 1949; MRCGP 1972. Prev: Med. Ref. DHSS S. Region Reading.

RYLEY, Helen Elizabeth 11 Royal Gardens, Bowdon, Altrincham WA14 3GX — MB BS Lond. 1984; MA (Hons.) Camb. 1985; DRCOG 1987; MRCGP 1988. GP Principle. Prev: Trainee GP Bradford VTS.

RYLEY, Jonathan Paul 1 Elwick Road, Ashford TN23 1PD Tel: 01233 204163 Fax: 01233 204165 Email: drp.ryley@ekentmht.nhs.uk — BM BCh Oxf. 1981; MA Camb. 1982; MRCPsych 1987. Cons. Psychiat. (Psychotherapist.) SE Kent HA. Specialty: Gen. Psychiat. Prev: Lecturer in Psychiatry, Univ. of Nottingham, 1987-1991.

RYLEY, Nicholas Gavin Department of Histopathology, Torbay Hospital, Lawes Bridge, Torquay TQ2 7AA — BM BCh Oxf. 1984; MA Camb. 1985; MRCPath 1991; FRCPath 1999. Cons. Path. S. Devon Healthcare NHS Trust. Specialty: Histopath. Prev: Cons. Path. King Edwd. VII Hosp. Midhurst; Clin. Lect. Nuffield Dept. Path. John Radcliffe Hosp. Oxf.

RYLEY, Simon Philip Berkeley Place Surgery, 11 High Street, Cheltenham GL52 6DA Tel: 01242 513975 — MB ChB Birm. 1981; MA Camb. 1979; DRCOG 1983; MRCGP 1985; DCH RCP Lond. 1985.

RYMAN, Ann Elizabeth South Tyneside Trust, 10/12 Franligton Place, Newcastle upon Tyne; Thorn Wood, Elm Bank Road, Wylam NE41 8HT — MB ChB Ed. 1986; BSc (Hons.) Ed. 1984; Cert. Family Plann. JCC 1990; MRCGP 1991; DRCOG 1991; MRCPsych 1994; Mphil. Univ. Of Edinb. 1997. Sen. Regist. (Psychiat.) Newc. & N. Region. Specialty: Gen. Psychiat. Prev: SHO/Regist. (Psychiat.) Lothian HB; Clin. Med. Off. N. Manch. HA; Trainee GP Langley Pk. Co. Durh. VTS.

RYMASZEWSKI, Olgierd (retired) 67 Lyndhurst Avenue, Hazel Grove, Stockport SK7 5LT Tel: 0161 483 5876 — MD Polish Sch. of Med. 1946.

RYMER, Janice Mary Department of Obstetrics & Gynaecology, 6th Floor, N. Wing, St Thomas Hospital, London SE1 7EU Tel: 020 7928 9292 Fax: 020 7620 1227; 56 Scott Sufferance Wharf, 5 Mill St, London SE1 2DE — MB ChB Auckland 1981; MRCOG 1987;

FRNZCOG 1989; MD Lond. 1994. Cons. & Sen. Lect. O & G GUY's, Kings, & St. Thomas Hosp.Lond. Specialty: Obst. & Gyn. Socs: Coun. Mem. RCOG.; Coun. Mem. Brit. Menopause Soc.

RYMER, Michael John Worthing Hospital, Lyndhurst Road, Worthing BN11 2DH — (St. Bart.) MB BS Lond. 1970; MRCS Eng. LRCP Lond. 1970; MRCOG 1984; FRCOG 1998. Cons. O & G Worthing HA. Specialty: Obst. & Gyn. Prev: Sen. Regist. (O & G) Poole Gen. Hosp.; Assoc. Specialist (O & G) W. Dorset Hosp. Dorchester.

RYMES, Nichola Lyndsay — MB ChB Bristol 1987; MRCP UK; MRCPath UK. Cons. Haematologist, Torbay Hosp., Torquay. Specialty: Haematology.

RYRIE, Gillian Elizabeth Carronbank Medical Practice, Denny Health Centre, Carronbank House, Denny FK6 6GD Tel: 01324 822382 Fax: 01324 826675; 241 Main Street, Larbert FK5 4RA Tel: 01324 553649 — MB ChB Glas. 1971; DObst RCOG 1974.

RYTINA, Edward Robert Charles Dept. of Histopathology, Addenbrookes Hospital, Hills Road, Cambridge CB2 2QQ; Rose Cottage, 36 Glinton Road, Helpston, Peterborough PE6 7DQ — MB BS Lond. 1984; MRCPath; BSc Lond. 1981; PhD Lond. 1994.

SA'ADU, Alfa Watford General Hospital, Care of Elderly Department, Vicarage Road, Watford WD18 0HB Tel: 01923 217227 Fax: 01923 217715; 2 Kendalmere Close, Muswell Hill, London N10 2DF Tel: 020 8444 4535 Fax: 020 8444 0919 Email: asaadu@btinternet.com — MB BS Lond. 1976 (Univ. Coll. Hosp.) BSc (Anat.) Lond. 1973; MRCP (UK) 1979; DTM & H RCP Lond. 1984; MSc Clin. Trop. Med. Lond. 1985; PhD (Immunol.) Lond. 1989; FRCP UK 1999. Cons. Phys. Watford Gen. Hosp.; Sen. Lect. UCL Med. Sch. 1995; 2nd Nat. Vice-Pres. Nigerian Med. Assn. Specialty: Care of the Elderly; Immunol. Prev: Cons. Phys. Gen. Hosp. Bida, Nigeria 1982-1984; Clin. Lect. & Sen. Regist. (Gen. & Geriat. Med.) Univ. Coll. Lond. Med. Sch. 1992-1994; Sen. Regist. (Clin. Immunol.) Clin. Research Centre Harrow 1988-1992.

SAAB, Mr Michael Bury General Hospital, Bury BL9 6PG — MB BCh BAO NUI 1984; FRCS Ed. 1994. Sen. Regist. (A & E) Stockport & Manch. Specialty: Accid. & Emerg. Prev: Regist. (A & E) St. Peters Hosp. Chertsey; SHO (Thoracic Surg.) Harefield Hosp.

SAAD, Adnan 41 Nathans Road, North Wembley, Wembley HA0 3RZ — MB BS Lond. 1996.

SAAD, El Sayed Mostafa Flat 28, Moss Manor, The Avenue, Sale M33 4SH — MB BCh Cairo 1954 (Kasr-El Aini) DTM & H Liverp. 1967; DIH Eng. 1967; DPM Eng. 1969; MRCPsych 1972; LMSSA Lond. 1975. Cons. Psychiat. Bridgwater Hosp. Manch. Specialty: Gen. Psychiat. Prev: Sen. Regist. (Psychiat.) W. Chesh. Hosp. & Moston Hosp. Chester; Regist. & SHO (Psychiat.) Carlton Hayes Hosp. NarBoro..

SAAD, Isam El Din Babiker Flat 2, Stratheden Place, Reading RG1 7BH — MB BS Khartoum, Sudan 1985; MRCP (UK) 1992.

SAAD, Karim Fouad Georgi The Caludon Centre, Clifford Bridge Rd, Walsgrave, Coventry CV2 2TE Tel: 024 76 602020 — MB ChB Alexandria 1985; MRCPsych 1992. Cons. (Old Age Psych). Specialty: Geriat. Psychiat.

SAAD, Mr Khalil Jabbour 2 Marchfield Avenue, Dumfries DG1 1GN — Lekarz Lodz, Poland 1971; FRCSI 1984. Assoc. Specialist in Orthop. Dumfries & Galloway Roy. Infirm. NHS Trust Dumfries. Specialty: Orthop.

SAAD, Mr Magdy Naguib The Princess Margaret Hospital, Osborne Road, Windsor SL4 3SJ Tel: 01753 743434 — (Alexandria) MB BCh Alexandria 1958; MRCS Eng. LRCP Lond. 1964; FRCS Ed. 1964; FRCS Eng. 1964. Hon. Cons. Plastic Surg. Heatherwood & Wexham Pk. Hosps. Trust. Specialty: Plastic Surg. Socs: Fell. Roy. Soc. Med. (Ex-Pres.) Plastic Surg. Sect.; (Ex-Pres.) Brit. Assn. Plastic Surgs.; (Ex-Pres.) Brit. Assn. Aesthetic Plastic Surgs. Prev: Sen. Regist. (Plastic Surg.) Odstock Hosp. Salisbury; Sen. Regist. (Plastic Surg.) Liverp. RHB & United Liverp. Hosps.; Regist. (Plastic Surg.) Mt. Vernon Hosp. Northwood.

SAAD, Marniza 22 Huntsmead Close, Thornhill, Cardiff CF14 9HY — MB BCh Wales 1997. Specialty: Gen. Med.

SAADA, Janak Norfolk and Norwich University Hospital, Colney Lane, Norwich NR4 7UY — MB BS Lond. 1987 (University College Hospital Medical School London) BSc (Hons.) Lond. 1984; MRCP (UK) 1990; FRCR 1994. Cons. Radiol. Norf. & Norwich Univ. Hosp. Specialty: Radiol. Prev: Sen. Regist. (Radiol.) Roy. Free Hosp. Hampstead NHS Trust.

SAADAH, El Sayed Mohamed Sussex Rehabilitation Centre, Brighton General Hospital, Elm Grove, Brighton BN2 3EX Tel: 01273 674391 Fax: 01273 605063; Montrose, 87 Woodland Drive, Hove BN3 6DF Tel: 01273 554333 — MB BCh Ain Shams 1967 (Ain Shams Med. Sch. Cairo) MSc Surrey 1979. Dir. Rehabil. & Cons. Rehabil. Med. Brighton Gen. Hosp. Specialty: Rehabil. Med.; Rheumatol. Prev: Regist. (Orthop.) Hull Roy. Infirm., Ipswich & Southend Gen. Hosps.

SAADAH, Mohga Ali Montrose, 87 Woodland Drive, Hove BN3 6DF Tel: 01273 554333 — MB BCh Ain Shams 1970; DA Eng. 1978. Clin. Med. Off. (Community Med. & Child Health) Mid Downs HA. Specialty: Community Child Health. Socs: Fac. Comm. Health; Brit. Assn. Community Drs in Audiol. Prev: Regist. (Anaesth.) Roy. Marsden Hosp. Sutton, Guildford Hosp. & Frimley Pk. Hosp. Camberley.

SAADEH, Imad PO Box 14235, Damascus, Syria Tel: 00 963 11 2245118; 10 Wonston Road, Lordwood, Southampton SO16 5JH — MD Damascus 1984; MRCPI 1993. Cons. Neurol. & Head Neurophysiol. Dept. Teshreen Hosp. Damascus, Syria. Specialty: Neurol. Socs: Collegiate Mem. Roy. Soc. Phys. Irel.

SAADIEN-RAAD, Maurice Halifax General Hospital, Free School Lane, Halifax HX1 2YP — MB BCh Witwatersrand 1974.

SAAFAN, Ahmed Amin Morsi Maindiff Court Hospital, Abergavenny NP7 8NF — MB BCh Ain Shams 1976.

SAAGANDI, Mr Francis Wee 18 Bryony Road, Harrogate HG3 2UQ; 31 Perseverance Road, Haleland Park, Maraval, Port of Spain, Trinidad, West Indies Tel: 809 629 3224 — MB BCh BAO NUI 1980 (Roy. Coll. Surgs. Irel.) MRCS Eng. LRCP Lond. 1980; LRCPI & LM, LRCSI & LM 1980; DTM & H Liverp. 1984; FRCS Ed. 1986; MPhil (Biol. Med. Sci.) Bradford 1993. Cons. Gen. Surg. Eric Williams Med. Scs. Comlpex Champs Fleurs, Trinidad, W. Indies; Assoc. Lect. (Surg.) Univ. W. Indies, St. Augustine, Trinidad. Specialty: Urol. Prev: Sen. Regist. (Gen. Surg.) Gen. Hosp., Port of Spain; Regist. (Gen. Surg.) Princess Roy. Hosp. Hull & Maidstone Gen. Hosp.

SAARY, Mihaly — MB BS Lond. 1964; MRCP (UK) 1971; FRCPath 1987, M 1976. Cons. Haemat. The Doctors Laborat., 55 Wimpole St., Lond. W1G 8LQ; Cons. Haemat. Cromwell Hosp. Lond. Specialty: Haematology. Socs: Brit. Soc. Haematol.; RSM. Prev: Cons. Haemat. Nat. Guard Hosp. Jeddah, Saudi Arabia & Corniche Hosp. Abu Dhabi; Sen. Regist. (Haemat.) St. Bart. Hosp. Lond.

SABA, George Yousef Saleh 9 Dee Court, Ribble Road, Liverpool L25 5PW — MB BS Jordan 1982; FRCA 1994.

SABA, Hisham Peter Tudor House Surgery, 43 Broad Street, Wokingham RG40 1BE Tel: 0118 978 3544 Fax: 0118 977 0420; 4 Stafford Close, Woodley, Reading RG5 4QZ — MB BS Lond. 1985; BSc Lond. 1982, MB BS 1985; DRCOG 1992; MRCGP 1993.

SABA, Tarek Sami Zahi 23 Abberbury Road, Iffley, Oxford OX4 4ET Tel: 01865 747771 — MB ChB Ed. 1992. Ho. Off. (Cas. & Anaesth.) Wansbeck Gen. Hosp. Ashington.

SABANATHAN, Kanagasabesan Norfolk & Norwich University Hospital, Colney Lane, Norwich NR4 7UZ — MB BS Ceylon 1972 (Colombo) MRCP (UK) 1981; FRCP (UK) 1994. Cons. Phys. (Geriat. Med.) Norwich Hosp.; Hon Senior Lecturer/ Skill Co-ordinator Medical School UEA. Specialty: Gen. Med. Prev: Sen. Regist. (Geriat. Med.) Leicester Gen. Hosp.; Regist. (Thoracic Med.) St. Thos. Hosp. Lond.

SABAR, Mansoor Ahmad 2 Wilderswood Close, Manchester M20 4XU; 7 rutland Road, Ellesmer parks, Eccles, Manchester M30 9FA Tel: 0161 789 8513 — MB ChB Manch. 1985 (Manch) FRCA 1994. Specialty: Anaesth.

SABAT, Atif Lotfy 31 Woodlands Park Road, London N15 3RU — MB BCh Assiut, Egypt 1980.

SABBAT, Jan Kazimierz Mikolaj 120 Worple Road, Wimbledon, London SW19 4JB — MB BS Lond. 1985; BSc Lond. 1979; MRCP (UK) 1989. Specialty: Pharmaceutical Medicine.

SABBAT, Jolanta Maria Merck, Sharp & Dohme Idea Inc., Warsaw Branch, Przasnyska Ga, Warszawa 01-756, Poland Tel: 00 48 22 639 7000 Fax: 00 48 22 639 7001; 38 Parkside, London SW19 5NB — MB BS Lond. 1980 (University College Hospital Medical School) BSc Lond. 1974; MRCPath 1988; MSc Lond. 1996. Director Healthcare Policy MSD Warsaw, Poland. Prev: WHO Liaison Off. (Pub. Health) Poland; Sen. Regist. (Chem. Path.) Roy. Free Hosp. Lond. & W. Middlx. Hosp.

SABETI, Hamid 53 Rossmore Court, Park Road, London NW1 6XY Tel: 020 7723 1897 — MD Tehran 1961; DLO RCS Eng. 1983. Clin. Asst. (ENT) Roy. Lond. & Bart. Hosps. Specialty: Otolaryngol. Prev: Assoc. Prof. (ENT) Univ. Teheran; Prof. (ENT) Univ. Teheran; Dean Razi Med. Sch. Univ. Teheran.

SABETIAN, Mr Manuchehr 27 Welbeck Street, London W1M 7PG Tel: 020 7224 2242 Fax: 020 7224 2493; 7 Boscastle Road, London NW5 1EE Tel: 020 7485 1888 — MB BS Durh. 1954; FRCS Ed. 1958; ChM Liverp. 1962; FRCS Eng. 1967. Cons. Surg. Lond. Welbeck Hosp. Specialty: Gen. Surg. Socs: Mem. World Assn. Hepato-pancreatico-biliary Surg.; BMA; Assoc. Mem. of B.A.U.S. (Brit.Ass of Urological Surg.s). Prev: Sen. Regist. (Surg.) Roy. North. Hosp. Lond.; Sen. Regist. St. Mark's Hosp. Lond.; Regist. (Surg.) Liverp. Roy. Infirm.

SABHARWAL, Mr Atul Jiwan Raj Yorkhill NHS Trust, Royal Hospital for Sick Children, Glasgow G3 8ST Tel: 0141 201 0000 Fax: 0141 357 3824 — MB ChB Aberd. 1990 (Univ. Aberd.) FRCS Glas. 1995. Specialist Regist. (Paediat. Surg.) Roy. Hosp. For Sick Childr., Glas. Specialty: Paediat. Surg. Prev: ECMO Clin. & Research Fell. Yorkhill Childr. Hosp. Glas.

SABHARWAL, Mrs Chander Kanta The Surgery, 19 Lancelot Road, Wembley HA0 3AL Tel: 020 8903 0609 — MB BS Jammu & Kashmir 1969 (Srinagar Med. Coll.) DObst RCOG 1971.

SABHARWAL, Narindar Nath The Surgery, 19 Lancelot Road, Wembley HA0 3AL Tel: 020 8903 0609 — MB BS Delhi 1965 (Maulana Azad Med. Sch.) DTM & H Liverp. 1967. Prev: Cas. Off. Plymouth Gen. Hosp. & Hertford Co. Hosp.; Ho. Off. (Gen. Med.) Lond. Jewish Hosp.

SABHARWAL, Nikant Kumar 19 Lancelot Road, Wembley HA0 2AL — BM BCh Oxf. 1996 (UMDS Oxf.) BSc Lond. 1993. Research Fell. (Cardiol.) Northwick Pk. Hosp. Middlx. Specialty: Gen. Med. Prev: SHO (Gen. Med.) Northwick Pk. Hosp. Middlx.

SABHARWAL, Mrs Sangeeta Department of Obstetrics and Gynaecology, Scunthorpe General Hospital, Cliff Gardens, Scunthorpe DN15 7BH — MB BS Delhi 1984; MRCOG 1989. Cons. O & G Scunthorpe Gen. Hosp. Specialty: Obst. & Gyn.

SABHARWAL, Mr Tarun Guy's and St Thomas' Hospital, London — MB BCh Wales 1990 (Cardiff) FRCSI 1994; FRCR 1997. Cons. (Interventional Radiol.) & Hon. Sen. Lect. Guy's & St Thomas' Hosp. Lond. Specialty: Radiol. Prev: Regist. (Radiol.) Char. Cross Hosp. Lond.; SHO (Orthop & Trauma & A & E) Morriston Hosp. Swansea; Demonst. (Anat.) Univ. Birm.

SABHERWAL, Peter 5/7 Ballyoran Hill, Portadown, Craigavon BT62 1DJ — MB BCh BAO Belf. 1989.

SABIH, Irfan 64 Bermuda Road, Nuneaton CV10 7HU — MB BS Karachi 1986.

SABIH, Mohammad Raouf Kingston Hospital, Galsworthy Road, Kingston upon Thames KT2 7QB Tel: 020 8546 7711 Fax: 020 8934 3318; 12 Ullswater Crescent, London SW15 3RQ Tel: 0208 549 2550 Fax: 0208 459 2550 — MB BCh Ain Shams 1972; DRCOG 1990. Staff Grade (O & G) Kingston Hosp. Surrey. Specialty: Obst. & Gyn. Prev: Regist. & Clin. Asst. (O & G) Kingston Hosp. Surrey.

SABIN, Mr Howard Ian Royal London Hospital, Department of Neurosurgery, Whitechapel, London E1 1BB Tel: 020 7377 7250 Fax: 020 7377 7024 — MB ChB Dundee 1981; BMSc (Hons.) Dund 1978; FRCS Eng. 1986; FRCS Ed. 1986. Cons. Neurosurg. St. Bart. Hosp. Lond. & Roy. Lond. Hosp.; NeroSurgic. Tutor, Roy. Coll. of Surg.s of Eng. Lond..; Co-Dir. Lond. Radiosurg. Cemtre, Gamma Knife Unit. Specialty: Neurosurg. Socs: Brit. Cervical Spine Soc.; Soc. Brit. Neurol. Surgs.; N. Amer. Skull Done Soc. Prev: Sen. Regist. (Neurol. Surg.) Qu. Sq. Lond.; Regist. (Clin. Neurosci.) West. Gen. Hosp. Edin.; Research Fell. Inst. Neurol. Qu. Sq. Lond.

SABIR, Abdul W St Davids Court Surgery, 1 St. Davids Court, 68a Cowbridge Road East, Cardiff CF11 9DU Tel: 029 2030 0266 Fax: 029 2030 0273.

SABIR, Azra Tanweer Waheed 3 Balmoral Close, Lisvane, Cardiff CF14 0EX — MB BS Bangalor 1972 (Bangalore Med. Coll.) MB BS Bangalore 1972; MRCPsych 1982. Cons. (Child & Family Psychiat.) Brynffynon Mid. Glam. Specialty: Child & Adolesc. Psychiat. Prev: Sen. Regist. (Child & Family Psychiat.) Cardiff; Regist. (Child Psychiat.) Roy. Hosp. Sick Childr. Glas.

SABIR, Hakimuddin Mohamedali (retired) The Mushrique, 38 Penycae Road, Port Talbot SA13 2EL Tel: 01639 882260 — MB BS Bombay 1948.

SABIR, Maryam Saba 34 Wheatlands Drive, Bradford BD9 5JJ — MB ChB Leic. 1994.

SABIR, Nadeem Murtaza 9 Berkeley Crescent, Moseley, Birmingham B13 9YD — MB BS Lond. 1996.

SABIR, Omeima Mohy Eldin 57 St Nicholas Street, Carlisle CA1 2EF — MB BS Khartoum Sudan 1986; DCH RCP Lond. 1991; MRCP (UK) 1992; DCCH RCP Ed. 1993.

SABIR, Mr Saleem 56 Holland Street, Hyson Green, Nottingham NG7 5DS — MB BS Punjab 1989; FRCS Eng. 1994.

SABISTON, Margaret Alison Castlehill Health Centre, Castlehill, Forres IV36 1QF Tel: 01309 672233 Fax: 01309 673445; Redcliffe, Prospect Terrace, Lossiemouth IV31 6JS Tel: 0134 381 3018 Email: nsabiston@aol.com — MB ChB Aberd. 1975; LFHom 1995. Clinic Spynie Hosp. Elgin.

SABISTON, Neil Laich Medical Practice, Clifton Road, Lossiemouth IV31 6DJ Tel: 01343 812277 Fax: 01343 812396; Redcliffe, Prospect Terrace, Lossiemouth IV31 6JS Tel: 0134 381 3018 — MB ChB Aberd. 1975; FRCGP 1995, M 1979.

SABNIS, Sushma — MB BS Bombay 1974; MSc Manch. 1992. Assoc. Specialist (Community Child Health & Paediatric Audiol.) Basildon PCT. Specialty: Audiol. Med.; Community Child Health.

SABOOR, Tariq Stirling Royal Infirmary, Livilands, Stirling FK8 2AU Tel: 01786 434000 Ext: 4464 Email: tariq.saboor@fvah.scot.nhs.uk — MB BS Punjab 1987 (King Edwd. Med. Coll. Lahore) FRCS Edin.; FRCOphth Lond. Cons. Ophthalmologist Stirling. Specialty: Ophth. Special Interest: Cataract Surg.; Med. Retina; Refractive Surg.

SABOURIN, Andrew Cole Hilary Cottage Surgery, Keble Lawns, Fairford GL7 4BQ Tel: 01285 712377 Fax: 01285 713084 — MB BS Lond. 1987; DCH RCP Lond. 1990; MRCGP 1991.

SABOURN, Paul William 11 Claremont Gardens, Whitley Bay NE26 3SF — MB BS Newc. 1983; MRCGP 1990.

SABRI, Kourosh Ophthalmology Dept, Leicester Royal Infirmary, Leicester LE2 7LX Tel: 0116 254 1414 — MB ChB Bristol 1994; FRCOphth 1999. Specialist Regist. (Ophth.) Leicester Roy Infirm. Leicester. Specialty: Ophth. Socs: FREphth.

SABRI, Reehan 82 Virginia Road, Thornton Heath, Croydon CR7 8EJ Email: rsabri@sghms.ac.uk — MB BS Lond. 1997 (St Geo.) MRCPsych. Specialty: Gen. Psychiat. Socs: MDU.

SABRINE, Nilofer 4 Lomond Place, Ladybridge, Bolton BL3 4PS — MB ChB Sheff. 1989 (Univ. Sheff.) MRCP (UK) 1994; DCH RCP Lond. 1994. Specialist Regist. (Neonat.) S. Cleveland Hosp. Middlesbrough. Specialty: Paediat.; Neonat.

SABROE, Ian Leukouyk Biology Section, Biomedical Sciences Division, Imperial College School of Medicine, London SW7 2AZ — MB BS Lond. 1989 (King's Coll.) AKC Lond. 1986; BSc Lond. 1986, MB BS 1989; MRCP (UK) 1992; PhD Lond. 1998. Research Fell., Imperial Coll. Specialty: Respirat. Med. Prev: MRC Clin. Train. Fell. (Appled Pharmacol.) Nat. Heart & Lung Inst.; Regist. & Acting Sen. Regist. (Respirat. Med.) Hammersmith Hosp. Lond.

SABUR, Riyazali Yusufali Lochthorn Medical Centre, Edinburgh Road, Heathhall, Dumfries DG1 1TR — MB BCh Wales 1981; Dip. Travel Med. Glas. 1998. GP Princip. Dumfries. Specialty: Gen. Pract. Special Interest: Minor Surg.; Travel Med. Prev: Trainee GP Dumfries; Trainee GP/SHO (Cas.) Roy. Aberd. Childr. Hosp.; Regist. Rotat. (Surg.) Aberd. Roy. Infirm.

SACCO, Dominic Francis 11 Primrose Gardens, Hatch Warren, Basingstoke RG22 4UZ — MB BS Lond. 1998; MB BS Lond 1998.

SACCO, Joseph 85 Hollins Road, Walsden, Todmorden OL14 6PG — MB BCh BAO NUI 1955; TDD Wales 1958; DPH Bristol 1970.

SACH, Mr Michael Accident and Emergency Department, West Suffolk Hospital, Hardwick Lane, Bury St Edmunds IP33 2QZ Tel: 01284 713024 Fax: 01284 713024 Email: michael.sach@wsh.nhs.uk — MB ChB Birm. 1974; FRCS Eng. 1981; FFAEM 1994. Cons. A & E W. Suff. Hosp. Bury St. Edmunds. Specialty: Accid. & Emerg. Special Interest: Med. Educat. Socs: Brit. Assn. of Accid. and Emergency Med.; Fell.of Fac. of Accid. & Emergencey Med.; Brit. Med. Assn. Prev: Cons. & Head of A & E Dept. Roy. Naval Hosp. Haslar; Higher Professional Trainee A & E Med. RN Hosp. & Affil. NHS Centres; Sen. Regist. (A & E) Soton Gen. Hosp.

SACHA, Mr Bhupinder Singh Hollycroft Medical Centre, Clifton Way, Hollycroft, Hinckley LE10 0XN Tel: 01455 234414 Fax: 01455 632110; 5 Lance Close, Burbage, Hinckley LE10 2NT — MB BS Rajasthan 1969; MS ENT Rajasthan 1975. GP Hinckley Leics.; Hosp. Practitioner (ENT). Prev: Assoc. Specialist (ENT) & Sen. Med. Off. (Audiol) N. Manch. Dist.; Regist. (ENT) N. Manch. Dist. (T); Clin. Tutor (ENT) S.M.S. Med. Coll. Hosp. Jaipur.

SACHAR, Amrit 59 Woodfield Road, Hounslow TW4 6LL — MB BS Lond. 1993.

SACHDEV, Arun Pal Singh 26 Albany Avenue, Eccleston Park, Prescot L34 2QW — MB BS Lond. 1998; MB BS Lond 1998.

SACHDEV, Bhavesh 36 Addington Road, South Croydon CR2 8RB — MB BS Lond. 1994.

SACHDEV, Roopinder Singh 26 Albany Av, Eccleston Park, Prescot L34 2QW — MB ChB Sheff. 1997.

SACHDEVA, Lalta Queens Road Surgery, 7 Queen's Road, Tunbridge Wells TN4 9LL Tel: 01892 520027 Fax: 01892 540833; Mankash, Tree Lane, Plaxtol, Sevenoaks TN15 0QH Tel: 01732 810082 — MB BS Delhi 1962. Prev: Regist. (Anaesth.) Falkirk & Dist. Roy. Infirm.

SACHDEVA, Rajiv First Floor Flat, 88 Oakley St., London SW3 5NP — MB BS Newc. 1988. PHO Stud. Imperial Coll. Roy. Marsden Hosp. Lond. Prev: SHO (A & E) Sunderland Dist. Gen. Hosp.; Ho. Off. (Surg.) Roy. Vict. Infirm. Newc. u. Tyne; Ho. Off. (Med.) Freeman Hosp. Newc. u. Tyne.

SACHDEVA, S K Queens Road Surgery, 7 Queen's Road, Tunbridge Wells TN4 9LL Tel: 01892 520027 Fax: 01892 540833 — MB BS Panjab 1962; MB BS Panjab 1962.

SACHS, John Andre (retired) Department of Immunology, St Bartholomew's and The Royal London School of Medicine, and Dentistry, West Smithfield, London EC1A 7BE; 4 Ashworth Mansions, Elgin Avenue, London W9 1JL Tel: 020 7289 0330 Fax: 020 7289 0330 — (Cape Town) MB ChB Cape Town 1961; Dip. Biochem. Lond 1965; PhD Lond. 1970; FRCPath 1990, M 1980. Emerit. Reader in Immunol. St. Bartholomews & Roy. Lond. Sch. of Med. Lond. Prev: Cons. Immunol. Roy. Lond. Trust.

SACHS, Martin (retired) Flat 2, 8 Palace Gardens Terr., London W8 4RP Tel: 020 7229 6867 — MB BS Sydney 1960; MRCOG 1966. Prev: Regist. (O & G) Hillingdon Hosp. Uxbridge.

SACKETT, Katherine Mary Park House, Park Road, Stroud GL5 2JG Tel: 01453 562100 Email: k.sackett@glospart.nhs.uk — MB ChB Birm. 1983; MRCPsych 1989. Cons in Gen. Psychiat. Stroud. Specialty: Psychother. Prev: Sen. Regist. (Psychother.) Bristol.

SACKEY, Adziri Harold Mid Cheshire Hospitals, Leighton Hospital, Crewe CW1 4QJ Tel: 01270 255141 Fax: 01270 273491 — MB ChB Univ. Ghana 1982 (Univ. Ghana Med. Sch.) MRCP (UK) 1990; FRCPCH 1997. Cons. Paediat. Mid Chesh. Hosps. Specialty: Paediat. Socs: BMA; FRCPCH. Prev: Cons. Paediat. W. Cumbria NHS Trust; Sen. Regist. (Paediat.) Hull Roy. Infirm.; Regist. Roy. Liverp. Childr.'s Hosp.

SACKIN, Paul Albert Alconbury and Brampton Surgeries, The Surgery, School Lane, Alconbury, Huntingdon PE28 4EQ Tel: 01480 890281 Fax: 01480 891787 — (Univ. Coll. Hosp.) BSc (Pharmacol.) Lond. 1966; MB BS Lond. 1970; MRCS Eng. LRCP Lond. 1970; DObst RCOG 1972; FRCGP 1987, M 1974. GP Huntingdon; Asst. Edr. Educat. for Gen. Pract.; VTS Course Organiser Camb. VTS. Socs: (Pres.) Balint Soc. (1996-99). Prev: Hon. Sec. Assn. Course Organisers; Tutor (Gen. Pract.) Huntingdon; Course Organiser Huntingdon VTS.

SACKS, Gavin Paul 79 Antrobus Road, London W4 5NQ; 294 Woodstock Road, Oxford OX2 7NW — BM BCh Oxf. 1992; BA (Hons.) Camb. 1989; DPhil Oxf. 1998; MRCOG 2000. Sen. Regist. O&G N. Thames. Prev: Clin. Research Asst. Nuffield Dept. O & G John Radcliffe Hosp. Oxf.; Sen. Reg. Sydney Australia; SHO (O & G) Rosie Matern. Hosp. Camb. & St. Jas. Hosp. Leeds.

SACKS, Gerald Edmund Manor Surgery, Osler Road, Headington, Oxford OX3 9BP Tel: 01865 762535; 25 Stone Meadow, The Waterways, Oxford OX2 6TD Tel: 01865 292950 — MB ChB Leeds 1967; MB ChB (Distinc.) Leeds 1967; MRCGP 1983. Hon. Vis. Fell Oxf. Brookes Univ.; Club Doctor Oxf. United Football Club; Mem. Green Coll. Oxf.

SACKS, Lisa Jennifer Plastic Surgery Department, North Bristol Trust, Frenchay, Bristol BS16 1LE Tel: 0117 975 3994 Fax: 0117 907 0086 — MB BCh Witwatersrand 1986; BSc Witwatersrand 1981; FCSC (Plast) Coll Med S Afr 1994; MMed (Plastic) Witwatersrand 1996; FRCS (Lond.) 1998. p/t Cons. Plastic Surg. Frenchay Hosp. Bristol. Specialty: Plastic Surg. Special Interest: Breast Surg.; Hand Surg. Socs: Brit. Assn. of Plastic Surgs.; Brit. Soc. Surg. Of the Hand; Brit. Assn. of Aesthetic Plastic Surg. Prev: Cons., Plastic Surg., Baragwanath Hosp. & Univ. of Witwatersrand; Locum Cons., Plastic Surg., Wexham Pk. Hosp., Slough.

SACKS, Mark David 20 Belsize Square, London NW3 4HT — MB ChB Cape Town 1991.

SACKS, Mr Nigel Philip Michael Royal Marsden Hospital, Fulham Road, London SW3 6JJ Fax: 020 7808 2782 Email: nigel.sacks@rmh.nthames.nhs.uk — MB BS Melbourne 1980 (Univ. Melbourne) MS Melbourne 1989; FRACS 1989; FRCS Eng. 1990. Cons. Surg. The Roy. Marsden & Hon Sen. Lect. Int. of Cancer Research Lond..; Hon. Cons. Surg. Roy. Brompton Hosp. Specialty: Gen. Surg.; Plastic Surg. Socs: Brit. Breast Gp.; BASO (Breast Gp.); Roy. Soc. Med. Prev: Sen. Lect. & Hons. Cons. Surg. Roy. Marsden Hosp. & Inst. of Cancer Research Lond.; Lect. & Hon. Sen. Regist. John Radcliffe Hosp. Oxf.; Sen. Regist. City Hosp. Nottm.

SACKS, Simon Lawrence The Montpelier Surgery, 2 Victoria Road, Brighton BN1 3FS Tel: 01273 328950 Fax: 01273 729767 — MB BS Lond. 1972; MRCGP 1980. Med. Off. Brighton & Hove Jewish Home for the Aged.

SACKS, Professor Steven Howard Renal Unit, Guy's Hospital, St Thomas St., London SE1 9RT Tel: 020 7955 4151 Fax: 020 7407 4909 — MB ChB Bristol 1975; BSc Bristol 1972, MB ChB 1975; MRCP (UK) 1978; PhD Camb. Univ. 1982; FRCP Lond. 1991. Head of Renal Med. Guy's King's & St. Thomas's Sch. Of Med., King's Coll. Lond. Specialty: Nephrol. Prev: Tutor (Med.) Nuffield Dept. Med. John Radcliffe Hosp. Oxf.; Regist. (Med.) Addenbrooke's Hosp. Camb.; MRC Fell. MRC Laborat. Molecular Biol. Camb.

SACKVILLE WEST, Jane Eleanor Kentish Town Health Centre, London NW5 2AJ Tel: 020 7530 4747 — MB BS Lond. 1989 (Roy.Free.Hosp) DCH RCP Lond. 1992; DRCOG 1992; MRCGP 1994. GP; Clin.Tutor.UCL.

SACKWOOD, Sidney (retired) 2 Fernhill Lane, Upper Hale, Farnham GU9 0JJ — MB BS Lond. 1954. Prev: Cons. A & E Dept. Frimley Pk. Hosp. Surrey.

SACOOR, Mahomed Hanif Allimahomed Silverstream, Hamm Court, Weybridge KT13 8YB — MB ChB Sheff. 1963; MRCP Lond. 1967.

SADABA, Mr Justo Rafael Dept. of Cardiothoracic Surgery, Leeds General Infirmary, Great George St., Leeds LS1 3EX Tel: 0113 293 6657 — LMS Basque Provinces 1991; LMS Basque Provincces 1991; FRCS Ed 1996. SpR (Cardiothor. Surg.) Leeds Gen. Infirm. Specialty: Cardiothoracic Surg. Socs: Eur. Assoc. of Cardiothor. Surg.; Soc. of Cardiothoracic Surgeons of Gt. Britain & Irel. Prev: Res. Fell. (Cardiothor. Surg.) Leeds Gen Infirm. Leeds.

SADANA, Mr Arvinder 18 Claremont Park, London N3 1TH — MB BS Lond. 1984; BSc Pharmacol. Lond. 1981; MRCP (UK) 1987; FRCS Ed. 1989. Cons. A & E Whipps Cross Hosp. Lond. Specialty: Accid. & Emerg. Prev: Sen. Regist. (A & E) Whipps Cross Hosp. Lond.; Regist. (A & E) Whittington Hosp. Lond.

SADDLER, John Mackay Department Anaesthetics, Royal Devon & Exeter Hospital, Barrack Road, Exeter EX2 5DW — MB ChB Zimbabwe 1981; LRCP LRCS Ed. LRCPS Glas. 1981; FRCA 1986. Specialty: Anaesth.

SADDLER, Nicola Jill 22 Ennerdale Road, Doncaster DN2 5QR — MB BS Lond. 1990.

SADEK, Rafik Ismail Mohammed 18 Rowan Park, Roundswell, Barnstaple EX31 3QR — MB BChir Camb. 1982; BA Camb. 1978, MB BChir 1982.

SADEK, Saher — MB BCh Ain Shams 1980; MSc (Obst. & Gyn.) Ain Shams 1985; MRCOG 1988; MD Leic. 1996. Cons. O & G Solihull Hosp. Birm. Specialty: Obst. & Gyn. Prev: Sen. Regist. (FetoMatern. Med.) Roy. Matern. Hosp. Belf.; Sen. Regist. Rosie Matern. Hosp. & Addenbrooke's Hosp. Camb.; Clin. Research Assoc. Univ. Leicester.

SADEK, Sami Alfons Queen Alexandra Hospital, Department of Surgery, Cosham, Portsmouth PO6 3LY Tel: 02392 286000 Ext: 6885 Email: sami.sadek@ntlworld.com — MB ChB Cairo Egypt 1974; FRCS Eng. 1982; PhD Dundee 1986. Cons. Surg. Upper GI Surg. Portsmouth NHS Trust Portsmouth. Specialty: Gen. Surg. Special Interest: Upper GI & Laparoscopic. Socs: Association of

Surgeons of GB & Ireland; Association of Upper GI Surgeons. Prev: Sen. Lect. Gen. Surg. Univ. of Leeds.

SADHEURA, Mohinder Kumar 44 St Albans Road, Ilford IG3 8NL — MB BS Lond. 1989.

SADHRA, Kesar Singh Manor Park Medical Centre, 2 Lerwick Drive, Slough SL1 3XU — MB BS Lond. 1981; DCH RCP Lond. 1987; MRCP (UK) 1987; MRCGP 1988; DRCOG 1989. GP Principle; Clin. Asst. (Gastroenterology & Upper GI Endoscopy).

SADIDEEN, Mr Munir 175 Express Drive, Goodmayes, Ilford IG3 9RD — MD Damascus 1973; FRCS Ed. 1981.

SADIEQ, Shamas Ahmed — MB ChB Dundee 1993 (Ninewells Hospital Medical School (Dundee)) Dip. Family Plann 1998. Vocationally Trained GP. Specialty: Gen. Pract. Socs: St. Paul.

SADIK, Sabah Rasoul West Kent NHS & Social Care Trust, 35 Kings Hill Avenue, Kings Hill, West Malling ME19 4AX — MB ChB Baghdad 1974 (Baghdad Med. Sch.) FRCPsych 1996, M 1982; DPM Eng. 1983. Cons. Psychiat. (Learning Disabl.) W. Kent NHS & Social Care Trust W. Malling; Med. Dir. W. Kent NHS & Social Care Trust W. Malling. Specialty: Gen. Psychiat. Socs: BMA; Fell. Roy. Soc. Med.; World Psychiat. Assn. Prev: Hon. Sen. Lect., Kent Uni.; Clin. Dir., Learning Disabilities; Med. Dir., Thames Gateway NHS Trust.

SADIK, Samir Monir Waterloo Medical Centre, 1 Dunkerley St., Ashton-under-Lyne OL7 9EJ Tel: 0161 330 7087 Fax: 0161 308 2788 — LRCP LRCS Ed. 1983; MB BS Khartoum 1977; LRCPS Glas. 1983. Clin. Asst. (c/o the Elderly). Specialty: Cardiol.

SADIK, Wallaa Bashar c/o Haematology Department, Walton Hospital, Rice Lane, Liverpool L9 1AE — MB ChB Baghdad 1973; MRCP (UK) 1987.

SADIQ, Farakh Jamil Hyde Park Surgery, 3 Woodsley Road, Leeds LS6 1SG Tel: 0113 295 1235 Fax: 0113 295 1220 — MB ChB Leeds 1992.

SADIQ, Mr Hafiz Asadullah 23 Rannoch Drive, Bearsden, Glasgow G61 2JJ Tel: 0141 577 9199 — MB BS Karachi 1985; FRCS Ed. 1992. Ent. Surgeon (Paed.) Roy. Hosp. Sick Childr. Glas. Specialty: Otolaryngol. Prev: Assoc. Specialist (Otolaryngol.) Roy. Hosp. Sick Childr. Glas.

SADIQ, Mohamed Najumudeen Mohamed 41 Egerton Gate, Shenley Brook End, Milton Keynes MK5 7HH — MB BS Ceylon 1965 (Colombo) DCH Sri Lanka 1976; DCH RCP Lond. 1981; MRCP (UK) Paediat. 1983. SCMO (Child Health) Milton Keynes Community NHS Trust. Specialty: Community Child Health. Prev: Paediat. Nawalapitiya Hosp. Sri Lanka; Regist. (Paediat.) Wycombe Gen. Hosp. High Wycombe; SHO (Paediat.) Pilgrim Hosp. Boston.

SADIQ, Mustafa 9 Talbot Road, Fallowfield, Manchester M14 6TA — MB ChB Dundee 1987.

SADIQ, Pervez Muhammad Hillside House, Hillside Road, Huyton, Liverpool L36 8BJ Tel: 0151 489 4539 — MB BS Punjab 1977; MRCP (UK) 1986; DGM RCP Lond. 1986.

SADIQ, Mr Saghir Ahmed Royal Eye Hospital, Oxford Road, Manchester M13 9WH Tel: 0161 276 1234 Fax: 0161 276 6618 — MB BS Lond. 1987; MRCOphth 1990; DO RCS Eng. 1990; FRCS Ed. 1992. Cons. (Ophth. Surg.) Roy. Eye Hosp. Manch. Specialty: Ophth. Prev: Regist. (Ophth.) Univ. Hosp. Nottm. & King's Mill Hosp. Mansfield; SHO (Ophth.) Kingston Hosp. Surrey & St. Geo. Hosp. Lond.

SADIQ, Syed Tariq 2 Long Walk, New Malden KT3 3EJ — BM Soton. 1989; MSc Lond. 1994; DTM & H 1994; MRCP 1996. Specialist Regist. HIV. Specialty: Genitourinary Medicine.

SADIQ, Miss Syeda Shaheena Qamar 70 Brynteg, Cardiff CF14 6TT Tel: 029 2061 8525; Department Radiology, University Hospital of Wales, Heath Park, Cardiff CF14 4XW Tel: 029 2074 7747 Fax: 01222 743838 — MB BS Lond. 1993 (Charing Cross & Westminster) BSc Pharmacology Lond. 1990; FRCS Lond 1998. Specialist Regist. (Diagnostic Radiol.) Univ. Hosp. Wales, Cardiff. Specialty: Radiol. Prev: Sen. SHO (Gen. Surg.) Princess of Wales Hosp. Bridgend; Sen. SHO Orthop. Cardiff Roy. Infirm.; Sen. SHO Gen. Surg. Llandough Hosp. Cardiff.

SADIQ, Zulfiqar Ali 75 Meltham Avenue, Withington, Manchester M20 1FE — MB ChB Sheff. 1993.

SADIQUE, Mr Tanveer Manor Hospital, Walsall NHS Trust, Moat Road, Walsall WS2 9PS Tel: 01922 721172 Ext: 7287 Fax: 01922 656836; 25 Canning Road, Park Hall, Walsall WS5 3HN Tel: 01922 625466 Fax: 01922 625466 — MB BS Karachi 1981; FRCS Ed. 1989; FRCS (Orth.) 1995. Cons. Orthop. & Trauma Surg. Walsall NHS Trust; Mem. RCS Fac. for Train. Basic Surgic. Skills; UK Mem. AO Instruc. Fac. Specialty: Orthop.; Trauma & Orthop. Surg. Special Interest: Jt. Replacement in Young Adults. Socs: BOA; AOUK. Prev: Sen. Regist. (Orthop. & Trauma) St Jas. Univ. Hosp. Leeds.

SADLER, Mr Andrew Geoffrey Department of Oral & Maxillofacial Surgery, County Hospital, Lincoln LN2 5QY — MB BS Lond. 1986; FRCS Ed. 1991.

SADLER, Anthony Peter Department of Obstetrics & Gynaecology, Torbay Hospital, Torquay TQ2 7AA Tel: 01803 614567; The Moorings, Berry Head Road, Brixham TQ5 9AA Tel: 01803 859965 — MB BS Lond. 1980 (Middlx.) BSc (Hons.) (Biochem.) Lond. 1974; MRCOG 1986. Cons. O & G Torbay Hosp. Torquay. Specialty: Obst. & Gyn. Socs: Roy. Coll. Obst. & Gyn. Prev: Sen. Cons. Specialist & Hon. Lect. (O & G) Univ. Witwatersrand, S. Afr.; Clin. Research Fell. (O & G) King's Coll. Hosp. Med. Sch. Lond.; Ho. Surg. The Middlx. Hosp. Lond.

SADLER, Carolyn Jane 9 Guildford Drive, Eastleigh SO53 3PR — BM BS Nottm. 1982; DCH RCP Lond. 1985; DRCOG 1986; MRCGP 1987. Specialty: Family Plann. & Reproduc. Health. Socs: Brit. Menopause Soc.; Fac. Fam. Plann. & Reproduc. Health Care. Prev: GP Chandlers Ford Retainer Scheme.

SADLER, Christopher Leslie The Royal London Hospital , Barts & The London NHS Trust, Whitechapel Road, London E1 1BB Tel: 0207 377 7787 Fax: 0207 377 7153 Email: Chris.sadler@bartsandthelondon.nhs.uk — MB BS Lond. 1991 (Univ. Coll. & Middlx. Sch. of Med., Univ. of Lond.) PhD (Physiol.) Lond. 1987; FRCA 1996. Cons. Anaesth., Barts & The Lond. NHS Trust, Lond.; Director, Barts & The Lond. Med. Simulation Centre, Barts & The Lond., NHS Trust, Lond. Specialty: Anaesth. Special Interest: Med. Simulation; Obst. Socs: Obstetric Anaesth. Assn.

SADLER, David William Department of Forensic Medicine, University of Dundee, Dundee DD1 4HN Tel: 01382 348020 Fax: 01382 348021 Email: d.w.sadler@dundee.ac.uk — MB ChB Sheff. 1986; FRCPath 1994; MD Dundee 1996. Sen. Lect. (Forens. Med.) Dundee Univ. Specialty: Forens. Path. Socs: Amer Acad of Forens Sci. Prev: Regist. (Histopath.) Northampton Gen. Hosp.

SADLER, Derek James (retired) 29 Clos Derwen, Roath Park, Cardiff CF23 5HT — MB BCh Wales 1958.

SADLER, Ethna Daisy Hill Hospital, Newry Mental Health Department, Newry BT35 8DR Tel: 028 3083 5012 — MB BCh BAO NUI 1975; DPM RCPSI 1979; MRCPsych 1982. Cons. Psychiat. Specialty: Gen. Psychiat. Special Interest: Old Age.

SADLER, George Dawson The Surgery, 85 St Quintin Avenue, London W10 6PB Tel: 020 8969 2563 020 8354 3836; 96 Boileau Road, London W5 3AJ Tel: 020 8997 5755 — MB ChB Birm. 1965; MRCS Eng. LRCP Lond. 1965; MRCP (UK) 1970.

SADLER, Gillian Mary Kent Cancer Centre, Maidstone Hospital, Hermitage Lane, Maidstone ME16 9QQ Tel: 01622 225041 Fax: 01622 225074 — MB BS Lond. 1986 (Guy's) MRCP (UK) 1990; FRCR 1994. Cons. (Clin. Oncol.) Mid-Kent. Oncol. Centre Maidstone. Specialty: Oncol.

SADLER, Mr Gregory Paul The John Radcliffe, General Surgery, Headley Way, Oxford OX3 9DU — MB BCh Wales 1982; FRCS Ed. 1988; FRCS Eng. 1988. Specialty: Gen. Surg. Prev: Regist. Univ. Hosp. of Wales.

SADLER, James Andrew Stonecrest House, Breach Hill Lane, Chew Stoke, Bristol BS40 8YA — MB ChB Leic. 1998; MB ChB Leic 1998.

SADLER, Jonathan Calvert The Health Centre, Banks Road, Haddenham, Aylesbury HP17 8EE Tel: 01844 291874 Fax: 01844 292344; Birch House, Rosemary Lane, Haddenham, Aylesbury HP17 8JS Tel: 01844 290210 — MB BS Lond. 1968 (St. Bart.) MRCS Eng. LRCP Lond. 1968; LMCC 1971; DObst RCOG 1972; DCH Eng. 1972; MRCGP 1978. Prev: Med. Off. St. Barnabas Miss. Hosp. Transkei, S. Africa; SHO (Paediat.) Bristol Roy. Hosp. Sick Childr.; Resid. Paediat. Univ. West. Ontario, Canada.

SADLER, Kevin Michael Northern General Hospital, Hessies Road, Sheffield S5 7AM Tel: 0114 243 4343/0114 271 4818 Email: kevin.sadler@sth.nhs.uk; 7 Church View, Middlewood, Sheffield S6 1TY Tel: 0114 232 0772 Email: kevin.sadler@virgin.net — MB ChB (Hons.) Ed. 1991; BSc (Hons.) Anat. Ed. 1989; MRCP (UK) 1995; FRCA 1997. Cons. Anaesth. Sheff. Teachg. Hosps. NHS Trust Sheff.; Sen. Lect. Anaesth. Sheff. Univ. Sheff. Specialty: Anaesth. Prev: Specialist Regist. (Anaesth.) Lothian Univ. Hosps. HNS Trust,

Edin.; Specialist Regist. (Anaesth.) Ninewells Hosp. Dundee; Clin. Res. Fell. (Transpl.. Anaesth. & Int. Care).

SADLER, Malcolm Glyn Queen Street Surgery, 9-11 Queen Street, Whittlesey, Peterborough PE7 1AY Tel: 01733 204611 Fax: 01733 208926; Stanground Surgery, Whittlesey Road, Stanground, Peterborough PE2 8RB Tel: 01733 568569 Fax: 01733 892419 — MB BS Lond. 1971 (Lond. Hosp.) MRCS Eng. LRCP Lond. 1971; DObst RCOG 1973; FRCGP 1989, M 1976. Chairm. LMC. Prev: Bd. Mem. P'boro. S. PCG.

SADLER, Martin John Morriston Hospital NHS Trust, Morriston, Swansea SA6 6NL Tel: 01792 702222 — MB BS Lond. 1991 (Guy's Hospital) BSc Birm. 1982; PhD Lond. 1986; MRCP (UK) 1994. Specialist Regist. (Neurol.). Specialty: Neurol. Prev: SHO Rotat. (Med.) St. Geo. Hosp. Lond.

SADLER, Mary Aaroon Roseburn Cottage, 40 Purdysburn Hill, Belfast BT8 8JY — MB BCh Wales 1986; BSc St. And. 1981; Dip Palliat Med 2003.

SADLER, Michael Andrew Eastleigh Health Centre, Newtown Road, Eastleigh SO50 9AG; 9 Guildford Drive, Eastleigh SO53 3PR — BMedSci Nottm. 1980, BM BS 1982; DCH RCP Lond. 1985; DRCOG 1985; MRCGP 1986.

SADLER, Michael Robin de Clifford Spindleberries, Chalbury Hill, Wimborne BH21 7EY Tel: 01258 840357 Fax: 01258 840357 Email: robmar.sadler@virgin.net — MB BChir Camb. 1967 (Camb. & St. Thos.) MA Camb. 1967; MRCP (UK) 1970; DObst RCOG 1973. p/t GP Specialist (Cardiol.) Bournmouth & Wimborne Hosps.; GP Locum. Prev: Regist. (Cardiac) King's Coll. Hosp. Lond.; Regist. (Med.) Poole Gen. Hosp.; GP Princip., Quarter Jack Surg., Wimborne.

SADLER, Paul 146 Lichfield Road, Four Oaks, Sutton Coldfield B74 2TF Tel: 0121 308 2389 — MB ChB Birm. 1959; MRCS Eng. LRCP Lond. 1959; DObst RCOG 1961; DCH Eng. 1962; MRCGP 1980; DFFP 1994. Diplomatic Family Plann. Birm. Prev: Ho. Surg. Childr. Hosp. Birm.; Ho. Phys. Roy. Hosp. Wolverhampton; Ho. Surg. (Obst.) St. Chad's Hosp. Birm.

SADLER, Paul James, Lt.-Col. RAMC Intensive Care Unit, Queen Alexandras Hospital, Soham, Portsmouth PO14 3UR Tel: 02392 286035 — MB ChB Sheff. 1988; FRCA 1994. Cons. (Intens. Care Med.) QAH Portsmouth; Head of Anaestetic Dept, Roy. Hosp. Haslar. Specialty: Anaesth.; Intens. Care. Socs: AAGBI; ICS; RCA. Prev: Sen. Regist. Leicester Rotat.; Sen. Regist. Camb. Milit. Hosp. Aldershot.; Regist. (Anaesth.) Guy's Hosp. Lond.

SADLER, Robert Owen Mildmay Court Surgery, Mildmay Court, Bellevue Road, Ramsgate CT11 8JX Tel: 01843 592576 Fax: 01843 852980; Willow cottage, Bromstone Road, Broadstairs CT10 2HT — MB BS Lond. 1979 (Charing Cross) DRCOG 1982; FRCGP 1999. Vice Chairm. E. Kent MC; Thonet GP Tutor. Specialty: Gen. Pract. Prev: Trainee GP Shere Gp. Pract.; SHO (O & G & Paediat.) St. Luke's Hosp. SW Surrey HA.

SADLER, Rory Stephen 79 St Anne's Way, Kirkstall, Leeds LS4 2SQ — MB ChB Dundee 1982.

SADLER, Stephanie Jane 40 Stallcourt Avenue, Cardiff CF23 5AN — MB BS Lond. 1987; MRCPsych 1994. Clin. Research Fell. & Hon. Sen. Regist. (Psychiat. Genetics) Univ. Wales Coll. Med. Cardiff. Specialty: Gen. Psychiat.

SADO, Graham David Belmont Health Centre, 516 Kenton Lane, Kenton, Harrow HA3 7LT Tel: 020 8427 1213; 18 Royston Park Road, Hatch End, Pinner HA5 4AE — MRCS Eng. LRCP Lond. 1976; BSc Lond. 1973, MB BS 1977; MRCGP 1984. Clin. Asst. (Endoscopy) St Marks Hosp. Harrow.

SADOW, Mr Geoffrey John (retired) 5 Pond Close, Walton-on-Thames KT12 5DR Tel: 01932 269947 Fax: 01932 269942 — (Univ. Coll. Hosp.) MB BS Lond. 1954; FRCS Eng. 1962. Prev: Sen. Cons. Orthop. Surg. Kingston Hosp. Surrey.

SADRANI, Pravin Jagjivandas Tile Hill Health Centre, Jardine Crescent, Coventry CV4 9PN Tel: 024 7647 4744 Fax: 024 7646 9891; 3 Heritage Court, Coventry CV4 7HD — MB BS Saurashtra 1972.

SADULLAH, Shalal Department of Haematology, Borders General Hospital, Melrose TD6 9BS; Oatlands House, Parsonage Road, Galashiels TD1 3HS Tel: 01896 758451 — MB BS Karachi 1982; MRCP (UK) 1987; MRCPath 1995. Cons. (Haemat.) Borders Gen. Hosp. Melrose Scotl. Specialty: Haematology. Prev: Leukaemia Research Fell. Soton. Univ. & Bournemouth Gen. Hosp.; Regist. (Haemat.) King's Coll. Hosp. Lond.; SHO (Gen. Med.) Roy. Vict. Hosp. Bournemouth.

SAED, Elrasheid Abdel-Hafiz Flat 19, Blcok D, Temple Bank Flats, Duckworth Lane, Bradford BD9 6TB — MB ChB Alexandria 1983.

SAEDI, Kamran (retired) Florence Nightingale Hospital, Edward House, 7 Lisson Grove N10 3PT Email: ksaedi@aol.com — MD Teheran 1968; FRCPsych 2000. Prev: Cons. Child & Adolesc. Psychiat. Hackney Child & Family Consultation Serv.

SAEED, Abdel Moneim Department of Genitourinary Medicine, Victoria Hospital, Whinney Heys Road, Blackpool FY3 8NR Tel: 01253 306925 Fax: 01253 306924; 10 Beach Street, Lytham St Annes FY8 5NS — MRCS Eng. LRCP Lond. 1972; MB BS Khartoum 1964; FRCOG 1989, M 1971; Dip. Ven. Soc. Apoth. Lond. 1978. Cons. Genitourin. Med. Blackpool & Preston Health Dists. Specialty: Genitourinary Medicine.

SAEED, Abdul, Maj. RAMC Baillie Street Health Centre, Baillie Street, Rochdale OL16 1XS Tel: 01706 622491; 10 King Street E., Rochdale OL11 3ST Tel: 01706 341303 — MB BS Punjab 1965 (Nishtar Med. Coll. Multan) MB BS Punjab (Pakistan) 1965; DA Eng. 1968. Princip. GP Rochdale. Prev: Regist. (Anaesth.) Withington Hosp. Manch.; Regist. (Anaesth.) Blackburn Roy. Infirm.; Regist. (Anaesth.) Vict. Hosp. Blackpool.

SAEED, Bakri Osman Department of Clinical Biochemistry, Whittington Hospital, London N19 5NF Tel: 0207 2885042 Fax: 0207 2883485 Email: saeedbakri@hotmail.com — MB BS Khartoum 1978; MD, PhD, FRCPath. Cons. in Clin. Biochem., Whittington Hosp. Lond.; Hon. Sen. Lect., Dept. of Med., Univ. Coll. of Lond. Specialty: Chem. Path. Special Interest: Endocrinol. Socs: BMJ; MDU; ACB. Prev: Consultant- Clin. Biochem., Qu. Eliz. Hosp., Gateshead.

SAEED, Ibtisam Thannoon Harold Wood Hospital, Gubbins Lane, Harold Wood, Romford RM3 0BE Tel: 01708 345533; 3 Oakwood Chase, Hornchurch RM11 3JT Tel: 01708 457211 Fax: 01708 477211 — MB ChB Baghdad 1974; FRCPath 1992, M 1982; FFPath RCPI 1986. Cons. Histopath. Harold Wood Hosp. Romford. Specialty: Histopath. Socs: Brit. Soc. Gastroenterol.; Brit. Soc. Of Cervical Cytol.; Assn. Of Clin. Path. Prev: Sen. Regist. (Histopath.) St. Geo. Hosp. Lond.; Regist. (Histopath.) King's Coll. Hosp. Lond.

SAEED, Iqbal 8 Queen Victoria Street, Rugby CV21 3SY Tel: 01788 561074 — LRCP LRCS Ed. 1986; MB BS Pakistan 1977; LRCP LRCS Ed. LRCPS Glas. 1986.

SAEED, Mr Mohammad 140 Elm Road, New Malden KT3 3HS — MB BS Karachi 1985; FRCS Glas. 1994.

SAEED, Nadeem Riaz 48 Leegate Road, Heaton Moor, Stockport SK4 4AX — MB BS Lond. 1996; BDS Lond. 1988; FDS RCS Eng. 1992.

SAEED, Naveed Riaz 9 Buckingham Road West, Heaton Moor, Stockport SK4 4AZ — MB BS Lond. 1992.

SAEED, Mr Nur Ashton New Road Surgery, 863 Ashton New Road, Clayton, Manchester M11 4PB Tel: 0161 370 7115/6 Fax: 0161 371 1548 — MB BS Pubjab 1983; FRCSI 1988.

SAEED, Riaz Ashton New Road Surgery, 863 Ashton New Road, Clayton, Manchester M11 4PB Tel: 0161 370 7115/6 Fax: 0161 371 1548; 48 Leegate Road, Heaton Moor, Stockport SK4 4AX Tel: 0161 432 9339 — MB BS Punjab 1961; MB BS Punjab (Pakistan) 1961.

SAEED, Mr Shakeel Riaz Manchester Royal Infirmary, Oxford Road, Manchester M13 9WL Tel: 0161 276 4426 Fax: 0161 276 5811; Greyroofs, Cliffside, Wilmslow SK9 4AF — MB BS Lond. 1985 (Guys Hospital and Kings College Hospital Medical Schools) FRCS Ed. 1989; FRCS (Orl.) Eng. 1990; FRCS Eng 1990; FRCS Eng 1996. Cons. Otolaryngologist & Neuro-otological Surg. Manch. Roy. Infirm & Hope Hosp. Salford; Hon. Clin. Lect. Univ. of Manch. Specialty: Otorhinolaryngol. Socs: Coun. N Engl. Otorminolaryngological Soc. Prev: Regist. (Otolaryngol.) Orsett Hosp. & Roy. Nat. Throat, Nose & Ear Hosp.; SHO (Otolaryng. & Gen. Surg.) Manch. Roy. Infirm.; Sen. Regist. (otolaryngol) Manch. Roy. Infirm.

SAEED, Tariq 17 Woodville Road, Birmingham B17 9AS — MB BS Punjab 1970.

SAEED, Mr Waseem Riaz — MB ChB Manch. 1987; BSc 1984; FRCS Ed. 1992; FRCS Plast. 1997; GMC spec.reg.plast.surg. 1999;

CCST 1999. Cons. Plast. Surg. St James Univ. Hosp. Leeds; Sen. Clin. Lect. Univ. Leeds. Specialty: Plastic Surg.

SAEED, Zahedah Pervin 17 Woodville Road, Harborne, Birmingham B17 9AS — MB ChB Manch. 1977.

SAEED-AHMAD, Sheikh Central Medical Centre, 42 St. Pauls Road, Coventry CV6 5DF Tel: 024 7668 1231 Fax: 024 7666 4935; 96 St. Martin Road, Finham, Coventry CV3 6ER — MB BS Punjab 1966; DTM & H Liverp. 1970.

SAETTA, Mr John Patrick Department of Accident & Emergency, Queen Elizabeth II Hospital, Howlands, Welwyn Garden City AL7 4HQ Tel: 01707 365094 Fax: 01707 391228 Email: jsaetta@msn.com — MRCS Eng. LRCP Lond. 1981 (Middlx. Hosp. Med. Sch.) FRCS Eng. 1986; FFAEM 1993. Clin. Dir. (A & E), OPD Clin. Servs., Clin Tutor & Cons. Qu. Eliz. II Hosp. Welwyn Garden City; Mem. Specialty Train. Comm. for A & E; Dir. of Educat. (A &E) N. Thames (W.). Specialty: Accid. & Emerg. Prev: Sen. Regist. (A & E) St. Geo. Hosp. Lond.; Regist. (Gen. Surg.) N. Middlx. Hosp. Lond.; Regist. (A & E) Leicester Roy. Infirm.

SAFDAR, Mr Muhammad 326 Old Bedford Road, Luton LU2 7EJ — MB BS Bahauddin Zakariya Univ. Pakistan 1985; MB BS Bahauddin Zakariya U. Pakistan 1985; FRCS Glas. 1993.

SAFE, Amir Fahim 36 Sunningdale Mount, Ecclesall, Sheffield S11 9HA — MB BCh Alexandria 1976; MS Alexandria 1981; MRCP (UK) 1985; MD Bristol 1993. Cons. Phys. & Gastroenterol. Barnsley Dist. Gen. Hosp. Trust. Specialty: Gastroenterol.

SAFE, George Beverley Lodge, Beverley Gardens, Cullercoats, North Shields NE30 4NS Tel: 0191 252 2065 — (Durh.) MB BS Durh. 1953, BDS 1949.

SAFFAR, Mr Nabil 30 Pershore Road, Halesowen B63 4QJ Tel: 0121 550 4178 — MB ChB Mousul 1971; FRCS Glas. 1987.

SAFFER, Clive Mitchell Windmill Health Centre, Mill Green, Leeds LS14 5JS Tel: 0113 273 3733 Fax: 0113 232 3202 — MB ChB Leeds 1983; BSc (1st cl. Hons.) Physiol. Leeds 1980; MRCGP 1987; DRCOG 1987; T(GP) 1991; DFFP 1996; Docc Med (Diploma in Occupational Medicine), Faculty of Occupational Medicine, 2001. Prev: Regist. (Infec. Dis.) Seacroft Hosp. Leeds; Ho. Phys. Profess. Med. Unit & Ho. Surg. Profess. Surg. Unit Leeds Gen. Infirm.

SAFFMAN, Charles Michael Eastfield Group Practice, 1 Eastway, Eastfield, Scarborough YO11 3LS Tel: 01723 582297 Fax: 01723 582528; Blue Bank, 543 Scalby Road, Scarborough YO13 0NW Tel: 01723 353046 Email: c.saffman@btinternet.com — MB ChB Liverp. 1986 (Liverpool) DA (UK) 1990; MRCGP 1994. GP Princip.; Bd. Mem. ScarBoro., Whitby & Ryedale PCG. Specialty: Anaesth. Prev: Trainee GP/SHO ScarBoro. VTS; Regist. (ITU) Fremantle, Austral.; SHO (Anaesth.) Whiston Hosp. Prescot.

SAFIR, Jeffrey Gerald Spitalfields Practice, 20 Old Montague Street, London E1 5PB Tel: 020 7247 7070 Fax: 020 7650 1920; 36 Crystal Palace Park Road, Sydenham, London SE26 6UG — MB ChB Bristol 1972. Prev: Ho. Surg. Mayday Hosp. Thornton Heath; Ho. Phys. St. Martin's Hosp. Bath.

SAFRANEK, Margaret Mary Schofield Dukes Avenue Surgery, 1 Dukes Avenue, London N10 2PS Tel: 020 8883 9149; 36 Dukes Avenue, London N10 2PU Tel: 020 8883 9556 — MB BS Lond. 1980 (St Thomas's) BA Oxf. 1956. Specialty: Gen. Pract.

SAFRANEK, Mr Peter Michael 15 The Paddock, Longworth, Abingdon OX13 5BX Email: peter.safranek@virgin.net — BM Soton. 1993; BSc (Hons.) Soton. 1992; FRCS (Eng.) 1997. SpR in Gen. Surg., Oxf. Region. Specialty: Gen. Surg. Socs: Affil. Fell. Assn. of Surg. of GB & Irel.; Associate Member of the Association of Upper Gastrointestinal Surgeons. Prev: Basic Surgic. Train. Rotat. (Cardiothoracic, Gen. & Orthop. Surg.) Wessex Region; SHO (Orthop. Surg. & A & E) Soton.; Research Fell. (Gen. Surg.) Soton.

SAFWAT, Sherif Moustafa Mohamed Flat 17, James Paget Hospital, Lowestoft Road, Gorleston, Great Yarmouth NR31 6LA Tel: 01493 452524; Fazakerley Hospital, Lower Lane, Liverpool L9 7AL Tel: 0151 529 2392 — MB ChB Alexandria 1981; MRCP (UK) 1988. Specialty: Gen. Med. Prev: Regist. (Med.) Derriford Hosp. Plymouth.

SAGAR, A Teehey Lane Medical Centre, 66-68 Teehey Lane, Bebington, Wirral CH63 2JN Tel: 0151 608 2519.

SAGAR, Mr Chintapalli Vidyasagar 10 Holiday Sq, Vicarage Road, Birmingham B15 B4A Tel: 0121 608 7860 Fax: 0121 628 0382 Email: vidya1950@aol.com — MB BS Andhra 1974 (Andhra Med. Coll. Visakhapatnam) FRCS Ed. 1978. Clin. Asst. (Gastroenterology) Solihull Hosp.; Police Surgeon W. Midlands; Dir. Kanaka Durga Nursing Home, Governorpet, India. Prev: Regist. (Gen. Surg.) N. Warks. AHA; Rotating SHO (Gen. Surg.) Kent AHA.

SAGAR, Daya (retired) 89 Plumptre Way, Eastwood, Nottingham NG16 3LQ; 21 North Street, Newthorpe NG16 2E Tel: 01773 710483 Email: dayasagar@hotmail.com — MB BS Osmania 1958 (Osmania Med. Coll.) DTM & H Ed. 1961.

SAGAR, Derrick Alan Centre for Medical & Dental Education, Pilgrim Hospital ULH Trust, Sibsey Road, Boston PE21 9QS Tel: 01205 364801 Fax: 01205 354395 Email: alan.sagar@ulh.nhs.uk — MB ChB Leeds 1976; ALS (Instruc); BSc Leeds 1973; FRCA 1981; Dip. ATLS RCS Eng. 1994. Cons. Anaesth. United Lincs. Hosps. Trust; Chairm. Lives Lincs. Integrated Volun. Basics Scheme Emerg. Serv.; Trustee Lincs and Notts Air Ambul.; Clin. Tutor, Pilgrim Hosp.; lead Clinician, Med. Educat., Leicester and Warwick Med. Schools. Specialty: Anaesth. Special Interest: paediatric ENT; Urology. Socs: Assn. Anaesth.; Intens. Care Soc.; BMA. Prev: Sen. Regist. Yorks. Rotat., Leeds.

SAGAR, Giselle Annette Old Brandon Road Surgery, Old Brandon Road, Feltwell, Thetford IP26 4AY Tel: 01842 828481 Fax: 01842 828172; Silver Birches, 2 The Grove, Mundford, Thetford IP26 5HF Tel: 01842 879164 — BM BS Nottm. 1987; DCH RCP Lond. 1991; DRCOG 1992; MRCGP 1993. Specialty: Family Plann. & Reproduc. Health. Prev: Clin. Asst. (Rheum.) Princess Margt. Hosp. Swindon; Trainee GP Plymouth HA VTS.

SAGAR, Professor Harvey James Thornbury Hospital, Fulwood Road, Sheffield S10 3BR Tel: 0114 266 1133 Fax: 0114 267 8730; Sycamore House, Cliff Lane, Calver, Hope Valley S32 3XD Tel: 01433 639215 Fax: 01433 639215 Email: harvpip@globalnet.co.uk — BM BCh Oxf. 1972; MRCP (UK) 1975; BA (Physiol.) Oxf. 1969, MA 1972, DM 1980; FRCP Lond. 1990. Cons. (Neurol.) Thornbury Hosp. Sheff.; Director, Medi-consult Ltd. Specialty: Neurol. Socs: Movem. Disorder Soc.; Amer. Acad. of Neurol. (Corr. Fell.); Assn. of Brit. NeUrol.s. Prev: Prof. Clin. Neurol. Univ. Sheff.; Cons. Neurol. Roy. Hallamsh. Hosp. Sheff.; Sen. Regist. (Neurol.) Radcliffe Infirm. Oxf.; Clin. & Research.

SAGAR, Jack (retired) 51 Rottingdean Place, Rottingdean, Brighton BN2 7FS — MB ChB Leeds 1949; MRCGP. (Occupat. Med.) T & N plc.

SAGAR, Jawahar Lal 45 Armroyd Lane, Elsecar, Barnsley S74 8ET Tel: 01226 743012 — MB ChB Glas. 1960. GP Trainer Barnsley VTS. Prev: SHO (Paediat.) & Ho. Off. (Med.) St. Margt. Hosp. Stratton st Margt.; Ho. Off. (Surg.) Poole Gen. Hosp.

SAGAR, Peter Jeremy The Surgery, 1 The Ridgway, Woodingdean, Brighton BN2 6PE Tel: 01273 307555 Fax: 01273 304861; 41 Gorham Avenue, Rottingdean, Brighton BN2 7DP Tel: 01273 309799 — MB BS Lond. 1980 (Char. Cross) MRCS Eng. LRCP Lond. 1980; DRCOG 1982; DCH RCP Lond. 1983; MRCGP 1984.

SAGAR, Prem Park House Surgery, 55 Higher Parr Street, St Helens WA9 1BP Tel: 01744 23705 Fax: 01744 454601 — MB ChB Liverp. 1984; DRCOG 1988.

SAGAR, Mr Samir Abdulla 31 Hollymead Close, Colchester CO4 5JU Tel: 01206 851913 — MB BCh Al Fateh 1982; FRCS Ed. 1986.

SAGAR, Mr Shanti Consultant Surgeon, Wirral Hospitals Trust, Clatterbridge, Hospital, Bebington Tel: 0151 482 7753 Fax: 0151 482 7759 — MB BS Osmania 1967; FRCS Ed. 1971; FRCS Eng. 1975. Cons. Surg., Wirral Hosps., Gen. & Upper GI Surg.; Clin. Lect. (Surg.) Univ. Liverp. Specialty: Gen. Surg. Special Interest: Gastroenterol. Socs: Brit. Laser Soc.; Brit. Soc. of Gastroenterol.; Assn. of Surg. Of Upper GI Surg.

SAGAR, Stephen Mark 31 Hillbury Road, Tooting Bec Common, London SW17 8JT Tel: 020 8675 1751 — MB BS Lond. 1981 (St. Geo.) BSc (Pharmacol.) Lond. 1978, MB BS 1981. Regist. (Med.) Greenwich Dist. Hosp. Prev: SHO (Med.) Roy. Marsden Hosp.; SHO (Med.) St. Jas. Hosp. Balham.

SAGAR, Sushila Daya Parkview Surgery, 89 Plumptre Way, Eastwood, Nottingham NG16 3LQ Tel: 01773 714414 Fax: 01773 533306.

SAGAR, William (retired) Carlton, 156 Barrier Bank, Cowbit, Spalding PE12 6AL Tel: 01406 380382 Fax: 01406380382 — (Manch.) MB ChB Manch. 1963; DObst RCOG 1965. Lincs. Br.

Med. Off. Brit. Red Cross Soc.; Med. Asst. Abbey. View. Pract. Crowland. Lincs. Prev: GP Boston.

SAGAY, Atiene Solomon 35 Seymour Gardens, London SE4 2DN — MB ChB Nigeria 1982; MRCOG 1994.

SAGE, Christopher Harrison Student Health Service, 25 Belgrave Road, Bristol BS8 2AA Tel: 0117 973 7716 Fax: 0117 970 6804; 61A Kingsdown Parade, Kingsdown, Bristol BS6 5UG Tel: 0117 942 2819 — MB BS Lond. 1973 (Middlx.) MRCS Eng. LRCP Lond. 1973; DRCOG 1978; MRCPsych 1984. Med. Off. Stud. Health Serv. Bristol Univ.

SAGE, Fiona Judith Dowstall Cottage, Angarrick, Mylor, Falmouth TR11 5NX — MB BS Lond. 1985; DRCOG 1988; DCH RCP Lond. 1990. Specialty: Community Child Health.

SAGE, Frederic Jean Anaesthetic Department, East Surrey Hospital, Canada Avenue, Redhill RH1 5RH — MD Paris 1988; FRCA Lond 1994. Cons. Anesthetist - E. Surrey Hosp. - Redhill RH1 5RH. Specialty: Anaesth.

SAGE, Hilary The Barn Surgery, Newbury, Gillingham SP8 4XS Tel: 01747 824201 Fax: 01747 825098; Innox Hill Cottage, 35 Innox Hill, Frome BA11 2LN Tel: 01373 467993 — MB BS Lond. 1985 (Roy. Free Hosp. Sch. Med.) DRCOG 1987; MRCGP 1995. Specialty: Gen. Pract. Prev: Trainee GP Welwyn Garden City.

SAGE, Martin Royal Gwent Hospital, Cardiff Road, Newport NP20 2UB Tel: 01633 234234 — MB BCh Wales 1964 (Cardiff) DObst RCOG 1966; FFA RCS Eng. 1969. Cons. Anaesth. Roy. Gwent Hosp. Newport. Specialty: Anaesth.

SAGE, Naomi Janet (retired) Heath House, Offley Brook, Eccleshall, Stafford ST21 6HA Tel: 01785 280318 — (St. Mary's) MB BS Lond. 1958; MRCS Eng. LRCP Lond. 1958; DObst RCOG 1960. Prev: Assoc. Specialist (O & G) Dist. Gen. Hosp. Stafford.

SAGE, Roger Edmund Maitland Parkbury House Surgery, St Peters Street, St Albans AL1 3HD; Old Post Office, Whipsnade, Dunstable LU6 2LL — MB BS Lond. 1978; BA Oxf. 1972; MRCS Eng. LRCP Lond. 1978; Cert. Family Plann. JCC 1980; DRCOG 1980; MRCGP 1990. Chair Exec. Comm., St. Albans & Harrendon PCT.

SAGE, Roger James Basildon Hospital, Nether Mayne, Basildon SS16 5NL Tel: 01268 533911 Fax: 01268 593020 — MB BS Lond. 1976; MRCP (UK) 1980; FRCPath 1996, M 1985. Cons. Med. Microbiol. Basildon Hosp. Specialty: Med. Microbiol.

SAGER, Jeremy Marshall Shadwell Medical Centre, 137 Shadwell Lane, Leeds LS17 8AE Tel: 0113 293 9999 Fax: 0113 293 0900; 9 Sandhill Grove, Leeds LS17 8ED Tel: 0113 269 2359 — MB ChB Leeds 1980; DRCOG 1984; MRCGP 1987.

SAGGAR, Anand Kumar St. Georges Hospital Medical School, Cranmer Terrace, London SW17 0RE Tel: 020 8672 1255 Fax: 020 8725 3444 — MB BS Lond. 1982 (St. Bart. Med. Coll. Hosp. Lond.) MRCP (UK) 1986. Cons. in Clin. Genetics & Gen. Phys. St. Geo. Hosp. Lond.; Hon. Sen. Lect. in Med., St. Geo.'s Hosp. Med. Sch. Specialty: Genetics; Gen. Med. Socs: Brit. Hypertens. Soc.; Internat. Soc. Nephrol.; Clin. Genetics Soc. (Gen. Sec.). Prev: Williams Fell. Univ. Lond. St. Geo. Med. Sch.; Research Fell. Karolinska Inst. Stockholm, Sweden; Regist. Liver Unit King's Coll. Hosp. Lond.

SAGGAR, Dharam Pal (retired) 115 Thurleigh Road, London SW12 8TY Tel: 020 8673 4746 — MB BS Calcutta 1952 (Lake Med. Coll. Calcutta) DCH Eng. 1962. Prev: GP Lond.

SAGGAR, Karam Dev 'Aashiana', 27 Albany Terrace, Dundee DD3 6HS — MB BS Punjab (India) 1954; MRCGP 1968.

SAGGAR, Surinder Nath, Lt.-Col. RAMC Stagecoach House, Gatherley Road, Brompton on Swale, Richmond DL10 7JT Tel: 01748 811095 — (Amritsar Med. Coll.) MB BS Panjab 1962; DA Eng. 1978; FFA RCS Eng. 1981. Cons. Anaesth. Roy. Hosp. Haslar, Gosport. Specialty: Anaesth. Socs: Assn. Anaesth.

SAGGU, Rajinder Singh 12 Fairholme Road, Ilford IG1 3QR — MB BS Newc. 1988; MRCGP 1995. Specialty: Gen. Pract.

SAGLANI, Sejal 4 Beaconsville Court, Beaconsville Road, London N11 3AF Tel: 020 8361 7807 Email: ssaglani@doctors.org.uk — MB ChB Leic. 1994 (Univ. Leic.) BSc Leic. 1992; MRCP 1997. Specialist Regist. (Paediat.) Qu. Eliz. II Hosp, Wellyn Garden City. Specialty: Paediat. Prev: SHO (Paediat.) Guy's Hosp. Lond.; SHO (Paediat.) St. Mary's Hosp. Lond.; SHO (Paediat.) Roy. Brompton Hosp.

SAGOE, Mr Kofi Bondzie Department of Accident & Emergency, Milton Keynes General Hospital NHS Trust, Eaglestone, Milton Keynes MK6 5LD Tel: 01908 660033; 54 Normandy Way, Bletchley, Milton Keynes MK3 7UW Tel: 01908 643830 — MB ChB Univ. Ghana 1976; FRCS Glas. 1994. Staff Grade Surg. (Accid & Emerg.) Milton Keynes Gen. Hosp. Specialty: Accid. & Emerg.

SAGOO, Mandeep S — MB BChir Camb. 1997; BSc Lond. 1992; PhD Camb. 1997. Specialist Regist. (Ophth.) N. Thames Rotat. Specialty: Ophth.

SAGOO, Raghbir Singh Newmains Health Centre, 17 Manse Road, Newmains, Wishaw ML2 9AX Tel: 01325 488075 — MB ChB Leeds 1969. GP Stockton-on-Tees; Hosp. Practitioner (Rheum.) Univ. Hosp. of N. Tees, Stockton on Tees. Socs: Brit. Soc. Rheumat.; Arthritis Care (Pres. N. Cleveland Div.).

SAGOO, Victor Singh 348 Chester Road N., Sutton Coldfield B73 6RP — MB BCh Wales 1992.

SAGOR, Mr Geoffrey Roland St Albans City Hospital, Department of Surgery, Waverley Road, St Albans AL3 5PN Tel: 01727 866122 Ext: 4519 Fax: 01727 897519; 53 Belsize Lane, London NW3 5AU Tel: 020 7431 6448 Fax: 020 7431 6420 — MB ChB Cape Town 1967; FRCS Eng. 1972; ChM Cape Town 1985. Cons. Surg. St Albans City Hosp. & Hemel Hempstead Gen. Hosp. Specialty: Gen. Surg. Special Interest: Colorectal Surg.; Laparoscopic Surg.; Upper GI Surg. Socs: Roy. Soc. Med.; Assn. Surg.; Brit. Soc. Gastroenterol. Prev: Sen. Regist. & Regist. (Surg.) Roy. Free Hosp. Lond.; Research Fell. Roy. Postgrad. Med. Sch. Hammersmith Hosp. Lond.

SAGOVSKY, Ruth Lucille van Geest Centre, Peterborough District Hospital, Peterborough PE3 6DA Tel: 01733 318142 — MB ChB Birm. 1974; MRCPsych 1979. Cons. Psychiat. P'boro. Health Dist. Specialty: Gen. Psychiat. Prev: Research Univ. Camb. Child Care & Developm. Gp.; Sen. Regist. Roy. Edin. Hosp.; Sen. Regist. Fulbourn Hosp. Camb.

SAH, Anita 9 Greyfriar Walk, Bradford BD7 4BD — MB ChB Sheff. 1996; MB ChB Hons Sheff. 1996. SHO (Med.) Kingston Hosp.; SHO Atkinson Morley Hosp.; SHO (Renal Med.) St Geo. Hosp. Lond. Prev: PRHO Roy. Hallamshire Hosp. Sheff.

SAHA, Ajoy Kumar 25 Menlove Avenue, Liverpool L18 2EH — MB BS Calcutta 1957 (R.G. Kar Med. Coll. Calcutta) DObst RCOG 1963; DPH Liverp. 1968. Med. Off. (Matern. & Child Welf.) Liverp. AHA (T). Prev: SHO O & G Roy. Infirm. Stirling.; Regist. (O & G) Wakefield, & Pontefract, Castleford & Goole Hosp. Gps.; Regist. (O & G) Sefton Gen. Hosp. Liverp.

SAHA, Anirban Romi 40 Highcliffe Gardens, Ilford IG4 5HR Tel: 020 8924 8265 — BM BCh Oxf. 1994 (Oxford University and John Radcliffe Hospital) MA Cantab 1991; MRCP (UK) 1997. Wellcome Clin. Research Train. Fell. Inst. of Psychiat. Lond.; Hon. Research Regist. (Neurol.) Kings Coll. Univ. Hosp. Lond. Specialty: Neurol.; Gen. Med.; Care of the Elderly. Prev: SHO Rotat. (Gen. Med.) Kings's Coll. Hosp. Lond.

SAHA, Mr Arabinda Department of Obstetrics & Gynaecology, Northern Lincolnshire and Goole Hospital NHS Trust, Scartho Road, Grimsby DN33 2BA Tel: 01472 874111 Fax: 01472 875452 Email: arabinda.saha@nlg.nhs.uk — MB BS Calcutta 1981; MRCOG 1989; FRCOG 2001. Cons. O & G NE Lincs. NHS Trust. Specialty: Obst. & Gyn. Special Interest: Minimal Access Surg.; Surg. for genital prolapse. Socs: Asst. Sec., BMA Grimsby Div.; Mem., Internat. Soc. of Gyn. endoscopist; Mem., Brit. Soc. of colposcopy and cervical Path. Prev: Lect. (O & G) St. Mary's Hosp. Manch.; Regist. (O & G) Basildon Hosp.; Research Fell. RCOG Med. Audit Unit.

SAHA, Bijan Kumar Lakeside Medical Centre, Todd Crescent, Church Milton, Sittingbourne ME10 2TZ Tel: 01795 424315; 1 The Crescent, Dollis Hill, London NW2 6HA Tel: 020 8208 1823 — (Sir S.M. Med. Coll. Univ. Dacca) MB BS Dacca 1968; DMRT (Eng.) 1974; LMSSA Lond. 1981; T(GP) 1989; DFFP 1995. Clin. Asst. (A & E) Medway Hosp. Gillingham; Med. Dir. Elvy Ct. Nursing Home Kent. Specialty: Oncol.; Radiother.; Nuclear Med.; Oral & Maxillofacial Surg. Socs: Fell. Roy. Soc. Med. Prev: Regist. (Radiother. & Oncol.) Roy. Free Hosp. Lond. & Roy. Marsden Hosp. Lond.; Sen. Clin. Research Fell. (Nuclear Med.) Roy. Free Hosp. Lond.

SAHA, Birendra Nath 7 Bramshott Court, South Bank, Surbiton KT6 6DD — MB BS Calcutta 1967.

SAHA, Dilip 2 Lauriston Close, Darlington DL3 8TU Tel: 01325 461057 Fax: 01325 743875 Email: dilip.saha@virgin.net — MB BS Calcutta India 1966; DA; FFARCSI. Cons. Anaesth. Darlington Memor. Hosp. Specialty: Anaesth. Socs: Intens. Care Soc.; Assn. Anaesth. GB & Irel.; Obst. Assn. Prev: Cons. Anaesth. Dubai Hosp.

SAHA, Mr Jibesh Ranjan 18 Shore Court, Shore Lane, Sheffield S10 3BW — MB BS Banaras Hindu, India 1981; FRCSI 1994.

SAHA, Minakshi Kennard Street Health Centre, 1 Kennard Street, North Woolwich, London E16 2HR Tel: 020 7473 1971 Fax: 020 7473 2042 — (Calcutta National Medical College) MB BS Calcutta 1971. GP. Specialty: Gen. Med.; Respirat. Med. Socs: BMA; Small Pract.s Assn.; Indian Med. Assn.

SAHA, Monika 46 Ruskin Park House, Champion Hill, London SE5 8TQ — MB BS Lond. 1998; MB BS Lond 1998.

SAHA, Nani Gopal 8 Forest Way, Fulwood, Preston PR2 8PR — MB BS Calcutta 1962.

SAHA, Mr Nirmal Kanti Royal Oldham Hospital, Rochdale Road, Oldham OL1 2JH — MB BS Calcutta 1967 (Calcutta Med. Coll.) DLO Eng. 1972; FRCS Ed. 1976; FRCS Eng. 1980. Cons. ENT Surg. Oldham & Dist. Gen. Hosp. Specialty: Otolaryngol. Prev: Sen. Regist. (ENT) Hallamshire Hosp. Sheff.; SHO Roy. Nat. Throat, Nose & Ear Hosp. Lond.; Sen. Regist. (ENT) Leicester Roy. Infirm.

SAHA, Pijush Kumar Tilbury Surgery, 4 Commonwealth House, Montreal Road, Tilbury RM18 7QX Tel: 01375 855755 Fax: 01375 857673; 25 Whitmore Close, Orsett, Grays RM16 3JE Tel: 01375 892724 — MB BS Dacca 1969 (Dhaka Medical College, Bangladesh) DTM & H Liverp. 1984. Specialty: Gen. Pract.; Diabetes; Gen. Med. Prev: Regist. Rotat. (Gen. Med.) Coronary Care Unit Colchester; SHO Rotat. (Gen. Med. & Chest Dis.) Coronary Care Unit Sunderland.

SAHA, Ranjan 12 Erica Grove, Marton Manor Park, Middlesbrough TS7 8RY — MB BS Lond. 1995.

SAHA, Sharmistha 2 Lauriston Close, Darlington DL3 8TU — MB ChB Manch. 1997.

SAHA, Mr Simal Chandra The Whitfield Practice, Hunslet Health Centre, 24 Church Street, Leeds LS10 2PE Tel: 0113 270 5194 Fax: 0113 270 2795 — MB BS Patna 1977; MS Patna 1981; FRCS Glas. 1991.

SAHA, Sisir Kanti (retired) 5 Pinfold Lane, Norton Canes, Cannock WS11 9PH Email: sisir@tiscali.co.uk — (Nilratan Sircar Med. Coll. Calcutta) MB BS Calcutta 1958. Prev: GP Cannock.

SAHA, Mr Sisir Kumar 41 Long Close, Bessacarr, Doncaster DN4 7PN Tel: 01302 537719 — MB BS Calcutta 1965 (R.G. Kar Med. Coll. Calcutta) FRCS Ed. 1975. Cons. Gen. Surg. Doncaster. Specialty: Gen. Surg.; Urol. Socs: BMA.; FRSM. (Lond.). Prev: Regist. (Surg.) Bronglais Gen. Hosp. Aberystwyth, Burnley Gp. Hosps. & Rotherham HA; Regist. (Urol.) Ballochmyle Hosp. Mauchline; SHO (Surg.) Hull Roy. Infirm.

SAHA, Mr Tapash Kumar 28 Charwood Drive, Pontprennau, Cardiff CF23 8NN — MB BS Dacca 1984 (Dhaka Medical College) MRCOG Lond. 1995. Cons. Obst. & Gynaecologist. Prev: Specialist Regist. (O & G).

SAHA, Mr Tushar Kanti c/o Mr K. Roy, 421 Ilford Lane, Ilford IG1 2PF — MB BS Calcutta 1965; MS Calcutta 1967.

SAHA, Professor Vaskar Department of Paediatric Haematology & Oncology, Royal London Hospital, London E1 1BB Tel: 020 7377 Ext: 7796 Fax: 020 7377 7796 Email: vaskar.saha@cancer.org.uk — MB BS India 1992 (Christian Med. Coll., Velcore, India) DCH 1985; MD 1989; FRCPCH 1997; PhD 1997. Prof. of Paediatric Oncology; Head Cancer Research UK Children's Cancer Group. Specialty: Paediat.

SAHADEVAN, Subramaniam Broadstairs Health Centre, The Broadway, Broadstairs CT10 2AJ Tel: 01943 861565 — MB BS Ceylon 1971; DFFP. GP.

SAHAI, Indu B Aberaman Surgery, Glamorgan Street, Aberdare CF44 6SR Tel: 01685 872006 Fax: 01685 875380.

SAHAI, Shesh Nandan Claypath Medical Practice, Glamorgan Street, Aberdare Tel: 01685 872006 Fax: 01685 875380 — MB BS Patna 1961; DTM & H Liverp. 1968; Dip Ven Liverp. 1971; DLO Eng. 1973. Gen. Practitioner. Prev: SHO (ENT) Frenchay Hosp. Bristol & Roy. Infirm. Sunderland; SHO (Cas.) Ingham Infirm. S. Shields.

SAHAL, Anoop Kumar 46 Sandringham Drive, Stockport SK4 2DE — MB ChB Manch. 1985.

SAHAR, Mohammad Ashraf c/o Dr S. M. Sulaiman, 49 Castle Road, Colne BB8 7AR — MB BS Pubjab 1957; MB BS Punjab 1957; MRCGP 1975.

SAHARAY, Mr Mrinal Old Chruch Hospital, Waterloo Road, Romford RM7 0BE Tel: 01708 708276 Fax: 01992 571383 Email: mrinal@ntlworld.com; 19 Regent Road, Epping CM16 5DL Tel: 01992 571383 Fax: 01992 571383 — MB BS Calcutta 1985 (Medical College Calcutta) FRCS RCS Ireland 1990; FRCS RCS England 1992; PhD London 1998. Cons. Surg. (Gastrointestinal & Endocrine) Oldch. Hosp. Romford. Specialty: Endocrinol.; Gen. Pract.; Medico Legal. Socs: Roy. Soc. Med.; Brit. Med. Assn.; Assn. of Coloproctology of Gt. Britain and Irel.

SAHARIA, Mrs Era Childrens Centre, City Hospitals Trust, Durham Road, Sunderland SR3 9AF Tel: 0191 565 6256 — MB BS Dibrugarh 1969 (Assam Med. Coll.) DCH Dibrugarh 1970; MRCP (U.K.) 1974. Cons. (Community Child. Health) City Hosps. Sunderland; Hon. Lect. Univ. Newc. Specialty: Community Child Health.

SAHATHEVARAJAN, Navaretnam (retired) The White Rose Surgery, Exchange St., South Elmsall, Pontefract WF9 2RD Tel: 01977 642190 — MB BS Ceylon 1955.

SAHAY, Prakash Kumar Mirfield Surgery, Scholars Gate, Lea Village, Birmingham B33 0DL Tel: 0121 789 7607 Fax: 0121 686 4542 — MB BS Ranchi 1975; MB BS Ranchi 1975.

SAHAY, Sandhya The Surgery, Wellington Road, Yate, Bristol BS37 5UY Tel: 01454 323366 Fax: 01454 323366 — LRCP LRCS Ed. LRCPS Glas. 1983.

SAHDEV, Anju 168 The Drive, Ilford IG1 3PP — MB BS Lond. 1991 (Char. Cross & Westm. Lond.) MRCP (UK) 1995; FRCR (Part 1) 1996. Cons. Radiologist Homerton & St. Bartholomews Hosps. Lond. Specialty: Radiol. Prev: Specialist Regist. (Radiol.) UCH Hosps. Lond.; Ho. Off. (Surg.) Char. Cross Hosp. Lond.; SHO (Gen. Med.) N. Middlx. Hosp. Lond.

SAHDEV, Ashok Kumar The Medici Practice, 37 Castle Street, Luton LU1 3AG Tel: 01582 726123 Email: aksahdev@hotmail.com; 185 Old Bedford Road, Luton LU2 7EH Tel: 01582 655353 — MB BS Lond. 1979; DRCOG 1981; MRCGP 1986. GP Tutor Luton; Trainer Luton & Dunstable Hosp. VTS. Specialty: Occupat. Health.

SAHEECHA, Behnam Saeed Harold Hill Health Centre, Gooshays Drive, Romford RM3 9SU Tel: 01708 343991 Fax: 01708 346795 — MB ChB Mosu 1968; MB ChB Mosu 1968.

SAHEED, Ahamed Hibishy 59 Carrington Road, Dartford DA1 1XN Tel: 01322 228370 — MB BS Ceylon 1951; DCH Ceylon 1958.

SAHGAL, Surender Mohan (retired) Friarwood Surgery, Carleton Glen, Pontefract WF8 1SU Tel: 01977 703235 Fax: 01977 600527; 5A Lowther Avenue, Garforth, Leeds LS25 1EP — MB BS Osmania 1971. Prev: GP Pontefract, W. Yorks.

SAHI, Mukesh Kumar 111 Hillcrest Road, Orpington BR6 9AG — MB BS India 1979; MD A. P. Singh, India 1979, MB BS (Hons.) 1976; MRCP (UK) 1982.

SAHIN, Ayse Newham General Hospital, Glen Road, Plaistow, London E13 8SL Tel: 020 8919 5555 Fax: 020 7476 4000; 25 Strood House, Staple St, London SE1 4LR Tel: 020 7407 5559 — LMSSA Lond. 1995; LRCS Eng. LRCP Lond. 1995. SHO (O & G) Newham Gen. Hosp. Prev: SHO (O & G) Gravesend Hosp.; Ho. Off. (Gen. & Respirat. Med.) Homerton Hosp. Lond.

SAHNI, Ajit Singh The Surgery, 3 Formby Avenue, Atherton, Manchester M46 0EX Tel: 01942 883044 Fax: 01942 888777; 5 High Bank, Atherton, Manchester M46 9HZ Tel: 01942 877416 — MB BS Panjab 1971 (Christian Med. Coll. Ludhiana) MB BS Panjab (India) 1971. Mem. Wigan LMC.

SAHNI, Dev Raj 15 High Street, Cheshunt, Waltham Cross EN8 0BX.

SAHNI, Mr Kamal Eye Department, Broglais General Hospital, Aberystwyth SY23 1ER Email: ksahni@mailcity.com — MB BS Delhi 1983; FRCS Ed. 1992. NHS Cons. Eye Surg. Specialty: Ophth.

SAHNI, Parmindar Pontllanfraith Health Centre, Blackwood Road, Pontllanfraith, Blackwood NP12 2YU — MB BS Panjab 1969.

SAHNI, Vikram Anik Singh 5 High Bank, Atherton, Manchester M46 9HZ — MB BS Lond. 1998; MB BS Lond 1998.

SAHOTA, Balbir Singh 16 Old Lindens Close, Streetly, Sutton Coldfield B74 2EJ — MB ChB Leeds 1992.

SAHOTA, Jesbir Kaur 7 Anthony Way, Coventry CV2 5LJ — MB ChB Leeds 1989.

SAHOTA, Kirpal Kaur 114 Elgin Avenue, London W9 2HD — MB ChB Sheff. 1989.

SAHOTA, Mandeep 220 City Way, Rochester ME1 2BN; 52 Steele Avenue, Greenhithe DA9 9PH — MB BS Lond. 1998; MB BS Lond 1998.

SAHOTA, Manpinder 52 Steele Avenue, Greenhithe DA9 9PH — MB BS Lond. 1994.

SAHOTA, Onkar Singh Family Health Practice, 20 Church Road, Hanwell, London W7 1DR Tel: 020 8579 7338 Fax: 020 8840 9928; 19 Thorncliffe Road, Norwood Green, Southall UB2 5RJ Tel: 020 8574 7337 — MB ChB Sheff. 1983; MRCS Eng. LRCP Lond. 1984; DRCOG 1988; MRCGP 1989. JP. Socs: Fell. Roy. Soc. Med.; BMA. Prev: Trainee GP St. Mary's Hosp. Med. Sch. Lond. VTS; Ho. Phys. Milton Keynes Gen. Hosp.; Ho. Surg. Roy. Hallamsh. Hosp. Sheff.

SAHOTA, Opinder Singh 4 Croxley Gardens, Nuthall, Nottingham NG16 1RR — MB ChB Dundee 1992; MRCP (UK) 1995; ILTM 1999; DM 2002. Cons. Phys., QMC, Univ. Hosp., Nottm. Specialty: Care of the Elderly. Prev: Lect. (Bone Metab.) & Hon. Specialist Regist. & (Gen.: & Geriat. Med.) Nottm. Univ.; Regist. Rotat. (Gen. Med. & Endocrinol.) Nottm.; SHO Nottm. City Hosp.

SAHOTA, Surinderpal Kaur — MB BS Lond. 1998.

SAHU, Debendra Nath 42 Worcester Crescent, Woodford Green IG8 0LU Tel: 020 8504 9580 — MB BS Lond. 1995 (Lond. Hosp. Med. Coll.) BSc (Path.) Lond. 1993; MRCO phth (Part 1) 1999. SHO (Ophth.) Sussex Eye Hosp. - Brighton. Specialty: Ophth. Prev: Ho. Off. (Med.) OldCh. Hosp. Romford; Hon. Demonst. (Anat.) Qu. Mary & Westfield Coll. Lond.; SHO (Neurosurg.) Kings Coll., Lond., SHO (Ophth.) Qu. Mary's Hosp., Sidcup.

SAHU, Jonathan 17 Denton Road, Wokingham RG40 2DX — MB ChB Manch. 1988; MRCP (UK) 1991. Fell. (Cardiovasc. Med.) Rush Presbyt.-St. Luke's Med. Center, Chicago, Illinois, USA. Specialty: Gen. Med.; Cardiol.

SAHU, Mr Rama Chandra 126A Burnley Road, Padiham, Burnley BB12 8SJ Tel: 01282 771525 — MB BS Utkal 1956; FRCS Ed. 1967. Assoc. Specialist (A & E Med.) Blackburn. Prev: Regist. (Gen. Surg.) St. John of God Hosp. Richmond; Regist. (Cas, Traum. & Orthop. Surg.) Batley & Plymouth & Tynemouth; SHO (Orthop.) Sedgefield Gen. Hosp. & SHO (Gen. Surg.) Gen. Hosp. W. Hartlepool.

SAHU, Surendra Prasad Pleck Health Centre, 16 Oxford Street, Pleck, Walsall WS2 9HY Tel: 01922 647660 Fax: 01922 629251 — MB BS Bihar 1966 (Darbhanga Med. Coll.) DTM & H Liverp. 1973.

SAHU, Upendra Nath Gants Hill Medical Centre, 63-65 Ethelbert Gardens, Ilford IG2 6UW Tel: 020 8504 9580 — MB BS Utkal 1965 (S.C.B. Med. Coll. Cuttack Orissa, India) DCH Dub. 1979. Specialty: Gen. Pract.

SAI SANKAR, Mr Nagamanickam c/o Mr. Sathyamoorthy, 85 Gladstone Avenue, Manor Park, London E12 6NR Tel: 020 8503 5236; 7 Frognal Staff Residences, Queen Mary's Hospital, Sidcup DA14 6LT Tel: 020 8302 2678 — MB BS Madras 1986; FRCS Glas. 1993. Staff Grade (A & E) Qu. Mary's Hosp. Sidcup. Specialty: Accid. & Emerg. Prev: SHO (Plastic Surg.) Odstock Hosp. Salisbury & Shotley Bridge Gen. Hosp.

SAICH, Andrew Jonathan 10 Hauxton Road, Little Shelford, Cambridge CB2 5HJ — MB BS Lond. 1993.

SAID, Abdul Crosswayws, 72 Upland Road, Sutton SM2 5JB Tel: 020 8661 9041; Health Centre, Robin Hood Lane, Sutton SM1 2RJ — MB BS Peshawar 1968 (Khyber Med. Coll. Peshawar)

SAID, Mr Ahmed Jamil 6 Alford Court, Bonchurch Close, Sutton SM2 6AY Tel: 020 8643 1017 Fax: 020 8643 1017 — MB ChB Baghdad 1972; FRCS Ed. 1983. Staff Paediat. Surg. Lewisham Hosp. Specialty: Paediat. Surg. Prev: Resid. Surg. Off. Westm. Childr. Hosp.

SAID, Joseph Raymond 5 South View, Evenwood, Bishop Auckland DL14 9QS Tel: 0388 832236 — MRCS Eng. LRCP Lond. 1979.

SAID, Wafa Al Din Khairi 8 Sandybed Lane, Scarborough YO12 5LH — MB ChB Alexandria 1970; MB ChB Alexandria, Egypt 1970.

SAID, Mr Walid Qasim 30 Hall Farm Close, Stocksfield NE43 7NL — MD Damascus 1967; FRCS Glas. 1978.

SAIDI, Samir Arif 26 Hinde Street, Manchester M40 5LW — MB ChB Manch. 1993; BSc St And. 1990.

SAIDIN, Dahlia 60 Stoddart House, Meadow Road, London SW8 1ND — MB BS Malaya 1986.

SAIF, Maha Rosa Water Lane Surgery, 48 Brixton Water Lane, London SW2 1QE Tel: 020 7274 1521 Fax: 020 7738 3258; 89 Balham Park Road, London SW12 8EB — MB BCh BAO NUI 1981; LRCPI & LM, LRCSI & LM 1981; MRCGP 1985. Store Doctor to Harvey Nichols Lond. Specialty: Community Child Health. Prev: SHO (Gyn.) Eliz. Garrett Anderson Hosp. Lond.; SHO (Obst.) Coventry Matern. Hosp.; SHO (Psychiat.) & Cas. Off. Ealing Hosp. Lond.

SAIFUDDIN, Asif 165 Uxbridge Road, Harrow Weald, Harrow HA3 6DG — MB ChB Manch. 1984; BSc (Hons.) Path. Manch. 1982; MRCP (UK) 1987; FRCR 1991; T(R) (CR) 1992. Cons. Diagn. Radiol. Roy. Nat. Orthop. Hosp. Stanmore. Specialty: Radiol. Prev: Regist. (Diag. Radiol.) Leeds West. HA.

SAIGAL, Rajkumar Hukumchand Elmfield Health Group, 18 Elmfield Road, Gosforth, Newcastle upon Tyne NE3 4BP Tel: 0191 285 1663 Fax: 0191 284 7015; 68 Beatty Avenue, High West Jesmond, Newcastle upon Tyne NE2 3QS Tel: 0191 285 7543 — MB BS Saurashtra 1975; FRCS (E) 1984 Ed. GP Newc.

SAIGAL, Sudhir Hollies Health Centre, Swan Street, Merthyr Tydfil CF47 8ET Tel: 01685 723363 Fax: 01685 350106 — MB BS Delhi 1974. GP Merthyr Tydfil.

SAIGOL, Maryam (retired) 6 Metchley Park Road, Edgbaston, Birmingham B15 2PG Tel: 0121 454 6999; 6 Metchley Park Road, Edgbaston, Birmingham B15 2PG Tel: 0121 454 6999 Fax: 0121 454 6999 — MB BS Punjab 1966 (Fatima Jinnah Lahore, Pakistan)

SAIGOL, Muhammad Younus The Surgery, 75-77 Cotterills Lane, Alum Rock, Birmingham B8 3RZ Tel: 0121 327 5111 Fax: 0121 327 5111; 6 Metchley Park Road, Edgbaston, Birmingham B15 2PG Tel: 0121 454 6999 — MB BS Punjab 1969 (King Edwd. Med. Coll. Lahore) BSc Punjab (Pakistan) 1965; DPM Eng. 1973. Affil. RCPsych. Specialty: Gen. Pract.

SAIGOL, Sara Maryam 4 Fairfax Mews, London E16 1TY — MB ChB Birm. 1996.

SAIKIA, Mr Adhita Nanda Consultant Orthopaedic Surgeon, Burnley General Hospital, Casterton Avenue, Burnley BB10 2PQ Tel: 01282 474431 Email: saikiaan@hotmail.com; 6 Woodlands Walk, Skipton BD23 1TZ — MB BS Gauhati 1978; LMSSA 1984; FRCS Ed. 1985; MCh (Ortho) Liverp. 1990; FRCS (Tr & Oth) Ed. 2000. Cons. (Orthop.) Burnley Gen. Hosp. Specialty: Trauma & Orthop. Surg. Special Interest: Lower Limb. Socs: MPS; Brit. Med. Assn.; Brit. Orthopaedic Assn. Prev: Regist. (Orthop.) Blackburn Roy. Infirm. & Airedale Gen. Hosp.; Regist. Hip Unit & Upperlimb Serv. Wrightington Hosp.; Specialist Regist. St James Univ. Hosp. Leeds.

SAIKIA, Bibhra Allendale, Six Acre Lane, Longton, Preston PR4 4SE Tel: 01772 614158 — MB BS Gauhati 1966 (Assam Med. Coll., India) DObst RCOG 1971. Med. Off. Preston Acute Trust. Specialty: Family Plann. & Reproduc. Health. Socs: Fac. Family Plann. Prev: GP Drumchapel, Glas.; Regist. & SHO (O & G) Redlands Hosp. Wom. Glas.

SAIKIA, Nripendra Kumar (retired) Preston Med.Ltd, 11 Moor Park Avenue, Preston PR1 6AS Tel: 01772 710232; Allendale, Six Acre Lane, Longton, Preston PR4 4SE Tel: 01772 614158 — MB BS Gauhati 1960; Dip. Ven. Liverp. 1966; PhD Glas. 1973. Prev: Cons. Dermat. Roy. Preston Hosp.

SAIKIA, Shyamodabhiram The Surgery, 1 Warstone Tower, Bromford Drive, Bromford, Birmingham B36 8TU Tel: 0121 747 9161; 8 Byford Way, The Oaks, Coleshill Road, Birmingham B37 7GH — MB BS Gauhati 1972.

SAIKIA-VARMAN, Nita Church Lane Medical Centre, 111 Church Lane, Stechford, Birmingham B33 9EJ Tel: 0121 783 2567 — MB BS Gujarat 1972; MB BS Gujarat 1972.

SAINI, Asha Rani Royal Marsden Hosptial, Fulham Road, London SW10 — MB BS Lond. 1985; MRCP (UK 1988; PhD Lond. 1995. Sen. Regist. (Med. Oncol.) Roy. Marsden Hosp. Lond. Specialty: Oncol. Prev: Research Fell. (Med. Oncol.) Imperial Cancer Research Fund.; Regist. (Med.) St. Mary's Hosp. Lond.; Hon. Sen. Regist. (Oncol.) Hammersmith Hosp.

SAINI, Avtar Singh Oakeswell Health Centre, Brunswick Park Road, Wednesbury WS10 9HP Tel: 0121 556 2114 Fax: 0121 505 1843; 59 Vernon Road, Edgbaston, Birmingham B16 9SQ Tel: 0121

454 1566 — MB ChB Glas. 1990; MRCGP 1995. Specialty: Gen. Pract. Socs: RCGP; Brit. Med. Accupun. Soc.

SAINI, Gurdev Singh Lynwood Medical Centre, Lynwood Drive, 2A-6 Collier Row, Romford RM5 3QL Tel: 01708 743244 Fax: 01708 736783; Aquatic Lodge, Robinson Road, Horndon-on-the-Hill, Stanford-le-Hope SS17 8PU Tel: 01375 360718 Fax: 01375 645366 — MB BS Punjab 1970 (Med. Coll. Amritsar) MB BS Punjab (India) 1970; MS Guru Nanak 1973; FICS 1982. GP; Chairm. GLK Healthcre LMD, Romford; Chairm. Nat. ME Centre, Romford. Specialty: Gen. Surg. Prev: Research Asst. (Surg.) V.J. Hosp. Amritsar, India; SHO (A & E) Lister Hosp. Stevenage; SHO Rotat. (Surg.) Roy. Salop Infirm. Shrewsbury.

SAINI, Mahesh 33 Roseville Avenue, Hounslow TW3 3TE — MB BS Lond. 1994. SHO (Paediat.) Roy. Lond. Hosp.

SAINI, Mandeep Singh 43 Woodend, Handsworth Wood, Birmingham B20 1EW — MB ChB Liverp. 1998; MB ChB Liverp 1998.

SAINI, Mohan Singh Soho Health Centre, Louise Road, Handsworth, Birmingham B21 0RY Tel: 0121 523 2343 Fax: 0121 507 1607; 16 The Russells, Moseley, Birmingham B13 8RT Tel: 0121 449 9307 — MB BS Poona 1971 (Armed Forces Med. Coll.) Univ. of Poona. GP Princip.; Clin. Med. Off. (Ophth.) Sandwell & Dudley HAs. Specialty: Gen. Pract. Prev: Trainee GP Sturry Canterbury VTS; SHO (Ophth.) Leeds Gen. Infirm.

SAINI, Sarvesh Ram 45 Ellington Road, Hounslow TW3 4HX — MB BS Lond. 1992.

SAINS, Parvinderpal Singh 241 Beaconsfield Road, Southall UB1 1DD Tel: 020 8574 7176 — MB ChB Birm. 1995; MRCS; ChB Birm. 1995. Specialty: Gen. Surg.

SAINSBURY, Alan David Port Isaac Practice, Hillson Close, Port Isaac PL29 3TR Tel: 01208 880222 Fax: 01208 880633; Springside Barn, Trewetha, Port Isaac PL29 3RU Tel: 01208 880231 — MB BS Lond. 1979; DRCOG 1982.

SAINSBURY, Clive Peter Quine Torbay Hospital, Lawes Bridge, Torquay TQ2 7AA Tel: 01803 614567 Fax: 01803 616334; 80 Walnut Road, Torquay TQ2 6HU Tel: 01803 605500 Fax: 01803 617174 — MB ChB Ed. 1972; MRCP (UK) 1977; FRCP Lond. 1996; FRCPH 1997. Cons. Paediat. Torbay Hosp. Specialty: Paediat. Socs: Roy. Coll. Paediat. & Child Health. Prev: Sen. Regist. (Paediat.) Dept. Child Health Univ. Hosp. Wales Cardiff; Research Fell. (Child Life & Health) Roy. Hosp. Sick Childr. Edin.; Sen. Resid. Hosp. Sick Childr., Toronto.

SAINSBURY, James 107 Ripple Road, Barking IG11 7NY Tel: 020 8594 1311 Fax: 020 8591 4686; 27 Meadow Way, Chigwell IG7 6LR — MB BCh BAO Dub. 1959; LAH Dub. 1958; DObst RCOG 1963.

SAINSBURY, Jane Anne Hednesford Street Surgery, 60 Hednesford Street, Cannock WS11 1DJ Tel: 01543 503121 Fax: 01543 468024; The Red House, 8 The Green, Milford, Stafford ST17 0UR Tel: 01785 661010 — MB ChB Birm. 1973.

SAINSBURY, Mr John Richard Cochrane Royal Free & University College London Medical School, Dept. Surgery, 2nd Floor, Charles Bell House,, Riding House Street, London W1W 7EJ Tel: 020 7679 9310 Fax: 020 7636 5176 — MB BS Newc. 1977; FRCS Eng. 1981; MD Newc. 1986. Sen. Lect. And Cons. Surg., Univ. Coll. Lond. Specialty: Gen. Surg. Prev: Cons. Surg. Huddersfield Roy. Infirm.

SAINSBURY, Matthew Charles Oxford Regional Health Authority, Old Road, Headington, Oxford OX3; 8 The Rookery, Kidlington OX5 1AW — MB BS Lond. 1983; Dip. IMC RCS Ed. 1990; FCAnaesth 1991. Sen. Regist. (Anaesth.) Oxf. RHA. Specialty: Anaesth. Prev: Research Regist. (Anaesth.) John Radcliffe Hosp. Oxf.; SHO (Anaesth.) Southmead Hosp. Bristol; SHO (Anaesth.) Roy. Devon & Exeter Hosp.

SAINSBURY, Olga Mary (retired) 50 Rookwood Park, Guildford Road, Horsham RH12 1UB Tel: 01403 255454 — MRCS Eng. LRCP Lond. 1942 (Lond. Sch. Med. Wom.) Prev: Sen. Resid. Med. Off. Roy. Free Hosp.

SAINSBURY, Paul Antony 34 Beechwood View, Leeds LS4 2LP — MB ChB Leeds 1994.

SAINSBURY, Wendy Alison Rickmansworth Road Surgery, 35 Rickmansworth Road, Watford WD18 7HD Tel: 01923 223232 Fax: 01923 243397 — MB BS Lond. 1981.

SAINT, Thomas Morris Campbell (retired) 1 Reid Park Close, Newcastle upon Tyne NE2 2EZ Tel: 0191 281 3308 — MB BS Durh. 1951.

SAINT-YVES, Ian Fleming Marie (retired) Dunvegan, School Brae, Whiting Bay, Brodick KA27 8PZ — MB ChB Glas. 1960; DTM & H Liverp. 1961; DObst RCOG 1962; MD Glas 1976; T(PHM) 1991. Prev: Head Scott. Clin. Coding Centre Edin.

SAINTEY, Patricia Anne, Maj. RAMC Northay Farmhouse, Northay, Chard TA20 3DN — MB BS Lond. 1984 (Westm.) Cert. Prescribed Equiv. Exp. 1990; MRCGP 1990. Med. Off. Alanbrooke Barracks, Germany. Socs: BMA. Prev: Cas. Off. Milit. Wing Musgrave Pk. Hosp. Belf.; SHO (Rehabil. & Rheum.) Headley Ct. Defence Servs. Med. Rehabil.; Unit Chessington; Families Med. Off. Roy. Milit. Acad. Sandhurst.

SAIR, Mark Derriford Hospital, Intensive Care Unit, Plymouth PL6 8DH Tel: 01752 763789 Email: mark.sair@phnt.swest.nhs.uk — MB ChB Bristol 1988; DA (UK) 1991; MRCP (UK) 1993; FRCA 1994; PhD Lond. 1998. Cons. In Intens. Care and Anaesth., Derriford Hosp. Plymouth. Specialty: Anaesth.; Intens. Care. Socs: Eur.Soc. Intens. Care Med.; Soc. Critical Care Med. USA. Prev: Specialist Regist., Hammersmith Hosp. Imperial Coll.; PICU Fell., St. Marys Hosp. Paddington; Clin. Research Fell. (Critical Care) Nat. Heart & Lung Inst. Lond. & Physiol. Flow Studies Gp. Imperial Coll. Sci., Technol. & Med.

SAIT, Christopher Lewis Sketty Surgery, De la Beche Road, Sketty, Swansea SA2 9EA Tel: 01792 206862; De-La-Beche House, 42 De-La-Beche Road, Sketty, Swansea SA2 9AR Tel: 01792 420109 Fax: 01792 291129 — MB BCh Wales 1971. Socs: BMA.

SAIT, Mr Mohammed Suhaib Darenth Valley Hospital, Orthopaedic Department, Darenth Wood Road, Dartford DA2 8DA Tel: 01322 428461 Fax: 01322 428470 Email: saitsuhaib@hotmail.com; Fawkham Manor Hospital, Manor Lane, Longfield DA3 8ND — MB BS Madras 1986 (Madras Medical) MSc (Orth); FRCS (Orth); FRCS Ed.; LLM. Cons. Orthop. Surg. Specialty: Orthop.; Sports Med.; Osteop. Special Interest: Shoulder & Hand Surg.; Upper Limb Surg. Socs: Brit. Orthopaedic Assn.; Brit. Elbow & Shoulder Soc.; Brit. Hand Soc.

SAITCH, Christopher David Wadebridge and Camel Estuary Practice, Brooklyn, Wadebridge PL27 7BS Tel: 01208 812222 Fax: 01208 815907 — MB BChir Camb. 1982 (Cambridge and St Georges) MB Camb. 1983, BChir 1982; MA Camb. 1983. Specialty: Gen. Pract. Prev: Trainee GP/SHO Cornw. & I. of Scilly HA VTS; Ho. Phys. St. Jas. Hosp. Lond.; Ho. Surg. Ashford Hosp. Middlx.

SAIZ, Ana Maria Benedicto 35 Crofton Avenue, Bexley DA5 3AS; 2A Foots Cray Lane, Sidcup DA14 4NR — LMS Basque Provinces 1982.

SAJID, Mr Mahmud Vale of Leven Hospital, North Main St., Alexandria G83 0UA; 42 Woodbank, Gdns., Alexandria G83 0SW — MB BS Pakistan 1986 (Nishtar) FRCS Glas. 1993; FRCS Irel. 1996; FRCS Ed. 1996. Staff Surg. Specialty: Gen. Surg. Prev: SHO (Gastnaval) Gen. Hosp. Glas.

SAJID, Mohammed 3 Careless Green, Stourbridge DY9 8XE — MB ChB Dundee 1997.

SAJID, Mr Syed Abdul Maryfield Lodge, Bankend Road, Dumfries DG1 4AN — MB BS Karachi 1983; FRCS Ed. 1991.

SAJJANHAR, Tina 85 Boyne Road, Lewisham, London SE13 5AN — MB BS Lond. 1987 (Guys Hospital) DRCOG 1990; DCH RCP Lond. 1991; MRCP (UK) 1993. Cons. Paediat. Lewisham Hosp. Specialty: Paediat. Prev: Sen. Regist. (Paediat.) St. Thos. Hosp. Lond.; Clin. Research Fell. (Paediat. Intens. Care) Guy's Hosp. Lond.; Regist. Lewisham Hosp.

SAJNANI, Dushant Kumar Sandwell General Hospital, 200/B Hallam Site, West Bromwich B71 4HJ — LMS La Laguna 1983; MRCOphth 1992. SHO (Ophth.) HM Stanley Hosp. St. Asaph. Specialty: Ophth.

SAKEL, Rezina 3 Glyncoli Close, Treorchy, Cardiff CF42 6SU — MB BS Lond. 1995.

SAKELLARIOU, Mr Anthony Firmley Park Hospital, Department of Orhopaedics, Portsmouth Road, Camberley GU16 7UJ Tel: 01276 604573 Fax: 01279 604457 — MB BS Lond. 1987 (Univ. Coll.) BSc Lond. 1980; FRCS Eng. 1992; FRCS (Orth.) 1996. Cons. Orth. Surg. Frimley Pk. Hosp. Camberley. Specialty: Trauma & Orthop. Surg. Special Interest: Foot & Ankle Surg. Prev: Clin. Fell. (Foot & Ankle Surg.) Vancouver Gen. Hosp. Canada; Vis. Fell. (Foot & Ankle

Surg.) Mayo Clinic Scottsdale Arizona, USA; SHO (Plastic Surg.) Mt. Vernon Hosp. Northwood Middlx.

SAKHRANI, Lavina Wessex Road Surgery, Wessex Road, Parkstone, Poole BH14 8BQ Tel: 01202 734924 — BM Soton. 1991. GP Princip. Poole. Specialty: Gen. Pract. Socs: MRCGP.

SAKHUJA, Jagdish Chandar (retired) Flat 5, Chesterton Court, Eaton Rise, London W5 2HJ Tel: 020 8566 7507 — (Rangoon & King Edwd. Med. Coll. Lahore) MB BS Panjab (India) 1944; DPM Eng. 1978. Prev: Clin. Asst. (Psychiat.) Severalls Hosp. Colchester.

SAKHUJA, Shashi Bala City Hospital NHS Trust, Birmingham B18 7HQ Tel: 0121 554 3801 — MB BS Madras 1980; MD Chandigarh 1983; FFA RCSI 1988. Cons. Anaesth. City Hosp. Birm. Specialty: Anaesth. Prev: Cons. Anaesth. Bolton Hosps. NHS Trust; Sen. Regist. (Anaesth.) Withington Hosp. Manch.; Regist. (Anaesth.) South. Gen. Hosp. Glas.

SAKKA, Mr Samir Akram Asad Orthopaedic Department, University Hospital, Lewisham, London SE13 6LH Tel: 020 8333 3167 Fax: 020 8333 3159 — MB BS Lond. 1985 (St. Geo. Hosp. Med. Sch. Lond.) FRCS Ed. 1990; FRCS (Orth) 1997. Cons. (Orthop. & Spinal Surg.) Lond.; Hon. Sen. Lect. KGT 1998. Specialty: Orthop. Prev: Sen. Spinal Fell. Roy. Orthop. Hosp. Birm.; Fell. Scoliosis Unit Roy. Nat. Orthop. Hosp. Stanmore; Career Regist. (Orthop.) NW Thames Region.

SAKKADAS, Ambrose 96 Station Road, London NW4 3SR — Ptychio Iatrikes Thessalonika 1994.

SAKLATVALA, Jacqueline Haywood Hospital X-ray Department 2, High Lane, Burslem, Stoke-on-Trent ST6 7 Tel: 01782 556239 Fax: 01782 813419; Highwood, Tower Road, Ashley Heath, Market Drayton TF9 4PU — MB ChB Dundee 1975; DA Eng. 1978; DMRD Eng. 1981; FRCR 1982. Cons. Radiol. (s/i Musculoskeletal Imaging) N. Staffs. Hosp. Trust Stoke-on-Trent. Specialty: Radiol. Socs: Roy. Coll. of Radiologists; Brit. Soc. of Skeletal Radiologists; Skeletal Dysplania Gp.

SAKLATVALA, Jeremy 71 Lonsdale Road, London SW13 9DA — MB BS Lond. 1968; MRCS Eng. LRCP Lond. 1968; MRCP (UK) 1970.

SAKSENA, Joyti 4 Cherry Hills, Little Oxmey Lane, Watford WD19 6DH Tel: 020 8428 6477 Fax: 020 8428 6477 — MB ChB Dundee 1995 (Dundee Univ.) BMSc Dund 1992; MRCS Lond. 1999. SHO Rotat. (Surg.) Bedford Hosp. Specialty: Gen. Surg.; Orthop.; Urol. Socs: BMA. Prev: SHO (Orthop.) Hillingdon Hosp. Hillingdon; SHO (A&E) Brisbane, Aust.

SAKSENA, M K Heath Road Medical Centre, 78 Heath Road, Runcorn WA7 5TJ Tel: 01928 565881 Fax: 01928 566748 — MB BS Agra 1973; MRCGP 1986; MICGP 1987.

SAKSENA, Shiv Chandra 85 Nursery Road, Edgbaston, Birmingham B15 3JU Tel: 0121 454 0116 — MB BS Lucknow 1950.

SAKSENA, Vinod Kumar, TD (retired) 9 Forest Grove, Eccleston Park, Prescot L34 2RY — MB BS Vikram 1961; DCH Delhi 1969. Locum GP.

SAKTHIBALAN, Maheswaralingam The Surgery, 167 Eastern Avenue, Redbridge, Ilford IG4 5AW Tel: 020 8550 4532 Fax: 020 8551 2199 — LRCP Ed. 1986; T.Gip (UK); LRCS Ed. LRCPS Glas. 1986.

SALA, Carmelo Department of Anaesthetics, North Middlesex Hospital, Sterling Way, Edmonton, London N18 1QX; 12 Lancaster Avenue, Hitchin SG5 1PB — State Exam Pisa 1984.

SALA, Mr Matthew John Northwick Park Hospital, Department of Orthopaedic Surgery, Level 5, Watford Road, Harrow HA1 3UJ Tel: 020 8869 3379 Fax: 020 8869 2469; 75A Kensington Gardens Square, Bayswater, London W2 4DJ Tel: 020 7727 3916 Fax: 020 7727 3916 — MB ChB Liverp. 1983; FRCS Eng. 1990; FRCS (Orth.) 1997. Cons. Orth. & Trauma Surg. NW Lond. Hosps. NHS Trust. Specialty: Orthop. Special Interest: Hip & Knee Arthroplasty; Shoulder; Sports Injury. Prev: Sen. Regist. Centr. Middlx. Hosp. Lond.; Sen. Regist. Qu. Eliz. II Hosp. Welling Gdn. City, Ealing & Char. Cross Hosp. Lond.

SALA TENNA, Adrianno Michele GFR, 6 South Oxford St., Edinburgh EH8 9QF — MB ChB Ed. 1996.

SALAH, Ibrahim Hussein Ibrahim Ansdell Road Surgery, 2-4 Ansdell Road, Blackpool FY1 5LX Tel: 01253 761293; 208 West Park Drive, Blackpool FY3 9LW — MB BCh Cairo 1973.

SALAH, Mr Magdy Mohammed Riad Mohammed c/o Mr Coleman, 42 Lavender Road, Holts Village, Oldham OL4 5NY — MB BCh Ain Shams 1977; FRCS Ed. 1987; FRCSI 1987.

SALAH, Mr Munzer Walid Flat 3, 36 Devonshire Place, London W1G 6JR Tel: 020 7935 4520 — MB BS Lond. 1966 (King's Coll. Hosp.) MRCS Eng. LRCP Lond. 1966; FRCS Eng. 1972. Socs: BMA; Fell. Roy. Soc. Med.; Fell. Hunt. Soc. Prev: Cons. Surg. Ladbroke Diag. Clinic; Regist. (Surg.) St. Thos. Hosp. Lond.; Sen. Regist. (Surg.) Hillingdon Hosp. Uxbridge.

SALAHUDDIN, Azam X-Ray Department, Basildon and Thurrock NHS Trust, Nethermayne, Basildon SS16 5NL Tel: 01268 795177 — MB BS Karachi 1963; BSc Karachi 1959; DMRD Eng. 1975. p/t Cons. Radiologist, Basildon and Brentwood; Private Pract., The Essex Nuffield Hosp., Brentwood. Specialty: Radiol. Special Interest: Nuclear Med.; Ultrsound. Socs: Roy. Coll. af Radiologists. Prev: Clin. Director, Cons. Radiologist.

SALAHUDDIN, Mobin The Surgery, 11 Thorpe Road, Staines TW18 3EA Tel: 01784 454965 Fax: 01784 441244 — MB BS Karachi 1983. Specialty: Gen. Med.

SALAHUDDIN, Mohamed — MB BS Bihar 1973; DA Bihar 1975.

SALAHUDDIN, Mohammad Old Chester Road Surgery, 241 Old Chester Road, Lower Tranmere, Birkenhead CH42 3TD Tel: 0151 645 2306 — MB BS Punjab 1971 (King Edwd. Med. Coll.) BSc, MB BS Punjab Pakistan 1971; MSc Ed. (Human Genetics) 1981; Dip. Pract. Dermat. Wales 1991.

SALAHUDDIN, Muhammad Junaid 63 Lee Road, Perivale, Greenford UB6 7DA Tel: 020 8991 1787 — MB ChB Mosul 1973. Assoc. Specialist (Plastic Surg.) City Hosp. Dudley Rd. Birm. Specialty: Plastic Surg. Prev: Craniofacial Fell. Qu. Eliz. Hosp. Birm.; Regist. (Plastic Surg.) St. And. Hosp. Billericay.

SALAKO, Abayomi Oluremilekn 171 Charlemont Road, London E6 6AG — MB BS Ibadan 1985; MRCP (UK) 1993.

SALAM, Imroz Department of Gastroenterology, West Wales General Hospital, Carmarthen NHS Trust, Dolgwili Road, Carmarthen SA31 2AF Tel: 01267 235151 Fax: 01267 227921 — MB BS Poona 1979 (Armed Forces Med. Coll. Pune, India) FRCPI 1997, M 1985. Cons. Gastroenterol. W. Wales Gen. Hosp. Carmarthen. Specialty: Gastroenterol. Socs: FEBG. Prev: Sen. Specialist (Gastroenterol.) Qu. Eliz. Milit. Hosp.; Cons. Gastroenterol. Daharan Med. Center, Saudi Arabia; Regist. (Med.) Ysbyty Gwynedd Bangor.

SALAM, Mr Mahmoud Abdel Mohamed El-Hosseiny The Ipswich Hospital NHS Trust, Heath Road, Ipswich IP4 5PD Tel: 01473 703503 Fax: 01473 703111; 145 The St, Rushmene St. Andrew, Ipswich IP5 1DG — MB BCh Ain Shams 1982; FRCS Ed. 1989; MD Ain Shams 1989; MSc War. 1995; FRCS (ORL.) 1996. Cons. Otolaryngologist (Head and Neck Surgery) Ipswich Hosp.; Cons. Otolaryngologist (Head and Neck Surgery), Nuffield Hosp. Ipswitch. Specialty: Otorhinolaryngol. Socs: BMA; BAOL - HNS; Europ. Rhinological Soc. Prev: Sen. Regist. Oxf. & Reading Rotat. (ENT); Regist. W. Midl. Rotat. (ENT) (Birm. Coventry & Warks.).

SALAM, Mohammad Abdus 100 Princes Road, Eastbourne BN23 6HH Tel: 01323 734827 — MB BS Dacca 1966; DO RCPSI 1979; MRCOphth 1989. Clin. Asst. (Ophth.) Hastings & Eastbourne HA's. Prev: SHO (Ophth.) Eastbourne HA, Colchester & Whipps Cross Hosps.

SALAM, Samia 17 Brookside Close, Caerphilly CF83 2RR — MB BCh Wales 1992.

SALAM, Souheir 87 Dudley Gardens, London W13 9LU — MB BS Lond. 1998; MB BS Lond 1998.

SALAMA, Alan David 41 Ramillies Road, London W4 1JW Tel: 020 8994 8689 — MB BS Lond. 1990; MRCP (UK) 1993; PhD Lond. 2001. Regist. (Gen. Med. & Nephrol.) Ealing & Hammersmith Hosp.

SALAMA, Amir Adib Kamel 4 Mill Court, City Hospital, Dudley Road, Birmingham B18 7QH — MB ChB Alexandria 1989.

SALAMA, Mr Fayek Dimitri Thoracic Department, The City Hospital, Hucknall Road, Nottingham NG5 1PB Tel: 0115 691169 — MB BCh Cairo 1958 (Ain Shams) FRCS Eng. 1969; FRCS Ed. 1969; LMSSA Lond. 1974. Cons. Thoracic Surg. Notts. AHA (T). Specialty: Cardiothoracic Surg. Socs: Soc. Thoracic & Cardiovasc. Surgs. Gt. Brit. & Irel. & BMA. Prev: Regist. Shotley Bridge Gen. Hosp. Consett; Sen. Regist. Westm. Hosp. & St. Geo. Hosp. Lond.

SALAMA, Nabel Doss The Surgery, 41 Ellers Lane, Auckley, Doncaster DN9 3HY Tel: 01302 770327 Fax: 01302 771302;

Orchard Grange, 89 Main St, Auckley, Doncaster DN9 3HJ — MB BCh Cairo 1966.

SALAMA, Mr Nabil Youssef c/o Postgraduate Medical Centre, Lewisham Hospital, High St., London SE13 6LH Tel: 020 8333 3000; Beaumanor, 23 Manor Way, Beckenham BR3 3LH Tel: 020 8658 3751 — MB BCh Cairo 1973 (Cairo Univ) FRCS Eng. 1980. Cons. ENT Lewisham NHS Trust; Hon. Sen. Lect. UMDS. Specialty: Otorhinolaryngol. Socs: Roy. Soc. Med.

SALAMA, Nadia Salama Ibrahim 52 Cornflower Lane, Shirley Oaks Village, Shirley, Croydon CR0 8XJ — MB BCh Cairo 1980.

SALAMAN, Professor John Redcliffe (retired) 5 Brooklyn Close, Rhiwbina, Cardiff CF14 6UT Tel: 029 2062 6539 Fax: 029 2065 5735 Email: j.salaman@doctors.org.uk — (Camb. & Lond. Hosp.) MB BChir Camb. 1963; MRCS Eng. LRCP Lond. 1963; MChir Camb. 1995, MA 1964; FRCS Eng. 1967. Prev: Prof. Transpl. Surg. Univ. Wales Coll. Med. Cardiff.

SALAMAN, Judith Helen Huddersfield Royal Infirmary, Acre Street, Lindley, Huddersfield HD3 3EA — MB BCh Wales 1989; FRCS Ed. 1993. Specialty: Gen. Surg.

SALAMAN, Patricia Faith (retired) 5 Brooklyn Close, Rhiwbina, Cardiff CF14 6UT Tel: 029 2062 6539 — MB BChir Camb. 1964 (Camb. & St. Thos.) MRCS Eng. LRCP Lond. 1963; MA Camb. 1964; FRCR 1979. Prev: Cons. Radiother. Velindre Hosp. Cardiff.

SALAMAN, Mr Robert Arthur Blackburn Royal Infimary, Bolton Road, Blackburn BB2 3LR — MB BCh Wales 1988; FRCS Eng. 1992. Specialty: Gen. Surg.

SALAMANI, Mr Murad Mohamed Hassan 29 The Baulk, Worksop S81 0HU — MB BCh Cairo 1972; FRCS Ed. 1987.

SALAMAT, Ahmed Ali 6 Adria Road, Sparkhill, Birmingham B11 4JN Tel: 0121 449 6074 — MB BCh Al Fateh Libya 1981; MSc Glas. 1989; MRCP (UK) 1992. Hon. Clin. Research Fell. (Haemat.) Qu. Eliz. Univ. Hosp. Birm. Specialty: Haematology. Prev: SHO (Haemat.) Glas. Roy. Infirm. & Whipps Cross Hosp. Lond.; SHO (Med.) Vict. Infirm. Glas.

SALAME, Mahomed Yazeed 81 Carlton Avenue E., Wembley HA9 8LZ Tel: 020 8904 7863 — BSc Basic Med. Scs. & Biochem. (Hons.) Lond. 1985, MB BS 1988; MRCP (UK) 1991. BHF Jun. Research Fell. & Hon. Regist. (Cardiol.) Glenfield Hosp. Leics. Prev: SHO (Med., Cardiol. & Neurol.) Addenbrooke's Hosp. Camb.; Ho. Surg. Char. Cross Hosp. Lond.; Ho. Phys. Westm. Hosp. Lond.

SALAMEH, Yasser Mohammad Mohammad Hassain 17 Atherstone Avenue, Peterborough PE3 9TT — MB BS Jordan 1993.

SALAMONSKI, John Henry The Surgery, 11 Main Street, Leuchars, St Andrews KY16 0HB Tel: 01334 839210 Fax: 01334 838770 — MB ChB Dundee 1989; BSc Hons. (Physiol.) St. And. 1984.

SALARIA, Dabeer Ahmad 20 Ensign Close, Staines TW19 7RF — MB BS Punjab 1986.

SALASA, Mohamed Hassan (retired) 37 Woodhouse Road, Finchley, London N12 9ET — MB ChB Cape Town 1967; MRCPsych 1972; DPM Eng. 1972. Prev: Cons. Psychiat. Hill End Hosp., St. Albans City Hosp. & St. Crispin Hosp. Northampton.

SALATHIA, Kulvir Singh 27 Greer Park Heights, Knockbreda, Belfast BT8 7YG — MB BS Jammu & Kashmir 1969.

SALATIAN, Miral Dunrowan Day Hospital, 37 Maggir Woods Loan, Falkirk FK1 5EH Tel: 01324 639009 Fax: 01324 626238; 62 Kenning Knowes Road, Stirling FK7 9JG Tel: 01786 465943 Fax: 01786 465943 — MD Vienna 1971 (Vienna Med. Sch. Austria) MD Vienna Austria 1971. Assoc. Specialist (Psychiat.) Forth Valley Primary Care - NHS Trust. Specialty: Gen. Psychiat.

SALCEDO, Aurelio Advincula 175 Clarence Road, London E5 8EE Tel: 020 8985 7096 — LAH Dub. 1966.

SALDANHA, Mr Clyde Bosco Raymond 72 Churston Drive, Morden SM4 4JQ — MB BS Lond. 1986; FRCS Ed. 1992. Regist. (Cardiothoracic Surg.) St. Bart. Hosp. Lond. Specialty: Cardiothoracic Surg. Prev: Research Fell. (Cardiovasc. Research) St. Thos. Hosp. Lond.

SALDANHA, Gerald Stephen Department of Histopathology, Level III, Phase III, Leicester Royal Infirmary, Leicester — MB ChB Leic. 1989; MRCP (UK) 1992. SHO (Histopath.) Leicester Roy. Infirm. Prev: SHO Rotat. (Med.) Leicester Hosps.

SALDANHA, Gerard Joseph Francis 182 Greenvale Road, London SE9 1PQ — MB BS Lond. 1989 (St. Thos. Hosp. Med. Sch.) BA (Hons.) Oxf. 1984; MRCP (UK) 1992. Research Regist. (Neurol.) Roy. Lond. Hosp. Specialty: Neurol. Prev: Regist. (Neurol.) Guy's Hosp. Lond.; Regist. & SHO (Neurol.) Brook Hosp.

SALDANHA, Luis Joseph The Surgery, 131 Thornbridge Avenue, Great Barr, Birmingham B42 2AP Tel: 0121 357 1286 Fax: 0121 505 3705 — MB ChB Birm. 1978.

SALDANHA, Maria Benicia Yvette Watling Medical Centre, 108 Watling Avenue, Burnt Oak, Edgware HA8 0NR Tel: 020 8906 1711 Fax: 020 8201 1283 — MB BS Lond. 1985; DCH RCP Lond. 1989; MRCGP 1995. GP Trainer. Prev: Trainee GP Edgware Gen. Hosp. Lond. VTS.

SALE, Andrew Colin Buchanan Staithe Road Surgery, Staithe Road, Ludham, Great Yarmouth NR29 5AB Tel: 01692 580880; Lankaster, Norwich Rd, Ludham, Great Yarmouth NR29 5QD Tel: 01692 678262 — MB BS Lond. 1991 (Guy's Lond. Med. Sch.) MA Camb. 1990; DRCOG 1994; MRCGP 1996.

SALE, John Philip Stoke Manderville Hospital, Aylesbury HP21 8AL; One Acre, Peters Lane, Whiteleaf, Princes Risborough, Aylesbury HP27 0LG Tel: 01844 345805 — MB BS Lond. 1977; FFA RCS Eng. 1982. Specialty: Anaesth.

SALE, Julian Edward M.R.C Laboratory of Molecular Biology, Cambridge CB2 2QH Tel: 01223 252941 Email: jes@mrc-lmb.cam.ac.uk; 3 Coniston Road, Cambridge CB1 7BZ Tel: 01223 572841 — MB BChir Camb. 1991 (Cambridge) MA Camb. 1993, BA 1989; MRCP (UK) 1994; PHD Camb. Uni. 1999. Gp. Ldr. MRC Laborat. of Molecular Biol. Camb.; Fell. Gonville & Caius Coll. Camb.; Director of Studies in Med., Gonville & Caius Coll. Camb.; Coll. Lecture in Path., Gonville & Caius Coll. Camb. Specialty: Research; Educat. Prev: Regist. (Gen. Med. & Hepatol.) Univ. Hosp. Qu. Med. Centre Nottm.; SHO Rotat. Addenbrooke's Hosp. Camb.; MRC Clinician Scientist, MRC Laborat. of Molecular Biol., Camb.

SALE, Steven Michael Department of Anaethesia, Bristol Royal Infirmary, Marlborough Street, Bristol BS2 8HW — MB ChB Bristol 1993. Specialty: Anaesth.

SALEEM, Amtul Karim Najma 15 St Anthonys Way, Haverfordwest SA61 1EL Tel: 01437 764545 — MB BS Punjab 1962; MRCPath 1979; FRCPath 1981. Cons. Haemat. Withybush Gen. Hosp. HaverfordW.. Specialty: Haematology. Prev: Sen. Regist. (Haemat.) Westm. Hosp. Lond.; Sen. Regist. (Haemat.) Co. Laborat. Dorchester; Regist. (Haemat.) Ninewells Hosp. Dundee.

SALEEM, Anneela 39 Cromwell Grove, Manchester M19 3QD — MB ChB Leeds 1994.

SALEEM, Mrs Asra Liverpool Women's Hospital, Crown St, Liverpool L8 Tel: 0151 708 9988; 24 Burder Road, Heswall, Wirral CH6U 2TY — MB BS Lond. 1990 (King's Coll. Sch. Med. Lond.) FRCS Ed. 1994; MRCOG 1997. SpR (O&G) Liverp. Wom.'s Hosp. Specialty: Obst. & Gyn. Prev: Regist. (O & G) Addenbrooke's Hosp. Camb.; Specialist Regist. (O & G) Ipswich Hosp.

SALEEM, Haris Royal Gwent Hospital, Cardiff Road, Newport NP9 2UB — MB BS Karachi 1987; MRCP (UK) 1993. Cons. Acute Phys. Gwent Healthcare NHS Trust. Specialty: Gen. Med.; Gastroenterol. Special Interest: Gastroenterol. Socs: BMA; MPS.

SALEEM, Ishrat 55 Ryfold Road, London SW19 8DF — MRCS Eng. LRCP Lond. 1979.

SALEEM, Mubashar Ahmad The Surgery, 158 Alcester Road South, Kings Heath, Birmingham B14 6AA Tel: 0121 444 1186 Fax: 0121 443 3252; 158 Alcester Road S., Kings Heath, Birmingham B14 6AA Tel: 0121 444 1186 Fax: 0121 443 3252 — MB BS Punjab 1973.

SALEEM, Muhammad 22 Ashmole Close, Lichfield WS14 9RS Tel: 01543 255539 — MB BS Punjab 1965 (Nishtar Med. Coll. Multan) MPS ST. Pauls. GP S. Staffs. HA. Specialty: Gen. Pract.

SALEEM, Muhammad Fayyaz Department Ophthalmology, Withybush General Hospital, Haverfordwest Tel: 01437 764545; Freshwinds, 15 St. Anthonys Way, Haverfordwest SA61 1EL Tel: 01437 766909 — MB BS Karachi 1966; DO RCPSI 1971; MRCOphth 1989. Specialist (Ophth.) Pembrokesh. NHS Trust HaverfordW. Specialty: Ophth. Prev: Regist. (Ophth.) Ophth. Inst. Glas., Ninewells Hosp. Dundee & Roy.N.. Hosp. Lond.

SALEEM, Muhammed Shiregreen Medical Centre, 492 Bellhouse Road, Sheffield S5 0RG Tel: 0114 245 6123 Fax: 0114 257 0964 — MB BS Karachi 1967.

SALEEM, Mrs Sabiha The Surgery, 141 Plumstead High Street, Plumstead, London SE18 1SE Tel: 020 8855 0052 Fax: 020 8855

7672; The Surgery, 253 Wickham Lane, London SE2 0NX Tel: 020 8317 8708 Fax: 020 8316 1239 — MB BS Osmania 1954.

SALEEM, Shahzadi 44 East Avenue, Oxford OX4 1XP — MB BS Lond. 1994.

SALEEM, Tausif 22 Ashmole Close, Lichfield WS14 9RS — MB BCh Wales 1993.

SALEEM-UDDIN, Moin Ahson Bristol Childrens Hospital, Childrens Renal Unit, Bristol BS2 8BJ Tel: 0117 342 8880 Email: m.saleem@bristol.ac.uk — MB BS Lond. 1986 (Royal Free) MRCP (UK) 1990; PhD 1997. Cons. Sen. Lect. in Paediatric Nephrol. Specialty: Paediat.; Nephrol. Special Interest: Renal Cell Biol. Prev: Lect. Paediat Nephrol, Gt. Ormond St. Hosp.; Research Fell., Gt. Ormond St. Hosp.; SHO Rotat. (Paediat.) City Hosp. Nottm.

SALEEMI, Mohammad Hussain Highfield Medical Centre, Highfield Road, Widnes WA8 7DJ Tel: 0151 424 3646 Fax: 0151 424 3646 — (King Edwd. Med. Coll. Lahore) MB BS Punjab (Pakistan) 1965; DA Eng. 1970. GP. Specialty: Anaesth.; Gen. Pract. Socs: Med. Protec. Soc.; Fell.Roy.Soc.Med.; Assoc. Mem. Roy. Coll. Gen. Pract.

SALEEMI, Sarfraz Ahmed 46 Montana Road, London SW17 8SN Tel: 020 8767 5214 — MB BS Punjab 1983; MRCP (UK) 1992.

SALEH, Mr Adnan Jamil Bronglais General Hospital, Aberystwyth SY23 1ER — LAH Dub. 1964; FRCS Ed. 1980.

SALEH, Ahmed Hosny Shoukry 31 Northfield, Swanland, North Ferriby HU14 3RG Tel: 01482 631987 Fax: 01482 632631 Email: asleh@compuserve.com — MB BCh Ain Shams 1978; DA (UK) 1984; FFA RCSI 1986. Cons. Anaesth. Castle Hill Hosp. Hull. Specialty: Anaesth. Prev: Cons. & Chief Resid. (Anaesth.) King Faisal Specialist Hosp., Riyadh; Assoc. Specialist Castle Hill Hosp. Hull; Sen. Regist. Riyadh Milit. Hosp., Saudi Arabia.

SALEH, Assil 12 Alfriston Avenue, Harrow HA2 7DZ — MB BS Lond. 1998; MB BS Lond 1998.

SALEH, Badie Tawfiec Scunthorpe General Hospital, Cliff Gardens, Scunthorpe DN15 7BH Tel: 01724 290148 Fax: 01724 290419 Email: badie.saleh@dsh.nhs.uk — (Assuit Univ.) MB BCh Assuit 1969; MRCPsych 1983; DPM RCPSI 1983. Cons. Psychiat. DASH Community Health Trust Scunthorpe; Clin. Med. Dir., Scunthorpe. Specialty: Gen. Psychiat. Socs: Roy. Coll. Psychiat.; Reg. Psychiat. Assn.; Med. Prot. Soc. Prev: Sen. Regist. (Psychiat.) Glas.; Regist. (Psychiat.) Bridgend S. Wales.

SALEH, Mr Farouq Awad Ali 129 Barley Lane, Goodmayes, Ilford IG3 8XH — Vrach Peoples Friendship U Moscow 1970; Vrach Peoples Friendship U, Moscow 1970; FRCS Glas. 1982.

SALEH, Isam Wenlock St Surgery, 40 Wenlock St, Luton LU2 0NN Tel: 01582 727094 — State Exam Med. Munich 1983; MD Tech. Univ. Munich 1985.

SALEH, Mehboobali Ismail School Health, Canterbury & Thanet Healthcare Trust, Little Bourne Road, Canterbury CT1 1TD Tel: 01227 459371; 1 Monkton Gardens, Cliftonville, Margate CT9 3HN Tel: 01843 223577 — State Exam Med Munster 1985; DCH RCP Lond. 1993; DRCOG 1993; DFFP 1996. Staff Grade (Community Paediat.) Canterbury & Thanet Community Healthcare Trust. Specialty: Community Child Health.

SALEH, Professor Michael Bridge Farm, Thurgarton, Norwich NR11 7HR Tel: 01263 768145 Fax: 01263 768145 Email: m.saleh@stumperlowe.demon.co.uk — MB ChB Sheff. 1975; FRCS Ed. 1980; FRCS Eng. 1980; MSc Biomed. Engineering Sci. Dundee 1982; HST RCS England 1986. p/t Hon. Prof. Orthop. Univ. Sheff.; Cons. Orthop. Surg. Specialty: Orthop. Special Interest: Amputation Surgery; Limb Reconstruction. Socs: Brit. Orth. Assn.; Brit. Limb Reconstruc. Soc. (Past Pres.); Brit. Trauma Soc. Prev: Sen. Regist. (Orthop.) Sheff. HA; Regist. (Orthop.) Tayside HB.

SALEH, Mohamed Salah Al Dean Abdul Hamead 101 The Park, Redbourn, St Albans AL3 7LT — MB BCh Ain Shams 1987; MRCOG 1995; MRCPI 1996.

SALEH, Noorolah Department of Obst. & Gyn., Hope Hospital, Eccles Old Road, Salford M6 8HD Tel: 0161 789 7373; 17 March Bank Drive, Cheadle SK8 1QY — MD Tehran 1972; MRCOG 1980. Assoc. Specialist (O & G) Hope Hosp. Salford. Specialty: Obst. & Gyn.

SALEH, Roy St Johns Medical Centre, St. Johns Road, Altrincham WA14 2NW Tel: 0161 928 8727 Fax: 0161 929 8550 — MB ChB Manch. 1973. Prev: SHO (Paediat.) Booth Hall Hosp. Manch.; SHO (Obst.) N. Manch. Gen. Hosp.; Ho. Off. (Surg.) Ancoats Hosp. Manch.

SALEH, Sanna St Julians Medical Centre, 13A Stafford Road, Newport NP19 7DQ Tel: 01633 251304 Fax: 01633 221977 — MB ChB Alexandria 1976; MB ChB Alexandria 1976; LRCP LRCS Ed. LRCPS Glas. Edinburgh & Glasgow 1980.

SALEH, Sion Fernclogh Surgery, 1 Tavistock Square, Manchester M9 5RD Tel: 0161 205 1638 Fax: 0161 205 1638 — MD Teheran 1974; Cert. Family Plann. JCC 1991. GP Manch. Specialty: Gen. Med.; Orthop.; Gen. Surg. Prev: Regist. Gen. Surg.; Reg. Orthop.

SALEK HADDADI, Ali Afraim 88 Truro Road, London N22 8DN — MB BS Lond. 1996 (St. George's London) Specialty: Gen. Med.

SALEM, Mr Fawzi Ahmed Ali (retired) — MB BCh Alexandria 1966; FRCS Ed. 1981. Cons. Neurosurg. Lam Wah Ee Hosp. 11600 Penang Malaysia. Prev: Cons. Neurosurg. OldCh. Hosp.

SALEM, Mr Hasan Abdel Majid Derbyshire Royal Infirmary, London Road, Derby DE1 2QY Tel: 01332 254698 Fax: 01332 254698 Email: hasan.salem@derbyhospitals.nhs.uk — MB BCh Ain Shams 1965. Cons. (Ophth. Surg.) Derbysh. Roy. Infirm. Specialty: Ophth. Special Interest: Oculo Plastics; Retina.

SALEM, Jack (retired) 7 Larch Rise, Prestbury, Macclesfield SK10 4UY Tel: 01625 829396 — MRCS Eng. LRCP Lond. 1942 (W. Lond. Hosp. & Paris) MRCGP 1957; FFCM 1978, M 1972. Prev: Area Med. Off. Trafford AHA.

SALEM, Naglaa 4 Elm Road, Ewell, Epsom KT17 2EU — MB BS Lond. 1985.

SALEM, Mr Richard John The Edinburgh Breast Unit, Western General Hospital, Crewe Road, Edinburgh BL1 4AP Tel: 0131 537 1000 — MB ChB Manch. 1967; DObst RCOG 1970; FRCS Eng. 1973. Cons. Surg. Fife Acute Hosp.s NHS Trust and Lothian Univ. NHS Trust. Specialty: Gen. Surg. Prev: Sen. Regist. (Surg.) Hammersmith Hosp. Lond. & Roy. Berks. Hosp. Reading; Wellcome Surg. Research Fell. Roy. Postgrad. Med. Sch. Lond.; Cons Surge. Bolton Hosp.s NHS Trust.

SALERNO, Javier Oscar Parkway Health Centre, 1 Parkway, New Addington, Croydon CR0 0JA Tel: 01689 841264; 7 Gravel Hill, Addington, Croydon CR0 5BG Tel: 020 8655 4013 Fax: 020 8655 2750 — Medico Cirujano Univ. Nat. Mayor de San Marcos Peru 1977 (San Marcos University, Lima, Peru) LRCP LRCS Ed. LRCPS Glas. 1985. Specialty: Cardiol.; Paediat.

SALERNO, Julie Anne Parkway Health Centre, New Addington, Croydon CR0 0JA Tel: 01689 841264 Fax: 020 8655 2750; 7 Gravel Hill, Addington, Croydon CR0 5BG — MB ChB Liverp. 1984 (Liverpool) Cert. Family Plann. JCC 1988. GP Croydon. Specialty: Gen. Pract.

SALES, David Rothwell — MB BS Lond. 1978; DRCOG 1982; MRCGP 1985; FRCGP 1997.

SALES, James Douglas Lochinvar, Dalginross, Comrie, Crieff PH6 2ED — MB ChB Glas. 1997.

SALES, Joanna Mary Flat 1 Pilgrims Court, Kidbrooke Grove, Blackheath, London SE3 0PQ — MB BS Lond. 1982; MRCPsych 1989. Sen. Regist. (Child Psychiat.) Hosp. for Sick Childr. Gt. Ormond St. Lond. Prev: Trainee Psychiat. St. Geo. Hosp. Lond.; Trainee GP Greenwich VTS; SHO (Psychiat.) Univ. Hosp. W. Indies Kingston, Jamaica.

SALES, Mr John Edward Lawson (retired) Brackenhurst, Orchehill Avenue, Gerrards Cross SL9 8QL — MB Camb. 1962; MChir Camb. 1973, MB 1962, BChir 1961; FRCS Eng. 1967. Cons. Surg. Hillingdon Hosp. Uxbridge & Mt. Vernon Hosp. Northwood; Regional Adviser Surg. N. W. Thames; Examr. Surg. Univ. Camb.; Mem. Ct. Examrs. RCS. Prev: Sen. Surg. Regist. St. Bart. Hosp. Lond.

SALES, Norman Ronald (Surgery) 2 Salisbury Road, Farnborough GU14 7AW; The Old Stables, 32 Chobham Road, Frimley, Camberley GU16 8PF Tel: 01276 22130 — MB BS Lond. 1953 (Univ. Coll. Hosp.) MRCS Eng. LRCP Lond. 1953; MRCGP 1966. Prev: Squadron Ldr. RAF Med. Br.; Med. Regist. Roy. Infirm. Bradford; Ho. Surg. Univ. Coll. Hosp.

SALES, Rebecca Clare 31A Blenheim Grove, London SE15 4QS — MB ChB Birm. 1990; ChB Birm. 1990.

SALES, Richard Andrew 4 Levylsdene, Guildford GU1 2RS — BM Soton. 1990.

SALES, Timothy Stephen 105 Anderton Park Road, Birmingham B13 9DS — MB ChB Liverp. 1994.

SALFIELD, Derek Julius (retired) c/o 19 Kenwyn Street, Truro TR1 3BU Tel: 01872 263170 — MD Med. Acad. Dusseldorf 1948 (Berlin Leipzig & Sheff.) BSc (Psychol.) Lond. 1942; MD Med. Acad. Duesseldorf 1948; DPM Lond. 1952; FRCPsych 1971; Cert. Psychiat./Psychother. Trier 1974; BA Studies Lond. 1988. Indep. Psychother. Truro. Prev: Med. Dir. Alcoholics Unit, Reinerzau, W. Germany.

SALFIELD, Nicolas Julian NHS Executive Trent, Fulwood House, Old Fulwood Road, Sheffield S10 3TH Tel: 0114 263 0300 Fax: 0114 282 0397; Moorlow Cottage, Moor Road, Great Longstone, Bakewell DE45 1UA Tel: 01629 640091 — MB BS Newc. 1978; MFCM RCP Lond. 1988; T(GP) 1991; T(PHM) 1991; FFPHM 1999. Cons. Pub. Health Med. NHS Exec. Trent, Sheff. Specialty: Pub. Health Med. Prev: Dir. Pub. Health N. Derbysh. HA; Cons. Pub. Health Med. Trent RHA; Sen. Regist. (Community Med.) Sheff. HA.

SALFIELD, Stephen Albert William (retired) Old Garden House, Main Street, Winster, Matlock DE4 2DJ Tel: 07885 478534 Email: steve.salfield@doctors.org.uk — (Newc.) FRCP (UK); FRCPCH; MB BS Newc. 1970; DObst RCOG 1972; DCH Eng. 1975; MRCP (UK) 1975. Prev: Cons. (Paediat.) Rotherham Dist. Gen. Hosp.

SALIB, Emad Hollins Park Hospital, Warrington WA2 8WA Tel: 01925 664123 Fax: 01925 664117; 18 Broughton Close, Appleton, Warrington WA4 3DR — MB ChB Alexandria 1969; MRCPsych 1975; MSc Manch. 1994; FRCPsych 1995; MRCPI 1998. Cons. Psychiat. Mersey RHA since 1997 Clincal Director of Psychiat., Warrington Community Trust; Chairm. Clin. Audit Quality & Research; Hon. Sen. Lect., Univ. of Liverp..; Roy. Coll. tutor - Psychiat. Hollins Pk. Hosp. Specialty: Geriat. Psychiat.

SALIB, Mr Nassif Rizk (retired) Plas-y-ffynnon, Maeshafn, Mold CH7 5LR — MB ChB Cairo 1951; LMSSA Lond. 1962; FRCS Ed. 1966.

SALIB, Sherine Shawky Eskander 9 Burdons Close, Birmingham B34 6ET — MB ChB Bristol 1993.

SALIB, Zaki Rizk, SBStJ Plas y Ffynnon, Maeshafn, Mold CH7 5LR — MRCS Eng. LRCP Lond. 1951 (Liverp.) DObst RCOG 1953; MRCGP 1965. Div. Surg. St. John Ambul. Brig.

SALIH, Abdel Rahman Mohd Mohd 2 Strafford Road, Twickenham TW1 3AE — MB BS Khartoum 1972.

SALIH, Abdel Raziq Mustafa Department of Rheumatology, Appleton Wing, Warrington Hospital, Lovely Lane, Warrington WA5 1QG Tel: 01925 662553 Fax: 01925 662284; 7 Farmleigh Gardens, Great Sankey, Warrington WA5 3FA — MB BS Khartoum 1980 (University of Khartoum) Mmed Khartoum, 1987; MRCP (UK) 1988; DGM RCP Lond. 1990; MD Keele Univ. 1996; FRCP Edinburgh 1999. Cons. Rheum. Warrington Gen. Hosp. NHS Trust. Specialty: Rheumatol. Socs: Brit. Soc. for Rheum. Prev: SCMO (Rheum.) Haywood Hosp. Stoke-on-Trent; Lect. Sch. Trop. Med. Univ. Liverp.; ARC Fell. Char. Cross & Westm. Med. Sch. Lond.

SALIH, Haluk 20 Cypress Avenue, Enfield EN2 9BZ Tel: 020 8363 4963 Fax: 020 8363 4963 — MB ChB Glas. 1988; BSc (Hons) Ed. 1985. Specialty: Gen. Pract.

SALIH, Isam Newcastle University, Wolfson Unit, Newcastle upon Tyne NE2 4HH — MB BS khartoum 1994. Specialist Regist. (Clin. Pharmaeology & GIM) Newc. Univ.

SALIH, Jasmine Elizabeth 21B Rivermount, Walton-on-Thames KT12 2PR — MB ChB Leeds 1995.

SALIH, Mr Khalid Mohummed 18 Roman Road, Ayr KA7 3SZ Tel: 01292 267900 — MB ChB Mosul 1970; FRCS Glas. 1986. Specialty: Orthop.

SALIH, Mohamed Ali St. Mary's Hospital, Newcroft, Newport PO30 5TG Tel: 01983 524081 Fax: 01983 825634; Berridale, Shanklin Road, Sandford, Ventnor PO38 3AJ Tel: 01983 840104 — MRCS Eng. LRCP Lond. 1974 (Khartoum) MB BS Khartoum 1962; DPM Eng. 1969; FRCPsych 1992, M 1972. Locum. Specialty: Gen. Psychiat.; Geriat. Psychiat. Socs: Fell. The Roy. Soc. of Med. Prev: Clin. Asst. Inst. Psychiat. Bethlem Roy. & Maudsley Hosps. Lond.; Jun. Specialist (Psychiat.) Clinic Nerv. Disorders Khartoum, Sudan; Sen. Regist. (Psychiat.) Kensington, Chelsea & Westm. AHA (T).

SALIM, Abdul Salford Medical Centre, 194 Langworthy Road, Salford M6 5PP Tel: 0161 736 2651 Fax: 0161 745 8955.

SALIM, Alena Royal Berkshire Hospital, London Road, Reading RG1 5AN — BM BS Nottm. 1993. Specialist Regist. (Dermat.) Churchill Hosp. Oxf. Specialty: Dermat. Prev: Staff Grade (Dermat.) Walegrave Hosp. Coventry; SHO (Gen. Med.) Walsgrave Hosp. Coventry; Ho. Off. (Surg.) Yeovil Dist. Hosp.

SALIM, Amer Falcon Road Surgery, 47 Falcon Road, Battersea, London SW11 2PH Tel: 020 7228 1619/3399 Fax: 020 7924 3375 — MB ChB Manch. 1988; MRCGP 1993; DRCOG 1993. Prev: Trainee GP Croydon VTS.

SALIM, Ferekh 16 Chiltern Rise., Brinsworth, Rotherham S60 5JT Email: fsalim@ukonline.co.uk — MB ChB Leic. 1992; MRCP Ed. 1996; FRCR 2000. SPR Radiol., Centr. Sheff. Uni. Hosp. Trust. Specialty: Radiol.

SALIM, Ghulam Murtaza 16 Brunel Close, Grimsby DN32 9FE Tel: 01472 597989 — MB BS Punjab 1962; DTM & H Liverp. 1967.

SALIM, Mohammad The Surgery, 157-159 Rotton Park Road, Edgbaston, Birmingham B16 0LJ Tel: 0121 454 0508 — MB BS Peshawar 1974; MB BS Peshawar 1974; LRCP LRCS Ed. LRCPS Glas. Edinburgh & Glasgow 1991.

SALIM, Rahuman 37B Ellesmere Road, Eccles, Manchester M30 9JH — MB ChB Manch. 1995.

SALIM, Rukhsana 16 Heatherbrae, Bishopbriggs, Glasgow G64 2TA — MB ChB Glas. 1995.

SALIM, Saima Namreen 44 Alexander Road, Birmingham B27 6HE — MB BS Lond. 1996.

SALIM, Mr Salaheddin Abdul-Razzak Royal National Throat, Nose and Ear Hospital, Gray's Inn Road, London WC1; 55 Chaseville Park Road, Winchmore Hill, London N21 1PE Tel: 020 8372 8022 — MB ChB Mosul 1977; FRCS Ed. (ENT) 1987; FRCS Eng. (Surg.) 1989. Cons. Roy. Nat. Throat Nose & Ear Hosp. Lond. Specialty: Otorhinolaryngol.

SALIM, Syeda Hamida 2 St John's Hill Grove, London SW11 2RG — MB BS Lond. 1993.

SALIMEE, Sultan Ghani Lambeth, Southwark and Lewisham Health Authority (LSLHA), 1 Lower Marsh, London SE1 7NT Tel: 020 716 7000 Ext: 7615; 83 High Street, Lewes BN7 1XN Tel: 01273 470723 — MD Kabul 1975; MSc London 1997; DMFPHA 2001. Specialist Regist. (SpR) Pub. Health Med., Lambeth, Southwark & Lewisham Health Auth., 1 Lower Marsh, Lond. SE1 7NT; Specialist Regist. Pub. Health Med., W. Surrey Health Auth., The Ridgewood Centre, Old Bailey Rd., Camberley, Surrey GU16. Specialty: Pub. Health Med.; Gen. Pract.; Gen. Med. Socs: Fell. of theRoy. Inst. of Pub. Health & Hyg. and The Soc. of Pub. Health of the UK (FRIPHH); Fac. of Pub. Health Med. of the Roy. Coll. of Phys.s of UK & Irel. (MFPHM). Prev: Specialist Regist. Pub. Health Med., E. Sussex, Brighton & Hove Health Auth., Lewes, E. Sussex, UK; Sen. Ho. Off. (SHO) - Pub. Health Auth., Brent & Harrow Health Auth., Lond.

SALINAS, Juan Carmarthen NHS Trust, West Wales General Hospital, Ophthalmology Department, Carmarthen SA31 2AF Tel: 01267 235151 Fax: 01267 227414; 24 Lon-y-Plas, Johnstown, Carmarthen SA31 3NJ Tel: 01267 221906 Fax: 01267 221906 — Medico y Cirujano Bolivia 1978 (University Of San Simon, Cochabamba-Boliva) MSc (Ophth.) Bristol 1990; MRCOphth 1995. Assoc. Specialist (Ophth.) W. Wales Gen. Hosp. Carmarthen; OMP Carmarthen. Specialty: Ophth. Socs: BMA; Amer. Acad. Ophth.; Coll. of Ophthalmol. Prev: Staff Grade (Ophth.) W. Wales Gen. Hosp. Carmarthen; Cons. Ophth. Hosp. Comibol, Catavi & Viedoma Cochabamba, Bolivia; Regist. & SHO (Ophth.) W. Wales Gen. Hosp. Carmarthen.

SALINSKY, John Victor Chalkhill Health Centre, Chalkhill Road, Wembley HA9 9BQ Tel: 020 8904 0911; 32 Wentworth Hill, Wembley HA9 9SG Tel: 020 8904 2844 Fax: 020 8904 2844 — BM BCh Oxf. 1965; MA Oxf. 1965; MRCP Lond. 1969; FRCGP 1989, M 1974. Gen. Sec. Internat. Balint Federat.; Course Organiser Whittington Hosp. GP VTS Lond.

SALISBURY, Amanda Jane Churchill Hospital, Department of Oncology, Old Road, Headington, Oxford OX3 7LJ Tel: 01865 225653 Fax: 01865 225660 Email: amadna.salisbury@orh.nhs.uk — BM BCh Oxf. 1989; BA (Hons.) Physiol. Scis. Oxf. 1986; MRCP (UK) 1992; FRCR 1997. Cons. (Clin. Oncol.) Oxf. Radcliffe NHS Trust; Nuffield Lect. (Clin. Med.) Linc. Coll. Oxf. Univ. Specialty: Oncol. Special Interest: Head & Neck Cancer; Skin Cancer. Prev: Clin. Research Fell. Weatherall Inst. Molecular Med. Oxf.

SALISBURY, Andrew John (retired) 59 Corby Avenue, Swindon SN3 1PR Tel: 01793 527080; 59 Corby Avenue, Swindon SN3 1PR

Tel: 01793 527080 — MB BS Lond. 1962 (St. Geo.) MRCS Eng. LRCP Lond. 1962; DObst RCOG 1965; DCH Eng. 1966; MRCP (UK) 1970; FRCP Lond. 1983. Prev: Cons. (Paediat.) Princess Margt. Hosp., Swindon.

SALISBURY, Anthony Kenneth Woodford Surgery, 29-31 Chantry Lane, Grimsby DN31 2LL Tel: 01472 342325 Fax: 01472 251739; White Cottages, Abbey Lane, North Ormsby, Louth LN11 0TJ Tel: 01472 840939 — MB BS Lond. 1989 (Roy. Free Hosp. Sch. Med. Lond.) BSc (1st cl. Hons.) Lond. 1986; T(GP) 1993; MRCGP 1996.

SALISBURY, Barbara Jean (retired) L'Iraugnie, Candie Road, St Peter Port, Guernsey GY1 1UP Tel: 01481 720232 — MB BS Lond. 1950 (Roy. Free) MRCS Eng. LRCP Lond. 1950; DCH Eng. 1953; DPM Eng. 1957; MRCPsych 1971. Prev: Cons. Psychiat. Guernsey Child Guid. Clinic.

SALISBURY, Christopher John Cotham House, Cotham Hill, Bristol BS6 6JL Tel: 0117 9546658 Fax: 0117 9546677 — MB ChB Bristol 1979; DRCOG 1982; MRCGP (Distinc.) 1984; MSc (Distinc.) Univ. Lond. 1989; FRCGP 1997; MD Bristol 1998. Reader (Primary Health Care) Univ. Bristol; GP William Budd Health Centre Bristol. Specialty: Gen. Pract. Prev: Cons. Sen. Lect. in GP Univ. of Bristol; GP Grovelands Med. Centre Reading; Sen. Lect. Imperial Coll. Lond.

SALISBURY, David Maxwell, CB Department of Health, Skipton House, 80 London Road, London SE1 6LH Tel: 020 7972 1522 Fax: 020 7972 5758; Pound Cottage, Bell Lane, Brightwell-cum-Sotwell, Wallingford OX10 0QD Tel: 01491 37209 — MB BS Lond. 1969; MRCP (UK) 1977; FRCP Lond. 1992; MFPHM RCP (UK) 1994; FRCPCH 1997. Princip. Med. Off. DoH Lond.; Hon. Sen. Lect. (Child Health) King's Coll. Lond. Specialty: Infec. Dis. Prev: Cons. Paediat. New Cross Hosp. Wolverhampton; Sen. Regist. Hosp. Sick Childr. Gt. Ormond St. & St. Bart Hosp. Lond.; Sir William Coxen Fell. & Regist. (Paediat.) Univ. Oxf. John Radcliffe Hosp. Oxf.

SALISBURY, Jennifer Ann 41 Crossways, Gidea Park, Romford RM2 6AJ Tel: 01708 726516 — MB BChir Camb. 1966 (Camb. & St. Thos.) FRCP London; MA; BChir 1965. Cons. Dermat. Specialty: Dermat. Prev: Sen. Regist. (Dermat.) Lond. Hosp.

SALISBURY, Jonathan Dept of Anaesthetics, Ninewells Hospital, Dundee DD1 9SY Tel: 01382 660111; Beech House, Foodieash, Cupar FY15 4PW — MB ChB Dundee 1997; MB ChB Dundee 1997 (Commendation). SHO (Anaesth.). Specialty: Anaesth.

SALISBURY, Jonathan Richard King's College Hospital, Department of Histopathology, Bessemer Road, London SE5 9RS Tel: 020 7346 3093 Fax: 020 7346 3670 Email: jon.salisbury@kingsch.nhs.uk/jonathan.salisbury@kcl.ac.uk; 84 Harbut Road, London SW11 2RE Tel: 020 7924 6495 — MB BS Lond. 1980 (Univ. Coll. Hosp.) MRCPath 1986; BSc (Hons.) Lond. 1977, MD 1993; FRCPath 1997. Cons. Histopath. Specialty: Histopath. Special Interest: Haematopathology, dermatopathology and musculo-skeletal Path. Socs: Europ. Soc. for Path.; Path. Soc. of Gt. Britain; Internat. Soc. for Cellular Oncol. Prev: Reader & Hon. Cons. Histopath. King's, Denmark Hill Campus, Lond.

SALISBURY, Mark Steven 7 Keld Road, Carlisle CA2 7QX — BM BS Nottm. 1997.

SALISBURY, Mrs Maxine Rina (retired) 81 Penrhyn Crescent, Beeston, Nottingham NG9 5PA — MB ChB Birm. 1957; AFOM RCP Lond. 1990. Prev: Clin. Asst. Renal Unit City Hosp. Nottm.

SALISBURY, Nigel Swinburne, TD, Maj. RAMC (retired) Church House, Westbury Leigh, Westbury BA13 3SQ — (St. Bart.) MB BS Lond. 1964; MRCS Eng. LRCP Lond. 1964; DObst RCOG 1966. CMP (Civil. Med. Practitioner). Prev: GP W.bury.

SALISBURY, Richard Sydney Thermoteknix Systems Ltd., Mount Pleasant House, Mount Pleasant, Cambridge CB3 0RN Tel: 01223 500777 Fax: 01223 500888 Email: r.salisbury@thermoteknix.com; Courtings, 301A Hills Road, Cambridge CB2 2QS Tel: 01223 502777 Fax: 01223 503778 Email: r.salisbury@attglobal.net — MB BS Lond. 1973 (The Lond. Hosp.) MRCP (UK) 1978. Managing Dir. Thermoteknix Systems Ltd. Cambs. Specialty: Rehabil. Med.; Rheumatol. Prev: Sen. Regist. (Rheum.) Hope Hosp. & Manch. Roy. Infirm.; Research Fell. & Hon. Sen. Regist. Addenbrooke's Hosp. Camb.; Regist. (Med.) Roy. Berks. Hosp. Reading.

SALISBURY, Robert David 72 Cwmfferws Road, Tycroes, Ammanford SA18 3UA — MB BCh Wales 1995.

SALKELD, David Victor, TD (Surgery) 5 Saville Place, Newcastle upon Tyne NE1 8DH Tel: 0191 232 4274; Threeplands, North Brunton, Newcastle upon Tyne NE3 5HD Tel: 0191 236 7691 — MRCS Eng. LRCP Lond. 1946 (Char. Cross) Socs: BMA. Prev: Med. Supt. North. Cos. Schs. for the Deaf; Maj. RAMC, TA; Ho. Surg. Fract. Clinic, Orthop. Dept. & ENT Dept. Char. Cross Hosp. Lond.

SALKELD, John Walton, TD (retired) 93 Cleadon Lea, Cleadon Village, Sunderland SR6 7TG Tel: 0191 537 4729 — MB BS Durh. 1949. DL Tyne & Wear. Prev: GP Co. Durh.

SALKELD, Judith Victoria Saville Medical Group, 7 Saville Place, Newcastle upon Tyne NE1 8DQ Tel: 0191 232 4274 Fax: 0191 233 1050 — MB BS Lond. 1978.

SALKELD, Susan Anne Portobello Medical Centre, 14 Codrington Mews, London W11 2EH Tel: 020 7727 5800/2326 Fax: 020 7792 9044; 39 Park View Road, London NW10 1AJ — MB BS Lond. 1982; MA Oxf. 1974; MRCGP 1986; Dip. Primary Care Lond. Therap. 1997.

SALKER, Mr Digamber Mangesh 45 Corringham Road, Wembley Park, Wembley HA9 9PX Tel: 020 8908 3443 — MB BS Bombay 1973; MS (Gen. Surg.) Bombay 1976, MB BS 1973; FRCS Ed. 1981; FRCS Glas. 1981. Sen. Regist. (Urol.) Armed Forces Hosp. Sultanate of Oman. Specialty: Urol. Prev: Regist. (Urol. & Surg.) Hackney Gen. Hosp. Lond.; Regist. (Gen. Surg.) Stafford Dist. Hosp.; SHO (Gen. Surg.) N. Devon Dist. Hosp.

SALKIN, Barry David 40 Quakers Lane, Potters Bar EN6 1RJ — MB BS Lond. 1994; BSc (Hons.) Manch. 1989. Prev: Ho. Surg. Middlx. Hosp. Lond.

SALKIN, Cyril 30 Siddall Street, Heywood OL10 2AS Tel: 01706 625098; 10 Elswick Green, Marshside, Southport PR9 9XT Tel: 01704 212451 — MB ChB Manch. 1957.

SALKIN, David Stephen Humberstone Park Surgery, 190 Uppingham Road, Leicester LE5 0QG Tel: 0116 276 6605 — MB ChB Manch. 1983; MRCGP 1992.

SALKIND, Professor Malvin Ronald 8 Heathfielde, Lyttelton Road, London N2 0EE Tel: 020 8455 7971 — MRCS Eng. LRCP Lond. 1950 (Univ. Coll. Hosp.) PhD Lond. 1973; FRCPsych 1980, M 1974; FRCGP 1975. Emerit. Prof. Gen. Pract. Univ. Lond. Specialty: Gen. Pract.; Gen. Psychiat. Prev: Prof. Jt. Acad. Dept. Gen. Pract. & Primary Care St. Bart. Med. Coll. & Lond. Hosp. Med. Coll.; Chairm. Med. Bds. DHSS; Research Fell. Acad. (Psychiat.) St. Bart. Hosp. Lond.

SALKIND, Susan Ruth 43 Cranley Gardens, London N10 3AB — MB ChB Birm. 1982; ChB Birm. 1982; DRCOG Lond. 1986.

SALLOMI, David Francis X-Ray Department, Eastbourne District General Hospital, Kings Drive, Eastbourne BN21 2UD — MB ChB Manch. 1988; FRCR 1995. Specialty: Radiol. Prev: Sen. Regist. (Radiol.) Guy's & St. Thos. Hosps. Lond.

SALMAN, Mansur Nasrideen 51 Haweswater, Huntingdon PE29 6TW — MB BS Ahmadu Bello, Nigeria 1983; MRCOG 1994.

SALMAN, Michael Sabah King's College Hospital, Denmark Hill, London SE5 9RS Tel: 020 7737 4000; 13 Knoll House, Carlton Hill, London NW8 9XD — MB BS Lond. 1990; BSc (Hons.) Lond. 1987; MRCP (UK) 1993; DCH RCP Lond. 1994. Lect. (Paediat. Neurosci.) King's Coll. Hosp. Lond. Specialty: Paediat. Prev: Regist. (Paediat. Neurol.) Gt. Ormond St. Hosp. for Childr. Lond.; Regist. (Paediat.) St. Helier Hosp. Jersey; SHO (Paediat.) Lewisham & Guy's Hosps. Lond.

SALMAN, Mr Saad Masud Rochdale Infirmary, Whitehall Street, Rochdale OL12 0NB — MB BS Karachi 1980; FRCSI 1990; FRCS Eng. 1993. Specialty: Gen. Surg.

SALMAN, Walid Daoud Burnley General Hospital, Casterton Avenue, Burnley BB10 2PQ; Robin Hill, 149 Wheatley Lane Road, Fence, Nelson BB9 6QN — MB ChB Baghdad 1973; DCPath Baghdad 1979; MRCPath 1984.

SALMASI, Abdul-Majeed Cardiac Department, The Central Middlesex Hospital, Acton Lane, London NW10 7NS Tel: 020 8453 2151 Fax: 020 8453 2145 — MB ChB Baghdad 1971; PhD Lond. 1979; FACA 1988; FHRS 1998; FHS 1999. Specialty: Cardiol. Prev: Asst. Dir. Irvine Cardiovasc. Laborat. St. Mary's Hosp. Lond.

SALMON, Andrew Howard John 18 Mymms Drive, Brookmans Park, Hatfield AL9 7AF — MB ChB Bristol 1998.

SALMON, Anthony James (retired) Past Field, 9 Rotherfield Road, Henley-on-Thames RG9 1NR Tel: 01491 573600 — MB BS Lond. 1949 (Guy's) DCH Eng. 1953; DObst RCOG 1955. Prev: Med. Off. Townlands Hosp. Henley-on-Thames.

SALMON, Anthony Peter 71 Kingsway, Hiltingbury, Chandlers Ford, Eastleigh SO53 1FH Tel: 023 8027 0437 — BM BS Nottm.

1980; MRCP (UK) 1983; FRCP Lond. 1993. Cons. Paediat. Cardiol. Wessex Regional Cardiac Thoracic Centre Gen. Hosp. Soton. Specialty: Cardiol. Prev: Sen. Regist. (Paediat. Cardiol.) Birm. Childr. Hosp.; Regist. Roy. Childr. Hosp. Melbourne, Austral.; SHO Nottm. Univ. Hosp.

SALMON, Cecil Roland (retired) Harvest House, Branch Lane, Chilham, Canterbury CT4 8DR — MB BS Lond. 1955 (Middlx.) MRCS Eng. LRCP Lond. 1955. Prev: GP Canterbury.

SALMON, Douglas Neil The Surgery, 190 Aston Lane, Handsworth, Birmingham B20 3HE Tel: 0121 356 4669 — MB ChB Birm. 1985.

SALMON, Geraldine Louise P&O Princess Cruises, Richmond House, Terminus Terrace, Southampton SO14 3PN — MB ChB Sheff. 1983; BMedSci Sheff 1982; DRCOG 1992; DA UK 1992. Ships Doctor P&O Princess Cruises Soton. Specialty: Gen. Pract. Prev: GP Tavistock; Staff Grade (Anaesth.) Weston Gen. Hosp. Weston super Mare; SHO (Anaesth.) Derriford Hosp. Plymouth.

SALMON, Miss Gillian Margaret 26B Frampton End Road, Frampton Cotterell, Bristol BS36 2JZ — MB ChB Birm. 1988; ChB Birm. 1988.

SALMON, Graham Bentley St Peters Surgery, 49-55 Portsmouth Road, Woolston, Southampton SO19 9RL Tel: 023 8043 4355 Fax: 023 8043 4511; Bay House, 56 Athelston Road, Bitterne, Southampton SO19 4DD Tel: 02380 227902 — MB ChB Bristol 1967; DCH Eng. 1970; MRCP (U.K.) 1973. Prev: SHO (Med.) Soton. Univ. Gp. Hosps.

SALMON, Haydn (retired) 1 Corwell Lane, Hillingdon, Uxbridge UB8 3DD Tel: 020 8573 0085 — MB BS Lond. 1952 (Westm.) Prev: Med. Adviser Brit. Red Cross (Lond. Br.).

SALMON, Mr John Dyster Woodridge, The Ridge, Woldingham, Caterham CR3 7AH Tel: 01883 653250 Fax: 01883 653250 — MB BChir Camb. 1954 (St. Bart.) FRCOPath; MA, MB Camb. 1954, BChir 1953; DObst RCOG 1957; FRCS Eng. 1967. Specialty: Ophth. Socs: Ophth. Soc. UK. Mem. Oxf. Ophth. Congr.; Christ. Med. Fellowsh. Prev: Cons. Eye Surg. Kent & Sussex Hosp. Tunbridge Wells; on Staff St. John Ophth. Hosp. Jerusalem; Regist. St. Bart. Hosp. Lond.

SALMON, Mr John Frank Oxford Eye Hospital, Radcliffe Infirmary, Woodstock Road, Oxford OX2 6HE Tel: 01865 224360 — MB ChB Pretoria 1976; FRCS Ed. 1984; FRCOphth UK 1988; MD Capetown 1993. Cons. Ophth., Oxf.; Sen. Lect. in Clin. Ophth., Oxf. Univ. Specialty: Ophth. Socs: Roy. Soc. of Med.; Glaucoma Soc. of UK. Prev: Cons. Ophth., Groote Schuur Hosp., Cape Town.

SALMON, John Geoffrey David Southmead Surgery, Southmead House, Blackpond Lane, Slough SL2 3ER Tel: 01753 643195 Fax: 01753 642157; 25 Crispin Way, Farnham Common, Slough SL2 3UD Tel: 01753 645962 Fax: 01753 642157 — MB ChB Manch. 1972 (Manchester) MRCP (UK) 1975. Partner in Gen. Pract.; Clin. Asst. (Upper Gastrointestinal Endoscopy) Slough. Prev: SHO Booth Hall Childr. Hosp. Manch. & Manch. Roy. Infirm.; Ho. Off. Manch. Roy. Infirm.

SALMON, John Richard (retired) Carlton House Surgery, 28 Tenniswood Road, Enfield EN1 3LL Tel: 020 8363 7575 Fax: 020 8366 8228 — MRCS Eng. LRCP Lond. 1964 (Char. Cross) Prev: Ho. Surg. Roy. E. Sussex Hosp. Hastings.

SALMON, Katherine Mary Lamb Cottage, 1 Swan Street, Sible Hedingham, Halstead CO9 3RE — MB BS Lond. 1997.

SALMON, Margaret May (retired) 58 Beechwood Road, Newport NP19 8AH Tel: 01633 271631 — MB BCh Wales 1954 (Cardiff) DObst RCOG 1956; DPH Wales 1971; FFCM 1988, M 1974; FFPHM 1989. Cons. Pub. Health Med. Gwent. Prev: Dist. Community Phys. S. Gwent Health Dist.

SALMON, Michael Vaughan (retired) 12 St Mary's Road, Harborne, Birmingham B17 0HA Tel: 0121 427 1708 — LMSSA Lond. 1948 (St. Mary's) MD (Path.) Lond. 1953, MB BS 1948; FRCPath 1974. Prev: Cons. Neuropath. Midl. Centre for Neurosurg.

SALMON, Morag Alison Jean 140 Woodsmoor Lane, Stockport SK3 8TJ — MB ChB Manch. 1982 (St Andrews/Manch)

SALMON, Nancy Jane Falcon Square Surgery, 9-10 Falcon Square, Castle Hedingham, Halstead CO9 3BY Tel: 01787 460436 Fax: 01787 462829; Church Farm House, Church Lane, Toppesfield, Colchester CO9 4DR — MB BS Lond. 1990 (St Mary's Paddington London) DRCOG; MRCP (UK) 1994. GP. Specialty: Gen. Pract. Prev: SHO (O & G) Essex.

SALMON, Nigel Paul Department Anaesthetics, Hereford Co. Hospital, Union Walk, Hereford HR1 2ER — BM BS Nottm. 1977; BMedSci 1975; FFA RCS Eng. 1981. Cons. Anaesth. Hereford. Specialty: Anaesth. Socs: BMA; Assn. Anaesth.

SALMON, Paul Raymond 80 Harley Street, London W1G 7HL Tel: 07802 873621 Fax: 020 7602 2562 Email: paulsalmon@btinternet.com — MB BS Lond. 1961 (Middlx.) BSc (Anat., 1st cl. Hons.) Lond. 1958; MRCS Eng. LRCP Lond. 1961; FRCP Ed. 1977, M 1966; FRCP Lond. 1978, M 1967. p/t Cons. Phys. & Gastroenterologist, Independ. Med. Pract. Specialty: Gastroenterol.; Gen. Med. Socs: Chelsea Clin. Soc. (Counc.); Brit. Soc. of Gastroenterol. Prev: Cons. Phys. & Sen. Clin. Lect. (Gastroenterol.) Middlx. Hosp. Lond.; Sen. Lect. (Med.) Univ. Bristol & Cons. Phys. Bristol HA (T); Lect. (Med.) Univ. Bristol.

SALMON, Ralph Paul Red House Surgery, 96 Chesterton Road, Cambridge CB4 1ER Tel: 01223 365555 Fax: 01223 356848; 14 Hills Avenue, Cambridge CB1 7XA Tel: 01223 248354 — MB BS Sydney 1980 (University of Sydney) Clin. Asst. Chesterton Hosp. Cambs.; Police Surg. Camb. Specialty: Care of the Elderly. Prev: Regist. (Med.) Stoke Mandeville Hosp. Aylesbury; Regist. (Med.) P. of Wales Hosp. Sydney, Austral.; Resid. Med. Off. Roy. N. Shore Hosp. Sydney, Austral.

SALMON, Robert William (retired) Carrington House Surgery, 19 Priory Road, High Wycombe HP13 6SL Tel: 01494 526029 Fax: 01494 538299; Copper Beeches, Beamond End, Amersham HP7 0QT Tel: 01494 713303 — MB BS Lond. 1961 (Guy's) LMSSA Lond. 1957; DObst RCOG 1962. Company Med. Off. Bucks. Cadet Bn. Roy. Green Jackets; Exam Med. Pract. DoH. Prev: Clin. Asst. (Path.) Wexham Pk. Hosp. Slough.

SALMON, Roland Laurance, SBStJ NPHS Wales Communicable Disease Surveillance Centre, Abton House, Wedal Road, Cardiff CF14 3QX Tel: 029 2052 1997 Fax: 029 2052 1987 Email: roland.salmon@nphs.wales.nhs.uk — MB BS Lond. 1980 (St Bart.) MA Camb. 1978, BA 1974; DRCOG 1982; MRCGP 1984; FFPHM RCP (UK) 1995, M 1989. Cons. Epidemiol. Nat. Pub. Health Serv. for Wales. Specialty: Epidemiol. Prev: Sen. Regist. (Community Med.) W. Midl. RHA.

SALMON, Rosemarie Philomena The Grove Medical Centre, Church Road, Egham TW20 9QJ Tel: 01784 433159 Fax: 01784 477208; The Grove Medical Centre, The Grove, Church St., Egham TW20 — MB BS Lond. 1980; DRCOG 1986. Prev: Ho. Surg. St. Geo. Med. Sch. Hosp. Lond.; SHO (Anaesth. & Gen. Med.) Pboro. Dist. Hosp.; SHO (O & G & Paediat.) St. Peter's Hosp. Chertsey.

SALMONS, Paula Hilary — MB ChB Birm. 1966; DCH Eng. 1969; FRCPsych 1987, M 1976. Vis. Cons. Altrincham Priory Hosp. Specialty: Gen. Psychiat. Prev: Cons. Psychiat. & Hon. Clin. Lect. Salford HA; Sen. Lect. (Psychiat.) Univ. Birm.

SALOM DE TORD, Ramiro 17 The Millars, Broomfield, Chelmsford CM1 7HJ — LMS Barcelona 1982.

SALOOJA, Nina Charing Cross Hospital, Fulham Palace Road, London W6 8RF Tel: 020 8846 7122 Fax: 020 8846 7111 — MB BS Lond. 1986 (Oxford) MA Oxf. 1983; MRCP (UK) 1989; MRCPath 1999; DM 2001; MILTHE 2002. p/t Cons. Haemat.; Sen. Lect. (Investigative Sci. Div.) Imp. Coll. Sci. Tech. & Med. Lond. Specialty: Haematology. Special Interest: Late Efffects Foll. Stem Cell Transplants.

SALPEKAR, Shashikar Dattatray The New Surgery, Old Road, Tean, Stoke-on-Trent ST10 4EG Tel: 01538 722323 Fax: 01538 722215 — MB BS Vikram 1964 (Gandhi Med. Coll. Bhopal) Prev: Ho. Off. (Obst.) Preston Roy. Infirm.

SALT, Alane St Mark's Dee View Surgery, Church Street, Connah's Quay, Deeside CH5 4AD Tel: 01244 812003 Fax: 01244 822609 — MB BS Lond. 1984; BA Camb. 1981; DRCOG 1988. Specialty: Community Child Health.

SALT, Brigid Deirdre Medical Advisers Office, Foreign & Commomwealth Office, Old Admiralty Building, The Mall, London SW1A 2PA Tel: 020 7008 0595 Fax: 020 7008 0622; 13 Grafton Square, London SW4 0DQ Tel: 020 7652 6381 — MB BS Lond. 1970 (St. Bart.) MRCS Eng. LRCP Lond. 1970; D.Occ.Med. RCP Lond. 1995. Sen. Med. Adviser Foreign & Commonw. Off. Lond. Specialty: Occupat. Health. Prev: GP Stockwell; Regist. (Radiol.) & SHO St. Bart. Hosp. Lond.

SALT, Eric Michael (retired) Alyn Lodge, Gun St., Rossett, Wrexham LL12 0HR Tel: 01244 570495 — MB ChB Birm. 1950;

DObst RCOG 1957; MRCGP 1971; Cert. JCC Lond. 1977. Prev: GP Rossett.

SALT, John Campbell 126 Harley Street, London W1N 1AH Tel: 020 7935 9409 Fax: 020 7224 2520; 13 Grafton Square, London SW4 0DQ Tel: 020 7622 6988 — MB BS Lond. 1970 (St. Bart.) MRCS Eng. LRCP Lond. 1970; FFA RCS Eng. 1976. Cons. Anaesth. Char. Cross Hosp. Lond. Specialty: Anaesth. Prev: SHO (Anaesth.) Roy. Berks. Hosp. Reading; Regist. (Anaesth.) Sheff. AHA (T); Sen. Regist. (Anaesth.) Brompton Hosp. Lond.

SALT, Melanie Jane Mayfield Surgery, 54 Trentham Road, Longton, Stoke-on-Trent ST3 4DW Tel: 01782 315547; 6 Bergamot Drive, Meir Park, Stoke-on-Trent ST3 7FD — BM Soton. 1990 (Southampton University) DRCOG 1994; MRCGP 1997. Partner. Specialty: Gen. Pract.

SALT, Michael John Glenfield Surgery, 111 Station Road, Glenfield, Leicester LE3 8GS; Spion Lodge, Links Road, Kirby Muxloe, Leicester LE9 2BP Tel: 0116 238 8291 — MB ChB Liverp. 1978 (Liverp) MRCP (UK) 1986. Princip. GP Leicester. Prev: Trainee GP Measham Med. Unit Burton on Trent; Regist. (Med. & Geriat.) Leicester Gen. Hosp.; Regist. (Med.) St. Albans City Hosp.

SALT, Nicola Jill The Surgery, 77 Thurleigh Road, Balham, London SW12 8TZ Tel: 020 8675 3521 Fax: 020 8675 3800 — MB BS Lond. 1987; MRCP (UK) 1991.

SALT, Patrick John Department of Anaesthetics, Charing Cross Hospital, Fulham Palace Road, London W6 8RF Tel: 020 8846 1234; 24 Archway Street, Barnes, London SW13 0AR — MB BChir Camb. 1975; PhD Camb. 1972; FFA RCS Eng. 1982; BA Camb. 1968, MA 1 9970. Cons. Anaesth. Char. Cross Hosp. Lond. Specialty: Anaesth. Prev: Cons. Anaesth. St. Jas. Univ. Hosp. Leeds.; Cons. (Anaesth.) St. Vincent's Hosp., Dub.; Sen. Lect. & Hon. Cons. (Anaesth.) Qu. Eliz. Hosp. Birm.

SALT, Paula Jane 126 Viceroy, Close, Edgbaston, Birmingham B5 7UY Tel: 0121 446 5035 — MB ChB Birm. 1993; ChB Birm. 1993; MRCP (UK) 1998. Specialist Regist. (Geriat. & Gen. Med.) City Hosp. Birm. Specialty: Care of the Elderly; Gen. Med. Prev: Regist. Barnet Hosp. Lond.; SHO Roy. Masele Hosp. Lond.

SALT, Robert William Richards and Partners, Llanfair Surgery, Llanfair Road, Llandovery SA20 0HY Tel: 01550 720648 Fax: 01550 721428; Ty Rhawg, 74A Broad St, Llandovery SA20 0AY Tel: 01550 721006 — MB BCh Wales 1980; DRCOG 1982. Specialty: Paediat.

SALT, Susan Douglas Calderdale Royal Hospital, Salter Hebble Hill, Halifax HX3 0PW Tel: 01422 222710 — MB BS Lond. 1989 (St. Mary's Hospital Medical School) BSc Lond. 1983; DRCOG 1993; MRCGP 1994. Specialist Reigst. (Palliat. Med.); Macmillan Cons. in Palliat. Care. Specialty: Palliat. Med.

SALTER, Adrian Gerard 55 The Shades, Knights Place, Rochester ME2 2UB — MB ChB Leic. 1990.

SALTER, Angela Lilian The Surgery, Manor Fam Road, Bere Regis, Wareham BH20 7HB — BM Soton. 1980; DRCOG 1983; MRCGP 1985; DCCH RCGP & FCM 1986. Asst. GP Bere Regis.; Clin. Asst. Community Paediat., Weymouth, Dorset. Prev: Trainee GP Portland.

SALTER, David Graham Welsh Office, Cathays Park, Cardiff CF10 3NQ Tel: 029 2082 5402 Fax: 029 2082 5175 Email: david.salter@wales.gsi.gov.uk; Woodpeckers, St Andrew's Road, St Andrew's Major, Dinas Powys CF64 4HB Tel: 029 2051 5093 — (Cardiff) MB BCh Wales 1967. Princip. Med. Off. Specialty: Civil Serv. Socs: Brit. Assn. Day Surg.; Cardiff Med. Soc. Prev: Sen. Med. Off. Welsh Office Cardiff.

SALTER, Derek Harold Rex (retired) 265 Chells Way, Stevenage SG2 0HN — MB BS Lond. 1957; MRCS Eng. LRCP Lond. 1957. Prev: Surg. Lt.-Cdr. RN.

SALTER, Donald McGovern Milton House, Pencaitland, Tranent EH34 5EP — MD Ed. 1990; BSc (Hons.) Ed. 1978, MD 1990, MB ChB 1981; MRCPath 1989. Sen. Lect. Dept. Path. Med. Sch. Univ. Edin.

SALTER, Edmund John Assertive Outreach & Early Intervention Team, Sutton Health Centre, New Street, Sutton-in-Ashfield NG17 1BW Tel: 01623 602551 — MB BChir Camb. 1969 (Guy's) MRCP (UK) 1973; DPM Eng. 1974; MRCPsych 1974. Cons. Psychiat. Millbrook King's Mill Notts. Specialty: Gen. Psychiat. Prev: Sen. Regist. (Psychiat.) Mapperley Hosp. Nottm.; Regist. (Psychiat.) St. John's Hosp. Aylesbury; Ho. Surg. & Ho. Phys. Wycombe Gen. Hosp.

SALTER, Hazel Anne Department Child Health, East Lodge Court, High St., Colchester CO1 1UJ — MB ChB Leic. 1980; DRCOG 1982. Specialty: Community Child Health.

SALTER, Mrs Helen Rosemary — MB ChB Leic. 1988; FRCS Ed. 1996; FFAEM 2002. Specialist Regist. A & E Homerton Hosp. Lond. Specialty: Accid. & Emerg. Prev: Specialist Regist. A & E Oldenuran Hosp. Romford.

SALTER, John Charles The Health Centre, Beeches Green, Stroud GL5 4BH Tel: 01453 763980; The Orchard, Keble Road, France Lynch, Stroud GL6 8LU — MB ChB Sheff. 1983; DRCOG 1986; MRCGP 1987.

SALTER, Jonathan Philip Hartley Parkwood, Parklane, Knebworth SG3 6PP — MB BS Lond. 1983; DA (UK) 1986; DRCOG 1988; MRCGP 1989. Overseas Recruitment Off. (BUPA). Prev: Trainee GP Worcs. VTS.; Dir. Montpellier Health Care Ltd.

SALTER, Mrs Katherine Elizabeth Urmston Kings Road Surgery, Mumbles, Swansea SA3 4AJ Tel: 01792 360933; Southbourne, Groves Avenue, Langland, Swansea SA3 4QF — MB BS Lond. 1965 (Roy. Free) MRCS Eng. LRCP Lond. 1965; DCH Eng. 1967; MFFP 1993. Prev: Ho. Surg. New End Hosp. Lond.; Ho. Phys. St. And. Hosp. Bow.

SALTER, Mark Steven East Wing, Homerton Hospital, Homerton Row, London E9 6SR — MB BS Lond. 1983; MRCPsych 1989.

SALTER, Mark William Arthur Philip CDSC-SW, Gloucester GL1 3NN — MB BS Lond. 1996; PhD Lond. 1991; MSc Lond. 2000; DLSHTM Lond. 2000.

SALTER, Mr Michael Charles Patrick 4 Chadwick Road, Westcliff on Sea SS0 8LS Tel: 01702 353181 Fax: 01702 353181 — MB BS Lond. 1976; MRCS Eng. LRCP Lond. 1976; FRCS Eng. 1980. Cons. Gen. & Vasc. Surg., Southend Gen. Hosp.; Cons. Breast & Vasc. Surg., Southend Gen. Hosp. Specialty: Gen. Surg. Prev: Sen. Regist. (Gen. Surg.) Yorks. RHA.

SALTER, Penelope Ann Balham Health Centre, 120 Bedford Hill, London SW12 9HS Tel: 020 8673 1720 Fax: 020 8673 1549; 28 Lyford Road, Wandsworth Common, London SW18 3LT Tel: 020 8874 9802 — MB BS Lond. 1962 (Roy. Free) MRCS Eng. LRCP Lond. 1962.

SALTER, Robin Hugh (retired) 13 Newfield Drive, Kingstown, Carlisle CA3 0AG Tel: 01228 515318 — (Lond. Hosp.) BSc Lond. 1957; MB BS Lond. 1961; FRCP Lond. 1978, M 1964; Dip Med Educat. Dund 1996. Prev: Clin. Tutor Cumbld. Infirm. Carlisle.

SALTER, Sandra Helen Dragons Pool, Peterchurch, Hereford HR2 0TE — BM BS Nottm. 1989; MRCPsych 1994. Regist. (Psychiat.) W. Midl. Specialty: Gen. Psychiat.

SALTER, Mr Timothy Charles Michael 83 Corfe Road, Stoborough, Wareham BH20 5AY — MB BCh Wales 1980; FRCS Ed. 1986; FRCS Eng. 1988. Specialty: Accid. & Emerg.

SALTERS, Mark 57 Old Forge Manor, Belfast BT10 0HY — MB BCh BAO Belf. 1983; DGM 1987; MRCGP 1989; DRCOG 1990.

SALUCCI, Gabriele Umberto North Berwick Health Centre, 54 St Baldreds Road, North Berwick EH39 4PU Tel: 01620 892169 Fax: 01620 897005 — MB ChB Ed. 1987; BSc (Hons) Ed. 1984; MRCGP 1993. Trainee GP E. Cumbria VTS. Socs: BMA; Assoc. Mem. RCGP. Prev: Ho. Off. (Med. Surg.); Trainee GP. Edin. VTS.

SALUJA, Balijeet Kaur — MB BS Ranchi 1978; DRCPath (Lond.). Primary Care.

SALUJA, Gurpinder Singh — MB BS Ranchi 1973; DCH; MD; MRCP. Gen. Pract. Princip.

SALUJA, R S The Saluja Clinic, 36A Northcote Avenue, Southall UB1 2AY Tel: 020 8574 5136 — MB BS Calcutta 1974; MB BS Calcutta 1974.

SALUJA, Ranjeet Kaur 9 Cloister Crofts, Leamington Spa CV32 6QG Tel: 01926 428321 — MB BS Rajasthan 1968 (S.M.S. Med. Coll. Jaipur) Family Plann. Med. Off. Warks. HA.

SALUJA, Surinder Singh (retired) 'Ashton House' Surgery, 15 George St., Leamington Spa CV31 1ET; 9 Cloister Crofts, Leamington Spa CV32 6QG Tel: 01926 428321 — MB BS Lucknow 1967 (G.S.V.M Med. Coll. Kanpur) Prev: SHO (ENT) Bridgend Gen. Hosp.

SALUJA, Tilak Raj c/o Mr. S. Madan, 31 Banstead Road S., Sutton SM2 5LG — MB BS Lucknow 1966.

SALUKHE, Tushar Vilas 24 More Close, London W14 9BN — MB BS Lond. 1998; MB BS Lond 1998.

SALUSBURY, Ceri Alison Beech House Surgery, Beech House, 69 Vale Street, Denbigh LL16 3AU Tel: 01745 812863 Fax: 01745 816574 — MB ChB Manch. 1984.

SALUSBURY-TRELAWRY, Joanna Mary Leighton Hospital, Middlewich Road, Leighton, Crewe CW1 4QJ — MB ChB Cape Town 1984 (Univ. Cape Town) MRCP (UK) 1988; MD Cape Town 1996; FRCP Ed. 1997. Cons. Phys. (cardiol) Leighton Hopital Crewe. Specialty: Cardiol. Socs: Roy. Coll. of Phys.s of Edin. - Fell.; Brit. Cardiac Soc. - Fell.; Brit. Echocardiography Soc. - Fell. Prev: Cons. Phys. (Cardiol.) Trafford Gen. Hosp. Manch.

SALVAGE, Mr David Roy Department of Radiology, Hull Royal Infirmary, Anlaby Road, Hull HU3 2JZ Tel: 01482 328541; Broomfleet House, Ponds Lane, Broomfleet, Brough HU15 1RG — MB BS Lond. 1985 (The London Hospital Medical College) FRCS Glas. 1990; FRCR 1994. Cons. Radiol. Hull Roy. Infirm. Specialty: Radiol. Prev: Sen. Regist. & Regist. (Radiol.) Leeds/Bradford Train. Scheme.

SALVAJI, Abhijeetha Pentyla, Pannar Lane, Pentwynmawr, Newbridge, Newport NP11 4GY — MB BCh Wales 1998.

SALVAJI, Chandra Shaker Newbridge Medical Centre, High Street, Newbridge, Newport NP11 4FW Tel: 01495 243409 Fax: 01495 243746 — MB BS Osmania 1967.

SALVARY, Ingrid Althea Department of Dermatology, James Paget Hospital, Lowestoft Road, Gorleston, Great Yarmouth NR31 6LA — MB BS West Indies 1993; FRCP; Dip Dermat (Distinc.) St. John's Inst. Dermatol Lond. 1995.

SALVESEN, Mr Douglas Ronald Lister Hospital, Stevenage SG1 4AB Tel: 01438 314333; 7 Cranborne Avenue, Hitchin SG5 2BS Tel: 01462 457720 — MD Lond. 1994 (St. Thomas' Hospital London) MB BS 1986; MRCOG 1994. Cons. (O & G) Lister Hosp. Stevenage. Specialty: Obst. & Gyn. Prev: Sen. Regist. (O & G) Qu. Charlotte's Hosp. Lond.; Regist. St. Thos. Hosp. Lond. & Pembury Hosp. Kent; Research Regist. King's Coll. Hosp. Lond.

SALVESEN, Theodore Michael Noel (retired) Easter Catter, Croftamie, Drymen, Glasgow G63 0EX Tel: 01360 660575 Fax: 01360 660065 — MB ChB Ed. 1950.

SALVI, Anthony Ettore Keith (retired) 12 Rothesay Road, Dorchester DT1 2DT Tel: 01305 264908 — (Guy's) MRCS Eng. LRCP Lond. 1935. Emerit. Cons. Geriat. W. Dorset Health Dist. Prev: Med. Supt. Douglas Ho. Sanat. W. Southbourne.

SALWEY, Michael Geoffrey 14 Green Road, Weston, Stafford ST18 0JA — LMSSA 1997; LMSSA Lond. 1997.

SALZ, Mr Michael The Nuffield Hospital, Derriford, Plymouth PL6 8BG Tel: 01752 761803; 144 Harley Street, London W1N 1AH Tel: 020 7935 0023 — (Camb. & Middlx.) MA Camb. 1943, BA 1937; MRCS Eng. LRCP Lond. 1940; FRCS Eng. 1948. Socs: Fell. BOA & Roy. Soc. Med. Prev: Regist. Surg.) Princess Eliz. Orthop. Hosp. Exeter & Mt. Gould Orthop. Hosp. Plymouth; Cons. Orthop. Surg. Mt. Gould Orthop. Hosp. Plymouth & Plymouth Gen. Hosp.

SALZMAN, Nicholas George Woodlands Medical Centre, Woodland Road, Didcot OX11 0BB Tel: 01235 511355 Fax: 01235 512808 — MRCS Eng. LRCP Lond. 1973; DObst RCOG 1975; DCH Eng. 1975. GP Didcot.

SALZMANN, Maurice Brooke Department of Clinical Chemistry, Royal Devon & Exeter Hospital (Wonfrod), Barrack Road, Exeter EX2 5DW Tel: 01392 402933 Fax: 01392 402919; 16 Miller Way, St Martins Gardens, Exminster, Exeter EX6 8TH Tel: 01392 824324 Email: salzmann_millerway@tinyworld.co.uk — MB BS Lond. 1982 (King's Coll. Hosp.) MSc Lond. 1989, BSc 1979; MRCPath 1993; FRCPath 2001. Cons. Chem. Path. Roy. Devon & Exeter Hosp. Specialty: Chem. Path. Socs: Assn. of Clin. Biochem.s Ordinary Mem. Prev: Sen. Regist. (Chem. Path.) Roy. Devon & Exeter Hosp.; Regist. (Chem. Path.) Northwick Pk. Hosp. Harrow.

SALZMANN, Maurice Michael (retired) 10 Birch Close, Farnham GU10 4TJ Tel: 01252 792174 — LRCP LRCS Ed. LRFPS Glas. 1944 (Univ. Ed.) DPM Lond. 1951; MRCPsych 1972. Hon. Cons. Psychiat. Basingstoke & N. Hants Health Dist. Prev: Cons. Psychiat. Pk. Prewett Hosp. Basingstoke.

SAM, George Joseph 3 St Luke's Houses, Armagh BT61 7PJ Tel: 01861 2381 — MB BCh BAO Belf. 1965. Prev: Assoc. Specialist (Psychiat.) St. Luke's Hosp. Armagh; Regist. Psychiat. Downshire Hosp.; Ho. Phys. Moyle Hosp. Larne.

SAM, Rachel Clare 147 Galton Road, Bearwood, Smethwick B67 5JT Email: drsam@compuserve.com — MB ChB Manch. 1996; MA Camb. 1997. SHO (Surg.) Birm. Heartlands Hosp. Specialty: Gen. Surg. Prev: SHO (A & E) City Hosp. NHS Trust Birm.

SAMA, Mr Anshul Dept. of Otorhinolaryngology, Queens Medical Centre, University Hospital, Nottingham NG7 2UH Tel: 0115 924 9924 Ext: 35113 — BM BS Nottm. 1988; BMedSci Nottm. 1986; FRCS Ed. 1993; FRCS Eng. 1994; FRCS Otol 1997. Cons. Otorhinolaryngologist, Univ. Hosp., Nottm. Specialty: Otolaryngol. Prev: SHO (ENT) Univ. Hosp. Nottm.; SHO (Gen. Surg.) Leicester, Grantham & Kesteven Gen. Hosps.; SHO (ENT) Leicester Roy. Infirm.

SAMAAN, Amir Alphonse Abdoh Diana Princess of Wales Hospital, Scartho Road, Grimsby DN33 2BA Tel: 01472 874111 — MB BCh Cairo 1975; FFA RCSI 1985. Cons. Anaesth. North. Lincs. & Goole Hosps. NHS Trust. Specialty: Anaesth. Special Interest: Acute Pain Managem.; Obstetric Anaesth. Socs: Obst. Anaesth. Assn.; BMA.

SAMAAN, Anahita Hull Royal Infirmary, Kingston upon Hull, Hull HU3 2JZ Tel: 01482 328451; 9 Cassbrook Drive, Fulstow, Louth LN11 0XR Tel: 01507 363718 — MB BS Delhi 1976; DA Eng. 1980; FFA RCS Eng. 1982. Cons. Anaesth. Hull Roy. Infirm. Specialty: Anaesth. Prev: Sen. Regist. (Anaesth.) Leeds Gen. Infirm.

SAMAAN, Mr Nady Mekhaiel 18 Hornton Street, Kensington, London W8 4NR Tel: 020 7937 0040 — MB ChB Assiut 1973; MRCOG 1992; FRCS Ed. 1993.

SAMAD, Abdul c/o Drive Q. Zaman, 56 Scott Road, Denton, Manchester M34 6FT — MB BS Peshawar, Pakistan 1979; MRCP (UK) 1990.

SAMAD, Essam Mohamed Abdel-Monem 50 Aylmer Road, Highgate, London N2 0PL Tel: 020 8442 7077 Fax: 020 8442 7078 — MB BCh Ain Shams 1969. Specialty: Anaesth.

SAMADI, Nasar Roxbourne Medical Centre, 37 Rayners Lane, South Harrow, Harrow HA2 0UE Tel: 020 8422 5602 Fax: 020 8422 3911; 3 Wakehams Hill, Pinner HA5 3AQ Tel: 020 8866 8702 — MB BS Lucknow 1963 (King Geo. Med. Coll.) DTCD Wales 1969. Specialty: Respirat. Med. Prev: Hosp. Pract. (Cardiorespirat.) Watford Gen. Hosp.

SAMADIAN, Samad St Helier Hospital, Wrythe Lane, Carshalton SM5 1AA Tel: 020 8296 2518 Fax: 020 8296 2421 — FRCP; MD. Cons. Phys., Care of the Elderly, St Helier Hosp., Carshalton. Specialty: Care of the Elderly.

SAMAK, Mahrous Aziz Rophael 21 Links Court, Colbert Avenue, Thorpe Bay, Southend-on-Sea SS1 3BW — MB BCh Ain Shams 1956.

SAMAL, Kamdev Birches Head Medical Centre, Diana Road, Birches Head, Stoke-on-Trent ST1 6RS Tel: 01782 286843 Fax: 01782 535291 — MB BS Utkal 1975 (Sriram Chandra Bhanj Medical College Cuttack Orissa, India) Princip. (Gen. Pract.) Stoke-on-Trent. Socs: Med. Protec. Soc.

SAMANI, Professor Nilesh Jayantilal Department of Cardiology, Glenfield General Hospital, Groby Road, Leicester LE3 9QP Tel: 0116 256 3236 Fax: 0116 287 5792 Email: njs@le.ac.uk — MD Leic. 1994; BSc (Med Sci) Leics. 1978; MB ChB Leics. 1981; MRCP UK 1984; FRCP Lond 1994; FACC 1998; FMedSci 2002. Prof. of Cardiol. & Hon. Cons. Cardiol. Univ. Leicester & Glenfield Hosp.; Head of Dept. of Cardiovasc. Sci., Univ. of Leicester. Specialty: Cardiol. Special Interest: Molecular genetics of Cardiovasc. Dis. Socs: Brit. Cardiac Soc.; Assn. of Phys.s; Brit. Hypertens. Soc. (mem. Exec. Com.). Prev: Lect. & Hon. Sen. Regist. (Med.) Univ. Leicester; MRC Train. Fell. Univ. Leic.; SHO (Med.) Hammersmith Hosp. Lond.

SAMANIEGO, Nicolas Carlos — MB ChB Sheff. 1993; MRCP (Lond.) 1997. Specialist Regist. Barnsley Dist. Gen. Hosp.; Cons & Hon. Sen. Clin. Lect. Gen Internal Med. & Health Care of the Elderly. Specialty: Gen. Med.; Care of the Elderly. Prev: SpR Roy. Hallowshire Hosp.; SpR N. Gen. Hosp. Sheff.; SHO (Neurol.) Sheff.

SAMANTA, Amal Kumar 15 Merrydale Avenue, Eccles, Manchester M30 9DS — MB BS Calcutta 1972; MD All India Med. Scs. 1977; T(GP) 1991.

SAMANTA, Ashok Kumar University Hospital of Leicester, Leicester Royal Infirmary, Leicester LE1 5WW Tel: 0116 254 1414; The Mount, Great Glen, Leicester LE8 9FL — MB BS All India Inst. Med. Scs. 1977 (AU India Inst. Med. Sci. New Delhi) MD All India Inst Med. Scs. 1980; MRCP (UK) 1981; MD Leic. 1988; FRCP Ed. 1994; FRCP (Lond.) 2000. Cons. Phys. Rheum. Leicester Roy. Infirm.; Clin. Tutor (Med.) Univ. Leicester. Specialty: Rheumatol. Prev: Pfizer Clin. Research Fell.; Sen. Regist. (Med.) Leics. HA.

SAMANTA, Asok Kumar 1-3 St John's Road, East Ham, London E6 1NW Tel: 020 8503 5783; 37 Cheyne Avenue, South Woodford, London E18 2DP Tel: 020 8989 6363 Fax: 020 8989 6363 — (Calcutta Med. Coll.) MB BS Calcutta 1956. GP Lond. Socs: BMA. Prev: Regist. (Surg.) Lond. Jewish Hosp.; Regist. (Orthop.) Qu. Mary's Hosp. & E. Ham Mem. Hosp. Lond.; Regist. (Orthop.) Princess Margt. Hosp. Swindon.

SAMANTA, Kamal The Health Centre, Commercial Road, Skelmanthorpe, Huddersfield HD8 9DA Tel: 01484 862239; Skelmanthorpe Health Centre, Commercial Road, Skelmanthorpe, Huddersfield HD8 9DA Tel: 01484 862239 — (R.G. Kar Medical College Calcutta, West Bengal) MB BS Calcutta 1967. SHO Med. for the Elderly St. James Hosp. Leeds. Specialty: Gen. Pract.; Gen. Med. Socs: Hudds. Med. Soc.; Ex-Pres. R. G. Kas Med. Coll.

SAMANTA, Nabagopal 4 Wakerfield Close, Nelmes Park, Hornchurch RM11 2TH Tel: 0140 24 42350 — MB BS Calcutta 1965 (N.R.S. Med. Coll.) DO Eng. 1972.

SAMANTA, Renuka The Health Centre, Commercial Road, Skelmanthorpe, Huddersfield HD8 9DA Tel: 01484 862239; Samanta, Samanta & Welch, Skelmanthorpe Health Centre, Commercial Road, Skelmanthorpe, Huddersfield HD8 9DA Tel: 01464 862239 — (R.G. Kar Medical College Calcutta) MB BS Calcutta 1967. SHO G&O Huddersfield; SHO G&O Dewbury; SHO Psychiat. Huddersfield; Clin. Med. Off. Huddersfield; GP Skelmanthorpe Huddersfield. Specialty: Family Plann. & Reproduc. Health; Obst. & Gyn.; Paediat. Socs: Hudds. Med. Soc.; Disp. Pract. Assn.; ODA.

SAMANTA-LAUGHTON, Manjir Flat 2, 3 Blackdown Close, London N2 8JF — MB BS Lond. 1997.

SAMARAGE, Lalith Hiran Jessop Hospital for Women, Leavygreave Road, Sheffield S3 7RE Tel: 0114 276 6333 — MB BS Sri Lanka 1982; MRCOG 1991.

SAMARAGE, Mr Shantha Upali Department of Obstetrics & Gynaecology, Friarage Hospital, Northallerton DL6 1JG Tel: 01609 779911 — MB BS Sri Lanka 1976 (Colombo) MS (Obst. & Gyn.) Sri Lanka 1982, MB BS 1976; MRCOG 1985. Staff Grade (O & G) Friarage Hosp. NHS Trust N.allerton. Specialty: Obst. & Gyn. Prev: Regist. (O & G) St. Mary's Hosp. & Newc. Gen. Hosp.

SAMARAJIWA, Harsha Kamalochana 16 Silver Birch Avenue, Fareham PO14 1SZ — MB BS Ceylon 1968; MRCP (UK) 1981; MRCS Eng. LRCP Lond. 1981; FRCP Ed. 1992.

SAMARANAYAKE, Bernadette Marina 14 The Hawthorns, Wakefield WF1 3TL — MB BS Ceylon 1967. Specialty: Haematology.

SAMARANAYAKE, Joseph James 14 The Hawthorns, Wakefield WF1 3TL Tel: 01924 871151 — MB BS Sri Lanka 1970; FFA RCS Eng. 1979. Specialty: Anaesth.

SAMARASINGHE, Anuji Madara 34 Fontaine Road, London SW16 3PA — MB BS Lond. 1997.

SAMARASINGHE, Chatra Rajiv 34 Fontaine Road, London SW16 3PA — MB BS Lond. 1997.

SAMARASINGHE, Dunisha Gayomi 34 Fontaine Road, London SW16 3PA — MB BChir Manch. 1991.

SAMARASINGHE, Ivan Leslie Perera (retired) 225 Malden Road, New Malden KT3 6AG Tel: 020 8942 3394 — MB BS Ceylon 1942; LMS Ceylon Med. Coll. 1942; FDS RCS Eng. 1956, LDS 1951; DOrth RCS Eng. 1957.

SAMARASINGHE, Kaluaratchige Percy Bertram 64 Dollis Hill Lane, London NW2 6JG; 64 Dollis Hill Lane, London NW2 6JG Tel: 020 8452 1853 — MB BS Ceylon 1959 (Ceylon Med. Coll.) DPhysMed Eng. 1971. Med. Practitioner, Lond., Rheumatologist. Specialty: Rehabil. Med.; Rheumatol.; Clin. Neurophysiol. Prev: Cons. Rheum. Manor Hse. Hosp. Lond.; Clin. Asst. Roy. Free Hosp. Lond.

SAMARASINGHE, Lionel The High Road Surgery, 391 High Road, Wood Green, London N22 8JB Fax: 020 8881 4372 Email: dchall@doctors.org.uk — MB BS Ceylon 1968; MRCOG 1977. Cons. Gyn. Brit. Pregn. Advis. Serv. Specialty: Gen. Pract. Socs: Fell. Roy. Soc. Med.

SAMARASINGHE, Louis Alwis Taplow Dixon Day Unit, Yardley Green Unit, East Birmingham Hospital, Yardley Green Road, Birmingham B9 5PX Tel: 0121 766 6611; 67 Pavenham Drive, Birmingham B5 7TN — MB BS Ceylon 1968 (Peradiniya) DPM Eng. 1978. Assoc. Specialist Asst. (Psychogeriat.) W. Midl. RHA. Prev: Regist. (Psychiat.) Hollymoor Hosp. Birm.

SAMARASINGHE, Nihal 21 High Drive, New Malden KT3 3UJ Tel: 020 8949 3102 — MB BS Ceylon 1972 (Colombo) DCH Eng. 1980; MRCP (UK) 1983. Assoc. Specialist Epsom and St Helier NHS Trust. Specialty: Community Child Health. Socs: BMA; Roy. Coll. of Paediat. and Child Health. Prev: Regist. (Paediat.) Brook Gen. Hosp. Lond.

SAMARASINGHE, Pulun Chandrika 21 High Drive, New Malden KT3 3UJ Tel: 020 8949 3102 — MB BS Sri Lanka 1976 (Colombo) Staff Grade (Anaesth.) Roy. Surrey Co. Hosp. Guildford. Specialty: Anaesth. Socs: Med. Protec. Soc.; Assn. Anaesth.; BMA. Prev: Regist. (Anaesth.) Princess Margt. Hosp. Swindon.

SAMARASINGHE, Sujith Rohantha 20 Woodbine Lane, Worcester Park KT4 8SZ — MB BS Lond. 1998 (Imperial Coll.) BSc (Hons.) Lond. 1995.

SAMARASINGHE, Wickramapala 5 The Pastures, Welwyn Garden City AL7 4PX — MB BS Sri Lanka 1966; DPM Eng. 1979; MRCPsych 1983. Med. Fac. (Univ. Colombo); Assoc. Specialist W. Herts. Community NHS Trust. Specialty: Gen. Psychiat. Prev: Regist. (Psychiat.) Qu. Eliz. II Hosp. Welwyn Gdn. City; Regist. (Psychiat.) Princess Alexandra Hosp. Harlow & Barnet Gen. Hosp.

SAMARASINGHE, Yohan Pradeep — MB BS Lond. 1994 (Char. Cross & Westm.) BSc (Hons.) Lond. 1992; MRCP Lond. 1999. SHO (Haemat. & Gen. Med.) Lewisham Hosp. Lond.; SpR (Clin. Pharmacol. & Gen. Internal Med.) Chelsea & Westm. Hosp. Specialty: Gen. Med. Prev: SHO (Cardiol. & Med.) Kingston Hosp.; SHO (Genitoryurin. Med. & HIV) Chelsea & Westm. Hosp.; SHO (Respirat. & Gen. Med.) Frimley Pk. Hosp.

SAMARATUNGA, Mr Ranasinhage Dayaratna c/o Albany House, 41 Judd Street, London WC1H 9QS — MB BS Ceylon 1957; DLO (Eng.) RCP Lond. 1963; FRCS Ed. 1973. Socs: BMA.

SAMARATUNGA, Varuna Sanjaya Taylor Joynson Garrett, Carmelite, 50 Victoria Embankment, Blackfriars, London EC4Y 0DX Tel: 020 7353 1234 Fax: 020 7936 2666; 34 Elmer Cottages, Guildford Road, Fetcham, Leatherhead KT22 9BU — MB BS Lond. 1990 (King's Coll.) BSc (Hons.) Immunol. Lond. 1987; AKC 1990; DFFP 1993; DGM RCP Lond. 1993; DRCOG 1994; MRCGP 1995; Dip (LLB) 1996; Dip. (Legal Practice) 1997. Lawyer. Specialty: Gen. Pract. Prev: Trainee GP Oxf.; SHO (Paediat.) Northampton Gen. NHS Trust; SHO (Geratol.) Radcliffe Infirm. Oxf.

SAMARAWICKRAMA, Mrs Padma Grace Purley Medical Practice, 73 Lansdowne Road, Purley CR8 2PE — MB BS Ceylon 1968; MRCP (UK) 1974. Clin. Asst. (Geriat.) Hither Green Hosp. Prev: GP Purley; Sen. Lect. (Clin. Pharmacol.) Fac. Med. Peradeniya, Sri Lanka.

SAMAVEDAM, Sam Microbiology, Western Infirmary, Dumbarton Road, Glasgow G11 6NT Tel: 0141 211 2246; 0/1 46 Clarence Drive, Glasgow G12 9TQ Tel: 0141 576 4431 — MB BS Andhra 1973. Staff Grade Microbiol. West. Infirm. Glas. Specialty: Med. Microbiol. Socs: BMA; Hosp. Infec. Soc.; Scott. Microbiol. Assn.

SAMBANDAN, Mr Sidheshwara Bonsai Surgery, Bowthorpe Health Centre, Wendene, Bowthorpe, Norwich NR5 9HA Tel: 01603 748255 Fax: 01603 740741; Sailands, 44 Brettingham Avenue, Cringleford, Norwich NR4 6XQ Tel: 01603 507070 Fax: 01603 506605 — MB BS Colombo 1972 (Colombo, Ceylon) MRCS Eng. LRCP Lond. 1978; FRCS Eng. 1981; MRCGP 1988; DFFP 1996; FRCGP 1997. GP CME Tutor Norwich Dist.; Clin. Asst. (Adult Psychiat.) Town Cl. Clinic & W. Norwich Hosp.; Hon. Sen. Lect. Univ. E. Anglia, Norwich. Specialty: Gen. Pract. Prev: Lect. (Orthop. Surg.) Traumatol. Univ. Malaya; Clin. Specialist Orthop. Surg. Univ. Hosp. Kuala Lumpur.

SAMBASIVA RAO, Mr Gundabolu Shotley Bridge Hospital, Consett DH8 0NB Tel: 01207 583583 Ext: 4317 — MB BS Andhra 1977 (Andhra India) FRCS Ed. 1984; T(S) 1993. Cons. Plastic & Reconstruct. Surg. Specialty: Plastic Surg.

SAMBATAKAKIS, Andreas Orthopaedic Department, Birmingham Heartlands Hospital, Bordesley Green E., Birmingham B9 5SS; 11 Graham Court, Graham Road, Sheffield S10 3DX — State Exam Med Erlangen 1973.

SAMBROOK, Andrew James Sycamore House, Oram Road, Brindle, Chorley PR6 8NT — MB ChB Manch. 1995.

SAMBROOK, Janice Helen 4 Garlands Road, Redhill RH1 6NT; 4 Garlands Road, Redhill RH1 6NT — MB ChB Sheff. 1992. Specialty: Gen. Pract.

SAMBROOK, Martin Gerard 49 Lenzie Road, Stepps, Glasgow G33 6BZ — MB BS Lond. 1992.

SAMBROOK, Michael Andrew 135 Palatine Road, Manchester M20 34A Tel: 0161 445 0332/01689 833735 Fax: 01625 584 5347; Southbarn, Whitebarn Road, Alderley Edge SK9 7AN Tel: 01625 590197 — MB ChB Birm. 1966; MRCP (UK) 1969; MD Birm. 1972; FRCP Lond. 1983. Indep. Med. Pract. Manch. Specialty: Neurol. Socs: Assn. Brit Neurol. Prev: Lect. (Neurol.) Univ. Manch.; Regist. (Neurol.) Nat. Hosp. Nerv. Dis. Qu. Sq. Lond.; Sheldon Research Fell. N. Staffs. Hosp. Centre Stoke-on-Trent.

SAMBROOK, Pauline Southbarn, Whitebarn Road, Alderley Edge SK9 7AN Tel: 01625 590197 — MB ChB Birm. 1967; DMRD Eng. 1979; FRCR 1981. Cons. Radiol. Univ. Hosp. S. Manch.; Lect. (Radiol.) Univ. Manch. Specialty: Radiol. Prev: Cons. Radiol. Stepping Hill Hosp. & Stockport Infirm.; Sen. Regist. (Diag. Radiol.) Manch. Roy. Infirm.

SAMEJA, S High Street Surgery, High Street, Pelsall, Walsall WS3 4LX Tel: 01922 694186 Fax: 01922 682644 — MB BS Karnatak 1977; MB BS Karnatak 1977.

SAMES, Mr Christopher Patrick (retired) Mamre, The High St, Norton St Philip, Bath BA2 7LH Tel: 01373 834547 — MB BS Lond. 1937 (St. Mary's) MRCS Eng. LRCP Lond. 1937; FRCS Eng. 1939; MS Lond. 1943. Hon. Cons. Surg. Bath Clin. Area. Prev: Asst. Dir. Surgic. Unit St. Mary's Hosp.

SAMES, Matthew Peter 28 Creslow Way, Stone, Aylesbury HP17 8YW — MB ChB Birm. 1987; FRCA 1995. Specialty: Anaesth.

SAMI, Ammed Sami Abd El Hamid The Bungalow, Llantrisant Road, Pontyclun CF72 8NJ — MB BCh Cairo 1972.

SAMI, Naweed 25 St Martins Road, Portland DT5 1JY — MB BS Punjab 1975.

SAMI, Mr Shahid Ahmed 7 Corcullentragh Road, Portadown, Craigavon BT62 4JB — MB BS Karachi 1982; FRCS Ed. 1989.

SAMI, Syed Z A St David's Street Surgery, St David's Street, Ton Pentre, Pentre CF41 7NE Tel: 01443 435846 Fax: 01443 431480.

SAMIEI, Haidar Reza 172C George Street, Aberdeen AB25 1HU — MB ChB Aberd. 1998; MB ChB Aberd 1998.

SAMJI, Faisal 18 Skipton Avenue, Chadderton, Oldham OL9 0QA — MB ChB Dundee 1981; DCH RCP Lond. 1983; DRCOG 1986.

SAMMES, Heidi Ruth Weston Cottage, 2 Crown Hill, Weston, Bath BA1 4DE — BM Soton. 1995. Socs: MPS; BMA.

SAMMON, Mr Alastair Macnaughton Department of Surgery, Gloucestershire Royal Hospital, Great Western Road, Gloucester GL1 3NN Tel: 01452 395643 Fax: 01452 395643 — MB ChB Glas. 1971 (Glasgow) Dobst RCOG 1973; FRCS Glas. 1978; MD (Hons.) Glas. 1992; MD Hons Glas. 1993. Cons. Breast Surg. Gloucester Roy. Hosp. Gloucester; Honarary Sen. Lect. in Surg. Univ. of Bristol. Specialty: Gen. Surg. Socs: Christ. Med. Fellowsh.; Brit. Assn. Surg. Oncol; Brit. Soc. Gastroenterol. Prev: Med. Off. i/c Chogoria Hosp., Kenya; Sen. Lect. & Princip. Surgic. Specialist Umtata Transkei, S. Afr.

SAMMON, Mr Douglas John Orthopaedic Department, Royal Hospital for Sick Children, Glasgow G3 8SJ Tel: 0141 201 0276; 10 Kidston Drive, Helensburgh G84 8QA Tel: 01436 675340 — MB ChB Glas. 1969; DObst RCOG 1971; FRCS Glas. 1974; FRCS Ed. (Orth) 1980. Cons. Orthop. Surg. Roy. Hosp. Sick Childr. Glas. Specialty: Orthop. Prev: Cons. Orthop. Surg. CrossHo. Hosp. Kumarnock.

SAMMON, Reverend Helen Mary Kirkman Windycot, Cranham, Gloucester GL4 8HS Email: helen.sammon@doctors.org.uk — MB ChB (Hons.) Bristol 1982; MA Camb. 1979; DCH RCP Lond. 1984; MRCGP 1997; DRCOG 1998. GP Retainer. Specialty: Gen. Pract. Prev: Palliat. Care Med. Off.; SHO (Obstetris & Gyn.); Med. Off. Chogoria, Kenya.

SAMMON, Paul Matthew 5 Chestnut Close, Summerwood Lane, Halsall, Ormskirk L39 8SY — MB ChB Aberd. 1950; DPH Aberd. 1953; MFCM 1974. Prev: DMO W. Lancs. HA, Lancs. CC & MOH Accrington Dists., Yorks. W. Riding CC & MOH Colne Valley Area.

SAMMONS, Helen Mary 214B Loughborough Road, West Bridgford, Nottingham NG2 7EE — MB ChB Birm. 1996.

SAMMUT, Mr Donald Paul The Hand Clinic, Oakley Green, Windsor SL4 4LH Tel: 01753 838431 Fax: 01753 832109; The Chesterfield Nuffield Hospital, 3 Clifton Hill, Bristol BS8 1BP Tel: 0117 973 5544 — MRCS Eng. LRCP Lond. 1980 (Char. Cross) FRCS Eng. 1984; FRCS (Plast) 1994. Cons. Hand Surg., The Hand Clinic,Windsor, The Chesterfield Nuffield, Bristol; Vis. Lect. / Hand Surg. Humanitas Hosp. Milan. Specialty: Plastic Surg. Socs: Of Counc.: Brit. Hand Soc.; Brit. Assn. of Plastic Surgeons. Prev: Cons. Plastic Surg. Frenchay Hosp. Bristol (1993-2003); Sen. Regist. (Plastic Surg.) Withington Hosp. Manch.; Regist. (Plastic Surg.) St. And. Hosp. Billericay.

SAMMUT, Mario Saviour Freeman Hospital, Freeman Road, High Heaton, Newcastle upon Tyne NE7 7DN Tel: 0191 284 3111 Fax: 0191 223 1180 — MD Malta 1984; LRCP LRCS Ed. LRCPS Glas. 1988; MRCP (UK) 1989; FRCA 1994; FFA RCSI 1994. cons. Anaesth. Freeman Hosp. New. u. Tyne. Specialty: Anaesth. Prev: Sen. Regist. (Anaesth.) North. Region.; Regist. Rotat. (Anaesth.) Newc. u. Tyne; SHO (Anaesth.) Roy. Vict. Infirm. Newc. u. Tyne.

SAMMUT, Robert St. Ann's Hopsital, St. Ann's Road, London N15 Tel: 020 8442 6000; 74 Jessel House, Judd St, London WC1H 9NX Tel: 020 7837 2040 — MB BCh BAO NUI 1983; MRCPsych 1988. Sen. Regist. Rotat. (Psychiat.) St. Bart. Hosp. Med. Sch. Lond.; Sen. Regist. (Psychiat.) St. Ann's Hosp. Lond. Specialty: Gen. Psychiat. Prev: Research Psychiat. TAPS Friern Hosp. Lond.; Regist. (Psychiat.) Friern Hosp. Lond.; SHO (Psychiat.) Whittington Hosp. Lond.

SAMMUT ALESSI, Carmel William Churchill Medical Centre, Clifton Road, Kingston upon Thames KT2 6PG Tel: 020 8546 1809 Fax: 020 8549 4297; 40 Cranes Park, Surbiton KT5 8AD Tel: 020 8399 5489 Fax: 020 8399 5489 — MRCS Eng. LRCP Lond. 1980. Vice-Chairm. Kingston & Richmond HA; Chairm. Kingston & Richmond Drug & Therap. Comm.; Non-Exec. Dir. Primary Care Agency. Specialty: Gen. Pract. Prev: Non-Exec. Dir. Kingston & Richmond FHSA; Assoc. Med. Dir. Kingston & Dist. Community Trust; Hosp. Pract. Kingston Hosp. Trust.

SAMPATH, Mr Raghavan — MB BS Madras 1986; FRCS Ed. 1990; FCOphth 1990. Cons. (Ophth. Surg.) Leicester Roy. Infirm.; Hon. Sen. Lect. Leicester Univ. Specialty: Ophth. Special Interest: Ophth. Plastics.

SAMPATH, Mr Shameem Anthony Carl Blackpool Victoria Hospital, Whinney Heys Road, Blackpool FY3 8NR Tel: 01253 303546 — MB BS West Indies 1980; FRCS Ed. 1987; MChOrth Liverp. 1991. Cons. Orthop. Surg. Specialty: Orthop.

SAMPEYS, Carolyn Susan Old Mill Farmhouse, Lettons Way, Dinas Powys CF64 4BY — BM Soton. 1982; DRCOG 1984; MRCPCH 1997. Assoc. Specialist (Community Paediat.) Cardiff Community Healthcare Trust. Specialty: Community Child Health. Prev: SCMO (Community Paediat.) S. Glam.

SAMPLE, Sally Obank (retired) Emberside House, Warkworth, Morpeth NE65 0XA Tel: 01665 711321 — (Dundee) MB ChB St. And. 1963; DObst RCOG 1965; DA Eng. 1966; DCH RCPS Glas. 1967. SCMO (Wom.s Health) & Clin. Asst. (Anaesth.) Northumberland HA.; CMO Family Plann. N.umbrid Health Care Trust. Prev: SCMO Wom.'s Health & Clin. Asst./Anaesth.

SAMPSON, Andreas The Park Lane Medical and Surgical Services, 625 Green Lane, Hornsey, London N8 0RE — MB BCh Wales 1974.

***SAMPSON, Anna Louise** — BM BCh Oxf. 1998; BM BCh Oxf 1998. Ho. Off. (Gen. Surg.), John Radcliffe Hosp. Prev: Ho. Off. (Gen. & Resp. Med.), Glos. Roy. Hosp.

SAMPSON, Christopher Stuart Beacon Surgery, Beacon Road, Crowborough TN6 1AF Tel: 01892 652233 Fax: 01892 668840 — MB BS Lond. 1974; DRCOG 1977; DCH Eng. 1978. Med. Off. Health Screening Clinic, Nuffield Hosp., Tonbridge Wells, Kent, TN2 4UL. Prev: Vis. Med. Off. Horder Centre for Arthritis CrowBoro.; Ho. Off. (Surg.) King's Coll. Hosp. Lond.

SAMPSON, Elizabeth Lesley — MB ChB Birm. 1993; MRCPsych 1999. Lect. Dept. Of Psychiat. & Behavioural Sci. Roy. Free Hosp. Pond St. Lond. NW3. Prev: SHO (Psychiat.) St. Mary's Hosp. Lond.; SHO (Psychiat.) Hill End Hosp. St. Albans; Resid. Med. Off. (Intens. Care & Trauma) Liverp. Hosp. Sydney.

SAMPSON, Gwyneth Ann (retired) Rampton Hospital, Retford DN22 0PD; Hanbury House, Main St, Ulley, Sheffield S26 3YD Tel: 0114 287 2150 — MB ChB Sheff. 1967; DPM Eng. 1970; FRCPsych 1991, M 1972. Mem. Parole Bd. Hon. Con. Rampton Hosp. Prev: Med. Dir. & Cons. Psychiat. Rampton Hosp. Retford.

SAMPSON, Harvey Charles Reginald Burnham Medical Centre, Love Lane, Burnham-on-Sea TA8 1EU Tel: 01278 795445 Fax:

01278 793024; Venture, 34 Rectory Road, Burnham-on-Sea TA8 2BZ Tel: 01278 795504 Email: hcrsampson@aol.com — MB BS Lond. 1976 (St Mary's) MRCS Eng. LRCP Lond. 1976. Chairm. - Som. LMC; Clin. Tutor Bristol Univ. Med. Sch.

SAMPSON, Mrs Jane Magretha c/o Kuswin Hospital, Kuswin, Pakistan; Copt. Hall Cottage, Little Wigborough, Colchester CO5 7RD Tel: 0120635 349 — BM BCh Oxf. 1950 (Oxf. & Middlx) MA; DTM & H 1988. Miss. Doctor Ch. of Pk.istan. Prev: Clin. Med. Off. Sch. Colchester.

SAMPSON, John Stephen Heathgate Surgery, The Street, Poringland, Norwich NR14 7JT Tel: 01508 494343; Woodton Grange, Woodton, Bungay NR35 2LP — BM Soton. 1978; DCH Eng. 1981; DCH Eng. 1981. Chairm. S. Norf., Primary Care Gp., S. Norf.

SAMPSON, Professor Julian Roy Institute of Medical Genetics, University of Wales College of Medicine, Cardiff CF14 4XN Tel: 029 2074 3922 Fax: 029 2074 7603 — MB BS Nottm. 1982; DM Nottm. 1990, BMedSci 1980; MRCP (UK) 1985; MSc Glas. 1987; FRCP 1996. Prof. Med. Genetics Univ. Wales Coll. Med.; Hon. Cons. Clin. Genetics. Specialty: Genetics.

SAMPSON, Kathleen (retired) Sandiway, Sir William Hill Road, Grindleford, Hope Valley S32 2HS Tel: 01433 630693 — MB ChB Sheff. 1949. Prev: Asst. Med. Off. (Insp. Nursing Homes) Sheff. HA.

SAMPSON, Keith MUBZKA and Partners, 1 North Street, Peterborough PE1 2RA Tel: 01733 312731 Fax: 01733 311447; 194 Broadway, Peterborough PE1 4DT — MB ChB Ed. 1974. JP.

SAMPSON, Madeleine Anne Department of Radiology, Southampton General Hospital, Tremona Road, Southampton SO16 6YD; 18 Olivers Battery Road North, Winchester SO22 4JA — MB ChB Leic. 1982; MRCP (UK) 1985; FRCR 1988; FRCP Lond. 1998. Cons. Radiol. Soton. Univ. Hosps. Trust. Specialty: Radiol. Special Interest: Musculoskeletal Disorders. Socs: RCR; BMA; BIR. Prev: Cons. Radiol. Roy. Hants. Co. Hosp. Winchester; Sen. Regist. (Radiol.) Northwick Pk. Hosp. Harrow Middlx.; Regist. (Radiol.) Hallamsh. Hosp. Sheff.

SAMPSON, Marianne Tove 35 Northover Road, Westbury on Trym, Bristol BS9 3LN — BChir Camb. 1996.

SAMPSON, Michael John Norfolk & Norwich University Hospital NHS Trust, Brunswick Road, Norwich NR1 3RS — MD Lond. 1992 (St Thomas' Hospital) BSc Lond. 1980, MD 1992, MB BS 1983; MRCP (UK) 1986; FRCP 1998. Cons. Phys. Norf. & Norwich Healthcare NHS Trust. Specialty: Diabetes; Endocrinol.; Gen. Med. Prev: Sen. Regist. (Diabetes & Endocrinol.) Middlx. & Univ. Coll. Hosps. & Whittington Hosp. Lond.; Research Fell. (Diabetes) King's Coll. Hosp. Lond.

SAMPSON, Peter William Sheringham Medical Practice, Health Centre, Cromer Road, Sheringham NR26 8RT Tel: 01263 822066 Fax: 01263 823890 — MB BS Lond. 1982 (St. Mary's) BSc (2nd cl. Hons.) Physiol. Lond. 1978; MRCS Eng. LRCP Lond. 1981; DRCOG 1985.

SAMPSON, Rena Dora 27 Oakleigh Park S., Whetstone, London N20 9JS — MB BCh Witwatersrand 1958; BSc Witwatersrand 1954; DCH Eng. 1961. Sen. Med. Off. (Community Med.) Enfield, Haringey & Barnet DHAs; Family Plann. & Psychosexual Counsellor. Specialty: Psychosexual Med.; Family Plann. & Reproduc. Health. Socs: MFFP; BSMDH; Inst. Psychosexual Med. Prev: Sen. Res. Med. Off. Belgrave Hosp. Childr. Lond.; Res. Med. Off. Qu. Eliz. Hosp. Childr. Lond.

SAMPSON, Rod Paul 3 Woodside Terrace, Raigmore Hospital, Inverness IV2 3UJ — MB ChB Aberd. 1996. GP Regist. on Inverness GP Scheme. Specialty: Gen. Pract.

SAMPSON, Sarah Ruth Muluskha Manali Cottage, Gilwern, Abergavenny NP7 0ER — MRCS Eng. LRCP Lond. 1983; DLO RCS Eng. 1986. GP Wimbledon. Prev: SHO (ENT, A & E & O & G) Roehampton Hosp.

SAMPSON, Stephen Andrew 7 Top Park, Beckenham BR3 6RU — MB BS Lond. 1986.

SAMRA, Gurdip Singh 50 Allendale Avenue, Southall UB1 2SW; 145 Oswald Road, Southall UB1 1HJ — MB BS Lond. 1986; BSc (Biochem.) Lond. 1983, MB BS 1986.

SAMRA, Jagbir Singh The Lodge, Chamberlains Lane, Penn, Wolverhampton WV4 5HT — MD Birm. 1992; MB ChB 1981; MRCOG 1986. Cons. O & G New Cross Hosp. Wolverhampton. Specialty: Obst. & Gyn. Prev: Sen. Regist. (O & G) Birm. Matern. Hosp. & Birm. & Midl. Hosp.; Regist. (O & G) Dudley Rd. Hosp. Birm.; Clin. Research Fell. Univ. Birm.

SAMRA, Mr Jaswinder Singh 21 Delbush Avenue, Headington, Oxford OX3 8EA — MB ChB Manch. 1988; FRCS Eng. 1992; FRCS Ed. 1993. Wellcome Research Regist. Univ. Oxf. Specialty: Gen. Surg.

SAMRA, Manjeet Kaur Penn Manor Medical Centre, Manor Road, Penn, Wolverhampton WV4 5PY Tel: 01902 331166 Fax: 01902 575078; The Lodge, Chamberlains Lane, Penn, Wolverhampton WV4 5HT — MB ChB Manch. 1982; MRCGP 1986; DRCOG 1986.

SAMRAI, Paramjit Singh Regional Medico-Legal Service, Pelham House, Peterborough District Hospital, Thorpe Road, Peterborough PE3 9NH Tel: 01733 875283 Fax: 01733 875003; 7 Green Lane, Warwick CV34 5BP Tel: 01926 497153 — (Med. Coll. St. Bart. Hosp. Univ. Lond.) MB BS Lond. 1986; LLB (Hons.) Sheff. 1991. Regional Medico-Legal Adviser. Prev: SHO (Anaesth.) Jas. Paget Hosp. Gt. Yarmouth; SHO (A & E) Colchester Gen. Hosp.; SHO (Med. & Med. for Elderly) Rochford Hosp. Essex.

SAMS, Virginia Ruth Norfolk and Norwich Hospital, Department of Histopathology, Colney Lane, Norwich NR4 7UY Tel: 01603 286013 Fax: 01603 286017 Email: virginia.sams@nnuh.nhs.uk — MB ChB Sheff. 1979; BSc (Hons.) Sheff. 1976; FRCS Ed. 1984; FRCPath 2000. Cons. (Histopath.) Norf. & Norwich Univ. Hosp.; Lect. UEA Med. Sch. Specialty: Histopath. Socs: Brit. Soc. of Gastroenterol.; Internat. Acad. of Path. Prev: Sen. Lect. (Histopath.) Univ. Coll. Lond.

SAMSAMI, Shahla Monireh 17 King's Avenue, Woodford Green IG8 0JD Tel: 020 8505 3211 Fax: 020 8559 1161 — (St. Mary's) MRCS Eng. LRCP Lond. 1969; MB BS Lond. 1969; DObst RCOG 1971.

SAMSON, Geoffrey John 9 Orchard Rise, Richmond TW10 5BX Tel: 020 8876 1684 — (St. Mary's) MRCS Eng. LRCP Lond. 1961; T(GP) 1991. Indep. GP Lond. Specialty: Gen. Pract. Socs: Fell. Roy. Soc. Med.; W Lond. M-C Soc.; BMA. Prev: Ho. Surg. & Ho. Phys. Harold Wood Hosp.

SAMSON, Hilarie Christine Stonydelph Health Centre, Ellerbeck, Tamworth B77 4JA; Idle Hollow, 71 South St, Atherstone CV9 1ED — MB ChB Birm. 1986; DCCH 1994. Staff Grade (Communiy Paediat.) Tamworth. Specialty: Community Child Health.

SAMSON, Jadhav Daniel Health Centre, Great James Street, Londonderry BT48 7DH Tel: 028 7137 8522; 51 Stoneypath, New Buildings, Victoria Road, Londonderry BT47 2AF Tel: 01504 312789 — (Christian Med. Coll. Ludhiana) MB BS Panjab (India) 1966; DCH Punjab (India) 1972. GP Lond.derry. Specialty: Gen. Psychiat. Prev: Regist. (Ment. Health) N. Irel. Hosps. Auth.

SAMSON, Margaret Noel (retired) 5 Millwood Rise, Overton, Wrexham LL13 0EL Tel: 01978 710335 — BM BCh Oxf. 1955 (Oxf. & King's Coll. Hosp.) MA, BM BCh Oxf. 1955. Prev: GP Overton, Wrexham.

SAMSON, Patricia Woraine The Old School House, Falls of Truim, Newtonmore PH20 1BE Tel: 01540 673011 — MB BS Sydney 1981; MA Melbourne 1964.

SAMSWORTH, Peter Raymond (retired) 26 Western Esplanade, Herne Bay CT6 8RW Tel: 01227 374364 — BM BCh Oxf. 1954; DObst RCOG 1959. Prev: GP Herne Bay.

SAMTANEY, Narendra Thaverdas Airedale General Hospital, Skipton Road, Steeton, Keighley BD20 6TD Tel: 01535 652511; 3 Oaklands, West Wood Drive, Ilkley LS29 9RE Tel: 01943 817797 — MB BS Gujarat 1975; MD Gujarat 1978; MRCOG 1985; MFFP 1994. Cons. O & G Airedale Gen. Hosp. Keighley. Specialty: Obst. & Gyn. Prev: Sen. Regist. North. Region.

SAMTANI, Akash The Surgery, 939 Green Lanes, Winchmore Hill, London N21 2PB Tel: 020 8360 2228 Fax: 020 9360 5702 — BM Soton. 1990; DFFP 1993; MRCGP 1994. Specialty: Gen. Pract. Prev: SHO (Paediat. A & E) Qu. Eliz. Hosp. Hackney.; Trainee GP Soton.; SHO (A & E) Soton. Gen. Hosp.

SAMTANI, Bhagwan Khushaldas, OBE Chatur Nivas, 158 Northampton Road, Kettering NN15 7JY — MB BS Bombay 1955 (G.S. Med. Coll.) FRCP Lond. 1977, M 1962. Private Med. Specialty: Gen. Med. Socs: BMA; Kettering Med. Soc.; N.ampton Med. Soc. Prev: Cons. Phys. Kettering HA; Sen. Regist. (Med.) Northampton Gen. & Assoc. Hosps.; Regist. (Med.) High Wycombe & Dist. Hosp. Gp.

SAMUDRI, Meheboob Fhakaruddin The Surgery, 33 Penrose Street, London SE17 3DW Tel: 020 7703 3677 — MB BS Karnatak 1971 (Karnatak Med. Coll. Hubli) MRCOG 1984, D 1980. GP Lond.; Clin. Asst. (Obst. & Gyn.) St. Thos. Hosp. Lond. Prev: Regist. (O & G) Roy. Infirm. Huddersfield; SHO (O & G) Cameron Hosp. Hartlepool; GP Trainee Lond.

SAMUEL, Mr Alan Warwick Baybridge Farm, Owslebury, Winchester SO21 1JN Tel: 01962 777515 — MB ChB Manch. 1970; FRCS Eng. 1976; FRCS Ed. 1976; MD 1981. Cons. Orthop. Surg. Roy. Hants. Co. Hosp. Specialty: Orthop. Socs: Mem. Brit. Orthopaedic Assn.; Mem. Brit. Orthopaedic Research Soc.; Mem. Brit. Soc. Surg. of the Hand. Prev: Sen. Regist. Manch. Roy. Infirm. & Hip Centre Wrightington Hosp.

SAMUEL, Anne Margaret EDF Energy, 134 Harley Street, London W1G 7JY Tel: 020 7486 3801 Fax: 020 7486 3804; 50 Clifton Hill, St. John's Wood, London NW8 0QG Tel: 020 7625 5697 — MB BS Lond. 1977; MRCP Lond. 1980; FFOM RCP Lond. 1993, MFOM 1988, AFOM 1984; MSc Lond. 1984; FRCP Lond. 1987. Occupat. Health Adviser Lond. Electric plc; Assessor for GMC Performance Procedures, 1998. Specialty: Occupat. Health. Socs: Fell. Roy. Soc. Med.; Soc. Occupat. Med. Prev: Sen. Employm. Med. Adviser Health & Safety Exec. N. Lond.

SAMUEL, Carolyn 29 Brynfield Road, Langland, Swansea SA3 4SX — MB ChB Manch. 1980; MRCGP 1984.

SAMUEL, Claire Amanda Laurel Bank Surgery, 216B Kirkstall Lane, Leeds LS6 3DS Tel: 0113 230 7474 Fax: 0113 230 2475; 7 The Cresent, Alwoodley, Leeds LS17 7LU — MB ChB Bristol 1981; MB ChB (Hon.) Bristol 1981; MRCGP 1985; DRCOG 1985.

SAMUEL, David Ponniah Royal Marsden Hospital, Department of Paediatric Oncology, Downs Road, Sutton SM2 5PT Email: dsamuel@doctors.org.uk; Apartment 2125N, 5500 Friendship Boulevard, Chevy Chase 20815, USA Tel: 00 1 301 6567664 — MB ChB Dundee 1989; BSc (Hons.) Med. Biol. St. And. 1984. Clin. Research Fell. Roy. Marsden Hopsital Sutton; Hon. Clin. Lect., Qu. Mary and Westfield Coll. Lond.; Specialist Regist., (Paediatric Neuro-Oncol.), Roy. Maisden Hosp., Sutton. Specialty: Paediat. Socs: Brit. Med. Assn.; Amer. Soc. of Paediatric Hemotolgy Oncol.; Amer. Assn. of Cancer Research. Prev: ICRF, Clin. Research Fell.; Paediatric Oncol., Barts and the Roy. Lond. Hosp., Lond.; Clin. Fell. Paediatric Oncol., Nat. Cancer Institue, USA.

SAMUEL, Iain Scott 85/4 East London Street, Edinburgh EH7 4BQ — MB ChB Aberd. 1998; MB ChB Aberd 1998. Specialty: Accid. & Emerg.

SAMUEL, Mr Jacob Department of Surgery, Central Middlesex Hospital, Park Royal, London NW10 7NS Tel: 020 8965 5733 Fax: 020 8453 2418 — MB BS Kerala India 1986; MS Kerala India 1989; FRCS Ed. 1995. Assoc. Specialist (General Surgery) Centr. Middlx. Hosp. Lond. Specialty: Gen. Surg.

SAMUEL, Janice Louise Grovemead Health Partnership, 67 Elliot Road, Hendon, London NW4 3EB Tel: 020 8203 4466 Fax: 020 8203 1682 — MB BS Lond. 1988.

SAMUEL, Leslie McGillivray Clinical Oncology Department, Aberdeen Royal Infirmary, Foresterhill, Aberdeen Fax: 01224 404495/01224 553499 — MB ChB Ed. 1989; BSc (Hons.) Glas. 1982; MSc Surrey 1984; MRCP (UK) 1992; FRCR 1997; FRCP Edin. 2002. MacMillan Cons. Oncologist, Aberd. Roy. Infirm. Specialty: Oncol.; Radiother. Prev: Regist. (Med. Oncol.) Auckland Hosp. NZ; SHO (Med.) Roy. Infirm. & East. Gen. Hosp. Edin.; Sen. Regist. (Oncol.) West. Gen. Hosp. Edin.

SAMUEL, Malcolm Clifford 14 Fearnley House, Vestry Road, London SE5 8JW — MB BS West Indies 1983.

SAMUEL, Malcolm Sajjad 4 Stubden Grove, Clifton Moor, York YO30 4UY — MB BS Punjab, Pakistan 1982.

SAMUEL, Mr Mark John Taff Vale Surgery, Duffryn Road, Rhydyfelin, Pontypridd CF37 5RW Tel: 01443 400940 Fax: 01443 492900 — MB BCh Wales 1978; FRCS Ed. 1983.

SAMUEL, Mary Baybridge Farm, Owslebury, Winchester SO21 1JN — MB ChB Manch. 1970; DObst RCOG 1972.

SAMUEL, Mary Harrow Road Surgery, 110 Harrow Road, Leytonstone, London E11 3QE Tel: 020 8519 5627 Fax: 020 8519 9879 — MB BS Colombo 1979; MB BS Colombo 1979.

SAMUEL, Memy 9 The Hermitage, Dunmurry, Belfast BT17 9NH — MB BS Panjab 1970.

SAMUEL, Michel Sadek Hayes Grove Priory Hospital, Prestons Road, Hayes, Bromley BR2 7AS Tel: 020 8462 7722; The Somerfield Hospital, London Road, Maidstone ME16 0DU Tel: 01622 686581 — MB BCh Ain Shams 1956; Dip. Med. Ain Shams 1965; DPM Ain Shams 1965; BA (Psych.) Ain Shams 1969; FRCPsych 1974. Hon. Cons. Psychiat. St. Thos. Health Dist. & Maidstone Invicta Community. Specialty: Gen. Psychiat. Socs: Fell. Roy. Soc. Med. Prev: Cons. Psychiat. Maidstone Health Dist.; Sen. Regist. St. Thos. Health Dist.

SAMUEL, Oliver Wilfred (retired) 24 Lancaster Grove, London NW3 4PB Tel: 020 7419 4624 — MB BCh BAO Dub. 1954; BA Dub. 1952; MB BCh BAO Dub, 1954; DObst RCOG 1958; FRCGP 1980, M 1965. Prev: Clin. Audit Advisor to RCGP 1990-94.

SAMUEL, Mr Peter Roger Ashmore Consulting Rooms, 2 Ashmore Terrace, Sunderland SR2 7DE Tel: 0191 514 0666 Fax: 0191 567 0356; Dalkeith Lodge, Aykley Heads Farm, Durham DH1 5AN Tel: 0191 386 5811 — MB ChB Ed. 1967; FRCS Ed. 1972. Cons. Otolaryngol. Sunderland, Durh. & S. Tyneside AHAs. Specialty: Otolaryngol. Socs: Roy. Soc. Med.; N. Eng. Otolaryngological Soc.; BMA. Prev: Sen. Regist. (ENT) Newc. Univ. Hosps.

SAMUEL, Roger de Koning Graham (retired) 39 Alexandra Road, Epsom KT17 4DA Tel: 01372 812747 — MB BS Lond. 1957; MRCS Eng. LRCP Lond. 1957; MRCP Lond. 1964; DMRD Eng. 1965; FFR 1969.

SAMUEL, Rohit Cherian 32 Westwick Road, Sheffield S8 7BT — MB ChB Manch. 1997.

SAMUEL, Ronald Aneurin (retired) Southway Surgery, Bampfylde Way, Southway, Plymouth PL6 6TA Tel: 01752 776650 Fax: 01752 770249; Bowlea, 20 Great Berry Road, Crownhill, Plymouth PL6 5AU Tel: 01752 777312 Fax: 01752 777312 — MB BCh Wales 1966 (Cardiff)

SAMUEL, Saramma Boyne Avenue Surgery, 57 Boyne Avenue, Hendon, London NW4 2JL Tel: 020 8203 2230 Fax: 020 8202 7900 — MB BS Madras 1972; MB BS Madras 1972.

SAMUEL, Thomas Wyn Uplands Surgery, 48 Sketty Road, Uplands, Swansea SA2 0LJ Tel: 01792 298554 / 298555 Fax: 01792 280416 — MB BS Lond. 1976; DA Eng. 1978; DRCOG 1980; MRCGP 1981.

SAMUEL-GIBBON, Andrew George Askwith Road, Saintbridge, Gloucester GL4 4SH Tel: 01452 500252 Fax: 01452 387844 — BM BCh Oxf. 1970 (Oxf. & Guy's) BA Oxf. 1967; MRCP (UK) 1973; DCH Eng. 1974; DObst RCOG 1974; DTM & H Liverp. 1975; MRCGP 1983. Socs: Soc. Orthopaedic Med. Prev: Govt. Med. Off. Malawi.

SAMUELS, Abigail Research Registrar, Rheumatology Unit, Bristol Royal Infirmary, Bristol BS2 8HW Fax: 01179 928 3841 Email: abigail.samuels@bris.ac.uk; 69 Old Park Riding, London N21 2ER — MB BS Lond. 1990; MRCP Lond. 1993. Clin. Research Fell. Rheum. Unit Bristol Roy. Infirm. Univ. Div. of Med. Bristol. Specialty: Rheumatol.

SAMUELS, Andrew Jonathan Laurie Park Road Health Centre, Park Road, Radyr, Cardiff CF15 8DF Tel: 029 2084 2767 Fax: 029 2084 2507 — MB BS Lond. 1987.

SAMUELS, Bernard Rosarden, 56A Waterloo Road, Hillside, Southport PR8 2LR Tel: 01704 66150 — MB ChB Manch. 1944. Prev: Res. Med. Off. North. Hosp. Manch. & City Gen. Hosp. Stoke-on-Trent; Res. Surg. Off. Eccles & Patricroft Hosp.

SAMUELS, Lisa Simone 7 Chaworth Road, West Bridgford, Nottingham NG2 7AE Tel: 0115 982 7239 — MB BS Lond. 1991; BSc Lond. 1988. Trainee GP Nottm. Train. Scheme.

SAMUELS, Martin Philip University Hospital of North Staffordshire, Academic Department of Paediatrics, Stoke-on-Trent ST4 6QG Tel: 01782 715444 Fax: 01782 713946 Email: martin.samuels@uhns.nhs.uk — MB BS Lond. 1981 (Guy's) MRCP (UK) 1984; FRCP 1992; FRCPCH 1992; BSc Lond. 1978, MD 1992. Cons. Paediat. Univ. Hosp. N. Staffs. Stoke-on-Trent; Sen. Lect. (Paediat.) Univ. Keele. Specialty: Paediat. Special Interest: APLS; Non-invasive Ventilation; Sleep Disorders. Socs: Brit. Paediatric Respirat. Soc.; Paediatric Intens. Care Soc. Prev: Lect. (Paediat.) Nat. Heart & Lung Inst. Roy. Brompton Hosp. Lond.; Research Fell. & Regist. (Paediat.) Roy. Brompton Hosp. Lond.; Regist. (Paediat.) Hillingdon Hosp. Uxbridge.

SAMWAYS, Diana Marjorie PO Box 52, Haslemere GU27 1JA Tel: 01428 643021 Fax: 01428 654850 — MB BS Lond. 1964 (Roy. Free) MRCS Eng. LRCP Lond. 1964. Indep. Cons. Addic. Disorders, Eating Disorders, Environm. Med. and Food and Inhalant Allergies, Surrey; Hon. Life Mem. (Exec. Comm.) Med. Counc. Alcoholism. Specialty: Alcohol & Substance Misuse. Socs: Soc. Occupat. Med.; Expert Witness Inst.; Treas. Brit. Soc. Allergy & Nutrit. Med. Prev: Cons. Addic. Dis. Unit Charter Clin. Chelsea Lond.; Ho. Surg. Roy. Free Hosp. Lond.; Ho. Phys. Hither Green Hosp. Lond.

SAMY, Mr Ahmed Kamal Eldin Mohamed North East Lincolnshire NHS Trust, Diana, Princess of Wales Hospital, Scartho Road, Grimsby DN33 2BA Tel: 01472 874111 Fax: 01472 875646 Email: aksamy@ntlworld.com — MB BCh Ain Shams 1978; FRCS Glas 1987; LRCP Ed. LRCS Ed. LRCPS Glas. 1987; FRCS Ed. 1987; MSc, Glas. 1991; FACA 1993; MD, Aberd. 1997. Cons. Gen. & Vasc. Surg. Diana, Princess of Wales Hosp.; Extern. Examr., Ismailia Univ. Med. Sch.; Examr., Roy. Coll. of Surg.s of Edin. Specialty: Gen. Surg. Socs: Vasc. Surg. Soc.; Assn. Surgs.; Brit. Assn. of Endocrine Surg.s. Prev: Cons. Surg. Dumfries & Galloway Acute NHS Trust Scotl.

SAMY, Mahmoud Alaa Eldin Diana Princess of Wales Hospital, Paediatric Department, Grimsby DN33 2BA — MB BCh Al-Azhar 1982; MSc (Paediat.) Al-Azhar 1989. Assoc. Specialist Paediat. Specialty: Neonat.; Gastroenterol. Socs: Assoc. Mem. Roy. Coll. Paediat. & Child Health; Yorks. Paediat. Soc.; Brit. Assn. Perinatal Med. Prev: Staff Grade Paediat.; Paediat. Regist.; Paediat. SSHO.

SAN, Suman Moira 20 Abingdon Drive, Reading RG4 6SD Tel: 01189 476944; 23 Joseph Conrad House, Tachbrook St, Pimlico, London SW1V 2NF Tel: 020 7821 0702 — MB BS Lond. 1990 (Royal Free Hospital) DRCOG; MRCGP. Asst. GP. Specialty: Gen. Pract. Prev: SHO (O & G) St. Thos. Hosp. Lond.; SHO (A & E) Chase Farm Hosp. Enfield; SHO (ENT) Luton & Dunstable Hosp.

SAN THEIN, Dr 52 Goddard End, Stevenage SG2 7ER — MB BS Rangoon 1956.

SANAGHAN, Sarah Ann 19 Kirkton Place, E. Kilbride, Glasgow G74 4HS — MB ChB Glas. 1991.

SANAI, Leyla Department of Anaesthetics, Western Infirmary, Dumbarton Road, Glasgow G11 6NT Tel: 0141 211 2069; 2nd Floor Left, 137 Hyndland Road, Glasgow G12 9JA Tel: 0141 339 4885 — MB ChB Ed. 1989 (Edinburgh) MRCP (UK) 1992; FRCA 1994. Cons. Anaesth., Western Infirm., Glas.; News Edr. Brit. Jl. Intens. Care; News Edr. Internat. Jl. Intens. Care; Freelance Contributor to Herald Newspaper. Specialty: Anaesth. Prev: Specialist Regist. Anaesth., Western Infirm. Glas.; Sen. Health Off. (Intens.r Care, Coronary Care & Gen. Med.) Western Gen. Hosp. Edin.; Sen. Health Off. (Anaesth.) Western Infirm. Glas.

SANATI, Mohammad 33 Templars Avenue, London NW11 0NU — MD Tehran 1970; MRCPsych 1983.

SANCHEZ, Efren German Churchgate Surgery, 119 Manchester Road, Denton, Manchester M34 3RA Tel: 0161 336 2114 Fax: 0161 320 7045; 33 Reddish Lane, Gorton, Manchester M18 7JH Tel: 0161 223 9438 — Medico Cirujano Peru 1975. GP Tameside FHSA. Prev: Trainee GP Tameside VTS; Regist. (Radiother.) Manch. HA; SHO (Gen. Med.) Bolton HA.

SANCHEZ, Maria-Jose Flat 2, 22 More Lane, Esher Green, Esher KT10 8AD — MB BS Lond. 1990.

SANCHEZ-ANDRADE BOLANOS, Jose Maria Royal United Hospital, Bernard Ireland Hospital, Flat 7-C, Bath BA1 3NG — LMS Santiago de Compostela 1988.

SANCHEZ-MOYANO LEA, Jose Manuel The Charlton Lane Medical Centre, Charlton Lane, Cheltenham GL53 — LMS Cadiz 1994.

SAND, Priscilla Rosemary 5 Selborne Road, Croydon CR0 5JQ — MB BCh BAO NUI 1966; DCH NUI 1968.

SANDALL, Deborah 3 Deans Walk, Durham DH1 1HA — BM Soton. 1993; Dip. Anaesth. 1997.

SANDARS, John Edward Cheadle Hulme Health Centre, Smithy Green, Cheadle Hulme, Cheadle SK8 6LU Tel: 0161 485 7233; Wilmslow Road Medical Centre, 166 Wilmslow Road, Handforth, Wilmslow SK9 3LF Tel: 01625 523102 — MB ChB Sheff. 1975; MB ChB (Hons.) Sheff. 1975; MRCP (UK) 1978; FRCGP 1994, M 1982; Cert. Family Plann. JCC 1987; Dip. Palliat. Med. Wales 1993. Lect. (Gen. Pract.) Univ. Manch.; Examr. & Exam Course Tutor RCGP; Vice-Chairm. Stockport Med. Audit Advis. Gp. Specialty: Gen. Med. Socs: BMA. Prev: Clin. Tutor (Gen. Pract.) Stepping Hill Hosp. Stockport; SHO (Paediat.) N. Staffs. Hosp. Stoke-on-Trent; SHO (O & G) Hope Hosp. Manch.

SANDBACH, Christopher Shaun 68 Killingworth Drive, Sunderland SR4 8QX — MB BS Newc. 1984.

SANDBERG, Michael Duncan Alexander Cadogan Place Practice, 29 Cadogan Place, London SW1X 9RX Tel: 020 7235 5850 Email: msandberg@cppractice.com — MB BS Lond. 1983 (Char. Cross) MRCGP 1994. GP Princip. In Private Pract.; Echocardiography, Lond. Clinic. Prev: Regist. (Cardiol. & Chest Med.) St. Mary's Hosp. Lond.

SANDBERG, Seija Unelma Tuulikki 131 Court Lane, London SE21 7EE — Lic Med. Turku, Finland 1970.

SANDBY-THOMAS, Mark Glynn 22 Malvern Road, Maida Hill, London NW6 5PP — MB BS Lond. 1996.

SANDE, Winston George Theodore Chanterlands Avenue Surgery, 149-153 Chanterlands Avenue, Hull HU5 3TJ Tel: 01482 343614; 149-153 Chanterlands Avenue, Hull HU5 3TJ Tel: 01482 43614 — MB BS Bangalore 1969; MRCS Eng. LRCP Lond. 1978.

SANDELL, Julian Mark — MB BS Lond. 1992 (Roy Free Hosp.) MRCPI 1997. Specialist Regist. (Paediat.) Basildon Hosp. N. Thames Deanery; Paediatric Accid. & Emerg. St. Mary's Hosp., Paddington, N. Thames Deanery. Specialty: Paediat. Socs: MDU; BMA; Assoc. Mem. RCPCH. Prev: SpR PICU, St. Mary's Hosp.; Specialist Regist. (Paediat.) Southend Hosp. N. Thames Deanery; Community Paediat. Sen. SHO Enfield Community Care Trust Chase Farm Hosp. Middlx.

SANDEMAN, Alison Peters East Riding, The Gardens, Sion Road, Bath BA1 2TJ — MB BS Lond. 1985 (Univ. Coll. Lond.) DMRD Liverp. 1990; FRCR 1993. Cons. Radiol. Roy. United Hosp. NHS Trust Bath. Specialty: Radiol. Prev: Sen. Regist. Rotat. (Radiol.) SW RHA; Regist. Rotat. (Radiol.) Mersey RHA; Regist. & SHO Rotat. (Med.) King's Coll. Hosp. Lond.

SANDEMAN, Mr David Robert Department of Neurosurgery, Frenchay Hospital, Bristol BS16 1LE Tel: 0117 975 3956 Fax: 0117 970 1161 Email: info@david-sandeman.com — MB BS Lond. 1979 (Westm.) BSc Lond. 1975, MB BS 1979; FRCS Ed. 1983. Cons. Neurosurg. Frenchay Hosp. Bristol. Specialty: Neurosurg. Socs: Soc. of Brit. Neurosurgeons; BMA; RSM. Prev: Regist. (Neurosurg.) Walton Hosp. Liverp.; Sen. Regist. (Neurosurg.) Manch. Roy. Infirm. & Hope Hosp. Salford.

SANDEMAN, Derek David Southampton University Hospital, Tremona Road, Southampton SO16 6YD Tel: 023 8079 8472; Merrie Orchard, Football Green, Minstead, Lyndhurst SO43 7FR — MB BS Lond. 1983; FRCP Lond. 1999. Cons. Endocrinologist, Soton. Univ. Hosps. Specialty: Endocrinol. Prev: Sen. Regist. (Diabetes & Endocrinol.) Univ. Hosp. Wales Cardiff.

SANDEMAN, James Meldrum Cruden Medical Group, The Surgery, Main St Hatton, Peterhead AB42 0QQ Tel: 01779 841208 Fax: 01779 841239; Gowanlea, Hatton, Peterhead AB42 0RX — MB ChB Aberd. 1972 (Aberdeen) DObst RCOG 1974; MRCGP 1976. GP. Specialty: Gen. Pract.

SANDEMAN, Mr John Charles (retired) Oak Lee, Pound Lane, Burley, Ringwood BH24 4EE; 72 Rodney Street, Liverpool L1 9AF — MB BCh Witwatersrand 1952; FCS (S. Afr.) 1963; FRCS Ed. 1963; FRCS Eng. 1963; MChOrth Liverp. 1964. Indep. Orthop. Pract. Liverp. Prev: Cons. Orthop. Surg. Arrowe Pk. & Clatterbridge Hosps.

SANDEMAN, John Graeme (retired) 153b Burton Road, Woodville, Swadlincote DE11 7JW — MB ChB Glas. 1954.

SANDER, Clare Rachel — BM BCh Oxf. 1997; MRCP 2000. Clin. Research Fell. Univ. of Oxf. Prev: SpR Respirat. Med. N. W. Thames Deanery.

SANDER, Professor Josemir Wanderley National Hospital for Neurology and Neurosurgery, Institute of Neurology, Queen Square, London WC1N 3BG Tel: 020 7837 3611 Fax: 020 7837 3941 Email: lsander@ion.ucl.ac.uk — Medico Federal U Parana Brazil 1981 (Faculdade de Medicina, U Parana) PhD Lond. 1994; MRCP Royal College of Physicians 2000. Prof. (Neurol.) Univ. Coll. Lond.; Cons. Neurol. Chalfont Centre, Chalfont St. Peter; Hon. Cons. Neurol. Nat. Hosp. for Neurol. & Neurosurg. Lond.; Mem. of the Managem. Comm. of the Internat. League Against Epilepsy. Specialty: Neurol. Socs: BMA; Fell. RSM. Prev: Sen. Regist. Chalfont Centre; Sen. Lect. (Neurol.), Inst. of Neurol., Lond.

SANDER, Peter Nicholas (retired) — MB BS Lond. 1973; Cert. Av. Med. 1983.

SANDERCOCK, Professor Peter Andrew Gale Department of Clinical Neurosciences, Western General Hospital, Edinburgh EH4 2XU Tel: 0131 537 2928 Fax: 0131 332 5150 — BM BCh Oxf. 1976; MRCP (UK) 1978; DM Oxf. 1985; FRCP Ed. 1991. Prof. (Neurol.) Univ. of Edin.; Hon. Cons. (Neurol.) Western Gen. Hosp., Edin. Specialty: Neurol. Socs: Assn. Brit. Neurols.; Brit. Atherosclerosis Soc.; Brit. Stroke Research Gp. Prev: Lect. (Neurol.) Walton Hosp. Liverp.; Research Sen. Regist. (Neurol.) Radcliffe Infirm. Oxf.; Regist. (Neurol.) N. Manch. Gen. Hosp. & Manch. Roy. Infirm.

SANDERCOTT, Anne Meryl A&E Department, Royal Berkshire Hospital, London Road, Reading RG1 5AN Tel: 01189 875111; Greenray Cottage, Sunnyside, Theale, Reading RG7 4BE Tel: 01189 302697 — MB ChB Ed. 1981; DA Eng. 1984. Clin. Asst. (A & E) Roy. Berks. Hosp. Reading.

SANDERS, Alison Jane 131 Penrhyn Road, Sheffield S11 8UP; 9 Westfield Road, Bengeo, Hertford SG14 3DL — MB ChB Sheff. 1995. SHO A+E. Specialty: Accid. & Emerg. Prev: SHO (Orthop. & A & E) Northern Gen. Hosp. Sheff.; Ho. Off. Rotherham Dist. Gen.

SANDERS, Anne Deborah Cadbury Heath Health Centre, Parkwall Road, Cadbury Heath, Bristol BS30 8HS Tel: 0117 980 5706 Fax: 0117 960 0164 — MB ChB Bristol 1989; DCH RCP Lond. 1994; DRCOG 1995; MRCGP 1996. Specialty: Gen. Pract.

SANDERS, Awena Ffowcs Royal Dundee Liff Hospital, Dundee DD2 5NF; The Old Bridge House, Douglastown, Forfar DD8 1TL — MB ChB Manch. 1992 (St Andrews and Manchester) BSc 1989; MRCPsych 1997. Specialist Regist. (Psychiat.) Roy. Dundee Liff Hosp. Specialty: Gen. Psychiat. Socs: BMA; MDU. Prev: SHO (Psychiat.) Roy. Dundee Liff Hosp.; SHO (Psychiat.) Corn Hill Hosp. Aberd.; SHO (Med.) Glan Clwyd Hosp.

SANDERS, Caroline Roberta The Queen Edith Medical Practice, 59 Queen Ediths Way, Cambridge CB1 8PJ Tel: 01223 247288 — MB BS London 1984 (UCH, London) MRCP (Glas.); BSc (Hons.) Biochemistry (Univ. Sussex) 1975; Research MPhil (Cambs.) 1977. Gen. Practitioner. Specialty: Gen. Pract.; Gen. Med.

SANDERS, David John 18 Sandwon Close, Downend, Bristol BS16 6SJ — BM BCh Oxf. 1985.

SANDERS, David Surendran Consultant Gastroenterologist, Gastroenterology & Liver Unit, Royal Hallamshire Hospital, Sheffield S10 2JF — MB ChB Glas. 1991; MRCP (UK) 1996; FACG 2003; MD 2003. Action Research Train. Fell. 1999-2001. Specialty: Gastroenterol. Prev: Specialist Regist. (Gastroenterol. & Internal Med.) Sheff. 1996; Action Research Training Fellow 1999-2001.

SANDERS, Donald Scott Anderson Dept. of Histopathology, Warwick Hospital, Warwick CU34 5BW Tel: 01926 495321 Email: scott.saunders@swh.nhs.uk — MB ChB Dundee 1983; MD; FRCPath; MRCPath Glas. 1990. Cons. Histopath. UHB NHS Trust Birm.; Hon. Cons. Path. Birm. Gen. Hosp. Specialty: Gastroenterol.; Histopath. Prev: Sen. Regist. (Histopath.) Ninewells Hosp. Dundee.

SANDERS, Eileen Mary The Hadleigh Practice, Hadleigh Lodge, 216A Warhem Road, Corfe Mullen, Wimborne BH21 3LN Tel: 01202 694721; 21 Sorrel Way, Wyke, Gillingham SP8 4TP Tel: 01747 826578 — BM Soton. 1986 (Southampton University) DRCOG 1990. GP; Med. Adviser W. Dorset Youth Advis. Serv. Specialty: Gen. Pract.

SANDERS, Eric Universyt Hospital of North Durham, North Road, Durham DH1 5TW Tel: 0191 333 2597 Fax: 0191 333 2747; 101 Thorntons Close, Pelton, Chester-le-Street DH2 1QJ Tel: 0191 370 2133 — MB BCh Wales 1971; MRCP (UK) 1974; FRCP Lond. 1990. Cons. Phys. Univ. Hosp. of N. Durh., Co. Durh. Specialty: Gen. Med.; Diabetes. Prev: Cons. Phys. W. Wales Gen. Hosp. Carmarthen; Lect. (Renal Dis.) Roy. Infirm. Cardiff; Hon. Regist. Research Fell. Inst. Renal Dis. Roy. Infirm. Cardiff.

SANDERS, Fiona Elizabeth Heron Practice, John Scott Health Centre, Green Lanes, London N4 2NU Tel: 020 7690 1172 Fax: 020 8809 6900 — MB BS Lond. 1986 (UCH/Middlesex) MRCGP 1991; DFFP 1991. GP Principle. Specialty: Gen. Pract.

SANDERS, Frances Louise 35 Lansdowne Road, Tonbridge TN9 1JD — MB BS Lond. 1998; MB BS Lond 1998.

SANDERS, Gillian Linda Tees Health Authority, Poole House, Stokesley Road, Nunthorpe, Middlesbrough TS7 0NJ Tel: 01642 320000; 178 Osborne Road, Jesmond, Newcastle upon Tyne NE2 3LE — MB BS Newc. 1973; FFPHM; MRCP (UK) 1976; MFPHM 1987; MD Newc. 1989; FRCP Ed. 1995. Dir. of Pub. Health. Specialty: Pub. Health Med. Prev: Cons. Epidemiol. North. RHA.; Sen. Lect./Cons. Pub. Health Med. Newc. & N. Tyneside HA.

SANDERS, Gillian Margaret 20 Bernard Gardens, London SW19 7BE — MB BS Lond. 1980; DCH RCP Lond. 1984; DRCOG 1985.

SANDERS, Mr Grant — MB BS Lond. 1992 (St Mary's Hosp.) FRCS 1997; MD plymouth 2003. Specialty: Gen. Surg.

SANDERS, John Carl 28 Orchard Road E., Manchester M22 4ER Tel: 0161 613 1965 — MB BS Lond. 1986; FRCA 1998. Specialty: Anaesth.

SANDERS, Jonathan Hume Lonsdale 18 Manor Drive, Newcastle upon Tyne NE7 7XN — MB BS Lond. 1990 (St. Geo.) MRCPsych 1996. Specialty: Geriat. Psychiat.

SANDERS, Judith Ann St Ann's Medical Centre, Effingham Street, Rotherham S65 1BL Tel: 01709 379283/364437; 1 Clifton Crescent N., Rotherham S65 2AS Tel: 01709 837656 — MB ChB Sheff. 1983 (Sheffield University) DCH RCP Lond. 1987; MRCGP 1990.

SANDERS, Julia 36 Home Park Road, London SW19 7HN — MB ChB Liverp. 1980; MRCPsych 1987; Dip. Human Sex Univ. Lond. 1991; Dip. Criminol. Lond. 1996.

SANDERS, Kenneth 20 Basing Hill, London NW11 8TH Tel: 020 8458 7809 — MB ChB Leeds 1951; MRCGP 1958; MD Leeds 1959. Specialty: Psychother. Socs: Brit. Psychoanal. Soc. Prev: Ho. Phys. & Ho. Surg. Wakefield Gen. Hosp.; Capt. RAMC.

SANDERS, Mr Kevin John Maxillofacial Unit, Wythenshawe Hospital, Southmoor Road, Manchester M23 9LT Tel: 0161 291 4995 Fax: 0161 291 4996; The Willows, 1 Hillside, Heaton, Bolton BL1 5DT Tel: 01204 845172 — MB BChir Camb. 1989; FRACDS 1982; FDS RCS Ed. 1984; MA Camb. 1989; FRCS Eng. 1992. Cons. Maxillofacial Surg. S. Manch. Univ. Hosps. NHS Trust. Specialty: Oral & Maxillofacial Surg.

SANDERS, Lewis Roger Tilehurst Surgery, Tylers Place, Pottery Road, Tilehurst, Reading RG30 6BW Tel: 0118 942 7528 Fax: 0118 945 2405 — MB BS Lond. 1966; MRCS Eng. LRCP Lond. 1966. GP Reading.

SANDERS, Mr Mark Nathan 49 Chiltern Crescent, Wallingford OX10 0PG — MB BS Newc. 1988; FRCS Eng. 1993; FRCS Ed. 1993; FRACS 2001. Cons. Surg. Whangarei Area Hosp.; Cons. Sen. Lect. Bristol Roy. Infirm. UK. Specialty: Gen. Surg. Prev: Regist. (Orthop Surg.) New Plymouth Hosp. New Zealand; Regist. (Orthop. Surg.) Invercargill Hosp. New Zealand; Sen. Regist. (Gen. Surg.) Auckland Hosp. New Zealand.

SANDERS, Mr Michael David (retired) National Hospital, Queen Square, London WC1 Tel: 020 7837 3611 Ext: 3382; Chawton Lodge, Chawton, Alton GU34 1SL — MB BS Lond. 1959 (Guy's) MRCS Eng. LRCP Lond. 1959; DO Eng. 1962; FRCP Lond. 1977, M 1964; FRCS Eng. 1967. Cons. Ophth. St James' Hosp. Lond.; Cons. Ophth. Nat. Hosp. Qu. Sq. Lond.; Civil Cons. (Ophth.) RAF. Prev: Ho. Off. Guy's Hosp. Lond.

SANDERS, Michael Samuel (retired) 104 Newland Park, Hull HU5 2DU Tel: 01482 342897 — MB ChB Leeds 1948; DObst RCOG 1950; FRCGP 1983, M 1961. Prev: Provost Humberside Fac. RCGP.

SANDERS, Neil Peter Westgate Surgery, 60 Westgate, Peterborough PE1 1RG Tel: 01733 562420 Fax: 01733 564081; 30 Thorpe Lea Road, Peterborough PE3 6BZ Tel: 01733 60821 — BM BCh Oxf. 1986; DCH RCP Lond. 1991. Specialty: Gen. Pract.

SANDERS, Paul Anthony University Hospital of South Manchester, Withington Hospital, West Didsbury, Manchester M20 2LR Tel: 0161 611 4285 Fax: 0161 445 5631; 21 Dean Road, Handforth, Wilmslow SK9 3AH — MB ChB Leeds 1979; MRCP (UK) 1982; MD Leeds 1989; FRCP Ed. 1998; FRCP Lond. 1998. Cons. Rheum. Univ. Hosp. S. Manch. & Stepping Hill Hosp., Stockport; Hon. Lect. Univ. of Manch. Specialty: Rheumatol. Socs: Brit. Soc. Rheum. Prev: Research Fell. Hope Hosp. Salford; Manch. Roy. Infirm. Sen. Regist. Rheum.; Tutor in Rheum., Manch. & Salford Hosps. (Hon. Regist.).

SANDERS, Robert Keith Morice (retired) 36 Grayston Close, Tewkesbury GL20 8AY Tel: 01684 293760 — MB ChB Bristol 1954; DObst RCOG 1956; MD Bristol 1963. Prev: Gen. Sen. Christian Med. Fellowship Lond.

SANDERS, Rosemary Susan (retired) Souldern Manor, Bicester OX27 7LF — MB BS Lond. 1977 (Univ. Coll. Hosp.) MA Oxf. 1978; FFA RCS Eng. 1982. Cons. Anaesth. Horton Gen. Hosp. Banbury.

SANDERS, Roshini 3 Cammo Brae, Edinburgh EH4 8ET Tel: 0131 339 4563; 28 Hillfoot Drive, Bearsden, Glasgow G61 3QF — MB ChB Glas. 1984; DO RCS Eng. 1988; FRCS Ed. 1990. Cons. Ophth. Qu. Margt. Hosp. Dunfermline. Specialty: Ophth. Prev: Sen. Regist. (Ophth.) Ninewells Hosp. Dundee.

SANDERS, Professor Roy Suite 1, 82 Portland Place, London W1N 3DH Tel: 020 7580 3541 Fax: 020 7436 2954 Email: roy.sanders@btclick.com; 77 Harley Street, London W1G 8QN Tel: 020 7935 7417 — (Char. Cross) BSc (Hons.) Anat. Lond. 1959; MB BS Lond. 1962; MRCS Eng. LRCP Lond. 1962; FRCS (Hons.) Eng. 1967. Cons. Plastic Surg. Mt. Vernon Hosp. N.wood; Dir. RAFT Inst. Plastic Surg. Specialty: Plastic Surg. Socs: (Sec.) Brit. Assn. Plastic Surgs. (Ex-Pres.); Roy. Soc. Med. (Pres. Plastic Surg. Sect.); Internat. Soc. Aesthetic Plastic Surg. Prev: Surg. i/c Rainsford Mowlem Burns Centre; Vis. Prof. Univ. Hong Kong 1988; Vis. Prof. Univ. Bombay 1988.

SANDERS, Stuart 22 Harmont House, 20 Harley St., London W1G 9PH Tel: 020 7935 5687 Fax: 020 7436 4387 Email: www.drsanders.net; 51 Springfield Road, London NW8 0QJ Tel: 020 7586 0175 Fax: 020 7586 0041 — MB ChB Leeds 1958; MRCS Eng. LRCP Lond. 1959; DObst RCOG 1960; DCH Eng. 1961; FRCGP 1996, M 1965. Indep. Primary Care Phys. & Corporate Doctor Lond.; Founder Mem. & Ex-Chairm. Indep. Doctors Forum; Med. Examr. Legal & Gen. & other Insur. Companies; Med. Adviser Grant Thornton, Lond. Clubs, Zurich Insurance & other Companies. Socs: Fell. Roy. Soc. Med.; (Past Chair.) InDepend. Doctors Forum; (Past Chair.) St Marylebone BMA Div. Prev: Ho. Phys. (Paediat.) Gen. Infirm. Leeds; Hon. Sen. Research Fell. Hosp. Sick Childr. Gt. Ormond St. Lond.; Resid. Path. Roy. Free Hosp. Lond.

SANDERS, Sureshini — MB ChB Glas. 1988 (Glasgow) DRCOG 1991; MRCGP 1992. Specialty: Gen. Pract.; Hospital Practitioner. Special Interest: Care of the Elderly. Socs: BMA; RCGP.

SANDERSON, Alan Lindsay 2 Caroline Close, London W2 4RW Tel: 020 7229 8533 Fax: 020 7229 8533 Email: sandersona@onetel.net.uk — (St. Thos.) MB BS Lond. 1954; MRCP Lond. 1959; DPM Eng. 1963; MRCPsych 1971. p/t Cons. Psychiat. in Private Pract. Specialty: Gen. Psychiat.; Hypnother. Socs: Scientif. & Med. Network; Fell. Roy. Soc. Med. Prev: Cons. Psychiat. S. Beds. Community Health Care Trust Leighton Buzzard.; Hon. Research Fell. (Psychiat.) Univ. Birm.; Sen. Regist. Maudsley Hosp. Lond.

SANDERSON, Andrea 96 Sunnyside, Underbank Old Road, Holmfirth, Huddersfield HD9 1AS — BM BS Nottm. 1991; MRCP (UK) 1995. Regist. Rotat. (Radiol.) Leeds & Bradford. Specialty: Radiol.

SANDERSON, Andrew Alexander Fleck Sanderson and Partners, Adan House Surgery, St. Andrews Lane, Spennymoor DL16 6QA Tel: 01388 817777 Fax: 01388 811700; Adan House, St. Andrew's Lane, Spennymoor DL16 6QA Tel: 01388 817777 Fax: 01388 811700 — MB BS Newc. 1969; MRCGP 1976; Cert. Family Plann. JCC 1980; Dip. Pract. Dermat. Wales 1992; MA 1998. Mem. Durh. LMC (Vice-Chairm.); Sedgefield PCT. Specialty: Pathology, General. Socs: Durh. Clin. Soc. Prev: Clin. Asst. (Ophth.) Dryburn Hosp. Durh.; SHO (Ophth.) Sunderland Eye Infirm.; SHO (Paediat.) Dryburn Hosp. Durh.

SANDERSON, Anthony John Xray Department, North Devon District Hospital, Raleigh Park, Barnstaple EX31 4JB Tel: 01271 322453; Hillpark House, Whitestone Lane, Knowle, Braunton EX33 2LT Tel: 01271 816033 — MB ChB Dundee 1981 (Dundee Univ.) MRCP (UK) 1986; FRCR 1993. Cons. Radiol. N. Devon Dist. Hosp. Raleigh Pk., Barnstaple N. Devon. Specialty: Radiol. Socs: Fell. Roy. Coll. Radiols. Prev: Sen. Regist. (Diag. Radiol.) Wessex Train Scheme.; Regist. (Diag. Radiol.) Soton.; Reserach Regist. (Med. & Cardiol.) Edin.

SANDERSON, Cara Jane 20 Taunton Drive, Aintree, Liverpool L10 8JW — MB ChB Sheff. 1997.

SANDERSON, Charles Hamilton, Maj. RAMC(V) — MB ChB Glas. 1987; Dip. Forens. Med. Glas 1996. Clin. Asst. Geriat. Med. Monklands Dist. Gen. Hosp. Specialty: Care of the Elderly. Socs: Ordinary Mem. Scott. Medio-Legal Soc. Prev: SHO (Psychiat. & Learning Disabil.) Roy. Scott. Nat. Hosp. Larbert; GP/Regist. Alva Med. Pract.; SHO (Anaesth.) Roy. Gwent Hosp. & Stirling Roy. Infirm.

SANDERSON, Charles Joseph (retired) Flat 1, 4 Queen's Park West Drive, Bournemouth BH8 9BX Tel: 01202 304632 — MRCS Eng. LRCP Lond. 1929 (St. Bart.) DPH Lond. 1935. Prev: Cas. Ho. Phys. St. Bart. Hosp.

SANDERSON, Mr Christopher John Whiston Hospital, Warrington Road, Prescot L35 5DR Tel: 0151 426 1600 Fax: 0151 608 1836; Lansdowne, Mountwood Road, Prenton, Birkenhead CH42 8NG Tel: 0151 608 1836 — MB ChB Liverp. 1971 (Liverpool) FRCS Eng. 1977 Gen Surr; MRCS Eng. LRCP Lond. 1971; FRCS Ed. 1976. Cons. Gen. Surg. St Helens Knawsley H.A. Clin. Dir. Surgic. Serv.s; Hon. Lect. Dept. Surg. Univ. Liverp. Specialty: Gen. Surg.; Gastroenterol. Socs: Assn. of Upper GI Surg.s; BMA; Assn. of Surg.s. Prev: Sen. Regist. (Surg.) Mersey RHA; Research Fell. Dept. Surg. Univ. Chicago, USA.

SANDERSON, David Andrew Essex Rivers Healthcare NHS Trust, Colchester General Hospital, Turner Road, Colchester CO4 5JL Tel: 01206 742977 Fax: 01206 742660; Plummers, Plummers Road, Fordham, Colchester CO6 3NP — MB BS Lond. 1985. Cons. O & G Colchester Gen. Hosp. Specialty: Obst. & Gyn. Prev: Cons. O&G Colchester Gen. Hosp.

SANDERSON, Eileen Patricia Blackshiels Frm., Blackshiels, Pathhead EH37 5SX Tel: 0187 533288 — MB ChB Ed. 1986; DRCOG 1990; MRCGP 1992.

SANDERSON, Evelyn — MB BS Lond. 1992 (St. Bart. Hosp. Med. Sch.) BA (Med. Scis.) Camb. 1983; MRCP (UK) 1995; FRCR 1999. Regist. (Radiol.) Guys' and St. Thomas' NHS Trust. Specialty: Radiol. Socs: BMA.

SANDERSON, Frances Nuffield Department Medicine, Level 7, John Radcliffe Hospital, Oxford OX3 9DU Tel: 01865 741166 Email: frances.sanderson@ndm.ox.ac.uk; 2 Caroline Close, London W2 4RW — BM BCh Oxf. 1987 (Camb. & Oxf.) MA Camb. 1986; MRCP (UK) 1990; PhD London 1996; MSC London 1998. Sen. Fell., Nuffield Dept. Med. John Radcliffe Hosp. Oxf.; SpR (Infec. Dis.s) W. Midl.s. Specialty: Infec. Dis.; Gen. Med. Prev: Sen. Regist. (Nephrol.) Hammersmith Hosp. & RPMS Lond.; Clin. Research Fell. Human Immunogenetics Laborat. Imperial Cancer Research Fund Lond.; Regist. (Med.) John Radcliffe & Churchill Hosp. Oxf.

SANDERSON, Gail Yew Tree Cottage Surgery, 15 Leyton Road, Harpenden AL5 2HX Tel: 01582 712126 Fax: 01582 462414; 69 Station Road, Harpenden AL5 4RL — MB BS Lond. 1989; DRCOG 1992; MRCGP 1993. Specialty: Gen. Pract.; Family Plann. & Reproduc. Health; Obst. & Gyn. Prev: Trainee GP St. Albans VTS.

SANDERSON, Graham Donald University of Bradford Health Centre, Laneisteridge Lane, Bradford BD5 0NH Tel: 01274 234979 Fax: 01274 235940 — MB ChB Liverp. 1984; DTM & H Liverp. 1985; MRCPsych 1990; MRCGP 1991; T(GP) 1991.

SANDERSON, Heather (retired) 9 Branksome Crescent, Heaton, Bradford BD9 5LD Tel: 01274 545779 — MB ChB Leeds 1955. Prev: Ho. Surg., Ho. Phys. & Jun. Receiv. Room Off. Leeds Gen. Infirm.

SANDERSON, Helen 10 Thistle Place, Dumfries DG1 3UT — MB ChB Manch. 1994. GP Regist. - Lochmaben Med. Gp. - Lochmaben. Specialty: Gen. Pract.

SANDERSON, Hilary (retired) 1 St Chads Grove, Leeds LS6 3PN Tel: 0113 275 5440 — MB ChB Sheff. 1955; BSc (Hons.) Leeds 1945; DPH Leeds 1963; DPM Leeds 1970; MD Sheff. 1975. Prev: Cons. Psychiat. Fieldhead Hosp. Wakefield.

SANDERSON, Hugh Francis Central South Coast Cancer Network, Oakley Rd, Southampton SO16 4GX Tel: 02380 725633; The Pebbles, 5 Stoney Lane, Winchester SO22 6DN Tel: 01962 883320 Email: hugh.sanderson@hiowha.nhs.uk — MB BS Lond. 1972 (St. Mary's) MSc (Social Med.) Lond. 1978, BSc 1969; MFCM 1979; FFPHM 1987. Cons. in Pub. Health/ Informat. Lead. Specialty: Pub. Health Med. Prev: Med. Director WInchester and Eastleigh Healthcare Trust; Dir. Nat. Casemix Off. IMG G Winchester; Cons. Pub. Health Med. Wessex RHA.

SANDERSON, Ian Antony 96 Sunnyside, Underbank Old Road, Holmfirth, Huddersfield HD9 1AS — MB ChB Manch. 1990; MRCP (UK) 1993; MRCGP 1996. Trainee GP Huddersfield VTS. Specialty: Gen. Pract.

SANDERSON, Professor Ian Rutherford Barts & The London NHS Trust, Adult & Paediatric Gastroenterology, Turner Street,

London E1 2AD Tel: 020 7882 7191 Fax: 020 7882 7192 Email: i.r.sanderson@qmul.ac.uk; 6 Markham Street, London SW3 3NP — MB BS Lond. 1979 (St. Bart.) MRCP (UK) 1982; BA Oxf. 1975, MSc, MA 1981, MD 1989; FRCPCH 1997; FRCP 2001. Prof. (Paediat. Gastroenterol.); Head Dept. of Adult & Paediatric Gastroenterol. Specialty: Paediat. Socs: Fell. Roy. Soc. Med.; Amer. Gastroenterol. Assn.; Brit. Soc. of Paediatric Gastroenterol., Hepat. & Nutrit. (President). Prev: Asst. Prof. Pediatrics Harvard Med. Sch.; Sen. Regist. Hosp. Sick Childr. Gt. Ormond St. Lond.; SHO Qu. Eliz. Hosp. Childr. Lond.

SANDERSON, Isabel Brenda (retired) 5 Winchester Close, Kingston Hill, Kingston upon Thames KT2 7JJ — MB BS Lond. 1943; MRCS Eng. LRCP Lond. 1941; DCH Eng. 1949; DA Eng. 1955; FFA RCS Eng. 1956. Prev: Cons. Anaesth. Kensington, Chelsea & Westm. AHA (T).

SANDERSON, Isabel Mary 66 Queens Road, Wimbledon, London SW19 8LR Tel: 020 8947 7806 — MB ChB Glas. 1968; MRCP (U.K.) 1972. Under-Sec. Med. Defence Union. Socs: Med. Legal Soc. Prev: Sen. Regist. (Gen. Med. & Gastroenterol.) St. Geo. Hosp. Tooting; Regist. St. Jas. Hosp. Lond.; Ho. Phys. Profess. Med. Unit Glas. Roy. Infirm.

SANDERSON, Janet Ulgham Grange Nurseries, Ulgham, Morpeth NE61 3AX — MB BS Durh. 1967.

SANDERSON, Jeremy David 93 Black Lion Lane, London W6 9BG — MB BS Lond. 1984; MD Lond. 1993; FRCP 1998. Cons. Gastroenterol. Guy's & St. Thos. Hosps. Trust Lond. Specialty: Gastroenterol. Prev: Sen. Regist. (Gastroenterol.) Guy's Hosp. Lond.; Clin. Research Fell. (Gastroenterol.) St. Geo. Hosp. Med. Sch. Lond.; Sen. Regist. (Gastroenterol.) St. Vincent's Hosp. Melbourne, Austral.

SANDERSON, Joel Harvey 10 Tumblewood Drive, Cheadle SK8 1JZ Tel: 0161 491 3597 & profess. 061 428 1731 — BM BCh Oxf. 1965; BSc Oxf. 1963, MA, BM BCh 1965; MRCP Lond. 1969; FFPM 1989. Proprietor MediMark Serv. Cheadle. Socs: Brit. Soc. Haemat. Prev: Med. Manager ICI Pharmaceut. (UK) Alderley Pk.; Head Haemat. Sect. ICI plc Centr. Toxicol. Laborat. Alderley Pk.; MRC Clin. Research Fell. Manch. Roy. Infirm.

SANDERSON, John Gilbert, MBE (retired) Little Berkeley, Rowhedge, Colchester CO5 7EL Tel: 01206 728060 — MB BS Lond. 1954 (St. Geo.) MRCS Eng. LRCP Lond. 1954; DObst RCOG 1956. Prev: Ho. Surg. & Resid. Obst. Asst. St. Geo. Hosp.

SANDERSON, Joseph Brian DDS Medicine Research LTD, Ninewells Hospital & Medical School, Dundee DD1 9SY Tel: 01382 646317 Fax: 01382 645606; 11 Wemyss Gardens, Broughty Ferry, Dundee DD5 3BX Tel: 01382 732604 Email: brian.sanderson@tesco.net — MB ChB Dundee 1986; MRCGP 1990. Dep. Med. Dir., DDS Med. Research. Specialty: Pharmacology; Gen. Pract.; Pharmaceutical Medicine. Prev: Clin. Research Phys. Inveresk Edin.; GP Lochgelly.

SANDERSON, Kirsty Jane Friarwood Surgery, Carleton Glen, Pontefract WF8 1SU Tel: 01977 703235 Fax: 01977 600527 — MB ChB Leeds 1994; DRCOG 1997. GP Princip. - Full Parity Partner. Specialty: Gen. Pract. Socs: BMA.

SANDERSON, Lynne Exmouth Health Centre, Claremont Grove, Exmouth EX8 2JF Tel: 01395 273001 Fax: 01395 273771; 14 Avondale Road, Exmouth EX8 2NQ Tel: 01395 277807 — MB BS Newc. 1985; BSc Newc. 1980; MRCGP 1989.

SANDERSON, Margaret Lily Trent View Medical Practice, 45 Trent View, Keadby, Scunthorpe DN17 3DR Tel: 01724 782209 Fax: 01724 784472 — MB ChB Leic. 1983; DRCOG 1987.

SANDERSON, Mark Richard The Spinney, Ramsey Road, St Ives PE27 3TP Tel: 01480 484000 Fax: 01480 356159; 4 Priors Road, Hemingford Grey, Huntingdon PE28 9BT Tel: 01480 469414 — MB BS Lond. 1986; BSc Lond. 1983; MRCP (UK) 1989; DPH Camb. 1994; MFPHM 1997; MRCGP 1999. Specialty: Pub. Health Med. Prev: Sen. Regist. (Pub. Health Med.) Camb. & Huntingdon Health Auth.; Regist. (Gen. Med. & Thoracic Med.) Guy's Hosp. Lond.; Regist. (Gen. Med.) Brook Gen. Hosp. Lond.

SANDERSON, Mary Christina (retired) 5 Alma Field, Castle Cary BA7 7JD — MB BS Lond. 1964; MRCS Eng. LRCP Lond. 1964.

SANDERSON, Mr Paul Lewis Freeman Hospital, High Heaton, Newcastle NE7 7DW Tel: 0191 233 6161 — MB ChB Manch. 1984; FRCS Ed. 1988; FRCS Orth. 1994. Cons. Orthop. Surg. Specialty: Orthop. Special Interest: Spinal. Prev: Tutor (Orthop. Surg.) Manch. Univ.; Sen. Regist. (Orthop.) N. Trent.

SANDERSON, Peter Mark Highclere, 11 Glencairn Park Road, Cheltenham GL50 2NA — MB ChB Ed. 1988; FRCA 1993. Cons. (Anaesth.) Glos. Roy. Hosp. Specialty: Anaesth.; Intens. Care. Socs: Soc. Anaesth. SW Region; Med. Protec. Soc.; BMA. Prev: Sen. Regist. (Anaesth.) Bristol & SW Region; Clin. Fell. (Paediat. Anaesth.) Brit. Columbia's Childr. Hosp. Vancouver, Canada; Regist. (Anaesth.) Bristol & SW Region.

SANDERSON, Peter William Guidepost Health Centre, North Parade, Guidepost, Choppington NE62 5RA Tel: 01670 822071 Fax: 01670 531068 — MB ChB Liverp. 1969. GP Choppington, N.d.

SANDERSON, Philip James 26 Chalcot Road, London NW1 8LN Tel: 020 7586 4442 — MB BS Lond. 1960 (Lond. Hosp.) BSc (Anat.) (1st. cl. Hons.) 1957; Dip. Bact. (Distinc.) 1964; PhD Lond. 1968; FRCPath 1983, M 1971. Microbiologist to the N. Lond. Nuffield Hosp., Enfield. Specialty: Med. Microbiol. Socs: Brit. Antimicrobiol. Chemother. Hosp. Infec. Soc. Prev: Cons. Microbiologist, Edgware & Barnet Hosp.s, Roy. Nat. Orthopaedic Hosp.,Lond.

SANDERSON, Richard Anthony The Surgery, 280 Havant Road, Drayton, Portsmouth PO6 1PA Tel: 023 9237 0422 Fax: 023 9261 8383 — MB Camb. 1973 (St. Mary's) BChir 1972; DCH Eng. 1977; MRCGP 1978.

SANDERSON, Robert Desmond Stuart The Farley Road Practice, 53 Farley Road, Selsdon, South Croydon CR2 7NG Tel: 020 8651 1222 Fax: 020 8657 9297 — MB Camb. 1977; BChir 1976. Socs: Camb. Med. Grad. Club.

SANDERSON, Mr Robert James Edinburgh Cancer Centre, Western General Hospital, Edinburgh EH4 2XU Email: sandtol@ukgateway.net; 48 Bonaly Road, Edinburgh EH13 0EQ — MB ChB Manch. 1984; FRCS Eng. 1988; FRCS Ed. 1988. Cons. Otolaryngol. West. Gen. Hosp. Edin. Specialty: Otolaryngol.

SANDERSON, Robert Louis, TD (retired) 1 Coleridge Court, Harpenden AL5 5LD Tel: 01582 462772 — MB ChB Ed. 1937 (Univ. Ed.) MRCGP 1966. Prev: Tutor (Community Med.) Newc. Univ.

SANDERSON, Rosalind Mary Fleck (retired) Newhouse Farm, Marstow, Ross-on-Wye HR9 6HF — MB BS Newc. 1967; DCH RCP Lond. 1970; DRCOG 1971; MRCGP 1976; Cert. Prescribed Equiv. Exp. JCPTGP 1996.

SANDERSON, Simon Peter — MB ChB Bristol 1989; MRCP (UK) 1992; DPH Camb. 1993; MFPHM 1996; MRCGP 1998. Med. Off., Aviat. Med., Qinetd. Specialty: Aviat. Med.

SANDERSON, Thomas Allan, OStJ, Col. late RAMC Retd. (retired) Ivy Cottage, 18 Main St., North Queensferry, Inverkeithing KY11 1JG Tel: 01383 419020 — (Ed.) MB ChB Ed. 1952; DObst RCOG 1956; DTM & H Eng. 1969; AFOM RCP Lond. 1981. Prev: Cdr. Med. Army HQ Scotl.

SANDFORD, Alison Elizabeth 2C Montford Gate, Darnley Road, Barrmead, Glasgow G78 2W — MB ChB Glas. 1995; DRCOG 1999; MRCGP 2001.

SANDFORD, Jeremy Mark Hampstead Group Practice, 75 Fleet Road, London NW3 2QU Tel: 020 7435 4000 Fax: 020 7435 9000 — MB BS Lond. 1982 (Middlesex Hospital Medical School) DRCOG 1986; MRCGP 1988. Clin. Asst. (A & E) Whittington Hosp. Lond.

SANDFORD, John Jennings Psychopharmacology Unit University of Bristol, School of Medical Sciences, University Walk, Bristol BS8 1TD Tel: 0117 925 3066 Fax: 0117 927 7057 — MB ChB Leic. 1990 (Leicester) DCH RCP Lond. 1992; MRCPsych 1996. Fromside Clinic Blackberry Hill Hosp. Manor Rd. Fishponds Bristol BS16 1TD; Long Fox Unit Weston Gen. Hosp. Upill, Weston Super Mare BS29 4TQ. Specialty: Forens. Psychiat.; Gen. Psychiat.; Medico Legal. Socs: Roy. Coll. Psychiat.; Brist. Assn. for Psychopharm.; Brit. Assn For Ment. Health and Law. Prev: Locum Cons. Forens. Psychiat., Fromside; Spr Forens. Psychiat., Butler Clinic; Spr Forens. Psychiat., Francis Clinic.

SANDFORD, Richard Nicholas Dept. of Medical Genetics, Cambridge Institute for Medical Research, Addenbrook's Hospital, Cambridge CB2 2XY Tel: 01223 762616 Fax: 01223 331206; Granby House, 11 Church Street, Haslingfield, Cambridge CB3 7JE Tel: 01223 871190 — MB BS Lond. 1985 (St. Thomas' Hospital, London) BSc Lond. 1982; MRCP (UK) 1988; PhD Cambridge 1995. Wellcome Trust Sen. Fell. in Clin. Research; Hon. Cons. Med. Genetics. Specialty: Genetics.

SANDFORD-HILL, Averil Mary Church Street Surgery, 15 Church Street, Calne SN11 0HY; Poona, Fieldside, Coate, Devizes SN10 3LE Tel: 01380 860080 — MB BS Lond. 1988; BSc (Hons.) Biochem. 1985; DRCOG 1991.

SANDFORD-HILL, Richard Charles Simon Market Lavington Surgery, 15 Church Street, Market Lavington, Devizes SN10 4DT Tel: 01380 812500 — MB BS Lond. 1988; MRCGP 1992.

SANDFORD-SMITH, Mr John Henry (retired) 14 Morland Avenue, Leicester LE2 2PE — MB Camb. 1962 (Middlx.) BChir 1961; FRCS Eng. 1967; DO Eng. 1967; FRCS Ed. 1968; FCOphth 1988. Cons. Ophth. Leic. Roy. Infirm. Prev: Sen. Regist. Bristol Eye Hosp.

SANDHAM, Patricia Ann Rosamar, Allanfauld Road, Kilsyth, Glasgow G65 9DE — MB ChB Glas. 1973; MSc (Health Informatics) Glas. 1993. Med. Edr. Informat. Servs. Gtr. Glas. NHS Bd. Prev: Project Doctor Resource Managem. Initiative Yorkhill NHS Trust Glas.

SANDHAR, Babinder Kaur Department Anaesthesia, Royal Devon & Exeter Hospital, Barrack Road, Exeter EX2 5DW Tel: 01392 402474 Fax: 01392 402472 — BM BS Nottm. 1980 (Nottingham University) FRCA London 1985. Cons. Anaesth. Roy. Devon & Exeter Hosp. Specialty: Anaesth. Socs: Assn. Paediatric Anaesthetists; Anaesthetic Research Soc.; Associaiton of Anaesthetists. Prev: Sen. Regist. Leicester Roy. Infirm.; Regist. Nuffield Dept. Anaesth. Oxf.; Research Fell., Foothills Hosp., Calgary, Canada.

SANDHER, Dilraj Singh 9 Crawford Close, Wollaton, Nottingham NG8 2AZ — MB ChB Manch. 1996.

SANDHU, Amandip Singh 18 Sackville Road, Sheffield S10 1GT — MB ChB Sheff. 1998; MB ChB Sheff 1998.

SANDHU, Mr Bachittar Singh Queen Elizabeth II Hospital, Welwyn Garden City AL7 4HQ Tel: 01707 328111; 3 Rectory Croft, Stevenage SG1 4BY Tel: 01438 353030 — (Med. Coll. Amritsar) MB BS Punjab (India) 1958; DO Eng. 1962; FRCS Eng. 1963; FRCOphth 1989. Cons. Ophth. Surg. Qu. Eliz. II Hosp. Welwyn Gdn. City & Lister Hosp. Stevenage; Mem. Oxf. Ophth. Congr. Specialty: Ophth. Socs: BMA. Prev: Sen. Regist. (Ophth.) St. Paul's Eye Hosp. Liverp.; Regist. (Ophth.) Leisham Gp. Hosps. & Derbysh. Roy. Infirm.

SANDHU, Professor Bhupinder Kaur Bristol Royal Hospital for Sick Children, St Michael's Hill, Bristol BS2 8BJ Tel: 0117 921 5411; 20 West Mall, Clifton, Bristol BS8 4BQ Tel: 0117 973 9278 — MD Lond. 1988 (University College London) MB BS 1974; MRCP (UK) 1978; FRCP 1996; FRCPCH 1997. Cons. Paediat. (Gastroenterol.) Roy. Hosp. Sick Childr. Bristol. Prof. of paediatric Gastroenterol.; Hon. Sen. Clin. Lect. Univ. Bristol; Vis. Prof. - Univ. of W. of Eng.. Specialty: Paediat.; Gastroenterol. Socs: Brit. Soc. Paediat. Gastroenterol.; Eur. Soc. Paediat. Gastroenterol. and Nutrit.; MRCPCH. Prev: Research Fell. Inst. Child Health Lond. & Hon. Sen. Regist. Hosp. Sick Childr. Lond.; Regist. (Paediat.) Middlx. Hosp. Lond.; Lect & Hon. Sen. Regist. Char. Cross & Westminster Med. Sch. & Westminster Childr.'s Hosp. Lond.

SANDHU, Caron 43 William Square, London SE16 5XJ — MB BS Lond. 1992; BSc (Hons.) Lond. 1989; MRCP (UK) 1995. Specialist Regist. (Radiol.) St. Geo. Hosp. Lond.

SANDHU, Mr Davinder Pal Singh Leicester General Hospital NHS Trust, Gwendolen Road, Leicester LE5 4PW Tel: 0116 249 0490; Winkadale, Uppingham Road, Bushby, Leicester LE7 9RP Tel: 0116 243 3018 — MB BS Lond. 1980 (Royal Free) FRCS Glas. 1986; FRCS Ed. 1986; FRCS (Urol.) 1991; MD Leic. 1994. Cons. Urol. Surg. Leicester Gen. Hosp. & Hon. Lect. Univ. Leicester; Assoc. Postgrad. Dean for Overseas Doctors. Specialty: Urol. Socs: Brit. Assn. Urol. Surgs.; Roy. Coll. Surgs. Edin.; Amer. Urol. Assn. Prev: Sen. Regist. (Urol.) City Hosp. Nottm. & Derbysh. Roy. Infirm.; Ho. Phys. Roy. Free Hosp. Lond.; Regist. (Urol.) Univ. Hosp. S. Manch.

SANDHU, Gurjinder Singh 42 Quaves Road, Slough SL3 7PA — MB BS Lond. 1998; MB BS Lond 1998.

SANDHU, Mr Gurpreet Singh ENT Department, Royal Glamorgan General Hospital, Ynys Maerdy, Llantrisant CF72 8XR — MB BS Lond. 1990 (Lond. Hosp. Med. Coll.) FRCS Eng. 1994; FRCS (Oto) 1996. Specialty: Otolaryngol.

SANDHU, Harjinder Singh Tower House Practice, St Pauls Health Centre, High Street, Runcorn WA7 1AB Tel: 01928 567404; 7 Granby Road, Walton, Warrington WA4 6PH — MB ChB Liverp. 1989; DRCOG 1994. GP Princip. Prev: GP Trainee, The Knoll, Frodsham; SHO (O & G & Paediat.) Warrington Gen. Hosp.

SANDHU, Harvinder Singh Flat 3, 49 Cavell St., London E1 2BP — MB BChir Camb. 1993.

SANDHU, Inderjit Kaur Horsenden Lane North Surgery, 2A Horsenden Lane North, Greenford UB6 0PA Tel: 020 8869 7910 Fax: 020 8869 7911; 64 High Beeches, Gerrards Cross SL9 7HY Tel: 01753 883640 — MRCS Eng. LRCP Lond. 1978. Socs: MDU; BMA.

SANDHU, Jagteswar Singh 8 Jackers Road, Coventry CV2 1PF — MB BCh Wales 1989.

SANDHU, Kanwaljit Singh 14 Pirie Close, Bradford BD2 1EP — MB BChir Camb. 1991; BA Camb. 1987, MA 1991; MRC (UK) 1995. Regist. (Renal & Gen. Med.) Roy. Sussex Co. Hosp. Brighton. Specialty: Nephrol. Prev: Regist. (Renal & Gen. Med.) St. Thos. Hosp. Lond.; Regist. (Renal) Guy's Hosp. Lond.; Regist. (Gen. Med.) Worthing.

SANDHU, Nirver Singh Alveley Health Centre, Alveley, Bridgnorth WV15 6NG Tel: 01746 780553 Fax: 01746 780976; 11 Beaconsfield, Tasley Park, Bridgnorth WV16 4RX Tel: 01746 761715 — MB ChB Manch. 1981; MRCGP 1988.

SANDHU, Param Jeet Singh Hammond Road Surgery, 95 Hammond Road, Southall UB2 4EH Tel: 020 8574 5057; 22 Bengeworth Road, Harrow HA1 3SE — MB BS Punjab 1972 (Govt. Med. Coll. Patiala) MB BS Punjabi 1972. GP Southall. Socs: Primary Care Rheum. Soc. (Mem. Steering Comm.). Prev: SHO (Comm. Dis.) S. Middlx. Hosp. Isleworth; SHO (Rheum.) W. Middlx. Univ. Hosp. Isleworth; SHO (Thoracic. Med.) Colindale Hosp.

SANDHU, Punam Winkadale, Uppingham Road, Bushby, Leicester LE7 9RP — MRCS Eng. LRCP Lond. 1987.

SANDHU, Ravinder Kaur Kingfisher Medical Centre, 65 Fisher Street, Willenhall WV13 2HT Tel: 01902 606303 — MB ChB Birm. 1997.

SANDHU, Ravinder Singh 138 Broadway W., Walsall WS1 4DN — MB ChB Birm. 1998.

SANDHU, Sandeep Singh 41 Kingsleigh Drive, Castle Bromwich, Birmingham B36 9SB — MB ChB Manch. 1997.

SANDHU, Saranjit Singh Flat D, 40 Hermon Hill, London E11 2AP — MB BS Lond. 1989.

SANDHU, Mr Sarbjinder Singh 128 Waye Avenue, Cranford, Hounslow TW5 9SF Tel: 020 8897 8394 — MB BS Lond. 1991 (Royal Free Hospital London) BSc (Hons.) Biochem. & Med. Sci. Lond. 1988; FRCS Eng. 1993; FRCS (Urol.) 2002. Specialist Regist. (Urol.) N. Thames Urol. Train. Scheme; Hon. Regist. (Urol.) Roy. Free Hosp. Lond. Specialty: Urol. Prev: Sen. Surg. SHO (Surg.) Swindon; SHO Acad. Dept. Surg. Roy. Marsden Hosp. Lond.; SHO (Urol.) St. Gen. Hosp. Lond.

SANDHU, Sharron Kaur Room 308 Biggart House, Broadway, Belfast BT12 6HG — MB BCh BAO Belf. 1994.

SANDHU, Swairaj 21 Arley Av, Manchester M20 2LQ — MB ChB Manch. 1997.

SANDHU, Virinderjit 2 Mornington Crescent, Hounslow TW5 9SS — BM Soton. 1993.

SANDIFER, Quentin Dudley Kent and Medway Strategic Health Authority, Preston Hall, Aylesford ME20 7NJ Tel: 01622 713055 Email: quentin.sandifer@kentmedway.nhs.uk; Rhiw Goed, Westra, Dinas Powys CF64 4HA Tel: 02920 515931 Fax: 02920 515898 Email: quentin-sandifer@supanet.com — MB BCh Wales 1985 (Univ. of Wales, Coll. of Med., Cardiff) MRCGP 1989; DRCOG 1989; MPH Wales 1995; MFPHM RCP (UK) 1997; FRCGP 2000; FFPHM 2004; MBA Columbia, NY 2005; MBA Lond. 2005. Specialty: Pub. Health Med. Socs: Past Chairm. SE Wales Fac. RCGP; Past Pres. Sect. Gen. Pract., Roy. Soc. Med.; Curr. Hon. Sec. Roy. Soc. Med. Prev: Director of Pub. Health (Swansea Local Health Board) and Cons. in Pub. Health Med., Nat. Pub. Health Serv. NHS Wales; Director of Pub. Health, Iechyd Morgannwg Health, Swansea; Sen. Regist. (Pub. Health Med.), Bro Taf HA, Cardiff.

SANDILAND, Arthur Cleave Ernest (retired) 6 Parkway, Orsett, Grays RM16 3HA Tel: 01375 891847 — MB BS Lond. 1948 (Lond. Hosp.) MRCS Eng. LRCP Lond. 1944.

SANDILANDS, Mr David George Douglas Burnley General Hospital, Casterton Avenue, Burnley B10 2PQ — MB ChB Manch. 1970; FRCS Eng. 1976; MD 1984. Specialty: Gen. Surg.

SANDILANDS, Mr David George Douglas Burnley General Hospital, Casterton Avenue, Burnley BB10 2PQ — MB ChB Manch.

1970; FRCS 1976; MD 1984. Cons. Gen. Surg., Breast & Colorectal Surg., E. Lancs. Health Care Trust.

SANDILANDS, David William Ian MacRae 19 Frederick Road, Edgbaston, Birmingham B15 1JN — MRCS Eng. LRCP Lond. 1955 (Camb. & St. Thos.) MA Camb. 1957; DObst RCOG 1957; DMJ Soc. Apoth. Lond. 1968; MB BChir Camb. 2955. Med. Adviser W. Midl.s Fire Serv. Specialty: Occupat. Health. Socs: Assn. Local Auth. Med. Adviser - Life Memer; Assn. Police Surg. - Life Memner. Prev: Ho. Surg. Essex Co. Hosp. Colchester; Ho. Phys. Hereford Co. Hosp.; Ho. Surg. (O & G) St. Thos. Hosp.

SANDILANDS, Gordon Arthur Hamilton (retired) 6 Sheraton Drive, Wollaton, Nottingham NG8 2PR — MB ChB Glas. 1944; DObst RCOG 1950. Prev: Maj. RAMC.

SANDISON, Mr Andrew James Paterson Department of Surgery, Conquest Hospital, The Ridge, St Leonards-on-Sea TN37 7RD — MB BS Lond. 1987; BA Camb. 1984; FRCS Eng. 1991; FRCS (Gen.Surg.) 1999. Cons. Surg., E. Sussex Hosps. NHS Trust. Specialty: Gen. Surg. Prev: Specialist Regist. SE Thames Higher Surg. Train Scheme.

SANDISON, Anita Louise 145 Itchen Stoke, Alresford SO24 0QZ — BM Soton. 1993.

SANDISON, Ann Department of Histopathology, Charing Cross Hospital, Fulham Palace Road, London SW6 8RF Tel: 020 8846 7139 Fax: 020 8846 1864 — MB ChB Ed. 1989 (Edinburgh) BSc (Hons.) Biol. Sc. E. Anglia 1978; MPhil Ed. 1984, MB ChB 1989; MRCPath 1996. Cons Histopath. Hammersmith Hosp.s NHS Trust (Char. Cross Hosp.0. Specialty: Histopath. Socs: Path. Soc. of GB & N. Irel.; Internat. Acad. of Pathol.; Roy. Soc. Med. Prev: Clin. Lect. (Histopath.) Univ. Coll. Lond. Med. Sch.; SHO (Histopath.) Med. Sch. Univ. Birm.; Cons. Hisopathologist RNOH Stanmore 1996-1999.

SANDISON, Donald Ross, MC (retired) 63 Learmonth Court, Edinburgh EH4 1PD — LDS RCS Ed. 1939; LRCP LRCS Ed. LRFPS Glas. 1939.

SANDISON, Ronald Arthur Parkview, 28 The Southend, Ledbury HR8 2EY Tel: 01531 631388 Email: sandy@intonet.co.uk — MB BS Lond. 1940 (King's Coll. Hosp.) MRCS Eng. LRCP Lond. 1940; DPM Eng. 1948; FRCPsych 1971. Specialty: Psychother. Socs: Gp. Analyt. Soc.; Fell. Roy. Soc. Med. Prev: Hon. Cons. Margt. Pyke Centre Soho Sq. Lond.; Cons. Psychiat. Shetland HB; Hon. Cons. Psychiat. Grampian HB.

SANDLAND, Richard Mark Maternity & Gynaecology Unit, Whiston Hospital, Prescot L35 5DR Tel: 0151 426 1600; 37 White Hart Gardens, Hartford, Northwich CW8 2FA — MB ChB Liverp. 1988; MRCOG 1995. Staff Grade (O & G) Whiston Hosp. Specialty: Obst. & Gyn. Prev: Specialist Regist. (O & G) Warrington Gen. Hosp.; Regist. (O & G) Liverp. Wom. Hosp., Countess of Chester Hosp. & Macclesfield Dist. Gen. Hosp.

SANDLE, Professor Geoffrey Ian St James's University Hospital, Molecular Medicine Unit, Clinical Sciences Building, Leeds LS9 7TF Tel: 0113 206 5686 Fax: 0113 244 4475 Email: g.i.sandle@leeds.ac.uk — MB ChB Leeds 1971; MRCP (UK) 1974; BSc (Hons.) Leeds 1968, MD 1980; PhD Manch. 1987; FRCP Lond. 1993. Prof. of Clin. Sci., Univ. of Leeds; Mem.Ct. of Examrs. RCS of Eng.; Mem Bd. of Examrs. RCP (Lond.). Specialty: Gastroenterol. Socs: Amer. Gastroenterol. Assn.; Brit. Soc. Gastroenterol.; Physiol. Soc. Prev: Nat. Foundat. for Ileitis & Colitis Sen. Research Fell. (Gastroenterol.) Yale Univ., USA; Sen. Lect. (Med.) Manch. Univ. & Hon. Cons. Phys. Hope Hosp. Salford; MRC Sen.Clin. Fell. & Hon. Cons. Phys. Hope Hosp. Salford.

SANDLE, Hugh John (retired) 18 Sharp Road, Bury St Edmunds IP33 2NB — MB BS Lond. 1983.

SANDLE, Lance Nigel Department of Chemical Pathology, Trafford General Hospital, Moorside Rd, Manchester M41 5SL Tel: 0161 746 2473 Fax: 0161 746 8545 Email: lance.sandle@trafford.nhs.uk — MB ChB (Distinc. Biochem.) Leeds 1978; BSc (Hons.) Leeds 1975; FRCPath 1996, M 1984. Cons. Chem. Path. Trafford HA; Hon. Clin. Teach. Fac. of Med. Univ. Manch.; Dep. Med. Director Trafford Healthcare NHS Trust. Specialty: Chem. Path. Socs: Assn. Clin. Pathol.; BMA; Assn. Clin. Biochem.s. Prev: Sen. Regist. (Chem. Path.) NW RHA; Resid. Clin. Path. Manch. Roy. Infirm.; Ho. Phys. Profess. Med. Unit St. Jas. Hosp. Leeds.

SANDLE, Linda Henrietta New Collegiate Medical Centre, 407 Cheetham Hill Road, Manchester M8 0DA Tel: 0161 205 4364 Fax: 0161 203 5511 — MB ChB Manch. 1982 (Manchester) DRCOG 1985; MRCGP 1986. Med. Mem. Indep. Trib. Serv. Socs: BMA. Prev: SHO N. Manch. VTS; Ho. Off. (Gen. Surg.) Hope Hosp. Salford; Ho. Off. (Gen. Med.) N. Manch. Gen. Hosp.

SANDLER, Bernard Maurice (retired) Flat No. 2, The Red House, Brick Kiln Lane, Limpsfield, Oxted RH8 0QG — MB BCh Witwatersrand 1946; FRCOG 1977, M 1954. Prev: Hon. Cons. (O & G) United Bulawayo Hosps. Zimbabwe & Zimbabwe Defence Forces & Zimbabwe Railways.

SANDLER, David Deparment of Geriatric Medicine, Birmingham Heartlands Hospital, Bordesley Green E., Birmingham B5 Tel: 0121 766 6611 Fax: 0121 753 0653 — MB ChB Glas. 1986; MRCP (UK) 1990; MSc 1997; FRCP 1999. Cons. Phys. (Geriat. Med.) Birm. Heartlands Hosp. Specialty: Gen. Med. Prev: Sen. Regist. (Med. eriat. & Diabetes); Career Regist. (Geriat.) Glas. Roy. Infirm.; Regist. (Gen. Med. & Diabetes) Glas. Roy. Infirm.

SANDLER, David Anthony Chesterfield & North Derbyshire Royal Hospital, Calow, Chesterfield S44 5BL Tel: 01246 277271 Fax: 01246 552613; 6 Brookfield Avenue, Brookside, Chesterfield S40 3NX — MB ChB Sheff. 1979; MRCP (UK) 1982; MD Sheff. 1986; FRCP Lond. 1996. Cons. Phys. Cardiol. Chesterfield & N. Derbysh. Roy. Hosp. Specialty: Cardiol. Socs: Brit. Cardiac Soc. Prev: Lect. (Med.) Univ. Hosp. Nottm.; Hon. Sen. Regist. Nottm. Hosps.; Research Fell. (Med.) Roy. Hallamsh. Hosp. Sheff.

SANDLER, Gerald Sunningdale, 185 Millhouses Lane, Sheffield S7 2HF Tel: 0114 236 6124 — MD Lond. 1959 (Middlx.) MB BS (Hons. & Gold Medal) 1952; FRCP Lond. 1973, M 1956. Cons. Phys. Barnsley Dist. Gen. Hosp.; Hon. Clin. Lect. in Med. Univ. Sheff. Specialty: Gen. Med. Socs: Brit. Cardiac Soc. & Assn. Phys. Prev: Sen. Med. Regist. United Sheff. Hosps.; Med. Regist. Profess. Therap. Unit Sheff. Roy. Infirm.; Regist. Sheff. Region Cardiovasc. Centre.

SANDLER, Laurence Melvyn Newlands, Bridle Lane, Loudwater, Rickmansworth WD3 4JH; Diabetes Centre, Wycombe General Hospital, High Wycombe HP11 2TI — MB ChB Cape Town 1974; MRCP (UK) 1977; MD Cape Town 1988; FRCP 1997. Cons. Phys. Wycombe Gen. Hosp. High Wycombe Bucks.; Cons. Phys. Chiltean Hosp. Gt. Missenden Bucks. Specialty: Gen. Med.; Diabetes; Endocrinol. Socs: Brit. Diabetic Assn.; Brit. Assn. Clin. Diabetologists; Nat. Osteoporosis Soc.

SANDLER, Mark Gerald The Surgery, 19 Amwell Street, Hoddesdon EN11 8TU Tel: 01992 464147 Fax: 01992 708698 — MB ChB Sheff. 1984; DRCOG 1989. Socs: BMA. Prev: Trainee GP Lond.; SHO (O & G) Lond. Hosp.; SHO (Anaesth.) St. Mary's Hosp. Lond.

SANDLER, Martin Solihull Hospital, Lode Lane, Solihull B91 2JL Tel: 0121 685 5315 Fax: 0121 685 5057; BUPA Parkway Hospital, Damson Parkway, Solihull B91 2PP Tel: 0121 704 1451 — MB ChB Glas. 1983; MRCP (UK) 1986; T(M) 1991. Cons. Phys. Solihull Hosp. Specialty: Gen. Med. Socs: Brit. Geriat. Soc. (Mem. Train. Comm.). Prev: Sen. Regist. Rotat. (Gen. & Geriat. Med.) W. Midl.; Regist. (Gen. Med. & Clin. Pharmacol.) Dept. Mat. Med. Stobhill Gen. Hosp. Glas.; Regist. & SHO Rotat. (Med.) Glas. Roy. Infirm.

SANDLER, Professor Merton 33 Park Road, Twickenham TW1 2QD Tel: 020 8383 3099 Fax: 020 8741 1948 Email: adept.lrs@btinternet.com; 33 Park Road, Twickenham TW1 2QD Tel: 020 8892 9085 Fax: 020 8891 5370 — (Manch.) MB ChB Manch . 1949; FRCP Lond. 1974, M 1955; MD Manch. 1962; FRCPath 1970, M 1963; FRCPsych 1986. Emerit. Prof. Chem. Path. Roy. Postgrad. Med. Sch. Univ. Lond.; Hon. Cons. Chem. Path. Qu. Charlotte's & Chelsea Hosp. Lond. Specialty: Chem. Path. Socs: (Pres.) Assn. for Postnatal Illness; (Ex-Pres.) Brit. Assn. Psychopharmacol.; (Ex-Pres.) Harv. Soc. Lond. Prev: Lect. (Chem. Path.) Roy. Free Hosp. Sch. Med.; Jun. Specialist (Path.) RAMC; Ho. Phys. Profess. Unit Roy. Manch. Childr. Hosp.

SANDLER, Rodney Michael (retired) 2 Breeze Mount, Prestwich, Manchester M25 0AH Tel: 0161 773 1200 — D(Obst) RCOG 1965 (Royal College of Obsterics & Gynaecology, London); MRCGP 1972(Royal College of General Practitioners) 1959; MB ChB Manchester 1959. Prev: Princip. in Gen. Pract. (Retd.).

SANDOE, Jonathan Ashley Torlot Craven Ridge House, Giggleswick, Settle BD24 0DY — MB ChB Manch. 1992.

SANDOZ, Maurice Douglas (retired) Neuchatel, Church Walk, Allesley, Coventry CV5 9ER Tel: 024 7640 2711 — M.B., Ch.B. Birm. 1928.

SANDRAMOULI, Mr Soupramanien Wolverhampton Hospitals NHS Trust, Wolverhampton WV10 0ZP Tel: 01902 307999 Fax: 01902 645019 — MB BS Madras 1987; FRCS Ed. 1994. Cons. Ophth. Wolverhampton & Midl. Counties Eye Inirm. Specialty: Ophth. Socs: Affil. Mem. Roy. Coll. of Ophth. Prev: Sen. Regist. Birm. Rotat.; SHO Watford & Mt Vernon NHS Trust.

SANDRASAGRA, Anton James Rajadurai Accident & Emergency Dept, Ashford St Peters Hospital, London Rd, Ashford TW15 3AA; 70A Royston Park Road, Hatch End, Pinner HA5 4AF — MB BS Sri Lanka 1976; MRCS Eng. LRCP Lond. 1990. A & E Ashford St Peters Hosp. Middlx.

SANDRASAGRA, Vasanti Westmount Surgery, 191 Westmount Road, London SE9 1XY Tel: 020 8850 1540 Fax: 020 8859 4737 — MB BS Sri Lanka 1973; MRCS Eng. LRCP Lond. 1980.

SANDRASEGARAN, Kumar Birmingham Heartlands NHS (Teaching) Trust, Bordesley Green E., Radiology Department, Birmingham B9 5SS Tel: 0121 766 6611 Ext: 4905 Fax: 0121 766 6919; 71 Sir Harrys Road, Edgbaston, Birmingham B15 2UX Tel: 0956 941062 Email: k_sandrasegaran@hotmail.com — MB ChB Zimbabwe 1985; MRCP (UK) 1990; MRCPI 1990; FRCR 1994. Cons. Radiol. Birm. Heartlands Hosp. Specialty: Radiol. Socs: BMA; RSNA. Prev: Sen. Regist. Rotat. (Radiol.) Leeds & Bradford.

SANDRESEGARAM, Mr Kasipillai 29 Larkspur Road, Marton Manor, Middlesbrough TS7 8RL Tel: 01642 319538 — MB BS Sri Lanka 1973; MRCS Eng. LRCP Lond. 1981; FRCS Eng. 1983.

SANDRY, Robert John (retired) Priory Cottage, Church Lane, Flax Bourton, Bristol BS48 3QF — (Bristol) MB ChB Bristol 1944; MD Bristol 1959; FRCPath 1975, M 1963. Prev: Cons. Path. Frenchay Hosp. Bristol.

SANDRY, Sheila Ann Priory Cottage, Church Lane, Flax Bourton, Bristol BS48 3QF — (Bristol) MB ChB Bristol 1957; FRCPath 1978, M 1966. Prev: Sen. Regist. Burden Neuropath. Laborat. Frenchay Hosp. Bristol; Sen. Regist. (Paediat. Path.) Roy. Hosp. Sick Childr. Edin.; Regist. (Path.) Southmead Hosp. Bristol.

SANDS, Amanda Melanie Lewisham Hospital, Paediatric Accident and Emergency, Lewisham High St., London SE13 6LH; 74 Barons Keep, Gliddon Road, London W14 9AU — MB BS Lond. 1992 (Lond. Hosp. Med. Coll.) DRCOG 1998. SHO (Paediat.) Lewisham Hosp. NHS Trust; GP Regist. Bradford Rd. Surg. Trowbridge Wilts. Specialty: Gen. Pract.; Obst. & Gyn. Prev: SHO (Psychiat.) SHO (Gen. Med. & Cas.); SHO (Paediat.).

SANDS, Andrew John 21 Antrim Road, Lisburn BT28 3ED Tel: 01846 664760 — MB BCh BAO Belf. 1992 (Qu. Univ. Belf.) MRCP Ed. 1995. Consultant (Paediat. & Cardiol.) Roy. Belf. Hosp. for Sick Childr. Specialty: Paediat. Cardiol.

SANDS, Caroline Jane Northland Surgery, 79 Cunninghams Lane, Dungannon BT71 6BX Tel: 028 87722137 Fax: 028 8772 7696; 22 Mullaghanagh Road, Dungannon BT71 7AY — MB BCh BAO Belf. 1983; DCH RCPS Glas. 1986.

SANDS, Fiona Mary Montalto Medical Centre, 2 Dromore Road, Ballynahinch BT24 8AY Tel: 028 9756 2929 — MB BCh BAO Belf. 1988; RCGP; DMH Belf. 1991; DRCOG 1992; DCH RCPSI 1992; MRCGP 1993; DFFP 1995. Socs: BMA.

SANDS, Keith Alexander John Pearl Diabetes Centre, King's Mill Hospital, Mansfield Rd, Sutton-in-Ashfield N617 4JL Tel: 01623 672289 Fax: 01623 672332 — MB ChB Manch. 1971; MRCP (UK) 1976; FRCP 1990. Cons.Endocrinologist & Gen. Phys., Kings M. U. Hosp., Mansfield. Specialty: Gen. Med.; Diabetes; Endocrinol. Prev: Sen. Regist. (Med.) Roy. Hallamsh. Hosp. Sheff.

SANDS, Mark James 46 Millbank, Headcorn, Ashford TN27 9RD — BM Soton. 1995. GP VTS William Harvey Hosp. Ashford. Specialty: Gen. Pract. Prev: RMO Rotat. Roy. Darwin Hosp. Darwin, Australia; Ho. Off. (Med.) Roy. S. Hants. Hosp. Soton.; Ho. Off. (Surg.) St. Mary's Hosp., Isle of Wight.

SANDS, Mary Grainne 23 Cleveden Road, Glasgow G12 0PQ — MB ChB Dundee 1992.

SANDS, Sandra Louise Lisburn Health Centre, Linenhall Street, Lisburn BT28 1LU Tel: 028 9260 3090 Fax: 028 9250 1310; 21 Antrim Road, Lisburn BT28 3ED — MB ChB BAO (Hons.) Belf. 1992 (Qu. Univ. Belf.) DRCOG 1994; DCH NUI 1994; MRCGP 1996; DFFP 1996. Specialty: Gen. Pract. Prev: GP/Regist. HillsBoro. Health Centre Co. Down.

SANDY, Mr Charles John North Hampshire Hospital, Aldermaston Road, Basingstoke RG24 9NA Tel: 01256 314719 — MB BS Lond. 1986 (Westm.) FRCOphth 1993. Cons. Ophth. Surg. N. Hants. Hosp. Basingstoke. Specialty: Ophth. Special Interest: Oculoplastic and Cataract Surg. Prev: Research Fell. (Ophth.) St Mary's Hosp. Lond.; Regist. (Ophth.) Moorfields Eye Hosp. Lond.

SANDY, Nigel Kirkham 15 Station Road, Verwood BH31 7PY Tel: 01202 825353 Fax: 01202 829697; 11 Motcombe Road, Branksome Park, Poole BH13 6DJ — MB BS Lond. 1981 (St. Geo.) MRCP (UK) 1984; DRCOG 1984; MRCGP 1986. Hosp. Practitioner (Chest Med.) Roy. Bournemouth. Hosp. Prev: GP with special interest in Cardiol. Wimborne Hosp. 2003; Trainee GP/SHO Scheme E. Dorset HA; SHO (A & E) Salisbury Gen. Hosp.

SANDYS, Rebecca Mary 16 Grove Road, Sheffield S7 2GZ — MB BS Lond. 1987; MRCGP 1993.

SANEHI, Om Parkash Dept. of Anaesth., Trafford General Hospital, Davyhulme, Manchester M41 5SL — MB ChB Ed. 1988. Cons. (Anaesth.) Trafford Gen. Hosp. Manch. Specialty: Anaesth. Prev: Roy. Nat. Throat, Nose & Ear Hosp.; Nat. Hosp. For Neurol. & Neurosurg.; Gt. Ormond St. Hosp. For Sick Childr.

SANFEY, John Joseph 21 April Street, Hackney, London E8 2EF — MB BCh BAO NUI 1983.

SANFORD, Henry Ayshford (retired) — MB BChir Camb. 1951 (St. Thos.) MA, MB BChir Camb. 1951; DPhysMed Eng. 1971. Sen. Lect. Cyriax Organisat. Internat. Courses. Prev: Assoc. Cons. Dept. Rheum. & Rehabil. St. Thos. Hosp. Lond.

SANFORD, Winifred (retired) 33 The Marlowes, Hastings Road, Bexhill-on-Sea TN40 2NS — MB BS Lond. 1956 (St. Barts.) Prev: Regist. Springfield Hosp. Lond., Psychiat.

SANGALA, Ann Vanessa Department of Reproductive & Sexual Health, Kings College Hospital, 100 Denmark Hill, London SE5 9RS Tel: 020 7346 5000 Email: vanessa.sangala@kingsch.nhs.uk — MB ChB Manch. 1972; MRCOG (Lond.) 1988; MFFP 1993; MA (Family Plann. Progr. Management) Exeter 1996; (Dip. In Genitourin. Med. & Venereol.) Liverpool 1999. Sen. Clin. Med. Off. Dept. Reproductive & Sexual Health, Kings Coll. Hosp. Specialty: Family Plann. & Reproduc. Health; Obst. & Gyn.; Genitourinary Medicine. Prev: Gen. Practitioner, Newport, Pembrokesh.; Reproductive Health Project Co-ordinator, Overseas Developm. Admin. Progr.; Obst./Gynaecologist, Malawi.

SANGAR, Sanjeev Kumar 1 Stewart Avenue, Upminster RM14 2AE — MB BS Lond. 1997.

SANGER, Julian Lorimer Field Lane Surgery, 42 Field Lane, Kessingland, Lowestoft NR33 7QA Tel: 01502 740203 Email: juliansanger@hotmail.com; The Vale House, Frostenden, Beccles NR34 7JA Tel: 01502 578327 — MB BChir Camb. 1976.

SANGER, Leslie Vincent (retired) Towcester Medical Centre, Link Way, Towcester NN12 6HH Tel: 01327 359339 Fax: 01327 358944 — MB BCh Wales 1968.

SANGHA, Marik Singh Flat 7 James Brindley Basin, Piccadilly Village, Great Ancoats St., Manchester M1 2NL — MB ChB Manch. 1992.

SANGHA, Rageni Kaur Flat 2, 18 Chesham Place, Brighton BN2 1FB — MB BCh Wales 1995.

SANGHA, Sukhdev Singh 5 Sledmore Road, Dudley DY2 8DY — MB ChB Birm. 1994.

SANGHA, Sukhjit — MB BChir Camb. 1991; BSc Lond. 1987. GP Princip., Rickmansworth. Socs: BMA & Med. Protec. Soc.

SANGHANI, Jagjivan Valji Abercynon Health Centre, Abercynon, Mountain Ash CF45 4YB Tel: 01443 740447 Fax: 01443 740228 — MB BS Panjab 1965 (Amritsar Med. Coll.) MB BS Panjab (India) 1965.

SANGHANI, Neelam 8 Alexandra Place, Abercynon, Mountain Ash CF45 4YA — MB BCh Wales 1993.

SANGHANI, Rajesh 8 Alexandra Palace, Abercynon, Mountain Ash CF45 4YA — MB BS Lond. 1994.

SANGHANI, Vinaychandra Valji Preferred Health Care Ltd, Avalon House, Rowley Lane, Barnet EN5 3HT Tel: 0845 890 1260 Fax: 0845 890 1261 — MB BS Lond. 1976; MRCS Eng. LRCP Lond. 1976.

SANGHERA, Juggit Singh Severn House Surgery, 96 Albert Road, Stechford, Birmingham B33 8AG Tel: 0121 784 0208 Fax: 0121 789 7351; Grange Farm, Bicken Hill, Solihull B92 0DR — MB ChB Birm. 1976.

SANGHERA, Paul The Lodge, Edgefields La, Stockton Brook, Stoke-on-Trent ST9 9NS — MB ChB Leeds 1997.

SANGHERA, Satinder Kaur Stanhope Health Centre, Dales Street, Stanhope, Bishop Auckland DL13 2XD Tel: 01388 528555; 35 Gateways, Bishop Auckland DL13 3HW — MB BCh Wales 1991; DRCOG. GP. Specialty: Family Plann. & Reproduc. Health; Gen. Pract.; Ment. Health.

SANGHERA, Sukhdev Singh Princess Royal Hospital, Apley Castle, Telford TF1 6TF Tel: 01952 641222 Email: davesanghera@doctors.org.uk; 40 Cubbington Road, Coventry CV6 7BN — MB ChB Manch. 1974; FFA RCS Eng. 1981. Cons. Anaesth. Princess Roy. Hosp. Telford. Specialty: Anaesth. Socs: Assoc. of Anaesthetics; Roy. Coll. Of Anaesthetist. Prev: Sen. Regist. Rotat. (Anaesth.) W. Midl. RHA.

SANGHERA, Sumayer 1A Douglas Way, London SE8 4AG — MB ChB Leeds 1994.

SANGHERA, Vichitar — MB BS Punjab, India 1992; DFFP.

SANGHI, Anita Royal London Hospital, Whitechapel, London E1 1BB Tel: 020 7377 7000; 9 Burnhill Court, Standish, Wigan WN6 0AN Tel: 01257 421161 Fax: 01257 421161 — MB BS Meerut 1980 (L.L.R.M. Medical College Meerut India) MD Meerut 1983; DObst RCPSI 1986; MRCOG 1987; MD Manch. 1995. Cons. Obst. & Gyanecology Roy. Lond. Hosp., Lond. Specialty: Obst. & Gyn. Socs: BMA; N. Eng. Obst. & Gyn. Soc.; Roy. Coll. Obst. & Gyn. Prev: Sen. Regist. (O & G) St. Mary's Hosp. Manch. (Flexible).; Regist. (O & G) Sharoe Green Hosp. Preston & Marston Green Hosp. Birm.; Sen. Reg (O & G) Roy. Bolton Hosp. (Flexible).

SANGHI, Pradeep Kumar Royal Albert Edward Infirmary, Wigan Lane, Wigan WN1 2NN Tel: 01942 244000 Fax: 01942 822340 — MB BS Delhi 1977; MD (Med.) Delhi 1981; MRCPI 1986. Assoc. Specialist (Med.) Roy. Albert Edwd. Infirm. Wigan. Specialty: Gastroenterol. Socs: Brit. Soc. Gastroenterol.; N. Eng. Gastroenterol. Soc. Prev: Regist. (Med.) Roy. Albert Edwd. Infirm. Wigan; Regist. (Gen. Med.) Bury Gen. Hosp.

SANGHVI, Mukesh Vadilal 86 Elgin Road, Seven Kings, Ilford IG3 8LN — MB BS Lond. 1985.

SANGOWAWA, Olugbenga Oluseun Aylesbury Partnership, Aylesbury Medical Centre, Taplow House, Thurlow Street, London SE17 2XE Tel: 020 7703 2205 — MB BS Ibadan 1985; DRCOG 1993; DFFP 1993; T(GP) 1994.

SANGRA, Meharpal Singh 26 Marchmont Crescent, Edinburgh EH9 1HG — MB ChB Ed. 1996.

SANGRA, Rai Ahmad Sadiq Gate Medical Centre, 120 Washwood Heath Road, Saltley, Birmingham B8 1RE Tel: 0121 327 4427; 8 Newmarsh Road, Sutton Coldfield B76 1XW Tel: 0121 351 6148 — MB BS Punjab 1965 (Nishtar Med. Coll.) DO RCS Eng. 1968.

SANGSTER, Graeme Department Medicine for the Elderly, Arrowe Park Wirral Hospital NHS Trust, Upton, Wirral CH49 5PE Tel: 0151 678 5111; 8 Wicks Gardens, Formby, Liverpool L37 3QS — MB ChB Ed. 1975; MRCP (UK) 1979; FRCP 1998. Cons. Phys. (Med. for Elderly) Arrowe Pk. Wirral Hosp. Merseyside. Specialty: Care of the Elderly.

SANGSTER, Pamela Jean (retired) 7A Valley Road, Stone ST15 0DQ Tel: 01785 815266 — MB ChB Birm. 1946. Prev: Clin. Asst., N. Staffs Roy. Infrimary Stoke on Trent.

SANGTANI, Mr Hargun Jairamdas Ortho Relief Hospital & Research Centre, Opposite Ramkrishna Mission, Dhantoli, Nagpur 440 012, India Fax: 00 91 712 543314; 44 Blackbird Close, Poole BH17 7YA — MB BS Nagpur 1978 (Govt. Medical College & Hospital, Nagpur, India) MS (Orthop.) Nagpur 1982; FRCS Glas. 1986; MChOrth Liverp. 1988. Cons. Orthop. Surg. Orth. Relief. Hosp. & Research Centre, Dhantoli, Nagpur, India. Specialty: Dentistry/Orthodontics; Orthop. Socs: Overseas Fell. BOA; Life Mem. Indian Orthop. Assn. Prev: Sen. Regist. Our Lady's Childr. Hosp. Dub.; Sen. Regist. Pool & ChristCh. Hosp.; Sen. Regist. (Orthop.) Wrightington Hosp. Wigan.

SANIKOP, Shrishail Basavanneppa Royal Gwent Hospital, Newport NP20 2UB Tel: 01633 234234; 12A Llyn Berwyn Close, Rogerstone, Newport NP10 9AU Tel: 01633 897365 — MB BS Karnatak 1978 (Karnatak Med. Coll. Hubli, India) MRCOG 1989; MFFP 1995. Assoc. Specialist (O & G) Roy. Gwent Hosp. Newport. Specialty: Obst. & Gyn. Prev: Staff Grade Pract. (O & G) Roy. Gwent Hosp. Newport; Regist. (O & G) Falkirk Roy. Infirm.; SHO (O & G) Qu. Pk. Hosp. Blackburn.

SANJEEV, Doraiswamy c/o 114 Cross Street, Nottingham NG5 7BY — MB BS Bangalor 1979; MB BS Bangalore 1979, DPM 1982; MRCPsych 1988. Sen. Psychiat. Yorkton Ment. Health Centre Saskatchewan, Canada.

SANJEEVA RAO, Veluvolu Earls House Hospital, Durham City, Durham DH1 5RE — MB BS Andhra 1972.

SANKAR, Deivanayagam 30 Hawthorne Road, Rochdale OL11 5JQ — MB BS Madras 1979.

SANKAR, Kanthimathinathan Newcastle General Hospital, Westgate Road, Newcastle upon Tyne NE4 6BE Tel: 0191 256 3256 Email: k.n.sankar@ncl.ac.uk — MB BS Sri Lanka 1977; MRCP (UK) 1983; FRCP Lond. 1996. Cons. Genitourin. Phys. Newc. Gen. Hosp.; Hon. Clin. Lect. Univ. Newc. Specialty: Genitourinary Medicine. Socs: Med. Soc. Study VD. Prev: Cons. Genitourin. Phys. E.& W. Cumbria; Sen. Regist. (Genitourin. Med.) Newc. Gen. Hosp.; Regist. in Genitourin Med., Roy. North. Hosp., Lond.

SANKAR, Ramkrishna Mayfield, Boldon Lane, Cleadon Village, Sunderland SR6 7RT Fax: 0191 454 2424 Email: ramkrishna1610@btinternet.com — MB BS Calcutta 1972. GP S. Shields.

SANKAR, Sachin 18 Cliftonville Court, Northampton NN1 5BY Tel: 01604 545195 Email: sachin.sankar@virgin.net — MB BS Osmania 1988. Locum Cons. (Psychiat. Child & Adolesc.). Specialty: Child & Adolesc. Psychiat. Special Interest: Risk Assesment in Childr.

SANKAR, Vengudi Swaminathan Fairfield General Hospital , Pennine Acute Hospitals NHS Trust, Department of Paediatrics, Bury BL9 7TD Tel: 0161 778 3866 — MB BS Madras 1983; MRCP (UK) 1992; FRCPCH 1997. Sen. Regist. (Paediat.) King's Coll. Hosp. Lond. Specialty: Paediat. Special Interest: Neonatology; Paediatric Diabetes. Socs: Life Mem. Indian Acad. Paediat.; Brit. Paediat. Assn. Prev: Sen. Regist. Rotat. (Paediat.) Roy. Alexandra Hosp. Sick Childr. Brighton; Clin. Fell. (Paediat. Intens. Care) Leeds Gen. Infirm.; Regist. (Med. Paediat.) Edin.

SANKARAN, Mohanan Department of Neurosurgery, North Staffordshire Royal Infirmary, Princes Road, Hartshill, Stoke-on-Trent ST4 7LN — MB BS Karnatak, India 1982.

SANKARAYYA, Nanju (retired) 30 Augustus Road, Edgbaston, Birmingham B15 3PQ Tel: 0121 454 3101 — MB BChir Camb. 1958 (Camb. & Birm.) MRCS Eng. LRCP Lond. 1958; MB BChir Camb. 1959; MA Camb. 1960; MRCGP 1976. Prev: Capt. RAMC.

SANKEY, Arthur Octavius (retired) 34 Stormont Road, London N6 4NP Tel: 020 8340 0133 — MRCS Eng. LRCP Lond. 1945 (St. Thos.) MRCOG 1956, DObst 1948. Hon. Cons. O & G Newham HA. Prev: Cons. (Obst.) Newham Matern. Hosp. Lond.

SANKEY, Elizabeth Ann Department of Histopathology, The Pilgrim Hospital, Sibsey Road, Boston PE21 9QS Tel: 01205 364801 — MB BS Lond. 1985 (Roy. Lond.) BSc (Hons.) Bristol 1977; PhD Camb. 1981; MRCPath 1993; FRCPath 2001. Cons. Path. (Histopath. & Cytopath.) Pilgrim Hosp. Boston. Specialty: Histopath. Socs: Assn. Clin. Path; Internat. Acad. Path. Prev: Cons. Path. (Histopath. & Cytopath.) Qu. Eliz. Hosp. King's Lynn; Cons. Path. (Histopath. & Cytopath.) Co. Hosp. Hereford.; Lect. & Hon. Sen. Regist. (Histopath.) Roy. Free Hosp.

SANKEY, Rowena Jane Alexandra Hospital, Woodrow Drive, Redditch B98 7UB Tel: 01527 503030 — MB ChB Liverp. 1977; MRCP (UK) 1981; FRCPCH 1998; FRCP Ed 1998; FRCP Lond. 1998. Cons. Paediat. Alexandra Hosp. Redditch.; Hon. Sen. Clin. Lect. Inst. Child Health Univ. Birm. Specialty: Paediat.

SANKEY, Sarah Jane Meadowbank Health Centre, Salmon Inn Road, Polmont, Falkirk FK2 0XF — MB ChB Ed. 1997 (Edin.) DRCOG; MRCGP; DFFP. GP Princip. Specialty: Paediat. Prev: SHO (Paed.) Forth Pk. Matern. Hosp. Fife.

SANKOH, Mohammed Abioseh (retired) Kirklees, 6 Linwood Grove, Darlington DL3 8DP Tel: 01325 381739 Fax: 01325 484479 — (University of Newcastle Upon-Tyne) MB BS Newcastle Upon-Tyne 1971; MB BS Newcastle Upon-Tyne 1971; DTM & H London School of Hygiene & Tropical Medicine 1973; MRCP London 1976; FRCP London 1998. Locum Cons.-Gen. Med. & chest Med., Medway Martine Hosp., Gillingham, Kent. Prev: Locum Cons. Elderly Med., ystradgynlais/Brewnshire War Memor. Hosp., Brecon, Wales.

SANKSON, Hayley Quarter Jack Surgery, Rodways Corner, Wimborne BH21 1AP Tel: 01202 848262 Fax: 01202 882368 — BM Soton. 1991.

SANMUGANATHAN, Philemon Sabapathy Dept of Cerebrovascular Medicine, Worcester Royal Hospital, Worcester WR5 1DD — MD Columbo 1992; MB BS Peradeniya 1986; MRCP UK 1995. Consultant Physician. Specialty: Gen. Med.; Vasc. Med.; Pharmacology. Socs: BMA; BPS- Brit. Pharmacol. Soc.; BASP- Brit. Assoc. of Stroke Phys.s. Prev: Hon.Specialist Regist.; Senior Lect. Uiniversity of Peradeniya; Lect. University of Sheffield.

SANSBURY, Michael Arthur University Health Centre, Fulton House, Singleton Park, Swansea SA2 8PR Tel: 01792 295321 Fax: 01792 295854 — MB ChB Ed. 1972; BSc Ed. 1969. GP Univ. Coll. Swansea. Specialty: Gen. Med. Socs: BMA; Hon Pres. Brit. Assn. Health Servs. in Higher Educat.2001. Prev: Med. Off. 188th Gen. Disp. US Army Bamberg; Trainee GP Gwynedd VTS.

SANSOM, Alison Elizabeth Anne 12 Monks Mead, Brightwell Cum Sotwell, Wallingford OX10 0RL — MRCS Eng. LRCP Lond. 1956.

SANSOM, Christine Dinah West Wirral Group Practice, 3 Brooze Meadow, Irby, Wirral CH61 4YS — MB ChB Liverp. 1980; DRCOG 1992; DTM & H Liverp. 1997. Specialty: Community Child Health; Gen. Med. Socs: Local Med. Comm.

SANSOM, David Thomas Royal Leamington Spa Rehabilitation Hospital, Heathcote Lane, Warwick CV34 6SR; 42 Tenbury Road, Kings Heath, Birmingham B14 6AH — MB BS Lond. 1982; MRCPsych 1987. Cons. Psychiat. S. Warks. Specialty: Ment. Health. Prev: Sen. Regist. (Ment. Retardation) Monyhull Hosp. Birm.; Regist. (Psychiat.) Northwick Pk. Hosp. Harrow.

SANSOM, Hugh Edward Royal Shrewsbury Hospital, Mytton Oak Road, Shrewsbury SY3 8XQ Tel: 01743 261000 — MB BS Lond. 1986; MRCP (UK) 1992; FRCR 1995. Cons. (Radiol.) Roy. Shrewsbury Hosp. Specialty: Radiol.

SANSOM, Jane Elizabeth Bristol Royal Infirmary, Department of Dermatology, Bristol BS2 8HW Tel: 0117 923 2770 — MB ChB Bristol 1984; MRCP (UK) 1988; FRCP 2001. Cons. (Dermat.) Bristol Roy. Infirm. Specialty: Dermat. Prev: Sen. Regist. (Dermat.) Bristol Roy. Infirm.; SHO (Med. & Neurol.) Frenchay Hosp. Bristol; Ho. Off. (Med.) Frenchay Hosp. Bristol.

SANSOM, Mr Julian Rupert Dale Farm, Thorpe-Next-Haddiscoe, Norwich NR14 6PY — MRCS Eng. LRCP Lond. 1965 (St. Thos.) FRCS Eng. 1973. Cons. (Gen. Surg.) Gt. Yarmouth & Waveney Health Dist. Specialty: Gen. Surg. Prev: Surg. Regist. Artific. Kidney Unit Qu. Eliz. Hosp. Birm.; Sen. Regist. Surg. Professional Unit Qu. Eliz. Hosp. Birm.

SANSOME, Alison Donald Community Child Health, Idu Darwin Hospital, Fulburn, Cambridge CB1 5EE Tel: 01223 884162 Fax: 01223 884161; Wimbish Manor, Fowlmere Road, Shepreth, Royston SG8 6QL — BM BCh Oxf. 1988; MA Camb. 1989, BA 1985. Cons. in Community Paediat. Specialty: Paediat. Socs: Wom.s Med. Fed. (Sec.Camb. Distict). Prev: Regist. (Paediat.) Hammersmith Hosp. Lond.; Clin. Research Fell. Hammersmith Hosp. Lond.; Regist (Paediat) Addenbrookes Hosp. Camb.

SANSOME, Andrew Jonathan Thomas Department of Anaesthesia, Southampton General Hospital, Tremona Road, Southampton SO16 6YD Tel: 023 8077 7222 — MB ChB Sheff. 1980; FRCA 1984. Cons. Anaesth. Soton. NHS Trust. Specialty: Anaesth. Socs: Vasc. Anaesth. Soc.; Intens. Care Soc. Prev: Sen. Regist. (Anaesth.) Soton. Gen. Hosp.

SANSOME, David Anthony Woodruff 11 Meadowcourt Road, Oadby, Leicester LE2 2PD Tel: 0116 271 2994 — MB ChB Sheff. 1956; MRCS Eng. LRCP Lond. 1956; DObst RCOG 1961; FRCGP 1984, M 1968; AFOM RCP Lond. 1981; T(GP) 1991. Med. Off. & Appt. Doctor EMAS to Alstom & Alstec Power Eng. Whetstone; Med. Off. SPS Technologies (T. J. Brooks). Specialty: Occupat. Health. Socs: (Ex-Pres.) Leic. Med. Soc.; BMA (Ex-Pres. Leics. & Rutland Div.).; Leic. Medico Legal Soc. Prev: GP Leicester; SHO (Surg.) Leicester Roy. Infirm.; Ho. Off. (Gyn. & Obst.) City Gen. Hosp. Leicester.

SANSOME, John Frederick (retired) Stonecroft, Post Office Lane, Lighthorne, Warwick CV35 0AP Tel: 01926 651424 Email: jsansome@doctors.org.uk — MB BS Lond. 1957 (Univ. Coll. Hosp.) DPH Lond. 1968. Prev: SCMO S. Warks. Health Care Trust.

SANSOME, Jonathan David Woodruff Weavers Medical Centre, 50 School Lane, Kettering NN16 0DH Tel: 01536 513494 Fax: 01536 416521 — MB ChB Leic. 1992 (Leicester) MRCGP.

SANT, Andrew Mark 39 Ash Hayes Drive, Nailsea, Bristol BS48 2LQ; Little Mill, Egremont CA22 2NN Tel: 01946 820056 — BM Soton. 1995. GP Regist. Anne Burrow Thomas Health Centre Workington Cumbria. Specialty: Gen. Pract. Socs: Med. Protec. Soc. Prev: SHO (Cardiol. & Neurol.) Poole Hosp. NHS Trust Poole; SHO (Med.) Roy. Bournemouth Hosp. Bournemouth.

SANT, Kathleen Elizabeth Monteagle Surgery, Tesimond Drive, Monteagle Park, Yateley GU46 6FE Tel: 01252 878992; 21 Crail Close, Wokingham RG41 2PZ — BM BCh Oxf. 1985 (Oxford) DCH RCP Lond. 1988; MRCGP 1989.

SANT, Keith Godfrey Cross Street Health Centre, Cross Street, Dudley DY1 1RN Tel: 01384 459044 Fax: 01384 232467 — MRCS Eng. LRCP Lond. 1968 (Manch.) Specialty: Gen. Pract. Prev: Ho. Off. (Obst.) Stepping Hill Hosp. Stockport.; Ho. Phys. Bury & Rossendale Gen. Hosps.; Ho. Surg. Withington Hosp. Manch.

SANTANA HERNANDEZ, Diego Jose ENT Department, City Hospital, Greenbank Drive, Edinburgh EH10 5SB Tel: 0131 536 6000 — LMS La Laguna 1988; DLO RCS Eng. 1995. Regist. (ENT) Roy. Infirm. Edin. NHS Trust. Specialty: Otorhinolaryngol. Prev: Career SHO (ENT) York Dist. Hosp.; SHO (ENT) Hull Roy. Infirm.

SANTANIELLO-NEWTON, Autilia 17 Lichfield Avenue, Hale, Altrincham WA15 8PG — State Exam Naples 1980.

SANTER, Mr Graham Julian Stoneleigh, Orient Drive, Liverpool L25 5NZ — MB ChB Liverp. 1957; DObst RCOG 1959; FRCS Eng. 1963. Socs: Liverp. Med. Inst. & BMA.

SANTER, Miriam Clare — MB BChir Camb. 1993; DFFP 1995; DRCOG 1995; MRCGP 1996. Higher Professional Train. Fell. Edin. Univ. Depart. Gen. Pract. Specialty: Gen. Pract.

SANTER, Patricia Maureen Strathbrock Partnership Centre, 189A West Mall Street, Broxburn EH52 5LH Tel: 01506 771800 Fax: 01506 771820; 9 Ravelrig Park, Balerno EH14 7DL Tel: 0131 449 5278 — MB BS Lond. 1970 (Lond. Hosp.) BSc (Physiol.) Lond. 1967; DObst RCOG 1972; Cert. FPA 1974; DA Eng. 1974; MRCGP 1976; Dip. Ven. Soc. Apoth. Lond. 1982; Cert. Family Plann. JCC (Instruc. Doctor's Cert.) 1982; MFFP 1993. Socs: Scott. Family Plann. Med. Soc. Prev: Co-ordinating Doctor Edin. Brook Advis. Centre; Clin. Asst. (Genitourin. Med.) Ipswich Hosp.; Clin. Asst. (Genitourin. Med.) Roy. Shrewsbury & Wrekin Hosp.

SANTHAKUMAR, Della 54 Somertrees Avenue, London SE12 0BY — MB BS Lond. 1996.

SANTHIAPILLAI, Domingo c/o Mrs Margaret Rajapakse, Red Wood Day Unit, St John's Hospital, Wood St., Chelmsford CM2 9BG — MB BS Ceylon 1968.

SANTINI, Mr Alasdair John Ario — MB ChB Sheff. 1992; FRCS Glas. 1997; FRCS Eng. 1997; FRCS ((Tr. and Orth.)) 2002. Mersey Deanery Specialist Regist. Rotat. (Orthop.) 1998. Specialty: Trauma & Orthop. Surg. Socs: Assoc. Fell. of Brit. Orthopaedic Assn. (BOA); Brit. Med. Assn.; Brit. Assn. for Surg. of the Knee. Prev: SHO Rotat. (Gen. Surg.) Roy. Hallamsh. Hosp. Sheff.; SHO & Demonst. (Anat.) Univ. Sheff.; SHO (Orthop. & A & E) Roy. Hallamsh. Hosp. Sheff.

SANTIS, Georghios 19 King's Avenue, London W5 — MB ChB Leic. 1983; MRCP (UK) 1986. Research Fell. Brompton Hosp. & Nat. Heart & Lung Inst. Lond.

SANTORI, Louise Bernadette Newtown Surgery, 147 Lawn Avenue, Great Yarmouth NR30 1QP Tel: 01493 853191 Fax: 01493 331861 — MB ChB Birm. 1991; ChB Birm. 1991; MRCGP 1996.

SANTOS, Joseph Pele Dos 33 Wellington Gardens, Victoria Way, London SE7 7PJ — MB BS Lond. 1996.

SANTOS, Sean Rice Anaesthetic Department, Furness General Hospital, Dalton Lane, St Helier, Jersey JE2 3QS Tel: 01224 870870 — MB BS Lond. 1987 (St. Geo. Hosp. Lond.) MA Camb. 1987, BA 1983. Staff Grade. (Anaesth.) FGH. Specialty: Anaesth. Socs: BMA; Assn. Anaesth. Prev: Regist. (Anaesth.) Gen. Hosp. St. Helier, Jersey; Regist. Rotat. (Anaesth.) St. Mary's Hosp. Lond.; SHO (Intens. Care) Middlx. Hosp. Lond.

SANTOS RAMON, Angel Guy's Hospital, IPTS York Clinic, 47 Weston Street, London SE1 3RR Tel: 020 7188 7018 Fax: 020 7188 7024 Email: angel.santos@slam.nhs.uk — LMS Autonoma Madrid 1989; MRCPsych 1995. Cons. (Psychiat. & Psychother.) Guys Hosp. Lond. Specialty: Gen. Psychiat.; Psychother. Special Interest: Personality Disorders; Theraputic Community. Socs: Assoc. Mem. Brit. Psychanalytical Soc. Prev: Sen. Regist. (Psychother.) N. Thames (W.) Regional Psychother. Train. Scheme; Regist. Rotat. N. Lond. Teachg. Hosp. UCH.

SANTOSH, Celestine Gnanamuthu Department of Neuroradiology, Middlesbrough General Hospital, Middlesbrough TS5 5AZ Tel: 01642 850850; Flat 3, Middlesbrough General Hosptial, Middlesbrough TS5 5AZ Tel: 01642 850850 — MB BS Poona 1983; FRCR 1990. Cons. Neuroradiol. Middlesbrough Gen. Hosp. Specialty: Radiol. Socs: BMA; Med. Protec. Soc.; Roy. Coll. Radiol. Prev: Lect. MRI Univ. Edin.; Asst. Prof. Radiol. (SLTMIST, India).

SANUSI, Mr Fatai Abegboyega Department of Obstetrics & Gynaecology, 60 Vicarage Road, Watford WD18 0HB Tel: 01923 244366; 37B Chaplin Road, Willseden, London NW3 5PP — MB BS Lagos 1986 (College of Med. Univ. Lagos) MRCOG 1992. Cons. Obst./ Gynaecologist, W.Herts. NHS Trust, Watford. Specialty: Obst. & Gyn. Socs: Feto-Matern. Med. Soc.; BSCCP. Prev: SpR -St Geo.'s Hosp.; Regist. Barnet & Edgeware Hosps.; SHO Pontefract & Dewsbury Hosps.

SANVILLE, Philip Roland 1 Croft Road, Wilmslow SK9 6JJ — MB BS Lond. 1982 (St. Geo.) DRCOG 1984; MRCGP 1986; DCH RCP Lond. 1986; MRCP (UK) 1988; FRCR Lond. 1991. Cons. Radiol. Stepping Hill Hosp. Stockport. Specialty: Radiol. Prev: Sen. Regist. Rotat. (Radiol.) Manch.; Cook Fell. Interven. Radiol.

SANYAL, Aparna 15 The Chase, Edgware HA8 5DW — MB ChB Bristol 1997.

SANYAL, Buddhadeb Kettering General Hospital, Rothwell Road, Kettering NN16 8UZ Tel: 01536 422000; 120 Brambleside, Kettering NN16 9BP Tel: 01536 519811 — MB BS Sambalpur 1968; DLO RCS Eng. 1980. Regist. (Otolaryngol.) Kettering Gen. Hosp. Specialty: Otolaryngol. Socs: Assoc. Mem. Brit. Assn. Otolaryngol. Prev: SHO (ENT) King's Coll. Hosp. Lond.; SHO (ENT) FarnBoro. Hosp.

SANYAL, Debasis Royal Manchester Childrens Hospital, Hospital Road, Pendlebury, Manchester M27 4HA — MD Manch. 1992; BSc Manch. 1980, MB ChB 1982; MRCPath 1989; Dip. Bact. Manch. 1989. Cons. Microbiol. Roy. Manch. Childr. Hosp. Specialty: Med. Microbiol. Socs: Hosp. Infec. Soc. & Brit. Soc. Antimicrob. Chemother. Prev: SHO. (Clin. Path.) Manch. Roy. Infirm.; Regist. (Microbiol.) Univ. Hosp. of Wales Cardiff.; Sen. Regist. (Microbiol.) Pub. Health Laborat. N. Gen. Hosp. Sheff.

SANYAL, Karuna Prasad 11 Oak Dene Close, Hornchurch RM11 1HD Tel: 0140 24 51675 — MB BS Calcutta 1959; DA Eng. 1968. Assoc. Specialist Anaesth. Dept. OldCh. Hosp. Romford. Socs: BMA. Prev: Cas. Off. Boston Gen. Hosp.; SHO (Anaesth.) Dryburn Hosp. Durh.; Regist. (Anaesth.) Burton-on-Trent Gen. Hosp.

SANZERI, Marcus 24 Rhodes Street, Hightown, Castleford WF10 5LL — MB ChB Liverp. 1990.

SAPERIA, Joseph (retired) Flat 5, Ambassador Court, Century Close, London NW4 2EE Tel: 020 8202 6263 — (Qu. Univ. Belf.) MB BCh BAO Belf. 1948; MRCGP 1955. Prev: Ho. Surg. Roy. Vict. Hosp. Belf.

SAPEY, Elizabeth Homelands, Magdalen Road, Tilney St Lawrence, King's Lynn PE34 4RE — MB BS Lond. 1998; MB BS Lond 1998.

SAPHERSON, David Andrew 120 High Street, Knaresborough HG5 0HN — MB ChB Sheff. 1980.

SAPHIER, Emanuel (retired) 20 The Vale, Ovingdean, Brighton BN2 7AB Tel: 01273 305240 — MRCS Eng. LRCP Lond. 1940 (Westm.) Prev: Flight Lt. R.A.F.V.R.

SAPPER, Helen 3 Boston Gardens, Chiswick, London W4 2QJ Tel: 020 8742 8313 Email: helensapper@hotmail.com — MRCS Eng. LRCP Lond. 1959 (Roy. Free) MSc Lond. 1992, MB BS 1959; FRCGP 1992, M 1973; DHMSA 1997. Chairm. Indep. Review Panel for Continuing Care Ealing, Hammersmith & Hounslow HA; Med. Qual. Tribunal Mem. Appeal Serv. Specialty: Gen. Pract.; Med. Publishing. Socs: Fell.Roy. Soc. of Med. Prev: GP Acton Health Centre Lond.; Clin. Asst. Ealing Child Guid. Centre; SHO (Path.) King Edwd. Memor. Hosp. Ealing.

SAPPER, Miriam Esho South Saxon House Surgery, 150A Bexhill Road, St Leonards-on-Sea TN38 8BL Tel: 01424 441361 Fax: 01424 461799 — MB ChB Baghdad 1966.

SAPRE, S Westway, Maghull, Liverpool L31 0DJ.

SAPSFORD, David John Department of Anaesthesia, Box 93 Level E4, Addenbrooke's Hospital, Cambridge CB2 2QQ Tel: 01223 217889 Fax: 01223 217223 — MB BS Lond. 1980; FFA RCS Eng. 1987. Sen. Lect. (Anaesth.) Univ. Camb.; Hon. Cons. Anaesth. Addenbrooke's Hosp. Camb. Specialty: Anaesth. Prev: Lect. (Anaesth.) Leeds Univ.

SAPSFORD, Derrick (retired) 1 Fir Court, Hythe Road, Willesborough, Ashford TN24 0QW Tel: 01233 626714 — MB ChB St. And. 1960; DObst RCOG 1963.

SAPSFORD, Mr Ralph Neville 20 Birkdale Road, London W5 1JZ; 66 Harley Street, London W1N 1AE Tel: 020 7631 4820 — MB ChB Cape Town 1962; FRCS Eng. 1967; FRCS Ed. 1967; ChM Cape Town 1976. Cons. & Sen. Lect. (Cardiothoracic Surg.) Hammersmith Hosp. & Roy. Postgrad. Med. Sch. Lond.; Hon. Cons. (Cardiothoracic Surg.) St. Mary's Hosp. & Med. Sch. Lond. Specialty: Cardiothoracic Surg. Prev: Sen. Regist. (Cardiothoracic Surg.) Hammersmith Hosp. Lond.

SAPSFORD, Robert Andrew Rectory Meadow Surgery, School Lane, Amersham HP7 0HG Tel: 01494 727711 Fax: 01494 431790 — MB ChB Otago 1976; DRCOG 1979; DCH Eng. 1979; MRCGP 1980. Clin. Asst. (Gastroenterol.) Amersham Hosp. Specialty: Gastroenterol. Socs: Chiltern Med. Soc.

SAPSFORD, Robert John St. James's University Hospital, Leeds LS9 7TF — MB BS Lond. 1990; BSc London 1996. Specialist Regist. Cons. Cardiol. St James Univ. Hosp. Leeds. Specialty: Cardiol.

SAPSFORD, Mr Wayne — (Roy. Lond. Hosp. Med. Coll.) BA(Hons) Camb. 1988; MA Camb. 1992; FRCS Eng. 1997. Research Fell.; Roy. Air Force Off. RAF Innsworth Gloucester. Specialty: Gen. Surg. Socs: Freeman Worshipful Soc. Apoths.; Assoc. of Surg. Of GB & I.

SAPUAY, Biennita Corpuz 65 Roxburgh Road, London SE27 0LE — MB BS Lond. 1995.

SAQIB, Mohammad Najum-Us 31 Maidencastle, Blackthorn, Northampton NN3 8EH Tel: 01604 414520 — MB BS Punjab 1987; MRCP (UK) 1992.

SAQIB, Najam Us Bassetlaw District General Hospital, Worksop S81 0BD Tel: 01909 502270 Fax: 01909 502273 — MB BS Karachi (Dow Med. Coll., Karachi) DA Eng.; FFARCSI. Cons. Anaesth. Specialty: Anaesth. Socs: BMA; Assn. of Anaesthetists of Gt. Britain and Irel.; Brit. Assn. of Day Surg. Prev: Cons. Anaesth., King Fahad Hosp., Riyadh, Saudi Arabia; Asst. Prof. Anaesthetics, Aga Khan Univ. Hosp., Karachi, Pakistan.

SARAF, Iftikhar Mahmood Lane End Medical Group, 25 Edgwarebury Lane, Edgware HA8 8LJ Tel: 020 8958 4233 Fax: 020 8905 4657 — MB ChB Liverp. 1976; DRCOG 1979; MRCGP 1982. GP; Hosp. Practitioner Chest Clinic Edgware Community Hosp.; GP Trainer Northwick Pk. VTS.

SARAF, Rajesh Alexandra Group Medical Practice, Glodwick Health Centre, 137 Glodwick Road, Oldham OL4 1YN Tel: 0161 909 8388 Fax: 0161 909 8414 — MB BS Delhi 1979.

SARAFIAN, Anthony Haig (retired) — MB BS Lond. 1961; DObst RCOG 1964.

SARAKI, Olubukola Adebisi Alabuwale 123A Ashley Gardens, Thirleby Road, London SW1P 1HL Tel: 020 7931 0654 Fax: 020 7233 7447 — MB BS Lond. 1988.

SARAN, Sudhir Springfield Farmhouse, Ercall Heath, Newport TF10 8NQ Tel: 01952 550654 Email: saran999@yahoo.com — MB BS Patna 1971.

SARANG, Amman — MB ChB Dundee 1991; FRCA 1996. Cons. Anaesth. Barts & the Lond. NHS Trust. Specialty: Anaesth. Special Interest: Cardio-respiratory Intens. Care; Cardiothoracic Anaesth. Socs: RSM; Intens. Care Soc.; BMA. Prev: Specialist Regist. Roy. Brompton Hosp.; Specialist Regist. Centr. Middx, W. Middx, Char. Cross & Roy. Marsden Hosps. Lond. & QEII Welwyn Garden City; Specialist Regist. (Anaesth.) St Mary's Hosp. Lond.

SARANG, Kavita 150 Runnymede Road, Ponteland, Newcastle upon Tyne NE20 9HN — MB ChB Manch. 1992.

SARANGAPANI, Mr Krishnamoorthi Department of Plastic Surgery, Middlesbrough General Hospital, Ayresome Green Lane, Middlesbrough TS5 5AZ Tel: 01642 854316; Cleveland Nuffield Hospital, Junction Road, Norton, Stockton-on-Tees TS20 1QB Tel: 01642 360100 Fax: 01642 556535 — MB BS Madras 1962 (Madras Med. Coll.) MS Madras 1967; FRCS Eng. 1970. Cons. Plastic Surg. S. Tees Acute Hosps. NHS Trust Middlesbrough; Hon. Cons. Plastic Surg. Newc. AHA (T). Specialty: Plastic Surg. Socs: Brit. Assn. Plastic Surg. & Brit. Assn. Aesthetic Plastic Surgs.; Assoc. Mem. Brit. Soc. Surg. Hand. Prev: Sen. Regist. & Regist. (Plastic

Surg.) Newc. AHA (T); SHO (Plastic Surg.) Liverp. Regional Centre Whiston Hosp. Prescot.

SARANGI, Bimal Behari Trafford General Hospital, Moorside Road, Davyhulme, Manchester M41 5SL Tel: 0161 748 4022; 6 Kilworth Avenue, Sale, Manchester M33 4SE Tel: 0161 282 6065 — MB BS Calcutta 1955; DA (UK) 1971. Assoc. Specialist (Anaesth.) Trafford Gen. Hosp. Manch. Specialty: Anaesth. Prev: Regist. (Anaesth.) Worthing & Pk. Hosp. Manch.

SARANGI, Kashyap Kumar 6 Kilworth Avenue, Sale M33 4SE — MB ChB Manch. 1993.

SARANGI, Mr Partha Pratim Department of Orthopaedic Surgery, Bristol Royal Infirmary, Marlborough St., Bristol BS2 8HW Tel: 0117 923 0000 — MB ChB Manch. 1984; FRCS Ed. 1988; FRCS Eng. 1988; FRCS (Orth.) 1994; MD Bristol 1995. Cons. Orthop. Surg. Bristol Roy. Infirm. Specialty: Orthop. Prev: Sen. Regist. (Orthop. Surg.) Bristol Roy. Infirm.; Career Regist. (Orthop. Surg.) Bristol Roy. Infirm.; Peri Fellowship Regist. (Surg.) Cardiff Roy. Infirm.

SARAOGI, Mr Krishna Kumar Kailash, Church Grove, Wexham, Slough SL3 6LF Tel: 01753 579732 Mob: 07951 157 5560 Fax: 01753 571913 — MB BS Calcutta 1962 (R.G. Kar Med. Coll. Calcutta) MS Patna 1966. JP. Socs: Windsor. Med. Soc; Active Rotarian. Prev: Regist. Orthop. Hammersmith Hosp. Lond. & Wexham Pk. Hosp. Slough.

SARASOLA LOPETEGUI, Jose Angel Royal London Homeopathic Hospital, Great Ormond St., London WC1N 3HR — LMS Basque Provinces 1993.

SARATHCHANDRA, Cuda Bandara Consultant Psychiatrist, Clacton and District Hospital, Tower Road, Clacton-on-Sea CO15 1LH Tel: 01255 253527 Fax: 01255 421767 — MB BS Sri Lanka 1975 (Univ. Sri Lanka, Peradeniya) MRCPsych 1985; FRCPsych 1999. Cons. Psychiat. Clacton Dist. Hosps. Essex. Specialty: Gen. Psychiat. Socs: Brit. Med. Assn.; Med. Protec. Soc.; Brit. Assn. of PsychoPharmacol. Prev: Cons. Psychiat. Yarmouth Regional Hosp. Nova Scotia, Canada.

SARATHCHANDRA, Sunila Felicia Community Mental Health Centre, Holmer Court, Essex St., Colchester CO3 3BT Tel: 01206 287270 Fax: 01206 287272; 12 Woodview Close, Colchester CO4 4QW Tel: 01206 854308 Fax: 01206 854308 — MB BS Sri Lanka 1976; Dip. Psychol. Med. RCSI 1995. Staff Psychiat. Community Ment. Health Centre Colchester. Specialty: Gen. Psychiat. Socs: Affil. Roy. Coll. Psychiats. Prev: Clin. Asst. (Psychiat.) NE Essex & Mid Essex Ment. Health Trusts; Regist. (Psychiat.) NE Essex Ment. Health Trust Colchester.

SARATHY, Partha Liversedge Health Centre, Valley Road, Liversedge WF15 6DF Tel: 01924 404900 — MB BS Bangalor 1967 (Bangalore Med. Coll.) MB BS Bangalore 1967; DTCD Wales 1974; DTM & H Liverp. 1975. Socs: BMA.

SARATHY, Shaefali 128 Ashlands Road, Northallerton DL6 1HD Tel: 01609 770471 — MB ChB Leic. 1989 (Univ. Leic.) BSc (Med. Sci.) Genetics Leic. 1986; MRCGP 1994; DRCOG 1994; DA (UK) 1995; FRCA (II) 1996. Specialist Regist. (Anaesth.) N. Deanery Rotat. Specialty: Anaesth. Prev: Trainee GP Northallerton VTS; SHO (O & G & Paediat.) Friarage Hosp.; SHO (Anaesth.) S. Tees Hosps. Middlesbrough.

SARAVANAMATTU, Karunathevy Victoria Road Health Centre, Victoria Road, Washington NE37 2PU Tel: 0191 415 4477; 33 Polwarth Drive, Brunton Park, Gosforth, Newcastle upon Tyne NE3 5NJ — MB BS Ceylon 1967. GP Washington, Tyne & Wear.

SARAVANAMUTHU, Jamnarathi 4 Imperial Way, Kenton, Harrow HA3 9SW — BM BS Nottm. 1986.

SARAVANAMUTTU, Kasilingham Manohara Ward 34, Newcastle General Hospital, Westgate Road, Newcastle upon Tyne NE4 6BE — MB BS Ceylon 1965.

SARAVANAN, Ketharanathan 70 Turnpike Link, Croydon CR0 5NY; 21 Minster Court, Liverpool L7 3QB — MB BS Lond. 1990; DCH RCP Lond. 1993; MRCP (UK) 1995. Regist. (Paediat.) Alder Hey Childr.'s Hosp. Specialty: Paediat. Prev: Regist. (Neonates) Liverp. Wom.'s Hosp.; Regist. (Paediat.) Arrowe Pk. Hosp. Wirral.

SARDA, Kailash Little Roseworth Surgery, Little Roseworthy, 22 Meadow Lane, Sudbury CO10 2TD Tel: 01787 310000 Fax: 01787 75245; 54 Friars Street, Sudbury CO10 2AG Tel: 01787 74252 — LM Rotunda 1969 (TC Dub.) BA, MB BCh BAO Dub. 1967; DObst RCOG 1973. Cons. Med. Off. Dixon-Harris Gp., Shear Chem., Johnson Mathie Gp.; Companies & Dell Gp. Nursing Homes Sudbury. Specialty: Occupat. Health. Prev: Clin. Asst. St. Leonard's Hosp. & Walnutree Hosp. Sudbury; Med. Off. Red Cross; SHO (O & G) Rotunda Hosp. Dub.

SARDAR, Sohail Aabud 12 Sutherland Avenue, Glasgow G41 4JH — MB ChB Glas. 1989.

SARDER, Md Osman Ghani The Surgery, 433 New Cross Road, London SE14 6TD — MB BS Dhaka 1967 (Sir Sallimullah Med. Coll.) DGM; DFFP; DTCD.

SARDESAI, Bina Suhrud c/o Drive Meena Prabhu, Ajantha, Walpole Gardens, Twickenham TW2 5SL — MB BS Poona 1985; MRCP (UK) 1987.

SARDESAI, Suhrud Hanmant c/o Dr Meena Prabhu, Ajantha, Walpole Gardens, Twickenham TW2 5SL — MB BS Poona 1982; MRCP (UK) 1986.

SARDI, Armando Health Care International, Beardmore St., Clydebank G81 4HX — Medico y Cirujano National Univ. 1980.

SARFRAZ, Azhir Manzur 43 Hillhouse Drive, Billericay CM12 0BA — MB BS Lond. 1994.

SARFRAZ, Manzur-Ul-Hassan South Green Surgery, 14-18 Grange Road, Billericay CM11 2RE Tel: 01277 651702 Fax: 01277 631894; 43 Hill House Drive, Billericay CM12 0BA Tel: 01277 651702 Fax: 01277 631894 — MB BS Lond. 1973.

SARFRAZ, Muhammad Aamer Portnalls Unit, Farnborough Hospital, Orpington BR6 8ND — MB BS Punjab 1987.

SARGAISON, Jane Melissa Elm Croft, Elm Grove, Berkhamsted HP4 1AE — MB BChir Camb. 1991; BA Camb. 1988, MB BChir 1991; MRCP Lond. 1994. Med. Co-ordinator Merlin, Rwanda. Prev: SHO (Endocrinol.) Ealing Hosp. NHS Trust; SHO (Renal) Guy's Hosp. Trust Lond.; SHO (Med.) Hammersmith Hosp. & Postgrad. Med. Sch. Lond.

SARGAISON, Mark Frederick Robert East Donnington Street Clinic, East Donnington Street, Darvel KA17 0JR Tel: 01560 320205 Fax: 01560 321643 — MB BCh BAO Belf. 1988; MB BCh Belf. 1988.

SARGANT, Nicholas Robert 61 Park Avenue, Eastbourne BN21 2XH — MRCS Eng. LRCP Lond. 1971; BSc (Biochem.) Lond. 1968, MB BS 1971; DCH Eng. 1973; DObst RCOG 1974.

SARGEANT, Christopher Frederick 52 Beaufort Avenue, Kenton, Harrow HA3 8PF — MB BS Lond. 1989; DRCOG 1994.

SARGEANT, Mr Ian David 9 Dowding Road, Biggin Hill, Westerham TN16 3BE Tel: 01959 573518 — MB BS Lond. 1986; FRCS Ed. 1992; DAvMed FOM RCP Lond. 1993; FRCS (Orth.) 1996. Cons. (Trauma & Orthop. Surg.) MDHU PeterBoro. Dist. Hosp. Specialty: Trauma & Orthop. Surg. Socs: Assoc. Mem. BOA; Milit. Surg. Soc. Prev: Sen. Regist. (Orthop. & Trauma) Qu.s Med. Centre Nottm.; Regist. (Orthop.) RAF Hosp. Wegburg & RAF Hosp. Halton & Ely; Unit Med. Off. RAF St. Athan.

SARGEANT, Ian Robert Dept of Gastoenterology, Lister Hospital, Correys Mill Lane, Stevenage SG1 4AB Tel: 01438 781245 Fax: 01438 781241; 3 Engel Park, Mill Hill, London NW7 2HE — MB BS Lond. 1994; FRCP (UK) 2001; BSc Lond. 1984 (Middlesex Hospital Medical School) MB BS 1983; MD 1994. Cons. (Gastroenterol. & Gen. Med.) Lister Hosp. Stevenage. Specialty: Gastroenterol. Socs: BMA; BSG; RCOP.

SARGEANT, Matthew Paul Wellfield Road Resource Centre, Wellfield Road, Carmarthen SA31 1DS — MB BS Lond. 1981 (Selwyn Coll. Camb. & Lond. Hosp.) MA Camb. 1982; MRCPsych 1987; FRCPC 1994. Cons. Psychiat. St. David's Hosp. Carmarthen. Specialty: Gen. Psychiat. Prev: Cons. Psych. Millbrook Psychiat. Unit Sutton in Ashfield; Chief of Psychiat. Chatham, New Brunswick; Cons. Psychiat. Merthyr Tydfil.

SARGEANT, Rhona Jean Psychological Therapies Service, Department of Psychiatry, Royal South Hants Hospital, Southampton Tel: 023 8082 5787 Fax: 023 8082 5672; 3 Bower Gardens, Salisbury SP1 2RL — MB ChB Sheff. 1989 (Univ. Sheff.) BMedSci Sheff. 1989; MRCPsych 1996; MMedSci 1998. Flexible Sen. Regist. (Psychother.) S. & W. RHA. Specialty: Psychother. Socs: MRCPsych. Prev: Regist (Psych) S&W RHA; Regist. (Psychiat.) W. Midl. RHA; SHO (Psychiat.) N. Birm. HA.

SARGEN, Frances Elizabeth Shelley Road Surgery, Shelley Road, Worthing BN11 4BS Tel: 01903 234844 — MB ChB Sheff. 1994; DRCOG 1996; DCH 1999; MRCGP 2000; DFFP 2000. Gen. Pract. Retainee; Clin. Asst., Family Plann., Centr. Clinic Worthing; Clin. Asst., Dematology, Worthing Gen. Hosp. Specialty: Gen. Pract.;

Family Plann. & Reproduc. Health; Dermat. Prev: GP Regist.; SHO Neonatology, Southampton; Sho Med., St Richards Hosp., Chichester.

SARGENT, Abigail Margaret Foster The Bedford Park Surgery, 55 South Parade, Chiswick, London W4 5LH; 33 Mount Park Road, London W5 2RS Tel: 020 8997 4695 Email: asargent@waitrose.com — MB ChB Bristol 1977; DRCOG 1980; DCH RCP Lond. 1981; MFOM RCP Lond. 1996, AFOM 1991. Specialty: Occupat. Health; Gen. Pract. Prev: GP N.olt; Dep. Head of Med. Serv. John Lewis Partnership.

SARGENT, Catherine Sarah 3 Steynings Way, London N12 7LN — BM BCh Oxf. 1998; BM BCh Oxf 1998.

SARGENT, Claire Blanche (retired) 8 Manse Road, Stoke Newington, London N16 7QD — MB BS Lond. 1984 (Char. Cross) BSc Lond. 1981; MB BS (Hons.) Lond. 1984. Prev: Regist. (Histopath.) Univ. Coll. Hosp. Lond.

SARGENT, David Edward (retired) The Tynings, Far Forest, Kidderminster DY14 9TR Tel: 01299 266297 — MRCS Eng. LRCP Lond. 1949 (St. Thos.) DObst RCOG 1950. Prev: Jun. Obst. Ho. Phys. St. Thos. Hosp.

SARGENT, Jenefer Caroline The Wolfson Centre, Gt Ormond St Hospital, Mecklenburgh Square, London WC1N 2AP Tel: 020 7837 7618 Fax: 020 7833 9469 — MB BChir Camb. 1992; MA Camb. 1988; MRCP (UK) 1994. p/t Cons. Paediatric Neurodisability The Wolfson Centre Gt. Ormond St. NHS Trust. Specialty: Paediat. Neurol. Socs: Roy. Coll. Paediat. & Child Health; BMA; Brit. Assn. of Community Child Health. Prev: Specialist Regist. Paediatric Neurodisablity. The Wolfson Centre, Gt. Ormond St NHS Trust; Sen. Regist. (Community Paediat.) City & Hackney Community Servs. NHS Trust; Regist. (Paediat.) Whipps Cross Hosp. Lond.

SARGENT, John Hector Philip Scott — MRCS Eng. LRCP Lond. 1971 (Guy's Hosp.) MSc (Rehabil.) Soton. 1997. Dir. Sandaire plc. Prev: Chairm. Nursing Home Servs. Ltd.; Chairm. Med. Screening Servs. Ltd.; Chairm. Kitnocks Hse. Ltd. & Pentree Hse. Rehabil. Ltd.

SARGENT, Peter Anthony University Department of Psychiatry, Warneford Hospital, Warneford Lane, Headington, Oxford OX3 7JX Tel: 01865 226676 Fax: 01865 793101 — MB ChB Birm. 1986; DCH RCP Lond. 1989; MRCPsych 1994. Clin. Tutor (Psychiat.). Specialty: Gen. Psychiat.

SARGENT, Philippa Mary The Old Rectory, Bighton, Alresford SO24 9RB Tel: 01962 732300 — MB BS Lond. 1974 (St. Thos.) DO Eng. 1978. Clin. Asst. (Ophth.) Soton. Gen. Hosp. Specialty: Ophth. Prev: Clin. Asst. Roy. Hants. Co. Hosp. Winchester; Ho. Phys. St. Thos. Hosp. Lond.; Ho. Surg. (Orthop.) Roy. Hants. Co. Hosp. Winchester.

SARGENT, Thomas Stewart Pitt The Richmond Practice, Health Centre, Dean Road, Bo'ness EH51 0DH Tel: 01506 822665 Fax: 01506 825939; 16 Grahamsdyke Road, Bo'ness EH51 9EG Tel: 01506 823302 Fax: 01506 825939 Email: tspsargent@blueyonder.co.uk — MB ChB Glas. 1969; BSc (Hons.) Physiol. Glas. 1967. GP Trainer Bo'ness. Prev: Regist. (Med.) Gartnavel Gen. Hosp. Glas.; Ho. Phys. & Ho. Surg. West. Infirm. Glas.

SARGENT, William 38 Polwarth Crescent, Edinburgh EH11 1HN — MB ChB Ed. 1997.

SARGINSON, John, TD 32 Hawthorn Road, Bamford, Rochdale OL11 5JQ Tel: 01706 643256 — MB BS Durh. 1954; DPH Dur. 1960; FFCM 1980, M 1974; FFPHM 1989; BA Open 1991. Med. Ref. Rochdale MBC. Specialty: Pub. Health Med. Prev: Dist. Med. Off. Rochdale HA; Dep. Co. Med. Off. N.ants. CC; Sen. Med. Off. Leics. CC.

SARGINSON, Richard Emsley Royal Liverpool Childrens Hospital, Department of Anaesthesia, Eaton Road, Liverpool Tel: 0151 252 5223 Fax: 0151 252 5460 Email: Richard.Sarginson@rlc.nhs.uk — MB ChB Bristol 1978; BSc Bristol (Physiol.) 1975; MRCGP 1982; DRCOG 1982; FRCA 1986. Cons.(Paediat Anaesth.) Roy Liverp Childr NHS Trust. Specialty: Anaesth.; Intens. Care. Prev: Regist. (Anaesth.) Roy. Devon & Exeter Hosp.

SARGISON, Mr Kenneth Duthie (retired) The Rockeries, 16 New Walk, Beverley HU17 7DJ Tel: 01482 868426 — MB ChB Aberd. 1955; FRCS Ed. 1963. Prev: Cons. Orthop. Surg. Hull Roy. Infirm.

SARHADI, Mr Nanak Singh 28 Ashdown Drive, Wordsley, Stourbridge DY8 5QY — MB BS Calcutta 1977; MS (Gen. Surg.) Calcutta 1980, MB BS 1977; FRCS Glas. 1986.

SARIDOGAN, Mr Ertan Elizabeth Garrett Anderson Hospital, Huntley Street, London WC1E 6AU Tel: 020 7380 9759 Fax: 020 7380 9600 Email: ertan.saridogan@uclh.org — Tip Doktoru Hacettepe 1985; MRCOG 1997; PhD Lond. 1998. Cons. (Reproductive & Minimal Access Surg.) Univ. Coll. Lond. Hosps.; Cons. Gynaecologist, The Portland Hosp. for Wom. and Childr., Lond. Specialty: Obst. & Gyn. Special Interest: Minimal Access Surg.; Reproductive Medicine.

SARIN, Mr Ganesh 45 St Leonards Road, Harrogate HG2 8NS — MB BS Bhagalpur 1984; MB BS Bhagalpur U 1984; FRCS Ed. 1992.

SARIN, Mr Rajesh Burnley General Hospital, Casterton Avenue, Burnley BB10 2PQ — MB BS Rajasthan 1981; MCh (Orthop.); MS (Orthop.). Cons. Orthop. Surg. Specialty: Orthop. Socs: BMA; Brit. Orthop. Assn. (BOA); Amer. Orthop. Assn.

SARIN, Rajiv Academic Unit of Radiotherapy OncolgyRoyal Marsden Hospital, Sutton SM2 5PT — MB BS Kanpur, India 1986; FRCR 1995.

SARIN, Mr Sanjeev PO Box 187, Northwood HA6 3TR Tel: 07771 924632 Fax: 01923 826554 Email: mail@sarin.uk.com — BM Soton. 1984 (Univ. Soton.) FRCS Eng. 1988; MS Soton. 1993; FRCS (Gen.) 1996. Cons. Gen. & Vasc. Surg. Watford Gen. Hosp. Specialty: Gen. Surg. Special Interest: Venous Dis., varicose veins.

SARIN, Sanjeev The Surgery, 352 College Road, Erdington, Birmingham B44 0HH Tel: 0121 603 9446; College Road Surgery, 352 College Road, Kingstanding, Birmingham B44 0HH Tel: 0121 373 1244 Fax: 0121 384 6670 — MB ChB Manch. 1991 (Manch. Univ.) DFFP 1995. GP Regist. Eldington, Birm. Specialty: Gen. Pract. Socs: MDU; MSS. Prev: SHO (Paediat., Special Care Baby Unit & O & G) Birm. Heartlands Hosp.; SHO (Geriat.) Sandwell Dist. Gen.

SARIN, Uma c/o Mr C. Sutton, Department Obstetrics & Gynaecology, Royal Surrey County Hospital, Eggerton Road, Guildford GU2 7XX — MB BS Delhi 1974.

SARJUDEEN, Michael Taijnaraine Melbourne House Surgery, 12 Napier Court, Queensland Crescent, Chelmsford CM1 2ED Tel: 01245 354370 Fax: 01245 344476; 26 Wilshire Avenue, Springfield, Chelmsford CM2 6QW Tel: 01245 494562 — MB BS Lond. 1983; DRCOG 1993. Prev: Trainee GP Norf.; SHO (O & G) Ipswich Hosp.; SHO (Psychiat.) Hellesdon Hosp.

SARKANY, Imrich (cons. rooms), 132 Harley St., London W1N 1AH Tel: 020 7935 3678 Fax: 020 7935 3678; 2 Romney Close, Hampstead Way, London NW11 7JD — MRCS Eng. LRCP Lond. 1952 (St. Thos.) FRCP Lond. 1968, M 1956. Cons. Dermat. Garden Hosp. Lond. Specialty: Dermat. Prev: Cons. Dermat. Roy. Free Hosp. Lond.; Cons. Dermat. Roy. Nat. Throat, Nose & Ear Hosp. Lond.; Sen. Regist. King's Coll. Hosp. Lond.

SARKANY, Robert Paul Edmond Mayday University Hospital, London Rd, Croydon CR7 7YE — MB BS Lond. 1986; BSc (Hons.) Lond. 1983; MRCP (UK) 1989; M.D Lond 1995. Cons.s (Dermat) Mayday Univ. Hosp., Croyden, Surrey; Hon. Cons. (Dermat) St. John's Inst. of Dermat., Lond. Specialty: Dermat. Prev: Regist. (Dermat.) Addenbrooke's Hosp. Camb.; Wellcome Research Fell. & Hon. Regist. (Med.) Addenbrooke's Hosp. Camb.; SHO (Neurol.) Nat. Hosps. Nerv. Dis. Lond.// Sen. Regist (dermat)Addenbrooke's Hosp.Camb.

SARKAR, Ajoy 18 Muchall Road, Penn, Wolverhampton WV4 5SE — MB ChB Manch. 1996.

SARKAR, Bhabendramohan 48 Athol Square, London E14 0NP Tel: 020 7531 1813 — MB BS Calcutta 1967 (Sir Nilratan Sircar Med. Coll.)

SARKAR, David Anthony Dept. of cardiology, St. Georges Hospital, Blackshaw Road, London SW17 — MB BS Lond. 1991; BSc (Hons.) Lond. 1988; MRCP (UK) 1994. SpR Cardial St. Geo.s Hosp. Lond.; SpR Cardial Roy. Surrey Co. Hosp. Guildford; Regist. St. Geo.s Hosp. Lond. Specialty: Cardiol. Prev: Research Fell. (Brit. Heart Foundat.) UCL & the Nat. Heart & Lung Inst.; Regist. (Cardiol.) St. Geo. Hosp. Tooting; Regist. (Cardiol.) Frimley Pk. Hosp.

SARKAR, Mr Debabrata Fairfield General Hospital, Rochdale Old Road, Bury BL9 7TD Tel: 0161 764 6081 — MB BS Calcutta 1959 (R.G. Kar Med. Coll.) BSc Calcutta 1954, MB BS 1959; FRCS Eng. 1970 FRCS Ed. 1967. Med. Asst. Orthop. & Accid. Dept. Bury AHA.

SARKAR, Debasish Raby Cottage, 85 Low Etherley, Bishop Auckland DL14 0EX — MB BS Calcutta 1964.

SARKAR, Dinabandhu Blundell Park Surgery, 142-144 Grimsby Road, Cleethorpes DN35 7DL Tel: 01472 699522 Fax: 01472

694652; 52 Humberston Avenue, Humberston, Grimsby DN36 4SS Tel: 01472 567963 Fax: 01472 590629 Email: drdsarkar@ntlworld.com — MB BS Calcutta 1972 (Calcutta Med. Coll.) MSc Calcutta 1972. Specialty: Gen. Pract.; Gen. Med. Socs: Fell. Roy. Soc. Med.; BMA; Overseas Doctors Assn.

SARKAR, Jagadis Chandra Crayford Medical Centre, 4-6 Green Walk, Crayford, Dartford DA1 4JL Tel: 01322 520100 Fax: 01322 520101 — MB BS Calcutta 1961.

SARKAR, Mr Jay Soorya 3 Tudor Close, Stevenage SG1 4DB Tel: 01438 367090 Fax: 01438 367090; 3 Tudor Close, Stevenage SG1 4DB Tel: 01438 367090 Fax: 01438 367090 — MB BS Delhi 1977; FRCS Glas. 1990; FRCS (Orth.) 1998. Specialist Regist. Orthop. Kings Coll. Hosp. Denmark Hill Lond.; Sen. Specialist Regist. (Orthopaed.) Greenwich Dist. Hosp. Lond. Specialty: Trauma & Orthop. Surg. Socs: MDU.

SARKAR, Jhumpa 11 Harleys Field, Abbeymead, Gloucester GL4 4RN — MB BS Lond. 1993.

SARKAR, Manjusri 2 Broughton Road, South Shields NE33 2RU — MB BS Calcutta 1959.

SARKAR, Paresh Nath (retired) 233 Millhouses Lane, Sheffield S11 9HW Tel: 0114 235 2960 — MB BS Calcutta 1955 (Calcutta Med. Coll.) DPM Eng. 1966; MRCPsych 1971. Cons. Psychiat. (Ment. Handicap) Maclesfield HA. Prev: Cons. Psychiat. Cranage Hall Hosp.

SARKAR, Paul Pallab 30 Thomson Street, Aberdeen AB25 2QQ — MB ChB Aberd. 1995.

SARKAR, Prabodh Kumar 52 Wood Road, Tettenhall Wood, Wolverhampton WV6 8NF — MB BS Calcutta 1977; MD (Gen. Med.) Calcutta 1981; MRCPI 1986. Cons. Phys & Head Dept. Med. King Faisal Hosp., Saudi Arabia. Specialty: Care of the Elderly; Gen. Med. Socs: Fell. Internat. Coll. Angiol. USA; Acupunc. Assn. India.; Brit. Geriat. Soc. Prev: Regist. (Med. & Cardiol.) Brighton HA; SHO (Med.) Grantham & Kesteven Gen. Hosp.

SARKAR, Mr Pradip Kumar 6 Torsway Avenue, Blackpool FY3 8JF — MB BS Calcutta 1969; FRCS Ed. 1981.

SARKAR, Pranab Kumar Burnley General Hospital, Casterton Avenue, Burnley BB10 2PQ Tel: 01282 474221 — MB BS Calcutta 1974 (Med. Coll. Calcutta) Cons. in Obst. and Gyn., E. Lancs. Hosps. Trust, Burnley. Specialty: Obst. & Gyn. Socs: BSCCP; Brit. Menopause Soc.; N. of Eng. Obst. and Gyn. Soc. Prev: Cons. in Obst. and Gyn., Highland Acute Hosps. Trust, Wick.

SARKAR, Prosanta Kumar Muchall Lodge, 18 Muchall Road, Wolverhampton WV4 5SE — MB BS Calcutta 1966.

SARKAR, Saibal Kumar 139 Wilton St., Top Left, Glasgow G20 6DQ Tel: 0141 946 9300 — MB BS Calcutta 1977; LRCP LRCS Ed. LRCPS Glas. 1982.

SARKAR, Mr Sandip Prasad 6A 36 Buckingham Gate, London SW1E 6PB — MB BS Lond. 1989 (St. Thos.) FRCS Eng. 1993; FRCS (Orth) 1999. Specialist Regist. Rotat. (Orthop. Surg.) Roy. Nat. Orthop. Hosp. Stanmore. Specialty: Trauma & Orthop. Surg. Socs: Fell. Roy. Soc. Med.; BMA. Prev: SHO (Cardiothorcic Surg.) St. Geo. Hosp. Lond.; SHO (A & E) Univ. Coll. Hosp. Lond.; SHO (Surg.) Roy. Marsden Hosp. Lond.

SARKAR, Santosh Kumar (retired) 6 Hammy Close, Shoreham-by-Sea BN43 6BL — MB BS Patna 1951; MRCP Ed. 1963. Prev: Regist. (Med.) Bridge of Earn Hosp. Perth.

SARKAR, Sharmila Helen 4 Wath Wood Drive, Swinton, Mexborough S64 8UW Tel: 01709 872388 — MB ChB Leic. 1998; MB ChB Leic 1998. GP Reg. Leics. Specialty: Gen. Pract. Prev: Ho. Off. Surg. Kettering Gen. Hosp; HO.med.Leics.Gen.Hosp.

SARKAR, Shyamal Kanti Ramsbottom Health Centre, Carr Street, Ramsbottom, Bury BL0 9DD Tel: 01706 824445 Fax: 01706 821196 — MB BS Calcutta 1964; DObst. 1967. Specialty: Obst. & Gyn.; Family Plann. & Reproduc. Health. Prev: Regist. (Psychiat.) Whittington Hosp. Preston; Regist. (Path.) Fazakerley Hosp. Liverp.; SHO (O & G) St. John's Hosp. Keighley.

SARKAR, Subhajit 32 Hawk Close, Abbeydale, Gloucester GL4 4WE — BChir Camb. 1995.

SARKAR, Subhendra Krishna (Surgery), 373 Hainton Avenue, Grimsby DN32 9QP Tel: 01472 357050 — MB BS Calcutta 1972.

SARKAR, Sucheta 4 Bessy Brook Close, Lostock, Bolton BL6 4EA — MB BS Calcutta 1972 (Nilratan Sarkar Med. Coll.) DA Eng. 1978.

SARKAR, Usharani (Surgery) 1 East Street, Rochdale Tel: 01706 39002; Darjeeling, 46 Linnet Hill, Bamford, Rochdale OL11 4DA Tel: 01706 59500 — MB BS Calcutta 1957. Prev: SHO (Psychiat.) Ashton-Under-Lyne Gen. Hosp.; Ho. Off. (Med.) Macclesfield Hosp.

SARKER, Debashis 2 Kinloch Drive, Bolton BL1 4LZ — MB ChB Liverp. 1997. SHO Gen. Med. Roy. Liverp. Univ. Hosp. Specialty: Gen. Med.

SARKER, Mohammed Abdul Khaleque Ryburn Surgery, 17/21 Ryburn Buildings, Sowerby Bridge HX6 3AH Tel: 01422 831924 — MB BS Dacca 1962. Socs: BMA. Prev: SHO (Paediat. Surg.) Nottm. Childr. Hosp.; Ho. Off. (Gen. Med.) Manor Hosp. Nuneaton; SHO City Hosp. Stoke-on-Trent.

SARKER, Prosenjit 5 Algernon Road, London SE13 7AU — MB BS Lond. 1992.

SARKER, Sabyasachi Knotty Ash Medical Centre, 411-413 East Prescot Road, Liverpool L14 2DE Tel: 0151 228 4369 Fax: 0151 252 0030 — MB BS Calcutta 1969. GP Liverp. Specialty: Gastroenterol.

SARKER, Mr Sudip Kumar 89 Cornwall Gardens, London SW7 4AX — MB ChB Glas. 1991; FRCS Glas. 1998. Specialist Regist. in Surg., Acad. Surgic. Unit, St Mary's Hosp. Lon. Specialty: Gen. Surg. Socs: ASGBI; ACPGBI; AESGBI. Prev: Clin. Research Fell. & SHO (Otolaryngol. & Paediat.) St. Mary's Hosp. Lond.; SHO Rotat (Surg.) St. Mary's Hosp. Lond.

SARKHEL, Rama Prosad Pashimtra, 10 Oaten Hill Place, Canterbury CT1 3HJ Tel: 01227 69246 — MB BS Calcutta 1962 (Nilratan Sircar Medical College, Calcutta) DGO 1963; MRCOG 1969, DObst 1969; FRCOG 1984; BA Open University 1996. Cons. (Genito-Urin. Med.) Canterbury & S.E. Kent Gp. Hosps. Specialty: Genitourinary Medicine. Socs: FRSH; Med. Soc. Study VD. Prev: Sen. Regist. (Genito-Urin. Med. & Gyn.) Addenbrooke's Hosp. Camb.

SARKHEL, Swantana Tanaya 158 New Dover Road, Canterbury CT1 3EJ — MB BS Lond. 1991 (Char. Cross & Westm.) BSc (Hons.) Lond. 1988. Regist. (Orthop.) Nambour Gen. Hosp. Queensland, Austral. Specialty: Orthop. Socs: Med. Defence Union; BMA. Prev: SHO Rotat. (Surg.) Roy. Sussex Co. Hosp. Brighton; SHO (Orthop. & Urol.) St. Richard's Hosp. Chichester.

SARKIES, Mr Nicholas Jonathan Courtenay Ophthalmic Department, Box 41, Addenbrooke's Hospital, Hills Road, Cambridge CB2 2QQ Tel: 01223 216427; Wistow, The Green, Hilton, Huntingdon PE28 9NB Tel: 01480 830412 Fax: 01480 831461 — MB BChir Camb. 1977; FRCOphth; FRCOphth; MRCP (UK) 1979; MRCP UK 1979; FRCS Eng. 1982; FRCS Eng. 1982. Cons. Ophth. Addenbrookes Hosp.Camb. Specialty: Ophth. Socs: Fell. Roy. Coll. Ophth. Prev: Sen. Regist. (Ophth.) St. Thos. Hosp. & Nat. Hosp. Nerv. Dis. Lond.; Resid. Surgic. Off. Moorfields Eye Hosp. Lond.; Ho. Phys. (Med.) Westm. Hosp. Lond.

SARKOZY, Vanessa Elizabeth 33 Ashton Avenue, Rainhill, Prescot L35 0QQ — MB ChB Birm. 1996; ChB Birm. 1996. SHO (Paediat.) Roy. Alexandra Hosp. For Sick Childr., Brighton. Specialty: Paediat. Prev: SHO (Paediat.) Good Hope Hosp. Sutton Coalfield; Ho. Off. (Surg.) Russells Hall Hosp. Birm.; Ho. Off. (Med.) Heartlands Hosp.

SARMA, Mr Asoke (retired) 8 Wayside Close, Harrogate HG2 8PJ — MB BS Calcutta 1955 (R.G. Kar Med. Coll.) FRCS Ed. 1972. Prev: Asst. (Accid. & Orthop.) Harrogate Dist. Hosp. & Bradford Roy.

SARMA, David Ian Mayday University Hospital Trust, Radiology Department, London Road, Croydon CRY 7YE Tel: 020 8401 3054; 14 Mill View Close, Ewell Village, Epsom KT17 2DW — MB ChB Liverp. 1989; MRCP (UK) 1992; DMRD Liverp. 1994; FRCR 1995. Cons. (Radiol.) Mayday Univ. Hosp. Trust Croydon. Specialty: Radiol. Special Interest: MRI; Uroradiology; Vasc. Prev: Sen. Regist. (Radiol.) King's Coll. Hosp. Lond.; Regist. (Radiol.) Roy. Liverp. Hosp. & Aintree Trust Hosp.; SHO Rotat. (Med.) Aintree Trust Hosps. Liverp.

SARMA, Jaydeep 8 Wayside Close, Harrogate HG2 8PJ — BChir Camb. 1992.

SARMA, Mr Kishori Mohan Malabar, 19 Woodlands Road, Cleadon Village, Sunderland SR6 7UD — MB BS Gauhati 1955 (Assam Med. Coll. Dibrugarh) FRCS Ed. 1968. Asst. Orthop. Surg. Orthop. & Accid. Unit, Qu. Eliz. Hosp. Gateshead. Socs: Brit. Orthop. Assn.; BMA. Prev: Orthop. Regist. Orthop. & Accid. Hosp. Sunderland.

SARMA, Mr Kundurty Purnananda 8 Mayfield Park S., Bristol BS16 3NG Tel: 0117 976 1491 — MD Bristol 1979; MB BS Calcutta 1959; FRCS Eng. 1963.

SARMA, Ramesh Chandra Regent's Park Clinic, 184 Gloucester Place, London NW1 6DS — MB BS Lond. 1996 (King's Coll. Lond.) MRCP (UK) 2001. p/t Marketing Dir.; Clin. Research Fell. (HIV Med.) Imp. Coll. Lond. Specialty: Genitourinary Medicine. Prev: SHO (Gen. Med.) Jas. Paget Hosp. Gt. Yarmouth.

SARMA, Tapan Chandra Bentinck Road Medical Centre, 2 Bentinck Road, Arthur's Hill, Newcastle upon Tyne NE4 6UT Tel: 0191 273 3919 Fax: 0191 273 6323 — MB BS Gauhati 1967. GP Newc.

SARMA, Umesh Chandra 177 Great Northway, Hendon, London NW4 1PP Tel: 020 8203 4380 Fax: 020 8203 4380 — MB ChB Ed. 1989 (Univ. Edin.) Specialty: Gen. Med. Socs: BMA. Prev: SHO (Cardiothoracic Surg.) Roy. Infirm. Edin.; Ho. Off. Chest Unit City Hosp. Edin.; Ho. Off. (Surg.) Westm. Gen. Hosp. Edin.

SARMAH, Amit Queen Elizabeth The Queen Mother Hospital, St Peters Road, Margate Tel: 01843 225544 Email: amit.sarmah@euht.nhs.uk — MB BS India; MRCP UK; DCH Lond.; FRCPCH UK. Cons. Paediat.; Hon. Cons. Paediat., Guys and St Thomas Hosp. Lond. Specialty: Paediat.

SARMAH, Anita 51 Green Pastures, Heaton Mersey, Stockport SK4 3RB; 8 Ashley House, Park Drive, The Park, Nottingham NG7 1DB — MB ChB Manch. 1991; FRCA 1997. Specialist Regist. Anaesth. Qus. Med. Centre Nottm. Specialty: Anaesth. Socs: Assn. Anaesth.; BMA.

SARMAH, Mr Bhupendra Dev Department Of Urology, Birmingham Heartlands Hospital NHS Trust (Teaching), Bordesley Green E., Birmingham B9 5SS Tel: 0121 766 6611 Fax: 0121 773 6897; Winchmore Oak, 19 Poundley Close, Castle Bromwich, Birmingham B36 9SZ — MB BS Gauhati 1971; FRCS Ed. 1980.

SARMAH, N N Chorlton Health Centre, 1 Nicolas Road, Chorlton, Manchester M21 9NJ Tel: 0161 860 4545 Fax: 0161 860 4565 — MB BS Gauhati 1962; MB BS Gauhati 1962.

SARMIENTO, Augusto Health Care International, Beardmore St., Clydebank G81 4HX — Medico y Cirujano National Univ. 1952.

SARMOTTA, Jagdish Singh Park View Surgery, 127 Station Road, Rainham, Gillingham ME8 7SP.

SARNA, Nirmal Rai Yeading Medical Centre, 18 Hughenden Garden, Northolt UBZ 6LD Tel: 020 8845 3434 Fax: 020 8841 8222 — MB BS Kanpur 1973 (GSVM Medical College Kanpur) DRCOG 1979; Cert. Family Plann. JCC 1980; Cert. Prescribed Equiv. Exp. JCPTGP 1981; AFOM RCP Lond. 1991. GP; Occupational Health Phys. Specialty: Occupat. Health. Socs: Soc. Occupat. Med.; BMA. Prev: Med. Off. Smith & Nephew; Med. Off. Thorne Poultry, Thorne Goole; Med. Off English Village salads.

SARNAIK, Bhoopal Sivasiddappa (retired) Annapoorna, Helmington Grange, Crook DL15 0SE — MB BS Karnatak 1963 (Kasturba Med. Coll. Mangalore) Prev: SHO (Orthop., A & E) Bishop Auckland Gen. Hosp.

SARNAIK, Nirmala Bhoopal Health Centre, Chapel Street, Willington, Crook DL15 0EQ Tel: 01388 646000 — MB BS Bombay 1964. GP Crook, Co. Durh.

SARNER, Martin Wellington Hospital, London NW8 9LE Tel: 020 7586 5959 Ext: 2572 Fax: 020 7483 0297 Email: m.sarner@ntlworld.com — MB BS Lond. 1959 (St. Mary's) MRCS Eng. LRCP Lond. 1959; FRCP Lond. 1976, M 1962. Cons. Pysician, Univ. Coll. Lond. Hosp.s. Specialty: Gastroenterol. Socs: Fell. Roy. Soc. Med. Prev: Cons. Phys. Portsmouth Gp. Hosps.; Sen. Regist. (Med.) St. Geo. Hosp. Lond.; Ho. Phys. (Med.) St. Mary's Hosp. Lond.

SARNICKI, Marek Anthony The Surgery, 321 Shirland Road, London W9 3JJ Tel: 020 8969 2626 Fax: 020 8964 0353; 321 Shirland Road, London W9 Tel: 020 8969 2626 — MB BS Lond. 1978.

SARNOBAT, Meenakshi S Bute Street Health Centre, 34 Bute Street, Treorchy CF42 6BS Tel: 01443 771728 Fax: 01443 772164.

SARNOBAT, Sudheer R Bute Street Health Centre, 34 Bute Street, Treorchy CF42 6BS Tel: 01443 771728 Fax: 01443 772164.

SARODIA, Usman Ahmed 25 Oswald Street, Blackburn BB1 7EF — MB ChB Leic. 1994.

SARRIS, Ioannis Block 5, Flat 1, St. Peter's Hospital, Guildford Road, Chertsey KT16 0PZ — Ptychio Iatrikes Thessalonika 1991.

SARSAM, Mr Soufian Abdul Ahad 14A Arterberry Road, London SW20 8AJ — MB ChB Baghdad 1965; FRCS Ed. 1978. Staff Grade Surg. Kingston Hosp.

SARSFIELD, Mr David Alan (retired) Vale Cottage, Hawkcombe, Porlock, Minehead TA24 8QW Tel: 01643 862616 — (Bristol) MB ChB Bristol 1943; FRCS Eng. 1948.

SARSON, Mr David 2 Belle Vue Drive, Holmelands Park, Sunderland SR2 7SF Tel: 0191 283240 — MB BS Lond. 1962; MRCS Eng. LRCP Lond. 1962; FRCS Eng. 1966. Cons. Surg. Sunderland Roy. Infirm. Specialty: Gen. Surg. Prev: Regist. (Surg.) Walton Hosp. Liverp.; Surg. Daboo Hosp., Ivory Coast; Sen. Regist. (Surg.) United Liverp. Hosps.

SARTORI, Josephine Eileen Kings Road Surgery, 2-6 Kings Road, Mumbles, Swansea SA3 4AJ Tel: 01792 360933 Fax: 01792 368930 — MB BCh Wales 1993.

SARTORI, Naldo Penbryn, 155 Vicarage Road, Morriston, Swansea SA6 6DT Tel: 01792 71115 — MB ChB Bristol 1952. Police Surg. S. Wales Police, Swansea. Prev: Sen. Cas. Off. Bristol Roy. Infirm.; Ho. Surg. ENT Dept. Bristol Roy. Hosp.; Sen. Ho. Off. Bristol Homoeop. Hosp.

SARTORI, Patricia Carmen Ermina 18 Lynfield Lane, Cambridge CB4 1DR Tel: 01223 312043 — MB BS Lond. 1983 (Guy's Hosp. Lond.) MRCP (UK) 1986; MD Bristol 1996. Sen. Regist. (Paediat. Oncol.) Addenbrooke's Hosp. Camb. Specialty: Paediat.

SARTORI, Rossano Alfredo 54 Over Lane, Almondsbury, Bristol BS32 4BW — MB ChB Cape Town 1993.

SARTORIS, Anthony Woodland View Surgery, Woodland View, West Rainton, Houghton-le-Spring DH4 6RQ Tel: 0191 584 3809 Fax: 0191 584 9177; School House, Leamside, Houghton-le-Spring DH4 6QR Tel: 0191 512 0533 — MB BS Newc. 1974 (Newcastle-upon-Tyne) MRCGP 1978. Prev: Trainer, Northumbria VTS Div. Gen. Pract. Univ. Newc., Newc.

SARTORY, Francis Bernard 12 Ferndale Road, Summersdale, Chichester PO19 6QJ Tel: 01243 527984 — MRCS Eng. LRCP Lond. 1950 (Guy's) LDS RCS Eng. 1943.

SARVA ISWERAN, Muttucumaru 49 Orchard Drive, Watford WD17 3DX Tel: 01923 29421 — MB BS Ceylon 1971; DCH Ceylon 1976; MRCPsych 1980; DPM Eng. 1980. Cons. Psychiat. Leavesden Hosp. Abbots Langley. Specialty: Gen. Psychiat. Prev: Sen. Regist. (Ment. Handicap) Leavesden Hosp. Abbots Langley; Regist. (Psychiat.) Warlingham Pk. Hosp.

SARVANANTHAN, Nagini Leicester Royal Infirmary, Infirmary Road, Leicester LE1 5WW Tel: 0116 254 1414 — MB BS Newc. 1992; MMedSci Newc. 1993. SpR (Ophth.) Leics. Specialty: Ophth.

SARVANANTHAN, Rajini 3 Woodlea Gardens, Meanwood, Leeds LS6 4SE — MB BS Newc. 1993; MRCP (UK) 1996. Specialist Regist. (Paediatiatrics) p/t. Bradford Roy. Infirm. & St. Luke's Hosp. Bradford. Specialty: Paediat. Socs: BMA; Med. Protec. Soc.; MRCPCH. Prev: SHO/Tutor (Paediat.) St. Jas. Univ. Hosp. Leeds; SHO (Paediat., Neonat. & Paediat. Neurol.) Leeds Gen. Infirm.; SHO (Paediat.) York Dist. Hosp.

SARVESVARAN, Joseph Shanker 19 Baliol Street, Woodlands, Glasgow G3 6UT — MB BS Lond. 1992.

SARVOTHAM, Racharla 15 Hill Side, Pen-y-Fai, Bridgend CF31 4BG — MB BS Osmania 1967 (Kakatiya Med. Coll.) DPM Eng. 1980.

SARWAR, Mohammad Iqbal Mohammad Flat D, 13 Printfield Terrace, Aberdeen AB24 4AL — MB ChB Aberd. 1998; MB ChB Aberd 1998.

SARWAR, Mohammad Naveed 40 Parkview Road, London W5 2JB — MB BS Lond. 1996.

SARWAR, Nadeem 21 Everton Road, Hunters Bar, Sheffield S11 8RY — MB ChB Sheff. 1995.

SARWAR, Naheed 106 Clayton Street, Nelson BB9 7PR — MB ChB Manch. 1992.

SARWAR, Sajjad 45 Treaford La, Birmingham B8 2UF — MB ChB Birm. 1997.

SARWAR, Shakeel 22 Causey Foot, Nelson BB9 0DR — MB ChB Leeds 1995.

SARWAR-E-ALAM, Abul Kalam Mohammad 26 Matlock Road, Ferndown BH22 8QU Tel: 01202 876703 Fax: 01202 876703; Dorset Health Care NHS Trust, Ringwood BH24 2RR Tel: 01202 895945 — MB BS Dacca 1966; DPH Punjab 1968; DTM & H 1973.

Clin. Asst. ElderlyMed.Dorset Health Care NHS Trust. Socs: Med. Protec. Soc.

SASADA, Kay 5 St Paul's Close, Lower Willingdon, Eastbourne BN22 0LT — MB BS Lond. 1984; DCH RCP Lond.; DRCOG 1987; MRCGP 1988.

SASADA, Martin Paul 4 Holmes Grove, Bristol BS9 4EE — MB BS Lond. 1983.

SASH, Leonard The Surgery, 80 Cambridge Gardens, London W10 6HS Tel: 020 8969 5517 Fax: 020 8964 4766; 71 Lansdowne Road, London W11 2LG Tel: 020 8969 5517 — MB BCh Witwatersrand 1954; DCH Eng. 1961; DPhysMed. Eng. 1969. Cons. Sports Med. St. Mary's Hosp. Lond.; Cons. Phys. (Med.) Arsenal Football Club.; Cons. Imperial Coll. in Sports Med. Specialty: Rehabil. Med.; Rheumatol. Prev: Assoc. Specialist (Rheum.) St. Chas. & St. Mary's Hosps. Lond.

SASHIDHARAN, Ratnasabapathy Department of Anaesthetics, Royal London Hospital, Whitechapel, London E1 1BB Tel: 020 7377 7793 Fax: 020 7377 7153; 5 Collard Place, Harmood St, London NW1 8DU Tel: 020 7482 1141 — MB BS Colombo 1983 (Faculty of Medicine, University of Colombo, Sri Lanka) DA (UK) 1988; FFA RCSI 1991; FRCA 1992. Cons. Anaesth. Roy. Hosp. St. Bartholomews, Roy. Lond. Hosp. & Lond. Chest Hosp. NHS Trust; Cons. Anaesth. St Bart. & the Roy. Lond. Hosps. Specialty: Anaesth. Prev: Hon. Cons. (Anaesth.) Homerton Hosp.; Sen. Regist. (Anaesth.), Roy. Lond. Hosp.

SASHIDHARAN, Professor Sivasankaran Pillay Northern Birmingham Mental Health Trust, Trust Headquarters, 71 Fentham Road, Erdington, Birmingham B23 6AL Tel: 0121 623 5861 Fax: 0121 623 5870 — MB BS Madras 1974 (Jawaharlal Inst. Med. Educat. Pondicherry) MRCPsych 1978; PhD Ed. 1986, MPhil 1980. Med. Dir., Northern Birm. Ment. Health Trust, Birm.; Cons. Psychiat., NBMNT; Director, Centre for Community Ment. Health NBMNT and Univ. of Centr. Eng. Specialty: Gen. Psychiat. Prev: Mem. Scientif. Staff MRC Unit Epidemiological Studies in Psychiat. Univ. Dept. Psychiat. Roy. Edin. Hosp.; Sen. Regist. (Psychiat.) Roy. Edin. Hosp.; Prof. of Community Psychiat. Univ. of Birm.

SASITHARAN, Nadrajah 63 Langland, King's Lynn PE30 4TH — MB BS Sri Lanka 1983; MRCOphth. 1993.

SASITHARAN, Thangaluxmy 35 Colney Heath Lane, St Albans AL4 0TG — MRCS Eng. LRCP Lond. 1979.

SASSE, William Michael Peter (retired) 421 Westleigh Lane, Leigh WN7 5PU Tel: 01942 883793 — MD Hamburg 1946.

SASSOON, Elaine Moira Dept of Plastic Surgery, NNU Hospital, Colney Road, Norwich NR4 7UY Tel: 01603 286286 Fax: 01603 288378 — MB BS Lond. 1983 (UCL) BA (Hons.) Biol. Harvard 1976; FRCS Ed. 1989; FRCS Eng. 1989; FRCS Plast 1998. Cons. Plastic Surg. Norf. & Norwich Univ. Hosp. & Cromer Hosp.; Cosmetic Surg. BUPA Hosp. Norwich; Aesthetic & Oculoplastic Fell. Atlanta Georgia USA. Specialty: Plastic Surg. Socs: BAPS; Aesthetic Soc. (USA). Prev: Cons. Plastic.Surg.W. norwich Hosp and aesthetic Surg.

SASSOON, Jeremy Howard 45 High Grove Road, Cheadle SK8 1NW Tel: 0161 428 4765 — MB BS Lond. 1988. Regist. Rotat. (Psychiat.) NW RHA. Specialty: Gen. Psychiat.

SASSOON, Sonia Miriam Helen The Surgery, 404 Honeypot Lane, Stanmore HA7 1JP Tel: 020 8204 1363 Fax: 020 8903 0286; 4 Barn Rise, Wembley Park, Wembley HA9 9NA Tel: 020 8904 5698 — MB BS Lond. 1978 (Roy. Free) MRCS Eng. LRCP Lond. 1977; DRCOG 1980.

SASTRE CABRER, Juan Antonio 50 Holland Road, London W14 8BB — LMS Barcelona 1987; LMS Autonoma Barcelona 1987.

SASTRULU, Kanakamedala 18 Hornby Lane, Liverpool L18 3HH — MB BS Andhra 1971; DTM & H Liverp. 1975.

SASTRY, M R Halling Medical Centre, Ferry Road, Halling, Rochester ME2 1NP Tel: 01634 240238 — MB BS Andhra 1965; MB BS Andhra 1965.

SASTRY, Sanjay Rajesh Vascular Studies Unit, South Manchester University Hospital, Nell Lane, Withington, Manchester M20 2LR Tel: 0161 291 4527; 102 Parkville Road, Withington, Manchester M20 4TZ Tel: 0161 445 9063 — MB ChB Manch. 1995; BSc St Andrews 1992; MRCP (UK) 1998. Specialty: Cardiol.

SATARASINGHE, Kathri Achchige Sandya 30 Heol Beili Glas, Swiss Valley, Llanelli SA14 8DS — MB BS Colombo, Sri Lanka 1985; LRCP LRCPS Ed. LRCPS Glas. 1994.

SATCHELL, Raoul Harold (retired) 5 Fishermans Wlak, Craigweil-on-Sea, Bognor Regis PO21 4BU Tel: 01243 268650 — MB BS Lond. 1947 (Char. Cross) Prev: Cas. Off. Watford & Dist. Peace Memor. Hosp.

SATCHELL, Simon Charles 5 Holland Avenue, Knowle, Solihull B93 9DW — MB BS Lond. 1992.

SATCHITANANDA, Muttucumarasamy 55 Gatcome, Great Holm, Milton Keynes MK8 9EA — MB BS Ceylon 1971; MRCP (UK) 1988.

SATCHITHANANDA, Dunwarakan Kirupanantha Papworth Hospital, Cambridge CB3 8RE; Flat 12, Livemore Court, Grove Park, Liverpool L8 0TL — MB ChB Liverp. 1991. Specialist Regist., Papworth Hosp. Camb. Specialty: Cardiol.; Transpl. Surg.

SATCHITHANANDA, Susan Jane — BChir Camb. 1995.

SATCHITHANANTHAN, Gnanarathy Whiston Hospital, Prescot L35 5DR Tel: 0151 430 1825 Fax: 0151 430 1823 — MB BS Ceylon 1968; MRCPath 1982. Cons. Haemat. Specialty: Haematology. Special Interest: Malignancies; Thrombotic Disorders. Socs: Brit. Soc. Haemat.; Assn. Clin. Path.

SATCHITHANANTHAN, N St James Health Centre, 29 Great George Square, Liverpool L1 5DZ Tel: 0151 709 1120.

SATCHITHANANTHAN, Sivakhami Stepaside, Brancote Road, Oxton, Birkenhead CH43 6TL — BChir Camb. 1995.

SATCHWELL, George Malcolm (retired) Trevarrick House, North Curry, Taunton TA3 6LX Tel: 01823 490262 — MB ChB St. And. 1965. Prev: GP Taunton.

SATCHWELL, Victoria Jane 122 New Penkridge Road, Cannock WS11 1HN — MB BS Lond. 1991.

SATHANANDAN, Mr Saiha-M Haroldwood Hospital, Consultant Obstetrician, Haroldwood, Romford RM3 0BE Tel: 01708 345533 Fax: 01708 708385 Email: m_saiha@hotmail.com — MB BS Sri Lanka 1973; MRCS Eng. LRCP Lond. 1979; FRCS- RCS Ed. 1980; MPhil Lond. 1989; T(OG) 1991; MFFP 1993; FRCOG (UK) 1994. Cons. (O & G); Hon. Sen. Lect. UCL & St. Bart. Med. Sch. Lond. Specialty: Obst. & Gyn.; Family Plann. & Reproduc. Health; Endocrinol. Special Interest: Endometriosis; Fertil.; Menopause. Socs: Brit. Menopause Soc.; Brit. Soc. Gyn. Endoscopy; Brit. Fertil. Soc. Prev: Clin. Director (Gyn.) BH & R Trust Hesselmind.

SATHANANDAN, Sankarakumaran Blenheim Chase Surgery, 9 Blenheim Chase, Leigh-on-Sea SS9 3BZ Tel: 01702 470336 Fax: 01702 476210 — MB BS Sri Lanka 1979; MRCS Eng. LRCP Lond. 1982; MRCGP 1985. GP Princip.

SATHANANTHAN, Dilakshini 24 Lazenby Grove, Darlington DL3 9QD — MB ChB Sheff. 1992.

SATHANANTHAN, Kanagaratnam Dept of Psychiatary, Mayday University Hospital, London Road, Croydon CR7 7YE Tel: 020 8401 3596 Fax: 020 8401 3577 — MB BS Ceylon 1964 (Univ. Ceylon) DPM Eng. 1970; MRCP (U.K.) 1971; MRCPsych 1972. S. Lond. & Maudsley (NHS) Trust; Med. Dir. Surrey Rest & Nursing Homes Ltd. Specialty: Gen. Psychiat. Prev: Sen. Regist. Bethlem Roy. & Maudsley Hosps. Lond.

SATHANANTHAN, Muttiah (retired) 20 Meadow Close, Farmoor, Oxford OX2 9NZ Tel: 01865 863698; 21 Field House, West Way, Oxford OX2 9JN Tel: 01865 726694 Email: msatha1031@aol.com — MB BS Ceylon 1952; DLO RCS Eng. 1962. Prev: ENT Cons. Sir Lankian Gov. Serv.

SATHANANTHAN, Niranjani 12 Sandybrook Close, Fulwood, Preston PR2 5QX — MB ChB Dundee 1993.

SATHANANTHAN, Roshanthi 30 Castlemaine Avenue, South Croydon CR2 7HQ — MB BS Lond. 1991; MRCP (UK) 1994.

SATHANANTHAN, Shobana 32 Dulverton Road, South Croydon CR2 8PG — MB BS Lond. 1993.

SATHANANTHAN, Yasodhara The Surgery, Rockleigh Court, 136 Hutton Road, Brentwood CM15 8NN Tel: 01277 223844 Fax: 01277 230136 — MB BS Sri Lanka 1976.

SATHE, Sharad Bhargav 11 The Brooks, St Helens WA11 7DY — MB BS Bombay 1963.

SATHI, Navtej 274 Barton Road, Manchester M32 9RD — MB ChB Manch. 1995.

SATHIA, Prabhati Julie 5 Dursley Drive, Cannock WS11 1TN — MB BS Lond. 1994.

SATHIA, Mr Pranab The Surgery, 24 Bideford Way, Cannock WS11 1QD Tel: 01543 571055 Fax: 01543 574930 — MB BS Utkal 1955 (S.C.B. Med. Coll. Cuttack) FRCS Glas. 1977.

SATHIA, U The Surgery, 24 Bideford Way, Cannock WS11 1QD Tel: 01543 571055 Fax: 01543 574930 — MB BS Utkal 1963; MB BS Utkal 1963.

SATHIA, Upali Leena 149A Melrose Avenue, London NW2 4NA — MB BS Lond. 1998; MRCP Dip Gum; MB BS Lond 1998.

SATHIYASEELAN, Subbiah Stretton Medical Centre, 5 Hatton Lane, Stretton, Warrington WA4 4NE Tel: 01925 730412 Fax: 01925 730960; 5 Fairways, Appleton, Warrington WA4 5HA Tel: 01925 264650 Fax: 01925 730960 — MB BS Mysore 1972 (Kasturba Med. Coll.) DIH Eng. 1980; Dip. Pract. Dermat. Wales 1993. Specialty: Accid. & Emerg. Socs: FRSH.

SATHYAN, Neena 24 Wheatsheaf Walk, Standish, Wigan WN6 0RH — MB BS Calicut 1989.

SATHYANANDHA, Mr Arunachalam 20 Ibsley Way, Cockfoster, Barnet EN4 9EY Tel: 020 8887 2303 — MB BS Peradeniya 1985; FRCS Ed. Staff Grade N. Middlx. Hosp. Lond. Specialty: Accid. & Emerg.

SATHYANARAYANA, Chakralvar Narasimhachar Department of Anaesthesia, Walsgrave Hospital, Clifford Bridge Road, Coventry CV2 2DX — MB BS Mysore 1973.

SATKUNANAYAGAM, Vaithianathan (retired) 10 Kendor Avenue, Epsom KT19 8RH Tel: 01372 813265 — MB BS Ceylon 1953; Acad. DPM Eng. 1963; FRCPsych 1980. Prev: Cons. Psychiat. Surrey Heartlands Care St. Ebbas Epsom.

SATKURUNATH, Gayathri 4 Wendover Road, Bromley BR2 9JX — MB BS Lond. 1998; MB BS Lond 1998.

SATKURUNATHAN, Saravanamuttu 48 Eton Avenue, New Malden KT3 5AZ Tel: 020 8942 1901 Fax: 020 8241 2146 Email: satkuru@aol.com — MB BS Ceylon 1951; MRCP Ed. 1959; FRCP Ed. 1979. Adjudicating Med. Pract. Benefit Agency Med. Servs. Sutton. Specialty: Gen. Med. Socs: Fell. Roy. Coll. Phys.; Brit. Med. & Geriat. Assn.; Ceylon Coll. Phys. Prev: Cons. Phys. (Geriat. Med.) Roy. Vic. Hosp. Dundee; Cons. Phys. (Geriat. Med.) Dorset Co. & Poole Gen. Hosps.; Cons. Phys. Wattala Hosp. & Wattala Hosp. Sri Lanka.

SATSANGI, Mr Prem Nath (retired) Belgrave Avenue Surgery, 233 Ongar Road, Brentwood RM15 9DZ Tel: 01277 223882 — MB BS Lucknow 1954 (K.G. Med. Coll.) MS Lucknow 1958, MB BS 1954; FRCS Ed. 1966; FRCS Eng. 1967.

SATTAR, Daoud Abdul Englefield Road Surgery, 8 Englefield Road, London N1 4LN Tel: 020 7254 1324 — MB ChB Baghdad 1962.

SATTAR, Mohammad High Green Surgery, High Green, Brooke, Norwich NR15 1JD Tel: 01508 50204 — MB BS Dacca 1964; MB BS Dacca 1964.

SATTAR, Professor Naveed Amjid Glasgow Royal Infirmary, Department of Pathological Biochemistry, Queen Elizabeth Building, Glasgow G31 2ER Tel: 0141 211 4312 Fax: 0141 553 2558 Email: nsattar@clinmed.gla.ac.uk — MB ChB Glas. 1990; PhD Glas. 1998; MRCPath 1998. Prof. in Metab. Med. and Hon. Cons. in Clin. Biochem. Specialty: Chem. Path. Special Interest: Inflammation; Insulin resistance; Cardiovasc. risk. Socs: Assn. Clin. Biochem.; Scott. Soc. Experim. Med.; HEART, UK.

SATTAR, Naweed 17 Broomieknowe Gardens, Bonnyrigg EH19 2JE — MB ChB Manch. 1992.

SATTAR, Nedal Bacup Health Centre, Yorkshire St., Bacup OL13 9RA Tel: 01706 875050 — MB ChB Basrah 1978; PhD Ed. 1989; DCH RCPS Glas. 1991; MSc Audiological Medicine Manchester 1998. Staff Grade (Paediat.) Burnley Health Care NHS Trust; Assoc. Specialist in Paediatric Audiol., Burnley Health Care NHS Trust. Specialty: Community Child Health; Audiol. Med. Socs: MRCPCH; Brit. Assn. Community Drs in Audiol.; Brit. Soc. Audiol. Prev: Clin. Med. Off. (Child Health) Argyll & Clyde HB Paisley; Regist. (Paediat.) Roy. Alexandra Hosp.; SHO (Paediat.) Roy. Hosp. Sick Childr. Glas.

SATTAR, Sanjida Ahmed 6 Bradshaw Close, Pogmor, Barnsley S75 2JN — MB ChB Manch. 1998; MB ChB Manch 1998.

SATTAR, Shaila Ahmed 6 Bradshaw Close, Barnsley S75 2JN — MB ChB Manch. 1992.

SATTARI, Mohsen 24 The Fairway, Westella, Hull HU10 7SB Tel: 01482 658632 — MD Tehran 1969 (Tehran Univ. Tehran/Iran) A/S Orthop. Surg. Hull Roy. Infirm. Specialty: Orthop. Socs: Brit. Orthop. Assn.; BMA.

SATTIANAYAGAM, Aiyadurai The Surgery, 1 Crawley Lane, Pound Hill, Crawley RH10 7DX — MB BS Ceylon 1970; FRCOG 1997, M 1979.

SATTIARAJAH, Appudurai Immanuel 5 Nodders Way, Biddenham, Bedford MK40 4BJ — MRCS Eng. LRCP Lond. Lond. 1977; MRCS LRCP Lond. 1977.

SATUR, Mr Christopher Michael Raymond 2 School Croft, Rothwell, Leeds LS26 0UQ Tel: 0113 288 7103 — MB BS Lond. 1982 (Lond. Hosp.) FRCS Eng. 1988; MS 1996; DRCOG 1997; DFFG 1999; DCH 1999. Specialist Regist. (Cardiothoracic Surg.). Specialty: Cardiothoracic Surg.; Gen. Pract. Socs: Soc. Cardiothoracic Surg.; CSRC. Prev: Regist. (Cardiothoracic Surg.) Birm Childr Hosp.

SATYA PRASAD, Koneru Westwood Clinic, Wicken Way, Peterborough PE3 7JW Tel: 01733 265535 Fax: 01733 264263; Srinivas, Church St, Alwalton, Peterborough PE7 3UU Tel: 01733 265535 Fax: 01733 264263 — MB BS Andhra 1974; DTM & H Liverp. 1979; DFFP 1994. GP P'boro. Specialty: Gen. Pract. Socs: Fell. Roy. Soc. Health; Accred. Mem. (Chairm.) Brit. Med. Acupunc. Soc.; Fell. Roy. Soc. Med.

SATYANARAYANA, Polubothu 10 Marywell, Kirkcaldy KY1 2RJ — MB BS Andhra 1973.

SATYAVADANAN, Mr Bangalore Sundaravadanan Darlington Memorial Hospital, Hollyhurst Road, Darlington DL3 6HX Tel: 01325 743110 Fax: 01325 743013 — (Madras Med. Coll.) MB BS Madras 1967; MS (Gen. Surg.) Madras 1971; FRCS Ed. 1976. Cons. Urol. Darlington Mem. Hosp. & S. Cleveland Hosp, Middlesbro'. Specialty: Urol. Socs: BAUS; Eur. Assn. Urol.; Assn. Surgs India. Prev: Urol. Surg. Qu. Eliz. Hosp. Gateshead; Regist. (Urol.) Kent & Canterbury Hosp., Walsgrave Hosp. Coventry, Leeds Gen. Infirm. & Bradford Roy. Infirm.

SAUDI, Mamdouh Nabil Said Abdel Rahman West Cumberland Hospital, Hensingham, Whitehaven CA28 8JG Tel: 01946 692347 Email: mamsaudi@hotmail.com — MB ChB Egypt 1980; FRCA UK 1997. Cons. Anaesth. - Lead Clinician in Obstetric Anaesth., W. Cumbld. Hosp., Whitehaven. Specialty: Anaesth.; Intens. Care. Special Interest: Obstetric Anaesth. Socs: Obstetric Anaesthetists Assn.; Intens. Care Soc.; Europ. Soc. of Anaesthesiologists. Prev: Locum Cons. in Anaesth. SITU - Southport and Ormskirk; Specialist Regist. in Anaesth. and ITU, Liverp. Womens Hosp.

SAUJANI, Arvind Vallabhdas Horn Lane Surgery, 156 Horn Lane, Acton, London W3 6PH Tel: 020 8992 4722 — MB BS Rajasthan 1971.

SAUJANI, Virendra Kumar Tulsidas 39 Huntsmans Way, Rusheymead, Leicester LE4 7ZG — MB BS Lond. 1979 (Middlx.) DRCOG 1982.

SAUL, Peter Anthony Spring House, 555 Chorley Old Road, Bolton BL1 6AF Tel: 01204 848411 Fax: 01204 849968 — MB ChB Manch. 1968; DObst RCOG 1971.

SAUL, Peter Damien Health Centre, Beech Avenue, Rhosllanerchrugog, Wrexham LL14 1AA Tel: 01978 845955 Fax: 01978 846757 — MB ChB Liverp. 1977; DCH Eng. 1979; DRCOG 1984; MRCGP 1984. Hosp. Pract. (Paediat.) Chester Gp. Hosps.

SAULSBURY, Nicola Kerry Gail Ambrose King Centre, Royal London Hospital, Whitechapel, London E1 1BB; St James' Vicarage, Arlington Square, Islington, London N1 7DS — MB BS Lond. 1992 (St. Mary's Hospital Medical School) Dip GUM (Distinction) Soc. Apoth; BSc (Psychol.) 1989; MRCP (UK) 1995. Specialist Regist. (Genitourin. & HIV Med.) Roy. Lond. & St. Bart. Hosp. Lond. Specialty: Genitourinary Medicine; HIV Med. Socs: BMA; Brit. HIV Assn.

SAUND, Narinder Singh Cross Street Surgery, 5 Cross Street, Hathern, Loughborough LE12 5LB Tel: 01509 646326 Fax: 01509 646098; 19 Linley Avenue, Shepshed, Loughborough LE12 9HJ Tel: 01509 507650 — MB BS Lond. 1986 (Guys Hosp.) DRCOG 1992; DFFP 1994. Prev: Clin. Asst. (Rheum.) Coalville Hosp.; Clin. Asst. (c/o Elderly) LoughBoro. Hosp.; Clin. Asst. (Dermat.) LoughBoro. Hosp.

SAUNDBY, Edith (retired) Persondy, Llangynidr, Crickhowell NP8 1NT Tel: 01874 730932 — MB ChB Bristol 1955; DObst RCOG 1957.

SAUNDBY, Robert Peter (retired) Persondy, Llangynidr, Crickhowell NP8 1NT Tel: 01874 730932 Email: peter.saundby@virgin.net — MB ChB Bristol 1956; MMedSci Nottm. 1981; MFOM 1981; FFPHM RCP (UK) 1992, M 1982; T(OM)

1991; T(PHM) 1991. Med. Tech. Off. Europe Air Sports; Med. Adviser, Brit. Gliding Assn.; Sec., Commiss. Internationale Medico-physiologique, Federat. Aeronautique Internationale. Prev: Air Commodore, Roy. Air Force.

SAUNDERS, Alan John Everest House Surgery, Everest Way, Hemel Hempstead HP2 4HY Tel: 01442 240422 Fax: 01442 235045 — MB BS Lond. 1964 (Univ. Coll. Hosp.) DObst RCOG 1966. Prev: Ho. Surg. & Ho. Phys. W. Suff. Gen. Hosp.; Ho. Surg. St. Helier Hosp. Carshalton.

SAUNDERS, Andrew James Selkirk Dept. Of Radiology, Guys Hospital, St Thomas St., London SE1 9RT — MB BS Lond. 1964; MRCP (U.K.) 1969; DMRD Eng. 1971; FFR 1972; FRCR 1975; FRCP Lond. 1984. Cons. Radiol. Guy's Hosp. Lond. Specialty: Radiol.

SAUNDERS, Andrew Paul Gregory 54 Dulwich Road, London SE24 0PA Tel: 020 7733 8360 — MB BChir Camb. 1979; MA, MB BChir Camb. 1979; MRCP UK 1982.

SAUNDERS, Anna Cleeve Lawn, 117 Hales Road, Cheltenham GL52 6ST Tel: 01242 702104 — MB BS Lond. 1979; DFFP Lond. 1998; LFHom (Med.) 2001. GP Locum, Cheltenham. Prev: Asst. GP Cheltenham.; Clin. Asst. (Ophth.) Cheltenham.

SAUNDERS, Anne Patricia Sunbury Health Centre Group Practice, Green Street, Sunbury-on-Thames TW16 6RH Tel: 01932 713399 Fax: 01932 713354 — MB BS Lond. 1981.

SAUNDERS, Arthur Courtenay Greenwood Medical Centre, 249 Sneinton Dale, Sneinton, Nottingham NG3 7DQ Tel: 0115 950 1854 Fax: 0115 948 4999; Melton Spinney Farm, Melton Spinney Road, Thorpe Arnold, Melton Mowbray LE14 4SB Tel: 01664 500 5057 Fax: 01664 500 5057 — (Liverp.) MB Ch Liverp. 1952; Dip. Clin. Hypn. Sheff. 1991. Cons. Hypnother. Nottm. Specialty: Disabil. Med. Socs: Roy. Soc. Med.; Brit. Soc. Med. & Dent. Hypn.; Brit. Soc. Experim. & Clin. Hypn. Prev: Hon. Med. Sec. Notts. Local Med. Comm.

SAUNDERS, Brian Paul Wolfson Unit For Endoscopy, St. Mark's Hospital, Watford Road, Harrow HA1 3UJ Tel: 020 8235 4225 Fax: 020 8423 3588; 50 Nightingale Road, Rickmansworth WD3 7DB Tel: 01923 721269 — MB BS Lond. 1988 (Univ. Coll. Hosp. Lond.) MRCP (UK) 1991; MD Lond. 1996. Cons. Phys. & Sen. Lect. (Endoscopy) St. Mark's Hosp. Lond.; Cons. Gastroenterol. & Endoscopist The Lond. Clinic. Specialty: Gastroenterol. Socs: (Treas.) St. Mark's Assn.; Roy. Soc. Med.; Brit. Soc. Gastroenterol. Prev: Sen. Regist. (Gastroenterol.) Guy's Hosp. Lond.; Sen. Regist. (Gen. Med. & Gastroenterol.) Lewisham Hosp. Lond.; Regist. (Med.) Darlington Memor. Hosp.

SAUNDERS, Caroline Scarborough Health Trust, Scarborough YO12 6QL; Key Green Farm House, Egton Grange, Whitby YO22 5AX — MB BS Lond. 1985 (Univ. Coll. Lond.) Dip. Occupat Med. Occupat. Health Off. ScarBoro. Trust. Specialty: Occupat. Health.

SAUNDERS, Christobel Mary Dept. Surgery VCL, 67-73 Riding House St., London W1P 7LD Tel: 020 7504 9314 Fax: 020 7636 5176; Seale House, 37 Dartford Road, Sevenoaks TN13 3TD — MB BS Lond. 1986; FRCS Eng. 1991. Sen. Lect. UCL; Hon. Cons. (Surg.) UCLH. Specialty: Gen. Surg.

SAUNDERS, Christopher John The Health Centre, Canterbury Way, Stevenage SG1 1QH Tel: 01438 357411 Fax: 01438 720523; 96 Astwick Road, Stotfold, Hitchin SG5 4BG — MB BS Lond. 1989 (University College Hospital London) BSc Loughborough 1983; MSc Lond. 1985; MRCGP 1993. Specialty: Gen. Pract. Prev: MRC Research Doctor Environm. Epidemiol. Unit Soton. Univ.; Trainee GP Stevenage VTS; SHO (Paediat., O & G & A & E) Lister Hosp. Stevenage.

SAUNDERS, Dame Cicely Mary Strode, OM, DBE (retired) St. Christopher's Hospice, 51-59 Lawrie Park Road, Sydenham, London SE26 6DZ Tel: 020 8778 9252 Fax: 020 8659 8680 — (St. Thos.) MA Oxf.; Hon. Dr. Law Univ. Camb. 1986; Hon. Dr. Law Univ. Oxf. 1986; Hon. FRCPsych. 1988; MB BS Lond. 1957; FRCP Lond. 1974, M 1968; Hon. DSc Yale 1969; Hon. Dr. Law Columbia Univ. 1979; Hon. Dr. Law Jewish Theolog. Seminary, New York 1982; Hon. DSc Univ. Lond. 1983; Hon. Dr. Med. Qu. Univ. Belf. 1984; FRCS 1986. Hon. Cons. St. Joseph's Hospice Hackney & St. Thos. Hosp. Lond.; Pres. St. Christopher's Hospice, Sydenham.

SAUNDERS, Daniel John Sandwell General Hospital, Lyndon, West Bromwich B71 4HJ — MB ChB Leic. 1996 (Leics.) BSc (Hons.) Leic. 1994; MRCP (UK) 2002. SHO Med. Rotat. Leicester; SHO Med. Rotat. Sandwell Gen. Hosp. Specialty: Gen. Med.; Oncol. Socs: Hon. Sec. - Gay and Lesbian Assoc. of Doctors and Dentists; Hon. Sec. - W. Midl.s Reg. Jun. Doctors Comm.; Dept. of Health Sexual Orientation Extern. Refer. Gp.

SAUNDERS, Dave Mark 38 Stanley Avenue, Birmingham B32 2HA — BM BS Nottm. 1989.

SAUNDERS, David Arthur, TD Department of Anaesthetics, Southampton General Hospital, Tremona Road, Southampton SO16 6YD; The Gatehouse, 2 Stag Gates, Exbury Road, Blackfield, Southampton SO45 1SR — MB ChB Leeds 1968; PhD Leeds 1979, BSc 1965, MB ChB 1968; FFA RCS Eng. 1975. Cons. Anaesth. Soton. Univ. Hosps. Trust. Specialty: Anaesth.

SAUNDERS, David Cameron (retired) Anthony House, 9 Vicarage Road, Penygraig, Tonypandy CF40 1HN — (Cardiff) BSc, MB BCh (Commend.) Wales 1949; DCH Eng. 1956; MRCGP 1958. Med. Ref. & Divisional Med. Off. Welsh Office. Prev: RAF.

SAUNDERS, David Clifford H. M. Stanley Hospital, St Asaph LL17 1UL Tel: 01745 589680 Fax: 01745 589770 — MB ChB Manch. 1986; DO Lond. 1989; FRCOphth Lond. 1991. Cons. (Ophth. Surg.) HM Stanley Hosp. St. Asaph. Specialty: Ophth.

SAUNDERS, Dawn Elizabeth Dept. of Radiology, King's College Hospital, Denmark Hill, London SE5 8RS Tel: 020 7346 3331 Fax: 020 7346 3445; 92 Horne Park Road, Wimbledon, London SW19 7HR Tel: 020 8879 1012 Email: desaund@aol.com — MB BS Lond. 1986 (King's Coll. Sch. Med. & Dent.) MRCP (UK) 1990; MD Lond. 1996. Sen. Regist. (Radiol.) Kings Coll. Hosp. Lond. Specialty: Radiol. Socs: Soc. Magenetic Resonance. Prev: Lect. (Magnetic Resonance) St. Geo. Hosp. Med. Sch. Lond.; Regist. (Thoracic Med.) Bromley Hosp. Kent & King's Coll. Hosp. Lond.; SHO (Cardiol.) Brook Hosp. Lond.

SAUNDERS, Douglas Robert Sinclair (retired) The Stables, 22 White St., West Lavington, Devizes SN10 4LP Tel: 01380 813648 — (Guy's) MB BS Lond. 1944; MRCP Lond. 1951. Prev: Surg. Lt. RNVR.

SAUNDERS, Elizabeth Hesling (retired) Swiss Cottage, Kitty Lane, Marton Moss, Blackpool FY4 5EG — MB ChB Manch. 1959.

SAUNDERS, Elizabeth Jane 149 Kinghsheath Avenue, Liverpool L14 2DQ Tel: 0151 283 4254 — MB BS Lond. 1987; DCH RCP Lond. 1991; MSc (Pub. Health) Lond. 1993. Paediat. Doctor (A & E)Roy. Liverp. Childrs. Hosp. NHS Trust (Alder Hey). Specialty: Paediat.

SAUNDERS, Elizabeth Mary Jane 23 Horseguards, Exeter EX4 4UU — MB ChB Bristol 1993; DRCOG; MRCGP; DFFP.

SAUNDERS, Elizabeth Rosemary May (retired) 7 Dan-y-Graig, Machen, Caerphilly CF83 8RF Tel: 029 2088 4439 — (Cardiff) MB BCh Wales 1960; DCH Eng. 1964; DObst RCOG 1964; MFCH 1989. Prev: SCMO Gwent HA.

SAUNDERS, Elizabeth Stewart Coniston Medical Practice, The Parade, Coniston Road, Bristol BS34 5TF Tel: 0117 969 5208 Fax: 0117 969 0456; 13 Russet Close, Olveston, Bristol BS35 4EE — MB ChB Bristol 1972; DObst RCOG 1974; DCH Eng. 1978; MRCP (UK) 1980. Gen. Practitioner.

SAUNDERS, Elizabeth Susanna West Sussex Health Authority, 1 The Causeway, Durrington, Worthing BN12 6BU Tel: 01903 708623 Fax: 01903 502684 Email: lizsaunders@tinyworld.co.uk — MB BS Lond. 1981 (Roy. Free) MFPHM RCP (UK) 1992. Cons. Pub. Health Med. W. Sussex HA and Crawley PCG. Specialty: Pub. Health Med. Prev: Sen. Regist. (Pub. Health Med.) Brighton DHA; Regist. (Community Med.) Medway Dist. HA; Research Regist. (Neuropsychiat.) MRC Neuropsychiat. Research Laborat. W. Pk. Hosp. Epsom.

SAUNDERS, Emily Jane 12 Royal Park Mount, Leeds LS6 1HL — MB ChB Leeds 1998.

SAUNDERS, Emma Jane 9 Welton Mount, Leeds LS6 1ET — MB ChB Leeds 1994.

SAUNDERS, Emma Jane 8 Farquhar Road E., Birmingham B15 3RD — MB BS Lond. 1990. Trainee GP/SHO Stoke Mandeville Hosp. Aylesbury VTS.

SAUNDERS, Fiona Margaret 15 Bryn Road, Mynydd Isa, Mold CH7 6UR — MB ChB Manch. 1989; DA (UK) 1994; FRCS Ed. 1995. Regist. (A & E Med.) NW RHA. Specialty: Accid. & Emerg. Socs: Assoc. Mem. Brit. Accid. & Emerg. Med. Soc.

SAUNDERS, Frank Coutts Inglehurst, Deaf Hill, Trimdon Station TS29 6DA — MB BS Newc. 1976.

SAUNDERS, Graham James Witton Street Surgery, 162 Witton Street, Northwich CW9 5QU Tel: 01606 42007 Fax: 01606 350659; 162 Witton Street, Northwich CW9 5QT Tel: 01606 42007 — MB ChB Manch. 1978; DRCOG 1983; MRCGP 1988.

SAUNDERS, Graham Peter York Medical Group, 199 Acomb Road, Acomb, York YO24 4HD Tel: 01904 342999 Fax: 01904 342990; Garden Cottage, Low Catton Lane End, Kexby, York YO41 5LE Tel: 01759 380695 — MB BS Lond. 1974 (St. Bart.)

SAUNDERS, Hilary Jane Parkgate Surgery, 28 St Helens Road, Ormskirk L39 4QR Tel: 01695 572561 — MB ChB Liverp. 1994; DFFP 1996; DRCOG 1996. GP Princip. Ormskirk. Specialty: Gen. Pract. Prev: Trainee GP/SHO Southport & Formby Dist. Gen. Hosp. VTS.

SAUNDERS, Ian Arthur — MB BS Lond. 1970 (St. Geo.) AKC; DFFP; MRCS Eng. LRCP Lond. 1970. Clin. Med. Off. Family Plann. Buxton; Med. Off. Buxton Lime Industs. Socs: N. Derbysh. LMC. Prev: Ho. Phys. Roy. Portsmouth Hosp.; Ho. Surg. Surgic. Unit St. Geo. Hosp. Lond.

SAUNDERS, Ian Michael The Surgery, 25 St Mary's Road, Tickhill, Doncaster DN11 9NA Tel: 01302 742503 — MB ChB Leeds 1983; BSc (1st cl. Hons. Chem. Path.) Leeds 1980; MRCGP 1988. Prev: Trainee GP Doncaster VTS.; SHO (A & E) Newham Gen. Hosp.; Ho. Off. (Gen. Med.) & (Gen. Surg.) Wharfedale Gen. Hosp. Otley.

SAUNDERS, Irene Gladys Gillian College Grove, 2 College Lane, Ripon HG4 4HE Tel: 01765 688306 — (Char. Cross) MB BS Lond. 1962; FRCPsych 1996, M 1977. Emerit. Cons. Psychiat. The Retreat York; Hon. Cons. Psychiat. St. Lukes Hosp. to the Clergy. Specialty: Gen. Psychiat. Prev: Cons. Psychiat. St. Luke's Hosp. Middlesbrough; Ho. Surg. Bromley Hosp.; Ho. Phys. Brook Hosp. Lond.

SAUNDERS, Jeremy Hugh Bannerman Bedford Hospital, Kempston Road, Bedford MK42 9DJ Tel: 01234 792271 Fax: 01234 792041; The Manor House, Felmersham, Bedford MK43 7JG Tel: 01234 781375 — (Roy. Free) MD Lond. 1981, MB BS Lond. 1969; MRCS Eng. LRCP Lond. 1969; MRCP (UK) 1973; FRCP Lond. 1989. Cons. Phys. Bedford Gen. Hosp. Trust; Med.Dir.Bedford Hosp.Trust. Specialty: Gastroenterol.; Gen. Med. Socs: Brit. Soc. Gastroenterol. Prev: Sen. Med. Regist. Dept. Therap. Ninewells Hosp. Dundee; Med. Regist. Qu. Alexandra Hosp. Cosham.; Wellcome Research Fell. Rigs Hosp.et Copenhagen, Denmark.

SAUNDERS, John Nevill Hall Hospital, Abergavenny NP7 7EG Tel: 01873 732432 Fax: 01873 732973 — (St Thomas's) Dip. Biochem. (Distinc.) Lond 1965; MB BS Lond. 1968; MRCP (UK) 1972; DCH Eng. 1974; MD Lond. 1980; MA Wales 1988; FRCP Lond. 1988. Cons. Phys. & Specialist (Endocrinol. & Diabetes); Hon. Prof., Centre for Philosophy, Humanities & Law in Healthcare, Univ. of Wales Swansea; Chairm., Comm. for ethical issues in Med., RoyColl PhycnLond; Chairm.,Multi-centre Research Ethics Comm. for Wales. Specialty: Gen. Med.; Diabetes; Endocrinol. Special Interest: Med. Ethics; Philosophy of Med. Socs: Wales Endocrine & Diabetes Society; Diabetes UK; Society of Physicians in Wales. Prev: Lect. (Med.) St. Thos. Hosp. Med. Sch. Lond.; Resid. (Paediat.) Univ. Brit. Columbia & Vancouver Childr. Hosp.; Regist. (Neurol.) Radcliffe Infirm. & Churchill Hosp. Oxf.

SAUNDERS, John Pendleside Medical Practice, Clitheroe Health Centre, Railway View Road, Clitheroe BB7 2JG Tel: 01200 422674 Fax: 01200 443652 — MB ChB Leeds 1978; DRCOG 1982; Cert. FPA 1982; MRCGP 1982; Dip. Sports Med. Lond 1994. GP Clitheroe; Sch. Med. Off. Stoneyhurst Coll. Univ. Wales Swansea. Specialty: Sports Med. Socs: Brit. Assn. Sport & Med.

SAUNDERS, John Alan (retired) Bede Cottage, Church Lane, Plummers Plain, Horsham RH13 6LU Tel: 01403 891368 — LMSSA Lond. 1958 (Oxf. & St. Geo.) MA Oxf. 1961, BA 1954; FRCGP 1978, M 1968. Prev: Hon. Sen. Regist. King's/Brook Family Plann. Dept. King's Coll. Hosp. Lond.

SAUNDERS, Mr John Harris Weston Area NHS Trust, Grange Rd, Uphill, Weston Super Mare BS23 4TQ Tel: 01934 647090 Fax: 01934647176 — MB ChB Glas. 1968; FRCS Glas. 1973; MBA Ed. 1989. Exec. Med. Dir. W. area NHS Health Trust. Specialty: Gastroenterol.; Gen. Surg. Prev: Cons. Surg. Gastrointestinal Unit West. Gen. Hosp. Edin.; Sen. Regist. (Surg.) Hammersmith Hosp. & Roy. Postgrad. Med. Sch. Lond.; Regist. & SHO Rotat. (Surg.) West. Infirm. Glas.

SAUNDERS, Judith Patricia 27 Chesterfield Grove, London SE22 8RP — MB ChB Leeds 1993.

SAUNDERS, Julia Mary Raleigh Unit, North Devon District Hospital, Barnstaple EX31 4JH Tel: 01271 322445 — MB ChB Bristol 1985; MRCGP 1989. Specialty: Care of the Elderly.

SAUNDERS, Kay Butetown Health Centre, Loudoun Square, Cardiff CF10 5UZ Tel: 029 2048 3126 Fax: 02920 471 879 — MB BCh Oxf. 1981; BM BCh Oxf. 1981; MA Camb. 1983; MRCGP 1985. Singlehanded GP Butetown Cardiff. Prev: GP Middlesbrough; Asst. GP Middlesbrough Doctors Retainer Scheme; Trainee GP Cleveland VTS.

SAUNDERS, Professor Kenneth Barrett 77 Lee Road, London SE3 9EN — MB BChir Camb. 1962 (Camb. & St. Thos.) FRCP Lond. 1978, M 1963; MA, MD Camb. 1966; DSc Lond. 1996. Emerit. Prof. Med. St. Geo. Hosp. Med. Sch. Lond. Specialty: Respirat. Med.; Gen. Med. Prev: Prof. Med. St. Geo. Hosp. Med. Sch. Lond.; Sen. Lect. & Reader (Med.) Middlx. Hosp. Med. Sch.; Dean Fac. Med. Univ. Lond.

SAUNDERS, Kenneth Michael (retired) 8 Little Gaddesden House, Little Gaddesden, Berkhamsted HP4 1PL Tel: 01442 842531 — MB BS Lond. 1949 (St. Thos.) Prev: Capt. RAMC (TA).

SAUNDERS, Lynette Jayne Montgomery House Surgery, Piggy Lane, Bicester OX26 6HT; 1 Blacksmith's Close, Church Road, Weston-on-the-Green, Bicester OX25 3FL — MB BS Lond. 1993 (St. Geo. Hosp. Med. Sch. Lond.) DRCOG 1996. Ass. GP under the Retainer Scheme. Specialty: Gen. Pract. Prev: Severn NHS Trust; E. Gloucs NHS Trust; Gloucs Roy. Hosp. NHS Trust.

SAUNDERS, Madeleine Iris Family Planning Clinic, Woking Community Hospital, Heathside Road, Woking GU22 7HS Tel: 01483 714160 — MB BS Lond. 1975 (King's Coll. Hosp.) MFFP; BSc (Hons. Biochem.) Sussex 1970. SCMO (Family Plann.) Woking PCT; Hospital Practitioner - Blanche Herriot Unit - St. Peter's Hosp. Gyn. Specialty: Family Plann. & Reproduc. Health; Genitourinary Medicine. Socs: Fac. Fam. Plann. Prev: Research Regist. (O & G) King's Coll. Hosp. Lond.; SHO (O & G) King's Coll. Hosp. Lond.

SAUNDERS, Marcus Lee Lake Road Health Centre, Nutfield Place, Portsmouth PO1 4JT Tel: 023 9282 1201 Fax: 023 9287 5658 — MRCS Eng. LRCP Lond. 1987; BSc Lond. 1983; DRCOG 1991.

SAUNDERS, Margaret Teresa Brookfields Hospital, Arthur Rank House, 351 Mill Road, Cambridge CB1 3DF Tel: 01223 723110 Fax: 01223 723111 Email: margaret.saunders@cambcity-pct.nhs.uk — MB BS Lond. 1978 (St. Geo.) MRCP (UK) 1982; FRCP UK 2001. Clin. Director Arthur Rank Ho. Specialist Palliat. Care Servs.; Cons. (Palliat. Med.) Papworth Hosp. Camb. Specialty: Palliat. Med.

SAUNDERS, Mark Gary Marton Medical Centre, 1 Glastonbury Avenue, Blackpool FY1 6SF Tel: 01253 761321 Fax: 01253 792701; 84 Arundel Drive, Poulton-le-Fylde FY6 7TR — MB ChB Dundee 1987; DA (UK) 1991; MRCGP 1993; T(GP) 1993. SHO (Psychiat.) Vict. Hosp. Blackpool. Prev: SHO (Gen. Surg., Geriat. & A & E) Auckland Gen. Hosp., NZ; SHO (Anaesth.) Vict. Hosp. Blackpool; Trainee GP Blackpool.

SAUNDERS, Mark Peter Department of Pharmacy, University of Manchester, Oxford Road, Manchester M13 9PL Tel: 0161 275 2428 — MB BS Lond. 1986; MRCP (UK) 1990; FRCR 1994. MRC Train. Fell. Univ. Manch. Specialty: Oncol.; Radiother. Socs: BACR; AACR; ACP. Prev: Clin. Research Fell. ICRF Churchill Hosp. Oxf.; Regist. (Clin. Oncol.) Churchill Hosp. Oxf.

SAUNDERS, Michael College Grove 2, College Lane, Ripon HG4 4HE Tel: 01765 588396 Fax: 01423 330688 — (Char. Cross) MB BS (Hons.) Lond. 1962; FRCP Ed. 1973, M 1965; FRCP Lond. 1978, M 1965. Emerit. Cons. Neurol. & Neuro-Rehabil. Newc. City Health NHS Trust & Nortallerton NHS Trust. Specialty: Neurol. Prev: Clin. Dir. Regional Rehabil. Centre Huntersmoor Hosp. Newc.

SAUNDERS, Michael Charles Little Morton, Tile Barn Lane, Brockenhurst SO42 7UE Tel: 01590 623376 Fax: 01590 623376 — MB BChir Camb. 1968 (St. Thos.) DA Eng. 1970; DObst RCOG 1971. Specialty: Anaesth.

SAUNDERS, Mr Michael Peter 51 Summerdown Road, Eastbourne BN20 8DR Tel: 01323 732504 Email: bowel.inspector@virgin.net — (Westm. Lond.) MB BS Lond. 1982; FRCS Ed. 1987; FRCS Eng. 1988; BSc Lond. 1979, MS 1995. Cons. Gen. Surg. Eastbourne Dist. Gen. Hosp. Specialty: Gen. Surg. Socs: Assn. Surg.; Brit. Soc. Gastroenterol.; Assn. Coloproctol. Prev: Sen. Regist. (Gen. Surg.) Guy's Hosp. Lond.

SAUNDERS, Mr Michael William 2 Russell Road, Westbury Park, Bristol BS6 7UB — MB ChB Bristol 1988; FRCS Eng. 1993.

SAUNDERS, Professor Michele Iris Marie Curie Research Wing, Centre for Cancer Treatment, Mount Vernon Hospital, Northwood HA6 2RN Tel: 01923 844533 Fax: 01923 844167 Email: mcrw@mtvern.co.uk — (Roy. Free) MRCS Eng. LRCP Lond. 1967; MB BS Lond. 1967; DMRT Eng. 1972; FRCR 1975; MD Lond. 1982; FRCP 1998. Cons. Radiother. & Oncol. Centre for Cancer Treatm. Mt. Vernon Hosp. Northwood; Prof. (Oncol.) Univ. Coll. & Middlx. Sch. of Med. Lond.; Director CRC Tumour Biol. & Radiat. Ther. Specialty: Oncol.; Radiother. Socs: Europ. Soc. Therapeutic Radiat. Oncol.; Brit. Oncol. Assn. Prev: Regist. Meyerstein Inst. Radiother. Middlx. Hosp. Lond.; Sen. Regist. St. Bart. Hosp. Lond. & Regional Radiother. Centre Mt. Vernon Hosp. N.wood.

SAUNDERS, Nancy Claire (retired) The Stables, 22 White St., West Lavington, Devizes SN10 4LP Tel: 01380 813648 — MB BS Lond. 1948 (Roy. Free) MRCS Eng. LRCP Lond. 1948. Prev: Sen. Med. Off. Borehamwood. St. Albans & Edgware Gen. Hosp. Family Plann. clinics.

SAUNDERS, Nicholas Charles 64 Peacock Lane, Brighton BN1 6WA — MB ChB Birm. 1992.

SAUNDERS, Nicholas Michael — MB BS Lond. 1998 (Univ. Coll. Hosp.) Specialty: Anaesth.

SAUNDERS, Mr Nigel James St George 146 Nottingham Street, Pitsmoor, Sheffield S3 9HL — MB ChB Manch. 1977; FRCS Ed. 1983; MRCOG 1983.

SAUNDERS, Pamela Wollaton Vale Health Centre, Wollaton Vale, Wollaton, Nottingham NG8 2GR Tel: 0115 928 2216 Fax: 0115 928 0590.

SAUNDERS, Paul Anthony 62 Rosemont Road, Aigburth, Liverpool L17 6DA — MB ChB Liverp. 1982.

SAUNDERS, Paul Richard Department of Anaesthesia, Royal Surrey County Hospital, Egerton Road, Guildford GU10 2LS Tel: 01483 464116 Email: p.saunderes@royalsurrey.nhs.uk; Stock Farm House, Tilford Road, Churt, Farnham GU10 2LS — MB BS Lond. 1982; FFA RCS Eng. 1987. Cons. Anaesth. And Intens. Care Roy. Surrey Co. Hosp. Guildford. Specialty: Anaesth.; Intens. Care. Socs: Brit. Med. Assn.; Roy. Soc. of Med.; Intens. Care Soc. Prev: Sen. Regist. (Anaesth.) Bristol Roy. Infirm.; Sen. Regist. Rotat. (Anaesth.) Derriford Hosp. Plymouth; Asst. Prof. Dept. Anaesth. Univ. Texas Med. Sch. Dallas, USA.

SAUNDERS, Peter Courtenay The Surgery, 577 Carlton Road, Nottingham NG3 7AF Tel: 0115 958 0415 Fax: 0115 950 9245; 9 Gordon Rise, Mapperley, Nottingham NG3 5GB Tel: 0115 956 1654 — MB BS Lond. 1987; DGM RCP Lond. 1990. Prev: GP Ashford; Trainee GP Ashford Kent VTS.

SAUNDERS, Mr Peter James Christian Medical Fellowship, 157 Waterloo Road, London SE1 8XN Tel: 020 7928 4694 Fax: 020 7620 2453; 86 Ladies Grove, St Albans AL3 5UB Tel: 01727 839157 Email: pjs@cmf.org.uk — MB ChB Auckland 1982 (Auckland, New Zealand) FRACS 1989. Stud. Sec. - Christian Med. Fellowship. Specialty: Gen. Surg. Socs: (Gen. Sec.) Christian Med. Fellowsh.; PRIME; ICTHES.

SAUNDERS, Peter Martin Donnington Health Centre, 1 Henley Avenue, Oxford OX4 4DH Tel: 01865 771313; 36 Argyle Street, Oxford OX4 1SS — MB ChB Sheff. 1980; DA (UK) 1986; MRCGP 1988. Prev: SHO (Anaesth.) Luton & Dunstable Hosp.; SHO (Trauma & Orthop.) Princess Margt. Hosp. Swindon; SHO (Anaesth.) Stoke Mandeville Hosp. Aylesbury.

SAUNDERS, Peter Warwick Brooklea Clinic, Wick Road, Bristol BS4 4HU Tel: 0117 971 1211 — MB ChB Manch. 1981; BSc St. And. 1978; MRCGP 1985; DRCOG 1985. Lead GP for Commissioning, Bristol S. & W. PCT. Specialty: HIV Med. Prev: Bd. Mem. S. E. Bristol PCG; GP Facilitator for HIV Avon.

SAUNDERS, Peter William Griffiths Newcastle General Hospital, Westgate Road, Newcastle upon Tyne NE4 6BE — MB ChB Bristol 1971; MRCPath 1977.

SAUNDERS, Philip Bernard Ridgacre House Surgery, 83 Ridgacre Road, Quinton, Birmingham B32 2TJ Tel: 0121 422 3111; 128 Bunbury Road, Northfield, Birmingham B31 2DN Tel: 0121 475 1303 — MB ChB Birm. 1991 (Birminngham) MRCGP 1995. GP Birm. Specialty: Gen. Pract.

SAUNDERS, Raymond Charles Oudot 26 Longdon Wood, Keston, Bromley BR2 6EW — MB BS Lond. 1946 (Lond. Hosp.) DA Eng. 1950; FFA RCS Eng. 1953. Cons. Anaesth. Orpington & Sevenoaks Hosp. Gp. Specialty: Anaesth. Prev: Asst. Lect. (Anaesth.) Univ. Glas.; Sen. Regist. Anaesth. Glas. Roy. Infirm.; Regist. Anaesth. Postgrad. Med. Sch. Lond.

SAUNDERS, Mr Richard Nigel — MB BChir Camb. 1995 (Addenbrooke's Hosp. Camb.) MA Camb. 1997; MRCS (Eng) 1998; MD (Leic.) 2003. S. Trent SpR Rotat. (Gen. Surg.). Specialty: Transpl. Surg.; Gen. Surg. Socs: MPS; BMA; Assn. Surgeons GB/Ireland. Prev: Research Regist. (Renal Transplant) Leicester Gen. Hosp.; SHO Surg. Rotat. Qu.'s Med. Centre Nottm.

SAUNDERS, Sarah Josephine 16 Melbourn Road, Crookes, Sheffield S10 1NS — MB ChB Sheff. 1989.

***SAUNDERS, Simon Andrew** 14 Ambassador Drive, Liverpool L26 6LT Tel: 0151 487 9552; 14 Ambassador Drive, Liverpool L26 6LT Tel: 0151 487 9552 — MB ChB Liverp. 1998 (L'pool) BSc (Hons) Liverp 1992; MB ChB Liverp 1998. Specialty: Gen. Med.

SAUNDERS, Mr Stephen Michael Francis 9 Cairns Close, St Albans AL4 0EA Tel: 01727 863109 Email: smfsaunders@rcsed.ac.uk; 6 Eversley Road, Sketty, Swansea SA2 9DA Tel: 01792 208789 Email: smfsaunders@hotmail.com — MB BS Lond. 1993 (Univ. Coll. Lond.) BSc (Hons.) Pharm. 1989 Lond.; MSc (Surgic. Sci.) Lond. 1988; FRCS Ed. 1997; FRCS (Gen. Surg.) Ed 2004. Specialist Regist. Gen. Surg. N. Thames; Sen. Specialist Regist. Gen. Surg. Roy. Glos. Hosp. Specialty: Gen. Surg. Prev: Clin. Teachg. Fell. (Gen. Surg.) Northwick Pk. Hosp. Harrow; Acting Regist. (Gen. Surg.) Roy. Surrey Co. Hosp. Guildford; Sen. SHO (Gen. Surg.) Roy. Surrey Co. Hosp. Guildford.

SAUNDERS, Mr Stuart Henry St George's Hospital, London SW17 Tel: 020 8336 0011 Fax: 020 8336 1800; Pinewood Manor, George Road, Kingston upon Thames KT2 7NR Tel: 020 8336 0011 Fax: 020 8336 1800 Email: stuarts@a4u.com — (Birm.) MB ChB Birm. 1964; MRCS Eng. LRCP Lond. 1964; FRCS Eng. 1971. Cons. ENT St. Geo. Hosp. Lond.; Hon. Sen. Lect. Univ. Lond. Specialty: Otolaryngol. Socs: Fell. Roy. Soc. Med.; Brit. Assn. Otol. Prev: Sen. Regist. (ENT) Radcliffe Infirm. Oxf.; Regist. (ENT) Char. Cross Hosp. Lond.; SHO (ENT) Lond. Hosp.

SAUNDERS, Timothy Hinton 1 Manorfields, Weston-on-the-Green, Bicester OX6 8FL Email: timsaunders@hotmail.com — MB BS Lond. 1994 (St Geos. Hosp.) FRCR Part1; BSc Lond. 1991; MRCP (UK) 1997. SHO (Neurol.) Qu. Med. Centre Nottm.; Regist. (Radiol.) John Radcliffe Hosp. Oxf. Specialty: Radiol. Prev: SHO Rotat. Princess Margt. Hosp. Swindon; SHO (Neurol.) Qu.s Med. Centr. Nottm.

SAUNDERS, Timothy Philip Heath Lane Medical Centre, Heath Lane, Chester CH3 5UJ Tel: 01244 348844 Fax: 01244 351057; Hollin Byre, Hollins Hill, Utkinton, Tarporley CW6 0JR Fax: 01829 752652 — MB ChB Liverp. 1983; BSc Liverp. 1980. GP Health La. Med. Centre; Vice Chair Professional Comm. Chesh. W. PCT; Primary Care Adviser, Centre for Ment. Health Serv. Developm. Prev: SHO (Opth.) St. Pauls Eye Hosp. Liverp.; Non Exec. Dir. S. Chesh. HA.

SAUNDERS, Westley Peter Penrhys Ty Isaf Farm Cottage, Pontygwaith, Ferndale, Ferndale CF43 3PW — MB BCh Wales 1996.

SAUNDERS, William Alyn Russells Hall Hospital, Dudley DY1 2HQ Tel: 01384 456111 — MB BCh Wales 1963 (Cardiff) MD Wales 1968; MRCP (UK) 1973; FRCP Lond. 1993. Cons. Phys. Dudley Gp. of Hosps.; Clin. Dir. (Med.) Dudley Gp. of Hosps.; Assoc. Prof. of Med., St. Geo.'s Univ., Grenada. Specialty: Gen. Med. Socs: Brit. Geriat. Soc. & W. Midl. Phys. Assn. Prev: Sen. Regist. (Geriat. Med.) Centr. Middlx. Hosp.; Regist. (Med.) Roy. Gwent Hosp. Newport; Asst. Lect. & Research Fell. in Pharmacol. Welsh Nat. Sch. Med. Cardiff.

SAUNDERS, William Anthony Meadow Cottage, Otterbourne, Winchester SO21 2EQ — (Middlx.) MA Camb. 1966; MB BChir Camb. 1966; DCH Eng. 1967; DPM Eng. 1970; FRCPsych 1989, M 1972. Cons. Psychiat Soton. Child & Family Guid. Serv.; Hon. Clin. Teach. Univ. Soton. Specialty: Child & Adolesc. Psychiat. Socs: (Ex-Chairm.) Assn. Profess. in Servs. for Adolesc. Prev: Cons. Psychiat. Leigh Hse. Adolesc. Units Chandlers Ford, Hants.; Sen. Regist. (Child Psychiat.) Bristol Roy. Hosp. Sick Childr.; Regist. Barrow Hosp. Bristol.

SAUNDERS, Yolande Hillingdon Hospital Trust, Department of Palliative Care, Pield Heath Road, Uxbridge UB8 3NN Tel: 01895 279412 — MB BS Lond. 1984; Cert. Family Plann. JCC 1988; MRCGP 1989. p/t Cons. (Palliat. Med.) Hilling Hosp. Uxbridge

Middlx. Specialty: Palliat. Med. Socs: Assn. Of Palliat. Med. Prev: SHO (Palliat. Med.) Isabol Hospice, Ou. Eliz. II Hosp. Welwyn Gdn. City; Specialist Regist. in Palliat. Med. N. Thames; GP Hillingdon.

SAUNDERSON, Eric Martin North Street Medical Centre, 274 North Street, Romford RM1 4QJ Tel: 01708 764477 Fax: 01708 757656; 43 Wakerfield Close, Hornchurch RM11 2TH Tel: 01708 472420 — MB ChB Ed. 1971 (Edinburgh) DObst RCOG 1975; FRCGP 1992, M 1976; MSc Lond. 1997. GP Romford; Dir. Educat. & Train. Barking & Havering HA. Specialty: Endocrinol. Socs: BMA. Prev: Chairm. Barking & Havering Med. Audit Advisory Gp.; Trainee GP Ilford & Dist. VTS.; Examr. RCGP.

SAUNGSOMBOON, Daranee 1 Claremont Court, Henleaze Park, Bristol BS9 4LR — MB BS Lond. 1989; FRCS Ed. 1994; FFAEM 2002. Locum Consultant (A&E) Bristol Roy. Infirmary. Specialty: Accid. & Emerg. Prev: Specialist Regist. (A & E) Frenchay Hosp. Bristol.; Specialist Regist. (A & E) Gloucs. Roy. Hosp.

SAUVAGE, Mr Alain Daniel Paul West Suffolk Hospital, Bury St Edmunds IP33 2QZ — MB ChB Aberd. 1984 (Aberdeen) FRCS Ed. 1992; FFAEM 2001. Cons. (A&E), W. Suff. Hosp., Bury St-Edmunds, Suff. Specialty: Accid. & Emerg. Prev: Sen. Regist. (A & E), Luton; Fell. (Retrieval Med.), Sydney, Australia; Sen. Reg. (A&E), Addenbrooke's Hosp, Camb.

SAUVAGE, Josephine Ann Maria City Road Medical Centre, 190 City Rd, London EC1V 2HQ Tel: 0207 530 2750 Fax: 0207 530 2755; 68 St John's Villas, London NI9 3EG Tel: 0207 272 2893 — MB BS Lond. 1988; BSc (Pharmacol.) Lond. 1985; DCH RCP Lond. 1994; MRCGP 1997. Princip. in Gen. Pract. Specialty: Gen. Pract.

SAUVE, Philip Stuart 1A Bassetts Close, Orpington BR6 7AQ — MB BS Lond. 1998; MB BS Lond 1998.

SAUVEN, Professor Paul David Broomfield Hospital, Department of Surgery, Chelmsford Tel: 01245 514073 Fax: 01245 514024 Email: paul.sauven@meht.nhs.uk; Badyngham's, Great Waltham, Chelmsford CM3 1DE — MB BS Lond. 1975; MRCS Eng. LRCP Lond. 1975; FRCS Eng. 1980; MS Lond. 1984. Prof. Surgic. Oncol. Broomfield Hosp. Chelmsford. Specialty: Gen. Surg. Special Interest: Breast Cancer. Socs: (Hon. Treas.) Brit. Assn. Surgic. Oncol. (1996-2001); Assn. Surg. GB & Irel.; RSM Sect. of Oncol. Pres. (2000 - 2001). Prev: Sen. Regist. (Surg.) St Mary's Hosp. Lond.; Hon. Fell. Memor. Sloan-Kettering Cancer Center NY, USA; Clin. Director Chelmsford & Colchester Breast Screening Progr. 1995-2002.

SAVAGE, Adam James Flat 3R, 27 Scott St., Dundee DD2 2AH — MB ChB Dund. 1998; MB ChB Dund 1998.

SAVAGE, Mr Adrian Paul Department of Surgery, Russells Hall Hospital, Dudley DY1 2HQ Tel: 01384 244093 Fax: 01384 244082 Email: asavage@compuserve.com; Langland House, 62 Salisbury Road, Moseley, Birmingham B13 8JT Tel: 0121 449 2249 — MB BChir Camb. 1978; FRCS Eng. 1982; MA, MChir Camb. 1988. Cons. Surg. Gen. Surg. Dudley Gp. Hosps. Specialty: Gen. Surg. Socs: Assn. Coloproctol.; Assn. Endoscopic Surgs.; Assn. Surg.s GB & I. Prev: Sen. Regist. John Radcliffe Hosp. Oxf.; Clin. Fell. Mass. Gen. Hosp. Boston, USA; Regist. Hammersmith Hosp. Lond.

SAVAGE, Aiden Piers 20 Ponthill Close, Shrewsbury SY3 8RR — BM BS Nottm. 1995; MRCGP.

SAVAGE, Alexandra Clare Clover Cottage, Station Road, Great Longstone, Bakewell DE45 1TS — MB BS Lond. 1992.

SAVAGE, Andrew William George 55 Huddleston Road, Tufnell Park, London N7 0AD — MB BS Lond. 1982. Med. Regist., Mt. Vernon Hosp.

SAVAGE, Ann (retired) Coddington Vineyard, Ledbury HR8 1JJ Tel: 01531 640668 Fax: 01531 640668 — MB BS Lond. 1962 (St. Bart.) MRCPath 1977. Cons. Path. Qu. Eliz. Hosp. Prev: Sen. Regist. (Path.) Southmead Hosp. Bristol.

SAVAGE, Barbara Frances 2 The Brontes, Sun St., Haworth, Keighley BD22 8AF — MB BS Newc. 1987.

SAVAGE, Professor Caroline Olive Sylvia Renal Immunobiology Group, Birmingham Centre for Immune Regulation, University of Birmingham, Birmingham B15 2TT Tel: 0121 414 7042 Fax: 0121 414 6840; Renal Unit, Queen Elizabeth University Hospital, Birmingham B15 2TT Tel: 0121 472 1311 — MB BS Lond. 1978 (The Royal London Hospital) PhD Lond. 1987, BSc (Hons.) 1975, MD 1989; FRCS Lond. 1996. Progr. Director, The Wellocme Trust, Clin. Research Facility in Birm. Specialty: Nephrol. Prev: MRC Clin. Scientist & Hon. Cons. Phys. Clin. Research Centre Harrow & Hammersmith Hosp. Lond.; MRC Trav. Fell. Harvard Med. Sch. & Brigham Wom. Hosp. Boston, USA; Sen. Regist. (Nephrol. & Gen. Med.) Hammersmith Hosp. Lond.

SAVAGE, Catherine 16 St Kingsmark Avenue, Chepstow NP16 5LY — MB BCh Wales 1994.

SAVAGE, Mr Christopher Smallwood (retired) Chimballs, High Easter, Chelmsford CM1 4RE Tel: 01245 231254 — (Camb. & Lond. Hosp.) MRCS Eng., LRCP Lond. 1941; FRCS Eng. 1948; MA Camb. 1943, MB BChir 1952. Prev: Cons. ENT Surg. Chelmsford Hosp. & Southend Hosp.

SAVAGE, David Anthony Lawson Road Surgery, 5 Lawson Road, Broomhill, Sheffield S10 5BU Tel: 0114 266 5180; 135 Walkley Bank Road, Walkley, Sheffield S6 5AN Tel: 0114 233 4035 — BM Soton. 1984; MRCGP (Distinc.); DRCOG 1988.

SAVAGE, Mr David Edmund Consulting Rooms, North London Nuffield Hospital, Cavell Dr., Uplands Park Road, Enfield EN2 7PR Tel: 020 8366 2122; The Wain House, 111 The Chine, Winchmore Hill, London N21 2EG Tel: 020 8360 4010 — MB BS Lond. 1946 (Char. Cross) FRCS Eng. 1950; FRCOG 1968, M 1954. Socs: Fertil. Soc. Lond. Prev: Cons. Gyn. Highlands Gen. Hosp. Lond.; Cons. Obstetr. Thorpe Coombe Matern. Hosp. Lond.; Cons. Gyn. Finchley Manor Hosp. Lond.

SAVAGE, Deirdre Mary Castlereagh Medical Centre, 220 Knock Road, Belfast BT5 6QD Tel: 028 9079 8308 Fax: 028 9040 3776 — MB BCh BAO Belf. 1986.

SAVAGE, Denis Christopher Lungley (retired) Coddington Vineyard, Ledbury HR8 1JJ Tel: 01531 640668 Fax: 01531 640668 Email: denissavage@aol.com — (Camb. & St. Bart.) MD Camb. 1975, MB 1959, BChir 1958; MRCS Eng. LRCP Lond. 1958; FRCP Lond. 1978, M 1962; DCH RCPS Glas. 1963; FRCPCH 1997. Prev: Cons. Paediat. & Endocrinol. Childr. Hosp. Bristol.

SAVAGE, Dereva Mary Fitzroy House, 4 Whiterock Road, Killinchy, Newtownards BT23 6PR — MB BCh BAO Belf. 1976.

SAVAGE, Douglas Saint Vincent Medical Centre, 77 Thorne Road, Doncaster DN1 2ET Tel: 01302 361318; 16 Avenue Road, Wheatley, Doncaster DN2 4AQ Tel: 01302 322541 — MB ChB Sheff. 1974; MRCGP 1978. GP Doncaster.

SAVAGE, George Crieff Health Centre, King Street, Crieff PH7 3SA Tel: 01764 652456 Fax: 01764 655756 Email: gsavage@crieff1.tayside.scot.nhs.uk; Fernbank, Ferntower Road, Crieff PH7 3DH Tel: 01764 652844 — MB ChB Glas. 1982; BSc Glas. 1979; MRCP (UK) 1986; MRCCIP 1987; FRCP 2000. Med. Off. to Arduredi School, Morrison's Acad.; Clin. Asst. Creft Hosp. Specialty: Gen. Pract.; Diabetes. Special Interest: Diabetics and Cardiol. Socs: Perth and Kinross Immediate Med. Care Soc. Prev: GP Edin.; Regist. & SHO (Med.) South. Gen. Hosp. Glas.; Community Phys. Stratheon.

SAVAGE, Henry (retired) Heathfield, 2 Thorngrove Drive, Wilmslow SK9 1DQ Tel: 01625 524777 — MB ChB Liverp. 1954 (Univ. Liverp.) DObst RCOG 1957; FRCP Lond. 1977, M 1964. Prev: Cons. Phys. Macclesfield Dist. Gen. Hosp.

SAVAGE, James Smallwood Staithe Road Surgery, Staithe Road, Ludham, Great Yarmouth NR29 5AB Tel: 01692 678611 Fax: 01692 678295; The Beeches, Horsefen Road, Ludham, Great Yarmouth NR29 5QG Tel: 01692 678615 — MB BS Lond. 1975 (Lond. Hosp.) DRCOG 1977; MRCGP 1981. Prev: Regist. (Med.) Launceston Gen. Hosp. Tasmania; SHO (O & G) Whipps Cross Hosp. Lond.; Ho. Surg. Lond. Hosp.

SAVAGE, Jane Rosemary Kennedy Way Surgery, Kennedy Way, Yate, Bristol BS37 4AA Tel: 01454 313849 Fax: 01454 329039; Bucklesbury, Engine Common, Yate, Bristol BS37 7PU — MB ChB Bristol 1971; MB ChB (Hons.) Bristol 1971; MRCGP 1977. Prev: SHO Southmead Hosp. Bristol; SHO Ham Green Hosp. Bristol; SHO Bristol Childr. Hosp.

SAVAGE, John (retired) 2 Christ Church Terrace, Thorne Road, Doncaster DN1 2HU Tel: 01302 323888 — MB ChB Glas. 1940; MD Glas. 1947. Prev: Cons. Vis. Dermatol. Roy. Infirm. Doncaster.

SAVAGE, Professor Joseph Maurice Department Child. Health, Royal Victoria Hospital, Belfast BT12 Tel: 01232 894743 Fax: 01232 236455; 10 Kensington Gardens S., Belfast BT5 6NN — MB BCh BAO Belf. 1971; DCH RCPSI 1973; FRCP Lond. 1989; FRCPCH 1994. Cons. Paediat. & Paediat. Nephrol. Roy. Belf. Hosp. Sick Childr.; Sen. Lect. (Child Health) Qu. Univ. Belf.; Prof. Paediat., Qu.s Univ., Belf.; Asst. Head of Med. Sch. (Educat.) and Director Med. Educat. Unit Qu.s Univ. Belf.. Specialty: Paediat.; Nephrol. Socs: Eur.

Soc. Paediat. Nephrol.; Brit. Paediat. Assn.; Renal Assn. Prev: Lect. (Child Health) Manch. Univ.; MRC Research Fell. Inst. Child Health Lond.

SAVAGE, Julie Elizabeth Evington Lodge, Tewkesbury Road, Coombe Hill, Gloucester GL19 4AS — MB BS Lond. 1982. Family Plann. Off. & Sch. Med. Off. Lond.

SAVAGE, Kathryn Jane Tain and Fearn Area Medical Practice, The Health Centre, Scotsburn Road, Tain IV19 1PR Tel: 01862 892759 Fax: 01862 892579 — MB BS Lond. 1992.

SAVAGE, Margaret 5 Savoy Gardens, Ulverston LA12 9LR — MB BChir Camb. 1957 (Camb. & St. Mary's) MB BChir Camb. 1958; BA Camb. 1958; DObst RCOG 1966.

SAVAGE, Margery Jane Peg House Farm, Slad Road, Stroud GL5 1RG — MB BS Lond. 1997.

SAVAGE, Marie Catherine Ysbyty Gwynedd, Bangor LL57 2PW — MB ChB Aberd. 1990; MRCPsych.

SAVAGE, Mark Edmund Regent House Surgery, 21 Regent Road, Chorley PR7 2DH Tel: 01257 264842 Fax: 01257 231387 — MB BS Lond. 1981; DRCOG 1989.

SAVAGE, Mark William Bury General Hospital, Walmersley Road, Bury BL9 6PG Tel: 0161 705 3315 Fax: 0161 705 3332; 36 Aire Drive, Bradshaw, Bolton BL2 3FX Email: savagemw@aol.com — MB ChB Manch. 1986; MD Manch. 1987; MRCP (UK) 1989. Cons. Phys. (Diabetes & Endocrinol.) Bury Gen. Hosp. Specialty: Endocrinol.; Diabetes; Gen. Med. Socs: Endocrine Soc.; Brit. Diabetic Assn. Prev: Sen. Regist. (Gen. Med. Diabetes & Endocrinol.) Liverp.; Research Fell. Univ. Liverp.; Regist. (Med. Endocrinol. & Diabetes) Hope Hosp. Salford.

SAVAGE, Professor Martin Oswald Paediatric Endocrinology Section, Department Endocrinolo, St. Bartholomew's Hospital, West Smithfield, London EC1A 7BE Tel: 020 7601 8468 Fax: 020 7601 8468 Email: m.o.savage@mds.qmw.ac.uk; 55 Doneraile Street, London SW6 6EW Tel: 020 7736 6413 — (St. Bart.) MD Camb. 1980, MA 1968; MB BChir Camb. 1969; MRCP (UK) 1972; FRCP Lond. 1986; FRCPCH 1997. Reader (Paediat Endocrinol.) & Hon. Cons. Paediat. St. Bart. Hosp. Lond. Specialty: Endocrinol. Socs: Roy. Soc. Med. (Mem. Endocrinol. & Paediat. Sects.); Sec. Europ. Soc. Paediat. Endocrinol. Prev: Sen. Regist. (Med.) Hosp. Sick Childr. Gt. Ormond St. Lond.; Clin. Lect. (Growth & Developm.) Inst. Child Health Lond.; Research Fell. (Paediat. Endocrinol.) Hôp. St. Vincent de Paul, Paris.

SAVAGE, Nigel Allen Rivermead Gate Medical Centre, 123 Rectory Lane, Chelmsford CM1 1TR Tel: 01245 348688 Fax: 01245 458800; 158 Wood Street, Chelmsford CM2 8BN — MB ChB Liverp. 1982; MFFP Liverp. 1982. GP Chelmsford. Med. Off. Family Plann. Prev: Asst. Prison Med. Off.

SAVAGE, Nigel John Twin Oaks Medical Centre, Ringwood Road, Bransgore, Christchurch BH23 8AD Tel: 01425 672741 Fax: 01425 674333 — MB BS Lond. 1987 (St. Geo. Hosp. Lond.) MRCGP 1992; T(GP) 1992. Specialty: Gen. Pract.

SAVAGE, Pamela 38 Runnymede Road, Twickenham TW2 7HF — MB BS Lond. 1976; DCH Eng. 1980. Complementary Pract. Middlx. Prev: Clin. Asst. NE Lond. Blood Transfus. Serv. Lond.; Regist. (Community Med.) SE Thames RHA; SHO (Path., Paediat. & O & G) Lewisham Hosp. Lond.

SAVAGE, Mr Paul Thwaites (retired) 7 Akenside Road, London NW3 5RA Tel: 020 7435 5305 — MB BS (Hons.) Lond. 1939 (Lond. Hosp.) MRCS Eng. LRCP Lond. 1939; FRCS Eng. 1947. Prev: Sen. Regist. (Surg.) Lond. Hosp. & W. Middlx. Hosp.

SAVAGE, Mr Peter Edmund Annesley (retired) 2 Lower Shapter Street, Topsham, Exeter EX3 0AT Tel: 01392 874983 Fax: 01392 874983 Email: peasavage@compuserve.com — (St. Mary's) MB BS Lond. 1960; FRCS Eng. 1964; MS Lond. 1972. Consg. Surg. Qu. Mary's Hosp. Sidcup. Prev: Med. Dir. Qu. Mary's Sidcup NHS Trust.

SAVAGE, Philip Edmund Stoke Mandeville Hospital, Department of Radiology, Aylesbury HP21 8AL Tel: 01296 316914 Email: philip.savage@smh.nhs.uk — MB BS Lond. 1976 (St. Bart.) MB BS (Distinc. Surg.) Lond. 1976; MRCS Eng. LRCP Lond. 1976; FRCS Lond. 1981; FRCS Ed. 1981; FRCR 1985. Cons. Radiol. Stoke Mandeville Hosp. Aylesbury. Specialty: Radiol. Special Interest: Diseases of the Breast; Spinal Injuries. Prev: Sen. Regist. & Regist. (Diagn. Radiol.) St. Geo. Hosp. Lond.

SAVAGE, Mr Philip Edward Warren Lodge, Kington Road, Thornbury, Bristol BS9 4RR — MB BS Lond. 1967 (St. Bart.) DObst 1969; FRCOG 1988, M 1975; FRCS Ed. 1976. Cons. (O & G) Southmead & Frenchay HA. Bristol.; Clin. Director, Wom.s Health, N. Bristol NHS Trust. Specialty: Obst. & Gyn. Prev: Cons. Sen. Lect. Dept. Obst. Univ. Bristol; Demonst. in Anat. Bristol Univ.; Sen. Ho. Surg. Bristol United Hosps.

SAVAGE, Philip Michael Velindre Hospital, Velindre Rd, Whitchurch, Cardiff CF14 2TS Tel: 029 2061 5888; 45 Northover Road, Wesbury on Trim, Bristol BS9 3LN Tel: 0117 904 4517 — MB ChB Bristol 1987; BSc Bristol 1982; PhD Lond. 1994; MRCP (UK) 1994; FRCP 2003. Cons. (Med. Oncol) Velindre Hosp Cardiff. Specialty: Oncol. Prev: Sen. Regist. (Med. Oncol.) Hammersmith & Char. Cross Hosps.

SAVAGE, Rachel Ann 14 Mount Pleasant Avenue N., Radipole, Weymouth DT3 5HW — MB BS Lond. 1996.

SAVAGE, Richard Anthony Stockwell Group Practice, 107 Stockwell Road, London SW9 9TJ Tel: 020 7274 3225 Fax: 020 7738 3005 — MB BS Lond. 1970 (St. Thos.) MRCS Eng. LRCP Lond. 1970; DObst RCOG 1972; FRCGP 1994, M 1975; MSc (Gen. Pract.) Lond. 1989; ILTM 2001. GP Lond.; Chairm. S. Lond. Organisation of VTS; Course Organiser Guys & St. Thos. Hosp. VTS. Specialty: Gen. Pract. Prev: RCGP Counc. Rep. S. Lond. Fac.; Hon. Clin. Tutor (Gen. Pract.) Guy's Hosp. Lond.; Vis. Med. Off. Home for Aged Jews Lond.

SAVAGE, Richard Henry 2 Richmond Road, Taunton TA1 1EW Tel: 01823 286251 — (Guy's) BSc Lond. 1968; MRCS Eng. LRCP Lond. 1970; MB BS Lond. 1971; DObst RCOG 1972; MFHom 1978. Clin. Fell. Bristol Homeopathic Hosp. Specialty: Homeop. Med. Special Interest: Holistic Counselling. Prev: GP St. Germans, Cornw.; SHO (Geriat.) Taunton & Som. Hosp. (Trinity Br.); SHO (Paediat.) Taunton & Som. Hosp. (MusGr. Pk. Br.).

SAVAGE, Mr Robert Royal Gwent Hospital, Cardiff Road, Newport NP20 2UB — MB BS Lond. 1976; MS Lond. 1991, MB BS 1976; FRCS Eng. 1981; FRCS Ed. (Orth.) 1989. Cons. Traum. & Orthop. Surg. (hand & upper limb) Roy. Gwent Hosp. Specialty: Orthop. Socs: Fell. BOA; BSSH. Prev: Sen. Regist. (Traum. & Orthop. Surg.) Cardiff Roy. Infirm.

SAVAGE, Robert Boundary House, Shields Road, Stobhill, Morpeth NE61 6LA Tel: 01670 516972; 70 Church Street, Kilwinning KA13 6BD — MB ChB Dundee 1991; FRCA 1996. Specialist Regist. (Anaesth.) Newc. u. Tyne. Specialty: Anaesth. Socs: BMA; Assn. Anaesth.; Intens. Care Soc. Prev: SHO (ImmunoDefic.) King's Cross Hosp. Dundee.

SAVAGE, Ronald Malcolm (retired) 44 Station Road, Cogenhoe, Northampton NN7 1LU — MB ChB Ed. 1956; DObst. RCOG 1962.

SAVAGE, Rosemary Anne Falcon Road Surgery, 47 Falcon Road, Battersea, London SW11 2PH Tel: 020 7228 1619/3399 Fax: 020 7924 3375 — MB BS Lond. 1981 (Char. Cross) MRCS Eng. LRCP Lond. 1981; DRCOG 1983; MRCGP 1985.

SAVAGE, Sandra Jill Dormer Cottage, 28 Deepdene Wood, Dorking RH5 4BQ Tel: 01306 889374 — MB ChB Bristol 1967; DObst RCOG 1971. Specialty: Pharmaceutical Medicine.

SAVAGE, Stephanie Jane — MB BCh BAO Belf. 1995 (Queen's Univ. Belf.) DRCOG Lond. 1997; DCH Dub. 1998; MRCGP 1999. GP Locum Northern Irel.; Doctor of Clin. Serv.s, Action Cancer, MarlBoro. Pk., Belf. Socs: Diplomates Assn. RCOG.

SAVAGE, Suzanne Jane The Surgery, St Andrews Hall, Guildersfield Road, London SW16 5LS Tel: 020 8765 4901; 53 Dalkeith Road, London SE21 8LT Tel: 020 8670 3334 — MB BS Lond. 1973 (St. Thos.) DObst RCOG 1974; FRCGP 1995, M 1979. Assoc. Dean (PostGrad. Gen. Pract. Educ.) Lond.

SAVAGE, Victoria Elizabeth 15 Atherton Lane, Brighouse HD6 3TJ — MB ChB Ed. 1990; MRCPsych.

SAVAGE, Professor Wendy Diane 19 Vincent Terrace, London N1 8HN Tel: 020 7837 7635 Fax: 020 7837 7635 Email: w.savage@qmw.ac.uk — MB BChir Lond. 1960 (Lond. Hosp.) MRCS Eng. LRCP Lond. 1960; FRCOG 1985, M 1971; MSc Public Health 1997; Hon. DSc Greenwich Univ. 2000. Hon. Vis. Prof. Middlx. Univ. Fac. Social Sci. Specialty: Obst. & Gyn. Socs: Elected Mem. Gen. Med. Counc. (1989, 1994, 1999, 2003); Fell. Roy. Soc. Med. (Mem. Forum Matern. & Newborn); BMA (Chairm. Local Div. Islington). Prev: Sen. Lect. (O & G) St Barts. & Roy. Lond. Sch. Med.; Hon. Cons. Roy. Lond. Hosp.; Specialist (Obst. Gyn. & Venereol.) Cook Hosp. Gisborne, NZ.

SAVANI, Alena Charlotta Konstancie Colne House Surgery, 99A Uxbridge Road, Rickmansworth WD3 7DJ Tel: 01923 776295 Fax: 01923 777744; 8 Meadow Way, Rickmansworth WD3 7NQ Tel: 01923 896301 — MRCS Eng. LRCP Lond. 1973 (Lond. Hosp.) Prev: SHO (O & G & Paediat.) & Ho. Phys. Lond. Hosp.

SAVANI, Narendra Yashlal Colne House Surgery, 99A Uxbridge Road, Rickmansworth WD3 7DJ Tel: 01923 776295 Fax: 01923 777744; 8 Meadow Way, Rickmansworth WD3 7NQ Tel: 01923 896301 — MB BS Mysore 1977 (Kasturba Med. Coll.) MRCS Eng. LRCP Lond. 1977; DRCOG 1977. Prev: SHO (Paediat. & Obst. Gyn.) Heatherwood Hosp. Ascot.; Ho. Off. (Surg.) Kent & Canterbury Hosp.; Ho. Phys. Ramsgate Dist. Hosp.

SAVANI, Ramesh Karsandas Manor Top Medical Centre, Ridgeway Road, Sheffield S12 2SS — MB BS Bombay 1963; MRCOG 1969.

SAVANI, U K Manor Top Medical Centre, Rosehearty, Ridgeway Road, Sheffield S12 2SS Tel: 0114 239 8324.

SAVE, Vicki Elaine Department of Histopathology, Level 5 Laboratory Block, Box 235, Addenbrooke's Hospital, Hills Road, Cambridge CB2 2QQ Tel: 01223 216041 Fax: 01223 216980; 8 Siskin Close, Royston SG8 7XX — MB ChB Glas. 1990; DRCPath 1996. Consultant Histopathologist, Addenbrook's Hospital, Cambridge. Specialty: Histopath. Socs: Assn. of Clin. Pathologists. Prev: Lect. & Hon Regist., Tayside Univ. Hosp Trust; Regist., Tayside Univ. Hosp Trust; STTO, Tayside Univ. Hosp Trust.

SAVEGE, Peter Beverley Enfield PCT, Holbrook House, Cockfosters Road, Barnet EN4 0DR Tel: 020 8272 5500 Fax: 020 8272 5700; 1 New House Park, St Albans AL1 1UA Tel: 01727 854870 — (St. Bart.) LMSSA Lond. 1964; DObst RCOG 1966; MSc (Community Med.) Lond. 1989. Head of Healthcare Servs.; Chair, Barnet, Enfield & Haringey Local Research Ethics Comm.; Advise, Enfield PCT & Haringey TPCT. Specialty: Gen. Pract.; Pub. Health Med. Socs: BMA. Prev: Asst. Director Pub. Health, Herts. Health Agency; Med. Dir. Kent FHSA; GP St. Albans.

SAVEGE, Timothy Michael (retired) — MB BS Lond. 1963 (Lond. Hosp.) MRCS Eng. LRCP Lond. 1963; FFA RCS Eng. 1968. Cons. (Anaesth.) Lond. Hosp. Prev: Sen. Lect. & Asst. Dir. Anaesth. Unit Lond. Hosp. Med. Coll.

SAVERIMUTTU, Ritar Kulasegaram (retired) Abercromby Health Centre, Grove Street, Edge Hill, Liverpool L7 7HG Tel: 0151 709 2806; Susanella, Chalfont Road, Allerton, Liverpool L18 9UP Tel: 0151 427 4853 Fax: 0151 427 4853 — MRCS Eng. LRCP Lond. 1964 (Liverp.) LMSSA Lond. 1961. Family Pract. Liverp. AHA (T). Prev: Hosp. Practitioner, Olive Mt. Childr. Hosp. Liverp. AHA (T).

SAVERYMUTTU, Sethna Hugo Broomfield Hospital, Broomfield, Chelmsford CM1 7ET — MB BS Lond. 1976; BSc (Hons.) Lond. 1973, MD 1989, MB BS (Hons.) 1976; MRCP (UK) 1978. Cons. Phys. Broomfield Hosp. Chelms. Specialty: Gen. Med. Socs: Brit. Assn. Liver Dis. Prev: Lect. (Med.) St. Geo. Hosp. Lond.; Regist. Hammersmith Hosp. Wellcome Research Fell.; Ho. Phys. King's Coll. Hosp.

SAVERYMUTTU, Therese Manel Cookley Surgery, 1 Lea Lane, Cookley, Kidderminster DY10 3TA Tel: 01562 850770 — MB BS Lond. 1976; MRCGP 1981; DRCOG 1981.

SAVIDGE, Geoffrey Francis Haemophilia Centre, St. Thomas Hospital, London SE1 7EH Tel: 020 7928 9292 Fax: 020 7401 3125 — MB BChir Camb. 1965; MB BChir Camb. 1966; Med. Lic. Scandinavia 1970; Specialist Accredit. Med. Path. Scandinavia 1977; MD Stockholm 1979; MA Camb. 1979. Dir. Haemophilia Refer. Centre; Sen. Lect. & Hon. Cons. Haemat. St. Thos. Hosp. Med. Sch. Lond.; Prof. Coagulation Med. 1997. Specialty: Haematology. Socs: Amer. Soc. Haemat.; NY Acad. Sc.

SAVIDGE, Malcolm John Gloucestershire Royal Hospital, Great Western Road, Gloucester GL1 3NN — MB BS Lond. 1989 (St Mary's) FFA RCSI 1996. Cons. (Anaesth.) Roy. Gloucester NHS Trust. Specialty: Anaesth. Special Interest: Acupunc.; Chronic Pain; Med. Ethics. Socs: Assn. Anaesth. of GB & Irel.; Pain. Soc and BMA. Prev: Specialist Regist. (Anaesth.) Wessex Sch. Anaesth. Soton.; Regist. (Anaesth.) Soton. Univ. Hosps. Trust; SHO (A & E) & Ho. Off. (Surg. & Urol.) Northwick Pk. Hosp.

SAVILL, Gary Alen Airedale General Hospital, Skipton Road, Steeton, Keighley BD20 6TD Tel: 01535 652511 Email: gary.savill@group.airedale.northy.nhs.uk — MB BCh Wales 1987 (University of Wales College of Medicine) BSc (Biochem.) Cardiff 1984; MRCP (UK) 1992. Cons. Paediat. Airedale Gen. Hosp. Specialty: Paediat. Socs: Roy. Coll. Paediat. & Child Health.

SAVILL, Guy (retired) 50 St Peter Street, Tiverton EX16 6NR Tel: 01884243907 — (Univ. Coll. Hosp.) MRCS Eng. LRCP Lond. 1940; DPhysMed. Eng. 1949. Prev: Cons. Rheum. & Rehabil. Soton. & I. of Wight Gps. Hosps.

SAVILL, Professor John Stewart College of Medicine and Veterinary Medicine, University of Edinburgh Medical School, Teviot Place, Edinburgh EH8 9AG Tel: 0131 650 3181 Fax: 0131 651 1754 — MB ChB (Hons.) Sheff. 1981; BA Oxf. 1978; MRCP (UK) 1984; PhD Lond. 1989; FRCP Lond. 1994; FMedSci 1998; FRCP Ed. 2000. Prof. (Med.) Univ. of Edin.; Head of Centre for Inflammation Research; Director of Univ. of Edin./Med. Specialty: Nephrol. Socs: (Comm. Phys.) Med. Research Soc.; Internat. Soc. Nephrol.; Founder Fell. Acad. of Med. Prev: Wellcome Trust Sen. research fell., Sen. Lect. & Hon. Cons. Renal Unit. Dept. of Med., Roy. Postgrad. Med. Sch. Lond.; Prof. (Med.) Univ. of Nottm.

SAVILL, Peter John 8 Churchward Gardens, Hedge End, Southampton SO30 2XP Tel: 01489 795552 — MB BS Lond. 1994 (Roy. Free Hosp. Sch. of Med. Univ. of Lond.) BSc (1st cl. Hons.) Lond. 1991, MB BS 1994. Specialty: Gen. Pract.

SAVILLE, Gillian Mary Trelake Cottage, Trelake Lane, Treknow, Tintagel PL34 0EW — MB ChB Bristol 1990.

SAVILLE, Mark Anthony Waterlooville Health Centre, Dryden Close, Waterlooville PO7 6AL Tel: 023 9225 7321 — MB BCh Wales 1987; DRCOG 1991; MRCGP 1993.

SAVILLE, Mark Jonathan 10 Moons Close, Ashingdon, Rochford SS4 3HA — MB BS Lond. 1997.

SAVILLE, Sheila Dorothy Devonshire Lodge Health Centre, Abbotsbury Gardens, Eastcote, Pinner Tel: 020 8866 0121 — MB BS Durh. 1966 (Newc.) Socs: BMA. Prev: SHO (O & G) Bensham Hosp. Gateshead; SHO (Paediat.) Qu. Eliz. Hosp. Gateshead.

SAVILLE, Stephanie 30 Oakhill Court, Edge Hill, London SW19 4NR Tel: 020 8946 4621 — MB BCh BAO Dub. 1949; DA Eng. 1953; FFA RCS Eng. 1954. Specialty: Anaesth. Socs: Assn. Anaesth. Prev: Sen. Regist. (Anaesth.) Westm. Hosp.; Regist. St. Bart. Hosp. Lond. & Albany Hosp. New York; Res. Anaesth. Bristol Roy. Infirm.

SAVIN, Garry Edward 8th Floor, The London Clinic, 149 Harley Street, London W1N 2DH Tel: 020 7935 4444 Ext: 3146 — MB BS Lond. 1988 (Roy. Free) DRCOG 1991; MRCGP 1993. Health Screening Doctor & Gen. Practitioner & Clin. Adviser to Nuffield Hosps. Health Screening. Specialty: Gen. Pract.

SAVIN, Helena Mary 11 Bedford Street, Iffley Fields, Oxford OX4 1SU Tel: 01865 245479 — MB BS Lond. 1989 (St. Geo.) DCH RCP Lond. 1991; MRCGP 1995. Specialty: Gen. Pract. Prev: Clin. Asst. (Gen. Pract.).

SAVIN, John Andrew The Royal Infirmary, Lauriston Place, Edinburgh EH3 9YW Tel: 0131 536 1000 Fax: 0131 337 7768; 86 Murrayfield Gardens, Edinburgh EH12 6DQ Tel: 0131 377 7768 Fax: 0131 337 7768 — (Cambridge and ST Thos.) MB BChir Camb. 1959; DIH Soc. Apoth. Lond. 1964; FRCP Lond. 1978, M 1965; FRCP Ed. 1979, M 1973; MA Camb. 1960, BA (1st cl. Hons.) 1956, MD 1978. Specialty: Dermat. Socs: (Ex-Pres.) Dowling Club; Roy. Soc. Med. (Ex-Pres. Sect. Dermat.); (Ex-Pres.) Brit. Assn. Dermat. Prev: Sen. Regist. (Dermat.) St. Thos. Hosp. Lond.; Sen. Regist. & Clin. Tutor St. John's Hosp. Dis. of Skin Lond.; Regist. Skin Dept. St. Geo. Hosp. Lond.

SAVIN, Paul Thomas Grove House Practice, St. Pauls Health Centre, High St, Runcorn WA7 1AB Tel: 01928 566561 Fax: 01928 590212; 54 Malpas Road, Runcorn WA7 4AJ — MB ChB Manch. 1978.

SAVINE, Rachel 26 Calton Gardens, Bath BA2 4QG — BM Soton. 1998.

SAVINE, Richard Laurence Edwin Flat 6, Forest Close, Chislehurst BR7 5QS — MB BS Lond. 1992.

SAVLA, Meenakshi Premchand Highfield Surgery, The Heights, Jupiter Drive, Hemel Hempstead HP2 5NU Tel: 01442 65322 Fax: 01442 256641; 57 Cedar Road, Berkhamsted HP4 2LB Tel: 01442 877682 — MB BS Newc. 1979; MA Oxf. 1974; DRCOG 1982; MRCGP 1983.

SAVLA, Navin Chandra Woodbury Unit, Department of Psychiatry for the Elderly, James Lane, Leytonstone, London E11 1NR Tel: 020 8535 6843 Fax: 020 8535 6829; 80 Overton Drive, Wanstead,

London E11 2NW Tel: 020 8989 0859 — MB BS Osmania 1967 (Gandhi Med. Coll. Hyderabad) DPM Eng. 1971; FRCPsych 1990, M 1972. Cons. Psych. Woodbury Unit; Clin. Dir. Ment. Health Forest Healthcare Trust; Hon. Sen. Lect. (Psychiat.) UCL; Examr., MRCPsy Part II. Specialty: Geriat. Psychiat. Socs: World Psych. Assn.; Overseas Doctors Assn.; Indian Med. Assn. Prev: Clin. Tutor (Psychiat.) Cherry Knowle Hosp. Ryhope; Sen. Regist. St. Crispin's Hosp. Northampton; Regist. St. John's Hosp. Lincoln & Cane Hill Hosp. Coulsdon.

SAVORY, Jane Catherine Northbay House, Balnabodach, Castlebay HS9 5UT — MB BS Lond. 1997.

SAVORY, Jonathan Nigel Church Close Surgery, 3 Church Close, Boston PE21 6NB Tel: 01205 311133 Fax: 01205 358986 — MB BS Lond. 1968; FRCGP 1988, M 1974.

SAVORY, Stephen John The Swineshead Medical Group, Church Lane, Swineshead, Boston PE20 3JA Tel: 01205 820204 Fax: 01205 359050; Jenny Hoolet House, South Road Tetford, Horncastle LN9 6QB, USA — MB BS Lond. 1991 (St. Geo. Hosp. Med. Sch.) MRCGP 1995; DFFP 1995; T(GP) 1995. GP Princip. Specialty: Gen. Pract. Prev: GP Princip., James St. Surg., Boston; GP/Regist. Birchwood Med. Pract. Lincoln; Trainee GP/SHO Lincoln Co. Hosp. VTS.

SAVUNDRA, Joseph Edward Hurst Farm Surgery, Chapel Lane, Milford, Godalming GU8 5HU Tel: 01483 415885 — MB BS Lond. 1980; BA Oxf. 1976; MRCS Eng. LRCP Lond. 1979; DRCOG 1985.

SAVUNDRA, Peter Aloysius Northwick Park Hospital, Watford Rd, Harrow HA1 3UJ Tel: 020 8869 2030; Burners Farm, Guildford Road, Pirbright, Woking GU24 0LW — BM BCh Oxf. 1976; MA; MRCPI 1988; MSc Lond. 1992; DCH RCP Lond. 1993; FRCP Lond. 2002. Cons. Phys. (Audiol.) Northwick Pk. Hosp. Lond.; Lect. Inst. Laryngol. & Otol. Univ. Lond. Specialty: Audiol. Med. Prev: Sen. Regist. (Neuro-Otol.) Nat. Hosp. for Neurol. & Neurosurg. Lond.; Hon. Sen. Regist. Hosp. Sick Childr. Lond.

SAVVA, Nicholas Flat 7, 11 Windsor Road, Poole BH14 8SF Email: nicholas_savva@hotmail.com — MB BS Lond. 1994; BMedSci; FRCS Eng.

SAVVAS, Michael King's College Hospital, Denmark Hill, London SE5 9RS Tel: 020 7737 4000 Email: mike.savvas@kingsch.nhs.uk — MB BS Lond. 1980; MRCOG 1986. Cons. Gynaecol. King's Coll. Hosp. Lond. Specialty: Obst. & Gyn. Socs: Roy. Soc. Med. (Counc. Mem. Sect. Obst. & Gyn.). Prev: Cons. O & G & Hon. Sen. Lect. Univ. Hosp. Lewisham; Sen. Regist. King's Coll. Hosp. Lond.; Regist. (O & G) Westm. Hosp. Lond.

SAVVAS, Savvakis 1 Western Road, Hailsham BN27 3DG — MB BS Lond. 1987; DCH; MRCGP; BSc (2nd cl. Hons.) Physiol. Lond. 1983.

SAVVIDOU, Louiza Kyrou 25B Thurlow Road, London NW3 5PP — MB BS Lond. 1988.

SAVY, Lloyd Edward 251 Petersham Road, Richmond TW10 7DA — MB BS Lond. 1985; BSc Lond. 1981, MB BS 1985; FRCR 1992. Cons. & Hon. Sen. Lect. in (NeuRd.iol.) Roy. Free. Hosp. & Roy. Nat. Throat, Nose & Ear Hosp. Lond. Specialty: Radiol. Prev: Sen. Regist. (Diag. Radiol.) Nat. Hosp. Lond.; Sen. Regist. (Diag. Radiol.) Roy. Lond. Hosp.; Regist. (Diag. Radiol.) Centr. Middlx. Hosp.

SAW LWIN AUNG, Dr 11 The Crescent, Lympsham, Weston Super Mare BS24 0BH — MB BS Med. 1968; MB BS Med. Inst. (II) Mingaladon 1968.

SAW MYINT, Dr 7 The Fletchers, Basildon SS16 5TU — MB BS Rangoon 1969; MB BS Med Inst (I) Rangoon 1969.

SAWANT, Nitin Hemant 1 Eastcroft, Slough SL2 1HT; 1 Eastcroft, Slough SL2 1HT Tel: 01753 643579 Email: sawant@lineone.net — MB BS Lond. 1998 (Imperial Coll.) BSc (Hons.) Lond. 1995. Specialty: Gen. Surg.

SAWAR, Mr Muhammad Omar 18A Le More, Four Oaks Road, Sutton Coldfield B74 2XY — MB BS Punjab 1982; FRCS Ed. 1987.

SAWCER, David 6 Bretts Cottages, Sandy Lane, Framfield, Uckfield TN22 5PX — MB ChB Birm. 1993; BSc Liverp. 1985.

SAWCZENKO, Andrew Bohdan Joseph 64 Mayfield Avenue, Orpington BR6 0AQ Email: a.s@i.am — BM Soton. 1987; MRCP (UK) 1991; MRCPCH 1997. Specialist Regist. Roy. Hosp. for Sick Childr. Bristol. Specialty: Paediat. Prev: Research Fell. Univ. Bristol; SHO (Paediat.) Hosp. for Sick Childr. Gt. Ormond St. Lond., Univ. Hosp. Nottm., Childr. Hosp. Birm. & Roy. Hosp. for Sick Childr. Glas.

SAWCZYN, Paul Gabriel Rosegarth Surgery, Rothwell Mount, Halifax HX1 2XB — MB BS Lond. 1982 (St. Bart.) DRCOG; Dip. Occ. Med.; MRCGP; DCH RCP Lond. 1988. Prev: SHO (Paediat. Nephrol.) Guy's Hosp. Lond.; SHO (Paediat.) Brook Gen., St. Thos. & Guy's Hosps. Lond.

SAWDAYEE-AZAD, Akram 5 Russell Grove, Mill Hill, London NW7 3QU Tel: 020 8959 4521 — MB BS Lond. 1973 (Middlesex Hospital Medical School London) MRCOG 1981. Specialty: Obst. & Gyn.

SAWDY, Robert John 9 Dryden Road, Enfield EN1 2PR Tel: 020 8364 0497 — MB BS Lond. 1988; BSc (Hons.) Experim. Path. Lond. 1985; MRCOG 1994. Research Fell. & Hon. Sen. Regist. Roy. Postgrad. Med. Sch. Hammersmith & Qu. Charlotte's Hosp. Lond. Specialty: Obst. & Gyn. Socs: Roy. Soc. Med. Prev: Lect. & Hon. Regist. (O & G) UMDS Guy's Hosp. Lond.

SAWEIRS, Manar Wilson — MB BS Newc. 1998; MB BS Newc 1998.

SAWEIRS, Walaa Wilson Matta Royal Infirmary of Edinburgh, Department of Renal Medicine, Edinburgh EH16 4SU Tel: 0131 536 1000 — MB ChB (Hons) Ed. 1994 (Edin.) BSc (Med. Sci.Hons.) Ed. 1992; MRCP (UK) 1997. SpR Nephrology/G(1)M. Edin. Roy. Infirm. Prev: SHO (ICU) Qu. Margt. Hosp. Dunfermline; SHO (Nephrol.) Churchill Hosp. Oxf.; Ho. Off. (Med. & Surg.) Roy. Infirm. Edin.

SAWEIRS, Wilson Matta Queen's Hospital, Belvedere Road, Burton-on-Trent DE13 0RB Tel: 01283 566333 Fax: 01283 593009; 18 Hillcrest Avenue, Burton-on-Trent DE15 0TZ Tel: 01283 537785 — (Cairo Univ.) MB ChB Cairo 1962; DM Ain. Shams 1966; MRCPI 1978; MRCP (UK) 1979; MRCS Eng. LRCP Lond. 1980; FRCP Lond. 1993. Cons. Phys. Burton Hosp. NHS Trust. Specialty: Care of the Elderly; Otorhinolaryngol. Socs: BMA; Brit. Geriat. Soc.; Fell. of The Roy. Coll. of Phys. Prev: Sen. Regist. (Gen. Med.) Selly Oak Hosp. Birm.; Sen. Regist. (Geriat. Med.) Birm. DHA (T); Regist. (Gen. Med.) W. Cumbld. Hosp. Whitehaven.

SAWERS, Alistair Henderson Department of Haematology, Worcester Royal Infimary NHS Trust, Ronkswood, Worcester WR5 1HN Tel: 01905 760636 Fax: 01905 760781 — MB ChB (Commend.) Glas. 1974; BSc (Hons.) Glas. 1972; MRCP (UK) 1977; FRCPath 1994, M 1982; FRCP Glas. 1989; FRCP Lond. 1995. Cons. Haemat. Worcs. Roy. Infirm. Specialty: Haematology. Socs: BMA & Brit. Soc. Haemat. Prev: Sen. Regist. (Haemat.) Manch. Roy. Infirm.; Regist. (Haemat.) Stobhill Gen. Hosp. Glas.

SAWERS, James Stewart Allison Cheltenham General Hospital, Cheltenham GL53 7AN — MB ChB Ed. 1973; MRCP (UK) 1975; FRCP Ed. 1990. Cons. Phys. Diabetes & Endocrinol. Specialty: Gen. Med.; Diabetes; Endocrinol. Prev: Cons. Phys. Angus Unit Tayside Health Bd.

SAWERS, Mr Robert Stewart 6 Carpenter Road, Birmingham B15 2JT — MB ChB Ed. 1969; BSc Ed. 1966; DObst 1972; MRCOG 1976; FRCOG 1993. Cons. Birm. Wom. Hosp.; Med. Dir. Fertil. Centre BMI Priory Hosp. Specialty: Obst. & Gyn. Socs: Brit. Fertil. Soc. Prev: Sen. Lect. (O & G) Univ. Birm.; Hon. Cons. Birm. Matern. Hosp. & Birm. & Midl. Hosp. Wom.; Lect. (O & G) Univ. Sheff.

SAWFORD, Raymond William Northville Family Practice, 521 Filton Avenue, Horfield, Bristol BS7 0LS Tel: 0117 969 2164 Fax: 0117 931 5743 — MB ChB Bristol 1971. Specialty: Gen. Pract. Prev: SHO (O & G) Dudley Rd. Hosp. Birm.; Ho. Surg. Qu. Alexandra Hosp. Portsmouth; Ho. Phys. Frenchay Hosp. Bristol.

SAWH, Breehaspaty Falls Road Practice, 181 Falls Road, Belfast BT12 6AF Tel: 028 9032 0547 Fax: 028 9024 9674 — MB BCh BAO Belf. 1962; Cert. JCC Lond. 1977. Socs: BMA; Brit. Med. Acupunct. Soc.

SAWHNEY, Bharat Bhushan Neurology Department, Royal Victoria Hospital, Belfast BT12 6BA — MB BS Panjab 1961 (Med. Coll. Amritsar) MB BS Panjab (India) 1961; DM (Neurol.) All India Inst. Med. Scs. 1972, MD (Gen. Med.) 1965. Cons. (Clin. Neurophysiol.) Roy. Vict. Hosp. Belf. Specialty: Clin. Neurophysiol. Prev: Asst. Prof. (Neurol.) Postgrad. Inst. Med. Educat. Chandigarh, India.

SAWHNEY, Inder Mohan Singh Morriston Hospital, Swansea SA6 6NL Tel: 01792 703851 Email: inder.sawhney@ntlworld.com.

SAWHNEY, Kamal Kumar Wycombe General Hospital, Queen Alexandra Road, High Wycombe HP11 2TT Tel: 01494 426602 Fax: 01494 425007 Email: kamal.sawhney@sbucks.nhs.uk — MB BS Meerut India 1980; DCH; FRCPCH. Paediat. Bucks Hosp. NHS Trust

High Wycombe. Specialty: Paediat. Special Interest: ADhD; Child Developm.; Neurol. Socs: BPA; BACCH.

SAWHNEY, Seema King Edward House, 27/30 King Edward Court, Windsor SL4 1TJ Tel: 01753 621904 Fax: 01753 621907 Email: ssawhney@rhms.co.uk; 40 Tangier Road, Richmond TW10 5DW — MB ChB Manch. 1991; BSc (Hons) Manch. 1988; MRCGP Lond. 1995; AFOM Lond. 2000. p/t Specialist Regist. (Occupat. Med.) RHMS, Windsor. Specialty: Occupat. Health.

SAWICKA, Elzbieta Halina Princess Royal University Hospital, farnborough Colonade, Orpington BR6 8ND Tel: 01689 865877 — MB BChir Camb. 1976 (Camb. & Univ. Coll. Hosp.) MRCP (UK) 1977; MA Camb. 1976, MD 1986; FRCP Lond. 1994. Cons. Phys. (Thoracic & Gen. Med.) Bromley Hosp. NHS Trust. Specialty: Gen. Med. Socs: Fell. Roy. Soc. Med.; Brit. Thorac. Soc. Prev: Sen. Regist. (Thoracic & Gen. Med.) Brompton & King's Coll. Hosps.; Doverdale Fell. & Hon. Regist. (Thoracic Med. & I.C.) Brompton Hosp.; Regist. (Gen. Med.) Univ. Coll. Hosp. & Whittington Hosp.

SAWICKI, Veronica Helena Laverton House, Fairford GL7 4AB Tel: 01265 711180 — MB BS Lond. 1982 (Roy. Free) GP. Specialty: Diabetes.

SAWIRES, Mona Ayad Awad The Willows, 54 North Road, Retford DN22 7XG — MB BCh Ain Shams 1978; DA (UK) 1985. Clin. Asst. (Anaesth.) Bassetlaw Dist. Gen. Hosp. Worksop. Specialty: Anaesth.

SAWITZKY, Christiane 15 Glen Iris Avenue, Canterbury CT2 8HP — State Exam Med Berlin 1993.

SAWLE, Guy Victor Division of Clinical Neurology, Queens Medical Centre, Nottingham NG7 2UH Tel: 0115 970 9792 Fax: 0115 970 9738 — BM BS Nottm. 1981; DM Nottm. 1991, BM BS 1981; MRCP (UK) 1984; FRCP 1998. Reader & Hon. Cons. Neurol. Qu. Med. Centre Nottm. Specialty: Neurol. Prev: Lect. & Sen. Regist. (Neurol.) Inst. Neurol. Roy. Postgrad. Med. Sch. Hammersmith Hosp.; Regist. (Neurol. & Med. Ophth.) St. Thos. Hosp. Lond.; Research Regist. Neurol.) Hammersmith Hosp. Lond.

SAWNEY, Philip Edward DWP Office of The Chief Medical Adviser, Room 638, Adelphi, 1-11 John Adam St., London WC2N 6HT Tel: 020 7962 8838 Fax: 020 7712 2330; 36 Manor Drive, Surbiton KT5 8NF — (Univ. Coll.) BSc (Hons.) Lond. 1978; MB BS (Hons.) 1983; Cert. Family Plann. JCC 1986; DGM RCP Lond. 1986; DRCOG 1986; MRCGP 1987; MBA (Distinc.) Kingston Univ. 1994. Med. Dir. DWP Lond. Specialty: Civil Serv. Socs: Assur. Med. Soc. Prev: GP Barnes; SCMO Richmond, Twickenham & Roehampton HA; GP Tutor Roehampton.

SAWTELL, Ivor James (retired) 100 Boston Place, London NW1 6EX — MB BS Lond. 1968 (Middlx.) Cert. CII 2003; MRCS Eng. LRCP Lond. 1968; MSc Lond. 1974; MFOM RCP Lond. 1980; BA (Hons.) 1998. p/t Med. Adviser; Med. Adviser Health Care Insur. Lond.

SAWYER, Adam Nicholas 1 Stagbury Avenue, Chipstead, Coulsdon CR5 3PA — MB BS Lond. 1981.

SAWYER, Christopher John 64 Taylor Street, Tunbridge Wells TN4 0DX — MB BS Lond. 1996.

SAWYER, Christopher Nicholas 48 Wimpole Street, London W1M 7DG Tel: 020 7935 4357 Fax: 020 7224 0625 Email: 113535.756@compuserve.com; 46a Belsize Square, London NW3 4HN Tel: 020 7431 6924 — MB BS Lond. 1981; MRCP (UK) 1985. Med. Cons. to Elf Oil UK Ltd & Bechtel Inc. & The Thomson Corpn. & Second Opinion UK Ltd. Specialty: Gen. Med.; Occupat. Health. Socs: Fell. Roy. Soc. Med.; Internat. Soc. Nephrol. Prev: Lect. (Nephrol.) Lond. Hosp. Med. Coll.

SAWYER, David Hugh 3 Deanston View, South Callander Road, Doune FK16 6AS Tel: 01786 841731 — MB BS Lond. 1966 (Guy's) MRCS Eng. LRCP Lond. 1966; AFOM RCP Lond. 1982. Med. Adviser Benefits Agency Med. Servs. Socs: BMA; Soc. Occupat. Med. Prev: Sen. Med. Off. Brit. Rail Scotl.; Ho. Surg. Ashford Hosp. Kent; Ho. Phys. WillesBoro. Hosp. Ashford.

SAWYER, James Philip Charles Baytree, Ombersley, Droitwich WR9 0JP — MB ChB Manch. 1989.

SAWYER, Martin Norman Carnau Mawr, Cilcennin, Lampeter SA48 8RG — MB ChB Manch. 1984.

SAWYER, Philip Edward Lawrence Parkbury House, St. Peters Street, St Albans AL1 3HD — MB BS Lond. 1994 (Roy. Free Hosp. Sch. Med.) BSc Lond. 1991; DFFP 1997; DRCOG 1997; MRCGP 1999.

SAWYER, Richard Hayes X-Ray Department, Wythenshawe Hospital, Southmoor Road, Manchester M23 9LT Tel: 0161 946 2105 Fax: 0161 946 2856 Email: richard.sawyer@man.ac.uk — MB Camb. 1983 (St. Thos.) BChir 1982; MRCP (UK) 1986. Cons. Radiol. Wythenshawe Hosp. Manch. Specialty: Radiol.

SAWYER, Richard John Doctor's Mess, West Suffolk Hospital, Bury St Edmunds IP33 2QZ — MB BCh Witwatersrand 1989.

SAWYERR, Afolabi Michael Whipps Cross Hospital, Whipps Cross Road, Leytonstone, London E11 1NR Tel: 020 8535 6414 — MB BCh Wales 1982; BSc Wales 1979; MRCP (UK) 1985; MD Wales 1994; FRCP 1999. Cons. Gastroenterol. Whipps Cross Hosp. Lond. Specialty: Gastroenterol. Prev: Lect. Univ. Edin.; Regist. Roy. Free Hosp. Lond.

SAWYERR, Caroline 20 Cotham Road S., Bristol BS6 5TZ — MB ChB Bristol 1985.

SAXBY, Katharine Maria Ordsall Health Centre, Regent Park Surgery, Belfort Drive, Salford M5 3PP Tel: 0161 872 2021 Fax: 0161 877 3592 — MB ChB Manch. 1993 (Manch. Med. Sch. & Univ. St. And.) DFFP 1996; DRCOG 1996; MRCGP 1997. GP Princip. Ordsal. Specialty: Gen. Pract. Socs: Roy. Coll. Gen. Pract. Prev: GP/Regist. Pendlebury Health Centre Swinton.

SAXBY, Mr Mark Fraser Department of Urology, General Hospital, Newcastle Road, Stoke-on-Trent ST4 6QG Tel: 01782 552167 Fax: 01782 553056 — MB BS Lond. 1983 (St. Mary's) FRCS Eng. 1988; BSc Lond. 1980, MD 1996; FRCS (Urol.) 1996. Cons. Urol. N. Staffs. Hosp. Specialty: Urol. Socs: Fell. Mem. Brit. Assn. Urol. Surgs.; Eur. Assn. of Urol. Prev: Sen. Regist. Rotat. (Urol.) W. Midl.; Research Regist. Wordsley Hosp.; Regist. Rotat. (Surg.) Dudley HA.

SAXBY, Norman Victor Redfern Health Centre, Shadycombe Road, Salcombe TQ8 8DJ; Redfern Health Centre, Salcombe TQ8 8DJ Tel: 0154 884 2284 — MB ChB Sheff. 1965. Prev: Ho. Phys. St. Helen's Hosp. Barnsley; Ho. Surg. Roy. Hosp. Sheff; Med. Off. Virol. Research Dept. Sandwich, Kent.

SAXBY, Mr Peter John Department of Plastic Surgery, Royal Devon & Exeter Hospital, Barrack Road, Exeter EX2; Nadder Farm, Nadderwater, Exeter EX4 2JQ Tel: 01392 430709 — MB ChB Ed. 1978; FRCS Eng. 1983; ChM 1991; FRCS (Plast) 1991. Cons. Plastic Surg. Exeter & N. Devon Hosps. Specialty: Plastic Surg. Socs: B. A. Plastic Surg.s; B. A. Aesthetic Plastic Surg.s; Examr. FRCS Plast. Prev: Sen. Regist. (Plastic Surg.) Char. Cross & Mt. Vernon Hosps.

SAXENA, Dolly Doctors Surgery, 7 Felhurst Crescent, Dagenham RM10 7XT Tel: 020 8592 2323 Fax: 020 8984 8732 — MB BS Agra 1958. Socs: BMA. Prev: JHMO St. Luke's Hosp. Rugby.

SAXENA, Indra Rani Richmond Medical Centre, 15 Upper Accommodation Road, Leeds LS9 8RZ Tel: 0113 248 0948 Fax: 0113 240 9898 — MB BS Lucknow 1971. GP Leeds.

SAXENA, Manoj Krishnan 54 Hill Road, Mitcham CR4 2HQ Tel: 020 8640 8328 — MB BChir Camb. 1994; BSc Lond. 1991.

SAXENA, Rajeev 26 Bader Drive, Heywood OL10 2QS; 26 Bader Drive, Heywood OL10 2QS — MB ChB Sheff. 1994; MB ChB Manch. 1994; MRCP (UK) 1997. Specialist Regist. (Med.) Liverp. Rotat. Specialty: Gen. Med.

SAXENA, Rajiv Narain The Conifers, Coedkernew, Newport NP10 8UD — MB BS Poona 1974.

SAXENA, Rema 26 Bader Drive, Hopwood, Heywood OL10 2QS — MB ChB Manch. 1997.

SAXENA, Sanjeev c/o Dr A. K. Bisaraya, 83B School Lane, Skelmersdale WN8 8PU — MB BS Jiwaji, India 1986.

SAXENA, Satish Chandra Sharrow Lane Surgery, 129 Sharrow Lane, Sheffield S11 8AN Tel: 0114 255 6600 — MB BS Lucknow 1967 (G.S.V.M. Med. Coll. Kanpur) DA Eng. 1971. Clin. Med. Off. Sheff. AHA. Prev: Clin. Asst. (Anaesth.) Roy. Hosp. Chesterfield.

SAXENA, Savita Sharrow Lane Surgery, 129 Sharrow Lane, Sheffield S11 8AN Tel: 0114 255 6600 — MB BS Rajasthan 1974 (S.P. Med. Coll. Bikaner) GP Sheff.; Ho. Off. (Chest Med., Infec. Dis. & Gen. Med.) Lodge Moor Hosp. Sheff. Prev: Ho. Off. (Accid. Surg. & Orthop.) North. Gen. Hosp. Sheff.

SAXENA, Sonia Krishna Dept. of General Practice and Primary Care, 6th Floor, Hunter Wing, St George's Hospital Medical School, Cranmer Terrace, London SW17 0RE — MB BS Lond. 1989 (St Barts Hosp. Med. School) DGM RCP Lond. 1994; MRCGP 1995; MSC Epidemiology 1999. Clin. Research Fell. S. Thames. Specialty: Gen. Pract.

SAXENA, Sunil Anaesthetics Department, St. Mary Hospital, Newport PO30 5TG; 68 Swanmore Road, Ryde PO33 2TG — MB BS Jiwaji 1987; DA (UK). Staff Grade (Anaesth.) St. Mary Hosp. Newport Isle of Wight. Specialty: Anaesth.; Intens. Care. Prev: Staff Grade St. Mary Hosp. Newport; Specialist Regist. St. Geo.'s Hosp. Lond.; Specialist Regist. Wexham Pk. Hosp.

SAXENA, Vinay Raj West Wales General Hospital, Carmarthen SA31 2AF — MB BS Hyderabad 1980; MRCPI 1989. Cons. (Paediat.) Carmanthenshire NHS Trust, W. Wales. Specialty: Paediat.

SAXSENA, Surya Prakash The Surgery, Basement Flat, 160 Gloucester Terrace, London W2 6HR Tel: 020 7706 2504 Fax: 020 7706 3870 — MB BS Vikram 1964; MB BS Vikram 1964.

SAXTON, Hugh Michael (retired) Ash House, Houghton Road, Stockbridge SO20 6LE Tel: 01264 811051 Fax: 01264 811052 — MB BS Lond. 1951 (St Mary's) FRCP Lond. 1972, M 1956; DMRD Eng. 1957; FFR 1960; FRCR 1975. Emerit. Cons. Radiol. Guy's Hosp. Lond. Prev: Cons. Radiol. Cheltenham Gen. Hosp.

SAXTON, John Christopher Robert East Cleveland Hospital, Alford Road, Brotton, Saltburn-by-the-Sea TS12 2FF Tel: 01287 676215 Fax: 01287 678121 — MB ChB Leic. 1987.

SAXTON, Julie Susan 1 East Terrace, Blennerhasset, Carlisle CA4 3QY — MB ChB Liverp. 1990. Trainee GP Carlisle VTS.

SAXTON, Tamsin Nicola 16 Connaught Road, Fleet GU51 3RA — BM Soton. 1995.

SAXTY, Patricia Sexual Health Service, Monkgate Health Centre, 31 Monkgate, York YO31 7WA Tel: 01904 630351 Fax: 01904 642116; 6 Aldwark, York YO1 7BU Tel: 01904 644666 — (Univ. Coll. Hosp.) MB BS Lond. 1964; DPM Leeds 1973; MFFP 1993. Cons. Family Plann. & Sexual Health York Health Servs. NHS Trust; Princip. Investigator/Hon. Research Assoc. Inst. Populat. Studies Univ. Exeter. Specialty: Family Plann. & Reproduc. Health. Socs: York Med. Soc. Prev: Ho. Phys. & Ho. Surg. Cossham Hosp. Bristol; Regist. (Psychiat.) Glenside Hosp. Bristol & Naburn Hosp. York.

SAY, Derek Thomas Kiveton Park Primary Care Centre, Kiveton Park Medical Practice, Chapel Way, Kiveton Park, Sheffield S26 6QU Tel: 01909 770213 Fax: 01909 510108; Peck Mill House, Ladyfield Road, Kiveton Park Station, Sheffield S26 6NR Tel: 01909 773969 — MB ChB Manch. 1980; DCH RCP Lond. 1982; DRCOG 1984; DGM RCP Lond. 1985; MRCGP 1987.

SAYAJI RAO, Mr Kaja Manor Hospital, Walsall WS2 9PS Tel: 01922 721172; 32 Redbourn Road, Bloxwich, Walsall WS3 3XT Tel: 01922 408332 — MB BS Osmania 1971; FRCS Glas. 1984. Regist. (Orthop. & Train.) Gen. Hosp. Walsall W. Midl.; Asst. Surg. (Orthop.) Manor Hosp. Walsall; Clin. Asst. (Orthop. & Trauma) Gen. Hosp. Walsall. Specialty: Trauma & Orthop. Surg. Prev: SHO (Orthop. & A & E) Burton Dist. Hosp.; SHO (Gen. Surg. & Urol.) Pk. Hosp. Manch.

SAYAL, Chandra (retired) Dera, 34 Fresco Drive, Littleover, Derby DE23 4EG Tel: 01332 515261 — MB BS Punjab 1950; MB BS Punjab (India) 1950; DCH Eng. 1952; DPH Lond. 1957; MFCM RCP (UK) 1974; FRSH 1987; MFPHM RCP (UK) 1989. Cons. Pub. Health Med. S. Derbysh.HA. Prev: Princip. Phys. (Social Servs. & Environm. Health) Camden & Islington AHA.

SAYAL, Kapil Sen Childrens Department, Maudsley Hospital, Denmark Hill, London SE5 8AF Tel: 020 7703 6333 — BM Soton. 1992; BSc Soton. 1991; MRCPsych 1996. Specialist Regist. (Child & Adolesc. Psychiat.) Bethlem & Maudsley Hosps. Lond. Specialty: Child & Adolesc. Psychiat. Prev: Regist. (Psychiat.) Bethlem & Maudsley Hosp.; SHO (Psychiat.) Oxf.

SAYANI, Mr Mohammed Irfan Royal Sussex County Hospital, Eastern Road, Brighton BN2 5BE Tel: 01273 696955; 146 Woodland Avenue, Hove BN3 6BN Tel: 01273 550969 — MB BS Osmania 1987; FRCS Glas. 1992; FRCS Ed. 1992. Staff Orthop. Surg. Roy. Sussex Co. Hosp. Brighton. Specialty: Orthop. Prev: Regist. (Orthop.) King Geo. Hosp. Ilford; Regist. (Orthop.) & Pre Fellowship SHO Rotat. N. Middlx. Hosp.

SAYCE, Graham Ewart (retired) Brunswick House, 63 New St., Wem, Shrewsbury SY4 5AE Tel: 01939 232814 — MB BChir Camb. 1951 (St. Thos.) MA, MB BChir Camb. 1951. Prev: Ho. Surg. W. Suff. Gen. Hosp.

SAYED, Gyasuddin Mohamed — MB BS Bombay 1969 (Grant Med. Coll.) DTM & H Liverp. 1973; Cert. Family Plann. JCC 1976; MRCGP 1977. Socs: Pakistan Med. Assn. - Exec. Counc. Mem.; Small Pract.s Assn. Bradford Chairm.; Brit. Med. Assn. Bradford Div., Pres.

SAYED, Mr Mohammed Aqeel 2 Taverners Road, Benskins Croft, Leicester LE4 2HZ — BM BS Nottm. 1992; FRCS Eng. 1996. Sen. SHO (Trauma) Selly Oak Univ. Hosp. Birm. Specialty: Orthop. Prev: SHO (Orthop. Surg.) Northampton Gen. Hosp.; SHO (Orthop. Surg.) Glenfield Hosp., Leicester.

SAYED, Saiqa 23 Norman Avenue, Nuneaton CV11 5NX — MB ChB Leic. 1998; MB ChB Leic 1998.

SAYED, Zakia Department of Family Planning & Women's Health, Central Clinic, Doncaster Gate, Rotherham S65 1DW Tel: 01709 824845; Bait-ul-Sayed, 67 Moorgate Road, Rotherham S60 2TP Tel: 01709 376005 — MB BS Karachi 1962 (Dow Med. Coll.) Accredit Gen. Paediat. with s/i in Community Child; Developm. Paediat. Cert. Leeds 1976; DCH RCPS Glas. 1980; Health RCP Lond. 1993; MFFP RCOG 1993; Spec. Accredit. Community Paediat. JCHMT 1993. Princip. Med. Off. (Child Health) Rotherham Priority Health Trust; Instruc. Family Plann. RCOG & RCGP. Specialty: Community Child Health. Socs: Pakistan Med. Assn. & BMA. Prev: Regist. Childr. Hosp. Karachi, Pakistan; SHO (Gen. Med. & Paediat.) Roy. Hosp. Wolverhampton; Med. Off. Health Dept. Sunderland Co. Boro.

SAYEED, (Abulfatah) Akram, OBE 352 East Park Road, Leicester LE5 5AY; Ramna, 2 Mickleton Drive, Leicester LE5 6GD Tel: 0116 241 6703 Fax: 0116 273 7443 — MB BS Dacca 1958; FRIPHH 1991; FRSH 1991; MRCGP 1992; FRCP Ed. 1994; FRCGP 1998. Sen. Partner & Princip.; Hon. Adviser. MoH Govt. Bangladesh (UK); Mem. Leics. LMC; Elected Mem., GMC, 1999-2004; Pres., Leiceister Med. Soc., 2001-2002. Socs: Fell. Roy. Soc. Med.; Leics. Med. Audit & Advis. Gp.; Fell. BMA. Prev: SHO (Ophth.) Leicester Roy. Infirm.; Rotat. Intern Monmouth Med. Center Long Br., USA; SHO (Ophth.) Dacca Med. Coll. Hosp.

SAYEED, Iqbal Ahmed 11 Pine Street, Woodley, Stockport SK6 1NN — MB BS Dacca 1968; MB BS Dacca Bangladesh 1968; FFA RCSI 1981. Assoc. Specialist (Anaesth.) Stockport NHS Trust. Specialty: Anaesth. Prev: Regist. (Anaesth.) Salop AHA.

SAYEED, Mr Rana Ahmed Papworth Hospital, Papworth Everard, Cambridge CB3 8RE Tel: 01480 830541 Email: r.a.sayeed@bioc.cam.ac.uk — BM BCh Oxf. 1991; MA Camb. 1992; FRCS Eng. 1995; MRCP (UK) 1995. Specialist Regis. In Cardiothoracic Surg. Specialty: Cardiothoracic Surg.

SAYEED-UZ-ZAFAR, Dr 89 Copsewood Way, Northwood HA6 2TX — MB BS Karachi 1964.

SAYEGH, Hanna Fouad Lincoln Road Practice, 63 Lincoln Road, Peterborough PE1 2SF Tel: 01733 565511 Fax: 01733 569230; 228 Fulbridge Road, Peterborough PE4 6SN Tel: 01733 575272 — MB BCh Cairo 1961; DTM & H Liverp. 1968; MRCP Lond. 1969; MRCS Eng. LRCP Lond. 1970. GP P'boro. Prev: Cons. Phys. Ender Clinic Tripoli, Libya; Regist. (Cardiol.) & Sen. Regist. Cardiac Unit Papworth Hosp. Papworth Everard.

SAYER, Antoine Richmond Green Medical Centre, 19 The Green, Richmond TW9 1PX — MB ChB Mid Delta U Tanta Egypt 1972; MB ChB Mid Delta U, Tanta Egypt 1972. Med. Off. Roy. Hosp. Neurodisabil. Lond. Specialty: Rehabil. Med. Socs: Brit. Soc. of Rehabil. Med.; Biol. Engin. Soc.

SAYER, Caroline Susan Adelaide Medical Centre, 111 Adelaide Road, London NW3 3RY Tel: 020 7722 4135 Fax: 020 7586 7558 — MB BS Lond. 1983 (Oxf. & Lond. Hosp.) MA Oxf. 1983; DCH RCP Lond. 1986; DRCOG 1987.

SAYER, Gabriel Leon Flat 5, 21 Pleshey Rd, London N7 0RA — MB BS Lond. 1993. Specialty: Gen. Surg.

SAYER, Jeremy William Princess Alexandra Hospital, Hamstel Road, Harlow CM20 1QX Tel: 01279 827584 Fax: 01279 827577 Email: jeremy.sayer@pah.nhs.uk; 30 Hollywood Way, Woodford Green IG8 9LQ Tel: 020 8527 9479 — MB BS Lond. 1987; BSc Lond. 1984; MRCP (UK) 1991; MD Lond. 2000. Cons. Cardiol., Princess Alexandra Hosp., Harlow; Cons. Cardiol., St Bartholomews Hosp., Lond. Specialty: Cardiol. Socs: Brit. Med. Assn.; Brit. Cardiac Soc.; Brit. Cardiac Interventional Soc. Prev: Regist. (Cardiol.) St. Bart. Hosp. Lond.; Regist. (Gen. Med.) Colchester Gen. Hosp.

SAYER, Joanna Mary Doncaster Royal Infirmary, Armthorpe Road, Doncaster DN2 5LT Tel: 01302 366666 — BM BCh Oxf. 1986; MA Oxf. 1986; FRCP (UK) 1989; M.D 1998. Cons. (Gen Med & Gastroenterol.). Specialty: Gen. Med.; Gastroenterol. Prev: Sen.

Regist. Countess of Chester Hosp. Chester; Sen. Regist. John Radcliffe Hosp. Oxf.

SAYER, John Bernard (retired) Ambleside, Courtlands Way, Goring-by-Sea, Worthing BN12 4BX — BM BCh Oxf. 1956 (Univ. Coll. Hosp.) BSc Oxf. 1955, MA 1956; DObst RCOG 1958. Prev: GP Worthing.

SAYER, Melissa Maria Ruth 90A Fortress Road, London NW5 2HJ — MB BS Lond. 1994.

SAYER, Nicholas John Furness General Hospital, Dalton Lane, Barrow-in-Furness LA14 4 Tel: 01229 870870; The School House, Scales, Ulverston LA12 0PE — MB ChB Birm. 1982 (Bristol University) DRCOG 1985; Cert. Family Plann. JCC 1985; MRCGP 1986; Dip. Palliat. Med. Wales 1993; MSc Palliative Medicine 1999. Cons. Palliat. Med. Furness Gen. Hosp. Cumbria; Med. Dir. St. Mary's Hospice Ulverston. Specialty: Palliat. Med. Prev: GP Dalton-in-Furness Cumbria & Buxton Derbysh.; Trainee GP SW Cumbria VTS.

SAYER, Mr Richard Earl Department of Cardiothoracic Surgery, St Georges Hospital, Blackshaw Road, London SW17 0QT Tel: 020 8725 3287 — MB BS Lond. 1969; FRCS Eng. 1974. Cons. Cardiothoracic Surg. St. Geo. Hosp. Lond. & King Edwd. VII Hosp. Midhurst. Specialty: Cardiothoracic Surg. Prev: Sen. Regist. St. Geo. Hosp. Lond. & Wessex Regional Cardiothoracic Unit Soton.; Fell. (Surg.) Washington Univ. St. Louis, USA.

SAYER, Timothy Robert Goudhurst, Maidenthorne Lane, North Waltham, Basingstoke RG25 2DD Tel: 01256 397781 — MD Aberd. 1992; MB ChB Aberd. 1981; MRCOG 1986. Cons. O & G Basingstoke Dist. Hosp. Specialty: Obst. & Gyn. Prev: Sen. Regist. (O & G) St. Mary's Hosp. Manch.

SAYERS, Brian Edward (retired) 17 Park Avenue, Wolverhampton WV1 4AH Tel: 01902 424748 Email: maltsayers@aol.com — (Oxf.) MA, Oxf. 1952, BM BCh 1955; DObst. RCOG 1958; MRCGP 1968.

SAYERS, Craig Lee 13 The Cresccent, Worsthorne, Burnley BB10 3LX — MB ChB Ed. 1993.

SAYERS, Donald Eric Gordon (retired) Little Croft, La Rue Du Froid Vent, St Saviour, Jersey JE2 7LJ Tel: 01534 726690 — MB BS Lond. 1948 (St. Thos.) MRCS Eng. LRCP Lond. 1948; FRCA 1954. Prev: Cons. Anaesth. Gen. Hosp. Jersey.

SAYERS, Ian Graham Holly House, 17 Murswell Lane, Silverstone, Towcester NN12 8UT — MB BS Lond. 1998; MB BS Lond 1998.

SAYERS, John Denton Welbeck Surgery, 481-491 Mansfield Road, Nottingham NG5 2JJ Tel: 0115 962 0932 — MB ChB Birm. 1974; DTM & H Liverp. 1978; MRCGP 1981; DRCOG 1981. Prev: Med. Miss. (Tear Fund) Thailand; Trainee Nottm. VTS; Project Dir. Dacca Camps & Dacope Thana Health Projects, HEED.

SAYERS, Mr Robert David Department of Surgery, Clinical Sciences Building, Leicester Royal Infirmary, Leicester Tel: 0116 2583142 Email: robert.sayers@uhl-tr.nhs.uk — MB ChB (Hons.) Birm. 1984; FRCS Ed. 1988; FRCS Eng. 1989; MD Leicester 1993. Cons. Vasc. Surg. Leicester Roy. Infirm.; Hon. Sen. Lect. (Surg.) Univ. Leics. Specialty: Gen. Surg. Special Interest: Endovascular Crewysn Repair. Prev: Research Fell. & Lect. (Surg.) Leic. Univ.; Regist. (Gen. Surg.) Leic. Hosp.

SAYERS, Robert David The Surgery, Cornerways, 145 George V Avenue, Worthing BN11 5RZ Tel: 01903 247740/241997 Fax: 01903 242110; 145 George V Avenue, Worthing BN11 5RZ — MB BCh BAO Belf. 1987 (Queen's University of Belfast) MRCGP; DCH RCP Lond. 1992. Specialty: Paediat. Socs: BMA. Prev: Trainee Gp Crawley; SHO (Paediat.) Addenbrookes Hosp. Camb.; Resid. Med. Off. Liverp. Hosp. Sydney, Austral.

SAYERS, Steven James c/o Mr & Mrs I Sayers, 79 Astley Rd, Seaton Delaval, Whitley Bay NE25 0DJ — MB ChB Ed. 1997.

SAYES, Rhys Morgan 3 Fron Heulog, Aberdovey LL35 0HF — MB BS Newc. 1975.

SAYNOR, Annette Marie Noelle 3 Sutherland Avenue, Broadstone BH18 9EB — MB BS Lond. 1977; DRCOG 1980.

SAYNOR, Caroline Elizabeth Harlestone Road Surgery, 117 Harlestone Road, Northampton NN5 7AQ Tel: 01604 751832 Fax: 01604 586065 — MB ChB Birm. 1976. GP N.ampton. Specialty: Gen. Pract.

SAYOUR, Samir 39 Juxon Street, London SE11 6NH — State Exam Med Greifswald 1993.

SAYWELL, James Humphrey (retired) 24 Fernhill Road, Moorhead, Shipley BD18 4SL — MB ChB St. And. 1967; DObst RCOG 1969.

SAYWELL, William Richard, Surg. Cdr. RN Department of Radiology, Yeovil District Hospital, Yeovil BA21 4AT Fax: 01935 707572 — BM BCh Oxf. 1978 (Oxford) MA Oxf. 1979, BM BCh 1978; FRCR 1987. Cons. Radiol. Yeovil Dist. Hosp. Specialty: Radiol. Socs: Brit. Inst. Radiol.; Roy. Soc. Med.; BMA. Prev: Cons. Radiol. RN Hosp. Plymouth; Sen. Lect. NMR Unit. RPMS Hammersmith; Sen. Regist. (Radiol.) Soton. Gen. Hosp.

SAYWOOD, Andrew Mason, Surg. Lt.-Cdr. RN 7 The Pastures, Duffield, Belper DE56 4EX Tel: 01332 840202 Fax: 01332 840101 Email: dr@saywood.f9.co.uk — MRCS Eng. LRCP Lond. 1976; DA (UK) 1976; MRCGP 1982; DFFP 1982; T(GP) 1991. Indep. Med. Cons.; Proprietor & Princip. Westminster Med. Ltd; Examg. Med. Practitioner, Benefits Agency; GP Locum; Tutor Medical Ethics and Law, Birmingham University; Forensic Physician for Medical Advice to Lawyers. Specialty: Gen. Pract.; Medico Legal. Socs: BMA; Expert Witness (UK Register) Lond.; Birm. Medico-Legal Soc. Prev: Cons. Forens. Phys. for Med. Advice to Lawyers; Princip. Police Surg.; Princip. GP Derbysh.

SAYYAH-SINA, Kamran The New Surgery, 387 Queens Road, London SE14 5JN Tel: 020 7635 2170 — MB ChB Birm. 1986. GP Princip. Prev: Trainee GP Kent; SHO (Gen. Med., Paediat. & O & G) William Harvey Hosp. Ashford.

SBANO, Hala 35 Dorset Drive, Edgware HA8 7NT Tel: 020 8951 3349 Fax: 020 8952 1136 — MB BS Lond. 1996 (Charing Cross and Westminster) BSc (Biochem. & Med. Sci.) Lond. 1994; MRCP Part 1 1999. SHO Rotat. Med. Harefield/Hillingdon. Specialty: Gen. Med. Socs: BMA; Med. Protec. Soc.; Med. Sickness Soc. Prev: Ho. Off. (Med.) Chelsea & Westminster Hosp. Lond.; Ho. Off. (Surg.) Bassetlaw Dist. Gen. Hosp. Lond.; SHO Rotat. (Med.) Chelsea & Westminster Hosp.

SCADDEN, John Edward Cartref Care Home, 10 East Back, Pembroke SA71 4HL — MB ChB Cape Town 1992.

SCADDING, Frank Haddow Coryton, 55 St Mary's Avenue, Northwood HA6 3AY Tel: 01923 821433 — MRCS Eng. LRCP Lond. 1937 (Middlx.) MD Lond. 1939, MB BS (Hnrs.) 1937; FRCP Lond. 1955, M 1939. Hon. Cons. Phys. Middlx Hosp. & Brompton Hosp. Lond.; Emerit. Cons. Phys. King Edwd. VII Hosp. Midhurst. Specialty: Respirat. Med. Socs: Brit. Thorac. Assn. & Med. Soc. Lond. Prev: Cons. Phys. Hounslow Hosp.; Hon. Cons. Chest Dis. to the Army; 1st. Asst. Brompton Hosp.

SCADDING, Glenis Kathleen Royal, National Throat, Nose & Ear Hospital Trust, Grays Inn Road, London WC1X 8DA Tel: 020 7915 1674 Fax: 020 7915 1674 Email: g.scadding@ucl.ac.uk; 143 Chevening Road, London NW6 6DZ — MB BChir Camb. 1973; MA Camb. 1973; MRCP UK 1975; MD Camb 1984; FRCP Lond. 1995. Cons. Phys. (Rhinol., Immunol. & Allergy) Nat. Throat, Nose & Ear Hosp. Lond.; Hon. Sen. Lect. (Immunol.) Univ. Coll. & Middlx. Hosp. Med. Sch. Lond.; Hon. Sen. Lect. (Clin. Immunol.) Roy. Free Hosp. Lond. Specialty: Allergy. Socs: Brit. Soc. Allergy & Clin. Immunol. (Chair ENT s/i Gp.); Assoc. Mem. RCPath; Roy. Soc. Med. (Ex-Pres. Sect. Immunol.). Prev: Sen. Regist. (Clin. Immunol.) Middlx. Hosp. Lond.; SHO Med. Unit Brompton Hosp. Lond.; Research Fell. Roy. Free Hosp. Lond.

SCADDING, John William The National Hospital for Neurology and Neurosurgery, Queen Square, London WC1N 3BG Tel: 020 7837 3611 — MB BS Lond. 1972; MD Lond. 1982, BSc (Anat.) 1969; FRCP Lond. 1988, M 1974. Neurol. Nat. Hosp. for Neurol. & Neurosurg. & Whittington Hosp. Lond.; Hon. Sen. Lect. Inst. Neurol. Lond.; Civil. Cons. Adviser Roy. Navy & Roy. Air Force; Hon. Cons. Neurol. Roy. Soc. of Musicians; Assoc. Dean, The Roy. Soc. of Med. Specialty: Neurol. Prev: Regist. Nat. Hosps. for Nerv. Dis. Lond.; Research Asst. (Neurol. Scs.) Roy. Free Hosp. & Dept. Anat. Univ. Coll. Lond.

SCADE, Thomas Paterson Riverview Medical Centre, 6/8 George St., Johnstone PA5 8SL Tel: 01505 20151; 38 Hillside, Houston, Johnstone PA6 7NT — MB ChB Glas. 1973; BSc (Hons. Path.) Glas. 1971; MRCP (UK) 1976; FRCP Glas. 1990.

SCAFFARDI, Roberto Agostino East Bridgford Medical Centre, 2 Butt Lane, East Bridgford, Nottingham NG13 8NY Tel: 01949 20216 Fax: 01949 21283 — BM BS Nottm. 1984; MRCGP 1988.

SCAGLIONI, Francesco Guiseppe Greenland Surgery, Greenland, Millbrook, Torpoint PL10 1DE Tel: 01752 822576 Fax: 01752 823155; (branch Surgery), York Road, Torpoint PL11 2LG Tel: 01752 812152 — MB BS Lond. 1985.

SCAHILL, Shaun James Hawkhill Medical Centre, Hawkhill, Dundee DD1 5LA Tel: 01382 669589 Fax: 01382 645526 — MB ChB Glas. 1988; BSc (Hons) Genetics Leeds 1977; PhD Ed. 1981.

SCAIFE, Bryan 3 Woodside, Stockton-on-Tees TS17 0ST — MB BS Lond. 1956 (King's Coll. Hosp.) MRCS Eng. LRCP Lond. 1956; DObst RCOG 1958; DCH RCPS Glas. 1976. Socs: BMA. Prev: Ho. Surg. & Ho. Phys. City Hosp. York; SHO (Paediat.) Co. Hosp. York.

SCALES, Alistair Hugh Westbourne Medical Centre, Milburn Road, Bournemouth BH4 9HJ Tel: 01202 752550 Fax: 01202 769700; 1 Powell Road, Parkstone, Poole BH14 8SG Tel: 01202 743758 — MB BS Lond. 1975; BSc Lond. 1972; MRCP (UK) 1978.

SCALES, Elizabeth Anna Newbyres Medical Group, Gorebridge Health Centre, 15 Hunterfield Road, Gorebridge EH23 4TP — MB ChB Dundee 1983; MRCGP 1987. Prev: Trainee GP Stewarton; Trainee GP Ayrsh. & Arran HB Train. Scheme.

SCALES, John Philip 63 Montgomery Crescent, Dunblane FK15 9FB — MB ChB Manch. 1993; DRCOG 1995; MRCGP 1998.

SCALES, Michael Frank Wellington House Surgery, Henrietta Street, Batley WF17 5DN Tel: 01924 470333 Fax: 01924 420981; 1 Park Avenue, Rutland Road, Upper Batley, Batley WF17 0LU — MB ChB Leeds 1983; MB ChB Leeds. 1983.

SCALLAN, Michael John Herbert Royal Brompton Hospital, Sydney St., London SW3 6NP Tel: 020 7352 8121 Fax: 020 7351 8524 — MB ChB Cape Town 1967; FFA (SA) 1973; FRCA 1983. Cons. Anaesth. Roy. Brompton Hosp. Lond. Specialty: Anaesth.

SCALLY, Bernard Gabriel (retired) 41 Andersonstown Road, Belfast BT11 9AF Tel: 02890 613463 — LRCPI & LM, LRSCI & LM 1948; LRCPI & LM, LRCSI & LM 1948; DPM RCPSI 1958; PhD Dub. 1966; FRCPsych 1981, M 1971; FRCPI 1980, M 1978. Hon. Cons. Muckamore Abbey Hosp. Prev: Mem. Ment. Health Commiss.

SCALLY, Catherine Mary 30 Barmouth Road, Castlerock, Coleraine BT51 4XG — MB BCh BAO Belf. 1982; MB BCh Belf. 1982; FRCS Ed. 1987.

SCALLY, John Department Medical Imaging, Leighton Hospital, Crewe CW14QJ Tel: 01270 255141; 3 The Acreage, Bunbury, Tarporley CW6 9NQ — MB ChB Liverp. 1980; DMRD Liverp. 1985; FRCR 1986. Cons. Radiol. Leighton Hosp. Crewe. Specialty: Radiol. Prev: Sen. Regist. Mersey RHA.

SCALLY, Marie Josephine 9 Brerton Crescent, Belfast BT8 6QD — MB BCh BAO Belf. 1973.

SCAMBLER, Peter James 29 Southfield Park, Harrow HA2 6HF Tel: 020 8248 9098 Fax: 020 7831 0488 — MB ChB Manch. 1982; BSc (1st cl. Hons. Med. Biochem.) Manch. 1979, MD 1986; MRCPath 1990; FRCPath 1998; FMedSci 2000. Prof. Molecular Med. Inst. Child Health Lond. Specialty: Genetics. Socs: Clin. Genetics Soc.; Amer. Soc. Human Genetics; Brit. Developm. Biol. Soc. Prev: Sen. Lect. (Med. Molecular Genetics) St. Mary's Hosp. Lond.

SCAMBLER, Sarah Miriam Lane End Medical Group, 25 Edgwarebury Lane, Edgware HA8 8LJ Tel: 020 8958 4233 Fax: 020 8905 4657; 29 Southfield Park, Harrow HA2 6HF — MB ChB Manch. 1982; MB ChB (Hons.) Manch. 1982; MRCGP 1985. Prev: GP Brent & Harrow FPC; Trainee GP Northwick Pk. VTS.

SCAMMELL, Alastair Michael The County Hospital, Greetwell Road, Lincoln LN2 5QY — MB BS Lond. 1977 (St. Thomas') FRCPCH; MRCP (UK) 1981. Cons. Paediat. Co. Hosp. Lincoln. Specialty: Paediat.

SCAMMELL, Brigitte Elfriede Department of Orthopaedics & Accident Surgery, University Hospital, Queen's Medical Centre, Nottingham NG7 2UH Email: b.scammell@nottingham.ac.uk — MB ChB Birm. 1982; FRCS Eng. 1987; FRCS Ed. 1987; FRCS (Orth.) 1994; DM Soton. 1995. Sen. Lect. & Hon. Cons. Orthop. Qu. Med. Centre & City Hosp. Nottm. Specialty: Trauma & Orthop. Surg.

SCANE, Andrew Christopher Department of Medicine, North Tees General Hospital, Hardwick, Stockton-on-Tees TS19 8PE Tel: 01642 617617 Fax: 01642 624922; 15 Ashville Avenue, Eaglescliffe, Stockton-on-Tees TS16 9AU Tel: 01642 659645 — BM BS Nottm. 1983 (Univ. Nottm. Med. Sch.) BMedSci Nottm. 1981; MRCP (UK) 1988; FRCP Ed 1998. Cons. Phys. (Geriat. Med.) N. Tees Gen. Hosp. Stockton-on-Tees. Specialty: Care of the Elderly. Prev: Clin. Fell. (Geriat. Med.) W.mead Hosp. Sydney, Austral.; Sen. Regist. (Geriat. Med.) North. & Yorks. RHA; Research Train. Fell. (Geriat.) Univ. Newc. u. Tyne.

SCANLAN, Christopher Mark Eversley, Devons Rd, Torquay TQ1 3PR Tel: 07970 806143 Email: cscanlan@doctors.org.uk — MB BCh Wales 1997; BSc (Hons) Wales 1994. SHO (Anaesth.) Nevue Hall Hosp. Abergavenny. Specialty: Anaesth.

SCANLAN, Judith 19 Eastfields Grove, Sughall, Chester CH1 6DA — BM Soton. 1992.

SCANLAN, Pascal Henry Taybank Medical Centre, 10 Robertson Street, Dundee DD4 6EL Tel: 01382 461588 Fax: 01382 452121 — MB BCh BAO NUI 1987.

SCANLON, Francesca Louise Child & Family Psychiatry, The Brow, Burgess Hill, Horsham — MB ChB Aberd. 1984. Assoc. Specialist (Child Psychiat.). Specialty: Child & Adolesc. Psychiat. Socs: BMA. Prev: Clin. Asst. Child & Family Psychiat.); Health Worker RePub. do Pequeno, Vendedor.; Regist. (Psychiat.) SW Thames.

SCANLON, Jacqueline Mary 96 Longmead Avenue, Bishopston, Bristol B57 8EF — MB ChB Leeds 1989. Specialist Regist. (O & G) Southmead Hosp. Bristol. Specialty: Obst. & Gyn. Prev: Regist. (O & G) Glos. Roy. Hosp.

SCANLON, John Edmond Milnes Department of Paediatrics, Worcester Royal Hospital, Charles Hastings Way, Worcester WR5 1DD Tel: 01905 760647 Fax: 01905 760588 Email: John.Scanlon@worcsacute.wmids.nhs.uk; 150 Battenhall Road, Worcester WR5 2BT — MB BS Lond. 1977 (The Lond. Hosp. Med. Sch.) MRCP (UK) 1980; DCH RCP Lond. 1983; FRCPCH 1996. Cons. Paediat. Worcs. Ac. Hosp. NHS Trust; Clin. Director Worcs. Ac. Hosp. NHS Trust; Hon. Sen. Lect., Univ. of Birm. Specialty: Paediat. Special Interest: Diabetes in Childr. Prev: Sen. Regist. (Paediat.) Wessex RHA; Regist. Childr.'s Hosp. Birm.

SCANLON, John Gerard Blackbrook Surgery, Lisieux Way, Taunton TA1 2LB Tel: 01823 259444 Fax: 01823 322715; The Cottage, Goosenford, Cheddon Fitzapaine, Taunton TA2 8LH Tel: 01823 412796 — MB BCh BAO NUI 1979; DCH Eng. 1981; MRCGP 1987. Prev: Regist. (Paediat.) Whitechapel Hosp. Lond.; Regist. (Paediat.) Som. HA; SHO (Paediat.) King's Coll. & Univ. Coll. Hosp. Lond.

SCANLON, John Joseph Oakwood House, St Mary Hospital, Kettering NN15 7PW Tel: 01536 493131 — MB BCh BAO NUI 1983; MRCPsych 1990. Cons. Psychiat. & Clin. Dir. (Adult Ment. Illness) N.ants. Specialty: Gen. Psychiat.

SCANLON, Professor Maurice Francis Department of Medicine, University of Wales College of Medicine, Heath Park, Cardiff CF14 4XN Tel: 029 2074 2182 Fax: 029 2074 4671 Email: scanlonmf@cf.ac.uk; 117 Pencisely Road, Llandaff, Cardiff CF5 1DL Tel: 029 2021 2651 Fax: 029 2074 4671 Email: scanlonmf@cf.ac.uk — MB BS Newc. 1973; MRCP (UK) 1975; BSc Newc. 1970, MD 1981; FRCP Lond. 1986. Prof. Endocrinol. & Cons. Phys. Univ. Wales Cardiff; Dir. of R&D Cardiff & Vale NHS Trust. Specialty: Endocrinol.; Gen. Med. Socs: Endocrine Soc. & Europ. Neuroendocrine Assn.; Assn. of Physicians (UK). Prev: Reader (Med.) & Cons. Phys. Univ. Wales Cardiff; Harkness Fell. Commonw. Fund of New York 1979-81.

SCANLON, Peter Henry 4 Haywards Road, Charlton Kings, Cheltenham GL52 6RH — MB BS Lond. 1977; MRCP (UK) 1980; DCH 1981; DRCOG 1983; DO RCS Eng. 1986; MCOphth 1988.

SCANLON, Thomas John Paul East Sussex, Brighton and Hove Health Authority, 36-38 Friars Walk, Lewes BN7 2PB; 1 Station Road, Horsham RH13 5EZ — MB ChB Aberd. 1984; DRCOG 1988; DCH RCP Lond. 1988; MRCGP 1989; MSc Lond. 1993; MFPHM 1996. Cons., Pub. health Med., E. Sussex, Brighton & Hone Health Auth..; Hon. Research Fell. Inst. Of Child Health. Lond.; Non-Princip. GP Horsham. Specialty: Pub. Health Med. Socs: BMA; Assn. PH. Prev: Regist. (Pub. Health Med.) SW Thames RHA; MSc Stud. Lond. Sch. Hyg. & Trop. Med.; Health Worker Repub. Do Pequeno Vendedor, Brazil.

SCANTLEBURY, Barbara Alexandra Surgery, 2 Wellington Avenue, Aldershot GU11 1SD Tel: 01252 332210 Fax: 01252 312490 — MB ChB Dundee 1974. Specialty: Family Plann. & Reproduc. Health.

SCARAVILLI, Professor Francesco Department of Neuropathology, Institute of Neurology, Queen Square, London WC1N 3BG Tel: 020 7837 3611 Fax: 020 7916 9546 — MD

Padua 1964; PhD Lond. 1978; FRCPath 1990, M 1985. Prof. Neuropath. & Hon. Cons. Inst. Neurol. Lond. Specialty: Neuropath. Socs: Brit. & French Neuropath. Soc.; Amer. Neuropath. Soc. Prev: Reader & Sen. Lect. (Neuropath.) Inst. Neurol. Lond.

SCARAVILLI, Nicoletta 4 Carver Road, London SE24 9LT — MB BS Lond. 1998; MB BS Lond 1998.

SCARBOROUGH, Helen — MB ChB Birm. 1996. SpR (Renal & GIM) Manch. N. W. Deanery. Specialty: Gen. Med.; Renal & General Internal Medicine.

SCARBOROUGH, Mark Andrew Falsgrave Surgery, 33 Falsgrave Road, Scarborough YO12 5EB Tel: 01723 360835 Fax: 01723 503220 — MB ChB Manch. 1983; MRCGP 1987.

SCARBOROUGH, Matthew Department of Physiology, Queen Mary & Westfield College, Mile End Road, London E1 4NS Tel: 020 7982 6379 — MB BCh BAO Belf. 1990; BSc Belf. 1988; MB BCh Belf. 1990. Clin. Lect. Qu. Mary & Westfield Coll. Lond.

SCARBOROUGH, Nigel Paul Barwell Medical Centre, 39 Jersey Way, Barwell, Leicester LE9 8HR Tel: 01445 842981 Fax: 01445 850065; Brungerley, 122 Leicester Road, Hinckley LE10 1LU Tel: 01455 618739 — MB ChB Manch. 1981; DRCOG 1983; FRCGP 1996, M 1985; Cert. Family Plann. JCC 1985. GP Princip. Barwell Leics.; Trainer (Gen. Pract.) & Course Organiser Leicester VTS; Clin. Teach. (Gen. Pract.) Univ. Leicester; Clin. Asst., Ophth., Hinckley & Dist. Hosp,. Specialty: Gen. Pract. Socs: BMA; Mem. of Fac. Bd., Leicester Fac. RCGP. Prev: Clin. Asst. (Ophth.) Hinckley & Dist. Hosp.; Med. Off. (Minor Surg.) Hinckley & Dist. Hosp.; Trainee GP Blackburn, Hyndburn & Ribble Valley HA VTS.

SCARBOROUGH, Sarah Ann Barbara Falsgrave Surgery, 33 Falsgrave Road, Scarborough YO12 5EB — MB ChB Manch. 1983. Gen. Pract. ScarBoro.. Specialty: Gen. Pract.

SCARFE, David Robert Marston Medical Centre, 24 Cherwell Drive, Headington, Oxford OX3 0LY Tel: 01865 761234 Fax: 01865 74406; 64 Picklers Hill, Abingdon, Oxford OX14 2BB Tel: 01235 201991 Fax: 01865 744066 — MB BS Lond. 1984; BSc Lond. 1981; DRCOG 1986; MRCGP 1988. Tutor (Pub. Health & Primary Care) Univ. Oxf.

SCARFE, Stephen Andrew Orchard 2000 Medical Centre, 480 Hall Road, Hull HU6 9BS Tel: 01482 854552 Fax: 01482 859900 — MB ChB Leeds 1978. Socs: Hull Med. Soc.

SCARFFE, Professor John Howard The Wellcome Trust, 183 Euston Road, London NW1 2BE Tel: 020 7611 8888 Fax: 020 7611 8545; Four Winds, Cinder Lane, Thelwall, Warrington WA4 3JL Tel: 01925 263549 Email: hscarffe@compuserve.com — (St. Bart.) MB BS Lond. 1970; MRCS Eng. LRCP Lond. 1970; MRCP (UK) 1973; MD Lond. 1980; FRCP Lond. 1986. Head Program.Career Schemes * Clin. Iniatives. Specialty: Oncol. Socs: BMA. Prev: Prof Reader, Sen. Lect. & Lect. (Med. Oncol.) Univ. Manch.

SCARGILL, Margaret Anne Ashville Medical Centre, 430 Doncaster Road, Barnsley S70 3RJ Tel: 01226 282280 Fax: 01226 216002 — MB ChB Leeds 1992 (St. Bart. & Leeds) BSc (Hons.) CNAA 1985; MPhil Sheff. 1989; MRCGP 1996. GP. Specialty: Gen. Pract. Socs: Med. Defence Union. Prev: SHO Barnsley VTS.

SCARISBRICK, Christopher David Queen Street Surgery, 9-11 Queen Street, Whittlesey, Peterborough PE7 1AY Tel: 01733 568569 Fax: 01733 892419; 9 Queen Street, Whittlesey, Peterborough PE7 1AY Tel: 01733 204611 Fax: 01733 208926 — MB BChir Camb. 1974; MA, MB Camb. 1974, BChir 1973; FRCGP 1993, M 1977. Vice Chairm. Cambs LMC.

SCARISBRICK, Douglas Arthur Spin Jenny, Main St., Norton Disney, Lincoln LN6 9JU Tel: 01522 788773 Fax: 01522 788773 — (Char. Cross) MB BS Lond. 1959; DIH Soc. Apoth. Lond. 1976; FFOM RCP Lond. 1985, MFOM 1978. Occupat. Phys. Specialty: Occupat. Health. Socs: Soc. Occupat. Med.; Fell.Roy.Soc.Med. Prev: Princip. Med. Off. Brit. Coal Corp.; Cons. Occupat. Med. Leics. HA; Sen. Employm. Med. Advis. Health & Safety Exec.

SCARISBRICK, Genevieve 63 Croslands Park, Barrow-in-Furness LA13 9LB Tel: 01229 30142 — MB ChB Manch. 1964; DTM & H (Milne Medal Trop. Med.) Liverp. 1965; DObst RCOG 1966; MRCGP 1972; DMRD Eng. 1975; FRCR 1977. Prof of Radiol. Sch. of Med. Sci.s UST Private Mailbag Kumasi Ghana. Specialty: Radiol. Prev: Cons. Radiologist, Furness Gen. Hosp., Barrow in Furness, Cumbria; Sen. Regist. (Radiol.) Withington Hosp. Manch.; GP Preston.

SCARISBRICK, Julia Jane St John's Hospital, St Thomas's Hospital, Lambeth Palace Road, Westminster, London SE1 7EH Tel: 020 7928 9292; 59 Klea Avenue, Clapham, London SW4 9HY — MB ChB Birm. 1994; ChB Birm. 1994; MRCP UK 1997. Research Regist. St Johns Inst. Dermat. Specialty: Dermat. Prev: SHO Rotat. (Gen. Med.) Roy. Berks. Hosp.

SCARISBRICK, Peter Hugh Princes Park Health Centre, Wartling Road, Eastbourne BN22 7PF Tel: 01323 744644 Fax: 01323 736094 — MB BS Lond. 1974 (Middlx.) DRCOG 1977; MRCGP 1978; DCH Eng. 1978. Prev: SHO (O & G) St. Helier Hosp. Carshalton; SHO (A & E) St. Helier Hosp. Carshalton; SHO (Paediat.) Qu. Mary's Hosp. Childr. Carshalton.

SCARISBRICK, Sally Ann (retired) London Road Surgery, 501 London Road, Thornton Heath CR7 6AR Tel: 020 8684 1172 Fax: 020 8665 5011; Chimneys, 130 Woodcote Valley Road, Purley CR8 3BF Tel: 020 8668 9541 — MB BS Lond. 1967 (Roy. Free)

SCARLAND, Michael Graham 24 Mather Avenue, Mossley Hill, Liverpool L18 5HS — MB ChB Leeds 1984.

SCARLE, Trevor John Brandon HMP Cardiff, Knox Road, Cardiff CF24 0UG Tel: 029 2049 1212 — MB BS Lond. 1972. Med. Off. Dept. Prison. Med. Servs. Cardiff. Prev: GP Gravesend/.

SCARLETT, Amanda Jane Newton Place Surgery, Newton Road, Faversham ME13; Oak Lodge, 161 The St, Boughton, Faversham ME13 9BH Tel: 01227 751246 — MB ChB Bristol 1988; DRCOG 1991; MRCGP 1992. Gen. Practioner, Faversham, Kent. Prev: Trainee GP S.sea VTS; SHO (Paediat. & Obst.) St. Mary's Hosp. Portsmouth.

SCARLETT, Clare Elizabeth 7 Jesmond Vale Terrace, Heaton, Newcastle upon Tyne NE6 5JT — MB BS Newc. 1994 (Newcastle upon Tyne) MA Centab 1979.

SCARLETT, James Frederick (retired) Stoneycroft, Field Broughton, Grange-over-Sands LA11 6HW — MB ChB Leeds 1949; DObst RCOG 1954; MRCGP 1977. Prev: GP Leeds.

SCARLETT, Nigel John David 16 North Lodge Close, Westleigh Avenue, Putney, London SW15 6QZ Tel: 020 8788 6657 Fax: 020 8788 6657 Email: nigel@scarlnett.demon.co.uk; Oak Tree Cottage, Burney Road, Westhumble, Dorking RH5 6AX Tel: 01306 883139 — MB BS Lond. 1988 (Char. Cross & Westm.) MA Camb. 1976; MRCGP 1996.

SCARLETT, Sheila Mary (retired) Stoneycroft, Field Broughton, Grange-over-Sands LA11 6HW Tel: 01395 36586 — MRCS Eng. LRCP Lond. 1953 (Leeds) SCMON. Yorks. (Harrogate) HA. Prev: Sen. MO N.Yorks (Harrogate) HA.

SCARPELLO, John Hugh Department of Diabetes and Endocrinology, City General Hospital, Stoke-on-Trent ST4 6QG Tel: 01782 553425 Fax: 01782 553427 — MB BCh Wales 1971; MRCP (UK) 1974; MD Wales 1978; FRCP Lond. 1989. Cons. Phys. City Gen. Hosp. Stoke-on-Trent; Sen. Lect. (Postgrad. Med.) Univ. Keele. Specialty: Gen. Med.; Diabetes; Endocrinol. Socs: Med. Scientif. Sect. Diabetes UK; Brit. Assn. of Hosp. Managers; Assn. of Brit. Clin. Diabetologists. Prev: Sen. Regist. (Med.) Roy. Hallamsh. Hosp. Sheff.; Postdoctoral Research Fell. Div. Endocrinol. & Metab. Univ. Michigan, Ann Arbor USA; Ho. Phys. Univ. Hosp. Wales. Cardiff.

SCARR, John Dargue (retired) 230 Benfleet Road, Hadleigh, Benfleet SS7 1QQ Tel: 01702 552169 — MB BChir Camb. 1970 (Camb. & St. Bart.) MA Camb. 1970. Prev: Gen. Practitioner Leigh on Sea.

SCARRATT, William Lawrence Herbert (retired) Robins Close, Kingston, Kingsbridge TQ7 4PL Tel: 01548 810786 — MB BS Lond. 1962 (Middlx.) FRCPath 1983, M 1970. Prev: Cons. Histopath. Plymouth Gen. Hosp.

SCARROW, George Davidson (retired) 20 Abbey Road, West Kirby, Wirral CH48 7EW Tel: 0151 625 6799 — MD Liverp. 1950; MB ChB 1941, MRad(D) 1948; DMRD Eng. 1948; FFR 1974. Prev: Cons. Radiol. Liverp. RHB.

SCARROW, Paul Larwood Surgery, Larwood, Worksop S81 0HH Tel: 01909 500233 Fax: 01909 479722; Lorelei, Old Blyth Road, Ranby, Retford DN22 8HZ — BM BS Nottm. 1982; BMedSci Nottm. 1980, BM BS 1982.

SCARSBROOK, Andrew Frederick 35a Rossett Avenue, Timperley, Altrincham WA15 6EU — BM BS Nottm. 1996.

SCARTH, Jennifer Clare North Tees General Hospital, Hardwick, Stockton-on-Tees TS19 8PE Tel: 01642 617617; 15 Brundon Avenue, Whitley Bay NE26 1SE Tel: 0191 252 6156 — MB BS Newc. 1993; MRCP (UK) 1996. Specialist Regist. Rotat. (Paediat.)

Northern Region. Specialty: Paediat. Socs: MRCPCH. Prev: SHO Rotat. (Paediat.) Newc. Teachg. Hosps.; SHO (Paediat.) N. Tees Gen. Hosp. Stockton & Roy. Vict. Infirm. Newc.

SCARTH, Leslie George (retired) 4 Beauchamp Road, Edinburgh EH16 6LQ Tel: 0131 658 1283 — MB BS Durh. 1964 (Newc.) DPM Eng. 1968; FRCPsych 1987, M 1978. Prev: Cons. Child & Family Psychiat. Roy. Hosp. Sick Childr. Edin.

SCASE, Anne Elizabeth Low Lane, Rocklands, Attleborough NR17 1TU — MB ChB Birm. 1987.

SCATCHARD, Katherine Mary Flat A, 106 Keslake Rd, Queen's Park, London NW6 6DG — MB BS Lond. 1994 (St Marys) BSc Hons 1991; MRCP 1997. Specialty: Oncol.

SCATCHARD, Michael Alva The Leeds Road Practice, 49/51 Leeds Road, Harrogate HG2 8AY Tel: 01423 566636 Fax: 01423 569208 — MB ChB St. And. 1968; Cert. Family Plann. JCC 1974; MRCGP 1975. Tutor (Gen. Pract.) Harrogate Dist. Hosp.; Hosp. Pract. (Dermat.) Harrogate Gen. Hosp. Socs: Brit. Inst. Med. Manipulation. Prev: Regist. (Dermat.) Dundee Teachg. Hosps.; Ch.ill Fell. 1980; Ho. Phys. (Prof.) Dundee Teachg. Hosps.

SCAWN, David Lionel, Maj. RAMC (retired) Health Centre, Bridge Street, Rothwell, Kettering NN14 6JW Tel: 01536 418518 Fax: 01536 418373 — LRCPI & LM, LRSCI & LM 1958; Sen. Med. Off. Chatham Dist; LRCPI & LM, LRCSI & LM 1958. Prev: Ho. Surg. & Ho. Phys. N. Staffs. Roy. Infirm. Stoke-on-Trent.

SCAWN, Nigel David Anthony The Liverpool Cardiothoracic Centre, Thomas Drive, Liverpool L14 3PE Tel: 0151 228 1616 Ext: 2202; 17 Bramhall Close, West Kirby, Wirral CH48 8BP — BM Soton. 1992; BPharm Lond. 1986; DA (UK) 1994; FCARCSI 1997; FRCA 1998. Cons. Cardiothoracic Anaesth. Specialty: Anaesth. Socs: Roy. Pharm. Soc. Prev: Specialist Regist. (Anaesth.) Mersey Deanery NW Region; SHO (Anaesth.) St. Jas. Univ. Hosp. Leeds & Roy. Liverp. Univ. Hosp.

SCERRI, Mr Godwin, Wing Cdr. RAF Med. Br. Consultant Plastic Surgeon, Department of Plastic & Reconstructive Surgery, Royal Hospital Haslar, Gosport PO12 2AA Tel: 023 9258 4255/023 9276 2481 Fax: 023 9276 2115 Email: godwscer@dsca.mod.uk — MRCS Eng. LRCP Lond. 1981 (Lond. Hosp. Med. Coll.) FRCS Eng. 1988; FRCS (Plast) 1995. Cons. Plastic Surg. Roy. Hosp. Haslar Gosport; Cons. Adviser (Plastic Surg.) Defence Med. Servs. Specialty: Plastic Surg. Socs: Brit. Assn. Plastic Surg.; Brit. Burns Assn.; Brit. Assn. Aesthetic Plastic Surgs. Prev: Sen. Regist. (Plastic Surg.) Addenbrooke's Hosp. Camb.; Sen. Regist. (Hand Surg.) Nuffield Orthop. Centre Oxf.; Regist. (Plastic Surg.) Canniesburn Hosp. Glas.

SCERRI, Joseph Juliet, Quarries Square, Msida, Malta; 5 Chalgrove Road, Sutton SM2 5JT Tel: 020 8642 7335 — MRCS Eng. LRCP Lond. 1981 (Westminster Medical School) DRCOG 1986; DGM 1986. Specialty: Gen. Pract.

SCHACHTER, Joan Parkside Clinic, 63-65 Lancaster Road, London W11 1QT — MB ChB Birm. 1971; MRCPsych 1976. Cons. Psychiat. (Psychother.) Parkside Clinic. Specialty: Psychother. Socs: Brit. Psychoanal Soc.

SCHACHTER, Michael Dept. Of Clinical Pharmacology, St. Mary's Hospital, London W2 1NY Email: m.schachter@ic.ac.uk; 71 Fortune Green Road, London NW6 1DR — MB BS Lond. 1974; BSc Lond. 1971; MRCP (UK) 1979. Sen. Lect. (Clin. Pharmacol.) Imperial Coll. Fac. of Med. Specialty: Pharmacology; Gen. Med. Socs: Fell. Roy. Soc. Med. Prev: BHF Sen. Research Fell. (Clin. Pharmacol.) St. Mary's Hosp. Med. Sch. Lond.; Research Regist. (Neurol.) King's Coll. Hosp. Lond.; Research Fell. MRC Unit & Univ. Dept. Clin. Pharmacol. Oxf.

SCHADY, Wolfgang Department of Neurology, Manchester Royal Infirmary, Oxford Road, Manchester M13 9WL — MRCS Eng. LRCP Lond. 1975; MRCP (UK) 1978; FRCP Lond. 1989. Sen. Lect. (Neurol.) Univ. Manch.; Hon. Cons. Neurol. Manch. Roy. Infirm.; Hon. Cons. Neurol. Hope Hosp., Salford; Hon.Cons. Neurol. Traffod Gen. Hosp.; Clin. Director, Gtr. Manchetser Neuro Sci. Centre. Specialty: Neurol.

SCHAEFER, Andrew Mark 55 Pickering Road, West Ayton, Scarborough YO13 9JE — MB ChB Leeds 1994; MRCP (UK) 1998.

SCHAEFER, Jennifer Ann Nailsea Health Centre, Somerset Square, Nailsea, Bristol BS48 1RR Tel: 01275 856611 Fax: 01275 857074 — MB ChB Bristol 1986; DCH RCPS Glas. 1988; MRCGP 1990; DRCOG 1991.

SCHAEFER, Wolfgang Cwm-Weeg, Dolfor, Newtown SY16 4AT Tel: 01686 628992 — State Exam Med Freiburg 1982. Specialty: Gen. Med.

SCHALLAMACH, Sarah 65 Shaftesbury Avenue, Roundhay, Leeds LS8 1DR — MB BS Newc. 1989; DRCOG 1993; MRCGP 1994.

SCHALLREUTER, Karin Chellow Grange, Malvern Road, Bradford BD9 6AP — State Exam Med Hamburg 1984; MD Hamburg 1985; Spec.Derm.Ven. 1992. Prof. Clin.Experim. Derm. Univ.Bradford; Dir. Inst. Pigmentaty Disorders. EM Arndt Univ. Germany. Specialty: Dermat.; Biochem. Socs: Brit. Assn. Derm.; Amer. Acad.Derm; Roy. Soc. Med.

SCHAMROTH, Alan Jeffrey Bounds Geen Group Practice, Bounds Green Group Practice, Gordon Road, New Southgate, London N11 2PF Tel: 020 8889 1961 Fax: 020 8889 7844; 19 Manor View, London N3 2ST Tel: 020 8346 1293 — BSc Lond. 1980, MB BS 1983; DRCOG 1986; DCH RCP Lond. 1987; MRCGP 1987; Dip PCR Bath 2002. Clin. Lect. (Primary Health Care) Whittington Hosp.; Princip. Lect. (Med. Ethics) Roy. Free Univ. Coll. Med. Sch. Prev: Trainee GP Northwick Pk. Hosp. VTS Harrow.

SCHAPIRA, Professor Anthony Henry Vernon University Department of Clinical Neurosciences, Royal Free and University College Medical School, UCL, Rowland Hill Street, London NW3 2PF Tel: 020 7830 2012 Fax: 020 7472 6829 Email: anthony.schapira@royalfree.nhs.uk; University Department of Clinical Neurosciences, Royal Free & University College Medical School, London NW3 2PF Tel: 020 7830 2012 Fax: 020 7472 6829 Email: anthony.schapira@royalfree.nhs.uk — MB BS Lond. 1979 (Westm.) MRCP (UK) 1982; BSc (Hons.) Lond. 1976, DSc 1994, MD 1988; FRCP Lond. 1992; DSc Lond. 1994; FMedSci 1999. Chairm. Clin. Neurosci. Roy. Free & Univ. Coll. Med. Sch. UCL & Prof. Clin. Neurol. Inst. Neurol. Qu. Sq. Lond.; Vis. Prof. Neurol. Mt. Sinai Med. Sch. NY, USA; Mem. Roy. Inst. Specialty: Neurol. Socs: Harveian Soc.; Lond. Med. Soc.; Amer. Neurol. Assn. Prev: Cons. Neurol. Roy. Free Hosp. & Nat. Hosp. Nerv. Dis. Lond.; Regist. & Sen. Regist. Nat. Hosp. Qu. Sq. Lond.

SCHAPIRA, Daniel John Meadow Barn, Hoddern Farm, Marping Hill, Peacehaven BN10 8AR Tel: 01273 587721 — MB BS Lond. 1979 (Middlx.) MRCGP; DRCOG 1980; DCH RCP Lond. 1981; MMedSc Birm. 1995; MSc Lond. 1996. Med. Locum; Indep. Multi-Media Cons. & Developer Lond.; Lect. (Computer Interface Design) Lond. Prev: GP Lond.

SCHAPIRA, Harry 16 Wide Way, Mitcham CR4 1BD Tel: 020 8764 7612; 4 Pollards Hill South, Norbury, London SW16 4LN — MRCS Eng. LRCP Lond. 1952 (Guy's)

SCHAPIRA, Kurt (retired) 4 Brookfield, Westfield, Newcastle upon Tyne NE3 4YB Tel: 0191 285 5678 — MB BS Durh. 1952; MD Durh. 1961; DPM Durham. 1963; FRCPsych 1975, M 1971; FRCP Lond. 1979, M 1973. Emerit. Cons. Psychiat. Newc. HA; Hon. Sen. Research Assoc. (Psychiat.) Univ. Newc. Prev: Sub Dean Roy. Coll Psychiats.

SCHAPIRA, Robert Clive 18 Millwell Crescent, Chigwell IG7 5HY — MB BS Lond. 1985.

SCHATZBERGER, Paul Maxim Upwell Street Surgery, 91 Upwell Street, Sheffield S4 8AN Tel: 0114 261 8608; 78 Carr Road, Sheffield S6 2WZ Tel: 0114 233 0523 — MB BS Lond. 1973 (Univ. Coll. Hosp.) DObst RCOG 1975; MRCGP (Distinc.) 1977; MFPHM RCP (UK) 1995. Specialty: Gen. Pract. Prev: Sen. Regist. (Pub. Health Med.) Barnsley HA; Regist. (Pub. Health Med.) Sheff. HA; GP Hampstead, Camden & Islington FPC.

SCHEEL, T A Trent Meadows Medical Centre, 87 Wood Street, Burton-on-Trent DE14 3AA Tel: 01283 845555 Fax: 01283 845222 — State Exam Med Freiburg 1987; State Exam Med Freiburg 1987.

SCHEELE, Kate Helene 218 Stannington View Road, Sheffield S10 1ST — MB ChB Sheff. 1998; MB ChB Sheff 1998.

SCHEEPERS, Bruce Duncan Meiring Developmental Neurosciences, Third Floor, London House, Hide Street, Stoke-on-Trent ST4 1NF Tel: 01782 427608 Fax: 01782 427642 Email: scheepers@supanet.com — MB ChB Stellenbosch 1984 (Stellenbosch (South Africa)) MRCPsych 1991. Cons. Neuropsychiat. N. Staffs Combined Healthcare NHS Trust; Sen. Clin. Lect. Dept. of Psychiat. Univ. Keele; Cons. Neuropsychiat. Transitional Rehabiliation Unit, Haydock. Specialty: Gen. Psychiat. Socs: Brit. Neuropsychiat. Assn.; Internat. League Against Epilepsy. Prev: Cons.

Neuropsychiat. Mid. Chesh. Hosp. NHS Trust, Crewe; Cons. Neuropsychiat. Chesh. Community Healthcare NHS Trust.

SCHEIMBERG SCHIFF, Irene Beatriz The Royal London Hospital, Whitechapel, London E1 1BB Tel: 020 7377 7347 Fax: 020 7377 7030; 19 Brockwell Park Gardens, London SE24 9BL — LMS U Complutense Madrid 1983; MRCPath 1994. Sen. Lect. & Hon. Cons. (Paediat. & Perinatal Path.) Roy. Lond. Hosp. Lond. Specialty: Histopath. Socs: MRCPath.; Paediatric Pathol. Soc.; Path. Soc. Prev: Lect. Gt. Ormond St. Hosp. for Childr.

SCHELLANDER, Fritz Gerhard 8 Chilston Road, Tunbridge Wells TN4 9LT Tel: 01892 543535 Fax: 01892 545160 — MD Vienna 1965; LMSSA Lond. 1974. Fell. St. John's Hosp. Dermat. Soc. Prev: Regist. Dept. Dermat. & Venereol. & Regist. Dept. Path. Univ. Vienna; Med. Sch., Austria; Research Fell. & Train. Fell. Inst. Dermat. Lond.

SCHELVAN, Christopher Selvam Keith 119B Dartmouth Road, London NW2 4ES — MB BS Lond. 1993 (St. Mary's) BSc Lond. 1990; MRCP (UK) 1997; FRCR 2000. Cons. Radiologist, St Mary's Hosp., Lond. Specialty: Radiol. Prev: SHO (Paediat. & Neonates) Northwick Pk. Hosp. Harrow; SHO (Paediat.) Qu. Eliz. Hosp. Childr. Lond.; SHO (A & E) Univ. Coll. Hosp. Lond.

SCHEMBRI, Joseph Anthony Lindley Village Surgery, Thomas Street, Lindley, Huddersfield HD3 3JD Tel: 01484 651403 Fax: 01484 644198 — MRCS Eng. LRCP Lond. 1981 (Univ. Leics.) D.Occ.Med. RCP Lond. 1995. Specialty: Occupat. Health.

SCHEMBRI WISMAYER, Franz 11 Chertsey Road, Redland, Bristol BS6 6NB — MB BS Lond. 1993.

SCHEMBRI WISMAYER, Joseph Liverpool Road Health Centre, 9 Mersey Place, Luton LU1 1HH Tel: 01582 22525 Fax: 01582 421602; 12 Montrose Avenue, Luton LU3 1HR Tel: 01582 23900 — MD Malta 1958. Hosp. Pract. (Orthop. & Accid.) Luton & Dunstable Hosp.

SCHENK, Christopher Paul Civil Aviation Authority, Gatwick Airport South, Gatwick RH6 0YR — MB BS Lond. 1986; DAvMED 1992; AFOM 2001.

SCHENK, Paul Michiel Fore Street Surgery, Fore Street, St Dennis, St Austell PL26 8AG — MB BS Lond. 1987 (King's Coll. Lond.) BSc Biochem. Lond. 1981. Specialty: Gen. Pract.

SCHER, Herschel Ward 5D, Hospital for Sick Children, Great Ormond St., London WC1N 3JH — MB ChB Cape Town 1983.

SCHER, Leslie Bernard (retired) 41 Albany, Manor Road, Bournemouth BH1 3EJ Tel: 01202 554362 — MB BCh BAO NUI 1942 (Cork) BDS 1944; FDS RCS Ed. 1955, HDD 1945; FFD RCSI 1964. Prev: Prof. Dent. Prosth.s, Univ. Coll. Cork.

SCHERF, Caroline Franziska Dept of Medicine, University of Wales College of Medicine, Cardiff CF4 4XX; 23 Chale Road, London SW2 4JD — State Exam Med. Berlin 1988. Res. Fell. (Gyn.) Uni. of Wales, Coll. of Med.

SCHERZINGER, Sabine Hilda Thorpe Health Centre, St. Williams Way, Norwich NR7 0AJ Tel: 01603 701212; 12 Chester Street, Norwich NR2 2AY Tel: 01603 617101 — MB ChB Cape Town 1992; BPharm S. Afr. 1985; MSc S. Afr. 1987. GP. Specialty: Gen. Pract. Socs: MDU 387678F. Prev: SHO (Gen. Med.) Norf. & Norwich Hosp.

SCHETRUMPF, Mr John Robert 17 Harley Street, London W1N 1DA Tel: 020 7637 5005 — MB BS Sydney 1964; FRCS Ed. 1969. Indep. Cosmetic Surg. Harley St. Lond. Specialty: Plastic Surg. Socs: Pres. Brit. Assn. Cosmetic Surg.; Allied Mem. Brit. Assn. Plastic Surgs. Prev: Dir. Regional Burns Unit Mt. Vernon Hosp. Northwood; Sen. Regist. & Burns Research Fell. Qu. Vict. Hosp. E. Grinstead; Sen. Regist. (Plastic Surg.) Hammersmith Hosp. Lond.

SCHEUER, Professor Peter Joseph 47 Northway, London NW11 6PB Tel: 020 8455 5459 Fax: 020 8455 4383 Email: scheuer@scheupj.demon.co.uk — (Roy. Free) MB BS Lond. 1954; DSc (Med.) Lond. 1986, MD 1962; FRCPath 1976, M 1963. Vice Chair., Brit. Liver Trust. Specialty: Histopath. Prev: Prof. Histopath. Univ. Lond.; Hon. Cons. Histopath. Roy. Free Hosp. Lond.

SCHEURMIER, Neil Ian Munro The Frome Medical Practice, Park Road, Frome BA11 1EZ Tel: 01373 301317 Email: nemesis@ukonline.co.uk — MB Camb. 1981; BSc Hons. (Physiol.) Dundee 1976; BChir 1980; JCPTGP 1985; Evidence Based Healthcare, (Oxford) 1988. GP Associate, Frome Medical Practice, Frome. Specialty: Gen. Med. Prev: GP Hayling Is.; Primary Care Med. Adviser, Wilts. Health Auth.

SCHEY, Stephen Arthur Department of Haematology, Guy's Hospital, St Thomas St., London SE1 9RT Tel: 020 7955 4003 Fax: 020 7955 4002 — MB BS Lond. 1974; MB BS. Lond. 1974; MRCP (UK) 1978; FRACP 1982; MRCPath. 1985; FRCP Lond. 1993. Hons. Cons. & Sen. Lect. (Haemat.) Guy's Hosp. Lond. Specialty: Haematology. Socs: Coun. Mem. Brit. Soc. of Haematol.; Sec. UK Myeloma Forum; Eur. Blood & Marrow Transpl.

SCHIERENBERG, Tai Seng Francis Department of Surgery, East Surrey Hospital, Canada Avenue, Redhill RH1 5RH Tel: 01958 349386 — MB BS Lond. 1992 (Char. Cross & Westm.) SHO (Gen. Surg.) E. Surrey Hosp. Surrey. Specialty: Gen. Surg. Socs: Fell. RCS. Prev: Regist. (Gen. Surg. & Trauma) Baragwanath Hosp. Soweto, Johannesburg, S. Afr.; SHO (Neurosurg.) Frenchay Hosp. Bristol; SHO (Orthop.) Ealing Hosp. Uxbridge.

SCHIESS, Fiona Jane Churchill Medical Centre, Clifton Road, Kingston upon Thames KT2 6PG; Westover 15C, St Albans Road, Kingston upon Thames KT2 5HQ — MB BS Lond. 1989; DRCOG 1992; T(GP) 1993.

SCHIFF, Anthony Adam 19 Whistley Close, Bracknell RG12 9LQ — MRCS Eng. LRCP Lond. 1963. Prev: Sen. Med. Adviser E.R. Squibb & Sons Ltd.

SCHIFFER, Gabriele Flat 2, Ridgway Court, London SW19 4SQ — State Exam Pisa 1992.

SCHILLER, Gillian Ida Gateway Consulting Group, 30 Paines Lane, Pinner HA5 3DB Tel: 020 8868 9898 Fax: 020 8898 3973 Email: lmosshrp@dircon.co.uk — MB BS Lond. 1979; DCH RCP Lond. 1983; MBA 1986.

SCHILLER, Klaus Frederick Richard The Mill, Cuddesdon, Oxford OX44 9HQ Tel: 01865 875174 Fax: 01865 872121 Email: kfr.schiller@virgin.net — BM BCh Oxf. 1951 (Oxf. & Lond. Hosp.) MA Oxf. 1953; FRCP Lond. 1977, M 1958; DM 1966. Cons. Gastroenterol.; Emerit. Cons. Phys. & Gastroenterol. St Peter's Hosp. Chertsey. Specialty: Gastroenterol. Socs: Hon. Mem. Brit. Soc. Gastroenterol. (Ex Vice-Pres. Endoscopy). Prev: Sen. Regist. (Med.) Radcliffe Infirm. Oxf.; Regist. (Med.), Ho. Phys. & Ho. Surg. Lond. Hosp.

SCHILLING, Christopher John 131 Eaton House, 38 Westferry Circus, London E14 8RN Tel: 020 7719 0444 Fax: 020 7719 0445 Email: schillcj@aol.com; 131 Eaton House, 38 Westferry Circus, London E14 8RN Tel: 020 7719 0444 Fax: 020 7719 0445 Email: schillcj@aol.com — (St. Thos.) BA Oxf. 1962; BM BCh Oxf. 1965; MRCP (UK) 1969; DIH Eng. 1981; MSc Lond. 1982; FFOM RCP Lond. 1988, MFOM 1984; T(OM) 1991. Princip. Med. Adviser Schilling & Schilling (Cons. in Occupat. Health). Specialty: Occupat. Health. Special Interest: Asbestos related chest disease; Health effects of exposure to radiofrequency radiation; Occupational dermatitis. Socs: Soc. Occupat. Med. Prev: Regional Speciality Adviser Occupat. Med. NE Thames RHA; Extern. Examr. DIH Lond.; Princip. GP Camden & Islington FPC.

SCHILLING, Richard John Cardiology Dept., St. Bartholomews Hospital, Dominion House, West Smithfield, London EC1A 7BE — MB BS Lond. 1989; MRCP (UK) 1992; MD London 1999. Cons. (Cardiol.) St Bartholomews Hosp. Lond. Specialty: Cardiol.

SCHINDLER, Jane Louise Chapelthorpe Medical Centre, Standbridge Lane, Chapelthorpe, Wakefield WF4 7EP Tel: 01924 255166 Fax: 01924 257653; 6 Claphouse Fold, Haigh, Barnsley S75 4BY Tel: 01924 830199 — MB ChB Sheff. 1986 (Sheffield) MRCGP 1990. GP; Eng. Wom. Rugby Team Med. Off. Specialty: Sports Med.

SCHINDLER, Margrid Brigitte The Intensive Care Unit, Hospital for Sick Children, Great Ormond St., London WC1N 3JH — MB BS New South Wales 1982; FANZCA 1990. Cons. Paediat. Intens. Care Gt. Ormond St. Hosp. Childr. Lond. Specialty: Paediat.; Intens. Care.

SCHIPPERHEIJN, Johanna Agnes Maria Edgware Community Hospital, Edgware Road, Edgware HA8 0AD — Artsexamen Amsterdam 1984; MRCPsych 1989. Cons. Psychiat. Specialty: Gen. Psychiat. Prev: Sen. Regist. Rotat. (Psychiat.) St. Mary's Lond.; Regist. (Psychiat.) Middlx. & Univ. Coll. Hosp. Lond.

SCHIRGE, Angelika Sigrid Fairfield House, c/o Accident & Emergency Department, Crawley Hospital, West Green Drive, Crawley RH11 7DH — MB ChB Stellenbosch 1996.

SCHIRRMACHER, Ulrich Otto Erich Davenal House Surgery, 28 Birmingham Road, Bromsgrove B61 0DD Tel: 01527 872008; 133

New Road, Bromsgrove B61 2LJ Tel: 01527 75954 — MB BS Lond. 1965 (St. Geo.) MRCS Eng. LRCP Lond. 1965.

SCHIZAS, Mr Constantin — MD Louvain 1986 (Universite Catholique de Louvain (Belgium)) MSc (Orthop.) Lond. 1994; Dip. Biomechanics, Strathclyde 1996; Qualification en Chirurgie Orthopedique, Paris 1996; FRCS (ed eundem) Lond. 2000. Cons. Orthop. Surg./Hon. Sen. Lectures, The Whittington Hosp. Lond. Specialty: Orthop. Socs: Fell. BOA; Federat. Medicorum Helveticorum.; Fell. Roy. Soc. Med. Prev: Cons. Orthop. Surg. Qu. Mary's Hosp., Sidcup; Oberarzt, Schulthess Hosp., Zurich; Sen. Regist. Roy. Nat. Orthop. Hosp. Stanmore.

SCHLECHT, Bernard Jean Marie Liverpool School of Trop. Medicine, Pembroke Place, Liverpool L3 5QA Tel: 0151 708 9393 Fax: 0151 708 5322; 33A Mauldeth Road, Withington, Manchester M20 4NF Tel: 0161 225 1383 — MD Paris 1974; MRCP (UK) 1979; MSc Manch. 1990; MFPHM 1990; T(PHM) 1991. Lect. (Epidemiol.) Liverp. Sch. Trop. Med. Specialty: Epidemiol. Prev: Sen. Regist. (Community Med.) N. West. RHA; ARC Med. Off. ARC Epidem. Research Unit Univ. Manch; Regist. (Gen. Med.) St. Martins Hosp. Bath.

SCHLESINGER, Antonia Jane 93 Eastern Way, Ponteland, Newcastle upon Tyne NE20 9RQ — MB ChB Leeds 1994.

SCHLESINGER, Mr Peter Ernst Department of Gynaecology, Princess Margaret Hospital, Okus Road, Swindon SN1 4JU Tel: 01793 536231; 6 The Beanlands, Wanborough, Swindon SN4 0EJ Tel: 01793 790265 Fax: 01793 790265 — MB BS Lond. 1975 (St. Bart.) MRCS Eng. LRCP Lond. 1975; FRCS Ed. 1981; MRCOG 1984; FRCOG 1997. Cons. O & G Princess Margt. Hosp. Swindon; Hon. Sen. Lect. Univ. Soton.; Assoc. Prof. Univ. of W. Indies. Specialty: Obst. & Gyn. Socs: Fell.Roy. Soc. Med.; Brit. Gyn. Cancer Soc.; Internat. Continence Soc. Prev: Sen. Regist. St. Bartholomews Hosp., N. Middlsex Hosp. Lond. & Roy. Marsden Hosp.; Regist. Kings Coll. & Char. Cross Hosp. Lond.; SHO Qu. Charlotte's & Samarit. Hosp. Lond.

SCHLEYPEN, Paulus Franciscus Hubertus Maria Josef Coldstream Health Centre, Kelso Road, Coldstream TD12 4LQ Tel: 01890 882711 Fax: 01890 883547; Hatfield, Duns Road, Coldstream TD12 4DR — Artsexamen Nijmegen 1986; T(GP) 1991; MRCGP 1991.

SCHLICHT, Justin Orchard Cottage, 23 Far Holme Lane, Sutton-on-Trent, Newark NG23 6PQ Tel: 01636 821081 — MRCS Eng. LRCP Lond. 1966; MSc (Soc. Med.) Lond. 1973, MB BS 1966; MRCPsych 1973. Cons. (Child. Adol. Psychiat.) Bassetlaw Hosp. & Community Servs. NHS Trust. Specialty: Child & Adolesc. Psychiat.; Psychother. Prev: Cons. (Child & Adolesc. Psychiat.) Göteborg; Cons. Psychother. Bethlem Roy. Hosp. & Maudsley Hosp. Lond.; Cons. Psychiat. Univ. Coll. Hosp. Lond.

SCHLIEN, Maren 19 Ivy Lane, Canterbury CT1 1TU — State Exam Med Marburg 1991.

SCHMID, Matthias Ludwig Department of Infection & Tropical Medicine, Newcastle General Hospital, Newcastle upon Tyne NE4 6BE Tel: 0114 271 1900 Fax: 0114 275 3061 Email: matthias.schmid@csuh.trent.nhs.uk; 27 Salt Box Grove, Grenoside, Sheffield S35 8SG Fax: 0114 275 3061 Email: matthiasschmid@hotmail.com — State Exam Med Ulm 1989 (Univ. Ulm) MD Ulm 1990; MRCP (UK) 1995; DTM & H Lond. 1996. Dept. of Infec. & Trop. Med. Newc..; Trav. Fell. Roy. Coll. Physic. & Surgs. Glas. Specialty: Infec. Dis.; Gen. Med. Socs: RCP (Lond.).

SCHMIDT, Annemarie Elizabeth 6 West Hill Court, Millfield Lane, London N6 6JJ — MB ChB Cape Town 1985.

SCHMIDT, Annette Catherine 55 The Crescent, Haversham, Milton Keynes MK19 7AW — MB ChB Bristol 1998.

SCHMIDT, Barbara Elisabeth Hunts Cross Group Practice, Hunts Cross Health Centre, 70 Hillfoot Road, Liverpool L25 0ND Tel: 0151 486 1428 Fax: 0151 448 0233 — State Exam Med Erlangen 1986; MD Erlangen 1990.

SCHMIDT, Jorg Ulverston Health Centre, Victoria Road, Ulverston LA12 0EW Tel: 01229 583732 — State Exam Med Wurzburg 1991. GP Ulverston, Cumbria.

SCHMIDT, Karl Ernst 3 Apple Close, Dowlish Wake, Ilminster TA19 0QG Tel: 01460 55270 — MD Graz 1954; MRCS Eng. LRCP Lond. 1953; DPM Manch. 1957; FRCPsych 1987, M 1971; FRANZCP 1983. Cons. Psych. NHS Yeovil Dist. Hosp.; Vis. Prof. Neurol. Psychiat. Hans Berger Inst. Friedrich Schiller Univ., Germany; Ment. Health Specialist i/c Ment. Health Serv. Med. Dept. Brunei. Specialty: Gen. Psychiat.; Alcohol & Substance Misuse. Socs: BMA; Assoc. World Federat. Ment. Health; Roy. Soc. Chem. Prev: Cons. Psychol. Med. Yeovil Dist. Hosp. & Tone Vale Hosp. Som.; Chief Adviser (Ment. Health) S. Pacific Commiss. Noumea New Caledonia; Cons. WHO (Geneva & India).

SCHMIDT, Paul Erald Flat 1, 7 Macaulay Road, London SW4 0QP Email: paul.schmitt.demon.co.uk — MB ChB Stellenbosch 1991 (Univ.Stellenbosch,South Africa) B.Med. Sci 1998. Assoc. Special. Med. Assessm. unit Qu. Alex. Hosp. Portsmouth. Specialty: Gen. Med. Prev: Reg.Gen.Med.Roy.Berks. & Battle hosps.Reading; med.Off.ITU Livingstone Hosp.port Eliz. SA; Ho. Off. Livingstone Hosp. Port Eliz. SA.

SCHMITGEN, Catja Foulds House, Briercliffe, Burnley BB10 3QY — State Exam Med Essen 1991 (University of Essen, Germany) Medical Doctorate Univ. Essen 1994.

SCHMITGEN, Gunther Burnley General Hospital, Casterton Avenue, Burnley BB10 2PQ Tel: 01282 474036 — State Exam Med Dusseldorf 1980 (University of Düsseldorf) Cons. Orthop. Surg. Specialty: Orthop.

SCHMULIAN, Charles Ealing Hospital NHS Trust, Uxbridge Road, Southall UB1 3HW; 8 Fpirus Road, London SW6 7UH Tel: 020 7610 1893 Fax: 020 7610 1893 — MB BCh Witwatersrand 1976. Ealing Hosp. NHS Trust. Specialty: Anaesth. Special Interest: ICU; Paediat.

SCHMULIAN, Lawrence Richard (retired) 36 Monreith Road, Glasgow G43 2NY — MB BS Newc. 1966; FRCP Glas. 1986; MRCP (UK) 19 7474. Prev: Med. Asst. Profess. Geriat. Unit Stobhill Hosp. Glas.

SCHNEELOCH, Brigitte Ferryhill Medical Practice, Durham Road, Ferryhill DL17 8JJ Tel: 01740 651238 Fax: 01740 656291; 8 Dunelm Court, South Street, Durham DH1 4QX Tel: 0191 384 2640 — MB BS Newc. 1978; DCH RCPS Glas. 1981; MRCGP Lond. 1982; DRCOG 1983; Dip. Therap. Newc. 1997. Specialty: Gen. Pract.

SCHNEIDAU, Andrea 66 Woodsome Road, London NW5 1RZ — MB BS Lond. 1975 (Middlx.) MRCS Eng. LRCP Lond. 1975; FRCR 1983. Cons. Breast Radiologist, St. George's Hosp., Lond.; Hon. Cons. Breast Radiologist Univ. Coll. Hosp. Lond.; Cons. Breast Radiol. Portland Hosp. Wom. & Childr.; Cons. Breast Radiologist,108 Harley St. Specialty: Radiol. Prev: Sen. Regist. & Regist. (Radiol.) Middlx. Hosp. Lond.; Cons. Radiol. Eliz. Garrett Anderson Hosp. & Soho Hosp. Wom. Univ. Coll. Hosp. Lond.

SCHNEIDER, Mr Harry Joseph The James Paget Hospital, Great Yarmouth NR31 6LA Tel: 01493 452452 Email: schneider_hank@hotmail.com — MB BS Lond. 1988 (Char. Cross & Westm.) FRCS Eng. 1994; FRCS (Gen Surg.) 2000. Cons. Gen. Surg. Specialty: Gen. Surg. Prev: Med. Off., Camb. Univ. Boat Club; Research Regist. Roy. Marsden Hosp. Lond.; Resid. (Gen. Surg.) Oregon Health Sci.s Univ. Portland, Oregon, USA.

SCHNEIDER, Vanessa 1F3 21 Rossie Place, Edinburgh EH7 5SD — MB ChB Ed. 1998; MB ChB Ed 1998.

SCHNEPEL, Bernd 24 Jenner House, Restell Close, London SE3 7UW — State Exam Med Essen 1992.

SCHNETLER, Mr Jeremy Fredrik Coenraad Department of Oral & Maxillofacial Surgery, Royal United Hospital, Bath BA1 3NG Tel: 01225 824267 Fax: 01225 824275 Email: jeremy.schnetler@ruh-bath.swest.nhs.uk — MB BS Lond. 1983; BDS Lond. 1975; FDS RCS Eng. 1986, L 1976; FRCS Ed. 1988. Cons. Oral Surg. Roy. United Hosp. Bath; Lect. (Oral Surg.) Univ. Bristol. Specialty: Oral & Maxillofacial Surg. Socs: Fell. Brit. Assn. Oral & Maxillofacial Surg.; BMA; Brit. Assn. of Head and Neck Oncologists. Prev: Sen. Regist. (Oral Surg.) John Radcliffe Hosp. Oxf.; Regist. (Oral Surg.) Guy's Hosp. Lond.; SHO (A & E) King's Coll. Hosp. Lond.

SCHNIEDEN, Vivienne 18 Hillcrest Road, Bramhall, Stockport SK7 3AE — MB BS Lond. 1986; MA Camb. 1987; MRCPsych 1990; FRANZCP 1996. Cons. Liaison Psychiat. & Dir. Train. P. of Wales Hosp. New S. Wales, Australia; Lect. Univ. NSW. Specialty: Gen. Psychiat. Prev: Anxiety Disorders Unit St. Vincents Hosp. NSW, Austral.

SCHOBER, Paul Carl Department of G. U. Medicine, Leicester Royal Infirmary, Leicester LE1 5WW Tel: 0116 258 6653 — MB BS Lond. 1977 (St. Thos.) BSc Lond. 1974; MRCP (UK) 1981. Cons. Genitourin. Med. Leicester Roy. Infirm. Specialty: Genitourinary

Medicine. Prev: Sen. Regist. (Genitourin. Med.) Univ. Coll. Hosp. Lond.

SCHOFIELD, Alison Marjorie 5 Manor Lane, Ettington, Stratford-upon-Avon CV37 7TE — MB BS Newc. 1998; MB BS Newc 1998.

SCHOFIELD, Mr Andrew Derek Reid Royal Shrewsbury Hospital, Department of Surgery, Mytton Oak Road, Shrewsbury SY3 8XQ Tel: 01743 261190 Email: andrew.schofield@rsh.nhs.uk — MB BS Lond. 1986 (St. Bart. Hosp. Lond.) BSc (Hons.) Lond. 1983; FRCS Ed. 1990; FRCS Eng. 1991; MS Lond. 1995; FRCS Gen. Surg. 1998. Cons. Gen. and Colorectal Surg., Roy. Shrewsbury Hosp., Shrewsbury; Cons. Gen. and Colorectal Surg., Princess Roy. Hosp., Telford; Cons. Gen. and Colorectal Surg., Robt. jones and Agnes Hosp., Oswestry; Cons. Gen. and Colorectal Surg., Shrops. Nuffield Hosp., Shrewsbury. Specialty: Gen. Surg. Socs: Assn. Surg.; Assn. Coloproctology Gt. Britain and Irel. Prev: RSO St. Mark's Hosp. Northwick Pk. & St. Mark's Hosps. NHS Trust; Sen. Regist. (Gen. Surg.) Chelsea & Westminster Hosp. Lond.

SCHOFIELD, Anne Dollar Gillespie 35 Lubnaig Road, Newlands, Glasgow G43 2RY Tel: 0141 632 8735 — MB ChB Ed. 1945 (Univ. Ed.) Prev: Res. Med. Off. Elsie Inglis Matern. Hosp. Edin.; Ho. Phys. Roy. Edin. Hosp. Sick Childr.; Sen. Ho. Phys. St. James' Hosp. Balham.

SCHOFIELD, Charles Basil Shaw (retired) 27 Woodlands, Gosforth, Newcastle upon Tyne NE3 4YN Tel: 0191 285 3659 — MD Durh. 1952 (Newc. upon Tyne) MB BS 1945; FRCP Ed. 1969, M 1959; FRCP Glas. 1974, M 1972. Prev: STD/AIDS Co-ordinator Ministries of Health Zanzibar & Mainland Tanzania.

SCHOFIELD, Christine Marie Clinical Oncology Unit, Royal Cornwall Hospital, Truro TR1 3JW Tel: 01872 250000 Fax: 01726 66421; Rosemullion, Kerley Downs, Chace Water, Truro TR4 8LA — MB ChB Leeds 1977; Dip. Therapeut Wales 1997. Clin. Med. Off., Clin. Oncol., Roy. Cornw. Hosp.; Research Fell. (Neurol.) Roy. Cornw. Hosps. (Treliske) Truro. Specialty: Oncol.; Palliat. Med. Socs: Inst. Health Educat. Prev: Clin. Asst. (Psychogeriat.) Penrice Hosps. St Austell; Lect. (Health Educat.) Open Univ. & Cornw. Coll. Further Educat.; Clin.Asst. (Palliat.Med.) Mt. Edgcumbe Hospice St Austell.

SCHOFIELD, Mr Christopher Brealey — MB BS Lond. 1979; FRCS Eng. 1984. Cons. Orthop. Surg. St. Peter's Hosp. Chertsey Surrey. Specialty: Orthop. Socs: Fell. BOA; BASS. Prev: Sen. Regist. (Orthop.) St. Geo. Hosp. Lond.; Lect. Orthop. Surg. Char. Cross & Westminster Med. Sch.; Jun. Lect. Dept. Anat. Lond. Hosp. Med. Coll.

SCHOFIELD, Christopher Ian Appleton Village Surgery, 2-6 Appleton Village, Widnes WA8 6DZ Tel: 0151 423 2990 Fax: 0151 424 1032 — MB ChB Liverp. 1986.

SCHOFIELD, Claire Elizabeth Eccleston House, The Old Warren, Broughton, Chester CH4 0EG — MB ChB Manch. 1997.

SCHOFIELD, Claire Elizabeth 58 Park View Road, Lytham St Annes FY8 4JF — MB ChB Leeds 1998.

SCHOFIELD, Clare Penelope 19 Devonshire Road, Bolton BL1 4PG — MB ChB Manch. 1993.

SCHOFIELD, David John (retired) The Abingdon Surgery, 65 Stert Street, Abingdon OX14 3LB Tel: 01235 523126 Fax: 01235 550625; Springfield, Hearns Lane, Gallowstree Common, Reading RG4 9DE Tel: 0118 972 1262 — MRCS Eng. LRCP Lond. 1966 (Sheff.) DObst RCOG 1968; MRCGP 1972. Prev: Clin. Tutor (Gen. Pract.) Dept. Pub. Health & Primary Care Univ. Oxf.

SCHOFIELD, Elisabeth Caroline 41 Armit Road, Greenfield, Oldham OL3 7LN — MB ChB Ed. 1986. Clin. Asst. (A & E) Roy. Oldham Hosp. Specialty: Accid. & Emerg.

SCHOFIELD, Emma Catherine 67 Devonshire Road, Westbury Park, Bristol BS6 7NQ — MB BChir Camb. 1990; DCH RCP Lond. 1993; MRCGP 1994. Specialty: Dermat.

SCHOFIELD, Emma Mary 15 Chaucer Mansions, Queen Club Gardens, London W14 9RF — MB BS Lond. 1996.

SCHOFIELD, Mr Graham Edward, Squadron Ldr. Retd. (retired) 35 Lubnaig Road, Newlands, Glasgow G43 2RY Tel: 0141 632 8735 — MB BS Lond. 1945 (Univ. Coll. Hosp.) FRCS Eng. 1952. Cons. Surg. Law. Hosp. Carluke. Prev: Sen. Regist. Vict. Infirm. Glas.

SCHOFIELD, Helen Claire — MB BS Newc. 1997 (Newcastle) Gen. Pract., Sunderland. Specialty: Gen. Pract.

SCHOFIELD, Hilda Marjorie Vane Cottage, 22 Cleveland Walk, Bath BA2 6JU Tel: 01225 465606 — MB ChB Liverp. 1942. Socs: Clin. Soc. Bath. Prev: Ho. Surg. (O & G) Roy. Infirm. Liverp.; Capt. RAMC.

SCHOFIELD, Ian James 10 Limes Avenue, Darwen BB3 2SG — MB ChB Manch. 1995.

SCHOFIELD, Ian Richard Alpine House Surgery, 86 Rothley Road, Mountsorrel, Loughborough LE12 7JU Tel: 0116 230 3062 Fax: 0116 237 4218; Quorn Lodge Farmhouse, Leicester Road, Loughborough LE12 8UE Tel: 01509 620727 — MB ChB Leic. 1982; DRCOG 1986; MRCGP 1986.

SCHOFIELD, Ian Stephen 12 Boundary Gardens, High Heaton, Newcastle upon Tyne NE7 7AA — MB BS Newc. 1978; BMedSc Newc. 1975; MRCP (UK) 1982; FRCP Lond. 1994. Cons. (Neurophysiol.) Newc. Gen. Hosp. Specialty: Clin. Neurophysiol. Prev: Sen. Regist. (Neurophysiol.) Newc. Gen. Hosp.; SHO (Med.) Roy. Vict. Infirm. Newc.

SCHOFIELD, Jarrod Four Acre Health Centre, Burnage Avenue, Clock Face, St Helens WA9 4QB Tel: 01744 819884 Fax: 01744 850382; 25 Cranshaw Avenue, Clock Face, St Helens WA9 4UR — MB ChB Liverp. 1992; DFFP. Specialty: Gen. Pract. Prev: Trainee GP Warrington Dist. HA.

SCHOFIELD, John (retired) Wyther Lodge, 185 Victoria Road W., Thornton-Cleveleys FY5 3PZ Tel: 01253 853166 — MB ChB Manch. 1933. Med. Off. Smith's Crisps, Fleetwood. Prev: Cas. Off. Roy. Salop Infirm. Shrewsbury.

SCHOFIELD, John Bellhouse Preston Hall Hospital, Cellular Pathology Department, Maidstone ME20 7NH Tel: 01622 224051 Fax: 01622 224061; 31 New Cross Road, London SE14 5DS — MB BS Lond. 1981 (St George's Hospital Medical School London) MRCPath 1990; FRCPath 1999. Cons. (Cellular Path.) Maidstone & Tunbridge Wells NHS Trust. Specialty: Histopath. Socs: Brit. Lymphoma Path. Gp.; Assn. ColoProctol. Prev: Sen. Regist. (Histopath.) Roy. Marsden & Hammersmith Hosp. Lond.; Regist. (Histopath.) Hammersmith Hosp. Lond.; Regist. (Histopath. & Cytopath.) St Stephens Hosp. Lond.

SCHOFIELD, John Gill Elsenham Surgery, Station Road, Elsenham, Bishop's Stortford CM22 6LA Tel: 01279 814730 Fax: 01279 647342; 18 Warwick Road, Bishop's Stortford CM23 5NN Tel: 01279 652783 — (King's Coll. Hosp.) MB BS Lond. 1969; MRCS Eng. LRCP Lond. 1969; DObst RCOG 1971. Assoc. Dean Lond. Deanery.

SCHOFIELD, Mr John Norman McMichael (retired) Greystones, Banbury St., Kineton, Warwick CV35 0JS Tel: 01926 640272 Fax: 01926 640272 — MB BS Lond. 1950 (Middlx.) DLO Eng. 1956; FRCS Ed. 1957; FRCS Eng. 1961. Prev: Cons. ENT Surg. Warneford, Leamington Spa, Warwick & Stratford-upon-Avon Hosps.

SCHOFIELD, Jules 66 St Leonards Road, Leicester LE2 1WR — MB ChB Leic. 1998; MB ChB Leic 1998.

SCHOFIELD, Julia Kathy Department of Dermatology, St Albans City Hospital, St. Albans & Hemel Hempstead NHS Hospitals Trust, Waverley Road, St Albans AL3 5PN Tel: 01727 897837 Fax: 01727 897837; 18 High Street, Rickmansworth WD3 1ER Tel: 01923 778279 — MB ChB Manch. 1979; DRCOG 1982; MRCP (UK) 1984; MRCGP 1986; FCRP 1999. Cons. Dermat. St. Albans & Hemel Hempstead NHS Hosps. Trust. Specialty: Dermat. Prev: Trainee GP Salford VTS; Sen. Regist. (Dermat.) Watford Gen. & Roy. Lond. Hosp.; Regist. (Dermat.) SW Herts. HA.

SCHOFIELD, Julian Paul 14 Tamar Close, St. Ives, Huntingdon PE27 3JE — MB ChB Leeds 1984; BSc (Hons.) Leeds 1981, MB ChB 1984; MRCP (UK) 1987; PhD Camb. 1991. Wellcome Advis. Train. Fell. Univ. Dept. Med. Addenbrooke's Hosp. Camb.; Hon. Sen. Regist. (Gen. Med.) Univ. Dept. Med. Addenbrooke's Hosp. Camb. Socs: Med. Res. Soc.

SCHOFIELD, Karen Patricia 8 Birches Farm Mews, Madeley, Crewe CW3 9TE — MD Sheff. 1992; MB ChB 1976; MRCP (UK) 1979; MRCPath 1986; PhD Manch. 1998. Specialty: Haematology.

SCHOFIELD, Lewis Paul 1 James Street S., Chadderton, Oldham OL9 9JA — MB BS Newc. 1997.

SCHOFIELD, Linda Elizabeth Gainsborough House, South St., Sherborne DT9 3LT — MB BS Lond. 1982; DRCOG 1986; MRCPsych 1991.

SCHOFIELD, Louise 12A Hawthorn Road, Alexandra Park, London N8 7NA Tel: 020 8347 5291 — MB BS Lond. 1994 (St. Bart. Hosp. Med. Coll.) BSc Lond. 1991; MRCP 1997. Specialist Regist. Palliat. Med., N. Thames. Specialty: Palliat. Med.

SCHOFIELD, Neil McCallum Nuffield Department of Anaesthetics, John Radcliffe Hospital, Headington, Oxford OX3 9DU Tel: 01865 741166 Fax: 01865 221593; Perrott's Farm, Bicester Road, Long Crendon, Aylesbury HP18 9BP Tel: 01844 201585 — MB BChir Camb. 1970 (Camb. & St. Thos.) BA Camb. 1966, MA 1970; FFA RCS Eng. 1974. Cons. Anaesth. Nuffield Dept. Anaesth. Oxf. Specialty: Anaesth. Socs: Assn. Anaesth.; Assn. Paediat. Anaesth.; Brit. Med. Assn.

SCHOFIELD, Olivia Marie Virginia Mine Department of Dermatology, Royal Infirmary Edinburgh, Edinburgh EH3 9YW Tel: 0131 536 2403 Email: olivia.schofield@luht.scot.nhs.uk; 109, Trinity Road, Edinburgh EH5 3JY Tel: 0131 551 1306 Email: jdwalker@mcmail.com — MB BS Lond. 1981; MRCP (UK) 1985. p/t Cons. Dermat. Roy. Infirm. Edin.; Med. Adviser Alopecia Help Scotl.; Director On the Bd. of Exzema Scotl. Specialty: Dermat. Socs: Brit. Assn. Dermat.; Brit. Soc. Paediat. Dermatol.; Scott. Dermatological Soc. Prev: Sen. Regist. (Dermat.) Roy. Infirm. Edin. & King's Coll. Hosp. Lond.

SCHOFIELD, Penelope Jane 1 Lesbury Road, Heaton, Newcastle upon Tyne NE6 5LB Tel: 0191 265 8898 — BM BCh Oxf. 1975; DRCOG 1980; MRCGP 1982.

SCHOFIELD, Peter Charles Hugh 12 Castle Town, Upper Beeding, Steyning BN44 3TR Tel: 01903 813378 — MB ChB Birm. 1965; BDS, LDS Manch. 1956; MRCS Eng. LRCP Lond. 1965; DA Eng. 1968. Prev: Ho. Phys. Barnet Gen. Hosp.; Ho. Surg. W. Herts. Hosp. Hemel Hempstead.

SCHOFIELD, Peter Marshall Papworth Hospital, Papworth Everard, Cambridge CB3 8RE Tel: 01480 364349 Email: peter.schofield@papworth.nhs.uk — MB ChB (Hons.) Manch.; FACC; FESC; MD; FRCP. Cons. Cardiol., Papworth Hosp. Specialty: Cardiol. Special Interest: Interventional Cardiol. Socs: Brit. Cardiac Soc.; Brit. Cardiovasc. Interven. Soc.

SCHOFIELD, Professor Philip Furness Longridge, The Dingle, Gee Cross, Hyde SK14 5EP Tel: 0161 368 2811 Fax: 0161 366 7338; (cons. rooms) 15 St John Street, Manchester M3 4DG Tel: 0161 834 7373 — MD Manch. 1966; FRCS Ed. 1962; FRCS Eng. 1963. Cons. Surg. Christie Hosp. Manch. (Hon); Vis. Prof. Univ. Manch. Specialty: Gen. Surg. Socs: Assn. Coloproctol. (Pres.).; Assn. Surg. Prev: Cons. Surg. Ashton, Hyde & Glossop Hosp. Gp.; Cons. Surg. W. Manch. Hosp. Gp.; John M. Wilson Memor Schol. Cleveland Clinic, Ohio.

SCHOFIELD, Philippa Jane New Southgate Surgery, Buxton Place, 91 Leeds Rd, Wakefield WF1 3JQ; 3 Lakeland Way, Walton, Wakefield WF2 6TG — MB ChB Leeds 1990; BSc (Hons) Physiology 1985. G.P. Specialty: Gen. Pract.; Family Plann. & Reproduc. Health. Socs: BMA; Diplomat Fac. Of Family Plann. + Reproductive Health Care.

SCHOFIELD, Roger Paul 35 Dalebrook Road, Sale M33 3LD — MB BS Lond. 1985; DRCOG 1988; MRCGP 1991. Specialty: Palliat. Med.

SCHOFIELD, Ronald (retired) 45 Hustler Road, Bridlington YO16 6RN Tel: 01262 675398 — (Manch.) MB ChB Manch. 1954; DCH Eng. 1958; DPH Manch. 1962; MD Manch. 1966; MFCM 1972. Prev: SCM E. Yorks. HA.

SCHOFIELD, Roy (retired) 29 Church Lane, Lincoln LN2 1QR Tel: 01522 528745 — MB ChB Manch. 1950; DObst RCOG 1954. Prev: Sen. Partner Drs Schofield, Sturton & Mallet Lincoln.

SCHOFIELD, Ruth (retired) 18 Deerswood Lane, Bexhill-on-Sea TN39 4LT — MB BS Lond. 1974 (Roy. Free) MRCS Eng. LRCP Lond. 1974.

SCHOFIELD, Sarah Florence The Ramblers, Long St., Wheaton Aston, Stafford ST19 9NF — MB BS Lond. 1998; MB BS Lond 1998.

SCHOFIELD, Sarah Patricia North Baddesley Surgery, Norton Welch Close, Fleming Avenue, Southampton SO52 9EP Tel: 023 8073 4523 Fax: 023 8073 0287; 9 Balmoral Way, Rownhams, Southampton SO16 8LL Tel: 02380 740776 Fax: 01703 740708 — MB ChB Leic. 1984 (Univ. Leic.) DCH RCP Lond. 1987; MRCGP 1988. Chairm. W. & Test PCG. Prev: Trainee GP Soton. VTS; SHO (A & E) Soton. Gen. Hosp.; Clin. Asst. A & E, Soton. Gen. Hosp.

SCHOFIELD, Sheila Farquharson (retired) 5 Manor Close, Bramhope, Leeds LS16 9HQ Tel: 0113 284 2875 — MB ChB Leeds 1944; DObst RCOG 1974, London; DCH Eng. 1944; DPH Glas. 1955. Prev: SCMO Bradford HA.

SCHOFIELD, Shona Jane Alice 32 Llanishen Street, Heath, Cardiff CF14 3QE; 5 Manor Lane, Ettington, Stratford-upon-Avon CV37 7TE Tel: 01789 740893 — MB BCh Wales 1996.

SCHOFIELD, Stephanie Ann Milton Park Surgery, 131 Goldsmith Avenue, Southsea PO4 8QZ — BM Soton 1978; BM Soton 1978.

SCHOFIELD, Stephen John Acomb Health Centre, 1 Beech Grove, Acomb, York YO26 5LD Tel: 01904 791094; 2A Knapton Lane, Acomb, York YO26 5PU Tel: 01904 798620 — MB ChB Manch. 1980; MRCP (UK) 1983; DRCOG 1985; MRCGP 1986.

SCHOFIELD, Mr Theo Legate (retired) Vane Cottage, 22 Cleveland Walk, Bath BA2 6JU Tel: 01225 465606 — MB ChB Liverp. 1942; MB ChB (Distinc. Surg.) Liverp. 1942; MRCS Eng. LRCP Lond. 1942; FRCS Eng. 1949; ChM Liverp. 1954.

SCHOFIELD, Theo Perry Calwell The Medical Centre, Badgers Crescent, Shipston-on-Stour CV36 4BD Tel: 01608 661845 Fax: 01608 663614; Dolphin Farm, Weatheroak Hill, Alvechurch, Birmingham B48 7EA Tel: 01564 826816 — BM BCh Oxf. 1968; MA Oxf. 1965; DObst RCOG 1970; MRCP (UK) 1972; FRCGP 1980, M 1974; FRCP 2002. Lect. (Gen. Pract.) Dept. Pub. Health & Primary Care Oxf. Prev: Ho. Off. (Gen. Med., Surg. & Obst.) & SHO (Gen. Med.) Radcliffe Infirm. Oxf.

SCHOFIELD, Thomas Charles 258 Milton Road E., Edinburgh EH15 2PG Tel: 0131 669 5676 — MB ChB Ed. 1979; DRCOG 1981; MRCGP 1984.

SCHOFIELD, William Norman The Castle, High St., Presteigne LD8 2BE — MB BCh Wales 1954 (Cardiff) BSc, MB BCh Wales 1954. Prev: Demonst. Anat. Univ. Manch.; Ho. Surg. & Ho. Phys. Aberystwyth Gen. Hosp.; Capt. RAMC.

SCHOFIELD, Zena June 18 Wilmot Street, London E2 0BS — MB BS Lond. 1998; MB BS Lond 1998.

SCHOLEFIELD, Charles (retired) — MB BS Lond. 1970; MRCS Eng. LRCP Lond. 1970; DA Eng. 1972; MRCPsych 1976. Prev: Sen. Regist. Rotat. (Adult Psychiat.) Yorks. VTS.

SCHOLEFIELD, Ida Mary (retired) Savernake, Bagatelle Road, St Saviour, Jersey JE2 7TZ Tel: 01534 35173 — MB ChB Leeds 1939.

SCHOLEFIELD, Jane Hazel Dinnington Group Practice, Medical Centre, New Street, Dinnington, Sheffield S25 2EZ — MB ChB Sheff. 1990.

SCHOLEFIELD, Professor John Howard Section of Surgery, University Hospital, Nottingham NG7 2UH Tel: 0115 970 9245 Fax: 0115 970 9428 — MB ChB Liverp. 1983; FRCS Ed. 1987; FRCS Eng. 1988; ChM Liverp. 1991. Prof. of Surg./Hon. Cons.. Univ. Hosp. Nottm. Specialty: Gen. Surg. Prev: Lect. (Surg.) Univ. Sheff.; Clin. Research Fell. ICRF Colorectal Unit, St. Mark's Hosp., Lond.; Regist. Rotat. (Surg.) Roy. Hallamsh. Hosp. Sheff.

SCHOLEFIELD, Robert Dean St Katherines Surgery, Market Street, Ledbury HR8 2AQ Tel: 01531 633271 Fax: 01531 632410 — MB BS Lond. 1970 (Guy's) MRCS Eng. LRCP Lond. 1969; DObst RCOG 1971; Cert. Family Plann. JCC 1976. Prev: SHO Heref. Hosp. Gp.

SCHOLES, Carol Fiona The Peace Hospice, Peace Drive, Watford WD17 3PH Tel: 01923 330349 Fax: 01923 330331 — MB BS Newc. 1988; MRCP (UK) 1993. Cons. in Palliat. Med. Dacorum Primary Care Trust; Med. Director Peace Hospice, Watford. Specialty: Palliat. Med. Prev: Sen. Regist. (Palliat. Med.) Mt. Vernon & Watford NHS Trust Hosps.; Regist. (Palliat. Med.) Mt. Vernon & Watford NHS Trust Hosp. & Camden & Islington NHS Trust.

SCHOLES, George Barrie 61 Wimpole Street, London W1M 7DE Tel: 020 7935 2617 Fax: 020 7224 1680; 17 Beaumont Street, London W1G 6DG Tel: 020 7935 8081 Fax: 020 7224 1925 Email: gbscholes@avnet.co.uk — MB ChB Dunedin, NZ 1959 (Univ. Otago, Dunedin NZ) FRCS Eng. 1966; Cert. Av. Med. 1993. Chief Med. Off. Unison Insur.; Med. Examr. (UK) Netherlands Min. Navigation; UK Maritime & Coastguard Agency. Socs: Assur. Med. Soc. Prev: Chief Exec. St. Martins Hosps. Ltd.; MRC Research Asst. & Hon. Sen. Regist. King's Coll. Hosp. Lond.; Dir. Foreign Hosp. Yokohama, Japan.

SCHOLES, Keith Turner Whalebridge Practice, Health Centre, Carfax Street, Swindon SN1 1ED Tel: 01793 692933; Rose Cottage, Queens Road, Hannington, Swindon SN6 7RP Tel: 01793 762515 — MB ChB Sheff. 1966; DObst RCOG 1968. Hosp. Pract. (Dermat.) Princess Margt. Hosp. Swindon. Specialty: Dermat.

SCHOLES, Mr Neville Edward, Surg. Cdr. RN (retired) 10 Coxfield Grove, Shevington, Wigan WN6 8DW — (Ed.) FFAEM; MB

ChB Ed. 1965; FRCS Ed. 1978. Prev: Cons. (A & E) Wigan & Leigh Health Servs. NHS Trust.

SCHOLES, Pauline Elizabeth Quine Manchester Road Surgery, 63 Manchester Road, Swinton, Manchester M27 5FX Tel: 0161 794 4343 Fax: 0161 736 0669 — MB ChB Manch. 1977. Socs: Fac. Fam. Plann.

SCHOLEY, Gareth Mark 74 Castle Lea, Caldicot, Newport NP26 4PJ — BM BCh Oxf. 1998; BM BCh Oxf 1998.

SCHOLEY, Julie Anne Brynderwen Surgery, Crickhowell Road, St. Mellons, Cardiff CF3 0EF Tel: 029 2079 9921 Fax: 029 2077 7740 — MB BCh Wales 1984; DRCOG 1987; MRCGP 1988.

SCHOLFIELD, David Peter Basset House, Hawksdown, Walmer, Deal CT14 7PJ — MB BS Lond. 1994.

SCHOLLER, Ingo Walter 220 Caerleon Road, Newport NP19 7GQ — MB ChB Cape Town 1990.

SCHOLTZ, Marthinus Christoffel The Annex, 67 Cupernham Lane, Romsey SO51 4LE — MB ChB Orange Free State 1995.

SCHON, Frederick Emanuel Gustav 97 Southwood Lane, London N6 5TB — MB BS Lond. 1977; PhD Camb. 1974; MRCP (UK) 1979. Cons. Neurol. Mayday Hosp. Croydon & Atkinson Morley Hosp. Wimbledon. Specialty: Neurol.

SCHONFIELD, Susan Department of Public Health, South East Regional Office, 40 Eastbourne Terrace, London W2 3QR Tel: 020 7725 2821 Fax: 020 7725 2666; 21 Wallingford Avenue, London W10 6QA Tel: 020 8969 2511 — MB BS Lond. 1983 (St. Mary's Hosp. Med. Sch. Lond.) BA Oxf. 1967; MSc Lond. 1987; MFPHM RCP (UK) 1995. Cons. (Pub. Health Med.) NHS Exec. S. E. Specialty: Pub. Health Med. Socs: Med. Wom. Federat. Prev: Sen. Regist. (Pub. Health Med.) N. Thames RHA; Hon. Regist. (Clin. Chem.) Hosp. Sick Childr. Gt. Ormond. St. Lond.; Regist. (Chem. Path.) Centr. Middlx. Hosp. Lond.

SCHOPP, Michael Jurgen 29 Solent Road, Hillhead, Fareham PO14 3LB — State Exam Med Heidelberg 1987.

SCHOTT, Geoffrey Dennis National Hospital for Neurology & Neurosurgery, Queen Square, London WC1N 3BG Tel: 020 7837 3611 Fax: 020 7419 1714 — (Camb. & Guy's) MB BChir CAmb. 1969; MD Camb. 1973, MA 1969; MRCP (UK) 1971; FRCP Lond. 1986; PhD (RCA) 1998. Cons. Neurol. Nat. Hosp. Neurol. & Neurosurg. Lond.& Roy. Nat. Orthop. Hosp. Lond. Specialty: Neurol. Socs: Assn. Brit. Neurol. & Internat. Assn. Study Pain. Prev: Sen. Regist. (Neurol.) King's Coll. Hosp. Lond. & Univ. Dept. Clin. Neurol. Nat. Hosp. Nerv. Dis. Lond.; Regist. (Neurol.) Nat. Hosp. Nerv. Dis. Lond. & Roy. Free Hosp. Lond.

SCHOTT, Jonathan Mark — MB BS Lond. 1996 (St. Mary's Hosp. Med. Sch.) BSc (Hons.) Lond. 1993; MB BS (Hons.) Lond. 1996; MRCP(UK) 1999. Clin. Research Fell. (Neurol.) Inst. Neurol. Lond. Specialty: Neurol. Prev: SHO (Neurol.) Roy. Free Hosp. Lond.; Med. SHO, Northwick Pk. Hosp.

SCHRAIBMAN, Mr Ivor Gerald (retired) 15 Beaufort Avenue, Sale M33 3WL Tel: 0161 973 7523 — MB BCh Witwatersrand 1953; FRCS Eng. 1960; FRCS Ed. 1960; MCh Witwatersrand 1970. Prev: Cons. Surg. Highfield Private Hosp. Rochdale.

SCHRAM, Catharina Maria Helena Queen's Park Hospital, Haslingden Road, Blackburn BB2 3HH Tel: 01254 687027 — Artsexamen Rotterdam 1984; MRCOG 1989; FRCOG 2001. Cons.(O & G) Blackburn, Hyndburn & Ribble Valley NHS Trust. Specialty: Obst. & Gyn. Special Interest: Feto-maternal Med. Prev: Sen. Regist. (O & G) St. Michael's Hosp. Bristol.

SCHRAM, Jennifer Ellen School Lane Surgery, Thetford IP24 2EP Tel: 01842 753115 Email: jennyschram@nhs.net — MB BS Lond. 1985 (St Thos.) DRCOG 1988; DCH RCP Lond. 1988; Dip. IMC RCS Ed. 1990; MRCGP 1991. Salaried GP Sch. La. Surg. Thetford; Clin. Tutor Camb. Grad. Course in Med.

SCHRAMM, Christopher John The Health Centre, Asher Green, Great Selford, Cambridge CB2 5EY — MB BS Tasmania 1993; DRCOG 1995; MRCGP 1998; DFFP 1999. GP Princip. Specialty: Gen. Pract. Prev: GP Regist. - Addenbrookes Hosp. Camb. VTS.

SCHRANZ, Mr Peter John Princess Elizabeth Orthopaedic Centre, Barrack Road, Exeter EX2 5DW Tel: 01392 403576 Fax: 01392 403505 — MRCS Eng. LRCP Lond. 1981; FRCS Ed. 1985; FRCS Ed. (Orth.) 1991. Cons. Orthop. Surg. Roy. Devon & Exeter Healthcare NHS Trust. Specialty: Orthop. Socs: Brit. Orthop. Assn. Prev: Cons. Orthop. RN Hosp. Haslar; Cons. Orthop. RAF; Sen. Regist. (Orthop.) Qu. Med. Centre Nottm.

SCHRECKER, Geoffrey Martin Kenneth Gleadless Medical Centre, 636 Gleadless Road, Sheffield S14 1PQ Tel: 0114 239 6475 Fax: 0114 264 2277 — MB BChir Camb. 1985; T(GP) 1981; MA Camb. 1986; MRCGP 1991. Specialty: Gen. Pract. Prev: Princip. Qu. Edith Med. Pract. Camb.

SCHREINER, Ms Annette Luise Darent Valley Hospital, Dartford DA2 8DA Tel: 01322 428 446 Fax: 01322 428 448 — State Exam Florence 1983. Specialty: Obst. & Gyn. Special Interest: Fetal Med.; Matern. Med. Socs: BMA; MDU; RSM.

SCHREUDER, Mr Frederik Brett 161 Mayals Road, Mayals, Swansea SA3 5HE; 161 Mayals Road, Mayals, Swansea SA3 5HE — MB ChB Witwatersrand 1991 (Med. Sch. Of the Univ. of Witwatersrand) FRCS (Eng) 1996. Specialist Regist. Morriston Hosp. Swansea. Specialty: Plastic Surg. Prev: Spec. Regist. Whiston Hosp. Liverp.; SHO Plastic Surg., Qu. Mary's Hosp., Roehampton.

SCHRIEBER, Victor Philip Northumberland House Surgery, 437 Stourport Road, Kidderminster DY11 7BL Tel: 01562 745715 Fax: 01562 863010; Apley House, 29 St. John's Avenue, Kidderminster DY11 6AU Tel: 01562 66457 Email: vschrieber@aol.com — MB BS Lond. 1972 (Middlx.) FRCGP 1996, M 1978. Course Organiser N. Worcs. VTS; Clin. Asst. (Rheum.) Kidderminster Health Care NHS Trust. Socs: BMA; Med. Action Global Security. Prev: Hosp. Pract. (Geriat. Med.) Kidderminster Gen. Hosp.; Regist. (Med.) Leicester Roy. Infirm. & Gen. Hosp.; SHO (Med. & Paediat.) Yeovil Dist. Hosp.

SCHROEDER, Harry Glynne (retired) Morlan Heights, 399 Redmires Road, Sheffield S10 4LE — MB ChB Birm. 1956; DA Eng. 1959; FFA RCS Eng. 1961. Cons. Anaesth. Sheff. DHA; Lect. in Clin. Anaesth. & Lect. Intens. Ther. & Resuscitat. Univ. Sheff; Lect. Sheff. Sch. Nursing. Prev: Sen. Regist. Anaesth. United Sheff. Hosps.

SCHROEDER, Kathryn Emma Maria 27 Hindsley Place, London SE23 2NF — MB BS Lond. 1989.

SCHROEDER, Ursula Elisabeth 110 Dudley Road, Manchester M16 8BR — State Exam Med Berlin 1986; State Exam Med. Berlin 1986.

SCHROVEN, Ivo Orthopaedic Department, Derbyshire Royal Infirmary, London Road, Derby DE1 2QY — MD Louvain 1988.

SCHRYER, Jeffrey Whittaker Lane Medical Centre, Daisy Bank, Whittaker Lane, Manchester M25 5EX Tel: 0161 773 1580; 18 Castleton Road, Salford M7 4GU Tel: 0161 795 4873 — MB ChB Manch. 1986; DRCOG 1989; MRCGP 1990. Specialty: Gen. Psychiat.

SCHUFF, Georg Heiner The Marlborough Family Service, 38 Marlborough Place, London NW8 0PJ — State Exam Med Berlin 1971 (Free Univ. Berlin) Dr Med Berlin 1975; MRCPsych 1978. Cons. (Psychiat.) CNWL Trust London. Specialty: Psychother. Prev: Sen. Regist. (Psychol. Med.) Hammersmith Hosp.; Regist. (Psychiat.) Maudsley Hosp. Lond.; Cons. Psychother. BKCW. Ment. Health NHS Trust.

SCHULENBURG, Mr Wilhelm Edmund 8 Upper Wimpole Street, London W1G 6LH Tel: 020 7486 2257 Fax: 020 7487 3764; 48 Stanhope Road, London N6 5AJ Tel: 020 8348 0026 — MB ChB Pretoria 1971; FRCS Eng. 1980. Cons. Ophth. Surg. Hammersmith Hosp. & Hon. Sen. Lect. Imperial Coll.; Cons. West. Ophth. Hosp. Lond. Specialty: Ophth. Socs: Roy. Soc. Med. (Counc. Mem. Ophth. Sect.).

SCHULGA, Alison 14 Batterflatts Gardens, Stirling FK7 9JU — MB ChB Ed. 1984; DCCH RCP Ed. 1989. Prev: Clin. Med. Off. Lothian HB.; GP Retainer scheme.

SCHULGA, John Department of Paediatrics, Stirling Royal Infirmary, Livilands, Stirling FK8 2AU Tel: 01786 434000 Fax: 01786 434199 Email: john.shulga@fvah.scot.nhs.uk — MB ChB Ed. 1984; MRCGP 1989; MRCPI 1992; FRCPCH 1997. Cons. Paediat. Forth Valley Acute Hosps. Trust, Stirling; Hon. Clin. Lect. in Child Health, Glas. Univ.; Hon. Cons. Paediat., Roy. Hosp. for Sick Childr., Glas. Specialty: Paediat.; Diabetes; Endocrinol. Socs: RCPCH. Prev: Sen. Regist. (Paediat.) Glas.; Research Fell. (Paediat. Endocrinol.) Glas.

SCHULLER, Ildiko Queen Mary's Hospital NHS Trust, Frognal Avenue, Sidcup DA14 6LT Tel: 0208 302 2678 Fax: 0208 308 3069 Email: ildiko.schuller@qms.nhs.uk — MB BS Lond. 1984; MRCPCH Lond. 1991; MRCP Lond. 1991; MA Lond. 1998; MSc Lond. 2001. Cons. Paediat. Specialty: Paediat.

SCHULTE, Alison Caroline 9 St Amand Drive, Abingdon OX14 5RQ — BM Soton. 1994.

SCHULTE, Anja Christina 33 Kings Quay, Chelsea Harbour, London SW10 0UX — State Exam Med Berlin 1991.

SCHULTE, Jane Frances Westgate House, Southmead Hospital, Bristol BS10 5NB — MB ChB Bristol 1981; FRCPCH; MRCP (UK) 1985. Cons. Paediat. Community Child Health North Bristol NHS Trust, Bristol. Specialty: Community Child Health.

SCHULTZ, Sabine Susanne 8 Whiterigg Court, Airdrie ML6 0RG — State Exam Med Mainz 1992.

SCHULZ, Ulrike Carola Lincluden Surgery, 53 Bellshill Rd, Glasgow G71 7PA Fax: 01698 813873 — State Exam Med Mainz 1992; MRCGP 2002. Gen. Pract. Princip. Specialty: Gen. Pract.

SCHUMAN, Andrew Nicholas New Chapel Surgery, High Street, Long Crendon, Aylesbury HP18 9AF Tel: 01844 208228 Fax: 01844 201906 Email: andrewschuman23@hotmail.com; 131 Magdalen Road, East Oxford, Oxford OX4 1RJ Tel: 01865 246393 Email: andrewschuman23@hotmail.com — MB BS Lond. 1993 (St. Thos. Hosp. Med. Sch.) BSc Lond. 1989; DRCOG 1996; DFFP 1998; MRCGP 2001. GP Locum, New Chapel Surg. Specialty: Gen. Pract. Prev: Trainee GP Angel Hill Surg. Bury St. Edmunds; SHO (Geriat. & O & G) W. Suff. Hosp. Bury St. Edmunds; SHO (Paediat.) Qu. Med. Centre Nottm.

SCHUMM, Barbara Alicia Fell Tower Medical Centre, Durham Road, Low Fell, Gateshead NE9 5EY Tel: 0191 487 6123; 57 Reid Park Road, Jesmond, Newcastle upon Tyne NE2 2ER — MB ChB Manch. 1972; MRCGP 1984.

SCHUPPLER, Philip Ernest Reinhardt Swanswell Medical Centre, 370 Gospel Lane, Acocks Green, Birmingham B27 7AL Tel: 0121 706 5676; 3 Alveley Close, Winyates W., Redditch B98 0JD — MB ChB Leeds 1982; MRCGP 1989. GP Tutor (CME) Birm. Heartlands Hosp.

SCHUR, Paul Edward Furlong Medical Centre, Furlong Road, Stoke-on-Trent ST6 5UD; Wiggo Cottage, 135 Main Road, Wynbury, Nantwich CW5 7LR — BM BCh Oxf. 1973; MA Oxf. 1973; DRCOG 1977; Cert JCC Lond. 1977; MSc Notts. 1999. Specialty: Gen. Pract. Socs: BASM.

SCHUR, Tripta Wiggo Cottage, 135 Main Road, Wybunbury, Nantwich CW5 7LR; Brookland House, 501 Crewe Road, Wistaston, Crewe CW2 6QP Tel: 01270 67250 — MB BS Rajasthan 1973 (S.M.S. Med. Coll. Jaipur) GP Chesh. Prev: SHO (Gen. Med.) Horton Gen. Hosp. Banbury.

SCHURR, Andrew Jaroslav Vlcek The Surgery, 23 The Square, Martlesham Heath, Ipswich IP5 3SL Tel: 01473 610028 Fax: 01473 610791; Pear Tree Farm, Clopton, Woodbridge IP13 6QE — MUDr Prague 1982; MRCS Eng. LRCP Lond. 1985. Trainee GP Hove. Specialty: Gen. Pract. Socs: Roy. Soc. Med. Prev: SHO (Gen. Med. & Paediat.) St. Richard's Hosp. Chichester; SHO (Cardiol.) Roy. Sussex Co. Hosp. Brighton.

SCHURR, Mr Peter Howel, CBE (retired) Brook House, High St., Ufford, Woodbridge IP13 6EQ Tel: 01394 460350 — (Camb. & Univ. Coll. Hosp.) MB BChir Camb. 1943; MRCP Eng. LRCP Lond. 1943; MA Camb. 1945; FRCS Eng. 1948. Prev: Emerit. Cons. Neurosurg. Guy's, Bethlem Roy. & Maudsley Hosps. Lond.

SCHUSTER, Raimund Orthopaedics Department, Southend Hospital, Prittlewell Chase, Westcliff on Sea SS0 0RY — State Exam Med. Munich 1992.

SCHUSTER BRUCE, Martin John Louis Critical Care Directorate, Royal Bournemouth Hospital, Castle Lane East, Bournemouth BH7 7DW — MB BS Lond. 1991 (Lond. Hosp. Med. Coll.) BSc (Hons.) Lond. 1988; MRCP (UK) 1994; FRCA 1997; Dip ICM 2000. Cons. Anaesth. and Intens. Care, Roy. Bournemouth Hosp. Specialty: Anaesth. Prev: SpR Rotation (Anaesth) Bristol; Regist. (Adult Intens. Care) Guy's Hosp. Lond.; SHO (Anaesth.) Roy. Lond. Hosp.

SCHUSTER BRUCE, Robert Maurice Charles — MB BS Lond. 1986; BSc (Hons.) Biochem. Human Dis. 1983; MRCP (UK) 1990; DRCOG 1991; MRCGP 1991; Dip Occupat. Med. 1996. Specialty: Occupat. Health. Prev: SHO Rotat. (Gen. Med.) Poole Gen. Hosp.; Ho. Phys. Char. Cross Hosp. Lond.; Ho. Surg. Roy. Hants. Co. Hosp. Winchester.

SCHUTT, Werner Heinrich (retired) 5 Grove Avenue, Coombe Dingle, Bristol BS9 2RN Tel: 0117 968 1181 Fax: 0117 968 1181; 5 Grove Avenue, Coombe Dingle, Bristol BS9 2RN Tel: 0117 968 1181 Fax: 0117 968 1181 — (Witwatersrand) MB BCh Witwatersrand 1953; DCH Eng. 1957; FRCP Ed. 1969, M 1958; FRCPCH 1997. Prev: Cons. Paediat. (Childh. Handicap.) Bristol Health Dist. (T) & Frenchay Health Dist.

SCHWAIBOLD, Mr Hartwig Bristol Urological Institute, Department of Urology, South Mead Hospital, Westbury-On-Trym BS10 5NB Tel: 0117 959 5146 Fax: 0117 959 5691 — State Exam Med Freiburg 1984; MD, Freiburg 1986; CCST Urol., Freiburg 1997. Cons. Urol. Surg., S. Mead Hosp., Bristol; Cons. Urol. Surg., Weston Gen. Hosp. Specialty: Urol. Special Interest: Andrology; Cancer. Prev: Jun. Cons. Dept. of Urol., Technical Univ. of Munich, Germany.

SCHWARTZ, Ellen Corine Institute of Ophthalmology, 11-43 Bath St., London EC1V 9EL — State Exam Med Bonn 1991; State Exam Med. Bonn 1991; MSc Lond. 1996. Specialty: Ophth.

SCHWARTZ, Jonathan Stephen St Georges Medical Centre, 7 Sunningfields Road, Hendon, London NW4 4QR Tel: 020 8202 6232 Fax: 020 8202 3906 — MB BS Lond. 1981 (Lond. Hosp.) MA Camb. 1982, BA 1978; DRCOG 1989. GP Lond. Prev: Trainee GP Borehamwood Herts.; Regist. (Gen. Med.) Newham Gen. Hosp. Lond.; SHO (Obst.) Newham Gen. Hosp. Lond.

SCHWARTZ, Martin Samuel St. George's Hospital, Department of Neurology, Atkinson Morley's Wing, Blackshaw Road, London SW17 0QT Tel: 020 8725 4632 Fax: 020 8725 4700 — MD Maryland 1965 (Univ. Maryland) MRCP (UK) 1994; FRCP Lond. 1995. Cons. Neurophysiol. Atkinson Morley's Hosp. Lond.; Hon. Cons. Neurol. St. Geo. Hosp. Lond. Specialty: Neurol.; Clin. Neurophysiol. Socs: Amer. Neurol. Assn.

SCHWARTZ, Morris The Surgery, Annie Prendergast Clinic, Ashton Gardens, Chadwell Heath, Romford RM6 6RT Tel: 020 8590 1461 & 081 599 2435 — MB BS Lond. 1945 (Char. Cross.) MRCGP 1960. Chairm. Barking & Havering LMC. Socs: Assur. Med. Soc. & Jewish Med. Soc. Prev: Maj. RAMC; Res. Obst. Off. & Ho. Surg. Gyn. Unit Char. Cross Hosp.; Res. Surg. Off. Leeds Matern. Hosp.

SCHWARTZ, Ruby Hazel Department of Paediatrics, Central Middlesex Hospital, Acton Lane, London NW10 4NS Tel: 020 8453 2121 Fax: 020 8453 2096 — MB BS Lond. 1972 (St. Geo.) DObst RCOG 1974; FRCP Lond. 1995; FRCPCH 1997. Cons. Paediat. Centr. Middlx. Hosp. Lond. Specialty: Paediat. Socs: Roy. Soc. Med.; Brit. Paediatric Neurol. Assn.; Roy. Coll. Phys.s. Prev: Sen. Regist. Northwick Pk. Hosp. Harrow & St. Chas. Hosp. Lond.; SHO (Paediat.) Hosp. Sick Childr. Gt. Ormond St.; Ho. Phys. St. Geo. Hosp. Lond.

SCHWARZ, Anthony Augustine (retired) 56 Monreith Road, Glasgow G43 2NZ — MB ChB Glas. 1950.

SCHWARZ, Professor Kurt 49 Grange Crescent, Chigwell IG7 5JD Tel: 020 8500 4815 — MB BCh Witwatersrand 1951; DPH Witwatersrand 1954; MRCP Lond. 1957; FFCM 1974; FRIPHH 1981; FFPHM 1989. Adviser & Tutor (Health Care Plann.) Univ. N. Lond. Specialty: Pub. Health Med. Socs: Fell. Roy. Soc. Med.; Vice-Pres. Internat. Federat. for Hyg. Prev. Med. & Social Med. Prev: Prof. & Head. of Dept. of Prev. & Community Med. ChristCh. Clin. Sch. Med. NZ; Hon. Cons. Canterbury Hosp. Bd. NZ.; Princip. Med. Off. Remploy.

SCHWARZ, Philip Anthony Rookwood House, Cimla Road, Neath SA11 3TL Tel: 01639 642736 — MB BS Lond. 1977 (St. Mary's) BSc Soton. 1968; MRCS Eng. LRCP Lond. 1976; FFA RCS Eng. 1982. Cons. Anaesth. Morriston Hosp. Swansea. Specialty: Anaesth. Prev: Cons. Anaesth. Neath Gen. Hosp.; Sen. Regist. (Anaesth.) Univ. Hosp. Wales Cardiff; Regist. (Anaesth.) Lond. Hosp. Whitechapel.

SCHWARZER, Andreas c/o Drive Chang, Christie Hospital, Wilmslow Road, Manchester M20 4BX — State Exam Med Leipzig 1986.

SCHWEIGER, Martin Steven 12 Montagu Place, Leeds LS8 2RG Tel: 0113 293 1604 Email: germbuster@schwefam.demon.co.uk — MB ChB Leeds 1972; DTM & H Liverp. 1981; MPH Leeds 1982; MFCM RCP (UK) 1984; FFPHM 1993; MA Leeds 1997. Cons. Communicable Dis. Control. Leeds HA; Hon. Lect. Univ. Leeds; Mem. Pub. Health Med. Enviromn. Gp. Specialty: Pub. Health Med. Socs: Med. Assn. Preven. of War; Soc. Social Med.; Leeds & W. Riding Medico-Legal Soc. Prev: Med. Adviser Rangpur Dinajpur Rehabil. Serv., Bangladesh; SHO (O & G) Airedale Gen. Hosp. Steeton; Med. Off. (Volun. Serv. Overseas) Concern Disp. Saidpur, Bangladesh.

SCHWEITZER, Mr Frank Austen Will The Guildford, Nuffield Hosp, Stirling Road, Guildford GU2 7RF Tel: 01483555860 Fax:

01483555862; Dunrozel, Farnham Lane, Haslemere GU27 1HD Tel: 01428 658301 Fax: 01428 643759 — (Guy's) MB BS Lond. 1962; MRCS Eng. LRCP Lond. 1962; FRCS Eng. 1966; MS Lond. 1972. Cons. Urol. Surg. Guildford Hosps.; Hon. Sen. Lect. Inst. Urol. Lond. Specialty: Urol. Socs: Fell. Roy. Soc. Med.; Brit. Assn. Urol. Surgs. Prev: Regional Specialist Advisor Eng.; Surg. Tutor RCS Eng.; Sen. Regist. (Urol.) & Ho. Off. Guy's Hosp. Lond.

SCHWENK, Achim Tl Coleridge Unit, North Middlesex Hospital, Sterling Way, London N18 1QX Tel: 020 8887 4236 Email: achim.schwenk@nmh.nhs.uk — State Exam Med Cologne 1987 (Med. Sch., Cologne, Germany) MD Cologne 1991; DTM & H Lond. 1997; MSc Lond. 1997. Cons. in HIV Med., N. Middlx. Hosp., Lond. Specialty: Infec. Dis.; HIV Med. Socs: RCP; BHIVA; ESCMID. Prev: Locum Cons. Infec. Diseases, Roy. Free Hosp., Lond.; Research Fell., St Georges Hosp. Med. Sch.

SCHWIGON, Sylvia Sabina Department of Psychiatry, Level 1 East, Crosshouse Hospital, Kilmarnock Road, Kilmarnock KA2 0BE — State Exam Med Kiel 1991.

SCIVIER, Annette Brookside Health Centre, Brookside Road, Freshwater PO40 9DT Tel: 01983 753433 Fax: 01983 753662 — BM Soton. 1987; DRCOG 1989; MRCGP 1991.

SCLARE, Goldwyn (retired) 58 Greenbank Crescent, Edinburgh EH10 5SW Tel: 0131 447 3752 — MB ChB Glasgow 1947 (Glas.) MD (Commend) Glas. 1959; MD Glas. 1959; FRCPath 1974, M 1963. Cons. Path. Bangour Gen. Hosp. Broxburn; Hon. Sen. Lect. (Path.) Univ. Edin. Prev: Lect. (Path.) Univ. Manch.

SCLARE, Helen Ground Floor Flat, 35 Woodford Bridge Road, Ilford IG4 5LL — MB ChB Glas. 1969; BSc Glas. 1964; Dobst RCOG Glas. 1971; DCH Eng. 1972; MRCP (U.K.) 1974.

SCLARE, Paul David 17 Rutland Avenue, Manchester M20 1JD — MB ChB Aberd. 1981.

SCOBBIE, Lisa Joanne — MB ChB Sheff. 1994.

SCOBIE, Brian Maybole Health Centre and Day Hospital, 6 High Street, Maybole KA19 7BY Tel: 01655 882278 Fax: 01655 889616; 2 Bolestyle Road, Kirkmichael, Maybole KA19 7PN — MB ChB Glas. 1976; DRCOG 1978; Dip. Pract. Dermat. Wales 1992. Med. Director, Ayr RFC. Specialty: Dermat.

SCOBIE, Mr Donald John Plane Tree, 4 Keil Crofts, Benderloch, Oban PA37 1QJ — MB ChB Glas. 1973; BSc Strathclyde 1968; FRCS Glas. 1978; FRCS Ed. 1979; FRCS Eng. 1980. Cons. Surg. Argyll & Clyde Health Bd. Specialty: Gen. Surg.

SCOBIE, Ian Neilson Diabetes Centre, Medway Maritime Hospital, Gillingham ME7 5NY Tel: 01634 830000 Fax: 01634 400484 — MB ChB Glas. 1973; MD Glas. 1988; FRCP Lond. 1995. Cons. Phys. & Endocrinol. Medway Maritime Hosp. Gillingham.; Hon. Sen. Lect. Guys, Kings and St Thomas Sch. of Med. Specialty: Gen. Med.; Diabetes; Endocrinol. Socs: Brit. Diabetic Assn.; Soc. Endocrinol. Prev: Lect. (Med.) St. Thomas's Hosp. Med. Sch. Lond.; Regist. (Gen. Med.) & Ho. Surg. Roy. Infirm. Glas.; Ho. Phys. W. Infirm. Glas..

SCOBIE, James Dinwoodie (retired) Iley Point Cottage, Keyhaven, Lymington SO41 0TR Tel: 01590 644982 Fax: 01590 644549 Email: james.scobie@btinternet.com — MB BChir Camb. 1960 (St. Bart.) MA, MB BChir Camb. 1960; FRCGP 1982, M 1975. Prev: GP Barnes Lond.

SCOBIE, Mr William Galbraith (retired) 133 Caiyside, Edinburgh EH10 7HR Tel: 0131 445 7404 Fax: 0131 445 7404 — MB ChB Glas. 1962; FRCS Ed. 1966; FRCS Glas. 1966. Prev: Cons. (Paedit. Surg.) Roy. Hosp. For Sick Childr. Edin.

SCOBLE, John Edward 38 South Park Road, London SW19 8SZ — MD Lond. 1987; MB BS 1978; MA Camb. 1979; MRCP (UK) 1980. Cons. Phys. & Hon. Sen. Lect. Kings Coll. Lond. Specialty: Nephrol. Prev: Sen. Regist. Roy. Free Hosp. Lond.; Renal Fell. Univ. Washington, St Louis, USA.

SCOBLE, Mr John Edward North Staffordshire Royal Infirmary, Princes Road, Hartshill, Stoke-on-Trent ST4 7LN — MB BS Lond. 1972; MRCS Eng. LRCP Lond. 1972; FRCS Eng. 1977; FRCR Eng. 1980. Cons. Radiother. N. Staffs. Roy. Infirm. Specialty: Oncol. Prev: Sen. Regist. (Radiotherp. & Oncol.) Velindre Hosp. WhitCh. Cardiff.

SCOFFIELD, Miss Julie Louise 6 Bloomfield Manor, 55 Abetta Parade, Belfast BT5 5LA Tel: 02890 225279 Email: juliescoffield@doctors.org.uk — MB BCh BAO Belf. 1994 (Qu. Univ. Belf.) FRCSI 1998. Specialist Regist. (Surg.)Ulster Hosp., Dundonald. Specialty: Gen. Surg. Socs: ASIT. Prev: Specialist Regist (Surg.) Roy. Vict. Hosp.; Specialist Regist.(Surg.) Craigavon Area Hosp.; Specialist Regist. (Surg.) Daisy Hill Hosp. Newry.

SCOFFINGS, Daniel James Flat 2, 324 Lordship Lane, London SE22 8LZ — MB BS Lond. 1998; MB BS Lond 1998.

SCOFFINGS, Katherine Anne — MB BS Lond. 1998.

SCOLDING, Kim Judith Penylan Surgery, 74 Penylan Road, Cardiff CF23 5SY Tel: 029 2049 8181 Fax: 029 2049 1507 — MB BCh Wales 1988; MRCGP 1992.

SCOLLAY, Gilbert 32 Brodick Avenue, Kilwinning KA13 6RL — MB ChB Ed. 1968.

SCOLLON, Derek Department of Thoracic Surgery, Hairmyres Hospital, East Kilbride, Glasgow Tel: 0141 220292; 2/5 Dalhousie Court, 42 West Graham St, Glasgow G4 9LH Tel: 0141 353 3656 — MB ChB Glas. 1994. SHO (Thoracic Surg.) Hairmyres Hosp. E. Kilbride.

SCONCE, Fiona Margaret West Norfolk PCT, St. James, Extons Road, King's Lynn PE30 5NU Tel: 01553 816200 Fax: 01553 770645; 4 Ravensway, Downham Market PE38 0DB — MB ChB St. And. 1972 (St. Andrews) T(GP) 1991; DFFP 1995. Assoc. Specialist Community Paediat., W. Norf. PCT, King's Lynn.; Family Plann. Med. Off. Specialty: Community Child Health; Family Plann. & Reproduc. Health. Prev: Staff Grade (Community Paediat.) N. W. Anglia Healthcare Trust Kings Lynn; GP Princip. N. Brink Pract. Wisbech.

SCONCE, Jonathan Charles Alexander The Howdale Surgery, 48 Howdale Road, Downham Market PE38 9AF Tel: 01366 383405 Fax: 01366 383433 — MB ChB St. And. 1972.

SCOONES, David James 1 Woodlands Walk, Stokesley, Middlesbrough TS9 5QG — MB BChir Camb. 1990; MA Camb. 1991, BA 1987; MRCPath 1997. Cons. Neuropath. Middlesbrough Gen. Hosp. Specialty: Neuropath. Prev: Sen. Regist. (Neuropath.) Newc. Gen. Hosp.; Regist. (Histopath.) Mt. Vernon & Harefield Hosps. Middlx. & Hammersmith Hosp. Lond.; SHO (Histopathol.) Qu. Eliz. Med. Centre Birm.

SCOONES, Francis Harold 83 Abbotsbury Road, London W14 8EP Tel: 020 7602 1942 — MRCS Eng. LRCP Lond. 1939 (Lond. Hosp.) FRCGP 1982, M 1953. Clin. Asst. W. Middlx. Hosp. Isleworth; JP. Socs: (Vice-Chairm.) Ealing Dist. Managem. Team; Harv. Soc.; BMA (Ex-Chairm. & Sec. Ealing Div.). Prev: Ho. Surg. Luton & Dunstable Hosp.; Asst. Med. Off. OldCh. Co. Hosp. Romford; Maj. RAMC 1940-46.

SCOOTE, Mark Cardiac Medicine, National Heart and Lung Institute, Imperial College, Dovehouse Street, London SW3 6LY — MB BS Lond. 1997.

SCOPES, Iliana 35 Deerhurst Close, Feltham TW13 7HU; 35 Deerhurst Close, Feltham TW13 7HU — Ptychio Iatrikes Thessalonika 1983.

SCORAH, Phillip John Swallownest Health Centre, Hepworth Drive, Aston, Sheffield S26 2BG Tel: 0114 287 2486 Fax: 0114 287 6045; 42 Hallam Road, Rotherham S60 3DA Tel: 01709 374393 — MB ChB Sheff. 1978.

SCORER, Harriet Jane Middleton Wyeth Consumer Healthcare, Huntercombe Lane S., Taplow, Maidenhead SL6 0PH Tel: 01628 414846 Fax: 01628 414870 — MB BS Lond. 1984; MA Camb. 1985; DRCOG 1987; Dip. Pharm. Med. RCP (UK) 1991; MFPM RCP (UK) 1993; FFPM RCP (UK) 1999. Med. Dir. Wyeth Consumer Healthcare, Maidenhead. Specialty: Pharmaceutical Medicine. Prev: Med. Servs. Manager Abbott Laborat.; Sen. Med. Adviser Abbott Laborat.; Regist. (O & G) St. Luke's Hosp. Guildford.

SCORER, Michael John Stephen (retired) The Little Wing, Loudwater House, Rickmansworth WD3 4HN Tel: 01923 776397 — MB Camb. 1958 (St. Bart.) BChir 1957.

SCORER, Rebecca Mowbray The Surgery, 1 Forest Hill Road, London SE22 0SQ Tel: 020 8693 2264 Fax: 020 8299 0200; 33 Montholme Rd, London SW11 6HX — MB BS Lond. 1984; DRCOG 1988.

SCORER, Richard Charles 163 Lake Road W., Roath Park, Cardiff CF23 5PL — MB BChir Camb. 1970 (Lond. Hosp.) MA Camb. 1970; MRCP (UK) 1972; MRCPsych 1976; DPM Eng. 1977; MSc (Hons.) Clin. Pyschother. Lond. 1985. Cons. (Psychiat.) Cardiff & Vale NHS Trust. Specialty: Gen. Psychiat. Prev: Hon. Sen. Regist. & Lect. (Psychol. Med.) Welsh Nat. Sch. Med. Cardiff; Regist. (Med.) Lond. Hosp. (Mile End); Cons. Psychiat. Llandough Hosp. & Community NHS Trust.

SCOREY, John (retired) Griffin Cottage, Woodrow, Amersham HP7 0QQ Tel: 01494 725851 — (Guy's) MB BS Lond. 1950. Prev: Med. Off. Equity & Law Life Assur. Soc. Ltd.

SCOREY, Phillipa Diana Eagle House Surgery, White Cliff Mill Street, Blandford Forum DT11 7DQ Tel: 01258 453171 — MB BS Lond. 1984 (Guy's) DRCOG 1986. GP Princip. Prev: Med. Off. 'Treads' Youth Advis. Clinic Blandford Forum; Resid. Med. Off. Roy. Newc. Hosp. NSW, Austral.; SHO Poole Gen. Hosp.

SCORGIE, Barbara McDonald The Cottage, 37 Main Road, Castlehead, Paisley PA2 6AN — MB ChB Glas. 1970; DObst RCOG 1972; FFA RCSI 1976. Cons. Anaesth. Roy. Alexandra Infirm. Paisley. Specialty: Anaesth. Prev: Sen. Regist. (Anaesth.) Vict. Infirm. Glas.; Regist. (Anaesth.) Wellington Hosp., NZ; SHO (Anaesth.) Roy. Alexandra Infirm. Paisley.

SCORGIE, Iain George Buckingham Terrace Medical Practice, 31 Buckingham Terrace, Glasgow G12 8ED Tel: 0141 221 6210 Fax: 0141 211 6232 — MB ChB Glas. 1975; DRCOG 1977; MRCGP 1979; DCH RCPS Glas. 1979.

SCOTCHER, Lilian Mary (retired) Chestnuts, Beresford Road, Goudhurst, Cranbrook TN17 1DN — MB ChB Aberd. 1951. Prev: GP Tonbridge.

SCOTCHER, Mr Stephen Michael The County Hospital, Victoria Eye Unit, Union Walk, Hereford HR1 2ER Tel: 01432 364460; Wye Valley Nuffield Hospital, Venns Lane, Hereford HR1 1DF Tel: 01432 355131 — MB ChB Bristol 1987; BSc (Hons.) Bristol 1984; MRCP (UK) 1990; FRCOphth 1993. Cons. Ophth. Surg. (Vict. Eye Unit) The Co. Hosp. Herefd. Specialty: Ophth. Special Interest: Cataract Surg.; Paediatric Ophth. & Strabismus. Prev: Specialist Regist. (Ophth.) Birm.; Exchange Regist. Brisbane, Austral.; SHO (Ophth.) Soton. Eye Hosp.

SCOTCHMAN, Frank George Vivian Garth, Welshmill Road, Frome BA11 2LA — MB BChir Camb. 1969 (St. Bart. Hosp. Lond.) MA, BChir Camb. 1968; MB Camb. 1969. Socs: Camb. Univ. Med. Soc.; Assoc. Mem. Brit. Inst. Radiol. Prev: SHO (Radiother.) Norf. & Norwich Hosp.; SHO (Radiother.) Glas. Inst. Radiother. Belvidere Hosp., West. Infirm. & Roy. Beatson Memor. Hosp.; SHO (Radiother.) Northampton Gen. Hosp.

SCOTHERN, Gillian Elizabeth 66 Ferres Way, Allestree, Derby DE3 2BB — MB ChB Leeds 1976; MRCOG 1982.

SCOTHORNE, Audrey Winifred Southerknowe, Friars Brae, Linlithgow Tel: 01506 842463 — MB ChB Leeds 1950; BSc (1st cl. Hons.) Leeds 1947, MB ChB 1950. Prev: Demonst. Anat. Univ. Glas.

SCOTHORNE, Catherine Louise Cookham Medical Centre, Lower Road, Cookham Rise, Maidenhead SL6 9HX Tel: 01628 524646 — MB Camb. 1982; MA Camb. 1983, MB 1982, BChir 1981; DRCOG 1985. Clin. Asst., Dept. Rheum., Wexham Pk. Hosp., Slought. Prev: Trainee GP Camb. VTS; SHO (Cas.) Wycombe Gen. Hosp.

SCOTHORNE, Professor Raymond John (retired) Southernknowe, Friars Brae, Linlithgow EH49 6BQ Tel: 01506 842463 — (Univs. Chicago & Leeds) FRSE; MD Chicago 1943; MB ChB (1st cl. Hons.) Leeds 1944; BSc (1st cl. Hons.) (Anat.) Leeds 1941, MD (Distinc.) 1951; FRCS Glas. 1962. Edr. (UK) Clin. Anat. Prev: Regius Prof. Anat. Univ. Glas.

SCOTLAND, Mr Alastair Duncan — MB ChB Aberd. 1975 (Univ. Aberd.) FRCS Ed. 1980; MFCM 1987; FFPHM 1993, M 1989; FRCP 1999. Specialty: Pub. Health Med. Socs: Fell. Roy. Soc. Med.; Scott. Soc. Experim. Med.; Brit. Assn. Med. Managers. Prev: Dir. Med. Educat. & Research Lond.; Cons. Pub. Health Med. NE Thames RHA; Trust Unit Med. Dir. NHS Exec. N. Thames.

SCOTLAND, Hugh William Fraser Ash Lodge Medical Centre, 73 Old Road, Chesterfield S40 2RA Tel: 01246 203138 Fax: 01246 231824; Wigley House, Wigley, Chesterfield S42 7JJ Tel: 01246 567020 — MB BS Lond. 1982 (St. Thos.) BSc (Hons.) Physiol. Lond. 1979; MRCP (UK) 1985; MRCGP 1989. Prev: Trainee GP Burton-on-Trent VTS.

SCOTLAND, Jennifer Jane 17 Marchbank Road, Bieldside, Aberdeen AB15 9DJ — MB ChB Ed. 1998; MB ChB Ed 1998.

SCOTLAND, Mr Thomas Robert 17 Marchbank Road, Bieldside, Aberdeen AB15 9DJ — MB ChB Ed. 1971; FRCS Ed. 1976. Cons. Orthop. Surg. Grampian Health Bd. Specialty: Orthop.

SCOTNEY, Amanda Jane The Granary, Back Lane, South Luffenham, Oakham LE15 9DG — MB ChB Leeds 1994.

SCOTSON, John Hector (retired) 5 Woodville Road, Altrincham WA14 2AN Tel: 0161 941 2712 — MB ChB Manch. 1956; MRCS Eng. LRCP Lond. 1957; DObst RCOG 1959; MRCGP 1974. Prev: GP Altrincham.

SCOTT, Mr Adam David Glenfield Hospital, Groby Road, Leicester LE3 9QP Tel: 0116 287 1471 — MB BS Lond. 1980 (St. Bart.) BSc (Hons.) 1976; MRCS Eng. LRCP Lond. 1980; FRCS Ed. 1985; FRCS Eng. 1986; MS Lond. 1990. Cons. Surg. Glenfield Hosp. Leicester; Clin. Lect. Univ. Leicester, Fac. Med. Specialty: Gen. Surg. Socs: Fell. Roy. Soc. Med.; Assn. Coloproctol.; Liveryman Worshipful Soc. Apoth. Prev: Lect. (Surg.) St. Bart. Univ. Lond.; Regist. (Surg.) Northampton Gen. Hosp.

SCOTT, Adrian Roy 36 George Road, West Bridgford, Nottingham NG2 7QG Tel: 0115 981 6975 — MB BS Lond. 1977 (Char. Cross) DCH RCP Lond. 1979; MRCP (UK) 1982; DM Nottm. 1988. Cons. Phys. Derby Roy. Infirm. Specialty: Diabetes; Endocrinol. Prev: Regist. Qu. Med. Centre Nottm.; Regist. Battle Hosp. Reading; Med. Off. Makiung Hosp. Tanzania.

SCOTT, Agnes Love Eastfield, Mauchline KA5 5EX Tel: 01290 50205 — MB ChB Glas. 1938; DPH 1940; FRCP Ed. 1960, M 1950; FRCPath 1963. Prev: Sen. Cons. Pathol. Roy. Infirm. Dumfries; Lect. Path. Univ. Glas.; Pathol. Roy. Infirm. Glas.

SCOTT, Ailsa Rayleigh House, Observatory, Eskdalemuir, Langholm DG13 0QW — MB ChB Ed. 1987.

SCOTT, Alan John The Health Centre, 68 Pipeland Road, St Andrews KY16 8JZ Tel: 01334 473441 Fax: 01334 466508 — MB ChB Glas. 1991; PhD Glas. 1986, BSc 1982, MB ChB 1991.

SCOTT, Alan Keith Gillygate Surgery, 28 Gillygate, York YO31 7WQ Tel: 01904 624404 Fax: 01904 651813; 15 Rawcliffe Lane, York YO30 6NP Tel: 01904 622349 — MB ChB St. And. 1963; FRCGP 1988, M 1978. Med. Adviser to York Minster & Glaziers Trust; Medico-Legal Examr. for Micrah Servs. Liverp.; for Expedia Servs. Bolton; for Medico-legal Reporting, Reading; for Doctors' Chambers, Windsor; for Albany Medico Legal, Peterlee. Socs: York Med. Soc. Prev: Med. Adviser Shepherd Building Gp.; Medico-Legal Examr. for Export Reports, Redditch; for LAB. Medico Legal Serv.s, Peterlee.; Ho. Phys. (Cardiol.) City & Co. Hosps. York.

SCOTT, Alan Richard Health and Safety Executive, The Pearson Building, 55 Upper Parliament, Nottingham NG1 6AU Tel: 0115 971 2875 Fax: 0115 971 2802 Email: alan.scott@hse.gsi.gov.uk; Nottingham Lane, Riddings, Alfreton DE55 4BT Tel: 01773 602483 — MB BS Lond. 1975 (St. Mary's) BSc (Physiol.) Lond. 1972; MRCS Eng. LRCP Lond. 1975; FFOM RCP Lond. 1993, M 1986; Specialist Accredit. Occupat. Med. JCHMT 1986. Sen. Med. Insp. Field Operats. Directorate. Health & Safety Exec.; Clin. Asst. (A & E) Univ. Hosp. Nottm. Specialty: Occupat. Health. Socs: Soc. Occupat. Med.; Nottm. Med. CH1 Soc. Prev: Lect. (Occupat. Health) Univ. Manch.; Sen. Regist. (Occupat. Med.) Brit. Coal, Boots plc. & Rolls-Royce Ltd.; Regist. (A & E Med.) Univ. Hosp. Nottm.

SCOTT, Alexander (retired) Quatrieme, Platte Saline, Alderney GY9 3XF — MB ChB Ed. 1944.

SCOTT, Alexander Douglas Alnbury, Silverdale Road, Brightons, Falkirk FK2 0TH Tel: 01324 713849 & profess. 0501 30432 — MB ChB Ed. 1962; LMCC 1964; DObst RCOG 1965; DPH Glas. 1966; DIH RCPS Glas. 1975; MFOM RCP Lond. 1978. Employm. Med. Adviser EMAS. Specialty: Occupat. Health. Socs: Soc. Occupat. Med. & Brit. Occupat. Hyg. Soc. Prev: Indust. Med. Off. Stewarts & Lloyds; Med. Off. Brit. Steel Corp. Scotl.; Med. Off. Govt. Train. Centre & Indust. Rehabil. Unit Bellshill.

SCOTT, Alexandra Jane Apartment 2, Weir Mill, 101 Mill St., East Malling, West Malling ME19 6DW — MB ChB Sheff. 1992.

SCOTT, Alexandra Kyle 9 Sunnybank Close, Whitchurch, Cardiff CF14 1EQ — MB BCh Wales 1979.

SCOTT, Aliçon Veronica (retired) 1 Highfield Drive, Upton, Macclesfield SK10 3DH Tel: 01625 618062 — MB ChB Liverp. 1955; DObst RCOG 1957; FRCOG 1980, M 1961. Prev: Cons. O & G Macclesfield Hosp. (W. Pk. & Dist. Gen. Hosp.).

SCOTT, Alison 20 Seton Place, Edinburgh EH9 2JT — MB ChB Dundee 1989; MRCOG 1994; MFFP 1995. Specialist Regist. (O & G) Roy. Infirm. Edin.; Locum Cons. Community Gynaecologist. Specialty: Obst. & Gyn. Prev: Research Regist. & SHO (O & G) Ninewells Hosp. Dundee; SHO III Aberd. Roy. Infirm.

SCOTT, Alison Margaret St. Albans Medical Group, Felling Health Centre, Stephenson Terrace, Gateshead NE10 9QG Tel: 0191 469

2316; 41 Norwich Road, Newton Hall, Durham DH1 5QA — MB BS Newc. 1973; MRCGP 1983. Occupat. Health Phys. Gateshead Gp. Hosps. Prev: Ho. Off. (Paediat. & Gen. Med.) Newc. Gen. Hosp.; SHO (Gen. Med.) Dryburn Hosp. Durh.; Regist. (Med.) Gateshead AHA.

SCOTT, Alison Marie-Louise 4 Bracklinn Road, Callander FK17 8EJ Tel: 01877 331001 Fax: 01877 331720; 3 Leighton Place, Callander FK17 8BG Tel: 01877 331725 — MB ChB Aberd. 1986; DRCOG 1992.

SCOTT, Alison Vivienne Drs Crosby, Steel, Rowe, Scott, The Ann Burrough Thomas Health Centre, South William Street, Workington CA7 8HA Tel: 01900 603985; Rosemount, Fellside, Caldbeck, Wigton CA7 8HA Tel: 016974 78674 Email: alisonscottso@hotmail.com — MB BS Lond. 1983; MRCGP 1998. GP, The Health Centre, Workington. Specialty: Pub. Health Med.; Gen. Pract. Prev: SR Pub. Health Med., N. Cumbria Health Auth.; Sen. Regist. (Community Med.) N. West. RHA.

SCOTT, Alister John 75 Clyde Road, London N22 7AD — MB ChB Aberd. 1985 (University of Aberdeen) MRCP (UK) 1988; MFOM RCP (Lond.) 1996; MBA Open Univ. 2000. Director, AON Health Solutions, Lond. Specialty: Occupat. Health.

SCOTT, Allan Ian Fraser Andrew Duncan Clinic, Royal Edinburgh Hospital, Edinburgh EH10 5HF Tel: 0131 537 6452 Fax: 0131 537 6116 Email: fiona.morrison@lpct.scot.nhs.uk — MB ChB Edin. 1980 (Edinburgh) BSc 1977; MRCPsych 1985; MPhil 1985; MD 1990; MBA 1995; FRCPsych 2003. Cons. Psychiat., Gen. Adult Psychiat., with particular Responsibil. for ECT. Specialty: Gen. Psychiat.

SCOTT, Althea Jane Department of Genitourinary Medicine, Clinic 1, Milne Centre, Bristol Royal Infirmary, Bristol BS2 8HW Tel: 0117 928 3010; Quakers Meet, Kingsweston Road, Bristol BS11 0UX Tel: 0117 982 2030 — (St. Bart.) MB BS Lond. 1962; MRCS Eng. LRCP Lond. 1962. Cons. Genitourin. Med. United Bristol Healthcare NHS Trust & Weston Area Health Trust. Specialty: Genitourinary Medicine. Socs: BMA & Med. Soc. Study VD. & AGUM. Prev: Sen. Regist. St. Thos. Hosp. Lond.; Ho. Off. St. Bart. Hosp. Lond.

SCOTT, Andrew Carr (retired) 43 Hampton Manor, Belfast BT7 3EL — MB BCh BAO Belf. 1953; DPH 1964. Prev: Med. Asst. (Geriat.) Braid Valley Hosp. Ballymena.

SCOTT, Andrew Kenneth Department of Medicine for the Elderly, Arrowe Park Hospital, Upton, Wirral CH49 5PE; 3 Fieldway, Heswall, Wirral CH60 1UP — MB ChB Aberd. 1976; MRCP (UK) 1978; BMedBiol Aberd. 1973, MD 1983; FRCP Lond. 1994. Cons. Phys. in Geriat. Med. Specialty: Care of the Elderly. Socs: Brit. Geriat. Soc.; Brit. Pharm. Soc.; Brit. Hypertens. Soc. Prev: Sen. Lect. (Geriat. Med.) Univ. Manch.; Sen. Lect. (Clin. Pharmacol.) Univ. Liverp.; Lect. (Therap. & Clin. Pharmacol.) Univ. Aberd.

SCOTT, Andrew Peter Blair (Surgery), Holman Way, Topsham, Exeter EX3 0EN Tel: 01392 874646 Fax: 01392 875261; The Coach House, Grove Hill, Topsham, Exeter EX3 0EG Tel: 01392 874296 — MB BS Lond. 1966 (Lond. Hosp.) MRCS Eng. LRCP Lond. 1966; DCH Eng. 1968; DObst RCOG 1969; DPM Eng. 1976; MRCGP 1978. Socs: Exeter Med. Soc.; (Counc.) Soc. Orthop. Med.

SCOTT, Andrew Raymond The Shrewsbury and Telford Hospital NHS trust, Head & Neck Centre, Royal Shrewsbury Hospital NHS Trust, Mytton Oak Road, Shrewsbury SY3 8XQ Tel: 01743 261499 — BM BS Nottm. 1992; FRCS Ed 1997; MPhil Keele 2003. Cons. ENT Surg. Specialty: Otorhinolaryngol. Socs: BMA; MPS; RSM.

SCOTT, Ann Armistead Child Development Centre, Broughty Ferry Rd, Dundee DD1 9SY Tel: 01382 660111 — MB ChB Dundee 1990 (Ninewells Hosp. Med. Sch. Dundee) BMSc (Hons.) Anat. Dund 1987; MRCP (UK) 1994. Paediat. Assoc. With s/i in child Developm. Specialty: Paediat. Socs: MRCP; MRCPCH.

SCOTT, Anne Ards Hospital, Church St., Newtownards BT23 4AS Tel: 028 9151 0106 — MB BCh BAO Belf. 1980; MRCPsych 1984. Cons. Psychiat. Ards Hosp. Co. Down. Specialty: Gen. Psychiat. Prev: Sen. Regist. Purdysburn Hosp. Belf.

SCOTT, Anne Marjory (retired) 9A East Mayfield, Edinburgh EH9 1SD Tel: 0131 667 6729 — MB ChB Ed. 1947; FRCS Ed. 1953. Prev: Med. Off. DHSS.

SCOTT, Anne Primrose (retired) The Old Rectory, Fornham All Saints, Bury St Edmunds IP28 6JX Tel: 01284 767177 — MB ChB Bristol 1959. Prev: GP Bury St. Edmunds.

SCOTT, Archibald Cunningham (retired) 22 Rocheid Park, Edinburgh EH4 1RU Tel: 0131 315 2720 — MD Glas. 1968; MB ChB 1955; FRCPath 1976, M 1964. Prev: Cons. Microbiol. Lothian HB.

SCOTT, Barbara The Surgery, Tennant Street, Stockton-on-Tees TS18 2AT Tel: 01642 613331 Fax: 01642 675612; Corner Ways, Brompton, Northallerton DL6 2RL — MB ChB Glas. 1977; FRCS Ed. 1981; DRCOG 1988; MRCGP 1988. Asst. Police Surg. Cleveland Constab. Prev: Surg. Arawa Gen. Hosp. North. Solomon Province, Papua New Guinea.

SCOTT, Barry Alexander St Martins Surgery, 378 Wells Road, Knowle, Bristol BS4 2QR Tel: 0117 977 5641 Fax: 0117 977 5490 — MB BS Lond. 1980 (Lond. Hosp. Med. Coll.) MRCGP 1995. GP St. Martins Surg. Bristol.

SCOTT, Betty Diana 18 Arden Road, London N3 3AN Tel: 020 8346 8531 Fax: 020 8346 8531 — (T.C. Dub.) MB BCh BAO Dub. 1944. Prev: Resid. Surg. Off. Kidderminster & Dist. Gen. Hosp.; Ho. Surg. Vict. Hosp. Blackpool; Resid. Med. Off. Finchley Memor. Hosp.

SCOTT, Brian Barry 9 Lee Road, Lincoln LN2 4BJ Tel: 01522 536829 — MRCS Eng. LRCP Lond. 1968 (St. Bart.) MD Lond. 1976, MB BS 1968; MRCP (UK) 1971; FRCP (Lond.) 1984. Cons. Phys. (Gen. Med. & Gastroenterol.) Lincoln Co. Hosp.; Clin. Teach. Nottm. Univ. Med. Sch. Specialty: Gastroenterol. Socs: Brit. Soc. Gastroenterol. & BMA. Prev: Sen. Regist. (Gen. Med.) Yorks. RHA; Research Fell. Dept. Med. Univ. Leeds; Regist. (Gen. Med. & Renal Med.) St. Jas. Hosp. Leeds.

SCOTT, Brian John The Greenlaw Practice, Northcroft Medical Centre, North Croft Street, Paisley PA3 4AD Tel: 0141 889 8465 — MB ChB Glas. 1991; MRCP (UK) 1994; MRCGP 1997; FRCGP ((by assessment)) 2003. GP Partner Greenlaw Pract., Paisley; Clin. Asst. Diabetic Centre, Gartnavel Gen. Hosp. Glas.; Clin. Tutor in Gen. Pract. Univ. of Glas.; Clin. Tutor in Communication Skills, Univ. of Glas. Specialty: Gen. Pract. Socs: Treas. - Alpha 91 Medics Year Club. Prev: SHO (Psychiat.) Gartnavel Roy. Hosp. Glas.; Med. Intern Amer. Hosp., Paris; SHO (Gen. Med.) West. Infirm. & Gartnavel Gen. Hosp. Glas.

SCOTT, Mr Brian William Dept. Orthopaedics, St James's University Hospital, Leeds LS9 7TF Tel: 0113 206 6940 — MB BS Newc. 1982; FRCS Ed. 1987; FRCS Eng. 1987; FRCS (Orth.) 1994. Cons. (Paediat. Orthop. Surg.) St James Univ. Hosp. Leeds. Specialty: Orthop.; Paediat. Socs: Brit. Orthopaedic Assn.; Fell. Roy. Coll. Surg.s.

SCOTT, Bridget Claire 8 Canon Frome Court, Canon Frome, Ledbury HR8 2TD — BM BCh Oxf. 1986.

SCOTT, Bryan Ogle (retired) 5 Dorchester Crescent, Abingdon OX14 2AH Tel: 01235 559252 — MRCS Eng. LRCP Lond. 1944 (Manch.) DPhysMed Eng. 1951; MA Oxf. 1967. Prev: Dir. & Cons. Phys. Rheum & Rehabil. Radcliffe Infirm. & Oxf. DHA.

SCOTT, Carol Marion 36 Parkstone Road, Poole BH15 2PG Tel: 01202 674344 Fax: 01202 660718; 14 Spur Hill Avenue, Lower Parkstone, Poole BH14 9PH Tel: 01202 731925 — MB ChB Ed. 1980 (Edin. Univ.) DRCOG 1986. GP.

SCOTT, Caroline Gillianne 6 Slades View Close, Diggle, Oldham OL3 5PE — MB ChB Leeds 1995.

SCOTT, Carolyn Angwin The Medical Centre, Forest, St Mary Church, Torquay TQ1 4QX Tel: 01803 325128 Email: carolyn.scott@gp-l83063.nhs.uk — (Lond. Hosp.) BA Camb. 1975; MB BChir Camb. 1979; DRCOG 1980; MRCGP 1982. Specialty: Gen. Pract.

SCOTT, Catherine Anne Turkey Cottage, Old Vicarage Lane, Sutton, Spalding PE12 9LU — MB BS Lond. 1992.

SCOTT, Catherine Jane Milton Surgery, 132 Mountcastle Drive South, Edinburgh EH15 3LL — MB ChB Ed. 1980; BA Hons. 1974; MRCGP 1988. GP Edin.

SCOTT, Cedric Mathieson, TD 9 Front Street, West Auckland, Bishop Auckland DL14 9HW Tel: 01388 832352 — MB BS Durh. 1949; MRCGP 1977. Med. Examr. MoD. Prev: Regional Med. Off. DoH; GP Co. Durh.

SCOTT, Charles Cameron 29 Trafalgar Road, Birkdale, Southport PR8 2HF — MB ChB Aberd. 1971; FFA RCS Eng. 1979. Cons. (A & E Med.) Southport Gen. Infirm. Specialty: Accid. & Emerg. Prev: Sen. Regist. (A & E) Yorks. RHA; Regist. (Anaesth.) Coventry AHA.

SCOTT, Charlotte Helene Rennie Roundal, Kinsteary, Auldearn, Nairn IV12 5HZ — MB ChB Aberd. 1997.

SCOTT, Christina Sui-Lin (retired) 8 Regents Drive, Keston, Bromley BR2 6BU Tel: 01689 51542 Fax: 01689 855512 Email: suiscott@classicfm.net — MB ChB Bristol 1967; FFA RCS Eng. 1974. Prev: Cons. (Anaesth.) Croydon Health Dist.

SCOTT, Christine Angela Downside, 48 Harnwood Road, Salisbury SP2 8DB Tel: 01722 336894 — MB BS Lond. 1969 (King's Coll. Hosp.) MRCS Eng. LRCP Lond. 1969; FRCPath 1988, M 1977. Cons. Dept. Path. Salisbury Dist. Hosp. Specialty: Histopath. Prev: Sen. Regist. Dept. Path. Roy. United Hosp. Bath; Regist. Dept. Path. Glas. Roy. Infirm.; Ho. Surg. Kilmarnock Infirm.

SCOTT, Christine Susan 9 Windsor Road, Teddington TW11 0SG — MB BS Newc. 1981; DCH RCP Lond. 1984; DCCH RCP Ed. 1984; MRCGP 1985; DRCOG 1985. Specialty: Gen. Pract.

SCOTT, Christopher Donald Queen Elizabeth Hospital, Sheriff Hill, Gateshead NE9 6SX Tel: 0191 487 8989 Email: christopher.scott@ghnt.nhs.uk — MD Manch. 1993; MB ChB 1984; MRCP (UK) 1990. Cons. Cardiol. & Gen. Med. Qu. Eliz. Hosp. Gateshead. Specialty: Cardiol. Prev: Research Regist. (Transpl.) Freeman Hosp. Newc.; 1st Asst. (Cardiol.) Univ. Newc. u. Tyne; Regist. (Cardiol.) Northwick Pk. Hosp.

SCOTT, Christopher John 1 Coverdale Drive, Scarborough YO12 5TP — MB ChB Leeds 1991.

SCOTT, Christopher John Woodend Hospital, Eday Road, Aberdeen AB15 6XS Tel: 01224 663131 Fax: 01224 404019; 51 Forest Road, Aberdeen AB15 4BN Tel: 01224 645886 — MB BS Newc. 1968; MRCP (UK) 1972; FRCP Ed. 1985; FRCP Lond. 1987; MBA Aberd. 1996; MBA 1997. Cons. Phys. (Geriat. Med. & Rehabil.) Woodend Hosp. Aberd. Specialty: Gen. Med.; Rehabil. Med. Socs: BMA; Brit. Assn. Med. Managers; Brit. Geriat. Soc. Prev: Sen. Regist. Longmore Hosp. Edin.; Regist. (Gen. Med.) Deaconess Hosp. Edin.; Ho. Phys. Hexham Gen. Hosp.

SCOTT, Christopher Linton Exmouth Health Centre, Claremont Grove, Exmouth EX8 2JF Tel: 01395 273001 Fax: 01395 273771 — MSc Birm. 1975, MB ChB 1980; DCH RCP Lond. 1984; MRCGP 1985; DRCOG 1986; DA (UK) 1990.

SCOTT, Claire Elizabeth 49 Kingsdale Park, Belfast BT5 7BZ — MB BCh BAO Belf. 1996.

SCOTT, Clifford Graham Jenner Health Centre, Turners Lane, Whittlesey, Peterborough PE7 1EJ Tel: 01733 203601 Fax: 01733 206210 — BM BCh Oxf. 1975; BA Oxf. 1972.

SCOTT, Colin Andrew The Health Centre, Dunning Street, Stoke-on-Trent ST6 5BE Tel: 01782 425834 Fax: 01782 577599 — MB BS Lond. 1986; DCCH RCP Ed. 1989; MRCGP 1990; Dip Palliat Med Card. 2002.

SCOTT, Colin Russell Medical Centre, 12 High Street, Fochabers IV32 7EP Tel: 01343 820247 Fax: 01343 820132 — MB ChB Dundee 1974.

SCOTT, Colin William David Pease Way Medical Centre, 2 Pease Way, Newton Aycliffe DL5 5NH — MB ChB Aberd. 1988; MRCGP 1995; DRCOG 1995; MSc Bath Univ. 2001. Specialty: Gen. Pract.; Sports Med.

SCOTT, Colin Wilson St Paul's Medical Centre, Dickson Road, Blackpool FY1 2HH Tel: 01253 623896 Fax: 01253 752818 — MB ChB Manch. 1989; MRCGP 1993. Prev: Trainee GP Lancs. VTS.

SCOTT, Daniel 59 Morris Lank, Kirkstall, Leeds LS5 3JD — MB ChB Leeds 1995.

SCOTT, Daphne Margaret Riverside Surgery, George Street, High Wycombe HP11 2RZ Tel: 01494 526500 Fax: 01494 450237; 64 Seeleys Road, Beaconsfield HP9 1TB Tel: 01494 676938 — MB BS Lond. 1965 (Roy. Free) MRCS Eng. LRCP Lond. 1965; DObst RCOG 1968; MRCGP 1980. Prev: SHO (Obst.) Perivale Matern. Hosp.; SHO (Paediat.) Preston Hosp. N. Shields; Ho. Surg. (Orthop.) Roy. Free Hosp. Lond.

SCOTT, Daphne Mary (retired) Fairbrook, Chichele Road, Oxted RH8 0AG Tel: 01883 714022 — MB ChB St. And. 1943; MRCP Lond. 1948; FRCS Eng. 1953. Prev: Med. Off. Family Plann. Assn. Clinics Croydon & Oxted.

SCOTT, David Gilbert 3 Malborough Court, Church Hill, Washingborough, Lincoln LN4 1EN Tel: 01522 791867 — MB BS Lond. 1954 (Westm.) MRCS Eng. LRCP Lond. 1954; MRCGP 1965.

SCOTT, Professor David Gordon Islay 443 Unthank Road, Norwich NR4 7QN Tel: 01603 259389 Fax: 01603 504101 — MB ChB Bristol 1973; MRCP (UK) 1977; MD Bristol 1982; FRCP Lond. 1994. Cons. Rheum. Norf. & Norwich University Hospital NHS Trust; Hon. Prof. Sch. of Med., Health Policy & Pract., Univ. of E. Anglia. Specialty: Rheumatol. Socs: Pres. Brit. Soc. For Rhuematology (2002-4). Prev: Cons. Rheum. Norf. & Norwich Health Care NHS Trust; Hon. Sen. Lect. (Rheum.) Roy. Lond. Hosp. Med. Coll. & Univ. E.Anglia; Lect. (Rheum.) Univ. Birm.

SCOTT, David Henry Thomson Royal Infirmary of Edinburgh, Department of Anaesthetics, Little France, Edinburgh EH16 4SU Tel: 0131 242 3188; 11 Granby Road, Edinburgh EH16 5NP Tel: 0131 667 4645 — MB ChB Ed. 1972; BSc Ed. 1969; FRCA 1976. Cons. Anaesth. Roy. Infirm. Edin. Specialty: Anaesth.; Intens. Care. Socs: Scott. Soc. Anaesth.; Assn. Cardiothoracic Anaesths.; Founding Mem. Expert Wittness Inst. Prev: Lect. Univ. Edin.; Research Fell. (Anaesth.) Roy. Infirm. Edin.

SCOTT, David John 16 Woodbine Avenue, Gosforth, Newcastle upon Tyne NE3 4EU — MB BS Durh. 1965; MRCPath 1972. Cons. Path. Newc. Gen. Hosp. & Roy. Vict. Infirm. Newc. Specialty: Pathology, General. Prev: Sen. Regist. (Path.) Newc. Gen. Hosp.

SCOTT, David John 39 The Spinney, Moortown, Leeds LS17 6SP — MB BS Newc. 1989; MRCP (UK) 1992. Regist. (Chest & Gastroenterol. Med.) Newc. u. Tyne. Specialty: Gastroenterol.

SCOTT, David John East Sussex Hospitals NHS Trust, Conquest Hospital, The Ridge, St Leonards-on-Sea TN37 7RD Tel: 01424 758049 Fax: 01424 757050 Email: david.scott@esht.nhs.uk; Rose Mount, 15 Laton Road, Hastings TN34 2ES Tel: 01424 442455 Fax: 01424 716007 Email: david@rose-mount.co.uk — MB BChir Camb. 1974 (Guy's) MB Camb. 1975, BChir 1974; MRCP (UK) 1976; DCH Eng. 1980; FRCP Lond. 1994; FRCPCH 1997, M 1996; MBA Keele 2000. Med. Dir. & Cons. Paediat. E. Sussex Hosps. NHS Trust; Hon. Cons. Paediat. Guy's Hosp. Lond. Specialty: Paediat. Socs: Fell. Roy. Soc. Med.; BMA. Prev: Cons. Paediat. RAF Hosp. Wegberg BFPO 40; Hon. Sen. Regist. (Paediat.) Brompton Hosp. & Guy's Hosp. Lond.

SCOTT, Mr David Julian Ashbridge Vascular Laboratory, Lincoln Wing, St James's Hospital, Beckett St., Leeds LS9 7TF Tel: 0113 206 5404 Fax: 0113 206 6746 — MB ChB Leic. 1981; FRCS Ed. 1985; FRCS Eng. 1986; MD Leic. 1991. p/t Cons. Vasc. Surg. St. Jas. Univ. Trust Hosp. Leeds; Examr., Europ. Bd. of Vasc. Surg.; Liason Mem. SAC Wales; Chairm. Educat. and Train. Comm. . VSSGBI; Examr. Roy. Coll. of Surgeons, Eng. Specialty: Surgery, Vascular. Special Interest: Abdom. Aortic Aneurysm; Varicose Veins; Peripheral Vasc. Dis. Socs: VSSGBI; ASSGBI; ESVS. Prev: Coll. Tutor, RCS Eng., Lond.; Comm. Mem. SRS; Director of Educat., Yorks. Sch. of Surg.

SCOTT, David Lindsay (retired) Ravelstone, Manley, Frodsham WA6 9ED Tel: 01928 740376 — MRCS Eng. LRCP Lond. 1942 (Lond. Hosp.) DA RCPSI 1948; FFA RCSI 1960. Indep. Hypnother. Chesh. Prev: Cons. Anaesth. Whiston & St. Helens Hosps.

SCOTT, Professor David Lloyd Kings College Hospital, Department of Rheumatology, Denmark Hill, London SE5 9RS Tel: 020 7346 1731 Fax: 020 7346 6475; Copperfield, 13 Ormonde Rise, Buckhurst Hill IG9 5QQ Tel: 020 8505 0175 — MB ChB (Hons.) Leeds 1975; MRCP (UK) 1978; BSc (Hons.) Leeds 1972, MD (Distinc.) 1982; FRCP Lond. 1990. Prof. Clin. Rheum. King's Coll. Hosp. Lond.; Hon. Cons. Rheum. King's Coll. Hosp. Lond. Specialty: Rheumatol. Socs: Brit. Soc. Rheum.; Roy. Soc. for Med. Prev: Reader (Rheum.) The Med. Coll. of St Batholomew's Hosp. Lond.; Lect. Rheum. Research Wing The Med. Sch. Birm.

SCOTT, Deborah Jane 6 King Charles Close, Willerby, Hull HU10 6LQ — MB ChB Leic. 1999.

SCOTT, Debra Ann c/o Medical Centre BFPO 47 — MB BS Tasmania 1989.

SCOTT, Debra Jayne 11 Beatty Close, Derriford, Plymouth PL6 6LJ — (Bristol) MB ChB Bristol 1987; DRCOG 1989; DCH RCP Lond. 1990; Cert. Family Plann. JCC 1990; MRCGP 1991; T(GP) 1991. GP Retainer Plymouth. Prev: Regist. Emerg. Dept. Concord Hosp. Sydney Austral.

SCOTT, Diana Margaret (retired) Cyprus Cottage, Broadway, Harwell, Didcot OX11 0HF Tel: 01235 221031 — MB BS Lond. 1950 (Roy. Free) MRCS Eng. LRCP Lond. 1950. Prev: Ho. Surg. Roy. Free Hosp. Lond.

SCOTT, Donald Fletcher (retired) 3 Weigall Rd, Lee, London SE12 8HE — MB ChB Ed. 1957; FRCP Lond. 1977, M 1960; MRCP Ed. 1960; DPM Lond. 1963. Prev: Cons. i/c EEG Dept. Lond. Hosp.

SCOTT, Dorothy Lilian (retired) Cringles, 130 Dynevor Road, Skewen, Neath SA10 6TH Tel: 01792 812106 — MB ChB Leeds 1948. Div. Med. Off. Brit. Red Cross Soc. Prev: Ho. Phys. St. Jas. Hosp. Leeds.

SCOTT, Edward Rupert 16 Livingstone Road, Portswood, Southampton SO14 6WN — BM Soton. 1998.

SCOTT, Elaine Christine Pentland Medical Centre, 44 Pentland View, Currie EH14 5QB Tel: 0131 449 2142 Fax: 0131 451 5855; 517 Lanark Road, Juniper Green EH14 5DQ Tel: 0131 453 3530 — MB ChB Ed. 1986; MRCGP 1990; DRCOG 1990. Specialty: Gen. Med. Prev: Trainee GP DunbLa. VTS; SHO (O & G) Falkirk Dist. Roy. Infirm.; SHO (Psychiat.) Livingston.

SCOTT, Miss Elaine Margaret Dept. of Obstetrics & Gynaecology, Royal Free Hospital, Pond St, London NW3 2QG Tel: 020 7794 0500 — MB BS Lond. 1984 (University College London) MD Lond. 1991; MRCOG 1993; CCST 1997. Cons./Hon. Sen. Lect. In Obst., Roy. Free Hosp. NHS Trust, Lond. Specialty: Obst. & Gyn. Socs: Roy. Soc. Med.; Brit. Matern. & Fetal Med. Soc.; Brit. Soc. Psychosomatic. Prev: Sen. Regist. Qu. Charlotte's Hosp. Goldhawk Rd, Lond.; Sen. Regist. Rotat. (O & G) Luton & Dunstable Hosp. NHS Trust & St. Mary's Hosp. Lond.; Clin. Lect. (O & G) Addenbrooke's Hosp. Camb.

SCOTT, Eleanor Margaret Academic Unit of Molecular Vascular Medicine, 6th Floor, Martin Wing, The General Infirmary, Leeds LS1 3EX; 30 Dam Lane, Saxton, Tadcaster LS24 9QF — BM BS Nottm. 1992 (Nottingham) BMedSci Nottm. 1990; MRCP (UK) 1995; MD Leeds 2000. Specialist Regist. Diabetes/Endocrinol/Gen. Med. St James Univ. Hosp. Leeds; Research Regist., St. James Univ. Hosp., Leeds; Sen. Lect. in Med.; Cons. in Diabetes and Endochrinology. Specialty: Diabetes. Socs: Brit. Diabetic Assn.; Brit. Endocrine Soc.; Roy. Coll. Phys. Prev: SHO (Med.) York Dist. Hosp.

SCOTT, Eleanor Roberta Moorfield, Ferry Road, Dingwall IV15 9QS Tel: 01349 863313; 8 Culcairn Road, Evanton, Dingwall IV16 9YT Tel: 01349 830388 Fax: 01349 830599 Email: eleanorsco@aol.com — MB ChB Glas. 1974; DCCH RCP Ed. 1986. SCMO Community Child Health Dingwall. Specialty: Community Child Health.

SCOTT, Elisabeth Beatrice Maria Cotlands, Horsham Road, Cowfold, Horsham RH13 8AH — MB ChB Bristol 1991.

SCOTT, Elizabeth Agnes Joyce 38 Queen's Crescent, Edinburgh EH9 2BA Tel: 0131 667 8417 Fax: 0131 667 8417 — MB ChB St. And. 1956. Mem. Disabil. Appeals Tribunal; Mem. Social Security Appeals Tribunal. Socs: GP Writers Assn. Prev: Sen. GP Edin.

SCOTT, Elizabeth Aline North Hall Moor, Shipton Lane, Wiggington, York YO32 2RQ — MB BS Lond. 1982; MSc Lond. 1987, MB BS 1982; MFCM 1988; FFPHM 1997. Dir. of Pub. Health Leeds HA; Hon. Sen. Clin. Lect. Univ. Leeds. Specialty: Pub. Health Med. Prev: Cons. Pub. Health Med. Yorks. Health.; Cons. Pub. Health Med. SW Herts DHA; Trainee (Community Med.) N.W. Thames RHA.

SCOTT, Elizabeth Amanda 96 East Street, Olney MK46 4DH — MB BS Lond. 1998; MB BS Lond 1998.

SCOTT, Elizabeth Anne Harvey Health Centre, Bank Street, Cupar KY15 4JN Tel: 01334 653478 Fax: 01334 657305; Ryvoan, 6 Hays Road, Newport-on-Tay DD6 8SJ — MB ChB Dundee 1976. Specialty: Gen. Pract.

SCOTT, Else Jane Beech Tree Surgery, 68 Doncaster Road, Selby YO8 9AJ — MB ChB Liverp. 1985.

SCOTT, Ewan Gilchrist Ca'd'Oro, Schlumberger, Gordon Street, Glasgow Tel: 0141 227 2300 Email: Escott@slb.com; 8 Atholl Place, Edinburgh EH3 8HP Tel: 0131 539 6136 Email: ewanscott@blueyonder.co.uk — MB ChB Ed. 1976; BSc Ed. 1973; DMRT Ed. 1982; DOccMed 2001. Occ. Health; Occupational Health Phys. Lothian Health OHS Astley Ainslie Hosp. Edin. Specialty: Occupat. Health. Socs: Soc. Occ. Med.

SCOTT, Fiona Margaret Dept. of Haemat., NineWells Hospital, Dundee — MB ChB Ed. 1984 (Univ. of Edin.) MRCP Edin 1987; MD 1997; MRCPath 1997. Cons. haematologist, Dept. of Haemat., Ninewells Hosp., Dundee. Specialty: Haematology. Special Interest: Blood Transfus.

SCOTT, Fiona Rosemary Department of Histopathology, Mount Vernon Hospital, Rickmansworth Road, Northwood HA6 2RN Tel: 01923 844210 Fax: 01923 844067 — MB ChB Leic. 1988 (Leicester Medical School) BSc (Med. Sci.) Leic. 1985; MRCPath 1997. Cons. Histopath. W.Herts NHS Trust. Specialty: Histopath. Socs: Assn. Clin. Path.; IAP. Prev: Regist. (Histopath.) Roy. Free Hosp.

SCOTT, Freya Elizabeth Hall Floor Flat, 10 Durdham Park, Redland, Bristol BS6 6XA — MB BS Newc. 1997.

SCOTT, Mr Gareth Orthopaedic Department, Royal London Hospital, Whitechapel, London E1 1BB Tel: 020 7377 7000; 54 Priests Lane, Brentwood CM15 8BY Tel: 01277 261841 — MB BS Lond. 1979 (Middlx.) FRCS Eng. 1985; FRCS Ed. 1985. Cons. Orthop. Roy. Lond. Hosp. Whitechapel; Hon. Sen. Lect. St. Bart & Roy. Lond. Sch. of Med. & Dent. Specialty: Orthop. Socs: Fell. BOA; Roy. Soc. Med. Prev: Sen. Regist. (Orthop.) Roy. Lond. Hosp., Roy. Nat. Orthop. Hosp. & Black Notley +Hosp.

SCOTT, Geoffrey Burnett (retired) Seaview House, 1 Loirston Road, Cove Bay, Aberdeen AB12 3NT — MB ChB Aberd. 1955; FRCPath 1976, M 1964. Prev: Sen. Lect. in Path. Univ. Aberd.

SCOTT, Geoffrey Laurence Department of Haematology, Bristol Royal Infirmary, Bristol BS2 8HW Tel: 0117 928 2655 Fax: 0117 928 2531; Quakers Meet, Kingsweston Road, Bristol BS11 0UX Tel: 0117 982 2030 — MB BChir Camb. 1962 (St. Bart.) FRCP Lond. 1979, M 1964; MD Camb. 1972. Cons. Clin. Haemat. United Bristol Healthcare Trust & Weston Healthcare Trust; Clin. Lect. Univ. Bristol. Specialty: Haematology. Socs: Brit. Soc. Haematol.; BMA. Prev: Sen. Lect. & Hon. Cons. (Haemat.) St. Thos. Hosp. Lond.; Regist. (Med.) & Ho. Phys. St. Bart. Hosp. Lond.

SCOTT, Geoffrey Malcolm Sikes 300 Earlsfield Road, London SW18 3EH Tel: 020 8874 9594 Fax: 020 7388 8514 — MB BS Lond. 1972 (Roy. Free) MRCS Eng. LRCP Lond. 1972; MRCP (UK) 1974; DTM & H Liverp. 1979; MD Lond. 1984; FRCPath 1996, M 1985; FRCP Lond. 1995. Cons. Microbiol. Univ. Coll. Hosp. Lond. & Lond. Sch. Hyg. Trop. Med.; Hon. Sen. Lect. UCL. Specialty: Med. Microbiol. Socs: Fell. Roy. Soc. Med.; Hosp. Infec. Soc.; BSAC. Prev: Scientif. Staff Div. Communicable Dis. MRC Clin. Research Centre & Hon. Sen. Regist. (Med. & Infec. Dis.) Northwick Pk. Hosp. Lond.; Regist. (Med.) Westm. Hosp. Lond.

SCOTT, George Walter Pantiles, Wilderness Road, Chislehurst BR7 5EZ Tel: 020 8467 5344 Email: scottpantiles@aol.com — MRCS Eng. LRCP Lond. 1949 (Guy's) MD Lond. 1952, MB BS 1949; FRCP Lond. 1968, M 1953. Cons. Phys. Emerit. Specialty: Gen. Med.; Respirat. Med. Socs: Fell. Thoracic Soc.; Fell. Assur. Med. Soc. Prev: Clin. Tutor & Med. Regist. Guy's Hosp.

SCOTT, Gillian Cwmfelin Medical Centre, 298 Carmarthen Road, Swansea SA1 1HW Tel: 01792 653941 — MB BS Lond. 1961 (Middlx.) DCH Eng. 1965; DObst RCOG 1966; MRCP (U.K.) 1971. GP Partner GP Cwmfelin Med. Centre Swansea. Specialty: Gen. Pract.

SCOTT, Gillian Kenmore Medical Centre, 60-62 Alderley Road, Wilmslow SK9 1PA Tel: 01625 532244 Fax: 01625 549024 — MB ChB Leic. 1988; DRCOG 1990.

SCOTT, Gillian Anne Mitchell and Partners, New Chapel Surgery, High Street, Aylesbury HP18 9AF Tel: 01844 208228 Fax: 01844 201906; 76 Sheerstock, Haddenham, Aylesbury HP17 8EX Tel: 01844 290860 — BM BS Nottm. 1984; MRCGP 1988.

SCOTT, Gillian Rachel Richmond Medical Centre, 462 Richmond Road, Sheffield S13 8NA — MB ChB Sheff. 1986; MRCGP 1990; DRCOG 1990; DFFP 2003. Specialty: Gen. Pract.

SCOTT, Gordon Wychwood Surgery, 62 High Street, Milton-under-Wychwood, Chipping Norton OX7 6LE Tel: 01993 830260 Fax: 01993 831867; The Doctors House, Shipton-under-Wychwood, Oxford OX7 6BQ Tel: 01993 830144 — MB Camb. 1970; BChir 1969.

SCOTT, Gordon James Luson Surgery, Fore Street, Wellington, Taunton TA21 8AB Tel: 01823 662836 Fax: 01823 660955 — MB BS Lond. 1976 (Lond. Hosp.) DRCOG 1978; Cert. Family Plann. 1981.

SCOTT, Gordon James Clelland Sighthill Health Centre, 380 Calder Road, Edinburgh EH11 4AU Tel: 0131 5377070; 79 Camus Avenue, Edinburgh EH10 6QY Tel: 0131 445 2529 — MB ChB Aberd. 1982 (Aberdeen) DCCH RCP Ed. 1986; MRCGP 1987. Specialty: Gen. Pract.

SCOTT, Gordon Robertson Department of Genitourinary Medicine, Lauriston Building, Edinburgh Royal Infirmary, Lauriston Place, Edinburgh EH3 9YW Tel: 0131 536 2103 Fax: 0131 536 2110; 26 Cherry Tree Gardens, Balerno EH14 5SP — MB ChB Ed.

1979; BSc (Med. Sci.) 1976; MRCP (UK) 1984; FRCP Ed. 1993. Cons. Genitourin. Med. Edin. Roy. Infirm. Specialty: Genitourinary Medicine.

SCOTT, Graham Alexander (retired) 5 EILDONBANK, EILDON, Melrose TD6 9HH Tel: 01895 824774 — MB ChB Ed. 1950, DPH 1957; FRCP Ed. 1979, M 1978; FFCM 1978. Prev: Dep. Chief Med. Off. Scott. Home & Health Dept.

SCOTT, Graham Ramsay Herd Prestonpans Health Centre, Preston Road, Prestonpans EH32 9QS Tel: 01875 810736 Fax: 01875 812979; 16 Kings Park, Longniddry EH32 0QL — MB ChB Dundee 1976.

SCOTT, Mr Gregor Ivan Department of Gynaecology, Leighton Hospital, Crewe Tel: 01270 612175 Fax: 01270 612176; Highlands, Crewe Road, Wistaston, Crewe CW2 6PS Tel: 01293 416604 — MB BS Lond. 1978 (St. Bart.) MRCOG 1986; FRCOG 1998. Cons. O & G Mid Chesh. Hosps. Trust. Specialty: Obst. & Gyn. Socs: Fell. Roy. Soc. Med.; Fell. North. Gyn. Soc.; Brit. Fertil. Soc. Prev: Sen. Regist. Westm. Hosp. Lond.; Research Regist. (Urodynamics) St. Bart. Hosp. Lond.; RMO Qu. Charlotte's Matern. Hosp. Lond.

SCOTT, Hazel R. Wishaw General Hospital, 50 Netherton St, Wishaw ML2 0DP Tel: 01698 366076 — MB ChB Glas. 1988; FRCP Glas 1998. Director Med. Educat. LAHT; Cons. Phys. Wishaw Hosp. Lanarksh.. Specialty: Gen. Med.; Respirat. Med. Prev: Postgrad.Tutor.

SCOTT, Heather Wynne Bethesda Medical Centre, Palm Bay Avenue, Cliftonville, Margate CT9 3NR Tel: 01843 209300 Fax: 01843 209301 — MB BS Lond. 1983; DRCOG 1985; DCH RCP Lond. 1985; MRCGP 1987. Prev: Med. Dir. U.S.P.G. Mission Hosp. Tanzania.; SHO (Paediat.) Gloucester Roy. Hosp.; SHO (Obst.) Addenbrooke's Hosp. Camb.

SCOTT, Helen Mary Bridgegate Surgery, 43 Bridgegate, Retford DN22 7UX Tel: 01777 702381; Forge Cottage, Town St., Askham, Newark NG22 0RS Tel: 01777 838028 — BM BS Nottm. 1996 (Nottingham) MRCGP 2000. Gen. Practitioner, Retford. Specialty: Gen. Pract. Prev: GP Regist., Lincoln.

SCOTT, Helena Clare Fenella Department of Anaestetics, 2nd Floor New Guy's House, Guy's Hospital, London SE1 Tel: 020 7955 4051 Email: hcfscott@hotmail.com — MB BChir Camb. 1988 (St. Mary's) FRCA 1993. Cons.(Anaesth) Guys Hosp. Londr. Specialty: Anaesth. Prev: Sen. Regist. (Anaesth.) St. Mary's Hosp. Lond.; Sen. Regist. (Anaesth.) Qu. Eliz. II Hosp. Welwyn Garden City; Regist. (Anaesth.) Edgware, Northwick Pk. & Hammersmith Hosps. Lond.

SCOTT, Hilary Marion West Suffolk Hospital NHS Trust, Hardwick Lane, Bury St Edmunds IP33 2QZ Tel: 01284 713748; The Gables, Rattlesden Road, Drinkstone, Bury St Edmunds IP30 9TL — MB BS Lond. 1967 (Guy's) FRCPCh; MRCS Eng. LRCP Lond. 1967; MRCP (UK) 1970; FRCPC 1976; FRCP Lond. 1989. Cons. Paediat. W. Suff. Hosp. Bury St. Edmunds. Specialty: Paediat. Special Interest: Epilepsy; Neonatology. Socs: Neonat. Soc.; Internat. Child Health. Prev: Sen. Regist. (Paediat.) Addenbrooke's Hosp. Camb.; Assoc. Resid. Hosp. Sick Childr. Toronto, Canada.

SCOTT, Howard Alan (retired) Newburn House, Newburn, Newcastle upon Tyne NE15 8LN Tel: 0191 267 1890 — MB BS Durh. 1946 (Newc.) Med. Off. Hexham Racecourse; Mem. Med. Bd. DSS. Prev: GP Newc.

SCOTT, Mr Humphrey James Mutton Farm House, Horsham Road, Abinger Hammer, Dorking RH5 6PW — MB BS Lond. 1983; FRCS Eng. 1987; MS Lond. 1991. Cons. Surg. (Gen. & Colorectal Surg.) St. Peter's Hosp. Chertsey. Specialty: Gen. Surg. Socs: Roy. Soc. Med.; Assn. Coloproctol.; Assn. Endoscopic Surgs. Prev: Sen. Regist. (Gen. Surg.) NW Thames RHA.; RSO St. Mark's Hosp. Lond.

SCOTT, Ian Gerard 17 Hillary Crescent, Liverpool L31 6BL — MB ChB Liverp. 1992.

SCOTT, Ian Graham Southside Road Surgery, 43 Southside Road, Inverness IV2 4XA Tel: 01463 710222 Fax: 01463 714072; Blar-Nan-Craubh, Lentran, Inverness — MB ChB Aberd. 1979; DRCOG 1981.

SCOTT, Mr Ian Hetherington Kenneth Ipswich Hospital NHS Trust, Heath Road, Ipswich IP4 5PD Tel: 01473 703507 Fax: 01473 702091; Three Corners, Witnesham, Ipswich IP6 9HZ Tel: 01473 785134 — MB BChir Camb. 1970 (Camb. & Guy's) FRCS Eng. 1975; MA Camb. 1972, MChir 1984. Cons. Coloproctol. Ipswich; Med. Dir. Ipswich Hosp. NHS Trust. Specialty: Gen. Surg. Prev: Cons. Surg. Ipswich Hosp.; Sen. Regist. (Gen. Surg.) Addenbrooke's Hosp. Camb.

SCOTT, Ian Victor 92 Belper Road, Derby DE1 3EQ — MB ChB Ed. 1966; FRCOG 1985, M 1972. Cons. O & G Derbysh. Hosp. Wom. Derby; Hon. Clin. Teach. Univ. Notts. Specialty: Obst. & Gyn. Prev: Sen. Regist. (O & G) Jessop Hosp. Wom. Sheff.; Lect. (O & G) Univ. Manch at Univ. Hosp. of S. Manch.; Withington.

SCOTT, Ian William Henderson (retired) 45 Lowton Road, Lytham St Annes FY8 3JG Tel: 01253 722667 — MB ChB Glas. 1956; DObst RCOG 1960. Prev: GP Blackpool.

SCOTT, James Gilbert Road Medical Group, 39 Gilbert Road, Bucksburn, Aberdeen AB21 9AN Tel: 01224 712138 Fax: 01224 712239; 45 Glenhome Gardens, Dyce, Aberdeen AB21 7FG Tel: 01224 723495 — MB ChB Aberd. 1980; MRCGP 1983.

SCOTT, James Andrew, TD Dr's ABBAS, ASH, ATTRUP and SCOTT, 85 Sykes Lane, Saxilby, Lincoln LN1 2NU Tel: 01522 702236 Fax: 01522 703132 — MB BChir Camb. 1972 (Camb. & St. Thos.) MA, MB Camb. 1972, BChir 1971; DObst. RCOG 1974; MRCGP 1978. Prev: Ho. Surg. (Obst.) Lambeth Hosp. Lond.; Ho. Phys. (Paediat.) St. Thos. Hosp. Lond.; Govt. Med. Off. Kitwe, Zambia.

SCOTT, James Angus NHS Forth Valley, Department of Ophthalmology, Stirling Royal Infirmary, Livilands, Stirling FK8 2AU — MB BS Lond. 1983 (Middlx.) BSc (Foetal Endocrinol. & Med. Physics) Lond. 1980; MRCOphth 1990; FRCS Glas. 1991; CCST 1998; FRCOphth Lond. 2005. Cons.(Opth.) Forth Valley Hosp. NHS Trust Stirling Roy. Infirm. Stirling FKL8 2AU. Specialty: Ophth. Socs: N. Eng. Ophth. Soc.; UK & Irel. Soc. of Cataract & Refractive Surg.; Scott. Ophth. Club. Prev: Corneal Fell. Singapore Nat. Eye Centre; Sen. Regist./ Hon, Lect. Aberd. Roy. Infirm.; Regist. (Ophth.) Merseyside Regional Ophth. Rotat. Roy. Liverp. Univ. Hosp. Liverp.

SCOTT, James Archibald (retired) 62 Leicester Lane, Leamington Spa CV32 7HF Tel: 01926 423620 — (Glasgow) MB ChB Glas. 1954; DIH Eng. 1977; MFOM RCP Lond. 1978. Prev: Sen. Med. Off. Minerva Health Managem. Redditch.

SCOTT, James Dudley (retired) 2 Capesthorne, Robins Way, Christchurch BH23 4AT — MB BChir Camb. 1948 (Guy's)

SCOTT, Mr James Empson The Lister Hospital, Chelsea Bridge Road, London SW1W 8RH Tel: 0207 2599216 Fax: 0207 2599221 Email: medleg@mailbox.co.uk — BM BCh Oxf. 1968 (Middlx.) MA Oxf. 1968; FRCS Eng. 1973. Cons. Orthop. Surg. Chelsea & Westm. Hosp. Lond. Specialty: Orthop. Socs: Fell. BOA & Roy. Soc. Med. Prev: Sen. Regist. (Orthop.) Middlx. Hosp. Lond. & Roy. Nat. Orthop. Hosp; Regist. Robt. Jones & Agnes Hunt Orthop. Hosp. OsW.ry.

SCOTT, James Gray (retired) 3 Hook Close, Ampfield, Romsey SO51 9DD Tel: 02080 253860 — (Glas.) MB ChB Glas. 1943. Prev: Ho. Surg. (Cas.) West. Infirm. Glas.

SCOTT, James Macdonald Calvert Cottage, Brindle, Chorley PR6 8NH Tel: 0125 485 2509 — MB ChB Ed. 1956; DObst RCOG 1960; FRCGP 1986. Exam. Med. Off. DHSS. Socs: BMA. Prev: Course Organiser (Gen. Pract.) Manch. Regional Counc. Postgrad. Med. Educat.; Clin. Asst. (Neurol.) Roy. Infirm. Preston & Clin. Tutor (Gen. Pract.) Preston; Ho. Phys. West. Gen. Hosp. Edin. & Ho. Surg. Roy. Infirm. Edin.

SCOTT, James Noel, TD Windsor House, City Hospital, Belfast BT9 7AB Tel: 02890 263923 Fax: 02890 263945 — MB BCh BAO Belf. 1973 (Queen's Belfast) MRCP (UK) 1977; MRCPsych 1979; FRCP Ed. 1992. Cons. Psychiat. Belf. City Hosp. Specialty: Geriat. Psychiat.; Gen. Psychiat. Prev: Sen. Lect. (Psychiat. of Old Age) Qu.'s Univ. Belf.; Research Fell. Roy. Vict. Hosp. Belf.; Sen. Regist. (Psychiat.) Purdysburn Hosp. Belf.

SCOTT, Professor James Steel (retired) Byards Lodge, Knaresborough HG5 0LT Tel: 01423 863353 — MB ChB Glas. 1946; FRCOG 1962, M 1953; FRCS Ed. 1959; MD Glas. 1959; FRCS Eng. 1986. Prev: Dean Fac. Med. & Prof. O & G Univ. Leeds.

SCOTT, James Thomas (retired) Winter's Lodge, Huish Champflower, Taunton TA4 2BZ Tel: 01984 624632 — (St. Mary's) MB BS Lond. 1949; MRCS Eng. LRCP Lond. 1949; FRCP Lond. 1968, M 1952; MD Lond. 1967. Hon. Cons. Phys. Char. Cross Hosp. Lond. Prev: Cons. Phys. Hammersmith Hosp. Lond.

SCOTT, Jane Frances Dartford West Health Centre, Tower Road, Dartford DA1 2HA Tel: 01322 223600 Fax: 01322 292282 — MB

ChB Liverp. 1985. Prev: SHO (Ophth., Geriat. Med. & O & G) Qu. Mary's Hosp. Sidcup.

SCOTT, Janet McGregor Lodgehill Clinic, Lodgehill Road, Nairn IV12 4RF Fax: 01259 769991; Woodlands, Cowdor Road, Nairn IV12 5EF Tel: 01667 454887 — MB ChB Ed. 1971. Asst. GP Lodgehill Clinic, Nairn. Specialty: Gen. Pract.

SCOTT, Professor Janine Linda Department of Psychological Medicine, Academic Centre, Gartnavel Royal Hospital, 1055 Great Western Road, Glasgow G12 0XH Tel: 0141 211 3937 Fax: 0141 357 4899 — MB BS Newc. 1979 (Newcastle) MRCPsych 1985; MD Newc. 1993; FRCPsych 1995. Prof. & Hon. Cons. (Psychiat.) Univ. of Glas. Specialty: Gen. Psychiat. Prev: Sen. Lect. & Cons. (Psychiat.) Univ. Newc.; Vis. Scientist John Hopkins, Baltimore Train. Fell., Centre for Cognitive Ther. Philadelphia.

SCOTT, Jason Albert 38 Gover Road, Southampton SO16 9BR Tel: 023 8086 2650 — MB BS Lond. 1994 (St. Bart. Hosp. Med. Coll.) Specialty: Anaesth.

SCOTT, Jean Mary (retired) Spring Court, Dockenfield, Farnham GU10 4EX Tel: 01252 794153 — MB ChB Birm. 1940; DCH Eng. 1965. Prev: Med. Asst. (Paediat.) St. Peter's Hosp. Chertsey.

SCOTT, Jean Mary, DStJ (retired) Tiriach, Clunie Bridge Road, Pitlochry PH16 5JX Tel: 01796 472403 — (Univ. Glas.) MB ChB (Commend.) Glas. 1944; MD (Commend.) Glas. 1948; FRCPath 1975, M 1963. Prev: Cons. Path. Glas. Roy. Matern. & Wom. Hosps. Asst. Pathol. Roy. Infirm., West. Infirm. & Roy. Matern. Hosp. Glas.

SCOTT, Jeremy Peter Dixon Trengweath Hospital, Redruth TR15 2SP; 2 Sarahs Gate, Little Petherick, Wadebridge PL27 7QT — MRCS Eng. LRCP Lond. 1968 (St. Geo.) DPM Eng. 1972; MRCPsych 1975. Cons. Psychiat. Trengweath Hosp. Specialty: Gen. Psychiat. Prev: Assoc. Specialist St. Lawrence's Hosp. Bodmin.

SCOTT, Jo Ann Vinette, Phildraw Road, Ballasalla IM9 3EG Tel: 01624 827220 Fax: 01624 827220 — MB ChB Sheff. 1987 (Sheffield) Cert. Family Plann. JCC 1991; DRCOG 1991.

SCOTT, Joan Elizabeth 5 Woodthorpe Gardens, Sandal, Wakefield WF2 6RA — MB ChB Leeds 1971; MB ChB Leeds. 1971; DPM Leeds 1975; BA (Hons.) Open 1989.

SCOTT, Joan Isabel G 0/2 12 Ripon Drive, Glasgow G12 0DX — MB ChB Glas. 1995.

SCOTT, John Adam (retired) 17 Trowlock Island, Teddington TW11 9QZ Tel: 020 8977 5175 — MB ChB Aberd. 1932. Prev: Maj. RAMC.

SCOTT, John Anthony Gerard 13 Turnoak Avenue, Woking GU22 0AJ — BM BCh Oxf. 1987; BA Camb. 1984; MRCP (UK) 1990. MSc Stud. Lond. Sch. Hyg. & Trop. Med. Specialty: Infec. Dis. Prev: Regist. (Infec. Dis.) Northwick Pk. Hosp.; SHO Hosp. for Trop. Dis. Lond.; SHO Rotat. (Gen. Med.) Newc.

SCOTT, Mr John Charles Richard Orthofix Ltd, The Guildway, Old Portsmouth Road, Guildford GU3 1LR Tel: 01483 468800 Fax: 01483 468829 Email: johnscott@orthofix.com; 54 Compton Avenue, Brighton BN1 3PS Tel: 01273 727732 Fax: 01273 738812 Email: jcrscott@easynet.co.uk — BChir 1967 (Univ. Coll. Hosp.) MB 1968; MRCS Eng. LRCP Lond. 1968; MA Camb. 1972; FRCS Eng. 1974. Med. Director Orthofix Gp. Specialty: Trauma & Orthop. Surg. Socs: Fell. Roy. Soc. of Med.; Internat. Soc. for Fract. Repair. Prev: Orthofix Gp. Med. Advisor Internat; GP Health Centre Univ. Sussex Brighton.

SCOTT, John Clelland (retired) 14 Pitcullen Terrace, Perth PH2 7EQ Tel: 01738 626266 — MB ChB Ed. 1954; DPM Eng. 1957; FRCP Ed. 1969, M 1961; FRCPsych. 1981, M 1972. Prev: Cons. Psychiat. Perth & Kinross.

SCOTT, Mr John David Eye Department, Box 41, Addenbrooke's Hospital, Hills Road, Cambridge CB2 2QQ Tel: 01223 245151 Fax: 01223 216701 — (St. Mary's) MB BS Lond. 1960; DO Eng. 1962; FRCS Eng. 1964. Cons. Vitreo-Retinal Surg. Specialty: Ophth. Socs: Club Jules Gonin. Prev: Sen. Regist. Moorfields Eye Hosp. Lond. (City Rd. Br.); Ho. Phys. (Med), Ho. Surg. & Sen Ho. Surg. Eye Dept. St. Mary's Hosp. Lond.

SCOTT, John Davie East Anglian Ambulance NHS Trust, Hospital Lane, Hellesden, Norwich NR6 5NA Tel: 01603 422701; 23 Coppice Avenue, Great Shelford, Cambridge CB2 5AQ Tel: 01223 843189 — MB ChB St. And. 1970; DA (Eng.) 1972; DObst RCOG 1973; Dip IMC RCS Ed. 1988; FIMC RCS Ed. 2002. Clin. Dir. E. Anglian Ambul. NHS Trust.

SCOTT, Mr John Eric Somerville (retired) 17 Stephenson Court, Wylam NE41 8LA Tel: 01661 853995 Fax: 01661 854140 Email: j.e.s.scott@ncl.ac.uk — MB BChir Camb. 1948 (Middlx. & Camb.) MA Camb. 1950; FRCS Eng. 1953; MD Camb. 1962. Sen. Lect. (Paediat. Surg.) Univ. Newc.; Hon. Sen. Research Assoc. Univ. Newc. Prev: Cons. Paediat. Surg. Newc. HA.

SCOTT, John Graham (retired) 8 Regent's Drive, Keston BR2 6BU Tel: 01689 55542 Email: johngscott@medix-uk.com — MB BS Lond. 1961 (St. Mary's) MRCS Eng. LRCP Lond. 1961; DA Eng. 1964; FFA RCS Eng. 1966. Prev: Cons. Anaesth. Bromley Health Dist.

SCOTT, Mr John James Law Hospital, Carluke ML8 5ER — MB BCh BAO Dub. 1983; DObst RCPI 1986; MRCGP 1990; Dip. IMC RCS Ed. 1991; FRCS Ed. 1993; FFAEM 1998. Cons. (A&E.) Law Hosp. Lanarksh..; Hon Sen Lect Glas Univ. Specialty: Accid. & Emerg.

SCOTT, John Michael 5 Tany Bonc, Valley Road, Llanfairfechan LL33 0ET — MB ChB Leic. 1988.

SCOTT, John Moffat 22 Brooke Way, Bushey Heath, Watford WD23 4LG — MB ChB Glas. 1976.

SCOTT, John Nicholas c/o Mrs Scott, 9 Emmott Drive, Rawdon, Leeds LS19 6PG — MB BChir Camb. 1989.

SCOTT, John Russell (retired) 17A Goldsmith Lane, London NW9 9AJ Tel: 020 8204 5233 — MB BChir Camb. 1955 (Middlx.) MB Camb. 1955, BChir 1954; MRCS Eng. LRCP Lond. 1954; MRCGP 1967.

SCOTT, John Simon Coleridge Carlisle House, 53 Lanegland Street, Poole BH15 1QD Tel: 01202 678484 Fax: 01202 660507; 22A Lower Golf Links Road, Broadstone BH18 8BH Tel: 01202 699362 — MB BS Lond. 1975 (St. Bart.) MRCS Eng. LRCP Lond. 1975.

SCOTT, John Walter Netheravon, Seaton Ross, York YO42 4LT — MB ChB Manch. 1989. Prev: Trainee GP Sheff.; SHO (A & E & Community Paediat.) Barnsley.

SCOTT, John Watson (retired) 11A Central Avenue, North Mount Vernon, Glasgow G32 9JP — MB ChB Glas. 1948. Prev: GP. Glas.

SCOTT, Jonathan Crispin Ealing Hammersmith & Fulham Trust, Uxbridge Road, Southall UB1 3EU Tel: 02083548012 Fax: 020 8354 8887 — BM BCh Oxf. 1986 (Oxford) MA Oxf. 1983; MRCPsych 1992. Cons. (Psychiat.) EHF Trust, Ealing Lond. Specialty: Gen. Psychiat.

SCOTT, Mr Jonathan Woodforde Merton Grange, Wheelers Lane, Bear Wood, Bournemouth BH11 9QJ Tel: 01202 573218 Fax: 01202 573218 — MB BS Lond. 1968 (Westm.) MRCS Eng. LRCP Lond. 1968; DObst RCOG 1970; FRCOG 1990, M 1978; FRCS Eng. 1974, M 1 9684. Cons. O & G Poole Gen. Hosp.; Hon. Sec. Nuffield Vis. Soc. Specialty: Obst. & Gyn. Socs: Fell. Roy. Soc. Med.; BMA. Prev: Sen. Regist. (O & G) Bristol Matern. Hosp.; Regist. (O & G) Westm. Hosp. Lond.; Res. Med. Off. Qu. Charlotte's Matern. Hosp. Lond.

SCOTT, Judith Kennedy The Health Centre, Aboyne AB34 5HQ; 8 Golf Palace, Aboyne, Aberdeen AB34 5GA Tel: 013 3988 6644 — MB BCh BAO Belf. 1980; DCH RCSI 1983; DRCOG Lond. 1984; MRCGP Lond. 1985. Socs: MRCGP.

SCOTT, Judy Monica Grimston Medical Centre, Congham Road, Grimston, King's Lynn PE32 1DW Tel: 01485 600341 Fax: 01485 601411 — MB ChB (Hons.) Leeds 1989; BSc (1st cl. Hons.) Leeds 1986; MRCP (UK) 1993; MRCGP 1997. Gen. Practitioner.

SCOTT, Karen-Anne 22 Stanley Road, Leicester LE2 1RE — MB ChB Leic. 1998; MB ChB Leic 1998.

SCOTT, Katherine Ann Department of Psychiatry, St George's Hospital, Cranmer Terrace, Tooting, London SW17 0RE; Flat 2, 10 Lawrie Park Crescent, London SE26 6HD — MB BS Lond. 1988; DGM RCP Lond. 1992. Regist. Rotat. (Psychiat.) St. Geo. Hosp. Lond. Prev: Regist. Rotat. (Psychiat.) Univ. Hosp. S. Manch.

SCOTT, Kathryn Cossart 46 North Road, Belfast BT5 5NH — MB BCh BAO Belf. 1990; MB BCh Belf. 1990.

SCOTT, Keith Wilson Holywood Arches Health Centre, Westminster Avenue, Belfast BT4 1QQ Tel: 028 9056 3354 Fax: 028 9065 3846; 35 Kensington Road, Belfast BT5 6NJ — MB BCh BAO Belf. 1980 (Univ. of Wales, Cardiff) DCH Dub. 1984; DRCOG 1985; MRCGP 1985; Dip. Palliat. Med. 1995. Clin. Asst. Beaconfield Marie Curie Centre Belf. Specialty: Palliat. Med.

SCOTT, Kenneth Garrion, 27 Forest View, Kildrum, Cumbernauld, Glasgow G67 2DB — MB ChB Glas. 1987.

SCOTT, Kenneth, OBE 31 Spencer Close, London N3 3TX Tel: 020 8346 1350 Fax: 020 8346 2399 — MB BS Lond. 1953 (Guy's) DObst RCOG 1955; FRCGP 1977, M 1968. Socs: Fell. Med. Soc. Lond.; BMA; (Pres.) Nat. Assn. Fundholding Pract.s. Prev: Ho. Surg. (O & G) St. Mary Abbot's Hosp. Kensington; Ho. Surg. & Ho. Phys. Qu. Mary's Hosp. Sidcup.

SCOTT, Kenneth Balfour (retired) Mansewood, Bonhill, Alexandria G83 9AS Tel: 01389 752112 — MB ChB Glas. 1952. Prev: Partner Scott. Pract.

SCOTT, Kenneth William (retired) 6 Dillon Heights, Armagh BT61 9HF Tel: 01861 523136 — MB BCh BAO Belf. 1958; FRCPI 1974, M 1963. Prev: Cons. Dermat. Craigavon Area Hosp. Portadown.

SCOTT, Kenneth William McKay Histopathology Department, New Cross Hospital, Wolverhampton WV10 0QP Tel: 01902 644810 Fax: 01902 644809; 18 Church Hill Road, Stockwell End, Tettenhall, Wolverhampton WV6 9AT Tel: 01902 753754 — MB ChB Glas. 1967; FRCPath 1986, M 1974; MD Glas. 1978. Cons. Path. Roy. Hosp. Wolverhampton. Specialty: Histopath. Socs: Coun. Roayl Coll. of Pathologists. Prev: Lect. (Path.) Univ. Sheff.; Regist. (Laborat. Med.) South. Gen. Hosp. Glas.; Home Office Pathologist.

SCOTT, Kim Michelle 9 Braemar Drive, Bridgehall, Bury BL9 7PF Tel: 0161 797 4243 — MB ChB Dundee 1981. Med. Asst. DSS Oldham. Prev: Princip. GP Marjory Lees Health Centre Oldham; Trainee GP Collegiate Med. Centre, Cheetham Hill, Oldham VTS; Asst. Pract. Marjory Lees Health Centre Oldham.

SCOTT, Kirsty Nina Lindsey Rosemount, 6 Forthill Road, Broughty Ferry, Dundee DD5 2JU — MB ChB Glas. 1996.

SCOTT, Leslie Gordon Trencrom, 17 Southcourt Avenue, Bexhill-on-Sea TN39 3AR Tel: 01424 212583 — MRCS Eng. LRCP Lond. 1939 (Guy's) MD Lond. 1951, MB BS 1940; FRCP Lond. 1969, M 1949; DCH Eng. 1949. Hon. Cons. Paediat. Hastings & Eastbourne Gp. Specialty: Paediat. Prev: Out-pat. Med. Regist. Hosp. Sick Childr. Gt. Ormond St.; Sen. Regist. Childr. Dept. Guy's Hosp.; Act. Squadron Ldr. RAFVR.

SCOTT, Leslie Thomas (retired) 14 Cove Road, Silverdale, Carnforth LA5 0RR Tel: 01524 701013 — BM BCh Oxf. 1941 (Oxf. & Univ. Coll Hosp.) BA, BM BCh Oxf. 1941; DA Eng. 1946; FFA RCS Eng. 1957. Prev: Cons. Anaesth. Lancaster Health Dist.

SCOTT, Liam Richard (retired) 33 Moira Drive, Bangor BT20 4RW Tel: 01247 454508 — MB BCh BAO Belf. 1970.

SCOTT, Lorna Isobel West Brook, 1 Finlays Road, Newtownards BT23 8SW — MB BCh BAO Belf. 1959; DCH Eng. 1962.

SCOTT, Louise Group Practice, Health Centre, Springfield, Stornoway HS1 2PS — MB ChB Dundee 1989; DRCOG 1994; MRCGP 1996. GP.

SCOTT, Louise Ann 139 Dunmow Road, Bishop's Stortford CM23 5HQ — MB BS Lond. 1990; DRCOG 1993; MRCGP 1994. GP Retainer, Bishops Stortford. Prev: Trainee GP Medway HA; Ho. Off. (Surg.) Joyce Green Hosp. Dartford; Ho. Off. (Med.) Brook Gen. Hosp. Greenwich.

SCOTT, Lucinda Valerie 44 Theberton Street, London N1 0QX — MB BCh BAO Dub. 1991.

SCOTT, Lucy Clare 26 Bawnmore Road, Belfast BT9 6LA — MB BCh BAO Belf. 1997.

SCOTT, Mairi Gray Browning Cairntoul Drive Surgery, 9 Cairntoul Drive, Glasgow G14 0XT Tel: 0141 959 5519 Fax: 0141 950 1028; 10 Marchmont Terrace, Glasgow G12 9LS — MB ChB Glas. 1977; Cert JCC Lond. 1978; FRCGP 1992, M 1981. GP Glas.

SCOTT, Malcolm Francis 49 Valiant House, Vicarage Crescent, London SW11 3LU Tel: 020 7228 5903 Fax: 020 7228 5903 — MB BS Lond. 1974 (Guy's) MRCS Eng. LRCP Lond. 1974. Med. Adviser Benefits Agency Lond.; GP Cromwell Hosp. Lond. Specialty: Disabil. Med. Prev: GP Lond. (NHS Princip.); Med. Off. Passage Day Centre for the Homeless Lond.; Company Med. Off. Ho. of Fraser plc.

SCOTT, Malcolm Peter Young 34A Church Road, Stoke Bishop, Bristol BS9 1QT — MB BS Lond. 1956 (Middlx.) MRCS Eng. LRCP Lond. 1956; DIH Soc. Apoth. Lond. 1959; MFOM RCP Lond. 1979. Gp. Med. Adviser Mardon Packaging Internat.; Med. Adviser St. Regis Gp. Bristol. Socs: Soc. Occupat. Med. Prev: Med. Adviser Nat. Cash Register Co. Ltd. Lond.; Asst. Med. Off. Stewarts & Lloyds Corby.

SCOTT, Margaret Christine (retired) 11 The Russets, Wakefield WF2 6JF Tel: 01924 259535 — MB ChB Ed. 1950.

SCOTT, Marianne Flat 211, 8 Govan Road, Glasgow G51 1HS — MB ChB Glas. 1997; DRCOG 1999. Specialty: Gen. Pract.

SCOTT, Mr Mark John Leonard Department Plastic & Reconstructive Surgery, Stoke Mandeville Hospital, Mandeville Road, Aylesbury HP21 8AL — MB BS Lond. 1986; FRCS Eng. 1990; FRCS (Plast) 1995. Cons. Plastic Surg. Stoke Mandeville Hosp. Aylesbury. Specialty: Plastic Surg. Socs: BMA; Brit. Assn. Plastic Surg.; Brit. Assn. Aesthetic Plastic Surgs. Prev: Sen. Regist. (Plastic Surg.) Qu. Mary's Univ. Hosp. Lond.; Regist. St. Jas. Univ. Hosp. Leeds.

SCOTT, Mary Links Medical Centre, 4 Hermitage Place, Edinburgh EH6 8BW Tel: 0131 554 1036 Fax: 0131 555 3995; 11 Granby Road, Edinburgh EH16 5NP — MB ChB Ed. 1973; BSc Ed. 1970, MB ChB 1973; Cert JCC Lond. 1976. Gen. Med. Pract.Links Med. Centre Edin. Prev: Med. Off. Brook Advis. Centre Edin.

SCOTT, Mary Caffyn Wright (retired) 13 Catherine Street, Gatehouse-of-Fleet, Castle Douglas DG7 2JD Tel: 01557 814000; 25 Park Gate, Blackheath, London SE3 9XF Tel: 020 8852 5267 — MB ChB Ed. 1951; FRCOG 1976, M 1960.

SCOTT, Mary Reid Nethertown Surgery, Elliot Street, Dunfermline KY11 4TF Tel: 01383 623516 Fax: 01383 624254 — MB ChB Aberd. 1970 (Aberdeen) DObst RCOG 1972; Cert. Family Plann. JCC 1976; MRCGP 1984; MFFP 1993.

SCOTT, Maureen Easton Portland Street Surgery, 101 Portland Street, Troon KA10 6QN Tel: 01292 313593 Fax: 01292 312020 — MB ChB Glas. 1970.

SCOTT, Maureen Jean — (Belf.) MD Belf. 1975, MB BCh BAO 1964; FFPHH (UK) 1990,M 1984; FFPHMI 1993, M 1987. Sen. Lect. (Epidemiol. & Pub. Health Med.) Qu. Univ. Belf.; Cons. Pub. Health Med. EHSSB. Specialty: Pub. Health Med. Socs: Fell. Ulster Med. Soc.; Soc. Social Med. Prev: Cons. Pub. Health Med. EHSSB; Friar Research Fell. (Community Med.) Qu. Univ. Belf.

SCOTT, Melanie Jane 217 Shawfield Road, Ash, Aldershot GU12 6SH — MB ChB Liverp. 1996 (Liverpool) BSc (Hons) Liverp. 1993. SHO (Gen. Surg.) Roy. Liverp. Univ. Hosp. Specialty: Gen. Surg. Prev: SHO (A & E) Roy. Liverp. Univ. Hosp. Liverp.; Ho. Off. Roy. Liverp. Univ. Hosp. Liverp.; SHO (Urol.) RLUH, SHO (Gen. Surg.) Warrington Gen. Hosp., SHO (Orthap) Univ. Hosp. Aintree.

SCOTT, Michael — MB BCh Belf. 1998. Specialty: Histopath. Socs: Ulster Med. Soc.; Christ. Med. Fellowsh.

SCOTT, Michael Andrew Briar Green, Adlington Road, Wilmslow SK9 2BN — BM BS Nottm. 1995.

SCOTT, Michael Edwin Newburn Road Surgery, 4 Newburn Road, Newcastle upon Tyne NE15 8LX Tel: 0191 229 0090 Fax: 0191 267 4830 — MB BS Newc. 1976; MRCGP 1980.

SCOTT, Michael Ernest (retired) Laurel Vale House, 121 Ballyskeagh Road, Dunmurry, Belfast BT17 9LL — (Belf.) MB BCh BAO (2nd cl. Hons.(Belf. 1963; FRCP Lond. 1980, M 1966; FRCPI 1975, M 1966; BSc (Anat. 1st cl. Hons.) Belf. 1960, MD 1969; FESC 1988. 25 Derryvolgie Avenue, Belf. BT9 6FN. Prev: Cons. Cardiol. Belf. City Hosp.

SCOTT, Mr Michael Hugh Whiston Hospital, Prescot L35 5DR Tel: 0151 430 1911 Fax: 0151 339 7765 Email: mhscott@dr-mike.co.uk; Springfield House, Margarets Lane, Childer Thornton, South Wirral CH66 5PF Tel: 0151 339 1366 Fax: 0151 339 7765 Email: mhscott@dr-mike.co.uk — MB ChB Liverp. 1978 (Liverpool) MRCS Eng. LRCP Lond. 1978; FRCS Eng. 1982; ChM Liverp. 1990. Cons. Gen. Surg. Whiston Hosp. Prescot. Specialty: Gen. Surg. Prev: Sen. Regist. Rotat. (Gen. Surg.) Merseyside HA; Surgic. Fell. Univ. Calif., San Diego, USA.; Sandoz Transpl. Fell. 1986-88.

SCOTT, Michael Joseph Brookeborough Surgery, Tanyard Lane, Brookeborough, Enniskillen BT94 4AB Tel: 028 8953 1225 Fax: 02889 531857 — MB BCh BAO Belf. 1984; DA (UK) 1986; DRCOG 1990; MRCGP 1990; DCH Dub. 1991. Specialty: Anaesth.

SCOTT, Mora Joan, MBE (retired) St. Michaels, Northfield Terrace, Elgin IV30 1NE Tel: 01343 543832 — MB ChB Aberd. 1940. DL. Prev: Ho. Surg. & Ho. Phys. Roy. Aberd. Hosp. Sick Childr.

SCOTT, Morna Catherine (retired) Grangemount, Alyth, Blairgowrie PH11 8NY Tel: 0182 832600 — MB ChB Aberd. 1941. Prev: Med. Off. City Fev. Hosp. Aberd. & Roy. Hosp. Sick Childr. Aberd.

SCOTT, Mr Nicholas Bruce 19 Bruce Road, Glasgow G41 5EE — MB ChB Aberd. 1979; FRCS Ed. 1985.

SCOTT, Nicholas Paul Department of Radiology, Jersey General Hospital, Gloucester Street, St Helier JE2 3QS Tel: 01534 622872 Email: drnce@doctors.org.uk — MB BS Lond. 1972 (Univ. of Lond.) FRCR 1984. Consultant Radiologist. Specialty: Radiol.

SCOTT, Nicola Christine 52 Warland Way, Corfe Mullen, Wimborne BH21 3NZ — BM Soton. 1988. Specialty: Gen. Pract.

SCOTT, Nicola Mary Sandborne, Clophill Road, Maulden, Bedford MK45 2AA — MB BS Nottm. 1982; MRCGP 1986; DRCOG 1986. Prev: Trainee GP Doncaster VTS.

SCOTT, Nigel Dept. of Pathology, St James University Hospital, Beckett Street, Leeds LS9 7TF Tel: 0113 206 5590 — MB ChB Sheff. 1985; MRCPath 1993; MD Sheff. 1995. Cons. Histopath. Leeds. Specialty: Histopath.

SCOTT, Mr Nigel Andrew Department of Surgery, Hope Hospital, Stott Lane, Salford M6 8HD Tel: 0161 787 5123 Fax: 0161 787 1276; The Knowle, Dalegarth Avenue, Heaton, Bolton BL1 5DW Tel: 01204 842970 — MB ChB Manch. 1979 (Manchester) MD Manch. 1988, BSc (Hons.) 1976; MB ChB (Hons.) Manch. 1979; FRCS Eng. 1983. Cons. Surg. Hope Hosp. Manch.; Hon. Sen. Clin. Lect. Univ. Manch. Specialty: Gen. Surg. Socs: Assn. Coloproctol. Prev: Sen. Lect. & Hon. Cons. (Surg.) Univ. Manch.; Lect. (Surg.) Univ. Wales Coll. Med.; Fell. Oncol. Mayo Clinic, USA.

SCOTT, Nigel William The Health Centre, Leypark Walk, Estover, Plymouth PL6 8UE Tel: 01752 784949; 190 Mannamead Road, Hartley, Plymouth PL3 5RE Tel: 01752 783493 — MB BChir Camb. 1989 (Univ. Camb.) MB BChir Camb. 1988; MA Camb. 1989; DRCOG 1991; MRCGP 1992.

SCOTT, Olive (retired) Byards Lodge, Boroughbridge Road, Knaresborough HG5 0LT Tel: 01423 863353 — MB ChB Sheff. 1948; FRCPCH (Hon); MRCS Eng. LRCP Lond. 1948; DCH . Lond. 1952; FRCP Lond. 1972, M 1955; MD Sheff. 1957. Cons. Paediat. Cardiol. Leeds Gen. Infirm. & Killingbeck Hosp. Leeds. Prev: Cons. Paediat. Roy. Liverp. Childr. Hosp.

SCOTT, Oliver Christopher Anderson (retired) 31 Kensington Square, London W8 5HH — (Camb. & St. Thos.) MD Camb. 1976, MB BChir 1946; MRCS Eng. LRCP Lond. 1946; FRCR (Hon.) 1998. Prev: Consult Inst. Cancer Research Lond.

SCOTT, Oliver John New House, Upper St., Leeds, Maidstone ME17 1RY Tel: 01622 861462 — BM BS Nottm. 1991; MRCGP (RCGP, Lond. 1997); Dip. Paediat. Auckland 1996; Dip. Obst. Auckland 1996. GP Regist. Maidstone; Locum GP. Specialty: Gen. Pract.

SCOTT, Oliver Lester Schreiner South Lodge, South Side, Wimbledon Common, London SW19 4TL Tel: 020 8946 6662 — MB BChir Camb. 1943 (Univ. Camb. St. Thos. Hosp. Lond.) MRCS Eng. LRCP Lond. 1942; MA Camb. 1943; FRCP Lond. 1964, M 1944. Chev. Nat. du Mérite (Rep. France); Hon. Cons. Dermat. Char. Cross Hosp. Lond., Roy. Surrey Co. Hosp. & St. Luke's Hosp Guildford; Vice-Pres. Roy. Med. Foundat. of Epsom Coll. Specialty: Dermat. Socs: Fell. (Ex-Hon. Treas.) Roy. Soc. Med.; Hon. Mem. (Ex-Pres.) Brit. Assn. Dermat.; St John's Hosp. Dermatol. Soc. Prev: Cons. Dermat. King Edwd. VII Hosp. for Offs. Lond.; Cons. Dermat. Dispensaire Francais Lond.; Vice-Dean Char. Cross. Hosp. Med. Sch.

SCOTT, Mr Patrick Damian Burnley General Hospital, Casterton Avenue, Burnley BB10 2PQ Tel: 01706 233142; 9 Braemar Drive, Bridge Hall, Bury BL9 7PF — MB ChB Manch. 1980; FRCS Ed. 1984; FRCPS Glas. 1984; MD Manch. 1992. Cons. Gen. Surg. Burnley Gen. Hosp. Specialty: Gen. Surg. Special Interest: Laparoscopic & Colorectal Surg. Socs: Oldham Med. Soc. Prev: Sen. Regist. (Surg.) NW Region.; Tutor (Gen. Surg.) Manch. Roy. Infirm.

SCOTT, Paul Primrose Mill Barn, Waste Lane, Kelsall, Chester CW6 0PE Tel: 01829 751409 Fax: 01829 751416; Primrose Mill Barn, Waste Lane, Kelsall, Chester CW6 0PE Tel: 01829 751409 Fax: 01829 751416 — MB ChB Leeds 1989; FRCA 1994. Cons. (Anaesth.) Warrington Hosp. NHS Trust. Specialty: Anaesth. Prev: Regist. (Anaesth.) Univ. Hosp. S. Manch.

SCOTT, Paul Habershon (retired) Park Cottage, 8, The Green, Royston SG8 7AD Tel: 01763 249974 — MB Camb. 1956 (Middlx.) BChir 1955; DObst RCOG 1958. Prev: Ho. Surg. Middlx. Hosp.

SCOTT, Paul James Bulley and Partners, Hamdon Medical Centre, Matts Lane, Stoke-sub-Hamdon TA14 6QE Tel: 01935 822236 Fax: 01935 826565 — MB BChir Camb. 1983; DRCOG 1987; DCH RCP Lond. 1987; MRCGP 1987. Prev: Trainee GP Kent & Canterbury Hosp. VTS.

SCOTT, Paul Meikle Flat 1, 6 Douglas Crescent, Edinburgh EH12 5BB — MB ChB Ed. 1993; MRCP (Ed.) 1997. Med. Regist. Borders Gen. Hosp. Melrose, Roxburghsh. Specialty: Gen. Med. Prev: SHO EGH Gen. Med. Edin. (E. Gen. Hosp.); SHO City Hosp. Infec. Dis. United; SHO Haemat. Unit Roy. Infirm. Edin.

SCOTT, Paul Robert David — MB BS Lond. (Barts) 1988 (St. Bart. Med. Coll.) DRCOG 1992; DFFP 1994; MRCGP 1995; Cert MDM 2003. LMC Member, Emergency Care Lead, GPSI Substance Misuse, GP Trainer; Triogl Lead and Counc. Mem., N. Staffs GP CoOperat.; Clin. Adviser, NHS Direct, Midl. Shires. Prev: Trainee GP Stafford VTS.

SCOTT, Mr Peter David Rankin 31 Mearns Road, Clarkston, Glasgow G76 7ES Tel: 0141 638 4396 — MB ChB Glas. 1967; FRCS Ed. 1971. Cons. Orthop. Surg. Vict. Infirm. Glas. Specialty: Orthop.

SCOTT, Mr Peter Douglas Campbell 71G Fitzjohns Avenue, London NW3 6PD Tel: 020 7431 2774 — MB BS Lond. 1991 (St. Barts. HMC) BSc Lond. 1988, MB BS 1991; DCH 1993; DRCOG 1994; MRCGP 1995; MRCOG 1999. Specialist Regist. (O & G) St. Barts. Hosp. Lond.; Specialist Regist. (Obst. & Gyn.) NE Thames. Specialty: Obst. & Gyn.

SCOTT, Peter Edward The Surgery, 406c Chester Road, Castle Bromwich, Birmingham B36 0LF Tel: 0121 770 3035; 31 Woodchester Road, Dorridge, Solihull B93 8EN Tel: 01564 773647 Fax: 0121 779 7109 — MB ChB Liverp. 1984; DRCOG 1986; Dip Occ Med 2002. Specialty: Gen. Pract. Special Interest: Acupunc.

SCOTT, Peter James Young (retired) Clifton College Santatorium, 83B Pembroke Road, Bristol BS8 3EA Tel: 0117 973 5642; Winnow Barn, Jasmine Lane, Claverham, Bristol BS49 4PY Tel: 01934 876640 — MRCS Eng. LRCP Lond. 1960 (St. Mary's) Med. Off. Clifton Coll. Bristol.

SCOTT, Peter John Castle Douglas Medical Group, Castle Douglas Health Centre, Academy Street, Castle Douglas DG7 1EE Tel: 01556 503888 Fax: 01556 504302; Chapel Place, Castle Douglas DG7 1EJ — MB ChB Ed. 1967. Clin. Asst. (Genitourin. Med.) Dumfries & Galloway Roy. Infirm.

SCOTT, Peter John Royal Bolton Hospital, Minerva Road, Farnworth, Bolton BL4 0JR Tel: 01204 390390; 1 Hillside, Off Chorley New Road, Bolton BL1 5DT — MB ChB Leeds 1984; MRCP (UK) 1987. Cons. Phys. (Cardiol.) Roy. Bolton Hosps. Specialty: Cardiol. Prev: Research Fell. (Cardiol.) Killingbeck Hosp. Leeds.

SCOTT, Mr Peter John (retired) Lady's Grace, Southcott, Westleigh, Bideford EX39 4NH Tel: 01273 475669 Email: pjs_dcs@ladysgrace.fsnet.co.uk — (St. Bart.) MB BS Lond. 1956; FRCS Eng. 1962; T(S) 1991. Prev: Cons. Orthop. & Traum. Surg. N. Devon Dist. Hosp.

SCOTT, Peter John Wellwood 12 Ancaster Drive, Glasgow G13 1ND — MD Glas. 1991; BSc (Hons.) Glas. 1971, MB ChB 1973; FRCP Glas. 1987. Cons. Phys. Gen. and Geriat. Med., Roy. Alexandra Hosp., Paisley PA2 9PN. Specialty: Gen. Med.

SCOTT, Mr Peter Milton The Old Vicarage, Babraham, Cambridge CB2 4AG — (Char. Cross) MB BS Lond. 1955; FRCS Eng. 1960; MA Camb. 1974. Specialty: Orthop. Socs: Fell. BOA; Fell. Roy. Coll. Surgs. Prev: Emerit. Cons. Orthop. Surg. Addenbrooke's NHS Trust Camb.; Sen. Regist. (Orthop.) Addenbrooke's Hosp. Camb. & Aberd. Roy. Infirm.; SHO (Surg.) Roy. Nat. Orthop. Hosp. Stanmore.

SCOTT, Peter William Bowen, OBE (retired) Wellfield, Bwlch, Brecon LD3 7RZ — (Middlx.) MB BS Lond. 1962; DObst RCOG 1964; DTM & H Eng. 1968; FRCPath 1989, M 1977, D 1971. Med. Dir.; Cons. Pathol. Nevill Hall Hosp. Abergavenny. Prev: Reader Pathol. Roy. Army Med. Coll. Lond.

SCOTT, Mr Philip Martyn John Poole Hospital NHS Trust, Longfleet Road, Poole BH15 2JB Tel: 01202 442459 Email: philip.se.dial.pipex.com — MB ChB Bristol 1984; FRCS 1989; FRCS (Orl) 1995. Cons. (ENT Surg.) Poole Gen. Hosp. Specialty: Otolaryngol.

SCOTT, Ralph Easdale (retired) The Old Rectory, Fornham All Saints, Bury St Edmunds IP28 6JX Tel: 01284 767177 — MB BChir Camb. 1956 (St. Thos.) MA Camb. 1956; DObst RCOG 1962. Prev: GP Bury St. Edmunds.

SCOTT, Ralph Platt Fisher Dept. of Anaesth. & Intens. Care, Salisbury Healthcare NHS Trust, Sailsbury District Hospital, Salisbury

SP2 8BJ Tel: 01722 425050 Fax: 01722 414143 — MB ChB Ed. 1978; FFA RCS Eng. 1982; BSc Ed. 1975, MD 1992. Cons. Anaesth. & Intens. Care, Salisbury Dist. Hosp.; Exam. Roy. Coll. Anaesth. Specialty: Anaesth. Special Interest: Intens. Care Med. Socs: Internat. Anaesth. Research Soc.; Anaes. Research Soc.; Assn. Anaesth. Of Gt. Britain & Irel. Prev: Director, Intens. Care Unit, Salisbury Dist. Hosp.

SCOTT, Raymond Deryck The Bridge Street Surgery, 30-32 Bridge Street, Downham Market PE38 9DH Tel: 01366 388888 Fax: 01366 383716; Carburton House, Ryston End, Downham Market Tel: 01366 388859 — MB BCh Wales 1975; DRCOG 1978; DCH Eng. 1978; MRCGP 1980.

SCOTT, Mr Richard John Holly Tree House, New Road, Swanmore, Southampton SO32 2PE — MB BS Lond. 1992 (United Medical and Dental Schools (Guy's)) FRCS Eng. 1998. Specialty: Orthop.

SCOTT, Richard McKerchar Queen Street Surgery, 9-11 Queen Street, Whittlesey, Peterborough PE7 1AY Tel: 01733 326834; 9 Queen St. Surgery, Whittlesey, Peterborough PE7 1AY Tel: 01733 204611 — MB ChB Leeds 1977; MRCGP 1982. Hosp. Pract. (Endoscopy) PeterBoro. Dist. Hosp.; Trainer Gen. Pract. Socs: Primary Care Soc. Gastroenterol. Prev: GP Trainee P'boro. VTS.

SCOTT, Ritchie Gibson Alexander Whyteman's Brae Hospital, Whyteman's Brae, Kirkcaldy KY1 2ND Tel: 01592 643355; 92 Balcarres Avenue, Glasgow G12 0QN — MB ChB Ed. 1996. SHO (Geriats.) Whyteman's Brae Hosp. Kirkcaldy. Prev: SHO (Psychiat.) Whyteman's Brae Hosp. Kirkcaldy; SHO (A & E) Vict. Hosp. Kirkcaldy.

SCOTT, Mr Robert (retired) Garrion, 27 Forest View, Kildrum, Cumbernauld, Glasgow G67 2DB Tel: 0123 67 22683 — MB ChB Glas. 1958; FRCS Glas. 1965; FRCS Ed. 1966; MD Glas. 1985. DL; Hon. Lect. Univ. Strathclyde. Prev: Cons. Urol. Roy. Infirm. Glas.

SCOTT, Mr Robert Adam Department of Emergency Medicine, Royal Brisbane Hospital, Herston Road, Brisbane 4061, Australia; 6 Moorside, Knutsford WA16 6EU — MB ChB Ed. 1982; MRCP (UK) 1987; FRCS Ed. 1992. Regist. (Emerg. Med.) Hope Hosp. Salford. Specialty: Accid. & Emerg. Socs: Brit. Assn. Accid. & Emerg. Med. & Emerg. Med. Research Soc.

SCOTT, Mr Robert Alastair Howie, Wing Cdr. University Hospital Brimingham NHS Trust, Royal Centre for Defence Medicine, Selly Oak Hospital, Birmingham B29 6JD Tel: 0121 627 8351 Fax: 0121 627 8922 Email: rob.scott@lineone.net — MB BS Lond. 1988 (St Thos.) FRCOphth 1993; FRCS Ed. 1993; DM (Ophth.) Nottm. 2005. Cons. (Ophth.) Royal Centre for Defence Med. Univ. Hosp. Birm.; Hon. Sen. Clin. Lect. Univ. Birm.; Roy. Air Force Cons. Adviser in Ophth.; Hon. Cons. Ophth. Birm. & Midl. Eye Centre. Specialty: Ophth. Special Interest: Aviat. Opthalmology; Cataract & Refractive Surg.; Vitreoretinal Surg. Socs: Brit & Eire Assoc. of Vitreoretinal Surgs.; Midl. Ophth. Soc.; Europ. Soc. Cataract & Refractive Surgeons. Prev: Sen. Regist. (Ophth.) Moorfields Eye Hosp. Lond.; Regist. (Ophth.) Princess Mary's RAF Hosp. Halton, Wendover; Sen. Regist. (Ophth.) Qu. Med. Centre Nottm.

SCOTT, Robert Baliol Lincoln County Hospital, Greetwell Road, Lincoln LN2 5QY — MB ChB Bristol 1978; FRCA Eng. 1983. Cons. Anaesth. Lincoln Co. Hosp. Specialty: Anaesth. Socs: BMA & Assn. Anaesth.

SCOTT, Robert Mackie The Medical Centre, 4 Bracklinn Road, Callander FK17 8EJ Tel: 01877 331001 Fax: 01877 331720; 3 Leighton Place, Callander FK17 8BG — MB ChB Aberd. 1987; DRCOG 1990; MRCGP 1991.

SCOTT, Robin Douglas Murray 23 Hemwood Road, Windsor SL4 4YX Tel: 01753 854169 — MB ChB Aberd. 1964; FRCP Ed. 1983, M 1968; FRCP Lond. 1984, M 1968. Cons. Phys. Heatherwood & Wexham Pk. Hosps. NHS Trust & E. Berks. Community Health NHS Trust. Specialty: Gen. Med.; Diabetes; Endocrinol. Socs: Brit. Diabetic Assn. (Med. & Scientif. Sect.). Prev: Dist. Clin. Tutor E. Berks.; Lect. (Med.) Univ. Edin.; Research Fell. Washington Univ. Sch. Med. St. Louis, USA.

SCOTT, Robin Ford West Gate Health Centre, Charleston Drive, Dundee DD2 4AD Tel: 01382 668189 Fax: 01382 665943; The Keepers Cottage, Redmyres Farm, Invergowrie, Dundee DD2 5LH — MB ChB Aberd. 1966; FRCGP 1982, M 1975. Regional Adviser (Gen. Pract.) Tayside HB. Socs: BMA. Prev: Terminable Lect. (Path.) Univ. Aberd.; Res. Med. Off. Aberd. Roy. Infirm.; Res. Surg. Off. Roy. Aberd. Hosp. Sick Childr.

SCOTT, Roderick John Leith Walk Surgery, 60 Leith Walk, Edinburgh EH6 5HB Tel: 0131 554 6471 Fax: 0131 555 4964; 34 Inverleith Gardens, Edinburgh EH3 5PR — MB ChB Ed. 1981; MRCGP 1986.

SCOTT, Roger William Station House Surgery, Kendal LA9 6SA Tel: 01539 722660 Fax: 01539 734845; 12 Cliff Terrace, Kendal LA9 4JR — MB ChB Manch. 1989 (Manchester) DRCOG 1993; MRCGP 1995. GP Kendal. Specialty: Gen. Pract.

SCOTT, Ronald Montalto Medical Centre, 2 Dromore Road, Ballynahinch BT24 8AY Tel: 028 9756 2929 — MB BCh BAO Belf. 1959; DObst RCOG 1962.

SCOTT, Rosemary Jane Department of Histopathology, University College Hospital, Medical School, London WC1E 6JJ — MB BChir Camb. 1980; MRCP (UK) 1983; MRCPath 1990. Sen. Lect. (Histopath.). Specialty: Histopath. Prev: Cons. Lect. Paediat. Path. Univ. Camb.; Sen. Regist. (Histopath.) Roy. Postgrad. Med. Sch. Lond. & Roy. Sussex Co. Hosp. Brighton.

SCOTT, Mr Roy Niblock Ross Hall Hospital, 221 Crookston Road, Glasgow G52 3NQ Tel: 0141 712266 Fax: 0141 760015; 17 Burnside Road, Burnside, Rutherglen, Glasgow G73 4RL Tel: 0141 569 6487 Email: roy.scott1@ntlworld.com — MB ChB Glas. 1981; FRCS Glas. 1985; MD Glas. 1990. Cons. Gen. & Vasc. Surg. Monklands Hosp. Airdrie; Monklands Hosp. Subdean, Univ. of Glas. Specialty: Gen. Surg. Socs: Vasc. Surg. Soc.; Assn. of Surg. of Gt. Britain & Irel. Prev: Sen. Regist. Vict. Infirm. Glas. & Glas. Roy. Infirm.

SCOTT, Sandra Loreen 22A Alexander Street, London W2 5NT — MB BS Lond. 1993.

SCOTT, Sandy Steel (retired) The Bartons, Perlethorpe, Newark NG22 9EH Tel: 01623 823504 — MB ChB Sheff. 1950; MRCGP 1968. AMP Bds. DSS. Prev: GP Mansfield.

SCOTT, Sara Elizabeth Barnard Medical Practice, 43 Granville Road, Sidcup DA14 4TA Tel: 020 8302 7721 Fax: 020 8309 6579; 145 Southborough Lane, Bromley BR2 8AP — MB BS Lond. 1985; DRCOG 1988; MRCGP 1989; DFFP 1994. GP Sidcup. Prev: Trainee GP Sidcup; SHO (A & E) Bromley Hosp.; SHO (O & G) FarnBoro. Hosp.

SCOTT, Sarah Theresa Dorset County Hospital, X-Ray Department, Williams Avenue, Dorchester DT1 2JY/01305 254484/4442 Fax: 01305 254136 Email: sally.scott@wdgh.nhs.uk; Merton Grange, Wheelers Lane, Bearwood, Bournemouth BH11 9QJ Tel: 01202 573218 Fax: 01202 573218 Email: sally@mertong.demon.co.uk — MB BS Lond. 1972 (Westm.) MRCS Eng. LRCP Lond. 1972; DMRD 1981; FRCR 1985. Cons. Radiol. W. Dorset Gen. Hosps. NHS Trust. Specialty: Radiol. Socs: BMA; Brit. Med. Ultrasound Soc.; Brit. Soc. Of Paediat. Radiol. Prev: Sen. Regist. (Radiol.) Soton. & Bristol Gen. Hosps.; Resid. Phys. Hosp. San José San Bernardo del Viento, Colombia.

SCOTT, Sharon Anne 21A The Nook, Anstey, Leicester LE7 7AZ Tel: 0191 384 6171 — MB BS Newc. 1987; DTM & H Liverp. 1989; DCH RCP Lond. 1991. Specialty: Gen. Pract. Prev: Asst. GP Leics.; Trainee GP Tyne & Wear; GP Partner, Durh.

SCOTT, Sheila Stewart (retired) 20 Glamis Terrace, Dundee DD2 1NA — MB ChB St. And. 1954; DPH St. And. 1963. Prev: Lect. (Med. Microbiol.) Univ. Dundee.

SCOTT, Shelagh Jean Falcon House Surgery, 17/19 Heaton Road, Newcastle upon Tyne NE6 1SA Tel: 0191 265 3361 Fax: 0191 224 3209; 76 Stuart Court, Kenton Bank Foot, Newcastle upon Tyne NE3 2SG — MB BS Newc. 1980; MRCP (UK) 1984; DRCOG 1988; MRCGP 1989. GP Newc.; Clin. Asst. Nephrol. Specialty: Nephrol. Prev: Research Regist. (Med.) Roy. Infirm. Sunderland.; Regist. (Med.) Roy. Infirm. Sunderland; SHO (Med.) Roy. Vict. Infirm. Newc.

SCOTT, Simon James Blackhorse Cottage, Lower End, Wavendon, Milton Keynes MK17 8AW; Flat 30, Princes Gardens, Highfield St, Liverpool L3 6LQ Tel: 0151 255 0429 Email: wiksyontour@hotmail.com — MB ChB Liverp. 1992 (Liverpool) FRCS Eng. 1997; MSc Cardiff 2001; FRCS (Tr & Orth) Eng. 2002. Specialist Regist. (Orthop.) Mersey Rotat.; Cons. in Orthopaedic Surg. Specialty: Orthop.

SCOTT, Stephen 4 Marian Way, South Shields NE34 8AL — MB BS Newc. 1992.

SCOTT, Stephen Basil Cuthbert 19 Danecroft Road, London SE24 9PA — MB BChir Camb. 1980; MRCP (UK) 1988; MRCPsych 1990.

SCOTT, Stephen James 10 Westminser Close, Charlton Kings, Cheltenham GL53 7QP Tel: 01242 522932 Email: stevescott.surfer@virgin.net — BM Soton. 1996 (Southampton) SHO (Med.); SpR Respirat. & Gen. Med. Specialty: Gen. Med. Socs: BMA; MDU. Prev: SHO (Med.); SHO (A & E); Ho. Off. (Med.).

SCOTT, Steven Fraser Owen Nunwell Surgery, 10 Pump Street, Bromyard HR7 4BZ Tel: 01885 483412 Fax: 01885 488739 Email: steven.scott@nhs.net; Jenks Cottage, The Downs, Bromyard HR7 4NU — MB ChB Bristol 1982; DA (UK) 1985; DCH RCP Lond. 1986. Specialty: Gen. Pract.

SCOTT, Stewart William Brewery Farm, Longburgh, Burgh by Sands, Carlisle CA5 6AF — MB ChB Bristol 1976; MRCPsych 1986. Cons. Child & Adolesc. Psychiat. Fairfield Centre Carlisle. Specialty: Child & Adolesc. Psychiat.

SCOTT, Mr Stuart Dalgleish BUPA Hospital Norwich, Old Watton Road, Colney, Norwich NR4 7TD Tel: 01953 600410 Fax: 01953 600410 Email: scottsurg@aol.com — MB ChB Ed. 1972; BSc Ed. 1969; FRCS Eng. 1981; MS Soton. 1987. Specialty: Gen. Surg. Special Interest: Breast and Endocrine. Socs: Brit. Assn. Surg. Oncol.; Brit. Soc. Antimicrob. Chemother.; BMA. Prev: Lect. (Surg.) Soton. Univ.; Regist. (Surg.) St. Thos. Hosp. Lond.; Lt. Col. RAMC Field Surg. Team Iraq, Kuwait Gulf War.

SCOTT, Stuart Thomas Holburn Medical Group, 7 Albyn Place, Aberdeen AB10 1YE Tel: 01224 400800 Fax: 01224 407777 Email: stuart.scott@nhs.net; 289 King's Gate, Aberdeen AB15 6AJ Tel: 01224 208237 — MB ChB Aberd. 1984. Clin. Director, Directorate of Health Informatics, NHS Grampian, Aberd.

SCOTT, Susan Christine Mary 2 Crookston Court, Crookston Road, Musselburgh EH21 7TR Tel: 0131 665 3159 — MB ChB Aberd. 1986; MRCOG 1992. Assoc. Specialist; RCOG/RCR Advanced Obst. Ultrasound 1995. Specialty: Obst. & Gyn. Socs: Ed. Obst. Soc.; BMA. Prev: Staff Grade (O & G) E. Gen. Hosp. Edin.; Regist. (O & G) East. Gen. Hosp. Edin.; SHO (O & G) East. Gen. Hosp. Edin.

SCOTT, Susan Joan Barnt Green Surgery, 82 Hewell Road, Barnt Green, Birmingham B45 8NF Tel: 0121 445 1704 Fax: 0121 447 8253; Wheeley House, Wheeley Road, Alvechurch, Birmingham B48 7DD Tel: 0121 445 1569 — MB BChir Camb. 1973; BA Camb. 1970, MB BChir 1973; MRCP (UK) 1976. GP Birm.

SCOTT, Sydney Cadzow Campbell (retired) 29 Piercing Hill, Theydon Bois, Epping CM16 7JW Tel: 01992 813164 Fax: 01992 813164 Email: scottbarrie@clara.co.uk — MB BS Lond. 1953 (Guy's) LMSSA Lond. 1952; DObst RCOG 1958; FRCGP 1991, M 1960; DCH Eng. 1966; MD Lond. 1974. Prev: Ho. Surg. (ENT) Guy's Hosp.

SCOTT, Tara Jane 26 Bawnmore Road, Belfast BT9 6LA — MB BCh BAO Belf. 1991.

SCOTT, Thomas Bell Greystoke Surgery, Kings Avenue, Morpeth NE61 1JA Tel: 01670 511393 Fax: 01670 503282 — MB BS Durh. 1966 (Newc.) DObst RCOG 1968; MRCGP 1973.

SCOTT, Mr Thomas Douglas 3 Lemon Villas, Truro TR1 2NX Tel: 01872 273689; Uplands, Kerley Downs, Chasewater, Truro TR4 8LA Tel: 01872 361702 — MB ChB Glas. 1975; BSc (Hons.) Glas. 1973; FRCS Glas. 1980; FRCS Ed. (Orth.) 1988. Cons. Orthop. Roy. Cornw. Hosp.. Truro. Specialty: Orthop. Socs: Fell. BOA; Brit. Soc. Surg. Hand; Roy. Soc. Med. Prev: Sen. Regist. (Orthop.) Princess Eliz. Orthop. Hosp. Exeter.

SCOTT, Thomas McMillan Grange Farmhouse, Grange Road, Dunfermline KY11 3DG — MB ChB Glas. 1970; DCH RCPS Glas. 1972; MRCP (U.K.) 1974.

SCOTT, Timothy Edward 25 Cherry Orchard, Highworth, Swindon SN6 7AU — MB BS Lond. 1998; MB BS Lond 1998.

SCOTT, Timothy Nigel Bradshaw 8 Nursery Gardens, Broadmeadows, South Normanton, Derby — MB ChB Sheff. 1987.

SCOTT, Valerie Anne Clackmannan and Kincardine Medical Practice, Health Centre, Main Street, Clackmannan FK10 4QX Tel: 01259 723725 Fax: 01259 724791; Kincardine Health Centre, 19 Kilbagie St, Kincardine, Alloa FK10 4QX — MB ChB Ed. 1985; DRCOG 1989; MRCGP 1990.

SCOTT, William c/o Smith, 117 Arkleston Road, Paisley PA1 3TY Tel: 020 8889 2977; 3437 - 111A Street, Edmonton Alb. T6J 3L1, Canada — (Glas.) LRCP LRCS Ed. LRFPS Glas. 1952. Prev: SHO Orthop. Unit, Kilmarnock Infirm.; Sen. Ho. Surg. Ingham Infirm. S. Shields; Sen. Ho. Surg. Thoracic Unit, East. Gen. Hosp. Edin.

SCOTT, Mr William Alexander 152 Harley Street, London W1G 7LH Tel: 020 7935 3834; 10 Handen Road, Lee, London SE12 8NP Fax: 020 8297 8955 Email: wscott@dircon.co.uk — MB BS Lond. 1972 (King's Coll. Hosp.) FRCS Eng. 1976. Cons. Orthop. Surg.Qu. Eliz. Hosp. Lond.; Hon. Cons. Blackheath Hosp. Lond. Specialty: Orthop.; Medico Legal. Socs: BMA; W Kent M-C Soc.; Brit. Orthop. Assn. Prev: Sen. Regist. (Orthop.) St. Mary's Hosp., Char. Cross Hosp. Lond. & Roy. Nat. Orthop. Hosp. Stanmore.

SCOTT, William Chisholm (retired) Muston Manor, Winterbourne Muston, Blandford Forum DT11 9BU — (St. Bart.) MB BS Lond. 1950; DMRD Eng. 1963; FFR 1966. Prev: Cons. Radiol. E. Dorset Health Dist.

SCOTT, William Edward, MBE (retired) 13 Hall Close, Kettering NN15 7LQ — (Glas.) MB ChB Glas. 1940; DIH Lond. 1952. Sen. Med. Off. Brit. Steel Corpn. Prev: Surg. Regist. Glas. Roy. Infirm.

SCOTT, William Gary 10 Swinburne Drive, Crewe CW1 5JE Tel: 01270 587601 — MB BCh BAO Belf. 1982; MB BCh Belf. 1982; DCH Dub. 1985.

SCOTT, William Semion (retired) Maryhill Health Centre, 41 Shawpark St., Glasgow G20 9DR Tel: 0141 946 7151; 29 Saint Kilda Drive, Glasgow G14 9LN Tel: 0141 959 4840 — MB ChB Glas. 1958.

SCOTT, William Sinclair Ayr Road Surgery, 69 Ayr Road, Douglas, Lanark ML11 0PX Tel: 01555 851226; Mansefield House, Weaver's Yards, Douglas, Lanark ML11 0QB Tel: 01555 851226 — MB ChB Glas. 1968. Socs: BMA. Prev: SHO (Gyn.) Law Hosp. Carluke; Ho. Off. (Obst.) Glas. Roy. Matern. Hosp. & Qu. Mother's Hosp. Glas.

SCOTT ANDREWS, Margaret Louise Pool Farm House, Mills Lane, Wroxton St Mary, Banbury OX15 6PY Tel: 01295 730486 — MB BS Lond. 1970 (Roy. Free) MRCS Eng. LRCP Lond. 1970; DObst RCOG 1972; MRCGP 1976. Clin. Med. Off. - family Plann. Specialty: Family Plann. & Reproduc. Health. Prev: Ho. Phys. (Paediat.) Hampstead Gen. Hosp.; Ho. Surg. (Gyn.) Roy. Free Hosp. Lond.; GP.

SCOTT-BARRETT, Sarah Department of Radiology, Norfolk & Norwich Healthcare Trust, Brunswick Road, Norwich NR1 3SR Tel: 01603 286286; South End House, Loddon, Norwich NR14 6DX Tel: 01508 520308 Fax: 01508 520308 — MB BS Lond. 1984 (Guy's Hosp. Med. Sch.) MRCP (UK) 1990; FRCR 1994. Cons. Radiol. Norf. & Norwich Hosp. Specialty: Radiol. Prev: Sen. Regist. (Radiol.) Char. Cross Hosp. Lond.; Regist. (Radiol.) Char. Cross Hosp. Lond.; SHO (Med.) St. Geo. Hosp. & Nat. Heart Hosp. Lond.

SCOTT-BROWN, Andrew William, Surg. Lt. RN Lake Road Health Centre, Nutfield Place, Portsmouth PO1 4JT Tel: 023 92 821201 — MB ChB Aberd. 1983 (Aberdeen) MRCGP; DRCOG. Hse. Med. Examr. Divers; MSA Med. Examr. Seafarers.

SCOTT-BROWN, Graham The Health Centre, Coxwell Road, Faringdon SN7 7EZ Tel: 01367 242407 — MB BChir Camb. 1955; FRCP Lond. 1973, M 1956.

SCOTT-BROWN, Mary Muriel Gosport War Memorial Hospital, Bury Road, Gosport PO12 3PW Tel: 023 9252 4611; Ythan Lodge, 2 Haddon Close, Fareham PO14 1PH Tel: 01392 823675 — MB ChB Aberd. 1983; MB ChB (Commend.) Aberd. 1983. Staff Grade Psychiat. Gosport War Memor. Hosp. Specialty: Geriat. Psychiat. Prev: Regist. (Psychiat.) St. Jas. Hosp. Portsmouth.

SCOTT BROWN, Nigel Myrie (retired) Orchard House, Low Street, Husthwaite, York YO61 4QA Tel: 01347 868173 — MB Camb. 1961 (St. Thos.) BChir 1960; DObst RCOG 1962; DA Eng. 1965.

SCOTT-BROWN, Sarah Ruth 152 Marlborough Road, Oxford OX1 4LS — MB BS Lond. 1994; MRCP UK 1997; DTM & H Liverp. 1999; MRCGP 2000.

SCOTT-COOK, Helen Ruth 78 Addison Road, Kings Heath, Birmingham B14 7EW Tel: 0121 444 6965 — MB ChB Bristol 1992. SHO (Orthop.) Selly Oak Hosp. Specialty: Orthop. Prev: Cas. Off. Birm. Heartlands Hosp.; Lect. (Anat.) Birm. Univ.

SCOTT-FLEMING, Mark Simon 13 Battersea Rise, London SW11 1HG — MB BS Lond. 1994.

SCOTT-JUPP, Claire Elizabeth — MB BS Lond. 1987.

SCOTT-JUPP, Robert Henry Salisbury District Hospital, Salisbury SP2 8BJ Tel: 01722 336262; 7 Church Lane, Lower Bemerton, Salisbury SP2 9NR Email: scottjupp@aol.com — MB BS Lond. 1980; DCH RCP Lond. 1983; MRCP (UK) 1986; FRCPCH 1997.

Cons. Paediat. Salisbury. Dist. Hosp. Specialty: Paediat. Prev: Lect. & Hon. Sen. Regist. (Child Health) Univ. Leicester; Regist. (Paediat.) Liverp. Hosps.; SHO (Paediat.) Bristol Hosps.

SCOTT-JUPP, Ruth Martha (retired) 17 Avon Run Road, Friars Cliff, Christchurch BH23 4DX Tel: 01425 275762 — MB BCh BAO Dub. 1949 (T.C. Dub.)

SCOTT-JUPP, Wendy Margaret Orchard Surgery, Christchurch Medical Centre, Purewell Cross Road, Christchurch BH23 3AF Tel: 01202 481902 Fax: 01202 486887 — BM Soton. 1978; DRCOG 1982.

SCOTT-KNIGHT, Victoria Catherine Elizabeth Bryn-y-Gwalia Hall, Llangedwyn, Oswestry SY10 9JW — MB BS Lond. 1977 (Roy. Free) MRCS Eng. LRCP Lond. 1977; FFA RCSI 1987. Cons. Anaesth. Wrexham Maelor Hosp. Specialty: Anaesth. Prev: Sen. Regist. Midl. Anaesth. Train. Scheme; Regist. (Anaesth.) Edgware Gen. Hosp. Middlx.; Ho. Phys. Roy. Free Hosp. Lond.

SCOTT-KNOX-GORE, Charles Leggett Kings Road Surgery, 67 Kings Road, Harrogate HG1 5HJ Tel: 01423 875875 Fax: 01423 875885 — MB BS Lond. 1972 (Middlx.) DObst RCOG 1975. Princip. GP N. Yorks. Family Pract. Comm. Prev: Trainee GP Harrogate VTS; Ho. Surg. Mt. Vernon Hosp. Northwood; Ho. Phys. Harrogate Gen. Hosp.

SCOTT-MACKIE, Pauline Lindsay Department of Radiology, Guy's Hospital, St Thomas St., London SE1 9RT Tel: 020 7955 5000 — MB BS Lond. 1989; MRCP (UK) 1993; FRCR 1996. Specialist Regist. (Radiol.) Guy's & St. Thos. NHS Trust Lond. Specialty: Radiol.

SCOTT-MONCRIEFF, Christina Mary Bristol Homoeopathic Hospital, Cotham, Bristol BS6 6JU Tel: 0117 973 1231 Fax: 0117 923 8759; 36 Gipsy Lane, Beckford Green, Warminster BA12 9LR Tel: 01985 846784 Fax: 01985 846784 — MB ChB Birm. 1975; MFHom 1987. Clin. Fell. Bristol Homoeop. Hosp. Specialty: Homeop. Med. Socs: Fell. Roy. Soc. Med.; BMA. Prev: SHO (Paediat.) Simpson Memor. Matern. Pavil. & Roy. Hosp. Sick Childr. Edin.

SCOTT-MONCRIEFF, Nigel Francis John, Surg. Cdr. RN 9 Devonshire Place, London W1 Tel: 020 7935 8425; 22 Sloane Avenue, London SW3 3JE — MB BS Lond. 1982 (The Lond. Hosp.) BSc (Hons.) Lond. 1982; MRCGP 1990. Indep. GP Lond.; Hon. Phys. to Westm. Abbey. Socs: Fell. Roy. Soc. Med.; Med. Soc. Lond. Prev: Princip. Med. Off. Her Majesty's Yacht Britannia; Princip. Med. Off. HMS St. Vincent (Lond.); Sen. Med. Off. Roy. Marines Sch. Music Deal.

SCOTT-PERRY, Stephen John 13 Borelli Mews, The Borough, Farnham GU9 7YZ — MB ChB Dund. 1985.

SCOTT-RUSSELL, Ann Margaret 49 Worrin Road, Shenfield, Brentwood CM15 8DH — MB BS Lond. 1995.

SCOTT-SAMUEL, Alex Jeremy Richard University of Liverpool, Department of Public Health, Whelan Building, Liverpool L69 3GB Tel: 0151 794 5569 Fax: 0151 794 5588 Email: alexss@liv.ac.uk; 218 Allerton Road, Liverpool L18 6JN — MB ChB Liverp. 1971; MCommH 1976; FFCM 1988; FFPHM 1989. Sen. Lect. (Pub. Health) Univ. Liverp.; Hon. Cons.Pub.Health Liverp. PCT. Specialty: Pub. Health Med. Prev: Cons. (Pub. Health) Liverp. HA; Sen. Regist. (Community Med.) Mersey RHA; Dept.al Med. Off. Liverp. City Counc..

SCOTT-SMITH, Wesley The Charter Medical Centre, 88 Davigdor Road, Hove BN3 1RF Tel: 01273 738070/770555 Fax: 01273 220 0883; 17 Woodland Avenue, Hove BN3 6BH Email: wesdoc@mcmail.com — MB BS Lond. 1979 (Guy's) MRCGP 1984; DRCOG 1984. Research Fell. Trafford Centre, Univ. Sussex.

SCOTT WARREN, David Noel Martin, CStJ (retired) Mont du Ouaisng, St Brelade, Jersey JE3 8AW Tel: 01534 742939 Mob: 07797 715417 — (Royal Lond. Hosp.) MRCS Eng. LRCP Lond. 1948. Prev: H.S. E.N.T. & General. Royal London Hospital.

SCOTTER, Betty (retired) 38 Gunton Drive, Lowestoft NR32 4QB Tel: 01502 574033 — MB BS Lond. 1947; MRCS Eng. LRCP Lond. 1946.

SCOTTON, Johanna Elizabeth 5 Filbert St. E., Leicester LE2 7JG — MB ChB Leic. 1997.

SCOTTON, Susan Johnson The Chantry, Dean St., Brewood, Wolverhampton Tel: 01902 850402; Maes y Haf, Porth Tocyn, Abersoch, Pwllheli Tel: 3377 — MB BS Lond. 1975; MRCS Eng. LRCP Lond. 1975. Assoc. Spacialist (Pallio) Compta Hospice Wolverhampton; Occupational Health Marks & Spencer plc. Specialty: Obst. & Gyn.

SCOUGAL, Isabel Jean Falkirk & District Royal Infirmary, Majors Loan, Falkirk FK1 5QE Tel: 01324 624000 Email: isabel.scougal@fvah.scot.nhs.uk; 3 Gardrum Place, Brightons, Falkirk FK2 0EX Tel: 01324 717394 — MB ChB Ed. 1985 (Ed. Univ.) BSc (Hons.) Ed. 1983; MRCP (UK) 1989; FRCP Edin. 2002. Cons. Phys. in Geriat. Med. Falkirk & Dist. Roy. Infirm. Specialty: Care of the Elderly; Diabetes. Socs: Brit. Geriat. Soc.; Diabetes UK. Prev: Sen. Regist. Gen. & Geriat. Med. Manch.; Clin. Lect. (Geriat. Med.) Univ. Manch.; Regist. (Endocrinol., Gen. Med. & Diabetic) Edin. Roy. Infirm.

SCOULAR, Anne Buchanan Department of Genitourinary Medicine, The Sandyford Initiative, Sandyford, Sauchiehall St, Glasgow G3 7NB Tel: 0141 211 8625 Fax: 0141 211 8609 — MB ChB Glas. 1978; DRCOG 1980; DCH RCPS Glas. 1981; MRCGP 1982; MRCP (UK) 1987; FRCP Glas 1997; FRCP Glas. 1997. Cons. Genitourin. Med. Greater Glas. Primary Care Trust. Specialty: Genitourinary Medicine. Prev: Sen. Regist. (Genitourin. Med.) Middlx. Hosp. Lond.

SCOULLER, Frances Elizabeth West Pottergate Health Centre, 137 West Pottergate, Norwich NR2 4BX Tel: 01603 628705 Fax: 01603 766789; The Wood Barn, Stoke Lane, Dunston, Norwich NR14 8QD Tel: 01508 471307 — MB BS Lond. 1982 (Univ. Coll. Lond.) BSc (Hons) Lond. 1979; MRCP (UK) 1985. Princip. GP. Specialty: Gen. Pract.

SCOURFIELD, Alan Edward Coalbrook Surgery, 18 Coalbrook Road, Pontyberem, Llanelli SA15 5HU Tel: 01269 870207 Fax: 01269 871314; Bryngwendraeth, Llanddarog, Carmarthen SA32 8PB Tel: 01267 275712 — MB BS Lond. 1979; MRCS Eng. LRCP Lond. 1979. Clical Asst. Orthopaedic, P. Philip Hosp., Llananelli, Carmarthen; Clin. Asst. Urol., P. Philip Hosp., Llanelli, Carmarthen.

SCOURFIELD, Alun James Scourfield and Partners, The Surgery, Oakfield Street, Hengoed CF82 7WX Tel: 01443 813248 Fax: 01443 862283; 3 Pen y Cae, Ystrad Mynach, Hengoed CF82 7FA — MB BS Lond. 1972; MRCS Eng. LRCP Lond. 1971. Hon. Lect. (Gen. Pract.) Univ. Wales.; CDP Coordinator Caerphilly, Univ. of Wales Coll. of Med. Prev: CME Tutor Rhymach Valley Postgrad. Centre.

SCOURFIELD, Derek Bennett (retired) Maes-y-Llwyn, Llanddarog, Carmarthen SA32 8BJ Tel: 01267 275718 Email: dbscourfield@maesyllwyn75.freeserve.co.uk — (Cardiff) BSc Wales 1947; MB BCh Wales 1950. Prev: SHO (Cas.) Cardiff Roy. Infirm.

SCOURFIELD, Dilys (retired) Maes-y-Llwyn, Llanddarog, Carmarthen SA32 8BJ Tel: 01267 275718 — (Cardiff) BSc Wales 1947; MB BCh Wales 1950. Prev: SHO (O & G) E. Glam. Hosp. Pontypridd.

SCOURFIELD, Ewan John Coalbrook Surgery, 18 Coalbrook Road, Pontyberem, Llanelli SA15 5HU Tel: 01269 870207 Fax: 01269 871314; Pennant, 29 Heol-y-Felin, Pontyberem, Llanelli SA15 5EH — MB BS Lond. 1981; MRCS Eng. LRCP Lond. 1981.

SCOURFIELD, Jane Department of Psychological Medicine, University of Wales College of Medicine, Heath Park, Cardiff CF14 4XN — BM BCh Oxf. 1988; MA Camb. 1988; MRCPsych 1994; MSc (Psychiat. Studies) Wales 1994; PhD Wales 2000. Sen. Clin. Research Fell. (Child and adolescant Psychiat.) Cardiff. Prev: Regist. (Psychiat.) Cardiff; M.R.C Train.Fell. Yale + Cardiff.; SpR child Psychiat.. Cardiff.

SCOVELL, Elizabeth Elaine Roseleat, 22 Middle St., Port Isaac PL29 3RH — MB ChB Dundee 1973; DMRD Eng. 1978.

SCOWEN, Beverley Manfordway Health Centre, 40 Foremark Close, Hainault, Romford Tel: 020 8500 3088 — MB BS Lond. 1992.

SCOWEN, Mark Kevin Health Centre, Handsworth Avenue, Highams Park, London E4 9PD Tel: 020 8527 0913 Fax: 020 8527 6597 — MB ChB Leeds 1980.

SCRAGG, Gillian Mary Cedars Medical Centre, 12 Sandbach Road South, Alsager, Stoke-on-Trent ST7 2AD Tel: 01270 882179 Fax: 01270 216330 — MB ChB Liverp. 1981; MRCGP 1985. GP. Prev: Partner in Gen. Pract.; Trainee GP Wirral VTS.

SCRAGG, Sheena Elizabeth Fife Palliative Care Service, Ward 16, Queen Margaret Hospital, Dunfermline KY12 0SG Tel: 01383 623623 Email: sheena.scragg@faht.scot.nhs.uk — MB ChB Ed. 1982 (Edinburgh) DRCOG 1984; MRCP (UK) 1986; FRCP Ed. 1995.

Cons. Palliat. Med. Fife Primary Care Trust Kirkcaldy. Specialty: Palliat. Med. Prev: Med. Off. MacMillan Serv. Fife.

SCRASE, Angela Mary Prospect Farm, Llanidloes SY18 Tel: 01978 122789 — MRCS Eng. LRCP Lond. 1965 (St. Thos.) DPM Eng. 1972.

SCRASE, Christopher David Paramor Cottage, 42 New Street, Chippenham, Ely CB7 5QF — MB BChir Camb. 1988; BA (Hons.) Camb. 1986; MA Camb. 1990; MRCP (UK) 1992; FRCR 1996; Cert Med Educat 2003. Macmillian Cons., Clin. Oncol., Ipswich Hosp. NHS Trust, Suff. Specialty: Oncol.; Radiother. Prev: Sen. Regist. (Clin. Oncol.) Nottm. City Hosp. NHS Trust; Regist. (Clin. Oncol.) Addenbrooke's Hosp. NHS Trust.

SCRASE, Edward Tuppin Prospect Farm, Llanidloes Tel: 01686 412789 — MB BChir Camb. 1966 (St. Mary's) MB Camb. 1966, BChir 1965; FFA RCS Eng. 1970; DObst RCOG 1972; DTM & H Liverp. 1989. Specialty: Anaesth.

SCREATON, Gavin Robert Field End, Bayswater Road, Headington, Oxford OX3 9RZ — BM BCh Oxf. 1987.

SCREATON, Nicholas John Field End, Bayswater Road, Oxford OX3 9RZ; 75 Norwich Street, Cambridge CB2 1ND Tel: 01223 354827 — BM BCh Oxf. 1990; BA Camb. 1987; MRCP (UK) 1993; FRCR 1997. Specialty: Radiol.

SCRIMGEOUR, John Beocher (retired) Cuilaluinn, Aberfeldy PH15 2JW Tel: 01887 820302 — MB ChB Ed. 1962; DObst 1964; FRCOG 1982, M 1968; FRCS Ed. 1987; FRCP Ed. 1993. Prev: Med. Dir. West. Gen. Hosps. Trust Edin.

SCRIMGEOUR, Karen Mathilda Agnes 47 Highcliffe Drive, Sheffield S11 7LT Tel: 0114 230 5757; 19 Shipley Road, Leicester LE5 5BX — MB ChB Sheff. 1992.

SCRIMINGER, Mark William 13 Elmtree Road, Teddington TW11 8SJ — MB BS Lond. 1992. Specialty: Gen. Pract.

SCRINE, Marion Department Community Paediatrics, Barham House, Wembley Centre for Health and Care, 116 Chaplin Road, Wembley HA0 4UZ Tel: 020 8795 6340 Fax: 020 8795 6350 — BM BCh Oxf. 1981; BA Oxf. 1981; DCH RCP Lond. 1985; MRCPI (Paediat.) 1986. Cons. Paediat. & Child Health, Brent Teaching PCT, Lond.; Cons. Paediat. Centr. Middlx. Hosp. NHS Trust. Specialty: Community Child Health. Prev: Sen. Regist. (Paediat.) W. Lond. Healthcare NHS Trust; Clin. Med. Off. Richmond, Twickenham & Roehampton HA; Lect. (Paediat. & Nephrol.) Roy. Free Hosp. Lond.

SCRIVEN, Anthony James 24 Haldane Road, London SW6 7EU — MB BS Lond. 1977.

SCRIVEN, Barrie Edward Leek Health Centre, Fountain Street, Leek ST13 6JB Tel: 01538 381022 Fax: 01538 398638; Bank House, Sandy Lane, Longsdon, Stoke-on-Trent ST9 9QQ Tel: 01538 399620 — MB ChB Birm. 1971; DObst RCOG 1973; DCH Eng. 1974; MRCGP 1976. Socs: BMA.

SCRIVEN, Jeanne Mary (retired) Anchorstone, Searle Road, Farnham GU9 8LU Tel: 01252 727378 — (Manch.) MB ChB Manch. 1941. Prev: Orthop. Ho. Surg. & Orthop. Regist. Manch. Roy. Infirm.

SCRIVEN, John Edward 30 Wolverton Gardens, London W6 7DY Tel: 020 8748 7612 — MB BS Lond. 1952 (Guy's) MRCGP 1970; MA (Med. Ethics & Law) Lond. 1992. Prev: Hosp. Pract. (Geriat.) W. Lond. Hosp.

SCRIVEN, John Kevin Littlecroft, 24 Elm Tree Square, Embsay, Skipton BD23 6RA Tel: 01756 797243 Email: jscriven@doctors.net — MB BS Lond. 1988 (Char. Cross & Westm.) DA (UK) 1992; FFA RCSI 1995. Cons. (Anaesth. & IC Med.) Airedale Gen. Hosp. Specialty: Anaesth.; Intens. Care. Socs: Intens. Care Soc.; Yorks. Soc. Anaesth.; Obst. Anaesth. Assn. Prev: SHO (Anaesth.) Bristol Roy. Infirm. & N. Devon Dist. Hosp. Barnstaple; Regist. (Anaesth.) Qu. Eliz. Hosp. Birm.

SCRIVEN, Mr John Mark 41 Sword Close, Glenfield, Leicester LE3 8SY — MB ChB Leic. 1989; BSc (Hons.) Leic. 1986; FRCS Eng. 1993; MD (Leic) 2000, FRCS (Gen. Surg) 2001. Specialty: Gen. Surg.

SCRIVEN, Mr Mark William Department of Surgery, Wrexham Maelor Hospital, Croesnewydd Road, Wrexham LL13 7TD Tel: 01978 725430 Fax: 01978 725418 Email: mark.scriven@new-tr.wales.nhs.uk — MB BS Lond. 1984 (Guy's) BSc (Hons.) Biochem. Lond. 1981, MS 1993, MB BS 1984; FRCS Eng. 1988. Cons. Surg. Wrexham Maelor Hosp. Specialty: Gen. Surg. Socs: Vasc. Surg. Soc. Prev: Advanced Surg. Trainee John Hunter Hosp. Newc., NSW, Austral.

SCRIVEN, Nicholas Andrew Calderdale Royal Hospital, Salterhebble, Halifax HY3 0PW Tel: 01422 357171 — MB ChB Leic. 1991 (Leicester) MRCP (UK) 1994. Cons. Phys., Claderdale Roy. Hosp., Halifax. Specialty: Respirat. Med.; Gen. Med. Socs: Brit. Thorac. Soc.; Yorks. Thoracic Soc. Prev: Sp. Reg. (Reg.) Nottm. City Hosp.

SCRIVEN, Patricia Mary Department of Anaesthesia, Russells Hall Hospital, Dudley Tel: 01384 456111; 87 Fitzroy Avenue, Harborne, Birmingham B17 8RH Tel: 0121 427 2940 — MB ChB Manch. 1970; FFA RCS Eng. 1978. Cons. Anaesth. Russells Hall Hosp. Dudley; Hon. Sen. Lect. Birm. Univ.; Assoc. Postgrad. Dean (W. Midl.s). Specialty: Anaesth.

SCRIVEN, Sharon Denise 41 Sword Close, Glenfield, Leicester LE3 8SY — MB ChB Leic. 1989; BSc Leic. 1986; FRCS Glas. 1994; MD 2000.

SCRIVEN, William Ashley Pendyffryn Medical Group, Ffordd Pendyffryn, Prestatyn LL19 9DH Tel: 01745 886444 Fax: 01745 889831 — MB BS Lond. 1980 (St. Mary's) BA Oxf. 1977; DRCOG 1985.

SCRIVENER, Sarah Louise Dept. Thoracic Medicine, Royal Bournemouth Hospital, Bournemouth BH7 7DW; Branksome House, 17 Nelson Road, Westbourne, Bournemouth BH4 9JA — BChir Camb. 1994 (Cambridge) BA (Hons) Cantab 1992; MB Camb. 1995; MA 1996; MRCP (UK) 1998. Specialist Regist. in Gen. and Respiratary Med., Roy. Bournemouth Hosp. Specialty: Gen. Med.; Respirat. Med. Socs: BMA. Prev: Ho. Off. (Thoracic Surg. & Gen. Surg.) Norf. & Norwich Healthcare NHS Trust; Ho. Phys. W. Suff. Hosp. Bury St. Edmunds; Res. Med. Off. Roy. N.shore & Manly Hosps. Sydney NSW, Australia.

SCRIVENS, James William Stour House, 11 Watery Lane, Shipston-on-Stour CV36 4BE; [New Address] — MB ChB Birm. 1991; MRCGP; ChB Birm. 1991.

SCRIVENS, Stuart Benjamin Flat 11, Tiffany Court, Albert Road, Leicester LE2 2AA — MB ChB Leic. 1997.

SCRIVINGS, Belinda Ann — BM Soton. 1985; DRCOG 1987; MRCGP 1991. Prev: SHO (Med. for Elderly) Southend HA; Ho. Off. (Med.) & Ho. Surg. St. Mary's Hosp. Portsmouth.

SCROGGIE, Brian McGregor Reith St Pauls Medical Centre, St Pauls Square, Carlisle CA1 1DG Tel: 01228 524354 Fax: 01228 616660 — MB ChB Ed. 1974; BSc Ed. 1971; MRCGP 1978. Prev: Trainee GP Highland VTS; Ho. Surg. Roy. North. Infirm. Inverness; Ho. Phys. Raigmore Hosp. Inverness.

SCRUTTON, Mark James Leslie 6 Pratt Walk, London SE11 6AR Tel: 020 7735 5228 — MB BS Lond. 1989 (St. Thos. Hosp. Lond.) FRCA 1993.

SCUDAMORE, John Anthony Bassett Road Surgery, 29 Bassett Road, Leighton Buzzard LU7 1AR Tel: 01525 373111 Fax: 01525 853767 — MB Camb. 1972; MA Camb. 1970, MB 1972, BChir 1971; MRCGP 1994. Clin. Governance Lead & Caldicott Guardian Chiltern Vale PCG; GP Trainer. Prev: SHO (Accid. & Orthop.) Battle Hosp. Reading; Ho. Off. & Resid. Accouch. Lond. Hosp.

SCUDAMORE, Joseph Henry (retired) Invermuick, Ballater AB35 5SQ — MB ChB Bristol 1951; FRCOG 1977, M 1963.

SCUDAMORE, Tom Osbert (retired) 58A Rutland Grove, Sandiacre, Nottingham NG10 5AQ Tel: 0115 939 7293 — MB BChir Camb. 1942 (Camb. & Lond. Hosp.) MRCS Eng. LRCP Lond. 1942; MA Camb. 1943; DObst RCOG 1948. Prev: Cas. Off. & Ho. Surg. Connaught Hosp. Lond.

SCUDDER, Claire Caroline The Chelsea Practice, Violet Melchett Clinic, 30 Flood Walk, London SW3 5RR — BM Soton. 1990; DFFP 1995; DRCOG 1995. Specialty: Gen. Pract.

SCULL, David Alan Kings Park Hospital, Gloucester Road, Boscombe, Bournemouth — MB ChB Bristol 1989; MRCPsych. Cons. Psychiat. Dorset Healthcare Trust Poole. Specialty: Gen. Psychiat.

SCULL, Judith Jane Land Orchard, Galhampton, Yeovil BA22 7AH Email: docscull@aol.com — MB ChB Sheff. 1991; DRCOG Oct 1998; DFFP 1999. Specialty: Gen. Pract.; Ophth. Prev: Fellowship Ophth. Path. McGill Univ. Montreal, Canada.

SCULL, Timothy James 133 Sundridge Park, Yate, Bristol BS37 4DH — MB ChB Dundee 1984.

SCULLIN, Paula 90 Moneysharvan Road, Maghera BT46 5PT — MB BCh BAO Belf. 1997.

SCULLION, Damian Francis 13 Ballyscullion Lane, Bellaghy, Magherafelt BT45 8NQ — MB BCh BAO NUI 1990. SHO (Anaesth.) Leicester Roy. Infirm.

SCULLION, Damian Michael The Surgery, 3 Glasgow Road, Paisley PA1 3QS Tel: 0141 889 2604 Fax: 0141 887 9039 — MB ChB Glas. 1974. GP Paisley, Renfrewsh.

SCULLION, David Anthony Department of Radiology, Harrogate District Hospital, Lancaster Park Road, Harrogate HG2 7SX Tel: 01423 553726 Email: david.scullion@hhc-tr.northy.nhs.uk — MB BS Lond. 1985; MRCP Lond. 1988; FRCR London 1994. Cons. Radiologist. Specialty: Radiol. Special Interest: Abdominal Imaging; Intervention.

SCULLION, Helen Clare 26 Glencairn Drive, Glasgow G41 4PW — MB ChB Glas. 1980. Cons. Cytopath. Inverurie Roy. Hosp. Greenock. Prev: Cons. Cytopath. Vale of Leven Dist. Gen. Hosp. Alexandria.

SCULLION, Mr James Edwin — MB BCh BAO Belf. 1969 (Queens Univ. Belf.) FRCS Ed. 1974. Cons. (Orthop.) Dundee. Specialty: Orthop.

SCULLION, Jane Christine 436 Mosspark Boulevard, Glasgow G52 Tel: 0141 882 5494; 2 Tudor Road, Jordanhill, Glasgow G14 9NJ Tel: 0141 959 2439 — MB ChB Glas. 1987; DCH RCPS Glas. 1990; DRCOG 1990; MRCGP 1991.

SCULLION, John Francis Easterhouse Health Centre, 9 Auchinlea Road, Glasgow G34 9HQ Tel: 0141 531 8180 Fax: 0141 531 8186 — MB ChB Glas. 1985; DRCOG 1988; MRCGP 1989.

SCULLION, Lynda Thérèse Balwherrie, 103 Strathern Road, West Ferry, Dundee DD5 1JU — MB ChB Glas. 1972; DObst RCOG 1974.

SCULLION, Michael The Surgery, 75 Bank Street, Alexandria G83 0NB Tel: 01389 752626 Fax: 01389 752169 — MB ChB Glas. 1979; MRCP (UK) 1983.

SCULLION, Regina 50 Kinross Avenue, Glasgow G52 3JB — MB ChB Glas. 1982.

SCULLION, Ursula Mary Elizabeth 13 Ballyscullion Lane, Bellaghy, Magherafelt BT45 8NQ — MB BCh BAO Belf. 1993.

SCULLION, William 3 Glenwood Avenue, Airdrie ML6 8RY — MB ChB Glas. 1981.

SCULLY, Anne Gabrielle Mill Hill Surgery, 111 Avenue Rd, Acton, London W3 8QH — MB BS Lond. 1992.

SCULLY, Crispian Michael, CBE Eastman Dental Institute for Oral Healthcare Sciences, University College London, 256 Grays Inn Road, London WC1X 8LD Tel: 020 7915 1038 Fax: 020 7915 1039 Email: c.scully@eastman.ucl.ac.uk — MB BS Lond. 1974; BDS Lond. 1968; BSc (Hons.) Lond. 1971; FDS Glas. 1979; PhD Lond. 1979; MD Bristol 1987; MDS Bristol 1988. Dean and Director of Studies and Research, Eastman Dent. Inst., UCL, Lond. Specialty: Oral & Maxillofacial Surg. Socs: Acad. of Med. Sci.; Europ. Assn. of Oral Med.; Roy. Soc. of Med. Prev: Prof. and Head of Dept., Dept. of Oral Med., Path. and Microbiol., Bristol Dent. Hosp.; Sen. Lect., Dept. of Oral Med. and Path., Glas. Dent. Hosp.

SCULLY, Marie Ann 102 Chatsworth Road, Cheam, Sutton SM3 8PN — MB BS Lond. 1993 (St Georges London) BSc (Hons.) 1990. Specialty: Haematology.

SCULLY, Patrick Gerard Main Street Surgery, 6 Main Street, Drumquin, Omagh BT78 Tel: 028 8283 223 — MB BCh BAO Dub. 1987.

SCULLY, Paul Joseph 38 Omagh Road, Drumquin, Omagh BT78 4QY — MB BCh BAO Dub. 1987; MRCPsych. Specialty: Gen. Psychiat.

SCUPLAK, Stephen Michael Basement Flat, 16A Westwick Gardens, London W14 0BU — MB BS Lond. 1987.

SCURLOCK, Hilary Jane Mental Health Unit, Chase Farm Hospital, The Ridgeway, Enfield EN2 8 Tel: 020 8366 6600 — (Middlx.) MB BS Lond. 1986; MRCPsych 1991. Cons. (Gen. Adult Psychiat.) Chase Farm Hosp. Enfield Middx. Specialty: Gen. Psychiat. Prev: Sen. Regist. Char. Cross Hosp. Lond.

SCURR, Andrew James 16 Grange Avenue, Totteridge Common, London N20 8AD Tel: 020 8445 7188 Fax: 020 7792 3236 — MB BS Lond. 1985 (Westm. Med. Sch.) FRCA 1991. Cons. Anaesth. & Cons. in Intens. Care, Newham Gen. Hosp. Lond. Specialty: Anaesth.; Intens. Care. Socs: Fell. Roy. Soc. Med.; Assn. Anaesth.; BMA. Prev: Sen. Regist. (Anaesth.) St Marys Hosp. Lond.; Sen. Regist. & Regist. (Anaesth.) Hammersmith Hosp. Lond.; SHO (Anaesth.) Northwick Pk. Hosp.

SCURR, Cyril Frederick, CBE, LVO 16 Grange Avenue, Totteridge Common, London N20 8AD Tel: 020 8445 7188 — MB BS Lond. 1942 (Westm.) MRCS Eng. LRCP Lond. 1941; DA Eng. 1947; FFA RCS Eng. 1953; FRCS Eng. 1974; Hon. FFA RCSI 1977; FRCA 1992. Specialty: Anaesth. Socs: Hon. Mem. Assn. Anaesth.; Roy. Soc. Med. (Ex-Pres. & Hon. Mem. Anaesth. Sect.); D'Honneur Sociéte Francaise D'Anaesth. et Reanimation. Prev: Emerit. Anaesth. Hosp. St. John & St. Eliz. Lond. Hon Cons. Anaesth. Westm. Hosp.; Dean Fac. Anaesth. RCS Eng. & Pres. Assn. Anaesth. GB & Irel.; Maj. RAMC.

SCURR, James University Hospital, Aintree, Longmoor Lane, Liverpool L9 7AL — MB BS Lond. 2000 (UCL) BSc (Hons.) Lond. 1997; MRCS Eng 2004. Surgic. Regist. (Gen. Surg.) Univ. Hosp. Liverp. Specialty: Gen. Surg.

SCURR, Mr John Henry The Lister Hospital, Chelsea Bridge Road, London SW1W 8RH Tel: 020 7730 9563 Fax: 020 7259 9938 Email: jscurr@uk-consultants.co.uk; 5 Balniel Gate, London SW1V 3SD Tel: 020 7834 5578 Fax: 020 7834 6315 — MB BS Lond. 1972 (Middlx.) BSc Lond. 1969; FRCS Eng. 1977. Sen. Lect. & Hon. Cons. Surg. Middlx. Hosp. & Univ. Coll. Hosp. Lond.; Cons. Surg. Margt. Pyke Family Plann. Centre Lond.; Hon. Cons. Surg. St. Luke's Hosp. for Clergy. Specialty: Gen. Surg. Socs: Fell. Roy. Soc. Med.; Surg. Research Soc.; Vasc. Surg. Soc. Prev: Sen. Regist. (Surg.) Westm. Hosp. Lond.; Lect. (Surg. & Physiol.) & Ho. Surg. Middlx. Hosp. Lond.

SCURR, Judith Ann The Great Western Hospital, Pathology Department, Marlborough Road, Swindon SN3 6BB Email: judy.scurr@smnhst.swest.nhs.uk; 57 Newland Mill, Witney OX28 3SZ — MB BS Lond. 1971; FRCPath 1989, M 1977; MSc Lond. 1977. Cons. Cytol. Gt. West. Hosp. Swindon. Specialty: Histopath. Prev: Cons. Cytol. Princess Margt. Hosp. Swindon; Lect. (Chem. Path.) Westm. Med. Sch. Lond.; Sen. Regist. (Chem. Path.) St Geo. Hosp. Lond.

SCURR, Martin John 121 Ladbroke Grove, London W11 1PN Tel: 020 7792 8060 Fax: 020 7792 3236 Email: martinscurr@nottinghillpractice.com — MB BS Lond. 1973; MRCS Eng. LRCP Lond. 1973; MRCP (UK) 1976; MRCGP 1977; FRCP 2002. Chairm. of Counc., Indep. Doctors Forum; Phys. Westm. Cathedral. Prev: Clin. Asst. (Otolaryngol.) Brompton Hosp.; Cons. Phys. Terminal Care Hosp. St. John & St. Eliz. Lond.; Ho. Phys. & Ho. Surg. Westm. Hosp. Lond.

SEABORNE, Lisa 101 Berberry Close, Bourneville, Birmingham B30 1TB — MB ChB Birm. 1991; MRCGP 1995.

SEABOURNE, Alice Ellen Bolton Mental Health Unit, Belmont Day Hospital, Minerva Road, Farnworth, Bolton BL4 0JR — MB ChB Ed. 1991; MRCPsych; BSc (Med. Sci.) Ed. 1989; CCST (Old Age Psych.) 1999. Cons. (Old Age Psychiat.) Bolton Ment. Health Unit Belmont Day Hosp. Bolton. Specialty: Geriat. Psychiat. Socs: Roy. Coll. Psychiat. Prev: Sen. Regist. (Old Age Psychiat.) Withington Hosp.; Regist. Rotat. (Psychiat.) NW Region; Ho. Off. Roy. Infirm. Edin.

SEABROOK, Jonathan Derek Wrightington Street Surgery, 1 Wrightington Street, Wigan WN1 2AZ Tel: 01942 231965 Fax: 01942 826427 — MB ChB Manch. 1990; MRCGP 1996. Specialty: Sports Med. Prev: Trainee GP Wigan & Leigh NHS Trust; SHO (A & E) Roy. Preston Hosp.

SEABROOK, Ruth Jayne 17 Fairfield Avenue, Cheadle Hulme, Cheadle SK8 6AF — MB ChB Liverp. 1986.

SEABURNE-MAY, Matthew Patrick Old Barn Cottage, Soames Lane, Ropley, Alresford SO24 0ER Email: seaburne@hotmail.com — MB BS Lond. 1998; MB BS Lond 1998. Specialty: Gen. Psychiat.

SEACOME, Mary Percival Silvester Barnwood Court W., Gloucester GL4 3AD Tel: 01452 66265 — (Oxf.) MA, BM BCh Oxf. 1947; DPH Bristol 1972; FFCM 1980. Prev: SCM (Health Care Plann. & Informat.) Glos. AHA.

SEAGER, Professor Charles Philip (retired) 9 Blacka Moor Road, Dore, Sheffield S17 3GH Tel: 0114 236 1925 Fax: 0114 236 2982 Email: pseager@btinternet.com — MB BCh Wales 1949 (Cardiff) DPM Eng. 1954; BSc Wales 1949, MD 1960; FRCPsych 1972. Cons. to SOVRN Project Sheff. Prev: Prof. Psychiat. Univ. Sheff.

SEAGER, Francis Geoffrey Maundrell (retired) The Old Garage, The Street, Roxwell, Chelmsford CM1 4PB Tel: 01245 248056 — MB BS Lond. 1953 (Lond. Hosp.) Specialist Accredit (Occupat. Med.)

RCP Lond; MRCS Eng. LRCP Lond. 1949; DObst RCOG 1954; DPH Lond. 1956; DIH Eng. 1957; MFOM RCP Lond. 1979. Prev: Med. Adviser Rank Xerox Ltd.

SEAGER, John Department of Paediatrics, Arrowe Park Hospital, Arrowe Park Road, Upton, Birkenhead CH49 5PE; 2 Waterford Road, Oxton, Prenton CH43 6UT — MD Liverp. 1976; MB ChB 1966; MRCP (U.K.) 1971; FRCP Lond. 1987; FRCPCH 1997. Cons. (Paediat.) Arrowe Pk. Hosp. Wirral. Clin. Director Wirral Serv.s for Child Health. Specialty: Paediat. Prev: Cons. Paediat. Childr. Hosp. Birkenhead & Clatterbridge Hosp. Wirral; Hon. Regist. Hosp. Sick Childr. Gt. Ormond St. Lond.; Research Fell. Inst. Child Health Lond.

SEAGER, Marian Catriona Northgate Hospital, Morpeth NE61 3AS — MB ChB Ed. 1990; MRCPSych 1996. Specialist Regist. (Psychiat.). Specialty: Ment. Health.

SEAGER, Matthew James Coedmor, Caswell Av, Caswell, Swansea SA3 4RU — MB BCh Wales 1997.

SEAGER, Sylvia Jeanne c/o Department of Anaesthetics, Glan Clwyd Hospital, Bodelwyddan, Rhyl LL18 5UJ Tel: 01745 583910 Fax: 01745 583143 — MB ChB Ed. 1972; FFA RCS Eng. 1977. Cons. Anaesth. Glan Clwyd Hosp. Bodelwyddan.; Asst. Med. Director; Conwy & Denbighsh. NHS Trust. Specialty: Anaesth. Socs: BMA; Sec. Welsh Advisory Sub-Comm. in Anaesth.; Soc. Anaesth. Wales. Prev: Cons. Anaesth. Grimsby Hosp.; Sen. Regist. (Anaesth.) Yorks. Region; Regist. St. Jas. Univ. Hosp. Leeds.

SEAGER-THOMAS, Robin Griffith (retired) Hafod Onen, 23 Gill Way, E. Beach, Sesley, Chichester PO20 0EX — (Westm.) MRCS Eng. LRCP Lond. 1948; DObst RCOG 1953. Prev: Surg. Lt.-Cdr. RNR.

SEAGGER, Robin Mark 22 Lansdown Park, Bath BA1 5TG — MB BS Lond. 1998; MB BS Lond 1998.

SEAGGER, Roger Alan 22 Lansdown Park, Bath BA1 5TG — MB BS Lond. 1965 (Westm.) MRCS Eng. LRCP Lond. 1965; FFA RCS Eng. 1970. Cons. Anaesth. Bath Health Dist. Specialty: Anaesth. Socs: Assn. Anaesths.; Brit. Assn. Immed. Care Schemes; Obst. Anaesth. Assn. Prev: SHO (Clin. Measurem.) & SHO (Anaesth.) Westm. Hosp. Lond.; Regist. (Anaesth.) Soton. Gen. Hosp.

SEAKINS, Elizabeth Claire 61 Winnie Road, Birmingham B29 6JU Tel: 0121 472 8922 Fax: 0121 472 8922 Email: eseakins@aol.com — MB ChB Birm. 1986; DRCOG 1994. Prev: Trainee GP Kidderminster; SHO Qu. Med. Centre Nottm.; Med. Off. Falkland Is.s.

SEAL, Anita Nicola 12 Shamrock Way, London N14 5RY — MB BS Lond. 1991.

SEAL, Arnab Kumar 8 Lawns Drive, New Farnley, Leeds LS12 5RJ — MB BS Calcutta 1988; MRCP (UK) 1993.

SEAL, David Venner 23 Charlton Place, Islington, London N1 8AQ — MRCS Eng. LRCP Lond. 1970; MD Lond. 1984, MB BS 1970; Dip Bact . Lond. 1975; MRCPath 1977; MIBiol 1983; FCOphth 1988. Hon. Sen. Lect. Dept. Path. Inst. Ophth. Lond. Prev: Cons. Microbiol. Northwick Pk. Hosp. & Clin. Research Centre Harrow & Soton. Gen. Hosp.

SEAL, Kenneth Stanley, OBE (retired) 44 Torr Lane, Hartley, Plymouth PL3 5NZ Tel: 01752 772816 — (Roy. Colls. Ed.) LRCP LRCS Ed. LRFPS Glas. 1939; DTM & H Eng. 1947; DPH Lond. 1957; MFPHM 1974. Prev: Rural Health Adviser MoH, E. Nigeria.

SEAL, Leighton John 12 Shamrock Way, London N14 5RY — MB BS Lond. 1992 (St. Bart. Hosp. Lond.) BSc Lond. 1990; MB BS (Hons.) Lond. 1992; MRCP (UK) 1995. Specialty: Endocrinol.

SEAL, Louise Ann (retired) The Vinery, Wellington, Hereford HR4 8AR — MB ChB Bristol 1965; DObst RCOG 1968; DA Eng. 1968.

SEAL, Martin Treharne The Old Vicarage, Cilcennin, Lampeter SA48 8RF — MB BCh Wales 1978; BDS 1972; FDS RCS Eng. 1980; Spec. Accredit. Oral Maxillofacial Surg. RCS Eng. 1992. Cons. Oral & Maxillofacial Surg. HM Armed Forces; Col. RADC. Specialty: Oral & Maxillofacial Surg. Socs: Fell. Dent. Surg. RCS Eng.; BMA; Brit. Assn. Oral & Maxillofacial Surg. Prev: Sen. Specialist (Oral & Maxillofacial Surg.) HM Armed Forces; Hon. Sen. Regist. Char. Cross Hosp. Lond.; GP Dyfed.

SEAL, Patrick James Longfleet Road Surgery, 117 Longfleet Road, Poole BH15 2HX Tel: 01202 676111 Fax: 01202 676111 — MB BS Lond. 1985; BA Camb. 1982, MA 1986; MRCGP 1990. Gen. Practitioner. Specialty: Dermat. Socs: BMA & Med. Protec. Soc.

SEAL, Paul Leonard 45 Wellington Square, Hastings TN34 1PN Tel: 01424 722366 — MB ChB Sheff. 1992; DCH RCP Lond. 1996; DRCOG Lond. 1997. Specialty: Gen. Pract.

SEAL, Mr Philip Victor Wye Valley Nuffield Hospital, Venns Lane, Hereford HR1 1DF Tel: 01432 355131 — MB ChB Manch. 1964; FRCS Eng. 1969. Cons. Orthop. & Traum. Surg. Hereford Gp. Hosps. Specialty: Orthop. Socs: Fell. BOA. Prev: Hon. Lect. (Orthop. Surg.) Univ. Hong Kong; Sen. Regist. (Orthop. & Traum. Surg.) Robt. Jones & Agnes Hunt Orthop. Hosp. & Birm. Accid. Hosp.

SEAL, Philippa Anne The Vinery, Wellington, Hereford HR4 8AR — MB BS Lond. 1996. Prev: SHO A & E Dunedin Pub. Hosp. New Zealand; SHO A & E Northampton Gen.; Ho. Off. Surgic. Qu. Alexandra Hosp. Portsmouth.

SEAL, Robert Harry (Surgery), Highfield Road, North Thoresby, Grimsby DN36 5RT Tel: 01472 840202; Roberts Farm, Third Lane, Ashby-Cum-Fenby, Grimsby DN37 0QU Tel: 01472 827934 — MB ChB Sheff. 1973. Prev: SHO (Obst.) Jessop Hosp. Wom. Sheff.; SHO (Accid. & Orthop.) Roy. Infirm. Sheff.

SEAL, Robert Leonard Beacon Medical Practice, Chuchill Avenue, Skegness PE25 2AN Tel: 01754 897000 Fax: 01754 761024; Fairfield House, Chapel Lane, Huttoft, Alford LN13 9RG Email: rlseal@aol.com — MB BChir Camb. 1980 (Camb. & St. Bart.) MA Camb. 1981; DRCOG 1987; MRCGP 1987. GP Princip.; Chairm. Lincs. LMC. Specialty: Gen. Pract. Special Interest: Orthopaedics/Rheumatology. Prev: Treas. Lincs. LMC.

SEAL, Roger Martin Ewart (retired) 3 Church Road, Penarth CF64 1AE; Swn-Y-Mor, Rock st, Newquay SA45 9PL Tel: 01545 560021 — MB BCh Wales 1945 (Cardiff) FRCP Lond. 1971, M 1949; FRCPath 1963. Cons. Path. Llandough Hosp. Prev: Ho. Phys. Roy. Infirm. Cardiff.

SEAL, Sarah Helen 5 The Close, Salisbury SP1 2EF — MB BS Lond. 1974. Clin. Med. Off. Community Health Salisbury HA.

SEALE, Anna Nancy Box Cottage, Shirenewton, Chepstow NP16 6LT — BChir Camb. 1994; MRCP (Paed.). Specialty: Paediat. Prev: SHO (Paediat.) Roy. Cornw. Hosp. Truro; SHO (Paediat.) Oxf. Paediat. Rotat.

SEALE, James Richard Cluxton Department of Haematology, Ysbyty Gwynedd, Bangor LL57 2PW Tel: 01248 384384 Fax: 01248 384505 Email: jim.seale@nww-tr.wales.nhs.uk — MB BS Lond. 1986 (Cambridge University & Guy's Hospital London) MA Camb. 1987; MRCP (UK) 1990; MD Camb 1997; MRCPath 1997; FRCP 2003. Cons. Haematologist Ysbyty Gwynedd Bangor. Specialty: Haematology. Special Interest: Haemostasis; Thrombosis. Socs: Brit. Soc. of Haemat. Prev: Sen. Regist. (Haemat.) Addenbrookes Hosp. Camb.; Regist. (Haemat.) Hammersmith Hosp. Lond.; SHO (Med.) Brighton Hosps.

SEALE, John Richard (retired) Southcombe House, Widecombe-in-the-Moor, Newton Abbot TQ13 7TU Tel: 01364 621365 — MB BChir Camb. 1951 (Camb., St. Thos. & Harvard) MA Camb. 1951, BA (1st cl. Nat. Sc. Trip. Pt. I) 1948, MD 1957, MB BChir 1951; MRCP Lond. 1953; MD 1957. Prev: Cons. Phys. Depts. Genitourin. Med. & Venereol. St. Thos. Hosp. & Middlx. Hosp. Lond.

SEALEY, Annie Robina (retired) 63 Rosemary Crescent W., Goldthorn Park, Wolverhampton WV4 5AN Tel: 01902 656015 — MB ChB Birm. 1959; DFFP 1994; MRCPCH 1997. Prev: Resid. Med. Off. Childr. Hosp. Birm.

SEALEY, Margaret Mary (retired) Queen Elizabeth Hospital, Edgbaston, Birmingham B15 2TH; 1 Millison Grove, Shirley, Solihull B90 4UN — MB ChB Birm. 1968; MRCS Eng. LRCP Lond. 1969; DA Eng. 1971; MA (OU) Nov. 2000; FFA RCSI 1976. Prev: Cons. Anaesth. Qu. Eliz. Hosp. Birm.

SEALEY, Sara Louise 5 Eden Road, West ENT, Southampton SO18 3QW Tel: 023 8046 6083 — BM Soton. 1995; DRCOG 1997. GP Regist. Portsmouth VTS. Specialty: Paediat.

SEAMAN, Alexander George (retired) 8 Oaklands, Lowestoft Road, Reydon, Southwold IP18 6RY Tel: 01502 724380 — (St. Thos.) MRCS Eng. LRCP Lond. 1941; MB BS Lond. 1946; MRCGP 1953. Prev: Clin. Asst. (Genitourin. Med.) Norf. & Norwich Hosp.

SEAMAN, Fiona Margaret Oliver & Partners, Millhill Surgery, 87 Woodmill Street, Dunfermline KY11 4JW Tel: 01383 621222 Fax: 01383 622862 — MB ChB Aberd. 1994.

SEAMAN, Fiona Margaret 43 Weaver's Way, Tillicoultry FK13 6BD Tel: 01259 752761 — MB ChB Glas. 1995. SHO (Psychiat.) Clackmannan Co. Hosp. Specialty: Gen. Psychiat. Socs:

BMA. Prev: SHO (O & G) Stirling Roy. Infirm. Livilands, NHS Trust; SHO (Paediat.) Stirling Ro.; SHO (A & E) Stirling Roy.

SEAMAN, Joan Lillias (retired) Glenuig, Dunshalt, Cupar KY14 7EU Tel: 01334 28647 — MB ChB Glas. 1947 (Univ. Glas.) Prev: Med. Off. E. Scotl. Blood Transfus. Serv.

SEAMAN, John Arthur Save The Children Fund (UK), 17 Grove Lane, London SE5 8RD Tel: 020 7703 5400; 2 Coppings Brook Cottages, Leigh, Tonbridge TN11 8PP Tel: 01732 463736 — MB BS Lond. 1967 (Lond. Hosp.) MRCS Eng. LRCP Lond. 1967; DCH Eng. 1971. Head Policy Developm. Unit Save the Childr. Fund (UK) Lond.; Hon. Sen. Lect. (Human Nutrit.) Lond. Sch. Hyg. & Trop. Med. Lond. Specialty: Trop. Med.

SEAMAN, Muriel Joan (retired) 21 Bailey Mews, Auckland Road, Cambridge CB5 8DR Tel: 01223 323535 — MB BS Lond. 1953 (Roy. Free) FRCPath 1976, M 1964. Prev: Cons. Haemat. Addenbrooke's Hosp. Camb.

SEAMAN, Robert Arthur John Larksfield Surgery, Arlesey Road, Stotfold, Hitchin SG5 4HB Tel: 01462 732200 Fax: 01462 730487 Email: rajseaman@aol.com — MB BS Lond. 1971 (St. Mary's) MRCS Eng. LRCP Lond. 1971; Dip Obst Auckland 1977. Socs: BMA. Prev: Resid. (Psychiat.) St. Brendan's Hosp. Bermuda; Regist. (Paediat.) Palmerston N. Hosp., NZ.

SEAMAN, Terence Frederick Central Surgery, Corporation Street, Rugby CV21 3SP Tel: 01788 574335 Fax: 01788 547693; 22 Beech Drive, Rugby CV22 7LT Tel: 01788 811778 — MB BS Lond. 1967 (St. Thos.) MRCS Eng. LRCP Lond. 1966. Med. Off. (Occupat. Health) Rugby NHS Trust. Specialty: Occupat. Health.

SEAMARK, Clare Jennifer The Surgery, Marlpits Lane, Honiton EX14 2NY Tel: 01404 41141 Fax: 01404 46621; 12 Oak Tree Close, Upottery, Honiton EX14 9QG Tel: 01404 861601 Fax: 01404 861304 — MB ChB Bristol 1980; DRCOG 1982; MRCGP 1985; MFFP 1993; MPhil (Med. Sci.) Exeter 1996; MD Bristol 2003. GP Honiton; Research Fell. Inst. Gen. Pract. Exeter Univ. Prev: Clin. Asst. (Med.) Roy. Devon & Exeter Hosp.; Clin. Med. Off. City & Hackney HA; Trainee GP Lond. Hosp. VTS.

SEAMARK, David Anthony The Surgery, Marlpits Lane, Honiton EX14 2NY Tel: 01404 41141 Fax: 01404 46621 Email: david.seamark@gp-l83002.nhs.uk; 12 Oak Tree Close, Upottery, Honiton EX14 9QG Tel: 01404 861601 Fax: 01404 861304 — MB BS Lond. 1985 (Lond. Hosp. Med. Sch.) MA Oxf. 1977; PhD Lond. 1980; DCH RCP Lond. 1988; MRCGP 1989. Lect. (Gen. Pract.) Univ. Exeter; Lead Research GP Honiton Research Pract. (NHS funded). Specialty: Gen. Pract. Socs: Fell. Roy. Soc. Med.; BMA (Treas. Exeter Div.); (Comm.) Community Hosp. Assn. Prev: Trainee GP Exeter VTS; Ho. Off. (Surg.) Roy. Devon & Exeter Hosp. Wonford Exeter; Ho. Off. (Med.) OldCh. Hosp. Romford.

SEAR, Mr Anthony James (retired) 1 Elms Drive, Colwall Green, Malvern WR13 6JE — MB ChB Birm. 1964; FDS RCS Eng. 1959, L 1953; BDS Birm. 1954. Cons. Oral & Maxillofacial Surg. S. & Mid. Worcs. Hosp. Gps. Prev: Lect. (Oral Surg.) Univ. Birm.

SEAR, Professor John William Nuffield Department of Anaesthetics, John Radcliffe Hospital, Headington, Oxford OX3 9DU Tel: 01865 221590 Fax: 01865 221593 Email: john.sear@nda.ox.ac.uk; 6 Whites Forge, Appleton, Abingdon OX13 5LG Tel: 01865 863144 Fax: 01865 221593 Email: john.sear@nda.ox.ac.uk — MB BS Lond. 1972 (Lond. Hosp.) MA Oxf. 1982, BSc (Hons.) Lond. 1969; DObst RCOG 1974; FFA RCS Eng. 1977; PhD Bristol 1981; FANZCA 1995. Prof. of Anaesth.; Hon. Cons. Anaesth. Oxford Radcliffe NHS Trust; Vice-Warden, Green College, Oxford. Specialty: Anaesth. Special Interest: Vasc. Anaesth. Socs: BMA; Assn. Anaesth.of GB & Irel.; Soc. of Intraveous Anaesth.; Immediate past Pres. (1999-2002). Prev: Lect. & MRC Train. Fell. Univ. Dept. Anaesth. & Biochem. Bristol; dir.Clin.Studies Univ.Oxf.; Non-Exec. Dir., Nuffield Orthop. Centre NHS Trust, Oxford.

SEARBY, Glenda Jean (retired) Bridge House, Bolton Road, Bradshaw, Bolton BL2 3EU Tel: 01204 300214 — MB BS Lond. 1966 (Roy. Free) MRCS Eng. LRCP Lond. 1966. Prev: SCMO (Family Plann.) Well Wom. & Young Peoples Serv. Salford Community Health Centre NHS Trust Salford.

SEARGEANT, Janet Muriel St Ann's Hospital, St. Ann's Road, Tottenham, London N15 3TH Tel: 020 8442 6000; 61 Fordington Road, Highgate, London N6 4TH — MRCS Eng. LRCP Lond. 1967; MB BS Lond. 1967; MRCPsych 1983. Cons. Psychiat. Haringey Healthcare Trust St. Ann's Hosp., St Ann's Rd., Lond. Specialty: Gen. Psychiat.

SEARL, Catherine Patricia 57 Bonaly Crescent, Edinburgh EH13 0EP Tel: 0131 441 5791 — MB ChB Manch. 1991; MRCP (UK) 1994. Specialist Regist. Anaes. & IC. Specialty: Anaesth. Prev: SHO (Cardiac Surg. & Cardiol.) Cardiff; SHO Rotat. (Med.) Tayside.

SEARLE, Mr Adam Eric The Royal Marsden Hospital, Fulham Road, London SW3 6JJ Tel: 020 7808 2782 Fax: 020 7808 2235; 30 Mayford Road, London SW12 8SD Tel: 020 8675 4689 Fax: 020 8675 4689 — MB BS Lond. 1985 (Guy's Hosp.) BDS 1979; FRCS Eng. 1989; FRCS (Plast) 1994. Cons. Plastic & Reconstruc. Surg. Roy. Marsden Hosp. Specialty: Plastic Surg. Socs: Brit. Assn. of Plastic Surgs.; Brit. Assn. of Aesthetic Plastic Surg.; Sec. Plastic Surg. Sect. of Roy. Soc. of Med. Prev: Sen. Regist. (Plastic Reconstruc.) Mt. Vernon Hosp. & Roy. Marsden Hosp.; Cons. Surg. Char. Cross Hosp.

SEARLE, Adrian Eric Derbyshire Royal Infirmary, London Road, Derby DE1 2QY Tel: 01332 347141; The Old Red House, 84 Main St, Etwall, Derby DE65 6LP Email: adrian@searle84.fsnet.co.uk — MB ChB Birm. 1979; FFA RCS Eng. 1986. Cons. Anaesth. & Pain Managem. Derbysh. Roy. Infirm. Specialty: Anaesth. Socs: Derby Med. Soc.; The Pain Soc.; Assn. of Anaethetists.

SEARLE, Clare Hilary Rickmansworth Road Surgery, 35 Rickmansworth Road, Watford WD18 7HD Tel: 01923 223232 Fax: 01923 243397 — MB ChB Leic. 1989; MRCGP 1994.

SEARLE, Rev. Dr John Francis, OBE 8 Thornton HillBelle Isle Lodge, Belle Isle Drive, Exeter EX2 4RY Tel: 01392 432153 Fax: 01392 216132 Email: johnlizex@aol.com — MB BS Lond. 1966 (Guy's) MRCS Eng. LRCP Lond. 1966; FRCA 1970. Cons. Anaesth. Exeter Health Care. Specialty: Anaesth. Socs: Vice-Pres. Assn. Anaesths.; Hewitt Lect. RCA 2001. Prev: Pres Hospiscare Exeter; Sen. Regist. (Anaesth.) Guy's Hosp. Lond.; Lect. (Anaesth.) Ghana Med. Sch. Accra Ghana.

SEARLE, Geoffrey Frank St Ann's Hospital, Haver Road, Canford Cliffs, Poole BH17 7LN — MB BS Lond. 1982; BSc (Pharmacol.) Lond. 1979. Cons. Psychiat. St Ann's Hosp. Poole.

SEARLE, Jane Margaret 15 Walgrove Road, Chesterfield S40 2DW — MB ChB Sheff. 1988.

SEARLE, John Stanley Teague (retired) Corner House, 18 Potacre St., Torrington EX38 8BL Tel: 01805 623263 — (Lond. Hosp.) MRCS Eng. LRCP Lond. 1945; MB BS Lond. 1949; DObst RCOG 1951; MRCGP 1965. Prev: Sqdn. Ldr. RAFVR.

SEARLE, Julie Michelle 232 Park Lane, Frampton Cotterell, Bristol BS36 2EN — BM Soton. 1995.

SEARLE, Martin Anthony Northlands Surgery, North Street, Calne SN11 0HH Tel: 01249 812091 Fax: 01249 815343; 37 Bremhill, Calne SN11 9LD — (Camb. & King's Coll.) BA 1979; MA Camb. 1980; BChir 1982; MB 1982; DCH RCP Lond. 1985; MRCGP 1987; DRCOG 1987. Prev: Trainee GP Epsom VTS; Ho. Surg. Brighton Gen. Hosp.; Ho. Phys. Dulwich Hosp.

SEARLE, Paul Jonathan Eaton Socon Health Centre, 274 North Road, Eaton Socon, Huntingdon PE19 8BB Tel: 01480 477111 Fax: 01480 403524 — MB ChB Aberd. 1975; Cert. Family Plann. JCC 1979. Specialty: Gen. Pract.; Dermat.; Medico Legal; Gen. Psychiat. Prev: Trainee GP Aberd. VTS; Ho. Phys. Woodend Gen. Hosp. Aberd.; Ho. Surg. (Thoracic) Roy. Infirm. Aberd.

SEARLE, Stella Margaret Church Farm, 17 Church St., North Cave, Brough HU15 2LJ — MB ChB Manch. 1969. Clin. Med. Off. Hull Health Auth.

SEARLE, Stephen John Occupational Health Service, Birmingham City Council, 137 Newhall St, Birmingham B3 1SF Tel: 0121 303 3300 Fax: 0121 303 4484 Email: stephen_searle@birmingham.gov.uk; 20 Marsett, Wilnecote, Tamworth B77 4QU Tel: 01827 896771 — MB BS Lond. 1971 (Roy. Free) MRCS Eng. LRCP Lond. 1971; MRCGP 1976; FFOM RCP Lond. 1993, MFOM 1985, AFOM 1983; DIH (Distinc.) Lond. 1983; MSc (Distinc. Occupat. Med.) Lond. 1985; Dip GU Med. Soc. Apoth. Lond. 1988; MBA Aston Univ. 1996. Director Ocupational Health; Hon. Sen. Lect. (Clin.) Inst. Occupat. Health Univ. Birm. Specialty: Occupat. Health. Socs: Fell. Roy. Soc. Med.; Soc. Occupat. Med. Prev: Regional Med. Off. Post Office Occupat. Health Serv. Lond. Postal Region; Ho. Surg. Roy. Free Hosp. Lond.; Ho. Phys. Noble's I. of Man Hosp. Douglas.

SEARLE, Wendy Helen Mill Lane, Cannington, Bridgwater TA5 2HB Tel: 01278 652335; Glebe House, Bridgwater TA5 2DF Tel: 01278 662523 — MB ChB Sheff. 1985; DObst. Auckland 1989; MRCGP 1991; T(GP) 1991. GP Som. Retainer Scheme. Prev: Trainee GP Som.; Regist. (Paediat.) & SHO (O & G) Waikato Hosp., NZ.

SEARLE-BARNES, Peter Gerald The Strand Practice, 2 The Strand, Goring-by-Sea, Worthing BN12 6DN Tel: 01903 243351 Fax: 01903 705804; 19 Third Avenue, Worthing BN14 9NZ Tel: 01903 237689 — MB BS Lond. 1980 (Guy's) MA Camb. 1981; DCH RCP Lond. 1982; DRCOG 1982; MRCGP 1984. Specialty: Gen. Pract.

SEARS, Andrew Fullerton Witley Surgery, Wheeler Lane, Witley, Godalming GU8 5QR Tel: 01428 682218 Fax: 01428 682218; Oaklee, Combe Lane, Wormley, Godalming GU8 5SX — MB BChir Camb. 1980; MA, MB Camb. 1980, BChir 1979; MRCP (UK) 1983; DRCOG 1986; FRCP 2001. Prev: Regist. (Med.) Roy. United Hosps. Bath; SHO (Med.) Leicester Roy. Infirm.; Ho. Phys. St. Thos. Hosp. Lond.

SEARS, Anna Louise 72 Church Road, Liversedge WF15 7LP — MB ChB Liverp. 1997.

SEARS, Antony Hammond (retired) 21 West Street, Chichester PO19 1QW Tel: 01243 785958; Mallards, Oak Meadow, Birdham, Chichester PO20 7BH Tel: 01243 785958 Fax: 01243 528081 — MB BChir Camb. 1956 (Guy's) MA, MB Camb. 1956, BChir 1955; LMSSA Lond. 1955; DObst RCOG 1960; FRCGP 1981, M 1972. Prev: Med. Adviser Electrolux & Autoliv.

SEARS, Charles Alistair Newton Grove House Surgery, 18 Wilton Road, Salisbury SP2 7EE Tel: 01722 333034 Fax: 01722 410308 — MB BS Lond. 1977 (Middlx.) MRCGP 1987; FRCGP 2003; FRIPHH 2005. Princip. GP Salisbury; Clin. Asst. (Learning Disabil.); Disabil. Partnership, Health Counc.; Comm. Safety Devices; RCGP Taskgroup of Disabil. - Chair; Vice Pres. Back Care (National Back Pain Association). Specialty: Rehabil. Med. Socs: Back Care (Nat. Back Pain Assn.) Vice Pres.; Brit. Inst. Musculo-Skeletal Med.; John Snow Soc. Prev: SHO Profess. Med. Unit Qu. Eliz. Hosp. Birm.; SHO (Neurosurg.) Whittington Hosp. Lond.; Ho. Off. Middlx. Hosp. Lond.

SEARS, Elizabeth Florence 3 Green's Court, St. Ann St., Salisbury SP1 2SX Tel: 01722 338817 — MB BS Lond. 1976 (St. Thos.) DCH Eng. 1980; MRCP (UK) 1981; Cert. Family Plann. JCC 1982; MRCGP 1983. GP Soton. Retainer Scheme. Socs: BMA; Salisbury Med. Soc. & Founder Mem. Trustee Pituitary Foundat. Prev: GP Princip. Med. Off. & Phys. Univ. Kent; SHO (Paediat.) Roy. Hosp. Sick Childr. Edin.; Ho. Phys. St. Thos. Hosp. Lond.

SEARS, Mr Richard Tankard Derwent Rise, 136 Edward's Lane, Nottingham NG5 3HU Tel: 0115 926 2168 — MB BChir Camb. 1948 (Camb. & Middlx.) MA Camb. 1948; DObst 1949; FRCOG 1968, M 1955; FRCS Eng. 1956. Specialty: Obst. & Gyn. Socs: Fell. Roy. Soc. Med.; Fell. N. Eng. & Birm. & Midl. Obst. & Gyn. Soc.; (Ex-Pres.) N. Eng. Obst. & Gyn. Soc. Prev: Sen. Regist. Jessop Hosp. Wom. Sheff.; Regist. City Hosp. Nottm.; Ho. Off. Middlx. Hosp.

SEARSON, James William Warrior Square Surgery, Marlborough House, 19-21 Warrior Square, St Leonards-on-Sea TN37 6BG Tel: 01424 430123/445644 Fax: 01424 433706 — MB BS Lond. 1963 (St. Geo.) MRCS Eng. LRCP Lond. 1965; DA Eng. 1968; DObst RCOG 1969.

SEARSON, John David Norwood Avenue Practice, 11 Norwood Avenue, Southport PR9 7EG — MB ChB Liverp. 1971.

SEARSON, John Joseph 14 Lowood Place, Revidge, Blackburn BB2 6JD Fax: 01254 667936; Meynell, 14 Lowood Place, Revidge, Blackburn BB2 6JD Tel: 01254 667936 — LAH Dublin 1948 (UCD) MB BCh BAO NUI 1949. Socs: BMA.

SEATH, Gillian Louise 56 Banchory Avenue, Inchinnan, Renfrew PA4 9PZ — MB ChB Glas. 1992.

SEATH, Kenneth Ross The Health Centre, 55 High Street, Great Wakering, Southend-on-Sea SS3 0EF Tel: 01702 218678 Fax: 01702 577853 — MB ChB Ed. 1972.

SEATON, Professor Anthony, CBE 8 Avon Grove, Cramond, Edinburgh EH4 6RF Tel: 0131 336 5113 Fax: 0131 336 2710 — (Camb. & Liverp.) MB BChir Camb. 1962; MRCS Eng. LRCP Lond. 1962; FRCP Lond. 1977, M 1964; BA Camb. 1959, MD 1972; FFOM RCP Lond. 1982, M 1980; FRCP Ed. 1985, M 1982; Fell. Acad. Med. Sci. 1998. Emerit. Prof. Environm. & Occupat. Med. Univ. Aberd. 1988; Sen. Cons., Inst. of Occupational Med., Edin. Specialty: Occupat. Health; Respirat. Med. Socs: Brit. Thorac. Soc. (Pres. 1999) & Brit. Soc. Occupat. Med.; Assn. Phys.GB and NI. Prev: Prof. Environm. & Occupat. Med. Univ. Aberd. 1988; Dir. Inst. Occupat. Med. Edin.; Cons. Phys. Respirat. Med. S. Glam. AHA (T).

SEATON, Anthony Trevor The Surgery, 27 Burges Road, East Ham, London E6 2BJ Tel: 020 8472 0421 Fax: 020 8552 9912; Seatoller House, Hermitage Walk, London E18 2BN Tel: 020 8989 0532 Fax: 020 8530 5332 — MB Camb. 1961 (St. Bart.) MA Camb. 1962, MB 1961, BChir 1960; DObst RCOG 1962. Clin. Asst. Roy. Nat. Throat, Nose & Ear Hosp. Lond.; Hosp. Pract. (Cardiol.) Lond. Chest Hosp. Socs: BMA. Prev: Ho. Phys. & Ho. Surg. Metrop. Hosp. Lond.; Ho. Surg. (O & G) Bromley Hosp.

SEATON, David Anderson (retired) 67 Swanston Avenue, Edinburgh EH10 7DA Tel: 0131 445 1899 — (Glas.) MD (Commend.) Glas. 1961, MB ChB 1950; MB ChB Glasgow 1950; DObst RCOG 1954; FRFPS Glas. 1957; FRCP Ed. 1967, M 1958; FRCP Glas. 1967.

SEATON, David George French Wymondham Medical Partnership, Postmill Close, Wymondham NR18 0RF Tel: 01953 602118 Fax: 01953 605313 — MB BChir Camb. 1973; MA 1974; MB Camb. 1974; Dip Obst Auckland 1976.

SEATON, Derek Norman (retired) Higher Collipriest, Tiverton EX16 4PT Tel: 01884 252018 Fax: 01884 252018 Email: seaton@collip.demon.co.uk — MB BChir Camb. 1945 (St. Thos.) MRCS Eng. LRCP Lond. 1945; MRCP Lond. 1955; DObst RCOG 1961. Prev: Med. Regist. Woolwich Hosp. Gp.

SEATON, Douglas King's Field, 23 Park Road, Ipswich IP1 3SX Tel: 01473 216671 — MB ChB Liverp. 1970; MRCS Eng. LRCP Lond. 1970; MRCP (UK) 1973; MD Liverp. 1978; FRCP Lond. 1988. Cons. Phys. The Ipswich Hosp. Specialty: Gen. Med. Socs: Brit. Thorac. Soc. Prev: Instruc. (Med.) Univ. W. Virginia, USA; Regist. (Cardiothoracic Med.), Ho. Phys. & Ho. Surg. Broadgreen Hosp. Liverp.

SEATON, Edward Douglas 23 Park Road, Ipswich IP1 3SX Tel: 01473 216671 Fax: 01473 212011 Email: seatons@compuserve.com — BM BCh Oxf. 1996; MA (Cambridge) 1997. SHO (Med.) Leeds Gen. Infirm. Specialty: Gen. Med. Prev: Ho. Off. Med. Oxf. Radcliffe Hosp.; Ho. Off. in Surg. York Dist. Hosp.

SEATON, James Michael Arno 18 Westlands Grove, Stockton Lane, York YO31 1EF — MB ChB Sheff. 1992.

SEATON, John Eric Vernon William Harvey Hospital, Ashford TN24 0LZ Tel: 01233 633331 — MB ChB Ed. 1990; MRCOG 1997. Cons., William Harvey Hosp., Ashford, Kent. Specialty: Obst. & Gyn. Prev: Specialist Regist. Norf. & Norwich Hosp.; Regist. (O & G) Addenbrooke's Hosp. & Rosie Matern. Hosp. Camb.; SHO (O & G) Roy. Infirm. Edin.

SEATON, John Stuart (retired) Dartford West Health Centre, Tower Road, Dartford DA1 2HA Tel: 01322 23600 — MRCS Eng. LRCP Lond. 1959 (Camb. & St. Geo.) DObst RCOG 1961.

SEAVERS, Janet Elizabeth Rosegrove Surgery, 225-227 Gannow Lane, Burnley BB12 6HY Tel: 01282 423295 Fax: 01282 832609; 6 Higham Road, Padiham, Burnley BB12 9AP Tel: 01282 72351 — MB ChB Manch. 1977; BSc (Med. Sci.) St. And. 1974.

SEAVERS, Peter Rosegrove Surgery, 225-227 Gannow Lane, Burnley BB12 6HY Tel: 01282 423295 Fax: 01282 832609; 6 Higham Road, Padiham, Burnley BB12 9AP Tel: 01282 72351 — MB ChB Manch. 1977; MRCGP 1982.

SEBAG-MONTEFIORE, David Joseph Yorkshire Centre for Clinical Oncology, Cookridge Hospital, Hospital Lane, Leeds LS16 6QB Tel: 0113 392 4244 Fax: 0113 392 4186 — MB BS Lond. 1983; MRCP (UK) 1986; FRCR 1990; FRCP 1999. Cons. Clin. Oncologist, Leeds Cancer Centre, Cookridge Hosp. Specialty: Oncol. Prev: Sen. Regist. (Radiother.) St. Bart. Hosp. Lond.; Regist. (Clin. Oncol.) Middlx. & Mt. Vernon Hosp. N.wood.

SEBAG-MONTEFIORE, Stephen Eric (retired) 34 Peninsula Square, Winchester SO23 8GJ Tel: 01962 856121 Fax: 01962 856121 — (Camb. & Middlx.) MB BChir Camb. 1950; MRCGP 1958; MD Camb. 1979. Prev: Clin. Asst. (Psychol. Med.) St. Bart. Hosp. Lond.

SEBAGH, Jean-Louis The French Cosmetic Medical Co Ltd, 25 Wimpole St., London W1M 7AD Tel: 020 7637 0548 Fax: 020 7637 5110 Email: doctor@frenchcosmetic.com — MD Paris 1982.

SEBARATNAM, Natalie Renuka 33A St Stephens Gardens, Twickenham TW1 2LT — MB BS Lond. 1993.

SEBARATNAM, Noeline Padmini 37 Cunningham Avenue, St Albans AL1 1JJ Tel: 01727 859614; 37 Cunningham Avenue, St Albans AL1 1JJ Tel: 01727 859614 — MB BS Ceylon 1960; DPM Eng. 1967; FRCPsych 1989, M 1972. Cons. (Psychiat.) W. Herts. Community Health Trust. Specialty: Gen. Psychiat. Prev: Cons. (Psychiat.) Cell Barnes Hosp. St. Albans; Med. Asst. Hill End Hosp. St. Albans; Regist. Cell Barnes Hosp. St. Albans.

SEBASTIAN, Joseph 13 Homer Row, 2nd Floor, London W1H 4AW — MB BS Karnatak 1960; LAH Dub. 1962.

SEBASTIAN, Thottacherry Chacko 51 Kaye Lane, Huddersfield HD5 8XP — MB BS Karnatak 1960.

SEBASTIANPILLAI, Chitra 17 Underne Avenue, London N14 7ND — MB BS Ceylon 1971 (Peradeniya)

SEBASTIANPILLAI, Francis Benedict Yohendiran 17 Underne Avenue, London N14 7ND — MB BS Ceylon 1971.

SEBASTIANPILLAI, Narishta Joanne 42 Michleham Down, Woodside Park, London N12 7JN Tel: 020 8445 5845 — MB BS Lond. 1994 (Roy. Free Hosp.) DCH RCP Lond. 1996. GP Regist. Specialty: Gen. Pract. Socs: BMA. Prev: SHO (Psychiat.); SHO (ENT); SHO (Paediat.).

SEBESTIK, Jan Paul NW Surrey Child and Adolescent Mental Health Service, Ashford & St Peter's NHS Trust, St. Peter's Hospital, Guildford Road, Chertsey KT16 0PZ Tel: 01932 722561 Fax: 01932 722563 Email: jan.sebestik@asph.nhs.uk — MB BS Lond. 1984; MRCPsych 1989. Cons. Child & Adolesc. Psychiat. St. Peter's Hosp. Chertsey. Specialty: Child & Adolesc. Psychiat.

SEBIRE, Neil James Great Ormond Street Hospital, Great Ormond Street, London WC1N — MB BS Lond. 1992 (St Mary's, London) MD London 1999; MRCPath 2002. Cons. (Paediat. Path.). Specialty: Histopath. Prev: SPR in Histopath., St Mary's, Lond.; Research Fell., Harris Birthright Unit, King's Coll. Lond.

SEBUGWAWO, Mr Silas Northamptonshire Health Authority, High Field, Northampton NN1 5DN Tel: 01604 615325 Fax: 01604 615146; 57 Berry Lane, Wootton, Northampton NN4 6JU — MB ChB Makerere 1975; MSc (Pharmacol.) Lond. 1979; FRCS Glas. 1984; MFPHM RCP (UK) 1993. Cons. Pub. Health Med. N.ants. HA. Specialty: Pub. Health Med. Prev: Sen. Regist. (Pub. Health Med.) S. West. RHA; Regist. (Neurosurg.) Univ. Hosp. Wales Cardiff & Morriston Hosp. Swansea; Regist. (Surg.) W. Fife Hosp. Dunfermline.

SECCOMBE, Martin Peter Jonathan 12 Lynmouth Road, Reading RG1 8DD Tel: 0118 951 1453 — MB BS Lond. 1993 (UMDS) SHO (Med.) Roy. Berks. Hosp. Reading. Specialty: Gen. Med. Prev: SHO (Paediat.) & Regist. (Med. & Emerg.); Waikato Hosp. Hamilton, NZ.

SECHIARI, Giles Pandely, TD, OStJ 42 Granville Park, Aughton, Ormskirk L39 5DU — MB BCh Witwatersrand 1957; FRCP Lond. 1977, M 1964. Cons. Phys. & Geriat. Ormskirk & Dist. Hosp. Gp. Specialty: Gen. Med. Prev: Lect. (Endocrinol.) Univ. Liverp.

SECKER, Christopher John 12 Northesk Street, Stone ST15 8EP — BM BS Nottm. 1988; FRCA 1994. Regist. (Anaesth.) Leicester Roy. Infirm. NHS Trust. Specialty: Anaesth.

SECKER WALKER, Jonathan University of Wales College of Medicine, Department of Clinical Governance, Heaty Park, Cardiff CF14 4XW Tel: 029 2074 5041; 40 Woodland Gardens, Muswell Hill, London N10 3UA Tel: 020 8444 9426 Fax: 020 8444 9426 Email: jonathansw@classicfm.net — MB BS Lond. 1967 (Univ. Coll. Hosp.) BSc Lond. 1964; MRCS Eng. LRCP Lond. 1967; FFA RCS Eng. 1972. Sen. Lect. Univ. Wales Coll. Med. Cardiff; Hon. Sen. Lect. (Anaesth.) UCL Med. Sch. Specialty: Anaesth. Socs: Roy. Soc. Med.; BAAM; Chelsea Clin. Soc. Prev: Gen. Manager UCL Hosps.; Cons. Anaesth. Univ. Coll. Hosp.; Sen. Regist. (Anaesth.) St. Thos. Hosp. Lond.

SECKL, Professor Jonathan Robert University of Edinburgh, Molecular Medicine Centre, Western General Hospital, Edinburgh EH4 2XU Tel: 0131 651 1035 Fax: 0131 651 1085 Email: j.seckl@ed.ac.uk — MB BS Lond. 1980 (Univ. Coll.) BSc London 1977; MRCP (UK) 1983; PhD Lond. 1989; FRCP Ed. 1993; F.Med.Sci 1999; FRSE 2002. Hon. Cons. Phys. (Endocrinol.) Lothian HB Edin.; Moncrieff-Arnott Prof. Molecular Med. Specialty: Endocrinol. Special Interest: Glucocorticoid Biol. Socs: Acad. of Med. Sci.s; Assn. of Phys.s; Soc. Endocrinol. Prev: Wellcome Trust Sen. Research Fell. Clin. Sci. West. Gen. Hosp. Edin.; Lect. (Med.) Univ. Edin. West. Gen. Hosp.; Prof. Endocrinol. Univ. Edin.

SECKL, Michael Julian 30 Fairmead Road, London N19 4DF — MB BS Lond. 1986; BSc (Immunol.) Lond. 1983; MRCP (UK) 1990; PhD Lond. 1995. Sen. Lect. & Hon. Cons. (Med. Oncol.) Char. Cross & Hammersmith Hosps. Lond. Specialty: Oncol. Socs: Fell. Roy. Soc. Med.; BMA. Prev: Clin. Research Fell. Imperial Cancer Research Fund Lond.; Hon. Sen. Regist. Roy. Free Hosp. Lond.; Regist. Rotat. (Gen. Med. & Oncol.) Char. Cross Hosp. Lond. & Lister Hosp. Stevenage.

SECRETT, Tracey Joanne Banchory Group Practice, Banchory AB31 5XS — MB BS Lond. 1996; DCH; DRCOG; MRCGP.

SEDANO BOCOS, Alberto c/o Dr D Santana-Hernandez, 82 Bootham Park Court, York YO31 8JT — LMS La Laguna 1992.

SEDAR, Mohammed Iqbal Mawbey Brough Health Centre, 39 Wilcox Close, London SW8 2UD Tel: 020 7411 5720 Fax: 020 7411 5775 — MB BS Sri Lanka 1975.

SEDDON, Anthony John The Penryn Surgery, Saracen Way, Penryn TR10 8HX Tel: 01326 372502; Killigarth House, Devoran, Truro TR3 6NE — MRCS Eng. LRCP Lond. 1972 (Westm.) MA, BM BCh Oxf. 1972; DObst RCOG 1974; DA Eng. 1977.

SEDDON, Beatrice Mary 114 Chestnut Grove, New Malden KT3 3JT — MB BS Lond. 1990 (St. George's) BSc Lond. 1987; MRCP (UK) 1994; FRCR 1998. Regist. (Clin. Oncol.) Roy. Marsden Hosp. Specialty: Oncol. Prev: Regist. (Clin. Oncol.) Ipswich Hosp.; SHO (HIV) Chelsea & Westm. Hosp. Lond.; SHO (Renal Med.) Guy's Hosp. Lond.

SEDDON, Daniel John 7-9 Civic Way, Ellesmere Port CH65 0AX — MB ChB Manch. 1981; DA (UK) 1986; MRCGP 1987; MPH Liverp. 1993; MFPHM RCP (UK) 1995. Director of Pub. Health. Specialty: Pub. Health Med. Prev: Cons. (Pub. Health Med.) Berks. HA; GP Sandbach, Chesh.; Cons. Pub. Health Med. S. Chesh. HA.

SEDDON, David James Health Care of The Elderly, Queens Medical Centre, University Hospital, Nottingham NG7 2UH Tel: 0115 924 9924 Fax: 0115 970 9496 — MB BChir Camb. 1979 (Oxf. & Camb.) MA Oxf. 1981, BA 1977; MRCP (UK) 1982; MD Camb. 1993; FRCP(L) 1999. Cons. Geriat. Med. Qu. Med. Centre Univ. Hosp. Nottm. & Nottm. Healthcare NHS Trust; Coll. Tutor, Qu.'s Med. Centre Nottm. Specialty: Care of the Elderly; Gen. Med.; Respirat. Med. Socs: Brit. Geriat. Soc.; BMA. Prev: Sen. Regist. (Gen. & Geriat. Med.) Oxf. & Anglia RHA; Research Fell. & Hon. Regist. (Med. & Nuclear Med.) Char. Cross Hosp. Lond.; Regist. (Med. & Thoracic Med.) Whipps Cross Hosp. Lond.

SEDDON, Geoffrey Boyd (retired) Kings Cottage, Barham Court, Melbourn, Royston SG8 6EW Tel: 01763 263320 — MB ChB Manch. 1956; DA Eng. 1963.

SEDDON, Ian Department of Histopathology, Essex Rivers NHS Trust, Chestnut Villa, Boxted Rd, Colchester CO4 5HG — MB ChB Manch. 1979; MRCPath 1986; FRCPath 1996. Cons. Histopath., Essex Rivers NHS Trust; Hon. (Path.) Univ. Manch. Specialty: Histopath. Socs: Assn. Clin. Paths.; Internat. Acad. of Path. Prev: Cons. Histopath., Roy. Oldham Hosp.; Lect. (Path.) Univ. Sheff.; Sen. Regist. (Histopath.) Roy. Hallamsh. Hosp. Sheff.

SEDDON, James Gideon Winstanley Plas Meddyg Surgery, Station Road, Ruthin LL15 1BP Tel: 01824 702255 Fax: 01824 707221; Bryn Awelon, Llangynhafal, Denbigh LL16 4LN — MB ChB Liverp. 1981; DRCOG 1984; MRCGP 1986.

SEDDON, Joanna Margaret Marshfield Surgery, 2 Back Lane, Marshfield, Chippenham SN14 8NQ Tel: 0117 937 2214 Fax: 0117 937 4692; The Lawn, 117 High St, Wick, Bristol BS30 5QQ — MB ChB Birm. 1978; DCH RCP Lond. 1981. Specialty: Pharmacology. Prev: SHO (ENT, Ophth., Derm. & Paediat.) Selly Oak Hosp. Birm.; SHO (Geriat.) & SHO (Supernum. Obst.) Plymouth; Trainee GP Plymouth.

SEDDON, Mr John Anthony 19 Rutland Avenue, Walton, Warrington WA4 6PB Tel: 01925 62859 — MB ChB Liverp. 1951; DObst RCOG 1957; ChM Liverp. 1965, MB ChB 1951, DPH 1958; FRCS Eng. 1961.

SEDDON, John David Middleton The Coach House, Clevedon Road, Nailsea, Bristol BS48 1HA — MB BS Lond. 1992.

SEDDON, Lesley Maswell Park Health Centre, Hounslow Avenue, Hounslow TW3 2DY Tel: 020 8321 3488 Fax: 020 8893 4368; 13 Murray Avenue, Hounslow TW3 2LQ Tel: 020 8894 5370 — MRCS Eng. LRCP Lond. 1981; BSc Lond. 1978, MB BS 1981.

SEDDON, Norman Ernest (retired) 6 Tarn Close, storth, Milnthorpe LA7 7HZ — MB ChB Manch. 1954.

SEDDON, Paul Christopher Royal Alexandra Hospital for Sick Children, Dyke Road, Brighton BN1 3JN Tel: 01273 328145 — MB ChB Manch. 1981; DCH RCP Lond. 1983; MRCP (UK) 1985. Cons. Paediat. Brighton Health Care. Specialty: Paediat. Socs: Brit. Thorac. Soc. Europ. Respirat. Soc. Prev: Research Fell. McGill Univ. Montreal, Canada; Sen. Regist. (Paediat.) S. West. RHA; Research Fell. Liverp. Univ.

SEDDON, Paul James, Wing Cdr. RAF Med. Br. Station Medical Centre, RAF Leuchars, St Andrews KY16 0JX Tel: 01334 839471; 1 Adam Close, Leuchars, St Andrews KY16 0LR — MB BS Newc. 1983; BSc Newc. 1978; DRCOG 1991; MRCGP 1992; DCH RCP Lond. 1995. Sen. Med. Off. RAF Leuchars. Specialty: Aviat. Med. Socs: BMA. Prev: Unit Med. Off. RAF Linton-on-Ouse; Regist. (Histopath.) Newc. Gen. Hosp.

SEDDON, Rebecca 7 Hillhead Terrace, Spital, Aberdeen AB24 3JE — MB ChB Aberd. 1996. GP VTS Aberd. Specialty: Gen. Pract. Prev: SHO (Surgic. Paediat.) Aberd.; SHO Aberd. Roy. Infirm.

SEDDON, Stephen John Meadowcroft, Sandyfields, Baldwins Gate, Newcastle ST5 5DW — MB ChB St. And. 1971; FFA RCS Eng. 1975. Cons. Anaesth. N. Staffs. RHA. Specialty: Anaesth.

SEDDON, Thomas Andrew Aspull Surgery, Haigh Road, Aspull, Wigan WN2 1XH Tel: 01942 831263 Fax: 01942 832065; 23 Avonhead Close, Horwich, Bolton BL6 5QD — MB BS Lond. 1987; MA Camb. 1987; MRCGP 1991.

SEDDON, Thomas Michael Winster, Hasty Brow Road, Slyne-with-Hest, Lancaster LA2 6AG Tel: 01524 410490 — MB ChB Aberd. 1962. Socs: BMA. Prev: Ho. Phys. & Ho. Surg., & SHO Cas. Vict. Hosp. Blackpool; SHO O & G W.mld. Co. Hosp. Kendal; Terminable Lect. Anat. Aberd. Univ.

SEDGWICK, Mr David Michael Tigh-A-Chiuil, Badabrie, Fort William PH33 7LX Tel: 01397 772035 — MB ChB Ed. 1980; BSc (Hons.) (Med. Sci.) St. And. 1977; FRCS Ed. 1984. Cons. Surg. Belford Hosp. Fort William. Specialty: Gen. Surg. Prev: Regist. (Gen. Surg.) West. Gen. Hosp. Edin.; Research Fell. (Gastroinestinal Laborat.) West. Gen. Hosp. Edin. Univ. & Edin. Med. Fac. Schol.; Regist. (Surg.) Dunfermline & W. Fife Hosp.

SEDGWICK, Professor Edward Michael (retired) Brackendale, 85 Lakewood Road, Chandlers Ford, Eastleigh SO53 5AD Tel: 023 8026 5073/023 8026 6647 Fax: 023 8026 3793 — MB ChB Bristol 1962; MD Bristol 1967, BSc 1959; MRCP (UK) 1992; FRCP Lond. 1994. Prev: Sen. Lect. (Physiol. & Biochem.) Univ. Soton.

SEDGWICK, Emma Child & Adolescent Mental Health Department, Chelsea & Westminster Hospital, Fulham Road, London SW10 9NH — MB BS Lond. 1993.

SEDGWICK, James Edward Charles Woodpeckers, Chilworth Old Village, Southampton SO16 7JP — MB BS Lond. 1993 (Lond. Hosp. Med. Coll.) BSc Lond. 1990; MRCP (UK) 1996. Specialty: Pub. Health Med.

SEDGWICK, John Maclaren Wylie (retired) Watermoor House, Watermoor Road, Cirencester GL7 1JR — MRCS Eng. LRCP Lond. 1941 (Camb. & Lond. Hosp.) Prev: Resid. Surg. Off. Rush Green Hosp. Romford.

SEDGWICK, John Philip 12 Finians Close, Uxbridge UB10 9NW — MB BS Lond. 1965; MRCS Eng. LRCP Lond. 1964; DA Eng. 1967. Sen. Occ. Health Phys. Grosvener Health; Director Med Servs. to Industry Ltd. Specialty: Occupat. Health. Socs: Fell. Roy. Soc. Med.; Med. Soc. Occupat. Med. Prev: Dir. Med. Serv. Brunel Univ.; Occ. Health Phys. Lond. Boro. Hillingdon & Hillingdon Hosp.; Med. Cons. to Coca-Cola Schweppes, Pioneer Hi-Fidelity & Others.

SEDGWICK, John Rich Hill Brow Road, Liss GU33 7LE; Longhill Cottage, Hillbrow Road, Liss GU33 7LH Tel: 01730 893258 — MB BS Lond. 1977 (St. Thos.) MRCS Eng. LRCP Lond. 1977; DRCOG 1979; MRCGP 1981. Hosp. Practitioner (ENT) Qu. Alexandra Hosp. Portsmouth. Specialty: Otolaryngol.

SEDGWICK, John Vincent King's College Hospital, Denmark Hill, London SE5 9RS; 2 Park Hill, Bickley, Bromley BR1 2JH — BM Soton. 1981; FFA RCS 1988. Cons. Anaesth. King's Coll. Hosp. Lond. Specialty: Anaesth. Socs: BMA & Assn. Pain Soc.

SEDGWICK, Mr Mark Accident & Emergency Department, Blackpool Victoria Hospital NHS Trust, Whinney Heys Road, Blackpool FY3 8NR Tel: 01253 303523 Fax: 01253 306668; 7 Forest Close, Meols, Wirral CH47 6BA Tel: 0151 632 1229 Fax: 01253 301984 — MB Camb. 1984 (Camb. & Guy's Hosp.) BA Camb. 1980; BChir Camb. 1983; MA Camb. 1988; MRCP (UK) 1988; FRCS Ed. 1990; FRCS Ed. (A&E Med. & Surg.) 1992; FFAEM, 1994; FRCP 2000. Cons. A & E Med. Blackpool Vict. Hosp. NHS Trust. Specialty: Accid. & Emerg.; Medico Legal. Socs: Brit. Assn. Accid. & Emerg. Med.; Brit. Med. Assn. (Pl. of Work Represen.).

SEDGWICK, Martin Leonard Countess of Chester Hospital, Liverpool Road, Chester CH2 1UL Tel: 01244 365000 Fax: 01244 366455 — MB ChB Leeds 1984; BSc (Hons.) Biochem. Leeds 1981; MRCP (UK) 1987; MD Leeds 1994; FRCP 2000. Cons. Phys. & Cardiol. Countess of Chester Hosp. Specialty: Cardiol. Socs: Brit. Cardiac Soc. Prev: Sen. Regist. (Cardiol.) West. Infirm. Glas.; Regist. (Cardiol.) Roy. Alexandra Hosp. Paisley & Glas. Roy. Infirm.; SHO (Gen. Med.) Seacroft Hosp. Leeds.

SEDGWICK, Paul Allan 26 Hawkeys Lane, North Shields NE29 0PN — MB ChB Liverp. 1993.

SEDLER, Mark Jonathan 37 Highwood Avenue, Leeds LS17 6EW — MB ChB Liverp. 1992.

SEDLER, Penelope Anne Susan Louise 46 Westwood Road, Sheffield S11 7EY — MB ChB Sheff. 1979.

SEDMAN, Mr Peter Charles Hull Royal Infirmary, Anlaby Road, Hull HU3 2JZ Tel: 01482 328541 Email: psedman@surgery.karoo.co.uk — MB ChB Leeds 1985; FRCS Ed. 1991; FRCS Eng. 1992; FRCS (Gen.) 1996. Cons. Upper Gastrointestinal & Gen. Surg. Roy. Hull Hosps. Specialty: Gen. Surg.

SEE CHYE HENG, Andrew 1 St Crispin's Close, London NW3 2QF — MB BS Singapore 1985.

SEEAR, Michael 86 Harley Street, London W1G 7HP Tel: 020 7580 3256 — MB BS Lond. 1969 (Westm.) MRCGP 1979; Diploma of Professional Psychotherapy 1985. Indep Complementary Med. Lond. Specialty: Psychother.; Hypnother. Socs: Fell. Med. Soc. Lond. (Ex. Mem. Counc.); Fell. Brit. Soc. Med. & Dent. Hypn. - Teach. of Hypnother.; Fell. Roy. Soc. of Med. Prev: RMO King Edwd. VII Hosp. for Off.s (Sister Agnes Founder) Lond.; SHO (Psychiat.) Guy's Hosp. Lond.; Vis. Phys. Bupa Med. Centre Lond.

SEED, Catherine Alison 52 Laverton Road, Fairhaven, Lytham St Annes FY8 1EN — MB ChB Ed. 1996.

SEED, Martin James Addenbrooke's Hospital, Department of Clinical Immunology, Box 109, Cambridge CB2 2QQ — MB ChB Leeds 1993; BSc Hons. (Chem. Path.) Leeds 1990; MRCP (UK) 1997. Specialist Regist. Clin. Immunol. Addenbrookes Hosp. Camb. Specialty: Immunol. Prev: SHO (Gen. Med.) Roy. Hallamsh. Hosp. Sheff.; SHO (Infec. Dis.) Roy. Hallamsh. Hosp. Sheff.; SHO (Renal Med.) St. Jas. Univ. Hosp. Leeds.

SEED, Mary (retired) Lipid Clinic, Private Out Patients, 15th Floor Charing Cross Hospital, Fulham Palace Road, London W6 8RF Tel: 020 8846 1148 Fax: 020 7221 4949; 15 St Olave's Court, St Petersburgh Place, London W2 4JY Tel: 020 7221 4949 Fax: 020 7221 4949 Email: drmaryseed@hotmail.com — BM BCh Oxf. 1961; MA Oxf. 1961, DM 1992; FRCPath 1996, M 1992; MRCP 2000. Hon. Consg. Phys. 15th Floor Char. Cross Hosp. Lond.; Cons. King. Edwd. VII Hosp. Midhurst; Cons. Lond. Woms. Clinic Lond. Prev: Resid. Fell. Metab. Unit St Mary's Hosp. Lond.

SEED, Peter Robinson (retired) 17 Milton Crescent, Cheadle SK8 1NT — MB ChB Birm. 1956 (Birmingham) MRCS Eng. LRCP Lond. 1956; DObst RCOG 1961; DCH Eng. 1973. Prev: Obst. Ho. Off. St. Mary's Hosp. Wom. & Childr. Manch.

SEED, Richard Gibson Francis Lloyd E230 Armed Forces Hospital, PO Box 7897, Riyadh 11159, Saudi Arabia Tel: 00 966 14777714 Fax: 00 966 14620625 Email: dicanjo@zajil.net; 18a Granville Road, Waltier, Deal CT14 7LS Tel: 01304 374344 Fax: 01304 374344 — MB BS Lond. 1960 (Middx.) FRCA 1967; FANZCA 1979; FFA RCSI 1995. Director (Anaesth.) Riyadh Armed Forces Hosp. Riyadh, Saudi Arabia. Specialty: Anaesth. Socs: Fell. Roy. Soc. Med.; Assn. Anaesth.; Austral. Soc. Anaesth. Prev: Director (Anaesth.) Roy. Perth Hosp., W. Austral.; Director, Sen. Lect. & Hon. Cons. Guy's Hosp. Lond.; Sen. Regist. & Research Asst. Roy. Postgrad. Med. Sch. Lond.

SEED, Professor William Anthony (retired) 15 St Olaves Court, St. Petersburgh Place, London W2 4JY; Department of Respiratory Medicine, Imperial College School of Medicine, Charing Cross Hospital, London W6 8RF Tel: 020 8846 7198 Fax: 020 8846 7170 — BM BCh Oxf. 1962; BSc Oxf. 1960, MA 1962; FRCP Lond. 1981, M 1965; PhD Lond. 1972. Emerit. Prof. (Med.) Imperial Coll. Sch. of Med. Prev: Cons. Phys. Char. Cross Hosp. Lond.

SEEDAT, Najib Ibrahim 60 Erskine Road, London E17 6RZ — MB ChB Birm. 1993.

SEEDHOUSE, Joanna Kate 5 The Beeches, Ebstree Road, Seisdon, Wolverhampton WV5 7EU — MB ChB Liverp. 1998; MB ChB Liverp 1998.

SEEHRA, Chatranjan Singh 64 Cantwell Road, Shooters Hill, London SE18 3LW; 17 Stanbridge Road, Downend, Bristol BS16 6AW Tel: 0117 957 3242 — MB ChB Glas. 1984; Cert. Family Plann. JCC 1987; DRCOG 1987; MRCGP 1989; DCH RCP Lond. 1990; MSc (Pub. Health) Lond. 2000. Sen. Regist. Pub. Health Med. S. Thames E. Lond. Specialty: Gen. Med. Prev: GP Princip. Bristol; SHO (ENT) Gartnavel Gen. Hosp. Glas.; SHO (Psychiat.) Bedford Gen. Hosp.

SEEHRA, Mr Harkiran 3 The Drive, Didsbury Village, Manchester M20 6HZ Tel: 0161 434 8444 Email: 100723.1726@compuserve.com — MB ChB Manch. 1986; FRCS Ed. 1992. Specialist Regist. (Gen. Surg.) Leighton Hosp. Crewe. Specialty: Gen. Surg. Prev: Regist. (Gen. Surg.) Whiston Hosp. Prescot; Regist. (Vasc. Surg.) Roy. Liverp. Univ. Hosp.; Research Fell. (Surg. Gastroenterol.) Univ. Manch.

SEEHRA, Kulwant Kaur 12 Abbey Road, Chertsey KT16 8AL — MB BS Jammu & Kashmir 1969 (Govt. Med. Coll. Srinagar) SHO Woolwich Memor. Hosp.

SEEHRA, Manjeet Singh The Surgery, High Street, Lowestoft NR32 1JE Tel: 01502 589151 Fax: 01502 566719 Email: manjeet.seehra@gp-d83023.nhs.uk — BM BS Nottm. 1982; BMedSci Nottm. 1980; DRCOG 1987. GP Princ.; Hosp. Practitioner (Renal Unit) James Paget Hosp. Gorleston. Specialty: Gen. Pract.

SEEHRA, Mohinderkaur 1 Thistledown Close, Streetly, Sutton Coldfield B74 3EE Tel: 0121 580 9597 — (Mahatma Gandhi Med. Coll. Indore) MB BS Vikram 1959. Deptm. Med. Off. Bexley Health Dist. Specialty: Community Child Health. Socs: BMA. Prev: Ho. Phys. & Ho. Surg. & Regist. (ENT) King Geo. VI Hosp. Nairobi; Kenya; Regist. Radiother. Dept. Roy. North. Hosp. Lond.

SEEHRA, Surinder Singh 49 Mayfair Avenue, Ilford IG1 3DJ — MB BS Lond. 1991.

SEEHRA, Taljit Kaur 64 Cantwell Road, Shooters Hill, London SE18 3LW — BM Soton. 1994. Specialty: Otolaryngol.

SEEL, Edward Hamer Wood Sorrel, Twyncyn, Dinas Powys CF64 4AS — BM Soton. 1998.

SEELEY, Anthony John Bridgnorth Medical Practices, Northgate House, 7 High Street, Bridgnorth WV16 4BU Tel: 01746 767121 Fax: 01746 765433 — MB ChB Manch. 1977; MRCGP 1981; DRCOG 1982; DFFP 1995. Princip. in Gen. Pract.; Trainer in Gen. Pract. & Family Plann. Socs: Counc. Mem. Brit. Menopause Soc.

SEELEY, Charles (retired) 27 Chesil Street, Winchester SO23 0HU Tel: 01962 860508 — LMSSA Lond. 1930 (St. Mary's) MD Lond. 1948, MB BS 1934; DPH Eng. 1938; FFCM 1974. Hon. Consg. Phys. St. Geo. Hosp.; Lect. Emerit. Social & Preven. Med. St. Geo. Hosp. Med. Sch.; Lect. St. Geo. Hosp. Sch. Nursing; Vis. Lect. Cornell Med. Coll. & Yale Med. Sch. USA; Examr. Univ. Lond, DPH Eng. & Gen. Nurs. Counc.; Mem. Bd. Studies (Social & Preven. Med.) Lond. Univ. Prev: Assoc. Phys. Social Med. & Comm. Care Radcliffe Infirm. Oxf. & United.

SEELEY, David Dearne Valley Health Centre, Wakefield Road, Scissett, Huddersfield HD8 9JL Tel: 01484 862793 Fax: 01484 866021 Email: david.seeley@gp-b85002.nhs.uk — MB ChB Sheff. 1984; BA (Physiol. Sci.) Oxf. 1981; MRCGP 1989.

SEELEY, David William 133 Nothfield Road, Sheffield S10 1QP — MB ChB Sheff. 1993.

SEELEY, Stephanie Kate Medical Centre, 20-22 Concord Way, Dukinfield SK16 4DB Tel: 0161 343 6382 — MB ChB Manch. 1993; BA (Hons) Birm. 1981; DRCOG 1998. GP Princ. Specialty: Paediat. Prev: SHO (Paediat.) Stockport.

SEELY, Martin Francis Victoria Medical Centre, 16-18 Victoria Parade, Urmston, Manchester M41 9BP Tel: 0161 799 2237; 16/18 Victoria Parade, Urmston, Manchester M41 9BP Tel: 0161 746 7086 Fax: 0161 746 7162 — MB ChB Manch. 1979; BA. GP; Forens. Med. Exam. Gtr. Manch. Police; Bd. Mem. Trafford N. PCG. Prev: Med. Examr. RAF Manch.

SEEMUNGAL, Barry Mitra 23 Lancaster Lodge, 83/85 Lancaster Road, London W11 1QH — MB BCh Wales 1993 (Cardiff) BSc (Physiol.) Wales Coll. Cardiff 1989; MRCP Ed. 1996. Specialist Regist. (Med.) Oxf. Deanery. Socs: Fell. Roy. Soc. Med.

SEENAN, Clare Frances 52 Crompton Avenue, Glasgow G44 5TH — MB ChB Glas. 1998; MB ChB Glas 1998.

SEENAN, Pamela Julie Wester Ross, Eglinton Ter, Skelmorlie PA17 5ER — MB ChB Glas. 1997.

SEENEY, Barbara Padiham Group Practice, Padiham Medical Centre, Burnley Road, Burnley BB12 8BP Tel: 01282 771298 Fax: 01282 777720; 1 Barley Green, Barley, Burnley BB12 9JU — MB ChB Liverp. 1983; BDS Liverp. 1975, MB ChB 1983; DRCOG 1985.

SEENI, Mr Kalm York District Hospital, York YO31 8HE Tel: 01904 631313 Fax: 01904 726879 Email: kseeni@lineone.net; The Purey Inst. Nuffield Hospital, Precentors Court, York YO1 7EL Tel: 01904 641571 — MB BS Malaya 1986 (University Malaya) FRCS 1990; PG Dip. Urol. Lond. 1992; FRCS (Urol III) 1994; MBA Leeds 2001. Cons. Urol. Specialty: Urol. Special Interest: Andrology; Endourology; Laparoscopy. Prev: Consultant Urologist,Friarage Hosp.Northallerton.

SEERAJ, Edwin Chandrabhose Lister Primary Care Centre, 101 Peckham Road, London SE15 5LJ Tel: 020 7708 5413 Fax: 020 771 3810 — LRCPI & LM, LRSCI & LM 1972; DObst RCOG 1976.

SEERY, J A Ward, Seery, Ahmad, Shakoor, Gardenia Surgery, 2A Gardenia Avenue, Luton LU3 2NS Tel: 01582 572612 Fax: 01582 494553 — MB BCh Witwatersrand 1976; MB BCh Witwatersrand 1976.

SEETULSINGH, Prema Saraspathy Department of Microbiology, Hemel Hempstead General Hospital, Hillfield Road, Hemel Hempstead HP2 4AD Tel: 01442 287834 Fax: 01442 287089; 34 Stewart Road, Harpenden AL5 4QB — MB BS Delhi 1986; MSc Lond. 1989; MRCPath 1994; FRCPath 2002. Cons. Microbiol. Hemel Hempstead Gen. Hosp. Herts. Specialty: Med. Microbiol. Socs: Hosp. Infec. Soc.; Brit. Soc. Antimicrob. Chemother.; Intern. Soc. of Travel med. Prev: Sen. Regist. (MicroBiol.) Qu. Mary's Univ. Hosp. Lond.; Sen. Regist. (Microbiol.) St. Geo.'s Hosp. Lond.; Fell. (Infec. Dis.) Houston, Texas, USA.

SEEVARATNAM, David Manoharan Department of Mental Handicap, Floor 'E', South Block, University Hospital, Queens Medical Centre, Nottingham NG7 2UH — MB BS Sri Lanka 1974; MRCPsych 1985. Lect. (Ment. Handicap) Qu. Med. Centre Nottm.

SEEVARATNAM, Mohan Surendra Top Flat, 310 Commercial Way, Peckham, London SE15 1QN; 46 Ventnor Drive, Totteridge, London N20 8BP — MB BS Lond. 1988; MRCGP 1993; DRCOG 1993. Asst. Gallions Reach Health Centre Lond. Prev: Trainee GP/SHO (O & G) Whitechapel Hosp. Lond. VTS; Ho. Surg. Kent & Sussex Hosp. Tunbridge Wells; Ho. Phys. Hither Green & Lewisham Hosp.

SEEVARATNAM, Nandini Shereen 46 Ventnor Drive, Totteridge, London N20 8BP — MB ChB Sheff. 1996.

SEEWOONARAIN, Kishore Santa Kumarsingh Runwell Hospital, Wickford SS11 7QE Tel: 01268 366000 Fax: 01268 570946 — MD Marseilles 1980; DTM & H Marseilles 1980; MRCPsych 1985; FRCPsych 2001. Cons. And Clin. Director Forens. Psychiat. Runwell Hosp. Wickford Essex. Specialty: Forens. Psychiat. Prev: Sen. Regist. (Forens. Psychiat.) Prestwich Hosp. Manch.

SEEX, Derek Michael Brooks Bar Medical Centre, 162-164 Chorlton Road, Old Trafford, Manchester M16 7WW Tel: 0161 226 7777 Fax: 0161 232 9963; 67 Church Road, Urmston, Manchester M41 9EJ Tel: 0161 748 7462 — MB ChB Leeds 1976; DRCOG 1979; MMedSc (Gen. Pract.) Leeds 1986; FRCGP 1997. Socs: Comm. Mem. Trafford Oncol. Soc. Prev: SHO (O & G & Paediat.) Staincliffe Gen. Hosp. Dewsbury; SHO (Psychiat) St. Lukes Hosp. Huddersfield.

SEFTON, Dominic Langham Place Surgery, 11 Langham Place, Northampton NN2 6AA Tel: 01604 38162 Fax: 01604 602457; 3 Holmfield Way, Weston Favell, Northampton NN3 3BJ Tel: 01604 786032 — BM BS Nottm. 1983; BMedSci Nottm. 1981.

SEFTON, Mr Graham Keith 473 Hotham Road, Hull HU5 — MB ChB Sheff. 1970; FRCS Ed. 1974. Cons. Orthop. Surg. Harrogate Dist. Hosp. Specialty: Transpl. Surg.

SEFTON, Sydney Lingwell Croft Surgery, Ring Road, Middleton, Leeds LS10 3LT Tel: 0113 270 4848 Fax: 0113 272 0030; 8 Sandmoor Avenue, Leeds LS17 7DW Tel: 0113 268 6794 — MB BCh BAO Belf. 1949; MRCGP 1966; MFFP 1994. Prev: SHO Ulster Hosp. Wom. & Childr. Belf.

SEFTON-FIDDIAN, Jill Link End Surgery, 39 Pickersleigh Road, Malvern WR14 2RP Tel: 01684 568466 Fax: 01684 891064 — MB ChB Birm. 1977.

SEFTON-FIDDIAN, Peter 5 Woodcroft Close, Blackwell, Bromsgrove B60 1DA — MB ChB Manch. 1978.

SEGAL, Professor Anthony Walter University College London Medical School, The Rayne Institute, 5 University St., London WC1E 6JF Tel: 020 7679 6175 Fax: 020 7679 0967; 48B Regents Park Road, London NW1 7SX Tel: 020 7586 8745 Fax: 020 7679 0967 — MB ChB Cape Town 1967; MRCP (UK) 1971; MD Cape Town 1974; PhD Lond. 1979, MSc 1972, DSc (Sci.) 1984; FRCP Lond. 1987; F Med Sci 1998; FRS 1998. Chas. Dent Prof. Med. Univ. Coll. & Middlx. Hosp. Med. Sch. Lond. Specialty: Gen. Med.; Biochem. Socs: Fell.Roy.coll.Phys.

SEGAL, Antony Maurice 98 Vine Lane, Hillingdon, Uxbridge UB10 0BE Tel: 01895 233034 — MB BS Lond. 1957 (St. Geo.) MRCS Eng. LRCP Lond. 1956; DObst RCOG 1960; DAvMed FOM RCP Lond. 1995. Specialty: Aviat. Med. Socs: Med. Adviser OSTIV SailpLa. Develop. Panel; Fell. Roy. Aeronaut. Soc. Prev: Ho. Surg. (Obst.) Soton. Gen. Hosp.; Ho. Phys. (Paediat.) Vict. Hosp. Childr. Chelsea; Ho. Surg. St. Margt. Hosp. Epping.

SEGAL, Brett Elliott Fabian — MB BS (Distinc. Surg.) Lond. 1998 (St Mary's) BSc Lond. 1995. SHO (Anaesth.) Belf. City Hosp. Socs: North. Irel. Soc. of Anaesthetists. Prev: Sen. Ships Phys. Carnival Cruise Lines, Miami, Fl. USA; SHO (A&E) St. Mary's Hosp. Lond.; Res. Med. Off. Logan Hosp. Queensland, Aust.

SEGAL, Dennis Selwyn SMA Nutrition, Huntercombe Lane S., Taplow, Maidenhead SL6 0PH Tel: 01628 660633 Fax: 01628 604949 — MB ChB Cape Town 1962; MFGP S. Afr. Coll. Med. 1974; MPharmMed Pretoria 1977. Dir. Nutrit. Div. Wyeth Laborat. Taplow Maidenhead. Prev: Sen. Dir. Clin. Affairs Sterling Research Gp. Europe; Med. Dir. Sterling Research Laborat. Guildford; Dir. Med. Servs. Boehringer Ingelheim Ltd. Bracknell.

SEGAL, Hanna Maria 38 Tetherdown, Muswell Hill, London N10 1NG Tel: 020 8883 3225; 44 Queens Avenue, London N10 3NU Tel: 020 8883 3348 — MB ChB Polish Sch. of Med. 1943; MB ChB Polish Sch. of Med 1943; FRCPsych 1972, M 1971. Socs: (Ex-Pres.) Brit. Psychoanal. Soc. Prev: Vice-Pres. Internat. Psychoanal. Assn.; Pres. Brit. Psychoanal. Soc.; Freud Prof. Univ. Coll. Lond.

SEGAL, Israel Michael (retired) 40 Cameron Road, Seven Kings, Ilford IG3 8LF Tel: 020 8590 1134; 26 Emerson Road, Gants Hill, Ilford IG1 4XA — MRCS Eng. LRCP Lond. 1939 (Univ. Coll. Hosp.) MRCGP 1953. Div. Med. Off. Brit. Red Cross Soc.; Lect. 1st Aid Newham Community Coll.

SEGAL, Jonathan Michael Lance The Verwood Surgery, 54 Manor Road, Verwood BH31 7PY Tel: 01202 825353 Fax: 01202 829697 — MB BS Lond. 1985; BA Oxf. 1982; DRCOG 1990. Clin. Asst. (Diabetes Mellitus) Roy. Bournemouth Hosp. Prev: Trainee GP Salisbury VTS; Maua Methodist Mission Hosp., Kenya.

SEGAL, Maximillian Peter Louis Doctor's House, 40 Cameron Road, Seven Kings, Ilford IG3 8LF Tel: 020 8590 1134 Fax: 020 8599 0282; 7 Lincoln Gardens, Ilford IG1 3NF — MB BS Lond. 1971 (Univ. Coll. Hosp.) DObst RCOG 1973. Lect. Redwood Coll. S. Bank Univ. Specialty: Obst. & Gyn. Socs: Fell. Roy. Soc. Med.; Eur. Soc. Human Reproduc. & Embryol.; Brit. Soc. Colpos. & Cerv. Path. Prev: Hosp. Pract. King Geo. Hosp. Ilford; SHO (O & G) Ilford Matern. Hosp.; SHO (A & E), Ho. Surg. & Ho. Phys. King Geo. Hosp. Ilford.

SEGAL, Norman Harold Oldfield Family Practice, 285 Greenford Road, Greenford UB6 8RA Tel: 020 8578 1914 Fax: 020 8575 6327; 6 Abinger Road, London W4 1EL Tel: 020 8747 1682 — MB ChB Leeds 1979; BSc (Hons.) Leeds 1976, MB ChB 1979; MRCGP 1983; DRCOG 1983; Cert Family Plann. 1983. L.M.O. Civil Serv. Med. Advis. Serv.; Approved Sect. 12 M.H.A. (1983); Med. Off. H.M. Y.C.C. Feltham Middlx. Prev: Hosp. Pract. Ealing Hosp. Lond.

SEGAL, Susan Melanie Oldfield Family Practice, 285 Greenford Road, Greenford UB6 8RA Tel: 020 8578 1914 Fax: 020 8575 6327; 6 Abinger Road, London W4 1EL Tel: 020 8747 1682 — MB ChB Leeds 1976; BSc (Hons.) (Pharmacol.) Leeds 1976, MB ChB (Hons.) 1979; DRCOG 1981; Cert. Family Plann. JCC 1981. Assoc. Specialist (Colposcopy) Hammersmith, Qu. Charlotte's & Chelsea Wom. Hosps. Lond. Prev: Trainer (Family Plann.) Qu. Charlotte's Matern. Hosp. Lond.; Clin. Asst. (Dermat.) Char. Cross. Hosp. Lond.

SEGAL, Terry Yvonne Great Ormond Street Hospital, Great Ormond Street, London WC1N 3HZ Email: tysegal@aol.com — MB ChB Bristol 1992; MRCPCH. Specialist Regist. (Paediat. Endocrin.) Gt. Ormond St. Hosp. & Middx. Hosp. Specialty: Paediat. Socs: MRCPCH. Prev: Specialist Regist. Barnet Healthcare; SHO (Paediat.) Guy's & Whittington Hosps. Lond.; SHO (A & E) Edgware Gen. Hosp.

SEGALL, Jacqueline Mandy 1 Manor House Drive, London NW6 7DE — MB BS Lond. 1986.

SEGALL, Jeffrey Joseph (retired) 308 Cricklewood Lane, London NW2 2PX Tel: 020 8455 5005 Fax: 020 8455 5005 — MB BS Lond. 1947 (Univ. Coll. Hosp.) MRCP (UK) 1972. Prev: Researcher (Clin. Physiol.) N. Middlx. Hosp. Lond.

SEGALL, Malcolm Maurice (retired) Institute of Development Studies, University of Sussex, Brighton BN1 9RE Tel: 01273 678450 Fax: 01273 621202 Email: m.segall@ids.ac.uk; 27 Wilbury Avenue, Hove BN3 6HS Tel: 01273 820041 Fax: 01273 820041 Email: ivanamalc@msegall.freeserve.co.uk — MB ChB Sheff. 1959; MRCP Lond. 1963. p/t Assoc. Inst. of Developm. Studies Univ of Sussex Brighton. Prev: Adviser to Dir. Gen., Dept. of Health Pretoria S. Africa.

SEGALL, Morris Sidney (retired) 31 Bishopsgate Street, Edgbaston, Birmingham B15 1EJ — MB ChB Glas. 1934.

SEGAR, Eric Philip Ear Nose and Throat Department, Conquest Hospital, The Ridge, St Leonards-on-Sea TN37 7RD; 1 Jubilee Square, Topsham, Exeter EX3 0JG — MB ChB Cape Town 1988.

SEGAR, Sian Lois Hulme Medical Centre, 175 Royce Road, Hulme, Manchester M15 5TJ Tel: 0161 226 0606 Fax: 0161 226 5644; 66 Brooklawn Drive, Withington, Manchester M20 3GZ — MB ChB Manch. 1990; DFFP 1993; DRCOG 1993; MRCGP 1994. GP Princip. Specialty: Gen. Pract.

SEGARAJASINGHE, John Saverimuttu Rohan 56 Discovery Walk, London E1W 2JG — MB ChB Manch. 1995.

SEGUI REAL, Bartolome 10 Oat Close, Aylesbury HP21 9LN — LMS Bilbao 1986.

SEHAT, Khosrow Rahbar 61 Ashton Lane, Sale M33 5PE — MB ChB Bristol 1996.

SEHDEV, Gautam 27 Fenmere Cl, Wolverhampton WV4 5EN — MB BCh Wales 1997.

SEHDEV, Rajesh Singh 5 Tudor Road, Southall UB1 1NY Tel: 07817 843264 — MB ChB Ed. 1990. Specialty: Alcohol & Substance Misuse.

SEHGAL, Nav Neet 7 Gideon Close, Belvedere DA17 6DR — MB ChB Manch. 1995.

SEHJPAL, Amarjit 125 Whitehall Road, Walsall WS1 4AT — MB ChB Birm. 1998; ChB Birm. 1998.

SEHMI, Shashi Kiran The Surgery, 356 Southborough Lane, Bromley BR2 8AA Tel: 020 8468 7081 — LRCPI & LM, LRCSI & LM 1973; DA Eng. 1976.

SEHRA, Ravi Tej Kennard Street Health Centre, 1 Kennard Street, North Woolwich, London E16 2HR Tel: 020 7473 1948 Fax: 020 7511 2040 — MB BS Panjab 1973.

SEIDELIN, Raymond (retired) Beech Hill, Owler Park Road, Ilkley LS29 0BG Tel: 01943 609042; 9 Woodland Grove, Bath BA2 7AT Tel: 01225 422619 — (Oxf. & Middlx.) MA Oxf. 1949, DM 1953, BM BCh 1947; FRCP Lond. 1974, M 1950; DPM Eng. 1962. Prev: Cons. Phys. Leeds W. Dist.

SEIDEN, Mr Zoheir Ahmed Salim Department of Surgery, Ealing Hospital NHS Trust, Uxbridge Road, Southall UB1 3HW — MB BCh Ain Shams 1975; FRCS Ed. 1984.

SEIF SAID, Vivian Kathlyn (retired) 48 Parkhurst Road, Torquay TQ1 4EP Tel: 01803 323011 — (Roy. Free) MB BS Lond. 1953; MRCS Eng. LRCP Lond. 1953; DObst RCOG 1955; DCH Eng. 1956. Prev: SCMO (Family Plann. Coordinator) S. Devon Healthcare Trust.

SEIFERT, Martin Howard The Hospital of St John & St Elizabeth, 60 Grove End Road, London NW8 9NH Tel: 0207 806 4062 Fax: 0207 806 4002; Rheumatology Department, St. Mary's Hospital, Praed St, London W2 1NY Tel: 0207 8861066 Fax: 0207 886 6083 — (Lond. Hosp.) MB BS Lond. 1964; MRCP (UK) 1971; FRCP Lond. 1980. Cons. Phys. Rheum. St. Mary's Hosp. Lond.; Hon. Sen. Lect. (Clin. Med.) Imperial Coll. Sch. Of Med. Lond. Specialty: Rheumatol. Socs: Fell. Roy. Soc. Med. (Ex.-Pres. Rheum. & Rehabil. Sect.); Chairm. SAC on Rheum.; Brit. Soc. Rheum. Mem. Of Counc. Prev: Cons. Rheum. The CharterHo. Rheum. Clinic Lond.; Fell. (Rheum.) Dept. Internal Med. Univ. Colorado Med. Center Denver, USA; Sen. Regist. (Rheum.) St. Thos. Hosp. Lond.

SEIFERT, Ruth (retired) 8 Upper Wimpole Street, London W1G 6LH Tel: 020 7226 1990 Fax: 020 7226 1990 — MRCS Eng. LRCP Lond. 1968; DPM Eng. 1972; MRCPsych 1975; FRCPsych 1988. Hon. Cons. Phys. St Barts Hosp. Lond.; Cons. Psychiat. Prev: Sen. Regist. Maudsley Hosp. Lond.

SEIGEL, Jonathan Fred Alrewas Surgery, Exchange Road, Alrewas, Burton-on-Trent DE13 7AS Tel: 01283 790316 Fax: 01283 791863; 170 Main Street, Alrewas, Burton-on-Trent DE13 7ED Tel: 01283 790379 Fax: 01283 792379 Email: 101604.1266@compuserve.com — MB ChB Cape Town 1975; DA Eng. 1982; MRCGP 1983. Hon. Clin. Lect. Keele Univ.; Course Organiser (Gen. Pract.) Staffs. VTS. Specialty: Gen. Pract. Prev: Med. Off. & Med. Supt. Chas. Johnson Mem. Hosp. Kwazulu S. Afr.; SHO (Anaesth.) Horton Gen. Hosp. Banbury.

SEIGER, Christine Paula Newlands House, Clock House Close, Byfleet, Weybridge — BM Soton. 1989.

SEIGER, Darin Guy Northampton Lane North Surgery, 120 Northampton Lane North, Moulton, Northampton NN3 7QP Tel: 01604 790108 Fax: 01604 670827 — MB ChB Dundee 1990; DRCOG 1993; MRCGP 1994; DFFP 1994. Prev: Trainee GP Northampton VTS.

SEIGLEMAN, Merton, OBE (retired) 1 Jackdaw Road, Greenmount, Bury BL8 4ER Tel: 01204 885434 Email: sunrayminor@easicom.com — MRCS Eng. LRCP Lond. 1954 (Manch.) DA Eng. 1959; BA Hons. (Open Univ.) 1997. Prev: Cons. Anaesth. Blackburn, Hyndburn, Ribble Valley HA.

SEILER, Edmund Ronald, TD University Health Service, 6 Bristo Square, Edinburgh EH8 9AL Tel: 0131 650 2777 Fax: 0131 662 1813; 30 Spylaw Bank Road, Edinburgh EH13 0JG Tel: 0131 441 1386 Fax: 0131 441 1386 — MB ChB Ed. 1959; DObst RCOG 1964; DCH Eng. 1965; FRCGP 1985, M 1968; FRCP Ed. 1996. Princip. Univ. Health Serv. Univ. Edin. Socs: BMA; (Treas.) M-C Soc. Edin.; Harv. Soc. Prev: Assoc. Regional Adviser (Gen. Pract.) Postgrad. Bd. Med. Educat. SE Scotl.; Lect. (Community Child Health) Edin.; Ho. Phys. Roy. Infirm. Edin.

SEIMON, Jayawardena Wickramaratna M S C 3 Mandeville Road, Northolt UB5 5HE — MB BS Lond. 1991.

SEIMON, Jayawardena Wickramaratne M D J Methley Cottage, Fulmer Road, Gerrards Cross SL9 7DT — BM Soton. 1993.

SEIMON, Jayawardena Wickramaratne M J B Mandeville Medical Centre, 3 Mandeville Road, Northolt UB5 5HB Tel: 020 8845 3275 Fax: 020 8845 1804 — MB BS Ceylon 1961.

SEIN, Edward Pe 32 Kenton Road, Newcastle upon Tyne NE3 4NA — MB BS Rangoon 1976.

SEIN WIN, Lim Chung Hwee Red House Surgery, 127 Renfrew Road, Hylton Red House, Sunderland SR5 5PS Tel: 0191 548 1269 Fax: 0191 549 8998 — MB BS Rangoon 1968; MRCS Eng LRCP Lond 1987; Dip Ther Newc. 1997; DCH Lond. 1999. GP Princip.; EMP (Examg. Med. Practitioner) for Disabil. Assessm., Med. Servs. Newc., Arden Ho., Regent Centre, Newc.-Upon-Tyne; Med. Practitioner, Nat. Slimming Centres, 31 Norf. St., Sunderland. Specialty: Community Child Health; Acupunc.; Dietetics/Nutrit. Prev: Dep.sing Doctor, Healthcall Med. Servs., Benton Ho., Newc.-Upon-Tyne.

SEINGRY, David Robert James Royal National Orthopaedic Hospital, Brockley Hill, Stanmore HA7 4LP — MB BS Lond. 1971; DA Eng. 1974; FFA RCS Eng. 1977. Specialty: Anaesth.

SEIVEWRIGHT, Helen Elizabeth The Poplars, Hawton, Newark NG24 3RL Tel: 01636 673591 Fax: 01636 673591; Department G.U. Medicine, King's Mill Hospital, Mansfield Road, Sutton-in-Ashfield NG17 4JL Tel: 01623 672260 Fax: 01623 672364 — MB ChB Leeds 1979; MRCGP 1983; DRCOG 1983; Dip. GU Med. Soc. Apoth. Lond. 1992. StaffGrade King's Mill Hosp., Sutton-in-Ashfield Notts.; Clin. Research Fell. Dept. Psychiat. Imperial Coll. Lond.; Clin. Asst. (Dermat.) Kingsmill Centre for Health Care Servs. Specialty: Genitourinary Medicine; Gen. Psychiat.; Dermat. Prev: GP Leicester; Clin. Asst. (Genitourin. Med.) Leicester Roy. Infirm.; Clin. Asst. (Genitourin. Med.) Roy. Oldham Hosp.

SEIVEWRIGHT, Nicholas Andrew — MB ChB Sheff. 1979; MRCPsych 1986; T(Psych) 1991; DM Nottingham 1999. Cons. Psychiat. (Subst. Misuse) Community Health Sheff. Specialty: Alcohol & Substance Misuse. Socs: Soc. for Study of Addic.; Internat. Soc. Study of Personality Disorders; Fell. Roy. Soc. Med. Prev: Sen. Lect. (Drug Depend.) Dept. Psychiat. Univ. Manch.; Cons. Drug Depend. N. W. Regional Drug Depend. Serv. Prestwich Hosp. Manch.; Sen. Regist. (Psychiat.) Mapperley Hosp. Nottm.

SEJRUP, Otto Roy Wallace (retired) 459 Chester Road, Woodford, Stockport SK7 1PR Tel: 0161 439 3296 — MB ChB Manch. 1947. Prev: SHO (Orthop.) Withington Hosp. Manch.

SEKHAR, Mr Cheemala John Raja Strouden Park Medical Centre, 2A Bradpole Road, Bournemouth BH8 9NX Tel: 01202 532253 Fax: 01202 548524; Maranatha, 10 Woodcocks Crescent, Bournemouth BH7 7JW, India — MB BS Andhra 1972 (Andhra Med. Coll. Visakhapatnam) MS (Orthop.) Andhra 1976, MB BS 1972; Cert. Family Plann. JCC 1985. Clin. Asst. (Orthop.) Poole Gen. Hosp. Specialty: Orthop. Prev: Trainee GP VTS; Regist. Orthop. Dept. Stirling Roy. Infirm.; SHO (Orthop.) Ashington Hosp.

SEKHAR, Mr Killathur Theperumal HM Walton Prison, Walton, Liverpool Tel: 0151 525 5971; 31 Widgeon Road, Altrincham WA14 5NP Tel: 0161 926 8630 — MB BS Madras 1974; FRCS Ed. 1984. Med. Off. Walton Prison Liverp. Specialty: Gen. Surg.

SEKHAR, Mallika West Middlesex University Hospital, Department of Haematology, Isleworth, Isleworth TW7 6AF Tel: 020 8565 5716 Fax: 020 8565 5516 Email: mallika.sekhar@umuh-tr.nthames.nhs.uk — MB BS Bombay 1982; MRCP UK 1989; MRCPath 1991; FRCPath 2000; FRCP 2002. Cons. Haemat. W. Middlx. Univ. Hosp.; Hon. Cons. & Hon. Sen. Lect. Hammersmith Hosp. & Imp. Coll. Sch. Med. Lond. Specialty: Haematology. Prev: Sen. Regist. Roy. Free Hosp. Lond.; Research Fell. NIH Bethesda USA.

SEKHAR, Palligondi Rudrappa Westbourne Surgery, Shiney Row, Houghton-le-Spring DH4 4QT Tel: 0191 385 2512; 41A Summerhill, East Herrington, Sunderland SR3 3TW Tel: 01783 528 0076 — MB BS Bangalor 1967 (Bangalore Med. Coll.) BSc (Nat. Sci.) Mysore 1958; MB BS Bangalore 1967. Exam. Med. Off. to DHSS Attendance & Mobility Allowances Units. Specialty: Cardiol. Prev: Res. SHO Vict. Hosp. Kirkcaldy; Res. SHO St. Michael's Hosp. Aylsham; Med. Regist. Roy. Bath Hosp. Harrogate.

SEKHAR, Ravi Furness General Hospital, Department of General Medicine, Barrow-in-Furness LA14 Tel: 01229 870870; 6 Rectory Close, Farnham Royal, Slough SL2 3BG Tel: 01753 642993 Email: drravisekhar@hotmail.com — MB BS Madras 1986; MRCP (UK) 1992. Cons. Phys. & Gastroenterologist. Specialty: Gen. Med.; Gastroenterol. Prev: Sen. Fell. (Gastroeneterol.) Wexham Pk. Hosp.

SEKHAWAT, Bijendra Singh Medical Centre, Farnham Road Hospital, Farnham Road, Guildford GU2 7LX — MB BS Rajasthan 1969.

SEKHON, Sanjit Singh Health Centre, Rodney Road, Walton-on-Thames KT12 3LB — MB BS Lond. 1989; Cert. Family Plann. JCC 1992; DRCOG 1992.

SEKWEYAMA, Silvanus Godfrey Galiwango Sekweyama and Pratt, 10 Trafalgar Avenue, London SE15 6NR Tel: 020 7703 9271 Fax: 020 7252 7209; 87 Newport Street, London SE11 6AH — MB BS Lucknow 1967.

SELBY, Andrew Mark Intensive Care Unit, Alder Hey Childrens Hospital, Eaton Road, Liverpool L12 2AP Tel: 0151 252 5241 Fax: 0151 252 5771 — MB BS Lond. 1983; MRCP (UK) 1986. Cons. Paediat. (Intens. Care) Alder Hey Childr Hosp. Liverp. Specialty: Intens. Care.

SELBY, Clive Singleton, TD (retired) The Health Centre, Hunter St., Briton Ferry, Neath SA11 2SF Tel: 01639 813272; 16 Rosewood Close, Brynoch, Neath SA10 7UL — MB BCh Wales 1958.

SELBY, Colin Derek Queen Margaret Hospital, Fife Acute Hospitals NHS Trust, Whitefield Road, Dunfermline KY12 0SU Tel: 01383 623623 Fax: 01383 627042 — BM BS Nottm. 1982 (Nottingham) MRCP (UK) 1985; BMedSci (Hons.) Nottm. 1980, DM 1992; FRCPE 1998. Cons. (Respirat. & IC) Qu. Margt. Hosp. Dunfermline. Specialty: Respirat. Med.; Intens. Care; Gen. Med. Socs: Brit. & Scott. Thoracic Socs.; Scott. Intens. Care Soc. Prev: Lect. (Respirat. Med.) Univ. Edin.; Hon. Sen. Regist. Roy. Infirm. Edin.

SELBY, Edward Michael Borough Road Surgery, 167a Borough Road, Middlesbrough TS4 2EL Tel: 01642 243668 Fax: 01642 222252; Greenlees, 59 Guisborough Road, Nunthorpe, Middlesbrough TS7 0JY Tel: 01642 317740 — MB BS Newc. 1979; MRCGP 1983; DRCOG 1983; DCCH RCP Ed. RCGP & FCM 1983. Socs: Assn. Brit. Cycling Doctors.

SELBY, Jonathan Neville Christmas Maltings Surgery, Camps Road, Haverhill CB9 8HF Tel: 01440 702010 Fax: 01440 714761; Hall Green Cottage, Great Wratting, Haverhill CB9 7HA Tel: 01440 783384 — MB BChir Camb. 1987; MA, MB BChir Camb. 1987; DRCOG 1991.

SELBY, Karen Fiona 12 Hallamshire Road, Sheffield S10 4FP — MB ChB Sheff. 1993.

SELBY, Kim 87 High Street, Newington, Sittingbourne ME9 7JJ — MB BS Lond. 1983. Clin. Med. Off. Medway HA.

SELBY, Leonard Milton 31 Queen Anne Street, London W1G 9HX Tel: 020 7636 5250 Fax: 020 7323 0349 — MB ChB Cape Town 1947. Socs: Fell. Roy. Soc. Med.; Roy. Coll. Gen. Pract. Prev: Med. Adviser J. Sainsbury Ltd.; Hon. Med. Off. Stellenbosch Hosp., S. Afr.

SELBY, Lesley Anne Benchill Medical Centre, 127 Woodhouse Lane, Benchill, Manchester M22 9WP Tel: 0161 998 4304 Email: lesley.selby@nhs.net; 22 Nevill Road, Bramhall, Stockport Sk7 3ET Tel: 0115 972 5243/0161 439 4735 — MB ChB Leeds 1985; MRCGP 1989. Asst. Gen. Practitioner, Benchill Med. Centre, Manch. Prev: Trainee GP Northumbria VTS.

SELBY, Louise Mary Prideaux Stonefield, St Patricks Lane, Liss GU33 7HQ — MB BS Lond. 1994.

SELBY, Miranda Ruth Brook Lane Surgery, 27 Brook Lane, Bromley BR1 4PX Tel: 020 8461 3333 Fax: 020 8695 5567; 9 Hawthorn Drive, West Wickham BR4 9EY Tel: 020 8462 3884 — BM BS Nottm. 1983 (Nottingham) BMedSci Nottm. 1981, BM BS 1983; MRCGP 1988. GP Bromley (job-share). Specialty: Gen. Pract. Prev: Trainee GP Finchley.

SELBY, Nicholas Michael Londonderry House, Low Pittington, Durham DH6 1BQ — BM BS Nottm. 1993; BM BS Nottm 1993.

SELBY, Pamela Ann 16 Lawn Road, Burley-in-Wharfedale, Ilkley LS29 7EU — MB ChB Leeds 1985; DRCOG 1987. GP, NW Leeds PCT Cancer Lead. Special Interest: Palliat. Care. Prev: Trainee GP Airedale VTS.

SELBY, Professor Peter John St. James's University Hospital, Leeds LS9 7TF Tel: 0113 244 2007 Fax: 0113 242 9886; 17 Park Lane, Roundhay, Leeds LS8 2EX — MB BChir Camb. 1975; MRCP (UK) 1976; MA 1980, MD Camb. 1980; FRCP Lond. 1990; FRCR 1994. Prof. Cancer Med., Cons. Phys & Dir. ICRF Cancer Med. Research Unit Leeds; Director of the Nat. Cancer Research Network. Specialty: Oncol. Socs: Pres. Brit. Oncol. Assn. Prev: Cons. Roy. Marsden Hosp. Lond.; Vis. Fell. (Med.) Ontario Cancer Inst. Toronto, Canada; Regist. (Med.) Univ. Coll. Hosp. Lond.

SELBY, Peter Leslie Manchester Royal Infirmary, Department of Medicine, Oxford Road, Manchester M13 9WL Tel: 0161 276 8917 Email: peter.selby@manchester.ac.uk — MB BChir Camb. 1978 (Camb. & Birm.) MD Camb. 1990 MA 1979; MRCP (UK) 1980; FRCP Lond. 1997. Cons. Phys. Centr. Manch. and Manch. Children's Univ. Hosps. NHS Trust; Hon. Sen. Lect., Univ. of Manch. Specialty: Gen. Med.; Endocrinol. Prev: Lect. (Med.) Univ. Manch.; Lect. (Med.) Univ. Newc. u Tyne; MRC Clin. Scientif. Staff Mineral Metab. Unit. Gen. Infirm. Leeds.

SELBY, Robin Leslie, Flight Lt. RAF Med. Br. — MB ChB Liverp. 1984.

SELBY, Roger Oldham (retired) 11 The Narrows, Harden, Bingley BD16 1HY — MB BChir Camb. 1954; DA Eng. 1958.

SELCON, Harold, OStJ (retired) Richmond House, Llandysul SA44 4DF Tel: 01559 363324 — MB ChB Manch. 1950. Prev: Exam. Med. Off. Benefits Agency.

SELF, Ann Elizabeth The Beeches, 67 Lower Olland Street, Bungay NR35 1BZ Tel: 01986 892055 Fax: 01986 895519; 4 Darrow Green Road, Denton, Harleston IP20 0AY Tel: 01986 788128 — MB BChir Camb. 1990 (Cambridge) BA (Hons.) Camb. 1987; DRCOG 1992; MRCGP 1993.

SELF, Colin Henry Department of Clinical Biochemistry & Metabolic Medicine, The Medical School, Framlington Place, Newcastle upon Tyne NE2 4HH Tel: 0191 222 6931 Fax: 0191 222 6227 — MB BChir Camb. 1980; PhD Leic. 1970, BSc 1966. Prof. Clin. Biochem. Univ. Newc. u. Tyne; Head Dept. Clin. Biochem. & Metab. Med. Univ. Newc.; Head Clin. Biochem. Diagn. Serv. Roy. Vict. Infirm. Newc. Specialty: Biochem. Prev: Sen. Regist. Roy. Postgrad. Med. Sch. Lond.

SELF, Frances Ruth 99 Bamfield, Whitchurch, Bristol BS14 0RB Tel: 0117 983 5005 — MB ChB Bristol 1981; DRCOG 1987; DFFP 1997.

SELF, Janet Elizabeth Chrisp Street Health Centre, 100 Chrisp St., London E14 6PG Tel: 020 7515 4860; 162 Albyn Road, St. Johns, London SE8 4JQ — MB BS Lond. 1981; DRCOG 1985; MRCGP 1986.

SELF, Mr John Bernard Orchard House, Cossington, Leicester LE7 4UX Tel: 01509 812377 — MB BChir Camb. 1949 (Camb. & St. Thos.) MA Camb. 1950; FRCS Eng. 1952; MChir 1962. Cons. Surg. Emerit. Leicester & LoughBoro. Hosps. Prev: Sen. Regist. (Surg.) Univ. Coll. Hosp. W. Indies; Sen. Regist. (Surg.) & Ho. Surg. &c. St. Thos. Hosp.

SELF, Mary Catherine 93 Shaftesbury Avenue, Blackpool FY2 9UZ — MB ChB Liverp. 1988; DA (UK) 1991.

SELF, Richard James 75 Liverpool Road, Chester CH2 1AW — MB ChB Liverp. 1989.

SELFRIDGE, David Ian Health Centre, Kersiebank Avenue, Grangemouth FK3 9EL Tel: 01324 471511 — MB ChB Glas. 1969.

SELIGMAN, Mr Stanley Albert (retired) 28 Bath Hill Court, Bath Road, Bournemouth BH1 2HP Tel: 01202 290463 — MRCS Eng. LRCP Lond. 1950 (Univ. Coll. Hosp.) MD Lond. 1965, MB BS 1950; FRCS Eng. 1955; FRCOG 1971, M 1959. Prev: Cons. O & G Luton & Dunstable Hosp. Gp.

SELIM, Mr Abobakr Mohamed Hazem 25 Oakwood Avenue, Paisley PA2 9NG — MB BCh Ain Shams 1978; DO RCS Eng. 1987; FRCS Glas. 1988; FRCOphth 1990. Cons. & Head Eye Unit Almana Gen. Hosp., Saudi Arabia. Specialty: Ophth.

SELIM, Samir Alphonse (retired) 14 Pendleton Avenue, Constable Lee Park, Rawtenstall, Rossendale BB4 8UX Tel: 01706 212916 — MB BCh Ain Shams 1956 (Ain Shams Univ. Cairo, Egypt) DPM Eng. 1981. Prev: Assoc. Specialist (Psychol. Med.) Qu. Pk. Hosp. Blackburn & NW RHA.

SELINGER, Mark Royal Berkshire Hospital, London Road, Reading RG1 5AN Tel: 0118 987 8910 — BM BS Nottm. 1976; DM Nottm. 1989, BMedSci 1974, BM BS 1976; MA Oxf. 1987; FRCOG 2000. Cons. Feto-Matern. Med. Roy. Berks. Hosp. Reading.; Hon. Lect. in O&G Univ. of Oxf. Specialty: Obst. & Gyn. Prev: Lect. (O & G) Nuffield Dept. O & G Univ. Oxf.

SELKON, Joseph Bernard, TD Microbiology Laboratory, John Radcliffe Hospital, Headington, Oxford OX3 9DU Tel: 01865 221226 Fax: 01865 764192; 4 Ethelred Court, Headington, Oxford OX3 9DA Tel: 01865 764098 — MB ChB Cape Town 1950; DCP Lond 1954; FRCPath 1977, M 1965. Hon. Cons. Microbiol. Oxf. Radcliffe NHS Trust; Hon. Lect. Dept. Microbiol. Univ. Oxf. Specialty: Med. Microbiol. Socs: Path. Soc. Gt. Brit. & Irel. & Brit. Soc. Antimicrobial Chemother. Prev: Dir. Oxf. Pub. Health Laborat.; Bacteriol. WHO Tuberc. Chemother. Centre Madras & MRC Unit For Research Into Drug Sensitivity in Tuberc.; Dir. Newc. Pub. Health Laborat.

SELL, Dorothy Mary (retired) 79 Calton Road, Gloucester GL1 5DT — MB BS Lond. 1952 (Roy. Free) Prev: Sen. Med. Off. (Child Health) Gloucester Health Dist.

SELL, John Norman The Stennack Surgery, The Old Stennack School, St Ives TR26 1RU Tel: 01736 796413 Fax: 01736 796245; Old Orchard Cottage, Church Road, Lelant, St Ives TR26 3LD Tel: 01736 752947 — MB ChB Bristol 1969; BSc (Hons.) Bristol 1966. Specialty: Gen. Pract. Prev: SHO Off. (Paediat.) Pembury Hosp. Tunbridge Wells; SHO (Psychiat.) Barrow Hosp. Bristol; Ho. Off. Bristol Roy. Infirm.

SELL, Louise Ann Alcohol & Drugs North W., Bolton, Salford &Trafford Mental Health Partnership, Bury New Road, Manchester M25 3BL Tel: 0161 773 9121 — MB BS Lond. 1987; MRCP (UK) 1990; MRCPsych 1992. Cons. Psychiat.Alcoholic & Drugs NW,Bolton, Salford & Trafford Ment. Health Partnership Servcs; Hon. Lect. Univ. Manch. 1998. Specialty: Gen. Psychiat. Prev: Clin. Lect. (Addic.) Inst. Psychiat. Lond.; Sen. Regist. Oxf. RHA; Regist. & SHO Oxon. DHA.

SELL, Mr Philip John Leicester General Hospital, Gwendolen Road, Leicester LE5 4PW — BM Soton. 1979; FRCS Eng. 1985; MSc Keele 1991. Cons. Spinal Surg., Univ. Hosp. Of Leicester & Qu.s Med. Centre, Nottm. Specialty: Gen. Surg.; Orthop. Socs: Sec. Brit. Assoc. Spine Surg.; Brit. Scoliosis Soc. & Brit. Orthop. Assn.

SELLAPPAH, Senathirajan The Surgery, 25 Mill Road, Erith DA8 1HW Tel: 020 8854 3736 Fax: 020 8854 3736; 379 Southborough Lane, Bromley BR2 8BQ Fax: 020 8295 0114 — MB

BS Sri Lanka 1973; MRCS Eng. LRCP Lond. 1980; MRCOG 1981; DA (UK) 1989; MRCGP 1990. Specialty: Accid. & Emerg.

SELLAR, Mr Peter William West Cumberland Hospital, Department of Ophthalmology, Whitehaven CA28 8JG Tel: 01946 693181 Fax: 01946 523553 — BM BS Nottm. 1980; BMedSci Nottm. 1978; FRCS Glas. 1988; FRCOphth 1993. Cons. Ophth. W. Cumbld. Hosp. Cumbria. Specialty: Ophth. Socs: Dutch Ophth. Soc.; N. Eng. Ophth. Soc.; Roy. Coll. Opth. (Fell.). Prev: Cons. Ophth. Maasziekenhuis, Boxmeer, Netherlands; Regist. (Ophth.) Roy. Vict. Hosp. Belf.

SELLAR, Robert John 82 Inverleith Place, Edinburgh EH3 5PA Tel: 0131 552 3393 Fax: 0131 552 8354 — MB BS Lond. 1975 (St. Thos.) BSc Lond. 1973; MRCP (UK) 1978; DMRD Ed. 1982; FRCR 1984; FRCP Lond. 1989; FRCS 2000. Cons. Neuroradiol. (Surg. Neurol.) Edin.; Sen. Lect. (Med. Radiol.) Univ. Edin. Specialty: Radiol. Socs: Brain Interface Gp.; UK Interven.al Neuroradiol. Gp.; Brit. Soc. of NeuroRadiol. Prev: Lect. (Radiol.) & Regist. (Cardiol.) Roy. Infirm. Edin.; SHO Roy. Brompton Hosp. Lond.

SELLAR, William Thomas Kynoch (retired) Murrayfield Medical Practice, 8 Corstorphine Road, Murrayfield, Edinburgh EH12 6HN Tel: 0131 337 6151 — MB ChB Ed. 1954; DCH RCPS Glas. 1961. GP Edin.; Asst. Chief Med. Off. Standard Life Assur. Co. Edin. Prev: Resid. (Fulbright Award) Pediat. Dept. Univ. Penna. Philadelphia, USA.

SELLARAJAH, Ariaratnam The Surgery, 115 Humberstone Road, Erdington, Birmingham B24 0PY Tel: 0121 351 3321 Fax: 0121 313 0919; Hollyhedge, 432 Jockey Road, Sutton Coldfield B73 5DQ Tel: 0121 355 1927 — MB BS Ceylon 1970 (Colombo)

SELLARS, Leslie Hull and East Yorkshire Hospitals NHS Trust, Anlaby Road, Hull HU3 2JZ Tel: 01482 674881 Fax: 01482 674998 Email: leslie.sellars@hey.nhs.uk — MB BS Newc. 1974; MRCP (UK) 1976; MD Newc. 1981; FRCP Ed. 1988; FRCP Lond. 1993. Cons. Phys. & Nephrol. Hull & E. Yorks. Hosp. NHS Trust. Specialty: Nephrol.; Gen. Med. Socs: Renal Assn.; Brit. Hypertens. Soc.; Europ. Renal Assn. Prev: 1st Asst. Med. (Nephrol.) Univ. Newc.

SELLARS, Naomi Anne London Chest Hospital, Bonner Road, London E2 9JX; 2 Winton Road, Farnham GU9 9QW — MB BS Lond. 1990. SHO (Chest.) Lond. Chest Hosp. Lond. Prev: SHO (Neurol.) Roy. Surrey Co. Hosp. Guildford; SHO (Endocrin.) Roy. Free Hosp. Lond.

SELLARS, Neil Robert Kingthorne Group Practice, 83A Thorne Road, Doncaster DN1 2EU Tel: 01302 342832 Fax: 01302 366995; Orchard House, Brockholes Lane, Branton, Doncaster DN3 3NH — MB ChB Sheff. 1986; MRCGP 1991.

SELLARS, Nigel Henry Leighton Goldsworth Park Health Centre, Denton Way, Woking GU21 3LQ Tel: 01483 767194 Fax: 01483 766042 — MB ChB Bristol 1982; DRACOG 1988. Clin. Asst. in Diabetes, St Peter's Hosp., Chertsey. Prev: Trainee GP Stroud; Regist. (Med.) Nepean Hosp. Penrith, NSW, Austral.

SELLATURAY, Rajini 55 Russell Road, Northwood HA6 2LP — MB BS Ceylon 1968. Staff Grade Doctor (Psychiat.) Barnet Health Care Trust Herts. Specialty: Geriat. Psychiat.

SELLATURAY, Selvaratnam 55 Russell Road, Northwood HA6 2LP — MB BS Ceylon 1965; FRCS Ed.; DLO Lond. Staff Grade (ENT) Wycombe Gen. Hosp. Specialty: Otolaryngol.

SELLEN, Elizabeth Mary Roper and Partners, Syston Health Centre, Melton Road, Leicester LE7 2EQ Tel: 0116 260 9111 Fax: 0116 260 9055; 6 Meadowcourt Road, Oadby, Leicester LE2 2PB Tel: 0116 271 2812 — MB ChB Leic. 1984; DRCOG 1988.

SELLENS, Graham Stuart Manchester Road Health Centre, 7-9 Manchester Road, Haslingden, Rossendale BB4 5SL Tel: 01706 212518; 1 Prospect House, Tanners St, Ramsbottom, Bury BL0 9ES Tel: 01706 821479 — MB ChB Sheff. 1985; DRCOG 1989.

SELLENS, Kathryn Fiona Bridge Surgery, St Peters Street, Stapenhill, Burton-on-Trent DE15 9AW Tel: 01283 563451 Fax: 01283 500896; Home Farm Cottage, Chilcote, Swadlincote DE12 8DQ — BM BCh Oxf. 1990 (Oxford) DRCOG 1992; DCH RCP Lond. 1992; MRCGP 1994. GP Princip. Bridge Surg. Stapenhill. Specialty: Gen. Pract.

SELLERS, Mr Jeffrey Irvin (retired) Crow's Nest, Pocklington, York YO42 1TS — MB ChB Birm. 1954; DO Eng. 1963; FRCS Eng. (Ophth.) 1964; FRCOphth 1988. Prev: Sen. Regist. United Sheff. Hosps.

SELLERS, John Wansbeck General Hospital, Woodhorn Lane, Ashington NE63 9JJ Tel: 01670 521212 Fax: 01670 529719; 37 Castle Street, Warkworth, Morpeth NE65 0UN Tel: 01665 711046 — (Univ. Coll. Hosp.) BSc Lond. 1965, MB BS 1968; MRCPath 1975; FRCPath 1998. Cons. Microbiol. Wansbeck Gen. Hosp.; Clin. Lect. (Microbiol.) Univ. Newc. Specialty: Med. Microbiol. Socs: Assn. Clin. Paths.; Hosp. Infec. Soc. Prev: Cons. Bact. Sundsvall Hosp. Sweden; Sen. Bact. Pub. Health Laborat. Oxf.; Regist. (Clin. Path.) United Bristol Hosps.

SELLERS, Susan Mary Level E, St Michael's Hospital, Southwell Street, Bristol BS2 8EG Tel: 0117 928 5250 — MB ChB Manch. 1972 (Univ. of Manch.) FRCOG 1994, M 1977; MD Manch. 1983. Cons. Obst., Matern. Med., Bristol; Mem. of Claims Comm., Counc. of Med. Protec. Soc. Specialty: Obst. & Gyn. Socs: Brit. Maternofetal Med. Soc. Prev: Cons. Obst. John Radcliffe Hosp. Oxf.

SELLERS, William Frederick Shiels Broadgate House, Broadgate, Great Easton, Market Harborough LE16 8SH — MB BS Lond. 1970; MRCS Eng. LRCP Lond. 1970; DObst RCOG 1975; FFA RCSI 1978; FFA RCS Eng. 1978. Cons. Anaesth. Kettering Gen. Hosp. Specialty: Anaesth. Prev: Sen. Regist. (Anaesth.) Avon AHA (T); Acting Instruc. Univ. Washington Seattle,USA; Regist. (Anaesth.) Glos. Roy. Hosp. & Cheltenham Gen. Hosp.

SELLEY, Carolyn Anne Royal South Hants Hospital, Southampton SO14 0YG Email: carryselley@hotmail.com — MB ChB Birm. 1972; MRCPsych 1976; MRCGP 1982; FRCPsych 2002. Specialty: Psychother.; Gen. Psychiat. Prev: Cons. Psychotherapist Roy. S. Hants. Hosp. Soton.; Sen. Regist. (Psychiat.) Roy. S. Hants. Hosp. Soton.

SELLEY, Peter John Fair Park Surgery, Fair Park, Bow, Crediton EX17 6EY Tel: 01363 82333; Fair Park, Bow, Crediton EX17 6EY — (King's Coll. Hosp.) MA 1976; DRCOG 1977; MRCGP 1980. Prev: Trainee GP Exeter VTS; Ho. Surg. King's Coll. Hosp. Lond.; Med. Off. St. Jude Hosp. Vieux-Fort St. Lucia.

SELLICK, Barry Christopher Apple Tree Cottage, Ridgway, Pyrford, Woking GU22 8PW — MB BS Lond. 1975; FFA RCS Eng. 1981. Cons. Anaesth. St. Peter's Hosp. Chertsey. Specialty: Anaesth.

SELLICK, Charles Steven Frome Valley Medical Centre, 2 Court Road, Frampton Cotterell, Bristol BS36 2DE Tel: 01454 772153 Fax: 01454 250078; Penrhys, Chaingate Lane, Iron Acton, Bristol BS37 9XJ Tel: 01454 228431 — (Middlx.) MB BS Lond. 1970; MRCS Eng. LRCP Lond. 1970; DObst RCOG 1974. Princip. GP. Specialty: Gen. Pract. Prev: SHO (Surg.) Kettering Hosp.; Ho. Phys. Harefield Hosp.; Ho. Surg. Middlx. Hosp.

SELLICK, Mr Richard James (retired) 10 Wodehouse Road, Hunstanton PE36 6JD Tel: 01485 532082 — MB BChir Camb. 1953 (Camb. & St. Thos.) FRCS Eng. 1961. Prev: Cons. ENT Surg. Norf. & Norwich Hosp.

SELLORS, Gareth Paul 2 Shrimpton Road, Knotty Green, Beaconsfield HP9 2AX — MB ChB Birm. 1995.

SELLORS, Jane Elizabeth 22 Lidgett Park Grove, Leeds LS8 1HW — MB ChB Sheff. 1990.

SELLS, Elizabeth Lucy (retired) Leith Hill Practice, The Green, Ockley, Dorking RH5 5TR Tel: 01306 711182 Fax: 01306 712751; Post Box House, Coldharbour, Dorking RH5 6HD Tel: 01306 712012 — MB BS Lond. 1965 (Univ. Coll. Hosp.) Prev: Regist. & SHO (Radiother.) St. Luke's Hosp. Guildford.

SELLS, Henry Department Of Urology, Southmead Hospital, Westbury-on-Trym, Bristol — MB BS Lond. 1991; FRCS.

SELLS, Martin Frank Lytton Eden Medical Group, Port Road, Carlisle CA2 7AJ Tel: 01228 24477 — MB BChir Camb. 1991 (Cambridge) MA; MRCGP 1996. GP Princip. Dr Raitt & Partners Carlisle. Specialty: Gen. Pract. Socs: Roy. Coll. Gen. Pract.; BMA. Prev: Staff Grade (A & E) Withybush Gen. Hosp. Haverfordshire; SHO (Ophth.) W. Wales Gen. Hosp.

SELLS, Professor Robert Anthony Royal Liverpool University Hospital, Prescot St., Liverpool L7 8XP Tel: 0151 708 0163 Fax: 0151 706 5819 Email: rsells@rlbuh-tr.nwest.nhs.uk — (Guy's) MRCS Eng. LRCP Lond. 1962; MB BS Lond. 1963; FRCS Ed. 1967; FRCS Eng. 1968; MA Camb. 1968. Cons. Surg. Gen. & Renal Transpl. Roy. Liverp. Hosp.; Hon. Prof. Surg. & Immunol. Univ. Liverp. Specialty: Gen. Surg.; Transpl. Surg. Socs: (Counc. & Vice-Pres.) Transpl. Soc. (Ex-Vice-Pres. & Ex-Counc.).; Brit. Transpl. Soc. (Ex-Pres.); Moynihan Chirurgical Club (Ex-Pres). Prev: Cons. Surg. &

Dir. Renal Transpl. Roy. Liverp. Hosp.; Lect. (Surg.) & Ho. Off. (Experim. Med.) Guy's Hosp. Lond.; MRC Fell. Harvard Univ. USA.

SELLS, Rupert William Blyth Lyngford Park Surgery, Fletcher Close, Taunton TA2 8SQ Tel: 01823 333355 Fax: 01823 257022; Longview, Buttsway, Milverton, Taunton TA4 1ND Tel: 01823 400349 — MB BS Lond. 1991 (Univ. Coll. Middlx. Sch. Med.) BSc Med. Microbiol. Lond. 1988; MRCGP 1996. GP Partner. Specialty: Gen. Pract.

SELLU, Mr David Patrick Department of Surgery, Hammersmith Hospital & Royal Postgraduate Medical School, Du Cane Road, London W12 0NN Tel: 020 8743 2030; Ealing Hospital, Department of Surgery, Uxbridge Road, Southall UB1 3HW Tel: 020 8967 5530 Fax: 020 8967 5530 — MB ChB Manch. 1973; FRCS Eng. 1979; FRCS Ed. 1979; ChM Manch. 1984 1984; MSc Lond. 1996. Cons. Surg. Ealing Hosp. Lond.; Sen. Lect. & Hon. Cons. Surg. Roy. Postgrad. Med. Sch. & Hammersmith Hosp Lond. Specialty: Gen. Surg. Socs: Assn. Surg. Gt. Britain & Irel.; Assn. of Endocrine Surg.; Assn. Coloproctol. Prev: Cons. Surg. Min. of Health, Oman; Ho. Phys. Hope Hosp. Salford; Ho. Surg. Manch. North. Hosp.

SELLWOOD, Karen 7 Tehidy Terrace, Falmouth TR11 2SZ — BM Soton. 1979.

SELLWOOD, Mark William 7 Evelyn Road, Ham, Richmond TW10 7HU Tel: 020 8948 3874 — MB BS Lond. 1990.

SELLWOOD, Mr Nigel Howard (retired) 7 Tehidy Terrace, Falmouth TR11 2SZ — MB BS Lond. 1974; MRCS Eng. LRCP Lond. 1974; FRCS Eng. 1978. Prev: Cons. A & E Roy. Cornw. Hosp. Truro.

SELLWOOD, Robert Binford (retired) Greenbanks, Agar Road, Truro TR1 1JU — MB Camb. 1961 (St. Geo.) BChir 1960; DMRD Eng. 1971; FFR 1973. Prev: Cons. Radiol. Roy. Cornw. Hosps.

SELLWOOD, William George Mid Staffordshire General Hospitals NHS Trust, Staffordshire General Hospital, Weston Road, Stafford ST16 3SA Tel: 01785 257731; Gobions, Brook Lane, Ranton Green, Stafford ST18 9JY Tel: 01785 823523 — MB ChB Manch. 1971; FFA RCS Eng. 1977. Cons. Anaesth. Mid Staff. Gerneral Hosps. Trust. Specialty: Anaesth.; Intens. Care. Socs: Mid Staffs. Med. Soc.

SELLY, Eryl William Montgomery County Infirmary, Llanfair Road, Newtown SY16 2DW — BChir Camb. 1975; MB 1976; MRCGP 1983. Staff Grade Old Age Psychiat.

SELMAN, Joanna Clare 7 Bereweeke Way, Winchester SO22 6BJ — MB ChB Liverp. 1994.

SELMAN, Mark Andrew 3 Dartside, Totnes TQ9 5HL Mob: 07718 017897 — BM BS Nottm. 1991; BMedSci. (Hons.) Nottm. 1989; DCH RCP Lond. 1995; DFFP 1996; MRCGP 1996. Specialty: Gen. Pract. Socs: Chairm. Torbay & S. Devon Non-Princip.s Gp.; Torbay PCG Clin. Governance Steering Comm.; GPC- Non-Princip.s SubComm. Prev: GP Princip. Taunton; GP/Regist. Torbay; SHO (Med.) Roy. Devon & Exeter Hosp. & Derriford Hosp. Plymouth.

SELMAN, Richard Michael 25 Ffordd Argoed, Bryn Awelon, Mold CH7 1LY Tel: 01352 55560 — MB ChB Liverp. 1988. Prev: Trainee GP/SHO (A & E) Warrington Dist. Gen. Hosp. VTS.

SELMAN, Tara Jayne — MB ChB Birm. 1998.

SELMES, Susan Elizabeth Empingham Medical Centre, 37 Main Street, Empingham, Oakham LE15 8PR Tel: 01780 460202 Fax: 01780 460283; 21 Foxhill, Whissendine, Oakham LE15 7HP Tel: 01664 474715 — MB ChB Ed. 1982 (Edinburgh) MRCGP 1986. GP Princip.

SELMI, Fahed 2 Palmer Avenue, Willerby, Hull HU10 6LJ — MB BS Karachi 1983.

SELMON, Mr Guy Philip Ford 6 Medebourne Close, Blackheath, London SE3 9AB Tel: 020 8318 6188 — MB BS Lond. 1992 (Guy's) FRCS 1997; FRCS (Tr. & Orth.) 2001. Specialist Regist. Rotat. (Trauma & Orthop.) S. E. Thames. Specialty: Orthop.

SELSBY, Daniel Sean 43 Leeds Road, Rawdon, Leeds LS19 6NW — MB ChB Bristol 1982; FRCA 1987. Cons. Anaesth. Leeds Gen. Infirm. Specialty: Anaesth. Prev: Regist. (Anaesth.) Leeds Gen. Infirm.; SHO (Anaesth.) Univ. Hosp. Nottm.; Cas. Off. Univ. Hosp. Nottm.

SELSON, Michael George (retired) 30 Lymister Avenue, Moorgate, Rotherham S60 3DD Tel: 01709 377332 — (Univ. Coll. Hosp.) MB BS Lond. 1952. Prev: GP Rotherham.

SELTZER, Abigail Ann — MB ChB Glas. 1979; MRCPsych 1984. Cons. (Psychiat.) Camden Islington Ment. Health & Social Care NHS Trust; Prin. Psychiat. Med. Foundat. for the Care of Victims of Torture. Specialty: Gen. Psychiat.

SELTZER, Basil (retired) 49 Aytoun Road, Glasgow G41 5HW — LRCP LRCS Ed. 1948 (Univ. Glas.) LRCP LRCS Ed. LRFPS Glas. 1948; MRCP Glas. 1952. Prev: Regist. (Med.) St. And. Hosp. Billericay.

SELTZER, Beverley Kim 8 Mansionhouse Gardens, Glasgow G41 3DP — MB ChB Glas. 1987.

SELTZER, Myer Solomon 5 Arran Drive, Giffnock, Glasgow G46 7NL Tel: 0141 638 6677 Fax: 0141 621 0395 Email: myersol1936@lineone.net — MB ChB Glas. 1958; DObst RCOG 1960; Cert JCC Lond. 1977. Socs: (Ex-Pres.) Brit. Soc. Med. & Dent. Hypn.; Life Mem. Glas. Univ. M-C Soc. Prev: Ho. Off. (Med.) South. Gen. Hosp. Glas.; Ho. Surg. Vict. Infirm. Glas.; SHO Belvidere Infec. Dis. Hosp. Glas.

SELVACHANDRAN, Mr Prince Selvadurai General Hospital, St Helier, Jersey Tel: 01534 71000 — MB BS Madras 1963; FRCS Ed. 1970; FRCS Eng. 1971.

SELVACHANDRAN, Mr Sithamparapillai Nadarajah Leighton Hospital, Crewe CW1 4QJ Tel: 01270 255141; 19 Hesketh Croft, Coppenhall, Crewe CW1 4RY Tel: 01270 582575 — MB BS Sri Lanka 1975; LRCP LRCS Ed. LRCPS Glas. 1982; FRCS Glas. 1985. Assoc. Specialist (Gen. Sug.) Leighton Hosp. Crewe. Specialty: Gen. Surg.

SELVADURAI, David Kishan St George's Hospital, Department of Otolaryngology, Garratt Lane, Tooting, London SW17 0QT; [New Address] — MB BS Lond. 1992; FRCS (OTO); FRCS (CSig); FRCS (ORL-HNS); MD. Cons. ENT Surg. Specialty: Otorhinolaryngol. Special Interest: Paediat. Otolaryngol.; Otol. Prev: Graham Fraser Memor. Fell. in Otol. Univ. Sydney.

SELVADURAI, Mrs Leila Rachel Nevins 8 Blenheim Court, Alsager, Stoke-on-Trent ST7 2BY Tel: 01270 877500 — MB BS Ceylon 1964 (Colombo) DMRD Eng. 1979; FFR RCSI 1983. Cons. Radiol. Leighton Hosp. Crewe. Specialty: Radiol. Socs: BMA; Roy. Coll. Radiol. Prev: Sen. Regist. (Radiodiag.) N. Staffs. Hosp. Centre; Regist. (Radiodiag.) Bristol Roy. Infirm.

SELVADURAI, Mary Ananthavathy Canterbury Way Surgery, 91A Canterbury Way, Stevenage SG1 4LQ Tel: 01438 316646 — MB BS Ceylon 1966.

SELVADURAI, Vasuki 20 Downsway, Shoreham-by-Sea BN43 5GN — MB BS Colombo 1985; LMSSA Lond. 1995.

SELVAKUMAR, Mr Sadasivam Lister Hospital, Coreys Mill Lane, Stevenage SG1 4AB — MB BS Madras 1983; FRCS Ed. 1988; FRCS (Gen.) 1997. Cons. Vasc. & Gen. Surg., Lister Hosp. Stevenage. Specialty: Gen. Surg. Special Interest: Carotid Artery Surg.; Laparoscopic Surg.

SELVAKUMAR, Shamugam Pillai 19 Bishops Avenue, Worcester WR3 8XA — MB BS Madurai Kamaraj, India 1978.

SELVAKUMARI, Navaneethakrishnan 39 Homebrook Drive, Horwich, Bolton BL6 6RH Tel: 01204 690877 Fax: 01204 690877 Email: selvakumari@yahoo.com — MB BS Madras 1986. Staff Grade (Obst. & Gyn.) Roy. Bolton Hosp. Specialty: Obst. & Gyn. Special Interest: Fetal Med.

SELVAM, Andiappan Chadmoor Medical Practice, 45 Princess St, Cannock WS11 2JT Tel: 01543 571650 Fax: 01543 462304 — MB BS Madras 1973 (Madras Med. Coll.) Prev: Regist. (Paediat. Surg.) E. Birm. Hosp.; SHO (Gen. & Paediat. Surg.) E. Birm. Hosp.

SELVAN, Subramaniyan Tamil Long Catlis Road Surgery, 119 Long Catlis Road, Parkwood, Rainham, Gillingham ME8 9RR Tel: 01634 360989 — MB BS Madras 1979; LRCP LRCS Ed. LRCPS Glas. 1981.

SELVANANTHAN, Mr Perampalam Prince Charles Hospital, Merthyr Tydfil CF47 9BT; 53 Ravensbrook, Morganstown, Cardiff CF15 8LT — MB BS Ceylon 1971 (Peradeniya) DO RCS Eng. 1981; FRCS Glas. (Ophth.) 1985. Regist. (Ophth.) P. Chas. Hosp. Merthyr Tydfil. Specialty: Ophth. Prev: SHO (Ophth.) Princess Margt. Hosp. Swindon, N.E. Essex HA & ScarBoro. Hosp.

SELVANATHAN, Esther Suganthaleela 9 Heath Park Drive, Bromley BR1 2WQ — MB BS Sri Lanka 1973. Specialty: Geriat. Psychiat. Socs: Med. Defence Union.

SELVANATHAN, Mr Gnanapragasam Anton Joseph Nightingdale Surgery, 2 Handen Road, Lewisham, London SE12 8NP Tel: 020 8692 1387; 9 Heath Park Drive, Bromley BR1 2WQ Tel: 020 8295 1696 — MB BS Sri Lanka 1973; FRCS Ed. 1983; LRCP LRCS Ed. LRCPS Glas. 1985. Specialty: Orthop. Socs: Med. Defence Union; BMA.

SELVARAJAH, David Thampoe Merefield, Mere Farm Road, Oxton, Birkenhead CH43 9TS — MB BS Ceylon 1970 (Colombo) DPM Eng. 1979; MRCPsych. 1982. Cons. Psychiat. Pk. Hosp., Rainhill Hosp. & Broadgreen Gen. Hosp. Liverp.; Sen. Regist. (Psychiat.) Univ. Liverp. & Roy. Liverp. Hosp.; Hon. Sen. Regist. (Psychiat.) Pk. La. Hosp. Liverp. Specialty: Gen. Psychiat. Prev: Sen. Regist. (Psychiat.) Winwick Hosp. Warrington; Sen. Regist. (Psychiat.) Rainhill Hosp. Liverp.; Regist. (Psychiat. & EEG) St. Francis Hosp. & Hurstwood Pk. Neurol. Centre Haywards Heath; .

SELVARAJAN, Bright Selvadurai Wandsworth Bridge Road Surgery, 29 Wandsworth Bridge Road, London SW6 2TA Tel: 020 7736 9341 Fax: 020 7384 1493 — MB BS Madras 1968.

SELVARAJAN, Mahadeva 268 Chadwell Heath Lane, Romford RM6 4YL — LRCP LRCS Ed. 1993; LRCP LRCS Ed. LRCPS Glas. 1993.

SELVARANGAN, Rengaswami Knoll Rise Surgery, 1 Knoll Rise, Orpington BR6 0EJ Tel: 01689 824563 Fax: 01689 820712 — MB BS Madras 1967.

SELVARATNAM, Murugesu Aiyampillai Stone House Hospital, Cotton Lane, Dartford DA2 6U Tel: 01322 622222; 27 Hollingbourne Avenue, Bexleyheath DA7 5ET Tel: 01322 440594 Fax: 01322 440881 — MB BS Ceylon 1972; DPM Eng. 1979; MRCPsych 1980. Cons. Psychiat., Gen. Psychiat., Stone Ho. Hosp., Dartford. Specialty: Gen. Psychiat.; Gen. Pract. Socs: BMA. Prev: Freelance Cons. Psychiat. & GP.

SELVARATNAM, Yamini 25 Listergate, 317 Upper Richmond Road, Putney, London SW15 6ST Tel: 020 8789 9989 Fax: 020 8789 9989 — MB BS Lond. 1994. GP Rotat. UMDS Lond. Specialty: Gen. Pract. Prev: SHO (A & E) St. Thos. Hosp. Lond.; SHO (Gen. Med.) Guy's Hosp. Lond.; SHO (O & G) St Thomas' Hosp.

SELVEY, David Morrish 41 Llanvair Drive, Ascot SL5 9LW — MB BCh Witwatersrand 1986.

SELWAY, Cedric Angus (retired) Coopers Brook, School Lane, Abbess Roding, Ongar CM5 0NY — MB BS Lond. 1958 (Char. Cross) DObst RCOG 1960; DCH Eng. 1961. Prev: GP Harlow.

SELWAY, Jennefer Rachel Department of Public Health, Bromley PCT, 11/12 Ashtree Close, Broadwater Gardens, Farnborough, Orpington BR6 7UA — MB BS Lond. 1988 (London) MRCGP 1993; DCH RCP Lond. 1993; Dip. Health Economics Aberd 1996; MFPHM 2001. Cons. (Pub. Health) Bromley PCT. Specialty: Pub. Health Med. Prev: Trainee GP Watford VTS.

SELWAY, Mr Richard Philip King's College Hospital, Department of Neurosurgery, Denmark Hill, London SE5 9RS — MB BChir Camb. 1989; MA Camb. 1990; FRCS Eng. 1994; MMed Sci (Distinc.) Keele 1998; FRCS (Neurosurg. Gold Medal) 1999; BSc (Maths) Open Univ. 2000. Cons. Neurosurg. King's Coll. Hosp. & Lond. Bridge Hosp. Lond. Specialty: Neurosurg. Special Interest: Surg. of the Cerebral Cortex for Tumours or Epilepsy. Socs: Soc. Brit. Neurol. Surgs.

SELWOOD, Amber 16 Holme Close, Woodborough, Nottingham NG14 6EX Tel: 0115 965 4298 — MB ChB Birm. 1995; ChB Birm. 1995. Specialty: Gen. Psychiat.

SELWOOD, David Peter 13 Banckside, Hartley, Longfield DA3 7RD — MB ChB Leeds 1996.

SELWOOD, Jane Elizabeth 1 Woodberry Avenue, Winchmere Hill, London N21 3LE Tel: 020 8886 2751; Flat 3, 15 Gentlemans Row, Enfield EN2 6PT Tel: 020 8366 5916 — MB BS Lond. 1981.

SELWYN, Alan Willow Tree Family Doctors, 301 Kingsbury Road, London NW9 9PE Tel: 020 8204 6464 Fax: 020 8905 0946 — MB BS Lond. 1982 (Roy. Free) DCH RCP Lond. 1985; MRCGP (Distinc.) 1986. Lect. Roy. Free Hosp. Sch. Med. Lond. Socs: Yeoman of Worshipful Soc. of Apoth. Prev: Trainee GP Edgware VTS.

SELWYN, Elaine Margaret Harnall Lane Medical Centre, Harnall Lane East, Coventry CV1 5AE Tel: 024 7622 4640 Fax: 024 7622 3859; 43 Rawnsley Drive, Kenilworth CV8 2NX Tel: 01926 850988 — MB BS Lond. 1977; DRCOG 1979; MFFP 1994. Clin. Med. Off. (Family Plann.) Leamington Spa. Specialty: Family Plann. & Reproduc. Health.

SELWYN, Jane Elizabeth Eborall and Partners, Fountain Medical Centre, Sherwood Avenue, Newark NG24 1QH Tel: 01636 704378/9 Fax: 01636 610875; Old Grange Farm, Sibthorpe, Newark NG23 5PN Tel: 01636 525092 — MB BS Lond. 1982 (St. Bart.) MRCP (UK) 1986; MRCGP 1989.

SELWYN, Mr Julian Ralph Merriman — MB BS Lond. 1981; MRCS Eng. LRCP Lond. 1981; FRCS Eng. 1989; MRCGP 1991.

SELWYN, Pamela Troed-y-Foel, Castle Road, Llangynidr, Crickhowell NP8 1NG — MB BCh Wales 1972 (Cardiff) Specialty: Family Plann. & Reproduc. Health; Gen. Pract. Prev: Ho. Off. (Gen. Med. & Gen. Surg.) Nevill Hall Hosp. Abergavenny.

SELWYN, Victor Graham Holly Park Clinic, Holly Park Road, London N11 3RA — MB BS Lond. 1969 (Middlx.) Cert Contracep. & Family Plann. RCOG, RCGP &; Mem. Brit. Med. Acupuncture Soc.; MRCS Eng. LRCP Lond. 1969; ECFMG Cert 1969; DObst RCOG 1971; Cert FPA 1975. Socs: BMA (Ex-Hon. Sec. Finchley & Barnet Br.). Prev: Clin. Asst. (ENT) Enfield Dist. Hosp.; Clin. Asst. (Obst.) Whittington Hosp. Lond.; SHO Centr. Middlx. Hosp. Lond.

SELZER, Mr Gunther Horst 12 Woodbury Close, Callow Hill, Redditch B97 5YQ Email: g@gselzer.freeserve.co.uk — State Exam Med Kiel 1990; FRCS Ed. 1997; MSc (Orthop. Engineering) 2002. Specialist Regist. W. Midl. Orthop. Rotat. Specialty: Orthop. Socs: Brit. Ortho. Train. Assoc.; BOA. Prev: SHO Rotat. (Surg.) Addenbrooke's Hosp. Camb.

SEMARK, Diane Wendy Ashcroft Road Surgery, 26 Ashcroft Road, Stopsley Green, Luton LU2 9AU Tel: 01582 722555 Fax: 01582 418145 Email: dianesemark@doctors.org.uk; The Shambles, 69 Bedford Road, Hitchin SG5 2TU Tel: 01462 432647 — MB BS Lond. 1966 (Roy. Free) MFFP; MRCS Eng. LRCP Lond. 1966; DObst RCOG 1969. GP; Sen. Clin. Med. Off. (Family Plann.) Bedford. Specialty: Family Plann. & Reproduc. Health. Socs: Brit. Med. Assn.; Brit. Menopause Soc. Prev: GP Sawtry; Phys. (Primary Care) King Faisal Specialist Hosp. Riyadh, Saudi Arabia; Clin. Med. Off. Beds AHA.

SEMBHI, Satvinder Kaur 7 Holmbury Gardens, Hayes UB3 2LU; Mental Health Liaison Team, Waterlow Unit, Whittington Hospital, London N19 5NF Tel: 020 7530 2216 — BM Soton. 1990; MRCPsych. Specialist Regist. N. Lond./UCLMS Train. Scheme. Specialty: Gen. Psychiat. Prev: Regist. Rotat. (Psychiat.) N. Lond.

SEMENIUK, Petro 221 Priory Road, Hull HU5 5RZ — MB ChB Manch. 1981; MRCGP 1987. GP Hull. Socs: Hull Med. Soc.; RCGP & BMA.

SEMENOV, Richard Arne Flat 1/3, Jacksons Lane, Highgate, London N6 5SR — MB BS Adelaide 1990. Specialty: Anaesth.

SEMERARO, David Histopathology Department, Derbyshire Royal Infirmary, London Road, Derby DE1 2QY Tel: 01332 47141 — MB ChB Bristol 1981; MRCPath 1990. Cons. Histopath. Derbysh. Roy. Infirm. Specialty: Histopath. Socs: Path. Soc.; Assn. Clin. Path. Prev: Sen. Regist. (Histopath.) Univ. Hosp. Wales.

SEMMENS, Jane Marjorie (retired) 32 Aldsworth Court, Goring St., Goring-by-Sea, Worthing BN12 5AG Tel: 01903 244515 Fax: 01903 244515 — (St. Mary's) MB BS Lond. 1955; DCH Eng. 1957; MD Lond. 1971. Nat. Co-ordinator Med. Wom. Internat. Assn. Prev: Cons. Paediat. Chichester & Worthing Health Dists.

SEMPA, Alexandra Vera 58 Vineyard Road, Northfield, Birmingham B31 1PR — MB ChB Bristol 1963.

SEMPLE, Alan James 3 Snowdon Place, Stirling FK8 2NH Tel: 01786 61715 — MB ChB Dundee 1979; FFA RCS Eng. 1983. Cons. Anaesth. Falkirk & Dist. Roy. Infirm. Specialty: Anaesth. Prev: Sen. Regist. (Anaesth.) Ninewells Hosp. Dundee.

SEMPLE, Andrew Best, CBE, VRD 433 Woolton Road, Liverpool L25 4SY Tel: 0151 428 2081 — (Univ. Glas.) MD (Commend.) Glas. 1947, MB ChB (Commend.) 1934; DPH 1936; FFCM 1974. Surg. Cdr. RNR; Fell. Soc. Community Med. Socs: FRSH (Exec. Vice-Pres. & Treas.). Prev: Hon. Phys. to H.M. The Qu.; Area Med. Off. Liverp. AHA (T); Prof. Community & Environm. Health Univ. Liverp.

SEMPLE, Colin Gordon 53 Tinto Road, Newlands, Glasgow G43 2AH — MB ChB Glas. 1977; FRCP (Glas., Ed., Lond.); MA, MD Glas. 1990, MB ChB 1977; MRCP (UK) 1980. Cons. Phys. Southern Gen. Hosp. Glas. Specialty: Endocrinol.; Gen. Med.; Diabetes. Socs: Hon. Sec. RCP & Surg. of Glas. 1998-2001; Chairm. Spec. Adv. Comm. on Gen. Internal Med. of Jt. Comm. Higher Med. Train.1999-2003.

SEMPLE, David Alexander — MB BChir Camb. 1989; MB BChir Camb. 1990; FRCA 1994. Cons. (Anaesth.) Roy. Infirm. Of Edin. Specialty: Anaesth.

SEMPLE, David Mark 13 Booths Hill Road, Lymm WA13 0DJ — MB ChB Glas. 1988; MRCOG 1994. Regist. Arrowe Pk. Hosp.

Wirral. Specialty: Obst. & Gyn. Prev: Regist. Rotat. (O & G) Liverp. Wom. Hosp.; Regist. Fazakerley Hosp. Liverp.

SEMPLE, Deborah Karon Comber Health Centre, 5 Newtownards Road, Newtownards BT23 5BA — MB BCh BAO Belf. 1987.

SEMPLE, Mr Graham Alan 16 Billendean Terrace, Spittal, Berwick-upon-Tweed TD15 2AX Tel: 01289 307773; 47 Bracklyn Court, Wimbourne St, Hackney, London N1 7EL Tel: 020 7490 1497 Fax: 020 7490 1497 Email: gsemple@compuserve.com — MB BS Lond. 1993 (Univ. Coll. & Middlx. Sch. Med.) BSc (Hons.) Lond. 1989; FRCS Eng. 1998. SHO (Orthop. Surg.) Barnet Gen. Hosp. Lond. Specialty: Orthop. Socs: BMA; Med. Protec. Soc.

SEMPLE, Iain Cameron Ovoca, 460 Didsbury Road, Heaton Mersey, Stockport SK4 3BT Tel: 0161 432 2032 Fax: 0161 947 9689 — MB ChB Manch. 1990; MRCGP 1994.

SEMPLE, Mr James Campbell 79 Harley Street, London W1G 8PZ Tel: 020 7224 0046 Fax: 020 7224 0082 Email: campbell@79harleystreet.co.uk; 34 Polwarth St, Glasgow G12 9TX Tel: 0141 339 5455 Fax: 0141 5769656 — (Glas.) MB ChB Glas. 1959; FRCS Glas. 1965; FRCS Ed. 1966. p/t Indep. Pract. (Hand & Surg.) Lond. & Glas. Specialty: Orthop.; Medico Legal. Prev: Cons. Hand Surg. West. Infirm. Glas.; Lect. Nuffield Dept. Orthop. Surg. Univ. Oxf.; Cons. Hand Surg. Sheff. RHB (Derby Area).

SEMPLE, Judith Mairi The Health Centre, 20 Duncan Street, Greenock PA15 4LY Tel: 01475 724477 Fax: 01475 727140 — MB ChB St. And. 1972; DCH Eng. 1975; MRCP (UK) 1977; FRCP Glas. 1994.

SEMPLE, Linsey Charlotte Drs Semple and Finney, 436 Mosspark Boulevard, Glasgow G52 1HX Tel: 0141 882 5494 Fax: 0141 883 1015 — MB ChB Glas. 1983; DRCOG 1985; MRCGP 1986.

SEMPLE, Malcolm G University of Liverpool, Institute of Child Health, Alder Hey, Eaton Road, Liverpool L12 2AP Tel: 0151 252 5440 Fax: 0151 293 3692 Email: m.g.semple@liv.ac.uk — BM BCh Oxf. 1995; PhD (Med.) Lond. 1995. Sen. Clin. Lect. & Clinician Scientist (Paediat.) Univ. of Liverp.; Hon. Specialist Regist. (Paediat. Respiritory Med.) Alder Hey Hosp. Liverp. Specialty: Paediat. Special Interest: Host defense to Respirat. Virus.

SEMPLE, Margaret Janet Epsom & St Helier NHS TrustDepartment of Haematology, Epsom General Hospital, Dorking Road, Epsom KT18 7EG Tel: 01372 735735 Fax: 01372 748802; 11 Redwoods, Alton Road, Roehampton, London SW15 4NL Tel: 020 8789 6248 — MB BS Lond. 1970 (StThomas) BSc (Hons. Special Physiol.) Lond. 1967; MRCP (UK) 1974; FRCPath 1989, M 1977; FRCP Lond. 1996. Cons. Haemat. Epsom Gen. Hosp. Specialty: Haematology.

SEMPLE, Margaret McIndoe Gowrie House, Royal Dundee Liff Hospital, Liff, Dundee DD2 5NF Tel: 01382 423046 — MB ChB Glas. 1979 (Univ. Glas.) DObst RCOG 1981; MRCPsych 1988. Cons. Psychiat. Roy. Dundee Liff Hosp. Liff Dundee. Specialty: Geriat. Psychiat. Prev: Sen. Regist. & Regist. (Psychiat.) Roy. Dundee Liff Hosp.; Cons. Psychiat. Hairmyres Hosp. E. Kilbride Lanarksh.

SEMPLE, Peter 8 North Park Grove, Roundary, Leeds LS8 1JJ Tel: 0113 240 0044 — BM Soton. 1984; DA (UK) 1986; FFA RCSI 1989; FCAnaesth 1990. Cons. Anaesth. St. Jas. Hosp. Leeds; Hon. Clin. Lect. Univ. Leeds. Specialty: Anaesth.

SEMPLE, Peter D'Almaine Inverclyde Royal Hospital, Larkfield Road, Greenock PA16 1JX Tel: 01475 633777 Fax: 01475 656142 Email: peter.semple@irh.scot.nhs.uk; High Lunderston, Inverkip, Greenock PA16 0DU Tel: 01475 522342 — MB ChB Glas. 1970; MRCP (UK) 1974; FRCP Glas. 1984; MD Glas. 1985; FRCP Ed. 1988; FRCP Lond. 1996. Cons. Gen. Med. & Respirat. Dis. Inverclyde Roy. Hosp. Greenock. Specialty: Gen. Med.

SEMPLE, Peter Ferguson Western Infirmary, Division of Cardiovascular and Medical Services, Glasgow G11 6NT Tel: 0141 211 2143 Fax: 0141 339 2800; 103 Southbrae Drive, Glasgow G13 1TU Tel: 0141 959 4462 Fax: 0141 959 4462 — MB ChB St. And. 1969; MRCP (UK) 1971; FRCP Glas. 1983. Sen. Lect. (Med.) W. Infirm. Glas.; Sub Dean Western Infirm. Glas. Specialty: Gen. Med. Socs: Assn. Phys. Prev: Cons. Pysician MRC Blood Pressure Unit Western Infirm.; Cons. Univ. Dept. Med. W. Infirm. Glas.; Regist. (Med.) Glas. Roy. Infirm.

SEMPLE, Stuart Mackenzie Mounthooly, Winchburgh, Broxburn EH52 6PY Tel: 01506 890357 — MB ChB Ed. 1962; LM Rotunda 1965; DObst RCOG 1965; FRCPath 1985, M 1972; MRCGP 1974; MFHom 1979; FFHom 1996. Specialty: Homeop. Med. Prev: Lect. Bact. Univ. Edin.; Regist. Clin. Path. Roy. Infirm. Edin.

SEMPLE, Verne Adrienne (retired) Larne House, 31 Buchanan St., Balfron, Glasgow G63 0TS Tel: 01360 440854 — MB ChB Glas. 1948. Prev: Ho. Phys. Vict. Infirm. Glas.

SEMPLE, William Gordon, SBStJ (retired) Larne House, 31 Buchanan St., Balfron, Glasgow G63 0TS Tel: 01360 440854 — (Glas.) MB ChB Glas. 1948. Prev: Squadron Ldr. RAF Med. Br.

SEMPLE, William John 7 Tothill Street, Minster-in-Thanet, Ramsgate CT12 4AG — MB BS Lond. 1963 (King's Coll. Hosp.) MRCS Eng. LRCP Lond. 1962; DA Eng. 1965; DObst. RCOG 1966.

SEMRAU, Ute 28 Ashley Road, London N19 3AF — State Exam Med Berlin 1992.

***SEN, Mr Aloke Srinath** — MB ChB Manch. 1998; MRCS Ed. 2002. SHO Ent., Fairfield General Hospital, Bury. Specialty: Otorhinolaryngol. Socs: MDU; BMA; RCS (Edinburgh).

SEN, Amitabha 19 The Chesters, West Denton, Newcastle upon Tyne NE5 1AF — MB BS Calcutta 1967. Specialty: Trauma & Orthop. Surg.

SEN, Anup Kumar (retired) 39 Station Road, Hemsworth, Pontefract WF9 4JW — MB BS Calcutta 1949 (R.G. Kar Med. Coll. Calcutta) DPH Eng. 1953, DIH 1953.

SEN, Arjune Four Oaks, 40 Russell Bank Road, Sutton Coldfield B74 4RQ — BM BCh Oxf. 1998; BM BCh Oxf 1998.

SEN, Mr Aruni Department of Accident & Emergency, N.E. Wales NHS Trust, Maelor Hospital, Croesnewydd Road, Wrexham LL13 7TD Tel: 01978 291100 Fax: 01978 725168 Email: aruni.sen@new-tr.wales.nhs.uk; 8 Chetwyn Court, Gresford, Wrexham LL12 8EG Tel: 01978 856068 Fax: 01978 856146 Email: thesens@msn.com — MB BS Calcutta 1982 (Med. Coll. Calcutta) MS (Surg.) Calcutta 1986; FRCS (Ed.) 1989; FRCS (Eng.) 1990; FFAEM 1996; Dip Med Educat Cardiff 2002. Cons. A & E Ysbyty Maelor Wrexham, N. E. Wales NHS Trust. Specialty: Accid. & Emerg.; Medico Legal; Educat. Prev: Sen. Regist. (A & E) West. Infirm. Glas.; Regist. (A & E) Vict. Infirm. Glas.

SEN, Asha The Surgery, 12 The Slade, Plumstead, London SE18 2NB Tel: 020 8317 3031 Fax: 020 8317 2536 — MB BS Indore 1970; MB BS Indore 1970.

SEN, Asim Kumar 6 Fallowfield, Shoeburyness, Southend-on-Sea SS3 8DF — MB BS Calcutta 1972.

SEN, Balarka (retired) Belmont, Sandheath Road, Beacon Hill, Hindhead GU26 6RU Tel: 01428 609299 — LMSSA Lond. 1967 (RCSI) Med. Asst. (Psychiat.) Geo. Eliot Hosp. Nuneaton. Prev: GP Nuneaton.

SEN, Mr Basav 19 Tankerville Terrace, Jesmond, Newcastle upon Tyne NE2 3AJ Tel: 0191 281 0859 — MB BS Bhagalpur 1984; FRCS Glas. 1989. Cons. (A&E) Head of Dept. Newcastle Gen. Hosp. Specialty: Accid. & Emerg. Prev: Cons. (A & E) Head of Dept. Roy. Vict. Infirm. Newc.

SEN, Mr Binayak 10 Ashville Croft, Halifax HX2 0QJ Tel: 01422 361381 — MB BS Calcutta 1981; FRCS Glas. 1989. Specialty: Gen. Surg.

SEN, Debajit 145 Roll Gardens, Gants Hill, Ilford IG2 6TL — MB BS Lond. 1993.

SEN, Debasish Grove House, Skerton Road, Manchester M16 0RB Tel: 0161 952 8200 Fax: 0161 952 8300 — MB BS Newc. 1980 (Newcastle upon Tyne) MRCGP 1986; DRCOG 1987; MFOM RCP Lond. 1996; FFOM RCP (Lond) 2003. Sen. Med. Insp. Health & Safety Exec.; Chief Examr. (AFOM), Fac.of Occ Med, RCP Lond.; Hon. Lect. Dept. of Pub. Health Med. Univ. of Liverp.; Hon. Lect. Centre for Occ. & Env. Health Univ. Manchester. Specialty: Occupat. Health. Socs: Soc. Occupat. Med.; MEDICHEM. Prev: Employm. Med. Adviser Health & Safety Exec.

SEN, Gurmeet 6 Fallowfield, Shoeburyness, Southend-on-Sea SS3 8DF — MB BS Delhi 1973; MRCPCH; DGO; MSc.

SEN, Indranil Victoria Road Health Centre, Victoria Road, Concord, Washington NE37 2PU Tel: 0191 417 3557 Email: i.sen@zen.co.uk; 60 Manor Gardens, Wardley, Gateshead NE10 8UZ Tel: 0191 469 0674 Email: i.sen@zen.co.uk — MB ChB Manch. 1996. GP Dr Fairs & Partners Pract. Vict. Rd. Health Centre Washington Tyne and Wear. Specialty: Gen. Pract. Prev: GP Regist., Bedlingtonshire Med. grp; SHO in Obst. and Gyn., Ashington; SHO in Psychiat. Cherry Knowle Hosp. Ryhope Sunderland.

SEN, Jon — MB BS (UCL) Lond. 1998 (Univ. Coll. Lond.) BSc (Hons. Anat. & Neurobiology) Lond. 1994; MRCS (i) Eng 2001; MSc (Clin. Neurosci., Distinc.) Lond. 2002. Research Fell. (PhD) Nat. Hosp. Qu. Sq. Special Interest: biomarkers of brain injury. Socs: MDU; Fell. Roy. Soc. Of Med. (Neurosciences Section); BMA. Prev: SHO (Neurosurgery) Derriford Hosp. Plymouth; SHO (Spinal) RD&E Hosp. Exeter; SHO (A&E ENT) Northwick Pk. Hosp. Harrow.

SEN, Julia Department of Ophthalmology, Royal Liverpool University Hospital, Prescot St., Liverpool L7 8XP Tel: 0151 706 2000; The Chimes, Glebe Lane, Gnosall, Stafford ST20 0ER Tel: 01785 822311 — MB ChB Leic. 1993. SHO (Ophth.) Roy. Liverp. Univ. Hosp. Specialty: Ophth. Socs: Med. Defence Union; BMA. Prev: SHO (Ophth.) P'boro. Dist. Hosp.; SHO (O & G) P'boro. Dist. Hosp.; SHO (Respirat. Med.) Glenfield Hosp. Trust Leicester.

SEN, Purnendu Kumar 18 Lime Grove, Littleborough OL15 8RP Tel: 01706 370579; 1 Bulwer Street, Rochdale OL16 2EU Tel: 01706 356422 — (Calcutta) MB BS Calcutta 1959; DA Calcutta 1969; DA Eng. 1975. GP Rochdale. Prev: Trainee GP Salford; SHO (Psychiat.) St. Mary's Hosp. Hereford; SHO (A & E) Gen. Hosp. Hereford.

SEN, Rabindra Nath (retired) 4 Snipe Close, Holymoorside, Chesterfield S42 7HD Tel: 01246 568292 — MB BS Calcutta 1958 (Calcutta Med. Coll.) DO Eng. 1965. Prev: Assoc. Specialist (Ophth.) Chesterfield & N. Derbysh. Roy. Hosp.

SEN, S K The Surgery, The Chantry, Coxwold, York YO61 4BB Tel: 01347 868426 Fax: 01347 868782 — MB BS Calcutta 1969; MB BS Calcutta 1969.

SEN, Salil Ranjan (Surgery), 96 Barnsley Road, Goldthorpe, Rotherham S63 9AB Tel: 01709 890686 Fax: 01709 888347 — DObst RLPI 1974 Dub; BSc Gauhati 1962; MB BS Gauhati 1967; FPA Lond. 1974; DRCOG Lond. 1979; Lic. AC Liverp. 1984; DFFP Lond. 1995; FRSM Lond. 1996; FRSH Lond. 1997; FRIPHH Lond. 1998. Princip. GP; Primary Care Gp. Bd. Mem. Specialty: Obst. & Gyn.; Paediat.; Diabetes. Socs: Med. Protec. Soc.

SEN, Sanjay Kumar 12 Hanworth Road, Feltham TW13 5AD Tel: 020 8890 2208; 9 Berwyn Avenue, Hounslow TW3 4ET. GP Feltham. Prev: SHO (Obst. & Psych.) Lister Hosp. Stevenage; SHO (Geriat.) St. Michaels Hosp. Enfield.

SEN, Sanjoy Anilkumar 97 Delaunays Road, Manchester M8 4RE Tel: 0161 795 4567 — MB BS Poona 1980; MRCOG 1987.

SEN, Sisir Kanti Crawley Road Medical Centre, 479 High Road, Leyton, London E10 5EL Tel: 020 8539 1880 Fax: 020 8556 1318; 66 Broadwalk, South Woodford, London E18 2DW Tel: 020 8989 7988 Fax: 020 8989 7988 Email: docssen@aol.com — MB BS Calcutta 1959 (NR Sircar Med. Coll.) DGO Calcutta 1961; MRCOG 1970; FRCOG 1997. GP. Specialty: Obst. & Gyn.; Oral & Maxillofacial Surg.; Diabetes. Socs: MPS; BMA; FMS.

SEN, Subhas Chandra The Surgery, Little London, Caldmore, Walsall WS1 3EP Tel: 01922 28280 Fax: 01922 23023; 32 Park Road, Walsall WS5 3JU Tel: 0121 357 1979 — MB ChB Birm. 1974.

SEN, Mr Subrata — MB BS Calcutta 1961 (Calcutta Med. Coll.) FRCS Eng. 1973. Specialty: Orthop.

SEN, Susmita 66 Broadwalk, London E18 2DW Tel: 020 8989 7988 — MB BS Calcutta 1960 (N.R. Sircar Med. Coll. Calcutta) DGO Calcutta 1962; MRCOG 1968; DA Eng. 1971; FRCOG 1998.

SEN GUPTA, Arup Kumar Abraham Cowley Unit, Holloway Hill, Lyne, Chertsey KT16 0AE — MB BS Ranchi 1973. Locum Cons. (Psychiat.). Specialty: Gen. Psychiat.

SEN GUPTA, Pinaki Summervale Medical Centre, Wharf Lane, Ilminster TA19 0DT Tel: 01460 52354 — MB BS Calcutta 1960.

SEN-GUPTA, Tapan Acocks Green Medical Centre, 999 Warwick Road, Acocks Green, Birmingham B27 6QJ Tel: 0121 706 0501 — MB BS Lond. 1989.

SENANAYAKE, Gamini Memorial Hospital, Darlington DH3 6HX Tel: 01325 380100; 47 Ancroft Garth, High Shincliffe, Durham DH1 2UD — (University of Ceylon, Peradeniya, Sri Lanka) MB BS Ceylon 1970; DO RCS Eng. 1984; MRCOphth 1990. Staff Grade (Ophth.) Memor. Hosp. Darlington.

SENANAYAKE, Hemantha Malinath 8 Winckley Close, Kenton, Harrow HA3 9QW — MB BS Sri Lanka 1978; MRCOG 1987.

SENANAYAKE, Indrani Pramilla International Planned Parenthood Federation, Regents College, Inner Circle, Regents Park, London NW1 4NS Tel: 020 7487 7852 Fax: 020 7487 7950; 22 Cavendish Avenue, St John's Wood, London NW8 9JE — MB BS Ceylon 1967; DTPH Lond 1971; PhD Lond. 1975. Asst. Sec. Gen. Internat. Planned Parenthood Federat.; Vice Chairm. Bd. Family Health Internat.; Div. Soc. Advancem. of Contracep. Specialty: Pub. Health Med. Socs: Fell. Roy. Soc. Health. Prev: Lect. (Pub. Health & Community Med.) Univ. Colombo, Sri Lanka; Epidemiol. WHO (Small Pox Eradication Progr.).

SENANAYAKE, Lakshman Felix Nonis Department of Radiotherapy & Oncology, Royal Free Hospital, Pond St., London NW3 2QG Tel: 020 7794 0500 Fax: 020 7830 2968; The Garden Flat, 24 Parliament Hill, London NW3 2TN — MB BS Ceylon 1965 (Colombo) DMRT Eng. 1973; MSc (Radiobiol.) Lond. 1974. Cons. & Dir. Radiother. & Oncol. Roy. Free Hosp. Lond. Specialty: Oncol.; Radiother. Socs: Chairm. Internat. Adjuvant Ther. Assn.; MRC Brain Tumour Working Party. Prev: Research Regist. Mt. Vernon Hosp. Northwood; Sen. Regist. Middlx. Hosp. Lond.; Regist. Roy. Free Hosp. Lond.

SENAPATI, Asha Queen Alexandra Hospital, Cosham, Portsmouth PO6 3LY Tel: 023 92 286000 Fax: 023 92 286710; Bunchfield, Lynchmere Ridge, Haslemere GU27 3PP Tel: 01428 658510 Fax: 01428 658516 — MB BS Madras 1976; MRCS Eng. LRCP Lond. 1978; FRCS Eng. 1979; PhD Lond. 1986. Cons. Surg. Qu. Alexandra Hosp. Portsmouth. Specialty: Gen. Surg. Socs: Roy. Soc. Med. (Mem. Surg. Sect. Mem. Sect. & Clin. Sect.Counc. & Mem.Coloproctol. Sect.). Prev: Cons. Surg. Mayday Univ. Hosp. Croydon.

SENAPATI, Mr Mihir Kumar (retired) Bunchfield, Lynchmere Ridge, Haslemere GU27 3PP Tel: 01428 652071 Fax: 01428 645304 — MB BS Patna 1948; FRCS Eng. 1957; FRCS Ed. 1957; FRACS 1984.

SENAPATI, Ranganayaki (retired) Bunchfield, Lynchmere Ridge, Haslemere GU27 3PP Tel: 01428 652071 Fax: 01428 645304 — MB BS Lucknow 1946.

SENARATH, Violet Lorraine Department of Radiotherapy & Oncology, Norfolk & Norwich Hospital, Norwich NR1 3SR Tel: 01603 286286; 39 Buckland Rise, Eaton, Norwich NR4 6EU Tel: 01603 505565 — MB BS Ceylon 1971 (Colombo) FRCR 1985. Staff Grade (Radiother.& Oncol.) Norf. & Norwich Hosp. Specialty: Oncol.; Radiother. Prev: Regist. (Radiother. & Oncol.) Norf. & Norwich Hosp.; SHO (Radiother.) Norf. & Norwich & Newc. Gen. Hosps.

SENARATH YAPA, Ranjith Sampath Wansbeck General Hospital, Woodhorn Lane, Ashington NE63 9JJ — MB BS Sri Lanka 1975; MRCP (UK) 1983; FRCP 1999.

SENARATH YAPA, Sarath Chandra Bury PCT Community Services, Talbot Grove, Bury BL9 6PH Tel: 0161 293 5512/0161 761 6793 — MB BS Sri Lanka 1976; MRCP UK. Princip. Clin. Med. Off. (Adult Health) Bury PCT Community Servs. Bury. Special Interest: Nutrit. of the Elderly; Young Disabled.

SENARATNE, Kollura Mudianselage Jayawickrama The New Surgery, Adwick Road, Mexborough S64 0DB Tel: 01709 590707 Fax: 01709 571986; 114 Carr Manor View, Moor Town, Leeds LS17 5AT Tel: 0113 269 5474 — LRCP Ed. 1987; LRCP LRCS Ed. LRCPS Glas. 1987; DGM RCP Lond. 1990.

SENATHIRAJAH, Dharmarajan 45 Oakwood Drive, Fulwood, Preston PR2 3LY — MB BS Ceylon 1968.

SENATHIRAJAH, Sinnatamby Sanmugam 314 Torbay Road, Harrow HA2 9QW — MB BS Ceylon 1960; FRCOG 1989, M 1969.

SENDALL, Katherine (retired) 36 Kew Gardens, Whitley Bay NE26 3LY Tel: 0191 252 2672 — MB BS Durh. 1963.

SENDEGEYA, Christina 62 Norseman Close, West Derby, Liverpool L12 5LS Tel: 0151 256 6177 — Ptychio Iatrikes Athens 1989; MRCP Lond. 1993.

SENDER, Helen 12 Gertrude Street, Chelsea, London SW10 0JN Tel: 020 7352 2411 — MB BCh Witwatersrand 1941; DPH 1943; DMRD Eng. 1954. Cons. Radiol. Bolingbroke Hosp., St. John's Hosp. & Tooting Bec Hosp. Lond. Specialty: Radiol. Socs: Brit. Inst. Radiol. & Fac. Radiols. Prev: Sen. Radiol. Regist. Roy. Marsden Hosp. & St. Helier Hosp.; Radiol. Johannesburg Gen. Hosp.

SENDER, Jerome Merrow Park Surgery, Kingfisher Drive, Guildford GU4 7EP Tel: 01483 503331 Fax: 01483 303457; 4 Coltsfoot Drive, Guildford GU1 1YH Tel: 01483 453138 — MB BS Lond. 1982 (St. Mary's) DCH RCP Lond. 1986; DRCOG 1986; MRCGP 1986; Dip Occ Med 1998. Clin. Asst. Migraine & Headache Clinic Guildford. Prev: Trainee GP Watford VTS.

SENDER, Simon Nathan 12 Gertrude Street, Chelsea, London SW10 0JN Tel: 020 7352 2411 — MB BCh Witwatersrand 1953; BA Pretoria 1930, LLB 1932; DMRD Eng. 1957; FFR 1967. Emerit. Cons. Radiol. St. Stephen's Hosp. Lond. Specialty: Radiol. Socs: Fell. Roy. Soc. Med.; FRCR. Prev: Sen. Radiol. Regist. Roy. Marsden Hosp. & St. Helier Hosp.; Radiol. Baragwanath Hosp. Johannesburg.

SENEVIRATNE, Gertrude Nimali 1 Sheerwater Road, London E16 3SU — MB BS Lond. 1992.

SENEVIRATNE, Kirihettige Boniface Clement 1 Sheerwater Road, London E16 3SU — MB BS Ceylon 1963; DCCH RCGP & FCM 1988. Staff Grade (Paediat.) Lond. Socs: Fac. Community Health. Prev: Clin. Med. Off. Tower Hamlets Health Dist.

SENEVIRATNE, Saaliya 39C Leyborne Avenue, London W13 9RA — MB ChB Sheff. 1987.

SENGUPTA, Anup 47 Heldhaw Road, Bury St Edmunds IP32 7ES — MBBS Bhopal India 1981; FRCPS Glas. 1992; FRCS Glas. 1992; MSc (Urol.) Lond. 1996. Staff Grade W. Suff. Hosp. Prev: Staff Grade Surg. E. Surrey Hosp.; Regist. (Surg.) Wycombe Gen. Hosp. High Wycombe.

SENGUPTA, Catherine Woodlands, 46 The Causeway, March PE15 9NX — BM BS Nottm. 1995; BMedSci (Hons.) Nottm 1993 BM BS 1995; MRCP 1999. SpR (Anaesthetics) Leeds Teachg. Hosps. Specialty: Gen. Med. Prev: SHO Rotat. (Gen. Med.) Kings Coll. Hosp. NHS Trust Lond.

SENGUPTA, Dibyendu Grafton Road Surgery, 11 Grafton Road, Solihull Lodge, Solihull B90 1NG Tel: 0121 474 4686 Fax: 0121 608 4900 — (Calcutta Nat. Med. Coll.) MB BS Calcutta 1966; DGO Calcutta 1967; DRCOG 1979.

SENGUPTA, Fergus Ranjan The Moorings, Falkirk Rd, Linlithgow EH49 7BQ — MB ChB Ed. 1997.

SENGUPTA, Gautam Essenden Road Surgery, 49 Essenden Road, St Leonards-on-Sea TN38 0NN Tel: 01424 720866 Fax: 01424 445580 — MB BS Lond. 1977; DRCOG 1981.

SENGUPTA, Nandita Turners Hill Surgery, 161 Turners Hill, Cheshunt, Waltham Cross EN8 9BH Tel: 01992 624696.

SENGUPTA, Partha Sarathi East Glamorgan Hospital, Church Village, Pontypridd CF38 1AB Tel: 01443 218218 Fax: 01443 217213 — MB BS Newc. 1987; MRCOG 1993. Regist. (O & G) E. Glam. Gen. Hosp. Pontypridd. Specialty: Obst. & Gyn.

SENGUPTA, Prasun Lister Hospital, Department of Anaesthetics, Coreys Mill Lane, Stevenage SG1 4AB Tel: 01438 781086; 10 Arnold Close, Stevenage SG1 4TR — MB BS Lond. 1976; MRCP (UK) 1980; FRCA 1982; FFA RCS Eng. 1982. Cons. Anaesth. East & North Herts. NHS Trust. Specialty: Anaesth.

SENGUPTA, Priyadarshi Geriatric Day Hospital, Royal Alexandra Hospital, Paisley Tel: 0141 887 9111; 44 Balgonie Woods, Paisley PA2 6HW Tel: 0141 884 3839 — MB BS Calcutta 1975; MD Patna 1980. Staff Grade Phys. (Geriat. Med.) Roy. Alexandra Hops. Paisley. Specialty: Care of the Elderly.

SENGUPTA, Mr Ram Prasad Newcastle General Hospital, Regional Neurosciences Centre, Westgate Road, Newcastle upon Tyne NE4 6BE Tel: 0191 233 6161 Fax: 0191 272 3231 Email: robin.sengupta@nuth.nhs.uk — MB BS Calcutta 1961 (national Medical College) FRCSE 1967; FRCS 1968; MSc 1976. Cons. Neurosurg., Regional Neurosciences Centre, Newcastle-Upon-Tyne. Specialty: Neurol. Special Interest: Pain Surg.; Vasc. Surg. Socs: Soc. of Brit. Neurol. Surg.; Assn. of Neurol. Surg.; Congr. of Neurol. Surg.

SENGUPTA, Sajalbaran Maerdy Surgery, North Terrace, Maerdy, Ferndale CF43 4DD Tel: 01443 733202 Fax: 01443 733730 — MB BS Calcutta 1963.

SENGUPTA, Shiuli 27 Ailsa Drive, Giffnock, Glasgow G46 6RJ — MB ChB Glas. 1998; MB ChB Glas 1998.

SENGUPTA, Swapan Kumar Castle Street Medical Centre, Castle Street, Bolsover, Chesterfield S44 6PP Tel: 01246 822983 — MB BS Ranchi 1969.

SENGUPTA, Tarun Kumar The Moorings, Falkirk Road, Linlithgow EH49 7BQ — (Assam Med. Coll.) MB BS Gauhati 1955. Socs: BMA. Prev: Asst. Surg. Kohima Civil Hosp., India; SHO Stirling Roy. Infirm.; Regist. Falkirk Roy. Infirm.

SENGUPTA, Usha Paediatric Ward, Crosshouse Hospital, Kilmarnock KA2 0BE Tel: 01563 521133; 44 Balgonie Woods, Paisley PA2 6HW Tel: 0141 884 3839 — MB BS Calcutta 1976; DCH RCP Lond. 1983. Staff Grade (Paediat.) CrossHo. Hosp. Kilmarnock. Specialty: Paediat.

SENHENN, Jane Susanne Almond Bourne Hall Health Centre, Spring Street, Ewell, Epsom KT17 1TG; 50 Gerard Road, Barnes, London SW13 9QQ Tel: 020 8748 5431 — MB BS Lond. 1982 (St. Bart.) Cert. Family Plann. JCC 1984; MRCGP 1986. Specialty: Gen. Pract. Prev: SHO (Paediat.) Mayday Hosp. Croydon; SHO (Psychiat.) S. West. Hosp. Lond.; SHO (O & G) & Cas. Off. St. Thos. Hosp. Lond.

SENIOR, Andrew Park Medical Centre, 164 Park Road, Petorborough, Peterborough PE1 2UF Tel: 01733 552801 — MB BS Lond. 1991.

SENIOR, Mr Andrew John Benbecula Medical Practice, Griminish Surgery, Griminish, Isle of Benbecula HS7 5QA Tel: 01870 602215 Fax: 01870 602630 — MB ChB Ed. 1978; FRCS Ed. 1984; MRCGP 1993.

SENIOR, Angus Dominic Tregarken, The Square, Tregony, Truro TR2 5RS — MB ChB Sheff. 1992. GP Princip. Polkyth Surg. St. Austell Cornw.

SENIOR, Colin James 6 Rushmoor Grove, Backwell, Bristol BS48 3BW — BM BS Nottm. 1998; BM BS Nottm 1998; MRCS Ed. 2002. Orthopaedic Regist., Wessex Rotat.

SENIOR, David 25A Eastgate S., Driffield YO25 6LW; Bridlington & District Hospital, Bessingby Road, Bridlington YO16 4QP Tel: 01262 606666 — MB ChB Leeds 1965; DObst RCOG 1969; DTM & H Liverp. 1970; MRCPsych. 1981. Cons. Psychiat. Bridlington & Dist. Hosp. N. Humberside. Specialty: Gen. Psychiat. Socs: BMA & World Federat. for Ment. Health. Prev: Sen. Regist. (Psychiat.) St. Bart. Hosp. Gp. Lond.; Sen. Regist. (Psychiat.) Goodmayes Hosp. Ilford; Med. Supt. Catherine Booth Mission Hosp., Zululand.

SENIOR, David Cedric (retired) Dunthwaite, Dark Lane, Barnsley S70 6RE Tel: 01226 205586 — MB ChB Leeds 1955. Prev: GP Barnsley.

SENIOR, David Frank 22 Parkside, Vanburgh Fields, Blackheath, London SE3 7QQ Tel: 020 8858 7570 — MB BS Lond. 1973; DA Eng. 1978.

SENIOR, Eileen Mary (retired) 11 Lyndhurst Grove, Allerton, Bradford BD15 7AS Tel: 01274 225792 — MB ChB Manch. 1965; DObst RCOG 1967; FRCOG 1991, M 1972. Prev: GP The Ridge Med. Pract. Bradford.

SENIOR, Emma Louise Littlewood House, 172 Poolbrook Road, Malvern WR14 3JG — BM BCh Oxf. 1997.

SENIOR, Fai Louise Dovedale, Old Woodhouses, Broughall, Whitchurch SY13 4EH — MB ChB Sheff. 1998; MB ChB Sheff 1998.

SENIOR, Jane Elizabeth Prospect Road Surgery, 22 Prospect Road, Ossett WF5 8AN Tel: 01924 274123 Fax: 01924 263350; 152 Shay Lane, Walton, Wakefield WF2 6LA Tel: 01924 257310 — MB ChB Manch. 1983; DCH RCP Lond. 1986; MRCGP 1987.

SENIOR, Michael Arthur 26 South Parade, Pudsey LS28 8NZ — MB ChB Leeds 1995; BChD Leeds 1984.

SENIOR, Nina Margaret The Health Centre, Central St., Countesthorpe, Leicester LE8 5QJ Tel: 0116 277 6336; Pine Garth, 6 Enderby Road, Blaby, Leicester LE8 4GD — MB ChB Leic. 1980; DRCOG 1983; Cert. Family Plann. JCC 1983; MRCGP 1986.

SENIOR, Peter Alexander 18 Hillside Terrace, Dundee DD2 1QS — MB BS Newc. 1993.

SENIOR, Robert Elvyn Senior and Partners, Morrab Surgery, 2 Morrab Road, Penzance TR18 4EL Tel: 01736 363866 Fax: 01736 367809 — MB ChB Sheff. 1961; DObst RCOG 1963.

SENIOR, Robert Simon 19 Navarino Road, London E8 1AD — MB BS Lond. 1977; BA Camb. 1974.

SENIOR, Roxy Northwick Park Hospital, Watford Road, Harrow HA3 0AX Tel: 020 8869 2547 Fax: 020 8864 0075; 23 Churchill Avenue, Harrow HA3 0AX Tel: 020 8907 9638 — MB BS Calcutta 1980; MD Cal 1983; DM Cal (Cardiology) 1987; MRCP (UK) 1990; FRCP(Lond) 1999; DESC 2001. Cons. Cardiol. Northwick Pk. Hosp. Harrow. Specialty: Cardiol. Socs: Brit. Cardiac Soc.; Brit. Soc. Echocardiogr.; Brit. Nuclear Cardiol. Soc. Prev: Hon. Sen. Regist. Northwick Pk. Hosp. Harrow.

SENIOR, Timothy Patrick Mansell 7 Ox Hey Close, Lostock, Bolton BL6 4BQ — BM BCh Oxf. 1997.

SENNETT, Karen Jane Killick Street Health Centre, 75 Killick Street, London N1 9RH Tel: 020 7833 9939 Fax: 020 7427 2740;

23 Langbourne Avenue, London N6 6AJ Tel: 020 8340 3739 — MB BS Lond. 1984 (Univ. Coll. Hosp.) MRCGP 1988; Dip. Addic. Behaviour Lond. 1992. GP Partner. Specialty: Gen. Pract. Prev: GP Som. Gdns. Health Centre; GP Facilitator for Homeless People Lond.; GP Hornsey Rise Health Centre Lond.

SENNIK, Avinash Kumar 15 Colombo Road, Ilford IG1 4RH — MB BS Rajasthan 1971 (S.P. Med. Coll. Bikaner) Off. i/c, US Army Health Clin., Bad Aibling W. Germany.

SENNIK, Surinder Kumar The Surgery, Briset Corner, 591 Westhorne Avenue, Eltham, London SE9 6JX Tel: 020 8850 5022 Fax: 020 8855 4970 — MB BS Bihar 1980 (Darbhanga) LRCP LRCS Ed. LRCPS Glas. 1984. GP Princip. Specialty: Gen. Pract.

SENOR, Concepsion Begona West Side Flat, Cleveland Lodge, Great Ayton, Middlesbrough TS9 6BT — LMS Cadiz 1989.

SENSIER, Alan Eric Sanderson and Partners, Adan House Surgery, St. Andrews Lane, Spennymoor DL16 6QA Tel: 01388 817777 Fax: 01388 811700; 54 Archery Rise, Nevilles Cross, Durham DH1 4LA Tel: 0191 384 2078 — MB BS Lond. 1983 (Cambridge and Middlesex Hospital Medical School) MA Camb. 1983; DRCOG 1987; MRCGP 1987. Prev: Trainee GP N.d. VTS.

SENSKY, Penelope Ruth 105 Julian Road, West Bridgford, Nottingham NG2 5AL — BM BCh Oxf. 1990; DRCOG 1993; MRCP (UK) 1994.

SENSKY, Thomas Ernest Lakeside Mental Health Unit, West Middlesex University Hospital, Isleworth TW7 6AF Tel: 020 8321 5179 Fax: 020 8321 6874 Email: t.sensky@imperial.ac.uk — MB BS Lond. 1979 (University College Hospital Medical School) BSc 1971; PhD Lond. 1975; M 1983; FRCPsych 1993. Prof. Psychol. Med., Imperial Coll.; Hon. Cons. Psychiat. W. Lond. Ment. Health NHS Trust. Specialty: Gen. Psychiat. Socs: Founding Fell. Acad. Cognitive Ther.; Fell. and President-elect, Intern. Coll. of Psychosomatic Med. Prev: Reader (Psychol. Med.) Imperial Coll. Of Sci., Technol. & Med.; Lect. & Hon. Sen. Regist. (Psychiat.) Char. Cross Hosp. Lond.; Sen. Regist. (Psychiat.) Hellingly Hosp. Hailsham & Bethlem Roy. & Maudsley Hosps. Lond.

SENTHIL KUMAR, Chitra Department of Gynaecology, Glasgow Royal Infirmary, Glasgow G4 0SF Tel: 0141 211 4000; 61 Moorfoot Way, Bearsden, Glasgow G61 4RL — MB BS Papua New Guinea 1989; MRCOG 1996. Staff Grade Gyn. Glas. Roy. Infirm. Specialty: Obst. & Gyn.

SENTHILKUMAR, Mr Chinnasamy Department of Orthopaedics, Glasgow Royal Infirmary, Glasgow G4 0SF Tel: 0141 211 5402; 61 Moorfoot Way, Bearsden, Glasgow G61 4RL — MB BS Madras 1986; FRCS Eng. 1992; FRCS (Tr. & Orth.) 1999. Cons. Orthopaedic Surg. Glas. Roy. Infirm. Specialty: Orthop.

SENTHILNATHAN, Mr Govindarajan 8 Maude Street, Darlington DL3 7PW — MB BS Madras 1986; FRCS Glas. 1994.

SENTHIRAMAN, Veeriah 9 Curtis Wood Park Road, Herne Bay CT6 7TY — MB BS Madras 1972; LMSSA Lond. 1988.

SENTHURAN, Sivagnanavel 282 Coombe Lane, London SW20 0RW — MB BS Lond. 1994.

SEPAI, Tehmton Meherwan The Surgery, 1 Hicks Road, Markyate, St Albans AL3 8LJ — MB ChB Sheff. 1983.

SEPHTON, Beryl Lindsay (retired) 18 Hargill Drive, Redmire, Leyburn DL8 4DZ — MB ChB Manch. 1955; DPH Manch. 1960; MFCM 1974; MFPHM RCP (UK) 1990. Prev: SCMO Blackburn Health Dist.

SEPHTON, Elizabeth Ann Cadbury Heath Health Centre, Parkwall Road, Cadbury Heath, Bristol BS30 8HS Tel: 0117 980 5700 Fax: 0117 980 5701 — MB ChB Bristol 1982; MB ChB (Hons.) Bristol 1982; MRCP (UK) 1985; DRCOG 1986; MRCGP 1988; MPhil (Cape Town) 2001. Specialty: Gen. Pract.

SEPHTON, Jean Edna 38 Old Wells Road, Glastonbury BA6 8EA — MB BS Lond. 1953 (Roy. Free) DObst RCOG 1964.

SEPHTON, Timothy James The Surgery, Madam's Paddock, Chew Magna, Bristol BS40 8PP Tel: 01275 332420 Fax: 01275 331355 — MB ChB Cape Town 1990; MRCGP 1996.

SEPHTON, Victoria Claire 12 Albury Close, The County Park, Liverpool L12 0NR Tel: 0151 283 8676 — MB ChB Leeds 1995; DFFP 1997. SHO (O & G) Liverp. Woms. Hosp. Liverp. Specialty: Obst. & Gyn. Socs: SHO Represent. Mersey Region Train. Comm. Prev: SHO (O & G) Bradford Roy. Infirm.; Ho. Off. Med. Huddersfield Roy.; Ho. Off. Surg. BRI.

SEPPELT, Ian Hugh 10 Cavendish Lodge, Cavendish Road, Bath BA1 2UD Tel: 01225 329273 — MA, MB BChir Camb. 1950 (Camb. & Univ. Coll. Hosp.) DPH Eng. 1955; MFCM 1974. Prev: Area Med. Off. Barnet AHA; MOH Lond. Boro. Ealing.

SEPPING, Paul (retired) Poole General Hospital, Longfleet Road, Poole BH15 2JB Tel: 01202 665511 Fax: 01202 661671 — MB BS New South Wales 1971 (University of New South Wales) BSc (Hons.) New South Wales 1968; DPM Eng. 1975; MRCPsych. 1976. Cons. Child & Adolesc. Psychiat. Poole Gen. Hosp.; Mem. Inst. Gp. Anal. Prev: Sen. Regist. Hosp. for Sick Childr. Gt. Ormond St. Gp. Lond.

SEQUEIRA, Jane Mary St Clare Hospice, Stone Barton, Hastingwood Road, Hastingwood, Harlow CM17 9JX Tel: 01279 435481; Ugley Hall, Bishop's Stortford CM22 6JB — MB BS Lond. 1979 (London) MRCPath 1987; FRCPath 1997. Clin. Asst. St Clare Hospice Essex. Specialty: Histopath.; Palliat. Med. Socs: Brit. Soc. Clin. Cytol.; Internat. Acad. Path. (Brit. Div.). Prev: Sen. Regist. & Lect. (Morbid Anat.) Lond. Hosp.; Cons. Cytopath. Bedford Hosp.

SERAFI, Sohel (Sam) Priory Hospital, Altrincham Rappax Road, Hale WA15 0NX Fax: 0161 904 0050 — MB BCh Cairo 1965 (Kasr El Eini, Cairo) Dip. Med. Cairo 1969; DPM Eng. 1973; MRCPsych 1975. Cons BUPA Regency Hosp. Macclesfield; Visinting Cons Priory Hosp. Hale. Specialty: Alcohol & Substance Misuse. Prev: Cons. Cornw. Ho. Clinic Sandy La. Staffs; Cons. Psychiat. (Alcoholism & Drug Addic.) Macclesfield Dist. Gen. Hosp.

SERAFINI, Franca 53 Tile House Road, London SW18 3EU — State DMS Padua 1984. Regist. (Anaesth.) Mayday Hosp. Croydon & St. Geo. Hosp. Lond. Specialty: Anaesth. Socs: Assn. Anaesth. Prev: Regist. (Anaesth.) Joyce Green Hosp. Dartford; SHO (Anaesth.) St. Heliers NHS Trust & St. Geo. Hosp. Lond.; SHO (Anaesth.) Westm. Hosp. Lond.

SERAJUDDIN, Mohammed 14 Hearnville Road, Balham, London SW12 8RR Tel: 020 8673 2949 — MB BS Rajshahi 1966 (Rajshahi Med. Coll.) DA Eng. 1969. Cons. Anaesth. Louth Co. Hosp. Specialty: Anaesth.

SERCOMBE, Karen Maria 3 Creek House, Russell Road, London W14 8HZ — MB BS Lond. 1996 (Char. Cross and Westm.) SHO (c/o the Elderly) Hillingdon Hosp. Lond. Specialty: Care of the Elderly. Prev: Ho. Off. (Med.) Kent & Canterbury Hosp.; Ho. Off. (Surg.) Hillingdon Hosp.

SERDESHMUKH, Waman 46 Quarry Lane, Sheffield S11 9EB Tel: 0114 255 6664 — MB BS Osmania 1954 (Osmania Med. Coll. Hyderabad, India) FICS 1987; FFAEM 1993. Cons. A & E N. Gen. Hosp. Sheff.; Hon. Clin. Lect. Univ. Dept. Surg. Sheff. Specialty: Accid. & Emerg. Socs: Fell. Roy. Soc. Med. (Accid. & Emerg. Sect.); Fell. Fac. Accid. & Emerg. Med.; Brit. Assn. Accid. & Emerg. Med. Prev: Regist. (Accid. & Orthop.) Mansfield & Dist. Gen. Hosp., Derby Roy. Infirm., Derby Childr. Hosp. & Nottm. Gp. Hosps.; SHO (Med.) & Med. Asst. Accid. & Orthop. Dept. North. Gen. Hosp. Sheff.

SERENYI, Anne Gwyneth The Riverside Surgery, Waterside, Evesham WR11 1JP Tel: 01386 40121 Fax: 01386 442615 — MB BS Lond. 1976 (Guy's) MRCS Eng. LRCP Lond. 1976; DRCOG 1978; DCH Eng. 1980.

SERGEANT, Howard Gordon Stanley 152 Harley Street, London W1G 7LH Tel: 020 7935 2477 Fax: 020 7224 2574 Email: howard@hgssergeant.demon.co.uk; 20 Well Walk, Hampstead, London NW3 1LD Tel: 020 7435 2308 Fax: 020 7435 2308 — MB BS Lond. 1957 (Char. Cross) MRCS Eng. LRCP Lond. 1957; DPM Lond. 1965; FRCP Ed. 1976, M 1965; FRCPsych 1978, M 1971. Hon. Cons. Psychiat. Roy. Free Hosp. Lond. Specialty: Gen. Psychiat.; Medico Legal. Special Interest: Negligence; Post-traumatic Stress Disorder; RTA Sequelae. Socs: Fell. Roy. Soc. Med. Prev: Cons. Psychiat. Roy. Free Hosp. Lond.; Cons. Psychiat. Roy. North. & Whittington Hosps. Lond.; Sen. Regist. Bethlem Roy. & Maudsley Hosps. Lond.

SERGEANT, Mr Robert James Nuffield Hospital, Kingswood Road, Tunbridge Wells Tel: 01892 512506; Stone House, Rocks Lane, High Hurstwood, Uckfield TN22 4BN — MB BS Lond. 1967 (Middlx.) MRCS LRCP 1967; FRCS Eng. 1973; FRCS Ed. 1976. Cons. ENT Surg. Maidstone & Tunbridge Wells NHS Trust. Specialty: Otolaryngol. Socs: Fell. Roy. Soc. Med.; Soc. Apoth.; Fell. Zool. Soc. Lond. Prev: Sen. Regist. Roy. Nat. Throat Nose & Ear Hosp. Lond.; Fell. Univ. Iowa, USA; Regist. Mt. Vernon Hosp. N.wood.

SERGI, Consolato St Michael's University Hospital, Department of Paediatric Pathology, Bristol BS2 8EG Tel: 0117 928 5234 — MD Genoa 1989. Cons. (Paediat. Path.). Specialty: Pathology, General. Special Interest: Paediatric Path.

SERHAN, Ergin The Royal Hospitals NHS Trust, New Cross Hospital, Wolverhampton WV10 0QP Tel: 01902 307999; Findon, Haughton Lane, Shifnal TF11 8HG Tel: 01952 460795 — MD Istanbul 1963; DCH Eng. 1968; LAH Dub. 1969. Specialist (Rheum.) New Cross Hosp. Wolverhampton. Prev: GP Shifnal; Regist. (Paediat.) & SHO (Orthop. & Paediat.) Wolverhampton Gp. Hosps.

SERHAN, Jonathan Timur Findon, Haughton Lane, Shifnal TF11 8HG — MB ChB Ed. 1998; MB ChB Ed 1998.

SERIES, Hugh George Warneford Hospital, Warneford Lane, Headington, Oxford OX3 7JX Tel: 01865 226263 — MB BS Lond. 1984; MA Oxf. 1984; MRCPsych 1990; DM Oxford 1996. Cons. Psychiat. (Old Age) Oxon. Ment. Healthcare NHS Trust. Specialty: Geriat. Psychiat. Prev: Sen. Regist. Rotat. Oxf.; Hon. Sen. Regist. (Psychiat.) Warneford Hosp. Oxf.; Wellcome Train. Fell. Univ. Johns Hopkins Baltimore, USA & Oxf.

SERIES, John Julian Dumbarton District Laboratory, Vale of Leven District General Hospital, Alexandria G83 0UA Tel: 01389 754121 — MB BChir Camb. 1981.

SERIGHT, Mr William (retired) The Oaks, 44 Rotchell Park, Dumfries DG2 7RJ Tel: 01387 252020 — (Glas.) MB ChB Glas. 1946; FRCS Ed. 1952; FRCS Glas. 1972. Prev: Sen. Cons. Surg. Dumfries & Galloway Roy. Infirm.

SERIKI, Dare Mutiyu 518 Claremont Road, Rusholme, Manchester M14 5WA — MB ChB Leeds 1995.

SERJEANT, Mrs Marion Keith (retired) Summerhill Cottage, Denhead, St Andrews KY16 8PA Tel: 01334 850211 — MB ChB Ed. 1940; DTM & H Eng. 1942. Prev: Welf. Off. Wom. & Childr. Mukalla, E. Aden.

SERLE, Elisabeth Christian Mission Hospital, Sarenea Village & Post Office, Sarenea, Bankura District, West Bengal 722150, India; 3 Oakfern Drive Stewartfield, East Kilbride, Glasgow G74 4UF Tel: 0135 526 5321 — MB ChB Aberd. 1980; MRCOG 1986; MD Aberd. 1994. Med. Off. in Obst & Gyn. Rural India. Specialty: Obst. & Gyn. Prev: Research fell. Jessop Hosp. Sheff.; Sen. Reg. Obst & Gyn. St Mary Hosp. Mans.

SERLIN, Matthew Jeremy 32 Westbourne Road, Birkdale, Southport PR8 2JA — MB ChB Birm. 1971; MD (Hons.) Birm. 1980 (Univ. Birm. MD Prize); MRCP (UK) 1974; FRCP Lond. 1991. Cons. Phys. Southport & Formby Dist. Gen. Hosp. Specialty: Respirat. Med. Socs: Brit. Thorac. Soc. Prev: Lect. (Clin. Pharmacol.) Univ. Liverp.; Hon. Sen. Regist. (Med.) Roy. Liverp. Hosp.

SERMIN, Nicola Hilary John Elliott Unit, Birch Hill Hospital, Rochdale OL12 9QB Tel: 01706 754305 — MB ChB Manch. 1984; MRCPsych 1991. Cons. of Psychiat. (Learning Disabil.) John Elliott Univ. Birch Hill Hosp. Rochdale. Specialty: Gen. Psychiat. Prev: Sen. Regist. & Regist. (Psychiat. Ment. Handicap) NW RHA.

SERPELL, Michael Graham University Department of Anasthesia, 30 Shelley Court, Gartnavel General, 1053 Great Western Road, Glasgow G12 0YN Tel: 0141 211 2069 Fax: 0141 211 3466 Email: mgserpell@cheerful.com; Dalarne, Pier Road, RHU, Helensburgh G84 8LJ Tel: 01436 820492 — MB ChB Dundee 1983; FRCA 1989. Sen. Lect. Univ. Dept. of Anaesth. Glas.; Lect. Sch. Podiatry Caladonian Univ. Specialty: Anaesth.; Research. Socs: Sec. N. Brit. Pain Assn. (Ex-Sec. & Counc. Mem.); W Scot. Pain Gp. (Ex-Sec. & Counc. Mem.); Roy. Soc. Med. Prev: Sen. Regist. (Anaesth.) Ninewells Hosp. & Med. Sch. Dundee.; Pain Fell. Dartmouth Hitchcock Med. Center Hanover, NH, USA.

SERRA MESTRES, Jordi Wodland Centre, Hillingdon Hospital, Pield Heath Road, Uxbridge UB8 3NN Email: jordi.serra-mestres@thh.nhs.uk — LMS U Autonoma Barcelona 1989; MRCPsych 1996. Specialist Regist. (Psychiat.) Char. Cross. Higher Psychiat. Train. Scheme Lond.; Hon. Research Asst. Dept. Neuropsychiat. Inst. Neurol. Lond. Specialty: Gen. Psychiat.; Geriat. Psychiat. Prev: Clin. Research Fell. (Neuropsychiat.) Qu. Mary & Westfield Coll. & Inst. Neurol. Lond.; SHO (Psychiat. & Regist.) Fulbourn Hosp. & Addenbrooke's NHS Trust Camb.

SERRANO GARCIA, Jose Antonio Department of Accident & Emergency, Conquest Hospital, The Ridge, St Leonards-on-Sea TN37 7RD — LMS Saragossa 1995.

SERRELL, Iain Robert Ash Lodge Medical Centre, 73 Old Road, Chesterfield S40 2RA Tel: 01246 203138 Fax: 01246 231824 — MB ChB Manch. 1977; DRCOG 1981; MRCGP 1982. Clin. Asst. Ment. Handicap. Socs: Roy. Coll. Gen. Pract.

SERVANT, Mr Christopher Terence Jackson Ipswich Hospital, Heath Road, Ipswich IP4 5PD — MB BS Lond. 1990 (St Bart.) BSc (Hons.) Lond. 1987; FRCS Eng. 1995; FRCS (Tr & Orth) 2002. Cons. (Orthop.) Ipswich Hosp. Specialty: Orthop. Socs: Assn. Mem. Brit. Orthop. Assn.; Brit. Trauma Soc.; Brit. Orthop. Sports Trauma Assn. Prev: Regist. (Orthop.) Roy. United Hosp. Bath; SHO (Orthop.) Roy. United Hosp. Bath; SHO (Gen. Surg.) Roy. Lond. Hosp.

SERVANT, John Byron Christmas Maltings Surgery, Camps Road, Haverhill CB9 8HF Tel: 01440 702010 Fax: 01440 714761; 60 Lion Meadow, Steeple Bumpstead, Haverhill CB9 7BY — MB ChB Dundee 1978. Specialty: Gen. Pract.

SERVICE, Elaine 8 Bleasdale Road, Bolton BL1 5QS — MB BS Lond. 1991; MRCPCH 1999. Specialist Regist. Paediat. Roy. Lancs. Infirm. Specialty: Paediat.

SERVICE, Margaret Ann Whittle Surgery, 199 Preston Road, Whittle-le-Woods, Chorley PR6 7PS Tel: 01257 262383 Fax: 01257 261019; 2 Juniper Croft, Clayton le Woods, Chorley PR6 7UF — MB ChB Manch. 1987; DCH RCP Lond. 1990; MRCGP 1991; DRCOG 1991.

SESHAPPA, Vasanth Bag Lane Surgery, 32 Bag Lane, Atherton, Manchester M46 0EE Tel: 01942 896489 Fax: 01942 888793 — MB BS Osmania 1971; MB BS Osmania 1971.

SET, Patricia Ai Khoon 6 Beaumont Crescent, Cambridge CB1 8QA — MB BS Lond. 1985; MRCP UK 1989; MRCP (UK) 1989; FRCR 1991; FRCR 1991; MA 2000. Cons. (Radiol.) New Addenbrooke's Hosp. Camb. Specialty: Radiol.

SETCHELL, Mr Marcus Edward (cons. rooms), 149 Harley St., London W1G 6DE Tel: 020 7935 4444 Fax: 020 7486 3446; 64 Wood Vale, London N10 3DN Tel: 020 8444 5266 — (Camb. & St. Bart.) MB Camb. 1968, BChir 1967; MRCS Eng. LRCP Lond. 1967; FRCOG 1984, M 1972; FRCS Ed. 1973; FRCS Eng. 1974. Surg. Gyn. to HM the Qu.; Cons. Obst. & Gyn Whittington Hosp., Lond. & Kiing Edwd. VII Hosp.; Examr. Univ. Lond., Univ. Camb. & RCOG. Specialty: Obst. & Gyn. Socs: Fell. (Past Counc. Mem.) Fell. Roy. Soc. Med.; Brit. Fertil. Soc.; Eur. Endoscopic Surg. Soc. Prev: Sen. Regist. (O & G) Soton. Gen. Hosp.; Regist. (Surg.) Torbay Hosp. Torquay; Ho. Surg. (Gyn.) Churchill Hosp. Oxf.

SETH, A K The Surgery, 142 Marshland Road, Moorends, Doncaster DN8 4SU Tel: 01405 740094 Fax: 01405 741063 — MB BS Calcutta 1967; MB BS Calcutta 1967.

SETH, Anil Department of Anaesthesia, Royal Preston Hospital, Sharoe Green Lane, Preston PR2 9HT Tel: 01772 716565 Fax: 01772 710162 — MB ChB Manch. 1975; FFA RCS Eng. 1982. Cons. Anaesth. Roy. Preston Hosp. Specialty: Anaesth. Socs: MRCAnaesth. & Assn. Anaesth. Prev: Sen. Regist. (Anaesth.) Mersey RHA; Regist. (Anaesth.) West. Infirm. Glas.

SETH, Ashok University Department of Cardiovascular Medicine, Queen Elizabeth Medical Centre, Edgbaston, Birmingham B15 2TH Tel: 0121 472 1311 — MB BS Aligarh 1979; MB BS Aligarh Muslim 1979; MRCP (UK) 1984; MRCPI 1986. Clin. Research Fell./Regist. Univ. Dept. Cardiol. Qu. Eliz. Med. Centre Birm. Specialty: Cardiol. Prev: Regist. (Gen. Med. & Cardiol.) Good Hope Gen. Hosp. Birm.; SHO (Med. Rotat.) Wordsley Hosp. Stourbridge.

SETH, Chhama Handsworth Medical Centre, 1 Fitzalan Road, Sheffield S13 9AW Tel: 0114 269 3044 — MB BS Lucknow 1969 (G.S.V.M. Med. Coll. Kanpur)

SETH, Harvansh Kishore (retired) 3 Ashton Close, Oadby, Leicester LE2 5WH Tel: 0116 271 4211 Fax: 0116 271 4984 — MB BS Lucknow 1952 (King Geo. Med. Coll.) DMRE Lucknow 1954. Prev: Phys. (Geriat. Med.) Leicester Gen. Hosp.

SETH, Kesho Nath Baker Street Surgery, Baker Street, Fenton, Stoke-on-Trent ST4 3AG Tel: 01782 45666; 9 Roe Lane, Newcastle ST5 3PL — MB BS Lucknow 1967.

SETH, Pearlita 69 Baring Road, London SE12 0JS — MB ChB Leic. 1983; DFFP 1993. Sessional Clin. Med. Off. Optimum Health Serv. NHS Trust Lond. Specialty: Family Plann. & Reproduc. Health.

SETH, Pramod Chandra Handsworth Medical Centre, 1 Fitzalan Road, Sheffield S13 9AW Tel: 0114 269 3044 — MB BS Lucknow 1967.

SETH, Priya Vallabh 58 Cecil Avenue, Barking IG11 9TF — BM Soton. 1976.

SETH, Ram Vallabh Hithergreen Hospital, Hithergreen Lane, London SE13 6RU Tel: 020 8698 4611 Fax: 020 8698 5655 — BM Soton. 1981; MRCPsych. 1987. Cons. Gen. Psychiat. Guy's & Lewisham Trust. Specialty: Gen. Psychiat. Socs: Brit. Assn. Psychopharmacol. Prev: Sen. Regist. Rotat. (Psychiat.) Maudsley Hosp. & St. Mary's Hosp Lond.; Regist. (Psychiat.) Char. Cross Hosp. Lond.

SETH, Ramendra Nath (retired) 592 Derby Road, Adams Hill, Nottingham NG7 2GZ Tel: 0115 978 6956; 592 Derby Road, Adams Hill, Nottingham NG7 2GZ Tel: 0115 978 6956 — (M.Azad Medical College, New Delhi, India) FRCS Edin. 1969; MB BS Delhi Univ. 1964. Surg. to the Family Plann. Assn.; Specialist in Erectile DysFunc. Prev: GP in Notts (Retd.).

SETH, Sarah Abigail 18 Hartington Place, Edinburgh EH10 4LE — MB ChB Ed. 1996.

SETH, Vir Royal Surrey County Hospital, Egerton Road, Guildford GU2 7XX Tel: 01483 571122 — MB BS Delhi 1972 (Maulana Azad Med. Coll.) MRCP (UK) 1977; FRCP Lond. 1995. Cons. Phys. Geriat. Med. SW Surrey Health Dist. Specialty: Care of the Elderly. Prev: Sen. Regist. (Geriat. Med.) Ipswich & E. Suff. Health Dist.; Regist. (Gen. Med.) Barnsley Dist. Gen. Hosp.

SETH-SMITH, Mr Alan Brian (retired) Les Merriennes, St Martin's, Guernsey GY4 6RN Tel: 01481 36811 — MB BS Lond. 1950 (Lond. Hosp.) FRCS Eng. 1956. Prev: Cons. Surg. Princess Eliz. Hosp. Guernsey.

SETHI, Amarjit Singh St Bartholomews Hospital, West Smithfield, London EC1A 7BE; 301 Brompton Park Crescent, Seagrave Road, Fulham, London SW6 1SP — MB BS Lond. 1992 (UMDS Guy's & St. Thos.) BSc Lond. 1989; MRCP (UK) 1995. Regist. Rotat. (Cardiol.) St. Bart. Hosp. Lond. Specialty: Cardiol. Socs: BMA; Roy. Soc. Trop. Med. & Hyg. Prev: Regist. King Geo. Hosp. Ilford; SHO (Med.) Lond. Chest Hosp.; SHO (Med.) Roy. Brompton Nat. Heart & Lung Hosp.

SETHI, Anthony Krishen (retired) 7 Park Avenue, Cheadle, Stoke-on-Trent ST10 1LZ Tel: 01538 755520 Fax: 01538 756825 — MB ChB Birm. 1962; DObst RCOG 1964. Prev: GP & Asst. Postgrad. Tutor Stoke-on-Trent.

SETHI, Mr Charanjit Singh 9 Lambourn Way, Chatham ME5 8PU; 91 Brompton Park Crescent, Seagrave Road, Fulham, London SW6 1SP Tel: 020 7610 1488 — MB BS Lond. 1994 (United Med. & Dent. Sch. Guy's & St. Thos. Hosp. Lond.) BSc (Hons.) Lond. 1991; FRCOphth. Lond. 1998. Vitreo-Retinal Research Regist. Moorfields Eye Hosp. Specialty: Ophth. Socs: Fell. Roy. Soc. Med.; BMA. Prev: SHO (Ophth.) Bristol Eye Hosp.

SETHI, Dinesh Health Policy Unit, London School Of Hygiene & Tropical Medicine, Kepple Street, London WC1E 7HT Tel: 020 7927 2122 Fax: 020 7637 5391; 43 St Helen's Gardens, London W10 6LN — MB ChB Liverp. 1990 (Liverpool) MD Liverp. 1990, MB ChB 1980; MRCP (UK) 1984; MSc (Lond. Sch. Hyg. & Trop. Med.) Lond. 1994; MFPHM 1996. Lect. Internat. Pub. Health & P.H. Med. Lon. Sch. Hyg. & Trop. Med. Specialty: Pub. Health Med. Socs: Fac. Pub. Health Med.; Renal Assn. Prev: Lect. Char. Cross Hosp. Lond.; Sen. Regist. (Pub. Health Med.) Wolfson Inst. Preven. Med. Lond.

SETHI, Gulshan 4 Cotman Drive, Marple Bridge, Stockport SK6 5DL — MB ChB Leeds 1997.

SETHI, Mr Inder Singh (retired) 30 Marchbank Drive, Cheadle SK8 1QY Tel: 0161 491 1142 Fax: 0161 428 5761 — MB BS Punjab, India 1955 (Med. Coll. Amritsar) FRCS Ed. 1966; FRCS Eng. 1966. Prev: Clin. Asst. (A & E) Stockport AHA.

SETHI, Jasbir Kaur Lordswood Health Centre, Sultan Road, Lordswood, Chatham ME5 8TJ Tel: 01634 666996; 9 Lambourn Way, Lordswood, Chatham ME5 8PU — MB BS Nagpur 1968 (Nagpur Med. Coll.) DCH Eng. 1976. Med. Off. (Child Health & Community Med.) Medway Health Dist. Specialty: Paediat. Socs: BMA; Fac. Community Health. Prev: SHO (Anaesth.) Middlesbrough Gen. Hosp.; SHO (Anaesth.) Roy. Halifax Infirm.; SHO (Paediat.) Gravesend & N. Kent Hosp.

SETHI, Jasminder Kaur Silver Birches, 53C Gordon Avenue, Stanmore HA7 3QN Tel: 020 8954 6743 Fax: 020 8537 8701 — MB BS Lond. 1981 (St. Thos.) Specialty: Obst. & Gyn.; Paediat.; Family Planning. Prev: Course Organiser Edgware Gen. Hosp. VTS.

SETHI, Krishna K 39 College Way, Hayes UB3 3DZ Tel: 0208 573 2365 — MB BS 1967 (Punjab University Amritsar, India) FRCOG 1999 Roy. Coll. of Obst. & Gyn., Lond.; MRCOG 1974 Roy. Coll. of Obst. & Gynacology, Lond.; LF Hom (Med) 1999. Specialty: Gen. Pract.; Homeop. Med.; Acupunc. Socs: Med. Protec. Soc.; Brit. Menopause Soc.; Nat. Osteoporosis Soc.

SETHI, Kulwant Bir Singh, OBE, TD, OStJ, Col. late RAMC Highwood, Endon, Stoke-on-Trent ST9 9AR Tel: 01538 385088 Fax: 01538 385088 — (Med. Coll. Amritsar, Punjab India) BSc Agra 1954; MB BS Punjab, India 1959; DLO Eng. 1964; FICS 1965; MRCGP 1977; FRCGP 1998. Trainer (Gen. Pract.) Stoke-on-Trent; DL Staffs. Specialty: Otolaryngol. Socs: Fell. Roy. Soc. Med. & Arts. Prev: Sen. Resid. NW Univ. Med. Sch. Chicago, USA; Co. 224 Field Ambul. RAMC (V); Hon. Col. RAMC.

SETHI, Padam Chand Child Guidance Clinic, 6 Southey Road, Worthing BN11 3HT; White Oaks, 4 Sea Drive, Ferring, Worthing BN12 5HD — MB BS Rajasthan 1968; DPM Ed. & Glas. 1972; MRCPsych 1973. Cons. Psychiat. Child & Adolesc. Psychiat. Child Guid. Clinic Worthing. Specialty: Child & Adolesc. Psychiat. Prev: Cons. Psychiat. Stratheden Hosp. Cupar; Sen. Regist. (Child & Adolesc. Psychiat.) Univ. Hosp. Wales Child & Family Centre Cardiff; Sen. Regist. (Psychiat.) Botleys Pk. Hosp. Chertsey.

SETHI, Permindar 62 Grange Park Avenue, London N21 2LL — MB BS Lond. 1996.

SETHI, Pradeep Pennine Acute Hospitals Trust, Fairfield Hospital, Rochdale Road, Bury BL9 7TD Tel: 0161 705 3873 Fax: 0161 705 3707; 29 Fairhaven Avenue, Whitefield, Manchester M45 7QG — MB BS Panjab 1977; MRCP (UK) 1982; FRCP 1999. Cons. Phys. (Geriat. Med.) Pennine Acute Hosps. Trust. Specialty: Gen. Med.; Care of the Elderly. Socs: BGS. Prev: Cons. Phys. (Geriat. Med.) Fairfield & Bury Gen. Hosps. Bury.; Sen. Regist. (Geriat.) & (Gen. Med. Rotat.) Manch. Gp. Hosps.

SETHI, Rohit Phoenix Surgery, 9 Chesterton Lane, Cirencester GL7 1XG Tel: 01285 652056 Fax: 01285 641562; Laverton House, Fairford GL7 4AB Tel: 01285 711180 Email: rohit@ciren44.freeserve.co.uk — BM BS Nottm. 1983; BMedSci Nottm. 1981, BM BS 1983; DA Eng. 1985; MRCGP 1988. Princip. GP; Doctor to Roy. Agricultural Coll.; Hosp. Pract. (Anaesth.) Cirencester Hosp.; Med. Dir. In Touch with Health. Specialty: Anaesth.

SETHI, Mr Tapan Deep Singh — MB BS Lond. 1999; MRCS Eng. 2003. Specialist Regist. Robt. Jones & Agnes Hunt Orthop. Hosp. Oswestry. Specialty: Trauma & Orthop. Surg. Socs: RSM. Prev: Spinal Research Fell. Univ. Hosp. N. Staffs.

SETHI, Tariq Jabbar 10 Queen's Gate Place, London SW7 5NX — MB BS Lond. 1983; BSc Lond. 1978; BA Camb. 1980, MA 1984; MRCPI 1989; MRCP (UK) 1989. Clin. Fell. Imperial Cancer Research Fund. Prev: SHO (Gen. Med.) Hammersmith Hosp. Lond.; Lect. (Gen. Med.) Guy's Hosp. Lond.; Regist. (Respirat. Med. & Cardiol.) St. Mary's Hosp. Lond.

SETHIA, Babulal Royal Brompton Hospital, Sydney Street, London SW3 6NP Tel: 020 7351 6550 Fax: 020 7351 3214 Email: b.sethia@rbh.nthames.nhs.uk — MB BS Lond. 1975 (St Thomas' Hosp., Univ. of Lond.) FRCS Eng. 1981. Cons. Cardiac Surg., Roy. Brompton Hosp., Lond. Specialty: Cardiothoracic Surg. Special Interest: Congen. heart Surg. Prev: Cons. Cardiac Surg., Birminham Childrens Hosp.

SETHIA, Mr Krishna Kumar Hedenham Hall Farm, Hedenham, Bungay NR35 2LG — MB BS Lond. 1979; FRCS Lond. 1984; DM Oxon. 1990. Cons. Urol. Norf. & Norwich Hosp. Specialty: Urol.

SETHNA, Edulji Rustumji (retired) 32 Little Sutton Lane, Sutton Coldfield B75 6PB Email: eddysethna@virgin.net — MB BS Bombay 1951; FRCP Lond. 1987, M 1956; DTM & H Liverp. 1958; DPM Eng. 1963; FRCPsych 1986, M 1971. Prev: Cons. Psychiat. Hollymoor Hosp. Birm. & Lyndon Clinic Solihull.

SETHU, Parayath Rosewood Medical Centre, 30 Astra Close, Hornchurch RM12 5NJ Tel: 01708 554557 Fax: 01708 554212 — MB BS Kerala 1968 (Med. Coll. Trivandrum) Specialty: Gen. Med. Prev: Regist. Rush Green Hosp. Romford.

SETHUGAVALAR, Chinnadurai 43 Sylvan Way, Redhill RH1 4DE — MB BS Mysore 1978; LRCP LRCS Ed. LRCPS Glas. 1981. SHO (O & G) Torbay Hosp. Torquay. Prev: SHO (Gyn.) St. Jas. Hosp. Lond.; SHO (O & G) Southmead Hosp. Bristol; SHO (O & G) Roy. Gwent Hosp. Newport.

SETHURAJAN, Anjana 38 Emlyn Road, Stamford Brook, London W12 9TD Tel: 020 8740 0192 — MB ChB Glas. 1991; DCH RCP Lond. 1994; DRCOG 1994; MRCGP 1995. Specialty: Gen. Pract.

SETHURAJAN, Shantha Grove Park Surgery, 95 Burlington Lane, Chiswick, London W4 3ET Tel: 020 8747 1549 Fax: 020 8995 9529; 40 Emlyn Road, London W12 9TD Tel: 020 8743 5294 — MB BS Lond. 1994; DCH; DRCOG; BSc Lond. 1991.

SETIA, Rama (Surgery), 143 Rookwood Avenue, Leeds LS9 0NL Tel: 0113 249 3011; The Manor, Manor House Lane, Leeds LS17 9JD Tel: 0113 269 7197 — MB BS Delhi 1965 (Maulana Azad Med. Coll.) DMRT Eng. 1971. Prev: Ho. Surg. (O & G) Irwin Hosp. New Delhi, India; Regist. (Radiother.) Regional Radiother. Centre Cookridge Hosp. Leeds; Clin. Med. Off. Leeds AHA (T).

SETIYA, Megharaj Sukharaj Marfleet Lane Surgery, 358 Marfleet Lane, Hull HU9 5AD Tel: 01482 781032 Fax: 01482 789180; 7 Northwood Drive, Tranby Park, Jenny Brough Lane, Hessle HU13 0TA — (B.J. Med. Coll. Pune, India) MB BS Bombay 1959; DLO RCS Eng. 1964; DObst.RCOG 1966. Mem. Disabil. Appeals Tribunal; Med. Adviser to Social Security Appeals Tribunals. Specialty: Care of the Elderly; Otorhinolaryngol.; Obst. & Gyn. Socs: Hull Med. Soc.; DRCOG. Prev: Clin. Asst. (Med. for Elderly) Hull; Clin. Asst. Matern. Hosp. Hull; Regist. (ENT) N. Staffs. Roy. Infirm. Stoke-on-Trent.

SETNA, Farokh Jal Department of Radiology, Arrowe Park Hospital, Arrowe Park Road, Upton, Wirral CH49 5PE Tel: 0151 678 5111 Fax: 0151 604 1068; 43 Manvers Road, Childwall, Liverpool L16 3NP Email: 106113.1540@compuserve.com — MB BS Punjab, Pakistan 1981 (King Edwd. Med. Coll. Lahore, Pakistan) BSc Punjab 1975; FFR RCSI (I) Dub. 1991. Staff Radiol. Arrowe Pk. Hosp. Wirral. Specialty: Radiol. Prev: Sen. Regist. (Radiol.) Arrowe Pk. Hosp. Wirral; Sen. Regist. (Radiol.) Whiston Hosp. Prescot, Aintree Hosp. Liverp., Warrington Gen. Hosp. & Roy. Liverp. Univ. Hosp.

SETON, Alexander (retired) 20 Horsemarket, Kelso TD5 7HA Tel: 01573 2531 — MB ChB Glas. 1930. Prev: Ho. Surg. Hartlepools Hosp.

SETON, Dorothy Lyall (retired) 15 Queen's Road, Aberdeen AB15 4YL Tel: 01224 322624 — MB ChB St. And. 1925.

SETT, Mr Pradipkumar Clinical Director, Northwest Regional Spinal Injuries Centre, Southport & Formby District General Hospital, Southport PR8 6NJ Tel: 01704 547471 Fax: 01704 543156 — MB BS Calcutta 1972; MS Calcutta 1976; FRCS Ed. 1978; FRCS (SN) 1988. Clin. Dir. NW Regional Spinal Injuries Centre Southport & Formby Dist. Gen. Hosp.; Hon. Lect. (Neurosci.) Univ. of Liverp. Specialty: Neurosurg.; Orthop. Socs: Soc. Brit. Neurosurgs.; Brit. Cervical Spine Soc.; Internat. Med. Soc. Paraplegia.

SETTATREE, Ralph Stewart Solihull Women's Unit, Solihull Hospital, Birmingham B91 2JL Tel: 0121 424 4392 Fax: 0121 424 5389 Email: ralph.settatree@heartsol.wmids.nhs.uk; Fox House, 14 Ashford Road, Cheltenham GL50 2QZ Tel: 01242 701166 Email: ralph.settatree@blueyonder.co.uk.com — (Guy's) MB BS Lond. 1969; MRCS Eng. LRCP Lond. 1969; FRCOG 1990, M 1977, DObst 1971. Cons. O & G Birm. Heartlands & Solihull NHS Trust. Specialty: Obst. & Gyn. Socs: BMA; (Ex-Treas.) Birm. & Midl. Obst. & Gyn. Soc.; (Conf. Comm.) Brit. Matern. and Fetal Med. Soc. Prev: Clin. Dir. Confidential Enquiry into Stillbirths & Deaths in Infancy; Director, W. Mids. Perinatal Audit.; MOH Dist. Hosp. Marsabit, Kenya.

SETTERFIELD, Jane Frances St. John's Institute of Dermatology, St. Thomas' Hospital, Lambeth Palace Road, London SE1 7EH Tel: 020 7928 9292 Fax: 020 7922 8232; 40 Roanalds Road, Highbury, London N5 1XG Tel: 020 7609 3749 — (Univ. Coll. Hosp.) BDS Lond. 1980; LDS RCS Eng. 1981; MB BS Lond. 1987; DCH RCP Lond. 1989; MRCGP 1991; DRCOG 1991; MRCP (UK) 1993. Specialist Regist. (Dermatol.) St John's Inst. Dermatol. St. Thos. & Guy's Hosp. Lond. Specialty: Dermat. Socs: Train. Mem. Brit. Assn. Dermat. Prev: Clin. Research Fell. St. John's Inst. Dermat. St. Thos. Hosp. Lond.; SHO (Dermat.) St. John's Inst. Dermat. St. Thos. Hosp. Lond.

SETTLE, Christopher David Department of Microbiology, Sunderland Royal Hospital, Kayll Road, Sunderland SR4 7TP — MB ChB Ed. 1990.

SETTLE, Frances Caroline 1 Meadow Way, Leeds LS17 7QY — MB ChB Sheff. 1991.

SETTLE, Paul 11 Old Hall Lane, Westhoughton, Bolton BL5 2HQ — MB ChB Manch. 1992.

SETTLE, Vera (retired) 56 Greenfield Road, Stafford ST17 0PU — MB ChB Manch. 1941; BSc Manch. 1938; DCH Eng. 1942. Prev: Asst. MOH (Matern. & Child Welf.) Manch.

SETTY, Guduthur Roopa 20 St Michael's Avenue, South Shields NE33 3AN — MB ChB Dundee 1995.

SETTY, Matta Venkataramanaiah S Stanhope Surgery, 85 Kildown Close, Stanhope, Ashford TN23 5SU Tel: 01233 636816 Fax: 01233 662188; 2 Summerhill Park, Hythe Road, Willesborough, Ashford TN24 0TG Tel: 01233 636816 Fax: 01233 503606 — MB BS Bangalor 1971 (Bangalore)

SETTY, Pathiyappa Hallur Raghavendra Countess of Chester Hospital, Liverpool Road, Chester CH2 1UL Tel: 01244 365000 Fax: 01244 365435; 19 Deva Lane, Upton, Chester CH2 1BN Tel: 01244 364766 Fax: 01244 375794 — MB BS Mysore 1972 (Govt. Med. Coll. Mysore) DA Eng. 1984. Cons. Anaesth. Co. of Chester Hosp. Chesh. Specialty: Anaesth. Prev: Assoc. Specialist Barnsley; Regist. Doncaster & Barnsley.

SETTY, Shubha 55 Wellington Avenue, Wavetree, Liverpool L15 0EH — MB ChB Liverp. 1996.

SEVAR, Raymond 26 Whiteclosegate, Carlisle CA3 0JD Tel: 01228 531691 — BSc St. And. 1976; MB ChB Manch 1979; DCH RCP Lond. 1981; MRCGP 1983; MFHOM 1994. Homoeop. Phys.; 1999 Med. Examr., Fac. of Homoeopathy. Specialty: Homeop. Med. Prev: 1994 Lect., Acad. Depts, Glas. Homoeop. Hosp.

SEVENOAKS, Michael Ron Old Cottage Hospital Surgery, Alexandra Road, Epsom KT17 4BL Tel: 01372 724434 Fax: 01372 748171 — MB BS Lond. 1989; BSc (Hons.) Lond. 1986; DRCOG 1993; DFFP 1994; MRCGP 1994.

SEVENOAKS, Tamsin Alexandra The Surgery, Tanners Meadow, Brockham, Betchworth RH3 7NJ Tel: 01306 631242 — MB BS Lond. 1989; DFFP 1994. GP Princip., Dr Kober and Partners.

SEVER, Peter Sedgwick Department of Clinical Pharmacology, NHLI at St Mary's Hospital, Imperial College of Science, Technology & Medicine, London W2 1NY Tel: 020 7886 1117 Fax: 020 7886 6145 — MRCS Eng. LRCP Lond. 1968 (Camb.) MB Camb. 1969, BChir 1968; MRCP (UK) 1971; PhD Lond. 1975; FRCP Lond. 1981. Prof. Clin. Pharmacol. & Therap. & Hon. Cons. Phys. St. Mary's Hosp. Lond. Specialty: Pharmacology. Socs: Fell. Europ. Soc. Cardiol.; (Ex-Pres.) Brit. Hypertens. Soc.; Pres. Elect Europ. Counc. High Blood Pressure & Cardiovasc. Res. Prev: Sen. Lect. (Med.) & Hon. Cons. Phys. St. Mary's Hosp. Lond.; Jun. Research Fell. Med. Research Counc.; Lect. (Med. & Pharmacol.) St. Marys Hosp. Med. Sch. Lond.

SEVERN, Alison Ninewells Hospital, Renal Unit, Dundee DD1 9SY Tel: 01382 660111 Email: alison.severn@tuht.scot.nhs.uk — MB BS Lond. 1983; MRCP (UK) 1986; PhD Lond. 1991; FRCP 2003. Cons. Nephrol. Ninewells Hosp. Dundee. Specialty: Nephrol. Special Interest: Diabetic Renal Dis.; Peritoneal Dialysis; Vasc. Access. Prev: Regist. (Renal Med.) Dulwich Hosp. Lond.; Regist. (Renal & Gen. Med.) Roy. Sussex Co. Hosp. Brighton; SHO (Renal Med.) Dulwich Hosp. Lond.

SEVERN, Andrew Moore Morcambe Bay Hospitals NHS Trust, Ashton Road, Lancaster LA1 4RP Tel: 01254 583528 Email: andrew.severn@rli.mbht.nhs.uk — MB BS Newc. 1981; MA Camb. 1982; FRCA 1987. Cons. Anaesth. Lancaster. Specialty: Anaesth. Socs: Age Anaestheisia Assn.; Pain Soc. Prev: Sen. Regist. (Anaesth.) Manch.

SEVERN, Michael (retired) Department of Microbiology, General Hospital, Northampton NN1 5BD — MB ChB Birm. 1961; FRCPath. 1982, M 1971. Prev: Asst. Bact. Pub. Health Laborat. Radcliffe Infirm. Oxf.

SEVERS, Professor Martin Peter Portsmouth Institute of Medicine Health & Social Care, St George's Building, 141 High Street, Portsmouth PO1 2HY Tel: 023 9284 5247 Fax: 023 9284 5326 — MB BS Lond. 1980 (St Mary's) MRCP (UK) 1984; FRCP Lond. 1992; FFPHM (Hon.) 1999. Prof. of Healthcare for Older People Univ. Portsmouth; Cons. Geriat. E. Hants. PCT. Specialty: Care of the Elderly; Educat.; Research. Special Interest: Health Informatics; Serv. Design & Developm. Socs: Brit. Geriat. Soc. Prev: Chairm. Roy. Coll. Phys. Med. Informat. Technol. Comm.; Chairm. Conf. of Med. Roy. Coll. & their Fac. in UK Informat. Advis. Gp.; Sen. Regist. & Lect. (Geriat. Med.) Portsmouth & Soton.

SEVERS, Paul Hirst 74 Skipton Road, Keighley BD20 9LL — MB BS Newc. 1977 (Newcastle) MFCH 1989; FRIPHH 1996. SCMO Airedale HA; Med Ref. to Skipton Cremat. Socs: SPH.(Fell). Prev: Clin. Med. Off. (Child Health) N.d. AHA; Clin. Med. Off. Newc. AHA (T); Trainee GP Northumbria VTS.

SEVILLE, Malcolm Heywood 6 Lansdowne Road, Bare, Morecambe LA4 6AL Tel: 01524 418871 — MB BS Lond. 1974 (St. Thos.) Prev: Clin. Asst. Dermat. Beaumont Hosp. Lancaster.; Clin. Asst. Ophth. Garnett Clinic Lancaster; SHO Path. Roy. Lancaster Infirm.

SEVITT, Lewis Howard 27 Devonshire Place, London W1G 6JF Tel: 020 7636 3979 Fax: 020 7487 4295; 14 Queen Annes Gardens, Bedford Park, London W4 1TU Tel: 020 8994 1493 — MB BCh BAO Dub. 1962 (T.C. Dub.) BA Dub. 1960, MB BCh BAO 1962; FRCP Lond. 1979, M 1965. Cons. Phys. (Gen. Med.) Hillingdon HA; Hon. Sen. Lect. Roy. Postgrad. Med. Sch. Lond.; Assoc. Teach. St. Mary's Hosp. Med. Sch. Lond. Specialty: Gen. Med. Prev: Hon. Cons. Phys. Hammersmith Hosp. Lond.; Clin. Tutor Hillingdon HA; Sen. Regist. Dept. Med. (Renal Unit); Hammersmith Hosp. Lond.; SHO Med. Profess. & Renal Units Roy. Free Hosp. Lond.

SEVITT, Michael Andrew 7 Upper Park Road, Kingston upon Thames KT2 5LB Tel: 020 8546 8825 — (Univ. Coll. Hosp.) MA; MB Camb. 1969, BChir 1968; MRCP (U.K.) 1971; MRCPsych 1975; MInstGA 1979. Specialty: Child & Adolesc. Psychiat. Socs: UK Counc. Psychother.; Inst. for Gp. Anal.; Assn. for family Ther. Prev: Sen. Regist. (Child & Adolesc. Psychiat.) Wessex Unit for Childr. & Parents Portsmouth; Lect. (Psychiat.) Soton. Gen. Hosp.; Cons. Psychiat. Woodside Adolesc. Unit W. Pk. Hosp. Epsom.

SEWARD, Christopher Frederic Milford Medical Centre, Sea Road, Milford-on-Sea, Lymington SO41 0PG Tel: 01590 643022 Fax: 01590 644950 Email: c.f.seward@btinternet.com; Hillbrow, West Road, Milford-on-Sea, Lymington SO41 0NZ Tel: 01590 645730 Fax: 01590 644950 — BM BCh Oxf. 1974 (Middlx.) MA Oxf. 1974; MRCS Eng. LRCP Lond. 1974; DObst RCOG 1975. GP. Socs: Roy. Soc. Med.; BMA. Prev: SHO (O & G) Westm. Hosp.; Ho. Surg. Middlx. Hosp.; Ho. Phys. St. Albans City Hosp.

SEWARD, Helen Clare Mayday University Hospital, 530 London Rd, Thornton Heath, Croydon CR7 7YE Tel: 020 8401 3127 Fax: 020 8401 3489 Email: helen.seward@mayday.nhs.uk; Shirley Oaks Hospital, Poppy Lane, Shirley Oaks Village, Croydon CR9 8AB Tel: 020 8655 2255 — MB BCh BAO NUI 1976; DO RCS Eng. 1980; FRCS Eng. 1981; FRCOphth 1990. Cons. Ophth. Surg. Croydon Eye Unit; Mem. (Audit Comm.) Roy. Coll. Ophth.; Mem. Oxf. Ophth. Congr. Specialty: Ophth. Socs: BMA; (Counc.) UK ISCRS. Prev: Sen. Regist. West. Eye Hosp. & Moorfields; Regist. (Ophth.) Croydon Eye Unit Surrey; SHO Regional Neurosurg. Servs. Brook Hosp. Lond.

SEWARD, William Percival Castle Road, 1 - 2 Castle Road, Chirk, Wrexham LL14 5BS Tel: 01691 772434 Fax: 01691 773840; Grove House, Pontyblew, Chirk, Wrexham LL14 5BH — MB BS Lond. 1971; DObst RCOG 1973.

SEWART, John Hunter (retired) Slanning's House, Trematon, Saltash PL12 4RT Tel: 01752 846434 Fax: 01752 846434 — MB BChir Camb. 1952 (Univ. Coll. & Camb.) BA Camb. 1952; DPH Lond. 1958; DTM & H Liverp. 1961; DIH Soc. Apoth. Lond. 1968; MFCM 1973; MFOM RCP Lond. 1979. Prev: SCMO (Environm. Health) Cornw. & I. of Scilly HA.

SEWELL, Amanda Claire 18B Victoria Road, Netley Abbey, Southampton SO31 5DG Tel: 01580 200187 Fax: 01580 201443 — BM (Hons.) Soton. 1996. Specialty: Anaesth.

SEWELL, Elizabeth 95 Hunters Way, Uckfield TN22 2BB — MB ChB Otago 1989 (Otago, NZ) Dip. Obst. Auckland 1992; MRCGP 1995; DFFP 1995. Acad. Asst. (Gen. Pract.) St. Geo. Med. Sch. Specialty: Gen. Pract. Prev: Assoc. GP ISL Health Commiss. VTS; Trainee GP Maidstone VTS.

SEWELL, Eric Mansfield (retired) 19 Hinderton Drive, West Kirby, Wirral CH48 8BN Tel: 0151 625 5899 — MB ChB Glas. 1940; DPH Glas. 1948. Prev: Sen. Asst. Med. Off. Regional Transfus. Serv. Liverp.

SEWELL, Professor Herbert Fitzgerald Department of Immunology, Queens Medical Centre, University Hospital, Nottingham NG7 2UH Tel: 0115 970 9123 Fax: 0115 970 9125; 75 Oakland Avenue, Leicester LE4 7SG — MB ChB Leic. 1983; PhD Birm. 1978, MSc (Immunol.) 1975, BDS 1973; FRCPath (Immunol.) 1992, M 1980; FRCP Glas. 1989. M 1987. Prof. & Hon. Cons. Immunol. Univ. Hosp. Qu. Med. Centre Nottm. Specialty: Immunol. Prev: Sen. Lect. & Hon. Cons. Immunopath. Univ. Aberd. Med. Sch.

SEWELL, Joanne Margaret Monksfield Surgery, 1 Wimbourne Place, Daventry NN11 5XY Tel: 01327 877770 Fax: 01327 310267; 24 Moreton Drive, Buckingham MK18 1JQ — MB BS Lond. 1987; BSc (Hons.) Lond. 1984; DRCOG 1990; DCH RCP Lond. 1992; MRCGP 1993. Prev: Trainee GP W. Middlx. Hosp. Lond.; GP Princip. N. End Surg. Buckingham.

SEWELL, John Martin Alexander Royal Glamorgan Hospital, Ynysmaerdy, Llantrisant Tel: 01443 443600 Fax: 01443 443468; 7 New Hill Villas, Goodwick SA64 0DS — MB BCh Cantab. 1976 (Lond. Hosp.) DRCOG 1978; DObst 1978; MRCGP 1981; LMCC 1982; DA Eng. 1984; FRCA 1985. Cons. Anaesth., Roy. Glam. Hosp., Ynysmaerdy, Llantrisant; Relate Counsellor Swansea. Specialty: Anaesth. Socs: Obst. Anaesth. Assn.; Brit. Holistic Med. Assn.; Brit. Med. Acupunct. Soc. Prev: GP Brecon, Powys.

SEWELL, John Robin The William Harvey Hospital, Kennington Road, Willesborough, Ashford TN24 0LZ Tel: 01233 633331 Fax: 01233 616118; Fairlight Corner, 138 North Road, Hythe CT21 4AT Tel: 01303 265657 — MB BChir Camb. 1971 (Camb. & St. Thos.) MA Camb. 1970, MB BChir 1971; MRCP (UK) 1972; FRCP Lond. 1989; FRCP (UK) 1990. Cons. Phys. Rheum. & Rehabil. The William Harvey Hosp & Buckland Hosp. Dover. Specialty: Gen. Med.; Rheumatol.; Rehabil. Med. Socs: Brit. Soc. Rheum. Prev: Hon. Sen. Regist. (Med.) Hammersmith Hosp. Lond.; Lect. Roy. Postgrad. Med. Sch. Lond.; Clin. & Research Asst. St. Thos. Hosp. Lond.

SEWELL, Matthew Stephen North Devon District Hospital, Raleigh Park, Barnstaple EX31 4JB Tel: 01271 22577; Hedna Cottage, Church Town, Parracombe, Barnstaple EX31 4RJ — MB BS Lond. 1981; MRCPsych 1986. Cons. Psychiat. (Special Responsibil. for Old Age Psychiat.) N. Devon Dist. Hosp. Specialty: Geriat. Psychiat.

SEWELL, Maxwell Stanley (retired) 145 Cranley Gardens, London N10 3AG Tel: 020 8883 4409 — MB ChB Leeds 1952. GP. Prev: Ho. Phys. (Dermat.) Newsham Gen. Hosp. Liverp.

SEWELL, Nigel Bernard 19 Cornaway Lane, Portchester, Fareham PO16 9DA — MB BS Lond. 1982.

SEWELL, Peter Francis John 32 Checkstone Avenue, Bessacarr, Doncaster DN4 7JX Tel: 01302 535766 — MB BS Lond. 1957 (Univ. Coll. Hosp.) BSc (Zool.) Lond. 1945, PhD 1949; FRCPath 1975, M 1963. Emerit. Cons. Doncaster Roy. Infirm. Specialty: Chem. Path. Socs: Hon. Mem. (Ex-Pres.) Assn. Clin. Biochem.; Emerit. Mem. Amer. Assn. Clin. Chem. Prev: Mem. Assn. Clin. Paths.; Vice-Chairm. Trent RHA; Cons. Clin. Chem. Doncaster HA.

SEWELL, Mr Peter Frederic Toyne Hinchingbrooke Hospital, Huntingdon PE18 8NT Tel: 01480 416416 — BA (Cantab.) 1966; BChir 1969; MB Camb. 1970; FRCS Ed. 1976. Cons. Orthop. Surg. Hinchingbrooke Hosp. Huntingdon. Specialty: Orthop. Socs: Brit. Hip Soc. Prev: Lt. Col. RAMC; Cons. Orthop. Surg. Princess Alexandra Hosp. Wroughton.

SEWELL, Rebecca Caroline Toyne Farthings, 10 Jeffs Close, Upper Tysoe, Warwick CV35 0TQ Tel: 01295 688051 — MB BS Lond. 1994 (Charing Cross & Westm. Hosps) MA Camb. 1995, BA 1991; MRCP (UK) 1998. SHO (Paediat.) Princess Alexandra Hosp. Haslow. Specialty: Paediat. Prev: SHO (Neonat.) Harold Wood Hosp. Romford; SHO (Paediat. Oncol.) St. Barts. Hosp. Lond.

SEWELL, Richard Norman Ash Trees Surgery, Market Street, Carnforth LA5 9JU Tel: 01524 720000 Fax: 01524 720110; Brooklands, 26 Hanging Green Lane, Hest Bank, Lancaster LA2 6JB Tel: 01524 823220 Fax: 01524 823220 — MB ChB Dundee 1982; DRCOG 1984; MRCGP 1986. Specialty: Occupat. Health.

SEWELL, Mr Robert Henry (retired) 4 Bayards, Warlingham CR6 9BP Tel: 01883 624343 — MB ChB Manch. 1943; MRCS Eng. LRCP Lond. 1943; FRCS Ed. 1948; BSc Manch. 1940, ChM 1949; FRCS Eng. 1950. Hon. Cons. Orthop. Surg. Greenwich Dist. Hosp. Prev: Sen. Regist. (Orthop.) Roy. Nat. Orthop. Hosp.

SEWELL, Ruth Alexandra Sewell Practice, 91 Kirkintilloch Road, Bishopbriggs, Glasgow G64 2AA Fax: 0141 762 3482; 16 Paterson Place, Bearsdon, Glasgow G61 4RU Tel: 0141 943 0729 — MB ChB Ed. 1979; DCH RCP Lond. 1983; T(GP) 1991. GP Partner. Specialty: Community Child Health. Prev: SHO (Paediat.) Soton. Gen. Hosp.; Trainee GP Aldermoor Soton.; Regist. (Paediat.) Falkirk & Stirling Roy. Infirms.

SEWELL, Stephen Peter Wroughton Health Centre, Barrett Way, Wroughton, Swindon SN4 9LW Tel: 01793 812221 Email: steve@westlecot.freeserve.co.uk; 38 Westlecot Road, Old Town, Swindon SN1 4HB Tel: 01793 497113 — BM Soton. 1990; DRCOG 1994; MRCGP 1995. Prev: GP/Regist. Wroughton; SHO (Paediat.) Princess Margt. Hosp. Swindon; SHO (Psychiat.) N. Birm. Hosp. Trust.

SEWELL, Professor William Arthur Carrock Path Links Immunology, Scunthorpe General Hospital, Scunthorpe DN15 7BH Tel: 01724 387820 Fax: 01724 865680 Email: carrock.sewell@nlg.nhs.uk — MB BS Newc. 1991; BMedSc (Hons.) Newc. 1988; MRCP (UK) 1994; DRCPath 1996; PhD UCL 2000; MRCPath 2001. Cons. Immunol. & Clin. Director Immunol.; Vis. Prof. of Immunol., Fac. of Life, Health & Social Sci., Univ. of Lincoln. Specialty: Immunol.; Allergy. Socs: Fell. Roy. Soc. Med.; Brit. Soc. Allergy & Clin. Immunol.; Assoc. Clin. Pathologists. Prev: Specialist Regist. (Immunol.) King's Coll. Hosp., St Bart's. Hosp. & Roy. Free Hosp. Lond.; Clin. Fell. in Knowledge Architecture, doctors.net.uk Ltd. & NeLH; Regist. (Clin. Immunol.) Oxf. Radcliffe Hosp. NHS Trust.

SEWELL, William Lawson (retired) Spetses, Neilston Walk, Kilsyth, Glasgow G65 9TF Tel: 01236 823298 — MB ChB Ed. 1946.

SEWNAUTH, Dev Kumar 8 Abercrombie Drive, Alderglen, Bearsden, Glasgow G61 4RR Tel: 0141 943 1720 — MB ChB Glas. 1972; FFA RCS Irel. 1978. Cons. Anaesth. Stobhill Gen. Hosp. Glas. Specialty: Anaesth. Prev: Cons. Anaesth. Inverclyde Roy. Hosp. Greenock.

SEXTON, John Patrick, OBE (retired) 3 Aldermoor Avenue, Storrington, Pulborough RH20 4PT Tel: 01903 742108 — MB ChB Ed. 1940; DTM & H Eng. 1942; DPH Ed. 1949; DMSA Ed. 1960; MFCM 1973. Prev: Exec. Dean Undergrad. & Postgrad. Studies, Fac. Med. Aberd. Univ.

SEXTON, Nicola Jane 209 Priests Lane, Shenfield, Brentwood CM15 8LE Tel: 01277 223739 — MB BS Lond. 1993 (Lond. Hosp.) BSc (Hons.) Hist. Med. Lond. 1989. Prev: Clin. Asst. (c/o Elderly) Broomfield Hosp. Chelmsford; SHO (A & E) Broomfield Hosp. Chelmsford.

SEXTON, Shaun Alan The Loaning, Station Road, Sunningdale, Ascot SL5 0QR — MB BS Lond. 1998; MB BS Lond 1998.

SEYAN, Rabinder Singh Atma Singh Seyan, Saffar and Rodin, The Health Centre, Robin Hood Lane, Sutton SM1 2RJ Tel: 020 8642 2010/3848 Fax: 020 8286 1010; 2 Morton, Tadworth Park, Tadworth KT20 5UA Tel: 01737 37321 — MB Camb. 1980 (Westm.) MA (Med. Sci.) Camb. 1976, MB 1980, BChir 1979; MRCGP 1983; DRCOG 1983. GP Tutor St Heliers Postgrad. Centre. Carshalton. Prev: Trainee GP/SHO Herts. & Essex VTS; Ho. Phys. St. Stephens Hosp. Lond.; Ho. Surg. Qu. Mary's Hosp. Roehampton.

SEYAN, Sirjit Singh Atma Singh Simpson House Medical Centre, 255 Eastcote Lane, South Harrow, Harrow HA2 8RS Tel: 020 8864 3466 Fax: 020 8864 1002; Silver Birches, 53C Gordon Avenue, Stanmore HA7 3QN Tel: 020 8954 6743 Fax: 020 8864 1002 — MB BChir Camb. 1974 (Westm.) MA Camb. 1974; DRCOG 1976; DCH Eng. 1977; MRCGP 1979. Prev: SHO Northwick Pk. Hosp. Harrow; Ho. Phys. & Ho. Surg. Gordon Hosp. Lond.

SEYFOLLAHI, Sonia 10 (IFL) East Norton Place, Edinburgh EH7 5DR — MB ChB Aberd. 1997.

SEYLER, Ina Beata Felicia Ridgeway Surgery, 6-8 Feckenham Road, Astwood Bank, Redditch B96 6DS Tel: 01527 892418 — Artsexamen Leiden 1973; MFFP (Member of the Faculty of Family Planning 1993); Cert. Family Plann. JCC 1984; Dip. Community Paediat. Warwick 1985; Certificate for Equivalent Experience JCTGP 1998. Gen. Practitioner Gen. Pract. Redditch Worcs.; Clin. Asst. Old Age Psychiat.; Clin. Med. Off. Family Plann. (Locum Sessions). Specialty: Gen. Pract.; Gen. Psychiat.; Family Plann. & Reproduc. Health. Socs: Fac. Family Plann. Prev: Clin. Med. Off. (Child Health & Family Plann.) Worcs. HA.

SEYMOUR, Alan Holt Dept. of Anaethetics, Birmingham Heartlands Hospital, Bordesley Green East, Birmingham B95SS Tel: 0121 424 2000 — MB ChB Birm. 1969; DObst RCOG 1971; DA Eng. 1972; FFA RCS Eng. 1975. Cons. Anaesth. Birm. Heartland Hosp. Specialty: Anaesth. Prev: Sen. Regist. (Anaesth.) Qu. Eliz. Hosp. Birm.; Regist. (Anaesth.) Bristol Roy. Infirm.; SHO (Anaesth.) N. Devon Infirm. Barnstaple.

SEYMOUR, Alexandra Louise Flat 19 Brunswick Place, Amersham Road, High Wycombe HP13 5AQ — MB BS Lond. 1998; MB BS Lond 1998.

SEYMOUR, Alison Louise 21 Chadacre Road, Epsom KT17 2HD — MB BS Lond. 1998; MB BS Lond 1998.

SEYMOUR, Andrew Heathville Road Surgery, 5 Heathville Road, Gloucester GL1 3DP Tel: 01452 528299 Fax: 01452 522959 — MB BS Lond. 1987; MRCGP 1991. Gen. Practitioner Princip. and Forens. Med. Examr. Prev: Trainee GP/SHO (Geriat.) W. Norwich Hosp.; SHO (O & G & Paediat.) Norf. & Norwich Hosp.

SEYMOUR, Miss Anne (retired) 35 The Lounen, South Shields NE34 8EQ — MB BS Lond. 1959; MRCS Eng. LRCP Lond. 1959; FRCS Eng. 1974.

SEYMOUR, Anne-Marie Frances Clinical Oncology Department, Guy's Hospital, London SE1 9RT — MB BCh BAO Dub. 1984; MRCPI 1987. ICRF Clin. Research Fell. Guy's Hosp. Lond. Specialty: Oncol.

SEYMOUR, Benjamin John Longmeadow, Burleigh La, Street BA16 0SL — MB ChB Manch. 1997.

SEYMOUR, Professor Carol Anne Office of Parliamentary & Health Service Ombudsman, 13th Floor, 30 Millbank, Millbank Tower, London SW1P Tel: 020 7217 4134 Fax: 020 7217 4035 — BM BCh Oxf. 1969; BA (Hons) Oxf. 1966; MA Oxf. 1970; MRCP (UK) 1972; MSc Lond. 1975; MA Camb. 1977; FRCP Lond. 1985; MRCPath 1991; LLDip/CPE 1998; FRCPath 1999. Prof. & Cons., Div. of Cardiological Sci. (Metab. Med.) St Geo.'s Hosp. Med. Sch., Lond.; Director for Clin. Advice to Parlimentary & Health Serv., Ombudsman, Lond.; Metab. Phys. Hepatol. Lond.; Prof. (Clin. Biochem. & Metab. Med.); Div. of Cardiological Sci.s (Metab. Med.), St. Geo.'s Hosp. Med. Sch. Lond. Specialty: Gastroenterol.; Endocrinol.; Civil Serv. Socs: Brit. Hyperlipidaemia Ass; Brit. Soc. of Gastroenterol.; Assoc. of Phys.s GB & I. Prev: Fell. & Dir. Med. Studies Trintiy Coll. Camb. & Fell. & Sen. Research Fell. Girton Coll. Camb.; Lect. & MRC Research Fell. Roy. Postgrad. Med. Sch. Lond.; Lect. (Med.) & Hon. Cons. Phys. Med. Addenbrooke's Hosp. Camb.

SEYMOUR, Professor David Gwyn Medicine for the Elderly, Foresterhill Health Centre, Westburn Road, Aberdeen AB25 2AY Tel: 01224 663131 Fax: 01224 840683 Email: d.g.seymour@abdn.ac.uk — (Birm.) MB ChB Birm. 1973; MRCP (UK) 1975; BSc Birm. 1970, MD 1988; FRCP Lond. 1994; FRCP Ed. 1995. Prof. c/o Elderly Univ. Aberd. Specialty: Care of the Elderly. Prev: Sen. Lect. (Geriat. Med.) Univ. Wales Coll. Med. & Rhymney Valley Health Dist. M. Glam.; Sen. Regist. (Geriat.) Roy. Vict. Hosp. Dundee; SHO (Med.) St. Luke's Hosp. Bradford.

SEYMOUR, Ernest John Racton, Breach Avenue, Emsworth PO10 8NB Tel: 01243 373608 — MB ChB Bristol 1958; DObst RCOG 1964. Socs: Brit. Med. Acupunct. Soc. Prev: Capt. RAMC.

SEYMOUR, Miss Felicity Kay — BChir Camb. 1998. Specialist Regist. N. Thames Region.

SEYMOUR, Hannah Mary White House Farm, Stokesley, Middlesbrough TS9 5LE — MB BS Lond. 1996.

SEYMOUR, Helen Rebecca 180 Balvernie Grove, London SW18 5RW; The Willows, Rectory Road, East Carlton, Norwich NR14 8HT — MB BS Lond. 1991; BSc Lond. 1989; MRCP (UK) 1995. Regist. (Radiol.) St. Geo. Hosp. Lond. Specialty: Radiol.

SEYMOUR, Ian Campbell, TD (retired) 9 Broadgait Green, Gullane EH31 2DW Tel: 01620 842677 — MB ChB Glas. 1948. Prev: Assoc. Specialist Spinal Inj. Clin. Philipshill Hosp. Busby.

SEYMOUR, Jean Elizabeth Ann 33 Hurst Close, Baldock SG7 6TL Tel: 01462 894830 — MB BS Lond. 1987. Retainer Scheme.

SEYMOUR, Jeremy Nether Edge Hospital, Brincliffe Road, Sheffield S11 9BF Tel: 0114 271 6018 Fax: 0114 271 8035 — MB BS Lond. 1982; DGM RCP Lond. 1985; MRCPsych 1989. Cons. Old Age Psychiat. Community Health Sheff.; Hon. Lect. Sheff. Univ. Specialty: Geriat. Psychiat. Prev: Tutor & Hon. Sen. Regist. (Old Age Psychiat.) Univ. Leeds; SHO (Med. for Elderly) Whipps Cross Hosp.; Regist. & SHO (Psychiat.) Sheff.

SEYMOUR, John Hyeyrie, Woodlands, The Narth, Monmouth NP25 4QT — MB ChB Bristol 1998.

SEYMOUR, Mr Keith c/o Mrs. Seymour, 208 Mowbray Road, South Shields NE33 3BE; Raby House, 15 North View, Hunwick, Crook DL15 0JR Tel: 01388 662559 — BM BS Nottm. 1991; FRCS Eng. 1996. Specialist Regist. (Surg.) Northern Region. Specialty: Gen. Surg.; Gastroenterol.

SEYMOUR, Lesley Katie 7 Mansion Street S., Accrington BB5 6SH — MB BCh Witwatersrand 1978.

SEYMOUR, Mary Virginia Wrangham (retired) Hollybank, 11 Seymour Drive, Plymouth PL3 5BG Tel: 01752 660694 — MB ChB Leeds 1960; DObst RCOG 1962.

SEYMOUR, Matthew Thomas Cookridge Hospital, Yorkshire Regional Centre for Cancer Treatment, Leeds LS16 6QB Tel: 0113 29244270113 3924427 Fax: 0113 292 4361 — MB BS Lond. 1984 (Qu. Coll. Camb. and The Lond. Hosp. M.C.) MA Camb. 1985; MRCP (UK) 1987; MD Lond. 1994; FRCP 1999. ICRF Sen. Lect. & Hon. Cons. Med. Oncol. Cookridge Hosp. & Leeds Gen. Infirm. Specialty: Oncol. Socs: Brit. Assn. Cancer Research; Assn. Cancer Phys.; Eur. Soc. Med. Oncol. Prev: Sen. Regist. (Med. Oncol.) Roy. Marsden Hosp. Lond. & St. Barts. Hosp. Lond.

SEYMOUR, Matthew Wadham Doctor's Mess, St Georges Hospital, 117 Suttons Lane, Hornchurch RM12 6RS — MB BS Lond. 1997.

SEYMOUR, Mr Michael Thomas James Clare House Practice, Clare House Surgery, Newport Street, Tiverton EX16 6NJ Tel: 01884 252337 Fax: 01884 254401 — MB BChir Camb. 1979 (Camb. & Middlx.) MA, MB Camb. 1979; FRCS Eng. 1982. Specialty: Gen. Pract. Prev: Regist. SW Thames Orthop. Train. Scheme; Demonst. (Anat.) Univ. Camb.; Ho. Surg. Middlx. Hosp. Lond.

SEYMOUR, Mr Neville (retired) 11 Seymour Drive, Mannamead, Plymouth PL3 5BG Tel: 01752 660694 Fax: 01752 660694 Email: neville@nevseymour.freeserve.co.uk — MB ChB Leeds 1957; FRCS Eng. 1962. Prev: Cons. Orthop. & Trauma Surg. Plymouth Health Dist.

SEYMOUR, Noel Richard Empingham Medical Centre, 37 Main Street, Empingham, Oakham LE15 8PR Tel: 01780 460202 Fax: 01780 460283; The Durham Ox, 6 Back Lane, South Luffenham, Oakham LE15 8NQ Tel: 01780 720112 — MB BS Lond. 1972 (Middlesex) DObst RCOG 1974; MRCGP 1977. Prev: Dist. Med. Off. Swansea Tasmania; Squadron Ldr. RAF Med. Br.; SHO (Paediat.) Essex Co. Hosp. Colchester.

SEYMOUR, Pamela Jane Consultant Community Paediatrician, WiSCH, Clatterbridge Hospital, Bebingham, Birkenhead CH63 4AY Tel: 0151 482 7273; Lansdowne, Mountwood Road, Prenton, Birkenhead CH42 8NG — MB ChB (Hons.) Liverp. 1970; MRCS Eng. LRCP Lond. 1970; DObst RCOG 1972; DCH Eng. 1973; MSc (Community Paediat.) Nottm. 1994; FRCPCH 1997. Specialty: Community Child Health. Prev: SCMO (Child Health) Wirral HA.

SEYMOUR, Richard Department of Radiology, Torbay Hospital, Lawes Bridge, Torquay TQ2 7AA Tel: 01803 655614 Fax: 01803 655638 — MB BChir Camb. 1990; MA Camb. 1989; MRCP (UK) 1992; FRCR 1995. Cons. (Diagn. Radio.) Torbay Hosp. Torquay. Specialty: Radiol. Prev: Sen. Regist. (Diagn. Radiol.) Univ. Hosp. Wales Cardiff; Regist. (Diagn. Radiol.) Univ. Hosp. Wales Cardiff; SHO (Med.) Northwick Pk. Hosp. Harrow.

SEYMOUR, Richard Nicholas Eagle Medical Practice (Dr Lyons), Oliver Court, Oliver Street, St Anne's, Alderney Tel: 01481 822494; La Tonnelle, Route de Pleinmont, Torteval, Guernsey GY8 0PA Tel: 01481 266327 — MB ChB Bristol 1963; DObst RCOG 1966. Assoc. Gen. Med. Practitioner Eagle Med. Pract. Alderney. Specialty: Accid. & Emerg. Prev: GP Sreet, Som.; SHO (O & G & Paediat.) Plymouth Gen. Hosp.

SEYMOUR, Ruth Department of Rehabilitation Medicine, Woodend Hospital, Eday Road, Aberdeen AB15 6XS Tel: 01224 663131 Fax: 01224 404019; Blair Lodge, Auchenblae Road, Stonehaven AB39 2NL Tel: 01569 766853 — MB ChB Dundee 1983; PhD Birm. 1975, BSc 1972; MRCP (UK) 1987; FRCP Ed. 1997. Cons. Rehabil. Med. Specialty: Rehabil. Med. Special Interest: Architectural design; Rehabil. Process.

SEYMOUR, Sarah-Jane 4 St Aubyn's Park, Tiverton EX16 4JG — MB Camb. 1983 (Camb. & Middlx.) MA Camb. 1983, MB 1983, BChir 1982. Prev: Med. Off. Tidcombe Hall Tiverton.

SEYMOUR, Sharon Christine 4 Collinbridge Court, Newtownabbey BT36 7UZ — MB BCh BAO Belf. 1993.

SEYMOUR, William Martin Vanbrugh Castle, Maze Hill, Greenwich, London SE10 8XQ Tel: 020 8853 2373 — MB BS Lond. 1963 (Lond. Hosp.) MRCS Eng. LRCP Lond. 1963; FRCP Lond. 1981, M 1965. Cons. Phys. Qu. Mary's Sidcup NHS Trust & Greenwich Health Care NHS Trust. Specialty: Gen. Med. Prev: Sen. Lect. Guy's Hosp. Med. Sch. Lond.; Sen. Regist. Chest & Gen. Med. Guy's Hosp. Lond.; Ho. Phys. Med. Unit. & Regist. (Med.) Lond. Hosp.

SEYMOUR, William Richard Dunham (retired) Abbeyfield, Ovens House, 57 Corn Street, Witney OX28 6BT Tel: 01993 778344 — (Qu. Univ. Belf.) MB BCh BAO Belf. 1939; MRCGP 1952. Prev: Ho. Surg. Childr. Hosp. Birm. & Coventry & Warw. Hosp.

SEYMOUR-JONES, Mr John Anthony Weald Cottage, 58 Warblington Road, Emsworth PO10 7HH Tel: 01243 372600 — MB BChir Camb. 1937 (Camb. & St. Thos.) MRCS Eng. LRCP Lond. 1935; FRCS Eng. 1940; DLO Eng. 1946. Cons. ENT. King Ed. VII Hosp. Midhurst; Emerit. Cons. ENT Surg. Portsmouth & SE Hants. Health Dist.; ENT Cons. DHSS. Socs: Fell. Roy. Soc. Med. (Mem. Sects. Laryng. & Otol. & Clin. Med.); BMA (Ex-Chairm. Portsmouth Div.).; (Ex-Chairm.) SW Laryngol. Assn. Prev: Cons. ENT Camb. Milit. Hosp. Aldershot; Regist. Portsmouth & South. Cos. Eye & Ear Hosp.; Ho. Surg. (ENT) St. Thos. Hosp. Lond.

SEYMOUR MEAD, Alison Margaret (retired) Pinley Rudding, Claverdon, Warwick CV35 8LU Tel: 01926 842428 — MB ChB Birm. 1972; DA (UK) 1974. Prev: SCMO W. Midl. Regional Transfus. Centre Birm.

SEYMOUR MEAD, Richard The Henley in Arden Medical Centre, Prince Harry Road, Henley in Arden, Solihull B95 5DD Tel: 01564 794311 Fax: 01564 793280; Pinley Rudding, Claverdon, Warwick CV35 8LU Tel: 0192 684 2428 — MB ChB Birm. 1972.

SEYMOUR-PRICE, Muriel, Capt. RAMC Retd. (retired) 32 Rheast Mooar Lane, Ramsey IM8 3LW Tel: 01642 2162 — (TC Dub.) MB BCh BAO Dub. 1948; BA Dub. 1948.

SEYMOUR-SHOVE, Ronald Nonsuch, Hunter's Lodge, 205 North Road, Yate, Bristol BS37 7LG — MB ChB Bristol 1954; DPM Eng. 1960; FRCPsych 1985, M 1972. Cons. Psychiat. i/c Rehabil. & Drug Addic. Treatm. Centre ScarBoro. Gen. Hosp.; Clin. Tutor Roy. Coll. Psych. Specialty: Alcohol & Substance Misuse. Socs: BMA. Prev: Sen. Regist. (Psychiat.) Liverp. United Hosps. & Deva & Moston Hosps. Chester; JHMO Glenside Hosp. Bristol.

SEYMOUR SMITH, Margaret Della 67 Rosemary Hill Road, Little Aston, Sutton Coldfield B74 4HH Tel: 0121 353 5765 — (Birm.) MB ChB Birm. 1947; DCH Eng. 1950.

SEYWRIGHT, Morag Mathews Department of Pathology, Inverclyde Royal NHS Trust, Greenock PA16 0XN Tel: 01475 633777 — MB ChB Glas. 1980 (Glas. Univ.) MRCPath. 1986. Cons. Path. Inverclyde Roy. Hosp. Greenock. Specialty: Histopath. Prev: Cons. Path. Dermat. West. Infirm. Glas.

SGOUROS, Mr Spyridon Birmingham Children's Hospital, Steelhouse Lane, Birmingham B4 6NH Tel: 0121 333 8075 Fax: 0121 333 8701 Email: s.sgouros@bham.ac.uk — Ptychio Iatrikes Athens 1985; FRCS Glas. 1992; FRCS SN 1997; MD Birm. 2000. Cons. Neurosurg. Specialty: Neurosurg. Socs: Soc. Brit. Neurol. Surg.; Internat. Soc. Paediat. Neurosurg.; Europ. Soc. Paediat. Neurosurg.

SGOUROS, Xenofon Greenfield Centre, Furlong Road, Tunstall, Stoke-on-Trent ST6 5UD Tel: 01782 425740 Fax: 01782 425741 Email: xenofon.sgouros@nsch-tr.wmids.nhs.uk — Ptychio Iatrikes Thessalonika 1991; Cert Med Educat. Cons. Psychiat. N. Staffs. Combined Healthcare NHS Trust. Specialty: Alcohol & Substance Misuse. Special Interest: Subst. Misuse.

SHA'ABAN, Mahir Abbas Jawad 7 Macneill Drive, East Kilbride, Glasgow G74 4TR — MB ChB Baghdad 1973; MB ChB Baghdad.

SHAATH, Nabeel Mohamed 12 Edinburgh Close, Sale M33 4EZ — MB BCh BAO NUI 1987; LRCPSI 1987; MRCP (UK) 1996; CCST 2001.

SHAATH, Mr Nebal Mohamed 12 Edinburgh Close, Sale M33 4EZ — MB BCh BAO NUI 1988; LRCPSI 1988; FRCSI 1994; MSc 1998. Specialist Regist. Lat. Specialty: Orthop.

SHABBO, Mr Fikrat Putrus Guy's and St Thomas' Hospital Trust, Lambeth Palace Road, London SE1 Tel: 020 7960 5812 Fax: 020 7922 8005; Manor Cottage, Manor Way, Leatherhead KT22 0HS Tel: 01372 844570 — MRCS Eng. LRCP Lond. 1977 (University of Baghdad Medical School) MB ChB 1968; FRCS Eng. 1975. Cons. Cardio-Thoracic Surg. St Thomas' Hosp. Specialty: Cardiothoracic Surg. Socs: Soc. Cardiovasc. Surg. & Brit. Cardiac Soc. Prev: Sen. Regist. Nat. Heart Hosp. & St. Bart. Hosp. Lond.

SHABDE, Ishita 17 Oaklands, Newcastle upon Tyne NE3 4YQ — MB ChB Leeds 1998.

SHABDE, Neela Community Child Health Department, Albion Road Clinic, Albion Road, North Shields NE29 0HG Tel: 0191 219 6657 Fax: 0191 219 6650; 17 Oaklands, Gosforth, Newcastle upon Tyne NE3 4YQ Tel: 0191 213 1155 — MB BS Ravishankar 1971; DCH Jabalpur 1974; DCCH RCP Ed. 1983; MRCPI 1987; FRCP Lond. 1996; FRCPCH 1997. Cons. Paediat. (Community Child Health) N. Tyneside Health Care NHS Trust; Hon. Clin. Lect. (Child Health) Univ. Newc. Specialty: Community Child Health. Prev: Sen. Regist. (Community Child Health) N. Tyneside HA.

SHABESTARY, Mr Shahrokh Moaddab Ilford Medical Centre, 61-63 Cleveland Road, Ilford IG1 1EE — MD Tabriz 1970; FRCS Ed. 1979.

SHABO, Gregory 17 Braziers Quay, Bishop's Stortford CM23 3YN — MD Louvain 1992 (Louvain, Belgium) SHO. (Gen Med.). Specialty: Gen. Med.; Gen. Pract. Prev: SHO, Gen. Med. Nobles, Isle of Man Hosp.; SHO, Gen. Med. Medway Hosp. Gillingham, Kent; SHO, Gen Med. Princess Alexandra Hosp. Essex.

SHABROKH, Pedram 12 Twyford Abbey Road, London NW10 7HG Tel: 020 8991 1168 Fax: 020 8991 1168 — MB ChB Sheff. 1990. Specialty: Gen. Pract.

SHACKCLOTH, Michael John 2 Sandwell Drive, Sale M33 6JL — MB ChB Manch. 1994.

SHACKEL, Geoffrey George Spinneys, Five Ashes, Mayfield TN20 6HH Tel: 01435 873113 — MB BChir Camb. 1964 (Camb. & St. Thos.) MA Camb. 1964; DObst RCOG 1965. Prev: Ho. Phys. (Paediat.) Whipps Cross Hosp. Lond.; Ho. Surg. (O & G) St. Thos. Hosp. (Lambeth Hosp.) Lond.; Ho. Phys. St. Helier Hosp. Carshalton.

SHACKELL, Margaret Mary Hillview Surgery, 179 Bilton Road, Greenford UB6 7HQ Tel: 020 8997 4661 Fax: 020 8810 8015 — MB BS Lond. 1971 (Roy. Free) MRCP (UK) 1976. Lect. (Gen. Pract.) St. Mary's Hosp. Med. Sch. Lond. Prev: Hon. Sen. Regist. (Med.) Whittington Hosp. Lond.; Regist. (Cardiol.) Papworth Hosp. Cambs.; Research Fell. (Cardiol.) Hillingdon Hosp. Uxbridge.

SHACKLES, David Alexander The Taymount Surgery, 1 Taymount Terrace, Perth PH1 1NU Tel: 01738 627117 Fax: 01738 444713 — MB ChB Ed. 1987; DCCH RCP Ed. 1990; MRCGP 1991. Prev: Ho. Off. (Med.) Roy. Infirm. Edin.

SHACKLETON, Clive David Eskdaill Medical Centre, Eskdaill Street, Kettering NN16 8RA Tel: 01536 513053 Fax: 01536 417572; 12 Queensberry Road, Kettering NN15 7HL Tel: 01536 416680 — MB BS Lond. 1984; DLO RCS Eng. 1986; MRCGP 1988. Clin. Asst. (ENT) Kettering Hosp. N.ants. Specialty: Gen. Pract.; Otolaryngol. Prev: SHO (ENT & A & E) Worthing Hosp.; Ho. Phys. Ealing Hosp. Lond.

SHACKLETON, David Andrew 1 Nursery View Cottages, Seven Sisters Lane, Ollerton, Knutsford WA16 8RL Tel: 01565 652993 — MB ChB Manch. 1990. Specialty: Gen. Pract.

SHACKLETON, David Barry Occupational Health Solutions Ltd., 6 Silk House, Park Green, Macclesfield SK11 7QJ Tel: 01625 430039 Email: admin@occhealth.co.uk — MB ChB Liverp. 1986; MRCP (UK) 1989; MFOM RCP Lond. 1994. Cons. Occupat. Phys. Manch. Specialty: Occupat. Health. Socs: Soc. Occupat. Med. Prev: Employm. Med. Adviser Health & Safety Exec. Manch.; Regist. (Med.) Macclesfield HA.

SHACKLETON, Geoffrey Ernest The Ridgeway Surgery, 71 Imperial Drive, North Harrow, Harrow HA2 7DU Tel: 020 8427 2470 — MB BS Lond. 1955 (St. Mary's) MRCGP 1975; DGM RCP Lond. 1985.

SHACKLETON, Janet Elizabeth — MB ChB Manch. 1987.

SHACKLETON, John Park (retired) Flat 38 Oak Tree Lodge, Harlow Manor Park, Harrogate HG2 0QH Tel: 01423 561042 — MRCS Eng. LRCP Lond. 1951 (Camb. & Leeds) Prev: Ho. Surg. Bradford Roy. Infirm.

SHACKLETON, John Robert St Marys Surgery, 37 St. Mary's Street, Ely CB7 4HF Tel: 01353 665511 Fax: 01353 669532 — MB Camb. 1973 (Lond. Hosp.) BChir 1972; DObst RCOG 1975.

SHACKLETON, Sara Elizabeth 24 Cranleigh, Standish, Wigan WN6 0EU — MB ChB Leeds 1980.

SHACKLETON, Sarah Caroline Newbury Street Practice, Newbury Street, Wantage OX12 7AY Tel: 01235 763451 — MB BS Lond. 1984; MRCGP 1988.

SHACKLEY, Mr David Clifford 97 Long Lane, Chadderton, Oldham OL9 8AZ — MB ChB Manch. 1992; FRCS Ed. 1996. Specialty: Urol.

SHACKLEY, Emma Caroline The Manor House, Lenchwick, Evesham WR11 4TG — BM BS Nottm. 1988; MRCGP; MRCP.

SHACKLEY, Fiona May 101 Hunter House Road, Hunters Bar, Sheffield S11 8TX — MB ChB Ed. 1989.

SHACKLEY, Timothy Richard 18 Radford Grove Lane, Radford, Nottingham NG7 5QB — BM BS Nottm. 1987.

SHACKMAN, Steven Gerson Northwood Health Centre, Acre Way, Northwood HA6 1TQ Tel: 01923 828488; The Surgery, Mount Vernon Hospital, Rickmansworth Road, Northwood HA6 2RN Tel: 01923 820626 — MB BS Lond. 1972 (Lond. Hosp.) MRCS Eng. LRCP Lond. 1972. N.wood, Pinner & Dist. Hosp.; Div. Police Surg. Herts. Constab. Prev: SHO Rotat. (Orthop. & Gen. Surg.) Roy. Surrey Co. Hosp. Guildford; SHO Thoracic Surg. Unit Milford Chest Hosp. Godalming; Regist. Regional Radiother. & Oncol. Centre St. Luke's Hosp.

SHAD, Mr Amjad Walsgrave Hospital, Department of Neurosurgery, Coventry CV2 2DX Fax: 01926 982602 Email: amjadshad@hotmail.com — MB BS Bahauddin Zakariya 1985 (Wishtal Med. Coll.) FRCS Edin. Cons. Neurosurg.

SHAD, Irshad Ahmad Swindon Health Centre, Carfax Street, Swindon SN1 1ED Tel: 01793 619955 Fax: 01793 533920; 88 Okebourne Park, Swindon SN3 6AJ Tel: 01793 692064 — MB BS Punjab, Pakistan 1968 (Nishtar Med. Coll. Multan) Clin. Asst., Accid. & Emerg., Princess Margt. Hosp., Swindon, Wilts., SN1 4JU.

SHAD, Mr Sujay Kumar Harefield Hospital, Harefield, Uxbridge UB9 6JY Tel: 01895 823737 Fax: 01895 828666 — MB BS All India Inst. Med. Sciences 1988 (India Inst. Med. Sci.) MB BS All India Inst. of Med. Sciences 1988; FRCS Glas. 1994. Specialist Regist. (Cardiothoracic Surg.) Harefield Hosp. Specialty: Cardiothoracic Surg. Special Interest: Valvular Heart Dis. Prev: Vis. Regist. Rotat. (Cardiothoracic Surg.) W. Midl.; Regist. (Cardiothoracic Surg.) Harefield Hosp.

SHADBOLT, Clair Louise Department of Diagnostic Radiology, Hammersmith Hospital, Du Cane Road, London W12 0NN — MB ChB Otago 1988.

SHADBOLT, Clemency Jane Quarry Street Surgery, 16-24 Quarry Street, Johnstone PA5 8EB Tel: 01505 321733 Fax: 01505 322181 — MB ChB Bristol 1986; DCH RCP Lond. 1990; MRCGP 1990; T(GP) 1991; DRCOG 1991. Princip. in GP Johnstone. Socs: BMA. Prev: GP Retainer Scheme Glas.; GP Bracknell; SHO (O & G) Perth Roy. Infirm.

SHADDICK, Rowland Allen 107 High Street, Southgate, London N14 6BP Tel: 020 8886 0388 — MRCS Eng. LRCP Lond. 1945 (Lond. Hosp.) DPhysMed. Eng. 1953. Sen. Lect. Rheum. & Orthop. Med. Brit. Sch. Osteopathy Lond. Socs: Brit. Soc. Rheum. Prev: Sen. Cons. Rheum. Enfield Dist. Hosps. & N.E. Regional Rheum. Centre; Regist. Dept. Phys. Med. & Rheum. Middlx. & Lond. Hosps.; Lect. Anat. & Histol. Lond. Hosp. & Univ. Coll. W. Indies.

SHADFORTH, Colin (retired) 12 Mulberry Court, Carr Hall Gardens, Ruswarp, Whitby YO21 1RW — MB BS Durh. 1950. Prev: Ho. Surg. (ENT) & Profess. Surg. Clinic Roy. Vict. Infirm. Newc. u. Tyne.

SHADFORTH, Michael Fletcher Rheumatology Unit, Haywood Hospital, High Lane, Burslem, Stoke-on-Trent ST6 7AG Tel: 01782 835721; The Beald, Heather Hills, Stockton Brook, Stoke-on-Trent ST9 9PS Tel: 01782 504258 — MB BS Newc. 1968; MRCP (UK) 1974. Cons. (Rheum.) Staffs. Rheum Centre, Haywood Hosp. Stoke-on-Trent; Hon. Research Fell. Univ. Birm. Specialty: Rheumatol. Socs: Brit. Soc. Rheum.; Midl. Rheum. Soc. Prev: Rotat. SHO Roy. Vict. Infirm. Newc.; Sen. Regist. Qu. Eliz. Hosp. Birm.; Arthritis & Rheum Counc. Trav.; Fell. Univ. Virginia Charlottesville, U.S.A.

SHADWELL, Richard Neil Highgate Wood Dental Practice, 14-15 Aylmer Parade, Highgate, London N2 0PE Tel: 020 8340 2455 — MB BCh Wales 1981; BDS Lond. 1986; LDS RCS Eng. 1987. Dent. Surg. Lond.

SHADWICK, Peter (retired) 11 Hilton Court, South Promenade, Lytham St Annes FY8 1LZ Tel: 01253 722610 Email: peter@shadwick.freeserve.co.uk — MB BS Durh. 1951. Prev: Sen. Med. Off. DSS Norcross Blackpool.

SHAEENA, Mr Petrous Roufa (retired) 73 Kenilworth Road, Coventry CV4 7AF Tel: 024 76 417515 — MB ChB Baghdad 1959; LMSSA Lond. 1968; FRCS Ed. 1969; FRCS Eng. 1970; DMJ Soc. Apoth Lond. 1980; ECFMG (USA) 1982. Police Surg. and Forens.

Expert 1972-1999, Retd. 1999. Prev: Regist. (Orthop.) Coventry & Warks. Hosp. & St. Cross Hosp. Rugby.

SHAFAFY, Masood — MB BS Lond. 1994 (St. Bartholomew's Hospital Medical College London) FRCS (Eng) 1998. Specialist Regist. (Trauma & Orthop.) Oldchurch Hosp. Specialty: Neurosurg.; Orthop.; Trauma & Orthop. Surg. Prev: Specialist Regist. (Trauma & Orthop.) The Roy. Lond. Hosp.; Specialist Regist. (Trauma & Orthop.) The Roy. Nat. Orthopaedic Hosp.; Specialist Regist. (Trauma & Orthop.) Whipps Cross Univ. Hosp. Lond.

SHAFAR, Susanne (retired) 58 Carr Hall Road, Barrowford, Nelson BB9 6PY Tel: 01282 613631 — MB ChB Glas. 1946; MB ChB (Commend.) Glas. 1946; DPM Eng. 1950; FRCPsych 1979, M 1971. Cons. Psychiat. N. Manch. Health Dist. Prev: Ho. Surg. Roy. Infirm. Glas.

SHAFFER, Jonathan Lionel Hope Hospital, Salford M6 8HD Tel: 0161 787 5145 Fax: 0161 787 5366 — MB BS Lond. 1972 (Univ. Coll. Hosp.) MRCP (UK) 1978; FRCP Lond. 1995. Cons. Phys. Hope Hosp. Salford; Clin. Dir. (Intestinal Failure Unit); Hosp. Dean for UnderGrad. Stud.s. Specialty: Gastroenterol. Prev: Lect. (Gastroenterol. & Clin. Pharmacol.) Univ. Manch.

SHAFFER, Joseph 156 Kennington Park Road, London SE11 4DJ Tel: 020 7735 0661 Fax: 020 7735 1194 — MB BS Lond. 1993 (United Med. & Dent. Sch. Lond.) BSc (Hons.) Lond. 1991; MRCP (UK) 1996. SHO (Dermat.) St. John's Inst. Dermat. Lond. Specialty: Dermat. Prev: SHO (Respirat. Med.) Roy. Brompton Hosp. Lond.; SHO (HIV & A & E) St. Mary's Hosp. Lond.; SHO (Gastroenterol.) Hammersmith Hosp. Lond.

SHAFFI, Siyana Herne Hill Group Practice, 74 Herne Hill, London SE24 9QP Tel: 020 7274 3314 Fax: 020 7738 6025 — MB BS Lond. 1994.

SHAFFORD, Elizabeth Ann 18 Hillhouse Close, Billericay CM12 0BB Tel: 01277 659953 — MB BS Lond. 1974 (Middlx.) DCH Eng. 1977; MRCP (UK) 1979. Staff Grade Palliat. Med. St. Luke's Hospice, Basildon. Specialty: Paediat. Prev: Clin. Research Fell.. (Paediat. Oncol.) St. Bart. Hosp. Lond.

SHAFFU, N G Westcotes Family Practice, 2 Westcotes Drive, Leicester LE3 0QR Tel: 0116 254 7887 — LRCP LRCS Ed. LRCPS Glas.; MB ChB Baghdad 1972; MB ChB Baghdad 1972.

SHAFI, Ghazala 13 Kenerne Drive, Barnet EN5 2NW — MB BS Lond. 1987; DCH RCP Lond. 1991; MRCGP 1992. GP Princip. Herts. Prev: Trainee GP Ealing.

SHAFI, Mahmood Iqbal Department of Gynaecology, Birmingham Women's Hospital, Edgbaston, Birmingham B15 2TG Tel: 0121 472 1377 Fax: 0121 627 2667 Email: mahmood.shafi@bwhct.nhs.uk — MB BCh Wales 1981 (Welsh National School of Medicine) DRCOG 1984; DA Eng. 1984; MRCOG 1987; MD Wales 1997; FRCOG 2002. Cons. (Gyn. Surg. & Oncol.) Birm. Wom.'s Hosp. Specialty: Obst. & Gyn. Prev: Sen. Lect. & Cons. O & G City Hosp. NHS Trust Birm.; Sen. Regist. (Subspecialty Trainee in Gyn. Oncol.) City Hosp. & Birm. Midl. Hosp. for Wom.; Research Fell. & Regist. (O & G) Dudley Rd. Hosp. Birm.

SHAFI, Miheengar Mohamad Lake Street Surgery, 20-22 Lake Street, Leighton Buzzard LU7 1RT Tel: 01525 851995 Fax: 01525 374783; Nishaat, Plantation Road, Leighton Buzzard LU7 3HU — (M.P.S. Med. Coll. Jamnagar, India) MB BS Gujarat 1966. Prev: Dist. Surg. Kashmir, India.

SHAFI, Mohammed Shujauddin PHL Department of Microbiology, Central Middlesex Hospital NHS Trust, Park Royal, London NW10 7NS Tel: 020 8965 1603 Fax: 020 8965 6071 — MB BS Osmania 1967 (Osmania Med. Coll. Hyderabad) FRCPath 1987, M 1975. Cons. Microbiol. Centr. Middlx. Hosp. Lond. Specialty: Med. Microbiol. Socs: Assn. Med. Microbiol. Hosp. Infec. Soc. Prev: Cons. Microbiol. Nat. Guard Hosp. Jeddah, Saudi Arabia; Sen. Regist. (Med. Microbiol.) Centr. Middlx. Hosp. Lond.; Lect. & Asst. Lect. Middlx. Hosp. Med. Sch. Lond.

SHAFI, Mushtaq Ahmed Clovelly, 176 Swallow St., Iver SL0 0HR — MB BS Ibadan 1980; MRCOG 1991.

SHAFI, Shafiq 51 Buxton Street, Leicester LE2 0FL — MB ChB Leic. 1991; DCH RCP Lond. 1994; DFFP 1995; MRCGP 1995; DRCOG Lond. 1996. GP Princip. Leicester. Specialty: Occupat. Health. Socs: Brit. Med. Acupunct. Soc. Prev: Ship's Doctor (P&O/P.ss Cruises); GP/Regist. Leicester.

SHAFIGHIAN, Mr Bijan Foscote Private Hospital, Foscote Rise, Banbury OX16 9XP Tel: 01295 229411 Fax: 01295 272877; Stonewalls, Hempton, Banbury OX15 0QS Tel: 01869 338439 — MD Iran 1974; FRCS Ed. 1986. Cons. Orthop. Surg. Horton Gen. Hosp. Banbury. Specialty: Orthop. Socs: Fell. BOA; BMA; Girdlestone Orthop. Soc. Prev: Research Fell., Sen. Regist. (Reconstruc. Surg.) & Regist. (Orthop. & Trauma) Mayday Univ. Hosp. Thornton Heath.

SHAFIK, Amina Mohamed University Hospital Lewisham, Department of Obstetrics & Gynaecology, Lewisham High Street, London SE13 6LJ Tel: 020 8333 3068 Fax: 020 8690 1963 — MB BCh Ain Shams 1979. Cons. (O & G) Univ. Hosp. Lewisham. Specialty: Obst. & Gyn.

SHAFQAT, Mr Syed Owais Scunthorpe General Hospital, Department of Orthopaedics, Cliff Gardens, Scunthorpe DN15 7BH Tel: 01724 290188; The Vicarage, 5 Paul Lane, Appleby, Scunthorpe DN15 0AR Tel: 01724 734905 — MB BS Karachi 1977 (Dow Medical) FRCS Glas. 1988. Cons. Trauma & Orthop. Surg.: Scunthorpe Gen. Hosp.; Goole & Dist. Hosp.; St Hugh's Hosp. Grimsby; BUPA Hosp. Hull & E. Riding Anlaby Hull; Pk. Hill Hosp. Doncaster. Specialty: Orthop. Socs: BMA; BOA; Brit. Soc. for Revision Surg.

SHAFQUAT, Mr Shahzad Guest Hospital, Dudley DY1 4SE Tel: 01384 456111 Ext: 5812 — FCPS, FRCS; MB BS Punjab 1985 (King Edwd. Med. Coll.) Cons. Ophth. Surg. Special Interest: Med. Retina. Socs: Med. Retina Gp.; Midl. Ophth. Soc.; Roy. Coll. of Ophth. Prev: Specialist Regist., Ophth. S. Thames Deanery, Lond.

SHAH, Professor Ajay Manmohan Guy's, King's & St Thomas' School of Medicine & Dentistry, Department of Cardiology, Bessemer Road, London SE5 9PJ Tel: 020 7737 4000 — MD Wales 1990 (Uni. Of Wales College of Medicine) MB BCh 1982; MRCP (UK) 1985; FESC 1997; FRCP 1998. Prof. (Cardiovasc. Med.) King's Coll., Brit. Heart Found. Specialty: Cardiol. Prev: MRC Sen. Clin. Fell. & Sen. Lect. (Cardiol.) Univ. of Wales Coll. Med. Cardiff.

SHAH, Ajazul Haq 1 Foxhome Close, Chislehurst BR7 5XT — MB BS Lond. 1997.

SHAH, Ajit Hirji The Primary Care Medical Centre, 475 Kenton Road, Kenton, Harrow HA3 0UN Tel: 020 8204 8228; 115 Elmsleigh Avenue, Kenton, Harrow HA3 8HY Tel: 020 8907 0923 — MB BS Bombay 1979 (Lokmanya Tilak Med. Coll. Bombay) DTM & H RCP Lond. 1984; MRCS Eng. LRCP Lond. 1988; DGM RCP Lond. 1988; MRCPI 1990; MRCGP 1996. Specialty: Care of the Elderly. Socs: Fell. Roy. Soc. Trop. Med. & Hyg.; BMA. Prev: Trainee GP Lond.; Regist. (Med. for Elderly) Edgware Gen. Hosp.; SHO (Med. for Elderly) Walton Hosp. Chesterfield.

SHAH, Ajit Kumar 49 Erlesmere Gardens, London W13 9TZ Tel: 020 8321 5443 Fax: 020 8321 5961 — MB ChB Liverp. 1984; MRCPsych 1989. Sen. Lect. & Hon. Cons. (Psychiat. of Old Age) Char. Cross & Westm. Med. Sch. Lond. Specialty: Geriat. Psychiat.

SHAH, Ambrish Kumar Goodmayes Medical Centre, 4 Eastwood Road, Goodmayes, Ilford IG3 8XB Tel: 020 8590 1169 Fax: 020 8590 1170 — MB BS India 1972 (J.N. Med. Coll.) BSc Aligarh Muslim, India 1965, MB BS 1972; MRCP (UK) 1978. Clin. Asst. (Med. & Rheum.) King Geo. Hosp. Ilford. Specialty: Gen. Med.; Rheumatol. Prev: Sen. Regist. (Med.) Walsgrave Hosp. Coventry; Regist. (Med. & Haemat.) Walsgrave Hosp. Coventry.

SHAH, Amrut Chunilal The Surgery, 188/189 Lewes Road, Brighton BN2 3LA Tel: 01273 603616 Fax: 01273 694101 — MB BS India 1968 (Indore) GP Brighton.

SHAH, Arunkumar Revulal New Invention Health Centre, 66 Cannock Road, Willenhall WV12 5RZ Tel: 01922 475100 Fax: 01922 712934 — MB BS Bombay 1972.

SHAH, Arvind Rasiklal 86 Bertram Road, Enfield EN1 1LS Tel: 020 8363 7650 — MB BS Poona 1979; MRCPI 1986.

SHAH, Ashia — MB BS Lond. 1998 (St Bart. & Roy. Lond. Hosp.) Ho. Off. (Gen. Med.) Newham Gen. Hosp. Lond. Specialty: Gen. Med. Prev: Ho. Off. (Gen. Surg.) Whipps Cross Hosp.

SHAH, Ashwin Mukund Stratford Village Practice, 50C Romford Road, London E15 4BZ Tel: 020 8534 4133 Fax: 020 8534 3860; 45 Gyllyngdune Gardens, Ilford IG3 9HJ — MB BS Gujarat 1975. GP. Specialty: Diabetes; Paediat.; Respirat. Med.

SHAH, Atta Ullah Khyber Surgery, 38 Havelock Road, Saltley, Birmingham B8 1RT Tel: 0121 328 1174 — MB BS Peshawar 1962 (Khyber Med. Coll. Peshawar) DA Eng. 1965.

SHAH, B J Mahavir Medical Centre, 10 Chestnut Way, East Goscote, Leicester LE7 3QQ Tel: 0116 260 1007 Fax: 0116 260

1008 — MRCS Eng. LRCP London; MB BS Mysore 1980; MB BS Mysore 1980.

SHAH, Bakhtiar Ahmed c/o Anaesthetic Department, Kent & Canterbury Hospital, Ethelbert Road, Canterbury CT1 3NG — MB BS Pershawar 1983; FFA RCSI 1988. Specialty: Anaesth.

SHAH, Miss Bareen Nusarrat 70 Wilson Gardens, Harrow HA1 4EA Tel: 020 8442 9889; 70 Wilson Gardens, Harrow HA1 4EA Tel: 020 8442 9889 — LMSSA Lond. 1986; FRCS (Eng) 1992. Specialist Regist. Gen. Surg. Hillingdon Hosp. Specialty: Gen. Surg. Socs: RSM; AS &BI.

SHAH, Bella Rupa 7A Temple Road, London W4 5NW — MB BS Lond. 1992.

SHAH, Bhagwandas Damodar 23 Challacombe, Southend-on-Sea SS1 3TY Tel: 01702 582066 — MB BS Newc. 1967; DMRD Eng. 1971; FRCR 1977. Cons. (Radiol.) Southend Health Dist. Specialty: Radiol. Prev: Sen. Regist. (Radiol.) Roy. Vict. Infirm. Newc.; Ho. Off. Qu. Eliz. Hosp. Birm.; Demonst. Anat. Med. Sch. Univ. Newc.

SHAH, Bharati Amritlal The Surgery, 20-22 Bannockburn Road, Plumstead, London SE18 1ES Tel: 020 8855 5540 Fax: 020 8855 4970; 120 Knights Way, Dartford DA1 5SP Tel: 279613 — LMSSA Lond. 1978 (Kasturba Med. Coll. Mangalore) GP. Prev: SHO (Psychiat.) Roy. Cornw. Hosp. (City) Truro; Ho. Surg. Roy. Cornw, Hosp. (Treliske) Truro; Ho. Phys. Joyce Green Hosp. Dartford.

SHAH, Bhupendra Keshavlal Oakview, Thornton Manor Drive, Ryde PO33 1PQ — MB BS Saurashtra 1971.

SHAH, Bindu Mohanlal 103 Springfield Road, Moseley, Birmingham B13 9NN — MB ChB Bristol 1985.

SHAH, Bipin Keshavlal (retired) 45 The Avenue, Ystrad Mynach, Hengoed CF82 8BA Tel: 01443 812066 — (Seth G.S. Med. Coll.) MB BS Bombay 1958. Prev: Clin. Asst. Ystrad Mynach Hosp.

SHAH, Bipinchandra Balvantlal The Surgery, 27 Clifton Rise, London SE14 6ER Tel: 020 8692 1387; 2 Wellands Close, Bickley, Bromley BR1 2AQ — MB BS Bombay 1966 (Grant Med. Coll. Bombay) DObst RCOG 1969; MRCOG 1972. Specialty: Obst. & Gyn. Prev: Regist. (Gyn. & Obst.) Lewisham Hosp. Lond.; SHO (O & G) Stepping Hill Hosp. Stockport & Huddersfield Roy. Infirm.

SHAH, Mr Chandrakant Hirachand 27 Filsham Road, St Leonards-on-Sea TN38 0PA Tel: 01424 428433 — MB BS Bombay 1953 (Grant Med. Coll. Bombay) FRCS Ed. 1966; DLO Eng. 1970. Cons. Surg. ENT Conquest Hosp. Hastings. Specialty: Otorhinolaryngol. Socs: Fell. Roy. Soc. Med.; Assn. Otorhinolaryngol. Prev: Cons. Surg. ENT Roy. E. Sussex Hosp. Hastings; Sen. Regist. (ENT) Singleton Hosp. Swansea Cardiff Roy. Infirm.

SHAH, Chandrakant Natverlal Houghton Regis Medical Centre, Peel Street, Houghton Regis, Dunstable LU5 5EZ Tel: 01582 866161 Fax: 01582 865483 — MB BS Bombay 1969 (Topiwala Nat. Med. Coll.) DRCOG 1977. SHO (O & G) Wordsley Hosp. Stourbridge. Specialty: Obst. & Gyn. Socs: Med. Defence Union.

SHAH, Mr Chandrakant Trambaklal Gulabchand ENT Department, St James's Hospital, James's Street, Dublin, Republic of Ireland Tel: 00353 1416 2677 Fax: 00353 1410 3464 Email: ctshah99@yahoo.com; 23 Beverington Close, Eastbourne BN21 2SB Email: ctshah99@yahoo.com — LMSSA Lond. 1986 (B. J. Med. Coll. Ahmedabad, India) MB BS Gujaret 1976; MS (ENT) Gujarat 1980; DLO RCS Eng. 1983; FRCS Ed. 1986; FRCS (ORL-HNS) Glasgow 2001. Cons. ENT Surg., Epsom Gen. Hosp.; Hon. Cons. ENT Surg. Hosp.; ENT Dept., Epsom Gen. Hosp., Dorking Rd, Epsom, KT18 8EG Tel: 01372 735735. Specialty: Otolaryngol.; Otorhinolaryngol. Socs: Assn. Otolaryngol. UK; Assn. Otorhinolaryng. India; Brit. Med. Laser Assn. Prev: Cons. ENT Surg. Pinderfield Gen. Hosp. Wakefield; Cons. ENT Surg. Roy. Liverp. Hosp. Liverp.; Cons. ENT Surg. Epsom Gen. Hosp. and St Mary's Hosp. for Childr. Epsom.

SHAH, Devang Kanubhai Mill Street Surgery, 439 Mill Street, Bradford, Manchester M11 2BL Tel: 0161 223 0637 Fax: 0161 220 7220 — MB ChB Manch. 1991; DRCOG 1995; MRCGP 1996. GP Princip. Specialty: Gen. Pract.

SHAH, Dharmesh Brentfield Medical Centre, 10 Kingfisher Way, Brentfield Road, London NW10 8TF Tel: 020 8459 8833 Fax: 020 8459 1374 — MB ChB Leeds 1992. Specialty: Gen. Pract.

SHAH, Dhiren Shantilal Canbury Medical Centre, 1 Elm Rd, Kingston upon Thames KT2 6HR Tel: 020 8549 8818 — MB BS Lond. 1993 (St. Mary's Hospital Medical School) BSc Lond 1991; DRCOG 1996; MRCGP 1997. GP. Specialty: Gen. Pract.

SHAH, Dilesh — MB ChB Manch. 1988; DRCOG 1992; MRCGP 1993. GP Watton at Stone Herts. Socs: MRCGP; DRCOG; FMA.

SHAH, Dilip Kumar Bousfield Health Centre, Westminster Road, Liverpool L4 4PP Tel: 0151 207 1468 Fax: 0151 284 6864; Sneheel, Woodlands Park, Liverpool L12 1ND — MB BS Rajasthan 1975 (R.N.T. Med. Coll. Udaipur)

SHAH, Dilip Kumar Liladhar Jaina House, 66 Arnos Grove, Southgate, London N14 7AR Tel: 020 8886 4035 Fax: 020 8882 7024 — MB BS Lond. 1978; DCH RCP Lond. 1981; DRCOG 1982; MRCGP 1983; Dip Med AC 1997.

SHAH, Dinesh Karmshi 39 Bourneside, Bedford MK41 7EQ — MB BS Vikram 1963; MS Vikram 1966. Assoc. Specialist Bedford Hosp. Trust. Specialty: Accid. & Emerg. Prev: Cons. Surg. Raipur, India.

SHAH, Dinesh Panachand 70 St Edmunds Drive, Stanmore HA7 2AU Tel: 020 8424 9974 — MB BS Saurashtra 1973.

SHAH, Dipak Vidhu Wenlock Street Surgery, 40 Wenlock Street, Luton LU2 0NN Tel: 01582 27094; 9 Cooks Meadow, Edlesborough, Dunstable LU6 2RP Tel: 01525 222349 — MB ChB Glas. 1984 (Univ. Glas.) Cert. Family Plann. JCC 1988; DRCOG 1989. Specialty: Family Plann. & Reproduc. Health. Prev: Trainee GP Leighton Buzzard; SHO (Accid. Serv., Orthop, Paediat., O & G, Psychiat. & Paediat.) Luton & Dunstable Hosp.

SHAH, Divyen 51 Park Crescent, Harrow Weald, Harrow HA3 6EU — MB ChB Manch. 1990.

SHAH, Farida 11 Long Leason, Selly Oak, Birmingham B29 4LT — MB ChB Leeds 1989; MB ChB (Hons.) Leeds 1989; MRCP (UK) 1992. Regist. (Dermat.) Skin Hosp. Birm. Specialty: Dermat. Prev: SHO Rotat. (Med.) Qu. Eliz. Hosp. & Gen. Hosp. Birm.; Ho. Off. Leeds Gen. Infirm.

SHAH, Fatima Noorain 142 Trinity Road, London SW17 7HS — MB BS Lond. 1996.

SHAH, Fozia Zafar 35 Queen's Road, Blackburn BB1 1QF — MB ChB Dund. 1996.

SHAH, Mr Hasmukh Vadilal Thorns Road Surgery, 43 Thorns Road, Quarry Bank, Brierley Hill DY5 2JS Tel: 01384 77524 Fax: 01384 486540; 4 Wigorn Lane, Redlake Drive, Pedmore, Stourbridge DY9 0TB Tel: 01562 886555 — MB BS Baroda 1957 (Med. Coll. Baroda) FRCS Eng. 1967. Prev: JHMO (Urol.) & Regist. (Urol.) Joyce Green Hosp. Dartford; Regist. (Gen. Surg.) Joyce Green Hosp. & W. Hill Hosp. Dartford.

SHAH, Hasmukhlal Kunvarji 4 Glynde Road, Bexleyheath DA7 4ET — MB BS Baroda 1957 (Med. Coll. Baroda) DLO 1960.

SHAH, Hasmukhlal Rajpal 93 Empire Avenue, London N18 1AR Tel: 020 8803 9944 — MB BS Bombay 1973.

SHAH, Mr Hasmukhlal Vadilal 3 Vista Rise, Radyr Cheyne, Llandaff, Cardiff CF5 2SD — MB BS Baroda 1972 (Med. Coll. Baroda) MS (ENT) Baroda 1975, MB BS 1972; DLO Baroda 1973; DLO Eng. 1978. GP Llwynypia.

SHAH, Hitesh Rasiklal 16 St Johns Villas, Friern Barnet Road, London N11 3BU — MB ChB Manch. 1982; MRCGP 1986.

SHAH, Imtiaz Maqbool 38 Annette Street, Glasgow G42 8EQ — MB ChB Glas. 1996; BSc (Hons) Glasgow 1991; MB ChB Glasgow 1996; MRCP Glasgow 1999. Sen. Health Off. (Med.) Western Infirm. Glas.; Research Fell., Western Infirm. Glas. Specialty: Gen. Med.; Pharmacology; Vasc. Med.

SHAH, Indira Shantilal Sunnybank Health Centre, Bryn Road, Cefn Fforest, Blackwood NP12 1HT Tel: 01495 224321 Fax: 01495 832156 — MB BS Gujarat 1965 (B.J. Med. Coll. Ahmedabad)

SHAH, Mr Indra Kumar Chimanlal 25 Manley Rd., Oldham OL8 1AU — MB BS Calcutta 1959; FRCS Glas. 1969.

SHAH, Irshad Ali Waterloo Medical Centre, 41 Dunkley Street, Wolverhampton WV1 4AN Tel: 01902 423559 — MB BS Punjab 1965.

SHAH, Jacques 10 Howberry Road, Cannons Park, Edgware HA8 6ST Tel: 020 8952 0874 — MRCS Eng. LRCP Lond. 1941; DTM & H Eng. 1942; MB BS Lond. 1943.

SHAH, Jaffar 67 Church Street, Darlaston, Wednesbury WS10 8DY Tel: 0121 526 2924; 21 Parkhall Road, Walsall WS5 3HF Tel: 01922 20608 — MB BS Peshawar 1962 (Khyber Med. Coll.) Prev: Regist. (Anaesth.) Roy. Albert Edwd. Infirm. Wigan; SHO (Anaesth.) City Gen. Hosp. Stoke-on-Trent.

SHAH, Jayantilal Chhaganlal The Drive Surgery, 90 The Drive, London NW11 9UL Tel: 020 8455 5901 Fax: 020 8731 9517 — MB BS Baroda 1965.

SHAH, Jayantilal Lakhamshi 15 St Denis Road, Selly Oak, Birmingham B29 4LN Tel: 0121 475 7789 — MB ChB Birm. 1961; DA Eng. 1963; FFA RCS Eng. 1969. Cons. Anaesth. Birm. AHA (T). Specialty: Anaesth.

SHAH, Mr Jayendra Kumar Raishi London Lane Clinic, Kinnaird House, 37 London Lane, Bromley BR1 4HB Tel: 020 8460 2661 Fax: 020 8464 5041 — MB BS Gujarat 1965 (M.P.S. Med. Coll. Jamnagar) FRCS Ed. 1970. Clin. Asst. (Surg.) Bromley Hosp.

SHAH, Jaymin Shantilal 2 The Pastures, Red Hill Grange, Wellingborough NN9 5YR — MB BS Lond. 1996.

SHAH, Joegy Kunjbihari Young and Partners, The Ryan Medical Centre, St Marys Road, Preston PR5 6JD Tel: 01772 335136 Fax: 01772 626701; 22 Fowler Close, Hoghton, Preston PR5 0DS — MB ChB Manch. 1987; BSc (Med. Sci) St. And. 1984; MRCGP 1993. Prev: Trainee GP Accrington.

SHAH, Jyotiben 28 Silkfield Road, London NW9 6QU — MB BS Lond. 1996 (Charing Cross of Westminster) BSc Lond. (Hons.) 1993. SHO Rotat. (Gen. Surg.), St Geo.'s Hosp. Lond. Specialty: Gen. Surg. Socs: MDU; BMA.

SHAH, Kaksha Oak Lodge Medical Centre, 234 Burnt Oak Broadway, Edgware HA8 0AP — MB ChB Leeds 1995; DCH 1997; DRCOG 1998; MRCGP 1999; DFFP 1999. GP Princip. at above professional adress. Socs: BMA; Med. Protec. Soc.

SHAH, Kantilal Devshi Ashcroft Road Medical Centre, 170 Ashcroft Road, Stopsley, Luton LU2 9AY — MB ChB Glas. 1964.

SHAH, Kantilal Rajpal (Surgery), 336 Uxbridge Road, Shepherds Bush, London W12 7LL Tel: 020 8743 5153 Fax: 020 8742 9070 — MB BS Saurastra 1971 (Univ. Saurastra, India) T(GP) 1991. GP. Specialty: Gen. Pract. Socs: Med. Protec. Soc. Prev: GP Kenya; Trainee GP Lond.

SHAH, Ketan Amritlal 43 Stilecroft Gardens, Wembley HA0 3HD — MB BS Bombay 1988; MRCPath 1994.

SHAH, Khalid (retired) 1-2 Felinheli Terrace, Port Dinorwic LL56 4JF — MB BS Peshawar 1965. Prev: GP Menai Bridge.

SHAH, Kinnari 73 Lakeside Gardens, Merthyr Tydfil CF48 1EW — MB ChB Manch. 1997.

SHAH, Kirtikumar Popatlal 71 Streatfield Road, Kenton, Harrow HA3 9BP — MB BS Bombay 1970.

SHAH, Kishorchandra Jatashanker (retired) 43 Gillhurst Road, Harborne, Birmingham B17 8PD Tel: 0121 427 1287 — MB ChB Birm. 1965; DMRD Eng. 1970; FFR 1972; FRCR 1975; T(R) (CR) 1991; FRCPCH 1997. Prev: Ho. Surg. St. Chad's Hosp. Birm.

SHAH, Kuntal Kunjvihari 3 Phillips Court, Whitchurch Lane, Edgware HA8 6QD — MB ChB Manch. 1995.

SHAH, Lalchand Devshi 22 Spencer Close, London N3 3TX — MB BS Bombay 1964 (Grant Med. Coll.)

SHAH, Madhvi 2 Rosemary Avenue, Finchley, London N3 2QN — MB BS Lond. 1991 (Kings College London) DCH RCP Lond. 1994; DGM RCP Lond. 1994; DRCOG 1995; MRCGP 1995. GP Princip. Specialty: Gen. Pract. Prev: Trainee GP Bounds Green Gp. Pract. Lond.; Trainee GP/SHO (Paediat.) N. Middlx. Hosp. VTS.

SHAH, Mahendra Popatlal 50 Elmcroft Crescent, London NW11 9SY Tel: 020 8455 6598 Fax: 020 8455 6598 — MB BS Baroda 1965. Clin. Asst. (Psychiat.) Napsbury Hosp. St. Albans. Specialty: Geriat. Psychiat.; Gen. Pract. Socs: Affil. Roy. Coll. Psychiat.; Diploma - Brit. Med. Acupunct. Soc. Prev: Asst. Gen. Pract.

SHAH, Mahesh Vasantlal Department of Anaesthetics, Leeds General Infirmary, Great George St., Leeds LS1 3EX; Longways, The Firs, Ling Lane, Scarcroft, Leeds LS14 3JH — MB BS Madras 1975 (Christian Med. Coll. & Hosp. Vellore) MRCS Eng. LRCP Lond. 1977; FFA RCS Eng. 1980; Dip. Amer. Bd. Anaesthesiol. 1986. Cons. Anaesth. Leeds Gen. Infirm.; Clin. Sen. Lect. (Anaesth.) Univ. Leeds. Specialty: Anaesth. Prev: Sen. Regist. (Anaesth.) S. Glam. HA; Vis. Asst. Prof. Oregon Health Scis. Univ. Portland Oregon, USA; Lect. (Anaesth.) Univ. Wales Sch. Med.

SHAH, Malati Rasikchandra 16 Fisher House, Ward Road, London N19 5EB Tel: 020 7272 0650 — MB BS Gujarat 1963 (B.J. Med. Coll. Ahmedabad) DGO Gujarat 1964; DA Eng. 1979. Socs: BMA & Assn. Anaesth. Prev: SHO (Anaesth.) Bethnal Green Hosp.; Regist. (Anaesth.) Qu. Eliz. Childr. Hosp. Lond. & Eliz. G.; Anderson Hosp. Lond.

SHAH, Manish Natverlal 16 Wyatts Drive, Southend-on-Sea SS1 3DH — MB BS Lond. 1993 (St. Bart. Hosp. Lond.) DCH RCP Lond. 1995; DFFP 1996; DRCOG 1996; MRCGP 1997.

SHAH, Mansukhlal Lakhamshi Paston Health Centre, Chadburn, Peterborough PE4 7DH Tel: 01733 572584 Fax: 01733 328131 — MB BS Gujarat 1980; LMSSA Lond. 1988; MRCS Eng. LRCP Lond. 1988. Specialty: Gen. Med.

SHAH, Mansukhlal Mohanlal — MB BS Gujarat 1970; DA Eng. 1978. Assoc. Specialist (Anaesth.). Specialty: Anaesth. Special Interest: Ophth. Anaesth.

SHAH, Mansukhlal Vershi Belsize Priory Health Centre, 208 Belsize Road, London NW6 4DX Tel: 0207 530 2666 Fax: 0207 372 2404 — MB ChB Sheff. 1974; T (GP); BDS Sheff. 1969; MRCS Eng. LRCP 1974.

SHAH, Manu Department of Dermatology, Dewsbury and District Hospital, Halifax Road, Dewsbury WF13 4HS Tel: 01924 816260 Fax: 01924 816286 — MB ChB Birm. 1988 (Birmingham) FRCP Lond.; MRCP (UK) 1993; MD (Birm.) 2000. Cons. Dermatol., Dewsbury & Dist. Hosp.; Hon. Sen. Lect. (University of Leeds). Specialty: Dermat. Socs: Brit. Associaton of Dermatologists.

SHAH, Mayank Ramanlal Grove Surgery, 103-105 Grove Road, Walthamstow, London E17 9BU Tel: 020 8521 2221 Fax: 020 8503 7773; 12 Michleham Down, Woodside Park, London N12 7JN Tel: 020 8445 1634 Fax: 020 8446 4614 — MB BS Lond. 1984 (Lond. Hosp.) DRCOG 1989. Dir. Lotus Healtcare 144 Harley St. Lond. W1G 7IA: health screening, medico-legal reports, primary care Phys. Socs: Chairm. Redbridge and Waltham LMC. Prev: Trainee GP St. Jas. Health Centre Lond. VTS.; SHO (Paediat.) Barking & K. Geo. Hosp. Essex; SHO (A & E) The Lond. Hosp.

SHAH, Mayur Ratilal 59 Ibstone Avenue, Bradwell Common, Milton Keynes MK13 8EB — MB BCh Wales 1983; DRCOG 1986; MRCGP 1987.

SHAH, Minaxi Central Surgery, 22 Cowley Hill Lane, St Helens WA10 2AE Tel: 01744 24849 Fax: 01744 456497 — MB ChB Leic. 1988. Specialty: Gen. Pract.

SHAH, Minesh J Bordesley Green Surgery, 143-145 Bordesley Green, Bordesley Green, Birmingham B9 5EG Tel: 0121 773 2170 — MB BS Gujarat 1969; MD Gujarat 1973.

SHAH, Minesh Khetshi Glan Clwyd Hospital, Bodelwyddan, Rhyl LL18 5UJ Tel: 01745 583910 Fax: 01745 583143 — BM BS Nottm. 1986; BMedSci (Hons.) Nottm. 1984. Staff Cardiol. Glan Clwyd Hosp. Bodelwyddan. Specialty: Cardiol. Prev: Regist. (Gen. Med.) Glan Clwyd Hosp. Bodelwyddan.

SHAH, Miranda Jane Selma, Winford Road, Chew Magna, Bristol BS40 8QQ — MB ChB Birm. 1997. Ho. Off. (Med.) Birm. Heartlands Hosp. Socs: BMA; MDU. Prev: Ho. Off. (Surg.) Kidderminster Gen. Hosp.

SHAH, Mrudula Vinodchandra 67 Malford Grove, South Woodford, London E18 2DY; 120 Hampton Road, Ilford IG1 2PR Tel: 020 8553 1774 — MB BS Gujarat 1969 (MP Shah Med. Coll. Jamnagar) Cert FPA. 1975. Trainer FPA Clinic City & E. Lond. AHA.

SHAH, Muhammad Akhtar Ali 42 Sandy Lane, Mitcham CR4 2HD — MB BS Punjab 1962.

SHAH, Mrs Mukta Prakash Hattersley Group Practice, Hattersley Road East, Hyde SK14 3EH Tel: 0161 368 4161 Fax: 0161 351 1989 — MD Nagpur 1976 (Govt. Med. Coll. Nagpur) MD (Gyn. & Obst.) Nagpur 1976, MB BS 1972; DGO Nagpur 1974. Ho. Off. (Med.) Dist. Gen. Hosp. Rotherham.

SHAH, Musharaf Motherwell Health Centre, 138-144 Windmill Street, Motherwell ML1 1TB Tel: 01698 265566 — MB BS Karachi 1963 (Dow Med. Coll.) BSc Peshawar 1957; DO RCPSI 1972. Socs: BMA. Prev: SHO (Paediat.) Roy. Hosp. Sick Childr. Glas.; Regist. (Neonat. Paediat.) Glas. Roy. Matern. Hosp.; Regist. (Ophth.) Glas. Eye Infirm.

SHAH, Nainal 4 Alliance Road, Glenfield, Leicester LE3 8SE — MB BS Baroda 1987.

SHAH, Najmul Hassan c/o General Office, Corbett Hospital, Stourbridge DY8 4JB — MB BS Peshawar 1986; MRCP (UK) 1994.

SHAH, Mr Nalin Damodar 3 Ville Franche, Bagatelle, St Saviour, Jersey JE2 Tel: 01534 59095 — MB BS Indore 1971; MS Gujarat 1974, DLO 1973; DLO RCS Eng. 1975; FRCS Eng. 1980. Cons.

Surg. ENT Gen. Hosp. St. Helier Jersey. Specialty: Otorhinolaryngol. Prev: Regist. (ENT) Roy. Berks. Hosp. Reading.

SHAH, Nalin Kantilal 40 Acacia Close, Stanmore HA7 3JR — MB BS Newc. 1964.

SHAH, Natvarlal Keshavlal (retired) 20 James Close, Woodlands, London NW11 9QX — MB BS Bombay 1957 (Grant Med. Coll. Bombay) Prev: SHO Anaesth. Roy. Infirm. Huddersfield.

SHAH, Natverlal Kantilal North Avenue Surgery, 332 North Avenue, Southend-on-Sea SS2 4EQ Tel: 01702 467215 Fax: 01702 603160 — MB BS Gujarat 1968 (B.J. Med. Coll. Ahmedabad) DObst RCOG 1972.

SHAH, Mr Navnit Shankerlal (retired) 80 Harley Street, London W1N 1AE Tel: 020 7580 3664; Sunnybank, 6 Holmdene Avenue, Mill Hill, London NW7 2LX Tel: 020 8959 3711 — (Seth G.S. Med. Coll.) MB BS Bombay 1958; Dip. Otorhinolaryng. 1959; DLO Eng. 1961; FRCS Eng. 1964. Hon. Cons. Surg. Roy. Nat. Throat, Nose & Ear Hosp. Lond.; Hon. Cons. Otol. Nuffield Hearing & Speech Centre Lond.; Hon. Prof. Portmann Foundat. Bordeaux, France. Prev: Dep. Dir. & Sen. Lect. Profess. Unit. Inst. Laryngol. & Otol. Lond.

SHAH, Nayankumar Chandrakant 8 Sarsfield Road, London SW12 8HN — MB BS Newc. 1986; DRACOG 1990; MRCGP 1991; DFFP 1993. Princip. GP Kent. Specialty: Gen. Pract. Socs: (Counc.) RCGP. Prev: Trainee GP N.d. VTS.

SHAH, Neil Kishore 43 Gillhurst Road, Birmingham B17 8PD Tel: 0121 427 1287 — BM BS Nottm. 1993. SHO (O & G) Nottm. City Hosp.

SHAH, Nicholas 34 Somerville Close, Bromborough, Wirral CH63 0PH — MB ChB Liverp. 1987.

SHAH, Nihar — MB BChir Camb. 1996; MA 1998; MRCP 2000.

SHAH, Nilofer 1 Foxhome Close, Chislehurst BR7 5XT — MB BS Punjab 1965 (Fatima Jinnah Med. Sch.) DA Eng. 1979. Assoc. Specialist (Anaesth.) Greenwich Dist. Hosp. Lond. Prev: Regist. (Anaesth.) Greenwich Dist. Hosp. Lond.; SHO (Anaesth.) Brook Gen. Hosp. Lond. & Qu. Mary's Hosp. Sidcup; Med. Off. Univ. Teach. Hosp. Lusaka, Zambia.

SHAH, Nimish Chhaganlal Addenbrookes NHS Trust, Hills Road, Cambridge CB2 2QQ — MB BS Lond. 1992; FRCS (Unl) 2002. Cons. Urol. Addenbrookes NHS Trust Camb. Prev: SHO (Gen. Surg.) Luton & Dunstable; SHO (Gen. Surg.& Orthop.) Watford Gen. Hosp.

SHAH, Nimish Shantilal Station Road Surgery, 15-16 Station Road, Penarth CF64 3EP Tel: 029 2070 2301 Fax: 029 2071 2048; Chruchfields, Village Farm, Bonvilston, Cardiff CF5 6TY Tel: 01446 781378 — MB BCh Wales 1987 (University of Wales) DRCOG 1992; MRCGP 1993. GP Princip. Specialty: Gen. Pract. Prev: Trainee GP Bridgend VTS.; SHO (Paediat.) Singleton Hosp. Swansea; Resid. (Med.) K. Edwd. VII Memor. Hosp. Paget, Bermuda.

SHAH, Nirmala Saresh 37 Churnfield, 6 Acres Est., Bigger Staff St., London N4 3LP — MB BS Saugar Univ. India 1975.

SHAH, Nisha Indu Flat 3, 113 Canfield Gardens, London NW6 3DY — MB BChir Camb. 1989.

SHAH, Nita 35 Central Avenue, Welling DA16 3AZ — MB BS Lond. 1992.

SHAH, Nitin Keshavlal 30 New Heath Close, New Cross Hospital, Wednesfield, Wolverhampton WV11 1XX — MB BS Baroda 1970.

SHAH, Padma Rashmi 11 Downes Court, Winchmore Hill, London N21 3PT Tel: 020 8886 5540 — MB BS Bombay 1965 (T.N. Med. Coll.) DObst RCOG 1969. Prev: Clin. Med. Off. Enfield & Haringey AHA; SHO (O & G) W. Middlx. Hosp. Isleworth; Ho. Off. (Psychiat.) Princess Alexandra Hosp. Harlow.

SHAH, Pallav Lalji Chelsea & Westminster Hospital, 369 Fulham Road, London SW10 9NH Tel: 020 8746 8063 Fax: 020 8746 8183; Royal Brompton Hospital, Sydney Street, London SW3 6NP Tel: 020 7351 8021 Fax: 020 7351 8085 — MB BS Lond. 1989 (Guy's) MD Lond. 1995; FRCP (UK) 2003. Cons. Phys. (Respirat. Med. & Gen Med.) Chelsea & Westm. Hosp. & Roy. Brompton Hosp.; Cons. Phys. (Respirat. Med.) Roy. Brompton Hosp. Lond.; Hon. Sen. Lect. (Respirat. Med.) Imperial Coll. Sch. Med. at Nat. Heart & Lung Inst. Lond. Specialty: Gen. Med.; Respirat. Med. Socs: Brit. Thoracic Soc., Roy. Soc. of Med. Prev: Sen. Regist. Rotat. (Gen. & Respirat. Med.) Roy. Brompton Hosp. & Chelsea & Westm. Hosp.; Regist. Rotat. (Gen. & Respirat. Med.) St. Mary's Hosp. Lond.; Research Fell. Roy. Brompton Hosp. & Nat. Heart & Lung Inst. Lond.

SHAH, Pankaj Ramniklal 227 Barrows Lane, Yardley, Birmingham B26 1RD — MB ChB Manch. 1991. Specialty: Community Child Health; Paediat.

SHAH, Pankaj S Pantglas Surgery, Aberfan Community Centre, Aberfan, Merthyr Tydfil CF48 4QE Tel: 01443 690382 Fax: 01443 690382.

SHAH, Parag 11 Downes Court, Wichmore Hill, London N21 3PT Tel: 020 8886 5540 Fax: 020 8886 5540 — MB BS Lond. 1991 (Charing Cross and Westminster) FRCS Pt. I. SHO (Neurosurg.). Specialty: Neurosurg.; Occupat. Health.

SHAH, Parag Jitendra 3 Woodend, Danras Hall, Newcastle upon Tyne NE20 9ES Tel: 0191 223 2226 — MB ChB Glas. 1991; MRCPsych 1977. Cons. (Child & Adolescent Forens. Psychiatrist) 3N's Ment. Health NHS Trust. Specialty: Child & Adolesc. Psychiat. Socs: BMA; Roy. Coll. Psychiat. Prev: Specialist Regist. (Child & Adolesc. Psychiat.) N. Manch. Health Care NHS Trust; Career Regist. (Psychiat.) Glas.

SHAH, Peter Moorfields Eye Hospital, City Road, London EC1V 2PD; 15 St. Denis Road, Selly Oak, Birmingham B29 4LN — MB ChB Leeds 1987; FRCOphth; BSc (Hons.) Leeds 1985, MB ChB 1987. Sen. Regist./Fell. Moorfields Eye Hosp. Lond. Specialty: Ophth. Prev: Regist. Birm. & Midl. Eye Hosp.; SHO (Neurosurg.) Midl. Centre Neurosurg. & Neurol. Birm.

SHAH, Mr Pir Julian Rabani Institute of Urology, 48 Riding House Street, London W1W 7EY Tel: 020 7679 9303 Fax: 020 7637 7076 Email: j.shah@ucl.ac.uk; King Edward VII Hospital, Emmanuel Kaye House, 37a Devonshire Street, London W1G 6QA Tel: 01923 286685 Fax: 01923 286687 Email: pjrshah@hotmail.com — MB ChB Leeds 1972 (Leeds Univ.) MRCS Eng. LRCP Lond. 1972; FRCS Eng. 1976. Sen. Lect. Inst. Urol. Univ. Coll. Lond.; Hon. Cons. (Urol.) St. Peter's Hosp. & UCL Hosps. Lond.; Cons. (Urol.) Roy. Nat. Orthop. Hosp. Stanmore. Specialty: Urol. Special Interest: Female Urol.; Neurourology; Reconstruction. Socs: Brit. Assn. Urol. Surg.; Corr. Mem. Amer. Urol. Assn.; Internat. Continence Soc. Prev: Sen. Regist. (Urol.) St. Peter's Hosp., Guy's & Middlx. Hosp. Lond.; Regist. (Urol.) Norf. & Norwich Hosp. Norwich; Ho. Surg. Profess. Surg. Unit Leeds Gen. Infirm.

SHAH, Piyush Ayrshire & Arran acute Hospitals NHS Trust, Dalmellington Road, Ayr KA6 6DX Tel: 01292 610555 Fax: 01292 614576; 10 Neward Crescent, Prestwick KA9 2JB Tel: 01292 75564 — MB BS Calcutta 1962 (Med. Coll. Calcutta) DOMS Calcutta 1968; DO Eng. 1970; MRCOphth 1989. Assoc. Ophth. Heathfield Hosp. Ayr. Specialty: Ophth. Socs: Ophth. Soc. UK; UK Intraocular Implant Soc.; Scott. Ophth. Circle. Prev: Regist. (Ophth.) Heathfield Hosp. Ayr; SHO (Ophth.) Princess Margt. Hosp. Swindon & Perth Roy. Infirm.

SHAH, Pradipkumar Rasiklal Shotley Bridge General Hospital, Consett DH8 0NB Tel: 01207 583583 Fax: 01207 586000 — MB BS Gujarat 1972. Staff Grade (Orthop.) Shotley Bridge Gen. Hosp., Co. Durh. Specialty: Orthop.

SHAH, Pratik Narendra Mayday University Hospital, London Road, Croydon CR7 7YE Tel: 020 8401 3158 Fax: 020 8401 3681 — MB BS Lond. 1985 (St. Geo.) MRCOG 1990; MD Lond. 1996. Cons. (O & G), Mayday Hosp. Specialty: Obst. & Gyn.

SHAH, Pravin Hiralal Hanford Clinic, New Inn Lane, Trentham, Stoke-on-Trent ST4 8EX Tel: 01782 642992 Fax: 01782 642992; 3 Fermain Close, Newcastle ST5 3EF — MB BS Gujarat 1967.

SHAH, Punita 19 Heatherbrook Road, Leicester LE4 1AJ — MB ChB Leic. 1994.

SHAH, Raj 16 Brendon Gardens, Harrow HA2 8NE — MB BS Lond. 1992; FRCS; BSc (Hons.) Lond. 1989, MB BS 1992. Research Regist. (Cardiothoracic Surg.) Inst. of Molecular Med. Oxf. Specialty: Cardiothoracic Surg.; Gen. Surg.

SHAH, Rajeev 5 Alma Farm Road, Toddington, Dunstable LU5 6BG — MB BChir Camb. 1998; MB BChir Camb 1998.

SHAH, Rajnikant Keshavlal 33 Pendle Fields, Fence, Near Burnley BB12 9HW Tel: 01282 694 426 Mob: 07976 329 404; 33 Pendle Fields, Fence, Burnley BB12 9HN Tel: 01282 694426 — MB BS Bombay 1973; DA, Bombay 1970; MD, Bombay 1973; FRCA Eng. 1977. Cosultant Anaesth. for Indep. Hosps. Gisburne, Beardwood, Highfield. Specialty: Anaesth. Special Interest: Obst.; Opthalm.; Orthopaedic Anaesth. Socs: Brit. Med. Assn.; Assn. of Anaesth. of Gt. Britain & Irel.; Europ. Soc. of Anaesth. Prev: Cons. Anaesth. Burnley Health Care NHS Trust Burnley Lancs.

SHAH, Ramanlal Bhikhabhai Grove Surgery, 103-105 Grove Road, Walthamstow, London E17 9BU Tel: 020 8521 2221 Fax: 020 8503 7773 — (Grant Med. Coll.) MB BS Bombay 1957; MRCS Eng. LRCP Lond. 1981. Socs: (Sec.) Walthamstow Med. Soc.; Akshar Health Comm.; Akshar Professional Gp. Prev: SHO (Geriat.) W. Middlx. Hosp.; Ho. Off. (Surg.) G.T. Hosp. Bombay, India; Ho. Off. (Med. & O & G) Methodist Miss. Hosp. Nadiad, India.

SHAH, Ramesh Shankerlal Yaikunth, 7 Crucible Close, Chadwell Heath, Romford RM6 4PZ — MB BS Gujarat 1970; MS Gujarat 1973.

SHAH, Rameshchandra Manilal Thorns Road Surgery, 43 Thorns Road, Quarry Bank, Brierley Hill DY5 2JS Tel: 01384 77524 Fax: 01384 486540 — MB BS Gujarat 1972 (B.J. Med. Coll. Ahmedabad) DPM Eng. 1981. Specialty: Gen. Psychiat. Socs: St Pauls. Prev: Assoc. Specialist Lea Castle Hosp. Kidderminster; Regist. (Psychiat.) St. Cadoc's Hosp. Newport.

SHAH, Ramnik Bhogilal 2 Glade Close, Coed Eva, Cwmbran NP44 4TF Tel: 0163 332839 — MB BS Gujarat 1959 (B.J. Med. Coll. Ahmedabad) DOMS Gujarat 1966; DO Eng. 1970; MCOphth 1990. Clin. Med. Off. & SCMO Eye Clinics Gwent Community Health Trust. Specialty: Ophth.

SHAH, Rashmi Chunilal 11 Downes Court, Winchmore Hill, London N21 3PT Tel: 020 8886 5540 — MB BS Bombay 1962 (T.N. Med. Coll.) DA Bombay 1965; DA Eng. 1966; FFA RCS Eng. 1970. Cons. Anaesth. N. Middlx. Hosp. Lond. Specialty: Anaesth. Socs: Assn. Anaesths.

SHAH, Rashmikant Rasiklal Croide Aaram, 28 Thames Ave, Perivale, Greenford UB6 8JL Tel: 020 8998 3493 — MRCS Eng. LRCP Lond. 1970 (St. Mary's) MD Lond. 1983, BSc (Hons.) 1967, MB BS 1970; MRCP (U.K.) 1976. Chief Internal Med. & Dir. Cardiol. King Fahad Hosp. Saudi Arabia. Prev: Hon. Sen. Regist. (Med.) St. Mary's Hosp. Paddington; Research Regist. (Cardiol.) St. Mary's Hosp. Lond.; Wellcome Research Fell. St. Mary's Hosp. Med. Sch. Lond.

SHAH, Reena 2 Warren Heights, Chafford Hundred, Grays RM16 6YH Tel: 01379 480578 Fax: 020 8538 1887 — MB ChB Leic. 1998. PRHO Surg. Newham Gen. Hosp. Plaistow, Lond. Specialty: Gen. Surg. Prev: PRHO Med. Basildon Gen. Hosp. Basildon, Essex.

SHAH, Reena Chhotalal 6 Wildcroft Gardens, Edgware HA8 6TJ — BM Soton. 1996.

SHAH, Rekha The Surgery, 114-116 Carden Avenue, Brighton BN1 8PD Tel: 01273 500155 Fax: 01273 501193; 10 Varndean Holt, Brighton BN1 6QX Tel: 01273 552383 Fax: 01273 552383 — MB ChB Dundee 1983; DRCOG 1986.

SHAH, Rimi Mansukhlal 32 Edgeworth Crescent, London NW4 4HG — MB BS Lond. 1994.

SHAH, Sachit 196 East Lane, Wembley HA0 3LF — MB ChB Manch. 1985; MRCGP 1990. Socs: Canad. Coll. Family Pract.

SHAH, Saima 38 Annette Street, Crosshill, Glasgow G42 8EQ — MB ChB Aberd. 1996.

SHAH, Samina Nuzhat 2 Beaulieu Place, London W4 5SY — MB BS Lond. 1998; MB BS Lond 1998.

SHAH, Samir Natvarlal 20 James Close, Woodlands, London NW11 9QX — MB ChB Sheff. 1984; MRCS Eng. LRCP Lond. 1984; MRCP (UK) 1987; Dip. Pharm. Med. RCP (UK) 1990. VP Corporate Marketing Serono,Geneva; Hon. Lect. (Med.) Dept. Kings. Coll. Hosp. Med. Sch. Lond. Specialty: Pharmacology. Prev: Sen. Med. Adviser Sandoz Pharmaceut. Camberley; SHO (Ophth.) Soton HA; SHO (Med.) Grampian Health Bd.

SHAH, Sandeep Sobhagchand 26 Valley View, Barnet EN5 2NY Tel: 07768 552224 — MB BS Lond. 1990 (Roy. Lond. Hosp. Med. Coll.) DFFP 1994; T(GP) 1994; MBA Imper. Coll. Lond. 1996. GP & Pharmaceut. Phys.; Vis. Lect. Westminster Univ.; Vis. Lect. Imperial Coll.; Counc. Mem. of ABHI (Assn. of Brit. Healthcare Industries). Specialty: Gen. Pract.; Pharmaceutical Medicine; Research. Socs: Fell. RSM; Fell. RSA; Brit. Assn. of Regulatory Affairs.

SHAH, Sangeeta 3 Woodlands Drive, Yarm TS15 9NU — MB ChB Leic. 1994. Trainee GP Leicester VTS. Specialty: Gen. Pract. Prev: Ho. Off. Walsgrave Hosp. Coventry; Ho. Off. Glenfield Gen. Hosp. & Leicester Gen. Hosp.

SHAH, Sanjay Hasmukhlal 4 Alliance Road, Glenfield, Leicester LE3 8SE — MB BS Baroda 1987.

SHAH, Sanjay Kantilal 79 Wychwood Avenue, Canons Park, Edgware HA8 6TQ — MB BS Calcutta 1987.

SHAH, Mr Sanjay Mulji Epsom & St Helier NHS Trust, The Roy Harfitt Eye Unit, Sutton Hospital, Cotswold Road, Sutton SM2 5NF Tel: 020 8296 4288 — MB BS Lond. 1983 (St Geo.) BSc (1st cl. Hons) Lond. 1980; MRCP (UK) 1986; FRCS Eng. 1988; DO RCS Eng. 1988; FRCOphth 1989. Cons. Ophth. Surg. Epsom & St Helier NHS Trust. Specialty: Ophth. Special Interest: Cataract Surgery; Glaucoma; Laser Surgery. Socs: BMA. Prev: Cons. Ophth. Surg. St Bart. & The Roy. Lond. Hosp. Lond.; Sen. Regist. (Ophth.) West. Eye Hosp. Lond.; Research Fell. (Ophth.) St Thos. Hosp. Lond.

SHAH, Sanjiv Suryakant Southend Hospital, Prittlewell Chase, Westcliff on Sea SS0 0RY; 50 Rodney Road, London E11 2DE — MB BS Lond. 1988.

SHAH, Saroj Sudhir Victoria Square, 134 Broad St., Hanley, Stoke-on-Trent ST1 4EQ — (M. P. Shah Medical College, India) MB BS.

SHAH, Shaheen Pravin Khimji 14 Windsor Court, Golders Green Road, London NW11 9PP — MB BS Lond. 1997.

SHAH, Shahnaz New Cross Hospital, Wednesfield, Wolverhampton WV11 1XX Tel: 01902 732255; 24 New Heath Close, Wolverhampton WV11 1XX — MB BS Punjab 1971; DGO TC Dub. 1980; MRCOG 1988.

SHAH, Shamsul Hudda 62 Craythorne Gardens, North Heaton, Newcastle upon Tyne NE6 5UL — MB BS Newc. 1996.

SHAH, Shantilal Hiralal Sunnybank Health Centre, Bryn Road, Cefn Fforest, Blackwood NP12 1HT Tel: 01495 224321 Fax: 01495 832156 — MB BS Gujarat 1962 (B.J. Med. Coll. Ahmedabad)

SHAH, Shantilal Mulchand Department of Histopathology, Pilgrim Hospital, Boston PE21 9DW Tel: 01205 364801; 46 Allington Gardens, Boston PE21 9DW Tel: 01205 363439 — MB BS Gujarat 1967 (B.J. Med. Coll. Ahmedabad) FRCPath 1992, M 1981. Cons. Histopath. Pilgrim Hosp. Boston. Specialty: Histopath. Socs: BMA; Assn. Clin. Path.; Internat. Assn. Path. Prev: Sen. Regist. (Histopath.) New Med. Sch. Manch. & Hope Hosp. Salford; Regist. (Path.) Withington Hosp. Manch.

SHAH, Shantilal Ramjibhai 28 Churchill Avenue, Harrow HA3 0AY Tel: 020 8909 2199 — MB BS Gujarat 1963. Prev: GP Nairobi, Kenya.

SHAH, Shashikant Zaverchand Pinn Medical Centre, 8 Eastcote Road, Pinner HA5 1HF Tel: 020 8866 5766 Fax: 020 8429 0251 — MB ChB Sheff. 1967; MRCGP 1976.

SHAH, Shobhna 41 Free Trade Wharf, 340 The Highway, London E1W 3ES Tel: 020 7790 2774 — MB BS Bombay 1977; DA (UK) 1978; Cert. Av. Med. 1986. Specialty: Anaesth.

SHAH, Snehal Sudhir 48 Meakin Avenue, Westbury Park, Clayton, Newcastle ST5 4EY — BM BS Nottm. 1998; BM BS Nottm 1998.

SHAH, Sobagchand Mepa 25 Ravenscraig Road, London N11 1AE — MB BS Gujarat 1965.

SHAH, Sobhagchandra Mohanlal Oakington Medical Centre, 41 Oakington Avenue, Wembley HA9 8HX Tel: 020 8904 3021; 30 Ashworth Mansions, Elgin Avenue, Maida Vale, London W9 1JP Tel: 020 7289 5401 — MB BS Saurashtra 1971 (M.P.S. Med. Coll. Jamnagar) Cert. Family Plann. JCC 1976. Clin. Asst. (Venereol.) Roy. N. Hosp. Lond. Prev: SHO (Gen. Surg. & A & E) Maidenhead Hosp.; Ho. Phys. (Gen. Med.) Rochford Gen. Hosp.; Ho. Phys. (Paediat.) Southend Gen. Hosp.

SHAH, Sonal Kantilal The Medical Centre, 45 Enderley Road, Harrow Weald, Harrow HA3 5HF Tel: 020 8863 3333 — MB ChB Manch. 1992.

SHAH, Sonia 126 Thornbury Road, Isleworth TW7 4NE — MB BS Lond. 1996.

SHAH, Suerekha Karstensen 19 Carcraig Place, Dalgety Bay, Dunfermline KY11 9ST — MB ChB Dund. 1996.

SHAH, Mr Sunil 20 Farquhar Road, Edgbaston, Birmingham B15 3RB — MB BS Lond. 1987; FRCS Ed. 1992; FRCOphth 1992. Regist. (Ophth.) Roy. Eye Hosp. Manch. Specialty: Ophth.

SHAH, Sunil Mulji — MB BS Lond. 1990 (St. Geo. Hosp. Med. Sch.) MSc (Informat. Sci.) City 1992, BSc 1987; MSc (Pub. Health) Lond. 1997; MFPHM, 1999. Cons., Pub. Health, E. Surrey HA. Specialty: Pub. Health Med. Prev: Sen. Regist. (pub.Health), Dept. of pub. Health Sci.s, St Geo.s Hosp. Med. Sch., Lond.; Regist. (Pub. Health) Croydon HA; Sen. Regist. (Pub. Health) E. Surrey HA.

SHAH, Surendra Chimanlal St George's Medical Centre, Field Road, New Brighton, Wallasey CH45 5LN Tel: 0151 630 2080 Fax: 0151 637 0370 — MB BS Gujarat 1968 (Ahmedabad, India) GP Wallasey; Mem. LMC. Specialty: Orthop. Prev: Sec. Wallasey Med. Soc.

SHAH, Susan Community Child Health, Child Development Centre, Crawley Hospital, Crawley RH11 7DH Tel: 01293 531951 — MB ChB Birm. 1974. Assoc. Specialist (Community Child Health) Surrey-Sussex Healthcare NHS Trust. Specialty: Community Child Health. Prev: Assoc. Specialist (Community Child Health) Crawley-Horsham Health Serv. NHS Trust.

SHAH, Syed A High Street Health Centre, High Street, Aberdare CF44 7DD Tel: 01685 874614 Fax: 01685 877485.

SHAH, Syed Azim Newbury Park Health Centre, 40 Perrymans Farm Road, Newbury Park, Ilford IG2 7LE — MB BS Lond. 1993; DFFP 2002.

SHAH, Syed Ghafoor 62 Craythorne Gardens, Newcastle upon Tyne NE6 5UL — MB ChB Sheff. 1992.

SHAH, Mr Syed Mohammad Ali 854 Great West Road, Isleworth TW7 5NG Tel: 020 8568 2466 Fax: 020 8655 3237; A. O. Clinic, Nazimabad No. 4, Karachi, Pakistan Tel: 009221 668 5564 Fax: 009221 668 5555 — MRCS Eng. LRCP Lond. 1977 (Dow Karachi) MBBS Karachi 1970; MRCS Eng LRCP Lond. 1977; FRCS Glas. 1979; FRCS Ed. 1979; LMSSA Lond. 1980. Cons. Orthop. Surg. A. O. Clinic Karachi. Specialty: Trauma & Orthop. Surg. Socs: Fell. Brit. Orthop. Assoc.

SHAH, Syed Mumtaz Ali Cardiology Department, Wythenshawe Hospital, Southmoor Road, Manchester M23 9LT — MB BS Peshawar 1987.

SHAH, Syed Nadir 17 Mornington Road, Norwich NR2 3NA — MB BS Peshawar 1987.

SHAH, Mr Syed Tariq Kazim Consultant Urologist, Bradford Teaching Hospitals NHS Trust, Urology Office, St. Luke's Hospital, Little Horton Lane, Bradford BD5 0NA Tel: 01274 365865 Fax: 01274 365877 Email: t.shah@dial.pipex.com; Willow House, 107 All Alone Road, Idle, Bradford BD10 8TR Tel: 01274 614229 — MB BS Karachi 1975 (Dow Medical College, University of Karachi) MRCS Eng. LRCP Lond. 1981; FRCS Glas. 1983. Cons. Urol. Bradford Hosps. Teachg. NHS Trust, Bradford; Cons. Urol., The Yorks. Clinic, Bradford. Specialty: Urol. Socs: Brit. Assn Urol. Surgs.; Amer. Urol. Assn.; Soc. Internat. Urologie.

SHAH, Syed Zabier Hussnan 3 Ridgewell Way, Colchester CO2 8NG — BM Soton. 1994.

SHAH, Tahir Hussain Saplings, Weir Road, Hanwood, Shrewsbury SY5 8LA — MB ChB Wales 1995.

SHAH, Tanja Maria Witley Surgery, Wheeler Lane, Witley, Godalming GU8 5QR Tel: 01428 682218 Fax: 01428 682218 — MB BS Lond. 1988; MRCGP 1993.

SHAH, Tanuja — BM BS Nottm. 1995; SpR Wessex; FRCA (Aanaesth.) 2001. Prev: SHO (Med.) Roy. Perth Hosp.; SHO (A&E) Northampton; PRHO (Surg.) Bath Roy. United.

SHAH, Tejshri Harivallabh 40 Woodbridge Lawn, Leeds LS6 3LU — MB ChB Leeds 1994.

SHAH, Tulsidas Haridas Galleries Health Centre, Washington Centre, Washington NE38 7NQ Tel: 0191 416 6130 Fax: 0191 416 6344; 23 Fatfield Park, Washington NE38 8BW Tel: 0191 416 8824 — MB ChB Glas. 1964; MSc Med. Sc. Glas. 1983. Clin. Asst. (Geriat. Med.) Sunderland AHA; Div.al Surg. St. John Ambul. Assn.; Bd Mem. Sunderland W. PCG. Specialty: Care of the Elderly. Socs: BMA. Prev: Ho. Phys. Gartloch Hosp. Gartlosh; SHO (Path.) Frenchay Hosp. Bristol; Clin. Asst. (Haemat.) Wolverhampton Gp. Hosps.

SHAH, Upma Willow Tree Family Doctors, 301 Kingsbury Road, London NW9 9PE Tel: 020 8204 6464 Fax: 020 8905 0946; 15 Totternhoe Close, Kenton, Harrow HA3 0HS — MB ChB Manch. 1990; DRCOG 1992; MRCGP 1994; DFFP 1994; Dip. Pract Dermat. 1999.

SHAH, Usha U The Surgery, 19 Chichele Road, London NW2 3AH Tel: 020 8452 3232 Fax: 020 8452 9812 — MB BS Gujarat 1969; MB BS Gujarat 1969.

SHAH, Uttamchand Raishi The Surgery, 19 Chichele Road, London NW2 3AH Tel: 020 8452 3232 Fax: 020 8452 9812; 28 Salehurst Close, Kenton, Harrow HA3 0UG Tel: 020 8204 5377 — MB BS Gujarat 1969 (B.J. Med. Coll. Ahmedabad)

SHAH, Varsha Minesh Bordesley Green Surgery, 143-145 Bordesley Green, Bordesley Green, Birmingham B9 5EG Tel: 0121 773 2170 — MB BS Gujarat 1969; MD Gujarat 1973; MRCPath U.K. 1985.

SHAH, Veena Suhas 35 The Croft, Euxton, Chorley PR7 6LH Tel: 01257 241039 — MB BS Bombay 1972; DA (UK) 1978. Specialty: Anaesth.

SHAH, Vibhuti Shantilal 5 Old Mill Avenue, Cannon Park, Coventry CV4 7DY — MB BS Bombay 1985; MRCP (UK) 1994.

SHAH, Mr Vikram 9 Park Lane, Aberdare CF44 8HN — MB BS Bombay 1960 (Grant Med. Coll.) DLO Eng. 1965; FRCS Ed. 1967. Dep. Med. Dir. Cons. ENT Surg.; Clin. Dir. Surg./Anaesth. Specialty: Otorhinolaryngol. Socs: Chairm. Welsh Assoc. OtorhinoLaryngol. Prev: Sen. Regist. & Hon. Clin. Tutor United Birm. Hosp.

SHAH, Vinaykumar Punja 59 Eversleigh Road, Finchley, London N3 1HY — LMSSA Lond. 1978.

SHAH, Vinit Navinchandra Department of Paediatrics, William Harvey Hospital, Kennington Road, Ashford TN24 0LZ Tel: 01233 633331 Ext: 6211 Fax: 01233 616139 Email: vinitshah@aol.com; 29 Canon Woods Way, Kennington, Ashford TN24 9QY Tel: 01233 629384 — MB BS Bombay 1984; MD (Paediat.) Bombay 1988; MRCP (UK) 1992; FRCPCH 1996; (FAM) Singapore 1999. Cons. Paediat. William Harvey Hosp. Ashford Kent; Hon. Cons. Paediatric Cardiol. Guy's Hosp. Lond. Specialty: Paediat.; Neonat.; Paediat. Cardiol. Socs: Roy. Coll. Paediat. & Child Health; Indian Acad. Paediat.; Fell.Roy. Coll. of Paediat. and Child Health.

SHAH, Vinodchandra Keshavlal (retired) (Surgery) 120 Hampton Road, Ilford IG1 1PR Tel: 020 8553 1774 Fax: 020 8514 4622; 67 Malford Grove, South Woodford, London E18 2DY — MB BS Gujarat 1966 (M.P. Shah Med. Coll.) Cert FPA 1972.

SHAH, Vinodkumar Bhogilal 11 The Hayfield, Beardwood Park, Blackburn BB2 7BP — MB BS Gujarat 1987.

SHAH, Waqaar Ali 89 Bennerley Road, London SW11 6DT — MB BS Lond. 1993.

SHAH, Yashwant Zaverchand Grahame Park Health Centre, The Concourse, Grahame Park Estate, London NW9 5XT Tel: 020 8205 2301 Fax: 020 8200 9173 — LRCPI & LM, LRSCI & LM 1958; LRCPI & LM, LRCSI & LM 1958.

SHAH, Yogeshkumar Bhagwatilal Silverdale Drive Health Centre, 6 Silverdale Drive, Thurmaston, Leicester LE4 8NN Tel: 0116 260 0640 Fax: 0116 260 1640 — MB BS Baroda 1973.

SHAH, Zaheer Hussain 1A Adria Road, Sparkhill, Birmingham B11 4JL — MB ChB Birm. 1994.

SHAH, Zaverchand Padamshi Anaesthetic Department, Queen Elizabeth II Hospital, Welwyn Garden City AL7 4HQ Tel: 01707 328111; 4 Russell Croft Road, Welwyn Garden City AL8 6QT Tel: 01707 321692 — (Topiwalla Nat. Med. Coll.) MB BS Bombay 1965; DA Eng. 1966; FFA RCS Eng. 1969. Cons. Anaesth. Qu. Eliz. II Hosp., Welwyn Garden City. Specialty: Anaesth. Socs: Assn. Anaesth. Gt. Brit. & Irel.; BMA. Prev: Sen. Regist. (Anaesth.) Gen. Infirm. Leeds; Regist. (Anaesth.) W. Middlx. Hosp. Isleworth; SHO (Anaesth.) Gen. Hosp. Burton-on-Trent.

SHAHA, Monica Rose 3 Normanhurst, Ormskirk L39 4UZ Tel: 01695 573370 Fax: 01695 573370 — MB ChB Manch. 1997.

SHAHAB, Khalid Latif The Surgery, 480 Footscray Road, New Eltham, London SE9 3UA; 3 Vogue Court, 107-109 Widmore Road, Bromley BR13AF Tel: 01358 721631 — (King Edwd. Med. Coll. Lahore) MB BS Punjab (Pakistan) 1964; DCH RCPSI 1969; DTM & H Eng. 1977. Specialty: Gen. Pract.

SHAHABDEEN, Mr Mohamed Mahir Maidstone Hospital, Hermitage Lane, Barming, Maidstone ME16 9QQ Tel: 01622 729000; 34 Chestnut Close, Kings Hill, West Malling ME19 4FP — MB BS Sri Lanka 1981; FRCS Eng. 1990. Staff Grade Surg. (Gen. Surg.) Maidstone Hosp. Specialty: Gen. Surg.

SHAHABUDDIN, Mr Mohammad Brandon Road Surgery, 108 Brandon Road, Binley, Coventry CV3 2JF Tel: 024 7645 3634 Fax: 024 7663 6886; 37 Asthill Grove, Coventry CV3 6HN Tel: 024 76 501101 — MB BS Rajshahi 1966 (Rajshahi Med. Coll.) FRCS Ed. 1978. GP Coventry.

SHAHBAZI, Syed Shah Abedul Haque 98 High Street, Golborne, Warrington WA3 3DA — MB BS Dacca 1969.

SHAHDADPURI, Vivek Dayal 5 St Stephens Close, 20 Avenue Road, London NW8 6DB — MB BS Lond. 1996.

SHAHEEN, Mr Ahmed Aly Mohamed ULH NHS Trust, Family Health Directorate, Dept. Obstetrics & Gynaecology, Pilgrim Hospital, Boston PE21 9QS — MB BCh Ain Shams 1973; Cert. Family Plann. JCC 1985; DObst RCPI 1985; FRCS Ed. 1992; DRCOG 1986, M 1992; MFFP 1993; MRCPI 1994; Diploma of advanced Train. in Obstetric ultrasound scan of Jt. Comm. of RCOG & RCR 2002. Cons. (O & G) Pilgrim Hosp. Lincs.; Boston Menopause Clinic at The Bostonian Private Wing Pilgrim Hosp. Specialty: Obst. & Gyn.; Gen. Surg.; Gen. Med. Socs: Brit. Soc. Colpos.; Brit. Menopause Soc.; Brit. Soc. of Obst.s. Prev: Sen. Regist. (O & G) The Princess Anne Hosp. Southampton Hants.; Sen Regist. (O & G) Roy Devon & Exeter Hosp. S. Devon & Torbay-Torque; Acting Registr. (O & G) Rochford Hosp. Southend-on-Sea.

SHAHEEN, Jenanne Sameera Omar 118-120 Stanford Avenue, Brighton BN1 6FE Tel: 01273 506361 — MB BS Lond. 1985; DRCOG 1991.

SHAHEEN, Mr Maas Abd El-Kader Beechlands, Elwick Road, Hartlepool TS26 0DN Tel: 01429 522509 — MB BCh Cairo 1971; FRCS Ed. 1976; FRCS Glas. 1976; MChOrth. Liverp. 1980.

SHAHEEN, Mr Omar Hassan (retired) Flat 3, 4 Shad Thames, London SE1 2YT Tel: 020 7403 3606 Fax: 020 7357 6172 — MB BS Lond. 1954 (Guy's) FRCS Eng. 1958; MS Lond. 1967; FRCS Ed. 1987. Prev: Cons. Surg. (Head & Neck Oncol. & ENT) Guy's Hosp. Lond.

SHAHEEN, Seif Omar Department of Public Health Sciences, GKT School of Medicine (Guy's Campus), King's College London, 5th Floor, Capital House, 42 Weston St., London SE1 3QD Tel: 020 7848 6635 Fax: 020 7848 6605 Email: seif.shaheen@kcl.ac.uk — MB BS Lond. 1984 (Cambridge & Guy's Hospital) MA Camb. 1985; MRCP (UK) 1987; MSc Epidemiol. Lond. 1993; PhD Epidemiol. Soton. 1996; DFPH 1999. Sen. Lect. In Clin. Epidemiol., Dept. Pub. Health Sci.s, GKT Sch. of Med. King's Coll. Lond. Specialty: Epidemiol.; Pub. Health Med. Special Interest: Role of diet & prenatal environment in Aetiol. of asthma; Early life origins of Respirat. Dis.; Respirat. Epidemiol. Socs: Amer. Thoracic Soc.; Europ. Respirat. Soc. Prev: Regist. (Med.) St. Richard's Hosp. Chichester; Wellcome Fell. (Clin. Epidemiol.) MRC Environm. Epidemiol. Unit Soton. Univ.; Lect. (Pub. Health Med) UMDS.

SHAHI, Abhishek 2 Rosslyn Avenue, Ackworth, Pontefract WF7 7QF — MB ChB Sheff. 1992.

SHAHID, Humma 106 Cairns Road, Bristol BS6 7TG Tel: 0117 942 2383 Email: humma@doctors.org.uk — BM BCh Oxf. 1998. SHO A&E St Geo.s Hosp. Lond. Specialty: Accid. & Emerg. Prev: Ho. Off. Cardiol.Gen.Med.Qu. Eliz. hosp.Birm; Ho. Surg.Plastic/Reconstruct.Surg.Gen Surg.John Radcliffe Hosp.Oxf.

SHAHID, Jamil 6 Birchlea, Altrincham WA15 8WF — MB BS Punjab 1968 (King Edwd. Med. Coll. Lahore) BSc DDS 1983; PDS Wales 1984; PhD (Derm.) Wales 1987. Cons. (Derm.) Roy. Preston Hosp. (North Lancs Teachg. Hospitals) Preston Lancs. Prev: Cons. (Derm.) (Locom) Burnley Gen. Hosp. Burnley Lancs; Assoc. Prof. F. J. Med. Coll. Lahore Pakistan; Asst. Prof. (Derm.) A.1 Med. Coll. Lahore Pakistan.

SHAHID, Manjoor 38 Cromwell Street, Burnley BB12 0DB — MB BS Lond. 1994.

SHAHID, Saiyed Zakaullah Deepdale Road Surgery, 228-232 Deepdale Road, Preston PR1 6QB Tel: 01772 555733 Fax: 01772 885406 — MB BS Bihar 1969; MB BS Bihar 1969.

SHAHIDULLAH, Begum Sara 170 Upper Road, Greenisland, Carrickfergus BT38 8RW — MB BCh BAO Belf. 1988; MB BCh Belf. 1988.

SHAHIDULLAH, Hossain 128 Station Road, Broughton Astley, Leicester LE9 6PW — BM BS Nottm. 1986; BMedSci Nottm. 1984, BM BS 1986; MRCP (UK) 1989. Cons. (Dermat.) Derbsh. Roy. Infirm. Specialty: Dermat. Prev: Sen. Regist. (Dermat.) Leicester Roy. Infirm.; Research Fell. (Dermat.) Roy. Infirm. Edin.; Regist. (Dermat.) Roy. Infirm. Edin.

SHAHIDULLAH, Mohammad (retired) 53 Knighton Road, Stoneygate, Leicester LE2 3HL Tel: 0116 270 8970 — (Dhaka Med. Coll.) MB BS Dacca 1958; PhD (Clin. Dermat.) St. And. 1969; DTM & H Liverp. 1970; Dip. Ven. Liverp. 1971. Locum Cons. in Genitourin. Med. Leicester Roy. Infirm. Prev: Cons. Genitourin Med. Lincoln Co. Hosp.

SHAHIN, Ghodsieh 47 Oakland Road, West Jesmond, Newcastle upon Tyne NE2 3DR — MB BS Newc. 1982; DCH RCPS Glas. 1986; MRCP (UK) 1990. Clin. Med. Off. (Child Health) N. Tyneside HA.

SHAHMANESH, Maryam Flat 1, 52 Salisbury Road, Moseley, Birmingham B13 8JT; Flat 1, (Ground Floor), 13 St Charles Square, London W10 6EF Tel: 020 7565 4243 Email: m.shahmanesh@internet.com — BChir Camb. 1993 (Cains College Cambridge) MRCP (Lond.) 1997.

SHAHMANESH, Mohsen Department of Genitourinary Medicine, Whittall Street Clinic, Whittall St., Birmingham B4 6DH Tel: 0121 237 5720 Fax: 0121 237 5729 — MB BS Lond. 1965; MRCS Eng. LRCP Lond. 1965; MRCP Lond. 1968; MD Bristol 1976; FRCP Lond. 1992. Cons. Genitourin. Med. Whittall St. Clinic Birm.; Edr. Sex Transm Inf. Med. Specialty: Genitourinary Medicine; HIV Med. Prev: Chairm. Specialist Advisory Comm Genitourin. Med.

SHAHNAWAZ, Ghausia 15 The Spinneys, St. Georges Road W., Bickley, Bromley BR1 2NT Tel: 020 8467 9556 — MB BS Punjab 1964; MRCOG 1969; LicAc, MBAcA 1986. GP/Acupunct. Bromley. Specialty: Obst. & Gyn.

SHAHRABANI, Rashid Majid Jafar 22 Westfields Road, Acton, London W3 0AX — MB ChB Baghdad 1971; MRCP (UK) 1979. Regist. (Cardiol.) Soton. Gen. Hosp. Specialty: Cardiol. Prev: Regist. (Cardiol.) Groby Rd. Hosp. Leic.; Regist. (Gen. Med.) Medway Health Dist.

SHAHRAD, Mr Bahram Somerfield Hospital, London Road, Maidstone ME16 0DU Tel: 01622 208000 Fax: 01622 674706 Email: bshahrad@virgin.net; Upton Gray, 119 Ashford Road, Bearsted, Maidstone ME14 4BT Tel: 01622 738896 — MD Teheran 1964; FRCS Ed. 1977. Cons. Orthop. Surg. Somerfield Hosp. Maidstone. Specialty: Orthop. Socs: Fell. BOA. Prev: Cons. Orthop. & Trauma Maidstone Gen. Hosp.

SHAHRAD, P Lindo Wing, St Mary's Hospital, South Wharf Road, London W2 1NY Tel: 020 7886 1607 Fax: 020 7286 6502; BUPA Hospital, Harpenden, Ambrose Lane, Harpenden AL5 4BP Tel: 01582 763191; 22 Harley Street, London W1N 1AP Tel: 020 7637 0491 Fax: 020 7286 6502 — MD Teheran 1968; Dip. Dermat. Lond. 1973. Board of Dermatology 1976 Tehran.

SHAHRIARI, Shahrokh 12 Huntly Gardens, Glasgow G12 9AT Tel: 0141 339 3113 — MB ChB Glas. 1967; DCP Lond 1971; MRCPath 1979. Cons. Haemat. N. Lanarksh. Gp. Hosps. Specialty: Haematology. Socs: Assn. Clin. Pathols.; Brit. Soc. Haemat. Prev: Sen. Regist. (Haemat.) Westm. Hosp. Med. Sch. Lond.

SHAIDA, Azhar Mohammed The Royal National Throat Nose and Ear Hospital, 330 Gray's Inn Road, London WC1X 8DA Tel: 020 7915 1672 Email: doctor@ent-doctor.co.uk — BM BCh Oxf. 1990; MA (Exp. Psychol.) Camb. 1991; FRCS (Gen. Surg.) Lond. 1994; FRCS (ENT) Lond. 1995; MD Lond. 2004. Cons. ENT Surg., Roy. Nat. Throat Nose and Ear Hosp., Lond. Specialty: Otorhinolaryngol. Prev: ENT Specialist Regist. E. Anglia Rotat.

SHAIDA, Wahid Asif Roxbourne Medical Centre, 37 Rayners Lane, South Harrow, Harrow HA2 0UE Tel: 020 8422 5602 Fax: 020 8422 3911 — MB BS Lond. 1991; DCH RCP Lond. 1995; DFFP Lond. 1997. GP Princip. Roxboune Med. Centre, S. Harrow; Primary Care Pract. A & E Whittington Hosp. Lond. Specialty: Gen. Pract.; Paediat. Prev: GP/Regist. Caversham Gp. Pract. Kentish Town, Lond.; SHO (Med. & Elderly Care) Edgware Gen. Hosp.; Trainee GP Univ. Hosp. Lond. VTS.

SHAIKH, Abdul Aleem Drummond Street Surgery, 94 Drummond Street, London W1 2HN Tel: 020 7387 4048 — MB BS Punjab 1962.

SHAIKH, Abdul Mannan Handsworth Grange Medical Centre, 432 Handsworth Road, Sheffield S13 9BZ Tel: 0114 269 7505 Fax: 0114 269 8535 — MB BS Karachi 1962 (Dow Med. Coll. Karachi) DTM & H Eng. 1963; MRCGP 1976. Socs: Soc. Occupat. Med. Prev: Clin. Asst. (Mass Radiogr.) Sheff.; Regist. (A & E) Doncaster Roy. Infirm.; SHO (Surg.) Doncaster Roy. Infirm.

SHAIKH, Amanullah Child & Family Consultation Service, 62 Maidstone Road, Grays RM17 6NF Tel: 01375 816900 Fax: 01375 816913; 359 Upper Rainham Road, Hornchurch RM12 4DB Tel: 01708 438997 Fax: 01708 438997 — MB BS Dacca 1969 (Dhaka) DPM Lond. 1977; MRCPsych 1980; T(Psych) 1991. Cons. Psychiat. Child & Family Consultation Serv. Grays, Essex. Specialty: Child & Adolesc. Psychiat.; Psychother.; Psychosexual Med. Socs: BMA; Amer. Acad. Child & Adolesc. Psychiat.; Bd. of Managem. - Nat.

Child Bureau. Prev: Clin. Dir. & Cons. Psychiat. Child Adolesc. & Family Servs. Lincoln.

SHAIKH, Amer 28 Manor Drive, Wembley HA9 8ED — MB BS Lond. 1991.

SHAIKH, Gazala 14 Wellwood Close, Bicton Heath, Shrewsbury SY3 5BP — BM BS Nottm. 1990.

SHAIKH, Ghulam Farid, Squadron Ldr. Retd. Regional Medical Centre, RAF Halton, Aylesbury HP22 5PG Tel: 01296 623535 — MB BS Karachi 1977 (Dow Med. Coll. Karachi, Pakistan) DTM & H RCP Lond. 1979; DFFP 1996. Civil. Med. Pract. RAF Halton Aylesbury. Specialty: Gen. Pract. Prev: Gen. Duty Med. Off. RAF; Regist. (Gen. Med.) Dumfries & Galloway Roy. Infirm. & StoneHo. Gen. Hosp.

SHAIKH, M Holderness Road Surgery, 1181 Holderness Road, Hull HU8 9EA Tel: 01482 784966 — MB BS Karachi 1968; MB BS Karachi 1968.

SHAIKH, Mohamad Guftar 39 Bright Street, Wolverhampton WV1 4AT — MB ChB Aberd. 1994.

SHAIKH, Muhammad Afzal (retired) 73 Atherstone Avenue, Peterborough PE3 9UG Tel: 01733 263681 — MB BS Sind 1961 (Liaquat Med. Coll.) DTM & H Eng. 1963.

SHAIKH, Muhammad Imtiaz Bedford Hospital, Kempston Road, Bedford MK42 9DJ Tel: 01234 355122 Fax: 01234 792106 Email: Muhammad.Shaikh@bedhos.anglox.nhs.uk — MB BS Karachi (Dow Med. Coll., Karachi) FRCR; DMRD. Cons. radiologist, Bedford Hosp., bedford; Cons. radiologist, manor Hosp., Biddenham, Bedford. Specialty: Radiol. Socs: Roy. Coll. of Radiologists; BMA; BAPR. Prev: Cons. Radiologist, Diana Princess of Wales Hosp., Grimsby; Sen. Regist. / Regist. Northwick Pk. Kings Coll. and St georges Hosps. Lond.

SHAIKH, Munawar Saleem Haymarket Health Centre, Dunning Street, Tunstall, Stoke-on-Trent ST6 5BE Tel: 01782 575730 Fax: 01782 575858 Email: munnu@bugs.fslife.co.uk — MB ChB Manch. 1987; GP Prin. Mental Health Acb Section 12(2) Approved.; BSc St. And. 1984; MRCGP 1991. GP Princip.; Clin. Asst. - c/o the Elderly. Special Interest: Psychiat. Socs: BMA. Prev: Trainee GP Blackpool Vict. Hosp. VTS.; Clin. Ass. In Gen. Psychiatry.

SHAIKH, Mr Naeemuddin Ahmed (Nicholas) Airedale General Hosptial, Department of Urology, Skipton Road, Keighley BD20 6TD Tel: 01535 652511 Ext: 3131 Fax: 01535 292952 Email: shaikhnick@hotmail.com; The Yorkshire Clinic (Private consultation), Bradford Road, Bingley Tel: 01274 560311 — MB BS Sind 1979 (Liaquat Med. Coll.. Hyderabad. Pakistan) FRCS Ed. 1984; PhD Lond. 1990. Cons. Urol. Airedale Gen. Hosp. Keighley. Specialty: Urol. Special Interest: Uro Oncol. Socs: Brit. Assn. Urol. Surgs.; BMA. Prev: Sen. Regist. (Urol.) Qu. Eliz. Hosp. Birm. & Walsgrave Hosp. Coventry; Regist. (Urol.) Dudley Rd. Hosp. Birm. & Hammersmith Hosp. Lond.

SHAIKH, Mr Nasiruddin 109 Victoria Road, Fallowfield, Manchester M14 6DA — MB BS Karachi 1975; MB BS Karachi Pakistan 1975; DO RCS Eng. 1982; FCOphth 1990; FRCSI 1990.

SHAIKH, Naveed Ahmed 9 Oaklands Road, London N20 8BA Tel: 020 8446 0925 — MB BS Lond. 1998 (Royal Free Hospital School of Medicine) MB BS Lond 1998. Newham Gen. Hosp., Lond. Basic Surgic. Train., Rotat.; Sen. SHO, Conquest Hosp., Hastings. Prev: Kings Coll. Hosp., Roy. Nat. Orthopaedic Hosp.

SHAIKH, Riaz Ahmed 18 Holcombe Road, Chatham ME4 5RU — MB BS Karachi 1982; FFA RCSI 1992.

SHAIKH, Shagufta Sophia Parchmore Medical Centre, 97 Parchmore Road, Thornton Heath, Croydon CR7 8LY — MB BS Lond. 1990; DRCOG 1992; MRCGP 1994; DFFP 1994.

SHAIKH, Shahina Akhtar 88 Turnpike Link, Croydon CR0 5NY — MB BS Lond. 1991.

SHAIKH, Shamsuddin The Surgery, 70 Minehead Road, Harrow HA2 9DS — MB BS SIND 1957; DCMT Lond. 1967; LMSSA Lond. 1976. Med. Off. Lond. Regional Transport. Socs: Fell. Roy. Soc. Trop. Med.; BMA. Prev: GP Rainham Kent.

SHAIKH, Taiyabur Rahman 23 Pear Tree Lane, Loose, Maidstone ME15 9QY — MB BS Dacca 1967.

SHAIKH, Zaheer Ahmed (Surgery), Tandon Medical Centre, Kent Street, Upper Gornal, Dudley DY3 1UX Tel: 01902 882243 — MB BS Karachi 1965.

SHAINE, Bruce Jay PO Box 79, Saunderton, High Wycombe HP14 4HJ Fax: 01494 567445/01985 847059; 28 Chaucer Street, Stoneygate, Leicester LE2 1HD Tel: 0116 254 6025 — MB ChB Leic. 1990; MA Lond. 1993; MA Sheffield 1999. Med. Adviser, Pharmaceutical Med., Janssen-Cilag Ltd, Bucks. Specialty: Pharmaceutical Medicine. Prev: Regist. (Pub. Health Med.) N. & Yorks. RHA.; SHO (Psychiat.) Nottm. Train. Scheme.

SHAIRP, Brian Edward 3 Carrick Drive, Sevenoaks TN13 3BA Tel: 01732 453289 — MB BChir Camb. 1948 (Camb. & St. Bart.) MRCS Eng. LRCP Lond. 1946. Prev: Ho. Surg. & Ho. Phys. North. Hosp. Winchmore Hill; Ho. Surg. High Wycombe War Memor. Hosp.

SHAJAHAN, Polash Mohammed 6 North Avenue, Carluke ML8 5TR — MB ChB Ed. 1989 (Edinburgh) MRCP (UK) 1993; MRCPsych 1996; MPhil 1997. Cons. (Psychiat.) Lanarksh. Primary Care Trust. Prev: Sen. Lect. & Cons. Psychiat. Univ. Of Newc. upon Tyne & Newc. Gen. Hosp.; Regist. Rotat. (Psychiat.) Lothian Train. Scheme; Clin. Scientist & Hon. Specialist Regist. MRC Brain Metab. Unit Roy. Edin. Hosp.

SHAKEEL, Mohamad Hasan Sandwell General Hospital, Lyndon, West Bromwich B71 4HJ Tel: 0121 553 1831 Fax: 0121 607 3133; Foxcroft, 42A Pk Road, Walsall WS5 3JU Tel: 0121 358 3767 — (Dow Med. Coll. Karachi) MB BS Karachi 1963; MRCP (UK) 1970; FRCP Lond. 1988. Cons. Phys. (Elderly Care) Sandwell Healthcare NHS Trust. Specialty: Gen. Med.; Care of the Elderly. Socs: BMA; W. Midl. Consulant and Specialist Comm.; Brit. Geriat. Soc. (Chairm. W. Midl. Br.). Prev: Sen. Regist. (Geriat.) Ipswich Gp. Hosps.; Regist. (Med.) Dist. & Gen. Hosp. W. Bromwich; SHO (Med.) N. Cambs. Hosp. Wisbech.

SHAKER, Adel Gamal Assisted Conception Unit, Ross Hall Hospital, 221 Crookston Road, Glasgow G52 3NQ — MB BCh Ain Shams 1978.

SHAKESPEARE, Carl Frederick Cardiac Department, Queen Elizabeth Hospital, Stadium Road, Woolwich SE18 4QH Tel: 0208 836 4349 Fax: 0208 836 4326 Email: carl.shakespeare@nhs.net — MB BS Lond. 1984 (Westm. Med. Sch.) BSc Lond. 1981, MD 1994; FRCP UK 2001. Cons. Cardiol., Med. & Cardiol., Greenwich Healthcare Trust, Woolwich; Hon. Cons., St Thomas Hosp., Lond. Specialty: Cardiol. Special Interest: Invasive Cardiol. Socs: Brit. Cardiac Soc. Prev: Sen. Regist., Roy. Lond. Hosp., Lond.

SHAKESPEARE, Mr David Terence Kimberley House, 3 Lillington Avenue, Leamington Spa CV32 5UF — BM BCh Oxf. 1975; FRCS Eng. 1979. Cons. Orthop. Surg. S. Warwicks. HA. Specialty: Orthop.

SHAKESPEARE, Emma Jane 19 Albert hill Street, Didsbury, Manchester M20 6RF — MB ChB Manch. 1993; MRCP 1997, Glasgow. Specialist Regist. in Paediat., N. W. Rotat. Specialty: Paediat.

SHAKESPEARE, John Ash Trees Surgery, Market Street, Carnforth LA5 9JU Tel: 01524 720000 Fax: 01524 720110; The White House, 1 Hatlex Hill, Heast Bank, Lancaster LA2 6ET — MB ChB Manch. 1968; DObst RCOG 1970; MRCGP 1974. Prev: SHO (O & G) Good Hope Hosp. Sutton Coldfield; Trainee GP Kettering VTS.

SHAKESPEARE, Judith Mary Summertown Group Practice, 160 Banbury Road, Oxford OX2 7BS Tel: 01865 515552 Fax: 01865 311237; 91 Bainton Road, Oxford OX2 7AG — BM BCh Oxf. 1975; MRCP (UK) 1977; MRCGP 1980; MFFP 1993.

SHAKESPEARE, Karen Maud Aylesford Medical Centre, Admiral Moore Drive, Royal British Legion Village, Aylesford ME20 7SE — MB BS Lond. 1980 (Guys) GP Partner. Specialty: Gen. Pract.

SHAKESPEARE, Ruth Marion 9 Barn Road, Broadstone BH18 8NH — (St. Geo.) BSc Lond. 1975, MB BS 1978; DCH RCP Lond. 1981; MRCP (UK) 1985; MFPHM 1989. Cons. Pub. Health Med. Soton. & SW Hants. DHA. Specialty: Pub. Health Med. Prev: Regist. (Community Med.) Wessex RHA.

SHAKESPEARE, William Martyn 199 Holdenhurst Road, Bournemouth BH8 8DE Tel: 01202 558337 Email: william.shakespeare@gp-J81024.nhs.uk — MB BS Lond. 1978 (St Geo.) DRCOG 1980; MRCGP 1983. GP Princip. Specialty: Gen. Pract.

SHAKIR, Ayad Abdul Kareem Anaesthetic Department, Pennine House, Burnley General Hospital, Burnley — MB ChB Baghdad 1972; FFARCSI 1982. Consultant in Pain Management and Anaesthetics, Burnley, East Lancs Heath Care Trust. Specialty: Anaesth. Socs: Brit. Med. Assn.; Roy. Coll. of Anaestatist; Pain Society. Prev: SpR in Anaesth., for N. W. Thames Region, 1996-1998.

SHAKIR, Irfan The Calderdale Royal Hospital, Halifax HX3 0PW Tel: 01422 357171 Email: irfan.shakir@cht.nhs.uk — BM BS Nottm. 1978; BMedSci Nottm. 1976; MRCP (UK) 1981; FRCP Lond 1995; FRCP Glas 1995. Cons. Phys. Elderly. Med. Calderdale and Huddersfield NHS Trust. Specialty: Gen. Med. Socs: BMA; Brit. Geriatric. Soc.; Brit. Assn. of Stroke Physicians. Prev: Sen. Regist. (Geriat. Med.) Stobhill Gen. Hosp. Glas.; Regist. (Med.) Leic. Gen. & P.boro. Dist. Hosps.; SHO. (Med.) Nottm. City Hosp.

SHAKIR, Nasaar Ahmad 26 Oswald Road, Southall UB1 1HW — MB ChB Sheff. 1990.

SHAKIR, Naseer Ahmad Bridge Lane Health Centre, 20 Bridge Lane, Battersea, London SW11 3AD Tel: 020 7978 6737 Fax: 020 7924 7385; 26 Oswald Road, Southall UB1 1HW — MB ChB Sheff. 1984. Socs: BMA.

SHAKIR, Raad Abdul Wahab Regional Neurosciences Centre, Charing Cross Hospital, Fulham Palace Road, London W6 8RF Tel: 020 8846 7489 Fax: 020 8846 7487 Email: r.shakir@ic.ac.uk; Central Middlesex Hospital, Acton Lane, Park Royal, London NW10 7NS Tel: 020 8453 2247 Fax: 020 8453 2246 — MB ChB Baghdad 1971; MSc Glas. 1978; MRCP (UK) 1979; FRCP Ed. 1987; FRCP Glas. 1987; FRCP Lond. 1989. Cons. Neurol. Char. Cross Hosp. & Centr. Middlx. Hosp.; Hon. Sen. Lect. Imperial Coll. Sch. Med.; Sec. Trop. & Geogr. Neurol. Research Gp. World Federat. of Neurol.; Mem. Educat. Comm. ILAE; Mem. (Pub. Relation Comm.) World Federat. of Neurol. Specialty: Neurol. Socs: Internat. League Against Epilepsy. Prev: Cons. Neurol. Middlesbrough; Assoc. Prof. & Acad. Vice-Dean Fac. of Med., Kuwait.

SHAKIR, Saad Abdul Wahab 38 Lorne Gardens, Shirley, Croydon CR0 7RY Tel: 020 8966 4641 Fax: 020 8662 1654 — MB ChB Baghdad 1976; LRCP LRCS Ed. LRCPS Glas. 1980; MRCP (UK) 1984; MRCGP 1988; FRCP Glas. 1994; FFPM RCP Lond. 1995; FRCP Ed. 1997. Dir. Drug Safety Research Unit Soton.; Vice-Chairm. Soc. Pharmaceut. Med.; Convenor Pharmacovigilance Gp. & Signal Generation & Eval. Gp. Specialty: Pharmaceutical Medicine; Epidemiol.; Gen. Pract. Socs: Soc. Pharmaceut. Med.; Internat. Soc. Pharmacoepidemiol.; Exec. Comm. Europ. Soc. of Pharmacovigilance. Prev: Vice Pres. Worldwide Pharmacovigilance & Pharmacoepidemiol. Rhone Polenc Rover; Head Safety Eval. Gp. Glaxo Wellcome Research & Developm.; Sen. Med. Off. Med. Control Agency.

SHAKIR, Sudad Abdul Wahab 7 Hoppers Way, Ashford TN23 4GP — MB ChB Baghdad 1973; FFA RCS Eng. 1981.

SHAKOKANI, Adel Abelmajid Flat 5 Addison Court, 2 Brondesbury Road, London NW6 6AS — LMS Saragossa 1972; MRCOG 1982.

SHAKOOR, Abdul 7 Claremont Road, Luton LU4 8LY — MB ChB Dundee 1997.

SHAKOOR, Sameena The Homoeopathic Hospital, South West Kent Primary Care, 41 Church Wells, Tunbridge Wells TN1 1JU Tel: 01892 539144 Fax: 01892 532585 Email: sameena.shakoor@swkentpct.nhs.uk; 3 Fernside, Bishops Down Road, Tunbridge Wells TN4 8XN Tel: 01892 526029 Email: sameena.shakoor@doctors.org.uk — MB BS Lond. 1986 (Oxford University & UCH/Middlesex, London) MA (Hons. Physiol. Sci.) Oxf. 1983; MRCP (UK) 1990; FRCPCH (UK) 1998. Cons. Paediat. Specialty: Community Child Health. Special Interest: Social Communication Disorders. Socs: Brit. Soc. Human Genetics; Brit. Assn. Community Child Health; Roy. Soc. Med. Prev: Sen. Regist. (Paediat.) Northwick Pk. Hosp. Harrow; Regist. Rotat. (Paediat.) Edgware & Middlx. Hosp. Lond.; SHO (O & G) St. Geo. Hosp. Lond.

SHAKOOR, Shaheena 19 North Avenue, Gosforth, Newcastle upon Tyne NE3 4DT — LMSSA Lond. 1991.

SHAKUR, Josephine 9 Monreith Road, Glasgow G43 2NX — MB ChB Aberd. 1992.

SHALDERS, Kerry 30 Newcomen Road, Dartmouth TQ6 9BN — BM BS Nottm. 1997.

SHALDON, Mr Cyril (retired) Robin Hill, Deepdene Park, Wonford Road, Exeter EX2 4PH Tel: 01392 431600 Email: seeshaldon@aol.com — MB BChir Camb. 1951 (Westm.) FRCS Eng. 1955; MChir Camb. 1959; MD Bristol 1962. Prev: Sen. Lect. (Surg.) Lond. Hosp.

SHALES, Carmel Ann Salisbury Road Surgery, 43 Salisbury Road, Plymouth Tel: 01752 665879; 32 Burnett Road, Crownhill, Plymouth PL6 5BH Tel: 01752 707127 — MB ChB Liverp. 1966. Freelance Non-Principal GP Salisbury Rd. Surg. Plymouth.

SHALET, Stephen Michael 3 Hulme Hall Avenue, Cheadle Hulme, Cheadle SK8 6LN Tel: 0161 485 1463 Fax: 0161 446 3772; Department of Endocrinology, Christie Hospital, Wilmslow Road, Manchester M20 4BX Tel: 0161 446 3667 Fax: 0161 446 3772 — (Lond. Hosp.) MB BS Lond. 1969; MRCS Eng. LRCP Lond. 1969; MRCP (UK) 1972; BSc (Hons.) Lond. 1966, MD 1979; FRCP Lond. 1984. Cons. Phys. & Endocrinol. Manch. S. Health Dist. (T); Prof. Med. Manch. Univ. Specialty: Endocrinol. Socs: Fell. Roy. Soc. Med. (Pres. Endocrine Sect.); (Counc.) Europ. Soc. Pediatric Endocrinol.; Soc. Endocrinol. Prev: Research Regist. (Endocrinol.) Univ. Manch.; Regist. (Med.) Bristol Roy. Infirm.; Ho. Phys. Med. Unit & Ho. Surg. Lond. Hosp.

SHALHOUB, John Toufic Perywick Farm, Brightling Road, Brightling, Robertsbridge TN32 5HB — MD Beirut 1968 (Amer. Univ. Beirut) BSc Amer. Univ. Beirut 1963; MRCOG 1977. Med. Dir. Coombe Private Med. Centre. Prev: Regist. King's Coll. Hosp. Lond. & Enfield Dist. Hosp.

SHALLAL, Salih Abdul Mahdi Al-Temimi 62 Hollybush Road, Kingston upon Thames KT2 5SE — MB ChB Baghdad 1960; DTM & H Liverp. 1970; DTCD Wales 1973; MRCS Eng. LRCP Lond. 1978.

SHALLCROSS, Timothy Mark Caithness General Hospital, Wick KW1 5NS Tel: 01955 605050 Fax: 01955 604606; Stirkoke Woods, Wick KW1 5SZ Tel: 01955 604323 — MB BS Lond. 1982 (St. Thos.) FCRP (Edin Glas); BSc Lond. 1979; MRCP (UK) 1986. Cons. Phys. Caithness Gen. Hosp. Wick. Specialty: Gen. Med.; Care of the Elderly. Socs: Fell. RCP Edin.& Glas.

SHALLEY, Mr Martin John 9 Kennet Close, Ash, Aldershot GU12 6NN — MB BS Lond. 1972 (Lond. Hosp.) MRCS Eng. LRCP Lond. 1972; FRCS Eng. 1977. Specialty: Accid. & Emerg.

SHALOM, Mr Albert Saimah (retired) 11 Stonehill Road, East Sheen, London SW14 8RR Tel: 020 8876 9006 Fax: 020 8876 9006 — (Univ. Coll. Hosp.) MB BS Lond. 1954; DLO Eng. 1959; FRCS (Orl.) Eng. 1961. Prev: Cons. ENT Surg. NW Surrey DHA.

SHALOM, Jane Isabel Kennedy (retired) 11 Stonehill Road, London SW14 8RR Tel: 020 8876 9006 Fax: 020 8876 9006 — BSc Wales 1950, MB BCh 1953; DObst RCOG 1956; DA Eng. 1957; FFA RCS Eng. 1963. Prev: SHO (Anaesth.) Qu. Charlotte's Matern. Hosp. & Chelsea Hosp. Wom.Lond.

SHALOM, Stephen David — MB BCh Wales 1980; DDAM; MRCP (UK) 1985. Med. Adviser Atos Origin Med. Servs. Specialty: Occupat. Health.

SHALTOT, Mohamed Adel Ali 47 Padnell Road, Cowplain, Waterlooville PO8 8EB Tel: 02392 262488 — MB ChB Alexandria 1964; Dip. Neurol. & Psychiat. Alexandria 1968; MRCP (U.K.) 1975; MRCS Eng. LRCP Lond. 1976; FRCR 1979; DMRD Eng. 1979. Cons. Radiol. St. Mary's & Qu. Alexandra Hosps. Portsmouth. Specialty: Radiol. Prev: Sen. Regist. (Radiol.) King's Coll. Hosp. Lond.; Regist. (Radiol.) King's Coll. Hosp. Lond.; Regist. (Neurol.) Hurstwood Pk. Hosp. Haywards Heath.

SHAM, Julian Ken Wai 433 Valley Road, Nottingham NG5 1HX — MB BS Lond. 1994.

SHAM, Pak Chung Department of Psychological Medicine, Institute of Psychiatry, Denmark Hill, London SE5 8AF — BM BCh Oxf. 1984; MRCPsych 1990; MSc Lond. 1991; PhD 2002. Prof. of Psychiatric and Statistical Genetics and Honourary Cons. Psychiat. Specialty: Gen. Psychiat.

SHAM, Sui-Yuen The Surgery, 108 Banbury Road, Northfield, Birmingham B31 2DN Tel: 0121 475 1050 — MB ChB Glas. 1980.

SHAM, Tasneem 21 Stratford Road, West Bridgford, Nottingham NG2 6AZ — MB ChB Birm. 1996.

SHAMAS-UD-DIN, Sakib Flat 10, 38 Ullet Road, Liverpool L17 3BP — MB ChB Liverp. 1996.

SHAMAS-UD-DIN, Sobia 43 Carrwood, Halebarns, Altrincham WA15 0EN — MB ChB Manch. 1997.

SHAMASH, Alan 33 Meadowbank, Primrose Hill, London NW3 3AY Tel: 020 7586 3542 — MRCS Eng. LRCP Lond. 1952 (Leeds) DA Eng. 1958. GP (semi-Retd.). Prev: Regist. (Anaesth.) Edgeware Gen. Hosp.; Ho. Off. (Paediat.) Whipps Cross Hosp. Lond.; Capt. RAMC.

SHAMASH, Jonathan KGV Building, Department of Medical Oncology, St Bartholomew's Hospital, London EC1A 7BE Tel: 020 7483 3673 Email: jonathan@jshamash.demon.co.uk; 14 Elliott

Square, London NW3 350 — MB ChB Ed. 1987; MRCP (UK) 1990; MD Ed. 1996. Sen. Lectures in Med. Oncol. St Bart. Hosp Lond. Specialty: Oncol. Special Interest: Hodgkin's Dis.; Managem. of refractory germ cell tumours. Socs: Assn. of Cancer Physicians; American Society of Clinical Oncology. Prev: Clin. Research Fell. (Med. Oncol.) St. Bart. Hosp. Lond.; Regist. (Gen. Med. & Endocrinol.) St. Mary's Hosp. Lond.; Regist. (Gen. Med.) Edgware Gen. Hosp.

SHAMASH, Kim Aldington Home, 35 New Church Road, Brighton BN3; 74 Peacock Lane, Brighton BN1 6WA — BM Soton. 1981; MRCPsych 1986. Cons. Old Age Psychiat., Clin. Director, Adult Ment. Health Servs. Specialty: Gen. Psychiat. Special Interest: Old Age Psychiat.

SHAMBROOK, Anthony St John Anaesthetic Department, Ysbyty Gwynedd, Penrhosgarnedd, Bangor Tel: 01248 384384 — MB ChB Liverp. 1980; DA (UK) 1987; FCAnaesth 1991. Cons. Anaesth. Ysbyty Gwynedd Bangor. Specialty: Anaesth. Prev: Sen. Regist. (Anaesth.) Ysbyty Gwynedd Bangor & Univ. Hosp. Wales Cardiff.; Regist. (Anaesth.) Blackburn Roy. Infirm. & Univ. Hosp. Wales Cardiff; Med. Off. (Anaesth.) ChristCh. Hosp., NZ.

SHAMEEM, Maheen 14 Malcolmson Cl, Birmingham B15 3LS — MB BCh Wales 1997.

SHAMI, Shukri Khalid Oldchurch Hospital, Waterloo Road, Romford RM7 9BE Tel: 01708 708474 Fax: 01708 708474; 14 Napier Road, Wembley HA0 4UA — MB BS Lond. 1977 (Char. Cross Hosp. Med. Sch.) MS, FRCS (Ed). Cons. Surg. BHRH. Specialty: Gen. Surg. Special Interest: Colorectal; laparoscopic Surg.; Vascular. Socs: Roy. Soc. of Med.; SRS. Prev: Clin. Director of Surg.

SHAMIL, Mr Abdul Shahib Abdul Raheem 54 Cambridge Avenue, Romford RM2 6QU — MB ChB Baghdad 1970; FRCSI 1990.

SHAMIM, Shamim Uddin 237 Tonbridge Road, Maidstone ME16 8ND Tel: 01622 729000 — MB BS Karachi 1968; DPM Eng. 1978.

SHAMLAYE, Conrad Francois 60A London Road, Kilmarnock KA3 7DD — MB ChB Glas. 1978.

SHAMOUN, Osman Sid Ahmed Mohamed Jubilee Maternity Ward, Belfast City Hospital, Lisburn Road, Belfast BT9 7AB — MB BCh Ain Shams 1979; MRCOG 1993.

SHAMPRASADH, Vinod The Oakley Surgery, Addington Way, Luton LU4 9FJ Tel: 08704 173989 Fax: 01582 561808 — MB BCh BAO NUI 1990; DFFP; MRCGP 1994.

SHAMSAH, Mohammed Ali 85 Goodwood, Newcastle upon Tyne NE12 6LX — MB BS Newc. 1993.

SHAMSEE, Muhammad Yusuf Saleem Elmwood Health Centre, Huddersfield Road, Holmfirth, Huddersfield HD9 3TR Tel: 01484 689111 Fax: 01484 689333 — MB ChB Leeds 1992.

SHAMSHAD, Sohail 70 Priestfields, Rochester ME1 3AB — MB BS Karachi 1975.

SHAMSI, Saghir Ahmad Health Clinic, Grindley Lane, Blyth Bridge, Stoke-on-Trent ST11 9JS Tel: 01782 395101 Fax: 01782 398183; Staffordshire Family Health Services Authority, Britania House, 6/7 Eastgate St, Stafford ST16 2NJ Tel: 01785 256341 Fax: 01785 57114 — (Dow Med. Coll. Karachi, Pakistan) MB BS Karachi 1962; DPath. Eng. 1972. Socs: Med. Protec. Soc. Prev: Clin. Asst. Histopath. Lond. Chest Hosp.

SHAMSUDDIN, Mr Altaf Badsha Flat 19, Orchard Court, Stonegrove, Edgware HA8 7SX — MB BS Madras 1972 (Madurai Med. Coll.) BSc Madras 1965; FRCS Glas. 1984. SHO (Gen. Surg.) Pontefract Gen. Infirm. Prev: SHO (Thoracic Surg.) Colindale Hosp. Lond.

SHAMSUDIN, Norashikin 155a O'Driscoll House, Du Cane Road, London W12 0UB — BM BS Nottingham 1997.

SHAN, Kesavan 40 Montreal Road, Gants Hill, Ilford IG1 4SH — MB BS Lond. 1990. SHO (A & E) St. Bart. Hosp. Specialty: Accid. & Emerg.

SHANAHAN, Anthony Pius City Walls Medical Centre, St Martin's Way, Chester CH1 2NR Tel: 01244 357800 Fax: 01244 357809 — MB ChB Manch. 1978 (Manchester) DA Eng. 1981; DRCOG 1981. Gen. Practitioner; Clin. Asst., Dermat. Dept., Countess of Chester Hosp., Chester. Specialty: Dermat.; Diabetes. Socs: Chester & N. Wales Med. Soc. Prev: G.P. Trainer, Univ. of Liverp.

SHANAHAN, Mr Donal BUPA Roding Hospital, Roding Lane South, Ilford IG4 5PZ Tel: 0208 5511100 — MB BS Lond. 1979 (Westm.) FRCS Eng. 1983; MS Lond. 1987. Sen. Lect. (Surg.) St. Bart. Hosp. Lond.; Cons. Surg. Homerton Hosp. Lond. Specialty: Gen. Surg. Socs: Roy. Soc. Med.; AESGBI. Prev: Sen. Regist. St. Geo. Hosp. Lond.

SHANAHAN, Mr Michael Denis Ghislain Department of Trauma and Orthopaedics, The Ipswich Hospital, Heath Road, Ipswich IP4 5PD Tel: 01473 702211 — MB ChB Bristol 1977; FRCS Eng. 1981. Cons. Orthop. Surg. Ipswich. Specialty: Orthop.; Trauma & Orthop. Surg. Prev: Cons. Orthop. Surg. Gwynedd Health Auth.; Lect. & Hon. Sen. Regist. (Orthop.) Univ. Sheff.; Regist. (Orthop.) Roy. Hallamsh. Hosp. Sheff.

SHANAHAN, Sarah Elizabeth Emma 28 Woodlands Gate, Woodlands Way, London SW15 2SY — MB BCh Witwatersrand 1995.

SHANAHAN, William John The Soho Treatment Centre, 4th Floor, 1 Frith Street, London W1V 5DH Tel: 020 7534 6700 Email: william.shanahan@nhs.net — MB BCh BAO Dub. 1980; DCH Dub. 1983; DObst. RCPI 1984; MRCPsych 1986; FRCPsych 2002. Cons. Psychiat. Subst. Misuse Serv., Centr. & NW Lond. MHT. Specialty: Alcohol & Substance Misuse. Prev: Sen. Regist. (Psychiat.) Gordon Hosp., St. Bernards Hosp. & Char. Cross Hosps. Lond.

SHANAZ, Mr Mohamed 18 Laleham Road, London SE6 2HT — MB BS Colombo 1982; MB BS Colombo Sri Lanka 1982; FRCS Eng. 1991.

SHAND, Alan George Gastrointestinal Unit, Western General Hospital, Edinburgh EH4 2XU Email: ashand@ed.ac.uk — MB ChB Aberd. 1992; MRCP (UK) 1995. Specialist Regist. Gastrointestinal Unit, Western Gen. Hosp. Edin. Specialty: Gastroenterol.

SHAND, Claudia Ruth Odiham Health Centre, Deer Park View, Odiham, Hook RG29 1JY Tel: 01256 702371 Fax: 01256 393111 — MB BS Lond. 1980 (King's Coll. Hosp.) LMSSA Lond. 1980; DRCOG 1986; MRCGP 1986. Prev: RAF Med. Br. 1982-1987.

SHAND, David St. Richards Hospital, Chichester PO19 6SE Tel: 01243 831478; Springwood, Pine Grove, Chichester PO19 3PN Tel: 01243 537249 Fax: 0709 223 5707 Email: davidshand@doctors.org.uk — MB ChB Manch. 1984; BSc (Med Sci) St. And. 1981; MRCGP 1990; Dip. Travel Med. Lond. 1996; MFOM RCP Lond. 1998. Cons. Occupat. Phys. Chichester & Portsmouth NHS Trust. Specialty: Occupat. Health. Socs: Soc. Occ. Med.; Internat. Soc. Travel Med.; Brit. Inst. Musculoskel. Med. Prev: Sen. Med. Off. Brit. Steel plc Teeside; Med. Off. Avesta Sheff. Ltd.; Regist. (Gen. Med.) Stepping Hill Hosp. Stockport.

SHAND, Gill 24 Oatlands Road, Boorley Green, Botley, Southampton SO32 2DE; Flat 1, 6 Kellett Road, London SW2 1EB — MB BS Lond. 1996. SHO Psychiat. (part of GP VTS), Newha, Healthcare, Lond.

SHAND, Ian Richard Osmaston Road Medical Centre, 212 Osmaston Road, Derby DE23 8JX Tel: 01332 346433 — MB ChB Leeds 1979; DRCOG 1982; MRCGP 1983.

SHAND, Jacqueline Dorothy The Old Manse, Dalriach Road, Oban PA34 5JE — MB ChB Glas. 1997.

SHAND, Jean Malcolm Bank Street Surgery, 46-62 Bank Street, Alexandria G83 0LS Tel: 01389 752419 Fax: 01389 710521 — MB ChB Aberd. 1980.

SHAND, John X-Ray Department, Stobhill Hospital, Balornook Road, Glasgow G21 3UW Tel: 0141 201 3625 Fax: 0141 201 3693 — MB ChB Glas. 1980; FRCR 1986. Cons. (Radiol.) Stobhill Gen. Hosp. Glas. Specialty: Radiol.

SHAND, Mr John Ewen Greig Street House, Westward, Wigton CA7 8AF — MB ChB Ed. 1973; FRCS Ed. 1977. Cons. Surg. Carlisle. Specialty: Gen. Surg.

SHAND, Lynne Margaret 14 Elrick Gardens, Newmachar, Aberdeen AB21 0PY — MB ChB Aberd. 1998; MB ChB Aberd 1998.

SHAND, Rebecca Mia — MB ChB Birm. 1998.

SHAND, Mr William Stewart (retired) Dan-Y-Castell, Castle Road, Crickhowell NP8 1AP Tel: 01873 810452 — MB BChir Camb. 1962 (Camb. & St. Bart.) MD Camb. 1970; FRCS Ed. 1970; FRCS Eng. 1970. Hon. Cons. Surg. St. Mark's Hosp. Lond.; Penrose May Teach. RCS Eng.; Hon. Consulting Surg. St. Bart. & Roy. Lond. Hosps. Prev: Cons. Surg. St. Bart. Hosp. Lond.

SHANDALL, Mr Ahmed Ahmed Abu El Futuh Royal Gwent Hospital, Cardiff Road, Newport NP20 0UB Tel: 01633 234124 Fax: 01633 656064; 10 Craig- Yr - Haul, Castleton, Cardiff CF3 2SA —

MB BCh Wales 1975; FRCS Eng. 1980; MCh Wales 1987. Cons. Surg. Roy. Gwent Hosp. Newport; Welsh Surg. Soc. Fellowship (USA); Fullbright Fellowship (USA) 1985-6. Specialty: Gen. Surg. Socs: Internat. Soc. of EndoVasc. Specialists; Vasc. Soc. & Welsh Surg. Soc.; Assoc. Surg.s GB Counc. Prev: Research Fell. Cardiff; Sen. Regist. (Surg.) Univ. Hosp. Wales, Cardiff & Roy. Gwent Hosp.; Vasc. (Clin.) Fell. Albany New York, USA.

SHANKAR, Ananth Gouri The Royal London Hospital, Department of Paediatric Oncology, 1st Floor Eva Luckes House, Whitechapel, London E1 1BB Tel: 020 7377 7000 Ext: 3928 Fax: 020 7377 7796 Email: a.shankar@cancer.org.uk — MB BS Calicut 1986; DCH 1987; MD 1990; MRCP, FRCPCH 1992. Cons., Paediat. Oncol., The Roy. Lond. Hosp.; Hon. Cons. in Paediat. Oncol., Guys' Hosp., Lond. Specialty: Paediat. Special Interest: BMT; Lymphomas. Socs: SIOP; BMA.

SHANKAR, Arun Nathan 11 Bedford Road, Willington, Bedford MK44 3PP — MB BS Newc. 1998; MB BS Newc 1998.

SHANKAR, Dorairaj Houghton Road Medical Centre, Welfare Road, Thurnscoe, Rotherham S63 0JZ Tel: 01709 894653 — MB BS Madras 1971.

SHANKAR, Mr Nanjappa Queen Elizabeth Hospital, Sheriff Hill, Gateshead NE9 6SX Tel: 0191 487 8989; 20 Barons Wood, Gosforth, Newcastle upon Tyne NE3 3UB Tel: 0191 285 2995 — MB BS Bangalore 1979; BSc Bangalore 1972; FRCS Ed. 1985; FRCS Glas. 1986; MChOrth Liverp. 1989. Cons. Orthop. Qu. Eliz. Hosp. Gateshead. Specialty: Orthop. Socs: BMA. Prev: Regist. (Orthop.) N. Tyneside Gen. Hosp.; Regist. (Orthop.) Basildon Hosp.; SHO (Orthop.) Warrington Gen. Hosp.

SHANKAR, Rajesh Kumar St Richards Hospital, Spitalfield Lane, Chichester PO19 4SE Email: ra2.shankar@rws-tr.nhs.uk; 20 Caledonian Road, Chichester PO19 7PH — MB BS Lond. 1985 (St. Bart. Hosp. Lond.) FRCA 1997. Cons. Anaesth. with an interest in Pain Managem., St Richards Hosp., Chichester. Specialty: Anaesth. Prev: Cons. Anaesth. with an interest in Pain Managem. Barts and The Lond. NHS Trust.

GOODWIN, Richard Geoffrey 26 The Rise, Llanshen, Cardiff CF14 0RD — MB BS Lond. 1994 (St Mary's) MRCP Lond. 1998. Cons. Dermatol., Gwent Healthcare NHS Trust; Cons. Dermatol., St Jospeh Hosp. Specialty: Dermat. Special Interest: Paediatric Dermat.; Skin Cancer; Skin Surg. Socs: Brit. Assn. of Dermat.; Brit. Soc. Dermat. Surg.

SHANKAR, Mr Sambasivan Tanglewood, 11 Bedford Road, Willington, Bedford MK44 3PP — MRCS Eng. LRCP Lond. 1976 (Roy. Free) BDS Madras 1964; FDS RCS Ed. 1970; LMSSA Lond. 1975; FRCS Ed. 1980; FFD RCSI 1982. Cons. (A & E Med.) Bedford Gen. Hosp.Clin. Dir. A & E Dept.; CHJ Comission for Health Imporovement - Med. Reviewer; Assesor Performance Precedures-A&E-GMC; Hon. Sec.-Sect. of A&E Med.- Roy. Soc. of Med. Specialty: Accid. & Emerg. Socs: Fell. Roy. Soc. Med.; Cas. Surgs. Assn. & BMA. Prev: Sen. Regist. (A & E Med.) Oxf. RHA; Regist. (Gen. Surg.) OldCh. Hosp. Romford & Harefield Hosp.; Regist. (Orthop.) Heatherwood Hosp. Ascot.

SHANKAR, Sonal Epsom General Hospital, Epsom KT18 Tel: 01372 735735; 406 Old Bedford Road, Luton LU2 7BP Tel: 01582 491661 — MB BS Lond. 1995 (UMDS Guy's & St. Thos. Hosps. Univ. Lond.) SHO (Gen. Med.) Epsom Gen. Hosp. Specialty: Gen. Med. Prev: SHO (A & E) Hammersmith Hosp. Lond.; Ho. Off. (Gen. Surg.) St. Peter's Hosp. Chertsey; Ho. Off. (Med.) Worthing Hosp.

SHANKAR, Yelandur Puttaveerappa Health Centre, Trethomas, Newport Tel: 029 2086 8011; 35 Mountain Road, Caerphilly CF83 1HH Tel: 029 2088 4241 — MB BS Mysore 1956. Socs: Med. Defence Union. Prev: Ho. Phys. Llanelli Hosp.; Regist. Merthyr & Aberdare Gp. Hosps. & St. Joseph's Hosp. Clonmel.

SHANKER, Mr Jai Shanker 5, Mornington Villas, Manningham Lane, Bradford BD8 7JX Tel: 01274 544 000 Fax: 01274 544 111 Email: jai_grace@hotmail.com — MB BS Madras 1977; FRCS, Dub. 1985; MChOrth, Liverp. 1991. Cons. Orthop. & Trauma, Bradford Roy. Infirm.; Cons. Orthop. Surg., Bradford Teachg. Hosps. NHS Trust. Specialty: Trauma & Orthop. Surg. Special Interest: Foot & Ankle Surg. Socs: Brit. Foot &b Ankle Soc.; Amer. Orthop. Foot & Ankle Soc.; Brit. Orthop. Assn.

SHANKER, Mr Jyoti 54 Dungannon Chase, Southend-on-Sea SS1 3NJ — MB BS Rajasthan 1960; FRCS Ed. 1968. Specialty: Orthop. Socs: Fell. BOA; BMA.

SHANKERNARAYAN, Munuswamy Govindarjula Saltley Health Centre, Saltley, Birmingham B8 1RZ Tel: 0121 327 3321 — MB BS Osmania 1967.

SHANKLAND, Catherine Ruth 36 Old Kiln Lane, Bolton BL1 5PD — MB ChB Sheff. 1997.

SHANKLAND, Lorna Jean (retired) 7 The Leas, Wallasey CH45 3HZ Tel: 0151 639 4931 — MB ChB Manch. 1950; DCH Eng. 1955. Prev: SCMO Liverp. Sch. Health Dept.

SHANKLAND, Pushpa Macfarlane (retired) 13 Bladon Close, London Road, Guildford GU1 9TY Tel: 01483 502814 — MRCS Eng. LRCP Lond. 1932 (Lond. Sch. Med. Wom.) LM Rotunda 1932; DCH Eng. 1943. Prev: Asst. Co. Med. Off. & Asst. Sch. Med. Off. E. Riding, Yorks.

SHANKS, Adrian Barton Department of Anaesthetics, Cumberland Infirmary, Newtown Road, Carlisle CA2 7HY Tel: 01228 814196; Beck House, Pow Maughan Court, Scotby, Carlisle CA4 8EG — MB BS Lond. 1979 (St. Thos.) BSc Lond. 1976; FFARCS Eng. 1984. Cons. Anaesth. & Pain Relief Carlisle Hosps. NHS Trust. Specialty: Anaesth. Socs: Assn. Anaesth. & Pain Soc.; Internat. Assn. Study of Pain. Prev: Sen. Regist. (Anaesth.) Yorks. RHA; Regist. (Anaesth.) N. Staffs. HA; Regist. (Anaesth.) Leic. HA.

SHANKS, Brian Larne Health Centre, Gloucester Avenue, Larne BT40 1PB Tel: 028 2826 1919 Fax: 028 2827 2561 — MB BCh BAO Belf. 1970; DCH RCPS Glas. 1973; DObst RCOG 1974.

SHANKS, Elizabeth Mary Crosslands Hospital, Kilmarnock KA2 0BE Tel: 01563 577368 Fax: 01563 577974 Email: drshanks@aaaht.scot.nhs.uk — MB ChB (Hons.) Dundee 1978; FRCS Ed. 1982. Cons. ENT Surg., Ayrsh. and Arran Acute Hosps. Trust, Kilmarnock. Specialty: Gen. Surg. Special Interest: Cochlear Implant; Otol.; Paediatric ENT. Socs: Roy. Soc. of Med.; Roy. Coll. of Surgeons of Edin.; Scott. Otolaryngological Soc.

SHANKS, Hazel Anne Campbell Department of Genitourinary Medicine, Falkirk & District Royal Infirmary NHS Trust, Major's Loan, Falkirk FK1; Brackenhirst, Glenmavis, Airdrie ML6 0PP Tel: 01236 763157 — (Glas.) MB ChB Glas. 1968. Staff Grade Doctor (Genitourin. Med.) Falkirk & Dist Roy. Infirm. NHS Trust; Clin. Asst. (Genitourin. Med. & Sexual Health) Lanarksh. Specialty: Genitourinary Medicine. Prev: Clin. Asst. (Genitourin. Med.) Glas. Roy. Infirm.; Cytopathol. Monklands Dist. Gen. Hosp. Airdrie; SHO (Anaesth.) & Ho. Phys. Law Hosp. Carluke.

SHANKS, Jean Mary 8 South Eaton Place, London SW1W 9JA Tel: 020 7730 3175 Fax: 020 7824 8174; Holywell Hall, Stamford PE9 4DT Tel: 01780 410665 Fax: 01780 410665 — (Middlx.) BA, BM BCh Oxf. 1950; Hon. FRCPath 1993. Dir. Chandos Clin. Research (CCR). Specialty: Pathology, General. Socs: Assn. Clin. Pathols.; (Liveryman) Soc. Apoth.; Lond. Med. Soc. Prev: Chairm. & Managing Dir. of JS Path. plc; Regist. (Path.) Hosp. Sick Childr. Gt. Ormond St.

SHANKS, John Edward Department of Public Health, Croydon Health Authority, 17 Addiscombe Road, Croydon CR0 6SR Tel: 020 8401 3951 Fax: 020 8401 3769 — MB ChB Glas. 1977 (Univ. Glas.) BSc (Hons.) Glas. 1973; MB ChB (Commend.) Glas. 1977; MRCPsych 1981; MFPHM RCP (UK) 1993. Dir. Pub. Health Croydon. Specialty: Pub. Health Med.; Gen. Psychiat. Prev: Cons. Pub. Health Med. Lambeth Southwark & Lewisham HA; Sen. Regist. St. Geo. Hosp. Lond.; Regist. Maudsley Hosp. Lond.

SHANKS, Jonathan Hugh Christie Hospital, Department of Histopathology, Wilmslow, Manchester M20 4BX Tel: 0161 446 8025 Fax: 0161 446 3300 Email: jonathan.shanks@christie-tr.nwest.nhs.uk; 59 Dalston Drive, Didsbury, Manchester M20 5LQ Tel: 0161 445 3772 — MB ChB Manch. 1987; BSc (Hons.) Manch. 1984; MD Belf. 1994; MRCPath 1995; FRCPath 2003. Cons. Histopath. Christie Hosp. Manch. Specialty: Histopath. Special Interest: Urological Path. Socs: Internat. Acad. Path.; Path. Soc.; Assn. Clin. Path. Prev: Sen. Regist. Rotat. (Histopath.) N. West. RHA; Regist. & SHO (Histopath.) Roy. Vict. Hosp. Belf.

SHANKS, Michael Fraser Royal Cornhill Hospital, Clerkseat Building, Cornhill Road, Aberdeen AB25 3ZH Tel: 01224 663131; 14 College Bounds, Old Aberdeen, Aberdeen AB24 3DS Tel: 01224 493838 — MB ChB Aberd. 1971; BMedBiol (Hons.) Aberd. 1968; FRCPsych 1995, M 1978; DPhil Oxf. 1980. Cons. Old Age Psychiat. Grampian Healthcare NHS Trust; Hon. Sen. Lect. Dept. of Psychol. and Ment. Health Univ. of Aberd. Specialty: Geriat. Psychiat. Socs: Brit. Assn. Psychopharmacol.; Brit. Neuropsychiatric Assn. Prev:

Cons. Psychiat. Highland HB; Sen. Lect. (Psychol. Med.) Univ. Glas.; Lect. Inst. Psychiat. Lond.

SHANKS, Michael Peter Severn Surgery, 159 Uplands Road, Oadby, Leicester LE2 4NW Tel: 0116 271 9042 — MB BChir Camb. 1979; MB Camb 1979, BChir 1978.

SHANKS, Nicholas Roland c/o Shanks, 7 Hollymount Avenue, Newtownards BT23 7DG — MB ChB Dundee 1995.

SHANKS, Oliver Edward Pattison (retired) 19 Derryvolgie Avenue, Belfast BT9 6FN — MB BCh BAO Belf. 1974; DCH NUI 1976; MRCP (UK) 1978; FRCPsych 1992, M 1980. Cons. Psychiat. (Learning Disabil.) Muckamore Abbey Hosp. Antrim. Prev: Sen. Regist. (Child Psychiat.) Roy. Belf. Hosp. Sick Childr.

SHANKS, Robert The Shrubbery, 65A Perry Street, Northfleet, Gravesend DA11 8RD Tel: 01474 356661 Fax: 01474 534542; 16 Orchard Avenue, Gravesend DA11 7NX — (Belf.) MB BCh BAO Belf. 1970. Police Surg.; Childr.'s Serv. Commissioner for PCG. Socs: BMA & Assn. Police Surgs. Prev: Ho. Off. Waveney Hosp. Ballymena; SHO Belf. City Hosp. & North. Irel. Radiother. Centre Belf.

SHANKS, Sheila Deborah 2 Bellfield Terrace, Inverness IV2 4ST — MB BCh BAO Belf. 1985 (Queens Univ. Belf.) DCH RCPI 1988; MRCP (UK) 1992. Cons. Paediat., Raigmore Hosp. Inverness, IV2 3UJ. Specialty: Paediat. Socs: MRCPCH.

SHANKS, Wilhelmina (retired) Ingham, Lincoln LN1 2XT Tel: 01522 730269 — MB BCh BAO Dub. 1949 (T.C. Dub.) BA, MB BCh BAO Dub. 1949. Prev: Asst. MOH Matern. & Child Welf. Lindsey CC.

SHANLEY, Michael Joseph The Linden Medical Group, The Health Centre, 97 Derby Road, Nottingham NG9 7AT Tel: 0115 939 2444 Fax: 0115 949 1751 — MB BCh BAO NUI 1986.

SHANMUGALINGAM, Mr Sinnathamboo Bronglais General Hospital, North Road Eye Clinic, North Road, Aberystwyth SY23 2EG Tel: 01970 636200 — MB BS Sri Lanka 1973; DO RCS Eng. 1981; FRCS Glas. 1985; FRCOphth 1988. Cons. Ophth. Bronglais Gen. Hosp. Specialty: Ophth. Prev: Assoc. Specialist (Ophth.) Kent Co. Hosp. Maidstone; Regist. (Ophth.) Roy. Surrey Co. Hosp. Guildford & Huddersfield Roy. Infirm.

SHANMUGALINGAM, Vathany 90 Alpine Rise, Styvechale, Coventry CV3 6NR — BM Soton. 1998.

SHANMUGANATHAN, Chellappah 146 Ridge Lane, Watford WD17 4WU Tel: 01923 235552 Email: vaani84@hotmail.com; 146 Ridge Lane, Watford WD17 4WH Tel: 01923 235552 Fax: 01923 235552 — (Colombo) MB BS Ceylon 1965; Dip. Ven. Soc. Apoth Lond. 1974; FRIPHH 1976; DPH Eng. 1977; DIH Eng. 1978; DTM & H Liverp. 1979. Indep. GP Watford. Specialty: Genitourinary Medicine; Gen. Pract. Socs: BMA. Prev: Regist. Char. Cross Hosp. Lond.; Med. Off. Gen. Hosp. Bandar Seri Begawan, Brunei; Dist. Med. Off. Kilinochi, Sri Lanka.

SHANMUGANATHAN, Mr Kathirithamby 31 Finmere Crescent, Bedgrove, Aylesbury HP21 9DQ — MB BS Ceylon 1963; FRCS Ed. 1967.

SHANMUGANATHAN, Manohari 31 Finmere Crescent, Bedgrove, Aylesbury HP21 9DQ — MB BS Ceylon 1967. Specialty: Gen. Psychiat.

SHANMUGANATHAN, Thevarayapillai Long Grove Hospital, Epsom KT19 8PU Tel: 01372 726200 — MB BS Madras 1971.

SHANMUGANATHAN, Vijay Anand Division of Ophthalmology & Visual Science, 3rd Floor, Eye & Ent Centre, Queens Medical Centre, Nottingham NG7 2UH — MB BS Lond. 1996 (UMDS) MRCPath 2001. Research Fell. (Ophthalmology & Visual Science) Univ. of Nottm. Specialty: Ophth. Prev: RMO St. Mary's Hosp. Bristol; SHO (Ophthalmology) Manch. Roy. Eye Hosp.

SHANMUGARAJU, Mr Palaniappa Gounder Mayday University Hospital, 530 London Road, Croydon CR8 5JH Tel: 020 8401 3331 Fax: 020 8401 3675 Email: palaniappa.raju@mayday.nhs.uk; 4 and 6 Abbots Lane, Kenley CR8 5JH Tel: 020 8645 9929 Fax: 020 8240 1044 — MB BS Madras 1978; LRCP LRCS Ed. LRCPS Glas. 1983; FRCS Ed. 1984; Dip. Urol. Lond 1988. Cons. Urol., Mayday Univ. Hosp., Croydon. Specialty: Urol.; Oncol. Socs: BAUS; RSM; AUA. Prev: Cons. Urol., Law Hosp., Carluke.

SHANMUGARATNAM, Kanagaratnam Bedford Hospital, Kempston Road, Bedford MK42 9DJ Tel: 01234 792146; The Pines, 8 Cryselco Close, Kempston, Bedford MK42 7TJ Tel: 01234 854355 — MB BS Sri Lanka 1978 (Colombo) FRCP; LRCP LRCS Ed. LRCPS Glas. 1985. Cons. Genitourin. Med. Bedford Hosp. Specialty: Genitourinary Medicine. Prev: Sen. Regist. (Genitourin. Med.) Newc. Gen. Hosp.; Regist. (Genitourin. Med.) Roy. North. Hosp. Lond.; SHO (Gen. Med.) Manch. Roy. Infirm.

SHANMUGASUNDARAM, Govindaraju (retired) 33 Cefn Coed, Bridgend CF31 4PH Tel: 01656 645098 — MB BS Madras 1973 (Madras Med. Coll.) Regist. (Psychiat.) Parc Hosp. Bridgend. Prev: Trainee GP S. Clwyd VTS.

SHANMUGASUNDARAM, Mr Obli 228 Newton Drive, Blackpool FY3 8NB Tel: 01253 391330 Fax: 01253 391330 — MB BS Madras 1973; FRCSI 1984; FRCS Ed. 1989; FFAEM 1993. Assoc. Specialist (Orthop.) Vict. Hosp. Blackpool. Specialty: Orthop.; Trauma & Orthop. Surg. Socs: Assoc. Mem. BOA; Brit. Assn. Accid. & Emerg. Med.; (Counc.) Brit. Assn. Sports Med. Prev: Assoc. Specialist (A & E) Vict. Hosp. Blackpool.

SHANN, Debra Jayne 10 Craigmore Dr, Ilkley LS29 8PG — MB ChB Dundee 1997.

SHANNON, Charles John 5 Old Rectory Close, Westbourne, Emsworth PO10 8UB — MB BS Lond. 1966 (St. Geo.) MRCS Eng. LRCP Lond. 1966; FFA RCS Eng. 1971. Cons. Anaesth. S.E. Hants. Gp. Hosps. Specialty: Anaesth. Prev: Regist. Nuffield Dept. Anaesth. Radcliffe Infirm. Oxf.; Sen. Regust. (Anaesth.) RiksHosp.er Oslo, Norway.

SHANNON, Claire Nicola 24 Solon Road, London SW2 5UY Tel: 020 7978 9493 — MB BS Lond. 1987; FRCA 1993. Sen. Regist. (Anaesth.) UCLH Lond. Specialty: Anaesth. Socs: Assn. Anaesth. Prev: Regist. (Anaesth.) Hosp. for Sick Childr. Gt. Ormond St. Lond.; Regist. Rotat. (Anaesth.) Greenwich Dist., Brook & King's Hosps. Lond.; SHO Rotat. (Anaesth.) Char. Cross & Barnet Gen. Hosps.

SHANNON, Elizabeth Gwendoline Mary Health Centre, John St., Rathfriland, Newry BT34 3JD Tel: 028 40630666; 26 Bishopswell road, Dromore BT25 1ST — MB BCh BAO Belf. 1983; DCH RCPSI 1985; DRCOG 1986; MRCGP 1987. GP Rathfriland. Socs: Ulster Med. Soc.; Med. Wom. Federat.

SHANNON, Ernest Nathaniel Lodge Health, 20 Lodge Manor, Coleraine BT52 1JX Tel: 028 7034 4494 Fax: 028 7032 1759 — MB BCh BAO Belf. 1974. Med. Off. Dhu Varren Childr. Home Portrush; Med. Off. Ulster Bus Ltd. Coleraine. Specialty: Care of the Elderly.

SHANNON, Gavin Michael Ground Floor Flat, 24 Solon Road, London SW2 5UY — MB BS Lond. 1988.

SHANNON, Gillian Elizabeth Mary 20 Magheraconluce Road, Dromore BT25 1EE — MB BCh BAO Belf. 1991; DMH Belf. 1994; DGM RCPS Glas. 1994; DRCOG 1995; MRCGP 1996; DFFP 1996.

SHANNON, Jason Lee 18 Ware Road, Caerphilly CF83 1SX — MB ChB Birm. 1996; ChB Birm. 1996.

SHANNON, Jeanetta Margaret 17 School Road, Newtownbreda, Belfast BT8 6BT — MB BCh BAO Belf. 1961; MB BCh Belf. 1961.

SHANNON, John Richard 48 Chestnut Grove, Coleshill, Birmingham B46 1AD — MB BCh BAO Dub. 1977 (TC Dub.) Med. Off. DHSS Birm. Specialty: Disabil. Med. Prev: SHO (Gen. Med.) N. Manch. Gen. Hosp.; SHO (Gen. Med./O & G) W. Pk. Hosp. Macclesfield; SHO (Nephrol./Geriat.) Withington Hosp. Manch.

SHANNON, Muriel Susan Department of Haematology, St George's Hospital, Tooting, London SW17 0QT Tel: 020 8725 5480 Email: m.shannon@sghms.ac.uk — MB ChB Glas. 1975 (Glasgow) FRCPath 1994, M 1982. Cons. (Haemat.) St Geo. Hosp. Lond. Specialty: Haematology. Socs: Brit. Soc. Haematol. Prev: Clin. Asst. (Haemat.) St. Geo. Hosp. Lond.; Clin. Research Fell. Imperial Cancer Research Fund Lond.; Sen. Regist. (Haemat.) Roy. Free Hosp. Lond.

SHANNON, Nora Letitia Clinical Genetics Unit, Birmingham Women's Hospital, Metchley Park Rd, Birmingham B!5 2TG — MB BS Lond. 1992 (St. Geo. Hosp. Med. Sch. Lond.) MRCP (UK) 1995. Cons. Clin. Geneticist, Clin. Genetics Unit, Birm. Wom.'s Hosp. Specialty: Genetics. Socs: Brit. Soc. For Human Genetics; The Cancer Genetics Grp.; The Skeletal Dysplasia Grp. Prev: Specialist Regist. (Clin. Genetics) Centre Human Genetics Sheff.

SHANNON, Paul Edington 16 Croft Drive, Tickhill, Doncaster DN11 9UL — MB ChB Leeds 1987; FRCA 1993. Cons. Anaesth. Doncaster Roy. Infirm. Specialty: Anaesth. Socs: Assn. Anaesth. & Obst. Anaesth. Assn. Prev: Regist. (Anaesth.) Sheff. HA; SHO (Paediat. & Anaesth.) Bradford Roy. Infirm.; SHO (A & E) Dewsbury Dist. Hosp.

SHANNON, Rosemary Susan 3 Llewellyn Court, Off Elmsleigh Avenue, Stoneygate, Leicester LE2 2DH — MB BCh BAO Dub. 1966 (T.C. Dub.) MA, MB BCh BAO Dub. 1966; DCH Eng. 1969; FRCP Lond. 1973. Cons. (Paediat.) Leicester Roy. Infirm. Specialty: Paediat. Prev: Sen. Regist. (Paediat.) Childr. Hosp. Birm.

SHANNON, Sarah White (Surgery) 27 Parkfield Road, Coleshill, Birmingham B46 3LD Tel: 01675 463165; 48 Chestnut Grove, Coleshill, Birmingham B46 1AD Tel: 01675 463255 — MB BCh BAO Dub. 1977; BSc Loughborough 1972; DCH RCPSI 1978; DRCOG 1982; MRCGP 1983; DCP Warwick 1989. Prev: SHO (Obst. & Neonat. Paediat.) St. Mary's Hosp. Manch.; SHO (Paediat.) Nat. Childr. Hosp. Dub. & Duchess of York Hosp. Manch.

SHANNON, Sian Eirian 5 Hollybush Close, Sevenoaks TN13 3XW — MB BS Lond. 1983; DRCOG 1986.

SHANNON, Thomas Edward (retired) Oakroyd, Foxholes Road, Horwich, Bolton BL6 6AS Tel: 01204 697883 — (Glas.) MB BCh BAO NUI 1942; DOMS Eng. 1946. Sen. Hosp. Med. Off. Roy. Eye Hosp. Manch. Prev: Cons. Ophth. Bolton Roy. Infirm.

SHANNON, Violet Courtney (retired) Garliebank, Brighton Road, Cupar KY15 5DQ — MB ChB St And. 1964; DObst RCOG 1966; DPM Ed. & Glas. 1968; MRCPsych 1972. Prev: Cons. Child Psychiat. Stratheden Hosp. Cupar Fife.

SHANSON, Barnett 1 Ravenscroft Court, 56 Ravenscroft Avenue, London NW11 8BA Tel: 020 8458 9221 — MRCS Eng. LRCP Lond. 1949 (Lond. Hosp.) MRCS Eng. LRCP Lond. 1932; DPhys. Med. Eng. 1949. LCC Certif. of Efficiency in VD; Clin. Asst. Roy. Nat. Throat, Nose & Ear Hosp. Lond. & Brit. Red Cross Clinic For Rheum. Peto Pl; Hon. Advis. Edr. Brit. Jl. Physical Med.; Research Asst. First Pulverisation of Caculi ref: Terrence Millin. Specialty: Rehabil. Med.; Rheumatol. Socs: Lond. Jewish Med. Soc.; Soc. Rheum.; Founder Mem. Heberden Soc. Prev: Researcher Coley, Fluid in Sarcoma of No Value; Ho. Surg. Roy. Albert Hosp. Plymouth; Hon. Dent. Anaesth. Qu. Mary's Hosp. Stratford.

SHANSON, David Charles 48 Middleway, London NW11 6SG Tel: 020 8455 8238 Email: davidsha87@hotmail.com — (Westm.) MB BS Lond. 1966; MRCS Eng. LRCP Lond. 1966; FRCPath 1986, M 1973. Cons. MicrobiolAPS/Unilabs Clin.Path.27 harley St. Lond; Emerit. Cons. Microbiol. Chelsea & Westminster Hosp. Specialty: Med. Microbiol. Socs: Fell. Roy. Soc. Med. (Prev. Pres. Path. Sect.); Past Chairm. Hosp. Infec. Soc. Prev: Sen. Lect. & Hon. Cons. Med. Microbiol. Char. Cross, Westm. Med. Sch. & W.m. Hosps. Lond.; Sen. Lect. & Hon. Cons. (Med. Microbiol.) Lond. Hosp.; Sen. Regist. (Microbiol.) Univ. Coll. Hosp. Lond.

SHANSON, Ronald Louis (Surgery) 8 Englefiled Road, Islington, London N1 4LN Tel: 020 7254 1324; 43 Essex Road, Islington, London N1 2SF Tel: 020 7226 8096 — MB BS Lond. 1968 (Univ. Coll. Hosp.) MRCS Eng. LRCP Lond. 1968. Prev: Regist. (Anaesth.) Hornsby Hosp. Sydney, Austral.; SHO (Anaesth.) Guy's Hosp. Lond.; Cas. Off. Lond. Jewish Hosp.

SHANTHA, A L Huyton Primary Care Resource Centre, Nutgrove Villa, Westmorland Road, Liverpool L36 6GA Tel: 0151 489 2276.

SHANTHAKUMAR, Ratnasingham Edward Department of Anaesthetics, Barnet and Chasefarm NHS Trust, Barnet General Hospital, Barnet EN5 3DJ Tel: 020 8216 4000 Fax: 020 8216 5297; 27 Leavesden Road, Stanmore HA7 3RQ Tel: 020 8954 7598 — MB BS Sri Lanka Peradeniya 1980; DA (UK) 1990; FFA RCSI 1992; FRCA 1993; EDICM 1996. Cons. Anaesth. Barnet Gen. Hosp. Specialty: Anaesth. Socs: BMA; Assn. Anaesth.; Intens. Care Soc. Prev: Fell. (Intens. Care) Univ. Hosp. Groningen, Netherlands; Sen. Regist. Hammersmith Hosp. Lond.

SHANTI RAJU, Kankipati Department of Gynaecology, St. Thomas' Hospital, Guys & St. Thomas' NHS Trust, Lambeth Palace Road, London SE1 7EH Tel: 0207 928 9292 Ext: 2068 — MB BS Andhra 1973; MD; DRCOG Lond.; DTCDHE 1986; FRCOG 1992. Cons. & Gyn. Oncol., St. Thos. Hosp. and NHS Trust. Specialty: Obst. & Gyn. Socs: Internat. Gyn. Cancer Soc.; Past Europ. Gyn. Cancer Soc.; Brit. Soc. of Colposcopy and Cervical Path. Prev: Sen. Lect., UMDS, Lond.; Lect. UMDS, Lond.; Lect. Roy. Marsden Hosp., Lond.

SHANTIR, Dauod Yosuf Abdul-Rahman Forest Road Medical Centre, 354-368 Forest Road, Walthamstow, London E17 5JG Tel: 020 8520 7115 Fax: 020 8923 1199 — MB BCh Ain Shams 1971.

SHAOUL, Doreen Diana Rachel Brook Green Medical Centre, Bute Gardens, London W6 7EG Tel: 020 8237 2800 Fax: 020 8237 2811; Compton Lodge, 140 Upper Richmond Road West, London SW14 8DS Tel: 020 8876 0632 — MB BS Lond. 1962. Prev: Ho. Phys. St. Geo. Hosp. Lond.

SHAOUL, Edward The Brook Green Medical Centre, Bute Gardens, London W6 7BE Tel: 020 8237 2800 Fax: 020 8237 2811; Compton Lodge, 140 Upper Richmond Road W., East Sheen, London SW14 8DS Tel: 020 8876 0632 — MB ChB Manch. 1958; DObst RCOG 1961; FRCGP 1981. Assoc. Dean (Gen. Pract.) N. Thames W. Region; Hon. Sen. Lect. (Gen. Pract.) Char. Cross & Westm. Med. Sch. Lond.

SHAPER, Professor Andrew Gerald (retired) 12 Greenholme Farm, Leather Bank, Burley in Wharfedale, Ilkley LS29 7HP Tel: 01943 865 675 Fax: 01943 865 675 Email: agshaper@wentworth.u-net.com — (Cape Town) MB ChB Cape Town 1951; DTM & H Liverp. 1953; FRCP Lond. 1969, M 1955; FRCPath 1976, M 1968; FFPHM 1972. p/t Emerit. Prof. Clin. Epidemiol. Roy. Free & Univ. Coll. Med. Sch. 1992-. Prev: Mem. Scientif. Staff, MRC Social Med. Research Unit 1970-1975.

SHAPER, Miss Katherine Rosamond Lees Luton & Dunstable Hospital, Lewsey Road, Luton LU4 0DZ — MB BS Lond. 1987 (Univ. Coll. Lond.) FRCS Eng. 1992; MS 1997; FRCS (Gen. Surg.) 2001. Cons. Coloproctol. Specialty: Gen. Surg.

SHAPER, Mr Nicholas Joel Bradford Royal Infirmary, Duckworth Lane, Bradford BD9 6RJ Tel: 01274 364782 Email: nick.shaper@bradfordhospitals.nhs.uk — MB BS Lond. 1987 (Roy. Free) BSc (Hons) Lond. 1982; FRCS Eng. 1992; FRCS (Gen.) 1999. Cons. Vasc. Surg., Bradford Teachg. Hosps. NHS Trust. Specialty: Surgery, Vascular. Socs: VSSGBI; ASGBI; RSM. Prev: Regist. (Gen. Surg.) SE Thames Higher Surgic. Train. Scheme.

SHAPERO, Jonathan Stewart NHS Milton Keynes Hospital Campus, Marlborough House Secure Unit, Standing Way, Milton Keynes MK6 5NG Tel: 01908 243049 Email: jonathan.shapero@bmh-tr.nhs.com; NHS Northants Community Forensic Mental Health Service, Campbell House, Campbell Square, Northampton NN1 3EB Tel: 01604 658985 Email: jonathan.shapero@nht.northants.nhs.uk; PO Box 6885, Market Harborough LE16 8WY Email: jshapero@aol.com — MB ChB Birm. 1978; MRCPsych 1982. Cons. Forens. Psychiat.; Vis. Psychiat. HM Young Offenders' Centre Glen Parva Leicester. Specialty: Forens. Psychiat. Socs: BMA. Prev: Cons. Forens. Psychiat. St. Andrews Hosp. Northampton; Cons. Forens. Psychiat. Leicester Ment. Health Trust; Vis. Psychiat. HMP Woodhill Milton Keynes.

SHAPIRO, Mr Andrew Mark James Surgical-Medical Research Institute, 1074 Dentistry-Pharmacy Building, University of Alberta, Edmonton T6G 2N8, Canada Tel: 00 1 403 4928822 Fax: 00 1 403 4310704; 12 Clifton Wood Crescent, Bristol BS8 4TU Tel: 01179 268381 — MB BS Newc. 1988; BMedSci. 1985; FRCS Eng. 1992. Specialty: Gen. Surg. Socs: Fell. (Liver Transpl.) Univ. Edmonton, Alberta, Canada; Fell. Paediat. Islet Research. Prev: Demonst. (Anat.) Univ. of Bristol; Regist. Profess. Surg. Unit Bristol Roy. Infirm.; Ho. Surg. Profess. Surgic. Unit Roy. Vict. Infirm. Newc. u Tyne.

SHAPIRO, Brian William Renfrew Health Centre, 103 Paisley Road, Renfrew PA4 8LL Tel: 0141 886 2455 Fax: 0141 855 0457; 23 Humbie Road, Eaglesham, Glasgow G76 0LX Tel: 013553 2976 — MB ChB Glas. 1977.

SHAPIRO, Emma Bernardine Awbery 34 Henry Gardens, Chichester PO19 3DL — MB BS Lond. 1991.

SHAPIRO, Frank Norman Strahaven Health Centre, The Ward, Strathaven ML10 6AS Tel: 01357 522993 — MB ChB Glas. 1976; DRCOG 1980; Cert FPA. RCOG 1980. Prison Med. Off. Dungavel Prison Drumclog; GP Strathaven.

SHAPIRO, Henry 24 Harewood Mews, Harewood, Leeds LS17 9LY Tel: 0113 288 6215 Fax: 0113 288 6183 Email: hshap0922@aol.com — (Leeds) MRCS Eng. LRCP Lond. 1947; MRCGP 1966; MFOM RCP Lond. 1982. Socs: Fell. Roy. Soc. Med.; BMA; Leeds & W. Riding M-C Soc. Prev: Hon. Clin. Asst. Coronary Preven. Clinic St. Jas. Unit Teach. Hosp. Leeds; Cons. Phys. Burton Gp. plc Lond. & Leeds; GP Leeds.

SHAPIRO, Joan Cree 23 Humbie Road, Eaglesham, Glasgow G76 0LX — MB ChB Glas. 1977.

SHAPIRO, Jonathan Abraham Health Services Management Centre, Park House, 40 Edgbaston Park Road, Birmingham B15 2RT Tel: 0121 414 7050 Fax: 0121 414 7051 Email:

j.a.shapiro@bham.ac.uk — MB ChB Birm. 1977; MA Camb. 1978; MRCGP 1981. Sen. Fell. (Health Servs. Managem.) Univ. of Birm. Prev: Indep. Med. Adviser Leics. RHSA; GP Bulkington N. Warks. FHSA; Ho. Phys. Med. Profess. Unit Qu. Eliz. Hosp. Birm.

SHAPIRO, Leonard Melvyn Papworth Hospital, Papworth Everard, Cambridge CB3 8RE Email: ims@ntlworld.com — MD Manch. 1981; BSc Manch. 1973, MD 1981, MB ChB 1976; MRCP (UK) 1978; FRCP Lond. 1993; FACC 1994. Cons. Cardiol. Papworth Hosp.; Cons. Cardiol. Addenbrooke's Hosp. Camb. Specialty: Cardiol. Special Interest: Athletes; Interventional Cardiol. Socs: British Cardiac Society; American College of Cardiology; British Cardiac Intervention Society. Prev: Assoc. Lect. Univ. Camb; Sen. Regist. Nat. Heart & Brompton Hosp.; Regist. Hammersmith Hosp. Lond.

SHAPIRO, Leslie (retired) 4 Windsor House, Regency Crescent, London NW4 1NW Tel: 020 8371 0569 — MB ChB Leeds 1952. Prev: Principal GP Leeds.

SHAPIRO, Linda Rae River Brook Medical Centre, 3 River Brook Drive, Stirchley, Birmingham B30 2SH Tel: 0121 451 2525 Fax: 0121 433 3214 — MB ChB Birm. 1975.

SHAPIRO, Steven Maurice 48 Kewferry Road, Northwood HA6 2PG — MB BS Lond. 1982; DRCOG 1986; MRCGP 1988.

SHAPIRO-STERN, Paul Rayd Church End Medical Centre, 66 Mayo Road, Church End Estate, Willesden, London NW10 9HP Tel: 020 8930 6262 Fax: 020 8930 6260; 1 Talbot Walk, Willesden, London NW10 9HU Tel: 020 8451 2401 — MB ChB Cape Town 1965.

SHAPLAND, John David (retired) Glen Mar, Longacre Rock, Wadebridge PL27 6LG — MB BS Lond. 1949 (Lond. Hosp.) MRCS Eng. LRCP Lond. 1949. Prev: Hosp. Pract. (Geriat.) Plymouth.

SHAPLAND, Judith Mary Cutlers Hill Surgery, Bungay Road, Halesworth IP19 8HP Tel: 01986 874136 — MB BS Lond. 1985; MRCGP 1991. Specialty: Gen. Pract.

SHAPLAND, Michael Courtenay (retired) — BM BCh Oxf. 1962 (Oxf. & Lond. Hosp.) MRCS Eng. LRCP Lond. 1961; MA Oxf. Prev: GP Oxf.

SHAPLAND, William David, Wing Cdr. — MB BS Lond. 1981 (Roy. Lond. Hosp.) DA (UK) 1984; DRCOG 1985; MRCPsych 1990; Cert. Cog. Ther Oxf. 1996. Cons. (Gen. Adult) Dept. of Community Psychiat. Marham. Specialty: Gen. Psychiat. Socs: BMA; Roy. Coll. of Psychiat.s. Prev: Hon. Clin. Fell. (Psychopharmacol) Bristol Roy. Infirm.; Regist. (Psychiat.) I. of Wight & Moorhaven Hosp. Ivybridge Devon; Hon. Sen. Regist. (Forens.) Fromeside Clinic Bristol.

SHAPLEY, Mark Wolstanton Medical Centre, Palmerston Street, Newcastle ST5 8BN Tel: 01782 627488 Fax: 01782 662313 — MB BS Lond. 1982; BA Oxf. 1979; DRCOG 1984; DCH RCP Lond. 1985; MRCGP 1986.

SHAPLEY, Roger West Bar Surgery, 1 West Bar Street, Banbury OX16 9SF Tel: 01295 256261 Fax: 01295 756848; The Old Forge, Main St, North Newington, Banbury OX15 6AF Tel: 01295 730466 — MB BS Lond. 1972; MRCP (U.K.) 1975; DObst RCOG 1976; MRCGP 1977; DCH Eng. 1977.

SHAR, Mohamed Bahgat Saddleton Road Surgery, 32 Saddleton Road, Whitstable CT5 4JQ Tel: 01227 272809 — MB BCh Cairo 1972.

SHARAF, Adnan 106 Lawton Road, Alsager, Stoke-on-Trent ST7 2DE — MB BS Lond. 1998; MRCP 2002; DTM & H 2003.

SHARAF, Loutfy Amin Mosa 7 Mountjoy Road, Edgerton, Huddersfield HD1 5QB Tel: 01484 311166 — MB ChB Alexandria 1964; DA Alexandria 1970; FFA RCSI 1975. Cons. Anaesth. Huddersfield Roy. Infirm. Specialty: Anaesth. Prev: Sen. Regist. Leeds Hosp.

SHARAF, Taher Fathi Ali 4 Shottfield Avenue, London SW14 8EA — MB BS Lond. 1998; MB BS Lond 1998.

SHARAF, Mr Usama Ibrahim 23 Hoel Ysgawen, Sketty, Swansea SA2 9GS — MB BCh Ain Shams 1979; FRCS Ed. 1990; FRCS Glas. 1990.

SHARAF-UD-DIN, Syed Kidsgrove Medical Centre, Mount Road, Kidsgrove, Stoke-on-Trent ST7 4AY Tel: 01782 784221 Fax: 01782 781703; The Rowans, 106 Lawton Road, Alsager, Stoke-on-Trent ST7 2DE — MB BS Karachi 1962 (Dow Med. Coll.) DCH RCPS Glas. 1965.

SHARAIHA, Mr Yousef Mitri Doctor's Residence, Prince Philip Hospital, Dafen, Llanelli SA14 8QF; Flat C, 30 Kempsford Gardens, London SW5 9LH Tel: 020 7244 6352 — MB BS Jordan 1988; BA (Psychol.) Univ. India 1983; FRCS Ed. 1994. Regist. (Gen. Surg.) P. Philip Hosp. Llanelli, Dyfed. Specialty: Gen. Surg. Prev: SHO Qu. Eliz. Hosp. King's Lynn; SHO Bradford Roy. Infirm.

SHARAN, Kalpana Springfield Farmhouse, Ercall Heath, Newport TF10 8NQ Tel: 01952 550654 Email: saran999@yahoo.com — MB BS Patna 1971; MB BS Patna 1976; MRCOG 1983; FRCOG 1998. Assoc. Specialist (O & G). Specialty: Obst. & Gyn.

SHARARA, Abdelmonem Mohammad Office of Jordan Military Naval and Air, 16 Upper Phillimore Gardens, London W8 7HE — MB BS Jordan 1980; MRCP (UK) 1988.

SHARARA, Mr Fawzi 35 Redclyffe Gardens, Helensburgh G84 9JJ Tel: 01436 678826 Email: drfawzisharara@aol.com — MB BCh Ain Shams 1967; FRCS Eng. 1979. Complementary Med. Practitioner Helensburgh. Specialty: Homeop. Med. Socs: Brit. Med. Acupunct. Soc.; Assoc. Mem. Fac. Homeop.; Mem. Brit. Med. & Den. Hypno. Soc. Scotland.

SHARD, Helen Mary 60 Eagle Brow, Lymm WA13 0LZ — MB BS Lond. 1990.

SHARDA, Arun Dev Stantonbury Health Centre, Purbeck, Stantonbury, Milton Keynes MK14 6BL Tel: 01908 316262 — MB BS Punjab 1973 (Govt. Med. Coll. Patiala) MB BS Punjabi 1973.

SHARDLOW, Mr David Lloyd 3 Pine Tree Close, Thorpe Willoughby, Selby YO8 9FP — MB BS Lond. 1989; FRCS (Eng) 1993; MSc (Eng) Leeds 1998. Specialist Regist. (Trauma & Ortho.) St. James Univ. Hosp. Leeds. Specialty: Trauma & Orthop. Surg. Socs: BOA; BORS; BOTA.

SHARE, Alison 14 Osbourne Road, Wolverhampton WV4 4AY — MB ChB Leeds 1989.

SHARE, Aubrey Ingram Sherwood 67 Sandmoor Lane, Leeds LS17 7EA Tel: 0113 268 4401 — MB ChB Leeds 1945; LDS Leeds 1948. JP. Prev: Ho. Surg. Gen. Infirm. Leeds.

SHAREEF, Syed Hasnain The Health Centre, Canterbury Way, Stevenage SG1 1QH Tel: 01438 357411 Fax: 01438 720523 — MB BS Dacca 1958. Socs: Med. Defence Union.

SHARER, Nicholas Montague Poole Hospital NHS Trust, Longfleet Road, Poole BH15 2JB Tel: 01202 448315 Fax: 01202 442996 Email: nsharer@poole-tr.swest.nhs.uk — BM Soton. 1986; BSc (Hons) Wales 1980; MRCP (UK) 1989; FRCP 2000; DM Soton 2003. Cons. Phys. & Gastroenterol. Poole Hosp. NHS Trust. Specialty: Gastroenterol.; Gen. Med. Prev: Regist. & Med. Co-ordinator (Pancreato-Biliary Serv.) Centr. Manch. HA; Regist. (Med.) Newc. u. Tyne Hosps.; SHO (Med.) Portsmouth.

SHARFUDDIN, Imtiaz 215 Sydney Road, London N10 2NL — MB BS Karachi 1981.

SHARIEF, Mohammad Kassim Department of Neurology, Medical School Building, Guy's Hospital, London SE1 9RT Tel: 020 7955 4398 Fax: 020 7378 1221; Department of Neurology, St. Thomas's Hospital, London SE1 7EH Tel: 020 7928 9292 Fax: 020 7922 8263 — MB ChB Baghdad 1980; PhD 1992, MPhil 1989; MRCP (UK) 1993. Sen. Lect. & Cons. Neurol. Lond. Specialty: Neurol.

SHARIEF, Nawfal Natheir Younis Basildon Hospital, Paediatric Department, Nether Mayne, Basildon SS16 5NL Tel: 01268 593979 Fax: 01268 593194 Email: doreen.roberts@btuh.nhs.uk — MB ChB Baghdad 1973; PhD Lond. 1980; MRCP (UK) 1983; DCH RCP Lond. 1983; FRCP Lond. 1996; FRCPCH 1997. Cons. Paediat. Basildon Hosp. Specialty: Paediat. Socs: BMA; Roy. Coll. Paediat. & Child Health; Brit. Assn. of Perinatal Med. Prev: Sen. Regist. (Paediat. Respirat. Dis. & Gastroenterol.) Qu. Eliz. Hosp.; Sen. Regist. (Developm. Paediat. & Neonat.) Qu. Eliz. & Homerton Hosps.

SHARIEFF, Sayeda Fouzia 19 Loughan Road, Coleraine BT52 1UB — MB BS Osmania 1973.

SHARIF, Ala Towfiq The Albany CLinic, 11 Station Road, Sidcup DA15 7EN Tel: 020 8300 4361 — MB ChB Baghdad 1973.

SHARIF, Mr Dhia George Elliot Hospital, Lewes House, College Street, Nuneaton CV10 7DJ Tel: 02476 865129.

SHARIF, Harpreet The Hetherington Group Practice, 18 Hetherington Road, London SW4 7NU Tel: 020 7274 4220 Fax: 020 7737 0205 — MB ChB Dundee 1988.

SHARIF, Jalal The Surgery, 62 Windsor Drive, Orpington BR6 6HD Tel: 01689 852204 Fax: 01689 857122 — MD Isfahan 1976. GP Chelsfield; Clin. Asst. (Cardiol.) FarnBoro. Hosp. Prev: Research Fell. (Cardiol.) Guy's Hosp. Lond.; Regist. (Med.) FarnBoro. Hosp.

SHARIF, Khaldoun Walid Said 22 Aboyne Close, Birmingham B5 7PQ — MB BCh Ain-Shams 1985; MRCOG 1991.

SHARIF, Mohammad c/o M. A. Nusrat, 9 Carew Road, Thornton Heath, Croydon CR7 7RF — MB BS Punjab 1961; MRCPSych 1973.

SHARIF, Mr Mohammed (retired) Flat 4 Newmount, 11 Lyndhurst Terrace, Hamstead, London NW3 5QA Tel: 020 7435 5721 — MB BS Bombay 1936 (Grant Med. Coll.) Dip. Genitourin. Surg. Inst. Urol. Lond. 1950; FRCS Eng. 1951; DAvMed. US Air Univ. 1956; DSc (Hon. Causa) Malta 1989. Prev: Dir.-Gen. (Health) & Jt. Sec. Min. Health Pakistan.

SHARIF, Mohammed Mahmood Kings Park Surgery, 274 Kings Park Avenue, Glasgow G44 4JE Tel: 0141 632 1824 Fax: 0141 632 0461 — MB ChB Glas. 1980. SHO Orthop. Dept. Glas. Roy. Infirm. Prev: Jun. Ho. Off. (Surg.) Duke St. Hosp. Glas.; Jun. Ho. Off. (Med.) Vict. Infirm. Glas.; Jun. Ho. Off. Gartnavel Gen. Hosp. Glas.

SHARIF, Mr Riadh Ali Mohamed Stoke Mandeville Hospital, Mandeville Road, Aylesbury HP21 8AL Tel: 01296 315773; 15 Creslow Way, Stone, Aylesbury HP17 8YN Tel: 01296 748323 — MB ChB Baghdad 1976 (Baghdad Iraq) FRCS Ed. 1983; FRCS 2000. Cons. Surg. Stoke Mandeville Hosp. Aylesbury. Specialty: Gen. Surg. Special Interest: Colorectal Surg. Socs: MDU; Colo-Proctol. Assn. of Britain & Irel.; Royal College of Surgeons (Edinburgh). Prev: Sen. Regist. Roy. Lond. and St Bart. NHS Trust, Univ. Hosp. 2000-01; Regist. Mid. Stafford Dist. Hosp.; Regist. Macclesfield Dist. Hosp.

SHARIF, Saba 273 Fullwell Avenue, Clayhall, Ilford IG5 0RE Tel: 020 8550 7793 — MB BS Lond. 1996 (UMDS) BSc Lond.; MRCP (Paediat.) 1999. SpR (Clinical Genetics) St. Mary's Hosp. Manch. Specialty: Paediat. Prev: SHO (Neurology/Neurosurgery) Gt. Ormond St.; SHO (Paediat.) UMDS Rotat.; Greenwich Ho. Surg.

SHARIFF, Abdul Ghaffar (retired) 78 The Park Paling, Cheylesmore, Coventry CV3 5LL Tel: 024 7650 2016 — MB BS Karachi 1962 (Dow Med. Coll.) BSc Karachi 1955, MB BS 1962; DA Eng. 1965. Clin. Asst. (Anaesth.) Geo. Eliot Hosp. Nuneaton; Clin. Asst. (Endocrinol.) Coventry Warks. Hosp.

SHARIFF, Amina Tazeen 4 hazelbourne Road, London SW12 9NS Tel: 0208 675 0703 — MB BS Lond. 1990 (St. Geo. Hosp.) FRCA 1996. Specialist Regist. (Anaesth.) King's Coll. Hosp. Lond. Specialty: Anaesth. Prev: SHO (Ananesth.) St. Richards Hosp. Chichester; SHO (Paediat.) St. Helier Hosp. Lond.; SHO (Anaesth.) Frimley Pk. Hosp. Surrey.

SHARIFF, Syed Yakub Queens Road Surgery, 17 Queens Road, Broadstairs CT10 1NU Tel: 01843 862648 Fax: 01843 860739 — MB BS Andhra 1966.

SHARIH, Gauhar 276A Uxbridge Road, Rickmansworth WD3 8YL Tel: 01923 710811; 276A Uxbridge Road, Rickmansworth WD3 8YL Tel: 01923 710811 — BM Soton. 1995; FRCA Lond. 2001. SPR (Aneasthetics)Birm. Childrens Hosp. Specialty: Anaesth. Socs: MDDUS. Prev: SHO Cas. Lister Hosp. Stevenage; SHO Geriat. Soton. Gen. Hosp.; SPR (Aneas) Russells Hall Hosp. Dudley.

SHARIH, Samina 12 Maxwell Road, Northwood HA6 2YF — MB BS Lond. 1991.

SHARKAWI, Eamon 23 Kenerne Drive, Barnet EN5 2NW — MB BS Lond. 1996.

SHARKEY, Annie Sonia The Surgery, High Street, Moffat DG10 9HL Tel: 01683 220062 Fax: 01683 220453; Pinewood Cottage, Chapelbrae, Moffat DG10 9SB — MB ChB Aberd. 1989; DRCOG 1993; MRCGP 1994. GP Moffat. Prev: Trainee GP Dumfries & Galloway HB VTS.

SHARKEY, Christina Irene — BM BS Nottm. 1998. Specialty: Gen. Med.

SHARKEY, Donald 27 Betony Close, Scunthorpe DN15 8PP — BM BS Nottm. 1998; BM BS Nottm 1998.

SHARKEY, James (retired) Elm Tree House, Wales Lane, Barton under Needwood, Burton-on-Trent DE13 8JF — (St. Thos.) BSc. (Physiol.) Lond. 1939; MB BS Lond. 1942; MRCS Eng. LRCP Lond. 1942; FRCP Lond. 1972, M 1944. Prev: Cons. Phys. S.E. Staffs. Health Dist.

SHARKEY, Mr James Anthony Mary Royal Victoria Hospital, Belfast BT12 6BA Tel: 0289 0240503 Ext: 3520; 619 Ormeau Road, Belfast BT7 3JD Tel: 01232 640077 — MB BCh BAO Belf. 1985 (Queens Univ., Belf.) FRCS Glas. 1989; FCOphth 1990. Cons. Opthalmic Surg., Roy. Vict. Hosp., Belf. Specialty: Ophth. Special Interest: Cataract Surg.

SHARKEY, John James Mary Avoca Ward, Knockbracken, Healthcare Park, Saintfield Road, Belfast BT8 8BH Tel: 01232 756 5480; 6 Thompsons Grange, Hillsborough Road, Carryduff, Belfast BT8 8TG — MB BCh BAO Belf. 1989; DMH Belf. 1991; DRCOG 1992; MRCPysch 1994. Specialist Regist. (Forens. Psychiat.) Knockbracken Healthcare Pk. Belf. Specialty: Gen. Psychiat. Prev: SHO (Psychiat.) Shaftesbury Sq. Hosp. Belf. & Gransha Hosp. Londonderry; SHO (Psychiat.) Dept. Psychother. Belf., Mater Hosp. Belf. & Muchamore Abbey Antrim.

SHARKEY, Patrick Joseph Carryduff Surgery, Hillsborough Road, Carryduff, Belfast BT8 8HR Tel: 028 9081 2211 Fax: 028 9081 4785 — MB BCh BAO Belf. 1984; MRCP (UK) 1987; DRCOG 1989; DCH RCPSI 1989; DMH 1990; MRCGP 1990.

SHARLAND, Desmond Edward (retired) Cecille Cottage, Church Path, Woodside Lane, London N12 8RH Tel: 020 8445 1214 — (Lond. Hosp.) MB BS Lond. 1953; MRCS Eng. LRCP Lond. 1953; DObst RCOG 1955; FRCP Lond. 1975, M 1960; BSc (Hons. Anat.) Lond. 1950, MD 1967. Lect. (Anat.) Univ. Coll. Lond. Prev: Cons. Phys. Whittington Hosp. Lond.

SHARLAND, Gurleen Kaur Department Fetal Cardiology, 15th Floor Guy's Tower, St Thomas St., London SE1 9RT Tel: 020 7407 3351 Fax: 020 7955 2637; 48 Palmerston Road, London SW14 7PZ — MD Lond. 1993; BSc (Physiol.) 1979, MB BS 1982; FRCP 1997. Sen. Lect. & Hon. Cons. Fetal & Paediat. Cardiol. Guy's Hosp. Lond. Specialty: Paediat. Cardiol. Prev: Lect. (Perinat. Cardiol.) Guy's Hosp. Lond.

SHARLAND, Michael Roy Paediatric Infectious Diseases Unit, 5th Floor Lanesborough Wing, St Georges Hospital, Cranmer Terrace, London SW17 0RE Tel: 020 872532632 Fax: 020 8725 3262 Email: m.sharland@sghms.ac.uk; 48 Palmerston Road, London SW14 7PZ — MB BS Lond. 1982; FRCPCH (UK) (Paediat.) 1986; BSc (Physiol.) Lond. 1979, MD 1991; DTM & H RCP Lond. 1994. Cons. Paediat. (Infec. Dis.) St. Geo. Hosp. Lond. Specialty: Infec. Dis. Socs: Convenor, Brit. Paediatric Allergy, Immunity and Infec. Gp. Prev: Lect. (Paediat. Infec. Dis.) St. Geo. Hosp. Lond.

SHARLAND, Roy John 19 Deepdene Road, London SE5 8EG Tel: 020 7274 2290 — (King's Coll. Hosp.) MB BS Lond. 1953, BDS 1946; FDS RCS Eng. 1951, LDS 1947. Socs: BDA & Brit. Soc. Study Orthodont. Prev: Ho. Phys. Dulwich Hosp.; Ho. Surg. ENT Dept. King's Coll. Hosp.; Sen. Hosp. Dent. Off. Middlx. Hosp. Lond.

SHARMA, A K Westminster Medical Centre, Aldams Grove, Liverpool L4 3TT Tel: 0151 922 3510 Fax: 0151 902 6071.

SHARMA, Abhishek 2 Manor House, Crawford Village, Upholland, Skelmersdale WN8 9QZ — MB ChB Manch. 1998; MB ChB Manch 1998.

SHARMA, Alka Central Health Clinic, 1 Mulberry Street, Sheffield S1 2PJ Tel: 0114 271 8153; 31 Bingham Park Road, Greytones, Sheffield S11 7BD Tel: 0114 268 5639 Email: alka@edincastle-freeserve.ci.uk — MB ChB Glas. 1989 (Glasgow) MRCOG 1997; OFFP 1998. Cons. Incommunity Gyn. & Reproductive Health Care. Specialty: Obst. & Gyn. Socs: RCOG; FFP; BMS. Prev: Specialist Regist. (O & G) SE of Scotl.; Spec. Regist. (O & G) SE of Scotl.

SHARMA, Mr Alok High Street Surgery, 77 High Street, Nantyffyllon, Maesteg CF34 0BT Tel: 01656 732217 Fax: 01656 730119 — MB BCh Wales 1994; FRCS Ed. (Ordocryngology) 1999. Specialist Regist. Otolocryngology, E. Anglia Deanery; Specialist Regist. Otolocryngology Peterbrough Hosp. Specialty: Otorhinolaryngol.

SHARMA, Amita 3 Patent House, 48 Morris Road, London E14 6NU — MB BS Lond. 1989; MRCP (UK) 1992.

SHARMA, Anand 3 Parkwood Road, Liverpool L25 4RJ — MB ChB Manch. 1993.

SHARMA, Anant 10 Inverclyde Gardens, Chadwell Heath, Romford RM6 5SJ — MB BChir Camb. 1987.

SHARMA, Angela 49 Green Pastures, Heaton Mersey, Stockport SK4 3RB Tel: 0161 431 6171 — MB ChB Manch. 1996; BSc (Hons.) 1993.

SHARMA, Mr Anil Soho Health Centre, Louise Road, Birmingham B21 0RY Tel: 0121 554 5151 Fax: 0121 515 2884; Richmond Park House, 1 Belgrove Close, Edgbaston, Birmingham B15 3RQ — MB BS Lond. 1980 (Charing Cross Hospital Medical School) MRCS LRCP Lond. 1981; FRCS Ed. 1985; MRCGP 1986. Specialty: Otorhinolaryngol.

SHARMA, Anil Kumar Fazakerley Hospital, Lower Lane, Liverpool L9 7AL Tel: 0151 529 3695 — MB BS Punjab 1968 (Amritsar Med. Coll.) MRCP (UK) 1976; FRCP Lond. 1992. Cons. Phys. Walton & Fazakerley Hosps. Liverp.; Hon. Clin. Lect. Univ. Liverp. 1980. Specialty: Care of the Elderly. Socs: Brit. Geriat. Soc. (Chairm. Mersey Br.). Prev: Sen. Regist. (Med.) Walton & Fazakerley Hosps.; Regist. Rotat. (Med.) Walton, Whiston & Roy. South. Hosps. Liverp.; SHO (Med.) Whiston Hosp.

SHARMA, Anil Kumar 70 Evelyn Grove, Southall UB1 2BS — MB ChB Leic. 1987 (Leicester) DGM RCP Lond. 1990; MRCOG 1996; MRNZCOG 1997. Specialist Regist. Roy. Gwent Hosp. Newport. Specialty: Obst. & Gyn. Prev: Regist. (O & G) Waikato Hosp. Hamilton, NZ; Specialist Regist. Univ. Hosp. Wales, Cardiff.

SHARMA, Anjla 103 Friary Road, Birmingham B20 1BA — MB ChB Birm. 1990; ChB Birm. 1990.

SHARMA, Mr Anup Kumar Department of Surgery, St Georges Hospital, Blackshaw Road, London SW17 0QT Tel: 020 8672 1255 Fax: 020 8725 3466 — MB BS Lond. 1985 (Middlesex Hospital Medical School) MS Lond. 1994, Bsc (Hons.) 1982, MB BS 1985; FRCS Eng. 1990; FRCS (Gen.) 1997. Cons. (Gen. Surg.) St. Geo.s Hosp. Lond. Specialty: Gen. Surg. Socs: BASO and BAES. Prev: Sen. Regist. Cardiff Hosps.; Research Regist. Cardiff.; Regist. (Surg.) Birm. Hosp.

SHARMA, Anuradha 13 The Byway, Sutton SM2 5LE; 13 The Byway, Sutton SM2 5LE — MB BS Lond. 1998 (CXWMS) BSc (Hons); MB BS Lond 1998. Socs: MDU; BMA.

SHARMA, Mr Arun Kumar c/o Renal Transplant Unit, The Royal Free Hospital, Pond St., London NW3 2QG — MB BS Agra 1974 (S.N. Med. Coll.) MS Agra 1977, BSc 1969, MB BS 1974; FRCS Ed. 1983; Dip. Urol. Lond 1986. SHO Renal Transpl. Unit Roy. Free Hosp. Lond. Prev: Regist. (Urol.) All India Inst. Med. Scs. New Delhi; SHO (Surg./Urol.) Oldham Roy. Infirm.; SHO (Paediat. Surg.) Gt. Ormond St. Hosp. Lond.

SHARMA, Arun Kumar 13 Singleton Close, Elm Park, Hornchurch RM12 4LT — BM BCh Oxf. 1988.

SHARMA, Asha The Grove Surgery, Farthing Grove, Netherfield, Milton Keynes MK6 4NG Tel: 01908 668453 Fax: 01908 695064 — MB BS Delhi 1978; MB BS Delhi 1978.

SHARMA, Asha Omkar 19 Demontfort Road, Streatham, London SW16 1NF Tel: 020 8769 1017 — MSc; DFP; DGO. Assonali Spec. Community Paediat., Epsom & St Helier NHS Trust.

SHARMA, Ashutosh 123 Robin Hood Lane, Chatham ME5 9NL — MB BS Lond. 1992 (St. Thos. Hosp. Lond.) BSc (Hons.) Lond. 1989; MRCP (UK) 1995. Specialty: Ophth.

SHARMA, Atma Dev (retired) Amatar House, Manor Road, Woodley, Stockport SK6 1RT Tel: 0161 494 6692 Fax: 0161 406 6752; 6/6 Sarva Priya Vihar, New Delhi, India Tel: 00 91 11 6856845 Fax: 00 91 11 6861203 Email: atma_dev@hotmail.com — MB BS Lucknow 1960 (King Georges Lucknow India) FRCP Glasg. 2000; DCH RCP Lond. 1964; MRCP Glas. 1969; MRCP (UK) 1970; T(M) 1990. Indep. Cons. Cardiol. & Specialist Phys. Prev: Cons. Phys. (Gen. Med.) Dennevirke Hosp. NZ.

SHARMA, Awadh Kishore Tennyson Avenue Medical Centre, Saltergate, Chesterfield S40 4SN Tel: 01246 232339; Staddle Stones, Old Brampton, Chesterfield S42 7JG Fax: 01246 209097 — MD Patna 1967, MB BS 1963; DCH RCPS Glas. 1970; MRCPI 1974; MRCP (UK) 1975. Trainer GP Chesterfield. Specialty: Community Child Health. Socs: Roy. Coll. Phys.; Brit. Paediat. Assn. Prev: Sen. Regist. (Paediat. & Developm. Med.) Northampton & Kettering Health Dists.; SHO (Paediat.) Roy. Liverp. Childr. Hosp.

SHARMA, Bal Krishna 1 Newheath Close, Wolverhampton WV11 1XX — MB BS Jiwaji 1971.

SHARMA, Mr Bhu Datt 2 Wisteria Lane, Carluke ML8 5TB Tel: 01555 70601 — MB BS Lucknow 1960 (King Geo. Med. Coll. Lucknow) BSc Agra 1954; FRCS Ed. 1964; MS Allahabad 1968. Cons. Orthop. Surg. Law Hosp. Carluke. Specialty: Orthop.

SHARMA, Bhupinder 149 Firs Drive, Hounslow TW5 9TB — BM Soton. 1993.

SHARMA, Mr Chandra Maulishwar Prasad (retired) 33 Ilston Way, West Cross, Swansea SA3 5LG Tel: 01792 403383 Fax: 01792 403383 — MB BS Patna 1958 (P.W. Med. Coll.) MS Patna 1962, MB BS 1958; FRCS Eng. 1965. Vist. Cons. Gen. Surg. Indraprastha Apollo Hosps. Prev: Cons. Gen. Surg. Nevill Hall Hosp. Abergavenny.

SHARMA, Davanand Chandranauth Inverclyde Royal Hospital, Larkfield Road, Greenock PA16 0XN Tel: 01475 633777 — MB ChB Manch. 1991; BSc (Med. Sci.) St. And. 1988; MRCP (UK) 1996. Staff Grade (Resp. Med.), Inverclyde Roy. Hosp., Greenock. Specialty: Respirat. Med. Prev: Regist. (Respirat. Med.) Vict. Infirm. NHS Trust, Glasg.; SHO (Med.) HCI Internat. Clydebank 1996; Regist. (Resp. Med.) Vict. Infirm. NHS Trust, Glas. 1997.

SHARMA, Deepak 99 Barclay Road, Bearwood, Smethwick B67 5JY — MB ChB Leic. 1998; MB ChB Leic 1998.

SHARMA, Devesh 12 Ravenswood Road, Strathaven ML10 6JB — MB ChB Glas. 1984; BSc (Hons. Biochem.) St. And. 1981. Lect. Anat. Glas. Univ. Prev: Jun. Ho. Off. Glas. Roy. Infirm.

SHARMA, Geeta Tennyson Avenue Medical Centre, 1 Tennyson Avenue, Chesterfield S40 4SN Tel: 01246 232339 Fax: 01246 209097; Staddle Stones, Old Brampton, Chesterfield S42 7JG— MB BS Agra 1964 (S.N. Med. Coll.) MRCOG 1974, DObst 1969; Cert. JCC Lond. 1980. Prev: Med. Asst. (O & G) Nether Edge Hosp. Sheff.

SHARMA, Gopal Krishan Fosse Medical Centre, 344 Fosse Road North, Leicester LE3 5RR Tel: 0116 253 8988 Fax: 0116 242 5178 — MB ChB Leic. 1987 (Leicester) BMedSci. Leic. 1985; Cert. Family Plann. JCC 1991. GP Princip.; Hosp. Pract. (Rheum.) Leicester; Sess. Med. Off. (Occupat. Health) Leicester Roy. Infirm.; Med. Off. Alliance & Leicester; Med. Off. Nestle UK Ltd. Specialty: Occupat. Health; Gen. Pract.

SHARMA, Harbinder Kumar 2 Glenmore Road, Leicester LE4 9GE — BM BS Nottm. 1991.

SHARMA, Indra Datt Treevale, 60 View Road, Rainhill, Prescot L35 0LS Tel: 0151 493 1741 — MB BS Agra 1967 (Sarojini Naidu Med. Coll.) Socs: Med. Protec. Soc. Prev: Trainee GP Liverp. VTS; SHO (Med.) Clwyd HA.

SHARMA, Jagdish Chander 87 Barrowby Road, Grantham NG31 8AB Tel: 01476 565646 — MB BS Punjab 1973 (Govt. Med. Coll. Patiala) MRCP (UK) 1981; FRCP Lond. 1994; FRCP Glas. 1995. Cons. Phys. Kings Mill Hosp Sutton in Ashfield Notts.; Sen. Regist. & Hon. Lect. (Geriat. Med.) Roy. Vict. Hosp. Dundee. Specialty: Gen. Med. Special Interest: Stroke & Parkinson's Dis. Socs: Europ. Stroke Counc.; Movement Disorders Soc.; Brit. Geriat. Soc. (Sec. PD Sect.). Prev: Cons. Phys. Geriat. Med. Hawtonville Hosp. Newark; Regist. (Gen. Med.) Harrogate Gen. & Dist. Hosps.; Regist. (Geriat. Med.) Centr. Middlx. Hosp. Lond.

SHARMA, Kalpana 1 Crosslands Avenue, Southall UB2 5QY Tel: 020 8574 1906 — MB BS Lond. 1982 (King's Coll. Hosp.) BSc Lond. 1979, MB BS 1982; DCH RCP Lond. 1985; DRCOG 1986; MRCGP 1987. GP S.all; Course Organiser W. Middlx. Hosp. GPVTS. Prev: Princip. GP N.olt.

SHARMA, Kalpana RHR Medical Centre, Calverton Drive, Strelley, Nottingham NG8 6QN Tel: 0115 975 3666 Fax: 0115 975 3888; Kia-Mena, Bilborough Road, Wollaton, Nottingham NG8 4DR — MB BS Utkal 1970 (S.C.B. Med. Coll. Cuttack) DObst RCOG 1976; MRCOG 1978. Mem. LMC. Socs: M-C Soc.; (Exec.) Overseas Doctors Assn. Prev: Clin. Asst. (O & G) Univ. Hosp. Nottm.; Clin. Med. Off. (Family Plann.) Nottm. Health Dist. (T); SHO (Anaesth.) Gen. Hosp. Nottm. & Nottm. City Hosp.

SHARMA, Kamal Kant Moorfields Eye Hospital, 162 City Road, London EC1V 2PD Tel: 020 7566 2041; 17 Foxglove Court, Vicars Bridge Close, Wembley HA0 1YG — MB BS Patiala 1976; DO RCS Eng. 1990; FRCS Ed. 1992. Assoc. Specialist (Ophth.) Moorfields Eye Hosp. Lond.; Cons. Med. Advis. Internat. Glaucoma Assn. Specialty: Ophth.

SHARMA, Kanika Flat 1, 28 Valentines Road, Ilford IG1 4SA; 1 Vaughan Gargeh, Ilford IG1 3PA — MB ChB Aberd. 1998; MB ChB Aberd 1998. GP VTS AT Chase Farm Hosp. Enfield Middlx. Socs: MDU; AMS (Aberd. Med. Soc.). Prev: PRHO in Surg. at Wrexham Maelor Gen. Hosp.; PRHO in Med. @ Aberd. Roy. Infirm.

SHARMA, Kiran — MB BS Lond. 1993 (United Med. & Dent. Schs. Guy's & St. Thos. Hosps.)

SHARMA, Kiran Kumari St. Barnabus Hospice, Columbia Drive, Worthing BN13 2QF Tel: 01903 264222 — MB BS Lond. 1988 (The Royal Lond. Hosp.) BSc Psych. 1985; DRCOG 1993; MRCGP 1994. Cons. (Pall. Med.) St. Barnabas Hospice; Hon. Cons. (Palliat. Med.) Worthing & Southlands Hosp. Trusts. Specialty: Palliat. Med. Socs: Assn. of Palliat. Med.

SHARMA, Krishan Kant 26 Coates Hill Road, Bromley BR1 2BJ — MB BS Panjab 1951; MB BS Panjab (India) 1951.

SHARMA, Mr Madan Mohan 50 Menzieshill Road, Dundee DD2 1PU Tel: 01382 642612 — (St. And.) MB ChB St. And. 1968; FRCS Ed. 1973. Cons. Dept. Orthop. & Traum. Surg. Ninewells Hosp. Dundee; Hon. Sec. Lect. Dept. of Orthop. & Trauma Surg., Univ. of Dundee. Specialty: Trauma & Orthop. Surg.; Orthop.

SHARMA, Madan Mohan Pendlebury Health Centre, Nelson Fold Medical Centre, 659 Bolton Road, Manchester M27 8HP Tel: 0161 950 4545 Fax: 0161 950 4546; 9 Thornway, Worsley, Manchester M28 1YS Tel: 0161 799 7115 — MB BS Calcutta 1972 (NRS Medical College Calcutta, India) BSc (Hons.) India 1965. GP; Clin. Asst. (Psychiat.) N. Manch. Gen. Hosp. Specialty: Gen. Pract.; Gen. Psychiat. Prev: SHO (Psychiat. & Gen. & Geriat. Med.) St. Lukes Hosp. Middlesbrough & S. Shields Gen. Hosp.

SHARMA, Malini Anuradha 23 Wedgwood Way, London SE19 3ES Tel: 020 8771 9921 — MB BS Lond. 1994 (UMDS London) BSc (Hons.) Biochem.) 1991; MRCOG 1998. SHO (O & G) St. Geo.'s Hosp. Lond. Specialty: Obst. & Gyn. Socs: MDU; BMA. Prev: SHO (O & G) St Peter's Chertsey; SHO (Geriat.) St. Geo.'s Hosp. Lond.; SHO (A & E) Guy's Lond.

SHARMA, Manju 1 The Paddock, Blackburn BB2 7QY — MB BS Indore 1973.

SHARMA, Manjula (retired) — MB BS Lucknow 1968 (GSVM Med. Coll. Kanpur, India) AFOM RCP Lond. 1993; MFFP 1993; MFCM 2000. Prev: Hon. Cons. Occupat. Med. Roy. Marsden Hosp. Lond. & Surrey.

SHARMA, Manu Shankar 4 Parkland Close, Mansfield NG18 4PR — MB ChB Birm. 1998.

SHARMA, Meenakshi Walsgrave Hospital, Clifford Bridge, Coventry CV2 2DX Tel: 024 7660 2020 — MB ChB Leic. 2000. Ho. Phys. Walsgrave Hosp. Coventry. Specialty: Gen. Med.

SHARMA, Mridula — MB BS Lond. 1995; BSc Lond. 1989; MB BS Lond. 1995. Specialty: Gen. Pract.

SHARMA, Narendra Kumar Compton Acres Medical Centre, West Bridgford, Nottingham NG2 7PA Tel: 0115 984 6767 Fax: 0115 945 5888; 8 Leigh Close, West Bridgford, Nottingham NG2 7TN Tel: 0115 982 2282 Fax: 0115 914 9383 — MB BS Punjab 1974 (Govt. Medical College, Punjab) GP Clin. Asst. Psychiat. of Old Age.

SHARMA, Mr Naresh Kumar Altnagelvin Hospital, Londonderry BT47 2SB — MB BS Punjab 1967 (Govt. Med. Coll. Patiala) MB BS Punjabi 1967; DO RCPSI 1976; FRCS Ed. 1979; PhD Belf. 1984. Cons. Ophth. Surg. Alinagelvin Hosp. Lond.derry. Specialty: Ophth.

SHARMA, Mr Narinder Kumar Milesgarth, Cawcliffe Road, Brighouse HD6 2HP — MB BS Punjab 1974 (Govt. Med. Coll. Patiala) FRCS Ed. 1981. Cons. Gen. Surg. Calderdale Royal Hosp. Specialty: Gen. Surg.

SHARMA, Narinder Kumar — MB BS Lond. 1994; DRCOG 1997; MRCGP 1998.

SHARMA, Naveen Kumar 2 Honeybourne Way, Willenhall WV13 1HN — MB ChB Birm. 1995.

SHARMA, Neel-Kumari Fosse Medical Centre, 344 Fosse Road North, Leicester LE3 5RR Tel: 0116 253 8988 Fax: 0116 242 5178 — MB ChB Leic. 1991.

SHARMA, Neha 23 Merstal Drive, Solihull B92 0PU Email: ns698@hotmail.com — MB ChB Birm. 1998; ChB Birm. 1998.

SHARMA, Nirmal Kumar 10 Weld Road, Southport PR8 2AZ Tel: 01704 68029 — MB BS Delhi 1967; DRCOG 1976; DTM & H 1977; MRCGP 1978.

SHARMA, Nitika 20 Norton Road, Tunbridge Wells TN4 0HE — MB BS Lond. 1994. Ho. Off. (Urol.) Mayday Hosp. Croydon. Prev: Ho. Off. (Gen. Surg.) Mayday Hosp.

SHARMA, Om Prakash Greenfields Medical Centre, 12 Terrace Street, Hyson Green, Nottingham NG7 6ER — MB BS Vikram 1969 (Gandhi Med. Coll. Bhopal) DOrth Kanpur 1971. GP Nottm.

SHARMA, Omkar Parmanand Medical Centre, 13/15 Barmouth Road, London SW18 Tel: 020 8874 4984; 19 Demontfort Road, Streatham, London SW16 1NF Tel: 020 8769 1017 — MB BS Bombay 1969.

SHARMA, P Ilford Avenue, 24 Ilford Avenue, Crosby, Liverpool L23 7YF Tel: 0151 931 3181.

SHARMA, Pankaj Hammersmith Hospitals NHS Trust, Fulham Palace Road, London W6 8RF Tel: 020 8846 1184 Fax: 020 8846 7487 — MB BS Lond. 1988 (Univ. Lond. & Lond. Hosp.) DHMSA 1989; MRCP (UK) 1991; PhD Cantab. 1998; MD Lond. 2003. Cons. Neurol. Hammersmith Hosps. Lond.; Hon. Sen. Lect. Imperial Coll. Lond. Specialty: Neurol. Special Interest: Vasc. Dis. & Vasc. Genetics. Prev: BHF Clinician Scientist & Fulbright Schol., Harv. Med. Sch. Boston, USA; Clin. Regist. (Pharmacol.) Univ. of Camb.; Regist. Nat. Hosp. for Neurol. & Neurosurg. Qu. Sq. Lond.

SHARMA, Paul 105 Ardleigh Green Road, Hornchurch RM11 2LE — MB BS Lond. 1991.

SHARMA, Peeyush c/o Liver Unit, Transplantation Centre, Freeman Hospital, High Heaton, Newcastle upon Tyne NE7 7DN — MB BS Jammu 1981.

SHARMA, Poonam Redhill Famils Practice, 11 Redhill, Chislehurst BR7 6DB Tel: 09756827160 — MB ChB Manch. 1987 (St. And. & Manch.) BSc (Med. Sci.) St. And. 1984; Cert. Family Plann. JCC 1990; Cert. Prescribed Equiv. Exp. JCPTGP 1991; MFHom 1996. Roy. Lond. Homoeop. Hosp. Lond. (Clin. Asst.); Gen. Pract. Specialty: Homeop. Med.; Gen. Pract.

SHARMA, Prabani Cliftonville Road Surgery, 59/61 Cliftonville Road, Belfast BT14 6JN Tel: 028 9074 7361 — MB BS Gauhati 1971.

SHARMA, Pradeep Wanstead Place Surgery, 45 Wanstead Place, Wanstead High Street, London E11 2SW Fax: 020 8532 9124 — MB BS Lond. 1979 (Char. Cross) BSc (Hons.) (Biochem.) Lond. 1976; MRCS Eng. LRCP Lond. 1979; DRCOG 1985.

SHARMA, Mr Pramod Kumar, Maj. RAMC Retd. West Suffolk Hospital, Bury St Edmunds IP33 2QZ Tel: 01284 31000 Ext: 66 — MB BS Delhi 1981 (Maulana Azad Med. Sch., Delhi) FRCS Ed. 1992; MCh Liverp. 1994. Staff Surg. (Orthop. & Trauma) W. Suff. Hosp. Specialty: Orthop. Socs: Assoc. Mem. BOA; MDU. Prev: Regist. (Orthop. & Trauma) Roy. Halifax & Huddersfield Roy. Infirms.

SHARMA, Praveen TR, 30 Falkland Street, Glasgow G12 9QY — MB ChB Glas. 1990.

SHARMA, Mr Prem Dayal 4 Barlow Fold Road, Romily, Stockport SK6 4LH Tel: 0161 494 1999 — MB BS Jammu & Kashmir 1970 (Govt. Med. Coll. Srinagar) MS (ENT) Delhi 1975; DLO Eng. 1976; FRCS Eng. 1979. Cons. ENT Surg. Tameside & Glossop HA. Specialty: Otolaryngol. Prev: Sen. Regist. (ENT) St. Bart. Hosp. Lond.; Sen. Regist. (ENT) N. Riding Infirm. Middlesbrough.

SHARMA, Priya 14 Bradley Road, Haslington, Crewe CW1 1PN; Flat 2, 2A Dunkraven Road, West Kirby, Wirral L48 4DS — MB ChB Liverp. 1996. VTS Trainee, Wirral NHS Trust. Specialty: Gen. Pract.

SHARMA, Mr Raj Kumar 13 Ryecroft Close, Wakefield WF1 2LW — LMSSA Lond. 1966; FRCS Ed. 1968; MCh Orth Liverp. 1972; MRCS Eng. LRCP Lond. 1975. Indep. Med. Practioner. Prev: Cons. Orthopaedic Surg. Huddersfield Roy. Infirm.

SHARMA, Raj Pal Chatham Street Surgery, 121 Chatham Street, Reading RG1 7JE Tel: 0118 950 5121 Fax: 0118 959 0545; 21 Squirrells Way, Earley, Reading RG6 5QT Tel: 0118 987 3650 — MB BS Rajasthan 1974 (S.P. Med. Coll. Bikaner) DCH RCPSI 1977. Specialty: Gastroenterol.

SHARMA, Rajan 3 Winifred Road, Dartford DA1 3BL — MB BS Lond. 1993.

SHARMA, Rajeev QE II Hospital, Howlands, Welwyn Garden City — MB BS Indore 1982; FRCS (Tr. & Orth.) Ed.; DNB (Orth.). Cons. Orthopaedic & Upper Limb Surg.

SHARMA, Rajendra Chandrakant 87 North Road, Parkstone, Poole BH14 0LT Tel: 01425 461740 Fax: 01428 727875 — MB BCh BAO NUI 1984 (Royal College of Surgeons Dublin) LRCPI & LM, LRCSI & LM 1984; MFHom 1994. Med. Dir. 101 Gp. Ltd.; Med. Dir. Hale Clinic, Lond. Specialty: Homeop. Med. Socs: Brit. Soc. Nutrit. Med.; Scientif. & Med. Network. Prev: Sen. Lect. Hahnemann Coll. Homeop.

SHARMA, Rajendra Prasad The Surgery, 20 North Sea Lane, Humberston, Grimsby DN36 4UZ Tel: 01472 211116 — MB BS Patna 1965.

SHARMA, Rajiv Amersham Hospital, Hale Acre Unit, Whielden Street, Amersham HP7 0JD Tel: 01494 724422 Fax: 01494 734506 — MB ChB Aberd. 1984; MRCPsych 1989. Cons. Psychiat.; Cons. Psychiat. Bucks. Mental Health NHS Trust. Specialty: Gen. Psychiat. Prev: Sen. Regist. (Psychiat.) Char. Cross Hosp. Lond.

SHARMA, Rajiv Sea Road Surgery, 39-41 Sea Road, Bexhill-on-Sea TN40 1JJ Tel: 01424 211616 Fax: 01424 733950; 72 Cowdray

Park Road, Bexhill-on-Sea TN39 4EZ Tel: 01424 846059 Fax: 01424 840335 — MB BS Lond. 1984.

SHARMA, Rakesh 41 Eyston Drive, Weybridge KT13 0XD — MB ChB Glas. 1989.

SHARMA, Ram Charan, TD 7 Signals Regiment Medical Centre, Javelin Barracks BFPO 35 Tel: 02432 893309 Fax: 02432 893309 Email: lomashram@hotmail.com; 8 Davidson Road, Croydon CR0 6DA Tel: 020 8656 4213 Email: lomashram@hotmail.com — MB BS Punjab 1972 (Govt. Med. Coll. Patiala, India) MB BS Punjabi 1972; T(GP) 1991; DFFP 1993. Sen. Med. Off. CMP MoD BAOR BFPO 35; Div.al Surg. St. John's Ambul. (Germany Div.). Specialty: Accid. & Emerg.; Obst. & Gyn. Special Interest: Aviation Med.; Travel Med.; Underwater Med. Socs: BMA (Full); British Medical Acupuncture Society (Full). Prev: GP Bracknell; SHO (O & G) Fairfield Gen. Hosp. Bury; SHO (A & E) Crawley Hosp.

SHARMA, Ramesh Chandra 23 Pages Hill, Muswell Hill, London N10 1PX Tel: 020 8883 2310 — MB BS Bangalor 1967 (Bangalore Med. Coll.) MB BS Bangalore 1967; MRCS Eng. LRCP Lond. 1981. Regist. (Orthop.) Manor Ho. Hosp. Lond. Specialty: Orthop.

SHARMA, Rashmi 14 Laurel Avenue, Twickenham TW1 4JA — MB ChB Leeds 1992; MRCP (UK) 1995.

SHARMA, Rewati Raman Department of Neurosurgery, Khoula Hospital, Mina Al Fahal, Muscat, Oman; 25 Clos Crucywel, Park Gwern Fadog, Cwmrhydyceirw, Morriston, Swansea SA6 6RD — MB BS Bombay 1978; MS (Neurosurg.) Bombay 1986. Regist. (Neurosurg.) Khoula Hosp. Muscat, Oman & Morriston Hosp. Swansea. Prev: Regist. (Neurosurg.) Roy. Preston Hosp.; Specialist (Neurosurg.) Khoula Hosp. Muscat, Oman; Lect. (Neurosurg.) Kem Hosp. Bombay, India.

SHARMA, Ricky Anupam University of Leicester, Leicester Royal Infirmary, Oncology Department, Leicester LE2 7LX Tel: 0116 223 1855/0116 254 1414 — MB BChir Camb. 1994 (Univ. Camb.) MA Camb. 1996; MRCP 1998; PhD Univ. Leic. 2001. Lect. & SpR (Oncology) Univ. Hosps. of Leicester Leicester. Specialty: Oncol. Socs: RCP; Fell. Roy. Soc of Med.; Brit. Assn. of Cancer Res. Prev: Clin. Res. Fell. Univ. Dept. of Oncol. Leic. Roy. Infrim.; SHO (Gen. Med.) Leicester Roy. Infirm.; Ho. Off. (Gen. Med.) Addenbrooke's Hosp. Camb.

SHARMA, Rita Institute of Health Sciences, Department of Primary Health Care, Oxford OX3 7LF — MB BS Lond. 1993. Clin. Lect. Oxf.

SHARMA, S S Manor Top Medical Centre, Rosehearty, Ridgeway Road, Sheffield S12 2SS Tel: 0114 239 8324.

SHARMA, Sangeeta 50 Cam Wood Fold, Clayton-Le-Woods, Chorley PR6 7SD — MB ChB Manch. 1996 (Manchester) Specialist Regist. (anaesthetics) N. W. Sch. of Anaethesia. Specialty: Anaesth. Socs: AAGBI; OAA; NDA. Prev: SHO (Anaesth.) Blackpool Vict. NHS Trust.

SHARMA, Sanjay 44 Minster Walk, London N8 7JS — MB ChB Leeds 1989.

SHARMA, Sanjay Wheatfield Surgery, 66 Wheatfield Road, Luton LU4 0TR Tel: 01582 601116; 38 West End, Brampton, Huntingdon PE28 4SD — MB BS Lond. 1986 (St. George's Hospital London)

SHARMA, Sanjeev Datt Southport and Ormskirk NHS Trust, Town Lane, Southport PR8 6PN Tel: 01704 704635 Fax: 01704 704636 Email: sanjeev.sharma@southportandormskirk.nhs.uk — MB BS Delhi (University College of medical Sciences, Delhi, India) MD; FRCOG. Cons. Southport; Postgrad. Clin. tutor, Univ. of Liverp. Specialty: Obst. & Gyn. Special Interest: Infertil.; Reproductive Endocrinol.

SHARMA, Sanjiv 46 Maswell Park Road, Hounslow TW3 2DW — MB BS Lond. 1996 (King's College London) BSc Lond. 1993. SHO (Paediat.) Kingston Hosp. Kingston-upon-Thames. Specialty: Paediat.

SHARMA, Sapna Devi 38 Tavistock Avenue, Greenford UB6 8AJ Tel: 020 8991 2032 Email: sapnasharma@email.com — MB ChB Aberd. 1992; DRCOG 1995; DFFP 1996; MRCGP 1998. Res. Fell. (Genetics) Harv. Med. Sch. Boston, USA. Prev: GP Regist. VTS Worthing Scheme; Ho. Off. (Med./ Renal Prof. Med.) Aberd. Roy. Infirm.

SHARMA, Saroj Bala 22 Lime Crescent, Marriott Grove, Sandal, Wakefield WF2 6RY Tel: 01924 252733 — MB BS Punjab 1972 (Govt. Med. Coll. Patiala) MB BS Punjabi 1972. SCMO Pontefract HA. Specialty: Community Child Health.

SHARMA, Sarojini Westfield Medical Centre, 2 St Martin's Terrace, Chapeltown Road, Leeds LS7 4JB Tel: 0113 295 4750 Fax: 0113 295 4755 — MB BS Osmania 1967. GP Leeds.

SHARMA, Satya Kishore 46 Pentwyn, Radyr, Cardiff CF15 8RE — MB BS Vikram 1963 (M.G.M. Med. Coll. Indore) DOMS Indore 1965; DO Eng. 1970. Clin. Asst. (Ophth.) Univ. Hosp. Wales Cardiff. Prev: Regist. (Ophth.) Gen. Hosp. Southend-on-Sea; Regist. (Ophth.) Singleton Hosp. Swansea.

SHARMA, Satya Vrat Bilston Health Centre, Prouds Lane, Bilston WV14 6PW Tel: 01902 405200 — MB BS Punjab 1973.

SHARMA, Satyapaul The Surgery, 68 The Drive, Ilford IG1 3PW Tel: 020 8554 3014 Fax: 020 8518 0863 — MB BS Rajasthan 1960 (S.M.S. Med. Coll. Jaipur) DIH Eng. 1974. Prev: Lect. Dept. Physiol. Maulana Azad Med. Coll. New Delhi, India; Chief Med. Off. Kakira Hosp. Uganda.

SHARMA, Seema The Surgery, 6 Queens Walk, Ealing, London W5 1TP Tel: 020 8997 3041 Fax: 020 8566 9100 — MB BS Bangalore 1988; MRCP (UK) 1994.

SHARMA, Shreekant 16 Nicholson Webb Close, Danescourt, Llandaf, Cardiff CF5 2RL Tel: 029 2055 1378 — MB BS Punjab 1983; MRCPsych 1982.

SHARMA, Siya Sharan Harold Wood Hospital, Department of Obstetrics and Gynaecology, Gubbins Lane, Harold Wood, Romford RM3 0BE Mob: 07814 620533 — MB BS Rajasthan 1989. Specialist Regist. (Obst. & Gyn.) Harold Wood Hosp. Romford.

SHARMA, Sobhna Room 4, Flat 1, Oklea House, Darlington Memorial Hospital, Hollyhurst Road, Darlington DL3 6HX — MB ChB Liverp. 1992.

SHARMA, Soorya Kant 24 Farmway, Leicester LE3 2XA — LRCP LRCS Ed. 1983; MB BS Panjab 1979; LRCP LRCS Ed. LRCPS Glas. 1983.

SHARMA, Srilakshmi Missula 55 Belsize Road, Harrow HA3 6JL — MB ChB Bristol 1998.

SHARMA, Subhash Chander c/o Drive Harshad Parikh, 9 Brookwood Close, Westbury Park, Clayton, Newcastle ST5 4HU — M.Phil. Leics. 1978, MB ChB 1982; DRCOG 1984; DCH RCP Lond. 1985; MRCGP 1987. GP Evington.

SHARMA, Sunil 70 Western Road, Crookes, Sheffield S10 1LA — MB ChB Dundee 1995.

SHARMA, Mr Sunil Dutt Edith Cavell Hospital, Bretton Gate, Peterborough PE3 9GZ — MB BS Agra 1983; FRCS Eng. 1990; FRCS Ed. 1990; FRCS (Urol.) 1996. Cons. (Urol.) Edith Cavell Hosp., Bretton Gate, P'boro. Specialty: Urol. Prev: Regist. Rotat. (Urol.) Norf. & Norwich Hosp.

SHARMA, Sunil Dutt — MB BS Lond. 1998; MB BS Lond 1998.

SHARMA, Suraj Prakash Stanley Medical Centre, 60 Stanley Road, Kirkdale, Liverpool L5 2QA Tel: 0151 207 1076 — MB BS Allahabad 1968.

SHARMA, Surendra Kumar David Medical Centre, 274 Barlow Moor Road, Chorlton, Manchester M21 8HA Tel: 0161 881 1681 Fax: 0161 860 7071; 49 Green Pastures, Heaton Mersey, Stockport SK4 3RB Tel: 0161 431 6171 — MB BS Rajasthan 1969; BSc Lucknow 1962. Prev: Clin. Asst. (A & E) Altrincham Gen. Hosp. Chesh.; Clin. Asst. (Plastic Surg.) Withington Hosp. Manch.

SHARMA, Sushil Roy Health Centre, Lydney GL15 5NQ Tel: 01594 842167 Fax: 01594 845550; Acre House, Pillowell, Lydney GL15 4QA — MB BCh Wales 1978; MA Camb. 1979.

SHARMA, Mrs Sushma 12 Ravenswood Road, Strathaven ML10 6JB — MB BS Punjab 1955; MB BS Punjab (India) 1955; DA Eng. 1963.

SHARMA, Tina 49 Green Pastures, Stockport SK4 3RB — MB ChB Manch. 1997.

SHARMA, Professor Tonmoy Clinical Neuroscience Research Centre, 7 Twisleton Court, Priory Hill, Dartford DA1 2EN Tel: 01322 286862 Fax: 01322 286861 — MB BS Dibrugarh 1986; MRCPsych 1991; MSc Lond. 1994. Director Clin. Neurosci. Research Centre Dartford. Specialty: Gen. Psychiat.; Forens. Psychiat. Socs: BMA; Brit. Assn. Psychopharmacol.; Brit. Neuropsychiat. Assn. Prev: Sen. Lect. (Psychol. Med.) Inst. Psychiat. Lond.; Regist. (Psychiat.) Univ. Coll. Hosp. Lond.; Clin. Lect. (Psychiat.) Inst. Psychiat. Lond.

SHARMA, Mr Umesh Chandra 12 Ravenswood Road, Strathaven ML10 6JB Tel: 01355 0827 — MB BS Nagpur 1955 (Med. Sch. Nagpur) FRCS Ed. 1967. Cons. Orthop. Surg. StoneHo. Hosp. Specialty: Orthop.

SHARMA, Vandana Princes Road Surgery, 51 Princes Road, Wimbledon, London SW19 8RA Tel: 020 8542 2827 Fax: 020 8296 9505 — MB BS, MRCGP (Lond.) (RNT Medical School Vdaipur (Rajasthan) India) GP. Specialty: Family Planning.

SHARMA, Veena Treevale, 60 View Road, Rainhill, Prescot L35 0LS Tel: 0151 493 1741 — MB BS Agra 1969 (Sarojini Naidu Med. Coll. Agra) DPM RCPSI 1987. Assoc. Specialist Psychiat. Merseyside. Specialty: Geriat. Psychiat. Prev: SHO & Regist. (Psychiat.) Rainhill Hosp. Liverp.

SHARMA, Venita Royal Victoria Infirmary, Newcastle upon Tyne NE1 4LP — MB ChB Glas. 1988; MRCGP 1992; MRCP (UK) 1993. Regist. (Paediat.) Roy. Vict. Infirm. Specialty: Paediat.

SHARMA, Vijay Hoylake Road Surgery, 314 Hoylake Road, Wirral CH46 6DE Tel: 0151 677 2425 Fax: 0151 604 0482; 66 Farndon Way, Oxton, Birkenhead — MB BS Saurashtra 1972 (M.P. Shah Med. Coll. Jamnagar) DRCOG 1978.

SHARMA, Vijay Narain 11 Fernbank, Chorley PR6 7BH Tel: 01257 274220 — (G.M. Med. Coll. Lucknow) BSc Aligarh 1945; MB BS Lucknow 1951; TDD Wales 1957; DPM Eng. 1970; MRCPsych 1972. Cons. Psychiat. Whittingham Hosp. Preston. Specialty: Gen. Psychiat. Prev: Dir. Nat. Tuberc. Servs. Min. of Health Accra, Ghana.

SHARMA, Vijayalaxmi 109 Dormers Wells Lane, Southall UB1 3JA Tel: 020 8574 8614 — MB BS Bhopal 1977; MRCPsych 1989.

SHARMA, Vikas 89 Little Green Lane, Chertsey KT16 9PS — MB BS Lond. 1996.

SHARMA, Vinod Kumar 373 Wanstead Park Road, Ilford IG1 3TT — MB BS Delhi 1971.

SHARMA, Vinod Kumar Omparkash 24 Kingcup Close, Leicester Forest Bar, Leicester LE3 3JU — MB BS Poona 1982; MRCPsych 1995.

SHARMA, Mr Virendar Lal ENT Consultant, The Royal Oldham hospital, Rochdale Road, Oldham OL1 2JH Tel: 0161 627 8262 Email: v.sharma1@btinternet.com — MB BS Punjabi U 1974; MS; DLO, RCS Lond.; FRCS Edin. p/t ENT Cons., The Roy. Oldham Hosp., Lancs. Specialty: Otolaryngol. Socs: BMLA; BMA; N. of Eng. Otolaryngol. Soc.

SHARMA, Virendra Kilsyth Medical Partnership, Kilsyth Health Centre, Burngreen Park, Kilsyth, Glasgow G65 0HU Tel: 01236 822081 Fax: 01236 826231 — MB BS Punjab 1966 (Govt. Med. Coll. Patiala) MB BS Punjabi Univ. 1966. Socs: BMA.

SHARMA, Vishwesh Chandra 70 Bank Street, Irvine KA12 0LP — MB BS Rajasthan 1970.

SHARMA, Mr Yogdutt 14 Ash Street, Bacup OL13 8AJ — MB BS West Indies 1981; FRCS Glas. 1994.

SHARMA, Yogendra Dutt Dulmer Drive Surgery, Fulmer Drive, Offerton, Stockport SK2 5JL Tel: 0161 483 3363 — MB BS Delhi 1972.

SHARMA, Kavindra Nath Springwell Medical Group, Alderman Jack Cohen Health Centre, Springwell Road, Sunderland SR3 4DX Tel: 0191 528 2727 Fax: 0191 528 3262; The Stables, Tunstall Lodge Farm, Burdon Lane, Sunderland SR3 2QB — MB BS Newc. 1981; BMedSc (Hons.) Newc. 1980; DRCOG 1985; DCCH RCP Ed. 1985; MRCGP 1985; Dip in Palliative Medicine (Cardiff) 2000. GP Sunderland; Trainer (Gen. Pract.) Sunderland; Examr. RCGP; McMillan Facilitator in Cancer for Sunderland; Course Organiser Northumbria Vocational Train. Scheme for Gen. Pract. Specialty: Palliat. Med. Prev: Chair Sunderland LMC; Co-Chairm. Sunderland Med. Audit Advis. Gp.

SHARMACHARJA, Gopa 20 Sparken Close, Crabtree Park, Worksop S80 1BN — MB BS Dhaka 1973; MB BS Dhaka, Bangladesh 1973.

SHARMACHARJA, N R Larwood Health Centre, 56 Larwood, Worksop S81 0HH Tel: 01909 500233 Fax: 01909 479722 — MB BS Dacca 1967; MB BS Dacca 1967.

SHARMAN, Andrew 21 Herbert Road, Kesgrave, Ipswich IP5 2XX; 21 Herbert Road, Kesgrave, Ipswich IP5 2XX — MB BS (Hons) Lond. 1997 (Univ. Coll.) BSc (Hons)KCL; MRCP. Aneas. Rotation Nottingham. Specialty: Gen. Med. Prev: Med. Norwich; Surg. Roy. Free, Lond.; A&E Leeds.

SHARMAN, Gail 44 Hillcrest Avenue, Edgware HA8 8PA — MB BS Lond. 1996.

SHARMAN, Michael Anthony 37 Downs View Road, Seaford BN25 4PU — MB ChB Manch. 1996.

SHARMAN, Michael John Hove Medical Centre, West Way, Hove BN3 8LD Tel: 01273 430088 Fax: 01273 430172 — MB BS Lond. 1963 (Guy's) MRCS Eng. LRCP Lond. 1963; DObst RCOG 1965.

SHARMAN, Robin Andrew Lockwood Surgery, 3 Meltham Road, Lockwood, Huddersfield HD1 3XH Tel: 01484 421580 Fax: 01484 480100; 24 Primrose Lane, Kirkburton, Huddersfield HD8 0QY — MB ChB Sheff. 1987.

SHARMAN, Sarah Louise 17 Foxcombe Road, Bath BA1 3ED — BM BCh Oxf. 1993.

SHARMAN, Vivian Laurence 11 Park Way, London NW11 0EX Tel: 020 8458 5154 Fax: 020 8458 5154 Email: jonsan@hotmail.com — MB BChir Camb. 1971 (Camb. & Lond. Hosp.) MA, MB Camb. 1971, BChir 1970; MRCP (UK) 1973; FRCP Lond. 1990. Cons. Phys. King Geo. Hosp. Goodmayes. Specialty: Gen. Med.; Nephrol. Prev: Cons. Phys. & Sen. Lect. (Nephrol.) St. Mary's Hosp. Portsmouth; Sen. Regist. (Renal Med.) Lond. Hosp.; Regist. (Med.) Harold Wood Hosp.

SHARMAN, William Angus (retired) The Barn, 25 Crow Lane, Thurley, Bourne PE10 0EZ Tel: 01778 422921 Fax: 01778 422921 — MB ChB Ed. 1960; FRCOG 1992, M 1973. Hosp. Pract. (O & G) Matern. Unit Kettering Gen. Hosp. Prev: SHO Simpson Memor. Matern. Pavil. Roy. Infirm. Edin.

SHARMAN, William Evans (retired) 9 Rowley Lane, Fenay Bridge, Huddersfield HD8 0JN Tel: 01484 602374 — MB ChB Sheff. 1953. Prev: Ho. Surg. & Ho. Phys. Roy. Hosp. Chesterfield.

SHARNAGIEL, Zbigniew Marian (retired) 249 Felmongers, Harlow CM20 3DR Tel: 01279 424888 — MB ChB Polish Sch. of Med. 1948. Prev: Ho. Phys. City Hosp. Edin.

SHARP, Mr Andrew John Hughdeburg South Wigston Health Centre, 80 Blaby Road, Wigston LE18 4SE — MB BS Lond. 1979; FRCS Ed. 1985; DRCOG 1988; MRCGP 1991.

SHARP, Andrew Lance Howard Richmond Surgery, Richmond Close, Fleet GU52 7US Tel: 01252 811466 Fax: 01252 815031; Park Hill, Fitzroy Road, Fleet GU51 4JH Tel: 01252 614126 — MB BS Lond. 1976 (Char. Cross) MRCS Eng. LRCP Lond. 1976; DObst. RCOG 1980; MRCGP 1982. Specialty: Gen. Pract. Prev: SHO (O & G) & (Anaesth.) Frimley Pk. Hosp.; Resid. Med. Off. (Gen. Med.) Roy. Perth Hosp., Australia; Resid. Med.; Off. (Gen. Surg.) Broken Hill & Dist. Hosp. N.S.W. Australia.

SHARP, Andrew Simon 14 The Gardens, Coach Road, Whitehaven CA28 7TG — MB ChB Ed. 1998; MB ChB Ed 1998.

SHARP, Benjamin Titus 3 Stapledon Lane, Ashburton, Newton Abbot TQ13 7AE — MB BS Lond. 1991; BSc Cellular Path. Lond. 1987. Prev: Ho. Off. (Gen. Surg.) Roy. Surrey Co. Hosp. Guildford; Ho. Off. (Cardiol. & Gen. Med.) Roy. United Hosp. Bath.

SHARP, Caroline Denton Turret Medical Centre, 10 Kenley Road, Slatyford, Newcastle upon Tyne NE5 2UY Tel: 0191 274 1840; 4 Elgy Road, Gosforth, Newcastle upon Tyne NE3 4UU Tel: 0191 284 6004 — MB BS Lond. 1985; BSc Lond. 1982, MB BS 1985; DCH RCP Lond. 1988; MRCGP 1990; Dip. Pract. Dermat. 1995. Socs: BMA.

SHARP, Christopher AWG plc, Anglian House, Ambury Road, Huntingdon PE29 3NZ Tel: 01480 326979 Fax: 01480 323011 — MB BS Lond. 1975 (Guy's) MRCS Eng. LRCP Lond. 1975; DCH RCP Lond. 1978; MRCP (UK) 1978; MRCGP 1980; DAvMed. RCP Lond. 1982; T(GP) 1991; MSc (Occupat. Health) Aberd. 1992; MFOM RCP Lond. 1994, AFOM 1992; T(OM) 1994; FRCP Lond. 1997. Gp. Med. Adviser; Cons. Internat. Atomic Energy Agency; Comm. 3, Internat. Comission on Radiological Protec.; Pres.-Elect Sect. of Ocupational Med., Roy. Soc. of Med. Specialty: Occupat. Health. Socs: Fell. Roy. Soc. Med.; Soc. Occupat. Med.; Amer. Coll. Occupat. & Environm. Med. Prev: Head Med. Dept. Nat. Radiol. Protec. Bd.; Hon. Sen. Clin. Lect. Oxf. Univ.; Off. Commanding RAF Aviat. Med. Train. Centre.

SHARP, Clifford William Huntleburn House, Melrose TD6 9BD Tel: 01896 827157 Fax: 01896 827154; The Knowe, 24 High Cross Avenue, Melrose TD6 9SU — MB ChB Ed. 1985; BSc Ed. 1982; MRCPsych 1990. Cons. Psychiat. Melrose; Chair of Clin. Bd. and Assoc. Med. Diretcor, NHS Borders. Specialty: Gen. Psychiat. Prev: Sen. Regist. Roy. Edin. Hosp.; MRC Clin. Sci. 1991-93; Regist. (Psychiat.) Roy. Edin. Hosp.

SHARP, David James 11 Banner Cross Road, Sheffield S11 9HQ — MB BS Lond. 1996.

SHARP, Mr David John Spinal Unit, Orthopaedic Department, Ipswich Hospital, Heath Road, Ipswich IP4 3PD Tel: 01473 702097 Fax: 01473 702094 Email: david.sharp@ipswichhospital.nhs.uk — MB BS 1972 (St. Mary's) FRCS Eng. 1979; MD Lond. 1991. Cons. Orthop. Surg. Ipswich Hosp. Specialty: Trauma & Orthop. Surg. Socs: Roy. Soc. Med.; Brit. Orthopaedic Research Soc.; Brit. Assn. of Spinal Surg.s. Prev: Sen. Regist. Rotat. (Orthop. Surg.) Northampton & Hammersmith; Regist. Rotat. (Orthop. Surg.) Roy. Orthop. Hosp. Birm. & Coventry.

SHARP, David Stanley (retired) Roselands, 4 Middleton Road, Higher Crumpsall, Manchester M8 5DS Tel: 0161 795 9111 Fax: 0161 795 3383; Lyndhurst, 44 Ridgeway Road, Timperley, Altrincham WA15 7EZ Tel: 0161 980 4984 — MB BS Lond. 1966 (St. Mary's) MRCS Eng. LRCP Lond. 1966; FRCOG 1989, M 1972. Prev: Clin. Dir. (O & G) N. Manch.

SHARP, Deborah Janette Taylor and Partners, Shirehampton Health Centre, Pembroke Road, Shirehampton, Bristol BS11 9SB Tel: 0117 916 2233 Fax: 0117 930 8246; 31 Fremantle Road, Cotham, Bristol BS6 5SX Tel: 0117 924 1998 Fax: 0117 924 1998 — BM BCh Oxf. 1977; MA Oxf. 1977; DRCOG 1980; PhD Lond. 1993; FRCGP 1995. Prof. Primary Health Care Univ. Bristol. Specialty: Gen. Pract. Prev: Sen. Lect. & Lect. (Gen. Pract.) UMDS Lond.; Trainee GP Oxf. VTS.; HON. S.L Inst of Psych. Lond.

SHARP, Deborah June Quayside Medical Practice, Chapel St., Newhaven BN9 9PW Tel: 01273 615000 Fax: 01273 611527; 13 Third Avenue, Newhaven BN9 9JA Tel: 01273 513222 — MB BS Lond. 1980 (Guy's) DRCOG 1983. Prev: Clin. Asst. (Accid & Emerg. Centre) Roy. Sussex Co. Hosp. Brighton; GP Brighton VTS.

SHARP, Miss Elizabeth Jean — MB BS Lond. 1983; FRCS Eng. 1988; MS Lond. 1995; FRCS (Gen) 1998. Cons. Surg. Qu. Eiiz. The Qu. Mother Hosp. Margate. Specialty: Gen. Surg.; Vasc. Med.

SHARP, Estelle 16 Mount Eden Park, Belfast BT9 6RA — MB BCh BAO Belf. 1948.

SHARP, Frank Clinical Sciences Centre, Northern General Hospital NHS Trust, Sheffield S5 7AU Tel: 0114 243 7988 Fax: 0114 244 1728; University of Sheffield, School of Medicine, Beech Hill Road, Sheffield S10 2RX Tel: 0114 271 2736 Fax: 0114 271 3960 — (Glas.) MB ChB Glas. 1962; DObst RCOG 1964; FRCOG 1979, M 1968; MD Glas. 1975. Hon. Cons. Obst. & Gyn. Centr. Sheff. Univ. Hosps. NHS Trust. Specialty: Obst. & Gyn. Socs: (Ex-Pres. Ex. Sec.) Brit. Soc. Colposcopy & Cervical Path.; (Foundat. Mem.) Brit. Gyn. Cancer Soc. Prev: Sen. Lect. Midw. Univ. Glas.; Hon. Cons. Obst. Qu. Mother's Hosp. Glas.; Hon. Cons. Gyn. West. Infirm. Glas.

SHARP, Geoffrey Mark GP Principal, Park Road Medical Practice, Park Road, Shepton Mallet BA4 5BP Tel: 01749 342350 Fax: 01749 346859; Long Barn, Shepton Montague, Wincanton BA9 8JB Tel: 01749 813760 — MB BS Lond. 1987; MA Camb. 1982; DCH RCP Lond. 1991; DRCOG 1991; MRCGP 1992. GP Princip. Pk. Med. Pract. Shepton Mallet; PEC Chair Mendip PCG. Specialty: Gen. Pract.; Orthop.; Sports Med. Socs: BMA.

SHARP, The Hon. Gordon Russell Forth Valley Health Board, Occupational Health Service, Central Unit, Stirling Royal Infirmary, Livilands Gate, Stirling FK8 2AU Tel: 01786 73151 — MD Glas. 1972; PhD Glas. 1970, MD 1972, MB ChB 1958; FRCP Glas. 1987, M 1985; FFOM RCP Lond. 1989. Cons. Occupat. Phys. & Dir. Occupat. Health Servs. Forth Valley HB.; Dir. Occupat. Health Servs. Scott. Health Serv., Common Servs. Agency; Hon. Clin. Lect. Glas. Univ. Specialty: Gen. Med. Prev: I.C.I. Research Fell. & Asst. Lect. Dept. Physiol. Univ. Glas.; Reader Aviat. Physiol. RAF; Cons. Aviat. Med. RAF.

SHARP, Graham Leith Marr Dept of GU Medicine and Sexual Health, The Sandyford Initiative, Sauchiehau Street, Glasgow G3 7NB Tel: 0141 211 8608 Fax: 0141 211 8609; 37 Monreith Road, Newlands, Glasgow G43 2NY Tel: 0141 632 0977 — MB ChB Aberd. 1972; FRCOG 1994, M 1979. Cons. Genitourin. Med. Gtr. Glas. Primary Care NHS Trust; Hon. Clin. Sen. Lect. (Med.) Univ. Glas. Specialty: Genitourinary Medicine. Socs: Med. Soc. Study VD; Brit. Soc. Colposc. & Cervic. Pathol.; Assn. for Genitourin. Med. Prev: Sen. Regist. (Genitourin. Med.) Bristol Roy. Infirm.; Regist. (O & G) Qu. Mother's Hosp. & West. Infirm. Glas.; Regist. (O & G) Newc., N.d. & N. Tyneside HAs.

SHARP, Guy Thomas Mount Edgcumbe Hospice, Porthpean Road, St Austell PL26 6AB Tel: 01726 65711 Fax: 01726 66421 — (St. Bart.) MB BS Lond. 1962; MRCS Eng. LRCP Lond. 1963; DObst RCOG 1965. Clin. Asst. Mt. Edgcumbe Hospice St. Austell. Specialty: Palliat. Med. Prev: GP Truro.

SHARP, Mr Henry Richard Ent Department, Guys Hospital, St Thomas' St., London SE1 9RT — MB BS Lond. 1990; FRCS Eng. 1995; FRCS (Oto.) 1996. Specialist Regist. (Otolaryngol.) Guys & St. Thos. Hosps. Lond. Specialty: Otorhinolaryngol. Prev: SpR (Otolaryngol.) Gt. Ormand St. Hosp. For Childr.; SHO (Otolaryngol.) Char. Cross Hosp. Lond.; Ho. Surg. & Cas. Off. St. Thos. Hosp. Lond.

SHARP, Hugh Culliford Torside, Coursing Batch, Glastonbury BA6 8BH Tel: 01458 832130 — (Guy's) MRCS Eng. LRCP Lond. 1968; MB BS Lond. 1969; DObst RCOG 1970; Dip. Sports Med. 1996. Specialty: Gen. Pract.; Sports Med. Socs: Med. Off.s of Sch.s Assn. Prev: SHO ENT & (Surg. & Gyn.) Wycombe Gen. Hosp.; Ho. Off. (Obst.) Radcliffe Infirm. Oxf.; Sch. Med. Off. Millfield.

SHARP, Jacquelyn The Smethwick Medical Centre, Regent Street, Smethwick, Warley B66 3BQ Tel: 0121 558 0105 Fax: 0121 555 7206 — MB ChB Liverp. 1979; DTM & H Liverp. 1982; DRCOG 1985; MRCGP 1985; DCH RCP Lond. 1986.

SHARP, James Frederick The Wycke, 25 Warwick Road, Walmer, Deal CT14 7JE; Church Lane Surgery, Church Lane, New Romney TN28 8ES — MB BS Lond. 1992.

SHARP, Janet Elizabeth 2A Whin Hill Road, Bessacarr, Doncaster DN4 7AE Tel: 01302 535040 — MRCS Eng. LRCP Lond. 1952 (Leeds.)

SHARP, Jennifer Mary Arran Surgery, 40 Admiral Street, Glasgow G41 1HU Tel: 0141 429 2626 Fax: 0141 429 2331 — MB ChB Glas. 1988; DRCOG 1992; MRCGP 1993.

SHARP, Mr Jeremy Frederick ENT Department, Derbyshire Royal Infirmary NHS Trust, London Road, Derby DE1 2QY Tel: 01332 254657; 77 Hazelwood Road, Duffield, Belper DE56 4AA — MB ChB Birm. 1984; MA Oxf. 1982; FRCS Ed. 1988. Cons. ENT Derbysh. Roy. Infirm. NHS Trust; ENT and head and Neck Cons. Surg., Derby Nuffield Hosp. Specialty: Otorhinolaryngol.; Otolaryngol. Socs: BMA; Brit. Assn. Otol.; Brit. Assn. of Head and Neck Surgeons. Prev: Sen. Regist. Rotat. (ENT) Qu. Eliz. Hosp. Birm.; Regist. (ENT) City Hosp. Edin.; SHO (ENT) Selly Oak Hosp. Birm.

SHARP, John 591 Kilmarnock Road, Newlands, Glasgow G43 2TH — MB ChB Glas. 1981; MRCGP 1986; MSc (Sports Medicine) 1999.

SHARP, John Clarkson Macgregor (retired) 6 Cammo Hill, Edinburgh EH4 8EY — MB ChB Ed. 1955; DPH Ed. 1958; FFCM 1980, M 1972; MRCP Glas. 1984. Prev: Cons. Epidemiol. Communicable Dis. (Scotl.) Unit Ruchill Hosp. Glas.

SHARP, John Richard Cowper (retired) Rossie Mills House, Rossie Braes, Montrose DD10 9TJ Tel: 07768 570574 — MB BS Lond. 1967 (Guy's) MRCS Eng. LRCP Lond. 1966. Prev: GP.

SHARP, Mrs June Rosemary (retired) 22 St Peters Road, Seaford BN25 2HP Tel: 01323 491162 — MB ChB Sheff. 1954. Prev: SCMO Jarvis Breast Screening Centre Guildford.

SHARP, Madeleine Agnes (retired) 49 Baginton Road, Coventry CV3 6JX Tel: 024 7641 4512 Fax: 024 7641 4512 — MB BS Durh. 1953; DSc (hon causa) Coventry 1995. Prev: Ho. Phys. Workington Infirm.

SHARP, Mr Malcolm (retired) (cons. rooms), St. Anthony's Hospital, Cheam, Sutton Tel: 020 8337 6691; 6 Grange Park Place, Thurstan Road, London SW20 0EE Tel: 020 8879 0669 — MB BS Lond. 1956 (Univ. Coll. Hosp.) MRCS Eng. LRCP Lond. 1956; FRCS Eng. 1961. Cons. ENT Surg. St. Helier Trust Carshalton; Cons. Ent. Surg. St. Geos., NHS Trust; Hon Cons. Surg. Head & Neck Unit Roy. Marsden Hosp. Lond. Prev: Sen. Regist. Roy. Nat. Throat, Nose & Ear Hosp. Lond.

SHARP, Michael Andrew 31 Orchardson House, Orchardson St., London NW8 8NN Tel: 020 7723 4014 — MB BS Lond. 1991 (St. Mary's Lond.) BSc Clin. Sci. Lond. 1989, MB BS 1991; FRCS Lond. 1995. Specialist Regist. (Gen. Surg.) Oxf. Specialty: Gen. Surg.

SHARP, Michael John Aubrey North Laine Medical Centre, 12-14 Gloucester Street, Brighton BN1 4EW Tel: 01273 601112 — MB BChir Camb. 1980.

SHARP, Michael Philip Downlands Medical Centre, 77 High Street, Polegate BN26 6AE Tel: 01323 482323/486449 Fax: 01323

488497 — MB BS Lond. 1988; DCH RCP Lond. 1992; MRCGP 1993.

SHARP, Michael William (retired) 2A Whin Hill Road, Bessacarr, Doncaster DN4 7AE Tel: 01302 535040; 77 Thorne Road, Doncaster DN1 2ET Tel: 01302 361318 — MB ChB Leeds 1950; DObst RCOG 1951. Prev: SHO (Obst.) St. Helen's Hosp. Barnsley.

SHARP, Nigel Stewart 3 Sutherland Avenue, Broadstone BH18 9EB — MB BS Lond. 1977. Garrison Med. Off. Blandford Camp Dorset.

SHARP, Olive Persica (retired) 76 Wessington Park, Calne SN11 0AX — MB BS Lond. 1958; MRCS Eng. LRCP Lond. 1958; DA Eng. 1961; DObst RCOG 1961. Prev: GP Calne Wilts.

SHARP, Patrick Stephen Northwick Park Hospital, Watford Road, Harrow HA1 3UJ Tel: 020 8869 2623 Fax: 020 8869 2961 — MB ChB Glas. 1977; MRCP (UK) 1980; MD Glas. 1987; FRCP 1996. Cons. Phys. (Endocrinol. & Gen. Med.) Northwick Pk. Hosp. Harrow. Specialty: Endocrinol.; Diabetes. Special Interest: Microvascular Complications.

SHARP, Rachel Jane Inish Fail, Orchard Close, E. Hendred, Wantage OX12 8JJ — MB ChB Sheff. 1990; DRCOG 1993; MRCGP 1994.

SHARP, Robert John 121A Hilmanton, Lower Earley, Reading RG6 4HJ; Frogs Meadow, Milton Combe, Yelverton PL20 6HL Tel: 01822 854926 Fax: 01822 854926 — MB BS Lond. 1992 (Lond. Hosp. Med. Coll.) Specialty: Orthop.

SHARP, Robert Jonathan c/o The Coach House, 25 North Park Parade, Harrogate — BM BCh Oxf. 1991.

SHARP, Robert Wylie (retired) 53 Hatton Park Road, Wellingborough NN8 5AQ Tel: 01933 222761 — MB ChB Glas. 1954; MRCOG 1964. Prev: GP WellingBoro. & Port Glas.

SHARP, Ronald Alexander Victoria Infirmary, Langside Road, Glasgow G42 9TY Tel: 0141 201 6000; 52 Castlehill Drive, Newton Mearns, Glasgow G77 5LB Tel: 0141 639 8840 — MB ChB Dundee 1974; MRCP UK 1978; FRCPath UK 1996; FRCP Edin. 2002. Cons. Haemat. Vict. Infirm. Glas.; Hon. Clin. Sen. Lect. Univ. Glas. Specialty: Haematology. Socs: Assn. Clin. Paths.; Brit. Soc. For Haemoatology. Prev: Sen. Regist. & Hon. Lect. (Haemat.) Ninewells Hosp. & Med. Sch. Univ. Dundee.

SHARPE, Andrew Paul Ashley Centre Surgery, Ashley Square, Epsom KT18 5DD Tel: 01372 723668 Fax: 01372 726796; 6 Woodcote Mews, 84 Worple Road, Epsom KT18 7AH — MB BS Lond. 1988 (St. Geos.) DRCOG 1992; MRCGP 1995. Chairm. New Epsom & Ewell Cottage Hosp.

SHARPE, Bruce David Magill Department of Anaesthesia, Chelsea & Westminster Hospital, 369 Fullham Road, London SW10 9NH — MB BS Monash 1977.

SHARPE, Cathleen Margaret Hollywell, Tile Barn, Woolton Hill, Newbury RG20 9XE Tel: 01635 253007 — MB ChB Leeds 1967; DObst RCOG 1969; DCH Eng. 1970. Staff Grade (Paediat.) N. Hants. Hosp. Trust Basingstoke. Specialty: Community Child Health. Socs: BMA. Prev: Community Med. Off. Basingstoke HA; GP Ealing; SHO (Paediat.) Warrington Gen. Hosp.

SHARPE, Christopher Erel West Suffolk Hospital, Hardwick Lane, Bury St Edmunds IP33 2QZ Tel: 01284 713000; 21 Collingwood Close, Steepletower, Hethersett, Norwich NR9 3QE — MB BS West Indies 1991 (Univ. of the WI) FRCA 1998. Specialist Regist. (Anaesth.) W. Suff. Hosp. Bury St. Edmunds. Specialty: Anaesth. Socs: BMA; Anaesth. Assoc. of GB & Ire. Prev: Specialist Regist. (Anaesth.) Norf. & Norwich Hosp.; SHO (Anaesth.) Mayday Univ. Hosp. Thornton Heath; SHO (Anaesth.) Kingston Pub. Hosp. Jamaica.

SHARPE, Christopher James Selkirk Health Centre, Viewfield Lane, Selkirk TD7 4LJ Tel: 01750 21674 Fax: 01750 23176; Easthill, Anderson Road, Selkirk TD7 4EB Tel: 01750 20546 — MB BS Lond. 1968; MRCP (U.K.) 1971; MRCGP 1978.

SHARPE, Coral Rosemary Woodbridge Road Surgery, 165-167 Woodbridge Road, Ipswich IP4 2PE Tel: 01473 256251 — MB BS Lond. 1961; MRCS Eng. LRCP Lond. 1961; DObst RCOG 1964.

SHARPE, Damian Patrick 6 Park Road, Exeter EX1 2HP — MB BCh BAO NUI 1984.

SHARPE, David Stephen Bellingham Green Surgery, 24 Bellingham Green, London SE6 3JB Tel: 020 8697 7285 Fax: 020 8695 6094 — MB BS Lond. 1990.

SHARPE, Elizabeth Ann Bryceson (retired) 23 Macclesfield Road, Buxton SK17 9AH — MB ChB Sheff. 1961. Prev: G.P. The Sq., Buxton.

SHARPE, Elizabeth Louise — MB BS Lond. 1998; MRCP 2001.

SHARPE, Evelyn Edith Oxleas NHS Trust, Charlton Cmht, 68 The Heights, London SE7 8JH Tel: 020 8921 2445 Fax: 020 8921 2427 Email: evelyn.sharpe@oxleas.nhs.uk — MB BCh BAO Belf. 1977 (Queen's University Belfast) MRCPsych 1985; BA (ICI Internat. Correspondence Inst.) 1990. p/t Cons. Psychiat. Oxleas NHS Trust; Cons. Psychiat. Interhealth Lond. Specialty: Gen. Psychiat. Socs: Ulster Med. Soc. Prev: Cons. Psychiat. Greenwich Dist. Hosp.

SHARPE, Fiona Margaret 7A Learmonth Terrace, Edinburgh EH4 1PQ — MB ChB Ed. 1993.

SHARPE, Geoffrey 5 Larch Close, West End, Southampton SO30 3RB — BM Soton. 1986; MRCP (UK) 1991; FRCR 1996; PhD Soton. 1998. Cons. (Clin. Oncol.) Wessex Cancer Centre, Soton. Specialty: Oncol.; Radiother. Prev: Sen. Regist. & Regist. (Radiother. & Oncol.) Roy. Marsden Hosp.; Clin. Research Fell. & Hon. Regist. (Med.) Univ. Soton.; Ho. Phys. & SHO (Med.) Soton. Univ. Hosp.

SHARPE, Geoffrey Frank Appleby Health Centre, Low Wiend, Appleby-in-Westmorland CA16 6QP Tel: 01768 351584 Fax: 01768 353375; Carleton Derrick, Carleton Derrick Drive, Penrith CA11 8LS — BM BS Nottm. 1980; MRCP Ed. 1983; MRCGP 1986.

SHARPE, Georgina Helen Maimie The Corner Surgery, 180 Cambridge Road, Southport PR9 7LW Tel: 01704 506055 Fax: 01704 505818 — MB BS Lond. 1976 (Guy's) MA Oxf. 1980; MRCGP 1981. Prev: Trainee GP Coventry VTS.

SHARPE, Gillian Anne 76 North Street, Caistor, Lincoln LN7 6QU — MB BS Lond. 1988.

SHARPE, Gordon Charles William (retired) 3 Shillingford Court, Shillingford, Wallingford OX10 7EP Tel: 01865 858345 — MB BS Lond. 1946 (Lond. Hosp.) DObst RCOG 1952; MRCGP 1978. Prev: Receiv. Room Off. Lond. Hosp.

SHARPE, Graeme Douglas Macgregor Dundee Teaching Hospitals NHS Trust, Directorate of Ophthalmology, Ninewells Hospital and Medical School, Dundee DD2 1YY; East Wing, Waterybutts Farm Steading, Grange by Errol, Perth PH2 7SZ — MB ChB Dundee 1990; BMSc (Hons.) Dund. 1987; MRCOphth 1995. Staff Grade (Ophth.). Specialty: Ophth.

SHARPE, Graham Richard Department of Dermatology, Royal Liverpool Hospital, Prescot St., Liverpool L7 8XP Tel: 0151 706 4030 Fax: 0151 706 5842 Email: grs@liv.ac.uk — MB ChB Leeds 1977; MRCP (UK) 1980; DTM & H Liverp. 1980; BA (Hons.) Open 1988; PhD Newc. 1994; FRCP Lond. 1996. Cons. Dermatol., Roy. Liverp. Univ. Hosp.; Alder Hey Childr. Hosp., Liverp. Specialty: Dermat. Special Interest: Paediatric Dermat.; Skin Cancer. Socs: Brit. Assn. of Dermatol.; The Brit. Soc. for Paediatric Dermat.; Brit. Soc. for Investigative Dermat.

SHARPE, Mr Ian Terence Princess Elizabeth Orthopaedic Centre, Royal Devon and Exeter Hospital, Barrcak Road, Exeter EX2 5AW Tel: 01392 403598 Fax: 01392 403505 — MB BS Lond. 1991 (St Mary's Paddington) BSc (Hons.) Lond. 1988; FRCS Eng. 1995; FRCS (TR&Orth) 2001. Cons. in Orthop. and Trauma. Specialty: Trauma & Orthop. Surg. Special Interest: Foot and Ankle; Paediatrics. Socs: BMA; BOFFS.

SHARPE, James Edward 48 Thornwood Terrace, Glasgow G11 7QZ — MB ChB Glas. 1992.

SHARPE, Julia Catherine (retired) Treberfydd, Bagshot Road, Egham TW20 0RS — MB BS Lond. 1989; BSc Lond. 1986. Regist. (Histopath.) Hammersmith Hosp.

SHARPE, Karen Tacye Appleby Health Centre, Low Wiend, Appleby-in-Westmorland CA16 6QP Tel: 01768 351584 Fax: 01768 353375 — MB BS Lond. 1984 (St. Bart.) MRCGP 1990. GP N. Cumbria HA.

SHARPE, Keryn Elizabeth 10 Tudor House, Heath Road, Weybridge KT13 8TZ — MB ChB Leic. 1993. Specialty: Gen. Pract.

SHARPE, Lawrence David 24 Neville Street, London SW7 3AS Tel: 020 7589 1562 — MB BS Lond. 1954 (Univ. Coll. Hosp.) DPM 1961; MRCPsych 1980. Asst. Prof. Columbia Univ. New York; Surg. Lt. RNR. Socs: Fell. Roy. Soc. Med. Prev: Instruc. in Paediat. & Psychiat. Johns Hopkins Hosp. Baltimore; Regist. Maudsley Hosp. & Bethlem Roy. Hosp. Lond.; Ho. Phys. & Ho. Surg. Highlands Hosp.

SHARPE, Mandy Sharon Rustlings Road Medical Centre, 105 Rustlings Road, Sheffield S11 7AB Tel: 0114 266 0726 Fax: 0114

267 8394; 2 Slayleigh Drive, Fulwood, Sheffield S10 3RD Tel: 0114 230 6658 — MB BS Lond. 1981; MRCP (UK) 1984; DRCOG 1987. Specialty: Gen. Pract.

SHARPE, Michael Christopher Royal Edinburgh Hospital , Kennedy Tower, Edinburgh EH10 5HF — MB BChir Camb. 1980; MA Oxf. 1979; MRCP (UK) 1984; MRCPsych 1987; MD Camb. 2002. Reader & Hon. Cons. (Psychol. Med.) Univ. Edin. Specialty: Gen. Psychiat. Prev: Clin. Tutor & Hon. Sen. Regist. (Psychiat.) Oxf. RHA.

SHARPE, Nicola Louise — MB ChB Manch. 1988; BSc St. And. 1985. Specialist Regist. Child & Adolesc. Psychiat. Acad. Unit, Pine Lodge, Chester; Flexible Trainee. Specialty: Child & Adolesc. Psychiat. Socs: MRCPsych.

SHARPE, Peter Carlisle Clinical Biochemistry, Craigavon Area Hospital, 68 Lurgan Road, Portadown, Craigavon BT63 5QQ Tel: 028 3861 2657 Fax: 028 3833 4582 Email: pcsharpe@cahgt.n-i.nhs.uk; 80 Old Kilmore Road, Moira, Craigavon BT67 0NA Tel: 028 9261 3762 — MB BCh BAO Belf. 1988; MRCP (UK) 1992; MD Belf. 1997; MRCPath 1997; FRCP Glas. 2003; FRCPath 2005. Cons., (Chem. Pathol.) Craigavon Area Hosp. Specialty: Chem. Path. Socs: Roy. Coll. Phys. & Surgs. Glas.; MRCPath.; Assn. Clin. Biochem.

SHARPE, Rodney Charles Brookside Group Practice, Brookside Close, Gipsy Lane, Reading RG6 7HG Tel: 0118 966 9222 Fax: 0118 935 3174; 32 Aldbourne Avenue, Earley, Reading RG6 7DB — MB BS Lond. 1977; BSc Lond. 1974, MB BS 1977; DRCOG 1982; DCH RCP Lond. 1984; MRCGP 1989. GP Trainer Reading VTS. Prev: Trainee GP York VTS; Med. Off. Ch. of Christ N. Nigeria; SHO (Obst.) Mothers Hosp. Lond.

SHARPE, Roger Malcolm 65 Rossendale Way, London NW1 0XB Email: rsharpe065@aol.com — MB BS Lond. 1986; BSc Lond. 1983; FRCA 1993. Cons. Anaesth. Northwick Pk. Hosp. Harrow. Specialty: Anaesth. Socs: Anaesth. Research Soc. Prev: Lect., Hon. Sen. Regist. & Regist. (Anaesth.) St. Mary's Hosp. Lond.; SHO (Anaesth.) Chelmsford; SHO (Gen. Med.) Colchester.

SHARPE, Ronald Albert Dipple Medical Centre, Wickford Avenue, Pitsea, Basildon SS13 3HQ Tel: 01268 555115; 163 Noak Hill Road, Billericay CM12 9UJ — MB ChB Bristol 1958; DObst RCOG 1960; MRCGP 1972. Prev: Govt. Med. Off. Bahamas; Ho. Phys. Southmead Hosp. Westbury-on-Trym.

SHARPE, Stephen William Adams and Partners, The Health Centre, Tavanagh Avenue, Portadown, Craigavon BT62 3BU Tel: 028 3835 1393; 19 The Avenue, Portadown, Craigavon BT63 5UJ — MB BCh BAO Belf. 1988; DCH RCPSI 1991; T(GP) 1992; MRCGP 1992; DRCOG 1992; DFFP 1993; DMH Belf. 1993. Specialty: Gen. Pract.

SHARPE, Thomas Daniel Emmett 19B Bridge Road, Helens Bay, Bangor BT19 1TT Tel: 01247 852534 — MB BCh BAO Belf. 1978; FFA RCSI 1983; MPhil (Law & Ethics) Belf. 1995. Cons. Anaesth. Roy. Vict. Hosp. Belf.; Lect. (Anaesth.) Univ. Calgary 1985. Specialty: Anaesth.

SHARPLES, Andrew Department of Paediatric Intensive Care, Manchester Children's Hospitals, NHS Trust, Royal Manchester Children's Hospital, Pendlebury, Manchester M27 4HA Tel: 0161 727 2468 Fax: 0161 727 2198; 22 Arkhome, Ellenbrook, Worsley, Manchester M28 1SJ Tel: 0161 790 1217 — MB BS Lond. 1983; DA (UK) 1985; FRCA 1990. Cons. Intens. Care & Anaesth. Manch. Childr. Hosp. NHS Trust. Specialty: Anaesth.; Intens. Care. Prev: Sen. Regist. (Anaesth.) NW RHA; Regist. (Intens. Care) Roy. Childr. Hosp. Melbourne, Austral.

SHARPLES, Anthony Church View Surgery, 30 Holland Road, Plymstock, Plymouth PL9 9BW Tel: 01752 403206 — MB BS Lond. 1979; MRCGP 1982.

SHARPLES, Claude Alwyn (retired) 3 Dalby Avenue, Bushby, Leicester LE7 9RE — (Univ. Coll. Hosp.) MA Camb. 1957, BA (Hnrs.) 1949, MB BChir 1952; DObst RCOG 1957. Prev: Mem. Leics. Area Local Med. Comm.

SHARPLES, David Lionel (retired) Pippins, Cemetery Road, Yeadon, Leeds LS19 7UR — MB ChB Liverp. 1947.

SHARPLES, Edward John 36 Southlands Avenue, Orpington BR6 9NZ — MB BS Lond. 1993.

SHARPLES, Peta Mary Department of Child Health, The Medical School, Framlington Place, Newcastle upon Tyne NE2 4 — MB BS Lond. 1978; DCH RCP Lond. 1982; MRCP (UK) 1983; PhD Newcastle Upon Tyne 1995; FRCP 1996; FRCPCH 1997. Cons. Paediatric NeUrol. and Sen. Lect., Bristol Roy. Hosp. Specialty: Paediat. Neurol. Socs: Brit. Paediat. Assn. & Brit. Paediat. Neurol. Assn. Prev: Hon. Sen. Regist. & Lect. (Paediat. Neurosci.) Univ. Newc. Upon Tyne; 1st Asst. in Paediatric Neurosci., Univ. of Newc. Upon Tyne; Regist. (Paediat.) John Radcliffe Hosp. Oxf.

SHARPLES, Philip Elwin (Surgery), 229 West Barnes Lane, New Malden KT3 6JD Tel: 020 8336 1773 Fax: 020 8395 4797 — MB BS Lond. 1983 (Westm.) MRCGP 1987; DRCOG 1989; Dip Occ Med. 1996. GP New Malden. Specialty: Gen. Pract. Prev: RMO 1 DERR Hong Kong; BMH Rinteln Germany; RMO Welsh Guards Germany.

SHARPLES, Philip James Duke Street Surgery, 4 Duke Street, Barrow-in-Furness LA14 1LF Tel: 01229 820068 Fax: 01229 813840 — MB ChB Manch. 1969; Dip. Occ. Med.; MRCGP 1977.

SHARPLES, Rachel Harriet 26 Woodkind Hey, Spital, Bebington, Wirral CH63 9JZ — MB BS Newc. 1997.

SHARPLEY, John Guy Department of Psychiatry, Royal Hospital Haslar, Gosport PO12 2AA Tel: 023 9276 2205 Fax: 023 9276 2257 — MB BChir Camb. 1990 (United Med. & Dental School (Guy's)) MRC Psych 1997. Cons. in Gen. Adult Psychiat. Specialty: Gen. Psychiat.

SHARPLEY, Oliver John Burford Surgery, 59 Sheep Street, Burford OX18 4LS Tel: 01993 822176 Fax: 01993 822885; Field House, Westhall Hill, Fulbrook, Burford OX18 4BJ Tel: 01993 822484 — MB BS Lond. 1972 (St. Thos.) MRCGP 1983. Specialty: Gen. Pract. Prev: Med. Off. (O & G) Addington Hosp. Durban, S. Afr.; Ho. Phys. St. Stephen's Hosp. Lond.; Ho. Surg. St. Thos. Hosp. Lond.

SHARPSTONE, Daniel Robert West Suffolk Hospital, Hardwick Lane, Bury St Edmunds IP33 2QZ Tel: 01284 713481 Fax: 01284 712877 — MB BS Lond. 1988 (King's Coll.) FRCP; MRCP (UK) 1991; MD Lond. 1997. Cons. Phys. (Gastroenterol.) W. Suff. Hosps. NHS Trust. Specialty: Gastroenterol. Prev: Sen. Regist. (Med.) Chelsea & Westm. Hosp. Lond.; Regist. (HIV) Chelsea & Westm. Hosp. Lond.; Regist. (Med.) Portsmouth HA & Soton. Gen. Hosp.

SHARPSTONE, Paul The Hove Nuffield Hospital, 55 New Church Road, Hove BN3 4BG Tel: 01273 779471 Fax: 01273 220919; 27 Warnham Court, Grand Avenue, Hove BN3 2NJ Tel: 01273 204752 — MB BS Lond. 1960 (King's Coll. Hosp.) MRCS Eng. LRCP Lond. 1960; FRCP Lond. 1977, M 1964. Cons. Phys. (Gen. & Renal Med.) Brighton Health Care. Specialty: Nephrol. Socs: Renal Assn.; Eur. Dialysis & Transpl. Assn. Prev: Lect. (Med.) King's Coll. Hosp. Med. Sch. Lond.; Regist. (Med.) King's Coll. Hosp. & Roy. North. Hosp. Lond.

SHARR, Mr Michael Maurice 11 Brimstone Close, Chelsfield, Orpington BR6 7ST Tel: 01689 861114 — MB BS Lond. 1965 (St. Geo.) MRCP Lond. 1969; FRCS Eng. 1971. Cons. Neurosurg. SE Thames Regional Neurosurgic. Unit King's Coll. Hosp. Lond. Specialty: Neurosurg. Prev: Cons. Neurosurg. Walton Hosp. Liverp. & Gwynedd AHA; Sen. Regist. (Neurosurg.) Wessex Neurol. Centre Soton.; Regist. (Neurosurg.) Hosp. Sick Childr. Gt. Ormond St.

SHARRARD, Gordon Anthony Wells (retired) 1 Cotswold Avenue, Hazel Grove, Stockport SK7 5HJ Tel: 0161 483 1893 — BM BCh Oxf. 1954 (Oxf. & Univ. Coll. Hosp.) DM Oxf. 1973, MA, BM BCh 1954; DLO Eng. 1958. Prev: Clin. Med. Off. (Audiol. Servs.) Tameside (Manch.) AHA.

SHARRARD, Helen Elizabeth — BM BS Nottm. 1982; BMedSci Nottm. 1980; MRCPsych 1988. p/t Cons. Learning Disabil. Banes Primary Care Trust, St. Martins Hosp. Specialty: Ment. Health. Prev: Sen. Regist. (Ment. Handicap) Fairleigh Hosp. & Brentry Hosp. Bristol; Regist. & SHO (Psychiat.) Frenchay HA.

SHARRARD, Mark Jonathan 205 Ringinglow Road, Sheffield S11 7PT — MB BS Lond. 1988; BA (Biochem.) Oxf. 1983. Cons. Paediat. Sheff. Childr. NHS Trust. Specialty: Paediat. Special Interest: Metab. Dis. Prev: Regist. Rotat. (Paediat.) Sheff. Childr. Hosp. NHS Trust.; SHO (Paediat.) Brompton Hosp.; SHO (Paediat.) Qu. Eliz. Hosp. Lond.

SHARRARD, Mr William John Wells (retired) 140 Manchester Road, Sheffield S10 5DL Tel: 0114 266 4918 — MB ChB Sheff. 1944; MB ChB (Hons.) Sheff. 1944; FRCS Eng. 1950; MD (Distinc.) Sheff. 1954, ChM (Commend.) 1966. Prof. Orthop. Surg. Univ. Sheff. Prev: Cons. Orthop. Surg. Roy. Hallamsh. & Childr. Hosps. Sheff.

SHARRATT, Michael, OBE 28 Stoatley Rise, Haslemere GU27 1AG — MB ChB Birm. 1967; BSc (Chem.) Lond. 1954; MSc 1958; PhD Birm. 1961; FFOM 1988, M 1980; FRCPath 1983, M 1980. Specialty: Occupat. Health. Prev: Toxicol. Adviser BP Occupat. Health Centre; Sen. Med. Off. (Toxicol.) DHSS; Chief Toxicol. Brit. Indust. Biol. Research Assn. Carshalton.

SHARROCK, John Kieran Clive The Fountains, Park Lane, Blunham, Bedford MK44 3NJ — MB BS Lond. 1997 (St. Bart's Lond.) BSc (Hons) 1994. GP Train., Chelsea & Westm. Hosp. Specialty: Gen. Pract.

SHARVILL, Nicholas John Balmoral Surgery, 1 Victoria Road, Deal CT14 7AU Tel: 01304 373444; 19 Cowper Road, Deal CT14 9TW Tel: 01304 360516 Email: rogi11111@aol.com — MB BS Lond. 1979 (King's Coll. Hosp.) DRCOG 1982; DCH RCP Lond. 1982; MRCGP 1983; Dip. IMC RCS Ed. 1991; Cert. Av. Med. 1992; Dip. Occ. Med. R.C.P. 1997. Trainer GP; GP with special interest in Cardiol. E. Kent PCT. Specialty: Gen. Pract.; Medico Legal. Special Interest: Primary Care Cardiol.; Travel Med. Socs: BMA; SE Thames Fac. RCGP. Prev: Clin. Asst. (Anaesth.) Deal Hosp.; Trainee GP Kings Lynn VTS; SHO (Anaesth.) Qu. Eliz. Hosp. Kings Lynn.

SHARWOOD-SMITH, Geoffrey Hugh Department of Anaestheitcs, Royal Infirmary, Edinburgh EH16 4SA — MB ChB St. And. 1969; DA Eng. 1972; FFA RCS Eng. 1974. Cons. Anaesth. Roy. Infirm. Edin. Specialty: Anaesth. Socs: BMA; OAA; WAS. Prev: Specialist Anaesth. RAF.

SHASHIDHARAN, Mr Maniamparampil 20C Victoria Drive E., Salisbury District Hospital, Salisbury SP2 8BJ — MB BS Osmania 1988; FRCS Ed. 1992.

SHASHIKANTH, Subramaniam 43 Ravensdale Mansions, Haringay Park, London N8 9HS — LMSSA Lond. 1994.

SHASTRI, Mr Keshav Devdatta 5 Beechgrove Heights, Magherafelt BT45 5EF; 5 Beechgrove Heights, Magherafelt BT45 5EF Tel: 028 7963 2918 Fax: 028 7963 2918 — (Grant Med. Coll.) BSc Bombay 1941; MB BS Bomaby 1946; FRCS Eng. 1953. Hon. Cons. Surg. Mid Ulster Hosp. Magherafelt. Specialty: Gen. Surg.; Gastroenterol. Socs: BMA; Mid Ulster Clin. Soc. Prev: Prof. & Head Dept. Surg. Ravindra Nath Tagore Med. Coll. Udaipur, India; Cons. Surg. Mid Ulster Hosp. Magherafelt.

SHASTRI, Mayank Mahendraprasad Shenley Green Surgery, 22 Shenley Green, Selly Oak, Birmingham B29 4HH Tel: 0121 475 7997 — MB BS Baroda 1971.

SHATA, Maged Mohamed Hassanin 3 Ackford Drive, Worksop S80 1YQ — MB ChB Alexandria 1982.

SHATHER, Nabil Aziz Bilston Street Surgery, 25 Bilston Street, Sidgley, Dudley DY3 1JA Tel: 01902 665700 Fax: 01902 688533; Longcroft, Lowe Lane, Kidderminster DY11 5QR — LMSSA Lond. 1986; MB ChB Baghdad 1972.

SHATTLES, Warren Geoffrey 8 Arthur Road, Horsham RH13 5BQ — MB BS New South Wales 1982; MRCP (UK) 1987.

SHATTOCK, Gillian Mary (retired) Morningwell Cottage, Piddletrenthide, Dorchester DT2 7QZ — MB BS Lond. 1955 (Roy. Free) DCH Eng. 1977. Prev: SCMO (Child Health) S.W. Surrey Health Dist.

SHATWELL, Beryl Lomax (retired) Bunbury House, Warfleet, Dartmouth TQ6 9BZ — MB ChB Liverp. 1951. Prev: GP Devon.

SHATWELL, Mr Michael Antony 32 Baroncroft Road, Woolton, Liverpool L25 6EH — MB ChB Liverp. 1974; MChOrth Liverp. 1981, MB ChB 1974; FRCS Eng. 1979. Hon. Sen. Regist. (Orthop.) Liverp. HA; Lect. (Orthop. & Accid. Surg.) Univ. Liverp. Specialty: Orthop. Socs: Liverp. Med. Inst.; Assoc. Mem. Brit. Orthop. Assn. Prev: Regist. (Orthop.) Alder Hey Childr. Hosp. Liverp. & Roy. Liverp. Hosp.

SHATWELL, William John X-ray Department, Walsgrave Hospital, Clifford Bridge Road, Walsgrave, Coventry CV2 2DX Tel: 02476 602020; 66 Windy Arbour, Coventry CV8 2BB — MB BChir Camb. 1979 (St. Geo.) MA Camb. 1974; MRCP (UK) 1986; FRCR 1990. Cons. Radiol Univ. Hosp.s Coventry and Warks. NHS Trust. Specialty: Radiol. Prev: Sen. Regist. & Regist. (Diagn. Radiol.) John Radcliffe Hosp. Oxf.; SHO (Gen. Med.) Kent & Canterbury Hosp. Canterbury.

SHAUKAT, Mohammed Naeem 16 Hartland Drive, Littleover, Derby DE23 1LU — MB ChB Manch. 1985.

SHAUNAK, Lok Nath 53 A/B Maidstone Road, Rainham, Gillingham ME8 0DP Tel: 01634 231423 Fax: 01634 261665 — MB BS Jiwaji 1973; BSc Punjab India 1966; MRCS Eng. LRCP Lond. 1982.

SHAUNAK, Rohit — MB BS Lond. 1987. GP Staines Health Centre Staines. Prev: SHO (Surg.) Rotat. St. Geo. Hosp. Lond.; Anat. Demonst. St. Geo. Hosp. Med. Sch. Lond.

SHAUNAK, Sunil Imperial College London, Hammersmith Hospital, Du Cane Road, London W12 0NN Tel: 020 8383 2301 Email: sshaunak@imperial.ac.uk — MB BS Lond. 1982 (St. Geo.) BSc (Hons.) 1979; MRCP UK 1985; PhD Lond. 1993; FRCP Lond. 1996; FRCP (Ed) 1999. Cons. Phys. (Infec. Dis.) Hammersmith Hosp. Lond.; Hon. Cons. Phys. Chelsea & Westm. Hosp. Lond.; Reader (Infec. Dis.) Imperial Coll. London at Hammersmith. Specialty: Infec. Dis.; HIV Med. Prev: MRC Train. Fell. & Hon. Sen. Regist. (Infec. Dis.) Roy. Postgrad. Med. Sch. Hammersmith Hosp. Lond.; Fell. (Infec. Dis.) Duke Univ., USA; SHO (Med.) Nat. Hosp. Lond., Hammersmith Hosp. Lond. & Roy. Infirm. Edin.

SHAUNAK, Vidosava 34 Grain Road, Wigmore, Gillingham ME8 0ND — MB ChB Leeds 1975; DCH Eng. 1977; DRCOG 1978; MRCGP 1979. Socs: Brit. Assn. Manip. Med.

SHAVE, Norman Rossen Bridge End Surgery, Chester-le-Street DH3 3SL Tel: 0191 388 3236 Fax: 0191 389 0989; 27 Warkworth Drive, Deneside View Estate, Chester-le-Street DH2 3JR Tel: 0191 388 3462 — MB BS Newc. 1985; DRCOG 1987; MRCGP 1990. Prev: Trainee GP Northumbria VTS.

SHAVE, Peter Adeane (retired) 1 Sadlers Way, Ringmer, Lewes BN8 5HG — (Guy's) DTM & H Eng. 1952; MB BS Lond. 1948, DPH 1966; MFCM 1972. Prev: SCM (Child Health) E. Sussex AHA.

SHAVE, Ruth Mary X-Ray Department, Russell's Hall Hospital, Dudley DY1 2HQ — MB ChB Sheff. 1981; FRCS Eng. 1987; FRCR 1993. Cons. Radiol. Dudley Gp. Hosps. NHS Trust. Specialty: Radiol. Prev: Sen. Regist. (Diagn. Radiol.) W. Midl. RHA.

SHAVREN, Ruth Elaine — MB BS Lond. 1990. Specialty: Gen. Psychiat.

SHAW, Adam Charles 32 Hargwyne Street, London SW9 9RG — BM Soton. 1996.

SHAW, Alastair Martin Eastmost Cottage, Old Huntly Hill, Stracathro, Brechin DD9 7PU Tel: 01356 622919 Email: amshaw@doctors.org.uk; The Steyne, Forest Road, Colgate, Horsham RH12 4TB — MB ChB Aberd. 1988; DRCOG 1993; DFFP 1993; MRCGP 1994; FRACGP 2000. Prev: SHO (Med.) Frenchay Hosp. Bristol; SHO (Obst, & Gyn.) Bedford Hosp.; SHO (Med.) Selly Oak Hosp. Birm.

SHAW, Alexander Duncan Hill House, Upper Allan St, Blairgowrie PH10 6HL Tel: 01250 872078 — MB ChB Glas. 1969; DObst RCOG 1971; MRCGP 1973; FRCCP 1997. Socs: BMA. Prev: Ho. Off. (Surg. & Med.) Glas. Roy. Infirm.; Trainee Gen. Pract., Glas. Vocational Train. Scheme.

SHAW, Alexander John (retired) The Steyne, Forest Road, Colgate, Horsham RH12 4TB — (King's Coll. Hosp.) MB Camb. 1957, BChir 1956. Prev: Ho. Surg. & Ho. Phys. King's Coll. Hosp.

SHAW, Allen Bernard (retired) 2 The Stables, Weeton Lane, Harewood, Leeds LS17 9LP Tel: 0113 288 6907 — MB BS Lond. 1961 (St Bart.) MRCS Eng. LRCP Lond. 1961; FRCP Lond. 1979, M 1965; MD Lond. 1972. Prev: Cons. Phys. Bradford Roy. Infirm. & St. Lukes Hosp. Bradford.

SHAW, Amanda Anaesthetic Department, Trafford General Hospital, Moorside Road, Davyhulme, Manchester M41 5SL Tel: 0161 748 4022 Fax: 0161 746 2287 Email: amanda.shaw@trafford.nhs.uk; 2A Boothstown Drive, Worsley, Manchester M28 1UF — MB ChB Birm. 1984; FRCA 1994. Cons. Anaesth. NHS. Specialty: Anaesth. Socs: Intens. Care Soc.

SHAW, Andrew James Flat 7A, 55 Balmoral Road, Westcliff on Sea SS0 7DB — MB BS Lond. 1993 (Univ. Lond., UMDS) BSc Lond. 1986. SHO (Genitourin. Med.) St. Thos. Hosp. Lond. Specialty: Obst. & Gyn. Prev: SHO (O & G) King's Coll. Hosp. Lond. & Roy. Sussex Co. Hosp. Brighton.

SHAW, Andrew John 38 Castlepark Drive, Fairlie, Largs KA29 0DG — MB ChB Manch. 1993.

SHAW, Andrew John Department Genitourinary Medicine, Northwick Park Hospital, Harrow HA1 3UJ Tel: 020 869 3143 Fax: 020 8869 3156 — MB BS Lond. 1991 (Kings Coll. Lond.) BSc (Hons.) Lond. 1988, MB BS 1991; MRCP (UK) 1995; Dip. GU Med. 1996. Cons., (GUM. & HIV) Northwick Pk. Hosp.; Cons., (GUM & HIV) Centr. Middlx. Hosp. Specialty: Genitourinary Medicine; HIV

Med. Socs: MSSVD; BHIVA (Brit. HIV Assn.). Prev: Sen. Regist., (GUM & HIV) Char. Cross Hosp.

SHAW, Angela Christine Darent Valley Hospital, Darenth Wood Road, Dartford DA2 8DA Tel: 01322 428732 Email: angela.shaw@dag-tr.sthames.nhs.uk; 36 Shearwater, Longfield DA3 7NL — MB BS Lond. 1980 (Oxf. Univ. & Guy's Hosp.) MA Oxf. 1981; MRCPath 1987; MSc (Immunol.) Lond. 1990. Cons. Microbiol. Darent Valley Hosp., Dartford; Cons. Microbiologist, Fawkham Manor Hosp., Fawkham, Kent (Private Hosp. Self-employed). Specialty: Med. Microbiol. Socs: Hosp. Infec. Soc.; Assn. Med. Microbiol. Prev: Sen. Regist. (Microbiol.) Centr. Middlx. Hosp. Lond.; Regist. (Microbiol.) St. Mary's Hosp. Lond.

SHAW, Anne Patricia Leslie 37 Sandy Lodge Road, Rickmansworth WD3 1LP Tel: 01923 827663 Fax: 01923 827663 — MB BS Lond. 1963; MRCS Eng. LRCP Lond. 1963; DA Eng. 1966. Specialty: Psychosexual Med. Socs: Inst. Psychosexual Med.; Fac. Fam. Plann. & Reproduc. Health Care. Prev: SCMO (Family Plann.) Harrow HA.

SHAW, Anthony Moorlands Surgery, 139 Willow Road, Darlington DL3 9JP Tel: 01325 469168 — MB ChB Liverp. 1977; MFHom 1996. Bd. Mem. and Ment. Health Lead, Darlington Primary Care Gp. Specialty: Gen. Pract.; Homeop. Med. Prev: SHO (Psychiat.) Fazakerley Hosp. Liverp.; SHO (O & G & Paediat.) Clatterbridge Hosp. Bebington.

SHAW, Anthony John, CB, CBE, CStJ, Maj.-Gen. late RAMC Retd. Standing Medical Board, Duchess of Kent Barracks, Aldershot GU11 2DW Tel: 0125 234152 Fax: 0125 284 2654; Plovers Moss, Winchfield, Hook RG27 8SN Tel: 0125 842 2645 Email: shawanthony@totadisc.co.uk — MB BChir Camb. 1955 (Camb. & Westm.) MRCS Eng. LRCP Lond. 1954; MA Camb. 1955; DObst RCOG 1957; DTM & H Eng. 1961; FFCM 1983, M 1972; FRCP Lond. 1989. Specialty: Pub. Health Med.; Gen. Pract. Socs: Fell. Med. Soc. Lond. Vice Pres. Prev: Dir. Gen. Army Med. Servs.; Cdr. Med. Svc UK Land Forces; Hon. Phys. to HM The Qu..

SHAW, Anthony John Carteknowle and Dore Medical Practice, 1 Carterknowle Road, Sheffield S7 2DW Tel: 0114 255 1218 Fax: 0114 258 4418; 30 Whitworth Road, Sheffield S10 3HD — MB ChB Sheff. 1984; MRCGP 1990.

SHAW, Antony Leonard 22 Woodhill Grove, Prestwich, Manchester M25 0AE — MB ChB Liverp. 1996.

SHAW, Ashley Scott 26 Lemox Road, West Bromwich B70 0QT — MB ChB Sheff. 1996. SHO (Gen. Med.) Barnet Gen. Hosp. Herts. Specialty: Accid. & Emerg.; Gen. Med.

SHAW, Aubrey Abraham Arnold 34 Albany Manor Road, Bournemouth BH1 3EN Tel: 01202 291385 — LRCPI & LM, LRSCI & LM 1948 (RCSI) LRCPI & LM, LRCSI & LM 1948. Med. Assessor DHSS Dorset; Med. Off. TA 1st Wessex Infantry. Prev: Ho. Phys. (Orthop.), Ho. Surg. & Asst. to Psychiat. Crumpsall Hosp.

SHAW, Brian Galbraith Queens Crescent Surgery, 10 Queens Cresent, Glasgow G4 9BL Tel: 0141 332 3526 Fax: 0141 332 1150 — MB ChB Glas. 1973.

SHAW, Bronwen Elizabeth 42A Ridley Road, London NW10 5UA — MB ChB Cape Town 1993.

SHAW, Caroline Department of Accident and Emergency, Norfolk and Norwich Hospital, Brunswick Road, Norwich NR1 3JR Tel: 01603 287324; 157 Mundesley Road, North Walsham NR28 0DD Tel: 01692 406075 — MB BS Lond. 1980 (St Barthelomews Hospital) Associate Specialist (A & E) Norf. & Norwich Hosp. Specialty: Accid. & Emerg. Socs: Brit. Assn. Accid. & Emerg. Med. Prev: SHO (A & E) Scunthorpe Gen. Hosp.; Trainee GP S. Humberside; Clin. Med. Off. (Child Health) Wrexham.

SHAW, Caroline Anne Garden City Practice, 11 Guessen Road, Welwyn Garden City AL8 6QW — MB BS Lond. 1989; DGM RCP Lond. 1991; MRCGP 1997. GP. Specialty: Gen. Pract. Prev: GP Asst.Brook Green.Lond; GP Townsville AU; SHO A&E Blue Mt.ains.Au.

SHAW, Catherine Ann The Whittington Hospital, Highgate Hill, London N19 5NF Tel: 020 7272 3070 Email: catherine.shaw@whittington.nhs.uk — MB BS Lond. 1989 (Lond. Hosp.) BSc (Hons.) Anat. Lond. 1986; FRCA 1994. Cons. Anaesth., Whittington Hosp. NHS Trust; Hon. Sen. Lect., Whittington Hosp. NHS Trust. Specialty: Anaesth. Special Interest: Orthop.; Paediat.; Trauma. Prev: Regist. (Anaesth.) Univ. Coll. Hosp. & Middlx. Hosp. Lond.

SHAW, Catherine Louise Elmfield, Moyallen Road, Portadown, Craigavon BT63 5JX — MB ChB Ed. 1992.

SHAW, Catherine Mary Department of Psychiatry, Tameside General Hospital, Fountain St., Ashton-under-Lyne OL6 9RW — MB BChir Camb. 1989; BA Camb. 1985, MB BChir 1989; MSc Lond. 1990; MRCPsych 1994. Clin. Research Fell. (Psychiat.) Manch. Roy. Infirm. Specialty: Gen. Psychiat. Prev: Regist. (Psychiat.) NW RHA; SHO (Psychiat.) S. & Centr. Manch. HAs.

SHAW, Catherine Susan c/o Kirkstone Unit, Westmorland General Hospital, Burton Road, Kendal LA9 7RG — MB BS Lond. 1978.

SHAW, Charles Drury Shaw Institute (Quality in Health Care), Roedean House, Brighton BN2 5RQ Tel: 01273 687938 Email: cdshaw@btopenworld.com; 77 Curzon Street, Calne SN11 0DW Tel: 01249 816100 Fax: 01249 816100 — MB BS Lond. 1969 (Middlx.) Dip. Health Care Organisat. & Managem. Canad. Hosp. Assn. 1977; PhD Wales 1986. Chairm. UK and European Accred. Forum. Lond. Specialty: Pub. Health Med. Socs: BMA; Scientif. Counc. ANAEs Paris; (Ex-Pres.) Internat. Soc. Quality in Health Care Melbourne, Austral. Prev: Dir. Med. Audit Progr. King's Fund Centre Lond.; Gen. Manager Cheltenham HA; Med. Dir. King Edwd. VII Memor. Hosp. Bermuda.

SHAW, Charles Stuart (retired) Netherbourne, New Farm Road, Alresford SO24 9QH Tel: 01962 732163 — MB BS Lond. 1946 (Guy's) DCH Eng. 1949; FRCP Lond. 1975, M 1951; FRCPath 1970. Cons. Chem. Pathol. Roy. Hants. Co. Hosp.

SHAW, Christine Jane The Surgery, Long Street, Topcliffe, Thirsk YO7 3RP Tel: 01845 577297 Fax: 01845 577128 — MB ChB Sheff. 1971; DObst RCOG 1973; Dip. Therap. Newc 1997. Specialty: Gen. Pract. Prev: SHO (Obst. & Gen. Med.) Doncaster Roy. Infirm.; SHO (Paediat.) N. Sheff. Univ. Gp. Hosps.

SHAW, Christopher David Strathmore Medical Practice, 26-28 Chester Road, Wrexham LL11 7SA Tel: 01978 352055 Fax: 01978 310689 — MB ChB Edinburgh 1984.

SHAW, Mr Christopher John Castle Hill Hospital, Castle Road, Cottingham HU16 5JQ Tel: 01482 623021 — BM BCh Oxf. 1985; MA Camb. 1986; FRCS Eng. 1989; FRCS (Orth.) 1995. Cons.Orthopaedic Surg., Castle Hill Hosp. Cottingham. Specialty: Orthop. Socs: Brit. Elbow & Shoulder Soc.

SHAW, Christopher Paul Westmorland General Hospital, Kirkstone Unit, Burton Road, Kendal LA9 7RG — MB ChB Birm. 1982; MRCGP 1988.

SHAW, Christopher Quentin 49 Church Road, Altofts, Normanton WF6 2NU Tel: 01924 893989 — MB ChB Sheff. 1987.

SHAW, Claire Elizabeth 33 West Busk Lane, Otley LS21 3LY — BM BS Nottm. 1995.

SHAW, Clare Elizabeth, Surg. Lt. RN (retired) 40 Ravenshead Close, Selsdon, South Croydon CR2 8RL; 2 The Orchard, Kington St Michael, Chippenham SN14 6JH Email: kingshaw@iee.org — MB ChB Sheff. 1992; DFFP 1994; MRCGP 1998; DRCOG 1998. GP Retainee.

SHAW, Clifford Hamer (retired) 7 Celandine Gardens, Sheffield S17 4JJ Tel: 0114 235 2729 — MB BS Lond. 1942 (St. Bart.) MRCS Eng. LRCP Lond. 1942; MD Lond. 1947; DPH Eng. 1947; DPA Sheff. 1949; FFCM 1972. Prev: MOH & Princip. Sch. Med. Off. City Sheff.

SHAW, Clive Henry Ringwood Surgery, Cornerways, School Lane, Ringwood BH24 1LG Tel: 01425 472515 Fax: 01425 470030 — MB BS Lond. 1984. GP Ringwood, Hants.

SHAW, Clive Richard Shaw & Partners, 30 Kingsway, Waterloo, Liverpool L22 4RQ Tel: 0151 928 8668 Fax: 0151 949 1117; 37 Elton Avenue, Blundellsands, Liverpool L23 8UW Tel: 0151 931 3365 — MB ChB Dundee 1981; MRCGP 1985. Co-Chair, Crosby & Maghull PCG.

SHAW, David (retired) 2 Chapel View, Cadney Lane, Bettisfield, Whitchurch SY13 2LU Tel: 01948 710882 — MB BCh Wales 1964 (Cardiff) MFOM RCP Lond. 1985, A 1981; DIH Eng. 1981. Prev: Occupat. Health Phys. Wrexham.

SHAW, Professor David Aitken, CBE (retired) The Coach House, 82 Moor Road N., Newcastle upon Tyne NE3 1AB Tel: 0191 285 2029 — MB ChB Ed. 1951; FRCP Ed. 1968, M 1955; FRCP Lond. 1976, M 1971. Hon. Cons. Neurol. Roy. Vict. Infirm. Newc. Prev: Prof. Clin. Neurol. & Dean of Med. Univ. Newc.

SHAW, David Barrington Cardiac Department, Royal Devon & Exeter Hospital, Barrack Road, Exeter EX2 5DW Tel: 01392 403973

Fax: 01392 402067; Bixley Haven, Woodbury, Exeter EX5 1NR Tel: 01395 232531 — MB BS Lond. 1952; MRCS Eng. LRCP Lond. 1952; FRCP Lond. 1973, M 1956; FRCP Ed. 1971, M 1956; MD Lond. 1959; T(M) 1991; FESC 1994. Hon. Cons. Phys. & Hon. Sen. Lect. Roy. Devon & Exeter Hosp. Exeter. Specialty: Cardiol. Socs: Brit. Cardiac. Soc. Prev: Sen. Regist. (Med.) Bristol Roy. Hosp. & Tutor (Med.) Bristol Univ.; Regist. (Med.) Postgrad. Med. Sch. Hammersmith; Clin. Asst. Brompton Hosp. Lond.

SHAW, Mr David Lyon Bradford Teaching Hospitals NHS Trust, Bradford Royal Infirmary, Bradford BD9 6RJ Tel: 01274 364061 Fax: 01274 366592 — MB ChB Leeds 1984; FRCS Ed. 1988; MSc Salford 1992; FRCS (Orth.) 1995. Cons. Orthop. & Trauma Surg. Bradford Roy. Infirm. Specialty: Orthop.; Trauma & Orthop. Surg. Special Interest: Hip and Knee Arthroplasty; Trauma. Socs: Brit. Orthop. Assn.; Brit. Research Assn.; Amer. Orthopaedic Assn. Prev: Amer. Orthop. Fell., USA.

SHAW, David Murray Ballnalargy, Dalby, Peel IM5 3BP Tel: 01624 844415 Email: dmjeshaw@advsys.co.uk — (St. Bart.) MB BS Lond. 1953; FRCP Lond. 1978, M 1957; PhD Lond. 1961; DPM Eng. 1967; FRCPsych 1979, M 1972. Prev: Hon. Sen. Lect. Univ. Hosp. Wales Coll. Med. Cardiff; Scientif. Off. Med. Research Counc.; Temp. Act. Surg. Lt. RNVR.

SHAW, David Robert New Park Medical Practice, 163 Robertson Road, Dunfermline KY12 0BL Tel: 01383 629200 Fax: 01383 629203; 120 Grieve Street, Dunfermline KY12 8DW Email: davrshaw@aol.com — MB ChB Ed. 1976; FRCGP; MRCGP 1980. Assoc. Dean(SHO Training) S.E.Scotland. Prev: Director of SHO Train. (S.-E. Scotl. Region).

SHAW, Davida Georgina Margaret 543 Yarm Road, Eaglescliffe, Stockton-on-Tees TS16 9BJ — MB BS Newc. 1979.

SHAW, Deborah Jane 11 Kirklees Close, Farsley, Pudsey LS28 5TF — MB ChB Leeds 1996.

SHAW, Dominick Edward Warwick Lodge, Piddington Lane, Piddington, High Wycombe HP14 3BD — MB ChB Liverp. 1998; MB ChB Liverp 1998.

SHAW, Donald George 37 Sandy Lodge Road, Rickmansworth WD3 1LP — BM BCh Oxf. 1962 (Oxf. & Univ. Coll. Hosp.) BA (1st cl. Hons.) 1958; BSc 1959; MA 1962; FRCP Lond. 1980, M 1965; DMRD Eng. 1968; FFR (Rohan Williams Medal) 1970; FRCR 1975; MSc Oxf. 1981. Radiol. Hosp. Sick Childr. Lond. Prev: Cons. Radiol. Univ. Coll. Hosp.; Med. Regist., & Ho. Off. Med. & Surg. Units Univ. Coll. Hosp. Lond.; Ho. Phys. Lond. Chest Hosp.

SHAW, Mr Donald Grant Forest Health Care, The Health Centre, Dockham Road, Cinderford GL14 2AN Tel: 01594 598030; Armada Lodge, Hope Mansell, Ross-on-Wye HR9 5TL Tel: 01989 750797 Email: dgsebs@globalnet.co.uk — BM Soton. 1980; FRCS Eng. 1985; DRCOG 1987; Cert. Family Plann. JCC 1990; MRCGP 1990. Specialty: Gen. Surg. Socs: Primary Health Care Specialist Computer Gp. & Assn. Gp. Community Hosps. Prev: Regist. Rotat. (Gen. Surg.) Northampton Gen. Hosp.; SHO (O & G) Bedford Gen. Hosp.; SHO (Gen. Surg.) Mayday Hosp. Croydon.

SHAW, Douglas (retired) Huntly Cottage, Castle Huntly Road, Longforgan, Dundee DD2 5HA Tel: 01382 360600 — MB ChB St. And. 1968; MD (Commend) Dundee 1974; MRCP (UK) 1978; FRCP Ed. 1985; BA (Hons.) Dund 1997. Cons. Phys. (Med. Rehabil.) & Hon. Sen. Lect. Tayside Health Bd. & Univ. Dundee. Prev: Cons. Phys. (Geriat. Med.) & Hon. Sen. Lect. Roy. Vict. Hosp. & Univ.

SHAW, Duncan 3 Elmbank Drive, Kilmarnock KA1 3AT Tel: 01563 25437 — MB ChB Glas. 1962; DObst RCOG 1964.

SHAW, Duncan Alastair Sinclair Firvale, Heatherlands Road, Chilworth, Southampton SO16 7JB — MB ChB Sheff. 1994.

SHAW, Edward Alan 64 Broom Lane, Salford M7 4RS — MB ChB Ed. 1958; DObst RCOG 1960; FFA RCS Eng. 1964. Hon. Cons. Anaesth., Centr. Manch. and Manch. Children's Univ. Hosps.; Hon. Lect. in Paediat. Anaesth. Univ. Manch. Specialty: Anaesth. Prev: Cons. Anaesth. Roy. Manch. Childr. Hosp. & St. Mary's Hosp. Manch.

SHAW, Elizabeth Jane The Three Swans Surgery, Rolkstone Street, East Grimstead, Salisbury SP1 — MB BS Lond. 1982 (Guy's) MRCS Eng. LRCP Lond. 1982; LMSSA Lond. 1982; DRCOG 1985; MRCGP 1986. GP Salisbury.

SHAW, Enid Hilary Park End Surgery, 3 Parkend, South Hill Park, Hampstead, London NW3 2SE Tel: 020 7435 7282; 55 Lanchester Road, London N6 4SX — (Roy. Free) MB BS (Hons.) Lond. 1955; Cert. Family Plann. JCC 1978. Socs: Balint Soc.

SHAW, Fabia Melanie Kilburn Park Medical Centre, 12 Cambridge Gardens, London NW6 5AY Tel: 020 7624 2414 Fax: 020 7624 2489 — (Lond. Hosp.) MB BS Lond. 1980; DRCOG 1981. Prev: Out-Pat. Off. Roy. Nat. Throat, Nose & Ear Hosp. Lond.; Teenage Family Plann. Clinic Doctor Haringey.

SHAW, Felicity Ruth Gosport Health Centre, Bury Road, Gosport PO12 3PN Tel: 023 9258 3344; 12 Garstons Close, Titchfield, Fareham PO14 4EN — BM Soton. 1984; DRCOG 1987; MRCGP 1989.

SHAW, Fiona Elisabeth Newcastle General Hospital, Department of Geriatric Medicine, Westgate Road, Newcastle upon Tyne NE4 6BE — MB ChB Ed. 1990; BSc Ed. 1987; MRCP (UK) 1994; PhD Newc. 2002. Cons. Phys. & Geriatrician Newc. Gen. Hosp. Specialty: Gen. Med.; Care of the Elderly. Special Interest: Dementia; Falls & Syncops.

SHAW, Frances Eleanor Black Lion Lodge, Kensington Gardens, Bayswater Road, London W2 4RU — MB BCh BAO Dub. 1971 (Trinity Coll. Dub.) BA Dub. 1971; DCH RCPSI 1973; MRCP (UK) 1977. GP. Specialty: Gen. Pract.

SHAW, Frederick Antony Bowden House, Market Harborough LE16 9HW Tel: 01858 4242 — MB ChB Sheff. 1960; DObst RCOG 1964. Clin. Tutor Dept. Gen. Pract. Leicester Univ. Med. Sch. Socs: BMA. Prev: Rotating Intern St. John's Gen. Hosp. Newfld.; SHO (O & G) Scarsdale Hosp. Chesterfield.

SHAW, Frederick Ernest (retired) Hawkridge, Chantry Crescent, Stanford-le-Hope SS17 — MB BS Lond. 1953(Lond. Hosp.) LDS RCS Eng. 1944; MRCS Eng. LRCP Lond. 1953; DObst RCOG 1955.

SHAW, Frederick Joseph Oak Tree Medical Centre, 273-275 Green Lane, Seven Kings, Ilford IG3 9TJ Tel: 020 8599 3474 Fax: 020 8590 8277; 24 Bressey Grove, South Woodford, London E18 2HU Tel: 020 8597 0921 Fax: 020 8590 8277 — MB BCh Wales 1967 (Cardiff) DA Eng. 1969. Clin. Asst. (Psychiat.) Claybury Hosp. Woodford Bridge.

SHAW, Gavin Brown, CBE (retired) 31 St Germains, Bearsden, Glasgow G61 2RS — (Univ. Glas.) MB ChB Glas. 1942, BSc Glas. 1939; FRCP Lond. 1965, M 1947; FRFPS Glas. 1950; FRCP Glas. 1964, M 1962; FRCP Ed. 1969, M 1964; Hon. FACP 1979; Hon. FRCPI 1980; Hon. FRCPsych 1980; Hon. FRCGP 1980. Hon. Cons. Phys. S. Gen. Hosp. Glas. Prev: Cons. Phys. & Cardiol. South. Gen. Hosp. Glas.

SHAW, George Frederick (retired) Hillcote W., First Raleigh, Bideford EX39 3NJ Tel: 01237 476189 — MB BCh BAO Dub. 1942 (T.C. Dub.) Prev: Capt. RAMC 1943-46 (mentioned in despatches).

SHAW, Gertraud Bullfer Grove, Gunthorpe, Melton Constable NR24 2PD — LMSSA Lond. 1972. Asst. GP Melton Constable.

SHAW, Grainne Marie 18 Station Road, Magherafelt BT45 5PD — MB BCh BAO Belf. 1997.

SHAW, Grant David 12 Garstons Close, Titchfield, Fareham PO14 4EN Tel: 01329 845134 Email: 100573.373@compuserve.com — BM Soton. 1984. Staff Grade (Orthop.) Qu. Alexandra Hosp. Cosham. Specialty: Orthop.

SHAW, Helen Jane Bleak House, Jubilee Lane, Milton-under-Wychwood, Chipping Norton OX7 6EW — MB BS Lond. 1991; MRCGP 1995.

SHAW, Helen Margaret Boots Healthcare International, BHI Headquarters D6, Nottingham NG90 6BH — MB ChB Leic. 1986. Head of Clin./Med. Affairs Boots Healthcare Intern. Nottm. Specialty: Pharmaceutical Medicine. Prev: Med. Manager Boots Healthcare Internat. Nottm.; Assoc. Med. Dir. Fisons UK Operats. Coleorton.

SHAW, Mr Henry Jagoe, VRD (retired) Lislee House, Tredenham Road, St Mawes, Truro TR2 5AN Tel: 01326 270223; 52 Winchester Court, Vicarage Gate, Kensington, London W8 4AE Tel: 020 7376 1260 — (Oxf.) BM BCh Oxf. 1945; MA Oxf. 1945; FRCS Eng. 1950; MD New York State, US 1958. Prev: Cons. ENT Surg. St. Mary's Hosp. Lond.

SHAW, Hilary Elizabeth Mill Lodge, Reading Road, Cholsey, Wallingford OX10 9HG — MB BS Lond. 1978 (St. Mary's) DRCOG 1980; MRCGP 1983.

SHAW, Hung Ming Albert 63 Westacre, Bucknall, Stoke-on-Trent ST1 6AF — MB BS Bangalore 1979.

SHAW, Ian Norfolk & Waveney Mental Health Partnership NHS Trust, Northgate Hospital, Northgate Street, Great Yarmouth NR30 1BU Tel: 01493 337643 Email: ishaw@doctors.org.uk — MB ChB Birm. 1981; DRCOG 1983; MRCPsych. 1988; DGM RCP Lond. 1992. Cons. Old Age Psychiat. Northgate Hosp. Gt. Yarmouth. Specialty: Geriat. Psychiat. Prev: Sen. Regist. Rotat. (Psychiat.) Devon & Som. Train. Scheme; Regist. (Psychiat.) Walsgrave Hosp. Coventry.

SHAW, Ian Charles Northern General Hospital, Herries Road, Sheffield S5 7AU Tel: 0114 243 4343 Ext: 4818 Email: ian.shaw@sth.nhs.uk — MB ChB Sheff. 1991; FRCA. Cons. Anaesth., The Northern Gen. Hosp., Sheff. Specialty: Anaesth. Socs: BMA; The Assn. of Anaesth.s; The Intens. Care Soc. Prev: SHO Rotat. (Med.) Hull Roy. Infirm.

SHAW, Ian Hewison — MB BChir Camb. 1982 (Camb.) BSc (Hons.) Pharmacol. Bradford 1974; PhD Camb. 1978; DA Eng. 1985; FRCA 1987. Cons. Anaesth. & Intens. Care Newc. Gen. Hosp.; Hon. Clin. Lect. Univ. Newc.; Examr., Final Fell.ship, Roy. Coll. of Annesthetists; Chairm., North. Region Rita Panel For Anaesth. Specialty: Anaesth.; Intens. Care. Socs: Assn. Anaesths.; BMA. Prev: Sen. Regist. (Anaesth. & Intens. Care) Newc. Gen. Hosp.; Regist. (Anaesth.) Nuffield Dept. Anaesth. Radcliffe Infirm. Oxf.; SHO (Gen Med.) Aberd. Roy. Infirm.

SHAW, Ian Stuart Gloucester Royal Hospital, Department of Gastroenterology, Gloucester GL1 3NN — MB ChB Bristol 1994 (University of Bristol) MRCP (UK) 1997. Cons Gastroenterol. Gloucester Roy. Hosp. Specialty: Gastroenterol.; Gen. Med.

SHAW, Imogen Clare Freshwell Health Centre, Wethersfield Road, Finchingfield, Braintree CM7 4BQ Tel: 01371 810328 Fax: 01371 811282 — MB BChir 1984; MA 1985; MRCGP 1988. Prev: SHO Heath Rd. Hosp. Ipswich.

SHAW, Jacqueline Frances South Wigston Health Centre, 80 Blaby Road, Wigston LE18 4SE; 9 Link Road, Leicester LE2 3RA — BM BS Nottm. 1984; BMedSci Nottm. 1982.

SHAW, James Alistair MacGregor Diabetes Research Laboratory, 4th Floor William Leeth Building, The Medical School, Tramlington Place, Newcastle upon Tyne NE2 4HH Tel: 0191 222 7019 Fax: 0191 222 0723 Email: jim.shaw@ncl.ac.uk; 40 New Street, Stonehaven AB39 2LE Tel: 01569 765177 — MB ChB Manch. 1990 (St. And. & Manch.) BSc (Hons.) St. And. 1987; MRCP (UK) 1993; PhD 2000; FRCP RCPE 2003. Sen. Fell. and Hon. Cons. Phys. Diabetes Research Gp. Newc. upon Tyne; MRC Train. Fell. Specialty: Diabetes; Endocrinol. Prev: Specialist Regist. (Diabetes & Endocrinol.) Aberd. Roy. Infirm.

SHAW, James Charlton Halliday Waynes Cottage, The Croft, Fairford GL7 4BD — (TC Dub.) BA Dub. 1942; MB BCh BAO Dub. 1944; DCH RCPS Dub. 1948; MA Dub. 1984. Prev: Med. Off. Cirencester Pk. Polo Club (Emerit.); Ho. Phys. Nat. Childr. Hosp. Dub.; Ho. Surg. Roy. I. of Wight Co. Hosp. Ryde.

SHAW, James William, TD (retired) The Rest, Albert St., Tayport DD6 9AR — MB BCh BAO Dub. 1970; FRCP Ed. 2000; BA Dub.; DMRD Ed. 1974. Cons. Radiol. Ninewells Hosp. Dundee.

SHAW, Janis 31 Broad Lane, Hale, Altrincham WA15 0DQ Tel: 0161 980 3024 — MB ChB Liverp. 1976; FRCA 1980. Cons. Anaesth. Manch. Roy. Infirm. Specialty: Anaesth.

SHAW, Jean Margaret Victoria Health Centre, Glasshouse Street, Nottingham NG1 3LW Tel: 0115 948 3030 Fax: 0115 911 1074 — MB BS Lond. 1983; BA Camb. 1977; DRCOG 1986; MRCGP 1987; DCH RCP Lond. 1987.

SHAW, Jennifer Jayne 7 Moor Park Avenue, Preston PR1 6AS Tel: 01772 886171; Home Farm, Clifton Hill, Forton, Preston PR3 0AR Tel: 01524 791313 — MB ChB Manch. 1982; MRCPsych 1987.

SHAW, Jeremy Francis (retired) 2 Bell Hill Ridge, Petersfield, Petersfield GU32 2DZ Tel: 020 7229 6165 — MB ChB Bristol 1957; DPM Eng. 1961; MRCPsych 1971. Prev: Sen. Regist. (Psychol. Med.) Univ. Coll. Hosp. Lond.

SHAW, Jeremy Nicholas The Health Centre, Manor Road, Beverley HU17 7BZ Tel: 01482 862733 Fax: 01482 864958; 15 New Walk, Beverley HU17 7AE — MB ChB St. And. 1970 (St. And. Dundee) Specialty: Gen. Pract. Prev: Regist. (Med.) Papworth Hosp. Camb.; SHO (Paediat.) Jenny Lind Hosp. for Childr. Norwich; SHO Rotat. Hull Roy. Infirm.

SHAW, Jessie Marion Anderson Ardblair Medical Practice, Ann Street, Blairgowrie PH10 6EF Tel: 01250 872033 Fax: 01250 874517; Hill House, Upper Allan St, Blairgowrie PH10 6HL Tel: 01250 872078 — MB ChB Glas. 1969; Cert FPA 1974. GP Blairgowrie. Socs: BMA.

SHAW, Joan Patricia Vivian (retired) 12c Murray Road, Northwood HA6 2YJ Tel: 01923 821811 — MB BS Lond. 1953 (Middlx.) Prev: GP Hatch End & Northwood.

SHAW, Joanna Louise 17 Broughton Road, Pedmore, Stourbridge DY9 0XP — MB ChB Birm. 1995.

SHAW, John 405 Thornaby Road, Thornaby, Stockton-on-Tees TS17 8QN — MB ChB Leeds 1995.

SHAW, John David Highfield Surgery, Holtdale Approach, Leeds LS16 7ST Tel: 0113 295 3600 Fax: 0113 295 3602 — MB ChB Leeds 1989.

SHAW, Mr John Dennis (retired) The Gables, Sandygate Road, Sheffield S10 5UE Tel: 0114 230 7784 Email: admin@jdshaw.co.uk — (Sheff.) MB ChB Sheff. 1962; FRCS Ed. 1967; FRCS Eng. 1969. Prev: Cons. ENT Surg. Roy. Hallamsh. Hosp. Sheff.

SHAW, Mr John Francis Longsdon Derriford Hospital, Plymouth PL6 8DH Tel: 01752 777111; Homefield, Grenofen, Tavistock PL19 9EW Tel: 01822 612435 — MB BS Lond. 1975 (Guy's) ChM Oxf. 1983, BA 1972; MRCS Eng. LRCP Lond. 1975; FRCS Eng. 1980. Cons. Surg. Derriford Hosp. Plymouth. Specialty: Gen. Surg.; Transpl. Surg. Socs: Surgic. Research Soc.; Brit. Transpl. Soc. Prev: Sen. Regist. (Surg.) Roy. Free Hosp. Lond.; Regist. & Research Fell. (Surg.) Addenbrooke's Hosp. Camb.; Ho. Phys. & Ho. Surg. Guy's Hosp. Lond.

SHAW, Mr John Fraser (retired) 6 Gamekeeper's Park, Edinburgh EH4 6PA Tel: 0131 336 2828 — MB BS Lond. 1945 (Guy's) FRCS Eng. 1954; FRCS Ed. 1965; FRCP Ed. 1982. Prev: Cons. Surg. Surg. Neurol. Roy. Infirm., West. Gen. Hosp. & Roy. Hosp. Sick Childr. Edin.

SHAW, John Herbert Thorndike Vine Cottage, Spode Lane, Mark Beech, Edenbridge TN8 7HG Tel: 01342 850592 — MB BS Durh. 1955. Exam. Med. Pract. Benefits Agency Med. Servs. Specialty: Disabil. Med. Prev: GP Edenbridge; Ho. Phys. (Paediat.) Southmead Hosp. Bristol; Ho. Surg. Maidenhead Hosp.

SHAW, John Humphrey Wilfred (retired) 10 The Mount Drive, Reigate RH2 0EZ Tel: 01737 226250 — (St. Bart.) MB BChir Camb. 1958; MA Camb. 1959; DObst RCOG 1959. Prev: SHO (O & G) & Ho. Phys. Ilford Matern. Hosp. & King. Geo. Hosp. Ilford.

SHAW, Johnstone Eskbridge Medical Centre, 8A Bridge Street, Musselburgh EH21 6AG Tel: 0131 665 6821 Fax: 0131 665 5488 — MB ChB Ed. 1979; MRCOG 1985; MRCGP 1986. GP Edin.

SHAW, Jonathan Conrad Lister 11 Grand Avenue, Muswell Hill, London N10 3AY Tel: 020 8883 4326 — BM BCh Oxf. 1962 (Univ. Coll. Hosp.) BA Oxf. 1959, BM BCh 1962; DCH Eng. 1965; FRCP 1979, M 1967. Specialty: Paediat. Socs: Neonat. Soc. & Europ. Soc. Paediat. Research. Prev: Cons. Neonat. Paediat. Univ. Coll. Hosp. Lond.

SHAW, Mr Jonathan Harvey — MB ChB Ed. 1991; DA RCA Lond. 1995; Dip IMC RCS Ed. 1996; MRCS Ed. 2000. Specialist Regist. A & E, N.W. (Manch.) Deanery. Specialty: Accid. & Emerg. Socs: Brit. Assn. Accid. & Emerg. Med.; Fac. Pre-Hosp. Care.

SHAW, Jonathan Patrick Tristram 88 Ethel Street, Benwell, Newcastle upon Tyne NE4 8QA Tel: 0191 273 8666 — MB Camb. 1977, BChir 1976; DCH RCP Lond. 1983; MRCGP 1983.

SHAW, Mr Joseph, RD, CStJ (retired) Monks Meadows, Church Road, Holywood BT18 9BZ — (Camb. & St. Bart.) MB BChir Camb. 1956; FRCS Ed. 1965; FRCSI 1983; FFAEM 1993. Civil. Cons. (A & E) RN; Surg. Capt. RNR. Prev: Cons. Surg. Ulster Hosp. Belf.

SHAW, Kanika 29 Hayley Bell Gardens, Bishop's Stortford CM23 3HA — BM Soton. 1988.

SHAW, Katharine Lisa Flat 6, 1 Mornington Crescent, London NW1 7RH — MB BS Lond. 1991.

SHAW, Katherine Nicola 37 Sandy Lodge Road, Rickmansworth WD3 1LP Tel: 019238 27663 — BM BS Nottm. 1994; BMedSci Nottm. 1992.

SHAW, Kathryn Campbell 3 Elmbank Drive, Kilmarnock KA1 3AT — MB ChB Glas. 1990; DRCOG 1992; MRCGP 1994; T(GP) 1995. Trainee GP Glas.

SHAW, Kenneth Ian Chessel Surgery - Bitterne Branch, 4 Chessel Avenue, Bitterne, Southampton SO19 4AA — MB BS Lond. 1975

(Lond. Hosp.) DRCOG 1978. Specialty: Gen. Pract. Prev: Trainee GP Bath VTS.

SHAW, Professor Kenneth Martin Castle Acre, Hospital Lane, Portchester, Fareham PO16 9QP — (Univ. Coll. Hosp.) MB BChir Camb. 1969; MRCP (UK) 1970; MA, MD Camb. 1979; FRCP Lond. 1985. Cons. Phys. & Dir. of Research & Developm. Portsmouth Hosps. NHS Trust; Vis. Prof. Postgrad. Med. Sch. Univ. Portsmouth; Hon. Clin. Teach. Soton. Univ. Med. Sch.; Edr. in Chief Jl. Pract. Diabetes Internat. Specialty: Gen. Med.; Diabetes; Endocrinol. Socs: Fell. Roy. Soc. Med.; Scientif. Fell. Zool. Soc.; Brit. Diabetic Assn. Prev: Resid. Asst. Phys. Univ. Coll. Hosp. Lond.; MRC Asst. Dept. Clin. Pharmacol. Univ. Coll. Hosp. Med. Sch. Lond.

SHAW, Keren Ann The Surgery, St Albans Road, Hersden, Canterbury CT3 4EX — MB BS Lond. 1984 (St. Mary's) GP Herne Bay. Prev: Regist. (Chem. Path.) Qu. Mary's Hosp. Lond.; Ho. Off. Ealing Hosp. Lond.

***SHAW, Kirsty** — MB ChB Aberd. 1998; MB ChB Aberd 1998.

SHAW, Kirsty Jane Dunvegan Medical Practice, Dunvegan, Isle of Skye IV55 8GU — MB ChB (Commend.) Dundee 1993; DRCOG 1995; DFFP 1995; MRCGP (Merit) 1998. GP Princip., Dunvegan Med. Pract. Isle of Skye.

SHAW, Laurence Marcus Alan Queen Elizabeth Queen Mother Hospital, St Peters Road, Margate CT9 4AN; Brabourne Suite, Chaucer Hospital, Nackington Road, Canterbury CT4 7AR Tel: 01227 721338 — MB BS Lond. 1978 (St. Bart.) MRCS Eng. LRCP Lond. 1979; DRCOG 1981; MRCOG 1984; FRCOG 1997. Cons. O & G E. Kent Hosps. NHS Trust. Specialty: Obst. & Gyn.; Gynaecology. Special Interest: Endometriosis; Menopause; Infertil. Socs: Fell. Roy. Soc. Med.; Liveryman Worshipful Soc. Apoth. Lond.; Brit. Fertil. Soc. Prev: Clin. Dir. Woms. & Childrs. Health Qu. Eliz. Qu. Mother Hosp.; Sen. Regist. (O & G) Westm. Hosp. Lond.; Regist. (O & G) Hammersmith Hosp. Lond.

SHAW, Lindsay Jane 141 Sefton Park Road, St. Andrews, Bristol BS7 9AW — MB ChB Bristol 1991; BSc Bristol 1988. Dermat. Specialist Regist., Bristol Roy. Infirm. Specialty: Dermat.; Paediat. Socs: Brit. Soc. of Paediatric Dermat. Prev: Paediat. Regist. Southmead Bristol; Paediat. Regist. Taunton & Som. Hosp.; Paediat. Regist. Roy. Childr.s Hosp. Melbourne.

SHAW, Lisa Clare 68 Culcheth Hall Drive, Culcheth, Warrington WA3 4PX — BM BCh Oxf. 1998; BM BCh Oxf 1998.

SHAW, Louise Johanna Royal United Hospital, Older People's Unit, Combe Park, Bath BA1 3NG — MB ChB Sheff. 1992; MRCP (UK) 1995. Cons. in Geriat. and Stroke Med. Specialty: Care of the Elderly.

SHAW, Mr Malcolm (retired) 1 Brown Road, Kirkcudbright DG6 4HP Tel: 01557 330900 — (Univ. Glas.) MB ChB Glas. 1938; MA Glas. 1938; DA Eng. 1946; FFA RCS Eng. 1954; FRCS Glas. 1962. Prev: Cons. Anaesth. Vict. Infirm. Glas. & Roy. Hosp. Sick Childr. Glas.

SHAW, Mr Malcolm Donald Macalister Walton Centre for Neurology & Neurosurgery NHS Trust, Lower Lane, Liverpool L9 7LJ Tel: 0151 529 5671/5533 Fax: 0151 529 5500 — BM BCh Oxf. 1966; MA Oxf. 1966; FRCS Eng. 1972. Cons. Neurosurg. & Med. Dir. Walton Centre; Lect. (Neurosurg.) Liverp. Univ.; Med. Director, Trust Bd., The Walton Centre for Neurol. and Neurosurg. NHS Trust, Liverp. Specialty: Neurosurg. Special Interest: Intracranial Surg.; Vasc. Surg. Socs: Oxf. Grads. Med. Club & Soc. Brit. Neurol. Surgs. Prev: Sen. Regist. (Neurosurg.) Inst. Neurol. Sc. South. Gen. Hosp. Glas.; Regist. (Neurosurg.) Radcliffe Infirm. Oxf.

SHAW, Marcia Susan 20 Adelaide St, Plymouth PL1 3JF Tel: 01803 313881 — MB BS Lond. 1974; MRCP (UK) 1977. Cons. Dermat. Derriford Hosp. Plymouth. Specialty: Dermat. Prev: Cons. Dermat. Torbay Hosp. Torquay.

SHAW, Margaret (retired) 65 Carter Knowle Road, Sheffield S7 2DW — MRCS Eng. LRCP Lond. 1958 (Sheff.) Prev: Ho. Phys. Mansfield Gen. Hosp. Ho. Surg. & SHO Anaesth. Roy. Infirm. Sheff.

SHAW, Maria Emilia Lourdes Cordeira (retired) Chimney Stones, off Leek Road, Stockton Brook, Stoke-on-Trent ST9 9NJ — LRCPI & LM, LRSCI & LM 1961. GP Stoke on Trent.

SHAW, Mark Christopher UMDS Department of Public Health Medicine, 5th Floor Capital House, 42 Weston St., London SE1 3QD Tel: 020 7955 5000 Ext: 6249 Fax: 020 7403 4602; Flat 10, Victoria Court, Victoria Road, Shoreham-by-Sea BN43 5WS Tel: 01273 884522 Email: markcs@mistral.co.uk — MB BS Lond. 1988. Hon. Lect. (Pub. Health Med.) UMDS. Specialty: Pub. Health Med. Prev: Sen. Regist. (Pub. Health Med.) E. Sussex HA; Regist. (Pub. Health Med.) E. Sussex & Maidstone HA; SHO (Med.) Worthing Hosp.

SHAW, Martin Bellamy Banks Medical Centre, 272 Wimborne Road, Bournemouth BH3 7AT Tel: 01202 512549 Fax: 01202 548534 — MB BS Lond. 1976 (Roy. Free) MRCS Eng. LRCP Lond. 1976; D.Occ.Med. RCP Lond. 1995. GP Princip. Bournemouth; Occupat. Health Phys.; GP Commr. Specialty: Gen. Pract.; Occupat. Health. Socs: Soc. Occupat. Med.

SHAW, Martin Whitney (retired) Manor Farm House, East Dean, Chichester PO18 0JA Tel: 01243 811207 — MB Camb. 1966 (St. Thos.) BChir 1965; DA Eng. 1968.

SHAW, Mary Kay (retired) 15 Hatt Close, Moulton, Spalding PE12 6PX — MRCS Eng. LRCP Lond. 1951 (Leeds) MRCS Eng. LRCP Lond. 1951.

SHAW, Matthew Benjamin Keeble 22 Brookfields, Netherton, Wakefield WF4 4NL — BM BCh Oxf. 1997.

SHAW, Matthew Byrom Brookside Group Practice, Brookside Close, Gipsy Lane, Reading RG6 7HG Tel: 0118 966 9222 Fax: 0118 935 3174 — MB ChB Bristol 1987.

SHAW, Matthew Jon 19 Glaisedale Grove, Willenhall WV13 1HB — MB BS Lond. 1998; MB BS Lond 1998.

SHAW, Matthew Philip MRC Laboratory, Fajar, PO Box 273, Banjul, Gambia; 8 Harlesden Gardens, London NW10 4EX Tel: 020 8961 3208 — MB BS Lond. 1986; BSc (Hons.) Sociol. Applied to Med. Lond. 1983; DCH RCP Lond. 1990; MRCGP 1992; MSc Lond. 1995. Research Fell. HIV Interven & Domestic Violence Health olicy Unit, Lond. Sch. of Hyg. & Trop. Medicines. Prev: GP Fell. (HIV) St Mary's Hosp. Lond.; Trainee GP St Mary's Hosp. Lond.; HIV Preven. Researcher. MRC, The Gambia.W. Africa.

SHAW, Melanie Sara Brunswick Xray, Norfolk and Norwich Hospital, Norwich NR1 3RR Tel: 01603 286523; The Maltings, South Walsham Road, Panxworth, Norwich NR13 6JG Tel: 01603 270471 Email: mleadbe@aol.com — MB BS Lond. 1989 (St Georges Hospital Medical School) BSc Lond. 1986; MRCP (UK) 1994; FRCR (UK) 1997. Cons. Pathologist, Norf. and Norwich HNS Health Care Trust. Specialty: Radiol. Prev: Regist. (Radiol.) Roy. Lond. Hosp.; SHO (Thoracic Med.) Lond. Chest Hosp.; SHO (Renal Med.) St. Bart. Hosp. Lond.

SHAW, Michael John St Georges Hospital, Morpeth, Birmingham NE61 2NU Tel: 01670 512121 — MB ChB Leeds 1990. Cons. (Adult Gen. Psychiat), Newc., N. Tyneside and N.d. Ment. Health (NHS) Trust, St Geo.s Hosp. Morpeth. Specialty: Gen. Psychiat. Socs: Roy. Coll. Psychiat.s. Prev: Regist. (Psychiat.) Mersey RHA.; Specialist Regist. (Adult Gen Psychiat.) Mersey RHA.

SHAW, Michael Maurice Bersted Green Surgery, 32 Durlston Drive, Bognor Regis PO22 9TD Tel: 01243 821392 Fax: 01243 842590 Email: michael.shaw@gp-h82016.nhs.uk — MB BS Lond. 1972 (Guy's) MRCS Eng. LRCP Lond. 1972; DObst RCOG 1974; DIH Soc. Apoth. Lond. 1976. Socs: BMA. Prev: Med. Off. Brit. Steel Corp. Lackenby; SHO (O & G & Cas.) St. Richard's Hosp. Chichester; Ho. Phys. St. Mary's Hosp. Newport I. of Wight.

SHAW, Muriel Kathleen 19 Upper Crofts, Alloway, Ayr KA7 4QX Tel: 01292 443785 — BM BS Nottm. 1977; FFA RCS (Eng.) 1981. Cons. Anaesth. CrossHo. Hosp. Kilmarnock. Specialty: Anaesth. Socs: BMA & Assn. Anaesth. Prev: Sen. Regist. (Anaesth.) Qu. Med. Centre Nottm.; Regist. (Anaesth.) Bristol Roy. Infirm.

SHAW, Neil Howard Po Box 121, Leeds LS16 8XH Tel: 0113 2817741 Fax: 0113 2817741 — MB ChB Leeds 1985; DRCOG 1989; Cert. Prescribed Equiv. Exp. JCPTGP 1989; MRCGP 1991; Afom RCP Lond 2002. Occupational hys., Leeds & W.Yorks. Specialty: Occupat. Health. Socs: Soc. Occupat. Med. Prev: Trainee GP Bradford VTS; Med. Off. Univ. Leeds Health Serv.; GP Prinncipal, Foundat. Med. Centre, Leeds.

SHAW, Nicholas Alastair Oxford Street Surgery, 20 Oxford Street, Workington CA14 2AJ; 20 Oxford Street, Workington CA14 3AL Tel: 01946 603302 — MB BChir Camb. 1978; MA Camb. 1979, MB BChir 1978; DRCOG 1981; MRCGP 1982. Prev: Regist. (Med.) Whakatane Hosp. New Zealand; Ho. Surg. Essex Co. Hosp. Colchester; Ho. Phys. Qu. Marys Hosp. Sidcup.

SHAW, Nicholas John University Hospital North Durham, North Road, Durham DH1 5TW — MB ChB Sheff. 1988; BSc Sheff. 1983;

MB ChB Sheff. 1988; FRCS Glas. 1992; FRSC (orthopaedics and Traumatology) 1998. Cons. Surg. and Traumatologist.

SHAW, Nicholas John — MB ChB Birm. 1978; DRCOG 1982; DTM & H (Liverp.) 1982; DCH RCP Lond. 1983; MRCP (UK) 1985; FRCPCH 1997. Cons. Paediat. Endocrinol. Birm. Childr. Hosp.; Hon. Sen. Lect. (Paediat.) Univ. Birm. Specialty: Endocrinol.; Paediat. Socs: Roy. Coll. Paediat. & Child Health; Amer. Soc. of Bone & Mineral Research; Eur. Soc. Paediat. Endocrinol. Prev: Sen. Regist. (Paediat. Endocrinol.) Birm. Childr. Hosp.; Lect. (Child Health) Alder Hey Childr. Hosp. Liverp.; Lect. (Paediat.) St. Jas. Univ. Hosp. Leeds.

SHAW, Nigel John — MB ChB Birm. 1980; FRCP; FRCPCH; MD; PGCLT.

SHAW, Mr Norman Carey Chestnut Byre, Rudham Road, Harpley, King's Lynn PE31 6TH Tel: 01485 520646 Email: carey.shaw@harpley.net — MB BS Lond. 1963 (Char. Cross) FRCS Eng. 1970. Specialty: Orthop. Prev: Cons. (Orthop. Surg. & Trauma) Qu. Eliz. Hosp. Kings Lynn. & N. Cambs. Hosp. Wisbech.; Sen. Regist. Roy. Nat. Orthop. Hosp. Stanmore; Sen. Regist. (Orthop.) Norf. & Norwich Hosp.

SHAW, Professor Pamela Jean Department of Neurology, Ward 11, Royal Victoria Infirmary, Newcastle upon Tyne NE1 4LP Tel: 0191 232 5131 Fax: 0191 227 5267; 20 Parklands, Hamsterley Mill, Rowlands Gill NE39 1HH Tel: 01207 543239 — MD Newc. 1988 (University of Newcastle-upon-Tyne) MB BS 1979; MRCP (UK) 1981; FRCP 1994. Wellcome Sen. Research Fell. (Clin. Sci.), Prof. Neurol. Med. & Hon. Cons. Neurol. Univ. Newc. u. Tyne. Specialty: Neurol.

SHAW, Paul Anthony Vernon Linton House, 50 Main St, Barkby, Leicester LE7 3QG — MB BChir Camb. 1980; MA Camb. 1982; MRCPath 1988. Cons. Cytopath. & Histopath. Leics. Roy. Infirm. Specialty: Histopath. Prev: Sen. Regist. (Histopath.) Leicester Roy. Infirm.

SHAW, Paul Hamelton 26 Tudor Hollow, Fulford, Stoke-on-Trent ST11 9NP — MB ChB Liverp. 1993.

SHAW, Penelope Jane 45 Hartington Road, Grove Park, Chiswick, London W4 3TS — MB BS Lond. 1977; MRCP (UK) 1980; FRCR 1983. Cons. Radiol. Univ. Coll. Hosp. Lond. Specialty: Radiol.

SHAW, Mr Peter Alan Field House, Sandy Lane, Newcastle ST5 0LZ Tel: 01782 630630 Fax: 01782 630630; Park House, Oakley, Market Drayton TF9 4AG — MB ChB Leeds 1965; BSc Lond. 1959; DO Eng. 1972; FRCS Ed. 1975. Cons. Ophth. N. Staffs. Roy. Infirm. Stoke on Trent. Specialty: Ophth. Socs: FRCOphth. Prev: Sen. Regist. (Ophth.) Leeds Gen. Infirm.; Regist. (Ophth.) Birm. & Midl. Eye Hosp.; Anat. Demonst. Bristol Med. Sch.

SHAW, Mr Peter Cosmo (retired) 8 Castlemaine Avenue, South Croydon CR2 7HQ — MB BS Lond. 1957 (Guy's) FRCS Ed. 1963; FRCS Eng. 1965. Prev: Cons. Orthop. Surg. Bromley Gp. Hosps.

SHAW, Peter John The Symons Medical Centre, 25 All Saints Avenue, Maidenhead SL6 6EL Tel: 01628 626131 Fax: 01628 410051; The Gables, 49 Whyteladyes Lane, Cookham, Maidenhead SL6 9LT Tel: 01628 522852 Email: shorkie@aol.com — MB BS Lond. 1985 (Char. Cross) DRCOG 1991. Specialty: Cardiol.; Gen. Psychiat. Special Interest: Migraine. Socs: Sec. Windsor & Dist. Med. Soc. Prev: GP Tutor E. Berks.; Edit. Bd. Psychiat. in Pract.; SHO (Cardiol. & Transpl. Med.) Harefield Hosp. Middlx.

SHAW, Peter Quentin Stirchley Medical Practice, Stirchley Health Centre, Stirchley, Telford TF3 1FB Tel: 01952 660444 Fax: 01952 415139; Mount Farm, Cruckton, Shrewsbury SY5 8PR — MB BS Lond. 1981 (Univ. Coll. Hosp.) BSc (1st cl. Hons.) Hist. Med. Lond. 1978; MRCP (UK) 1984; DCH RCP Lond. 1984; DRCOG 1989; MRCGP (Distinc.) 1989. Specialty: Gen. Pract.

SHAW, Mr Reginald Ernest (retired) Glebe Cottage, Horn Hill, Barford-St.-Michael, Banbury OX15 0RQ — MB BS Lond. 1943; FRCS Eng. 1948; DRCOG 1964; FRCSC 1968; DA (UK) 1970.

SHAW, Mr Richard Emmott (retired) 1 Enright Close, Old College Park, Leamington Spa CV32 6SQ Tel: 01926 882985 — MRCS Eng. LRCP Lond. 1940 (Leeds) ChM Leeds 1949, MB ChB 1940; FRCS Eng. 1947. Prev: Cons. Urol. Coventry Hosp. Gp.

***SHAW, Richard John** Flat Top Right, 19 Highburgh Road, Glasgow G12 9YF — MB ChB Glas. 1998 (Glasgow) BDS (Bristol) 1990; FDS RCS Eng 1993; MB ChB Glas 1998. Sen. Health Off., Roy. Alexander Infirm., Paisley. Specialty: Oral & Maxillofacial Surg. Socs: BMA; BAUMS. Prev: Regist. in Oral & Maxillofacial Surg., RAF Hosp., Wrougton; Sen. Health Off. in Oral Maxillofacial Surg., Monklands DGH; Monklands DGH.

SHAW, Robert Frederick Holsworthy Medical Centre, Dobles Lane, Holsworthy EX22 6GH Tel: 01409 253692 Fax: 01409 254184; Holsworthy Health Centre, Well Park, Holsworthy EX22 6DH Tel: 01409 253692 — MB ChB Leic. 1991. Specialty: Gen. Pract.

SHAW, Robert Logan Radiology Department, Southern General Hospital, 1345 Govan Road, Glasgow G51 4TF Tel: 0141 201 1100 Email: robert.shaw@sgh.scot.nhs.uk — MB ChB Glas. 1982; BSc Glas. 1980; FRCS Glas. 1986; FRCR 1990. Cons. Radiologist,South Glas. Univ. Hosps. Trust. Specialty: Radiol. Prev: Sen. Regist. (Radiol.) Northwick Pk. Hosp. Harrow.

SHAW, Professor Robert Wayne Derby City General Hospital, Academic Division Obstetrics & Gynaecology, Clinical Sciences Building, Uttoxeter Road, Derby DE22 3NE — MB BCh Birm. 1969; MB ChB (Hons.) Birm. 1969; MD (Hons.) Birm. 1975; FRCOG 1993, M 1977; FRCS Ed. 1978. Prof. (Obst. & Gyn.) University of Nottingham. Specialty: Obst. & Gyn. Special Interest: Reproductive Med. Socs: (Ex-Chairm.) Blair Bell Research Soc. 1986-89; Pres. World Endornetriosis Soc. 2002-05. Prev: Chairm. Matern. & Child Health Research Consortium - Confidential Enquiry into Stillbirth (CESDI); Postgrad. Dean East. Deanery Camb.; Prof. Head Acad. Dept. O & G Roy. Free Hosp. Sch. Med.

SHAW, Robin Richard 3 Pendorlan Road, Penrhyn Bay, Llandudno LL30 3PS — MB ChB Manch. 1987.

SHAW, Roderick John McIntosh, Gourlay and Partners, Stockbridge Health Centre, 1 India Place, Edinburgh EH3 6EH Tel: 0131 225 9191 Fax: 0131 226 6549 — MB ChB Manch. 1985; MRCGP 1989.

SHAW, Roderick Watson Kingsway Medical Practice, 12Kingsway Court, Glasgow G14 9SS Tel: 0141 959 6000 Fax: 0141 954 6971; 18 Corbie Place, Milngavie, Glasgow G62 7NB Tel: 0141 956 3685 — MB ChB Glas. 1980; DRCOG 1981; MRCGP 1983. GP Trainer Glas.; Undergrad. Tutor. Glas. Univ. Specialty: Rehabil. Med.; Rheumatol. Socs: BMA; Primary Care Rheum. Soc.; Christ. Med. Fellowsh. Prev: Hosp. Pract. S. Gen. Hosp.; SHO (O & G) Stobhill Hosp. Glas.; SHO (Paediat.) Monklands & Dist. Gen. Hosp. Airdrie.

SHAW, Professor Rory James Swanton Hammersmith Hospital, Du Cane Road, London W12 0HS Tel: 020 8383 3370 — MB BS Lond. 1977 (St. Bart.) MRCP (UK) 1979; BSc (1st cl. Hons.) Lond. 1974, MD 1985; T(M) 1991; FRCP Lond. 1993; MBA Univ. Lond. 1995. Prof., Cons. Phys. (Respirat. Med.), Med. Dir. Hammersmith Hosps. Trust Lond.; Chairm. of the Nat. Pat. Safety Agency. Specialty: Respirat. Med. Socs: Brit. Thorac. Soc.; Amer. Thorac. Soc. Prev: MRC/Lilly Trav. Fell. & RCP Prophit Sch. Nat. Jewish Centre for Immunol. & Respirat. Med. Denver Co., USA; Cons. Phys. St Mary's Hosp. Lond. & Dir. of Med. Educat. Unit Imperial Coll. Sch. of Med.

SHAW, Rosaleen Amanda Crumlin Road Health Centre, 130-132 Crumlin Road, Belfast BT14 6AR — MB BCh Dublin 1988.

SHAW, Ruth Elizabeth — BM BS Nottm. 1993; BMedSci Nottm. 1991.

SHAW, Sally Anne Old Hall Surgery, 26 Stanney Lane, Ellesmere Port, South Wirral CH65 9AD Tel: 0151 355 1191 Fax: 0151 356 2683; 29 Whitegates Crescent, Willaston, South Wirral CH64 2UX Tel: 0151 327 6706 — MB BS Lond. 1980; MRCP Ed. 1985; MRCGP 1988. GP Ellesmere Port. Specialty: Gen. Pract. Prev: Med. Dir. Hospice of Good Shepherd Chester; Regist. (Radiother.) Clatterbridge Hosp. Wirral; Regist. (Med.) Sheff.

SHAW, Samantha Jane 26 Lewisham Park, London SE13 6QZ — MB ChB Leic. 1994.

SHAW, Samuel MacKay Dufftown Medical Group, Health Centre, Stephen Avenue, Keith AB55 4FJ Tel: 01340 820888 Fax: 01340 820593 — MB ChB Aberd. 1985; MRCGP 1989.

SHAW, Sarah 55 Old Park Avenue, Enfield EN2 6PJ — MB BS Lond. 1996; BA (Hons.) Oxf. 1992.

SHAW, Sheila Joan Drs Angior, Shaw & Owen, Pemberton PCRC, Sherwood Drive, Pemberton, Wigan WB5 9QX — MB ChB Manch. 1981; T(GP) 1991.

SHAW, Simon Alexander 24 Bressey Grove, London E18 2HU — MB BS Lond. 1996.

SHAW, Simon Andrew Holly House, Smithy Lane, Bardsey, Leeds LS17 9DT — BM BCh Oxf. 1997; MA (Hons.) Camb. 1994. Res. Med. Off. Roy. Perth Hosp. Perth, Australia. Specialty: Gen. Surg.

Socs: BMA (Sec. Yorksh. JDS 1997-98). Prev: Ho. Off. (Med. & Surg.) York Dist. Hosp.

SHAW, Simon John Geoffrey Street Health Centre, Geoffrey Street, Preston PR1 5NE Tel: 01772 401760 Fax: 01772 401766 — BM BCh Oxf. 1986 (Cambridge 1980-83; Oxford 1983-86) MA Camb. 1990, BA 1983. GP Princip. Prev: Trainee GP Sandbach; SHO Rotat. Leighton Hosp. Crewe VTS.

SHAW, Simon Nicholas Mental Health Dept., Lerwick Health Centre, South Road, Lerwick ZE1 0RB Tel: 01595 743006 Fax: 01595 646559 Email: simon.shaw@shb.shetland.scot.nhs.uk; 10 Seaton Road, Uppingham, Oakham LE15 9QX — MB ChB Ed. 1988; BSc Liverp. 1981; MRCPsych 1993; MPhil. Psychiat. Ed. 1997. Cons. Community Phsychiatrist NHS Shetland; Postgrad. Tutor & Assoc. Adviser in Gen. Pract. NHS Educat. for Scotl.; Clin. Teach. (Fac. of Med.) Univ. Leicester; Hon. Cons. Psychiat. St. Luke's Hosp. for the Clergy Lond. Specialty: Gen. Psychiat. Special Interest: Post Traum. Stress. Prev: Sen. Regist. (Psychiat.) Leics.; Cons. Gen. Psychiat. Leics. & Rutland Healthcare NHS Trust; Clin. Dir.; Regist. (Psychiat.) Fife Train. Scheme.

SHAW, Stephen Douglas Department of Anaesthesia, Aintree Hospitals NHS Trust, Fazakerley Hospital, Longmoor Lane, Liverpool L9 Tel: 0151 529 2565; 79 Meols Drive, West Kirby, Wirral CH48 5DF — MB ChB Liverp. 1983; FRCA. 1991. Cons. Anaesth. Aintree Hosps. NHS Trust. Specialty: Anaesth.; Intens. Care. Prev: Sen. Regist. Rotat. (Anaesth.) Mersey Regional Train. Scheme.

SHAW, Stephen Hirst The Moorings, 100 Selby Road, West Garforth, Leeds LS25 1LW Tel: 01132 862617 — (Leeds) MB ChB Leeds 1967; DPM Leeds 1970; DMJ (Clin.) Soc. Apoth. Lond. 1972; MRCPsych 1972; FRCPsych 1997; MA 1998. cons. Neuropsychiat.; Hon. Lect. (Psychiat.) Leeds Univ. Specialty: Gen. Psychiat. Socs: World Psychiat. Assn.; Brit. Acad. Forens. Sci. Prev: Sen. Regist. (Forens. Psychiat.) United Leeds Hosps.; SHO (Psychiat.) St. Jas. Hosp. Leeds; Regist. (Psychiat.) Scalebor Pk. Hosp. Burley-in-Wharfedale.

SHAW, Stephen Hywel Dalzell Chippenham Surgery, Monnow Street, Monmouth NP25 3EQ Tel: 01600 713811 Fax: 01600 772652 — BM BCh Oxf. 1974; DRCOG 1980; MRCGP 1985.

SHAW, Stephen Rodney 9 Boston Drive, Marton, Middlesbrough TS7 8LZ — MB ChB Dundee 1990.

SHAW, Stuart Antony Graham Harwood Medical Centre, Hough Fold Way, Bolton BL2 3HQ Tel: 01204 521094 — MB BS Lond. 1980 (Westm.) DRCOG 1983; MRCGP 1984, GP Bolton; Clin. Asst. Dept. Genito-Urin. Med. Bolton HA. Specialty: Genitourinary Medicine.

SHAW, Mr Stuart John 7 Moor Park Avenue, Deepdale, Preston PR1 6AS Tel: 01772 886171 Fax: 01772 886181 Email: sjshaw@dial.pipex.com — MB ChB Manch. 1982; FRCS Ed. FRCS (Orth.). Cons. Trauma & Orthopaedic Surg. Preston & Chorley HHS Trust Roy. Preston Hosp., Preston. Specialty: Orthop.; Sports Med.

SHAW, Stuart Lawson Colhook Cottage, London Road, Petworth GU28 9NB — MB BS Lond. 1996 (UMDS) BSc (Hons) Lond. 1991. Med. Off. Roy. Navy.

SHAW, Susan Christine Department of Experimental Psychopathology, Institute of Psychiatry, De Crespigny Park, London SE5 8AF Tel: 020 7919 3363 Fax: 020 7740 5244 — MB BS Lond. 1992 (University College Hospital and Middlesex School of Medicine) BSc Lond. 1989; MRCPsych 1996. Specialist Regist. in Old Age Psychiat.; Hon. Specialist Regist. Specialty: Geriat. Psychiat. Socs: RCPsych. Prev: Clin. Lect. (Psychother.) Inst. of Psychiat. Lond.; Clin. Research Inst. of Psychiat. Lond.; Regist. Rotat. (Psychiat.) Roy. Free Hosp. Lond.

SHAW, Susan Elizabeth Battersea Fields Practice, 3 Austin Road, Battersea, London SW11 5JP; 52 Burnbury Road, London SW12 0EL — MB ChB Manch. 1985; MRCGP 1996. Specialty: Gen. Pract. Prev: Trainee GP Lond.; SHO (Med. & Rheum.) Trafford Gen. Hosp.; SHO (A & E) Stockport Infirm.

SHAW, Susan Patricia Bootham Park Hospital, Bootham Park, York YO30 7BY Tel: 01904 610777 Fax: 01904 453794 — MB BCh BAO Dub. 1977 (TC Dub.) MRCPsych 1981; MMedSci Clin. Psychiat. Leeds 1984. Cons. Psychiat. Bootham Pk. Hosp. York. Specialty: Gen. Psychiat.

SHAW, Therese Bridget St Anne's Hospital, St Anne's Road, London N15 3TH — MB BS Lond. 1986; MRCPsych 1993. Specialty: Geriat. Psychiat.

SHAW, Thomas (retired) Woodlands, May Lodge Drive, Rufford, Newark NG22 9DE Tel: 01623 822379 — (Birm.) MB ChB Birm. 1959.

SHAW, Thomas James Iain 24B Moorbank Road, Sandygate, Sheffield S10 5TR Tel: 0114 230 6723 — MB ChB Sheff. 1972; FFA RCS Eng. 1976. Cons. Anaesth. Chesterfield Roy. Hosp. Specialty: Anaesth. Socs: Assn. Anaesths.; Obst. Anaesth. Assn. Prev: Sen. Regist. & Regist. (Cardiothoracic Anaesth.) Sheff. AHA (T); Staff Anaesth. Univ. Hosp. Groningen, Netherlands.

SHAW, Thomas Raymond Dunlap Department Cardiology, Western General Hospital, Edinburgh EH4 2XU; 29 Merchiston Park, Edinburgh EH10 4PW — MB ChB Glas. 1968; MRCP (UK) 1972; BSc Glas. 1966, MD 1983; FRCP Ed. 1986; FRCP Glas. 1992; FESC 1993. Specialty: Cardiol. Socs: Brist. Cardiac Soc.; Brist. Cardiovasc. Interven. Soc. Prev: Sen. Regist. (Cardiol.) Edin. Hosps.; Hon. Regist. (Cardiol. Dept.) St. Bart. Hosp. Lond.; SHO (Gen. Med.) Roy. Infirm. Edin.

SHAW, Timothy John 3 Church Avenue, Norwich NR2 2AQ Email: 100603.726@compuserve.com — BChir Camb. 1994; MA Camb. 1996; MRCP 1998. Specialty: Respirat. Med.; Gen. Med.

SHAW, Valerie Jane Eleanor 13 Dundela Gardens, Belfast BT4 3DH Tel: 01232 654902 — MB BCh BAO Belf. 1983; DCH RCPI 1987; MRCGP 1988. GP Belf. Retainer Scheme. Socs: Roy. Coll. Gen. Pract. Prev: Trainee GP Belf. VTS.

SHAW, Victoria Marie Diana Nicoresti (retired) 3 Meadsway, 8 Staveley Road, Eastbourne BN20 7LH Tel: 01323 638860 — MB ChB Leeds 1943; DObst RCOG 1945; DPH Eng. 1949; MFCM 1972. Prev: Specialist Community Med. (Social Servs.) Hillingdon AHA.

SHAW, W A Burncross Surgery, 1 Bevan Way, Chapeltown, Sheffield S35 1RN Tel: 0114 246 6052 Fax: 0114 245 0276.

SHAW, Wendy Alison Newbold Surgery, 3 Windemere Road, Newbold, Chesterfield S41 8DU Tel: 01246 277381 — MB BS Lond. 1991 (St. Geo. Hosp. Med. Sch.) BSc (Hons.) Lond. 1988; DRCOG 1993; DCH RCP Lond. 1994; DFFP 1995; MRCGP 1996. Asst. GP Newbold Surg. Chesterfield. Specialty: Gen. Pract. Prev: Trainee GP Warwick, SHO (Geriat. Med.) Northampton Hosp.; SHO (Paediat. & Neonat.) Birm. Heartlands Hosp.

SHAW, Yvonne Pearl Alexandra Gardens Day Hospital, Old See House, 603 Antrim Road, Belfast BT15 4DR — MB BCh BAO Belf. 1974; MRCPsych. 1981. Specialty: Gen. Psychiat.

SHAW-BINNS, Stephanie 10 McKendrick Villas, North Fenham, Newcastle upon Tyne NE5 3AB — MB BS Newc. 1989; MRCGP 1994; DRCOG 1994.

SHAW DUNN, Gilbert Leverndale Hospital, Crookston Road, Glasgow G52 7TU Tel: 0141 211 6400 — MB ChB Glas. 1973 (Glasgow) BSc (Path.) Glas. 1971, MB ChB 1973; MRCP (UK) 1978; MRCPsych 1981; FRCP Glasgow 1990. Cons. Psychiat. Leverndale Hosp. Glas. And Southern Gen. Hosp. Glas.. (Cons. in Psychiat. of old age). Specialty: Geriat. Psychiat. Prev: Sen. Regist. (Psychiat.) Roy. Ed. Hosp.; Regist. (Psychiat.) East. Glas. Health Dist.; SHO (Med.) Glas. Roy. Infirm.

SHAW-SMITH, Charles James 36 High Street, Stetchworth, Newmarket CB8 9TJ — BM BCh Oxf. 1989; MRCP (UK) 1992; PhD 2000. Clin. Lect. (Medical Genetics) Addenbrookes Hosp. Camb. Specialty: Gastroenterol. Prev: Wellcome Research Fell. Gastroenterol. Unit Hammersmith Hosp. Lond.; Regist. (Med.) Hammersmith Hosp. & Ealing Hosp. Lond.; SHO (Med.) Qu. Med. Centre Nottm.

SHAWCROSS, Carol Joan Totley Rise Medical Centre, 96 Baslow Road, Sheffield S17 4DQ Tel: 0114 236 5450 Fax: 0114 262 0942 — MB ChB Sheff. 1976; BSc (Hons.) (Physiol.) Sheff. 1971, MB ChB 1976; DRCOG 1978. Prev: SHO (Obst.) N. Gen. Hosp. Sheff.; Ho. Phys. Roy. Hosp. Sheff.; Ho. Surg. North. Gen. Hosp. Sheff.

SHAWCROSS, Charles Richard Gosport War Memorial Hospital, Bury Road, Gosport PO12 3PW Tel: 02932 524611 Fax: 02932 580360 Email: charles.shawcross@ports.nhs.uk — MB ChB (Hons.) Bristol 1976; BSc (Hons.) Bristol 1973; FRCPsych (1997), MRCPsych. 1980. Cons. Psychiat. Gosport War Memor. Hosp. Specialty: Gen. Psychiat. Prev: Sen. Regist. Mapperley Hosp. Nottm.; Regist. & SHO (Psychiat.) Barrow Hosp.; Ho. Phys. & Ho. Surg. Bristol Roy. Infirm.

SHAWCROSS, Colin Stuart Firth Park Road Surgery, 400 Firth Park Road, Sheffield S5 6HH Tel: 0114 242 6406; 6 Riverdale Road, Sheffield S10 3FA Tel: 0114 662073 — MRCS Eng. LRCP Lond. 1974. Med. Adviser to Kvaerner Metals (Sheff.) Ltd., UCAR

Carbon Ltd.; Clin. Asst. (Endoscopy) Roy. Hallamshire Hosp. Sheff. Prev: SHO (Anaesth.) Centr. (Sheff.) Health Dist. (T); Ho. Surg. & Ho. Phys. Roy. Hosp. Sheff.

SHAWCROSS, Deborah Lindsay John Radcliffe Hospital, Headley Way, Oxford OX3 9DU Tel: 01865 741166; Tudor Lodge, Franklin Road, North Fambridge, Chelmsford CM3 6NF Tel: 01621 742194 — MB BS Lond. 1996 (St. Mary's Hospital) BSc (Hons) Lond. 1993; MRCP 1998, Part 1 1998, Part 2, 1999. SHO (Gen. Med.) Rotat. John Radcliffe Oxf. Specialty: Gen. Med. Prev: Mem. BMA; Mem. MPS.

SHAWCROSS, Joanna Hillside Hospice, 2-4 Mill Gap Road, Eastbourne BN21 2HJ Tel: 01323 644500; Pond Cottage, Friston Place, Eastbourne BN20 0AL Tel: 01323 422422 — MB BS Lond. 1976; DRCOG 1979; Dip. Palliat. Med. 1996. Cons. in Palliat. Care; Asst. GP Sussex. Specialty: Palliat. Med.

SHAWE, Deirdre Jill North Hampshire Hospital, Aldermaston Road, Basingstoke RG24 9NA Tel: 01256 313650 Email: djshawe@aol.com — MB BS Lond. 1978 (Char. Cross) DCH 1981; MRCP (UK) 1982; MRCGP 1984. Cons. (Rheum.) N. Hants. Hosp. Basingstoke. Specialty: Rheumatol. Prev: Sen. Regist. (Rheum.) Northwick Pk. Hosp. Middlx.

SHAWE, Elizabeth Alison 28 Chestwood Grove, Hillingdon, Uxbridge UB10 0EN — MB BS Lond. 1981 (Char. Cross Lond.) FFA RCS Eng. 1988; FFA RCS I 1988. Sen. Regist. (Anaesth.) NW Thames. Specialty: Anaesth. Prev: Regist. (Anaesth.) St. Geo. Hosp. Lond.; Regist. & SHO (Anaesth.) Hillingdon Hosp. Middlx.

SHAWIS, Mr Rang Noory Sadeek Sheffield Children's Hospital, Western Bank, Sheffield S10 2TH Tel: 0114 271 7000 Fax: 0114 276 8419 — MB ChB Mosul 1973; FRCS Ed. 1979; M Ed Sheffield 2001. Cons. (Paediat. Surg.) Sheff. Childr.s Hosp.; Hon. Lect. Med. Sch. Sheff. Univ.; Hon. Sen. Lect. Med. Sch. Sheff. Univ.; Examr., Intercollegiate Bd. for Paediatric Surg. Specialty: Paediat. Surg.; Gastroenterol.; Neonat. Socs: Counc. Mem. BAPS; Brit. Assn. Paed. Gastro. & Nutrit..; BAPES (Brit. Assn. Paed. Endoscopic Surg.). Prev: Cons. (Paediat. Surg.) Tawam Hosp. Alain UAE; Sen. Regist. (Paediat. Surg.) Westm. Childr.s Hosp.; Alder Hey Childr.s Hosp. L'pool.

SHAWIS, Teshk Nouri 10 Westchester House, Seymour St., London W2 2JG — MB ChB Leeds 1989; MRCP (UK) 1994. Cons (Phys.) Colchester Gen Hosp. Specialty: Care of the Elderly. Socs: BMA; Brit. Geriat. Soc. Prev: Sen. Regist. (Geriat. Med.) Qu. Alexandra Hosp. Portsmouth; Regist. (Geriat.) Burnley Gen. Hosp.; Regist. (Diabetic & Gen. Med.) Blackburn Roy. Infirm.

SHAWKET, Saffana Abdul Jabbar 17 Meadowcourt Road, Leicester LE2 2PD — MB ChB Baghdad 1974; FFA RCSI 1984; MSc Camb. 1992. Cons. Anaesth. Geo. Eliot Hosp. Nuneaton. Specialty: Anaesth. Socs: Eur. Soc. Regional Anaesth.; Obst. Anaesth. Assn.; Brit. Soc. of Orthopaedic Anaesth.s. Prev: Sen. Regist. (Anaesth.) Trent RHA; Research Fell. (Clin. Pharmacol.) Camb. Univ. Med. Sch. Addenbrooke's Hosp.

SHAXTED, Edward John Kingswood, 75 The Avenue, Clifftonville, Northampton NN1 5BT Tel: 01604 632309 Fax: 01604 632351 Email: edshax@btinternet.com; 10 Favell Way, Weston Favell, Northampton NN3 3BZ Tel: 01604 403490 — MB BS Lond. 1970 (Lond. Hosp.) DObst 1972; FRCOG 1989, M 1977; DM Nottm. 1982. Cons. O & G Northampton Gen. Hosp.; Vis. Prof. Cranfield Univ. Specialty: Obst. & Gyn.; Medico Legal. Socs: (Counc.) Brit. Soc. Gyn. Endoscopy. Prev: Sen. Regist. (O & G) Nottm. Univ. Hosp.; Hon. Sen. Lect. (Obst. & Gyn.) Birm. Univ.; Regist. (O & G) Addenbrooke's Hosp. Camb.

SHAYLOR, Jane Margaret (retired) Bluebell House, Poplar Avenue, Norwich NR4 7LB — MB BS Lond. 1967 (Westm.) MRCS Eng. LRCP Lond. 1967; MRCP (UK) 1981; FRCP 1999. Prev: Cons. in Repiratory Med. Norf. and Norwich Hosp.

SHAYO, Simon Daniel 114 Eden Close, Slough SL3 8TZ — MB BS Makerere 1974.

SHEA, Mr Frederick William (retired) New Place, 9 Newall Mount, Otley LS21 2DY Tel: 01943 465379 — MB BS Melbourne 1948 (Melb.) MChOrth Liverp. 1953; FRCS Ed. 1956. Prev: Cons. Orthop. Surg. St. Jas. Univ. Hosp. & Wharfedale Gen. Hosp.

SHEA, Mr John Gordon Dewsbury & District Hospital, Halifax Road, Dewsbury WF13 4HS Tel: 01924 512000 — MB BS Lond. 1966 (Char. Cross) MRCS Eng. LRCP Lond. 1966; FRCS Eng. 1974. Cons. Orthop. Surg. Dewsbury Dist. Hosp. Specialty: Orthop. Prev: Sen. Regist. (Orthop.) E. Berks. (Windsor) Health Dist.; Sen. Regist. (Orthop.) Roy. Free Hosp. Lond.; Regist. (Gen. Surg.) Mt. Vernon Hosp. N.wood.

SHEAFF, Michael Timothy Morbid Anatomy Department, Royal London Hospital, Whitechapel, London E1 1BB — MB BS Lond. 1990; BSc Lond. 1988, MB BS 1990; MRCPath 1996. Cons./Hon. Sen. Lect. (Histopath. & Cytopath) Barts and the Lond. NHS Trust. Specialty: Histopath. Prev: Regist. & SHO (Histopath.) Roy. Lond. Hosp.

SHEALS, David Gordon Royal Albert Edward Infirmary, Wigan Lane, Wigan WN1 2NN; Royal Lancaster Infirmary, Ashton Road, Lancaster LA1 4RP — MB ChB Liverp. 1977; DMRD Liverp. 1981; FRCR 1983. Cons. Radio. Morecambe Bay. Specialty: Radiol. Prev: Cons. Radiol. Wigan HA.

SHEALS, Gail Summerdale House, Cow Brow, Lupton, Carnforth LA6 1PE — MB BCh Wales 1976; DMRD Liverp. 1981; FRCR 1983. Specialty: Radiol. Prev: Cons. Radiol. Ormskirk & Dist. Gen. Hosp.

SHEARD, Alan Varley (retired) 7 Northfield, Swanland, North Ferriby HU14 3RG Tel: 01482 633971 Email: gilalsrd@fish.co.uk — MB ChB Leeds 1956; DObst RCOG 1962; DPH Lond. 1967; MFCM 1972. Prev: Dir. Pub. Health E. Yorks. HA.

SHEARD, Jonathan Daniel Henry Green Gates, 10 St Georges Road, Formby, Liverpool L37 3HH — MB ChB Liverp. 1987; MRCPath 1993; MD Liverp. 1997. Cons. Histopath. & Cytopath. Fazakerley Hosp. Liverp. Specialty: Histopath. Prev: Sen. Regist. Rotat. (Histopath.) Mersey.

SHEARD, Lucy Doris (retired) 5 West Parklands Drive, North Ferriby HU14 3EX Tel: 01482 634744 — MB ChB Leeds 1958. Prev: GP S. Cave.

SHEARD, Peter Hubert Walker (retired) Stroud House, Freshwater PO40 9JA — MB BChir Camb. 1957 (Camb. & Guy's) MRCS Eng. LRCP Lond. 1956; MA Camb. 1957. Prev: GP Freshwater, I. of Wight.

SHEARD, Richard Michael Royal Hallamshire Hospital, Glossop Road, Sheffield S10 2JF Tel: 0114 271 1900 — MB BChir Camb. 1993; BA (Hons.) Camb. 1991; FRCOphth 1998. Specialty: Ophth.

SHEARD, Simon Charles BMI Health Services, Grey Friars, 10 Queen Victoria Road, Coventry CV1 3PJ Tel: 01204 844943/02476 500705 Email: ssheard@bmihs.co.uk; Malt House Farm House, 8 Grange Avenue, Kenilworth CV8 1DD Tel: 01926 864452 Email: saschrel@aol.com — MB ChB Bristol 1982; DAvMed FOM RCP Lond. 1988; MMedSci Birm. 1991; MFOM RCP Lond. 1992; FFOM (RCP) Lond. 2000. Director Clin. Developm. Specialty: Occupat. Health. Prev: Roy. Navy Med. Off.

SHEARD, Timothy Andrew Boyd Division of Psychiatry, 41 St Michael's Hill, Bristol BS2 8PL Tel: 0117 928 2342 Fax: 0117 928 3865 — BChir Camb. 1980; MB 1981. CAT Psychotherapist; Clin. Research Fell. Univ. Bristol. Specialty: Psychother. Prev: Cancer Research Campaign Train. Fell. Bristol Oncol. Centre.; Phys. Cancer Help Centre Bristol; McMillan Fell. St. Peter's Hospice Bristol.

SHEARD, Timothy Simon Rawdon Surgery, 11 New Road Side, Rawdon, Leeds LS19 6DD Tel: 0113 295 4234 Fax: 0113 295 4228; 66 Broadgate Lane, Horsforth, Leeds LS18 4AG Tel: 0113 258 4401 — MB ChB Leeds 1983; DRCOG 1987. GP. Socs: Brit. Assn. Sport & Med. Prev: Mem. Leeds LMC; BCG Bd. Mem.; NW Leeds PCG.

SHEARER, Alexander Charles Iain Four Oaks Medical Centre, Carlton House, Mere Green Road, Sutton Coldfield B75 5BS Tel: 0121 308 2080 Fax: 0121 323 4694; Charter House, Church St, Appleby Magna, Swadlincote DE12 7AN Tel: 01570 270257 — MB ChB Birm. 1971; BSc (1st cl. Hons.) St. And. 1960; PhD Birm. (Exp. Path.) 1965. Specialty: Gen. Pract.

SHEARER, Alexander Fleming 5 Fonthill Terrace, Aberdeen AB11 7UR — MB ChB Aberd. 1971.

SHEARER, Alfred James Department of Anaesthesia, Ninewells Hospital, Dundee DD1 9SY Tel: 01382 660111 Fax: 01382 644914; 10 Graystane Road, Invergowrie, Dundee DD2 5JQ Tel: 01382 562444 — MB ChB Aberd. 1971; FFA RCS Eng. 1976. Cons. Anaesth. & Intens. Care, Tayside Univ. Hosps. Specialty: Anaesth.; Intens. Care. Prev: Sen. Regist. & Regist. (Anaesth.) Aberd. Teach. Hosps.; Regist. (Anaesth.) Hosp. Sick Childr. Gt. Ormond St.

SHEARER, Donald (retired) Loch Na Moighe, Culloden Moor, Inverness IV2 5EE Tel: 01463 790676 — (Ed.) MB ChB Ed. 1947;

DPH Ed. 1956; MRCGP 1959; FFPHM RCPI 1988, M 1978. Prev: Cons. Pub. Health Med. & Community Med. Specialist Highland HB.

SHEARER, Euan Sinclair 22 Lingfield Road, Liverpool L14 3LA — MB ChB Liverp. 1982; DA Eng. 1985.

SHEARER, Hamish Lawrie 93 Towerhill Avenue, Cradlehall, Inverness IV2 5FX — MB ChB Glas. 1993.

SHEARER, James Holmes (retired) 4 Dunavon Park, Strathaven ML10 6LP Tel: 01357 521589 — MB ChB Glas. 1952. Prev: Ho. Surg. Vict. Infirm. Glas.

SHEARER, James Malcolm Latham (retired) Grey's Cottage, Maldon Road, Kelvedon, Colchester CO5 9BD — MB BChir Camb. 1948 (King's Coll. Hosp.) FRCGP 1996, M 1977. Prev: Regist. (Med.) Chelmsford Hosp. Gp.

SHEARER, Professor John Robertson Wessex Nuffield Hospital, Woodside House, Winchester Road, Chandlers Ford, Eastleigh SO53 2DW Tel: 023 8027 5478 Fax: 023 8027 5479; Greystoke, Heatherlands Road, Chilworth, Southampton SO16 7JD Tel: 023 8076 8815 — MB ChB Aberd. 1966; PhD Aberd. 1975, MB ChB 1966; FRCS Ed. 1971. Prof. (Orthop. Surg.) Univ. Soton.

SHEARER, Katrina Helen 63 Clepington Road, Dundee DD4 7BQ — MB ChB Glas. 1994.

SHEARER, Kenneth Bowland Road, 52 Bowland Road, Baguley, Manchester M23 1JX Tel: 0161 998 2014 Fax: 0161 945 6354 — MB ChB Manch. 1970; MRCGP 1980. Hosp. Pract. (Cardiol.) Wythenshawe Hosp. Manch.

SHEARER, Kieran Springfield Road Surgery, 26 Springfield Road, Belfast BT12 7AG — MB BCh BAO Belf. 1982; DRCOG 1986.

SHEARER, Lesley Margaret Flat 3, 1 Hamilton Drive, Kelvinbridge, Glasgow G12 8DN Tel: 0141 337 1262 — MB ChB Glas. 1996. SHO (Med. for the Elderly) Mansion Ho. Unit Vict. Infirm. Glas. Specialty: Care of the Elderly; Gen. Med. Prev: SHO (A & E) CrossHo. Ho. Kilmarnock; SHO (Surg.) Hairmyres Hospita Lanarksh.; SHO (Med.) CrossHo. Kilmarnock.

SHEARER, Mr Michael George Dumfries & Galloway Royal Infirmary, Bankend Road, Dumfries DG1 4AP — MB ChB Glas. 1977; FRCS Glas. 1981; BSc (Hons.) Glas. 1975, MD 1992. Cons. Urol. Dumfries & Galloway Roy. Infirm. Specialty: Urol.

SHEARER, Pauleen Elizabeth Cathcart Practice, 8 Cathcart Street, Ayr KA7 1BJ Tel: 01292 264051 Fax: 01292 293803; 23 Forehill Road, Ayr KA7 3DU — MB ChB Glas. 1985.

SHEARER, Raymund Michael Springfield Road Surgery, 26 Springfield Road, Belfast BT12 7AG — MB BCh BAO Belf. 1954; MD Belf. 1966.

SHEARER, Mr Robert John (retired) Royal Marsden Hospital, Fulham Road, London SW3 6JJ Tel: 020 7351 2166 Fax: 020 7376 7163; Kentsleigh, Broadenham Lane, Winsham, Chard TA20 4JF Tel: 01460 30306 Email: robertshearer@kentsleigh.demon.co.uk — (St. Bart.) MB BS Lond. 1962; FRCS Eng. 1967. Prev: Cons. Urol. St. Jas. Hosp. Lond. & St. Geo. Hosp. Lond.

SHEARER, Simon Andrew Devonshire Road Surgery, 467 Devonshire Road, Blackpool FY2 0JP Tel: 01253 352233; 258 Blackpool Road, Poulton-le-Fylde FY6 7QU — MB ChB Manch. 1980; DRCOG 1983; MRCGP 1984. Specialty: Gen. Med. Socs: BMA.

SHEARES, Karen Kwie Kay Respiratory Medicine Unit, Box 157, Addenbrooke's NHS Trust, Cambridge CB2 2QQ Tel: 01223 762007 — BM BCh Oxf. 1993; MA oxf. 1995; MRCP (UK) 1996. Specialty: Pharmacology; Respirat. Med.

SHEARING, Laura Jane 29 Thyme Way, off Lincoln Way, Beverley HU17 — MB ChB Leeds 1988.

SHEARMAN, Anthony John Village Surgery, Gillett Road, Talbot Village, Poole BH12 5BF Tel: 01202 525252 Fax: 01202 533956; 16 Sandecotes Road, Parkstone, Poole BH14 8NX — BM Soton. 1986.

SHEARMAN, Professor Clifford Paul Department of Vascular Surgery, Southampton General Hospital, Southampton SO16 6YD Tel: 023 8089 8801 Fax: 023 8082 5565 — MB BS Lond. 1979 (Guy's) FRCS Eng. 1983; BSc Lond. 1976, MS 1989. Prof. of Vasc. Surg./Hon. Cons. Vasc. Surg., Southampton Univ.; Hon. Sen. Lect. Univ. Soton. Specialty: Gen. Surg. Socs: Vasc. Soc. GB & Irel.; Eur. Soc. Vasc. Surg. Prev: Sen. Lect. & Hon. Cons. Surg. Birm. Univ.; Cons. Vasc. Surg. Soton. Univ. Hosps. Trust.

SHEARMAN, Jeremy David Department of Gastroenterology, Warwick Hospital, Lakin Road, Warwick CV34 5BW Tel: 01926 495321 Fax: 01926 482601 Email: jeremy.shearman@swh.nhs.uk — MB ChB Leeds 1988; BSc (Hons.) Path. Leeds 1988; MRCP (UK) 1991; DPhil 1996. Cons. Gastroenterologist Warwick Hosp. Specialty: Gastroenterol.; Gen. Med. Socs: Brit. Soc. of Gastrenterology; Brit. Assn. for the Study of Liver; American Gastroenterological Association. Prev: Regist. (Gen. Med.) Oxf. RHA; SHO Rotat. (Oncol., Endocrine & Gen. Med.) Oxf. RHA; SHO (Neurol. & Renal.) Univ. Hosp. Wales Cardiff.

SHEARN, Christopher Anthony Health Centre, Windmill Avenue, Hassocks BN6 8LY Tel: 01273 844242 Fax: 01273 842709; New Close Farm House, London Road, Hassocks BN6 9ND Tel: 01273 846639 — MB BS Lond. 1977 (Kings College) DRCOG 1980; MRCGP 1981. Sen. Part. Gen. Pract.; Chairm. W. Sussex MAAG. Specialty: Gen. Pract. Prev: Clin. Asst. (Clin. Med. for Elderly) Cuckfield Hosp.; GP Tutor Mid. Downs - Base Unit.

SHEARS, Daniel 69D Bushey Grove, Bushey, Watford WD23 2GJ — MB BS Lond. 1991.

SHEARS, Deborah Jane 1 Warren Road, Ickenham, Uxbridge UB10 8AA — MB BS Lond. 1990 (Oxford University/St Bartholomew's) BA Oxon. 1987; MRCP (UK) 1993. Clin. Research Fell. (Clin. Genetics) Inst. of Child Health Lond. Specialty: Genetics.

SHEARS, Mary-Rose Byars Seaford Health Centre, Dane Road, Seaford BN25 1DH Tel: 01273 679434; 3A Southdowns Avenue, Lewes BN7 1EL Tel: 01273 472585 — MB BS Lond. 1986; BA (Hons.) Oxf. 1983; MRCGP 1990; DRCOG 1990. Prev: Ho. Surg. Roy. E. Sussex Hosp. Hastings; Ho. Phys. Roy. Sussex Co. Hosp. Brighton & Brighton Gen. Hosp.

SHEARS, Paul Department of Medical Microbiology, Royal Liverpool Hospital, Prescott St., Liverpool L7 8XP — MD Liverp. 1991; MB BS Lond. 1980; FRCPath 1996. Sen. Lect. & Cons. Dept. Med. Microbiol. Roy. Liverp. Childr.'s Hosp. and Dept Trop Med Liverp. Sch Trop Med. Specialty: Med. Microbiol. Prev: Clin. Lect. & Sen. Regist. Dept. Med. Microbiol. Univ. Liverp.; Refugee Health Co-ordinator Oxfam Med. Unit; SHO (Paediat.) John Radcliffe Hosp. Oxf.

SHEARSTONE-WALKER, Christopher George Tuxford Medical Centre, Faraday Avenue, Tuxford, Newark NG22 0HT — BM BS Nottm. 1992.

SHEAVES, Richard Michael The London Clinic, 145 Harley Street, London W1G 6BJ Tel: 020 7616 7713 Fax: 020 7790 7603 — BM BCh Oxf. 1988; Dphil Oxf. 1980; MRCP Lond. 1991; FRCP Lond. 1999. Cons. (Endocrin. & Dermat.) The Lond. Clin. Specialty: Endocrinol.; Diabetes; Gen. Med. Socs: FRCP; Fell. Amer. Endoc. Soc. Prev: Cons. (Phys.) Singapore; Lect. (Endocrin.) St. Bart's Hosp. Lond.; Cons. (Phys.) Jersey.

SHEDDEN, Mr Ronald George 37 Burdon Lane, Cheam, Sutton SM2 7PP Tel: 020 8643 9763 — MD Manch. 1976; MB ChB Manch. 1963; DCH Eng. 1965; FRCS Eng. 1970. Cons. Orthop. Surg. Croydon AHA. Specialty: Orthop.

SHEDDEN, William Ian Hamilton (retired) Beachamwell House, Beachamwell Road, Swaffham PE37 8BF Tel: 01760 724126 Fax: 01760 724135 Email: ian.shedden@ukgateway.net — (Ed.) BSc (1st cl. Hons.) Ed. 1957; MB ChB Ed. 1959; MD Birm. 1967; FIBiol 1970; FRCP Lond. 1991, M 1976; FRCP Ed. 1983, M 1980; FACP 1981; FFPM RCP (UK) 1990. Prev: Cons. Phys. Institut Henri Beaufour, Paris.

SHEE, Charles Damien Queen Mary's Hospital, Sidcup DA14 6LT Tel: 020 8302 2678; Park Farm House, Otford, Sevenoaks TN14 5PQ Tel: 01959 522036 — MD Lond. 1987 (St. Thos.) MB BS Lond. 1974; MRCP (UK) 1976; FRCP Lond. 1995. Cons. Phys. Qu. Mary's Hosp. Sidcup. Specialty: Gen. Med. Socs: Assn. Palliat. Med.; Brit. Thorac. Soc. Prev: Sen. Regist. (Med.) Lond. Chest Hosp.; Regist. & Lect. (Med.) St. Thos. Hosp. Lond.

SHEEHAM, Margaret — MB BCh N U Irel. 1987. Cons. (Path.) Aberd. Roy. Infirm. Specialty: Histopath. Special Interest: Breast; Gastrointestinal Tract; Liver.

SHEEHAN, Anna Loraine Department of Histopathology, Doncaster Royal Infirmary, Armthorpe Road, Doncaster DN2 5LT Tel: 01302 553130 Fax: 01302 553264 Email: lorraine.sheehan@dbh.nhs.uk — MB BS Lond. 1983; MRCPath 1991; FRCPath 2000. Cons. Histopath. Doncaster Roy. Infirm. Specialty: Histopath. Prev: Sen. Regist. (Histopath.) Glos. Roy. Hosp. & Bristol Hosps.; Regist. (Histopath.) Roy. Berks. Hosp. Reading.

SHEEHAN, Mr Anthony John, Wing Cdr. RAF Med. Br. Retd. 9 Ballard Close, Poole BH15 1UH — MB BS Lond. 1960 (St. Mary's) DLO Eng. 1965; FRCS Ed. 1976. Prev: Cons. in Otorhinolaryng. RAF; Ho. Surg. (ENT & Plastic Surg.) St. Mary's Hosp. Lond.; SHO (Cas. & ENT) Roy. North. Hosp. Lond. SHO (ENT) Roy. Devon &.

SHEEHAN, Barbara Eimear 11 Lennys Road, Derryadd, Craigavon BT66 6QS — MB BCh BAO Belf. 1987; DRCOG 1992; Dip Soc. Learning Theory 1997. Staff Grade Paediat. Cupar St Belf. Prev: Trainee GP Ayrsh.; Clin. Med. Off. (Community Paediat.) Belfast.

SHEEHAN, Bartholomew David Department of Old Age Psychiatry, Maudsley Hospital, Denmark Hill, London SE5 8AZ — MB BCh BAO Dub. 1991.

SHEEHAN, Brendan David Castle Surgery, 1 Prince of Wales Drive, Neath SA11 3EW Tel: 01639 641444 Fax: 01639 636288 — MB BCh BAO NUI 1973.

SHEEHAN, Denise Jane Exeter Oncology Centre, Royal Devon & Exeter Hospital, Barrack Road, Exeter EX2 5DW Tel: 01392 210 2114 Fax: 01392 310 2112 Email: denise.sheehan@rdehc.tr.west.nhs.uk — MB BCh Wales 1986 (Univ. of Wales Coll. of Med.) FRCR 1999. Cons. Clin. Oncologist, Exeter Oncol. Centre, Roy. Devon & Exeter Hosp., Exeter; Cons. Clin. Oncologist, N. devon Dist. Hosp. Barnstaple. Specialty: Oncol. Special Interest: Colorectal and Anal malignancies; Urological malignancy. Prev: Regist. (Clin. Oncol.) Roy. Berks. Hosp.; Specialist Regist., Clin. Oncol., Roy. Berks Hosp.; Specialist Regist. Clin. Oncol., Churchill Hosp., Oxf.

SHEEHAN, Georgina Eveline Mary Gloucestershire Health Authority, Victoria Warehouse, The Docks, Gloucester GL1 2EL Tel: 01452 300222; 26 Hyde Avenue, Thornbury, Bristol BS35 1JA — MB ChB Manch. 1977; MFPHM; MFCM 1987. Cons. Pub. Health Med. Glos. HA. Specialty: Pub. Health Med. Prev: SCM SW RHA.

SHEEHAN, Gerard Patrick (retired) Four Seasons, Black Lion Road, Capel Hendre, Ammanford SA18 3SD Tel: 01269 844351 — MB BCh BAO NUI 1948 (Cork) Prev: Orthop. & Gen. Ho. Surg. Grimsby & Dist. Gen. Hosp.

SHEEHAN, Jennifer Mary Woodbridge Road Surgery, 165-167 Woodbridge Road, Ipswich IP4 2PE; 11 Mayfield Road, Ipswich IP4 3NE — MB BS Lond. 1973 (Lond. Hosp.) BSc (Hons.) Lond. 1970.

SHEEHAN, John, MC (retired) 18 Dovedale Road, Stoneygate, Leicester LE2 2DJ Tel: 0116 270 1785 — MB BCh BAO NUI 1941 (Cork) MRCGP 1953. Prev: Ho. Surg. Shotley Bridge Hosp.

SHEEHAN, John Patrick (retired) 50 Carmarthen Avenue, Cosham, Portsmouth PO6 2AQ Tel: 023 9238 1607 — MB BCh BAO NUI 1958 (Cork)

SHEEHAN, Leslie James Services for the Elderly, Ipswich Hospital, Ipswich IP4 5PD Tel: 01473 704137 — MB BS Lond. 1972 (Lond. Hosp.) MRCP (UK) 1980; FRCP Lond. 1994. Cons. Phys. Ipswich Hosp. NHS Trust. Specialty: Care of the Elderly. Prev: Sen. Regist. (Geriat. Med.) St. Geo. Hosp. Lond.; Regist. (Med.) Lond. Hosp. Whitechapel.

SHEEHAN, Nicholas John The Edith Cavell Hospital, Rheumatology Department, Bretton Gate, Peterborough PE3 9GZ Tel: 01733 875143 Fax: 01733 875633 Email: njsheehan@doctors.org.uk; 52 Casewick Lane, Uffington, Stamford PE9 4SX Tel: 01780 757597 Fax: 01780 480038 Email: njsheehan@doctors.org.uk — MB ChB Sheff. 1973 (Univ. of Sheff.) MRCP (UK) 1977; DPMSA 1982; MD Sheff. 1990; FRCP Lond. 1994. p/t Cons. Rheum. PeterBoro. NHS Trust. Specialty: Rheumatol. Special Interest: Inflammatory Jt. Dis. Socs: Pres. of Sect. Rheumatol. & Rehab. Roy. Soc. Med.; Chairm. of the E. Anglian Soc. for Rheum.; Hon. Past Brit. Soc. Rheumatol. (Ex-Hon. Treas.). Prev: Sen. Regist. St. Thos. Hosp. Lond.; Regist. Roy. Hosp. Sheff.

SHEEHAN, Mr Patrick Zaid North Manchester General Hospital, Delaunays Road, Crompsal, Manchester M8 5RB Tel: 0161 720 2847 Fax: 0161 720 2228 Email: patrick.sheehan@pat.nhs.uk; Manchester Children's University Hospitals, Booth Hall Childrens Hospital, Charlestown Road, Blackley, Manchester M9 7AA Tel: 0161 220 5039 Email: patrick.sheehan@cmmc.nhs.uk — MB BCh BAO NUI 1987; LRCPI&SI 1987; FRCS Ed. 1994; FRCSI 1994; FRCS(ORL-HNS) 1997. Cons. ENT Surg. and Paediatric Otolarygologist, Manch.; Cons. Paediatric Otolaryngologist, Roy. Manch. Childrens Hosp.; Cons. Paediatric Otolaryngologist, Booth Hall Children's Hosp. Specialty: Otolaryngol. Special Interest: Paediatric Otolaryngology; Voice disorders; ENT problems in Down syndrome. Socs: Brit. Assn. of Otolayrngology - Head and Neck Surgeons; Brit. Assn. of Paediatric Otolayrngologists; Brit. Voice Assn.

SHEEHAN, Pauline Barbara (retired) 63 Wellwood, Llanedeyrn, Cardiff CF23 9JR Tel: 029 2073 6905 — MB BCh Wales 1966 (Cardiff) Prev: Ho. Off. (Neurol. & ENT) Cardiff Roy. Infirm.

SHEEHAN, Richard Timothy (retired) The Doctor's House, Victoria Road, Marlow SL7 1DN — MB BCh BAO NUI 1941 (Univ. Coll. Dub.) DPH 1947. Prev: Ho. Surg. Roy. Infirm. Worcester.

SHEEHAN-DARE, Robert Alexander Leeds Centre for Dermatology, Leeds General Infirmary, Great George St., Leeds LS1 3EX Tel: 0113 392 2295 Fax: 0113 392 3565 — MB ChB Leeds 1982; MRCP (UK) 1985; FRCP 1999. Cons. Dermat. Gen. Infirm. Leeds & Hon. Sen. Lect. Univ. Leeds. Specialty: Dermat. Socs: FRCP.

SHEEHY SKEFFINGTON, Francis Eugene Denis (retired) 3 Blenheim Road, Wakefield WF1 3JZ Tel: 01924 377358 — MB BCh BAO Dub. 1973 (Trinity College University of Dublin) DCH NUI 1975 DObst RCOG 1975; MRCP (UK) 1978. Prev: Cons. Community Paediat. Barnsley Community & Priority Servs. NHS Trust.

SHEELA SRIDHAR, Kunjuveetil 594 Howlands, Welwyn Garden City AL7 4ET — MB BS Bangalor 1984; MB BS Bangalore 1984; FRCS Ed. 1994.

SHEEN, Aali Jan 5 Cotford Road, Thornton Heath, Croydon CR7 8RB — MB ChB Dundee 1993; FRCS Eng. 1998.

SHEEN, Michael 33 Lynton Court, Century Wharf, Cardiff CF10 5NF Tel: 029 2093 0499 — MB ChB Bristol 1974; DRCOG 1977.

SHEERAN, Ellen Brosna, 180 Liverpool Road, Great Crosby, Liverpool L23 0QW — MB BCh BAO NUI 1951 (Galw.) Prev: Cas. Off. Maidenhead Gen. Hosp.; Ho. Surg. Mile End Hosp. Lond.; Ho. Surg. & Ho. Phys. Noble's Hosp. Douglas.

SHEERAN, Margaret Rachael Mary 5 Marino Villas, Marino Park, Holywood BT18 0AN; 213 Sutton Passey's Crescent, Nottingham NG8 3AE — MB ChB Leeds 1992; PhD Liverp. 1987. SHO (Histopath.) City Hosp. Nottm. Specialty: Gen. Med. Prev: SHO (Gen. Med.) Pinderfield Hosp. Wakefield.

SHEERAN, Padraig Bernardine Majella Brosna, 180 Liverpool Road, Crosby, Liverpool L23 0QW — MB ChB Liverp. 1983. SHO (Anaesth.) Ealing Hosp. Lond. Prev: SHO (Med. Rotat.) Roy. Liverp. Hosp.; SHO (A & E) Ealing Hosp. Lond.; Ho. Phys. & Surg. Mersey RHA.

SHEERBOOM, Derek John (retired) Casa Mia, Halliford Drive, Barnham, Bognor Regis PO22 0AB — MB BS Lond. 1948 (Guy's) LMSSA Lond. 1948; DPH Bristol 1958; MFCM 1972; DIH Soc. Apoth. Lond. 1975. Prev: Employm. Med. Adviser EMAS.

SHEERIN, Declan Finnian Department of Child & Family Psychiatry, Yorkhill NHS Trust, Glasgow G3 8SJ — MB BCh BAO NUI 1982; MRCPsych 1987; MMedSc (Psychotherap.) NUI 1988. Cons. Child & Adolesc. Psychiat. Yorkhill NHS Trust Glas. Specialty: Child & Adolesc. Psychiat. Prev: Sen. Regist. (Child & Adolesc. Psychiat.) Young People's Unit Roy. Edin. Hosp.

SHEERIN, Neil Stephen 41 Holbrook Road, Leicester LE2 3LG — MB BS Lond. 1990; BSc Lond. 1987, MB BS Lond. 1990. SHO (Thoracic Med.) Roy. Brompton Nat. Heart & Lung Hosp. Lond.

SHEERIN, Sheila Mary Stepaside, 32 Manor Park Avenue, Princes Risborough HP27 9AS Tel: 01844 345353 — MB BCh BAO Dub. 1969 (TC Dub.) FRCPath 1993, M 1981. Cons. Haemat. Stoke Mandeville Hosp. Aylesbury. Specialty: Haematology. Prev: Sen. Regist. (Haemat.) Oxf. RHA; Ho. Surg. Westm. Childr. Hosp. Lond.; Ho. Phys. St. Mary Abbot's Hosp. Lond.

SHEERMAN-CHASE, Gaye Lynn Craven Road Medical Centre, 60 Craven Road, Leeds LS6 2RX Tel: 0113 295 3530 Fax: 0113 295 3542 — MB ChB Leeds 1987.

SHEERS, Geoffrey (retired) 1 Barton Bridge Close, Raglan NP15 2JW — MB BChir Camb. 1938 (Camb. & St. Thos.) MRCS Eng. LRCP Lond. 1937; MA, MD Camb. 1951. Prev: Cons. Chest Phys. Plymouth Gen. Hosp.

***SHEERS, Helen** Fron Vox, Llandyrnog, Denbigh LL16 4HR — MB ChB Manch. 1998; MB ChB Manch 1998.

SHEERS, Roger Fron Vox, Llandyrnog, Denbigh LL16 4HR — MB BS Lond. 1970 (St. Thos.) MRCP (UK) 1974; FRACP 1978. Cons.

Phys. & Gastroenterol. Glan Clwyd Hosp. N. Wales. Specialty: Gastroenterol. Prev: Sen. Med. Regist. Broadgreen Hosp. Liverp.; Regist. (Med.) Burton-on-Trent Gen. Hosp.; Sen. Med. Regist. Roy. Adelaide Hosp. S. Austral.

SHEFFIELD, Dennis Gerard, MC (retired) Apple Cottage, Lt. Mongeham, Deal CT14 0HP Tel: 01304 372697 — MRCS Eng. LRCP Lond. 1938 (St. Thos.) MB BS 1939; MD Lond. 1950; MRCGP 1953.

SHEFFIELD, Edward Alexander Frenchay Hospital, Department of Cellular Pathology, Frenchay, Bristol BS16 1LE Tel: 0117 970 1212 Fax: 0117 956 9284 Email: edward.sheffield@north-bristol.swest.nhs.uk — BM Soton. 1980; MRCPath 1986; MD Soton. 1990; FRCPath 1996. Cons. Histopath. N. Bristol Healthcare Trust; Cons. (Path) North Bristol NHS Trust. Specialty: Histopath. Special Interest: Head & Neck; Thyroid. Socs: Association of Clinical Pathologists; International Academy of Pathologists. Prev: Hon. Cons. (Path.) United Bristol Hosps. Trust; Sen. Regist. (Path.) Brompton Hosp. Lond. & Roy. Berks. Hosp. Reading; Sen. Lect. Bristol Univ.

SHEFFIELD, Jonathan Paul Department of Pathology, East Somerset NHS Trust, Yeovil District Hospital, Yeovil BA21 4AT Tel: 01935 707314 — MB ChB Dundee 1981; MRCPath 1991. Cons. Histopath. E. Som. NHS Trust. Specialty: Histopath. Socs: Brit. Soc. Gastroenterol.; Path. Soc. Prev: Clin. Research Fell. (Path.) Imperial Cancer Research Fund St. Mark's Hosp. Lond.; Regist. (Histopath.) Nottm. Hosps.; SHO (Path.) Leicester Roy. Infirm.

SHEFFRIN, Stanley (retired) 7 Alwoodley Chase, Harrogate Road, Leeds LS17 8ER Tel: 0113 266 9846 — MB ChB Leeds 1950; BSc Leeds 1947; MRCGP 1962; MFOM RCP Lond. 1982, AFOM 1979. Hon. Med. Off. Amateur Swimming Assn.; Local Med. Off. Civil Serv. Occupat. Health Serv. Prev: Cons. Med. Adviser Tibbett & Britten plc.

SHEFLER, Alison Gail Paediatric Intensive Care Unit, Oxford Radcliffe Hospital, Headley Way, Oxford OX3 9DU Tel: 01865 741166 Fax: 01865 222061 — MD Toronto 1984 (Univ. Toronto) Cons. Paediat. Paediat. Intens. & Critical Care Radcliffe Hosp. Oxf. Specialty: Paediat. Socs: Fell. Roy. Coll. of Paediat. & Child Health; Fell. Roy. Coll. Phys. & Surg. Canada.

SHEFRAS, Julia c/o David Shefras, 12 Aldenholme, Ellesmere Road, Weybridge KT13 0JF — BChir Camb. 1990.

SHEHAB, Abdullah Mohammed Abdullah 20 The Vale Edgbaston, Birmingham B15 2PR — MB ChB Dundee 1995; MB ChB Dundee 1995; MRCP UK 1998; Dip ME, Dundee, 2000; Mmed Dundee 2002.

SHEHADE, Suhail James Cook University Hospital, Marton Road, Middlesbrough TS4 3BW Tel: 01642 854709 Fax: 01642 854763 Email: suhail.shehade@stees.nhs.uk — MB ChB Glas. 1976; MRCP (UK) 1983; FRCP (Ed.) 1995. Cons. Dermat. Specialty: Dermat. Special Interest: Laser Ther. . Melanoma . PDT. Socs: BMA; N. Eng. Dermatol.s Soc.; Brit. Assn. of Dermat. Prev: Sen. Regist. (Dermat.) NW Eng. RHA; Regist. (Dermat.) W. Midl. RHA; Regist. (Med.) E. Cumbria HA.

SHEHADEH, Emil Saleem 253 Albany Road, Roath, Cardiff CF24 3NW Tel: 029 2049 5959 — MB ChB Glas. 1988; MSc Glas. 1984; BSc (Hons.) Glas. 1983, MB ChB 1988; T(GP) 1993. Prev: Lect. (Psychol.) Cardiff Univ.

SHEHU, Abdullahi Department of Neurology, Walsgrave Hospital NHS Trust, Clifford Bridge Road, Coventry CV2 2DX Tel: 024 76 538954 — MB BS Nigeria 1983; Dip. Clin. Neurol. Lond 1987; MRCP (UK) 1991. Cons. Neurol. Walsgrave Hosp. Specialty: Neurol.

SHEHU, Tijjani Halton General Hospital, Department of Medicine/Cardiology, Hospital Way, Runcorn WA7 2DA; 97 Oaklands Avenue, Saltdean, Brighton BN2 8PD Email: drtshehu@hotmail.com — MB BS Ahmadu Bello Univ. Zaria, Nigeria 1984; MRCPI 1998; DGM RCP Lond. 1999; MSc (Cardiology) Sussex 2001. Staff Phys. (Cardiol.) Halton Gen. Hosp. Runcorn; Regist. (Gen. Med.) Princess Roy. Hosp. Haywards Heath. Specialty: Cardiol. Prev: Regist. (Cardiol.) Dorset Co. Hosp. Dorchester; Locum Regist. (Med.) Crawley Hosp.

SHEIK HOSSAIN, Saddeck Mohammed 399 Carlton Hill, Carlton, Nottingham NG4 1HW — BM BS Nottm. 1994.

SHEIKH, Abdul Jawad Department of Psychiatry, Solihull Hospital, Lode Lane, Solihull B91 2JL Tel: 0121 678 4833 Fax: 0121 678 4828 Email: jawad1984@aol.com; 107 Dovehouse Lane, Solihull B91 2EQ Tel: 0121 682 4664 — MB BS Karachi 1978 (Dow Med. Coll. Karachi) Dip. Psychiat. Lond. 1986; DGM RCP Lond. 1986; MRCPsych 1987; MMedSc Birm. 1996. Cons. Psychiat. Solihull Hosp./Newington Centren & Woodbourne Hosp./BUPA Baukingy Hosp.; Med. Mem. Ment. Health Review Tribunial; Examr. MRCPsych Part II Roy. Coll. of Psychiat.; Second Opinion Assessm. Doctor (SOAD) for Ment. Health Comm.; Review for Commisiion for health improvements (CHI) 2001; Hon. Sen. Clin. Lect. Univ. of Birm. 1997. Specialty: Gen. Psychiat. Socs: BMA; MDU; W.Midlands Inst. Psychother. Prev: Sen. Regist. (Psychogeriat.) Edwd. St. Hosp. W. Bromwich; Sen. Regist. (Adult Psychiat.) All St.s Hosp. Birm. & Midl. Nerv. Hosp. Birm.; Lead Clinician, Business team NHS Trust.

SHEIKH, Abdul Qayyum Queens Road Surgery, 48 Queens Road, Walthamstow, London E17 8PX Tel: 020 8520 2625 Fax: 020 8925 4195 — MB BS Punjab 1965 (Nishtar Med. Coll.) Nat. Chairm. Pakistan Med. Soc. UK.

SHEIKH, Afzal Ahmed 17 Stepney Drive, Scarborough YO12 5DP — MB BS Punjab 1971; MB BS Punjab, Pakistan 1971.

SHEIKH, Aijaz Ahmed Holbrook Surgery, Bartholomew Way, Horsham RH12 5JL Tel: 01403 755900 Fax: 01403 755909 — MB BS Pakistan 1970; DRCOG (Lond) 1986; DTM & H (London) 1987; DCCH Ed 1989; DPD (Wales) 1997. Clin. Asst. Dermat. E. Surrey Hosp. Redhill Surrey. Specialty: Gen. Pract.; Dermat.; Trop. Med. Socs: Primary Care Dermat. Soc.; Brit. Travel Health Assoc.; BMA. Prev: GP Horsham, W. Sussex; Clin. Asst. Dermat., Princess Roy. Hosp., W. Sussex 1995-1998.

SHEIKH, Amer 77 Southwood Avenue, Knaphill, Woking GU21 2EZ — MB ChB Aberd. 1991; MRCGP 1995.

SHEIKH, Asme Kings College Hospital, Denmark Hill, London SE5 9RS — BM Soton. 1990; DCH (Eng.) 1992; FRCA 1996. Cons. Anaesth.; With interest in Paediatric Anaesth. Specialty: Anaesth.

SHEIKH, Azhar Zia Medical Centre, Chesterfield Road, North Wingfield, Chesterfield S42 5ND Tel: 01246 851035 — MB BS Sind 1964 (Liaquat Med. Coll.) Socs: BMA. Prev: Regist. (Anaesth.) Sunderland Gp. Hosps.; SHO Gen. Surg. Salop Roy. Infirm. Shrewsbury; SHO Psychiat. Barnsley Hall Hosp. BromsGr..

SHEIKH, Professor Aziz Division of Community Health Sciences, University of Edinburgh, General Practice Section, 20 West Richmond Street, Edinburgh EH8 9DX Tel: 0131 651 4151 Fax: 0131 650 9119 Email: aziz.sheikh@ed.ac.uk — MB BS Lond. 1993 (Univ. Coll. & Midddlx. Sch. Med.) BSc Lond. 1990; DRCOG 1995; MRCP 1996; DCH 1996; MRCGP 1997; DFFP 1997; MSc Lond. 2001; MD Lond. 2002. Prof. Primary Care R & D Div. Community Health Sci. GP Sect. Uni. Edin.; GP Adviser, BMJ Internat. Edit. Advis. Bd. JRSM. Specialty: Gen. Pract. Socs: Roy. Coll. Gen. Pract.; BSACI; GPIAG. Prev: Nat. Primary Care Doc. Fell. St. George's Hosp. Med. Sch.; GP Asst. Harrow, Middlx.; NHS Research & Developm. Nat. Primary Care Train. Fell. (Gen. Pract.) Imperial Coll. of Sci., Technol. & Med. Lond..

SHEIKH, Haleema Fatima 3 Lord Chancellor Walk, Kingston upon Thames KT2 7HG — MB BS Lond. 1998; MB BS Lond 1998.

SHEIKH, Idris 9 Winchfield Way, Rickmansworth WD3 4DL — MRCS Eng. LRCP Lond. 1977.

SHEIKH, Ijaz Hussain Winwick Hospital, Winwick, Warrington WA2 8RR — MB BS Punjab 1965.

SHEIKH, Imran 51 Beech Hall Road, London E4 9NJ — MB BS Lond. 1998; MB BS Lond 1998.

SHEIKH, Iram Safia 5 Birkbeck Gardens, Woodford Green IG8 0SA — MB BS Lond. 1996.

SHEIKH, Javed Hassan — MB BCh Cairo 1978; BSc Karachi 1973; MRCS Eng. LRCP Lond. 1988; LMSSA Lond. 1988; MSc Pain Management Cardiff 2001. Socs: BMA & Assoc. Mem. RCGP.; Freedom Soc. Apoth. Prev: Civil. Med. Pract. Roy. Engineers 12 RSME Regt. Chattenden Barracks Rochester.

SHEIKH, Javed Younus Kenmore Medical Centre, 60-62 Alderley Road, Wilmslow SK9 1PA — MB ChB Liverp. 1996; MRCGP.

SHEIKH, Mohammad Yunus Trafford General Hospital, Davyhulme, Manchester M41 5SL Tel: 0161 748 4022; 20 The Avenue, Sale M33 4PD Tel: 0161 962 1976 — MB BS Punjab 1963; BSc Punjab 1957, MB BS 1963; DPath Eng. 1970. Cons. (Histopath.) Trafford Gen. Hosp. Manch. Specialty: Histopath. Socs: BMA & NW Represen. Nishtarian Med. Soc. (UK). Prev: SHO (Path.) Bury Gen. Hosp.; Regist. (Clin. Path.) United Sheff. Hosps.; Temp. Sen. Lect. Path. Univ. Edin.

SHEIKH, Mohammed Anwar Parkview Clinic, 60 Queensbridge Road, Birmingham B13 8QE Tel: 0121 243 2000 Fax: 0121 243 2010 — MB BS Punjab (Pakistan) 1962 (Nishtar Med. Coll. Multan) DPM Eng. 1972; FRCPsych 1991, M 1973. Locum Cons. (Psychiat. Child & Adolesc.) Heart of Birm. CAMHS. Specialty: Child & Adolesc. Psychiat. Socs: Assn. Child Psychol. & Psychiat. Prev: Cons. (Child & Adolesc. Psychiat.) Coventry Healthcare NHS Trust; Clin. Co-ordinator CAMHS; Chairm. Child & Adolesc. Sub-Sect. Midl. Div. Roy. Coll. Psychiat.

SHEIKH, Muhammad Nadeem 118 Glen Road, Oadby, Leicester LE2 4RF — MB BCh Wales 1989.

SHEIKH, Munir Ahmad Old Orchard, Manor Way, Ratton, Eastbourne BN20 9BL Tel: 01323 508729 — MB BS Punjab 1961 (King Edwd. Med. Coll. Lahore) MB BS Punjab Pakistan 1961; DPM Eng. 1972. Cons. Psychiat. Ment. Handicap Eastbourne & Hastings HA's. Specialty: Ment. Health. Socs: BMA & Overseas Doctors Assn. Prev: Sen. Regist. (Psychiat.) Mersey RHA.

SHEIKH, Mushkoor Ellahie, Squadron Ldr. RAF Bentley Health Centre, Askern Road, Bentley, Doncaster DN5 0JX Tel: 01302 820494 Fax: 01302 820496; Old School House, Village St, Adwick-le-Street, Doncaster DN6 7AA — MB ChB Aberd. 1984; Cert. Family Plann. JCC 1986; Cert. Av Med. 1986. Specialty: Aviat. Med. Prev: Station Med. Off. RAF Honington; SHO (O & G) Princess of Wales Hosp. Ely; SHO (A & E) RAF Hosp. Ely.

SHEIKH, Nargis Fatima 7 Raphael Drive, Watford WD24 4GY — MB BS Punjab, Pakistan 1971.

SHEIKH, Nassar Seema, Llanvair Drive, Ascot SL5 9LW Tel: 01344 25152; B-2 Belle View Apartments, FL-6 Block &, Clifton, Karachi, Pakistan Tel: 534762 — MB BS Karachi 1986; MRCP (UK) 1991. Regist. (Thoracic Med.) Char. Cross Hosp. Lond. Specialty: Respirat. Med. Prev: Regist. (Med.) Ashford Hosp. Middlx.; Regist. (Gen. & Thoracic Med.) St. Margt. Hosp. Epping.

SHEIKH, Nissar Ahmad 8 Corone Close, Folkestone CT19 5LJ Tel: 01303 275847 — MB BS Punjab 1960; MRCP (UK) 1974. Specialty: Gen. Med.; Care of the Elderly. Socs: Brit. Med. Assn.; Overseas Doctors Assn. Prev: Free Lance Cons. Phys.

SHEIKH, Raian Rahmat Orchard Medical Practice, Innisdoon, Crow Hill Drive, Mansfield NG19 7AE Tel: 01623 400100 Fax: 01623 400101 — MB BS Lond. 1986.

SHEIKH, Saeed Ahmed Sheikh, 91 St. Peters Road, Leicester LE2 1DJ Tel: 0116 254 3003 Fax: 0116 270 0743; 14 Sycamore Close, Oadby, Leicester LE2 2RN Tel: 0116 270 0743 — MB BS Karachi 1967 (Dow Med. Coll.) BSc Karachi 1961.

SHEIKH, Mr Saghir Hussain 88 Wordsworth Way, Bothwell, Glasgow G71 8QS — MB BS Sind 1978; FRCSI 1987.

SHEIKH, Mr Shahid Aziz 252 Bridgwater Road, Wembley HA0 1AS — MB BS Punjab 1982; FRCS Ed. 1992.

SHEIKH, Shahida Bokhari 14 Sycamore Close, Oadby, Leicester LE2 2RN Tel: 0116 270 0743 — MB BS Karachi 1970 (Dow Med. Coll.) GP. Special Interest: Counselling; Psychiat.

SHEIKH, Turabali Badruddin Noorbhai The Clinic, Charles St., Neyland, Milford Haven SA73 1AS Tel: 01646 600268 Fax: 01646 602080 — MRCS Eng. LRCP Lond. 1973; DRCOG 1978. Specialty: Obst. & Gyn.

SHEIKH, Zahid Inayat York District Hospital, Wigginton Road, York YO31 8HE Tel: 01904 631313; 2 Doe Park, York YO30 4UQ — Vrach Lvov Med Inst. USSR 1985; Vrach Lvov Med Inst, USSR 1985.

SHEIKH-SAJJAD, Adina Rihab 49 Sharman Close, Penkhull, Stoke-on-Trent ST4 7LS — LMSSA 1996; LMSSA Lond. LRCS Eng LRCP Lond. 1996.

SHEIKH-SOBEH, Mohammed Vascular Unit, Department of Surgery, The Royal London Hospital, London E1 1BB Tel: 020 7377 7695 Fax: 020 7377 7675 — MB ChB Bristol 1983; MRCS Eng. LRCP Lond. 1982; FRCS (Eng) 1988; FRCS (Gen) 1997. Cons. in Gen. Vasc. & Transpl. Surg. Specialty: Gen. Surg.; Transpl. Surg.

SHEIL, Louise Jane Mount Florida Medical Centre, 183 Prospecthill Road, Glasgow G42 9LQ Tel: 0141 632 4004 Fax: 0141 636 6036; 61 Braidpark Drive, Giffnock, Glasgow G46 6LY — MB ChB Manch. 1984; DRCOG 1986; MRCGP 1990. Specialty: Gen. Pract. Socs: BMA & Med. Wom. Federat. Prev: SHO (Med.) Manch. Roy. Infirm.

SHEIL, Patrick Alan The Health Centre, 80 Main Street, Kelty KY4 0AE Tel: 01383 831281 Fax: 01383 831825; 24 Ross Avenue, Dalgety Bay, Dunfermline KY11 9YN — MB ChB Dundee 1989; RCOG; MRCGP. Specialty: Gen. Pract.

SHEILL, Michael John Cambridge Court, 37 Cambridge Road, Hastings TN34 1DJ — MB BCh BAO NUI 1985; LRCPI & LM LRCSI & LM 1985.

SHEIN, Ilana Gabi 4 Downside Crescent, London NW3 2AP — MB BCh Witwatersrand 1991.

SHEINMAN, Bryan David North Middlesex Hospital, Stirling Way, London N18 1QX; Consulting Suite, Wellington Hosp, Wellington Place, London NW8 9LE Tel: 020 7794 0664 — MB BS Lond. 1976 (St. Bart.) MD (Lond.) 1987, BPharm (Hons.) 1971; MRCP (UK) 1980. Cons. Phys. in Respirat. & General Med., N. Middlx. Hosp. Specialty: Respirat. Med. Socs: Brit. Thorac. Soc.; Brit. Soc. Allergy & Clin. Immunol.; Worshipful Soc. Apoth. Prev: Regist. Roy. Free Hosp.; Research Fell. St. Bart. Hosp. Lond.; Lect. Nat. Heart & Lung Inst. Lond.

SHEK, Fanny Wai-Tsing Flat 3, 10 Roxborough Avenue, Harrow HA1 3BU Tel: 020 8423 9735 — BM BS Nottm. 1993; MRCP UK 1996. Specialist Regist. (Gastroenterol.) Princess Margt. Hosp. Swindon. Specialty: Gastroenterol. Prev: Specialist Regist. (Gastroenterol.) Dorset Co. Hosp. Dorchester.

SHEK, Kwei-Chuen 41 Gloucester Road, Walsall WS5 3PL — MRCS Eng. LRCP Lond. 1982.

SHEK, Rosa Jenny 21 Cuerden Close, Bamber Bridge, Preston PR5 6BX — MB ChB Ed. 1994.

SHEKAR, Chandra Minden Medical Centre, 2 Barlow Street, Bury BL9 0QP Tel: 0161 764 2651 Fax: 0161 761 5967 — MB BS Mysore 1972 (Mysore Med. Coll.) Clin. Asst. (Chest Med.) Bury Gen. Hosp. Prev: Regist. (Med.) Bury Gen. Hosp.

SHEKAR, Saraswathy c/o Mr Allern Braganza, 345 Strone Road, Manor Park, London E12 6TW — MB BS Madras 1987; FFA RCSI 1995.

SHEKELTON, Frances Anne 35 Oakwood Lane, Bowdon, Altrincham WA14 3DL — MB ChB Sheff. 1991.

SHEKERDEMIAN, Lara Sevanne Great Ormond Street, Great Ormond St., London WC1N 3JN; Flat C, 22 St Anns Villas, Holland Park, London W11 4RS — MB ChB Birm. 1990; MRCP (UK) 1993; MD Birm. 1997. Paediat. Gt Ormond St Hosp. Lond. Specialty: Intens. Care. Prev: Research Regist. (Paediat. Cardiol.) Roy. Brompton Hosp. Lond.

SHEKHAR, Satish Scunthorpe General Hospital, Scunthorpe DN15 7BH Tel: 01724 282282 Fax: 01724 290151; 11 Chaffinch Close, Scunthorpe DN15 8EL Tel: 01724 343108 Fax: 01724 343109 — MB BS Magadh 1980; DCH Patna 1983; MD (Paediat.) Ranchi 1986; MRCP (UK) 1990. Cons. Paediat. Scunthorpe Gen. Hosp.; Hon. Clin. Lect. (Paediat.) Sheff. Univ. Sheff. Specialty: Paediat.; Neonat. Socs: Fell. Roy. Coll. Paediat. and Child Health; Roy. Coll. Phys. Prev: Staff Grade (Paediat.) E. Glam. Gen. Hosp. Pontypridd; Regist. (Med.) Roy. Hosp. Sick Childr. Glas.

SHEKHAWAT, Fateh Singh 11 Cheltenham Drive, Kingswinford DY6 9XH — MB BS Rajasthan 1974.

SHELAT, Chandrika Chandramauli c/o Mr P. D. Patel, 30 Audley Road, Hendon, London NW4 3EY Tel: 020 8202 0229 — MD Gujarat 1973 (B.J. Med. Coll. Ahmedabad) MD (Obst. & Gyn.) Gujarat 1973, MB BS 1970; DGO Gujarat 1972.

SHELBOURN, Kevin Richard 58 Harlaxton Road, Grantham NG31 7AJ — BM BS Nottm. 1997.

SHELDON, Ailsa Jane Lindsaye Linkylea House, Haddington EH41 4PE — MB ChB Aberd. 1997.

SHELDON, Christopher David Department of Respiratory Medicine, Royal Devon & Exeter Hospital, Barrack Road, Exeter EX2 5DW Tel: 01392 402132 Fax: 01392 402828 — BM Soton. 1981; MRCP (UK) 1984; T(M) 1992; DM Soton. 1993; FRCP 1998. Cons. Phys. (Respirat. Med.) Roy. Devon & Exeter Hosp.; Dir. Adult Cystic Fibrosis Care; Cystic Fibrosis Consortium. Specialty: Respirat. Med.; Gen. Med. Socs: Brit. Thoracic Soc.; Amer. Thoracic Soc. Prev: Sen. Regist. (Gen. & Thoracic Med.) Lond. Hosp. Whitechapel & Lond. Chest Hosp.; Research Fell. Cystic Fibrosis Brompton Hosp. Lond.; Regist. (Med.) Lond. Chest Hosp. & Whittington Hosp. Lond.

SHELDON, David Maxwell The Pease Way Medical Centre, 2 Pease Way, Newton Aycliffe DL5 5NH Tel: 01325 301888 — MB BS Newc. 1978; MRCGP 1986; BSc 2001. Specialty: Cardiol. Prev: GP Newton Aycliffe; GP Consett Co. Durh.; Clin. Research Phys. Merck, Sharp & Dohme Ltd.

SHELDON, Debra Elizabeth Barbara — MB BCh BAO Belf. 1986 (Qu. Univ. Belf.) Cert. Family Plann. JCC 1991. Retainer Gen. Pract. Specialty: Gen. Pract. Socs: BMA.

SHELDON, Helen Elizabeth Dept. Clinical Psychology, Royal Bolton Hospital, Minerva Road, Farnworth, Bolton BL4 0JR Tel: 01204 390675; 12 Raynham Avenue, Didsbury, Manchester M20 6BW — MB BS Lond. 1973. Adult Psychother. Dept. Clin. Psychol. Roy. Bolton Hosp.

SHELDON, John Victor (retired) Eastontown House, Horn Blotton, Shepton Mallet BA4 6SG Tel: 01963 240288 — MRCS Eng. LRCP Lond. 1940 (King's Coll. Lond. & Westm.) DOMS Eng. 1948; LMCC 1957; BA Toronto 1961. Prev: Chief of Ophth. Oshawa Gen. Hosp. Canada.

SHELDON, Jonathan Howard The Keats Group Practice, 1B Downshire Hill, London NW3 1NR Tel: 020 7435 1131 Fax: 020 7431 8501 Email: jsheldon@fonthill.demon.co.uk — MB BChir Camb. 1988 (Camb. Lond.) BA Camb. 1985; MA Camb. 1989; DCH RCP Lond. 1990; DRCOG 1991; MRCGP RCGP 1992. GP Princip. Lon.; SMO Univ. Coll. Sch. Lon. Specialty: Gen. Pract. Prev: CFP USA.; SHO Whittington Hosp. Lond. GP VTS; Ho. Phys. N. Middlx. Hosp.

SHELDON, Jonathan Westmacott Sirr Queens Hospital, Belvedere Road, Burton-on-Trent DE13 0RB Tel: 01283 566333 Email: jonathan.sheldon@burton-tr.wmids.nhs.uk; Crossfield Mews, Cross Lane, Rolleston on Dove, Burton-on-Trent DE13 9EB Tel: 01283 813355 Fax: 01283 593129 — MB BS Lond. 1973 (St. Thos.) MRCS Eng. LRCP Lond. 1973; MRCP (UK) 1976; FRCP Lond. 1991. Cons. Phys. (Respirat. Med.) Qu. Hosp. Burton on Trent. Specialty: Respirat. Med. Socs: Brit. Thorac. Soc. Prev: Cons. Phys. Burton Dist. Hosp. Burton on Trent; Lect. (Med.) St. Thos. Hosp. Med. Sch. Lond.; Sen. Regist. Lond. Chest. Hosp.

SHELDON, Judith Claire Shillingford Lodge, Shillingford Abbot, Exeter EX2 9QQ Tel: 01392 832222 — BM Soton. 1981; DRCOG 1984; Dip. Occ. Med. 1997. Clin. Asst. Occupat. Med. Roy. Devon & Exeter Hosp. Specialty: Occupat. Health. Prev: SHO (Geriat. & O & G) Guy's Hosp. Lond.; SHO (Paediat.) Alder Hey Hosp. Liverp.

SHELDON, Kenneth Mark Mountain (retired) 10 Borrins Way, Baildon, Shipley BD17 6NP — (Camb. & Lond. Hosp.) MA, MB BChir Camb. 1937; MRCS Eng. LRCP Lond. 1937. Prev: Ho. Phys. St. Luke's Hosp. Bradford.

SHELDON, Kenneth Paul Idle Medical Centre, 440 Highfield Road, Idle, Bradford BD10 8RU Tel: 01274 771999 Fax: 01274 772001 — MRCS Eng. LRCP Lond. 1966. Prev: Ho. Surg. Lond. Hosp. Annexe Brentwood; Ho. Phys. Sheppey Gen. Hosp. Minster; Jun. Accouch. All St.s' Hosp. Chatham.

SHELDON, Laurence Alan Priory Hospital North London, The Bourne, Southgate, London N14 6RA Tel: 07947 762995 Fax: 02084 478138 — MB BS Lond. 1982 (Royal Free Hospital School of Medicine, Lond.) BSc (Hist. Med.) 1979; MRCPsych. 1989; DCH RCP Lond. 1992. Cons. in Child and Adolesc. Psychiat., Priory Hosp.,N. Lond.; Honarary Cons. in Child & Adolesc. Psychiat. St Geo.'s Hosp. Lond. Specialty: Child & Adolesc. Psychiat. Prev: Sen. Regist. (Child & Adolesc. Psychiat.) Lond; Med. Off. Prof. Dept. Med. Baragwanath Hosp. Soweto, S. Afr.; Regist. (Paediat.) Kenepuru Hosp., NZ.

SHELDON, Michael Graham The Mission Practice, 208 Cambridge Heath Road, London E2 9LS Tel: 020 8983 7303 Fax: 020 8983 6800; 23 Lancaster Drive, Isle of Dogs, London E14 9PT Tel: 020 7538 2375 Fax: 020 7538 1551 — MB BS Lond. 1964 (Middlx.) FRCGP 1982, M 1973; BA Open 1994. Hon. Sen. Lect. (Gen. Pract.) St. Bart. & The Roy. Lond. Hosp. Lond. Univ.; Mem. Med. Practs Comm. Specialty: Gen. Pract. Socs: Irish Coll. GP's. Prev: Sen. Lect. (Primary Care & Gen. Pract.) Univ. Nottm. Med. Sch.; Lect. (Cardiac Surg.) St. Thos. Hosp. Lond.; Ho. Phys. & Ho. Surg. Middlx. Hosp.

SHELDON, Nicholas Hanson Holmwood Corner Surgery, 134 Malden Road, New Malden KT3 6DR Tel: 020 8942 0066 Fax: 020 8336 1377 Email: Nicholas.Sheldon@gp-H84042.nhs.uk; Osborne Villa, 29 Bellevue Road, Kingston upon Thames KT1 2UD — MB BChir Camb. 1976 (St. Thoma's Hospital) MA Camb. Senior Partner in General Practice; Vis. Med. Off. Mary Mt. Internat. Sch. Kingston Hill; Clinical Lead in Mental Health, Kingston PCT. Prev: Med. Adv. (Occupat. Health) Kingston Hosp. Trust.

SHELDON, Paul Burnett 6 Tieranan Terrace, Murgon 4605, Australia; 33 St. Andrews Drive, Lowfell, Gateshead NE9 6JU — MB ChB Leeds 1986.

SHELDON, Peter John Herbert Schalscha 42 Holmfield Road, Leicester LE2 1SA Tel: 0116 270 6817 Email: pjs@le.ac.uk; Department of Microbiology & Immunology, Medical Sciences Building, University Road, Leicester LE1 9HN Tel: 0116 252 2953 — MD Birm. 1987; MB ChB 1963; MRCP (UK) 1969; FRCP Lond. 1991. Clin. Sen. Lect. (Immunol.) Univ. Leicester; Hon. Cons. Rheum. Leicester Roy. Infirm. Specialty: Rheumatol. Socs: Brit. Soc. Immunol. & Brit. Soc. Rheum. Prev: Sen. Regist. (Rheum.) Middlx. Hosp. Lond.; Mem. Scientif. Staff MRC Rheum. Unit Taplow.

SHELDON, Philip Watson Eadon (retired) Rockley Farm House, Cumnor, Oxford OX2 9QH Tel: 01865 862123 — MB ChB Manch. 1944; DMRD Eng. 1949; FFR 1953; MA Oxf. 1964; FRCR 1975. Cons. Neuroradiol. Radcliffe Infirm. Oxf.; Clin. Lect. Radiol. Univ. Oxf. Prev: Regist. Dept. Radiol. & Ho. Phys. Roy. Infirm. Manch.

SHELDRAKE, John Hobson Good Hope Hospital NHS Trust, Rectory Road, Sutton Coldfield B75 7RR Tel: 0121 378 2211; Tadorna, 117 Sherifoot Lane, Four Oaks, Sutton Coldfield B75 5DU Tel: 0121 323 3128 — MB ChB Birm. 1981; BA (Hons.) Oxf. 1976; FRCA 1987. Cons. Anaesth. Good Hope Hosp. Sutton Coldfield. Specialty: Anaesth. Prev: Sen. Regist. (Anaesth.) W. Midl. RHA.

SHELDRAKE, Lynn Joy Ashfield Surgery, 8 Walmley Road, Sutton Coldfield B76 1QN Tel: 0121 351 3238; Tadorna, 117 Sherifoot Lane, Four Oaks, Sutton Coldfield B75 5DU — MB ChB Birm. 1981; DRCOG 1984; MRCGP 1986.

SHELDRICK, Caroline Mary 72 Lexden Road, Colchester CO3 3SP — MB BS Lond. 1983; DO RCPS Glas. 1988; MCOphth. 1989. Clin. Asst. Ophth. Colchester. Prev: SHO (Ophth.) Norwich HA; SHO (Ophth.) Blackpool, Wyre & Fylde HA.; Clin. Asst. Leicester.

SHELDRICK, Mr James Harry — MB BS Lond. 1984; BSc (Physiol.) Lond. 1981, MB BS 1984; DO RCS Eng. 1988; FRCS Glas. (Ophth.) 1989; FCOphth. 1989. Lect. (Ophth.) Leic. Univ.

SHELDRICK, Michael Day (retired) 55 Beauchamp Avenue, Leamington Spa CV32 5TB Tel: 01926 426255 — MB ChB Bristol 1952. Examg. Med. Off. for the Benefits Agency; Clin. Asst. in Psychiat. S. Warw. Hosp. Gp.; Reserve Mem. Coventry Appeal Tribunal. Prev: O & G Ho. Surg. Warneford Hosp. Leamington.

SHELLEY, Donald Frederick 7 Vyne Meadow, Sherborne St John, Basingstoke RG24 9PZ Tel: 01256 850573 — MB BS Lond. 1969 (Guy's) MRCP (UK) 1975; DMRD Eng. 1977; FRCR 1978. Cons. Radiol. N. Hants. Hosp. Specialty: Radiol. Prev: Sen. Regist. (Radiol.) Guy's Hosp. Lond.

SHELLEY, Frederick Charles 7-27 Heathside, Avalon, Poole BH14 8HT Tel: 01202 707510 — MB BS Lond. 1952 (Guy's) MRCS Eng. LRCP Lond. 1952; DA Eng. 1960; FRCA Eng. 1961. Barrister (Gray's Inn). Prev: Secretariat Med. Defence Union.

SHELLEY, James Charles 94 Brandon Street, London SE17 1AL Mob: 07720 433230 — MB BS Lond. 1997 (Guy's and St Thomas') BSc (Hons) Lond 1995; DTM & H, Liverp 1999; MRCP (UK) 2000. SpR (Dermatology) Wessex Rotat.

SHELLEY, Joanna Catherine College Clinic Ltd, PO Box 517, Regal House, Queensway, Gibraltar, Gibraltar Tel: 00 350 77777 Fax: 00 350 72791 Email: jshelley@collegeclinic.gi; Thatch Farm, Glaston, Oakham LE15 9BX — MB BS Lond. 1987 (Cambridge, Charing Cross and Westminster) BA Camb. 1984, MA 1991. p/t Private Pract., Coll. Clinic, Gibraltar; Aviat. Med. Examr., Civil Aviat. Auth.; Approved Doctor, Maritime & Coastguard Agency; Port Health Off., Gibraltar. Specialty: Occupat. Health. Socs: Roy. Soc. Med.; BMA. Prev: Police Surg. Roy. Gibraltar Police.

SHELLEY, John Richard, Bt South Molton Health Centre, 10 East Street, South Molton EX36 3BZ Tel: 01769 573101 Fax: 01769 574371 — (St. Mary's) MB BChir Camb. 1967; MA Camb. 1967; DObst RCOG 1969; MRCGP 1978. Socs: BMA; Treas. N. & E. Devon. LMC; RCGP. Prev: Ho. Phys. Qu. Eliz. II Hosp. Welwyn Garden City; Ho. Surg. Salisbury Gen. Hosp.; Ho. Surg. (Obst.) Princess Margt. Hosp. Swindon.

SHELLEY, Katherine Elizabeth 6 Lostock Hall Road, Poynton, Stockport SK12 1DP — MB ChB Manch. 1994.

SHELLEY, Mrs Rosemary Anne Meneage Street Surgery, 100 Meneage Street, Helston TR13 8RF Tel: 01326 435888 Fax: 01326 563310; Tilly Whim, Poldown, Breage, Helston TR13 9NN — MB

BCh Wales 1976 (Welsh Nat. Sch. of Med.) MRCGP 1980. GP Helston. Specialty: Gen. Med.

SHELLEY, Simone Avril 59 The Drive, Edgware HA8 8PS — MB BS Lond. 1983; DRCOG 1987; MRCGP 1988.

SHELLIM, Arthur Jonathan 125 Carlton Towers, North St., Carshalton SM5 2EH; (Surgery) 41 Streatham Road, Mitcham CR4 2AD Tel: 020 8648 2611 — MRCS Eng. LRCP Lond. 1971 (Guy's) DObst RCOG 1973. Prev: Ho. Off. (Gen. Surg. & Gen. Med.) Orpington Hosp. Kent; Div. Surg. St. John Ambul. Brig.

SHELLIM, Maurice Arthur 76 Boydell Court, St. John's Wood Park, London NW8 6NG Tel: 020 7722 7598 — MRCS Eng. LRCP Lond. 1939 (Guy's) Socs: BMA. Prev: Regist. (Dermat.) Guy's Hosp. Lond.; Capt. RAMC, Graded Dermatol.

SHELLING, David North Cardiff Medical Centre, Excalibur Drive, Thornhill, Cardiff CF14 9BB Tel: 029 2075 0322 Fax: 029 2075 7705 — MB BCh Wales 1967 (Cardiff) Fact. Med. Off. Amersham Internat. Prev: SHO (A & E) Unit Roy Gwent Hosp. Newport; Ho. Surg. (Obst.) St. David's Hosp. Cardiff.; Med. Off. Roy. Ordnance Fact. Cardiff.

SHELLOCK, Alison Jane 4 Milton View, Hitchin SG4 0QD — BM Soton. 1996.

SHELLY, Maire Patricia Acute Intens. Care Unit, Wythenshawe Hosp., Southmoor Rd., Manchester M23 9LY — MB ChB Birm. 1979 (Univ. Birm. Med. Sch.) FRCA 1985. Cons. in Anaesth. & Intens. Care Wythenshawe Hosp.; Hon. Clin. Lect. Univ. Manch.; Assoc. Postgrad. Dean, NW Region; Chair, Emerg. & Critical Care Gp., Gtr. Manch. Workforce Developm. Confederation. Specialty: Anaesth.; Intens. Care.

SHELLY, Martin Anthony 1 Suffolk Court, Yeadon, Leeds LS19 7JN — MB ChB Leeds 1980; MRCGP 1985; DRCOG 1985.

SHELLY, Mr Richard William 111 Dunvegan Drive, Lordswood, Southampton SO16 8DB — BM Soton. 1989; BSc (Hons.) Pharmacol. Liverp. 1982; FRCS Ed. 1994.

SHELOCK, Columba Fionnuala McDonagh 99 South Side, Clapham Common, London SW4 9DN — MB BCh BAO NUI 1948 (Galw.)

SHELSWELL, Anthony Eric (retired) Moorways, Ashover Road, Kelstedge, Chesterfield S45 0DT — MB ChB Manch. 1946. Prev: SHO (Anaesth.) N. & Mid-Chesh. Hosp. Gp.

SHELTON, Diana Mary Chest Clinic, Lewisham Hospital, Lewisham High Street, London SE13 6LH Tel: 020 8690 4311; Mycrobacterium Reference Unit, Dulwich Hospital, London SE22 8QF — MB ChB St. And. 1967; MRCP (UK) 1972. Assoc. Specialist (Respirat. Med.) Lewisham Trust; Assoc. Specialist (PHLS) Dulwich Hosp. Lond. Specialty: Respirat. Med. Socs: Brit. Thorac. Soc. Prev: Sen. Regist. (Respirat. Med.) SE Thames RHA; Regist. (Respirat. & Gen. Med.) New Cross Hosp. Lond.; Hon. Clin. Lect. Cardiothoracic Inst. Lond.

SHELTON, Fiona Carol 112 Teignmouth Road, Selly Oak, Birmingham B29 7AY — MB ChB Birm. 1993 (Birmingham) DRCOG 1995; MRCGP 1997. Specialty: Gen. Pract. Socs: DRCOG; MRCGP.

SHELTON, Peter John Millwood Surgery, Bradwell, Great Yarmouth NR31 8HS Tel: 01493 661549 Fax: 01493 440187 — MB ChB Sheff. 1984; DRCOG 1988; MRCGP 1989; FPCert 1998. Prev: Trainee GP Failsworth Health Centre; SHO (Psychiat. & A & E) N. Manch. Gen. Hosp.

SHELTON, Rhidian John Easter Cottage, 25 Low Way, Bramby, Wetherby LS23 6QT — MB ChB Sheff. 1998; MB ChB Sheff 1998.

SHEMBEKAR, Madhuri Vithal Section of Gene Function, CRC Section of Cell and Molecular Biology, Chester Beatty Laboratories, Fulham Road, London SW3 6JB — MB BChir Camb. 1992; BA Camb. 1988; DRCPath 1997. Clin. Research Fell. (Gene Func. & Regulat.) Chester Beatty Laboratories Lond. Specialty: Histopath. Socs: Assn. Clin. Path.; Internat. Acad. Path. (Brit. Div.); Path. Soc. Prev: Sen. Regist. St Thomas' Hosp.; Sen. Regist. Lewisham Hosp.; Regist. (Histopath.) W. Middlx., Char. Cross & Westm. Med. Sch. Lond.

SHEMILT, John Christopher 12 Wykeham Road, Glasgow G13 3YT Tel: 0141 954 9885 — MB ChB Ed. 1975; MPhil. Ed. 1982, BSc (Med. Sc.) Hons. 1972; MRCPsych. 1979. Specialty: Child & Adolesc. Psychiat.; Psychother. Socs: Fell. (Ex-Pres.) Roy. Med. Soc. Edin.; Chair. Of Reg. Dev. Comm. Brit. Psychoanalyt. Soc.; Scott. Assn. Psychoanalyt. Psychother. Prev: Hon. Clin. Sen. Lect. Univ. Glas.

SHEMILT, Mr Philip (retired) 20 The Close, Salisbury SP1 2EB Tel: 01722 336000; 42 Darby Lane, Burton Bradstock, Bridport DT6 4QX Tel: 01308 897050 — (St. Thos.) MB BS Lond. 1938; MRCS Eng. LRCP Lond. 1938; FRCS Eng. 1947. Prev: Cons. Surg. Salisbury Hosp. Gp.

SHEN, Richard Nanyang 232 Noak Hill Road, Billericay CM12 9UX — MB BS Punjab 1984; MRCP (UK) 1990.

SHENDEREY, Kenneth David The Medical Centre, 143 Rookwood Avenue, Leeds LS9 0NL Tel: 0113 264 7278; 8 Ring Road, Shadwell, Leeds LS17 8NJ Tel: 0113 265 6550 — MB BS Lond. 1969 (Middlx.) Cert. FPA 1971; Cert. JCC Lond. 1976. Prev: Ho. Off. Middlx. Hosp.; Ho. Off. Whittington Hosp.; Med. Off. Family Plann. Assn.

SHENFIELD, Francoise 55 Frognal, London NW3 6YA Tel: 020 7380 9435 Fax: 020 7380 9600 Email: mfi@easynet.co.uk — MRCS Eng. LRCP Lond. 1975 (King's Coll. Lond. & St. Mary's) DCH Eng. 1977; MA (Med. Law & Ethics) Lond. 1993. Clin. Lect. (O & G & Infertil.) Middlx. Hosp. Lond. & Univ. Coll. Hosp. Lond.; Fertil. Specialist Lond. Woms. Clinic. Specialty: Obst. & Gyn. Socs: (Comm.) Brit. Fertil. Soc.; Eur. Soc. Human Reproduc. & Embryol.; Scientif. Comm. Condiwater SIG Ethics & Law.

SHENFINE, Claire (retired) 10 Denewell Avenue, Gateshead NE9 5HD Tel: 0191 487 8229 — MB BS Durh. 1961 (Newcastle) Prev: Retd. GP.

SHENFINE, Jonathan Flat 1A Eslington Terrace, Jesmond, Newcastle upon Tyne NE2 4RJ Tel: 0191 281 2246 — MB BS Newc. 1993. SHO Rotat. (Surg.) Newc. Specialty: Orthop.

SHENFINE, Sharon Diane 1A Esslington Terrace, Jesmond, Newcastle upon Tyne NE2 4RJ — MB BS Newc. 1993.

SHENG, Morgan Hwa-Tze 30 Wykeham Road, London NW4 2SU — MB BS Lond. 1982.

SHENKIN, Professor Alan The University Department of Clinical Chemistry, 4th Floor Duncan Building, Daulby Street, Liverpool L69 3GA Tel: 0151 706 4232 Fax: 0151 706 5813 Email: shenkin@liverpool.ac.uk; 10 Rockbourne Green, Liverpool L25 4TH — MB ChB 1969; BSc (Hons.) 1965; PhD Glas. 1974; FRCPath 1990, M 1987; FRCP Glas. 1990; FRCP 1993. Prof. Clin. Chem. Univ. Liverp.; Hon. Cons. Chem. Path. Roy. Liverp. Univ. Hosp. Specialty: Chem. Path. Special Interest: Clin. Nutrit. Socs: Counc. Mem. Nutrit. Soc.; Europ. Soc. for Parenteral & Enteral Nutrit.; Assn. Clin. Biochem. Prev: Cons. Dept. Path. Biochem. Glas. Roy. Infirm.; Lect. (Biochem.) Univ. Glas.; Roy. Soc. Europ. Exchange Fell. Karolinska Inst. Stockholm.

SHENKIN, Ian Richman Cleveland Clinic, 12 Cleveland Road, St Helier, Jersey JE1 4HD Tel: 01534 722381/734121 — MB BS Durh. 1967.

SHENKMAN, John Joseph The Surgery, Stowe Drive, Southam, Leamington Spa CV47 1NY Tel: 01926 812577; Mynyddislwyn, Church Road, Long Itchington, Rugby CV23 Tel: 0192 681 2731 — MRCS Eng. LRCP Lond. 1961 (St. Mary's) MB Camb. 1962, BChir 1961; DObst RCOG 1963. Socs: (Treas.) Gen. Practs. Writers Assn. & BMA. Prev: Ho. Surg. & Ho. Phys. Amersham Gen. Hosp.; Ho. Off. (Paediat.) St. Mary's Hosp. Lond.; Ho. Off. (Obst.) Warneford Hosp. Leamington Spa.

SHENNAN, Andrew Hoseason St Thomas's Hospital, Lambeth Palace Road, London SE1 7EH — MB BS Lond. 1985; MRCOG 1991. Prof. (Obst.) Guy's, King's & St Thos. Sch. Med. Lond. Specialty: Obst. & Gyn. Socs: Roy. Soc. Med. Prev: Hon. Sen. Regist. & Lect. Qu. Charlotte's & Chelsea Hosp. Lond.; Regist. (O & G) Qu. Charlotte's & Chelsea Hosp. Lond.; Regist. (O & G) Baragwanath Hosp. Johannesburg, S. Afr.

SHENNAN, Douglas Hoseason (retired) 9 Hardwick Green, Ealing, London W13 8DN Tel: 020 8997 4363 — MB ChB Cape Town 1950; DPH Lond. 1954; MD Cape Town 1956. Prev: Chief Med. Off. (Tuberc.) Transkei DoH.

SHENNAN, Jill Catherine Flat 9, Summertown House, Banbury Road, Oxford OX2 7QZ — MB ChB Dundee 1985.

SHENNAN, Mr John Millward BUPA Murrayfield Hospital, Holmwood Drive, Thingwall, Wirral CH61 1AU Tel: 0151 929 5182 — MB ChB (Hons.) Liverp. 1963; FRCS Ed. 1967; FRCS Eng. 1968. Cons. Surg., BUPA Murrayfield Hosp., Wirral.; Hon. Lect. In Surg. Univ. Liverp. Specialty: Gen. Surg. Socs: Assn. of Surg. GB & Irel.; Brit. Assn. Surg. Oncol.; Brit. Assn. of Breast Surg. Prev: Cons. Gen.

Surg. Wirral Hosp.NHS Trust; Cons. Gen. Surg. Whiston & St. Helens Hosps.; Cons. Gen. Sur. Wirral NHS Trust Hosp.

SHENNAN, William John Shankland Medical Centre, 3 Edinburgh Road, Perth PH2 8AT — MB ChB Dundee 1980.

SHENOLIKAR, Mr Aneil Huddersfield Royal Infirmary, Lindley, Huddersfield HD3 3EA Tel: 01484 342457; 100 Sturthes Hall Lane, Kirkburton, Huddersfield HD8 0PT Tel: 01484 606109 Email: a.shenolikar@virgin.net — MB ChB Dundee 1986; BMSc Dund 1983; FRCS Glas. 1990; FRCS Orth. 1997. Cons. (Orthop. Surg.) Huddersfield Roy. Infirm. Specialty: Trauma & Orthop. Surg. Socs: Brit. Orthopaedic Assn.; Brit. Orthopaedic Foot Surg. Soc.; FRCPSG. Prev: Sen. Regist. (Trauma & Orthop.) S. Wales; Regist. Rotat. (Orthop.) Morriston Hosp. Swansea, W. Wales Gen. Hosp. Carmarthen & Cardiff Roy. Infirm.; Regist. Rotat. (Surg.) Aberd. Roy. Infirm.

SHENOLIKAR, Mr Balwant Kashinath (retired) Aneil-Sarita, 164 Lower Morden Lane, Morden SM4 4SS — MB Calcutta 1947 (Carmichael Med. Coll. Calcutta) FRCS Ed. 1955; FRCS Eng. 1957; FBIM 1982. Prev: Sen. Med. Off. Dept. Health & Social Security.

SHENOLIKAR, Vindra Y Gilfach Glyd, Plascadwgan Road, Ynystawe, Swansea SA6 5AG; Y Gilfach Clyd, Plas Ladwian Road, Ynystawe, Swansea SA6 5AG Tel: 01792 845705 — MB ChB Aberd. 1992. Ho. Off. (Gen. Surg.) E. Glam. Hosp. Prev: Ho. Off. (Med.) Morriston Hosp. Swansea.

SHENOUDA, Mr Nabil Adib (retired) 31 Whitethorn Gardens, Enfield EN2 6HF Tel: 020 8366 0194 — MB BCh Cairo 1965 (Kasr El-Aini) Dip. Gen. Surg. Cairo 1968; Dip. Orthop. Surg. Cairo 1970; FRCS Ed. 1979. Prev: Clin. Asst. (Orthop. Surg.) Harold Wood Hosp.

SHENOY, Ashok Narayan 39 Goodwin Gardens, Waddon Way, Croydon CR0 4HS Tel: 020 8681 5633 — MB BS Mysore 1978; MD (Anaesth.) Bangalore 1984; DA (UK) 1988; FRCA. 1992. Regist. (Anaesth.) St. Thos. Hosp. Lond. Specialty: Anaesth.

SHENOY, Kudpi Krishnakantha 16 Abbotsbury Way, Nuneaton CV11 4GB Email: shnink@hotmail.com — MB BS Mysore 1974; DObst RCPI 1984; DRCOG 1984; Dip. Gen. Psychiat. Keele 1991. Locum Cons. Old age Psychi. St. Martins' Hosp. Bath. Specialty: Gen. Psychiat. Prev: Staff Psychiat. N. Warks. NHS Trust, Nuneaton.

SHENTON, Antony Frank 39 Aylmer Grove, Newton Aycliffe DL5 4NF — MB BS Newc. 1977.

SHENTON, Frederick George Alan Bybridge, 142 Percy Road, Twickenham TW2 6JG Tel: 020 8894 6888 — MRCS Eng. LRCP Lond. 1953 (Univ. Coll. Hosp.) MA Camb. 1952. Socs: MRCGP; BMA. Prev: GP Hounslow; Ho. Surg. & Ho. Phys. City Gen. Hosp. Stoke-on-Trent; Med. Off. RAMC.

SHENTON, Geoffrey Alister 37 Toyne Street, Sheffield S10 1HH — MB ChB Sheff. 1995.

SHENTON, Karyn Clare 15 Keele Road, Newcastle ST5 2JT — MB BS Lond. 1990; FRCS Eng. 1995. Specialist Regist., SW Thames Rotat., Gen. Surg. Specialty: Gen. Surg. Prev: Research Regist. (Breast Surg.) St. Geo. Hosp. Lond.

SHENTON, Mark Irving Stowhealth, Violet Hill House, Violet Hill Road, Stowmarket IP14 1NL Fax: 01449 776005 Email: mark.sair@phnt.swest.nhs.uk — MB BS Newc. 1989.

SHENTON, Paul Adrian Maswell Park Health Centre, Hounslow Avenue, Hounslow TW3 2DY Tel: 020 8321 3488 Fax: 020 8893 4368; 7 Tring Court, 60 Waldegrave, Twickenham TW1 4TH — MB BS Lond. 1980 (University College Hospital, London) DRCOG 1985; MRCGP 1986. Socs: BMA. Prev: Trainee GP Middlx. VTS.; Ho. Surg. & Ho. Phys. Northampton Gen. Hosp.

SHEPARD, Clare Louise 19 Limes Way, Shabbington, Aylesbury HP18 9HB — BM Soton. 1996.

SHEPARD, Mr Gordon James Department of Orthopaedics, Manchester Royal Infirmary, Manchester; 10 Wrenswood Drive, Worsley, Manchester M28 7GS Tel: 01204 390390 — MB ChB Leic. 1990 (Leicester) FRCS Ed. 1995. Specialist Regist. NW Region. Specialty: Trauma & Orthop. Surg. Socs: BOSTA; BTS; Assoc. Mem. BOA. Prev: Regist. (Orthop.) Roy. Liverp. Hosp., Whiston Hosp. Prescot & Arrowe Pk. Hosp. Wirral.

SHEPHARD, Mr Edmund 10 Harley Street, London W1N 1AA Tel: 020 7467 8300; Grove Lodge, Hunton, Maidstone ME15 0SE Tel: 01622 820318 — MRCS Eng. LRCP Lond. 1940 (Oxf. & St. Bart.) BM BCh Oxon. 1942; FRCS Eng. 1951. Hon. Cons. Orthop. Surg. SE Thames RHA. Specialty: Orthop. Socs: Sen. Fell. BOA; Emerit. Fell. Internat. Soc. Orthop. & Accid. Surg; Medico-Legal Soc. Prev: Chief Asst. (Orthop.) St. Bart. Hosp.; Maj. RAMC Surg. Specialist; Ho. Surg. (Orthop.) Hosp. Oswestry.

SHEPHARD, Edmund Peter 80 Harley Street, London W1G 7HL Tel: 020 7637 4962 Fax: 020 7637 4963 Email: drpete1@attglobal.net — MB BS Lond. 1970; BA (1st cl. Hons. Physics) Oxf. 1964; MRCP UK 1972; MD Lond. 1979; T(M) 1991. Hon. Research Fell. Univ. Coll. Lond.; Hon. Cons. Phys. St Luke's Hosp. for the Clergy. Specialty: Gen. Med.; Diabetes; Endocrinol. Prev: Research Fell. (Nuclear Physics) Ecole Polytechnique Paris & CERN, Geneva; Sen. Regist. & Chief Asst. (Med. Profess. Unit) St. Bart Hosp. Lond.

SHEPHARD, Elizabeth Anne 2 Heron Court, 53 Alexandra Rd, Epsom KT17 4HU Tel: 01372 749130 — MB ChB Glas. 1979; DRCOG 1982; DCH RCPS Glas. 1983; MRCGP 1984. Asst. GP Crieff. Prev: Asst. Br. Med. Off. Brit. Red Cross Soc. Perth & Kinross.

SHEPHARD, Elizabeth Ruth St. Helier Hospital, Wrythe Lane, Carshalton SM5 1AA Tel: 020 8296 2926 Email: rshephard@sthelier.sghms.ac.uk — MB ChB Bristol 1990 (Bristol Univ.) MRCP (UK) 1994; DRCOG 1995. Cons. Neonatologist, St. Helier Hosp., Wrythe La., Charshalton, Surrey, SM5 1AA. Specialty: Paediat. Prev: SpR Neonat. Medicare, Kings Coll. Hosp.; SpR Neonat. Medicare Mayday Univ. Hosp.; SpR Neonat. Medicare St Geo.'s Hosp.

SHEPHARD, Graham David Hopper (retired) Brook Cottage, Walton Cardiff, Tewkesbury GL20 7BL — MB BChir Camb. 1953; MA Camb. 1954; DObst RCOG 1954. Prev: on Staff Tewkesbury Hosp.

SHEPHARD, John Andrew 4 The Green, Horrabridge, Yelverton PL20 7QP — MB BS Lond. 1991.

SHEPHARD, John Neville Pinehurst, 12 Bassett Row, Southampton SO16 7FS — MB BS Lond. 1985. Sen. Regist. (Anaesth.) Shackleton Dept. of Anaesth. Soton. Gen. Hosp. Specialty: Anaesth. Socs: Fell. Roy. Coll. Anaesth.

SHEPHARD, Neville Wilson Peterscroft, Stuckton, Fordingbridge SP6 2HG — MB ChB Sheff. 1953; DObst RCOG 1958; FFPM RCP (UK) 1990. Dir. Med. Sci. Research Buckingham. Specialty: Pharmaceutical Medicine. Socs: Fell. Roy. Soc. Med.; Brit. Pharm. Soc. Prev: Med. & Research Dir. Ortho Pharmaceut. Ltd. Saunderton; Head, Clin. Research Roussel Laborats.

SHEPHARD, Mr Reginald Harry The Oaks, 776 Wollaton Road, Wollaton, Nottingham NG8 2AP Tel: 0115 928 5602 — MB BS Lond. 1945 (Univ. Coll. Hosp. & Yale Univ.) MD Yale 1943; MRCS Eng. LRCP Lond. 1944; FRCS Eng. 1950. Emerit. Cons. Neurosurg. Derby & Leicester Hosp. Gps. Specialty: Neurosurg. Socs: Soc. Brit. Neurol. Surgs.; Past Pres. Derby. Med. Soc; Leics.Med.Soc. Prev: Sen. Regist. Neurosurg. Lond. Hosp. & Maida Vale Hosp. Nerv. Dis.; Surg. Regist. Univ. Coll. Hosp.

SHEPHEARD, Antony Charles Westbyfleet Health Centre, Madeira Road, West Byfleet KT14 6DH Tel: 01932 336933 Fax: 01932 355681; The Hoyte, Woodham Lane, Woodham, Weybridge KT13 3QA Tel: 01932 34839 — BM BCh Oxf. 1971.

SHEPHEARD, Mr Brian George Frank Parkfield, Park Lane, Greenfield, Oldham OL3 7DX Tel: 0145 773257 — MB BS Lond. 1962 (Lond. Hosp.) BSc Lond. 1959, MB BS 1962; FRCS Eng. 1969. Cons. Urol. Oldham AHA. Specialty: Urol. Socs: Assoc. Mem. Brit. Assn. Urol. Surgs. Prev: Sen. Regist. Roy. Marsden Hosp. Lond.; Sen. Regist. St. Peters' Hosps. Lond.; Surg. Regist. Lond. Hosp.

SHEPHERD, Alan Neill The Knowe, 43 Queen St., Perth PH2 0EJ — MB ChB Dundee 1975; BSc (Med. Sci.) St. And. 1972; MRCP (UK) 1978; FRCP Ed. 1989; FRCPS 1990. Cons. Phys. Perth Roy. Infirm.; Hon. Sen. Lect. Univ. Dundee. Specialty: Gen. Med. Prev: Lect. (Hon. Sen. Regist.) Univ. Dept. Med. Ninewells Hosp. & Med.; Sch. Dundee; Regist. Univ. Dept. Mat. Med. Stobhill Hosp. Glas. & Univ. Dept. Med. W. Infirm. Glas.

SHEPHERD, Alison Judith — MB ChB Leeds 1995; BSc (Psychol.) Leeds Univ. 1992; Dip Dermat Cardiff 2003. Salaried GP. Specialty: Gen. Pract. Prev: GP Regist. Leeds VTS; Ho. Off. (Surg.) Airedale Gen. Hosp.; Ho. Off. (Med.) N. Allerton Hosp.

SHEPHERD, Alistair John Newbolt National Blood Service Liverpool Centre, West Derby St., Liverpool L7 8TW Tel: 0151 551 8800 Fax: 0151 551 8895 Email: alistair.shepherd@nbs.nhs.uk; 28 Bath Street, Liverpool L22 5PS Tel: 0151 920 7189 — MB ChB Liverp. 1967; FRCPath 1989, M 1977; DOccMed. 1998. Cons. Haemat. Nat. Blood Serv. Liverp. Centre Liverp. Specialty: Blood

Transfus. Special Interest: Transfus. Microbiol. Socs: Assn. Clin. Path.; Liverp. Med. Inst.; Soc. Occupat. Med. Prev: Sen. Regist. (Haemat.) Liverp. AHA (T); Regist. (Haemat.) Nottm. City Hosp.; SHO (Haemat.) St. Thos. Hosp. Lond.

SHEPHERD, Mr Allister Frederick Irwin Elm Cottage, Craggs Lane, Tunstall, Richmond DL10 7RB — MB BCh BAO Belf. 1973; FRCS Ed. 1978. Cons. Surg. MOD Hosp. Unit Friarage Hosp. Northallerton; Command Off. MOD Hosp. Unit Friarage Hosp. Northallerton. Specialty: Gen. Surg. Socs: Roy. Soc. Med. & Milit. Surg. Soc.; Assn. Surg. Prev: Sen. Regist. (Surg.) Canterbury & Margate Hosps.; Cons. Surg. BMH, Hong Kong; Cons. Surg. Milit. Wing Musgrave Pk.

SHEPHERD, Andrew David Heaton Moor Medical Centre, 32 Heaton Moor Road, Stockport SK4 4NX Tel: 0161 432 0671; 5 Styperson Way, Poynton, Stockport SK12 1UJ Tel: 01625 858840 Fax: 01625 858840 — MB ChB Manch. 1971; DObst RCOG 1973.

SHEPHERD, Andrew James 40 Wylde Green Road, Sutton Coldfield B72 1HD — MB ChB Bristol 1998.

SHEPHERD, Angela Mary Urodynamic Unit, Southmead Hospital, Bristol BS10 5NB Tel: 0117 959 5181 Fax: 0117 950 2229; Pine Cottage, Old Down, Tockington, Bristol BS32 4PP Tel: 01454 416466 — (Bristol) MB ChB Bristol 1968; FRCOG 1988, M 1974; MD Bristol 1980. Clin. Dir. Urodynamic Unit Southmead Hosp. Bristol. Specialty: Urol. Socs: Chartered Soc. Physiother.; Bristol M-C Soc.; Internat. Urogyn. Assn. Prev: Research Fell. (Urol.) Ham Green Hosp. Bristol; Regist. (O & G) Roy. Free Hosp. Lond.; SHO (Obst. & Paediat.) Harari Hosp., Zimbabwe.

SHEPHERD, Annie McLeod 8 St Clair Terrace, Edinburgh EH10 5NW Tel: 0131 447 6647 — MB ChB Ed. 1950; BSc Ed. 1945, MB ChB 1950. Socs: Med. Wom. Federat.

SHEPHERD, Barbara Catherine Green End Surgery, 58 Green End, Comberton, Cambridge CB3 7DY Tel: 01223 262500 Fax: 01223 264401; 4 Eltisley Avenue, Cambridge CB3 9JG Tel: 01223 365571 — MB BChir Camb. 1990; MA Camb. 1990; DRCOG 1991; DCH RCP Lond. 1993; MRCGP 1993. GP Camb.

SHEPHERD, Beryl Mary 1 Forgan Way, Newport-on-Tay DD6 8JQ — MB ChB St. And. 1969; MRCPsych 1985. Cons. Psychiat. Roy. Dundee Liff Hosp. Specialty: Gen. Psychiat.

SHEPHERD, Caroline West Grove, 420 Blackness Road, Dundee DD2 1TQ Tel: 01382 68313 — MB ChB Aberd. 1980; DRCOG 1984; DCCH RCP Ed. 1984; MRCGP 1985.

SHEPHERD, Carolyn Deborah Seaside Medical Centre, 18 Sheen Road, Eastbourne BN22 8DR Tel: 01323 725667 Fax: 01323 417169; Goldrings, PrideAUX Rd, Eastbourne BN21 2ND — MB BS Lond. 1983.

SHEPHERD, Charles Bernard Friars Cottage Surgery, Queens Square, Chalford Hill, Stroud GL6 8EH Tel: 01453 885462 Fax: 01453 885462 — MB BS Lond. 1974 (Middlx.) Cons. Med. to UK ME Assn. & Clin. Adviser Media Resource Servs. (CIBA Foundat.). Specialty: Gen. Med.; Neurol.; Medico Legal; Research. Socs: Med. Adviser to ME Assn. of S. Afr.; BMA & Campaign Against Health Fraud. Prev: Resid. Med. Off. Cirencester Memor. Hosp.; SHO (Sexually Transm. Dis.) Middlx. Hosp. Lond.; SHO (Paediat.) Princess Margt. Hosp. Swindon.

SHEPHERD, Charles William 44 Mullahead Road, Tandragee, Craigavon BT62 2LA — MB BCh BAO Belf. 1979; MRCP (UK) 1984; MD Belf. 1995. Cons. Paediat. Craigavon Area Hosp. Specialty: Paediat. Prev: Sen. Regist. (Paediat.) Roy. Hosp. for Sick Childr. Glas.; Regist. (Paediat.) Ulster Hosp. Dundonald, Baragwanath Hosp. Johannesburg & Belf. City Hosp.

SHEPHERD, Christopher Michael Filey Surgery, Station Avenue, Filey YO14 9AE — MB BChir Camb. 1988. GP. Specialty: Gen. Pract.

SHEPHERD, Daniel Tobias Sherrington Randmoor Cottage, Robins Lane, Coppice Row, Theydon Bois, Epping CM16 7DS — MB BS Lond. 1996.

SHEPHERD, David Brynne 5 Spout Spinney, Stannington, Sheffield S6 6EQ — MB ChB Leeds 1985; FRCA 1993. Regist. (Anaesth.) Sheff. Specialty: Anaesth.

SHEPHERD, David Christian (retired) Rosehaven, 490 Pilgrims Way, Wouldham, Rochester ME1 3RB Tel: 01634 861416 Fax: 01634 861416 — MB ChB Aberd. 1965; DObst RCOG 1968.

SHEPHERD, Mr David Francis Charles Royal Bournemouth Hospital, Castle Lane, Bournemouth BH7 7DW Tel: 01202 704113 Fax: 01202 704035 Email: david.shepherd@rbc-tr.swest.nhs.uk — MB BChir Camb. 1970; FRCS Eng. 1974; FRCR Eng. 1979. Cons. Radiol. (Interventional & Gastrointestinal) Roy. Bournemouth Hosp. Specialty: Radiol. Special Interest: Interventional & Gastrointestinal Radiol. Socs: Europ. Soc. Gastrointestingal & Interventional Radiol.; CIRSE; BSIR. Prev: Sen. Regist. (Radiol.) Soton. Gen. Hosp.; Regist. (Gen. Surg.) Peace Memor. Hosp. Watford.

SHEPHERD, David James Saffron Group Practice, 509 Saffron Lane, Leicester LE2 6UL Tel: 0116 244 0888 Fax: 01162 831405 — BM BCh Oxf. 1985; MRCGP 1989; DRCOG 1989. Socs: BMA. Prev: Med. Off. Berega Hosp., Tanzania.

SHEPHERD, David Richard Thompson Level 8, Belfast City Hospital, 93 Lisburn Road, Belfast BT9 7AB Tel: 02890 329241; 17 Richmond Court, Lisburn BT27 4QU Tel: 02892 665305 — MB BCh BAO Belf. 1971; MRCP (UK) 1976; MRCGP 1977; FRCP Lond. 1994. Cons. Phys. Belf. City Hosp. Specialty: Respirat. Med.

SHEPHERD, Deborah Anne 71 Hornhill Road, Rickmansworth WD3 9TG — MB BS Lond. 1990.

SHEPHERD, Debra Joy 3 Park Terrace, Loftus, Saltburn-by-the-Sea TS13 4HU — MB BS Lond. 1996.

SHEPHERD, Elizabeth Helen 38 Colchester Avenue, Pen-y-Lan, Cardiff CF23 9BP — BM Soton. 1996.

SHEPHERD, Francis George Graham (retired) 308 North Deeside Road, Cults, Aberdeen AB15 9SB Tel: 01224 868721 — MB ChB Aberd. 1948; FRCGP 1978.

SHEPHERD, Gillian Helen Harrogate District Hospital, Lancaster Park Road, Harrogate HG2 7SX Tel: 01423 885959; Spring Close, 25 Rossett Drive, Harrogate HG2 9NS — MB ChB Leeds 1979; MB ChB (Hons.) Leeds 1979; FRCS Ed. 1989; FRCOphth. 1989. Assoc. Specialist Ophth. Harrogate. Specialty: Ophth. Prev: Regist. (Ophth.) Harrogate Dist. Hosp.

SHEPHERD, Gillian Louise 4 Netherton Road, St. Margarets, Twickenham TW1 1LZ — MB BS Lond. 1976 (Univ. Coll. Hosp.) MRCP (UK) 1980; MD Lond. 1984; MRCGP 1985. Specialty: Cardiol. Prev: Clin. Director in Cardiovasc. Clin. Developm., Glaxo; Regist. (Med.) Hammersmith Hosp. Lond.; Mem. Clin. Pharmacol. Subcomm. Roy. Coll Phys.

SHEPHERD, Gordon Andrew Allison Ark Occupational Health, 6 BonAccord Cres Lane, Aberdeen AB11 6DF Tel: 01224 584584 Fax: 01224 584567/01722 334011 — MB ChB Glas. 1973; AFOM RCP Lond. 1991. Occupat. Phys. Specialty: Occupat. Health. Socs: Soc. Occupat. Med. Prev: Research Fell. (Clin. Biochem. & Metab. Med.) Roy. Vict. Infirm. Newc.; Resid. (Endocrinol. & Metab.) Univ. West. Ontario & Assoc. Hosps., Canada; Regist. (Med.) Raigmore Hosp. Inverness.

SHEPHERD, Henry Robert, DSC (retired) 4 The Glade, Enfield EN2 7QH Tel: 020 8363 3677 — MB ChB Liverp. 1942. Mem. Enfield HA; Mem. Enfield & Haringey FPC. Prev: O & G Ho. Surg. Liverp. Roy. Infirm.

SHEPHERD, Hilary Jean 4 Troon Drive, Bridge of Weir PA11 3HF Tel: 01505 614155 — MB ChB Glas. 1965. Prev: Ho. Phys. Stobhill Hosp. Glas.; Ho. Surg. Roy. Alexandra Infirm. Paisley.

SHEPHERD, Hugh Arkwright Flexford House, Flexford Road, North Baddesley, Southampton SO52 9DF — MB BChir Camb. 1976; BA (Hons.) Camb. 1972, MA, MB 1976, BChir 1975; MRCP (UK) 1978; MD 1985. Cons. Phys. (Gen. Med. & Gastroenterol.) Roy. Hants. Co. Hosp. Winchester. Specialty: Gastroenterol. Socs: Brit. Soc. Gastroenterol. Prev: Research Fell. Gastroenterol. Unit Radcliffe Infirm. Oxf.

SHEPHERD, Professor James Department of Biochemistry, Royal Infirmary, Glasgow G4 0SF Tel: 0141 552 0689 Fax: 0141 553 1703; 17 Barriedale Avenue, Hamilton ML3 9DB Tel: 01698 428259 Fax: 01698 286281 Email: jshepherd@gri-biochem.org.uk — MB ChB Glas. 1968; PhD Glas. 1972, BSc 1965. Prof. Path. Biochem. Univ. Glas. & Hon. Consult. Path. Biochem. Glas. Roy. Infirm. Specialty: Chem. Path. Socs: Fell. Roy. Coll. Path; Fell. Roy. Coll. Phys. of Glas. Prev: Reader (Path. Biochem.) Univ. Glas.; Asst. Prof. (Med.) Baylor Coll. Med. & Methodist Hosp. Houston, USA; Vis. Prof. (Med.) Cantonal Hosp. Geneva, Switz.; Vis. Specialist Mehlati Hosp & Univ. Helsinki Finland.

SHEPHERD, James Baikie Moir 90 Thorne Road, Doncaster — MB BChir Camb. 1963 (Guy's) MA, MB BChir Camb. 1963; DTM & H Eng. 1964. Res. Med. Off. Samarit. Hosp. Wom. Lond. Socs: Fell.

Roy. Soc. Trop. Med. & Hyg. Prev: Res. Obstetr. & Gyn. Ho. Surg. Guy's Hosp. Lond.; Res. Obstetr. Qu. Charlotte's Hosp. Lond.

SHEPHERD, Jane Caroline 38 Mayfield Road, Sutton SM2 5DT — MB BS Lond. 1991; BA (Chem.) Open 1985; MSc (Biochem.) 1988.

SHEPHERD, Jane Ellen Elizabeth Foxcote, Harberton Mead, Headington, Oxford OX3 0DB — MB BS Lond. 1979; FFA RCS Eng. 1983. Cons. Anaesth. St. Mary's Hosp. Lond. Specialty: Anaesth. Prev: Sen. Regist. St. Mary's Hosp. Lond.; Regist. (Anaesth.) Kings Coll. Hosp. Lond.

SHEPHERD, Jennifer Hazel Legatesden Farm, Pitcaple, Inverurie AB51 5DT — MB ChB Aberd. 1979; DRCOG 1984. GP Brimmond Med. Gp., Bucksburn, Aberd.; DRS Cardiol., Aberd. Roy. Infirm. Prev: GP Inverurie; SHO (Obst.) Paisley Matern. Hosp.; SHO (Surg.) Bradford Roy. Infirm.

SHEPHERD, Professor John Henry Department of Gynaecological Oncology, St. Bartholomew's Hospital, West Smithfield, London EC1 7BE Tel: 0207 601 7180 Fax: 0207 601 7182 Email: johnshepherd@bartsandthelondon.nhs.uk; Pickwick Cottage, 31 College Road, Dulwich, London SE21 7BG Tel: 020 8693 6342 Fax: 020 8299 0453 — MB BS Lond. 1971 (St. Bart.) MRCS Eng. LRCP Lond. 1971; FRCS Eng. 1976; MRCOG (Gold Medal) 1978; FRCOG 1996, M (Gold Medal) 1978; FACOG 1981; T(OG) 1991. Cons. Gyn. (Surg. & Oncol.) St. Bart. Hosp. & The Lond. NHS Trust, The Roy. Marsden Hosp. NHS Trust Lond..; Prof. Surgic. Gyn. St Bars & Roy. Lond. Clinic of Med. and Dent.; Cons. Surg., The Roy. Marsden Hosp., Fulham Rd., Lond. Specialty: Obst. & Gyn. Socs: Fell. Roy. Soc. Med.; Fell. Soc. Pelvic Surgs. (Vice-Pres. 1999); Soc. Gyn. Oncol. Prev: Cons. Surg. Chelsea Hosp. for Wom. Lond.; Gyn. Oncol. Cancer Fell. Univ. S. Florida, USA; Vis. Prof. Univ. Monash, Melbourne, Austral., 1994.

SHEPHERD, John Moncrieff Occupational Health Service, Boots Company plc, PO Box 94, Nottingham NG2 3AA Tel: 01159 492484 Fax: 01159 492600 — MB ChB Manch. 1977; BSc St. And. 1974; AFOM RCP Lond. 1993; MFOM RCP Lond. 1997. Occupat. Phys. The Boots Company. Specialty: Occupat. Health. Socs: Soc. Occupat. Med.

SHEPHERD, John Steven (retired) 28 Barton Road, Cambridge CB3 9LF Tel: 01223 313058 — MB ChB Ed. 1954; DCH Eng. 1959. Prev: GP Kirkby Stephen.

SHEPHERD, Mrs Juliet Sarah Upton Road Surgery, 30 Upton Road, Watford WD18 0JS Tel: 01923 226266 Fax: 01923 222324; 37 Mount View, Rickmansworth WD3 7BB — MB BS Lond. 1965 (St. Bart.) DA Eng. 1970. Prev: SHO (Anaesth.) N. Middlx. Hosp. Lond.; Ho. Surg. Whipps Cross Hosp. Lond.; Ho. Phys. St. Bart. Hosp.

SHEPHERD, Malcolm Cameron Flat 1 Left, 72 Lauderdale Gardens, Glasgow G12 9QW — MB ChB Glas. 1993; BSc (Hons) Glas. 1991; MRCP 1997. Clin. Lect. Univ. Glas.; Hon Specialist Reg Respirat. Med W. of Scotl. Prev: SpR Med Stirling Roy. Infirm.

SHEPHERD, Matthew James 16 Adel Vale, Adel, Leeds LS16 8LF Tel: 0113 245 0340 Email: DrShep1@msn.com — MB ChB Leeds 1995. SHO Rotat. (Med.) Leeds Gen. Infirm. Specialty: Gen. Med. Prev: SHO (A & E) Leeds Gen. Infirm.; Ho. Off. (Surg.) St Jas. Univ. Hosp. Leeds; Ho. Off. (Med.) Leeds Gen. Infirm.

SHEPHERD, Michael Anthony Walsham Warrior Square Surgery, Marlborough House, 19-21 Warrior Square, St Leonards-on-Sea TN37 6BG Tel: 01424 430123/445644 Fax: 01424 433706 — MB BS Lond. 1972 (Middlx.) MRCS Eng. LRCP Lond. 1972; DObst RCOG 1974; DCH Eng. 1975; DFFP 1993; FRNZCGP 1998. GP St Leonards on Sea. Socs: BMA; NZ Med. Assn. Prev: GP Wellington, NZ; Regist. (Med.) Wellington Hosp., NZ; Ho. Phys. Middlx. Hosp.

SHEPHERD, Nancy Jane The Barn, Grove Place, Nursling, Southampton SO16 0XY — MB BS Lond. 1963 (Middlx.) DA Eng. 1965.

SHEPHERD, Professor Neil Anthony Department of Histopathology, Gloucestershire Royal Hospital, Great Western Road, Gloucester GL1 3NN Tel: 01452 395263 Fax: 01452 395285; Department of Histopathology, Cheltenham General Hospital, Sandford Road, Cheltenham GL53 7AN Tel: 01242 274073 Fax: 01242 274078 — MB BS Lond. 1979 (St. Bart.) FRCPath 1995, M 1985. Cons. Histopath. Glos. Roy. Hosp.; Vis. Prof., Univ. of Cranfield. Specialty: Histopath. Socs: Hon Sec. Brit. Div. of Int. Acad. of Pathol.; Assn. Clin. Paths.; Brit. Soc. Gastroenterol. Prev: Sen. Lect. & Hon. Cons. (Histopath.) St. Bart. Hosp., St. Mark's Hosp. & ICRF Colorectal Cancer Unit Lond; Lect. (Histopath.) St. Bart. Hosp. & St. Mark's Hosp. Lond.; Regist. (Histopath.) & Ho. Surg. St. Bart. Hosp. Lond.

SHEPHERD, Nicholas Ironside Glover Street Medical Centre, 133 Glover Street, Perth PH2 0JB Tel: 01738 639748 Fax: 01738 635133; Denwood, Strathview Place, Methven, Perth PH1 3PP Tel: 01738 840729 Email: nishep@globalnet.co.uk — MB ChB Dundee 1980 (Univ. Dundee) BMSc (1st cl. Hons.) Pharmacol. Dund 1977; DRCOG 1982; MRCGP 1984.

SHEPHERD, Patricia Carolyn Anne Western General Hospital, Department of Haematology, Edinburgh EH4 2XU Tel: 0131 537 1633 Fax: 0131 537 2552 Email: pat.shepherd@luht.scot.nhs.uk; 53A Fountainhall Road, Edinburgh EH9 2LH Tel: 0131 667 9530 — MB BCh BAO Belf. 1972; MRCP (UK) 1979; Amer. Bd. Internal. Med. 1979; MRCPath 1987; FRCPath 1997; FRCP Ed. 2002. Cons. (Haemat.) W. Gen. Hosp. Edin. & St. Johns Hosp. Howden. Specialty: Haematology. Special Interest: Chronic Myeloid Leukaemia; Myeloproliferative disorders. Socs: Brit. Soc. of Haemat.; Europ. Haemat. Assoc.; EBMT. Prev: Lect. (Haemat.) W. Gen. Hosp. Edin.; Staff Grade Haemat. W. Gen. Hosp. Edin. & St. Johns Hosp. Howden.; Assoc. Special. (Haemat.) W. Gen. Hosp. Edin.& St Johns Hosp.

SHEPHERD, Paul Richard Park Practice, 12 Brodrick Close, Hampden Park, Eastbourne BN22 9NQ Tel: 01323 502200/503240 Fax: 01323 500527 — MB BS Lond. 1980; MRCGP 1984. GP Eastbourne.

SHEPHERD, Paul Robert 2 Colepike Hall, Lanchester, Durham DA7 0RW — MB BS Newcastle 1977; MRCGP 1981. GP Durh.; Med. Off. in Psychosexual Med. Newc.-Upon-Tyne. Socs: RCGP.

SHEPHERD, Peter Douglas Warwick 49 The Avenues, Norwich NR2 3QR Tel: 01603 250441 Email: peterdwshepherd@btinternet.com — MRCS Eng. LRCP Lond. 1944 (Middlx.) MB BS Lond. 1946, DPM 1951; MRCPsych 1971. Specialty: Gen. Psychiat. Prev: Cons. Psychiat. Rauceby Hosp. Sleaford; SHMO Shenley Hosp.; Ho. Phys. Middlx. Hosp. Lond.

SHEPHERD, Philip George 1 Huntersbuoy, Larne BT40 2HH — MB BCh BAO Belf. 1983 (Queen's University Belfast) MRCP (UK) 1986; DCH Glas. 1986; DRCOG 1986; MRCGP 1987. Socs: BMA.

SHEPHERD, Philip Stephen Department of Immunology, MS3, Guy's Hospital Medical School, UMDS, London Bridge, London SE1 9RT Tel: 020 7955 4656 Fax: 020 7955 2317; 187 Banstead Road, Carshalton Beeches, Carshalton SM5 4DP Tel: 020 8642 2975 Fax: 020 8642 2975 — MB ChB Birm. 1970; MSc Birm. 1975, MB ChB 1970; MRCP (UK) 1974; FRCP Lond. 1994. Sen. Lect. & Hon. Cons. Immunol. UMDS Guy's Hosp. Lond.; Head Clin. Immunol. Serv. Guys & St Thos. Trust. Specialty: Immunol. Socs: Brit. Soc. Immunol. & Brit. Nuclear Med. Soc. Prev: Clin. Research Fell. Inst. Cancer Resarch Sutton, Surrey.

SHEPHERD, Richard Ian 1 Bronte Old Road, Thornton, Bradford BD13 3HN — MB ChB Manch. 1993.

SHEPHERD, Richard Julian Ash House, Ball La,, Caton, Lancaster LA2 9QN Tel: 01524 770476 — MB ChB Liverp. 1969; MRCOG 1974, DObst 1972. Cons. (O & G) Roy. Lancaster Infirm. Specialty: Obst. & Gyn. Prev: Sen. Regist. (O & G) Hammersmith Hosp. Lond.; Sen. Regist. St. Mary's Hosp. Portsmouth; Regist. (O & G) St. Mary's Hosp. Manch.

SHEPHERD, Richard Thorley PO Box 2, Peel IM99 9XF Email: r.shepherd@sghms.ac.uk — MB BS Lond. 1977 (St. Geo.) BSc (Hons.) Lond. 1974; DMJ Path.) Soc. Apoth. Lond. 1984; MRCPath 1986; FRCPath 1996. Sen. Lect. & Hon. Cons. Forens. Med. St. Geo. Hosp. Med. Sch. Lond. Specialty: Forens. Path. Socs: Medico-Legal Soc.; Fell. And Pres. Elect Brit. Assn. Forens. Med.; Pres., Clin. Legal and Forens. Sect. of The Roy. Soc. of Med. Prev: Sen. Lect. & Lect. (Forens. Med.) Guy's Hosp. Lond.; Lect. (Forens. Med.) St. Geo. Hosp. Lond.

SHEPHERD, Robert Barry 70 Shields Road, Sunderland SR6 8JN — MB BS Newc. 1997.

SHEPHERD, Robert Cameron Royal Alexandra Hospital, Corsebar Road, Paisley PA2 9PN Tel: 0141 887 9111 Fax: 0141 580 4207; 4 Troon Drive, Bridge of Weir PA11 3HF Tel: 01505 614155 — (Glas.) MB ChB Glas. 1965; DCH RCPS Glas. 1967; FRCP Glas. 1980, M 1969; FRCPCH 1996. Cons. Paediat. Roy. Alexandra Hosp. Paisley & Inverclyde Roy. Hosp. Greenock; Hon.Sen. Lect. Univ. Glas.

Child Health; Hon.Sen. Lect. Univ. Dundee Child Health. Specialty: Paediat. Prev: Sen. Regist. Roy. Hosp. Sick Childr. Glas.; SHO Glas. Roy. Infirm.

SHEPHERD, Robert John (retired) Ty Gwyn, 37 Ashfield Road, Stoneygate, Leicester LE2 1LB Tel: 0116 270 7029 Fax: 0116 270 8438 — MB ChB Liverp. 1968; MRCP (UK) 1975; FRCP Ed. 1992; FRCP Lond. 1995; FRCP Glas. 1997. Prev: Sen. Regist. (Med.) Radcliffe Infirm. Oxf.

SHEPHERD, Mr Rolf Carter (retired) Church Villa, Morden, Wareham BH20 7DS Tel: 01929 459265 — MB BChir Camb. 1950 (St. Thos.) FRCS Eng. 1955; MChir Camb. 1960. Hon. Surg. Poole Gen. Hosp. Prev: Res. Asst. Surg. St. Thos. Hosp. Lond.

SHEPHERD, Simon Tobias The Clapham Park Surgery, 72 Clarence Avenue, London SW4 8JP Tel: 020 8674 0101 Fax: 020 8674 2941 — MB ChB Birm. 1974; MRCGP 1981.

SHEPHERD, Stanley George Lawrence Hill Health Centre, Hassell Drive, Lawrence HIll, Bristol BS2 0AN — MB ChB Bristol 1979; BSc Bristol 1967, MB ChB 1979; DRCOG 1982. Socs: Assoc. MRCGP. Prev: GP Bristol.

SHEPHERD, Stephen Francis Gloucestershire Oncology Centre, General Hospital, Sandford Road, Cheltenham GL53 7AN Tel: 08454 224316 Fax: 08454 223506 Email: stephen.shepherd@glos.nhs.uk — MB ChB (Gold Medallist) Leic. 1987; MRCP (UK) 1990; FRCR 1994; MD 2004. Cons. Clin. Oncol. GloucestershireOncol.Centre Cheltenham Gen. Hosp. Specialty: Oncol.; Radiother. Socs: Fell.of Roy. Coll. of Radiologists; UK Assn. Head and Neck Oncol. Prev: Sen. Regist. (Clin. Oncol. & Radiother.) Roy. Marsden NHS Trust Lond. & Sutton; Research Fell. (Stereotactic Radiother.) Roy. Marsden Hosp. Lond.; Regist. Rotat. (Clin. Oncol.) Roy. Marsden Hosp. Lond. & Sutton.

SHEPHERD, Stephen John Dove River Practice, Gibb Lane, Sudbury, Ashbourne DE6 5HY Tel: 01283 812455; 13 Duncan Close, Belper DE56 1FS — MB ChB Birm. 1990.

SHEPHERD, Susan (retired) Flat 19, Spice Court, Asher Way, London E1W 2JD — MB ChB Bristol 1980.

SHEPHERD, Terence Patrick 16 Larch Grove, Sidcup DA15 8WJ — MB BS Lond. 1990.

SHEPHERD, Thomas Huw, Surg. Capt. RN Retd. Constantia, 168 West Street, Portchester, Fareham PO16 9XG Tel: 023 9232 6388 Fax: 023 9232 6388 — MB BS Lond. 1971 (Middlx. Hosp.) LLM Wales 1994. Medico Legal Adviser to Med. Dir. Gen. (Naval) & MOD (Navy). Prev: Medico Legal Adviser Med. Dir. Gen. (Naval); Med. Off i/c Roy. Naval Hosp., Gibraltar.

SHEPHERD, William Clyne (retired) 8 St Clair Terrace, Edinburgh EH10 5NW Tel: 0131 447 6647 — MB ChB Ed. 1950; Dip. Community. Med. 1975. Cons. Pub. Health Med. Lothian HB. Prev: Sec. Presbyt. Med. Bd. & Med. Supt. Presbyt. Hosps., Nigeria.

SHEPHERD, William Frederick Ian Deloraine Cottage, Greenend, Longnewton, St Boswells, Melrose TD6 9ES Tel: 01835 823074 MB BCh BAO Belf. 1969; DO RCPSI 1974; FRCS Ed. 1976. Cons. Ophth. Borders Gen Hosp. Melrose. Specialty: Ophth. Prev: Cons. (Ophth. Surg.) Roy. Vict. Hosp. Belf.; Hayward Fell. & Sub-Warden St. John Ophth. Hosp. Jerusalem, Israel; Fell. (Anterior Segment Surg.) Moorfields Eye Hosp. Lond.

SHEPHERD, William Henry Thompson (retired) 4 Tudor Oaks, Holywood BT18 0PA Tel: 01232 423050 — MD Belf. 1950; MB BCh BAO 1939; DMRD Eng. 1946; FFR RCSI 1962; FFR 1965; FRCR 1975. Prev: Cons. Radiol. Roy. Vict. Hosp. & Roy. Matern. Hosp. Belf.

SHEPHERDSON, David Hempton House, Hempton Lane, Almondsbury, Bristol BS32 4AR — MRCS Eng. LRCP Lond. 1963 (Char. Cross) DA Eng. 1968. Socs: Canad. Med. Assn. & Coll. Family Pract. Canada. Prev: SHO (Cas. & Anaesth.) W. Lond. Hosp.; Orthop. & Trauma Ho. Surg., Ho. Phys. & Ho. Surg. Ashford Hosp.; Middlx.

SHEPPARD, Adam Peter Lupset Surgery, off Norbury Road, Wakefield WF2 8RE Tel: 01924 376828 Fax: 01924 201649; 19 Ash Grove, Stanley, Wakefield WF3 4JY — MB ChB Leeds 1987; Cert Family Plann JCC 1992. Prev: SHO (Anaesth.) Pinderfields Gen. Hosp. Wakefield VTS; Ho. Surg. Harrogate Dist. Hosp.; Ho. Phys. Leeds Gen. Infirm.

SHEPPARD, Carol Ann 18 Rivers Street, Bath BA1 2QA — BM Soton. 1990.

SHEPPARD, Cathryn Jane 3 Lulworth Crescent, Bristol BS16 6SB Tel: 0117 956 1470 — BM Soton. 1990; MRCGP 1997. GP Non Princip. Specialty: Gen. Pract. Prev: GP Regist. Totnes Devon; Regist. (Palliat. Care) Gosford Hosp. NSW, Austral.; SHO (O & G) Torbay Hosp.

SHEPPARD, Clive Thomas The Bridge Street Surgery, 30-32 Bridge Street, Downham Market PE38 9DH Tel: 01366 388888 Fax: 01366 383716 — MB Camb. 1983; BA Camb. 1980, MB 1983, BChir 1982; MRCGP 1987. Princip. GP Downham Market. Prev: Cas. Off. Heatherwood Hosp. Ascot; Ho. Surg. New Addenbrookes Hosp. Camb.; Ho. Phys. James Paget Hosp. Gt. Yarmouth.

SHEPPARD, David Alan Harley Street Medical Centre, Harley Street, Hanley, Stoke-on-Trent ST1 3RX Tel: 01782 212066 Fax: 01782 201326 Email: daveshep@tinyworld.co.uk; Old Spring House, 51 Dilhorne Road, Forsbrook, Stoke-on-Trent ST11 9DJ Tel: 01782 396919 Fax: 01782 393510 — MB BS Lond. 1979 (Lond. Hosp.) BSc (Hons.) Lond. 1976; DRCOG 1983; DCH RCP Lond. 1984; MRCGP 1986; DMJ(Clin) Soc. Apoth. Lond. 1995. Police Surg. N. Staffs. Socs: Assn. Police Surg. Prev: Trainee GP N. Staffs. VTS; Ho. Off. & Cas. Off. Lond. Hosp.; Ho. Surg. Epsom Dist. Hosp.

SHEPPARD, Emma Jane — MB BS Newc. 1992 (Newcastle upon Tyne) DRCOG 1994; MRCGP 1997. Specialty: Gen. Pract.

SHEPPARD, Geoffrey Edward The Lodge, 230 Manchester New Road, Alkrington, Middleton, Manchester M24 1NP Tel: 0161 643 4340 — LRCP LRCS Ed. 1966 (RCSI) LRCP LRCS Ed. LRCPS Glas. 1966. Hosp. Pract. (ENT) Ancoats Hosp. Manch. Specialty: Otorhinolaryngol. Prev: GP Manch.; Ho. Off. (Med. & Surg.) N. Manch. Gen. Hosp.; Clin. Asst. (ENT) Ancoats Hosp. Manch.

SHEPPARD, Harvey William Westberts priority Care Trust, 5 Craven Road, Reading RG1 5LE Tel: 01189 862277 Fax: 01189 750297; North View House, Farm Road, Goring-on-Thames, Reading RG8 0AA Tel: 01491 872184 — MRCS Eng. LRCP Lond. 1966 (Camb. & Lond. Hosp.) MA Camb. 1966; MRCPsych 1980; DPM Eng. 1980. Specialty: Child & Adolesc. Psychiat. Prev: Sen. Regist. (Child Psychiat. & Ment. Handicap) BoroCt. Hosp. Reading; Regist. (Med. & Paediat.) St. Mary's Hosp. Plaistow; Regist. (Paediat.) Roy. Hosp. Sick Childr. Edin. & Area Serv. Ment.

SHEPPARD, Ian James 24 Hardcastle Gardens, Bradshaw, Bolton BL2 4NZ — MB ChB Leic. 1986.

SHEPPARD, John Midland Road Surgery, Midland Road, Thrapston, Kettering NN14 4JR Tel: 01832 734444 Fax: 01832 734426 — MB BS Lond. 1978 (St. Geo.) BSc (Hons.) Lond. 1974.

SHEPPARD, Leyland Curtis Fermoy Unit, Queen Elizabeth Hosp, Gayton Royal, King's Lynn PE30 4ET Tel: 01553 613613 Fax: 01223 359062; 42 Rathmore Road, Cambridge CB1 7AD Tel: 01223 246275 Email: isheppard@onetel.net.uk — MB ChB Dundee 1988; MRCP (UK) 1991; BMSc (Hons.) Dund 1985, MD 1994; MRCPsych 1995. Wellcome Research Train. Fell. & Hon. Sen. Regist. (Psychiat.) Addenbrooke's NHS Trust; Sen. Regist. Gen. Adult Psychiat.; Qu. Eliz. Hosp. Kings Lynn. Specialty: Gen. Psychiat. Prev: Sen. Regist. (Psychiat.) Maudsley Hosp.; Regist. (Psychiat.) Camb. HA & Maudsley Hosp.; SHO (Med.) Freeman NHS Trust.

SHEPPARD, Louise (retired) 3 Drummond Close, Pitsford, Northampton NN6 9BA — MB BS Lond. 1959 (Guy's) MRCS Eng. LRCP Lond. 1959; DObst RCOG 1961; DCH Eng. 1961; DMRD Eng. 1969; FFR 1971. Prev: Cons. Radiol. Kettering Gen. Hosp.

SHEPPARD, Mary Noelle Department of Pathology, Royal Brompton Hospital, Sydney St., London SW3 6NP Tel: 020 7351 8424 Fax: 020 7351 4883; Longcourt House, 46 The Drive, South Woodford, London E18 2BL Tel: 020 8530 7758 — MD NUI 1984 (Univ. Coll. Cork) BSc NUI 1979, MD 1984, MB BCh BAO 1977; MRCPath 1986. Sen. Lect. & Cons. Path. Roy. Brompton Heart & Lung Hosp. Lond. Specialty: Pathology, General. Socs: Fell. Roy. Soc. Med.; Path. Soc. Prev: Sen. Lect. & Cons. Path. Roy. Lond. Hosp.; Sen. Regist. Univ. Coll. & Middlx. Hosps. Lond.; Regist. & Research Fell. Hammersmith Hosp. Lond.

SHEPPARD, Professor Michael Charles Department of Medicine, Queen Elizabeth Hospital, Edgbaston, Birmingham B15 2TH Tel: 0121 627 2380 Fax: 0121 627 2384 Email: m.c.sheppard@bham.ac.uk — MB ChB Cape Town 1971; MRCP (UK) 1974; PhD Cape Town 1979; FRCP Lond. 1985; F med Sci 1998. Prof. Med. Univ. Birm. & Hon. Cons. Phys. Qu. Eliz. Hosp. Birm. Specialty: Endocrinol. Socs: Assn. Phys.; RCP (Censor); Soc. Endocrinol. (USA). Prev: Wellcome Trust Sen. Lect. Univ. Birm. &

Hon. Cons. Phys. Qu. Eliz. Hosp. Birm.; Sen. Regist. (Gen. Med. & Endocrinol.) Qu. Eliz. Hosp. Birm.

SHEPPARD, Reginald Gilbertson (retired) 18 Bolton Crescent, Windsor SL4 3JQ Tel: 01753 865820 — (Lond. Hosp.) MRCS Eng. LRCP Lond. 1941; MB BS Lond. 1943; DA Eng. 1943; FCA Eng. 1954. Prev: Cons. (Anaesth.) E. Berks Hosps.

SHEPPARD, Robin Francis (retired) 3 Drummond Close, Pitsford, Northampton NN6 9BA — MB BS Lond. 1958 (Middlx.) FRCPath M 1969. Prev: Cons. Haemat. Northampton Gen. Hosp.

SHEPPARD, Sally Christine Morris, Harker, Bleiker and Partners, Ivybridge Health Centre, Station Road, Ivybridge PL21 0AJ Tel: 01752 690777 Fax: 01752 690252 — BM Soton. 1988 (Univ. Soton.) DRCOG 1993; MRCGP 1994. Specialty: Gen. Pract.

SHEPPARD, Sheila (retired) 8 Kelvin Court, Petitor Road, Torquay TQ1 4QE Tel: 01803 314196 — MB ChB Leeds 1950. Prev: Sen. Research Fell. Dept. Paediat. & Child Health Leeds Univ.

SHEPPARD, Timothy John Harwood Trevaine, King Charles Road, Newbridge, Newport NP11 4HF — MB BS Lond. 1986.

SHEPPERD, Mr Harold Walter Henry, RD (retired) 68 Osborne Park, Belfast BT9 6JP Tel: 02890 665911 — (Belf.) FRCSI 1980 (Ad Eundem); MB BCh BAO Belf. 1947; DLO Eng. 1952; FRCS Eng. 1954. Prev: Cons. Surg. (Otorhinolaryng.) Roy. Vict. Hosp. Belf.

SHEPPERD, Margaret Joyce (retired) Pennance, Port Navas, Falmouth TR11 5RJ Tel: 01326 340275 — (K. C. H. London & Maudsley) MRCS Eng. LRCP Lond. 1940; DPM Eng. 1965. Prev: Cons. Psychiat. Hersham Child Guid. Clinic S.W. Metrop. RHA.

SHEPPERD, Rosemary Allison The Child and Family Clinic, The Clockhouse, 22-26 Ock Street, Abingdon OX14 5SW Tel: 01235 205425 — MB BS Lond. 1984; BSc (Hons.) Lond. 1981; DRCOG 1986; DCH RCP Lond. 1987; MRCGP 1988; MRCPsych 1991. Cons. (Child & Adolesc. Psychiat.). Specialty: Child & Adolesc. Psychiat. Prev: Sen. Regist. (Child Psychiat.) Oxf. Region Higher Train. Scheme; Regist. (Child Psychiat.) Tavistock Centre Lond. & Watford Child & Family Clinic.

SHEPPEY, Marie Claire 106 Kingswood Avenue, Bromley BR2 0NP — MB BS Lond. 1992.

SHEPSTONE, Basil John Department of Radiology, University of Oxford, Radcliffe Infirmary, Woodstock Road, Oxford OX2 6HE Tel: 01865 24679 Fax: 01865 816315; Oxfordsh. Health Authority Breast Care Unit, The Churchill Hospital, Headington, Oxford OX3 7LJ Tel: 01865 25319 Fax: 01865 225978 — MD Cape Town 1977; BSc (Hons.) Orange Free State 1957, BSc 1956; DSc Orange Free State 1960, MSc 1958; MA Oxf. 1978, DPhil 1964, BM BCh 1968; MRCS Eng. LRCP Lond. 1969; DMRD Eng. 1975; BA (Econ.) Univ. S. Afr. 1982; FRCR Eng. 1984. Univ. Lect. (Radiol.) & Head Dept. Univ. Oxf. & Hon. Cons. Nuclear Med. & Radiol. Oxf. HA; Clin. Dir. Oxf. HA Breast Care Unit. Specialty: Radiol. Socs: Fell. & Dean of Degrees Wolfson Coll. Oxf.; Brit. Inst. Radiol.; Brit. Nuclear Med. Soc. Prev: Dir. (Clin. Studies) Oxf. Univ. Clin. Med. Sch.; Clin. Lect. (Radiol.) Univ. Oxf.; Head Dept. Nuclear Med. Groote Schuur Hosp. & Univ Cape Town, S. Africa.

SHER, Carmel 36 Clovelly Road, London N8 7RH — BM BS Nottm. 1993.

SHER, Mr Joel Lester East Molesden House, Molesden, Morpeth NE61 3QF Tel: 0167 075380 — MB BCh Witwatersrand 1972; BSc Witwatersrand 1968; FRCS Eng. 1980. Cons. Traum. & Orthop. Surg. Ashington Hosp.; Hon. Clin. Lect. Traum. & Orthop. Surg. Univ. Newc. Specialty: Orthop. Socs: Brit. Orthop. Assn. & Brit. Soc. Surg. of Hand. Prev: Sen. Orthop. Regist. North. RHA.

SHER, Karnail Singh Birstall Medical Centre, 4 Whiles Lane, Birstall, Leicester LE4 4EE Tel: 0116 267 5255; 51 Rectory Road, Wanlip, Leicester LE7 4PL Tel: 0116 267 5425 Fax: 0116 267 5425 Email: ksher85768@aol.com — MB BS Guru Nanak Dev 1974; FRCPI 1995, M 1986. Hosp. Pract. (Gastroenterol.) Leicester Gen. Hosp.; Clin. Tutor (Gen. Pract.) Leicester Univ. Specialty: Gastroenterol. Socs: BMA & Med. Defence Union. Prev: Hosp. Pract. (Rheum.) Leicester Roy. Infirm.; Regist. (Med.) Orsett Gen. Hsop. & Leicester Gen. Hsop.

SHERAFAT, Hooman 18 Mount View, Mount Avenue, London W5 1PR — MB BS Lond. 1992 (St. George's Hosp. Med. Sch.) FRCOphth. Lond. 1997. Res. Fell. (Ophth.) Bris. Eye Hosp. Specialty: Ophth. Socs: BMA; MDU. Prev: Specialist Regist. Moorfields Eye Hosp. Lond.; Sen. Hse. Off. Rotat. The Roy. Free Hosp. Lond.

SHERATON, Tei Elizabeth 88 Newfoundland Road, Cardiff CF14 3LD — MB BCh Wales 1993. Specialty: Anaesth.

SHERBURN, Vincent England (retired) Cogolin, High Meadow, Bawtry, Doncaster DN10 6LT Tel: 01302 710107 — MB ChB Manch. 1946; MRCS Eng. LRCP Lond. 1946; MFOM RCP Lond. 1986, AFOM 1978. Prev: Sen. Med. Off. Med. Bd.ing Centre (Respirat. Dis.) Sheff.

SHERE, Michael Henry Breast Care Centre, Frenchay Hospital, Bristol BS16 1LE Tel: 0117 956 2036 Fax: 0117 975 3767 — MB BS Lond. 1979; MRCS Eng. LRCP Lond. 1979. Clin. Asst. Breast Surg. Fenchey Hosp. Bristol. Socs: Assoc. of Breast Clinics. Prev: SHO (Surg.) Roy. Devon & Exeter Hosp. Exeter.; SHO (Surg.) Gt. Yarmouth Dist. Gen. Hosp. & Plymouth Hosps.; Regist. Ho. Surg. Watford Gen. Hosp.

SHERGILL, Bhavneet Singh 218 Balfour Road, Ilford IG1 4JA — MB BS Lond. 1996.

SHERGILL, Mr Gurd Salisbury District Hospital, Odstock Rd, Salisbury SP2 8BJ Tel: 01722 336262 — MB BS Lond. 1989 (Univ. Coll. Middlx.) FRCS Eng. 1994; FRCS (Orth.) 2000. Orthop. Cons., Salisbury Dist. Hosp., Salisbury. Specialty: Orthop. Special Interest: Cartilage Transplantation; Shoulder Surg. Socs: Assoc. BOA. Prev: Specialist Regist., Roy. Nat. Orthop. Hospial, Starmore.

SHERGILL, Mr Nilam Singh 79 Kenilworth Road, Coventry CV4 7AF — MB ChB Leeds 1982; FRCS Ed. 1989; FRCS Eng. 1990.

SHERGILL, Shubhinder Singh 32 Chandos Avenue, London N14 7ET Tel: 020 8886 6336 — MB BS Lond. 1995; BSc (Hons.) Physiol. Lond. 1991. SHO (Psychiat.) Maudsley Hosp. Lond. Specialty: Gen. Med. Socs: MDU; BMA. Prev: Ho. Phys. Joyce Green Hosp. Dartford; Ho. Surg. Derriford Hosp. Plymouth.

SHERGILL, Sukhpal SINGH 62 Ward Avenue, Grays RM17 5RW Tel: 07970 259975; Hillview Surgery, 179 Bilton Road, Perivale, Greenford UB6 7HQ Tel: 020 8997 4661 — MB ChB Leic. 1994 (Leicester) DRCOG 1998; DCH 1999; DFFP 1999. Princip. GP. Specialty: Gen. Pract. Prev: SHO (O & G, Paediat. & A & E) Greenwich.

SHERGILL, Sukhwidner Singh 44 Grange Road, Gravesend DA11 0EU — MB BS Lond. 1991; BSc (Hons.) Lond. 1988, MB BS 1991. Regist. (Psychiat.) Univ. Coll. Hosp. Lond. Specialty: Gen. Surg. Prev: Research Regist. Univ. Coll. Lond. Med. Sch.; SHO Univ. Coll. Hosp.

SHERIDAN, Anthony John Glenburn, 5 Elmsway, Hale, Altrincham WA15 0DZ — MB ChB Liverp. 1977; DMRD Liverp. 1982; FFR RCSI 1985. Cons. Radiol. Warrington Gen. Hosp. Specialty: Radiol.

SHERIDAN, Cyril Henry (retired) 1 Stanhope Road, Highgate, London N6 5NE Tel: 020 8340 3773; 1 Stanhope Road, Highate, London N6 5NE Tel: 0208 340 3773 — MB BS Lond. 1951 (St. Geo.) MRCS Eng. LRCP Lond. 1951. Med. Ref. Crusader, Co-op. & Pearl Insur. Cos. Prev: Clin. Asst. Radiother. Roy. N. Hosp. Lond.

SHERIDAN, Professor Desmond John Academic Cardiology Unit, NHLI Imperial College of Medicine, St Mary's Hospital, London W2 1NY Tel: 020 7886 6129 Fax: 020 7886 6732; 14 Dukeswood Drive, Gerrards Cross SL9 7LR — MD Dub. 1974; MB BCh BAO 1971; MRCP (UK) 1974; PhD Newc. 1982; FRCP Lond. 1987. Prof. Clin. Cardiol. & Hon. Cons. St. Mary's Hosp. Lond. W2. Specialty: Cardiol. Prev: Sen. Lect. (Cardiol.) & Hon. Cons. Welsh Nat. Sch. Med. Cardiff; Research Fell. Div. Cardiovasc. Med. Washington Univ. St. Louis, USA; Sen. Regist. (Cardiol.) Newc. Gen. & Freeman Hosp. Newc. u. Tyne.

SHERIDAN, Eamonn Gerard 103 Moss Park Road, Stretford, Manchester M32 9HN — MB ChB Manch. 1985.

SHERIDAN, Edward Ashley Parkstone Health Centre, Mansfield Road, Poole BH14 0DJ Tel: 01202 741370 Fax: 01202 730952 — MB BS Lond. 1985; DRCOG 1990; MRCGP 1990. Specialty: Gen. Pract.; Sports Med. Prev: Sen. Ships Phys. P & O Lines.

SHERIDAN, Elizabeth Anne Department of Medical Microbiology, Royal London Hospital, London Tel: 020 7377 7251 — MB BS Lond. 1994 (St. Bart. Hosp.) BA Camb. 1991; MSc (Medical Microbiology) QMW London 1998; Dip RCPath 2001. Regist. (Microbiol.) St. Bart. and the Lond. Hosp. Lond. Specialty: Med. Microbiol.

SHERIDAN, Jacqueline Susan Park Lane Surgery, 8 Park Lane, Broxbourne EN10 7NQ Tel: 01992 465555; 46 Fairley Way, West Cheshunt, Waltham Cross EN7 6LG Tel: 01992 642523 — MB BS

Lond. 1990 (University College London) DFFP 1994; MRCGP 1994. Specialty: Gen. Pract. Prev: Trainee GP Harlow; Trainee GP/SHO Whipps Cross Hosp. Lond.

SHERIDAN, James Anthony Brinsley (retired) 30 Stanbury Close, Barnsley S75 2QX Tel: 01226 282163 — LRCPI & LM, LRSCI & LM 1945; LRCPI & LM, LRCSI & LM 1945.

SHERIDAN, John Hugh Sampford Peverell Surgery, 29 Lower Town, Sampford Peverell, Tiverton EX16 7BJ Tel: 01884 820304 Fax: 01884 821188; 1 Caumont Close, Uffculme, Cullompton EX15 3XY — MB BS Lond. 1978 (Oxf. & Lond. Hosp.) BA (Physiol. Sci.) Oxf. 1975; MRCGP 1983. Specialty: Gen. Med.

SHERIDAN, John Joseph Department of Radiology, The Royal Bournemouth Hospital, Castle Lane E., Bournemouth BH7 7DW — MB BCh BAO NUI 1979; FRCS Eng. 1985; FRCR 1989. Cons. Radiol. Roy. Bournemouth Hosp. Specialty: Radiol.

SHERIDAN, Linda Mary Lucia 45 Bury Green, Wheathampstead, St Albans AL4 8DB — MB BCh BAO Dub. 1977 (TC Dub.) MSc London Sch. Of Hygiene & Tropical Med.; BA Dub. 1977; Cert JCC Lond. 1980; DCH Dub. 1980; DRCOG 1981; MRCGP 1983; DM (Diploma Health Management) Keele 1998. Specialist Regist. In Pub. Health Med. N.Lond.; Pub. Health Train. Progr., based at Herts. Health Auth. Specialty: Pub. Health Med.; Gen. Pract. Prev: GP Bedford; SHO Bedford Gen. Hosp. Ho. Phys. & Ho. Surg. St. Jas. Hosp. Dub.; Primary Care Med. Adviser, Beds. Health Auth. ('93-'97).

SHERIDAN, Maria Bernadette Department of Clinical Radiology, St James's University Hospital, Leeds Teaching Hospitals Trust, Beckett Street, Leeds LS9 7TF — MB ChB Manch. 1984 (Manchester) MRCP Manchester; FRCR Manchester.

SHERIDAN, Mark Christopher 37 Saul Road, Downpatrick BT30 6PA — MB BCh BAO Belf. 1990; MB BCh Belf. 1990.

SHERIDAN, Michael Charles 24 Castlehill Drive, Newton Mearns, Glasgow G77 5JZ — MB ChB Glas. 1997.

SHERIDAN, Paul John 16 Botanical Road, Botanical Gardens, Sheffield S11 8RP — MB ChB Sheff. 1996.

SHERIDAN, Peter Seacroft Hospital, York Road, Leeds LS14 6UH Tel: 0113 206 3481; Tanglewood House, 16 Grove Lane, Leeds LS6 2AP Tel: 0113 274 0765 — (Guy's) MRCS Eng. LRCP Lond. 1965; MRCP (U.K.) 1971; FRCP Lond. 1987. Cons. Phys. Seacroft Hosp. Leeds and St Jas. Univ. Hosp. Leeds; Sen. Clin. Lect. Univ. of Leeds. Specialty: Gen. Med.; Endocrinol.; Diabetes. Prev: Hon. Cons. Phys. St. Jas. Hosp. Leeds; Sen. Regist. (Research) Roy. Devon & Exeter Hosp.

SHERIDAN, Peter John North Central London Health Protection Unit, Holbrook House, Cockfosters Road, Barnet EN4 0DR Tel: 020 8272 5553 Fax: 020 8272 5582 Email: peter.sheridan@enfield.nhs.uk; 45 Bury Green, Wheathampstead, St Albans AL4 8DB Tel: 01582 834804 — MB ChB Bristol 1977; DRCOG 1980; DCH Dub. 1980; Cert JCC Lond. 1980; MRCGP 1983; MSc London 1993; MFPHM RCP (UK) 1995; FFPHM 2002. Cons. In Communicable Disease Control, Health Protection Agency. Specialty: Pub. Health Med. Prev: GP Bedford; Consultant in Public Health Medicine, Enfield & Harringey HA; Director of Public Health, Enfield PCT.

SHERIDAN, Philip Gerard 15 Gleneagles Park, Bothwell, Glasgow G71 8UT — MB ChB Glas. 1976; MRCGP 1980.

SHERIDAN, Raymond Paul Glenfields, Sladacre Lane, Blagdon, Bristol BS40 7RP — MB ChB Bristol 1993; BSc (Hons), MRCP.

SHERIDAN, Mr Richard Jonathan Watford General Hospital, Vicarage Road, Watford WD18 0HB Tel: 01923 217935 Fax: 01923 217939; Ferndale, Church Lane, Sarratt, Rickmansworth WD3 6HN Tel: 01923 270451 Fax: 01923 260943 — (Guy's) MB BS Lond. 1979; LMSSA Lond. 1979; FRCS Ed. 1985; FRCOG 1998. Cons. O & G Watford Gen. Hosp. Vicarage Rd. Watford WD1 8HB. Specialty: Obst. & Gyn. Socs: Roy. Soc. Med (Vice-Pres. Obst. & Gyn. Branch); Gyn. Res. Soc. Prev: Sen. Regist. (O & G) St. Mary's Hosp. & Samarit. Hosp. for Wom. Lond.; Regist. (O & G) Guy's Hosp. Lond.; SHO Qu. Charlottes Matern. Hosp. Lond.

SHERIDAN, Mr William Gerard John Department of Surgery, West Wales General Hospital, Carmarthen SA31 2NE Tel: 01267 235151 Email: wgsheridan@aol.com — MB BCh BAO Dub. 1977 (University of Dublin Trinity College) MCh Dub 1989, MB BCh BAO 1977; FRCSI 1981; FRCS Eng. 1985; MA Dub 1995. Cons. Surg. W. Wales Gen. Hosp. Carmarthen; Cons. Surg., Werndale Private Hosp. Banctfelin, Carmarthen. Specialty: Gen. Surg. Socs: Assn. Surg.; Assn. Coloproctol.; Welsh Surg. Trav. Club. Prev: Sen. Regist. (Surg.) Univ. Hosp. Wales Cardiff & Singleton Hosp. Swansea; Research Fell. (Surg.) Univ. Hosp. Wales Cardiff.

SHERIF, Mr Ahmed Helmy Mohamed Broadview, North Orbital Road, Chiswell Green, St Albans AL2 2AB Tel: 01727 67331; (surgery) Wrafton House, 24 The Common, Hatfield AL10 0NB — MRCS Eng. LRCP Lond. 1978 (Ein Shams) MB BCh Ein Shams 1969; FRCS Ed. 1976. Prev: Regist. (Orthop.) Broomfield Hosp. Chelmsfield, Black Notley Hosp.; Braintree & Tameside Gen. Hosp. Ashton-under-Lyne.

SHERIF, Ali Sherif Adel Department of Cytology, Royal Gwent Hospital, Cardiff Road, Newport NP20 2UB; c/o Mr. K. Mohamed, 7 Gascony Avenue, West Hampstead, London NW6 4NB — MB BCh Cairo 1979; MRCPath (UK) 1992. Specialty: Histopath.

SHERIF, Tag El Baha'a Ahmed Fathi Brondesbury Medical centre, 279 Kilburn High Road, London NW6 7JQ Tel: 020 7624 9853 Fax: 020 7372 3660 — MRCS Eng. LRCP Lond. 1978 (Ein Shams) MB BCh Ein Shams 1971; DA Eng. 1975. Socs: Med. Protec. Soc. Prev: GP Hatfield; Clin. Asst. (Cas.) Clacton & Dist. Hosp.; Clin. Asst. (Anaesthetics) Colchester Health Dist.

SHERIF, Tayyaba GP Direct, 5/7 Welback Road, West Harrow, Harrow HA2 0RH Tel: 020 8515 9300 Fax: 020 8515 9300 — MRCS Eng. LRCP Lond. 1980.

SHERIFF, Shafiqa 14 Ruxley Lane, Ewell, Epsom KT19 0JA — MB BS Punjab 1949 (King Edwd. Med. Coll. Lahore) MB BS Punjab (Pakistan) 1949; DCH RCPS Glas. 1961; DObst RCOG 1966. GP Ruxley La. Ewell Surg. Socs: Pakistan Med. Assn. & BMA. Prev: Sessional Med. Off. Merton, Sutton & Wandsworth AHA; Regist. (O & G) Sobhraj Matern. Hosp. Karachi, Pakistan & United Christian Hosp. Lahore, Pakistan; SHO (O & G) WillesBoro. Hosp. Ashford.

SHERIFI, James (retired) 30 Strickmere, Stratford St Mary, Colchester CO7 6YG Tel: 01206 322218 — MB ChB Dundee 1975; BSc St. And. 1972; DRCOG 1979; Dip. Occ Med 1996. Prev: Regist. (Med. & Paediat.) Yeovil Hosp.

SHERIL, David Brian Surgery, 343 Ripple Road, Barking IG11 7RJ Tel: 020 8594 2770 — MB BS Lond. 1979 (Middlx.) MB BS (Hons.) Lond. 1979; DRCOG 1981; LLB Lond. 1990; AFOM RCP Lond. 1993. Socs: BMA; Brit. Med. Acupunct. Soc.; Ilford Med. Soc.

SHERLALA, Khaled Hussain X-Ray Department, Walsgrave General Hospital, Clifford Bridge Road, Coventry CV2 2DX — MB BCh Al-Fateh 1986; MRCP (UK) 1991.

SHERLAW, John Andrew The Surgery, 157-159 Reservoir Road, Erdington, Birmingham B23 6DN — MB BS Lond. 1976 (Westm.) BSc Lond. 1973; DCH RCP Lond. 1981; MRCGP 1982; DRCOG 1983.

SHERLAW, Shirley Rachel 11 New Church Road, Sutton Coldfield B73 5RT Tel: 0121 354 9132 — MB ChB Birm. 1978; BSc (Hons.) Birm. 1975; DCH RCP Lond. 1981; MRCGP 1982; DRCOG 1983.

SHERLEY-DALE, Andrew Charles Magnolia House Practice, Magnolia House, Station Road, Ascot SL5 0QJ Tel: 01344 637800 Fax: 01344 637823 — BM BCh Oxf. 1986; MA Camb. 1987; DCH RCP Lond. 1988; DRCOG 1990; MRCGP 1990. Prev: Trainee GP Ipswich Hosp. E. Suff. VTS.

SHERLOCK, Alexander (retired) 58 Orwell Road, Felixstowe IP11 7PS Tel: 01394 284503 — MB BS Lond. 1945 (Lond. Hosp.) MB BS (Hnrs.) Lond. 1945. Mem. Europ. Parliament. Prev: Barrister At Law Grays Inn 1961.

SHERLOCK, Clive Reginald Francis PO Box 4, Chipping Norton OX7 3XP Tel: 01865 308700 — MB BS Lond. 1972 (Char. Cross) MRCPsych 1978. Counsellor. Specialty: Psychother.

SHERLOCK, Mr David James Department of Surgery, North Manchester Healthcare NHS Trust, Delaunays Road, Manchester M8 5RL Tel: 0161 720 2612 Fax: 0161 720 2228; BUPA Hospital Manchester, Russells Road, Whalley Range, Manchester M16 8AJ Tel: 0161 226 0112 Fax: 0161 232 2255 — MB BS Lond. 1977 (King's Coll. Hosp.) FRCS Ed. 1981; FRCS Eng. 1982; MS Lond. 1986. Cons. Surg. N. Manch. Gen. Hosp.; Cons. Surg. Christie Hosp. Manch. Specialty: Gen. Surg. Socs: Assn. Surg.; Brit. Soc. Gastroenterol. Prev: Sen. Lect. (Surg.) Kings Coll. Hosp. Lond.; Sen. Regist. W. Midl. RHA; Chef du Clinique Hosp. Paul Brousse, Villejuif, Paris.

SHERLOCK, Julie Doreen The Peel Medical Practice, Peel Croft, 2 Aldergate, Tamworth B79 7DJ Tel: 01827 50575 Fax: 01827 62835 — MB ChB Bristol 1979; DRCOG 1984; MRCGP 1985.

SHERLOCK, William 8 Deans Park, South Molton EX36 3DY — MB ChB Sheff. 1995.

SHERMAN, David Ian Nicholas Department of Gastroenterology & Nutrition, Central Middlesex Hospital, Acton Lane, London NW10 7NS Tel: 020 8453 2202 Fax: 020 8453 2201 Email: david.sherman@nwlh.nhs.uk; 83 Burlington Lane, Chiswick, London W4 3ET — MB BS Lond. 1984 (Char. Cross) MRCP (UK) 1987; MD Lond. 1997; FRCP 2000. Cons. Phys. & Gastroenterol. Centr. Middlx. Hosp. Lond. Specialty: Gastroenterol.; Gen. Med. Special Interest: Alcoholic Liver Dis. & Gen. Hepat.; Endoscopy; Inflammatory Bowel Dis. Socs: Brit. Assn. for the Study of Liver; Amer. Gastroenterol. Assn. Prev: Sen. Regist. (Gastroenterol.) Qu. Eliz. Hosp. Birm. & Inst. Liver Studies King's Coll. Hosp. Lond.; Clin. Research Fell. Liver Unit & (Clin. Biochem.) King's Coll. Hosp. Lond.; Regist. (Med. & Gastroenterol.) Char. Cross Hosp. Lond. & W. Middlx. Univ. Hosp.

SHERMAN, Mr Ian Walter Wirral Hospital, Arrowe Park, Upton, Wirral CH49 5PE Tel: 0151 678 5111 — BM Soton. 1985; FRCS Eng. 1989; FRCS (Orl.) 1994. Cons. ENT Surg. Wirral Hosp. Specialty: Otorhinolaryngol. Prev: Sen. Regist. Rotat. (Otorhinolaryngol.) W. Midl.; Regist. (Otorhinolaryngol.) Roy. Liverp. Hosp. & Roy. Liverp. Childr. Hosp.

SHERMAN, Jane (retired) 43A Harrow Road, Linthorpe, Middlesbrough TS5 5NT Tel: 01642 828562 — MB BS Durh. 1953. Prev: Hon. Cons. & Cons. Phys. Geriat. Med. N. Manch. AHA (T).

SHERMAN, Janet Mary The Health Centre, 11 Hull Road, Hessle HU13 9LU — BM BCh Oxf. 1977; MA Camb. 1978; DRCOG 1979; MRCGP 1984. GP Hessle. Prev: Trainee GP Oxf. VTS.

SHERMAN, Mr Jeremy Alan Dept. of Oral & Maxillofacial Surgery, Queen Elizabeth II Hospital, Howlands, Welwyn Garden City Email: jasherman@doctors.org.uk — MB ChB Manch. 1990 (Kings College, Manchester) BDS Lond. 1981; FDS RCS Eng. 1992; FRCS Ed. 1993; FRCS (Max Fae) 1998. Cons. In O & M Surg., Qu. Eliz. II Hosp., Welwyn Garden City; Cons. In O & M Surg., Lister Hosp., Stevenage. Specialty: Oral & Maxillofacial Surg. Socs: Brit. Assoc. of Head & Neck Oncologists; Brit. Assn. Oral & Maxillofacial Surg. (Jun. Fell.); BMA. Prev: Career Regist. (Maxillofacial Surg.) Roy. Surrey Co. Hosp. Guildford; Sen. Regist. (Maxillofacial Surg.) Guy's & St Thomas' Hosp.; Sen. Regist. (Maxillofacial Surg.) Ipswich Hosp.

SHERMAN, Mr Kevin Paul 21 Albion Street, Hull HU1 3TG Tel: 01482 20088; The Elms, Nunburnholme Avenue, North Ferriby HU14 3AW Tel: 01482 631552 — BM BCh Oxf. 1975; MA Camb. 1975; FRCS Eng. 1979. Cons. Orthop. Yorks. RHA. Specialty: Trauma & Orthop. Surg. Socs: Brit. Orthop. Assoc. Prev: Sen. Regist. (Orthop.) Oxf..

SHERMAN, Laurence Howard Greyland Medical Centre, 468 Bury Old Road, Prestwich, Manchester M25 1NL — MB ChB Manch. 1982; MRCGP 1988; Cert. Family Plann. JCC 1988; DCH RCP Lond. 1988. GP Prestwich; Clin. Asst. (Psychiat.) Prestwich Hosp. Manch.; Dep. Police Surg. Rochdale.

SHERMAN, Lionel Maurice Bounds Geen Group Practice, Bounds Green Group Practice, Gordon Road, London N11 2PF Tel: 020 8889 1961 Fax: 020 8889 7844; 36 Arlow Road, London N21 3JU — MB Camb. 1983; BChir 1982. Socs: Brit. Med. Acupunct. Soc.

SHERMAN, Mark Andrew Psychiatric Unit, Derby City General Hospital, Uttoxeter Road, Derby DE22 3NE Tel: 01332 624554; 2 Wilson Close, Mickleover, Derby DE3 5DT — MB BS Lond. 1981 (St. Bart.) MRCPsych 1987. Cons. Psychiat. S. Derbysh. Ment. Health Trust. Specialty: Gen. Psychiat. Prev: Research Regist. (Psychiat.) MRC Units W.Pk. Hosp. Epsom; SHO & Regist. (Psychiat.) Univ. Coll. & Middlx. Hosp. Lond.

SHERMAN, Richard William 16 Acorn bank, West Bridgford, Nottingham NG2 7SH — MB ChB Sheff. 1991. Specialty: Anaesth.

SHERMAN, Yael Clare House, St. George's Hospital, Blackshaw Road, London SW17 0QT; 13 Talbot Avenue, London N2 0LS — MB BCh Witwatersrand 1958; DCH Witwatersrand 1973. Sen. Med. Off. Camden & Islington AHA (T); Princip. Phys. (Child Health) Wandsworth HA. Socs: BMA & Soc. Community Med. & Brit. Paediat. Assn. Prev: Med. Off. & Regist. (Paediat.) Transvaal Memor. Hosp.; esburg, S. Africa; Regist. (Paediat.) Baragwanath Hosp. Johannesburg, S. Africa.

SHERON, Nicholas Clive Department of Medicine, Level D, South Path / Lab Block, Southampton General Hospital, Tremona Road, Southampton SO16 6YD — MB ChB Sheff. 1982.

SHERPA, Tsilden Phutarkey St. Mary's Hospital, Newport PO30 5TG Tel: 01983 524081 Fax: 01983 534720; 106 Earisbrooke Rd, Newport PO30 1DB Tel: 01983 529443 — MB BS Shivaji 1977; DA (UK) 1986. Staff Grade Anaesth. I. of. Wight HA. Prev: Regist. (Anaesth.) Plymouth Gen. Hosp.; Regist. (Anaesth.) Dumfries & Galloway Roy. Infirm.

SHERRARD, Elizabeth Sarah May (retired) 5 North Circular Road, Belfast BT15 5HB Tel: 01232 779082 — (Qu. Univ. Belf.) MB BCh BAO Belf. 1945; DObst RCOG 1948; DPH Belf. 1952. Med. Off. (Community Health) E. Health & Social Servs. BD.

SHERRARD, Jacqueline Susan Radcliffe Infirmary NHS Trust, Woodstock Road, Oxford OX2 6HE — MB BS Lond. 1986; MRCP (UK) 1989. Cons. Genitourin. Med. Radcliffe Infirm. Oxf. Specialty: Genitourinary Medicine.

SHERRARD, Kieran Edward Dublin Road Surgery, 4 Dublin Road, Castlewellan, Newcastle BT31 9AG; 30 Bryansford Avenue, Newcastle BT33 0LG Tel: 03967 23495 — MB BCh BAO Belf. 1973; MRCGP 1977. Prev: GP Bedlington; Trainee GP Newc. VTS; Ho. Phys. & Ho. Surg. Altnagelvin Hosp. Lond.derry.

SHERRATT, Margaret The Surgery, Johnson St., Teams, Gateshead NE8 2PJ Tel: 0191 460 4239; 21 Albert Drive, Low Fell, Gateshead NE9 6EH — MB BS Newc. 1978; DRCOG 1981; MRCGP 1982.

SHERRATT, Margaret Trafford (retired) 4 Carlton Close, Newcastle upon Tyne NE3 4SA Tel: 0191 285 4115 Email: stan@sherratts.fsnet.co.uk — MB ChB Birm. 1951; DObst RCOG 1954; DPH Liverp. 1959.

SHERRATT, Reginald Michael Luton & Dunstable Hospital, Lewsey Road, Luton LU4 0DZ Tel: 01582 497069 Fax: 01582 497326 — BM BCh Oxf. 1970; MA Oxf. 1970; MRCP (UK) 1973; FRCP Lond. 1992. Cons. Clin. Neurophysiol. Roy. Free Hosp. Lond. & Luton & Dunstable Hosp.; Emerit. Cons. Chelsea & Westm. Hosp. Lond. Specialty: Clin. Neurophysiol. Socs: Assn. Brit. Neurol.; Brit. Soc. Clin. Neurophysiol. Prev: Research Fell. Inst. Neurol. Lond.; Sen. Regist. (Clin. Neurophysiol.) Nat. Hosp. for Nerv. Dis. Lond.

SHERRET, Ian Ritchie Lyndhurst, West Park Road, Cupar KY15 Tel: 01334 52466 — MB ChB Glas. 1954; DPM Eng. 1960; FRCPsych 1986. Specialty: Gen. Psychiat. Prev: Cons. Psychiat.Stratheden Hosp.; Sen. Regist. (Psychiat.) South. Gen. Hosp. Glas.; Regist. Hawkhead Ment. Hosp. Glas.

SHERRIFF, David 52A Main Street, Bushby, Leicester LE7 9PP — MB ChB Dund. 1998; MB ChB Dund 1998.

SHERRIFF, Elizabeth Ann 15 Parkfields, Putney, London SW15 6NH — MB BS Lond. 1981 (St. Thos.) MRCOG 1989; FRCOG 2001. p/t Cons. (O & G) St. Helier Hosp. Carshalton. Specialty: Obst. & Gyn. Special Interest: Reproductive Med. Socs: British Fertility Society. Prev: Clin. Research Fell. & Hon. Sen. Regist. Hammersmith Hosp. Lond.; Sen. Regist. (O & G) St. Helier Hosp. Carshalton.

SHERRIFF, Mr Howard Munro, OStJ Accident Service Box 87, Addenbrooke's Hospital, Cambridge CB2 2QQ Tel: 01223 217117 Fax: 01223 217057; 11 Lynfield Lane, Cambridge CB4 1DR Tel: 01223 357559 Fax: 01223 357559 — (St. And.) MB ChB St. And. 1966; FRCS Ed. 1974. Cons. Accid. Addenbrooke's Hosp. NHS Trust Camb.; Cons. A & E Camb. & Huntingdon HA. Specialty: Accid. & Emerg. Socs: Brit. Assn. Emerg. Med.; BASICS (Mem. Research Comm. & Chairm. Educat. Managem. Comm.). Prev: Cons. Orthop. Surg. RAF Med. Br.; Wing Cdr. RAF Med. Br.; Sen. Regist. (Orthop.) Addenbrooke's Hosp. Camb. & Newmarket Gen. Hosp.

SHERRIFF, Richard James Kennedy Way Surgery, Kennedy Way, Yate, Bristol BS37 4AA; 35 Canterbury Close, Rectory Meadow, Yate, Bristol BS37 5TL Tel: 01454 311559 — MB ChB Bristol 1976; BSc (Hatfield) 1971; MRCGP 1981; DRCOG 1981. Specialty: Diabetes; Educat.; Gen. Pract. Prev: Trainee GP Yate; SHO (Obst.) Bristol Matern. Hosp.; SHO (A & E), SHO & Regist. (Path.) Bristol Roy. Infirm.

SHERRIFF, Robert George Greenways, Weydown Road, Haslemere GU27 1DT — MB BS Lond. 1987.

SHERRINGHAM, Paul Edward Charles Well Lane Surgery, Well Lane, Stow on the Wold, Cheltenham GL54 1EQ Tel: 01451 830625 Fax: 01451 830693 — MB ChB Bristol 1993; BSc (Hons) Bristol 1990; Dip IMC RCS Ed. 1997; DRCOG 1998. SHO (Paediat.) Cheltenham Gen. Hosp. Specialty: Gen. Pract. Socs: BMA; MDU; BASICS.

SHERRINGTON, Charles Robert Greater Manchester Neurosciences Centre, Hope Hospital, Stott lane, Salford; 4 The Hollies, Didsbury, Manchester M20 2GD — MB ChB Liverp. 1988; MRCP (UK) 1991; MD Liverp. 2003. Cons. Nerologist Hope Hosp., Salford; Vis. Neurologist, Tameside Hosp., Ashton-under-Lyne; Private Neurologist, Highfield Hosp., Rochdale and Pennine Ho. Ashton. Specialty: Neurol.; Medico Legal. Special Interest: Stroke medicine. Socs: Brit. Assn. of Stroke Physicians; Assn. of Brit. Neurologists; Roy. Coll. of Physicians Lond. Prev: Specialist Regist. (Neurol.) Manch. Roy. Infirm.; Research Fell. (Neurol.) St. Jas. Hosp. Leeds & Univ. Leeds; Regist. (Neurol.) St. Jas. Hosp. & Leeds Gen. Infirm.

SHERRINGTON, Jean Maria Sussex West & Downs NHS Trust, The Old Court House, Grange Road, Midhurst GU29 9LT Tel: 01730 811300 Fax: 01730 817512 — MB ChB Bristol 1981 (Bris.) MRCPsych 1990. Cons. (Psychiat.). Specialty: Gen. Psychiat. Prev: Sen. Regist. (Psychiat.) Graylingwell Hosp. Chichester.

SHERRINGTON, Joanne Marie Wychall Lane Surgery, 11 Wychall Lane, Kings Norton, Birmingham B38 8TE Tel: 0121 628 2345 Fax: 0121 628 8282 — MB ChB Liverp. 1989; DCH; MRCGP. GP Princip. Specialty: Gen. Pract.

SHERRINGTON, Lesley Jane 53 Cumnor Hill, Oxford OX2 9EY — MB ChB Leeds 1995.

SHERRY, Barclay John (retired) 116 Old Road, Headington, Oxford OX3 8SX — MB ChB Glas. 1951.

SHERRY, Colin Campbell (retired) Kennelling Cottage, Kennelling Road, Charing, Ashford TN27 0HF — LMSSA Lond. 1951 (King's Coll. Hosp.) DPM Eng. 1962; FRCPsych 1990, M 1971. Prev: Vis. Psychiat. HM Prison Holloway Lond.

SHERRY, Eoin Niall Department of Anaesthesia, Guy's Hospital, London SE1 9RT Tel: 020 7976 5151 — MB BCh BAO NUI 1982; DCH RCP Lond. 1984; FRCA 1988. Cons. Anaesth. Guy's Hosp. Lond. Specialty: Anaesth.

SHERRY, Kathleen Mary Northern General Hospital NHS Trust, Herries Road, Sheffield S5 7AU Tel: 0114 243 4343; 27 Taptonville Road, Broomhill, Sheffield S10 5BQ Tel: 0114 266 0479 Fax: 0114 266 5552 — MB BS Lond. 1975; FFA RCS Eng. 1981. Cons. (Anaesth.) Northern Gen. Hosp. NHS Trust, Sheff.; Anaesth. Coodinator at Nat. Confidential Enquiry into PeriOperat. Deaths (NCEPOD), Lond. Specialty: Anaesth.

SHERRY, Mary Kathleen 46 Cumberland Street, London SW1V 4LZ Tel: 020 7834 0767 Fax: 020 7834 0767 — MB BS Lond. 1984 (St. Geo.) BSc (1st cl. Hons.) Lond. 1981; MRCP (UK) 1988; MFOM RCP Lond. 1999; FFOM 2004. Indep. Cons. in Ocupational Med. Specialty: Occupat. Health. Socs: Roy. Soc. Med.; Soc. Occupat. Med.; Brit. Occupat. Hyg. Soc. Prev: Regist. (Radiol. Sci.) Guy's Hosp. Lond.; SHO (Med.) St. Geo. Hosp. Lond.; Ho. Surg. St. Geo. Hosp. Lond.

SHERRY, Mr Paul Gordon North Cheshire NHS Trust, Lovely Lane, Warrington WA5 1QG Tel: 01925 662383 Fax: 01925 662211 Email: paul_sherry@nch.nhs.uk; Hunters Moon, Hollins Lane, Antrobus, Northwich CW9 6NL Tel: 01565 777572 — MB BS Lond. 1983 (St. Barths.) BSc Lond. 1988; FRCS Eng. 1988. Cons. Trauma & Orthop. Warrington Hosp. NHS Trust. Specialty: Orthop. Socs: Fell. BOA.

SHERRY, Simon Norwood Medical Centre, 360 Herries Road, Sheffield S5 7HD Tel: 0114 242 6208 Fax: 0114 261 9243; 27 Taptonville Road, Sheffield S10 5BQ — MB BS Lond. 1975.

SHERRY, Susan Jane 12 Adria Road, Didsbury Village, Manchester M20 6SG — MB ChB Manch. 1987.

SHERRY, Vincent Francis (retired) 17 Herondale Avenue, London SW18 3JN Tel: 020 8874 8588 — MB BCh BAO NUI 1942; LM Coombe 1942. Prev: Res. Surg. Off. Roy. Masonic Hosp. Lond.

SHERRY-DOTTRIDGE, Florence Gertrude (retired) 15 Westfield Road, Beaconsfield HP9 1EG Tel: 0149 464205 — MB ChB Manch. 1920; DPH Camb. 1923. Hon. Cons. Dermat. King Edw. VII Hosp. Windsor. Prev: Cons. Dermatol. Lond. Skin Hosp & N.W. Metrop. RHB.

SHERSKI, Leonard Adrian The Groves Medical Centre, 72 Coombe Road, New Malden KT3 4QS Tel: 020 8336 2222 Fax: 020 8336 0297; 3 Coombe House Chase, New Malden KT3 4SL Tel: 020 8336 2233 — MB BCh BAO Belf. 1959 (Queens University Belfast) DObst RCOG 1961; DCH Eng. 1962. Prev: Regist. Roy. Hosp. Sick Childr. Belf.; Regist. Roy. Vict. Hosp. Belf.

SHERSTON-BAKER, Professor Arthur Joseph Percy (retired) 3 Olden Lane, Purley CR8 2EH Tel: 020 8645 9395 — MB BS Lond. 1944; MRCS Eng. LRCP Lond. 1943; DPM Lond. 1949; MD Lond. 1951; FRCPsych 1971. Prev: Cons. Psychiat. Guy's Hosp. Gp. Lond.

SHERVEY, Christopher Sydney James Watledge Surgery, Barton Road, Tewkesbury GL20 5QQ Tel: 01684 293278; High Gables, Aston-on-Carrant, Tewkesbury GL20 8HL Tel: 01684 773269 — MB ChB Bristol 1972; DA Eng. 1974; MRCGP 1981. Specialty: Gen. Pract. Socs: BMA. Prev: SHO (Paediat.) Glos. Roy. Hosp.; SHO (Anaesth.) Cheltenham Health Dist.; SHO (A & E) Frenchay Hosp. Bristol.

SHERVINGTON, Mr Peter Charles (retired) Vinesend House, Vinesend, Near Cradley, Malvern WR13 5NH Tel: 01886 880775 Fax: 01826 880775; Vinesend House, Vinesend, Malvern WR13 5NH Tel: 020 86 880775 — MRCS Eng. LRCP Lond. 1961 (St. Mary's) FRCOG 1979, M 1967, DObst 1964. Cons. O & G Worcester Roy. Infirm. Prev: Sen. Regist. (O & G) Hammersmith Hosp. Lond. & St. Helier Hosp. Carshalton.

SHERWELL, David 18 Coombe Gardens, Wimbledon, London SW20 0QU Tel: 020 8879 1152 Email: dsherwell@x-stream.co.uk — BM BCh Oxf. 1996; BA Oxf. 1993. GP Regist. Surrey. Prev: SHO (Psychiat.) E. Surrey Hosp.; SHO (A&E) St. Geo.'s Hosp.; Ho. Off. (Gen. Surg.) John Radcliffe Oxf.

SHERWIN, James Robert Alexander 12 Orchard Road, Bardsea, Ulverston LA12 9QN — MB BS Lond. 1994.

SHERWIN, Julie Deborah University Hospitals, Coventry & Warwickshire NHS Trust, Walsgrave Hospital, Clifford Bridge Road LE3 8EH Tel: 02476 602 020 — MB BCh Wales 1982 (Welsh Nat. Sch. of Med.) FFARCSI; DA, United Kingdom 1985. Cons. Anaesth., Specialising in Obst., Coventry. Specialty: Anaesth.

SHERWIN, Karen Elizabeth 12 Orchard Road, Bardsea, Ulverston LA12 9QN — MB BChir Camb. 1992; MRCP (UK) 1995. Specialist Regist. (Clin. Oncol.) Addenbrooke's Hosp. Camb. Specialty: Oncol.; Radiother.

SHERWIN, Nicholas John Peter Batgells, Sandford Orcas, Sherborne DT9 4RP — MB BS Lond. 1998; MRCGP 2003.

SHERWOOD, Andrew Nicholas St James House Surgery, County Court Road, King's Lynn PE30 5SY Tel: 01553 774221 Fax: 01553 692181 — MB BS Lond. 1976; DRCOG 1979; DA (UK) 1980; MRCGP 1983.

SHERWOOD, Anthea Joy Department of Histopathology, Derriford Hospital, Derriford Road, Plymouth PL6 8DH Email: anthea.sherwood@phnt.swest.nhs.uk — MB BS Lond. 1973 (Univ. Coll. Hosp.) BSc Lond. 1970; FRCPath 1992, M 1980. Cons. Histopath. Derriford Hosp. Plymouth. Specialty: Histopath. Special Interest: Gastro-intestinal Path. Socs: Assn. Clin. Path. (Mem. Counc. 1988-91); Internat. Acad. Path. (Brit. Div.).; Brit. Med. Assn. Prev: Lect. (Morbid Anat.) Univ. Coll. Hosp. Med. Sch. Lond.; Lect. (Histopath.) Inst. Child Health Gt. Ormond St.; Cons. Histopath., Torbay Hosp.

SHERWOOD, Benedict Thomas Hedgewick, Station Road, Rock, Kidderminster DY14 9UA — BM BS Nottm. 1998; BM BS Nottm 1998.

SHERWOOD, Graham John Park Road Medical Centre, 44 Park Road, Guiseley, Leeds LS20 8AR — MB ChB Leeds 1978; BA (Hons. Chem.) York 1965; MPhil (Med. Eng.) Leeds 1974, MB ChB (Hons.) 1978; DRCOG 1980; MRCGP 1983. GP Princip. Prev: SHO (Infec. Dis.) Seacroft Hosp. Leeds; Ho. Off. Leeds Gen. Hosp, York Dist. Hosp. & Leeds Matern. Hosp.

SHERWOOD, Helen The Ashgrove Surgery, Morgan Street, Pontypridd CF37 2DR Tel: 01443 404444 Fax: 01443 480917; 12 Cyn Coed Ave, Cardiff CF23 6SU — BM BS Nottm. 1991; DRCOG 1994; MRCGP 1995. Specialty: Gen. Pract.

SHERWOOD, Julie Isabella 328 Cregagh Road, Belfast BT6 9EX — MB BCh BAO Belf. 1991 (Qu. Univ. Belf.) DRCOG 1994; DCH RCPSI 1994; MRCGP 1995. Specialty: Gen. Pract.

SHERWOOD, Kathryn Elizabeth West Wyke Farm, Wyke Lane, Ash, Aldershot GU12 6EE — BM BS Nottm. 1998; BM BS Nottm 1998.

SHERWOOD, Mr Mark Brian 4935 North West 51st Place, Gainesville FL 32653, USA; c/o G. J. Sherwood, 4 Key Thorpe, 27 Manor Road, Eastcliffe, Bournemouth BH1 3ER — MB ChB Manch. 1976; MB ChB (Hons.) Manch. 1976; MRCP (UK) 1979; FRCS Eng. 1982; FRCOphth 1989. Prof. & Chairm. (Ophth.) Univ. Florida Gainesville, USA. Specialty: Ophth.

SHERWOOD, Martin Paul 2nd Floor, 2 Devonshire Place, London W1G 6HJ Tel: 020 7580 4691 Fax: 020 7224 2832 — MRCS Eng. LRCP Lond. 1942 (Westm.) DA Eng. 1944; MA, MB BChir Camb. 1955; FFA RCS Eng. 1955. Specialty: Physiother. Prev: Cons. SW & SE Regional HBs.

SHERWOOD, Naomi — MB ChB Ed. 1990; DRCOG 1992; MRCP 1994; DTM & H Liverp. 1995. Regist. Rotat. (Paediat.) Manch. Specialty: Paediat.

SHERWOOD, Nicholas Alexander Department of Anaesthesia, City Hospital NHS Trust, Birmingham B28 0H Tel: 0121 554 3801 — MB ChB Birm. 1987; DA (UK) 1989; FRCA 1993. Cons., Clin. Director, Critical Care Serv.s. Specialty: Anaesth. Socs: RCA; BMA; MPS. Prev: Regist. (Anaesth.) S. Midl. Train Scheme; SHO (Neonat. & Intens. Care) Walsgrave Hosp. Coventry; SHO (Anaesth.) Selly Oak Hosp. Birm.

SHERWOOD, Paul Victor Department of Gastroentebology, Northampton General Hospital, Cufton Ville, Northampton NN1 5BD Tel: 01604 545149 Fax: 01604 545149 — MB ChB Leeds 1991; MRCP (UK) 1994; DM (Nottingham) 2001. Cons. Gastro. Northampton Gen. Hosp. Specialty: Gastroenterol.; Gen. Med. Socs: BMA; BSG.

SHERWOOD, Simon Michael Woodgrange Medical Practice, 40 Woodgrange Road, Forest Gate, London E7 0QH Tel: 020 8250 7585 Fax: 020 8250 7587 — MB ChB Manch. 1991.

SHERWOOD, Thomas (retired) 19 Clarendon Street, Cambridge CB1 1JU — (Guy's) MB BS Lond. 1960; DCH Eng. 1962; FRCP Lond. 1979, M 1964; DMRD Eng. 1966; FFR 1968; FRCR 1975; MA Camb. 1978. Prev: Clin. Dean Univ. Camb.

SHERWOOD, William James 4 The Moorlands, Kidlington OX5 2XX — MB BS Lond. 1996.

SHERWOOD-JONES, David Mark Occupational Health Service, Laurie House, Colyear Street, Derby DE1 1LJ Tel: 01332 868851 Email: david.sherwood-jones@derwentsharedservices.nhs.uk; 4 Abney Close, Mickleover, Derby DE3 9DZ — MB BS Lond. 1976 (St Thos.) MRCS Eng. LRCP Lond. 1976; MRCP (UK) 1980; DIH Soc. Apoth. Lond. 1983; FFOM RCP Lond. 1995, MFOM 1986. Cons. Occupational Med. Specialty: Occupat. Health. Socs: Soc. Occupat. Med.; Nat. Back Exchange. Prev: Hon. Sec. E. Midlands Gp. Soc. Occupational Med.; Med. Insp. Health & Safety Exec. Midls. Div.; Dep. MO Nat. Coal Bd. S. Yorks. Area.

SHESHGIRI, Mr Jitendra Basavanneppa Accident & Emergency Department, Frenchay Hospital, Frenchay, Bristol BS16 1LE Tel: 0117 970 1212 Fax: 0117 957 2335; 148 Frenchay Park Road, Stapleton, Bristol BS16 1HB Tel: 0117 965 7529 Fax: 0117 965 7529 — MB BS Karnatak 1980; FRCS Glas. 1988. Assoc. Specialist (A & E) Frenchay Healthcare Trust Bristol. Socs: Assoc. Mem. Brit. Assn. Accid. & Emerg. Med. Prev: Regist. (Cardiothoracic Surg.) Univ. Hosp. Wales Cardiff; Regist. (Surg.) Bishop Auckland Gen. Hosp. Co. Durh.

SHETH, Bipin Chandra Ramniklal 31 Briar Dene close, East Herrington, Sunderland 5R3 3RU Fax: 0191 528 1506 Email: bipincr@lycos.com — MB BS Ranchi 1969. GP Sunderland; Mem. Sunderland LMC. Specialty: Orthop.; Accid. & Emerg.; Rheumatol. Socs: Fell.Roy. Soc. of Med.; Roy. Soc. of Health.

SHETH, Gyandev Punyadev 63 Ealing Road, Wembley HA0 4BN Tel: 020 8902 7135 — MB BS Indore 1968 (M.G.M. Med. Coll.) MS (Ophth.) Gujarat 1971, DO 1970.

SHETH, Himanshu 68A West Park Road, Maidstone ME15 7AG — MB BS Gujarat 1975.

SHETH, Hiten Gyandev 16 Scotia Building, Atlantic Wharf, The Highway, London E1W 3WA Email: hiten@doctors.org.uk — MB BS Lond. 1997; BSc Lond. 1994; MRCOphth Lond. 2003. Specialist Regist. (Ophth.) St Thomas' Hosp. Lond. Specialty: Ophth.

SHETH, Jyotika Gyandev The Surgery, 131 Dartmouth Road, London NW2 4ES Tel: 020 8450 0403 Fax: 020 8450 3355; 63 Ealing Road, Wembley HA0 4BN Tel: 020 8902 7135 Fax: 020 8902 7135 — MB BS Gujarat 1970 (BJ Med. Coll. Ahmedabad) DCH Bombay 1973; DCH RCP Lond. 1989; Dip. Pract. Dermat. Wales 1992; MFFP 1993. Family Plann. Doctor Ealing HA; Trainer (Family Plann.) Lond.; Examr. Red Cross; Med. Examr. DSS. Specialty: Dermat. Socs: BMA; Med. Protec. Soc.; Fac.Fam.Plann.

SHETH, Pradip Kumar Shantilal c/o Mrs Rama G. Sheth, 24 Hood Road, London SW20 0SR — MB BS Indore 1973.

SHETH, Tanay Rajnikant 114 Albert Road, Epsom KT17 4EL — MB BS Lond. 1994; MA Camb. 1995.

SHETTAR, Chanabasappa Kuruvatteppa 111A Wood Lane, Isleworth TW7 5EG — MB BS Bombay 1956 (Grant Med. Coll.) Socs: BMA. Prev: Res. Surg. Off Roy. North. Hosp. Lond.; Surg. Regist. Gateshead Hosp. Gp.; SHO (Orthop.) Vict. Infirm. Glas.

SHETTY, Ajeya Krishna 24 Wrenn House, Harrow Village, Trinity Church Road, Barnes, London SW13 8NN — MB ChB Glas. 1993; MRCP (UK) 1997.

SHETTY, Arun Apple Tree Medical Practice, 4 Wheatsheaf Court, Burton Joyce, Nottingham NG14 5EA — MB ChB Manch. 1987; MRCP (UK); BSc (Hons.); MRCGP. Special Interest: Lipid Managem. & Cardiovasc. Med.

SHETTY, Mr Asode Anantharam Medway Hospital, Gillingham ME7 5NY; 6 Barncroft Drive, Hampstead, Gillingham ME7 3TJ — MB BS Karnatak 1982; FRCS Ed. 1989.

SHETTY, Bola Krishna Kishore Pallion Health Centre, Hylton Road, Sunderland SR4 7XF Tel: 0191 657 1319 — MB BS Mysore 1976. GP Sunderland.

SHETTY, Manjaya Kaliyur The Surgery, 997 Romford Road, Manor Park, London E12 5JR Tel: 020 8478 2711 Fax: 020 8553 4696 — MB BS Karnatak 1965 (Kasturba Med. Coll.)

SHETTY, Muniyal Aravinda Shettleston Health Centre, Shettleston Health Centre, 420 Old Shettleston Road, Glasgow G32 7JZ Tel: 0141 531 6250 Fax: 0141 531 6216 — MB BS Mysore 1970 (Mysore Med. Coll.) GP Glas.

SHETTY, Narendra Vithal Bridge Street Surgery, 48 Bridge Street, Newton-le-Willows WA12 9QS Tel: 01925 225755 — MB BS Bombay 1966.

SHETTY, Padubidri Ramanand Northowram Hospital, Northowram, Halifax HX3 7SW Tel: 01422 201101; 5 Savile Lea, Halifax HX1 2DD Tel: 01422 252462 — MB BS Bangalore 1972 (Bangalore Med. Coll.) DPM RCPSI 1995. Assoc. Specialist (Psychiat.) Calderdale HA. Specialty: Gen. Psychiat. Prev: Clin. Asst. (Psychiat.) Calderdale HA; Regist. (Psychiat.) Calderdale HA.

SHETTY, Mr Thimmangoor Thimmappa 50 Larch Drive, Stanwix, Carlisle CA3 9FL — MB BS Mysore 1979; DO RCPSI 1987; FRCS Glas. 1987. Assoc. Specialist (Ophth.) Cumbld. Infirm. Carlisle. Specialty: Ophth.

SHEVILLE, Eli 11 Stone Hall Road, Winchmore Hill, London N21 1LR Tel: 020 8360 6621 — (Glasgow University) MB ChB Glas. 1951; DMRD RCS Eng. 1957; FFR Lond. 1962; FRCR Lond. 1975. Specialty: Radiol. Prev: Cons. Radiol. Qu. Eliz. II Hosp. Welwyn Gdn. City; Med. Dir. Herts. Magnetic Imaging Campus Qu. Eliz. II Hosp.; Sen. Regist. (Radiol.) Hosp. Sick Childr. Gt. Ormond St. & Roy. Free Hosp.

SHEVKET, Mehmet 57 Woodland Road, Northfield, Birmingham B31 9AB — MB BS Lond. 1996; MRCGP.

SHEVLIN, Bernard Anthony The New Surgery, Old Road, Tean, Stoke-on-Trent ST10 4EG Tel: 01538 722323 Fax: 01538 722215 — MB BCh Wales 1968; LMCC 1970; DObst RCOG 1972; MRCGP 1976.

SHEVLIN, Peter Vincent Hawthorn Surgery, Wilfrid Terrace, Branch Road, Leeds LS12 5NR Tel: 0113 295 4770 Fax: 0113 295 4771 — MB ChB Leeds 1983.

SHEVLIN (LEECH), Anne Bridget (retired) 12 West End Drive, Ilkeston DE7 5GG Tel: 0115 917 7324 — MB ChB Ed. 1963 (Edinburgh University) DObst RCOG 1966; FRCGP 1993, M 1976. Prev: Research Regist. (Geriat.) Dryburn Hosp. Durh.

SHEWAN, David Michael 5 St Botolph's Close, Saxilby, Lincoln LN1 2PS Tel: 01522 702097 Fax: 01522 702097 — MB ChB Ed. 1963 (Camb. & Ed.) BA Camb. 1960; FFA RCS Eng. 1968. Cons. Anaesth. Lincoln Co. Hosp. Specialty: Anaesth. Prev: Sen. Regist. (Anaesth.) Edin. Roy. Infirm.; SHO (Anaesth.) Edin. City Hosp.; SHO (Anaesth.) & Ho. Phys. West. Gen. Hosp. Edin.

SHEWAN, Doreen Baxter (Surgery), Kidlington Health Centre, Kidlington, Oxford OX44 7SS; 19 Stanley Road, Oxford OX4 1QY Tel: 01865 725203 — MB ChB Aberd. 1970; DObst. RCOG 1975; MRCGP 1976. Socs: BMA. Prev: SHO (O & G) Raigmore Hosp. Inverness; Ho. Off. (Med.) & Ho. Off. (Surg.) Qu. Eliz. Hosp. Barbados; Resid. (Paediat.) Kingston Gen. Hosp., Canada.

SHEWARD, Jonathan Christopher — MB ChB Ed. 1985; MRCGP 1993. Gen. Practitioner Maybole H.C.; Clin. Asst. (Geriat. Med.) Ayrsh.; Chairm. Carrick & Doon LHCC. Socs: MRCGP.

SHEWELL, Mr Peter Charles The White House, Didley, Wormbridge, Hereford HR2 9DA Tel: 01981 570233 Fax: 01981 570233 — MB ChB Birm. 1984; MSc Birm. 1989; FRCS Ed. 1989; FRCS (Orth.) 1995. Cons. Orthop. Surg. Hereford Gen. Hosp. Specialty: Orthop.

SHEWELL, Phyllida Kathleen Royal Devon and Exeter Hospital, Barrack Road, Exeter EX2 5DW; Western Cottage, Church St, Kenton, Exeter EX6 8LU — MB BS Lond. 1973; BSc Lond. 1971; MRCS Eng. LRCP Lond. 1973; DGM RCP Lond. 1987. Clin. Asst. (Elderly Med.) Roy. Devon & Exeter Hosp.; Clin. Asst. (Elderly Care) Exeter & Dist. Community Health Trust. Specialty: Care of the Elderly.

SHEWRING, Mr David Joseph Department of Orthopaedics, University Hospital of Wales, Heath Park, Cardiff CF4 4XN Tel: 029 2074 7747; 62 Victoria Road, Penarth CF64 3HZ Tel: 029 2070 8384 — MB BCh Wales 1984 (Welsh National School of Medicine) FRCS Ed. 1989; FRCS (Orth.) 1994; Dip Hand Surg (Europe) 1996. Cons. (Orthop. & Hand Surg.) Univ. Hosp. Wales NHS Healthcare Trust; Hon. Lect. Univ. of Wales Coll. of Med. Specialty: Orthop. Socs: Brit. Soc. Surg. Hand; Brit. Orthop. Assn.

SHEWRING, John Ignatius Llanedeyrn Health Centre, Maelfa, Llanedeyrn, Cardiff CF23 9PN Tel: 029 2073 1671 Fax: 029 2054 0129 — MB BCh Wales 1991 (Univ. Wales Coll. Med.) DRCOG 1995; MRCGP 1998. Co-Dir. E. Cardiff Co-op. Specialty: Gen. Pract. Socs: (Sec.) Welsh Assn. GP Regist.s. Prev: GMSC Regist.s Commiss. (Welsh Represen.).

SHEWRING, Paul Michael Lisson Grove Medical Centre, 3-5 Lisson Grove, Mutley, Plymouth PL4 7DL Tel: 01752 205555 Fax: 01752 205558; 288 Fort Austin Avenue, Crownhill, Plymouth PL6 5SR Tel: 01752 701345 — MB BS Lond. 1973; MRCS Eng. LRCP Lond. 1973; DCH Eng. 1976; DRCOG 1979; MRCGP 1980.

SHEWRING, Sarah Anne The Emergency Unit, University Hospital of Wales, Heath Park, Cardiff CF14 Tel: 029 2074 7747 — MB BCh Wales 1993 (Univ. Wales Coll. Med.) DRCOG 1995; DFFP 1996; MRCGP 1998. Middle Grade A & E. Specialty: Accid. & Emerg.

SHEWRY, Sylvia Mary 8 Kings Road, North Luffenham, Oakham LE15 8JH Tel: 01780 720893 Fax: 01780 720893 — (Newc.) MB BS Newc. 1970; DObst RCOG 1972; DA Eng. 1974; DCH Eng. 1975.

SHEYBANY, Shiva Stonewalls, Hempton, Banbury OX15 0QS Tel: 01869 338439 — MD Tehran 1974; MRCOG 1976. Sen. Regist. (O & G) Northampton Gen. Hosp. & John Radcliffe Hosp. Oxf. Specialty: Obst. & Gyn. Socs: CCST 1998. Prev: Sen. Regist. & Clin. Lect. John Radcliffe Hosp. Oxf.

SHIA, Gilbert Tsai-Wei 109 Bloxham Road, Banbury OX16 9JT — MB BChir Camb. 1988 (Cambridge) BSc (Hons.) Lond. 1980; MSc Oxf. 1983; DCH 1991; DRCOG 1991. Specialty: Gen. Pract. Socs: BMA.

SHIBU, Mr Mohamed Meh Plastic Surgery Department, Barts and The London Hospital Trust, Whitechapel, London E1 1BB Tel: 020 7377 7192 Fax: 020 7377 7447 Email: mohamed.shibu@barstandthelondon.nhs.uk — MB BCh Al Fateh 1981; FRCS Ed. 1988.

SHICKLE, Darren Arthur Public Health, Scharr, University of Sheffield, Regent Court, 30 Regent St., Sheffield S1 4DA Tel: 0114 222 0818 Fax: 0114 222 0798 Email: d.shickle@sheffield.ac.uk; 262 Abbeydale Road S., Totley Rise, Sheffield S17 3LL — MB BCh Wales 1988; MPH Wales 1994; MFPHM 1995; MA Wales 1996. Clin. Sen. Lect. (Pub. Health Med.) Univ. Sheff. Specialty: Pub. Health Med.

SHIDRAWI, Ray George Acad. Dept. of Med. and Surgic. Gastroenterol., Homerton University Hospital, Homerton Row, London E9 6SR Tel: 020 8510 7473 Fax: 020 8510 7378 Email: ray.shidrawi@homerton.nhs.uk — MB BS Lond. 1987; MRCP Lond. 1990; MD Lond. 1996; FRCP 2004. Cons. Phys. and Gastroenterologist. Specialty: Gen. Med.; Gastroenterol. Special Interest: Interventional Endoscopy; Liver Diseases. Socs: Brit. Soc. of Gastroenterol.; Brit. Assn. for the Study of Liver Diseases; Med. Counc. for Alcohol. Prev: Sen. Regist. in Gen. Med. and Gastroenterol., Centr. Middlx. Hosp. 1999-2000; Sen. Regist. in Gen. Med. and Gastroenterol., Chelsea and Westm. Hosp. 1997-1999; Sen. Regist. in Gen. Med. and Gastroenterol., W. Middlx. Univ. Hosp. 1996-1997.

SHIEFF, Mr Colin Louis The Royal Free Hospital, London NW3 2QG Tel: 020 7830 2097 Fax: 020 7830 2560 Email: colin.shieff@royalfree.nhs.uk — MB ChB Liverp. 1973; FRCS Ed. 1979. Cons. Neurosurg. Roy. Free. Hosp. Lond.; Hon. Cons. Neurosurg., Nat. Hosp. for Neurol. + Neurosurg. Lond.; Lt Col RAMC (V). Specialty: Neurosurg.; Medico Legal. Socs: World Soc. Sterotactid & Funct. Neurosurg.; Roy. Soc. of Med.; Europ. Soc. Stereotactic & Funct. Neurosug. Prev: Sen. Regist. (Neurosurg.) Midl. Centre for Neurosurg. & Neurol., Birm.; Fell. Duke Univ. Med. Centr. Durh. N. Carolina; Regist. Atkinson Morley's Hosp. Lond.

SHIEL, Deborah Anne Hillview Medical Centre, 3 Heathside Road, Woking GU22 7QP Tel: 01483 760707 — MB BCh BAO NUI 1986 (Univ. Coll. Galway) DMH Belf. 1990; DRCOG 1991; MRCGP 1996; Cert. in Diabetes Care (Warwick) 2003. Gen. Pract. Trainer. Socs: BMA; RCGP.

SHIEL, Julian Iannis 26 Southway, Lewes BN7 1LY — MB BCh BAO NUI 1990.

SHIELD, John Edwin Hamilton 93 Kingweston Avenue, Shirehampton, Bristol BS11 0AH Tel: 0117 982 2548 — MB ChB Bristol 1959.

SHIELD, Julian Paul Hamilton Institute of Child Health, St. Michaels Hill, Bristol BS2 8BJ Email: j.p.h.shield@bristol.ac.uk — MB ChB Bristol 1985; FRCPCH (1998); MRCP (UK) 1988; MD Bristol 1997. Cons. Sen. Lect. Dept. of Child Health Univ. of Bristol. Specialty: Paediat.

SHIELD, Michael James Botts Furlong, Stone, Aylesbury HP17 8PR Tel: 01296 747054 — MB BS Lond. 1973 (Middlesex) MRCPath 1979; MFPM 1990; FRCPath 1991. Sen. Director, Europ. Med. Operat.s, Searle; Hon. Research Fell. Dept. Med. Physics Univ. of Exeter. Specialty: Pharmaceutical Medicine; Med. Microbiol. Socs: BMA; Fell. Roy. Coll. Pathol.; Fac. Pharmaceut. Med. Prev: Med. Dir. G.D. Searle & Co. High Wycombe; Dir. Clin. Research (Europe) G.D. Searle & Co. High Wycombe; Sen. Lect. & Hon. Cons. (Bacteriol.) St. Mary's Hosp. Med. Sch. Lond.

SHIELD, Nigel Boyd Ringwood Health Centre, The Close, Ringwood BH24 1JY Tel: 01425 478901 Fax: 01425 478239; The Greenaway, 13 Warren Close, Ringwood BH24 2AJ Tel: 01425 477079 — MB BS Lond. 1972 (Middlx.) DObst RCOG 1976; Cert. Family Plann. JCC 1976. Prev: Trainee GP Salisbury VTS.

SHIELDS, Mr David Alan The County Hospital, Union Walk, Hereford HR1 2ER Tel: 01432 355444; Bank House, Perton, Hereford HR1 4HP — MB ChB Liverp. 1981; FRCS Eng. 1989; MD Liverp. 1995. Cons. Surg., Hereford Co. Hosp., Union Walk, Hereford, HR1 2ER. Specialty: Vasc. Med. Prev: Locum Cons. Surg., Norf. & Norwich Hosp.; Sen. Surgic. Regist., Norf. & Norwich Hosp.; Research Fell. (vasc. Surg.), Middlx. Hosp., Lond.

SHIELDS, Erica Glynis 59 Lyndhurst Parade, Belfast BT13 3PB — MB BCh BAO Belf. 1993.

SHIELDS, Gavin Graham Primrose Hill, Draycote, Rugby CV23 9RB — MB ChB Birm. 1989.

SHIELDS, Gillian Leigh c/o 77 Mullahead Road, Tandragee, Craigavon BT62 2LB — MB BCh BAO Belf. 1988; MB BCh (Hons.) BAO Belf. 1988; DRCOG 1991; DMH Belf. 1992; MRGCP 1993. Socs: BMA.

SHIELDS, Jean May (retired) de Bathe Cross, North Tawton, Okehampton EX20 2BB Tel: 01837 82218 — MB BS Lond. 1953 (Middlx.) MRCS Eng. LRCP Lond. 1953; DObst RCOG 1955. Prev: G.P. Princip., Okehampton, Devon.

SHIELDS, Jennifer Law Medical Group Practice, 9 Wrottesley Road, London NW10 5UY Tel: 020 8903 4848; 66 The Avenue, London NW6 7NP — MB BS Lond. 1976 (Oxford University and Westminster University) BA (Hons.) Oxf 1973; MRCP (UK) 1980; MRCGP 1983.

SHIELDS, Martin Oliver 15 Beechmount Park, Newry BT34 1LA — MB BCh BAO Belf. 1997.

SHIELDS, Mary Frances The Health Centre, Park Drive, Stenhousemuir, Falkirk; 40 The Quadrant, Clarkston, Glasgow G76 8AG — MB ChB Glas. 1983; MRCGP 1987. Prev: SHO (Psychiat.) Woodilee Hosp. Lenzie; Ho. Off. Roy. Alexandra Infirm. Paisley; Ho. Off. Stobhill Hosp. Glas.

SHIELDS, Michael Anthony (retired) Brora, Springfield Court, Gresford, Wrexham LL12 8HY — MB ChB Aberd. 1954; DObst RCOG 1958.

SHIELDS, Mr Michael David Pinderfields Hospital, Aboyon Road, Wakefield WF1 4EE Tel: 01924 201688 Fax: 01924 214147; The Dower House, Heath, Wakefield WF1 5SL Tel: 01924 382361 — BSc (Anat.) Lond. 1965, MB BS 1968; MRCS Eng. LRCP Lond. 1968; FRCS Eng. 1973; FRCOG 1989, M 1975. Cons. (O & G) Wakefield Gp. Hosps. Specialty: Obst. & Gyn. Socs: BMA. Prev: Sen. Regist. Middlx. Hosp. Lond.; Regist. (O & G) Westm. Hosp. Lond.; SHO (O & G) Qu. Charlotte's Metern. & Chelsea Hosps. for Wom.

SHIELDS, Michael David Department of Clinical Health, The Queens University of Belfast, Grosvenor Road, Belfast BT12 6BJ Tel: 01232 240503 Fax: 01232 236455 — MB ChB Bristol 1979; MRCP (UK) 1982; MD Bristol 1988; FRCP Lond. 1996; FRCPCH 1997. Cons. & Sen. Lect. (Respirat. Paediat.) Nuffield Dept. Child Health Qu.s Univ. Belf. Specialty: Paediat. Prev: Sen. Regist. Roy. Belf. Hosp. for Sick Childr.; Research Fell. Sick Childr. Hosp. Toronto.

SHIELDS, Michael Leslie Priory Cottage, 14 Northgate, Cottingham HU16 4HH — MB ChB Leeds 1983; MRCP (UK) 1989; MRCPath 1994. Cons. Haemat. Hull Hosps. NHS Trust. Specialty: Haematology. Prev: Sen. Regist. Rotat. (Haemat.) St. Geo. Hosp. Lond.

SHIELDS, Noel Peter (retired) 21 Mount Street, Taunton TA1 3QF — (St. Bart.) MRCS Eng. LRCP Lond. 1938; MA Camb. 1946; MRCGP 1956. Prev: Ho. Surg. St. Bart. Hosp.

SHIELDS, Penny Alice Aspley Medical Centre, 511 Aspley Lane, Aspley, Nottingham NG8 5RW Tel: 0115 929 2700 Fax: 0115 929 8276 — MB ChB Bristol 1987; BSc Hons. Leeds 1976; PhD Lond. 1982; MRCGP 1996. Trainee GP Nottm. VTS. Prev: SHO (A & E) Kingston Hosp. Surrey; SHO (O & G) Mayday Univ. Hosp. Croydon; Ho. (Surg.) Mayday Univ. Hosp. Croydon.

SHIELDS, Sir Robert, Deputy Lt. 81 Meols Drive, West Kirby, Wirral CH48 5DF Tel: 0151 632 3588 Fax: 0151 632 5613 Email: r.shields@rcsed.ac.uk — MB ChB Glas. 1953; M.B., Ch. B. 1953 (Glas.) FRCS Ed. 1959; MD (Hons.) Glas. 1965; FRCS Eng. 1966; Hon. DSc Wales 1990; Hon. FCS (SA) 1991; Hon. FACS 1991; FRCPS 1993; Hon. FCS HK 1995; Hon. FRCSI 1996; FRCP Ed 1997; Hon. FRACS 1997. Cons. Surg. Emerit. Roy. Liverp. Univ. Hosp. & Prof. Surg. Emerit. Univ. Liverp. Specialty: Gen. Surg.; Gastroenterol. Socs: Pres., Trav. Surigical Soc.; Regent & Past Pres. RCSEd; (Ex-Pres.) Surgic. Research Soc. & Assoc. of Surgs. Prev: Dean Fac. Med. Univ. Liverp.; Reader (Surg.) & Cons. Surg. Welsh Nat. Sch. Med.; Lect. (Surg.) & Sen. Regist. West. Infirm. Glas.

SHIELDS, Robert Hay 14 Oxwich House, Burton Pidsea, Hull HU12 9AF — MB BS Durh. 1952 (Newc.) Prev: Ho. Phys. Walkergate Hosp. Newc.; Ho. Surg. Princess Mary Matern. Hosp. Newc.

SHIELDS, Robert Stuart David 25 Balmoral Road, Andover SP10 3HY — MB ChB Liverp. 1991; MRCGP 1995.

SHIELDS, Rodger Park (retired) 38 Connaught Way, Tunbridge Wells TN4 9QL Tel: 01892 531577 — (St. Mary's) MRCS Eng. LRCP Lond. 1945; MB BS Lond. 1946; DTM & H Eng. 1947. Prev: Med. Off. Angolan Refugee Med. Relief (Congo Protestant Relief Agency.

SHIELDS, Sheila Deirdre Allesley Park Medical Centre, Whitaker Road No.2, Coventry CV5 9JE Tel: 024 7667 4123 Fax: 024 7667 2196; Health Centre, University of Warwick, Coventry CV4 7AL Tel: 024 76 523523 — MB BCh BAO Dub. 1958. Prev: Anaesth. Regist. Coventry & Warw. Hosp.

SHIELDS, Simon Alexander Norfolk & Norwich University Hospital, Colney Lane, Norwich NR4 7UY Tel: 01603 286286 Email: simon.shields@nnuh.nhs.uk — BM BCh Oxf. 1992; MRCP (UK) 1995. Specialist Regist. Neurol., Nat. Hosp. (Lond.) & Addenbrookes (Camb.). Specialty: Neurol. Prev: Regist. (Med. & Cardiol.) Camb.; SHO Lond. & Camb.; MRC Clin. Train. Fell. (Camb. Centre Brain Repair).

SHIELDS, Stephanie Anne 33 Stamperland Av, Clarkston, Glasgow G76 8EX — MB ChB Glas. 1997.

SHIELL, Kate Ann 5 Lomas Close, Stannington, Sheffield S6 6EU — MB ChB Sheff. 1994.

SHIELLS, Gordon McIntyre The Park Medical Group, Fawdon Park Road, Newcastle upon Tyne NE3 2PE Tel: 0191 285 1763 Fax: 0191 284 2374 — MB BS Newc. 1983. SHO (Paediat.) Bishop Auckland Gen. Hosp. W. Durh. HA. Socs: BMA. Prev: Ho. Off. (Gen. Med.) Newc. Gen. Hosp.; Ho. Off. (Gen. Surg.) Ashington Hosp.

SHIELLS, Linda Ann Fleet Medical Centre, Church Road, Fleet GU51 4PE Tel: 01252 613327 Fax: 01252 815156 — MB ChB Dundee 1995.

SHIELLS, William Arnott (retired) Elm Tree Farm, Farnham, Saxmundham IP17 1JZ Tel: 01728 602695 — MB BS Durh. 1951.

SHIELS, Aine Maria Kathryn 28 Dorchester Park, Malone Road, Belfast BT9 6RJ — MB BCh BAO Belf. 1991; MB BCh Belf. 1991.

SHIELS, Annette Martina 132 Englefield Road, London N1 3LQ Tel: 020 7226 2547 — MB ChB Birm. 1989; MRCP (UK) 1993. Specialty: Gen. Med.; Nephrol.

SHIELS, Rachel Mary 46 Howden Hall Road, Edinburgh EH16 6PJ — MB ChB Ed. 1991.

SHIER, Deborah Lucy John Scott Health Centre, Green Lanes, London N4 2NU; 10 St Pauls Road, Islington, London N1 2QN Tel: 020 7359 4518 — MB BS Lond. 1984 (St. Thos.) LMSSA Lond. 1983. GP. Specialty: Gen. Pract. Prev: Ho. Surg. Qu. Alexandra's Hosp. Portsmouth; Ho. Phys. Medway Hosp. Gillingham.

SHIER, Dermot Ievers (retired) Beach House, 10 Trevallion Park, Feock, Truro TR3 6RS Tel: 01872 865385 Fax: 01872 865385 Email: dermot@dishier.freeserve.co.uk — (T.C. Dub.) MB BCh BAO Dub. 1968; DCH Eng. 1972; DObst RCOG 1974. p/t Locum GP. Prev: Med. Off. Labrador W. Med. Clinic Labrador City Canada.

SHIERS, Caroline Essex Rivers Health Care Trust, Child Health Department, Clacton Hospital, Freeland Road, Clacton-on-Sea CO15 1LH Tel: 01255 201654; 25 Holmbrook Way, Frinton-on-Sea CO13 9LW Tel: 01255 673032 — (St. Mary's) MB BS Lond. 1968. Clin. Med. Off. Essex Rivers Health Care Trust Colchester. Specialty: Community Child Health.

SHIERS, David Edward Leek Health Centre, Fountain Street, Leek ST13 6JB Tel: 01538 381022 Fax: 01538 398638 — MB ChB Manch. 1974; MRCP (UK) 1977. Prev: Regist. (Gen. Med.) North. Gen. Hosp. Sheff.; SHO (A & E) & Regist. (Gen. Med.) Pk. Hosp. Manch.

SHIEW, Chun Ming Flat 7, Ashdown, 36 Camborne Road, Sutton SM2 6RE Tel: 020 8642 8460 Email: mshiew@aol.com — MB BS Lond. 1996 (St. Geos.) Specialty: Anaesth.

SHIEW, Marianne May Foon No.7 Ashdown, 36 Cambourne Road, Sutton SM2 6RE — MB BS Lond. 1995. Specialty: Ophth.

SHIFFMAN, Ellen Mali (retired) 16 Primrose Road, Calderstones, Liverpool L18 2HE Tel: 0151 280 3051 — LRCP LRCS Ed. LRFPS Glas. 1948 (Roy. Colls. Ed.) LRCP LRCS Ed., LRFPS Glas. 1948; FRCGP 1980. Prev: Hosp. Pract. (Psychiat.) Sefton Gen. Hosp. Liverp.

SHIFFMAN, Ian Felix Ellergreen Medical Centre, 24 Carr Lane, Norris Green, Liverpool L11 2YA — MB ChB Liverp. 1979; MRCS Eng. LRCP Lond. 1979; DRCOG 1983. Prev: Trainee GP Liverp. AHA VTS; SHO (Cardiol.) Sefton Gen. Hosp.; Ho. Surg. Broadgreen Hosp. Liverp.

SHIFFMAN, Kenneth 31 Rodney Street, Liverpool L1 9EH Tel: 0151 703 2907 Fax: 0151 703 2924; 16 Primrose Road, Liverpool L18 2HE Tel: 0151 280 3051 — (Liverp.) MRCS Eng. LRCP Lond. 1952; FRCGP 1980. Socs: Brit. Geriat. Soc.; Med. Assn. Soc.; Liverp. Med. Inst. Prev: Hosp. Pract. (Geriat. Med.) Pk. Hosp. Liverp.; Ho. Phys. Broadgreen Hosp. Liverp.

SHIKOTRA, Bharat Keshavji The Surgery, 612 Saffron Lane, Leicester LE2 6TD Tel: 0116 291 1212 Fax: 0116 291 0300; 12 Kingswood Avenue, Leicester LE3 0UN — MB ChB Manch. 1985; DCH RCP Lond. 1989; Cert. Family Plann. JCC 1990; DRCOG 1990; T(GP) 1992. GP Leicester. Specialty: Gen. Pract.; Gen. Med. Prev: Trainee GP Leicester VTS; SHO (Geriat.) Leicester Gen. & Groby Rd. Hosp.; SHO (O & G) Chase Farm Hosp. Enfield.

SHIKOTRA, Kishan Keshavji 22B Strathern Road, Glenfrith, Leicester LE3 9RY — MB BS Lond. 1997.

SHILLAM, Geoffrey Norman Eastfield House Surgery, 6 St. Johns Road, Newbury RG14 7LW Tel: 01635 41495 Fax: 01635 522751

— MB ChB Bristol 1975; DCH Eng. 1980; DRCOG 1981; MRCGP 1982. Gen. Pract. in Newbury Berks.

SHILLIDAY, Ilona Ruth Renal Unit, Monkands Hospital, Monkscourt Avenue, Airdrie ML6 0JS — MB ChB Ed. 1984 (Edinburgh) MRCP Ed. 1987; MD Ed. 1998. Sen. Cons. Nephrologist and Phys., Monklands Hosp., Airdrie. Specialty: Nephrol.; Gen. Med. Prev: Staff Grade (Gen. Med.) Falkirk & Dist. Roy. Infirm.; Research Fell. (Med.) Univ. Glas.; Regist. (Renal) Roy. Infirm. Glas.

SHILLIDAY, Peter Frame 11 Thorpe Avenue, Peterborough PE3 6LA — MB ChB Manch. 1990.

SHILLING, Mr John Stanley St. Thomas' Hospital, Lambeth Palace Road, London SE1 7EH; Blackheath Hospital, 40-42 Lee Terrace, Blackheath, London SE3 9UD Tel: 020 8318 7722 — MB BS Lond. 1965 (St. Thos.) DO Eng. 1969; FRCS Eng. 1972. Cons. Ophth. Surg. St. Thos. Hosp. Lond. & Greenwich Hosp. Specialty: Ophth.

SHILLING, Rosemary Suhasini Solihull Hospital, Department of Anaesthetics, Lode Lane, Solihull B91 2JL Tel: 0121 711 4455 Fax: 0121 685 5476; 168 St. Bernards Road, Solihull B92 7BL — MB BS Madras 1975 (Vellore India) FFA RCS Eng. 1985. Cons. Anaesth. W. Midl. RHA. Specialty: Anaesth. Socs: BMA; MDUUS; RCA.

SHILLINGFORD, Michael John Pulborough Medical Group, Barnhouse Surgery, Barnhouse Close, Pulborough RH20 2HQ Tel: 01798 872815 Fax: 01798 872123; Highfield, Codmore Hill, Pulborough RH20 1BA Tel: 01798 872710 Fax: 01798 875947 — MB BS Lond. 1972 (St. Mary's) MRCS Eng. LRCP Lond. 1972. Socs: Fell. Roy. Soc. Med.; Fell Amer. Coll. of Phys.; Soc. Gen. Internal Med. Prev: SHO (Gen. Med.) Roy. W. Sussex Hosp. Chichester; Ho. Surg. St. Mary's Hosp. Lond.

SHILLINGLAW, Catherine Lily 39 The Glade, Langley, Southampton SO45 1ZP — BM Soton. 1993. Trainee GP Poole Hosp. VTS.

SHILLINGLAW, David 2 Knoll Croft, Styvechale, Coventry CV3 5BZ Tel: 024 76 62318 — MB ChB Glas. 1962; DObst RCOG 1965. Prev: SHO (Gyn.) & Res. Surg. Roy. Infirm. Glas.; SHO (Obst.) East. Dist. Hosp. Glas.

SHILLINGTON, Rosemary Kathleen Alexandra 43 Ballykeel Road, Hillsborough BT26 6NN — MB BCh BAO Belf. 1971; MB BCh Belf. 1971.

SHILLITO, Michael The Manford Way Health Centre, 40 Foremark Close, Hainault, Ilford IG6 3HS; Norlands, 2 Chigwell Park, Chigwell IG7 5BE — MB BS Lond. 1956 (King's Coll. Hosp.) DObst RCOG 1958. Clin. Asst. (Genitourin. Med.) Herts & Essex Hosp.

SHILLITO, Robert Nigel 1 Bryn Githw, Moel Fammau, Llanferres, Mold CH7 5ST — MB ChB Liverp. 1984; BSc Liverp. 1981, MB ChB 1984.

SHILLITO, Tina Jayne Anne 18 The Valley, Alwoodley, Leeds LS17 7NL Tel: 0113 261 1733; University Department of Obstetrics and Gynaecology, Leeds General Infirmary, Leeds LS2 9NS Tel: 0113 243 2799 Fax: 0113 292 6021 — MB ChB Leeds 1988; MRCOG 1994. Lect. O & G Leeds Univ. Leeds Gen. Infirm. Specialty: Obst. & Gyn. Prev: Research Regist. St. Jas. Hosp. Leeds.; Regist. York Dist. Hosp. & St. Jas. Hosp. Leeds; SHO (O & G) Huddersfield Roy. Infirm.

SHILLITO, Wendy Elizabeth 1 Bryn Eithin, Moel Fammau Road, Llanferres, Mold CH7 5SJ Tel: 01352 85394 — MB ChB Liverp. 1984; DObst. 1986.

SHIMI, Mr Sami Mahmoud Ninewells Hospital, Dundee DD1 9SY — MB ChB Dundee 1983; BSc (Hons.) Dundee 1979; FRCS Glas. 1987. Specialty: Gen. Surg. Prev: Regist. (Surg.) Stobhill Gen. Hosp. Glas.; Regist. (Vasc. Surg.) Stobhill Gen. Hosp. Glas.; Regist. (Plastic Surg.) Canniesburn Hosp. Glas.

SHIMMIN, Hilary Joyce 3 Little Dene, Lodore Road, Newcastle upon Tyne NE2 3NZ — MB BChir Camb. 1952 (Camb. & St. Bart.) DObst RCOG 1954.

SHIMMINGS, Kenneth Ian (retired) 13 Penrith Road, Boscombe Manor, Bournemouth BH5 1LT Tel: 01202 309098 — MB BS Lond. 1954 (St. Thos.) DA Eng. 1957; DObst RCOG 1960; FFA RCS Eng. 1962. Prev: Cons. Anaesth. Princess Margt. Hosp. Swindon.

SHIN, Christian Young-Myoung Sheet Street Surgery, 21 Sheet Street, Windsor SL4 1BZ Tel: 01753 860334 Fax: 01753 833696 — MB BChir Camb. 1989.

SHINA, Alfred Gourji Plender Street Surgery, 67 Plender Street, London NW1 0LB Tel: 020 7387 1929 Fax: 020 7387 1929 — MB BS Lond. 1979 (Oxf. & Westm.) MRCS Eng. LRCP Lond. 1978; MA Oxf. 1979; DRCOG 1981; MRCGP 1982.

SHINDE, Samantha Frenchay Hospital, Frenchay, Bristol BS16 1LE Tel: 0117 970 1212 — MB BS Lond. 1989; BSc (Hons.) Lond. 1986; FRCA 1994. Cons. Anaesth., Frenchay Hosp. Bristol. Specialty: Anaesth. Socs: AAGBI; RCA; BMA.

SHINDLER, Elizabeth (retired) 13 Corringway, Ealing, London W5 3AB Tel: 020 8998 3660 — MB BS Lond. 1960 (Lond. Hosp.) MB BS (Hnrs.) Lond. 1960; MRCS Eng. LRCP Lond. 1960. Prev: Staff Med. Off. Lond. Boro. Ealing.

SHINE, Alison Mary Esher Green Surgery, Esher Green Drive, Esher KT10 8BX Tel: 01372 462726; 3 Manor Road S., Esher KT10 0PY Tel: 020 8398 3528 — MB BS Lond. 1983; DRCOG 1987; MRCGP 1988.

SHINE, Brian Sean Francis Clinical Biochemistry, John Radcliffe Hospital, Oxford OX3 9DU Tel: 01865 220475 Fax: 01865 220348 Email: brian.shine@orh.nhs.uk — MB ChB Birm. 1974; FRCPath 1994, M 1982; MD Birm. 1985; MSc Lond. 1992. Cons. Chem. Pathologist, Chem. Path., Oxf. Radcliffe Hosps., Oxf. Specialty: Chem. Path.; Endocrinol. Socs: Fell. Roy. Soc. Med.; Fell. Roy. Statistical Soc. Prev: Sen. Lect. (Chem. Path.) Inst. Ophth. Lond.; Cons. Chem Path. Stoke Mandeville Hosp. Aylesbury.

SHINE, David Francis 34 The Firs, Kenilworth Road, Coventry CV5 6QD Tel: 024 76 73078 — MB ChB Birm. 1962; MRCP (U.K.) 1972.

SHINE, Ian Basil 35 Bryanston Square, London W1H 2DZ — MD Camb. 1966; MA Camb. 1963, MB 1958, BChir 1957 (Univ. Coll.; Hosp.).

SHINEBOURNE, Elliot Anthony Royal Brompton Hospital, Sydney St., London SW3 6NP Tel: 020 7351 8541 Fax: 020 7351 8544; 45 Larkhall Rise, London SW4 6HT Tel: 020 7498 9878 — (St. Bart.) MB BS (Hons.) Lond. 1963; MRCS Eng. LRCP Lond. 1963; FRCP 1979, M 1965; MD Lond. 1970; FRCPCH 1997. Cons. Paediat. (Cardiol.) Roy. Brompton Hosp.; Sen. Lect. Nat. Heart & Lung Inst. Specialty: Paediat. Cardiol. Socs: Brit. Cardiac Soc.; Brit. Paediat. Assn.; Assn. of Europ. Cardiol.s. Prev: MRC Clin. Research Fell. Inst. Cardiol. Nat. Heart Hosp. Lond.; Brit. Heart Foundat./Amer. Heart Assn. Trav. Fell. (Cardiovasc.) Univ. Coll. San Fransisco, USA; Ho. Phys. St. Bart. Hosp. Lond.

SHINER, Robert Joseph Herzliya Medical Centre, 7 Ramot Yam Street, Herzliya Pitvach 46851, Israel; Hammersmith Hospital, Department of Respiratory Medicine, Du Cane Road, London W12 0NN Tel: 020 8383 3269 Fax: 020 8743 9733 Email: r.shiner@imperial.ac.uk — (Middlx.) MRCS Eng. LRCP Lond. 1974; FRCPC 1982. p/t Cons. Phys. Herzliya Med. Centre Israel; Lect. (Med.) Tel-Aviv Univ. Med. Sch.; Hon. Sen. Lect. & Cons. (Respirat. Med.) Imperial Coll. Sch. Med. Lond. Specialty: Respirat. Med. Socs: Eur. Respirat. Soc.; Brit. Thorac. Soc.; Amer. Thorac. Soc. Prev: Cons. Phys. (Clin. Respirat. Physiol.) Chaim Sheba Med. Centre Tel-Hashomer, Israel; Resid. Respirat. Dis. McGill Univ., Montreal, Canada; Vis. Cons. Brompton Hosp. Lond.

SHINEWI, Fadha Fakhri East Surrey Hospital, Gynaecology Department, Canada Avenue, Redhill RH1 5RH Tel: 01737 231809 Fax: 01737 231727 — MB ChB Mosul 1970; Diploma Psychosexual Med., Lond. 1985; DRCOG, Lond. 1986. Cons. Family Plann., Reproductive Health Care, E. Surrey Hosp. Specialty: Family Plann. & Reproduc. Health. Special Interest: Colposcopy; Gen. Family Plann.; Menopause. Socs: Brit. Soc. of Colposcopy & Cervical Path.; Brit. Menopause Soc.; Lond. Soc. Family Plann. Doctor.

SHINGADIA, Delane Vanraj Royal London Hospital, Academic Child Health, Whitechapel, London EC1 1BB — MB ChB Zimbabwe 1987; MRCP (UK) 1992; DTM & H RCP Lond. 1995; MSc (Public Health) Univ. of Lond. 2000; FRCPCH 2001. Sen. Lect in Paediat. Infec.s Dis., St Barts & Roy. Lond. Med. & Dent. Sch.; Hon. Cons. At Barts & The Lond. NHS Trust, Gt. Ormond St. Hosp. NHS Trust. Specialty: Infec. Dis.; Paediat. Socs: RCPCh.; BMA; Brit. Immunol. & Infec. Dis. Gp. Prev: Sen. Regist. Gt. Ormond St. Hosp. Lond.; Fell. in Paediatric Infec. Dis.s; Childr.s Memor. Hosp. Chicago, USA; Regist. (Paediat.) St. Geo. Hosp. Lond., St. Helier Hosp. Carshalton & St. Peter's Hosp. Chertsey.

SHINH, Naval 7 Churchfield, Cringleford, Norwich NR4 6UP — LMSSA Lond. 1991.

SHINKFIELD, Mr Mark Noel Forsyth Department of General Surgery, St. Mary's Hospital, Newport PO30 5TG — MB BS Lond.

1982 (Roy. Free) BSc (Hons.) Lond. 1979; FRCS Eng. 1986. Cons. Gen. Surg. St. Mary's Hosp. Newport. I. of Wight. Specialty: Gen. Surg. Socs: Brit. Assn. Surgic. Oncol.; Assn. Surg.; BMA.

SHINKWIN, Mr Charles Antony 19 Balcaskie Close, Edgbaston, Birmingham B15 3UE — MB BCh BAO NUI 1984; FRCSI 1989; FRCS Eng. 1992.

SHINKWIN, Mary Patricia 39 Severn Road, Porthcawl CF36 3LN — MB BCh Wales 1979.

SHINN, Christopher Philip West Yorkshire Police, PO Box 9, Wakefield WF1 3QP Tel: 01924 292727; Lily Green Farm, Greenhow Hill, Harrogate HG3 5JL — MB ChB Leeds 1975; BSc (Pharmacol.) Leeds 1973. Force Med. Off. W. Yorks. Police.; Hon Sen. Clin. Lect. Leeds Univ. Med. Sch. Specialty: Occupat. Health.

SHINNAWI, Ahmed Kamal 45 Montagu Court, Gosforth, Newcastle upon Tyne NE3 4JL — LMSSA Lond. 1966; MRCP Glas. 1966.

SHINNER, Guy Anaesphetic Dept, Royal Orthopaedic Hospital, Bristol Road South, Northfield, Birmingham B31 2AP — MB BS Lond. 1990; FRCA; MB BS (Hons) Lond. 1990. Cons. (Anagith) Roy Orthop. Hosp Birm. Specialty: Anaesth.

SHINTON, Margaret (retired) 22 Winterbourne Road, Solihull B91 1LU Tel: 0121 705 0732 — (Leeds) MB ChB Leeds 1950. Prev: Clin. Asst. (Med.) Coventry & Warwick Hosp.

SHINTON, Professor Neville Keith 22 Winterbourne Road, Solihull B91 1LU Tel: 0121 705 0732 — MB ChB Birm. 1947; MRCS Eng. LRCP Lond. 1948; FRCP Lond. 1972, M 1952; MD Birm. 1961; FRCPath 1970, M 1963. Convener, Internat. Standards Organisation (ISO) In Vitro Med. devices. Specialty: Haematology; Pathology, General. Socs: (Ex-Pres.) Brit. Soc. Haematol.; (Ex-Pres.) Assn. Clin. Path. Prev: Dir. & Prof. Sch. Postgrad. Med. Educat. Univ. Warwick; Cons. Path & Haemat. Coventry Hosps.

SHINTON, Roger Anthony Birmingham Heartlands Hospital, Department of Medicine for the Elderly, Birmingham B9 5SS Tel: 0121 424 3768 Fax: 0121 753 0653 Email: r.shinton@bham.ac.uk — MB BChir Camb. 1980 (King's Coll. Hosp.) MD Camb. 1992, MA 1980; MSc Lond. 1988; FRCP 1999. Cons. Phys. (Med. for the Elderly) Birm. Heartlands Hosp. & Hon. Sen. Lect. Univ. Birm. Specialty: Gen. Med.; Vasc. Med.; Care of the Elderly. Special Interest: Stroke Preven. Socs: Brit. Geriat. Soc. (Sec W. Midl.s Br. 1998-1999); W. Midlands Physician's Assn. (Hon Sec 2003-); BMA (Chairman Solihull Div. 2003-05, Sec 1994-97). Prev: Hon. Sen. Regist. (Med.) Dudley Rd. Hosp. Birm.; SHO Rotat. (Med.) E. Birm. Hosp.; Ho. Phys. Kings Coll. Hosp. Lond.

SHIP, Rebecca Harriet Eisner, Goldman and Ship, Shipley Health Centre, Alexandra Road, Shipley BD18 3EG Tel: 01274 589153 Fax: 01274 770882 — BM Soton. 1985; BA Bristol 1972. Specialty: Gen. Pract. Prev: Ho. Off. (Surg.) Dorset Co. Hosp. Dorchester; Ho. Off. (Med.) Newmarket Gen. Hosp.

SHIPLEY, Michael Edward Centre for Rheumatology, The Middlesex Hospital, Mortimer Street, London W1N 8AA Tel: 020 7380 9035 Fax: 020 7380 9278 Email: mike.shipleypa@uclh.org; 70 The Lexington, 40 City Road, London EC1Y 2AN — MA Camb. 1974, MD 1983 (King's Coll. Hosp.) MB BChir Camb. 1973; MRCP (UK) 1976; FRCP Lond. 1988. Cons. Rheum. Univ. Coll. Lond. Hosps.; Hon. Cons. Rheum. King Edwd. VII Hosp. Lond. Specialty: Rheumatol. Socs: Fell. Roy. Soc. Med.; Brit. Soc. Rheum.; BMA.

SHIPLEY-ROWE, Ann Patricia Fernville Surgery, Midland Road, Hemel Hempstead HP2 5BL Tel: 01442 213919 Fax: 01442 216433; Avalon, 35 Grange Road, Bushey, Watford WD23 2LQ Tel: 01923 229288 — MB ChB Manch. 1984. Specialty: Gen. Pract.

SHIPMAN, Anthony John — MRCS Eng. LRCP Lond. 1978; MFPM RCP (UK) 1990. Freelance Privat. Phys. Specialty: Gen. Med. Socs: Fac. Pharmaceut. Med. Prev: Med. Dir. Pharmaco UK Ltd. Lond.; Med. & Managing Dir. J. S. Clin. Research; Head Med. Dept. Roche Products Ltd. Welwyn Gdn. City.

SHIPMAN, James Andrew Jonathan 12 Wetmore Road, Burton-on-Trent DE14 1SL Tel: 01283 564848 Fax: 01283 569416 Email: jajs@doctors.org.uk — MB ChB Leeds 1989; MRCGP 1993; DGM RCP Lond. 1993; T(GP) 1993; DFFP RCOG Lond. 1994; Dip Occ Med Lond. 1998. GP; GP Trainer (2 sessions); Company Doctor (1 session); PEC Member for PCT (2 Sessions). Specialty: Gen. Pract. Socs: Soc. of Occupat.al Med. Prev: SHO (Paediat.) Leeds Gen. Infirm.; SHO (Cas.) Bradford Roy. Infirm.; Ho. Off. (Gen. Surg.) Chapel Allerton Hosp. Leeds.

SHIPMAN, Paul Adrian Marc Hawkesley Health Centre, 375 Shannon Road, Kings Norton, Birmingham B38 9TJ Tel: 0121 486 4200 Fax: 0121 486 4201 — MB ChB Birm. 1977; BSc Birm. 1974, MB ChB 1977; DRCOG 1980; MRCGP 1981.

SHIPOLINI, Mr Alex Rudolf 25 Grange Avenue, London SE25 6DW — MB BS Lond. 1985. Specialty: Cardiothoracic Surg.

SHIPP, Phillida Ann 6 Dale Lane, Delph, Oldham OL3 5HY Tel: 01457 875171 Email: phillida@shipp.org — BM BCh Oxf. 1967 (Oxf. & Westm.) MA Oxf. 1967; MFFP 1993. Clin. Asst., GUM clinic, Tameside & Glossop PCT; Family Planning Dr. Tameside & Glossop PCT. Specialty: Family Plann. & Reproduc. Health; Genitourinary Medicine. Prev: Sen. Clin. Med. Off. (Child Health), Tameside & Glossop Community & Priority Serv.s NHS Trust; SCMO (sexual health) Tameside & Glossop Community & Priority Trust.

SHIPPEY, Benjamin John Mudcroft Farm, Newton in the Isle, Wisbech PE13 5HF — BM BS Nottm. 1995. SHO (Gen. Med.) Northampton Gen. Hosp. Specialty: Gen. Med. Prev: Ho. Off. (Surg.) Qu. Med. Centre Nottm.; Ho. Off. (Gen. Med.) Northampton Gen. Hosp.

SHIPSEY, Catherine Mary 4 Parklands Road, Chichester PO19 3DT — MB BS Lond. 1981; DRCOG 1986.

SHIPSEY, Dean 120 Grosvenor Road, Newcastle upon Tyne NE2 2RQ — MB ChB Ed. 1993. SHO (Orthop.) N. Tyneside Gen. Hosp. N. Shields. Prev: SHO (Cardiothoracic Surg.) Roy. Infirm. Edin.; SHO (A & E) Hull Roy. Infirm.; SHO (Gen. Surg.) East. Gen. Hosp. Edin.

SHIPSEY, Edward Mervyn (retired) 3 Manor Way, Beckenham BR3 3LH — MB BS Lond. 1950 (Middlx.) FRCGP 1977, M 1960. Hosp. Pract. (Orthop.) Bromley AHA. Prev: Ho. Surg. Radcliffe Infirm. Oxf. & Churchill Hosp. Oxf.

SHIPSEY, Margaret Mary (retired) Fairview Cottage, Ham Manor Way, Angmering, Littlehampton BN16 4JQ Tel: 01903 776015 — MB BCh BAO NUI 1953; DCH Eng. 1955.

SHIPSEY, Mary Josephine (retired) 3 Manor Way, Beckenham BR3 3LH — MB BCh BAO NUI 1952. Prev: Ho. Phys. Mater Miser. Hosp. Dub.

SHIPSEY, Maurice Mary Anthony (retired) Fairview Cottage, Ham Manor Way, Angmering, Littlehampton BN16 4JQ Tel: 01903 776015 — MB BCh BAO NUI 1953. Prev: Capt. RAMC. Jun. Surg. Specialist.

SHIPSEY, Mr Maurice Richard Lime Tree Surgery, Lime Tree Avenue, Findon Valley, Worthing BN14 0DL Tel: 01903 264101 Fax: 01903 695494 — MB BCh BAO Dub. 1981 (TC Dub.) FRCS Ed. 1985; MRCGP 1988; DRCOG 1988. Prev: Resid. Med. Off. King Edwd. VII Hosp. for Offs. Westm.

SHIPSEY, Sarah Jane Russell's Hall Hospital, Dudley DY1 2HQ Tel: 01384 456111; 28 Bond Street, Stirchley, Birmingham B30 2LA Tel: 0121 458 4481 — BM BCh Oxf. 1988; MRCP (UK) 1991. Regist. (Cardiol.) Russell's Hall Hosp. Dudley. Specialty: Cardiol. Prev: Regist. (Cardiol.) Qu. Eliz. Hosp. Birm.; Regist. (Gen. Med.) Salisbury Infirm.; Ho. Off. (Gen. Med.) John Radcliffe Hosp. Oxf.

SHIPSTON, Alison Mary 28 Wellington Road, Timperley, Altrincham WA15 7RE — MB ChB Manch. 1988; DRCOG 1991; MRCGP 1992.

SHIPSTON, James Edward 28 Wellington Road, Timperley, Altrincham WA15 7RE — MB ChB Manch. 1988; DRCOG 1991; MRCGP 1992.

SHIPSTONE, A V 14 Waterbridge Court, Appleton, Warrington WA4 3BJ Tel: 01925 601640 Fax: 01925 262701 Email: shipstonev@yahoo.com — (SMS Medical College, Jaipur, Rajasthan, India) MB BS Rajasthan 1969. Gen. Pract., Clin. Asst., M.I. Unit, Halton Gen. Hosp., Runcorn WA7 2DA. Specialty: Accid. & Emerg. Socs: D.F.F.P. (Family & Reproductive Diplomate Med.). Prev: Clin. Med. Off.

SHIPSTONE, Mr David Peter Alder Cottage, 19 Myddlewood, Myddle, Shrewsbury SY4 3RY — MB ChB Aberd. 1988; FRCS Eng. 1994. SHO Rotat. (Surg.) N. Staffs. HA.; Specialist Regist. (Urol.) Sheff. Specialty: Urol. Prev: Research Regist. (Urol.) Roy. Shrewsbury Hosp.; SHO (A & E) Leics. Demonst. (Anat.) Univ. Leics.

SHIPTON, Beryl Maude (retired) Virginia House, Shipton Gorge, Bridport DT6 4LL Tel: 01308 897391; Virginia House, Shipton Gorge, Bridport DT6 4LL Tel: 01308 897391 — MB ChB Bristol 1953; DObst RCOG 1956. Prev: Clin. Off. Surrey AHA.

SHIPTON, Peter Francis Croft Medical Centre, Calder Walk, Leamington Spa CV31 1SA Tel: 01926 421153 Fax: 01926 832343 — MB BS Lond. 1978; DRCOG 1981; MRCGP 1985.

SHIRALKAR, V M Twickenham Drive Surgery, 64 Twickenham Drive, Leasowe, Wirral CH46 1PF Tel: 0151 677 8882 Fax: 0151 604 0122.

SHIRAZ, Mahfel The Surgery, 80 Bickersteth Road, London SW17 9SJ Tel: 020 8682 0521 Fax: 020 8672 6532; 62 Woodcote Avenue, Wallington SM6 0QY Tel: 020 8669 6845 — MB BS Dacca 1975; DTM & H Liverp. 1984; MRCP (UK) 1985. Specialty: Gen. Med. Socs: Med. Protec. Soc.

SHIRAZI, Hussein Assadallah The Surgery, Riversley Road, Nuneaton CV11 5QT; The Surgery, 123 Pallett Drive, St. Nicolas Park, Nuneaton CV11 6JT — MB ChB Cairo 1958; LMSSA Lond. 1968.

SHIRAZI, Jane Elizabeth 13 The Park, Hampton Park, Hereford HR1 1TF Tel: 01432 351578 — MB BS Lond. 1986 (St. Bart.) MA Oxf. 1984.

SHIRAZI, Tarek Everglades, Shore Road, Wemyss Bay PA18 6AR — MB BS Lond. 1989.

SHIRBHATE, Naresh Champatrao 20 North Lodge, Chester-le-Street DH3 4AZ — MB BS Nagpur 1974; FFR RCSI 1982.

SHIRE, Catherine Mary Elizabeth The Grange Medical Centre, Dacre Banks, Harrogate HG3 4DX Tel: 01423 780497; Dacre Hall, Dacre, Harrogate HG3 4ET Tel: 01423 780497 — MB BS Newc. 1982; MRCGP 1986; DRCOG 1986. Socs: BMA. Prev: GP Stocksfield, N.ld.; SHO (Community Paeidat.) N.d.; Trainee GP Northallerton VTS.

SHIREHAMPTON, Teresa Ann Pewsey Surgery, High Street, Pewsey SN9 5AQ Tel: 01672 563511 Fax: 01672 563004 — MB BS Lond. 1973 (St. Bart.)

SHIRES, Kirsty Michelle 23 Lynwood Close, Willenhall WV12 5BW — MB ChB Leeds 1998.

SHIRES, Susan Elizabeth Elms Farm, Wimbish, Saffron Walden CB10 2PP — MB BS Lond. 1986; DRCOG 1988; DCH RCP Lond. 1989; MRCGP 1991; DPH Camb. 1995. Prev: Trainee GP OldCh. Hosp. Romford VTS.

SHIRLAW, Herbert Anthony Douglas (retired) 13 Well Cross Road, Up Holland, Skelmersdale WN8 0NU Tel: 01695 622745 — (Liverp.) MB ChB Liverp. 1950; DObst RCOG 1954.

SHIRLAW, Norman Alan 12 Crowland House, Springfield Road, London NW8 0QU Tel: 020 7624 3917 — LRCPI & LM, LRSCI & LM 1966 (Guy's & RCSI) LRCPI & LM, LRCSI & LM 1966; DObst RCOG 1968. Prev: SHO (Psychol. Med.) Roy. Free Hosp. Lond.; Ho. Surg. Roy. Sussex Co. Hosp. Brighton; Ho. Phys. Southlands Hosp. Shoreham-by-Sea.

SHIRLEY, Denise Susanna Lilian — MB BCh BAO Belf. 1995; AFRCSI Belfast 1995; MD Belfast 1995.

SHIRLEY, Isabel Mary Department of Clinical Radiology, The Hillingdon Hospital, Pield Heath Road, Uxbridge UB8 3NN Tel: 01895 279866 Fax: 01895 279865 Email: diz.shirley@thh.nhs.uk; 6 Waldron Road, Harrow HA2 0HU Tel: 020 8422 6381 Email: diz@farman.com — MB ChB Glas. 1969 (Glasgow) DObst RCOG 1971; DMRD Eng. 1982; FRCR 1984. Cons. Radiol. Hillingdon Hosp. Middlx.; Caldicot Guardian, Hillingdon Hosp.; Assoc. Med. Director Hillingdon Hosp. Specialty: Radiol. Socs: Fell. Roy. Soc. Med.; Brit. Med. Ultrasound Soc.; BMA. Prev: Clin. Dir. (Radiol.) Hillingdon Hosp.; Div.al Director (Clin. Support), Hillington Hosp.; Sen. Regist. & Regist. (Radiol.) & Clin. Asst. (Ultrasound) Univ. Coll. Hosp. Lond.

SHIRLEY, Janet Ann The Royal Surrey County Hospital NHS Trust, Egerton Road, Guildford GU2 7XX Tel: 01483 464122 Fax: 01483 464072; Everley Cottage, Wych Hill Lane, Woking GU22 0AH Tel: 01483 766423 Fax: 01483 766423 Email: shirleyjanet@hotmail.com — MB BS Lond. 1971 (Roy. Free) DCH Eng. 1974; FRCPath 1990, M 1978; Dip. Hlth. Mgt. Keele 1995. Cons. Haematologist, Roy. Surrey Co. Hosp., Guildford, Assoc. Med. Director, Roy. Surrey Co. Hosp., Guildford. Specialty: Haematology. Socs: Brit. Soc. Haematol.; BMA; (Bd.) Brit. Assn. Med. Managers. Prev: Cons. Haematologist & Med. Dir. King dwd. VII Hosp.; Cons. Haemat. & Clin. Dir. (Path.) Frimley Pk. Hosp. NHS Trust; Sen. Regist. (Haemat.) St. Thos. Hosp. Lond.

SHIRLEY, John Craig Nevis Surgery, Belford Road, Fort William PH33 6BU Tel: 01397 702947 Fax: 01397 700655 — MB ChB Sheff. 1977; MRCGP 1984. GP Fort William.

SHIRLEY, Robert Alan Bluebell Medical Centre, 356 Bluebell Road, Sheffield S5 6BS Tel: 0114 242 1406 Fax: 0114 261 8074; 23 Stainton Road, Sheffield S11 7AX Tel: 0114 268 7588 — MB ChB Bristol 1986; DGM RCP Lond. 1988; DCH RCP Lond. 1989; DRCOG 1991; MRCGP 1992.

SHIRLEY-QUIRK, Kathryn Jane The Mill House, Pangbourne, Reading RG8 7BB — MB BS Lond. 1985; DCH RCP Lond. 1987; MRCGP 1989. Garden Designer. Prev: GP Goring.

SHIRREFFS, Gordon Chisholm Jubilee Hospital, Huntly AB54 8EX Tel: 01466 792116; 2 Glamourhaugh Avenue, Huntly AB54 8AS Tel: 01466 2357 — MB ChB Aberd. 1957; DA Eng. 1962. Prev: Sen. Ho. Off. & Ho. Surg. & Ho. Phys. Aberd. Roy. Infirm.

SHIRREFFS, Murdoch John Gilbert Road Medical Group, 39 Gilbert Road, Bucksburn, Aberdeen AB21 9AN Tel: 01224 712138 Fax: 01224 712239; 72 Gray Street, Aberdeen AB10 6JE Tel: 01224 321998 Fax: 01224 315615 — MB ChB Aberd. 1970; DObst RCOG 1973; FRCGP 1992, M 1974; MF Hom 1996; Homeopathic Specialist 2000. GP Med. Homoeopath. & Hypnother. Aberd.; Specialist i/c of NHS Grampian Homepathy Serv. Specialty: Gen. Med. Socs: Hon. Sec. Grampian Div.; Brit. Soc. Med. & Dent. Hypn. Prev: Trainee GP Aberd. VTS; Ho. Off. Aberd. Roy. Infirm.

SHIRRIFFS, George Geddes 19 Richmondhill Place, Aberdeen, Aberdeen AB15 5EN Tel: 01224 311044 Fax: 01224 627159; 19 Richmondhill Place, Aberdeen AB15 5EN — MB ChB Aberd. 1963; FRCGP 1982, M 1974; MEd Aberd. 1989. Clin. Sen. Lect. (Gen. Pract.) Univ. Aberd.; Nat. Co-ord. Higher Prof. Fell. Specialty: Gen. Pract. Prev: Research Fell. (Pharmacol. & Therap.) Univ. Aberd.

SHIRSALKAR, Anand Madusudhan King George Hospital, Barley Lane, Ilford IG3 8YB Tel: 020 8970 8071 Fax: 020 8970 8175 — MB BS Osmania 1988; DCH 1990; MRCP UK 1994. Cons. Paediat., King Geo. Hosp., Ilford, Essex; Clin. Lead Neonalotology BHR Hosps. NHS Trust. Specialty: Paediat. Prev: Roy. Coll. Tutor, 1998-2001.

SHIRT, Dominic John Walter Sloan Practice, 251 Chesterfield Road, Sheffield S8 0RT Tel: 0114 255 1164 Fax: 0114 258 9006 — MB BS Newc. 1992.

SHIU, Kin Yee 11 Elizabeth Mews, London NW3 4TL — MB BS Lond. 1997.

SHIU, Man Fai Walsgrave Hospital, University Hospitals Coventry & Warwickshire NHS Trust, Cliffordbridge Road, Coventry CV2 2DX Tel: 02476 538930 Fax: 02476 535105 Email: man-fai.shiu@uhcw.nhs.uk — MD Lond. 1979; MB BS 1970; MRCP (UK) 1972; FRCP Lond. 1986. Cons. Cardiol. UHCW Clin. Director, Cardiol. Directorate; Vis. Cons. Cardiol. S. Warks. Hosp. Lakin Rd. Warwick. Specialty: Cardiol. Special Interest: Acute Interven. for Acute Myocardial Infec.; Coronary Angioplasty & Stent Implantation. Socs: PastChairm. Mem. Brit. Cardiol. Vasc. Interven. Soc.; Brit. Cardiac Soc. (Ex-Counc. Mem.). Prev: Sen. Lect. (Cardiol.) Qu. Eliz. Hosp. Birm.; Sen. Regist. (Paediat. Cardiol.) Birm. Childr. Hosp.; Regist. (Cardiac) St. Thos. Hosp. Lond.

SHIV SHANKER, Mr Vaidyanathan 8 Transom Close, London SE16 7FH — MB BS Madras 1986; FRCS Ed. 1992.

SHIVANATHAN, Sivasubramaniam 62 South Hill Road, Bromley BR2 0RT Tel: 020 8460 8461 — MB BS Ceylon 1953; DTM & H Ceylon 1956; DPH Lond. 1963; DCH Eng. 1966; DPM Eng. 1974. Cons. Psychiat. (Ment. Handicap) Lifecare NHS Trust Caterham. Specialty: Ment. Health. Prev: Cons. Psychiat. (Ment. Handicap & Child Developm.) Qu. Marys Hosp. Childr. Carshalton & St. Ebbas Hosp. Epsom; Sen. Regist. (Psychiat.) Qu. Mary's Hosp. Childr. Carshalton; Regist. (Child Psychiat. & Ment. Handicap) Qu. Marys Hosp. Childr. & Child Guid. Clin. Croydon.

SHIVAYOGI, Mahantinamath 51 Wellington Road, Sandhurst, Sandhurst GU47 9AW — MB BS Mysore 1972 (Mysore Med. Coll.) MSc (Neurosci.) Lond. 1993. Assoc. Specialist Broadmoor Hosp. Berks.

SHIWANI, Mr Muhammad Hanif Barnsley General Hospital, Gawber Road, Barnsley S75 2EP — MB BS Karachi 1986 (DOW Med. Coll. Karachi Pakistan) FRCSI 1991; FRCSI (Gen. Surg.) 2000; FRCS Eng. 2003; FRCS Glas. 2003. Cons. Barnsley Gen. Hosp. and Hon Sen. Clin. Lect. Univ. Sheff. Specialty: Gastroenterol.; Laparoscopy. Special Interest: Laparoscopic Surg.; Upper GI Surg.

SHLOSBERG, Charles Benjamin Charlotte Keel Health Centre, Seymour Road, Easton, Bristol Tel: 0117 951 2244 — MB BS Lond. 1978; BA Oxf. 1975; MRCP (UK) 1982; DRCOG 1987; DCH RCP Lond. 1993.

SHLOSBERG, David St Bees Surgery, 34-36 St. Bees Close, Moss Side, Manchester M14 4GG Tel: 0161 226 7615 Fax: 0161 226 0413 — MA Camb.; MRCS Eng. LRCP Lond. 1960; MRCGP 1996. Occupat. Health Phys. Hope Hosp.; Lect. (Gen. Pract.) Univ. Manch. Specialty: Gen. Pract.; Occupat. Health.

SHLUGMAN, David Neuro ITU, Radcliffe Infirmary, Oxford OX2 6HE Tel: 01865 311188 Email: david.shlugman@orh.nhs.uk; 4 Bullsmead, Sunningwell, Abingdon OX13 6RL Tel: 01865 326150 Fax: 01865 736813 — MB ChB Cape Town 1974; FRCA 1981. Cons. Anaesth. Radcliffe Infirm. Oxf.; Cons. Neuro ITU. Specialty: Anaesth. Socs: BMA; Neuroinaesth. Soc.; Assoc. of Anaesth. GB & Irel.

SHMUELI, Ehoud Integrated Surgical Centre, Northampton General Hospital, Northampton NN1 5BD Tel: 01604 545937; 3 Penfold Drive, Breat Billing, Northampton NN3 9EQ Tel: 01604 469961 — MB ChB Bristol 1984; MRCP (UK) 1987; MD Newc. 1993. Cons. Phys. & Gastroenterol., Northampton Gen., Northampton. Specialty: Gen. Med. Prev: Hon. Sen. Regist.; John Radcliffe Hosp., Oxf.; MRC Research Train. Fell.

SHNEERSON, Anne The Burwell Surgery, Newmarket Road, Burwell, Cambridge CB5 0AE Tel: 01638 741234 Fax: 01638 743948; 129 North Street, Burwell, Cambridge CB5 0BB Tel: 01638 741393 — MB BS Lond. 1971 (St. Thomas') MRCP (UK) 1974; MRCGP 1976. Prev: SHO (Neurol.) St. Thos. Hosp. Lond.; SHO Brompton Hosp. Lond. & St. Mary's Hosp. Portsmouth.

SHNEERSON, John Michael Papworth Hospital, Papworth Everard, Cambridge CB3 8RE Tel: 01480 830541 Fax: 01480 830620 — BM BCh Oxf. 1971 (Oxf.Univ./St Mary's Lond) MRCP (UK) 1973; MA, DM Oxf. 1977; FRCP Lond. 1986; MD Camb. 1987. Cons. Phys. Papworth & Newmarket Hosps.; Dir. Respirat. Support & Sleep Centre, Papworth Hosp.; Assoc. Lect. Univ. Camb. Specialty: Respirat. Med. Socs: Brit. Scoliosis Res. Found.; Fell. Amer. Coll. Chest Phys.; Brit. Sleep Soc. - Comm. Mem. Prev: Sen. Regist. Westm. Hosp. & Brompton Hosp. Lond.; Regist. (Med.) Whipps Cross Hosp. Lond.; SHO (Neurol.) St. Mary's Hosp. Lond.

SHNYIEN, Naif Kadem 2 Redlodge, Park View Road, Ealing, London W5 2JB Tel: 020 8998 8033 — MB ChB Mosul 1965.

SHOAIB, Asim 297 Park Road, Oldham OL4 1SF — MB ChB Manch. 1995.

SHOAIB, Taimur Plastic Surgery Unit, Jubilee Building, Royal Infirmary, Glasgow G4 0SF Email: t.shoaib@doctors. org.uk; 7C Hughenden Gardens, Hyndland, Glasgow G12 9XW — MB ChB Glas. 1992; FRCS Ed. 1997; DMI RCS Ed. 2001; MD 2003. Research Registrar. (Plastic Surg.). Specialty: Plastic Surg.

SHOAIBI, Asfia Taskeen 1 Wheatcroft Road, Yardley, Birmingham B33 8HH — MB BS Lond. 1998; MRCP 2004.

SHOBAN, Bandi Krishnarao Huntly Grove Practice, Princes Street, Peterborough PE1 2QP Tel: 01733 551771 — MB BS Dibrugarh 1980; LRCP LRCS Ed. LRCPS Glas. 1985.

SHOBOWALE, Folasade Oluyemisi Woodcote Group Practice, 140 Chipstead Valley Road, Coulsdon, Purley CR8 3EE Tel: 020 8660 1304 Fax: 020 8660 0721 — MB ChB Nigeria 1987; MRCGP UK 2000.

SHOEB, Ismail Hani Abdel-Hakim Surrey Hants. Borders NHS Trust, Farnham Road Hospital, Guildford GU5 5LX Tel: 01483 443660 Fax: 01483 799445 Email: ishoeb@shb-tr.nhs.uk — MB ChB Ain Shams 1974; MRCPsych 1983. Cons. Psychiat. Roy. Surrey Hants. Borders Hosp. Guildford; Cons. Liasian Psychiat., Roy. Surrey Co. Hosp., Guildford, Surrey. Specialty: Gen. Psychiat. Special Interest: Liasion Psychiat. Prev: Cons. Psychiat. Abha Psychiat. Hosp., Saudi Arabia; Cons. Psychiat. Lister Hosp. Stevenage, Herts.

SHOENBERG, Elisabeth (retired) 22 Stanley Crescent, London W11 2NA Tel: 020 7727 0454 — (King's Coll. & W. Lond.) MA Camb.; MRCS Eng. LRCP Lond. 1947; DPM Eng. 1953; FRCPsych 1973, M 1971. Prev: Cons. Psychiat. Claybury Hosp. Woodford Bridge & Lond. Sch. Hyg. & Trop. Med. MRC Social Med. Unit.

SHOENBERG, Peter Jacques Flat E, 30 Pembridge Villas, London W11 3EL; Flat E, 30 Pembridge Villas, London W11 3EL — MA Camb. 1970 (Univ. Camb. & Middlx. Hosp.) BChir 1969; MRCP (UK) 1972; MRCPsych 1975; FRCPsych 1998. Cons. Psychother. Univ. Coll. Hosp. Trust (for Camden & Islington Ment. Health Servs. NHS Trust); Hon. Sen. Clin. Lect. The Roy. Free and Univ. Coll. Sch. of Med. Specialty: Psychother. Socs: Brit. Assn. Psychother.; St. Marks Assn. Prev: Cons. Psychother. Claybury Hosp. Woodford Bridge, Essex.

SHOESMITH, David John Mayfield Medical Centre, 4 Glenholme Park, Clayton, Bradford BD14 6NF Tel: 01274 880650 Fax: 01274 883256; 11 Beechwood Grove, Moorhead, Shipley BD18 4JS Tel: 01274 591984 — MB BS Lond. 1976 (St. Bart.) MRCGP 1983. GP; Med. Off. Civil Serv. Specialty: Gen. Pract.

SHOESMITH, Mr John Harrop (retired) 21 Sandhill Lane, Leeds LS17 6AJ Tel: 0113 268 8186 — MB ChB Leeds 1948; MB ChB (Hnrs.) Leeds 1948; FRCS Eng. 1952. Gen. Surg. Gen. Infirm. Leeds & Cons. Surg. Chapel Allerton Hosp. Leeds. Prev: Sen. Surg. Regist. & Thoracic Surg. Regist. Leeds Gen. Infirm.

SHOHET, Naim Ishac Aboudi 1/12 Nitza Boulevard, Netanya, Israel; Red Bank Health Centre, Unsworth St., Radcliffe, Manchester M26 3GH Tel: 0161 723 2624 — MRCS Eng. LRCP Lond. 1945 (St. Bart.) Prev: Res. Surg. Off. Castleford Hosp.; Orthop. Ho. Surg. & Dep. Res. Surg. Off. War Memor. Hosp. Scunthorpe; Ho. Surg. St. Mary Islington Hosp.

SHOHETH, Joseph Raymond (retired) 75 Shortwood Crescent, Plymstock, Plymouth PL9 8TL Tel: 01752 401432 — MB BS Calcutta 1954; DTM & H Calcutta 1956; DLO Eng. 1961. Prev: Regist. (ENT) Gen. Hosp. Nottm., Dudley Rd. Hosp. Birm. & Plymouth Gen. Hosp.

SHOKAR, Navkiran Kaur 4 Stoneleigh Close, Luton LU3 3XE — BM BCh Oxf. 1992. Trainee GP Horton Gen. Hosp. VTS.

SHOKER, Balvinder Singh 24 Inglewood, Liverpool L12 0NP — MB ChB Liverp. 1991.

SHOLAPURKAR, Shashikant Laxman Department of Obstetrics & Gynaecology, Royal United Hospital, Coombe Park, Bath BA1 3NG — MB BS Poona 1984; MRCOG 1993. Staff Grade Doctor. Specialty: Obst. & Gyn.

SHOLL, Penelope Pat Hawkinge Health Centre, 74 Canterbury Road, Hawkinge, Folkestone CT18 7BP Tel: 01303 892434; 122 Cheriton Road, Folkestone CT19 5HQ Tel: 01303 259596 — MB BS Lond. 1977; AKC 1977; DCH Eng. 1979; DRCOG Lond. 1980; MRCGP 1983. GP Asst.

SHOME, Chittendra 8 Beadnell Drive, Penketh, Warrington WA5 2EG — MB BS Gauhati 1969.

SHONE, Mr Geoffrey Richard ENT Department, University Hospital of Wales, Heath Park, Cardiff CF14 4XW Tel: 029 2074 7747; 12 Pen Y Dre, Cardiff CF14 6EP — MB BChir Camb. 1979; MA, MB Camb. 1979, BChir 1978; FRCS Eng. 1983. Cons. Otolaryngol. Univ. Hosp. Wales Cardiff. Specialty: Otolaryngol.

SHOO, Estomih Elikaney Tameside General Hospital, Fountain St., Ashton-under-Lyne OL6 9RW Tel: 0161 331 6000 — MRCPCH; MB ChB Makerere 1971; DTCH Liverp. 1980; DCH RCP Lond. 1983; MRCP Dub. 1987; RC Paed. UK 1992. Assoc. Specialist (Paediat.) Tameside Gen. Hosp. Ashton-under-Lyne. Specialty: Paediat. Socs: BMA & Brit. Paediat. Assn. Prev: Regist. (Paediat.) Maelor Gen. Hosp. Wrexham & Tameside Gen. Hosp.; SHO (Paediat.) Roy. Liverp. Childr. Hosp. & Roy. Liverp. Childr. Hosp.

SHOOTER, Jean (retired) Eastlea, Back Edge Lane, Edge, Stroud GL6 6PE Tel: 01452 812408 — (Bristol) MB ChB Bristol 1942. Prev: Surg. Lt. RNVR.

SHOOTER, Michael Stanhope Ty Bryn Adolescent Unit, St Cadoc's Hospital, Lodge Road, Caerlon, Newport NP18 3XQ Tel: 01633 436831 Fax: 01633 436834; Ty Boda, Upper Llanover, Abergavenny NP7 9EP Tel: 01873 880093 Fax: 01873 880293 — MB Camb. 1976 (Cambridge) MA Camb. 1973, MB 1976, BChir 1975; FRCPsych 1994, M 1980. Cons. Child & Adolesc. Psychiat.Gwent Healthcare NHS Trust, Clin. Dir., Child & Adolesc. Ment. Health Serv.; Regist. Roy. Coll. Psychiat. Specialty: Child & Adolesc. Psychiat. Prev: Clin. Dir. S. Glam. Child & Adolesc. Psychiat. Serv.

SHOOTER, Professor Reginald Arthur, CBE (retired) Eastlea, Back Edge Lane, Edge, Stroud GL6 6PE Tel: 01452 812408 — (Camb. & St. Bart.) MB BChir Camb. 1940; MRCS Eng. LRCP Lond. 1940; MA Camb. 1941, MD 1945; FRCP Lond. 1968, M 1961; FCPath 1963; FRCS Eng. 1977. Prev: Prof. Med. Microbiol. Univ. Lond.

SHORA, Basharat Saleem Dartford West Health Centre, Tower Road, Dartford DA1 2HA Tel: 01322 280272 — MB BS Jammu 1972; DTM & H. GP, W. Kent Health Auth. Specialty: Gen. Pract.

SHORE, Mr Darryl Francis 148 Woodlands Road, Ashurst, Southampton SO40 7AQ — MB ChB Sheff. 1971; FRCS Eng. 1976.

SHORE, David James The Surgery, Barr Lane, Brinklow, Rugby CV23 0LU Tel: 01788 832994 Fax: 01788 833021; Fairfield House, Coventry Road, Brinklow, Rugby CV23 0NE — MB ChB Birm. 1984; MRCGP 1998. GP Brinklow.

SHORE, Eleanor Mary Custom House Surgery, 16 Freemasons Road, London E16 3NA Tel: 020 7476 2255 Fax: 020 7511 8980 Email: helshore@aol.com — MB BS Lond. 1981.

SHORE, Elizabeth Catherine, CB (retired) 23 Dryburgh Road, London SW15 1BN — (Camb. & St. Bart.) MRCS Eng. LRCP Lond. 1951; DObst RCOG 1953; FFCM 1972; FRCP Lond. 1984, M 1973. Prev: Dep. Chief Med. Off. DHSS.

SHORE, Hannah Ruth The Lodge, 34 Brighton Road, Purley CR8 3AD; 29 Charlotte Road, Stirchley, Birmingham B30 2BT Tel: 0121 433 4097 — MB ChB Birm. 1996; ChB Birm. 1996. SHO (Paediat.). Specialty: Paediat.

SHORE, Irene Medical Wing RTMC, Chetwynd Barracks, Chilwell, Nottingham WG9 5HA — MB ChB Liverp. 1975; DRCOG 1979; MRCGP 1982.

SHORE, John Hubert (retired) 11 Angmering Lane, East Preston, Littlehampton BN16 2TA Tel: 01903 782356 — MD Lond. 1952 (Char. Cross) MB BS 1947; FRCPath 1969, M 1964. Prev: Cons. Pathol. Worthing Hosp. Gp.

SHORE, Kathryn Margaret Demontfort Medical Centre, Burford Road, Bengeworth, Evesham WR11 3HD Tel: 01386 443333 Fax: 01386 422884 — MB BS (Distinc. Clin. Pharmacol. & Therap.) Lond. 1989 (Charing Cross and Westminster) MA Oxf. 1987; DRCOG 1991; DCH RCP Lond. 1992; MRCGP 1993; T(GP) 1993; DFFP 1995. Prev: Trainee GP Worcester; Ho. Off. (Surg.) Wycombe Gen. Hosp.; Ho. Off. (Med.) Stoke Mandeville Hosp.

SHORE, Peter Michael Heathfielde, Lyttlelton Road, London N2 0EE Tel: 020 8458 9262 Fax: 020 8455 0165 — MB BS Lond. 1952 (Char. Cross) Prev: Ho. Surg. Wembley Hosp.

SHORE, Susannah Louise Top Forge Cottage, Wortley, Sheffield S35 7DN — MB ChB Liverp. 1997.

SHORES, John Gresham Clifton House Medical Centre, 263-265 Beverley Road, Hull HU5 2ST Tel: 01482 341423; 43 Low Street, North Ferriby HU14 3DD Tel: 01482 631473 — LMSSA Lond. 1960 (W. Lond.) Clin. Asst. De la Pole Hosp. Willerby; Co. Surg. St. John Ambul. Humberside. Socs: BMA. Prev: SHO Vict. Hosp. Sick Childr. Hull.

SHOREY, Mr Brian Alexander (retired) Northwood Consulting Rooms, 7 Greenhill Court, Green Lane, Northwood HA6 2UZ Tel: 01923 826948 Fax: 01923 835794; 41 Sandy Lodge Way, Northwood HA6 2AR Tel: 01923 821297 — (St. Bart.) MS Lond. 1978, MB BS 1964; FRCS Eng. 1969. Cons. Surg. Hillingdon Hosp. Uxbridge. Prev: Hon. Cons. Bristol Childr. Hosp.

SHOREY, Greta Marion Arkley, 39 Hathaway Green Lane, Stratford-upon-Avon CV37 9HX — MB ChB Birm. 1976; DRCOG 1979; DCH Eng. 1980; DTM & H Liverp. 1981; MRCGP 1983; FMGEMS 1988. Med. Dir. (Gen. Pract., Trauma & Disaster Relief) Mexican Red Cross Delegacion ISCA Mujeres. Socs: BMA.

SHORLAND, Jean Eva (retired) Apple Garth, Knowle Gardens, Sidmouth EX10 8HR — MB BS Lond. 1965 (Westm.) BSc (Physiol.) Lond. 1962; FRCP Lond. 1984, M 1968. Prev: Sen. Regist. Dept. Child Health Univ. Hosp. Cardiff.

SHORNEY, Janet Susan Chiddenbrook Surgery, Threshers, Crediton EX17 3JJ Tel: 01363 772227 Fax: 01363 775528; 18 Thornton Hill, Exeter EX4 4NS Tel: 01392 258494 — MB BChir Camb. 1978; MRCGP 1983; DRCOG 1983.

SHORNEY, Neil Mark 22 Okefield Road, Crediton EX17 2DN — MB BS Lond. 1980; FFARCS Eng. 1984.

SHORROCK, Christopher John Blackpool Victoria Hospital NHS Trust, Whinney Heys Road, Blackpool FY3 8NR Tel: 01253 303711 Fax: 01253 306936 Email: dr.shorrock@bfwhospitals.nhs.uk — MB ChB Manch. 1980; BSc St. And. 1977; MRCP (UK) 1984; MD Manch. 1991; FRCP 1996. Cons. Phys. / Gastroenterologist Blackpool Vict. Hosp. Specialty: Gastroenterol.; Gen. Med. Special Interest: Endoscopy; Liver Dis. Socs: Member British Society of Gastroenterology; Member American Gastroenterological Society. Prev: Regist. (Gen. Med./Gastroenterol.) Univ. Dept. Med. Hope Hosp. Manch.; Lect. (Med.) Qu. Eliz. Hosp. Birm.; Regist. Regional Dept. Cardiothoracic Med. Wythenshawe Hosp. Manch.

SHORROCK, Kenneth Medioco Legal Centre, Watery Street, Sheffield S3 7ES Tel: 01142 738721 Fax: 01142798942 — MB ChB Sheff. 1978; FRCS Eng. 1982; MD Sheff. 1989; FRCPath 1991; LLB Leeds Metropolitan 1999. Sen. Lect. in Forens. Path. Univ. of Sheff. Cons. Pathologist to the Home Office. Specialty: Histopath. Socs: Internat. Acad. Path.; Brit. Assn. Forens. Med. Prev: Lect. (Histopath.) Univ. Leicester; Regist. (Histopath.) Nottm. HA; Cons. Pathologist Healthcare NHS Trust.

SHORROCK, Peter (retired) Oak House, Moss Lane, Leyland, Preston PR25 4SE Tel: 01772 422373 — MB ChB Manch. 1961 (Lond.) Cert Av Med. MoD (Air) & CAA 1975. Approved Examr. Civil Aviat. Auth. Prev: Ho. Off. Manch. Roy. Infirm. & Bolton & Dist. Gen. Hosp.

SHORT, Aidan Dominic 26 Willow Hey, Liverpool L31 3DL — MB ChB Sheff. 1997.

SHORT, Alasdair Ian Kennedy Broomfield Hospital, Chelmsford CM1 7ET Tel: 01245 440761 Fax: 01245 514060 — MB ChB Ed. 1975; MRCP (UK) 1977; FRCPC 1982; FRCP Ed. 1986; FRCP Lond. 1992. Cons. Phys. Intens. Care Unit Broomfield Hosp. Chelmsford. Specialty: Gen. Med.; Intens. Care; Nephrol.

SHORT, Andrew Worcestershire Royal Hospital, Charles Hastings Way, Worcester WR5 1DD Tel: 01905 760736 Fax: 01905 760584 Email: andrew.short@worcsacute.wminds.nhs.uk; Stedefield, Church Lane, Flyford Flavelc, Worcester WR7 4BZ Email: andrew@stedefield.fsnet.co.uk — MB ChB Aberd. 1981; FRCPCH; MRCP (UK) 1987. Cons. Paediat. Worcester Roy. Hosp. Specialty: Paediat. Prev: Cons. Paediat. Huddersflield Roy. Infirm.; Sen. Regist. (Paediat.) Leeds & Bradford Hosps.; Regist. (Paediat.) St. Lukes Hosp. Bradford.

SHORT, Andrew Keith Renal Unit, Walsgrave Hospital, Clifford Bridge Road, Coventry CV2 2DX; 3 Rowan Drive, Warwick CV34 5JS — MB ChB Manch. 1984; BSc (Hons.) Manch 1981; MRCP (UK) 1987; PhD Camb. 1994. Cons. Phys. & Nephrologist, Walsgrave Hosp., Coventry. Specialty: Nephrol.; Gen. Med. Prev: Research Sen. Regist. Sch. Clin. Med. Addenbrooke's Hosp. Camb.; Regist. (Renal Med.) St. Mary's Hosp. Lond.; SHO Univ. Hosp. S. Manch.

SHORT, Bernard Priory View Medical Centre, 2a Green Lane, Leeds LS12 1HU Tel: 0113 295 4260 Fax: 0113 295 4278 — MRCS Lond 1973 (London) MRCS Eng LRCP Lond 1973; LMCC (Camb.) 1979. GP Leeds. Specialty: Gen. Pract. Socs: BMA; MDU. Prev: GP Comox Brit. Columbia Canada.

SHORT, Clare Anna Ground Floor, 11 Miles Road, Clifton, Bristol BS8 2JN — MB ChB Bristol 1986.

SHORT, Colin David Manchester Royal Infirmary, Department of Renal Medicine, Oxford Road, Manchester M13 9WL Tel: 0161 276 6593 Fax: 0161 276 8022 Email: colin.short@cmmc.nhs.uk; 3 Homelands Road, Sale M33 4BJ — MB ChB Manch. 1975; BSc Hull 1970; MRCP (UK) 1979; MD Manch. 1990; FRCP Lond. 1995. Cons. Nephrologist, Renal Med., Manch. Roy. Infirm., Manch. Specialty: Nephrol. Special Interest: Glonerular Dis.; Hypertens.; Renal Transpl. Socs: Renal Assn.; Internat. Soc. Nephrol.; Brit. Transpl. Soc.

SHORT, David Hugh Dartford West Health Centre, Tower Road, Dartford DA1 2HA Tel: 01322 223600 Fax: 01322 292282; Brambles, Common Lane, Wilmington, Dartford DA2 7BA — MB BS Lond. 1984 (St Mary's Hospital, London) DRCOG 1986. GP; Sector GP for Bartford Town sector of PCG. Prev: Trainee GP Dartford VTS; Ho. Phys. St. Mary's Hosp. Eastbourne; Ho. Surg. Worthing Hosp.

SHORT, David James (retired) 12 Whitesfield Road, Nailsea, Bristol BS48 2DT Tel: 01275 855294 — MRCS Eng. LRCP Lond. 1973; MSc 1977; DIH Eng. 1977; MFOM RCP Lond. 1987, AFOM 1982; DAvMed RCP Lond. 1990. Cons. Occupat. Phys. Frenchay Hosp. Bristol. Prev: Sen. Med. Off. RAF.

SHORT, Professor David Somerset 48 Victoria Street, Aberdeen AB10 1PN Tel: 01224 645853 Email: short@dircon.co.uk — MB BChir Camb. 1942 (Bristol) FRCP Lond. 1964, M 1943; MA Camb. 1944, MD 1948; PhD Lond. 1957; FRCP Ed. 1970, M 1964. Emerit. Clin. Prof. Med. Univ. Aberd.; Hon. Cons. Phys. Aberd. Roy. Infirm. Specialty: Cardiol. Socs: Aberd. M-C Soc. (Ex-Pres.). Prev: Phys. to

HM the Qu. in Scotl.; Lect. (Med.) Middlx. Hosp. Med. Sch. Lond.; Chief Asst. (Cardiac) Lond. Hosp.

SHORT, Deborah Jill Midlands Centre for Spinal Injuries, Robert Jones & Agnes Hunt Hospital, Oswestry SY10 7AG — MB ChB Leeds 1978; MRCP (UK) 1981. Cons. in Spinal Injuries Rehabil. Med. Specialty: Gen. Med.; Rehabil. Med. Prev: Sen. Regist. Nat. Spinal Injuries Centre Stoke Mandeville.; Cons. Rehabil. Med., Haywood Hosp., Burslem, Stoke on trent.

SHORT, Diane Claire 86 Peveril Road, Sheffield S11 7AR Tel: 0114 268 1428 — MB ChB Liverp. 1996; MRCPCH.

SHORT, Donald Harry, RD (retired) Ballacree, West End, Somerton TA11 6RW Tel: 01458 272408 — MB BS Lond. 1955 (Lond. Hosp.) FFA RCS Eng. 1964. Prev: Cons. Anaesth. Bristol & West. HA.

SHORT, Edward Somerset (retired) The Manse, Yatton Keynell Road, Castle Combe, Chippenham SN14 7HD Tel: 01249 782629 — MB ChB Bristol 1944 (Bristol.) Prev: Supt. Bethesda Leprosy Hosp. Narsapur, India.

SHORT, Gerard Peter 101 Dunvegan Drive, Southampton SO16 8DB — MB BS Lond. 1992. SHO (Gen. Med.) Roy. Bournemouth Hosp.

SHORT, Jane Hyslop (retired) 7 Lochside, Bearsden, Glasgow G61 2SB Tel: 0141 943 1496 — MB ChB Glas. 1942; FRFPS Glas. 1945; BSc 1938, MD (Commend.) Glas. 1949; FRCP Glas, 1980, M 1962; DMRT Eng. 1975. Prev: Med. Asst. Inst. Radiother. Glas.

SHORT, Jennifer Mary Department Infection & Tropical Medicine, Hearlands Hospital, Bordesley Green East, Birmingham B9 5SS — MB ChB Liverp. 1990; MRCP UK 1994; DTM & H Liverp. 1995; MRCPath 2003. Cons. Phys., Dept. Infec. & Trop. Med., Heartlands Hosp., Birm. Specialty: Med. Microbiol. Prev: SHO (Infec. Dis.s) City Hosp. Edin.; SHO (Med.) Northampton Gen. Hosp. & Countess of Chester Hosp.; Specialist Regist. (MicroBiol.) John Radcliffe Hosp. Oxf.

SHORT, Mrs Joan Anne (retired) 48 Victoria Street, Aberdeen AB10 1PN Tel: 01224 645853 — MB BCh Wales 1948 (Cardiff) BSc Wales 1945. Prev: GP Aberd.

SHORT, Judith Alison 19 Twentywell Road, Bradway, Sheffield S17 4PU — BM BS Nottm. 1991; BMedSci (Hons.) Nottm. 1989; FRCA 1997. Regist Rotat. (Anaesth.) N. Trent Train. Scheme Sheff. Specialty: Anaesth. Socs: BMA; Fell. Roy. Coll. Anaesth.; Assn. Anaesth.

SHORT, Laura Clare Penleigh, 2 Melrose Crescent, Bishop Monkton, Harrogate HG3 3SW — BM BS Nottm. 1998; BM BS Nottm 1998.

SHORT, Lindsay Crawford Airbles Road Centre, 59 Airbles Road, Motherwell ML1 2TP — MB ChB Sheff. 1992; DFFP 1996; JCPTGP-Jt. Comm. Cert. for Post Grad. Traning in Gen. Pract. 1997. Airbles Rd. Centre Airbles Rd. Motherwell ML1 2TP, Lanarksh. Prim. Care NHS Trust. Prev: GP Regist. The Surg. 24 Quarry St. Johnstone; SHO (Med. for Elderly) Roy. Alexandra Hosp. NHS Trust Paisley.

SHORT, Lindsay Jane 133 Gardner Road, Formby, Liverpool L37 8DF — MB ChB Manch. 1995.

SHORT, Lindsay Margaret 2/L, 72 Lauderdale Gardens, Glasgow G12 9QW — MB ChB Glas. 1988; MRCP (UK) 1993. Sen. Regist. (Genitourin. Med.) Sandyford Initiative Glas. Specialty: Genitourinary Medicine. Prev: Regist. Rotat. (Genitourin. Med., Gen. Med. & Infec. Dis.) Newc. Gen. Hosp.; SHO Rotat. (Med.) West. Infirm. & Gartnavel Gen. Hosp. Glas.

SHORT, Matthew Adam The Barn Surgery, Newbury, Gillingham SP8 4XS Tel: 01747 824201 Fax: 01747 825098 Email: matthew.short@gp-j81081.nhs.uk — BM Soton. 1978 (Southampton) DRCOG 1983. GP Princip. Specialty: Gen. Pract. Prev: Trainee GP Netheravon; SHO (O & G, Orthop. & A & E) Salisbury HA.

SHORT, Norton Lynn, MBE Dartford East Health Centre, Pilgrims Way, Dartford DA1 1QY Tel: 01322 274211 Fax: 01322 284329; Keepers, St. Vincents Lane, Addington, Maidstone ME16 5BW — MB BS Lond. 1958 (St. Geo.) DObst RCOG 1961; MRCGP 1969; DPM Eng. 1972; MA Wales 1989. Prev: Ho. Surg. St. Geo. Hosp. Lond.; Ho. Phys. Ashford Hosp. Kent; Ho. Surg. (Obst.) All St.s' Hosp. Chatham.

SHORT, Penelope Anne Anaesthetic Department, Salisbury District Hospital, Salisbury SP2 8BJ Tel: 01722 425050; 3 Hillside Close, Mere, Warminster BA12 6LB — BM Soton. 1977; DA (UK) 1984. Staff Grade Anaesth. Salisbury Health Care. Specialty: Anaesth. Prev: SHO (Anaesth. & Orthop.) Salisbury HA; SHO (A & E) I. of Wight HA.; SHO (Paediat. Surg.) Soton.

SHORT, Peter Lemon Street Surgery, 18 Lemon Street, Truro TR1 2LZ Tel: 01872 73133 Fax: 01872 260900; 3 Tremorvah Crescent, Truro TR1 1NL Tel: 01872 42254 — MB BS Lond. 1984; DCH RCP Lond. 1989; DRCOG 1990; MRCGP 1994. Prev: Trainee GP Truro.

SHORT, Peter McLay Grove Medical Practice, Shirley Health Centre, Grove Road, Shirley, Southampton SO15 3UA Tel: 023 8078 3611 Fax: 023 8078 3156; 457 Coxford Road, Lordswood, Southampton SO16 5DA Tel: 02380 739513 — MB ChB Aberd. 1978; DRCOG 1982; MRCGP 1982. GP Shirley.

SHORT, Peter Richard David The Stewart Medical Centre, 15 Hartington Road, Buxton SK17 6JP Tel: 01298 22338 Fax: 01298 72678; The Barn, 91 Green Lane, Buxton SK17 9DJ — MB ChB Birm. 1983; DRCOG 1986; MRCGP 1988. Prev: SHO (Paediat.) Good Hope Gen. Hosp. Birm.; SHO (O & G) & (Med.) Doncaster Roy. Infirm.; SHO (A & E) Selly Oak Hosp. Birm.

SHORT, Miss Rachel Marian Crosshouse Hospital, Kilmarnock KA2 0BE — BM BS Nottm. 1986; FRCS (Orth) 1997. Cons. Orthop. Surg., CrossHo. Hosp., Kilmarnock. Specialty: Orthop.

SHORT, Stephanie Patricia Minfor Surgery, Park Road, Barmouth LL42 1PL Tel: 01341 280521 Fax: 01341 280912 — MB BS Lond. 1980; DCH RCP Lond. 1982; DRCOG 1984; MRCGP 1985.

SHORT, Stephen Mansel Peterborough District Hospital, Thorpe Road, Peterborough PE3 6DA Tel: 01733 874000 — MB BS Lond. 1979 (St. Geo.) FFA RCS Eng. 1983. Cons. Anaesth., P'boro. Hosps. NHS Trust. Specialty: Anaesth. Special Interest: Intens. Care. Socs: Roy. Coll. of Anaesth.; Assn. of Anaesth.; Intens. Care Soc. Prev: Lect. (Anaesth.) Chinese Univ., Hong Kong.; Cons. Anaesth. Lister Hosp. Stevenage.

SHORT, Stuart David Cobbs Garden Surgery, West St, Olney MK46 5QG; 22A West End, Stevington, Bedford MK43 7QU — MB BS Lond. 1990 (Roy. Free Med. Sch. Lond.) DFFP 1995. GP Cobbs Gdn Surg. Olney Bucks; Clin. Asst. Rheum. Bedford Hosp. Bedford. Specialty: Gen. Pract. Prev: SHO (Paediat. & O & G) Northampton Gen. Hosp.

SHORT, Susan Christine 40 Field Way, Rickmansworth WD3 7EJ Tel: 01923 711498 — MB BS Lond. 1989 (King's Coll. Lond.) BSc Lond. 1986, MB BS 1989; MRCP (UK) 1992; FRCR (UK) 1996. Specialty: Oncol.; Radiother.

SHORT, William John (retired) South Lodge, Lennox Castle Hospital, Lennoxtown, Glasgow G66 7LB Tel: 0141 329200 — LRCP LRCS Ed. LRCPS Glas. 1964. Acting Cons. Psychiat. Lennox Castle Hosp. Lennoxtown. Prev: SHO Paisley Matern. Hosp.

SHORT, William Robert, CB, CStJ, Maj.-Gen. late RAMC PHC Ltd., Talbot House, Green End, Whitchurch SY13 1AJ Tel: 01948 664452 Fax: 01948 666116 Email: robin.short@virgin.net; Beeswing, 26 Orchard Road, Farnborough GU14 7PR Tel: 01252 513328 Fax: 01252 653696 — (Glas.) FRCP Glas.; MB ChB Glas. 1967. Operat.s Dir., PHC Ltd. Special Interest: PTSD in Ex Servicemen. Prev: Dir. Gen. Army Med. Servs.

SHORTALL, Delia Ann 3 Clarendon Road W., Chorlton, Manchester M21 0RN — MB BS Lond. 1984; MRCPsych 1991; MSc Manch. 1995; DFFP 1995. Cons. Child & Adolesc. Psychiat. Roy. Centr. Manch. Childrens Hosp. NHS Trust. Specialty: Child & Adolesc. Psychiat.

SHORTALL, Myles Thomas Meadowlands Surgery, Monaghan Street, Newry BT35 6BW Tel: 028 3026 7534 — MB BCh BAO Belf. 1964 (Qu. Univ. Belf.) DObst RCOG 1966. Specialty: Gen. Pract.

SHORTALL, Therese Nicholette Newton Medical Centre, 14/18 Newton Road, London W2 5LT Tel: 020 7229 4578 Fax: 020 7229 7315; 31 Buckingham Close, Queens Walk, Ealing, London W5 1TS — MB BCh BAO NUI 1970; MPH NUI 1986. Specialty: Gen. Pract.

SHORTEN, John Benjamin 13 Tonsley Place, London SW18 1BH — MB BS Lond. 1992.

SHORTEN, Penelope Jane Houghton Health Centre, Church St., Houghton-le-Spring DH4 4DN; 20 Deneside Avenue, Low Fell, Gateshead NE9 6AD — MB BS Newc. 1969. SCMO City Hosps. Wearside. Specialty: Community Child Health.

SHORTEN, Wilson William John Lisburn Health Centre, Linenhall Street, Lisburn BT28 1LU Tel: 028 9260 3090 Fax: 028 9250 1310

— MB BCh BAO Belf. 1983; MB BCh BAO Belf. 1980; DRCOG 1982; DCH RCPI 1983; MRCGP 1984; Cert. Family Plann. JCC 1984.

SHORTHOSE, Kathryn Victoria c/o Corme-Ecluse, Main Street, Ravenfield, Rotherham S65 4NA — MB ChB Bristol 1996.

SHORTHOUSE, Mr Andrew John Royal Hallamshire Hospital, Glossop Road, Sheffield S10 2JF Tel: 0114 271 3143 Fax: 0114 271 3143; 36 Riverdale Road, Sheffield S10 3FB Tel: 0114 266 1781 Fax: 0114 267 9662 Email: shorthouse@doctors.org.uk — MB BS Lond. 1971 (St. Mary's) FRCS Eng. 1976; BSc (Hons.) Lond. 1968, MS 1981. Cons. Surg. (Colorectal Surg.) Roy. Hallamsh. Hosp. Sheff. Specialty: Gen. Surg. Socs: Hon. Sec. Assn. Coloproctol 1996-99; Hon. Sec. Europ. Assn. Coloproctol 1999-02; President-in-waiting Assn. Coloproctol 2003-04.

SHORTLAND, Betty Elisa (retired) 9 Westergate House, 30 Portsmouth Road, Kingston upon Thames KT1 2NE Tel: 020 8549 9439 — MB BS Lond. 1945 (Lond. Sch. Med. Wom.) MRCS Eng. LRCP Lond. 1945; DTM & H Eng. 1950; DPH 1962; MFCM 1974. Prev: Specialist (Community Med.) Lambeth, S.wark, Lewisham & Bromley HA.

SHORTLAND, David Barry Poole Hospital, Longfleet Road, Poole BH15 2JB Email: david.shortland@poole.nhs.uk — MB ChB Bristol 1979; MRCP (UK) 1982; DCH RCP Lond. 1982; MD Bristol 1992. Cons. Paediat. Poole Gen. Hosp. Specialty: Paediat. Socs: Brit. Paediat. Soc.; Neonat. Soc. Prev: Sen. Regist. & Regist. (Paediat.) Univ. Hosp. Nottm.; SHO (Paediat.) Hosps. for Sick Childr. Gt. Ormond St. Lond. & Bristol.

SHORTLAND, Graham John c/o Department of Child Health, University Hospital of Wales, Heath Park, Cardiff CF14 4XW — BM Soton. 1983 (University of Southampton) DCH RCP Lond. 1987; FRCP Lond. 1997; FRCPCH 1997. Cons. Paediat. Univ. Hosp. Wales Cardiff. Specialty: Paediat.; Neonat. Prev: Lect. & Hon. Sen. Regist. Univ. Wales Coll. Med.; Ho. Surg. Roy. S. Hants. Hosp. Soton; Ho. Phys. Roy. Hants. Co. Hosp. Winchester.

SHORTLAND-WEBB, Susan Caroline 40 Tilehouse Green Lane, Knowle, Solihull B93 9EY — MB BCh Wales 1989.

SHORTLAND-WEBB, William Richard (retired) 40 Tile House, Green Lane, Knowle, Solihull B93 9EY — MB ChB Birm. 1961; FRCPath 1982, M 1971. Cons. Path. City Hosp. NHS Trust.

SHORTRIDGE, Mr Richard Thomas John ENT Department, New Cross Hospital, Wednesfield, Wolverhampton WV10 0QP Tel: 01902 644911 Email: dickshortridge@doctors.org.uk — (Sheff.) MB ChB Sheff. 1970; FRCS Eng. 1976. Cons. Surg, ENT, The Roy. Wolverhampton Teachg. Hosps. NHS Trust; Chair HSTC Otolaryngol., W. Midlands. Specialty: Otorhinolaryngol. Socs: The Roy. Soc. of Med.; Midl. Inst. of Otorhinolaryng.; Brit. Med. Assn.

SHORTT, Alan Martin Drs. O'Leary, Shortt and Littlewood (University Practice), The Health Centre, Level 5, C S Building, University of Huddersfield, Huddersfield HD1 3DH Tel: 01484 430386 Fax: 01484 473085 — MB ChB Leeds 1988; T(GP) 1993; MRCGP 1994.

SHORTT, Edward Philip Hugh (retired) 41 Lenten Street, Alton GU34 1HE Tel: 01420 83118 — MB BChir Camb. 1947. Prev: Res. Obstetr. Guy's Hosp.

SHORTT, Michael Whitfield Dept of Orthopaedics, Charing Cross Hospital NHS Trust, Twickenham Rd, London W6 8RF Tel: 020 88461234 Email: mshortt@doctors.org.uk — MB BS Lond. 1997. SHO (Orthop.) W.Middlx. Hosp.; Clin. Research Fell. Char. Cross Hosp. Specialty: Orthop. Socs: Assoc. Mem. MSS; Assoc. Mem. MPS. Prev: SHO (A & E) Kingston Hosp. Kingston-upon-Thames; Ho. Off. (Upper GI Surg. & Urol.) Ealing Hosp. Lond.; Ho. Off. (Gen. Med. & Endocrinol.) St. Mary's Hosp. Paddington Lond.

SHORTT, Nicholas Lee — MB ChB Ed. 1996; MRCS Ed. 2001.

SHORTT, Stephen John The Health Centre, Gotham Lane, East Leake, Loughborough LE12 6SG Tel: 01509 852181 Fax: 01509 852099; 17 Meeting House Close, East Leake, Loughborough LE12 6HY Tel: 01509 853578 — BM BS Nottm. 1986; BMedSci Nottm. 1984; MRCGP 1991; DRCOG 1992. Clin. Tutor Univ. Nottm.

SHORVON, Philip John Department of Radiology, Central Middlesex Hospital North West London Hospitals NHS Trust, Acton Lane, London NW10 7NS Tel: 020 8453 2270 Fax: 020 8453 2511 Email: philip.shorvon@cmh-tr.nthames.nhs.uk; 27 Stamford Brook Road, London W6 0XJ Tel: 020 8748 0233 Email: phils@intonet.co.uk — MB BS Lond. 1976 (St. Thos.) MA Camb. 1975; MRCP (UK) 1979; FRCR 1986. Cons. Radiol., N. W. Lond. Hosps. NHS Trust, Lond.; Clin. Director, Radiol., Centr. Middlx. Hosp., Lond. Specialty: Radiol. Special Interest: GI Radiol. Socs: Eur. Soc. of Gastrointestinal and Abdom. Radiol. (ESGAR); Brit. Inst. of Radiol. (BIR); Roy. Coll. of Radiol. (RCD).

SHORVON, Professor Simon David National Hospital for Neurology & Neurosurgery, Institute of Neurology, Queen Square, London WC1N 3BG Tel: 020 7837 3611 Fax: 020 7676 2193 Email: s.shorvon@ion.ucl.ac.uk; The Brook Studio, 27A Stamford Brook Road, London W6 0XJ — MB BChir Camb. 1974 (St Thos.) MRCP (UK) 1975; MA Camb. 1974, MD 1983; FRCP Lond. 1990. Prof. Clin Neurol. Inst. Neurol. Lond.; Cons. Neurol. Nat. Hosp. Neurol. & Neurosurg. Lond. Specialty: Neurol. Special Interest: Epilepsy. Socs: (Exec. Comm.) Internat. League Against Epilepsy. Prev: Chairm. Clin. Neurol.; Sen. Regist. & Regist. Nat. Hosp. Nerv. Dis. Qu. Sq. Lond.; SHO (Clin. Neurol.) Univ. Oxf.

SHOTBOLT, John Paul 62 Howards Wood Drive, Gerrards Cross SL9 7HW — MB BS Lond. 1996.

SHOTLIFF, Kevin Peter — MB BS Lond. 1987 (St Geo. Hosp. Med. Sch. Lond.) DCH RCP Lond. 1989; DCH RCP Lond. 1989; MRCP (UK) 1991; MRCP (UK) 1991; MD Lond. 1995; MD Lond. 1995. Cons. (Diabetes & Endocrinol.) Chelsea & Westminster Hosp. Specialty: Endocrinol.; Diabetes. Prev: Sen. Regist. (Diabetes & Endocrinol.) St. Geo.'s Hosp. Lond.; Research Fell. (Diabetic Retinop.) Roy. Postgrad. Med. Sch. Hammersmith Hosp. Lond.; Cons. Kingston Hosp.

SHOTT, Claire Helen Flat 3/2, 5 Caird Drive, Glasgow G11 5DZ — MB ChB Glas. 1994; DRCOG 1998. Specialty: Gen. Pract.

SHOTTON, Mr John Carr Kent & Sussex Hospital, Tunbridge Wells TN4 8AT Tel: 01622 226209 Fax: 01622 226191 Email: j.c.shotton@btinternet.com; 7 Holmewood Ridge, Langton Green, Tunbridge Wells TN3 0BN Tel: 01892 862361 Email: j.c.shotton@btinternet.com — MB BCh Wales 1980; FRCS Eng. (ENT) 1986; FRCS Ed. (ENT) 1986. Cons. Otolaryngol. Maidstone Tunbridge Well NHS Trust; Hon. Cons. Regional Plastic Surg. Unit Qu. Vict. Hosp. E. Grinstead. Specialty: Otorhinolaryngol. Prev: Sen. Regist. (Otolaryngol.) SE Thames RHA, Kings Coll. Hosp.; Janet Nash Fell.; Skull Base/ OTO Neurosurg., Zurich 1990.

SHOTTS, Alan (retired) 3 Scotch Common, West Ealing, London W13 8DL Tel: 020 8997 6500 — MRCS Eng. LRCP Lond. 1951 (Guy's) LDS RCS Eng. 1947.

SHOTTS, Nina (retired) 12 Woodville Road, Ealing, London W5 2SF Tel: 020 8997 5671 Fax: 020 8997 5671 Email: nina@padwickshotts.freeserve.co.uk — (Roy. Free) MRCS Eng. LRCP Lond. 1958; FDS RCS Eng. 1963. Prev: Indep. Specialist Lond.

SHOULER, Mr Philip James, MBE Vale of Leven District General Hospital, Alexandria G83 0UA Tel: 01389 54121 — MB BS Lond. 1974; MRCS Eng. LRCP Lond. 1973; FRCS Eng. 1979; FRCPS Glas. 1991. Cons. Surg. Vale of Leven Dist. Gen. Hosp. Specialty: Gen. Surg. Socs: Brit. Soc. Gastroenterol.; Assn. Surg.; BMA. Prev: Cons. Surg. Roy. Naval Med. Serv.

SHOULS, Jennie Christine 63 The Lynch, Winscombe BS25 1AR — MB ChB Bristol 1994.

SHOULTS, Clare — MB BS Lond. 1998.

SHOUSHA, Mohamed Sami Mahmoud Department of Histopathology, Charing Cross Hospital, Fulham Palace Road, London W6 8RF Tel: 020 8846 7144 Fax: 020 8846 1364 Email: s.shousha@imperial.ac.uk — (Faculty of Medicine, Cairo University) MB BCh Cairo 1964; MD Cairo 1971; MRCPath 1976. Sen. Lect. & Hon. Cons. Char. Cross Hosp. & Imperial Coll. Sch. of Med. Lond. Specialty: Histopath. Special Interest: Breast, Liver and Gastrointestinal Path. Socs: Brit. Div. of Internat. Acad. of Path.; US and Canad. Acad. of Path.; Path. Soc. of Gt. Britain and Irel. Prev: Lect. Roy. Free Hosp. & Sch. of Med.

SHOVE, Mr David Colquhoun 17 Highpoint, North Hill, Highgate, London N6 4BA Tel: 020 8340 9154 — MB ChB Otago 1960; BA Auckland 1954; FRCS Ed. 1967; FRCPA 1973. Cons. (Path.) Barnet Gen. Hosp. Specialty: Pathology, General.

SHOVE, Roy Frederick (retired) 10 Priory Close, Pevensey BN24 6AD Tel: 01323 769490 — MRCS Eng. LRCP Lond. 1944 (Univ. Coll. Hosp.) FRCGP 1973. Prev: Orthop. Hosp. Pract. Kent & Sussex Hosp. Tunbridge Wells.

SHOVLIN, Claire Louise Imperial College of Medicine, National Heart and Lung Institute, Hammersmith Hospital, Du Cane Road,

London W12 0NN Tel: 020 8383 3269 Fax: 020 8743 9733 — MB BChir Camb. 1987. Sen. Lect. & Hon. Cons. (Respirat. Med.).

SHOVLIN, William Mathieson (retired) Stourton House, 67 Oakham Road, Dudley DY2 7TH Tel: 01384 253405 — (Glas.) MB ChB Glas. 1952.

SHOWELL, Daniel Gareth Leslie 68 Gaywood Road, King's Lynn PE30 2PT — MB BS Lond. 1992 (Royal Free School of Medicine London) DTM & H Liverp. 1995; DCH RCP Lond. 1995. Specialty: Gen. Pract.

SHOWGHI, Samina The Harley St. General Practice, 73 Harley St., London W1G 8QJ Tel: 020 7486 6011 Fax: 020 7224 6853 — MB BS Lond. 1993 (UCMSM) DCH RCP Lond. 1995; DRCOG Lond. 1996; MRCGP Lond. 1997. Specialty: Gen. Pract. Socs: BMA; RSM; IDF, Chelsea Clin. Soc.

SHRANK, Alan Bruce (retired) 20 Crescent Place, Town Walls, Shrewsbury SY1 1TQ Tel: 01743 362469 Email: alan.shrank@freeuk.com — BM BCh Oxf. 1956 (Oxf. & Middlx.) MA Oxf. 1956; FRCP Lond. 1977, M 1961. Mem. Med. Appeal Tribunals 1988-. Prev: Cons. Dermat. Shropsh. HA.

SHRAVAT, Mr Brijendra Pratap Victoria Hospital, Blackpool FY3 8NR Tel: 01253 34111 — MB BS Allahabad 1973 (M.L.N. Med. Coll.) MS (Orthop.) Allahabad 1977; DA (UK) 1986; FRCS Ed. 1992. Staff Surg. (A & E) Vict. Hosp. Blackpool. Specialty: Accid. & Emerg.

SHREEVE, David Randal 16 St John Street, Manchester M3 4EA Tel: 0161 834 1100 Fax: 0161 835 1465; Rough Meadow, 4 Gipsy Lane, Rochdale OL11 3HA — MB ChB Manch. 1961; FRCP Ed. 1980, M 1966; FRCP Lond. 1979, M 1966. Cons. Phys. N. Manch. HA Retd. From NHS Oct 2000. Specialty: Gastroenterol. Socs: Fell. Manch. Med. Soc.; Brit. Soc. Gastroenterol. & Diabetes UK. Prev: Sen. Regist. United Manch. Hosps.; Tutor (Med.) Univ. Dept. Med. & SHO (Med.) Manch. Roy. Infirm.

SHRESTHA, Badri Man Northern General Hospital, Sheffield Kidney Institute, Herries Road, Sheffield S5 7AU — MB BS Dibrugarh 1979. Specialty: Gen. Surg.

SHRESTHA, Basant Kumar The Maples Medical Centre, Barnfield Close, Staveley, Chesterfield S43 3UL Tel: 01246 472309 Fax: 01246 470546; 23 Elm Tree Drive, Wingerworth, Chesterfield S42 6QD Tel: 01246 276173 — MB BS Lucknow 1963 (King Geo. Med. Coll. Lucknow) MRCP (UK) 1977; FRCP (Lond.) 1998. Specialty: Gen. Pract. Socs: (Chairm.) Nepalese Doctors Assn. UK. Prev: Regist. (Med.) King's Mill Hosp. Sutton-in-Ashfield; Cons. Phys. Thapathali Kathmandu, Nepal.

SHRESTHA, Keshar Lal 74 Castlefields, Bournmoor, Houghton-le-Spring DH4 6HJ — MB BS Calcutta 1968 (Nilratan Sircar Med. Coll. Calcutta) FRCPsych 2001. Cons. Psychiat. Cherry Knowle Hosp. Sunderland. Specialty: Gen. Psychiat.

SHRESTHA, Rekha Department of Obstetrics & Gynaecology, Derriford Hospital, Plymouth PL6 8DH Tel: 01752 245281 Fax: 01752 763721 Email: rekha.shrestha@phnt.swest.nhs.uk; 10 Cheshire Drive, Tamerton Foliot, Plymouth PL6 6SQ — MB BS Bangalore 1980 (St Johns Med. Coll., Bangalore, India) MRCOG 1987; Dip Obst 2000; FRCOG Lond. 2002. Cons. In Obst. and Gyn., Derriford Hosp., Plymouth; Cons. In Obst. and Gyn., Plymouth Nuffield Hosp. Specialty: Obst. & Gyn. Special Interest: Adolescent / Paediatric Gynaecology; Gynaecology Ultrsound; menopause. Socs: Roy. Coll. of Obstetricians and Gynaecologists; Paediatric Gyn. Soc.; Brit. Menopause Soc. Prev: Staff Grade Doctor Plymouth HA.; Regist. (O & G) Southmead Hosp. Bristol, Freedom Fields Hosp. Plymouth & St. Jas. Hosp. Leeds; locum Cons. In Obst. and Gyn.

SHRESTHA, Subarna Man Oakwood Surgery, Church Street, Mansfield Woodhouse, Mansfield NG19 8BL Tel: 01623 633111 Fax: 01623 423480; 26 North Park, Mansfield NG18 4PB Tel: 01623 621336 — MB BS Lucknow 1963.

SHRIBMAN, Andrew Joseph Lane End Farm, Beat Lane, Rushton Spencer, Macclesfield SK11 0QY Tel: 01260 226304 Email: andrew@laneendfarm.freeserve.co.uk — MB BS Lond. 1977 (Roy. Lond. Hosp. Med. Coll.) FRCA 1981. Cons. Anaesth. E. Chesh. NHS Trust Macclesfield. Specialty: Anaesth. Socs: Assn. Anaesth. of GB & Irel.; BMA. Prev: Sen. Regist. (Anaesth.) Leic. HA; Clin. Instruc. (Anaesth.) Med. Coll. Virginia Richmond, USA; Regist. (Anaesth.) Bristol Roy. Infirm.

SHRIBMAN, Jonathan Howard Levitts Surgery, Levitts Road, Bugbrooke, Northampton NN7 3QN Tel: 01604 830348 Fax: 01604 832785; 3 Harrison Court, Bugbrooke, Northampton NN7 3ET Tel: 01604 830380 Fax: 01604 832785 Email: ghs@bugdoc.powernet.co.uk — MB BS Lond. 1975; MRCP (UK) 1977; DCH RCP Lond. 1983; MRCGP 1984; DRCOG 1985. GP Trainer N.ants. Prev: Trainee GP Moulton Northampton; Regist. Rotat. (Med.) St. Geo. Hosp. Lond.; SHO (O & G) Northampton Gen. Hosp.

SHRIBMAN, Sheila Joan Medical Director's Office, Northampton General Hospital NHS Trust, Cliftonville, Northampton NN1 5BD Tel: 01604 545868; Stonegables, 3 Harrison Court, Bugbrooke, Northampton NN7 3ET Tel: 01604 830380 — (Cambridge University Girton College) BChir 1975; MA, MB Camb. 1976; FRCP Lond. 1993; FRCP Lond. 1993. Med. Director Northampton Director Northampton Gen. Hosp. NHS Trust Cliftonville Northampton NN! 5BD. Specialty: Paediat. Socs: Roy. Coll. Paediat. & Child Health; College Registrar (Hon Sec). Prev: Sen. Regist. (Paediat.) Northampton Gen. Hosp.; Sen. Regist. Qu. Mary's Hosp. Carshalton & St. Geo. Hosp.; Clin. Lect. (Paediat. & Pharmacol.) Cardiothoracic Inst. Lond. Rotat.

SHRIDHAR, Sanjiv Wistaston Sugery, Brookland House, 501 Crewe Road, Wistaston, Crewe CW2 6QP; 140 Colleys Lane, Willaston, Nantwich CW5 6NU Tel: 01270 623507 — MB ChB Dundee 1988; MRCGP 1992; MBA (Masters in Business Administration) 1996. Prev: Trainee GP/SHO Rotat. N. Staffs. Roy. Infirm. VTS; Ho. Off. (Surg.) Leicester Teach. Hosp.; Ho. Off. (Med.) Dundee Teach. Hosps.

SHRIDHAR, Sunita 81 Old Park Avenue, Enfield EN2 6PN; 24 Gelligaer Street, Cathays, Cardiff CF24 4LA — MB BCh Wales 1994.

SHRIMAN NARAYAN, Mr Ramanthan Harrogate District Hospital, Lancaster Park Road, Harrogate HG2 7SX Tel: 01423 885959; 2 St. Ronans Road, Harrogate HG2 8LE Tel: 01423 886575 — MB BS Delhi 1980; MS (Orthop.) Delhi 1983; FRCS Glas. 1990. Sen. Staff Orthop. Surg. Harrogate Dist. Hosp. Prev: Regist. (Orthop.) Grimsby & Newport, Gwent; SHO (Gen. Surg.) Louth.

SHRIMPTON, Anna Ruth Leicester Royal Infirmary, Department of Immunology, Leicester LE1 5WN — MB BChir Camb. 1995; MA Cantab. 1993; MRCP Lond. 1999. Specialist Regist. (Immunol.) Leics. Roy. Infirm. Specialty: Gen. Med.

SHRIMPTON, Grant Russell 6 South Ash, Steyning BN44 3SJ — MB ChB Otago 1991.

SHRIMPTON, Helen Diane Worvell Cottage, Knole Pit Lane, Knole, Langport TA10 9JD — MB BChir Camb. 1992. Specialty: Gen. Pract.; Dermat.

SHRIMPTON, Miranda Kate 31 Alisa Avenue, Twickenham TW1 1NF — MB BS Lond. 1995.

SHRIMPTON, Simon Philip 3 Ashdown House, 17 Rydens Road, Walton-on-Thames KT12 3AB — MB BS Lond. 1989.

SHRIMPTON, Susan Bronwen Glaxosmithkline, New Frontiers Science Park, Third Avenue, Harlow CM19 5AW Tel: 020 8913 4784 Fax: 020 8913 4492 Email: susan_b_shrimpton@gsk.com; Clamber Cottage, Northchurch Lane, Ashley Green, Chesham HP5 3PD — MB BChir Camb. 1988; BA (Path.) Camb. 1984; Dip. Pharm. Med. RCP (UK) 1995; AFPM 1996; MFPM 2002; FFPM 2003. Clin. Director, Global Safety Eval. and Risk Managem. Specialty: Pharmaceutical Medicine. Socs: Brit. App.; BrAPP. Prev: Dir. Medical Renewal Group; Clin. Director, Europ. Med. Affairs, Respirat. Med.; Director of Clin. Developm., UK.

SHRINATH, Madhukar c/o Drive Sunil Sinha, Gunnergate Lane, Marton, Middlesbrough TS7 8JA — MB BS Patna 1985; MRCP (UK) 1994.

SHRIVASTAVA, Anupam Departmnt of Paediatrics, Coonsultant Paediatrician, Southend Hospital, Southend-on-Sea SS0 0RY Tel: 01702 221239 Fax: 01702 221252; 140 Barnstaple Road, Thorpe Bay, Southend-on-Sea SS1 3PW Tel: 01702 585122 — MB BS Calcutta 1983 (Calcutta National Medical College, Calcutta) FRCPCH; M.D(1987); MRCP (UK) 1991. Cons. Paediat. Specialty: Paediat.; Rheumatol. Socs: RCPCH; Fell.; Neonat. Soc.

SHRIVASTAVA, Mr Madhur Deokinandan 52 Rothwell Drive, Solihull B91 1HG Tel: 0121 733 8589 — MB BS Bhopal 1976; MB BS Bhopal, India 1976; FRCS Glas. 1989. Specialty: Trauma & Orthop. Surg.

SHRIVASTAVA, Om Prakash The Surgery, Photopia, Limesway, Rotherham S66 8JF Tel: 01709 812714 — MB BS Lucknow 1968.

SHRIVASTAVA, Mr Raj Kumar William Harvey Hospital, Ashford TN24 0LZ Tel: 01233 633331 — MB BS Indore, India 1979; FRCS Ed. 1985; FRCS Glas. 1986; MCh Liverp. 1988; FRCS (Orth.) 1995. Cons. Orthop. Surg. William Harvey Hosp. Ashford. Specialty: Orthop.

SHRIVASTAVA, Rani The Surgery, Photopia, Limesway, Rotherham S66 8JF Tel: 01709 812714 — MB BS Lucknow 1968 (G.S.V.M Med. Coll. Kanpur) DGO Delhi 1973.

SHRIVASTAVA, S K Caerau Lane Surgery, Ely, Cardiff CF5 5HJ Tel: 029 2059 1855 Fax: 029 2059 9739; The Surgery, Caeura Lane, Ely, Cardiff CF5 5 Tel: 01222 591855 — MB BS Ranchi 1972 (MGM Med. Coll. Jamshedpur) Clin. Asst. (Orthop. & Traum. Surg.) Roy. Gwent Hosp. Newport; Clin. Asst. (Traum. & Orthop. Surg.) Univ. Hosp. of Wales Cardiff. Specialty: Orthop. Prev: FICS (Orth.).

SHRIVASTVA, Dwarka Prasad Buckland Medical Centre, 24 Gamble Road, Portsmouth PO2 7BN Tel: 023 9266 0910 Fax: 023 9267 8175 — MB BS Vikram 1967; MB BS Vikram 1967.

SHROFF, Behram Jehangir (retired) Holly Bank, Vicarage Road, Halling, Rochester ME2 1BQ Tel: 01634 241896 — MB BS Karachi 1952; LRCP LRCS Ed. LRFPS Glas. 1962.

SHROFF, Katy Jamshed c/o Mrs M. Mountford, 26 Westbourne Park Road, London W2 5PH — MB BS Punjab 1976; MFFP 1993. Chief Technical Adviser - Romania United Nations Populat. Fund & World Health Organisation (Regional Office for Europe). Specialty: Family Plann. & Reproduc. Health. Prev: Assoc. Dir. Servs. for Wom. Parkside Health Trust Lond.

SHROFF, Rekha Whitegates, Maldon Road, Witham CM8 1HU — BM Soton. 1997.

SHROFF, Sandip Brunswick Health Centre, Hartfield Close, Manchester M13 9YA Tel: 0161 273 4901 Fax: 0161 273 5952 — MB ChB Manch. 1989; BDS Dundee 1981; DRCOG 1992; MRCGP 1993.

SHROTRIA, Ms Sunita — MB BS 1982; MS 1985; FRCS 1989. Cons. Gen. Surg. with an interest in Breast. Ashford Hosp., Lond. Rd.. Middlx YW15 3AA. Specialty: Gen. Surg.; Plastic Surg. Socs: Surg. Research Soc.; Brit. Assoc. of Surgic. Oncologists.

SHROUDER, Raymond David 3 School Lane, Old Somerby, Grantham NG33 4AH — MB ChB Leic. 1992.

SHROUFI, Mr Shamsi St. Mary's, Craig Road, Dumfries DG1 4EU Tel: 01387 2732 — MD Istanbul 1960; FRCS Glas. 1981. Orthop. Regist. Dumfries & Galloway Health Bd. Specialty: Orthop.

SHRUBB, Valerie Ann Ashurst Child & Family Centre, Lyndhurst Road, Ashurst, Southampton SO40 7AR Tel: 023 8074 3038 Fax: 023 8074 3033; 27 Westbroke Gardens, Fishlake Meadows, Romsey SO51 7RQ — MB BS Lond. 1975 (King's Coll. Hosp.) MRCS Eng. LRCP Lond. 1975; MRCP 1979; FRCP Lond. 1994; FRCPCH 1997. Cons. (Paediat. Community Child Health) Ashurst Child & Family Health Centre Soton. Specialty: Community Child Health. Special Interest: Physical Disabilities. Socs: Brit. Assn. Community Child Health. Prev: Cons. (Paediat. Community Child Health) Soton. Community Health Servs. Trust; Hon. Sen. Lect. (Community Paediat.) UMDS Guy's & Thos. Hosps. Lond.; Cons. (Paediat. Community Child Health) Lewisham & Southwark HA.

SHUAIB, M Swanlow Medical Centre, 60 Swanlow Lane, Winsford CW7 1JF Tel: 01606 862868 — MB BS Punjab 1965; MB BS Punjab 1965.

SHUBHAKER, Undinti David Cranbrook Road Surgery, 700 Cranbrook Road, Barkingside, Ilford IG6 1HP Tel: 020 8551 2341 Fax: 020 8551 1479 — MB BS Osmania 1965.

SHUBHAKER, Urmila Cranbrook Road Surgery, 700 Cranbrook Road, Barkingside, Ilford IG6 1HP Tel: 020 8551 2341 Fax: 020 8551 1479 — MB BS Osmania 1971.

SHUBSACHS, Alexander Philip Woolf Marlborough House Regional Secure Unit, Milton Keynes Hospital Campus, Standing Way, Eaglestone, Milton Keynes MK6 5NG Tel: 01908 243050 — MB BS Lond. 1980 (St. Mary's) BSc (Hons.) Psychol. Manch. 1968; MRCPsych 1986. Med. Dir. & Cons. Forens. Psychiat. MarlBoro. Hse. Regional Secure Unit Bucks.Ment. Health NHS Trust Milton Keynes Hosp. Campus, Milton Keynes. Specialty: Forens. Psychiat. Socs: BMA; Roy. Coll. Psych. (Forens. Psych. Div.); Fell.Roy. Soc. of Med. Prev: Clin. Dir. & Cons. Forens. Psychiat. Rampton Hosp.; Lect. & Hon. Sen. Regist. (Forens. Psychiat.) Univ. of Edin.; Regist. Roy. Edin. Hosp.

SHUCKSMITH, Mary Richardson (retired) 9 Nichols Way, Wetherby LS22 6NB Tel: 01937 581896 — MB ChB Leeds 1945. Prev: SCMO Leeds AHA (T).

SHUFFLEBOTHAM, Jonathan Quinn 4 Berne Avenue, Newcastle ST5 2QJ — MB ChB Leeds 1996.

SHUI, Elizabeth Margaret Yee-Lai Athena Medical Centre, 21 Atherden Road, Clapton, London E5 0QP Tel: 020 8985 6675 Fax: 020 8533 7775; 21 Rolls Park Road, Chingford, London E4 9BH — MB ChB Sheff. 1980; DRCOG 1983; MRCGP 1984. GP Hackney; Med. Adviser Hackney Chinese Community Servs. Specialty: Pub. Health Med. Prev: Ho. Surg. & Ho. Phys. Roy. Hosp. Chesterfield; Trainee GP Chesterfield VTS.

SHUJAAT, Rosina Yorkhill NHS Trust, Yorkhill, Glasgow G3 8SJ; 1FR 102 Dorcester Avenue, Kelvindale, Glasgow G12 0EB Tel: 0141 339 3414 — MB ChB Ed. 1997. Specialty: Paediat.

SHUJJA-UD-DIN, Omar Sadeeq 3 Tadcaster Road, Copmanthorpe, York YO23 3UL — MB ChB Sheff. 1997.

SHUKER, John Philip The Yard House, 20A The Green, Garsington, Oxford OX44 9DF — MB ChB Birm. 1997.

SHUKER, Mr Makki Tawfeeq 32 Clarewood Court, Seymour Place, London W1H 2NL Tel: 020 7724 6410 — MB ChB Mosul 1969; MSc Manch. 1980; FRCS Ed. 1990.

SHUKLA, Avinash Chandra 3 Patent House, 48 Morris Road, London E14 6NU — MB BS Lond. 1989.

SHUKLA, Chitranjan Jitendrarai 33 Peters Close, Stanmore HA7 4SB — MB BS Lond. 1998; MB BS Lond 1998.

SHUKLA, Dolarrai Keshavlal (retired) 20 Lawrence Crescent, Edgware HA8 5PD Tel: 020 8952 8741 — LAH Dub. 1960.

SHUKLA, Mr Kamal Kant 84 North End Road, West Kensington, London NW11 7SY Tel: 020 7603 7901 Fax: 020 7602 7167 — MB BS Banaras Hindu 1975; MB BS Banaras Hindu Univ. India 1975; FRCS Glas. 1980. Clin. Asst. (ENT) W. Middlx. Hosp. Isleworth. Prev: Regist. (ENT) Northwick Pk. Hillingdon & Mt. Vernon Hosp. Watford.

SHUKLA, Mr Rajendra Balkrishna Dukes Medical Centre, 1 Lankers Drive, North Harrow, Harrow HA2 7PA Tel: 020 8868 5268; 140 Streatfield Road, Harrow HA3 9BU Tel: 020 8206 0263 Fax: 020 8206 0263 Email: shukla_dr@yahoo.com — LRCP LRCS Ed. 1980; MS Gujarat 1976, MB BS 1972; FRCSI 1979; LRCP LRCS Ed. LRCPS Glas. 1980. Surg. Regist. Roy. Free Hosp. Lond.; GP. Specialty: Gen. Pract. Socs: Med. Mem. Disabil. Appeal Tribunal; Local Med. Comm. Mem. Prev: Regist. (Gen. Surg.) Guy's & King's Coll. Hosp. Lond.; Regist. (Surg.) St. Vincent's Hosp. & Jas. Connolly Memor. Hosp. Dub.; Lect. (Surg.) Cancer Research Inst. Ahmedabad India.

SHUKLA, Rashmita Eastern Leicester Primary Health Trust, Mansion House, 41 Guildhall Lane, Leicester LE1 5FR — BM Soton. 1984; MRCP (UK) 1988; MFPHM RCP (UK) 1993; FFPHM 2001. Cons. (Pub. Health Med.) Eastern Leicester PCT. Specialty: Pub. Health Med. Prev: Cons. (Communicable Dis. Control) Leics. Health; Sen. Regist. (Pub. Health Med.) Trent RHA; Regist. (Pub. Health Med.) Trent RHA.

SHUKLA, Yashwant Prataprai H.M.Y.O.I Lancaster Farms, Far Moor Lane, Stone Row Head, Off Quernmore Road, Lancaster LA1 3QZ Tel: 01524 848745 Fax: 01524 849308 — MB BS Gujarat 1974; DPM RCP Lond. 1981. Med. Off. HM Young Offenders Inst. Lancaster. Prev: Clin. Asst. Psychiat. Roy. Albert Hosp. Lancaster; Regist. (Psychiat.) Parkside Hosp. Macclesfield & Cranage Hall Hosp.

SHUKRALLA, Zekiya Amin 13 Hookstone Wood Road, Harrogate HG2 8PN — MB ChB Baghdad 1967; DObst. RCPI Dub. 1976; (DGO)TC Dub. 1976; MRCOG Lond. 1992. Cons. (O & G) New Mowasat Hosp. Kuwait Hosp. Kuwait. Specialty: Obst. & Gyn. Socs: Fell. Amer. Med. Soc. (Obst. & Gyn.) Vienna Univ. 1985; Pan Amer. Assn. 1997. Prev: Clin. Asst. (GU Med.) Maelori Hosp.; Clin. Asst. (O & G) Warrington Hosp.

SHULMAN, Caroline Esther London School of Tropical Medicine, Keppel St., London WC1 7HT; 64 Old Park Road, Palmers Green, London N13 4RE Tel: 020 8886 8411 — MB BS Lond. 1984; DCH RCP Lond. 1986; DRCOG 1988; DTM & H Liverp. 1989; MRCGP 1989; MSc Lond. 1992; PhD Amsterdam 2001.

SHUM, Chau Ming Walderslade Village Surgery, 62A Robin Hood Lane, Walderslade, Chatham ME5 9LD Tel: 01634 687250; 10 Barncroft Drive, Hempstead, Gillingham ME7 3TJ — MB BS Lond. 1988; DRCOG 1991; DCH RCP Lond. 1992; T(GP) 1993; MRCGP 1993. Partner GP Princip.; Research Assoc. UMDS. Specialty: Cardiol.

SHUM, Kid Wan Department of Dermatology, Royal Hallamshire, Glossop Rd, Sheffield S10 2JF Tel: 0114 271 1900 Fax: 0114 271 3763 — MB BChir Camb. 1994; MA Camb. 1995, BA 1991; MRCP Lond. 1997. Specialty: Dermat. Socs: Roy. Coll. of Phys.s, Lond.; Trainee Mem. Brit. Assn. Dermatol.s; Brit. Soc. of Paediat. Dermat.

SHUM, Poh Lin 17 Burnview Drive, Carryduff, Belfast BT8 8DD Tel: 02890 814546 — MB BCh BAO Belf. 1987 (Queen's University Belfast) Specialist Regist. (Radiother. & Oncol.). Specialty: Oncol.; Radiother. Socs: Irish Assn. Cancer Research; Mem. Roy. Coll. Radiol.

SHUM, Wing Kwan FLat 31 The Quadrangle, London W2 2RN — MB BChir Camb. 1980; BSc Lond. 1972; PhD Camb. 1975, MB BChir 1980. Socs: Brit. Pharmacol. Soc.

SHUMSHERUDDIN, Dean Mohammed 61 Newlands Road, Stirchley, Birmingham B30 2SA — MB ChB Birm. 1981.

SHUN-SHIN, Mr Georges Adrien Wolverhampton & Midland Counties Eye Infirmary, Compton Road, Wolverhampton WV3 9QR Tel: 01902 645025 Fax: 01902 645018 — MB BS Lond. 1978 (Guy's) FRCS (Ophth.) Glas. 1982; DO RCS Eng. 1982; FRCOphth Lond. 1990. Cons. Ophth. Wolverhampton & Midl. Counties Eye Infirm.; Cons Ophth. Manor Hosp. Walsall. Specialty: Ophth. Socs: (Treas.) Assn. Eye Research. Prev: Clin. Lect. & Hon. Sen. Regist. Oxf. Eye Hosp.; Research Fell. (Ophth.) Nuffield Laborat. Ophth. Oxf.; Regist. (Ophth.) Roy. Vict. Hosp. Bournemouth.

SHUR, Eric The Priory Hospital, Priory Lane, Roehampton, London SW15 5JJ Tel: 020 8392 4201/ 876 8261 Fax: 020 8876 4015 Email: ericshur@prioryhealthcare.com; 10 Harley Street, London W1G 9PF Tel: 020 7467 8300 — MB BCh Witwatersrand 1973; MRCPsych 1979; MPhil (Psych.) Lond. 1981; FRCPsych 1996. Dep. Med. Dir. Priory Hosp. Roehampton;; Hon. Research Fell. Char. Cross Med. Sch. Lond. Specialty: Gen. Psychiat. Prev: Cons. Psychiat. Westm. Hosp. Lond.; Sen. Lect. (Psychiat.) Char. Cross Med. Sch. Lond.; Clin. Tutor, Priory Hosp., Roehampton.

SHURMER, David Milne The Stannington Health Centre, Uppergate Road, Stannington, Sheffield S6 6BX Tel: 0114 234 8779 Fax: 0114 285 4778 — MB ChB Sheff. 1986. Specialty: Gen. Med.

SHURZ, Alison Mary Lucy 44A Harmer Green Lane, Welwyn AL6 0AT Tel: 01438 714632 — MB ChB Bristol 1962; DCH Eng. 1965; FRCP Lond. 1987; FRCPCH 1997. p/t Cons. Paediat. Luton & Dunstable NHS Trust; Cons. Paediat. BUPA Hosp. Harpenden; Cons. Paediat. The Rivers Hosp. Sawbridgeworth. Specialty: Paediat. Special Interest: Allergies & Food Intolerances; Asthma; Epilepsy & Seizure Disorders. Socs: Amer. Epilepsy Soc.; RSM. Prev: Prof. (Paediat.) Kigezi Internat. Sch. of Med. Camb.; Clin. Dir. & Cons. Paediat. Qu. Eliz. II Hosp. Welwyn Gdn. City; Sen. Regist. (Paediat.) St Mary's Hosp. Lond.

SHUTE, Jennifer Catherine Hill Cyder House, Newcastle, Monmouth NP25 5NT Tel: 01600 750249 — BM BCh Oxf. 1974; MA Oxf. 1974. GP Doctors Retainer Scheme Caerleon. Prev: Regist. (Anaesth.) St. Thos. Hosp. Lond.

SHUTE, Mr Kenneth 6 Church Street, Caerleon NP18 1AW Tel: 01633 423744 Fax: 01633 238539 Email: ken.shute@gwent.wales.nhs.uk — MB BS Lond. 1968; FRCS Eng 1972; MS Lond. 1978. Cons. Gen. Surg. Roy. Gwent Hosp. Newport. Specialty: Gen. Surg. Prev: Sen. Regist. (Gen. Surg.) Nottm. Gen. Hosp.; Wellcome Research Fell. & Lect Surg. St. Thos. Hosp. Lond.; Regist. St. Thos. Hosp. Lond.

SHUTE, Pauline Ericka Childrens Centre, Worthing Hospital, Worthing BN11 2DH Tel: 01903 286702 Fax: 01903 286701 Email: pauline.shure@wash.nhs.uk; Windmill House, 11 Mill Hill, Shoreham-by-Sea BN43 5TG Tel: 01273 463420 — MB BS Lond. 1975 (Roy. Free) MRCS Eng. LRCP Lond. 1975; DRCOG 1979; MSc Univ. Lond. 1991; DCH RCP Lond. 1991; FRCPCH 1998. Cons. Community Paediat., Worthing and Southlands NHS Trust. Specialty: Community Child Health. Special Interest: Adoption and Fostering; Child Protec.; Childr. with Disabil. Socs: Brit. Assn. Community Child Health; Roy. Coll. of Paediat. and Child Health.

SHUTE, Philip Alan Barton Surgery, Lymington House, Barton Hill Way, Torquay TQ2 8JG Tel: 01803 323761 Fax: 01803 316920; Court Barton Farm Cottage, Coffinswell, Newton Abbot TQ12 4SS Tel: 01803 872736 — MB BS Lond. 1980 (St. Mary's Hospital University of London) MRCGP 1984; DRCOG 1985.

SHUTES, Jonathan Charles Blackwell Woodcock Road Surgery, 29 Woodcock Road, Norwich NR3 3UA Tel: 01603 425989 Fax: 01603 425989; Gildencroft, 56 Norwich Road, Horsham St. Faith, Norwich NR10 3AE Tel: 01603 891495 — MB BS Lond. 1972; MRCS Eng. LRCP Lond. 1972; DRCOG 1975; DA Eng. 1977; Dip Pall Med (UCW) 2001. Prev: Staff Grade Palliat. Care Norf. & Norwich Univ. Hosp.; Clin. Asst. (Anaesth.) Norf. & Norwich Hosp.

SHUTKEVER, Martin Paul Station Lane Medical Centre, Station Lane, Featherstone, Pontefract WF7 6JL Tel: 01977 600381 Fax: 01977 600776 — MB ChB Leeds 1980; DRCOG 1982; MRCGP 1984; LLM Cardiff Univ. 1997. Gen. Practitioner, Featherstone; Professional Exec. CTTE Mem., East. Wakefield PCT. Specialty: Medico Legal. Socs: Law Soc. Checked Expert Register. Prev: Chief Resid. K. Edwd. VII Memor. Hosp. Bermuda; SHO (A & E) St. Jas. Hosp. Leeds; Ho. Off. (Surg.) ScarBoro. Hosp.

SHUTT, Mr Adrian Michael COU Kisiizi Hospital, PO Box 109, Kabale, Uganda Fax: 00871 761 587166 Email: kisiizi@bushnet.net; 12 Blackbrook Close, Walkhampton, Yelverton PL20 6JF Tel: 01822 854653 — MB BS Lond. 1986 (St. Mary's Hosp. Lond.) FRCS Eng. 1991; DTM&H 1999. Chief Surg., COU Kissizi Hosp. Kabale, Uganda. Specialty: Gen. Surg. Prev: Specialist Regist. (Surg.) Soton. Gen. Hosp.; Specialist Regist. (Surg.) Qu. Alexandra Hosp. Portsmouth; Regist. (Surg.) Wessex PostFellowsh. Train. Scheme.

SHUTT, Leslie Ernest St Michaels Hospital , Department of Anaesthesia, Saltwell Street, Bristol BS2 8EG Tel: 0117 928 5203; Dyrham House, 1 Dyrham Close, Henleaze, Bristol BS9 4TF — MB ChB Sheff. 1969; FFA RCS Eng. 1973. Cons. Anaesth.and Pain Managem. United Bristol Health Care NHS Trust; Hon. Cons. Sen. Lect., Univ. of Bristol. Specialty: Anaesth. Special Interest: Regional Anaesth., Obstetric Anaesth. and Analgesia, Pain Managem. Socs: Assn. Anaesth. GB & Irel. & Soc. Anaesth. S. West. Region. Prev: Sen. Regist. (Anaesth.) Avon AHA (T); Vis. Asst. Prof. (Anaesth.) Univ. Virginia Med. Center, USA; Regist. (Anaesth.) United Sheff. Hosps.

SHUTTE, Helen Anna Neale Rookwood, Rushmere Lane, Denmead, Waterlooville PO7 6HA — MB BS Lond. 1998; MB BS Lond 1998.

SHUTTLEWORTH, Barbara Joyce (retired) Linden House, Northbrook Avenue, Winchester SO23 0JW Tel: 01962 861142 — (Oxf.) MA Oxf. 1948, BM BCh 1945; DObst RCOG 1949; DPH Manch. 1954. Prev: Clin. Asst. (Psychiat.) Basingstoke Dist. Hosp.

SHUTTLEWORTH, Caroline Angela Rose — MB BS Lond. 1990; BA Oxf. 1987; DFFP 1992. Community Med. Off. Croydon Community Health. Specialty: Family Plann. & Reproduc. Health.

SHUTTLEWORTH, David Essex County Hospital, Lexden Road, Colchester CO3 3NB Tel: 01206 744435 Fax: 01206 744756; Cattles Barn, Chappel Road, Fordham, Colchester CO6 3LT Tel: 01206 241428 Email: davidsderm@aol.com — MB BS Lond. 1977 (Univ. Coll. Hosp.) MRCP (UK) 1980. Cons. Dermat. Essex Rivers Healthcare. Specialty: Dermat.

SHUTTLEWORTH, Doris Kathleen (retired) 44 West Street, Scarborough YO11 2QP Tel: 01723 72308 — MRCS Eng. LRCP Lond. 1922 (Leeds)

SHUTTLEWORTH, Garry Neil Singleton Hospital, Sketty, Swansea SA2 8QA Tel: 01792 205666 Fax: 01792 208647 Email: gary.shuttleworth@swansea-tr.wales.nhs.uk — MB BS Lond. 1991; FRCOphth 1994; BSc 1998. Cons. Ophth. Swansea NHS Trust Swansea. Specialty: Ophth. Special Interest: Oculoplastics; Strabismus; Gen. Ophth. Cataract/ Glaucoma. Socs: S. W. Ophth. Soc.

SHUTTLEWORTH, Herbert John (retired) 2 Galloway House, West Burton, Leyburn DL8 4JW Tel: 01969 663460 — (Liverp.) MB ChB Liverp. 1939. Prev: Cas. Off. Liverp. Stanley Hosp.

SHWEIKH, Mr Amir Musa Diana Princess of Wales Hospital, Accident & Emergency Department, Scartho Road, Grimsby DN33 2BA — MB ChB Baghdad 1974; FFAEM; FRCS Glas. 1984. Cons. A&E Diana Princess of Wales.Hosp. Specialty: Accid. & Emerg. Socs: BMA; Brit. Assn. A&E. Med; Fell.Fac.A&E.Med.

SHYAM SUNDAR, Ananthaiah University Hospital of North Tees, North Tees & Hartlepool NHS Trust, Hardwick, Stockton-on-Tees TS19 8PE Tel: 01624 624948/01642 624194/01642 642195 Fax: 01642 624948 Email: ananthaiah.shyam-sundar@nth.northy.nhs.uk; 26 Hemingford Gardens, Yarm TS15 9ST Tel: 01642 789435 — MB BS Bangalore 1981 (Bangalore Med. Coll.) MRCP (UK) 1992; T(M) 1995; FRCP Ed. 1998; FRCP London 2000. Cons. Phys. (Cardiol.) N. Tees Gen. Hosp. & Hon. Cons. Cardiol. S. Cleveland Hosp. S.Tees Acute Hosps. NHS Trust. Specialty: Cardiol. Socs: Brit. Cardiac Soc.; Brit. Cardiac Interven. Soc.; Eur. Soc. Cardiol. (Mem. Working Gp. Coronary Circ.). Prev: Career Sen. Regist. (Cardiol.) & Sen. Research Fell. Roy. Infirm. Edin.; Regist. (Cardiol.) Univ. Hosp. Wales Cardiff; Regist. (Cardiol.) All India Inst. Med. Sci. New Delhi, India.

SHYAMAPANT, Sanjay 7 Silverbirch Close, Little Stoke, Bristol BS34 6RL — MB BCh Wales 1995.

SHYAMSUNDAR, Mr Srinivasan 23 Dunleady Park, Dundonald, Belfast BT16 — MB BS Madras 1992. Specialist Regist. (Trauma & Orthop.) Ulster Hosp. Belf. Specialty: Orthop.

SIALA, Maria-Danuta Beeches Surgery, 9 Hill Road, Carshalton Beeches, Carshalton SM5 3RB Tel: 0208 647 6608 Email: dana53@blueyonder.co.uk; 33 Manor Way, South Croydon CR2 7BT Tel: 0208 681 7825 — MB ChB Bristol 1964; DObst RCOG 1966; Cert. Family Plann. JCC 1981; Cert. Prescribed Equiv. Exp. JCPTGP 1981. GP Carshalton Beeches. Socs: Polish Doctors Med. Soc. Prev: Regist. (Paediat.) INAS Hosp. Tripoli.

SIAN, Surinder Singh Spinney Hill Medical Centre, 143 St. Saviours Road, Leicester LE5 3HX Tel: 0116 251 7870 Fax: 0116 262 9816 — MB ChB Dundee 1989.

SIANI, Nanjit Mavji Argyll Road Surgery, 48 Argyll Road, Westcliff on Sea SS0 7HN Tel: 01702 432040 — MB BS Sri Venkateswara 1976; JCPTGP 1985; Cert. Family Plann. JCC 1985. Clin. Asst. (Genitourin. Med.) Southend Gen. Hosp. Specialty: Genitourinary Medicine; Cardiol.; Gen. Med. Prev: Regist. & SHO (Gerontol.) Univ. Hosp. Wales & St. Davids Hosp. Cardiff; Clin. Asst. (Geriat. Med.) Llandough Hosp. Cardiff; SHO (Psychiat.) E. Glam. Gen. Hosp. Pontypridd.

SIANN, Tanya Linda Audit Co-ordinator, Audit Resource & Training Centre, Kirklands Hospital, Fallside Road, Bothwell, Glasgow G71 8BU Tel: 0141 854637 Fax: 0141852517; 5 Wheatland Drive, Lanark ML11 7QG — MB ChB Aberd. 1983; MRCGP 1988; MPH Glas. 1990. Clin. Audit. Co-ordinator Lanarksh. HB. Prev: Sen. Regist. (Pub. Health Med.) Lanarksh. HB.

SIAS, Alessandro 31 Downleaze, Sneyd Park, Bristol BS9 1LU — State Exam Cagliari 1993.

SIBBALD, Barbara (retired) Ashiestiel, 42 Drumcross Road, Bathgate EH48 1AR Tel: 01506 652745 — MB ChB Ed. 1956. Prev: GP Bathgate.

SIBBALD, David Stewart (retired) Ashiestiel, 42 Drumcross Road, Bathgate EH48 1AR Tel: 01506 652745 — MB ChB Ed. 1956. Prev: GP Bathgate.

SIBBALD, Robert (retired) 10 Meadow View, Barwick-in-Elmet, Leeds LS15 4NZ — MB ChB Manch. 1961; FRCPath. 1981, M 1969. Prev: Cons. Pathol. Pontefract Gen. Infirm.

SIBBALD, Robert James Inglis (retired) Prospect Lodge, 38 Dean Hill, Plymstock, Plymouth PL9 9AD Tel: 01752 402146 Fax: 01752 480312 — MB BChir Camb. 1963 (St. Thos.) MRCS Eng. LRCP Lond. 1962; MA Camb. 1963; DObst RCOG 1964; DCH Eng. 1968; FRCGP 1981, M 1970; RCGP 2002. Provost, Tamar Faculty. Prev: GP Princip. Plymouth 1965-98.

SIBBERING, Mr David Mark Derby City General Hospital, Uttoxeter Road, Derby DE22 3NE Tel: 01332 625537 Fax: 01332 625696; 4 Hargreaves Close, Littleover, Derby DE23 4YH Tel: 01332 523851 Email: mark.sibbering@sdah-tr.trent.nhs.uk — MB BS Lond. 1986 (St. Thos. Hosp. Med. Sch.) FRCS Ed. 1991. Cons. Surg. (Breast Dis.) Derby City Gen. Hosp. Specialty: Gen. Surg. Prev: Lect. (Surg.) Univ. Nottm.; Hon. Sen. Regist. Mid. Trent Higher Surgic. Train. Scheme; Research Fell. (Breast Dis.) Profess. Unit. Surg. Nottm. City Hosp.

SIBELLAS, Mary (retired) Banjo Lodge, Common Road, Great Wakering, Southend-on-Sea SS3 0AG Tel: 01702 217458 — MRCS Eng. LRCP Lond. 1957 (Roy. Free) MD Lond. 1975, MB BS 1957; DTM & H Liverp. 1966; FFCM 1985, M 1977; T(PHM) 1991. Prev: Dir. (Pub. Health) S. Essex HA.

SIBERRY, Hazel Margaret Liffock Surgery, 69 Sea Road, Castlerock, Coleraine BT51 4TW Tel: 028 7084 8206 Fax: 028 7084 9146 — MB BCh BAO Belf. 1975; MRCGP 1980.

SIBERT, Professor Jonathan Richard — (Camb. & Univ. Coll. Hosp.) MD Camb. 1977, MA 1967; MB BChir Camb. 1967; DObst RCOG 1969; MRCP (UK) 1971; DCH Eng. 1971; FRCP Lond. 1986; FRCPCH 1997, MRCPCH 1996. Prof. Child Health Univ. Wales Coll. Med. Specialty: Paediat.; Community Child Health. Special Interest: Community Child Health. Socs: (Prev. Chairm.) Brit. Assn. Comm. Child Health; Fell. Roy. Coll. Paediat. & Child Health; Nat. Commiss. Preven. Child Abuse.

SIBERY, Ashley James 11 Enstone, Skelmersdale WN8 6AW — MB ChB Manch. 1997.

SIBLEY, Mr Gary Neil Andrew Department of Urology, Bristol Royal Infirmary, Bristol BS2 8HW — BM BCh Oxf. 1975; BSc (Anat. Hons.) Bristol 1972; MCh Oxf. 1985, DM 1985, BM BCh 1975; FRCS Eng. 1979. Cons. Urol. Surg. Bristol Roy. Infirm. Specialty: Urol. Prev: Clin. Lect. (Urol.) Addenbrooke's Hosp. Camb.; Surgic. Regist. Radcliffe Infirm. Oxf.; Research Fell. Urol. Churchill Hosp. Oxf.

SIBLEY, Yvonne Diane Leslie (retired) 15 Weylands Grove, Salford M6 7WX — BM BCh Oxf. 1971; BSc Bristol 1968; FRCS Eng. 1977. Prev: Cons. Paediat. Cardiol. Roy. Manch. Childr. Hosp.

SIBLEY-CALDER, Ian Clifford Eastgate Medical Group, 37 Eastgate, Hornsea HU18 1LP Tel: 01964 532212 Fax: 01964 535007; Westfield, Westwood Avenue, Hornsea HU18 1EE Tel: 01964 534925 Email: sibcald@aol.com — MB BS Lond. 1983 (St. Bart.) Cert. Family Plann. JCC 1985; DRCOG 1986; DCCH RCGP & FCM 1986. Med. Off. Child Developm. Clinic Hornsea; Mem. (Comm.) UK Sport Diving Med. Comms.; HSE Approved for Commercial Diving Med. Exams. Specialty: Gen. Pract.; Occupat. Health.

SIBLY, Mr Thomas Franklin Wye Valley Nuffield Hospital, Venns Lane, Hereford HR1 1DF Tel: 01432 265184 Fax: 01432 265184 — MB BS Lond. 1982 (Univ. Coll. Hosp.) MA Oxf. 1979; FRCS Eng. 1986. Cons. Orthop. Surg. Gen. Hosp. Hereford. Specialty: Orthop. Socs: Assoc. Mem. Brit. Soc. Surg. Hand; Brit. Orthop. Assn. Prev: Sen. Regist. (Orthop.) Harlow Wood Orthop. Hosp. & Derbysh. Roy. Infirm.; Regist. (Orthop.) Newc. u. Tyne; N.. Region Research Fell. Durh. Univ. Dept. Bioengin.

SIBSON, Mr Derek Edmund (retired) 24 Poplars Farm Road, Barton Seagrave, Kettering NN15 5AF Tel: 01536 512376 — MB Camb. 1961 (St. Bart.) BChir 1960; BA Camb. 1957, MB 1961; DObst RCOG 1962; FRCS Eng. 1966. Prev: Lect. (Surg.) St. Bart. Hosp. Lond.

SIBSON, Keith Richard 24 Poplars Farm Road, Barton Seagrave, Kettering NN15 5AF — MB ChB Sheff. 1995 (Sheffield) MRCP (UK). Paediat. Reg. (Haemat. & Oncol.) Gt Ormond St. Specialty: Paediat. Prev: Paediat. Reg. Barnet; SHO paediat.Gt.Ormond.St.Hosp.; SHO Community.Paediat.Camden & Islington.

SIBTHORPE, Elsie Margaret (retired) Flat 2, Hetton Lodge, 6 Ferndale, Tunbridge Wells TN2 3RU — (Roy. Free) MD Lond. 1953, MB BS 1945; FRCOG 1966, M 1951. Prev: Cons. Gynaecol. Mildmay Miss. Hosp.

SIBTHORPE, John Oliver (retired) Ansteys, New Road, Hemingford Abbots, Huntingdon PE28 9AB — MB BS Lond. 1958 (King's Coll. Hosp.) MRCS Eng. LRCP Lond. 1958; DObst RCOG 1960; DO Eng. 1963. Clin. Asst. (Ophth.) Addenbrooke's Hosp. Camb. Prev: SHO (Ophth.) Qu. Eliz. Hosp. Birm.

SIBTHORPE, Richard John 58B Ritherdon Road, London SW17 8QG — MB BS Lond. 1984.

SICHA, Marenka Anna Northgate Surgery, Church Street, Uttoxeter ST14 8AG Tel: 01889 562010 Fax: 01889 568948; 3 Milverton Drive, Uttoxeter ST14 7RE Tel: 01889 563739 — MB ChB Birm. 1984; DRCOG 1987; MRCGP 1988.

SICHEL, Gerald Robert Mackenzie (retired) 1 Groomsland Drive, Billingshurst RH14 9HA Tel: 01403 786905 — MB BS Lond. 1943 (Guy's) MRCS Eng. LRCP Lond. 1942; MRCGP 1973; FFCM 1978, M 1974. Prev: DMO Tunbridge Wells Health Auth.

SICHEL, John Henry Sylvester Beaumont Street Surgery, 28 Beaumont Street, Oxford OX1 2NP Tel: 01865 311811 Fax: 01865 310327; 13 Park Town, Oxford OX2 6SN Tel: 01865 515636 — MB BS Lond. 1975 (Middlx. Hosp.) Hosp. Practitioner Young Adult

Diabetic Clinic; Med. Off. Oxf. Univ. Boat Club; Med. Off. New Coll. Hartford Coll. Templeton Coll. Socs: Ex-Sec. Oxf. Coll. Doctors Assn.; Ex-Pres. Oxf. Med. Soc. Prev: Clin. Asst. Young Adult Diabetic Clinic John Radcliffe Hosp. Oxf.; Regist. (Gen. Med. & Nephrol.) St. Helier Hosp. Carshalton; SHO (Cardiol.) Papworth Hosp. Camb.

SICS, Martin Richard The Cottage, Upper Tankersley, Barnsley S75 3DQ Tel: 01226 744966 — MB ChB Liverp. 1976; MRCGP 1992. Prev: Clin. Asst. (Respirat. Med.) Barnsley Dist. Hosp.; Audit Facilitator Barnsley MAAG; Clin. Governance Lead, Barnsley E. PCG.

SIDA, Elizabeth Clare West Kirby Health Centre, Grange Road, Wirral CH48 4HZ Tel: 0151 625 9171 Fax: 0151 625 9171 — MB ChB Leeds 1981; DRCOG 1984; MRCGP 1985.

SIDANA, Sangat Singh The Surgery, 167 Bridge Road, Grays RM17 6DB Tel: 01375 373322 Fax: 01375 375329; 600 London Road (Branch Surgery), West Thurrock, Grays RM20 Tel: 01708 865444 — MB BS Rajasthan 1961 (S.M.S. Med. Coll. Jaipur) DO Eng. 1969. Vice Chairm. Small Practs Assn. Specialty: Ophth. Prev: Adviser GP Strategic Advis. Comm.; Chairm. GP Locality Forum.

SIDAT, Imtiaz Ahomed Gulam Mahomed 555 Chorley Old Road, Bolton BL1 6AF Tel: 01204 848411 Fax: 01204 849968 — MB ChB Zimbabwe 1985 (Godfrey Huggins) MRCP (UK) 1994; MRCGP 1997. GP Bolton. Prev: GP Regist. Halliwell Surg. Bolton; SHO (O & G) Roy. Bolton Hosp.; SHO (O & G) Roy. Bolton Hosp.

SIDAWAY, Muriel Elizabeth 70 Harley Street, London W1 1AE Tel: 020 7580 3383 Fax: 020 7636 6902; 1 Stanhope Road, Highgate, London N6 5NE Tel: 020 8340 3773 — MRCS Eng. LRCP Lond. 1949 (Camb. & Birm.) MA, MB BChir Camb. 1949; FRCP Ed. 1971, M 1956; MRCP Lond. 1956; DMRD Eng. 1958; FFR 1960; FRCR 1975. Cons. Radiol. Harley St. Lond. Specialty: Radiol. Socs: Fell. Roy. Coll. Radiol.; Brit. Inst. Radiol. Prev: Sen. Regist. (Radiol.) Univ. Coll. Hosp. Lond. & Hosp. Sick Childr. Gt. Ormond St.; Regist. (Radiol.) St. Bart. Hosp.; Ho. Phys. Gen. Hosp. Birm.

SIDAWAY, Steven Foley Minster Practice, Greenhill Health Centre, Church Street, Lichfield WS13 6JL Tel: 01543 414311 Fax: 01543 418668 — MB ChB Birm. 1984. SHO (Med.) Russells Hall Hosp. Dudley. Socs: BMA. Prev: Ho. Off. (Med.) E. Birm. Hosp.; Ho. Off. (Surg.) Stafford Dist. Gen. Hosp.

SIDDAL, Miss Jane Nerrol Department Obsterics, Royal Berkshire Hospital, London Road, Reading RG1 5AN Tel: 0118 987 8117 — MB BS Lond. 1984 (Roy. Free, Univ. Lond.) MRCOG 1989; DHMSA 1992; MFFP 1993. Cons. in Feto-Matern. Med. Roy. Berks Hosp. Reading. Specialty: Obst. & Gyn. Socs: BMA; Reading Path. Soc. Prev: Sen. Regist. (O & G) Wexham Pk. Hosp. Slough; Lect. (O & G) St. Mary's Hosp. Med. Sch. Lond.; Regist. (O & G) Wexham Pk. Slough.

SIDDALL, Barbara Lesley 8 Penmaes, Pentrych, Cardiff CF15 9QS — MB BCh Wales 1977.

SIDDALL, Howard Scott Charles The Stennings, Brill, Constantine, Falmouth TR11 5UR — MB ChB Bristol 1975; MRCP (UK) 1978.

SIDDALL, William Jegon Wellard (retired) Moor Tang, Two Mile Oak, Newton Abbot TQ12 6DF Tel: 01803 813434 — MB BS Lond. 1958 (Guy's) MRCS Eng. LRCP Lond. 1957; DA Eng. 1960; FRCA Eng. 1964. Prev: Cons. Anaesth. Torbay Hosp. Torquay.

SIDDEEQ, Mohamed Usman Abbas and Siddeeq, Clifford Coombs Health Centre, 70 Tangmere Drive, Castle Vale, Birmingham B35 7QX Tel: 0121 747 4633 Fax: 0121 747 1587 — MB BS Madras 1962. Specialty: Gen. Pract. Prev: Regist. (Geriat. Med.) Worthing Hosp.; SHO (Med.) Roy. Hosp. Weston-Super-Mare; Asst. Phys. Vict. Hosp. Bangalore, India.

SIDDIG, Mohamed Ahmed Nasr Royal Cornwall Hospital (Treliske), Truro TR1 3LJ Tel: 01872 74242; 11 Penair VIew, Truro TR1 1XR Tel: 01872 223294 — MD Debrecen, Hungary 1977; MD (Obst. & Gyn.) Budapest 1985; MRCOG 1992. Socs: Arab Bd. Obst. & Gyn. Jordan 1991.

SIDDINS, Mark Threlkeld Baker Flat 1, Emerson Bainbridge House, 47 Cleveland St., London W1T 4JQ — MB BS Monash 1983.

SIDDIQ, Mirza Azher Luqman Medical Centre, 75 Countess Street, Walsall WS1 4JZ Tel: 01922 621659 Fax: 01922 621702 — MB ChB Sheff. 1992.

SIDDIQI, Afsar Ghouse 'Olive Quill', 52 Nottingham Road, Ravenshead, Nottingham NG15 9HH Tel: 01623 797882 — MB BS Marathwada 1972.

SIDDIQI, Asma Flat 1, 80 Fitzjohns Avenue, London NW3 5LS — MB BS Lond. 1994.

SIDDIQI, Mashood Ali Ingle House, Margaret Road, Crosby, Liverpool L23 6TR Tel: 0151 931 3108 Fax: 0151 931 3202 — MB BS Patna 1968; MRCPI 1989; DGM RCP Lond. 1989; FRCP(1) 2002. Cons. Phys. Univ. Hosp. Aintree, Liverp. Specialty: Care of the Elderly.

SIDDIQI, Mr Midhat Nafis Queen Elizabeth Hospital, Stadium Road, Woolwich, London SE18 4QH Tel: 020 8836 5484 Fax: 020 8836 5436 — MB ChB Bristol 1983; FRCS Eng. 1988; FRCS Glas. 1988; FRCS Ed. 1988; FRCS (Gen. Surg.) 2000. Cons. Surg. Specialty: Gen. Surg. Special Interest: Gastro-oesophagal Reflux Dis. Socs: Assn. Surg. GB & Irel. Prev: Regist. (Paediat. Surg.) St Thos. Hosp. Lond.; Regist. (Gen. Surg.) Mt. Vernon Hosp. Northwood.

SIDDIQI, Mohd Anwar The Medical Centre, Gun Lane, Strood, Rochester ME2 4UW Tel: 01634 290644; 9 Harlech Close, Strood, Rochester ME2 3QP — MB BS Dacca 1965 (Chittagong Med. Coll.) DTM & H Liverp. 1968; MRCP (UK) 1972; LMSSA Lond. 1974. Prev: Regist. (Med.) & SHO (Gen. Med.) Medway Hosp. Gillingham; Ho. Off. (Gen. Surg.) N. Cambs. Hosp. Wisbech.

SIDDIQI, Naveed Iqbal 174 Dorset House, Gloucester Place, London NW1 5AH — MB BS Lond. 1989.

SIDDIQI, Mr Nusrat Jamal "Crestar", 6 Pentland Close, Hazel Grove, Stockport SK7 5BS Tel: 0161 456 4556 Fax: 0161 456 4556 — MB BS Lond. 1987 (United Guys/St Thomas) BDS; FRCS 1997; FDS 1999. Reg.Oral.Surg.; Specialist Regist., Oral and Maxillofacial Surg., Derrifield Hosp., Plymouth. Specialty: Oral & Maxillofacial Surg. Socs: Roy. Coll. of Surg.s, Eng.; BDA; BMA. Prev: Basic.Surg.Train.Rotat.leeds.Univ.hosp.

SIDDIQI, Shafia "Crestar", 6 Pentland Close, Hazel Grove, Stockport SK7 5BS Tel: 0161 456 4556 — MB BS Dacca 1963 (Dacca Med. Coll., Dacca Univ.) DRCOG 1970; MRCOG 1997; FRCOG 1997. Gen. Practitioner, Stockport; Princip. Gen. Practitioner, Stockport PCT. Socs: Roy. Coll. of Obst.s and Gynaecologists; BMA; MPS.

SIDDIQI, Shahab Ahmad 102 Pirbright Road, London SW18 5NA — MB BS Lond. 1993 (St. Geo. Hosp.) BSc Lond. 1992; FRCS Eng. 1997. SpR N. E. Thames. Specialty: Gen. Surg. Prev: Lect. (Gen. Surg.) Roy. Lond. Hosp.; SHO (Gen. Surg.) York Dist. Hosp.; SHO (Cardiothoracic Surg.) Guy's & St. Thos. Hosps.

SIDDIQI, Shareen Claire The Coach House, Vicarage Lane, Allithwaite, Grange-over-Sands LA11 7QN; The Coach House, Vicarage Lane, Allithwaite, Grange-over-Sands LA11 7QN — MB ChB Leic. 1998.

SIDDIQUE, Abdul Quayum Minsmere House, Heath Road Wing, Ipswich Hospital, Ipswich IP4 5PD Tel: 01473 704203; 3 Cecil Road, Ipswich IP1 3NW — MB BS Dacca 1966 (Dacca Med. Coll.) MCPS Pakistan (Med.) 1969; DPM Eng. 1975; MRCPsych 1977; MSc Leic. 1979. Cons. Psychiat. Old Age St. Clement's Hosp. & Ipswich Hosp. Specialty: Geriat. Psychiat. Socs: Brit. Geriat. Soc.; Fell. of the Roy. Soc. of Med. Prev: Cons. Psychiat. Lynfield Mt. Hosp. Bradford; Sen. Regist. Birm. AHA (T).

SIDDIQUE, Abul Basher Mohammad 14 Alleyn Road, London SE21 8AL — MB BS Dacca 1968.

SIDDIQUE, Farooque Hayder Denmark Hill, London SE5 9RS — MB BS Calcutta 1958 (Lond.) MFFP 1998 RCOG; DObst RCOG 1964. GP in NHS & Privat. Pract. Specialty: Gen. Surg. Socs: Med. Protec. Soc. Prev: King's Coll. Hosp.; Clin. Asst. (Gyn.) Dulwich Hosp. Lond.

SIDDIQUE, Haroon Aqeel 28 Tyrone Road, Thorpe Bay, Southend-on-Sea SS1 3HF — MB BS Lond. 1989.

SIDDIQUE, Mr Muhammad Farooq 12 Avon Close, Taunton TA1 4SU — MB BS Pakistan 1975; DLO RCS Eng. 1982; FRCSI 1990.

SIDDIQUE, Neelam 9A North Terrace, Claremont Road, Newcastle upon Tyne NE2 4AD — MB BS Punjab 1977; MRCP (UK) 1992.

SIDDIQUE, Tariq Ben 3 Waverley Street, York YO31 7QZ — MB ChB Leeds 1989.

SIDDIQUE, Yaseen 156 Headley Drive, Ilford IG2 6QJ — MB ChB Manch. 1991; DCH RCP Lond. 1998. Specialty: Gen. Pract.

SIDDIQUI, Abdul Majeed Gransha Hospital, Londonderry BT47 6TF Tel: 01504 860261; 10 The Beeches, Drumahoe, Londonderry BT47 3XS Tel: 01504 301653 — BSc Agra 1951, MB BS 1957; DTCD Wales 1972; DMH Belf. 1989. Assoc. Specialist in Psychiat. WHSS Bd. Gransha Hosp. Lond.derry. Socs: Fell. Overseas Doctors Assn. Prev: Med. Off. Karachi Municip. Corp.; Med. Off. Karachi Electric Supply Corp.; Sen. Med. Off. PIDC Karachi, Pakistan.

SIDDIQUI, Adnan Rasheed The Surgery, 6 Galpens Road, Thornton Heath, Croydon CR7 6EA Tel: 020 8684 3450 Fax: 020 8683 0439 — BM BS Nottm. 1991 (Univ. Nottm.) BMedSci Nottm. 1989; MRCGP 1997. GP Asst. Thornton Heath; GP Princip. Thornton Heath. Specialty: Gen. Pract. Socs: Fell. Roy. Soc. Med. Prev: SHO (c/o Elderly) St. Helier Hosp. Carshalton; SHO (Psychiat. & O & G) E. Surrey Hosp. Redhill; SHO (A & E) Ealing Hosp. S.all.

SIDDIQUI, Ahmad Sayeed The Health Centre, Marmaduke Street, Hessle Road, Hull HU3 3BH Tel: 01482 323449 Fax: 01482 610920 — MB BS Karachi 1980; LMSSA Lond. 1986. Regist. (Geriat.) Hull Roy. Infirm. & Kingston Gen. Hosp. Specialty: Care of the Elderly. Prev: Regist. (Geriat.) York. Dist. Hosp. & Ipswich Hosp.

SIDDIQUI, Arifa Moin Carisbrooke Road Surgery, 41 Carisbrooke Road, Walthamstow, London E17 7EE Tel: 020 8520 8284 Fax: 020 8520 7077; 15 Broadwalk, London E18 2DL — MB BS Karachi 1966.

SIDDIQUI, Asim Ali 338 Birkby Road, Huddersfield HD2 2DB — MB ChB Leeds 1993.

SIDDIQUI, Asra Sabena 86 Swakeley's Drive, Ickenham, Uxbridge UB10 8QG — MB BCh Wales 1993.

SIDDIQUI, Ayesha Saleem Flat No1, 80 Fitzjohn Avenue, London NW3 5LS — MB BS London 1989.

SIDDIQUI, Farah 27 Copeland Avenue, Leicester LE3 9BT — MB ChB Dundee 1996.

SIDDIQUI, Miss Frah Najeeba 21 Albany Mews, Gosforth, Newcastle upon Tyne NE3 4JW — MB BS Newc. 1994. Specialty: Paediat. Prev: SHO (Paediat.) Tyneside Hosp. S. Shields, Tyne & Wear; SHO (Geriat.) Sunderland Dist Gen. Hosp., Sunderland, Tyne & Wear.

SIDDIQUI, Ghazna Khalid 41 Pymmes Green Road, London N11 1DE — MB BS Lond. 1996.

SIDDIQUI, Hameeduddin 112 Conway Drive, Fulwood, Preston PR2 3ER Tel: 01772 787602 — (Sind) MB BS Sind Pakistan 1959; DTM & H Eng. 1965; DPH Liverp. 1969; DPM Eng. 1978. Assoc. Specialist (Psychiat.) Whittingham Hosp. & Roy. Preston Hosp. Specialty: Gen. Psychiat. Socs: Med. Ethical Soc. Prev: Regist. (Psychiat.) Whittingham Hosp.; SHO (Infec. Dis.) Fazakerley Hosp. Liverp.; SHO (Gen. Med.) Newsham Gen. Hosp. Liverp.

SIDDIQUI, Mr Kamran Haider Tameside General Hospital, Fountain Street, Ashton-under-Lyne OL6 9RW Tel: 0161 331 6000 Email: kamran.siddiqui@tgh.nhs.uk — MB BS Punjab 1982; FRCS Ed. 1990; FRCS Glas. 1990. Cons. Surg. (Gen. & Colorectal) Tameside Gen. Hosp. Specialty: Gen. Surg. Special Interest: Colorectal Surg.

SIDDIQUI, Khairuddin Department of Urology, Doncaster Royal Infirmary, Armthorpe Road, Doncaster DN2 5LT Tel: 01302 366666 Fax: 01302 553267 — MB BS India 1970; FCPS Bombay 1973; FRCS Glas. 1987; Dip Urol 1989. Cons. Urol., Doncaster Roy. Infirm. Specialty: Urol. Prev: Cons. Urol., York Dist. Hosp.; Cons. Urol., Leicester Gen. Hosp.; Cons., Doncaster Roy. Infirm.

SIDDIQUI, Mohammad Farooq 12 Balmoral Avenue, Glenmavis, Airdrie ML6 0PY Tel: 01236 761832 — MB ChB Manch. 1994; BSc (Med. Sci.) St. And. 1991.

SIDDIQUI, Mohammad Fouad 12 Balmoral Avenue, Glenmavis, Airdrie ML6 0PY — MB BS Lond. 1996.

SIDDIQUI, Mr Mohammad Mutiy Fayaz Bristol Childrens Hospital, Peadiatric Surgery, Bristol BS2 Tel: 0117 923 0000 Email: siddiquimmf@yahoo.co.uk — MB BS Univ. Sind 1991. (Paedia. Surg.) Bristol Childr. Hosp. Specialty: Paediat. Surg.

SIDDIQUI, Mohammed Akhtar Jawed 34 Greaves Avenue, Walsall WS5 3QG Tel: 01922 23788 — MB BS Punjab 1966; MB BS Punjab (Pakistan) 1966; DMRD Eng. 1971.

SIDDIQUI, Mohammed Lutfur Rehman Walnut Way Surgery, 21 Walnut Way, Ruislip HA4 6TB Tel: 020 8845 4400 Fax: 020 8845 4403 — MB BS Osmania 1967.

SIDDIQUI, Nadeem 69 Fulmer Road, Beckton, London E16 3TE — BChir Camb. 1996.

SIDDIQUI, Naila 15 Lincoln Road, Harrow HA2 7RQ — MB BS Karachi 1989.

SIDDIQUI, Nasim Ahmed 68 Aberford Road, Wakefield WF1 4AL — MB BS Karachi 1966.

SIDDIQUI, Mr Raheel 1 Leeses Close, Telford TF5 0NN — MB BS Karachi 1985; FRCS Ed. 1993.

SIDDIQUI, Sabina 51 Brighton Grove, Manchester M14 5JG — MB ChB Leic. 1994.

SIDDIQUI, Shaukat Ali Mel Valley, 338 Birkby Road, Huddersfield HD2 2DB Tel: 01484 531856 — MB BS Punjab 1964 (Nishtar Med. Coll.) MB BS Punjab Pakistan 1964; FFA RCS Eng. 1980 DA Eng. 1978. Cons. Anaesth. Calderdale Health Dist. Halifax. Specialty: Anaesth. Socs: Yorks. Anaesth. Soc.; BMA & Assn. Anaesth. UK & N.Irel. Prev: Sen. Regist. RAF Halton Bucks.; SHO & Regist. (Anaesth.) Huddersfield Roy. Infirm.; Fac. Anaesth. Dallas Texas, USA.

SIDDIQUI, Sughrat 2 Boyce Street, Walkley, Sheffield S6 3JS — MB ChB Sheff. 1998; MB ChB Sheff 1998.

SIDDIQUI, Syeda Vajiha Akmal Royal Albert Edward Infirmary, Christopher Home Eye Unit, Wigan Lane, Wigan WN1 2NN — MB ChB Manch. 1984 (Manchester) MRCS Eng. LRCP Lond. 1984; DO RCS Eng. 1989; FRCOphth 1989. Cons. Ophth., Roy. Albert Edwd. Infirm. Specialty: Ophth. Prev: Regist. (Ophth.) Manch. Roy. Eye Hosp. & Alder Hey Hosp. Liverp.; SHO. (Ophth.) Kingston Gen. Hosp. & Leeds Gen. Infirm.; Sen. Regist. Roy. Liverp. Univ. Hosp.

SIDDIQUI, Tariq Nadim 19 Briksdal Way, Lostock, Bolton BL6 4PQ — MB ChB Manch. 1998; MB ChB Manch 1998.

SIDDIQUI, Usma Shaukat 338 Birkby Road, Huddersfield HD2 2DB — MB ChB Manch. 1994. SHO (Anaesth.) N. Manch. Gen. Hosp. Specialty: Anaesth. Prev: SHO (Geriat. Med.) Withington Hosp. Manch.; Ho. Off. (Surg.) N. Manch. Gen. Hosp.; Ho. Off. (Med.) Roy. Oldham Hosp.

SIDDIQUI, Uzair Ahmad Summerfold House, 152 Leylands Road, Burgess Hill RH15 8JE Tel: 01444 257248 Fax: 01444 257265 — MB BS Sind 1960; DPM Eng. 1968; MRCPsych 1972. Cons. Psychiat. Mid Sussex NHS Trust; Chairm. & Lead Clin. Specialty: Rehabil. Med. Prev: Cons. Psychiat. Co. Hosp. Durh.

SIDDIQUIE, Shazia 6 Sarazen Court, Motherwell ML1 5TW — MB ChB Glas. 1998; MB ChB Glas 1998.

SIDDLE, David Ralph (retired) 41 Mount Crescent, Thornes Road, Wakefield WF2 8QG Tel: 01924 374921 — LRCP LRCS Ed. LRFPS Glas. 1957. Prev: Ho. Surg. Clayton Hosp. Wakefield.

SIDDLE, Stephen Geoffrey (retired) 57 Cedar Drive, Chichester PO19 3EH Tel: 01243 782624 — MD Durh. 1947 (Newc.) MB BS 1944; MRCGP 1954.

SIDDONS, Elizabeth Mary 9 Haywood Close, Evington, Leicester LE5 4JZ Fax: 0116 241 6284 Email: lizsid@aol.com — MB ChB Sheff. 1993.

SIDE, Christopher Douglas Siam Surgery, Sudbury CO10 6JH Tel: 01787 370444; 13 Bridgewater Road, Berkhamsted HP4 1HN Tel: 01442 874744 Email: chris@c-s-side.demon.co.uk — BM BCh Oxf. 1975 (Oxford) BSc Lond. 1969. Specialty: Gen. Pract. Prev: Clin. Asst. (Diabetes) Hemel Hempstead Hosp.; SHO (O & G), Ho. Phys. & Ho. Surg. Northampton Gen. Hosp.

SIDE, Lucy Elizabeth Department of Clinical Genetics, The Churchill Hospital, Old Road, Headington, Oxford OX3 7LJ — MB ChB Bristol 1988; MRCP (UK) 1991; MD Bristol 2002. Specialist Regist. in Clin. Genetics, Oxf. Radcliffe NHS Trust.

SIDEBOTHAM, Charles Francis The Perranporth Surgery, Perranporth TR6 0PS Tel: 01872 572255 — MRCS Eng. LRCP Lond. 1979 (Guy's) BSc Lond. 1976, MB BS 1979; MRCGP 1983; DRCOG 1984; DCH RCP Lond. 1986. Syntex Award 1984. Socs: BMA. Prev: Ho. Phys. Torbay Hosp.; Ho. Surg. Kent & Canterbury Hosp.

SIDEBOTHAM, Miss Emma Louise 59 Ribbesford Avenue, Wolverhampton WV10 6DU — MB ChB Bristol 1994; FRCS Eng. 1998. SHO (Surg.).

SIDEBOTHAM, Peter David Community Child Health, King Square House, King Square, Bristol BS2 8EF Tel: 0117 900 2353 Fax: 0117 900 2370 Email: peter.sidebotham@ubht.swest.nhs.uk — MB ChB Bristol 1987; MRCP (UK) 1991; MSc Bath 2000. Cons. Paediat. Community Child Health Bristol. Specialty: Community Child Health. Socs: BMA; Fell. Roy. Coll. Paediat. and Child Health. Prev: Lect.

(Community Child Health) Univ. Soton.; Regist. (Paediat.) Roy. Gwent Hosp. Newport; Lect. (Community Child Health) Bath.

SIDEBOTTOM, Eric 27 Hayward Road, Oxford OX2 8LN Tel: 01865 53023 Fax: 01865 53023 — BM BCh Oxf. 1963 (Oxf. & St. Bart.) DPhil Oxf. 1969, MA 1963. Indep. Cons. Med. Educat. & Research Oxf. Socs: Oxf. Med. Soc.; Oxf. Med. Alumni. Prev: Asst. Dir. Research ICR Fund; Univ. Lect. (Experim. Path.) Univ. Oxf.; Nuffield Research Fell. & Tutor (Med.) Lincoln Coll. Oxf.

SIDEBOTTOM, Paul 27 Hayward Road, Oxford OX2 8LN — MB BS Lond. 1994; BSc Lond. 1993. SHO (Med.) Sir Geo. Gairdner Hosp. Perth. Prev: SHO (A & E) Frimley Pk. Hosp.; Ho. Off. Qu. Eliz. Hosp. King's Lynn; Ho. Off. Char Cross Hosp. Lond.

SIDERY, John Charles Gurnett Cottage, Blakes Road, Wargrave, Reading RG10 8LA; Redwood House, Canon Lane, Maidenhead SL6 3PH — MB Camb. 1977; MA Camb. 1976, BA 1973, MB 1977, BChir 1976; DCH RCP Lond. 1981; DRCOG 1983; Dip. Occ. Med. RCP Lond. 1996. GP Berks. HA.

SIDES, Anne Pamela St. Johns House, 12 Station Road, Cullingworth, Bradford BD13 5HN — MB ChB Leeds 1978.

SIDES, Brian Arthur (retired) — MB ChB Manchester 1959; DObst RCOG 1961; FRCGP 1996, M 1972.

SIDES, Christopher Andrew — MB ChB Leeds 1978; FRCA 1983. Cons. Anaesth. Bradford Roy. Infirm. Specialty: Anaesth.

SIDES, Jeremy Robert Flat 2, 51 Mill Hill Road, Norwich NR2 3DR Tel: 01603 764344 Fax: 01603 764344 — MB BS Lond. 1973 (The London Hospital) BSc (Hons.) (Biochem.), MB BS Lond. 1973; DObst RCOG 1976; DCH Eng. 1978. Staff Grade Old Age Psychiat. Julien Hosp. Norwich; Blood Transfus. Session. Off. E. Anglian Blood Centre Cambs; Clin.Med.Off.ADAPT Diana Princess of Wales Trat.Centre.Mundesley Norf. Specialty: Geriat. Psychiat.; Blood Transfus.

SIDES, Kathleen Margaret (retired) Derrygonnelly, Enniskillen BT93 6HW; Cashel, Blaney, Enniskillen BT93 7AU Tel: 013656 41208 — (Belf.) MB BCh BAO Belf. 1941. Med. Off. Ely Disp.

SIDEY, Margaret Clare (retired) 2 Ferrings, Dulwich, London SE21 7LU Tel: 020 8693 8106 Fax: 020 8693 8106 — MB ChB New Zealand 1954 (Otago) MRCP Lond. 1959. Prev: Clin. Asst. Chelsea & Westm. Hosp. Lond.

SIDFORD, Kenneth Iain, RD St. Stephens Surgery, Adelaide St., Redditch B97 4AL Tel: 01527 65444 Fax: 01527 69218 Email: iainsidford@doctors.org.uk; 44 Salop Road, Redditch B97 4PS Tel: 01527 65444 Fax: 01527 69218 — MB ChB Birm 1977 (Birm.) BSc Lond. 1963; M.Med.Educat. Dundee 1995. GP Redditch; Lect. Med. Educat. Wolverhampton Univ. Specialty: Gen. Pract. Prev: Ho Phys. Dudley Rd. Hosp. Birm.; Ho Surg. Qu. Eliz. Hosp. Birm.; Surg. Lt.-Cdr RNR.

SIDHOM, Atef Tawfik Mikhail Ladywood Surgery, 35 Morville Street, Ladywood, Birmingham B16 8BU Tel: 0121 454 3774 Fax: 0121 456 5713; 93 Augustus Road, Birmingham B15 3LT — MB ChB Alexandria 1972. GP Edgbaston; Clin. Asst. (Accid. & Trauma) Birm. Gen. Hosp. Specialty: Orthop.; Acupunc.

SIDHU, Balwinder Singh The Surgery, Chancery Lane, Chapel End, Nuneaton CV10 0PB Tel: 024 7639 4766 Fax: 024 7639 6870; 129 Tresillian Road, Exhall, Coventry CV7 9PP Tel: 02476 315966 — MB BCh Wales 1982; BSc (Hons.), MB BCh Wales 1982; MRCPI 1984; MRCGP 1986. Prev: Regist. (Med.) Dudley HA; Regist. (Med.) Edgware Lond.

SIDHU, Davinder Singh 64 Metcalf Road, Ashford TW15 1EZ — MB BS Lond. 1996.

SIDHU, Gurpreet Singh North London Nuffield Hospital, Cavell Drive, Enfield EN2 7PR Tel: 020 8366 2122 — MB BS Lond. 1987 (Middlx. Hosp. Med. Sch.) DRCOG 1990; MRCGP 1991. Indep. GP Middlx.; In Flight Doctor (Aviat. Med.) Middlx. Specialty: Aviat. Med.

SIDHU, Harmini Kaur 31 Grove Hill Road, Moira, Craigavon BT67 0PP — MB BCh BAO Belf. 1985; MRCOG 1990. Regist. (O & G) Belf. City Hosp. Specialty: Obst. & Gyn. Socs: BMA & Ulster Med. Soc.

SIDHU, Jagdip Singh 68 Sherington Avenue, Pinner HA5 4DT — MB BS Lond. 1994; MB BS (Distinc.) Lond. 1994; MRCP (UK) 1997. SHO (Med.) Harefield & Hillingdon Hosps.; Specialist Regist. (Cardiol.) Harefield Hosp. Specialty: Cardiol. Socs: BMA. Prev: Ho. Off. (Surg.) Northwick Pk. Hosp. Lond.; Ho. Off. (Gen. Med.) Ealing.

SIDHU, Kamlesh Queen Square Surgery, 2 Queen Square, Lancaster LA1 1RP Tel: 01524 843333 Fax: 01524 847550; 7 Peacock Lane, Hest Bank, Lancaster LA2 6EN Tel: 01524 824437 — MB ChB Manch. 1983 (Manchester) MRCGP 1988. Specialty: Dermat.

SIDHU, Paul Singh Department of Diagnostic Radiology, Kings College Hospital, Denmark Hill, London SE5 9RS Tel: 020 7346 3063 Fax: 020 7346 3061 Email: paulsidhu@compuserve.com — MB BS Lond. 1982 (St. Mary's) BSc Lond. 1979; MRCP (UK) 1987; DTM & H RCP Lond. 1988; FRCR 1994. Cons. Diagn. Radiol. King's Coll. Hosp. Lond. Specialty: Radiol. Socs: Fell. Roy. Soc. Trop. Med. & Hyg.; Radiol. Soc. N. Amer.; Brit. Med. Ultrasound Soc. Prev: Cons. HCI (Internat.) Hosp. Clydebank; Regist. (Diagn. Radiol.) Hammersmith Hosp Lond.; Lect. Univ. Malaya Kuala Lumpur, Malaysia.

SIDHU, Shireen Kaur Flat 1/3, Jackson's Lane, Highgate, London N6 5SR — MB BS Adelaide 1990. Specialty: Dermat.

SIDHU, Sukhdev Singh 3 Lower Calderbrook, Littleborough OL15 9NW — MB BS Ranchi 1980.

SIDHU, Virinder Singh — MB BCh Wales 1982; MRCP (UK) 1985; FRCA 1989. Cons. Anaesth. St. Mary's Hosp. Lond. Specialty: Anaesth. Socs: Intens. Care Soc.; Assn. Anaesth.; Assn. Cardiothoracic Anaesth. Prev: Sen. Regist. Univ. Coll. Lond. Hosps., Gt. Ormond St. Hosp. Sick Childr. & Roy. Brompton Nat. Heart Hosp.

SIDIKI, Sikander Sandro c/o Southern General Hospital NHS Trust, 1345 Govan Road, Glasgow G51 4TF Tel: 0141 201 1583; 10 West Chapelton Drive, Bearsden, Glasgow G61 2DB — MB ChB Glas. 1989 (Univ. Glas.) BSc Miami 1984; FRCOphth 1996. SHO (Ophth.) South. Gen. Hosp. Glas. Specialty: Ophth. Socs: BMA. Prev: SHO (Ophth.) Gartnavel Gen. Hosp. Glas.; SHO (Geriat.) Vict. Geriat. Unit. Glas.; SHO (Neurosurg.) South. Gen. Hosp. Glas.

SIDKY, Kamla Hassan Ismail Histopathology Department, Arrowe Park Hospital, Arrowe Park Road, Upton, Wirral L49 5PE Tel: 0151 678 5111 Ext: 2563 Fax: 0151 604 1733 Email: sidky@doctors.org.uk — MB ChB; FRCPath. Cons. Histopath. and Cytopathologist, Wirral Hosp. NHS Trust. Socs: Brit. Soc. for Clin. Cytol.; Assn. of Clin. Pathologists.

SIDNEY, James Alexander 3 St James Close, Thorpe Thewles, Stockton-on-Tees TS21 3LH — MB ChB Bristol 1998.

SIDRA, Losil Moris 17 Brackenwood Close, Royton, Oldham OL2 5DE — State Exam Med Sofia 1986; MRCOG 1994.

SIDRA, Mr Rushdi Shafiq Highfield Health Centre, 2 Proctor Street, off Tong Street, Bradford BD4 9QA Tel: 01274 227700 Fax: 01274 227900 — MB BS Khartoum, Sudan 1969; FRCS Eng. 1976.

SIDWELL, Ian Philip 63 Redlake Drive, Taunton TA1 2RU — MB BS Lond. 1986. Specialty: Anaesth.

SIDWELL, Rachel Ursula Charnwood House, Dalby Road, Melton Mowbray LE13 0BJ — MB ChB Bristol 1990; DFFP 1994; DA Lond. 1996; MRCPCH Lond. 1997; MRCP Lond. 1997. SHO (Paediat.) Guy's Hosp. Lond. Specialty: Paediat. Socs: BMA & Med. Protec. Soc. Prev: SHO (Paediat.) Chelsea & Westm. Hosp.; SHO (O & G) Lister Hosp. Stevenage.

SIE, Adrian Hian Ing 89 Millbrae Road, Glasgow G42 9UP — MB ChB Sheff. 1995; MRCP 1999; DTM & H 1999.

SIE, Thwan Hwie Hospital Residences, Block B, Manthorpe Road, Grantham NG31 8DW — Artsexamen Amsterdam 1991.

SIEBER, Frederick Alexander Furlong Medical Centre, Furlong Road, Tunstall, Stoke-on-Trent ST6 5UD Tel: 01782 577388 Fax: 01782 838610 — MB ChB Dundee 1982; DA (UK) 1988.

SIEFF, Ivor Flat 8, The White House, Suffolk Road, Altrincham WA14 4QX Tel: 0161 929 0956 — (Manch.) MB ChB Manch. 1949.

SIEGLER, David Ivor Maurice Luton & Dunstable Hospital, Lewsey Road, Luton LU4 0DZ Tel: 01582497236; 8 Barton Road, Luton LU3 2BB Tel: 01582 597544 — (Univ. Coll. Hosp.) MB BS Lond. 1966; MRCS Eng. LRCP Lond. 1966; FRCP Lond. 1986, M 1969; MD Lond. 1977. Cons. Phys. (Gen. & Thoracic Med.) Luton & Dunstable Hosp. Specialty: Respirat. Med. Socs: Brit. Thorac. Soc.; Assn. Palliat. Med. Prev: Sen. Regist. (Med.) Roy. Free & Brompton Hosps. Lond.; Regist. (Med.) Univ. Coll. Hosp. Lond.

SIEGLER, Mr Joseph 31 Rodney Street, Liverpool L1 9EH Tel: 0151 709 8522 Fax: 0151 722 7538 Email: j.siegler@talk21.com; 4 Aldbourne Close, Liverpool L25 6JD Tel: 0151 722 1000 Fax: 0151 722 1000 Email: j.siegler@talk21.com — (St. Bart.) MB BS Lond. 1944; FRCS Eng. 1950; DLO Eng. 1954. Emerit. Cons.

Otorhinolaryng. United Liverp. Hosps. & Liverp. RHB; Emerit. Clin. Lect. (Otol.) Univ. Liverp. Specialty: Otolaryngol. Socs: Fell. Roy. Soc. Med.; Liverp. Med. Inst.; Life Mem. BMA. Prev: Cons. ENT Surg. to the Home Off. at Walton Jail; Sen. Regist. (Otolaryng.) United Liverp. Hosps.; Regist. Roy. Nat. Throat, Nose & Ear Hosp.

SIEGLER, Sarah Anne Peel Health Centre, Angouleme Way, Bury BL9 0BT Tel: 0161 763 7613 Fax: 0161 763 9625 — MB ChB Manch. 1979.

SIEGRUHN, Gert Cornelius (retired) 25 Arlington Square, London N1 7DP Tel: 020 7226 3456 Fax: 020 7226 3456; 25 Arlington Square, London N1 7DP Tel: 020 7226 3456/0208 421 0454 Fax: 020 7226 3456 Email: gert.siegruhn@which.net — MB ChB Pretoria 1958; MSc (Community Med.) Lond. 1971; MFCM RCP (UK) 1988; FFPHM RCP (UK) 1990. Prev: DMO Redbridge.

SIENKOWSKI, Ian Kazimierz Adelaide Medical Centre, 111 Adelaide Road, London NW3 3RY Tel: 020 7722 4135 Fax: 020 7586 7558 — MB BS Lond. 1974 (Westm.) MRCS Eng. LRCP Lond. 1974.

SIERADZAN, Katarzyna Aleksandra Frenchay Hospital, Department of Neurology, Frenchay Park Road, Bristol BS16 1LE — Lekarz Warsaw 1984; PhD (Neurosc.) Polish Acad. Sc. 1990; MRCP UK 1994; FRCP Lond. 2003. Cons. Neurol. Frenchay Hosp. Bristol. Specialty: Neurol. Special Interest: Epilepsy; Movement Disorders. Socs: Assn. Brit. Neurol.; SW Eng. Neuro. Assn. Prev: Clin. Lect. (Neurol.) Univ. Manch.

SIERATZKI, Jechil Harry Flat 39, Parkside, Knightsbridge, London SW1X 7JP — State Exam Med Giessen 1979.

SIEVERS, Paul Frederick St Marys Road Surgery, St. Marys Road, Newbury RG14 1EQ Tel: 01635 31444 Fax: 01635 551316; Crestholme, Well Meadows, Shaw, Newbury RG14 2DS Tel: 01635 42170 — MB BS Lond. 1962 (Guy's) MRCS Eng. LRCP Lond. 1962; DObst RCOG 1966; DCH Eng. 1966. Hosp. Practitioner & Clin. Asst. (Paediat.) Berks.; Med. Off. Vodaphone Gp., Quantel & Electrolux. Specialty: Gen. Pract. Socs: Newbury Med. Soc. Prev: SHO (Paediat.) Pembury Hosp.

SIEVERT, Julia Vale of Leven District General Hospital, Alexandria G83 0UA — State Exam Med Munich 1990.

SIEW TU, Chooye-Ling 8 Fern Avenue, Flixton, Manchester M41 5RZ Tel: 0161 746 9730 — MB ChB Manch. 1984.

SIFMAN, Morris (retired) 47 The Ridgeway, London NW11 8QP Fax: 020 8731 6276 — (Witwatersrand) MB BCh Witwatersrand 1952. Med. Off. Initiation Soc. GB. Prev: SHO St. Benidicts Hosp. Tooting.

SIGGERS, Benet Richard Charles, Surg. Lt.-Cdr. RN 1 Invincible Road, Seafield Park, Hillhead, Fareham PO14 2AZ — MB ChB Bristol 1994; Dip IMC RCS (Ed); FRCA 2003. SpR (Anaesth.) Soton. Gen. Hosp. Specialty: Accid. & Emerg. Prev: SHO (A & E) Frimley Pk. Hosp. Surrey; RMO (Primary Care) 29 Commando Regt. RA Plymouth; Ho. Off. (Surg. & Orthop.) CMH Aldershot.

SIGGERS, Diana Joan Eastleigh Surgery, Station Road, Westbury BA13 3JD Tel: 01373 822807 Fax: 01373 828904; Portway, Bratton, Westbury BA13 4SZ Tel: 01380 830894 — MB BS Lond. 1966 (Guy's) MRCS Eng. LRCP Lond. 1966; DObst RCOG 1976. Specialty: Gen. Pract.

SIGGERS, Georgina Rosemary North Star Farm, Beech Road, Mereworth, Maidstone ME18 5QJ Tel: 01622 813794; 6 Mast Court, 1 Boat Lifter Way, London SE16 7WH Tel: 020 7231 8970 Email: gsiggers@aol.com — MB BS Lond. 1993 (UMDS) MRCPCH; BSc (Hons.) Lond. 1990; MRCP (UK) 1997. Specialist Regist. (Paediat.) Qu. Mary's Hosp. Sidcup. Specialty: Paediat. Prev: SHO (Paediat.) Pembury Hosp. Tunbridge Wells.

SIGGERS, Stephen Henton Southbroom Surgery, 15 Estcourt Street, Devizes SN10 1LQ Tel: 01380 720909; Upper Coneygar, Northgate Gardens, Devizes SN10 1JY Tel: 01380 725924 — MRCS Eng. LRCP Lond. 1968 (Guy's)

SIGGINS, Paul Charles The Green Man Medical Centre, 1 Hanbury Drive, Leytonstone, London E11 1HR Tel: 020 8989 2936 Fax: 020 8530 8540 — MB BS Lond. 1981 (Lond. Hosp. Med. Coll.) MRCGP 1986.

SIGNY, Charles Michael Doctors Surgery, Great Melton Road, Hethersett, Norwich NR9 3AB Tel: 01603 810250 Fax: 01603 812402; Northfield Lodge, Barnham Broom Road, Wymondham NR18 0RN Tel: 01953 602196 — MB BS Lond. 1960 (St. Geo.) MRCS Eng. LRCP Lond. 1960; DObst RCOG 1963. Prev: Ho. Surg. (O & G) St. Mary Abbot's Hosp. Lond.; Ho. Surg. (Orthop.) & Ho. Phys. St. Geo. Hosp. Lond.

SIGNY, Mark Worthing Hospital, Cardiac Department, Lyndhurst Road, Worthing BN11 2DH Tel: 01903 205111 Ext: 5580 Fax: 01903 285011 — MB BS Lond. 1978 (Oxf. & St. Thomas's.); MA Oxf. 1979, BA (Physiol. Sc.) 1975; MRCP (UK) 1980; FRCP Lond. 1994. Cons. (Cardiol.) Worthing and Southlands Hosps.; Hon. Cons. Cardiol. St. Thos. Hosp. Lond.; Hon. Cons. Cardiol. Roy. Sussex Co. Hosp. Brighton. Specialty: Cardiol. Special Interest: Interventional Cardiol.; Ischaemic Heart Dis., Acute Coronary Syndromes. Socs: Brit. Cardiac Soc.; (Ex.-Pres.) Jun. Cardiac Club; Scientif. Fell. Zool. Soc. Prev: Sen. Regist. (Med. & Cardiol.) Medway & St. Thos. Hosp.; Regist. (Cardiac) St. Tho. Hosp. Lond.; SHO (Cardiac) Brompton Hosp. Lond.

SIGSTON, Paul Edmund St. Bartholomews Hospital, West Smithfield, London EC1A 7BE Tel: 020 7601 7518; 8 Priory Gardens, London SW13 0JU — MB ChB Ed. 1987; DA (UK) 1992; MRCP (UK) 1993; FRCA 1994. Sen. Regist. (Anaesth.) St. Bart. Hosp. Lond. Specialty: Anaesth. Prev: Regist. (Anaesth.) Gt. Ormond St. Hosp. & St. Bart. Hosp. Lond.; SHO (Med.) Chester; SHO (Anaesth.) Edin.

SIGSWORTH, Elisabeth Rome Crofton Elvington Medical Practice, Church Lane, Elvington, York YO41 4AD Tel: 01904 608224; Sycamore Cottage, Newton Road, Tollerton, York YO61 1QX — MB BS Lond. 1980 (Roy. Free Hosp. Sch. of Med.) DRCOG 1983; MRCGP 1987; DFFP 2001. GP Elvington Med. Pract. Specialty: Family Planning. Prev: GP Retainer Easingwold.

SIGURDSSON, Audun Svavar 11 Kelton Court, Carpenter Road, Edgbaston, Birmingham B15 2JX Tel: 07801 106542; 11 Kelton Court, Carpenter Road, Edgbaston, Birmingham B15 2JX Tel: 07801 106542 — Cand Med et Chir Reykjavik 1983 (Univ. of Iceland) FRCS 1991; FRCS (Gen) 1997. Specialty: Gen. Surg. Socs: Assn. Endoscopic Surgs.; BMA.

SIGURDSSON, Mr Helgi Helgason Hammersmith Hospital, Du Cane Road, London W12 0NN Tel: 020 8743 2030; Flat 7, 15 Girdlers Road, London W14 0PS Tel: 020 7602 8066 Fax: 020 7602 8066 — Cand Med et Chir Reykjavik 1988; FRCS Eng. 1992; FRCS Ed. 1992. Career Regist. (Surg.) Hammersmith Hosp. Lond. Specialty: Gen. Surg. Prev: Career Regist. (Surg.) Ashford Hosp. Middlx.

SIGURDSSON, R G The Park Surgery, 116 Kings Road, Herne Bay CT6 5RE — MD St Georges U 1990; MD St Georges U 1990.

SIGWART, Ulrich (retired) Royal Brompton National Heart & Lung Hospital, Sydney St, London SW3 6NP Tel: 020 7351 8615 Fax: 020 7351 8614 — State Exam Med Freiburg 1967; MD Freiburg 1967; MRCP (UK) 1992; FRCP Lond. 1993. Prof. Med. Univ. Dusseldorf; Hon. Sen. Lec. Nat. Heart & Lung Inst. Univ. Lond. Prev: Cons. Cardiol. Roy. Brompton Nat. Heart & Lung Hosp.

SIHOTA, Jagroop Singh Telfer Road, 190 Telfer Road, Coventry CV6 3DJ Tel: 024 7659 6060 Fax: 024 7660 1607; 31 Whitefield Close, Westwood Heath, Coventry CV4 8GY — MB ChB Birm. 1978. Prev: Trainee GP Coventry AHA VTS; Ho. Phys. St. Chad's Hosp. Birm.; Ho. Surg. Walsgrave Hosp. Coventry.

SIHRA, Bhupinder Singh Colchester General Hospital, Turner Road, Colchester CO4 5JL Tel: 01206 742158 Fax: 01206 742795 Email: bsihra@hotmail.com — BM Soton. 1984; MRCP (UK) 1989; FRCPCH 2004. Cons. (Gen. & Respirat.& Allergy Paediat.) Colchester Gen. Hosp.; Hon. Cons. (Paediatric Allergy) Guy's Hosp., Lond. Specialty: Paediat. Socs: MRCP; BSACI. Prev: Regist. (Paediat.) May Day Hosp. Croydon & St. Geo. Hosp. Tooting.; Specialist Regist. (Paediat.) King's Coll. Hosp. Lond.; Clin. Research Fell. (Allergy & Clin. Immunol.) Roy. Brompton Nat. Heart & Lung Inst. Lond.

SIHRA, Perminder Kaur Larkfield Resource Centre, Garngable Avenue, Greenock G66 3UG — MB ChB Glas. 1988. Staff Grade: General Adult Psychiatry. Specialty: Forens. Psychiat. Socs: Inceptor Roy. Coll. Psychiats. Prev: Staff Grade (Forens. Psychiat.) Rampton Hosp. Retford, Notts.; Rotat. Psychiat. Hartwood Shotts.; Psychiat. Bellsdyke Hosp. Larbert.

SIKA, Mr Mounir 1 St Ronan's Crescent, Woodford Green IG8 9DQ Tel: 020 8504 8767 — MB BCh Cairo 1959; DLO Ain Shams 1964; FRCS Eng. 1978. Assoc. Specialist (ENT) Centr. Middlx. Hosp. Lond. Prev: Regist. (ENT) P. of Wales Gen. Hosp. Lond.; Regist. (ENT) Centr. Middlx. Hosp. Lond.

SIKANDER, Nasreen Jarvis House Surgery, Jarvis Street, Oldham OL4 1DT Tel: 0161 2728 Fax: 0161 628 8876; 95 Fredrick Street, Oldham OL8 1RD — MB BS Punjab 1965; DA RCPSI 1977. Socs: Med. Defence Soc.

SIKDAR, Atindra Nath Teynham Medical Centre, The Surgery, 72 Station Road, Sittingbourne ME9 9SN Tel: 01795 521948 Fax: 01795 520785; Managing Director, Bengal Medical Research, 34/4 Patuatola Lane & 63/2B Surja Sen St, Calcutta 700009, India Tel: 00 91 33 2418210 Fax: 00 91 33 4643072 — MB BS Calcutta 1962 (R.G. Kar Med. Coll. Calcutta India) DGO Calcutta 1972; Cert. JCC Lond. 1974. Med. Adviser Bengal Med. Research Calcutta & Calcutta Med. Centre. Specialty: Biochem. Socs: Med. Protec. Soc. Prev: SHO (Neurosurg.) Morriston Hosp. Swansea; Sen. Health Off. (Anaesth.) Roy. Hosp. Wolverhampton; Ho. Off. (O & G) St. Davids Hosp. Bangor N. Wales.

SIKDAR, N Dartford West Health Centre, Tower Road, Dartford DA1 2HA Tel: 01322 291636/292001 — MB BS Gauhati 1961; MB BS Gauhati 1961.

SIKKA, Chander Kiran Tollgate Health Centre, 220 Tollgate Road, London E6 5JS — MB BS Lond. 1989. Trainee GP/SHO (O & G) Essex.

SIKKA, Charanpal Singh Oakswell Health Centre, Brunswick Park Road, Wednesbury WS10 9HP Tel: 0212 556 2114 Email: sikka@doctors.org.uk — MB BCh Wales 1993 (UWCM) MRCGP; DRCOG 1997; DCH 1997; DFFP 1997. GP Princip. Specialty: Gen. Pract.; Medico Legal.

SIKKA, Jangbir Singh Manor Hospital, Moat Road, Walsall WS2 9PS — MB BS Panjab 1962 (Med. Coll. Patiala) MS Panjab, India 1968. Assoc. Specialist (A & E) Manor Hosp. Walsall.

SIKKA, Mr Om Prakash (retired) 5 Scartho Road, Grimsby DN33 2AB Tel: 01472 878779 — MB BS Lucknow 1952 (King Geo. Med. Coll. Lucknow) DOMS Lucknow 1954; FRCS Eng. (Ophth.) 1963; FCOphth 1988. Prev: Cons. Ophth. Surg. Grimsby Gen. & Assoc. Hosps.

SIKKA, Swadesh 5 Scartho Road, Grimsby DN33 2AB Tel: 01472 78779 — MB BS Lucknow 1957; DCH Eng. 1961. Clin. Med. Off. Comm. Health Grimsby HA. Specialty: Community Child Health. Socs: Med. Protec. Soc. Prev: Clin. Asst. (Dermat. & Psychiat.) Grimsby HA; Regist. (Infec. Dis.) Leeds Rd. Hosp. Bradford.

SIKLOS, Paul William Leopold West Suffolk Hospital, Hardwick Lane, Bury St Edmunds IP33 2QZ Tel: 01284 713406 Fax: 01284 713406 Email: paul.siklos@wsh.nhs.uk; 58 Hardwick Lane, Bury St Edmunds IP33 2RB Tel: 01284 768043 Email: pasik@anglianet.co.uk — MB BS Lond. 1972 (Middlx.) BSc Lond. 1969; MB BS (Hons. Surg.) Lond. 1972; MRCP (UK) 1975; MA Camb. 1979; FRCP Lond. 1991. Cons. Phys. (GIM) W. Suff. Hosps. NHS Trust Bury St. Edmunds; Assoc. Clin. Dean, Univ. of Camb.; Director, Camb. Grad. Course in Med. Specialty: Gen. Med. Prev: Assoc. Clin. Dean Camb. Univ; Director of Camb. Grad. Course in Med.; Clin. Lect. Univ. Camb.

SIKORA, Professor Karol 79 Harley Street, London W1G 8PZ Tel: 020 7935 7700 Ext: 541 Fax: 020 7935 2719 Email: karolsikora@hotmail.com — MB BChir Camb. 1972 (Middlx.) PhD 1975; FRCR 1979; FRCP 1980. p/t Dean, Univ. of Buckingham Med. Sch.; Prof. of Cancer Med. Hammersmith Hosp. Lond.; Scientif. Director Med. Solutions Plc. Specialty: Oncol.; Radiother. Prev: Chairm. Cancer Futures Internat.; Strategic Adviser Cancer Servs. HCA Internat.; Chief WHO Cancer Progr. Geneva 1997-99.

SIKORSKI, Andrew David Alexander 41 Church Road, Tunbridge Wells TN1 1JU; Westley, Hackwood, Robertsbridge TN32 5ER — MB BS Lond. 1988 (Char. Cross & Westm. Hosp. Lond.) MRCGP 1997; MFHom 1999. Homoeop. Acupunc. Specialty: Homeop. Med.; Hypnother.; Acupunc. Socs: Brit. Holistic Med. Assn.; Fac. Homoeop. -S.E. Eng. Mem. Rep. Prev: GP/Regist. Glastonbury Som.; GP, Robt.s Bridge, E.Sussex; GP Locum, Marylebourne Health Centre, Lond.

SIKORSKI, James Jan Sydenham Green Group Practice, 26 Holmshaw Close, London SE26 4TH Tel: 020 8676 8836 Fax: 020 7771 4710 — MB BS Newc. 1978; MRCP (UK) 1980; MRCGP 1982; DRCOG 1983. Princip. GP Sydenham Green Health Centre Lond.

SIKORSKI, Mr Jerzy Marian 24 Woodfield Avenue, London W5 1PA — MB BS Lond. 1969; FRCS Eng. 1974.

SIL, Ajoy Kumar Horden Group Practice, The Surgery, Sunderland Road, Peterlee SR8 4QP Tel: 0191 586 4210 Fax: 0191 587 0700 — MB BS Calcutta 1966; DA Eng. 1979.

SIL, Bijoykumar (retired) 67 Ashness Gardens, Greenford UB6 0RW Tel: 020 8902 6533 — MB Calcutta 1947 (Calcutta Med. Coll.) DA Eng. 1956. Prev: Cons. Anaesth. Head Dept. Anaesth. & Hon. Lect. UTH Lusaka, Zambia.

SIL, Mr Samir Kumar Burbage Surgery, Tilton Road, Burbage, Hinckley LE10 2SE Tel: 01455 634879; Highcliffe, Shilton Road, Barwell, Leicester LE9 8 Tel: 01455 842313 — MB BS Calcutta 1960 (N.R.S. Med. Coll. Calcutta) FRCS Ed. 1967. Edr. & Sec. Jl. Dispensing Doctors Assn. Socs: BMA. Prev: Med. Asst. (A & E) Manor Hosp. Nuneaton; Regist. Roy. Infirm. Lancaster; Regist. W. Cumbld. Hosp. Whitehaven.

SILAS, Aaron Michael 7 St Mary's Avenue, Wanstead, London E11 2NR Tel: 020 8989 3766 — MB BS Calcutta 1959 (Calcutta Med. Coll.) DPhysMed. Eng. 1970; MRCP (UK) 1977; T(M) 1991. Specialty: Rehabil. Med.; Rheumatol. Socs: Brit. Soc. Rheum. Prev: Cons. Rheum. & Rehabil. OldCh. & Rushgreen Hosps. Romford; Sen. Regist. (Rheum. & Rehabil.) Univ. Coll. Hosp. Lond., Whittington Hosp. Lond. & Med. Rehabil. Centre Lond.; Regist. (Orthop) Brighton Hosp. Gp.

SILAS, Joseph Hyam Cardiovascular Department, Arrowe Park Hospital, Wirral CH49 5PE Tel: 0151 678 5111 Fax: 0151 604 7220 — MB ChB Sheff. 1970; MRCP (UK) 1972; MD Sheff. 1979; FRCP Lond. 1988. Cons. Phys. (Cardiol.) Arrowe Pk. Hosp. Wirral. Specialty: Cardiol. Prev: Cons. Phys. (Cardiol.) Clatterbridge Hosp. Bebington, Wirral.

SILBERGH, Alexander Edward, MBE (retired) Ashvale, Midmar St., Buckie AB56 1BJ Tel: 01542 831030 — MA Aberd. 1949, MB ChB 1956. Prev: SHO (O & G) Qu. Vict. Hosp. Morecambe.

SILBIGER, Catherine Anne 12 Kingston Way, Nailsea, Bristol BS48 4RA — MB ChB Ed. 1996.

SILBURN, Janice Nancy Lagmhor Surgery, Little Dunkeld, Dunkeld PH8 0AD Tel: 01350 727269 Fax: 01350 727772 — MB ChB Ed. 1968; DObst RCOG 1971; MRCGP 1975. GP Dunkeld, Perthsh. Prev: Cas. Off. Whittington Hosp. Lond.

SILBURN, Michael David William Lagmhor Surgery, Dunkeld PH8 0AD Tel: 0135 02 269; Torwood House, St. Mary's Road, Birnam, Dunkeld PH8 0BJ Tel: 0135 02 255 — MB Camb. 1971; BChir 1970; DObst RCOG 1972.

SILCOCK, John Gerard The Endoscopy Centre, South Cleveland Hospital, Middlesbrough TS4 3BW Tel: 01642 854865 — MB BS Newc. 1986; MRCP (UK) 1989. Cons. Gastroenterologist, S. Cleveland Hosp., MiddlesBoro. Specialty: Gastroenterol. Prev: Cons. Phys. (Gen. Med. & Gastroenterol.) Sunderland Dist. Gen. Hosp.; Sen. Regist. (Gen. Med. & Gastroenterol.) Roy. Vict. Infirm. Newc. & Middlesbrough Gen. Hosp.; Research Fell. (Virol.) Med. Sch. Newc. u. Tyne.

SILCOCKS, Paul Benet Stevens Trent Institute for Health Services Research, Room B39, School of Community Health Sciences, University of Nottingham Medical School, Nottingham NG7 2UH Tel: 0115 970 9765 Fax: 0115 970 9766 Email: paul.silcocks@nottingham.ac.uk; Wingates, Shatton Lane, Bamford, Hope Valley S33 0BG — BM BCh; MSc, FRCPath, FFPH, Cstat. Clin. Sen. Lect. Univ. Nottm.; Asst. Director Trent Cancer Registry. Specialty: Epidemiol. Socs: BMA; Assn. Clin. Pathol. Prev: Sen. Lect. (Pub. Health Med.) Univ. Sheff.; Research Fell. ICRF Cancer Epidemiol. Unit Radcliffe Infirm. Oxf.; Lect. (Epidemiol.) St. Geo. Med. Sch. Lond.

SILGRAM, Vasiliki Vicky Grace — MB ChB Stellenbosch 1992.

SILHI, Ranweer Baldevdutt Canterbury Street Surgery, 511 Canterbury Street, Gillingham ME7 5LH Tel: 01634 573020 Fax: 01634 281287 — MB BS Nagpur 1969 (Med. Coll. & Hosp. Nagpur, India) DTD Nagpur 1972. GP Hypnother. Gillingham; Mem. Kent LMC; Cancer Lead, Medway Dist. for Breast and Urol. Socs: Med. Defence Union. Prev: Mem. Rainham and Gillingham PCG.

SILK, David Baxter Department of Gastroenterology, Central Middlesex Hospital, Acton Lane, London NW10 Tel: 020 8453 2205; Division of Surgery, Anaesthetics and Intensive Care, Imperial College, London — MB BS Lond. 1968 (Guy's) MRCS Eng. LRCP Lond. 1968; MRCP (UK) 1970; MD Lond. 1974; FRCP Lond. 1983. p/t Cons. Phys. & Gastroenterol. & NutrutionHosp. Lond. Specialty: Gen. Med.; Gastroenterol. Special Interest: Functional

Gastrointestinal Disorders; Inflammatory Bowel Disease; Nutritional Support. Socs: Brit. Assn. Parenteral & Enteral Nutrit. (Past Pres); Brit. Soc. Gastroenterol.; Assn. Phys. Prev: Sen. Lect. & Cons. Phys. (Liver Unit) King's Coll. Hosp. Lond.; Vis. Assoc. Prof. Univ. Calif., USA.

SILK, Mr Frederick Fendley (retired) 9 Broom Road, Kinross KY13 8BU Tel: 01577 864150 — MB ChB Ed. 1948; FRCS Ed. 1959; MChOrth Liverp. 1960. Prev: Cons. Orthop. Surg. United Leeds Hosps.

SILK, Mr John 18 Rowben Close, London N20 8QR — MB ChB Mosul 1969; FRCSI 1984.

SILK, Nicholas Brownfields, Midhurst Road, Petersfield GU31 5AT Tel: 01730 263822 Fax: 01730 233750 — MRCS Eng. LRCP Lond. 1968 (Oxf. & St. Thos.) BSc, MA Oxf., BM BCh 1968; DObst RCOG 1970; DCH Eng. 1971.

SILKE, Carmel Mary Whiston Hospital, Warrington Road, Prescot L35 5DR — MB ChB Liverp. 1996.

SILKOFF, Benjamin Joseph (retired) 24 Grange Park Road, Leyton, London E10 Tel: 020 8539 2962 — MB BS Lond. 1948 (Guy's) MRCS Eng., LRCP Lond. 1948. Prev: GP Leyton, Lond.

SILL, Peter Richard Ashington Hospital, West View, Ashington NE63 0SA — MB ChB Liverp. 1978; MRCOG 1983; FRCOG 1996. Cons. O & G Northumbria Healthcare NHS Trust. Specialty: Obst. & Gyn. Prev: Lect. (O & G) Univ. Papua New Guinea.

SILLAH, Abdul Karim Warrington Hospital, Lovely Lane, Warrington WA5 1QG — MB BS Shanghai 2000. Surgic. Rotat. Mersey Deanery.

SILLARS, Joanne 103 Briarhill Road, Prestwick KA9 1HZ — MB ChB Aberd. 1995.

SILLENDER, Mark 31 Cottage Road, Leeds LS6 4DD — MB ChB Ed. 1993. SHO (O & G) York Dist. Hosp. Specialty: Obst. & Gyn.

SILLER, Catherine Sandra 15 Peterborough Road, Liverpool L15 9HN — MB ChB Liverp. 1996.

SILLERS, Mr Barrie Royston 111 Harley Street, London W1G 6AW Tel: 020 7258 8877 Fax: 020 7258 8876 — MB ChB Leeds 1964; BChD LDS Leeds 1960; FICOI 1992. Cons. Dent. Surg. Humana Hosp. Lond. Specialty: Oral & Maxillofacial Surg. Socs: BMA; BAOMS; ADI.

SILLETT, Rachel Eileen Wellesley (retired) 12 Town Mill, Marlborough SN8 1NS Tel: 01672 515044 — (Birm.) MB ChB (Hons.) Birm. 1941; DPH Lond. 1954; MD Birm. 1956; MFCM 1973. Prev: Med. Ref. DHSS.

SILLICK, Jennifer Mabel Walton Health Centre, Rodney Road, Walton-on-Thames KT12 3LB Tel: 01932 228999 Fax: 01932 225586 — MB BChir Camb. 1983 (Camb. & St. Thos.) MA Camb. 1984. Princip. in Gen. Pract. Specialty: Gen. Pract. Socs: Assoc. Mem. Roy. Soc. Med. Prev: SHO (A & E) St. Geo. Hosp. Lond.; SHO Rotat. (Med. & Paediat.) St. Peter's Hosp. Chertsey; SHO (O & G) St. Helier Hosp. Carshalton.

SILLIFANT, Kate Louise 72 Buckingham Way, Royston, Barnsley S71 4SL — MB ChB Leic. 1988.

SILLINCE, Claire Cheadle Royal Hospital, 100 Wilmslow Road, Cheadle SK8 3US — MB ChB Birm. 1975; MRCP (UK) 1977; FRCPsych 1996, M 1980. Cons. Psychiat. Cheadle Roy. Hosp. Specialty: Gen. Psychiat. Prev: Cons. Psychiat. Halton HA; Sen. Regist. (Psychiat.) NW RHA; Regist. (Psychiat.) Manch. HA (T).

SILLINCE, David Norman Holts Health Centre, Watery Lane, Newent GL18 1BA Tel: 01531 820689; Cothers, Moat Lane, Taynton, Gloucester GL19 3AR Tel: 01452 790504 — MB BS Lond. 1972 (Char. Cross) MRCGP 1989.

SILLITOE, Antony Thomas 2 Hawthorn Road, Roby, Huyton, Liverpool L36 9TT — MB ChB Liverp. 1996.

SILLITOE, Claire 1 Hopgarden Cottages, Filston Lane, Shoreham, Sevenoaks TN14 7SX — MB ChB Sheff. 1997.

SILLS, David John (retired) 58 The Gardens, Watford WD17 3DW Tel: 01923 243560 — MB BS Lond. 1955 (Med. Sch. Guy's Hosp.) MRCS Eng. LRCP Lond. 1955; DObst RCOG 1959; DCH Eng. 1960. Prev: GP Watford.

SILLS, David William Queensway Surgery, 75 Queensway, Southend-on-Sea SS1 2AB Tel: 01702 463333 Fax: 01702 603026 — MB BChir Camb. 1977.

SILLS, Jennifer Anne Birmingham Childrens Hospital, Birmingham B16 8ET; 58 The Gardens, Watford WD17 3DW — MB BS Lond. 1988; DCH RCP Lond. 1990; DRCOG 1992; MRCP (UK) 1996. Regist. (Paediat.) Birm. Childr. Hosp. Specialty: Paediat. Prev: SHO (Paediat.) Leicester Roy. Infirm.; SHO (O & G & Paediat.) Roy. Berks. Hosp.; SHO (Paediat. & A & E) Milton Keynes Gen. Hosp.

SILLS, John Anthony 23 Knowsley Park Lane, Prescot L34 3NA; Royal Liverpool Childrens Hospital, Alder Hey, Liverpool L12 2AP Tel: 0151 252 5541 Fax: 0151 252 5928 — (Camb. & St. Bart.) MB Camb. 1969, BChir 1968; DCH Eng. 1972; MRCP (UK) 1973; FRCP Lond. 1988; FRCPCH 1997. Cons. (Paediat.) Alder Hey Childr. Hosp. Liverp. & Whiston Hosp. Prescot. Specialty: Paediat.; Rheumatol. Prev: Sen. Regist. Roy. Hosp. Sick Childr. Edin.; Regist. Roy. Liverp. Childr. Hosp.

SILLS, Michael Alfred 27 Le Marchant Avenue, Lindley, Huddersfield HD3 3DF — MB Camb. 1974, BChir 1973; DCH RCPS Glas. 1975; DObst RCOG 1975; MRCP (UK) 1978. Cons. (Paediat.) Huddersfield Roy. Infirm. Specialty: Paediat. Prev: Regist. (Med.) Roy. Gwent Hosp. Newport; Regist. (Paediat.) Gen. Infirm. Leeds; Sen. Regist. (Paediat.) Yorks. RHA.

SILLS, Michael David Goodinge Health Centre, Goodinge Close, North Road, London N7 9EW Tel: 020 7530 4940 — MB BS Lond. 1984.

SILLS, Oliver Anthony (retired) 128 Cambridge Road, Barton, Cambridge CB3 7AR Tel: 01223 263612 — (St. Bart.) MRCS Eng. LRCP Lond. 1944; MRCGP 1954. Prev: Hosp. Pract. (Psychiat.) Addenbrooke's Hosp. Camb.

SILLS, Philip Radcliffe The Old Rectory Surgery, 18 Castle Street, Saffron Walden CB10 1BP Tel: 01799 522327 Fax: 01799 525436 — MB ChB St. And. 1972.

SILLS, Richard Oliver c/o 48 Carisbrooke Drive, Mapperley Park, Nottingham NG3 5DS — MB BS Lond. 1984.

SILLS, Susan Catherine Johan Hardwicke House Surgery, Hardwicke House, Stour Street, Sudbury CO10 2AY Tel: 01787 370011 Fax: 01787 376521 — MB ChB Ed. 1972; DPM Eng. 1978. Socs: W Suff. Postgrad. Assn.; Brit. Med. Assn.; Sudbury Med. Soc.

SILMAN, Harry 6 Sandmoor Mews, Leeds LS17 7SA Tel: 0113 680880 — MRCS Eng. LRCP Lond. 1935 (Leeds) BSc (Hons. Physiol.) Leeds 1932, MB ChB 1935.

SILMAN, Robert Edward 83 Highgate West Hill, London N6 6LU Tel: 020 7252 2541 Fax: 020 7394 7180 Email: r.e.silman@mds.qmw.ac.uk — MB BS Lond. 1971 (Middlx.) LèsL Paris 1964; BSc (1st cl. Hons.) Lond. 1968, MB BS 1971; PhD Lond. 1980. Sen. Lect. & Hon. Cons. Dept. O & G/Reproduc. Physiol. Lond. Hosp. Specialty: Obst. & Gyn. Prev: Wellcome Trust Sen. Lect. & Hon. Cons. Dept. Reproduc. Physiol. St. Bart. Hosp. Lond.; Ho. Phys. Med. Profess. Unit & Ho. Surg. (Neurosurg.) Middlx. Hosp. Lond.

SILOVE, Eric Dale Birmingham Childrens Hospital, Ladywood, Middleway, Birmingham B16 8ET Tel: 0121 333 9439 Fax: 0121 333 9441; 19 Hintlesham Avenue, Edgbaston, Birmingham B15 2PH Fax: 0121 243 9941 Email: e.silove@btinternet.com — MB BCh Witwatersrand 1958; FRCPCH; FRCP Ed. 1975, M 1963; FRCP Lond. 1979, M 1964; MD Witwatersrand 1976. Cons. Paediat. Cardiol. Birm. Childr. Hosp.; Clin. Sen. Lect. Univ. Birm. Specialty: Paediat. Cardiol. Socs: (Ex-Pres.) Brit. Paediat. Cardiac Assn.; (Counc.) Brit. Cardiac Soc.; (Pres.) Assn. Europ. Paediat. Cardiol. (Counc. Scientif. Sect.). Prev: Sen. Research Fell. & Hon. Cons. Hosp. Sick Childr. Gt. Ormond St.; Asst. Prof. Med. Mt. Sinai Hosp. Sch. of Med., NY, USA; Research Fell. (Cardiol.) Univ. Colorado Med. Center Denver, USA.

SILOVE, Yvonne Margaret Flat 5, 25 Avenue Road, London NW8 6BS — MB BChir Camb. 1994.

SILOVSKY, Karol Haven Health Surgery, Grange Farm Avenue, Felixstowe IP11 2FB Tel: 01394 670107 Fax: 01394 282872 — MB ChB Leic. 1988 (Leics.) T(GP) 1992.

SILSBY, Joseph Francis 138 South Street, Taunton TA1 3AG — MB ChB Bristol 1996.

SILVA, Daya The Bayswater Surgery, 46 Craven Road, London W2 3QA Tel: 020 7402 2073 Fax: 020 7723 8579; Flat 1, 4 and 5 Hyde Park Place, London W2 2HL — (Univ. Ceylon) MB BS Ceylon 1962. Socs: RSM.

SILVA, Edward Paul Clarence The Langdale Unit, Guild Park, Whittingham, Preston PR3 2JH — MB ChB Liverp. 1992.

SILVA, Francisco Briones Longmead Surgery, Norman Colyer Court, Hollymoor Lane, Epsom KT19 9JZ Tel: 01372 743432 Fax: 0372 817595; Greenhills, 102 Kingsmead Avenue, Worcester Park KT4 8UT Tel: 020 8395 3728 Fax: 020 8330 6244 Email: alwyn.s@virgin.net — MD Univ. East Philippines 1969.

SILVA, Kottoruge Gilbert Stoneleigh Avenue Surgery, 98A Stoneleigh Avenue, Longbenton, Newcastle upon Tyne NE12 8NT Tel: 0191 266 2271 — MB BS Ceylon 1970. GP Newc.

SILVA, Lakshman Upali Meads End, Forewood Lane, Crowhurst, Battle TN33 9AB Tel: 0142 483388 — MB BS Ceylon 1962; FFA RCS Eng. 1966. Specialty: Anaesth.

SILVA, Liyanage Francis Adolphus Fieldhead Hospital, Ouchthorpe Lane, Wakefield WF1 3SP Tel: 01924 375217 — MB BS Ceylon 1961 (Colombo) DPH Liverp. 1972; DPM Eng. 1978; MRCPsych 1982. Cons. Psychiat. Fieldhead Hosp. Wakefield. Specialty: Gen. Psychiat. Prev: Sen. Regist. Lea Castle Hosp. Kidderminster; SHO (Psychiat.) Hosp. St. Cross Rugby; Regional Med. Off. Leprosy Control S. Ceylon.

SILVA, Mark Timothy Gloucestershire Royal Hospital NHS Trust, Great Western Road, Gloucester GL1 3NN Tel: 01452 394410 Fax: 01452 394499 — MB BCh Wales 1988; PhD; BSc Wales 1985; MRCP (UK) 1991. Cons. Neurologist, Golucestershire Hosps. NHS Trust; Cons. Neurologist, Gloucestershire Roy. Hosp.; Cons. Neurologist, Cheltenham Gen. Hosp. Specialty: Neurol. Special Interest: Movement Disorders. Socs: Roy. Soc. Med.; Assn. of Brit. neurologists; Roy. Coll. of Physicians. Prev: Research Regist. (Neurol.) Inst. Neurol. Lond.; Regist. (Neurol.) St. Thos. Hosp. Lond.; SHO Rotat. (Med.) Bristol & Weston HA.

SILVA, Obadage Sarath Gamini 145 Canterbury Road, Harrow HA1 4PA — MB BS Sri Lanka 1974; MRCS Eng. LRCP Lond. 1979; FFA RCS Eng. 1980. Specialty: Anaesth.

SILVA, Punsiri Sanjeev 43d Anerley Park, London SE20 8NQ — MB BS Lond. 1997.

SILVA, Therese Savitri Swarnamalie — MB BS Colombo 1979; DA (UK) 1982; FFA RCSI 1986.

SILVER, Mr Alan Jonathan Shieldfield Health Centre, Stoddart Street, Shieldfield, Newcastle upon Tyne NE2 1AL Tel: 0191 232 4872; 98 The Wills Building, Coast Rd, Newcastle upon Tyne NE7 7RG — MB BS Newc. 1975; FRCS Eng. 1979; DRCOG 1983; MRCGP 1983; DFFP 1998. Clin. Asst. (Endoscopy) Freeman Rd. Hosp. Newc.; Vasectomy Surg. Marie Stopes Organisation. Prev: GP Trainee N.ld. VTS; Regist. (Gen. Surg.) Cheltenham Gen. Hosp.; Demonstr. (Anat.) Bristol Med. Sch.

SILVER, Christopher Patrick (retired) 25 Primrose Hill Road, London NW3 3DG — BM BCh Oxf. 1942; DM Oxf. 1954, MA, BM BCh 1942; FRCP Lond. 1972, M 1948. Prev: Cons. Geriat. Lond. Hosp. & Tower Hamlets HA.

SILVER, David Anthony Trevor Colestocks House, Colestocks EX14 3JR Email: david.silver@rdehc-tr.swest.nhs.uk — MB BS Lond. 1985 (St Barts. Hosp. Med. Coll.) BSc Lond. 1983; MRCP (UK) 1989; FRCR 1993. Cons. Musculoskeletal Radiol. Roy. Devon & Exeter Hosp.; Hon. Sen. Lect. Univ. Bristol. Specialty: Radiol. Socs: Brit. Med. Ultrasound Soc.; RCR; Brit. Soc. of Skeletal Radiol. Prev: Fell. (Radiol.) Princess Alexandra Hosp. Brisbane, Austral.; Regist. (Med.) Soton. Gen. Hosp.; Ho. Surg. St. Bart. Hosp. Lond.

SILVER, Deborah Miriam Staines Health Centre, Knowle Green, Staines TW18 1XD — MB ChB Dundee 1986; MRCP (UK) 1992. Prev: Regist. (Paediat.) Addenbrooke's Hosp. Camb.

SILVER, Gary Alexander Green Lane Cottage, Green Lane, Stanmore HA7 3AB — MB BS Lond. 1995.

SILVER, Hyman (retired) Shearwater, Smithy Lane, Down Holland, Ormskirk L39 7JS Tel: 01704 840106 Fax: As above — MB ChB Liverp. 1951; MRCS Eng. LRCP Lond. 1950. Prev: Hosp. Pract. (Paediat.) Fazakerley & Walton Hosps. Liverp.

SILVER, Jack 52 Upper Montagu Street, London W1H 1SJ Tel: 020 722249905 Fax: 020 7224 9907 — MB BCh Witwatersrand 1957; DA (UK) 1961; FFA RCS Eng. 1967. Specialty: Anaesth. Prev: Cons. Anaesth. Greenwich Healthcare Trust Lond.; Sen. Regist. Guy's & Lewisham Hosp. Lond.

SILVER, John Russell The Chiltern Hospital, Great Missenden HP16 0EN Tel: 01494 890250; 8 High Street, Wendover, Aylesbury HP22 6EA Tel: 01296 623013 Fax: 01296 623020 — (Middlx.) MB BS Lond. 1954; FRCP Ed. 1978, M 1962; FRCP Lond. 1980. Emerit. Cons. Spinal Injuries Centre Stoke Mandeville Hosp. Aylesbury. Specialty: Orthop. Socs: Fell. Inst. Sports Med.; Cervical Spine Soc.; Brit. Assn. Neurol. Prev: Cons. Spinal Injuries Stoke Mandeville Hosp.; Cons. i/c Liverp. Regional Paraplegia Centre (Lect. Surg.); Regist. (Neurol.) Middlx. Hosp. Lond.

SILVER, Lisa Rebecca McWhirter, Barton and Silver, The Surgery, Wanbourne Lane, Henley-on-Thames RG9 5AJ Tel: 01491 641204 Fax: 01491 641162; 38 St Andrews Road, Henley-on-Thames RG9 1JB Tel: 01491 571072 Email: drlisasilver@hotmail.com — MB ChB Manch. 1988; BSc (Hons.) Aberd. 1983; Dip. MedSci. St. And. 1985. GP Oxon.

SILVER, Michael Ellman Fore Street Surgery, 234 Fore Street, Edmonton, London N18 2LY Tel: 020 8803 6705 Fax: 020 8884 2065 — MB BS Lond. 1961 (St. Geo.) MRCS Eng. LRCP Lond. 1961; DObst RCOG 1963; AFOM 1978. Specialty: Occupat. Health. Prev: Employm. Med. Adviser EMAS; Ho. Surg. & Ho. Phys. St. Geo. Hosp. Lond.; Resid. Obst. Off. Cheltenham Matern. Hosp.

SILVER, Nicholas Charles Walton Centre for Neurology & Neurosurgery, Lower Lane, Fazakerley, Liverpool L9 7LJ Tel: 0151 529 5420 Email: n.silver@ion.ucl.ac.uk/ Nicholas.Silver@thewaltoncentre.nhs.uk — MB BS Lond. 1989 (St Geo.) MRCP (UK) 1992; PhD Lond. 2001. Cons. Neurol. Walton Centre Neurol. & Neurosurg. Liverp.; Hon. Clin. Lect., Univ. of Liverp. Specialty: Neurol. Special Interest: Headache; Magnetic Resonance Imaging; Multiple Sclerosis. Socs: Assn. Brit. Neurol.; Brit. Assn. Neuro; Brit. Neuropsychiat. Assn. Prev: Specialist Regist. Nat. Hosp. Neurol. & Neurosurg. Lond.; Research Fell. (Neurol.) Inst. Neurol. Lond.; Regist. Rotat. (Med.) Char. Cross. Lond.

SILVER, Simon Nathan Waldron House, Hoovers Lane, Lea, Ross-on-Wye HR9 5TX — MB BS Newc. 1978; MRCGP 1982. Course Organiser Gloucester & Cheltenham VTS.

SILVER, Trevor 4 Deveraux Close, Beckenham BR3 3GW Tel: 020 8639 0410 Fax: 020 8639 0410 — MB BS Durh. 1949; FRCGP 1973, M 1960; DA Eng. 1962. Hon. Sen. Lect. (Gen. Pract.) St. Geo. Hosp. Lond. Socs: Hon. Fell. BMA; Fell. Roy. Soc. Med.; Fell. BMA. Prev: Regional Adviser Gen. Pract. SW Thames RHA; Regist. (Anaesth.) & SHO (O & G) Sunderland Hosp. Gp.

SILVERDALE, Montague Adam 15 Larchfield Avenue, Newton Mearns, Glasgow G77 5PW — MB ChB Glas. 1995.

SILVERMAN, Andrew James Niden Manor Estate, Moreton Pinkney, Daventry NN11 3SJ — MB ChB Dundee 1991; BMSc (Hons.) Dund 1988.

SILVERMAN, Ann Marisa 34 Fawnbrake Avenue, Herne Hill, London SE24 0BY Tel: 020 7274 6222 — BM BCh Oxf. 1972; BA Oxf. 1969, BM BCh 1972; MRCPsych 1977. Cons. Psychiat. King's Coll. Hosp. Lond. & Cane Hill Hosp. Coulsdon. Specialty: Gen. Psychiat. Prev: Sen. Regist. (Psychiat.) Bethlem Roy. & Maudsley Hosp.; SHO Northwick Pk. Hosp. Harrow; Regist (Psychiat.) Bethlem Roy. & Maudsley Hosps. Lond.

SILVERMAN, Barbara Helen Cloptons, 23 Green Lane, Linton, Cambridge CB1 6JZ Tel: 01223 892107 — BM BCh Oxf. 1977; BA (Hons.) Oxf. 1974; DRCOG 1980; MRCGP 1980. Assoc. Spec. (Rheum.) Addenbrookes Hosp. Cambs. Specialty: Rehabil. Med.; Rheumatol. Prev: Trainee GP Newc. VTS; Ho. Phys. Radcliffe Infirm. Oxf.

SILVERMAN, Jonathan David Linton Health Centre, Coles Lane, Linton, Cambridge CB1 6JS Tel: 01223 891456 Fax: 01223 890033; Cloptons, 23 Green Lane, Linton, Cambridge CB1 6JZ Tel: 01223 892107 Email: js355@medschl.cam.ac.uk — BM BCh Oxf. 1977; BA (Hons.) Oxf. 1974; DRCOG 1979; FRCGP 1995, M 1980. Assoc. Clin. Dean Sch. Clin. Med. Camb. Uni. Prev: Trainee GP Newc. VTS; Ho. Phys. Radcliffe Infirm. Oxf.; Course Organizer Camb. VTS.

SILVERMAN, Leon Stanley 393 Green Street, Upton Park, London E13 9AU Tel: 020 8552 8784 — MB BS Lond. 1971 (Middlx. Hospital, London) Association of Medical Advisers in Pharmaceutical Industry Cert. 1974; Family Plan Association Cert 1975; Cert. Family Plann. RCOG & RCGP 1977; Cert. Prescribed Equiv. Exp. JCPTGP 1981. GP Lond. Specialty: Gen. Pract. Socs: Fell. Roy. Soc. Med.; BMA. Prev: Clin. Research Med. Adviser Schering Chem.s Ltd., (Pharmaceut.; Div.) Burgess Hill; SHO (Venereol.) & Ho. Phys. (Dermat. & Gen. Med.) & Ho. Surg.

SILVERMAN, Maurice (retired) Apartment 5, The Hollows, 9 Ringley Road, Whitefield, Manchester M45 7LD Tel: 0161 766 3576 — (Leeds) MB ChB Leeds 1943; DPM Eng. 1947; MD Leeds 1952;

FRCPsych 1971. Prev: Mem. Standing Ment. Health Advis. Comm. Centr. Health Servs. Counc.
SILVERMAN, Professor Michael Department of Child Health, University of Leicester, Clinical Sciences Building, Leicester Royal Infirmary, Leicester LE2 7LX Tel: 0116 252 3262 Fax: 0116 252 3282 Email: ms70@le.ac.uk — MD Camb. 1973 (Camb. & St. Geo.) MB 1968, BChir 1967; MRCP (UK) 1970; DCH Eng. 1972. Prof. Child Health Univ. Leicester. Specialty: Paediat. Socs: Brit. Paediat. Assn. & Brit. Thoracic Soc. Prev: Prof. Paediat. Respirat. Med. Roy. Postgrad. Med. Sch. Lond.; Lect. (Child Health) Univ. Bristol; Lect. (Paediat.) Ahmadu Bello Univ. Zaria, Nigeria.
SILVERMAN, Sharon Ruth 17 Links Road, Wilmslow SK9 6HQ — BM BS Nottm. 1993.
SILVERMAN, Mr Stanley Harry City Hospital, Sandwell & West Birmingham Hospitals NHS Trust, Dudley Road, Birmingham B18 7QH Tel: 0121 507 4283 Fax: 0121 507 4816; 92 Moorcroft Road, Moseley, Birmingham B13 8LU Tel: 0121 449 1831 Email: stanleysilverman@blueyonder.co.uk — MB ChB Birm. 1977 (Univ. Birm. Med. Sch.) FRCS Ed. 1981; FRCS Eng. 1982; MD Birm. 1988. Cons. Surg. General/Vascular Surgery/SWB4 NHS Trust, Birm.; Divisional Director of Surgery. Specialty: Gen. Surg. Socs: BMA; VSSGBI; ESVS. Prev: Cons. Surg. Wordsley Hosp. Stourbridge; Lect. (Surg.) Univ. Birm.
SILVERSTON, Neville Arnold, MBE (retired) Chapters, 6b Babraham Road, Cambridge CB2 2RA Tel: 01223 249911 Fax: 01223 246862 Email: nevillesilverston@btopenworld.com — MB ChB Manch. 1954 (Manchester University) MRCS Eng. LRCP Lond. 1954; FRCGP 1979, M 1965. Prev: Sen. Med. Resid. Jewish Hosp. Med. Center, Cincinnati, USA.
SILVERSTON, Paul Philip Oakfield Surgery, Vicarage Road, Newmarket CB8 8JF Tel: 01638 662018 Fax: 01638 660294; The Manor House, Little Wilbraham, Cambridge CB1 53Y Tel: 01223 811310 Fax: 01223 811310 — MB ChB Bristol 1985; BA (Hons.) 1977, MB ChB 1985. Co-ordinator Camb. Pre Hosp. Trauma Life Support Course & Mem. Internat. Fac. Socs: Fac. Pre Hosp. Care. Prev: Trainee GP Addenbrooke's Hosp. VTS.
SILVERSTONE, Mr Anthony Charles The Portland Hospital, 209 Gt Portland St., London W1W 5AH Tel: 020 7383 7884; 77 King Henry's Road, London NW3 3QU — MB ChB Birm. 1969; FRCS Eng. 1976; FRCS Ed. 1976; FRCOG 1992, M 1978. Cons. Univ. Coll. Lond. Hosps. Specialty: Obst. & Gyn. Prev: Sen. Regist. (O & G) John Radcliffe Hosp. Oxf.; Resid. Surg. Off. Chelsea Hosp. Wom. & Qu. Charlotte's Matern. Hosp. Lond.
SILVERSTONE, Elizabeth Jane Wrexham Maelor Hospital, North East Wales NHS Trust, Wrexham LL13 7TD Tel: 01978 291100 Fax: 01978 725440 — MB BCh Wales 1977; MRCP (UK) 1981; FRCR 1984. Cons. Wrexham Maelor Hosp. Clwyd. Specialty: Radiol.
SILVERT, Barry David Stonehill Medical Centre, Piggott St., Farnworth, Bolton BL4 9QZ Tel: 01204 573445 Fax: 01204 791633 — MB ChB Manch. 1966. Prev: Ho. Surg. Manch. Vict. Memor. Jewish Hosp.; Ho. Phys. Crumpsall Hosp. Manch.
SILVERTON, Kathryn Leigh 20 Bramley Avenue, Coulsdon CR5 2DP — BM Soton. 1998.
SILVERTON, Nicholas Paul Cardiac Department, Airedale General Hospital, Steeton, Keighley BD20 6TD Tel: 01535 292017 Fax: 01535 292019; The Yorkshire Clinic, Bradford Road, Bingley BD16 1TW Tel: 01274 560311 Fax: 01274 551247 — MB BS Lond. 1974 (Middlx.) MRCP (UK) 1977; MD Lond. 1985; FRCP Lond. 1992. Cons. Cardiol. Airedale HA; Hon. Cons. Cardiol. N. Gen. Hosp. Sheff. & Leeds Gen. Infirm. Specialty: Cardiol. Prev: Lect. (Cardiovasc. Studies) & Hon. Sen. Regist. (Cardiol.) Univ. Leeds; Regist. (Cardiol.) Leeds Gen. Infirm.
SILVESTER, Katharine Mary 33 Dorsington Close, Hatton Park, Warwick CV35 7TH — MB BS Lond. 1986; BSc (Hons.) Lond. 1983, MB BS 1986; FCOphth 1992, M 1991. Specialty: Ophth. Prev: SHO (Ophth.) Cheltenham Dist. Gen. Hosp.; SHO (Ophth.) Univ. Hosp. Wales Cardiff.
SILVESTER, Mr Keith Charles Morriston Hospital, Morriston, Swansea SA6 6NL Tel: 01792 703670 Fax: 01792 703068 Email: kcsilv@globalnet.co.uk; Brynderw, 117 Rhydypandy Road, Rhydypandy, Morriston, Swansea SA6 6PB Tel: 01792 844044 — MB BS Lond. 1985; BDS Lond. 1976; FDS RCS Eng. 1983; FRCS Ed. 1989. Cons. Oral & Maxillofacial Surg. Morriston Hosp. Swansea; Vis. Cons., Glangwili Hosp., Camarthen Bronglais Hosp., Aberystwyth. Specialty: Oral & Maxillofacial Surg. Prev: Sen. Regist. (Oral & Maxillofacial Surg.) Roy. Lond. Hosp.; Regist. (Oral & Maxillofacial Surg.) Eastman Dent. Hosp. & Univ. Coll. Hosp. Lond.; SHO Qu. Vict. Hosp. E. Grinstead.
SILVESTER, Neil William Hugh West End Cottage, West End Road, Norton, Doncaster DN6 9EF — MB ChB Leeds 1979; MRCPsych 1983. Cons. (Psychiat.) Doncaster Roy. Infirm. Specialty: Gen. Psychiat.
SILVESTER, Richard Donald Beaumont Street Surgery, 19 Beaumont Street, Oxford OX1 2NA Tel: 01865 240501 Fax: 01865 240503 — MB BChir Camb. 1991 (Lond. Hosp. Med. Coll.) MA Camb. 1990; DRCOG 1995; MRCGP 1996.
SILVESTRI, Miss Giuliana Royal Victoria Hospital, Eye and Ear Clinic, Grosvenor Road, Belfast BT12 6BA Fax: 028 9033 0744 Email: g.silvestri@qub.ac.uk — MD Belf. 1994; MB BCh BAO 1983; FRCP (1997), MRCP (UK) 1987; ECFMG 1987; FRCS Ed. 1989; FRCOphth 1990. Head of Depart. Roy. Vict. Hosp. Belf. Specialty: Ophth. Special Interest: Med. Retina; Ophth. Genetics. Socs: ARVO; BOSU (Com.); Oxf. Congr. (Exec. Com.). Prev: Sen. Lect. & Cons. Ophth. Surg. Roy. Vict. Hosp. Belf.
SILVEY, Hugh Stuart Sea Mills Surgery, 2 Riverleaze, Sea Mills, Bristol BS9 2HL Tel: 0117 968 1182 Fax: 0117 962 6408 — MB ChB Bristol 1972.
SILVEY, Stuart John (retired) Denewood, 16 Westbury Lane, Bristol BS9 2PE Tel: 0117 968 1577 — MB ChB Bristol 1939; MRCGP 1952. Prev: Pres. Bristol M-C Soc.
SIM, Alan James The Surgery, 142 Manse Road, Ardersier, Inverness IV2 7SR Tel: 01667 62240; 34 Blackthorn Road, Culloden, Inverness IV2 7LA — MB ChB Aberd. 1988. Trainee GP Inverness. Prev: SHO (Psychiat.) Craig Dunain Hosp. Inverness.
SIM, Mr Andrew John Wyness Western Isles Hospital, Macauley Road, Stornoway — MB BS Lond. 1971; FRCS Glas. 1975; MS Lond. 1988. Specialty: Gen. Surg. Socs: Nutrit. Soc.; Surgic. Research Soc. Prev: Prof. Surg. UAE Univ., Al Ain; Asst. Director Acad. Surg. Unit St Mary's Hosp. Med. Sch. Lond.; Sen. Regist. Roy. Infirm. Glas.
SIM, Angus James Wyness 14D South Mount Street, Aberdeen AB25 4TB — MB ChB Aberd. 1996.
SIM, Charles Gordon (retired) 22 Coniscliffe Road, Hartlepool TS26 0BT Tel: 01429 274785 — (Univ. Ed.) MB ChB Ed. 1946.
SIM, Colville Graeme (retired) Ashcroft, Haltwhistle NE49 0DA Tel: 01434 20079 — MB BS Durh. 1943; MA 1934, MB BS Durh. 1943.
SIM, David Anthony James Daisy Hill Hospital, Hospital Road, Newry BT35 8DR Tel: 028 303 5000 Fax: 028 3026 8285; Cranmore, 143 Dublin Road, Loughbrickland, Banbridge BT32 3NT Tel: 028 4062 2822 — MB BCh BAO Belf. 1980 (Qu. Univ. Belf.) MRCOG 1986; MD Belf. 1991; FRCOG 1999. Cons. O & G Daisy Hill Hosp. Newry, Co. Down. Specialty: Obst. & Gyn.
SIM, David Morrice Longshut Lane West Surgery, 24 Longshut Lane West, Stockport SK2 6SF Tel: 0161 480 2373 Fax: 0161 480 2660; Lothlorian House, Carrwood Road, Bramhall, Stockport SK7 3LR Tel: 0161 486 1213 — MB ChB Aberd. 1963; MRCGP 1972. Med. Off. Brit. Boxing Bd. of Control. Specialty: Medico Legal; Alcohol & Substance Misuse. Prev: Ho. Surg. Roy. Aberd. Hosp. Sick Childr.; Ho. Phys. Newsham Gen. Hosp. Liverp.; SHO Obst. Preston Roy. Infirm.
SIM, David Robert (retired) 13/6 South Oswald Road, Edinburgh EH9 2HQ Tel: 0131 662 0447 — (University of Edinburgh) MB ChB Ed. 1951.
SIM, Mr David William St John's Hospital, Howden Road West, Livingston EH54 6PP Tel: 01506 419666 — MB ChB Glas. 1982; MSc Glas. 1985; DLO RCS Eng. 1987; FRCS Ed. 1987; FRCS (Orl.) 1991. Cons. Otolaryngol. Head & Neck Surg. Edin. Specialty: Otorhinolaryngol. Special Interest: Skullbase Surgery. Prev: Sen. Regist. (Otolaryngol.) Edin.; Lect. (Otolaryngol.) Univ. Edin.
SIM, Douglas William (retired) Tanglewood, Broad Campden Road, Chipping Campden GL55 6DJ Tel: 01386 841509 — (Manch.) MB ChB Manch. 1951. Prev: Gen. Practitioner, Merton.
SIM, Ewen — MB ChB Ed. 1990 (Edin.) BSc (Hons.) Anat. Ed. 1987; Dip Health Mgt Keele 2002. p/t GP - Birkenhead; GP - Arrowe Pk. Hosp. - Primary Care Assessm. Unit. Specialty: Gen. Pract.; Histopath.; Civil Serv. Socs: Fell. (Ex-Pres.) Roy. Med. Soc. Edin.; Postgrad. Med. Educat. and Train. Bd.; BMA GPC.

SIM, Fiona Marion Barnet Healthcare NHS Trust, Colindale Hospital, Colindale Avenue, London NW9 5HG Tel: 020 8200 1555 Fax: 020 8200 9499; 111 Newberries Avenue, Radlett WD7 7EN Tel: 01923 852524 — (Lond.) MSc (Community Med.) Lond. 1982, BSc (Hons.) 1975, MB BS 1978; MFCM RCP (UK) 1984; FFPHM RCP (UK) 1992. Med. Dir. Barnet Healthcare NHS Trust. Specialty: Pub. Health Med. Prev: Dir. Pub. Health Barnet HA.

SIM, Gordon Duns Medical Practice, The Knoll, Station Road, Duns TD11 3EL Tel: 01361 883322 Fax: 01361 882186; Dingleside, Clouds, Duns TD11 3BB Tel: 01361 882578 — MB ChB Aberd. 1988. SHO (Geriat.) Kingston Gen. Hosp. Hull. Prev: SHO (Paediat.) Hull Roy. Infirm.

SIM, Hok Gwan 59 Redlane, Claygate, Esher KT10 0ES — MD Cologne 1967; State Exam. Med. Cologne 1965; LMSSA Lond. 1971; MRCOG 1978, DObst 1973. Prev: Sen. Regist. (O & G) Caritas Med. Centre Kowloon, Hong Kong; Regist. (O & G) Profess. Unit Welsh Nat. Sch. Med. Cardiff & Vale of Leven Dist. Gen. Hosp. Alexandria.

SIM, Ian Stuart George (retired) 18 Ashfield Road, Compton Road W., Wolverhampton WV3 9DP Tel: 01902 755149 — MB BS Lond. 1955 (Univ. Coll. Hosp.) MRCS Eng. LRCP Lond. 1954. Prev: GP Wolverhampton.

SIM, Ivor John Ardblair Medical Practice, Ann Street, Blairgowrie PH10 6EF Tel: 01250 872033 Fax: 01250 874517 — MB ChB Dundee 1977; MRCGP 1983.

SIM, John Wilson The Health Centre, High St., Snaith, Goole DN14 9HJ Tel: 01405 860217 Fax: 01405 862580; 6 Manor Close, Camblesforth, Selby YO8 8HP Tel: 01757 618395 — MB ChB Aberd. 1964. Socs: BMA. Prev: Ho. Off. Aberd. Roy. Infirm. & Bridge of Earn Hosp. & Ayrsh. Centr. Matern. Hosp.

SIM, Juliet Claire 26B Hunterhill Road, Paisley PA2 6ST — MB ChB Glas. 1994.

SIM, Justein Sarah Noble Royal infirmary of Edinburgh, Laviston place, Edinburgh EH3 9YN; 368 Perth Road, Dundee DD2 1EN — MB ChB Dundee 1992; BSc (Hons.) Dund 1990; MRCP (UK) 1995. SpR Cardiol. Lothian Univ. Hosps. NHS trust. Specialty: Cardiol.; Gen. Med. Prev: Regist. (Cardiol.) Dundee Trust Hosps.; Research Fell. Dept. of Clin. Pharmocology.

SIM, Kuan Tzen 23 Dogfield Street, Cardiff CF24 4QJ — MB BCh Wales 1997.

SIM, Man Fai Victor Llandough Hospital, Penlan Road, Llandough, Penarth CF64 2XX Tel: 029 2071 5653 Email: victor.sim@cardiffandvale.wales.nhs.uk — MB BCh Wales 1985; MRCP (UK) 1990; DRCOG 1991; DGM RCP Lond. 1994; MRCGP 1996. Cons. Phys. Gen. Med. and Care of Elderly, Llandough Hosp. Specialty: Gen. Med.; Care of the Elderly. Special Interest: Chronic Heart Failure.

SIM, Natalie Alexis 175 Machanill, Larkhall — MB ChB Aberd. 1996.

SIM, Pamela Georgina Esplanade Surgery, 19 Esplanade, Ryde PO33 2EH Tel: 01983 611444 Fax: 01983 811548; Fairlight, Playstreet Lane, Ryde PO33 3LJ Tel: 01983 566040 — MB ChB Birm. 1966; DObst RCOG 1968. GP.

SIM, Richard James Fairlight, Playstreet Lane, Ryde PO33 3LJ — MB ChB Birm. 1994; ChB Birm. 1994; MB ChB Birmingham 1994. SHO (Ent.) Radcliffe Infirm. Oxf. Specialty: Otolaryngol.

SIM, Sheila Margaret Langton Field, Hardens Road, Duns TD11 3NS Tel: 01361 882578 — MB ChB Glas. 1988. Prev: SHO (O & G) Hull Matern. Hosp.

SIM, Yen Tai Basement Flat, 55A Union St., Greenock PA16 8DR — MB ChB Dundee 1994.

SIMANOWITZ, Milton David (retired) Evergreen, 7 The Avenue, Radlett WD7 7DG Tel: 0192 765007 — MD Cape Town 1971; MB ChB 1958; FRCOG 1979, M 1965. Prev: Lect. Westm. Med. Sch. Lond.

SIMCOCK, Antony David 7 Passage Hill, Mylor, Falmouth TR11 5SN Tel: 01326 374026 Fax: 01326 374026 — MB BS Lond. 1967 (Lond. Hosp.) MRCS Eng. LRCP Lond. 1967; FFA RCS Eng. 1971. Hon. Cons. Anaesth. Roy. Cornw. Hosps. Truro. Specialty: Anaesth. Prev: Lect. & Demonst. BASICS; Sen. Regist. (Anaesth.) United Bristol Hosps.; Regist. & SHO (Anaesth.) Lond. Hosp.

SIMCOCK, David Ewart 7 Passage Hill, Mylor Bridge, Falmouth TR11 5SN Tel: 01326 374026 — MB BS Lond. 1997 (Guy's & St. Thomas's Hosps.) MRCP Lond. 2000. Specialist Reg. Thoracic Medicine, Lond. Specialty: Gen. Med.; Anaesth. Prev: Ho. Off. (Med.) Guy's Hosp. Lond.; Ho. Off. (Surg.) Eastbourne Dist. Gen. Hosp.; SHO (Med.) Frimley Pk. Hosp.

SIMCOCK, Lolita Anne 29 Park Street, Brighton BN2 2BS Tel: 01273 699767 Email: rich.lol@virgin.net — MB BS Lond. 1994 (UMDS) BSc Lond. 1992; DRCOG 1998; MRCGP Lond. 2000. GP Retainer. Specialty: Gen. Pract. Prev: Gen. Pract.; SHO (Paediat.); SHO (O & G).

SIMCOCK, Paul David — MB ChB Birm. 1997; MRCP 2000.

SIMCOCK, Mr Peter Reginald 4 Manston Terrace, Exeter EX2 4NP Tel: 01392 434141 Fax: 01392 435301 Email: p.r.s@btconnect.com; Whitley Cottage, 8 Northview Road, Budleigh Salterton EX9 6BZ Email: psimcock@hotmail.com — MB ChB Leic. 1983 (Leicester) DO RCS Eng. 1987; FRCS Eng. 1988; MRCP (UK) 1990; FRCOphth 1990. Cons. Ophth. Surg. Roy. Devon & Exeter Hosp. Specialty: Ophth. Prev: Fell. (Vitreoretinal) Manch. Roy. Eye Hosp.; Sen. Regist. Char. Cross Hosp. & Moorfields Eye Hosp. Lond.; Regist. (Ophth.) Manch. Roy. Eye Hosp.

SIMCOCK, Richard Alexander John Radiotherapy Department, St. Thomas' Hospital, London SE1 7EU — MB BS Lond. 1993 (UMDS) MRCP Ireland 1997; FRCR Lond. 2001. Specialist Regist. (Clin. Oncol.) Guys & St. Thomas' NHS Trust Lond. Specialty: Oncol.

SIME, David Patterson (retired) Summerlea, Manse Lane, Portree IV51 9QR Tel: 01478 613612 Fax: 01478 612421 Email: summerlea@lineone.net — MB ChB Glas. 1965; DObst RCOG 1967; FRCGP 1999.

SIME, Joanne Lesley 46 Parkgrove Gardens, Edinburgh EH4 7QS — MB ChB Ed. 1997.

SIME, Linda Anne Alloa Health Centre, Marshill, Alloa FK10 1AB Tel: 01259 212088 Fax: 01259 724788 — MB ChB Aberd. 1984; DCH RCPS Glas. 1986; DRCOG 1986; MRCGP 1988.

SIMENACZ, Mark Anthony 4A Paul Gardens, Croydon CR0 5QL — MB ChB Leeds 1990.

SIMENOFF, Charles Julius Oak Leigh Medical Centre, 58 Ash Tree Road, Crumpsall, Manchester M8 5SA Tel: 0161 740 1226 Fax: 0161 795 8611 Email: charles.simenoff@zoom.co.uk — MB ChB Ed. 1978 (Edin.) BSc Ed. 1975; DRCOG 1981; MRCGP 1982. Chairm. Manch. LMC.; Mem. Gen. Pract. Comm. Of BMA. Specialty: Gen. Pract.; Medico Legal. Socs: BMA - GPC; BMA (Mem. Gen. Med. Servs. Comm.). Prev: Trainee GP Unsworth Med. Centre Bury.

SIMHACHALAM, Dharmana 22 Humberston Avenue, Humberston, Grimsby DN36 4SP — MB BS Andhra 1975.

SIMHADRI, Nanduri Gloucester Centre, Morpeth Close, Orton Longueville, Peterborough PE2 7JU — MB BS Andhra 1968.

SIMISON, Mr Alastair John McIvor Arrowe Park Hospital, Upton, Wirral CH49 5PE; 7 Belmont Road, West Kirby, Wirral CH48 5EY — MB ChB Ed. 1973; BSc (Hons.) Ed. 1970; FRCS Ed. 1978; MChOrthop Liverp. 1984; FRCS Ed. (Orth.) 1984. Cons. Orthop. Surg. Arrowe Pk. & Clatterbridge Hosps. Specialty: Orthop.

SIMISTER, John Michael (retired) 80 King Street, Seahouses NE68 7XS — MB BChir Camb. 1952 (Camb. & St. Bart.) MA Camb 1959. Prev: Med. Dir. Lundbeck Ltd. Luton.

SIMKISS, Douglas Eric Birmingham Specialist Community NHS TrustTrust, BCCC, 61 Bacchus Road, Winson Green, Birmingham B18 4QY Tel: 0121 507 9508 Fax: 0121 507 9533 Email: douglas.sinkiss@southbirminghampct.nhs.uk — MB ChB Sheff. 1988; BMedSci Sheff. 1987; MRCP (UK) 1991; DCH RCP Lond. 1991; DTM & H Liverp. 1992; MSc Warwick 1997; MRCPCH UK 1997. Cons. (Paediat.) Birm. Specialist Community NHS Trust; Hon. Sen. Clin. Lect., Birm. Univ.; Hon. Cons. (Paediat.) City Hosp. Birm.; Hon. Cons. (Paediat.) Childrens Hosp. Birm. Specialty: Community Child Health. Special Interest: Epilepsy; Social Paediat. Socs: MRCPCH. Prev: Sen. Regist. (Community Child Health) N. Birm. Community NHS Trust; Regist. Rotat. Birm. Childr. Hosp.; SHO (Paediat.) Birm. Childr. Hosp., Walsgrave Hosp. & Gt. Ormond St. Hosp. Lond.

SIMLER, Nicola Ruth Wythenshawe Hospital, North West Lung Research Centre, Southmoor Road, Manchester M23 9LT Tel: 0161 291 5054 Fax: 0161 291 5054 Email: nsimler@aol.com — MB ChB Manch. 1993; MRCP Royal College of Physicians London 1996 July. Specialist Regist. in Respirat. Med. Specialty: Respirat. Med.; Intens. Care. Socs: Brit. Thoracic Soc. Prev: Research Regist. Respirat. Med. N. W. Lung Centre Wythenshawe Hosp.

SIMM, Francis 3 Mount Avenue, Bare, Morecambe LA4 6DJ — MRCS Eng. LRCP Lond. 1951 (King's Coll. & St Geo.) Asst. Div. Med. Off. Lancs. CC. Socs: Fell. Soc. MOH.; Fell. RSM; Life Mem. BMA. Prev: Asst. MOH & Sch. Med. Off. Co. Boro. Warrington.

SIMM, Janet Margaret Allerton Medical Centre, 6 Montreal Avenue, Leeds LS7 4LF Tel: 0113 295 3460; 6 Montreal Avenue, Leeds LS7 4LF Tel: 0113 295 3460 Fax: 0113 295 3469 — MB ChB Leeds 1973.

SIMMONDS, Anthony James Wood Farmhouse, Hasketon, Woodbridge IP13 8JJ Tel: 0147 335521 — MRCS Eng. LRCP Lond. 1960 (Lond. Hosp.) DObst RCOG 1962. Socs: BMA.

SIMMONDS, Anthony John Preston Grove Medical Centre, Preston Grove, Yeovil BA20 2BQ Tel: 01935 474353 Fax: 01935 425171; Michaelmas Cottage, North Lane, Hardington Mandeville, Yeovil BA22 9PF Tel: 01935 862078 — MB ChB Liverp. 1969; DObst RCOG 1973. S. Som. PCG Bd. Mem. and Hi MP Lead. Socs: Brit. Assn. Sport & Med. Prev: Clin. Asst. (A & E) Yeovil Hosp. Som.; Ho. Phys. & Ho. Surg. David Lewis North. Hosp. Liverp; Flight Lt. RAF Med. Br.

SIMMONDS, Edward John 121 Beechwood Avenue, Earlsdon, Coventry CV5 6FQ; University Hospitals, Coventry and Warwicleshire NHS Trust, Clifford Bridge Road, Walsgrave, Coventry CV2 2DX Tel: 01203 602020 — (Sheff.) MB ChB Sheff. 1982; B. Med. Sci. Shef. 1985; MRCP (UK) 1987; MD Sheff. 1994. Cons. Paediat. Walsgrave Hosps. NHS Trust. Specialty: Paediat. Prev: Clin. Research Fell. (Cystic Fibrosis) St. Jas. Univ. Hosp. Leeds.

SIMMONDS, Jeffrey Philip 65 Trafalgar Road, Birkdale, Southport PR8 2NJ — MB BS Lond. 1971 (Char. Cross) MRCS Eng. LRCP Lond. 1971; MRCP (UK) 1974; FRCP Lond. 1991. Cons. Phys. Southport Dist. Gen. Hosp. Specialty: Gen. Med. Prev: Sen. Regist. (Med.) Leicester Roy. Infirm.; Med. Regist. Westm. Hosp. Lond. & King Edwd. VII Hosp. Windsor.

SIMMONDS, Katherine Anne 27 The Parade, St. Helier, Jersey JE2 3QQ — MB BS Lond. 1993 (Char. Cross & Westm.) BSc (Hons.) Anat. Lond. 1990; DRCOG 1997; DFFP 1998; MRCGP 1999. GP Non-Princip., Jersey; Clin. Asst. Dermat. Specialty: Gen. Pract. Prev: GP/Regist. Torbay Hosp. Torquay VTS.

SIMMONDS, Mark Kenneth — MB ChB Bristol 1984; Cert. Family Plann. JCC 1987; MRCGP 1990; DA (UK) 1990; FRCA 1996; CCST (Anaesth.) 2000. Clin. Research Fell., Dept. Anaesthesiology & Pain Med., 3B2.32 Walter Mackenzie Health Sci. Centre, Univ. of Alberta, Edmonton, Canada T6G 2B7. Tel: 001 780 407 3552. Specialty: Anaesth. Prev: GP Springdale Newfld. Canada; Doctors/Ldr. Rambler Holidays (UK) Nepalese Himalaya; Trainee GP N. Devon Dist. Hosp. Barnstaple VTS.

SIMMONDS, Martin John, TD 54 St. Augustines Road, Bedford MK40 2NA — MB BS Lond. 1964 (Westm.) MRCS Eng. LRCP Lond. 1964; AKC Lond. 1964; DObst RCOG 1969. Prev: GP Luton; SHO Obst. Orsett Hosp. Grays; Ho. Surg. Qu. Mary's Hosp. Roehampton.

SIMMONDS, Martin Richard 2 Cairn Close, Nailsea, Bristol BS48 2UT; 29 St Mary's Close, Nailsea, Bristol BS48 4NQ — MB BS Lond. 1989. Neonat. Research Fell. St Michaels Hosp. Bristol. Specialty: Paediat.; Neonat.

SIMMONDS, Michael Norman (retired) 1 Emily Place, Camp Road, Clifton, Bristol BS8 3ND Tel: 0117 973 1087 Fax: 0117 973 6953 — MB ChB Bristol 1951; DObst RCOG 1959.

SIMMONDS, Nicola Jane Luton & Dunstable Hospital, Lewsey Road, Luton LU4 0DZ Tel: 01582 491122 Email: nicola.simmonds@ldh.tr.anglox.nhs.uk — BM BCh Oxf. 1984; MA Camb. 1985; FRCP (UK) 1987; DM Oxf. 1993; FRCP 2000. Cons. Phys. (Gen. Med. & Gastroenterol.) Luton & Dunstable Hosp. NHS Trust. Specialty: Gastroenterol. Prev: Sen. Regist. (Med. & Gastroenterol.) Roy. Hants. Co. Hosp. & Soton. Gen. Hosp.; Lect. (Gastroenterol.) Lond. Hosp. Med. Coll.; Regist. (Med.) Whittington Hosp. Lond. & Univ. Coll. Hosp. Lond.

SIMMONDS, Peter Damien Cancer Research UK Oncology Unit, Southampton General Hospital, Southampton SO16 6YD Tel: 02380 798476 Fax: 02380 795176 Email: p.d.simmonds@soton.ac.uk — MB BS (Hons.) Melbourne 1985 (Monash Univ., Melbourne, Australia) FRACP 1993. Cons. Med. Oncologist, Soton. Univ. Hosps. NHS Trust; Hon. Sen. Lect. in Med. Oncol., Univ. of Soton.; Hon. Cons. Med. Oncologist, Portsmouth Hosps. NHS Trust; Hon. Cons. Med. Oncologist, Poole Hosps. NHS Trust. Specialty: Oncol. Special Interest: Bone and Soft tissue Sarcomas; Breast Cancer; testicular cancer. Socs: Europ. Soc. of Med. Oncol.; Amer. Soc. of Clin. Oncol.; Assn. of cancer Physicians. Prev: Sen. Lect. in Med. Oncol., Univ. of Soton.; Clin. research Fell. and Hon. Sen. Regist. in Med. Oncol. - Univ. of Soton.

SIMMONDS, Robert Canterbury Health Centre, 26 Old Dover Road, Canterbury CT1 3JH Tel: 01227 780437 Fax: 01227 784979 — MB ChB Leeds 1980; DRCOG 1983; MRCGP 1984. Clin. Asst. (Endoscopy) Kent & Canterbury Hosp.; Trustee of Candoc Chestfield. Specialty: Gen. Pract. Socs: BMA; RCGP; BSG.

SIMMONDS, Sally-Jane The Tower, Victoria Road, Aldeburgh IP15 5EG — BM Soton. 1987.

SIMMONS, A Louise E Hunter Health Centre, Andrew Street, East Kilbride, Glasgow G74 1AD Tel: 01355 906643 — MB ChB Glas. 1972.

SIMMONS, Adrian Victor 47 Whinfield, Adel, Leeds LS16 7AE Tel: 0113 267 4033 Fax: 0113 267 4033 Email: avsimmons@doctors.org.uk — MB ChB Manch. 1962; BSc (Hons. Physiol.) Manch. 1960, MB ChB 1962; DObst RCOG 1964; FRCP Lond. 1980, M 1967. Specialty: Gen. Med.; Medico Legal. Socs: Brit. Soc. Of Gastroenterol. Prev: Cons. Phys. St. Jas. Univ. Hosp. Leeds; Sen. Med. Regist. United Leeds Hosps.; Med. Regist. Univ. Coll. Hosp. Lond.

SIMMONS, Andrea Jacqueline 64 Ladbrooke Drive, Potters Bar EN6 1QW — MB ChB Manch. 1994.

SIMMONS, Catherine Mary Howdenhall Surgery, 57 HowdenHall Road, Edinburgh EH16 6PL Tel: 0131 664 3766 Fax: 0131 672 2114 — MB ChB Aberd. 1968. GP Edin.

SIMMONS, Mr Clifford Alan (retired) 21 Heath Rise, Kersfield Road, Putney, London SW15 3HF Tel: 020 8789 2166 — BM BCh Oxf. 1942; BA Oxf. 1939; MA Oxf. 1944; FRCS Eng. 1950; FRCOG 1964, M 1952. Hon. Cons. Gyn. Roy. Marsden Hosp. Lond., Mt. Vernon Hosp. & Radium Inst.

SIMMONS, Damon John 42 Coroners Lane, Widnes WA8 9JB — MB ChB Liverp. 1994. SHO (Orthop.) S. Manch. Univ. Hosps. NHS Trust. Specialty: Orthop.

SIMMONS, David Alastair Ross (retired) 21 Dougalston Avenue, Milngavie, Glasgow G62 6AP Tel: 0141 956 3900 — MB ChB St. And. 1951; MD (Hons.) St. And. 1957; FRCPath 1976, M 1963; DSc Glas. 1972. Prev: Sen. Lect. Bact. & Immunol. Univ. Glas.

SIMMONS, Gillian Sandra (retired) 70 Abercorn road, Mill Hill, London NW7 1JT Tel: 020 8346 4412 Mob: 07836 556213 Email: gilsimmons@aol.com — MB ChB Liverp. 1964; MRCS Eng. LRCP Lond. 1964; DObst RCOG 1966; MFPHM 1973. Prev: GP Wembly (Brent & Harrow HA).

SIMMONS, Grace 262 Hardhorn Road, Poulton-le-Fylde FY6 8DW — MB ChB Manch. 1995 (Manchester) DCH (London 1998); DFFP 2001. Specialty: Gen. Pract.

SIMMONS, Heather Olive Kent Forensic Psychiatry Service, Trevor Gibbens Unit, Maidstone ME16 9QQ Tel: 06122 723187 — MB BS Lond. 1986 (St. George's Hospital Medical School London) Locum Cons. (Psychiat.) Forens. Servs. W. Kent NHS & Social Care Trust. Specialty: Alcohol & Substance Misuse. Prev: Staff Grade (Psychiat.) Addic. Servs. Thames Gateway Trust.

SIMMONS, Helen 130 St William's Way, Thorpe, Norwich NR7 0AR Tel: 01603 433428 — BM BCh Oxf. 1992; MA Oxf. 1997, BA 1992; MRC Psych 1999. Regist. Maudsley Hosp. Lond. Specialty: Child & Adolesc. Psychiat. Socs: Med. Defence Union; BMA. Prev: SHO Roy. Free Hosp. NHS Trust Lond. VTS; SHO (A & E) St. Geo. Healthcare NHS Trust.

SIMMONS, Ian Geoffrey c/o 102 Kenwood Drive, Beckenham BR3 6RA — MB ChB Manch. 1990.

SIMMONS, Joanna Top Flat, 31 Rye Hill Park, London SE15 3JN Tel: 020 7358 1940 — MB BS Lond. 1993. SHO (Psychiat.) Goodmayes Hosp. Ilford. Socs: BMA.

SIMMONS, John Alexander School House, Muddles Green, Chiddingly, Lewes BN8 6HN — MB BS Lond. 1996.

SIMMONS, Jonathan David Royal Berkshire Hospital, Gastroenterology Department, London Road, Reading RG1 5AN — BM BCh Oxf. 1990; MA Oxf. 1993; MRCP (UK) 1993; DM Oxf. 2002. Cons. Gastroenterologist, Roy. Berks. and Battle Hosp. NHS Trust Reading. Specialty: Gastroenterol. Special Interest: Inflammatory Bowel Dis.; Nutrition. Socs: BSG. Prev: Specialist Regist. and Research Fell., Oxf. Radcliffe Hosp.

SIMMONS, Katherine Leah 1A Grove Cottages, Falconer Road, Bushey, Watford WD23 3AE — MB ChB Liverp. 1992.

SIMMONS, Margaret Elizabeth Shelcote Brow, Montford Bridge, Shrewsbury SY4 1EG Tel: 01743 850430 — MB ChB Sheff. 1962; FRCP Lond. 1980, M 1966. Cons. Phys. Roy. Shrewsbury Hosp. Specialty: Gen. Med. Socs: Brit. Cardiac Soc.; Brit. Pacing & Electrophysiol. Gp. Prev: Sen. Regist. (Med.) Univ. Coll. Hosp. Lond.; Sen. Regist. (Research) Bristol Gen. Hosp.; Regist. (Med.) Bristol Roy. Infirm.

SIMMONS, Margaret Rose (retired) Vales Court, Vales Road, Budleigh Salterton EX9 6HS — MB ChB Ed. 1967.

SIMMONS, Mark Andrew 47 Whinfield, Adel, Leeds LS16 7AE — BM BCh Oxf. 1993; FRCS (Oto) London 1999. SpR Otolaryngol. Northwest Deanery.

SIMMONS, Maureen Helen 5 Fishpond Lane, Egginton, Derby DE65 6HJ — BM Soton. 1985.

SIMMONS, Michael David Welsh Assembly Government, Cathays Park, Cardiff CF10 3NQ Tel: 029 2082 3505 Email: mike.simmons@wales.gsi.gov.uk — MB ChB Liverp. 1976; MSc Lond. 1983; MRCPath 1986; FRCPath 1996; MFPH 2002. Sen. Med. Off., Welsh Assembly Govt. Specialty: Med. Microbiol.; Pub. Health Med. Prev: Director, Pub. Health Laborat., Carmarthen.

SIMMONS, Michael George (retired) Hatt Farm, Hatt Common, Newbury RG20 0NJ Tel: 01635 253408 — BM BCh Oxf. 1940 (Oxf. & St. Thos.) MA, BM BCh Oxf. 1940. Prev: Flight Lt. RAFVR.

SIMMONS, Michael John (retired) 22 Reading Road, Wallingford OX10 9DS — MB BS Lond. 1968 (St. Bart.) MRCS Eng. LRCP Lond. 1968; DMRD Eng. 1973; FRCR 1975. Cons. Radiol. Roy. Berks. Hosp. & W. Berks. Health Dist. Prev: Sen. Regist. (Diag. Radiol.) St. Bart. Hosp. & Hosp. Sick Childr. Gt.

SIMMONS, Michael Richard Lewis The Surgery, 34 Raymond Road, Upper Shirley, Southampton SO15 5AL Tel: 023 8022 7559; 32 Hickory Gardens, West End, Southampton SO30 3RN Tel: 023 8047 3183 — MB ChB Bristol 1962; DObst RCOG 1965. Specialty: Gen. Pract. Prev: Med. Off. i/c Govt. Hosp. Leribe, Lesotho; Ho. Off. Southmead Hosp. Bristol & Soton. Gen. Hosp.

SIMMONS, Moira 21 Dougalston Avenue, Mmilngavie, Glasgow G62 6AP — MB ChB Glas. 1983; FFA RCS Eng. 1987. Sen. Regist. (Anaesth.) Ninewells Hosp. Dundee. Specialty: Anaesth.

SIMMONS, Norman Alan, CBE (retired) 64 Ladbrooke Drive, Potters Bar EN6 1QW Tel: 01707 653369 Fax: 01707 646871 Email: nasimmons@doctors.org.uk — (St. Mary's) MB BS Lond. 1958; MRCS Eng. LRCP Lond. 1958; FRCPath 1977, M 1965. Emerit. Cons. Microbiol. Guy's & St. Thos. Hosp. Trust; Hon. Sen. Lect. (Microbiol.) Lond. Hosp. Med. Coll. Prev: Cons. Clin. Microbiol. Guy's Hosp. Lond.

SIMMONS, Paul Douglas (retired) 98 Thomas More House, Barbican, London EC2Y 8BU Tel: 020 7588 5583 — (Univ. Leeds) MB ChB Leeds 1971; FRCP Lond. 1992, M 1976; DFFP 1993. Prev: Cons. Genitourin. Phys. St. Bart. Hosp. Lond.

SIMMONS, Peter Hamilton (retired) 1 Queens Road, Barnet EN5 4DH Tel: 020 8449 4130 — (St. Bart.) MB BS Lond. 1950; DA Eng. 1952; FFA RCS Eng. 1954. Hon. Cons. Anaesth. Roy. Free Hosp., N. Middlx. Hosp. Edmonton & Roy. N. Hosp. Lond. Prev: Hon. Cons. Anaesth. Lond. Chest Hosp.

SIMMONS, Peter Michael High Street Surgery, 87 High Street, Abbots Langley WD5 0AJ Tel: 01923 262363 Fax: 01923 267374; 125 Mobcroft Cottages, Bragmans Lane, Flaunden, Hemel Hempstead HP3 0PL Tel: 01442 832632 — MB BS Lond. 1973 (St. Thos.) DRCOG 1976. Prev: Trainee GP Watford VTS; Ho. Surg. Lambeth Hosp. Lond.; Ho. Phys. Shrodells Hosp. Watford.

SIMMONS, Philip Arthur Circuit Lane Surgery, 53 Circuit Lane, Reading RG30 3AN Tel: 0118 958 2537 Fax: 0118 957 6115 Email: phil.simmons@gp-k81067.nhs.uk; 33 Honey End Lane, Reading RG30 4EL Tel: 0118 957 5157 Email: suesimmons33@yahoo.co.uk — MB ChB Bristol 1973; BSc (Hons.) (Anat.) Bristol 1970; DObst RCOG 1975; MRCGP 1980. Specialty: Homeop. Med.

SIMMONS, Richard Lewis Laurence 40 Parkhill Road, Bexley Village, Bexley DA5 1HU Tel: 01322 522056 — MRCS Eng. LRCP Lond. 1966 (St. Mary's) MRCOG 1974; MRCGP 1975. Clin. Asst. (Gyn.) Lond. Hosp. Socs: Fell. Roy. Soc. Med.; Brit. Soc. Med. & Dent. Hypn. Prev: Regist. (O & G) Lond. Hosp.; Resid. (O & G) Foothills Prov. Gen. Hosp. Calgary, Canada.

SIMMONS, Roger Eric The Surgery, Kinloch Rannoch, Pitlochry PH16 5PR Tel: 01882 632216 — MB ChB Ed. 1974 (Edinburgh) BSc (Hons.) Ed. 1971; DCH RCPS Glas. 1977; MRCP (UK) 1978; MRCGP 1980; FRCP Ed. 1993. GP Princip. Specialty: Gen. Pract. Prev: Sen. Med. Off. (Primary Care) Scott. Off. Edin.; GP & Trainer N. Berwick.

SIMMONS, Sheila (retired) 11 Roecliffe Grove, Stockton-on-Tees TS19 8JU Tel: 01642 618880; 11 Roecliffe Grove, Stockton-on-Tees TS19 8JU Tel: 01642 618880 — MB BS Durh. 1949 (Newc.) Prev: Clin. Med. Off. SW Durh.

SIMMONS, Sir Stanley Clifford (retired) 23 Chapel Square, Virginia Park, Virginia Water GU25 4SZ Tel: 01344 844029 Fax: 01344 844067 — (St. Mary's) Hon. F.Inst.Obst.RCP Irel.; MB BS Lond. 1951; DObst 1953; FRCS Eng. 1957; FRCOG 1971, M 1960; Hon. FRACOG 1991; Hon. FACOG 1992; Hon. FRCS Ed. 1994. Prev: Cons. O & G Heatherwood Hosp. Ascot & King Edwd. VII Hosp. Windsor.

SIMMONS, Stephen 77 Bedford Road, Southport PR8 4HU — MB ChB Glas. 1983; MRCPsych 1989.

SIMMONS, Valerie Elizabeth Eli Lilly & Company Ltd., Lilly Research Centre, Erl Wood Manor, Sunninghill Road, Windlesham GU20 6PH Tel: 01276 853320 Fax: 01276 853325 Email: simmons_valerie@lilly.com; 28 Clarendon Road, Ealing, London W5 1AB — MB BS Lond. 1979. Dir. Global Pharmacovigilance, Eli Lilly & Company (Erl Wood). Specialty: Pharmaceutical Medicine. Socs: Fac. Pharmaceut. Med. Prev: Dir. Internat. Product Safety & Pharmacovigilance Glaxowellcome Research & Developm. Greenford; Sen. Research Phys. Glaxo Gp. Research Ltd. Greenford; Med. Adviser Janssen Pharmaceut. Ltd. Wantage.

SIMMONS, William Busby Road Surgery, 75 Busby Road, Clarkston, Glasgow G76 7BW Tel: 0141 644 2669 Fax: 0141 644 5171; Brucefield, 11 Otterburn Drive, Giffnock, Glasgow G46 6PZ Tel: 0141 638 4070 — MB ChB Glas. 1973; MRCGP 1979; DRCOG 1980; DFM Glas. 1989; MPhil. Glas. 1992.

SIMMONTE, Muriel Gwyneth Prestonpans Health Centre, Preston Road, Prestonpans EH32 9QS Tel: 01875 810736 Fax: 01875 812979; 16 Cotlands Avenue, Longniddry EH32 0QU — MB ChB Ed. 1979; DCH RCP Lond. 1981; DRCOG 1982; MRCGP 1983.

SIMMS, Caryn Margaret 7 Lennox Avenue, Glasgow G14 9HF — MB ChB Glas. 1994; DRCOG 1996; DFFP 1996. GP Regist. South. Gen. Hosp. Glas. Specialty: Gen. Pract. Socs: BMA. Prev: SHO (O & G & Med.) South. Gen. Hosp. Glas.; Ho. Off. (Surg.) Inverclyde Roy. Hosp.

SIMMS, Mr John Michael Chesterfield & North Derbyshire Royal Hospital, Chesterfield S44 5BL; 4 Slayleigh Drive, Sheffield S10 3RD — MD Sheff. 1985; MB ChB Glas. 1974; FRCS Eng. 1979. Cons. (Gen. Surg.) N. Derbysh. HA. Specialty: Gen. Surg. Prev: Lect. (Surg.) Roy. Hallamsh. Hosp. Sheff.; Regist. Roy. Infirm. Sheff.; Ho. Surg. Roy. Infirm. Glas.

SIMMS, Katharine Claire The Gables Medical Centre, 45 Waveney Road, Ballymena BT43 5BA Tel: 028 2565 3237 Fax: 028 2564 0754 — MB BCh BAO Belf. 1986; Cert. Family Plann. JCC 1989; DCH RCPSI 1990; DMH Belf. 1990; DRCOG 1990; MRCGP 1991.

SIMMS, Mr Malcolm Harold Quarry Cottage, 80 Quarry Lane, Northfield, Birmingham B31 2PY — MB BS Lond. 1969 (St. Geo.) FRCS Eng. 1974. Cons. Surg. (Vasc. Interest) Selly Oak Hosp. Birm. Specialty: Gen. Surg. Prev: Lect. (Surg.) Univ. Birm. Med. Sch; Regist. (Renal Transpl.) & Research Fell. (Renal Transpl.) Qu. Eliz.; Hosp. Birm.

SIMMS, Matthew Stewart 42 Gestrade Rd, Nottingham NG2 5BY — MB ChB Sheff. 1993; FRCS (Eng) 1997; DM Univ. of Nottm. 2002.

SIMMS, Rosemary Jane 4 Slayleigh Drive, Sheffield S10 3RD — MB ChB Sheff. 1980. Prev: Regist. (Psychiat.) North. Gen. Hosp. Sheff.; Ho. Off. Roy. Hallamshire Hosp. Sheff.

SIMON, Adam Stuart 10 Holmfield Avenue, Prestwich, Manchester M25 0BH — MB BS Lond. 1993.

SIMON, Chantal Anne Else 7 The Rampart, Lymington SO41 9FR — BM BCh Oxf. 1990; MA Camb. 1992; DRCOG 1992; Cert. Fam. Plann. JCC 1992; MRCGP 1994.

SIMON, Dominic William Neil 88 Dalling Road, London W6 0JA — MB BS Lond. 1996.

SIMON, Ellis Julian Department of Anaesthetics, Critical Care and Pain Medicine, Royal Infirmary, Lauriston Place, Edinburgh EH3 9YW Tel: 0131 536 3651; 100 Findhorn Place, Edinburgh EH9 2NZ Tel: 0131 662 4321 Fax: 0131 662 9506 Email: e.simon@ed.ac.uk — MB ChB Ed. 1984; FFA RCSI 1990; FRCA 1991. Cons. (Anaesth.) Roy. Infirm. Edin. Specialty: Anaesth. Prev: Clin. Fell. Transport of The Critically Ill West. Infirm. Glas.

SIMON, Gowry Raji 23 Woodcote Road, Tettenhall, Wolverhampton WV6 8LP — MB BS Bombay 1980; FFA RSCI 1992.

SIMON, Jacob (retired) 143 Hammerson House, The Bishop's Avenue, London N2 0BE Tel: 020 8455 3648 — MRCS Eng. LRCP Lond. 1935 (Lond. Hosp.) Hon. Maj. RAMC. Prev: Sen. Ho. Surg. LoW.oft & N. Suff. Hosp.

SIMON, John Wingate 21 Hinstock Close, Farnborough GU14 0BE Tel: 01295 516425 — MRCS Eng. LRCP Lond. 1974; MA, BM BCh Oxf. 1974; MRCP (UK) 1982.

SIMON, Patrick Dorairaj The Surgery, 119 Sheldon Heath Road, Sheldon, Birmingham B26 2DP Tel: 0121 784 5465 Fax: 0121 789 6707 — MB BS Bangalor 1973; MB BS Bangalore 1973.

SIMON, Raji Idicula 23 Woodcote Road, Tettenhall, Wolverhampton WV6 8LP — MB BS Bombay 1980; MRCOG 1994.

SIMON, Ron David Ben 9 Mary Street, London N1 7DL — MB BS Lond. 1991; BSc (Hons) Chem. Lond. 1984.

SIMON, Sacha Dominic 84 Ivy Lane, Headington, Oxford OX3 9DY — MB BS Lond. 1996 (Char. Cross & Westm.) BSc (Biochem.) Lond. 1994. Ho. Off. (Surg.) King Edwd. VII Hosp. Midhurst; SHO (A & E) Ealing Hosp.; SHO (Paediat. Surg.) John Radcliffe Hosp. Specialty: Paediat. Prev: Ho. Off. (Med.) Char. Cross Hosp. Lond.

SIMON, Sybil 57 Stanley Road, Broughton Park, Salford M7 4FR — MB ChB Manch. 1965; DCH RCP Lond. 1968. Dir. Manch. Tay-Sachs Screening Progr. Roy. Manch. Childr. Hosp. Socs: Fell. Manch. Med. Soc. Prev: Cas. Off. Booth Hall Hosp. Childr. Manch.; MRC Schol. in Med. Genetics; Ho. Off. (Paediat. Med.) Duchess of York Hosp. Babies Manch.

SIMONDS, Anita Kay Royal Brompton & Harefield NHS Trust, Sydney St., London SW3 6NP Tel: 020 7351 8911 Fax: 020 7351 8911 — MB BS Lond. 1979; MRCP (UK) 1983; MD Lond. 1988; FRCP Lond. 1994. Cons. Respirat. Med. Roy. Brompton Hosp. Specialty: Respirat. Med. Prev: Sen. Regist. N. Tees & Newc. Hosps. Gp.; Doverdale Fell. Brompton Hosp. Lond.

SIMONDS, Mr Geoffrey Walter (retired) Pear Tree Farm, Loversall, Doncaster DN11 9DD Tel: 01302 852554 — MB BS Lond. 1960 (Char. Cross) MRCS Eng. LRCP Lond. 1960; FRCS Eng. 1966; MChOrth Liverp. 1968. Prev: Cons. Orthop. Surg. Doncaster Roy. Infirm.

SIMONIS, Mr Robert Brand Norfolk Lodge, 7 Farmhouse Close, Pyrford, Woking GU22 8LR Tel: 01932 351427 Email: simonis7@hotmail.com — MB BS Lond. 1967 (Univ. Coll. Hosp.) MRCS Eng. LRCP Lond. 1967; FRCS Ed. 1974. Cons. Orthop. St. Peter's Hosp. Chertsey; Hon. Cons. St. Thos. Hosp. Lond. Specialty: Orthop. Special Interest: Non-union fractures. Socs: BLRS; Fell. BOA; Fell. Soc. Surg. of Hand. Prev: Sen. Regist. (Orthop.) St. Thos. Hosp. Lond.; Vis. Assoc. Prof. Orthop. Albert Einstein Coll. Med. New York, USA.

SIMONOFF, Emily Ann Department of Child and Adolescent Psychiatry, Institute of Psychiatry, De Crespigny Park, London SE5 8AZ Tel: 020 7703 5411 — MD Harvard 1983; MRCPsych 1986.

SIMONS, Mr Adrian William Lawn Cottage, Shrewsbury St., Hodnet, Market Drayton TF9 3NS — MB BS Lond. 1990; BSc (Hons.) Lond. 1987, MB BS 1990; FRCS (Tr. & Orth.) (Eng.) 1994. Specialist Regist. Orthop. & Trauma- stroke- Oswestry Rotat.; Cons. Orthopaedic Surg., New Cross Hosp., Wolverhampton, WV10 0QP. Specialty: Orthop.

SIMONS, Dawn Margaret 216 The Avenue, Acocks Green, Birmingham B27 6NR — MB ChB Sheff. 1987.

SIMONS, Eric Gregory Cromwell Hospital, Cromwell Road, London SW5 0TU Tel: 020 7460 5713 Fax: 020 7460 5726; 12 Saracens Wharf, Ferry Stratford, Milton Keynes MK2 2AL Tel: 01908 630579 Fax: 01908 630579 — MB ChB Pretoria 1961; FRCOG 1983, M 1970. Cons. Gyn. (IVF); Hon Cons. Singleton Hosp. Swansea. Specialty: Obst. & Gyn. Socs: Fell. Roy. Soc. Med. & Roy. Soc. Obst. & Gyn.; BMA. Prev: Cons. O & G Harare, Zimbabwe; Cons. Obst. IVF Unit Humana Hosp. Lond.; Cons. O & G Internat. Hosp. Bahrain.

SIMONS, Gregory Donald North End Surgery, High St., Buckingham MK18 1NU Tel: 01280 813239 Fax: 01280 823449; 5 Huntingdon Crescent, Bletchley, Milton Keynes MK3 5NT Tel: 01908 379539 — MB BCh BAO NUI 1988; LRCPSI 1988; DFFP 1993; MRCGP 1995. GP Princip. Specialty: Gen. Pract. Prev: Med. Off. 4th Field Ambul., 22 Field Hosp. RAMC & 212 Field Hosp. (v).

SIMONS, Henry Roy (retired) 14 Moorend Lane, Thame OX9 3BQ Tel: 01844 261005 — MB BS Lond. 1955 (Middlx.) DPM Eng. 1970; FRCPsych. 1982, M 1972. Prev: Cons. Psychiat. (Ment. Health of Elderly) Aylesbury & High Wycombe Clin. Area.

SIMONS, Mary Ann Prudence 4 Greensleeves, Hartopp Road, Sutton Coldfield B74 2QE; City Hospital NHS Trust, Dudley Road, Birmingham B18 7QH Tel: 0121 507 4906 — MB BS Newc. 1974; MRCP (UK) 1979; FRCP 1998. Cons. Phys. (Geriat. Med.) W. Birm. HA; Hon. Sen. Lect. (Geriat. Med.) Univ. Birm. Specialty: Gen. Med. Prev: Lect. & Hon. Sen. Regist. (Geriat. Med.) Univ. Birm.; Regist. Newc. Gen. Hosp.

SIMONS, Phillip Stuart Willow Surgery, Coronation Road, Downend, Bristol BS16 5DH Tel: 0117 970 9500 Fax: 0117 970 9501 — MB ChB Manch. 1992; BSc (Hons) Manch. 1990; DCH 1995; DRCOG 1997; MRCGP 1997; DFFP 1998. GP Princip. Bristol. Specialty: Gen. Pract.

SIMONS, Mr Richard Michael (retired) 42 Somerville Road, Sutton Coldfield B73 6HH Tel: 0121 354 6537 — MB BChir Camb. 1959 (St. Bart.) MRCS Eng. LRCP Lond. 1958; MA Camb. 1959; FRCS Eng. 1967. Prev: Cons. ENT. Surg. E. Birm. Hosp. Gp.

SIMONS, Robert Stuart, QHP c/o Department Anaesthesia, Royal Free Hospital, Pond St., London NW3 2QG Tel: 020 7794 0500 Fax: 020 7830 2245 — MB ChB Otago 1967; FANZCA 1972; FRCA 1980. Cons. Anaesth. Roy. Free Hosp. Lond.; Hon. Sen. Lect. (Anaesth.) Roy. Free Hosp. Sch. Med. Lond. Specialty: Anaesth. Socs: (Exec.) Resucit. Counc.; Intens. Care Soc. Prev: Sen. Regist. (Anaesth.) Hammersmith Hosp. Lond.; Regist. (Anaesth.) Westm. Hosp. Lond.; Regist. (Anaesth.) Auckland Hosp., N.Z.

SIMONS, Steven Edward Danbolt Square Medical Centre, High Street, Godalming GU7 1AZ Tel: 01483 415141 Fax: 01483 414881 — MB BS Lond. 1989 (Middlx. Hosp. Lond.) DA (UK) 1992; DFFP 1996; MRCGP 1996. Med. Off. Meath Home Godalming. Specialty: Gen. Pract. Socs: Roy. Coll. Gen. Pract.; Fac. of family plann. and reproduct. Health c/o RCOG.

SIMONSEN, Helen Flat 2B, 42 West Port, Dundee DD1 5ER — MB ChB Dundee 1997.

SIMONTON, Hilary Frances Diamond Medical Centre, Magherfelt — MB ChB Manch. 1985; BSc (Hons.) St. And. 1982; DRCOG 1990. Specialty: Gen. Pract. Socs: Roy. Coll. Gen. Pract.

SIMOYI, Tirivanhu 25 Mountserrat Road, Bromsgrove B60 2RU Tel: 0121 704 9202 — MRCPath 1989; FRCPath 1989.

SIMPKIN, Paul 2 Upper Wimpole Street, London W1G 6LD Tel: 020 7935 5614 — MB BS Lond. 1970 (St. Thos.) MRCP (U.K.) 1974; AFOM RCP Lond. 1982. Cons. Occupat. Health Phys.; Occupat. Health Adviser to Various Pub. Bodies & Cos. Specialty: Occupat. Health. Prev: Med. Adviser Lond. Residuary Body; Cons. Phys. Gtr. Lond. Counc.; Regist. (Med.) & Hon. Clin. Asst. Chest Dept. St. Thos. Hosp. Lond.

SIMPKINS, Howell Grant 78 Pastoral Way, Sketty, Swansea SA2 9LY — MB BCh Wales 1998.

SIMPKINS, Keith Charles (retired) The Mount, Main St., Kirk Deighton, Wetherby LS22 4EB Tel: 01937 582661 — MB BS Lond. 1956 (Char. Cross) DTM & H Liverp. 1961; FRCP Lond. 1982, M 1964; FRCP Ed. 1982, M 1964; DMRD Eng. 1966; FFR (Rohan Williams Medal) 1968; FRCR 1975; FRACR (Hon.) 1985. Hon. Sen. Lect. (Radiol.) Univ. Leeds. Prev: Cons. Radiol. Leeds Gen. Infirm.

SIMPKISS, Michael John (retired) 41 Western Road, Branksome Park, Poole BH13 6EP — (Univ. Birm.) MB ChB Birm. 1947; FRCP Lond. 1972, M 1951. Hon. Sen. Lect. Inst. Child Health Lond.; Hon. Cons. (Paediat.) Hosp. Sick Childr. Lond.; Hon. Clin. Teach. Child Health Soton. Univ. Med. Sch. Prev: Cons. (Paediat.) E. Dorset Health Dist.

SIMPSON, Mr Alasdair Hamish Robert Wallace Department of Orthopaedics, University of Edinburgh, Edinburgh Royal Infirmary, Edinburgh EH16 4SU Tel: 0131 242 6464 (Secretary)/0131 242

6465 Fax: 0131 242 6467 Email: hamish.simpson@ed.ac.uk — BM BCh Oxf. 1981; MA Camb. 1981; FRCS Eng. 1985; FRCS Ed. 1985; DM Oxf. 1993. Prof. of Orthop. and Trauma, Univ. of Edin.; Pres. Brit. Orthopaedic Research Soc. Specialty: Trauma & Orthop. Surg. Special Interest: Bone and Joint Infection; Limb Lenghtening; Trauma Reconstruction. Socs: Brit. Orthop. Research Soc.; (Educat. Sec.) Brit. Limb Reconstruction Soc.; BOA. Prev: Sen. Regist. (Orthop.) John Radcliffe Hosp. Oxf.; Research Fell. Brit. Orthop. Assn.; Prof. of Orthop. Oxf. Univ.

SIMPSON, Mr Alexander Lilly Research Centre, Erlwood Manor, Windlesham GU20 6PH Tel: 01276 483892 Fax: 01276 483782 — MB ChB Ed. 1979; BSc (Med. Sci.) Ed. 1976; FRCS Ed. 1983; Dip Pharm Med RCP (UK) 1989; MFPM 1990; FRCP Ed. 1997; FFPM 2001. Europ. Team Ldr. Endocrinol. Specialty: Pharmaceutical Medicine. Socs: Fell. Roy. Med. Soc. Edin.; Fell. Roy. Soc. Med. Prev: Med. Dir. Eli Lilly & Co. Ltd UK & Irel.; Med. Dir. Eli Lilly & Co Ltd. Nordic Area.

SIMPSON, Mr Alexander Ian 17 Smith Drive, Elgin IV30 4NE — MB BS Durh. 1960; FRCS Ed. 1966; DMRD Eng. 1969.

SIMPSON, Amanda Maxine Church Street Surgery, 4 Church Street, Wingate TS28 5AQ Tel: 01429 838217; 5 Church Close, Peterlee SR8 5QT Tel: 0191 586 8996 — MB ChB Leic. 1981.

SIMPSON, Mr Andrew Donald James Paget Hospital NHS Trust, Lowestoft Road, Gorgleston on Sea, Great Yarmouth NR31 6LA Tel: 01493 453180; 3 Ferrier Court, Barleycroft, Hemsby, Great Yarmouth NR29 4NS Tel: 01493 730272 — MB BS Lond. 1987 (St Bartholomew) MA Cambridge 1987; MB BS London 1987; FRCS Eng 1992; FRCS (Urol) 1998. Cons. (Urol.) James Paget Hosp. NHS Trust. Specialty: Urol. Prev: Regist. (Urol.) Camb. & Addenbrooke's NHS Trust; Regist. (Urol.) Ipswich Hosp.

SIMPSON, Andrew Hugh Portglenone Road Surgery, 23 Portglenone Road, Ahoghill, Ballymena BT42 1LE; Casaloma, 3 Carnearney Road, Ahoghill, Ballymena BT42 2QR Tel: 01266 871303 — MB BCh BAO Dub. 1957.

SIMPSON, Mr Andrew Neil University Hospital of Hartlepool, Accid. & Emerg. Dept, Holdforth Road, Hartlepool TS24 9AH Fax: 01429 522755; 15 Hillston Close, Naiseberry Park, Hartlepool TS26 0PE — MB BS Lond. 1988 (Roy. Free Hosp. Sch. Of Med., Univ. of Lond.) FRCS Ed. 1993; DCH RCP Lond. 1994; FFAEM 1998. Cons.(A&E.) Univ. Hosp. of Hartlepool. Specialty: Accid. & Emerg. Socs: Fac. of A&E Med. (Fell); BAAE; BPAE. Prev: Regist. (A & E) Sheff. Childr. Hosp.

SIMPSON, Andrew Paul Forsythe Marlow and Partners, The Surgery, Bell Lane, Stroud GL6 9JF Tel: 01453 883793 Fax: 01453 731670 — MB ChB Bristol 1991; Dip. IMC RCS Ed. 1994; DRCOG 1994; MRCP (UK) 1995; DCH RCP Lond. 1996; MRCGP 1997. GP Partner Minchinhampton Surg. Specialty: Gen. Pract. Socs: Co-ordinator Stroud PostGrad. Centre. Prev: GP Regist. Minchinhampton; SHO (Paediat.) Glos. Roy. Hosp.; SHO Rotat. (Med.) Frenchay Hosp. Bristol.

SIMPSON, Angela Trafford General Hospital, Trafford, Manchester M41 5SL; 14 Fletcher Drive, Bowdon, Altrincham WA14 3FZ — MB ChB Manch. 1991; BA Oxf. 1988; MRCP (UK) 1994; MD Manchester 2000. Specialist Regist. (Respirat. & Gen. Med.) NW Region. Specialty: Respirat. Med. Socs: Brit. Thorac Soc.; Manch. Med. Soc.; Roy. Coll. of Phys.s. Prev: Research Fell., N. Wing Key Centre, Wythslave Hosp. Manch.

SIMPSON, Ann Isabella (retired) 2 Addison Road, Broughty Ferry, Dundee DD5 2NB Tel: 01382 75546 — MB ChB Ed. 1959; CIH Dund 1983.

***SIMPSON, Anna Christine** 34 High Street, Bassingbourn, Royston SG8 5LD Tel: 01763 243350 — MB ChB Sheff. 1998; DCH; DFFP; DRCOG. GP VTS Notts. Specialty: Gen. Pract.

SIMPSON, Anna Louise 2 St Hilary Close, Bristol BS9 1DA — BM BS Nottm. 1997.

SIMPSON, Anne Brigid 7 The Common, Ealing, London W5 3TR Tel: 020 8567 7140 — MB ChB Otago 1980; MRCGP 1993. Specialty: Gen. Pract.; Ment. Health.

SIMPSON, Anne Jennifer Grahame Walnut Tree House, 15 The Pingle, Woodhouse Road, Quorn, Loughborough LE12 8AJ — MB BS Lond. 1977; MRCS Eng. LRCP Lond. 1977. Specialty: Community Child Health.

SIMPSON, Anthony Noel Brace Spring Gardens Health Centre, Providence Street, Worcester WR1 2BS Tel: 01905 681781 Fax: 01905 681766; The Sycamores, Old Rectory Gardens, Leigh, Worcester WR6 5LD — MB ChB Birm. 1969; DObst RCOG 1971; DCH Eng. 1972.

SIMPSON, Archibald Craig Cathcart Practice, 8 Cathcart Street, Ayr KA7 1BJ Tel: 01292 264051 Fax: 01292 293803; 47 Midton Road, Ayr KA7 2SQ Tel: 01292 263738 — MB ChB Glas. 1972 (Glasgow) MRCP (UK) 1978; MRCGP 1979; FRCP Glas. 1994. GP Trainer.

SIMPSON, Barbara Jean (retired) The Oaks, 1 Penfold Way, Dodleston, Chester CH4 9NL Tel: 01244 661041 — MRCS Eng. LRCP Lond. 1962; FRCOG 1991, M 1968, DObst 1964. Prev: MO & Instruc. Doctor Family Plann., Ante Natal & Well Wom. Servs. Clwyd HA.

SIMPSON, Beulah Llandudno General Hospital, Llandudno LL30 1LB; 16 Hafod Road E., Penrhyn Bay, Llandudno LL30 3NH — (Birm.) PhD Birm. 1955, BSc (Hons.) 1952, MB ChB 1970; DTM & H Liverp. 1972; DCH Eng. 1972; MRCP (UK) 1975; FRCP Lond. 1987. Emerit. Cons. Geriat. Med. Gwynedd HA. Specialty: Care of the Elderly. Socs: Brit. Geriat. Soc. Prev: Cons. Phys. (Geriat. Med.) Llandudno Gen. Hosp.; Sen. Regist. (Geriat. Med.) Ipswich Hosp.; Regist. (Gen. Med.) Caerns. & Anglesey Gen. Hosp. Bangor.

SIMPSON, Brian (retired) Inglewood, Eva Grove, Clayton, Newcastle-under-Lyme ST5 4DF — MB ChB Birm. 1965; AFOM RCP Lond. 1986. Prev: Sen. Med. Off. Benefits Agency Med. Serv.s, Blackpool.

SIMPSON, Mr Brian Arthur Department of Neurosurgery, University Hospital of Wales, Heath Park, Cardiff CF14 4XW Tel: 029 2074 2708 Fax: 029 2074 2560 — MB Camb. 1974 (Lond. Hosp.) BChir Camb. 1973; MA Camb. 1974; FRCS Eng. 1978; MD Camb. 1984. Cons. Neurosurg. Univ. Hosp. of Wales Cardiff. Specialty: Neurosurg. Socs: Internat. Neuromodulation Soc. Past Pres. Prev: Sen. Regist. Neurosurg. Lond. Hosp.

SIMPSON, Bruce, Col. late RAMC Retd. (retired) Tall Trees, Rhinefield Road, Brockenhurst SO42 7SQ Tel: 01590 623655 — MB ChB Ed. 1956; MA Ed. 1950; FRCP Ed. 1975, M 1961. Prev: Cons. Phys. Army Med. Servs. & Al Qassimi Hosp. Sharjah, United Arab Emirates.

SIMPSON, Carolyne Alexandra 11 Dreghorn Loan, Edinburgh EH13 0DF — MB ChB Aberd. 1998; MRCGP 2002.

SIMPSON, Christine Helen Burscough Health Centre, Stanley Court, Lord Street, Ormskirk L40 4LA Tel: 01704 892254 Fax: 01704 897182 — MB ChB Aberd. 1983; DA (UK) 1987.

SIMPSON, Christopher Guy Borril — MB BS Lond. 1973 (Char. Cross) BSc Lond. 1970; MRCPath 1981; FRCPath 1994. Cons. Histopath. Bronglais Gen. Hosp. Aberystwyth. Specialty: Histopath. Socs: Assn. Clin. Path.; Internat. Acad. Path. Prev: Lect. (Path.) Newc. Gen. Hosp. & Char. Cross Med. Sch.

SIMPSON, Christopher Jack Friarage Hospital, Northallerton DL6 1JG Tel: 01609 779911 — MB BS Lond. 1980; MRCPsych 1984; MPhil Lond. 1986; FRCPsych 1997; Dip. Health Serv. Management 1997. Cons. Psychiat. Friarage Hosp. N.allerton. Specialty: Gen. Psychiat.; Geriat. Psychiat. Prev: Sen. Regist. (Psychiat.) N. West. HA; Regist. (Psychiat.) St. Geo. Hosp. Lond.

SIMPSON, Claire Linda 2 Clarendon Road, Alderbury, Salisbury SP5 3AS — MB BS Lond. 1980.

SIMPSON, Constance Cowan 20 Whittingehame Drive, Glasgow G12 0XX Tel: 0141 339 0504 — MB ChB Glas. 1967.

SIMPSON, David 25 Dunkirk Avenue, Fulwood, Preston PR2 3RY — MB ChB Sheff. 1993.

SIMPSON, David Alexander Medway Hospital, Anaesthetic Department, Windmill Road, Gillingham ME7 5NY Tel: 01634 830000 Email: davidsimpson@nhs.net — MB BS Lond. 1977 (St. Bart.) FFA RCS (Eng.) 1982. Cons. Anaesth. Medway HA. Specialty: Anaesth.; Intens. Care. Prev: Sen. Regist. (Anaesth.) Kings Coll. Hosp. Lond.; Regist. (Anaesth.) Char. Cross Hosp. Lond.; SHO (Anaesth.) Roy. Sussex Co. Hosp.

SIMPSON, Mr David Charles ENT Department, Stobhill Hospital, Balornock Road, Glasgow G21 3UW; 20 Treemain Road, Lower Whitecraigs, Glasgow G46 7LB Tel: 0141 638 9518 — MB ChB Bristol 1979; MRCS Eng. LRCP Lond. 1979; FRCS Ed. 1984. Cons. ENT Stobhill Hosp. Glas. Specialty: Otolaryngol.

SIMPSON, David Creffield The Surgery, New Street, Stockbridge SO20 6HG Tel: 01264 810524 Fax: 01264 810591; Greenways, School Lane, Broughton, Stockbridge SO20 8BZ — MB BCh Wales

1980; DRCOG 1982; DCH RCP Lond. 1984; MRCGP 1986. Prev: Trainee GP/SHO Neath Gen. Hosp. VTS.

SIMPSON, Professor David Ian Hewitt Department of Microbiol. & Immunol., Queens University Belfast, Grosvenor Road, Belfast BT12 6BN Tel: 01232 240503 Fax: 01232 247895; 129 Ballylesson Road, Belfast BT8 8JU Fax: 01232 439181 — MD Belf. 1971 (Qu. Univ. Belf.) MB BCh BAO 1959; FRCPath 1983, MRCPath 1971. Prof. Microbiol. & Immunobiol. Qu.s Univ. Belf. Specialty: Med. Microbiol. Socs: Fell. Roy. Soc. Trop. Med. & Hyg. Prev: Cons. Dir. Special Pathogens Ref. Laborat., PHLS Centre for Applied Microbio. & Research Porton Down; Sen. Lect. (Med. Microbiol.) Lond. Sch. Hyg. & Trop. Med.; Research Off. E. Afr. Virus Research.

SIMPSON, David Laurence 22 Summerside Street, Edinburgh EH6 4NU — MB ChB Ed. 1976; FFA RCS Eng. 1982. Specialty: Anaesth.

SIMPSON, David Stewart 9 Windsor Place, Stirling FK8 2HY — MB ChB Glas. 1971; FFA RCS Eng. 1975. Specialty: Anaesth.

SIMPSON, Deborah Susan Westhaven Community Mental Health Unit, Radipole Lane, Weymouth DT4 0QE Tel: 01305 786905 — MB ChB Aberd. 1986; MRCPsych 1990; MSc Manch. 1993. Cons. (Gen. Adult & Rehabil. Psychiat.) N. Dorset Primary Care NHS Trust Furston Clinic Dorchester. Specialty: Gen. Psychiat. Socs: BMA. Prev: Cons. (Gen. Adult & Rehabil. Psychiat.) Wet Dorset Community Health Trust Weymouth; Sen. Regist. Rotat. (Psychiat.) Manch.; Regist. Rotat. (Psychiat.) Manch.

SIMPSON, Derek (retired) 94 St James Road, Bridlington YO15 3PQ Tel: 01262 424158 — (Ed.) MB ChB Ed. 1945. Prev: Clin. Asst. Anaesth. Huntingdon Co. Hosp.

SIMPSON, Douglas Bowie Clydebank Health Centre, Clydebank G81 Tel: 0141 952 2080 — MB ChB Glas. 1978. GP Glas.

SIMPSON, Mr Edmond (retired) 24 Perries Mead, Folkestone CT19 5UD Tel: 01303 259094 — MB BS Durh. 1961; DO RCS Eng. 1969; FRCS Eng. 1972; FRCOphth 1989. Cons. Ophth. S. Kent NHS Trust. Prev: Sen. Regist. (Ophth.) Roy. Free Hosp. & Maida Vale Hosp. Lond.

SIMPSON, Elizabeth Davis Liken (retired) 9 Boyne Terrace Mews, Holland Park, Kensington, London W11 3LR — MB BCh BAO Dub. 1941 (Univ. Dub.) BA 1939; DOMS Eng. 1944; FRCS Eng. 1952. Hon. Ophth. Surg. St. Jas. Hosp. Balham, St. Geo. Hosp. Tooting & S. Lond. Hosp. Wom. Prev: Ophth. Surg. Qu. Mary's Hosp. Childr. Carshalton.

SIMPSON, Professor Elizabeth Margaret Murray (retired) 42 St Aidans Road, Carlisle CA1 1LS Tel: 0191 285 2029; Lanecost House, Berkley Grange, Carlisle CA2 7PW Tel: 01228 522912 Email: cavie@one-name.org — MB ChB Aberd. 1937.

SIMPSON, Elizabeth Marguerite Hood (retired) 87 Glencairn Drive, Glasgow G41 4LL Tel: 0141 423 2863 — MB ChB Ed. 1948. Prev: Med. Off. Glas. Family Plann. Centre.

SIMPSON, Emily — MB ChB Pretoria 1991; DA (UK) 1995; FRCA 1999. Cons. (Anaesth.) Southend Hosp. Specialty: Anaesth. Prev: SHO (Anaesth.) Broomfield Hosp. Chelmsford; SHO (Anaesth.) Kent & Sussex Hosp. Tunbridge Wells.

SIMPSON, Emma Katherine 46 Bridge Street, Godalming GU7 1HL Tel: 01483 414147 Fax: 01483 414109 — MB BS Lond. 1994.

SIMPSON, Eric Walter The Village Surgery, 24-28 Laughton Road, Thurcroft, Rotherham S66 9LP Tel: 01709 542216 Fax: 01709 702356; 23 High Street, Laughton-en-le-Morthen, Sheffield S25 1YF Tel: 01909 567018 Fax: 01909 565263 — MB ChB Sheff. 1974; DA Eng. 1981. GP Rotherham Family Pract. Comm. Mem. RCS; Mem. Rottherham LMC. Specialty: Gen. Pract. Prev: Trainee GP Barnsley; Regist. (Anaesth.) Rotherham & Sheff. AHA (T).

SIMPSON, Fiona Mary Fontana and Partners, Silsden Health Centre, Elliott Street, Silsden, Keighley BD20 0DG Tel: 01535 652447 Fax: 01535 657296; Old Quarry, Borgue Road, Kirkcudbright DG6 4SA — MB ChB Aberd. 1981; DRCOG 1986; MRCGP 1987.

SIMPSON, Francis Vivian (retired) Nutgrove, 498 Scalby Road, Scalby, Scarborough YO13 0RA Tel: 01723 360726 Fax: 01723 360726 — MB BChir Camb. 1952 (Camb. & Univ. Coll. Hosp.) MA Camb. 1952; MRCGP 1974; BA (Music) Leeds 1999. Prev: Capt. RAMC.

SIMPSON, Frank Anthony (retired) Stabekk, Hough Lane, Norley, Frodsham, Warrington WA6 8JZ Tel: 01928 788577 — MB ChB Liverp. 1957.

SIMPSON, Gary Taylor High Pastures, 138 Liverpool Road North, Maghull, Liverpool L31 2HW; 138 Liverpool Road N., Maghull, Liverpool L31 2HW Tel: 0151 526 2161 — MB ChB Aberd. 1980; MRCGP 1987.

SIMPSON, Gavin David 9 Windsor Pl, Stirling FK8 2HY — MB ChB Ed. 1997.

SIMPSON, Gavin John Stuart (retired) Oulder Hill House, Oulder Hill Drive, Rochdale OL11 5LB Tel: 01706 630301 — MB ChB Ed. 1956; DPM Eng. 1967; MRCPsych 1973. Prev: Cons. Child Psychiat. Rochdale DHA.

SIMPSON, Graeme Kenneth Department of Medicine for Elderly, Royal Alexandra Hospital, Paisley PA2 9PN Tel: 0141 887 9111; Weybridge, 18 Stanely Drive, Paisley PA2 6HE Tel: 0141 884 2760 — MB ChB Ed. 1980; BSc Med. Sc. Ed. 1978; MRCP (UK) 1983; FRCP Ed. 1995; FRCP Glas. 2001. Cons. Phys. Geriat. Med. Roy. Alexandra Hosp. Paisley. Specialty: Gen. Med. Socs: Life Mem. Roy. Med. Soc. Prev: Sen. Regist. (Gen. & Geriat. Med.) North. RHA.

SIMPSON, Professor Hamish 24/2 Rothesay Terrace, Edinburgh EH3 7RY Tel: 0131 226 2370 — MD Ed. 1973; MB ChB 1957; DCH Eng. 1962; DObst RCOG 1962; FRCP Ed. 1971, M 1964; FRCP Lond. 1986. Emerit. Prof. Child Health Univ. Leicester. Prev: Cons. & Sen. Lect. (Child Life & Health) Univ. Edin.

SIMPSON, Helen Anne 34 Banknowe Drive, Tayport DD6 9LN — MB ChB Ed. 1991.

SIMPSON, Helen Louise Flat 2, Wilton Court, Cavell St., London E1 2BN — MB BS Lond. 1993.

SIMPSON, Howard Keith North Hampshire Hospital, Aldermaston Road, Basingstoke RG24 9NA — BM Soton. 1990; FRCS Ed. 1996; FFAEM 2000; Dip IMC RCS Ed. 2003. Emerg. Care Cons. (A & E) North Hants. Hosp. Specialty: Accid. & Emerg. Special Interest: Immediate Care; Prehospital Care.

SIMPSON, Hugh Cameron — MB ChB Glas. 1982 (Univ. Glas.) BSc Glas. 1982; MRCGP 1986. Unit Med. Off. RAF Markham Norf. Specialty: Gen. Pract. Prev: Sen. Med. Off. (RAF) Sek Kong Med. Recep. Station, Hong Kong; Sen. Med. Off. RAF Gatow Berlin, Germany.

SIMPSON, Hugh Charles Rowell Laurel Cottage, Rotten Row, Bradfield, Reading RG7 6LL Tel: 0118 974 4418 — MB BS Lond. 1973 (St. Bart.) MRCS Eng. LRCP Lond. 1973; MRCP (UK) 1977; MD Lond. 1984; FRCP Lond. 1993. Cons. Phys. Roy. Berks. Hosp. Reading. Specialty: Gen. Med.; Diabetes; Endocrinol. Socs: Brit. Hyperlipid. Assn.; Roy. Soc. Med.; Diabetes UK (Med. & Scientif. Sect.). Prev: Lect. (Diabetes & Endocrinol.) Univ. Soton.; Regist. (Endocrinol. & Gen. Med.) St. Geo. Hosp. Lond.; Research Regist. (Diabetes) Radcliffe Infirm. Oxf.

SIMPSON, Professor Hugh Walter University Department of Surgery, Royal Infirmary, Glasgow G4 0SF Tel: 01540 651280 Fax: 01540 651013 Email: simpsonhwsimpson@aol.com; 7 Cleveland Crescent, Glasgow G12 0PD Tel: 0141 357 1091 Fax: 0141 5779 4224 — (Ed.) MD Ed. 1959, MB ChB 1954; PhD Glas. 1965; FRCPath 1981, M 1967; FRCP Glas. 1987, M 1986. Hon. Sen. Research Fell. (Surg.) Glas. Roy. Infirm.; Prof. (Path.) Roy. Infirm. Glas.; Exec. Edr. Internat. Jl. Chronobiol.; Vis. Prof. (Path. & Laborat. Med.) Univ. Minnosota USA. Specialty: Pathology, General; Histopath. Special Interest: Breast Cancer Histopath. Socs: Path. Soc. Prev: Cons. & Head (Univ. Div. & NHS Dept. Path.) Roy. Infirm. Glas.; Vis. Prof. Path. Univ. Minnesota USA; Vis. Scientist Hypertens.-Endocrine Br. Nat. Inst. Health Bethesda, USA.

SIMPSON, Iain Alastair Wessex Cardiothoracic Centre, Southampton General Hospital, Tremona Road, Southampton SO16 6YD Tel: 023 8079 6648 Fax: 023 8079 6352 Email: ias@cardiology.co.uk — MB ChB Glas. 1980; MRCP (UK) 1983; MD Glas. 1987; FRCP Glas. 1993; FACC 1994; FRCP Lond. 1996. Cons. Cardiol. Wessex Regional Cardiac Centre. Specialty: Cardiol. Prev: Sen. Regist. (Cardiol.) Roy. Brompton Nat. Heart & Lung Hosp. St. Geo. Hosp. Lond.; Brit. Heart Foundat. Research Fell. Univ. Calif. San Diego, USA.

SIMPSON, Ian Grahame Mackintosh House, 120 Blythswood St., Glasgow G2 4EA Tel: 0141 221 5858 Fax: 0141 228 1208 Email: isimpson@mddus.com; 25 Lynedoch Street, Glasgow G3 6AA Email: ian.g@simpson4207.fslife.co.uk — MB ChB Aberd. 1966; Dip. Soc.

Med. Ed. 1970; MRCGP 1998; FRCP Ed. 2000. Chief Exec. & Sec. Med. & Dent. Defence Union Scotl. Socs: Fell. Roy. Soc. Med.; BMA; Fell. Roll. Soc. Arts. Prev: Under Sec. MDU Lond.; Dist. Med. Off. S. Grampian Health Dist.; Specialist (Community Med.) Grampian HB.

SIMPSON, Ian John Phoenix Surgery, 9 Chesterton Lane, Cirencester GL7 1XG Tel: 01285 652056 Fax: 01285 641562; The Coach House, Cranhams Lane, Cirencester GL7 1TZ Tel: 01285 651264 — MB ChB Bristol 1975; MRCGP 1982. Hosp. Pract. (Orthop.) Cirencester Hosp. Specialty: Orthop.

SIMPSON, Ian Macdonald (retired) 13 Dundee Road W., Stannergate, Dundee DD4 7NY — MB ChB Ed. 1949 (Univ. Ed.) Prev: Gen. Pratitioner.

SIMPSON, Ian Robert (retired) 1 Kingston Way, Whitley Bay NE26 1JL Tel: 0191 252 4955 — (Glas.) MB ChB Glas. 1943. Prev: Ho. Surg. Clackmannan Co. Hosp. Alloa.

SIMPSON, Ian Taylor Ellon Group Practice, Health Centre, Schoolhill, Ellon AB41 9JH Tel: 01358 720333 Fax: 01358 721578; 32 Craigpark Circle, Ellon AB41 9FH — MB ChB Aberd. 1977; MRCGP 1981.

SIMPSON, James (retired) 17 Woodlands Road, Motherwell ML1 2PX Tel: 01698 263454 — MB ChB Glas. 1944 (Univ. Glas.) Prev: Ho. Surg. Greenock Roy. Infirm. & Bellshill Matern. Hosp.

SIMPSON, James Donald The Calverton Practice, 2A St. Wilfrids Square, Calverton, Nottingham NG14 6FP Tel: 0115 965 2294 — MB BS Lond. 1966 (Westm.) MRCS Eng. LRCP Lond. 1966; MRCGP 1972. Specialty: Gen. Pract. Prev: Squadron Ldr. RAF Med. Br.

SIMPSON, James Oliver 9 York Road, Strensall, York YO32 5XT — BM BS Nottm. 1998; BM BS Nottm 1998.

SIMPSON, Janice 19 Beechwood Drive, Mossley, Ashton-under-Lyne OL5 0QJ — MB ChB Ed. 1977.

SIMPSON, Jason Trevor 3 Claragh Crescent, Strathfoyle, Londonderry BT47 6XQ — MB ChB Glas. 1998; MB ChB Glas 1998.

SIMPSON, Jennifer Ann 8 Aubery Crescent, Largs KA30 8PR — MB ChB Aberd. 1993.

SIMPSON, Jennifer Linda 1 Hungry Lane, Bradwell, Hope Valley S33 9JD — MB ChB Manch. 1976; DCH Eng. 1979. Regional Head of Resource Managem. Mersey RHA Liverp. Socs: Amer. BMA Coll. Phys. Exec. Prev: Resource Managem. Project Manager Sheff. Childr. Hosp.

SIMPSON, Joanna Elizabeth 29 Vyner Street, York YO31 8HR — MB ChB Sheff. 1993.

SIMPSON, Joanna Kate Sussex Cancer Centre, Royal Sussex County Hospital, Brighton BN2 5BE Tel: 01273 696955 Fax: 01273 623312 Email: joanna.simpson@bsuh.nhs.uk; 10 Lucastes Road, Haywards Heath RH16 1JL — MB BS Lond. 1987 (Univ. Coll. Lond. Hosps..) MRCP (UK) 1991; FRCR Lond. 1996. Cons. Clin. Oncologist, Brighton and Sussex Univ. Hosps. Specialty: Oncol.; Radiother. Special Interest: Head and Neck Cancer; Lung Cancer; Lymphoma. Socs: Brit. Assn. of Head and Neck Oncologists; Brit. Oncological Soc.

SIMPSON, John Department of Surgery, Queens Medical Centre, Nottingham NG7 2UH — MB ChB Leeds 1994.

SIMPSON, John Alexander Daisy Hill Hospital, Mental Health Department, 5 Hospital Road, Newry BT35 8DR — MB BCh BAO Belf. 1981; MRCPsych 1986. Cons. Psychiat. and Clin. Director, Newry Ment. Health Dept. Specialty: Gen. Psychiat.

SIMPSON, John Alexander 87 Glencairn Drive, Glasgow G41 4LL Tel: 0141 423 2863; 87 Glencairn Drive, Glasgow G41 4LL Tel: 0141 423 2863 — MB ChB Glas. 1944 (Univ. Glas.) FRSE; MB ChB (Commend.) Glas. 1944; FRCP Lond. 1964, M 1949; FRFPS Glas. 1950; FRCP Ed. 1961, M 1958; FRCP Glas. 1964, M 1962; MD (Hons. Bellahouston Medal) Glas. 1964; DSc Ed. 1992; DSc Glas. 1993. Emerit. Prof. Neurol. Univ. Glas. Specialty: Neurol.; Clin. Neurophysiol. Socs: Assn. Phys.; (Ex-Pres.) Assn. Brit. Neurol.; Amer. Acad. Neurol. Prev: Phys. (Neurol.) Inst. Neurol. Sc., South. Gen. Hosp. & West. Infirm. Glas; Reader (Neurol.) Univ. Edin.; Hon. Cons. Neurol. Brit. Army, Scott. Command.

SIMPSON, John Cameron 32 Oakley Avenue, Ealing, London W5 3SD Tel: 020 8992 6171 — MB BS Lond. 1962 (Guy's) MRCS Eng. LRCP Lond. 1962; DA Eng. 1965; FFA RCS Eng. 1966. Hon. Cons. Anaesth. Roy. Brompton & Harefield NHS Trust. Specialty: Anaesth. Socs: Intens. Care Soc. & Assn. Cardiothorac. Anaesth.; Anaesthetic Research Soc. Prev: Hon. Sen. Lect. Imperial Coll. Sch. of Med.; Cons. Anaesth. Roy. Brompton & Warefield Hosps. NHS Trust; Sen. Regist. (Anaesth.) St. Thos. Hosp. Lond. & Hosp. Sick Childr. Gt. Ormond St. Lond.

SIMPSON, John Derek Smithfield Medical Centre, 7 Smithfield Place, Ballymena BT43 5HB Tel: 028 2565 2301 Fax: 028 2563 0869; Carnearney House, Ahoghill, Ballymena Tel: 02825 871526 — MB BCh BAO Belf. 1965; FRCGP 1987, M 1971.

SIMPSON, Mr John Ernest Peter London Implementation Group, 40 Eastbourne Terrace, Paddington, London W2 3QR Tel: 020 7725 2500; 31 Hillbrow, Richmond Hill, Richmond on Thames, Richmond TW10 6BH Tel: 020 8940 0935 — BM BCh Oxf. 1967 (St. Thos.) MA, BM BCh Oxf. 1967; FRCS Eng. 1972; MFPHM 1990. Med. Adviser Lond. Implementation Gp. Socs: Fell. Roy. Soc. Med.; BMA; (Counc.) Brit. Assn. Day Surg. Prev: Regional Med. Off. Mersey RHA; Tutor King's Fund Coll. Lond.; Ho. Surg. & Lect. (Community Med.) St. Thos. Hosp. Lond.

SIMPSON, Professor John Gruer University of Aberdeen, Department of Pathology, Foresterhill, Aberdeen AB25 2ZD Tel: 01224 552848 Fax: 01224 663002 Email: j.g.simpson@abdn.ac.uk; Fae-Me-Well, Cothal, Fintray, Aberdeen AB21 0HU Tel: 01224 722500 Fax: 01224 722066 Email: j.g.simpson@abdn.ac.uk — MB ChB Aberd. 1965; MB ChB (Hons.) Aberd. 1965; FRCPath 1986, M 1973; PhD Aberd. 1975; FRCP Ed. 1995; ILTM 2000. Head of Dept. (Path) Univ Aberd., Ass. Dean (Med. Educat.) Univ Aberd; Hon. Cons. Aberd. Grampian Univ. Hosp. NHS Trust. Specialty: Histopath. Prev: Vis. Prof. Univ. Michigan, USA; MRC Jun. Research Fell. (Med.) Univ. Aberd.; Ho. Off. Aberd. Roy. Infirm.

SIMPSON, John Harold (retired) 2 Salutary Mount, Heavitree, Exeter EX1 2QE Tel: 01392 273815 — (Camb. & Middlx.) MRCS Eng. LRCP Lond. 1942; MB BChir Camb. 1943; MD Camb. 1952, MA 1943; FRCP Lond. 1969, M 1949. Prev: Cons. Phys. Exeter Clin. Area.

SIMPSON, John Mark Wallace M.I.S. House, 23 St Leonards Road, Eastbourne BN21 3PX Tel: 01323 724889 Fax: 01323 721161; 13 De Roos Road, Eastbourne BN21 2QA Tel: 01323 643824 — MB BChir Camb. 1982; BSc (Hons.) St. And. 1979; DRCOG 1985; MRCGP 1987; AFOM 1997; MIOSH 1998; MFOM 1998. Med. Dir. Health Support Div. PPP Healthcare; Managing Director AXA PPP Occupational Health Servs. Specialty: Occupat. Health. Socs: Soc. Occupat. Med.; Assur. Med. Soc.; Fac. Of Occupat. Med.

SIMPSON, John Munro Department of Paediatric Cardiology, Guy's Hospital, London Bridge, London SE1 9RT Tel: 020 74073351 Fax: 020 7955 2637 Email: john.simpson@gstt.sthames.nhs.uk — MB ChB Ed. 1987 (Edin.) MD 2000, Univ. Lond; BSc (Hons.) Ed. 1985; MRCP (UK) 1990. Cons. (Fetal & Paediat. Cardiol.) Guy's Hosp. Lond. Specialty: Paediat. Cardiol.; Paediat. Socs: Brit. Paediat. Cardiac Assn.; Brit. Cardiac Soc.; Internat. Soc. of Ultrasound in Obst. & Gynaecol. Prev: Fell. (Fetal & Paediat. Cardiol.) Guy's Hosp. Lond.; Fell. (Paediat. Cardiol.) Univ. of Calif., San Francisco, USA.

SIMPSON, John Roger (retired) Stacks, Priest Hill, Hailey, Witney OX29 9TT Tel: 01993 704549 — (Oxf.) BM BCh Oxf. 1964; MA Oxf. 1964. Prev: GP Long HanBoro. & Eynsham.

SIMPSON, Jonathan Christian Gerard Dept. Respiratory Medicine, Manchester Royal Infirmary, Oxford Road, Manchester M13 9WL Tel: 0161 276 1234; 14 Fletcher Drive, Bowdon, Altrincham WA14 3FZ — MB ChB Manch. 1989 (St Andrews & Manchester) BSc (Med. Sci.) St. And. 1986; MRCP (UK) 1992; AFOM RCP Lond. 1995; MD 1996; FRCP 2003. Cons. (Respirat. & Gen Med.) Manch. Roy. Infirm., Manch. Specialty: Respirat. Med.; Gen. Med. Socs: Brit. Thorac. Soc.; Manch. Med. Soc.; Roy. Coll. of Phys.s (Lond.). Prev: Cons. (Respirat. & Gen. Med.) Stepping Hill Hosp. Stockport; Sen. Regist. (Respirat. Med.) Wythenshawe Hosp. Manch.; Clin. Lect. (Respirat. Med.) Manch. Roy. Infirm.

SIMPSON, Judith Christina Bellshill Clinic, Main Street, Bellshill, Glasgow ML4 1AB — MB BS Newc. 1972; DCCH RCP Ed. 1989. Sen. Clin. Med. Off. (Community Paediat.) Bellshill. Socs: Fac. Comm. Health; MRCPCH. Prev: Clin. Med. Off. (Community Child Health) Bellshill.

SIMPSON, Judith Helen 37a Aytoun Road, Glasgow G41 5HW Tel: 0141 424 0173 — MB ChB Ed. 1989 (Edinburgh) DRCOG 1992; DCH 1993; MRCGP 1994; MRCP (UK) 1996. Specialist Regist. in Paediat. Specialty: Paediat.; Neonat.

SIMPSON, Judy Hope Gibson Court Medical Centre, Gibson Court, Boldon Colliery NE35 9AN Tel: 0191 519 0077 Fax: 0191 537 3559 — MB BS Newc. 1982; DRCOG 1985; MRCGP 1986.

SIMPSON, June Margaret (retired) Marliam, Guards Road, Lindal, Ulverston LA12 0TN — MB BS Durh. 1962 (Newc.) Prev: SCMO S. Cumbria Health Auth.

SIMPSON, Karen 23 Riverpark, Nairn IV12 5SP — MB ChB Ed. 1996.

SIMPSON, Karen Hilary Pain Management Service, St. James's University Hospital, Beckett St., Leeds LS9 7TF Tel: 0113 206 4001 Fax: 0113 206 4001; Glebe House, Scholes Lane, Scholes, Leeds LS15 4NE — MB ChB Leeds 1979; FRCA Eng. 1983. Cons. Pain Managem. & Anaesth. St. Jas. Univ. Hosp. Leeds. Specialty: Anaesth.

SIMPSON, Karen Louise 53 Fairfield Road, Newcastle upon Tyne NE2 3BY Tel: 0191 281 6229 — MB BS Newc. 1991; FRCA 1998. SHO Anaesth. Freeman Newc. Specialty: Anaesth. Prev: Ho. Off. (Gen. Med.) S. Cleveland Hosp.; Ho. Off. (Gen. Surg.) S. Tyneside Dist. Hosp.

SIMPSON, Kathryn Lisa 46 Wentworth Road, Dronfield Woodhouse, Sheffield S18 8ZU — MB ChB Leeds 1991; DRCOG 1995; MRCGP 1996. Prev: GP/Regist Windsor.

SIMPSON, Kathryn Rose 71 Lochmaben Road, Glasgow G52 3NG — MB ChB Glas. 1998; MB ChB Glas 1998.

SIMPSON, Kenneth 6 Springfield Road, Leicester LE2 3BA Tel: 0116 270 7968 — MD Lond. 1951 (Guy's) MB BS 1948; FRCP Lond. 1974, M 1951. Emerit. Cons. Paediat. Leicester Area. Specialty: Paediat. Socs: Brit. Paediat. Assn. Prev: Sen. Regist. Bristol Roy. Hosp. Sick Childr.; Regist. St. Thos. Hosp.; Ho. Phys. Hosp. Sick Childr. Gt. Ormond St.

SIMPSON, Kenneth James Royal Infirmary, Scottish Liver Transplantation Unit, Edinburgh EH13 4SA — MB ChB (Hons.) Dundee 1983; BMSc (Hons.) Dundee 1980; MRCP (UK) 1986; MSc Lond. 1988; MD Dundee 1990; PhD Edin. 1997; FRCS Ed. 2000. Sen. Lect.(Hepat.), Div. of Clin. & Surgic. Servs., Univ. Edin.; Hon. Cons. Phys., Scott. Liver Transpl.ation Unit, Roy. Infirm., Edin. Socs: Brit. Assn. of Study of the Liver; Europ. Assn. of Study of the Liver; Amer. Assn. of Study of the Liver. Prev: MRC Trav. Fell. Univ. of Michigan, Michigan, USA; Sen. Regist. and Lect. in Med., Roy. Infirm., Edin.; Regist., Liver Unit, Kings Coll. Hosp. Lond.

SIMPSON, Kenneth Malcolm 62 Hillfield Court, Belsize Avenue, London NW3 4BG — MB BS Lond. 1958; MRCS Eng. LRCP Lond. 1958.

SIMPSON, Kirsty Elizabeth 14 Kingsmeadows Gardens, Peebles EH45 9LB — MB ChB Glas. 1998; MB ChB Glas 1998.

SIMPSON, Linda The Surgery, Bissoe Road, Camon Downs, Truro TR3 6LD — MB BS Newc. 1991 (Univ. of Newc. Upon Tyne) DRCOG 1994; MRCGP 1995; DFFP 1995; MSc Univ. Glasgow 1999. Retained Gen. Practitioner, 18 Lemon St, Truro. Specialty: Gen. Pract.

SIMPSON, Lynsey Nicola Flat 2 Right, 75 Queen Margaret Drive, Glasgow G20 8PA — MB ChB Glas. 1991.

SIMPSON, Mari Rebecca (retired) 53 Elms Road, Stoneygate, Leicester LE2 3JD Tel: 0116 270 5661 — MRCS Eng. LRCP Lond. 1947 (Camb. & Bristol) MA Camb. 1945, MB BChir 1947. Assoc. Specialist Neurol. Leicester Roy. Infirm. & Derby Roy. Infirm. Prev: Sen. Med. Off. Family Plann. Assn. (Leicester Br.).

SIMPSON, Marie Patricia Alexandria Medical Centre, Bank St., Alexandria G83 0LS Tel: 01382 756029; 99 Drymen Road, Bearsden, Glasgow G61 3RP Tel: 0141 942 6243 — (University of Glasgow) MB ChB Glas. 1968; DObst RCOG 1970; MFFP 1993. Prev: SCMO Domiciliary Family Plann. Glas.

SIMPSON, Marion Lordswood House, 54 Lordswood Road, Harborne, Birmingham B17 9DB Tel: 0121 426 2030 Fax: 0121 428 2658; 55 Wentworth Road, Harborne, Birmingham B17 9SS Tel: 0121 427 2945 — MB ChB Birm. 1971. Specialty: Paediat.

SIMPSON, Mark David Charles 6 Cambridge Road, Middlesbrough TS5 5NQ — MB ChB Dundee 1990. SHO (Gen. Surg.) Darlington Memor. Hosp. Prev: SHO (A & E) Leicester Roy. Infirm.; SHO (Orthop. & Trauma) Northampton; Ho. Off. (Gen. Med.) Cleveland.

SIMPSON, Mark James The Surgery, Lorne Street, Lochgilphead PA31 8LU Tel: 01546 602921 Fax: 01546 606735; (resid.) Drimlussa, Kilduskland Road, Ardrishaig, Lochgilphead PA30 8EQ Tel: 01546 3297 — (Ed.) BSc Ed. 1976, MB ChB 1979; DCH Glas. 1982; DRCOG 1983; MRCGP 1986. Prev: GP Trainee Pembs. VTS; Ho. Phys. & Ho. Surg. at Roy. Infirm Edin.

SIMPSON, Mary Bradford Hopefield, Wannock Road, Polegate BN26 5EA Tel: 01323 483851 — MB ChB Glas. 1956; DA Eng. 1962; DPH Eng. 1967; MFCM 1979; DHMSA 1993.

SIMPSON, Maureen June Townhead Practice, Links Health Centre, Montrose DD10 8TR; St Monans, 3 Hayshead Road, Arbroath DD11 5AZ Tel: 01241 879184 — MB ChB Aberd. 1986; DRCOG 1990; MRCGP 1993. Locum GP, Queensland, Australia. Prev: GP, Gibraltar; Long-term Locum GP Dargaville, New Zealand; Assoc. GP I. of Mull.

SIMPSON, Michael Menzies (retired) Birch Hill, Backies, Golspie KW10 6SE Tel: 01408 633414 — MB ChB Ed. 1959; DObst RCOG 1962; FRCGP 1993, M 1980. Prev: Clin. Asst. (Geriat.) Cambusavie Unit Golspie.

SIMPSON, Mr Michael Thomas Lonach, 8A Bushmead Avenue, Bedford MK40 3QL Tel: 01234 214998 Fax: 01234 214998 — MB BS Lond. 1981; BDS 1973; MRCS Eng. LRCP Lond. 1981; FFD 1984. Cons. Oral & Maxillofacial Surg. Milton Keynes Hosp., Bedford Gen. Hosp. & Lister Hosp. Stevenage; Cons. to various private Hosp.s. Specialty: Oral & Maxillofacial Surg. Socs: BMA; BDA; Brit. Assn. Hand and Neck Oncologists. Prev: Sen. Regist. St. Geo. Hosp.; Sen. Regist. Chichester Hosp. St Richards; Sen. Regist. (Oral & Maxillofacial Surg.) St. Thos. Hosp. Lond.

SIMPSON, Moira-Jane Mackay 15 Suffolk Road, Edinburgh EH16 5NR Tel: 0131 667 2614 — MB ChB Aberd. 1995. Specialty: Gen. Pract.

SIMPSON, Neil 64 Moorside S., Fenham, Newcastle upon Tyne NE4 9BB — MB ChB Leeds 1987.

SIMPSON, Neil 60 Meadowbank Road, Kirknewton EH27 8BS — MB ChB Ed. 1993. SHO (Med.) Roy. Infirm. Edin. Prev: SHO (Cas.) Roy. Infirm. Edin.; SHO (Surg.) St. Johns Hosp. Livingston; SHO (Med.) West. Gen. Hosp. Edin.

SIMPSON, Neill John Gartnavel Royal Hospital , Greater Glasgow Primary Care NHS Trust, The West House, 1055 Great Western Road, Glasgow G12 0XH Tel: 0141 211 3530 Email: neill.simpson@glacomen.scot.nhs.uk — MB ChB Ed. 1977; MRCPsych 1982; MSC Psych. Manch. 1984; PhD 1999; FRCPsych 2003. Cons. Psychiat. (Learning Disabil.) Gartnavel Roy. Hosp. Glas.; Hon. Sen. Clin. Lect. Univ. Glas. Specialty: Ment. Health. Prev: Cons. Psychiat. (Learning Disabil.) Borders Primary Care NHS Trust; Cons. Psychiat. (Learning Disabil.) Centre Manch. Healthcare Trust; Hon. Clin. Lect. (Psychiat.) & Hon. Research Fell. Univ. of Manch.

SIMPSON, Nicholas Barry Department of Dermatology, Royal Victoria Infirmary, Newcastle upon Tyne NE1 4LP Tel: 0191 282 4597 Fax: 0191 227 5058 Email: nick.simpson@ncl.ac.uk — MB BCh Wales 1971; MD Wales 1981; FRCP Glas. 1990; FRCP Lond. 1992. Cons. Dermat. Roy. Vict. Infirm. Newc. u. Tyne. Specialty: Dermat. Prev: Sen. Lect. & Cons. Dermat. Roy. Vict. Infirm. Newc. u Tyne; Cons. Dermat. Glas. Roy. Infirm.; Sen. Regist. (Dermat.) Leeds Gen. Infirm.

SIMPSON, Mr Nicholas Harold Randell Barrow Health Centre, 27 High Street, Barrow on Soar, Loughborough LE12 8PY Tel: 01509 413525 Fax: 01509 620664; Walnut Tree House, 15 The Pingle, Woodhouse Road, Quorn, Loughborough LE12 8AJ Tel: 01509 621078 — MB BS Lond. 1976 (St. Mary's Hosp. Med. Sch.) MA Oxf. 1977; FRCS Eng. 1981; DRCOG 1982.

SIMPSON, Mr Nigel Alastair Buist Leeds General Infirmary, Academic Division of Obstetrics & Gynaecology, D Floor, Clarendon Wing, Belmont Grove, Leeds LS2 9NS Tel: 0113 392 3901 Fax: 0113 392 6021 Email: n.a.b.simpson@leeds.ac.uk — MB BS Lond. 1986 (St Thomas's Hosp. Med. Sch.) MRCOG 1993. Sen. Lect. & Hon. Cons. in Obst. & Gyn., Leeds Gen. Infirm. Specialty: Obst. & Gyn. Prev: Lect. & Hon. Sen. Regist., St. James Univ. Hosp., Leeds 1996-99; Reseach Fell. Div. of Perinatology, Ottawa Gen. Hosp., Ottawa 1993-96; 3) Regist., St Bart. Hosp., Lond., 1991-93.

SIMPSON, Mr Nigel Shaun 6 Greenstone Place, Dundee DD2 4XB — MB BCh BAO Belf. 1984; FRCS Ed. 1988.

SIMPSON, Noel Robert Wyndham (retired) 53 Elms Road, Stoneygate, Leicester LE2 3JD — MB BS Lond. 1946 (St. Mary's) MRCS Eng. LRCP Lond. 1942; DPhysMed. Eng. 1948. Prev: Cons. (Rheum. & Rehabil.) Leics. AHA (T).

SIMPSON, Patricia Hill Crest, Wigan Road, Leyland, Preston PR25 2UD Tel: 01772 424571 Fax: 01772 424571 Email: alpat@btinternet.com — MB ChB Manch. 1966; DA Eng. 1968; MSc (Audiol. Med.) Manch. 1992. Specialty: Paediat.; Audiol. Med. Socs: FRCPCH. Prev: SCMO Wigan HA; Cons. Paediat. (Community Audiol.) Wigan & Leigh Health Servs. NHS Trust.

SIMPSON, Paul David Station House Surgery, Station Road, Kendal LA9 6SA Tel: 01539 722660 Fax: 01539 734845; Oak Bank Mill, Skelsmergh, Kendal LA8 9AQ Tel: 01539 720764 — MB BS Newc. 1986; MRCGP 1990; Cert. Family Plann. JCC 1990. Prev: GP Windermere.

SIMPSON, Peter Butler (retired) 8 High Drive, New Malden KT3 3UG Tel: 020 8942 7472 — MB ChB Leeds 1954. Med. Off. Health Control Unit Heathrow Airport Lond. Prev: GP Kuala Lumpar.

SIMPSON, Peter Jeffery Frenchay Hospital, Department of Anaesthetics, Frenchay, Bristol BS16 1LE Tel: 0117 970 2020 Fax: 0117 904 8725; 2 St Hilary Close, Stoke Bishop, Bristol BS9 1DA Tel: 0117 968 1537 Fax: 0117 904 8725 Email: psimpson@blueyonder.co.uk — MB BS Lond. 1970 (St Bart.) MRCS Eng. LRCP Lond. 1970; FFA RCS Eng. 1975; MD Lond. 1978. Cons. Anaesth. Frenchay Hosp. Bristol; Sen. Clin. Lect. (Anaesth.) Univ. Bristol.; Pres. Roy. Coll. Anaesth. Specialty: Anaesth. Special Interest: Neuroanaesthesia; Neuro-radiology. Socs: Assn. Anaesth.; RSM.

SIMPSON, Peter Michael (retired) 28 Elwyn Road, Sutton Coldfield B73 6LB Tel: 0121 321 3284 — MB ChB Birm. 1961 (Birmingham) DObst RCOG 1966; FRCA Eng. 1975. Prev: Cons. Anaesth. Solihull Hosp. & Marston Green Hosp. Birm.

SIMPSON, Peter Michael Andrew Bodmin Road Health Centre, Bodmin Road, Ashton on Mersey, Sale M33 5JH Tel: 0161 962 4625 Fax: 0161 905 3317 — MB ChB Manch. 1980; DRCOG 1983; MRCGP 1984.

SIMPSON, Philip Millbrook, Guelles Road, St Peter Port, Guernsey GY1 2DB — MB ChB Manch. 1978; MRCP (UK) 1982.

SIMPSON, Rachael Joanne 80 Wroxham Road, Norwich NR7 8EX Tel: 01603 410523 — MB ChB Leeds 1994. SHO (Orthop.) Sheff. Childr. Hosp. & N. Gen. Hsop. Sheff. Specialty: Orthop. Prev: Demonst. (Anat.) Leeds; SHO (Transpl. Surg.) St. Jas. Hosp. Leeds.

SIMPSON, Mr Ralph Nelson Robert Springbank Surgery, York Road, Green Hammerton, York YO26 8BN Tel: 01423 330030 Fax: 01423 331433; 6 Springfield Rise, Great Ouseburn, York YO26 9SE Tel: 01423 331410 Email: ralph.simpson@virgin.net — MB BS Newc. 1980 (Newcastle u Tyne) FRCS Ed. 1985; DRCOG 1987; Cert Family Plann 1987; MRCGP 1987. Specialty: Gen. Pract.

SIMPSON, Rhian Margaret Clinical Gerontology, University of Cambridge, School of Clinical Medcine, Addenbrooke's Hospital, Cambridge CB2 2QQ; 45 Rathmore Road, Cambridge CB1 7AB — MB BS Lond. 1990; MRCP (UK) 1993; MPhil Camb. 1995. Clin. Research Assoc. (Gerontol.) Addenbrooke's Hosp. Camb. Specialty: Care of the Elderly. Prev: Regist. (Geriat. & Gen. Med.) P'boro. Hosp.

SIMPSON, Richard Alistair Peter House Surgery, Captain Lees Road, Westhoughton, Bolton BL5 3UB Tel: 01942 812525 Fax: 01942 813431; 305 Wigan Lane, Wigan WN1 2QY Tel: 01942 496635 Email: ras@doctors.net.uk — MB ChB Manch. 1985; DRCOG 1988; MRCGP 1989; Dip. Oca. Med. 2000. Specialty: Gen. Pract.; Occupat. Health. Socs: Bolton Med. Soc. Prev: Trainee GP Salford VTS.

SIMPSON, Robert Anthony (retired) 23 Larkhill, Rushden NN10 6BG Tel: 01933 314952 — (Newc.) MB BS Durh. 1951. Prev: Clin. Asst. Electromyog. N. Staffs. Roy. Infirm. Stoke-on-Trent.

SIMPSON, Robert Arthur Hyem (retired) 37 Tartane Lane, Dymchurch, Romney Marsh TN29 0LJ Tel: 01303 872052 — MRCS Eng. LRCP Lond. 1940 (St. Bart.) Prev: Temp. Surg. Lt. R.N.V.R. 1940-46.

SIMPSON, Robert Burgoyne Royal Alexandria Hospital, Corsebar Road, Paisley PA2 9PN Tel: 0141 887 9111 — MB ChB Glas. 1991; BSc (Hons.) Glas. 1988; FRCA Lond. 1995. Cons. Anaestetist, RAM, Paisley. Specialty: Anaesth. Socs: Glas. W. of Scot. Soc. of Anaesth.; BMA; MDDUS. Prev: SHO (Anaesth.) Roy. Alexandra Hosp. Paisley; Specialist Regist. (Anaesth.) Vict. Infirm. Glas.

SIMPSON, Robert Cyril North Street Surgery, 22 North Street, Ilminster TA19 0DG Tel: 01460 52284 Fax: 01460 57233 — MB BCh BAO Dub. 1960; MRCGP 1972.

SIMPSON, Robert David 5 Church Farm Lane, Sidlesham, Chichester PO20 7RE Tel: 01243 641321 Fax: 01243 641321 — MB BChir Camb. 1965 (St. Mary's) MA Camb. 1970, BA 1962; MRCP (UK) 1970; FRCP Lond. 1990. Cons. Phys. St. Richards Hosp. Chichester.; Clin. Teach. St. Mary's Hosp. Paddington. Specialty: Diabetes; Endocrinol.; Gen. Med. Socs: Brit. Diabetic Assn.; Brit. Endocrine Soc.; Eur. Assn. Study Diabetes. Prev: Lect. Metab. Unit St. Mary's Hosp. Paddington; Sen. Regist. (Med.) Radcliffe Infirm. Oxf.; Regist. (Med.) St. Mary's Hosp. Paddignton.

SIMPSON, Mr Robert Gavin 20 Whittingehame Drive, Glasgow G12 0XX Tel: 0141 339 0504 — MB ChB Glas. 1967; FRCS Ed. 1972.

SIMPSON, Robert Ian Dyer (retired) Dean Wood House, Woodcote, Reading RG8 0PL Tel: 01491 681593 — (St. Bart.) Cert. Contracep. & Family Plann. RCOG, RCGP &; MB BS Lond. 1958; MRCS Eng. LRCP Lond. 1958; DObst RCOG 1960; MRCGP 1968; Cert FPA 1975. Prev: Ho. Phys., Ho. Surg. & Sen. Obst. Intern. St. Bart. Hosp. Lond.

SIMPSON, Robert Loudon, TD (retired) 105 Brierton Lane, Owton Manor, Hartlepool TS25 5DW Tel: 01429 274724 — MB ChB Ed. 1949. Prev: Ho. Phys. Roy. Infirm. Edin.

SIMPSON, Robert McDonald Paediatric Department, Dumfries and Galloway Royal Infirmary, Bankend Road, Dumfries DG1 4AP Tel: 01387 246246 Fax: 01387 241831 — MB ChB Ed. 1973 (Edinburgh) DCH Eng. 1976; MRCGP 1978; FRCP Ed. 1990; FRCPCH 1998. Cons. (Paediat.) Dumfries & Galloway HB; Post Grad. tutor, Dumfries and Galloway Roy. Inf. Specialty: Paediat. Prev: Sen. Regist. (Paediat.) Aberdeen.

SIMPSON, (Robert) Neil Child Health Department, Newbridge Hill, Bath BA1 3QE Tel: 01225 731500 Email: neil.simpson@banes-pct.nhs.uk; 19 Fairfield Park Road, Bath BA1 6JW — MB BS Lond. 1988 (St. Bartholomews) DCH RCP Lond. 1991; MRCP (UK) 1992; DRCOG 1993; MSc- Health Policy, Planning and Financing, Lond. 1998; FPHM Part 1, U.K 1998. Cons. Paediat. Community Child Health, Bath. Specialty: Paediat. Socs: MRCPCH.

SIMPSON, Robin Gordon, Col. L/RAMC SO 1 Med, Primary Care, Army Medical Directorate, The Former Staff College, Slim Road, Camberley GU15 4NP — MB ChB Aberd. 1983; MRCGP 1987; DRCOG 1990; MFFP 1995; FRCCP 2000; D Occ Med 2001; MSc 2003. Regional Clin. Director Primary Care Lond. & SE Eng.; MRCGP Examr. & Mem. Oral Developm. Gp. Prev: SO1 Med Primary Care Army Med. Directorate; Regional Clin. Director MRS Fennelgan; Sen. Med. Off. EPIS KOPI BFPU 53.

SIMPSON, Roderick Howard Wallace Royal Devon & Exeter Hospitals, Area Department of Pathology, Church Lane, Heavitree, Exeter EX2 5DY Tel: 01392 402941 Fax: 01392 402964 Email: roderick.simpson@virgin.net — MB ChB Dundee 1974; BSc St. And. 1972; MMed (Anat. Path.) Stellenbosch 1981; FRCPath 1996, M 1983. Cons. Histopath., Roy. Devon and Exeter Hosp., Exeter. Specialty: Histopath. Socs: Sec., Europ. Soc. of Path. Prev: Cons. & Sen. Lect. Histopath. Roy. Devon & Exeter Hosp. & Univ. Exeter.; Cons. & Sen. Lect. (Histopath. & Neuropath.) Univ. Witwatersrand Johannesburg, S. Africa; Regist. (Anat. Path.) Tygerberg Hosp. Cape Town, S. Africa.

SIMPSON, Roger James South Cheshire Health Authority, 1829 Building, Countess of Chester, Health Park, Liverpool Road, Chester CH2 1UL Tel: 01244 650342 Fax: 01244 650341 — MB ChB Manch. 1981; MFCM 1987; FFPHM 1997, MFPHM 1989; MPhil Bath 1990. Dir. Pub. Health S. Chesh. HA; Hon. Lect. Liverp. Univ. Specialty: Pub. Health Med. Socs: Treas. Assn. Directors of Pub. Health; Chester & N. Wales Med. Soc. Prev: Dir. Pub. Health Chester & Wirral HAs; Cons. Pub. Health Med. W. Berks. HA; Sen. Regist. (Community Med.) Wessex RHA.

SIMPSON, Roland Lee Brook House Surgery, 98 Oakley Road, Shirley, Southampton SO16 4NZ Tel: 023 8077 4851 Fax: 023 8032 2357 — BM Soton. 1981; DCH RCP Lond. 1985; DRCOG 1987; MRCGP 1988. Prev: SHO (O & G) King's Mill Hosp. Mansfield; SHO (Geriat. & Paediat.) Nottm. Univ. Hosp.; Clin. Med. Off. (Community Paediat.) Nottm.

SIMPSON, Ronald Duncairn Gardens Surgery, 36 Duncairn Gardens, Belfast BT15 2GH — MB BCh BAO Belf. 1980.

SIMPSON, Rosalind Margaret Brook House Surgery, 98 Oakley Road, Shirley, Southampton SO16 4NZ Tel: 023 8077 4851 Fax: 023 8032 2357; 59 Brookvale Road, Highfield, Southampton

SO17 1QS Tel: 02380 900640 Fax: 01703 900650 — BM Soton. 1981; DRCOG 1985; Cert. Family Plann. JCC 1985; MRCGP 1987. Clin. Asst. (Rheum.) Soton.; Med. Attendants Alcohol Unit & Homeless Unit Soton. Specialty: Gen. Pract. Prev: Trainee GP Nottm. VTS.

SIMPSON, Ruth 22 Norrishill Drive, Heaton Norris, Stockport SK4 2NN — MB ChB Aberd. 1986; FRCS Eng. 1990. Regist. Rotat. (Gen. Surg.) S. Manch. HA. Specialty: Gen. Surg. Prev: SHO Rotat. (Gen. Surg.) S. Manch. HA.

SIMPSON, Seonaid Anne The Surgery, Grove Street, Petworth GU28 0LP Tel: 01292 476626; 4 Grey Gables, Southwood Road, Troon KA9 1UR — MB ChB Aberd. 1982; DRCOG 1984; MRCGP 1986.

SIMPSON, Sheelagh Margaret (retired) Kingsbridge, 32 Silverdale Road, Gatley, Cheadle SK8 4QS — MB ChB Manch. 1954; DObst RCOG 1956; MFFP 1993. Prev: Med. Off. Manch. & Dist. & Wilmslow & Dist. Family Plann. Clinics.

SIMPSON, Sheila Anne Clinical Genetics, Argyll House, Foresterhill, Cornhill Road, Aberdeen AB25 2ZR Tel: 01244 552120 Fax: 01244 559390 Email: s.a.simpson@abdn.ac.uk — MB ChB Aberd. 1974; DObst RCOG 1976; DCH RCPS Glas. 1977; BSc (Hons.) Aberd. 1987; MD Aberd. 1992. Assoc. Specialist in Clin. Genetics, Grampian Univ. Hosp. Aberd. Specialty: Clinical Genetics. Special Interest: Huntington's Dis.; Med. Ethics. Socs: Brit. Soc. Human Genetics; World Federat. Neurol. HD Research Gp.; Chair, Grampian Research Ethics Comm.

SIMPSON, Stephen William Department of Old Age Psychiatry, Forston Clinic, Dorchester DT2 9TB — MB ChB Aberd. 1987; MRCPsych 1992. Sen. Regist. (Psychiat.) Manch. Roy. Infirm. Specialty: Geriat. Psychiat. Prev: Lect. (Psychiat.) & Hon. Sen. Regist. Withington Hosp.; Sen. Regist. (Neuropsychiat.) MRI Manch.; Regist. (Forens. Med.) St. Brendan's Hosp. Bermuda.

SIMPSON, Thomas David — MB ChB Bristol 1977; BSc (Hons.) Bristol 1974; FRCP Ed. 1997, M (UK) 1981; MRCPsych 1983; T(Psych) 1991; FRCPsych 1999. Cons. (Child & Adolesc. Psych) Tavistock Clinic Lond.; Private Prac. (Psycho-Anal.); Hon. Sen. Lect. (Child & Adolesc. Psychiat.) Roy. Free Hosp. Lond. Specialty: Child & Adolesc. Psychiat. Socs: Mem. Brit. Psychoanalyt. Soc. Prev: Cons. (Child & Adolesc. Psychiat.) Watford Child & Family Clinic; Cons. (Child & Adolesc. Psychiat.) Barnet Healthcare Trust; Sen. Regist. Maudsley Hosp. Lond.

SIMPSON, Thomas James Peter Department of Anaesthesia, Royal United Hospital, Coombe Park, Bath BA1 3NG Tel: 01225 825057 Email: tom.simpson@ruh.swest.nhs — MB BS Lond. 1991 (St. Mary's Hosp. Lond.) BSc Lond. 1988; FRCA 1996. Cons. Anaesth., Roy. United Hosp., Bath. Specialty: Anaesth.; Paediat. Prev: Specialist Regist. (Anaesth.) SW Region, Bristol.

SIMPSON, Thomas William Old Machar Medical Practice, 526 King Street, Aberdeen AB24 5RS Tel: 01224 480324 Fax: 01224 276121; 147 Blenheim Place, Aberdeen AB25 2DL Tel: 01224 641623 — MB ChB Aberd. 1964; DA Eng. 1968. Prev: Regist. (Anaesth.) NE RHB (Scotl.); Ho. Phys. Dumfries Roy. Infirm.; Ho. Surg. (Thoracic Surg.) Woodend Hosp. Aberd.

SIMPSON, Victoria Margaret Anne Fernlea, West End Lane, Henfield BN5 9RA — MB BS Lond. 1997; BSc; MRCP.

SIMPSON, William (retired) Glen Cottage, Glen Road, Dunblane FK15 0DJ Tel: 01786 823248 — MB ChB Glas. 1958 (Univ. Glas.) Prev: Ho. Surg. & Ho. Phys. Roy. Infirm. Glas.

SIMPSON, William 64 Moorside S., Newcastle upon Tyne NE4 9BB — MB ChB Ed. 1958; DMRD Eng. 1964; FFR 1966; FRCR 1975. Cons. Radiol. Newc. Gen. Hosp. Specialty: Radiol. Prev: Sen. Regist. Roy. Vict. Infirm. Newc.; Ho. Phys. Edin. Roy. Infirm.; Capt. RAMC.

SIMPSON, Mr William Alasdair Cumming (retired) Stirling Royal Infirmary, Livilands, Stirling FK8 2AU Tel: 01786 73151 — MB BS Lond. 1974 (Guy's) FRCOphth.; BSc Toronto 1969; MRCS Eng. LRCP Lond. 1974; FRCS (Ophth.) Ed. 1981. Cons. Ophth. Stirling Roy. Infirm., Falkirk & Dist. Roy. Infirm.; Cons. Ophth. King's Pk. Hosp. Stirling. Prev: Hon. Sen. Regist. & Fell. Moorfields Eye Hosp. Lond.

SIMPSON, William Allan (retired) Flat 15, Craiglockhart Court, 75 Lockharton Avenue, Edinburgh EH14 1BD Tel: 0131 443 1326 — (Univ. Ed.) MB ChB Ed. 1951; DPH Ed. 1955; MFCM 1972. Prev: MOH Co. W. Lothian.

SIMPSON, William George Salisbury House, Queen Street, Ballymena BT42 2BD — MB BCh BAO Belf. 1962. Apptd. Fact. Doctor. Specialty: Gen. Pract.

SIMPSON, William Gordon Aberdeen Royal Infirmary, Department of Clinical Biochemistry, Aberdeen AB25 2ZD Tel: 01224 681818 Ext: 54620 Fax: 01224 694378 Email: w.g.simpson@arh.grampian.scot.nhs.uk — MB ChB Glas. 1984; MRCPath 1994; FRCPath 2002. Cons. (Clin. Biochem.ry) Grampian Univ. Hosps. Trust. Specialty: Chem. Path. Prev: Sen. Regist. (Clin. Biochem.ry) Grampian HB.

SIMPSON, William Scott Health Centre, The Glebe, Kirkliston EH29 9AS Tel: 0131 333 3215 Email: drscottsimpson@totalise.co.uk — MB ChB Edinburgh 1978; MRCGP 1982. GP Kirkliston, W. Lothian.

SIMPSON-WHITE, Robert (retired) The Old Rectory, English Bicknor, Coleford GL16 7PQ Tel: 01594 861113 — MB ChB Bristol 1947; FRCGP 1979, M 1955. GP. Prev: Hosp. Pract. (Psychogeriat.) Moorhaven Hosp. Ivybridge.

SIMPSON-WHITE, Robert William Carroll 2 Boyce Street, Sheffield S6 3JS Tel: 0114 233 9645 — MB ChB Sheff. 1998; MA Cantab 1997; MRCS Ed. 2003. Ho. Off. Rotherham Dist. Gen. Specialty: Gen. Med.

SIMS, Adrian John 951 Manchester Road, Bury BL9 8DN Tel: 0161 766 3255 — MB BS Lond. 1951 (St. Bart.) MRCS Eng. LRCP Lond. 1951; DA Eng. 1953; FFA RCS Eng. 1956. Cons. Anaesth. Bury & Rossendale Hosp. Gp. & Sch. Dent. Serv. Lancs. CC. Specialty: Anaesth. Prev: Capt. RAMC, Jun. Specialist Anaesth.; Anaesth. Regist. Chelmsford Hosp. Gp.; Sen. Ho. Off. (Anaesth.) S.E. Essex Hosp. Gp.

SIMS, Professor Andrew Charles Petter Division of Psychiatry, St. James's University Hospital, Leeds LS9 7TF Tel: 0113 206 5646 Fax: 0113 243 5053 — (Westm.) MB BChir Camb. 1963; MRCS Eng. LRCP Lond. 1963; DObst RCOG 1965; DPM Eng. 1969; FRCPsych 1979, M 1971; MA Camb. 1964, MD 1974; MD Lambeth 1995; FRCP Ed. 1993, Lond. 1997. Prof. Psychiat. Univ. Leeds; Cons. Psychiat. St. Jas. Univ. Hosp. Leeds. Specialty: Gen. Psychiat. Socs: Fell. Roy. Soc. Med.; Christ. Med. Fellowsh.; Assn Europ. Psychiat. Prev: Pres. & Deans Dir., Continuing Professional Developm. Roy. Coll. Psychiat.; Cons. Psychiat. & Sen. Lect. Qu. Eliz. Hosp. Birm. & Univ. Birm.; Cons. Psychiat. All St.s' Hosp. Birm.

SIMS, Brian Alexander (retired) 2 Orchard Hill, Gracehill, Ballymena BT42 1JP Tel: 028 2564 3463 — MB BCh BAO Belf. 1964; MD Belf. 1968; MRCP (UK) 1970; FRCP 1987. Prev: Cons. Phys. Antrim Area Hosp. & Waveney Hosp. Ballymena.

SIMS, Charles David Petter Child and family unit, Hillbrook, Mayfield Road, Keighley BD20 6LD Tel: 01535 661531 — MB BChir Camb. 1990; MA Camb. 1991. Specialty: Child & Adolesc. Psychiat. Socs: Roy. Coll. Psychiat.

SIMS, Mr Colin David 82 Harley Street, London W1G 7HN Tel: 020 7636 2766 Fax: 020 7631 5371; Huntley Cottage, 29 The Downs, Wimbledon, London SW20 8HG Tel: 020 8946 1978 — (Westm.) MB Camb. 1963, BChir 1962; FRCS Ed. 1969; FRCOG 1987, M 1973. Cons. Gyn. Char. Cross & Chelsea & Westm. Hosp. Lond.; Cons. O & G Qu. Charlotte's & Chelsea Hosp. for Wom. Lond. Retd.

SIMS, Diana Elizabeth Barton Surgery, Barton, Horn Lane, Plymouth PL9 9BR Tel: 01752 407129 Fax: 01752 482620 — MB ChB Liverp. 1969; DA Eng. 1973. Prev: Regist. (Anaesth.) Plymouth Gen. Hosp.; Ho. Phys. & Surg. St. Bernards Hosp. Gibraltar; Ho. Phys. & Surg. Whiston Hosp. Prescot.

SIMS, Don Graham 45 Glenmore Drive, Kings Norton, Birmingham B38 8YR — MB ChB Birm. 1996.

SIMS, Douglas Gordon (retired) St Mary's Hospital, Hathersage Rd, Manchester M13 0JH Tel: 0161 276 6543 Fax: 0161 276 6536 — MB ChB Bristol 1966; DObst RCOG 1968; MRCP (UK) 1972; FRCP Lond. 1987; FRCPCH 1997. Cons. Neonatologist. St. Mary's Hosp. Manch. (Retired). Prev: Sen. Regist. (Paediat.) St. Mary's Hosp. Manch.

SIMS, Eliot Craig Department of Radiotherapy, Oldchurch Hospital, Waterloo Road, Romford RM7 0BE Tel: 01708 708317 Fax: 01708 737690 — MB BChir Camb. 1993; MA Camb. 1994; MRCP 1996; FRCR 1999; MD 2003. Cons. Clin. Oncologist, Old Ch. Hosp., Rumford and King Geo. Hosp., Goodmayes; SpR Oncol., St

Bartholomew's Hosp., The Middlx. Hosp. Specialty: Oncol. Special Interest: Breast Cancer; CNS Tumours.

SIMS, Enoch Harrington, Surg. Cdr. RN Retd. (retired) The Mill, Swinbrook, Burford OX18 4DY Tel: 01993 823108; The Mill, Swinbrook, Burford OX18 4DY Tel: 01993 823108 — MB ChB Sheff. 1954; FRCP Ed. 1982, M 1968. Prev: Surg. Cdr. RN.

SIMS, Gwyneth Maclean (retired) 19 Milton Road, Ickenham, Uxbridge UB10 8NH Tel: 01895 633007 — MB BCh Wales 1942 (Cardiff) BSc Wales 1939, MD 1954; FRCPath 1970, M 1963. Prev: Cons. Path. Harefield & Northwood Gp. Hosps.

SIMS, Hemalini North End Medical Centre, 211 North End Road, London W14 9NP; 21 Cherrywood Drive, London SW15 6DS Tel: 020 8789 4989 — MB BS Lond. 1992; DRCOG 1996; DFFP 1996; MRCGP 1997. Specialty: Care of the Elderly. Prev: Clin. Asst. (Genitourin. Med.) Chelsea & Westm. Hosp.

SIMS, Justine Shirley Portchester Health Centre, West Street, Portchester, Fareham PO16 9TU — MB BCh Wales 1992; DRCOG 1994; DFFP 1994; MRCGP 1995. GP Princip. -Portsmouth and SE Hants.

SIMS, Michael Andrew Dipple Medical Centre, Wickford Avenue, Pitsea, Basildon SS13 3HQ Tel: 01268 555115 Fax: 01268 559935 — MB BS Lond. 1991.

SIMS, Miss Pamela Frances Hexham General Hospital, Hexham NE46 1QJ Tel: 01434 655655 Fax: 01434 655347; Ivy Cottage, Lowgate, Hexham NE46 2NN Tel: 01434 606700 Fax: 01434 606700 — (Cardiff) MB BCh Wales 1969; FRCS Eng. 1979; FRCOG 1994, M 1981. Vis. Cons. Roy. Vict. Infirm. Specialty: Obst. & Gyn. Socs: Brit. Soc. Colpos. & Cerv. Path. Prev: Sen. Regist. Rotat. (Obst & Gyn.) Newc. HA; Regist. (O & G) Hammersmith Hosp. Lond. & Luton & Dunstable Hosp.

SIMS, Professor Peter Anthony Maynes Orchard, Silver Street, Braunton EX33 2EN Tel: 01271 814933 Email: p.sims@sosi.net — MB BS Lond. 1969 (Guys) MSc (Social Med.) Lond. 1975, BSc (Hons.) Physiol. 1962; LDS RCS Eng. 1965; BDS Lond. 1965; MRCS Eng. LRCP Lond. 1969; MFCM 1976; MRCGP 1982; FFPHM RCP (UK) 1991. Consultancy work in Papua New Guinea and UK. Specialty: Pub. Health Med.; Gen. Pract. Socs: Fac. Comm. Health (Fell.). Prev: Prof. of Pub. Health Med., Div. of Pub. Health, The Sch. of Med., Papua New Guinea; Prof. Community Med. Univ. Zambia, Lusaka; Director Pub. Health N. Devon.

SIMS, Peter Justin 46 Pemdevon Road, Croydon CR0 3QN — MB BS Lond. 1992.

SIMS, Rebecca Jane Alexandra Catesby Lodge Farm, Catesby, Daventry NN11 6LB — BM BS Nottm. 1998 (Nottingham) BMedSci Nottm 1996; BM BS Nottm 1998. SHO (A&E) Addenbrookes - Camb. Specialty: Accid. & Emerg.; Gen. Med. Prev: SHO (Medicine) Queens Med. Centre Nottm. & South. Derbysh. NHS Trust; Research Regist. Renal Med. Nottm. City Hosp.

SIMS, Roy Thomas (retired) 7 Chestnut Close, Grayshott, Hindhead GU26 6LN — (Char. Cross) BSc Lond. 1952, MD 1967, MB BS 1955; MA Camb. 1957; MFCMI 1978.

SIMS, Ruth Marie Church Farm House, Bridgwork, Shropshire WV15 6ND Tel: 01746 780469 Fax: 01746 780469; Kidderminster Treatment Centre, Sawdley Road, Kidderminster Tel: 01562 823424 Ext: 53459 — LMSSA 1983 (Cambridge) MA Camb. 1967, MB BChir 1983; MRCPsych 1988; M.Psychotherapy 1992. Cons. Child & Adolesc. Psychiat. Specialty: Child & Adolesc. Psychiat.; Psychother. Socs: BMA; MDU; Assoc. of Family Therapists. Prev: Cons. Child and Adolesc. Psychiat., Wakefield, and Pontefract Community NHS Trust.

SIMS, Stanley Robert (retired) 5 St Peter's Close, Horton, Ilminster TA19 9RW — (St. Geo.) MB BS Lond. 1946. Prev: Asst. Chest Phys. P'boro. & Huntingdon Chest Clinic Areas.

SIMS WILLIAMS, Heather Gillian The Family Practice, Western College, Cotham Road, Bristol BS6 6DF Tel: 0117 946 6455 Fax: 0117 946 6410 — MB ChB Bristol 1970.

SIMSON, Mr Jay Nicholas Litton St. Richard's Hospital, Department of Colorectal Surgery, Spitalfield Lane, Chichester PO18 4SE Tel: 01243 831538 Fax: 01243 831683 Email: jnlsimson@rws-tr.nhs.uk — MB BChir Cantab. 1974; MA Cantab. 1973; MRCP (UK) 1976; FCS (SA) 1977; FRCS Eng. 1980; MChir Cantab. 1982; FRCP Lond. 2003. Cons. (Gen. & Colorectal) Surg. St. Richard's Hosp. Chichester; Cons. (Gen. & Colorectal) Surg. Chichester Nuffield Hosp. King Edwd. VII Hosp. Midhurst. Specialty: Gen. Surg. Socs: Roy. Soc. Med.; Assn. Surg.; Assn. Coloproctol. Of GB & Irel. Prev: Research Fell. Harvard Univ.; Sen. Regist. St. Mark's Hosp. Lond. & Guy's Hosp. Lond.

SIN, Julie Pui Yee — MB ChB Manch. 1990.

SINANAN, Rabindra Druva Kenneth 137 Strensall Road, Earswick, York YO32 9SJ — MB BCh BAO Belf. 1976; Dip Psych; DMPsych. Sen. Cons. Psychiat. - Learning Disabilities.

SINASON, Michael David Adrian Forest House Psychotherapy Clinic, Thorpe Coombe Hospital, 714 Forest Road, London E17 3HP Tel: 020 8535 6899 Fax: 020 8535 6849 — MB BS Lond. 1974 (Univ. Coll. Hosp.) BSc (Hons. Psychol.) Lond. 1971; MRCPsych 1979; T(Psych.) 1991. Private psychoanalytic pract. Lond.; Locum Cons. (Psychother.) Forest Hse. Psychother. Clinic Thorpe Coombe Hosp. Lond. Specialty: Psychother. Prev: Cons. Psychother. Willesden Centre for Psychol. Treatm. Willesden Hosp. Lond.; Cons. Psychother. Shenley Hosp.; Sen. Regist. Psychother, Maudsley Hosp., Lond.

SINCLAIR, Aisla Mary Robertha 9 Clarendon Place, Stirling FK8 2QW — MB BCh BAO Dub. 1970. Clin. Med. Off. Forth Valley Health Bd.; Med. Off. (Occupat.) Health Serv. Forth Valley HB. Specialty: Community Child Health. Prev: Regist. (Gen. Med.) Stoke Mandeville Hosp. Aylesbury; Ho. Off. Dr. Steevens' Hosp. Dub.; SHO (Gastroenterol.) Sir P. Dun's Hosp. Dub.

SINCLAIR, Alan George Huntly Health Centre, Jubilee Hospital, Bleachfield Street, Huntly AB54 8EX Tel: 01466 792116 Fax: 01466 794699; The Beeches, Deveron Road, Huntly AB54 8DU Tel: 01466 793625 — MB ChB Aberd. 1972; DA Eng. 1974; DObst RCOG 1975; MRCGP 1977; Cert. Family Plann. JCC 1981; ATLS 1995. Hosp. Practitioner Jubilee Community Hosp. Huntly.

SINCLAIR, Alan James University Department of Geriatric Medicine, Cardiff Royal Infirmary, Cardiff CF24 0SZ Tel: 029 2049 2233; Glenholm, Bradford Place, Penarth CF64 1AF — MB BS Lond. 1979 (St. Bart.) BSc (1st cl. Hons.) Lond. 1976, MD 1993, MB BS 1979; MRCS Eng. LRCP Lond. 1979; MRCP (UK) 1985; T(M) 1992. Sen. Lect. (Geriat. Med.) Univ. Wales Coll. of Med. Specialty: Care of the Elderly. Socs: Brit. Geriat. Soc.; Brit. Diabetic Assoc. Prev: Research Fell. & Regist. (Med.) St. Barts Hosp. Lond.; Lect. (Geriat. Med.) Univ. Birm.; Med. Regist. (Geriat.) Hammersmith Hosp. Lond.

SINCLAIR, Alison Alexandra McKenzie Medical Centre, 20 West Richmond Street, Edinburgh EH8 9DX Tel: 0131 667 2955; 27 Ormidale Terrace, Edinburgh EH12 6DY Tel: 0131 337 7693 — MB ChB Ed. 1982; DRCOG 1984; DCH RCP Lond. 1986; DCCH RCP Ed. 1986; MRCGP 1987. Clin. Lect. (Gen. Pract.) Univ. Edin. Specialty: Gen. Pract.

SINCLAIR, Alistair (retired) 9 Ash Grove, Messingham, Scunthorpe DN17 3QY — MB ChB Aberd. 1955; DIH Soc. Apoth. Lond. 1962; FFOM RCP Lond. 1985, M 1980. Prev: Chief Med. Off. Brit. Steel.

SINCLAIR, Allan (retired) Glendale, 13 Glasgow Road, Uddingston, Glasgow G71 7AU Tel: 01698 813578 — MB ChB Glas. 1952; DPM Eng. 1958; FRFPS Glas. 1960; FRCP Glas. 1976, M 1962; FRCPsych 1987, M 1971. Prev: Cons. Psychiat. Hartwood Hosp. Shotts & Monklands Dist. Gen. Hosp. Airdrie.

SINCLAIR, Allan Alexander Darwen Health Care 2000, Union Street, Darwen BB3 0DA Tel: 01254 778366 Fax: 01254 778367 — MB ChB Manch. 1988; BSc St. And. 1985; DGM RCP Lond. 1990; MRCGP 1993; Cert. Prescribed Equiv. Exp. JCPTGP 1993.

SINCLAIR, Amanda Susan The Surgery, 22 Shenley Green, Selly Oak, Birmingham B29 4HH Tel: 0121 475 7997 Fax: 0121 475 9239; Old Barn, Old Birmingham Road, Alvechurch, Birmingham B48 7TQ Tel: 0121 447 7206 Fax: 0121 447 7206 — MB ChB Birm. 1987; MRCGP 1991. Prev: Trainee GP BromsGr. & Redditch VTS.

SINCLAIR, Andrew Michael 199 Farley Road, Croydon CR2 7NP — MB BS Lond. 1998; MB BS Lond 1998.

SINCLAIR, Anne Department of Ophthalmology, Queen Margaret's Fife Acute Hospitals Trust, Whitefield Road, Dunfermline KY12 0SU Tel: 01383 623623 Fax: 01383 624156 — MB ChB Ed. 1979; DO Eng. 1981; FRCS Ed. 1992. Assoc. Specialist (Ophth.) Fife Acute Hosps. Trust. Specialty: Ophth. Prev: Staff Grade (Ophth.) Fife HB.

SINCLAIR, Anne-Marie 25 Garrygall, Castlebay HS9 5UH — MB ChB Glas. 1987.

SINCLAIR, Barbara Jane Higher Hewish, Muddiford, Barnstaple EX31 4HH — MB ChB Sheff. 1986; MRCGP 1990; DRCOG 1990.

GP Retainer Scheme Barnstaple. Prev: GP Clin. Asst. (Genitourin. Med.) Roy. Gwent Hosp. Newport; Trainee GP Doncaster VTS.

SINCLAIR, Barbara Louise 30 Lochinver Crescent, Dundee DD2 4UA — MB ChB Aberd. 1981.

SINCLAIR, Beatrice Margaret (retired) Kilkerry, 105 Beach Road, Hartford, Northwich CW8 3AB Tel: 01606 74335 — LRCP LRCS Ed. 1950; LRCP LRCS Ed. LRFPS Glas. 1950.

SINCLAIR, Beryl Euman (retired) 5 The Grove, Harrogate HG1 5NN — MB ChB Ed. 1948.

SINCLAIR, Catherine Margaret 66 Southlands Avenue, Standish, Wigan WN6 0TT — BM BS Nottm. 1998; BM BS Nottm 1998.

SINCLAIR, Catriona Jane 33 Runnymede, Nunthorpe, Middlesbrough TS7 0QL — MB ChB Dundee 1991.

SINCLAIR, Christopher Chalmer Ross Laundry Cottage, Habyn, Rogate, Petersfield GU31 5HS — MB BS Lond. 1982.

SINCLAIR, Colin David Calsayseat Medical Group, 44 Powis Place, Aberdeen AB25 3TS Tel: 01224 634345 Fax: 01224 562220; Newhills House, Newhills, Aberdeen AB21 9SQ Tel: 01224 714439 — MB ChB Aberd. 1971. Prev: Jun. Ho. Off. Stracathro Hosp. Brechin; SHO Aberd. Roy. Infirm.

SINCLAIR, Colin John 'Mazoe', 2 Grange Road, Ballymena BT42 2DS Tel: 028256 42743 — MB BCh BAO Belf. 1966 (Belf) DMRD Eng. 1970; FRCR 1972. Cons. Radiol. Waveney Hosp. & Mid Ulster Hosp. Specialty: Radiol.

SINCLAIR, Colin John Department of Anaesthetics, The Royal Infirmary of Edinburgh, Lauriston Place, Edinburgh EH3 9YW Tel: 0131 536 3706 Fax: 0131 229 0659 Email: colin.sinclair@ed.ac.uk; Viewforth, Broomieknowe, Lasswade EH18 1LN Tel: 0131 663 8868 — (Edinburgh) BSc 1973; MBChB 1976; FRCA 1980. Cons. Anaesth., Cardiothoracic Unit, Roy. Infirm. of Edin. Specialty: Anaesth.

SINCLAIR, Professor David Cecil (retired) Apartment 3, Netherby, 1 Netherby Road, Cults, Aberdeen AB15 9HL Tel: 01224 867151 — MB ChB St. And. 1937; MD St. And. 1947; DSc (Univ. West. Austral.) 1965; FRCS Ed. 1966. Prev: Emerit. Prof. Univ. W. Austral.

SINCLAIR, David Graeme Torbay Hospital, Torquay TQ2 7AA Tel: 01803 654888 Email: david.sinclair@nhs.net — MB ChB Birm. 1981; MRCP (UK) 1987; MD Birm. 1996; FRCP (Lond.) 1998. Cons. Phys. (Respirat. & Intens. Care Med.) Torbay Hosp. Specialty: Respirat. Med.; Intens. Care. Socs: Brit. Thorac. Soc.; Intens. Care Soc. Prev: Hon. Sen. Lect. (Critical Care) Nat. Heart & Lung Inst. Lond.

SINCLAIR, David James Jubilee Surgery, Barrys Meadow, High St Titchfield, Fareham PO14 4EH Tel: 01329 844220 Fax: 01329 841484 — MB BCh BAO Dub. 1975 (Trinity College, Dublin) DCH Dub. 1977; MRCPI 1983; MRCGP 1984. Hosp. Pract. (Cardiol.) St. Mary's Hosp. Portsmouth. Specialty: Cardiol.

SINCLAIR, David John MacGregor South Cleveland Hospital, Marton Road, Middlesbrough TS4 3BW Tel: 01642 850850; Highfield West End, Hutton Rudby, Yarm TS15 0DJ — MB ChB Aberd. 1971; MRCP (UK) 1974; FRCP Lond. 1988; FRCP Ed. 1989. Cons. Phys. Gen. & Respirat. Med. S. Cleveland Hosp. Middlesbrough. Specialty: Respirat. Med.

SINCLAIR, David Maxwell The Health Centre, Victoria Road, Leven KY8 4ET Tel: 01333 425656 Fax: 01333 422249 — MB ChB Ed. 1976; BSc (Med. Sci.) Ed. 1973, MB ChB 1976; DRCOG 1978; MRCGP 1980. Trainer (Gen. Pract.) Leven; Clin. Asst. Colposcopy Clinic N. Pk. Hosp. Kirkcaldy; Civil. Med. Pract. Army Careers Office Leven. Specialty: Obst. & Gyn. Socs: BMA & Anglo-French Med. Soc. Prev: Regist. (Gen. Med.) Vict. Hosp. Kirkcaldy; SHO (O & G) West. Gen. Hosp. Edin.; Ho. Phys. Leith Hosp. Edin.

SINCLAIR, Mr David William Division Biomedical Sciences (School of Biology), University of St Andrews, Bute Medical Buildings, St Andrews KY16 9TS Tel: 01334 463169 Fax: 01334 462144; 26 Drumcarrow Road, St Andrews KY16 8SE Tel: 01334 474349 — MB ChB St. And. 1972 (Univ. of St. Andrews) FRCS Ed. 1982; Dip. Med. Educat. Dund 1993. Sen. Lect. (Anat.) Div. of Med. Sci. Sch. Of Biol. Univ. St Andrews; Pro-Dean (Med. Sci.) Univ. St Andrews; Examr. (Anat.) RCS Edin. Specialty: Anat. Socs: Fell. Brit. Assn. Clin. Anat.; Anat. Soc. Prev: Regist. (Surg.) Lothian Health Bd.; Ho. Surg. Profess. (Surg. Unit) Dundee Roy. Infirm.; Demonst. (Human Morphol.) Univ. Nottm.

SINCLAIR, Derek Urquhart (retired) Royal Scottish National Hospital, Larbert FK5 4SD — MB ChB Glas. 1964; MA (Hons.) Glas. 1970; DPM Ed. & Glas. 1973; MRCGP 1975. Prev: Med. Dir. Centr. Scotl. Healthcare NHS Trust.

SINCLAIR, Donald Henderson (retired) 19 Welbeck Avenue, Kirk Hallam, Ilkeston DE7 4NL — LRCP LRCS Ed. 1945; LRCP LRCS Ed. LRFPS Glas. 1945.

SINCLAIR, Donald Ian — MB ChB Bristol 1986; MRCP (UK) 1990; MSc (PH) 1998; MFPHM 2001. Director of Pub. Health Slough PCT Upton Hosp. Albert St. Slough.

SINCLAIR, Mr Donald Malcolm (retired) Achnacree, Tighnabruaich PA21 2EB Tel: 01700 811382 — MB ChB Glas. 1944 (Univ. Glas.) BSc Glas. 1941, MB ChB 1944; FRFPS Glas. 1948; FRCS Ed. 1956; FRCS Glas. 1962. Prev: Cons. Surg. Glas. Roy. Infirm.

SINCLAIR, Douglas Neil (retired) Tablehurst, Lindfield Road, Ardingly, Haywards Heath RH17 6TS Tel: 01444 892693 — (Lond. Hosp.) MRCS Eng. LRCP Lond. 1952; DObst RCOG 1954; MRCGP 1956. Prev: Surg. Lt. RNVR.

SINCLAIR, Elizabeth Anne The Surgery, 409 Kings Road, Chelsea, London SW10 0LR Tel: 020 7351 1766 Fax: 020 7352 2240 — MB BS Lond. 1990 (Char. Cross & Westm.) Specialty: Gen. Pract.

SINCLAIR, Elizabeth Morton 26 Drumcarrow Road, St Andrews KY16 8SE Tel: 01334 474349 — MB ChB Dundee 1975; BSc (Med. Sci.) St. And. 1972. Clin. Asst. Meds. Research DDS LTD, Dundee; Blood Transfus. Serv. E Scotl. Specialty: Pharmaceutical Medicine. Socs: Assn. Anaesth. Gt. Brit. Prev: Regist. (Anaesth.) Tayside Health Bd.; Regist. (Med.) Tayside Health Bd.; Demonst. (Physiol.) Univ. St. And.

SINCLAIR, Elizabeth Romana Tunnel Road Surgery, 24 Tunnel Road, Beaminster DT8 3BN Tel: 01308 862225; Greenway Cottage, Ryall, Bridport DT6 6EN Tel: 01297 489519 Fax: 01297 489139 — MB ChB Bristol 1973.

SINCLAIR, Fiona Margaret Knebworth Surgery, Station Road, Knebworth SG3 6AP Tel: 01438 812494 — MB ChB Sheff. 1986 (Sheffield) MRCGP 1990; T(G)) 1991; DRCOG 1991; DFFP 1996. p/t FCS GP. Specialty: Gen. Pract. Prev: Clin. Asst., Breast Clinic, Hertford Co. Hosp., Hertford; GP Non-Princip., Letchworth.

SINCLAIR, Flora Margaret 59A Lockharton Avenue, Edinburgh EH14 1BB — MB ChB Glas. 1985. Prev: Ho. Off. (Med.) South. Gen. Hosp. Glas.; Ho. Off. (Surg.) Vale of Leven Hosp. Alexandria.

SINCLAIR, Gillian Winifred Royal Berkshire Hospital, Reading RG1 5AN — BM Soton. 1987; DA (UK) 1990.

SINCLAIR, Gordon Burton Croft Surgery, 5 Burton Crescent, Leeds LS6 4DN Tel: 0113 274 4777 Fax: 0113 230 4219 — MB ChB Leeds 1986; DCH RCP Lond. 1991; MRCGP 1993.

SINCLAIR, Hilary Deborah North Middleton Hospital, Sterling Way, London N18 1QX Tel: 020 8887 2698 — MB BS Lond. 1980 (St. Geo.) MRCP (UK) 1983; BSc Lond. 1977, MD 1995; FRCP 1998. Cons. Rheum. N. Middlx. Hosp. Specialty: Rheumatol. Socs: BMA; Brit. Soc. Rheum. Prev: Sen. Regist. Roy. Free Hosp. Lond.; Research Fell. Univ. Coll. & Middlx. Sch. Med. Lond.; Research Assoc. Duke Univ. Med. Centre Durh., N. Carolina, USA.

SINCLAIR, Janet Carolyn West Hampshire NHS Trust, Adult Mental Health Services, Park Way Centre, Park Way, Havant PO9 1HH Tel: 0239 247 1661 Fax: 0239 249 8291 — MB BS Lond. 1982 (Char. Cross) MRCPsych 1987. Cons. Gen. Adult Psychiat., W. Hants NHS Trust, Havant. Specialty: Gen. Psychiat. Special Interest: Adult Psychiat.

SINCLAIR, Janet Isobel The Taymount Surgery, 1 Taymount Terrace, Perth PH1 1NU Tel: 01738 627117 Fax: 01738 444713 — MB ChB Glasgow 1950 (Aberdeen) DCH, DRCOG 1977. GP Perth.

SINCLAIR, Mr John 7 Bridgegait, Milngavie, Glasgow G62 6NT Tel: 0141 956 3247 — MB ChB Ed. 1965; FRCS Ed. 1969. Cons. (Urol.) South. Gen. Hosp. Glas. Specialty: Urol. Prev: Sen. Regist. (Urol.) Glas. Roy. Infirm.; Surg. Regist. Lewis Hosp. Stornoway & South. Gen. Hosp. Glas.

SINCLAIR, John Alfred George 17 Flodden Way, Billingham TS23 3LF — MB BS Newc. 1992.

SINCLAIR, John Fraser Yorkhill NHS Trust, Glasgow G3 8SJ Tel: 0141 201 0000 — MB ChB Aberd. 1980. Specialty: Anaesth.; Intens. Care.

SINCLAIR, John Maxwell (retired) 4 Manderlea Court, Links Road, Lundin Links, Leven KY8 6AT Tel: 01333 320438 — MB ChB Glas. 1944 (Univ. Glas.) Prev: Maj. RAMC.

SINCLAIR, John Meehan (retired) Fairhurst, The Avenue, Fairlight, Hastings TN35 4DE — MB ChB Leeds 1957; MFHom 1972. Prev: Asst. Dir. of Health Care HM Prison Serv.

SINCLAIR, John Raymond Royal Cornwall Hospital Trust (Treliske), Truro TR1 2XN Tel: 01872 74242 — MB ChB Wales 1979; FFA RCS Eng. 1984. Cons. Anaesth. & Intens. Care. SW RHA. Specialty: Anaesth. Prev: Sen. Regist. (Anaesth.) S. West. RHA; Lect. (Anaesth.) Univ. Zambia, Lusaka; Regist. (Anaesth.) King's Coll. Hosp. Lond.

SINCLAIR, Mr John Stephen Plastic Surgery Dept., The Ulster Hospital, Dundonald BT16 1RH Tel: 028 90 484571 — MB BCh BAO Belf. 1987; FRCSI 1991; FRCS (Plast.) 1997; MD 1999. Cons. Plastic Surg., The Ulster Hosp., Belf. Specialty: Plastic Surg. Socs: BMA; Brit. Assn. Of Plastic Surg.; Brit. Assn. of Aesthetic Plastic Surg.

SINCLAIR, Julia Margaret Anne — MB BS Lond. 1994.

SINCLAIR, Keith Gareth Alexander Buen, Crowborough Hill, Crowborough TN6 2HJ Tel: 01892 663911; 126 Volunteer Drive, Somerset KY 42501-1926, USA Tel: 00 1 606 678 5602 Fax: 00 1 606 679 9308 Email: keithsinclair@yahoo.com — MB BS Lond. 1982 (Middlx.) BSc Psychol. & Pharmacol. Manch. 1975. Attend. Surg. Lake Cumbld. Regional Hosp. Som. KY, USA. Specialty: Gen. Surg. Socs: BMA; Fell. Amer. Coll. Surgs. Prev: Resid. Gen. Surg. Univ. of Florida; SHO (Cardiothoracic Surg.) Oxf. HA; Demonstr. (Human Anat.) Oxf. Univ.

SINCLAIR, Kenneth (retired) 2 Kirk Cottages, High St., Aberdour, Burntisland KY3 0SR Tel: 01383 860073 — MB ChB Ed. 1946; FRCP Ed. 1965, M 1951; MRCP Lond. 1956. Prev: Cons. Phys. Head Of Med. & Clinics, Abdulla Fouad Hosp. Dammam, Saudi Arabia.

SINCLAIR, Leonard 152 Harley Street, London W1G 7LH Tel: 020 7935 3834 Fax: 020 7224 2574; 34 Armitage Road, London NW11 8RD Tel: 020 8458 6464 Fax: 020 8905 5433 — MB BS Lond. 1954 (Middlx.) BSc Physiol. (Hons.) Lond. 1952; DCH Eng. 1957; FRCP Lond. 1974, M 1960; FRCPCH 1998. Emerit. Cons. Paediat., Chelsea & Westm. Hosp., Lond. SW10. Specialty: Paediat. Socs: Fell. Roy. Soc. Med. (Mem. Counc. & Ex-Sec. Sect. Paediat. & Mem.; Soc. Study of Inborn Errors of Metab.; Mem. of BHA. Prev: Sen. Regist. (Paediat.) Westm. Hosp. & W.m. Childr. Hosp.; Regist. (Med.) Qu. Eliz. Hosp. Childr. Lond.; New Health Trust Clin. Research Fell. Qu. Eliz. Hosp. Childr. Lond.

SINCLAIR, Margaret (retired) 4 Manderlea Court, Links Road, Lundin Links, Leven KY8 6AT Tel: 01333 320438 — MB ChB Glas. 1944 (Univ. Glas) Prev: Clin. Med. Off. Fife Health Bd.

SINCLAIR, Margaret Ann 9 Newmill Gardens, St Andrews KY16 8RY — MB ChB Aberd. 1993.

SINCLAIR, Mr Martin Thomas Ipswich Hospital, Department of Surgery, Heath Road, Ipswich IP4 5PD — MB ChB Glas. 1991; FRCS Glas. 1996; FRCS Ed. 1996; FRCS (Gen. Surg.) 2001. Cons. Surg. Ipswich Hosp. Specialty: Gen. Surg. Socs: BMA; Pancreatic Soc.; Roy. Coll. Phys.s & Surg. Glas.

SINCLAIR, Michael Edward 104 Southmoor Road, Oxford OX2 6RB Tel: 01865 559496 — MB ChB Bristol 1976; FFARCS Eng. 1981. Cons. Cardiothoracic Anaesth., Nuffield Dept. Anaesth., Oxf. Specialty: Anaesth. Prev: Sen. Regist. & Lect. Nuffield Dept. Anaesth., Oxf.; Sen. Lect. Univ. Hosp. Geneva; SHO Rotat. (Anaesth.) Bristol Roy. Infirm.

SINCLAIR, Michelle 6 Swan Drive, Aldermaston, Reading RG7 4UZ Tel: 01189 713351 — MB BS Lond. 1992; DRCOG Nov 1995; DFFP 1995; MRCGP July 1997.

SINCLAIR, Neil Edward 1A Baptist Gardens, London NW5 4ET — MB BS Lond. 1998; MB BS Lond 1998.

SINCLAIR, Niall Mackay The Surgery, High Street, Epworth, Doncaster DN9 1EP Tel: 01427 872232 Fax: 01427 874944; 1 Mill Lane, Westwoodside, Doncaster DN9 2AF Tel: 01427 752193 — MB ChB Ed. 1971; BSc (Med. Sci.) Ed. 1968; DObst RCOG 1974; FRCGP 1995, M 1975. Course Organiser Doncaster VTS. Socs: Anglo-French Med. Soc. Prev: Trainee GP Doncaster VTS.

SINCLAIR, Paul 126 Blenheim Place, Aberdeen AB25 2DN; Waratah Apartments, 24/71 Victoria St, Potts Point, Sydney 2011, Australia Tel: 00 61 2 3573870 — MB ChB Dundee 1989. Specialty: Anaesth.

SINCLAIR, Penelope Mace Bradford University Health Centre, Bradford BD7 1DP; 16 Oakburn Road, Ilkley LS29 9NN — BM Soton. 1984; MRCGP 1988; DRCOG 1988.

SINCLAIR, Mr Peter Kemp East Cheshire NHS Trust, Macclesfield District General Hospital, Victoria Road, Macclesfield SK10 3BC Tel: 01625 421000 Fax: 01625 661644; Bon Vista, 89 High St, Bollington, Macclesfield SK10 5PF Tel: 01625 573379 Fax: 01625 573379 — MB ChB Glas. 1969; FRCS Glas. 1974; FRCS Eng. 1976; FRCR Eng. 1983. Cons. Radiol. Macclesfield Dist. Gen. Hosp. Specialty: Radiol.

SINCLAIR, Robert Gillies (retired) Inchmahome, Arbuthnot Est., Dorrator Road, Camelon, Falkirk FK1 4BN Tel: 01324 623202 — MB ChB Glas. 1949; DObst RCOG 1954; FRCGP 1974, M 1958. Prev: Hospice Med. Cons. Strathcarrow Hospice Denny.

SINCLAIR, Robin Douglas 141 Whyteleaf Road, Caterham CR3 — MRCS Eng. LRCP Lond. 1964 (Camb. & Guy's) MB Camb. 1965, BChir 1964. Prev: Ho. Surg. Obst., Cas. Off. & Ho. Phys. W. Middlx. Hosp. Isleworth.

SINCLAIR, Ronald Kilpatrick (retired) Westgarth, Garelochhead, Helensburgh G84 0AT Tel: 01436 810542 Fax: 01436 810542 — MB ChB Glas. 1965; DObst RCOG 1967. Prev: SHO (Obst.) Rankin Memor. Hosp. Greenock.

SINCLAIR, Ruth Margaret Flat 2, Rosemont, 80/81 Mount Ephram, Tunbridge Wells TN4 8BU — MB ChB Glas. 1985; FFA RCSI 1994. Staff Grade (Anaesth.) Monklands & Bellshill Hosps. Lanarksh. Prev: Career Regist. (Anaesth.) Glas. Roy. Infirm.

SINCLAIR, Shona Stanley Medical Centre, 43 Shielhill Place, Stanley, Perth PH1 4NN Tel: 01738 828294; 22 Duchess Street, Stanley, Perth PH1 4NG — MB ChB Dundee 1984; MBLLB 1984 Dundee; DRCOG 1988; DRCOS 1988. Clin. Asst. Murray Roy. Hosp. Perth.

SINCLAIR, Simon Chester-le-StreetCMHT, Chester-le-Street — MB BS Lond. 1977; MA Oxf. 1977; PhD Lond. 1996, MSc 1992, MB BS 1977; DTM & H RCP Lond. 1983; MRCPsych 1987. Cons. Psychiat.s, Co. Durh. and Darlington Priority Servs. NHS Trust, Chester-li-St.; Hon. Fell., Dept. of Anthropol. Specialty: Gen. Psychiat. Prev: Field Doctor Brit. Nepal Med. Trust, Bhojpur, E. Nepal.; Sen. Regist. Oxf. Ment. Healthcare NHS Trust.

SINCLAIR, Siobhan Alexandra University Hospital of North Durham, North Rd, Durham DH1 2UD — MB ChB Ed. 1988; MRCP (UK) 1994. Cons. Dermatol., Univ. Hosp. of N. Durh. Specialty: Dermat. Socs: BAD; BAD; BSDP. Prev: SHO (Med. & Dermat.) S. Cleveland. Hosp.; SHO (A & E) Middlesbrough Gen. Hosp.

SINCLAIR, Susan Isabelle Grace 39 Eburne Road, Finsbury Park, London N7 6AU — MB BS Lond. 1985.

SINCLAIR, Tessa Annemarie Lewis 6 Haverfield Gardens, Kew, Richmond TW9 3DD — MB BS Lond. 1989.

SINCLAIR, Thomas (retired) 67 Chew Valley Road, Greenfield, Oldham OL3 7JG Tel: 01457 873100 Fax: 01457 873100 Email: tomsinclair@doctors.org.uk; 67 Chew Valley Road, Greenfield, Oldham OL3 7JG Tel: 01303 851220/01457 873100 Email: nagesh.rao@virgin.net/tomsinclair@doctors.org.uk — MB BS Durh. 1961 (Newc.) Cert Av Med MoD (Air) & CAA; DObst RCOG 1966; Aviat. Auth. 1977. Authorised Med. Examr. Uk Civil.Aviat.Auth.Jt. Aviat.Auth. Prev: Teach. (Gen. Pract.) Univ. Manch.

SINCLAIR, Torquil Macleod (retired) West Lodge, Longridge Towers, Berwick-upon-Tweed TD15 2XQ Tel: 01289 307499 — MB ChB Ed. 1954.

SINCLAIR, William Yuille (retired) 5 Southfield Close, Blackwood ML11 9YZ Tel: 01555 894317 — MB BS Durh. 1959 (Newc.) FRCOG 1977, M 1963. Prev: Clin. Lect. (Obst. & Gyn.) Univ. Newc.

SINDALL, Fiona Mary Putneymead Medical Centre, 350 Upper Richmond Road, Putney, London SW15 6TL — BM Soton. 1986; DA 1988. GP Retainer Putneymead Med. Centre Lond. Specialty: Gen. Pract. Prev: GP Trainee; SHO (O & G) Princess Anne Hosp. Soton.; SHO (Anaesth.) Soton Gen. Hosp.

SINDEN, Lada Y — Med. Dipl. Kiev med Inst 1997.

SINDEN, Mark Peter Maidstone & Tunbridge NHS Trust, c/o Anaesthetics Department, Kent & Sussex Hospital, Mount Ephraim, Tunbridge Wells Tel: 01982 526111 Ext.2529; Bridge House, Summerhill, Goudhurst, Cranbrook TN17 1JT Tel: 01580 211388 Email: mpsinden@btinternet.com — MB BS Lond. 1985 (Guy's

Hospital, London University) DCH RCP Lond. 1989; T(GP) 1990; DA (UK) 1993; DFFP 1993; FRCA 1996. p/t Cons. Anaesth. Specialty: Anaesth. Socs: Obst. Anaesth. Assn.; Difficult Airway Soc.; Assn. of Anaesth. GB & Irel. Prev: Sp REG (Anaesth.) Guy's Hosp., Lond.; Regist. (Anaesth.) Eastbourne DGH Sussex; Regist. (Anaesth.) E. Grinstead Qu. Vict. Hosp.

SINFIELD, Karen Elizabeth The Laurels Medical Practice, 28 Clarendon Road, St Helier, Jersey JE2 3YS Tel: 01534 733866 Fax: 01534 769597 — MB BS Lond. 1979.

SINGAL, Ajay Greenbank Surgery, 1025 Stratford Road, Hall Green, Birmingham B28 8BG Tel: 0121 777 1490 Fax: 0121 778 6239; 6 Brampton Crescent, Solihull B90 3SY — MB BS Newc. 1986; DRCOG 1988; MRCGP 1990.

SINGAL, Arun Kumar Northgate Medical Centre, Anchor Meadow Health Centre, Aldridge, Walsall WS9 8AJ Tel: 01922 450900 Fax: 01922 450910; 26 Newick Avenue, Little Aston, Sutton Coldfield B74 3DA — MB BS Newc. 1984; DRCOG 1987; MRCGP 1988.

SINGAL, Ashish Kumar 70 Launceston Road, Walsall WS5 3EE — MB BS Newc. 1992.

SINGANAYAGAM, Jeyakumar Queens Hospital, Department of Radiology, Burton Hospital NHS Trust, Belvedere Road, Burton-on-Trent DE13 0RB Tel: 01283 566333 Fax: 01283 593013 — MB BS Peradeniya 1981 (university of Peradeniya, Sri Lanka) FRCS Ed. 1987; FRCR 1993. Cons. Radiol. Qu.s Hosp. Burton Hosp. NHS Trust Burton-upon-Trent. Specialty: Radiol. Prev: Sen. Regist. (Radiol.) N. Staffs. Hosp. Centre Stoke on Trent; Regist. (Radiol.) N. Staffs. Hosp. Centre Stoke-on-Trent; Regist. (Surg.) Dumfries & Galloway Roy. Infirm.

SINGANAYAGAM, Selvadorai Faifield General Hospital, Bury — (Univ. of Ceylon) MB BS Ceylon; FRCR; MRCP UK; DMRD. Cons. Radiologist, Fairfield Gen. Hosp.; Cons. radiologist, Highfield Hosp. (BMI) Rochdale. Specialty: Radiol. Prev: Chair of Audit - Bury Health Trust; Clinical Director Radiology, Bury.

SINGARAYER, Chandrakumar 24 St Andrews Avenue, Sudbury, Wembley HA0 2QD — MB BS Lond. 1994 (Royal Free Hosp. Sch. Of Med.) BSc Lond. 1991; Board Certified by the American Board of Internal Medicine 1999. Cons., Internal Med., Memor. Hosp., N. Conway, New Hants., USA; Clin. Fell. (Med.) Harvard Med. Sch. Specialty: Gen. Med. Socs: Mass. Med. Soc.; Amer. Med. Assn. Prev: SHO (A & E) Qu. Eliz. II Hosp. Welwyn Bdn. City; Ho. Off. (Med.) Roy. Free Hosp. Lond.; Ho. Off. (Gen. Surg. & Orthop.) Lister Hosp. Stevenage.

SINGARAYER, Karen Naomi Montcalm, 11 Lankaster Gardens, London N2 9AZ — MB BS Lond. 1993.

SINGER, Mr Adolf 16 Manor Court, Aylmer Rd, Finchley, London N2 0PJ Tel: 001 631 287 2561/020 8348 8448 Fax: 001 631 287 2561; 191 Herrick Road, Southampton, New York 11968, USA Tel: 001 631 283 9531 Fax: 001 631 287 2561 — MB BS (Hons) London 1951 (Univ. Coll. Hosp., London) FRCS 1956; FACS 1964; MD New York 1979. Assoc. Clin. Prof (Surg.), Albert Einstein Coll. Of Med., New York; 16 Manor Ct., Aylmer Rd, Fingale, Lond, N20 0PJ, Tel: 0208 348 8448. Specialty: Vasc. Med. Socs: Sen. Mem. NY Surg. Soc.; Fell. Emerit. Amer. Coll. Angiol.; Sen. Mem. Internat. Cardiovasc. Soc. Prev: Emerit. Attend., N.Y. Hosp. Med. Centre Qu.; Hon. Attend. Long Is. Jewish. Hosp.; Hon. Attend. N. Shore Univ. Hosp.

SINGER, Professor Albert Department of Women's Health, Whittington Hospital NHS Trust, London N19 5NF Tel: 020 7288 5409 Fax: 020 7288 5066 Email: albert.singer@whittington.nhs.uk; (cons. rooms), 212-214 Great Portland St, London W1N 5HG Tel: 020 7390 8442 Fax: 020 8458 0168 Email: albert.singer@nhs.uk.com — MB BS Sydney 1962; DGO Sydney 1967; FRCOG 1980, M 1967; PhD Sydney 1972; DPhil Oxf. 1973. Cons. O & G Whittington Hosp. Lond.; Vis. Prof. Dept. Molecular Pathol. UCL; Prof. Gyn. Research Univ. Lond. Specialty: Obst. & Gyn. Special Interest: Colposcopy; Gyn.; Med. Gyn. Socs: Brit. Soc. for Colposcopy and Cervical Path. (BSCCP) - Trustee.; Europ. Research Organisation on Genital Infec.s and Neoplasia (EROGEN) - Exec. Comm..; Brit. Soc. of Gyn. Oncol. Prev: Reader (O & G) Univ. Sheff.; Cons. O & G Jessop Hosp. Sheff.; Research Fell. & Clin. Lect. Nuffield Dept. O & G Univ. Oxf.

SINGER, Mr Brian Robert Perth Royal Infirmary, Perth PH1 1NX Tel: 01738 474480 Fax: 01738 473990 Email: brian.singer@tuht.scot.nhs.uk — MB ChB Aberd. 1983; FRCS Eng. 1988; FRCS (Orth.) 1994; FRCS Ed. 2001. Cons. Orthop. Surg. Perth Roy. Infirm. Specialty: Orthop. Special Interest: Hip and knee arthroplasty; Young adult hip. Prev: Orthop. Surg. Roy. Hosp. Haslar Princess Margt. Rose Orthop. Hosp.; Orthop. Surg. Qu. Eliz. Milit. Hosp. London.

SINGER, Charles Robert John Department of Haematology, Royal United Hospital, Bath BA1 3NG Tel: 01225 824760 Fax: 01225 461044 Email: charles.singer@ruh-bath.swest.nhs.uk; 40 Garstons, Bathford, Bath BA1 7TE Tel: 01225 859396 Email: crjsinger@crjsbath.demon.co.uk — MB ChB Glas. 1977; BSc (Hons.) Glas. 1975; MB ChB (Commend.) Glas. 1977; MRCP (UK) 1980; MRCPath 1987; FRCP Glas. 1990; FRCP Lond. 1996; FRCPath 1997. Cons. Haemat. Roy. United Hosp. Bath; Postgrad. Clin. Tutor Bath. Specialty: Haematology. Socs: Brit. Soc. for Haemat., (Comm. Mem. 1998-2000), Treas. 2000; Amer. Soc. Hematology, 1998. Prev: Lect. (Haemat.) Univ. Coll. & Middlx. Sch. of Med. Lond.; Regist. (Haemat. & Gen. Med.) Glas. Roy. Infirm.

SINGER, Professor Donald Robert James University of Warwick Medical School, Clinical Sciences Research Institute, Clifford Bridge Road, Coventry CV2 2DX Tel: 024 7696 8649 Fax: 024 7696 8653 Email: mdscaf@warwick.ac.uk; University Hospitals - Walsgrave, Clifford Bridge Road, Coventry CV2 2DX Tel: 02476 535 004 — MB ChB Aberd. 1978 (Univ. of Aberd.) BMedBiol Aberd. 1975; MRCP 1981; MD Aberd. 1995; FRCP 2000. Prof. of Clin. Pharmacol.; Head of Clin. Sci. Specialty: Pharmacology; Gen. Med. Special Interest: Blood Pressure; Pharmacogenetics; Vascular Biology. Socs: Brit. Microcirculation Soc.; Europ. Federat. of Internal Med.; Europ. Counc. for Blood Pressure and Cardiovasc. Research. Prev: Hon. Cons. Phys. Walsgrave Hosp.; Reader (Clin. Pharmacol.) & Hon. Cons. Phys. St Geo. Hosp. Med. Sch. Lond.; Hon. Sen. Lect. Imperial Coll. Nat. Heart & Lung Inst. Heart Sci. Centre, Harefield.

SINGER, Mr Gian Charles Heatherwood and Wexham District Hospirtals NHS Trust, London Road, Ascot SL5 8AA Tel: 01344 877184 Fax: 01344 877843 Email: giansinger@aol.com — MB BS Lond. 1985; FRCS (Orth); FRCS Eng. 1990. Cons. Orthopaedic and Trauma Surg. Specialty: Trauma & Orthop. Surg. Special Interest: Hip Resurfacing; Minimal Invasive Hip Replacement; Revision Hip Surgery. Socs: Brit. Hip Soc.

SINGER, Helen Grant Bramhall Health Centre, 66 Bramhall Lane South, Bramhall, Stockport SK7 2DY Tel: 0161 439 8213 Fax: 0161 439 6398 — MB ChB Glas. 1971; DObst RCOG 1973.

SINGER, Iain Ogilvie Flat 2/3, 170 Elmbank St., Glasgow G2 4NY Tel: 0141 332 5195 Email: iain@ioscm.demon.co.uk — MB ChB Glas. 1987; BSc (Hons.) Immunol. Glas. 1984, MB ChB 1987; MRCP (UK) 1991; MRCPath 1997. Career Regist. (Haemat.) Stobhill Gen. Hosp. Glas.; Specialist Regist. Stobhill NHS Trust Glas. Specialty: Haematology. Prev: SHO (Med.) Monklands Dist. Gen. Hosp. Airdrie; Ho. Off. (Med.) Glas. Roy. Infirm.; Ho. Off. (Surg.) South. Gen. Hosp. Glas.

SINGER, Jack Donald Academic Department of Child Health, Chelsea & Westminster Hospital, 369 Fulham Road, London SW10 9NH Tel: 020 8746 8627; 73 Harley Street, London W1N 1DE Tel: 020 7935 2023 Fax: 020 7935 3857 — MD Washington Univ. 1962; Lic. Newfld. Med. Bd. 1975; T(M) (Paediat.) 1991; FRCPCH 1997. Hon. Sec. Lect. (Child Health) Chelsea & Westm. Hosp. Lond. Specialty: Paediat. Socs: Brit. Paediat. Assn. & Clin. Genetics Soc. Prev: Sen. Lect. & Hon. Cons. Human Genetics King's Coll. Hosp. & Med. Sch. Lond.; Med. Off. P. Philip Research Laborat. Paediat. Research Unit Guy's Hosp. Med. Sch.; Sen. Regist. (Paediat.) Guy's Hosp. Lond.

SINGER, Jonathan 11 Newcombe Park, London NW7 3QN — MB BCh Witwatersrand 1974.

SINGER, Julian Mark 16 Canonbury Park N., London N1 2JT Tel: 020 7226 8933 — MB BS Lond. 1984 (Roy. Lond. Hosp. Med. Coll.) MRCP (UK) 1988; FRCR 1993. Cons. Clin. Oncologist, Princess Alexandra Hosp., Harlow; Cons. Clin. Oncologist, N. Middlx. Hosp., Lond. Specialty: Oncol. Special Interest: Breast cancer; Lung Cancer. Prev: Research Regist. (Oncol.) Middlx. Hosp. Lond.; Sen. Regist. (Clin. Oncol.) Hammersmith Hosp. Lond.

SINGER, Juliet Amanda 23 Cocksheadhey Road, Bollington, Macclesfield SK10 5QZ; Flat 3 16 Marlborough Road, London N19 4NB Tel: 020 7272 7266 — MB BCh Wales 1993. SHO Rotat. (Psychiat.) Roy. Free Hosp. Lond.

SINGER, Jutta (retired) 17 Schonfield Square, Lordship Road, London N16 0QQ Tel: 020 8800 0406 — ((Lond. Sch. of Med. for Wom.) Roy. Free Hosp.) MRCS Eng. LRCP Lond. 1946; BA (Hons.) Psychol. Lond. 1952; DTM & H RCP Lond. 1955; Cert. Family Plann. JCC 1955. Prev: Regist. (Path.) St. Peter's Hosp., Eliz. Garret. Anderson Hosp. & Roy. North. Hosp.

SINGER, Lawrence Lydia House Surgery, 8 Sutherland Boulevard, Leigh-on-Sea SS9 3PS Tel: 01702 552900 Fax: 01702 553474; 1809 London Road, Leigh-on-Sea SS9 2ST — MB ChB Manch. 1967; DObst RCOG 1969. GP Leigh-on-Sea. Socs: BMA & N. Lond. Gp. Anaesths. Prev: Regist. (Anaesth.) P. of Wales Hosp. Tottenham; SHO (O & G) St. Mary's Hosp. Manch.

SINGER, Mervyn University College London Medical School, Mortimer Street, London W1T 3AA Tel: 020 7679 9666 Fax: 020 7679 9660; 16 Coppice Walk, Totteridge, London N20 8BZ — MB BS Lond. 1981. Prof. (Intens. Care Med.) UCL. Specialty: Intens. Care. Prev: Sen. Lect. (Intens. Care Med.) UCL Med. Sch.

SINGER, Paul Ashley Liverpool Road Health Centre, 9 Mersey Place, Liverpool Road, Luton LU1 1HH Tel: 01582 31321 — MB ChB Liverp. 1984. GP Computing Facilitator Beds. FHSA. Prev: Trainee GP Milton Keynes VTS.

SINGER, Ralph 1 Latimer House, Morning Lane, London E9 6HE Tel: 020 8985 2249; 3 Thornton Way, London NW11 6RY Tel: 020 8458 7929 — MRCS Eng. LRCP Lond. 1944 (St. Bart.) DCH Eng. 1949. Prev: Ho. Off. (Obst.) St. And. Hosp. Bow; Regist. Pk. Hosp. Hither Green; Ho. Phys. (Paediat.) Whipps Cross Hosp.

SINGER, Ronald Victor Julius The Health Centre, 2A Forest Road, Edmonton, London N9 8RZ Tel: 020 8804 0121 — MB BChir Camb. 1973; MRCGP 1987.

SINGER, Ruth Snaefell Avenue Surgery, 14 Snaefell Avenue, Liverpool L13 7HA Tel: 0151 228 2377; Parkview, Allerton Road, Liverpool L18 3JU Tel: 0151 724 5160 — MRCS Eng. LRCP Lond. 1963 (Univ. Coll. Lond. & Liverp.) BSc (Physiol) Lond. 1960. Prev: Med. Off. St. Helens Co. Boro. & Liverp. Educat. Comm.

SINGFIELD, Catherine Jane 182 Grace Way, Stevenage SG1 5AG Tel: 01438 359249 — MB BS Lond. 1991.

SINGH, Ajai Pratap 21 Moorcroft Road, Fulwood, Sheffield S10 4GS — MB BS Lucknow 1972 (King Geo. Med. Coll. Lucknow) DA Agra 1974. Assoc. Specialist Regional Transfus. Centre Sheff.

SINGH, Ajit Glan Yr Afon Surgery, Shop Row, Tredegar NP22 4LB Tel: 01495 722460 Fax: 01495 724410 — MB BS Panjab 1962 (Govt. Med. Coll. Patiala) DPM Eng. 1973. Sen. Regist. Cheadle Roy. Hosp. Prev: Regist. Hellesdon Hosp. Norwich, S.H.M.S. Hosp. Srinagar, India & Claybury Hosp. Woodford Bridge.

SINGH, Amarendra Kumar 5 Netherfield Road, London N12 8DP — MB BS Patna 1958; PhD Lond. 1968; FFPath (RCPI - Dub.) 1997. Sen. Lect. & Cons. Dept. Haemat. St. Thos. Hosp. & Med. Sch. Lond.; Assoc. Prof. (Haemat.) Med. Sch. Hazall Zimbabwe March 1997. Specialty: Haematology.

SINGH, Amarjeet 6 Forest Close, Pinders Heath, Wakefield WF1 4TL — MB BS Ranchi 1976; MRCPI 1984.

SINGH, Amarjit (retired) — MB BS Punjab 1961 (Govt. Med. Coll. Amritsar) MB BS Punjab (India) 1961; DO Eng. 1969. Hosp. Pract. (Ophth.) Leigh Infirm. Prev: Hosp. Pract. (Ophth.) Hope Hosp. Salford.

SINGH, Amrik Marine Surgery, 29 Belle Vue Road, Southbourne, Bournemouth BH6 3DB Tel: 01202 423377 Fax: 01202 424277; 37 Keswick Road, Boscombe Manor, Bournemouth BH5 1LR — MB ChB Manch. 1976. GP Bournemouth. Specialty: Homeop. Med. Socs: Assoc. Mem. Brit. Med. Acupunc. Soc.; Assoc. Mem. Fac. Homeop. Lond.

SINGH, Amrit Bir Royal Shrewsbury Hospital, Shelton, Bicton Heath, Shrewsbury SY3 8DN Tel: 01743 261296; 12 Highridge Way, Radbrooke Green, Shrewsbury SY3 6DJ Tel: 01743 369123 — MB BS Punjab 1977; BSc Punjab 1969, MB BS 1977; DPM Eng. 1980; MRCPsych 1982.

SINGH, Anirudh Prasad St Peters Hospital, Guildford Road, Chertsey KT16 0PZ — MB BS Patna 1973.

SINGH, Mr Anoop Kumar 30 Nursey Road, Rainham, Gillingham ME8 0DS; 320 Applewood Drive, Slidell 70461, USA Tel: 001 985 7817903 Fax: 001 985 7817904 Email: anoopks@bellsouth.net — MB BS Poona 1978; FRCS Ed. 1983; MRCS Eng. LRCP Lond. 1985; Dip. Biomechanics Strathclyde 1990; MPhil (Bioengineering) Strathclyde 1993. Asst. Prof. in Emerg. Med., Louisiana State Univ. Baton Rouge, LA, USA. Specialty: Orthop.; Accid. & Emerg.; Research. Socs: Assoc. Mem. BOA; Internat. Soc. Biomech. Prev: Regist. (A & E) St. Peters' Hosp. Chertsey; Research Fell. Univ. Calif., Los Angeles; Regist. (Orthop.) Medway Hosp. Gillingham & Odstock Hosp. Salisbury.

SINGH, Arun Kumar Wynyard Road Surgery, 35-37 Wynyard Road, Hartlepool TS25 3LB Tel: 01429 223195 Fax: 01429 296007; 14 Endeavour Close, Hartlepool TS25 1EY Tel: 01429 236682 — MB BS Panta 1974; MS (ENT) Panta 1979; DLO RCS Eng. 1981.

SINGH, Ashok Nandan — MB BS Mithila 1978; MD Patna 1985. Cons. (Psychiat.) Lincolnshire Partnership Trust. Specialty: Gen. Psychiat. Special Interest: Sexual Dysfunction. Prev: Cons. Psychiat. Rauceby Hosp. Sleaford; Staff Psychiat. Westm. Hosp. Lond.; Regist. St. Brigid's Hosp. Ardee.

SINGH, Avtar St Pauls Surgery, 36-38 East Street, Preston PR1 1UU Tel: 01772 252409 Fax: 01772 885509.

SINGH, Baldev Malkit Wolverhampton Diabetes Centre, New Cross Hospital, Wolverhampton WV10 0QP Tel: 01902 643035 Fax: 01902 642864 — MB BS Lond. 1979; MRCP (UK) 1982; MD Lond. 1988; FRCP 1998. Cons. Phys. (Diabetes Endocrinol.) Wolverhampton; Reader in Diabetic Med. Univ. of Wolverhampton; Assoc. Dean, W. Midlands Deanery. Specialty: Diabetes; Endocrinol.; Gen. Med.

SINGH, Baljit 9 Pennant Road, Burbage, Hinckley LE10 2LA — BM BCh Oxf. 1992 (Oxf. Univ.) BA (Physiol. Sci.) Oxf. 1989; FRCS (Irel.) 1997; FRCS (Eng.) 1997; Royal College of Surgeons of England Research Felolowship 1998. SHO Rotat. (Gen. Surg.) Leics. Specialty: Gen. Surg.

SINGH, Bhawna Holton Grange, Station Road, Holton-le-Clay, Grimsby DN36 5HT — MB ChB Leic. 1998; MB ChB Leic 1998.

SINGH, Bijendra Narayan Garden Street Surgery, 28A Garden Street, Brompton, Gillingham ME7 5AS Tel: 01634 845898 Fax: 01634 817823; 29 Barleymow Close, Walderslade, Chatham ME5 8JZ Tel: 01634 316841 — MB BS Bihar 1971; MD (Mlthila) 1978.

SINGH, Bikram Jit Flat 2, 79 Lancefield Quay, Glasgow G3 8HA — LRCP LRCS Ed. 1984; LRCP LRCS Ed. LRCPS Glas. 1984.

SINGH, Binod Kumar City hospital NHS Trust, Dudley Road, Birmingham B18 7QH Tel: 0121 507 5482 Fax: 0121 507 5483.

SINGH, Binoy Kumar Avicenna Medical Practice, 14 Institute Road, Eccleshill, Bradford BD2 2HX Tel: 01274 637417 Fax: 01274 776511 — MB BS Ranchi 1967 (Rajendra Med. Coll.) BSc Bihar 1961; MB BS Ranchi India 1967.

SINGH, Bir Bahadur Hillside Health Centre, Tanhouse Road, Tanhouse, Skelmersdale WN8 6DS Tel: 01695 726888 Fax: 01695 556330 — MB BS Patna 1973; MB BS Patna 1973.

SINGH, Bishnu Deo Narayan 164 Melwood Drive, Liverpool L12 4XH — MB BS Patna 1974.

SINGH, Boota Fairwinds, Highrigg Drive, Broughton, Preston PR3 5LJ Tel: 01772 862054 — MB BS Lucknow 1968. GP. Specialty: Gen. Pract.; Paediat.; Diabetes. Special Interest: Diabetes. Prev: Med. Off., Rainfall Agency.

SINGH, Brijindera Balbir Ridgecrest, 9 Foxlands Avenue, Penn, Wolverhampton WV4 5LX Tel: 01902 336861 — MB BS Lond. 1980; DCH RCP Lond. 1984; DRCOG 1984; MRCGP 1985.

SINGH, Bulu Deepdale Road Surgery, 98 Deepdale Road, Preston PR1 5AR Tel: 01772 821069; Fairwinds, High Rigg Drive, Broughton, Preston PR3 5LJ Tel: 01772 862054 Fax: 01772 862054 — MB BS Lucknow 1968 (King Geo. Med. Coll.) DFFP. GP; Clin. Asst. (Genitourin. Med. & O & G).

SINGH, Bupinder Ashingdon Medical Centre, 57 Lascelles Gardens, Ashingdon, Rochford SS4 3BW Tel: 01702 544959 Fax: 01702 530160 — MB BS Jammu & Kashmir 1972.

SINGH, Mr Chandra Bhan Springfield Hospital, Lawn Lane, Chelmsford CM1 7GU Tel: 01245 359038 Fax: 01245 280616 Email: cbsinghent@hotmail.com — MB BS Vikram 1961 (Gajra Raja Med. Coll. Gwalior) FRCS Eng. 1970; DLO Eng. 1970. Specialty: Otorhinolaryngol. Special Interest: Microsurgery of Middle Ear; Rhinoplasty. Socs: BMA; Brit. Assn. of Otolaryngologists; The Hosp. Consultants and Specialists Assn. Prev: Sen. Regist. (Otorhinolaryng.) Notts HA; Cons. Surg. (Otorhinoloaryng.) Mid Essex Hosp. Trust.

SINGH, Chandra Deo Prasad 4 Overton Place, West Bromwich B71 1RL — MB BS Bihar 1961.

SINGH, Clare Antonia 57 Cork Road, Bowerham, Lancaster LA1 4AY — MB ChB Leeds 1993.

SINGH, Dave Gobin 1 Hayes Barton, Thorpe Bay, Southend-on-Sea SS1 3TS Tel: 01702 585455 — MD Odessa Med. Inst. USSR 1969.

SINGH, Davendra Park Grove Surgery, 124-126 Park Grove, Barnsley S70 1QE Tel: 01226 282140 Fax: 01226 213279 (Call before faxing) — (Nat. Med. Inst. Calcutta) MB BS Calcutta 1966; DTM & H Liverp. 1968; Dip. Ven. Liverp. 1968. Specialty: Gen. Psychiat. Socs: Fell. Roy. Soc. Trop. Med. & Hyg.; BMA. Prev: Ho. Off. (Gen. Surg.) & Resid. Ho. Off. (Med.) Safder Jung Hosp. New Delhi, India; Resid. SHO (ENT) St. Hilda's Hosp. Hartlepool; Resid. SHO (Obst.) Stirling, Falkirk & Alloa Gp. Hosps.

SINGH, Dev Raj 10 Garrett Close, Maiden Bower, Crawley RH10 7UP Tel: 01293 885516 — MB BS Panjab 1972; MD Delhi 1975; MRCOG 1982; FRCOG 1997.

SINGH, Devendra Rockview Health Centre, Rockview Place, Helmsdale KW8 6LF Tel: 01431 821225 Fax: 01431 821567 — MB BS Rajasthan 1970; Cert. Family Plann. JCC 1983; DFFP 1994. GP Highland HB. Socs: Assoc. Mem. RCGP. Prev: Civil Asst. Surg. Govt. Rajasthan; Med. Off. Govt. Hosp. Weir, Rajasthan.

SINGH, Dhinesh PRN Medical Agency, c/o Martyn Fenwick, 42 Theobalds Road, London WC1X 8NW — MB BCh Witwatersrand 1993.

SINGH, Dhruva Narayan Prasad Peartree Medical Centre, 159 Pear Tree Road, Derby DE23 8NQ Tel: 01332 360692 Fax: 01332 368181 — MB BS Bihar 1973.

SINGH, Mr Dishan Royal National Orthopaedic Hospital, Stanmore HA7 4LP Tel: 020 8909 9314 Email: dishansingh@aol.com/ sheard@londondeanery.ac.uk — MB ChB Manch. 1983; FRCS Eng. 1988; FRCS (Orth.) 1995. Cons. Roy. Nat. Orthop. Hosp. Stanmore; Hon. Sen. Lect. Univ. of Lond. Specialty: Trauma & Orthop. Surg. Socs: Fell. BOA; Brit. Orthop. Foot Surg. Soc.; Amer. Orthop. Foot & Ankle Soc. Prev: Sen. Regist. (Orthop.) Roy. Nat. Orthop. Hosp. Lond.; Regist. (Orthop.) Roy. Lond. Hosp.

SINGH, Gautam Kumar Department of Paediatric Cardiology, Southampton General Hospital, Tremona Road, Southampton SO16 6YD Tel: 023 8077 7222 — MB BS Ranchi 1978; MD (Paediat.) 1982; DCH RCP Lond. 1987; MRCP (UK) 1988. SHO (Paediat. Cardiol.) Soton. & S. W. Hants. HA. Socs: Med. Protect. Soc. Prev: SHO (Paediat. Cardiol.) Hosp. Sick Childr. Gt. Ormond St.; Regist. (Paediat) St. Peter's Hosp. Chertsey; SHO (Paediat. Nephrol.) E. Birm. Hosp.

SINGH, Gian Beechdale Centre, Edison Road, Walsall WS2 7EZ Tel: 01922 775200 Fax: 01922 775203; 15 Sydney Close, West Bromwich B70 0SR — LMSSA Lond. 1992; DFFP; MB BS Panjab 1987. Specialty: Gen. Pract.

SINGH, Gurbachan (Surgery), 26 Rough Road, Kingstanding, Birmingham B44 0UY Tel: 0121 354 8213 — MB ChB Birm. 1953; MRCS Eng. LRCP Lond. 1953. Prev: Ho. Surg. Solihull Hosp.; Ho. Off. Obst. Burton-on-Trent Gen. Hosp.

SINGH, Gurcharan Collington Surgery, 23 Terminus Road, Bexhill-on-Sea TN39 3LR Tel: 01424 217465/216675 Fax: 01424 216675; 121 Cooden Drive, Bexhill-on-Sea TN39 3AJ — MB BS Lond. 1986; BSc (Hons.) Path. Lond. 1985. Clin. Asst. (Rheum.) E. Sussex. Specialty: Rehabil. Med.; Rheumatol. Prev: Trainee GP Lond.

SINGH, Gurdeep Department of GU Medicine, Central Outpatients, University Hospital of North Staffordshire, Hartshill, Stoke-on-Trent ST4 7PA Tel: 01782 554144 Fax: 01782 846660 Email: gurdeep.singh@uhns.nhs.uk — MB BS Delhi 1978; FRCPI. Cons. in GU Med., Univ. Hosp. of N. Staffs., Stoke on Trent. Specialty: Genitourinary Medicine; HIV Med.; Gen. Pract. Special Interest: HIV; HPV; Recurrent Genital Herpes. Socs: BASHH; BHIVA; BMA.

SINGH, Gurminder Pal Oakwood Surgery, Glenhow Rise, Leeds LS8 4AA Tel: 0113 295 1515 Fax: 0113 295 1500 — MB BS Delhi 1975 (Maulana Azad Med. Coll. New Delhi) LRCP LRCS Ed. LRCPS Glas. 1981; DRCOG 1982; MRCGP 1985. GP Leeds. Socs: BMA. Prev: GP WSI Vasectomy & Minor Surg.

SINGH, Gurmit 15 Regency House, Newbold Terrace, Leamington Spa CV32 4HD Tel: 01926 33774 — MB ChB Manch. 1987. Specialty: Accid. & Emerg.

SINGH, Mr Gurpreet Consultant Urologist, Southport & Ormskirk Hospital, Southport PR8 6PN Tel: 01704 704025 Fax: 01704 704518 Email: gurpreet.singh@southportandormskirk.nhs.uk; 18 Westbourne Road, Southport PR8 2JA — MB BS Delhi 1981; FRCS Glas. 1985; FRCS Ed. 1985; FRCS (Urology) 1997. Cons. Urol., Southport; Cons. Neurologist, Southport; Hon. Cons. Neurologist, Walton Hosp. Specialty: Urol.; Neurol. Socs: Brit. Assn. of Urol. Surg.s; BMA; Roy. Soc. of Med. Prev: Sen. Regist. (Urol.), Sheff.; Lect. (Urol.), Sheff.; Regist. (Urol.), Canterbury.

SINGH, Gyan Prakash 1 Holly Court, Hyde SK14 3DF — MB BS Patna 1973.

SINGH, H K Halifax Crescent Surgery, 4 Halifax Crescent, Thornton, Liverpool L23 1TH Tel: 0151 924 3532 Fax: 0151 924 3171.

SINGH, Harbhajan Shah G Pendlebury Health Centre, The Lowry Medical Centre, 659 Bolton Road, Manchester M27 8HP Tel: 0161 793 8686 Fax: 0161 727 8011.

SINGH, Hardeep 11 Glenesk Road, London SE9 1AG — MB BS Lond. 1993.

SINGH, Hardev Fishergate Hill Surgery, 50 Fishergate Hill, Preston PR1 8DN Tel: 01772 254484 Fax: 01772 881835; 50 Fishergate Hill, Preston PR1 8DN Tel: 01772 54484 — MB ChB Manch. 1977; MRCGP 1981. Specialty: Gen. Med. Socs: Brit. Med. Acupunct. Soc.

SINGH, Hardev Calfaria Surgery, Regent Street, Treorchy CF42 6PR Tel: 01443 773595 Fax: 01443 775067 — MB BS Panjab 1971 (Govt. Med. Coll. Amritsar) MB BS Panjab (India) 1971. SHO (Orthop. & Trauma) Singleton Hosp. Swansea. Prev: SHO (Orthop. & Trauma) Neath Gen. Hosp.

SINGH, Hardial Department of Cardiology, Walsgrave Hospital, UHCW NHS Trust, Clifford Bridge Road, Coventry CV2 2DX Tel: 024 7653 8932; Priors Close, 24a Birchges Lane, Kenilworth CV8 2AD — MB ChB Ed. 1973; MRCP (UK) 1976; MD Ed. 1986; T(M) 1991; FRCP Lond. 1993. Cons. Cardiol. Walsgrave Hsop. Coventry. Specialty: Cardiol. Socs: Brit. Cardiac Soc.; Brit. Cardiac Interven. Soc.; BMA. Prev: Lect. (Cardiol.) Univ. Wales Coll. Med.; Regist. (Cardiol.) Hammersmith Hosp. & Gt. Ormond St. Lond.

SINGH, Hari B Clare Road Medical Centre, 150 Clare Road, Grangetown, Cardiff CF11 6RW Tel: 029 2023 1109 Fax: 029 2034 2122.

SINGH, Harikrishna 28 Hospital Close, Evington, Leicester LE5 4WP — MB BS W. Indies 1990.

SINGH, Harinandan Prasad 12 Leander Close, Littleover, Derby DE23 1TN — MB BS Patna 1973.

SINGH, Harjit 53 Mighell Avenue, Redbridge, Ilford IG4 5JP — MB BS Lucknow 1964 (King Geo. Med. Coll.) BSc Allahabad 1959. Socs: BMA. Prev: Ho. Phys. Walton Hosp. Liverp.; SHO Barrowmore Hosp. Gt. Barrow; Med. Regist. Colindale Hosp. Lond.

SINGH, Harjit Eccles Health Centre, Corporation Road, Eccles, Manchester M30 0EL Tel: 0161 788 7337 Fax: 0161 707 0504 — MB BS Panjab 1971. GP Princip. Specialty: Gen. Pract.

SINGH, Harjit Manor Court Surgery, 5 Manor Court Avenue, Nuneaton CV11 5HX Tel: 024 7638 1999 Fax: 024 7632 0515 — MB BS Lucknow 1964.

SINGH, Hem Chandra Springwell House Surgery, Durham Road, North Moor, Sunderland SR3 1RN Tel: 0191 528 3251 Fax: 0191 528 3100 — MB BS Bihar 1969; MS. Sunderland Tyne & Wear T.P.C.T. Special Interest: Surg., Orhtopaedics, Sports Med.

SINGH, Himani 53 Hope Park, Bromley BR1 3RG Tel: 020 8464 8633 Email: suveer.singh@ic.ac.uk — (UMDS Lond.) LMSSA Lond. 1995. Specialty: Gen. Pract.

SINGH, Hiralal Bendasari 23A Four Oaks Road, Sutton Coldfield B74 2XT Tel: 0121 308 1855 — LRCP LRCS Ed. 1951; LRCP LRCS Ed. LRFPS Glas. 1951. Prev: GP W. Midl.

SINGH, Inder Pal 98 Seamons Road, Altrincham WA14 4LB — MB BS Ranchi 1980.

SINGH, Inder Pal Health Centre, Great James Street, Londonderry BT48 7DH Tel: 028 7137 8500 — MB BS Allahabad 1971. GP Londonderry.

SINGH, Inderjit 3 The Bantocks, West Bromwich B70 0PA — MB BS Lond. 1994.

SINGH, Mr Inderjit 7 Wykeham Hill, Wembley Park, Wembley HA9 9RY Tel: 020 8904 6119 — MB BS Lucknow 1973 (King Geo. Med. Coll. Lucknow) MRCS Eng. LRCP Lond. 1978; DO Eng. 1978; FRCS (Ophth.) Eng. 1980. Res. Surg. Off. Moorfields Eye Hosp. Lond. Prev: Regist. Dept. Ophth. Westm. Hosp. Lond.

SINGH, Mr Inderjit Drumchapel Health Centre, 80 Kinfains Drove, Drumchapel, Glasgow G15 6EG Tel: 0141 211 6090 — MB BS Medical College, Amritsar 1971; FRCS Glas. 1979. Gen. Pract., Drumchapel Health Centre, Glas.; Hosp. Practitioner Grade, ENT, Hairmyers Hosp., E. Kilbridge, G76. Specialty: Gen. Pract.; Otolaryngol.; Allergy. Socs: Gen. Med. Counc.; Overseas Doctor's Assoc.; SIKH Doctor's Assoc. OPU.K.

SINGH, Iqbal Hillingdon Hospital, Field Heath Road, Uxbridge UB8 3NN; 7 Grovewood Close, Chorleywood, Rickmansworth WD3 5PU Tel: 01923 282663 — MB BS Punjab 1974; FRCPsych 1995, M 1983. Cons. Psychiat. Hillingdon Hosp. Middlx. & Horizon NHS Trust Herts.; Vis. Cons. Psychiat. HM Prison Psychiat. Servs. Specialty: Gen. Psychiat. Prev: Cons. Psychiat. Leavesden Hosp. Abbots Langley & Hillingdon Hosp. Middlx.; Sen. Regist. Rotat. (Psychiat.) Leavesden & Char. Cross Hosp. Lond.; Regist. Rotat. Princess Alexandra Hosp. Harlow & St. Bart. Hosp. Lond.

SINGH, Irengbam Mohendra Kensington Street Health Centre, Whitefield Place, Girlington, Bradford BD8 9LB Tel: 01274 499209 — MB BS Agra 1962 (S.N. Med. Coll. Agra) BSc Agra 1957, MB BS 1962; MRCGP 1977.

SINGH, Mr Jagmohan University Hospital of North Staffordshire, Department of Neurosurgery, Princes Road, Stoke-on-Trent ST4 7LN — MB BS Poona 1975; FRCS Glas. 1987. Cons. (Neurosurg.). Specialty: Neurosurg.

SINGH, Jasbir — MB BS Panjab 1967; MRCPsych 1980. Specialty: Geriat. Psychiat.; Forens. Psychiat.

SINGH, Jasminder Kaur 52 Eamont Court, Shannon Place, London NW8 7DN — MB BS Lond. 1997.

SINGH, Jaswant Peter Hodgkinson Centre, Greetwell Road, Lincoln LN2 5UA Tel: 01522 512512 — MB BS Bangalor 1973; MRCPsych 1986. Cons. Psychiat. (Gen. Adult & Rehabil.) Peter Hodgkinson Centre Lincoln. Specialty: Gen. Psychiat. Special Interest: Forens. Psychiat. Prev: Sen. Med. Off. HM Prison Lincoln; Cons. Psychiat. Rampton Hosp.

SINGH, Mr Jaswinder 68 Comiston Drive, Edinburgh EH10 5QS — MB ChB Glas. 1986 (Glasgow) BSc Hons. (St. And.) 1982; MSc St. And. 1983; FRCS Ed. 1992. Cons. (Ophth.) Princess Alexandra Eye Pavilion Edin.; Hon. Sen. Lect., Univ. of Edin.; Examr. for Roy. Coll. of Surg.s of Edin. Specialty: Ophth.

SINGH, Jillian Kaur St Pauls Surgery, 36-38 East Street, Preston PR1 1UU Tel: 01772 252409 Fax: 01772 885509 — MB BS Delhi 1969; MB BS Delhi 1969.

SINGH, Joginder Paul 12 Bellevue Terrace, Southampton SO14 0LB — MB ChB Glas. 1974.

SINGH, John Lawrence Shaftesbury Medical Centre, 480 Harehills Lane, Leeds LS9 6DE Tel: 0113 248 0392 Fax: 0113 235 1585 — MB BS Vikram 1963. GP Leeds.

SINGH, John Pratap (retired) Pondfield House, Bellingdon, Chesham HP5 2XL — MRCS Eng. LRCP Lond. 1962 (Nagpur) BSc Nagpur 1947, MB BS 1952; LMSSA Lond. 1960; DA Eng. 1960; FFA RCS Eng. 1965. Indep. Cons. Anaesth. Herts. Prev: Cons. Anaesth. Centr. Middlx. Hosp. Lond.

SINGH, Joy Carmelina Indira 38 Newport Road, London E10 6PJ — MB BS Lond. 1994.

SINGH, Mr Juswant c/o Orthopaediac Department, Princess Royal Hospital, Telford TF1 6TF — MB BS Lond. 1979; FRCS Ed. 1986. Staff Orthop. Surg. Princess Roy. Hosp. Telford. Specialty: Orthop. Prev: Regist. (Orthop.) N. Middlx. Hosp. Lond.; SHO Rotat. (Surg.) Worcester Roy. Infirm.; SHO Princess Eliz. Orthop. Hosp. Exeter.

SINGH, Jyoti Prakash Barkerend Health Centre, Bradford BD3 8QH Tel: 01274 661341 Fax: 01274 775880 — MB BS Patna 1973. GP Bradford, W. Yorks.

SINGH, K The Surgery, 14a Norheads Lane, Bigginhill, Westerham TN16 3XS Tel: 01959 574488.

SINGH, Kamala Pati 32 Waldorf Road, Cleethorpes DN35 0QD Tel: 01472 812002 — MB BS Bihar 1967; DCH RCPI 1981.

SINGH, Kamaljit 5 Chestnut Drive, Bushby, Leicester LE7 9RB Tel: 0116 241 8252 — MB ChB Leeds 1990; BSc (Hons.) Physiol. Leeds 1987; MRCGP 1995. Princip. GP, Thurmaston Med. Centre. Specialty: Gen. Pract. Prev: Regist. Leics. VTS; SHO (Haemat.) Leicester Roy. Infirm.; Ho. Off. (Med. & Surg.) Leeds Gen. Infirm.

SINGH, Kanimbakam Rameshwari Lynwood, 33 Danygraig Drive, Talbot Green, Pontyclun CF72 8AQ — MB BS Osmania 1965 (Osmania Med. Coll. Hyderabad) DPM Eng. 1973. Clin. Asst. Ely Hosp. Cardiff.

SINGH, Karan Vir Sides Medical Centre, Moorside Road, Swinton, Manchester M27 0EW Tel: 0161 794 1604 Fax: 0161 727 3615 — MB ChB Manch. 1975.

SINGH, Karen Jit 93 Whitehall Road, Gateshead NE8 4ER — MB BS Lond. 1994; BSc Lond. 1991. SHO (A & E) N. Tyneside. Prev: Ho. Off. (Med.) Croydon.

SINGH, Karnail 21 Ferry Road, Eastham, Wirral CH62 0AJ — MB ChB Liverp. 1974.

SINGH, Mr Kaushlendra Narayan Department of Orthopaedics, Hillingdon Hospital, Pield Heath Road, Uxbridge UB8 3NN Tel: 01895 238282 Fax: 01895 811687; 80 Harlington Road, Uxbridge UB8 3EY Tel: 01895 462720 Fax: 01895 462720 Email: kaushal@postmaster.co.uk — MB BS Bhagalar 1981 (Bhagalpur & Patna) MB BS Bhagalar, India 1981; Dip. Orthop. Patna 1983; MS (Orthop.) Patna 1985. Staff Orthop. Surg. Hillingdon Hosp. Uxbridge. Specialty: Orthop. Socs: BMA. Prev: Regist. Rotat. Roy. Orthop. Hosp. Birm.

SINGH, Mr Kewal 10 Abingdon Close, Uxbridge UB10 0BU — MB BS Delhi 1978; FRCS Eng. 1990.

SINGH, Kirpal 184 Lady Margaret Road, Southall UB1 2RW — MB BS Jammu & Kashmir 1967.

SINGH, Krishna Ballabh Prasad Coatbridge Health Centre, 1 Centre Park Court, Coatbridge ML5 3AP Tel: 01236 421434 — MB BS Patna 1974.

SINGH, Mr Krishna Kumar Worthing Hospital, Lyndhurst Road, Worthing BN11 2DH — MB BS Poona 1986; FRCS Glas. 1989. Specialty: Gen. Surg.

SINGH, Krishna Mohan 201 Rochford Gardens, Slough SL2 5XD — MB BS Patna 1973.

SINGH, Kuljinder — MB ChB Glas. 1989; MRCGP 1994. GP. Specialty: Gen. Pract.

SINGH, Kulvinder The Medical Centre, 10A Northumberland Court, Shepway, Maidstone ME15 7LN Tel: 01622 753920 Fax: 01622 692747; Saran-Nivas, Queens Avenue, Maidstone ME16 0EN Tel: 01622 670495 Fax: 01622 675475 — MB BS Delhi 1978; LRCP LRCS Ed. LRCPS Glas. 1983.

SINGH, Mr Kulwant (retired) 21 Lushington Road, Eastbourne BN21 4LG Tel: 01323 410441 Fax: 01323 410978 — MB BS Calcutta 1959; BSc Punjab 1953; DLO RCS Eng. 1964; FRCS Ed. 1969. Prev: Cons. ENT Surg. Eastbourne Hosps. NHS Trust.

SINGH, Kumar Himanshu Prasad Elizabeth Ash Road, Hartley, Longfield DA3 8HA — MB BS Bihar 1966.

SINGH, Kumar Sitaram Prasad Narain The Medical Centre, Keldholme Lane, Alvaston, Derby DE24 0RY Tel: 01332 571677 — MB BS Patna 1973 (P. of Wales Med. Coll.) GP Derby; Capt. RAMC (V). Prev: SHO (Accid., Emerg. & Orthop.) Ashington Hosp.; Trainee GP Lincoln VTS; GP Co. Durh.

SINGH, Kumari Kavita 38 Longdon Wood, Keston BR2 6EW Tel: 01689 853303 — LMSSA Lond. 1975; MD (Paediat.) Jabalpur 1970, MB BS 1967; DCH Jabalpur 1969; MRCP (U.K.) 1974. SCMO Oxleas NHS Trust. Specialty: Community Child Health. Socs: Brit. Paediat. Assn. Prev: Regist. (Paediat.) Whipps Cross Hosp. Lond.; SHO Roy. Belf. Hosp. Sick Childr.; Clin. Med. Off. Ealing HA.

SINGH, Lehmbar Millfield Medical Centre, 63-83 Hylton Road, Sunderland SR4 7AF Tel: 0191 567 9179 Fax: 0191 514 7452; October House, 18 Silksworth Hall Drive, Sunderland SR3 2PG — MB ChB Manch. 1986; DCH RCP Lond. 1989; MRCGP 1990; DRCOG 1990.

SINGH, Linda Nalini Department of Histopathology, St. Helier Hospital, Wrythe Lane, Carshalton SM5 1AA Tel: 020 8644 4343 — MB BS Madras 1975; MRCPath 1984.

SINGH, Madan Mohan Department of Obstetrics & Gynaecology, Leazes Wing, Royal Victoria Infirmary, Queen Victoria Road, Newcastle upon Tyne NE1 4LP — MB ChB Aberd. 1965.

SINGH, Mahendra Pratap 9 Coniston Gardens, Ashby-de-la-Zouch LE65 1FB — MB BS Kanpur 1970.

SINGH, Mala Basudeo 2 Moatlands House, Cramer St., London WC1H 8DF — MB ChB Baghdad 1982.

SINGH, Maneesha 2 The Sidings, Worsley, Manchester M28 2QD — MB BS Lond. 1995.

SINGH, Mr Manmeet (retired) Holly House Hospital, High Road, Buckhurst Hill IG9 5HX Tel: 020 8559 2339 Fax: 020 8559 2339; 97 Hainault Road, Chigwell IG7 5DL Tel: 020 8500 6137 — MB BS Lond. 1960 (Lond. Hosp.) FRCS Eng. 1966. Cons. Urol. Surg. Whipps Cross Hosp.; Hon. Sen. Lect. Inst. Urol. Univ. Lond. Prev: Sen. Lect. (Urol.) Lond. Hosp. Med. Coll.

SINGH, Mehar M O Wallis & Partners, 5 Stanmore Road, Stevenage SG1 3QA Tel: 01438 313223; 28 Gibson Close, Hitchin SG4 0RS Tel: 01462 438465 Email: mehar1960@hotmail.com — MB BS Guru Nanak Dev India 1985 (Govt. Med. Coll., Amritsar, India) DOrth Amritsar (India) 1987. G.P. M.O. Wallis & Partners Stevenage. Specialty: Gen. Pract.; Orthopaedics. Special Interest: Back Pain. Prev: Trust Specialist (Trauma & Orthop.) P. Chas. Hosp. Merthyr Tydfil.

SINGH, Mira 17 Bank Street, Horbury, Wakefield WF4 6LN — MB BS Mithila, India 1975.

SINGH, Mohan Bhadoor Arrow Lodge Medical Centre, Kinwarton Road, Alcester B49 5QY Tel: 01789 763293; Arrow Lodge, Alcester B49 5QY Tel: 01789 763293 — MB BS Patna 1967. Hosp. Pract. Alcester Hosp. Prev: Sen. Med. Off. McCord Zulu Miss. Hosp. Durban S. Africa; Regist. Surg. R.K. Khan Hosp. Durban; Med. Asst. Accid. Dept. Watford Gen. Hosp. (Peace Memor. Wing.).

SINGH, Monica Fairwinds, Highrigg Drive, Durton Lane, Broughton, Preston PR3 5LJ — MB BS Lond. 1996.

SINGH, Mreenal Nandan 15 Riplingham Road, Kirkella, Hull HU10 7TS — MB BCh Wales 1993.

SINGH, Mukhtar 5 Park Avenue, Goldthorn Park, Wolverhampton WV4 5AL — MB ChB Glasg. 1986.

SINGH, Nandita Woodcroft, Barnet Wood Road, Bromley BR2 8HJ — MB BS Lond. 1994.

SINGH, Narayani Prasad Dinas Lane Medical Centre, 149 Dinas Lane, Huyton, Liverpool L36 2NW Tel: 0151 489 2298 — MB BS Allahabad 1968; MD Allahabad 1976.

SINGH, Narendra 38 Colne Road, Burnley BB10 1LG Tel: 01282 448244 Fax: 01282 448282; Edge End Hall, Edge End Lane, Nelson BB9 0PR Tel: 01282 611008 Fax: 01282 690808 — MB BS Rajasthan 1963 (Sawai Man Singh Med. Coll. Jaipur) Prev: SHO Dept. Dermat. Roy. Vict. Infirm. Newc.; Ho. Off. Glos. Roy. Hosp. Gloucester; Ho. Off. (Med.) Roy. Vict. Hosp. Boscombe.

SINGH, Narendra Pal Singh and Reddy, 44 Grimsby Road, Cleethorpes DN35 7AB Tel: 01472 342763 Fax: 01472 344490 — BSc Agra Univ. India 1965 (Agra Univ. India & Kanpur Medical College, India) MB BS Kanpur Medical Coll. India 1970. GP, NHS, Grimsby; Clin. Asst., Family Plann. & Sexual Health. Specialty: Family Plann. & Reproduc. Health; Community Child Health; Orthop. Prev: Regist. Orthapaedic Surg., Scunthorpe Gen. Hosp. Scunthorpe.

SINGH, Nitish Kumar Blackburn Road Medical Centre, Birstall, Batley WF17 8PL Tel: 01924 478285 — MB BS Lond. 1998; MB BS Lond 1998.

SINGH, Nivedita St Helier Hospital, Carshalton SM5 1AA — MB BS Lond. 1992; MRCP 1996; MD 2002.

SINGH, Padm Deo Narayan c/o Barclays Bank, Haverfordwest SA61 2DA Tel: 01793 30045 — MD Bihar 1957 (Darbhanga Med. Coll.) MB BS 1954; MRCP (U.K.) 1971. Cons. Phys. Princess Margt. & St. Margt. Hosps. Swindon. Specialty: Gen. Med. Prev: Cons. Phys. St. Jas. Hosp. Leeds; Sen. Regist. (Med.) Singleton Hosp. Swansea; Cons. Geriat. Phys. Hartlepool Gen. Hosp.

SINGH, Padma Nand 18 Woodcourt Close, Sittingbourne ME10 1QT — MB BS Bihar 1961 (Darbhanga Med. Coll.) DTM & H Ed. 1970.

SINGH, Param Jit Daybrook Health Centre, Salop Street, Daybrook, Nottingham NG5 6HP.

SINGH, Parminder Jit 43 Barnes Heath Road, Rowlatts Hill, Leicester LE5 4LB — MB BS Lond. 1996.

SINGH, Parvinder 27 Alexander Road, Hounslow TW3 4HW Email: drpsnarang@yahoo.com — (Maulana Azad Medical College Delhi) MB BS Delhi 1980, DCH 1982; DCH Eng. 1984; MRCP (UK) 1986. Regist. (Community Paediat.) Centr. Middlx. Hosp. Lond. Specialty: Paediat.; Gastroenterol.; Neonat. Prev: SHO (Paediat. Gastroenterol.,Metos. Dis.) Gt. Ormond St. Lond.; Regist. (Paediat.) Maidstone Gen. Hosp.

SINGH, Phulwantjit c/o Barclays Bank Ltd, Clapham Common Branch, PO Box 4038, London SW12 9YB — LRCP LRCS Ed. LRCPS Glas. 1983.

SINGH, Pradeep Kumar Fryerns Medical Centre, Peterborough Way, Basildon SS14 3SS Tel: 01268 532344 Fax: 01268 287641 — MB BS Calcutta 1974. Specialty: Gen. Pract.

SINGH, Pradip Department of Gastroenterology, Staffordshire General Hospital, Stafford ST16 3SA Tel: 01785 230959 Fax: 01785 230771; High Trees, Inglewood, Rowley Avenue, STAFFORD ST17 9FN Tel: 01785 223951 Email: psingh56@doctors.org.uk — MB BS Banaras Hindu 1980; MD Med. Banaras Hindu 1983; MD Med. Banaras Hindu 1993; DM Soton. 1993. Cons. Gastroenterologist. Specialty: Gastroenterol.

SINGH, Prashant Kishore 125 Hatherton Road, Cannock WS11 1HH — BM BS Nottm. 1997.

SINGH, Prem 2 Weaver Avenue, Birmingham B26 3AA — MB BCh Wales 1990.

SINGH, Priya Darshani Arrow Lodge, Alcester B49 5QY — MB ChB Leic. 1990.

SINGH, Raj Pal The Health Centre, High Street, Dodworth, Barnsley S75 3RF Tel: 01226 203881 — MB BS Kanpur 1972 (G.S.V.M. Med. Coll.) DCH RCPSI 1979.

SINGH, Rajendra Kumar Maypole Road Surgery, Maypole Road, Tiptree, Colchester CO5 0EN Tel: 01621 816119 — MB BS Patna 1959; MD Patna 1965; DCH Patna 1966. Socs: Med. Protec. Soc.

SINGH, Rajinder 43 Barnes Heath Road, Leicester LE5 4LB — MB BS Lond. 1995.

SINGH, Rajinder 8A Beech Road, London N11 2DA Tel: 020 8888 5157 — MB BS Poona 1977; DMedRehab. RCP Lond. 1986; MRCS Eng. LRCP Lond. 1989. SHO (O & G) N. Middlx. Hosp. Lond. Prev: SHO (Geriat., A & E) Middlx. Hosp. Lond.

SINGH, Rajiv Kumar 55 Craigour Avenue, Edinburgh EH17 7NH — MB ChB Ed. 1992; MA Camb. 1993; MRCP (UK) 1995. SHO Roy. Infirm. Edin.

SINGH, Rakesh Kumar 2 Rosslyn Ave, Ackworth, Pontefract WF7 7QF — MB BS Patna 1986.

SINGH, Ram Chandra Prasad Robins Hill, Bent Lane, Colne BB8 7AA — MB BS Patna 1962; MRCP (UK) 1971.

SINGH, Ram Karan Queen Elizabeth Hospital, Gateshead Health NHS Trust, Gateshead NE9 6SX; 38 Baronswood, Gosforth, Newcastle upon Tyne NE3 3UB — MB BS L.N. Mithila, India 1983; FRCA 1992; FFA RCSI 1992. (Anaesth.) Qu. Eliz. Hosp. Gateshead. Specialty: Anaesth. Special Interest: Trauma Anaesthetics.

SINGH, Rama Shanker South Tyneside Hospital, South Shields ME34 0DL Tel: 0191 959 8888 Fax: 0191 202 4049 Email: von.singh@sthct.nhs.uk — MB BS; FRCS; FFAEM; MS. Cons. in Accid. and Emerg. Specialty: Accid. & Emerg. Special Interest: Orthopaedic Surgery; Sports Injuries; Trauma. Socs: GMC; BMA; MDU.

SINGH, Rameet Whipps Cross Hospital, Leytonstone, London E11 1NR Tel: 020 8539 5522 Fax: 020 8558 8115; 19 Lansdowne Road, South Woodford, London E18 2AZ Tel: 020 8530 4370 — MB BS Lond. 1972 (Lond. Hosp.) DA Lond. 1980. Assoc. Specialist (Anaesth.) Whipps Cross Hosp. Lond. Specialty: Anaesth. Socs: Fell. Roy. Soc. Med.; Assn. Anaesth.; BMA. Prev: GP Lond.

SINGH, Ramnandan County Hospital, ENT Department, Union Walk, Hereford HR1 2ER Tel: 01432 355444 — MB BS Patna 1974. Staff Grade (ENT) Co. Hosp. Hereford.

SINGH, Miss Rashmi Department of Surgery, St. Georges Hospital, Blackshaw Road, Tooting, London SW17 0QT Tel: 020 8672 1255; Flat 8, Clockhouse Place, Lytton Grove, Putney, London SW15 2EL Tel: 020 8789 6533 — MB BS Lond. 1994 (UMDS Guy's & St. Thos.) BSc (Hons.) Genetics Lond. 1991; FRCS (Eng) 1998. Clin. Res. Fell. (Urol.) Roy. Marsden Hosp. Lond. Specialty: Urol. Socs: Wom. Surgic. Train.; Med. Protec. Soc. Prev: SHO (Urol.) Roy. Marsden; SHO Rotat. (Surg.) St. Geo. Hosp. Lond.; SHO (A & E) St. Thos. Hosp. Lond.

SINGH, Rashmi Kumari 6 Leigham Drive, Osterley, Isleworth TW7 5LU Email: rashmi_singh@doctor.com — MB BS Lond. 1997; DRCOG 2001; DFFP 2001.

SINGH, Ravi Kumar 1 Deepdale Drive, Burnley BB10 2SD — MB BCh Wales 1994; MRCP (UK) 1998. SHO (Clin. Cardiol.) Glenfield Hosp. Leicester. Prev: SHO (Gen. Med.) Doncaster Roy. Infirm.

SINGH, Ravinder 76 Townley Road, Bexleyheath DA6 7HN — MB BS Lond. 1996. SHO (Trauma & Orthop.) Kent & Canterbury Hosp. Specialty: Orthop. Prev: SHO (Accid.) Emerg.) Kent & Canterbury

Hosp.; Ho. Off. (Surg.) Wartling Hosp.; Ho. Off. (Med.) Qu. Mary's Hosp. Sidcup.

SINGH, Rema 28 Charlbert Court, Charlbert St., London NW8 7BX — MB BS Lond. 1993; MA Camb. 1994. SHO (Respirat. Med.) Roy. Brompton Hosp. Lond.

SINGH, Roger Rambaran 42 Epping Close, Mawyneys, Romford RM7 8BH; 205 Henley Road, Ilford 1G1 2TP Tel: 020 7924 5271 — (Royal London Hospital, Whitechapel) MB BS Lond. 1996. SHO in Psychiat. Specialty: Gen. Psychiat. Prev: Ho. Off. Surg. Roy. Lond. Hosp.; Ho. Off. Surg. King Geo. Hosp.; SHO Psychiat. Goodmayes Hosp.

SINGH, Rudolph Bickram (retired) 10 Princes Avenue, Petts Wood, Orpington BR5 1QS — (Glas.) BSc (Hons.) Glas. 1965; MB ChB (Commend.) Glas. 1969; MSc Ed. 1982. Prev: Sen. Med. Off. DoH.

SINGH, S The Surgery, 14a Norheads Lane, Bigginhill, Westerham TN16 3XS Tel: 01959 574488.

SINGH, S Townsend Lane Surgery, 263 Townsend Lane, Clubmoor, Liverpool L13 9DG Tel: 0151 226 1358.

SINGH, S 104 Tarbock Road, Huyton, Liverpool L36 5TH.

SINGH, S B P 4 Halifax Crescent, Thornton, Liverpool L23 1TH.

SINGH, Mr Sadmeet 46 Redcliffe Road, Nottingham NG3 5BW Tel: 0115 9624925 Email: sadmeet@yahoo.com — BM BS Nottm. 1993; BMedSci Nottm. 1991; FRCS (Eng) 1998; DM 2004.

SINGH, Mr Sakaldip 1 The Chenies, Orpington BR6 0ED — MB BS Patna 1959; MS Patna 1966; FRCS Ed. 1977. Cons. A & E Med. Greenwich Dist. Hosp. Lond. Specialty: Accid. & Emerg. Socs: BMA; W Kent M-C Soc.; Brit. Assn. Accid. & Emerg. Med. Prev: Cons. A & E Brook Gen. Hosp. Lond.

SINGH, Salil 42 Druids Park, Liverpool L18 3LJ — MB ChB Ed. 1997.

SINGH, Sandip 10 Girdlers Close, Coventry CV3 6LS — MB ChB Liverp. 1987; Dip. Amer. Bd Anesthesiol 1997. Specialty: Anaesth.; Intens. Care. Prev: Fell. (Critical Care Med.) Univ. of Texas at Houston USA; Resid. (Anesthesiology) Univ. of Texas at Houston USA; Resid. (Internal Med.) Univ. of Connecticut USA.

SINGH, Mr Sanjay Kumar James Paget Hospital, Lowestoft Rd,, Gorleston, Great Yarmouth NR31 6LA Tel: 01493 452620 Fax: 01493 452061; Peddars Croft, Main Road, Rollesby, Great Yarmouth NR29 5EQ Tel: 01493 748739 Fax: 01493 748068 — MB BS Delhi 1985; MS (Gen. Surg.) Delhi 1990; FRCSI 1994. Assoc. Specialist (Gen. Surg.) Jas. Paget Hosp. Gt. Yarmouth. Specialty: Gen. Surg. Prev: Regist. (Gen. Surg.) Jas. Paget Hosp. Gt. Yarmouth.

SINGH, Santokh 13 Mellor Street, Rochdale OL12 6XD — MB ChB Manch. 1985.

SINGH, Mrs Sarla St. Peters Hospital, Chertsey KT16 0PZ; Dorin Lodge, 6 Dorin Court, Woking GU22 8PS Tel: 01932 347950 Fax: 01932 347950 — MB BS Jiwaji 1971; MS (Obs & Gynae) Jiwaji 1973; MRCOG 1981; FRCOG 1997. Staff O & G St. Peter's Hosp. Guildford Rd. Chertsey. Specialty: Obst. & Gyn. Prev: Specialist (O & G) Dammam Matern. Hosp. Dammam, Saudi Arabia.

SINGH, Satish Shankar Medicine Control Agency, Market Towers, 1 Nine Elms Lane, London SW8 5NQ Tel: 020 7273 0420; Dorin Lodge, 6 Dorin Court, Pyrford, Woking GU22 8PS — MB BS Banaras Hindu 1969 (Inst. Med. Scs. Varanasi) MD (Gen. Med.) Banaras Hindu 1974, MB BS 1971; MRCP (UK) 1978; FRCP Ed. 1992. Sen. Med. Off. Med. Control Agency Lond. Specialty: Cardiol. Prev: Cons. Cardiol. Dammam Centr. Hosp. Saudi Arabia; Regist. (Cardiol.) Regional Adult Cardiac Centre Broadgreen Gen. Hosp. Liverp.; Regist. (Gen. Med.) Middlesbrough Gen. Hosp.

SINGH, Satpal Harvey House Surgery, 13-15 Russell Avenue, St Albans AL3 5HB Tel: 01727 831888 Fax: 01727 845520 — MB BS Delhi 1968.

SINGH, Satwant Ahluwalia 4 Gledhow Wood, The Chase, Kingswood, Tadworth KT20 6JQ Tel: 01737 833783 — LRCP LRCS Ed. 1952; MB BS Panjab 1949; LRCP LRCS Ed. LRCPS Glas. 1952; FRCP Ed. 1982, M 1952.

SINGH, Mr Sewa Surgical Directorate, Doncaster Royal Infirmary, Armthorpe Road, Doncaster DN2 5LT Tel: 01302 553225 Fax: 01302 553266; 56A Sunderland Street, Tickhill, Doncaster DN11 9QJ — MB ChB Sheff. 1983; FRCS Ed. 1988; MD Sheff. 1992. Cons. Surg. Doncaster Roy. Infirm.; Roy. Coll. of Surg.s Tutor.

SINGH, Shambhu Nath Queens Drive Surgery, 73 Queens Drive, Mossley Hill, Liverpool L18 2DU Tel: 0151 733 2812 — MB BS Patna 1973.

SINGH, Shareen Royal Hospitals Trusts, Royal Victoria Hospital, Department Of Anaesthetics, Grosvenor Rd, Belfast BT12 6BA — MB ChB Univ. of Natal Med. Sch. 1992 (Univ. of Natal Med. Sch., Durban, S. Africa) Diploma in Anaesth. (DA, SA) Coll. of Med. of SA, Fac. of Anaesthetists 1995; Primary FFARCSI, Fac. of Anaesthetists, Roy. Coll. of Surgeons of Irel. 1998. Staff Grade, Anaesthetics, Roy. Vict. Hosp., Belf. Specialty: Anaesth. Socs: N. Irel. Soc. of Anaesth.s; Assn. of Anaesth.s of GB & Irel.; Roy. Coll. of Anaesth.s. Prev: Sen. Ho. Off. Anaesthetics, Belf. City Hosp.; Sen. Ho. Off. Anaesthetics, Ulster Hosp., Belf.; Sen. Ho. Off. Anaesthetics, Craigavon Hosp., Craigavon, North. Irel.

SINGH, Shatrughna Prasad Singh, Craven Park Health Centre, Shakespeare Crescent, London NW10 8XW Tel: 020 8965 0151 Fax: 020 8965 4921 — MB BS Patna 1960.

SINGH, Mr Shiva Dayal 206 Emblem House, London Bridge Hospital, 27 Tooley St., London SE1 2PR Tel: 020 7935 3763 Fax: 020 7403 2523 Email: shivasingh@aol.com — MB BS Kanpur 1970; FRCS Eng. 1975; FRCS Ed. 1975. Cons. Surg. Lond. Bridge Hosp. & Highgate Private Hosp. Lond.; Vis. Cons. Surg. N. Downs Hosp. Caterham; Cons. Surg. Devonsh. Hosp. Lond. & Suttons Manor Clinic Stapleford Tawney; Vis. Cons. Surg. Hosp. of St. John & St. Eliz. Nuffield Hse. Guy's Hosp. & Med. Sch. Lond. Specialty: Gen. Surg. Socs: Fell. Assn. Surgs.; Fell. Med. Soc. Lond.; BMA. Prev: Chief Surg. Nat. Iranian Oil Company Hosp. Aghajari & Oil Fields; Regist. (Cardiothoracic) Freeman Hosp. Newc. u. Tyne; Regist. (Surg.) Stepping Hill Hosp. Stockport.

SINGH, Shree Krishna Department of Medicine (General Medicine), Burnley General Hospital, Casterton Avenue, Burnley BB10 2PQ Tel: 01282 425071 Fax: 01282 474607 — MB BS Patna 1971; DTM & H Liverp. 1983; Dip. Cardiol. Lond 1985. Locum Cons. (Physician) Dept. Of Med. Burnley Gen. Hosp. Burnley. Specialty: Gen. Med. Prev: Assoc. Specialist (Med.) Burnley Gen. Hosp. Burnley; Assoc. Specialist (Med. Elderly) Burnley Gen. Hosp.; Regist. (Gen. & Geriat Med.) Burnley Gen. Hosp.

SINGH, Shyam Pratap 101 Westfield Road, Edgbaston, Birmingham B15 3JE Tel: 0121 454 5943 — (King Geo. Med. Coll. Lucknow) MB BS Lucknow 1954; FRCP Ed. 1971, M 1959. Hon. Cons. Cardiol. City Hosp. Univ. Dept. of Med. Birm.; Sen. Fell. Univ. Birm.; Examr. MRCP (UK). Specialty: Cardiol. Socs: Brit. Cardiac. Soc. & Assn. Europ. Paediat. Cardiols.; Working Gp. Grown Up Congen. Heart Dis.; Eur. Soc. Cardiol. Prev: Director Cardiac Thoracic Unit, Birm. Childr.s Hosp. 1990-1983; Sen. Clin. & Research Fell. (Med.) Mass. Gen. Hosp. Harvard Univ., USA; Vis. Sci. Mayo Clinic USA.

SINGH, Mr Subhash Chandra Kensington House, Lodge Lane, Kingswinford DY6 9XE — MB BS Ranchi 1980; FRCS Glas. 1989. Specialty: Urol.

SINGH, Sudarshan Springhill Medical Centre, Arley, Coventry CV7 8FD; 34 Bulkington Lane, Nuneaton CV11 4SA — MB BS Punjab 1956; MB BS Punjab (India) 1956; DTM & H Liverp. 1965; MRCP Ed. 1967. Hosp. Pract. Gulson Hosp. Coventry; Hosp. Pract. Med. OPD Geo. Eliot Hosp. Nuneaton. Socs: Overseas Doctors Assn. & BMA. Prev: Clin. Asst. High View Hosp. Exhall; Med. Regist. Geo. Eliot Hosp. Nuneaton; Jun. Ho. Phys., Sen. Ho. Phys. & Cas. Med. Off. Rajendra Hosp.

SINGH, Sujaan Flat 1, Victoria Hospital, Thursby Road, Burnley BB10 3HP — MB BS Delhi 1975.

SINGH, Sukh Dave 4 Oaks Drive, Colchester CO3 3PR — MB BChir Camb. 1992.

SINGH, Sukhbinder University Hospital NHS Trust, Queen Elizabeth Hospital, Edgbaston, Birmingham B15 2TH Tel: 0121 472 1311; 132A Rosemary Hill Road, Sutton Coldfield B74 4HN Email: sukhbinder.singh@virgin.net — BM Soton. 1991 (Soton) MRCP Roy. Coll. Psychiat. 1995; DA Roy. Coll. Anaesth. 1997; FRCA 1999. Specialist Regist. Anaesth & Intens. Care Med. Uni. Hosp. NHS Trust. Birm. FT. Specialty: Anaesth.; Psychother. Socs: RCA; Brit. Intens. Care Soc.; Brit. Pain Soc. Prev: SHO Anaesth & Inten. Care Med.; SHO Med.

SINGH, Sukhdev Department Gastroenterology, Good Hope Hospital, Rectory Road, Sutton Coldfield B75 7RR — MB ChB Leeds 1986; BSc (1st cl. Hons. Physiol.) Leeds 1983; MB ChB (Hons.)

Leeds 1986; MRCP (UK) 1989; MD Leeds 1995. Hon. Cons. & Sen. Lect. Univ. of Birm. Specialty: Gen. Med.; Gastroenterol. Socs: Brit. Soc. Gastroenterol. Prev: MRC Train. Fell. Univ. Birm.; SHO Rotat. (Med.) Leicester Gen. Hosp.

SINGH, Sukhdev Bellevue Medical Group Practice, 6 Bellevue, Edgbaston, Birmingham B5 7LX Tel: 0121 446 2000 Fax: 0121 446 2015 — MB ChB Dundee 1984; MRCGP 1988; Cert. Family Plann. JCC 1988. Med. Off. Woodbourne Clinic Edgbaston. Specialty: Gen. Pract.

SINGH, Sukhdev Sanghera 5 Rectory Close, Exhall, Coventry CV7 9PA — MB ChB Manch. 1975.

SINGH, Mr Sukhpal Frimley Park Hospital NHS Trust, Portsmouth Road, Frimley, Camberley GU16 7UJ Tel: 01276 604604; Puckridge, Crooksbury Lane, Seale, Farnham GU10 1ND Tel: 01252 781849 Fax: 01252 783929 — MB BS Lond. 1983 (Guy's) FRCS Ed. 1987; FRCS Eng. 1988; MS Lond. 1993; FRCS (Gen.) 1995. Cons. Surg. Specialty: Gen. Surg. Prev: Sen. Regist. Qu. Alexandra Hosp. Portsmouth, Roy. Surrey Co. Hosp., St. Geos. Hosp. & St. Thos. Hosp.; Regist. (Surg.) Roy. Surrey Co. Hosp. Guildford & Qu. Mary's Hosp. Roehampton.

SINGH, Surendra Prasad Steps to Health, Mental Health Directorate, Wolverhampton City PCT, Showell Circus, Law Hill, Wolverhampton WV10 9TH — MB BS India (King Georges Medical College, India) MD. Gen. Adult Psychiat.; Hon. Reader in Ment. Health, Univ. of Wolverhampton. Specialty: Gen. Psychiat. Special Interest: Bipolar Effective Disorder; genomics of Psychiatric disorders. Prev: S.C.M.D. Regist.

SINGH, Surendra Pratap The Surgery, 69 Stockingate, South Kirkby, Pontefract WF9 3PE — MB BS Patna 1974. GP Pontefract, W. Yorks.

SINGH, Sureshwar Prasad 146A Griffin Road, London SE18 7QA — MB BS Bihar 1954.

SINGH, Surinder Waldron Health Centre, Stanley Street, London SE8 4BG — BM Soton. 1982; DGM RCP Lond. 1985; DRCOG 1985; MRCGP 1986; FRCGP 2003. Lead Partner in Gen. Pract.; Community Med. Off. W. Lambeth HA.; Lect. (Department of Primary Care and Popular Sci.) Roy. Free and Univ. Coll. Med. Sch. Lond. Specialty: Gen. Pract. Socs: BMA; EAGA; Independant Advis. Gp. on Sexual Health and AIDS. Prev: Princip. Med. Off. Lond.; Community AIDS Fell. St. Stephens Hosp. Lond.; Princip. Med. Off. Lond.

SINGH, Surinder 44/46 Wyresdale Road, Bolton BL1 4DN Tel: 01204 494133 Fax: 01204 848919; 77 Timberbottom, Bradshaw, Bolton BL2 3DQ — MB ChB Glas. 1984; DRCOG 1988; MRCGP 1989; LF Hom. 1995. GP. Specialty: Homeop. Med. Prev: SHO (Paediat.) Seafield Hosp. Ayr; SHO (A & E) Hairmyres Hosp. E. Kilbride; SHO (Obst.) Bellshill Matern. Hosp.

SINGH, Mr Surjait Malhi Queen Elizabeth Hospital, Gayton Road, King's Lynn PE30 4ET Tel: 01553 613697; Mansfield House, 14 Sandringham Hill, Dersingham, King's Lynn PE31 6LL Tel: 01485 544577 — MB ChB Leeds 1980; FRCS Glas. 1985; FRCS Eng. 1986; ChM (Commend.) Leeds 1991. Cons. Surg. King's Lynn & Wisbech NHS Trust. Specialty: Gen. Surg. Socs: Assn. Surg.; BMA; Vasc. Surg. Soc. Prev: Sen. Regist. Yorks. RHA; Regist. E. Anglia RHA.

SINGH, Suveer Chelsea & Westminster Hospital, 369 Fulham Road, London SW10 9NH Tel: 020 8746 8472/8063 Fax: 020 8746 8547/8183 — MB BS Lond. 1992 (Guy's & St Thomas' Hospitals (UMDS)) BSc (Hons.) Lond. 1989; MRCP (UK) 1995; PhD Lond. 2000; EDIC Lond. 2002; BDICM Lond. 2002. Cons. Respirat. Med. & Intens. Care Med.; Clin. Sen. Lect. Imperial Coll. Sch. of Med., Lond. Specialty: Respirat. Med.; Intens. Care; Gen. Med. Special Interest: Critical care outreach; ICU follow up; Non-invasive ventilation. Socs: BMA; MDU; BTS.

SINGH, Swaran Preet Department of Psychiatry, B Floor, South Block, Queens Medical Centre, Nottingham NG7 2UH Tel: 01159 249924 Fax: 01159 709706 — MB BS Jammu India 1985; MD 1990; MRCPsych 1993. Cons. Psychiat. (Gen. Adult Psychiat.) Nott. Healthcare NHS Trust; Clin. Teach. Univ. of Nottm. Specialty: Gen. Psychiat. Socs: BMA; Indian Psychiat. Soc.; MRCPsych. Prev: Lect. & Hon. Sen. Regist. (Psychiat.) Univ. Nottm.

SINGH, Tara 35 Warren Road, London E11 2LX — MB BS Lond. 1994.

SINGH, Tej Narayan Johnstone Health Centre, 60 Quarry Street, Johnstone PA5 8EY Tel: 01505 324348 Fax: 01505 323710 — MB BS Bihar 1961. GP Johnstone, Renfrew.

SINGH, Tejinder Gurmit Stanley Corner Medical Centre, 1-3 Stanley Avenue, Wembley HA0 4JF Tel: 020 8902 3887 — MB BS Panjab 1969. Princip., G.P.; Clin. Assist. Dermatol., Hillingdon Hosp., Hillingdon, Middx. Specialty: Dermat.; Family Plann. & Reproduc. Health; Acupunc. Socs: BMA; Brit. Med. Accupuncture Soc.

SINGH, Tejwant 10 Girdlers Close, Stivichall Grange, Coventry CV3 6LS Tel: 024 76 411742; 190 Telfer Road, Coventry CV6 3DR Tel: 024 76 596060 — MB BS Vikram 1960 (G.M. Med. Coll. Bhopal)

SINGH, Thakur Hari Hensol Hospital, Pontyclun CF7 8YS Tel: 01443 237373 Fax: 01443 238284; Lynwood, 33 Danygraig Drive, Talbot Green, Pontyclun CF72 8AQ — MB BS Osmania 1965 (Gandhi Med. Coll. Hyderabad) DPM Eng. 1971; FRCPsych 1989, M 1973. Cons. (Psychiat.) Hensol Hosp. Pontyclun. Specialty: Gen. Psychiat. Prev: SHO & Regist. (Psychiat.) Penyval & Maindiff Ct. Hosps. Abergavenny; Rotat. Regist. (Psychiat.) Barrow Hosp. Bristol & SW Hosp. Bd.; Sen. Regist. (Psychiat.) St. Clement's Hosp. Ipswich.

SINGH, Thakur Sukdeo Harold Street Surgery, 2 Harold Street, Sheffield S6 3QW Tel: 0114 233 5930 — MB BS Agra 1964 (S.N. Med. Coll. Agra) DObst RCOG 1968; DA Eng. 1970. Gen. Practitioner. Socs: Med. Practitioner Soc. Prev: Cas. Off. Birm. Gen. Hosp.; ENT Regist. Burnley Gen. Hosp.

SINGH, Thangjam Man Ridvan, Etterby, Carlisle CA3 9QS — MB BS Gauhati 1963 (Assam Med. Coll. Dibrugarh) MRCP (UK) 1972; MRCPsych 1973; DPM Eng. 1973. Cons. Psychiat. (Ment. Illness) Monklands Dist. Gen. Hosp. Airdrie. Specialty: Gen. Psychiat. Prev: Cons. Psychiat. (Ment. Illness) E. Cumbria Health Dist.; Sen. Regist. (Psychiat.) St. John's Hosp. Stone; Hon. Sen. Regist. (Psychiat.) Oxf. Univ.

SINGH, Upendra Birleywood Health Centre, Birleywood, Skelmersdale WN8 9BW Tel: 01695 728073 Fax: 01695 556172 — MB BS Bihar 1969; MB BS Bihar 1969.

SINGH, Valishti Malini Mahani C43 Musgrave House, Royal Bolton Hospital, Minerva Road, Farnham, Bolton DL4 0JR — MB BS W. Indies 1996.

SINGH, Vatsala Institute Road Surgery, 14 Institute Road, Eccleshill, Bradford BD2 2HX Tel: 01274 637417 Fax: 01274 776511 — MB BS Ranchi 1967 (Rajendra Med. Coll.) DA Eng. 1971; DObst RCOG 1973. SCMO Bradford AHA.

SINGH, Mr Vijay — MB BS Himachal Pradesh 1981; DLO RCS Eng. 1990; FRCS Ed. 1991; FRCS (ORL-HNS) 1999. Specialty: Otolaryngol.

SINGH, Vijoy Kumar Highfield Surgery, 25 Severn Street, Leicester LE2 0NN Tel: 0116 254 3253 — MB BS Patna 1971.

SINGH, Vinod Kumar 1 Kingsdown Road, Northfield, Birmingham B31 1AJ Tel: 0121 685 6053 Fax: 0121 685 6086 Email: vinod.singh@bsmht.nhs.uk — MB BS Delhi 1979 (Maulana Azad Med. Coll. Delhi Univ.) BSc- MD; MRCPsych. Cons. (Psychiat.) & Director (Clinical Trials Unit) N. Birm. Ment. Health Trust; Progr. Director (Home Treatm.); Director (Clin. Trials Unit). Specialty: Gen. Psychiat. Special Interest: Home Treatm.; Psychopharmacology.

SINGH, Vivian 2 Southgate Road, Warsop, Mansfield NG20 0QZ Tel: 01623 842864; 18 Ampthill Road, Aigbirth, Liverpool L17 9QW Tel: 0151 728 9625 — MB ChB Liverp. 1992; MB ChB (Hons.) Liverp. 1992. Demonst. (Anat.) Univ. Liverp. Prev: Ho. Off. Walton Hosps.

SINGH, Yadavindra Shah 3 Glenart, Ellesmere Park, Eccles, Manchester M30 9HT — MB BS Lond. 1997.

SINGH, Yashwant Westminster Medical Centre, Aldams Grove, Liverpool L4 3TT Tel: 0151 922 3510 Fax: 0151 902 6071 — MB BS Patna 1971.

SINGH BACHRA, Permjit Queens Medical Centre, Derby Rd, Nottingham NG7 2UH Tel: 0115 924 9924 — MB ChB Birm. 1984; DA (UK) 1988; FRCA 1992. Cons. Anaesth. Qu. Med. Centre Nottm. Specialty: Anaesth. Prev: Sen. Regist. Rotat. (Anaesth.) E. Midl.

SINGH JOSSON, Kashmir Monsoon, Minffordd, Bangor LL57 4DR — MB BS Punjab 1976; MRCOG 1985.

SINGH KHANNA, Harmohan Dayal 3 Pinewood Avenue, Edwinstowe, Mansfield NG21 9JS — MB BS Punjab 1966; MRCGP 1971.

SINGH-NIJJER, Bhajan 1A Field Street, Willenhall WV13 2NY — MB ChB Manch. 1990.

SINGH-RANGER, Deepak 28 Circle Gardens, London SW19 3JU — MB BS Lond. 1994.

SINGH-RANGER, Gurpreet 28 Circle Gardens, London SW19 3JU — MB BS Lond. 1997 (UMDS) BSc (Hons) 1994. Specialty: Gen. Surg.

SINGH RANGER, Ravinderpal Department of General Surgery, Royal United Hospital, Bath BA1 3NG Tel: 01225 428331; 28 Circle Gardens, London SW19 3JU — MB BS Lond. 1991 (Middlx. & Univ. Coll. Med. Sch.) BSc (Hons.) Lond. 1988; FRCS Eng. 1995. Research Fell. (Vasc.) Univ. Coll. Lond. Specialty: Gen. Surg. Prev: Specialist Regist. (Surg.) Wessex Region; SHO (Surg.) Broomfield Hosp. Chelmsford; Prosector (Anat.) & SHO (A & E) Univ. Coll. Hosp. Lond.

SINGHA, Mr Hiran Sirikantha Kirthi Department of Genito-Urin. Medicine, Royal South Hampshire Hospital, Brinton's Terrace, off St Mary's Road, Southampton SO14 0AJ — MB BChir Camb. 1951; MChir Camb. 1963, MB BChir 1951; FRCS Eng. 1955; FRCS Ed. 1955. Sen. Lect. (Genitourin. Med.) Univ. Soton.; Cons. Genitourin. Med. Soton. & S.W. Hants. HA. Specialty: Genitourinary Medicine. Prev: Prof. Surg. Univ. Ceylon.

SINGHAI, Satyen 28 Prior Avenue, Sutton SM2 5HY — MB ChB Manch. 1995.

SINGHAI, Soumit 13 Ranelagh Gardens Mansions, Ranelagh Gardens, London SW6 3UG — MB BS Lond. 1995.

SINGHAL, Arun Kumar Hillside Road Surgery, 30 Hillside Road, Huyton, Liverpool L36 8BJ Tel: 0151 480 4205 Fax: 0151 489 2204 — MB BS Allahabad 1973 (M.L.N. Med. Coll.) Dip. Orthop. Surg. Allahabad 1975; MS (Orthop.) Allahabad 1977. Prev: Police Surg. Liverp.

SINGHAL, Atul 13 Bure Close, North Brickhill, Bedford MK41 7TX — MB BS Lond. 1986; DCH RCP Lond. 1988; MRCP (UK) 1989. Specialty: Paediat.

SINGHAL, Mr Hemant 15 Furrowfelde, Basildon SS16 5HB Tel: 01268 521035 — MB BS Delhi 1984; MS New Delhi 1989, MB BS 1984; FRCS Ed. 1989.

SINGHAL, Mr Keshav RHIWAU, Old Port Road, Wenvoe, Cardiff CF5 6AL — MB BS Jiwaji 1985; MS (Orthop.) Jiwaji 1987; MCh Liverp. 1990; FRCS Eng. 1999. Consultant Orthopaedic Surgeon, Princess of Wales Hospital, Bridgend. Specialty: Orthop. Prev: Regist. (Orthop.) Chester Roy. Infirm.; SHO (Orthop.) Broadgreen Hosp. Liverp.

SINGHAL, Saket 7 Gilchrist Drive, Edgbaston, Birmingham B15 3NG Tel: 0121 684 1236 — BM BCh Oxf. 1991 (Univ. Oxf.) BA (Hons.) Oxf. 1988; MRCP (UK) 1994. Specialist Regist. Birm. Heartland Hosp. Specialty: Gastroenterol.

SINGHAL, Shradha Nand The Alexandra Hospital, Woodrow Drive, Redditch B98 7UB Tel: 01527 503030; 3 Finlarigg Drive, Edgbaston, Birmingham B15 3RH — MB BS Lucknow 1964; MRCP (UK) 1972; FRCP Lond. 1989. Cons. Phys. Geriat. & Gen. Med. The Alexandra Hosp. Redditch. Specialty: Care of the Elderly.

SINGHAL, Sumeet 3 Finlarigg Drive, Edgbaston, Birmingham B15 3RH — MB ChB Manch. 1996.

SINGHAL, Mr Virender Kumar 36 Chichester Road, Street BA16 0QX Tel: 01458 45867; 15 Davenport Avenue, New York 10805, USA Tel: 914 654 1249 — MB BS Delhi 1978; FRCS Ed. 1985; MRCS Eng. LRCP Lond. 1986.

SINGLETON, Carol Dorothy North Derbys. Health, Scarsdale, Newbold Road, Chesterfield S41 7PF Tel: 01246 231255 Fax: 01246 277919; Highfields, 41 Eversleigh Rise, South Darley, Matlock DE4 2JW Tel: 01629 733642 — BM BS Nottm. 1981; DRCOG 1983; Cert. Family Plann. JCC 1983; MRCGP 1985; MFPHM RCP (UK) 1993. Dir. of Pub. Health & Health Policy Northern Derbysh. Health. Specialty: Pub. Health Med. Prev: Cons. in Pub. Health N. Derbysh. Health Chesterfield; Dep. Dir. Of Pub. Health Southern Derbys. Health.

SINGLETON, Christine Dora Attenborough Surgery, Bushey Health Centre, London Road, Bushey, Watford WD23 2NN Tel: 01923 231633 Fax: 01923 818594 — MB ChB Manch. 1975.

SINGLETON, Geoffrey John (retired) Ancroft, Elvaston Pk Road, Hexham NE46 2HT Tel: 01434 605361 — MB BS Lond. 1972 (St. Mary's) DCH Eng. 1975; DRCOG 1976; MRCGP 1977. Med. Adviser Dept. Educat. & Employm. Darlington. Med.Dir. GS Med. Adviser. Prev: GP N.d.

SINGLETON, Nicholas Andrew Talbot Court Medical Practice, The Delamere Centre, Stretford, Manchester M32 0AF Tel: 0161 864 0200 — MB ChB Manch. 1982. Prev: SHO (Cas.) War Memor. Hosp. Wrexham; SHO (O & G & Geriat.) Leighton Hosp. Crewe.

SINGLETON, Nicola Jane 72 Milton Street, Fleetwood FY7 6QS — MB ChB Liverp. 1998; MB ChB Liverp 1998.

SINGLETON, Stephen James Bolam House, Rothbury, Morpeth NE65 7UA — MB ChB Leeds 1979; MRCGP 1985; MSc Newc. 1992; MFPHM RCP (UK) 1993; FFPHM 1998. Dir. (Pub. Health) N.d. HA; Lect. (Epidemiol. & Pub. Health) Univ. of Newc. Specialty: Pub. Health Med.

SINGTON, James Daniel The John Radcliffe Hospital, Headly Way, Oxford OX3 9DU Tel: 01865 741166 — MB ChB Sheff. 1998; MB ChB Sheff 1998.

SINHA, Abhijit 10 The Circuit, Manchester M20 3RA — MB ChB Sheff. 1992; DA (UK) 1995. Cons. (Anaesth.) Roy. Bolton Hosp. Specialty: Anaesth. Prev: SHO (Anaesth.) Manch. Roy. Infirm.; SHO (Emerg. Med.) Gosford Hosp., Austral.; SHO (Paediat.) Qu. Mary's Hosp. Childr. Carshalton.

SINHA, Ajay Consultant Ophthalmologist, Broomfield Hospital, Court Road, Chelmsford CM1 7ET Tel: 01245 514899 Fax: 01245 514898; Fairwood, Coppins Close, Chelmsford CM2 6AY Tel: 01245 264731 — MB BS Delhi 1976; MD Delhi 1978; FRCOphth 1990. Cons. Ophth. Specialty: Ophth. Socs: MRCOphth.; BMA; All India. Ophth.

SINHA, Mr Alokmoy 8 Belgrave Close, Abergavenny NP7 7AP — MB BS Calcutta 1967; FRCS Eng. 1973 (Nat. Med. Inst. Calcutta). GP Abergavenny & Hon. Clin. Asst. (Gen. Surg.) Neville Hall Hosp. Abergavenny. Socs: Med. Protec. Soc. Prev: Resid. Surgic. Off. Staffs. Gp. Hosps.; Regist. (Neurosurg.) N. Staffs. Gp. Hosps.; Regist. (Gen. Surg.) Nevill Hall Hosp. Abergavenny.

SINHA, Amar Krishna (retired) 45 Parkers Road, Sheffield S10 1BN Tel: 0114 266 8394 — MB BS Bihar 1958 (Darbhanga Med. Coll.) DTM & H Eng. 1968; DPM Eng. 1972; MRCPsych 1974. Hon. Clin. Lect. Sheff. Univ. Prev: Cons. Psychiat. (Learning Disabil.) Community Health Sheff. NHS Trust.

SINHA, Mr Amit Glan Clwyd Hospital, Department of Orthopaedics, Rhyl LL18 5UJ Tel: 01745 583910 Fax: 01745 534997 Email: amit.sinha@cd-tr.wales.nhs.uk — MB BS (Hons.) Ranchi 1980, MS Orth 1983; FRCS, Glas. 1988; MChOrth, Liverp. 1991; FRCS Tr & Orth, Edin. 1999. Cons., Orthop. Conwy & Denbighsh. NHS Trust, RHYL. Specialty: Trauma & Orthop. Surg. Special Interest: Elbow; Knee Liagment Surgery; Shoulder. Socs: Brit. Orthop. Assn.; Brit. Med. Assn.

SINHA, Anant Kumar Cheriton Medical Centre, Cheriton Crescent, Portmead, Swansea SA5 5LB Tel: 01792 561122 — MB BS Ranchi 1969 (Ranandra Med. Coll. Hosp. Ranchi) Specialty: Cardiol.

SINHA, Aparna — MB ChB Birm. 1998.

SINHA, Arun Kumar Greenmount Surgery, 25 Church Road, Caerau, Cardiff CF5 5LQ Tel: 029 2059 3003 Fax: 029 2059 1771; 8 Knightswell Close, Culverhouse Cross, Cardiff CF5 4NA Tel: 029 2059 3284 Fax: 01222 593284 — MB BS Patna 1980 (Patna Med. Coll. Patna (India)) LRCP LRCS Ed. LRCPS Glas. 1984. GP Princip. Caerau La. Surg. Cardiff. Specialty: Ophth. Socs: Assoc. Mem. RCGP. Prev: SHO (Geriat.) Arrowe Pk. Hosp. Upton; SHO (Ophth.) Gloucester Roy. Hosp.; SHO (A & E) P. Chas. Hosp. Merthyr Tydfil.

SINHA, Ashok Kumar (Surgery), 16 Rosslyn Road, Longton, Stoke-on-Trent ST3 4JD Tel: 01782 599822 — MB BS Patna 1974.

SINHA, Mr Ashok Kumar North West Wales NHS Trust, Ysbyty Gwynedd, Bangor LL57 2PW Tel: 01248 384670 Fax: 01248 384935; Na-nog, Penrhosgarnedd, Bangor LL57 2SX — MB BS Patna 1986; MS (Orth); FRCS (Tr & Orth); FRCS Glas. 1992. Cons. Orthopaedic Surg., N. W. Wales NHS Trust. Specialty: Otolaryngol. Socs: BMA; BOA.

SINHA, Aswinee Kumar (Surgery), 258 Westborough Road, Westcliff on Sea SS0 9PT Tel: 01702 348800; 33 Kilworth Avenue, Southend-on-Sea SS1 2DS — MB BS Calcutta 1957 (N.R.S. Med. Coll. Calcutta) BSc Calcutta 1951; DTM & H Liverp. 1966; DCH Eng. 1966. GP Southend-on-Sea. Socs: Fell. Roy. Soc. Trop. Med. &

Hyg.; Assoc. of Internat. Fed. of Sports Med.; BMA. Prev: Med. Off. Sierra Leone Developm. Co. Ltd. Freetown & Nat. Diamond Mining Company Ltd. Yengema, Sierra Leone; Regist. W. Hendon Hosp. Lond.

SINHA, Avinash Kumar 36 Mortain Road, Rotherham S60 3BX — MB ChB Manch. 1993.

SINHA, B K Bigdale Drive, Kirkby, Liverpool L33 6XJ.

SINHA, Baij Nath West Cheshire District General Hospital, Liverpool Road, Chester CH1 3SS — MB BS Bihar 1957 (Darbhanga Med. Coll.) DCH Calcutta 1960. Prev: SHO (Geriat.) & SHO (Infec. Dis.) W. Norwich Hosp.; SHO (Psychol. Med.) Hellesdon Hosp. Norwich.

SINHA, Bharat Prasad Sinha, 56 Western Avenue, Acton, London W3 7TY Tel: 020 8743 4133; 6 Highway Avenue, Maidenhead SL6 5AF Tel: 01628 771515 Fax: 01628 771515 — MD Patna 1978 (P. of Wales Med. Coll.) MB BS 1969; DTM & H Liverp. 1976. Specialty: Gen. Pract. Socs: BMA. Prev: GP Maidenhead.; visit.med.Off.Subst. misuse .E. Berks.

SINHA, Bhupendra Kumar Birchdale Road Medical Centre, 2 Birchdale Road, London E7 8AR Tel: 020 8472 1600 Fax: 020 8471 7712 — MB BS Patna 1964 (Patna Med. Coll.) Prev: SHO (Cas. & Orthop.) Hackney Hosp. Lond.; SHO (Orthop.) OldCh. Hosp. Romford; SHO (Gen. Surg.) German Hosp. Lond.

SINHA, Birendra Kumar Edge Hill Health Centre, Crosfield Road, Liverpool L7 5QL Tel: 0151 260 2777 — MB BS Patna 1973; DTCD Wales 1976; MRCP (UK) 1980; MRCPI 1980.

SINHA, Chitra 26 The Crayke, Bridlington YO16 6YP; Bridlington Hospital, Bridlington YO16 4QP Tel: 01262 607187 — MB BS Jodhpur, India 1981; LRCP LRCS Ed. LRCPS Glas. 1984; DObst RCPI 1989; DRCOG 1990; MRCOG 1995. Specialist Regist. (O & G) York Dist. Hosp. Socs: Obst. & Gyn. Soc. Prev: Regist. (O & G) W. Wales Gen. Hosp. Carmarthen; SHO (O & G) Warnford Hosp. Roy. Lamington Spa, Hosp. St. Cross Rugby & Dudley Rd. Hosp. Birm.

SINHA, Gauri Hatfield Road Surgery, 61 Hatfield Road, St Albans AL1 4JE Tel: 01727 853079.

SINHA, Gopal Chandra Grove Park Surgery, 116 Sutton Road, Maidstone ME15 9AP Tel: 01634 201877; Grove Park Surgery, 116 Sutton Road, Maidstone ME15 9AP Tel: 01622 753211 — LRCP LRCS Ed. LRCPS Glas. 1983; T (GP) 1991; MFFP 1994. GP Sessional Family Plann. M.O. Specialty: Gen. Pract. Socs: FRSH; Soc. Occupat. Med.; Fac. Fam. Plann. Prev: Med. Off. HM Prison Serv.

SINHA, Guria 27 Nursery Avenue, Ormskirk L39 2DY — MB ChB Manch. 1998; MB ChB Manch 1998.

SINHA, Gyanranjan Prasad Manor Hospital, Department of Paediatrics, Moat Road, Walsall WS2 9PS Tel: 01922 656547 Fax: 01922 656742 — MB BS Patna 1973; MD (Patna Univ.) 1977; DCH (RCPS of Irel.) 1984; MRCP (UK) 1990; FRCPCH 1993; FRCP Glas. 1999. Cons. Paediat. Manor Hosp. Walsall; Hon. Sen Clin. Lect. (Paediat.) Univ. Birm.; Cons. Paediat. Nuffield Hosps. Birm & Wolverhampton & BUPA Hosp. Sutton Coldfield. Specialty: Paediat. Special Interest: Neonates; Neurodisability. Socs: BMA; Med. Protec. Soc.; W Midl. Paediat. Soc.

SINHA, Jaisi 52 Corporation Road, Newport NP19 0AW — MB BS Lond. 1996.

SINHA, Jayanta Kumar 54 Codicote Drive, Garston, Watford WD25 9QY Tel: 01923 673974 — MB BS Calcutta 1967; DPH Lond. 1983; DIH Lond. 1984. Regional Med. Off. BT Lond. Centr. Specialty: Occupat. Health. Socs: Soc. Occupat. Med.; Internat. Soc. Travel Med. Prev: Sen. Regist. (Occupat. Med.) Clwyud HA; SHO (Gen. Med.) Tynemouth Infirm. Clwyd HA; Regist. (Infec. Dis.) Benghazi Univ. Hosp.

SINHA, Mr Joydeep Department of Orthopaedics, King's College Hospital, Denmark Hill, London SE5 9RS Tel: 020 7346 3463 Fax: 020 7346 3497 Email: joydeep.sinha@btinternet.com — (University of Manchester) BSc (Hons.) (Pharmacol.) Manch. 1982; MB ChB Manch. 1985; FRCS Ed. 1989; FRCS Eng. 1990; FRCS (Orth.) 1995. Cons. (Orthop. Surg.) King's Coll. Hosp. Lond. Specialty: Orthop.; Trauma & Orthop. Surg. Socs: Fell. BOA; Fell. Brit. Elbow and Shoulder Soc.; Fell. Brit. Soc. Surg. Hand. Prev: Sen. Regist. (Orthop. & Trauma) King's Coll. Hosp. Lond.; Fellowship Train. USA (Seattle & NY).

SINHA, Mr Kunja Madhab 26 Lighcliffe Road, London N13 5HD Tel: 020 8882 4271 — MB BS Calcutta 1961 (R.G. Kar Med. Coll.) BSc Calcutta 1955, MB BS 1961; FRCS Ed. 1973; FRCS Glas. 1973. Prev: Regist. Dept. Gen. Surg. R. G. Kar Med. Coll. Hosps. Calcutta, India; Resid. Div. Gen. Surg. Wesley Med. Center Wichita, U.S.A. & St.; Joseph's Hosp. Phoenix, U.S.A.

SINHA, Leena 30 Springdale Court, Mickleover, Derby DE3 9SW — MB BCh Wales 1993.

SINHA, Manas Kumar St George's Hospital, Atkinson Morley Wing, Blackshaw Road, London SW17 0QT Tel: 020 86721255 Ext: 1225 Email: msinha@sghms.ac.uk; 142 Brudenell Road, Tooting, London SW17 8DF Tel: 020 8767 3933 Email: manas@msinha.freeserve.co.uk — MB BS Lond. 1994 (St. Geo. Hosp.) BSc (Hons.) Med. Sci. & Clin. Pharmacol. Lond. 1991; MRCP (UK) 1997; MD Univ. of Lond. 2004. Specialist Regist. in Cardiol., St George's Hosp., Lond. Specialty: Gen. Med.; Cardiol. Prev: Specialist Regist. (Cardiol), E. Surrey Hosp., Rehill, Surrey; Clin. Research Fell. (Cardiol), St Georges Hosp. Med. Sch.; Specialist Regist. (Cardiol), Basildon and Thurrock Hosps.

SINHA, Mr Mukesh The Surgery, 28 Church Road, Aston, Birmingham B6 5UP Tel: 0121 327 2348; 17 Hainfield Drive, Solihull B91 2PL Tel: 0121 705 2802 — MB BS Bihar 1980; FRCS Ed. 1984; Cert. Family Plann. JCC 1989; MRCGP 1990. Hosp. Pract. (Surg.) Solihull Hosp.; Provision of Minor Surg. (including Vasectomy) mainly for Fundholding GPs. Specialty: Paediat. Surg. Socs: MDU. Prev: Regist. (Gen. Surg.) E. Birm. Hosp.; Regist. (Paediat. Surg.) E. Birm. Hosp.; SHO Rotat. (Gen. Surg./Urol./Thoracic Surg./Trauma) E. Birm. Hosp.

SINHA, Murli Pleck Health Centre, 16 Oxford Street, Pleck, Walsall WS2 9HY Tel: 01922 647660 Fax: 01922 629251 — MB BS Patna 1971 (Patna India) MS (Gen. Surg.) Patna 1975. GP Walsall Clin. Asst. (Psychiat.). Specialty: Accid. & Emerg. Socs: BMA; ODA.

SINHA, N K Aintree Road Practice, 2 Aintree Road, Bootle L20 9DW Tel: 0151 922 1768.

SINHA, Miss Prabha Conquest Hospital, The Ridge, St Leonards-on-Sea TW37 7TH Tel: 01424 755255 Ext: 6434 Fax: 01424 758086 Email: prabha.sinha@esht.nhs.uk — MB BS Patna 1980; Dip Mgmt Open Univ.; DGO 1981; MRCPI 1999; FRCOG 2003. Cons. (O & G) E. Sussex Hosp. NHS Trust; Hon. Cons. St Thos. Hosp. Lond. Specialty: Obst. & Gyn. Special Interest: Adolescent Gynaecology; Menopause; Ultrasound Scan. Socs: BMA; MDU. Prev: Locum Cons. (O & G) Jessop Hosp. Sheff.

SINHA, Prithwiraj Wingate Surgery, Medical Centre, Front West Street, Wingate TS28 5PZ Tel: 01429 838203 Fax: 01429 836928 — MB BS Calcutta 1968.

SINHA, Rabindra Nath c/o Drive R. P. Yadava, 40 Caverstral Road, Blyth Bridge, Stoke-on-Trent ST11 9BG — MB BS Patna 1968.

SINHA, Raghavendra Prasad 41 Reedfield, Reedley, Burnley BB10 2NJ Tel: 01282 696006; 90 Worsley Road N., Walkden, Worsley, Manchester M28 3QW Tel: 01204 791409 — MD Patna 1979 (Patna Med. Coll.) MB BS Patna 1974. GP Worsley. Prev: SHO (Psychiat.) Oldham & Dist. Gen. Hosp.; SHO (Geriat. Med.) Grantham & Kesteven Gen. Hosp.; SHO (Gen. Med.) Stracathro Hosp. & Arbroath Infirm. Brechin.

SINHA, Raj Kumar 35 Staveley Way, Rugby CV21 1TP — MB BS Ranchi, India 1980.

SINHA, Rajeshwar Prasad Rainbow Medical Centre, 265 Dunstable Road, Luton LU4 8BS — MB BS Bihar 1972.

SINHA, Rama Shankar Kumar Bridlington District Hospital, Bridlington YO16 4QP Tel: 01262 607034; The Crayke, Bridlington YO16 6YP — MB BS Ranchi 1973; DTM & H Liverp. 1986. Staff Grade (A & E) Bridlington Hosp. E. Yorks. Socs: Fell. Roy. Soc. Trop. Med.

SINHA, Ranjan Kumar 16 Lime Close, Crawley RH11 7NN — MB BS Calcutta 1984; MRCOG 1990. Clin. Research Fell. (O & G) Roy. Lond. Hosp. & Newham Gen. Hosp. Lond. Specialty: Obst. & Gyn. Prev: Regist. (O & G) Luton & Dunstable Hosp. & Roy. Lond. Hosp.

SINHA, Ravi Nandan 4 Poplar Drive, Milton of Campsie, Glasgow G66 8DZ — MB ChB Manch. 1987.

SINHA, Ritendra Nath The Health Centre, Lawson Street, Stockton-on-Tees TS18 1HX Tel: 01642 676520 Fax: 01642 614720; The Gables, 607 Yarm Road, Eagescliffe, Stockton-on-Tees TS16 9BN — MB BS Patna 1969.

SINHA, S K Aintree Road Practice, 2 Aintree Road, Bootle L20 9DW Tel: 0151 922 1768.

SINHA, Sanjay Alexandra Park Health Centre, 2 Whitswood Close, Manchester M16 7AW Tel: 0161 226 3620 — MB BChir Camb. 1988; BA (Hons.) Physiol. Camb. 1985; MRCP (UK) 1992. MRC Clin. Train. Fell. Univ. Manch. Specialty: Cardiol. Prev: Regist. (Cardiol. & Gen. Med.) Castlehill Hosp. Cottingham; SHO (Gen. Med.) Wythenshawe Hosp. Manch. & Hope Hosp. Salford.

SINHA, Sanjay Kumar 8 Gordonsfield, Ackworth, Pontefract WF7 7QN — MB BS Bihar, India 1984.

SINHA, Sankarprasad Department of Radiology, George Eliot Hospital, College Street, Nuneaton CV10 7DJ Tel: 024 7686 5392 Fax: 024 7686 5095 Email: sankar.sinha@geh.nhs.uk; 20 Falstaff Close, Whitestone, Nuneaton CV11 6FB Tel: 024 7637 5142 Fax: 024 7673 6806 — MB BS Calcutta 1987 (R. G. Kar Med. Coll. Calcutta, India) DMRD Calcutta 1991; DNB (Radiodiagnosis) New Delhi 1992; FRCR 1996; MBA (Health Exec.) Keele 2002. p/t Cons. Radiol. Geo. Eliot Hosp. Nuneaton. Specialty: Radiol. Special Interest: Interventional Radiol.; Magnetic Resonance Imaging. Socs: BMA; MDU; The Brit. Inst. of Radiol. Prev: Specialist Regist. (Radiol.) Roy. Liverp. Univ. Hosp. Eng.; Specialist Regist. (Radiol.) Alder Hey Childr. Hosp. Liverp.; Specialist Regist. (Radiol.) Whiston Hosp. Prescot, Merseyside.

SINHA, Santosh Vidya Medical Centre, 12 Charnwood Street, Derby DE1 2GT Tel: 01332 345406 Fax: 01332 345863 — MB BS Bihar 1964 (Darbhanga Med. Coll. Laheriasarai) Prev: SHO (Obst.) Lincoln Co. Hosp.; SHO (Geriat.) Castle Hill Hosp. Cottingham; SHO (Gen. Surg.) Hull Roy. Infirm.

SINHA, Sarla 2 Gilescroft Avenue, Northwood, Kirkby, Liverpool L33 9TW Tel: 0151 546 3396 — MB BS Delhi 1961 (Lady Hardinge Med. Coll.)

SINHA, Saurabh 3 St Marys Close, Hessle HU13 0KY — BM BCh Oxf. 1994; BA (Hons.) Oxf. 1991; FRCS Ed. 1999.

SINHA, Seema 32 Corporation Road, Cardiff CF11 7YA — MB BS Newc. 1989; BSc Chem. (Hons.) 1984; DRCOG 1993; MRCGP 1994.

SINHA, Shashi Kiran Balfour Road Surgery, 92 Balfour Road, Ilford IG1 4JE Tel: 020 8478 0209 Fax: 020 8220 8777 — MB BS Patna 1966.

SINHA, Shirley 10 Knoll Avenue, Uplands, Swansea SA2 0JN — BM Soton. 1986.

SINHA, Shivendra Manor Hospital, Walsall WS2 9PS Tel: 01922 656449 Email: shivendrasinha@aol.com — MB BS Patma 1961. Cons. (Care of the Elderly) Manor Hosp. Walsall. Specialty: Care of the Elderly. Special Interest: Parkinson's Dis.

SINHA, Shobha Brookfield Park Surgery, 2 Brookfield Road, London NW5 1ER Tel: 020 7485 7363 — MB BS Patna 1971.

SINHA, Shubhada 37 Hills Avenue, Cambridge CB1 7UY — BChir Camb. 1992.

SINHA, Shyama Withybush Hospital, Fishguard Road, Haverfordwest SA61 2PZ; 9 Heritage Park, Haverfordwest SA61 2QF Tel: 01437 768722 — MB BS Patna 1982; MRCOG 1992, D 1992. Staff Grade (O & G) Withybush Hosp. HaverfordW. Specialty: Family Plann. & Reproduc. Health.

SINHA, Subrata Glan Yr Afon Surgery, Shop Row, Tredegar NP22 4LB Tel: 01495 722630 Fax: 01495 726173 — MB BS Calcutta 1965. Clin. Asst. (Elderly Care) Nevill Hall & Dist. NHS Trust. Specialty: Care of the Elderly.

SINHA, Sudhir Kumar Brookfield Park Surgery, 2 Brookfield Road, London NW5 1ER Tel: 020 7485 7363 — MB BS Patna 1971.

SINHA, Suman Kumar 2 Clare Close, Bury BL8 1XN — MB BS Bihar 1973.

SINHA, Sunil Kumar Alderney Hospital, Ringwood Road, Poole BH12 4NB Tel: 01202 735537 Fax: 01202 730657 — MB BS Ranchi 1978; MB BS Ranchi. 1988. Assoc. Specialist Old Age Psychiat., Alderney Hosp., Poole. Specialty: Geriat. Psychiat. Prev: Trainee GP Broadstone.

SINHA, Professor Sunil Kumar — MB BS Patna (P. of Wales Med. Coll., Patna, India) MD; MRCP; PhD Manch.; FRCPCH. Cons. Paediat., James Cook Univ. Hosp., Middlesborough; Hon. Prof. of Paediat., Univ. of Durh. Specialty: Paediat. Socs: Brit. Assn. of Paediat.; BMA.

SINHA, Supriya Kumar 4 Havisham Place, London SE19 3HN — MB BS Lond. 1995.

SINHA, Vineeta 62 Green Lane, Stockport SK4 3LH — MB ChB Manch. 1993; BSc St And. 1990. Demonst. (Anat.) Univ. Dundee. Prev: Ho. Off. (Surg. & Med.) Manch. Roy. Infirm.

SINHA, Vishwambhar Nath Prasad Crane Park Medical Centre, 748 Hanworth, Hounslow TW4 5NT Tel: 020 8893 4567 Fax: 020 8893 8026 — MB BS Patna 1974.

SINHA ROY, Amarendra Nath Lakeside Surgery, Church St., Langold, Worksop S81 9NW Tel: 01909 540488 Fax: 01909 540477; 'Moonrakers', 77 Thievesdale Lane, Worksop S81 0PG Tel: 01909 472616 — MB BS Calcutta 1960. Prev: Med. Protec. Soc.

SINNAMON, Sarah Edith 90 Harberton Park, Malone, Belfast BT9 6TU — MB BCh BAO Belf. 1979.

SINNATAMBY, Mr Chummy Sundararaja Royal College of Surgeons of England, 35-43 Lincoln's Inn Fields, London WC2A 3PE Tel: 020 7405 3474 Fax: 020 7869 6329 Email: csinnatamby@rcseng.ac.uk; 17 Granta Leys, Linton CB1 6YT Tel: 01223 890264 — MB BS Ceylon 1960; FRCS Eng. 1965. Head Teach. Dept. Educat. RCS Eng.; Surgical Anatomy Tutor RCS Eng.; Anatomy Tutor, University of Cambridge. Specialty: Anat. Socs: Fell. Brit. Assn. Clin. Anat. Prev: Prof. Surg. Univ. Colombo, Sri Lanka.

SINNATAMBY, Ruchira Department of Radiology, Addenbrooke's Hospital, Cambridge CB2 2QQ Email: ruchi.sinnatamby@addenbrookes.nhs.uk — MB BChir Camb. 1988 (Univ. Camb.) BA (Hons.) Camb. 1986; MRCP (UK) 1991; FRCR 1994. Fell. & Coll. Lect. (Anat.) & Dir. Studies of Clin. Med. New Hall Univ. Camb. Specialty: Radiol.

SINNATAMBY, Mrs Selvadevi Northwick Park Hospital, Watford Road, Harrow HA1 3UJ Tel: 020 8869 2309; 11 Meadowcroft, St Albans AL1 1JD Tel: 01727 850027 — MB BS Ceylon 1961; DA Eng. 1964; PhD Lond. 1973; MRCPsych 1987. Cons. Psychiat. Northwick Pk. Hosp. Harrow. Specialty: Geriat. Psychiat. Prev: Clin. Asst. Shenley Hosp. Radlett; Sen. Lect. (Pharmacol.) Univ. Colombo, Sri Lanka.

SINNATHAMBY, Subothini Wendy 13 Stradbrooke Grove, Ilford IG5 0DN — MB BS Lond. 1994.

SINNERTON, Mr Richard Jacob Woking Nuffield Hospital, The Orthopaedic Centre, Shores Road, Woking GU21 4BY Tel: 01483 765880 Fax: 01483 750664 Email: enquires@theorthocentre.com — MB BS Lond. 1988 (St. Thos.) FRCS Eng. 1992; FRCS (Orth.) 1998. Cons. (Orthop. Surg.) Ashford & St. Peters Hosp. Specialty: Orthop. Special Interest: Shoulder & Elbow. Prev: Regist. Rotat. (Orthop.) St. Mary's Hosp. Lond.

SINNERTON, Timothy John L'Aumone and St. Sampsons Practice, L'Aumone Surgery, Castel, Guernsey GY5 7RU Tel: 01481 256517 Fax: 01481 255190 — MB BS Lond. 1988 (St. Thos. Hosp. Med. Sch. (Lond.)) DRCOG 1993; MRCGP 1995. Specialty: Gen. Pract.

SINNETT, Mr Hugh Dudley Department Surgery, Charing Cross Hospital, Fulham Palace Road, London W6 8RF Tel: 020 8846 7303 Fax: 020 8846 1617; 6 Wilbury Avenue, Cheam, Sutton SM2 7DU Tel: 020 8770 3806 Fax: 020 8770 3806 — MB BS Lond. 1972 (Char. Cross) FRCS Eng. 1976; MS Lond. 1984. Cons. Surg. Char. Cross Hosp. Lond.; Mem. Ct. Examrs. RCS Eng. Specialty: Gen. Surg. Prev: Sen. Lect. & Hon. Cons. Surg. Roy. Marsden Hosp. Lond.; Sen. Regist. (Surg.) St. Bart. Hosp. Lond.

SINNETT, Kate Joanne 90 Squires Gate, Rogerstone, Newport NP10 0BQ — MB BCh Wales 1998.

SINNIAH, Anton Ravindra Department of Chest Medicine, Fairfield General Hospital, Rochdale Old Road, Bury BL9 7TD Tel: 0161 778 2652 — MB BS Lond. 1989 (St. Geo. Hosp. Med. Sch.) MRCP (UK) 1992; Dip. Trop. Med. RCSI 1995. Cons. (Thoracic & Gen Med.) Bury Gen Hosp. Manc. Specialty: Respirat. Med.; Gen. Med. Prev: Regist. (Thoracic & Gen. Med.) Char. Cross Hosp. Lond.; Regist. (Thoracic, ICU, Neurol. & Gen. Med.) Centr. Middlx. Hosp. Lond.; Regist. (Thoracic & Transpl. Med.) Harefield Hosp. Uxbridge.

SINNIAH, Arulrajah Thiruchelvam North London Nuffield Hospital, Cavell Drive, Enfield EN2 7PR Tel: 020 8366 2122; Shalimar, 9 Greenway, Totteridge, London N20 8EE Tel: 020 8445 4472 Fax: 020 8446 5491 — MB BS Punjab 1960 (Manch. & Ludhiana) MB BS Punjab. (India) 1960; MRCP Ed. 1967; FRCP Ed. 1994. Cons. Phys. N. Lond. Nuffield Hosp. Specialty: Gen. Med. Socs: BMA. Prev: Cons. Phys. Highlands Hosp. Lond.; Cons. Phys. Dept. Geriat. Med. High Wycombe & Dist. Hosp. Gp. Bucks. CC.

SINNOTT, Anthony David Imperial Road Surgery, 8 Imperial Road, Matlock DE4 3NL Tel: 01629 583249 — MB ChB Sheff. 1983; DRCOG 1987. Specialty: Gen. Pract.

SINNOTT, Brendon Simon Broomhill House, 1 Broomhill Park, Belfast BT9 5JB; Broomhill House, 1 Broomhill Park, Belfast BT9 5JB Tel: 01232 209962 — MB BCh BAO NUI 1985; LRCPI & LM, LRCSI & LM 1985; BSc 1987; FRCSI 1991; FFAEM 1996. Cons. (A & E) Down Lisburn Trust Lagan Valley Hosp. Lisburn Co. Antrim. Specialty: Accid. & Emerg. Socs: BMA; BAEM.

SINNOTT, Claire Rose 7 Sutherland Grove, Teddington TW11 8RP — MB BChir Camb. 1985; MRCP (UK) 1989.

SINSON, John Denis (retired) 10 Avondale Court, Shadwell Lane, Leeds LS17 6DT Tel: 0113 268 7862 — MB BS Durh. 1948 (Newc. u. Tyne) FRCGP 1977, M 1969. Prev: Med. Dir. St. Gemma's Hospice Leeds.

SINTLER, Mr Martin Peter 131 Beamont Road, Bournville, Birmingham B30 1NT — MB ChB Birm. 1993; FRCS (Eng) 1998; MMedSci 2002. Specialty: Gen. Surg.

SINTON, Miss Janet Elizabeth Altnagelvin Hospital, Department of Ophthalmology, Glenshane Road, Londonderry BT47 6SB Email: jsinton@alt.n-i.nhs.uk — MB BCh BAO Belf. 1988 (Queens Univ. Belf.) FRCOphth 1992. Cons. (Ophth.) Altnagelvin Hosp. Londonderry N. Irel. Specialty: Ophth. Special Interest: Cataracts; Corneal Disease; Ext. Eye Disease.

SINTON, John Roger Wardlaw (retired) Meadowfield Cottage, 32 Ramsey's Lane, Wooler NE71 6NY Tel: 01668 281944 — MB BS Durh. 1947.

SINTON, Richard Ian Rae Department of Anaesthesia, Kingston Hospital, Galsworthy Road, Kingston upon Thames KT2 7QB; Hungerdown Barn, Brittens Lane, Fontwell, Arundel BN18 0ST Tel: 01243 544094 Fax: 01243 544094 — MB BChir Camb. 1960 (Westm. Hosp. Lond.) FRCA 1967. p/t Cons. Anaesth. Kingston. Hosp.Kingston on Thames. Specialty: Anaesth. Special Interest: Anaesth. for Head and Neck Surg.; Regional Anaesthesia. Prev: Attend. Anaesth. Highline Hosp. Seattle, USA; Asst. Prof. Anesthesiol. Univ. Washington Seattle, USA.

SINTON, William Srigley (retired) Flat 2, Westfield House, Cote Lane, Westbury on Trym, Bristol BS9 3UL Tel: 0117 949 4802 — MB BS Lond. 1953 (Lond. Hosp.) DObst RCOG 1955. Prev: Ho. Surg. Lond. Hosp.

SINUFF, Syama Hamid Flat 3, 275A Fulwood Road, Broomhill, Sheffield S10 3BD — MB ChB Sheff. 1997.

SIODLAK, Mr Martyn Zbyszek ENT Department, The General Hospital, St Helier, Jersey Tel: 0151 529 4691 — MB BS Lond. 1979 (Char. Cross) MRCS Eng. LRCP Lond. 1979; FRCS Lond. 1984; T(S) 1991. Cons. Otolaryngol. Head & Neck Surg. Gen. Hosp. St. Helier. Specialty: Otolaryngol. Prev: Cons. Otolaryngol. Head & Neck Surg. Walton Hosp. & Ormskirk Dist. Gen. Hosp.; Sen. Regist. (ENT Surg.) Mersey Regional Rotat. Scheme; Clin. Research Fell. (Otorhinolaryngol.) Univ. Liverp.

SIOW, Wenchee 45 Broadley Terrace, London NW1 6LG — MB BS Lond. 1998 (St Bart.) PRHO, Gen. Med. Newham Gen. Plaistow, Lond. Specialty: Gen. Med. Prev: PRHO, Gen Surg. Eastbourne.

SIPPERT, Alan Flat 3, Lesley Court, 23/33 Strutton Ground, London SW1P 2HZ Tel: 020 7222 7264 — MB ChB Manch. 1950; DPH Manch. 1960; FFPHM 1979, M 1972; FRCPsych 1984, M 1974. Socs: BMA.

SIPPLE, Mr Mushtaq Ahmad 135 Glebe Farm Road, Birmingham B33 9NE Tel: 0121 784 4228 — MB BS Punjab 1956 (Nishtar Med. Coll.) MS (Neurosurg.) Punjab Pakistan 1964, MB BS 1956; DPM Eng. 1975; MRCPsych 1979. Cons. Psychiat. St. Matthew's Hosp. Walsall. Specialty: Gen. Psychiat. Socs: World Psychiat. Assn. Prev: Neurosurg. Specialist Pakistan Army Med. Corp.; Cons. Neurosurg. Centr. Hosp. Riyadh, Saudi Arabia; Sen. Regist. (Adult Psychiat.) St. Jas. Univ. Hosp. Leeds.

SIRCAR, Manisha Lynwood Medical Centre, Lynwood Drive, 2A-6 Collier Row, Romford RM5 3QL Tel: 01708 743244 Fax: 01708 736783 — MB BS Calcutta 1964 (N.R. Sircar Med. Coll.) DA Eng. 1968; MRCOG 1972. Prev: Regist. Dept. O & G Romford Gp. Hosps.

SIRCUS, Wilfred (retired) Easter Flisk, Blebo Craigs, Cupar KY15 5UQ Tel: 01334 850064 — MB ChB (Silver Medal Pub. Health) Liverp. 1943; FRCP Lond. 1965, M 1948; MD Liverp. 1949; PhD Sheff. 1956; FRCP Ed. 1961, M 1958. Reader (Med.) Univ. Edin.; Cons. Phys. West. Gen. Hosp. Edin. Prev: Sen. Research Regist. Sheff. Roy. Infirm.

SIRELING, Lester Ian Barnet Hospital , Barnet Enfield and Haringey Mental Health NHS Trust, Barnet Psychiatric Unit, Wellhouse Lane, Barnet EN5 3DJ Tel: 020 8216 4616 Fax: 020 8216 4082 Email: lester.sireling@beh-mht.nhs.uk; 999 Medical Centre, 999 Finchley Road, London NW11 7HB Email: sireling@msn.com — MB BS Lond. 1974 (Guy's) MRCS Eng. LRCP Lond. 1974; MRCPsych 1979; FRCPsych 2000. Cons. Psychiat. Barnet and Edgware. Hosps. Specialty: Gen. Psychiat. Socs: Mem., Brit. Assn. for PsychoPharmacol..; Hon. Off. Lond. Regional Psychiatric Comm. Prev: Sen. Regist. & Lect. (Psychiat.) St. Geo. Hosp. Lond.; Clin. Research Fell. (Adult Psychiat.) St. Geo. Hosp. Med. Sch. Lond.

SIRIMANNA, Mr Kusum Sekera Consultant Audiological Physician, Great Ormond Street Hospital for Children, Great Ormond St., London WC1N 3JH; 17 Garthland Drive, Arkley, Barnet EN5 3BB Tel: 020 8441 3171 Email: sirimt@gosh.nhs.uk — MB BS Sri Lanka 1977; MSc (Audiological Med.); DLO RCS Eng. 1983; FRCS Ed. 1985; MS Sri Lanka 1987. Cons. Audiol. Phys. Gt. Ormond St. Hosp. for Childr. Lond.; Hon. Sen. Lect. (Clin. Sci.) Inst. Child Health Univ. Lond. Specialty: Audiol. Med. Socs: Brit. Assn. of Audiol. Phys.; Internat. Assn. Phys. in Audiol.; Internat. Soc. Audiol. Prev: Cons. Audiol. Phys. Northwick Pk. Hosp. Harrow; Sen. Regist. (Audiol. Med.) Univ. Hosp. Wales Cardiff; Cons. ENT Surg. Base Hosp. Matara, Sri Lanka.

SIRIPURAPU, Mr Ankaiah (retired) 4 Dunhugh Park, Londonderry BT47 2NL Tel: 028 7134 8994 — MB BS Andhra 1966 (Andhra med.Coll) BSc Andhra 1960; DLO 1973; MS Banaras 1975; FRCS Ed. 1979. Prev: Cons. Otolaryngol. Altnagelvin Area Hosp. Londonderry.

SIRISENA, Liyana Arachchige Premachandra Crosshouse Hospital, Kilmarnock KA2 0BE Tel: 01563 521133 Fax: 01563 577774; 46 Bathurst Drive, Alloway, Ayr KA7 4QY Tel: 01292 443253 Email: 106270.3676@compuserve.com — MB BS Ceylon 1968; DPM Eng. 1979; MRCPsych 1983. Cons. Psychiat. CrossHo. Hosp. Kilmarnock. Specialty: Gen. Psychiat. Prev: Assoc. Specialist (Psychiat.) Alisa Hosp. Ayr; Cons. Psychiat. Bendigo Vict., Austral.

SIRISENA, Udawattage Nihal Harischandra 3 Sefton Avenue, Mill Hill, London NW7 3QB; 36 Christchurch Avenue, Harrow HA3 8NJ — MB BS Ceylon 1976; DA (UK) 1986; DRCOG 1992; DFFP 1993.

SIRISENA, Walpita Gamage 27 St George's Avenue, Grays RM17 5XB Tel: 01375 78840 — (Topiwala Nat. Med. Coll.) MB BS Bombay 1953; DTM & H Ceylon 1962. Med. Off. Health Dept. Basildon & Thurrock Health Dist. Prev: SHO (Geriat.) & SHO (Accid. & Orthop.) W. Suff. Gen. Hosp. Bury St.; Edmunds.

SIRIWARDANA, Nimmilee Chandanee Piyadasni Earls House Hospital, Lanchester Road, Durham DH1 5RE; 9 St Oswalds Drive, Durham DH1 3TE — MB BS Peradeniya 1979; MB BS Peradeniya Sri Lanka 1979; MRCPsych 1992.

SIRIWARDENA, Mr Ajith Kumar Department of Surgery, Manchester Royal Infirmary, Oxford Road, Manchester M13 9WL Fax: 0161 276 4530 Email: ajith@mri3.cmht.nwest.nhs.uk — MB ChB Manch. 1982 (University of Manchester) FRCS Ed. 1986; FRCS Eng. 1988; MD (Gold Medal) Manch. 1991; FRCS (Gen) 1995. Cons. Surg. & Hon. Sen. Lect. In Surg., Manchster Roy. Infirm. Specialty: Gen. Surg. Prev: Sen. Regist. (Gen. Surg.) N. West. RHA; Sen. Lect. & Cons. Surg. Edin. Roy. Infirm.

SIRIWARDENA, Aloysius Niroshan The Minster Practice, Cabourne Court, Cabourne Avenue, Lincoln LN2 2JP Tel: 01522 568838 Fax: 01522 546740; North Dene, Langworth Road, Scothern, Lincoln LN2 2UP Tel: 01522 568838 — MB BS Lond. 1984 (St. Bart. Hosp. Lond.) DRCOG 1988; MRCGP 1989; DCH RCP Lond. 1989; MMedSci Nottm. 1995; FRCGP 1998.

SIRIWARDENA, Miss Dilani Krishni 42 Limehouse Court, 46 Morris Road, Poplar, London E14 6NQ — MB BS Lond. 1992; FRCOphth 1997. MRC Research Fell. Moorfields Eye Hosp. Lond. Specialty: Ophth.

SIRIWARDENA, Mr Goigodagamage Jewendra Ariyathilaka DHSS Artificial Limb & Appliance Centre, Oak Tree Lane, Moseley, Birmingham B29 6JA Tel: 0121 472 5343; 57 Moorcroft Road, Moseley, Birmingham B13 8LT — MB BS Ceylon 1957; FRCS Ed. 1967. Hon. Cons. (Prosth.s & Orthotics) W. Midl. RHA; Hon. Sen.

Lect. Univ. Birm.; Med. Off. DHSS Artific. Limb & Appliance Centre Birm.; Fell. Scientif. Counc. Internat. Coll. Angiol. Socs: Internat. Soc. Prosthetists & Orthotists. Prev: Regist. (Surg.) Crewe & Dist. Memor. Hosp.; Surg. Accid. Serv. Colombo, Ceylon; Surg. Gen. Hosp. Chilaw, Sri Lanka.

SIRIWARDENE, Seetha Kaushalyani (retired) 9 Hartland Close, Winchmore Hill, London N21 2BG — MB BS Ceylon 1957; DCH Eng. 1965; MFCM 1974. GP Dudley FPC. Prev: SCMO Dudley AHA.

SIRIWARDHANA, Shyrana Abeysinghe 191 Anson Road, London NW2 4AU — MRCS Eng. LRCP Lond. 1979. Prev: Ho. Surg. St. Andrews Hosp. (T) Lond.; Ho. Phys. Fazakerley Gen. Hosp. (T) Liverp.; SHO (A & E) St. Helier Hosp. (T) Carshalton.

SIRKER, Alexander Avijit 37 Fontmell Close, St Albans, St Albans AL3 5HU — BChir Camb. 1996.

SIROTAKOVA, Maria 51 Lampern Crescent, Billericay CM12 0FE; Timravinaz, Bratislava 81106, Slovak Republic Tel: 00 427 5312077 — MUDr Komensky Univ. Czech. 1973; MUDr Komensky U Czechoslovakia 1973. Clin. Asst. (Plastic Surg.) S. And. Hosp. Billericay. Specialty: Plastic Surg.

SIRR, Hubert Clement Ritchie 7 Shannon Road, Stubbington, Fareham PO14 3RL Tel: 01329 667150 — MB BCh BAO Dub. 1973 (TC Dub.) MRCGP 1980. Prev: Maj. RAMC; SHO SHAPE BFPO 26.

SIRRI, Teoman Necati 336 St Ann's Road, London N15 3TA — MRCS Eng. LRCP Lond. 1981 (St. Mary's) BSc (Hons.) Phys. & Biochem. 1974; MSc. (Dist.) Pharmacol. Lond. 1976. Clin. Asst. (Dermat.) Enfield & Haringey HA; Vis. Prof. Bursa Med. Fac. Turkey. Specialty: Dermat. Prev: Regist. (Psychiat.) St. Ann's Hosp. Lond.; SHO (Psychiat., O & G, Geriat. & A & E) N. Middlx. Lond.

SISODIA, Neelam Psychiatric Unit, Derbycity General Hospital, Uttoxeter Rd, Derby DE22 3NE Tel: 01332 623874 — MB BS Newc. 1983; MRCPsych 1994; MA Uni.Lond. 1997. Cons. (gen. Adult Psychiat.). Specialty: Gen. Psychiat. Prev: Sen. Regist. (Gen. Adult Psychiat.) Univ. Hosp. Nottm.

SISODIYA, Sanjay Mull Institute of Neurology, Queen Square, London WC1N 3BG — MB BChir Camb. 1989; MRCP (UK) 1991; PhD London 1996. Specialty: Neurol.

SISSON, Jennifer 7 St Saviours Place, Leas Road, Guildford GU1 4QN — MB BS Western Australia 1991.

SISSONS, Angela Mary — MB BS Durh. 1967.

SISSONS, Clifford Ernest Grosvenor Nuffield Hospital, Wrexham Road, Chester CH4 7QP Tel: 01244 680444; Cintra, Hillock Lane, Gresford, Wrexham LL12 8YL Tel: 01978 855565 Fax: 01978 854014 — (Liverp.) MB ChB Liverp. 1958; MRCP (UK) 1966; FRCP Lond. 1977. Cons. PhysBUPA Yale Hosp.Wrexham; Cons.Phys.Grosvenor Nuffield Hosp.Chester. Specialty: Gen. Med.; Cardiol. Socs: BMA; Brit. Soc. Echocardiogr.; Brit. Hyperlipid. Assn. Prev: Cons. Phys. Wrexham Mealor Hosp. NHS Trust; Sen. Regist. (Med.) Sefton Gen. Hosp. Liverp.; Regist. Profess. Med. Unit. Liverp. Roy. Infirm.

SISSONS, David Ashley The Pines, Kinnerton Lane, Higher Kinnerton, Chester CH4 9BG — MB ChB Liverp. 1973; MRCS Eng. LRCP Lond. 1973.

SISSONS, Guy Richard James Radiology Department, Countess of Chester Hospital, Liverpool Road, Chester CH2 1BQ Tel: 01244 366712 Fax: 01244 366728 Email: g.sissons@coch.nhs.uk — MB ChB Birm. 1982; MRCP (UK) 1985; FRCR 1989; T(R) (CR) 1991. Cons. Diagn. Radiol. Countess of Chester Hosp. Specialty: Radiol. Socs: Brit. Inst. Radiol.; Brit. Soc. Interven. Radiol. Prev: Sen. Regist. (Radiol.) Univ. Hosp. Wales & Flinders Med. Centre Adelaide, S. Austral.

SISSONS, Helen Margaret Rysseldene Surgery, 98 Conway Road, Colwyn Bay LL29 7LE Tel: 01492 532807 Fax: 01492 534846 — (Univ. Coll. Hosp.) BSc (Pharmacol.) Lond. 1976, MB BS 1979; DCH RCP Lond. 1982; MRCGP 1983; DRCOG 1984. Prev: SHO Bronglais Hosp. Aberystwyth; Ho. Surg. Univ. Coll. Hosp. Lond.; Ho. Phys. Treliske Hosp. Truro.

SISSONS, Professor John Gerald Patrick Department of Medicine, University of Cambridge Clinical School, Addenbrooke's Hospital, Hills Road, Cambridge CB2 2QQ Tel: 01223 336849 — MB BS Lond. 1968; MRCP (UK) 1970; MD Lond. 1977; FRCP Lond. 1983; FRCPath 1996. Prof. Med. Univ. Camb. Specialty: Infec. Dis.; Gen. Med. Prev: Prof. Infec. Dis. Roy. Postgrad. Med. Sch. Lond.; Wellcome Sen. Lect. (Med.) Roy. Postgrad. Med. Sch. Lond.; Asst. Mem. Research Inst. Scripps Clinic La Jolla, Calif., USA.

SISSONS, John Peter The Orchard House, 61 Links Lane, Rowlands Castle PO9 6AF — MB BS Lond. 1997.

SISSONS, Mark Christopher John The Grange, Grange Road, Hambleton, Poulton-le-Fylde FY6 9DB — MD Birm. 1988; MB ChB 1980; MRCPath 1987. Cons. Histopath. Blackpool Vict. Hosp. Specialty: Histopath. Prev: Lect. (Path.) Univ. Liverp.

SISSONS, Michael Paul Spire Hill Cottage, Fairmead Road, Saltash PL12 4QE — MB ChB Leeds 1995.

SISSONS, Paula Jane The Grange, Grange Road, Hambleton, Poulton-le-Fylde FY6 9DB — MB ChB Birm. 1980; MRCP (UK) 1983. Med. Off. DSS Blackpool.

SISSOU, Panikos 9 Belgrave Gardens, Oakwood, London N14 4TS Tel: 020 8360 7193 — MB BS Lond. 1990; BSc (Hons.) Lond. 1989, MB BS 1990.

SITARAS, Dimitrios 44 Vulcan Way, London N7 8XP — Ptychio Iatrikes Thessalonika 1968.

SITHAMPARANATHAN, Shamini 56 Compton Road, London SW19 7QD — MB BS Lond. 1998; MB BS Lond 1998.

SITHAMPARANATHAN, Thuraiappah The Surgery, 191 Westmount Road, London SE9 1XY Tel: 020 8850 1540 Fax: 020 8859 4737 — MB BS Sri Lanka 1974; MRCS Eng. LRCP Lond. 1986.

SITHAMPARAPILLAI, Sivaja 67 Hayes Chase, West Wickham BR4 0HX — MB BS Lond. 1997.

SITHIRAPATHY, Sivakumary Taara, Avenue Road, Bray, Maidenhead SL6 1UG Tel: 01628 676675 — MRCS Eng. LRCP Lond. 1987 (Univ. Colombo, Sri Lanka) DRCOG 1995; MRCOG 1996. Gen. Practitioner, Slough. Specialty: Gen. Pract. Prev: GP/Regist. Cookham, Berks.; Regist. (O & G) Hemel Hempstead Herts.; SHO (O & G) Centr. Middlx. Hosp. Lond.

SITJES LLADO, Narciso 134 Woodway Lane, Coventry CV2 2EJ — LMS Barcelona 1994; LMS Autonoma Barcelona 1994.

SITLANI, Pushpa Kishin Cherry Trees, 17 Pownall Avenue, Bramhall, Stockport SK7 2HE Tel: 0161 439 6050 — MB BS Osmania 1961; FRCPath 1981, M 1969. Cons. Haemat. Gp. Laborat. Stepping Hill Hosp. Stockport & N. Derbysh. Health Dist. Specialty: Haematology. Socs: Assn. Clin. Pathol. Prev: Sen. Regist. (Haemat.) St. Geo. Hosp. Lond. & S. Lond. Transfus. Sutton;Centre; Regist. (Path.) S. Lond. Hosp. Wom.

SITTAMPALAM, Ganeshwaran 18 Wycherley Crescent, New Barnet, Barnet EN5 1AR — MB BS Lond. 1998; MB BS Lond 1998.

SITTAMPALAM, Lara Winifred Eastcote Health Centre, Devonshire Lodge Practice, Abbotsbury Gardens, Pinner HA5 1TG — BM Soton. 1991; DFFP 1994; DRCOG 1994; MRCGP 1995. GP Retainer. Special Interest: Obst. & Gyn. Prev: Research in Pharm. Med. Mt. Vernon Hosp.; SHO (Paediat.) Portsmouth; Trainee GP Lordshill.

SITWELL, Isla Ashley Hurt Sitwell and Partners, Little Common Surgery, 82 Cooden Sea Road, Bexhill-on-Sea TN39 4SP Tel: 01424 845477 Fax: 01424 848225 — (Camb. & St. Bart.) MB BChir Camb. 1969.

SIU, Simon Kai Leung 34A Seafield Road, Dundee DD1 4NP — MB ChB Dund. 1998; MB ChB Dund 1998.

SIUDA, Zbigniew Edmund 20A West End, Swanland, North Ferriby HU14 3PE — (Poznan) Med. Dipl. Poznan 1936. Prev: Res. O & G Asst. Gen. Hosp. Chorzow.

SIVA, Roshan 2 Bourne Drive, Ravenshead, Nottingham NG15 9FN — MB BS Lond. 1996.

SIVA PRAKASH, Pappali Gopalan G C P Systems Ltd., Director, 222 Metro Central, 119 Newington Causeway, London SE1 6BW Tel: 020 79678 760 — MB BS Kerala 1975 (Kottam Med. Coll., Kerala) MSc Computer Studies S. Glam.; DTCD Delhi; DRM Delhi; DMRT Eng.; MB BS Kerala, India 1975. Company Dir. G.C.P. Systems Lond. Prev: IT Cons. Centr. Health Outcodes Unit, Dept. of Health, Lond.

SIVABALAN, Ponnudurai Edge Hill Health Centre, Crosfield Road, Liverpool L7 5QL Tel: 0151 260 2777 — MB BS Sri Lanka 1979; DGM RCP Lond. 1987.

SIVABALAN, Thambimuthu 57B Days Lane, Biddenham, Bedford MK40 4AE — MB BS Ceylon 1971; MRCOG 1983.

SIVABALASINGHAM, Suganya 1 Evelyn Mansions, Queen's Club Gardens, London W14 9RQ — MB BS Lond. 1997 (St Bart's Lond.) BSc Lond. 1994. SpR Clin. Oncol. Specialty: Gen. Med. Prev: SHO Rotat. (Med.).

SIVAGAMASUNDARI, Umapathy 5 Cooper Close, Langstone, Newport NP18 2LD Tel: 01633 413962 — MB BS Madras 1976; MRCPsych 1989. Cons. Psychiat. Gwent Community NHS Trust. Specialty: Gen. Psychiat. Prev: Sen. Regist. Phoenix Trust Bristol.

SIVAGNANAM, Chelliah (Surgery), 137 Greenwich South St., Greenwich, London SE10 8PP Tel: 020 8691 8999; 3 Papillons Walk, London SE3 9SF — MB BS Ceylon 1955.

SIVAGNANAM, Thamotharampillai Royal Infirmary, Blackburn Tel: 01254 687235; 20 Bosburn Drive, Mellor Brook, Blackburn BB2 7PA Tel: 01254 813281 — MB BS Sri Lanka 1972; FFA RCS Eng. 1982. Cons. Anaesth. & Pain Relief Roy. Infirm. Blackburn. Specialty: Anaesth. Socs: Assn. Anaesth.; Pain Soc.; NW Pain Soc. & Palliat. Med.

SIVAGNANASUNDARAM, Sivasundaram Winlaton Surgery, 139 Winlaton Road, Bromley BR1 5QA Tel: 020 8698 1810 — MB BS Sri Lanka 1978 (Colombo, Sri Lanka) LMSSA Lond. 1989. Socs: Med. Protec. Soc.

SIVAGNANAVEL, Sarathadevi 34 Leamington Avenue, Morden SM4 4DW Tel: 020 8542 7608 — MB BS Ceylon 1966.

SIVAGURU, Arulmaran 5 Maclean Avenue, Loughborough LE11 5XX — MB ChB Leeds 1991.

SIVAJI, Mr Chellappan 55 Nelson Road, Leigh-on-Sea SS9 3HX — MB BS Madurai Kamaraj Univ. India 1986; FRCS Eng. 1992.

SIVAKUMAR, Branavan 7 Gossington Close, Chislehurst BR7 6TG — MB BS Lond. 1998; MRCS (Eng) 2001.

SIVAKUMAR, Kanagaratnam Department Genitourinary Medicine, Queen Elizabeth Hospital, Gayton Road, King's Lynn PE30 4ET Fax: 01553 613833; 3 Old Kiln, West Winch, King's Lynn PE33 0EG Tel: 01553 841975 — MB BS Colombo 1980; LRCP LRCS Ed. LRCPS Glas. 1985; FRCP 1998, MRCP 1986. Cons. Phys. (Genitourin. Med.) Qu. Eliz. Hosp., King's Lynn & Dist. Hosp. PeterBoro. Specialty: Genitourinary Medicine. Prev: Sen. Regist. (Genitourin. Med.) Bournemouth & Soton. Gp. Hosps.

SIVAKUMAR, Kandiah Invicta Community Care NHS Trust, Priority House, Hermitage Lane, Maidstone ME16 9PH Tel: 01622 725000 Fax: 01622 725290; 7 Gossington Close, Chislehurst BR7 6TG Tel: 020 8468 7181 — (University of Ceylon, Colombo) MB BS Ceylon 1970; DPM Eng. 1979; MRCPsych 1979; FRCPsych 1996. Cons. (Psychiat.) Invicta Community Care NHS Trust; Hon. Cons. (Psychiat.) KCH; Hon. Sen. Lect. Div. of Psychiat. Guys Hosp. Lond. Specialty: Gen. Psychiat.

SIVAKUMAR, Mr Muthuthamby Queen Elizabeth, Queen Mother Hospital, Margate CT9 4AN Tel: 01803 225549 — MB BS Colombo 1983; FRCS Ed. 1992. Staff Surg. Specialty: Gen. Surg. Prev: Sur. Regist. Jersey Gen. Hosp. CI.; SHO, Surg. Thanet Dist. Gen. Hosp.

SIVAKUMAR, Paramasivam Luton & Dunstable Hospital, Lewsey Road, Luton LU4 0DZ Tel: 01582 491122 Fax: 01582 497280; 273 Luton Road, Harpenden AL5 3LN Tel: 01582 461695 — MB BS Sri Lanka 1979; MRCS Eng. LRCP Lond. 1986; DCH RCP Lond. 1987; MRCP (UK) 1989. Cons. Paediat. Luton & Dunstable Hosp. Specialty: Paediat.

SIVAKUMAR, Ranjesthanayakey 55 Elm Drive, St Albans AL4 0EH — MB BS Colombo 1977.

SIVAKUMAR, Sinnathamby 13 Petrel Close, Bamford, Rochdale OL11 5QT — MB BS Sri Lanka 1978; LMSSA Lond. 1990. Staff Grade(Ophth.) Birch Hill Hosp. Rochdale. Specialty: Ophth.

SIVAKUMAR, Thaiman Queens Avenue Surgery, 46 Queens Avenue, Muswell Hill, London N10 3BJ Tel: 020 8883 1846 Fax: 020 8365 2265; 2 Larkfield Avenue, Harrow HA3 8NF Tel: 020 8907 5616 — MB BS Sri Lanka 1975; MRCOG 1987. GP. Specialty: Obst. & Gyn.

SIVAKUMARAN, Muttuswamy Peterborough District Hospital, Thorpe Road, Peterborough PE3 6DA — MB BS Peradeniya, Sri Lanka 1979; LRCP LRCS Ed. LRCPS Glas. 1983; MRCP (UK) 1986; MRCPath UK 1993; PhD Leeds 1996; MSc (Hons.) 1998. Cons Haematol. P'boro. Dist. Hosp.

SIVAKUMARAN, Shantha Ruweena 182 Holmes Chapel Road, Congleton CW12 4QB — BChir Camb. 1996.

SIVAKUMARAN, Vijayasegaram 72 Rhydydefaid Drive, Skeety, Swansea SA2 8AN — MB BS Sri Lanka 1975; MRCS Eng. LRCP Lond. 1982.

SIVALINGAM, Thiyagarajan Royal Bolton Hospital, Consultant Anaesthetist, Department of Anaesthetist, Farnworth, Bolton BL4 0JR Tel: 01204 390 762 Fax: 01204 390 640 — MB BS Madras India 1972 (Jipmer Pondicherry S. India) MD Madurai India 1975; FRCA Lond. 1982. Cons. Anaesth. Roy. Bolton Hosp. Bolton; Beaumont Hosp. (private) Lostock Bolton. Specialty: Anaesth. Special Interest: Blood Transfus.; Overseas Doctors Train. Scheme. Socs: Bolton Medical Society; British International Doctors' Association.

SIVALOGANATHAN, Malathy 15 Verulam Avenue, Purley CR8 3NR — MB BS Lond. 1994.

SIVALOGANATHAN, Sampanthanathan 15 Verulam Avenue, Purley CR8 3NR — MB BS Ceylon 1967.

SIVALOGANATHAN, Saraswathy 15 Verulam Avenue, Purley CR8 3NR — MB BS Ceylon 1967; MRCPsych 1980; T(Psych) 1991.

SIVANANDAN, Manoranjini 4 Tollgate Drive, London SE21 7LS — MB BS Sri Lanka 1978; FFA RCSI 1987.

SIVANANTHAN, Anushtayini Elderly Mental Health Directorate, West Cheshire Hospital, Liverpool Road, Chester CH2 1UL Tel: 01244 364158 — MB ChB Liverp. 1991 (L'pool) MRCPsych 1995; DGM 1997. Cons. (Elderly Ment. Health). Specialty: Geriat. Psychiat.

SIVANANTHAN, Nadarajah Quedgeley Clinic, Quedgeley Health Campus, St. James, Gloucester GL2 4WD Tel: 01452 728882 — MB BS Sri Lanka 1975 (Univ. Ceylon, Colombo-Sri Lanka) LRCP LRCS Ed. LRCPS Glas. 1982; MRCP (UK) 1982. Specialty: Gen. Pract. Socs: Collegiate Mem. RCP Lond. Prev: Regist. Rotat. (Med.) Dudley HA; Regist. (Med.) Leighton Hosp. Crewe.

SIVANANTHAN, Nalliah Alexandra Surgery, 125 Alexandra Park Road, London N22 7UN Tel: 020 8888 2518; 279 Stradbroke Grove, Clayhall, Ilford IG5 0DH Tel: 020 8924 9512 — MB BS Ceylon 1972; MRCOG (UK) 1982. Specialty: Obst. & Gyn. Socs: Med. Inst. of Tamil.

SIVANANTHAN, Uduvil Mohanaraj Cardiac MRI Unit, D Floor, Jubilee Wing, Leeds General Infirmary, Great George Street, Leeds LS1 3EX Tel: 0113 392 5691 — MB BS Colombo 1979; MRCP (UK) 1984; DMRD Lond. 1987. Director Cardiac MRI Unit Leeds Gen. Infirm.

SIVANESAN, Ratnam (Surgery), 6 Townsend Road, Southall UB1 1EX Tel: 020 8574 2794 — MB BS Ceylon 1978; MRCP (UK) 1978; DCH Lond. 1978; DRCOG Lond. 1980. Specialty: Paediat. Neurol.

SIVANESAN, Vaithilingam Nagalingam Brereton Surgery, 88 Main Street, Brereton, Rugeley WS15 1DU Tel: 01889 575560 Fax: 01889 575560 — MB BS Ceylon 1971.

SIVAPALAN, Sivagnanam Department of Genitourinary Medicine, North Staffs Hospital NHS Trust, Hartshill Road, Stoke-on-Trent ST4 7PA Tel: 01782 554135 Fax: 01782 846660 — MB BS Sri Lanka 1974 (Colombo Med. Sch. Univ. Ceylon) MRCOG 1986. Cons. Genitourin. Med. N. Staffs. HA. Specialty: Genitourinary Medicine. Prev: Sen. Regist. (Genitourin. Med.) E. Dorset HA; Regist. (O & G) Clwyd HA.

SIVAPATHASUNDARAM, Paraneetharan 1 Percival Road, Hornchurch RM11 2AH — MB ChB Sheff. 1997.

SIVAPATHASUNDARAM, Mr Vythilingam Royal London Hospital, Whitechapel Road, London E1 1BB Tel: 020 7377 7240; 18 Highcliffe Gardens, Redbridge, Ilford IG4 5HR Tel: 020 8924 7950 — MB BS Ceylon 1967; MRCOG 1981; FRCOG 1995. Cons. O & G Roy. Lond. Hosp. Specialty: Obst. & Gyn. Socs: Fell. Roy. Soc. Med.

SIVAPATHASUNTHARAM, Logeswary 317 Dunchurch Road, Rugby CV22 6HT Tel: 01788 522548 — MB BS Ceylon 1972.

SIVAPRAGASAM, Mr Sinnathamby Worcestershire Acute Hospitals NHS Trust, Alexandra Hospital, Woodrow Drive, Redditch B98 7UB — MB BS Sri Lanka 1974 (Colombo, Sri Lanka) FRCS Ed. 1986; MRCS Eng. LRCP Lond. 1986; FRCS Eng. 1989. Specialty: Gastroenterol.; Vasc. Med.; Gen. Surg. Socs: BMA; Hosp. Cons. & Spec. Comm. (HCSC); Fell. ASGBI.

SIVARAJAN, Kandiah 89 Broadwater Road, Tooting, London SW17 0DY Tel: 020 8767 1134 — MB BS Sri Lanka 1972.

SIVARAJAN, Sweeta Carrfield Medical Centre, Carrfield Street, Sheffield S8 9SG; 24 Selby Close, Walton, Chesterfield S40 3HA — MB BS Kerala 1972 (Kottayam Med. Coll.)

SIVARAJAN, Vivek 24 Selby Close, Walton, Chesterfield S40 3HA — MB ChB Ed. 1997.

SIVARAMALINGAM, Thillaiampalam Ravishanker 75 Oaklands Road, London W7 2DT Tel: 020 8579 3319 — MB BS Lond. 1988 (Char. Cross & Westm.) DRCOG 1996; DCH 1996; MRCGP 1997; DFFP 1997.

SIVARDEEN, Gani Mathul Fawzia Cromartie Street Surgery, 39 Cromartie Street, Longton, Stoke-on-Trent ST3 4LG Tel: 01782 329488 — MB BS Ceylon 1963 (Colombo) DO Eng. 1977; MCOphth 1989. GP Stoke-on-Trent; Med. Pract. (Ophth.) Stoke-on-Trent & Stafford.

SIVARDEEN, Mr Khawaja Ashraff Ziali 11 Meliden Way, Stoke-on-Trent ST4 5DZ — BM BS Nottm. 1994. Specialty: Orthop.

SIVASANKER, Kemraj 5 Oakleigh Avenue, Edgware HA8 5DT Tel: 020 8952 0058 — MB BS Patna 1969 (P. of Wales Med. Coll.) MD (Paediat.) Patna 1974. Community Paediat. (Audiol. & Adopt.) Middlx. Specialty: Audiol. Med. Socs: Fell. Roy. Inst. Pub. Health & Hyg.; Fac. Comm. Health. Prev: Regist. (Paediat.) Chester City Hosp. & W. Chesh. Hosp. Matern. Wing Chester; SHO (Paediat.) Hemel Hempstead Gen. Hosp.

SIVASINMYANANTHAN, Kathiravellupillai The Surgery, 326 Philip Lane, Tottenham, London N15 4AB Tel: 020 8808 0322 — MB BS Sri Lanka 1974; LRCP LRCS Ed. LRCPS Glas. 1984; DPD 1998. Specialty: Dermat.; Rheumatol. Socs: BMA. Prev: Clin. Asst. (Rheum.) Chase Farm Hosp. Enfield; SHO (Rheum.) Devonsh. Roy. Hosp. Derby; SHO (Geriat.) P'boro Hosp. Lond.

SIVATHASAN, Sivadevi 303 Hempstead Road, Hempstead, Gillingham ME7 3QJ — MB BS Ceylon 1970; FFA RCS Eng. 1980. Specialty: Anaesth.

SIVATHASAN, Sivalingam 60 Central Hill, Upper Norwood, London SE19 1DT Tel: 020 8670 7117 Fax: 020 8670 1671; 90 Malmains Way, Park Langley, Beckenham BR3 6SF Tel: 020 8663 6668 — MB BS Sri Lanka 1978 (Faculty of Medicine University of Colombo, Sri Lanka) MRCS Eng. LRCP Lond. 1987; MRCOG 1991; DRCOG 1991. GP. Specialty: Obst. & Gyn.; Family Plann. & Reproduc. Health; Gastroenterol. Socs: Med. Protec. Soc.; Roy. Coll. Obst. & Gyns. Prev: Regist. (O & G).

SIVAYOHAM, Narani 5 Copperfield Court, 146 Worple Road, Wimbledon, London SW20 8QA — MB ChB Liverp. 1992; BSc (Hons.) Liverp. 1989; MRCP (UK) 1996. Specialist Regist. Rotat. (A & E Med.) St. Geo. Hosp. Lond. Specialty: Accid. & Emerg. Prev: SHO Rotat. (Med.) S. Cleveland Hosp. Middlesbrough.

SIVAYOHAM, Sabapathy — MB BS Ceylon 1961; DTPH 1972; DIH Eng. 1973; MFCM 1974; MD Colombo 1981; MFPHM RCP (UK) 1990. Cons. Communicable Dis. Control & Pub. Health Med. S. Lancs. HA Eccleston, Chorley. Specialty: Infec. Dis.; Pub. Health Med. Socs: Manch. Med. Soc. (Pres. Pub. Health Sect.). Prev: Dir. of Pub. Health Chorley & S. Ribble HA; Specialist (Community Med.) S. Cumbria HA.

SIVAYOKAN, Ponniah Department of Anaesthetics, General Hospital, Bishop Auckland DL14 6AD — MB BS Ceylon 1970; DA Eng. 1980; FFA RCS Eng. 1983. Cons. Anaesth. Gen. Hosp. Bishop Auckland. Specialty: Anaesth. Prev: Regist. (Anaesth.) PeterBoro. Dist. Hosp.; Sen. Regist. (Anaesth.) Addenbrooks Hosp. Camb.; Sen. Regist. (Anaesth.) City Gen. Stoke on Trent.

SIVES, Deirdra Ann 41 Glendevon Park, Winchburgh, Broxburn EH52 6UF — MB ChB Ed. 1990.

SIVITER, Gretchen 59 Acres Road, Chorlton, Manchester M21 9EB Tel: 0161 881 2809 — MB ChB Manch. 1992. Specialty: Anaesth.

SIVORI, Robert Emmanuel 14 Hollybank Road, Mossley Hill, Liverpool L18 1HP — MB ChB Liverp. 1997.

SIVRIDIS, Anestis Rampton Hospital, Retford DN22 0PD — Ptychio Iatrikes Thessalonika 1977.

SIVYER, Janet Elizabeth Regent Street Surgery, 73 Regent Street, Stonehouse GL10 2AA Tel: 01453 822145 Fax: 01453 821663; Woodfield Cottage, 157 Slad Road, Stroud GL5 1RD — MB ChB Sheff. 1981; DRCOG 1984.

SIX, Serge Pembroke Surgery, 9 Eldon Square, Reading RG1 4DP; 11 Allcroft Road, Reading RG1 5HJ Tel: 01734 872550 — MD Brussels 1977. Hon. Sec. BMA W. Berks. Div. Socs: BMA (Chairm. Oxf. Regional Counc.).

SIXSMITH, Andrew Milton 15 South Row, Horsforth, Leeds LS18 4AA — MB ChB Leeds 1994.

***SIXSMITH, Clare** 6 Cliff Castle, Castle Hill, Seaton EX12 2QW — BM BCh Oxf. 1998; BM BCh Oxf 1998. Specialty: Gen. Med.

SIXSMITH, Dona Jeromi Inoka 15 Melyd Avenue, Prestatyn LL19 8RN — MB ChB Leeds 1995.

SIXSMITH, Mark 39 Antonine Way, Houghton, Carlisle CA3 0LG — MB ChB Manch. 1994.

SIZER, Angela Jane 1 Quayside Walk, Marchwood, Southampton SO40 4AH — MB BS Lond. 1996.

SIZER, Bruce Francis 23 Guithavon Street, Witham CM8 1BJ — MB ChB Birm. 1983; ChB Birm. 1983.

SIZER, Elizabeth 119 Dunvegan Road, London SE9 1SD — MB BS Lond. 1993.

SIZER, Jeremy Mark 1 Riverside View, Milton Ernest, Bedford MK44 1SG — MB BS Lond. 1985 (Kings) DCH RCP Lond. 1988; FCAnaesth 1990. Cons. (Anaesth.) Bedford Hosp. NHS Trust. Specialty: Anaesth.; Intens. Care.

SIZER, Karen Ann 28 Hillmead Gardens, Bedhampton, Havant PO9 3NL — BM Soton. 1978.

SIZMUR, Fiona Margaret Meadow Cottage, Forest Road, Burley, Ringwood BH24 4DQ; 21 Chaworth Road, Ottershaw, Chertsey KT16 0PF — MB ChB Liverp. 1989. Regist. (O & G) Bournemouth Hosp. Specialty: Obst. & Gyn. Prev: Regist. (O & G) Leicester Gen. Hosp.; SHO (O & G) Leicester Roy. Infirm.

SJOLIN, Mr Soren Upton West Suffolk Hospital, Hardwick Lane, Bury St Edmunds IP33 2QZ Tel: 01284 712551 Fax: 01284 712551 — MD Odense 1981 (Odense, Denmark, 1981) FRCS (Orth.) 1996. Cons. Orthop. Surg. W. Suff. Hosp. Bury St Edmunds. Specialty: Trauma & Orthop. Surg. Socs: Brit. Orthopaedic Assn.; Brit. Elbow and Shoulder Soc.; Danish Orthopaedic Soc. Prev: Sen. Regist. Roy. Infirm. Edin.

SKAIFE, Paul Gerard Patrick 21 Towers Road, Liverpool L16 8NT — MB ChB Leeds 1990.

SKAILES, Geraldine Elizabeth Phyllis Cancer Services Directorate, Royal Preston Hospital, Sharoe Green Lane N., Fulwood, Preston PR2 9HT Tel: 01772 522984 Fax: 01772 522955 Email: geraldine.skailes@lthtr.nhs.uk — MB BS Lond. 1988; MRCP (UK) 1991; FRCR 1995. Cons. (Clin. Oncol.) Lancs. Teachg. Hosps. NHS Trust. Specialty: Oncol. Special Interest: Lung, Gynae and Breast Cancer.

SKALICKA, Anna Elizabeth Ave Group Practice, 2 Elizabeth Avenue, London N1 3BS Tel: 020 7226 6363 — MB ChB Leeds 1973; MRCP (U.K.) 1975; MRCGP 1977; DCH Eng. 1977.

SKAN, Delia Ida Mary 7 Notting Hill, Belfast BT9 5NS — MB BCh BAO Belf. 1975; MB BCh BAO (Hons.) Belf. 1975; DCH RCPSI 1977; MRCP (UK) 1980; MRCGP 1982; MFOM RCPI 1992, AFOM 1987. Occupat. Physic., Employ. Med. Advis. Serv. DHSS.

SKAN, John Phillip 20 Penrhyn Road, Hunters Bar, Sheffield S11 8UL Tel: 0114 266 0793 — MB ChB Sheff. 1981.

SKANDEROWICZ, Mr Andrew George 2 Wentworth Drive, Lichfield WS14 9HN Tel: 01543 257454 — MB BS Lond. 1974 (St. Bart.) MRCS Eng. LRCP Lond. 1974; FRCS Eng. 1979. Socs: BACS.

SKARBEK, Count Andrew Charles (retired) 26 Belsize Square, London NW3 4HU Tel: 020 7794 6857 — MRCS Eng. LRCP Lond. 1954 (St. Mary's) PhD Lond. 1969, MB BS 1954; FRCPsych 1983, M 1971. Prev: Assoc. Prof. Psychiat. Univ. Ottowa.

SKARIA, Joseph Hillcrest Medical Centre, Pryce Street, Mountain Ash CF45 3NT Tel: 01443 473783 Fax: 01443 477420; Pukkunnel, 1 Ynys y Coed, Llandaff, Cardiff CF5 2LU — MD Banaras Hindu 1975; MB BS 1971. Specialty: Gen. Med. Socs: Soc. Occupat. Med., Assur. Med. Soc. & Christian Med. Fellowsh.

SKARROTT, Pauline Helen Ling House Surgeries, 49 Scott Street, Keighley BD21 2JH Tel: 01535 605747 Fax: 01535 602901 — MB ChB Birm. 1979.

SKARSTEN, Anders Roy Hargrave Bracton Clinic, Bexley Hospital, Old Bexley Lane, Bexley DA5 2BW Tel: 01322 294300 Fax: 01322 293595; 43 Codicote Road, Welwyn AL6 9TT Tel: 0374 892164 Fax: 020 7787 0739 Email: skarsten@dircon.co.uk — MB BS Lond. 1990; BSc (Pharmacol.) Lond. 1987. Forens. Research Fell.

Bracton Clinic UMDS Dept. Psychiat. Guy's Hosp. Lond. Specialty: Forens. Psychiat.

SKEA, George Keillor 15 The Shires, Gilwern, Abergavenny NP7 0EX — MB ChB Glas. 1984. SHO (Anaesth.) Leicester Roy. Infirm.

SKEATES, Stuart John North Baddesley Surgery, Norton Welch Close, Fleming Avenue, Southampton SO52 9EP Tel: 023 8073 4523 Fax: 023 8073 0287; 55 Cherville Street, Romsey SO51 8FB Tel: 01794 522192 — MB BS Lond. 1974; MA (Mathematics) Camb. 1972; DRCOG 1978; MRCGP 1980. Course Organiser Soton.

SKEATH, Thalia Helen Somerset Partnership NHS and Social Care Trust, Holly Court, Summerlands, 56 Preston Road, Yeovil BA20 2BX Tel: 01935 428420 Fax: 01938 411612 — MB ChB Leeds 1986; MRCPsych 1996. Staff Grade (Psychiat.) Som. Partnership NHS & Social Care Trust. Prev: Clin. Med. Off. (Psychiat.) Avalon Trust Som.; Regist. (Psychiat.) Avalon Trust Som.; Regist. (Psychiat.) Norwich HA.

SKEATS, Christina Jane 42 Morris Road, South Nutfield, Redhill RH1 5SA — MB ChB Sheff. 1987.

SKEAVINGTON, John Reginald Birnam House, Stone Lane, North Wheatley, Retford DN22 9DF Tel: 01427 880759 Fax: 01427 881686 Email: gbdr2538@doctors.org.uk — MB ChB Sheff. 1960; MRCP Lond. 1968. Socs: BMA.(1960-2000); Med. Charitable Soc. of the W. Riding of the Co. of York. Prev: Gen. PRACTITIONER Princip.; Med. Regist. Derbysh. Roy. Infirm. Ho. Surg. Dept. Neurol. Surg. Roy.; Infirm. Sheff.

SKEENS, Erwine Mary (retired) 8 North Street, Fowey PL23 1DD — MRCS Eng. LRCP Lond. 1954.

SKEENS, Esmond Courtenay (retired) Amity House, 8 North St., Fowey PL23 1DD — MB ChB Bristol 1955.

SKEET, William Anthony George 2A Sydervelt Road, Canvey Island SS8 9EG — MB ChB St. And. 1962; DObst RCOG 1966; Dip. Pract. Dermat. Wales 1992. Specialty: Dermat.

SKEGGS, David Bartholomew Lyndon Radiotherapy Department, Cromwell Hospital, London SW5 0TU Tel: 020 7460 2000 Fax: 020 7460 5622; The Coach House, Barnes Common, London SW13 0HS Tel: 020 8876 7929 Fax: 020 8876 7929 — BM BCh Oxf. 1952 (Oxf. & St. Bart.) FRCR; MA Oxf. 1952; DMRT Eng. 1961; FFR 1964. Hon. Cons. Radiother. Roy. Free Hosp. Lond.; Hon. Cons. Radiother. Roy. N. Hosp. Lond.; Chairm. Pract. Privileges Cromwell Hosp. Specialty: Oncol.; Radiother. Prev: Dir. (Radiother.) Roy. Free Hosp. Lond.; Sen. Regist. (Radiother.) St. Bart. Hosp. Lond.; Chairm. Bd. Examrs. Part 1 FRCR.

SKEGGS, Peter Lyndon (retired) Valley House, Preston Candover, Basingstoke RG25 2DN — (St. Bart.) MA, BM BCh Oxf. 1945; FRCPath (Hon.) 1994. Prev: Local Treasury Med. Off.

SKEHAN, John Douglas Glenfield NHS Trust, Groby Road, Leicester LE3 9QP Tel: 0116 256 3888 Fax: 0116 231 4751; 87 Chaveney Road, Quorn, Loughborough LE12 8AB Tel: 01509 620325 — MB BS Lond. 1977 (Lond. Hosp.) BSc (Hons.) Lond. 1974, MB BS 1977; MRCP (UK) 1980; FRCP (UK) 1996. Cons. Cardiol. Glenfield NHS Trust Leics.; Clin. Director, CardioRespirat. Directorate, Univ. Hosp.s Leicester Trust. Specialty: Cardiol. Socs: Brit. Cardiac Soc.; (Counc. Mem.) Brit. Pacing & Electrophysiol. Gp.; BMA. Prev: Jun. Research Fell. Brit. Heart Foundat. Lond. Hosp.; Sen. Regist. Cardiac Dept. Lond. Hosp. Whitechapel; Regist. (Med.) OldCh. Hosp. Romford & Lond. Hosp.

SKEHAN, Paul Francis John 5 Orchard Gate, Larkhall ML9 1HA — MB BCh BAO NUI 1982.

SKELDON, Ian 4 Staveley Road, Ashford TW15 1TF — MB ChB Bristol 1977.

SKELKER, Miriam Hilary Windmill Medical Practice, 65 Shoot Up Hill, London NW2 3PS Tel: 020 8452 7646 Fax: 020 8450 2319 — MB BS Lond. 1985; MRCGP; BA.

SKELLERN, Elizabeth PM (retired) Snailscroft Farm, Waytown, Bridport DT6 5LF — MB BS Lond. 1975. Clin. Asst. (Rheum.) Bridport. Prev: GP Whitehaven & Egremont.

SKELLERN, Mr George Skellern and Partners, Bridport Medical Centre, North Allington, Bridport DT6 5DU Tel: 01308 421109 Fax: 01308 420869; Snailscroft Farm, Waytown, Bridport DT6 5LF Tel: 01308 488498 — MB BS Lond. 1974 (Roy. Free) MRCS Eng. LRCP Lond. 1974; FRCS Eng. 1979. Clin. Asst. (Gen. Surg. & Orthop.) Dorset.

SKELLETT, Sophie Clare Christina Little Heath House, Kent Hatch Road, Limpsfield Chart, Oxted RH8 0SZ — MB BChir Camb. 1990 (Camb. Univ. & Guy's Hosp.) MA Camb. 1990; MRCP (UK) 1995. Paediat. Regist. Guy's Hosp. Specialty: Paediat. Prev: Regist. (Paediat.) FarnBoro. Hosp.; SHO (Paediat.) Hammersmith & Qu. Charlottes Hosps.; SHO Rotat. (Paediat.) Guy's & Lewisham Hosps.

SKELLY, Cecil Michael Prebend Street Surgery, 15 Prebend Street, London N1 8PG Tel: 020 7226 9090 Fax: 020 7354 3330 — MB BCh BAO NUI 1970; MICGP.

SKELLY, Florence Joan (retired) 2 Thorny Road, Douglas IM2 5ED — MB ChB Leeds 1947. Prev: Assoc. Specialist Hortham Hosp. Almonsbury & Brentry Hosp. Bristol.

SKELLY, Robert Henry 58 Green Lane, Ockbrook, Derby DE72 3SE — MB BS Lond. 1989; MRCP (UK) 1993.

SKELLY, Roderick Thomas Dept of Surgery, Royal Victoria Hospital, Belfast BT12 6BJ — MB BCh BAO Belf. 1995; FRCSI Dublin 1999.

SKELLY, William John 18 Sussex Place, Slough SL1 1NS Tel: 01753 26478 — MB BCh BAO Belf. 1951 (Qu. Univ. Belf.) Socs: Brit. Med. Acupunc. Soc.

SKELTON, Carol Elizabeth Fife Rehabilitation Service, Cameron Hospital, Windygates, Leven KY8 5RR — MB BCh BAO Belf. 1985; DRCOG 1989; MRCGP 1990. Staff Grade (Rehabil. Med.) Fife Rehabil. Serv. Cameron Hosp. Windygates Fife. Specialty: Cardiol. Prev: Regist. (Rehabil. Med.) Astley Ainslie Hosp. Edin.

SKELTON, David Andrew Wingfield South Road Medical Centre, 40 South Road, Kingswood, Bristol Tel: 0117 967 5135; High Croft, Bury Hill, Winterbourne Down, Bristol BS36 1AD — MRCS Eng. LRCP Lond. 1964; DObst RCOG 1967.

SKELTON, Janina Beth Chestnut Lodge, Chestnut Grove, Nottingham NG3 5AD — MB ChB Birm. 1991; ChB Birm. 1991.

SKELTON, Marie Lilian 178 Charlton Road, London SE7 7DW — MB ChB Bristol 1941.

SKELTON, Martin Oliver (retired) 178 Charlton Road, London SE7 7DW Tel: 020 8856 1170 — MB ChB Bristol 1941; FRCPath 1963. Prev: Pathol. Gp. Laborat. Lewisham.

SKELTON, Philip Edmund The Maltings Surgery, 8-10 Victoria Street, St Albans AL1 3JB Tel: 01727 853296 Fax: 01727 862498 — MB BS Lond. 1976 (St. Geo.) Prev: Trainee GP Luton & Dunstable VTS; Ho. Phys. St. Albans City Hosp.; Ho. Surg. Luton & Dunstable Hosp.

SKELTON, Ruth Elizabeth Leeds General Infirmary, Belmont House, Belmont Grove, Leeds LS9 2NS Tel: 0113 3926106 Email: Ruth.SKELTON@Leedsth.nhs.uk — BM BS Nottm. 1985; RCPCH; DRCOG 1987; MRCP (UK) 1989. Cons. Paediat. Leeds Gen. Infirm. Specialty: Child Protection. Socs: Roy. Coll. Paediat. & Child Health. Prev: Neonat. Hull Roy. Infirm.; Lect. (Paediat.) Leeds Univ. & Leeds Gen. Infirm.; Fell. (Neonat..) King Geo. V Hosp. Sydney.

SKELTON, Vanessa Ann — MB BS Lond. 1991 (Guy's Hospital) FRCA 1996. Cons. Anaesthetics, King's Coll. Hosp. Lond. Specialty: Anaesth.

SKENE, Mr Anthony Iain Royal Bournemouth Hospital, Castle Lane East, Bournemouth BH7 7DW Tel: 01202 704070 Fax: 01202 704069 — BM Soton. 1981 (Univ. Soton. Med. Sch.) FRCS Ed. 1986; MS Soton. 1990. Cons. Surg. Roy. Bournemouth Hosp. Specialty: Gen. Surg. Socs: Brit. Assn. Surgs. Oncol.; Brit. Assn. Endocrine Surgs.; Assn. Surg. Prev: Sen. Regist. & Regist. (Surg.) Chelsea Westm. Hosp. Lond.; Regist. (Surg.) Roy. Marsden Hosp. Lond.; SHO Rotat. (Surg.) Basingstoke Dist. Hosp.

SKENE, Christopher Graham (2F2) 6 Roseneath Terrace, Edinburgh EH9 1JN — MB ChB Ed. 1997.

SKENE, John Robert, QHS, OStJ, TD (retired) Russets, Honiton Road, Staplehay, Taunton TA3 7HT Tel: 01823 251275 — MB ChB Aberd. 1962; DObst RCOG 1964. Prev: Col. Late RAMC (TA).

SKENSVED, Henrik 61 Chalcot Road, London NW1 8LY — MD Aarhus 1983; T(OG) 1994.

SKEOCH, Charles Hugh 21 Burnside Road, Rutherglen, Glasgow G73 4RW — MB ChB Manch. 1978.

SKEOCH, Helen Mary Craigallian Avenue Surgery, 11 Craigallian Avenue, Cambuslang, Glasgow G72 8RW Tel: 0141 641 3129 — MB ChB Manch. 1978.

SKEOCH, Jill Elizabeth Cill Chuimein Medical Practice, Fort Augustus PH32 4BN Tel: 01320 366216 Fax: 01320 366649 —

BM Soton. 1982; DRCOG 1987; MRCGP 1987. Specialty: Gen. Pract.

SKERRETT, Francis David (retired) The Surgery, Rawlings Lane, Fowey PL23 1DT Tel: 01726 832464 — MB ChB Bristol 1958; DObst RCOG 1960. Prev: Ho. Off. (Paediat.) Southmead Hosp. Bristol.

SKERRITT, Mrs Ethel (retired) 24 Clarendon Court, Carr Bank Lane, Sheffield S11 7FN — MRCS Eng. LRCP Lond. 1918 (Sheff.) MD Sheff. 1933, MB ChB 1918; DPH Manch. 1924. Prev: Cas. Off. & Ho. Surg. Sheff. Roy. Hosp.

SKERROW, Beverley Anne The Health Centre, Coronation Road, Peterculter AB14 0RQ Tel: 01224 733535; 17 The Meadows, Milltimber AB13 0JT — MB BS Lond. 1980 (St. Geo.) MB BS (Hons. Path.) Lond. 1980; DCH RCP Lond. 1983; DRCOG 1984; MRCGP 1986. Prev: Princip & Trainer (Gen. Pract.) Epsom.

SKERRY, Caroline Anne Leedham Ward, Pembury Hospital, Pembury, Tunbridge Wells TN2 4QJ Tel: 01892 823535 — MB BS Lond. 1982; DRCOG 1985; Cert. Family Plann. JCC 1986. Staff Grade (Psychiat.) Pembury Hosp. Tunbridge Wells. Specialty: Geriat. Psychiat. Prev: Trainee GP Tunbridge Wells HA VTS; SHO (Psychiat.) Hellingly Hosp. Eastbourne; SHO (A & E) Qu. Eliz. Hosp. King's Lynn.

SKEW, Barbara Lesley Southmead Hospital, Fertility Clinic, Monks Park Avenue, Westbury on Trym, Bristol BS10 5NB Tel: 0117 959 5102; 22A Somerset Street, Kingsdown, Bristol BS2 8LZ Tel: 0117 924 7152 — MB BS Lond. 1970 (Westm.) MRCS Eng. LRCP Lond. 1970; DObst RCOG 1974. Staff Grade (Gyn.) Southmead Hosp. Bristol; Med. Dir. Tower Ho. Clinic Bristol; HFEA Licensed Fertil. Clinic. Socs: BMA; Brit. Fertil. Soc.; Brit. Soc. Colpos. & Cerv. Path. Prev: Clin. Asst. (Gyn.) Roy. United Hosp. Bath & Southmead Hosp. Bristol; SHO (O & G) St. Martins Hosp. Bath; SHO (Radiother.) Westm. Hosp. Lond.

SKEW, Peter Graeme — MB BS Lond. 1976 (Westm.) Dip MS Med Soc. Apoth. Lond.; MRCS Eng. LRCP Lond. 1976. Special Interest: Musculoskeletal Med. Socs: (Pres.) Brit. Inst. Musculoskeletal Med.; (Exec. Off.) BackCare.; FRSM. Prev: Indep. GP Northwood & Specialist (Musculoskeletal Med.); Specialist (Musculoskeletal Med.) N. Middlx. Hosp.; Princip. GP Harrow Health Care Centre.

SKEWES, David Garland Royal Marsden Hospital, Fulham Road, London SW3 6JJ Tel: 020 7352 8171; 90 Grange Road, Ealing, London W5 3PJ Tel: 020 8579 7477 Fax: 020 8840 9560 — MB BS Melbourne 1971 (Melb.) FFA RCS Eng. 1977. Cons. Anaesth. Roy. Marsden Hosp. Lond. Specialty: Anaesth. Socs: Assn. Anaesth. & Intens. Care Soc. Prev: Sen. Regist. Roy. Marsden Hosp. Lond. & Hammersmith Hosp. Lond.; Lect. Lond. Hosp.

SKIA, Barbara 42 Cissbury Ring N., London N12 7AH Tel: 020 8445 4827 — Ptychio Iatrikes Thesslonika 1988; FRCS 1994; MSc Lond. 1996. Specialty: Otolaryngol.

SKIDMORE, David James 53 Slayleigh Lane, Sheffield S10 3RG — MB ChB Sheff. 1969; DObst RCOG 1971; DMRD Eng. 1974; FRCR 1977.

SKIDMORE, Mr Frederic David, OBE London Bridge Hospital, 27 Tooley Street, London SE1 2PR — MB BChir Camb. 1964 (Camb. & Birm.) MD Camb. 1974, MA 1965; FRCS Ed. 1968; FRCS Eng. 1971. Hon. Sen. Lect. Roy. Free Univ. Coll. Med. Sch.; Cons. Surg. (Oncol.) Lond. Bridge Hosp. Lond. Specialty: Gen. Surg. Socs: Fell. Roy. Soc. Med.; Brit. Assn. Surg. Oncol.; Assn. of Surg.s of Gt. Britain & Irel. Prev: Brit. Heart Foundat. Research Fell. Camb. UK and Baltimore USA; Registar Cariothoracic Surgey Harefield Hosp.; Registar Cariothoracic Surgey Papworth Hosp.

SKIDMORE, James Richard The Surgery, Limes Avenue, Alfreton DE55 7DW Tel: 01773 832525 — MB BS Newc. 1977; MRCGP 1981; DRCOG 1981.

SKIDMORE, Jennifer Ruth Centre for Learning Anatomical Sciences, University of Southampton, Biomedical Sciences Building, Bassett CrescentE., Southampton SO16 7PX — MB ChB Leic. 1980; PhD Soton. 1996. Sen. Lect. (Anatomical Sciences) & Admissions Tutor School of Medicine, Soton. Univ.

SKIDMORE, Richard Bryan Duncan Health Centre, Hunter St., Briton Ferry, Neath SA11 2SF Tel: 01639 812270 — MB BS Lond. 1959 (St. Mary's) MRCS Eng. LRCP Lond. 1959. Prev: Ho. Phys. & Ho. Surg. Morriston Hosp. Swansea; Ho. Off. (O & G) Neath Hosp.

SKILBECK, Anthony Bernard Kingswinford Medical Practice, Standhills Road, Kingswinford DY6 8DN Tel: 01384 271241 Fax: 01384 297530 — MB ChB Birm. 1974; Dip. Occ. Med. RCP Lond. 1997. Sen. Partner in a Gen. Pract. in Kingswinford W. Midl. Specialty: Occupat. Health.

SKILBECK, Bethel 4A Pippins Close, Deeside CH5 1PE Tel: 01244 831079 — MB ChB Liverp. 1992; DRCOG 1995; T(GP) 1996. Specialty: Gen. Pract. Socs: Assoc. Mem. RCGP; BMA. Prev: Trainee GP Sutton Med. Centre S. Wirral; Trainee GP/SHO N. Staffs. Hosp. Centre VTS; Ho. Off. (Med.) Wirral Hosp. NHS Trust.

SKILLERN, Laurence Howard Department Obstetrics & Gynaecology, St. George's Hospital Medical School, London SW17 0RE Tel: 020 8672 1255; 20B Ravenswood Road, Balham, London SW12 9PS Tel: 020 8675 4509 — MB BS Lond. 1986; BSc Lond. 1983, MB BS 1986; DRCOG 1989. Research Fell. (O & G) St. Geo. Hosp. Med. Sch. Lond.

SKILLMAN, Joanna Margaret 21 St Stephen's Road, Cheltenham GL51 3AB Email: joskillman@hotmail.com; 20A Bridge Street, Pinner HA5 3EH Tel: 020 8426 1175 — BM BCh Oxf. 1996 (Cambridge and Oxford) BA (Hons) Cantab. SHO (Plastic Surg.). Prev: Regist. (Surg.) St. Vincent's Hosp. Sydney; SHO Dryburn Hosp. Durh.; SHO John Radcliffe Hosp. Oxf.

SKILTON, Guy Henry Stewart Weeping Cross Health Centre, Bodmin Avenue, Weeping Cross, Stafford ST17 0HF Tel: 01785 665125 Fax: 01785 661064 — MB BS Lond. 1988; T(GP) 1992.

SKILTON, Juliet Ann The Surgery, Hazeldene House, Great Haywood, Stafford ST18 0SU Tel: 01889 881206 Fax: 01889 883083 — MB BS Lond. 1963. GP Gt. Haywood Surg. Mid Staffs HA.

SKILTON, Roger William Howard 28 Hewitt Street, Hoole, Chester CH2 3JD — MB BS Lond. 1983; MRCP (UK) 1987; Cert. Family Plann. JCC 1990; FRCA 1994. Sen. Regist. (Anaesth.) Frenchay Hosp. Bristol; Vis. Instruct. Univ. Michigan Med. Centre. Specialty: Anaesth.

SKIMING, Judith Anne — BM BCh Oxf. 1998; MA Cantab. 1999. Specialist Regist. (Paediat.).

SKINGLE, Ian Stewart The Surgery, Kingsmount, 444 Kingstanding Road, Kingstanding, Birmingham B44 9SA Tel: 0121 373 1734 — MB ChB Birm. 1981; DCH RCP Lond. 1986.

SKINNER, Adam John Winterton Surgery, Russell House, Westerham TN16 1RB Tel: 01959 564949 — MB BS Lond. 1980; DRCOG 1983.

SKINNER, Adam Victor 2nd Floor Flat, 17 Caledonia Place, Clifton, Bristol BS8 4DJ Tel: 01179 730967 — MB ChB Bristol 1994; BSc (Hons.) Bristol 1991; MRCP (UK) 1998. SHO (anaesth.) Cheltenham Gen. Hosp. Specialty: Anaesth. Prev: SHO Phys. (Med.) MusGr. Pk. Hosp. Taunton; SHO (A & E) Bristol Roy. Infirm.; Ho. Phys. (Med.) Roy. United Hosp. Bath.

SKINNER, Alyson Margaret Mary Department of Paediatrics, City Hospital NHS Trust, Winson Green, Birmingham B18 8QH — MB BCh BAO NUI 1981 (Univ. Coll. Dub.) MRCP (UK) 1985; DCH RCP Lond. 1987; M.D. (NUI) 1994. Cons. Paediat. City Hosp. NHS Trust Birm. Specialty: Paediat. Socs: Fell. Roy. Coll. Paediat. & Child. Health; Brit. Soc. Prenatal Med. Prev: Clin. Fell. B.C. Childs. Hosp. Vancouver, Canada; Sen. Regist. (Paediat.) Univ. Hosp. Wales Cardiff.

SKINNER, Andrew Charles Summerfield, Windmill Lane, Preston on the Hill, Warrington WA4 4AZ Tel: 0151 430 1267 Fax: 0151 430 1155 Email: skinner_doc@compuserve.com — BM BS Nottm. 1978 (Nottingham) BMedSci (Hons.) Nottm. 1976; FFA RCS Eng. 1983. Cons. Anaesth. St. Helens & Knowsley Hosps. Trust; Dir. of Educat. & Train., St Helens & Knowsley Hosps. Trust. Specialty: Anaesth. Prev: Sen. Regist. (Anaesth.) Mersey RHA; Regist. (Anaesth.) Nottm. Hosps.; SHO (Anaesth.) Gen. Hosp. Nottm.

SKINNER, Benjamin Charles 1 Pinefield Glade, Livingston EH54 9JX — MB ChB Dund. 1998; MBChB (Hons.); MRCP; MB ChB Dund 1998.

SKINNER, Celia Jean Ambrose King Centre, Royal London Hospital, Whitechapel Road, London E1 1BB Tel: 020 7377 7308 Fax: 020 7377 7648 — MB ChB Birm. 1987; FRCP; MRCP (UK) 1991. Cons. Phys. Genitourin. Med. & HIV Roy. Lond. Hosp. Specialty: Genitourinary Medicine. Prev: Sen. Regist. (GUM/HIV) Roy. Lond.

SKINNER, Charles Peter Robin Rock Cottage, Mill Lane, Furners Green, Uckfield TN22 3RN — MB ChB Bristol 1998.

SKINNER, Clare Maria — MB BS Lond. 1993 (St. Bart's Lond.) FRCA Part I 1996; FRCA Part II 1998; FRCA Part III 2000. Specialist Regist. (Anaesth.) Oxf.

SKINNER, Craig 305 Blossomfield Road, Solihull B91 1TE — MB ChB (Hons.) Aberd. 1965; MRCP (UK) 1970; FRCP Lond. 1983. Chairm., Heartlands Educat. Centre Ltd; Regional Respirat. Adviser, Atos Origin IT Servs. Internat. Specialty: Gen. Med.; Respirat. Med. Special Interest: Med. Managem., Quality Assur., Tuberc. Socs: Brit. Thorac. Soc. (Chairm. Jt. TB Comm.); Pres. Midl. Thoracic Soc. Prev: Cons. Phys.& Med. Dir. Birm. Heartlands & Solihull NHS Trust; Sen. Clin. Lect. Med. Univ. Birm.

SKINNER, Mr David Victor Northcott, Chiltern Road, Chesham Bois, Amersham HP6 5PH Tel: 01494 431652 — MB BS Lond. 1975 (Roy. Free) MRCS Eng. LRCP Lond. 1974; FRCS Ed. 1981; FRCS Eng. 1990; FRCS Glas. 1993. Clin. Dir. (A & E) John Radcliffe Hosp. Oxf. Specialty: Accid. & Emerg. Socs: Brit. Assn. Accid. & Emerg. Med. Prev: Cons. A & E St. Bart. & Homerton Hosps. Lond.; Lect. (Anat.) Kings Coll. Hosp. Lond.; Regist. (A & E) Northwick Pk. Hosp. Harrow.

SKINNER, Mr Derek William Department of Otolaryngology, Royal Shrewsbury Hospital NHS Trust, Mytton Oak Road, Shrewsbury SY3 8XQ Tel: 01743 261000; Albany House, Butler Road, Shrewsbury SY3 7AJ Tel: 01743 243501 Fax: 01743 356212 Email: dwskinner@mac.com — MB ChB Dundee 1978; FRCS (Gen. Surg.) Ed. 1983; FRCS (Orl.) Eng. 1985; Hon. FCSHK 1995. Cons. Otolaryngol. Eye, Ear & Throat Hosp. Shrewsbury.; Post Grad. Clin. Tutor, Roayl Shrewsbury Hosp. Shrewsbury; Progr. Director, W. Midl.s HST OtorhinoLaryngol. W. Midl.s. Specialty: Otorhinolaryngol. Prev: Regist. (ENT) Univ. Hosp. Wales Cardiff; Sen. Regist. (ENT) Nottm. & Leicester Hosps.; Vis. Lect. Chinese Univ., Hong Kong.

SKINNER, Evelyn George (retired) 2A Coniston Road, Basingstoke RG22 5HS Tel: 01256 323199 — MB BS Lond. 1962 (Middlx.) MA Camb. 1952; MRCS Eng. LRCP Lond. 1962. Prev: SHO Soton. Childr. Hosp.

SKINNER, Fiona Margaret Leith Mount, 46 Ferry Road, Edinburgh EH6 4AE Tel: 0131 554 0558 Fax: 0131 555 6911 — MB ChB Ed. 1971 (Edinburgh University) MRCGP 1975; DCH RCPS Glas. 1975. Managem. Gp. Mem. N-E Edin. LHCC. Prev: Clin. Med. Off. (Community Paediat.) Lothian HB; Trainee GP (N..) VTS.

SKINNER, Geoffrey Besley (retired) 57 Portland Avenue, New Malden KT3 6BB Tel: 020 8942 0157 — MB BS Lond. 1952 (Guy's) MRCS Eng. LRCP Lond. 1952; DPath Eng. 1960; FRCPath 1975, M 1964. Prev: Cons. Path. St. Helier Gp. Laborat.

SKINNER, Gordon Robert Bruce Harborough Banks, Old Warwick Road, Lapworth, Solihull B94 6LD — MB ChB Glas. 1965; FRCOG 1984, M 1972; DSc Birm. 1989, MD (1st cl. Hons.) 1975; FRCPath 1989, M 1988. Director & CEO Vaccine Internat. PLC; Chairm. Vaccine Research Trust 1983; Private Practitioner, Specialist interests in Endocrinol. and Sexually Transm. Dis.; Director HIV-Vac Inc. Specialty: Genitourinary Medicine. Socs: Soc. Gen. Microbiol.; Birm. and Midl.; Obst.al Soc. Prev: Dir. Vaccine Research Foundat. Ltd.; Med. Research Internat. Ltd.; Private Pract. Vaccine Research Scientist Birm.Vaccine Research Inst.

SKINNER, Howard David 18 Wentworth Drive, Stretton, Burton-on-Trent DE13 0YJ Tel: 01282 544523 — MB BS Lond. 1991 (Univ. Coll. Lond.) BSc (Psych.) Lond. 1988; DRCOG 1995; DFFP 1996; MRCGP 1996. Trainee GP/SHO (Paediat.) Burton Dist. Hosp. VTS; GP. Specialty: Cardiol. Prev: SHO P'boro. Dist. Hosp.

SKINNER, James Allan Tain and Fearn Area Medical Practice, Health Centre, Scotsburn Road, Tain IV19 1PR Tel: 01862 892759 Fax: 01862 892579 — MB ChB Aberd. 1969.

SKINNER, Jane Garforth Medical Centre, Church Lane, Garforth, Leeds LS25 1ER — MB BS Lond. 1959 (King's Coll. Hosp.) MRCS Eng. LRCP Lond. 1959. Prev: Ho. Phys. King's Coll. Hosp.

SKINNER, Jane Sarah Ward 49 Office, Royal Victoria Infirmary, Queen Victoria Road, Newcastle upon Tyne NE1 4LP Tel: 0191 232 5131 Fax: 0191 261 8505 — MB BS Newc. 1985 (Newcastle upon Tyne) BSc (Hons.) Lancaster 1980; MB BS (Hons.) Newc. 1985; DRCOG 1988; MRCP (UK) 1990; MD 1997. Cons. Community Cardiol. Roy. Vict. Infirm. Newc. Specialty: Cardiol. Socs: BMA; Brit. Cardial Soc. Prev: Cons. Phys. (Cardiol.) Bishop Auckland Gen. Hosp.

SKINNER, Jennifer Mary Murdishaw Health Centre, Gorsewood Road, Murdishaw, Runcorn WA7 6ES Tel: 01928712061; Summerfield, Windmill Lane, Preston on the Hill, Warrington WA4 4AZ Tel: 01928 716883 — BM BS Nottm. 1978; BMedSci (Hons.) Nottm. 1976, BM BS 1978; MRCGP 1982. Prev: Clin. Med. Off. Penketh Warrington; Clin. Med. Off. Selby N. Yorks. & Heanor Derbysh.

SKINNER, Mr John Andrew McInnes Thrombosis Research Instutute & Department of Orthopaedic Su, King's College Hospital, Denmark, London SE5 9PJ Tel: 020 7326 3015; Waterloo Lane, Trowell, Nottingham NG9 3QQ — MB BS Lond. 1988; FRCS Eng. 1992. Research Fell. & Hon. Regist. (Orthop.) King's Coll. Hosp. Lond. Specialty: Orthop.

SKINNER, John Bernard Department of Anaesthetics, The Ipswich Hospital NHS Trust, Heath Road, Ipswich IP4 5PD Tel: 01473 703435 — MB BS Lond. 1971 (St. Marys) FRCA 1977. Cons. Anaesth. & Pain Managem. Ipswich Hosp. NHS Trust. Specialty: Anaesth.

SKINNER, John Malcolm Orwell House, 22 Station St., Swaffham PE37 7LH Tel: 01760 723978 Fax: 01760 723703 Email: malcolm.skinner@nhs.net — (St. Bart.) MB BS St. Bart. Lond. 1969. PEC Chair W. Norf. PCT; Hon. Med. Adviser Swaffham & Watton Br. Far E. Prisoner of War Assn; Police Surg. Norf. Constab. Specialty: Orthop. Socs: Mem. Norf. LMC. Prev: Commitee Mem. Swaffham and Litcham Home Hospice; Director Olive Tree Projects (Domestic Violence); Hosp. Pract. (Orthop. Surg.) N. Cambs. Hosp. Wisbech & Qu. Eliz. Hosp. Kings Lynn.

SKINNER, Joyce Isobel (retired) 18G John Spencer Square, London N1 2LZ — MRCS Eng. LRCP Lond. 1959 (Ed.) MA Ed. 1945; MRCPath 1970.

SKINNER, Laura Jane 3 Allenstyle Drive, Yelland, Barnstaple EX31 3DY — MB ChB Bristol 1996. GP VTS Bath. Specialty: Gen. Pract. Prev: SHO (Med.) Trafford Gen. Hosp.; SHO (Paediat.) Roy. United Hosp. Bath; SHO (A & E) Weston Super Mare.

SKINNER, Lesley Phyllis Howden Health Centre, Howden West, Livingston EH54 6TP Tel: 01506 423800 Fax: 01506 460757; 6 Murrayfield Drive, Edinburgh EH12 6EB Tel: 0131 337 5185 — MB ChB Ed. 1985; DRCOG 1989; MRCGP 1990; DCCH RCP Ed. 1991; FRCGP 1999. Assoc. Adviser, SCPMDE, SE Scotl. Socs: Fell. RCGP. Prev: Trainee GP W. Lothian VTS; Ho. Off. (Gen. Med.) Bangour Gen. Hosp. W. Lothian; Ho. Off. (Gen. Surg.) Freeman Hosp. Newc.

SKINNER, Michael David 41A Sneyd Avenue, Newcastle ST5 2PZ — MB ChB Sheff. 1969; DMRD Eng. 1976; FRCR 1977. Cons. Radiol. N. Staffs. Roy. Infirm. Specialty: Radiol.

SKINNER, Michael Patrick 7 Edward Road, Clarendon Park, Leicester LE2 1TF — MB BS Lond. 1994.

SKINNER, Mr Paul Patrick 695 Manchester Road, Sheffield S10 5PS — MB ChB Sheff. 1988; FRCS Eng. 1992. Career Regist. Rotat. (Surg.) N. Trent. Specialty: Gen. Surg.

SKINNER, Mr Paul William Orthopaedic Department, Kent & Sussex Hospital, Mount Ephraim, Tunbridge Wells TN4 8AT — MB BS Lond. 1977 (Middlx.) FRCS Eng. 1981. Cons. Orthop. Surg. Kent & Sussex Hosp. Tunbridge Wells; lead Clinician Orthop., Maidstone and Tunbridge Wells NHS Trust. Specialty: Orthop. Socs: Fell. BOA; Fell. Roy. Soc. Med.; Brit. Elbow and Shoulder Surgeons Soc. Prev: Sen. Regist. (Orthop.) King's Coll. Hosp. Lond.

SKINNER, Peter John Newport Pagnell Medical Centre, Queens Avenue, Newport Pagnell MK16 8QT Tel: 01908 611767 Fax: 01908 615099 — MB BS Lond. 1972 (Guy's) MRCS Eng. LRCP Lond. 1972.

SKINNER, Peter Victor (retired) Ramhurst Oast, Powder Mill Lane, Leigh, Tonbridge TN11 9AS Tel: 01732 832244 — (Guy's) MA Oxf. 1953, BM BCh 1951; DObst RCOG 1955. Prev: Resid. Obst. Roy. Hants. Co. Hosp. Winchester.

SKINNER, Phillip James St James Medical Centre, St James Street, Taunton TA1 1JP Tel: 01823 285400 Fax: 01823 285405 — MB Camb. 1977; BChir 1976; MRCGP 1983; MSc Univ. of Lond. 2001. GP Princip. Specialty: Gen. Med.

SKINNER, Richard Osmond, Capt. RAMC (retired) Minton House, Staplehurst, Tonbridge TN12 0AS Tel: 01580 893358 — (The Lond. Hosp.) MB BS Lond. 1958; DObst RCOG 1960; Da RCP LmdeRCSEng 1971; MA Open University 2000. Prev: Ho. Phys. Roy. Vict. Hosp. Folkestone.

SKINNER, Roderick Sir James Spence Institute of Child Health, Royal Victoria Infirmary, Queen Victoria Road, Newcastle upon Tyne NE1 4LP Tel: 0191 202 3025 Fax: 0191 202 3060 Email: roderick.skinner@ncl.ac.uk — MB ChB (Hons.) Birm. 1983 1983 (Birm.) BSc (Hons.) Birm. 1980; MRCP (UK) 1986; DCH RCP Lond. 1987; PhD Newc. 1995; FRCPCH 1997. Specialty: Paediat. Special Interest: Childh. aplastic anaemia; Childh. leukaemia; Late effects of Treatm. for Childh. cancer. Socs: UK Childr. Cancer Study Gp.; Eur. Gp. Blood & Marrow Transpl.; Brit. Soc. of Haemat. Prev: MRC Train. Fell. (Child Health) Newc. u. Tyne Med. Sch.; Ho. Phys. Qu. Eliz. Hosp. Birm.

SKINNER, Roger Keith Alwyn Morgan Food Standards Agency, 125 Kingsway, London WC2B 6NH Tel: 020 7276 8984 Fax: 020 7276 8910 Email: roger.skinner@foodstandards.gsi.gov.uk; 66 Dartmouth Park Road, London NW5 1SN Tel: 020 7267 4791 — MB BS Lond. 1969; MRCS Eng. LRCP Lond. 1969; FRCPath 1991, M 1980; MSc (Epidemiol.) Lond. 1988, MSc Biochem, Lond. 1973, MD 1980. Head of MicroBiol. Safety Div. (Princip. Med. Off.) Food Standards Agency Lond. Specialty: Civil Serv. Socs: Fell. Roy. Soc. Med. Prev: Sen. Med. Off. DHSS Richmond Hse. Lond.; Lect. (Chem. Path.) Roy. Free Hosp. Sch. Med. Lond.; Sen. Regist. (Chem. Path.) St. Geo. Hosp. Lond.

SKINNER, Rory Robert 69 Ifield Road, London SW10 9AU — MB BS Lond. 1987.

SKINNER, Rosalind Scottish Executive Health Department, St Andrews House, Regent Road, Edinburgh EH1 3DE Tel: 0131 244 2296 Fax: 0131 244 2683 Email: rosalind.skinner@scotland.gov.uk; 19 Comely Bank, Edinburgh EH4 1AL Tel: 0131 332 8435 — MB BS Lond. 1969 (Lond. Hosp.) MD Lond. 1975; Cert. Family Plann. JCC 1976; MSc Ed. 1986; MFPHM 1988; FRCP Ed. 1995; FFPHM 1998. Princip. Med. Off. Scot. Exec. Health Dept. Specialty: Genetics; Pub. Health Med. Socs: Clin. Genetics Soc. Prev: Lect. (Human Genetics) Univ. Edin.; Sen. Regist. (Community Med.) Lothian HB; Resid. Clin. Pathol. St. Mary's Hosp. Lond.

SKINNER, Terence Alan, Wing Cdr. RAF Med. Br. Department of Anaesthetics, The Royal Hospital, Haslar, Gosport PO12 2AA Tel: 023 9258 4255 Fax: 023 9276 2555 Email: anaesthetics@haslib.demon.co.uk; 35 Barton Drive, Bradley Barton, Newton Abbot TQ12 1PD — MB BS Lond. 1982; DA (UK) 1986; FRCA 1990. Cons. Anaesth. RAF; Dir. Pain Servs. Specialty: Anaesth. Prev: Sen. Regist. Frenchay Hosp. Bristol.

SKINNER, Terence Gordon (retired) 124 Thurlow Park Road, West Dulwich, London SE21 8HP Tel: 020 8670 3538; Copperfield, 8 Dickens Wood Close, London SE19 3LA Tel: 020 8679 4188 — MB BS Lond. 1954 (St. Mary's) DObst RCOG 1957. GP (Private Pract.). Prev: SHO (Surg.) WillesBoro. Hosp. Kent.

SKIPP, David Gordon Park Surgery, Albion Way, Horsham RH12 1BG Tel: 01403 01403 217100 Fax: 01403 214639 — MB BS Lond. 1974 (Char. Cross) MRCS Eng. LRCP Lond. 1974; DRCOG 1976; Cert. JCC Lond. 1977; MRCGP 1979. Dep. Coroner W. Sussex. Prev: Trainee GP Mid-Sussex VTS; Ho. Phys. & Ho. Surg. Char. Cross Hosp. Lond.; Trainer SW Thames Region.

SKIPP, Helen Joyce Beech Community Clinic, Horsham Hospital, Hurst Road, Horsham RH12 2DR Tel: 01403 227012; 48 Grebe Crescent, Horsham RH13 6ED Tel: 01403 253306 — MB BS Lond. 1974 (Char. Cross) MRCS Eng. LRCP Lond. 1974; Cert JCC Lond. 1977; MFFP 1996. SCMO Horsham & Crawley Family Plann.; CMO Haywards Heath Family Plann. Specialty: Family Plann. & Reproduc. Health. Prev: Ho. Phys. & Ho. Surg. Char. Cross Hosp. Lond.

SKIPPER, Colin Doctor's Corner, Aldborough, Norwich NR11 7NR Tel: 01263 761512 — MB ChB Leeds 1957. Prev: Clin. Asst. Southlands Hosp. Shoreham by Sea & Littlehampton Hosp.; Ho. Phys. (Paediat.) St. Jas. Hosp. Leeds; Ho. Surg. (Obst.) Manygates Matern. Hosp. Wakefield.

SKIPPER, Mr David Bedford Hospitals NHS Trust, Kempston Road, Bedford MK42 9DJ Tel: 01234 792319 Fax: 01234 795840 — MB BS Lond. 1978; MA Camb. 1979; FRCS Eng. 1984; MS Soton. 1989. Cons. Surg. Bedford Hosp. Trust. Specialty: Gen. Surg.

SKIPPER, Mr John Joseph, Group Capt. RAF Med. Br. ENT Department, The Royal Hospital, Haslar, Gosport PO12 2AA Tel: 023 9258 4255 Ext: 2180/023 9276 2506 — MB BCh Wales 1979; FRCS Ed. 1985; T(S) 1991. Cons. Adviser OtoLaryngol. Defence Med. Servs.; Cons. Otolaryngologist Roy. Hosp. Haslar Gosport.; Cons. Otalaryngologist, Portsmouth NHS Trust. Specialty: Otorhinolaryngol. Socs: Fell. Roy. Soc. Med.; BMA; Brit. Assn. Otol. Prev: Cons. Otolaryngologist RAF Halton; Cons. Otolaryngologist RAF Akrotiri; Hon. Sen. Regist. (Ear, Nose & Throat) Leicester Roy. Infirm.

SKIPSEY, Ian Gerald Department Anaesthetics, Raigmore Hospital, Inverness Tel: 01463 704000 Fax: 01463 711322; 69 Drumsmittal Road, North Kessock, Inverness IV1 3JU Tel: 01463 731734 — MB ChB Manch. 1984; FRCA 1989. Cons. Anaesth. Raigmore Hosp. Inverness. Specialty: Anaesth.

SKIRROW, Martin Bingham Gloucestershire Royal Hospital , Microbiology Department, Gloucester GL1 3NN Tel: 01452 305334; Western Lodge, Hanley Swan, Worcester WR8 0DL Tel: 01684 310343 Email: martin.skirrow@camdenmusic.com — MB ChB Birm. 1952; DTM & H Liverp. 1962; PhD Liverp. 1963; FRCPath 1979, M 1967. p/t Hon. Emerit. Cons. Microbiol. Helath Protec. Agency Glos. Roy. Hosp. Specialty: Med. Microbiol. Special Interest: Campylobacter Infec. Socs: Brit. Infec. Soc. Prev: Cons. Med. Microbiol. Worcester Roy. Infirm.; Sen. Regist. (Path.) Childr. Hosp. Birm.; Lect. (Trop. Med.) Univ. Ibadan, Nigeria.

SKITT, Robin Charles Greenmeadow Surgery, Greenmeadow Way, Cwmbran NP44 3XQ Tel: 01633 864110 Fax: 01633 483761; Grasmoor, 6 Brechfa Close, Ponthir, Caerleon, Newport NP18 1GY — MB ChB Bristol 1977; DRCOG 1979. GP Cwmbran.

SKIVINGTON, Michael Anthony (retired) 34 Ravine Road, Boscombe, Bournemouth BH5 2DU Tel: 01202 432936 — (Char. Cross) MB BS Lond. 1961; FFA RCS Eng. 1966. Prev: Cons. Anaesth. Roy. Bournemouth & ChristCh. NHS Trust.

SKLAR, Eric Maurice, MBE Medical Centre, 144-150 High Road, London NW10 2PT Tel: 020 8459 5550 Fax: 020 8451 7268; 32 Sidmouth Road, London NW2 5HJ Tel: 020 8459 5550 Fax: 020 8451 7268 — MRCS Eng. LRCP Lond. 1949 (St. Geo.) FRCGP 1985, M 1953. Chairm. N. Thames (W.) GP Postgrad. Comm. Specialty: Dermat. Socs: Balint Soc. & BMA. Prev: Sen. Lect. (Gen. Pract.) Middlx. Hosp. Med. Sch. & Univ. Coll. Lond Sch. Med.; Capt. RAMC; Paediat. Hadassah Childr. Hosp. Israel.

SKLAR, Ian David The Surgery, 38 Cockington Road, Bilborough, Nottingham NG8 4BZ Tel: 0115 928 2231 Fax: 0115 928 4917 — MB BS Lond. 1981.

SKLAR, Jonathan 21 Church row, Hampstead, London NW3 6UP Tel: 020 7794 1085 Fax: 020 7433 1056 Email: jonathan@sklar.co.uk — MB BS Lond. 1974 (Roy. Free) MRCS Eng. LRCP Lond. 1973; MRCPsych 1977; TQAP Tavistock 1983. Train., Lond. Specialty: Psychother. Socs: Brit. Psychoanal. Soc.; Train. Analyst. Mem. Brit. Psychoanal. Soc. Prev: Cons. Psychother. Addenbrooke's & Fulbourn Hosps. Camb.; Sen. Regist. (Psychother.) Adult Dept. Tavistock Clinic Lond.; Vis. Prof. Arhus Univ. Psychiat. Hosp. Riskov, Denmark.

SKOGSTAD, Helga 52 Glasslyn Road, London N8 8RH — State Exam Med. Wurzburg 1979.

SKOGSTAD, Wilhelm Herbert The Cassel Hospital, 1 Ham Common, Richmond TW10 7JF Tel: 020 8237 2965 Fax: 020 8237 2996 Email: wilhelm.skogstad@ulmht.nhs.uk — State Exam Med Munich 1978; State Exam Psychother. & Psychoanal. 1986; State Exam Psych. 1991; Psychoanalyst 2001; MRCPsych 2001. Cons. Psychother. Cassel Hosp. Richmond; Private Pract. as Psychoanalyst 75 Cromwell Av Lond. N6 5BS. Specialty: Psychother.; Gen. Psychiat. Socs: Roy. Coll. of Psychiat.s; Brit. Psycho-Analyt. Soc. (Assn. Mem.). Prev: Psychiat. Ment. Hosp. Haar, Munich.

SKOLAR, Peter Justin Brunswick Medical Centre, 53 Brunswick Centre, London WC1N 1BP Tel: 020 7837 3811 Fax: 020 7833 8408; 7 Greenhalgh Walk, Hampstead Garden Suburb, London N2 0DJ Tel: 020 8455 1652 — MB Camb. 1969 (Camb. & Middlx.) BChir 1968. Chairm. Camden & Islington LMC. Specialty: Care of the Elderly. Socs: GMSC (NE Thames Region). Prev: Ho. Surg. Forest Gate Matern. Hosp.; Ho. Surg. St. Mary's Hosp. Plaistow; Ho. Phys. Middlx. Hosp.

SKOYLES, Julian Robert 5 Ennerdale Close, Leicester LE2 4TN Tel: 0116 271 2193 — MB BS Lond. 1984; BSc (Hons.) Lond. 1981, MB BS 1984; DA (UK) 1986; FCAnaesth. 1990. Sen. Regist. Leicester Roy. Infirm.; Research Fell. (Anaesth.) North. Gen. Hosp. Sheff. Specialty: Anaesth. Prev: Regist. (Anaesth.) Roy. Hallamsh. Hosp. Sheff.; SHO Intens. Care Unit Char. Cross Hosp. Lond.

SKRINE, Ruth Lister (retired) Castanea House, Sham Castle Lane, Bath BA2 6JN Tel: 01225 465440 Email: rskrine@compuserve.com

— MB ChB Bristol 1953; MRCGP 1979. Prev: Sen. Lect. (Family Plann. & Psychosexual Med.) Univ. Bristol.

SKRZYPIEC-ALLEN, Alan Irvin 53 Mersey Road, Sale M33 6LF Tel: 0161 973 8528 — MB ChB Manch. 1978; DRCOG 1986.

SKUCE, Angela Margaret South Lambeth Road Practice, 1 Selway House, 272 South Lambeth Road, London SW8 1UL Tel: 020 7622 1923 Fax: 020 7498 5530 — MB BCh BAO Dub. 1988; DCH RCPSI 1991; MRCGP 1992; MICGP 1992; DFFP 1994.

SKUES, Mark Alastair Threefield House, Mannings Lane, Hoole Bank, Chester CH2 4ET — BM BS Nottm. 1980; BMedSci (Hons.) Nottm. 1978, BM BS 1980; FFA RCS Eng. 1986. Rotat. Regist. (Anaesth.) Bristol Gp. Hosps. Specialty: Anaesth. Prev: Tutor/Specialist (Anaesth.) Waikato Hosp. Hamilton, New Zealand.

SKULL, Angela Jane 39 Albermarle, Parkside, London SW19 5NP Tel: 020 8785 9261 — MB BS Lond. 1991; FRCS 1996. Regist. (Gen. Surg.) SW Thames Rotat. Specialty: Gen. Surg. Prev: SHO (Ost. & Gyn.) St. Geo. Hosp. Lond.

SKULL, Mr Jonathan Douglas The Jessop Wing,Sheffield Teaching Hospitals NHS Trust , Centre for Reproductive Medicine and Fertility, Tree Root Walk, Sheffield S10 2SF Tel: 0114 226 8050 Fax: 0114 226 8052 Email: jonathan.skull@sth.nhs.uk; 9 Bristol Road, Sheffield S11 8RL Tel: 0114 266 2913 Email: jonathanskull@tiscali.co.uk — MB ChB Bristol 1988; MRCOG 1994. Cons. in Reprod. Med. Sheff. Teach. Hosp. NHS Trust. Specialty: Obst. & Gyn. Special Interest: Endometriosis; Infertil.; Minimal Access Surg. Socs: BMA; BFS. Prev: Clin. Lect. Dept. (O & G) Jessop Hosp. for Wom. Sheff.; Hon. Sen. Regist. & Research Regist. IVF Unit Hammersmith Hosp. Lond.; Specialist Regist. (O & G) Bassetlan Hosp. Worksop.

SKUSE, Professor David Henry Behavioural & Brain Sciences Unit, Institute of Child Health, University of London, 30 Guilford St., London WC1N 1EH Tel: 020 7831 0975 Fax: 020 7831 7050 Email: dskuse@ich.ucl.ac.uk; 53 The Avenue, Kew, Richmond TW9 2AL — MB ChB Manch. 1973; MRCP (UK) 1976; M 1978; FRCPsych 1991; FRCP Lond. 1993; MD 1995; FRCPCH 1997. Prof. Behavioural & Brain Scis. Inst. Child Health Lond.; Hon. Cons. Hosp. for Sick Childr. Gt. Ormond St. Lond. Specialty: Child & Adolesc. Psychiat. Special Interest: Autism Spectrum Disorders; Turner Syndrome; Velocardiofacial Syndrome. Socs: Brit. NeuroPsychiat. Assn., (Treas.); Assn. for Child Psychol. & Psychiat., (former Treas.). Prev: Sen. Lect. (Child Psychiat.) Inst. Child Health; Lect. (Child Psychiat.) Inst. Psychiat. Lond.; SHO Rotat. (Med.) United Oxf. Hosps.

SKYERS, Paul Andrew 21 Larkspur Gardens, Luton LU4 8SA — MD Yale, USA 1990.

SKYRME, Andrew David 116 Kidbrooke Park Road, Blackheath, London SE3 0DX — MB BS Lond. 1993.

SKYRME, Manon Llwyd 82 Heol Y Deri, Rhiwbina, Cardiff CF14 6HJ — MB BCh Wales 1993; DCH 1996; DObst 1997; MRCGP 1997. Specialty: Paediat.

SKYRME, Robert John 82 Heol Y Deri, Rhiwbina, Cardiff CF14 6HJ — MB BCh Wales 1993.

SKYRME-JONES, Rex Andrew Paul Guy's and St. Thomas NHS Trust, Lambeth Palace Rd, London Tel: 020 8928 9292 Fax: 020 8852 3709; 101 Quentin Road, London SE13 5DG Email: andrew@skyrmej.fsnet.co.uk — MB ChB Bristol 1989; BSc Bristol 1986; MRCP (UK) 1993. Specialist Regist., Cardiol. Specialty: Cardiol.; Gen. Med. Prev: Interven.al Fell., Monash Med. Centre Melbourne, Australia; Research Fell., Monash Med. Centre, Melbourne, Australia; Regist., John Radcliffe Hosp., Oxf.

SLACK, Andrew John Ham Meadow, Northway, Halse, Taunton TA4 3JL — MB BS Lond. 1998; MB BS Lond 1998.

SLACK, Carole Bernadette Therese 366 Rochdale Road, Middleton, Manchester M24 2GJ — MB ChB Manch. 1986; BSc (Hons.) Manch. 1983, MB ChB 1986; MSc Open 1992; MRCGP 1995; BsMDH 2000; Dip Med Acu 2000; Dip Phyt 2001. Specialty: Gen. Pract. Socs: Brit. Holistic Med. Assn.; Manch. Med. Soc.; MNIMH. Prev: Lect. (Gen. Pract.) Univ. Manch.; Regist. (Pub. Health Med.) N. Manch.

SLACK, Mr Christopher John 588 Bury Road, Bamford, Rochdale OL11 4AU Tel: 01706 32828 — MB ChB Manch. 1969; FRCS Eng. 1977.

SLACK, Graeme Barrie Friarwood Surgery, Carleton Glen, Pontefract WF8 1SU Tel: 01977 703235 Fax: 01977 600527 — MB ChB Leeds 1979. GP Pontefract, W. Yorks.

SLACK, Janet Elizabeth Lovemead Group Practice, Roundstone Surgery, Polebarn Circus, Trowbridge BA14 7EH Tel: 01225 752752 Fax: 01225 776388; The Old Farm House, Ashley Road, Bradford-on-Avon BA15 1RT Tel: 01225 867658 — MRCS Eng. LRCP Lond. 1984 (Middlx.) BA (Hons.) Lond. 1973; DRCOG 1991; MRCGP 1995. Socs: BMA. Prev: SHO John Radcliffe Hosp. Oxf.; SHO Stoke Mandeville Hosp. Aylesbury.; GP Princip. Edwd.s Partners Aylesbury.

SLACK, Lady Joan (retired) Hillside Cottage, Tower Hill, Stawell, Bridgwater TA7 9AJ Tel: 01278 722719 Fax: 01278 722719 — BM BCh Oxf. 1949 (St. Bart.) DM Oxf. 1972, BA; DCH Eng. 1952; MFCM 1974; FRCP Lond. 1979. Prev: Cons. Clin. Genetics St. Mark's Hosp. Lond.

SLACK, Malcolm Charles 35 Station Road, Felsted, Dunmow CM6 3HD — MB BS Lond. 1974.

SLACK, Margaret Mary (retired) Oaklynn, Keighley Road, Laneshaw Bridge, Colne BB8 7HL — MB ChB Aberd. 1963; DPM Leeds 1971; FRCPsych 1988, M 1972. Prev: Cons. Child & Adolesc. Psychiat. Burnley Health Dist.

SLACK, Mark Clifford Ermine House, Post St., Godmanchestr, Huntingdon PE29 2BA — MB BCh Witwatersrand 1980; MRCOG 1992.

SLACK, Martin Harry 4 Grosvenor Drive, Winchester SO23 7HF Tel: 01962 852597 — MB BChir Camb. 1994; MRCP (UK) 1996. Specialist Regist. (Paeds.) - St Mary's Hosp. - Portsmouth. Specialty: Paediat. Prev: SHO Rotat. (Paediat.) Soton. Hosps.; SHO (Paediat.) St. Mary's Hosp. Portsmouth; SHO (A & E) Roy. Hants. Co. Hosp. Winchester, Specialist Regist. (Paediat.) Roy. Hants Co. Hosp. Winchester.

SLACK, Mary Paulina Elizabeth Bacteriology Department, Level 6/7, John Radcliffe Hospital, Oxford OX3 9DU Tel: 01865 220859 Fax: 01865 220890; Hampden House, Clifton Hampden, Abingdon OX14 3EG — MB BChir Camb. 1973 (King's Coll. Hosp.) MB BChir Camb. (Distinc. Path.) 1973; MA (1st cl. Hons.) Camb. 1974; MA Oxf. 1976, BM BCh 1977; FRCPath 1991, M 1979. Univ. Lect. (Bacteriol.) Oxf. Univ.; Dir. PHLS Haemophilus Refer. Unit John Radcliffe Hosp. Oxf.; Hon. Cons. (Bact.) John Radcliffe Hosp. Oxf.; Hon. Cons. Pub. Health Laborat. Serv.; Supernum. Fell. Green Coll. Oxf.; PHLS Refer. Expert on Haemophilus Influenzae. Specialty: Med. Microbiol. Prev: Demonst. (Path.) King's Coll. Hosp. Lond.; Ho. Surg. King's Coll. Hosp.; Ho. Phys. Brook Gen. Hosp. Lond.

SLACK, Nicola Frances 23 Redland Grove, Redland, Bristol BS6 6PT — MB ChB Birm. 1976; FRCR 1982. Cons. Radiol. Frenchay Hosp. Bristol. Specialty: Radiol. Prev: Sen. Regist. (Ultrasound & Nuclear Med.) Roy. Marsden Hosp. Lond.; Sen. Regist. (Radiol.) Bristol HA.

SLACK, Patricia Mary 5 Magdala Road, Mapperley Park, Nottingham NG3 5DE Tel: 0115 960 5940 Email: tishslack@hotmail.com — MB BS Lond. 1969 (St Mary's) MRCS Eng. LRCP Lond. 1969; DCH Eng. 1972; MRCPsych 1984. Specialty: Psychother. Prev: Ho. Phys. (Paediat.) Unit St. Mary's Hosp. Lond.; Scientif. Off. Div. Communicable Dis. Clin. Research Centre, Harrow.; Cons. Psychotherapist Nottm. Psychother. Unit.

SLACK, Rachel Olivia 106 Long Road, Cambridge CB2 2HF — BM BS Nottm. 1996. SHO (Paediat.) Guys/St. Thomas' Hosp. Lond. Specialty: Paediat. Socs: MRCPCH.

SLACK, Richard Charles Bewick Nottingham Health Protection Unit, Standard Court, Park Row, Nottingham NG1 6GN Tel: 0115 912 3344 Fax: 0115 912 3351 Email: richard.slack@nott.ac.uk; 5 Magdala Road, Mapperley Park, Nottingham NG3 5DE — (Camb. & St. Mary's) MB BChir Camb. 1969; DObst RCOG 1970; MRCPath 1977; FFPH 1999; FRCPath 2002. Cons. Communicable Dis. Control Nottm. HA; Sen. Lect. (Microbiol.) Univ. Nottm. Specialty: Med. Microbiol.; Pub. Health Med. Socs: Past-Pres. Assn. Med. Microbiol.; Fell. Roy. Inst. of Pub. Health; President Pub. Health Med. Env. Group. Prev: Lect. (Path.) Univ. Nairobi, Kenya; Temp. Lect. (Path.) Middlx. Hosp. Med. Sch. Lond.; Ho. Surg. St. Mary's Hosp. Lond.

SLACK, Richard Francis Yeardsley Pump Cottage, 3 New Way Lane, Threshers Bush, Harlow CM17 0NT Tel: 01279 641122; Pump Cottage, 3 New Way Lane, Threshers Bush, Harlow CM17 0NT Tel: 01279 641122 — MB BS Lond. 1992. Princip. Med. Off. (A. & E.) Cairns Base Hosp. Cairns Queensland Australia. Specialty: Accid. &

Emerg. Prev: Clin. Asst. (A & E) Roy. Free Hosp. Lond.; SHO (A & E) Roy. Free Hosp. Lond.; Sen. Ho. Off. (Med.) King Geo. Hosp. Ilford Essex.

SLACK, Robert Alexnder Mendip, Hawks Hill, Bourne End SL8 5JQ — MB BS Lond. 1994.

SLACK, Mr Robert William Talbot The Bath Clinic, Claverton Down, Bath BA2 7BR Tel: 01225 835555 Fax: 01225 825466 — MB ChB Bristol 1977; BSc Lond. 1974; FRCS Ed. 1981; FRCS Eng. 1984. Cons. ENT Surg. Roy. United Hosp. Bath.; Elected Mem. of Gen. Med. Counc.1999-present. Specialty: Otorhinolaryngol. Socs: Counc. Mem. Sect. of Laryngol. Roy. Soc. Med. Prev: Sen. Regist. (ENT Surg.) Bristol & Bath HA; Regist. Roy. Nat. Throat Nose & Ear Hosp. Lond.; SHO (ENT & Gen. Surg) Bristol United Hosp.

SLACK, Roger Dutton (retired) Sycamore Cottage, Hellesvean, St Ives TR26 2HG Tel: 01736 795067 — (Camb. & Middlx.) BA Camb. 1940, MB BChir 1942; MRCS Eng. LRCP Lond. 1942.

SLACK, Stephen James Highbury New Park Surgery, 49 Highbury New Park, London N5 2ET Tel: 020 7354 1972 — MB BS Lond. 1987 (Lond. Hosp. Med. Sch.) MRCGP 1995. Specialty: Gen. Pract. Socs: BMA.

SLACK, Mrs Susanna Elizabeth 4 Grosvenor Drive, Abbotts Barton, Winchester SO23 7HF Tel: 01962 852597 — BM BCh Oxf. 1992; MA Camb. 1993; FRCS Eng. 1997. Specialist Regist. (A & E) Qu. Alexandra Hosp. Portsmouth. Specialty: Accid. & Emerg. Prev: SHO (A & E) Qu. Alex. Hosp. Portsmouth; SHO (Gen. Surg.) Roy. Hants. Co. Hosp. Winchester; SHO (Orthop.) Roy. Hants. Co. Hosp. Winchester.

SLACK, Walter Kenneth (retired) Pump Cottage, 3 New Way Lane, Threshers Bush, Harlow CM17 0NT Tel: 01279 641122 Fax: 01279 441496 — (King's Coll. Hosp.) MRCS Eng. LRCP Lond. 1949; DA Eng. 1954; Cert. Av. Med. 1979; FFA RCS Eng. 1986; FRCA. 1992. Hon. Cons. Anaesth. Whipps Cross Hosp. Lond. Prev: Cons. Anaesth. Whipps Cross & Wanstead Hosps. Lond. & Cons. i/c Regional Hyperbaric Oxygen Unit Whipps Cross Hosp. Lond.

SLACK, Sir William Willatt, KCVO Hillside Cottage, Tower Hill, Stawell, Bridgwater TA7 9AJ Tel: 01278 722719 Fax: 01278 722719 — BM BCh Oxf. 1950; MA Oxf. 1950, MCh 1961, BM BCh 1950; FRCS Eng. 1955. Emerit. Surg. Middlx. Hosp.; Hon. Fell. UCL. Socs: Fell. Roy. Soc. Med. Prev: Sgt. Surg. to HM the Qu.; Dean Univ. Coll. & Middlx. Sch. Med. Lond.; Ex-Pres. Sect. Proctol. Roy. Soc. Med.

SLADDEN, Christopher Simon 43 Hurst Road, Hinckley LE10 1AB — MB ChB Wales 1992; BSc Wales 1985, MB ChB 1992.

SLADDEN, David Kerrison Lawrence (retired) 5 Drayton Grove, Norwich NR8 6PU Tel: 01603 869334 Email: dklsladden@btinternet.com — (King's Coll. Hosp.) MRCS Eng. LRCP Lond. 1948; DObst RCOG 1948; MMSA Lond. 1959. Prev: Med. Off. Rehabil. Centre Norf.

SLADDEN, Jonathan Michael Drs COTTERELL,PFEIFFER & PTNRS, College Way Surgery, Comeytrowe Centre, Taunton TA1 4TY Tel: 01823 259333 Fax: 01823 259336; 6 Stone Close, Comeytrowe, Taunton TA1 4YG — MB ChB Sheff. 1978; MRCGP 1983. GP Taunton.

SLADDEN, Michael Joseph Department of Dermatology, Leicester Royal Infirmary, Leicester LE1 5WW Tel: 0116 258 5162 Fax: 0116 258 6792 — MB ChB Leic. 1985 (Univ. of Leicester) MRCGP 1989; DRCOG 1989; FRACGP 1992; Master Appl. Epidemiol. Austral. Nat. Univ. 1996; MRCP UK 2001. Specialist Regist., Dermat., Leicester Roy. Infirm. Specialty: Dermat.; Epidemiol.; Pub. Health Med. Socs: Brit. Med. Assn.; Brit. Assn. of Dermatol. Prev: Sen. Lect., Gen. Pract., Univ. of Tasmania, Mobart; GP, Mobart, Tasmania; Trainee GP Leic. VTS.

SLADDEN, Robert Arthur (retired) 7 Peninsula Square, Winchester SO23 8GJ Tel: 01962 850297 — (Oxf.) BSc Oxf. 1954, DM 1953, BM BCh 1944; DTM Liverp. 1946; FRCPath 1968, M 1964. Prev: Cons. Histopath. Northampton Gen. Hosp.

SLADE, Alistair Kenneth Bannerman Department of Cardiology, Royal Cornwall Hospitals Trust, Treliske Hospital, Truro TR1 3LJ Tel: 01872 252517 Fax: 01872 252877 Email: alistair.slade@rcht.cornwall.nhs.uk; Trevean, 11 St Johns Terrace, Devoran, Truro TR3 6NE Tel: 01872 864568 Email: alistairslade@lycos.co.uk — MB BS Lond. 1984 (Middlx.) BA Camb. 1981; MRCP (UK) 1988. Cons. Cardiol. Roy. Cornw. Hosp. Trust Treliske Hosp. Truro Cornw. Specialty: Cardiol. Socs: BMA; Brit. Pacing & Electrophysiol. Gp.; Brit. Cardiac Soc. Prev: Lect. & Hon. Sen. Regist. (Cardiol. Sci.s) St. Geo. Hosp. Med. Sch. Lond.; Brit. Heart Foundat. Research Fell. (Cardiol. Sci.s) St. Geo. Hosp. Med. Sch. Lond.; Regist. (Cardiol.) Bournemouth & Roy. Brompton & Nat. Heart Hosp.

SLADE, Andrew Mark c/o 170 Burden Road, Beverley HU17 9LN — MB ChB Liverp. 1993.

SLADE, Dawn Elizabeth 28 Llanberis Cl, Tonteg, Pontypridd CF38 1HR — MB ChB Leic. 1997.

SLADE, Diana Elizabeth Marianne 22 Ashmeads Way, Wimborne BH21 2NZ — MB BS Lond. 1993 (Charing Cross/Westminster) BSc 1990; FRCS Eng 1997. SHO Plastic Surg. Specialty: Plastic Surg. Socs: BMA; Roy. Soc. Med.; RCS (Eng.). Prev: SHO surg.Rotat.; SHO plast.surg.

SLADE, Mr Dominic Alexander James Manchester Royal Infirmary, Department of General Surgery, Oxford Road, Manchester; 163 Oldfield Road, Altrincham WA14 4HY Tel: 0161 941 5462 Email: dom.slade@virgin.net — MB ChB Birm. 1992 (Univ. of Birm.) FRCS (Eng.) 1997. Specialist Regsitrar. Specialty: Gen. Surg. Socs: Assn. of Surgeons in Train.; Assn. of Coloproctology; Assn. of Surgeons of Gt. Britain & Irel. Prev: Research Regist. (Dept. Surg. Univ. Manch.).

SLADE, Guy Malcolm (retired) 46 Roslin Road S., Bournemouth BH3 7EG Tel: 01202 510243 Fax: 01202 510243 — (Guy's) MRCS Eng. LRCP Lond. 1960; DObst RCOG 1962.

SLADE, Joanna Margaret 69 Home Farm Lane, Bury St Edmunds IP33 2QL — MB BCh Oxf. 1985; MRCPCH; MRCP (UK) 1994. Regist. (Paediat.) Oxf. & E. Anglia RHA. Specialty: Paediat. Prev: Clin. Med. Off. (Community Paediat.) Soton. Area HA; Resid. Med. Off. (Cas.) Childr. Hosp. Adelaide, S. Austral.; SHO (Paediat.) Soton. Gen. Hosp.

SLADE, John Michael Department of Anaesthetics, West Suffolk Hospital, Bury St Edmunds IP33 2QZ Tel: 01284 713330 — BM BCh Oxf. 1984; FCAnaesth. 1989. Cons. Anaesth. W. Suff. Hosp. Bury St. Edmunds. Specialty: Anaesth. Socs: Pain Soc.; Soc. Computing & Technol. in Anaesth. Prev: Sen. Regist. (Anaesth.) Soton. Gen. Hosp.; Sen. Regist. (Anaesth.) Roy. Adelaide Hosp., Austral.; Research Off. Univ. Hosp. Wales Cardiff.

SLADE, Karen 20 Penygraig, Aberystwyth SY23 2JA — BM Soton. 1997.

SLADE, Mark Gaisford Oxford Centre for Respiratory Medicine, Churchill Hospital, Old Road, Headington, Oxford OX3 7LJ Tel: 01865 225252 Fax: 01865 225221 Email: mark.slade@orh.nhs.uk — MB BS Lond. 1991 (Guy's & St Thos.) MRCP UK 1994; FRACP Sydney 1998. Cons. in Respirat. and Gen. Internal Med., Churchill Hosp., Oxf. Specialty: Respirat. Med. Special Interest: Interventional Bronchoscopy; Lung Cancer. Socs: Brit. Thoracic Soc.; Amer. Thoracic Soc.; Amer. Coll. of Chest Physicians.

SLADE, Paul Jonathan Baker Irnham Lodge Surgery, Townsend Road, Minehead TA24 5RG Tel: 01643 703289 Fax: 01643 707921 — MRCS Eng. LRCP Lond. 1974; DRCOG 1977; MRCGP 1980. Clin. Asst. (Ophth.); Clin. Asst. Som. Drug Serv. Prev: SHO Kent & Canterbury Hcsp.; Med. Off. RAF Med. Br.

SLADE, Paul Martin Bristol-Myers Squibb, 3 rue Joseph Monier, Rueil-Malmaison 92506, France Email: paul.slade@bms.com — MB BChir Camb. 1991 (Univ. Camb. & St. Mary's Hosp. Lond.) MA Camb. 1991; MRCP (UK) 1996; MFPM 2000; MBA (Lond. Business Sch.) 2004. Europ. Med. Lead, Bristol-Myers Squibb. Specialty: Infec. Dis.; Pharmaceutical Medicine. Prev: Med. Advisor (Anti-infectives) Bristol-Myers Squibb; Hon. Clin. Asst. St. Mary's Hosp. Lond.; Acad. Regist. (Communicable Dis.) St. Mary's Hosp. Lond.

SLADE, Philip Herbert Eastoft, 249 Normanby Road, South Bank, Middlesbrough TS6 6TB Tel: 01642 453457 — LRCP LRCS Ed. 1948 (Newc.) LRCP LRCS Ed. LRFPS Glas. 1948. Prev: Ho. Phys. & Res. Obst. Off. Bensham Gen. Hosp. Gateshead-on-Tyne.

SLADE, Mr Philip Ridd Helyar (retired) 6 Rockleaze, Bristol BS9 1NE — ChM Bristol 1955, MB ChB 1939; FRCS Eng. 1947. Prev: Cons. Thoracic Surg. Groby Rd. Hosp. Leicester.

SLADE, Richard 28 Glenbarry Close, Chorlton-Cum-Medlock, Manchester M13 9XR Tel: 0161 273 8481 — (Univ. Aberd.) MB ChB Aberd. 1980; DRCOG 1985; MRCGP 1986; MRCPsych 1989; T(GP) 1991. Specialty: Geriat. Psychiat.

SLADE, Mr Richard John Hope Hospital, Stott Lane, Salford M6 8HD Tel: 0161 789 7373 — MB ChB Leic. 1984 (Leicester) FRCS RCPS Glas. 1989; MRCOG 1991. Cons. O & G Hope Hosp. Salford; Cons. Gyn. Surg. Christie Hosp. Manch. Specialty: Obst. & Gyn. Socs: Brit. Gyn. Cancer Soc. Prev: Sen. Regist. (O & G) Univ. Hosp. Wales Cardiff & St. Davids Hosp. Bangor; Regist. (O & G) John Radcliffe Hosp. Oxf.; SHO (O & G) Bristol Gen. Hosp. & Leicester Roy. Infirm.

SLADE, Robert Rodney Trust Headquarters, Southmead Hospital, Westbury-on-Trym, Bristol BS10 5NB Tel: 0117 959 5206 Fax: 0117 959 1102 Email: robertslade@north-bristol.swest.nhs.uk — MB BS Lond. 1973; BSc (Biochem.) Lond. 1968; MRCP (UK) 1976; FRCPath (Haemat.) 1993, M 1980; FRCP Lond. 1993. Dir. Path. Southmead Hosp. Univ. Bristol; Med. Dir. WTE, N. Bristol NHS Trust; Cons. Haematologist. Specialty: Haematology. Prev: Clin. Dean & Cons. Haemat. Southmead Hosp. Univ. Bristol.

SLADE, Valerie Jane Copse Cottage, Church Lane, Brook, Godalming GU8 5UQ Tel: 01428 683866 — MB ChB Bristol 1988 (Bristol University) FRCA 1994. Cons. Anaesth., Frimley Pk. Hosp. Camberley. Specialty: Anaesth. Socs: Intens. Care Soc.; BMA; Assn. Anaesth.

SLADEN, Gordon Edward George (retired) Anchor Oast, Rochester Road, Aylesford ME20 7EA Tel: 01622 882395 — BM BCh Oxf. 1960 (Oxf. & Middlx.) FRCP Lond. 1975, M 1963; MA Oxf. 1961, DM 1970. Prev: Cons. Phys. (Gastroenterol.) Guy's Hosp. Lond. 1976-1994.

SLADER, Christopher John Llangennech Surgery, Llangennech, Llanelli SA14 8YR — MB ChB Sheff. 1969; BSc Lond. 1964; MRCP (U.K.) 1973; MRCGP 1981. Llanelli VTS Course Organiser.

SLADER, Marian Isabel Llangennech, Llanelli SA14 8YB — MB ChB Sheff. 1972. Prev: Clin. Asst. (Psychiat.) Dyke Bar Hosp. Paisley.

SLAFFER, Simon Neil Les Saisons Surgery, 20 David Place, St Helier JE2 4TD Tel: 01534 720314 Fax: 01534 733205 — MB BS Lond. 1972 (St. Bart.) MRCS Eng. LRCP Lond. 1973; MRCGP 1979; DRCOG 1980; ATLS RCS Eng. 1991. Specialist (Musculoskeletal Med.) Jersey; Lect. (Orthop. Med.) Internat. 1990; Hon. Lect. Jersey Wildlife Preservation Trust 1994; Maj. Incident Med. Off. Jersey; Certified Mem. Cyriax Foundat. (Exam. 1985). Specialty: Orthop. Socs: (Pres.) Jersey Med. Soc.; BMA (Chairm. Jersey Br.); Brit. Inst. Musculoskeletal Med. Prev: SHO Worcester Roy. Infirm.; Ho. Surg. St. Bart. Hosp. Lond.; Maj. RAMC.

SLANE, Frank 43A Roman Road, Bearsden, Glasgow G61 2QP Tel: 0141 943 0597 — LRCP LRCS Ed. LRFPS Glas. 1951; DPH Glas. 1958.

SLANE, Peter Wright Erskine Practice, Arthurstone Medical Centre, Arthurstone Terrace, Dundee DD4 6QY Tel: 01382 458333 Fax: 01382 461833 Email: peter.w.slane@tuht.scot.nhs.uk; 8 Arbuthnott Loan, Balgillo Park, Broughty Ferry, Dundee DD5 3TN — MB ChB Dundee 1983; MRCP (UK) 1986; MRCGP 1990; DRCOG 1990.

SLANEY, Charlotte Julia 455 Chester Road, Hartford, Northwich CW8 2AG — BM BCh Oxf. 1998; BM BCh Oxf 1998.

SLANEY, Sir Geoffrey, KBE Hill Crest, Collins Green, Knightwick, Worcester WR6 5PT Tel: 01886 822024 — MB ChB Birm. 1946; Hon. FACS 1985 Birm.; MB ChB Birm. 1947; FRCS Eng. 1953; MSc (Surg.) Illinois 1956; ChM Birm. 1961; Hon. FRCSI 1984; Hon. FRACS 1984; Hon. FRCA 1986; Hon. FRCSC 1986. Emerit. Prof. Surg. Univ. Birm.; Hon. Cons. Surg. Qu. Eliz. Hosp. Birm. Specialty: Gen. Surg. Socs: Fell. Assn. Surgs.; Fell. Amer. Surg. Assn. Prev: Pres. Roy. Coll. Surg. Eng.; Barling Prof. Dept. Surg. Univ. Birm.; Cons. Surg. Qu. Eliz. Hosp. Birm.

SLANEY, Mark West Hampshire NHS Trust, Cannon House, 6 Cannon Street, Shirley, Southampton SO15 5PQ; 18 Plantation Road, Tadley RG26 4QU — MB BS Lond. 1983; MA Oxf. 1984; DRCOG 1987; Cert. Prescribed Equiv. Exp. JCPTGP 1989; MRCPsych 1989; T(GP) 1991; T (Psychiat.) 1993. Locum Cons. Gen. Adult Psychiat., W. Hants. NHS Trust, Soton. Specialty: Gen. Psychiat. Socs: BMA. Prev: Locum Cons. Psychiat., Frankston Hosp. Melbourne, Vict.; Locum Cons. Gen. Adult Psychiat. Portsmouth Healthcare NHS Trust; Locum Cons. Psychiat. Loddon NHS Trust, Basingstoke.

SLANEY, Penelope Louise Radiology Department, Ronkswood Hospital, Worcester Royal Infirmary NHS Trust,, Newtown Road, Worcester WR1 5HN Tel: 01905 763333 Fax: 01905 760774 — MB ChB Birm. 1983; FRCS Ed. 1989; FRCR 1994. Cons. Radiol. Worcester Roy. Infirm. NHS Trust. Specialty: Radiol. Socs: BMA; BSIR; CIRSE. Prev: Sen. Regist. (Diagn. Radiol.) Russells Hall Hosp. Dudley; Regist. (Radiol.) Bristol Roy. Infirm.; SHO (Urol. & Gen. Surg.) Roy. Shrewsbury Hosp.

SLANN, Hilary Elizabeth Rose 27 Glasgow Road, Denny FK6 5DW — MB ChB Glas. 1990; MRCGP 1994. Specialty: Gen. Pract.

SLAPAK, Gabrielle Isabelle Abbey House, Itchen Abbas, Winchester SO21 1BN — MB BS Lond. 1988.

SLAPAK, Mr Maurice, CBE, Maj. RAMC World Transplant Games Federation, Highcroft, Winchester Tel: 01962 840767 Ext: 3 Email: wtgf@wtgf.demon.co.uk; Abbey House, Itchen Abbas, Winchester SO21 1BN Tel: 01962 779233 Fax: 01962 779673 Email: mslapak@compuserve.co — MB BChir Camb. 1957 (Westm.) FRCS Eng. 1963; FRCS Canada 1966; MChir Camb. 1967; FACS 1970. Cons. Surg. Cromwell Hosp. Lond.; Cons. Gen. Surg. Qu. Alexandra's Hosp. Cosham; Sen. Lect. Soton. Univ. Specialty: Gen. Surg. Socs: Transpl. Soc.; Eur. Soc. Organ Transpl. (Ex-Vice-Pres.); Roy. Soc. Med. (Ex.Pres. Transpl. Sect.). Prev: Sen. Surg. Wessex Regional Transpl. Unit St. Mary's Hosp. Portsmouth; Asst. Prof. Surg. Harvard Med. Sch. Boston, USA; Sen. Asst. Surg. Camb. Univ.

SLATER, Alan Brooklands, Durton Lane, Broughton, Preston PR3 5LD — MB BCh Liverp. 1961; DObst RCOG 1963. Socs: BMA.

SLATER, Alan John Clatterbridge Centre for Oncology NHS Trust, Bebington, Wirral CH63 4JY Tel: 0151 482 7827 Fax: 0151 482 7675 Email: alan.slater@ccotrust.nhs.uk; 5 Burlingham Avenue, West Kirby, Wirral CH48 8AJ Tel: 0151 625 9868 — MB ChB Birm 1972; FRCR 1980; BA Open 1988. Cons. Clin. Oncol. Clatterbridge Centre for Oncol NHS Trust Wirral; Hon. Clin. Lect. Univ. Liverp. Specialty: Oncol. Socs: BMA. Prev: Clin. Sci. MRC Clin. Oncol. & Radiother. Unit Addenbrooke's Hosp. Camb.; Resid. (Radiat. Oncol.) Princess Margt. Hosp. Toronto; MRC Clin. Assoc. Leukaemia) & Hon. Lect. (Haemat.) Univ. Hosp. Wales Cardiff.

SLATER, Alan Martin 2 Lovelace Close, Hurley, Maidenhead SL6 5NF — MB BS Lond. 1997.

SLATER, Alison Margaret 19 Station Road, Whyteleafe CR3 0EP Tel: 01883 624181; 65 Hartley Hill, Purley CR8 4EQ Tel: 020 8645 0275 — MB BS Lond. 1983; DRCOG 1986; MRCGP 1987. GP Princip. Prev: Trainee GP Croydon VTS; SHO (O & G & Geriat.) Mayday Hosp. Croydon; SHO (ENT/Paediat.) Bangour Gen. Hosp.

SLATER, Andrew 16 Colwell Drive, Headington, Oxford OX3 8XD — MB ChB Birm. 1996; BSc (Hons.) Birm. 1994; MRCP Lond. 1999; FRCR Lond. 2002.

SLATER, Andrew James 4 Ely Cl, Amersham HP7 9HS — MB ChB Manch. 1997.

SLATER, Anne Rose Cottage, Troston Road, Honington, Bury St Edmunds IP31 1RD — MB ChB Sheff. 1988.

SLATER, Anne Christine Southbank Road Surgery, 17-19 Southbank Road, Kirkintilloch, Glasgow G66 1NH Tel: 0141 776 2183 Fax: 0141 777 8321 — MB ChB Ed. 1967. GP Kirkintilloch. Prev: Ho. Off. (Paediat.) Falkirk Dist. Roy. Infirm.; Ho. Phys. Vict. Hosp. Kirkcaldy; Ho. Surg. Falkirk & Dist. Roy. Infirm.

SLATER, Anne Jennifer Rivington, Little Pluckets Way, Buckhurst Hill IG9 5QU — MB BS Lond. 1974 (Char. Cross Hosp. Med. Sch.) MRCS Eng. LRCP Lond. 1974.

SLATER, Mr Barry Joseph North Tyneside General Hospital, Rake Lane, North Shields NE29 8NH Tel: 0191 293 2527 Email: barry.slater@northumbria-healthcare.nhs.uk — MB ChB Manch. 1987; FRCS Ed. 1992; FRCS Eng. 1992; FRCS Gen Surg. 1999. Cons. Surg. N. Tyneside Gen. Hosp., Tyne and Wear. Specialty: Gen. Surg.

SLATER, Basil Crandles Smith, OBE (retired) 2/2 East Suffolk Road, Edinburgh EH16 5PH Tel: 0131 667 5964 — (Ed.) MD Ed. 1964, MB ChB 1952; FRCGP 1970, M 1960; FFCM 1989, M 1980; FRCP Ed. 1988, M 1984. Prev: Cons. Pub. Health Med. Edin. Roy. Infirm.

SLATER, Camilla Jane Silver Stream, Hackney Road, Melton, Woodbridge IP12 1NN — MB BS Lond. 1996.

SLATER, Catherine Brooklands, D'Urton Lane, Broughton, Preston PR3 5LD — BChir Camb. 1990.

SLATER, Catriona Susan 4 Tatton View, Withington, Manchester M20 4BU — MB ChB Manch. 1995; BSc Med Sci 1993. SHO (Gen.

Med.) Manch. Roy. Infirm.; Flexible Trainee. Specialty: Gen. Med. Prev: Clin. Fell. Wythenshawe Hosp. Manch.

SLATER, Charles Bell Longbarn Lane Surgery, 22 Longbarn Lane, Reading RG2 7SZ Tel: 0118 987 1377 Fax: 0118 975 0375 — MRCS Eng. LRCP Lond. 1981.

SLATER, Clare 36 Great Barrington, Burford OX18 4UR — MB BS Lond. 1983 (Char. Cross) MA (Chem.) Oxf. 1981; MRCP (UK) 1990; MSc (Epidemiol.) Lond. 1992; DFFP 1995; MRCGP 1998.

SLATER, Colin Anthony Ann Burrow Thames Health Centre, South William St., Workington CA14 2ED Tel: 01900 602244 Fax: 01900 871131 — MB BS Lond. 1975 (St. Thos.) BSc (Physiol.) Lond. 1972, MB BS 1975; DCH RCP Lond 1983. SCMO W. Cumbria Primary Care Trust & Audiol. Childr. Serv. Specialty: Community Child Health; Otorhinolaryngol. Prev: Clin. Med. Off. Cornw. & Is. Scilly HA.

SLATER, David Neil Floor E Histopathology, Royal Hallamshire Hospital, Glossop Road, Sheffield S10 2JF Tel: 0114 271 3378 Fax: 01142712200 Email: david.slater@sth.nhs.uk — MB ChB Sheff. 1971 (Sheffield) BMedSci Sheff. 1968; FRCPath 1990, M 1978. Cons. Dermatopathologist, Histopath. Dept., Roy. Hallamshire Hosp., Sheff.; Hon. Clin. Sen. Lect (Path) Sheff. Univ.; Directror of Dermatopathology Train. Centre; QA Dir. for East Midlands NHSCSP. Specialty: Histopath.; Dermat. Socs: Internat. Acad. Path. & Assn. Clin. Paths.; British Soc. Dermpath; Brit. Soc. for Clin. Cytol. Prev: CCons. Path. Rotherham NHS Hosps. Trust; Sen. Lect. (Path.) Sheff. Univ.; SHO Nottm. Gp. Hosps.

SLATER, David Richard Royal Crescent Surgery, 25 Crescent Street, Weymouth DT4 7BY Tel: 01305 774466 Fax: 01305 760538 — MB ChB Leeds 1974; DRCOG 1977.

SLATER, Edna Valerie (retired) Taney, Green Lane, West Clandon, Guildford GU4 7UR — (T.C. Dub.) MB BCh BAO Dub. 1960; MA Dub. 1964. Prev: Clin. Asst. (Geriat. Med.) Beechcroft Hosp. Woking.

SLATER, Edwin Antony Work (retired) Suleskerry, Ryanview Crescent, Stranraer DG9 0JL Tel: 01776 703903 — MB ChB Ed. 1961; DObst RCOG 1963; FRCGP 1994, M 1972. Prev: GP Stranraer.

SLATER, Elinor Margaret 58 Paisley Crescent, Edinburgh EH8 7JQ Tel: 0131 661 5137 Email: elcapitarn@geocities.com — MB ChB Aberd. 1990; LLB Ed. 1994; Primex Examination 1998. Gen. Pract. Locum. Specialty: Gen. Pract.

SLATER, Elizabeth 3F1 18 Montaigne Street, Edinburgh EH8 9QX — MB ChB Ed. 1998; MB ChB Ed 1998.

SLATER, Mr Eric George Winston (retired) Holly House Hospital, High Road, Buckhurst Hill IG9 5HX Tel: 0208 505 6423 — (The London Hospital) MB BS Lond. 1966; FRCS Eng. 1975. Cons. Surg. in Private Pract. Prev: NHS Cons. in Breast, Thyroid and Colo-Rectal Surg.

SLATER, Eva Marie Cleveland Clinic, 12 Cleveland Road, St Helier, Jersey JE1 4HD Tel: 01534 722381/734121 — MB ChB Glas. 1983.

SLATER, Geoffrey Dowell New Southgate Surgery, Buxton Place, off Leeds Road, Wakefield WF1 3JQ Tel: 01924 334400 Fax: 01924 334439; Oakland House, 16 Oxford Road, St Johns., Wakefield WF1 3LB Tel: 01924 201034 — MB ChB Leeds 1968; DPM Leeds 1972. Prev: Regist. High Royds Hosp. Menston; Ho. Off. (Gen. Surg.) Chapel Allerton Hosp. Leeds; Ho. Off. (Gen. Med.) St. Jas. Hosp. Leeds.

SLATER, Mr Guy Haining Minimal Access Therapy Training Unit, Royal Surrey County Hospital, Guildford GU2 7XX — MB BS Lond. 1990; FRCS Eng. 1994. Regist. (Gen. Surg.) Roy. Surrey Co. Hosp. Guildford. Specialty: Gen. Surg. Prev: Regist. St Thos. Hosp. Lond.; Regist. Frimley Pk. Hosp.; Regist. Mayday Univ. Hosp.

SLATER, Henry Bertram (retired) 63 Meltham Avenue, Withington, Manchester M20 1FE Tel: 0161 445 1294 — MB ChB Manch. 1936; MRCS Eng. LRCP Lond. 1936. Prev: Cons. Phys. (Chest) Tameside & Manch. AHAs.

SLATER, Ian (retired) Taney, Green Lane, West Clandon, Guildford GU4 7UR Tel: 01483 222775 Email: docianslater@aol.com — MB BCh BAO Dub. 1960 (T.C. Dub.) MA Dub. 1964. Prev: Regist. (Psychiat.) St. Patrick's Hosp. Dub.

SLATER, Jane Bodriggy Health Centre, 60 Queens Way, Bodriggy, Hayle TR27 4PB Tel: 01736 753136 Fax: 01736 753467 — MB BS Lond. 1984; DRCOG 1988; MRCGP 1993. Trainer (Gen. Pract.) Cornw. Prev: SHO DHCE City Hosp. Nottm.; SHO (O & G) Roy. Cornw. Truro; SHO (Orthop. & A & E) Northwick Pk. Hosp. Middlx.

SLATER, John David Eliot 40 Poplar Road, Botley, Oxford OX2 9LB — MB ChB Bristol 1989; MA Camb. 1979, BA 1976; Postgrad. Cert. Leeds 1977; MRCGP 1993; MPH Birmingham University 1999; MRCPsych 1999. Specialist Regist. Rehabil. Med.; Locum GP. Prev: Trainee in Psychiat. Oxf. Rotat.; Res. Fell. Birm. Univ.; GP RAF Cramwell.

SLATER, John Edward St Lawrence Medical Centre, 4 Bocking End, Braintree CM7 9AA Tel: 01376 552474 Fax: 01376 552417 — MB ChB Manch. 1982; DRCOG 1985; MRCGP 1986. Prev: Trainee GP Stockport VTS.

SLATER, John Norman Botley Medical Centre, Elms Road, Botley, Oxford OX2 9JS Tel: 01865 248719 Fax: 01865 728116; 43 Yarnells Hill, Botley, Oxford OX2 9BE Tel: 01865 248134 — MB ChB Aberd. 1971; DCH Eng. 1976.

SLATER, Jonathan Charles Cobb Cottage, 7 Park Farm, Croun Lane, Farnham GU9 9JP — MB BS Lond. 1997; MRCGP.

SLATER, Kerry Elizabeth Dept of Community Paediatrics, Wycombe General Hospital, High Wycombe HP11 2TT — MB BS Queensland 1972 (Queensld.) LF Hom.

SLATER, Laurence Billingsley 15 Brook Green, London W6 7BL Tel: 020 7603 7563; 2 Hartswood Gardens, Stamford Brook, London W12 9NR Email: drl@slater.org.uk — MB BS Lond. 1982; DCH RCP Lond. 1990; MRCGP 1991. IT lead for Hammersmith & Fulham Primary Care Trust; Mem. of Confidentiality Requirements Advis. Gp. (NPfIT); Mem. of Health Informatic Standing Gp. (RCGP); Mem. of GP Advis. panel (IDX). Specialty: Gen. Med.; Gen. Pract.; Medical Informatics. Socs: BMA. Prev: Hammersmith PCG Bd. Mem.; Computer Fell. (EHH Health Agency); Regist. (Paediat.) Greenwich Dist. Hosp. Lond.

SLATER, Lindsay Kay Townsend House Medical Centre, 49 Harepath Road, Seaton EX12 2RY Tel: 01297 20616 Fax: 01297 20810; Higher Bolshayne Barn, Whitwell Lane, Colyton EX24 6HS Tel: 01297 552102 — MB BS Lond. 1982; BSc Hons. Lond. 1976; DCH RCP Lond. 1984; DRCOG 1985; MRCGP 1985. Prev: Trainee GP Ealing VTS.

SLATER, Lorna Kay 41 Hatfield Road, Ainsdale, Southport PR8 2PE — MB ChB Sheff. 1996.

SLATER, Margaret (retired) 18 Trefonwys, Belmont Road, Bangor LL57 — (Liverp.) MB ChB Liverp. 1944; CPH Eng. 1947; DCH Eng. 1947; MFCM 1973. Prev: Princip. Sen. Med. Off. Child Health Serv. Gwynedd AHA.

SLATER, Mark Stephen Watford General Hospital, Shrodells Unit, Vicarage Road, Watford WD18 0HB Tel: 01923 811605 Fax: 01923 811601 Email: markslater@fastpsych.co.uk; Bowden House Clinic, London Road, Harrow-on-the-Hill, Harrow HA1 3JL Tel: 0870 600 2800 Fax: 0870 600 2801 Email: consultants@med-law.co.uk — MB ChB Otago 1983; MRCPsych 1989. Cons. Psychiat., Herts. Partnership NHS Trust. Specialty: Gen. Psychiat.; Medico Legal. Special Interest: Ment. Health Act (assessments and Indep. Tribunal reports); Ment. capacity; psychiatric aspects of personal injury litigation; psychiatric aspects of Family Ct. Proc. Socs: W Herts. & Watford Med. Soc.; BMA (Hon. Sec., W. Herts Division); Royal Society of Medicine. Prev: Sen. Regist. (Psychiat.) Roy. Lond. Hosp.; Regist. (Psychiat.) Bethlem Roy. & Maudsley Hosps. Lond.; SHO (Psychiat.) Middlx. Hosp. Lond.

SLATER, Michele Anne Brixton Hill Group Practice, 22 Raleigh Gardens, Brixton Hill, London SW2 1AE — MB ChB Glas. 1987; MRCGP 1992.

SLATER, Mr Nicholas Desmond 1 Wilton Villas, London N1 3DN Tel: 020 7354 3507 — MB BS Lond. 1977 (Guy's Hosp. Lond.) MRCS Eng. LRCP Lond. 1977; FRCS Eng. 1982; MS Lond. 1990. Cons. Surg. Lewisham Hosp. Lond. Specialty: Gen. Surg. Prev: Sen. Regist. St. Bart. Hosp. Lond.

SLATER, Nicolas Gilbert Pasternak (retired) 85 Balfour Road, London N5 2HE Tel: 020 7359 2287 Fax: 020 7503 6827 Email: nicolasslater@email.com — (Middlx.) MA Oxf. 1965; Dip. Biochem. Lond 1967; MB BS Lond. 1970; FRCP Lond. 1993, M 1973; FRCPath 1990, M 1978. Prev: Sen. Lect. & Hon. Cons. (Haemat.) United Med. & Dent. Sch. St. Thos. Hosp. Lond.

SLATER, Noel Arthur John 100 Poplar Avenue, Edgbaston, Birmingham B17 8ES Tel: 0121 429 4237 — MB ChB Birm. 1961;

DObst RCOG 1964; DA Eng. 1964; FFA RCS Eng. 1978. Specialty: Anaesth.

SLATER, Peter Forrester (retired) 5 Bede Court, College Grove Road, Wakefield WF1 3RW Tel: 01924 373077 — MB ChB St. And. 1954.

SLATER, Peter John (retired) 14 Rowan Crescent, Lenzie, Kirkintilloch, Glasgow G66 4RE — MB ChB Glas. 1965; MRCOG 1970, DObst 1967; FFA RCS Eng. 1975. Cons. Anaesth. Stobhill Hosp. Glas.

SLATER, Philip Denis Falmouth Health Centre, Trevaylor Road, Falmouth TR11 2LH Tel: 01326 317317; Timminoggy, 20 Boscawen Road, Falmouth TR11 4EN — MB BS Lond. 1970 (St. Mary's) MRCS Eng. LRCP Lond. 1970.

SLATER, Mr Richard Northern General Hospital , Department of Coloproctology, Herries Road, Sheffield S5 7AU Tel: 0114 2434343 — BM BS Nottm. 1993 (Nottingham) BMedSci (Hons.) Nottm. 1991; FRCS (Eng) 1998. SpR Gen. Surg. Specialty: Gen. Surg. Socs: Fell. Of Roy. Coll. of Surg. Of Eng.

SLATER, Mr Robert Neil Summers Department of Orthopaedic Surgery, The Maidstone Hospital, Hermitage Lane, Maidstone ME16 9NN Tel: 01622 729000; 1 Clare Wood Drive, West Malling, West Malling ME19 6PA Tel: 01732 875292 — MB BChir Camb. 1984; MB Camb. 1984; FRCS Ed. 1987; FRCS (Orth.) 1992. Cons. Orthop. Surg. Maidstone Hosp. Specialty: Orthop. Socs: Fell. Roy. Soc. Med. (Orthop. Sect.); Brit. Orthop. Assn. Prev: Sen. Regist. (Orthop.) Guy's & St. Thos. Hosp. Lond.

SLATER, Roger Martin Department of Anaesthesia, Manchester Royal Infirmary, Oxford Road, Manchester M13 9WL Tel: 0161 276 4551; 41 Eyebrook Road, Bowdon, Altrincham WA14 3LQ — MB BCh Manch. 1979 (St Andrews and Manchester Medical School) BSc (Med. Sci.) 1976; MB ChB Manch. 1979; MRCP (UK) 1982; FFA RCS Eng. 1984. Cons. Anaesth. Manch. Roy. Infirm. Specialty: Anaesth.; Intens. Care. Socs: BMA; Assn. Anaesth.; Intens. Care Soc. Prev: Cons. Anaesth. Univ. Hosp. Nottm.; Sen. Regist. (Anaesth.) N. West. RHA.

SLATER, Mr Ronald MacCallum Westward, 39 Sheridan Drive, Helens Bay, Bangor BT19 1LB Tel: 01247 852373 — MB BCh BAO Belf. 1955; DObst RCOG 1957; FRCS Ed. 1964. Cons. Plastic Surg. Ulster Hosp. Dundonald. Roy. Vict. Hosp. & Belf. Hosp. Sick Childr. Specialty: Plastic Surg.

SLATER, Sarah Elizabeth — MB BS Lond. 1989 (St. Barts.) MRCP 1993; MD 2000; CSST Medical Oncology 2001. Specialist Regist. (Med. Oncol.) & Hon. Lect. St. Barts. Hosp. Lond. Specialty: Oncol. Prev: Clin. Res. Fell. ICRF.

SLATER, Stefan Daniel (retired) 80 Whitehouse Road, Cramond, Edinburgh EH4 6PD Email: avowood@hotmail.com — MB ChB Glas. 1963; MRCP (UK) 1969; MD (Hons.) Glas. 1975; FRCP Glas. 1978; FRCP Lond. 1990; FRCP Ed 1998. Locum Cons. Phys. Work; Examr., Roy. Col. Prev: Hon. Sec. RCPS Glas. 1995-8.

SLATER, Susan Denise 10 Woodside Road, Beaconsfield HP9 1JG — MB BS Lond. 1987; MSc Lond. 1989, MB BS 1987; MRCPath 1996. Cons. Wexham Pk. Hosp. Slough. Specialty: Pathology, General. Prev: Cons. & Hon. Sen. Lect. Univ. Coll. Hosp. Lond.; Clin. Lect. (Histopath.) Univ. Coll. Hosp. Lond.; Regist. (Histopath.) Roy. Marsden Hosp. Lond.

SLATER, Victoria Margaret Anne 14 Rowan Crescent, Lenzie, Glasgow G66 4RE; 283 Crow Road, 3rd Floor Left, Glasgow G33 7BQ Tel: 0141 357 1279 — MB ChB Glas. 1993. GP Regist. Specialty: Gen. Pract. Prev: SHO (Neonat. Med.) Irvine Centr. Hosp.; SHO (Gen. Paediat.) CrossHo. Hosp. Kilmarnock; SHO (O & G) Monklands & Beushin NHS Trust.

SLATER, Wendy Jane Ardroy, Westpark Road, Blairgowrie PH10 6EL — MB ChB Glas. 1994.

SLATFORD, Kenneth Royal Edinburgh Hospital, Morningside Park, Edinburgh EH10 5HF Tel: 0131 537 6000 — MB ChB Glas. 1978 (Glasgow) BSc (Hons.) Glas. 1976; MRCPsych 1987; MPHil Ed. 1992; FRCP 1998; FRCPsych 2003. Cons. Gen. Psychiat. Roy. Edin. Hosp.; Hon. Sen. Lect. Univ. Edin. Specialty: Gen. Psychiat. Socs: Fell. Roy. Coll. Phys. Edin. Prev: Cons. Psychiat. Rosslynlee Hosp.; Sen. Regist. (Psychiat.) Roy. Edin. Hosp.

SLATOR, David Anthony Assynt Med. Centre, Main St., Lochinver, Lairg IV27 4JZ Tel: 01571 844755 — BM BCh Oxf. 1977; MA, BM BCh Oxf. 1977; MRCGP 1982.

SLATOR, James (retired) 20 Cromer Road, Holt NR25 6DX Tel: 01263 712129 — BM BCh Oxf. 1947; FRCP Ed. 1979.

SLATOR, Rona Caroline The Children's Hospital, Steelhouse Lane, Birmingham B4 6NH Tel: 0121 333 8132 Fax: 0121 333 8131 — MB BS Lond. 1984; DPhil Oxf. 1982; FRCS 1989; FRCS (Plast) 1995. Cons. Plastic Surg. Childr. Hosp. Birm. Specialty: Plastic Surg.

SLATTER, Elaine (retired) St. Fillans, 8 Woodham Road, Woking GU21 4DL — (Roy. Free) MB BS Lond. 1965; MRCS Eng. LRCP Lond. 1965. Prev: Med. Off. Surrey AHA.

SLATTER, Kenneth Hubert (retired) Hinderton Hall Farm, Chester High Road, Neston, South Wirral CH64 7TU Tel: 0151 336 1781 — (Liverp.) MB ChB Liverp. 1943; FRCP Lond. 1971, M 1951; MD Liverp. 1957. Prev: Emerit. Cons. Neurol. (Med. & Surg. Neurol.) Walton Hosp. Liverp.

SLATTER, Mary Anne Newcastle General Hospital, Westgate Road, Newcastle upon Tyne NE4 6BE Tel: 0191 273 8811 Fax: 0191 273 0183; 15 Harley Terrace, Newcastle upon Tyne NE3 1UL — MB ChB Bristol 1987; MRCP (UK) 1993. Assoc. Spec. Paediat. Childr.s Bone Marrow Transpl.ation; Paediat.,Nyankunde, democratic rePub. of Cango. Specialty: Paediat. Prev: SHO (Paediat.) Southmead Hosp. Bristol; Regist. Community Paediat., Leeds.

SLATTERY, David Antony Douglas, MBE (retired) 99 South Quay, Wapping Dock, Liverpool L3 4BW Email: david@slatt30.freeserve.co.uk — MB BS Lond. 1953 (St Thomas Lond) DIH Soc. Apoth. Lond. 1961; FFOM RCPI 1977; FFOM RCP Lond. 1981; FRCP Lond. 1986. Hon. Civil Cons. (Occupat. Med.) RAF. Prev: Adviser Occupat. Health Policy Mersey RHA 1992-94.

SLATTERY, Maria Anna Preston Park Surgery, 2A Florence Rd, Brighton BN1 6DJ Tel: 01273 559601 Fax: 01273 507746 — MB BS Lond. 1994; DRCOG 1997; MRCGP 1999; DFFP 2000. GP Princip. Preston Pk. Surg. Brighton. Specialty: Gen. Pract. Prev: Clin. Asst. in Psychiat. Priory Clinic, Hove.

SLATTERY, Michael Anthony Orford Lodge Surgery, 100 Bancroft, Hitchin SG5 1ND Tel: 01462 432042 Fax: 01462 436505 — MB BCh BAO NUI 1976; DRCOG 1978; MRCGP 1980; DCH Dub. 1981; Dip. In Primary Care Therap., Imperial Coll. Of Sci. Techn. & Med. 2000. GP Hitchin.

SLATTERY, Zoë Taschereau (retired) The Limes, The Street, Walsham Le Willows, Bury St Edmunds IP31 3AZ Tel: 01359 259422 — MB BS Lond. 1948 (Roy. Free) DCH Eng. 1951; FRCPsych 1985, M 1974. Prev: Cons. Psychiat. W. Suff. Gen. Hosp. Bury St. Edmunds.

SLAVIK, Zdenek Paediatric Intensive Care Unit, Royal Brompton Hospital, Sydney Street, London SW3 6NP Tel: 020 7352 8121 Fax: 020 7351 8547 — MD Prague 1982; MD Charles U Prague 1982; DM Soton. 1998. Cons. Paediatric Cardiol., Intens. Care, Roy. Brompton Hosp., Lond. Specialty: Paediat. Cardiol.; Paediat. Prev: Vis. Prof., Chas. U Pilsen 2000; Cons. Paediat. Cardiol./Intens. Care Hosp. Harefield Harefield.

SLAVIN, Brenda Mary (retired) 8 Normanhurst Park, Darley Dale, Matlock DE4 3BQ Tel: 01629 375644 — MB ChB Ed. 1957; BSc Witwatersrand 1953; FRCPath 1984, M 1972; MCB Roy. Inst. Chem. 1972. Prev: Prof. Path. Al Quds Univ. Jerusalem.

SLAVIN, Brendan Michael 1 Yeats Close, Newport Pagnell MK16 8RD Tel: 01908 617371 — BSc Lond. 1982; MB BS Lond. 1985; FRCA 1992. Cons. Anaesth. Milton Keynes Gen. Hosp. Specialty: Anaesth. Socs: Assn. Anaesth. GB & Irel.; Obst. Anaesth. Assn. Prev: Sen. Regist. W. Midl. Anaesth. Train. Scheme; SHO (Anaesth.) Oxon. HA; Ho. Phys. Roy. Free Hosp. Lond.

SLAVIN, Professor Gerard (retired) 8 Normanhurst Park, Darley Dale, Matlock DE4 3BQ Tel: 01629 735644 Email: gsbms@darleyd.fsnet.co.uk — MB ChB Ed. 1957; FRCP Glas. 1979, M 1963; DPath Eng. 1964; FRCPath 1979, M 1967; FGS 2000; BSc Lond. 2001. Emerit. Prof. Histopath. St. Bart. Med. Coll. Lond. Prev: Prof. Histopath. St. Bart. Hosp. Med. Coll. Lond.

SLAVIN, James Andrew Hunter Health Centre, Andrew Street, East Kilbride, Glasgow G74 1AD Tel: 01355 906655 — MB ChB Glas. 1988; MRCGP 1994. Gen. Med. Practitioner Princip. Hunter Health Centre E. Kilbridge.

SLAVIN, Mr John Patrick Department of Surgery, Mid Cheshire Hospital, NHS Trust, Leighton Hospital, Crewe CW1 4QJ Tel: 01270 612 441 Fax: 01270 612 046 Email: j.slavin@mcht.nhs.uk — MB BS (Distinc.) Lond. 1984; FRCS Eng. 1984; BSc (1st cl. Hons.) Lond. 1981, MS 1995. Cons. Gen. Surg., NHS Hosps. Trust, Chesh.

Specialty: Gen. Surg. Special Interest: ERCP; GI Surg. Socs: Assn. of Upper GI Surgeons; Assn. of Surg., Gt. Britain & Irel. Prev: Sen. Regist. (Surg.) Roy. Liverp. Univ. Hosp.; Regist. (Surg.) Westm. Hosp. & Mersey RHA; Research Fell. (Surg.) Univ. Calif., San Francisco, USA.

SLAVOTINEK, Anne Michele c/o Department of Clinical Genetics, Churchill Hospital, Old Road, Oxford OX3 7LJ; 8 Barrett Street, Osney, Oxford OX2 0AT Tel: 01865 248002 — MB BS Adelaide 1987. Specialty: Genetics.

SLAWSON, Jane Ann Frinton Road Medical Centre, 68 Frinton Road, Holland-on-Sea, Clacton-on-Sea CO15 5UW Tel: 01255 421778 Fax: 01255 812384 — MB ChB Leic. 1985; DGM RCP Lond. 1987; DRCOG 1989; MRCGP 1991.

SLAWSON, Keith Brian (retired) 27 Craigmount View, Edinburgh EH12 8BS Tel: 0131 339 4786 Email: brianslawson@blueyonder.co.uk — MB ChB Ed. 1958; BSc Ed. 1955; FRCA 1962; Dip. Sports Med. 1997. Prev: Cons. Anaseth. E. Gen. Hosp. Edin.

SLAYMAKER, Ann Elizabeth Leeds General Infirmary, Great George St., Leeds LS1 3EX; The Gables, 8 Old Vicarage Lane, Monk Fryston, Leeds LS25 5EA — MB ChB Leeds 1990; FRCA 1996. Specialist Regist. (Anaesth.) Leeds. Gen. Infirm. Specialty: Anaesth. Prev: Regist. & SHO (Anaesth.) Leeds Gen. Infirm.

SLEAP, Angela Gillian The Surgery, Evercreech, Shepton Mallet BA4 6JY; Oak cottage, Kingsdon, Somerton TA11 7JU — BM Soton. 1978. GP Assoc. Specialty: Gen. Pract.

SLEAP, Peter Guy Frederick Oak Cottage, Kingsdon, Somerton TA11 7JU — MB ChB Ed. 1971. Staff Grade (Anaesth.) Yeovil Dist. Hosp. Som. Specialty: Anaesth. Prev: GP Anaesth. Shell Petroleum Port HarCt., Nigeria.

SLEATH, Jonathan Duncan The Surgery, Kingstone, Hereford HR2 9HN Tel: 01981 250215 Fax: 01981 251189; The Villa, Kingstone, Hereford HR2 9ET — BM BCh Oxf. 1985; MA Camb. 1986; DRCOG 1988; MRCGP 1990. Socs: BMA. Prev: Med. Asst. St. Michael's Hospice Hereford; SHO Dr. MacKinnon Memor. Hosp. Isle-of-Skye; Ho. Surg. John Radcliffe Hosp. Oxf.

SLEATOR, Alexandra Moira Gay Fynescourt, Boundary Road, Grayshott, Hindhead GU26 6TX — MB BCh BAO Dub. 1972.

SLEATOR, David John Douglas West Surrey Health Authority, The Ridgewood Centre, Old Bisley Road, Camberley GU16 9QE Tel: 01276 671718 Fax: 01276 605491 — MB BCh BAO Dub. 1972; BA Dub. 1970; MSc 1998. Head of Clin. Developm. W. Surrey Health Auth. Camberley. Prev: Med. Adviser Surrey FHSA Surbiton; GP Hindhead Surrey; Ho. Phys. & Ho. Surg. Sir P. Dun's Hosp. Dub.

SLEE, Mr Gerald Charles Lindley House, Hinton Road, Hereford HR2 6BN Tel: 01432 272827 Fax: 01432 272827 Email: gerald.slee@zen.co.uk — MB ChB Liverp. 1947; FRCS Eng. 1953; MChOrth Liverp. 1955. Medico-Legal Pract. (Orth. & Traum.). Specialty: Orthop. Socs: Girdlestone Orthopaedic Soc.; Brit. Soc. Surg. of Hand.; Fell. Brit. Orthop. Assn. Prev: Cons. Robt. Jones & Agnes Hunt Orthop. Hosp. Oswestry & Hereford Hosps.; Sen. Regist. Roy. Infirm. Edin. & Princess Margt. Rose Orthop.; Regist. Accid. Serv. Radcliffe Infirm. Oxf.

SLEE, Ivor Patterson 9 Salamander Quay, Lower Teddington Road, Hampton Wick, Kingston upon Thames KT1 4JB Tel: 020 8977 5616 Fax: 020 8977 5616 Email: steamlaunch@amserve.com — MB BS Lond. 1960 (St. Thos.) FFA RCS Eng. 1966. Cons. Anaesth. Char. Cross Hosp. Lond. Specialty: Anaesth. Socs: Roy. Soc. Med.; Med. Sect. of Roy. Photographic Soc. Prev: Sen. Regist. St. Geo. Hosp. Lond.; Regist. (Anaesth.) & Ho. Off. (Orthop. & Plastic Surg.) St. Thos. Hosp. Lond.

SLEEMAN, Martin Lamont Derwent Practice, Norton Road, Malton YO17 9RF Tel: 01653 600069 Fax: 01653 698014; Paddock House, Swinton Grange, Malton YO17 6QP Tel: 01653 694168 — MB ChB Liverp. 1973; DObst RCOG 1976.

SLEEP, Tamsin Joanna Stoke, West Pentire, Crantock, Newquay TR8 5SE Email: tsleep@compuserve.com — BM BCh Oxf. 1993; BA (Hons.) Oxf. 1990; FRCOphth Lond. 1997. Specialist Regist. (Ophth.) Wessex Rotat. Specialty: Ophth. Prev: SHO (Ophth.) Qu. Med. Centre Nottm.

SLEET, Rodger Arthur (retired) Green Shutters, The Spinney, Bassett, Southampton SO16 7FW Tel: 023 8076 7310 — MB ChB Ed. 1959; FRCGP 1981, M 1968; FRCP Ed. 1987; FFAEM 1993. Prev: Cons. (A & E) Soton Univ. Hosps.

SLEGGS, John Hedworth Victoria Cross Surgery, 168/9 Victoria Road, Swindon SN1 3BU Tel: 01793 535584 Fax: 01793 497526; 11 Stratton Heights, Cirencester GL7 2RH Tel: 01285 651919 Email: johnsleggs@hotmail.com — MB ChB Manch. 1971; MRCP (UK) 1974; DTM & H Liverp. 1981; MRCGP 1988. Specialty: Gen. Med. Socs: Christ. Med. Fellowsh. Prev: Chief of Med., Patan Hosp., Kathmandu, Nepal 1997-1999; Specialist (Med.) Thimphu Gen. Hosp. Bhutan, 1981-1984; Hosp. Pract. (Med.) Cirencester Hosp. 1986-1997.

SLEIGH, Gillian Cheyne Child Development Service, Chelsea & Westminster Hospital, 369 Fulham Road, London SW10 9NH Tel: 020 8846 1286 Fax: 020 8846 1284; 1 Walton Crescent, Oxford OX1 2JG Tel: 01865 510206 Fax: 01865 510206 — (Roy. Free) MB BS Lond. 1963; DCH Eng. 1966; MRCP (UK) 1985. Cons. Paediat. (Community Child Health) Chelsea & Westm. Hosp. Lond. Specialty: Community Child Health. Socs: Brit. Paediat. Neurol. Assn.; Brit. Paediat. Assn.; Brit. Assn. for Community Child Health. Prev: Cons. Paediat. (Community Child Health) Univ. Hosp. Wales; SCMO Hugh Ellis Paediat. Assem. Centre Oxf.; Med. Dir. Princess Eliz. Centre Physically Handicap. Childr. Trinidad, W. Indies.

SLEIGH, John (retired) Bodran, St. Mary's Road, Monmouth NP25 3JE Tel: 01600 712899 — (St. And. & Aberd.) MB ChB Aberd. 1940; DPH Ed. 1946; BA Open 1984. Prev: Med. Off. Health S. Herefordsh. Co. Dists.

SLEIGHT, Claire Leila Wrangling Green, Castle Hill, Brenchley, Tonbridge TN12 7BX; Flat 5 Berrylands Lodge, 2 The Avenue, Surbiton KT5 8JQ Tel: 020 8287 5754 — MB BS Lond. 1996 (Charing Cross & Westminster London) Specialty: Gen. Pract.

SLEIGHT, Elizabeth (retired) Flat 4, 41 Sunderland Road, London SE23 2PS — MB ChB Sheff. 1987; DCH RCP Lond. 1991; MRCP (UK) 1992.

SLEIGHT, Mrs Gillian (retired) Wayside, 32 Crown Road, Wheatley, Oxford OX33 1UL Tel: 01865 872491 Fax: 01865 874169 — MB BS Lond. 1953 (St. Bart.) MRCS Eng. LRCP Lond. 1953. Prev: SCMO Community Health Oxon. HA.

SLEIGHT, Professor Peter Cardiovascular Medicine Dept, Level 5, John Radcliffe Hospital, Oxford OX3 9DU Tel: 01865 760564 Fax: 01865 768844; Wayside, 32 Crown Road, Wheatley, Oxford OX33 1UL Tel: 01865 872491 Fax: 01865 874169 — MB BChir Camb. 1953 (Camb. & St. Bart.) Hon. MD Univ. Pernambuco; DM Oxf. Stet; FRCP Lond. 1969, M 1957; MD Camb. 1965; MD Hon University of Gdansk 2000. Hon Cons. Cardiol., John Radcliffe Hosp.; Chairm. Isis Trials Gp; Emerit. Fell. Exeter Coll. Oxf.; Field Marshal Alexander Emerit. Prof. Cardiovasc. Med. Univ. Oxf. John Radcliffe Hosp Oxf. Specialty: Cardiol.; Gen. Med. Socs: (Ex-Pres.) Brit. Hypertens. Soc.; (Vice-Pres.) Action on Smoking & Health; (Ex-Counc.lor) Europ. Soc. Cardiol. Prev: Civil Cons. Med. RAF; Warren McDonald Fell. & Vis. Prof. Hallstrom Inst. Cardiol. Univ. Sydney; Cons. Phys. Cardiol. Radcliffe Infirm. Oxf.

SLEIGHT, Peter James Torbay Hospital, Lawes Bridge, Torquay TQ2 7AA Tel: 01803 614567 x 5516 Fax: 01803 616334; Old Vicarage, Orley Road, Ipplepen, Newton Abbot TQ12 5SA — (St. Bart.) MRCP UK 1977; MBBS Lond. 1973, MSc 1980; FRCP 1994. Specialty: Gen. Med.; Stroke Medicine.

SLEIGHT, Simon Paul Bridleway, 9 Woodrough Copse, Bramley, Guildford GU5 0HH — MB BS Lond. 1996.

SLEIGHT, Vivien Pamela (retired) Derrydown, Pouchen End Lane, Hemel Hempstead HP1 2SA Tel: 01442 876152 Fax: 01442 876151 Email: vsleight@doctors.org.uk — MB BS Lond. 1977 (Univ. Coll. Hosp.) MRCS Eng. LRCP Lond. 1977; LLM 1998.

SLEIGHTHOLM, Marcus Alexander Seacroft Hospital, York Road, Leeds LS14 6UH Tel: 0113 264 8164 — MD Liverp. 1988; MB ChB Liverp. 1979; MRCP (UK) 1983; FRCP 2001. Cons. Phys. Interest in Elderly Seacroft Hosp. Leeds; Sen. Lec. (Med.) Leeds Univ. Specialty: Gen. Med.

SLEMP, Margaret Christine Boundary House Surgery, Boundary House, Mount Lane, Bracknell RG12 9PG Tel: 01344 483900 Fax: 01344 862203; 5 Lawrence Grove, Bracknell RG42 4BL — MB BCh Wales 1975.

SLESENGER, Joseph Phillip Baronsmere Road Surgery, 39 Baronsmere Road, East Finchley, London N2 9QD Tel: 020 8883 1458 Fax: 020 883 8854 — MB ChB Manch. 1986; DGM RCP Lond. 1989; DCH RCP Lond. 1989; MRCGP 1990; DRCOG 1990. Prev: Trainee GP VTS.

SLESSOR, Ian Munro (retired) 2 Birch Tree Walk, Nascot Wood, Watford WD17 4SH Tel: 01923 236430 — MB ChB Aberd. 1956 (Aberd) MRCGP 1968; MSc CNAA 1978; FFPM RCP Lond. 1991. Prev: Med. Dir. Informat. Glaxo Gp. Research Ltd. Greenford.

SLEVIN, Maurice Louis 149 Harley Street, London W1G 6BN Tel: 020 7224 0685 Fax: 020 7224 1722 — MB ChB Cape Town 1973; MRCP (UK) 1978; MD Cape Town 1984; FRCP Lond. 1989. Cons. Phys. (Med. Oncol.) St Bart. Hosp. Lond. Specialty: Oncol. Prev: Lect. & Hon. Sen. Regist. (Med. Oncol.) St. Bart. Hosp. Lond.; Regist. (Med.) Groote Schuur Hosp. Cape Town; Regist. (Med. Oncol.) St. Bart. Hosp. Lond.

SLEVIN, Nicholas John Christie Hospital, Wilmslow Road, Manchester M20 4BX Tel: 0161 446 3361 — MB ChB Birm. 1978; MRCP (UK) 1981; FRCR 1987; FRCP 1998. Cons. Clinical Oncol. Christie Hosp. Manch. Specialty: Radiother.; Oncol. Special Interest: Non- Surgic. Managem. of Head & Neck Cancer. Prev: Sen. Regist. (Radioth. & Oncol.) Christie Hosp. Manch.; Regist. (Med.) ChristCh. Hosp., NZ.

SLEVIN, Paul Gerard Latham House Medical Practice, Sage Cross Street, Melton Mowbray LE13 1NX Tel: 01664 854949 Fax: 01664 501825 — MB BCh BAO NUI 1987 (Univ. Coll. Dub.) MRCOG 1995; DFFP 1995.

SLIBI, Mr Mahmoud 132 Woodway Lane, Coventry CV2 2EJ — MD Damascus 1986; FRCS Glas. 1994.

SLIGHT, Robert David 11 Boreland Park, Inverkeithing KY11 1ES — MB ChB Aberd. 1996.

SLIM, Jacqueline Margaret The Health Centre, Beeches, Green, Stroud GL5 4BH Tel: 01453 764471; Woodlands, South Woodchester, Stroud GL5 5EQ Tel: 01453 872158 — MB ChB Bristol 1987; DA (UK) 1991. GP Stroud Retainer Scheme. Specialty: Gen. Pract.

SLIMMINGS, Peter George The Surgery, 4 Stoke Road, Bishops Cleeve, Cheltenham GL52 8RP Tel: 01242 672007; Ivybank, Lye Lane, Cleeve Hill, Cheltenham GL52 3QD — MB ChB Birm. 1972; DObst RCOG 1975. Trainer GP Cheltenham VTS; Hosp. Pract. (Dermat.) Cheltenham Gen. Hosp. Specialty: Dermat. Prev: Ho. Surg. Qu. Eliz. Hosp. Birm.; Ho. Phys. & SHO (Gen. Med. & Infec. Dis.) E. Birm. Hosp.

SLINGER, Barry Christopher 14 The Grove, Shipley BD18 4LD — MB ChB St. And. 1971; DObst RCOG 1974; Dip Occ Med 1998.

SLINGER, Keith Michael Aldren Newton Lea, Westnewton, Wigton CA7 3NX Tel: 01697 320018 — MB ChB St. And. 1966; DA Eng. 1969.

SLINGSBY, Andrew John 49 Elmwood Close, Retford DN22 6SL — MB BS Lond. 1994 (Roy. Free Hosp.) DRCOG 1997. Prev: SHO (O & G) St. Richards Hosp. Chichester; SHO (ENT) Qu. Alexandra Hosp. Cosham; SHO Orthop. Epsom Gen. Hosp.

SLINN, Rebecca Mary Crichton Royal Hospital, Bankend Road, Dumfries DG2 0UX — MB BS Lond. 1991 (St Barts.) MRCPsych 1996. Cons. (Old Age Psychiat.) Stewartry & Wigtonsh. Specialty: Geriat. Psychiat. Special Interest: Dementia.

SLOAN, Barbara Elizabeth Horton Bank Practice, 1220 Great Horton Road, Bradford BD7 4PL Tel: 01274 410666 Fax: 01274 521605; 11 Paternoster Lane, Bradford BD7 3DS Tel: 01274 410666 Fax: 01274 521608 — MB ChB Leeds 1977; DRCOG 1979; Cert. Family Plann. JCC 1981; DCH RCP Eng. 1981; MRCGP 1981. Clin. Asst. (Obst.) St. Luke's Hosp. Bradford. Specialty: Gen. Pract.

SLOAN, Catherine Emma Linda 5 Hyde Close, Bromsgrove, Worcester B60 2RF — MB ChB Birm. 1996 (Birmingham) GP Retainer Worcs & Warwks. Specialty: Otolaryngol. Prev: ENT; A&E; Orthop.

SLOAN, David John Barking & Havering FHSA, St. Georges Hospital, Suttons Lane, Hornchurch RM12 6SD Tel: 014024 72011; 5 Elrington Road, Hackney, London E8 3BJ Tel: 020 7249 2471 — MB BChir Camb. 1972 (Camb. & St. Bart.) MA, MB Camb. 1972, BChir 1971; MRCP (UK) 1975; DRCOG 1977; MRCGP 1978. Med. Adviser Barking & Havering FHSA. Prev: SHO (Paediat.) Qu. Eliz. Hosp. Childr. Lond.; Princip GP. Hackney; Ho. Off. Poole Gen. Hosp.

SLOAN, David John (retired) 48 Main Street, Ballycarry, Carrickfergus BT38 9HH — MB BCh BAO Belf. 1954 (Qu. Univ. Belf.) DPH Eng. 1967; FFCM RCPI 1985, M 1978; MFCM 1985. Prev: Dep. Chief Med. Off. DHSS N. Irel.

SLOAN, David Robert (retired) Flat 4, Marlborough House, Marlborough Hill, Kingsdown, Bristol BS2 8EZ Tel: 0117 929 1781 — MB ChB Glas. 1938 (Univ. Glas.) Prev: Ho. Surg. Dorset Co. Hosp.

SLOAN, Felicity Jane Family Planning Clinic, St. Paul's Wing, Cheltenham General Hospital, Sandford Road, Cheltenham GL53 7AN Tel: 01242 272375; Mulberry House, Cleeve Hill, Cheltenham GL52 3QE Tel: 01242 241290 Fax: 01242 571292 — MB BS Lond. 1972 (St. Mary's) MFFP 1995 Fac. of Fam. Planning RCOG; Dobst RCOG 1974. Head of Family Plann. Reproductive Health E. Glos. NHS Trust; Clin. Asst. Pregn. Advis. Clinic Cheltenham Gen. Hosp. Specialty: Family Plann. & Reproduc. Health; Obst. & Gyn. Prev: Clin. Med. Off. (Child Health) Glos. HA.; GP Princip.

SLOAN, Geoffrey Drew 7 Montrose Avenue, West Didsbury, Manchester M20 2LA Tel: 0161 434 0256 — MB ChB Ed. 1996 (Edinburgh) BSc (Hons) 1993. SHO (A & E) Manch. Specialty: Accid. & Emerg.

SLOAN, Herbert Hill, TD (retired) Glenwherry, Blackburn Old Road, Great Harwood, Blackburn BB6 7UW Tel: 01254 885070 Fax: 01254 885070 Email: herbiesloanh@aol.com — MB BCh BAO Belf. 1947. Prev: GP.

SLOAN, James Martin Pathology Department, Royal Victoria Hospital, Grosvenor Road, Belfast BT12 6BL — MB BCh BAO Belf. 1964; DObst RCOG 1966; MD Belf. 1969; FRCPath 1984, M 1972. Cons. (Path.) Roy. Vict. Hosp. Belf. Specialty: Histopath. Prev: Reader (Path.) Qu. Univ. Belf. & Cons. Path. Roy. Vict. Hosp. Belf.; Lect. (Path.) Univ. Sheff.; Path. ICI Pharmaceut. Div. Macclesfield.

SLOAN, John Bankier Hunter Health Centre, Andrew Street, East Kilbride, Glasgow G74 1AD Tel: 01355 906639 Email: john.sloan@hunter.lanpct.scot.nhs.uk — MB ChB Glas. 1987 (Glasgow) MRCGP 1991; DGM RCP Glas. 1992; DRCOG 1994; LFHom RCP Lond. 1995; MBA Open Univ. 2001. Specialty: Gen. Pract.

SLOAN, Mr John Peter 357 Street Lane, Moortown, Leeds LS17 6RU Tel: 0113 293 5628 Fax: 0113 266 5924 — BM BS Nottm. 1978; BMedSci Nottm. 1976; FRCS Glas. 1982; FRCS Ed. 1985; FFAEM 1994. Cons. A & E Gen. Infirm. Leeds; Sen. Clin. Lect. (Surg.) Univ. Leeds. Specialty: Accid. & Emerg. Socs: Brit. Assn. Accid. & Emerg. Med.; Emerg. Med. Research Soc. Prev: Sen. Regist. (A & E) Univ. Hosp. Nottm. & Roy. Infirm. Derby.

SLOAN, Kathleen — MB ChB Aberd. 1993; MRCGP. SHO (O & G) Glas. Roy. Matern. Hosp. Specialty: Obst. & Gyn. Prev: SHO (A & E) Vale of Leven Dist. Gen. Hosp.; SHO (Oncol.) Beatson Oncol. Centre; SHO (O & G) Llandough Hosp. NHS Trust.

SLOAN, Linda Margaret Sloan Practice, 251 Chesterfield Road, Sheffield S8 0RT Tel: 0114 255 1164 Fax: 0114 258 9006 — MB ChB Leeds 1977; DRCOG 1980.

SLOAN, Lorna Doris Elspeth — MB BCh BAO Belf. 1979 (Queens University of Belfast) DA (S. Afr.) 1982; DTM & H Liverp. 1983; DRCOG 1984; MRCGP 1985; Dip. Occ. Med. 1996.

SLOAN, Lucy Malcolm Drs Gillies, Gillies & Crosby, 6 Church Place, Moffat DG10; Glendale, Lochmaben, Lockerbie DG11 1RF — MB ChB Ed. 1984; DRCOG 1986. Retainer GP Moffat. Prev: Trainee GP Dumfries VTS; Retainer GP Lockerbie.

SLOAN, Marian Kathleen Department of Anaesthetics, Belfast City Hospital, Belfast; 29 Malone Meadows, Belfast BT9 5BG — MB BCh BAO Belf. 1978. Staff Grade (Anaesth.) Belf. City Hosp. Specialty: Anaesth.

SLOAN, Marion Edith Sloan Practice, 251 Chesterfield Road, Sheffield S8 0RT Tel: 0114 255 1164 Fax: 0114 258 9006 — MB ChB Leeds 1975; MB ChB (Hons.) Leeds 1975; MRCP (UK) 1978; MRCGP 1982. Teach. Gen. Pract. Dept. Community Med. Univ. Sheff. Med. Sch.; Clin. Asst. Dept. Gastroenterol. Roy. Hallamsh. Hosp. Sheff.

SLOAN, Mark Anthony Regent House Surgery, 21 Regent Road, Chorley PR7 2DH Tel: 01257 264842 Fax: 01257 231387 — MB BS Lond. 1984; MRCGP 1990.

SLOAN, Melanie Gail Rose Isle, Aldie Crescent, Darnick, Melrose TD6 9AY — MB ChB Glas. 1997; DRCOG 2000; MRCGP 2001.

SLOAN, Morag Elizabeth Holland House, 31 Church Road, Lytham, Lytham St Annes FY8 5LL Tel: 01253 794999 Fax: 01253 795744 — MB ChB Aberd. 1986; MRCGP 1992. Police Surg.

Preston. Prev: Trainee GP Gt. Eccleston; SHO (Geriat.) Lancaster HA; SHO (Med., Haemat. & A & E) Blackpool & Wyre HA.

SLOAN, Myra Caroline Spencer Place Medical Practice, Chapeltown Health Centre, Spencer Place, Leeds LS7 4BB Tel: 0113 240 9090 Fax: 0113 249 8480; 357 Street Lane, Moortown, Leeds LS17 6RU Tel: 0113 266 5924 — BM BS Nottm. 1978; BMedSci Nottm. 1976. GP Princip. Leeds. Specialty: Gen. Pract. Prev: Trainee GP Nottm. VTS.

SLOAN, Peter John McLean Haslucks Green Road Surgery, 287 Haslucks Green Road, Shirley, Solihull B90 2LW Tel: 0121 744 6663 Fax: 0121 733 6895 — MB ChB Sheff. 1977; MRCP (UK) 1980. Princip. GP Solihull.

SLOAN, Richard Davidson Craigshill Health Centre, Craigshill Road, Livingston EH54 5DY Tel: 01506 432621 Fax: 01506 430431; South Lodge, Kirknewton EH27 8DA Tel: 01506 880286 Email: richard_kelsey@compuserve.com — BM BS Nottm. 1984; BMedSci (Hons.) Nottm. 1982, BM BS 1984; DRCOG 1989; MRCGP 1990; DFFP 1996; DPD 1997. Clin. Asst. in Diabetes St. John's Hosp. Livingston BUPA Health Screening Edin.

SLOAN, Richard Ernest George Tieve Tara, Rear of Park Dale, Airedale, Castleford WF10 2QT Tel: 01977 552360 Fax: 01977 603470 — MB BS Lond. 1969; PhD (Med.) Lond. 1976, BSc (Anat.) 1966, MB BS 1969; MRCGP 1984; FRCGP 2002. Assoc. Director of Postgrad. Gen. Pract., Yorks. Deanery. Prev: Lect. (Physiol.) Lond. Hosp. Med. Coll.; Ho. Phys. Mile End Hosp. (Lond. Hosp.); Ho. Surg. Lond. Hosp.

SLOAN, Richard Herbert 4 Southwalks Road, Dorchester DT1 1ED — MB BS Lond. 1976 (St. Mary's) MRCS Eng. LRCP Lond. 1976; DA Eng. 1978; DRCOG 1980; MRCGP 1983. Med. Dir. Joseph Weld Hse. Hospice-Respite Centre Dorchester; Hon. Cons. Palliat. Med. W. Dorset Gen. Hosps. NHS Trust. Specialty: Palliat. Med. Prev: Regist. (Palliat. Med.) St. Christopher's Hospice Lond.; GP W.way Med. Centre Merseyside; Sen. Lect. (Gen. Pract.) Univ. Liverp.

SLOAN, Robert Lance Fife Rehabilitation Service, Sir George Sharp Unit, Cameron Hospital, Cameron Bridge, Windygates, Leven KY8 5RR Tel: 01592 712472 Fax: 01592 715851; Berwyn, James Place, Cupar KY15 5JT Tel: 01334 652564 — MB ChB Aberd. 1981 (University of Aberdeen) MRCP (UK) 1986; FRCP Ed 1998. Cons. Rehabil. Med. Fife Primary Care NHS Trust. Specialty: Rehabil. Med. Socs: Soc. Research Rehabil. & Brit. Soc. Rehabil. Med. Prev: Sen. Regist. (Rehabil. Med.) Astley Ainslie Hosp. Edin.; Regist. Profess. Rheum. Dis. Unit North. Gen. Hosp. Edin.; Regist. Rotat. (Med.) The Lond. Hosp.

SLOAN, Rosemary 1 Shanlieve Court, Hilltown, Newry BT34 5YP — MB BCh BAO Belf. 1994.

SLOAN, Samantha Anne 18 Sandyknowes Drive, Newtownabbey BT36 5DF — MB BCh BAO Belf. 1994.

SLOAN, Samuel, SBStJ 25 Dunmurry Lane, Dunmurry, Belfast BT17 9RP Tel: 01232 301934 — MB BCh BAO Belf. 1945. Apptd. Fact. Med. Off. Falls Flax Spinning Co. Ltd. Belf. & Irish Linen Mills Ltd. Belf.; Co. Surg. St. John Ambul. Brig. (Cadets). Socs: Roy. Coll. Gen. Pract.; BMA & Belf. Postgrad. Soc. Prev: Teach. Domicilary Midw. Roy. Matern. Hosp. Belf.

SLOAN, Sara Barbara Sloan Practice, 251 Chesterfield Road, Sheffield S8 0RT Tel: 0114 255 1164 Fax: 0114 258 9006; 73 Ranmoor Road, Sheffield S10 3HJ — MB ChB Leeds 1980; DRCOG 1983; MRCGP 1984; DCCH RCP Ed. 1985; DTM & H Liverp. 1987.

SLOAN, Stanley Buchanan (retired) 63 Cricketers Lane, Herongate, Brentwood CM13 3QB — (T.C. Dub.) MB BCh BAO Dub. 1949; MA Dub. 1949; MRCGP 1970; Cert. Family Plann. JCC 1974. Prev: Med. Pract. 1950-85.

SLOAN, Stephanie Caroline 22 Balmoral Av, Belfast BT9 6NW — MB BCh BAO Belf. 1997.

SLOCOMBE, Gareth Wynne 39 Sutton Road, Shrewsbury SY2 6DL — MB BS Lond. 1977; BSc Lond. 1974, MB BS 1977; MRCP (UK) 1980; MRCPath 1983. Cons. Haemat. Princess Roy. Hosp. Telford. Specialty: Haematology. Prev: Sen. Regist. (Haemat.) Lond. Hosp.

SLOCOMBE, Robert Leslie Wymondham Medical Practice, Postmill Close, Wymondham NR18 0RF Tel: 01953 602118 Fax: 01953 605313; 21 Hawthorn Close, Spixwoth, Norwich NR10 3RD Tel: 01603 891563 Fax: 01603 891563 — MB BChir Camb. 1986; MRCGP 1991; DFFP 2000. p/t Asst. GP. Specialty: Gen. Pract. Prev: Trainee GP W. Suff. HA.

SLOCZYNSKA, Christine Wanda Specialist Community Childrens Services, Azalea Ward, Whipps Cross University Hospital, Whipps Cross Road, Leytonstone, London E11 1NR Tel: 020 8535 6705; 3 Ashbourne Avenue, South Woodford, London E18 1PQ Tel: 020 8989 7212 — MB ChB Ed. 1976 (Univ. Ed.) DCH RCP Eng. 1979; MRCPCH 1996. Cons. Community Paediat., Waltham Forest Primary Care Trust. Specialty: Community Child Health. Socs: RCPCH; BACCH; BASPCAN. Prev: SCMO (Child Health) Forest Healthcare Trust.

SLOKA, Richard Anthony 30 Broadmead, Heswall, Wirral CH60 1XD — MB ChB Liverp. 1974; DMRD Liverp. 1978; FRCR 1981. Cons. Radiol. Countess of Chester Hosp. Chester. Specialty: Radiol.

SLOLEY, Lorna Jane The Hole in the Wall, Bosham Lane, Bosham, Chichester PO18 8HG — MB BS Lond. 1997.

SLOME, John Joseph 146 Walm Lane, London NW2 4RU Tel: 020 8452 1973 — MRCS Eng. LRCP Lond. 1952 (St. Geo.) MB BS Lond. 1954; DObst RCOG 1956; DIH Eng. 1959, DCH 1957; DPH Lond. 1958.

SLOMINSKI, Henryk Bronislaw Mere Green Surgery, Carlton House, Mere Green Road, Sutton Coldfield B75 5BS Tel: 0121 308 0918/0121 308 2137 — MB ChB Birm. 1975.

SLOMKA, Henryk Withycombe Lodge Surgery, 123 Torquay Road, Paignton TQ3 2SG Tel: 01803 525525 Fax: 01803 550314 — BM BS Nottm. 1975; BMedSci Nottm. 1973, BM BS 1975. Princip. GP Devon.

SLOPER, Constance Myra Louise 46 New Park Road, Newgate Street Village, Hertford SG13 8RF — BM BCh Oxf. 1973 (University of Oxford & Royal London Hospital) MRCP (UK) 1983; DO RCPSI 1991; FRCOphth 1992. Locum Cons., The Nat. Hosp. for Neurol. & Neurosurg., Lond.. Specialty: Ophth. Special Interest: Immuno-suppression. Prev: Sen. Regist. (Med. Ophth.) Univ. Hosp. Nottm.; Research Fell. Univ. Hosp. Nottm.; SHO Oxf. Eye Hosp.

SLOPER, Irene Mary Susan (retired) 43 Sandy Lodge Road, Rickmansworth WD3 1LN Tel: 01923 823100 — MB BChir Camb. 1945 (King's Coll. Hosp.) MRCS Eng. LRCP Lond. 1945; DObst RCOG 1947. Prev: Assoc. Specialist Matern. Unit Watford Gen. Hosp.

SLOPER, Mr John Jenvey — BM BCh Oxf. 1975; DPhil Oxf. 1978; DO RCS Eng. 1989; FRCS Ed. 1990; FRCOphth 1991. Cons. Strabismus & Paediat. Servs. Moorfields Eye Hosp. Specialty: Ophth. Prev: Sen. Regist. (Ophth.) Univ. Hosp. Nottm.; Regist. (Ophth.) Roy. Vict. Hosp. Belf.; Roy. Soc. Research Fell. Univ. Oxf.

SLOPER, Katherine Susan Department of Paediatrics, Ealing Hospital NHS Trust, Southall UB1 3HX Fax: 020 8967 5445 — BM BCh Oxf. 1973; MRCP (UK) 1976; MA, DM Oxf. 1989; FRCP Lond. 1995; FRCPH 1998. Cons. Paediat. Ealing Hosp. NHS Trust Lond.; Hon. Clin. Sen. Lect., Imperial Coll. Sch. Med., Lond. Specialty: Paediat. Prev: Hon. Sen. Lect. Roy. Postgrad. Med. Sch. Lond.; Sen. Regist. (Paediat.) Centr. Middlx. Hosp. & Brompton Hosp. Lond.; Regist. (Paediat.) Middlx. Hosp. Lond.

SLOPER, Philip 46 New Park Road, Newgate St Village, Hertford SG13 8RF — MB BS Lond. 1998; MB BS Lond 1998.

SLOPER-AITCHISON, Marguerite Lucy (retired) Bod Awen, 19 Bridge Street, Llandeilo SA19 6BN Tel: 01558 822874 Email: margaret8@lineone.net — MB BS Lond. 1953 (St. Thos.) MRCS Eng. LRCP Lond. 1953.

SLORACH, Charles Cameron Stuart Hunter Health Centre, Andrew St., East Kilbride, Glasgow G74 1AD; (surgery) 126 Westwood Square, East Kilbride, Glasgow G75 8JQ — MB ChB Glas. 1953; DObst RCOG 1957. Prev: Sen. Ho. Phys. West. Dist. Hosp. Glas.; Flight Lt. RAF Med. Br.

SLORACH, Colum Alasdair Edinburgh Royal Infirmary, Old Dalkeith Road, Edinburgh EH16 4SU — MB ChB Glas. 1996; FRCA Lond. 2004. Specialist Regist. (Anaesth.) Edin. Roy. Infirm. Specialty: Anaesth.

SLORACH, John 58 Leicester Road, Narborough, Leicester LE19 2DG Tel: 0116 286 3169 — MB ChB Aberd. 1937; BSc Aberd. 1929, MB ChB 1937; DPM Eng. 1942. Cons. Emerit. Carlton Hayes Hosp. NarBoro.. Prev: Mem. Sheff. Region Ment. Health Rev. Tribunal; Dep. Phys. Supt. Pk. Prewett Hosp. Basingstoke; Assoc. Chief Asst. Skin (Psychosomatic) Dept. St. Bart. Hosp.

SLORACH, Marc 3 Stratford Close, Killingworth, Newcastle upon Tyne NE12 6GU — MB ChB Aberd. 1990; DRCOG 1995; DA (UK) 1995; MRCGP 1996. Specialty: Gen. Pract.

SLOSS, Gordon Alexander Sannox Farm, Sannox, Brodick KA27 Tel: 01770 81230 — MB BCh Wales 1989; BSc (Hons.) St. And. 1985; MRCPsych 1996. Specialist Regist. St. Mary's Hisher Psychiat. Train. Scheme Lond. Specialty: Gen. Psychiat. Prev: Regist. Rotat. (Psychiat.) St. Mary's Hosp. Lond.; SHO Rotat. (Psychiat.) Roy. United Hosp. Bath; Ho. Off. (Med. & Gen. Surg.) Univ. Wales Hosp. Cardiff.

SLOSS, John Dario Gregorio Grant The Old Vicarage, Crosthwaite, Kendal LA8 8BP — MB BS Lond. 1990.

SLOSS, John Murray Dept of Microbiology, Pathology Laboratory, Darlington Memorial Hospital, Darlington DL3 6HX Tel: 01325 743241 Fax: 01325 743622; 33 Wells Green, Barton, Richmond DL10 6NH Tel: 01325 339061 Fax: 01325 339061 — MB BS Lond. 1977 (St. Bart.) MSc Lond. 1989, BSc (Hons.) 1974; FRCS Ed. 1986; FRCPath 2000. Cons Med. Microbiol S. Durh. NHS Trust. Specialty: Med. Microbiol. Socs: Assn. Clin. Path.; Hosp. Infec. Soc.; Dales Microbiol. Audit Gp. Prev: Cons. Path. (Med. Microbiol.) BMH Rinteln BFPO 29; Cons. Path. (Med Microbiol.) Duchess of Kent Hosp. Catterick Garrison; Cons Path (Med Microbiol) MDHU Northallerton.

SLOT, Michael Joseph William Blackmore Health Centre, Blackmore Drive, Sidmouth EX10 8ET Tel: 01395 512601 Fax: 01395 578408 — MB ChB Bristol 1980; MB ChB Bristol 1980.

SLOTOVER, Mr Max Leonard (retired) 28 Arlington House, Arlington Street, London SW1A 1RL Tel: 020 7495 1870 Fax: 020 7495 6132; Le Roccabella, 24 Avenue Princess Grace, Monte Carlo, Monaco Fax: 00 377 9325 4975 — LRCPI & LM, LRSCI & LM 1934 (RCSI) LM Rotunda; FRCS Ed. 1939. Prev: Resid. Obst. Off. Withington Hosp. Manch.

SLOVAK, Andrej Jan Michal British Nuclear Fuels plc, Hinton House, Risley, Warrington WA6 3AS Tel: 01925 832890 Fax: 01925 835864; 102 Market Street, Ashby-de-la-Zouch LE65 1AP — MB BS Lond. 1970; MRCS Eng. LRCP Lond. 1970; DIH Soc. Apoth. Lond. 1976; FFOM RCP Lond. 1991; MD Lond. 1996; FRCP Lond. 1996. Chief Med. Off. Brit. Nuclear Fuels plc; Sen. Lect. Centre Occupat. Health Manch. Univ. Med. Sch. Specialty: Occupat. Health.

SLOVICK, David Ian Southend Hospital, Department of Medicine for the Elderly, Prittlewell Chase, Westcliff on Sea SS0 0RY Tel: 01702 221203 Fax: 01702 221377; 6 The Ridgeway, Westcliff on Sea SS0 8NT Tel: 01702 711115 — MB BS Lond. 1979 (Middlx.) MA Oxf. 1977; PhD Lond. 1977; MRCP (UK) 1983; FRCP Lond. 1999. Cons. Phys. Southend Health Care NHS Trust. Specialty: Care of the Elderly; Gen. Med. Socs: Fell. Roy. Soc. Med.; Brit. Geriat. Soc. Prev: Sen. Regist. (Gen. & Geriat. Med.) Hammersmith Hosp. Lond.; Sen. Med. Off. DoH Lond.; Ho. Phys. (Med.) Middlx. Hosp. Lond.

SLOVICK, Sidney 143 Sydenham Hill, London SE23 3PH Tel: 020 8693 3169 — MRCS Eng. LRCP Lond. 1947 (Univ. Coll. Hosp.) MRCGP 1959. Med. Examr. Pruden. Assur. Co. & United Friendly Insur. Co.; Mem. S.wark, Lambeth & Lewisham Family Pract. Comm. & Local Med. Comms. Socs: Brit. Assn. Manipulat. Med.; BMA (Ex-Chairm. Camberwell Div.). Prev: Flight Lt. RAF; Ho. Surg. Co. Hosp. FarnBoro. (Kent); Orthop. Ho. Surg. & Cas. Off. Roy. North. Hosp.

SLOWE, Michael Robert Ian Rookery Medical Centre, Rookery House, Newmarket CB8 8NW Tel: 01638 665711 Fax: 01638 561280; Wilwyn Cottage, 4 Hamilton Road, Newmarket CB8 0NQ — MB BS Lond. 1980 (Char. Cross) DRCOG 1982; MRCGP 1989. Clin. Asst. (Gastrointest. Endoscopy) W. Suff. Hosp. Prev: GP Hadlow, Kent; GP Trainee Tunbridge Wells VTS.

SLOWEY, Heather Frances Department of Anaesthetics, Singleton Hospital, Swansea SA2 8QA — MB BS Lond. 1976 (St. Mary's) MRCS Eng. LRCP Lond. 1976; FFA RCS Eng. 1981. Cons. Anaesth. (p/t), Singleton Hosp. Swansea. Specialty: Anaesth. Prev: Lect. (Anaesth.) Univ. Hosp. Wales Cardiff; Regist. (Anaesth.) Univ. Hosp. Wales Cardiff; SHO (Anaesth.) Nottm. Gen. Hosp.

SLOWIE, Dominic Francis 42 Warwick Street, Heaton, Newcastle upon Tyne NE6 5AQ — MB BS Newc. 1991. SHO (O & G) S. Cleveland Hosp. Middlesbrough. Prev: SHO (Med. Oncol.) Regional Radiother. Unit Newc. Gen. Hosp.

SLOWTHER, Christine Mary 1 Pembroke Close, Warwick CV34 5JA — MB ChB Manch. 1986.

SLUGLETT, Max (retired) 3 Dinard Drive, Glasgow G46 6AH Tel: 0141 633 1206 — MB ChB Glas. 1942.

SLY, Ian Leslie Colin The Meads Surgery, Grange Road, Uckfield TN22 1QU Tel: 01825 765777 Fax: 01825 766220; Lilac Cottage, Chillies Lane, High Hurstwood, Uckfield TN22 4AA — MB BS Lond. 1971 (Char. Cross) MRCS Eng. LRCP Lond. 1971; DCH Eng. 1974; MRCP (UK) 1977; MRCGP 1979. Prev: Regist. (Med.) Wycombe Gen. Hosp. High Wycombe; Regist. (Med.) High Wycombe AHA; SHO (Obst.) Derby City Hosp.

SLY, Janet Mary James Fisher Medical Centre, 4 Tolpuddle Gardens, Bournemouth BH9 3LQ Tel: 01202 522622 Fax: 01202 548480 — MB BS Newc. 1977; DRCOG 1981; MRCGP 1982. GP Bournemouth.

SLYNE, Denis Joseph 36 Ernest Street, Merthyr Tydfil CF47 0YP — MB BCh BAO NUI 1979; DRCOG 1983.

SMAHLIOUK, Petros c/o Ophthalmic Secretaries, Mayday University Hospital, London Road, Croydon CR7 7YE — Ptychio Iatrikes Thessalonika 1988.

SMAIL, Joanna Kathryn Frimley Park Hospital, Portsmouth Rd, Flimley, Camberley GU16 7UJ Tel: 01276 604604; 46 Dan-y-Bryn Avenue, Radyr, Cardiff CF15 8DD Tel: 01276 843230 — BM BCh Oxf. 1997; DCH 1999. Pre-Registration Ho. Off. (Gen. Surg.) Plymouth (February 1998). Specialty: Care of the Elderly. Prev: Pre-Registration Ho. Off. Gen. Med. Oxf. (August 1997).

SMAIL, Peter James Royal Aberdeen Children's Hospital, Aberdeen AB25 2ZG Tel: 01224 681818 Fax: 01224 550704 Email: p.smail@arh.grampian.scot.nhs.uk; 36 Ashley Gardens, Aberdeen AB10 6RQ Tel: 01224 325597 — (Oxf.) BM BCh Oxf. 1968; MA Oxf. 1968; DObst RCOG 1971; DCH RCPS Glas. 1974; FRCP Lond. 1987; FRCP Ed. 1995; FRCPCH 1997. Clin. Gp. Coordinator Combined Child Health Serv. Grampain Universities Hosps. Specialty: Paediat. Socs: Eur. Soc. Paediat. Endocrinol. Prev: Lect. (Child Health) Dundee Univ.; Fell. Health Sci. Centre Winnipeg; Regist. (Med.) Roy. Cornw. Hosp. (Treliske) Truro.

SMAIL, Professor Simon Andrew School of Postgraduate Studies, University of Wales College of Medicine, Heath Park, Cardiff CF14 4XN Tel: 029 2074 3927 Fax: 029 2075 4966 Email: postgrad@cardiff.ac.uk; 46 Dan-y-Bryn Avenue, Radyr, Cardiff CF15 8DD — BM BCh Oxf. 1970; MA Oxf. 1970; DRCOG 1973; DCH Eng. 1974; Cert. Family Plann. JCC 1975; FRCGP 1984 M (Distinc.) 1975; ILTM 2001. Dean & Dir. Sch. of Postgrad. Med. and Dent. Educat. Specialty: Educat.; Gen. Pract. Prev: Dir. Postgrad. Edu. For GP, Univ. Wales,Cardiff; Sen. Lect. (Gen. Pract.) Univ. Wales Coll. Med. Cardiff; Chairm. UK Conf. Postgrad. GP Adviser.

SMAILES, Catherine Mary 2 Ballard Close, Milton, Cambridge CB4 6DW — MB BS Lond. 1996.

SMAILES, June The Hollies Medical Centre, 20 St. Andrews Road, Sheffield S11 9AL Tel: 0114 255 0094 Fax: 0114 258 2863 — MB ChB Sheff. 1981; DCH RCP Lond. 1985; DRCOG 1986. Specialty: Gen. Pract.

SMAILES, Robert Andrew 10 Cobthorne Drive, Allestree, Derby DE22 2SY — MB ChB Leeds 1979; DA Eng. 1984.

SMAJE, Laurence Hetherington Medicine, Society & History Division, The Wellcome Trust, 183 Euston Road, London NW1 2BE Tel: 020 7611 8425 Fax: 020 7611 8526 — (Univ. Coll. Hosp.) PhD Lond. 1967, BSc 1958; MB BS Lond. 1961. Dir. Med., Soc. & Hist. Div., The Wellcome Trust. Socs: Physiol. Soc.; Roy. Soc. Med.; Brit. Microcirculat. Soc. Prev: Prof. & Head Phys. Dept. Char. Cross & Westm. Med. Sch.; Sen. Lect. (Physiol.) Univ. Coll. Lond.; Ho. Phys. & Ho. Surg. Univ. Coll. Hosp. Lond.

SMALDON, David Leslie 15 Chepstow Rise, Croydon CR0 5LX — MB BCh Wales 1970.

SMALE, Elisabeth Mary (retired) 7 Maclarens, Wickham Bishops, Witham CM8 3XE — MB ChB Manch. 1963; DObst RCOG 1965. Non Exec. Director of Mid Essex Hosp. Services Trust, Broomfield Ct., Pudding Wood La., Chelmsford, Essex, CM1 7WE. Prev: Sch. Med. Off. & Asst. MOH Southend-on-Sea.

SMALE, Simon Jonathan 68 Whitelake Road, Tonbridge TN10 3TJ — BM BS Nottm. 1992.

SMALES, Charles Hull & E. Yorkshire Hospitals, Anlaby Road, Hull HU3 2JZ Fax: 0148 267 4371 — MB ChB Leeds 1968; FFA RCS Eng. 1973. Cons. Anaestetist, Hull & E. Yorks. Hosps. Specialty: Anaesth. Prev: Ho. Phys. & Ho. Surg. Harrogate Gen. Hosp.

SMALES, Jeanne Rachael Breast Screening Unit, York District Hospital, York YO31 8HE — MB ChB Leeds 1976; DRCOG 1980.

SMALES, Keith Anthony Lovemead Group Practice, Roundstone Surgery, Polebarn Circus, Trowbridge BA14 7EH Tel: 01225 752752 Fax: 01225 776388 — MB BS Lond. 1970; MRCS Eng. LRCP Lond. 1970; MRCP (UK) 1975; DObst RCOG 1976.

SMALING, Alan Peter (retired) Stag Medical Centre, 162 Wickersley Road, Rotherham S60 4JW; Park Hill, 224 Doncaster Road, Thrybergh, Rotherham S65 4NU Tel: 01709 850101 — (Manch.) MB ChB Manch. 1968; DObst RCOG 1970.

SMALL, Barry John 11 Elmoor Avenue, Welwyn AL6 9PG — MB BS Lond. 1992.

SMALL, Christina Mary 55 Holyrood Crescent, St Albans AL1 2LY Tel: 01727 30097 — MB BS Lond. 1940; DPH Eng. 1947.

SMALL, Cormac 8 Kensington Gardens, Belfast BT5 6NP — MB BCh BAO Belf. 1996.

SMALL, David Gordon 1 North Place, Oxford OX3 9HX — BM BCh Oxf. 1965; MRCP (UK) 1971. Hon. Cons. (Clin. Neurophys.) Nat. Hosp. Nerv. Dis. Qu. Sq.; Hon. Cons. Dept. Clin. Neurol. Radcliffe Infirm. Oxf. Specialty: Neurol. Prev: Cons. (Clin. Neurophys.) & Sen. Lect. Dept. Neurol. Nat. Hosp. Nerv., Dis. Qu. Sq.; Regist. & Hon. Sen. Regist. Dept. Clin. Neurol. Churchill Hosp. Oxf.

SMALL, David James Accident and Emergency Department, Bedford Hospital, South Wing, Kempston Road, Bedford MK42 9DJ — MB ChB Bristol 1983.

SMALL, Feline Majella 26 Ravensdene Park, Ravenhill Road, Belfast BT6 Tel: 01232 641439; 25 Drummiller Lane, Gilford, Craigavon BT63 6BS Tel: 01762 831466 — MB BCh BAO Belf. 1989.

SMALL, Gillian 26 Hatchet Lane, Stonely, Huntingdon PE19 5EG — MB BS Lond. 1988; DCH 1992; DRCOG 1992; MRCP 1995. Specialty: Paediat.

SMALL, Mr Gordon Ian, Colonel L/RAMC Retd. (retired) 48 Dartford Road, Bexley DA5 2AT Tel: 01322 528758 — MB BS Lond. 1952 (St. Bart.) FRCS Eng. 1962. Prev: Cons. Orthop. Surg. Dartford & Gravesham HA.

SMALL, Helen Jane St Woolds Hospital, Stow Hill, Newport NP20 4SZ Tel: 01633 238237; The Cross, School Road, Hanbury, Bromsgrove B60 4BS — MB BCh Wales 1987; DRCOG 1991; DGM RCP Lond. 1996. Staff Grade Pract. (Geriat. Med.) St Woolos Hosp. Newport. Specialty: Rehabil. Med.; Care of the Elderly. Prev: Clin. Asst. (Rheum. & Geriat. Med.) & Trainee GP/SHO (Anaesth.) Roy. Gwent Hosp.

SMALL, Hellen Mary Muir Ravenscraig Hospital, Greenock PA16 9HA Tel: 01475 633777; Craiglyn Kirn, Dunoon PA23 8HH — MB ChB Glas. 1968. Assoc. Specialist (Psychiat.) Ravenscraig Hosp. Greenock. Specialty: Gen. Psychiat.

SMALL, Iain Robert Peterhead Group Practice, The Health Centre, Peterhead AB42 2XA Tel: 01774 474841 Fax: 01774 474848; Landfall, 1 Arran Avenue, Peterhead AB42 1PZ — MB ChB Dundee 1983; MRCGP 1987.

SMALL, Mr James Oliver The Ulster Independent Clinic Ltd, Stranmillis Road, Belfast BT9 5JH Tel: 01232 661212 — MB BCh BAO NUI 1976; FRCSI 1980. Cons. (Plastic Surg.) Temple St. & St Master Hosps. Dub. Specialty: Plastic Surg. Socs: Full Mem. Brit. Assn. of Plastic Surgs.; Full Mem. Brit. Assn. of Aesthetic Plastic Surgs.; Full Mem. Brit. Soc. for Surg. of the Hand. Prev: Sen. Regist. (Plastic Surg.) E. Health & Social Serv. BD. N. Irel.; Regist. (Plastic Surg.) Qu. Mary's Hosp. Roehampton.; Cons. (Plastic Surg.) E. Health & Social Serv. Bd. N. Irel.

SMALL, Jeremy Hugh Department of Radiology, Royal Bournemouth Hospital, Castle Lane E., Bournemouth BH7 7DW Tel: 01202 704894; 6 Middle Lane, Ringwood BH24 1LE — MB BS Lond. 1983 (Middlx. Hosp. Med. Sch.) MRCP (UK) 1988; FRCR 1993. Cons. Radiol. Roy. Bournemouth Hosp. Specialty: Radiol. Prev: Sen. Regist. (Radiol.) Addenbrooke's Hosp. Camb.

SMALL, Laura Louise Whiteabbey Health Centre, 95 Doagh Road, Newtownabbey BT37 9QN — MB BCh BAO Belf. 1980; DRCOG 1983; MRCGP 1984. GP Newtownabbey.

SMALL, Mandy Jayne 39 Caiystane Terrace, Edinburgh EH10 6ST — MB ChB Aberd. 1988.

SMALL, Margaret Lilian Forrester, Bowman and Rowlandson, Berry Lane Medical Centre, Berry Lane, Preston PR3 3JJ Tel: 01772 783021 Fax: 01772 785809 — MB ChB Glas. 1975; DRCOG 1977; MRCGP 1979.

SMALL, Mrs Margaret Smith Stuart (retired) 26 Bell Place, Edinburgh EH3 5HT Tel: 0131 332 6591 — MB ChB Glas. 1945; DPM Eng. 1948; MRCPsych 1972. Prev: Cons. Argyl & Clyde Health Board.

SMALL, Mary Jane Children's Services, Leicester City West PCT, Bridge Park Plaza, Bridge Park Road, Thurmaston, Leicester LE4 8PQ Tel: 0116 2256742 — BM Soton. 1989 (Soton. Univ.) MRCP (UK) 1995. Cons. Paediat. in Community Child Health. Specialty: Paediat. Socs: MRCPCH. Prev: Lect. (Paediat.) Univ. Hosp. Kuala Lumpur, Malaysia; SHO (Cardiol., Paediat., Gen. Med. & Neurol.) Soton. Gen. Hosp.; Sp. Regist. Paediat., Newc. Rotat.

SMALL, Michael (retired) 5 The Oriels, 146 Kingston Road, Wimbledon, London SW19 3NB Tel: 020 8287 3180 — MB BS Lond. 1951 (St. Mary's) FRCP Lond. 1971, M 1959. Prev: Cons. NeUrol.

SMALL, Mr Michael Higher Alston, Preston Road, Ribchester, Preston PR3 3XL Tel: 01254 878130 — MB ChB Glas. 1977; FRCS Glas. 1981. Cons. ENT Surg. Roy. Preston Hosp. Specialty: Otorhinolaryngol. Prev: Sen. Regist. (Otolaryngol.) Edin. Roy. Infirm. & City Hosp. Edin.

SMALL, Michael Gartnavel General Hospital, 1053 Great Western Road, Glasgow G12 0YN — MD Glas. 1986 (Glasgow) MB ChB 1978; MRCP (UK) 1980; FRCP Glas. 1988; FRCP Ed. 1991. Cons. Phys. Gartnavel Gen. Hosp. Glas. Specialty: Gen. Med.; Diabetes.

SMALL, Nicolas Mark Warren 102 Mollison Way, Edgware HA8 5QT — MB BS Lond. 1987; BSc Lond. 1983, MB BS 1987. Ho. Off. (Urol. & Gen. Surg.) Northwick Pk. Hosp. Harrow. Prev: Ho. Off. (Med.) Bedford Gen. Hosp.

SMALL, Mr Peter Kenneth Sunderland Royal Hospital, Department of General Surgery, Kayll Road, Sunderland SR4 7TP Tel: 0191 565 6256; 3 Eastfields, Whitburn, Sunderland SR6 7DA Tel: 0191 529 2275 — MB ChB Ed. 1982; BSc (Med. Sci.) Ed. 1979; FRCS Ed. 1989; MD Ed. 1996; FRCS Ed. (Gen.) 1997. Cons. Gen. Surg. Sunderland Roy. Hosp. Specialty: Gen. Surg.

SMALL, Philip George XRay Department, University Hospital Trust, Queens Medical Centre, Nottingham NG7 2UH Tel: 0115 942 1421 — MB ChB Sheff. 1962; DObst RCOG 1965; DMRD Eng. 1967; FFR 1969; FRCR 1975. Cons. Radiol. (Paediat.) Univ. Hosp. Trust Nottm.; Managing Edr. Paediat. Radiol.; Hon. Clin. Tutor Univ. Nottm. Specialty: Radiol. Socs: Eur. Soc. Paediat. Radiol.; Centr. Manpower Comm.; BMA (POWAR).

SMALL, Ramsay George (retired) 46 Monifieth Road, Broughty Ferry, Dundee DD5 2RX Tel: 01382 778408 — MB ChB St. And. 1954; DPH St. And. 1958; FFCM RCP (UK) 1978, M 1972; MRCP (Ed.) 1984; FRCP Ed. 1987. Prev: Chief Admin. Med. Off. Tayside HB.

SMALL, Robert George Dennis (retired) High Walls, North Lane, South Harting, Petersfield GU31 5NW — MB BChir Camb. 1954 (Middlx.) DObst RCOG 1955. Prev: Ho. Surg. & Ho. Off. (O & G) Middlx. Hosp.

SMALL, Rosemary Byers Holywood Arches Health Centre, Westminster Avenue, Belfast BT4 1NS Tel: 02890 563350 — MB BCh BAO Belf. 1977; DRCOG Lond. 1980; MRCGP 1982. Gen. Practitioner; Mem. of DLA Tribunal Panel.

SMALL, Una Roisin 28 Drumnaconagher Road, Crossgar, Downpatrick BT30 9JQ — MB BCh BAO NUI 1991; DRCOG 1994; DMH 1994; MRCGP 1995; DCH 1996. Princip. GP Downpatrick Co. Down.

SMALL, Yvette Jean 33 Fairmile Lane, Cobham KT11 2DL Tel: 01932 862557 — MB BS Lond. 1977; MRCS Eng. LRCP Lond. 1977. SCMO (Occupat. Health) Wandsworth HA & Lond. Boro. Richmond u. Thames. Prev: SCMO (Occupat. Health) Richmond, Twickenham & Roehampton HA.

SMALLBONE, David Frank Foxlow Grange, Harpur Hill, Buxton SK17 9LU Tel: 01298 24507 Fax: 01298 73011 — MB ChB Birm. 1961; MRCS Eng. LRCP Lond. 1962. Specialty: Gen. Med.; Endocrinol. Socs: Fell.Roy.Soc.Med; Fac. Homoeop.

SMALLCOMBE, Gerald William (retired) 35 Wychwood Crescent, Earley, Reading RG6 5RA Tel: 01734 987 1739 — MB BChir Camb. 1952 (St. Mary's) BSc (Reading) 1952, MA 1952. Prev: SHO Peppard Chest Hosp.

SMALLDRIDGE, Ann Oswald Medical Centre, 4 Oswald Road, Chorlton, Manchester M21 9LH Tel: 0161 881 4744 Fax: 0161 861 7027; 22 Langham Road, Bowdon, Altrincham WA14 3NN Tel: 0161 928 1752 — BM BS Nottm. 1981; DRCOG 1982; DCH RCP Lond. 1984; MRCGP 1991. Prev: GP Lond.

SMALLDRIDGE, Jacqueline 618 Wells Road, Knowle, Bristol BS14 9BD; 18 Anglesea Street, Posonby, Auckland, New Zealand — MB BS Lond. 1986; DObst Auckland 1989; MRCOG 1991. Regist. (O & G) Nat. Wom. Hosp. & Wellington Hosp. NZ. Specialty: Obst. & Gyn. Prev: SHO (Gyn.) Bloomsbury HA; SHO (Obst.) Nat. Wom. Hosp. Auckland NZ; Regist. (Paediat.) Princess Mary Hosp. Auckland NZ.

SMALLEY, Andrew Dennis Rose Dean Surgery, 8 Dean Street, Liskeard PL14 4AQ Tel: 01579 343133 Fax: 01579 344933 — MB BS 1987 (Guys) BSc (1st cl. Hons.) Lond. 1984, MB BS 1987; DCH RCP Lond. 1990; DGM RCP Lond. 1990; MRCGP 1991. GP Trainer.

SMALLEY, Christine Angela Central Health Clinic, East Park Terrace, Southampton SO14 0YL Tel: 023 8090 2562 Fax: 023 8090 2602 — MB ChB Sheff. 1969; DCH Eng. 1971; MRCP (UK) 1973; FRCP Lond. 1988; FRCPCH 1997. Cons. Paediat. Community Child Health Soton. City PC. Trust. Specialty: Paediat. Prev: Cons. Paediat. S. Birm. HA.; Sen. Regist. (Paediat.) Birm. AHA (T); Research Fell. (Clin.) Inst. Child Health Birm. Univ.

SMALLEY, David Simon Nuffield House Surgery, The Stow, Harlow CM20 3AX Tel: 01279 425661 Fax: 01279 427116 — BSc Lond. 1979, MB BS 1982; MRCGP (Distinc.) 1985; DCH RCP Lond. 1985; DRCOG 1985; FRCGP 2001. Examr. RCGP.; Hon. Sec. Essex RCGP.

SMALLEY, Dorothy Mary Wilson Street Surgery, 11 Wilson Street, Derby DE1 1PG Tel: 01332 344366 Fax: 01332 348813; 11 Oak Road, Thulston, Derby DE72 3EW Tel: 01332 574259 Fax: 01332 574259 — (Sheff.) MB ChB Sheff. 1969; MRCGP 1976. Prev: Med. Off. Stud. Health Serv. Sheff. Univ.; SHO (Gen. Med.) Doncaster Roy. Infirm.; Ho. Phys. & Ho. Surg. United Sheff. Hosps.

SMALLMAN, Lesley Ann Alexandra Hospital, Worcestershire Acute Hospitals NHS Trustq, Woodrow Drive, Redditch B98 7UB Tel: 01527 512008 Ext: 35156 Fax: 01527 512007; Pint Bar Cottage, Foredraught Lane, Tibberton, Droitwich WR9 7NH Tel: 01905 345259 Fax: 01905 345601 — MB ChB Birm. 1978; MB ChB (Hons.) Birm. 1978; FRCPath 1996, M 1985. Cons. Pathologist Alexandra Hosp., Worcs. Acute Hosp.s NHS Trust; Adviser (Path.) J. Laryngol. & Otol; Mem. Ct. Examrs MRCS RCS Eng.; Hon. Sen. Lect. Med. Sch. Univ. Birm.; Extern. Examr. Cardiff Dent. Sch. Specialty: Histopath. Socs: Assn. Clin. Pathol.; Brit. Soc. Clin. Cytol.; Internat. Acad. Path. Prev: Sen. Lect. & Hon. Cons. Path. Med. Sch. Univ. Birm. & Gen. Hosp. Birm.; Lect. Path. Med. Sch. Univ. Birm.

SMALLMAN, Robert Ian Bulling Lane Surgery, Bulling Lane, Crich, Matlock DE4 5DX Tel: 01773 852966 Fax: 01773 853919; Hollins Grove, Little London, Holloway, Matlock DE4 5AZ — MB ChB Birm. 1982; MRCGP 1986; DRCOG 1986. Prev: Trainee GP S. Warks. VTS.

SMALLPEICE, Mr Christopher John North Staffordshire Royal Infirmary, Princes Road, Hartshill, Stoke-on-Trent ST4 7LN Tel: 01782 554249 Fax: 01782 554830 — MB BS Lond. 1972 (King's Coll. Hosp.) MRCS Eng. LRCP Lond. 1972; FRCS Eng. 1978. Cons. Cardiothoracic Surg. N. Staffs. Health Dist. Stoke-on-Trent. Specialty: Cardiothoracic Surg. Prev: Sen. Regist. (Cardiothoracic Surg.) W. Midls. RHA; Regist. (Cardiothoracic Surg.) King's Coll., Brook & Guy's Hosp.; Lond.

SMALLSHAW, John Kendall (retired) 2 Stagbury Close, Chipstead, Coulsdon, Croydon CR5 3PH Tel: 01737 552512 — MRCS Eng. LRCP Lond. 1960 (Guy's) Prev: Med. Off. Roy. Alfred Seamen's Soc. & Banstead Pl. Qu. Eliz. Foundat.

SMALLWOOD, Bernard Henry Turning Cottage, Garway, Hereford HR2 8RJ Tel: 01600 750411 — MB ChB Birm. 1973; DObst RCOG 1976. Specialty: Gen. Pract. Prev: GP Kingstone Herefordsh.

SMALLWOOD, Diana Margaret 9 Ribblesdale Drive, Ridgeway, Sheffield S12 3XB — MRCS Eng. LRCP Lond. 1972; DObst RCOG 1975.

SMALLWOOD, Elizabeth Helen Oaksworth House, Long Bottom Lane, Beaconsfield HP9 2UL — MB BS Lond. 1990 (Char. Cross & Westm.) DCH RCP Lond 1994; DRCOG 1994. Retainer scheme. Specialty: Gen. Pract.

SMALLWOOD, Mr James Anthony Department of Surgery, E-Level, West Wing, Southampton General Hospital, Tremona Road, Southampton SO16 6YD; Whispers, Hadrian Way, Chilworth, Southampton SO16 7HX Tel: 01703 768543 — MB BS Lond. 1976 (St. Bart.) MRCS Eng. LRCP Lond. 1975; FRCS Eng. 1980; MS Soton. 1986. Cons. Gen. Surg. (Surg. Oncol.) Soton. Gen. Hosp. Specialty: Gen. Surg. Socs: (Vice-Pres.) Europ. Surgic. Research Soc. Prev: Research Fell. Breast Cancer Soton.; Regist. (Surg.) Crawley Hosp.; SHO (Surg.) Char. Cross Hosp. Lond.

SMALLWOOD, Neil Nicholas Barnfield Hill Surgery, 12 Barnfield Hill, Exeter EX1 1SR Tel: 01392 432761 Fax: 01392 422406; 4 Lower Summerlands, Exeter EX1 2LJ Tel: 01392 496955 — MB ChB Bristol 1985; DCH RCP Lond. 1989; MRCGP 1991.

SMALLWOOD, Robert Ingamar Larsen Parkside Hospital, 53 Parkside, London SW19 5NE Tel: 020 8946 4202; 86 Marryat Road, London SW19 5BN — MRCS Eng. LRCP Lond. 1947 (St. Bart.) DObst RCOG 1951. Med. Ref. Various Insur. Cos.; Authorised Examr. Bd. Civil Aviat. Auth. Br. Socs: Med.-Leg. Soc. Prev: RAF; Intern. Gyn. Dept. St. Bart. Hosp.; Sen. Res. Obst. Off. Luton & Dunstable Hosp.

SMALLWOOD, Stephen Hugh Wickham Surgery, Station Road, Wickham, Fareham PO17 5JL Tel: 01329 833121 Fax: 01329 832443; Westwood, Droxford Road, Swanmore, Southampton SO32 2PY — MB BS Lond. 1973 (St. Thos.) BSc (Biochem. Hons.) Lond. 1970, MB BS 1973; DCH Eng. 1975; MRCP (UK) 1979; Dip. IMC RCS Ed. 1991. Prev: Regist. (Paediat.) St. Peter's Hosp. Chertsey; Regist. (Gen. Med.) Mayday Hosp. Thornton Heath; SHO (Neonat.) Hammersmith Hosp. Lond.

SMARASON, Alexander Kristinn Nuffield Department of Obstetrics and Gynaecology, University of Oxford, John Radcliffe Hospital, Oxford OX3 9DU Tel: 01865 221021; 27 Walkers Close, Freeland, Witney OX29 8AY Tel: 01993 883686 — Cand Med et Chir Reykjavik 1987; DPhil. Oxf. 1994; MRCOG 1997. Clin. Lect. (Obstretrics & Gyn.) Univ. of Oxf. Specialty: Obst. & Gyn. Socs: BMA; MDU.

SMART, Amanda Lucy Whitby Group Practice, Spring Vale Medical Centre, Whitby YO21 1SD Tel: 01947 820888 Fax: 01947 603194 — MB ChB Leeds 1985.

SMART, Andrew Galloway Weir Keston, 78 Muirs, Kinross KY13 8AY — MB ChB Ed. 1979.

SMART, Anna Rachel Theresa Isadora 4 Cairnaquheen Gardens, Aberdeen AB15 5HJ — MB ChB Aberd. 1998.

SMART, Mr Christopher James Department of Urology, Southampton General Hospital, Southampton SO16 6YD Tel: 023 8077 7222; The Old Vicarage, Emery Down, Lyndhurst SO43 7EA Tel: 01421 282000 Fax: 01421 282000 — MB BS Lond. 1965 (St. Bart.) FRCS Eng. 1971. Cons. Urol. & Gen. Surg. Soton. & SW Hants. Health Dist. (T). Specialty: Urol.

SMART, Christopher Jeremy Northwood Medical Centre, 10/12 Middleton Hall Road, Kings Norton, Birmingham B30 1BY Tel: 0121 458 5507 — MB ChB Birm. 1967; DObst RCOG 1970; DA Eng. 1970; MRCGP 1972; DMJ Soc. Apoth. Lond. 1983. Hosp. Pract. (Geriat. Med.) W. Heath Hosp. Birm.; Div. Police Surg. W. Midl. Police. Socs: Counc. Mem. Assn Police Surgs. Gt. Brit.; Fell. Roy. Soc. Med.; Clin. Forens. Med. (Counc.).

SMART, Mr Colin Campbell Queen Mary's Sidcup NHS Trust, Frognal Avenue, Sidcup DA14 6LT Tel: 020 8302 2678 Fax: 020 8302 3155 — MB ChB Glas. 1985; FRCS (Tr. & Orth. 1999); FRCS Glas. 1991; Dip Biomech. 1996. Cons. Orthopaedic Surg., Qu. Mary's Sidcup NHS Trust, Sidcup. Specialty: Orthop.; Trauma & Orthop. Surg.

SMART, David James Garfield Hanway Road Surgery, 2 Hanway Road, Buckland, Portsmouth PO1 4ND Tel: 023 9281 5317 Fax: 023 9289 9926 — MB Camb. 1981; MA Camb. 1981, MB 1981, BChir 1980; DRCOG 1983; MRCGP 1984. Clin. Asst. (Ophth.) Qu. Alexandra Hosp. Portsmouth. Prev: Trainee GP Portsmouth VTS.

SMART, David John Leicester Terrace Health Care Centre, 8 Leicester Terrace, Northampton NN2 6AL Tel: 01604 633682 Fax: 01604 233408 — MB ChB Leic. 1985 (Leicester) MRCGP 1990. Trainee GP Kettering VTS.; GP Trainer. Specialty: Gen. Psychiat.

SMART, David Keith Archibald 117 Dane Road, Sale M33 2BY — MB ChB Manch. 1996.

SMART, David Wilson Dunelm Medical Practice, 1-2 Victor Terrace, Bearpark, Durham DH7 7DF Tel: 0191 373 2077 Fax: 0191

373 6216; Kelvin House, 1/2 Victor Terrace, Bearpark, Durham DH7 7DR — MB ChB Glas. 1981; DRCOG 1983; MRCGP 1985.

SMART, Donald McGregor (retired) 14 Framers Court, Lane End, High Wycombe HP14 3LL — MRCS Eng. LRCP Lond. 1944 (Middlx.) Prev: GP Hayes Middlx.

SMART, Felicity Anne Llanilar Health Centre, Llanilar, Aberystwyth SY23 4PA Tel: 01974 241556 Fax: 01974 241579; Fairview, Penyfron, Llanbadarn Fawr, Aberystwyth SY23 3QU — MB ChB Birm. 1976; MRCGP (Distinc.) 1982; DCH RCP Lond. 1982.

SMART, George Edward Beechcroft, 24 Cramond Road N., Cramond, Edinburgh EH4 6JE Tel: 0131 312 8499 Email: george@smart8.fsnet.co.uk; Royal Infirmary of Edinburgh, Lauriston Place, Edinburgh EH3 9YW Tel: 0131 536 1000 Fax: 0131 536 4254 — MB ChB Ed. 1960; FRCOG 1979, M 1967; FRCS Ed. 1968. Cons. O & G Simpson Memor. Matern. Pavil. & Roy. Infirm. Edin.; Hon. Sen. Lect. Univ. Edin. Specialty: Obst. & Gyn. Prev: Cons. Sen. Lect. O & G Univ. Bristol & Hon. Cons. Southmead Hosp. & United Bristol Hosps.; Sen. Fell. Gyn. Oncol. State Univ. New York Downstate Med. Center Brooklyn, USA.

SMART, Hazel Elizabeth Linlithgow Health Centre, 288 High Street, Linlithgow EH49 7ER Tel: 01506 670027; 20 Kettilstoun Grove, Linlithgow EH49 6PP — MB ChB Ed. 1988; DRCOG 1992; MRCGP 1994.

SMART, Howard Leighton Royal Liverpool Broadgreen University Hospitals NHS Trust, Prescot St., Liverpool L7 8XP Tel: 0151 706 3557 Fax: 0151 706 5832 — MB BS Lond. 1979 (St. Bart.) MRCP (UK) 1982; DM Nottm. 1988; FRCP Lond. 1996. Cons. Phys. (Gastroenterol.) Roy. Liverp. & Broadgreen Univ. Hosps. NHS Trust; Clin. Lect. (Med.) Univ. Liverp. Specialty: Gastroenterol. Socs: Brit. Soc. Gastroenterol.; Brit. Assn. for the Study of the Liver. Prev: Lect. (Med.) Univ. Sheff.; Research Fell. (Med.) Univ. Hosp. Nottm.; Regist. (Med.) City Hosp. Nottm.

SMART, Iain Seymour Mackintosh Bonnyrigg Health Centre, High Street, Bonnyrigg EH19 2DA Tel: 0131 663 7272 — MB ChB St. And. 1967; DObst RCOG 1967; MRCGP 1976. Socs: BMA. Prev: SHO (O & G) Dundee Roy. Infirm.; SHO (Gen. Surg.) & (Gen. Med.) Falkirk Roy. Infirm.

SMART, Isobel Alice (retired) Holmwood, Holt, Wimborne BH21 7DQ Tel: 01202 841943 — (Newc.) MB BS Durh. 1961.

SMART, James Anderson Crossways, 39 Windson Rd, Radyr, Cardiff CF15 8BQ — MB ChB Leic. 1994.

SMART, James Finlayson Union Street Surgery, 75 Union Street, Larkhall ML9 1DZ Tel: 01698 882105 Fax: 01698 886332 — MB ChB Glas. 1969.

SMART, James Matthew The Old Vicarge, Emery Down, Lyndhurst SO43 7EA — MB ChB Leic. 1992.

SMART, John Charles Woodbury Cottage, Chatley, Ombersley, Droitwich WR9 0AP Tel: 01905 621088; Woodbury Cottage, Chatley, Ombersley, Droitwich WR9 0AP Tel: 01258 837251/01905 621088 — MB ChB Birm. 1948; DObst RCOG 1950. JP. Socs: Fell. Roy. Soc. Med.; Nat. Chairm. Brit. Soc. Med. & Dent. Hypn. Prev: Ho. Surg. & Ho. Phys. Gen. Hosp. Birm.; Ho. Surg. (Obst.) Birm. Matern. Hosp.

SMART, Kieran 45 Laurel Drive, Penperlleni, Pontypool NP4 0BQ Tel: 0966 508220 — MB ChB Bristol 1992; BA Open Univ. 1987; MRCGP 1987. Socs: Aerospace Med. Assn.

SMART, Lesley Newbattle Group Practice, Mayfield, Dalkeith E22 4AD Tel: 0131 663 1051; 6 Ancrum Bank, Dalkeith EH22 3AY — MB ChB Glas. 1979; DRCOG 1981; MRCGP 1983. Clin. Med. Off., Family Plann. and Reproductive Health, Edin.

SMART, Lesley Margaret St. John's Hospital at Howden, Livingston — MB ChB Ed. 1982; BSc (Hons.) (Med. Sc.) Ed. 1979, MB ChB 1982; MRCP (UK) 1985; FRCR 1989. Cons. Radiol. St. John's Hosp. at Howden. Livingston. Specialty: Radiol. Prev: Sen. Regist. & Regist. (Radiol.) Lothian HB.

SMART, Louise Mary Pathology Department, Medical School Building, Foresterhill, Aberdeen AB25 2ZD Tel: 01224 552836 Fax: 01224 663002 — MB ChB Aberd. 1984; MD Aberd. 1991; MRCPath 1992. Cons. Cytopath. Aberd. Roy. Hosp. Specialty: Histopath. Prev: Sen. Regist. (Path.) Aberd. Roy. Hosp.

SMART, Lynda Kay 41 Melville Avenue, South Croydon CR2 7HZ — MB BS Lond. 1984; DRCOG 1987. GP Lond.

SMART, Michael Alan Brent House Surgery, 14 King Street, Bridgwater TA6 3ND Tel: 01278 458551 Fax: 01278 431116 — BM Soton. 1985; MRCGP 1989.

SMART, Neil Gow — MB ChB Glas. 1984; BSc (Hons.) Glas. 1981; DA (UK) 1986; FFA RCSI 1989; MBA 2002. Cons. (Anaesth.) Glas. Roy. Infirm. Specialty: Anaesth. Prev: Regist. (Anaesth.) Glas. Roy. Infirm.; SHO Dept. of Anaesth. Glas. Roy. Infirm.; Jun. Ho. Phys. Stobhill Gen. Hosp. & West. Infirm. Glas.

SMART, Mr Paul James Gregory (retired) Hockhams House, Martley, Worcester WR6 6QR — (St. Bart.) MS Lond. 1968, MB BS 1955; DObst RCOG 1957; FRCS Eng. 1962. Prev: Cons. Surg. Worcester Roy. Infirm.

SMART, Peter Charles 5 The Oaks, Vicarage Road, Blackwater, Camberley GU17 9BE Tel: 01276 33844 Fax: 01276 33844 — MB BS Lond. 1953 (St. Geo.) MRCS Eng. LRCP Lond. 1953; DA Eng. 1955. Police Surg. Winchester Div. Hants. Constab. Socs: BMA. Prev: Clin. Tutor (GP) St. Geo. Hosp. Lond.; SHO (Anaesth.) St. Geo. Hosp. Lond.

SMART, Peter Donald (retired) 'Holmcroft', 2 The Knoll, Ellington Village, Morpeth NE61 5LQ Tel: 01670 862941 — MB BS Durh. 1954. Prev: Res. Med. Off. Preston Hosp. N. Shields.

SMART, Peter Howard La Route Du Fort Surgery, 2 La Route Du Fort, St Helier, Jersey JE2 4PA Tel: 01534 31421 Fax: 01534 280776; D'Eaudeville, La Pouquelaye, St. Helier, Jersey JE2 3GF — MB BCh Wales 1973 (Univeristy College Cardiff & Welsh National School Medicine) MRCS Eng. LRCP Lond. 1973; Cert. Av Med. MoD (Air) & Civil Av Auth. 1977; MRCGP 1978; DRCOG 1979. Specialty: Aviat. Med.

SMART, Philip John Edward 10 Langstrath Drive, West Bridgford, Nottingham NG2 6SD — MB BS Lond. 1994; MA Camb. 1987.

SMART, Rosemary Ann The Surgery, Worcester Road, Great Witley, Worcester WR6 6HR Tel: 01299 896370 Fax: 01299 896873; Hockham's House, Martley, Worcester WR6 6QR Tel: 01886 812276 — MB ChB Ed. 1967. Specialty: Accid. & Emerg. Prev: Hosp. Pract. (A & E) Worcester Roy. Infirm.

SMART, Russell George 37 Eton Wick Road, Eton Wick, Windsor SL4 6LU — MB BS Lond. 1984.

SMART, Simon Jeremy The Chase, Watery Lane, Weatheroak, Birmingham B48 7JN — MB BS Lond. 1996.

SMART, Victoria Mary Eve Hill Medical Practice, 29-53 Himley Road, Dudley DY1 2QD Tel: 01384 254423 Fax: 01384 254424 — MB ChB Birm. 1984; DCH RCP Lond. 1988; MRCGP 2003. Prev: Ho Surg. Gen. Hosp. Birm.; Ho. Phys. Dudley Rd. Hosp.; Trainee GP Dudley VTS.

SMEATON, Nicola Clare Mill Practice, Arthurstone Terrace, Dundee DD4 6QY Tel: 01382 456700 — MB ChB Dundee 1986.

SMEDLEY, Mr Frank Herbert Wildwood, Cudham Lane South, Cudham, Sevenoaks TN14 7QA — MB BS Lond. 1978; FRCS Eng. 1983; MS Lond. 1987. Specialty: Gen. Surg.

SMEDLEY, Mr Geoffrey Thomas (retired) Flat 16 Bishops Court, Bishops Down Road, Tunbridge Wells TN4 8XL — (Westm.) MB BS Lond. 1949; FRCS Eng. 1953; FRCOG 1972, M 1957. Prev: Cons. O & G Salisbury Hosp. Gp.

SMEDLEY, Howard Martin c/o Department of Radiotherapy, Kent & Canterbury Hospital, Ethelbert Road, Canterbury CT1 3NG — MB BS Lond. 1977 (Univ. Coll. Hosp.) FRCR 1982. Cons. Radiother. & Oncol. Kent & Canterbury Hosp.; Clin. Tutor Kent Postgrad. Med. Centre. Specialty: Oncol.; Radiother. Prev: Clin. Scientist & Hon. Sen. Regist. Ludwig Inst. Cancer Research Camb.; Sen. Regist. (Radiother. & Oncol.) Addenbrooke's Hosp. Camb.

SMEDLEY, Julia Carol Occupational Health Department, Southampton General Hospital, Tremona Road, Southampton SO16 6YD Tel: 023 8079 4156 Fax: 023 8079 4324 Email: julia.smedley@doctors.org.uk — BM BS Nottm. 1985 (Nottm. Univ.) BMedSci Nottm 1983; DM Soton 1999; FFOM 2002; FRCP 2002. Cons. Occupat. Phys. Soton. Univ. Hosps. NHS Trust Soton. Specialty: Occupat. Health. Socs: Soc. Occupat. Med.; Assoc. of NHS Occupat. Phys. (ANHOPS). Prev: Sen. Regist. (Occupat. Med.) Soton.; Regist. (Haemat.) King Coll. Hosp.; SHO (Gen. Med.) Soton. Gen. Hosp.

SMEED, Richard Charles Kenneth Church Cottage, Claypit Lane, Ledsham, South Milford, Leeds LS25 5LP Mob: 07713 202371 — MB ChB Leeds 1975; AFOM RCP Lond. 1995. Med. Advis. Yorks.

Water, Harrogate NHS Trust & others; Clin. Asst. (Care of Elderly) Castleford. Specialty: Occupat. Health. Socs: Soc. Occupat. Med. Prev: GP Kippax & Garforth Leeds.

SMEETH, Liam Keats Group Practice, 1B Downshire Hill, London NW3 1NR — MB ChB Sheff. 1990 (Sheffield) DCH 1994; MRCGP 1995; DRCOG 1996; MSc Lond. Sch. of Hyg. & Trop. Med. 1998. GP; Clin. Lect. Dept. of Primary Care & Populat. Sci. Roy. Free & UCL Med. Sch. Specialty: Gen. Pract.

SMEETON, Anthony Keith Hereford House, Clifton Park, Clifton, Bristol BS8 3BP Tel: 0117 974 5232 — MB ChB Bristol 1961. Police Surg. Avon & Som. Constab. Socs: BMA; Assn. Police Surg. Prev: Ho. Phys. Ham Green Hosp. Bristol; Ho. Surg. (Cas. & Orthop.) Bristol Roy. Infirm.; Ho. Surg. (Obst.) Roy. United Hosp. Bath.

SMEETON, Fiona Janet 6 Long Acre E., Bingham, Nottingham NG13 8BY — MB BS Lond. 1996 (Charing Cross & West Minster) BSc Lond 1993; MRCP June 1999. SpR (Diabetes & Endocrinol.) S. W. Thames. Specialty: Gen. Med. Prev: SHO Med., St Helier Hosp., Carshalton.

SMEETON, Richard James Chilham House, 5 The Spinney, Thurnby, Leicester LE7 9QS — (Univ. Coll. Hosp.) DObst RCOG 1970; MRCGP 1975. Indep. Occupat. Health Phys.; Med. Off. & Police Surg. Leics. Constab. Socs: BMA. Prev: GP Leicester.

SMELLIE, Alexander James (retired) Roselea, Victoria Road, Brookfield, Johnstone PA5 8TZ Tel: 01505 320266 — MB ChB Glas. 1955; DObst RCOG 1959. Prev: Ho. Surg. Roy. Alexandra Infirm. Paisley.

SMELLIE, Anne Stephen 62 Gough Way, Cambridge CB3 9LN Tel: 01223 352035 — MB BS Lond. 1957 (St. Thos.)

SMELLIE, Janet Helen (retired) Queen Victoria Park, Inchmarlo, Banchory AB31 4AL — (Liverp.) MB ChB (Hons.) Liverp. 1947; MB ChB 1947; DCH Eng. 1949. Prev: Ho. Phys. Liverp. Roy. Infirm. & Roy. Childr. Hosp. Liverp.

SMELLIE, Jean McIldowie 23 St Thomas' Street, Winchester SO23 9HJ Tel: 01962 852550 Fax: 01962 852550 — (Oxf. & Univ. Coll. Hosp.) BM BCh Oxf. 1950; DCH Eng. 1953; FRCP Lond. 1975, M 1954; MA Oxf. 1951, BA 1947, DM 1981; Hon. FRCPCH 1996. Emerit. Cons. Paediat. Univ. Coll. Lond. Hosps.; Hon. Cons. (Paediat.) Hosp. Sick Childr. Lond; Scientif. Adviser, Internat. Reflux Study in Childr. 1982-. Specialty: Paediat.; Nephrol. Socs: Hon Mem. Brit. Assn. for Paed. Nephrol.; Europ. Soc. for Paediatric Nephrol.; Hon Mem. Amer. Urological Assn. Prev: Sen. Lect. (Paediat.) Univ. Coll. Lond. Med. Sch.; Hon. Cons. (Paediat.) Guy's Hosp. Lond.; Hon. Sen. Clin. Lect. (Community Child Health) Univ. of Soton.

SMELLIE, Maida Kelly Reid 25 Earls Way, Doonfoot, Ayr KA7 4HF — MB ChB Ed. 1975; BSc Ed. 1972; MPH Glas. 1982; MFCM 1985. Specialty: Pub. Health Med.

SMELLIE, Vivien Rachel 4 Stoke road, Bishops Cleeve, Cheltenham GL52 8RP Tel: 01242 672007 — MB BS Lond. 1992 (Univ. Coll. and Middlx. Hosp. Med. Sch.) BSc (Hons.) KQC 1989 (Lond.); DCH 1995; DRCOG 1996; DRCOG 1996.

SMELLIE, Mr William Alastair Buchanan (retired) 62 Gough Way, Cambridge CB3 9LN Tel: 01223 352035 — MB Camb. 1958 (Camb. & St. Thos.) BA Camb. 1954, MChir 1966, MB 1958, BChir 1957; FRCS Eng. 1962. Cons. Surg. Addenbrooke's Hosp. Camb.; Assoc. Lect. Univ. Camb; Examr. (Surg.) Univs. Oxf., Camb. & Lond.; RCS Regional Adviser in Surg. E. Anglia; Hon Col. RAMC. Prev: Res. Asst. Surg. St. Thos. Hosp. Lond.

SMELLIE, Mr William James Buchanan Chelsea & Westminster Hospital, 369 Fulham Road, Chelsea, London SW10 9NH Tel: 020 8746 8463 Fax: 020 8746 8282 — MB BChir Camb. 1988; BA Camb. 1985; FRCS 1992; MD Camb. 1998. Cons. Gen. and Endocrine Surg., Chelsea and Westm. Hosp.; Cons. to the Lister, Cromwell and Princess Grace Hosps.; Hon. Cons., Brompton and Harefield NHS Trust. Specialty: Gen. Surg. Prev: Sen. Regist. (Endocrine Surg.) Hammersmith Hosp. Lond.; Regist. (Gen. Surg.) St Thos. Hosp. Lond.; Regist. (Gen. Surg.) St Geo. Hosp. Lond.

SMELLIE, William Stuart Adams Bishop Auckland Hospital, Cockton Hill Road, Bishop Auckland DL14 6AP Tel: 01388 454064; Morely Farm, Morley Lane, Brancepeth, Durham DH7 8DS Tel: 0191 373 9416 Fax: 0191 373 9417 Email: info@smelli.com — BM BCh Oxf. 1985; MA Camb. 1986; MRCP (UK) 1989; MRCPath 1994; DM Oxf. 1996. Cons. Bishop Auckland NHS Trust. Specialty: Chem. Path. Prev: Sen. Regist. Glas. Roy. Infirm.

SMELT, Mr Graham Jonathan Casterton ENT Department, The Royal Infirmary, Lindley, Huddersfield HD3 3EA Tel: 01484 342693 Fax: 01484 342147 — MB BS Lond. 1976 (St. Thos.) BSc Lond. 1973; FRCS Ed. 1982; LMCC 1985. Cons. ENT Surg. Calderdale & Huddersfield NHS Trusts. Specialty: Otolaryngol. Socs: N. Eng. Otol. Soc. Prev: Sen. Regist. Nottm. & Leics. HAs; Regist. St. Bart. Hosp. Lond.

SMERDON, Anthony William Stockbridge Village Health Centre, Leachcroft, Waterpark Drive, Stockbridge Village, Liverpool L28 1ST Tel: 0151 489 9924; 16 Brooke Road W., Liverpool L22 7RW Tel: 0151 920 9246 — MB ChB Liverp. 1967; MSc Liverp. 1990, MB ChB 1967; MRCGP 1975.

SMERDON, Mr David Laurence James Cook University Hospital, Marton Road, Middlesbrough TS4 3BW Tel: 01642 854069; Hazel Grove, Whorl Hill, Faceby, Middlesbrough TS9 7BZ Tel: 01642 700013 — MB ChB Dundee 1978; FRCS Ed. 1983; FRCOphth 1989. Cons. Ophth. Surg. & Hon. Clin. Sen. Lect. Ophth. James Cook Univ. Hosp. Middlesbrough; Chairm. Update N. Specialty: Ophth. Socs: Treas. Oxf. Ophth. Congr.; Sec. UKISCRS; Hon Treas Enter. Prev: Cons. Ophth. Surg. N. Riding Infirm. Middlesbrough; Chairm. of Ocular Tissue Advisary Gp. of U.K. Transpl.; Sen. Regist. (Ophth.) Birm. & Midl. Eye Hosp.

SMERDON, Geoffrey Hugh, MBE (retired) Maleme Roseland, Liskeard PL14 3PQ Tel: 01579 343460 — (Lond. Hosp.) MB BS Lond. 1949; MRCS Eng. LRCP Lond. 1949; FRCGP 1980, M 1953; DObst RCOG 1955; DCH Eng. 1959.

SMERDON, Geoffrey Thomas (retired) The White Cottage, 190 Wivenhoe Road, Alresford, Colchester CO7 8AH Tel: 01206 822055 — BM BCh Oxf. 1950; MA Oxf. 1950; MFOM RCP Lond. 1978. Prev: Civil. Med. Pract. Med. Reception Centre, Sennelager 1979-81.

SMERDON, George Robert The Spinney Surgery, The Spinney, Ramsey Road, St. Ives, Huntingdon PE27 37P Tel: 01480 492501 Fax: 01480 356159 — MB BS Lond. 1969 (St. Thos.) DObst RCOG 1973; MRCGP 1975; FRCGP 1989.

SMEREKA, Adam Kazimierz Church Street Medical Centre, 11B Church Street, Eastwood, Nottingham NG16 3BP Tel: 01773 712065 Fax: 01773 534295 — MB BCh BAO NUI 1964.

SMETHURST, Dominic Paul Dermatology Unit, University of Nottingham, Queen's Medical Centre, Nottingham NG7 2UH — BChir Camb. 1996 (Cambridge) Research Fell. Univ. of. Nottm. Specialty: Gen. Med. Prev: SHO (Gen. Med.) Qu.'s Med. Nottm.; Pre-Regist. Ho. Off. (Gen. Surg.) Milton Keynes; Pre-Regist. Ho. Off. (Gen. Med.) Addenbrookes.

SMETHURST, Fraser Andrew 22 Kingsmead Road N., Oxton, Birkenhead CH43 6TB Tel: 0151 652 3470 — BM BCh Oxf. 1987; DMRD Liverp. 1982; FRCR 1984; BA (Hons.) Oxf. 1984. Cons. Radiol. Aintree Hosp. Trust. Specialty: Radiol. Prev: Sen. Regist. (Radiol.) Fazakerley Hosp. Liverp.

SMETHURST, John Roderic (retired) 4 Warren Drive, Dorridge, Solihull B93 8JY Tel: 01564 776387 Fax: 01564 776387 — (Birm.) MB ChB Birm. 1959; FFA RCS Eng. 1966; FRCA 1992. Sen. Clin. Lect. Univ. Birm. Prev: Cons. Anaesth. Birm. Centr. Health Dist. (T).

SMETHURST, Marianne 62 Leamington Street, Crookes, Sheffield S10 1LW — MB ChB Sheff. 1995.

SMETHURST, Marion Elizabeth West Kirby Health Centre, Grange Road, Wirral CH48 4HZ Tel: 0151 625 9171 Fax: 0151 625 9171 — BM BCh Oxf. 1987; BA (Hons.) Oxf. 1984; DRCOG 1990. GP. Specialty: Gen. Pract. Prev: Trainee GP/SHO (O & G) Horton Gen. Hosp. Banbury.

SMETHURST, Meera Elizabeth The Surgery, St Peters Close, Cowfold, Horsham RH13 8DN Tel: 01403 864204 Fax: 01403 864408 — BM BCh Oxf. 1985; MA Camb. 1986; DRCOG 1988. GP Cowfold, Horsham.

SMEULDERS, Naima 3 The Nursery, Sutton Courtenay, Abingdon OX14 4UA — BChir Camb. 1994.

SMEYATSKY, Norman Raphael St. Michael's Hospital, St. Michael's Road, Warwick CV34 5QW Tel: 01926 406789; 15 Willes Terrace, Leamington Spa CV31 1DL Tel: 01926 831702 — MB BCh Witwatersrand 1979; BSc Witwatersrand 1975; MRCPsych 1985. Cons. Old Age Psychiat. St. Michael's Hosp. Warwick. Specialty: Geriat. Psychiat.; Gen. Psychiat.

SMIBERT, George McMillan (retired) 44 Mount Road, Penn, Wolverhampton WV4 5SW Tel: 01902 341574 — MB ChB Ed. 1946 (Univ. Ed.)
SMIBERT, Mr John Graham Yeovil District General Hospital, Yeovil — MB BS Lond. 1976; FRCS Lond. 1980; FRCS Ed. 1980. Cons. Orthop. Yeovil Dist. Gen. Hosp. Specialty: Orthop. Prev: Sen. Regist. Rotat. (Orthop.) Kings Coll. Hosp. Lond.
SMILEY, Elita Gartnavel Royal Hospital, 1055 Great Western Road, Glasgow G12 0XH Tel: 0141 211 3600; 7 Brierie Hills Court, Crosslee, Houston, Johnstone PA6 7DU — MB ChB Glas. 1993. SHO (Psychiat.) Gartnavel Roy. Hosp. Glas. Specialty: Gen. Psychiat.
SMILLIE, Dorothy Clair River Place Health Centre, Essex Road, London N1 2TS Tel: 020 7226 1473 — MB ChB Dundee 1974. Socs: BMA. Prev: SHO (Gen. Med.) Stracathro Hosp. Brechin; Med. Edr. Med. News; SHO (Paediat.) Edgware Gen. Hosp.
SMILLIE, Jane Fiona Riversdale Surgery, Riversdale House, Merthyrmawr Road, Bridgend CF31 3NL Tel: 01656 766866 Fax: 01656 668659 — MB ChB Bristol 1981; MRCGP 1985; MRCPsych 1988; Dip. Palliat. Med. Wales 1991. GP Bridgend.
SMILLIE, Martin Watt (retired) The Surgery, Union Road, Camelon, Falkirk FK1 Tel: 01324 22854 — MB ChB Glas. 1956; DObst RCOG 1961. Prev: Resid. Stobhill Gen. Hosp. & Glas. Roy. Infirm.
SMIRK, Thomas Winfield Haslington Surgery, Crewe Road, Haslington, Crewe CW1 5QY Tel: 01270 581259 Fax: 01270 257958; 336 Crewe Road, Winterley, Sandbach CW11 4RP — MB BS Newc. 1974.
SMIRL, Jeanine Elizabeth The Miller Practice, 49 Highbury New Park, London N5 2ET Tel: 020 7354 1972 — MB BS Lond. 1987; DCH RCP Lond. 1990; DRCOG 1991. GP Trainer. Specialty: Gen. Pract. Prev: SHO (O & G) Lond. Hosp.; SHO (Paediat.) King Geo. Hosp. Ilford.; SHO (A & E) Broomfield Hosp. Chelmsford.
SMIT, Ian David 6 Gatton Close, Sutton SM2 5QL — MB ChB Pretoria 1968.
SMITH, Mr Adam Neil (retired) 2 Ravelston House Park, Edinburgh EH4 3LU Tel: 0131 332 4077 — MB ChB Glas. 1948; FRCS Ed. 1956; MD (Hons.) Glas. 1959; FRSE 1982; FRCP Ed. 1988; DSc Ed. 1995. Prev: Wade Prof. Surg. Studies Roy. Coll. Surg. Edin.
SMITH, Adrian Curtis 58 Hargreaves Road, Oswaldthistle, Accrington BB5 4RN — MB ChB Manch. 1983.
SMITH, Adrian David 20 Whitworth Street, London SE10 9EN — MB BS Lond. 1991.
SMITH, Adrian Grenville 301 Court Lane, Erdington, Birmingham B23 5JS — MB ChB Birm. 1984; MB ChB (Hons.) Birm. 1984; MRCP (UK) 1988. Regist. (Haemat.) Selly Oak Hosp. Birm. Specialty: Haematology.
SMITH, Adrian Henry Lampard Nethergreen Road Surgery, 34-36 Nethergreen Road, Sheffield S11 7EJ Tel: 0114 230 2952; 133B Tom Lane, Sheffield S10 3PE Tel: 0114 230 9625 — MB ChB Sheff. 1985; DRCOG 1989; MRCGP 1990; DFFP 1994. Prev: Trainee GP Sheff. VTS.
SMITH, Alan Douglas Forensic Psychiatry Service, (Box 175) S3, Addenbrooke's Hospital, Cambridge CB2 2QQ Tel: 01223 216442 Fax: 01223 217941 — MB ChB Glas. 1990; BSc (Hons.) Glas. 1987; MRCPsych 1994; MPhil Ed. 1996. Cons. (Forens. Psychiat.) Addenbrooke's Hosp. Cambs. Specialty: Forens. Psychiat. Socs: Parole Board for England and Wales. Prev: Lect. (Forens. Psychiat.) Inst. Of Psychiat. & Maudsley Hosp. Lond.; Lect. & Sen. Regist. (Forens. Psychiat.) Univ. Camb. & Norvic Clinic Norwich; Regist. & SHO (Psychiat.) Roy. Edin. Hosp.
SMITH, Alan Inglis Murrayfield Medical Practice, 13B Riversdale Crescent, Edinburgh EH12 5QX Tel: 0131 337 6151 Fax: 0131 313 3450 — MB ChB Ed. 1983.
SMITH, Mr Alan Malcolm (retired) 29 Sunningdale Close, Birmingham B20 1LH — BM BCh Oxf. 1954 (Univ. Coll. Hosp.) MA Oxf. 1954; BM BCh Oxf. 1954; MA Oxf. 1954; DObst 1956; FRCS Ed. 1963; M 1969; FRCOG 1973; FRCP Ed. 1979; BSc Open 1998. Prev: Cons. O & G Wolverhampton Gp. Hosps. & W. Bromwich Hosp. Gp.
SMITH, Alan Mark 125 Cholmley Gardens, London NW6 1AA — MB ChB Leeds 1993.
SMITH, Alan McGregor Kenilworth Medical Centre, 1 Kennilworth Court, Glasgow G67 1BP Tel: 01236 727816 Fax: 01236 726306; Hollybank, 2A Mill Road, Riggend, Airdrie ML6 7ST Tel: 01236 830031 — MB ChB Ed. 1961 (Edin. Univ.) DObst RCOG 1963; MRCGP 1980.
SMITH, Alan Peter Watson Health Centre, Balmellie Road, Turriff AB53 4DQ Tel: 01888 562323 Fax: 01888 568682 — MB ChB Aberd. 1978.
SMITH, Alan Robert 5 Crimond Court, Fraserburgh AB43 9QW — MB ChB Aberd. 1997.
SMITH, Mr Alan Robert Clifton Wrythe Green Surgery, Wrythe Lane, Carshalton SM5 2RE Tel: 020 8669 3232/1717 Fax: 020 8773 2524 — MB BS Lond. 1983; FRCS Eng. 1989. Prev: Trainee GP Crawley VTS; Regist. Rotat. SW Thames; Cas. Off. & SHO St. Geo. Hosp. Lond.
SMITH, Alan William McIntosh (retired) 29 Links Road, Lundin Links, Leven KY8 6AT Tel: 01333 320221 — MB ChB Ed. 1950; MB ChB (Hons.) Ed. 1950; FRCP Ed. 1962, M 1952. Hon. Sen. Lect. (Med.) Univ. Edin. Prev: Cons. Phys. Vict. Hosp. Kirkcaldy & E. Fife Gp. Hosps.
SMITH, Alastair Gordon Haematology Department, Southampton General Hospital, Southampton SO16 6YD Tel: 023 8079 4438 Fax: 023 8079 4134; 24 Oakenbrow, Sway, Lymington SO41 6DY Tel: 01590 683484 — MB ChB Glas. 1974; BSc (Hons.) Glas. 1972; MRCP (UK) 1976; MRCPath 1981; FRCP Glas. 1988; FRCP Lond. 1994. Cons. Haemat, Clin. Director, Clin. Soton. Univ. Hosps.; Hon. Clin. Sen. Lect. Soton. Univ. Specialty: Haematology. Socs: Brit. Soc. Haematol.; Amer. Soc. Haemat. Prev: Sen. Regist. (Haemat.) West. Infirm. Glas.; Regist. (Haemat.) Stobhill Hosp. Glas.; SHO (Med.) Stobhill Hosp. Glas.
SMITH, Alastair William, MBE, OStJ (retired) Wayside, Birkett Hill, Bowness-on-Windermere, Windermere LA23 3EZ Tel: 015394 43658 — LRCP LRCS Ed. LRFPS Glas. 1942. Prev: Clin. Asst. Glas. Roy. Infirm.
SMITH, Albert Edward Centre for Occupational Health & Environmental, University of Manchester, C Block, Humanities Building, Manchester M13 9PL, Switzerland Tel: 0161 275 5202 Fax: 0161 275 5625 Email: ted.smith@clara.net; North Wing, Harewood Lodge, Broadbottom, Hyde SK14 6BB Tel: 01457 762665 Email: ted.smith@clara.net — MB BS Lond. 1966 (Univ. Coll. Hosp.) BSc Lond. 1963; DObst RCOG 1968; MRCGP 1974; DIH Eng. 1979; FFOM RCP 1992, MFOM 1983, AFOM 1981. Sen. Clin. Fell. Centre Ocupational Health Univ. Manch.; Cons. Occupat. Phys. Roy. Oldham Hosp. Specialty: Occupat. Health. Socs: BMA; Soc. Occup. Med.; Brit. Occup. Hyg. Soc. Prev: Corporate Ocupational Phys. Novartis Internat.; Gp. Ocupational Phys. Ciba-Geigy UK; Head Med. Serv. UK Atomic Energy Auth. Dounreay Nuclear Power Developm. Estabm.
SMITH, Alexander David Stuart 18 Craigleith View, Edinburgh EH4 3JZ — MB ChB Manch. 1976; BSc (Hons.) St. And. 1969. Med. Adviser Semaslumberger. Specialty: Disabil. Med. Prev: Sen. Regist. (Clin. Biochem.) Glas. Roy. Infirm.; Med. Adviser Benefits Agency.
SMITH, Alexander Gordon Lochhead (retired) 6 Bishops Close, Old Coulsdon, Coulsdon CR5 1HH Tel: 01737 554576 — MB ChB Ed. 1958; DObst RCOG 1961; DFFP 1993. Prev: SHO (O & G) Buchanan Hosp. St. Leonards-on-Sea.
SMITH, Alexander James (retired) Foxstones, 29 Friar Crescent, Brighton BN1 6NL Tel: 01273 506566 — MB ChB Aberd. 1953. Prev: Med. Off. RAF Med. Br.
SMITH, Alexander John (retired) The Manor House, Stretton-on-Dunsmore, Rugby CV23 9NA Tel: 024 7654 2718 — (Guy's) MB BS Lond. 1952; MRCS Eng. LRCP Lond. 1952; DPath Eng. 1960; FRCPath 1972, M 1963. Prev: Cons. Path. Hosp. St. Cross Rugby,Warwick Hosp.Coventry.
SMITH, Mr Alexander McEwen, VRD (retired) 46 Lichfield Lane, Mansfield NG18 4RZ Tel: 01263 465845 — (Univ. Ed.) MB ChB Ed. 1939; FRCS Ed. 1948. Prev: Cons. Surg. Mansfield Gen. Hosp. & King's Mill Hosp. Sutton in.
SMITH, Alexander Peter (retired) Holmview, Penyturnpike, Dinas Powys CF64 4HG Tel: 029 2051 3231 — MD Sheff. 1976; MB ChB 1965; FRCP Lond. 1984, M 1968. Prev: Lect. (Med.) & Sen. Regist. King's Coll. Hosp. Lond.
SMITH, Alfred Leonard Gordon (retired) 125 Caldercliffe Road, Taylor Hill, Huddersfield HD4 7RH Tel: 01484 532332 — (Glas.) MB ChB Glas. 1947; DPM RCPSI 1950; FRCPsych 1971. Prev: Med.

Supt. Storthes Hall Hosp. & Cons. Psychiat. St. Luke's Hosp. Huddersfield.

SMITH, Alison Church View Surgery, School La, Collingham, Wetherby LS22 5BQ Tel: 01937 573848 Fax: 01937 574754; Shrewton House, Harewood Road, Collingham, Wetherby LS22 5BY Tel: 01937 572280 — MB ChB Ed. 1967; MRCP (UK) 1970; DObst (NZ) 1973; DCH RCP Lond. 1974.

SMITH, Alison Doreen Northbourne Medical Centre, Eastern Avenue, Shoreham-by-Sea BN43 6PE; Magnolia House, 49 Southwick St, Southwick, Brighton BN42 4TH Tel: 01273 593963 Fax: 01273 593963 — MB ChB Birm. 1978; DRCOG 1980; MRCGP 1984; DFFP 1993. Specialty: Dermat. Prev: Prof. Exec. Comm. Chair. For Adur. Arun & Worthing PCT.

SMITH, Alison Duff Craig Nevis Surgery, Belford Road, Fort William PH33 6BU Tel: 01397 702947 Fax: 01397 700655 — MB ChB Dundee 1985.

SMITH, Alison Elisabeth Exwick Health Centre, New Valley Road, Exwick, Exeter EX4 2AD Tel: 01392 270063 Fax: 01392 431884 — MB ChB Sheff. 1985; MRCGP 1990. GP Princip. Specialty: Gen. Pract.

SMITH, Alison Jane Westerhope Medical Group, 377 Stamfordham Road, Westerhope, Newcastle upon Tyne NE5 2LH Tel: 0191 243 7000 Fax: 0191 243 7006; 29 First Avenue, Newcastle upon Tyne NE6 5YE — MB BS Newc. 1987; MRCGP 1991; DRCOG 1991. Prev: Trainee GP/SHO (Psychiat.) St. Geo. Hosp. N.d.; Trainee GP/SHO (A & E) Qu. Eliz. Hosp. Gateshead.

SMITH, Alison Jane Dept Anaesthesia, Weston General Hospital, Grange Road, Weston Super Mare BS23 4TQ Tel: 01934 647162 — MB BS Lond. 1988; BSc Lond. 1985; DA (UK) 1990; FRCA 1993. Cons. (Anaesth.) Weston Gen Hosp. Specialty: Anaesth.

SMITH, Alison Jane 8 Huddersfield Road, New Mill, Huddersfield HD9 7JU — MB ChB Glas. 1997.

SMITH, Alison Kay A & E Department, Barnsley District General Hospital, Gawber Road, Barnsley S75 2EP Tel: 01226 730000 — MB ChB 1990; MB ChB Sheff. 1990; MRCP (UK) 1995; FFAEM 1999. Cons. Emergengy Med., Barnsley Dist. Gen. Hosp. Specialty: Accid. & Emerg.

SMITH, Alison Lindsay Church View Surgery, 14 Church View, Dundrum, Newcastle BT33 0NA; 50 Sunningdale Drive, Newcastle BT33 0QJ Tel: 013967 23983 — MB ChB Ed. 1982; BSc (Hons.) Ed. 1979, MB ChB 1982. Trainee GP Newc. VTS. Prev: SHO (Psychiat., Geriat & Cas.) Roy. Vict. Hosp. Edin.

SMITH, Alistair Fairley Department of Clinical Biochemistry, Royal Infirmary, Edinburgh EH3 9YW Tel: 0131 536 2758 Fax: 0131 229 3543; 38 Cammo Road, Edinburgh EH4 8AP Tel: 0131 339 4931 Fax: 0131 339 9113 — MB BChir Camb. 1961 (Lond. Hosp.) FRCP Ed. 1973, M 1965; FRCPath 1979, M 1967; MA Camb. 1957, MD 1971. Sen. Lect. (Clin. Biochem.) Roy. Infirm. Edin. Specialty: Biochem. Prev: Ho. Phys. Lond. Hosp. & Addenbrooke's Hosp. Camb.; Jun. Asst. Path. Univ. Camb.

SMITH, Allison Lucy Blair Schopwick Surgery, Everett Court, Romeland, Borehamwood WD6 3BJ Tel: 020 8953 1008 Fax: 020 8905 2196; 77 Upper Paddock Road, Watford WD19 4DY — (Royal Free Hospital School of Medicine) BSc 1982; MB BS London 1987; MB BS London 1987; MRCGP 1993.

SMITH, Amanda 79 Farquhar Road, Edgbaston, Birmingham B15 2QP — MB ChB Leic. 1983; DA (UK) 1985; MBA 1993.

SMITH, Amanda Elizabeth Rachel Saltegate Health Centre, Chesterfield S40 15X — MB BS Lond. 1987 (Guy's) DRCOG 1992; DFFP 1993; MFFP 2000. Sen.Clin. Med. Off. (Family Plann. & Wom.'s Health) Chesterfield & Mansfield. Specialty: Family Plann. & Reproduc. Health; Genitourinary Medicine. Socs: British Menopause Soc.; FFPRHC. Prev: Asst. GP Chesterfield; Clin. Asst. (Genitourin. Med.) Redford; Clin. Med. Off. (Family Plann & Reprod. Health) Chesterfield & Mansfield.

SMITH, Amanda Jean The Garth Surgery, Rectory Lane, Guisborough TS14 7DJ Tel: 01287 632206 Fax: 01287 635112; 15 Weardale, Pinehills, Guisborough TS14 8JL — MB BS Lond. 1982 (Royal Free) DRCOG 1985; MRCGP 1986. GP Tutor Longbourgh PCT. Socs: Primary Care Rheum. Soc.; Local Med. Comm. Prev: Clin. Asst. Carter Bequest Hosp. Middlesboro.; Trainee GP/SHO (Med.) Middlesbrough Gen. Hosp.; Trainee GP/SHO (O & G) N. Tees Hosp.

SMITH, Andrew 23 Aynsley Court, St Helens WA9 5GE — MB ChB Liverp. 1987. Trainee GP/SHO (Cas.) Whiston Hosp.; GP Princip., St. Helens, Merseyside. Prev: Ho. Off. (Med. & Surg.) Roy. Liverp. Hosp.

SMITH, Andrew Medway Hospital, Windmill Road, Gillingham ME7 5NY Tel: 01634 830000 — MB BS Lond. 1990; BSc (Hons.) 1987; MRCP (UK) 1994. Regist. (Diabetes, Endocrinol. & Gen. Med.) Medway Hosp. Gillingham.

SMITH, Andrew Combe Down Surgery, Combe Down House, The Avenue, Combe Down, Bath BA2 5EG Tel: 01225 832226 Fax: 01225 840757 — MB BS Lond. 1989 (Univesity College London) BSc Lond. 1986; DCH RCP Lond. 1993; DRCOG 1995; MRCGP 1995. GP. Specialty: Gen. Pract. Prev: Non Princip. GP Bath; Sen. Med. Off. Aboriginal Med. Serv. Carnarvon, Western Australia; GP Regist. Bath VTS.

SMITH, Andrew Edward Rodney The Old Rectory Surgery, 18 Castle Street, Saffron Walden CB10 1BP Tel: 01799 522327 Fax: 01799 525436 — MB BS Lond. 1972 (Westm.) BSc (Anat.) Lond. 1969; MRCS Eng. LRCP Lond. 1972; DObst RCOG 1976. Specialty: Gen. Med. Prev: Trainee GP Camb. VTS; SHO Auckland Pub. Hosp. Auckland, NZ; Ho. Off. (Med.) W. Middlx. Hosp. Isleworth.

SMITH, Andrew Fairley Royal Lancaster Infirmary, Department of Anaesthesia, Ashton Road, Lancaster LA1 4RP Tel: 01524 583517 Fax: 01524 583519 — MB BS Newc. 1988; MRCP (UK) 1991; FRCA 1994. Cons. Anaesth. Morecambe Bay Hosps. NHS Trust; Hon. Sen. Lect. Lancaster Sch. Postgrad. Med. & Health. Specialty: Anaesth. Special Interest: Ophth. Anaesth.; Paediatric Anaesth. Socs: Fell. Manch. Med. Soc.; Assn. Anaesth.; Assn. for Study of Med. Educat. Prev: Sen. Regist. (Anaesth.) NW RHA; SHO (Gen. Med.) Stepping Hill Hosp. Stockport; Ho. Phys. Freeman Hosp. Newc. u Tyne.

SMITH, Andrew George Department of Dermatology, Central Outpatients Department, Univ. Hosp. of N. Staffs., Stoke-on-Trent ST4 7PA Tel: 01782 554265 Fax: 01782 554233 — MB BChir Camb. 1970 (Camb. & St. Mary's) MD Camb. 1982; FRCP Lond. 1989. Cons. Dermatol., Univ. Hosp. of N. Staffs. Specialty: Dermat. Special Interest: Dermatopathology.

SMITH, Andrew Gourdie Path House Medical Practice, Path House, 7 Nether Street, Kirkcaldy KY1 2PG Tel: 01592 644533 Fax: 01592 644550; 20 Townsend Crescent, Kirkcaldy KY1 1DN — MB ChB Ed. 1977. Prev: Trainee GP W. Lothian VTS; Ho. Phys. Bangour Gen. Hosp. Broxburn; Ho. Surg. Peel Hosp. Galashiels.

SMITH, Andrew Gregory College Surgery Partnership, College Rd, Cullompton EX15 1TG Tel: 01884 831300 Fax: 01884 831313 Email: andy.smith@gp-l83092.nhs.uk — MB ChB Bristol 1991; BSc (Microbiol.) 1988; DRCOG 1995; DCH 1996; MRCGP 1997. GP Cullompton, Devon. Specialty: Gen. Pract.

SMITH, Andrew James Barrow Hospital, Barrow Gurney, Bristol BS48 3SG — MB BS Lond. 1987. SHO (Geriat. Med.) St. Stephens Hosp. Lond.

SMITH, Mr Andrew Malvern — MB BS Lond. 1991 (St. Mary's Hospital) BSc (Hons.) Lond. 1989; FRCS Eng. 1995; DM Nottm. 1999. Lect. (Surg.) Univ. of Hull; Hon. Specialist Regist. (Gen. Surg.) Mid-Trent Rotat.; Specialist Regist. (Gen. Surg.). Specialty: Gen. Surg. Socs: Surg. Research Soc.; Assn. Surg. Train.; Assn. of Upper Gastrointestinal Surg.s. Prev: Research Fell. & Hon. Regist. (Surg.) Univ. Nottm.; SHO Rotat. (Surg.) Leicester; Lect. (Surg.) Univ. of Nottm.

SMITH, Andrew Michael Flat 9, 1-2 Percival Terrace, Brighton BN2 1FA — MB BS Lond. 1993.

SMITH, Andrew Neil Leigh View Medical Centre, Bradford Road, Tingley, Wakefield WF3 1RQ Tel: 0113 253 7629 Fax: 0113 238 1286 — MB ChB Leeds 1984; MRCGP 1991. Prev: Trainee GP/SHO (A & E) Dewsbury Dist. HA VTS.

SMITH, Mr Angus 42 Kenilworth Road, Bridge of Allan, Stirling FK9 4RP Tel: 01786 833455 — MB ChB Glas. 1976; BSc (Hons.) Glas. 1974; FRCS Glas. 1981; FRCS Ed. 1993. Cons. Surg. Stirling Roy. Infirm. Specialty: Gen. Surg.

SMITH, Mr Angus Cameron (retired) 1103 Aikenhead Road, Cathcart, Glasgow G44 5SL — MB ChB Glas. 1950; DLO Eng. 1954; FRFPS Glas. 1961; FRCS Glas. 1962. Prev: Cons. ENT Surg. Vict. Infirm. Glas. & S. Gen. Hosp. Glas.

SMITH, Anina Mary Brindley 34 Rugby Road, Bulkington, Nuneaton — MB ChB Manch. 1975.

SMITH, Anna Elizabeth Clark Kirkhall Surgery, 4 Alexandra Avenue, Prestwick KA9 1AW Tel: 01292 476626 Fax: 01292 678022 — MB ChB Aberd. 1973; DRCOG 1977.

SMITH, Anna Mary Louise Merchiston Surgery, Highworth Road, Swindon SN3 4BF Tel: 01793 823307 Fax: 01793 820923 — MB BS Lond. 1990; DFFP 1994; MRCGP 1994; DRCOG 1994.

SMITH, Annabelle Toni Maria 185 Barnfield Avenue, Kingston upon Thames KT2 5RQ Tel: 020 8549 9003 — MB BS Lond. 1993. Specialty: Paediat. Prev: SHO (paed) St Geo.'s Hosp.; SHO (Paediat.) Chelsea & Westminster Hosp.

SMITH, Anne Helen Walmsley Carseview Centre, Dundee Medipark, Dundee DD2 1NH Tel: 01382 878712 Email: anne.smith@tpct.scot.nhs.uk — MB ChB St. And. 1969; DPM 1972; MRCPsych 1974. Cons. Psychiat. Tayside NHS Trust; Hon. Sen. Lect., Univ. of Dundee. Specialty: Gen. Psychiat. Special Interest: Psychiat. of Learning Disabil. Prev: Lect. in Psychiat. Univ. Dundee.

SMITH, Anne Louise 45 Conduit Road, Stamford PE9 1QL Tel: 01780 762940 — MB ChB Leic. 1992 (Leicester) MRCP (UK) 1996. Regist. (Paediat.) P'boro. Dist. Hosp. Specialty: Paediat. Socs: Roy. Soc. Med. Prev: SHO (Paediat. Cardiol.) Glenfield Hosp. Leicester; SHO (Paediat.) P'boro. & Leicester Roy. Infirm.

SMITH, Anne Patricia Mary 15 Station Road East, Peterculter, Aberdeen AB21 7BA — MB ChB Aberd. 1977; DRCOG 1984; MD Aberd. 1994. Assoc. Specialist (Ultrasonics & Colposcopy) & Hon. Lect. (O & G) Aberd. Matern. Hosp. Specialty: Obst. & Gyn. Socs: Brit. Med. Ultrasound Soc. (Counc. & Scientif. Educat. Advis. Comm.).

SMITH, Anne Vera 6 The Crescent, Longbenton, Newcastle upon Tyne NE7 7ST Tel: 0191 215 0268 Email: anne.smith@btinternet.com — MB BS Newc. 1966. p/t SCMO (Psychosexual Med.) Dept. Reproductive Med. and Sexual Health Newc. Gen. Hosp., Newc. Upon Tyne. Specialty: Psychosexual Med. Socs: Inst. Psychosexual Med. Prev: Sen. Partner, Gen. Pract., Newc. Upon Tyne.

SMITH, Anthony Bernard Upton Group Practice, 32 Ford Road, Wirral CH49 0TF Tel: 0151 677 0486 Fax: 0151 604 0635; Roseneath, Arno Road, Oxton, Prenton CH43 5UX Tel: 0151 652 1108 — MB ChB Leeds 1984; BSc (Hons.) Leeds 1981; DRCOG 1987; MRCGP 1989; DFFP 1993. Specialty: Gen. Pract. Prev: Trainee GP Burnley Gen. Hosp. VTS; SHO (Clin. Path.) Roy. Hallamsh. Hosp. Sheff.

SMITH, Anthony Clive Mill House, Higher Wych, Malpas SY14 7JR — MB ChB Manch. 1998; MB ChB Manch 1998.

SMITH, Anthony David Addison Derby Psychotherapy Unit, Temple House, Mill Hill Lane, Derby DE23 6SB Tel: 01332 364512; 59 South Avenue, Darley Abbey, Derby DE22 1FB — MB BS Newc. 1976; MRCPsych 1981; Dip. Psychother. Leeds 1985. Cons. Psychother. (Community Psychiat. Servs.) South. Derbysh. HA. Specialty: Gen. Psychiat. Prev: Sen. Regist. (Psychother.) St. Jas. Hosp. Leeds.

SMITH, Anthony Derek Kinmylies Medical Practice, Assynt Road, Kinmylies, Inverness IV3 8PB Tel: 01463 239865 Fax: 01463 711218 — MB ChB Ed. 1971; DCH RCPS Glas. 1974; MRCP (UK) 1980; FRCP Ed. 1997; MRCPCH 1998. Assoc. Adviser in Gen. Pract. N. Scotl.; Hosp. Pract. GUM.; Med. Adviser Highland Counc.; Police Surg. Specialty: Gen. Pract. Socs: Div.al Hon. Sec. BMA; SACCH; Pres. Highland Med. Soc. 2000.

SMITH, Mr Anthony Mighell (retired) Gillrock House, Main Road, Sellindge, Ashford TN25 6AQ — MB BChir Camb. 1963 (Camb. & St. Geo.) MA Camb. 1963; DObst RCOG 1964; FRCS Ed. 1972; T(M) 1990; Cert. Med. Educat. Univ. of Dundee 1998. Prev: Dir. of Studies St. Christopher's Hospice Sydenham.

SMITH, Anthony Richard The Surgery, Chilton Place, Ash, Canterbury CT3 2HD Tel: 01304 812227 Fax: 01304 813788 — MB BS Lond. 1981; DRCOG 1987.

SMITH, Anthony Ross Broadhurst The Warrell Unit, St Mary's Hospital, Manchester M13 0JH Tel: 0161 276 6750 Fax: 0161 276 6140 Email: anthony.smith@cmmc.nhs.uk; 23 Anson Road, Victoria Park, Manchester M14 5BZ Tel: 0161 248 2027 Fax: 0161 248 2034 — MB ChB Manch. 1977; BSc St. And. 1974; FRCOG 1995, M 1982; MD Manch. 1985. Cons. Gyn. St Mary's Hosp. Manch. Specialty: Obst. & Gyn. Special Interest: Endoscopic Surg.; Pelvic floor failure; Urin. incontinence. Socs: Pres. Brit. Soc. Gyn. Endoscopy - 2001; Brit. Soc. of Gyn. Prev: Lect. Jessop Hosp. Sheff.; Research Regist. (O & G) St. Mary's Hosp. Manch.; Regist. (O & G) St. Mary's Hosp. Manch.

SMITH, Mr Antony Langley Robert Jones and Agnes Hunt Orthopaedic Hospital, Oswestry SY10 7AG Tel: 01691 404385 — MB ChB Ed. 1989 (Edin.) FRCS Ed. 1995; FRCS Eng. 1995; FRCS (orth) 2000. Cons. Orthopaedic and Trauma Surg. Robt. Jones & Agnes Hunt Orthop. Hosp. OsW.ry. And Wrexham Maelor. Specialty: Trauma & Orthop. Surg. Socs: Brit. Orthopaedic Soc.; Brit. Assn. of Surg. of The Knee. Prev: Maj RAMC.

SMITH, Archibald Brian (retired) Cove Villa, 83 Hecklegirth, Annan DG12 6HL Tel: 01461 203250 Fax: 01461 203250 Email: archie@covevilla.freeserve.co.uk — MB ChB St. And. 1969.

SMITH, Arthur Hopper Low Reins Gill, Middleton-in-Teesdale, Barnard Castle DL12 0RY Tel: 01833 640502 — MB BS Durh. 1955. Locum Gen. Practitioner. Specialty: Accid. & Emerg.; Gen. Med.

SMITH, Arthur Thomas Stockton Heath Medical Centre, The Forge, London Road, Stockton Heath, Warrington WA4 6HJ Tel: 01925 604427; 36 Kildonan Road, Grappenhall, Warrington WA4 2LJ — MB BCh Wales 1971; MRCGP 1978. Prev: Ho. Phys. & Ho. Surg. Roy. Alexandra Hosp. Rhyl.

SMITH, Ashley Lee Nicola Flat 5, 4 Wandle Road, Morden SM4 6AH — MB BS Lond. 1996.

SMITH, Audrey Christine 116 Ainsworth Road, Bury BL8 2RX — MB ChB Liverp. 1997.

SMITH, Augustine Martin James 37 Church Road, Hayes UB3 2LB — MB BCh BAO NUI 1993; LRCPSI 1993.

SMITH, Mr Austen Thornton Head & Neck Unit, Royal Hallamshire Hospital, Glossop Road, Sheffield CF24 4QY Tel: 0114 271 7946 Email: austensmith@shef.ac.uk — MB BCh Wales 1988; BDS Wales 1980; FRCS Ed. 1991. Consultant, Maxillofacial Surg., Sheff. Teachg. Hosps. NHS Trust, Barnsley Dist. Gen. Hosp. NHS Trust; Hon. Sen. Clin. Lect., Univ. of Sheff. Specialty: Oral & Maxillofacial Surg. Special Interest: Head & Neck Cancer; Reconstruc. Surg. including Microvascular Transfer. Socs: BMA; BAOMS; BAHNO.

SMITH, Barbara Anne New Cumnock Surgery, 67 Afton Bridgend, New Cumnock, Cumnock KA18 4BA Tel: 01290 338242 Fax: 01290 332010 — MB ChB Glas. 1982; BSc Glas. 1979, MB ChB 1982. SHO (Gyn.) CrossHo. Hosp. Kilmarnock. Socs: BMA; Inceptor of Roy. Coll. Psychiat. Prev: Jun. Ho. Off. (Med. & Surg.) Glas. Roy. Infirm.; SHO (Psychiat.) Woodilee Hosp. Gtr. Glas. Health Bd.; Regist. (Psychiat.) Woodilee Hosp. Gtr. Glas. Health Bd.

SMITH, Barrie Stanley 104 Kingsbury Road, Erdington, Birmingham B24 8QU Tel: 0121 373 6740 — MB ChB Birm. 1956; MRCS Eng. LRCP Lond. 1956; FRCP Lond. 1978, M 1964. Med. Off., Aston Villa FC. Specialty: Gen. Med.; Sports Med. Prev: Cons. Phys. Sandwell Dist. Gen. Hosp. (Retd.); Ho. Phys. Qu. Eliz. Hosp. Birm.; Cons. Phys. W. Bromwich Hosp. Gp.

SMITH, Barry Sabden & Whalley Medical Group, 42 King St., Whalley, Clitheroe BB7 9SL Tel: 01254 823273 Fax: 01254 824891; The Old Vicarage, Mitton, Whalley, Blackburn BB6 9PH Tel: 01254 826473 — MB ChB Manch. 1962; DObst RCOG 1964; FRCGP 1990, M 1970; Cert Contracep. & Family Plann. RCOG & RCGP 1974.

SMITH, Barry Arthur Charles, TD Whitehouse Farm, Miles Green, Stoke-on-Trent ST7 8LQ — MB ChB Birm. 1975; FRCA 1980. Cons. Anaesth. N. Staffs. Hosp. NHS Trust. Specialty: Anaesth. Socs: Midl. Anaesth. Soc.; Anaesth. Soc. Prev: Asst. Prof. Univ. Texas Med. Sch. Houston, USA; Sen. Regist. (Anaesth.) Midl. Train. Scheme.

SMITH, Basil John 13A Rawlinson Road, Oxford OX2 6UE — MB BS Lond. 1978 (St. Bart.) BSc Lond. 1961; DPhil Oxf. 1964; MRCP (UK) 1981; FRCR 1986. Cons. Clin. Oncol. New Cross Hosp. Wolverhampton. Specialty: Oncol.; Radiother. Prev: Sen. Regist. (Radiother. & Oncol.) Univ. Coll. Hosp. Lond.; Regist. (Radiother. & Oncol.) Westm. Hosp.; SHO Nuffield Dept. Med. John Radcliffe Hosp. Oxf.

SMITH, Benjamin John 15 (2Fl) Gladstone Terrace, Edinburgh EH9 1LS — MB ChB Ed. 1994.

SMITH, Blair Hamilton Department of General Practice & Primary Care, University of Aberdeen, Foresterhill Health Centre, Westburn Road, Aberdeen AB25 2AY Tel: 01224 553972 Email:

blairsmith@abdn.ac.uk; North Arnybogs, Methlick, Ellon AB41 7BT — MB ChB Glas. 1987; MRCGP 1993; DFFP 1993; MEd. Aberdeen 1998; MD Aberdeen 2000. Sen. Lect.(Gen. Pract.) Univ. Aberd.; GP Deveron Med. Pract. Banff; Surg. Lt. Cdr. Roy. Naval Reserve, HMS Scotia Rosyth. Specialty: Gen. Pract.; Epidemiol. Socs: Assn. of Univ. Dept.s of Gen. Pract.; Internat. Epidemicological Assn. Prev: SHO (Endocrinol. & Infertil.) Jessop Hosp. for Wom. Sheff.; SHO (O & G) North. Gen. Hosp., Aberd. Roy. Infirm. & Jessop Hosp. Sheff.; GP Trainee, Aberd.

SMITH, Brendan Edward The Berrow Hill Medical Centre, Berrow Hill, Feckenham, Redditch B96 6QS — MB ChB Sheff. 1977; FFA RCS Eng. 1984. Specialty: Anaesth.

SMITH, Brendon Glenn Timperley Health Centre, 169 Grove Lane, Timperley, Altrincham WA15 6PH — MB ChB Manch. 1980; Cert. Family Plann. JCC 1982; DRCOG 1982; DCH RCP Lond. 1983; MRCGP 1984. Princip. GP Timperley.

SMITH, Brent Charles Howden Well Close Square Surgery, Well Close Square, Berwick-upon-Tweed TD15 1LL Tel: 01289 356920 Fax: 01289 356939 — MB ChB St. And. 1970; LMCC 1972; DObst RCOG 1974; DA Eng. 1977. Hosp. Pract. (Anaesth.) Berwick Infirm. Specialty: Anaesth. Socs: Coll. Phys. & Surg. Brit.; Columbia & Fac. Anaesth. RCS Eng.

SMITH, Mr Brian David (retired) 38 Fiskerton Road, Cherry Willingham, Lincoln LN3 4AP Tel: 01522 751603 Fax: 01522 751603 — MB ChB St. And. 1957; FRCS Eng. 1967. Prev: Cons. Mem. Med. Appeals Tribunal Nottm.

SMITH, Brian Hall (retired) 26 Metchley Park Road, Edgbaston, Birmingham B15 2PG Tel: 0121 454 6538 — (Birmingham) MB ChB Birm. 1948; MRCS Eng. LRCP Lond. 1948; FRCA 1954. Prev: Cons. Anaesth. Qu. Eliz. Hosp. Birm.

SMITH, Brian James 43 West Bank, Abbotts Park, Chester CH1 4BD — MB ChB Birm. 1987.

SMITH, Brian Leslie Wexham Park Hospital, Slough SL2 4HL Tel: 01753 633000 Fax: 01753 634460; Fairview, River Road, Taplow, Maidenhead SL6 0BG Tel: 01628 674321 Fax: 01628 621845 — (St. Mary's) MB BS Lond. 1962; MRCS Eng. LRCP Lond. 1962; DObst RCOG 1963; FRCA. 1970. Clin. Dir. Anaesth. Heatherwood & Wexham Pk. Hosp. Trust. Specialty: Anaesth. Socs: Assn. Anaesths., B.M.A., H.C.S.A. Prev: Sen. Regist. (Anaesth.) Middlx. Hosp. Lond.; Asst. Anaesth. S.well Hosp. (Kuwait Oil Co.) Ahmadi, Kuwait; Asst. Prof. Anaesth. Univ. Calif. San Francisco, USA.

SMITH, Brian Spencer (retired) LongFriday Fieldhouse, Canon Pyon Road, Hereford HR4 7SL Tel: 01432 263498 — (Middlx.) MB BS Lond. 1955; MRCS Eng. LRCP Lond. 1955. Prev: Gen. Pract. Ross-on-Wye.

SMITH, Brigid Teresa Mary Abbey Medical Practice, Abbey Street, Londonderry BT48 9DN Tel: 028 7136 4016 — MB BCh BAO Belf. 1981; DRCOG 1984; MRCGP 1986; FRCGP 1997.

SMITH, Bruce Alexander Murison (retired) 197 Millhouses Lane, Sheffield S7 2HF Tel: 0114 361870 — MB ChB Leeds 1956; FRCPCH; DCH Eng. 1959; DObst RCOG 1960; FRCP Ed. 1978, M 1962. Prev: Cons. Paediat. North. Gen. Hosp. Sheff.

SMITH, Cameron Cairns 198 Rullion Road, Penicuik EH26 9JF — MB ChB Aberd. 1991.

SMITH, Carlyle Wilhelm Ernst 213 Northdown Park Road, Margate CT9 3UJ — MB BS Ceylon 1958 (Colombo) FRCP Lond. 1981, M 1968. JP; Cons. Phys. (Geriat.) I. of Thanet & Canterbury Hosp. Gp. Specialty: Care of the Elderly. Socs: Brit. Geriat. Soc.; BMA. Prev: Regist. (Med.) Croydon Gen. Hosp.; Cons. Chest Phys. Canterbury Hosp. Gp.

SMITH, Carol Ann Woodeside Health Centre, Barr Street, Glasgow G20 7LR Tel: 0141 531 9570 Fax: 0141 531 9572 — MB ChB Glas. 1970.

SMITH, Carol Jane 31 Crosslet Vale, Greenwich, London SE10 8DH Tel: 020 8691 9642 — MB BS Lond. 1992 (Kings College, London University) Staff Grade (Community Paediat.) Community Health S. Lond. NHS Trust. Specialty: Paediat. Prev: Clin. Med. Off. (Community Paediat.) W. Lambeth.

SMITH, Caroline Anne 103 Station Rd., Hampton TW12 2BD — MB BS Lond. 1993; FRCS (Eng.); BSc (Hons.).

SMITH, Caroline Anne 84 Reservoir Road, Solihull B92 8AR — BM BS Nottm. 1997.

SMITH, Caroline Donna 3 Chaldon Close, Redhill RH1 6SX — MB BS Newc. 1994. SHO (Oncol.) Derbysh. Roy. Infirm. Derby. Specialty: Oncol.; Radiother.

SMITH, Caroline Eunice Department of Anaesthetics, Warrington District Hospital, Lovely Lane, Warrington WA5 1QG Tel: 01925 635911 — MB ChB Manch. 1988; FFA RCSI 1992; FRCA 1993. Cons. Anaesth. Warrington Hosp. Specialty: Anaesth.

SMITH, Caroline Frances 28 Okefield Road, Crediton EX17 2DL — MB BS Newc. 1990. SHO (Psychiat.) Barrow Hosp., Flexible Trainee, Psychiat. Wonford Ho. Hosp.,Exeter. Prev: Trainee GP Backwell, Avon.; Flexible Traniee; Psychiat. Bristol.

SMITH, Caroline Margaret Dumbledore Surgery, High Street, Handcross, Haywards Heath RH17 6BN — MB BS Lond. 1984 (Univ. Lond. & Char. Cross) MRCGP 1991. Socs: BMA. Prev: Trainee GP Lightwater, Surrey; Asst. GP E. Grinstead.

SMITH, Carolyn Margaret Braehead, St. Margaret's Drive, Dunblane FK15 0DP — MB ChB Glas. 1983; DRCOG 1986; MRCP (UK) 1989; FFA RCS Eng. 1994. Staff Grade (Anaesth.) Falkirk NHS Trust. Specialty: Anaesth.

SMITH, Carolyn Sarah Northville Family Practice, 521 Filton Avenue, Horfield, Bristol BS7 0LS Tel: 0117 969 2164 Fax: 0117 931 5743 — MB BCh Wales 1983.

SMITH, Carolyne Dawn Meadowside Family Health Centre, 30 Winchcombe Road, Solihull B92 8PJ Tel: 0121 743 2560 — MB ChB Birm. 1990; DRCOG 1993; MRCGP 1996. GP Meadowside Surg. Solihull; Clin. Asst. Dermatol. Solihull Hosp. Specialty: Dermat.; Diabetes; Family Planning. Socs: BSMDH. Prev: Trainee GP/SHO E. Birm. Hosp. VTS; Ho. Off. Dudley Rd. & Goodhope Hosps.

SMITH, Mrs Catharine Elizabeth (retired) 19 Moira Road, Ashby-de-la-Zouch LE65 2GB Tel: 01530 415287 — MB BS Lond. 1945 (King's Coll. Hosp.) MRCS Eng. LRCP Lond. 1944. Prev: SCMO Leics. HA.

SMITH, Catherine 7 Holford Way, Newton-le-Willows WA12 0BZ — MB ChB Manch. 1998; MB ChB Manch 1998.

SMITH, Catherine Anne Dunlule, 1 Ben Rhydding Drive, Ilkley LS29 8AY — MB ChB Dund. 1998; MB ChB Dund 1998.

SMITH, Catherine Gaynor St. Luke's (Cheshire) Hospice, Grosvenor House, Queensway, Winsford CW7 4AW Tel: 01606 551246 Fax: 01606 861129; 33 Rushton Drive, Middlewich CW10 0NJ Tel: 01606 737108 — MB ChB Manch. 1982; DRCOG 1986; MRCGP 1990; Dip. Palliat. Med. Wales 1991. Med. Dir. St. Luke's Hospice Chesh.; Hon. Cons. (Palliat. Med.) Mid Chesh. Hosps. Trust. Specialty: Palliat. Med.

SMITH, Catherine Howard Department of Dermatology, University Hospital Lewisham, Lewisham High St., London SE13 6LH Tel: 020 8333 3000 Fax: 020 8333 3096 — MB BS Lond. 1986; MRCP (UK) 1989; MD Lond. 1994; FRCP 2001. Cons. & Sen. Lect. (Dermat.) Univ. Hosp. Lewisham. & St. John's Inst. Dermat. St. Thos. Hosp. Lond. Specialty: Dermat. Prev: Sen. Regist. St. John's Inst. Dermat. St. Thos. Hosp. Lond.; Regist. Guy's Hosp. Lond.

SMITH, Catherine Louise 62 Fentiman Road, London SW8 1LF — MB BS Lond. 1993.

SMITH, Cecilia Catherine Mary 143 Rochdale Road, Abbey Wood, London SE2 0UR — MB BS Lond. 1976; MRCS Eng. LRCP Lond. 1976; DCH Eng. 1979.

SMITH, Charles Christopher Wards 25/26 and the Infection Unit, Aberdeen Royal Hospitals NHS Trust, Aberdeen Royal Infirmary, Foresterhill, Aberdeen AB25 2ZN Tel: 01224 681818; Lynston Park, Maryculter, Aberdeen AB12 5GJ Tel: 01224 732878 Fax: 01224 840919 — MB ChB Ed. 1963; MRCP (UK) 1967; FRCP Ed. 1977; FRCP Lond. 1994. Cons. Phys. & Head of Serv. Infec. & Trop. Med. Infec. Unit Aberd. Roy. Infirm.; Clin. Sen. Lect. (Med). Univ. Aberd.; Examr. MB Finals, MRCP (UK), PLABS, LRCP & S (UK); Extern. Examr. MB Univ. Dundee, M.Med Malaysia & MRCP Hong Kong & Malaysia; Mem. UEB. Specialty: Gen. Med. Socs: Assn. Phys.; Brit. Soc. Infec. & Antimicrob. Chemother. Prev: Sen. Regist. (Infec. Dis.) City Hosp. Edin. & (Med. & Therap.) Roy. Infirm. Edin.; Regist. Univ. Dept. Med. & Thoracic Med. Edin.; Invited Lect. Hong Kong, Singapore, Malaysia, Zimbabwe, Kenya, Saudi Arabia, Irel. & S. Afr.

SMITH, Mr Charles William (retired) 21 Shipton Road, York YO30 5RE Tel: 01904 653500 — MB BS Lond. 1948 (St. Thos.) MRCS Eng. LRCP Lond. 1947; DLO Eng. 1950; FRCS Eng. 1954.

Mem. Ct. Examrs. RCS Eng. Prev: Hon. Cons. Surg. (ENT) York Hosps.

SMITH, Charles William Lauder (retired) 74 Twyford Avenue, London N2 9NN Tel: 020 8883 6868 — MB BS Lond. 1963 (Lond. Hosp.) MRCS Eng. LRCP Lond. 1962; DObst RCOG 1964; MRCGP 1973.

SMITH, Christine Anne (retired) 23/7 Clarence Street, Edinburgh EH3 5AE Tel: 0131 556 5515 Email: c.a.smith@ukgateway.net — MB ChB St. And. 1959; DA Eng. 1963. Prev: GP Stranraer Health Centre.

SMITH, Christine Mary Lee Department of Neuropathology, Royal Hallamshire Hospital, Glossop Road, Sheffield S10 2JF Tel: 0114 271 2949 Fax: 0114 271 2200; 10 Moorbank Close, Sheffield S10 5TP — BA Oxf. 1966; MB ChB Sheff. 1969; FRCPath 1986. Cons. Neuropath. Roy. Hallamsh. Hosp. Sheff. Specialty: Neuropath.

SMITH, Christine Pamela (retired) Rolleston, Oaksway, Heswall, Wirral CH60 3SP Tel: 0151 342 2094 — MB ChB Birm. 1967. Prev: Regist. (Anaesth.) United Sheff. Hosps.

SMITH, Christine Rosemary Aylmer Lodge Surgery, Broomfield Road, Kidderminster DY11 5PA Tel: 01562 822015 Fax: 01562 827137 — MB ChB Birm. 1971.

SMITH, Christopher Department of Anaesthetics, St. Richards Hospital, Chichester PO19 6SE Tel: 01243 788122 Email: chris1smith@compuserve.com; The Old School House, School Lane, North Mundham, Chichester PO20 6LA Tel: 01243 530874 — MB BS Lond. 1983 (Lond. Hosp. Med. Coll.) FRCA 1989. Cons. Anaesth. St. Richard's Hosp. Chichester. Specialty: Anaesth. Socs: BMA; Assn. Anaesth.; MRCAnaesth. Prev: Sen. Regist. (Anaesth.) Midl. Train. Scheme; Regist. Rotat. (Anaesth.) Whipps Cross & Lond. Hosps.; Vis. Assoc. (Anaesth.) Duke Univ. Med. Centre N. Carolina, USA.

SMITH, Christopher David 47 Murrayfield Drive, Willaston, Nantwich CW5 6QF — MB BCh Wales 1998.

SMITH, Christopher Eric Timothy Frimley Park Hospital, District Laboratory, Portsmouth Road, Frimley, Camberley GU16 7UJ — MB BS Lond. 1980 (St. Geo.) MA Camb. 1981; MRCPath 1988. Cons. Histopath. & Cytopath. Frimley Pk. Hosp. Surrey. Specialty: Histopath. Prev: Sen. Regist. (Histopath.) North. Gen. Hosp. Sheff.

SMITH, Christopher John The Surgery, 66 Crown Road, Twickenham TW1 3ER Tel: 020 8892 2543 Fax: 020 8744 3055 — MB BChir Camb. 1982; MRCGP 1986.

SMITH, Christopher John 20 Gatley Gate, Sale M33 2RQ — MB BS Newc. 1988. SHO (Psychiat.) St. Luke's Hosp. Middlesbrough.

SMITH, Christopher John Peel House, 18 Peel Road, Mansfield NG19 6HB — MB ChB Leeds 1998.

SMITH, Christopher Michael Meadowcroft Surgery, Jackson Road, Aylesbury HP19 9EX Tel: 01296 25775 Fax: 01296 330324 — MB ChB Bristol 1984; MRCGP 1989; FRCGP 2000. GP Trainer.

SMITH, Christopher Michael Dodds Aylmer Lodge Surgery, Broomfield Road, Kidderminster DY11 5PA Tel: 01562 822015 Fax: 01562 827137 — MB ChB Birm. 1971; BSc (Hons.) Birm. 1968, MB ChB 1971.

SMITH, Claire Blomfield House Health Centre, Looms Lane, Bury St Edmunds IP33 1HE Tel: 01284 775271 — MB ChB Birm. 1972; DObst RCOG 1974; MFFP 1993. Cons. in Family Plann. & Reproductive Healthcare, Local Health Partnership NHS Trust Suff. Specialty: Family Plann. & Reproduc. Health.

SMITH, Claire Percival East Lancashire Hospitals NHS Trust, Queens Park Hospital, Haslingden Road, Blackburn BB2 3HH Tel: 01254 293750; Weaver's Cottage, 43 Cross Lane, Holcombe, Ramsbottom, Bury BL8 4LY Tel: 01706 828291 — MD Lond. 1990 (The London Hosp.) MB BS Lond. 1977; MRCP (UK) 1980; FRCP 1997; FRCPCH 1997. Cons. Paediat. Qu.s Pk. Hosp. Blackburn. Specialty: Paediat. Socs: Brit. Diabetic Assn.; Brit. Soc. Paediat. Endocrinol. Prev: Cons. (Paediat.) Booth Hall Childr.s Hosp. Manch.; Sen. Regist. Roy. Manch. Childr. Hosp.; Research Fell. (Childh. Diabetes) Qu. Eliz. Hosp. for Childr. & St. Bart. Hosp. Lond.

SMITH, Clare Elizabeth South Kensington & Chelsea Mental Health Centre, 1 Nightingale Place, London SW10 9NG — BM BCh Oxf. 1987; BA Camb. 1984; MRCPsych 1991. Specialty: Gen. Psychiat. Socs: BMA; Roy. Coll. Psychiats. Prev: Clin. Lect. & Hon. Sen. Regist. (Psychiat.) John Radcliffe Hosp. Oxf.

SMITH, Clare Elizabeth 86 Bates Street, Crrokes, Sheffield S10 1NQ Email: clare.adrian@ic24.net — MB ChB Sheff. 1995. SHO (Anaesth.). Specialty: Anaesth.

SMITH, Clare Hilda Child & Family Service, Newtown Hospital, Newtown Road, Worcester — MB ChB Sheff. 1986; DFFP 1993. Specialty: Child & Adolesc. Psychiat.

SMITH, Clare Joanne Marion 24 Millsmead Way, Loughton IG10 1LR — BM BS Nottm. 1994.

SMITH, Clare Margaret Magnolia Cottage, 1 Risborough Road, Stoke Mandeville, Aylesbury HP22 5UP Tel: 01296 612839; Brickwall Farm, Susans Hill, Woodchurch, Ashford TN26 3RG — MB BS Lond. 1986; MRCGP 1991; T(GP) 1991.

SMITH, Clare Nicola 54 Spring Lane, Fordham Heath, Colchester CO3 9TG — MB ChB Leeds 1998.

SMITH, Clifford Corbett, OStJ Thatcham Medical Practice, Bath Road, Thatcham RG18 3HD Tel: 01635 867171 Fax: 01635 876395 Email: clifford.smith@gp-k81073.nhs.uk; 36 Fylingdales, Thatcham RG19 3LB Tel: 01635 864903 — MB BS Lond. 1971 (Char. Cross) MRCS Eng. LRCP Lond. 1971; DCH Eng. 1973; DObst RCOG 1974; MRCGP 1975; Cert. FPA 1975. GP Princip.; Co. Commissioner St John Ambul. Roy. Berks. Specialty: Gen. Pract. Socs: Assn. BRd.casting Doctors. Prev: SHO (Obst.) Northwick Pk. Hosp. Harrow; SHO (Paediat.) Char. Cross Hosp. Fulham; SHO Profess. Dept. Paediat. Hammersmith Hosp. Lond.

SMITH, Colin (retired) Farthing Piece, Oddingley, Droitwich WR9 7NE Tel: 01905 773548; Farthing Piece, Oddingley, Droitwich WR9 7NE Tel: 01905 773548 — MB BS Durh. 1963; MRCGP 1977.

SMITH, Colin Haigh (retired) 6 Shorts Lane, Beaminster DT8 3BD Tel: 01308 862440 — (Oxf. & Guy's) BM BCh Oxf. 1958; MA Oxf. 1963; DCH Eng. 1967; FRCGP 1988, M 1976; MSc Lond. 1988. Prev: Asst. Regional Adviser Audit.

SMITH, Colin Lunn Southampton General Hospital, Southampton SO16 6YD Tel: 023 8079 6737 — MD Leeds 1978; BSc Leeds 1960, MD 1978, MB ChB 1962; FRCP Lond. 1980, M 1965; Fmed.Sci. 1998. Sen. Lect. Med. & Gastroenterol. & Cons. Phys. Univ. Soton. & Soton. Gen. Hosp. Specialty: Gastroenterol. Socs: Brit. Soc. Gastroenterol. Prev: Lect. Med. Gen. Infirm. Leeds; Asst. Prof. Med. (Gastroenterol.) Univ. Cincinnati, U.S.A.

SMITH, Colin Stanley (retired) 94 Saughall Massie Lane, Upton, Wirral CH49 6ND Tel: 0151 677 6674 — MB ChB Liverp. 1964; FRCP Lond. 1981, M 1969. Prev: Sen. Lect. Child Health Univ. Liverp.

SMITH, Constance Frances — MB BS Lond. 1990 (St. Mary's Hosp. Med. Sch.) BSc Biochem. Lond. 1985; DFFP 1993; DCH RCP Lond. 1993; MRCGP 1994; DRCOG 1996.

SMITH, Craig Manderson The Chilterns, The Old Road, Leavenheath, Colchester CO6 4QB — MB ChB Dundee 1990.

SMITH, Damian Michael 1 Elliot Drive, Giffnock, Glasgow G46 7NT — MB ChB Glas. 1996.

SMITH, Daniel Joseph 71 Orchardville Gardens, Finaghy, Belfast BT10 0JU — MB ChB Ed. 1996.

SMITH, Daniel Kenneth Sunnybank, Cutmere, Tideford, Saltash PL12 5JU Tel: 01752 851850 — MB ChB Bristol 1982; DA (UK) 1985; DCH RCPS Glas. 1987; MRCGP 1989. Specialty: Gen. Psychiat.

SMITH, Danielle Joanne 10 Cousley Close, Gloucester GL3 3RN — MB BS Lond. 1992 (Guy's Hosp Med School) DRCOG Lond 1995; MRCGP (LOND) July 1997; DFFP (Lond) 1998. GP Locum. Specialty: Gen. Pract.

SMITH, Darren Jeffrey 115 Rivington Drive, Burscough, Ormskirk L40 7RW — MB ChB Liverp. 1998; MB ChB Liverp 1998.

SMITH, Darron Eufryn Brynteg Surgery, Brynmawr Avenue, Ammanford SA18 2DA Tel: 01269 592058 — MB BCh Wales 1991.

SMITH, David (retired) Headway, 8 Church Hill, Hensingham, Whitehaven CA28 8NE Tel: 01946 693018 — (Manchester) MB ChB Manch. 1956; DPath Eng. 1962; FRCPath 1977, M 1965. Prev: Cons. Pathol. W. Cumbld. Hosp. Whitehaven.

SMITH, David Great Harwood Health Centre, Water Street, Great Harwood, Blackburn BB6 7QR Tel: 01254 885764 Fax: 01254 877360 — MB ChB Manch. 1981; DRCOG 1983.

SMITH, David Alistair Locking Hill Surgery, Stroud GL5 1UY Tel: 01453 764222; Woolpack Cottage, Rodborough Lane, Butterrow,

Cheltenham GL54 2LH Tel: 01453 762513 — BM BCh Oxf. 1994; MA Oxf. 1996; DRCOG 1996; DFFP 1997; MRCGP 1998. GP Princip.; Med. Off. Cheltenham Town F.C. Specialty: Gen. Pract. Prev: GP Regist. Brockworth Glos.; SHO Elderly Care Delancy Hosp. Cheltenham; SHO (O & G) Gloucester Roy. Hosp.

SMITH, David Andrew The Grove Surgery, Trinity Medical Centre, Thornhill Street, Wakefield WF1 1PG Tel: 01924 372596 Fax: 01924 200913 — MB ChB Birm. 1985; DRCOG 1988; MRCGP 1989. Specialty: Accid. & Emerg.

SMITH, David Andrew Hammersmith Hospital, Du Cane Road, London W12 0HS Tel: 020 8383 1000 Ext: 9299 Email: voiseysmith@talk21.com — BM Soton. 1993; MRCP UK 1997; MD Lond. 2005. Interventional Fell. Specialty: Cardiol. Socs: BMA; Brit. Cardiac Soc.; Brit. Cardiovasc. Interven. Soc. Prev: Specialist Regist. (Cardiol.) Univ. Hosp. of Wales; Research Fell. & Hon. Lect. in Cardiol. St. Geo. Hosp. Med. Sch.; Regist. (Cardiol.) Roy. Bournemouth Hosp.

SMITH, David Anthony Wansbeck General Hospital, Woodhorn Lane, Ashington NE63 9JJ Tel: 01670 521212; Blackfords, Jesmond Park E., Newcastle upon Tyne NE7 7BT Tel: 0191 281 6128 — MB BChir Camb. 1975; MA, MB Camb. 1975, BChir 1974; MRCP (UK) 1979; MRCPath 1985. Cons. Histopath. Wansbeck Gen. Hosp. Ashington. Specialty: Histopath. Prev: Sen. Regist. (Histopath.) King's Coll. Hosp. Lond.; SHO (Gen. Med.) Northwick Pk. Hosp.; Ho. Off. Univ. Coll. Hosp. Lond.

SMITH, David Balfour 284 Telegraph Road, Heswall, Wirral CH60 7SG — MD Ed. 1988; MB ChB 1978; MRCP (UK) 1981. Cons. Med. Oncol. Clatterbridge Centre for Oncol. Wirral. Specialty: Oncol. Prev: Sen. Regist. (Med. Oncol.) Char. Cross Hosp. Lond.; Regist. (Med.) Roy. Lancaster Infirm.; Research Fell. (Med. Oncol.) Christie Hosp. Manch.

SMITH, David Charles Department of Anaesthesia, Southampton General Hospital, Southampton SO16 6YD Tel: 023 8079 6135 Fax: 023 8079 4348; Little Herons, Heron Lane, Timsbury, Southampton SO51 0ND Tel: 01794 367134 — BM BS Nottm. 1980; BMedSci Nottm. 1978; FFA RCS Eng. 1985; DM Nottm. 1996. Cons. & Sen. Lect. (Anaesth.) Soton. Gen. Hosp. Specialty: Anaesth. Socs: Assn. of Cardiothoracic Anaestetists, Comm. Mem.; Soc. of Cardiovasc. Anaesthesiologists; Europ. Assn. of Cardiothoracic Anaesthesiologists. Prev: Cons. Anaesth. West. Infirm. Glas.

SMITH, Mr David Cunningham 333 Albert Drive, Glasgow G41 5HJ Tel: 0141 423 2801 Fax: 0141 423 5117 — MB ChB Glas. 1966; FRCS Glas. 1970; FRCS Eng. 1971. Cons. Surg. Vict. Infirm. Glas.; Hon. Clin. Sen. Lect. (Surg.) Univ. Glas. Specialty: Gen. Surg. Socs: Glas. S.ern Med. Soc., Pres. (1999-2000); Roy. Coll. of Phys.s & Surg.s of Glas., Vice Pres. (Surgic. 2000-2002). Prev: Regist. (Orthop. & Gen. Surg.), Ho. Surg. & Ho. Phys. West. Infirm. Glas.

SMITH, David Dow Oxford Terrace Medical Group, 1 Oxford Terrace, Gateshead NE8 1RQ Tel: 0191 477 2169; 9 Swinburne Place, Newcastle upon Tyne NE4 6EA — MB BS Newc. 1979; MRCGP 1984.

SMITH, Mr David Flett (retired) 52 Moor Crescent, Gosforth, Newcastle upon Tyne NE3 4AQ Tel: 01632 851694 — MB ChB Aberd. 1935; FRCS Ed. 1938; FRCOG 1961, M 1949. Prev: Sen. Obst. Gyn. Gateshead AHA.

SMITH, David Frank Walton Centre, Liverpool L9 7LJ Tel: 0181 529 5707 Fax: 0151 529 5513 Email: dave.smith@doctors.org.uk — MB ChB Aberd. 1983; MRCP (UK) 1987; MD Aberd. 1993; FRCP 2001. Cons. Neurologist Walton Centre Liverp.; Hon. Sen. Lect. (Neurosci.) Univ. Liverp. Specialty: Neurol. Special Interest: Epilepsy. Socs: Assn. Brit. Neurol.; Internat. League Against Epilepsy. Prev: Research Regist. (Neurosci.) Walton Hosp. Liverp.

SMITH, David Geoffrey Malagay Barn, Church Road, West Tilbury, Grays RM18 8UB — MB ChB Ed. 1969.

SMITH, David Gordon Brookland House, 501 Crewe Road, Wistaston, Crewe CW2 6QP Tel: 01270 567250 Fax: 01270 665829; 4 Mill Race Drive, Wistaston, Crewe CW2 6XG Tel: 01270 668195 — MB ChB Dundee 1988; MRCGP 1994. Specialty: Gen. Pract.

SMITH, David Ian Andrew 27 Fiskerton Road, Cherry Willingham, Lincoln LN3 4LA — MB BS Lond. 1983.

SMITH, David Ian Hamilton Rosegarth Surgery, Rothwell Mount, Halifax HX1 2XB; Upper Greystones, Manor Heath Road, Halifax HX3 0EE — MB BS Lond. 1978; MRCGP 1982; DCH RCP Lond. 1982. Clin. Asst. (A & E.) Roy. Halifax Infirm.; Hon. Hosp. Pract. (Gastroenterol.) Roy. Halifax Infirm. Prev: Trainee GP Calderdale AHA VTS; Ho. Phys. Epsom Dist. Hosp.; Ho. Surg. Roy. Cornw. Hosp. Truro.

SMITH, David Keith Flat 3, 45 Cavendish Road, London NW6 7XS — MB BS Lond. 1997.

SMITH, David Lindsey Department of Medicine, Frenchay Hospital, Frenchay Park Road, Bristol BS16 1LE Tel: 0117 970 1212 Fax: 0117 957 3075 — BM Soton. 1982 (Univ. Soton.) MRCPI 1986; MRCP (UK) 1986; DM Soton. 1995; FRCP 2000. Cons. Phys. (Respirat. & Gen. Med.) Frenchay Hosp. Bristol. Specialty: Respirat. Med. Socs: Brit. Thorac. Soc.; Amer. Thoracic Soc.; Europ. Respirat. Soc. Prev: Sen. Regist. Glenfield Hosp. Leicester; Sen. Regist. Chelsea & Westm. Hosp. Lond.; Clin. Tutor Brompton Hosp. Lond.

SMITH, David Mark Haresfield House Surgery, 6-10 Bath Road, Worcester WR5 3EJ Tel: 01905 763161 Fax: 01905 767016; The Mount, Red Hill Lane, Worcester WR5 2JL — MB ChB Manch. 1976; DRCOG 1979; MRCGP 1980.

SMITH, Mr David Monro The Friarage, 4 Little Causeway, Forfar DD8 2AD — MB ChB Ed. 1983; FRCS Ed. 1987; MD Ed. 1993. Cons. Surg. Ninewells Hosp. Dundee. Specialty: Gen. Surg. Prev: Sen. Regist. (Surg.) Ninewells Hosp. Dundee.

SMITH, Mr David Neal Wirral Hospital NHS Trust, Arrowe Park Hospital, Arrowe Park Road, Wirral CH49 5PE Tel: 0151 678 5111; 12 Oaksway, Heswall, Wirral CH60 3SP Tel: 0151 342 2094 — MB ChB Birm. 1967; FRCS Ed. 1973. Cons. (Orthop. Surg.) Wirral Hosp. NHS Trust. Specialty: Orthop. Socs: Fell. BOA; BMA. Prev: Sen. Regist. (Orthop.) Birm. AHA; Regist. (Neurosurg.) Roy. Infirm. Sheff.; Regist. (Surg.) United Birm. Hosps.

SMITH, David Phillip c/o Barnsoul Farm, Irongray, Dumfries DG2 9SQ — MB ChB Leeds 1966; BSc (Hons. Pharmacol.) 1968; PhD Leeds 1973; MRCPath 1977.

SMITH, David Ross Sutherland 20 Herefordshire Drive, Durham DH1 2DQ — MB BS Newc. 1967; DObst RCOG 1971; DCH Eng. 1973; MRCP (UK) 1974; FRCP Lond. 1990; FRCPCH 1997. Cons. Paediat. Univ. Hosp. of N. Durh. Specialty: Paediat. Socs: BMA & Brit. Paediat. Assn. Prev: Sen. Regist. (Paediat.) Middlx. Hosp. Lond.; Research Fell. Hosp. Sick Childr. Toronto, Canada; Regist. (Paediat.) Brompton Hosp. Lond.

SMITH, David Trevor Mitchell 4 South Mill Close, Amesbury, Salisbury SP4 7HS Tel: 01980 623207 Fax: 01980 623207 — MB BS Lond. 1961 (Guy's) MRCS Eng. LRCP Lond. 1961. Assitant Salisbury Indep. Med. Pract.; Med. Off. Commision Bd. Westbury; Med. Off. HQ Land Command Wilton. Prev: Dep. MOH & Port Med. Off. Grimsby RD.; Sen. Parnter Baracroft Pract.; Med. Off. Pains Wessex Salisbury.

SMITH, David Ward (retired) The Knowltons, Podington, Wellingborough NN29 7HX Tel: 01933 353306 — MB BChir Camb. 1951; DObst RCOG 1956; MRCGP 1971. Prev: Ho. Surg. Middlx. Hosp.

SMITH, David Ward Lawson (retired) Warlaby House, Warlaby, Northallerton DL7 9JS Tel: 01609 774812 Fax: 01609 783720 — MB ChB St And. 1965.

SMITH, David William, Brigadier late RAMC Clifton Lodge, Banff Road, Keith AB55 5ET Tel: 01542 882617 — MB ChB Aberd. 1971; DObst RCOG 1976; FRCGP 1987. Dir. Army Gen. Pract. Specialty: Gen. Pract. Prev: Com.MedGP Brit. Army, Germany; Command. Med. Adviser Brit. Forces, Cyprus; Course Organiser SW Dist. HM Armed Forces.

SMITH, Dawn Ann Crownhall Medical Group, Felling Health Centre, Stephenson Tce, Gateshead NE10 9QJ Tel: 0191 469 2311 Fax: 0191 438 4661 — MB BS Newc. 1987; DRCOG 1990; MRCGP 1991.

SMITH, Deborah Anne Leeds Student Medical Practice, 4 Blenheim Court Walk, Leeds LS2 9AE Tel: 0113 295 4488 — MB BS Lond. 1980 (Guy's Hosp. Lond.) DRCOG 1985; DCH RCP Lond. 1985; MRCGP 1986; DFFP 1998. GP Leeds Stud. Med. Pract. Specialty: Family Plann. & Reproduc. Health. Prev: CMO (Family Plann.) Leeds Community & Ment. Health Trust; GP Westfield Med. Centre Leeds.

SMITH, Deborah Jane 16 Brompton Avenue, Sefton Park, Liverpool L17 3BU — MB ChB Liverp. 1993.

SMITH, Deborah Jane 31 Crofters Fold, Galgate, Lancaster LA2 0RB — MB ChB Leic. 1995.

SMITH, Debra Ellen Harrogate District Hospital, Lancaster Park Road, Harrogate HG2 7SX Tel: 01423 885959; 28 Scriven Road, Knaresborough HG5 9EJ — MD Camb. 1992; MA Camb. 1981, MD 1992, MB BChir 1979; MRCP (UK) 1985. Cons. Paediat. Harrogate HA. Specialty: Paediat.

SMITH, Dena Alexandra 76 Cunningham Drive, Bromborough, Wirral CH63 0JZ — MB ChB Manch. 1990; DRCOG 1995; MRCGP 1995. Specialty: Gen. Pract.

SMITH, Dennis Gutteridge Carrington House Surgery, 19 Priory Road, High Wycombe HP13 6SL Tel: 01494 526029; Mountjoys Retreat, Plomer Green Lane, Downley, High Wycombe HP13 5XN — MB BS Lond. 1974 (St. Geo.) DRCOG 1977; DCH Eng. 1979. GP High Wycombe. Prev: SHO (Paediat.) Worcester Roy. Infirm. (Ronkswood Br.); SHO (Med.) Battle Hosp. Reading; SHO (O & G) Heatherwood Hosp. Ascot.

SMITH, Desmond James Lawrence Berkley Laboratories, Building 74-174, 1 Cyclotron Road, University of California, Berkeley CA 94720, USA Tel: 00 1 510 4865090 Fax: 00 1 510 4866746; 72 Ormesby Way, Kenton, Harrow HA3 9SF Tel: 020 8204 0081 — BA Oxf. Physics (1st cl. Hons.) & Prize Distinc. 1981, BM BCh; PhD Camb. 1986; MA Oxf. 1987. Prev: Ho. Off. (Surg.) John Radcliffe Hosp. Oxf. Univ.; Ho. Off. (Med.) Wycombe Gen. Hosp. High Wycombe.

SMITH, Desmond Murray Brenkley Avenue Health Centre, Brenkley Avenue, Shiremoor, Newcastle upon Tyne NE27 0PR Tel: 0191 251 6151; 34 King Edward Road, Tynemouth, North Shields NE30 2RP — MB BS Newc. 1977.

SMITH, Diane Elizabeth Croft Cottage, 29 Langton Road, Tunbridge Wells TN4 8XA — MB ChB Birm. 1989.

SMITH, Dianne Elizabeth Glodwick Health Centre, 137 Glodwick Road, Oldham OL4 1YN Tel: 0161 909 8370; Goldturf Pits, Moorside, Oldham OL4 2NA — MB ChB Manch. 1987 (Manchester) DRCOG 1990; MRCGP 1991.

SMITH, Dominic Paul York Hospital, Wigginton Road, York YO31 8HE — BM BS Nottm. 1993; MRCPCH; MRCP; MMed Sc.

SMITH, Donald (retired) 9 Monastery Avenue, Dover CT16 1AB Tel: 01304 206366 Fax: 01304 306366 — (King's Coll. Newc.) MB BS Durh. 1948. Prev: Asst. Dir.-Gen. AMD 3.

SMITH, Donald (retired) 'Windygates', 13 Crosbie Road, Troon KA10 6HE — MB ChB Glas. 1958; FRCOG 1978, M 1964; BA (Hons.) 1994; BSc 2000. Prev: Cons. Obstetr. & Gynaecol. Ayrsh. Centr. Hosp. Irvine & Assoc. Hosps.

SMITH, Donald Angus (retired) 12 Sutcliffe Court, Anniesland, Glasgow G13 1AP Tel: 0141 954 3971 — MB ChB Glas. 1948.

SMITH, Donald Fitzroy, SBStJ, RD Adult & Elderly Medicine, Countess of Chester Hospital, Liverpool Road, Chester CH2 1BQ; Trenance, 57 Mill Lane, Upton-by-Chester, Chester CH2 1BS Tel: 01244 380422 Fax: 01244 380422 — MB ChB Liverp. 1974; MRCP (UK) 1979; MD Liverp. 1995; FRCP 2003. Cons. Phys. (c/o Elderly) Countess of Chester Hosp. Specialty: Care of the Elderly; Gen. Med. Socs: Liverp. Med. Inst.; Brit. Geriat. Soc. Prev: Sen. Regist. (Gen. & Geriat. Med.) Frenchay Hosp. Bristol & Derriford Hosp. Plymouth; Research Fell. Univ. West. Ontario, Lond., Canada.

SMITH, Donalda Matheson (retired) 6 Field Lane, Willersey, Broadway WR12 7QB Tel: 01386 852628 — MB ChB Ed. 1950; DObst RCOG 1954; DIH Soc. Apoth. Lond. 1972; FFOM RCP Lond. 1986, MFOM 1979. Prev: Sen. Employm. Med. Adviser EMAS, Marches Area.

SMITH, Dorothy Lindsay (retired) 15 Mansionhouse Road, Edinburgh EH9 1TZ Tel: 0131 667 4665 — FRCP 1988; MD Ed. 1980, MB ChB 1954.

SMITH, Dorothy Mary Agnes (retired) 17 Knapp Close, Ledbury HR8 1AW Tel: 01531 634620 — MB ChB Aberd. 1942; DObst RCOG 1953.

SMITH, Douglas Harrison Kerr 14 Lakeside Road, Raith Lake, Kirkcaldy KY2 5QJ Tel: 01592 266503 — MB ChB Ed. 1963; DMRD Ed. 1970; FFR 1973; FRCR 1975; MRCP Ed. 1987; FRCP Ed. 1994. Cons. Radiol. Vict. Hosp. Kirkcaldy; Hon. Sen. Lect. St. And. Univ. Specialty: Nuclear Med. Socs: Fell. Roy. Med. Soc. Prev: Sen. Regist. (X-Ray) Roy. Infirm. Edin.; Regist. (Med.) Vict. Hosp. Kirkcaldy.

SMITH, Douglas Peter Quance (retired) Ryecroft, 54 Cross Road, Tadworth KT20 5ST Tel: 01737 812037 — MB BS Lond. 1951 (St. Bart.) MRCS Eng. LRCP Lond. 1951; DObst RCOG 1953. Prev: Resid. Med. Off. St. And. Hosp. Dollis Hill.

SMITH, Douglas Robert Walter 15 Hugh Mill, Shepherds Loan, Dundee DD2 1UN — MB ChB Dundee 1996.

SMITH, Drew Dept. of Anaesth., Walton Building, Glasgow Royal Infirmary, Castle St., Glasgow G4 0SF Tel: 0141 211 4620 Fax: 0141 211 4622 — MB ChB Glas. 1989 (Glas. Univ.) FRCA 1995. Cons. (Anaesth.) Glas. Roy. Infirm. Glas. Specialty: Anaesth. Special Interest: Obstetric Anaesth.; Hepatic / colorectal anaesth. Prev: Specialist Regist. (Anaesth.) Glas. Roy. Infirm.; SHO (Anaesth.) Glas. Roy. Infirm. & Law Hosp. Carluke.

SMITH, Edward Baxter Owen, VRD (retired) The Manor House, Ewelme, Wallingford OX10 6HQ Tel: 01491 36036 — (St. Thos.) MB BS Lond. 1953, DPM 1962; FRCP Ed. 1972, M 1964; FRCPsych 1975, M 1971. Prev: Emerit. Civil. Advisor RN.

SMITH, Mr Edward Ernest John Cardiothoracic Unit, St George's Hospital, Blackshaw Road, London SW17 0QT Tel: 020 8725 3551 Fax: 020 8946 3130 Email: eejmss@supanet.com; Homewood, 4A Drax Avenue, Wimbledon, London SW20 0EH Tel: 020 8946 1893 Fax: 020 8946 3130 Email: eejmss@supanet.com — MD Camb. 1991; MB BChir 1974; FRCS Eng. 1978. Cons. Cardiothoracic Surg. St. Geo. Hosp. Lond. & Roy. Surrey Co. Hosp. Guildford. Specialty: Cardiothoracic Surg. Prev: Regist. (Surg.) Hammersmith Hosp. Lond.; Cas. Off. & Ho. Surg. St. Thos. Hosp. Lond.

SMITH, Edward Maxim Moor Park Surgery, 49 Garstang Road, Preston PR1 1LB Tel: 01772 252077 Fax: 01772 885451 — MB ChB Ed. 1970.

SMITH, Eileen Dorothy (retired) — MB BS Lond. 1970 (Roy. Free) MRCS Eng. LRCP Lond. 1961; FRCPsych. 1988, M 1973; DPM Eng. 1973. Med. Mem. Ment. Health Review Tribunal. Prev: Cons. Psychiat. Salford AHA (T).

SMITH, Elaine Caroline Consultant Rheumatologist, North West London Hospitals NHS Trust, Northwick Park & Central Middlesex, London Tel: 020 8864 3232 Fax: 020 8864 2009 — MB BS Lond. 1985 (St. Bart. Hosp. Lond.) MRCP (UK) 1989; MD 1997. Cons. Rheum. Northwick Pk. and Centr. Middlx. Hosp.s, Lond.; Editorial Bd. of the Druga nd Therap. Bull. since 1998. Specialty: Rheumatol. Socs: Brit. Soc. Rheum.; Mem. for Sect. Rheumatol. and Rehabil. Roy. Soc. Med.; Edr.ial Bd. Drugs and Therap. Bull. 1998-2001. Prev: Staff Phys., Dubbo Base Hosp., NW Australia; Locum Cons. (Rheum.) Guy's Hosp. Lond.; Sen. Regist. (Rheum.) King's Coll. Hosp. Lond.

SMITH, Elaine Nicola Keepers Cottage, Raycombe Lane, Coddington, Ledbury HR8 1JH Tel: 01531 2409 — MB BS Lond. 1975; MRCS Eng. LRCP Lond. 1975; DRCOG 1978.

SMITH, Elaine Paula 1 Grange Drive, Manchester M9 7AJ Tel: 0161 740 9434 — MB ChB Manch. 1994; BSc (Med. Sci.) St. And. 1991. SHO (Cardiothoracic Med.) Wythenshawe Hosp. Manch. Specialty: Cardiol. Prev: Ho. Off. (Gen. Med. & Renal Med.) Hope Hosp. Salford; Ho. Off. (Gen. & Vasc. Surg. & Urol.) Univ. Hosp. S. Manch.

SMITH, Eleanor Grace Birmingham Public Health Lobaratory, Heartlands Hospital, Birmingham B9 5SS — MB BS Lond. 1979 (St. Thomas) BSc (Hons.) Lond. 1976; MRCP (UK) 1982; FRCPath 1998; FRCP 2000. Cons. Microbiologist Birm. Pub. Health Laborat. Birmington Heartlands Hosp. Specialty: Med. Microbiol.

SMITH, Elizabeth Margaret Musters Medical Practice, 214 Musters Road, West Bridgford, Nottingham NG2 7DR Tel: 0115 981 4124 Fax: 0115 981 3117; 40 St Helens Road, West Bridgford, Nottingham NG2 6EX Tel: 0115 923 1144 — BM BS Nottm. 1986, BMedSci 1984; MRCGP 1990; DCH RCP Lond. 1990; DRCOG 1991.

SMITH, Elizabeth Robin 46 Fitzroy Road, London NW1 8TY — MB BS Lond. 1996.

SMITH, Elizabeth Sheila Highfield Surgery, Holtdale Approach, Leeds LS16 7RX Tel: 0113 230 0108 Fax: 0113 230 1309; 63 Otley Old Road, Lawnswood, Leeds LS16 6HG Tel: 0113 261 4118 — MB ChB Ed. 1974; DCH RCPS Glas. 1977; MRCGP 1978. Prev: Trainee GP Lothian HB VTS; Ho. Phys. (Infec. Dis. Unit) City Hosp. Edin.; Ho. Surg. (Profess. Surg. Unit) Roy. Infirm. Edin.

SMITH, Ellen (retired) 704 Kings Court, Ramsey IM8 1LW Tel: 01624 814554 — (W.Lond.) MB BChir Camb. 1949; MRCS Eng.

LRCP Lond. 1949; DObst RCOG 1950. Prev: Clin. Asst. (Dermat.) Birm. Gen. & Birm. Skin Hosps.
SMITH, Elliot Jonathan 133 High Lane, Whitefield, Manchester M45 7WH — MB BS Lond. 1994.
SMITH, Elvet Edward Walson Suite, Rochdale Infirmary, Whitehall Street, Rochdale OL12 0NB Tel: 01706 517086 Email: elvet.smith@pat.nhs.uk — MB ChB Bristol 1971; MRCP (UK) 1974; FRCP Lond. 1991; BA (Open) 1996. Cons. Rheum. & Rehabil. Rochdale HA. Specialty: Rheumatol.; Rehabil. Med. Socs: Brit. Soc. Rheum.; Brit. Soc. Rehab. Med.; Fell. Roy. Soc. Med. Prev: Sen. Regist. (Rheum. & Rehabil.) Manch. Roy. Infirm. & Withington Hosp.; Research Regist. ARC Field Unit Epidemiol. Dept. Community Med. Univ. Manch.; Ho. Phys. Prof. Med. Unit Bristol Roy. Infirm.
SMITH, Emmanuel Ademola (retired) 14 Aina Eleko Street, Onigbongbo, Maryland, Ikeja POBOX616, Nigeria Tel: 00234 1 4961145; 33 Radley House, Gloucester Place, London NW1 6DP Tel: 020 7724 6481 — MRCS Eng. LRCP Lond. 1961 (London School Hygiene; Tuzare-London; Guy's; W. London Hosp.) DPH Lond. 1966; MS (Hyg.) Talune 1971. Assoc. Lect. Univ. Lagos, Nigeria; Med. Dir. Ademola Smith Holdings Nigeria Ltd. Charity Clinic Maryland Ikeja, Nigeria. Prev: Director Pub. Health Servs. Nigeria.
SMITH, Eric Ernest (retired) The Garth, Windmill End, Epsom KT17 3AQ — MB BS Lond. 1956 (Guy's) MRCS Eng. LRCP Lond. 1956.
SMITH, Eric Harry (retired) Ty'n Llechwedd, Dinbren, Llangollen LL20 8EB Tel: 0131 667 9087/01987 869364 — MB ChB Ed. 1963; DCH Eng. 1968; MRCP (UK) 1971; FRCPCH 1997; FRCP Lond. 1988; LLM (Cardiff) 1999. Prev: Cons. (Paediat.) Kettering Gen. Hosp.
SMITH, Eric John Queens Road Medical Practice, The Grange, St. Peter Port, Guernsey GY1 1RH Tel: 01481 724184 Fax: 01481 716431; Les Lohiers, La Grande Lande, St. Saviours, Guernsey GY7 9 — MB BS Lond. 1970.
SMITH, Eric Leslie (retired) Erradale, 2 Ladies Walk, Inverness Iv2 4tb Tel: 01463 237295 — MB ChB Aberd. 1959; FRCP Ed. 1978, M 1964. Prev: Head of Dept. Dermat./Venereol./ Med. Educat. Dept. King Khaled Hosp. Jeddah.
SMITH, Professor Ernest Alwyn, CBE Plum Tree Cottage, Silverdale Road, Arnside, Carnforth LA5 0AH Tel: 01524 761976 — MB ChB Birm. 1952; PhD Birm. 1955; DPH (Distinc.) Lond. 1956; FRCP Glas. 1971, M 1967; MSc Manch. 1971; FFCM 1972; FRCGP 1973; FRCP Ed. 1981; FRCP Lond. 1983. Emerit. Prof. Epidemiol. & Social Oncol. Univ. Manch. Specialty: Epidemiol. Socs: (Ex-Pres.) Fac. Pub. Health Med.; Soc. Social Med. Prev: Prof. Community Med. Univ. Manch.; Sen. Lect. i/c Social Paediat. Research Gp. Univ. Glas.; Med. Statistician Scott. Home & Health Dept.
SMITH, Rev Dr Felicity Ann 14 Oakwood Grove, Warwick CV34 5TD Tel: 01926 492452 Fax: 01926 747449 — MB ChB Bristol 1963; DObst RCOG 1965; MFFP 1993. Specialty: Family Plann. & Reproduc. Health.
SMITH, Francesca Clare 42 Cambrian Avenue, Redcar TS10 4HF — MB BS Lond. 1997.
SMITH, Francis Herbert Nixon (retired) Turnstones, Perrancoombe, Perranporth TR6 0HX Tel: 01872 573324 — (Birm.) MB ChB Birm. 1947; MRCS Eng. LRCP Lond. 1948; DObst RCOG 1951. Prev: Sch. Med. Off. Newquay Area.
SMITH, Francis Robert Highcroft, Wessex Deanery, Romsey Road, Winchester SO22 5DH Tel: 01962 863511 Fax: 01962 877211 Email: fsmith@doh.gsi.gov.uk — MB ChB Birm. 1974; MB ChB (Hons.) Birm. 1974; MRCP (UK) 1977; FRCGP 1996, M 1984; MSC 1998. Dir. of Postgrad. GP Educat. Specialty: Gen. Pract. Prev: Sen. Lect. (Gen. Pract. & Primary Care) St. Geo. Hosp. Med. Sch. Lond.; Ment. Health Fell. TPMDE S. Thames (W..); GP Caterham, Surrey.
SMITH, Francis William Woodend Hospital, Eday Road, Aberdeen AB15 6XS Tel: 01224 556040 Fax: 01224 556232; 7 Primrosehill Road, Cults, Aberdeen AB15 9ND Tel: 01224 868745 — MD Aberd. 1987 (Aberdeen) MB ChB 1970; DMRD Aberd. 1975; FFR RCSI 1978; Dip. Sports Med. Scotl. 1992; FRCP Ed. 1992; FRCR 1997. Cons. Radiol. Grampian Univ. Hosp. NHS Trust; Prof. of Health Sci.s, The Robt. Gordon Univ. Aberd.. Specialty: Radiol.; Nuclear Med.; Sports Med. Socs: Scott. Inst. Sports Med. & Sports Sci.; Internat. Soc. Magnetic Resonance in Med.; Brit. Inst. Radiol. Prev: Cons. Nuclear Med. Aberd. Roy. Hosp. NHS Trust.
SMITH, Mr Frank Charles Theodore University Department of Surgery, Level 7, Bristol Royal Infirmary, Bristol BS2 8HW Tel: 0117 9272 696; The Old Halt, Downleaze, Sneed Park, Bristol BS9 1NA — MB ChB Birm. 1984; BSc (Hons. Pharmacol.) Birm. 1981; FRCS Glas. 1989; FRCS Ed. 1989; FRCS Eng. 1990; MD Birm. 2000. Cons. Sen. Lect. (Gen. & Vasc. Surg.) Univ. Bristol Bristol Roy. Infirm.; Vis. Cons. (Vasc. Surg.) Weston Gen. Hosp. Specialty: Gen. Surg. Socs: Surgic. Research Soc.; Eur. Soc. Vasc. Surg.; Vasc. Surgic. Soc. Prev: Sen. Regist. Rotat. (Gen. & Vasc. Surg.) SW RHA; Career Regist. Rotat. (Surg.) W. Midl. RHA; Research Fell. (Vasc. Surg.) Qu. Eliz. Hosp. Birm.
SMITH, Frederic M S (retired) Fairview, 176 Stony Lane, Burton, Christchurch BH23 7LD Tel: 0135 48 485375 — MRCS Eng. LRCP Lond. 1939 (Westm.) Prev: GP Dorset.
SMITH, Mr Frederick 37 Broadsway, Morecambe LA4 5BQ Tel: 01524 410096 — DObst RCOG 1960; MD Manch. 1968, MB ChB 1951, DPH 1962; DCH Eng. 1959, DIH 1964; FRCS Ed. 1978; MRCP (UK) 1984; FRCGP 1985. Socs: Fell. Manch. Med. Soc.; Manch. Med. Soc. Prev: Asst. Div. Med. Off. Lancs. CC; Rotating Intern Northampton Gen. Hosp; Nuffield Research Fell. Manch. Univ.
SMITH, Frederick Duncan X-Ray Department, Derbyshire Royal Infirmary, London Road, Derby DE1 2QY — MB ChB Sheff. 1976; MRCP (UK) 1979; FRCR 1985. Cons. Radiol. South. Derbysh. HA. Specialty: Radiol.
SMITH, Frederick George Mammatt 10 Park Crescent, Merthyr Tydfil CF47 0EU — MB ChB Glas. 1943 (Univ. Glas.) DObst RCOG 1949. Prev: Regist. Luton Matern. Hosp.; Ho. Surg. Co. Lanark Matern. Hosp. Bellshill; Ho. Phys. Stobhill Hosp. Glas.
SMITH, Freya Marion Pollokshaws Doctors Centre, 26 Wellgreen, Glasgow G43 1RR Tel: 0141 649 2836 Fax: 0141 649 5238 — MB ChB Ed. 1978; DRCOG 1981; MRCGP 1982; MPhil Glas. 1994. Specialty: Gen. Med.
SMITH, Gareth David Phelps Neurology Department, Royal Cornwall Hospital, Truro TR1 3LJ Tel: 01872 250000 — MB BCh Wales 1984; MRCP UK. 1988; MD 1996. Cons. Neurol. Roy. Cornw. Hosp. Specialty: Neurol. Socs: Assn. Brit. NeUrol.s. Prev: Cons. Neurol. Taunton and Som. NHS Trust; Cons. Neurol. Yeovil NHS Trust.; Sen. Regist. (Neurol Bristol).
SMITH, Gareth Lindsay 31 Regent Park Square, Glasgow G41 2AF — MB ChB Aberd. 1992.
SMITH, Garry Michael 100 St Richards Road, Deal CT14 9LD — BM Soton. 1998.
SMITH, Professor Gary Brian c/o Department of Critical Care, Queen Alexandra Hospital, Portsmouth PO6 3LY Tel: 023 9228 6844 Fax: 023 9228 6967 — BM Soton. 1977; FRCA 1981; FCRP 2000; Cert Med Educat Dundee 2004. Cons. in Intens. Care Med., Portsmouth Hosp. NHS Trust; Vis. Prof., Univ. of Bournemouth; Hon. Sen. Lect., Univ. of Portsmouth. Specialty: Intens. Care. Socs: Assn. Anaesth.; Resuscitation Council (UK); Euro. Soc. Intensive Care Med. Prev: Sen. Regist. (Anaesth.) Soton. Gen. & Portsmouth Hosps.; Instruc. (Anaesth.) Yale Univ., USA; Regist. (Anaesth.) Bristol Roy. Infirm.
SMITH, Gemma Elizabeth Catherine 41 St Helens Way, Adel, Leeds LS16 8LP — MB ChB Leeds 1997; MRCP.
SMITH, Geoffrey Barry, OStJ, TD (retired) Lutterworth, The Square, South Harting, Petersfield GU31 5PZ Tel: 01730 825336 — MB BS Lond. 1957 (Lond. Hosp.) MRCS Eng. LRCP Lond. 1957; DA Eng. 1959; FFA RCS Eng. 1963. Prev: Cons. Anaesth. Moorfields Eye Hosp. Lond.
SMITH, Geoffrey Charlton (retired) 16 Kelsey Close, Hunstanton PE36 6HL Tel: 01485 532955 Fax: 01485 532955 Email: jgsmith@btinternet.com — MRCS Eng. LRCP Lond. 1957 (Middlx.) DObst RCOG 1961. Prev: Pres. Med. Commiss. Internat. Water Ski Federat.
SMITH, Geoffrey Francis (retired) 5 Eastmead Lane, Stoke Bishop, Bristol BS9 1HW — MB ChB Manch. 1951; DObst RCOG 1953; DIH Soc. Apoth. Lond. 1958; FFOM RCP Lond. 1985. Prev: Regional Med. Off. S.W. Brit. Telecom.
SMITH, Professor Geoffrey Harry Stable House, Main St., Great Longstone, Bakewell DE45 1TZ Tel: 01629 640143 Fax: 01629 640852 — MB BS Lond. 1961 (St. Mary's) MB BS (Hons.) Lond. 1961 Distinction in Surgery; MRCS Eng. LRCP Lond. 1961; FRCS Eng. 1965. Med. Advisor Brit. Counc. Specialty: Cardiothoracic Surg. Socs: Soc. Cardiothoracic Surgs. GB & Irel.; Eur. Assn.

Cardiothoracic Surg. Prev: Vis. Prof. Cardiac Surg. Norrlands Univ. Sweden; Prof. Cardiac Surg. Univ. Sheff.; Sen. Regist. (Surg.) Hosps. For Dis. of Chest.

SMITH, Geoffrey John Medical Centre, The Grove, Rowlands Gill NE39 1PW Tel: 01207 542136 Fax: 01207 543340; 6 Greenhead Terrace, Chopwell, Newcastle upon Tyne NE17 7AH Tel: 01207 562227 — MB ChB Aberd. 1983; MRCGP 1988. Prev: Regist. (Gen. Med.) Rockhampton Base Hosp. Qu.sland., Austral.

SMITH, Geoffrey Keay 70 New Wokingham Road, Crowthorne RG45 6JJ — MB ChB Birm. 1993.

SMITH, Geoffrey Leighton Woodlands Surgery, Woodland Terrace, Caerau, Maesteg CF34 0SR; 50 Parc Tynywaun, Llangynwyd, Maesteg CF34 9RG — MB BS Lond. 1993 (St. George's Hosp. Med. Sch.) GP. Specialty: Gen. Pract. Prev: Trainee GP Bridgend VTS.

SMITH, Geoffrey Paul 4 Bowes Lyon Place, Lytham St Annes FY8 3UE — MB BS Lond. 1994.

SMITH, Geoffrey Taylor Worcester Royal Infirmary, Castle St., Worcester WR1 3AS Tel: 01905 25238; Tutnall House, Claines Lane, Claines, Worcester WR3 7RN — MB ChB Sheff. 1975; MRC Path. 1981. Cons. Histopath. Worcester Roy. Infirm. Specialty: Histopath.

SMITH, Geoffrey Vincent Department of Gastroenterology, Middlesex Hospital, Mortimer Street, London W1 Tel: 020 7882 7203 Fax: 020 7882 7192 Email: g.v.smith@qmul.ac.uk — MB BS Lond. 1993 (Lond. Hosp. Med. Coll.) MRCP (UK) 1997. Specialist Regist. (Gastroenterol. & Gen. Internal Med.) NE Thames. Specialty: Gastroenterol. Prev: SHO (High Dependency Med.) St. Thos. Hosp. Lond.; SHO (Haemat. & Oncol.) St. Bart. Hosp. Lond.; SHO Rotat. (Med.) Roy. Lond. Hosp.

SMITH, George Intensive Therapy Unit, Aberdeen Royal Infirmary, Foresterhill, Aberdeen AB25 2ZN Tel: 01224 552970 Fax: 01224 840724 — MB ChB Aberd. 1970; DObst RCOG 1973; DA Eng. 1973; FFA RCS Eng. 1977. Cons Anaesth. & Intens. Care Med.Aberd Roy. Infirm. Specialty: Anaesth.; Intens. Care. Socs: BMA; Intens. Care Soc.; Scott. Intens. Care Soc. Prev: Sen. Regist. (Anaesth.) Nottm. City Hosp. Derbysh. Roy. Infirm. & The Groby Rd. Hosp. Leicester; Squadron Ldr. (Rtd.) RAF Med. Br.

SMITH, George Dobbie Ninewells Hospital and Medical School, Department of Pathology, Dundee DD1 9SY Tel: 01382 660111 32548 Email: george.d.smith@tuht.scot.nhs.uk; 1 County Place, Kilspindie, Perth PH2 7RX Tel: 01821 670315 — MB ChB Glas. 1977; BSc (Hons.) Glas. 1973; MRCPath 1983; Dip. Forens. Med. Glas. 1990; FRCPath 1995. Cons. Path. Ninewells Hosp. & Med. Sch. Dundee (Tayside Univ. Hosp. NHS Trust). Specialty: Histopath. Socs: Path. Soc.; Assn. Clin. Path.; Internat. Acad. of Path. Prev: Cons. Path. Admin. Charge Stobhill Gen. Hosp. Glas.; Lect. (Path.) Univ. Edin.; Hon. Sen. Regist. (Path.) Lothian HB.

SMITH, George Lindsay (retired) Creag Ruadh, 13 Balfour Crescent, Milnathort, Kinross KY13 9TA Tel: 01577 864911 — (Glas.) MB ChB Glas. 1950; DObst RCOG 1954. Prev: Clin. Asst. (Community Med.) Fife HB.

SMITH, George William (retired) 6 Hop Gardens, Henley-on-Thames RG9 2EH — (St. Geo.) MRCS Eng. LRCP Lond. 1950. Prev: Clin. Asst. (Dermat.) Heatherwood Hosp., King Edwd. VII Hosp., Windsor.

SMITH, Georgina Ann 42 Hyde Terrace, Newcastle upon Tyne NE3 1AT — MB BS Newc. 1997.

SMITH, Gerald Halfway House, Upper Maund, Bodenham, Hereford HR1 3JD Tel: 01568 797460 Fax: 01568 707077 Email: oldrec@clara.co.uk — MB ChB Birm. 1968; FFOM RCP Lond. 1993, MFOM 1990, AFOM 1988; MSc (Occupat. Med.) Lond. 1989. Dir. (Occupat. Health) Occupat. Health Care (Railways) Ltd. Specialty: Occupat. Health. Socs: Fell. Roy. Soc. Med.; Soc. Occupat. Med. Prev: Dep. Chief Med. Adviser Post Office; Med. Off. Atomic Weapons Estab. Aldermaston; Surg. Cdr. RN MoD Lond.

SMITH, Gerald Martin 26 Abercorn Place, St. John's Wood, London NW8 9XP Tel: 01895 232102 Fax: 01895 235969 — MB BS Lond. 1983.

SMITH, Gerald Norman Haematology Department, Guys Hospital, St Thomas St., London SE1 9RT Tel: 020 7955 4609 Fax: 020 7955 4002; 23 Burlington Road, Chiswick, London W4 4BQ Tel: 020 8995 9008 — (St. Mary's) PhD Lond. 1976, BSc 1961; MB BS Lond. 1964; FRCPath 1986, M 1975. Cons. Haemat. Guy's & St. Thos. Trust. Specialty: Haematology. Prev: Cons. Haemat. Northwick Pk. Hosp. Harrow; Sen. Regist. (Haemat.) St. Thos. Hosp. Lond.; on Scientif. Staff MRC Haemat. Unit St. Mary's Hosp. Med. Sch.

SMITH, Gilbert Reginald The Birmingham Medical Clinic, 69-71 Whitehead Road, Aston, Birmingham B6 5EL Tel: 0121 327 2255 Fax: 0121 327 2255; 79 Farquhar Road, Edgbaston, Birmingham B15 2QP Tel: 0121 454 6969 — MB ChB Birm. 1954. Indep. GP Birm. Socs: Sands Cox Soc. Birm. Grad.s.

SMITH, Giles Rowan Grove Surgery, Grove Lane, Thetford IP24 2HY Tel: 01842 752285 Fax: 01842 751316 — MB ChB Birm. 1971; MRCP (UK) 1975.

SMITH, Gillian Brindle 35 Milbourne Lane, Esher KT10 9EB — MB ChB Liverp. 1972; FFA RCS Eng. 1977. Cons. Anaesth. Kingston Hosp. Kingston upon Thames. Specialty: Anaesth. Socs: Intractable Pain Soc. Prev: Sen. Regist. Dept. Anaesth. Westm. Hosp. Lond.

SMITH, Gillian Dawn 69 Prince George Avenue, Southgate, London N14 4TL — MB BCh Wales 1989; FRCS Ed. 1994. Specialist Regist. (Plastic Surg.) Selly Oak Hosp. Birm.; Clin. Hand Fell., Gt. Ormond St. Hosp., Lond. Specialty: Plastic Surg. Prev: SPR (Plastic Surg.) City Gen. Hosp., Stoke-on-Trent; SPR (Plastic Surg.) Birm. Childr.'s Hosp.; SPR (Plastic Surg.) Selly Oak Hosp., Birm.

SMITH, Gillian Deborah Longfleet House Surgery, 56 Longfleet Road, Poole BH15 2JD Tel: 01202 666677 Fax: 01202 660319; 7 Greenwood Avenue, Lilliput, Poole BH14 8QD — BM (Hons.) Soton. 1983. Specialty: Dermat.

SMITH, Gillian Lesley Ferguson Department of Oral Medicine, Glasgow Dental Hospital & School, 378 Sauchiehall St., Glasgow G2 3JZ Tel: 0141 211 9600 Email: gill.smith@northglasgow.scot.nhs.uk — MB ChB Ed. 1996; BDS Ed. 1982; PhD Ed. 1985; FDS RCS Ed. 1990; Intercollegiate Diploma Oral Med. 1999; FDS RCPS Glasgow 2003. Cons./Hon. Sen. Lect. Oral Med., Glas. Dent. Hosp. & Sch. Socs: BMA; Brit. Soc. Oral Med. Prev: Regist. (Oral Med.) Glas. Dent. Hosp. & Sch.; Preregistration Ho. Off. (Med.) (W.. Gen. Edin.) & Surg. (E. Gen. Edin.); Lect. Oral Med. Dent. Sch. Edin.

SMITH, Miss Gillian Louise — MB BS Lond. 1990; MA Oxf. 1993, BA 1987; FRCS Ed. 1994; FRCS Eng. 1995; FRCS (Urol.) Lond. 2002; MD Lond. 2003. Specialty: Urol.

SMITH, Gillian Margaret — MB BCh BAO Belf. 1977; MRCPsych 1982; Med. Dipl. (Clinical Hypnosis) 2002. Cons. Psychiat. Specialty: Gen. Psychiat. Prev: SCMO (Adult Psychiat.) Bexhill-on-Sea.

SMITH, Gladys Honeyman 325A Albert Drive, Glasgow G41 5EA — MB ChB Glas. 1962.

SMITH, Godfrey William Thomas 106 Warwick Road, Bounds Green, London N11 2ST Tel: 020 8361 2127 — MB BChir Camb. 1976 (Middlx.) MB Camb. 1976, MA, BChir 1975; MRCP (UK) 1979. Lect. (Med. Microbiol.) Roy. Free Hosp. Lond. Socs: Fell. Roy. Soc. Med. Prev: Resid. Med. Off. Nat. Heart Hosp. SHO (Neurol.) Radcliffe Infirm.; Oxf.; SHO (Thoracic Med.) Brompton Hosp. Lond.

SMITH, Mr Gordon Western General Hospital, Crewe Road, Edinburgh EH4 2XU; 137 Mayfield Road, Edinburgh EH9 3AN Tel: 0131 668 3683 Fax: 0131 668 3683 — MB ChB Ed. 1976; FRCS Glas. 1981. Cons. Urol. West. Gen. Hosp. Trust Edin. Specialty: Urol.

SMITH, Professor Gordon Campbell Sinclair Department of Obstetrics & Gynaecology, Rosie Hospital, Robinson Way, Cambridge CB2 2SW Tel: 01223 336871 Fax: 01223 763889 Email: bmh24@cam.ac.uk — MB ChB Glas. 1987; BSc (1st cl. Hons.) Physiol. Glas. 1987; MD 1995; MRCOG 1995; PhD 2001. Prof. (Obst. & Gyn.) Univ. Camb. Specialty: Obst. & Gyn. Socs: Roy. Coll. of Obst. & Gynaecologists; Perinatal Research Soc. (USA); Soc. for Gynecologic Investig. (USA) (Assoc. Mem.). Prev: Sub-Specialist Trainee Matern. Fetal Med., Glas.

SMITH, Gordon Francis Nelson Department of Anaesthetics, Victoria Hospital, Hayfield Road, Kirkcaldy KY2 5AH Tel: 01592 643355; 1 Silverbank, Leslie Road, Scotlandwell, Kinross KY13 9JE Tel: 01592 840484 — MB ChB Glas. 1971; FFA RCS Eng. 1976. Cons. Anaesth. Vict. Hosp. Kirkcaldy, Fife Acute Hosps. NHS Trust.; Clin. Director, Theatre & Anaesthetics, Fife Acute Hosps. NHS Trust. Specialty: Anaesth. Socs: BMA; Assn. of Anaesth.; Scott. Soc. Anaesth.

SMITH, Mr Gordon Graham (retired) Mullagrach, Polbain, Achiltibuie, Ullapool IV26 2YW — MB ChB Glas. 1966; CIH Dund

1974; FRCS Glas. 1978. Cons. ENT Surg. Vict. Hosp. Kirkcaldy. Prev: Ho. Off. (Surg. & Med.) Glas. Roy. Infirm.

SMITH, Gordon Stirling 9 St Mary's Court, Porthcawl CF36 5SD — MB ChB Sheff. 1970.

SMITH, Graeme Murray Dept. of Haematology, Leeds General Infirmary, Great George St., Leeds LS1 3EX Email: graemes@pathology.leeds.ac.uk — (Guy's) MD Lond. 1992, MB BS 1980; FRCP (UK) 1997; FRCPath 1998. Cons. Haemat. Leeds Gen. Infirm. & Wharfedale Gen. Hosp. Otley. Specialty: Haematology. Socs: Brit. Soc. Haematol. Prev: Sen. Regist. (Haemat.) Yorks. RHA; Hon. Regist. (Haemat.) E. Birm. Hosp.; Regist. (Chest & Gen. Med.) Walsgrave Hosp. Coventry.

SMITH, Graham (retired) 95 Kingsmills Road, Inverness IV2 3PE Tel: 01463 239144 — MB BS Durh. 1954. Prev: Ho. Surg. & Ho. Phys. Newc. Gen. Hosp.

SMITH, Professor Graham University Department of Anaesthesia, Leicester Royal Infirmary, Leicester LE1 5WW Tel: 0116 258 5291 Fax: 0116 285 4487; 12 Sycamore Close, Oadby, Leicester LE2 2RN — MRCS Eng. LRCP Lond. 1966 (Guy's) BSc Lond. 1963, MD 1972, MB BS 1966; FRCA. 1969. Prof. Anaesth. Univ. Leicester; Hon. Cons. (Anaesth.) Leicester DHA; Edr. Brit. Jl. Anaesth.; Acad. Europ. Acad. Anaesth. Specialty: Anaesth. Socs: (Counc.) Roy. Coll. anaesth.; Hon. Mem. Amer. Assn. Univ. Anaesthesiol. Prev: Sen. Lect. (Anaesth.) Univ. Glas.; Cons. Anaesth. West. Infirm. Glas.; MRC Trav. Fell. (Anaesthesiol.) Univ. Washington, USA.

SMITH, Graham Colin Kruf Children's Kidney Centre, University Hospital of Wales, Cardiff CF14 4XN Tel: 029 2074 3310 Fax: 029 2074 4822 Email: smithgc@cardiff.ac.uk — MB BS Lond. 1986 (London) FRCPCH; MA Camb. 1985; MRCP (UK) 1989. Cons. Paediat. Nephrol. Univ. Hosp. of Wales. Specialty: Paediat. Socs: Brit. Assn. Paediat. Nephrol.; Fell. Roy. Coll. Paediat. and Child Health; Eur. Soc. Paediat. Nephrol. Prev: Sen. Regist. (Paediat.) Roy. Hosp. Sick Childr. Glas.; Fell. (Paediat. Nephrol.) Hosp. Sick Childr. Toronto, Canada; Research Fell. (Paediat. Nephrol.) Birm. CHildr. Hosp.

SMITH, Graham Douglas Guardian Street Medical Centre, Guardian Street, Warrington WA5 1UD Tel: 01925 650226 Fax: 01925 240633 — MB ChB Liverp. 1970.

SMITH, Graham Lawrence Rainbow Medical Centre, 333 Robins Lane, St Helens WA9 3PN Tel: 01744 811211; 35 Ashton Avenue, Rainhill, Prescot L35 0QQ — MB ChB Liverp. 1978; DRCOG 1982.

SMITH, Graham Michael 46 Quarry Street, Leeds LS6 2JU — MB ChB Leeds 1994.

SMITH, Mr Graham Munro (retired) 1 Sycamore Close, Knighton Rise, Oadby, Leicester LE2 2RN Tel: 0116 270 8304 — MB ChB Glas. 1960; DObst RCOG 1961; FRCOG 1980, M 1967. Cons. O & G Gen. Hosp. Leicester. Prev: Sen. Regist. Nottm. Hosp. Wom. & Jessop Hosp. Wom. Sheff.

SMITH, Graham Nicholas Community Mental Health Unit, St. Charles Hospital, Exmoor St., London W10 6DZ — MB BS Lond. 1986. Clin. Asst. (Psychiat.) St. Chas. Hosp. Lond. Prev: SHO (Psychiat.) Princess Alexandra Hosp. Harlow; Ho. Off. (Med.) S. Cleveland Hosp. Middlesbrough; Ho. Off. (Surg.) St. Helier Hosp. Carshalton.

SMITH, Graham Thomas Hexworthy House, Lawhitton, Launceston PL15 9PE Tel: 01566 777024 — (St. Geo.) BM BCh Oxf. 1962; MA Oxf. 1962.

SMITH, Graham Yates Govanhill Health Centre, 233 Calder St., Glasgow G42 7DR Tel: 0141 424 3003; 19 Rozelle Avenue, Newton Mearns, Glasgow G77 6YS — MB ChB Glas. 1983; DRCOG 1986; MRCGP 1987.

SMITH, Grahame Bower 12 Almondbury Close, Almondbury, Huddersfield HD5 8XX — MB ChB Manch. 1966; MRCP (U.K.) 1971. Cons. Phys. (Geriat. Med.) Bradford AHA. Specialty: Gen. Med. Prev: Cons. Phys. (Geriat. Med.) Doncaster AHA. Late Sen. Regist . North.; Gen. Hosp. Sheff.

SMITH, Grahame David Northgate Surgery, Northgate, Pontefract WF8 1NG Tel: 01977 703635 Fax: 01977 702562; 54 Carleton Road, Pontefract WF8 3NF Tel: 01977 600880 — MB BS Lond. 1968 (Univ. Coll. Hosp.) DObst RCOG 1970; DA Eng. 1973; Dip. Clin. Hypn. Sheff. 1991. Local Med. Off. Civil Serv. Med. Advis. Serv. Specialty: Gen. Pract.; Psychother. Socs: Accredit. Mem. Brit. Soc. Med. & Dent. Hypn. Prev: Hosp. Pract. (Anaesth.) Pontefract & Wakefield; Med. Off. i/c Governm. Hosp. Mankayane, Swaziland; SHO (Paediat.) Worcester Roy. Infirm.

SMITH, Mr Guy St John Tristram — MB BS (Hons.) Lond. 1994 (St Thos.) BSc (Hons.) 1991; FRCOphth 1998. Cons. Ophth. Gt. West. Hosp. Swindon. Specialty: Ophth. Socs: Undersea & Hyperbaric Med. Soc.; Amer. Acad. Ophthalmologists; Europ. Soc. Cataract & Refractive Surgeons.

SMITH, Gwendoline (retired) St. Monance, Coggins Mill, Mayfield TN20 6UL Tel: 01435 2301 — MRCS Eng. LRCP Lond. 1926 (Univ. Coll. Hosp.) MD Lond. 1930, MB BS 1926; FRCS Eng. 1929. Prev: Surg. S. Lond. Hosp. Wom. & Childr.

SMITH, Harold Rubislaw Terrace Surgery, 23 Rubislaw Terrace, Aberdeen AB10 1XE Tel: 01224 643665 Fax: 01224 625197 — MB ChB Aberdeen 1973; MB ChB Aberdeen 1973.

SMITH, Harry Charles Thomson (retired) 12 Avondale Road, Ponteland, Newcastle upon Tyne NE20 9NA Tel: 01661 823636 Fax: 01661 823636 — MB ChB St. And. 1951; DPH Glas. 1956; DPA Glas. 1960. Prev: SCM (EnviroMent. Health) Gateshead HA.

SMITH, Harry Napier Far Lane Medical Centre, 1 Far Lane, Sheffield S6 4FA Tel: 0114 234 3229; 10 Moorbank Close, Sheffield S10 5TP — MB ChB Sheff. 1969; DObst RCOG 1971; MRCGP 1977.

SMITH, Harvey Ronald 19 Arlington Place, Gordon Road, Winchester SO23 7TR — MB BS Lond. 1990.

SMITH, Heather Jane 2 Norfolk Hill Croft, Greoside, Sheffield S35 8SE — MB BS Lond. 1991; MRCGP 1995.

SMITH, Heather Joy Macklin Street Surgery, 90 Macklin Street, Derby DE1 1JX Tel: 01332 340381 Fax: 01332 345387; 36 South Avenue, Littleover, Derby DE23 6BA Tel: 01332 765020 — BM BS Nottm. 1988; BMedSci Nottm. 1986; MRCGP 1993. Clin. Asst. (Palliat. Med.) Nightingale Continuing Care Macmillan Unit, Derby. Specialty: Palliat. Med. Prev: Trainee GP Derby VTS; SHO/Macmillan Fell. Hayward Hse. Nottm. City Hosp.

SMITH, Heather Lesley Department of Paediatrics, The General Hospital, Bishop Auckland DL14 6AD Tel: 01388 455189 — MB BS Lond. 1979; MRCS Eng. LRCP Lond. 1979; FRCP (UK) 1997, MRCP 1982; DCH RCP Lond. 1982; FRCPCH 1997; Cert Med Educat Univ. Newc. upon Tyne 2001. Cons. Paediat. Bishop Auckland Gen. Hosp. Specialty: Paediat.; Gastroenterol. Socs: Brit. Soc. Paediat. Gastroenterol. & Nutrit.; Fell. Roy. Coll. Paediat. & Child Health; Fell. Roy. Coll. of Phys. Prev: Sen. Regist. (Paediat.) S. Cleveland Hosp. Middlesbrough; Clin. Research Fell. Inst. Child Health Univ. Birm.; Regist. (Paediat.) Leicester Roy. Infirm.

SMITH, Helen Elizabeth Brighton and Sussex Medical School, Mayfield House, Village Way, Falmer, Brighton BN1 9PH Tel: 01273 644192 Fax: 01273 644440 Email: h.e.smith@bsms.ac.uk; Clevelands, 72 Westwood Road, Southampton SO17 1DP Tel: 023 8058 4459 — BM BS Nottm. 1981 (Nottingham) DM Nottm. 1996, BMedSci 1979; DCH RCP Lond. 1983; MSc (Comm. Med.) Lond. 1988; MFPHM RCP Lond. 1989; FFPHM RCP Lond. 1996; MRCGP RCP Lond. 2000. Prof. of Primary Care, Brighton and Sussex Med. Sch. Specialty: Gen. Pract.; Pub. Health Med. Socs: Soc. Social Med.; WONCA; SAPC. Prev: Vis. Sc. Univ. Brit. Columbia Health Care & Epidemiol. Vancouver; Sen. Regist. (Pub. Health Med.) W. Midl. RHA; Regist. (Community Med.) SW Thames RHA.

SMITH, Helen Jane 79 Bower Mount Road, Maidstone ME16 8AS Email: drhjsmith@hotmail.com — MB ChB Birm. 1996; DRCOG 1998. Specialty: Gen. Pract.

SMITH, Helen Leisa 27 King Edgar Close, Ely CB6 1DP Tel: 01353 612149 Fax: 01353 669175 — MB BS Lond. 1989 (University College London) DA (UK) 1991; FRCA 1993. Cons. (Anaesth.) Addenbrookes's Hosp. Camb. Specialty: Anaesth. Socs: Train. Mem. Assn. AnE.h. Prev: Regist. (Anaesth.) Addenbrooke's Hosp. Camb.; SHO (Anaesth.) Hammersmith Hosp. & Edgware Gen. Hosp. Lond.

SMITH, Helen Mary Ash-View, Tamworth Rd, Corley, Coventry CV7 8BQ — MB ChB Birm. 1990; ChB Birm. 1990.

SMITH, Helen Patricia 590 King Street, Aberdeen AB24 5SQ — MB ChB Aberd. 1997.

SMITH, Helena Rebecca 133 Higher Lane, Whitefield, Manchester M45 7WH — MB ChB Liverp. 1991.

SMITH, Hilary Maltings Surgery, 8 Victoria Street, St Albans AL1 3JB Tel: 01727 855500 Fax: 01727 845537; 4 Faircross Way,

St Albans AL1 4SD — MB BS Lond. 1976 (Univ. Coll. Hosp.) MRCGP Lond. 1981. GP Trainer W. Herts. HA.

SMITH, Miss Hilary Margaret (retired) — MB BS Lond. 1967 (Lond. Hosp.) DA Eng. 1970; FRCOG 1986, M 1974, DObst 1970. Prev: Cons. (O & G) MusGr. Pk. Hosp.

SMITH, Hilary Royle 1 Railway Path, Ormskirk L39 4TR — MB ChB Dundee 1987.

SMITH, Hillas George 24 Oakleigh Avenue, Whetstone, London N20 9JH Tel: 020 8445 1876 — MB BCh BAO Dub. 1951 (T.C. Dub.) BA Dub. 1948, MA, MD 1961, MB BCh BAO 1951; FRCP Lond. 1975, M 1964. Cons. Phys. Roy. Free Hosp., Dept. Infec. Dis. Coppetts Wood Hosp.; Lister Unit Northwick Pk. Hosp. Harrow; Emerit. Edr. Jl. Infec. Specialty: Gen. Med. Prev: Leverhulme Research Schol. Middlx. Hosp.; Ho. Off. Char. Cross Med. Unit, Mt. Vernon Hosp. Northwood & Adelaide; Hosp. Dub.

SMITH, Hillas Rodney St Andrews Medical Practice, 50 Oakleigh Road North, Whetstone, London N20 9EX Tel: 020 8445 2352 Fax: 020 8446 0179; 49 Crescent W., Hadley Wood, Barnet EN4 0EQ Tel: 020 8440 4774 — MB BS Lond. 1981; BSc (Hons.) Lond. 1978; DRCOG 1984; MRCGP 1986. GP. Specialty: Dermat. Prev: Whipps Cross Hosp. VTS; Trainee Highgate Gp. Pract. Lond.; Clin. Asst. (Dermat.) Barnet Gen. Hosp.

SMITH, Mr Howard Duncan (retired) 42 Hayes Road, Bromley BR2 9AA — (Char. Cross) MB BS Lond. 1961; FRCS Eng. 1967. Prev: Sen. Regist. (Orthop.) St. Bart. Hosp. Lond.

SMITH, Howard George 61 Stafford Place, Weston Super Mare BS23 2QZ Fax: 01934 627300 — MB ChB Bristol 1966; DPM Eng. 1972; MRCPsych 1975.

SMITH, Howard Stephen anaesthetics Dept, Peterborough District Hospital, Thorpe Road, Peterborough PE3 6DA Tel: 01733874000 Email: howard.s.smith@tesco.net — MB BS Lond. 1972 (Lond. Hosp.) MRCS Eng. LRCP Lond. 1972; FFA RCS Eng. 1980. Cons. (Anaesth. & IC) PeterBoro. Dist. Hosps. PeterBoro., Camb. Specialty: Intens. Care. Prev: Sen. Regist. Cambs. AHA (T); Sen. Specialist (Anaesth.) RAF.

SMITH, Hugh Norman, MC (retired) 9 Harvey Orchard, Beaconsfield HP9 1TH Tel: 01494 673830 — MRCS Eng. LRCP Lond. 1942 (Camb. & Univ. Coll. Hosp.) MA Camb. 1946. JP.; Maj. RAMC TARO. Prev: GP Beaconsfield.

SMITH, Iain David Gartnavel Royal Hospital, 1055 Great Western Road, Glasgow G12 0XH — MB ChB Glas. 1983; BSc (Hons.) Glas. 1980, MB ChB 1983; MRCPsych 1987. Cons. & Hon. Sen. Clin. Lect. Gartnavel Roy. Hosp. Specialty: Gen. Psychiat. Prev: Lect. (Psychol. Med.) Univ. Glas.; Regist. (Psychiat.) Argyll & Bute Hosp. Lochgilphead; Regist. (Psychiat.) Dykebar Hosp. Paisley.

SMITH, Iain James 19 Fortis Way, Huddersfield HD3 3WW — MB ChB Ed. 1974; MPH Leeds 1990; MBA Leeds 1994; FRCPCH 1996; FRCP Ed. 1996. Sen. Lect. (Health Servs. Research) & Hon. Cons. Child Health N. Yorks. HA & N. & Yorks. Regional Exec. Specialty: Paediat. Prev: Project Manager Yorks. Health; Lect. (Paediat.) Univ. Leeds.

SMITH, Ian Afton Shiel, 8 North Deeside Road, Bieldside, Aberdeen AB15 9AJ Tel: 01224 867799 — MB ChB Aberd. 1961; DObst RCOG 1963; FFA RCS Eng. 1969. Cons. Anaesth. Aberd. Roy. Infirm. Specialty: Anaesth. Prev: Obst. Ho. Surg. Dundee Roy. Infirm.; Paediat. Ho. Phys. Inverness Hosp. Gp.; Staff Anaesth. Toronto Gen. Hosp.

SMITH, Ian Directorate of Anaesthesia, North Staffordshire Hospital, Newcastle Road, Stoke-on-Trent ST4 6QG Tel: 01782 553054 Fax: 01782 719754 Email: damsmith@btinternet.com — MB BS Lond. 1984 (Westm.) BSc Lond. 1981; FRCA Eng. 1988. Cons. & Sen. Lect. N. Staffs. Hosps. Stoke-on-Trent; Vis. Asst. Prof. Univ. Texas S.W.. Med. Center Dallas, Texas. Specialty: Anaesth. Socs: Coun. Mem. - Brit. Assn. of Day Surg.; Chairm. Ambulatory Anaesthetics Subcomm.of the Europ. Soc. of Anaesthosiolists; Coun. Mem. Midl. Soc. of Anaesth.s. Prev: Sen. Regist. (Anaesth.) Midl. Anaesth. Train. Scheme Birm.; Research Fell. Washington Univ. St. Louis, USA; Regist. (Anaesth.) E. Birm. Hosp.

SMITH, Ian Charles Sheringham Medical Practice, Health Centre, Cromer Road, Sheringham NR26 8RT Tel: 01263 822066 Fax: 01263 823890 — BM BS Nottm. 1985; DRCOG 1992; DCH 1992.

SMITH, Mr Ian Christopher Evanson Abergele Hospital, Llanfair Road, Abergele LL22 8DP Tel: 01745 832295 Ext: 3483 Email: ian.smith@cd-tr.wales.nhs.uk — MB BS Lond. 1987 (St Georges Lond.) FRCS Eng. 1992; FRCS (Tr. & Orth.) 2000. Cons. Orthopaedic Surg., Abergele Hosp. Specialty: Trauma & Orthop. Surg.; Orthop. Prev: SHO (Orthop. & Trauma) Rowley Bristow Orthop. Unit St. Peter's Hosp. Chertsey; SHO (Paediat. & Gen. Surg.) St. Geo. Hosp. Lond.; Spec.regist, (trauma & Orthop) Welsch Train. scheme.

SMITH, Ian Douglas Department of Anaesthesia, Princess Margaret Hospital, Okus Road, Swindon SN1 4JU Tel: 01793 536231 — MB BS Lond. 1981; DRCOG 1985; FRCA 1990. Cons. Anaesth. Princess Margt. Hosp. Swindon. Specialty: Anaesth. Prev: Sen. Regist. Trent RHA; Lect. (Anaesth.) Univ. Hong Kong; Regist. NW Thames RHA.

SMITH, Ian Duncan 12 Woodmansterne Road, Carshalton Beeches, Sutton SM5 4JL Tel: 020 8643 4122 Fax: 020 8643 4122; 12 Woodmasterne Road, Carshalton Beeches, Carshalton SM5 4JL Tel: 020 8643 4122 Fax: 020 8643 4122 — MB BS Lond. 1955 (King's Coll. Hosp.) MRCS Eng. LRCP Lond. 1955; MRCGP 1968. Indep. GP Carshalton; Examr. Scott. Widows & Legal & Gen. Assur. Soc.; Hon. Sec. Sutton & Distance Med. Soc.; Expert Witness. Socs: BMA; Indep. Doctors Forum; Sutton Med. Soc. Prev: Ho. Off. Paediat. & Ho. Off. Surg. (O & G) King's Coll. Hosp. Gp.; HOPhysican St JamesHosp. Lond.

SMITH, Ian Edward The Respiratory Support & Sleep Centre, Papworth Hospital, Papworth Everard, Cambridge CB3 8RE Tel: 01480 830541 Fax: 01480 830620 Email: ian.smith@papworth.nhs.uk; 69 Hurst Park Ave, Cambridge CB4 2AB Tel: 01223 368976 — MB BS Lond. 1987 (Caius College Cambridge (Pre-Clinical); Royal London Hospital Medical College) MA Camb. 1988, BA 1984; MRCP (UK) 1990; MD Camb. 1997; FRCP (UK) 2001. Cons. (Chest Med.) Respirat. Support & Sleep Centre Papworth Hosp. Camb., Addenbrookes Hosp. Camb. & Bedford Hosp.; Assoc. Lect., Univ. of Camb. Specialty: Respirat. Med. Socs: Brit. Thorac. Soc.; Brit. Sleep Soc. Prev: Sen. Clin. Fell. (Chest Med.) Respirat. Support & Sleep Centre Papworth Hosp. Camb.; Regist. (Chest Med.) Papworth & Addenbrooke's Hosps. Camb.; SHO (Cardiol.) Brook Hosp. Lond.

SMITH, Professor Ian Edward Royal Marsden Hospital - London/Surrey, Fulham Road, London SW3 6JJ Tel: 020 8661 3280 Fax: 020 8643 0373 Email: ian.smith@rmh.nthames.nhs.uk — MB ChB 1971 (Ed.) BSc (Hons.) Ed. 1968; MRCP UK 1973; MD 1978; FRCP (Ed.) 1984; FRCP Lond. 1988. Prof. of Cancer Med. Inst. of cancer research. Specialty: Oncol. Socs: Amer. Soc. Clin. Oncol. & Brit. Assn. Cancer Phys.; Past Chairm. Assn. Cancer Phys.; Chairm.NCRI Lung Cancer Clin. Studies Gp. Prev: Hon. Sen. Lect. Inst. Cancer Research Lond.; Lect. (Med.) Roy. Marsden Hosp. Sutton; Research Fell. Inst. Cancer Research Sutton.

SMITH, Ian Fairley (retired) 13 The Drive, Kilner Park, Ulverston LA12 0DT Tel: 01229 582144 — MB BChir Camb. 1952 (Lond. Hosp.) MA Camb. 1952; MRCS Eng. LRCP Lond. 1952; DObst RCOG 1955; DCH Eng. 1956. Prev: Ho. Off. (O & G) Wom. Hosp. Wolverhampton.

SMITH, Ian Geoffrey Synexus Ltd, Sandringham House, Ackhurst Park, Chorley PR7 1NY Tel: 01257 230723 Fax: 01257 231981 Email: ian.smith@synexus.com; Woodside of Tulliemet, Tulliemet, Pitlochry PH9 0NZ Tel: 01796 482304 — MB ChB Manch. 1974; BMedSc (Hons.) Dundee 1971. Med. Director, Synexus Ltd.; Hon. Research Fell. (Clin. Chem.) Univ. Liverp.; Hon. Research Fell. (Nuclear Med.) Guy's Hosp. Lond. Specialty: Pharmaceutical Medicine. Prev: Partner in Gen. Pract.

SMITH, Ian Inglis (retired) 15 Mansionhouse Road, Edinburgh EH9 1TZ Tel: 0131 667 4665 — PhD Ed. 1974, MB ChB 1954. Cons. Pathol. Roy. Hosp. Sick Childr. Edin.

SMITH, Ian Lennox Taylor Merstow Green Medical Practice, Merstow Green, Evesham WR11 4BS Tel: 01386 765600 Fax: 01386 446807; 16 Andrews Drive, Evesham WR11 6JN — MB ChB Birm. 1982; BSc Chem. Glas. 1974. Socs: BMA. Prev: Regist. (O & G) Qu. Eliz. Hosp. Barbados; SHO (Paediat.) Worcester Infirm.; Ho. Off. (Surg.) Worcester Infirm.

SMITH, Ian Mark 41 St. Helen's Way, Adel, Leeds LS16 8LP Email: ian.smith165@virgin.net — MB ChB Leeds 1997; BDS Birm. 1988; FDS RCS Eng. 1992; MSc Leeds 1996; FRCS Ed. 1999; FRCS Eng. 1999. Specialty: Gen. Surg.

SMITH, Ian Mark Andrew The New Surgery, Hillyfields Way, Winscombe BS25 1AF Tel: 01934 842211; Hunters Lodge, Cooks Lane, Banwell, Weston Super Mare BS24 0AD Tel: 01934 824135

— MB BS Lond. 1987; MRCP (UK) 1992; DFFP 1994; T(GP) 1994. GP Princip. Winscombe, Som. Prev: Med. Off. Bethesda Hosp. Kwazulu, RSA.; CMO (Obst. & Paediat.) Maitland Hosp. NSW, Austral.; Trainee GP Cinderford, Glos.

SMITH, Ian Michael 22 Hazel Grove, Stotfold, Hitchin SG5 4JZ — MB ChB Leeds 1986.

SMITH, Mr Ian Michael ENT Department, Royal Cornwall Hospital (Treliske), Truro TR1 3LJ Tel: 01872 253401/ 2 Fax: 01872 253406; Treveth, Kea, Truro TR3 6AJ Tel: 01872 862805 — MB ChB Dundee 1981; BDS Dundee 1975; FRCS Ed. 1983; MD Dundee 1993. Cons. ENT Surg. Roy. Cornw. Hosp. (Treliske) Truro. Specialty: Otorhinolaryngol. Prev: Sen. Regist. St. Michael's Hosp. Bristol.

SMITH, Ian Robertson Culduthel Road Health Centre, Ardlarich, 15 Culduthel Road, Inverness IV2 4AG Tel: 01463 712233 Fax: 01463 715479; Dromard, 43 Midmills Road, Inverness IV2 3NZ Tel: 01463 236741 — MB ChB Glas. 1968; DObst RCOG 1970; FRCGP 1991, M 1975. Ness Doc.; Highland Hospice Dir. Socs: Past Pres. Highland Med. Soc.; Past Chairm. N. Scotl. Fac. RCGP. Prev: Ho. Phys. Roy. Alexandra Infirm. Paisley; Ho. Surg. Roy. North. Infirm. Inverness; Ho. Off. (Obst.) Raigmore Hosp. Inverness.

SMITH, Mr Ian Stanley Ashford, 16 Albert Drive, Bearsden, Glasgow G61 2PF Tel: 0141 942 7452 Fax: 0141 942 7452 — MB ChB Glas 1962; Dobst RCOG 1964; FRCS Ed. 1967; FRCS Glas. 1981. Cons. (Surg.) Ross Hall Hosp. Glas. Specialty: Gen. Surg. Special Interest: Gastrointestinal Surg. Prev: Cons. (Surg.) Vict. Infirm. Glas.

SMITH, Ian Stewart The Department of Clinical Neurophysiology, The General Infirmary at Leeds, Gt George St, Leeds LS1 3EX Tel: 0113 392 3530 Fax: 0113 392 6337 — MB Camb. 1974 (Univ. Coll. Hosp.) BChir 1973; MRCP (UK) 1975; FRCP Lond. 1995. Cons. Clin. Neurophysiol. Leeds Gen. Infirm. Specialty: Clin. Neurophysiol. Prev: Sen. Regist. (Clin. Neurophysiol.) Qu. Eliz. Hosp. Birm.; Research Asst. (EEG) Nat. Hosp. Qu. Sq. Lond.; Regist. (Neurol.) Roy. Free Hosp. Lond.

SMITH, Ian William The Surgery, 14 Queenstown Road, Battersea, London SW8 3RX Tel: 020 7622 9295 Fax: 020 7498 5206; Flat 3, 3 Leinster Square, London W2 4PL — MB BS Lond. 1984; BSc Lond. 1981; DRCOG 1988; MRCGP 1988.

SMITH, Ini Akpan 23 The Charter Road, Woodford Green IG8 9RE — BM BCh Nigeria 1977.

SMITH, Irene Graham Dumfries & Galloway Royal Infirmary, Bankend Road, Dumfries DG1 4AP — MB ChB Aberd. 1985; DRCOG 1987; MRCGP 1990. Staff Grade (Geriat. Med.) Dumfries & Galloway Roy. Infirm. Specialty: Care of the Elderly.

SMITH, Mr Irvine Battinson 3 Holland Park, Barton under Needwood, Burton-on-Trent DE13 8DU Tel: 01283 712734 Fax: 01283 712734 — MB BChir Camb. 1947 (Camb. & Univ. Coll. Hosp.) MRCS Eng. LRCP Lond. 1944; MA Camb., MD 1959, MB BChir 1947; FRCS Eng. 1949. Prev: Cons. Urol. SE Staffs. Health Dist.; Research Fell. Mayo Foundat. USA; Mem. Counc. Brit. Assn. Urol. Surg.

SMITH, Isabel 23 Burlington Road, Chiswick, London W4 4BQ Tel: 020 8995 9008 — (St. Mary's) BSc Lond. 1962; MB BS Lond. 1965; DCH Eng. 1968; MRCP (UK) 1969; FRCP Lond. 1984; FRCPCH 1997. Cons. Hosp. Sick Childr. Gt. Ormond St. Lond.; Hon. Sen. Lect. Inst. Child Health Lond. Specialty: Paediat. Socs: MRCPCH; FRCP.

SMITH, Isabel Frances Anaesthetics, Bromley Hospital, Bromley BR2 9AJ — MB BS Lond. 1994. Specialty: Anaesth.

SMITH, Isabella Marshall c/o Drive Peter Illingworth, Department of Obstetrics & Gynaecology, Westmead Hospital, Westmead NSW 2145, Australia; 11 Belgrave Place, Edinburgh EH4 3AW — MB ChB Glas. 1980; MRCGP 1988; MPH Dundee 1990; MFPHM RCP (UK) 1993. Med. Dir. & Cons. Pub. Health Med. Nat. Servs. Div. Edin. Specialty: Pub. Health Med. Prev: Regist. (Pub. Health Med.) Tayside HB.

SMITH, Mr Ivo (retired) 229 Princes Gardens, London W3 0LU Tel: 020 8992 0939 — (Camb. & St. Mary's) MA Camb. 1960, BA 1954, MChir 1965, MB, BChir 1957; FRCS Eng. 1960. Indep. Surg. Lond.; Mem. Med. Appeals Tribunals; Med. Chairm. Pens. Appeal Tribunals. Prev: Cons. Surg. Guy's & Lewisham Trust.

SMITH, Jaclyn Ann 57 Longford Road W., Stockport SK5 6EU — MB ChB Manch. 1992.

SMITH, Jacqueline Cos Lane Medical Practice, Woodside Road, Glenrothes KY7 4AQ Tel: 01592 752100 Fax: 01592 612692; 5 The Row, Letham, Cupar KY15 7RS Tel: 01337 810404 — MB ChB Dundee 1988; DRCOG 1991; MRCGP 1992. Specialty: Gen. Med.

SMITH, Jacqueline Sarah 148 Campbell Drive, Cardiff CF11 7TQ — MB BCh Wales 1995.

SMITH, James Core Sorbie (retired) 4 Fullarton Drive, Troon KA10 6LE Tel: 01292 314256 Email: jcss@omne.uk.net — MB ChB Glas. 1957; DObst RCOG 1961; DMRD Eng. 1968; FFR 1970; FRCR 1975. Cons. Radiol. CrossHo. Hosp. Kilmarnock. Prev: Ho. Off. (Obst.) Stobhill Hosp. Glas.

SMITH, James George Elder, CStJ Tristans, Grandfield Crescent, Radcliffe-on-Trent, Nottingham NG12 1AN Tel: 0115 933 3920 — LRCP LRCS Ed. LRFPS Glas. 1950 (Ed.) DIH Soc. Apoth. Lond. 1971; FFOM RCP Lond. 1988, M 1978. Indep. Cons. Nottm. Specialty: Occupat. Health. Socs: Fell. Roy. Med. Soc. Edin.; (Ex-Chairm.) Soc. Occupat. Med.; Brit. Occupat. Hyg. Soc. Prev: Princip. Med. Off. (York.) Brit. Coal Doncaster; Area Med. Off. Boots Co. Ltd. Nottm.; Ho. Surg. & Ho. Off. (O & G) Dist. Gen. Hosp. Bolton.

SMITH, James Hogg (retired) 3 Mains of Dun Cottages, Montrose DD10 9LQ Tel: 01674 810274 — MB ChB Glas. 1956; MRCGP 1965. Prev: Relief Med. Off. U.K.A.E.A. Chapelcross.

SMITH, James Mark Perry 175 Victoria Road, Lockwood, Huddersfield HD1 3TT — BM BCh Oxf. 1980. Regist. Community Med. Norwich Health Auth. Specialty: Pub. Health Med.

SMITH, Mr James Michael (retired) Court View Surgery, Rosemary Street, Mansfield NG19 6AB Tel: 01623 623600 Fax: 01623 635460 — MB ChB Sheff. 1969; FRCS Ed. 1975; FRCS Eng. 1975; MRCGP 1988. GP Mansfield. Prev: Rotating Orthop. Regist. Battle Hosp. Reading & Nuffield Orthop.

SMITH, James Michael Beth-Shalom, Laxton, Newark NG22 0PA — MB ChB Leeds 1993.

SMITH, James Murray The Surgery, 2 Heathcote Street, Newcastle ST5 7EB Tel: 01782 561057 Fax: 01782 563907 — MB ChB Glas. 1961; BA Open Univ. 1979. Prev: Ho. Surg. & Ho. Phys. Ballochmyle Hosp.

SMITH, James Neil (retired) c/o 9 Wellington Drive, Grantham NG31 7HU — MB ChB Leeds 1957; DObst RCOG 1961. Prev: GP Grantham.

SMITH, Mr James Richard The Lister Hospital, Chelsea Bridge Road, London SW1W 8RH Tel: 020 7730 0431 Fax: 020 7730 6861; The Garrochty, Kingarth, Rothesay PA20 — MB ChB Glas. 1982 (Glasgow) MRCOG 1988; MD 1992; FRCOG 2000. Cons. Gyn. Chelsea & Westm. Hosp. Lond.; Hon. Sen. Lect. Imperial Coll. Sch. of Med.; Hon. Cons. Gyn. RMH; Adjunct Assoc. Prof. New York Univ. Med. Center New York USA; Hon. Cons. O & G RBH; Cons. Gyn. Hammersmith Hosp. Lond. Specialty: Obst. & Gyn. Socs: Fell. Roy. Soc. Med.; Brit. Gyn. Cancer Soc.; Med. Soc. Study VD. Prev: Sen. Lect. & Cons. O & G Char. Cross & Westm. Med. Sch., Chelsea & W.m. Hosp. Lond.; Research Fell. (O & G & Genitourin. Med.) St. Mary's Hosp. Lond.; Lect. (O & G) Char. Cross & Westm. Med. Sch. Lond.

SMITH, Jane Elizabeth Dean Terrace Centre, 18 Dean Terrace, Edinburgh EH4 1NL Tel: 0131 332 7941/7705 Fax: 0131 332 2931; 34A Dundas Street, Edinburgh EH3 6JN Tel: 0131 557 0186 — MB ChB Bristol 1978; BSc (1st cl. Hons.) Anat. Bristol 1975; MFFP 1993. SCMO (Family Plann. & Psychosexual Med.) Lothian Primary Care NHS Trust, Edin. Specialty: Psychosexual Med.; Family Plann. & Reproduc. Health. Socs: Brit. Assn. Sexual & Marital Ther.; Scott. Family Plann. Med. Soc. Prev: Research Fell. Roy. Soc. Univ. Edin.; Postdoctoral Research Fell. Univ. Chicago & Univ. Texas, Houston.

SMITH, Jane Katharine Wolverhampton Eye Infirmary, Compton Road, Wolverhampton WV3 9QR Tel: 01902 307999 Fax: 01902 564019; 15 Waterdale, Compton, Wolverhampton WV3 9DY Tel: 01902 710564 — MB BCh Wales 1977; BSc (Physiol. & Biochem.) Soton 1972; DO RCS Eng. 1982; MCOphth 1990. Clin. Asst. Wolverhampton & Cos. Eye Infirm. Specialty: Ophth.

SMITH, Jane Louise Mansfield Medical Centre, 56 Binley Road, Coventry CV3 1JB Tel: 024 7645 7551 Fax: 024 7644 2250; 6 Montpellier Close, Styvechale, Coventry CV3 5PL — BM BS Nottm. 1986; DRCOG 1990; MRCGP 1991. Specialty: Gen. Pract. Prev: Trainee GP Walsgrave Hosp. Coventry VTS.

SMITH, Janet Elizabeth Wykeham, Score Lane, Blagdon, Bristol BS40 7RX — MB BS Lond. 1998; MB BS Lond 1998.

SMITH, Janet Linda The Surgery, Station Road, Bridge of Weir PA11 3LH Tel: 01505 612555 Fax: 01505 615032; Rosslyn, Bonar Crescent, Bridge of Weir PA11 3EH — MB ChB Aberd. 1981; DRCOG 1983. GP Bridge of Weir.

SMITH, Janet Marie Bristol Royal Hospital for Sick Children, St. Michaels Hill, Bristol BS2 8BJ Tel: 0117 929 4530; Lower Flat, 8 Cowper Road, Redland, Bristol BS6 6NY — MB ChB Bristol 1983; MRCPsych 1991. Locum Cons. Child Psychiat. Childr.s Hosp., Bristol (P/T). Specialty: Child & Adolesc. Psychiat. Prev: Sen. Regist. (Child Adolesc. Psychiat.) SW RHA.

SMITH, Janet Urquhart Abernethy 39 Colwyn Road, Bramhall, Stockport SK7 2JG — LRCP LRCS Ed. 1951; LRCP LRCS Ed. LRFPS Glas. 1951; DObst RCOG 1954.

SMITH, Jason Edward The Park Medical Group, Shopping Centre, Fawdon Park Road, Newcastle upon Tyne NE3 2PE Tel: 0191 285 1763 Fax: 0191 284 2374 — MB BS Newc. 1992 (Newcastle upon Tyne) MRCP Lond. 1998. GP Newc.

SMITH, Mr Jason John Charing Cross Hospital, Dept. of Vasculas Surgery, Fulham Palace Road, London W6 8RP Tel: 020 8846 7320 Fax: 020 8846 7330 Email: jj.smith@ic.ac.uk; Greenways, Nags Head Lane, Great Missenden HP16 0HD Email: jason@smithfrcs.freeserve.co.uk — MB BS Lond. 1992 (Roy. Free Hosp. Lond.) FRCS Eng. 1996. Specialist Regist. (Gen. Surg.). Specialty: Gen. Surg. Socs: Fell. Roy. Soc. Med.; Affil. Mem. Vasc. Surg. Soc. of GB & Irel.; Jun. Mem. Europ. Soc. Vasc. Surg. Prev: Research Fell. & Regist. (Vasc. Surg.) Char. Cross Hosp. Lond.

SMITH, Jayne Mary 9 Hayhouse Road, Earls Colne, Colchester CO6 2PD — MB ChB Leeds 1976.

SMITH, Jean Mendip Country Practice, Coleford, Bath BA3 5PG Tel: 01373 812244 — BM BS Nottm. 1975; DRCOG 1978; MRCGP 1979.

SMITH, Jean Hamilton Lang (retired) Hollybank, 2A Mill Road, Riggend, Airdrie ML6 7ST Tel: 01236 830640 Fax: 01236 830640 — MB ChB Glas. 1961; DObst RCOG 1963.

SMITH, Jeanne Amelia Cranberry, 23A Percy Road, Winchmore Hill, London N21 2JA Tel: 020 8360 6129 Email: doctorajeanne@connectfree.co.uk — MB BS (Hons. Obs & Gyn, Clin. Pharm & Therapeutics) Lond. 1968 (Middlx.) BSc (Hons. Biochem.) Lond. 1968; MRCP (UK) 1973; FRCP Glas. 1986. Locum Cons. Phys. & Endocrinol. Specialty: Gen. Med.; Diabetes; Endocrinol. Socs: Soc. Endocrinol.; Fell. Roy. Soc. Med. Prev: Cons. Phys. & Endocrinol. Saudi Arabia; Cons. Phys. Law Hosp. Carluke; Regist. (Med.) Glas. Roy. Infirm.

SMITH, Jeannette Alexandra (retired) 50 Endcliffe Hall Avenue, Sheffield S10 3EL Tel: 0114 266 1722 — MB ChB Liverp. 1959.

SMITH, Jenifer Ann Evelyn South West Cancer IntelligenceService, Highcroft, Romsey Road, Winchester SO22 5DH Tel: 01962 863511 Fax: 01962 878360; 8 Portersbridge Street, Romsey SO51 8DJ — MB BS Lond. 1980 (Charing Cross Hospital) MRCP (UK) 1985; MSc Lond. 1987; FFPHM 1997, M 1990. Dir. S. W. Region Cancer Intelligence Serv., Winchester. Specialty: Pub. Health Med.; Epidemiol. Prev: Cons. Pub. Health Med. Soton. & SW Hants. DHA; Sen. Regist. (Community Med.) Oxf. RHA; Regist. (Gen. Med. & Rheum.) Univ. Hosp. Wales Cardiff.

SMITH, Jennifer Catherine 16 Priory Farm Close, Liverpool L19 3RS Tel: 0151 494 9647 — MB ChB Leeds 1989; BSc (Hons. Path.) Leeds 1985; MRCP (Edin.) 1997. Specialist Regist. In Palliat. Med., Mersey Region. Specialty: Palliat. Med. Socs: RCP(Ed.); Assn. Palliat. Med.; Roy. Soc. Med. Prev: SHO (Palliat. Med.), Liverp., Marie Curie Centre; SHO (Neurol.) St. Jas. Hosp. Leeds; SHO (Oncol.) St James' Hosp. Leeds.

SMITH, Jennifer Jane Mary Directorate of Obstetrics & Gynaecology, Cygnet Wing, South Wing Hospital, Bedford MK42 9DJ Tel: 01234 355122; Standalone Farm, Sutton Road, Potton, Sandy SG19 2DT Tel: 01767 260248 Fax: 01767 262440 Email: dpsmith4@aol.com — MB ChB Birm. 1966; DRCOG 1979; MFFP 1993. Hosp. Pract. (O & G) Bedford Hosp. NHS Trust; Senior Clin. Med. Off. & Instruc. Doctor Family Plann. Luton PCT. Specialty: Family Plann. & Reproduc. Health; Obst. & Gyn. Special Interest: Colposcopy; Family Plann.; Ultrasound-Gynaecology and Early Pregn. Socs: Registered Colposcopist; BMA; Brit. Menopause Soc. Prev: Ho. Surg. (O & G) & Ho. Phys. (Med.) Bedford Gen. Hosp.

SMITH, Jennifer Marie (retired) 61 Melbreck Road, Allerton, Liverpool L18 9SF Tel: 0151 494 9656 & profess. 051 706 2000 — MB ChB Sheff. 1959; DObst RCOG 1964; DCH Eng. 1962, DA 1965; FFA RCS Eng. 1970. Cons. (Anaesth.) Mersey RHA & Liverp. AHA (T). Prev: Ho. Phys. Gen. Hosp. & Baragwanath Hosp. Johannesburg, S. Africa.

SMITH, Jenny 22 Horn Lane, Woodford Green IG8 9AA — MB ChB Manch. 1994.

SMITH, Jeremy David 13 Spunhill Avenue, Great Sutton, South Wirral CH66 2HT Tel: 0151 348 1149 — MB BS Calcutta 1967 (Nat. Med. Coll. Calcutta) Clin. Asst. (Psychogeriat.) St. Catherine's Hosp. Birkenhead. Specialty: Palliat. Med.

SMITH, Jeremy Edward 4 Barne Close, Nuneaton CV11 4TP — MB ChB Birm. 1998.

SMITH, Jeremy Vaughan 17 The Lea, Kidderminster DY11 6JY — MB ChB Leic. 1993.

SMITH, Jill Elaine The Park Medical Group, Fawdon Park Road, Newcastle upon Tyne NE3 2PE Tel: 0191 285 1763 Fax: 0191 284 2374 — MB BS Lond. 1989.

SMITH, Jillian Beverley Flat 18, Lexham House, Lexham Gardens, London W8 5JT — MB BCh Wales 1967 (Cardiff) FFA RCS Eng. 1972. Cons. Anaesth. St. Mary's Hosp. Lond. Specialty: Anaesth. Prev: Regist. (Anaesth.) Hosp. Sick Childr. Gt. Ormond St. Lond. & St.; Thos. Lond.; Rotating Sen. Regist. (Anaesth.) Hosp. Sick Childr. Gt. Ormond St. & The Lond. Hosp.

SMITH, Joanna Claudia Somerton House Surgery, 79A North Road, Midsomer Norton, Bath BA3 2QE Tel: 01761 412141 Fax: 01761 410944 — (Univ. Coll. Lond.) BSc Lond. 1986, MB BS 1989; MRCGP 1995.

SMITH, Joanna Kathreen Royal Edinburgh Hospital, Morningside Terrace, Edinburgh EH10 5HF Tel: 0131 537 6000; 72 Falcon Avenue, Edinburgh EH10 4AW Tel: 0131 447 6326 — MB ChB Aberd. 1996. SHO (Psychiat.) Edin. Lothian & Fife Rotat. Specialty: Gen. Psychiat. Socs: BMA.

SMITH, Joanne Deborah 25 Ashley Drive, Belfast BT9 7BE Tel: 01232 683153 — MB BCh BAO Belf. 1994. Specialty: Gen. Pract.

SMITH, Joanne Louise 25 Glengarry Gardens, Wolverhampton WV3 9HX — MB ChB Bristol 1998.

SMITH, Joanne Marie 19 Chynance, Portreath, Redruth TR16 4NJ — MB ChB Manch. 1991.

SMITH, John The Surgery, Upper Carloway, Isle of Lewis HS2 9AG Tel: 01851 73333; 9 Holm Village, Stornoway HS1 OAE — MB ChB Aberd. 1968; FRCGP 1994, M 1975. Specialty: Pub. Health Med.

SMITH, John, OBE, TD (retired) 5/10 Oswald Road, Edinburgh EH9 2HE Tel: 0131 667 5617 — (Camb. & Glas.) FFPHM 1989 (FFCM 1972); MB BChir Camb. 1938; MB ChB Glas. 1938; MA Camb. 1943; FRCP Glas. 1967, M 1965; FRCP Ed. 1969. Prev: Dep. Chief Med. Off. Scott. Home & Health Dept.

SMITH, John St. Mary's Hospital, I.O.W. Healthcare Trust, Newport PO30 5TG Tel: 01983 524081 Ext: 4808/4859 Fax: 01983 825437; Ashlake House, Ashlake Copse Road, Fishbourne, Ryde PO33 4EY Tel: 01983 882497 — BM BCh Oxf. 1965 (Leeds & Oxf.) BSc (Hons. Anat.) Leeds 1962; DCP Lond 1972; FRCPath 1988, M 1976. Cons. Chem. Path. & Metab. Med. St. Mary's Hosp. Newport I. of Wight; Hon. Clin. Teach. Univ. Soton. Med. Sch. Specialty: Chem. Path. Socs: Assn. Clin. Biochems.; BMA; Nat. Osteoporosis Soc. Prev: Cons. Chem. Path. Inst. Path. & Trop. Med. RAF Halton Aylesbury; Cons. Clin. Path. RAF Hosp. Wegberg W. Germany; Wing Cdr. RAF Med. Br.

SMITH, Mr John Allan Raymond Northern General NHS Trust, Herries Road, Sheffield S5 7AU Tel: 0114 243 4343 Fax: 0114 256 0472; 4 Endcliffe Grove Avenue, Sheffield S10 3EJ Tel: 0114 268 3094 Fax: 0114 267 0295 — MB ChB Ed. 1966; FCRS ED 1972; FRCS Eng. 1972; PhD Aberd. 1979. Cons. Surg. N. Gen. Hosp. Sheff.; Chairm. Jt. Comm. Higher Surgic. Train. Specialty: Gastroenterol. Socs: Brit. Soc. Gastroenterol. & Assn. Surgs. Prev: Sen. Lect. (Surg.) Univ. Sheff. & Hon. Cons. Surg. Roy. Hallamsh. Hosp. Sheff.; Sen. Regist. (Surg.) S. Grampian (Aberd.) Health Dist.; Ho. Phys. & Ho. Surg. Roy. Infirm. Edin.

SMITH, John Anthony (retired) The Old Rectory, Great Massingham, King's Lynn PE32 2EY Tel: 01485 520806 Fax: 01485

520806 Email: john.smith35@which.net — MB BS Durh. 1956 (Newc.) DTM & H Liverp. 1960. Med. Examr. Benefts Agy. Prev: Hon. Surg. Newc. Gen. Hosp.

SMITH, John Anthony James 81 Thurlow Park Road, London SE21 8JL Tel: 020 8670 6610 — MB BChir Camb. 1952 (Camb. & Guy's) MRCS Eng. LRCP Lond. 1951.

SMITH, John Dawson Lochmaben Medical Group, The Surgery, 42-44 High Street, Lockerbie DG11 1NH Tel: 01387 810252 Fax: 01387 811595 — MB ChB Aberd. 1977; MRCGP 1981; DRCOG 1981. GP Stonehaven. Prev: Trainee GP Dumfries & Galloway Roy. Infirm. VTS.

SMITH, John Eric 9 Dunedin Drive, Barnt Green, Birmingham B45 8HZ Tel: 0121 445 1431 — MB ChB Liverp. 1969; FFA RCS Eng. 1979. Cons. Anaesth. Univ. Hosp. Birm. Specialty: Anaesth.

SMITH, John Francis Boucher Little Broich, Kippen, Stirling FK8 3DT — MB ChB St. And. 1962; MRCP Lond. 1967; FRCP Glas. 1986. Working in Independent Practice; Sen. Med. Officer, Prudential Insurance Company. Specialty: Gen. Med. Prev: Cons. Phys. Stirling Roy. Infirm.

SMITH, John Francis Ferguson, VRD 42 Kelvin Court, Glasgow G12 0AE — MB ChB Glas. 1944 (Univ. Glas.) Cons. Dermatol. Vict. Infirm. Glas., & Dumfries & Galloway Hosps. & Corp. of Glas. & Co. of Renfrew Sch. Health Servs.; Hon. Phys. to HM the Qu.; Surg. Capt. RNR. Specialty: Gen. Med. Prev: Sen. Regist. Dept. Dermat. & Ho. Surg. West. Infirm. Glas.; Asst. Regist. Dept. Dermat. Univ. Coll. Hosp. Lond.

SMITH, John Glyn (retired) 48 Lime Tree Avenue, Retford DN22 7BA Tel: 01777 703837 — MB ChB Sheff. 1966; DObst RCOG 1968; DCH Eng. 1969; MRCGP 1978. Prev: SHO (Paediat. Med.) Childr. Hosp. Sheff.

SMITH, Professor John Graham Department of Haematology, Royal United Hospital, Combe Park, Bath BA1 3NG Tel: 01225 824731 Fax: 01225 461044; Crinan, Miller Walk, Bathampton, Bath BA2 6TJ Tel: 01225 460358 Fax: 01225 461044 — MB ChB Glas. 1977; MRCP (Glas.) 1980; FRCPath 1996, M 1984; BSc (Hons.) Immunol. Glas. 1975, MD 1985; FRCP Lond. 1994. Cons. Haematologist Roy. United Hosp. Bath; Prof. Haemat. Univ. W. Eng. Bristol 1997; Designated AIDS Phys. Bath; Med. Dir. Roy. United Hosp. Specialty: Haematology. Socs: Fell. Internat. Soc. Haematol.; Brit. Soc. Haematol. & Assn. Clin. Path.; (Chairm.) BCSH Clin. Haematol. Task Force. Prev: Sen. Regist. (Haemat.) W. Infirm. Glas.; Clin. Dir. (Path.) Roy. Univ. Hosp.; Clin. Dir. (Med.) Roy. United Hosp.

SMITH, John Harry 96 Harley Street, London W1G 7HY Tel: 020 7935 9904 Fax: 020 7486 5770 — MB BChir Camb. 1978 (St. Thos. & Camb.) MD Camb. 1990, MA 1978; MRCOG 1983. Cons. O & G St. Mary's Hosp. Lond. Specialty: Obst. & Gyn. Prev: Sen. Regist. St. Mary's Hosp. Lond.; Research Fell. John Radcliffe Hosp. Oxf.; Regist. (O & G) Pembury Hosp. & SE Thames.

SMITH, John Henry Wilfred (retired) c/o Coutts & Co., Adelaide Branch, 440 The Strand, London WC2R 0QS — MB ChB Leeds 1947; DA Eng. 1949; FFA RCS Eng. 1954. Prev: Cons. Anaesth. Leic. Roy. Infirm. & Rutland Memor. Hosp.

SMITH, John Herbert Frederick Department of Histopathology, Royal Hallamshire Hospital, Sheffield S10 2JF Tel: 0114 2713728 Fax: 0114 2712200 — MB BS (Hons.) Lond. 1977 (Middlx.) BSc (Hons.) Lond. 1974; FRCPath 1996, M 1985. Cons. Histopath.Roy. Hallamshire Hosp; Dir. Sheff. Cytol. Train centre. Specialty: Histopath. Socs: Brit. Div. Internat. Acad. Path. & Assn. Clin. Path.; Brit. Soc. Clin. Cytol.(Hon. Asst. secetary 1992-95); Internat. Acad. of Cytol. Prev: Sen. Regist. (Histopath.) Southmead & Frenchay Hosps. Bristol & Bristol Roy. Infirm.; Lect. (Toxicol.) St. Bart. Hosp. & DHSS Toxicol. Unit.

SMITH, John Joseph 6 West Lawn, Ashbrooke, Sunderland SR2 7HW — MB BCh BAO Belf. 1941. Prev: Res. Surg. Off. Birm. Accid. Hosp. & Doncaster Roy. Infirm.

SMITH, John Joseph 1-3 Church Street, Ballymena BT43 6DD Tel: 01266 630588 Fax: 01266 630696 Email: eyespec@hotmail.com — MB BCh BAO Belf. 1990; BSc Biochem. (Hons.) Belf. 1987, MB BCh BAO 1990; MRCOphth 1994; FRCS (Ophth) 1996. Staff Grade Ophth. Dept. of Ophth. Roy. Vict. Hosp. Belf.; Lect. (Ophth.) Univ. of Ulster Coleraine N. Irel.; Dir. of Waveney Eye Care Ltd. Specialty: Ophth. Socs: Irish Coll. Ophth.; Brit. Contact Lens Assn.

SMITH, John Lister (retired) Ravelston Cottage, 16 Ravelston Dykes Road, Edinburgh EH4 3PB Tel: 0131 332 9541 — MB ChB Ed. 1954. Prev: Ho. Surg. Princess Margt. Rose Hosp. Edin.

SMITH, Mr John Robert (retired) The Anchorage, Alves, Elgin IV30 8UY Tel: 01343 850274 — (Glas.) MB ChB Glas. 1945; FRCS Ed. 1952. Prev: Cons. Surg. Dr. Gray's Hosp. Elgin.

SMITH, John Simon Kettering & District General Hospital, Rothwell Road, Kettering NN16 8UZ Tel: 01536 492000 Fax: 01536 492567 Email: john.smith@dsnpct.nhs.uk; 34 Poplars Farm Road, Barton Seagrave, Kettering NN15 5AG Tel: 01536 513786 — MB BS Lond. 1970; DObst RCOG 1972; FRCGP 1991, M 1977. Cons. Palliat. Med. Daventry & S. Northants NHS Trust, Cransley Hospice, Kettering & Dist. Gen. Hosp. & Cynthia Spencer Hospice Northampton. Specialty: Palliat. Med. Prev: Ho. Surg. Middlx. Hosp. Lond.

SMITH, John Taylor (retired) 252 Elwick Road, Hartlepool TS26 0EL Tel: 01429 274570 — (Glas.) MB ChB Glas. 1947. Prev: Clin. Asst. Dept. Psychiat. Gen. Hosp. Hartlepool.

SMITH, John Warner (retired) Crow End, Graveley, Hitchin SG4 7LX Tel: 01438 353248 — BM BCh Oxf. 1940 (Middlx.) BA 1937, BM BCh Oxf. 1940. Prev: Med. Regist. Metrop. Hosp.

SMITH, John Weston The Secret House, 101 Main Road, Wiggington, Tamworth B79 9DU Tel: 01827 69283 — MB ChB Birm. 1944; DObst. RCOG 1946; DA Eng. 1954; MRCGP 1968. Anaesth. & Med. Off. Tamworth Hosps.; Clin. Asst. Psychother. Uffculme Clinic Birm. Socs: Fac. Anaesths. Prev: Gyn. Regist. Dudley Rd. Hosp. Birm; Regist. Roy. Hosp. Wolverhampton; Obst. Ho. Surg. Birm. United Hosps.

SMITH, Jonathan Harvey — MB BS Lond. 1993 (Univ. Coll. Lond.) BSc Lond. 1990; FRCA 1999. Cons. Anaesth. Specialty: Anaesth.

SMITH, Jonathan Hayden Freeman Hospital, Department of Cardiothoracic Anaesthesia, High Heaton, Newcastle upon Tyne NE7 7DN Tel: 0191 284 3111 Fax: 0191 223 1175; Chapel Cottage, Halton Shields, Corbridge NE45 5PZ — MB ChB Leeds 1982; MRCP (UK) 1986; FRCA 1989. Cons. Paediat. (Cardiothoracic Anaesth. & Intens. Care) Freeman Hosp. Newc. u. Tyne. Prev: Instruc. (Paediat. Anaesth.) CS Mott Childr. Hosp. Ann Arbor Michigan, USA; Regist. (Anaesth.) Our Lady's Hosp. for Sick Childr. Dub.; Anaesthesiol. Project Orbis.

SMITH, Jonathan Kenneth Laing Glenridding Health Centre, Glenridding, Penrith CA11 0PD Tel: 017684 82297; Stanley House, 89 Preston Old Road, Freckleton, Preston PR4 1HD — MB ChB Ed. 1979; MRCGP 1983; DRCOG 1983. GP Penrith. Prev: GP Lytham; South Lothian Vocational VTS.

SMITH, Jonathan Mark 31 Forest Hills Drive, Talbot Green, Pontyclun CF72 8JB — MB BCh Wales 1986; MRCPsych 1992. Cons., Old Age Psychiat., E. Glam. Hosp. Prev: Regist. (Psychiat.) S. Glam. HA.

SMITH, Jonathan Neil 30 Downs Side, Sutton SM2 7EQ — BM Soton. 1992; DRCOG 1996; DCH 1997; MRCP 1999. Specialist Regist. (A&E) Qu.'s Med. Centre, Nottm. Specialty: Accid. & Emerg.

SMITH, Jonathan Paul 5 Meadow Court, Ponteland, Newcastle upon Tyne NE20 9RA — BChir Camb. 1992.

SMITH, Jonathan Timothy 69 Leicester Road, Fleckney, Leicester LE8 8BG — MB ChB Manch. 1995.

SMITH, Mr Joseph Colin, OBE (retired) Church Lane House, Yarnton, Oxford OX5 1PY Tel: 01865 460005 Fax: 01865 460062 Email: jo-smith@ntlworld.com — (Univ. Coll. Hosp.) MB BS Lond. 1954; MRCS Eng. LRCP Lond. 1954; FRCS Eng. 1958; MS Lond. 1966. Prev: Cons. Urol. Surg. Oxf.

SMITH, Joseph Donald Robert (retired) 106 Kenton Lane, Newcastle upon Tyne NE3 3QD — MB BS Durh. 1948.

SMITH, Sir Joseph William Grenville (retired) 95 Lofting Road, London N1 1JF — MB BCh Wales 1953 (Cardiff) Dip. Bact. Lond 1960; FRCPath 1975, M 1963; MD Wales 1966; FFPHM 1976, M 1972; FRCP Lond. 1987; Hon. Dip. HIC 1996. Chairm. WHO Global Poliomyelitis Commiss. Prev: Dir. Pub. Health Laborat. Serv.

SMITH, Julia Rosemary Gladstone Imaging Department, Queen Elizabeth Hospital, Stadium Rd, Woolwich, London SE18 4QH Tel: 020 8836 6000 Fax: 020 8228 6109 — MB BS Lond. 1977; MRCP (UK) 1981; FRCR 1984. Cons. Radiol. Qu. Eliz. Hosp., Woolwich. Specialty: Radiol. Prev: Greenwich Dist. Hosp.; Cons. Radiol. Brook Gen. Hosp. Lond.

SMITH, Julian Abel 4 Aston Road, Chipping Campden GL55 6HR — MB BS Lond. 1996.

SMITH, Julian Harold Joshua Grove House, Skerton Road, Manchester M16 0RB Tel: 0161 952 8363 Fax: 0161 952 8300 Email: julian.smith@hse.gsi.gov.uk — MB ChB Dundee 1984; MFOM Lond. 2000; MBA Open Univ. 2002. Med. Inspector Health & Safety Exec. Specialty: Occupat. Health. Special Interest: Diving Med. Socs: SOM. Prev: Med. Adviser, Post Office Occupational Health Serv., Manch.; Cons. Occupational Health Phys., Medigold Ltd, Manch.

SMITH, Julie Carol 5 Imperial Avenue, Beeston, Nottingham NG9 1EZ — BM BCh Oxf. 1993; MA Camb. 1990; MRCP (UK) 1996. Specialist Regist. (Paediat.) Univ. Hosp. Nottm. Specialty: Paediat.

SMITH, Julie Elizabeth The Bull Ring Surgery, 5 The Bull Ring, St. John's, Worcester WR2 5AA Tel: 01905 422883 Fax: 01905 423639; The Mount, Red Hill Lane, Worcester WR5 2JL — MB ChB Birm. 1978; DRCOG 1980.

SMITH, Juliet Ann 51 Kennedy Road, Kingsland, Shrewsbury SY3 7AA — MB BS Lond. 1991.

SMITH, June Mary (retired) Ava Cottage, 46 The Butts, Chippenham SN15 3JS Tel: 01249 652675 — MB ChB Bristol 1949; MB ChB (Hnrs.) Bristol 1949; MRCS Eng. LRCP Lond. 1949; DObst. RCOG 1951; DCH Eng. 1953.

SMITH, Justin Deval 50 Langdale Grove, Bingham, Nottingham NG13 8SS Tel: 01949 875899 — MB BCh Wales 1993; DCH 12/97 RCP.; DCH RCP Lond. 1997. SHO (O & G) (GP Regist). Specialty: Gen. Pract. Prev: SHO (Psychiat.); SHO (Acc. & Emerg.); SHO (Med.).

SMITH, Justin Michael Alaric Royal Eye Unit, Kingston General Hospital, Galsworthy Road, Kingston upon Thames KT2 7QB; 20 Glebeland Gardens, Shepperton TW17 9DH — MB ChB Bristol 1988; MRCP (UK) 1992; FRCOphth 1995. Med. Retina Clin. Research Fell. (Ophth.) Moorfields Eye Hosp. Specialty: Ophth. Prev: Specialist Regist. Rotat. (Ophth.) SW Thames; SHO (Ophth.) Chelsea & Westm. Hosp. Lond., Frimley Pk. Hosp. & Cheltenham Gen. Hosp.; SHO Rotat. (Gen. Med.) Bristol & Weston HA.

SMITH, Justine Lydia 101 Hailgate, Howden, Goole DN14 7SX Tel: 01430 431449 — MB ChB Manch. 1994; BA (Hons.) Oxf. 1990. SHO Med. Rotat. - Hull Roy. Infirm.

SMITH, Karen 56 Grampian Way, Bearsden, Glasgow G61 4RW — MB ChB Glas. 1993.

SMITH, Karen Patricia Brunswick House Medical Group, 1 Brunswick St., Carlisle CA1 1ED Tel: 01228 515808; Fellend, Heads Nook, Carlisle CA8 9DA — MB BS Newc. 1986; MRCGP 1990; DRCOG 1990.

SMITH, Katharine Alison Fulbrook Centre, Warneford Hospital, Churchill Hospital, Oxford OX3 7JU — BM BCh Oxf. 1990; DM Oxford 2000. Specialist Regist. in Psychiat. of oold age, fulbrook centre, Churchill Hosp., Oxf.. Specialty: Geriat. Psychiat.; Gen. Psychiat. Prev: Clin. Lect., Univ. Dept of Psychiat. Oxf. welcome Train. Fell., Iniv. Dept of Psychiatr. Oxf..

SMITH, Katherine — BM BCh Oxf. 1994; DRCOG. 1996; MRCGP. 1998. GP Retainer W. Kirby. Specialty: Gen. Pract. Socs: BMA.

SMITH, Kathleen 11 Castle Court, Elveston, Derby DE72 3GZ — BM BS Nottm. 1992. SHO (Med.) Derbysh. Roy. Infirm. Specialty: Gen. Med.

SMITH, Kathleen Lilley 19 Wheatley Lane, Winshill, Burton-on-Trent DE15 0DX Tel: 01283 42745 — (Univ. Coll. Hosp.) MB BS Lond. 1945.

SMITH, Kathleen Mary (retired) The Ragged School, 51 Roxburgh St., Kelso TD5 7DS Tel: 01573 226009 Fax: 01573 225134 — MB ChB Ed. 1952.

SMITH, Kathryn Jane 17 Newton Road, Torquay TQ2 5DB — MB ChB Bristol 1984.

SMITH, Kathryn Shauna Minsmere House, Heath Road, Ipswich IP4 5PD Tel: 01473 704203 — BM Soton. 1988; DA (UK) 1992. Staff Grade (Psychiat. of Old Age) E. Suff. Local Health Servs. Trust, Ipswich. Specialty: Geriat. Psychiat. Prev: Clin. Med. Off. in Psychiat. of Old Age E. Suff. Local Health Servs. Trust Ipswich; SHO (Psychiat.) St. Clements Hosp. Ipswich; Trainee GP Ipswich.

SMITH, Katrina 24 Windmill Way, Kegworth, Derby DE74 2FA — MB ChB Ed. 1996.

SMITH, Katrina Louise 14 Chaddesley Road, Kidderminster DY10 3AD — BM BCh Oxf. 1996.

SMITH, Kay 1 Castle Street, Stogursey, Taunton TA1 3DY — MB BS Lond. 1970 (Lond. Hosp.) MRCS Eng. LRCP Lond. 1970; DObst RCOG 1973; Dip. Clin. Bact. Lond 1983. Staff Grade (c/o Elderly) Taunton & Som. NHS Trust; Clin. Asst. St. Margt. Hospice Som. Specialty: Care of the Elderly.

SMITH, Kay Louise Northern Centre for Cancer Treatment, Newcastle general Hospital, Westgate Road, Newcastle upon Tyne NE4 6BE Tel: 0191 285 2025; 123A Craig Walk, Bo'ness LA23 3AX Tel: 01539 446813 Email: 113200.3552@compuserve.com — MB ChB Manch. 1991. Specialist Regist. (Clin. Oncol.) Northern Centre for Cancer Treatm.; Attachment at S. Cleveland. Specialty: Oncol. Prev: SHO (Med.) King Edwd. VII Hosp. Midhurst & Shotley Bridge Gen. Hosp.; SHO (A & E) Wythenshawe & Withington Hosps. Manch.; Ho. Off. (Med.) Qu. Eliz. Hosp. Gateshead.

SMITH, Keay Gordon — MB BCh Witwatersrand 1965 (Witwatersrand) DIH Lond. 1982; MFOM RCP Lond. 1987. Princip. Occupat. Health Off. Lond. Boro. Ealing; Cons. Occupat. Phys. Wycombe Gen. Hosp. High Wycombe Bucks. Specialty: Occupat. Health. Socs: Soc. Occupat. Med.; Assn. Local Auth. Med. Advisers.; BMA. Prev: Occupat. Phys. Hants. Fire & Rescue Serv.; Med. Adviser Hants. CC; Sen. Med. Off. Brit. Airways Health Servs. Heathrow.

SMITH, Mr Kenneth Halstead — MB ChB Manch. 1943; MRCS Eng. LRCP Lond. 1943; FRCS Eng. 1952. Specialty: Gen. Surg. Prev: Emerit. Cons. Surg. Gwynedd HA.; Cons. Accid. Surg. Gen. Hosp. Northampton; Res. Surg. Off. Ancoats Hosp. Manch.

SMITH, Kerry Marie Handsworth Wood Medical Centre, 110 Church Lane, Handsworth Wood, Birmingham B20 2ES; 42 Sandyacre Way, Stourbridge DY8 1JD — MB ChB Birm. 1988.

SMITH, Kevin John 4 Rufford Close, Birmingham B23 5YZ — MB BS Lond. 1994.

SMITH, Mr Kevin Robert Hodson Well Work Ltd, Westbrook House, Allendale Road NE46 2DE Tel: 01920 461243 Fax: 01920 462997 — MB ChB Birm. 1988; BSc (Hons.) Anat. Birm. 1985; FRCS Eng. 1993; DTM & H Liverp. 1995. Specialty: Gen. Surg.; Occupat. Health. Socs: Fell. Roy. Soc. Trop. Med. & Hyg.; Med. Protec. Soc.; MDDUS. Prev: SHO (O & G) Walsall Manor Hosp.; SHO Rotat. (Surg.) Dudley Rd. Hosp. Birm.

SMITH, Kirsten Teresa Elizabeth 1 Appleton Court, Thornton, Bradford BD13 3TD — BM Soton. 1998.

SMITH, Laura Jane Anderson 10 Hindon Square, Vicarage Road, Edgbaston, Birmingham B15 3HA — MB ChB Leeds 1991. Specialty: Gen. Pract.

SMITH, Lesley-Ann 71 Harriet Street, Cardiff CF24 4BW — MB BCh Wales 1998.

SMITH, Lesley Anne Abbey Medical Centre, Lonend, Paisley PA1 1SU Tel: 0141 889 4088; 1 Victoria Gardens, Kilmacolm PA13 4HL Tel: 01505 874884 — MB ChB Glas. 1985 (Univ. Glas.) DRCOG 1988. Gen. Asst., Merchiston Hosp., Brookfield by Johnstone.

SMITH, Leslie David Rosslyn Cardiac Department, Royal Devon & Exeter Hospital, Wonford, Exeter EX2 5DW Tel: 01392 402276 Fax: 01392 402276; 26 Salutary Mount, Exeter EX1 2QE — MB BS Lond. 1977; BSc Lond. 1974, MB BS 1977; MRCP (UK) 1980; FRCP 1996. Cons. Cardiol. Roy. Devon & Exeter Hosp. Specialty: Cardiol. Socs: Sec. of the Brit. CardoVasc. Interven. Soc. Prev: Sen. Regist. (Cardiol.) St. Thos. Hosp. Lond.; Regist. (Cardiol.) Brompton Hosp. Lond.

SMITH, Leslie Ernest (retired) 4 Conifer Close, Botley, Oxford OX2 9HP Tel: 01865 724316 — MRCS Eng. LRCP Lond. 1939. Prev: Asst. Med. Off. Lambeth Hosp.

SMITH, Leslie Ronald Nimmo North Avenue Surgery, 18 North Avenue, Cambuslang, Glasgow G72 8AT Tel: 0141 641 3037 Fax: 0141 646 1905; 82 Stewarton Drive, Glasgow G72 8DJ — MB ChB Glas. 1977; DRCOG 1979; MRCGP 1981.

SMITH, Leslie Stuart Premier Occupational Healthcare, Shearway Business Park, Shearway Road, Folkestone CT19 4RH Tel: 0870 444 1399 Fax: 0870 444 2908 Email: doclsmith@premierohc.co.uk; Milestone Lodge, Canterbury Road, Elham, Canterbury CT4 6UE Tel: 01303 840149 Email: doclsmith@aol.com — MB ChB Manch. 1975; Cert AU Med; MIOSH; MFOM; MRCGP 1982. Med. Director Premier Occupational Healthcare; Med. Adviser to Eon UK. Specialty: Occupat. Health. Special Interest: Populat. Health Managem.; Wellbeing Managem. Socs: Soceity Occupational Med.; Roy. Soceity Med.; Assn. Aviat. Med. Examiners. Prev: Med. Director

Business Heath; Regional Med. Adviser Brit. Rail; Chief Med. Off. Scottishpower Gp. PLC.

SMITH, Linda — MB ChB Dundee 1998.

SMITH, Mrs Lindsay 18 Telford Street, Gateshead NE8 4TT — MB BS Durh. 1951; DObst RCOG 1953.

SMITH, Lindsay Frederick Paul Westlake Surgery, High Street, West Coker, Yeovil BA22 9AH Tel: 01935 840207 Fax: 01935 840002 — MB ChB Bristol 1982; MRCP (UK) 1985; FRCGP 1996, M 1987; Cert. Family Plann. JCC 1987; DRCOG 1988; BSc Bristol 1979, MD 1996. Hon. Cons. Sen. Lect. Qu. Mary & Westfield Coll. Univ. Lond. Specialty: Gen. Pract. Socs: Chairm. Clin. Network RCGP; Edit. Bd. Brit. Jl. Gen. Pract.; Assn. for Community Based Matern. Care. Prev: RCGP Train. Fell.

SMITH, Lindsey Fiona Fraser Moorfields Eye Hospital, 162 City Rd, London EC1V 2PD Tel: 020 7251 4835 — MB ChB Sheff. 1987 (Univ. Sheff. Med. Sch.) BMedSci (Hons.) Sheff. 1985; FRCOphth 1993. Specialist Regist. Ophth. Moorfields eye Hosp. Specialty: Ophth. Prev: Regist. (Ophth.) Univ. Hosp. Nottm.; Demonst. (Anat.) Univ. Coll. Lond.; SHO (A & E) Univ. Coll. Hosp. Lond.

SMITH, Lorna Katherine Ritchie Smith and Partners, South Park Surgery, 250 Park Lane, Macclesfield SK11 8AD Tel: 01625 422249 Fax: 01625 502169; 114 Prestbury Road, Macclesfield SK10 3BN — MB ChB Liverp. 1975; DRCOG 1977; MRCGP 1980.

SMITH, Malcolm Dunlop 155 West Princess Street, Helensburgh G84 8EZ — MB ChB Glas. 1991; DA (UK) 1995; FRCA 1996. Specialist Regist. (Anaesth.) West. Infirm. Glas. Specialty: Anaesth. Socs: BMA; Glas. & W. Scot. Soc. Anaesth.

SMITH, Malcolm Gavin 18 Beechgrove Place, Aberdeen AB15 5HF — MB ChB Aberd. 1997.

SMITH, Malcolm John Whickham Health Centre, Rectory Lane, Whickham, Newcastle upon Tyne NE16 4PD Tel: 0191 488 5555 Fax: 0191 496 0424 — MB BS Newc. 1976; DRCOG 1978; MRCGP 1980.

SMITH, Malcolm Joseph The Gainsborough Practice, Warfield Green Medical Centre, Whitegrove, Bracknell RG42 3JP Tel: 01344 428742 Fax: 01344 428743 — MB BChir Camb. 1977; MA Camb. 1977; DRCOG 1979; MRCGP 1981; DFFP 1993; Dip. Sports Med. RCS Ed. 1994. Clin. Asst. (Sports Med.) Heatherwood & Wexham Pk. Hosps. Trust. Socs: Brit. Assn. Sport & Exercise Med.; UKADIS.

SMITH, Marcus Cooke 8 Greystoke Drive, Bolton BL1 7DW — MB ChB Liverp. 1988. SHO (Anaesth.) S. Manch. HA.

SMITH, Margaret 7 Elm Walk, Bearsden, Glasgow G61 3BQ Tel: 0141 942 3134 — MB ChB Glas. 1976; MRCPsych 1981. Cons. Geriat. Psychiat. Dykebar & Roy. Alexandra Hosps. Paisley. Specialty: Geriat. Psychiat. Prev: Cons. Geriat. Psychiat. Stobhill & Woodilee Hosps. Glas.

SMITH, Margaret Albertha Elder 25 Turnberry Road, Glasgow G11 5AH Tel: 0141 339 7400 — MB ChB Glas. 1946; FRCPsych 1979, M 1973. Indep. Cons. Forens. Psychiat. Glas. Specialty: Forens. Psychiat. Prev: Cons. Psychiat. Douglas Inch Centre for Forens. Psychiat. Glas.; Hon. Clin. Lect. (Postgrad. Med. Educat.) Glas. Univ.; Regist. (Psychol. Med.) E. Dist. Hosp. Glas.

SMITH, Margaret Anne Norton Brook Medical Centre, Cookworthy Road, Kingsbridge TQ7 1AE Tel: 01548 853551 Fax: 01548 857741 — MB ChB Glas. 1986; DCH RCPS Glas. 1988; DRCOG 1990; MRCGP 1994. Prev: Trainee GP Salcombe.

SMITH, Margaret Baillie 38 Ralston Road, Bearsden, Glasgow G61 3BA Tel: 0141 942 0670 — (Glas.) MB ChB Glas. 1953; DObst RCOG 1955. Socs: Fac. Comm. Health. Prev: Clin. Asst. Canniesburn Hosp. Glas.; SCMO Community Health Glas.

SMITH, Margaret Campbell (retired) 2 Easter Ferrygate Park, Abbotsford Road, North Berwick EH39 5DB — MB ChB Ed. 1948; DObst RCOG 1953. Prev: Ho. Phys. Stracathro Hosp. Brechin.

SMITH, Margaret Catherine Govan Health Centre, 5 Drumoyne Road, Glasgow G51 4BJ Tel: 0141 531 8400 Fax: 0141 531 8404 — MB ChB Glas. 1974; MRCGP 1978. GP Glas..

SMITH, Margaret Fisher 2/4 Littlefield Lane, Grimsby DN31 2LG Tel: 01472 342250 Fax: 01472 251742; Lichfields, 63A Bargate, Grimsby DN34 5AA Tel: 01472 70794 — MB ChB Manch. 1959. Prev: SHMO (Cas.) Grimsby Gen. Hosp.; Ho. Phys. Lincoln Co. Hosp.; Ho. Surg. Salisbury Gen. Infirm.

SMITH, Margaret Isabella Abernethy (retired) Summerfield, Bronygarth, Weston Rhyn, Oswestry SY10 7LY — LRCP LRCS Ed. 1950 (Roy. Colls. Ed.) LRCP LRCS Ed. LRFPS Glas. 1950; DObst RCOG 1953. Prev: Clin. Med. Off. Shrops. HA.

SMITH, Margaret Lothian (retired) 2 Willow Road, Grange Est., Kilmarnock KA1 2HL Tel: 01563 525251 — MB ChB St. And. 1944; DObst 1949; MRCOG 1958. Prev: Assoc. Specialist (O & G) Ayrsh. & Arran HB.

SMITH, Margaret Mary (retired) Park Lodge, Ripley, Harrogate HG3 3DN — MB BS Lond. 1957 (Roy. Free)

SMITH, Margaret Nancy (retired) 6 Westbrook Park, Weston, Bath BA1 4DP Tel: 01225 424795 — (Leeds) MB ChB Leeds 1942, DPH (Distinc.) 1947. Prev: Ho. Surg. Leeds Matern. Hosp.

SMITH, Margaret Rebecca 22 Cull's Road, Normandy, Guildford GU3 2EP — MB BS Lond. 1980; FFA RCS Eng. 1987. Specialty: Anaesth.

SMITH, Margaret Ruth The Surgery, 1 Church St., Newtownards BT23 Tel: 028 9181 6333 — MB BS Lond. 1991 (Roy. Lond. Hosp.) MRCGP Lond. 1997 RCGP; DGM RCPS Glas. 1994; DCH Dub. 1995; DRCOG 1995; DFFP 1997. GP Retainee. Specialty: Gen. Pract. Prev: GP Regist. Bangor Co. Down; Trainee GP Ulster, N. Downs & Ards Hosp. Trust Belf.; SHO (Med., A & E & O & G & Paediat.) Ulster Hosp. Belf.

SMITH, Margaret Whyte Little Broich, Kippen, Stirling FK8 3DT — MB ChB St. And. 1963; DPM Ed. 1967; MRCPsych 1985.

SMITH, Marguerita Reid Portosy Medical Practice, 16 Seafield Terrace, Portsoy, Banff AB45 2GB — MB ChB Glas. 1993; DRCOG; DFFP. GP.

SMITH, Marguerite Elizabeth (retired) 36 Eton Court, Eton Avenue, London NW3 3HJ Tel: 020 7722 6316 — (St. Bart.) MB BS Lond. 1956; DCH Eng. 1961; FRCP Lond. 1991, M 1964; FRCPCH 1997. Prev: Sen. Med. Off. DoH Lond.

SMITH, Marie Clare Lee Cottage, Slade Lane, Mubberley, Knutsford WA16 7QP — BM BCh Oxf. 1989.

SMITH, Marie Linda Department of Nuclear Medicine, Royal Liverpool & Broadgreen University Hospital Trust, Prescot St., Liverpool L7 8XP — MB ChB Glas. 1978; BSc (Hons.) Glas. 1975; MRCP (UK) 1980; FRCP Glas. 1992; FRCP Lond. 1996. Specialty: Nuclear Med.

SMITH, Marilyn Jane c/o 24 Victoria Road, Hartlepool TS26 8DD Tel: 01429 234324 — MB BS Lond. 1963 (Roy. Free) MRCS Eng. LRCP Lond. 1963; MRCPsych 1981; FRCPsych 1996; MD 1998. Specialty: Gen. Psychiat. Prev: Cons. Psychiat. N. Tees Gen. Hosp. Stockton-on-Tees.

SMITH, Marion Jane — MB BS Lond. 1992 (Kings College London) DCH 1997; DFFP 1999. Specialty: Gen. Pract. Prev: SHO Obstetics & Gyn. Whiltington Horp 1998; SHO Neonates Qu. Charlottes Hosp. 1997; SHO Paediatics, Greenwich Hosp. 1996.

SMITH, Mark Anthony 32 Larden Road, Acton, London W3 7SU — MB BS Lond. 1988; DA (UK) 1990; FRCA 1994. Cons. Hillingdon Hosp. Specialty: Anaesth.; Intens. Care. Prev: SHO (Anaesth.) Hillingdon Hosp., Univ. Coll. Hosp. & Middlx. Hosp. Lond.

SMITH, Mark Antony Lane End Surgery, 2 Manor Walk, Benton, Newcastle upon Tyne NE7 7XX Tel: 0191 266 5246 Fax: 0191 266 6241 — MB ChB Leeds 1986. GP Newc.

SMITH, Mark Boraston Abbeystone Barn, Moss Lane, Thurnham, Lancaster LA2 0AY — MB BS Lond. 1980; FFA RCS Eng. 1985. Cons. Anaesth. Lancaster HA. Specialty: Anaesth. Prev: Sen. Regist. Rotat. (Anaesth.) Addenbrooke's Hosp. Camb. & P'boro.; Vis. Asst. Prof. Anaesthiol. Oklahoma Univ., USA.

SMITH, Mark Charles 36B Surrey Road, Bournemouth BH4 9BX — MB BS Lond. 1996.

SMITH, Mark Christopher Sullivan Way Surgery, Sullivan Way, Scholes, Wigan WN1 3TB Tel: 01942 243649 Fax: 01942 826476 — MB ChB Manch. 1981.

SMITH, Mark Edward Jaunty Springs Health Centre, 53 Jaunty Way, Gleadless, Sheffield S12 3DZ; 48A Boundary Road, West Bridgford, Nottingham NG2 7BZ — BM BS Nottm. 1983.

SMITH, Mr Mark Eric Ballacurn, Ballaugh, Kirk Michael IM4 2HR Tel: 01624 7577 — MB BS Lond. 1959 (St. Thos.) BA Oxf. 1954; MRCS Eng. LRCP Lond. 1959; DO Eng. 1964; FRCS Eng. 1968. Socs: Fell. Roy. Soc. Med. Prev: Cons. Ophth. Surg. Chelmsford Hosp. Gp.; Sen. Regist. St. Bart. Hosp. Lond.; Regist. St. Thos. Hosp. Lond.

SMITH, Mark Ernest Fitzgerald Department Histopathology, Plymouth Hospitals NHS Trust, Derriford Hospital, Derriford Road, Plymouth PL6 8DH — MB ChB Leeds 1981; MRCP (UK) 1984; PhD Lond. 1990; MRCPath 1991. Cons. Histopath. Derriford Hosp. Plymouth. Specialty: Histopath. Prev: Sen. Lect. (Histopath.) Univ. Coll. Med. Sch. Lond.
SMITH, Mark Patrick 25 Adam and Eve Mews, Kensington, London W8 6UG — MB ChB Otago 1985.
SMITH, Mark Paul Blackbrook Surgery, Lisieux Way, Taunton TA1 2LB Tel: 01823 259444 Fax: 01823 250200 — MB ChB Bristol 1986; DRCOG 1992; MRCGP 1993. GP; Police Surg. Prev: SHO (O & G) Brit. Milit. Hosp. Iserlohn FRG; SHO (Psychiat.) Brit. Milit. Hosp. Hannover.
SMITH, Mark Peart Astrazeneca, Alderley House, Alderley Park, Macclesfield SK10 4TF Tel: 01625 517986 Fax: 01625 590913; 103 Bollington Road, Turner Heath, Bollington, Macclesfield SK10 5EL Tel: 01625 572274 — MB ChB Birm. 1982; MRCP (UK) 1987. Head of Oncol. & Immunol. Research Sandoz Pharmaceut. Ltd. Surrey.; Global Product Dir. (Oncol.) at Astrazeneca, Alderley Pk., Macclesfield. Specialty: Pharmaceutical Medicine. Prev: Pharmaceut. Phys. Farmitaila Carlo Erba Ltd. St Albans; Regist. (Med.) Walsgrave Hosp. Coventry; Lect. & Regist. (Haemat.) Univ. Coll. Hosp. Lond.
SMITH, Mark Stephen Haley Department of Gastroenterology, Royal Shrewsbury Hospital, Mytton Oak Road, Shrewsbury SY3 8XQ Tel: 01743 261065 Fax: 01743 261066 — MB BS Lond. 1985 (Univ. Lond.) MD Lond. 1995; FRCP (UK) 2001. Cons. (Phys. & Gastro.) Roy. Shrewsbury Hosp. Specialty: Gastroenterol.; Gen. Med. Socs: Brit. Soc. Gastroenterol.; Midl. Gastroentoological Soc., W.Midl.s Phys.s Assn. Prev: Sen. Regist. (Gastroenterol. & Gen. Med.) N. Staffs. Hosp. Stoke-on-Trent; Regist. (Med.) Roy. Free Hosp. Hampstead.
SMITH, Martin Tavistock Surgical ITU, National Hospital for Neurology & Neurosurgery, Queen Square, London WC1N 3BG Tel: 020 7837 3611 Fax: 020 7829 8734 — MB BS Lond. 1980 (Roy. Free) FFA RCS Eng. 1985. Cons. Anaesth. Nat. Hosp. for Neurol. & Neurosurg. Lond.; Hon. Sen. Lect. (Anaesth.) Univ. Coll. Lond. Specialty: Anaesth.; Intens. Care. Socs: Fell. Roy. Soc. Med.; Assn. Anaesth.; Intens. Care Soc. Prev: Sen. Regist. (Anaesth.) St. Thos. Hosp. Lond.; Jules Thorn Research Fell. (Med.) The Middlx. Hosp. Lond.; Lect. (Human Anat.) Stanford Univ. Sch. Med. Calif., USA.
SMITH, Martin Clive 40 New Road, Little Kingshill, Great Missenden HP16 0EZ — MB ChB Birm. 1979; DCH RCP Lond. 1983.
SMITH, Martin Daniel Swallowfield Medical Practice, The Street, Swallowfield, Reading RG7 1QY Tel: 0118 988 3134 Fax: 0118 988 5759; Wayside, Brunces Shaw Rd, Farley Hill, Reading RG7 1UU — MB Camb. 1971; BChir 1970.
SMITH, Martin David Arrandene, 60 Bank Crescent, Ledbury HR8 1AE — MB ChB Birm. 1984; DA (UK) 1987. Clin. Anaesth. Dudley Gp. Hosps. NHS Trust. Specialty: Anaesth. Prev: Regist. Rotat. (Anaesth.) W. Midl. RHA.
SMITH, Martin Graham Milner 12 Clandon Road, Guildford GU1 2DR Tel: 01483 531825 Fax: 01483 829184 Email: martingsmith@btinternet.com; 12 Clandon Road, Guildford GU1 2DR Tel: 01483 531825 Fax: 01483 829184 Email: martingsmith@btinternet.com — MB Camb. 1967 (St. Thos.) BChir 1966; FRCP Lond. 1982, M 1969. Cons. Phys. Roy. Surrey Co. Hosp. Specialty: Gen. Med.; Gastroenterol. Socs: (Ex-brit. Represen) Internat. Soc. Internal Med.; Brit. Soc. Gastroenterol.; (Ex Sec.) Harv. Soc. Prev: Sen. Regist. (Med.) King's Coll. Hosp. Lond.; Regional Adviser (Med.) RCP Lond.; MRCP Examr. RCP.
SMITH, Martin Nicholas 5 Espland Close, Newton Reigny, Penrith CA11 0AR — MB ChB Ed. 1989; FRCS Ed. (A&G); FFAEM.
SMITH, Martin Richard 6 Eastfield Road, Benton, Newcastle upon Tyne NE12 8BD — MB BS Newc. 1992; MRCP 1996. SHO (Med.) Newc. Gen. Hosp.; Regist. Paediat. Roy. Vict. Infirm. Newc. Specialty: Paediat.
SMITH, Martin Robert Salisbury District Hospital, Department of Medicine, Odstock Road, Salisbury SP2 8BJ Tel: 01722 336262 Ext: 4229 Fax: 01722 332606 Email: martin.smith@salisbury.nhs.uk; Capio New Hall Hospital, Bodenham, Salisbury SP5 4EY — MB BS Lond. 1992 (Char. Cross & Westm. Med. Sch.) BSc Lond. 1989; MRCP (UK) 1995. Cons. Phys. and Endocrinologist. Specialty: Endocrinol.; Diabetes. Special Interest: Insulin Resistance; Thyroid Dis.; Polycystic Ovary Syndrome. Socs: Soc. for Endocrinol.; Brit. Thyroid Assn.; Diabetes UK. Prev: Locum Cons. (Endocrinol.) Kingston Gen. Hosp.; Specialist Regist. (Diabetes & Endocrinol.) St. Mary's Hosp. Lond.; Regist. Chelsea & Westminster Hosp.
SMITH, Martyn Vernon Kiddrow Lane Health Centre, Kiddrow Lane, Burnley BB12 6LH Tel: 01282 426840 Fax: 01282 433252 — MB BChir Camb. 1972 (King's Coll. Hosp.) MA Camb. 1972; DObst RCOG 1973. Prev: SHO (A & E) St. Jas. Hosp. Leeds; SHO (Paediat.) St. Luke's Hosp. Bradford; Ho. Off. (Gen. Surg., Gen. Med. & O & G) King's Coll. Hosp.
SMITH, Mary Burnside Cottage, Edlingham, Alnwick NE66 2BL Tel: 01665 74280 — MB BS Durh. 1945.
SMITH, Mary Jane Yeovil District Hospital, Higher Kingston, Yeovil BA21 4AT Tel: 01935 475122 Fax: 01935 384208 — MB ChB Manch. 1972; DCH Eng. 1974; MRCP (UK) 1976. Cons. Paediat. E. Som. NHS Trust Yeovil. Socs: FRCP (Lond.); FRCPCH.
SMITH, Mary Neville (retired) 39 Wimbledon Close, The Downs, Wimbledon, London SW20 8HL — MB BS Lond. 1953 (Char. Cross) DCH Eng. 1957; Hon. FRCPCH 1998. Prev: Hon. Assoc. Specialist (Paediat.) Kingston Hosp.
SMITH, Matthew Guy 14 Cowesby Street, Manchester M14 4UG — MB ChB Manch. 1997.
SMITH, Matthew Leonard 11 Highroyd Lane, Huddersfield HD5 9DN — MB ChB Leeds 1989.
SMITH, Matthew Liam Walker 12 Julien Road, Coulsdon CR5 2DN — MB BS Lond. 1994 (Kings Coll. Med. Sch.) MRCP Lond. 1997. Specialist Regist./Lect. (Haemat.) Roy. Lond. Hosp. & St. Bart. Hosp., Lond. Specialty: Haematology.
SMITH, Maureen Hanretty The Health Centre, Port Glasgow — MB ChB Glas. 1978; DRCOG 1982.
SMITH, Maurice Anthony Department Medicine of The Elderly, Harold Wood Hospital, Gubbins Lane, Romford RM3 0BE Tel: 01708 708257 Fax: 01708 708283 — MB ChB Liverp. 1979; FRCP Lond. 1998. Cons Phys Geriatric Med., Highwood Hosp. Brentwood; PostGrad. Acad. Organiser, Harold Wood Hosp. Romford Essex; Cons Geriatitian Nuffield Hosp. Brentwood Essex. Socs: BMA & Brit. Geriat. Soc. Prev: Sen. Regist. Middlx. Hosp. & Univ. Coll. Hosp. Lond.; Sen. Regist. Northwick Pk. Hosp. Harrow; Regist. (Med.) Roy. Liverp. Hosp.
SMITH, Maurice Raymond Mather Avenue Practice, 584 Mather Avenue, Liverpool L19 4UG Tel: 0151 427 6239 Fax: 0151 427 8876 — MB ChB Manch. 1986; DRCOG 1988; MRCGP 1990; Dip. Occ. Med. 1997. GP Princip.; Occupat. Phys.; Occupat. Phys. for Type Talk Liverp. Specialty: Gen. Med. Socs: Soc. Occupat. Med.
SMITH, Megan 3F2/ 4 Merton Place, Edinburgh EH11 1JZ Tel: 0131 229 3002 — MB ChB Ed. 1998 (Edinburgh) BSc (Hons) 1995; MB ChB Ed 1998. JHO.Qu Margt. Hosp. Dunfermline. Specialty: Gen. Med.
SMITH, Megan Rachel Birmingham Children's Hospital, Steelhouse Lane, Birmingham B4 6NH Tel: 0121 333 9652; 20 Hursthead Walk, Brunswick, Manchester M13 9UT Tel: 0161 274 4807 — MB ChB Manch. 1994 (Univ. Manch.) MRCPCH; MRCP (UK) 1997. Specialist Regist. (Paediatric Intens. Care) Birm. Childr.'s Hosp. Specialty: Paediat. Prev: SpR Paediat. - N.W.; SHO (Neonat. Med.) St. Mary's Hosp. Manch.; Ho. Off. Manch. Roy. Infirm.
SMITH, Melanie Jane 26 Marmion Road, Liverpool L17 8TX — MB BS Adelaide 1980.
***SMITH, Melissa Ann** 15 Vine Avenue, Sevenoaks TN13 3AH — MB ChB Bristol 1998 (Bris.) BSc (Hons) 1995. Specialty: Gen. Med.
SMITH, Michael Arthur (retired) 19 St Clare Road, Colchester CO3 3SZ Tel: 01206 574592 — BM BCh Oxf. 1952; DObst RCOG 1954; DM Oxf. 1958; FRCP Lond. 1976, M 1958. Prev: Dermatol. Colchester & Dist. Gp. Hosps.
SMITH, Mr Michael Clive Franklyn ENT Department, County Hospital, Union Walk, Hereford HR1 2ER Tel: 01432 364074 Fax: 01432 364149; Urdimarsh Farm, Marden, Hereford HR1 3HB Fax: 01432 359893 Email: mikesmith@urdimarsh.freeserve.co.uk — MB BS Lond. 1977 (St. Mary's) MRCS Eng. LRCP Lond. 1976; DLO Eng. 1980; FRCS (Otol.) Eng. 1985; T(S) 1991. Cons. ENT. Co. Hosp. Hereford, & Roy. Infirm., Worcester. Specialty: Otorhinolaryngol. Socs: Indian Assn. Otolaryngols.; Indian Soc. Otol.; Nepal Med. Assn. Prev: Cons. ENT West. Regional Hosp. Pokhara, Nepal; Sen. Regist. (ENT) Freeman Hosp. Newc. u. Tyne; Regist. (ENT) Warwick Gen. Hosp.

SMITH, Michael Colin George 19 Counting House Road, Disley, Stockport SK12 2DB — MB ChB Birm. 1988.

SMITH, Michael David Department of Microbiology, Taunten and Somerset Hospital, Taunton TA1 5DA — BM Soton. 1979; MRCP (UK) 1984; MRCPath 1990. Cons. Microbiol. Specialty: Med. Microbiol. Prev: Sen. Clin. Lect. Wellcome - Mahidol Univ. Oxf. Trop. Med. Research Progm. Mahidol Univ. Bangkok, Thailand.

SMITH, Mr Michael Fleming, TD Falkirk & District Royal Infirmary, Department of Urology, Falkirk FK1 5QE Tel: 01786 634000; Dunardoch, St. Margaret's Drive, Dunblane FK15 0DP Tel: 01786 824261 Fax: 01786 824261 Email: michael.smith@btopenworld.com — (Univ. Camb. & Univ. Ed.) MB ChB Ed. 1970; MA Camb. 1971; FRCS Ed. 1975; MRCOG 1975; ChM Ed. 1980; T(S) 1991. Cons. (Urol.) Forth Valley Acute Hosps. NHS Trust. Specialty: Urol. Special Interest: Childrens Urol.; Endoscopic Stone Surg. Prev: Cons. (Urol.) Stirling Roy. Infirm. & Falkirk & Dist. Roy. Infirm.; Cons. (Urol.) Law Hosp. Carluke; Sen. Regist. (Urol. Surg.) Roy. Infirm. Edin.

SMITH, Michael Francis The Ryegate Childrens Centre, The Childrens Hospital, Tapton Crescent Road, Sheffield S10 5DD Tel: 0114 267 0237 — MB BS Lond. 1972 (Lond. Hosp.) MRCP (UK) 1978; FRCP Lond. 1991; FRCPCH 1998. Cons. Paediat. Ryegate Childr. Centre; Cons. Paediat. Jessop Hosp. for Wom.; Clin. Tutor (Paediat.) Univ. Sheff. Specialty: Paediat. Socs: Brit. Paediat. Neurol. Assn.; Neonat. Soc.; Brit. Assn. for Perinatal Med. Prev: Sen. Regist. Sheff. Childr. Hosp.; Regist. & Research Regist. St. Thos. Hosp. Lond.

SMITH, Michael Graham 94 Hayclose Road, Kendal LA9 7ND — MB BS Lond. 1991 (St. Mary's Hosp. Med. Sch.) BSc (Microbiol. & Immunol.) Lond. 1988; MRCP (UK) 1994. GP/Regist. Poplars Surg. Birm. Specialty: Diabetes. Prev: SHO (O & G) Good Hope Hosp. Sutton Coldfield; SHO Rotat. (Med.) Dudley Rd. Hosp. Birm.

SMITH, Mr Michael Hanby 38 Billy Bunns Lane, Wombourne, Wolverhampton WV5 9BP Tel: 01902 893140 — MB BS Lond. 1971; FRCS Ed. 1977.

SMITH, Michael Inglis Bank House Surgery, The Health Centre, Victoria Road, Hartlepool TS26 8DB Tel: 01429 274386 Fax: 01429 860811 — MB ChB Ed. 1985; BSc (Hons.) Ed. 1983, MB ChB 1985; DRCOG 1990; MRCGP 1991.

SMITH, Michael John 22 Southwell Road, Benfleet SS7 1JB Tel: 01268 751728 — MRCS Eng. LRCP Lond. 1960.

SMITH, Michael John Heatherwood Hospital, Department of Medicine, London Road, Ascot SL5 8AA Tel: 01344 877186 Fax: 01344 877620 Email: mike.smith@hwph-tr.nhs.uk; Windsor Chest Clinic, King Edward VII Hospital, St Leonards Road, Windsor SL4 3DP Tel: 01753 636459; Moorlands, Coronation Road, Ascot SL5 9HF — MD Manch. 1986 (Manchester) MB ChB 1973; MRCP (UK) 1977; FRCP Lond. 1994. Cons. Gen. & Respirat. Med. Heatherwood Hosp. Ascot. Specialty: Gen. Med.; Respirat. Med. Socs: Brit. Thoracic Soc.; Roy. Coll. of Physicians; Europ. Respirat. Soc. Prev: Sen. Regist. (Thoracic & Gen. Med.) Brompton Hosp. Lond.; Clin. Lect. & Hon. Regist. Cardiothoracic Inst. Brompton Hosp. Lond.; Regist. (Med.) Qu. Mary's Hosp. Roehampton.

SMITH, Michael John The Royal Surrey County Hospital, Egerton Road, Guildford GU2 7XX Tel: 01483 571122; 13 Fairway, Merrow, Guildford GU1 2XQ Tel: 01483 38053 Fax: 01483 574508 — MB BS Durh. 1957 (Newc.) FRCP Lond. 1977, M 1962. Cons. Phys. Guildford & Godalming Gp. Hosps.; Sen. Lect. (Biochem.) Univ. Surrey. Specialty: Endocrinol. Socs: Fell. Roy. Soc. Med.; BMA; Brit. Diabetic Assn. Prev: Regist. Postgrad, Med. Sch. Hammersmith; Research Fell. NIH, Univ. South. Calif. USA; 1st Asst. Univ. Dept. Med. Roy. Vict. Infirm. Newc.

SMITH, Michael John Moon Borough Medical Centre, 1-5 Newington Causeway, London SE1 6ED Tel: 020 7407 4248 Fax: 020 7234 0849 Email: michael_johnsmith@hotmail.com; 41 Manor Road N., Hinchley Wood, Esher KT10 0AA — (Univ. Coll. Hosp.) MB BChir Cantab. 1950.

SMITH, Michael Joseph Department of Psychological Medicine, Gartavel Royal Hospital, 1055 Great Western Road, Glasgow G12 0XH Tel: 0141 211 3908 Fax: 0141 357 4899 — MB ChB Liverp. 1990; BSc (Hons.) Liverp. 1987; MRCGP 1994; MRCPsych 1996. Cons. Psychiat., Dykebar Hosp., Paisley; Sen. Research Fell.. (Psychol. Med.) Univ. Glas. Specialty: Gen. Psychiat. Prev: Specialist Regist. (Psychiat.) Gartnavel Roy. Hosp. Glas.

SMITH, Michael Lawson 8 Priestthorpe Lane, Bingley BD16 4EE Tel: 01274 510268 — MB ChB St. And. 1971; DRCOG 1973; MRCP (UK) 1976; FRCP Ed. 1990; FRCPCH 1996. Med. Dir. Bradford NHS Trust; Hon. Sen. Lect. (Paediat.) Leeds Univ. Specialty: Paediat. Prev: Cons. Paediat. Bradford DHA; Sen. Regist. (Paediat.) Derbysh. & Notts. (T) AHAs; Regist. (Paediat.) Ninewells Teach. Hosp. Dundee.

SMITH, Michael McDonald The Health Centre, Clitheroe Tel: 01200 25201 — MB ChB St. And. 1960; DObst RCOG 1962; FRCGP 1984, M 1969; Assoc. Fac. Occupat. Med. RCP Lond. 1980. Socs: Soc. Occupat. Med.

SMITH, Michael Ralph Dolly Barn, Ash Lane, Etwall, Derby DE65 6HT — MB BCh Wales 1962 (Cardiff) DObst RCOG 1964; FRCOG 1980, M 1967. Cons. O & G Burton Hosps. NHS Trust. Specialty: Obst. & Gyn. Socs: BMA. Prev: Cons. O & G E. Anglia RHA; Sen. Regist. Plymouth Gen. Hosp.; Surg. Cdr. RN.

SMITH, Michael Robert Paddock House, 7 Orchard View, Skelton, York YO30 1YQ — MB ChB Leeds 1995.

SMITH, Michael Robert 23 Blenheim Avenue, Liverpool L21 8LN — MB ChB Sheff. 1998; MB ChB Sheff 1998.

SMITH, Michael Stuart Checkley Lodge, Checkley, Nantwich CW5 7QA — MB ChB Liverp. 1974.

SMITH, Michael Victor 38 East Sheen Avenue, London SW14 8AS Tel: 020 8876 1570 Email: enquiries@drmikesmith.com — MB BS Lond. 1963 (Guy's) MRCS Eng. LRCP Lond. 1963; DObst RCOG 1964; DPH Lond. 1967; MFPHM 1989, MFCM 1972. Indep. Med. Author & Broadcaster. Socs: Hon. Fell. Nat. Assn. Family Plann. Doctors; Med. Journalists Assn (MJA). Prev: Chief Med. Off. Family Plann. Assn.; Research Assoc. GP Research Unit Guy's Hosp. Lond.; Dir. (Pub. Health) Kingston & Esher HA.

SMITH, Michael William 4 Burlingham Avenue, West Kirby, Wirral CH48 8AP — MB ChB Liverp. 1975; FCAnaesth. 1989. Regist. Rotat. (Anaesth.) Mersey RHA. Specialty: Anaesth.

SMITH, Myles Gerard 22A Ipswich Road, Woodbridge IP12 4BU Tel: 01394 385600 — MB BS Lond. 1974; FFA RCS Eng. 1979. Cons. Anaesth. Ipswich Hosp. Ipswich. Specialty: Anaesth.

SMITH, Nancy Heron (retired) 1 Edge Point Close, Knights Hill, London SE27 0QS Tel: 020 8670 6475 — MB ChB (Hons.) Leeds 1945; DObst RCOG 1948; MRCGP 1960. Prev: Ho. Surg.Birm.Accid..Hosp.

SMITH, Naomi The Farmhouse, Hillhead, Portlethen, Aberdeen AB12 4QP Tel: 01224 783778 — MB ChB Dundee 1996; BMSc (Hons.) 1993; DRCOG RCOG. 1998; DFFP RCOG. 1998. SHO GP VTS Aber. Roy. Infirm.; Paediat. Roy. Aberd. Child. Hosp. Specialty: Gen. Pract. Prev: SHO A & E Abdn. Roy. Infirm; SHO (O & G) Aber. Roy. Infirm.; Jun. Ho. Off. (Surg.) Roy. Infirm. Shirley.

SMITH, Neil Andrew Montague Health Centre, Oakenhurst Road, Blackburn BB2 1PP Tel: 01254 268436 Fax: 01254 268440 — MB ChB Manch. 1990; MB ChB (Hons.) Manch. 1990; MRCP (UK) 1992; MRCP Ed. 1992; DRCOG 1993; DFFP 1993. Trainee GP Chesh. Prev: Trainee GP/SHO Trafford Gen. Hosp.

SMITH, Neil Andrew Leighton Silsden Health Centre, Elliott Street, Silsden, Keighley BD20 0DG Tel: 01535 652447 Fax: 01535 657296 — MB BS Lond. 1982 (St. Tos.) DRCOG 1985; MRCGP 1986; Dip Occ Med RCP Lond. 1995; AFOM 2001. NHS Occupat. Health Phys. Specialty: Occupat. Health. Socs: BMA; Soc. of Occupat. Med.; ANHOPS.

SMITH, Neil Anthony Birmingham Heartlands and Solihull Trust, Bordesley Green East, Birmingham B15 2SQ Tel: 0121 424 2000 — MB ChB Birm. 1979; MRCP (UK) 1984; MRCPath 1994. Cons. Haemat, Birm. Heartlands and Solihull NHS Trust. Specialty: Haematology.

SMITH, Neil Jonathan Flat 5, 4 Wandle Road, Morden SM4 6AH — MB BS Lond. 1996.

SMITH, Neil Robert Ling House Surgeries, 49 Scott Street, Keighley BD21 2JH Email: nsmith@bradford-ha.nhs.uk — MB BS Lond. 1983; MRCP (UK) 1986. Partner in Gen. Pract.

SMITH, Neville Vincent (retired) Department of Medicine, University Hospital, Queens Medical Centre, Nottingham NG7 2UH; 9 Beeston Fields Drive, Beeston, Nottingham NG9 3DB — MB ChB Sheff. 1963; MRCS Eng. LRCP Lond. 1966; MRCP (UK) 1994. Hon. Clin. Asst. Gen. Med. Dept. Med. Univ. Hosp. Nottm.

SMITH, Niall Cameron 33F Herbert Street, Glasgow G20 6NB — MB ChB Glas. 1993; DRCOG 1996; MRCGP 1997.

SMITH, Nicholas 17 Colliery Green Drive, Little Neston, South Wirral CH64 0UA Tel: 0151 336 7452 — MB ChB Liverp. 1979; FRCS Ed. 1986; DMRT 1997. Assoc. Spec. Thoracic Oncol. Clatterbridge Hosp. Bebington Wirral. Specialty: Oncol.; Radiother.

SMITH, Nicholas Anthony Gould Danks, Smith, Sykes and Farrell, 134 Beeston Road, Beeston Hill, Leeds LS11 8BS Tel: 0113 276 0717 Fax: 0113 270 3727 — MB ChB Leeds 1976; DRCOG Lond. 1981. GP Leeds. Prev: Trainee GP Aylesbury VTS.

SMITH, Mr Nicholas Charles 19 Old Brickfields, Broadmayne, Dorchester DT2 8UX — BM Soton. 1978; FRCS Ed. 1983; FRCR 1987. Cons. Radiol. W. Dorset Gen. Hops. NHS Trust. Specialty: Radiol. Prev: Sen. Regist. (Diag. Radiol.) W. Midl. Region. HA.

SMITH, Nicholas James 62 New Hall Lane, Bolton BL1 5LG — MB ChB Manch. 1981; FRCA. Specialty: Anaesth.

SMITH, Nicholas Peter 49 Preston Down Road, Paignton TQ3 2RR Tel: 01803 557038; Flat 2, 31 Corfton Rd, Ealing, London W5 2HP Tel: 020 8998 0682 — MB BS Lond. 1991. Regist. (HIV & Genitourin. Med.) St. Stephens Clinic Chelsea & Westm. Healthcare Lond. Specialty: HIV Med.; Genitourinary Medicine; Gen. Med.

SMITH, Nicholas Stephen Borcharot Medical Centre, 62 Whitchurch Road, Withington, Manchester M20 1EB Tel: 0161 445 5907 Fax: 0161 448 0466; 14 Salisbury Road, Chorlton-Cum-Hardy, Manchester M21 0SL — MB ChB Manch. 1990; MRCGP 1994; DFFP 1994. GP Manch.

SMITH, Nicholas William Patrick 175 Whitham Road, Broomhill, Sheffield S10 2SN — MB ChB Sheff. 1995.

SMITH, Nicola Aileen The West London Centre for Sexual Health, Charing Cross Hospital, Fulham Palace Road, London W6 8RF Tel: 0208 846 1568 Fax: 0208 846 7582 Email: nicola.smith@chelwest.nhs.uk — MB BS Lond. 1989 (St. George's Hosp., Lond.) Cert of Completion of Specialist Training 1997 (Genitourinary Medicine); BSc Lond. 1986; MRCP (UK) 1992; DFFP 1994. Cons., Genitorurinary Med., Chelsea & Westm. NHS Trust. Specialty: Genitourinary Medicine. Special Interest: NHV 8 Infection; HIV 2 Infection. Socs: Brit. HIV Assn.

SMITH, Nicola Lisbeth Whaddon Way Surgery, 293 Whaddon Way, Bletchley, Milton Keynes MK3 7LW Tel: 01908 375341 Fax: 01908 374975 — MB ChB Leic. 1989.

SMITH, Nigel Ian Bromley House, Ormes Lane, Tettenhall Wood, Wolverhampton WV7 3QG — MB ChB Liverp. 1976; Dip Occ Med 1995.

SMITH, Nigel Jollyon Clinical Neurophysiology (EEG) Department, University Hospital, Nottingham NG7 2UH; The Grange, Bunny, Nottingham NG11 6QX — MB BChir Camb. 1972 (St. Thos.) LMSSA Lond. 1971; MA Camb. 1972; MRCP (UK) 1975; FRCP Lond. 1996. Cons. Clin. Neurophysiol. Univ. Hosp. Nottm. & Derbysh. Roy. Infirm.; Clin. Teach. Univ. Nottm. Specialty: Clin. Neurophysiol. Socs: Fell. Roy. Soc. Med.; (Ex-Pres.) Electrophysiol. Tech. Assn.; (Ex-Mem. Counc.) Brit. Soc. Clin. Neurophysiol. Prev: Sen. Regist. (Clin. Neurophysiol.) Wessex Neurol. Centre; Regist. (Neurol.) Derbysh. Roy. Infirm.; Regist. (Neurosurg.) Nat. Hosp. Qu. Sq. Lond.

SMITH, Nigel Kenneth Gladstone 33 Lambley Lane, Burton Joyce, Nottingham NG14 5BG — MB BS Newc. 1976; MRCP (UK) 1979; DM Nottm. 1994; FRCP Lond. 1995. Cons. Phys. (Med. for Elderly) Nottm. City Hosp. Specialty: Gen. Med. Prev: Cons. Phys. (Med. for Elderly) Leicester Gen. Hosp.; Cons. Phys. (Health c/o Elderly) Univ. Hosp. Nottm.

SMITH, Noel Howard (retired) Waldron Health Centre, Stanley Street, London SE8 4BG Tel: 020 8692 2314; 41 Manor Way, Blackheath, London SE3 9XG Tel: 020 8852 5823 — MB BCh BAO NUI 1956; DCH 1960; DObst RCOG 1961. Med. Off. Tunnel Refineries Greenwich.

SMITH, Norman Charles Aberdeen Maternity Hospital, Cornhill Road, Aberdeen AB25 2ZL Tel: 01224 553904 — MD Aberd. 1983; MB ChB 1974; FRCOG 1991, M 1979. Cons. Obst & Gyn. i/c Fetal Med. Aberd. Matern. Hosp. Specialty: Obst. & Gyn. Prev: Lect. (O & G) Dept. Midw. Qu. Mother's Hosp. Glas.

SMITH, Oladimeji Omabegho William Harvey Hospital, Department of Paediatrics, Kennington Road, Ashford TN24 0LZ Tel: 01233 616295 Fax: 01233 616139 Email: osmith@ekht.nhs.uk — MB BS Benin, Nigeria 1990; MRCPCH 1995; MRCP (UK) 1995; DCH RCP Lond. 1996. Cons. Paediat. Specialty: Paediat. Special Interest: allergy & Respirat. Paediat. Socs: Brit. Paediat. Assn.; BMA. Prev: Specialist Regist. Rotat. (Paediat.) Sheff. Childr. Hosp. NHS Trust; Specialist Regist. (Paediat.) North. Gen. Hosp. Sheff. & Pembury Hosp. Tunbridge Wells, Kent; SHO (Neonatol.) Hammersmith Hosp. Lond.

SMITH, Pamela Jane 3 Siskin Green, Liverpool L25 4RY — MB ChB Liverp. 1990. SHO (Med.) Southport & Formby NHS Trust.

SMITH, Patricia Ann Park Road Group Practice, The Elms Medical Centre, 3 The Elms, Liverpool L8 3SS Tel: 0151 727 5555 Fax: 0151 288 5016; 23 Court Hey Drive, Bowring Park, Liverpool L16 2NB Tel: 0151 489 4742 — MB ChB Liverp. 1978; MRCS Eng. LRCP Lond. 1978; DA Eng. 1984; MRCGP 1992. GP Liverp.

SMITH, Patricia Anne Fields Farm, Alt Hill Lane, Ashton-under-Lyne OL6 8AP Tel: 0161 330 5413 Fax: 0161 339 0763 — BM BS Nottm. 1981; BMedSci Nottm. 1979; MRCP (UK) 1984; Dip. Pharm. Med. RCP (UK) 1989. Indep. Pharmaceut./Healthcare Cons. Ashton-under-Lyme. Specialty: Pharmaceutical Medicine.

SMITH, Patricia Elizabeth (retired) The Rea House, Neenton, Bridgnorth WV16 6RL Tel: 01746 784254 — MB ChB Birm. 1946; MRCS Eng. LRCP Lond. 1946. Prev: Paediat. Regist. Jessop Hosp. Sheff.

SMITH, Patricia Jane City General Hospital, Stoke-on-Trent ST4 6QG Tel: 01782 715444 — MB BCh BAO Dub. 1976 (T.C. Dub.) BA 1976; MRCP (UK) (Paediat.) 1982; FRCP 1997; FRCPCH 1997. Cons. Paediat. (Endocrinol. & Diabetes) City Hosp. Stoke on Trent. Specialty: Paediat. Socs: Brit. Paediat. Assn.; Brit. Soc. Paediat. Endocrinol.; Eur. Soc. Paediat. Endocrinol. Prev: Cons. Paediat. (Endrocrinol. & Diabetes) Roy. Vict. Infirm. Newc.; Research Regist. (Paediat. Endocrinol.) Middlx. Hosp. Lond.; Sen. Regist. Yorkhill Childr. Hosp. Glas.

SMITH, Patricia Joyce 3 Oakfield Road, Didsbury, Manchester M20 6XA — MB ChB Manch. 1969; MRCP (UK) 1971; FRCP Lond. 1989. Cons. Rheum. Blackburn Health Dist. Specialty: Rheumatol. Socs: Fell. Manch. Med. Soc. Prev: Sen. Regist. (Rheum.) Manch. RHB; Regist. (Cardiol.) Baguley Hosp. Manch.; SHO (Med.) Withington Hosp. Manch.

SMITH, Patrick (retired) Heathfields, Forest Hill, Mansfield NG18 5BQ Tel: 01623 465821 — MB BS Lond. 1960.

SMITH, Mr Patrick Joseph Bradshaw Litfield House, Clifton, Bristol BS8 3LS Tel: 01179 731323 Fax: 01179 733303 — (Bristol) ChM Bristol 1970, MB ChB 1962; FRCS Eng. 1967. Cons. Urol. Surg. Bristol Roy. Infirm. Specialty: Urol. Prev: Cons. Urol. Surg. United Bath Hosps. SHO Gen. Surg. Bristol Roy.; Infirm.; SHO (Urol.) United Bristol Hosps.

SMITH, Paul Ainsdale Village Surgery, 2 Leamington Road, Southport PR8 3LB Tel: 01704 577866 Fax: 01704 576644; 11 Clinning Road, Birkdale, Southport PR8 4NU Tel: 01704 565355 — MB ChB Liverp. 1983.

SMITH, Paul Andrew 5 Banklands Avenue, Silsden, Keighley BD20 0JL — MB ChB Leeds 1996.

SMITH, Paul Dominic Elmhirst, Ninelands Road, Hathersage, Hope Valley S32 1BJ — MB ChB Bristol 1985; FRCA 1992. Lect. (Anaesth.) Univ. Leeds. Specialty: Anaesth. Prev: Regist. Rotat. (Anaesth.) Univ. Hosp. S. Manch.; SHO (Anaesth.) Univ. Hosp. S. Manch.

SMITH, Mr Paul John Bishopswood Hospital, Rickmansworth Road, Northwood HA6 2JW Tel: 01923 828100 Fax: 01923 844849; Kimble Farm, Fawley, Henley-on-Thames RG9 6JP — MB BS Newc. 1968; FRCS Glas. 1974. Cons. Plastic Surg. Hosp. for Childr. Gt. Ormond St., Mt. Vernon Hosp. N.wood, St. Albans City Hosp. Specialty: Plastic Surg. Socs: (Past Counc. Mem.) Brit. Soc. Surg. Hand.; Brit. Assn. Aesth. Plastic Surg.; Brit. Assn. Plastic Surg. Prev: Vis. Prof. Dept. Plastic Surg. Salt Lake City; Christine Kleinert Fell. Hand Surg. Louisville, USA; Resid. & Clin. Instruc. (Plastic Surg.) Duke Univ. USA.

SMITH, Paul Jonathan — MB ChB Leeds 1992.

SMITH, Paul Kirkel Woodwiss Westfield Surgery, Radstock, Bath BA3 3UJ Tel: 01761 436333 Fax: 01761 433126 Email: paul.smith@gp-l81132.nhs.uk — BM BS Nottm. 1975; BMedSci (Hons.) Nottm. 1973; DRCOG 1978; MRCGP 1979. GP Bath. Specialty: Gen. Pract. Prev: Trainer & Tutor GP Bath VTS; Trainee GP Exeter VTS; GP Mem. Avon PCAG.

SMITH, Paul Mapleston Woodside, Park Road, Dinas Powys CF64 4HJ Tel: 029 2051 4127 — MB BS Lond. 1959 (St. Thos.) FRCP Lond. 1978, M 1964; MD Lond. 1969. Cons. Phys. BUPA

Hosp., Cardiff. Specialty: Gastroenterol. Socs: (Ex-Pres.) Cardiff Med. Soc.; (Ex-Pres.) Brit. Soc. Gastroenterol.; (Ex-Pres.) Soc. Phys in Wales. Prev: Hon. Lect. (Med.) King's Coll. Hosp. Lond.; Research Fell. Boston Univ. Sch. Med., USA; Cons. Phys., Llandough Hosp., Penarth.

SMITH, Paul Robert Diabetes Centre, Ward 24, Birmingham Heartlands Hospital, Bordeley Green E., Birmingham B9 5SS; 132 Rectory Road, Sutton Coldfield B75 7RS Tel: 0121 311 1694 Email: p.r.smith@bham.ac.uk — MB ChB Leeds 1988; BSc (Hons.) Psychol. in relation to Med. Leeds 1985; MRCP (UK) 1992. Lect./Hon. Specialist Regist. (Gen. Med., Diabetes & Endocrinol.)Birm. Heartlands Hosp. Specialty: Diabetes; Endocrinol.; Gen. Med. Prev: Lect./Hon. Specialist Regist. (Gen. Med., Diabetes & Endocrinol.) Qu. Eliz. Hosp. Birm.; Research Fell. Dept. Med. Univ. Birm.; Regist. (Gen. Med., Diabetes & Endocrinol.) Birm. Heartlands Hosp.

SMITH, Paul Stevenson (retired) Easdon Hill Cottage, Manaton Road, North Bovey, Newton Abbot TQ13 8QX Tel: 01647 221318 — MB BS Lond. 1960 (Middlx.) BSc (Hons.) Lond. 1957; MB BS (Hons.) Lond. 1960; MRCGP 1985. Prev: GP Sandhurst.

SMITH, Paula Jane Rudgwick Medical Centre, Station Road, Rudgwick, Horsham RH12 3HB Tel: 01403 822103; 15 Grange Park, Cranleigh GU6 7HY Tel: 01483 271042 — MB BS Lond. 1986; MA Camb. 1983; MRCGP 1993. Princip. GP Rudgwick, W. Sussex. Prev: GP Windsor; Trainee GP Tadworth Surrey VTS; Regist. (Gen. Med.) King Edwd. VII Hosp. Windsor.

SMITH, Penelope Ann Dept. Of Anaesthesia, Dewsbury & District Hospital, Halifax Rd, Dewsbury WF13 4HS Tel: 01924 816038; Cherry Garth, 43 Birkdale Road, Dewsbury WF13 4HH — MB ChB Leeds 1974; FFA RCS Eng. 1979. Cons. Anaesth. Dewsbury Dist. Hosp. Specialty: Anaesth.

SMITH, Penelope Frances Litchdon Medical Centre, Landkey Road, Barnstaple EX32 9LL Tel: 01271 323443 Fax: 01271 325979; Hannaford House, Landkey, Barnstaple EX32 0NY Tel: 01271 830271 — MB BS Lond. 1976; MRCS Eng. LRCP Lond. 1976; MRCP (UK) 1979; MRCGP 1985.

SMITH, Penelope Susan 14 Montagu Drive, Leeds LS8 2PD Tel: 0113 240 2987 — MB BS Lond. 1984; MA (Cantab) 1981; DA (UK) 1987. SpR Anaesthetics N. & W. Yorks. Deanery. Specialty: Anaesth. Prev: Clin. Asst. (Anaesth.) Leeds Gen. Infirm.

SMITH, Mr Peter 17 Fortwilliam Drive, Belfast BT15 4EB — MB BCh BAO Belf. 1960; FRCS Ed. 1966; FRCOG 1979, M 1966.

SMITH, Peter 12 Shepherds Avenue, Worksop S81 0JA — MB ChB Bristol 1977.

SMITH, Peter Andrew University Department of Pathology, Duncan Building, Daulby St., Liverpool L69 3GA Tel: 0151 706 4495 Fax: 0151 706 5859 Email: peter.smith@rlbuh-tr.nwest.nhs.uk — MB BS Lond. 1976 (Char. Cross) BSc (Anat.) Lond. 1974; MRCS Eng. LRCP Lond. 1976; FRCPath 1996, MRCPath 1984. Cons. Cytopath. Roy. Liverp. Univ. Hosp.; Hon. Lect. Univ. Liverp. Specialty: Histopath. Socs: (Pres.) Brit. Soc. Clin. Cytol.; Internat. Acad. of Cytol. Prev: Cons. Histopath. Roy. Liverp. Hosp. & Wom. Hosp. Liverp.; Lect. (Histopath.) Char. Cross & Westm. Med. Sch. Lond.; Regist. (Histopath.) Sir Chas. Gairdner Hosp. Perth, W. Austral.

SMITH, Peter Campbell 33 Tithebarn Street, Poulton-le-Fylde FY6 7BY — MB ChB Manch. 1987.

SMITH, Peter David Frederick Wolverhampton Road Surgery, 13 Wolverhampton Road, Stafford ST17 4BP Tel: 01785 258161 Fax: 01785 224140; March Cottage, Whitgreave Lane, Great Bridgeford, Stafford ST18 4SJ — MB BS Lond. 1982.

SMITH, Peter Donald 34 Goldsmith Lane, Kingsbury, London NW9 9AH Tel: 020 8204 2029 — MB BS Lond. 1980 (Char. Cross) MRCS Eng. LRCP Lond. 1980; DRCOG 1985. Family Plann. Doctor Brook Advis. Center Lond. Specialty: Family Plann. & Reproduc. Health. Socs: BMA. Prev: Natural Growth Project Co-Worker Med. Foundat. c/o Victims of Torture; SHO (Neonat. Paediat.) Whittington Hosp. Lond.; Regist. (O & G) St. Bart. Hosp. Lond.

SMITH, Peter Gareth David Yelverton Surgery, Westella Road, Yelverton PL20 6AS Tel: 01822 852202 Fax: 01822 852260 — MB BS Lond. 1983; MA Camb. 1983; DRCOG 1985; DCH RCP Lond. 1986; MRCGP 1987. Specialty: Gen. Pract. Prev: Med. Off. Princess Alice Hospice Esher; Trainee GP Camb. VTS; Ho. Phys. (Gen. Med.) Guy's Hosp. Lond.

SMITH, Peter George (retired) Landyke, Ton Lane, Lowdham, Nottingham NG14 7AR — MB BS Lond. 1956 (Lond. Hosp.) FRCPath 1977, M 1965. Prev: Cons. Histopath. Univ. Hosp. Nottm.

SMITH, Peter Henry 11 St John Street, Manchester M3 4DW Tel: 0161 832 9999; Harwood Lodge, Harwood, Bolton BL2 4JA Tel: 01204 387085 Fax: 01204 382637 — MB ChB Manch. 1963; FRCP Lond. 1982, M 1967. Hon. Clin. Lect. Rheumatol. Manch. Univ. Specialty: Rheumatol. Prev: Cons. Rheum. N. Manch. Gen. & Ancoats Hosps.

SMITH, Peter Hubert (retired) 1A Woodlands Way, Middleton, Manchester M24 1WL Tel: 0161 643 4604 — MRCS Eng. LRCP Lond. 1944 (Sheff.) Treasury Med. Off. Prev: Dep. Med. Off. Jericho EMS Hosp. & Inst. Bury.

SMITH, Peter James 28 Elmdale Close, Warsash, Southampton SO31 9RX — BM Soton. 1992. GP Fareham. Socs: Fareham Med. Soc. Prev: GP Regist. Lyndhurst; SHO (Psychogenat.) Moorgreen; SHO (Paediat.) Soton. Gen. Hosp.

SMITH, Peter John Roland Hillview Medical Centre, 3 Heathside Road, Woking GU22 7QP Tel: 01483 760707 — MB BS Lond. 1977; DRCOG 1981; MRCGP 1984. Hosp. Practitioner (Cardiol.) St. Peter's Hosp. Chertsey. Prev: Clin. Asst. (Cardiol.) St. Peters Hosp. Chertsey.; GP Trainee Frimley Pk Hosp. VTS.

SMITH, Peter Karl Edward Kent House Surgery, 36 Station Road, Longfield DA3 7QD Tel: 01474 703550; 65 Redhill Wood, New Ash Green, Longfield DA3 8QP Tel: 01474 874292 — BM BCh Oxf. 1975; MA. Specialty: Gen. Med.

SMITH, Mr Peter Lincoln Chivers Hammersmith Hospital, Cardiothoracic Unit, Du Cane Road, London W12 0HS Tel: 020 8383 3125 Fax: 020 8383 2034 Email: plsmith@hhnt.org — MB BS Lond. 1975 (St Bartholemews Hosp Med School) FRCP 1997, M 1978; FRCS Eng. 1980. Cons. Cardiothoracic Surg. Hammersmith Hosps. Trust Lond. Specialty: Cardiothoracic Surg. Socs: Soc. Thoracic & Cardiovasc. Surg. GB & Irel.; Eur. Assn. Cardiothoracic Surg.; Eur. Soc. Cardiol. Prev: Sen. Regist. (Cardiothoracic Surg.) Hammersmith, Harefield & Middlx. Hosps. Lond.; Regist. (Cardiothoracic Surg.) Harefield Hosp. Lond.; Resid. Surg. Off. (Cardiothoracic Surg.) Brompton Hosp. Lond.

SMITH, Peter Robin 232 Milton Road, Weston Super Mare BS23 8AG Tel: 01934 625022 Fax: 01934 612470 Email: peter.smith@gp-l81058.nhs.uk; Elmhurst, Eastertown, Lympsham, Weston Super Mare BS24 0HP Tel: 01934 750041 Email: peterrobin.smith@btinternet.com/peterrobinsmith@hotmail.com — MB BS Lond. 1976 (Middlx.) DRCOG 1980; Dip. Occ. Me. 1997. Occupat. Med. Adviser (Occupat. Med. Serv.) Weston super Mare; LMC Represen. for N. Som., Avon LMC; Professional Exec. Comm. Mem., N. Som. PCT; Bd. Director, N. Som. (Out-of-Hours) Primary Care. Specialty: Occupat. Health. Prev: Caldicott Guardian (Data Protec.); Lead Clinician (Clin. Governance).

SMITH, Peter Samuel Churchill Medical Centre, Clifton Road, Kingston upon Thames KT2 6PG Tel: 020 8546 1809 Fax: 020 8549 4297 — MB ChB Sheff. 1983; Cert. Family Plann. JCC 1987. Socs: Assoc. Mem. Fac. Homoeopath; Brit. Med. Accupunc. Soc.

SMITH, Peter Stewart Haxby Health Centre, The Village, Wiggington, York — MB ChB Liverp. 1975; DCH Eng. 1979; DRCOG 1980; MRCGP 1981. Prev: SHO (Med.) Walton Hosp. Liverp.; SHO (Paediat.) York Dist. Hosp.

SMITH, Peter Stuart (retired) Keepers Lodge, Hadley Heath, Droitwich WR9 0AR Tel: 01905 620897 — (Camb. & Birm.) MB BChir Camb. 1943; MRCS Eng. LRCP Lond. 1943. Prev: Princip. Gen. Pract.

SMITH, Peter Thomas Lanes Farm, Marlborough Road, Wootton Bassett, Swindon SN4 7SA — MB BS Lond. 1997.

SMITH, Philip Eric Main 3 Fordwell, Cardiff CF5 2EU — MB ChB Liverp. 1979 (Univ. Liverp.) MRCP (UK) 1982; MD Liverp. 1988. Cons.Neurol. Cardiff. Specialty: Neurol. Prev: Cons. Neurol. Roy. Cornw. Hosp.; Sen. Regist. (Neurol.) Cardiff HA; Regist. (Neurol.) Newc. HA.

SMITH, Philip George Huthwaite Health Centre, New Street, Huthwaite, Sutton-in-Ashfield NG17 2LR — MB BS Lond. 1990 (Lond. Hosp.) BSc (Hons.) Lond. 1987, MB BS 1990; MRCGP 1994. GP Notts. HA. Socs: Roy. Soc. Med.; BMA. Prev: Trainee GP/SHO Kings Mill Hosp. Sutton-in-Ashfield.

SMITH, Philip George Lock The Ridgeway, 46A Main St., Repton, Derby DE65 6FB — MB ChB Manch. 1979.

SMITH, Philip Harold Thie Plaish, Glen Road, Colby, Castletown IM9 4NX Tel: 01624 832226 — MB ChB Manch. 1973.

SMITH, Mr Philip Henry BUPA Hospital, Jackson Avenue, Leeds LS8 1NT Tel: 0113 269 3939 Fax: 0113 268 1340; 2 Creskeld Lane, Leeds LS16 9AW Tel: 0113 267 3616 Fax: 0113 261 9748 — MB ChB Leeds 1957; FRCS Eng. 1960. Specialty: Urol. Socs: Brit. Assn. Urol. Surgs.; Internat. Soc. Urol. Prev: Med. Dir. St. Jas. Hosp. Leeds; Cons. i/c Dept. Urol. St. Jas. Hosp. Leeds.

SMITH, Philip Malcolm The Surgery, 18 Fouracre Road, Bristol BS16 6PG Tel: 0117 970 2033 — MB ChB Bristol 1975; MRCGP 1986.

SMITH, Philip Russell Beccles Medical Centre, 7-9 St Marys Road, St Marys Road, Beccles NR34 9NQ Tel: 01502 712662 Fax: 01502 712906; Castanea, Staithe Court, Beccles NR34 9EA Tel: 01502 714923 — MB BS Lond. 1972; MRCP (U.K.) 1975; DRCOG 1977; DA Eng. 1978. Hosp. Pract. (Anaesth.) Gt. Yarmouth & Waveney HA; Med. Adviser Sanyo (UK) LoW.oft. Specialty: Occupat. Health. Prev: Regist. (Gen. Med.) Newmarket Gen. Hosp.; SHO (Obst.) Mill Rd. Matern. Hosp. Camb.

SMITH, Phillip Alexander Litfield House, Clifton Down, Bristol BS8 3LS Tel: 0117 973 1323 Fax: 0117 973 3303; Druids Mead, Shirehampton Road, Stoke Bishop, Bristol BS9 1BL Tel: 0117 968 1894 Email: pasmithgyn@aol.com — MB BS Lond. 1976 (Lond. Hosp.) FRCOG 1994, M 1981. Cons. O & G Southmead Hosp. Bristol. Specialty: Obst. & Gyn. Socs: Fothergill Club; Gyn. Res. Soc.; Gynaecological Visiting Society. Prev: Sen. Regist. The Lond. Hosp.; Resid. Fell. King's Coll. Hosp. Lond.; Resid. Qu. Charlotte's & Chelsea Hosp. Lond.

SMITH, Phillip Hywel St Isan Road Surgery, 46 St. Isan Road, Heath, Cardiff CF14 4LX Tel: 029 2062 7518 Fax: 029 2052 2886 — MB BCh Wales 1981; MRCGP 1984.

SMITH, Priscilla Claire Conamore Raymede Clinic, St Charles Hospital, Exmoor St., London W10 6DZ Tel: 020 8962 4450 Fax: 020 8962 4451 — MB BS Lond. 1976; MFFP 1994. Dir. Servs. for Wom. Parkside Health NHS Trust; Cons. Family Plann. & Reproductive Health Care. Specialty: Family Plann. & Reproduc. Health. Socs: Chairm. (Clin. Advisory Comm.) Family Plann. Assn. Prev: Cons. to Clin. Effectiveness Comm. Fac. of Family Plann. & Reproductive Health.

SMITH, Rachel 48 Llwyn Castan, Cardiff CF23 7DA — MB BCh Wales 1997.

SMITH, Rachel Bland 3 Lodge Cottage, Main St., Staveley, Knaresborough HG5 9NJ; 3 Lodge Cottage, Main St., Staveley, Knaresborough HG5 9NJ — MB BS Newc. 1994; MRCGP 2000. Clin. Asst. Palliatice Care, St. Leonards Hospice, York. Specialty: Gen. Pract. Socs: Med. Protec. Soc.; BMA; RGCP.

SMITH, Rachel Hurndall — MB ChB Manch. 1992; BSc (Med. Sci.) St. And. 1989; FRCA 1999. Specialist Regist. (Anaesth.) N.W. Rotat. Specialty: Anaesth. Socs: BMA; MRCAnaesth.; Assn. Anaesth.

SMITH, Rachelle Victoria 53 Augusta Road, Birmingham B13 8AE — MB ChB Aberd. 1998; MB ChB Aberd 1998.

SMITH, Raymond Ernest (retired) 6 Owlswick Close, Littleover, Derby DE23 7SS Tel: 01332 517621 — MB ChB Sheff. 1953. Prev: Obst. Ho. Surg. Derby City Hosp.

SMITH, Mr Raymond Malcolm Department of Orthopaedic Surgery, Chancellors Wing, St James' University Hospital, Beckett St., Leeds LS9 7TF Tel: 0113 243 3144 Fax: 0113 206 5156 — MB ChB Leeds 1979; FRCS Glas. 1983; FRCS Eng. 1984; MD Leeds 1988. Cons. Trauma & Orthop. St. Jas. Univ. Hosp. Leeds; Sen. Clin. Lect. Univ. Leeds. Specialty: Trauma & Orthop. Surg. Socs: Brit. Trauma Soc. (Ex-Comm. 94-97) Pres. 200-2002; Orthopaedic Trauma Assoc.; Edr.ial Bd. Jl. of Bone Jt. Surg. Prev: Fell. (Orthop. Surg.) Univ. Harvard Boston Mass.; Clin. Lect. (Orthop. Surg.) Univ. Oxf.; Sen. Lect. (Orthop. & Trauma) Univ. Leeds.

SMITH, Raymond Stephen Wordsley Hospital, Renal Unit, Stourbridge DY9 0RL Tel: 01384 456111 Fax: 01384 244543 Email: rs.smith@dudleygoh-tr.wmids.nhs.uk — MB ChB Birm. 1973; MRCP (UK) 1977; MD Birm. 1985; FRCP Lond. 1995. Cons. Nephrologist Dudley Hosps. NHS Trust. Specialty: Nephrol. Socs: Renal Assn.; RCP. Prev: Lect. (Renal Med.) N. Staffs. Roy. Infirm.

SMITH, Raymond Thomas Department of Anaesthesia, St. James University Hospital, Beckett St., Leeds LS9 7; 2 Ash View, Whinney Lane, Harrogate HG2 9LY Tel: 01423 508994 — MB ChB Leeds 1988; MRCP (UK) 1992; FRCA 1994. Sen. Regist. (Anaesth.) St. Jas. Hosp. Leeds. Prev: Regist. (Anaeth.) Leeds Gen. Infirm.; SHO (Anaesth. & Renal Med.) St. Jas. Hosp. Leeds.

SMITH, Rebecca Louise Sheffield Childrens Hospital, Western Bank, Sheffield GL5 3RT; Lynthorpe, Rodborough Hill, Stroud GL5 3RT — MB ChB Sheff. 1997. SHO. (A&E.) Sheff. Childr Hosp. Specialty: Paediat. Prev: SHO.(Gen Paediat.) Rotherham Dist Hosp.; PRHO. (Orthop Surg.) Barnsley Dist Hosp.

SMITH, Rebekah Alison 4 Kentsford Drive, Radcliffe, Manchester M26 3XX — MB ChB Manch. 1996.

SMITH, Mr Redmond John Hamilton (retired) 9 Birkdale Road, London W5 1JZ Tel: 020 8998 1883 — (St. Mary's) MS Lond. 1956, MB BS 1946; DO Eng. 1950; FRCS Eng. 1952. Hon. Cons. Ophth. Surg. St. Mary's Hosp. & West. Eye Hosp. Lond.; Hon. Cons. Moorfields Eye Hosp. Lond. Prev: Edr. Brit. Jl. Ophth.

SMITH, Rhona Gail c/o Victoria Geriatric Unit, Victoria Infirmary, Mansions House Road, Glasgow G42 9TY; 56 Kierhill Road, Cumbernauld, Glasgow G68 9BH — MB ChB Glas. 1993.

SMITH, Richard, Squadron Ldr. RAF Med. Br. Retd. Park Surgery, 2 Oark Road North, Middlesbrough TS1 3LF Tel: 01642 247008 Fax: 01642 245748; Ashton House Farm, Kirry Sigston, Northallerton DL6 3TE Tel: 01609 883727 Fax: 01609 883105 — MB ChB Sheff. 1984 (Shiff. Univ. Med. Coll.) DCH RCP Lond. 1989. GP Princip.; Police Surg. N. Yorks. Police. Specialty: Gen. Pract. Socs: Assn. of Police Surg. Prev: Med. Off. RAF Leeming N. Yorks.

SMITH, Richard Anthony 4 Westway, Chellow Dene, Bradford BD9 6AZ — MB ChB Leeds 1977.

SMITH, Richard Barry (retired) Bright Boss Ltd, The Beehive, Station Road, Goring-on-Thames, Reading RG8 9HB Tel: 01491 871621 Fax: 01491 875326 — (Manch.) MB ChB Manch. 1965; BSc (Hons. Anat.) Manch. 1962, MD 1969; Dip. Pharm. Med. RCP (UK) 1976; FFPM RCP (UK) 1989. Dir. Brightboss Ltd Reading. Prev: Med. Adviser ICI Ltd. Pharmaceut. Div. Macclesfield.

SMITH, Mr Richard Daron Nut-Tree Cottage, Littlefield Green, White Waltham, Maidenhead SL6 3JN Email: daron@discon.co.uk — BM BCh Oxf. 1994 (Camb. & Oxf. Univ.) MA Camb. 1994; FRCS (Eng) 1998. Research Fell. (Urol.), Northwick Pk. Inst. of Med. Research. Specialty: Urol. Prev: SHO Rotat. (Surg.) Northwick Pk. & St. Mark's NHS Trust; Demonst. (Anat.) Camb. Univ.; Resid. Med. Off. St. Edmunds Hosp. Bury St. Edmunds.

SMITH, Richard Dennis (retired) Furahi, 64 Horsham Road, Crawley RH11 8PA Tel: 01293 521644 — MB BS Lond. 1957 (Guy's) DObst RCOG 1959. Prev: Ho. Surg., Ho. Phys. & Resid. (Obst.) Guy's Hosp. Lond.

SMITH, Richard Edward Wallice Huddersfield Royal Infirmary, Lindley, Huddersfield HD3 3EA Tel: 01484 422191 Fax: 01484 422191; Rest Harrow, Cleeve Road, Goring-on-Thames, Reading RG8 9BH Tel: 01491 875283 — MB ChB Leeds 1995; BSc Leeds 1992. SHO Rotat. (Gen. Med.) Huddersfield Roy. Infirm. Huddersfield. Specialty: Gen. Med. Prev: Ho. Off. (Gen. Med.) St. Jas. Univ. Hosp. Leeds; SHO Rotat. (Gen. Med.) Princess Alexandra Hosp. Brisbane, Austral.

SMITH, Mr Richard Geoffrey Department of Ophthalmology, Stoke Mandeville Hospital, Mandeville Road, Aylesbury HP21 8AL Tel: 01296 315033 Fax: 01296 314893 — MB ChB Birm. 1982; DO RCS Eng. 1985; FRCS Eng. 1986; FRCOphth 1988. Cons. Ophth. Stoke Mandeville Hosp. Aylesbury & Hemel Hempstead Gen. Hosp. Specialty: Ophth. Socs: Internat. Soc. Clin. Electrophysiol. of Vision. Prev: Sen. Regist. Roy. Berks. Hosp. Reading & Moorfields Eye Hosp. Lond.; Regist. Qu. Med. Centre Nottm.; SHO Birm. & Midl. Eye Hosp.

SMITH, Richard Graham Morant Wem and Prees Medical Practice, New Street, Wem, Shrewsbury SY4 5AU — MB ChB Birm. 1978; DRCOG Lond. 1981. Specialty: Gen. Pract.

SMITH, Richard Ian Eller Yew, Sweden Bridge Lane, Ambleside LA22 9EX Tel: 015394 32560 — MB ChB Liverp. 1953; DObst RCOG 1955; MRCGP 1963. Socs: BMA.

SMITH, Richard James Wellside Surgery, 45 High Street, Sawtry, Huntingdon PE28 5SU Tel: 01487 830340 Fax: 01487 832753 — BM BS Nottm. 1990; MRCGP 1996. Princip. in GP. Specialty: Gen. Pract. Prev: Trainee GP P'boro. VTS.

SMITH, Richard Mark 13 Rockleaze Road, Sneyd Park, Bristol BS9 1NF; Academic Renal Unit, Southmead Hospital, Bristol BS10 5NB Tel: 0117 959 5438 Email: richard.smith@bris.ac.uk —

BM BCh Oxf. 1986; MRCP (UK) 1990; PhD (Cambridge) 1995. Lect. Renal Med. Univ. Bristol. Specialty: Nephrol.

SMITH, Richard Naylor Parkstone Health Centre, Mansfield Road, Poole BH14 0DJ Tel: 01202 741370 Fax: 01202 730952 — MB BS Lond. 1983.

SMITH, Richard Nicholas Evans Birchwood Medical Practice, Jasmin Road, Lincoln LN6 0QQ Tel: 01522 699 999 Fax: 01522 682793 — MB ChB Leeds 1988; BSc Leeds 1985; DRCOG 1991; MRCGP 1992; MSc 1996. Prev: Clin. Research Fell. Centre for Research Primary Care Univ. Leeds.

SMITH, Mr Richard Paul Powell St Michael's Hospital, Department of Obstetrics & Gynaecology, Southwell Street, Bristol BS2 8EG Tel: 0117 921 5411 — MD ChB Birm. 1992; MRCOG 1998 (Prize Medal); PhD (Fetal Physiol.) Imperial Coll., Lond. 2003. Subspecialty trainee in Matern. and fetal Med. Specialty: Obst. & Gyn. Prev: Specialist Regist. Rotat. (O & G) E. Anglian.

SMITH, Richard Spalding Portsonachan, Meadle, Aylesbury HP17 9UD Tel: 0184 444096 — MRCS Eng. LRCP Lond. 1942 (Middlx.) DMRD Eng. 1949. Cons. Radiol. Roy. Bucks. Co. Hosp. Aylesbury, High Wycombe Memor. Hosp. & Stoke Mandeville Hosp. Aylesbury. Specialty: Radiol. Prev: Cas. Off. Roy. Sussex Co. Hosp. Brighton; Ho. Surg. Kingston Co. Hosp.; Regist. Radiodiag. Dept. Middlx. Hosp.

SMITH, Richard William Milton Keynes General NHS Trust, Standing Way, Eaglestone, Milton Keynes MK6 5LD Tel: 01908 660033; Copper Beeches, Heath Lane, Aspley Heath, Woburn Sands, Milton Keynes MK17 8TN Tel: 01908 584449 — MB ChB Dundee 1980; MRCP (UK) 1985; FRCP 1999. Cons. Phys. & Rheum. Milton Keynes Hosp. Specialty: Gen. Med.; Rheumatol. Prev: Cons. Phys. & Rheum. Derriford Hosp. Plymouth.

SMITH, Robert (retired) Department of Obstetrics & Gynaecology, Ninewells Hospital, Dundee DD1 9SY — MB ChB St. And. 1969; MRCOG 1975. Cons. O & G Ninewells Hosp. Dundee. Prev: MRC Fell. Univ. Aberd.

SMITH, Robert Aidan Rodney University Health Centre, 9 Northcourt Avenue, Reading RG2 7HE Tel: 0118 987 4551 — MB Camb. 1980 (Westm.) MA Camb. 1979, MB 1980, BChir 1979; DRCOG 1982; MRCGP 1983. Asst. Phys. Reading Univ. Health Serv.

SMITH, Robert Andrew Lisanelly Lodge, 9 Gortin Road, Omagh BT79 7DH — MB BCh BAO Belf. 1990; DRCOG 1993; DGM RCPS Glas. 1994.

SMITH, Robert Andrew 67 Hayling Rise, Worthing BN13 3AG — MB BS Lond. 1993.

SMITH, Robert Antony 128 Tadcaster Road, Dringhouses, York YO24 1LU — MD Wales 1990; MB BCh 1982; MRCP (UK) 1985. Cons. Paediat. York Dist. Hosp. Specialty: Paediat. Socs: Brit. Paediat. Assn. Prev: Sen. Regist. (Paediat.) Newc.; Research Fell. Inst. Med. Genetics Cardiff; Regist. (Paediat.) Newc.

SMITH, Robert Benjamin Hereford County Hospital, Department of Obstetrics & Gynaecology, Union Walk, Hereford HR1 2ER Tel: 01432 364125 Fax: 01432 364169 Email: rob.smith@hhtr.nhs.uk — MB BCh Wales 1981; MRCOG 1991. Cons. (Obstet. & Gyn.) Hereford Co. Hosp. Specialty: Obst. & Gyn. Socs: Brit. Menopause Soc.; Welsh Obst. & Gynaecologists Soc. Prev: Sen. Regist. (O & G) Llandough Hosp., Cardiff; Sen. Regist. (O & G) Wrexham Maelor Hosp.; Clin. Research Fell. (O & G) Univ. Wales Coll. Med. Cardiff.

SMITH, Mr Robert Cameron Falkirk & District Royal Infirmary, Major's Loan, Falkirk FK1 5QE Tel: 01324 624000 Email: robert.smith@fvah.scot.nhs.uk; 2 Windsor Place, Kings Park, Stirling FK8 2HY Tel: 01786 446791 Email: robcamsmith@btopenworld.com — MB ChB Ed. 1970; FRCS Ed. 1974; ChM Ed. 1983. Cons. Gen. Surg. Falkirk & Dist. Roy. Infirm.; Hon. Clin. Teach. Univ. Edin. Specialty: Gen. Surg. Socs: Scott. Thoracic Soc.; BMA.

SMITH, Robert Chad Jubilee Healthcare, 41 Westminster Road, Coventry CV1 3GB Tel: 024 7622 3565 Fax: 024 7623 0053; Ash View, Tamworth Road, Corley, Coventry CV7 8BQ Tel: 01676 540555 — MB ChB Birm. 1964; MRCS Eng. LRCP Lond. 1964; DA Eng. 1966. Socs: BMA. Prev: SHO (Anaesth.) Dudley Rd. Hosp. Birm.; Ho. Phys. Aberystwyth Gen. Hosp.; Ho. Surg. (O & G) St. Chad's Hosp. Birm.

SMITH, Robert Charles (retired) 8 Belmont, Shrewsbury SY1 1TE Tel: 01743 232360 — MB ChB Birm. 1957; DObst RCOG 1960. Prev: GP Shrewsbury.

SMITH, Robert Gladstone The Thatched Cottage, 53 Woodcote Avenue, Wallington SM6 0QU Tel: 020 8647 4636 — (King's Coll. Hosp.) MB BS Lond. 1951; MRCS Eng. LRCP Lond. 1951; DObst RCOG 1957; DA Eng. 1961; MRCGP 1967. Socs: BMA & Assur. Med. Soc.; RCGP. Prev: Med. Off. & Clin. Asst. (Anaesth.) Carshalton, Beddington & Wallington Dist. War Memor. Hosp.; Ho. Surg., Jun. Anaesh. & Cas. Off. (ENT Dept.) King's Coll. Hosp. Lond.; Ho. Surg. (Obst.) St. Jas. Hosp. Lond.

SMITH, Robert Houghton 21 Lancaster Place, Great South West Road, Hounslow TW4 7NE — MB BS Lond. 1954 (Middlx.)

SMITH, Robert John 17 Orlingbury Road, Pytchley, Kettering NN14 1ET Tel: 01536 790602 — MB BS Lond. 1964 (King's Coll. Hosp.) MRCS Eng. LRCP Lond. 1964; FRCOG 1984, M 1971. Cons. (O & G) Kettering & Dist. Gen. Hosp. Specialty: Obst. & Gyn. Prev: Sen. Regist. (O & G) Kings Coll. Hosp. Lond.

SMITH, Mr Robert Kennedy Sandwell Hospital, Sandwell & West Birmingham Trust, Lyndon, West Bromwich B71 4HJ Tel: 0121 607 3243 — MB ChB Otago 1970 (Otago Univ.) Cons. Gyn. (Onocology), Sandwell & W. Birm. Trust, W. Bromwich, W. Midlands. Specialty: Obst. & Gyn. Special Interest: Gyn. Oncol. Socs: Brit. Soc. of Gyn. Cancer.

SMITH, Robert Malcolm Christie Castle Road, 1 - 2 Castle Road, Chirk, Wrexham LL14 5BS Tel: 01691 772434 Fax: 01691 773840; Hillside, Pont-y-Blew, Chirk, Wrexham LL14 5BH Tel: 01691 773487 — BM BCh Oxf. 1979; BA Camb. 1976; DRCOG 1982; DCH RCP Lond. 1982; MRCGP 1985.

SMITH, Robert Newton New England Cottage, London Road, St Ippolyts, Hitchin SG4 7NG Tel: 01462 437362 Fax: 01462 437364 Email: robert.n.smith@btinternet.com — MB ChB Birm. 1958; BSc (1st cl. Hons.) Birm. 1955, MD 1969, MB ChB 1958; DObst RCOG 1960; FRCP Ed. 1983, M 1967; FFPM 1989; FRCP Lond. 1991. Edit. Advis. Bd. Int. J. Pharm. Med. Specialty: Pharmaceutical Medicine. Socs: Fell. Roy. Soc. Med. & Fac. Pharm. Med.; BMA & Med. Res. Soc. Prev: Med. Dir. Glaxo Gp. Research Ltd. Greenford; Dir., Clin. Research & Drug Developm. Hoffmann-La Roche Basel; Sen. Lect. (Clin. Pharm. & Therap.) & Cons. Phys. Sheff. Univ. & Roy. Infirm.

SMITH, Robert Norman Frankley Health Centre, 125 New St., Frankley, Rubery, Rednal, Birmingham B45 0EU Tel: 0121 453 8211 Fax: 0121 457 9690 — MB ChB Manch. 1964.

SMITH, Robert Reekie Currie Road Health Centre, Currie Road, Galashiels TD1 2UA Tel: 01896 752476; Hiltons Hill, St Boswells, Melrose TD6 0DL Tel: 01835 823281 — MB ChB Ed. 1980 (Edinburgh) BSc (Med. Sci.) Ed. 1977; MRCGP 1984. Gen. Practitioner, Galashiels. Specialty: Gen. Pract.; Gen. Med. Socs: Mem. of the Soc. of Orthopaedic Med.; Mem. of the Brit. Inst. of Musculoskeletal Med.; Mem. of the Primary Care Rheum. Soc.

SMITH, Robert Russell The Health Centre, 2 Kirkland Road, Kilbirnie KA25 6HP Tel: 01505 683333 Fax: 01505 684098; Carrick, 96 Milton Road, Kilbirnie KA25 7HY Tel: 01505 683223 — MB ChB Glas. 1959; DObst RCOG 1961; MRCGP 1971. Local Treasury Med. Off. Socs: BMA. Prev: Ho. Surg. & Ho. Phys. Kilmarnock Infirm.; Ho. Off. Braeholm Matern. Hosp. Helensburgh & Overtoun Matern. Hosp. Dumbarton.

SMITH, Robin Frederick Arthur 55 Palmer Road, Plaistow, London E13 8NU Tel: 020 7474 2455 — MB BS W. Indies 1985.

SMITH, Robin Pierre Department of Chest Medicine, Victoria Hospital, Kirkcaldy KY2 5AH Tel: 01592 643355 Fax: 01592 647090; 33 High Street, Auchtermuchty, Cupar KY14 7AP — MB ChB Ed. 1988; MRCP (UK) 1992. Cons. Phys. Vict. Hosp. Kirkcaldy. Specialty: Respirat. Med. Prev: Sen. Regist. (Respirat. Med.) Frenchacy Hosp. & Bristol Roy. Infirm.; Research Fell. (Respirat. Med.) Grenoble, France; Regist. (Respirat. Med.) King's Cross Hosp. Dundee.

SMITH, Robin Wellesley Ancrum Medical Centre, 12-14 Ancrum Road, Dundee DD2 2HZ Tel: 01382 669316 Fax: 01382 660787 — MB ChB Dundee 1981.

SMITH, Roderick Andrew Balmore Park Surgery, 59A Hemdean Road, Caversham, Reading RG4 7SS Tel: 0118 947 1455 Fax: 0118 946 1766; 7 Jefferson Close, Emmer Green, Reading RG4 8US Tel: 01734 473587 — MB BChir Camb. 1973 (Camb. and Middlx. Hosp.) MA Camb. 1973; DObst RCOG 1976; FRCGP 2000.

SMITH, Rodney Stewart J D Lansdowne and Partners, Helston Medical Centre, Trelawney Road, Helston TR13 8AU Tel: 01326 572637 Fax: 01326 565525 — MRCS Eng. LRCP Lond. 1968.

SMITH, Roger Nuffield Orthopaedic Centre, Headington, Oxford OX3 7LD Tel: 01865 741155; 6 Southcroft, Elsfield Road, Old Marston, Oxford OX3 0PF Tel: 01865 790800 — (Univ. Coll. Hosp.) MB BChir Camb. 1956; MD Camb. 1960; FRCP Lond. 1974, M 1963; PhD Lond. 1971. Cons. Phys. & Cons. Metab. Med. Nuffield Orthop. Centre Oxf.; Emerit. Fell. Green Coll. Oxf. Specialty: Gen. Med. Socs: Assn. Phys.; Med. Res. Soc. Prev: Fell. Nuffield Coll. Oxf.; Clin. Reader & Cons. Phys. Nuffield Depts. Med. & Orthop. Surg. Oxf.; Sen. Wellcome Research Fell. Med. Unit & Hon. Sen. Lect. & Cons. Univ. Coll. Hosp.

SMITH, Roger The Saltscar Surgery, 22 Kirklfatham Street, Redcar TS10 1UA — MB ChB Leeds 1986; DFFP 1990. Hon. Med. Asst., Roy. Nat. Lifeboat Inst., Redcar & Teesmouth Stations. Specialty: Gen. Pract. Socs: Brit. Assn. of Immidiate Care.

SMITH, Mr Roger Abbey The Old Hall, Somerton TA11 7NG — MB ChB Liverp. 1940; FRCS Ed. 1943; MCh Liverp. 1948; FRCS Eng. 1971.

SMITH, Mr Roger Battersby 11 Moor Park Avenue, Preston PR1 6AS Tel: 01772 251507 Fax: 01772 881975 Email: rbsmith@uk-consultants.co.uk — (St. Geo.) MRCS Eng. LRCP Lond. 1970; BSc (Anat.) Lond. 1967, MB BS 1970; FRCS Eng. 1975. Cons. Orthop. Surg. Roy. Preston Hosp. Specialty: Orthop. Socs: Fell. BOA; Edit. Sec. BASK. Prev: Sen. Regist. (Orthop.) Gen. Infirm. & St. Jas. Hosp. Leeds; Regist. (Surg.) Roy. Infirm. Edin.; Regist. (Orthop.) Bristol Roy. Infirm.

SMITH, Roger Charles The Surgery, Grove St., Petworth GU28 0LP Tel: 01798 342248 Fax: 01798 343987 — MB BS Lond. 1966 (Univ. Coll. Hosp.) MRCS Eng. LRCP Lond. 1966. Med. Off. Seaford Coll. Petworth.

SMITH, Roger Galbraith (retired) 56 Alnwickhill Road, Edinburgh EH16 6LW Tel: 0131 664 1745 — MB ChB Ed. 1966; MRCP (UK) 1971; DObst RCOG 1973; FRCP Ed. 1980; FCRP Lond. 1989; FRCPS Glas. 1991. Prev: Cons. Phys. Geriat. Med. Roy. Vict. Hosp. Edin.

SMITH, Roger Hugh Norfolk House, 4 Norfolk St., Sheffield S1 2JB Tel: 0114 226 1844 Fax: 0114 226 1845; Flat 2, 27 Collegiate Crescent, Sheffield S10 2BJ Tel: 0114 268 6924 — MB BS Lond. 1967 (Westm.) Specialty: Alcohol & Substance Misuse.

SMITH, Roger Huntington University Hospital of North Tees, Stockton-on-Tees TS19 8PE — MB ChB Ed. 1969; BSc (Physiol.) (Hons.) Ed. 1966; MRCP (UK) 1972; FRCP Ed. 1983; FRCP Lond. 1987. Cons. Phys. & Cardiol. Univ. Hosp. of N. Tees; Cons. Phys. (Gen. Med. & Cardiol.) & Clin. Dir. (Med.) N. Tees NHS Trust. Specialty: Cardiol. Special Interest: Cardiol. Socs: Fell. (Ex-Sen. Pres.) Roy. Med. Soc. Edin.; Vice Pres. Roy. Coll. of Physicians Edin.; Roy. Coll. of Physicians Lond. Prev: Research Fell. (Cardiol.) Freeman Hosp. Newc.; Sen. Regist. (Med.) Newc. HA; Regist. (Cardiol.) West. Gen. Hosp. Edin.

SMITH, Roger Macleod Laing Mount Farm Surgery, Lawson Place, Bury St Edmunds IP32 7EW — MB ChB Ed. 1977.

SMITH, Roger Nigel John Queen Marys Hospital, Frognal Avenue, Sidcup DA14 JO85 Tel: 020 8308 3085 Email: roger.smith@qms.nhs.uk; 43 Camden Road, Sevenoaks TN13 3LU Tel: 01732 453098 Email: rnjs@boltblue.com — MB ChB Manch. 1983; MRCP 1987; MRCOG 1990. Consultant, Gynaecology and Obstetrics, Queen Mary's Hospital, Sidcup, Kent; Cons. Gynaecologist, Chelsfield Pk. Hosp., Orpington, Kent; Cons. Gynaecologist, the Blackheath Hospital,, Lond. Specialty: Obst. & Gyn.

SMITH, Roger Philip Roy 4 Manor Close, Lincoln LN2 1RL; 4 Manor Close, Lincoln LN2 1RL — MB ChB Sheff. 1987; Dip. Obst. Auckland 1990; FRCA 1997. Consultant Anaestetist, Macclesfield District General Hospital. Specialty: Anaesth. Socs: Manch. Med. Soc.; Anaesth Socs.; Intens. Care Soc. Prev: Specialist Regist. Anaesth.

SMITH, Mr Roger Philip Sutherland Eye Department, Cumberland Infirmary, Carlisle CA2 7HY; Holcombe House, Irthington, Carlisle CA6 4NJ — MB BS Newc. 1975; MA Camb. 1974; DO Eng. 1978; FRCS Ed. 1979; FCOphth. 1989. Cons. Ophth. N. RHA; Mem. Oxf. Ophth. Congr. Specialty: Ophth. Socs: Life Mem. Camb. Univ. Med. Soc. Prev: Sen. Regist. (Ophth.) Gen. Infirm. Leeds.

SMITH, Mr Roger William Queen Victoria Hospital, Holtye Road, East Grinstead RH19 3DZ Tel: 01342 410210 Fax: 01342 317959 Email: rwsmith@uk-consultants.co.uk — MB BChir Camb. 1978; FRCS Eng. 1982; BA Camb. 1974, MChir Camb. 1987; T(S) 1991. p/t Cons. Plastic & Reconstruc. Surg. Qu. Vict. Hosp. E. Grinstead; Vis. Cons. Plastic & Reconstruc. Surg. to Maidstone & The Dartford Hosp. Gp. Specialty: Plastic Surg. Special Interest: Breast Reduction & Non-Oncological Breast Surg.; Head & Neck Surg. Socs: BAPS; BAAPS; RSM. Prev: Sen. Regist. (Plastic & Reconstruc. Surg.) Frenchay Hosp. Bristol.

SMITH, Ronald Bertram 8 Fletchers, Basildon SS16 5TU Tel: 01268 45228 — MB BS Lond. 1963 (Univ. Coll. Hosp.) MRCS Eng. LRCP Lond. 1962; DObst RCOG 1964; MRCGP 1975. Socs: BMA. Prev: Ho. Off. (Med.) & Ho. Off. (Surg.) Southend Gen. Hosp.; Ho. Off. (Obst.) Rochford Gen. Hosp.

SMITH, Ronald Campbell Department of Child Health, Postgraduate Medical School, University of Exeter, Church Lane, Exeter EX2 5SQ Tel: 01392 403144 Fax: 01392 403158 Email: r.c.smith@ex.ac.uk; 35 Rosebarn Avenue, Exeter EX4 6DY Tel: 01392 254034 — MB BS Lond. 1975 (L.H.M.C.) MRCP (UK) 1981; DRCOG 1982; FRCPCH 1996. Cons. Paediat. Roy. Devon & Exeter NHS Trust; Lect. Univ. Exeter. Specialty: Paediat.; Community Child Health. Socs: Brit. Paediat. Assn.; Brit. Assn. Community Child Health. Prev: Cons. Paediat. (Community Child Health) Banbury & Oxon. HA; Sen. Regist. Newc. HA; Research Fell. Univ. Exeter Paediat. Research Unit.

SMITH, Ronald Clifford (retired) 28 Thorney Green Road, Stowupland, Stowmarket IP14 4AB — MB BS Lond. 1952 (Guy's) DObst RCOG 1953.

SMITH, Ronald Mitchell (retired) 140 Kinghorn Road, Burntisland KY3 9JU Tel: 01592 873304 — MB ChB Ed. 1961. Prev: Med. Adviser Benefits Agency Edin.

SMITH, Rosemary Helen 136A Southbrae Drive, Glasgow G13 1TZ — MB ChB Glas. 1971. Regist. (Bacteriol.) Roy. Infirm. Glas. Specialty: Med. Microbiol. Prev: Lect. Anat. Univ. Manch.; Ho. Phys. West. Infirm. Glas.; Ho. Surg. South. Gen. Hosp. Glas.

SMITH, Rosemary Rose Yew Tree Medical Centre, 100 Yew Tree Lane, Solihull B91 2RA Tel: 0121 705 8787 — MB ChB Birm. 1983 (Birmingham) DRCOG 1986; DCH RCP Lond. 1987; MRCGP 1988. GP; Clin. Asst. Dermat., Solihull Hosp. Socs: MDU.

SMITH, Rowena Elizabeth 27 Hillside Road, Cheam, Sutton SM2 6ET — MB ChB Manch. 1984; BSc St. And. 1980. Sen. Regist. (Histopath.) Char. Cross Hosp. Lond. Specialty: Histopath.

SMITH, Rowland Michael Hamilton Spring Gardens Health Centre, Providence Street, Worcester WR1 2BS Tel: 01905 681681 Fax: 01905 681699; 52 Beech Avenue, Worcester WR3 8PY — MB BS Lond. 1975; ARCS 1970; BSc Lond. 1970, MB BS 1975; DCH Eng. 1979; DRCOG 1979; MRCGP 1980. GP Worcester.

SMITH, Rupert Alexander Department of Oncology, ICI Pharmaceuticals, Macclesfield; 1 Broomfield Road, Broomfield Villas, Heaton Moor, Stockport SK4 4NB — MB ChB Liverp. 1976; DCH Eng. 1979; MRCP (UK) 1980. Research Fell. & Hon. Sen. Regist. Univ. Oxf. Childr. Cancer Research Gp.; Med. Adviser ICI Pharm. Chesh.

SMITH, Rupert Alistair Four Elms Medical Centre, 103 Newport Rd, Roath, Cardiff CF24 0AF — MB BCh Wales 1997 (UWCM) GP Princip. Four Elms Med. Centre, Cardiff. Specialty: Gen. Pract. Socs: BMA; MDU. Prev: GP Reg., Portway PCE, Porthcawl; GP Registra Woodlands Surg. Masteg.; SHO (A & E) Princess of Wales Hosp., Bridgend.

SMITH, Rupert Noel Flat 1-1, 170 Lochee Road, Dundee DD2 2NH — MB ChB Dund. 1998; MB ChB Dund 1998.

SMITH, Russell Edward Ashleigh Good Hope Hospital, Rectory Road, Sutton Coldfield B75 7RR Tel: 0121 378 6188 Ext: 2370 Fax: 0121 378 6095; 8 Foxes Meadow, Walmley, Sutton Coldfield B76 1AW — MB BS Lond. 1984; FRCP; MRCP (UK) 1988; BSc (1st cl. Hons.) Lond. 1981, MD 1992. Cons. Phys. (Cardiol.) Good Hope Hosp. Sutton Coldfield; Hon. Cons. Univ. Hosp. Birm. Specialty: Cardiol. Socs: Fell. Roy. Soc. Med.; BMA; Brit. Cardiac Soc. Prev: Lect. & Hon. Sen. Regist. (Med. & Cardiol.) King's Coll. Sch. Med. & Dent. Lond.; Research Regist. (Cardiol.) Kings Coll. Hosp. Lond.; Regist. & SHO Rotat. (Med.) The Lond. Hosp.

SMITH, Ruth Alice Griffin House, Appledore Heath, Ashford TN26 2BA Tel: 01233 758564 — MB ChB Manch. 1976. GP Dymchurch. Prev: Clin. Med. Off. (Community Child Health) SE Kent HA.; Med. Off. Transkei Health Serv., SE Africa.; Community Med. Off. (Child Health) Camberwell HA.

SMITH, Sally Agnes Culver The Surgery, Highwood Road, Brockenhurst, Lymington SO41 7RY Tel: 01590 622272 Fax: 01590 624009; The Surgery, Station Road, Sway, Lymington SO41 6BA Tel: 01590 682617 Fax: 01590 682226 — MB ChB Glas. 1973; DObst RCOG 1975; MRCGP 1977. Hon. Clin. Lect. Soton. Univ. Med. Sch. Specialty: Gen. Pract. Prev: Trainee GP Glas. (S. Gen. Hosp.) VTS; Clin. Asst. (Geriat. Med.) Lymington Hosp.; Ho. Off. (Med.) & Ho. Off. (Surg.) South. Gen. Hosp. Glas.

SMITH, Sally Jane Manford Way Health Centre, 40 Foremark Close, Hainault, Ilford IG6 3HS Tel: 020 8500 3088 Fax: 020 8559 9355 — (Royal London Hospital Medical College) BSc Lond. 1986, MB BS 1989; MRCGP 1994. Hon. GP Tutor.

SMITH, Sally Megan 6 Cragg Terrace, Rawdon, Leeds LS19 6LF — MB ChB Leeds 1992; MRCGP 1996; MRCP (Paed.) 1998. Specialist Regist. St James Univ. Hosp. Leeds. Specialty: Paediat.

SMITH, Samantha Joanne The Coach House, Clevedon Road, Nailsea, Bristol BS48 1HA — BM Soton. 1995.

SMITH, Samuel David Coulter 10 Highgate Spinney, Crescent Road, London N8 8AR — MB BCh BAO NUI 1986; LRCPSI 1986.

SMITH, Samuel McCall (retired) Cornerstones, Oulston Road, Easingwold, York YO61 3PR Tel: 01347 823319 Fax: 01347 823319 — MB ChB Ed. 1950; DMRD 1958. Prev: Cons. Radiol. Peel Hosp. Galashiels.

SMITH, Samuel Peter Helsby Health Centre, Lower Robin Hood Lane, Helsby, Warrington WA6 0BW Tel: 01928 723676 Fax: 01928 725677 — MB Camb. 1978; BChir 1977.

SMITH, Sara Henry Lautch Centre, Bushey Fields Hospital, Bushey Fields Road, Dudley DY1 2LZ — MB ChB Liverp. 1994; BClinSci (Hons.) Liverp. 1993; MRCPsych 2000. Cons. Psychiat. Specialty: Gen. Psychiat. Prev: Specialist Regist. (Psychiat.), W. Midl.s Rotat.

SMITH, Sara Joanna 63 Park Street, Swinton, Manchester M27 4UN — MB ChB Leic. 1989.

SMITH, Sara Melody Linda Buchanan Llys Meddyg, Manthrig Lane, Caersws SY17 5EX Tel: 01686 688225 Fax: 01686 688344; CEFN, Trefeglwys, Caersws SY17 5QT Tel: 01686 430508 — BM Soton. 1980; DRCOG 1983; MRCGP 1984; DFFP 1994; Dip. Pract. Dermat. Wales 1996. Specialty: Dermat. Prev: Trainee GP E. Lond. VTS; Ho. Surg. Basingstoke Dist. Hosp.; Ho. Phys. Brook Gen. Hosp. Lond.

SMITH, Sarah Alexandra (retired) 2 River Row, Blowing House, Redruth TR15 3AT Tel: 01209 218555 — MB BS Lond. 1986.

SMITH, Sarah Alexandra 10 Blakebrook, Kidderminster DY11 6AP — MB BS Lond. 1998; MB BS Lond 1998.

SMITH, Sarah Ann Rhianfa, The Highway, Croesyceiliog, Cwmbran NP44 2HE — MB ChB Bristol 1998.

SMITH, Sarah Carolyn The Surgery, 10 Compayne Gardens, London NW6 3DH Tel: 020 7624 5883 Fax: 020 7328 8670; Flat 2, 17 Adamson Road, London NW3 3HU — MB BS Lond. 1986; DRCOG 1988; MRCGP 1990; T(GP) 1991.

SMITH, Sarah Catherine Dept. of Clinical Geratology, Radcliffe Infirmary, Woodstock Road, Oxford OX2 6HE — MB BS Lond. 1994 (St. Mary's Hosp. Med. Sch. Lond.) BSc Lond. 1990; MRCP Lond. 1997. Cons. (Geratology & Gen. Med.) Oxf. Radcliffe Hosps. Specialty: Care of the Elderly; Gen. Med. Prev: Specialist Regist. (Geratology & Gen. Med.) Oxf. Region; SHO Intens. Care Sussex Co. Hosp. Brighton.

SMITH, Sarah Jane Dr N R Williams and Partners, Egginton Road, Etwall, Derby DE65 6NB — MB ChB Leic. 1994 (Leicester) DCH 1996; DRCOG 1998; MRCGP 1998. GP Principal. Prev: GP non-Princip.

SMITH, Sarah Jane 50 Langdale Grove, Bingham, Nottingham NG13 8SS Email: sarahsmith@innotts.co.uk — MB BCh Wales 1993; MRCP (UK) 1997. Locum Grade (Paediat.) Grantham & Dist. Hosp. Specialty: Paediat. Prev: SHO (Paediat.) Community Paediat.; SHO (Paediat.) Qu. Med. Centre Nottm.

SMITH, Sarah Napier 10 Moorbank Close, Sheffield S10 5TP — MB ChB Bristol 1994; MRCP (Lond.) 1998. Med. SHO Roy. Devon & Exeter Healthcare Trust. Specialty: Gen. Med. Socs: BMA.

SMITH, Sarah Nicola Gloucester Road Medical Centre, Tramway House, 1a Church Road, Horfield, Bristol BS7 8SA — MB ChB Birm. 1992; DFFP 1995; DRCOG 1995; MRCGP 1998. GP Asst. Specialty: Gen. Pract. Prev: GP Asst. Norwich; GP Locum Northampton.

SMITH, Mrs Saraswati 32 Long Buftlers, Harpenden AL5 1JE Tel: 01582 761313 — MB BS Bihar 1958; MS Bihar 1963; MRCOG 1969; MFFP 1993. Sen. Med. Off. S. (Beds.) Health Dist.

SMITH, Scott Mackenzie 45 Colinhill Road, Strathaven ML10 6HF — MB ChB Aberd. 1996.

SMITH, Selwyn Trevor 23 Albion Avenue, Blackpool FY3 8NA Tel: 01253 38473 — MB ChB Manch. 1963.

SMITH, Sharon Janet Taverham Surgery, Sandy Lane, Taverham, Norwich NR8 6JR Tel: 01603 867481 Fax: 01603 740670 — MB BS Lond. 1980; DCH RCP Lond. 1986. Gen. Practitioner Clin. Med Off (Family Plann.).

SMITH, Sheila Gordon (retired) David Place Medical Practice, 56 David Place, St Helier, Jersey JE1 4HY Tel: 01534 33322; Glen Isla, Elizabeth Avenue, St Brelade, Jersey JE3 8G Tel: 01534 44083 — MB ChB Aberd. 1977. Prev: GP Jersey.

SMITH, Sheila Margaret 23 Dundonald Road, Kilmarnock KA1 1RU — MB ChB Glas. 1972. Paediat. (Child Protec.) Ayrsh. Specialty: Paediat. Prev: Clin. Med. Off. Community Child Health Ayrsh. Centr. Hosp. Irvine; Regist. (Med.) Kilmarnock Infirm.; SHO (Anaesth.) Glas. Roy. Infirm.

SMITH, Shelagh Jean MacSorley The National Hospital for Neurology & Neurosurgery, Department of Clinical Neurophysiology, Queen Square, London WC1N 3BG Tel: 020 7676 2039 Fax: 020 7713 7743 — MB ChB Birm. 1981; BSc Birm. 1978; MRCP (UK) 1984; FRCP Lond. 1995. Cons. Clin. Neurophysiol. Nat. Hosp. Lond., Nat. Soc. for Epilepsy & Chalfont Centre for Epilepsy Bucks. Specialty: Clin. Neurophysiol. Special Interest: EMG in obstetric brachial plexopathy; Investig. of epilepsy; Video EEG monitoring. Socs: (Counc.) Brit. Soc. Clin. Neurophysiol.; Assn. Brit. Neurol.; Assn. Brit. Clin. Neurophysiol. Prev: Sen. Regist. (Clin. Neurophysiol.) Nat. Hosp. Lond.

SMITH, Shubulade Mary Eniola 2E Abbeville Road, London SW4 9NJ Tel: 020 8673 7125; Institute of Psychiatry, 103 Denmark Hill, Camberwell, London SE5 8AZ — MB BS Lond. 1991 (Guy's Hospital) MRCPsych 1995. Research Fell. (Psychol. Med.) Inst. of Psychiat.) Lond.; Hon. Sen. Regist. Maudsley Hosp. Lond. Specialty: Gen. Psychiat. Prev: S. Thames Research Train. Fell. Inst. of Psychiat.; Hon. Sen. Regist.; Regist. Rotat. Maudsley Hosp.

SMITH, Simon Fordingbridge Surgery, Bartons Road, Fordingbridge SP6 1RS Tel: 01425 652123 Fax: 01425 654393 — MB BS Lond. 1987; MRCGP 1993; DRCOG 1994; DCH RCP Lond. 1994. Specialty: Gen. Pract. Socs: Wessex Educat.al Trust; BMA. Prev: Trainee GP Guildford VTS; Clin. Med. Off. Bournemouth Health Trust; Ho. Off. (Orthop. & Gen. Surg.) St. Stephens Hosp.

SMITH, Simon David Longton Hall Surgery, 186 Longton Hall Road, Blurton, Stoke-on-Trent ST3 2EJ Tel: 01782 342532; 2 Post Office Terrace, Fulford, Stoke-on-Trent ST11 9QS Email: simonsmith@talk21.com — MB BS Lond. 1990 (Lond. Hosp. Med. Coll.) BSc (1st cl. Hons.) Biochem. Lond. 1987; DRCOG 1992; MRCGP 1994; DFFP 1996. GP Stoke-on-Trent; Med. Off. Macmillan Hospice Stoke-on-Trent. Specialty: Gen. Pract.; Palliat. Med. Prev: Lect. (Primary Care) Univ. Soton.; Trainee GP/SHO Soton. VTS; Ho. Surg. Princess Margt. Hosp. Swindon.

SMITH, Simon Donald South Shropshire CMHT, 25 Corve Street, Ludlow SY8 1DA Tel: 01584 878167 Fax: 01584 878187 Email: simon.smith@shropcomm.wmids.nhs.uk — MB ChB (Hons.) Birm. 1987; MRCPsych 1991; MMedSci (Birm.) 1993. Cons. Adult Psychiat. Shrops. Co. PCT; Med. Director, Shrops. Co. PCT. Specialty: Gen. Psychiat. Prev: Cons. Psychiat. Shrops.'s Community & Ment. Health Servs. NHS Trust.

SMITH, Mr Simon Duncan 56 Buckingham Road, London E18 2NJ — MB ChB Aberd. 1985; FRCS Glas. 1989; FRCS (Orth.) 1997. Sen. Regist. (Orthop.) Norf. & Norwich Hosp. Specialty: Orthop. Prev: Sen. Regist. (Orthop.) Lond. Hosp.; Regist. Holly Hse. Hosp. Essex; Regist. (Orthop.) Bury St. Edmonds.

SMITH, Simon George Twyman 26 Ruthein Road, Blackheath, London SE3 7SH Tel: 020 8853 0308 Email: s.g.t.smith@ic.ac.uk — MB BS Lond. 1993 (St Marys) BSc (Hons.) Neurosci. Lond. 1990, MB BS 1993; FRCS Eng. 1997. Surg. Clin./Research Fell. (St Marys Minimal Access Surgic. Unit) Imperial Coll. Sch. of Med. St Marys

Hosp. Lond.; Specialist Regist. (Gen. Surg.) NW Thames. Specialty: Gen. Surg. Socs: Roy. Soc. Med.; Assn. Surg. Train. Prev: SHO Rotat. (Surg.) St Mary's Hosp. Lond.; Ho. Phys. Wexham Pk. Hosp. Slough; Ho. Surg. St Mary's Hosp. Lond.

SMITH, Simon Guy Weston Department of Pathology, Conquest Hospital, The Ridge, St Leonards-on-Sea TN37 7RD Tel: 01424 755255 — MB BChir Camb. 1983; MA Camb. 1983; FRCPath 2001; FRCP 2002. Cons. Haemat. Conquest Hosp. Hastings; Hon. Sen. Lect. (Med.) UMDS Lond. Specialty: Haematology. Prev: Lect. (Haemat.) UMDS St. Thos. Hosp. Lond.

SMITH, Simon Leslie The Ipswich Hospital NHS Trust, Department of Imaging, Heath Road, Ipswich IP4 5PD Email: simon.smith@ipsh-tr.anglox.nhs.uk; Wanda Cottage, Ipswich Road, Pettaugh, Ipswich IP14 6DN Tel: 01332 517016/01473 890844 Email: simonsmith@ukonline.co.uk — BM BS Nottm. 1991; BMedSci (Hons.) Nottm. 1989; MRCP (UK) 1995; FRCR 1998. Cons. Radiol. Specialty: Radiol. Prev: Regist. (Radiol.) Nottm. Univ. Hosps.; SHO Rotat. (Med.) Ipswich Hosp.

SMITH, Simon Paul Lanner Vean Barns, Porthleven, Helston TR13 0RQ — MB BS Lond. 1992.

SMITH, Mr Simon Robert Gray University Hospital Birmingham NHS Trust, Raddlebarn Road, Birmingham B29 6JD Tel: 0121 627 1627 Email: simon.smith@uhb.nhs.uk; 14 Barlows Road, Edgbaston, Birmingham B15 2PL — MB BS Lond. 1971 (St. Bart.) MRCS Eng. LRCP Lond. 1971; FRCS Eng. 1977; MS Lond. 1988. Cons. Surg. (Gen. & Vasc.) Univ. Hosp. Birm. NHS Trust; Hon. Cons. Surg. (Vasc.), B'ham Children's Hosp. Specialty: Gen. Surg. Socs: Vasc. Soc. GB & Irel.; Assn. Surg. Prev: Sen. Regist. St. Mary's Hosp. Lond.; Regist. Char. Cross Hosp. Lond.; Regist. St. Albans City Hosp.

SMITH, Simon Timothy Christmas Maltings Surgery, Camps Road, Haverhill CB9 8HF Tel: 01440 702203 Fax: 01440 712198 — MB BS Lond. 1980 (St. Thos.) BSc Lond. (Pharmacol.) 1977; FFA RCS Eng. 1985; DA (UK) 1985; DRCOG 1987; MRCGP 1988. Specialty: Anaesth.

SMITH, Stanley (retired) 15 Waxwell Lane, Pinner HA5 3EJ Tel: 020 8429 4316 — MB ChB Leeds 1942; MD Leeds 1947; FRCP Lond. 1968, M 1949; DPM Lond. 1951; FRCPsych 1971. Mem. (Ex-Chairm.) Lancs. HA. Prev: Med. Supt. Lancaster Moor Hosp.

SMITH, Stephanie Anne Paediatric Emergency Dept., University Hospital, Clifton Boulevard, Nottingham NG7 2UH Tel: 0115 924 9924 Email: stephanie.smith@mail.qmcuh-tr.trent.nhs.uk; Ashwick, 13 Shop Lane, Nether Heage, Belper DE56 2AR Tel: 01773 852482 Email: docsmithharvey@aol.com — BM BS Nottm. 1983; MRCP (UK) 1989. p/t Cons. Emerg. Paediat. Univ. Hosp. Nottm. Specialty: Paediat. Socs: FRCPCH; BAEM. Prev: Sen. Regist. & Regist. (Paediat.) Trent RHA.

SMITH, Stephanie Jane Evans Abington Park Surgery, Christchurch Medical Centre, Ardington Road, Northampton NN1 5LT Tel: 01604 630291 Fax: 01604 603524 — BM BCh Oxf. 1987; MA Camb. 1984; DRCOG 1989; MRCGP 1991.

SMITH, Stephen 7 Knowles Street, Widnes WA8 6QX — MB ChB Ed. 1996.

SMITH, Stephen Andrew Birmingham Heartlands and Solihull Hospital Trust, Bordesley Green East., Birmingham B9 5ST Tel: 0121 424 2156 Email: steve.smith@heartsol.wmids.nhs.uk; Vernon House, 26, Vernon Road, Edgbaston, Birmingham B16 9SH Tel: 0121 454 3411 — MB ChB Bristol 1978; MRCP (UK) 1981; MD Bristol 1989; FRCP 1997. Clin. Dir. Renal Servs. & Cons. Gen. Med. & Nephrol. Birm. Heartlands Hosp. Specialty: Nephrol. Special Interest: Provision of Haemodialysis facilities; Non dialysis care of ESRF. Socs: Pres. Brit. Renal Soc. Prev: Sen. Regist. (Nephrol.) St. Helier Hosp. Carshalton; Trav. Fell. Brit. Heart Found, Adelaide.

SMITH, Stephen Charles Department of Histopathology, Taunton and Somerset NHS Trust, Musgrove Park Hospital, Taunton TA1 5DA Tel: 01823 333444 — MB BS Lond. 1973 (London Hospital Medical College) BSc Lond. 1970, MB BS 1973; FRCPath 1994. Cons. Histopath. MusGr. Pk. Hosp. Taunton. Specialty: Histopath. Prev: Lect. (Path.) Med. Sch. Univ. Nottm.; Lect. (Human Morphol.) Med. Sch. Univ. Nottm.; Lect. (Anat.) Lond. Hosp. Med. Coll. Univ. Lond.

SMITH, Stephen Cullum 29 Joseph Conrad House, Tachbrook St, London SW1V 2NF — MB BS Lond. 1990; BSc 1987; MRCP 1995.

SMITH, Stephen Edward 38 Oakfield Gardens, Dulwich Wood Avenue, London SE19 1HQ — BM BCh Oxf. 1953; DA Eng. 1955; PhD Lond. 1960; MA Oxf. 1954, DM 1974. Socs: Brit. Pharm. Soc.; Roy. Soc. Med. Prev: Emerit. Prof. Applied Pharmacol. & Therap. Univ. Lond.; Resid. Anaesth., Ho. Phys. & Cas. Off. St. Thos. Hosp. Lond.

SMITH, Stephen John Astley Ainslie Hospital, 133 Grange Loan, Edinburgh EH9 2HL Fax: 0131 537 9030 Email: sj.smith@ipct.scot.nhs.uk — MB BCh Leeds 1977; BSc Hons 1974; MD 1981; FRCPE 2001. Cons. in Rehabil. Med. for NHS Lothian, in Edin.; Hons Clin. Tutor, Univ. of Edin. Specialty: Rehabil. Med. Special Interest: Brain Injury; MS; Spasticity Managem. Socs: Brit. Soc. of Rehabil. Med.; Scott. Soc. of Rehabil.; Soc. for research in Rehabil. Prev: Sen. Lect. in Rehabil. Med., Liverp. Univ.

SMITH, Professor Stephen Kevin University of Cambridge Clinical School, Department of Obstetrics & Gynaecology, The Rosie Maternity Hospital, Robinson Way, Cambridge CB2 2SW Tel: 01223 336871 Fax: 01223 248811 Email: sks1000@cam.ac.uk; 14 Hertford Street, Cambridge CB4 3AG Tel: 01223 357736 — MB BS Lond. 1974 (Westm.) F.I.Biol.; MRCS Eng. LRCP Lond. 1974; MRCOG 1979; MD Lond. 1983; MA Camb. 1993; FRCOG 1997. Prof. Dept. O & G Univ. Camb. Clin. Sch.; Hon. Cons. Obst. & Gyn. Addenbrooke's Hosp. Camb. Specialty: Obst. & Gyn. Socs: Eur. Assn. Obst. & Gyn. (Scientif. Comm.); FIGO; Euop. Soc. Human Reproduc. & Embryol. Prev: Cons. MRC Reproduc. Biol. Unit Centre for Reproduc. Biol. Edin.; Hon. Cons. Simpson Memor. Matern. Pavil. & Roy. Infirm. Edin.; Lect. (O & G) Univ. Sheff. & Jessop Hosp. Wom.

SMITH, Stephen Mark 58 Avenue Road, London N6 5DR — MB BS Newc. 1990; BMedSc. Newc. 1984; PhD Newc. 1987. SHO (Neurol.) Nat. Hosp. Neurol. Lond.

SMITH, Stephen Michael Vincent Windrush Health Centre, Welch Way, Witney OX28 6JS Tel: 01993 702911 Fax: 01993 700931 — MB BS Lond. 1990 (St. Barts) DRCOG 1994; MRCGP 1995; DFFP 1995. GP Partner. Specialty: Gen. Pract.

SMITH, Stephen Patrick 88 Station Road, Greenisland, Carrickfergus BT38 8UP — MB BCh BAO Belf. 1990; MB BCh Belf. 1990.

SMITH, Stephen Richard Torbay Hospital, Department of Haematology, Lawes Bridge, Torquay TQ2 7AA Tel: 01803 655236 Fax: 01803 655244 — MB ChB Liverp. 1982; MRCP (UK) 1985; MD Liverp. 1990; MRCPath 1993; FRCP 2000. Cons. Haemat. Torbay Hosp. S. Devon Healthcare. Specialty: Haematology. Prev: Sen. Regist. (Haemat.) Centr. Newc. Hosps.; Research Fell. MRRC Univ. Liverp.; Regist. (Haemat.) Roy. Liverp. Hosp.

SMITH, Stephen Rolf Horton General Hospital, Oxford Radcliffe NHS Hospitals Trust, Oxford Road, Banbury OX16 9AL Tel: 01295 275500 — MB ChB Birm. 1975 (Birmingham) MRCP (UK) 1978; BSc (Hons.) Birm. 1972, MD 1982; FRCP Lond. 1994. Cons. Phys. (Gen. & Respirat. Med.) Horton Gen. Hosp Oxf. Radcliffe NHS Hosp.s Trust. Specialty: Gen. Med. Prev: Sen. Regist. (Med.) Qu. Eliz. Hosp. Birm.

SMITH, Steven Evans (retired) Moorlands Friar's Gate, Crowborough TN6 1XF — BLitt, MA Oxf. 1946, BM BCh 1954.

SMITH, Steven Jonathan Croft Hall Medical Practice, 19 Croft Road, Torquay TQ2 5UA Tel: 01803 298441 Fax: 01803 296104 — MB ChB Manch. 1977.

SMITH, Steven Mark 2 Hepburn Gardens, Bromley BR2 7HL — MB BS Lond. 1984.

SMITH, Steven Michael — MB ChB Liverp. 1977; MRCGP 1985; T(GP) 1991. GP Locum. Specialty: Gen. Pract. Socs: BMA. Prev: Trainee GP Bury HA; Med. Off. Brit. Antarctic Survey Camb.

SMITH, Stuart Leslie Balintore Farmhouse, Kirkhill, Inverness IV5 7PX Tel: 01463 831337 Fax: 01463 831337 Email: stuartsmith@doctors.org.uk — MB ChB Aberd. 1991; MRCP (UK) Ed. 1995; DFFP 1997; DRCOG 1997; MRCGP 2000. GP non Princip.

SMITH, Mr Stuart Lindley 19 Chantrey's Drive, Elloughton, Brough HU15 1LH Tel: 01482 665660 Fax: 01482 665660 — BM BCh Oxf. 1975 (University of Oxford) MA Oxf. 1975; FRCS Eng. 1981. Cons. Dept. Otolaryngol. Roy. Hull. Hosps. Trust. Specialty: Otolaryngol. Prev: 1st Asst. Dept. Surg. Newc.; Regist. (ENT) Radcliffe Infirm. Oxf.; SHO (Neurosurg. & Accid.) Radcliffe Infirm. Oxf.

SMITH, Stuart Nicholas 161 Horbury Road, Wakefield WF2 8BG — MB BS Lond. 1985.

SMITH, Susan 52 Shaftesbury Road, Bournemouth BH8 8ST — BM Soton. 1985.

SMITH, Susan Elizabeth Nelson Health Centre, Cecil St., North Shields NE29 0DZ Tel: 0191 257 1191 — MB BS Newc. 1984; MRCGP 1988. GP N. Shields, Tyne & Wear Trainee GP Northumbria VTS.

SMITH, Susan Jane Norwich Road Surgery, 199 Norwich Road, Ipswich IP1 4BX Tel: 01473 289777 Fax: 01473 289545; 11 Tuddenham Road, Ipswich IP4 2SH Tel: 01473 258968 — BM BCh Oxf. 1986 (Oxford) MA Camb. 1986; MRCGP 1990. GP Trainer Ipswich.

SMITH, Susan Jane Amy Evans Centre, 190 Holton Road, Barry CF63 4HN Tel: 01446 420953; 3 Bryn Calch, Morganstown, Cardiff CF15 8FD Tel: 029 2084 4466 Email: suespaul@tinyworld.co.uk — MB BCh Wales 1988 (Univ. of Wales) MRCPsych 1993. Cons. Psychiat. (Gen. Adult & Perinatal Psychiat.) Cardiff & Vale NHS Trust. Specialty: Gen. Psychiat.

SMITH, Miss Susan Joy 1 St Thomas Street, London Bridge, London SE1 9RY Tel: 020 7403 3363 Fax: 020 7403 8552 — MB BS Lond. 1977 (St Mary's) MRCOG 1983. Dep. Med. Dir. Bridge Fertil. Centre Lond. Specialty: Obst. & Gyn.

SMITH, Susan Maree c/o 45 Ailesbury Road, Dublin 4, Republic of Ireland; 9 Grenfell Road, Didsbury, Manchester M20 6TG — MB BCh BAO Dub. 1987 (Trinity Coll. Dub.) MRCPI 1989; DCH RCPI 1990; MRCGP 1992; MSc (Econ.) Wales 1994. SHO (Palliat. Med.) St. Ann's Hospice Manch. Specialty: Gen. Pract.

SMITH, Susan Margaret 39 Egerton Road, Bishopston, Bristol BS7 8HN — MB ChB Liverp. 1991. Staff Grade (Psychiat. of the Elderly) Avonmead, Southmead Hosp. Bristol. Specialty: Gen. Psychiat.

SMITH, Susan Margaret St Pancras Hospital, Occupational Health Service, Ground Floor South Wing, 4 St Pancras Way, London NW1 0PE Tel: 020 7530 3450 Fax: 020 7530 3451 Email: sue.smith@camdenpct.nhs.uk; 63 Connaught Gardens, London N10 3LG Tel: 0208 444 9491 — MB BS Lond. 1976 (St. Bart.) BSc Lond. 1973; DCH Eng. 1978; AFOM RCP Lond. 1992. SCMO (Occupat. Health) Camden PCT. Specialty: Occupat. Health. Socs: BMA; Soc. Occupat. Med.; Fac. Occupat. Med. Prev: Clin. Asst. (Occupat. Health) Islington HA; Clin. Med. Off. (Family Plann.) Haringey HA; SHO (Paediat.) St. Stephen's Hosp. Lond.

SMITH, Susan Mary Durrington Health Centre, Durrington Lane, Worthing BN13 2RX Tel: 01903 264151 — MB BCh Wales 1975. Cons. Family Plann. & Reproduc. Health Care Worthing. Specialty: Family Plann. & Reproduc. Health; Psychosexual Med. Socs: Fac. Fam. Plann. & Reproduc. Health Care; Inst. Psychosexual Med.

SMITH, Susan Penelope Anaesthetic Department, Cheltenham General Hospital, Sandford Road, Cheltenham GL53 7AN Tel: 01242 274143 Fax: 01242 273405 Email: susan.smith@egnhst.org.uk — MB BS Lond. 1980; BSc Lond. 1977; FFA RCS Eng. 1985; MRCP (UK) 1985; FRCP 1999. Cons. Anaesth. & Dir. Intens. Care Cheltenham Gen. Hosp. Specialty: Anaesth.; Intens. Care. Prev: Gen. Profess. Train. (Anaesth.) Guys & Lewisham Hosps. Lond.; Sen. Regist. (Anaesth. & Intens. Care) Reading & Oxf.

SMITH, Sydney 1 Bowgreen Mews, Bowgreen Road, Bowdon, Altrincham WA14 3LX Tel: 0161 941 1632 — MB BCh BAO Belf. 1943; MRCGP 1952. Exam. Med. Off. Min. of Pens. & Nat. Insur. Prev: Hosp. Pract. (Surg.) Withington Hosp. Manch.; Res. Surg. Off. Eccles & Patricroft Hosp.; Ho. Phys. & Cas. Off. Vict. Memor. Jewish Hosp. Manch.

SMITH, Sydney James (retired) 1 Keble Close, Bishopthorpe, York YO23 2TE Tel: 01904 704787 — (Char. Cross) MRCS Eng. LRCP Lond. 1943. Prev: Ho. Surg. Char. Cross Hosp.

SMITH, Tanya Lillipot Surgery, Elmj Avenue, Poole BH14 8EE Tel: 01202 739122; Elysian, Wimborne Road, Lytchett Matravers, Poole BH16 6DH Tel: 01202 624352 — BM Soton. 1986 (Southampton) MRCGP 1994; Dip. Of Pall. Med. 1998. GP Lillipot Poole Dorset. Specialty: Gen. Pract.; Cardiol.; Oncol. Prev: Med. Off. Joseph Weld Hospice Dorchester; GP BRd.stone. Poole.

SMITH, Tasha Judine 38 Granada Close, Waterlooville PO8 9AU — BM Soton. 1997.

SMITH, Thomas Connal Gemmell The Croft, Poundland, Pinwherry, Girvan KA26 0RU Tel: 01465 841643 Fax: 01465 841643 — (Birm.) MB ChB Birm. 1962; Dip. Pharm. Med. RCP (UK) 1976. Med. Jl.ist Columnist Sunday Mail, Bradford Telegraph, Argus & The News Portsmouth; Adviser Jl. Dist. Nursing. Specialty: Pharmaceutical Medicine. Socs: BMA; Med. Jl.ists Assn. Prev: Ho. Surg. & Ho. Phys. Dudley Rd. Hosp. Birm.; Ho. Phys. Childr. Hosp. Birm.

SMITH, Thomas John Tyndall Top Floor Flat, 18 Bellevue, Bristol BS8 1DB — MB ChB Bristol 1995.

SMITH, Thomas Keith 23 Meadway, Liverpool L15 7LY — MB ChB Liverp. 1986.

SMITH, Thomas Scott 2 Little Hame, Milton Keynes Village, Milton Keynes MK10 9AN — MB BS Lond. 1998; MB BS Lond 1998.

SMITH, Mr Thomas William David Cleveland House, 3 Whitworth Road, Sheffield S10 3HD Tel: 0114 230 8398 Fax: 0114 230 9091 Email: t.w.smith@sheffield.ac.uk — MB Camb. 1964 (Camb. & St. Mary's) BChir 1963; MA MB (Distinc. Pharm. & Therap.) Camb. 1964; FRCS Ed. 1967; FRCS Eng. 1968. p/t Cons. Orthop. Surg. N. Gen. Hosp. & Sheff. Childs. Hosp. NHS Trusts; Exec. Edr. The Foot; Edr. Foot & Ankle Surg.; Hon. Sen. Lect. Univ. of Sheff. Specialty: Orthop. Socs: Fell. BOA; S. Yorks. Medico-Legal Soc. (Ex-Pres.); Brit. Orthopaedic Foot Surgic. Soc. (Ex-Pres.). Prev: Sen. Regist. (Orthop. Surg.) United Sheff. Hosps. & Sheff. RHB; Regist. (Orthop.) Nuffield Orthop. Centre Oxf.; Ho. Surg. & Cas. Surg. St. Mary's Hosp. Lond.

SMITH, Timothy Charles Department of Anaesthesia, Alexandra Hospital, Woodrow Drive, Redditch B98 7UB — MB ChB Birm. 1984; FRCA 1989; MD Birm. 1994. Cons. Anaesth. Alexandra Hosp. Redditch. Specialty: Anaesth.

SMITH, Timothy David Department of Anaesthetics, Royal Gwent Hospital, Newport NP20 2UB — MB BCh Wales 1994.

SMITH, Timothy Donald Weston Latham House Medical Practice, Sage Cross Street, Melton Mowbray LE13 1NX Tel: 01664 854949 Fax: 01664 501825 — MB ChB Birm. 1975; DRCOG 1977; MRCGP 1980. GP Melton Mowbray; Lect. (Community Med.) Univ. Leicester.

SMITH, Timothy Gervase Cloudesley (retired) Streams, West Kington, nr. Chippenham, Chippenham SN14 7SE — MB BS Lond. 1968 (St. Bart.) MRCS Eng. LRCP Lond. 1968; DObst RCOG 1970; DA Eng. 1972; FFA RCS Eng. 1974. Cons. (Anaesth.) Roy. Berks. Hosp. Reading.

SMITH, Timothy James Scott Top Floor Flat, 1 Albyn Place, Edinburgh EH2 4NG — MB ChB Ed. 1996.

SMITH, Tracey Glen Dr H. J. Dobson & Partners, Mere House, West Avenue, Weston, Crewe CW2 5LY Tel: 01270 582685; 4 Millacre Drive, Wistaston, Crewe CW2 6XG Tel: 01270 668195 — MB ChB Dundee 1988 (Univ. Dundee) Specialty: Gen. Pract. Prev: GP Regist. Chesh.; Trainee GP/SHO (Geriat.) Leighton Hosp. Crewe VTS.

SMITH, Tracy Amanda Smith, Niemczuk, Puuirajasingham, 279-281 Mill Road, Cambridge CB1 3DG Tel: 01223 247812 Fax: 01223 214191; Hope Cottage, 10 Brook Lane, Coton, Cambridge CB3 7PY Tel: 01223 211183 — MB BS Lond. 1983 (St. Mary's Hosp.)

SMITH, Trevor 14 Longlands Glade, Worthing BN14 9NR — BChir Camb. 1958; MA Camb. 1960, BChir 1958, MB 1959; DPM Eng. 1960; MFHom 1975. Cons. Phys. Winchester Clinic Winchester. Specialty: Gen. Med. Socs: Fac. Homoeop.; Brit. Homoeop. Assn. Prev: Sen. Regist. Tavistock Clinic.

SMITH, Trevor Allan PMI Health Group, The Courtyard, Hall Lane, Wincham, Northwich CW9 6DG Tel: 01606 354089 Fax: 01606 351330 — MB ChB Manch. 1978; BSc St And. 1975; MRCP 1981; AFOM Lond. 1984; MFOM Lond. 1986; FFOM RCP Lond. 2000; FRCP Lond. 2001. Specialty: Occupat. Health. Prev: Chief Med. Off. Rank Hovis McDougall Ltd; Div. Med. Off. Fisons Pharmaceut. Div. Loughboro.; Sen. Med. Off. Brit. Steel Corpn. Tubes Div. Corby.

SMITH, Ursula Magdalena (retired) 26 Metchley Park Road, Edgbaston, Birmingham B15 2PG Tel: 0121 454 6538 — (Bonn) MD Bonn. 1952; DA Eng. 1957; LAH Dub. 1958.

SMITH, Valerie Mary Elmhurst Surgery, Elmhurst Road, Aylesbury HP20 2AH Tel: 01296 431515 Fax: 01296 399597 — MB BS Lond. 1973; DObst RCOG 1975; DCH Eng. 1976.

SMITH, Vaughan Pearson 41 Peile Drive, Taunton TA2 7SZ Tel: 01823 353061 Email: vsmith1951@aol.com — BM BCh Oxf. 1975 (Oxford) BA (1st cl. Hons.) Oxf. 1972; MA Oxf. 1977; MRCGP 1978; DCH Eng. 1978; FRCGP 1993; DMS Med. Soc. Apoth. Lond.

1994; MLCOM 1994; MSc (Distinc.) Lond. 2001. Freelance GP; Registered Osteop. Som.; Lect. (Osteop.) Oxf. Brookes Univ. Specialty: Gen. Pract.; Osteop.; Acupunc. Special Interest: Musculoskeletal Med.; Osteopathy; Acupunc. Socs: Fell. Roy. Soc. Med.; Soc. Orthop. Med.; Brit. Med. Acupunct. Soc. Prev: Trainee GP Gt. Yarmouth VTS.

SMITH, Vaughn Leslie The Priory Hospital, Rappax Road, Hale, Altrincham WA15 0NX Tel: 0616 904 0050; 15 Yoxall Avenue, Hartshill, Stoke-on-Trent ST4 7JJ Tel: 01782 44692 — MB ChB Birm. 1971. Clin. Asst. Altringham Priory Hosp. Specialty: Alcohol & Substance Misuse; Gen. Psychiat.

SMITH, Vernon (retired) 34 Springkell Avenue, Glasgow G41 4AB Tel: 0141 423 1968 Email: v.smith@btinternet.com — (Leeds) MB ChB Leeds 1941. Prev: GP Glas.

SMITH, Victoria Clair Flat 48, Queens Court, Queens Road, Richmond TW10 6LB — MB BS Lond. 1992.

SMITH, Victoria Helen Hillcrest, Booth Road, Waterfoot, Rossendale BB4 9BP — MB ChB Birm. 1998.

SMITH, Victoria Jane Hawthorn Cottage, Seven Sisters Lane, Ollerton, Knutsford WA16 8RL — MB ChB Liverp. 1983.

SMITH, Victoria Jane Department of Psychiatry, Rannsle Building, Mancester Royal Infirmary, Hathersage Road, Manchester M13 9WL; 43 Austin Drive, Manchester M20 6FA — MB BCh Wales 1992.

***SMITH, Warren Emerson David** 196 Cambridge Road, Great Shelford, Cambridge CB2 5JU Tel: 01223 841529 — BChir Camb. 1991.

SMITH, Wayne Richard (retired) 9 Harding Road, Abingdon OX14 1SF Tel: 01235 521994 — (King's Coll. Hosp.) BSc (Hons) Lond. 1967; MB BS Lond. 1970; MRCS Eng. LRCP Lond. 1970; Cert. Family Plann. JCC 1973; DObst RCOG 1973; MRCGP 1975. Prev: SHO (Psychol. Med.) Guy's Hosp. Lond.

SMITH, Professor William Cairns Stewart Department of Public Health Medical School, Foresterhill, Aberdeen AB25 2ZD Tel: 01224 553802 Fax: 01224 550925 Email: w.c.s.smith@abdn.ac.uk — MB ChB Aberd. 1974; MFCM 1982; MPH Dundee 1982; MD Aberd. 1986; FFPHM RCP (UK) 1989; PhD Dundee 1990; FRCP Ed. 1992. Prof. (Pub. Health) Aberd.; Hon. Cons. Pub. Health Med. Grampian HB. Prev: Assoc. Prof. Nat. Univ. Singapore; Epidemiol. (Cardiovasc. Epidemiol. Unit) Dundee Univ.; Sen. Regist. (Community Med.) Tayside HB.

SMITH, William Cletus Bridge Medical Centre, Wassand Close, Three Bridges Road, Crawley RH10 1LL Tel: 01293 526025 — MB BS Lond. 1963; DObst RCOG 1965.

SMITH, William Denis Ashley, OBE (retired) 11 Moorland Drive, Leeds LS17 6JP Tel: 0113 268 4220 — MB BS Lond. 1952 (St. Mary's) DA Eng. 1956; FFA RCS Eng. 1961; MD Lond. 1969. Prev: Reader (Anaesth.) Leeds Univ.

SMITH, William Duncan (retired) 7 Adelaide Terrace, Dundee DD3 6HW Tel: 01382 225880 — MB ChB St. And. 1956; DObst RCOG 1958; MRCGP 1965. Prev: GP Dundee.

SMITH, Rev. William Ernest 3 Inglenook, East Keswick, Leeds LS17 9EU — MRCS Eng. LRCP Lond. 1944 (Leeds) MA (Hnrs. Philos.) Leeds 1934. Med. Off. Barnbow Ordnance Fact. Leeds. Socs: Leeds Regional Psychiat . Assn. Prev: Res. Med. Off. Pontefract Gen. Infirm.

SMITH, William Gerard St. Ann's Hospital, St Ann's Road, London N15 3TH Tel: 0208 442 6455 Ext: 6000 Fax: 0208 442 6354 — MB ChB Cape Town 1969; FRCPsych 1975; DPM Eng. 1975; MRCPsych 1976. Cons. Crisis Assessments and Home Treatments; Hon. Sen. Lect. Roy. Free Med. Sch.; Dir. Med. Educat. St. Geo. Grenada W. I. Specialty: Gen. Psychiat. Prev: Cons. Psychiat., 22 years, St. Anne Hosp., Gen. Adult Psychiat.

SMITH, William Homer Bedruthran House, The Royal Cornwall Hospital, Truro TR1 3LJ — MB BS Lond. 1970 (Guy's) MRCS Eng. LRCP Lond. 1970; DMRD Eng. 1974; FRCR 1977. Cons. Radiol. Roy. Cornw. Hosp.; Med. Dir. Roy. Cornw. Hosp., Truro. Specialty: Radiol. Prev: Cons. Radiol. RAF Hosp. Ely; Cons. Advisor Radiol. to RAF; Cons. Radiol. RAF Hosp. Nocton Hall Lincoln.

SMITH, William Homer (retired) Tanglin, Meavy Lane, Yelverton PL20 6AP Tel: 01822 852851 — MB BS Lond. 1943 (Guy's) MRCS Eng. LRCP Lond. 1943; DMRD Eng. 1950. Prev: Cons. Radiol. Plymouth HA.

SMITH, William Howard Thornton 373 Ring Road, Moortown, Leeds LS17 8NP Email: medws@leeds.ac.uk — MB BChir Camb. 1994 (Addenbrooke's Cambridge) MA Camb. 1995, BA 1991, MB BChir 1994; MRCP 1996. Research Fell. Inst. for Cardiovasc. Research Univ. of Leeds. Specialty: Cardiol.

SMITH, William Marcus Victor Pepper Arden Hall, Pepper Arden, Northallerton DL7 0JF Tel: 01325 378548; Pepper Arden Hall, Pepper Arden, Northallerton DL7 0JF Tel: 01325 378548 — MB BS Lond. 1969 (Lond. Hosp.) MRCGP 1974. Locum GP.

SMITH, William Merson 11 Bankside Close, Upper Poppleton, York YO26 6LH Tel: 01904 790307 — (Aberd.) MB ChB Aberd. 1969; MRCGP 1977. Sen. Medico-Legal Adviser Med. Protec. Soc., Leeds.

SMITH, Mr William Philip Maxillofacial Unit, Northampton General Hospital, Northampton NN1 5BD Tel: 01604 544579; Maxillofacial Unit, Kettering General Hospital, Kettering NN16 8UZ Tel: 01536 492597 — MB BS Lond. 1987 (The London Hospital) BDS (Hons.) Bristol 1980; FDS RCS Eng. 1985; FRCS Eng. 1997, Ed. 1990. Cons. Maxillofacial Surg. Northampton & Kettering Gen. Hosp. NHS Trust. Specialty: Oral & Maxillofacial Surg. Socs: Fell. Brit. Assn. Oral & Maxillofacial Surg. Prev: Sen. Regist. (Oral & Maxillofacial Surg.) Roy. Surrey Co. Hosp. Guildford; Regist. (Oral & Maxillofacial Surg.) Poole Gen. Hosp.; SHO (A & E, Med & Orthop.) St. Richards Hosp. Chichester.

SMITH, William Russell The Medical Centre, 7 Hill Place, Arbroath DD11 1AE Tel: 01241 431144 Fax: 01241 430764 — MB ChB Glas. 1973; DObst RCOG 1976; MRCGP 1977.

SMITH, William Thomas Malcolm Lour Road Group Practice, 3 Lour Road, Forfar DD8 2AS Tel: 01307 463122 Fax: 01307 465278; Kisimul, Welton Corner, Kingsmuir Road, Forfar DD8 2RQ — MB ChB Ed. 1978; BSc Ed. 1975, MB ChB 1978; DRCOG 1982; MRCGP 1983.

SMITH, Yuriko 26 Strath, Gairloch IV21 2DA — MB ChB Liverp. 1996.

SMITH, Yvette Louisa Osmond South Hermitage Medical Practice, Belle Vue, Shrewsbury SY3 7JS Tel: 01743 343148 — MB BS Lond. 1987; DGM RCP Lond. 1989; MRCGP 1991.

SMITH-HOWELL, Michael Arnold 5A Norton Road, Loddon, Norwich NR14 6JN — MB ChB Leic. 1995.

SMITH-LAING, Gray Farthing Green Farm, New Barn Road, Hawkenbury, Staplehurst, Tonbridge TN12 0EE — MB BS Lond. 1973; MRCP (UK) 1975; MD Lond. 1983; FRCP Lond. 1993. Cons. Phys. & Gastroenterol. Medway Hosp. Gillingham. Specialty: Gastroenterol. Prev: Sen. Regist. (Gastroenterol.) St. Mary's Hosp. Lond.; Research Fell. Med. Unit Roy. Free Hosp. Lond.

SMITH-MOORHOUSE, Grahame Peter Holme House, Luddenden, Halifax HX2 6TG Tel: 01422 842333 — MB ChB Leeds 1969.

SMITH-STANLEIGH, Pamela Field House, Field House Drive, Meole Brace, Shrewsbury SY3 9HL — BM BCh Oxf. 1973.

SMITH-WALKER, Malcolm Thomas South Meadow Surgery, 3 Church Close, Eton, Windsor SL4 6AP Tel: 01753 833777 Fax: 01753 833689; Bucks, 25 York Road, Windsor SL4 3NX Tel: 01753 833372 Fax: 01753 833372 — MB BS Lond. 1966 (St. Bart.) MRCS Eng. LRCP Lond. 1965; DObst RCOG 1969. Socs: Windsor Dist. Med. Soc.; Assoc. Mem. Brit. Med. Acupunc. Soc.; Fell.The Roy. Soc. Med.

SMITHARD, David Graeme Health Care of Older People,, William Harvey Hospital, Kennington Road, Ashford TN24 0LZ Tel: 01233 632331 Fax: 01233 616222 — MB BS Lond. 1986 (Roy. Lond. Hosp. Med. Coll.) BSc (Biochem.) Lond. 1983; MRCP (UK) 1989; MD Lond. 1997; FRCP 1998. Cons. Phys. (Elderly & Stroke Med.) E. Kent Hosp.; Vis. Lect. Roehampton Inst.; Dir. Of Research & Dev., E. Kent Hosp. Specialty: Care of the Elderly. Socs: Brit. Geriat. Soc.; BMA; Brit. Assoc. Stroke Phys. Prev: Cons. Phys. (Elderly & Stroke Med.) Qu. Mary's Sidcup; Sen. Regist. (Geriat. & Gen. Med.) St. Thos, Hosp. Lond.; Regist. (Geriat. Med.) Univ. Hosp. S. Manch.

SMITHARD, David John Renal Unit, Birch Hill Hospital, Rochdale OL12 9QB Tel: 01706 754673 Fax: 01706 754388 Email: dr.smithard@pat.nhs.uk — MB ChB 1970; MRCP (UK) 1974; MD 1980; FRCP Lond. 1991. Cons. Renal Phys., Pennine Acute Hosps. NHS Trust. Specialty: Nephrol. Special Interest: Diabetic Nephropathy. Socs: Internat. Soc. Peritoneal Dialysis; Europ. Renal Assn. Prev: Sen. Regist. (Med.) Manch. AHA; Research Fell. (Med.) Dept. Therap. Univ. Nottm.; Regist. (Med.) Glas. Roy. Infirm.

SMITHERS, Andrew John Bennetts Road North Surgery, 2 Bennetts Road North, Keresley End, Coventry CV7 8LA Tel: 024

7633 2636 Fax: 024 7633 7353; Fradley, Tamworth Road, Corley, Coventry CV7 8BX — MB BS Lond. 1984 (St. Bart.) Cert. Family Plann. JCC 1989. Network Co-ordinator Profiad Ltd. Socs: Brit. Menopause Soc.; ACRPI. Prev: SHO (Psychiat.) Centr. Hosp.; SHO (O & G) Warnford Hosp.; Trainee GP Bertie Rd. Surg. Kenilworth VTS.

SMITHERS, Deborah Anne Back O November, Donkey Lane, Burton, Bradstock, Bridport DT6 4QB — MB ChB Liverp. 1990; MRCP CH 1999. Specialist Regist. (Paediat.) W. Sussex Rotat. Specialty: Paediat. Prev: PICU Fell. Bristol Childr.s Hosp.

SMITHIES, Alison, OBE 1 De Vaux Place, Salisbury SP1 2SJ Tel: 01722 329505 — MB BS Lond. 1954 (Univ. Coll. Hosp.) DObst RCOG 1956; MD Lond. 1977; FRCPath 1988. Socs: Fell. Roy. Soc. Med. Prev: Regional Cons. Primary Med. Care Wessex RHA; Princip. Med. Off. DoH; Med. Asst. (Cytol.) Northwick Pk. Hosp. Harrow.

SMITHIES, Joan Mary Agnes 3 Silverdale Road, Southampton SO15 2NG — MB BS Lond. 1977; MRCS Eng. LRCP Lond. 1977; MRCPsych 1984; DGM RCP Lond. 1985. Sen. Regist. (Psychogeriat.) Moorgreen Hosp. Soton. Specialty: Geriat. Psychiat. Prev: Regist. (Psychiat.) Roy. S. Hants. Hosp.

SMITHIES, Mark Nicholas University Hospital of Wales, Heath Park, Cardiff CF14 4XW Tel: 029 2074 3084 Fax: 029 2074 3799; 34 Lake Road E., Roath Park, Cardiff CF23 5NN — MB BS Lond. 1981; MRCP (UK) 1984. Dir. Intens. Care Univ. Hosp. Wales Cardiff; Clin. Director, Critical Care, Cardiff NHS Trust. Specialty: Intens. Care. Prev: Cons. Intens. Care Guy's Hosp. Lond.

SMITHSON, Carolyn Jane 25 Seagers, Hall Road, Great Totham, Maldon CM9 8PB — MB ChB Sheff. 1998; MB ChB Sheff 1998.

SMITHSON, Donald Laurence Carisbrooke, 625 Dawsheath Road, Hadleigh, Benfleet SS7 2NH Tel: 01702 559056 — MB BS Lond. 1954 (Guy's) MRCS Eng. LRCP Lond. 1954. Prev: Orthop. Ho. Surg. Guy's Hosp.; Paediat. Ho. Phys. & O & G Ho. Surg. FarnBoro. Hosp.

SMITHSON, Edel Frances 8 St Patricks Av, Weymouth DT4 9EQ — MB BCh Wales 1997.

SMITHSON, Jacquelyn Anne Jane Department of Gastroenterology, Hull Royal Infirmary, Anlaby Road, Hull HU3 2JZ Tel: 01482 674862 Fax: 01482 675033 — MB BS Lond. 1987; MRCP (UK) 1992; FRCP 2000. Cons. and Sen. Lecuturer, Hull Roy. Infirm. Specialty: Gastroenterol. Prev: Sen. Regist. (Gastroenterol. & Gen. Med.) Hull Roy. Infirm.; Research Fell. (Gastroenterol. & HIV) Chelsea & Westm. Hosp. Lond.; Regist. (Gen. & AIDS Med.) Westm. Hosp. Lond.

SMITHSON, John Edmund Southmead Hospital, Department of Medicine, Bristol BS10 5NB Tel: 0117 959 5369 Email: johnesmithson@aol.com — MB ChB Bristol 1986; BSc (Hons. 1st cl. Anat.) Bristol 1983, MB ChB 1986; MRCP (UK) 1989; MD Bristol 1995. Cons. Phys. and Gastroenterologist N. Bristol NHS Trust. Specialty: Gastroenterol.; Gen. Med. Prev: Regist. (Gen. Med.) Southmead Hosp. Bristol; SHO Nat. Heart & Chest Hosps.; Ho. Off. Profess. Units of Med. & Surg. Bristol Roy. Infirm.

SMITHSON, Jonathan Michael 2 Yeo Vale Road, Barnstaple EX32 7AB Tel: 01271 321548 — MB ChB Liverp. 1996 (L'pool) Dip. Trop Med. & Hyg 1997. Specialty: Accid. & Emerg.

SMITHSON, Nicola 40 Clopton Gardens, Hadleigh, Ipswich IP7 5JG — MB ChB Birm. 1993; BSc (Hons.) Birm. 1992; MB ChB (Hons.) Birm. 1993. Prev: Ho. Off. (Med.) Selly Oak Hosp. Birm.; Ho. Off. (Surg.) Heartlands Hosp. Birm.

SMITHSON, Nicola Jane 3 West Preston Street (Flat 2F1), Newington, Edinburgh EH8 9PX — MB ChB Ed. 1996.

SMITHSON, Philippa District Health Centre, Palmalmal Pomio District, East New Britain, Papua New Guinea; 1 Beech Avenue, Northenden, Manchester M22 4JE — MB ChB Liverp. 1994 (Univ. Liverp.) Dip of Tropical Medicine and Hygiene (DTM&H), University of Liverpool, DEC, 1998; MRCEP, 1998. Specialty: Gen. Pract. Prev: GP Regist., Lancaster.

SMITHSON, Richard David Western Health & Social Services Board, 15 Gransha Park, Clooney Road, Londonderry BT47 1TG — MB ChB Birm. 1981; MFPHM 1989. Cons. Communicable Dis. Control & Pub. Health Med. WHSSB. Specialty: Pub. Health Med.

SMITHSON, Sarah Elizabeth The Robert Darbishire Practice, Rusholme Health Centre, Walmer Street, Manchester M14 5NP Tel: 0151 236 4620 — MB BChir Camb. 1989; MRCP (UK) 1993; MRCGP 1995. Assoc. GP (Primary Care Initiative) NW RHA.

SMITHSON, Sarah Francesca St Michael's Hospital, Department of Genetics, Southwell Street, Bristol BS2 8EG Tel: 0117 928 5653; 5 York Gardens, Clifton, Bristol BS8 4LL Tel: 0117 317 9447 — MB ChB Bristol 1986; BSc Bristol 1983; DCH RCP Lond. 1988; MRCP (UK) 1989; MD Bristol 1996. Cons. (Clin. Genetics) & Hon. Sen. Lect. in Clin. Genetics. Specialty: Genetics. Special Interest: Dysmorphology. Socs: Clin. Genetics Soc.; Brit. Soc. Clin. Genetics; Skeletal Dispatia Gp. for Teachg. Research. Prev: Sen. Regist. (Clin.. Genetics) Gt. Ormond St. Hosp; Research Fell. In Genetics, Oxf.; Regist. in Clin. Genetics, Oxf.

SMITHSON, Simon Richard Pallion Health Centre, Hylton Road, Sunderland SR4 7XF Tel: 0191 567 4673; 24 Underhill Road, Cleadon, Sunderland SR6 7RS — MB BS Newc. 1980; DRCOG 1983; MRCGP 1984. Prev: Trainee GP N.ld. VTS.

SMITHSON, William Henry The Surgery, Escrick, York YO4 19LE Tel: 01904 728243 Fax: 01904 728826 Email: henry.smithson@gp-B82018.nhs.uk — MB ChB Dundee 1976 (Univ. of Dundee) DRCOG 1980; FRCGP 1997, M 1985; MSc 2000. Princip. GP; Hon. Sen. Clin. Lect. Hull York Med. Sch.; GP Trainer York GP VTS. Specialty: Gen. Pract. Prev: RCGP/NSE P. of Wales Educat. Fell. in Epilepsy 1996-98.

SMITHURST, Helen Jane 5 Buck Lane, Ashton on Mersey, Sale M33 5WF — MB ChB Birm. 1989; MRCP (UK) 1993. Regist. Rotat. (Diabetes & Endocrinol.) Trafford Pk. Manch. Specialty: Gen. Med. Prev: Regist. (Med., Diabetes & Endocrinol.) Wythenshawe Hosp. Manch.; Regist. (Endocrinol.) Hope Hosp. Salford.

SMITS, Margaretha Maria Englefield House, 23 Highgale High Street, London N6 3ST — MD Copenhagen 1983. GP Lond.

SMOLLETT, Margaret Amelia Newton Craig, 99 Ayr Road, Prestwick KA9 1TF Tel: 01292 78166 — MB ChB Glas. 1977.

SMOUT, Arthur John Russell (retired) Little Baileys, 57 Henwood Green Road, Pembury, Tunbridge Wells TN2 4LH Tel: 01892 822031 — MB ChB Birm. 1958; DA Eng. 1968. Prev: Clin. Asst. (Psychogeriat.) Hastings HA & (Ment. Health for Elderly) St. Helens Hosp. Hastings.

SMOUT, Susan Mary Stonelands, 2 South Road, Newton Abbot TQ12 1HL — MB BS Lond. 1987.

SMULDERS, Thomas Cornelis MEDACS Professional Recruitment plc, High Street House, New Market St., Skipton BD23 2HU — Artsexamen Amsterdam 1993.

SMURTHWAITE, Glyn Jonathon Folly Bank Farm, Goodshaw Lane, Rossendale BB4 8DW — MB ChB Leeds 1985; BSc (Hons.) Leeds 1982; DA (UK) 1988; FFA RCSI 1991; FRCA 1992. Cons. Anaesth. Hope Hosp. Univ. Manch. Specialty: Anaesth. Prev: Sen. Regist. (Anaesth.) NW RHA.

SMURTHWAITE, William Aston, MC (retired) 6 Normandy Court, West Parade, Worthing BN11 3QY Tel: 01903 230304 — (St. Thos.) MRCS Eng. LRCP Lond. 1942; DMRD Eng. 1963; MB BS Lond. 1964; FRACR 1987, M 1968; FFR 1968; MRACR 1968; FRCR 1975. Prev: Regist. (Radiol.) Westm. Hosp. Lond.

SMYE, Richard Anthony Somerville Medical Practice, 64 Gorsey Lane, Wallasey CH44 4AA Tel: 0151 638 9333 Fax: 0151 637 0291; 41 Gayton Road, Lower Heswall, Wirral CH60 8QE — MB ChB Liverp. 1981.

SMYK, Darren The Family Practice, Western College, Cotham Road, Bristol BS6 6DF Tel: 0117 946 6455 Fax: 0117 946 6410 — MB ChB Bristol 1990.

SMYLIE, Ann Hillsborough Medical Practice, Hillsborough Health Centre, Ballynahinch Street, Hillsborough BT26 6AW Tel: 028 9268 2216 Fax: 028 9268 9721 — MB BCh BAO Belf. 1969; DObst RCOG 1971; DCH RCPSI 1972; FRCGP 1991, M 1974. Specialty: Occupat. Health. Socs: Ulster Med. Soc.; Soc. Occupat. Med.

SMYLIE, Carol Anne The Dower House, Chestnut Lea, Mont A L'Abbe, St Helier, Jersey JE2 3HA — MB BS Lond. 1982.

SMYLLIE, Hugh Curle (retired) 30 Whin Hill Road, Bessacarr, Doncaster DN4 7AF Tel: 01302 535673 — MB BS Lond. 1950 (King's Coll. Hosp.) FRCP Lond 1972, M 1953; MD Lond. 1959. Prev: Cons. Phys. with Special Duties in Chest Dis. Doncaster Roy. Infirm.

SMYLLIE, John Hugh Dewsbury District Hospital, Healds Road, Dewsbury WF13 4HS Tel: 01924 816179 — MB BS Lond. 1980; MRCP (UK) 1985; MD Lond. 1994. Cons. Cardiol. Dewsbury Dist. Hosp.; Hon. Cons. Cardiol. Yorks. Heart Centre Leeds Gen. Infirm. Leeds. Specialty: Cardiol. Socs: Brit. Cardiac Soc.; Brit. Cardiac.

Interven. Soc. Prev: Sen. Regist. (Cardiol.) Leeds; Research Fell. Thoraxcentre Erasmus Univ. Rotterdam; Regist. (Cardiol.) Soton.

SMYLY, Philip Adrian Jocelyn Woosehill Surgery, Emmview Close, Woosehill, Wokingham RG41 3DA Tel: 01491 612455; Woosehill Surgery, Emmview Close, Wokingham RG41 3DA Tel: 0118 978 8266 Fax: 0118 979 3661 — MB ChB Birm. 1978 (Birm. Univ.) DRCOG 1980; MRCGP 1983. GP Woosehill Surg. Wokingham, Berks. Socs: BMA; Med. Protec. Soc. Prev: GP Watlington, Oxon.; Govt. Med. Off. Elim Hosp., Zimbabwe Seconded by Oxfam (UK).

SMYRNIOU, Nedi Nicou Benchill Medical Practice, 127 Woodhouse Lane, Benchill, Wythenshawe, Manchester M22 9WP Tel: 0161 998 4304 Fax: 0161 945 4028; 23 Pine Road, Didsbury, Manchester M20 6UY — MB ChB Manch. 1982; MRCP (UK) 1985. Prev: Trainee GP Wythenshawe; SHO (Gen. Med.) Oldham & Dist. Gen. Hosp.; SHO (Cardiothoracic Med.) Wythenshaw Hosp. Manch.

SMYTH, Alan Robert Department of Paediatrics, Nottingham City Hospital, Hucknall Road, Nottingham NG5 1PB Tel: 0115 969 1169 Ext: 46475 Fax: 0115 9620564 — MB BS Lond. 1987; MA Camb. 1988; MRCP (UK) 1990; MD Liverp. 1995; FRCPCH 1996. Cons. Paediat. Respirat. Med. Nottm. City Hosp. Nottm.; Special Sen. Lect. in Child Health, Univ. Nottg. Specialty: Paediat. Socs: Brit. Thorac. Soc.; FRCPCh. Prev: Regist. (Paediat.) Roy. Liverp. Childr. Hosp. Alder Hey; SHO (Paediat.) Bristol Roy. Hosp. Sick Childr.; SHO (Paediat.) Leicester Roy. Infirm.

SMYTH, Alan Theodore (retired) 72 Fentham Road, Hampton-in-Arden, Solihull B92 0AY Tel: 01675 443506 — MB ChB Birm. 1951. Prev: GP Solihull.

SMYTH, Anita Elizabeth 18 Tullyhirm Road, Derrynoose, Armagh BT60 3DU — MB BCh BAO Belf. 1991; MB BCh Belf. 1991.

SMYTH, Anthony Shanroe House, Mullabawn, Newry BT35 9RD Tel: 028 3088 8042 Fax: 028 3088 8977 — MB BCh BAO Belf. 1952; DCH RCPSI 1962; FRCGP 1984. Hosp. Pract. (Paediat.) Daisy Hill Hosp. Newry; Mem. South. Health & Social Serv. Bd. Specialty: Cardiol. Socs: Irish Racecourse Med. Off. Assn.; BMA; Ulster Med. Soc. Prev: Clin. Asst. (Paediat.) Daisy Hill Hosp. Newry; Ho. Surg. & Cas. Off. Mater. Infirm. Hosp. Belf.

SMYTH, Mr Brian Turbett (retired) Tree Tops, Vicarage Close, Stoke Gabriel, Totnes TQ9 6QT Tel: 01803 782806 — MB BCh BAO Belf. 1945; FRCS Eng. 1952. Prev: Cons. Paediat. Surg. Roy. Belf. Hosp. Sick Childr. & Ulster Hosp. Dundonald.

SMYTH, Caroline Carmel Anne 5 Ryder Crescent, Aughton, Ormskirk L39 5EY Tel: 01695 423867 — MB ChB Liverp. 1996. SHO (Anaesth.)roy.Liverp.Univ.Hosp. Specialty: Anaesth.

SMYTH, Caroline Lucy Flat 2, 32 Princes Square, London W2 4NJ — MB BS Lond. 1993.

SMYTH, Colin Michael 5 Ryder Crescent, Ormskirk L39 5EY — MB ChB Dundee 1991.

SMYTH, Desmond Alcorn (retired) Bedmond, New Barn Road, Longfield DA3 7JF Tel: 01474 702560 — MB BS Durh. 1942; MFPH 2003; DPH Durh. 1948; MFCM 1972. Prev: Dist. Community Phys. Dartford & Gravesham Health Dist.

SMYTH, Diane Patricia Lesley Child Development and Neurology Service, St. Mary's Hospital, London W2 1NY Tel: 020 7886 1545 Fax: 020 7886 6952; Austins, Warners Hill, Cookham Dean, Maidenhead SL6 9NU Tel: 01628 482533 Fax: 01628 481439 — MB BS Lond. 1966 (St. Bart.) MRCS Eng. LRCP Lond. 1967; DCH RCPS Glas. 1968; MRCP (UK) 1971; MD Lond. 1980; FRCP Lond. 1990; FRCPCH 1997. Cons. Paediat. (Child Developm. & Neurol.) St. Mary's Hosp. Lond. Specialty: Paediat. Neurol. Socs: Standing Comm. on Disabil. (Chair) Roy. Coll. Paediat and Child Health; Child Developm. & Disabil. Gp. Roy. Coll. Paediat. & Child Health. Prev: SCMO Wycombe HA; Lect. (Child Health) Qu. Eliz. Hosp. Childr. Lond.; Sen. Regist. (Neurol.) Nat. Hosp. Nerv. Dis. & Hosp. Sick Childr. Gt. Ormond St. Lond.

SMYTH, Edward Francis 134 Monlough Road, Saintfield, Ballynahinch BT24 7EU — MB BCh BAO Belf. 1997.

SMYTH, Edward Thomas Martin Department of Bacteriology, The Royal Hospitals, Belfast BT12 6BA Tel: 02890 314043 Fax: 02890 314043 Email: edward.smyth@hisc.n-i.nhs.uk/ etms@etms13.demon.co.uk; 13 Glenshane Park, Jordanstown, Newtownabbey BT37 0QN — MD Belf. 1993; MB BCh BAO 1976; FRCPath. 1995, M 1983; Hon. FFP RCPI 1985; Hon. FRCPI 2003. Cons. Bact. Roy. Hosps. Belf.; Director North. Irel. Healthcare Assoc. Infec. Surveillance Centre (HISC). Specialty: Med. Microbiol. Socs: Hosp. Infec. Soc.; Soc. for Healthcare Epidemiol. of Amer.; Brit. Infec. Soc.

SMYTH, Fiona 28 Massey Court, Belfast BT4 3GJ — MB BCh BAO Belf. 1981; DRCOG 1983.

SMYTH, Frederick Brian CDSC (NI), McBrien Building, Belfast City Hospital, Belfast BT9 7AB Tel: 02890 263765 Fax: 02890 263511 Email: bsmyth@phls.org.uk; The Old Manse, 25 Dreen Road, Cullybackey, Ballymena BT42 1EB — MB BCh BAO Belf. 1978; MRCP (UK) 1982; MSc Community Med. Ed. 1985; MFCM 1988; FFPHM RCP (UK) 1997, M 1989; FRCP Ed. 1994; FRCP(L) 1998. Reg. Epidemiolog. Communicable Dis. Surveillance Centre, Belf. Hosp.; Honorary Lecturer, Dept. Epidemiology and Public Health, Queens University, Belfast 1999. Specialty: Pub. Health Med. Socs: Fell. Ulster Med. Soc. Prev: Cons. Pub. Health Med. & Communicable Dis. Control, N. Health Bd.

SMYTH, Mr George Thomas Chase Malago Surgery, 40 St. Johns Road, Bedminster, Bristol BS3 4JE Tel: 0117 966 3587 Fax: 0117 963 1422; 25 Montague Hill, Kingsdown, Bristol BS2 8ND Tel: 0117 942 1238 — MB BS Lond. 1975; FRCS Eng. 1980; DRCOG 1982; MRCGP 1983. GP Princip.; GP Clin. Tutor. Prev: Resid. Surg.Off. Manch. Roy. Infirm.; Surgic. Regist. Groote Schuur Hosp., Cape Town.

SMYTH, Gerald Vincent 'Craggets Lodge', Craggets Lane, Church St., Henfield BN5 9NS — LRCPI & LM, LRSCI & LM 1937 (RCSI) LRCPI & LM, LRCSI & LM 1937. Prev: Chairm. Bd. Dept. of Health & Social Security (S.E. Region) & War; Pens. S.E. Region; Mem. Brighton & Sussex M-C Soc.

SMYTH, Gerard Paul 2 Brownhills Gardens, St Andrews KY16 8PY — MB ChB Aberd. 1991.

SMYTH, Heather Jane 3 Kilburn Crescent, Woodburn Park, Waterside, Londonderry BT47 5PZ — MB BCh Belf. 1998; MB BCh Belf 1998.

SMYTH, James Harold Smyth Care Homes, 108-100 Cambridge Road, Churchtown, Southport PR9 9RZ Tel: 01704 25717 — LRCPI & LM, LRSCI & LM 1956; LRCPI & LM, LRCSI & LM 1956. Prev: Ho. Surg. Jervis St. Hosp. Dub.; Ho. Phys. Southport Infirm.

SMYTH, Professor John Fletcher University of Edinburgh, Cancer Research Centre, Crewe Road South, Edinburgh EH4 2XR Tel: 0131 777 3512 Fax: 0131 777 3520 Email: john.smyth@cancer.org.uk; 18 Inverleith Avenue South, Edinburgh EH3 5QA — MB BChir Camb. 1970 (St Bart.) BA Camb. 1967; MRCP (UK) 1973; MSc Lond. 1975; MA Camb. 1971, MD 1976; FRCP Ed. 1981; FRCP Lond. 1983; FRCS Ed. 1993; FRSE 1996; FRCR 1996. Prof. Med. Oncol. Univ. Edin.; Dir. Cancer Research Centre Edin. Specialty: Oncol. Special Interest: Developm. of Experim. Therap. of Cancer; Malig. Melanoma; Ovarian Cancer. Socs: (Ex-Pres.) Europ. Soc. Med. Oncol.; (Treas.) Federat. Europ. Cancer Socs. Prev: Sen. Lect. Inst. Cancer Research Lond.; Hon. Cons. Phys. Roy. Marsden Hosp. Sutton; Vis. Fell. Nat. Cancer Inst., USA.

SMYTH, John Seymour 21 Lucerne Parade, Strawmills, Belfast BT9 5FT — MB BCh BAO Belf. 1993.

SMYTH, Mr John Vincent Ward Manchester Royal Infirmary, Department of Vascular Surgery, Oxford Road, Manchester M13 9WL Tel: 0161 276 4525 — MB BS Lond. 1986 (Roy. Free Hosp.) FRCS Eng. 1990. Specialty: Gen. Surg. Socs: Assn. Surg. Train.; Vasc. Surg. Soc. (Rouleaux Club); BMA. Prev: Specialist Regist. (Vasc.) Manch. Roy. Infirm.; Regist. (Gen. Surg.) Roy. Albert Edwd. Infirm. Wigan; Research Fell. (Vasc. Surg.) Manch. Roy. Infirm.

SMYTH, John Walter 1 The Grange, Off Dobb Brow Road, Westhoughton, Bolton BL5 2AZ — MB ChB Manch. 1990.

SMYTH, Joseph Ernest Cookstown Health Centre, 52 Orritor Road, Cookstown BT80 8BN Tel: 028 8676 2995 Fax: 028 7976 1383 — MB BCh BAO Belf. 1973.

SMYTH, Mr Julian Michael 27 Kennington Palace Court, Sancroft Street, London SE11 5UL Tel: 020 7735 4866 Email: smyth27kpc@yahoo.co.uk — MB Camb. 1964 (St. Mary's) MA Camb. 1957, BChir 1963, VetMB 1958; FRCS Eng. 1972. Specialty: Palliat. Med. Prev: Cons. Palliat. Med. St. Josephs Hospice Lond.; Ho. Phys. Med. Unit St. Mary's Hosp. Lond.; Med. Off. St. Raphaels Hospice N. Cheam.

SMYTH, Katherine Lorna — MB ChB Liverp. 1989; MB ChB (Hons.) Liverp. 1989. Consultant (Ophtalmologist) Roy. Bolton Hosp. Specialty: Ophth.

SMYTH, Margaret Gavina Stewart (retired) Halycon House, Cable St., Formby, Liverpool L37 7DH Tel: 0170 48 74078 — MRCS Eng. LRCP Lond. 1937 (King's Coll. Hosp.) Prev: Med. Off. Family Plann. Assn. Liverp.

SMYTH, Mark Gordon 3 Eden Park, Bothwell, Glasgow G71 8SL — MB ChB Glas. 1991; DRCOG 1993. Specialty: Gen. Pract. Prev: Trainee GP South. Gen. Hosp. Glas. Train. Scheme.

SMYTH, Martin 27 Coleville Road, Farnborough GU14 8PY — MB BS Lond. 1988.

SMYTH, Mr Michael David Laurence Castlefields Health Centre, Chester Close, Castlefields, Runcorn WA7 2HY Tel: 01928 566671 Fax: 01928 581631; Stane Brae, Hall Park, Scotforth, Lancaster LA1 4SH Tel: 01524 37252 Email: thesmyths@compuserve.com — MB ChB Liverp. 1986; FRCS Ed. 1991; MRCGP 1993. Med. Adviser Morecombe Bay HA. Specialty: Pharmaceutical Medicine. Prev: Assoc. Phys. NW Primary Care Initiative.

SMYTH, Michael Gerard Maguires Bridge Surgery, The Surgery, Maguiresbridge, Enniskillen BT94 4PB Tel: 028 6772 1273 Fax: 028 6772 3303; Dr M. Smyth, Drumgoon, Maguiresbridge, Enniskillen BT94 4PB Tel: 01365 722528 Fax: 01365 723303 — MB BCh BAO Belf. 1981; DRCOG 1984; MRCGP 1986. GP Maguiresbridge Co. Fermanagh; Med. Assessor, Indep. Tribunal Serv. Socs: BMA; Ulster Med. Soc. Prev: SHO (Med. & Cas.) Erne Hosp. Enniskillen; SHO (Obst.) Altnagelvin Hosp. Derry; SHO (Psychiat.) Tyrone & Fermanagh Hosp. Omagh.

SMYTH, Michael James Wards Medical Practice, 25 Dundonald Road, Kilmarnock KA1 1RU Tel: 01563 526514 Fax: 01563 573558 — MB ChB Glas. 1974; DRCOG 1977; DCH RCPS Glas. 1978; FFA RCS Eng. 1980. Specialty: Anaesth.

SMYTH, Nigel Wesley 6 Innishowen Park, Ballymena BT43 5NE — MB ChB Glas. 1998; MB ChB Glas 1998.

SMYTH, Patrick Joseph Evanson St Johns Road Surgery, 10 St. Johns Road, Newbury RG14 7LX Tel: 01635 40160; Orchard Cottage, Adbury Park, Newbury RG20 4HB — MB BS Lond. 1971 (Guy's) MRCS Eng. LRCP Lond. 1971; DA Eng. 1974. Prev: Regist. (Anaesth.) Guy's Hosp.

SMYTH, Patrick Robert Francis Long Lane Farmhouse, Long Lane, Wimborne BH21 7AQ — MB BS Lond. 1972 (St. Bart.) DA Eng. 1974; FFA RCS Eng. 1979. Cons. (Anaesth.) Poole Gen. Hosp. Specialty: Anaesth. Prev: Sen. Regist. (Anaesth.) Westm. Hosp. Lond.; Regist. (Anaesth.) Roy. Devon & Exeter Hosps.; Med. Off. Britain Nepal Med. Trust.

SMYTH, Paul William John (retired) Stone Cottage, Mill Lane, Chideock, Bridport DT6 6JS — MB BS Lond. 1959 (St. Geo.) Apptd. Fact. Doctor.

SMYTH, Robert Andrew Colhoun Broadway Medical Centre, 65-67 Broadway, Fleetwood FY7 7DG Tel: 01253 874222 Fax: 01253 874448 — MB ChB Manch. 1988 (Manchester University) DRCOG 1991; MRCGP 1992. Specialty: Gen. Pract. Prev: SHO (Med. & O & G) N. Manch. Gen. Hosp.; SHO (Paediat.) Booth Hall Hosp.

SMYTH, Rosalind Jane 41 Crafordsburn Road, Newtownards BT23 4EA — MB BCh BAO Belf. 1996.

SMYTH, Professor Rosalind Louise University of Liverpool, Institute of Child Health, Alder Hey Children's Hospital, Liverpool L12 2AP Tel: 0151 252 5693 Fax: 0151 252 5456; Wexford Lodge, Noctorum Lane, Oxton, Prenton CH43 9UE — MB BS Lond. 1983; MRCP (UK) 1986; MA Camb. 1984, MD 1993. Brough Prof. of Paedriatric Med., Univ. of Liverp. Specialty: Paediat. Prev: Cons. Paediat. (Respirat. & Infec. Dis.) Roy. Liverp. Childr. Hosp.; Sen. Regist. (Paediat.) Mersey Region.

SMYTH, Rosemary Ballysillan Group Practice, 321 Ballysillan Road, Belfast BT14 6RD Tel: 028 9071 3689/7843 Fax: 028 9071 0626 — MB BCh BAO Belf. 1983; DRCOG 1990. Specialty: Gen. Med.

SMYTH, Sheila Catherine Douglas Street Surgery, 1 Douglas Street, Hamilton ML3 0DR Tel: 01698 286262; 3 Eden Park, Bothwell, Glasgow G71 8SL Tel: 01698 854546 — MB ChB Glas. 1991; DRCOG 1994; MRCGP 1995. Specialty: Gen. Pract.

SMYTH, Ursula Rachel (retired) 72 Fentham Road, Hampton in Arden, Solihull B92 0AY Tel: 01675 443506 — MB ChB Birm. 1952. Prev: Ho. Phys. & Ho. Surg. Qu. Eliz. Hosp. Birm.

SMYTH, William Randall 1 Church Road, Ballynure, Newtownabbey BT36 9UF — MB BCh BAO Belf. 1980; DRCOG 1992.

SMYTHIES, John Raymond 8 East Mount Road, York YO24 1BD — MD Camb. 1955; MB BChir 1945; DPM Eng. 1952. Emerit. Irel. Prof. Univ. Alabama, USA.; Vis. Schol. Dept. Philosophy Univ. Stanford, USA. Prev: Reader Psychiat. Univ. Edin.; Sen. Regist. Maudsley Hosp. Lond.

SNAITH, Alan Harrison (retired) Haddeo House, Upton, Taunton TA4 2HU Tel: 01398 371297 — (Durh) MD Durh. 1961, MB BS 1947; DPH Eng. 1961; FRCPath 1963; FFCM 1973.

SNAITH, Michael Linton Fircliffe, Whitworth Road, Darley Dale, Matlock DE4 2HJ Tel: 01629 732910 Email: michael.snaith@w3z.co.uk.co.uk — MB BS Newc. 1965; FRCP Lond. 1980, M 1968; MD Newc. 1973. Hon. Sen. Lect. (Rheum.) Molecular & Genetic Med. Fac. Med. Sheff. Univ. Specialty: Rheumatol. Special Interest: Connective Tissue Disorders; Gout. Socs: Brit. Soc. Rheum.; BMA; Amer. Coll. Rheum. Prev: Hon. Cons. Rheum. Sheff.; Cons. Rheum. Univ. Coll. & Middlx. Hosp. Lond.; Cons. Rheum. St. Stephens & Westm. Hosps. Lond.

SNAITH, Rosemary Jane 9 Kersland Drive, Milngavie, Glasgow G62 8DG — MB ChB Glas. 1998; MB ChB Glas 1998.

SNAPE, Catherine Jane The Gillygate Surgery, 28 Gillygate, York YO31 7WQ Tel: 01904 624404 Email: cjsnape@yahoo.com — MB BS Newc. 1982; MRCGP 1986; DRCOG 1987; MMed Sc Leeds 2001.

SNAPE, Elizabeth Elaine Bridge Lane Health Centre, 20 Bridge Lane, Battersea, London SW11 3AD Tel: 020 7585 1499 Fax: 020 7978 4707 — MB ChB Ed. 1981; DRCOG 1984; MRCGP 1987.

SNAPE, Olivia Jayne 35 Oathall Avenue, Haywards Heath RH16 3ES — MB BS Lond. 1989 (St. Thos. Hosp. Lond.) MRCGP 1995. Specialty: Genitourinary Medicine.

SNAPE, Peter Evans 6 Rubislaw Terrace, Aberdeen AB10 1XE Tel: 01224 622440 Fax: 01224 646612; 206 King's Gate, Aberdeen AB15 6DQ Tel: 01224 311209 Fax: 01224 322810 — MB ChB Aberd. 1975; BMedBiol 1972; AFOM RCP Lond. 1991. Indep. Occupat. Health Phys. Specialty: Occupat. Health. Socs: Soc. Occupat. Med. Prev: GP Aberd.

SNAPE, Sarah Louise Dept Anaesthetics, Bedford Hospital, Kemptston Road, Bedford MK42 9DJ; Honeystone, 22a West End, Stevington, Bedford MK43 7QU — MB BS Lond. 1988 (Roy. Free Hosp.) BSc Lond. 1985; BSc Lond. 1985; FRCA 1993; FRCA 1993. Cons. Anaestetist Bedford Hosp. Specialty: Anaesth. Prev: Regist. John Radcliffe Hosp. Oxf.; SHO (Anaesth.) Northampton Gen. Hosp. Cliftonville; SR John Radcliffe Oxf.

SNAPE, Simon Richard Orleton Surgery, Millbrook Way, Orleton, Ludlow SY8 4HW Tel: 01584 831300 — MB BS Lond. 1962 (St. Thos.) MRCS Eng. LRCP Lond. 1962. GP Herefordsh. Prev: Cas. Off. St. Thos. Hosp. Lond.; Med. Regist. Hereford Hosp. Gp.

SNAPE, Sonya Louise Pinehurst, Patshill Road, Pattingham, Wolverhampton WV6 7BG — MB ChB Birm. 1996.

SNASHALL, David Charles 2 Charity Cottages, Petsoe End, Emberton, Olney MK46 5JL Tel: 01234 711072 — (Ed.) MB ChB 1968; MRCP (UK) 1972; DIH Lond. 1979; MSc Lond. 1979; DTM & H RCP Lond. 1980; FFOM RCP Lond. 1987, MFOM 1983; FRCP Lond. 1993; LLM Cardiff 1996. Hon. Head of Service. (Occupat. Health) Guy's & St. Thos. NHS Trust; Principal. Adviser Health & Safety Exec.; Sen. Lecturer (Occupational Med.) GKT School of Med. Specialty: Occupat. Health. Socs: Internat. Commiss. Occupat. Health; Soc. Occupat. Med. Prev: Med. Adviser Hse. of Commons Lond.; Chief Med. Adviser Foreign & Commonw. Office.

SNASHALL, Phillip Douglas 4 Copeland Court, Archery Rise, Durham DH1 4LF — (Char. Cross) MRCS Eng. LRCP Lond. 1967; MB BS (Hons.) Lond. 1967; MRCP (UK) 1970; BSc (Hons.) Lond. 1964, MD 1974; FRCP Lond. 1986; FRCP Ed. 1995. Harold Macmillan Prof. Med. Univ. Newc. u. Tyne; Hon. Cons. Phys. N. Tees Gen. Hosp. Stockton-on-Tees; Sub-Dean (Teeside Div.) Fac. Med. Univ. Newc. Specialty: Gen. Med.; Respirat. Med. Socs: Brit. Thorac. Soc.; Amer. Thoracic Soc.; Assn. for Med. Educat. Prev: Asst. Dean (Med. Educat.) Char. Cross & Westm. Med. Sch.; Sen. Lect. (Med.) Char. Cross Hosp. Lond.; Sen. Research Fell. Wellcome Trust.

SNASHALL, Susan Elizabeth St. George's Hospital, Blackshaw, Tooting, London SW17 0QT Tel: 020 8725 1886 Fax: 020 8275

1874; 18A Beech Lane, Guildford GU2 4ES Tel: 01483 571615 — MB BS Lond. 1966 (Char. Cross. Hosp. Lond.) MRCS Eng. LRCP Lond. 1966; MD Lond. 1995. Cons. Audiological Phys. St. Geo. Hosp. Lond. & St. Helier's Hosp. Carshalton; Mem. (Chairm.) Pan Thames Speciality Train. Comm. Audiol. Med. Specialty: Audiol. Med. Socs: Brit. Assn. Audiol. Phys. Prev: Cons. Audiological Phys. Roy. Surrey Co. Hosp. Guildford.

SNEAD, Alan Roger (retired) Ty'n Llain, Mynedd Mechell, Amlwch LL68 0TN Tel: 01407 711302 — (Birm.) MB ChB Birm. 1957; DObst RCOG 1961. Prev: GP Newport, Shrops.

SNEAD, David Robert John Department of Histopathology, Walsgrave Hospital, Clifford Bridge Road, Walsgrave, Coventry CV2 2DX Tel: 024 76 538855; Wellington Cottage, Bourton-on-Dunsmore, Rugby CV23 9QS Tel: 01926 633754 — MB BS Lond. 1989 (St Thomas's Hospital) MRCPath 1995. Cons. Histopath. Walsgrave Hosp. Coventry. Specialty: Histopath. Prev: Sen. Regist. Nottm.; Regist. (Histopath.) Bristol Roy. Infirm. & Frenchay Hosp.; SHO (Histopath.) Nottm.

SNEAD, Mr Martin Paul Vitreoretinal Service, Addenbrooke's Hospital, Box 41, Hills Road, Cambridge CB2 2QQ Tel: 01223 216701 Fax: 01223 217968 — MB BS Lond. 1984 (St. Thos. Hosp. Med. Sch) DO Lond. 1988; FRCS Eng. 1989; FRCOphth 1989; MD Lond. 1996. Cons. Ophth. Surg. Addenbrooke's NHS Trust Camb. Specialty: Ophth. Socs: FRSM. Prev: Vitreo-Retinal Fell. Addenbrooke's NHS Trust; Oxf. Ophth. Research Sholarsh. Molecular Genetics Laborat. Camb.

SNEAD, Mrs Shirley Margaret (retired) Tyn Llain, Mynydd Mechell, Amlwch LL68 0TN Tel: 01407 711302 Fax: 01407 711302 — MB BCh BAO Dub. 1957 (TC Dub. & Birm.) BA Dub. 1957; MRCS Eng. LRCP Lond. 1957; DObst RCOG 1958. Clin. Asst. (Psychosexual) Shrops. HA. Prev: Med. Off. (Psychosexual Med.) Wolverhampton & Mid. Staffs. Has.

SNEARY, Michael Alfred Brinson (Surgery), 141 Brigstock Road, Thornton Heath, Croydon CR7 7JN Tel: 020 8684 1128 Fax: 020 8689 3647; Silwood, 129 Pollards Hill S., Norbury, London SW16 Tel: 020 8679 6966 — MB BS Lond. 1960 (Guy's) MRCS Eng. LRCP Lond. 1960; DObst RCOG 1962; MRCGP 1977.

SNEATH, Paula Epsom General Hospital, Dorking Road, Epsom KT19 7EG Tel: 01372 735735 Fax: 01372 735261 Email: paula.sneath@epsom-sthelier.nhs.uk; Berrow End, Downs Avenue, Epsom KT18 5HG Tel: 01372 722286 Fax: 01372 726933 — (St. Mary's) MRCS Eng. LRCP Lond. 1968; MB BS Lond. 1968; DCH Eng. 1970; MRCP (U.K.) 1972; FRCP (UK) 1996; FRCPCH 1998. Cons. Community Paediat. Epsom Health Care Trust. Specialty: Paediat. Special Interest: Autistic Spectrum Disorders; Childr. with Special needs. Prev: SCMO (Child Health) Tower Hamlets Health Dist. (T); Lect. (Child Health) Acad. Unit Qu. Eliz. Hosp. Childr. Lond., St.; Bart. & Lond. Hosps. Med. Schs.; Resid. MO Westm. Childr. Hosp. Lond.

SNEATH, Peter Henry Andrews c/o Midland Bank, 3 North St., Bourne PE10 9AE — MRCS Eng. LRCP Lond. 1947 (Camb. & King's Coll. Hosp.) MD Camb. 1959, MB BChir 1948; Dip. Bact. Lond 1953. Emerit. Prof. Microbiol. Univ. Leicester. Specialty: Med. Microbiol. Prev: Prof. Microbiol. Univ. Leicester; Dir. MRC Microbiol. Systematics Unit, Univ. Leicester; Demonst. (Path.) King's Coll. Hosp. Med. Sch.

SNEATH, Mr Robert James Saville 55 Monument Lane, Rednal, Birmingham B45 9QQ Email: rsneath@hotmail.com — MB BS Lond. 1991 (The London Hospital Medical College) FRCS (Eng) 1995. Orthop. on the N. W. thames Rotat. (Specialist Regist.). Specialty: Orthop.

SNEATH, Mr Rodney Saville (retired) Heatherfield, 55 Monument Lane, Rednal, Birmingham B45 9QQ Tel: 0121 453 3113 — MB ChB Sheff. 1957; MRCS Eng. LRCP Lond. 1948; FRCS Eng. 1958. Prev: Cons. Orthop. Surg. Roy. Orthop. Hosp. Birm.

SNEDDEN, Ann Elizabeth Department of Child & Family Psychiatry, Possilpark Health Centre, 85 Denmark St., Glasgow G22 5EG Tel: 0141 531 6106 Fax: 0141 531 6106; 4A Prince Albert Road, Dowanhill, Glasgow G12 9JX — MB ChB Glas. 1983 (University of Glasgow) Cert. Family Plann. JCC 1985; DRCOG 1985; MRCGP 1987; MRCPsych 1990. Cons. Child & Adolesc. Psychiat.; Hon. Sen. Lect. Specialty: Child & Adolesc. Psychiat. Socs: Roy. Coll. Psychiat.

SNEDDON, Alasdair James Cameron Muiredge Surgery, Merlin Crescent, Buckhaven, Leven KY8 1HJ Tel: 01592 713299 Fax: 01592 715728 — MB ChB Manchester 1981; MB ChB Manch. 1981. GP Leven, Fife.

SNEDDON, David Thomas Castlehill Health Centre, Castlehill, Forres IV36 1QF Tel: 01309 672233 Fax: 01309 673445 — MB ChB Aberd. 1976; DRCOG 1978; MRCGP 1980.

SNEDDON, Derek John Crawford The Pentlands Medical Centre, 44 Pentland View Court, Currie, Edinburgh EH14 5QB Tel: 0131 449 2142 Fax: 0131 451 5855; Lane Edge, Nisbet Road, Gullane EH31 2BQ Tel: 01620 842815 — MB ChB Ed. 1959; FRCGP 1980, M 1974. Specialty: Gen. Pract. Socs: Roy. Coll. Gen. Pract. (SE Scotl. Fac.); BMA; Ed. Clin. Club. Prev: Ho. Surg. Roy. Infirm. Edin.; Ho. Phys. Chalmers Hosp. Edin.

SNEDDON, Frances Elizabeth — MB BS Lond. 1987; BSc Lond. 1984; MRCP (UK) 1992; MRCGP 1995. GP Crowborough. Prev: GP Surrey.; Regist. (Med.) Greenwich Dist. Hosp.; SHO (Med.) St. Geo. Hosp. Lond.

SNEDDON, James Findlay East Surrey Hospital, Department of Cardiology, Canada Avenue, Redhill RH1 5RH Tel: 01737 768511 — MB BS Lond. 1983; MRCP (UK) 1986. Cons. Cardiol. & Phys. Surrey & Sussex Healthcare NHS Trust. Specialty: Cardiol. Prev: Cons. Phys. Cardiol. Crawley Health Serv. Trust; Research Fell. St Geo. Hosp. Lond.

SNEDDON, James John St Peters Hill Surgery, 15 St. Peters Hill, Grantham NG31 6QA Tel: 01476 590009 Fax: 01476 570898; 110 Barrowby Road, Grantham NG31 8AF Tel: 01476 62221 — MB ChB St. And. 1965; DA Eng. 1969. Prev: Regist. (Anaesth.) Dundee Roy. Infirm.; Demonst. (Physiol.) Univ. Dundee.; SHO (Obst.) Maryfield Hosp. Dundee.

SNEDDON, Mr Kenneth James The Queen Victoria Hospital, Holtye Road, East Grinstead RH19 3DZ Tel: 01342 414303 Email: ken.sneddon@quh.nhs.uk — MB BS Lond. 1991; BDS (Hons.) Lond. 1983; FDS RCS Eng. 1989; FRCS Eng. 1994. Cons. Maxillofacial Surg. Specialty: Oral & Maxillofacial Surg. Special Interest: Facial and Orbital Trauma; Orthognathic Surg. Socs: BMA; Brit. Assn. of Oral and Maxillofacial Surgeons; Craniofacial Soc. Prev: Sen. Regist. (Oral & Maxillofacial Surg.) Qu. Vict. Hosp. E. Grinstead; Regist. (Maxillofacial Surg.) Canniesburn Hosp. Glas.; Regist. (Oral & Maxillofacial Surg.) Qu. Vict. Hosp. E. Grinstead.

SNEE, Kevin North Derbyshire DHA, Scarsdale Hospital, Newbold Road, Chesterfield S41 7PF Tel: 01246 231255; 332 Bolton Road W., Ramsbottom, Bury BL0 9QY — MB ChB Liverp. 1982; MRCGP 1986; MSc Manch. 1991; MFPHM RCP (UK) 1992. Cons. Pub. Health Med. Scarsdale Hosp. Chesterfield. Specialty: Pub. Health Med. Prev: Lect. (Pub. Health) Univ. Liverp.; Regist. (Pub. Health Med.) Mersey Region.

SNEEDEN, Arthur Elvin Townsend (retired) Ladywood, 2 Wester Boghead, Lenzie, Glasgow G66 4SR Tel: 0141 775 2091 — MB ChB Glas. 1944; MRCGP 1968.

SNELL, Anthony David Birmingham and The Black Country Strategic Health Authority, St Chads Court, 213 Hagley Road, Edgbaston, Birmingham B16 9RG Tel: 0121 695 2247 Fax: 0121 695 2446 Email: tony.snell@bbcha.nhs.uk — MB ChB Liverp. 1977 (Liverpool) MRCGP 1983; DRCOG 1985. Med. Director Birm. & Black Country SHA Birm.; GP Retainee, Birm. Specialty: Gen. Pract. Special Interest: Medico Legal. Prev: Med. Adviser & Dep. Dir. Performance Managem. (Developm.); Dir. of Primary Care Barnet Health Agency; GP Colchester.

SNELL, Barbara Jean The Old Schoolhouse, Pishill, Henley-on-Thames RG9 6HJ — MRCS Eng. LRCP Lond. 1972 (St. Bart.) BSc (Hons.) (Physiol.) Lond. 1969, MB BS 1972; DO Eng. 1976; MRCOphth. 1993. Med. Off. Eye Unit Roy. Berks. Hosp. Reading. Specialty: Ophth. Socs: Med. Contact Lens Assn. Prev: Ho. Phys. Edgware Gen. Hosp.; Ho. Surg. Wycombe Gen. Hosp.; SHO (Ophth.) Roy. Berks. Hosp. Reading.

SNELL, Caroline Jane Holmes 46 Coniston Av, West Jesmond, Newcastle upon Tyne NE2 3HA — MB BS Newc. 1997.

SNELL, Eric Saxon (retired) 4 Flintcombe Square, Poundbury Village, Dorchester, Dorchester DT1 3GG Tel: 01305 261942 Email: eric@snell.gp-plus.net — (St. Mary's) MB BS Lond. 1948; FRCP Lond. 1973, M 1952; MA Oxf. 1961; MD Lond. 1967. Prev: Dir. Med. & Scientif. Affairs Assn. Brit. Pharmaceut. Indust.

SNELL, Jeffrey Kennard (retired) Highbury, Compton, Chichester PO18 9EX — MRCS Eng. LRCP Lond. 1954 (King's Coll. Hosp.) MA Camb. 1955, BA 1950, MB BChir 1953; DObst RCOG 1960. Prev: Ho. Surg. ENT Dept. King's Coll. Hosp.
SNELL, Jennifer Anne Fieldhead Surgery, 65 New Road Side, Horsforth, Leeds LS18 4JY Tel: 0113 295 3410 Fax: 0113 295 3417; 4 Redbeck Cottages, Woodbottom, Horsforth, Leeds LS18 4GQ Tel: 01132 503402 — MB ChB Leeds 1978; DRCOG 1981. Gen. Practitioner.
SNELL, Louise Rebecca 62 The Stray, South Cave, Brough HV15 2AL — MB ChB Leeds 1996.
SNELL, Margaret Jane (retired) The Lodge, Lower End, Layer-de-la-Haye, Colchester CO2 0LE Tel: 01206 734698 — MB BS Lond. 1959 (St. Mary's) MRCS Eng. LRCP Lond. 1959; DCH Eng. 1962. Prev: Community Med. Off. N. Essex HA.
SNELL, Noel James Creagh Respiratory Infection Firm, Royal Brompton Hospital, Sydney Street, London SW3 6NP Tel: 07880 782327 — MB BS Lond. 1972 (St. Bart.) MRCS Eng. LRCP Lond. 1971; DObst RCOG 1973; DA Eng. 1977; FRCP Lond. 1997, M 1977; Dip. Pharm. Med. RCP (UK) 1985; FIBiol. 1995, M 1985; FFPM RCP Lond. 1995, M 1989. Global Clin. Expert (Respir. Med.) AstraZeneca R. & D. Charnwood; Co-Ed. Int. Jl. Pharmaceut. Med.; Hon. Sen. Fell. Nat. Heart & Lung Inst.; Hon. Clin. Asst. Roy. Brompton Hosp. Specialty: Pharmaceutical Medicine; Respirat. Med. Socs: Brit. Thorac. Soc.; Brit. Assn. for Lung Research (Ex-Chairm.); Roy. Soc. Med. (Pres. Respir. Med. Sec.). Prev: Dir. Global Clin. Strategy (Resp.) Bayer Pharma; Assoc. Med. Dir. GlaxoWellcome UK; Clin. Scientist MRC Tuberc. & Chest Dis. Unit.
SNELL, Paul Heath, OBE (retired) Hope House, Saltergate Lane, Bamford, Hope Valley S33 0BE Tel: 01433 651533 Fax: 01433 651533 Email: phsnell@onetel.net.uk — BM BCh Oxf. 1962; MA Oxf. 1962; FRCP Lond. 1982, M 1966; DTM & H RCP Lond. 1971; FFPHM RCP (UK) 1990, M 1985. Prev: Dir. Policy & Pub. Health Sheff. Health & Hon. Clin. Lect. Univ. Sheff.
SNELL, Robert Olufemi Lionel Hilltop, Bicknoller, Taunton TA4 4ES — MB ChB Birm. 1990; ChB Birm. 1990.
SNELL, Theodore Peter (retired) Manali Cottage, Maesgwartha, Gilwern, Abergavenny NP7 0ET Tel: 01873 831033 — BM BCh Oxf. 1956. Prev: Sen. Lect. Christian Med. Coll. Ludhiana, India.
SNELL, Wendy Margaret 22 Abbey Gardens, London NW8 9AT; City Healthcare, 36 Moorgate, London EC2 Tel: 020 7638 4988 — MB BS Lond. 1983; DCH RCPS Glas. 1987; DGM RCP Lond. 1988; DRCOG 1990.
SNELLING, Tristram Henry 9 West Hill, South Croydon CR2 0SB — MB BS Lond. 1994.
SNELSON, Edward John 66 Slinn Street, Crookes, Sheffield S10 1NX — MB ChB Sheff. 1996. SHO (Med.). Specialty: Gen. Med.; Gen. Pract. Socs: BMA; Catholic Doctors Guild.
SNELSON, Michael Geoffrey Glenbourne, Morlax Drive, Derriford, Plymouth PL6 5AF Tel: 01752 763131 Fax: 01752 763133 — MB ChB Liverp. 1971; DPM Eng. 1975; MRCPsych 1976; FRCPsych 2002. Cons. Psychiat. Plymouth Community Servs. NHS Trust. Specialty: Gen. Psychiat.
SNEYD, Fiona Mary Catherine South Coldrenick, Menheniot, Liskeard PL14 3RQ Tel: 01503 240316 Fax: 01503 240885 — MB ChB Birm. 1980; DRCOG 1983; T(GP) 1991. GP Retainer, Rosedean surg. Liskeard. Specialty: Gen. Pract. Prev: Clin. Med. Off. Wandsworth HA; Community Med. Off. (Child Health) Macclesfield HA.
SNEYD, Professor John Robert Peninsula Medical School, C310, Portland Square, Drake Circus, Plymouth PL4 8AA Tel: 01752 238040 — MB BChir Camb. 1981; BA Camb. 1978; MA Camb. 1979; FRCA 1985; MD Camb. 1989; T(Anaesth.) 1992. Assoc. Dean Peninsula Med. Sch. Specialty: Anaesth. Special Interest: Neuroanaesthesia. Socs: Assn. Anaesth.; Physiol. Soc. Prev: Reader (Anaesth.) Univ. Plymouth; Instruc. (Anaesth.) Univ. Michigan Med. Sch. Ann Arbor, USA; Sen. Regist. (Anaesth.) Univ. Hosp. S. Manch.
SNODGRASS, Christine Averil (retired) 15 Moor Lane, Darras Hall, Ponteland, Newcastle upon Tyne NE20 9AD — (Univ. of Ed.) MB ChB Ed. 1958; DObst RCOG 1960; FRCOG 1976, M 1963; MD (Commend.) Ed. 1968; MA (Hons.) Ed. 1997. Prev: Cons. O & G Roy. Vict. Infirm. Newc.
SNODGRASS, Graeme John Anthony Inglis Department of Child Health, Royal London Trust, Whitechapel, London E1 1BB Tel: 020 7377 7428 Fax: 020 7377 7759 Email: g.j.a.snodgrass@mds.qmw.ac.uk; 42 Newark Street, London E1 2AA Tel: 020 7375 2417 — (Ed.) MB ChB Ed. 1958; DCH Eng. 1960; FRCP Ed. 1976, M 1964; FRCPCH 1997. Cons. Paediat. & Sen. Lect. Paediat. Lond. Hosp. Specialty: Paediat. Prev: Sen. Lect. Child Health Guy's Hosp. Med. Sch. Lond.; Sen. Regist. (Paediat.) Char. Cross Hosp. Lond.; Paediat. Regist. Qu. Eliz. Hosp. Childr. Lond.
SNODGRASS, Marjory Black (retired) 26 Garngaber Avenue, Lenzie, Glasgow G66 4LL Tel: 0141 776 1600 — MB ChB Glas. 1946; DOMS Eng. 1949; FRCP Glas. 1980. Sen. Hosp. Med. Off. Stirling Roy. Infirm. Prev: Asst. Ophth. Surg. Stirling Roy. Infirm.
SNOOK, Jonathon Anthony Poole Hospital NHS Trust, Longfleet Road, Poole BH15 2JB Tel: 01202 442357 — BM BCh Oxf. 1982; DPhil. Oxf. 1990, MA 1987, BM BCh 1982; MRCP (UK) 1985; FRCP 1997. Cons. Phys. Poole Gen. Hosp. Specialty: Gastroenterol. Prev: Sen. Regist. (Med. Gastroenterol.) Roy. Hants. Co. Hosp. Winchester & Soton. Gen. Hosp.; Research Fell. (Gastroenterol.) Radcliffe Infirm. Oxf.; Regist./SHO (Med.) Soton. Gen. Hosp.
SNOOK, Nicola Jane Little Bretons, Swan St., Chappel, Colchester CO6 2EE; Hillside Cottage, 1 Sandy Lobby, Old Pool Bank, Pool in Wharfedale, Otley LS21 1EL — MB ChB Leeds 1988; FRCA 1994. Regist. (Anaesth.) St. Jas. Univ. Hosp. Leeds. Specialty: Anaesth.
SNOOK, Roger Norman Neston Medical Centre, 14-20 Liverpool Road, Neston, South Wirral CH64 3RA Tel: 0151 336 4121 Fax: 0151 353 0151; 16 Kirby Park, West Kirby, Wirral CH48 2HA Tel: 0151 625 5390 — MB ChB Liverp. 1970. Prev: SHO (O & G & Paediat.) Clatterbridge Hosp. Bebington.
SNOOK, Simon 9 Ellerslie Close, Charminster, Dorchester DT2 9QQ — MB ChB Birm. 1996.
SNOOKS, Mr Steven James King George Hospital, Barley Lane, Goodmayes, Ilford IG3 8YB Tel: 020 8983 8000 Fax: 020 8970 8001; 27 Lindsey Street, Epping CM16 6RB Tel: 01992 572185 — (Middlx.) MB BS Lond. 1978; FRCS Eng. 1982; MD Lond. 1985. Cons. Gen. Surg. King Geo. Hosp. Ilford. Specialty: Gen. Surg. Socs: Assn. Coloproctol.; Assn. Surg.; BASO. Prev: Sen. Regist. (Gen. Surg.) St. Bart., N. Middlx. & Whipps Cross Hosps. Lond.; Sir Alan Pk.'s Research Fell. St. Mark's Hosp. Lond.
SNOW, Adele Louise — MB ChB Manch. 1995; MRCGP; DFFP; DRCOG.
SNOW, Alice Frances Culloden Medical Practice, Keppoch Road, Culloden, Inverness IV2 7LL Tel: 01463 793777 Fax: 01463 792143; The Old Mill House, Culcairn, Evanton, Dingwall IV16 9XS — MB ChB Aberd. 1990; BMed Biol. Aberd. 1987; MRCGP 1995. Specialty: Gen. Pract. Prev: Trainee GP Raigmore Hosp. Inverness VTS.
SNOW, Andrew Richard Station Approach Health Centre, Station Approach, Bradford-on-Avon BA15 1DQ Tel: 01225 866611 — MB BS Lond. 1969; MRCS Eng. LRCP Lond. 1969; DObst RCOG 1971; DCH Eng. 1973.
SNOW, David James Hampton Lodge, Hampton Avenue, St Marychurch, Torquay TQ1 3LA — MB ChB Leic. 1985; FRCA 1992. Specialty: Anaesth.
SNOW, David Martyn — MB ChB Ed. 1997.
SNOW, Howard David John Astraleneca, Mereside, Macclesfield SK10 4TG — MB BS Lond. 1994; MRCGP, MFFP.
SNOW, Janet Ann Wrington Vale Medical Practice, Station Road, Wrington, Bristol BS40 5NG Tel: 01934 862532 Fax: 01934 863568 — MB BCh Witwatersrand 1990.
SNOW, Mr John Thornton Greenlands, Greenhills, Barham, Canterbury CT4 6LE Tel: 01227 831756 — MB BS Lond. 1955 (St. Bart.) DO Eng. 1961; FRCS Ed. 1967. Cons. BMI Chaucer Hosp. Canterbury & BUPA St. Saviours Hosp. Hythe. Specialty: Ophth. Socs: Fell. Roy. Coll. Ophth.; UK Introcular Implant Soc. Prev: Hon. Cons. Ophth. SE Kent, Canterbury & Thanet Health Dists.; Sen. Regist. Kent Co. Ophth. & Aural Hosp. Maidstone; Asst. Lect. (Ophth.) Manch. Univ.
SNOW, Michael Harry Newcastle General Hospital, Department of Infection and Tropical Medicine, Newcastle upon Tyne NE4 6BE Tel: 0191 273 8811 Fax: 0191 273 0900 Email: michael.snow@nuth.northy.nhs.uk — MB BS Newc. 1969 (Newcastle Upon Tyne) MRCP (UK) 1973; FRCP Lond. 1985. Cons. Phys. (Gen. Med. & Infec. Dis.) Newc. Gen. Hosp. And Roy. Vict. Infirm., Newc.; Sen. Lect. (Med.) Univ. Newc. u. Tyne. Specialty: HIV Med.; Infec. Dis.; Trop. Med. Special Interest: HIV Med.; Imported

Infec. Socs: Brit. Soc. Antimicrob. Chemother.; Brit. Soc. Study of Infec.; Brit. HIV Assn.

SNOW, Percy John Deryk, OBE (retired) 4 Fairlea Avenue, Didsbury, Manchester M20 6GN — MB ChB Manch. 1948; MRCS Eng. LRCP Lond. 1948; FRCP Lond. 1970, M 1950; MD (Commend.) Manch. 1955. Prev: Cons. Phys. Bolton Roy. Infirm. & Bolton Gen. Hosp.

SNOW, Philip John Abergwdi, Brecon LD3 8NA — MB BS Lond. 1962; MRCS Eng. LRCP Lond. 1962; DObst RCOG 1964; DA Eng. 1965; FFA RCS Eng. 1969; MRCGP 1979. Specialty: Anaesth. Socs: BMA. Prev: Ho. Off. Roy. Hants. Co. Hosp. Winchester; Gen. Med. Off. Lesotho Govt.; Regist. (Anaesth.) Southmead Hosp. Bristol.

SNOW, Robert Geoffrey (retired) The Manor House, Town Ditch, Rossett, Wrexham LL12 0AN — (Birm.) MB ChB Birm. 1950; FFA RCS Eng. 1958. Prev: Cons. Anaesth. Chester & Centr. Wirral Hosp. Gps.

SNOW, Ronald Edward, CB, LVO, OBE, Surg. Rear-Admiral c/o Naval Secretary, Victory Building, HM Naval Base, Portsmouth PO1 3LS — MB BCh BAO Dub. 1960; MA Dub. 1960; LMCC 1963; DA RCPSI 1965; MFOM RCPI 1980. Prev: Phys. to HM the Qu.; Surg. Rear-Admiral (Operat. Med. Servs.) & (Support Med. Servs.); Fleet Med. Off. Cdr.-in-Chief Fleet & Med. Adv. Cdr.-in-Chief Channel & East. Atlantic.

SNOW, Stella Ray (retired) Abergwdi, Ffrwdgrech, Brecon LD3 8NA Tel: 01874 624045 Email: ray@abergwdi.force9.co.uk — MB BCh Wales 1962 (Cardiff) Dip. Palliat. Med. Wales 1993. Honorary Medical Officer to Usk House Day Hospice Brecon. Prev: Assoc.Special. c/o the elderly Bronllys. Hosp.

SNOWDEN, Ann Elizabeth Alice Kings Lane Medical Practice, 100 Kings Lane, Bebington, Wirral CH63 5LY; 52 Covertside, West Kirby, Wirral CH48 9UL — MB ChB Manch. 1973; BSc (Hons.) (Med. Biochem.) Manch. 1973.

SNOWDEN, Christopher Paul Freeman Hospital, Freeman Road, High Heaton, Newcastle upon Tyne NE7 7DN Email: c.p.snowden@ncl.ac.uk; The Coach House, 26 Adderstone Crescent, Jesmond, Newcastle upon Tyne NE2 2HH — MB BS Newc. 1989 (Newcastle upon Tyne) FRCA; B.Med.Sci. (Hons.) Newc. 1987. Cons. (Anaesth.) Freeman Hosp. Newc.; Sen. Lect. (Newc. upon Tyne). Specialty: Anaesth.; Intens. Care.

SNOWDEN, Geoffrey 78 Tranby Lane, Anlaby, Hull HU10 7DU — MB ChB Leeds 1940; DLO Eng. 1944. Assoc. Specialist ENT Dept. Roy. Infirm. Hull.

SNOWDEN, Howard Neil North Manchester General Hospital, Manchester M8 5RL Tel: 0161 720 2602; 8 Springdale Gardens, Didsbury, Manchester M20 2GX Email: neil@snowdenshome.freeserve.co.uk — MB Camb. 1984; BChir 1983; MRCP (UK) 1986; MRCPath 1996; FRCP 2001. Cons. (Rheum.) N. Manch. Gen. Hosp. Specialty: Rheumatol.; Immunol.

SNOWDEN, John (retired) Barnes Close Surgery, Barnes Close, Sturminster Newton DT10 1BN Tel: 01258 474500 Fax: 01258 471547 — BM BCh Oxf. 1972 (St. Geo.) MA.

SNOWDEN, Karen Alison Vaines 24 Stainsby Street, Thornaby, Stockton-on-Tees TS17 6HP — MB BS Newc. 1997.

SNOWDEN, Katharine Louise — MB ChB Dundee 1997.

SNOWDEN, Peter Richard Department of Forensic Psychiatry, Edenfield Centre, Salford Mental Health Trust, Bury New Road, Manchester M25 3BL Tel: 0161 772 3681 Fax: 0161 772 3446 — MB ChB Liverp. 1976; BSc (Hons.) (Biochem.) Liverp. 1973; FRCPsych 1995, M 1980. Cons. Forens. Psychiat. N. West. HA & Home Office; Hon. Clin. Lect. (Forens Psychiat.) Univ. Manch.; Mem. Home Secretaries Advis. Bd. on Restricted Pat.s. Specialty: Forens. Psychiat. Prev: Sen. Regist. (Forens. Psychiat.) Pk. La. Hosp. Liverp.; Hon. Lect. & Regist. (Psychiat.) Liverp. Univ.

SNOWDEN, Susan Ann 77 Sydenham Hill, London SE26 6TQ — MB ChB Liverp. 1968. Clin. Asst. Renal Unit King's Coll. Hosp. Lond.

SNOWDON, Brian Armstrong Society of Analytical Psychology, 1 Daleham Gardens, London NW3 5BY Tel: 020 7435 7696 — MB ChB Manch. 1957; DPM Lond. 1965; FRCPsych 1988, M 1972. Specialty: Psychother. Socs: Profess. Mem. Soc. Analyt. Psychol. Prev: Dir. C.G. Jung Clinic Lond.; Cons. Psychiat. Middlx. Hosp. Lond. & Social Serv. Dept. City Westm.; Sen. Regist. Tavistock Clinic Lond.

SNOWDON, Colin Maxwell Harbury Surgery, Mill Street, Harbury, Leamington Spa CV33 9HR Tel: 01926 612232 Fax: 01926 612991 — MB ChB Birm. 1986.

SNOWDON, Derek Vernon 173 Woodford Road, Woodford, Stockport SK7 1QE — MB ChB Manch. 1966. Specialty: Disabil. Med. Socs: BMA. Prev: Clin. Asst. (Gastroenterol.) Stockport AHA; Clin. Asst. (Anaesth.) Stockport AHA; Asst. Lect. (Physiol.) Univ. Manch.

SNOWDON, Jennifer Claire 131 Binley Road, Coventry CV3 1HX — MB BS Lond. 1984.

SNOWDON, Richard Lewis 112 Greenloons Drive, Formby, Liverpool L37 2LR — MB ChB Liverp. 1996; MRCP 1999. SHO (Cardiol.) L'pool. Specialty: Cardiol.; Gen. Med. Prev: SHO Rotat. Roy. L'pool & Broadgreen Univ. Hosps. NHS Trust.

SNOWISE, Neil Gabriel 1-3 Iron Bridge Road, Stockley Park, Uxbridge UB11 1BT — BM BCh Oxf. 1980; BA Oxf 1977; MA Oxf. 1980; Cert Family Planning (JCC) 1984; DA Eng. 1984; MRCGP 1985; DRCOG 1985. Pharmaceutical Phys.; Hon. Clin. Fell. (Respirat. Med.) Roy. United Hosp. Bath. Socs: BMA & Clin. Soc. Bath. Prev: SHO (Anaesth.) Roy. United Hosp. Bath; SHO (Med.) Roy. Cornw. Hosp. (Treliske) Truro; Primary Care Research Phys. Roy. Nat. Hosp., Rheumatic Dis.

SNYDER, Melvyn Ellergreen Medical Centre, 24 Carr Lane, Norris Green, Liverpool L11 2YA Tel: 0151 256 9800 Fax: 0151 256 5765 — MB ChB Liverp. 1964; MRCGP 1977.

SO, Elizabeth 5 Stafford House, Maida Avenue, London W2 1TE — MB BS Lond. 1993; DRCOG 1998. Locum GP & Family Planning.

SOAR, Beverley Anne 11 Banks Av, Pontefract WF8 4DL — MB ChB Leeds 1997.

SOAR, Jasmeet Southmead Hospital, Anaesthetics Department, Bristol BS10 5NB Tel: 0117 959 5114 Fax: 0117 959 5075 — MB BChir Camb. 1990; FRCA London 1994. Cons. Anaesthetic & Intens. Care N.Bristol NHS Trust; Director Intens. Care, Southmead Hosp., Bristol. Specialty: Anaesth.; Intens. Care. Special Interest: Resusc.; CPR; Critical Care.

SOAR, Noreen Mary The Surgery, Low Moor Road, Kirkby in Ashfield, Nottingham NG17 7BG Tel: 01623 759447 Fax: 01623 750906; 14 Parkside, Nottingham NG8 2NN — MB BCh BAO NUI 1979.

SOARES, Ann-Marie Rose Mount Chambers Surgery, 92 Coggeshall Road, Braintree CM7 9BY Tel: 01376 553415 Fax: 01376 552451 — MB BS Lond. 1991.

SOARES, Philip Orlando Bosco Longwood Gardens Surgery, 150 Longwood Gardens, Clayhall, Ilford IG5 0BE Tel: 020 8550 6362 — MB ChB Birm. 1987.

SOBALA, George Michael John 2 Occupational Road, Lindley, Huddersfield HD3 3AZ — BM BCh Oxf. 1983; MA (Camb.) 1984; MRCP (UK) 1986. Cons. Gen. Med. & Gastroenterol. Huddersfield NHS Trust. Specialty: Gastroenterol. Socs: Brit. Soc. Gastroenterol. Prev: Sen. Regist. (Gen. Med. & Gastroenterol.) Yorksh. Region; Tutor (Med.) Univ. Leeds.

SOBHANI, Sarfaraz 9 Martindale Close, Royton, Oldham OL2 6PR — MB ChB Manch. 1998.

SOBHI, Nabil Hanna Tyr Meddyg, 67a Crymlyn Road, Skewen, Neath SA10 6EG; The Poplars Surgery, 28 Vivian Park Drive, Port Talbot SA12 6RT Tel: 01639 890730 Fax: 01639 882082 — MB BCh Cairo 1968. GP Princip., The Poplars Surg. Port Talbot. Specialty: Anaesth.; Rheumatol. Prev: GP Neath, W. Glam.

SOBO, Abayomi Olusola 39 Beech Court, Ponteland, Newcastle upon Tyne NE20 9NE — MD Newc. 1970; MB BS Durh. 1960; DMRT Ed. 1965; MFCM 1985. S.C.M. (Environm. Health) Gateshead HA; WHO Represen. Freetown Sierra Leone. Prev: S.C.M. (Capital Plann.) Northern RHA Newc.-u-Tyne.

SOBOLEWSKI, Olek Andrew Hilly Fields Medical Centre, 172 Adelaide Avenue, London SE4 1JN Tel: 020 8314 5552 Fax: 020 8314 5557 — MB BS Lond. 1993; BSc (Hons.) Sociol. Applied to Med. Lond. 1990. Trainee GP/SHO Chelsea & Westm. Hosp. VTS. Specialty: Gen. Pract.

SOBOLEWSKI, Stanislaw 32 Linden Way, Boston PE21 9DS Tel: 01205 51655 — MRCS Eng. LRCP Lond. 1977 (Med. Acad. Bialystok) MB BS Bialystok 1967; MRCPath 1979; PhD Bradford 1987. Cons. Haemat. Trent RHA & Pilgrim's Hosp. Boston. Specialty: Haematology. Socs: Assn. Clin. Pathols. & Brit. Soc. Haemat. Prev: Sen. Regist. (Haemat.) Leeds & Bradford HAs; SHO

(Rheum.) Roy. Bath Hosp. Harrogate; Regist. (Clin. Haemat.) Centr. Sheff. HA(T).

SOBONIEWSKA, Krystyna Maria Teresa The Portland Road Practice, 16 Portland Road, London W11 4LA Tel: 020 7727 7711 Fax: 020 7226 6755 — MB BCh BAO NUI 1965; DObst RCOG 1968. Socs: BMA. Prev: Ho. Phys. & Ho. Surg. Dreadnought Seamen's Hosp. Lond.; Ho. Surg. O & G St. Mary Abbot's Hosp. Lond.

SOBOWALE, Adetokunbo Oluyomi 7 Garswood Close, Maghull, Liverpool L31 9PF Tel: 0151 531 0196 — MB BS Ibadan 1981; MRCOG 1993.

SOBTI, Anil Kumar Post Office Occupational Health Services, 9th Floor, Commerial Union House,, 24 Martineau Square, Birmingham B2 4UU Tel: 0121 233 7206; Mockley Manor Nursing Home, Forde Hall Lane, Ullenhall, Solihull B95 5PS Tel: 01564 741841 — MB BS Delhi 1972. Specialty: Occupat. Health.

SOBTI, Upender K The Surgery, 5 Brampton Road, Kingsbury, London NW9 9BX Tel: 020 8204 6919 Fax: 020 8206 0883 — (Meerut U.P., India) MB BS Meerut 1975; MB BS Meerut 1975. Specialty: Family Plann. & Reproduc. Health.

SOCKALINGAM, Mahendra Clent Grange, Clent, Stourbridge DY9 9RL — MB ChB Bristol 1974; DRCOG 1976; DCH Eng. 1978; MRCGP 1981.

SOCKALINGAM, Roger Rajendra Kenilworth Medical Centre, 1 Kenilworth Court, Greenfaulds, Cumbernauld, Glasgow G67 1BP Tel: 01236 727816 Fax: 01236 726306 — MB BS Lond. 1972 (The London Hospital Medical college)

SOCKALINGHAM, Inthuvathany North Herts NHS Trust, Lister Hospital, Correys Mill Lane, Stevenage SG1 4AB Tel: 01438 314333 — MB BS Sri Lanka 1983; DA (UK) 1988; FRCA 1992; FFA RCSI 1992. Specialty: Anaesth.

SOCKETT, Gareth John Peter Oral and Maxillofacial Department, Royal Surrey County Hospital, Egerton Road, Guildford GU2 7XX Tel: 01483 571122; Broomsqures, Thursley Road, Eutfad, Godalming GU8 6ED Tel: 01252 703917 — MB ChB Dundee 1982; BDS Liverp. 1974; FDS RCS Ed. 1978. Cons. Oral & Maxillofacial Surg. Roy. Surrey Co. Hosp. Guildford & Frimley Pk. Hosp. Specialty: Oral & Maxillofacial Surg. Prev: Sen. Regist. Yorks. RHA.

SOCOLOVSKY, Merav 12 Hinton Avenue, Cambridge CB1 7AS — MB BS Lond. 1986; MRCP (UK) 1989.

SOCRATES, Mr Antony North Devon District Hospital, Barnstaple EX31 4JB Tel: 01271 322577 Fax: 01271 311696; 42 West Yelland, Barnstaple EX31 3HF Tel: 01271 860819 Email: asocrates@onetel.net.uk — MB BChir Camb. 1982; MA Camb. 1983, BA 1979, MB BChir 1982; DO RCS Eng. 1985; FCOphth. Lond. 1990, M 1989; FRCS Eng. 1990. Assoc. Specialist (Ophth.) N. Devon Dist. Hosp. Barnstaple. Specialty: Ophth. Socs: Fell. Roy. Coll. Of Ophth.; Fell. Roy. Coll. Of Surgs. Prev: Lect. (Ophth.) Univ. Hosp. Kuala Lumpar; Regist. (Ophth.) Roy. Vict. Eye Hosp. Bournemouth.; SHO (Neurol. & Neurosurg.) Midl. Centre for Neurosurg. & Neurol.

SODEN, Frank Benjamin Wyatts Close, Sibford Gower, Banbury OX15 5RT — MB ChB Liverp. 1998.

SODERA, Mr Vija Kumar White Lodge Clinic, 37 Gossamer Lane, Aldwick, Bognor Regis PO21 3BX Tel: 01243 266248 — MB ChB Sheff. 1975; FRCS Ed. 1980. Indep. Surg. White Lodge Clinic. Prev: Cas. Surg. Bognor Regist. War Memor. Hosp. W. Sussex.

SODHI, Hardeep Kaur (retired) 67 Sunnymede Drive, Barkingside, Ilford IG6 1LD Tel: 020 8550 1186 — MB BS Bombay 1958 (Grant Med. Coll. Bombay) Prev: Intern P. Geo. Co. Hosp. Cheverly, MD.

SODHI, Mr Mahinder Singh The Clementine Churchill Hosp. (cons. rooms), Sudbury Hill, Harrow HA1 3RX Tel: 020 8872 3872; 119 Woodcock Hill, Kenton, Harrow HA3 0JW Tel: 020 8907 3356 — MB BS Calcutta 1957; FRCS Eng. 1967. Cons. Surg. Clementine Churchill Hosp. Harrow. Specialty: Gen. Surg. Socs: Assoc. Mem. BAUS; Assn. Coloproctol. Prev: Sen. Regist. (Surg.) Luton & Dunstable Hosp.; Urol. Resid. New York Univ. Med. Centre, USA; Regist. (Surg.) St. Nicholas' Hosp. Lond.

SODHI, Rajveen Kaur Rajsheel, Onslow Road, Sunningdale, Ascot SL5 0HW — MB BS Lond. 1993.

SODHI, Satnam Mahinder 2 Windover, London Road, Harrow on the Hill, Harrow HA1 3JQ — MB BS Lond. 1992.

SODHI, Sukhdev Singh Bridge Street Health Centre, Bridge Street, Ebbw Vale NP23 6EY Tel: 01495 302268 Fax: 01495 305169 — MB BS Punjab (India) 1962; DCH Eng. 1972. Prev: Asst. Clin. Dermat. Nevill Hall Hosp. Abergavenny.; Ho. Off. (Med.) St. Woolos Hosp. Newport; SHO Med. Nevill Hall Hosp. Abergavenny.

SODHI, Sundeep Paul Singh 5 Pantyfforest, Ebbw Vale NP23 5FR — MB BCh Wales 1995.

SODIPO, Joseph Oladeinde c/o Royal Overseas House, Park Place, St James's, London SW1A 1LR — LRCPI & LM, LRSCI & LM 1957; LRCPI & LM, LRCSI & LM 1957; FFA RCS Eng. 1964. Specialty: Anaesth.

SODIPO, Julius Adebiyi Junior Park Hospital, Moorside Road, Davyhulme, Manchester M41 5SL; 54 Arundel Avenue, Flixton, Urmston, Manchester M41 6NG — MB BCh BAO Dub. 1979; MRCS Eng. LRCP Lond. 1979.

SODSAI NATHAN, Mr Subra Maniyam West Middlesex University Hospital, Twickenham Road, Isleworth TW7 6AF Tel: 0208 321 5910 — MB BS Peradeniya 1982; FRCS (Ed) 1988; FRCS (Ed Orth.) Edin. 1997. Cons. Orthopaedic Surg. (Foot & Ankle, Gen. Orthopaedia, Trauma). Specialty: Orthop. Special Interest: Foot & Ankle. Socs: BOA; BOFFS.

SOE AUNG, Dr 10 Chenotrie Gardens, Birkenhead CH43 9WU Tel: 0151 652 0097 — MB BS Mingaladon 1974; MRCP (UK) 1994.

SOE THAN MYINT, Dr Chorley General Hospital, Preston Road, Chorley PR7 1PP Tel: 01257 261222; 16 Orchard Drive, Whittle-le-Woods, Chorley PR6 7JZ Tel: 01257 249968 — MB BS Rangoon 1976; MB BS Med Inst. Rangoon 1976; DA (UK) 1995. Staff Grade (Anaesth.) Chorley Hosp. Specialty: Anaesth.

SOEKARJO, Damayanti Dorothea Humares Ltd., 55-57 Tower St., Winchester SO23 8TA — Artsexamen Utrecht 1994.

SOFAER, David 94A Northend House, Fitzjames Avenue, London W14 0RY Tel: 020 7603 9172 — MB BS Lond. 1944 (Lond. Hosp.) MRCS Eng. LRCP Lond. 1944; MRCP Lond. 1946. Hotel Doctor Cunard Internat. Hotel Ltd. & other Hotels; Med. Dir. Spodefell Ltd.; Flight Personnel Med. Off. Singapore Airlines; Chairm. Med. Bd. Dept. Health & Social Security; Med. Adviser Brit. Vending Industries.

SOFAT, Mr Ajit 44 Greenacres, Leverstock Green, Hemel Hempstead HP2 4NA Tel: 01442 257579; 22 Waterslea Drive, Heaton, Bolton BL1 5FJ — MB ChB Manch. 1982; FRCS Ed. 1988; FRCS (SN) 1996. Cons. (Neurosurg.) Hope Hosp. Salford. Specialty: Neurosurg. Prev: Sen. Regist. (Neurosurg.) King's Coll. Hosp.; Research Fell. Inst. Neurol. Lond.; Regist. (Neurosurg.) Roy. Preston Hosp.

SOFAT, Nidhi 10 Paines Lane, Pinner HA5 3DQ — MB BS Lond. 1996 (Univ. Coll. Lond. Med. Sch.) BSc (Immunol. with Basic Med. Scis.) 1993. SHO (Gen. Med.) Char. Cross & Hammersmith Hosps. Specialty: Gen. Med.

SOFI, Mr Mohamad Abdullah Flat 5, 80 Fitzjohns Avenue, London NW3 5LS — MD Patna 1973; MRCPI 1980; MRCP (UK) 1981; FRCS Ed. 1990; FRCP Lond. 1991; FRCP Ed. 1991.

SOFOLUWE, George Oluwole 35 Danta Way, Baswich, Stafford ST17 0BA Tel: 01785 49487 — MB ChB St. And. 1957; DPH 1961, DIH 1965. Prof. & Head Dept Community Health & Prof. Occupat. Health Univ. Benin, Nigeria; Dir. Gen. Inst. Occupat. Health Ibadan, Nigeria. Socs: (Pioneer Pres.) Nigerian Soc. Occupat. Health Phys.; (Pres.) African Region. Assn. Occupat. Health. Prev: Region. Med. Advis. World Health Organisations; WHO Prof. Comm. & Occupat. Health, Univ. Lusaka, Zambia; Specialist Comm. Phys. Environ. Health, Birm. AHA.

SOFOLUWE, Grahame Oluwole Billericay Health Centre, Stock Road, Billericay CM12 0BJ Tel: 01277 658071 Fax: 01277 631892 — MB BS Ibadan 1984; MRCS Eng. LRCP Lond. 1992; MRCGP 1993; DCH RCP Lond. 1993; DRCOG 1994; AFOM 2001. Specialty: Gen. Pract.; Occupat. Health. Socs: Soc. of Occupat.al Med.

SOGLIANI, Franco Blackpool Victoria Hospital, Whinney Heys Road, Blackpool FY3 8NR Tel: 01253 303770 Fax: 01253 655528; 18 Walsingham Gardens, Stoneleigh, Epsom KT19 0LU Tel: 020 8393 3791 Fax: 020 8393 3791 — State Exam Turin 1987; Dip. Card Surg 1992; FRCSI Dub 1998. Specialist Regist. Middx Hosp. Lond. Specialty: Cardiothoracic Surg. Socs: EACTS; Soc. of CT Surg. UK & Irel.; ASIT. Prev: Specialist Regist. (Cardiothoracic Surg.) St Geo.'s Hosp. Lond.; Sen. Regist. (Cardiothoracic Surg.) St. Mary's Hosp. Lond.; Regist. St. Mary's Hosp. Lond.

SOH, Joo Kim 20 Abbey Court, Abbey Road, St John's Wood, London NW8 0AU Tel: 020 7625 5303 — MB BS Singapore 1987.

SOH, Vicky Ai Leen 25 Thorpe Way, Cambridge CB5 8UJ — MB BS Lond. 1994.

SOHAIB, Syed Azfer Aslam Radiology Dept, Roayl Marsden Hospital, Downs Road, Sutton SM2 5PT — MB BS Lond. 1990; BSc Lond. 1987; MRCP (UK) 1993; FRCR 1996. Cons. Radiologist Radiol. Dept Roy. Marsden Hosp. Sutton Surrey. Specialty: Radiol.

SOHAIL, Rashid 100 Birkby Hall Road, Huddersfield HD2 2TN — MB ChB Aberd. 1989.

SOHAIL SAHIBZADA, Mr Ahmed Department of Orthopaedics, Dundee Royal Infirmary, Barrack Road, Dundee DD1 9ND — MB BS Peshawar 1978; FRCS Ed. 1987; FRCSI 1987.

SOHAL, Aneel Singh 21 Roger Drive, Wakefield WF2 7NE Tel: 01924 219502 — MB BS Rajasthan 1976; MRCPath 1985; MSc Med. Microbiol. Surrey 1986. Cons. Microbiol. Pinderfields Gen. Hosp. Wakefield. Specialty: Med. Microbiol. Prev: Sen. Regist. Dept. Clin. Bacteriol. & Virol. Guy's Hosp. Lond.

SOHAL, Hardip 17 Petworth Way, Elm Park, Hornchurch RM12 4LR — MB ChB Leeds 1996.

SOHAL, Mamta 267 Rochford Gardens, Slough SL2 5XH — BM BS Nottm. 1993.

SOHI, Dalbir Kaur 113B Dartmouth Road, London NW2 4ES Email: dsohi@hotmail.com — MB ChB Glas. 1998; BSc (Hons.) Lond. 1996; MRCPCH 2001.

SOHI, Malvinder Singh The Surgery, 57 Gladstone Avenue, Manor Park, London E12 7NR Tel: 020 8471 4764 Fax: 020 8472 3378; Cedar Medical Centre, 4 Granville Road, Ilford IG1 4JY Tel: 020 8270 0040 Fax: 020 8270 0042 — MB BS Punjab 1969 (Govt. Med. Coll. Patiala) DOMS Punjab 1970. Specialty: Gen. Pract. Socs: Newham Med. Soc.

SOHN, Leslie Flat 1, 17 Prince Albert Road, London NW1 7ST — MB ChB Cape Town 1944; DPM Eng. 1949; FRCPsych. 1977, M 1972. Sen. Tutor & Hon. Cons. Psychother. Dept. Maudsley Hosp. Lond. Socs: Brit. Psycho-Anal. Soc. Prev: Cons. Psychother. Shenley Hosp. St. Albans; Regist. Maudsley Hosp.

SOILE, David Olayiwola 7 Haredon Close, London SE23 3TG — MB BS Ibadan, Nigeria 1985.

SOILLEUX, Elizabeth Jane Department of Histopathology, (Box 235), Addenbrookes Hospital, Hills Rd, Cambridge CB2 2QQ Tel: 01223 217 163 Fax: 01223 216 980 Email: ejs17@cam.ac.uk; 22 Fromont Close, Fulbourn, Cambridge CB1 5HS Tel: 01223 473954 Email: ejs17@cam.ac.uk — BChir Camb. 1996 (Cambridge) BA Cantab. 1994; MA Cantab. 1998; PhD Cantab. 2002. Specialist Regist. (Histopath.) Camb.; Teachg. Fell. in Path. Ch.hill Coll. Camb. Univ. Specialty: Histopath. Socs: BMA - (Past Sec.BMA, E. Anglian Regional Jun. Doctors' Comm. 1997-1998); MDU. Prev: Research Regist. (Histopath.) Camb. + MRC Clin. Train. Fell., Univ of Camb.; SHO (Histopath.) Camb.; PRHO (Gen. Surg.) Milton Keynes.

SOIN, Bob — MB BChir Camb. 1992; MA 1995; FRCS (Gen. Surg.) 2002; MD 2002.

SOIN-STANLEY, Simon Anthony John Tower Medical Centre, 129 Cannon Street Road, London E1 2LX Tel: 020 7488 4240 Fax: 020 7702 2443 — MB BS Lond. 1982; DCH RCP Lond. 1989.

SOINNE, Nicolle 24 Victoria Gardens, Kilmacolm PA13 4HL — MB ChB Glas. 1988.

SOJITRA, Nilesh Mavji 53 Hailes Gardens, Edinburgh EH13 0JH — MB ChB Ed. 1997.

SOJKA, Yves Jan Franciszek 24 Park Way, Ruislip HA4 8NY Tel: 018956 32858 — MB ChB Sheff. 1950. Prev: Orthop. Ho. Surg. Roy. Hosp. Sheff.; Ho. Phys. Wharncliffe Hosp. Sheff.

SOKAL, Michael Peter Jacob Wieselberg — MB ChB Sheff. 1970; MRCP (UK) 1974; FRCR 1978; FRCP Lond. 1991. Cons. (Radiother. & Oncol.) City Hosp. Nottm. Specialty: Oncol.; Radiother. Prev: Sen. Regist. (Radiother. & Oncol.) Roy. S. Hants. Hosp. Soton.; Regist. (Radiother. & Oncol.) Roy. Marsden Hosp. Lond.

SOKHI, Jasminder Singh O'Colmain and Partners, Fearnhead Cross Medical Centre, 25 Fearnhead Cross, Warrington WA2 0HD Tel: 01925 847000 Fax: 01925 818650; 17 Edward Gardens, Martinscroft, Warrington WA1 4QS Tel: 01925 485641 — MB ChB Liverp. 1978. Specialty: Gen. Surg.; Diabetes. Socs: BMA (Treas. Warrington Br.). Prev: SHO (Orthop.) Warrington HA.

SOKOL, Robert Josef (retired) 14 Harley Road, Ecclesall, Sheffield S11 9SD — MB ChB Shef. 1968; FRCPath 1986, M 1974; PhD Sheff. 1984, DSc 1992, MD 1979; FRCP Ed 1997.

SOLAN, Chantal Leigh 73 Kippington Road, Sevenoaks TN13 2LN — MB ChB Cape Town 1992.

SOLAN, Katharine Jane 55 Marine Drive, West Wittering, Chichester PO20 8HQ — MB BS Lond. 1994 (St. Barts. Hosp. Med. Sch.) Roy. Hosps. Trust Anaesth. SHO. Specialty: Anaesth.

SOLAN, Nerith Lindsay 29A Astonville Street, London SW18 5AN Tel: 020 8870 2619 — MB ChB Cape Town 1990; DCH Lond. 1993; DRCOG Lond. 1996; DFFP Lond. 1997; MRCGP Lond. 1997. Socs: Med. Protec. Soc.

SOLANGI, Mr Bashir Ahmed Northern Area Armed Forces Hospital, PO Box 10018, Hafar Al Batin 31991, Saudi Arabia Tel: 00 966 3 7871777; 7 Torquay Gardens, Redbridge, Ilford IG4 5PU Tel: 0208 550 6774 Fax: 0208 550 6774 — MB BS Sind 1970 (Liaquat Med. Coll.) FRCS Ed. 1984. Cons. Urol. North. Area Armed Forces Hosp., Saudi Arbia. Specialty: Urol. Prev: Regist. & SHO (Gen. Surg. & Urol.) OldCh. Hosp. Romford; SHO (Orthop.) Harold Wood Hosp.; Assoc. Prof. Surg. Dow Med. Coll. & Hosp. Karachi, Pakistan.

SOLANKI, Dharmendra Amarshi 160 Manor Dr N., Worcester Park KT4 7RU — MB BS Lond. 1997.

SOLANKI, Mr Guirish Arquissandas Department of Surgical Neurology, The National Hospital for Neurology & Neurosurgery, Queen Square, London WC1N 3BG Tel: 020 7837 3611 Fax: 020 7813 1138; 42 Finland Street, The Lakes, Rotherhithe, London SE16 7TP Tel: 020 7237 3048 Fax: 020 7237 3048 Email: 106055.361@compuserve.com — MB BS Bombay 1988 (Goa Med. Coll.) FRCSI 1991. Spinal Research Fell. (Surgic. Neurol.) & Sen. Regist. (Neurosurg.) Nat. Hosp. for Neurol. & Neurosurg. Lond. Specialty: Neurosurg. Socs: Brit. Cervical Spine Research Soc.; Soc. Brit. Neurol. Surgs. Prev: Career Regist. Rotat. (Neurosurg.) Roy. Lond. Hosp. & OldCh. Hosp.; Sen. Regist. (Neurosurg.) Humana Hosp. St. Johns Wood, Lond.; Regist. (Neurosurg.) Roy. Free Hosp.

SOLANKI, Jitendra Uttam — MB ChB Birm. 1993; DRCOG May 1997 (RCOG); DCH 1998 June; DFFP 1998; MRCGP 2000. Med. Advisor.- Pharmacia, Milton Keynes. Specialty: Gen. Pract.; Pharmaceutical Medicine.

SOLANKI, Pragna The Centre Surgery, Health Centre, Hill Street, Hinckley LE10 1DS — BM Soton. 1993.

SOLANKI, Tarunkumar Gordhandas Musgrove Park Hospital, Taunton TA1 5DA Tel: 01823 333444 Fax: 01823 344747 Email: tarun.solanki@tst.nhs.uk — MB BCh Wales 1984; FRCP; BSc (Hons.) Wales 1981; MSc Lond. 1994. Cons. Phys. special responsibil. Elderly MusGr. Pk. Hosp. Taunton; Clincial Director Community & Primary Care Directorate; Taunton & Som. NHS Trust. Specialty: Care of the Elderly. Socs: Brit. Geriat. Soc.; BMA. Prev: Sen. Regist. (Gen. & Geriat. Med.) W. Midl. Regional Train. Scheme; Regist. (Gen. Med. & Nephrol.) St. Mary's Hosp. Portsmouth.

SOLARI, John Ruddock Alvechurch Medical Centre, 5-6 The Square, Alvechurch, Birmingham B48 7LB Tel: 0121 445 1084; 52 Grassmoor Road, King's Norton, Birmingham B38 8BU Tel: 0121 458 4480 — MB ChB Birm. 1958; BSc Physiol. (1st cl. Hons.) Birm. 1958, MB ChB 1961; DObst RCOG 1964; MRCGP 1969. Hosp. Pract. Sheldon Geriat. Hosp. Rednal; Med. Dir. GP Deputising Serv.; Treas. Birm. Local Med. Comm.; Mem. St. John Ambul. Aeromed. Serv. Socs: BMA. Prev: Clin. Asst. (Geriat.) Sheldon Geriat. Hosp. Rednal; Ho. Surg. (O & G) Dudley Rd. Hosp. Birm.; Ho. Phys. & Ho. Surg. Qu. Eliz. Hosp. Birm.

SOLARI, Timothy John Robinson, Ashton, Leung, Solari and Thompson, James Preston Health Centre, 61 Holland Road, Sutton Coldfield B72 1RL Tel: 0121 355 5150 — MB ChB Birm. 1986.

SOLDI, Donatella Francesca Dept of Child & Adolescent Health, St. Leonards Primary Care Centre, Nuttall St., London N1 5LZ — MB ChB Manch. 1990 (Manchester) BA (Econ.) Hons. Manch. 1978; SRN UKCC 1982; DCH RCP Lond. 1994. Staff Grade (Community Child Health) City & Hackney PCT. Specialty: Community Child Health. Prev: SHO (Paediat. & Neonat.) Whittington Hosp. Lond.; SHO (Infec. Dis.) Monsall Hosp. Manch.; SHO (Med.) Monsall Hsop. Manch & N. Manch. Gen. Hosp.

SOLDINI, Marcus John Francesco — BM Soton. 1986; DGM RCP Lond. 1987; MRCGP 1996.

SOLE, Mr Graham Martin Southbourne, Dinmore, Hereford HR1 3JR Tel: 01432 355444 — MB BS Lond. 1976 (Univ. Coll. Hosp.) FRCS Eng. 1980; BSc Lond. 1973, MS 1986. Cons. Urol. Hereford Co. Hosp. Specialty: Urol. Prev: Sen. Regist. Rotat. (Urol.)

Leeds & Bradford; Regist. (Urol.) Qu. Eliz. Hosp. Birm.; Regist. (Surg. & Urol.) Dudley Rd. Hosp. Birm.

SOLE, Peter Wallis (retired) 17 Craigweil Lane, Aldwick, Bognor Regis PO21 4AN Tel: 01243 821809 — MB BChir Camb. 1950 (Camb. & Westm.) MA Camb. 1950.

SOLEBO, Junaid Oluseyi Kings George Hospital, Barley Lane, Ilford IG3 8 Tel: 020 8983 8000 — MB BS Lagos 1977 (College of medicine - University of Hagos - Nigeria) DCH RCPS Glas. 1984. Staff Grade (Paediat.) King Geo. Hosp. Ilford Essex. Specialty: Paediat. Prev: Regist. (Paediat.) Lewisham Hosp. Lond.; SHO (Paediat.) Watford Gen. Hosp.; SHO (Paediat.) Roy. Hosp. Chesterfield, SHO (Paed) Kettering Hosp.

SOLEIMANI, Mr Behzad Cardiothoracic Unit, The A Block, Hammersnith Hospital, Ducane Road, London W12 0HS Tel: 020 8383 3944 Fax: 020 8383 2725 — MB BChir Camb. 1994; MA 1995, BA (Hons.) Camb. 1991; FRCS Eng. 1997. Specialist Regist. (Cardiothor. Surg.) Hammersmith Hosp. Lond. Specialty: Cardiothoracic Surg. Socs: BMA. Prev: SHO (Gen. Surg.) Ealing Hosp. Lond.; SHO (Orthop.) Ealing Hosp. Lond.; SHO (Cardiothorac. Surg.) Hammersmith Hosp. Lond.

SOLESBURY, Kathryn Anne St. Martins Grate Surgery, Providence Street, Worcester WR1 2BS Tel: 01905 681781 Fax: 01905 681766; Brock Hall, Suckley, Worcester WR6 5DJ Tel: 01886 884192 — MB ChB Birm. 1983; MFFP; DCH RCP Lond. 1986; DRCOG 1987; MRCGP (Distinc.) 1987; MFFP 1995. Gen. Practitioner Worcester. Prev: Trainee GP Worcester VTS.

SOLIMAN, El Sayed Queen's Park Hospital, Blackburn BB2 3HH — MB ChB Alexandria 1965; MRCP (UK) 1978; LRCP LRCS Ed. LRCPS Glas. 1980. Cons. Phys. (Geriat. Med.) N. West. RHA. Specialty: Gen. Med. Socs: BMA; Brit. Geriat. Soc. Prev: Rotat. Sen. Regist. (Geriat. Med.) & Hon. Clin. Tutor Sheff. Med.; Sch.; Regist. (Geriat. Med.) Gwent AHA; SHO (Psychiat.) St. Nicholas Hosp. Gt. Yarmouth.

SOLIMAN, Mohamed Ossama Amin Mohamed Hanley Health Centre, Upper Huntbach Street, Hanley, Stoke-on-Trent ST1 2BN Tel: 01782 202422 — MB BCh Cairo 1964.

SOLIMAN, Soliman Mikhail Mohsen (cons. rooms), 29 Devonshire Place, London W1 Tel: 020 7935 9973 Fax: 020 8653 9628; (Surgery), 86 Woodland Road, London SE19 1PA Tel: 020 8670 3689 Fax: 020 8653 9628 — MB BCh Cairo 1956; LMSSA Lond. 1968; Cert. Family Plann. JCC 1976. Specialty: Family Plann. & Reproduc. Health. Socs: Fell. Roy. Soc. Med. Prev: Hosp. Pract. Beckenham Hosp.; Community Health Pract. (Child Health) Bromley Schs.

SOLIS REYES, Carlos Flat 1, Glebedale Court, Clebedale Road, Stoke-on-Trent ST4 3LT — LMS La Laguna 1987.

SOLJAK, Michael Anthony Ealing, Hammersmith & Hounslow Health Authority, 1 Armstrong Way, Southall UB2 4SA — MB ChB Auckland 1976; FRACP 1984; FAFPHM 1988; MFPHM RCP (UK) 1993. Dir. of Strategy & Health Gain Ealing, Hammersmith & Hounslow HA. Specialty: Pub. Health Med. Socs: FAFPHM 1988.

SOLLIS, Maria Emma 1 Maes Glas, Ynysawdre, Tondu, Bridgend CF32 9JZ — MB BS Lond. 1992.

SOLMAN, Nicola Seymour House Surgery, 154 Sheen Road, Richmond TW9 1UU Tel: 020 8940 2802 Fax: 020 8332 7877; 37 Larkfield Road, Richmond TW9 2PG — MB BS Lond. 1986; DRCOG 1990.

SOLOFF, Neville 16 Chartwell Avenue, Northampton NN3 6NT Tel: 01604 644378 — MB ChB Leeds 1959; DPH Leeds 1970; AFOM RCP Lond. 1982. Sen. Med. Off. N.ants. HA. Specialty: Pub. Health Med. Socs: Fac. Community Health; Soc. Occupat. Med.; Soc. Pub. Health. Prev: Med. Off. Repat. Dept., S. Austral.; Squadron Ldr. RAF Med. Br.

SOLOMKA, Bohdan Theodore 13 Stalham Road, Hoveton, Norwich NR12 8DG — BM BS Nottm. 1988.

***SOLOMON, Andrew Martin** 12 Chestnut Av, Edgware HA8 7RA — BM BCh Oxf. 1997; MRCP.

SOLOMON, Anthony Leopold Salop Road Medical Centre, Salop Road, Welshpool SY21 7ER Email: wmc@doctors.org.uk; Elmhurst, Severn Road, Welshpool SY21 7AR Tel: 01938 552744 Email: anthony.solomon@lineone.net — MB ChB Birm. 1969; DObst RCOG 1971. Prev: Med. Off. Brit. Solomon Isles Protectorate; Ho. Surg. Childr. Hosp. Birm.; Ho. Phys. Med. Profess. Unit Qu. Eliz. Hosp. Birm.

SOLOMON, Belinda 6 Aintree Drive, Rochdale OL11 5SH — MB BS Lond. 1998.

SOLOMON, Cedric Matthew Queens Walk Surgery, 69 Queens Walk, Ruislip HA4 0NT Tel: 020 8842 2991 Fax: 020 8842 2245; 54 Oakleigh Park N., London N20 9AS — MB BS Lond. 1981; MRCGP 1985; DCH RCP Lond. 1985; DGM RCP Lond. 1985.

SOLOMON, Christine Lorraine Medical Research Council, Environmental Epidemiology Unit, University of Southampton, Southampton General Hospital, Southampton SO16 6YD Tel: 023 8072 5537 Fax: 023 8072 5509 Email: cls@mrc.soton.ac.uk; Beulah, 71 Station Road, Netley Abbey, Southampton SO31 5AE Tel: 023 8056 1217 — BM BCh Oxf. 1985 (Camb. & Oxf.) MA Camb. 1986; DCH RCP Lond. 1987; Cert. Family Plann. JCC 1988; DGM RCP Lond. 1988; DRCOG 1988; MRCGP 1989; MFPHM Lond. 1998. p/t Consultant Research Fellow MRC Southampton. Specialty: Pub. Health Med.; Epidemiol.; Gen. Pract. Prev: Regist. (Pub. Health Med.) SE Thames RHA and S&W RHA; Clin. Fell. (Continuing c/o Elderly) Riverside HA; Trainee GP Davenport Hse. Harpenden VTS.

SOLOMON, Frank Stuart Blossoms Inn Medical Centre, 21 Garlick Hill, London EC4V 2AU Tel: 020 7606 6159 Fax: 020 7489 1134; 8 Millfield Lane, Highgate, London N6 6JD Tel: 020 8340 2376 Email: 101707.2436@compuserve.com — MB ChB Cape Town 1971; MB ChB (Hons.) Cape Town 1971; MRCP (UK) 1977. Neurol. Northwick Pk. Hosp. & City of Lond. Migraine Clinic; Chief Med. Off. ERC Francona Re, Legal & Gen. Specialty: Gen. Pract.; Neurol. Socs: Brit. Assoc. for Study of Headache; Assur. Med. Soc. Prev: Sen. Regist. (Neurol.) Groote Schur Hosp. S. Afr.; Clin. Fell. Nat. Hosp. Qu. Sq.

SOLOMON, George The Black Country Family Practice, Neptune Health Park, Sedgley Road West, Tipton DY4 8PX Tel: 0121 607 6448 — MB ChB Glas. 1978; DRCOG 1984. Prev: SHO/Trainee GP Som. VTS; SHO (Surg.) Taunton & Som. Hosps. Taunton; SHO (Surg. Specialties) West. Infirm. Glas.

SOLOMON, Jacob Israel Queens Walk Surgery, 69 Queens Walk, Ruislip HA4 0NT Tel: 020 8842 2991 Fax: 0161 868 8853 — MB BS Lond. 1980 (Univ. Coll. Hosp.) BSc (Immunol.) Lond. 1977; DCH RCP Lond. 1983; MRCGP 1984; Cert. Family Plann. JCC 1985; D Occ. Med. RCP Lond. 1999. Chairm. NW Thames Region GP Trainee Represen. Comm.; Med. Edr. Pulse Young Practitioner; Vice-Chairm. Hillingdon MAAG; Edit. Bd. Mem. Prescriber Magazine & Brit. Jl. Med. Economics; Bd. Mem. N. Hillingdon PCG; Med. Adviser Barnet Enfield & Haringay HA; Physician to The Royak Society, 6-9 Carlton House Terrace, London; Occupational Health Physician to Budgens Stores. Specialty: Occupat. Health. Prev: Trainee GP Northwick Pk. Hosp. Harrow; Ho. Surg. (Thoracic, Gen. & Orthop. Surg.) Univ. Coll. Hosp. Lond.; Ho. Phys. (Cardiol.) Hillingdon Hosp. Uxbridge.

SOLOMON, Laurence Richard Royal Preston Hospital, PO Box 66, Sharoe Green Lane, Preston PR2 4HT Tel: 01772 716565; 2 Oakwood Drive, Fulwood, Preston PR2 3LX — MB BChir Camb. 1973; MRCP (UK) 1974; MA Camb. 1973, MD 1988; FRCP Lond. 1994. Cons. Gen. Phys. (Renal Med.) Preston HA. Specialty: Gen. Med.; Nephrol. Socs: Renal Assn.; Internat. Soc. Nephrol. Prev: Lect. (Geriat. Med.) Univ. Liverp.; Tutor (Renal Med.) Manch. Roy. Infirm.; Lect. (Med.) Univ. Manch. & Withington Hosp. Manch.

SOLOMON, Lemke Solent Department of Urology, St Mary's Hospital, Milton Road, Portsmouth PO3 6AD Tel: 023 9228 6000 — MB BCh BAO NUI 1989; LRCPSI 1989. Specialty: Urol.

SOLOMON, Louis (retired) Pleasant, 32 Barcombe Heights, Paignton TQ3 1PT Tel: 01803 550156 — (TC Dub.) BA (Hons.) Dub. 1938, MA 1941, MB BCh BAO 1940; LM Rotunda 1946; DPH Lond. 1947; DCH Eng. 1949; MFCM 1974. Founder Med. Offs. Audiol. Gp. Prev: Dep. Controller Community Servs. Torbay Co. Boro.

SOLOMON, Professor Louis Department of Orthopaedic Surgery, Bristol Royal Infirmary, Bristol BS2 8HW Tel: 0117 973 3953 Fax: 0117 973 3953 Email: louis.solomon@btinternet.com; 7 Cotham Road, Cotham, Bristol BS6 6DG Tel: 0117 973 3953 Fax: 0117 973 3953 — MB ChB Cape Town 1951; FRCS Ed. 1958; FRCS Eng. 1959; MD Cape Town 1963. Emerit. Prof. Orthop. Surg. Univ. Bristol; Hon. Cons. Bristol Roy. Infirm. Specialty: Orthop. Socs: Fell. BOA; Internat. Hip Soc. Prev: Prof. Orthop. Surg. Univ. Witwatersrand, Johannesburg.

SOLOMON, Patricia 6 Aintree Drive, Bamford, Rochdale OL11 5SH — MB ChB Ghana 1974; FRCR 1984. Cons. (Radiol.) Roy. Oldham Hosp. Specialty: Radiol. Socs: BMA; Brit. Inst. Radiol.; Roy. Coll. Radiol. Prev: Cons. (Radiol.) Barnsley Dist. Hosp.

SOLOMON, Ruth Anne Willow House, Littlemore Hospital#Littlemore, Oxford OX4 4XN Tel: 01865 223148146 — MB ChB Dundee 1981; MRCPsych 1985. Cons. Psychiarist. Specialty: Rehabil. Med. Prev: Regist. (Psychiat.) (Rotat.) Oxon. HA.

SOLOMON, Samuel Appiah Department of Adult Medicine, Royal Oldham Hospital, Rochdale Road, Oldham OL1 2JH Tel: 0161 627 8479 Fax: 0161 627 8694 Email: samuel.solomon@oldham-tr.nwest.nhs.uk; 6 Aintree Drive, Bamford, Rochdale OL11 5SH — MB ChB Ghana 1974 (Univ. Ghana Med. Sch.) MRCP (UK) 1981; MRCP (UK) 1981; FRCP (Lond) 1999; FRCP (Lond) 1999. Cons. Phys. Roy. Oldham Hosp. Specialty: Care of the Elderly; Gen. Med. Socs: BMA; Brit. Geriat. Soc. Prev: Sen. Regist. Rotat. (Med. & Geriat.) Manch.; Research Fell. Roy. Hallamsh. Hosp. Sheff.; Regist. Rotat. (Med.) Liverp.

SOLOMON, Stephen Maxwell Ernest 79 Grays Inn Road, London WC1X 8TP Tel: 020 7405 9360 Fax: 020 7831 1964 — MB BS Lond. 1979 (University College Hospital London) DRCOG 1983; Cert. Family Plann. JCC 1984. GP Partner; Occupat. Phys. Brit. Gas plc; Forens. Med. Examr.; Occupat. Phys. Transco Plc. Specialty: Occupat. Health. Socs: (Counc.) Assn. Police Surgs.; Roy. Soc. Med. (Clin. Forens. Med. Sect.); Brit. Acad. Forens. Sci.

SOLOMON, Sylvia Nunes 4 Briardene Crescent, Kenton Park, Newcastle upon Tyne NE3 4RY — MB ChB Manch. 1945; MRCP Lond. 1949; DCH Eng. 1950; MRCGP 1968; BA Open Univ. 1988; BA (Hons.) Open Univ. 1991. Clin. Asst. Newc. BTS. Specialty: Paediat. Prev: M. O. Tshilidzini Hosp. Vendaland; Princip. GP Paediat. Regist. Leeds.

SOLOMON, Terence A The Farmhouse, 1 Gatehill Road, Northwood HA6 3QB Tel: 01923 825067 — MB BS Calcutta 1945; DObst RCOG 1948. Socs: Fell. Roy. Soc. Med. (Mem. Obst. Sect.); Fell. Amer. Coll. Sexol.; Life Mem. New York Acad. Sc. Prev: Ho. Surg. (Gyn.) Derbysh. Roy. Infirm.; Resid. Obst. Off. Bearsted Memor. Hosp.; Capt. RAMC 1945-48.

SOLOMON, Thomas Department of Neurological Science, University of Liverpool, Walton Centre for Neurology & Neurosurgery, Lower Lane, Liverpool L9 7LJ Tel: 0151 529 5460 Fax: 0151 529 5465 — BM BCh 1990; BA (Hons.) Phys. Scis. Oxf. 1987; MRCP UK 1993; DCH RCP Lond. 1994; DTM & H Liverp. 2000; PhD Op. Univ. 2000. Wellcome Trust Career Developm. Fell.; Lecturer in Neurolgy; Hon Lect. in Med. Microbiol. & Trop. Med. Specialty: Infec. Dis.; Neurol. Socs: Osler Club Lond.; Hist. Med. Soc. Prev: Vis. Scientist & Hon. Assoc. Prof. Univ. Texas Med. Br. Galveston; Clin. Research Fell. & Hon. Regist. Wellcome Trust, Vietnam; Regist. (Med.) City Hosp. Nottm.

SOLOMON, Winston Christadoss Asir St Clement's Surgery, 38 Bathurst Road, Ilford IG1 4LA Tel: 020 8554 1371 Fax: 020 8491 3345 — MB BS Madras 1975; FRCS Ed. 1985; FRCS Glas. 1985; DCH RCP Lond. 1990; DRCOG 1991. Specialty: Gen. Pract.

SOLOMONS, Bethel Eric Robert 7 Wimpole Street, London W1G 9SN Tel: 020 7584 1580 — MB BCh BAO Dub. 1940 (Dub. & Middlx.) MA Dub. 1955, MD 1944; FRCPI 1951, M 1947. Hon. Cons. Dermat. Chelmsford & Essex Gen. Hosp. Specialty: Dermat. Socs: Fell. (Mem. Dermat. Sect.) Roy. Soc. Med.; Brit. Assn. Dermat.

SOLOMONS, Carole Ann — MB BS Lond. 1981 (Univ. Coll. Hosp.) BSc (Hons.) Lond. 1976; DRCOG 1984; MRCGP 1985; Cert. Family Plann. JCC 1985; Dip. Psychosexual Med. 1994. Tutor (Gen. Pract.) Roy. Free Hosp. Med. Sch. Specialty: Gen. Pract. Socs: Inst. Psychosexual Med.; RCGP. Prev: Trainee GP Chesham; SHO (Paediat.) Amersham Gen. Hosp.; SHO (Obst. & Psychiat.) Wycombe Gen. Hosp.

SOLOMONS, Gary Elliott White Thorns, South Hill Avenue, Harrow on the Hill, Harrow HA1 3NZ — MB BS Lond. 1996.

SOLOMONS, Neil 39 Woodland Gardens, London N10 3UE — MB BS Lond. 1991.

SOLOMONS, Mr Neil Barry Mount Alvernia Hospital, Harvey Road, Guildford GU1 3LX Tel: 01483 451473 Fax: 01483 454286 Email: solomonsn@lasermebeautiful.com — MB ChB Cape Town 1979 (Univ. of Cape Town) FRCS Eng. 1984; FRCS Ed. 1987. p/t Consulatnt Surg. Otolaryngol. - Facial Plastic and Laser Surg., Roy. Surrey Co. Hosp., Guildford; Cons. Otolaryngol. Head & Neck Surg. St. Peter's Hosp. Chertsey & Roy. Surrey Co. Hosp. Guildford. Specialty: Otolaryngol.; Otorhinolaryngol. Special Interest: Facial Plastic, Laser & Skin Surg. Socs: Brit. Assn. of Otolaryngol. - Head and Neck Surg.; Europ. Acad. of facial Plastic Surg.; Amer. Soc. for Laser Med. and Surg. Prev: Sen. Regist. (Otolaryngol.) Roy. Free Hosp. Lond. & Roy. Surrey Co. Hosp. Guildford; Regist. (Otolaryngol.) Glos. Roy. Hosp.; Regist. (Otolaryngol.) Groote Schuur Hosp., Cape Town.

SOLOMONS, Richard Edgar Bethel Ling House Medical Centre, 49 Scott Street, Keighley BD21 2JH Tel: 01535 605747 Fax: 01535 672576 Email: richard.solomons@bradford.nhs.uk — MB BS Lond. 1977 (Middlesex) BSc Lond. 1974; MSc (Community Health in Developing Countries) Lond. 1982; DRCOG 1983; MRCGP 1984.

SOLOMONS, Stanley (retired) — BM BCh Oxf. 1953; MA Oxf. 1953; MRCGP 1971. Prev: Med. Off. Coll. of NW Lond.

SOLOMONSZ, Mr Francis Allistair Kilton Hill, Worksop S81 0BD Tel: 01909 500 990; Sheriwill, 131A Melton Road, West Bridgford, Nottingham NG2 6FG Tel: 0115 945 2668 — MB BS Sri Lanka 1975; MRCOG 1983; DFFP 1991. Specialty: Obst. & Gyn. Socs: Brit. Med Assoc.; Brit. Fert. Soc.; Brit. Soc. For Colposcopy & Cervical Path.

SOLTANI, Hassan — MB ChB Sheff. 1997.

SOLTANPOUR, Mr Abbas (retired) 58 Rosecroft Gardens, Twickenham TW2 7PZ Tel: 020 8 898 2870; 58/2 Alvand Avenue, Tehran 15168, Iran Tel: 00 98 21 8888868 — MD Teheran, Iran 1959; FRCS Ed. 1972. Prev: Asst. Prof. Orthop. Tehran Univ.

SOMAIYA, Rupin Suresh Fiveways Stores, Sturt Road, Charlbury, Chipping Norton OX7 3SX — MB BCh Wales 1993.

SOMALINGAM, Ramalingam 26 Orleans Road, Upper Norwood, London SE19 3TA — MB BS Ceylon 1963.

SOMAN, Vijay Bhaskarrao Church Lane Surgery, 77 Church Lane, Harpurhey, Manchester M9 1BA Tel: 0161 205 2714 Fax: 0161 205 2716 — MB BS Poona 1966 (B.J. Med. Coll.) DOMS CPS Bombay 1968. GP Manch. Prev: SHO (Ophth.) Roy. Eye Hosp. Manch.; SHO (Ophth.) Singleton Hosp. Swansea & Newc. Gen. Hosp.

SOMANATHAN, Lakshman Hill Croft, Green Lane, Chessington KT9 2DS; 43 Alwyne Road, Wimbledon, London SW19 7AE Tel: 020 8879 3900 Fax: 020 8879 3900 — MB BS Lond. 1994 (Charing Cross & Westm.) FRCS Eng. 1996. SHO (Surg.) Char. Cross Hosp. Lond. Specialty: Orthop. Prev: SHO (Surg.) W. Middlx.

SOMANI, Mr Nandkishor Radhakishan West Dorset Hospital, Damers Road, Dorchester DT1 2JY Tel: 01305 251150 — MB BS Marathwada 1965; MS (ENT) Bombay 1969; FCPS (ENT) Bombay 1969. Assoc. Specialist ENT, W. Dorset Hosp. Dorchester.

SOMANI, Neeta 32 Maiden Castle Road, Dorchester DT1 2ES; 32 Maiden Castle Road, Dorchester DT1 2ES — (St George's Hospital Medical School) MB BS Lond. 1994. GP Non Princip. Specialty: Gen. Pract. Prev: SHO Paediat. Penbury Hosp. Tunbridge Wells Kent; SHO c/o the Elderly Penbury Hosp. Tunbridge Wells Kent; SHO O & G Penbury Hosp. Tunbridge Wells Kent.

SOMANI, Rizwan 2 Lyndhurst Avenue, Twickenham TW2 6BY — MB ChB Leeds 1988. Trainee GP Hastings HA VTS.

SOMARATNE, Mr Dammearachchi Anuja 3 Kynance Gardens, Stanmore HA7 2QJ — MB BS Sri Lanka 1976; FRCS Ed. 1984. Specialist Regist. (Surg.) W. Middlx. Univ. Hosp. Specialty: Gen. Surg. Socs: Coll. Surg. Sri Lanka; Roy. Coll. Surg. of Ed.

SOMASEGARAM, Priya Dharshini 69 Wansunt Road, Bexley DA5 2DJ — MB BS Lond. 1998.

SOMASUNDARA-RAJAH, Jegatheswary Moseley Medical Centre, 21 Salisbury Road, Moseley, Birmingham B13 8JS Tel: 0121 449 0122 Fax: 0121 449 6262 — MB BS Ceylon 1967.

SOMASUNDARA-RAJAH, Kandiah Moseley Medical Centre, 21 Salisbury Road, Moseley, Birmingham B13 8JS Tel: 0121 449 0122 Fax: 0121 449 6262 — MB BS Calcutta 1966; MB BS Calcutta 1966; FRCS (Glas.) 1970; FRCS (Edin.) 1970.

SOMASUNDARAM, Anna Anbu 48 Claverdale Road, London SW2 2DP — MB ChB Dundee 1997; MRCP Lond. 2001.

SOMASUNDARAM, Veerappapillai Cleland House, Rm. 301, Page St., London SW1P 4LN Tel: 020 7217 6678 Fax: 020 7217 6345; 25 The Ridings, Epsom KT18 5JQ Tel: 01372 721488 — MB BS Madras 1968 (Tanjore Med. Coll.) DPM Eng. 1982; MRCPsych 1986. Health Care Adviser. Specialty: Gen. Psychiat. Prev: Sen. Med.

Off. HMP Brixton; Med. Off. HM Prison Wandsworth; Regist. W. Pk. Hosp. Epsom.

SOMASUNDERAM, Balakrishnan Leighton Hospital, Crewe CW1 4QJ Tel: 01270 612026 Fax: 01270 273455; 32 Copperfield Road, Cheadle Hulme, Cheadle SK8 7PN Tel: 0161 440 9533 — MB BS Ceylon 1968 (Colombo) DPM Eng. 1982; MRCPsych 1986. Cons. Old Age Psych. N. Warks. NHS Trust, The Manor, 6 Manor Ct. Av, Nuneaton CV11 5HX. Specialty: Geriat. Psychiat. Socs: BMA; Pres. Sri-Lankan Psychiat.s Assn. (UK); Internal PsychoGeriat..Assn. Prev: Cons. in Old Age Psychiat., St Michaels Hosp. Lichfield, Staffs; Cons. in Old Age Psychiat., Thameside Gen. Hosp., Ashton Under Lyne; Cons. in Old Age Psychiat., Fairfield Gen. Hosp., Bury Lancs.

SOMAUROO, John Deelun The Countess of Chester Health Park, Liverpool Road, Chester CH2 1UL Tel: 01244 365000 — BM BS Nottm. 1989 (Univ. Nottm.) MB BS.(Nottm) 1989; MRCP (UK) 1994. Cons. Cardiol. and Gen. Phys., Countess of Chester Hosp. NHS Trust, Chester; Lect. at Univ. Coll. Chester. Specialty: Cardiol. Socs: BMA; Britiah Soc. of heart Failure; Roy. Coll. of Physicians of Lond.

SOMER, Kenneth Gordon Ross (retired) The Old Oast House, 72 The Hill, Littlebourne, Canterbury CT3 1TD Tel: 01227 728347 — MB BS Lond. 1956 (King's Coll. Hosp.) MRCS Eng. LRCP Lond. 1956; DObst RCOG 1958; DCH Eng. 1960; Cert. Family Plann. JCC 1976; DHMSA 1994. Prev: GP Canterbury.

SOMERFIELD, David James South Devon Healthcare, Chadwell Bay Hospital, Torquay Road, Paignton TQ3 2DW Tel: 01803 559163 Fax: 01803 559163 — MB ChB Sheff. 1989; MRCPsych 1995. Cons. (Psychiat.) Torbay Hosp. Specialty: Geriat. Psychiat. Prev: Sen. Regist. (Psychiat.) Barrow Hosp. Bristol.

SOMERS, Henry Benedict Anton (retired) 2 Walnut Garth, Reepham, Lincoln LN3 4FF — MB Lond. 1956; LRCPI & LM, LRCSI & LM 1960; DPM Eng. 1966; MRCPsych 1971. Hon. Cons. Psychiat. Scunthorpe Community Health NHS Trust. Prev: Cons. Psychiat. Co. Hosp. Lincoln.

SOMERS, John Michael Nottingham City Hospital, Department of Radiology, Hucknall Road, Nottingham NG9 1PB Tel: 0115 969 1169 Email: jsomers@ncht.trent.nhs.uk — MB ChB Liverp. 1981; MRCP (UK) 1984; FRCR 1989. Cons. Paediat. Radiol. Nottm. City Hosp. NHS Trust & Univ. Hosp. NHS Trust.; Divisional Clin. Director Nottm. City Hosp. Nottm. Specialty: Radiol. Special Interest: Paediat. Socs: BSPR; RSNA; BMUS.

SOMERS, Lisa Jane 57 Berrylands Road, Surbiton KT5 8PB Tel: 020 8399 0264 Fax: 020 8399 7733 — MB BS Lond. 1993 (Char. Cross & Westm. Lond.) MRCP UK 1997. Specialist Regist. (A&E) S. E. Thmaes. Specialty: Accid. & Emerg.

SOMERS, Mr Shaw Stefano Department of Surgery, Queen Alexandra Hospital, Cosham, Portsmouth PO6 3LY — MB ChB Leeds 1986; FRCS Eng. 1992; BSc (Hons.) Leeds 1983, MD 1993. Cons. Surg. (Gen. Surg.) Qu. Alexandra Hosp. Portsmouth. Specialty: Gen. Surg. Socs: Assoc. of Surg.s of Gt. Britain & Irel.; Brit. Soc. of Gastroenterol. Prev: Sen. Lect. St James Univ. Hosp. Leeds; Assoc. Prof. Surg. P. of Wales Hosp. Shatin, Hong Kong; Hunt. Prof. RCS Eng. 1994-5.

SOMERS, Stanley Abram (retired) 10 Wedgewood Court, North Park Avenue, Leeds LS8 1DD Tel: 0113 266 6649 — MB ChB Leeds 1944. Prev: Anaesth. Seacroft Hosp. Leeds.

SOMERS HESLAM, Judith 64A Glebe Road, Cambridge CB1 7SZ — Artsexamen Amsterdam 1993; DRCOG 1996. GP Regist. E. Barnwell Health Centre Camb. Specialty: Gen. Pract. Socs: Med. Protec. Soc. Prev: SHO (Gen. Med.) Huntingdon; SHO (Paediat.) Ipswich Hosp.; SHO (O & G) Ipswich Hosp.

SOMERSET, Alison Mary Annandale Surgery, Mutton Lane, Potters Bar EN6 2AS Tel: 01707 64451; 30 Potters Road, New Barnet, Barnet EN5 5HW Tel: 020 8441 7154 — MB BS Lond. 1991 (Royal Free) MRCGP 1997; DRCOG 1998. GP Retainer Potters Bar Herts. Specialty: Gen. Pract. Prev: SHO (O & G) UCH Lond.; GP Regist. Potters Bar Herts.

SOMERSET, David Alan Dept. of Foetal Medicine, 3rd Floor, Birmingham Women's Hospital, Birmingham B15 2TG — BM Soton. 1992 (Southampton) DM Birmingham 2001. Lect. in Obst. & Gyn., Birmingha Wom.'s Hosp.; Specialist Regist. (O & G) W. Midl. Deanery. Specialty: Obst. & Gyn. Socs: Roy. Coll. of Obst. & Gynaecologists.

SOMERSET, Robert Birley (profess.) 26 Oakwood Road, Birmingham B11 4HA Tel: 0121 777 3082; 33 Grove Avenue, Birmingham B13 9RX Tel: 0121 449 1530 — MB ChB Birm. 1957; DObst RCOG 1961. GP Birm. Prev: SHO Wom. Hosp. Wolverhampton; Capt. RAMC; Ho. Surg. Gen. Hosp. Birm.

SOMERVAILLE, Tim Charles Plomer 12 Old Coppice, Lyth Hill, Shrewsbury SY3 0BP — MB BS Lond. 1993 (St. Mary's Hosp. Med. Sch.) BSc (Lond. 1990; MRCP (UK) 1996. Regist. (Haemat.) Univ. Coll. Hosp. Lond. Specialty: Haematology. Prev: Regist. (Haemat.) Mt. Vernon & Watford Hosps. NHS Trust; SHO (Respirat. Med.) Roy. Brompton Hosp. Lond.; SHO (Nephrol.) Middlx. Hosp. Lond.

SOMERVELL, David Howard (retired) Hap Cottage, Lynch Road, France Lynch, Stroud GL6 8LT Tel: 01453 886224 — MRCS Eng. LRCP Lond. 1955 (Middlx.) DObst RCOG 1966. Prev: GP Glos.

SOMERVELL, Mr James Lionel (retired) 3 Orchard Close, Cressage, Shrewsbury SY5 6BZ Tel: 01952 510755 — (Camb. & Univ. Coll. Hosp.) MB BChir Camb. 1951; MRCS Eng. LRCP Lond. 1951; FRCS Eng. 1960. Prev: Cons. Surg. Walsall Hosp. Gp.

SOMERVILLE, Deborah Ruth Thatched Cottage, Eridge Rd, Eridge Green, Tunbridge Wells TN3 9JU — MB ChB Birm. 1997. GP VTS, Maidstone Kent.

SOMERVILLE, Douglas Mark 6 Woods Lea, Hillside, Chorley New Road, Bolton BL1 5DU — MB ChB Manch. 1951; DO Eng. 1961. Cons. Ophth. Blackburn Roy. Infirm. Specialty: Ophth.

SOMERVILLE, Mr Douglas William 28 Island Bank Road, Inverness IV2 4QS — MB ChB Glas. 1976; FRCS Ed. 1983. Cons. Orthop. Surg. Raigmore Hosp. Inverness. Specialty: Orthop. Prev: Cons. Orthop. Surg. Roy. Naval Hosp. Haslar Gosport.

SOMERVILLE, Elizabeth Mary 15/2 Braehead Avenue, Barnton, Edinburgh EH4 6AU — MB ChB Aberd. 1948.

SOMERVILLE, Eric Townshend, SBStJ North Brink Practice, 7 North Brink, Wisbech PE13 1JR Tel: 01945 585121 Fax: 01945 476423; River Bend, 64 North Brink, Wisbech PE13 1LN Tel: 01945 585756 Fax: 01945 476423 — MB BS Lond. 1966 (St. Mary's) MRCS Eng. LRCP Lond. 1966; DObst RCOG 1969. Prev: SHO (Obst.) Zachary Merton Matern. Hosp. Rustington; Ho. Phys. St. Mary's Hosp. Lond.; Ho. Surg. Bolingbroke Hosp. Lond.

SOMERVILLE, Froma 31 Wilmington Square, London WC1X 0EG — MB BS Lond. 1954 (Westm.) MRCS Eng. LRCP Lond. 1954; DO Eng. 1958. Med. Asst. Moorfields Eye Hosp. Lond.

SOMERVILLE, Gordon, Col. late RAMC Retd. (retired) — MB ChB Glas. 1959; DTM & H Eng. 1975. Prev: Comd. Med. HQ Wales.

SOMERVILLE, Graham Waterson (retired) 2 Chapel Mews, Elloughton, Brough HU15 1HQ Tel: 01482 668463 — MB ChB Ed. 1960. Prev: GP Hull.

SOMERVILLE, Irene Dione The Calderdale Royal Hospital, Salter Habble, Halifax HX3 0PW Tel: 01422 357171 Fax: 01422 220478 Email: anaesthesia@calderdale.nhs.uk; The Gables, Linden Road, Halifax HX3 0BS Tel: 01422 341997 — MB BCh BAO Dub. 1970 (Trinity College Dublin) DA RCSI 1972; FFA SA 1980. Cons. Anaesth. The Calderdale Roy. Hosp. Specialty: Anaesth. Prev: Sen. Regist. (Anaesth.) Leeds Gen. Hosp.; Sen. Regist. (Anaesth.) King. Edwd. VIII & King Geo. V Hosp. Durban, SA.

SOMERVILLE, Jennifer Elizabeth Histopathology & Cytopathology Department, Belfast City Hospital, Lisburn Road, Belfast BT9 7AB Tel: 02890 263669 Fax: 02838 612690 — MB BCh BAO Belf. 1986; BSc Belf. 1983; MRCPath 1992. Cons. Path. Belfast City Hosp. Specialty: Histopath.

SOMERVILLE, Jonathan Mark 4 Irwell Close, Chandlers Ford, Southampton — MB BS Lond. 1989 (Charing Cross and Westminster) FRCA 1997. Specialty: Anaesth.

SOMERVILLE, Mr Julian John FitzGerald Calderdale Royal Hospital, Department of Urology, Salterhebble, Halifax HX3 0PW Tel: 01422 222474; The Gables, Linden Road, Halifax HX3 0BS Tel: 01422 341997 — MB BCh BAO Dub. 1970 (Trinity Coll. Dub.) MD Dub. 1974; MA Dub. 1974; FRCS Ed. 1976. Cons. Urol. Calderdale & Huddersfield NHS Trust, Halifax. Specialty: Urol. Socs: BMA; Brit. Assn. Urol. Surgs.; Internat. Soc. Urol. Prev: Sen. Regist. & Regist. (Urol.) Leeds HA; Sen. Regist. & Regist. (Urol.) King Edwd. VIII Hosp. Durban, S. Afr.

SOMERVILLE, Kevin William 33 Oxhey Road, Oxhey, Watford WD19 4QG Fax: 020 7204 3544 Email: kevin.somerville@swissre.com/kevin_somerville@swissre.com — MB ChB Auckland 1976 (Auckland, New Zealand) BSc Auckland 1973;

FRACP 1981; DM Nottm. 1990; FRCP 1995. Div. Cons. Phys. to Swiss Re Life & Health Lond.; Clin. Asst. Neuro-Ophth. Moorfields Eye Hosp. Lond. Specialty: Gen. Med.; Care of the Elderly; Epidemiol. Socs: Amer. Geriat. Soc.; Brit. Geriat. Soc.; Assur. Med. Soc. Prev: Sen. Lect. & Hon. Cons. Phys. (Geriat. Med.) St. Bart. Hosp. Lond.; Cons. Phys. Middlemore Hosp. Auckland, NZ; Sen. Regist. Oxf. RHA.

SOMERVILLE, Margaret South & West Devon Health Authority, The Lescaze Offices, Shinner's Bridge, Dartington, Totnes TQ9 6JE Tel: 01803 866665 Fax: 01803 861853; Willow Barn, Pitt Hill, Ivybridge PL21 0JJ — MB BS Newc. 1978 (Newcastle-upon-Tyne) MRCP (UK) 1981; MD Newc. 1990; MPH Liverp. 1992; MFPHM RCP (UK) 1994. Cons. Pub. Health Med. S. & W. Devon HA. Specialty: Pub. Health Med. Prev: Sen. Regist. (Pub. Health Med.) S. & W. RHA.

SOMERVILLE, Melanie Jane Flat 2/R, 17 Dalnair Street, Yorkhill, Glasgow G3 8SD — MB ChB Glas. 1994.

SOMERVILLE, Neil Alexander McCrie (retired) Sydenham House, Boulevard, Hull HU3 2TA Tel: 01482 326818 Fax: 01482 218267; Helensburgh, 6 Manor Fields, Westella, Hull HU10 7SG Tel: 01482 658659 Fax: 01482 658659 — MB ChB Ed. 1956; DCH RFPS Glas. 1960; FRCGP 1980, M 1965; Cert. Family Plann. JCC 1974. Med. Adviser P & O N. Sea Ferries; Med. Examr MCA UKOOA Indep. Med. SMES. Prev: Ho. Surg. (O & G) W.wood Hosp. Beverley.

SOMERVILLE, Nicola Suzanne 3 Brockhill Road, Hythe CT21 4AB — MB BS Lond. 1993 (St Geo.) DA (Lond.) 1995; DCH RCP Lond. 1998; FRCA Lond 1999. Specialist Regist. Rotat. St Geo. Lond. Specialty: Anaesth. Prev: SHO (Anaesth.) QA Portsmouth; SHO (Anaesth.) Frimley Pk. Hosp. Camberley; SHO (Paeds & Neonates), Brighton.

SOMERVILLE, Mr Philip Graham (retired) Chandos Lodge, 50 Paddockhall Road, Haywards Heath RH16 1HW Tel: 01444 413495 — MB BChir Camb. 1943 (Camb. & St. Geo.) MChir Camb. 1953, MA, MB BChir 1943; MRCS Eng. LRCP Lond. 1944; FRCS Eng. 1945; FACS 1983. Ct. Examrs. RCS Eng.; Exmar. Primary FRCS Eng. Prev: Cons. Surg. Roy. Sussex Co. Hosp. Brighton & Cuckfield Hosp. Mem.

SOMERVILLE, Simon James The John Kelso Practice, Park Medical Centre, Ball Haye Road, Leek ST13 6QR Tel: 01538 399007 Fax: 01538 370014 — MB BS Lond. 1987; DCH RCP Lond. 1990; DFFP 1991; MRCGP 1991; T(GP) 1991. Research Fell. N. Staffs. GP Research Network Keele Univ. Prev: Trainee GP P'boro. Dist. Hosp. VTS.

SOMERVILLE, Walter, CBE (retired) Flat 30, York House, Upper Montagu St., London W1H 1FR Tel: 020 7262 2144 Fax: 020 7724 2238 — MD NUI 1940 (Univ. Coll. Dub.) MB BCh BAO 1937; FRCP Lond. 1957, M 1940; FACC 1972. Hon. Phys. (Cardiac) Middlx. Hosp. Lond.; Hon. Lect. (Cardiol.) Middlx. Hosp. Med. Sch.; Hon. Cons. (Cardiol.) to The Army & RAF; Assn. RN Offs. & King Edwd. VII Convalesc. Hosp. Offs. Osborne; Edr. Brit. Heart Jl.; Trustee Brit. Assn. Performing Arts Med. Prev: Cons. Cardiol. Thoracic Surgic. Unit Harefield Hosp.

SOMERVILLE, Wendy Watford General Hospital, Vicarage Road, Watford WD18 0HB Tel: 01923 244366/217614 Fax: 01923 217715 — MB ChB Auckland 1976; MSc (Hons.) Auckland 1973; FRACP 1981; FRCP 1996. Cons. Phys. (Geriat. Med.) W. Herts Hosp.s Trust Eastern Region. Specialty: Care of the Elderly; Gen. Med. Socs: Brit. Geriat. Soc.; Amer. Geriat. Soc.; Alzheimers Dis. Soc. Prev: Cons. Geriat. Med. Nottm. & Newark, Trent RHA; Cons. Geriat. Med. Auckland HB, NZ.

SOMJEE, Miss Shehnaz — MB BS Karachi 1979; DLO RCS Eng. 1986; FRCS Eng. 1989; LLB (Hons.) Liverp. John Moores 1998. Specialty: Otolaryngol.; Medico Legal. Socs: Liverp. Med. Inst. & BMA (Hon. Treas. Liverp. Div. 1989-92). MWF; Brit. Assn. of Ocorhino-Laryngol./Head & Neck Surg.s; Founder & Chairm. Locum Doctors' Assn. (June 1997 to date).

SOMMERFIELD, Andrew John 178 Park Road, Timperley, Altrincham WA15 6QW — MB ChB Ed. 1996.

SOMMERFIELD, Joanne Flat 12, Bloomfield Court, Bourdon St., London W1K 3PU — MB BS New South Wales 1976.

SOMMERLAD, Mr Brian Clive The Old Vicarage, 17 Lodge Road, Writtle, Chelmsford CM1 3HY Tel: 01245 422477 Fax: 01245 421901 Email: brian@sommerlad.co.uk — MB BS Sydney 1966; FRCS Eng. 1971; FRCS Ed. (Hon) 2000. Cons. Plastic Surg. Broomfield Hosp. Chelmsford, Hosp. for Childr. Gt. Ormond St. & Roy. Lond. Hosp. Specialty: Plastic Surg. Special Interest: Cleft Lip & Palate & Other Congen. Abnormalities; Skin Cancer. Socs: Fell. Roy. Soc. Med. (Ex-Pres. Plastic Surg. Sect.); Brit. Assn. Plastic Surgs. (Pres. 1998); Craniofacial Soc. GB (Pres.1996-97). Prev: Sen. Regist. (Plastic Surg.) NE Thames RHA; Regist. (Surg.) Univ. Coll. Hosp. Lond.; Resid. Med. Off. Sydney Hosp., Austral.

SOMMERLAD, Marian Gwyneth The Old Vicarage, 17 Lodge Road, Writtle, Chelmsford CM1 3HY Tel: 01245 422477 — MB BS Lond. 1972 (Univ. Coll. Hosp.) MRCS Eng. LRCP Lond. 1972. Clin. Asst. Broomfield Hosp. Chelmsford. Prev: Clin. Asst., Ho. Phys. & Ho. Surg. Barnet Gen. Hosp.

SOMMERS, Andrew James 28 Church Street, Bramcote, Beeston, Nottingham NG9 3HD — MB ChB Leic. 1994.

SOMMERS, Stephanie Marguerite 28 Church Street, Bramcote, Beeston, Nottingham NG9 3HD — MB ChB Leic. 1993.

SOMMERVILLE, Garth Paul 4 Kensington Gardens, Portsmouth Road, Kingston upon Thames KT1 2JU — MB BCh Witwatersrand 1990.

SOMMERVILLE, Gordon Peter Westlands Medical Centre, 20B Westlands Grove, Portchester, Fareham PO16 9AE Tel: 023 9237 7514 Fax: 023 9221 4236 — MB BS Lond. 1979 (St. Thos.) BSc (Hons.) Lond. 1976; DRCOG 1981; MRCGP 1984.

SOMMERVILLE, James Gardner (retired) 2 Lentune Way, Lymington SO41 3PF Tel: 01590 673351 — (Ed.) MB ChB Ed. 1943; MD (Commend.) Ed. 1958; FRCP Lond. 1978, M 1969. Cons. Adviser Med. Rehabil. Centre, Univ. Coll. Hosp., St. Geo. Hosp. Lond. & Qu. Eliz. Foundat. for Disabled People Leatherhead, Surrey; Cons. Adviser Roy. Brit. Legion, Churchill Rehabil Centre Kent; Hon. Sen. Clin. Lect. Dept. Med. Univ. Lond.; Governor Qu. Eliz. Foundat. Disabled Leatherhead; Mem. Advis. Panel Disabled Living Foundat. Prev: Med. Dir. Med. Rehabil. Centre Lond.

SOMMERVILLE, John MacLeod Portland Road Surgery, 31 Portland Road, Kilmarnock KA1 2DJ Tel: 01563 522118 Fax: 01563 573562; 18 Howard Street, Kilmarnock KA1 2BP Tel: 01563 537915 — MB ChB Glas. 1975; MRCP (UK) 1979; MRCGP 1984. GP Princip. Prev: Regist. (Med.) Stobhill Gen. Hosp. Glas.; Regist. (Med.) Roy. Alexandra Infirm. Paisley.

SOMMERVILLE, Julia Anne 2 Brownhills Gardens, St Andrews KY16 8PY — MB ChB Aberd. 1991.

SOMMERVILLE, Mary Josephine Blantyre Health Centre, Victoria Street, Blantyre, Glasgow G72 0BS Tel: 01698 828868 Fax: 01698 823678 — MB ChB Glas. 1984; DRCOG 1987; MRCGP 1991; DFFP 1992; Dip FM 1994. GP Glas. Socs: Brit. Soc. Med. & Dent. Hypn.; Brit. Med. Acupunc. Soc.

SOMMERVILLE, Robert Gardner (retired) Monkmyre, Myreriggs Rd, Coupar Angus, Blairgowrie PH13 9HS — MD Glas. 1960; MB ChB 1950; FRCPath 1972; FRCP Glas. 1974. Prev: Prof. (Med. Microbiol.) Sultan Qaboos Univ. Muscat.

SOMMERVILLE, William Taylor 35 Whitemoss Road, E. Kilbride, Glasgow G74 4JB Tel: 01355 220717 — MB ChB Glas. 1953; DObst RCOG 1957. Insur. Panel Doctor; Fact. Med. Off. Socs: (Ex-Pres. & Ex-Hon. Sec.) E. Kilbride Med. Soc. Prev: Jun. Hosp. Med. Off. (Obst.) Lennox Castle Matern. Hosp. Glas.; Ho. Surg. West. Infirm. Glas.; Ho. Phys. Stobhill Gen. Hosp. Glas.

SOMNER, Alan Robert (retired) 88 The Rise, Ponteland, Newcastle upon Tyne NE20 9LQ Tel: 01661 23769 — MD Ed. 1951; MB ChB 1946; FRCP Ed. 1961, M 1952. Cons. Phys. Preston Hosp. N. Shields. Prev: Ho. Phys. Roy. Infirm. Edin.

SOMNER, Joan 88 The Rise, Ponteland, Newcastle upon Tyne NE20 9LQ Tel: 01661 23769 — MB ChB Ed. 1950. Asst. Med. Off. Community Med. N. Tyneside Health Auth. Specialty: Community Child Health. Prev: Asst. Dept. Med. Univ. Edin.; Ho. Surg. Roy. Infirm. Edin.; Ho. Phys. Roy. Hosp. Sick Childr. Edin.

SOMORIN, Adolphus Owolabi 57 Osborne Road, London E7 0PJ — MRCS Eng. LRCP Lond. 1965.

SOMPER, John Dennis 18 Wimpole Street, London W1M 7AD Tel: 020 7637 1113; 160 Fishpool Street, St Albans AL3 4RZ Tel: 01727 856440 — (St Mary's Hospital Paddington London W2) MB BS Lond. 1952; MFHom 1969. Specialty: Homeop. Med.

SONANIS, Mr Sanjay Valmikrao Airedale General Hospital, Orthopaedic Department, Skipton Road, Steeton, Keighley BD20 6TD Tel: 01535 652511 Fax: 01535 292098; 1 Teal Court, Steeton, Keighley BD20 6UW Tel: 01535 657632 Fax: 01535

657632 Email: svsonanis@aol.com — MB BS Bombay 1985; MSOrth (Bombay) 1989; MChOrth. 1997. Assoc. Specialist (Orthop.) Airedale NHS Trust; Hon. Lect. (Engineering) Univ. Bradford. Specialty: Orthop. Special Interest: Jt. Replacements & Revision; Managem. of Polytrauma; Research & AutoCAD Designing & Patenting Ideas. Socs: Indian Orthop. Soc.; Asian Assn. Dynamic Osteosynthesis; Brit. Orthop. Assn. Prev: Specialist Regist. (Orthop.) York; Lect. (Orthop.) Bombay, India.

SONDHEIMER, Josef 16A Westbourne Grove, London W2 5WG — MB BS Lond. 1939 (Lond. Hosp.) MRCP Lond. 1945. Itinerant Cons. Phys. UK. Specialty: Gen. Med. Prev: Clin. Asst. & Ho. Phys. Lond. Hosp.; Regist. (Med.) Univ. Coll. Hosp.; Sen. Regist. (Med.) Roy. Gwent Hosp. Newport.

SONDHI, Ravindra Portland Medical Centre, 184 Portland Road, London SE25 4QB Tel: 0208 662 1233 Fax: 0208 662 1223 — MB BS Lond. 1984 (St George's Medical School) BSc (Hons.) Lond. 1981; MBA City University 2000. Clin. Asst. in Gastroenterol. and Endoscopy, Mayday Hosp. Lond. Rd, Thornton Heath; Clin. Asst. in Urol.; Med. Director, Croydon, Doctors on call; Primary Care Practitioner in Accid. & Emerg., Kings/ Lewisham/ St Thomas's. Prev: Clin. Asst. Rheum.; Lect. Kings Coll. for UnderGrad.s.

SONEYE-VAUGHAN, Felicia Temitayo 31 Birch Court, Sherman Gardens, Chadwell Heath, Romford RM6 4AX — LRCPI & LM, LRSCI & LM 1969; LRCPI & LM, LRCSI & LM 1969; FFR RCSI 1976.

SONG, Fiona Mary 56 Dedworth Road, Windsor SL4 5AY Tel: 01753 860136 Fax: 01753 860136 — MB ChB Sheff. 1988. Specialty: Rehabil. Med.

SONG, Soon Hoo Diabetes Research, University Dept of Medicine, Western General Hospital, Crewe Road, Edinburgh EH4 2XU Tel: 0131 537 3074 Fax: 0131 537 1709; 43 Barclay Place, Edinburgh EH10 4HW Tel: 0131 228 4615 — MB ChB Ed. 1992; MRCP (UK) 1996. Clin. Research Fell. (Diabetes) Diabetes Research Univ. Dept. Med. West. Gen. Hosp. Edin. Specialty: Diabetes. Socs: BMA; Brit. Diabetic Assn. Prev: Med. SHO - Vict. Hosp., Kirkcaldy; Med. SHO - Sunderland City Hosp.; Ho. Off. (Med. & Surg.) Roy. Infirm. Edin.

SONGHURST, Lorice Zaki The Laurels, Lynch Close, London SE3 0RN — MB BCh Cairo 1968; FFA RCS Eng. 1977.

SONGO-WILLIAMS, Rosie AF c/o 10 Algernon Road, Lewisham, London SE13 7AT Tel: 020 8692 7832 — MD Berne 1974 (University of Berne Switzerland) DRCOG RCPSI; Dip. Arzt 1973; DCH RCPSI 1976; DObst RCPSI 1978; DTM & H Liverp. 1978; MRCP(I) 1984. Specialty: Paediat. Socs: MRCPCH; Fell. of the Roy. Soc. Of Med.

SONGRA, Ashok Kumar 1 Dorset Drive, Edgware HA8 7NT — MB BS Newc. 1994 (Univ. Newc.) BSc (Hons.) 1983; BDS Wales 1986; FFDRCSI Irel. 1996. Specialist Regist (Oral & Maxillofacial Surg.) Roy. Lond. Trust. Hosp. Socs: BMA; Brit. Oral and Maxillofacial Surg. Assn. Prev: SHO (ENT) Qu. Eliz. Hosp. Birm.; SHO (Gen. Surg.) Sunderland DG Hosp.; SHO (A&E) Sunderland DG Hosp.

SONI, Mr Bakulesh Madhusudan Spinal Injuries Centre, Southport & Formby District General Hospital, Town Lane, Southport PR8 6PN Tel: 01704 547471 Fax: 01704 543156; 10 Rutland Road, Southport PR8 6PB Tel: 01704 546276 — MB BS Gujarat 1974 (Ahmedabad India) Ms Neurosurg. 1977. Cons. (Spin. Injury) Dist. Gen. Hosp. Southport Town La. Southport PR8 6PN UK. Specialty: Rehabil. Med. Socs: BMA; Internat. Med. Soc. Paraplegia. Prev: Assoc. Specialist (Spinal Injury) DGH Southport; Sen. Regist. (Neurosurg.) Walton Hosp. Liverp.; Regist. (Neurosurg.) Walton Hosp. Liverp.

SONI, Neil Cranson 164 Court Lane, Dulwich, London SE21 7ED — MD Lond. 1993; MB ChB Bristol 1976; FANZCA 1982; FFICANZCA 1983; FRCA 1991. Sen. Lect. Anaesth. Westm. Char. Cross Med. Sch.; Cons. Chelsea & Westm. Hosp. 1999; Hon. Sen. Lect., Imperial Coll. Specialty: Anaesth.

SONI, Raj 19 Lombard Road, Merton, London SW19 3RH — MB BS Delhi 1960 (Lady Hardinge Med. Coll. New Delhi) DA Eng. 1977; MRCOG 1978.

SONI, Ram Kripal 24 Kingscliffe Road, Grantham NG31 8ET — LRCP LRCS Ed. 1982; LRCP LRCS Ed. LRCPS Glas. 1982; Mch (Orthop.) Liverp. 1984. Locum Cons. Orthopaedic Surg. Bedford Hosp. Specialty: Orthop. Prev: Locum Cons. Orthopaedic Surg. Scunthorpe Gen. Hosp.; Regist. (Orthop.) Merseyside HA.

***SONI, Sarita** 7 Lichfield Rd, Cambridge CB1 3SP — MB ChB Manch. 1997.

SONI, Saroj Meadowbrook, Department of Psychological Medicine, Stott Lane, Salford M6 8HG Tel: 0161 787 5700 Fax: 0161 787 5707; 79 Carrwood, Hale Barns, Altrincham WA15 0ER Tel: 0161 980 4341 Fax: 0161 980 4341 — MB BS Bombay 1964 (Grant Med. Coll. Bombay) MRCOG 1969; DPM Eng. 1976; FRCPsych 1989, M 1978. Cons. Psychiat. (Ment. Handicap) Salford Community Healthcare NHS Trust; Hon. Assoc. Lect. Univ. Manch. Specialty: Ment. Health.

SONI, Somdatta Gurudatta Cromwell House, Community Mental Health Centre, Cromwell Road, Eccles, Manchester M30 0QT Tel: 0161 787 8496 Fax: 0161 787 8560; 79 Carrwood, Hale Barns, Altrincham WA15 0ER Tel: 0161 980 4341 — MD Poona 1966; FRCP Ed. 1983, M 1968; DPM Ed. & Glas. 1970; PhD Belf. 1970; FRCPsych 1981, M 1972; MRCS Eng. LRCP Lond. 1973. Cons. Psychiat. (Ment. Health Servs.) Salford; Hon. Assoc. Lect. Univ. Manch. Specialty: Gen. Psychiat. Prev: Research Fell. Qu. Univ. Belf.

SONI, Virendra Kumar Bedford General Hospital, South Wing, Kempston Road, Bedford MK42 9DJ; 29 Donnelly Drive, Bedford MK41 9TT — MB BS Punjab 1968 (Govt. Med. Coll. Patiala) MS (Ophth.) Agra 1969; DO RCS Eng. 1975; DTM & H Liverp. 1978; MCOphth 1991; MRC Ophth 1991; MRCPCH 1996; FRCS (Ed.) Ophth. 2000. Sen. Med. Off. (Ophth.) N. Beds. HA. Specialty: Ophth. Socs: BMA; MRCPCH; MRCPCH. Prev: Regist. Dept. Ophth. Pinderfields Gen. Hosp. Wakefield.

SONIGRA, Hasmukh Karsan 4 Trent Gardens, London N14 4PY Tel: 020 8 441 6175 Email: hsonigra@hotmail.com; 2 Cale Street, Cale Green, Stockport SK2 6SW — MB ChB Manch. 1997; BSc (Hons). SHO (Cardiorespirat. Med.) Wythenshawe Hosp. Manch. Specialty: Gen. Med. Prev: Ho. Off. (Surg.) Hope Hosp. Manch.; Ho. Off. (Med.) Hope Hosp. Manch.

SONKSEN, Camilla Jane X-Ray Department, Royal Sussex County Hospital, Eastern Road, Brighton BN2 5BE Tel: 01273 696955; 3 Park Road, Lewes BN7 1BN — MB BS Lond. 1985; MRCP (UK) 1989; FRCR 1993; FRCP 2002. Cons. Radiol. Roy. Sussex Co. Hosp. Specialty: Radiol. Prev: Sen. Regist. (Radiol.) King's Coll. Hosp. Lond.; SHO (Med.) Roy. Sussex Co. Hosp.; SHO (Paediat.) Southlands Hosp. Shoreham by Sea.

SONKSEN, Julian Richard Anaesthetic Dept, Russells hall Hospital, Dudley DT1 2HQ — MB ChB Birm. 1988 (Birmingham) ChB Birm. 1988; FRCA 1994. Cons. Anaesth. Russells Hall Hosp. Dudley. Specialty: Anaesth.

SONKSEN, Patricia Mary (retired) The Wolfson Centre, Institute of Child Health, Mecklenburgh Square, London WC1N 2AP; 1 Pipe Passage, Lewes BN7 1YG Tel: 01273 476597 Fax: 01273 476597 — MB BS Lond. 1960 (Middlx.) DObst RCOG 1961; MD Lond. 1979; MRCP (UK) 1992; FRCP 1995; FRCPCH 1997. Hon. Sen. Lect. Inst. Child Health UCLH. Prev: Sen. Lect. (Neurol. & Developm. Paediat.) Inst. Child Health Lond.

SONKSEN, Professor Peter Henri Department of Medicine, St. Thomas' Hospital, London SE1 7EH Tel: 020 7928 9292 Fax: 020 7928 4458; East Wing, Preshaw House, Preshaw, Upham, Southampton SO32 1HP Tel: 01962 771029 Fax: 01962 771029 — (Middlx.) MB BS Lond. 1960; FRCP Lond. 1976, M 1963; MD Lond. 1968. Hon. Cons. Phys. Guy's & St. Thos. Hosp. Trust; Prof. Endocrinol. Guy's, King's Coll. & St Thomas' Hosps. Med. & Dent. Sch. Lond.; Mem. Med. Commiss. & Sub. Commiss. of 10C Doping & Biochem. in Sport (Internat. Olympic Comm.); Edr. in Chief Growth Hormone & IGF Research; Chairm. EASD Study Gp. Do It. Specialty: Endocrinol. Socs: EASD; Brit. Diabetic Assn.; Brit. Endocrine Soc. Prev: Edr. Clin. Endocrinol.; Harkness Fell. Harvard Med. Sch., USA; Chairm. Div. of Med. UMDS.

SONNABEND, Joseph Adolph 30 Hamilton Terrace, London NW8 9UG Tel: 020 7289 0932 — MB BCh Witwatersrand 1956; MRCP Ed. 1961.

SONNENBERG, Miss Sabine — State Exam Med Cologne 1991; MD 1992; FRCS 1997. Specialist Regist. Crawley & Horsham Hosp. Specialty: Gen. Surg. Prev: Specialist Regist. (Gen. Surg.) St. Thomas's Hosp. Lond.; SpR Frimley Pk. Hosp.

SONNEX, Christopher Addenbrooke's Hospital, Hills Rd, Cambridge CB2 2QQ Tel: 01223 217141 — MB BS Lond. 1978 (Middlx. Hosp., Univ. of Lond.) MRCP (UK) 1984; FRCP Lond. 1995. Cons. Phys. (Genitourin. Med.) Addenbrooke's Hosp. Camb. Specialty: Genitourinary Medicine. Special Interest: Genital Dermat.; Vulva Dis. Socs: Brit. Soc. Study of Vulval Dis.; British Association for Sexual Health & HIV. Prev: Clin. Lect. Acad. Dept. Genitourin. Med. Middlx. Hosp. Lond.

SONNEX, Timothy Stephen Purdis Hall, Foxhall, Ipswich IP10 0AD — MRCS Eng. LRCP Lond. 1975 (Middlx.) BSc (Hons.) Lond. 1972, MD 1988, MB BS 1975; MRCP (UK) 1979. Sen. Regist. St. John's Hosp. Dis. Skin Lond.

SONODA, Luke Ienari 11 Barrie House, 29 St Edmund's Terrace, St John's Wood, London NW8 7QH Tel: 020 7586 7410 Fax: 020 7586 7410 Email: luke@sonoda.co.uk; Christ's College, University of Cambridge, Cambridge CB2 3BU Tel: 01223 334900 — MB BChir Camb. 1994; BA Camb. 1990; MA Camb. 1993; PhD London 2003. SpR Radiol. Addenbrooke's Health NHS Trust Camb. Specialty: Radiol.; Orthop. Special Interest: Breast Cancer; MRI. Socs: Fell. Roy. Soc. Med.; Assn. of Surgs.; Brit. Assn. Surg. Oncol. Prev: Lect. (Surg.) Addenbrooke's Health NHS Trust Camb.; Lect. (Anat.) UMDS Guy's & St. Thos. Hosps. Univ. Lond.; SHO (Orthop. Surg.) Addenbrooke's Health NHS Trust Camb.

SONTHALIA, Vijay Bihari Hunter Health Centre, Andrew Street, East Kilbride, Glasgow G74 1AD Tel: 01355 906633 Fax: 01355 906639 Email: vijay.sonthalia@hunter.lanpct.scot.nhs.uk — MB BS. GP. Specialty: Cardiol.; Gastroenterol.; Gen. Med. Socs: Out of hours Co-op Assoc.; Local Med. Comm.; Aeromed. Comm.

SONTHEIMER, Hemantee Devi Talangerstrasse 5, 82152 Krailling, Germany; 76 Yew Tree Avenue, Lichfield WS14 9UA — MB ChB Leeds 1986.

SOO, Julia Kay — MB BS Lond. 1998 (Guy's & St Thos.) Specialist Regist. (Dermat.) St Geo. Hosp. Lond. Specialty: Gen. Med.; Dermat. Prev: SHO Med. Gloucestershire Roy. Hosp.

SOO, Kooi Guat 3 Elms Avenue, Great Shelford, Cambridge CB2 5LN Tel: 01223 2265 — LMS King Edwd. VII Coll. 1949; LMS King Edwd. VII Coll. Med. Singapore 1949.

SOO, Shiu-Ching Luton & Dunstable Hospital, Lewsey Road, Luton LU4 0DZ — MB BChir Camb. 1988 (Univ. of Camb.) MA Camb. 1989; MRCP (UK) 1990. Cons. Diabetes & Endocrinol. & Gen. Med., Luton & Dunstable Hosp. Specialty: Diabetes; Endocrinol.; Gen. Med.

SOO, Shiu-Shing Department Microbiology, Nottingham City Hospital, Hucknall Road, Nottingham NG5 1PB Tel: 0115 969 1169 Email: ssoo@neht.trent.nhs.uk — MB BChir Camb. 1987 (Camb. Univ.) MA Camb. 1987; MRC Path 1994; PhD 1999. Cons. Microbiologist, Dept. of Microbiol., Nottm. City Hosp., Nottm. Specialty: Med. Microbiol. Socs: Amer. Soc. for Microbiologists. Prev: Regist. (Microbiol.) Addenbrookes Hosp. Camb.

SOO, Sze Shun The Princess Street Group Practice, 2 Princess St., Elephant and Castle, London SE1 6JP Tel: 020 7928 0253 Fax: 020 7261 9804 — MB BCh BAO NUI 1990; LRCPSI 1990; MRCGP 1995.

SOOD, Anil Kumar Maples Family Medical Practice, 35 Hill Street, Hinckley LE10 1DS Tel: 01255 506451 — MB ChB Birm. 1987; MRCGP 1991; DRCOG 1991.

SOOD, Archana 1(b) The Green, Twickenham TW2 5TU Tel: 020 8894 6870 — MB ChB Glas. 1990 (Glasgow) DFFP 1993; T(GP) 1994; MRCGP 1994. GP Twickenham. Specialty: Family Plann. & Reproduc. Health; Dermat. Prev: Trainee GP StoneHo. Hosp. VTS; GP asst. W. Lond.

SOOD, Arvind Flat 2, 2 Victoria Crescent Road, Glasgow G12 9DB — MB ChB Glas. 1994.

SOOD, Harish Chandra 19 The Cloverlands, The Hawthorns, Nottingham NG2 7TF — MB BCh Wales 1986; MRCGP 1990. Specialty: Gen. Psychiat.

SOOD, Kamal Kumar Abington Park Surgery, Christchurch Medical Centre, Ardington Road, Northampton NN1 5LT Tel: 01604 630291 Fax: 01604 603524; 45 Thorburn Road, Weston Favell, Northampton NN3 3DA Tel: 01604 401426 — MB BS Lond. 1981; BSc Lond. 1978, MB BS 1981; MRCP (UK) 1984; DRCOG 1988; MRCGP 1989.

SOOD, Loopinder 20 Duncryne Place, Bishopbriggs, Glasgow G64 2DP — MB ChB Glas. 1986 (Glas. Univ.) BSc (Hons) Glas. 1983. Trainee Psychiat. Specialty: Paediat. Neurol.

SOOD, Mr Manoj Kumar 8 Brabourne Heights, Marsh Lane, Blackheath, London NW7 4NU Email: manojsood@yahoo.com — MB BS Lond. 1992; BSc (Hons.) Lond. 1989; FRCS Eng. 1996. Specialist Regist. (Orthop. & Trauma) RNOH Rotat. Specialty: Orthop. Socs: BOTA; Assoc. BOA; Roy. Soc. of Med. (Fell.). Prev: Sen. SHO (Orthop. & Trauma) Whipps Cross Hosp. Lond.; SHO (Plastic & Hand Surg.) Wexham Pk. Hosp. Slough; Surgic. SHO Rotat. King's Healthcare Lond.

SOOD, Manu Raj 103 Friary Road, Handsworth Wood, Birmingham B20 1BA — MB BS Himachal Pradesh, India 1987; MRCP (UK) 1994.

SOOD, Naresh Chander Family Medical Centre, 171 Carlton Road, Nottingham NG3 2FW Tel: 0115 504068 Fax: 0115 950 9844.

SOOD, Mr Rajinder Kumar Shanti-Nivas, 9 Longhill Avenue, Alloway, Ayr KA7 4DY — MB BS Bombay 1962; FRCS Ed. 1971; MRCS Eng. LRCP Lond. 1978. Cons. ENT Surg. Ayr Co. Hosp. Specialty: Otolaryngol.

SOOD, Ram Parkash (retired) — MB BS Bombay 1960 (Nat. Med. Coll. Bombay) DTM & H Liverp. 1962; DPH Eng. 1962. Prev: Regist. (Med.) Ransom Hosp. Rainworth & Peppard Hosp.

SOOD, Ravinder Nath 17 Ranford Drive, Leeds L517 7PJ Tel: 0113 2888252 — (King Geo. Med. Coll. Lucknow) BSc Lucknow 1958; MB BS Lucknow 1965; DLO Lucknow 1966; DObst RCOG 1971. GP Horsforth. Prev: East Leeds PCT.

SOOD, Mr Sanjai Department ENT, Bradford Teaching Hospitals, Duckworth Lane, Bradford BD9 6RJ Tel: 01274 364469 Fax: 01274 366549 Email: sanjaisood@aol.com — MB ChB Leic. 1991 (Leicester) FRCS (Surg.) Ed 1995; FRCS (Otol) Ed 1997; FRCS (Orl-Hns) 2001. Cons. Otolaryngologist, Head and Neck Surg., Bradford Teachg. Hosps.; Cons. Surg., Leeds Nuffield Hosp., Leeds; Cons. ENT Surg., Yorks. Clinic, Bingley, W. Yorks. Specialty: Otorhinolaryngol. Special Interest: Head and Neck Cancer; Rhinology. Socs: Fell. Roy. Coll. Of Surgs. Of Edin.; Assoc. Brit. Assoc. Otol. Head & Neck Surgs; BMA. Prev: SpR Otolaryngol., Yorks. Deanery; Fell. in Head and Neck Surg., Rhinology, Roy. Adelaide Hosp., Australia.

SOOD, Mr Satish Chandra 130 Harley Street, London W1N 1AH Tel: 020 7935 4000 — LRCPI & LM, LRCSI & LM 1962; DTM & H Liverp. 1965; FRCS Ed. 1972. Cons. Plastic Surg. Whittaker Life Sci. Corpn.; Clin. Director, Twenty 1st Century Helthcare Ltd. Specialty: Plastic Surg. Socs: Fell. Roy. Soc. Med. & Internat. Coll. Surgs. (Plastic Surg.); Counc. & Cons. Plastic Surg. Ramana Health Foundat. Prev: JIC Davis Research Fell. Univ. Liverp.; Sen. Regist. Hosp. Sick Childr. Gt. Ormond St. & Guy's Hosp. Lond.

SOOD, Sunil Heston Health Centre, Cranford Lane, Heston, Hounslow TW5 9ER Tel: 020 8321 3410 Fax: 020 8321 3409 — MB ChB Glas. 1984. GP Princip. Hounslow. Specialty: Gen. Pract. Socs: BMA; Med. Protec. Soc. Prev: SHO (O & G) Chase Farm Hosp. Enfield; SHO (Orthop. & Accid & Emerg.) Law Hosp. Carluke; SHO (Geriat. Med.) St. Michael's Hosp. Aylsham.

SOOD, Tara Suman 5 Tocil Croft, Coventry CV4 7DZ Tel: 024 76 415885 — MB ChB Bristol 1997; BSc 1994. SHO A&E John Radcliffe Hosp.Oxf. Specialty: Accid. & Emerg. Socs: BMA.

SOOD, Ved Brat Springcliffe Surgery, 42 St. Catherines, Lincoln LN5 8LZ Tel: 01522 520443 Fax: 01522 543430; Isben House, 13 Lincoln Road, North Hykeham, Lincoln LN6 8DL Tel: 01522 681885 — MB BS Delhi 1965 (M.A. Med. Coll. Delhi) DO Aligarh 1967; Cert JCC Lond. 1976. Socs: Mem. Overseas Doctor Assn. Prev: Regist. (Clin. Path.) Lond. Chest Hosp.; Regist. (Haemat. & Bact.) Nat. Hosp. Nerv. Dis. Qu. Sq. Lond.; Regist. (Haemat.) Lond. Hosp. (Whitechapel).

SOODEEN, David Elliott Charlotte Keel Health Centre, Seymour Rd, Easton, Bristol BS2 — MB BCh Wales 1993.

SOODEEN, Patricia Inez (retired) 19 Downs Hill, Beckenham BR3 5HA — MB BS Bombay 1956 (Grant Med. Coll. Bombay) DObst RCOG 1967. Prev: GP Lond.

SOODEEN, Sally Jane Hartcliffe Health Centre, Hareclive Road, Hartcliffe, Bristol BS13 0JP — MB BCh Wales 1993.

SOOKLALL, Conrad Richard Suresh 37 Wadbrough Road, Sheffield S11 8RF — MB ChB Sheff. 1995.

SOOKUR, Dharmendra 47 Lawnswood Drive, Swinton, Manchester M27 5NH — MB ChB Manch. 1994.

SOOLE, Martin John High Street Surgery, 26 High Street, Wanstead, London E11 2AQ Tel: 020 8989 0407 Fax: 020 8518 8435; 46 Preston Road, London E11 1NN — MB BS Lond. 1986; DRCOG 1988; MRCGP 1994.

SOOLTAN, Abdool Rajack The Surgery, 179 York Road, Leeds LS9 7RD Tel: 0113 248 0268 Fax: 0113 248 8490 — MB ChB

Leeds 1972; ECFMG Cert 1975; DObst RCOG 1975; MRCGP 1976; DCH Eng. 1977.

SOOLTAN, Mohammed Ali 49 Ridgeway, Leeds LS8 4DD Tel: 0113 265 9190 — MRCS Eng. LRCP Lond. 1964 (Leeds) DTM & H Liverp. 1968; MRCP (U.K.) 1973. Regist. (Med.) Pontefract Gen. Hosp.

SOOLTAN, Yasmin 67 Shortridge Terrace, Jesmond, Newcastle upon Tyne NE2 2JE Tel: 0191 281 3907 — MB BS Newc. 1991. Trainee GP Newc. u. Tyne.

SOOMAL, Rabinder Singh Academic Unit of Radiotherapy,Orchard House, Royal Marsden Hospital NHS Trust, Downs Rd, Sutton SM2 5PT Tel: 020 8642 6011 Fax: 020 8661 3127 Email: rubin.soomal@rmh.nthames.nhs.uk — MB BS Lond. 1992 (Char. Cross. & Westm.) BSc Hons. Physiol. Lond. 1989; MRCP Lond. 1995; FRCR Lond. 1999. Specialist Regist. (Clin. Oncol.) Roy. Marsden Hosp. NHS Trust Lond. Specialty: Oncol. Socs: BMA; Roy. Coll. Radiol.; Roy. Coll. Phys.s. Prev: Specialist Regist. (Clin. Oncol.) Guys & St. Thos. NHS Trust Lond.; SHO (Med.) Brighton.

SOOMRO, Ghulam Mustafa Springfield Hospital, London SW17 7DJ; 4 Twickenham Close, Beddington, Croydon CR0 4SZ Tel: 020 8680 1346 — MB BS Sind 1979; Dip. Psychiat. Lond. 1986; MRCPsych 1993; Dip. Systematic Reviews, Lond. 1999; Dip. E Divence Based Med. Oxford 2000; MSc Social Research Surrey 2001. Specialty: Gen. Psychiat.

SOOMRO, Irshad Nabi Department of Histopathology, Nottingham City Hospital, Huckhall Road, Nottingham NG5 1PB Tel: 0115 969 1169 Ext: 46870 Fax: 0115 840 5883 Email: isoomro@ncht.trent.nhs.uk — MB BS (Hyderabad) FRCPath; PhD. Cons. Histopath., Nottm. City Hosp. Specialty: Histopath. Prev: Asst. Prof., Dept. of Path., The Aga Khan Univ. Karachi, Pakistan.

SOON, Christine Cheng Young 2 Kingston Av, Sutton SM3 9TZ — BM Soton. 1997.

SOON, Sing Yang 15/8 East Parkside, Edinburgh EH16 5XL — MB ChB Ed. 1997.

SOON, Su Yang Flat 2, 44 Limehill Road, Tunbridge Wells TN1 1LL; PO Box 151, Sibu 96007, Sarawak, Malaysia — BM BS Nottm. 1992; MRCP (UK). Specialist Regist. (Gastroenterol.) Kent & Sussex Hosp. Specialty: Gastroenterol.; Gen. Med.

SOON, Ying 25 Priory Road, Newbury RG14 7QS — MB BS Lond. 1985.

SOON, Yuen 79 Grosvenor Road, Harborne, Birmingham B17 9AL — MB BS Lond. 1991.

SOONG, Mr Chee Voon — MB BCh BAO Belf. 1985; MB BCh Belf. 1985; FRCSI 1989; FRCS(Gen) 1997; MD 1997. Cons. Surg. Belf. City Hosp. Specialty: Gen. Surg.

SOOPRAMANIEN, Anbananden Salisbury District Hospital, Salisbury SP2 8BJ Tel: 01983 565356 Email: asoopraman@aol.com — MD Amiens 1985; FRCP; PhD (Toulouse) 1977; MB BCh (Bordeaux) 1982; MD (Amiens) 1985. Cons. (Spinal Injuries & Rehabil. Med.), Salisbury. Specialty: Orthop.; Rehabil. Med. Socs: Internat. Spinal Cord Soc.; Roy. Coll. of Physicians. Prev: Cons. (Rehabil. Med.) Lincoln.

SOOR, Sajjan Singh (retired) 44 Newlands Lane, Heath Hayes, Cannock WS12 5HH Tel: 01543 279975 — MB BS Lond. 1960 (St. Geo.) Prev: Ho. Phys. Huddersfield Roy. Infirm.

SOORAE, Mr Ajaib Singh The Cardiothoracic Centre NHS Trust, Thomas Drive, Liverpool L37 2YS Tel: 0151 293 2398 Fax: 0151 293 2254 Email: ajaib.soorae@ctc.nhs.uk — MB BS Punjab 1966 (Glancy Medical College, Amritsar) Glancy Med. Coll. Amritsar); MRCP Eng.; FRCS Ed. 1971; FRCS Eng. 1975; LRCP (UK) 1975; T(S) 1991. Cons. Cardio-Thoracic Surg. The Cardiothoracic Centre NHS Trust Liverp.; Dep. Med. Director, The Cardiothoracic Centre NHS Trust, Liverp. Specialty: Cardiothoracic Surg. Socs: Soc. Thoracic & Cardiovasc. Surgs. Gt. Brit. & Irel. & Med.; Europ. Assn. for Cardiothoracic Surg. Prev: Sen. Regist. (Cardiothoracic Surg.) Roy. Vict. Hosp. Belf.; Regist. (Cardiothoracic Surg.) Walsgrave Hosp. Coventry; SHO (Gen. Surg.) St. Annes Hosp. Lond.

SOORAE, Sarabjit Singh Ashfield Surgery, 8 Walmley Road, Sutton Coldfield B76 1QN Tel: 0121 351 7955 Fax: 0121 313 2509 — MB ChB Birm. 1994; ChB Birm. 1994.

SOORIAKUMARAN, Mr Sellaiah Queen Mary's University Hospital, Roehampton Lane, London SW15 5PR Tel: 020 8355 2725 Fax: 020 8355 2952; 50 High Drive, New Malden KT3 3UB Tel: 020 8949 4234 — MB BS Sri Lanka 1974; MRCS Eng. LRCP Lond. 1981; FRCS Eng. 1982; FRCS Glas. 1983; FRCS Ed. 1983; FRCP 2000. Cons. Rehabil. Qu. Mary's Univ. Hosp. Lond. Specialty: Rehabil. Med. Socs: RCS; BMA; Roy. Soc. Med. Prev: Med. Off. & Sen. Regist. DSC Qu. Mary's Univ. Hosp. Lond.; Regist. (Gen. Surg.) Dewsbury & Staincliffe Gen. Hosps.

SOORIAKUMARAN, Velaiuthar 260 Prittlewell Chase, Westcliff on Sea SS0 0PR — MB BS Sri Lanka 1973; LMSSA 1983; MRCGP 1986. GP Leigh-on-Sea.

SOORMA, Mr Akbar Maidstone Hospital, Hermitage Lane, Maidstone ME16 9QQ Tel: 01622 729000 Ext: 4216 Fax: 01622 224600 — MB BS Karachi, Pakistan 1982; FRCS Glas. 1994; FFAEM 1996. Cons. A & E Med. Maidstone Hosp. Kent. Specialty: Accid. & Emerg. Socs: Brit. Assn. Accid. & Emerg. Med.; Med. Protec. Soc.; BMA. Prev: Sen. Regist. Rotat. (A & E Med.) S. Thames (W.); Cons. A & E Med. Newham Gen. Hosp. Lond.

SOOSAY, Geraldine Nirmala Department of Histopathology, King George Hospital, Barley Lane, Goodmayes, Ilford IG3 8YB Tel: 020 8970 8419 — MB BS Lond. 1982; MSc Lond. 1986, MB BS 1982; MRCPath 1990. Cons. Histopath. King Geo. Hosp. Goodmayes. Specialty: Histopath.

SOOTHILL, James Stephen Department of Medical Microbiology, 2nd Floor, Clinical Sciences Building, Manchester Royal Infirmary, Oxford Road, Manchester M13 9WL Tel: 0161 276 8830 Fax: 0161 276 8826 — MB BS Lond. 1985 (Guy's Hospital Medical School London) MD Lond. 1993; MRCPath 1997. Lect. Med. MicroBiol. Specialty: Med. Microbiol.

SOOTHILL, Professor Peter William Department of Obstetrics & Gynaecology, University of Bristol, St Michaels Hospital, Southwells St., Bristol BS2 8EG Tel: 0117 928 5277 Fax: 0117 928 5683 Email: peter.soothill@bristol.ac.uk — MB BS Lond. 1982 (Guy's) BSc Lond. 1979, MD 1987; MRCOG 1989. Cons. (Matern. & Fetal Med.) St Michael's Hosp. Bristol. Specialty: Obst. & Gyn. Prev: Prof. Matern. & Fetal Med. & O & G Univ. Bristol; Sen. Lect. & Cons. O & G Univ. Coll. Lond.; Lect. & Sen. Regist. (O & G) King's Coll. Hosp. Lond.

SOPER, Frederick Robert Charles 1 Mackie Place, Aberdeen AB10 1PF — MB ChB Aberd. 1957; Cert. Family Plann. JCC 1978; LMCC 1980; MCFPC 1981; MFCM 1986. Comm. Med. Specialist Grampian Health Bd. Prev: Sen. Med. Off. Bonavista Hosp.; Ho. Phys. St. Woolos Hosp. Newport; Ho. Surg. Aberd. Roy. Infirm.

SOPER, James William (retired) White Horses, Sycamore Close, Milford on Sea, Lymington SO41 0RY Tel: 01590 642227; White Horses, Sycamore Close, Milford on Sea, Lymington SO41 0RY Tel: 01590 642227 Fax: 01590 642227 — MB BChir Camb. 1958 (St. Thos.) DObst RCOG 1959; MA Cantab. 1959; DA Eng. 1961. Prev: GP Lymington.

SOPER, Richard Henry Victoria Surgery, Victoria Street, Bury St Edmunds IP33 3BD Tel: 01284 725550 Fax: 01284 725551; Cobbs Hall, Great Saxham, Bury St Edmunds IP29 5JN Tel: 01284 755123 — (St. Bart.) MB BS Lond. 1968; MRCS Eng. LRCP Lond. 1968; DA Eng. 1971; DObst RCOG 1971.

SOPHER, Brian Joseph Unsworth Medical Centre, Parr Lane, Unsworth, Bury BL9 8JR Tel: 0161 766 4448 Fax: 0161 767 9811; 35 Upper Park Road, Salford M7 4JB Tel: 0161 795 7834 — MB ChB Manch. 1977; BSc St. And. 1974; MRCGP 1981. Occupat. Health Phys. Bolton Metrop. Local Auth. Specialty: Occupat. Health. Socs: Soc. Occupat. Med.; Assn. Police Surg. Prev: Clin. Asst. (Obst.) St. Mary's Hosp. Manch.; SHO (O & G & Paediat.) St. Mary's Hosp. Manch.; Ho. Surg. N. Manch. Gen. Hosp.

SOPHER, David Moses (retired) Chester House, Clarendon Place, London W2 2NP Tel: 020 7402 4005 Fax: 020 7262 4007 — MB BS Bombay 1954 (Grant Med. Coll.) DGO Bombay 1954; DObst RCOG 1958. Prev: Regist. (O & G) King Edwd. Memor. Hosp. Ealing & Hillingdon Hosp.

SOPHER, Solomon Mark 22 Lower Belgrave Street, London SW1W 0LN — MB BS Lond. 1990; BSc Basic Med. Sci. & Physiol. 1st cl. Hons. Lond. 1987; MB BS (Distinc.) Lond. 1990; MRCP (UK) 1993. Research Fell. (Cardiol. Sci.s) St. Geo. Hosp. Med. Sch. Lond. Specialty: Cardiol. Prev: SHO Nat. Hosp. Qu. Sq. Lond.; SHO Hammersmith Hosp. Lond.; SHO (ITU) St. Thos. Hosp. Lond.

SOPPET, Pamela Elizabeth Rose 1 Great Wheatleys Road, Rayleigh SS6 7AL — MB Camb. 1975; BChir 1974; DCH Eng. 1977.

SOPPITT, Richard William Orchard House, 17 Church Street, St Peters, Broadstairs CT10 2TT — MB ChB Birm. 1989; MRCPsych 1995; MMedSci 1997. Cons. E. Kent Hosp. Trust; Hon. Sen. Lect. KIMS. Specialty: Child & Adolesc. Psychiat. Prev: Cons. Solihull.

SOPWITH, Arthur Marcus Lorantis Limited, 410 Cambridge Science Park, Cambridge CB4 0PE Tel: 01223 702500 Fax: 01223 702599 Email: mark.sopwith@lorantis.com — MB BChir Camb. 1976; MRCP (UK) 1978; MD Camb. 1983; MFPM RCP (UK) 1996. Specialty: Pharmaceutical Medicine. Prev: Pfizer Centr. Research; Celltech R&D.

SORAGHAN, Pauline Gertrude 9 Stirling Drive, Bearsden, Glasgow G61 4NX — MB BCh BAO NUI 1980.

SORAPURE, John Boileau 14 Caledon Road, Parkstone, Poole BH14 9NN Tel: 01202 722947 — MB BS Lond. 1958 (Lond. Hosp.) MRCS Eng. LRCP Lond. 1958; DObst RCOG 1960. Specialty: Gen. Pract. Socs: BMA & Bournem. Med. Soc. Prev: Clin. Asst. (Paediat.) Roy. Vict. Hosp. Boscombe; Ho. Surg. St. And. Hosp. Dollis Hill; Ho. Phys. & Ho. Surg. (Obst.) Lond. Hosp.

SORBY, Nicholas Geoffrey Dare Parklands Hospital, Basingstoke RG24 9RH Tel: 01256 376355 Fax: 01256 376452 — MB BS Lond. 1979 (Middlx.) FRCPsych 2001. Cons. Psychiat. Surrey Hants. borders NHS Trust. Specialty: Gen. Psychiat.

SOREFAN, Oomar Mia Ayoob 27 St Stephens Court, Canterbury CT2 7JP Tel: 01227 66253 — MB ChB Sheff. 1981; MRCPI 1984; MRCGP 1988; DGM RCP Lond. 1989. SHO (O & G) OldCh. Hosp. Romford. Prev: SHO Rotat. Kent & Canterbury Hosp.; Trainee GP Canterbury Health Centre.

SOREN, Dhuni Boarijore, 33 Longmeadow Road, Knowsley, Prescot L34 0HN — MB BS Patna 1963.

SORENSEN, Michael Harry Berwyn House Surgery, 13 Shrubbery Avenue, Worcester WR1 1QW Tel: 01905 22888 Fax: 01905 617352; 2 Nash Close, Worcester WR3 7YD — MB ChB Bristol 1975. Specialty: Gen. Pract.

SORENSEN-POUND, David John Plowright Surgery, Market Place, Swaffham PE37 7LQ Tel: 01760 722797 Fax: 01760 720025; Pear Tree Farm, Southburgh, Thetford IP25 7TE Tel: 01362 821403 Email: peartree11@yahoo.com — MB BS Lond. 1983; DA (UK) 1985; DRCOG 1987; MRCGP 1988. Prev: Med. Off. Oman; GP Shipdham Norf.; Med. Off. Tristan Da Cunha.

SORIA, Andres 4 The Woodlands, Puddingwood Lane, Broomfield, Chelmsford CM1 7ES — LMS U Complutense Madrid 1992.

SORNALINGAM, Chelliah Crossways Surgery, Crossways, Addington, South Croydon CR2 8JL Tel: 01689 848939; 54 Kendall Avenue S., South Croydon CR2 0QQ Tel: 020 8660 3604 — MB BS Ceylon 1958; MRCOG 1975, DObst 1973. GP S. Croydon.

SORNALINGAM, Narendra Alexandra Surgery, 39 Alexandra Road, London SW19 7JZ Tel: 020 8946 7578 Fax: 020 8944 5650; 19 Fir Grove, New Malden KT3 6RH — (Univ. Coll. & Middl. Hosp.) DFFP 1996 (RCOG); MSBS Lond. 1991; DRCOG RCOG 1995. GP Princip. Wimbledon, Lond. Specialty: Gen. Pract.

SOROOSHIAN, Khodayar Central Health Centre, North Carbrain Road, Cumbernauld, Glasgow G67 1BJ Tel: 0141 731738; Tower House, Luggiebank, Cumbernauld, Glasgow G67 4AB — MB ChB Glas. 1958. Prev: Regist. Orthop. & Accid. Lister Hosp. Hitchin; Regist. in Orthop. Lord Mayor Treloar Hosp. Alton; SHO Path. Roy. Hants. Co. Hosp. Winchester.

SOROUR, Gillian Ann 34C Edbrooke Road, London W9 2DG — MB BCh Witwatersrand 1993.

SORRELL, Jennifer Anne Portfields, Port Lane, Rugeley WS15 3DX — MB BS Lond. 1969; MSc Manch. 1976. Chief Exec. S. Staffs. HA. Prev: Dir. (Pub. Health) SE Staffs.; Specialist Community Med. (Health Care Plann.) Derbysh. AHA; Specialist Community Med. (Plann. & Informat.) Trafford AHA.

SORRELL, John Eric, OStJ M K Occupational Health Ltd., 12 Vincent Avenue, Crownhill Industrial Centre, Milton Keynes MK8 0AB Tel: 01908 262464 Email: mkochealth@aol.com; Border Green, 81 Hartwell Road, Hanslope, Milton Keynes MK19 7BY — MRCS Eng. LRCP Lond. 1971 (St. Bart.) BSc (Hons.) Lond. 1968, MB BS 1971; DObst RCOG 1973; DCH Eng. 1975; MRCGP 1976; MFOM Lond. 2000. Med. Dir. MKOHS Ltd. Specialty: Occupat. Health. Socs: Fell.Roy.Soc.Med. Prev: GP Trainer Oxf. Region, Milton Keynes Scheme; G.P. Bucks.

SORRIE, George Strath, CB (retired) 30 Irvine Crescent, St Andrews KY16 8LG Tel: 01334 474510 — MB ChB Aberd. 1957; DObst RCOG 1962; DPH (Distinc.) Lond. 1963; DIH Dund 1976; FFOM RCP Lond. 1982. Prev: Med. Adviser to Civil Serv. & Dir. Civil Serv. Occupat. Health Serv.

SORSBIE, Leigh Firth Park Road Surgery, 400 Firth Park Road, Sheffield S5 6HH Tel: 0114 242 6406 — MB ChB Sheff. 1990.

SORUNGBE, Akanni Olufemi Olakunle 10 Gratton Terrace, London NW2 6QE Tel: 020 8450 6015 Fax: 020 8450 6015 — MB BS Lond. 1960; MCRS Eng. LRCP Lond. 1960; DPH Eng 1974; FRIPHH 1985. Specialty: Pub. Health Med. Socs: BMA; Roy. Soc. Trop. Med. & Hyg.; Fell. Roy. Inst. Pub. Health & Hyg.

SOSIN, Michael David — MB ChB Birm. 1998; MRCP 2000. Specialist Regist. (Cardiol.) Nottm. City Hosp. Specialty: Gen. Surg.

SOSKIN, Michelle Anne Anaesthetic Department, 1 Watford General Hospital, Vicarage Road, Watford WD18 0HB Tel: 01923 244366 — MB ChB (Hons) Manch. 1987; FRCA 1993. Cons. (Anaesth. & Intens. Care) Watford Gen. W. Herts Trust. Specialty: Anaesth.; Intens. Care. Socs: Intens. Care Soc.; Assn. Anaesth. Prev: Sen. Regist. Rotat. (Anaesth. & Intens. Care) Roy. Free Hosp.; Regist. Middlx. & Univ. Coll. Hosps.

SOSNOWSKI, Marcin Andrzej 54 Dumbleton Avenue, Leicester LE3 2EG — MB ChB Leeds 1992.

SOTHERAN, Wendy Justine 14 West Street, Titchfield, Fareham PO14 4DH — MB BS Lond. 1990 (St. Mary's Hosp. Lond.) BSc Lond. 1987; FRCS Eng. 1995. Guernsey Research Fell. Univ. Soton. Specialty: Gen. Surg.

SOTHI, Sharmila 46 Charles Road, Solihull B91 1TS — MB BS Lond. 1990; MRCP (UK) 1993; FRCR 1998. Regist. (Clin. Oncol.) Birm. Oncol. Centre. Specialty: Oncol.; Radiother. Prev: SHO Rotat. (Med.) Brighton.

SOTIRIOU, Sotirios 22 Lyveden Road, London SE3 8TP — Ptychio Iatrikes Athens 1994.

SOTT, Miss Andrea Helene 5 Cavendish Court, Cavendish Road, Weybridge KT13 0JN Email: cbusch9965@aol.com — State Exam Med Bochum 1991 (Germany) FRCS (Eng.) 1995. Specialist Regist. Rotat. (Orthop.) SW Thames Kingston Hosp. Specialty: Orthop.

SOUBERBIELLE, Bernard Eric 88 Egmont Road, Sutton SM2 5JS — MD Paris 1984. Wellcome Research Fell. Univ. St. And.; Lect. Kings Coll. Lond. Specialty: Immunol. Prev: SHO (Path.) Selly Oak Hosp. Birm.

SOUCEK, Sava St Mary's Hospital, ENT Department/Audiology, Praed Street, London W2 1NY Tel: 020 7886 6028 — MUDr Prague 1959 (Charles Univ.) PhD Lond. 1987. Cons. Audiol. Phys. St Mary's Hosp. Lond. Specialty: Audiol. Med. Socs: Internat. Soc. Audiol.; BMA; Brit. Assn. Audiol. Phys. (Social Sec.). Prev: Sen. Regist. (Audiol. Med.) Roy. Nat. Throat, Nose & Ear Hosp. Lond.; Sen. Regist. (ENT) Chas. Univ. Prague.

SOUFLAS, Pauline Rampton Hospital, Woodbeck Road, Retford DN22 0PD — MRCS Eng. LRCP Lond. 1982 (Sheff.) MRCPsych 1989; Dip. Forens. Psych. Lond. 1995. Cons. Forens. Psychiat. Specialty: Child & Adolesc. Psychiat.; Forens. Psychiat. Special Interest: Forens. Psychother. Socs: Internat. Assn. Forens. Psychother.; Assn. Child Psychol. & Psychiat. Prev: Cons. Child Psychiat., Marsden St. Chesterfield; Sen. Regist., Child Psychiat., Manch..

SOUKIAS, Nikolaos 2 Roundwood Close, Cyncoed, Cardiff CF23 9HH — Ptychio Iatrikes Thessalonika 1985.

SOUKOP, Michel 2nd Floor Administration, St Mungo Institute, Link Corridor, Glasgow Royal Infirmary, Glasgow G4 0SF Tel: 0141 211 1160 Fax: 0141 211 0515; 15 Cleveden Gardens, Glasgow G12 0PU Tel: 0141 357 1455 — MB ChB St. And. 1971; MRCP (UK) 1974; FRCP Glas. 1986; FRCP Ed. 1991; FRCP Lond. 1994. Cons. Phys. & Med. Oncol. Glas. Roy. Infirm.; Hon. Sen. Lect. Glas. Univ.; Represen. Jt. Counc. RCP & RCR in Oncol.; Sec. to the SAC in Med. Oncol. Specialty: Oncol.; Gen. Med. Socs: Assn. Cancer Phys.; BMA (Chairm. GCHMS & Represen. to SCHMS & CCSC). Prev: Vis. Lect. (Human Oncol.) Univ. Wisconsin, Madison, USA; Sen. Regist. & Research Fell. (Med. Oncol.) Glas. Univ. & Gartnavel Gen. Hosp. Glas.

SOUL, Mrs Anne Rosemary Knowle House Surgery, 4 Meavy Way, Crownhill, Plymouth PL5 3JB Tel: 01752 771895 Fax: 01752 766510 — MB BS Lond. 1972 (Guy's) MRCS Eng. LRCP Lond. 1969; DRCOG 1986.

SOUL, Mr John Oliver, Surg. Capt. RN Retd. Trevenevow, Crapstone Road, Yelverton PL20 6BT Tel: 01822 854923 — (Guy's)

LMSSA Lond 1970; MRCS Eng. LRCP Lond. 1970; MB BS Lond. 1971; FRCS Eng. 1976. Freeman Worshipful Soc. Apoth. Lond. Specialty: Gen. Surg. Prev: Cons. Surg. RN Hosp. Plymouth; Hon. Sen. Regist. (Thoracic Surg.) E. Birm. Hosp.

SOUL, Jonathan David Marfleet Group Practice, 350 Preston Road, Hull HU9 5HH Tel: 01482 701834; Swallownest, 15 Bond St, Hedon, Hull HU12 8NY Tel: 01482 890308 — MB ChB Sheff. 1990. Prev: Trainee GP Bassetlaw VTS.

SOULBY, Georgina Carol Raigmore Hospital, Children's Services, Terrapin Building, Inverness IV2 3UJ Tel: 01463 701305 Email: georgina.soulby@hpct.scot.nhs.uk — MB ChB Dundee 1975; FRCP (UK) 1978; DCH RCP Lond. 1982; FRCPCH 1997; FRCP Ed. 1998. Cons. (Community Paediat.) Highland PCT. Specialty: Community Child Health. Prev: Cons. Community Paediat. Airedale NHS Trust; SCMO Leeds Community & Ment. Health Servs. Trust; Clin. Med. Off. Wakefield HA.

SOULIOTI, Alexia Maria Angeliki 49 Shrewsbury House, Cheyne Walk, London SW3 5LW — MRCS Eng. LRCP Lond. 1975; BSc Lond. 1971; DCH Eng. 1978; FFA RCS Eng. 1979; MRCP (UK) 1982. Specialty: Anaesth.

SOULSBY, Niel Warren 3 Hunters Lodge, The Green, Wallsend NE28 7ES — MB BS Newc. 1992.

SOULSBY, Miss Rachel Emma — MB BS Lond. 1998; MRCS 2002.

SOULSBY, Ruth Helen Rosemary — MB ChB Sheff. 1989; FRCS Ed. 1995.

SOULSBY, Thomas Peter 22 High Street, Liverpool L25 7TE — MB ChB Liverp. 1986; MRCP (UK) 1990; DA (UK) 1994.

SOUNDARARAJAN, Portonovo Chockalingam North Gate Hospital, Morpeth NE61 3BP Tel: 01670 394000 Fax: 01670 394004 — MB BS Madras 1966 (Thanjavur Med. Coll.) DPM Eng. 1978; MRCPsych 1981. Cons. N.gate Hosp. Morpeth; Lect. (Psych. Med.) Univ. Newc. u. Tyne. Specialty: Gen. Psychiat.

SOUNDY, Victoria Clare Department of Histopathology, Gloucestershire Royal Hospital, Great Western Road, Gloucester GL1 3NN Tel: 01452 395262; 5 Wallbank House, Denmark Road, Gloucester GL1 3HZ — MB BS Lond. 1993 (Char. Cross & Westm.) BSc (Hons. Path.) Lond. 1990. Specialist Regist. (Histopath.) Gloucester/Bristol. Specialty: Histopath. Socs: Med. Defence Union; Train. Mem. Assn. Clin. Path. Prev: Specialist Regist. (Histopath.) Univ. Coll. Hosp. Lond.; SHO (Histopath.) John Radcliffe Hosp. Oxf.; SHO (A & E) Chelsea & Westm. Hosp. Lond.

SOUPER, Dorothy Kilner (retired) 154 Christchurch Road, Norwich NR2 3PQ Tel: 01603 54126 — MB BChir Camb. 1939 (Camb. & Univ. Coll. Hosp.) MA, MB Camb. 1939, BChir 1933; DOMS Eng. 1940. Mem. Oxf. Ophth. Congr. Prev: Ho. Surg. Cheltenham Eye Hosp.

SOUPER, Katharine 18 Fulmer Road, Sheffield S11 8UF; Yule Cottage, Upham St, Upham, Southampton SO32 1JA Tel: 0148 96 225 — MB BS Lond. 1990; BSc Lond. 1987; MRCP (UK) 1993.

SOURIAL, Amoun Sity Aziz Flat 57, 6/9 Charterhouse Square, London EC1M 6EU Tel: 020 7251 1106 — MB BCh Cairo 1978. Med. Adviser to Ecotherm (UK) Ltd. Basildon. Socs: Soc. Occupat. Med. Prev: Med. Adviser to Callenders Ltd. Basildon, Vulcanite Ltd., Wakefield, Flat Bed J. V. Chester & Laybond Products Chester, PUR Systems Glossop.; Occupat. Med. Adviser Med. & Indust. Servs. Ltd. Eastbourne.

SOUSSI, Mr Ahmad Chafic 8 Rowallan Gardens, Glasgow G11 7LJ — MB ChB Cairo 1972; FRCS Glas. 1987.

SOUSTER, Howard (retired) Norwood, 14 Park Road, Ipswich IP1 3ST Tel: 01473 720170 — (Lond. Hosp.) MRCS Eng. LRCP Lond. 1941. Prev: Med. Ref. Methodist Homes For The Aged.

SOUTAR, Alastair James (retired) Firdene, Redlynch, Salisbury SP5 2PR Tel: 01725 510210 — MB ChB Aberd. 1944.

SOUTAR, Alice Lindsay Duncan Kilsyth Medical Partnership, Kilsyth Health Centre, Burngreen Park, Glasgow G65 0HU — MB ChB Dundee 1986; DRCOG 1988; DCH RCPS Glas. 1990; MRCGP 1991. GP Princip. Kilsyth Med. Partnership, Kilsyth. Prev: GP Retainee Kirkintilloch & Bishopbriggs, Glas.; GP Princip. Woodside Med. Pract., Aberd.

SOUTAR, Sir Charles John Williamson, KBE, Air Marshal RAF Med. Br. (retired) Oak Cottage, 57 High St., Aldeburgh IP15 5AU Tel: 01728 452201 — MB BS Lond. 1945; LMSSA Lond. 1945; DPH Lond. 1959; DIH Eng. 1960; FFCM 1979, M 1974. Prev: Dir.-Gen. Med. Servs. RAF.

SOUTAR, Colin Andrew Institute of Occupational Medicine, 8 Roxburgh Place, Edinburgh EH8 9SU Tel: 0131 667 5131; 8 Ravelston Rise, Edinburgh EH4 3LH Tel: 0131 337 2104 — MB BS Lond. 1966 (Guy's) MRCS Eng. LRCP Lond. 1966; MRCP (UK) 1969; MD Lond. 1977; FRCP Ed. 1989; FFOM RCP Lond. 1994. Chief Exec. Inst. Occupat. Med. Edin.; Hon. Sen. Lect. Univ. Edin. Specialty: Occupat. Health. Prev: Head Med. Br. Inst. Occupat. Med. Edin.; Asst. Prof. of Med. (Pulm.) Univ. Illinois Med. Centre Chicago, USA; Hon. Cons. Phys. City Hosp. Edin.

SOUTAR, Mr David Strang The Glasgow Nuffield Hospital, Beaconsfield Road, Glasgow G12 0PJ Tel: 0141 334 9441 Fax: 0141 339 1352; Raheen, 7 Chesters Road, Bearsden, Glasgow G61 4AQ Tel: 0141 942 4175 — MB ChB Aberd. 1972; FRCS Ed. 1977; FRCS Glas. 1983; ChM Aberd. 1987. Cons. Plastic Surg. W. Scotl. Regional Plastic & Oral Surg. Unit Canniesburn Hosp. Glas.; Hon. Clin. Sen. Lect. Univ. Glas.; Chariman- Div. of Trauma and Related Serv.s N. Glas. Univ NHS Trust. Specialty: Plastic Surg. Socs: Brit. Assn. Plastic Surg.; Brit. Assn. Aesthetic Plastic Surgs.; Brit Assn. Head and Neck Oncologists. Prev: Sen. Regist. W. Scotl. Regional Plastic & Oral Surg. Unit Canniesburn Hosp. Glas.; Regist. (Gen. Surg.) Grampian HB.

SOUTAR, Ian 79 Slateford Road, Edinburgh EH11 1QW Tel: 0131 313 2796; 15 Douglas Crescent, Edinburgh EH12 5BA Tel: 0131 225 4593 — MB ChB Glas. 1956; DObst. RCOG 1961.

SOUTAR, Richard Lewis Western Infirmary, Haematology & Transfusion Medicine, Dumbarton Road, Glasgow G11 6NT Tel: 0141 211 2156 — MB ChB Dundee 1986; BMSc (Hons.) Dundee 1983; MRCP (UK) 1989; MRCPath 1994, D 1993; MD Dundee 1996; FRCPath 2002; FRCP Ed. 2002. Cons. Haemat. & Transfus. Med. West. Infirm. Glas.; Cons. Haemat. & Transfus. Med. Scott. Blood Transfus. Serv.; Hon. Sen. Lect. Glas. Univ. Specialty: Haematology. Socs: Brit. Soc. Haematol.; Scott. Soc. of Experim. Med.; Roy. Coll. Phys. Edin. Prev: Cons. Haemat. Monklands Dist. Gen. Hosp. Airdrie; Sen. Regist. (Haemat.) Aberd. Roy. Infirm.; Resid. (Haemat.) McMaster Univ. Hamilton, Ontario.

SOUTER, Andrew John Department of Anaesthesia, Royal United Hospital, Combe Park, Bath BA1 3NG Tel: 01225 825056 Fax: 01225 825061; 2 Cedric Close, Weston, Bath BA1 3PQ Tel: 01225 424393 — MB ChB Ed. 1986; FRCA 1992. Cons. Anaesth. Roy. United Hosp. Bath. Specialty: Anaesth. Socs: Obst. Anaesth. Assn.; Pain Soc.; Assn. Anaesth. Prev: Sen. Regist. & Regist. (Anaesth.) Nuffield Dept. Anaesth. Oxf.; Vis. Asst. Prof. Univ. Texas, Dallas, USA.

SOUTER, Keith Moray New Southgate Surgery, Buxton Place, off Leeds Road, Wakefield WF1 3JQ Tel: 01924 334400 Fax: 01924 334439; 106 Manygates Lane, Sandal, Wakefield WF1 7DP Tel: 01924 256201 Fax: 01924 256201 — MB ChB Dundee 1976; MRCGP 1981; DSc Colombo 1993; MIPsi Med 1998; FRCGP 1998; Dip Med Stats 1999; MFHom 2002. Hon Tutor (Gen. Pract.) Univ. Leeds. Socs: Brit. Soc. Med. & Dent. Hypn. & Brit. Med. Acupunc. Soc.

SOUTER, Michael James Institute of Neurological Sciences, Southern General Hospital, 1345 Govan Road, Glasgow G51 4TF Tel: 0141 201 1100; 7 Gloucester Place, Edinburgh EH3 6EE Tel: 0131 225 2974 — MB ChB Ed. 1984 (Edinburgh) DA (UK) 1990; FRCA. 1992. Cons. (Neuroanaesth. & Neuro-IC) Inst. of Neurol. Sci.s Southern Gen. Hosp. Glas.; Sen. Lect. (Anaesth.) Univ. Glas. Specialty: Anaesth.; Intens. Care. Prev: Lect. (Anaesth.) Edin.; Sen. Regist. (Anaesth.); MRC Clin. Res. Fell. (Clin. Neurosci.) Univ. of Edin.

SOUTER, Mr Robin Graham Milton Keynes Hospital NHS Trust, Standing Way, Eaglestone, Milton Keynes MK6 5LD Tel: 01908 243291 Fax: 01908 665947; 10 Cottisford Crescent, Great Linford, Milton Keynes MK14 5HH Tel: 01908 666196 Fax: 01908 665947 — MD Glas. 1981; MB ChB Glas. 1971; FRCS Glas. 1976; FRCS Eng. 1977; FRCS Edinb. 2001. Cons. Gen. Surg. Milton Keynes Hosp.; Lead Clinician Cancer Servs.; Chair Oxf. Regional Surg. Professional Developm. Comm.; Examr. Roy. Coll. of Surg.s of Glas. Specialty: Gen. Surg. Socs: Assn. of Surg.s of Gt. Britain & Irel.; Vasc. Surgic. Soc.; Brit. Assn. of Surgic. Oncol. Prev: Lect. Nuffield Dept. Surg. John Radcliffe Hosp. Oxf.

SOUTER, Mr William Alexander (retired) Old Mauricewood Mains, Penicuik EH26 0NJ Tel: 01968 672609 Email: wasouter@ukgateway.net — (Ed.) MB ChB (Hons.) Ed. 1957; FRCS Ed. 1960. Hon. Research Cons. Orthop. Surg. New Edin. Roy. Infirm. - Little France. Prev: Cons. (Orthop.) Princess Margt. Rose Orthop. Hosp. Edin.

SOUTER, William Angus (retired) Ardlui, 7 Iain Road, Bearsden, Glasgow G61 4LX Tel: 0141 942 3787 — MB ChB Glas. 1940; MRCOG 1950; FRCOG 1998.

SOUTH, Alison Louise 3 Central Av, Greenfield, Oldham OL3 7DH — MB ChB Leeds 1997.

SOUTH, David The Mede, Cotheridge, Worcester WR6 5LZ — MB ChB Birm. 1964; FFA RCS Eng. 1972; DMRD Eng. 1974; FRCR 1980. Cons. Radiol. Worcester HA. Specialty: Radiol. Prev: Sen. Regist. (Radiol.) Birm. AHA (T); SHO (Med.) King Edwd. VII Memor. Chest Hosp.; Ho. Off. (Med.) Roy. Hosp. Wolverhampton.

SOUTH, Mrs Elizabeth Ann (retired) Neville Cottage, Warren Rise, New Malden KT3 4SJ Email: south@warrenrise.freeserve.co.uk — MB ChB Manch. 1962. Prev: SCMO Merton & Sutton HA.

SOUTH, Joanna Pirians Tilt, Aviary Road, Pyrford, Woking GU22 8TH Tel: 01932 346876 — MB BS Lond. 1960; MRCS Eng. LRCP Lond. 1960; MRCOG 1967, DObst 1961; DA Eng. 1962.

SOUTH, Mr John Roger Neville Cottage, Warren Rise, New Malden KT3 4SJ — MB ChB Manch. 1961; FRCS Eng. 1967. Prev: Sen. Lect. & Cons. Neurosurg. Chinese Univ. Hong Kong; Sen. Regist. Nat. Hosp. & Atkinson Morley's Hosp. Lond.

SOUTH, Leah Marie Pullen Barn, Staplehurst Road, Frittenden, Cranbrook TN17 2EE Tel: 0158 080332 — MB BS Lond. 1968 (St. Bart.) FRCS Eng. 1973; MS Lond. 1979. Cons. Gen. & Vasc. Surg. Maidstone Hosp. Specialty: Gen. Surg. Socs: Fell. Roy. Soc. Med.; Vasc. Soc. GB & Irel. Prev: Sen. Regist. (Gen. Surg. & Urol.) St. Geo. Hosp. Lond.; Sen. Regist. (Surg.) St. Jas. Hosp. Balham; Bernard Sunley Research Fell. RCS Eng.

SOUTH, Peter John Pullen Barn, Staplehurst Road, Frittenden, Cranbrook TN17 2EE Tel: 01580 852332 — MB BS Lond. 1968 (St. Bart.) MRCP (UK) 1971; MRCGP 1977. Prev: Regist. (Med.) Hastings Gp. Hosps.; Regist. (Gen. Med. & Cardiol.) St. Stephen's Hosp. Lond.; Ho. Phys. (Chest Dis.) Lond. Chest Hosp.

SOUTH, Richard Paul 43 Lateward Road, Brentford TW8 0PL — MB ChB Liverp. 1987. Director (Malaria Progr.s & Treatm. Access) Global Community Partnerships. Specialty: Pharmaceutical Medicine. Prev: Scientif. Manager, Hoechst Marion Roussel.

SOUTHALL, Edward Mayfield Medical Centre, 37 Totnes Road, Paignton TQ4 5LA Tel: 01803 558257 Fax: 01803 663353 Email: ed.southall@nhs.net — MB BS Lond. 1975 (St. Geo.) MRCP (UK) 1979; Cert. Family Plann. JCC 1983. Hosp. Pract. (Cardiol.) Torbay Hosp. Torquay. Specialty: Cardiol. Socs: Brit. Soc. Echocardiogr. Prev: Regist. (Med. Cardiol. & Med. Gastroenterol.) Roy. United Hosp. Bath; Regist. (Med.) Torbay Hosp. Torquay.

SOUTHALL, Graham John Westgate Practice, Greenhill Health Centre, Church Street, Lichfield WS13 6JL Tel: 01543 414311 Fax: 01543 256364; 4 Park Road, Alrewas, Burton-on-Trent DE13 7AG — MB BS Lond. 1972 (Roy. Free) DObst RCOG 1975; DCH Eng. 1976; DA Eng. 1978; MRCGP 1978. Prev: GP Trainee Coleshill Warks.; Med. Off. Shining Hosp. Pokhara, Nepal.

SOUTHALL, Joseph Gerard Anthony St Peters Hill Surgery, 15 St. Peters Hill, Grantham NG31 6QA Tel: 01476 590009 Fax: 01476 570898 — MB ChB Leeds 1988; MRCGP 1995. Specialty: Gen. Pract.

SOUTHALL, Peter James Pathology Laboratory, The General Hospital, Gloucester St., St Helier, Jersey JE2 3QS Tel: 01534 59000 Fax: 01534 59805 — MB BS Lond. 1977 (St. Bart.) MRCPath 1988. Cons. Histopath. & Cytopath. Jersey Gen. Hosp. Specialty: Histopath. Prev: Cons. Histopath. & Cytopath. Aintree Hosps. Liverp.; Research Fell. & Hon. Sen. Regist. (Path.) Char. Cross & Westm. Med. Sch. Lond.; Regist. & Hon. Lect. (Path.) Bristol Roy. Infirm.

SOUTHALL, Philippa Helen Porking Barn, Clifford, Hereford HR3 5HE — M.B., Ch.B. Birm. 1947.

SOUTHALL, Tonya Ruth 21a Gloucester Avenue, London NW1 7AU Tel: 020 7267 0292; 316 Knightsfield, Welwyn Garden City AL8 7NQ — BM BS Nottm. 1994; BMedSci Nottm. 1992. GP Reg. Lond. Specialty: Gen. Pract. Prev: Ho. Off. (Surg.) Salisbury; Ho. Off. (Med.) Qu. Med. Centre Nottm.; SHO (O & G) Univ. Coll. Lond.

SOUTHAM, Mr John Armitage (retired) South Lodge, 49 Paul's Place, Ashtead KT21 1HN Tel: 01372 274452 — MB ChB Manch. 1953; FRCS Ed. 1961; FRCS Eng. 1961. Hon. Cons. Surg. Epsom Health Care NHS Trust. Prev: Mem. Med. Appeal Tribunals SE Eng.

SOUTHAM, Professor John Chambers (retired) 13 Corstorphine House Avenue, Edinburgh EH12 7AD Tel: 0131 334 3013 — MB BChir Camb. 1958; BChD, LDS Leeds 1962; FRCPath 1983, M 1971; FDS RCS Ed. 1981; MD Camb. 1981. Prev: Vice-Dean & Sec. Fac. Dent. Surg. RCS Ed.

SOUTHAM, Richard John CAPAL Medical Practice, 95 Goodrest Avenue, Halesowen B62 0HP; 9 Oakdene Drive, Barnt Green, Birmingham B45 8LQ — MB ChB Birm. 1983; DRCOG 1985; MRCGP 1988; D.OCC.Med. 2001. GP W. Midl.; Occupational Phys.

SOUTHAN, Adam Warwick 107 New Road, Gellinedd, Pontardawe — MB BCh Wales 1994 (Cardiff) DRCOG 1997. GP Princip. Port Talbot. Specialty: Gen. Pract. Prev: GP Regist.

SOUTHCOTT, Anne Marie Interstitial Lung Disease Unit, NHLI, Emmanuel Kaye Building, Manresa Road, London SW3 6LR — MB BS Adelaide 1984; FRACP 1991.

SOUTHCOTT, Barbara Maud Creswick Department of Radiotherapy & Oncology, Charing Cross Hospital, Fulham Palace Road, London W6 8RF Tel: 020 8846 1731 Fax: 0208 746 8429; 29 Melville Avenue, South Croydon CR2 7HZ Tel: 020 8688 2393 — MB BS Lond. 1967; MRCS Eng. LRCP Lond. 1966; DMRT Eng. 1971; FFR 1974; FRCR 1975. Sen. Lect. & Hon. Cons. Radiother. & Oncol. Char. Cross Hosp. Lond.; Hon. Cons. Oncologist, W. Middlx. Hosp. And Roy. Marsden Hosp.; Hon. Cons. Radiother. & Oncol. Mayday Hosp. Thornton Heath & Ealing Hosp. Chelsea & Westm. Hosp. Lond. Specialty: Oncol.; Radiother. Socs: Brit. Inst. Radiol. & Brit. Oncol. Assn.; Brit. Radiol. Soc.; Rad. Soc. Prev: Sen. Regist. (Radiother. & Oncol.) Char. Cross Hosp. Lond.; SHO (Path.) Lewisham Hosp. Lond.

SOUTHCOTT, Michael Robert Pytchley Court Health Centre, 5 Northampton Road, Brixworth, Northampton NN6 9DX Tel: 01604 880228 Fax: 01604 880467 — MB BS Lond. 1975; MRCS Eng. LRCP Lond. 1975; DRCOG 1977; DCH 1980; MRCGP 1981.

SOUTHCOTT, Mr Roy David Creswick 29 Melville Avenue, South Croydon CR2 7HZ Tel: 020 8688 2393 — MB BS Lond. 1956 (Guy's) MB BS (Hons.) Lond. 1956; MRCS Eng. LRCP Lond. 1956; DTM & H Eng. 1961; FRCS Eng. 1964. Hon. Cons. Urol. E. Surrey Hosp.; Lt.-Col. RAMC (V). Specialty: Urol. Socs: Assoc. Mem. BAUS; Brit. Prostate Gp. Prev: Cons. Surg. Mayday Hosp. Croydon; Sen. Regist. Roy. Free Hosp. Lond.; Ho. Off. Guy's Hosp. Lond.

SOUTHERN, David Andrew 1 Bracken Rise, Ellesmere SY12 9ET Email: dasouthern@doctors.org.uk — MB ChB Glas. 1988; BSc (Hons.) Glas. 1985; DA (UK) 1991; FRCA 1993; Dip IMC Edin. 2002. Cons. Anaesth. & Intens. Care, Wrexham Maeler Hosp. Specialty: Anaesth. Socs: BMA & Assn. Anaesth. Prev: Sen. Regist. (Anaesth.) Soton. Gen. Hosp.; Sen. Regist. & Regist. (Anaesth.) Townsville Gen. Hosp. Queensland, Austral.; Regist. (Anaesth.) Glan Clwyd Hosp. Wales & Univ. Hosp. Wales Cardiff.

SOUTHERN, Keith John Harold Health Centre, Fareham PO16 7ER Tel: 01329 823456; Ash House, Lee Ground, Fareham PO15 6RP Tel: 01329 844618 — MB ChB Liverp. 1963; DObst RCOG 1968.

SOUTHERN, Kevin William Dept of Paediatrics, University of Leeds Infirmary, Leeds LS2 9NS Tel: 0113 283 6999 Fax: 0113 283 6999; 21 Rochester Terrace, Headingley, Leeds LS6 3DF Tel: 0113 275 5054 — MB ChB Leeds 1987; PHD Leeds 1998. Lect. Univ of Leeds.; MRC Clin. Research Fell. St. Jas. Hosp. Leeds. Specialty: Paediat. Socs: Roy. Coll. Paediat. & Child Health; Yorks. Regional Paediat. Soc. Prev: SHO (Paediat.) Leeds West. HA; Ho. Off. (Med.) Seacroft Leeds; Ho. Off. (Paediat.) Clarendon Wing Leeds.

SOUTHERN, Lee Patricia Tarleton Group Practice, The Health Centre, Tarleton, Preston PR4 6UJ — MB ChB Birm. 1990 (Univ. Birmingham) DFFP 1995; LFHom 2000. GP Princip. Prev: Trainee GP Wroughton; SHO Centr. Birm. VTS; Princip., Jubilee Field Surg.

SOUTHERN, Paul Brian St. James's University Hospital, Beckett St., Leeds LS9 7TF Tel: 0113 243 3144; 15 Sandringham Way, Moortown, Leeds LS17 8BX Tel: 0113 269 1244 — MB ChB Leeds 1996. SHO (Integrated Med.) Seacroft Hosp. Leeds. Specialty: Gen. Med. Prev: SHO (Diabetes & Gen. Med.) St Jas. Leeds; PRHO (Diabetes & Gen. Med.) Airedale Gen. Reighley; PRHO (Surg. (Endocrine)) St. James' Leeds.

SOUTHERN, Peter John Dicconson Terrace Surgery, Dicconson Terrace, Wigan WN1 2AF Tel: 01942 239525 Fax: 01942 826552 — MB BS Lond. 1983; DRCOG 1987.

SOUTHERN, Robert John Cunliffe (retired) Cardunneth, Corby Hill, Carlisle CA4 8PJ Tel: 01228 560596 — MB ChB Ed. 1943; MRCP (UK) 1950; FRCP Ed. 1993. Prev: Cons. Chest Phys. Carlisle & E. Cumbria.

SOUTHERN, Mr Stephen James — MB BS Lond. 1987; FRCS (Plast); FRCS Ed. 1992. Cons. Plastic, Reconstruc. and Hand Surg. Specialty: Plastic Surg.

SOUTHERTON, Joanne Warden Lodge Surgery, Albury Ride, Cheshunt, Waltham Cross EN8 8XE Tel: 01992 622324 Fax: 01992 636900 — MB ChB Leic. 1985 (Leicester) DRCOG 1990.

SOUTHEY, Trevor James The William Fisher Medical Centre, High Street, Southminster CM0 7AY Tel: 01621 772360 Fax: 01621 773880 — MB BS Lond. 1974; DRCOG 1977; MRCGP 1978; DGM RCP Lond. 1997. GP Princip.; Clin. Asst. (Geriat.) Chelmsford.

SOUTHGATE, Brian Andrew (retired) Watersmeet, Churchill Way, Appledore, Bideford EX39 1PA Tel: 01237 477062 — MB BS Lond. 1953 (St. Bart.) DAP & E Lond. 1965; FFPHM 1980, M 1974. Prev: Sen. Lect. (Trop. Hyg.) Lond. Sch. Hyg. & Trop. Med.

SOUTHGATE, Clive Jonathan The Riverside Health Centre, Station Road, Manningtree CO11 1AA — MB BS Lond. 1984 (Guy's) Cert. Family Plann. JCC 1985. Specialty: Gen. Pract. Prev: Clin. Asst. (ENT) Essex Co. Counc. Colchester.; Trainee GP Colchester VTS.; SHO (O & G) Beverley N. Humberside.

SOUTHGATE, Crispin Robert William The Coach House, Woodlands Close, Cople, Bedford MK44 3UE — MB BCh Wales 1996.

SOUTHGATE, Mr George William Town Farmhouse, Old Weston, Huntingdon PE28 5LL — MB ChB Liverp. 1973; FRCS Eng. 1979. Cons. Orthop. Surg. Hinchingbrooke Hosp. Huntingdon. Specialty: Orthop. Prev: Sen. Regist. (Orthop.) Leeds Gen. Infirm.; Regist. (Orthop. & Gen. Surg.) Liverp. Postgrad. Train. Prog.; Regist. Orthop. Train. Prog. Soton. Gen. Hosp.

SOUTHGATE, Herbert John Old Stile, 179 Middleton Road, Middleton-on-Sea, Bognor Regis PO22 6DF — MRCS Eng. LRCP Lond. 1976; BSc (Hons.) Lond. 1973, MB BS Lond. 1976; MRCP (UK) 1983; MRCPath 1984.

SOUTHGATE, Mr Jeremy James Royal Bournemouth Hospital, Castle Lane, Bournemouth BH7 7DW Tel: 01202 303626; Manor Farmhouse, Old Ham Lane, Little Canford, Wimborne BU21 7LP — MB BS Lond. 1986 (The London Hosp. Med. College) FRCS Eng. 1991; FRCS (orth) 1997. Specialty: Orthop. Socs: BOA; Brit. Assn. for Surg. of the Hand. Prev: Regist. (Orthop.) Winchester & Portsmouth Hosps. Wessex Train. Progr.; Sen. Regist. Southampton Wessex Rotat.; Hand Fell. Sydney & St Luke's Hosp. Australia.

SOUTHGATE, Professor Lesley Jill, DBE University College London Medical School, Centre for Health Informatics & Multiprofessional Education, Whittington Hospital, Archway Road, London N19 3UA Tel: 020 7288 5209 Fax: 020 7288 3322 Email: l.southgate@chime.ucl.ac.uk — MB ChB Liverp. 1967; FRCGP 1985, M 1974; MClinSci. Univ. West. Ontario 1980; FRCP 1997. Prof. Univ. Coll. Lond. Med. Sch. Whittington Hosp. Specialty: Gen. Pract. Socs: BMA. Prev: Prof. Gen. Pract. & Primary Care St. Bart. Hosp. Med. Coll. Lond.; GP Hoddesdon; W.K. Kellog Fell. (Family Med.) West. Univ. Ontario, Canada.

SOUTHGATE, Matthew John Lower Road Medical Health Centre, Lower Road, Cookham Rise, Maidenhead SL6 9HX Tel: 01628 524646 Fax: 01628 810201; Tanglewood, Dean Lane, Cookham Dean, Maidenhead SL6 9BG Tel: 01628 890290 — BM BCh Oxf. 1975 (Oxford) BA Oxf. 1970, BM BCh 1975. Clin. Asst. (Obst.) St. Mark's Hosp. Maidenhead. Socs: Windsor & Dist. Med. Soc. & Soc. Med. & Dent. Hypn.; Roy. Soc. Med. Prev: Ho. Off. (Med.) Wycombe Gen. Hosp.; Ho. Off. (Surg., Obst. & Paediat.) Canad. Redr. Hosp. Taplow.

SOUTHWARD, Catherine Gwendolyn (retired) Braye Cottage, Sandwith, Whitehaven CA28 9UP Tel: 01946 693740 — MB ChB Ed. 1955; DObst RCOG 1958. Hosp. Pract. W. Cumbld. Hosp. Whitehaven.

SOUTHWARD, Nigel Ralph (retired) Drokesfield, Bucklers Hard, Beaulieu, Brockenhurst SO42 7XE Tel: 01590 616252 — (Middlx.) MB BChir Camb. 1965; MA Camb. 1966; MRCP Lond. 1969. Prev: Apoth. to HM the Qu. & HM Household & Households of Princess Margt. Countess of Snowdon, Princess Alice & Duke & Duchess of Gloucester.

SOUTHWARD, Mr Robert Dougal Accident & Emergency Dept., University Hospital of Hartlepool, Holdforth Road, Hartlepool — MB BS Newc. 1990 (Univ. Newc. u. Tyne) FRCS Eng. 1996; FFAEM RCS, London 2000. Cons., Accid. & Emerg. Dept., Univ. Hosp. of Hartlepool. Specialty: Accid. & Emerg. Prev: SHO (Anaesth.) Qu. Eliz. Hosp. Gateshead; Demonst. (Anat.) Univ. Newc. u. Tyne; Specialist Regist. (A & E) Northern Deanery Rotat.

SOUTHWARD, Stephen Paul Sea Road Surgery, 39-41 Sea Road, Bexhill-on-Sea TN40 1JJ Tel: 01424 211616 Fax: 01424 733950; 7 Collington Grove, Bexhill-on-Sea TN39 3UB Tel: 01424 842454 Email: steve@southward35.freeserve.co.uk — MB BS Lond. 1986 (St Bartholomews) Specialty: Gen. Pract.

SOUTHWELL, Arthur Gerrard William Street Surgery, 87 William Street, Lurgan, Craigavon BT66 6JB Tel: 028 3832 2509 Fax: 028 3834 7673 — MB BCh BAO NUI 1979; BSc (Hons.) Belf. 1971, MSc (Clin. Psychol.) 1973; DRCOG 1981; MRCGP 1984.

SOUTHWELL, Katherine Fiona Forest House Surgery, 25 Leicester Road, Shepshed, Loughborough LE12 9DF Tel: 01509 508412 — MB BS Lond. 1990 (St. Bart.) BSc Basic Med. Scs. & Physiol. Lond. 1987; MRCGP 1995. Specialty: Gen. Pract. Prev: Trainee GP Leics. VTS.

SOUTHWOOD, Margaret Carleton (retired) 1 Aldwick Avenue, Bognor Regis PO21 3AQ Tel: 01243 823073 — MB ChB Ed. 1954; DA Eng. 1957; FFA RCS Eng. 1959. Prev: Cons. Anaesth. Roy. United Hosp. Bath & United Bristol Hosps.

SOUTHWOOD, Professor Taunton Ray Department of Rheumatology, University of Birmingham, Birmingham B15 2TT Tel: 0121 414 6784 Fax: 0121 414 6794 Email: t.r.southwood@bham.ac.uk — BM BS Flinders 1980 (Flinders University South Africa) FRACP 1987; FRCPA 1989; FRCP Lond. 1994; FRCPCH 1997. Prof. (Paediat. Rheum.) University Birm.; Cons. & Clin. Dir. (Paediat. & Rheum.) Birm. Childr. Hosp. NHS Trust; Head of Acad. Dept. of Paediat. Specialty: Paediat. Socs: Fellow of Royal College of Paediatrics and Child Health; Fellow of Paediatric Rheumatology European Society. Prev: Clin. Research Fell. Brit. Columbia's Childr.s Hosp. Vancouver, BC, Canada.

SOUTHWOOD, Timothy Michael Tower House Medical Centre, Stockway South, Nailsea, Bristol BS48 2XX Tel: 01275 866700 — MB BS Lond. 1981 (St Georges) BDS 1975; DRCOG 1986; DGM RCP Lond. 1987; MRCGP 1988; DFFP 1993. Socs: Christian Med. Fellowsh.; BMA; Bristol M-C Soc. Prev: Regist. (Maxillofacial Surg.) Roy. Lond. Hosp.

SOUTHWORTH, Stephen Andrew 38 Willow Tree Road, Altrincham WA14 2EG — MB ChB Aberd. 1980.

SOUTTER, Andrew Peter Lena Peat Resource Centre, 33-34 Sydenham Road, Croydon CR2 2EF Tel: 020 8700 8700; 3 Crossway, Bush Hill Park, Enfield EN1 2LA — MB BS Lond. 1984; MRCPsych 1989. Cons. Psychother. Croydon. Specialty: Psychother. Prev: Sen. Regist. (Adult Psychother.) NE Thames RHA; Regist. Rotat. (Psychiat.) N. Lond. Train. Scheme; Clin. Lect. (Psychiat.) Univ. Coll. Hosp. Lond.

SOUTTER, Catherine Isabel (retired) 5 Old Kirk Place, Dunfermline KY12 7ST Tel: 01383 726231 — MB BS Lond. 1955 (Roy. Free) DObst RCOG 1958; DCH Eng. 1959; DPM Eng. 1972.

SOUTTER, Douglas Alistair Fraser Street Surgery, 10/14 Fraser Street, Largs KA30 9HP Tel: 01475 673380 Fax: 01475 674149 — MB ChB Glas. 1984.

SOUTTER, Frances Anne Edinburgh Royal Infirmary, 1 Lauriston Place, Edinburgh EH3 9YW; 9 Leithen Cresent, Innerleithen EH44 6JL — MB ChB Dundee 1980; DCH RCP Glas. 1983; DRCOG 1986. Clin. Asst. Specialty: Diabetes.

SOUTTER, Linda Patricia 48 Goodrich Road, London SE22 9EQ Tel: 020 8693 8604 — MB BS Lond. 1981; MRCP (UK) 1985; DCH RCP Lond. 1985. Cons. Paediat. (Community Child Health) Medway NHS Trust. Specialty: Community Child Health.

SOUTTER, Peter George 3-5 Bounds Green Road, Wood Green, London N22 8HE; 9 Queen Annes Grove, Bush Hill Park, Enfield EN1 2JP Tel: 020 8360 5261 — MB BS Lond. 1959 (Westm.) MRCS Eng. LRCP Lond. 1961; DObst RCOG 1961. Socs: BMA. Prev: Ho. Surg. Westm. Hosp.; Ho. Phys. St. Stephen's Hosp. Fulham.

SOUTTER, Robert Ian Currie Road Health Centre, Currie Road, Galashiels TD1 2UA Tel: 01896 754833 Fax: 01896 751389 — MB

ChB Glas. 1981 (Glasgow) DRCOG 1983; MRCGP 1985. GP Galashiels.

SOUTTER, William (retired) 56 Cranford Road, Aberdeen AB10 7NL — MB ChB Aberd. 1951. Prev: Civil Med. Pract. MoD Arborfield Garrison.

SOUTTER, Mr William Patrick 2nd floor Hammersmith House, Department of Gynaecological Oncology, Imperial College School of Medicine, Hammersmith Hospital, Du Cane Road, London W12 0HS Tel: 020 8383 3267 Fax: 020 8383 8065 Email: p.soutter@ic.ac.uk — MB ChB Glas. 1967; DObst RCOG 1969; FRCOG 1988, M 1975; MSc Glas. 1972, MD 1979. Reader Gyn. Oncol., Imperial Sch. Med. Specialty: Gynaecology. Special Interest: colposcopy. Socs: British Gynaecological Cancer Society, member. & past hononary secretary; British Society for Colposcopy & Cervical Pathology; International Gynaecological Cancer Society. Prev: Sen. Lect. (O & G) Univ. Sheff.; Lect. (Midw.) Qu. Mother's Hosp. Glas.; Med. Off. (Gyn.) King Edwd. VIII Hosp. Durban.

SOUTZOS, Theodore Baudon House Clinic, 3 London Road, Harrow-on-the-Hill, Harrow HA1 3JL Tel: 0705 009 7936 Fax: 020 8864 6092 Email: drs@psg.org — MB BS Lond. 1990; BSc; MRCPsych. Cons. Psychiat. Specialty: Gen. Psychiat.

SOUYAVE, Janet Rawdon Surgery, 11 New Road Side, Rawdon, Leeds LS19 6DD — MB ChB Leeds 1977; DRCOG 1979; MRCGP 1981.

SOUZA FARIA, Frederick Philip Bromsgrove B61 0Dd Tel: 01527 488282 — MB BS Bombay 1984; MRCPSych 1992. Cons. Psychiat. Brookhaven Princess of Wales Community Hosp. Worcs. Specialty: Gen. Psychiat. Prev: Regist. Rotat. Birm.

SOWAH, Adjei 4 Lister Close, Lister Hospital, Coreys Mill Lane, Stevenage SG1 4AB Tel: 01438 781184 — MB ChB Ghana 1984; MB ChB U Ghana 1984; MRCOG 1992.

SOWARD, Katherine Margaret 24 Wandsworth Road, Heaton, Newcastle upon Tyne NE6 5AD Tel: 0191 265 2542 — BM BS Nottm. 1994. Specialty: Paediat.

SOWDAGER, Ahsan 128 Southgate Road, London N1 3HX — LMSSA Lond. 1996.

SOWDEN, David Stewart 18 Tower Gardens, Ashby-de-la-Zouch LE65 2GZ — MB ChB Leeds 1979; DRCOG 1981; DCH RCPS Glas. 1982; FRCGP 1991, M 1983. Dir. Postgrad. Gen. Pract. Ed. S. Trent. Specialty: Gen. Pract.

SOWDEN, Gareth Richard North Devon District Hospital, Barnstaple EX31 4JB — MB BS Lond. 1973; MRCS Eng. LRCP Lond. 1973; FFA RCS Eng. 1978; DABA 1981. Cons. Anaesth. N. Devon Dist. Hosp. Barnstaple. Specialty: Anaesth. Socs: Eur. Resusc. Counc.; Assn. Anaesth. Prev: Sen. Regist. (Anaesth.) Bristol Roy. Infirm.; Ho. Phys. Med. Unit King's Coll. Hosp. Lond.; Instruc. Anaesth. Harvard Univ., USA.

SOWDEN, Helen 5 Boroughs Partnership NHS Trust, Hollins Park Hospital, Hollins Lane, Winwick, Warrington WA2 8WA Tel: 01925 664432 Email: Helen.Sowden@5boroughspartnership.nhs.uk — MB BS Lond. 1991; MRCPsych 1998; PGDip CT 2001. Cons. Psychiat. Specialty: Psychother. Special Interest: Main modality CBT.

SOWDEN, Jonathan Mark Dermatology Dept, Wrexham Hospital, Wrexham LL13 7TD Tel: 01978 725 5688 — BM BS Nottm. 1983; BMedSci Nottm. 1981; FRCP (UK) 1988. Cons. Dermat. Wrexham Maelar Hosp. Specialty: Dermat. Prev: Sen. Regist. (Dermat.) Univ. Hosp. Nottm.; Regist. (Dermat.) N. Staffs. Hosp. Centre Stoke-on-Trent; Regist. & SHO (Med.) Glan Clwyd Hosp.

SOWDEN, Lesley Margaret, Surg. Lt. RN 69 Frensham Road, Southsea PO4 8AE Tel: 023 9286 4092 — MB ChB Manch. 1994 (Manchester) Gen. Duties Med. Off. Roy. Navy. Specialty: Gen. Pract. Prev: Surg. Roy. Navy.

SOWDEN, Matthew Charles 34 Lancaster Avenue, Kirk Sandall, Doncaster DN3 1NG — MB ChB Manch. 1993.

SOWDEN, Penelope Anne The Surgery, 66 Crown Road, Twickenham TW1 3ER Tel: 020 8892 2543 Fax: 020 8744 3055 — BM BS Nottm. 1987; BMedSci Nottm. 1985; DRCOG 1991; MRCGP 1991. Specialty: Obst. & Gyn. Prev: SHO Nottm. VTS.

SOWEMIMO, George Morounfolu 1 Warwick Terrace, Lea Bridge Road, London E17 9DP Email: georgesowemimo@aol.com — MB BS Ibadan 1979; MB BS Ibadan 1979; FRCS (RPCS Glasgow) 1984; Dip Urol UCL 1990.

SOWERBUTTS, John George (retired) Upton Forge, Upton Magna, Shrewsbury SY4 4UD Tel: 01743 709330 — MB BS Lond. 1949 (St. Mary's) MRCS Eng. LRCP Lond. 1949; DMRD Eng. 1954; FRCR 1957; FRCP Ed. 1971, M 1958. Prev: Cons. Radiodiag. E. Surrey. Hosp. Redhill.

SOWERBY, Emma Louise 12 Fortescue Chase, Thorpe Bay, Southend-on-Sea SS1 3SS Tel: 01702 586982 — MB ChB Manch. 1996. SHO (O & G) Wythenshawe Hosp. Manch. Specialty: Obst. & Gyn.

SOWERBY, Howard Anthony Staffa Health Centre, 3 Waverley Street, Tibshelf, Alfreton DE55 5NU Tel: 01773 872252 Fax: 01773 591712; Ellenborough House, 95 High St., Stonebroom, Alfreton DE55 6JY Tel: 01773 874315 Fax: 01773 591703 Email: ros@hsowerby.funet.co.uk — MB BChir Camb. 1973; MA Camb. 1973. Prev: Regist. (Med.) W. Suff. Hosp. Bury St. Edmunds; Ho. Phys. & Ho. Off. (Paediat.) Guy's Hosp. Lond.

SOWERBY, Mary Kathleen Jane The Surgery, 29 High Stile, Leven, Beverley HU17 5NL Tel: 01964 542155 Fax: 01964 543954; Four Views, Grange Road, North Frodingham, Driffield YO25 8LN — MB BS Newc. 1991 (Univ. Newc. u. Tyne) DCH RCP Lond. 1994; DFFP 1994; MRCGP 1995. Specialty: Gen. Pract.

SOWERBY, Peter Redmore Bladeley House, Buckland Newton, Dorchester DT2 7BS — MB BS Lond. 1950 (Guy's) MRCS Eng. LRCP Lond. 1950; FRCGP 1976, M 1963. Socs: 1987, Founder:Egton Med. Informat. Systems Ltd.

SOWERBY, Rachel The Woodland Medical Practice, Jasmin Road, Birchwood, Lincoln LN6 0QQ Tel: 01522 683590 Fax: 01522 695666; 19B Drury Lane, Lincoln LN1 3BN — MB ChB Dundee 1987; DCH RCPS Glas. 1990; MRCGP 1991; DRCOG 1991.

SOWERBY, Roger Fielding 2 Troon Close, Bedford MK41 8AY Tel: 01234 214045 Fax: 01234 214045; 2 Troon Close, Bedford MK41 8AY Tel: 01234 214045 Fax: 01234 214045 — MB ChB Liverp. 1957; MRCGP 1966; DAvMed Eng. 1970; MFOM RCP Lond. 1980; T(OM) 1991. Med. Examr. Civil Aviat. Auth. & Europ. Ft. Aviat. Auth.; Cons. Occupat. Med. Bedford. Specialty: Aviat. Med.; Occupat. Health. Prev: Gp. Capt. RAF Med. Br.; Ho. Off. (Orthop.) & Med. Profess. Unit Liverp. Roy. Infirm.

SOWERBY, Roy George Rowton Grange E., Whitchurch Road, Rowton, Chester CH3 6AF — MB ChB Manch. 1969; DCH Eng. 1971.

SOWINSKA, Elzbieta 11 Hill Cliffe Road, Walton, Warrington WA4 6NX — MB ChB Manch. 1979.

SOWLER, Elisabeth Mary Kay (retired) Scottish Eecutive Health Department, St. Andrews House, Edinburgh EH1 3DG Tel: 0131 244 2827 Fax: 0131 244 2069; 19 Avondale Place, Edinburgh EH3 5HX Tel: 0131 332 6526 — (Ed.) MB ChB Ed. 1969, BSc (Med. Sci.) 1966; DA Eng. 1975; DObst RCOG 1975; MRCPsych 1983. Princip. Med. Off. Scott. Exec.Health.Dept.

SOWRAY, Professor John Herbert (retired) 44B Sutton Court Road, Chiswick, London W4 4NJ Tel: 020 8995 5999 Email: jhsowray@aol.com — MRCS Eng. LRCP Lond. 1959 (Roy. Dent. Hosp. & St. Geo.) BDS Lond. 1953; FDS RCS Eng. 1963, LDS 1953; FRCS Ed. 1986. Prev: Prof. Oral & Maxillofacial Surg. (Univ. Lond.) King's Coll. Hosp. Med. Sch.

SOWTER, Emma Mai 5 Holmes Close, Wokingham RG41 2SG Tel: 01734 782691 Fax: 01734 782691 — BM Soton. 1986. Specialty: Forens. Psychiat. Prev: SHO (Psychiat.) Heatherwood & Wexham Pk. Hosp. Trust Slough.; Ho. Phys. Medway HA; Ho. Surg. Wycombe HA.

SOWTER, Martin Christopher Department of Obstetrics and Gynaecology, National Womens Hospital, Claude Road, Epsom, Auckland, New Zealand Tel: 00 64 9 638 9919 Fax: 00 64 9 630 9858; First Floor Flat, 46 Arley Hill, Cotham, Bristol BS6 5PP — MB ChB Birm. 1988 (Birmingham) BSc Path 1987; ChB Birm. 1988; MRCOG 1994; MRNZCOG 1996. Research Fell. Univ. of Auckland. Specialty: Obst. & Gyn. Socs: Brit. Fertil. Soc.; Austral. Fertil. Soc.; Internat. Gyn. Endoscopy Soc.

SOWTON, John Victor (retired) Charman Cottage, Nutfield Marsh Road, Nutfield, Redhill RH1 4EU Tel: 01737 643488 Fax: 01737 644195 — MB BS Lond. 1956 (King's Coll. Hosp.) MRCS Eng. LRCP Lond. 1956; DObst RCOG 1963; FRCGP 1990. Chief Med. Off. Friends Provident Life Off. Dorking. Prev: GP Redhill.

SOWTON, Timothy James Seascale Health Centre, Gosforth Road, Seascale CA20 1PN Tel: 019467 28101 — MB BS Camb. 1990 (Char. Cross & Westm.) MA Camb. 1985; DGM RCP Lond. 1993; DCH RCP Lond. 1994; MRCGP 1994; DTM & H RCP Liverp. 1995;

Dip Palliat Med Wales 2002. GP Princip. Cumbria; Macmillan GP Facilitator in Palliat. Care N. Cumbria. Specialty: Palliat. Med. Prev: Médecins sans Frontiéres, Holland; Trainee GP/SHO Redhill VTS; Clin. Asst. (Palliat. Med.) W. Cumbld. Hosp. Whitehaven.

SOYE, Jonathan Albert 10 Lester Avenue, Lisburn BT28 3QD — MB BCh Belf. 1998.

SOYEMI, Adeoya Olakumle 92 Ashridge Way, Morden SM4 4ED — MB BS Lond. 1972; MRCOG 1979.

SOYER, Jacques Anthony Kailash, Centre of Oriental Medicine, 7 Newcourt St., St Johns Wood, London NW8 7AA Tel: 020 7722 3939 Fax: 020 7722 7878; 19 Chepstow Crescent, London W11 3EA — MB BS Sydney 1981.

SOYSA, Priyantha Naomal Chiswick Health Centre, Fishers Lane, London W4 1RX Tel: 020 8994 4482 Fax: 020 8742 7816 — MB BS Ceylon 1970; FRCOG 1991, M 1978; MRCP (UK) 1981.

SOYSA, Mr Shanti Mahendra Royal Berkshire Hospital, London Road, Reading RG1 5AN Tel: 01189 877012 Fax: 01189 878662 Email: shantsoysa@aol.com; 2 Lincoln Close, Winnersh, Wokingham RG41 5SZ Tel: 0118 977 4820 Fax: 0118 978 8209 — MB BS Ceylon 1970 (Colombo) FFAEM; FRCS Ed. 1979; FRCS Eng. 1979. Cons. Surg. (A & E) Roy. Berks. Hosp. Reading; Cons. i/c, Minor injuries unit, Newbury Dist. Hosp.; Cons. i/c, minor injuries unit, Townlands Hosp., Henley on Thames. Specialty: Accid. & Emerg. Special Interest: Burns; Soft tissue injuries; Trauma. Socs: BMA; BAAEM; FAEM. Prev: Sen. Regist. (A & E) Soton. Gen. Hosp.; Regist. (Surg.) Soton. Gen. Hosp. & Roy. Liverp. & Alder Hey Hosps.

SPACKMAN, David Derek Sibford Surgery, Sibford Gower, Banbury OX15 5RQ Tel: 01295 780213; 1 Folly Court, Sibford Ferris, Banbury OX15 5RH Tel: 01295 780734 — MB BS Lond. 1981 (Char. Cross Hosp.) DRCOG 1984; MRCGP 1986; Dip. Occupat. Med. 1996. Specialty: Gen. Pract.

SPACKMAN, David Robert 160 Culford Road, London N1 4HU Tel: 020 7254 6922 — MB BS Lond. 1988; FRCA 1994. Cons. Anaesth. St. Thomas' Hosp. Lond. Specialty: Anaesth. Socs: Assn. Anaesths.; Assn. Cardiothoracic Anaesths.

SPAFFORD, Peter John Douglas Child Health Nithbank, Dumfries DG1 2SD Tel: 01387 244000 Fax: 01387 244564; Banks O'Troqueer, Troqueer Road, Dumfries DG2 7DF Tel: 01387 247229 — MB ChB Cape Town 1984. Staff Grade (Community Paediat.) Nithbank. Specialty: Community Child Health.

SPAGNOLI, Erio Aldo Pawaroo and Partners, The Old Forge Surgery, Pallion Pk, Sunderland SR4 6QE Tel: 0191 510 9393 Fax: 0191 510 9595; 4 Grassholm Meadows, Tunstall, Sunderland SR3 1PZ — MB ChB Dundee 1981; DRCOG 1986; MRCGP 1987. GP Sunderland; Duty Crowd Dr. Sunderland FC. Specialty: Dermat.

SPAIN, John Robert Grange Medical Centre, Dacre Banks, Harrogate HG3 4DX Tel: 01423 780436 Fax: 01423 781416; 4 Holly Villas, Dacre Banks, Harrogate HG3 4EG Tel: 01423 780313 — MB BS Newc. 1982 (Newcastle) MRCGP 1986. Prev: Trainee GP Newc. VTS; SHO (Cardiol.) Freeman Hosp. Newc.; SHO (Gen. Med. & Paediat.) Dryburn Hosp. Durh.

SPAINE, Mr Lloyd Ayodeji 15 Ruddle Way, Langham, Oakham LE15 7NZ — MB BCh BAO NUI 1984; FRCS Ed. 1988.

SPALDING, Anne Elizabeth The Surgery, Worsley Road, Immingham, Grimsby DN40 1BE — MB ChB Sheff. 1985; DGM RCP Lond. 1988; DRCOG 1989; MRCGP 1989; Dip Occ Health & Safety Lond. 1999.

SPALDING, Duncan Richard Castell 19 Newfound Drive, Norwich NR4 7RY — MB ChB Birm. 1989.

SPALDING, Elizabeth De Carteret (retired) 4 The Old Stables, St Andrews Lane, Old Headington, Oxford OX3 9DP Tel: 01865 761509 — MB BS Lond. 1944 (Univ. Coll. & W. Lond.) DCH Eng. 1945; MRCP Lond. 1947. Prev: Instruc. Doctor Family Plann. Serv. Oxon AHA (T).

SPALDING, Elizabeth Margaret 309 Cressex Road, High Wycombe HP12 4QF Tel: 01494 426925 Fax: 01494 426852 — MB BS Lond. 1971 (Middlx.) DCH Eng. 1973; DTM & H Eng. 1974; DObst RCOG 1974; MRCPsych 1984. Cons. Learning Disabil. & Child Psychiat. S. Bucks. NHS Trust. Specialty: Ment. Health. Socs: BMA; MWF; NHSCA. Prev: Sen. Regist. (Ment. Handicap.) Kidderminster HA.

SPALDING, John Anthony Boyer (retired) 5 Curzon Road, Weybridge KT13 8UW Tel: 01932 843422 — (Char. Cross) MB BS Lond. 1954; DCH Eng. 1958; MRCGP 1966. Prev: Princip. GP Lond.

SPALDING, John Michael Kenneth 4 The Old Stables, St. Andrews Lane, Old Headington, Oxford OX3 9DP Tel: 01865 761509 — BM BCh Oxf. 1946; MA Oxf. 1944; FRCP Lond. 1964, M 1951; DM Oxf. 1952. Cons. & Research Neurol. United Oxf. Hosps. Specialty: Neurol. Socs: Assn. Brit. Neurols. & Physiol. Soc. Prev: Sen. Regist. (Med.) Maida Vale Hosp. Nerv. Dis.; Ho. Phys. (Paediat.) Radcliffe Infirm. Oxf.

SPALDING, John Philip The Surgery, Hemming Way, Chaddesley Corbett, Kidderminster DY10 4SF Tel: 01562 777239 Fax: 01562 777196; 30 Hill Grove Crescent, Kidderminster DY10 4RY — MB ChB Birm. 1982; MRCGP 1986.

SPALDING, Mr Timothy John Wallis, Surg. Cdr. RN Retd. Orthopaedic Department, Coventry and Warwickshire Hospital, Stoney Stanton Rd, Coventry CV1 4FH — MB BS Lond. 1982 (Charing Cross Hospital London) FRCS Ed. 1988; FRCS (Orth.) 1994. Cons. Orthop. Surg.Coventry & Warks. Hosp., Coventry. Specialty: Trauma & Orthop. Surg.; Sports Med.; Orthop. Prev: Fell. (Orthop. & Arthritics) Toronto, Canada; Regist. (Helicopter Emerg. Med. Serv.) Lond. Hosp. Whitechapel; Cons. Roy. Navy.

SPALTON, Mr David John Eye Department, St Thomas Hospital, London SE1 7EH Tel: 020 7935 6174 Fax: 020 7467 4376 Email: dspalton@hotmail.com — (Westm.) MRCS Eng. LRCP Lond. 1970; MB BS Lond. 1970; MRCP (UK) 1973; DO Eng. 1975; FRCS Eng. 1975; FRCOphth 1989; FRCP Lond. 1990. p/t Cons. Ophth. Surg.St. Thos. Hosp. Lond.; Hon. Cons. Ophth. Surg. Roy. Hosp. Chelsea Lond.; Ophth. Surg. King Edwd. VII Hosp. for Offs. Lond.; Hon. Sen. Lect. (Ophth.) UMDS Lond.; Ophth. Adivser to Metrop. Police. Specialty: Ophth. Prev: Cons. Ophth. Surg. Char. Cross Hosp. Lond.; Sen. Regist. (Ophth.) St. Thos. Hosp. Lond.; Resid. Surg. Off. Moorfields Eye Hosp. Lond.

SPANKIE, Alison Claire 8 Highgate West Hill, London N6 6JR — MB BS Lond. 1982.

SPANNER, Rebekah Mair Family Planning Department, Heathfield Family Centre, 131-133 Heathfield Road, Handsworth, Birmingham B19 1HL Tel: 0121 255 7587; 96 Woodlands Farm Road, Erdington, Birmingham B24 0PQ Tel: 0121 240 0555 — MB BS Lond. 1980 (Royal Free Hospital School of Medicine) DRCOG 1984. SCMO (Family Plann. & Wom. Health) N. Birm. Community Trust. Specialty: Pub. Health Med. Prev: GP Birm.; Staff Med. Off. Across, Juba, S. Sudan; Trainee GP Enfield & Haringey FPC.

SPANNUTH, Frank Kingsfield Medical Centre, 146 Alcester Road South, Kings Heath, Birmingham B14 6AA Tel: 0121 444 2054 Fax: 0121 443 5856 — State Exam Med Tubingen 1986; State Exam Med Tubingen 1986.

SPANSWICK, Christopher Charles Manchester & Salford Pain Centre, Hope Hospital, Stott Lane, Salford M6 8HD Tel: 0161 789 7373; 33 Cartier Close, Bridle Chase, Old Hall, Warrington WA5 8TD — MB ChB Manch. 1973; FFA RCS Eng. 1978. Cons. Pain Managem. & Anesth.; Hon. Clin. Lect. (Anaesth.) Hope Hosp. Salford. Specialty: Anaesth. Socs: Internat. Assn. Study of Pain; Assn. Anaesths.; (Hon. Asst. Treas.) Pain Soc. Prev: Cons. Anaesth. Trafford AHA.

SPANSWICK, Robert 36 Chaucer Road, Crowthorne RG45 7QN — MB BS Lond. 1988.

SPANTON, Ian Dale Alexander 3 Burdett Avenue, London SW20 0ST — MB BS Lond. 1996.

SPARE, John Turner (retired) 2 Gordon's Close, Shoreditch Road, Taunton TA1 3DA Tel: 01823 284822 — (Middlx.) MB BS Lond. 1941; MRCS Eng. LRCP Lond. 1942. Prev: Obst. Ho. Surg. Roy. United Hosp. Bath.

SPARE, Timothy John West Walk Surgery, 21 West Walk, Yate, Bristol BS37 4AX Tel: 01454 272200; The Old Farm House, Holly Hill, Iron Acton, Bristol BS37 9XZ Tel: 01454 228257 — MB BS Lond. 1972 (Middlx. Hosp.) MRCS Eng. LRCP Lond. 1972; DObst RCOG 1975; D Occ Med 2000. GP Princip. Bristol. Prev: Sen. Med. Off. Solomon Is. Govt.

SPAREY, Colette 15 Lyndhurst Avenue, West Jesmond, Newcastle upon Tyne NE2 3LJ — MB ChB Manch. 1987; MRCOG 1993. Sen. Regist. (O & G) Roy. Vict. Infirm. Newc. u. Tyne. Specialty: Obst. & Gyn. Prev: Research Fell (O & G) Countess of Chester Hosp.; Regist. Rotat. (O & G) Mersey RHA.

SPARGO, Anne Elizabeth The Surgery, Whitminster Lane, Frampton on Severn, Gloucester GL2 7HU; Ashleigh House, The St, Frampton-on-Severn, Gloucester GL2 7ED Tel: 01452 741147 —

MB BChir Camb. 1977; DRCOG 1979. Gen. Practitioner; Clin. Asst. G.U.M. Dept, Gloucester Roy. Hosp.

SPARGO, James Robert 4 Shannon Close, Willaston, Nantwich CW5 6QG — MB ChB Sheff. 1992.

SPARGO, John Barnes (retired) 22 Southview Gardens, Worthing BN11 5JA — MB BChir Camb. 1950 (St Mary's) MA, MB BChir Camb. 1950. Prev: Resid. Med. Off., Ho. Phys. & Ho. Surg. Nat. Temperance Hosp.

SPARGO, Paul Michael Southampton General Hospital, Department of Anaesthetics, Tremona Road, Southampton SO16 6YD Tel: 02380 796720 Fax: 02380 794348 Email: paul.spargo@suht.swest.nhs.net — MB BS Lond. 1977 (St. Mary's) MRCP (UK) 1982; FFA RCS Eng. 1984. Cons. Anaesth. Soton. Univ. Hosp. Trust. Specialty: Anaesth. Special Interest: Paediatric Anaesth. Prev: Sen. Regist. (Anaesth.) Soton HA; Instruc. Dept. Anesthesiol. Univ. Michigan Ann Arbor, USA; Regist. (Med.) Roy. Berks. Hosp. Reading.

SPARGO, Mr Peter John Ralph The Surgery, Whitminster Lane, Frampton on Severn, Gloucester GL2 7HU Tel: 01452 740213 Fax: 01452 740989; Ashleigh House, The St, Frampton-on-Severn, Gloucester GL2 7ED Tel: 01452 741147 Fax: 01452 740989 — MB BChir Camb. 1977; MA Camb. 1976; FRCS Ed. 1982; FRCS Eng. 1982; MRCGP 1989. Prev: Med. Supt. Bonda Mission Hosp., Zimbabwe.

SPARK, Evelyn Diana 36 Ashley Park, Ashley Heath, Ringwood BH24 2HB Tel: 01425 475193 — MB BS Lond. 1966 (Middlx.) DObst RCOG 1968; DA Eng. 1969; FFA RCS (Eng.) 1981. Specialty: Anaesth.

SPARK, Mr James Ian 88 Elton Road, Darlington DL3 8NA Tel: 01325 480964 — MB ChB Leeds 1988 (Leeds University) FRCS Eng. 1992; MD Leeds 2000; FRCS FRCS (Gen.Surg.) 2001. Cons. Vasc. Surg. St. James Univ. Hosp. Leeds. Specialty: Gen. Surg. Prev: Cons. Vasc. Surg. The Qu. Eliz. Hosp. Adelaide S. Australia; SpR (Surg.) Leeds Gen. Infirm.; Research Regist. (Vasc. Surg.) St. Jas. Univ. Hosp. Leeds.

SPARK, Michael Gallwey (retired) West House, 19 Meadow Lane, Beadnell, Chathill NE67 5AJ Tel: 01665 720255 — MB BS Durh. 1956; DObst RCOG 1958. Prev: GP Gateshead.

SPARKE, Paul Berthon (retired) St Giles Mount, Stratton Road, Winchester SO23 0JQ — (Middlx.) MB BS Lond. 1950; MRCS Eng. LRCP Lond. 1950; DObst RCOG 1954. Prev: GP W. Kingdown, Kent.

SPARKES, David John 31 Nettlecombe Avenue, Southsea PO4 0QW — MB BS Lond. 1993.

SPARKES, Julian Malcolm Shilpa Medical Centre, 1C Ashfield Avenue, Kings Heath, Birmingham B14 7AT — MB ChB Birm. 1979; DRCOG 1988.

SPARKS, Mr Michael John Whitaker 38 Oak Avenue, South Wootton, King's Lynn PE30 3JQ Tel: 01553 672372 — MB BS Lond. 1979; FRCS Ed. 1989; FRCR 1994. Cons. Radiol. Qu. Eliz. Hosp. King's Lynn. Specialty: Radiol.

SPARKS, Richard Alfred Cardiff Royal Infirmary, Newport Road, Cardiff CF24 0SZ Tel: 029 2033 5206 Fax: 029 2048 7096 Email: richard.sparks@cardiffandvale.wales.nhs.uk — MB BCh Wales 1967 (Cardiff) DObst RCOG 1970; Cert. Family Plann. FPA 1972; FRCOG 1989, M 1973; Dip. GU Med. Soc. Apoth. Lond. 1979; MFFP 1993. Cons. Genitourin. Med. Cardiff Roy. Infirm. & Clin. Teach. (Genitourin.) Univ. Wales Coll. Med. Specialty: Genitourinary Medicine. Socs: Brit. Assn. for Sexual Health & HIV. Prev: Sen. Lect. (Genitourin. Med.) Univ. Birm.; Cons. Genitourin. Med. Manch. Roy. Infirm.; Research Fell. (Human Reproduc.) Univ. Soton.

SPARKS, William Benjamin (retired) Corner House, Perrin Close, Temple Cloud, Bristol BS39 5LR Tel: 01761 452636 — (St. Thos.) MB BS Lond. 1951. Prev: Hosp. Pract. (ENT) Char. Cross Hosp. Lond.

SPARROW, Geoffrey Edward Alan Station Road Surgery, Station Road, Stalbridge, Sturminster Newton DT10 2RG Tel: 01963 362363 Fax: 01963 362866 Email: geoff@stalbridgesurgery.co.uk; Stayners Farm, Lydlinch, Sturminster Newton DT10 2JA Tel: 01258 473136 Email: geoff@stalbridgesurgery.co.uk — MB BS Lond. 1975 (Guy's) MRCS Eng. LRCP Lond. 1975; MRCP (UK) 1978; FRCP 2001. Gen. Practitioner, Stalbridge; Trainer (Gen. Pract.) Dorset; Assoc. Specialist Yeovil Dist. Hosp. Specialty: Gen. Med.; Oncol. Prev: Lect. (Med. Oncol.) Guy's Hosp. Lond.; Regist. (Gen. Med.) & SHO (Med. & Paediat.) Yeovil Dist. Hosp.

SPARROW, Ian Michael McNulty and Partners, Torkard Hill Medical Centre, Farleys Lane, Nottingham NG15 6DY Tel: 0115 963 3676 Fax: 0115 968 1957.

SPARROW, Ian Robert Christopher Balmoral Surgery, 1 Victoria Road, Deal CT14 7AU Tel: 01304 373444 — MB BS Lond. 1985 (St. Thos. Hosp. Med. Sch.) DCH RCP Lond. 1989; DRCOG 1990; MRCGP 1992. Specialty: Pharmacology. Prev: Trainee GP/SHO William Harvey Hosp. Ashford VTS; Ho. Surg. St. Thos. Hosp. Lond.; Ho. Phys. William Harvey Hosp. Ashford.

SPARROW, Michael Anthony Lifton Surgery, North Road, Lifton PL16 0EH Tel: 01566 784788 — MB BS Lond. 1981.

SPARROW, Nigel James Newthorpe Medical Practice, Eastwood Clinic, Nottingham Road, Nottingham NG16 3HB Tel: 01773 760202 Fax: 01773 710951; 1 Rectory Gardens, Wollaton Village, Nottingham NG8 2AR — MB ChB Bristol 1979; BSc (Hons.) Bristol 1976; DRCOG 1983; MRCGP 1984; FRCGP 1999. Hosp. Pract. (Colposc.) Qu. Med. Centre Nottm.; Lect. (Gen. Pract.) Univ. Nottm.; Mem. Notts. MAAG.; Associate Director Post Grad. GP Univ. Nottm. Specialty: Cardiol. Socs: RCGP (Vale of Trent Fac. Bd.); PEC Member Broxtowe & Hucknall PCT. Prev: SHO (Med.) Univ. Hosp. Nottm.; Ho. Phys. Southmead Hosp. Bristol; Ho. Surg. Leicester Roy. Infirm.

SPARROW, Mr Owen Charles Neurosurgery Department, Wessex Neurological Centre, Southampton General Hospital, Southampton SO16 6YD Tel: 023 8079 6791 Fax: 023 8079 8793 — MB BCh Witwatersrand 1974 (Univ. of The Witwatersrand) RCSEd 1980; FRCS Ed. 1980; FCS (SA) (Neurological Surgery) 1982; MMed (Neurosurg.) Witwatersrand 1986; FRCS 2000. Cons. Neurosurgeon. Specialty: Neurosurg. Prev: Sen. Lect. & Hon. Cons. Neurosurgeon, Roy. Lond. Hosp. & Med. Coll.; Cons. Neurosugeon & Hon. Lect. Baraguranath Hosp. & Univ. of The Witwatersrand, Johannesburg.

SPARROW, Pamela Marian (retired) Miranda Lodge, Broadlands Road, Brockenhurst SO42 7SX — MB BS Lond. 1954 (St. Mary's) MRCS Eng. LRCP Lond. 1953. Prev: Ho. Surg. & Ho. Phys. St. Chas. Hosp.

SPARROW, Robert Andrew 5 Long Row, The Sreen, Kingston-on-Soar, Nottingham NG11 0DA — BM BS Nottm. 1980.

SPARROW, Sally Angela La Route Du Fort Surgery, 2 La Route Du Fort, St Helier, Jersey JE2 4PA Tel: 01534 31421 Fax: 01534 280776 — MB ChB Sheff. 1974; BSc. (Hons) Sheff. 1969.

SPATHIS, Anna Olga — MB BChir Camb. 1992; MRCP 1996; MRCGP 1999.

SPATHIS, Gerassimos Spyros (retired) 20 Mount Carmel Chambers, Dukes Lane, Kensington, London W8 4JW Email: spathis@doctors.org.uk — (Oxf. & Guy's) DM Oxf. 1971, MA, BM BCh 1960; FRCP Lond. 1977, M 1963. Prev: Regist. (Med.) Middlx. Hosp. Lond., Addenbrooke's Hosp. Camb. & St. Thos. Hosp. Lond.

SPAUL, Kerrie Alice Juniper 6 The Croft, Kirby Muxloe, Leicester LE9 2AR Tel: 0116 241 4083 — MB ChB Sheff. 1991; MRCGP 1995. Assoc. GP Glenfield Surgery, Glenfield, Leicester. Specialty: Gen. Pract. Socs: BMA. Prev: SHO (O & G) URI NHS Trust; SHO (Psychiat) Bassetlaw NHS Trust; GP/Regist. Dunnington Gp. Pract.

SPEAK, Nigel James Manor Practice, James Preston Health Centre, 61 Holland Road, Sutton Coldfield B72 1RL Tel: 0121 354 2032 Fax: 0121 321 1779; 59 Somerville Road, Sutton Coldfield B73 6HJ — MB ChB Birm. 1982; DCH RCP Lond. 1985; MRCGP 1986; DRCOG 1986.

SPEAKE, John Graham The Medical Centre, The Medical Centre, Fore Street, St Marychurch, Torquay TQ1 4QX Tel: 01803 325123 Fax: 01803 322136 — MB BS Newc. 1976; FFA RCSI 1984. Specialty: Anaesth. Prev: Regist. (Anaesth.) Univ. Hosp. Wales Cardiff & Torbay Hosp.; SHO (Anaesth.) Qu. Eliz. Med. Centre Birm.

SPEAKE, Malcolm Douglas (retired) Dockyard, Kettlebaston, Ipswich IP7 7QA Tel: 01449 740254 Fax: 01449 740903 — MB ChB Leeds 1965. Prev: Research Asst. Univ. Leeds.

SPEAKE, William James Dockyard, Kettlebaston, Ipswich IP7 7QA — MB ChB Leeds 1994. SHO (Accid. & Emerg.) Leeds Gen. Infirm. Specialty: Gen. Surg. Socs: BMA; Med. Protec. Soc. Prev: Ho. Off. (Gen. Surg. & Orthop.) ScarBoro.; Ho. Off. (Med.) Huddersfield.

SPEAKMAN, Alice Rosie 130 Dicconson Street, Wigan WN1 2BA — MB ChB Manch. 1979.

SPEAKMAN, Mr Christopher Thomas More Norfolk and Norwich University Hospital, Colney Lane, Norwich NR4 7UY Tel:

01603 287947 Fax: 01603 287896 Email: chris.speakman@nnuh.nhs.com — MB BS Lond. 1983; FRCS Ed. 1988; MD Lond. 1993. Cons. Gen. Surg. Norf. & Norwich Hosp.; Hon. Sen. Lect. Univ. E. Anglia. Specialty: Gen. Surg. Socs: St. Mark's Assn.; Assn. Coloproctol.; Assn. Surg. Prev: RSO St. Marks Hosp. Lond.; Sen. Regist. (Surg.) Char. Cross Hosp. Lond.; Sir Alan Pk.s Research Fell. St. Marks Hosp. Lond.

SPEAKMAN, Helen Mary Anne 10 High Street, Edlesborough, Dunstable LU6 2HS — MB BS Lond. 1989.

SPEAKMAN, John Kenneth Wordsley Green Health Centre, Wordsley Green, Wordsley, Stourbridge DY8 5PD Tel: 01384 277591 Fax: 01384 401156; Broom Barn, Redhall Lane, Broome, Stourbridge DY9 0EZ — MB ChB Birm. 1990; DRCOG 1994. Prev: SHO (Med.) Russells Hall Hosp. Dudley.; Dip. Pall. Med. 2001 also at Marn Stevens Hospice, Stourbridge.

SPEAKMAN, Mr Mark Joseph Taunton & Somerset NHS Trust, Musgrove Park, Taunton TA1 5DA Tel: 01823 343571; Greenfield, Wild Oak Lane, Trull, Taunton TA3 7JS Tel: 01823 257891 Fax: 01823 257891 Email: speakmanmj@aol.com — MB BS Lond. 1978 (Char. Cross) MRCS Eng. LRCP Lond. 1978; FRCS Eng. 1983; MS Lond. 1988. Cons. Urol. & Director of Research & Developm. Taunton & Somserset NHS Trust; Mem. Counc. Brit. Assn. Urol. Surgs. Specialty: Urol. Socs: BMA; Brit. Assn. Urol. Surgs.; Roy. Soc. of Med. (Fell.). Prev: Research Regist. (Urol.) (MRC) Churchill Hosp. Oxf.; Regist. (Surg.) John Radcliffe Hosp. Oxf.; Sen. Regist. (Urol.) West. Infirm. Glas.

SPEAKMAN, Melanie Jane 13 Hardwick House, Harlington Square, London NW1 2JH — MB ChB Leic. 1993.

SPEAKMAN, Philip Frank Roseneath Medical Practice, The Health Centre, Padeswood Road, Buckley CH7 2JL Tel: 01224 550555 Fax: 01224 545712; Grassmere, Tram Road, Buckley CH7 3NH Tel: 01244 545889 — MB ChB Liverp. 1973; DObst RCOG 1975; DCH Eng. 1976; MRCGP 1978. Co. Staff Off. St. John Ambul. Brig.; Phys. Clwyd Mt.ain Rescue Team. Prev: SHO Pk. Psychiat. Day Hosp. Liverp., Mill Rd. Matern. Hosp. & Alder; Hey Childr. Hosp. Liverp.

SPEAR, Brian Scott Edenbridge Medical Practice, West View, Station Road, Edenbridge TN8 5ND Tel: 01732 864442 Fax: 01732 862376 — MB BS Lond. 1973 (Lond. Hosp.) DRCOG 1976; DCH Eng. 1978; MRCGP 1984. Fraser Rose Medal RCGP 1984; GP Edenbridge; Jt. Sec. Edenbridge Hosp. Clin. Soc.; Hosp. Pract. (Gastroenterol.) Kent & Sussex Hosp. Specialty: Gastroenterol. Socs: Primary Care Soc. Gastroenterol. Prev: Ho. Phys. & Ho. Surg. Lond. Hosp.; SHO Sydenham Childr. Hosp.

SPEAR, David William Shiphay Manor, 37 Shiphay Lane, Torquay TQ2 7DU Tel: 01803 615059 Fax: 01803 614545; Laurel Place, The Woods, Higher Lincombe Road, Torquay TQ1 2HS Tel: 01803 290673 Fax: 01803 290673 — MB BS Lond. 1989 (Middlesex Hospital & University College London) BSc Physiol. Lond. 1986; DRCOG 1993; DFFP 1993; MRCGP 1994. Prev: Trainee GP/SHO (Paediat.) Torbay Hosp. Torquay.

SPEAR, Frank Graham 326 Ecclesall Road S., Sheffield S11 9PU Tel: 0114 236 6766 Fax: 0114 236 6766 — (Bristol) MB ChB Bristol 1954; DPM Eng. 1958; MD Bristol 1964; FRCPsych 1974, M 1971. Specialty: Gen. Psychiat.; Medico Legal. Prev: Cons. Psychiat. Sheff. Ment. Illness Serv.; Lect.(Psychiat.) Univ. Sheff.; Vis. Psychother. HM Prison Wakefield.

SPEAR, George Edwin (retired) 39 The Empire, Grand Parade, Bath BA2 4DF Tel: 01225 313409 — MB BChir Camb. 1940 (St. Thos.) BA Camb. (Nat. Sc. Trip. Pt. I, cl. 1) 1937; MB BChir Camb. 1940; MRCS Eng. LRCP Lond. 1940; MRCP Lond. 1949. Prev: Sen. Regist. (Med.) Essex Co. Hosp. Colchester.

SPEARS, Frances Dorothy Dept of Anaestetics, Luton and Dunstable Hospital NHS Trust, Lewsey Road, Luton LU4 0DZ — MB ChB Dundee 1985; FRCA 1992. Cons. Anaesth. Luton & Dunstable Hosp. NHS Trust Luton. Specialty: Anaesth.

SPEARS, John Robert (retired) 32 Roxwell Road, Chelmsford CM1 2NB Tel: 01245 354173 — MRCS Eng. LRCP Lond. 1948 (Lond. Hosp.) DA Eng. 1953; FFA RCS Eng. 1954; FRCA 1992. Prev: Hon. Cons. Anaesth. Mid-Essex HA.

SPEARS, Joseph (retired) 8 Guards Road, Lindal-in-Furness, Ulverston LA12 0TN — MB ChB Glas. 1937; MD Glas. 1946; DCH Eng. 1951; FRCGP 1971, M 1964. Prev: Late. Act. Squadron Ldr. RAFVR.

SPECK, Mr Edward Holmes Rannoch, 50 Woodgates Lane, North Ferriby HU14 3JY Tel: 01482 634201 — MB BS Lond. 1968 (Middlx.) FRCOG 1988, M 1975; FRCS Ed. 1976. Cons. (O & G) Hull Health Dist. Specialty: Obst. & Gyn. Prev: Sen. Regist. (O & G) Leeds & Bradford AHAs; Regist. (Gen. Surg.) Orsett Hosp. Grays Thurrock; Regist. (O & G) Jessop. Hosp. Wom. Sheff.

SPECK, Eirlys (retired) Dolphin House, Glyn Garth, Menai Bridge LL59 5PF Tel: 01348 713515 — (Roy. Colls. Ed.) LRCP LRCS Ed. LRFPS Glas. 1948.

SPECTOR, Professor Roy Geoffrey Guys Drug Research, United Medical Schools, 6 Newcomen St., London SE1 1YR Tel: 020 7910 7700 Fax: 020 7910 7800; 3 St. Kilda Road, Orpington BR6 0ES Tel: 01689 810069 — (Leeds) MB ChB Leeds 1956; FRCP Ed. 1971, M 1959; FRCP Glas. 1972, M 1962; MD Leeds 1962; PhD Lond. 1964; FRCPath 1976, M 1965; Dip. Biochem. (Distinc.) Lond. 1966. Hon. Cons. Guy's Hosp. Lond.; Emerit. Prof. Applied Pharmacol. Univ. Lond. Specialty: Pharmacology. Socs: Brit. Pharm. Soc.; Med. Res. Soc. Prev: Vis. Prof. Clin. Pharmacol. W. China Med. Univ., Chengdu; Lect. (Experim. Path.) & Sen. Lect. (Experim. Biol.) Paediat. Research Unit. Guy's Hosp. Med. Sch. Lond.; Prof. Applied Pharmacol. Univ. Lond.

SPECTOR, Timothy David Twin Research Genetic Epidemiology Unit, St. Thomas' Hospital, London SE1 7EH Tel: 020 7960 5557 Fax: 020 7922 8234; 22 Aberdeen Road, London N5 2UH — MD Lond. 1989 (St. Bartholomews) MSc Lond. 1986, MD 1989, MB BS 1982; FRCP 1997, MRCP 1985. Cons. Rheum. St. Thos. Hosp. Lond.; Dir. Twin Research & Genetic Epidemiol. Unit; Hon. Prof., Genetic Epidemiol. SGHMS. Specialty: Rheumatol.; Genetics. Prev: Hon. Sen. Lect. MDS; Lect. (Epidemiol.) & Sen. Regist. (Rheum.) St. Bart. Hosp. Lond.; Wellcome Research Fell. Dept. Clin. Epidemiol. Lond. Hosp.

SPEDDING, Anne Valerie Department of Histopathology, Queen Alexandra Hospital, Southwick Hill Road, Cosham, Portsmouth PO6 3LY Tel: 023 92 286458 — MB ChB Manch. 1985; FRCPath 2001. Cons. Histopath. Qu. Alexandra Hosp. Portsmouth. Specialty: Histopath.

SPEDDING, Ruth Lynn Accident and Emergency, Warrington Hospital, Lovely Lane, Warrington WA5 1QG Tel: 01925 635911 Fax: 01925 662184 — MB BCh BAO Belf. 1988; MRCP (UK) 1992; FRCS Ed. 1993; FFAEM 1997. Cons. (A & E) Warrington Hosp. Warrington Chesh. Specialty: Accid. & Emerg. Prev: Altnagelvin Hosp. Derry Co. Londonderry; Belf. Regist. Rotat. (A & E).

SPEDDING, Sheila Margaret (retired) The Great Barn, Moot Lane, Downton, Salisbury SP5 3JP Tel: 01725 510319 — MRCS Eng. LRCP Lond. 1974; BSc Manch. 1953; MRCPsych 1979; T(Psych) 1991. Prev: Cons. Child Psychiat. Marchwood Priory Hosp.

SPEDEN, Deborah Jane The Royal Oldham Hospital, Rochdale Road, Oldham OL12JH Tel: 0161 6240420 — MB BS Tasmania 1990; FRACP 1998; PhD Bath 2003. Cons. Rheum. Specialty: Rheumatol. Socs: Brit. Soc. Rheum.; Fell.of RACP.

SPEECHLY-DICK, Marie Elsya The Middlesex Hospital, Mortimer St., London W1N 3AA — MB BChir Camb. 1987; BSc (Hons.) St. And. 1984; MRCP (UK) 1989; MD Camb. 1996. Cons. (Cardiol.) Univ. Coll. Lond. Hosps. & The Heart Hosp. NHS Trust. Specialty: Cardiol. Prev: Sen. Lect. & Hon. Cons. (Cardiol.) Univ. Coll. Lond. Hosps. NHS Trust; Clin. Regist. (Cardiol.) Univ. Coll. Hosp. NHS Trust; Research Fell. (Cardiol.) Middlx. & Univ. Coll. Hosp. Lond.

SPEED, Catherine Anne The Staddles, Prinsted Lane, Emsworth PO10 8HS — BM BS Nottm. 1989; BMedSci (Hons.) 1987. SHO (Med.) Newc. HA.

SPEED, Dorothy Elizabeth Maud — (Univ. Liverp.) MB ChB Liverp. 1956; DFFP 1960. Mem. Parole Bd. Specialty: Forens. Psychiat. Socs: Affil. Mem. Roy. Coll. Psychiat.; Fell. Counc. Europ.; Fell. Roy. Soc. Med. & Galton Inst. Prev: Princip. Med. Off. Directorate Prison Med. Servs. Home Office; Hon. Cons. Phys. Roy. Marsden Hosp. & Sen. Lect. Inst. Cancer Research Lond. Hosp.; Dir. Populat. Control (Mauritius: Min. Overseas Developm.).

SPEED, Henry Peter (retired) 30 Ballalough, Andreas, Ramsey IM7 4HS Tel: 01624 880428 — MRCS Eng. LRCP Lond. 1944 (Liverp.) Prev: Clin. Asst. St. Lawrence's Hosp. Bodmin.

SPEED, Katharine Mary — MB BCh Wales 1997.

SPEED, Kevin Ralph 6 Northumberland Close, Grimsby DN34 4TE — MB BS Lond. 1974 (St. Geo.) MSc Lond. 1979, MB BS 1974; MRCPath 1982. Cons. (Haemat.) Grimsby Dist. Gen. Hosp.

Specialty: Haematology. Prev: Lect. (Haemat.) St. Geo. Hosp. Med. Sch. Lond.

SPEED, Mary Allison Widcombe Surgery, 3-4 Widcombe Parade, Bath BA2 4JT Tel: 01225 310883 Fax: 01225 421600 — MRCS Eng. LRCP Lond. 1980.

SPEED-ANDREWS, Shonagh Carol 6 Glen Road, Ings Lane, Rochdale OL1Z 7DY — MB ChB Glas. 1985; DFFP 2000; MRCGP 2001. Clin. Asst. (Genitourin. Med.). Prev: Clin. Asst. (Dermat.) Cumbria; Trainee GP Cumbria VTS; Clin.. Asst. A & E Med.

SPEEDIE, Catherine Alison Chadmoor Medical Practice, 45 Princess St, Cannock WS11 2JT Tel: 01543 571650 Fax: 01543 462304 — MB BCh BAO Belf. 1984; MB BCh Belf. 1984.

SPEERS, Alan Gordon Heatherdene, 1 Bramblewood Place, Fleet GU51 4EF — MB BS Lond. 1997.

SPEIDEL, Brian David (retired) 224 Cranbrook Road, Redland, Bristol BS6 7QX Tel: 0117 949 5789 — (Oxf.) BA Oxf. 1962; BM BCh Oxf. 1965; FRCP Lond. 1982, M 1969; DCH Eng. 1971; MD Bristol 1976; FRCPCH 1997. Prev: Cons. Paediat. (Neonat. Med.) Southmead Hosp. Bristol & St. Michael's Hosp. Bristol.

SPEIGHT, Arthur Nigel Podmore University Hospitals of North Durham, Department of Paediatrics, Durham DH1 5TW Tel: 0191 333 2333 Fax: 0191 333 2327; Southlands, Gilesgate, Durham DH1 1QN Tel: 0191 384 7727 Fax: 0191 384 7727 Email: speightuk@yahoo.co.uk — MB BChir Camb. 1967 (Univ. Coll. Hosp.) MA, 1967; DCH Eng. 1976; FRCP Lond. 1986; FRCPCH 1997. Cons. Paediat. N. Durh. Acute NHS Trust; Hon. Sen. Lect. Univ. of Newc. Upon Tyne. Specialty: Paediat. Socs: BMA & Roy. Coll. Paediat. & Child Health & NHS Cons. Assn. Prev: 1st Asst. (Child Health) Roy. Vict. Infirm. Newc.; Lect. Med. Univ. Dar es Salaam, Tanzania; Sen. Regist. (Paediat.) Newc. Gen. Hosp.

SPEIGHT, Emma Lucy Department of Dermatology, Royal Victoria Infirmary, Newcastle upon Tyne NE1 4LP — MB BS (Hons. Path.) 1984; MA Camb. 1985; MRCP (UK) 1988; MD Lond. 1994. Cons. Dermatol. Roy. Vict. Infirm. Newc.-upon-Tyne. Specialty: Dermat. Prev: Sen. Regist. (Dermat.) Univ. Hosp. Nottm.; Research Fell & Regist. (Dermat.) Roy. Vict. Infirm. Newc.

SPEIGHT, Julian Michael Combe House, Throop Road, Templecombe — MB BS Lond. 1993; BSc (Hons.) Lond. 1990. Phys. Prosector & SHO (A & E) Som. Specialty: Accid. & Emerg.

SPEIGHT, Lenka 34 Ritchie Street, London N1 0DG Tel: 020 7837 1663 Fax: 020 7837 3656; 105 Gloucester Avenue, London NW1 8LB — MRCS Eng. LRCP Lond. 1971.

SPEIGHT, Martyn Bryan Grovegarth Cottage, Whitehouses Lane, Fellbeck, Pateley Bridge, Harrogate HG3 5EN Tel: 01423 712490 Fax: 01423 712490 — MB ChB Sheff. 1993. Specialty: Sports Med.

SPEIGHT, Michael David — MB ChB Ed. 1989; MA Camb. 1988. Specialty: Gen. Pract.

SPEIGHT, Robert Glynn The Park End Surgery, 3 Park End, Hampstead, London NW3 2SE Tel: 020 7435 7282; 105 Gloucester Avenue, London NW1 8LB — MB BS Lond. 1972; MRCS Eng. LRCP 1971; BA (Fine Arts) Lond. 1978.

SPEIRS, Alastair Thomas Orr (retired) 2l Glengarry Way, Friars Cliff, Christchurch BH23 4EH Tel: 01425 279528 — (King's Coll. Hosp.) MRCS Eng. LRCP Lond. 1939; DOMS Eng. 1948. Prev: Princ. GP 1948-1986.

SPEIRS, Alexander Logan, OBE (retired) 8 John Murray Drive, Bridge of Allan, Stirling FK9 4QH — MB ChB Aberd. 1943; FRCPCH; FRCP Lond. 1971, M 1949; DCH Eng. 1952; MD Aberd. 1954; FRCP Glas. 1971, M 1967. Prev: Cons. Paediat. Roy. Hosp. Sick Childr. Glas., Stirling Roy. Infirm. & Falkirk & Dist. Roy. Infirm.

SPEIRS, Christopher James 82 Lower Road, Fetcham, Leatherhead KT22 9NG — MB ChB Liverp. 1970; MRCP (UK) 1973; MSc (Epidemiol.) Lond. 1990; FFPM RCP (UK) 1993, M 1991. Specialty: Pharmacology; Pharmaceutical Medicine. Socs: Roy. Soc. Med.

SPEIRS, Colin Fairholme Medicines Control Agency, Market Towers, 1 Nine Elms Lane, London SW8 5NQ Tel: 020 7273 0460 Fax: 020 7273 0170; 3 Heathpark Drive, Windlesham GU20 6JA Tel: 01276 473744 — MB ChB Ed. 1961; FRCP Ed. 1974, M 1965; FFPM RCP (UK) 1989; FRCP Lond. 1994. Sen. Med. Off. Med. Control Agency Lond. Specialty: Pharmaceutical Medicine. Socs: Liveryman Worshipful Soc. Apoth. Lond.; Fell. Roy. Soc. Med. Prev: Head Europ. Med. Servs. Lilly Research Centre Ltd. Windlesham; Sen. Regist. (Infec. Dis.) City Hosp. Edin.; Regist. (Med.) Gardiner Inst. West. Infirm. Glas.

SPEIRS, Gail Elisabeth Department of Pathology, Level 1, North Devon District Hospital, Barnstaple EX31 4JB Tel: 01271 322798 Fax: 01271 322328 Email: gail.speirs@ndevon.swest.nhs.uk — MB ChB Birm. 1982 (Birmingham University) MRCPath 1989; FRCPath 1997. p/t Cons. Med. Microbiol. N. Devon Dist. Hosp. Barnstaple. Specialty: Med. Microbiol. Socs: Hosp. Infec. Soc.; Brit. Soc. Animicrobial Chemother. Prev: Sen. Regist. (Clin. Microbiol.) N. Devon Dist. Hosp. Barnstaple & Southmead Hosp. Bristol; Sen. Regist. (Clin. Microbiol.) Addenbrooke's Hosp. Camb.; Regist. (Clin. MicroBiol.) Addenbrooke's Hosp. Camb.

SPEIRS, Jean Marion The Priory Hospital, Priory Lane, London SW15 5JJ Tel: 020 8876 8261 Fax: 020 8392 2632 Email: jeaniespeirs@prioryhealthcare.com — MB BS Lond. 1973 (Guy's) MRCS Eng. LRCP Lond. 1972; MRCPsych 1977. Cons. Psychiat. Priory Hosp. Lond. Specialty: Gen. Psychiat. Socs: Marce.Soc. Prev: Regist. (Psychiat) Westm. Hosp. Lond.

SPEIRS, Mhairi Wilson — MB ChB Glas. 1990. Cons. Anaesth., John Radcliffe Hosp. Specialty: Anaesth. Socs: Intens. Care Soc. Prev: SHO (Anaesth.) Wycombe Gen. Hosp.; Specialist Regist. (Anaesth.) John Radcliffe Hosp. Oxf.

SPEIRS, Norma Isabelle Royal Surrey County Hospital, Guildford GU2 7XX; The Cedars, Maori Road, Guildford GU1 2EL Tel: 01483 567242 — MB ChB Ed. 1977; MSc Lond. 1998. Staff Grade Doctor Guildford. Specialty: Paediat. Prev: SCMO Havant Hants.; GP Bristol.

SPEIRS, Norman Thomas (retired) 24 Liberton Place, Edinburgh EH16 6NA Tel: 0131 672 2662 — (Univ. Ed.) BSc Ed. 1946; MB ChB Ed. 1947; DMRD Ed. 1953. Prev: Cons. Radiol. Roy. Vict. Disp. Chest Clinic Edin., Roy. Edin. Ment. Hosp. & Roodlands Hosp. Haddington.

SPEIRS, Richard Bradley Abbey Health Centre, East Abbey Street, Arbroath DD11 1EN Tel: 01241 870307 Fax: 01241 431414; 1 Fraserfield, Arbroath DD11 2LW Tel: 01241 890384 Fax: 01241 431414 — MB ChB St. And. 1968. Socs: Dundee Med.Soc.

SPEIRS, Robert Craig (retired) 99 South Street, Greenock PA16 8QN Tel: 01475 722577 Email: docspiers99south@adl.com — MB ChB Glas. 1962; DObst RCOG 1964. Prev: SHO Rankin Memor. Hosp. & Gateside Hosp. Greenock.

SPEIRS, William McArthur (retired) Ard Mara, 7 Laxdale, Lane, Stornoway HS2 0DR Tel: 01851 702019 — MB ChB Glas. 1953; DObst RCOG 1957; DA Eng. 1958. Prev: Cons. Anaesth. Lewis & Co. Hosps. Stornoway.

SPELDEWINDE, Deirdre Catherine Mary 10 Plymouth Wharf, Saunderness Road, London E14 3EL — MB BCh BAO NUI 1991 (Galway) Regist. (Paediat.) Princess Mgt. Hosp. Perth, WA, Australia. Specialty: Paediat.

SPELINA, Karel Rudolf Department of Anaesthetics, Wexham Park Hospital, Slough SL2 4HL Tel: 01753 633185 Fax: 01753 634460 — MD Prague 1967; MRCS Eng. LRCP Lond. 1972; FFA RCS Eng. 1976. Cons. in Anaesthetics, Heatherwood (Ascot) and Wexham Pk. Hosps. (Slough). Specialty: Anaesth. Special Interest: Chronic Pain; Regional Anaesth. Prev: Specialist Anaesth. Klinik Sonnenhop Berne.

SPELLER, Christopher John Learning Disability Service, Beaver House, Victoria Road, Swindon SN1 3BU Tel: 01793 644900 — MB ChB Bristol 1982; MRCPsych 1991. Cons. (Psychiat. in Learning Disabil.) Wilts. & Swindon Trust. Specialty: Ment. Health. Prev: Sen. Regist. (Psychiat. Ment. Handicap) Hanham Hall Hosp. Bristol.; Regist. (Psychiat.) Glenside Hosp. Bristol; SHO (Psychiat.) Bristol & Weston HA.

SPELLER, David Charles Endersby 9 Dowry Road, Bristol BS8 4PR Tel: 0117 929 8425 Email: dspeller@blueyonder.co.uk — (Oxf.) BM BCh Oxf. 1961; MA Oxf. 1961; FRCP Lond. 1981, M 1965; FRCPath. 1982, M 1970. Emerit. Prof. (Clin. Bact.) Univ. Bristol. Specialty: Med. Microbiol. Socs: (Ex-Pres.) Hosp. Infec. Soc.; Hon. Mem. (Ex-Pres.) Brit. Soc. for Antimicrobial. Chemother.; Hon. Mem. Brit. Soc. Med. Mycology. Prev: Head of Antibiotic Ref. Unit. Centr. Pub. Health Laborat. Lond.

SPELLER, Jeremy Clive West Devon CMHT, The Quay, Plymouth Road, Tavistock PL19 8AB — MB ChB Manch. 1981; MRCPsych 1986. Cons. Gen. Adult Psychiat.. Devon Partnership NHS Trust. Specialty: Gen. Psychiat. Prev: Cons. Gen. Psychiat. Avalon Som.

NHS Trust; Cons. Gen. Psychiat. Plymouth HA.; Clin. Research Fell. (Psychiat.) Char. Cross Hosp. Med. Sch. Lond.

SPELLER, Peter Joslin (retired) Limebank, Quantock Rise, Kingston St Mary, Taunton TA2 8HH — (Bristol) MB ChB Bristol 1949; DPH Bristol 1955; MFCM 1973. Prev: SCM (Dist. Support) Bristol & Weston HA.

SPELMAN, John Francis St James Surgery, 8-9 Northampton Buildings, Bath BA1 2SR Tel: 01225 422911 Fax: 01225 428398; 9 Sunny Bank, Lyncombe Vale, Bath BA2 4NA — MB ChB Birm. 1981; DRCOG 1984; MRCGP 1986.

SPENCE, Alan Kerr (retired) Brook Cottage, The Sallies, Kinnersley, Hereford HR3 6QE Tel: 01544 327721 — MB BCh BAO Dub. 1961; MA Dub. 1968, MB BCh BAO 1961; DPH Liverp. 1966; DCH NUI 1967; FFCM 1981, M 1972. Prev: Chief Admin. Med. Off. & Dir. Pub. Health Med. Powys HA.

SPENCE, Professor Alastair Andrew, CBE University Department Anaesthetics, Royal Infirmary, Little France, Edinburgh EH3 9YW Tel: 0131 242 3236 Fax: 0131 242 3138; Harewood, Broomvale Road, Kilmacolm PA13 4HX Tel: 01505 87 2962/01505 87 3575 — MB ChB Glas. 1960; MD Glas. 1976; FRCP Glas. 1980; FCAnaesth 1984; FRCS Ed. 1991; FRCP Ed. 1993; FDS RCS Eng. (Hons.) 1994; FRCS Eng. 1994. Prof. Anaesth. Univ. Edin. Specialty: Anaesth. Socs: Pres. RCAnaesth. Prev: Hunt. Prof. RCS Eng.; Prof. & Head Univ. Dept. Anaesth. West. Infirm. Glas.; Edr. Brit. Jl. Anaesth.

SPENCE, Mr Alexander James (retired) The Gables, Shore Road, Aberdour, Burntisland KY3 0TU Tel: 01383 860120 Fax: 01383 860120 — MB ChB Aberd. 1943; FRCS Eng. 1950; FRCS Ed. 1968. Cons. Surg. E. & W. Fife Health Dists. & Princess Margt. Rose Orthop. Hosp. Edin. Prev: Sen. Regist. & Res. Surg. Off. Roy. Nat. Orthop. Hosp. Stanmore.

SPENCE, Alexander Stewart (retired) Woodlea, Forres IV36 0DN Tel: 01309 672692 — MB ChB Aberd. 1938.

SPENCE, Colin Stanley Tramways Medical Centre, Farmley Road, Newtownabbey BT36 7XX Tel: 028 9034 2131 Fax: 028 9083 9111; 124 Circular Road, Jordanstown, Newtownabbey BT37 0RH — MB BCh BAO Belf. 1982; DCH Dub. 1986; Cert. Family Plann. JCC 1987; MRCGP 1987; DRCOG 1988. Socs: Brit. Assn. Sport & Med.; BMA. Prev: Ho. Off. (A & E) Belf. City Hosp. & Ulster Hosp.; Ho. Off. (Med.) Tyrone Co. Hosp.; Ho. Off. (Paediat.) Belf. City Hosp.

SPENCE, David George HCI International Medical Centre, Beardmore St., Clydebank G81 4HX Tel: 0141 951 5908 Fax: 0141 951 5869; 28 Hughenden Gardens, Glasgow G12 9YH Tel: 0141 357 4119 — MB ChB Glas. 1973; BSc (Hons.) (Path.) Glas. 1971; MRCP (UK) 1976; FRCPath 1992, M 1980; FRCP Ed. 1991. Chief of Haemat. Dir. BMT Program. HCI Internat. Med. Centre, Clydebank. Specialty: Haematology. Socs: Assn. Clin. Path. & Brit. Soc. Haemat. Prev: Sen. Cons. Haemat. King Fahd Nat. Guard Hosp. Riyadh, Saudi Arabia; Staff Haemat. (Oncol.) King Faisal Specialist Hosp. & Research Centre Riyadh, Saudi Arabia; Cons. Haemat. Tayside HB & Sen. Lect. Univ. Dundee.

SPENCE, David Peter Saunders Maynooth Hall, Knayton, Thirsk YO7 4AU — MB ChB Leic. 1983; MRCP (UK) 1987; MD Leic. 1993. Cons. Respirat. & Gen. Phys. Friarage Hosp. Northallerton. Specialty: Gen. Med.

SPENCE, David Stephen Bristol Homoeopathic Hospital, Cotham Hill, Bristol BS6 6JU Tel: 0117 973 1231 Fax: 0117 923 8759 Email: david.spence@ubht.swest.nhs.uk — MB BS Lond. 1969 (St. Geo.) MRCS Eng. LRCP Lond. 1969; DObst RCOG 1971; FFHom 1987, MFHom 1978. Cons. Homoeop. Phys. United Bristol Healthcare (NHS) Trust; Clin. Dir. Directorate of Homoeop. Med. Specialty: Homeop. Med. Socs: Fell. Roy. Soc. Med.; Fell. (Ex-Pres.) Fac. Homoeop. Prev: Regist. (Med.) Mt. Vernon Hosp. Northwood; Ho. Phys. St. Geo. Hosp. Lond.

SPENCE, Deborah Jane The Vyne, 35 Ellis Avenue, Worthing BN13 3DY — BM Soton. 1979. Prev: SHO (Psychiat., O & G & A & E) & Trainee GP Felpham & Middleton Health Centre.; Ho. Surg. (Gen. Surg.) & Ho. Phys. (Gen. Med.) Princess Margt. Hosp. Swindon.

SPENCE, Derek Wilson 33 Dore Road, Sheffield S17 3NA Tel: 0114 235 2508 — MB BCh BAO Belf. 1972 (Queen's Belfast) DCH RCP Lond. 1974; DObst RCOG 1975; DA (UK) 1976; FRACGP 1978; FRACMA 1982. Managem. Cons. Prev: Chair Regional Specialities Trent RHA; Supra Regional Contracts Gp. Mem.; Chief Exec. & Med. Dir. Princess Margt. Hosp. Childr. Perth, West. Austral.

SPENCE, Desmond Frederick Maryhill Health Centre, 41 Shawpark Street, Glasgow G20 9DR Tel: 0141 531 8811 Fax: 0141 531 8808 — MB ChB Glas. 1990. Prev: Trainee GP/SHO (Geriat.) Vict. Infirm. Glas.; SHO (A & E) Stobhill Hosp. Glas.

SPENCE, Eileen Margaret (retired) 14 Cairnlee Road, Bieldside, Aberdeen AB15 9BN Tel: 01224 861891 — MB ChB Aberd. 1949; MRCP Lond. 1955.

SPENCE, Elizabeth 5 Links View, Larkhall ML9 2JT — MB ChB Glas. 1998.

SPENCE, Fiona Mary University Medical Practice, University of Aberdeen, Block E, Taylor Buildings, Old Aberdeen, Aberdeen AB24 3UB Tel: 01224 272410 Fax: 01224 272394; 111 Brighton Place, Aberdeen AB10 6RT Tel: 01224 312078 — MB ChB Aberd. 1980; DGM RCPS Glas. 1991; MRCGP 1994. Gen. Practitioner, Univ. Med. Pract., Grampian Primary Care Trust, Aberd. Specialty: Gen. Pract.

SPENCE, Gary Mervyn 25 Mount Royal, Lisburn BT27 5BF — MB BCh BAO Belf. 1994.

SPENCE, Gerald George Shettleston Health Centre, 420 Old Shettleston Road, Glasgow G32 7JZ Tel: 0141 531 6220 Fax: 0141 531 6206 — MB ChB Aberd. 1978.

SPENCE, Imogen Pamela Westwater 2 Bramway, Bramhall, Stockport SK7 2AP — MB ChB Manch. 1989.

SPENCE, Joanna Rosalie The Shrubbery, 26 High Street, Eynsham, Witney OX29 4HB Tel: 01865 881385 Fax: 01865 881342 — MB BS Lond. 1973 (Roy. Free) Prev: Ho. Phys. Roy. Free Hosp. Lond.; Ho. Surg. Lister Hosp. Stevenage; Ho. Surg. (O & G) Roy. Sussex Co. Hosp. Brighton.

SPENCE, John Cameron 67 Gilbertfield Street, Glasgow G33 3TU; Stable End, 1A Middlemuir Road, Lenzie, Kirkintilloch, Glasgow G66 4NA Tel: 0141 774 5987 — MB ChB Glas. 1977; MRCGP 1989.

SPENCE, John Couper (retired) 116 Elizabeth Road, New Oscott, Sutton Coldfield B73 5AS Tel: 0121 355 6717 Email: ioannes@globalnet.co.uk — MB ChB Glas. 1958 (Glasgow) DObst RCOG 1965; MRCGP 1980. Prev: SHO (Med. & Cardiol.), Ho. Phys. & Ho. Surg. Vict. Infirm. Glas.

SPENCE, John Edward Waterside Health Centre, Glendermott Road, Londonderry BT47 6AU Tel: 028 7132 0100 Fax: 028 7132 0117; 3 West Lake, Londonderry BT47 6WE Tel: 028 7186 1650 — MB BCh BAO NUI 1983.

SPENCE, John Mountfort (retired) The Well House, Spa Close, Brill, Aylesbury HP18 9RZ Tel: 01844 237639 Fax: 01844 238568 — MB BS Lond. 1956 (Univ. Coll. Hosp.) MRCS Eng. LRCP Lond. 1956; DObst RCOG 1958. Prev: GP Aylesbury.

SPENCE, Joyce Sylvia Angulus Iste, Cotmaton Road, Sidmouth EX10 8ST — MRCS Eng. LRCP Lond. 1939 (Bristol) Prev: Ho. Surg. Bristol Roy. Infirm. & Nottm. Childr. Hosp.; Ho. Phys. Salisbury Gen. Infirm.

SPENCE, Kenneth Archibald Edmund, TD, SBStJ (retired) The Stables, 26 High Street, Eynsham, Witney OX29 Tel: 01865 881385 — MRCS Eng. LRCP Lond. 1951 (Guy's) Maj. RAMC, RARO. Prev: Ho. Phys. (Paediat.) Worthing Gen. Hosp.

SPENCE, Magnus Peter (retired) The Oast House, Wardsbrook Road, Ticehurst, Wadhurst TN5 7DR Tel: 01580 201084 — (Camb. & Middlx.) MB BChir Camb. 1947; FRCP Lond. 1975, M 1948. Prev: Cons. Phys. St. Albans City Hosp. & Qu. Eliz. II Hosp. Welwyn Gdn.

SPENCE, Margaret Ruth Coppins, Elm Green Lane, Danbury, Chelmsford CM3 4DR — MB BS Lond. 1984 (Guy's) MRCGP 1989; DRCOG 1989. GP Retainer Chelmsford. Socs: (Region. Rep.) Christian Med. Fell.ship. Prev: GP Retainer Maldon; Trainee GP Chelmsford VTS.

SPENCE, Martin Terence Wigan & Bolton Health Authority, Bryan House, 61 Standishgate, Wigan WN1 1AH Tel: 01942 772825 Fax: 01942 772769; 24 Tennyson Close, Briarsmount, Heaton Mersey, Stockport SK4 2ED — MB BCh BAO Belf. 1981; MFPHM RCP (UK) 1995. Cons. Pub. Health Med. Wigan & Bolton HA. Specialty: Pub. Health Med. Socs: Manch. Med. Soc.; Ulster Med. Soc.

SPENCE, Peter Johnson 6 Lisburn Road, Moira, Craigavon BT67 0JP — MB BCh Belf. 1998.

SPENCE, Richard William Spence Group Practice, Westcliffe House, 48-50 Logan Road, Bristol BS7 8DR Tel: 0117 944 0701; Birchwood, Eastfield, Westbury-on-Trym, Bristol BS9 4BE Tel: 01179 628848 — (St. Bart.) MB BChir Camb. 1970; MRCS Eng. LRCP Lond. 1970. Hosp. Pract. (Gastroenterol.) Frenchay Hosp. Bristol. Specialty: Gastroenterol. Socs: (Mem. Steering Comm.) Primary Care Soc. Gastroenterol. Prev: SHO (Respirat. & Infec. Dis.) Unit Ham Green Hosp. Bristol; Research Regist. (Gastroenterol.) & SHO (Gen. Med.) Frenchay Hosp. Bristol.

SPENCE, Robert Nicholas Francis The Strand Practice, 2 The Strand, Goring-by-Sea, Worthing BN12 6DN Tel: 01903 243351 Fax: 01903 705804; 35 Ellis Avenue, Worthing BN13 3DY — MB BChir Camb. 1975 (Guy's Hosp. Lond.) MA Camb. 1975; DRCOG 1983.

SPENCE, Professor Roy Archibald Joseph Belfast City Hospital, Lisburn Road, Belfast BT9 7AB Tel: 01232 329241 Fax: 01232 326614 Email: roy.spence@beh.n-i.nhs.uk; 7 Downshire Crescent, Hillsborough BT26 6DD Tel: 01846 682362 Fax: 01846 682418 — MB BCh BAO Belf. 1977 (Queens University Belfast) MB BCh BAO (Hons.) Belf. 1977; FRCS Ed. 1981; FRCSI 1981; MD Belf. (Hons.) 1984; MA Belf. 1997. Cons. (Surgey) Belf. City Hosp.; Hon. Lect. (Surg.) Qu.s Univ. Belf.; Arris & Gale Lect. RCS Eng.; Hon. Lect. (Anat.); Hon. Lect. (Oncol.); Hon. Prof. Univ. of Ulster. Specialty: Gen. Surg. Socs: Fell. Assn. Surgs.; Brit. Soc. Gastroenterol.; Moynihan Club. Prev: Cons. (Surgey) Groote Schuur Hosp., Cape Town; Exec. Dir. Belf. City Hosp. Trust Bd. (1993-1997); Vis. Prof. Cleveland Clinic Ohio, USA 1993.

SPENCE, Sinclair Dick Ballykennedy House, Nutt's Corner, Belfast — MB BCh BAO Belf. 1967.

SPENCE-JONES, Mr Clive 149 Harley Street, London W1G 6DE Tel: 020 7935 4444 Fax: 020 7486 2580 — MB BS Lond. 1981; FRCS Ed. 1986; MRCOG 1988. Cons. O & G Whittington Hosp. Lond. Specialty: Obst. & Gyn.

SPENCE-SALES, Dorothy (retired) 41 Christchurch Road, London SW14 7AQ — MA New Zealand 1932, BSc 1933 (Otago) MB ChB New Zealand 1938; DA Eng 1953; FFA RCS Eng. 1953. Prev: Cons. & Sen. Lect. Roy. Postgrad. Med. Sch. Lond.

SPENCELEY, James Howard (retired) Gairnshiel, 22 Beaufort Road, Inverness IV2 3NP — MB ChB Ed. 1967; FFA RCS Eng. 1972. Cons. Anaesth. Raigmore Hosp. Inverness.

SPENCELEY, Jane Elizabeth Occupational Health, Nestlé Rowntree, York YO91 1XY Tel: 01904 602343 — BM BCh Oxf. 1990; DFFP 1996; MRCGP 1996; DRCOG 1997; AFOM 2001. Specialist Regist. in Occupat. Health, Nestle Rowntree York. Specialty: Occupat. Health. Socs: Oxf. Med. Soc.; Roy. Coll. Gen. Pract.; Soc. of Occupat.al Med.

SPENCELEY, Judith Anne Gairnshiel, 22 Beaufort Road, Inverness IV2 3NP — MB ChB Ed. 1967; DObst RCOG 1970.

SPENCELEY, Kenneth Reid Merton Lodge Surgery, West Street, Alford LN13 9DH Tel: 01507 463262 Fax: 01507 466447 — MB ChB Glas. 1973; MRCGP 1977; DRCOG 1978.

SPENCELEY, Neil Campbell c/o Spenceley, 22 Beaufort Road, Inverness IV2 3NP — MB ChB Ed. 1993.

SPENCELEY, Simon Richard The Surgery, 162 Long St., Dordon, Tamworth B78 1QA — MB ChB Birm. 1986.

SPENCER, Alfred George, GM (retired) High Gate, Rock, Wadebridge PL27 6JZ — MRCS Eng. LRCP Lond. 1939 (Univ. Coll. Hosp.) MD Lond. 1947, MB BS (Hnrs.) 1940; FRCP Lond. 1962, M 1947. Prev: Cons. Phys. St. Bart. & Univ. Coll. Hosps.

SPENCER, Alison Catherine 10 Blandford Drive, Macclesfield SK11 8WB — MB ChB Manch. 1991.

SPENCER, Amanda Jane Bellowswood House, Ballinger, Great Missenden HP16 9LF — MB ChB Liverp. 1993.

SPENCER, Anne Elizabeth The Surgery, Earby Colne, Colne BB18 6QT Tel: 01282 843407; 35 York Fields, Barnoldswick, Colne BB18 5DA — MB ChB Leeds 1981.

SPENCER, Brian Trevor Holmside Medical Group, 142 Armstrong Road, Benwell, Newcastle upon Tyne NE4 8QB Tel: 0191 273 4009 Fax: 0191 273 2745; 20 Willow Way, Darras Hall, Ponteland, Newcastle upon Tyne NE20 9RJ — (St. Geo.) BSc (Special, Pharmacol.) Lond. 1967, MB BS 1970; MRCP (UK) 1975; MRCGP 1976.

SPENCER, Bryan John ThE Elizabeth Courtauld Surgery, Factory Lane West, Halstead CO9 1EX Tel: 01787 475944 Fax: 01787 474506; 30 Chapel Street, Halstead CO9 2LS Tel: 01787 473535 — MB BS Lond. 1974; BSc (Physiol.) Lond. 1971; MRCS Eng. LRCP Lond. 1974; MRCGP 1978.

SPENCER, Caroline Melanie 10 Beechwood Rise, Manor Park, Plymouth PL6 8AP — MB BS Lond. 1985 (Roy. Free) DRCOG 1987; Cert. Family Plann. JCC 1987; MRCGP 1994. Specialty: Cardiol. Socs: Assoc. Mem. BMA; Assoc. Mem. RCGP. Prev: Asst. GP Bath & Oxf.

SPENCER, Charles Guy Chapman High Gate, Rock, Wadebridge PL27 6JZ; Mid Staffordshire General Hospital NHS Trust, Princes Road, Stoke-on-Trent ST4 7LN — MB BS Lond. 1990; MRCP (UK) 1994. Cons. Cardiol., Mid, Staffs. Hosp. Specialty: Cardiol. Prev: Specialist Regist. (Cardiol.) Sandwell Healthcare NHS Trust, W. Bromwich; Regist. (Cardiol.) Univ. Hosp. Birm.; Regist. (Cardiol.) Birm. Heartlands Hosp.

SPENCER, Christopher Peter 60 Playford Road, Ipswich IP4 5RG Email: cpspencer@doctors.org.uk; 27 Royal Crescent, London W11 4SE Tel: 020 7602 6152 — MB BChir Camb. 1985 (Univ. of Camb.) MD; MRCOG. Cons. Obst. and Gynaecologist, NHS Ipswich. Specialty: Obst. & Gyn. Special Interest: Fertil.; Gynae. Endcrinology; Menopause. Socs: MPS; BMS; BFS.

SPENCER, Clifford Michael Ruddington Medical Centre, Church Street, Ruddington, Nottingham NG11 6HD Tel: 0115 921 1144 Fax: 0115 940 5139; Bradmere Barn, Loughborough Road, Bradmore, Nottingham NG11 6PA Tel: 0115 984 6333 — MB ChB Sheff. 1977; DRCOG 1981; MRCGP 1993. Trainer Nottm. VTS Scheme; Clin. Asst. (ENT) Nottm. Univ Hosp.; Clin. Tutor (Community Med.) Univ. Nottm.

SPENCER, Colin Wigmore The Marches Medical Practice, Mill Lane Surgery, 46 Mill Lane, Buckley CH7 3HB Tel: 01224 550939 Fax: 01224 549592 — MB ChB Liverp. 1967; BDS 1961; MRCGP 1977.

SPENCER, David Anthony Regional Cardiothoracic Centre, Freeman Hospital, Newcastle upon Tyne NE7 7DN Tel: 0191 284 3111 Fax: 0191 213 2167; Low House, Berwick Hill, Newcastle upon Tyne NE20 0BJ Tel: 01661 821354 — MB BS Lond. 1981 (Royal Free London) MRCP (UK) 1985; MD Lond. 1992; FRCPCH 1997. Cons. Respirat. Paediat. Freeman Hosp. Newc. u. Tyne. Specialty: Paediat.; Respirat. Med. Socs: Brit. Thorac. Soc.; Amer. Thoracic Soc.; Eur. Respirat. Soc. Prev: Cons. Respirat. Paediat. Birm. Childr. Hosp.; Sen. Regist. (Paediat.) W. Midl. RHA; Research Fell. (Thoracic Med.) King's Coll. Hosp. Lond.

SPENCER, David John Oakhaven Hospice, Lower Pennington Lane, Lymington SO41 8ZZ Tel: 01590 670346 Fax: 01590 679624; 280 Burley Road, Bransgrove, Christchurch BH23 8DQ Tel: 01425 672927 — MB BS Lond. 1970 (St. Geo.) DObst RCOG 1973; DCH Eng. 1973; MRCGP 1974; MSc (Social Med.) Lond. 1978. Cons. Palliat. Med. Oakhaven Hospice Lymington. Specialty: Palliat. Med. Socs: Assn. Palliat. Med.; (Founder) Mind and Mortality. Prev: Cons. Palliat. Med. & Clin. Dir. Prospect Hospice Swindon; Cons. Phys. St. Barnabas' Hospice Worthing.

SPENCER, Douglas Anthony (retired) 25 Standing Stones, Great Billing, Northampton NN3 9HA Tel: 01604 414825 — MB ChB Ed. 1956; DPM Leeds 1962; FRCPsych 1982, M 1971. Prev: Phys. Supt. & Cons. Psychiat. Meanwood Pk. Hosp. Leeds, Wharfe Grange Hosp. Wetherby & Crooked Acres Hosp. Leeds.

SPENCER, Elizabeth Mary Department of Anaesthetics, Gloucester Royal Hospital, Great Western Road, Gloucester GL1 3NN — BM Soton. 1981; FFA RCS Eng. 1988; DM Soton. 1992; Cert Med Educat Bristol 2003. Cons. Anaesth. & Intens. Care Gloucester Roy. Hosp.; Director of Med. Educat. Specialty: Intens. Care. Socs: Assn. Anaesth.; Intens. Care Soc.; Assn. of Med. Educat. in Europe. Prev: Sen. Regist. (Anaesth.) Plymouth & Bristol; Research Fell. Intens. Ther. Unit Bristol Roy. Infirm.; Regist. (Anaesth.) Derby & Nottm.

SPENCER, Emma Freda Anne (retired) 6 The Plateau, Piney Hills, Belfast BT9 5QP — (Belf.) MB BCh BAO Belf. 1961. Prev: Clin. Asst. Gastroenterol. Belf.

SPENCER, Geoffrey Stuart Bideford Medical Centre, Abbotsham Road, Bideford EX39 3AF Tel: 01237 476363 Fax: 01237 423351 — MB BS Lond. 1986; MRCGP 1992; T(GP) 1992.

SPENCER, Geoffrey Tallent, OBE 40 Cleaver Square, London SE11 4EA Tel: 020 7735 9357 — MB BS Lond. 1954 (St. Thos.) FFA RCS Eng. 1960. Cons. Anaesth. & Consult. i/c Respirat. Unit St.

Thos. Hosp. Lond.; Hon. Cons. Brompton Hosp. Lond.; Hons Cons. REFRESH. Specialty: Anaesth.; Intens. Care; Disabil. Med. Prev: Vis. Prof., Childr.s Med Hosp. Chicago USA; Cons. W.H.O.

SPENCER, Mr George Robert The Health Centre, Langholm DG13 0JY — MB ChB Ed. 1973; BSc (Med. Sci.) Ed. 1970; FRCS Ed. 1978; LMCC 1985. Chief of Staff St. Therese Hosp. St. Paul Alberta, Canada. Specialty: Gen. Surg.

SPENCER, Gillian Mary North Hampshire Primary Care Trust, Harness House, Aldermaston Road, Basingstoke RG24 9NB Tel: 01256 312250 — MB BS Lond. 1981; MRCPsych 1986; MFPHM RCP (UK) 1991; FFPHM 2002. Cons. Pub. Health Med. N. Hants. PCT. Specialty: Pub. Health Med. Prev: Sen. Regist. (Community Med.) Sheff. HA; Regist. (Community Med.) Trent RHA.

SPENCER, Glenn MacDonald Front Drive Offices, Oldchurch Hospital, Waterloo Road, Romford RM7 0BE Tel: 01708 708285 Fax: 01708 708285 — MB BS Lond. 1988 (St. Geo.) BSc Basic Med. Scs. & Physiol. (Hons.) Lond. 1985; MRCP (UK) 1991. Cons. Phys. & Gastroenterol., Barking, Havering & Redbridgeps. NSH Trust, Old Ch. Hosp., Romford. Specialty: Gen. Med.; Gastroenterol. Socs: BMA. Prev: Lect. (Gastroenterol.) Middlx. Hosp. Lond.; Regist. Rotat. (Med.) Ipswich Hosp.; SHO Rotat. (Med.) Derby Roy. Infirm.

SPENCER, Graeme Thomas Russell — MB ChB Liverp. 1989; DRCOG 1991; DFFP 1993; MRCGP 1993; T(GP) 1993. General Practioner, Crewe. Prev: SHO (A & E Paediat. & O & G) Leighton Dist. Gen. Hosp. Crewe; SHO (c/o the Elderly) Leighton Dist. Gen. Hosp. Crewe; Gen. Practitioner, Nelson.

SPENCER, Greg Bushey Fields Hospital, Bushey Fields Road, Dudley DY1 2LE Tel: 01384 244957 — MB ChB Aberd. 1991; MRCPsych 1995. Cons. in Old Age Psychiat. Bushey Fields Hosp., Dudley W. Midl.s. Specialty: Geriat. Psychiat. Socs: Roy. Coll. Psychiat. (Fac. Old Age Psychiat.); BMA; W Midl. Assn. Old Age Psychiatr. Prev: Sen. Regist. Rotat. (Old Age Psychiat.) W. Midl.; Regist. (Child Psychiat.) Selly Oak Hosp. Birm.; Regist. (Old Age Psychiat.) Highcroft Hosp. Birm.

SPENCER, Hal Lloyd Cruck Barn, Stocksbridge, Sheffield S36 4GH — MB BS Lond. 1993 (Lond. Hosp./Camb. Univ.) MA Camb. 1993; MRCP (UK) 1997. Regist. (Gastroenterol.), Sheff. Teachg. Hosp.s. Specialty: Gastroenterol. Prev: SHO (Gen. Med.) City Hosp. Nottm.; Ho. Off. (Gen. Surg.) S. Warwicks Hosp.; Ho. Off. (Med.) Roy. Lond. Hosp.

SPENCER, Heather Dawn 11 Upper High Royds, Mapplewell, Barnsley S75 5FB — MB ChB Leeds 1992.

SPENCER, Helen 446 Pinhoe Road, Exeter EX4 8EW — MB ChB Manch. 1993; DCH RCP Lond. 1995. SHO (Paediat.) S. Manch. Trust Hosps. Prev: SHO (A & E) Blackpool; Ho. Off. (Med.) Chester; Ho. Off. (Surg.) Blackpool.

SPENCER, Helen Amanda 9 Southlands, Town Close, Horsforth, Leeds LS18 5BR — MB BS Lond. 1980 (Roy. Free) DCH RCP Lond. 1984; DRCOG 1984; FFARCS Eng. 1988. Cons. Anaesth. St. Jas. Univ. Hosp. Leeds. Specialty: Anaesth. Socs: Assn. Anaesth.; Eur. Soc. Regional Anaesth. Prev: Sen. Regist. Rotat. (Anaesth.) Leeds; Post-Fellowsh. Regist. (Anaesth.) Middlx. Hosp. Lond.; Regist. (Anaesth.) Roy. Free Hosp. Lond.

SPENCER, Helen Frances The Spinney, Chapel Lane, Bruera, Chester CH3 6EW — BM BCh Oxf. 1977; MA Oxf. 1982. Socs: Chester & N. Wales Med. Soc. Prev: Trainee GP Brighton; Ho. Surg. Radcliffe Infirm. Oxf.

SPENCER, Helen Janet Greenview Surgery, 129 Hazeldene Road, Northampton NN2 7PB Tel: 01604 791002 Fax: 01604 721822; 70 Glenfield Drive, Great Doddington, Wellingborough NN29 7TE — BM BS Nottm. 1987; BMedSci Nottm. 1985; DRCOG 1990; MRCGP 1991. Prev: Trainee GP/SHO (Psychiat.) Lincoln VTS.

SPENCER, Helen Margaret Radula Scott The Lindley Village Surgery, Thomas Street, Lindley, Huddersfield HD3 3JD Tel: 01484 651403 Fax: 01484 644198; Radula, 21A Hopton Hall Lane, Upper Hopton, Mirfield WF14 8EA Tel: 01924 506684 — MB ChB Leeds 1975. Sen. Partner, Gen. Pract. Socs: Huddersfield Med. Soc. Prev: Clin. Asst. (A & E) Huddersfield Roy. Infirm.

SPENCER, Hilary Susan South Tyneside District Hospital, Harton Lane, South Shields NE34 0PL Tel: 0191 454 8888 Email: hilary.spencer@eem.sthct.northy.nhs.uk; 5 Park Head Road, Newcastle upon Tyne NE7 7DH — MB BS Newc. 1979; MRCP (UK) 1982; FRCR 1986. Cons. Radiologist S. Tyneside Healthcare NHS Trust. Specialty: Radiol.

SPENCER, Ian Newcastle & North Tyneside Health Authority, Benfield Road, Newcastle upon Tyne NE6 4PF Tel: 0191 219 6000 Fax: 0191 219 6084 Email: ian.spencer@nant-ha.northy.nhs.uk — MB BS Newc. 1974; MSc (Pub. Health Med.) Newc. 1992. Head of Primary Care Developm. Newc. & N. Tyneside HA. Specialty: Gen. Pract. Socs: DURG. Prev: Trainee (Pub. Health Med.) N. RHA; GP Ferryhill Co. Durh.; Demonst. (Path.) Univ. Newc.

SPENCER, Ian, Group Capt. RAF Med. Br. Retd. 3 Leazes Court, Durham DH1 1XF Tel: 0191 386 0799 — MRCS Eng. LRCP Lond. 1971; DObst RCOG 1974; FRCA 1980. Cons. Anaesth. Dryburn Hosp. Durh. Specialty: Anaesth. Socs: NESA; Assn. Anaesth.; BMA. Prev: RAF Cons. Adviser in Anaesth.; Hon. Sen. Regist. Frenchay Hosp. Bristol; SHO (Anaesth., O & G) N. Manch. Hosp.

SPENCER, Jason Richard Flat 26d, South Residence, King George Hospital, Barley Lane, Ilford IG3 8YB — MB BS Lond. 1992.

SPENCER, Jean Elizabeth Dept. of Psychiatry, Royal South Hants Hospital, Southampton SO14 0YG; Oakwood, Park Lane, Carhampton, Minehead TA24 6NL — MB BS Lond. 1979 (St. Bart.) MRCPsych 1984; DIP Clin. HYP. 1998. Specialist Regist. (Psychiat.) Roy. S. Hants Hosp., Soton. Specialty: Gen. Psychiat. Socs: Fell. RSM; Brit. Soc. Med. Dent. Hypn. Prev: Clin. Asst. (Psychiat.) Southmead Hosp. Bristol.; Regist. (Psychiat.) Mapperley Hosp. Nottm.

SPENCER, John 19 Station Road, South Cave, Brough HU15 2AA — MB BS Durh. 1962.

SPENCER, John Andrew Adelaide Medical Centre, Adelaide Terrace, Benwell, Newcastle upon Tyne NE4 8BE Tel: 0191 219 5599 Fax: 0191 219 5596; 38 Moorside S., Fenham, Newcastle upon Tyne NE4 9BB Tel: 0191 226 0585 Email: john@moorside38@demon.co.uk — MB ChB Ed. 1973 (Edinburgh) DA Eng. 1976; FRCGP 1991, M 1979. Sen. Lect. (Primary Health Care) Sch. of Health Sci. Univ. Newc. u. Tyne; Princip. in Gen. Pract.; Sen. Tutor for Professional Developm., Fac. of Med. Univ. of Newc. Prev: Princip. GP Gateshead.

SPENCER, John Anthony — MB BChir Camb. 1983 (Camb. & Westm.) MB (Hons. Distinc. Med.) Camb. 1983, BChir 1982; MRCP (UK) 1985; FRCR 1988; MA Camb. 1983, MD 1996. Cons. Radiol. St. Jas. Univ. Hosp. Leeds. Specialty: Radiol. Socs: Fell. Roy. Soc. Med.; Radiol. Soc. N. Amer.; Internat. Cancer Imaging Soc. Prev: Vis. Asst. Prof. Radiol. Thos. Jefferson Univ. Hosp. Philadelphia, USA; Regist. (Radiol.) John Radcliffe Hosp. Oxf.; SHO Hammersmith Hosp. Lond.

SPENCER, Mr John Anthony David Department Obstetrics & Gynaecology, Northwick Park & St Mark's NHS Trust, Watford Road, Harrow HA1 3UJ Tel: 020 8869 2861 Fax: 020 8869 2864 Email: john.spencer@nwlh.nhs.uk; 33 Eastbury Road, Northwood HA6 3AJ Tel: 01923 822991 Fax: 01923 822168 Email: jadspencer@msn.com — MB BS Lond. 1976 (St. Geo.) BSc (Hons.) Lond. 1973; FRCOG 1993, M 1981. Cons. O & G Northwick Pk. & St. Mark's NHS Trust, Harrow; Hon. Sen. Clin. Lect. UCL Med. Sch. Lond. Univ.; Hon.Sen. Clin. Lect. Imperial Coll. Med. Sch., Lond. Specialty: Obst. & Gyn. Special Interest: Fetal monitoring. Obstetric causation of cerebral palsy. Socs: (Ex-Hon. Sec. 1991-1994) Blair Bell Research Soc.; Neonat. Soc.; (ex.Exec. Comm.) Brit. Assn. Perinatal Med. Prev: Sen. Clin. Lect. UCL Med. Sch. Lond. Univ.; Sen. Lect. Inst. O & G Univ. Lond.; Clin. Lect. John Radcliffe Hosp. Oxf.

SPENCER, John Dalby (retired) The Elms, 4 West End, Beeston, Nottingham NG9 1GL — MB BS Lond. 1958 (Univ. Coll. Hosp.) Prev: Ho. Surg. N. Middlx. Hosp. Lond.

SPENCER, Mr John Derek Guy's Nuffield House, Newcomen Street, Guy's Hospital, London SE1 1YR Tel: 020 7955 4752 Fax: 020 7955 4754; Cloverley, 110B King George Street, Greenwich, London SE10 8PX Tel: 020 8425 1800 — (Guy's) MRCS Eng. LRCP Lond. 1967; MB BS Lond. 1967; MRCP Lond. 1971; FRCS Eng. 1974; MS Lond. 1988. Specialty: Orthop. Socs: Fell. BOA; Brit. Soc. Surg. Hand; Fell. Roy. Soc. Med. Prev: Emeritus Cons. Orthopaedic & Trauma Surg. Guys & St Thomas' Hosp. Lond.; Reader Trainer Guy's & St Thomas' Hosps. Lond.; Exchange Prof. Guy's Hosp. & John Hopkins Baltimore, USA 1992.

SPENCER, John Gordon Spring Hall Group Practice, Spring Hall Medical Centre, Spring Hall Lane, Halifax HX1 4JG Tel: 01422 349501 Fax: 01422 323091 — MB ChB St. And. 1967. Socs: BMA.

SPENCER, Jonathan OHSAS, 1 Edward St., Dundee DD1 5NS Tel: 01382 346030 Fax: 01382 346040; Landalla House, Kirkton of Glenisla, Blairgowrie PH11 8PH Tel: 01575 582213 — MB ChB Ed. 1977 (Edinburgh) BSc (Hons.) Ed. 1974; DIH Eng. 1982; MSc Occupat. Med. Lond. 1983; FFOM RCP Lond. 1995, MFOM 1984. Cons. Ocupational Phys. OHSAS, Dundee. Specialty: Occupat. Health. Socs: Soc. Occupat. Med. Prev: Manager Occupat. Med. BP Gp. Occupat. Health Centre; Med. Off. MoD Roy. Aircraft Estab. FarnBoro.; Med. Off. MoD Army Personnel Research Estab. FarnBoro.

SPENCER, Jonathan Patrick Greer King's College Hospital, Department of Occupational Health & Safety, Denmark Hill, London SE5 9RS Tel: 020 7346 4919 Fax: 020 7346 3601 Email: jonathan.spencer@kingsch.nhs.uk; 11 Woodland Way, Caterham CR3 6ER Tel: 01883 340867 Email: jonathan.spencer@btinternet.com — MB ChB Ed. 1978; DRCOG 1980; MRCGP 1982; MSc (Occupational Med.) Lond. 1986; DAvMed Lond. 1988; AFOM RCP Lond. 1990; MFOM RCP Lond. 1998; MSc (Organisational Psychol.) Lond. 2004. Cons. Occupat. Phys. King's Coll. Hosp. Lond. Specialty: Occupat. Health. Socs: Soc. Occupat. Med.; Assn. Aviat. Med. Examrs. Prev: Occupat. Phys. BAA Gatwick & Stansted Airports; Med. Off. Civil Aviat. Auth. Gatwick; Occupat. Phys. St Bart. Hosp. Lond.

SPENCER, Judith Vivien Calabar, Pica, Workington CA14 4PZ — MB BCh Wales 1979.

SPENCER, Keith Paul Dawley Medical Practice, Doseley Road, Dawley, Telford TF4 3; 9 Lees Farm Drive, Madeley, Telford TF7 5SU — MB BS Lond. 1976 (St. Bart.) DA Eng. 1979; DRCOG 1981. Socs: BMA (Sec. Salop. Div.). Prev: Chairm. W. Midl. Regional Hosp. Jun. Staff Comm.

SPENCER, Li Lian Lonsdale Medical Centre, 24 Lonsdale Road, London NW6 6RR Tel: 020 7328 8331 Fax: 020 7328 8630; 180 Goldhurst Terrace, London NW6 3HN — MB ChB Birm. 1968. Prev: Med. Off. City of Birm. Pub. Health Dept.; SHO (Anaesth.) Dudley Rd. Hosp. Birm.

SPENCER, Lisa Graham 33 Cromwell Road, Stretford, Manchester M32 8GH — MB ChB (Hons.) Leeds 1995; BSc (Hons. Physiol.) Manch. 1990; MRCP (UK) 2000. Specialty: Gen. Med.

SPENCER, Maria Jadwiga Melford Lodge, 16 Beech Drive, London N2 9NY Tel: 020 8883 8888 Fax: 020 8883 8888 — Lekarz Warsaw, Poland 1965 (Med. Acad. Warsaw) ECFMG 1969; MD Poland 1975. Clin. Asst. (Cardiol.) Roy. Free Hosp.; Hosp. Pract. (Cardiol.) Ealing Hosp. Lond.; Patent Holder for Frozen Display & Cardiac Arrest Timer. Specialty: Cardiol. Socs: BMA; Polish Med. Assn.; Brit. Cardiac Soc. Prev: Dir. Polish Clinic Lond.; Managing Dir. Cardiac Recorders Ltd. Lond.; Research Regist. (Cardiol.) St. Mary's Hosp.

SPENCER, Mark Mount View Practice, London Street Medical Centre, London Street, Fleetwood FY7 6HD Tel: 01253 873312 Fax: 01253 873130 — MB BS Lond. 1986; DRCOG 1987; MRCGP 1990. GP Fleetwood.

SPENCER, Mary Elizabeth Market Street Clinic, 20 Market St., Woolwich, London SE18 6QR Tel: 020 8317 9415; 56 Brooklands Park, London SE3 9AJ Tel: 020 8852 0394 — MB BS Lond. 1968 (Guy's) MRCS Eng. LRCP Lond. 1968; DObst RCOG 1969; DCH Eng. 1970; MFFP 1993. SCMO (Head Dp Family Plann.) Greenwich PCT. Specialty: Pub. Health Med.; Community Child Health; Family Plann. & Reproduc. Health. Socs: Inst. Psychosexual Med.; Pres. W. Kent Med-Chi. Soc.; Lond. Soc. FP Drs.

SPENCER, Michael Anthony Saxonbury House, Croft Road, Crowborough TN6 1DL Tel: 01892 652266 Fax: 01892 668607 — MB BS Lond. 1978 (King's Coll. Hosp.) MA Camb. 1969; DRCOG 1980; MRCGP 1982; DFFP 1997. GP CrowBoro.; Tutor Eastbourne Annual GP Refresher Course. Prev: Trainee GP Frome; Trainee GP Bath VTS; Ho. Phys. (Profess. Med. Unit) King's Coll. Hosp. Lond.

SPENCER, Michael Anthony Patrick (retired) North End Surgery, High Street, Buckingham MK18 1NU Tel: 01280 813239 Fax: 01280 823449 — MB BS Lond. 1968 (St. Bart.) MRCS Eng. LRCP Lond. 1968; DObst RCOG 1973. Prev: SHO (Cas.) Char. Cross Hosp. Lond.

SPENCER, Michael Charles Charity House, Church St., Finedon, Wellingborough NN9 5NA — MB BS Lond. 1968 (Middlx.) MRCS Eng. LRCP Lond. 1968; DObst RCOG 1971.

SPENCER, Michael Charles (retired) 8 Dolphin Close, Chichester PO19 3QP Tel: 01243 789938 — BM BCh Oxf. 1949 (Middlx.) MA, BM BCh Oxf. 1949; DTM & H Antwerp 1952; MRCGP 1974. Prev: GP Leiston.

SPENCER, Mr Michael Grant Department of Otolaryngology, Countess of Chester Hospital, Liverpool Road, Chester CH2 1UL Tel: 01244 366322; The Spinney, Chapel Lane, Bruera, Chester CH3 6EW — BM BCh Oxf. 1975 (University of Oxford) MA Oxf. 1975; FRCS Eng. 1982. Cons. Otolaryngol. Countess of Chester Hosp. Specialty: Otorhinolaryngol. Socs: Fell. Roy. Soc. Med.; Europ. Acad. Facial Surg.; Brit. Rhinological Soc. Prev: Sen. Regist. St. Thos. Hosp. Lond.; Ho. Surg. Nuffield Dept. Surg. Radcliffe Infirm. Oxf.; Demonst. (Human Anat.) Univ. Oxf.

SPENCER, Michael Richard Welbeck Road Surgery, 1A Welbeck Road, Bolsover, Chesterfield S44 6DF Tel: 01246 823742; 18 The Pinfold, Glapwell, Chesterfield S44 5PU Tel: 01632 810136 — MB ChB Aberd. 1978 (Aberdeen) MRCGP 1982. VTS Tutor Nott. Univ.

SPENCER, Murdoch Harris 11 Torrington Avenue, Giffnock, Glasgow G46 7LH Tel: 0141 638 8484 — LRCP LRCS Ed. 1951; LRCP LRCS Ed. LRFPS Glas. 1951.

SPENCER, Naomi Marydell Stapenhill Surgery, Fyfield Road, Stapenhill, Burton-on-Trent DE15 9QD Tel: 01283 565200 Fax: 01283 500617; Ridgeway, 64 Burton Road, Repton, Derby DE65 6FN — BM BS Nottm. 1984.

SPENCER, Professor Nicholas James School of Postgrad. Medical Education, University of Warwick, Coventry CV4 7AL Tel: 024 76 523167 Fax: 024 76 524415 Email: n.j.spencer@warwick.ac.uk; 5 Castle Road, Kenilworth CV8 1NG Tel: 01926 512436 — (Sheffield) FRCPCH; MRCS Eng. LRCP Lond. 1969; DCH Eng. 1973; MRCP (UK) 1975; MPhil. Nottm. 1980; FRCP Ed 1990. Prof. of Child Health Univ. of Warwick; Hon. Cons. Paediat. Coventry Healthcare NHS Trust. Specialty: Community Child Health. Socs: MRCPCH.

SPENCER, Nicholas James Blakey — MB ChB Leeds 1987; MRCP (UK) 1991; FRCR 1994. Cons. (Radiol.) Mid Yorkshire Hospitals NHS Trust Wakefield. Specialty: Radiol. Prev: Regist. (Radiol.) Nottm. HA.

SPENCER, Nigel George (retired) Church Close Surgery, 3 Church Close, Boston PE21 6NB Tel: 01205 311133 Fax: 01205 358986; Lynton House, 35 Sibsey Road, Boston PE21 9QY — MB ChB Birm. 1966. Prev: GP Boston.

SPENCER, Pamela Mary (retired) High Gate, Rock, Wadebridge PL27 6JZ — MB BS Lond. 1950 (Univ. Coll. Hosp.) MRCS Eng. LRCP Lond. 1950; FRCOG 1973, M 1960, DObst 1952; FRCS Eng. 1957. Prev: Cons. O & G Eliz. G. Anderson Hosp. & Whittington Hosp. Lond.

SPENCER, Paul Andrew Stephen Department Medical Imaging, Rotherham Hospital Trust, Moorgate Road, Rotherham S60 2UD Tel: 01709 304413 — MB BS Lond. 1978 (St. Mary's) BSc (Hons.) Lond. 1975; MRCS Eng. LRCP Lond. 1978; MRCP (UK) 1982; FRCR 1988. Cons. Radiol. Rotherham Gen. Hosp. Trust; Hon. Lect. Univ. Sheff. Specialty: Radiol. Prev: Cons. Radiol. Rotherham Dist. Hosp. & Hon. Lect. Sheff. Univ.

SPENCER, Pauline Westgate Surgery, Westgate, Otley LS21 3HD Tel: 01943 465406 Fax: 01943 468363; Thorne Croft, Burras Lane, Otley LS21 3EW Tel: 01943 465906 — MB ChB Leeds 1977; BSc (Hons.) Leeds 1974; Dip.Ther 2000. Clin. Asst. Minor Injuries Unit Wharfedale Gen. Hosp. Otley. Specialty: Accid. & Emerg. Socs: Whafedale Med. Soc. Prev: SHO (A & E) Leeds Gen. Infirm.; Ho. Off. Wharfedale Gen. Hosp. Otley.

SPENCER, Mr Peter John West Suffolk Hospitals NHS Trust, Hardwick Lane, Bury St Edmunds IP33 2QZ Tel: 01284 713405; 111 Westley Road, Bury St Edmunds IP33 3SA Tel: 01284 706133 — MB BChir Camb. 1970 (Camb. & St. Thos.) MA Camb. 1970; MRCOG 1978, DObst 1972; FRCS Eng. 1976; FRCS Ed. 1976; FRCOG 1990. Cons. O & G, W. Suff. Hosp., Bury St. Edmunds. Specialty: Obst. & Gyn. Socs: Brit. Soc. Colposcopy & Cervical Path.; Pres. NE. Anglian Obst. & Gyn. Soc. Prev: Clin. Lect. Dept. O & G Univ. Cam. Clin. Sch. Addenbrooke's Hosp.; Sen. Regist. (O & G) Norf. & Norwich Hosp; Regist. (O & G) Birm. & Midl. Hosp. Wom. & Birm. Matern. Hosp.

SPENCER, Philip Mark Doctors Surgery, Friar Row, Caldbeck, Wigton CA7 8DS Tel: 01697 478254 Fax: 01697 478661 — MB

ChB Bristol 1990; PhD Soton. 1986, BSc 1983; Dip. IMC RCS Ed. 1994; MRCGP 1994; DRCOG 1994; Dip. Ther. Newc. 1995.

SPENCER, Rachel May Leeds Road Practice, 49-51 Leeds Road, Harrogate Tel: 01423 885959; High Green, Burton Leonard, Harrogate HG3 3RW — MB ChB Leeds 1989. GP Retainee Harrogate. Specialty: Paediat. Prev: Staff Paediat. Harrogate Gen. Hosp.

SPENCER, Richard Wellesley (retired) 2 Elliscombe Park, Higher Holton, Wincanton BA9 8EA Tel: 01963 824427 — (Birm.) MB ChB Birm. 1944; FRCP Lond. 1975, M 1951; FRCPath 1972, M 1964. Prev: Cons. Chem Path. Cornw. & I. of Scilly DHA.

SPENCER, Robert Christopher Public Health Laboratory, Level 8, Bristol Royal Infirmary, Marlborough St., Bristol BS2 8HW Tel: 0117 928 2879 Fax: 0117 929 9162; 18 Lavender Close, Thornbury, Bristol BS35 1UL Tel: 01454 416454 Fax: 01454 850486 — MB BS Lond. 1970 (St. Mary's) MSc Lond. 1977; FRCPath 1989, M 1977; Hon.DipHIC 1999; FRCPG 1999. Cons. Med. Microbiol. Bristol PHL; Sen. Clin. Lect. Bristol Univ.; Asst. Edr. Jl. Hosp. Infec.; Edr. Jl. Antimicrob. Chemother. Specialty: Med. Microbiol. Socs: Brit. Soc. Antimicrobiol. Chemother.; Hosp. Infec. Soc.; Assn. Clin. Path. Prev: Cons. Bacteriol. Roy. Hallamsh. Hosp. Sheff.; Reader (Experim. & Clin. Microbiol.) Sheff. Univ.

SPENCER, Ruth Elizabeth 41 Old Park Avenue, Enfield EN2 6PJ Tel: 020 8366 6825; Top Floor Flat, 3 Redland Park, Bristol BS6 6SA Tel: 0117 973 7800 — MB ChB Bristol 1988; MRCP (UK) 1992; DTM & H Liverp. 1995; FRCA 1999; CCST (Anaesthesia) 2002. SpR Anaesthetics, Bristol Rotation. Specialty: Anaesth.; Intens. Care. Prev: Clin. Research Fell. (IC) Bristol Roy. Infirm.; SHO (Anaesth.) Southmead Hosp. Bristol; Regist. (Cardiol.) Hereford Co. Hosp.

SPENCER, Ruth Mary — MB ChB Ed. 1988. GP, Homeless Health Serv., Glas. Prev: GP Galston, Ayrsh.; Med. Off. Homeless Addic. Team, Galsgow; GP Parkhead Health Centre, Galsgow.

SPENCER, Sabina Anna 6 Queens Walk, Stamford PE9 2QE — BChir Camb. 1990.

SPENCER, Miss Sarah Elizabeth 39 Gloucester Road, Maidenhead SL6 7SN — MB BS Lond. 1994; FRCS (Eng) 1999.

SPENCER, Seymour Jamie Gerald (retired) 13 Victoria Court, 5 London Road, Headington, Oxford OX3 7SP Tel: 01865 434471 Fax: 01865 434715 Email: sjgspencer@aol.com — (Oxf.) BM BCh Oxf. 1943; DPM Lond. 1951; DM Oxf. 1958; FRCPsych 1975, M 1971. Hon. Cons. Psychiat. Oxf. HA; Sub-Edr. & Contributor Catholic Med. Quarterly. Prev: Clin. Lect. (Psychiat.) Univ. Oxf.

SPENCER, Simon Paul 16 William Peck Road, Spixworth, Norwich NR10 3QB — MB BS Lond. 1998.

SPENCER, Stephen Andrew University Hospital of North Staffordshire (NHS) Trust, Neonatal Unit, Newcastle Road, Stoke-on-Trent ST4 6QG Tel: 01782 552450 Fax: 01782 552481 Email: andy.spencer@uhns.nhs.uk — BM BS Nottm. 1976; DM Nottm. 1983, BMedSci 1974; MRCP (UK) 1979; FRCPCH 1997. Cons. Paediat. Univ. Hosp. N. Staffs.; Hon. Reader (Neonatal Medicine) Univ. Keele. Specialty: Paediat.; Neonat. Socs: Neonat. Soc. Prev: Lect. (Child Health) Nottm. Univ.; Sen. Regist. W. Birm. RHA.

SPENCER, Stephen John Wellesley Worcester Royal Hospital, Charles Hastings Way, Worcester WRS 1DD — MB BS Lond. 1983; BSc Lond. 1980, MD 1993; MRCP (UK) 1986 Fell. 2000. Cons. Phys. & Nephrol. Worcester Roy. Infirm. Specialty: Gen. Med. Prev: Sen. Regist. (Med. & Nephrol.) Soton. Univ. Hosp. Trust.

SPENCER, Stephen Mark Uxbridge Road Surgery, 337 Uxbridge Road, Acton, London W3 9RA Tel: 020 8993 0912; 136 Meadvale Road, Ealing, London W5 1LS Tel: 020 8933 4849 Email: mark.spencer@nhs.net — MB BS Lond. 1984 (Char. Cross & Westm.) DRCOG 1987; MRCGP 1995; FRCGP 2004. GP Adviser to Commissioning and Pub. Health; GP Trainer; Mem. Ealing PCT PEC. Prev: Trainee GP/SHO Hammersmith Hosp. VTS.

SPENCER, Mr Stephen Ralph Calderdale Royal Hospital, Halifax HX3 0PW; Huddersfield Royal Infirmary, Huddersfield HD3 3EA; 28 Lower Mill Lane, Holmfirth, Huddersfield HD9 2JB — MB BS Newc. 1979; DO RCS Eng. 1983; FRCS Eng. 1984; FRCOphth 1989. Cons. Ophth. Calderdale & Huddersfield NHS Trust. Specialty: Ophth. Prev: Sen. Regist. (Ophth.) Yorksh. RHA; Regist. (Ophth.) St. Thos. Hosp. Lond. & Newc. Gen. Hosp.; Research Regist. (Ophth.) Roy. Vict. Infirm. Newc.

SPENCER, Susan Frances Overgate Hospice, 30 Hullenedge Rd, Elland HX5 0QY Tel: 01422 379151; Upper Greystones, Manor Heath Road, Halifax HX3 0EE Tel: 01422 367643 — MB BS Lond. 1978 (St Bartholomew's Hospital) MRCS Eng. LRCP Lond. 1978. Med. Off. (Palliat. Med.) Overgate Hospice Elland. Specialty: Care of the Elderly; Palliat. Med.; Gen. Pract. Prev: Med. Dir. Overgate Hospice, Elland; Trainee GP VTS Calderdale AHA; Clin. Asst. Northowram Hosp. Halifax.

SPENCER, Susan Mary Almondbury Surgery, Westgate, Almondbury, Huddersfield HD5 8XJ Tel: 01484 421391 Fax: 01484 532405 — MB BS Newc. 1979 (Newcastle-upon-Tyne) MRCGP 1983; DRCOG 1983.

SPENCER, Teresa Marian 13 Oakhill Court, Edge Hill, London SW19 4NR — MB ChB Manch. 1955. Prev: Ho. Phys. Roy. Lancaster Infirm.

SPENCER, Mr Timothy Smedley c/o Woking Nuffield Hospital, Shores Road, Woking GU21 4BY Tel: 01483 762897 Fax: 01483 763687; Overmead, 26 Mayfield Road, Weybridge KT13 8XB Tel: 01932 829647 — (Guy's) MRCS Eng. LRCP Lond. 1962; MRCS Eng. LRCP Lond. 1962; MB BS Lond. 1963; MB BS Lond. 1963; FRCOG 1981, M 1968, DObst 1964; FRCOG 1981, M 1968, DObst 1964; FRCS Ed. 1969; FRCS Ed. 1969. Cons. O & G St. Peter's Hosp. Chertsey; Hon. Sen. Lect. St Geo. Hosp. Med. Sch. Specialty: Obst. & Gyn. Socs: Nat. Comm. Anglo French Med. Soc.; Brit. Assn. Med. Managers; Brit. Assn. Med. Managers. Prev: Sen. Regist. Middlx. Hosp., Hosp. Wom. Soho Sq. & Centr. Middlx. Hosp. Lond.; Regist. Middlx. Hosp., Hosp. Wom. Soho Sq. & St Luke's Hosp. Guildford.

SPENCER HAMMON, Catherine Anne — MB ChB Ed. 1997.

SPENCER JONES, Christopher John Wiltshire Health Authority, Southgate House, Pans Lane, Devizes SN10 5EQ Tel: 01380 733764 Fax: 01380 722443; 1 Cranhill Road, Bath BA1 2YF — MB ChB Bristol 1986; MRCGP 1990; MSc Pub. Health Med. Lond. 1992; MFPHM RCP Lond. 1995. Cons. Pub. Health Med. Wilts. HA. Specialty: Pub. Health Med. Prev: Primary Care Med. Adviser Soton. & SW Hants HA; Sen. Regist. (Pub. Health Med.) NW Thames RHA; Trainee GP Exeter VTS.

SPENCER-JONES, Julia Mary Tutbury Health Centre, Monk Street, Tutbury, Burton-on-Trent DE13 9NA Tel: 01283 812210 Fax: 01283 815810; Sandalwood, 34 Church Road, Rolleston-on-Dove, Burton-on-Trent DE13 9BE Tel: 01283 813433 — MB BChir Camb. 1973 (Cambridge & St. Bartholomew's London) MA Camb. 1974, MB BChir 1973; DObst RCOG 1975; DCH Eng. 1976; MRCGP 1977. Princip. in Gen. Pract. Specialty: Gen. Pract. Prev: Trainee Gen. Pract. Northampton Vocational Train. Scheme.

SPENCER-JONES, Roland Godfrey Tutbury Health Centre, Monk Street, Tutbury, Burton-on-Trent DE13 9NA Tel: 01283 812210 Fax: 01283 815810; 1 Callow End Cottages, Mappleton, Ashbourne DE6 2AB Tel: 01335 350455 — MB BChir Camb. 1974 (Camb. & St. Thos.) MA Camb. 1974; DObst RCOG 1975; MRCP (UK) 1976; MRCGP 1977. Med. Educat.; Co-Founder 'Scaling the Heights'. Specialty: Gen. Pract. Prev: Trainee GP Northampton VTS.

SPENCER-PALMER, Caroline Mary Colne Health Centre, Market Street, Colne BB8 0LJ Tel: 01282 862451 Fax: 01282 871698; 5 Woolpack, off Lenches Road, Colne BB8 8HQ Tel: 01282 870718 — MB BS Lond. 1979 (Lond. Hosp.) DRCOG 1982; MRCGP 1984. Gen.ist - Specialist to Community Drug Team, Burnley. Socs: Balint Soc. Prev: SHO (Pychiat.) Burnley Gen. Hosp.; Paediat. Save The Childr. Fund; SHO (Hospice Home Care Team) St. Josephs Hospice Lond.

SPENCER-SILVER, Professor Peter Hele Barclays Bank, Jewry St., Winchester SO23 8RG — (Middlx.) PhD (Anat.) Lond. 1952, MB BS 1945; MRCS Eng. LRCP Lond. 1945. Emerit. Prof. Anat. Univ. Lond. Socs: Anat. Soc. & Physiol. Soc. Prev: S.A. Ct.auld Prof. Anat. Univ. Lond.; Prof. Embryol. Univ. Lond.; Sub-Dean Middlx. Hosp. Med. Sch.

SPENCER-SMITH, Elizabeth Margery (retired) 71 Bell Barn Road, Stoke Bishop, Bristol BS9 2DF Tel: 0117 968 3148 — MB ChB Bristol 1949; FRCGP 1978, M 1951. Prev: Mem. Southmead Dist. HA Dist. Managem. Team.

SPENCER-SMITH, Maxwell Ocean Medical, 19/23 Canute Road, Southampton SO14 3FJ Tel: 023 8022 3546 Fax: 02380 228446 — MB BS Lond. 1967 (Middlx. Hosp. Med. Sch.) MRCS Eng. LRCP Lond. 1967; DRCOG 1970; MRCGP 1980; T(GP) 1991; AFOM RCP

Lond. 1992. Cons. Occupat. Phys. Ocean Med. Serv. Specialty: Occupat. Health; Gen. Pract. Socs: Soc. Occupat. Med.; Fac. Occupat.al Helpline; Internat. Maritine Health Assn. Prev: Regional Med. Off. Gen. Counc. of Brit. Shipping; Sen. Phys. King Faisal Specialist Hosp. & Research Centre, Riyadh, Saudi Arabia.

SPENDER, Quentin Wynn Child and Family Service for Mental Health, Orchard House, 9 College Lane, Chichester PO19 6PQ Tel: 01234 815514 Fax: 01234 815499 Email: quentin.spender@swdnhst.thenhs.com; 16 Hemingford Road, Sutton SM3 8HG Tel: 020 8644 8245/0208 644 9009 Email: quentin.spender@btinternet.com — MB BS Lond. 1979 (Roy. Free) DCH RCP Lond. 1981; MRCP (UK) 1983; MRCPsych 1990; Dip Family Ther (IFT) 1996; FRCPCH 2002. Cons. & Sen. Lect. W. Sussex Health & Social Care NHS Trust; Sen. Lect. St. Geo. Hosp. Med. Sch. Lond. 1995; Hon. Cons. St Georges and SW Lond. NHS Trust. Specialty: Child & Adolesc. Psychiat. Socs: Child Psychiat. Research Soc. Scientif. & Med. Network. Prev: Regist. Rotat. (Psychiat.) Oxf. Train. Scheme; Exchange Regist. Childr. Hosp. Philadelphia Pennsylvania, USA; Regist. (Paediat.) Hosp. Sick Childr. Gt. Ormond St. Lond.

SPENS, Fiona Jane Whitethorn House, 2 Perth Road, Milnathort, Kinross KY13 9XU — MB BS Newc. 1983; DRCOG 1987; MRCGP 1987. GP Principal Bannockburn, Stirlingshire.

SPENS, Heather Julie Royal Infirmary of Edinburgh, Department of Anaesthetics, Little France Crescent, Edinburgh EH16 4SA Tel: 0131 536 3652 — MB ChB Ed. 1986; FRCA 1991. Cons. Anaesth. Roy. Infirm. Edin. Edin. Specialty: Anaesth. Prev: Sen. Regist. (Anaesth.) Lothian Area Train. Scheme.

SPENSLEY, Charis Anne Dartford West Health Centre, Tower Road, Dartford DA1 2HA — MB ChB Leeds 1989; MRCP (UK) 1995. Specialty: Gen. Pract.

SPENSLEY, Kathryn Margaret Ruby 14 Old School Court, Lewes Road, Lindfield RH16 2LD — BM BS Nottm. 1997.

SPENSLEY, Paul James 6 Conisbord Way, Caversham Heights, Reading RG4 7HT — BM BS Nottm. 1997.

SPERBER, Galia 8 Freston Park, London N3 1UP — MB ChB Liverp. 1998.

SPERRING, Steven Jeffrey 2221 Old Hickory Boulevard, Nashville TN 37215, USA; Norley House, 1 Furness Road, Eastbourne BN21 4EX Tel: 01323 647392 — MB BS Lond. 1978 (Guy's) FFA RCS Eng. 1982. Fellowship Prize Fac. Anaesth. RCS 1982; Staff Anaesthesiol. Hermann Hosp. Houston, USA; Asst. Prof. Univ. Texas Med. Sch. Houston. Specialty: Anaesth. Socs: Obst. Anaesth. Assn. Prev: Staff Anesthesiol. Beth Israel Hosp. Boston, USA; Instruct. Anesthesiol. Harvard Med. Sch. Camb., USA; Regist. (Anaesth.) Guy's Hosp. Lond.

SPERRY, Lynn Margaret 41 Norman Avenue, Abingdon OX14 2HJ — MB BS Lond. 1987; BSc Lond. 1984, MB BS 1987.

SPERRY, Tanya Lesley Helen Humberstone Park Surgery, 190 Uppingham Road, Leicester LE5 0QG Tel: 0116 276 6605 — MB ChB Leic. 1981; MRCGP 1985; DRCOG 1985. GP Leicester.

SPIBY, Jacqueline Global House, Hayes, Bromley BR2 7EH Tel: 020 8462 2211; Heathside, 15 The Meadow, Chislehurst BR7 6AA — MB BS Lond. 1978; FFPHM RCP (UK) 1994. Dir. Pub. Health Bromley HA. Specialty: Pub. Health Med.

SPICE, Claire Louise Royal Hampshire County Hospital, Winchester SO22 5DG — BM Soton. 1993. Specialty: Care of the Elderly.

SPICER, Alan John, Col. late RAMC Occupational Health Unit, Kent Police Headquaters, Maidstone ME15 9BZ Tel: 01622 690690 — MB BS Lond. 1959 (King's Coll. Hosp.) MRCS Eng. LRCP Lond. 1959; FRCP Lond. 1983, M 1968; DCH Eng. 1970; DTM & H Eng. 1973; MD Lond. 1979. Sen. Occupat. Phys. Kent Police Force. Specialty: Gen. Med. Socs: Fell. Roy. Soc. Health.; Soc. Occupat. Med. Prev: Cons. Phys. Camb. Milit. Hosp. Aldershot; Cons. Phys. Brit. Milit. Hosp. Rinteln; Cons. Phys. Qu. Eliz. Milit. Hosp. Lond.

SPICER, Dominic David Mark Barths and the London NHS Trust, London E1 1BB — MB BS Lond. 1989; FRCS 1994; FRCS (Orth.) 2000. Cons. (Ortho. Surg.) Barts & Lond. NHS Trust.

SPICER, John Edmund Andrew Woodside Health Centre, 3 Enmore Road, South Norwood, London SE25 5NS Tel: 020 8656 5790 Fax: 020 8656 7984 Email: jspicer@sghms.ac.uk — MB BS Lond. 1977 (Middlesex) DFFP 1982; MRCGP 1984; MA 1999; FRCGP 2001. Assoc. Director, S. E. Sector, Lond. Deanery; Clin. Tutor in Med. Law & Ethics, St Georges Hosp. Med. Sch.

SPICER, Nicholas Adrian Albert Nunwell Surgery, 10 Pump Street, Bromyard HR7 4BZ Tel: 01885 483412 Fax: 01885 488739; The Old Rectory, Malvern Road, Stanford Bishop, Worcester WR6 5TT Tel: 01886 884058 Fax: 01886 884734 — MB ChB Birm. 1977.

SPICER, Nicola Ann Joy Kingsley Withycombe Lodge Surgery, 123 Torquay Road, Paignton TQ3 2SG Tel: 01803 525525; Darracott, Jubilee Rd, Totnes TQ9 5BW Tel: 01803 864124 — MB BS Lond. 1985 (Kings Coll. Sch. of Med. and Dent., Lond.) DRCOG 1987; MRCGP 1989. Gen. Practitioner Princip.

SPICER, Mrs Rachel Faith Elizabeth Haughton, OBE (retired) 31 Aberdeen Park, London N5 2AR; Cave Cottage, West Wycombe Hill Road, High Wycombe HP14 3AH Tel: 01494 524573 — (W. Lond.) MB BS Lond. 1944. Prev: Dir. Lond. Youth Advis. & Med. Dir. Brook Advis. Centres.

SPICER, Ranald John Waverley Medical Centre, Dhrymple Street, Stranraer DG9 7DW — MB ChB Aberd. 1976; MRCGP 1980; DA Eng. 1985; FFA RCSI 1986. Cons. Anaesth. Garrick Hosp. Stranraer; Regist. (Anaesth.) W. Infirm. & S. Gen. Hosp. Glas. Specialty: Anaesth. Prev: SHO (Anaesth.) Dumfries & Galloway Infirm.; Ho. Phys. (Gen. Med.) & Ho. Surg. (Gen. Surg.) Raigmore Hosp.; Inverness.

SPICER, Mr Richard Dudley Department of Paediatric Surgery, Bristol Children's Hospital, St Michael's Hill, Bristol BS2 8BJ Tel: 0117 928 5708 Fax: 0117 928 5701 — MB BS Lond. 1968 (Guy's) MRCS Eng. LRCP Lond. 1968; DCH Eng. 1973; FRCS Eng. 1974; FRCPCH 1997. Cons. Paediat. Surg. Bristol Childr. Hosp.; Sen. Clin. Lect. (Paediat. Surg.) Univ. Bristol. Specialty: Paediat. Surg. Socs: (Sec. & Hon. Treas.) Soc. Paediat. Surgic. Oncol.; (Exec.) Brit. Assn. Paediat. Surgs.; Société Internat. D'Oncol. Paediat. Prev: Cons. Paediat. Surg. Leeds; Cons. Paediat. Surg. Muscat, Oman.

SPICKETT, Gavin Patrick Regional Department of Immunology, Royal Victoria Infirmary, Queen Victoria Road, Newcastle upon Tyne NE1 4LP Tel: 0191 282 5517 Fax: 0191 282 5070 — BM BCh Oxf. 1980 (Oxford) DPhil. Oxf. 1983, MA 1981; MRCP (UK) 1985; MRCPath 1990; T(Path) 1991; T(M) 1991; FRCP Lond. 1995; FRCPath 1999; FRCPE 2003. Cons. & Sen. Lect. Immunol. Roy. Vict. Infirm. Specialty: Immunol.; Gen. Med. Socs: Brit. Soc. Allergy & Clin. Immunol.; Brit. Soc. Immunol. Prev: Clin. Scientist & Hon. Sen. Regist. Clin. Research Centre Harrow; Regist. (Med.) The Ipswich Hosp.; Mary Goodger Research Schol. MRC Cellular Immunol. Research Unit Oxf.

SPIEGLER, William John The Surgery, 30 North Street, Ashby-de-la-Zouch LE65 1HS Tel: 01530 417415 — MB ChB Birm. 1978 (Birmingham Medical School) DRCOG 1982; MRCGP 1983. Clin. Teach. (Gen. Pract.) Fac.

SPIER, Adolph 24 Merryfield Gardens, Marsh Lane, Stanmore HA7 4TG Tel: 020 8954 6612 — MD Lyon 1940 (Dijon)

SPIER, Gareth Walter City Medical Services Ltd., 17 St.Helen's Place, London EC3A 6DG Tel: 020 7638 7090 Fax: 020 7256 5295 Email: gspier@citymedical.co.uk; 106 Kenilworth Court, Lower Richmond Road, London SW15 1HA Tel: 020 8785 2452 Fax: 020 8788 7265 — MB ChB Liverp. 1965. Med. Dir. City Med. Servs. Lond.; Non-Exec. Dir. Lond. Ambul. Serv. NHS Trut. Specialty: Gen. Med.; Occupat. Health; Sports Med. Socs: Fell.Roy.Coll.Med; Soc. Occupat. Med.; Amer. Occupat. Med. Assn. Prev: Ho. Phys. & Ho. Surg. Clatterbridge Hosp. Bebington; Sen. Ho. Surg. (Orthop.) & Cas. Off. Liverp. Roy. Infirm.

SPIER, Sarah Joanne Redwood House Practice, Redwood House, Cannon Lane, Maidenhead SL6 3PH Tel: 01628 826227 Fax: 01628 829426; Ellums, Cockpole Green, Wargrave, Reading RG10 8NT Tel: 0118 940 3849 — MB ChB Manch. 1991. Specialty: Gen. Pract. Socs: Windsor Med. Soc.; Roy. Soc. Med.

SPIERS, Alexander S D Royal Devon & Exeter Hospital, Barrack Road, Exeter EX2 5DW Email: alexander.spiers@rdehc-tr.swest.nhs.uk — BM BCh Oxf. 1986; BA Oxon 1983; MRCP Lond. 1989; FRCR Lond. 1993. Const (Radiol.) Roy. Devon & Exeter Hosp. Specialty: Radiol. Special Interest: Cross-sectional imaging.

SPIERS, David Ronald Raleigh Surgery, 33 Pines Road, Exmouth EX8 5NH Tel: 01395 222499 Fax: 01395 225493; 39 Regents Gate, Exmouth EX8 1TR Tel: 01395 275562 Fax: 01395 266882 Email: drs@davidspiers.free-online.co.uk — MB ChB Leic. 1983

(Leicester) MRCGP 1988. GP; Cons. Pharmaceut. Med. DRS Servs. Exmouth. Specialty: Pharmaceutical Medicine. Socs: BMA. Prev: Head of UK CVS Research E. Merck Pharmaceut.; Med. Adviser SmithKline & French; SHO (Chest Med.) Warwick Hosp.

SPIERS, Diana Patricia Jockey Road Medical Centre, 519 Jockey Road, Sutton Coldfield B73 5DF Tel: 0121 354 3050 Fax: 0121 355 1840; 33 Beech Hill Road, Sutton Coldfield B72 1BY — MB ChB Birm. 1978.

SPIERS, Elizabeth May Lubnaig, 442 Blackness Road, Dundee DD2 1TQ Tel: 01382 667547 — MB BS Lond. 1966 (Middlx.) MRCP (UK) 1971. Assoc. Specialist (Immunol.) Ninewells Hosp. Dundee. Specialty: Immunol. Prev: Regist. (Haemat.) Univ. Hosp. Wales Cardiff & Ninewells Hosp. Dundee.

SPIERS, James Martin Mill Bank Surgery, Water Street, Stafford ST16 2AG Tel: 01785 258348 Fax: 01785 227144 — BM BS Nottm. 1984; MRCGP 1989. Prev: Trainee GP Pembrokesh. VTS.

SPIERS, Martin Richard Harrogate Road Surgery, 23 Harrogate Road, Bradford BD2 3DY Tel: 01274 639857 Fax: 01274 627006 — MB ChB Leeds 1973; DObst RCOG 1975. Prev: SHO (O & G) St. Jas. Hosp. Leeds; SHO (Infec. Dis.) Seacroft Hosp. Leeds.

SPIERS, Richard John Stepping Stones Medical Practice, Stafford Street, Dudley DY1 1RT Tel: 01384 459966 Fax: 01384 459885 — MB ChB Leeds 1977; DRCOG 1981.

SPIERS, Richard Jonathan Greater Peterborough Primary Care Partnership, Town Hall, Peterborough Email: richard.spiers@nhs.net; Windmill Cottage, 8 Tinwell Road, Stamford PE9 2QQ Email: richard@windmill3.demon.co.uk — MB BS Lond. 1975 (St. Mary's) MRCS Eng. LRCP Lond. 1975; MRCGP 1982; DAvMed FOM RCP Lond. 1985; Dip. Pharm. Med. RCP (UK) 1992; MFPM 2002. Gen. Practitioner. Specialty: Pharmaceutical Medicine; Gen. Pract. Special Interest: Primry care Respirat. Med. Prev: Med. Dir. 3M Health Care UK & Irel..; Wing Cdr. RAF Med. Br.

SPIERS, Stanley Paule (retired) 15 Welland Road, Barrow upon Soar, Loughborough LE12 — MB BS Lond. 1952 (Char. Cross) DObst RCOG 1958; BA (Law) CNAA 1982.

SPIES, John Anthony (retired) Priory Medical Practice, 48 Bromham Road, Bedford MK40 2QD Tel: 01234 262040 Fax: 01234 219288; Mistletoe Cottage, Grange Road, Felmersham, Bedford MK43 7HJ Tel: 01234 782088 — (St. Geo.) MB BS Lond. 1963; DCH Eng. 1966; MRCP Lond. 1969; MSc (Social Med.) Lond. 1972. Prev: Lect. (Community Paediat.) St. Mary's Hosp. Med. Sch. Lond.

SPIKKER, Angela Claire Wilhelmina 44 Wellmeadow Lane, Uppermill, Oldham OL3 6DX — LRCPI & LM, LRSCI & LM 1971; LRCPI & LM, LRCSI & LM 1971; DCH NUI 1973; DObst RCPI 1974.

SPILG, Edward George Gartnavel General Hospital, Department of Medicine for the Elderly, 1053 Great Western Road, Glasgow G12 0YN Tel: 0141 211 3166/0141 211 3465 Email: ed.spilg@northglasgow.scot.nhs.uk — MB ChB (Hons.) Glas. 1990; MRCP UK 1993; FRCP Glas. 2001. Cons (Ger. Med.) Garnavel Gen. Hosp. Glas.; hon. Clin. Sen. Lect Univ Glas. Specialty: Care of the Elderly. Prev: Career Regist. (Geriat. Med.) Roy. Infirm. Glas.; Sen. Regist. (Geriat. Med.) Gartnavel Gen. Hosp. Glas.; Sen. Regist (Gen Med) Vict. Inf. Glas.

SPILG, Sandra Jane Pollokshaws Doctors Centre, 26 Wellgreen, Glasgow G43 1RR Tel: 0141 632 8883 Fax: 0141 636 0654 — MB ChB Glas. 1988; DRCOG 1991; MRCGP 1992. Socs: S.. Med. Soc. & BMA. Prev: Trainee GP Glas.

SPILG, Walter Gerson Spence 4B Newton Court, Newton Grove, Newton Mearns, Glasgow G77 5QL Tel: 0141 639 3130 Fax: 0141 616 2190 — (Glas. Univ.) MB ChB (Hons.) Glas. 1964; FRCPath 1982, M 1970; MRCP (Glas.) 1986; FRCP Glas. 1988. Specialty: Histopath. Socs: Assn. Clin. Path.; BMA; Internat. Acad. Path. Prev: Cons. Path. i/c Glas. Vict. Infirm. & Assoc. Hosps. (1972-99); Hon. Clin. Sen. Lect. Univ. Glas.; Lect. (Path.) West. Infirm. Glas.

SPILLANE, Kathleen Department of Clinical Neurophysiology, Ninewells Hospital, Dundee DD1 9SY — MB BCh Wales 1988; PhD Leeds 1982, BSc (Hons.) 1979; MRCPI 1996. Cons. Clin. Neurophysiol. Ninewells Hosp., Dundee; Hon. Sen. Lect. Univ. Dundee. Specialty: Clin. Neurophysiol. Socs: BSCN. Prev: Cons. (Neurophysiol.) St James' Univ. Hosp. Leeds; Sen. Regist. (Neurophysiol.) St. Bart. Hosp. Lond.; SHO (Gen. Med.) Qu. Eliz. Hosp. & Gen. Hosp. Birm.

SPILLER, Jayne Elizabeth Greenmeadow Farm, Llangynwyd, Maesteg CF34 9RU — MB BCh Wales 1994.

SPILLER, Juliet Anne Marie Curie Hospice Edinburgh, Frogston Road West, Fairmilehead, Edinburgh EH10 7DR Tel: 0131 470 2201 Fax: 0131 470 2200 Email: juliet.spiller@mariecurie.org.uk — MB ChB Aberd. 1993; BMedSci Aberd. 1993; MRCP Edin. 1997. Cons. in Palliat. Med., Marie Curie Hospice, Edin.; Cons. in Palliat. Med., W. Lothian Integrated Trust. Specialty: Palliat. Med. Socs: Assn. of Palliat. Med.; Palliat. Care Research Soc.; Brit. Psychosocial Oncol. Soc. Prev: SHO (Infec. Dis.s, Palliat. Med. & Psychol. Med.); Specialist Regist., Palliat. med.

SPILLER, Penelope Anne St. Mary's Hospice, 176 Raddlebarn Road, Birmingham B29 7DA Tel: 0121 472 1191; The Parsonage, Sambourne Lane, Sambourne, Redditch B96 6PA Tel: 01527 892372 — MB BS Lond. 1972 (Royal Free Hospital School of Medicine) MRCS Eng. LRCP Lond. 1972; DCH Eng. 1977; DRCOG 1978; Dip. Palliat. Med. Wales 1996. Clin. Asst. (Palliat. Med.) St. Mary's Hospice Birm. Specialty: Palliat. Med. Prev: GP Warks..

SPILLER, Richard Wallace The Health Centre, 10 Gresham Road, Oxted RH8 0BQ Tel: 01883 832850 Fax: 01883 832851 — MB BS Lond. 1973; MRCP (UK) 1976.

SPILLER, Professor Robin Charles Wolfson Digestive Diseases Centre, C Floor, South Block, University Hospital, Nottingham NG7 2UH Tel: 0115 924 9924 Ext: 35077/44548 Fax: 0115 942 2232 — MB BChir Camb. 1975 (Univ. Coll. Hosp.) FRCP; MRCP (UK) 1977; MD Cantab. 1985. Prof. Gastoenterology & Hon. Cons. Phys. Univ. Hosp. Nottm. Specialty: Gastroenterol. Special Interest: Functional bowel Dis.; Neurogastroenterology. Prev: Cons. Physician, Univ. Hosp. 1988-1998; Sen. Regist. (Gastroenterol.) Centr. Middlx. & St. Mary's Hosps. 1985-1987.

SPILLING, Roy Alfred Eadie 160 Banbury Road, Oxford OX2 7BS Tel: 01865 515552 — BM BCh Oxf. 1968 (Oxf. & Lond. Hosp.) MA Oxf. 1969, BM BCh 1968; DObst RCOG 1970; DCH Eng. 1971; MRCGP 1976. Prev: Dep. Res. Med. Off. Qu. Eliz Hosp. Childr. Lond.; Sen. Res. Accouch. & Ho. Surg. Orthop. Unit Lond. Hosp.

SPILLMAN, Ian David Macclesfield District General Hospital, Victoria Road, Macclesfield SK10 3BL Tel: 01625 661302 Fax: 01625 663055 Email: ian.spillman@echeshire-tr.nwest.nhs.uk; 138 Prestbury Road, Macclesfield SK10 3BN — MB BS Lond. 1978 (Roy. Free) DA Eng. 1981; DCH RCP Lond. 1982; DTM & H RCP Lond. 1984; MRCP (UK) 1985; FRCPCH 1994. Cons. Paediat. Macclesfield Dist. Gen. Hosp.; Clin. Lect. Liverp. Univ. Specialty: Paediat. Socs: Christ. Med. Fellowsh.; FRCPCH; Brit. Paediatric Respirat. Soc. Prev: Sen. Regist. (Paediat.) Luton & Dunstable Hosp.; Med. Supt. Kisiizi Hosp. SW Uganda; Tutor (Child Health) Qu. Eliz. Hosp. for Childr. Lond.

SPILSBURY, Bernard Gwilym (retired) The Gables, Church Lane, Thrumpton, Nottingham NG11 0AW Tel: 0115 983 1020 — MB ChB Birm. 1951. Prev: Med. Off. RAF.

SPILSBURY, Richard Adrian (retired) Steeplechase, Horse & Groom Lane, Galleywood, Chelmsford CM2 8PJ — MB BS Lond. 1962 (King's Coll. Hosp.) MRCS Eng. LRCP Lond. 1962; DA Eng. 1965; FFA RCS Eng. 1967. Cons. Anaesth. Chelmsford Hosp. Gp. Prev: Sen. Regist. (Anaesth.) Lond. Hosp.

SPINCER, John Lister House Surgery, Lister House, 53 Harrington Street, Pear Tree, Derby DE23 8PF Tel: 01332 271212 Fax: 01332 271939; Post Office Farm, 18 Rectory Lane, Breadsall Village, Derby DE21 5LL — MB ChB Leeds 1976; PhD Leeds 1969, BSc 1966; DRCOG 1981; MRCGP 1981. GP Derby; Tutor GP Derby; Sen. Phys. (Occupat. Health) S. Derby Community Trust; Clin. Asst. Nightingale McMillan Unit Derby; Princip. Police Surg. Derbysh. Constab. Specialty: Occupat. Health. Socs: Derbysh. Med. Soc. Prev: Capt. RAMC; Med. Off. 3rd Bn. Light Infantry Catterick Garrison.

SPINDLER, Kim Danielle — MB ChB Manch. 1997.

SPINK, Carina Elizabeth Ann Rose, Spink, Smith and Walker, Spring Terrace Health Centre, Spring Terrace, North Shields NE29 0HQ Tel: 0191 296 1588 Fax: 0191 296 2901 — MB ChB Manch. 1981 (Manchester) DRCOG 1986; DCCH RCGP & FCM 1989; MFHom 1997. GP Princip. Specialty: Gen. Pract.; Homeop. Med. Prev: SHO (Community Paediat.) NW Durh.; Clin. Med. Off. SW Surrey HA; SHO (Paediat.) Bolton HA.

SPINK, Farley Richard Mead House, Wheelers Lane, Brockham, Betchworth RH3 7HJ Tel: 01737 842848 — MB BChir Camb. 1954; MFHom 1959; FFHom 2001. Specialty: Homeop. Med.

SPINK, John Douglas (retired) Timmins, Henley Road, Marlow SL7 2BZ Tel: 01628 483678 — (King's Coll. Hosp.) MB BS Lond. 1955; MRCS Eng. LRCP Lond. 1955. Prev: Med. Off. HM Young Offender Inst. Finnamore Wood Marlow.

SPINK, Malini Farnham Health Centre, Brightwells, East Street, Farnham GU9 7SA Tel: 01252 723122 Email: ros_goddard@hotmail.com — MB ChB Bristol 1981; DRCOG 1985; MRCGP 1985; DA (UK) 1987. Prev: Trainee GP/SHO Chase Farm Hosp. Enfield VTS; SHO (A & E & Anaesth.) Weston-Super-Mare Gen. Hosp.

SPINK, Margaret 3 Castle Drive, Berwick-upon-Tweed TD15 1NS — MB BS Durh. 1955.

SPINK, Mrs Prudence (retired) The Finches, Brancaster Staithe, King's Lynn PE31 8BW — MRCS Eng. LRCP Lond. 1940 (Lond. Sch. Med. Wom.)

SPINK, Spencer Charles Euan (retired) Barnholm, Back Lane, Easingwold, York YO61 3BW Tel: 01347 821562 Fax: 01347 821562 — MB ChB Ed. 1956; DA Eng. 1962. Prev: GP York.

SPINKS, Brian Christopher Department of Radiology, Chorley & South Ribble District General Hospital, Preston Road, Chorley PR7 1PP Tel: 01257 245868 Fax: 01257 247130; Whinfell, 767 Belmont Road, Bolton BL1 7BY Tel: 01204 309109 Fax: 01204 596718 Email: chris.spinks@lineone.net — MB ChB Dundee 1980 (Univ. Dundee) FRCR 1988. Cons. Radiol. Chorley & S. Ribble Dist. Gen. Hosp. Specialty: Radiol. Socs: BMA. Prev: Ho. Off. & SHO Hull Roy. Infirm. & W.wood Hosp. Beverley; Regist. (Radiol.) Northwick Pk. Hosp. & Clin. Research Centre Harrow; Sen. Regist. Rotat. (Radiol.) N. Manch. Gen. Hosp. & Hope Hosp. Salford.

SPINKS, Joanne 32 Heathermount Dr, Crowthorne RG45 6HN — BM Soton. 1997.

SPINKS, Julian Thomas William Court View Surgery, 2A Darnley Road, Strood, Rochester ME2 2HA Tel: 01634 290333 Fax: 01634 295131; 7 Keefe Close, Bluebell Hill, Chatham ME5 9AG — MB BS Lond. 1984 (St. Geo.) BSc (Hons.) Lond. 1981; DGM RCP Lond. 1986. Bd. Mem. Rochester & Strood PCG. Specialty: Diabetes. Socs: (Sec.) Medway Fundholders Assn.; GP Writers Assoc. Prev: Trainee GP Rochester VTS; Ho. Surg. St. Bart. Hosp. Rochester; Ho. Phys. St. Helier Hosp. Carshalton Surrey.

SPINKS, Margaret Jane Woodhouse Medical Centre, 5 Skelton Lane, Woodhouse, Sheffield S13 7LY Tel: 0114 269 2049 Fax: 0114 269 6539 — MB ChB Manch. 1982; DRCOG 1985; MRCGP 1986.

SPINOZA, Marc Howard 18 Cuffley Hill, Goff's Oak, Cheshunt, Waltham Cross EN7 5EU — MB BS Lond. 1994.

SPINTY, Stefan 57 Carr Manor Drive, Leeds LS17 5AP — State Exam Med Hamburg 1991.

SPIRA, Michael Ashcroft Road Surgery, 26 Ashcroft Road, Stopsley Green, Luton LU2 9AU Tel: 01582 722555 Fax: 01582 418145; North Limbersey Farm, Maulden, Bedford MK45 2EA Tel: 01525 841381 Fax: 01525 841387 — (St. Bart.) MRCS Eng. LRCP Lond. 1967; MB BS Lond. 1968. Med. Cons. Weight Managem. UK Ltd. Socs: Brit. Soc. Med. & Dent. Hypn.; Assn. Study Obesity; NLP Certified Practitioner. Prev: Phys. Inst. of Dir.s & BUPA Med. Centre, Lond.; SHO (O & G) St. Margt.'s Hosp. Epping; Ho. Surg. Eye Dept. St. Bart. Hosp. Lond.

SPIRES, Robert Christopher Stewart Davenal House Surgery, 28 Birmingham Road, Bromsgrove B61 0DD Tel: 01527 872008 — MB ChB Birm. 1965; DObst RCOG 1967. Prev: SHO O & G Nottm. City Hosp.; SHO Clin. Path. Birm. Gen. Hosp.; Ho. Surg. City Gen. Hosp. Stoke-on-Trent.

SPIRO, David Michael Cavendish Health Centre, 53 New Cavendish Street, London W1G 9TQ Tel: 020 7487 5244 Email: david.spiro@nhs.net; 120 West Heath Road, London NW3 7TX Email: dms@dspiro.com — MB BChir Camb. 1982 (Cambridge) MA Camb. 1982; DRCOG 1984; Cert. Family Plann. JCC 1986; MRCGP 1995. GP. Specialty: Gen. Pract. Socs: Fell. Roy. Soc. Med.

SPIRO, Jonathan Gabriel Capita Health Solutions, B220.28, Harwell Business Centre, Didcot OX11 0RA Tel: 01235 434077 Fax: 01235 435297; The Granary, E. Challow, Wantage OX12 9SS Tel: 01235 763180 — MB BS Lond. 1979 (Westm.) MA Camb. 1979; MRCP (UK) 1982; MFOM Lond. 1997. Sen. Occupat. Phys. Occupat. Health, Capita Health Solutions. Specialty: Occupat. Health. Socs: Soc. Occupat. Med.; BMA. Prev: Regist. Roy. Vict. Infirm. Newc., Sunderland Roy. Infirm. & Luton & Dunstable Hosp.

SPIRO, Mr Martin (retired) The Red House, Epping Road, Toothill, Ongar CM5 9SQ Tel: 01992 522402 Email: spirotoothill@talk21.com — MB BChir Camb. 1955 (King's Coll. Hosp.) MA Camb. 1955, MChir 1967, MB BChir 1955; FRCS Eng. 1964; FRCS Ed. 1964. Prev: Cons. Gen. & Periph. Vasc. Surg. Barking HA.

SPIRO, Martin (retired) 18A Hendon Avenue, London N3 1UE Tel: 020 8346 1559 — (Newc.) MB BS Durh. 1945; DMRD Eng. 1948. Prev: Cons. Radiol. Manor Hse. Hosp. Lond.

SPIRO, Professor Stephen George The Middlesex Hospital, Dept of Respiratary Medicine, Mortimer Street, London W1M 8HA Tel: 020 7380 9004; 66 Grange Gardens, Pinner HA5 5QF Tel: 020 8868 1815 — (Manch.) BSc (Hons. Anat.) Manch. 1964, MD 1975, MB ChB 1967; FRCP (UK) 1981, M 1969. Cons. Phys. Gen. & Thoracic Med. Univ. Coll. Lond. Hosps. Trust; Hon. Sen. Lect. Univ. Lond.; Prof. Respirat. Med.; Clin. Director, Med. Serv.s UCLH. Specialty: Respirat. Med. Socs: Past Pres. Europ. Respirat. Soc.; Prog. Comm. Amer.Thoracic Soc.; Pres. Brit. Thoracic Soc. 2004. Prev: Cons. Phys. Roy. Brompton Hosp. Lond.; Exec. Edr. Thorax; Pres. Europ. Respirat. Soc.

SPITERI, Hector Paul Cameron Road Surgery, 40 Cameron Road, Seven Kings, Ilford IG3 8LF Fax: 020 8599 0282 — MRCS Eng. LRCP Lond. 1982 (Lond. Hosp.) FRCGP 2001 DFFP; MRCGP 1987; T(GP) 1991. GP Ilford; Clin. Asst. (Neurol.) King Geo. Hosp. Ilford; Clin. Governance Lead Redbridge PCG; Chairm. Redbridge GP on Call (Out of Hours CoOperat.); Bd./Exec. Comm. Mem., Redbridge. Socs: BMA (Former Chairm. Redbridge & Stratford Div.); Redbridge & Waltham Forest Local Med. Comm.(former Chairm.); Ilford Med. Soc. (Vice Pres.).

SPITTAL, Murray James Anaesthetic Department, Pilgrim Hospital, Sibsey Road, Boston PE21 9QS — MB ChB Leeds 1983; DA (UK) 1987; FRCA 1989. Head of Serv., Anaesthetic Dept. Specialty: Anaesth. Socs: MDU & Assn. Anaesth.; UHMS; ICS. Prev: Cons. Anaesth.TPMH, RAF Alcrotiri; Cons. Anaesth. Princess Alexandra Hosp. RAF Wroughton; Hon. Sen. Regist. (Anaesth.) Bristol Roy. Infirm.

SPITTLE, Margaret Flora, OBE Meyerstein Institute of Oncology, The Middlesex Hospital, Mortimer Street, London W1T 3AA Tel: 020 7380 9090 Fax: 020 7436 0160; The Manor House, Beaconsfield Road, Claygate, Esher KT10 0PW Tel: 01372 465540 Fax: 01372 470470 — (Westm.) AKC 1963; MRCS Eng. LRCP Lond. 1963; MB BS Lond. 1963; DMRT Eng. 1966; FRCR 1968; MSc (Radiobiol.) Lond. 1969; FRCP Lond. 1995. Cons. Clin. Oncol. Meyerstein Inst. Oncol. Middlx. Hosp. Lond.; Cons. Radiother. St. John's Centre Dis. Skin St. Thos. Hosp. Lond.; Hon. Cons. Radiother. Roy. Nat. Throat, Nose and Ear Hosp.. Lond.; Chairm. UK AIDS Oncol. Gp. Specialty: Oncol.; Radiother.; Oncol.; Radiother. Special Interest: Breast cancer; Head & neck cancer; Skins & Gen. Oncol. Socs: (Pres..Open Sect.) Roy. Soc. Med.; (Library Comm.) Brit. Inst. Radiol.; Chair UK AIDS Onc. Gp. Prev: Sen. Regist. (Radiother.) Westm. Hosp. Lond.; Instruc. Stanford Univ. Med. Center, USA; Dean Roy. Coll. Radiol.

SPITTLE, Martin Charles Homecroft Surgery, Voguebeloth, Illogan, Redruth TR16 4ET Fax: 01209 843707; Mill Cottage, Menadarva, Kehelland, Camborne TR14 0JH Tel: 01209 716465 — MB ChB Birm. 1983. Specialty: Gen. Pract. Prev: Trainee GP Pool Cornw.; SHO (Med., Surg. & Paediat.) Cornw. & I. of Scilly HA.

SPITTLEHOUSE, Kenneth Ernest (retired) 36 Waldron Road, Broadstairs CT10 1TB Tel: 01843 862127; Stable Cottage, Parsonage Farm, Church Lane, Nackington, Canterbury CT4 7AD Tel: 01227 763903 — (Sheff.) MD Sheff. 1956, MB ChB 1949; FRCPath 1970, M 1964. Hon. Cons. (Chem. Path.) Canterbury & Thanet HA.

SPITZ, Professor Lewis Institute of Child Health, 30 Guilford St., London WC1N 1EH Tel: 020 7242 9789/829 8691 Fax: 020 7404 6181 Email: l.spitz@ich.ucl.ac.uk — MB ChB Pretoria 1963; FRCS Ed. 1969; PhD (Med.) Witwatersrand 1980; FRCS Eng. 1981; FAAP, (hons) amer. Acad of Ped 1986; FRCPCH 1997; MD (Hons) Sheffield 2002. Nuffield Prof. Paediat. Surg. Inst. Child Health Lond.; Cons. Paediat. Surg. Gt. Ormond St. Hosp. for Childr. Lond.; Neonat. Surg. Univ. Coll. Hosp. Lond. Specialty: Paediat. Surg. Socs: (Pres.) Brit. Assn. Paediat. Surg. (Specialist Advis. Comm. & Train. & Teach. Comm.); (Acad. Bd.) Brit. Paediat. Assn.; Past Pres. BAPS. Prev: Sen. Paediat. Surg. Baragwanath & Transvaal Memor. Hosps. Johannesburg & Childr. Hosp. Sheff.

SPITZER, Joseph The Surgery, 62 Cranwich Road, London N16 5JF Tel: 020 8802 2002 Fax: 020 8880 2112; 66 Rostrevor Avenue, London N15 6LP Tel: 020 8802 4104 — MB BS Lond. 1981 (King's Coll. Hosp.) Cert. FPA 1984; DRCOG 1984; DCCH RCGP & FCM 1984; MRCGP 1985. Hon. Sen. Lect. (Gen.) Med. Coll. St. Bart. & Roy. Lond. Hosps. Specialty: Gen. Pract. Socs: Fell. Roy. Soc. Med.; BMA. Prev: CMO (Child Health) Islington HA; Trainee GP N.d. VTS; Ho. Off. Sunderland Roy. Infirm.

SPITZER, Robert John Southend Hospital, Prittlewell Chase, Westcliff on Sea SS0 0RY Tel: 01702 221238 Fax: 01702 221234; 59 Fairleigh Drive, Leigh-on-Sea SS9 2HZ Tel: 01702 710395 — MB BS Lond. 1959 (St. Mary's) Cons. Genitourin. Phys. Southend Health Care NHS Trust. Specialty: Genitourinary Medicine. Socs: BMA & Med. Soc. Study VD. Prev: Ho. Surg. Childr. Hosp. Paddington; Cas. Off. Lambeth Hosp.; JHMO Dept. Venereol St. Thos. Hosp. Lond.

SPIVEY, Mr Christopher John Kings Road Private Consulting Rooms, 151A Kings Road, Westcliff on Sea SS0 8PP Tel: 01702 476650 Fax: 01702 711787; 61 Warren Road, Leigh-on-Sea SS9 3TT Tel: 01702 558318 Fax: 01702 558318 — (Lond. Hosp.) MRCS Eng. LRCP Lond. 1960; MB BS Lond. 1960; FRCS Eng. 1966. Hon. Cons. Orthop. Surg. Southend Health Dist.; Cons. Orthop. Surg. BUPA Wellesley Hosp. Southend-on-Sea. Specialty: Orthop. Socs: Fell. BOA; Fell.Hunt. Soc.; Fell. Roy. Soc. Med. Pres. Sect. of Orthop. 2000/01. Prev: Sen. Orthop. Regist. Lond. Hosp.; Surg. Regist. St. Margt.'s Hosp. Epping; Jun. Surg. Regist. Lond. Hosp.

SPIVEY, Michael Hugh Hollybank, 126 London Road, Westerham TN16 1GR — BM BS Nottm. 1997.

SPIVEY, Rosemary Sarah The Brow, 96 Cumnor Hill, Oxford OX2 9HY Tel: 01865 862132 — (St. Bart.) MFFP; MB BS Lond. 1963; MRCS Eng. LRCP Lond. 1963. Research Asst. Diabetic Research Laborat. Radcliffe Infirm. Oxf.; Sen. Clin. Med. Off. (Family Plann.) Oxon. HA; Clin. Asst. (Obst. & Gyn.) John Radcliffe Hosp. Oxf. Specialty: Diabetes; Family Plann. & Reproduc. Health; Endocrinol. Socs: Fac. Fam. Plan.; Brit. Menopause Soc.; Wom.s Med. Fed. Prev: Med. Off. John Radcliffe Hosp. Oxf.; Ho. Phys. N. Staffs. Roy. Infirm. Stoke-on-Trent; Ho. Surg. N. Middlx. Hosp. Lond.

SPOFFORTH, Peter Ash Surgery, 1 Ashfield Road, Liverpool L17 0BY Tel: 0151 727 1155 Fax: 0151 726 0018 — MB ChB Liverp. 1988. Specialty: Gen. Pract.

SPOKES, Ernest George Sutherland Leeds General Infirmary, Great George St., Leeds LS1 3EX Tel: 0113 292 3296 Fax: 0113 292 6337 — MB ChB Leeds 1972; MRCP (UK) 1975; BSc Leeds 1969, MD 1979; FRCP Lond. 1989. Cons. Neurol. Leeds Gen. Infirm. Specialty: Neurol. Prev: Cons. Neurol. York Dist. Hosp.; Dir. Neuropsychiat. Unit Bootham Pk. Hosp. York.

SPOKES, Gillian Ann 40 Baginton Road, Coventry CV3 6JW — MB ChB Birm. 1969; DObst RCOG 1971.

SPOKES, Jonathan Mark Market Hill House, Market Hill, Medon, Hull HY12 8JD Tel: 01482 899111 — MRCS Eng. LRCP Lond. 1982; MRCGP 1986; DRCOG 1988.

SPOKES, Robert Michael Spokes and Partners, Phoenix Family Care, 35 Park Road, Coventry CV1 2LE Tel: 024 7622 7234 Fax: 024 7663 4816 — MB ChB Birm. 1966; DObst RCOG 1969; MRCGP 1974.

SPOLTON, Elizabeth Mary Somers Town Health Centre, Blackfriars Close, Southsea PO5 4NJ Tel: 023 9285 1202 Fax: 023 9229 6380; 52 Southleigh Road, Havant PO9 2QH Tel: 023 9248 4904 — MB BCh Wales 1972; DObst RCOG 1975; MRCGP 1976.

SPOLTON, Mr Michael William Surrey & Sussex Health Care Trust, Redhill Tel: 01737 768511 — MB BS (St. Thomas's) MB; FRCS; FRCOphth; BSc; DO. Cons. Ophth., Lead Clinician in Ophth. Specialty: Ophth.

SPONG, Ambrose Henry Rowan (retired) Sunny Bank, Staveley, Kendal LA8 9PH Tel: 01539 822027 — (Lond. Hosp.) MB BS Lond. 1957; FFA RCS Eng. 1963. Prev: Cons. Anaesth. Lincoln Hosp. Gp.

SPOONER, Andrew Lawrence Grosvenor Medical Centre, Grosvenor Street, Crewe CW1 3HB Tel: 01270 256340 Fax: 01270 250786; Gresty Brook Medical Centre, Brookhouse Drive, Crewe CW2 6NA Tel: 01270 650012 — MB BS Newc. 1983 (Newc. u. Tyne) MRCGP 1987; FRCGP, 1998. Hon. Fell. Nat. Primary Care Research And Developm. Centre. Specialty: Ophth. Prev: Chairm. Mersey Regional Assn. Fundholding Pract.; Assoc. Med. Dir. Chesh. Community Health Care Trust; Trainee GP E. Cumbria VTS.

SPOONER, Catherine Ann The White House, 14 Park Avenue, Dronfield, Dronfield S18 2LQ — MB ChB Liverp. 1990; MRCGP 1995.

SPOONER, David 9 St Bernards Road, Sutton Coldfield B72 1LE — MB ChB Birm. 1973; BSc Birm. 1970; MRCP (UK) 1975; FRCR 1979; FRCP Lond. 1993. Cons. Clin. Oncol. Qu. Eliz., Dudley Rd., Sandwell & Childr. Hosps. Birm. Specialty: Oncol.; Radiother. Socs: Fell. RCP. Prev: Sen. Regist. (Radiother.) Roy. Marsden Hosp. Sutton & Lond.; Lect. (Radiother.) Inst. of Cancer Research Lond.; Regist. (Med.) Selly Oak Hosp. Birm.

SPOONER, John Bradley 5 Beaconsfield Road, Claygate, Esher KT10 0PX — MB Camb. 1963 (Middlx.) BChir 1962. Specialty: Pharmaceutical Medicine.

SPOONER, Laurel Loveday Rosemary North Station Road Surgery, 78 North Station Road, Colchester CO1 1SE Tel: 01206 574483 Fax: 01206 767558; 5 Ireton Road, Colchester CO3 3AT Tel: 01206 573860 — MB BChir Camb. 1979; MA Camb. 1979; DRCOG 1982; Cert. Family Plann. JCC 1982; DCH RCP Lond. 1983; MRCP (UK) 1983; MRCGP 1983. GP Colchester; Chairm. Colchester PCG. Specialty: Gen. Pract.

SPOONER, Louise 17 Armthorpe Road, Sheffield S11 7FA — MB BS Lond. 1987.

SPOONER, Monica Anne (retired) 30 South Oswald Road, Edinburgh EH9 2HG Tel: 0131 667 2555 Fax: 0131 668 2121 — MB BS Lond. 1964 (Westm.) MRCS Eng. LRCP Lond. 1964; DObst RCOG 1967; DCCH RCP Ed. RCGP & FCM 1986. Prev: Clin. Med. Off. Lothian HB.

SPOONER, Shirley Mildred 406 Uppingham Road, Leicester LE5 2DP Tel: 0116 243 2951 Fax: 01162 418740 — MB BS Lond. 1960 (Roy. Free) MRCS Eng. LRCP Lond. 1960.

SPOONER, Simon Jonathan 33 Cheltenham Road, Manchester M21 9GL — MB BCh Wales 1995.

SPOONER, Stephen Francis Department of Obstetrics & Gynaecology, Rotherham District General Hospital, Moorgate Road, Rotherham S60 2UD; 27 Moor Oaks Road, Sheffield S10 1BX — MB BChir Camb. 1977 (Cambridge/St Thomas London) FRCOG 1998. Cons. O & G Rotherham Hosp. Specialty: Obst. & Gyn.

SPOONER, Veronica Josephine Lensfield Medical Practice, 48 Lensfield Road, Cambridge CB2 1EH Tel: 01223 352779 Fax: 01223 566930; 11 Barton Close, Cambridge CB3 9LQ — MB BS Lond. 1978 (St. Mary's Hospital London) DRCOG 1982; MRCGP 1983.

SPOOR, Kathleen Mary 15 Burnhouse Road, Wooler NE71 6BJ Tel: 01688 281575 Fax: 01688 282442; East Longstone House, Church Hill, Chatton, Alnwick NE66 5PY — MB BS Newc. 1982; DCCH RCP Ed. 1986; MRCGP 1987. GP Wooler, N.d.

SPORIK, Richard Bernard 196 Battersea Park Road, London SW11 4ND — BM Soton. 1980; DCH RCP Lond. 1983; DRCOG 1984; MRCP (UK) 1986; DM Soton. 1994.

SPORTON, Simon Charles Edwin Department of Cardiology, Middlesex Hospital, Mortimer St., London W1T 3AA Tel: 020 7636 8333; 1 Pike End, Stevenage SG1 3XA Tel: 01438 358326 — MB BS Lond. 1991; BSc Lond. 1988; MRCP (UK) 1994. Specialist Regist. (Cardiol.) NE Thames. Specialty: Cardiol. Prev: Clin. Research Fell. (Cardiol.) Univ. Coll. Lond.; Regist. Rotat. (Med.) SW Thames; SHO Rotat. (Med.) Seacroft & Killingbeck Hosps. Leeds.

SPOTO, Giuseppe Department of Psychiatry, Crawley Hospital, West Green Drive, Crawley RH11 7DH Tel: 01293 600300 Fax: 01293 600411 Email: gspoto@cwcom.net; 101 Camberwell Grove, London SE5 8JH Tel: 020 7703 3228 Fax: 020 7703 3228 Email: gspoto@cwcom.net — MD Pisa 1972 (Italy) MRCPsych 1982. Cons. (Psychiat. Psychother.) Crawley & Horsham NHS Trust; Med. Mem. Ment. Health Review Tribunal. Specialty: Gen. Psychiat.; Psychother. Socs: Soc. Psychother. Research; Soc. Psychosomatic Research; Roy. Soc. Med. Prev: Sen. Regist. (Psychiat.) & Hon. Clin. Lect. Univ. Coll. Hosp.; Regist. (Child Psychiat.) Child Guid. Train. Centre Lond.; Regist. Roy. Free Hosp. Lond.

SPOTSWOOD, Valerie Janet Villiers House, Tolworth Hospital, Red Lion Road, Surbiton KT6 7QU Tel: 020 8990 0102 — (King's Coll. Hosp.) MB BS Lond. 1963; MRCS Eng. LRCP Lond. 1963; DPM Eng. 1972; MRCPsych 1973. Cons. Gen. Psychiat. Tolworth Hosp. Specialty: Gen. Psychiat. Prev: Cons. Psychiat. (Elderly) Long Gr. Hosp. Epsom; Sen. Regist. (Psychiat.) Lond. Hosp.; Regist. (Psychiat.) St. Mary's Hosp. Lond.

SPOUDEAS, Helen Alexandra London Centre for Paediatric Endocrinology, 3rd Floor Dorville House, Middlesex Hospital, Mortimer St., London W1T 3AA Tel: 020 7380 9455 Fax: 020 7636 2144 Email: h.spoudeas@uclh.nhs.uk — MB BS Lond. 1981 (St. Bart. Hosp. Lond.) DRCOG Lond 1983; MRCP (UK) 1985; MD Lond. 1995; FRCPCH 1999; FRCP Lond 2000. p/t Cons. Paediatric Endocrinol., Neuroendoc. & Late Effects of Childh. Malignancy, Lond. Centre of Paediat. Endocrin. at Univ. Coll. & Gt. Ormond St. Hosp. Lond.; Vice Chairm. Of Fundraising Comm. RMBF.; Dep. Regional Adviser, N. Centr. Thames RCPCH; Mem. of Managem. Team, Nat. Counselling Serv. for Sick Doctors; Hon. Sen. Lect. (Paediat. Endocrin.) UCL & Inst. Of Child Health; Volun. RMBF rep on Nat. Counc. Servs. for sick. Specialty: Paediat.; Endocrinol.; Oncol. Socs: Eur. & Brit. Socs. Paediat. Endocrinol.; Fell., Roy. Coll. Of Phys.; UK Childr.'s Cancer Study Gp. Prev: Sen. Regist. (Paediat. Endocrinol.) Middlx. Hosp. Lond.; Research Fell. (Paediat. Endocrinol.) Middlx. Hosp. Lond.; Regist. Rotat. (Paediat.) Char. Cross Hosp. Lond.

SPOULOU, Vassiliki Institute of Child Health, Department Of Immunology, 30 Guildford St., London WC1N 1EH Tel: 020 7405 9200 — Ptychio Iatrikes Athens 1985.

SPOWAGE, Paul Martin The Surgery, Queens Road, Earls Colne, Colchester CO6 2RR Tel: 01787 222641 — MB BS Lond. 1986; DCH RCP Lond. 1989; DRCOG 1990. GP Earls Colne. Specialty: Gen. Pract.

SPOWART, Keith John Morrison Queen Mothers Hospital, Yorkhill NHS Trust, Glasgow G3 8SJ — MB ChB Glas. 1983; BSc (Hons.) (Pharmacol.) Ed. 1978; MRCOG 1989; FRCOG 2002. Cons. Obst. and Gynaecologist, Qu. Mothers Hosp. and West. Infirm., Glas. Specialty: Obst. & Gyn. Special Interest: Early Pregn. loss; Hysteroscopy/One stop clinics. Socs: Glas. Obst. & Gyn. Soc.; Brit. Menopause Soc. Prev: Cons. Obst. and Gynaecologist Hairmyres and Withshaw Gen. Hosps. Lanarksh.

SPRACKLING, Margaret Ellen (retired) 6 Hillbrow, Richmond Hill, Richmond TW10 6BH Tel: 020 8948 3517 — MB BS Lond. 1958 (Middlx.) MRCS Eng. LRCP Lond. 1958; MRCP (UK) 1970; FRCP Lond. 1987. Prev: Emerit. Cons. Phys. (Geriat. Med.) City Hosp. Nottm.

SPRACKLING, Peter Dennis Derby Road Health Centre, 292 Derby Road, Nottingham NG7 1QG Tel: 0115 947 4002; Flat 2, 25 Park Valley, The Park, Nottingham NG7 1BS — MB BS Lond. 1958 (Middlx.) DObst RCOG 1960; FRCGP 1978, M 1972. Prev: Regional Adviser (Gen. Pract.) Trent RHA. Lect. Dept. Community Health Med. Sch. Nottm. Univ.; Ho. Off. (Obst.) Hammersmith Hosp. Lond.; Ho. Surg. & Ho. Phys. Roy. Berks. Hosp. Reading.

SPRAGGETT, David Thomas The Castle Medical Centre, 22 Bertie Road, Kenilworth CV8 1JP Tel: 01926 857331 Fax: 01926 851070; 12 Elizabeth Way, Kenilworth CV8 1QP — MB ChB Birm. 1981; DRCOG 1984; MRCGP 1985; DCH RCP Lond. 1986. Prev: Ho. Surg. Walsall Manor Hosp.; Ho. Phys. Good Hope Hosp. Sutton Coldfield.

SPRAGGINS, Debra The Health Centre, Laindon, Basildon SS15 5TR Tel: 01268 546411 Fax: 01268 491248 — MB ChB Manch. 1991; DFFP. Specialty: Gen. Pract.

SPRAGGS, Mr Paul David Robert ENT Department, Northamptonshire Hospital, Aldermaston Road, Basingstoke Tel: 01256 313525 — MB BS Lond. 1987; FRCS Eng. 1991; FRCS 1996. Cons. Otolaryngol., N. Hants. Hosp. Basingstoke; Cons. Otolaryngol. Hants. Clinic, Old Basing. Specialty: Otolaryngol.

SPRAGUE, Daphne Sharpe (retired) 14 Stephenson Terrace, Wylam NE41 8DZ Tel: 01661 852719 — MB BS Durh. 1948 (Newc.) Prev: SCMO (Family Plann.) S. Shields.

SPRAGUE, Nigel Bond 14 Stephenson Terrace, Wylam NE41 8DZ Tel: 01661 852719 — MB BS Durh. 1945; DA Eng. 1971. Assoc. Specialist (Anaesth.) Newc. HA. Prev: Ex-Pres. Newc. on Tyne & North. Counties Med. Soc.; Ho. Phys. Dryburn Hosp. Durh.; Ho. Surg. Newc. Gen. Hosp.

SPRAKE, Caroline Mary Lane End Surgery, 2 Manor Walk, Benton, Newcastle upon Tyne NE7 7XX Tel: 0191 266 5246 Fax: 0191 266 6241 — MB BS Newc. 1986; MB BS (Hons.) Newc. 1986, BMedSci (Hons.) 1983; MRCP (UK) 1989; MRCGP 1991.

SPRANGEMEYER, Dawn — MRCS Eng. LRCP Lond. 1971; MRCPCH; BSc Lond. 1967, MB BS 1971; DCCH Adelaide 1985; MA Child Protec. & Family Support (Tavistock Centre & E.London U.) 1999. Named Doctor for Child Protec., Thanet Community Child Health Servs., E.Kent NHS Trust. Prev: Med. Off. Child Health Servs. Townsville, Qu.sland.; SCMO & PMO Thanet Community Child Health Servs.; Sen. Regist. in Paediat. Roy. Childrens Hosp. Brisbane.

SPRATLEY, Terence Arthur (retired) Mount Zeehan Unit, St. Martin's Hospital, Littlebourne Road, Canterbury CT1 1TD Tel: 01227 761310; 253 Old Dover Road, Canterbury CT1 3ES Tel: 01227 455125 — MRCS Eng. LRCP Lond. 1961; MPhil Lond. 1969, MB BS 1961; MRCP Lond. 1966; MRCPsych 1973. Cons. Psychiat. St. Martins Hosp. Canterbury.

SPRATT, Henry Clifford General Hospital, St Helier, Jersey JE1 3QS Tel: 01534 622000 Fax: 01534 622895; La Falaise, Le Hocq, St. Clement, Jersey JE2 6FQ Tel: 01534 855256 Fax: 01534 851169 — (TC Dub.) MD Dub. 1974, MB BCh BAO 1969; MRCP (UK) 1973; FRCP Lond. 1986; FRCPCH 1997. Cons. Paediat. Gen. Hosp. St. Helier Jersey. Specialty: Paediat. Socs: RCPCH. Prev: Lect. (Paediat.) McGill Univ. Montreal, Canada.

SPRATT, James Samuel 59 Ballyquin Road, Limavady BT49 9EY; Flat 3F1, 29 Falcon Gardens, Morningside, Edinburgh EH10 4AR — MB ChB Manch. 1993; MRCP (UK) 1996; BSc MedSci Edin. 1998. Specialist Regist. (Cardiol.) Western Gen. Hosp. Edin. Specialty: Cardiol. Prev: Res. Fell. (Clin. Pharma.) Univ. of Edin.

SPRATT, Jonathan Daunton — MB BChir Camb. 1992 (Univ. Hosp. of N. Durh.) MA Camb 1992; FRCS Eng. 1996; FRCS Glas. 1997; FRCR 1999. Specialty: Radiol.

SPRAY, Christine Helen The Gastroentgrology Department, The Children's Hospital, Steelhouse Lane, Birmingham B4 6NH; Flat 2, 31 Wentworth Road, Harborne, Birmingham B17 9SN Tel: 0121 427 2600 — MB ChB Liverp. 1987. Clin. Lect. (Paediat., Gastroenterol. & Hepat.) Childr. Hosp. Liverp. Specialty: Gastroenterol. Prev: Clin. Research Fell. (Paediat. Hepat.) & Regist. Newc.

SPRAY, Rowland John (retired) 2 Sandringham Road, Swindon SN3 1HP Tel: 01793 537502 — MB BChir Camb. 1952 (Camb. & Univ. Coll. Hosp.) MA Camb. 1953, BA 1949; MRCGP 1968; DCH Eng. 1969; DObst RCOG 1970. Prev: GP Swindon.

SPREADBURY, Kate Victoria Hansford — BM (Hons. Distinc. Clin. Med.) Soton. 1994; DRCOG 1998; MRCGP (Distinc.) 1999. GP Locum; SHO (A & E). Prev: SHO (Psychiat.); Trainee GP Taunton VTS.

SPREADBURY, Peter Lawrence Little Oaks, 218 Stakes Hill Road, Waterlooville PO7 5UJ Tel: 0170 143336 — MB BS Lond. 1966 (Lond. Hosp.) DA Eng. 1969; FFA RCS Eng. 1973. Cons. Anaesth. Portsmouth & S.E. Hants. Health Dist. Specialty: Anaesth. Prev: Anaesth Sen. Regist. Soton. Univ. Hosp.

SPREADBURY, Thomas Hugh (retired) 52 Bridge End, Warwick CV34 6PB — MB Camb. 1961; BChir 1960; DA Eng. 1966; FFA RCS Eng. 1968. Prev: Cons. Anaesth. Warwick.

SPRECKLEY, Debra Elizabeth 12 Waterside Avenue, Marple, Stockport SK6 7LZ — MB ChB Birm. 1996; MB ChB (Hons.) Birm. 1996.

SPRIGG, Alan Department of Radiology, Sheffield Childrens Hospital, Western Bank, Sheffield S10 2TH Tel: 0114 271 7201 Fax: 0114 271 7514 — MB ChB Manch. 1978; DCH Eng. 1980; DRCOG 1981; DMRD Eng. 1983; FRCR 1985; FRCPCH 1997. Cons. Paediat. Radiol. Sheff. Childs. Hosp. NHS Trust; Cons. Radiol. Jessop Wing of Hallamshire Hosp., Sheff. Specialty: Radiol. Prev: Cons. Paediat. (Radiol.) Mersey RHA; Fell. (Radiol.) Hosp. Sick Childr., Toronto.

SPRIGG, Nikola 12 Sackville Road, Sheffield S10 1GT — MB ChB Sheff. 1995.

SPRIGG, Sandra Jane 105 Rustlings Road, Sheffield S11 7AB Tel: 0114 266 0726 — MB ChB Manch. 1978; DRCOG 1981; DCH RCP Lond. 1983; MRCGP 1985. GP Retainer Scheme Sheff. Prev: Regist. & Clin. Med. Off. Sheff. Childr. Hosp.; SHO (Cas.) Sheff. Childr. Hosp.

SPRIGGE, John Squire Arrowe Park Hospital, Department of Anaesthesia, Upton, Wirral CH49 5PE Tel: 0151 678 5111 — MB BChir Camb. 1969 (Westm.) BA Camb. 1969; MRCS Eng. LRCP Lond. 1972; FFA RCS Eng. 1976. Cons. (Anaesth.) Arrowe Pk. Hosp. Wirral; Clin. Tutor Arrowe Pk. Hosp. Specialty: Anaesth. Prev: Clin. Tutor Wirral Hosp.; Sen. Regist. (Anaesth.) Hammersmith Hosp.; Regist. (Anaesth.) Liverp. AHA (T).

SPRIGGS, Arthur Ivens (retired) 1 Gozzards Ford, Abingdon OX13 6JH Tel: 01865 390618 — BM BCh Oxf. 1943; FRCP Lond. 1968, M 1944; BA Oxf. 1941, DM 1952; FRCPath 1973, M 1964. Prev: Cons. Cytol. Oxon HA.

SPRING, Colin Department Anaesthesia, Worthing Hospital, Lyndhurst Road, Worthing BN11 2DH Tel: 01903 205111 Ext: 5151 Fax: 01903 285045; Pine Lodge, Fir Tree Lane, West Chiltington, Pulborough RH20 2RA Tel: 01903 815514 — MB BS Lond. 1987 (St George's Hospital Medical School) MRCGP 1991; FRCA 1995. Clin. Director,Cons. Anaesth Cons. Intens. Care. Worthing & Southlands Hosp. W. Sussex. Specialty: Anaesth.; Intens. Care. Prev: Regist. Rotat. (Anaesth.) Bristol & S. W.; Regist. (Anaesth.) Roy. Hobart Hosp. Tasmania, Austral.; Regist. (Anaesth.) MusGr. Pk. Hosp. Taunton.

SPRING, Jane Elizabeth Department of Obstetrics, Heatherwood Hospital, Lond. Road, Ascot SL5 8AA — MB BS Lond. 1978; DCH RCP Lond. 1983; MRCOG 1984; MRCP (UK) 1985. Cons. O & G Heatherwood Hosp. Ascot. Specialty: Obst. & Gyn. Prev: Sen. Regist. (O & G) Guy's Hosp. Lond.

SPRING, Jennifer Thea Manor Way Surgery, 27 Manor Way, Borehamwood WD6 1QR Tel: 020 8953 3095 — MB BS Lond. 1967 (St. Bart.) BSc Nottm. 1962; MRCS Eng. LRCP Lond. 1967; DObst RCOG 1969. Prev: Ho. Off. City of Lond. Matern. Hosp.; Ho. Surg. St. Albans City Hosp.; Ho. Phys. St. Paul's Hosp. Hemel Hempstead.

SPRING, Linford Craig Schumberger-Sema Medical Services, Sutherland House, 29-37 Brighton Road, Sutton SM2 5AN; 3 Horley Row, Horley RH6 8DN — MB BS Adelaide 1979. Med. Adviser Schumberger-Sema Med. Servs. Sutton. Specialty: Disabil. Med. Socs: BMA. Prev: GP Crawley & Horley; SHO (O & G) Guy's Hosp. Lond.; SHO (Paediat.) New Ealing Hosp. Southall & Perivale Hosp. Greenford.

SPRING, Mark William Department of Metabolic Medicine, Kingston Hospital, Galsworthy Road, Kingston upon Thames KT2 7QB Tel: 020 8546 7711 Ext: 2745 Fax: 020 8934 3276 — MB BS Lond. 1990 (UMDS Guy's) BSc (Hons.) Lond. 1987; MRCP (UK) 1993; FRCP 2003. Cons. (Diabetes Endocrinolory & Gen Med) Kingston & Qu. Mary's Hosps. Specialty: Diabetes; Endocrinol.; Gen. Med. Prev: Cons. Gen.Med Guy's Hosp. Lon; Sen. Regist. (Metab. & Gen Med) Guy's Hosp; Regist & Sho (MED) St. Geo Hosp, Lon.

SPRING, Robert David Leslie Presteigne Medical Centre, Lugg View, Presteigne LD8 2RJ Tel: 01544 267985 Fax: 01544 267682 — MB BS Lond. 1982; BA Oxf. 1979; MRCP (UK) 1985.

SPRINGALL, Christopher James 20 Woodgreen Road, Oldbury, Oldbury B68 0DF — MB ChB Liverp. 1978.

SPRINGALL, Mr Roger Graham 149 Harley Street, London W1G 6BN Tel: 020 7486 7927 Fax: 020 7486 7927 Email: rgspringal@aol.com; Oak End Mill, Amersham Road, Gerrards Cross SL9 0PU Tel: 01753 882880 — MB ChB Liverp. 1973; FRCS Eng. 1977; ChM 1984. Cons. Surg. (Gastrointestinal & Oncol. Surg.) Char. Cross Hosp. Lond.; Cons. Surg. King Edwd. VII Hosp. for Offs. Lond.; Hon. Cons. Surg. St. Luke's Hosp. for the Clergy Lond. Specialty: Gen. Surg. Socs: Fell. Roy. Soc. Med.; Assn. Coloproctol.; Fell. Assn. Surg. Prev: Resid. Surgic. Off. St. Mark's Hosp. Lond.; Sen. Regist. (Surg.) St. Bart. Hosp. Lond.; Demonst. (Anat.) Univ. Camb.

SPRINGER, Adele Leona Cynthia 1 Scoonie Court, Leven KY8 5TH — MB ChB Aberd. 1988.

SPRINGER, Heath Weston 4 Pembroke Road, Ilford IG3 8PH; 106 Cambridge Road, Ilford IG3 8LY — MB BS Lond. 1992.

SPRINGER, Jana Department of Ophthalmology, King's College Hospital, Denmark Hill, London SE5 9RS; 12 Deepdene Road, London SE5 8EG Tel: 020 7733 1024 — Promovany Lekar Chas. Univ. Prague 1959. Asst. Specialist (Ophth.) King's Coll. Hosp. Lond. Specialty: Ophth. Socs: BMA & Soc. Ophth. Surgs. Prev: Asst. Specialist (Ophth.) St. Thos. Hosp. Lond. & Kingston Hosp. Surrey.

SPRINGER, Susan Elizabeth 32a Chalsey Road, London SE4 1YW — MB ChB Manch. 1992.

SPROAT, Lois Mary Elizabeth Castle Douglas Medical Group, Castle Douglas Health Centre, Academy Street, Castle Douglas DG7 1EE; Strathmore, Abercromby Road, Castle Douglas DG7 1BA — MB ChB Dundee 1976; DRCOG 1980.

SPROSON, Janet Christine Ros-an-Dinas, Lamorna, Penzance TR19 6NY — MB ChB Manch. 1974.

SPROSTON, Antony Raymond Mark Flat 4 Rosewood Gardens, Hart Avenue, Sale, Manchester M33 2JS Tel: 0161 976 1609 — MB ChB Manch. 1985; MRCOG 1991. Clin. Research Fell. (Experim. Radiat. Oncol.) Paterson Inst. Cancer Research Christie Hosp. Manch. Specialty: Obst. & Gyn. Prev: SHO (O & G) Wythenshawe Hosp. Manch.; Regist. (O & G) Arrow Pk. Hosp. & Wom. Hosp. Liverp.

SPROTT, Margaret Mary 26 Claremont Gardens, Marlow SL7 1BS — MB BS Lond. 1983.

SPROTT, Veronica Mary Alexandra 24 Andover Road, Southsea PO4 9QG — MB BS Lond. 1983; BSc Lond. 1980 (Charing Cross Hospital London) MRCP (UK) 1986; MRCGP 1989. GP Asst. Prev: GP Soton; Regist. (Med.) Gen. Hosp. Soton. HA; Regist. (Med.) Qu. Alexandra's Hosp. Portsmouth.

SPROULE, Michael William Flat 1/R, 28 Gray Street, Kelvingrove, Glasgow G3 7TY Tel: 0141 334 5770 — MB ChB Ed. 1988; MRCP (UK) 1992; FRCR 1996. Sen. Regist. (Radiol.) Glas. Roy. Infirm. Specialty: Radiol. Socs: RCP Edin.; BMA; Roy. Coll. Radiol. Prev: Career Regist. (Radiol.) Glas. Roy. Infirm.; SHO (Gen. Med.) Roy. Shrewsbury Hosp.

SPROULE, William Bradley (retired) 23 Antrim Road, Lisburn BT28 3ED Tel: 028 9266 2080 Fax: 028 9266 2080 — (Dub.) BA Dub. 1964, MD 1975, MB BCh BAO 1964; FRCOG 1982, M 1969. Prev: Ho. Off. Dr. Steevens' Hosp. Dub.

SPRUCE, Barbara Ann Ninewells Hospital and Medical School, Department of Surgery and Molecular Oncology, University of Dundee, Dundee DD1 9SY — MB BS Newc. 1979; MRCP (UK) 1981; PhD Lond. 1990. Wellcome Sen. Research Fell. (Clin. Sci.) Univ. Dundee.

SPRUELL, David Andrew Forest End Surgery, Forest End, Waterlooville PO7 7AH; 10 The Fairway, Rowlands Castle PO9 6AQ Tel: 01705 413279 — MB ChB Dundee 1977; DRCOG 1979; MRCGP 1981.

SPRUNT, Deirdre Catriona Caoirtiona 17 Claremount Drive, Bridge of Allan, Stirling FK9 4EE Tel: 01786 833607 — MB ChB Aberd. 1957. Assoc. Specialist Histopath. Forth Valley Health Bd. Prev: SHO Aberd. Roy. Infirm.; Med. Off. Glas. Blood Transfus. Serv.; Ho. Off. (Med. & Orthop.) Bridge of Earn Hosp. Perth.

SPRUNT, Elizabeth Mary 100 Randolph Road, Glasgow G11 7EE — MB ChB Aberd. 1955. Assoc. Specialist E. Scotl. Blood Transfus. Serv. Prev: Trainee Gen. Pract. Dundee & Perth Vocational Train. Scheme; Med. Off. Health Dept. City Dundee; SHO (Anaesth.) Dundee Gen. Hosp.

SPRUNT, John William Ellis Otaki Medical Centre, 2 Aotaki St., Otaki, New Zealand Tel: 00 64 6364 8555; c/o 418 Crow Road, Glasgow G11 7EA Tel: 0141 357 1637 — MB ChB Dundee 1983; MRCGP 1989; Dip. Sports Med. Lond 1996. Specialty: Sports Med. Socs: Brit. Assn. Sport & Med.; NZ Federat. of Sports Med. Prev: Clin. Asst. (Accid. & Emerg.) S. Tyneside Dist. Gen. Hosp.; Asst. GP. St. Anthony's Med. Centre Newc. u. Tyne.

SPRUNT, Mr Thomas Glassford (retired) 17 Claremont Drive, Bridge of Allan, Stirling FK9 4EE — MB ChB St. And. 1951 (Dundee) FRCS Ed. 1959. Cons. Orthop. Surg. Stirling & Falkirk Roy. Infirm. Prev: Sen. Regist. (Orthop. Surg.) Aberd. Roy. Infirm.

SPRY, Professor Christopher John Farley (retired) 97 Ridgway, Wimbledon, London SW19 4SX Tel: 020 8946 6176 Email: cspry@cspry.co.uk — MB BChir Camb. 1965 (Camb. & Oxf.) FESC 1988; MA Camb. 1965; FRCP Lond. 1984, M 1967; DPhil Oxf. 1971; FRCPath. 1985, M 1980. Prev: Prof. Cardiovasc. Immunol. Univ. Lond.

SPURGEON, Jane The Medical Centre, Kingston Avenue, East Horsley, Leatherhead KT24 6QT Tel: 01483 284151 Fax: 01483 285814 — BM Soton. 1992; DRCOG 1997; DFFP 1997; DRCOG 1997; DGM 1998; MRCGP 1998; DPD 1999. GP Princip. Specialty: Gen. Pract. Socs: Roy. Coll. Gen. Pract.

SPURGIN, Hilary Margaret Kirkhouse Rozel, Round St., Cobham, Gravesend DA13 9BA — MB BS Lond. 1949 (Univ. Coll. Hosp.) MRCS Eng. LRCP Lond. 1949.

SPURLING, Basil Martin Elm Hayes Surgery, High Street, Paulton, Bristol BS39 7QJ Tel: 01761 413155 Fax: 01761 410573; Meadgate House, Camerton, Bath BA2 0NL Tel: 01761 470496 — MRCS Eng. LRCP Lond. 1971.

SPURLING, Susan Gisela Meadgate House, Meadgate West, Camerton, Bath BA3 1NL Tel: 01761 70496 — MB BS Lond. 1971.

SPURLOCK, Christina Jane Banks Street Surgery, 7 Banks Street, Willenhall WV13 1SP Tel: 01902 8624 Fax: 01902 602280 — MRCS Eng. LRCP Lond. 1969.

SPURR, David Westgarth, 56 Albert Road W., Heaton, Bolton BL1 5HG — BM BCh Oxf. 1969; MRCP (UK) 1973; FRCP Lond. 1990. Cons. Phys. Bolton Gen. Hosp. Specialty: Gen. Med.

SPURR, James Irving Stanhope Health Centre, Dale St., Stanhope, Bishop Auckland DL13 2XD Tel: 01388 528555 Fax: 01388 526122 — MB BS Newc. 1964.

SPURR, Jennifer June (retired) 1 Mayfield Road, Bickley, Bromley BR1 2HB Tel: 020 8467 9358 — (Middlx.) MB BS Lond. 1957; MRCS Eng. LRCP Lond. 1957. Assoc. Specialist in Rheum. Tunbridge Wells NHS Trust. Prev: Med. Asst. (Physical Med. & Rheum.) Sevenoaks & Orpington Hosps.

SPURR, Michael Jeremy Towson and Partners, Juniper Road, Boreham, Chelmsford CM3 3DX Tel: 01245 467364 Fax: 01245 465584; Boreham Manor, Church Road, Boreham, Chelmsford CM3 3EJ Tel: 01245 464195 Email: spurr.family@lineone.net — MB BS Lond. 1981 (St. Thos. Hosp. Med. Sch. Lond.) LMSSA Lond. 1980; DRCOG 1984; Dip. Occ. Med. 1998. GP; Occupat. Health Phys. Chelmsford. Specialty: Gen. Pract. Prev: Princip. Dist. Med. Off. Mulanje Dist. Hosp. Malawi, Afr.

SPURRELL, John Richard Roworth 334 Dyke Road, Brighton BN1 5BB Tel: 01273 507049 — BM BCh Oxf. 1959 (Guy's) MA, BM BCh Oxf. 1959; FRCP Lond. 1979, M 1963. Cons. Phys. Brighton & Lewes & Mid Sussex Hosp. Gps. Specialty: Gen. Med.

SPURRELL, Philip Anthony Roworth 334 Dyke Road, Brighton BN1 5BB — MB BS Lond. 1993.

SPURRELL, Roworth Adrian John 84 Harley Street, London W1G 7HW Tel: 020 7079 4222 Fax: 020 7079 4223 — MRCS Eng. LRCP Lond. 1960; BSc (Physiol.) Lond. 1962, MD 1974, MB BS 1966; FRCP Lond. 1979, M 1969; FACC 1975. Emer. Sen. Cons. Cardiac Dept. St. Bart. Hosp. Lond. Specialty: Cardiol. Socs: Brit. Cardiac Soc. Prev: Sen. Regist. (Cardiol.) Guy's Hosp. Lond.; Regist. (Cardiol.) St. Geo. Hosp. & Nat. Heart Hosp. Lond.

SPURRIER, Peter David Maywood Surgery, 180 Hawthorn Road, Bognor Regis PO21 2UY Tel: 01243 829141 Fax: 01243 842115; 6 A'Beckets Avenue, Aldwick Bay, Bognor Regis PO21 4UL Tel: 01243 265292 Fax: 01243 842115 Email: docspur@aol.com — BM Soton. 1980; DRCOG 1984; MRCGP 1986. Specialty: Diabetes.

SPURRING, Richard Drew Lyndon (retired) Garth, Beech Way, Selsdon, South Croydon CR2 8QR Tel: 020 8657 2273 — MB BS Lond. 1957 (Westminster Hospital)

SPYCHAL, Mr Robert Thomas 249 Spies Lane, Halesowen B62 9SN — MB BS Newc. 1982; FRCS Ed. 1986; MD Newc. 1991. Cons. Gen. Surg. City Hosp. Birm. Specialty: Gen. Surg.

SPYER, Ghislaine Department of Diabetes & Vascular Health, Royal Devon & Exeter Hospital, Barrack Road, Exeter EX2 5DW Tel: 01392 402281; 59 Long Fallow, Chiswell Green, St Albans AL2 3ED Tel: 01727 867150 — MB BS Lond. 1993 (Char. Cross. & Westm.) BSc (Med. Biochem.) Birm. 1988; MRCP (UK) 1997. Specialist Regist. Diabetes & Endocrin. Roy. Devon & Exeter Hosp. Specialty: Diabetes; Endocrinol.

SPYRANTIS, Niki 1 Podsmead Road, Manchester M22 1UZ — State Exam Med Berlin 1992.

SPYRIOUNIS, Petros Northern General Hospital, Plastic Surgery Department, Herries Road, Sheffield S5 7AU — Ptychio Iatrikes Thessalonika 1988.

SPYROU, Mr George — Ptychio Iatrikes Thessalonika 1988 (Aristotelian Univ. Thessaloniki) FRCS Ed. 1996. Specialist Regist. (Plastic Surg.) Leeds Gen. Infirm. Specialty: Plastic Surg. Special Interest: Breast & Plastic Surg. Prev: SHO (Plastic Surg.) Wordsley Hosp. W. Midl.; SHO Rotat. (Gen. Surg.) Roy. Devon & Exeter Hosp.

SPYROU, Nicolaos Royal Berks & Battle Hospital, Cardiology Department, Oxford Road, London RG1 Tel: 0118 963 6363 Fax: 0118 963 6622; 44 Burntwood Grange Road, London SW18 3JX — MB BS Lond. 1986; BSc Lond. 1983; MRCP (UK) 1990; MD 2000; FRCP (UK) 2004. Cons. Cardiol., Roy. Berks & Battle Hosp. Trust, Reading; Cons. Cardiol., Heart/ UCLH Lond. Specialty: Cardiol.; Gen. Med. Special Interest: Interventional Cardiol. Socs: Roy. Coll. of Phys.; Brit. Cardiac Soc.; Brit. Cardiac Internat. Soc. Prev: Sen. Regist., Cardiol., Hammersmith Hosp., Lond.; Sen. Regist., St. Mary's Hosp., Lond.

SQUIER, Marian Valerie Department of Neuropathology, Radcliffe Infirmary, Oxford OX2 6HE Tel: 01865 224932 Fax: 01865 224508 Email: waney.squier@clneuro.ox.ac.uk — MB ChB Leeds 1972; BSc Leeds 1969; MRCP (UK) 1974; FRCPath 1993, M 1981; FRCP 2003. Cons. & Clin. Lect. (Neuropath.) Radcliffe Infirm. Oxf. Specialty: Neuropath. Special Interest: Birth Asphixia; Cerebral Palsy; Disorders of Brain Developm. Socs: Brit. Neuropath. Soc.; French Neuropath. Soc.; Brit. Paediat. Neurol. Assn. Prev: Sen. Regist. (Neuropath.) Inst. Psychiat. Lond.; Lect. (Histopath.) Inst. Child Health Lond.

SQUIRE, Andrea Jane Boxwell Road Surgery, 1 Boxwell Road, Berkhamsted HP4 3EU — MB ChB Sheff. 1992; DRCOG; MRCGP; DFFP.

SQUIRE, Mr Benjamin Roly Department of Paediatric Surgery, St. James University Hospital, Leeds LS9 7TF Tel: 0113 243 3144 Fax: 0113 283 7059; Scott Hill House, 72 Main St, Thorner, Leeds LS14 3BU Tel: 0113 289 2537 — MB BS Lond. 1977 (St. Mary's) MRCS Eng. LRCP Lond. 1977; DCH Eng. 1981; FRCS Eng. 1982; FRCS (Paediat.) 1992. Cons. Paediat. Surg. St. Jas. Univ. Hosp. Leeds & Leeds Gen. Infirm.; Hon. Sen. Lect. Univ. Leeds. Specialty: Paediat. Surg. Prev: Sen. Regist. (Paediat Surg.) Hosp. for Sick Childr. Gt. Ormond St. Lond.; Regist. (Surg.) Roy. Manch. Childr. Hosp.; Research Fell. (Paediat Surg.) Childr. Hosp. Buffalo, USA.

SQUIRE, Christopher Michael Squire and Partners, Market Place, Hadleigh, Ipswich IP7 5DN Tel: 01473 822961 Fax: 01473 824895; Langdale, The St, Aldham, Ipswich IP7 6NH Tel: 01473 823026 — MRCS Eng. LRCP Lond. 1968 (St. Mary's) LMSSA Lond. 1967; DCH Eng. 1972. Prev: Clin. Asst. (Paediat.) St. Geo. Hosp. Lond.; Squadron Ldr. RAF Med. Br.; SHO (O & G) Ipswich Hosp.

SQUIRE, Iain Leicester Royal Infimary, Department of Medicine & Therapeutics, Clinical Sciences Building, Leicester LE2 7LX Tel: 0116 252 3125 Fax: 0116 252 3108 Email: is11@le.ac.uk — MB ChB Glas. 1987 (Glasgow) BSc Strathclyde 1982; MRCP (UK) 1990; MD Glasgow 1997; FRCP England 2002. Sen. Lect. in Med. & Therap., Univ. of Leicester; Hon. Cons. Phys., Leicester Roy. Infirm. Specialty: Pharmacology; Cardiol. Special Interest: natriuretic peptides; Epidemiol. of heart failure. Socs: Brit. Pharmacological Soc.; Brit. Soc. for Heart Failure; Heart Failure Assn. of the Europ. Soc. of Cardiol. Prev: Lect. in Clin. Pharmacol., Univ. of Leicester; Lect. in Med. & Therap., Univ. of Glas.; Clin. Research Fell. Univ. of Glas.

SQUIRE, Janet Katherine Sue Ryder Care Centre, Thorpe Hall, Longthorpe, Peterborough PE3 6LW Tel: 01733 330060 Fax: 01733 269078; Rushton Manor, Rushton, Kettering NN14 1RH Tel: 01536 711451 — MB BS Lond. 1971 (Middlx.) DObst RCOG 1973; Dip. Palliat. Med. Wales 1995. Med. Dir., Sue Ryder Care Centre, Thorpe Hall, PeterBoro.; Hon. Cons. Palliat. Med. P'boro Hosps. Trust. Specialty: Palliat. Med. Prev: Clin. Asst. (Palliat. Med.) Cynthia Spencer Hse. Manfield Hosp. N.ants.

SQUIRE, John Walter (retired) Squirrels, Cagefoot Lane, Henfield BN5 9HD Tel: 01273 492254 Email: johnsquire@doctors.org.uk — (Camb. & St. Bart.) MRCS Eng. LRCP Lond. 1942; DObst RCOG 1949; FRCGP 1969. Prev: Hon. Antenatal Off. Sussex Matern. Hosp. Brighton.

SQUIRE, June Mary (retired) Rose Cottage, Church Oakley, Basingstoke RG23 7LJ Tel: 01256 780225 — MB BS Lond. 1959 (Guy's) MRCS Eng. LRCP Lond. 1959; FFA RCS Eng. 1966. Cons. Anaesth. Basingstoke & Dist. Hosp. & Lord Mayor Treloar's Hosp. Alton. Prev: Sen. Regist. (Anaesth.) St. Geo. Hosp. Lond.

SQUIRE, Philip Legh Brinsmead St James Medical Centre, St. James Street, Taunton TA1 1JP Tel: 01823 285400 Fax: 01823 285405 — MB BS Lond. 1977 (The Royal London) MRCGP 1982. GP Taunton; Med. Off King's Coll & King's Hall, Taunton & Som. CCC. Specialty: Gen. Pract. Prev: Clin. Governance Lead & Bd. Mem., Taunton & Area PCG.

SQUIRE, Ruth Anne Ladyhope House, Mill Lane, Broomfield, Chelmsford CM1 7BQ — MB ChB Leic. 1983; DCH RCP Lond. 1985; MRCGP 1991. GP Tutor for Mid Essex. Specialty: Gen. Med. Socs: BMA. Prev: GP Norwich; Chief Resid. (Family & Community Med.) Univ. Missouri, USA.

SQUIRE, Stephen Bertel Liverpool School of Tropical Medicine, Pembroke Place, Liverpool L3 5QA Tel: 0151 708 9393 Fax: 0151 708 8733; Salisbury House, 18 Nicholas Road, Blundellsands, Liverpool L23 6TU Tel: 0151 932 0819 Fax: 0151 932 0936 — MB BChir Camb. 1984; BSc Lond. 1982; MRCP (UK) 1988; MD Camb.

1995. Wellcome Trust Fell. (Virol.) Roy. Free Hosp. Lond. Specialty: Immunol. Prev: Clin. Research Fell. (HIV/AIDS) Dept. Thoracic Med. & Virol. Roy. FreeHosp. Lond.; Regist. (Gen. Med.) OldCh. Hosp. Romford.

SQUIRES, Mr Benjamin 15 Fremantle Road, Cotham, Bristol BS6 5SY Tel: 0117 946 6188 — MB BS Lond. 1990; FRCS Eng. 1995; FRCS (Tr. & Orth.) 2000. Bristol Specialist Regist. Orthop. Rotat. Specialty: Trauma & Orthop. Surg. Prev: SHO Rotat. (Surg.) Bristol Roy. Infirm.; Ho. Phys. Kent & Canterbury Hosp.; Demonst. (Anat.) Sheff. Univ.

SQUIRES, Julian Patrick Teign Estuary Medical Group, Glendevon Medical Centre, Carlton Place, Teignmouth TQ14 8AB Tel: 01626 770955 Fax: 01626 772107 Email: julian.squires@nhs.net; Riverside Surgery, Albion St, Shaldon, Teignmouth TQ14 0D Tel: 01626 873331 — MB BCh Wales 1986 (Univ. Wales Coll. Med.) MRCGP 1990; DRCOG 1990; LLM Wales 2000. Clin. Asst. (Med.) S. Devon Healthcare; Mem. S. & W. Devon LMC. Specialty: Gen. Pract.; Medico Legal. Prev: Trainee GP Torbay VTS; SHO (O & G & Paediat.) Torbay HA; SHO (Clin. Oncol.) Exeter HA.

SQUIRES, Michael Jackson 30 Grove Road, Eastbourne BN21 4TR Tel: 01323 720140 — MB BS Lond. 1946 (King's Coll. Lond. & St. Geo.) MRCS Eng. LRCP Lond. 1946; DOMS Eng. 1949. Assoc. Specialist (Ophth.) E. Sussex. Specialty: Ophth. Socs: BMA; Medico-Legal Soc. Prev: Sen. Med. Off. West. Ophth. Hosp.; Designated Aviat. Med. Examr. Govt. Austral.; Ophth. Adviser Unilever.

SQUIRES, Neil Frederick Department for International Development, 1 Palace Street, London SW1E 5HE Tel: 020 7023 0405 Email: n-squires@dfid.gov.uk; 62 Stanford Avenue, Brighton BN1 6FD — MB ChB Sheff. 1986; MPH Liverp. 1993; MFPHM Lond. 1995. Sen. Health & Popul. Advisor, Dept. for Int. Devel. Specialty: Pub. Health Med. Prev: Specialist (Pub. Health) Dept. for Internat. Developm. Lond.; Cons. (Pub. Health) Liverp. Health Auth.

SQUIRES, Richard Charles (retired) Old Church House, Priory Road, Wantage Tel: 012357 2785 — MRCS Eng. LRCP Lond. 1962 (St. Thos.) Prev: Ho. Surg. Southlands Hosp. Shoreham-by-Sea.

SQUIRES, Stephen John, Surg. Cdr. RN Retd. Queen Victoria Hospital NHS Trust, Holtye Road, East Grinstead RH19 3DZ — MB BS Lond. 1979 (St. Geo.) FFA RCS Eng. 1984. Cons. Anaesth. Qu. Vict. Hosp. E. Grinstead; Director of Surg. Care Gp. Specialty: Anaesth. Special Interest: Burns & Plastic Surg. Socs: Brit. Burns Assn.; Assn. Anaesth. UK & Irel.; Intens. Care Soc. Prev: Cons. Anaesth. Burns Unit Qu. Vict. Hosp. E. Grinstead; Cons. Anaesth. RN Hosps. Haslar, Plymouth & Gibraltar; Sen. Regist. (Anaesth.) Bristol Roy. Infirm.

SQUIRRELL, David Michael 6 Ryegate Road, Sheffield S10 5FA — MB ChB Sheff. 1995.

SREEDARAN, Elayathamby 5 Denvale Walk, Goldsworth Park, Woking GU21 3PF — MB BS Peradeniya, Sri Lanka 1985.

SREEDHARAN, Kamprath Brunswick Health Centre, Hartfield Close, Manchester M13 9YA Tel: 0161 273 4901 Fax: 0161 273 5952; 6 Green Pastures, Stockport SK4 3RA — MB BS Kerala 1971.

SREEHARAN, Nadarajah New Frontiers Science Park, Third Avenue, Harlow CM19 5AW Tel: 01438 762602 Email: n.sree.haran@gsk.com — MB BS Ceylon 1970; MD Colombo 1974; MRCP (UK) 1976; PhD Leeds 1979; FRCP Glas. 1985; FRCP Ed. 1986; FRCP Lond. 1986; FFPM 1992; FACP 1994. Sen. Vice. Pres GSK R & D; Counc. Mem. and Mem. of Bd. of Examiners, FPM,RCP(Lond). Specialty: Pharmaceutical Medicine; Gen. Med. Prev: Vis. Prof. Cardiol. Univ. Alberta, Canada.; Prof. & Head of Dept. Med. Univ. Jaffna Sri Lanka.

SREEHARI RAO, Singu Amington Surgery, 130 Tamowrth Road, Amington, Tamworth B77 3BZ Tel: 01827 54777 Fax: 01827 59539; Wigginton Grange, 163 Gillway Lane, Tamworth B79 8PN — MB BS Andhra 1971; DA RCSI 1974; DObst RCPI 1979; FFA RCSI 1981. Specialty: Anaesth.

SREEKANTA, Gopalarao Edward Street Day Hospital, Edward St., West Bromwich B70 8NJ Tel: 0121 553 7676 Fax: 0121 607 3576; 11 Holly Wood, off White Crest, Great Barr, Birmingham B43 6EH Tel: 0121 357 2703 — MB BS Bangalor 1971 (Govt. Med. Coll. Bangalore, Karnataka, India) MB BS Bangalore 1971; Dip. Clin. Psychiat. RCP&S of Ire. 1997. Clin. Asst. (Pychogeriats.) Edwd. St. Day Hosp. W. Bromwich. Specialty: Geriat. Psychiat. Socs: Med. Protec. Soc. Prev: Regist. (Psychiat.) Pastures Hosp. Mickleover, Derby & St. Geo. Hosp. Stafford; SHO Carlton Hayes Hosp. Leicester.

SREENIVASA RAO, Col. L Pavar Madhavarao, Col. L/RAMC Consultant Advisor HIV & GU Medicine, Defence Medical Service, Frimley Park Hospital, Camberley GU16 5UJ Tel: 01276 604069 Fax: 01276 604297; 2 Silverdale Drive, London SE9 4DH Tel: 020 8851 2259 Fax: 020 8697 2920 Email: spavar@yahoo.com — MB BS Madras 1971 (Jipmer, India) MRCOG 1979; MD Madras 1980; Dip. Ven. Liverp. 1983; FRCOG 2003. Cons. Adviser (HIV & Genitourin. Med.) Defence Med. Serv. Frimley Pk. Hosp. Surrey. Specialty: Genitourinary Medicine. Socs: BMA, Soc. Study of VD., AGUM, BHIVA. Prev: Sen. Regist. (Genitourin. Med.) Roy. Liverp. Hosp.; Regist. (Genitourin. Med.) Chester & Arrowe Pk. Hosps.; Regist. (O & G) Walton & Fazakerley Hosp. Liverp. & Lister Hosp. Stevenage.

SREETHARAN, Maharojani St Ebba's Hospital, Hook Road, Epsom KT19 8QJ Tel: 020 8657 0018; 1 Balmoral Gardens, South Croydon CR2 0HN — MB BS Ceylon 1971 (Colombo) DPM Eng. 1980. Staff Grade Practitioner. Prev: Clin. Asst. Epsom.

SREETHARAN, Mathiaparanam Sai Medical Centre, 17B Balham Park Road, Balham, London SW12 8DT; Mathura, 1 Lupin Close, Shirley Oaks Village, Croydon CR0 8XZ — MB BS Ceylon 1971 (Colombo)

SREEVALSAN, santha K Oakwood Surgery, 380 Bishops Drive, Oakwood, Derby DE21 2DF Tel: 01332 281220 Fax: 01332 677150; 19 Gleneagles Close, Mickleover, Derby DE3 9YB Tel: 01332 514244 — MB BS Kerala 1966. Socs: Med. Protec. Soc.

SREEVALSAN, Mrs Santha Kumari Oakwood Surgery, 380 Bishops Drive, Oakwood, Derby DE21 2DF Tel: 01332 281220 Fax: 01332 677150 Email: santhasreevalsan@hotmail.com — MB BS Kerala 1966; MRCOG London 1978. Specialty: Family Planning; Obst. & Gyn. Socs: Med. Protec.-Full; Gen. Med. Counc.; Roy. Coll. of Obst. & Gynaecologists.

SRI GANESHAN, Moothathamby 107B Grand Drive, London SW20 9EB Tel: 020 8542 1369; 26 Marlings Park Avenue, Chislehurst BR7 6QW Tel: 01689 824780 Fax: 01689 813748 — MB BS Ceylon 1973; MRCOG 1987. GP Shewsbury Rd., Health Centre Lond. Specialty: Gen. Pract.; Obst. & Gyn. Socs: Roy. Coll. Obst. & Gyns. Prev: Regist. (Obst. & Gyna.) Barking Hosp.

SRI KRISHNA, Mudumbi The Surgery, 76 Herbert Road, London SE18 3PP Tel: 020 8854 3964 Fax: 020 8317 8512 — MB BS Osmania 1961.

SRI KRISHNA, Rama The Surgery, 76 Herbert Road, London SE18 3PR Tel: 020 8854 3964 Fax: 020 8317 8512 — MB BS Osmania 1961; MB BS Osmania 1961.

SRIDHAR, Janga Department of Anaesthesia, Tameside General Hospital, Fountain St., Ashton-under-Lyne OL6 9RW — MB BS Sri Venkateswara 1977; FFA RCSI 1986.

SRIDHAR, Mangalam Kumaraswasmy — MB BS Madras 1986; MRCP (UK) 1989; PhD Glas. 1996; FRCP Ed 1999; FCCP USA 1999; FRCP Lond. 2000. Cons. Phys. Hammersmith Hosps. NHS Trust, Lond.; Hon. Sen. Lect., NHLI Div., Fac. of Med. Imperial Coll. of Sci., Technol. of Med. Specialty: Respirat. Med.; Gen. Med. Socs: Brit. Thorac. Soc. Prev: Research Fell. (Med. & Human Nutrit.) Univ. Glas.; Regist. (Respirat. Med.) Glas. Roy. Infirm.; Cons. Phys., Mid-Staffs. NHS Trust.

SRIDHAR, Subbaramiah 9 Stirling Drive, Gourock PA19 1AH — MB BS Mysore 1979; MRCP (UK) 1987.

SRIDHARAN, Ganapathyagraharam Venkatanarayana 4 Peaslake Close, Romiley, Stockport SK6 4JX — MB BS Madras 1975; MRCPI 1983.

SRIEMEVAN, Amirthalingam Peterborough District Hospital, Thorpe Road, Peterborough PE3 6DA — MD Minsk. Cons. Opstetrician and Gynaecologist. Specialty: Obst. & Gyn. Special Interest: Colposcopy; High Risk Obst.; menstrual problems. Socs: RCOG; Fetal Med. Foundat.; BSCCP.

SRIKANTHARAJAH, Indradevi 52 Regal Way, Harrow HA3 0RY — LRCP LRCS Ed. 1982; LRCP LRCS Ed. LRCPS Glas. 1982.

SRINIVAS, Ranjit Kandadai 6 Warwick Close, Bexley DA5 3NL — MB ChB Manch. 1986.

SRINIVAS, Mr Subrahmanyam Accident & Emergency Department, Kent & Canterbury Hospital, Ethelbert Road, Canterbury CT1 2NG — MB BS Madras 1986; FRCS Glas. 1993.

SRINIVASA, Kanabur 46 Millers Walk, Pelsall, Walsall WS3 4QS — MB BS Bangalore 1971; T(GP). Locum (Psychiat.).

SRINIVASA MURTHY, Mr Lakkur Nagappa 184 Osborne Road, Newcastle upon Tyne NE2 3LE — MB BS Mysore 1965 (Bangalore Med. Coll.) FRCS Eng. 1970; DMRD Eng. 1982; FRCR 1983. Cons. Radiol. Freeman Hosp. Newc. u. Tyne. Specialty: Radiol. Prev: Surg. Hosp. Dr. Baski Gonbad-e-Qabus Iran; Surg. Shanthi Surg. Nurs. Home Bangalore, India; Regist. & Sen. Regist. Univ. Dept. Radiol. Newc. u. Tyne.

SRINIVASAN, Arul Malar Broomfield Hospital, Coourt Road, Chelmsford CM1 7ET Tel: 01245 515231 Fax: 01245 515207 — MB BS Madras 1977; LMSSA Lond. 1986; DGM RCP Lond. 1989; MRCP (UK) 1990. Cons. (Rheum.), Broomfield Hosp., Chelmsford. Specialty: Rheumatol. Socs: Memb. Of The Brit. Soc. For Rheum.; Memb. Of The Brit. Med. Assn. Prev: Regist. (Gen. Med.) Stoke Mandeville Hosp. Aylesbury; Regist.Rheumatogy stoke Mandeville Hosp., Aylesbury; SHO (Geriat.) Wythenshawe Hosp. Manch.// Sen.Reg. RNOHT of HOMERTON.

SRINIVASAN, Janaki Siambar Wen, Llanfair Road, Abergele LL22 8DL — MB BS Madras 1986.

SRINIVASAN, Mr Kuntrapaka 15 Dingle Road, Abergavenny NP7 7AR — MB BS Sri Venkateswara 1981; FRCS Glas. 1994.

SRINIVASAN, Mr Makaram Blackburn Royal Infirmary, Bolton Road, Blackburn BB2 3LR.

SRINIVASAN, Ramaiah Salisbury House, Lake St., Leighton Buzzard LU7 1RS Tel: 01525 373139; 12 Cooks Meadow, Cow Lane, Edlesborough, Dunstable LU6 2RP Tel: 01525 222284 Fax: 01525 853006 — MB BS Bangalor 1972; MB BS Bangalore 1972; DCH Dub. 1977.

SRINIVASAN, Singanayagam c/o Mrs V. Sivoyothy, 156 Balfour Road, Ilford IG1 4JB — MB BS Ceylon 1964 (Colombo) Socs: BMA.

SRINIVASAN, Sujatha The Surgery, 20 Southwick St., Southwick, Brighton BN42 4TE Tel: 01273 596077 — MB BS Lond. 1992; DRCOG 1995; DFFP 1996; MRCGP 1997. GP Princip. Specialty: Gen. Pract.

SRINIVASAN, Thottuvai Ramaiyer 2 Hall Drive, Burley in Wharfedale, Ilkley LS29 7LL — MB ChB Leeds 1971; BSc (Hons.) (Biochem.) Leeds 1971, MB ChB Leeds 1974; MRCP (UK) 1978; FRCP Lond. 1992. Cons. Phys. Dept. Geriat. St. Jas. Univ. Hosp. Leeds.; Hon. Sen. Lect. (Med.) Since 1991. Specialty: Gen. Med.

SRINIVASAN, Usha Princess of Wales Hospital, Bridgend CF31 1RQ Tel: 01656 752825 Fax: 01656 752821 — MB BCh BAO NUI 1988 (Nat. Univ. of Irel., Univ. Coll., Dub.) Cons. Rhematologist, Princess of Wales Hosp., Bridgend. Specialty: Rheumatol. Socs: BSR; NOS. Prev: Cons. Rheumatologist, Gwent Healthcare NHS Trust; Specialist Regist. in Rheum., Univ. Hosp. of Wales, Cardiff.

SRINIVASAN, Mr Vaikuntam Glan Clwyd Hospital, Bodelwyddan, Rhyl LL18 5UJ Tel: 01745 583910 Fax: 01745 583143; Siamber Wen, Llanfair Road, Abergele LL22 8DL Tel: 01745 832071 Fax: 01745 832071 Email: mrvsrini@aol.com — MB BS Madurai 1979; MS (Gen. Surg.) Madurai 1982; FRCS Ed. 1986; Dip. Urol. Lond 1988. Cons. Urol. Glan Clwyd Hosp. Bodelwyddan Rhyl. Specialty: Urol. Socs: Brit. Assn. Urol. Surgs.; Welsh Urol. Soc.; Corres. Mem. Amer. Urol. Assn. Prev: Regist. (Urol.) Edith Cavell Hosp. P'boro.

SRIPURAM, Sudhakara Gupta Broadway Surgery, 9 The Broadway, Whitehawk Road, Brighton BN2 5NF Tel: 01273 600888 Fax: 01273 605664; 16 Martyns Close, Ovingdean, Brighton BN2 7BU — MB BS Andhra 1975; DO Bangalore 1978. GP. Specialty: Gen. Pract.

SRIRAM, Sujata 9 Jackson Drive, Glasgow G33 6GE Tel: 0141 779 4161 — MB BS Bombay 1986 (Grant Med. Coll., Bombay) MD Bombay 1989; MRCP (UK) 1995. Assoc. Specialist Gartnavel Gen. Hosp. Glas. Specialty: Respirat. Med.; Gen. Med. Socs: Roy. Coll. Phys. & Surgs. Glas.; Brit. Thorac. Soc.; BMA. Prev: Staff Grade Phys. Gartnavel Gen. Hosp. Glas.

SRIRAMULU, Venkataramanappa Grimethorpe Surgery, Dorbren House, Cemetery Road, Barnsley S72 7JB Tel: 01226 716809 — MB BS Bangalore 1974. GP Grimethorne, Barnsley.

SRIRANGALINGAM, Sivaneshwary Medical Centre, Grosvenor Terrace, Trimdon Colliery, Trimdon Station TS29 6DH Tel: 01429 880284 Fax: 01429 881405; Medical Eye Centre, Willowfield House, Trimdon Station TS29 6DH Tel: 01429 880284 Fax: 01429 881405 — MB BS Ceylon 1967 (Colombo) DO Lond. 1973; Dip. Ven. Liverp. 1982. Ophth. Med. Pract. Trimdon Station.

SRIRANGALINGAM, Thambiya Sivagurunathan Sellam (Surgery), Willowfield House, Trimdon Station TS29 6DU — MB BS Ceylon 1966 (Colombo) MRCOG 1980; Dip. Venereol. Liverp. 1981.

SRIRANGAM, Shalom Justus Blackburn Royal Infirmary, Infirmary Rd, Blackburn BB2 3LR; 93 Cromwell Road, Stretford, Manchester M32 8QL — MB ChB Manch. 1997 (Manchester) SHO (A&E) BRI., Blackburn. Specialty: Accid. & Emerg. Socs: BMA; MDU. Prev: SHO. (Orthop.) BRI, Blackburn; Ho.Off.(Surg.) Hope Hosp. Salford; Ho. Off. (Med.) Stepping Hill Hosp. Stockport.

SRISKANDAN, Kumar Rookery Medical Centre, Rookery House, Newmarket CB8 8NW Tel: 01638 665711 Fax: 01638 561280; Durleigh, Falmouth Avenue, Newmarket CB8 0NB — MB BChir Camb. 1983 (Cambridge) MA, MB Camb. 1983, BChir 1982; DRCOG 1987; DCH RCP Lond. 1989; MRCGP (Distinc.) 1989. Specialty: Gen. Pract. Prev: Trainee GP Greenwich & Brook VTS.

SRISKANDAN, Shiranee Department of Infectious Diseases, Faculty of Medicine, Imperial College of Science, Technology and Medicine, Hammersmith Hospital, Du cane Road, London W12 0NN Tel: 020 8383 2065 Fax: 020 8383 3394 Email: s.sriskandan@ic.ac.uk — MB BChir Camb. 1988; MA Camb. 1985, MB BChir 1988; MRCP (UK) 1991; PhD (Lond.) 1997; FRCP 2001. Sen. Lect./Hon. Cons.Infec.dis.Fac. of Med., Imperial Coll., Hammersmith Hosp.. Lond. Specialty: Infec. Dis. Prev: MRC Clinican Scientist (infect. Dis), ICSM.

SRITHARAN, Sathasivam Department of Anaesthetics, Maidstone Hospital, Hermitage Lane, Maidstone ME16 9NN Tel: 01622 729000 Fax: 01622 723061; Shree-Rangham, 203 Willington St, Maidstone ME15 8EE Tel: 0850 666543 — MB BS Sri Lanka 1972; DA Eng. 1980; LMSSA Lond. 1985; FFA RCS Eng. 1985. Cons. Anaesth. Maidstone Hosp. Specialty: Anaesth.; Intens. Care.

SRIVASTAVA, Anand Swarup 33 Keynell Covert, Kings Norton, Birmingham B30 3QT Tel: 0121 458 2619; Anand Villa, 99 Bells Lane, Kings Heath, Birmingham B14 5QJ Tel: 0121 458 5432 — MB BS Lucknow 1958 (King Geo. Med. Coll.) DCP Baroda 1966. Socs: Med. Protec. Soc. Prev: Clin. Asst. (A & E) Selly Oak Hosp. Birm. & Corbett Hosp. Stourbridge; Regist. (Path.) Accid. Hosp. Birm.

SRIVASTAVA, Anil Kumar Brookside Medical Centre, Heol Afon Taf, Troedyrhiw, Merthyr Tydfil CF48 4DT Tel: 01443 692647 Fax: 01443 693255; Madhushala, 11 Hill Top Crescent, The Common, Pontypridd CF37 4AD Tel: 01443 406232 Fax: 01443 693255 — MB BS Ranchi 1966 (Rajendra Med. Coll.) BSc Ranchi 1966; Dip. Palliat. Med. Wales 1993; Cert. Med. Law Glas. 1996; Dip. Therapeut. Wales 1997; Mse (Paed) Glamorgan 1998. Clin. Asst. (Renal Med.) Merthyr Tydfil; GP CME Tutor Merthyr Tydfil; Clin. Asst. (Acc. & Emerg.) Llwnypia Hosp. Specialty: Nephrol.; Palliat. Med.; Accid. & Emerg. Socs: MRSH; Fell. Roy. Soc. Trop. Med. & Hyg.; Fell. Internat. Coll. Angiol. Prev: Resid. St. John's Hosp. St. John Canada; SHO (Orthop.) St. David's Hosp. Cardiff; Regist. Velindre Hosp. WhitCh.

SRIVASTAVA, Arun Kumar (retired) — (Madras Medical College) MB BS Madras 1955. Prev: Med. Asst. (A & E Dept.) Rotherham Hosp.

SRIVASTAVA, Emmanuel Devaprasad Department of Medicine, Royal Gwent Hospital, Newport NP20 2UB — MD Lond. 1992; MB BS 1984; MRCP (UK) 1987. Cons. Phys. Gen. Med. & Gastroenterol. Roy. Gwent Hosp. Newport. Specialty: Gastroenterol. Prev: Sen. Regist. (Gen. Med. & Gastroenterol.) North. RHA Newc. u. Tyne; Regist. (Gastroenterol.) Univ. Hosp. Wales Cardiff; Research Fell. Univ. Hosp. Rotterdam, Netherlands.

SRIVASTAVA, Geeta South Norwood Hill Surgery, 21B South Norwood Hill, London SE25 6AA Tel: 020 8653 0635 Fax: 020 8771 8013 — MB BS Lucknow 1974.

SRIVASTAVA, Krishna Kumar The Smethwick Medical Centre, Regent Street, Smethwick, Warley B66 3BQ Tel: 0121 558 0105 Fax: 0121 555 7206 — MB BS Lucknow 1967.

SRIVASTAVA, Madhu Shivam, 5 Dorcas Close, Thornhill, Nuneaton CV11 6XL Tel: 01203 372809 — MB BS Kanpur 1976; FRCA 1997. Specialist Regist. (Anaesth.) Cov. Sch. Of Anaesth. Specialty: Anaesth.

SRIVASTAVA, Prabodh Kumar North Park Health Centre, 290 Knowsley Road, Bootle L20 5DQ Tel: 0151 922 3841 Fax: 0151

933 7335; Ganano Que, Burbo Bank Road, Blundellsands, Liverpool L23 6TQ Tel: 0151 931 1980 Fax: 0151 933 7335 — MB BS Osmania 1971 (Osmania Med. Coll. Hyderabad) Prev: SHO Birkenhead Gen. Hosp., W. Suff. Hosp. Bury St. Edmunds & Norf. & Norwich Gen. Hosp.

SRIVASTAVA, Mr Pramod Kumar c/o Drive R.C. Prasad, 8 Hilderthorpe, Nunthorpe, Middlesbrough TS7 0PT Tel: 01642 317825 — MB BS Banares Hindu India 1978; FRCS 1990.

SRIVASTAVA, Prasima 63H Richmond Street, Aberdeen AB25 2TS Tel: 01224 643226; 178 Culduthel Road, Inverness IV2 4BH — MB ChB Aberd. 1993; BSc (Med. Sci.) (Hons.) Aberd. 1991; MRCP (UK) 1997. SHO (Med.) Aberd. Roy. Infirm.; Research Fell. (Respirat. Med.) Dept. of Childhealth Med. Sch. Aberd. Roy. Trust Hosp. Specialty: Respirat. Med. Prev: Ho. Off. (Surg.) Raigmore Hosp. Inverness; Ho. Off. (Med.) Aberd. Roy. Infirm.

SRIVASTAVA, Satya Prakash 28 Earnshaw Way, Beaumont Park, Whitley Bay NE25 9UN Tel: 0191 253 3886 Fax: 0191 253 3886 — MB BS Lucknow 1966 (G.S.V.M. Med. Coll. Kanpur) FRCR Lond.; MSc Allahabad 1960; DMRE Lucknow 1967; DMRD Eng. 1972. Cons. Radiol. Northumbria Health Care NHS Trust, N. Shield. Specialty: Radiol. Socs: BMA & Roy. Coll. Radiols. Prev: Sen. Regist. Midl. Centre for Neurol. & Neurosurg. Smethwick; Sen. Regist. (Radiol.) & Regist. (Radiol.) Selly Oak Hosp. Birm.; Trainee Regist. (Radiol.) United Birm. Hosps.

SRIVASTAVA, Mr Shekhar George Eliot Hospital, College Street, Nuneaton CV11 6XL Tel: 024 7686 5428 — MB BS Kanpur 1973; MS Kanpur 1976; FRCS Eng. 1981; FRCS Ed. 1981; FRCS (Plast) 1996. Cons. Plastic Surg. Geo. Eliot Hosp. Nuneaton Warks. Specialty: Plastic Surg. Socs: Assoc. Mem. Brit. Assn. Plastic Surgs.; Assoc. Mem. BSSH. Prev: Regist. (Plastic Surg.) Wordsley Hosp. Stourbridge.

SRIVASTAVA, Shobha (retired) South Tyneside District Hospital, Harton Lane, South Shields NE34 0PL Tel: 0191 454 8888; 35 St. George's Avenue, South Shields NE33 3DU Tel: 0191 455 8146 — (King Geo. Med. Coll. Lucknow) MB BS Lucknow 1955; MD (Physiol.) Lucknow 1961; MS (Anaesth.) Bihar 1964; FFA RCSI 1977; FFA RCS Eng. 1978. Examr. Fac. Anaesth. RCS Irel. Prev: Cons. Anaesth. S. Tyneside Dist. Hosp. S. Shields.

SRIVASTAVA, Sunil Kumar Richmond Medical Centre, 15 Upper Accommodation Road, Leeds LS9 8RZ Tel: 0113 248 0948 Fax: 0113 240 9898 Email: dr_sunil@madasafish.com; 6 Sandmoor Avenue, Leeds LS17 7DW — (GSVM Med. Coll. Kanpur) MB BS Kanpur 1970; DTCD Kanpur 1974; DTM & H Liverp. 1976. Socs: Assoc. Inst. Psychosexual Med. Lond; Soc. Occupat. Med.

SRIVASTAVA, Mr Suresh Prasad Arnold Medical Centre, 204 St. Annes Road, Blackpool FY4 2EF Tel: 01253 346351 Fax: 01253 400244; 18 Cotswold Road, Blackpool FY2 0UH Tel: 01253 55974 — MB BS Agra 1963 (S.N. Med. Coll. Agra) MS Lucknow 1967; FRCS Ed. 1974.

SRIVATSA, Surath Sanjay 23 Oaklands Avenue, Romford RM1 4DB — MB BChir Camb. 1988.

SRIWARDHANA, Kamala Bandumathie ENT Department, Gwynedd District General Hospital, Penrhos Garnedd, Bangor Tel: 01248 370007; 11 Coed-y-Castell, Bangor LL57 1PH — MB BS Ceylon 1967 (Colombo) DLO Eng. 1978; FRCS Glas. 1983. Assoc. Specialist (ENT Surg.) Gwynedd Dist. Gen. Hosp. Prev: Regist. (ENT) Gwynedd Gen. Hosp.; Regist. (ENT) Monkland Dist. Gen. Hosp.; SHO (ENT) Leicester Roy. Infirm.

SRODON, Mr Paul Damian 28 Tamworth Road, Coventry CV6 2EL Tel: 024 76 333253 — MB ChB Birm. 1988; FRCS Eng. 1992; MD Birm. 1997. Specialist Regist. Roy. Lond. Hosp. and St. Bart. Hosp. Lond. Specialty: Gen. Surg. Prev: Specialist Regist. UCL Hosps. Lond.; Lect. (Surg.) Med. Coll. of St. Bart. Hosp. Lond.

ST. BLAIZE-MOLONY, Ronald Thomas (retired) The Oak House, Westham, Pevensey BN24 5LP Tel: 01323 769784 — MB BCh BAO NUI 1952 (Univ. Coll. Dub.) LAH Dub. 1952; DPM Eng. 1959; MRCPsych 1971. Prev: Cons. Psychiat. St. Thos. Hosp. Lond.

ST. CLAIR, Mr David Malcolm Clinical Research Centre, Royal Cornhill Hospital, Aberdeen AB25 2ZH — BM BCh Oxf. 1975; FRCS Eng. 1978; MRCPsych 1984; DM Oxf. 1994. Sen. Lect. (Med.) Univ. Aberd. Specialty: Gen. Psychiat.

ST JOHN, Andrew Frank Robert Fairlawn, Lutterworth Road, Dunton Bassett, Lutterworth LE17 5LF Tel: 0116 277 1705 — MB BS Lond. 1969 (St. Bart.) MRCS Eng. LRCP Lond. 1969; DObst RCOG 1971. Prev: SHO (Anaesth. & O & G) Harold Wood Hosp. Essex.

ST. JOHN, Hanny Elizabeth Ward 36, Royal Infirmary of Edinburgh, 1 Lauriston Place, Edinburgh EH3 9YW; 11/2 Torpichen Street, Edinburgh EH3 8HX — MB ChB Ed. 1992 (Edinburgh) BSc Ed. 1987; MRCOG 1997. Specialist Regist. (O & G) Roy. Infirm. Edin. Specialty: Obst. & Gyn. Socs: BMA; MPS. Prev: SHO (O & G & Gen. Surg.) Roy. Infirm. Edin.; SHO (O & G & Gynae. Surg.) Roy. Infirm. Edin.

ST. JOHN, Janet Isabella (retired) 31 Upper Oldfield Park, Bath BA2 3JX Tel: 01225 334331 — (Edinburgh) MB ChB Ed. 1949.

ST. JOHN, Joan Mary 65 Wyverne Road, Chorlton-cum-Hardy, Manchester M21 0ZW — MB ChB Birm. 1982; DRCOG 1986; MRCGP 1987; DCH RCP Lond. 1989.

ST JOHN, Michael Arthur Farnham Stepney Health Centre, 79 Ben Jonson Road, London E1 4SA Tel: 020 7790 1059; 79 Lyal Road, Bow, London E3 5QQ — MB BS Lond. 1976 (St Bart.) Partner. Socs: MDU.

ST. JOHN JONES, Lima Siljan Harpscot, Slaugham Lane, Warninglid, Haywards Heath RH17 5TH — MB BCh BAO Dub. 1969; FFA RCS Eng. 1978. Cons. Anaesth. Crawley Horsham NHS Trust. Specialty: Anaesth.

ST. JOHN SMITH, Paul Barnet Psychiatric Unit, Barnet General Hospital, Wellhouse Lane, Barnet EN5 3DJ Tel: 020 8216 4400 — BM BCh Oxf. 1979; MA Oxf. 1980; MRCPsych 1990. Cons. (Psychiat.) Barnet Gen. Hosp. Lond. Specialty: Gen. Psychiat. Socs: Roy. Coll. Psychiat. Prev: Clin. Research Phys. (Psychopharmacol.) Roche Products Ltd., Welwyn Gdn. City.

ST. JOHNSTON, Charles Fisher Pinhoe Surgery, Pinn Lane, Exeter EX1 3SY Tel: 01392 469666 Fax: 01392 464178 — MB BS Lond. 1965 (Lond. Hosp.) DA Eng. 1973. Prev: Ho. Off. Lond. Hosp.

ST. JOSEPH, Anne Vivien Creffield Road Surgery, 19 Creffield Road, Colchester CO3 3HZ Tel: 01206 570371 Fax: 01206 369908; Mell Farm, Tollesbury, Maldon CM9 8SS — BM BCh Oxf. 1983; DRCOG 1986; MRCGP 1987. GP Colchester. Specialty: Ophth.

ST. LEGER, Sarah Ann Brunswick House, 299 Glossop Road, Sheffield S10 2HL Tel: 0114 271 6890 — MB ChB Sheff. 1989. Saff grade in Psychiat.

ST ROSE, Alison Jean 106 Crown Lane, Horwich, Bolton BL6 7QN — MB ChB Dundee 1988.

STABILE, Mrs Isabel 3086 Waterford Drive, Tallahassee FL 32308, USA Tel: 00 1 904 8933601 Fax: 00 1 904 5746704; Flat 7, Rowan, 48-50 Muswell Road, London N10 2BY Tel: 020 8883 5087 — MRCS Eng. LRCP Lond. 1981; PhD Lond. 1988; MRCOG 1989. Research Scientist Center for Biomed. Research Florida State Univ., USA; Prof. & Dir. Program Environm. Health Educat. & Train. Univ. Florida Gainsville, Florida USA. Prev: Regist. & Research Fell. Acad. Unit Obst. & Gyn. Lond. Hosp.

STABLEFORTH, Carol Frances 6 Arlington Park Mansions, Sutton Lane N., Chiswick, London W4 4HE; 17 Springfield Road, Wimbledon, London SW19 7AL Tel: 020 8879 3448 — MB ChB Bristol 1988; FRCA 1995. Cons. Anaesth., Dept. Anaesthetics, Kingston Hosp., Galsworthy Rd. Kingston Upon Thames Surrey KT2 7QB. Specialty: Anaesth.

STABLEFORTH, David Edward Birmingham Heartlands Hospital, Bordsley Green E., Birmingham B9 5ST Tel: 0121 424 2000 Fax: 0121 772 0292 Email: david.stableforth@heartsol.wmids.nhs.uk; Tower House, Spencers Lane, Berkswell, Coventry CV7 7BZ Tel: 01676 533279 — MB BChir Camb. 1968 (St. Mary's & Camb.) MA Camb. 1968; FRCP (UK) 1983, M 1970. Cons. Phys. (Gen. & Thoracic Med.) Heartlands Hosp. Birm.; Hon. Sen. Lect. Univ. Birm. Specialty: Respirat. Med. Socs: Brit. Thorac. Soc. & Europ. Respirat. Soc.; Midl. Thoracic Soc. Prev: Sen. Regist. (Med.) Brompton Hosp. Lond.; Sen. Regist. (Med.) St. Jas. Hosp. Balham; Regist. (Med.) Univ. Coll. Hosp. Lond.

STABLEFORTH, Mr Paul Godwin (retired) — MB BS Lond. 1957 (Middlx.) FRCS Eng. 1965. Cons. Traum. Orthop. Surg. United Bristol Hosps. Prev: Sen. Regist. Orthop. Serv. Edin.

STABLEFORTH, Penelope Jane Penny Tower House, Spencers Lane, Berkswell, Coventry CV7 7BZ — MB BS (Hnrs.) Lond. 1968 (St. Mary's) FRCPath 1977. Cons. Haemat. Sandwell Hosp. Specialty: Haematology. Prev: Sen. Regist. (Haemat.) Roy. Free Hosp. Lond.

STABLEFORTH, William David 4 Tamar Terrace, Saltash PL12 — MB BCh Wales 1997.

STABLER, Jacqueline Marcelle Hollies Medical Practice, Tamworth Health Centre, Upper Gungate, Tamworth B79 7EA Tel: 01827 68511 Fax: 01827 51163; Dryden House, 5 Comberford Road, Tamworth B79 8PB Tel: 01827 68382 — MB BS Newc. 1968; DObst RCOG 1971. Med. Asst. Sir Robt. Peel Hosp. Tamworth. Specialty: Obst. & Gyn. Prev: Ho. Phys. & Ho. Surg. Roy. Vict. Infirm. Newc.; SHO (Paediat.) Sunderland Childr. Hosp.; SHO (O & G) Dryburn Hosp. Durh.

STABLER, Robert John Department of Radiology, The Queen Elizabeth Hospital, Gayton Road, King's Lynn PE30 4ET Tel: 01533 613613 Fax: 01533 613838 — BM BCh Oxf. 1963; BA Oxf. 1960; DMRD Eng. 1966; FRCR 1968. p/t Cons. Radiol. King's Lynn & Wisbech Hosps NHS Trust. Specialty: Radiol. Prev: Cons. Radiol. Gateshead HA; Cons. Radiol. & Sen. Regist. (Radiol.) Roy. Vict. Infirm. Newc.

STABLES, Alison Barbara Jane Lime Tree Surgery, 38 Cann Hall Road, Leytonstone, London E11 3HZ Tel: 020 8519 9914 Fax: 020 855 7109; 189 Twickenham Road, Leytonstone, London E11 4BQ Tel: 020 8556 7872 — MB BS Lond. 1980 (Lond. Hosp.) DRCOG 1984. Prev: Princip GP Sixpenny Handley; Trainee GP W. Essex VTS.

STABLES, Gareth — MB ChB Liverp. 1998.

STABLES, Graeme Ian Department of Dermatology, Leeds General Infirmary, Leeds LS1 3EX; 7 Hollin Mews, Leeds LS16 5QP — MB ChB Leeds 1986; MRCP (UK) 1989; MD Leeds 2001; FRCP 2003. Cons. Dermatol. Leeds Gen. Infirm., Leeds. Specialty: Dermat. Special Interest: Mohs Micrograpitic Surgery. Socs: Brit. Assn. of Dermatologists; Brit. Soc. for Dermatological Surg.; Amer. Acad. of Dermat. Prev: Tutor & Hon.Sen. Regist. (Dermat.) Leeds Gen. Infirm.; YCRC Clin. Research Fell., Tutor (Dermat.) & Hon. Sen. Regist. Leeds Univ.; Regist. (Dermat.) West. Infirm. Glas.

STABLES, Philippa Rosemary Joan 40A St George's Drive, London SW1V 4BP — MB ChB Bristol 1988.

STABLES, Rodney Hilton, TD Cardiothoracic Centre, Thomas Drive, Liverpool L14 3PE Tel: 0151 293 2489 Email: rod.stables@ctc.nhs.uk — BM BCh Oxf. 1985; MA Camb. 1985; MRCP (UK) 1989; DM Oxf. 2000; FRCP (UK) 2003. Cons. Cardiol. Cardiothoracic Centre, Liverp. Specialty: Cardiol. Socs: Brit. Cardiac Soc. Prev: Regist. (Cardiol.) Roy. Brompton & John Radcliffe Oxf.; Sen. Regist. (Cardiol.) Roy. Brompton & Harefield NHS Trust.

STACEY, Andrew Robert Microbiology Department, Royal Berkshire Hospital, London Road, Reading RG1 5AN Tel: 0118 987 5111 — MB BS Lond. 1978 (Char. Cross) MRCS Eng. LRCP Lond. 1978; FRCPath 1996, M 1984. Cons. (Microbiol.) Roy. Berks. Hosp. Reading. Specialty: Med. Microbiol. Prev: Sen. Regist. Microbiol. Dept. St. Mary's Hosp. Lond.; Regist. (Microbiol.) Char. Cross Hosp. Lond.

STACEY, Anne Geraldine Lower Addiscombe Road Surgery, 188 Lower Addiscombe Road, Croydon CR0 6AH — MB BS Lond. 1970 (Univ. Coll. Hosp.) DObst RCOG 1972.

STACEY, Anthony Cedric Elvin Aon Health Solutions, 5 London Wall Buildings, Finsbury Circus, London EC2M 5NS Tel: 0207 6380909 Fax: 0207 6389211 — MB BS Lond. 1975 (Roy. Free Hosp. Sch. Med.) MRCS Eng. LRCP Lond. 1975; DCH Eng. 1979; MRCGP 1980; DRCOG 1981; DAvMed. 1982; DFFP 1996; Dip. Occ. Med. 1997. Private GP. Specialty: Aviat. Med.; Occupat. Health. Socs: Roy. Aeronautical Soc. (Med. Gp.); Soc. Occup. Med. Prev: Regional Med. Off. Foreign & Commonw. Office, Warsaw, Poland; Regional Med. Off. New Delhi, India; Company Med. Off. Anglo-Amer. Corpn. Zambia.

STACEY, Anthony Nicholas — MRCS Eng. LRCP Lond. 1981 (Sheff.) DRCOG 1984; DFFP 1995; MDCH 1998. Gen. Practitioner. Prev: Resid. Med. Off. St. Brendan's Hosp., Bermuda; Dist. Med. Off. Grenfell Regional Health Servs. Newfld., Canada; Trainee GP Torbay VTS.

STACEY, Bernard Stephan Frank Southampton General Hospital, Mailpoint 47, Tremona Road, Southampton SO16 6YD — MB ChB Bristol 1990; MRCP (UK) 1995. Cons. Phys. & Gastroenterol. Soton Gen. Hosp. Specialty: Gastroenterol. Special Interest: Oesoph. Cancer. Socs: Brit. Soc. Gastroenterol. Prev: Specialist Regist. (Gastroenterol.) Roy. United Hosp. Bath; Regist. (Gastroenterol.) Princess Mgt. Hosp. Swindon; Regist. (Gastroenterol.) Roy. Hosp. Haslar Gosport.

STACEY, Carolyn Mary Women and Young Peoples Services, St Leonards Primary Care Centre, Nuttall St, London N1 5LE — MB BS Lond. 1980; MRCOG 1989. Cons. Community Gyn. - St Leonards Primary Care Centre and Homerton Hosp. Specialty: Obst. & Gyn.

STACEY, Cheika Sian 71 St Cenydd Road, Caerphilly CF83 2TA — BM BS Nottm. 1994. Specialty: Radiol.

STACEY, David John Longlands, Westbourne Drive, Lancaster LA1 5EE Tel: 01524 34331 Fax: 01524 842556 — MB ChB Manch. 1981 (St And. & Manch.) BSc (Hons.) St. And. 1977; DRCOG 1983; MRCGP 1985; Cert. Family Plann. JCC 1987; DCCH RCGP & FCM 1989. Cons. Community Paediat. Lancaster. Specialty: Community Child Health. Socs: Fell. Roy. Coll. Paediat. & Child Health; Roy. Coll. Gen. Pract. Prev: SCMO (Child Health) Lancaster.

STACEY, Louise Tanworth Lane Surgery, 2 Tanworth Lane, Shirley, Solihull B90 4DR Tel: 0121 744 2025 Fax: 0121 733 6890 — BM BS Nottm. 1989; DRCOG 1992; MRCGP 1993.

STACEY, Mark Reginald William Department Anaesthetics, Llandough Hospital, Cardiff Tel: 029 2071 6860 Fax: 029 2070 2435; 67 Heol Don, Whitchurch, Cardiff CF14 2AS Tel: 029 2061 8100 — MB BChir Camb. 1987; MA Camb. 1988; FCAnaesth 1992. Cons. Anaesth. Llandough Hosp. Cardiff. Specialty: Anaesth. Prev: Sen. Regist. & MSc Lect. (Anaesth.) Univ. Hosp. Wales; Regist. (Anaesth.) Univ. Hosp. Wales; SHO (Anaesth.) Bristol Roy. Infirm. & Withy Bush Hosp. HaverfordW.

STACEY, Richard Grant Willson Kingston Hospital, Galsworthy Road, Kingston upon Thames KT2 7QB Tel: 020 8546 7711 — MB BS Lond. 1983 (Char. Cross Hosp. Med. Sch.) DA (UK) 1987; FFA RCS Eng. 1988. Cons. Anaesth. Kingston Hosp. Specialty: Anaesth. Socs: Assn. Obst. Anaesth. Prev: Cons. Anaesth. W. Middlx. Univ. Hosp.; Sen. Regist. St. Geo. Hosp. & Brompton Hosp. Lond.; Regist. (Anaesth.) Hammersmith & Roy. Marsden Hosps. Lond.

STACEY, Robert Kevin High Melton, Oakwood Road W., Rotherham S60 3AB — MB BS Lond. 1972; MRCS Eng. LRCP Lond. 1972; DObst RCOG 1974; FFA RCS Eng. 1977. Specialty: Anaesth.

STACEY, Sheila Margaret Cornwall House, Cornwall Avenue, London N3 1LD Tel: 020 8346 1976 Fax: 020 8343 3809; 23 Clifton Avenue, London N3 1BN — MB BChir Camb. 1969 (Camb. & Westm.) MA Camb. 1970, MB BChir 1969; DObst RCOG 1971; MRCGP 1983.

STACEY, Simon 63 Nelthorpe Street, Lincoln LN5 7SJ — MB ChB Manch. 1994. Specialty: Care of the Elderly; Gen. Med.

STACEY, Simon Gareth — MB BS Lond. 1990 (St. Mary's Hosp. Lond.) FRCA 1995. Cons. (Anaesth.) Barts and the Lond. NHS Trust. Specialty: Anaesth.; Intens. Care.

STACEY, Simon John 44 Corporation Street, London E15 3HD — MB BS Lond. 1994.

STACEY, Susan Ese — MB BS Lond. 1990 (St Mary's) DRCOG 1994; DCH RCP Lond. 1994; MRCGP 1995; MSc (Sports Med.) Lond. 1996; LFHom (Med) 1999. GP Retainer. Lond. Specialty: Sports Med.; Gen. Pract.; Haematology; Educat. Socs: BMA; RCGP; Brit. Assn. Sports Med. Prev: Fell. (Sports Med.) Childr.'s Hosp. Inst. Sports Med. (CHSM) Roy. Alexander Hosp. Childr. Sydney, Australia.

STACEY-CLEAR, Mr Adam Surrey & Sussex NHS Trust, Canada Avenue, Redhill RH1 5RH Tel: 01737 768511 — MB BS Lond. 1978; FRCS Eng. 1983; BSc (Anat.) Lond. 1974, MS 1989. Cons. Surg. (Breast & Endrocrinol.) E. Surrey Hosp. Redhill. Specialty: Gen. Surg. Socs: Brit. Assn. Surgic. Oncol.; Brit. Assn. Endrocrin. Surg.; Assn. Surg. Of GB & Irel. Prev: Sen. Regist. (Surg.) St. Thos. Hosp. Lond.; Fell. (Surg.) Harvard Med. Sch. Mass. Gen. Hosp., USA.

STACK, Bryan Hilleary Rowan Respiratory Medicine Unit, Level 6, Gartnaval General Hospital, Great Western Road, Glasgow G12 0YN Tel: 0141 211 3247 Fax: 0141 211 3464; 8 West Chapelton Crescent, Bearsden, Glasgow G61 2DE Tel: 0141 942 3921 Fax: 0141 211 3464 Email: wosacfc@hotmail.com — MB ChB Ed. 1960; FRCP Ed. 1975, M 1963; FRCP Lond. 1980, M 1963; FRCP Glas. 1982, M 1979; MD Ed. 1982; FRCPI 1999. Cons. Phys. Respirat. Dis. West. Infirm. & Gartnavel Gen. Hosp.; Dir. W. Scotl. Adult Cystic Fibrosis Centre; Hon. Sen. Lect. (Med.) Glas. Univ. Specialty: Respirat. Med. Socs: Brit. Thorac. Soc. & Scott. Thoracic Soc.; Scott. Soc. Phys. Prev: Sen. Regist. City Hosp. Edin.; Sen. Regist. Univ. Coll. Hosp. Lond.; Regist. Respirat. Dis. Unit North. Gen. Hosp. Edin.

STACK, Charles Graham Sheffield Children's Hospital, Western Bank, Sheffield S10 2TH Tel: 0114 271 7000 Fax: 0114 271 7195;

6 Clumber Road, Ranmoor, Sheffield S10 3LE Tel: 0114 230 8696 — MB BS Lond. 1980 (Middlx.) BSc Lond. 1977; FFA RCS Eng. 1985. Cons. Anaesth. & Dir. Paediat. Intens. Care Sheff. Childr. Hosp. Specialty: Anaesth.; Intens. Care. Socs: Hon. Sec. Paediat. Intens. Care Soc. Prev: Cons. Anaesth. Birm. Childr. Hosp.; Sen. Regist. (Anaesth.) Nottm. & E. Midl. Higher Prof. Train. Scheme; Regist. (Anaesth.) Hosp. for Sick Childr. Gt. Ormond St. Lond.

STACK, Mary Monica Jenner House Surgery, 159 Cove Road, Farnborough GU14 0HH Tel: 01252 373738 Fax: 01252 373799; 49 Nethervell Mead, Church Crookham, Aldershot, Fleet GU52 0YQ Tel: 01252 816163 — MB BCh BAO NUI 1983; DCH RCPSI 1987; DObst RCPI 1988. Specialty: Aviat. Med.

STACK, Mr Michael Maurice Milltop House, Leicester Road, Swadlincote DE12 7HF — MB BCh BAO NUI 1979; LRCPI & LM, LRCSI & LM 1979; FRCSI 1983.

STACK, William Alphonsus 29 Alford Road, West Bridgford, Nottingham NG2 6GJ — MB BCh BAO NUI 1987.

STACK, Winifred Clemence Oxford Terrace Medical group, 1 Oxford Terrace, Bensham, Gateshead NE8 1RQ — MB BS Newc. 1985; MRCP (UK) 1988; MA (Human Resource Managem.) Newc. 1992; MRCGP 1994. Gen. Practitioner (PMS). Specialty: Gen. Pract. Prev: Sen. Regist. (Genitourin. Med.) Newc. Gen. Hosp.(1991-1992).

STACKHOUSE, John Richard Cricketfield Surgery, Cricketfield Road, Newton Abbot TQ12 2AS Tel: 01626 208020 Fax: 01626 333356 — MRCS Eng. LRCP Lond. 1972; DObst RCOG 1974; DA Eng. 1976; MRCGP 1980.

STACPOOLE, Harold Adam Westover Surgery, Western Terrace, Falmouth TR11 4QJ Tel: 01326 212120 — MB BCh Wales 1986. Socs: BMA.

STACPOOLE-RYDING, Frank (retired) 21 Percy Road, Broadstairs CT10 2BJ — MRCS Eng. LRCP Lond. 1952 (St. Thos.) BA Open 1990.

STAFANOUS, Sabah Naeim Royal Hospital, Chesterfield S44 5BL Tel: 01246 277271 Ext: 3135 Fax: 01246 512687 Email: sstafanous@yahoo.com.

STAFF, Anthony, Flight Lt. RAF Med. Br. Retd. Island Cottage, Fore St., Looe PL13 2EZ Tel: 01503 4765 — MRCS Eng. LRCP Lond. 1983; BA Open 1975; Cert. Family Plann. JCC 1986. Indep. Med. Pract. Caradon Clinic Cornw. Prev: GP RAF Chivenor Devon; GP RAF St. Mawgan Cornw.; Trainee GP Afcent, Netherlands.

STAFF, Catherine Jayne — MB BS Lond. 1991; BSc (Hons.); MRCPsych; MSc. Cons. (Psychiat.) E. Glam. Ment. Health Unit Ch. Village.

STAFF, David Malcolm 24 Isham Road, Orlingbury, Kettering NN14 1JD — MB ChB Leeds 1971; MB ChB (Hons.) Leeds 1971; DObst RCOG 1973; MRCGP 1975. Prev: Trainee Gen. Pract., Wakefield Vocational Train. Scheme; SHO (O & G), Ho. Phys. & Ho. Surg. Huddersfield Roy. Infirm.

STAFF, Mr William Glenville 1 Queens Square, Lancaster LA1 1RN Tel: 01524 63080; The Birks, Silverdale Road, Arnside, Carnforth LA5 0EH Tel: 01524 761381 — MD Manch. 1970; MB ChB 1960; FRCS Eng. 1965. Cons. Urol. Surg. Lancaster DHA & S. Cumbria DHA. Specialty: Urol. Prev: Sen. Regist. (Urol.) United Manch. Hosps. & Manch. RHB; Sen. Regist. United Cardiff Hosps.; Regist. (Surg.) United Sheff. Hosps.

STAFFORD, Anthony James Mansion House Surgery, Abbey Street, Stone ST15 8YE Tel: 01785 815555 Fax: 01785 815541 — MB ChB Sheff. 1986 (Sheff. Univ.) BMedSci Sheff. 1985; DRCOG 1991; MRCGP 1992. Specialty: Gen. Pract. Socs: RCGP.

STAFFORD, Caroline Jane 179 Hemingford Road, London N1 1DA — MB BChir Camb. 1993.

STAFFORD, Deborah Mary Hartshill Surgery, 1 Longheld Road, Hartshill, Stoke-on-Trent ST4 6QN — MB ChB Birm. 1987; DRCOG 1990; DCH 1991. p/t Princ. GP. Specialty: Gen. Pract. Prev: Trainee GP City Gen. Hosp. Stoke-on-Trent VTS.; Retainor Scheme - Gen. Pract.

STAFFORD, Doreen Muriel (retired) Four Winds, Court Road, Newton Ferrers, Plymouth PL8 1DD Tel: 01752 872483 — MB ChB Birm. 1945. Prev: Clin. Asst. (Orthop. Med.) Mt. Gould Hosp. Plymouth.

STAFFORD, Eric John Highfield, 14 Stamford Road, Colsterworth, Grantham NG33 5JD Tel: 01476 860712 — MB BS Lond. 1949 (Guy's) LMSSA Lond. 1948. Prev: RAMC; Ho. Phys. & Ho. Surg. Croydon Gen. Hosp.

STAFFORD, Mr Francis William Department of Otolarysgowgy & Head and Neck Surgery, Freeman Hospital, Freeman Road, Newcastle upon Tyne NE2 1ZP Tel: 0191 231 6161 Email: frank.stafford@nuth.northy.nhs.uk; 22 Granville Road, Jesmond, Newcastle upon Tyne NE2 1TP Tel: 01912095186 Fax: 01912095186 — MB BS Newc. 1978 (Newcastle upon Tyne) FRCS Ed. 1982; FRCS Eng. 1984. Cons. Otolaryngol. & Head and Neck Surg., Newc. u. Tyne; Newcastle Nuffield Hosp., Newcastle upon Tyne; Washington Hosp., Washington, Tyne & Wear; Freeman Hosp. Newcastle upon Tyne. Specialty: Otolaryngol.; Otorhinolaryngol. Socs: Brit. Assoc. O.R.C and Head & Neck; Brit. Assoc. Head & Neck Oncologists; Brit. Assoc. Paed. Otolaryngology. Prev: Cons. Otolaryngol. Sunderland Roy. Hosp.; Cons. Otolaryngol. Aberd. Roy. Inf.

STAFFORD, Heather Gay The Surgery, 25 Greenwood Avenue, Beverley HU17 0HB Tel: 01482 881517 Fax: 01482 887022 — MB ChB Leeds 1978; BSc Leeds 1976. Prev: GP Muswell Hill, Lond.; Trainee GP Whittington Hosp. VTS.

STAFFORD, Helena Mary c/o Mrs Stafford, Southfields House, St Pauls St., Stamford PE9 2BQ — BM Soton. 1998.

STAFFORD, Ilva Cruddas Park Surgery, 178 Westmorland Road, Cruddas Park, Newcastle upon Tyne NE4 7JT — MB BS Newc. 1967; MRCP (U.K.) 1970.

STAFFORD, James West Cumberland Hospital, Whitehaven CA28 8JG Tel: 01946 693181 — MB BS Lond. 1969 (Univ. Coll. Hosp.) MRCS Eng. LRCP Lond. 1969; FRCOG 1990,M 1978. Cons. O & G W. Cumbld. Hosp. Whitehaven. Specialty: Obst. & Gyn.

STAFFORD, John (retired) Uplands, 9 Mill Hill, Shoreham-by-Sea BN43 5TG Tel: 01273 452545 — MRCS Eng. LRCP Lond. 1945 (Westm.) MRCGP 1966. Prev: Clin. Asst. (Dermat.) Southlands Hosp. Shoreham-by-Sea.

STAFFORD, Mary Teresa 37 Bristol Gardens, London W9 2JQ — MB BCh BAO NUI 1983; LRCPI & LM, LRCSI & LM 1983; MRCOG 1989; MRCGP 1991.

STAFFORD, Michael Alfred 3 Cricklewood Park, Londonderry BT47 5QU — MB BCh BAO Belf. 1993.

STAFFORD, Michael Anthony Department of Anaesthesia, Royal Victoria Infirmary, Queen Victoria Road, Newcastle upon Tyne NE1 4LP Tel: 0191 232 5131 — MB BChir Camb. 1974; MA, MB Camb. 1974, BChir 1973; MSc (Computing Sc.) Lond. 1977; FFA RCS Eng. 1980. Cons. Anaesth. Roy. Vict. Infirm. Newc. u. Tyne. Specialty: Anaesth. Prev: 1st Asst. & Sen. Lect. (Anaesth.) Univ. Newc.; Regist. (Anaesth.) Avon HA.

STAFFORD, Michael Keith Dept of Gynaecology, Chelsea & Westminster Hospital, 369 Fulham Road, London SW10 9NH Tel: 020 8746 8218 Fax: 020 8846 7998; 70 Thames St, Sunbury-on-Thames TW16 6AF — MB BS Lond. 1987; MRCOG 1993; MD 1998. Cons. Chelsea &W.minster.Hosp. Specialty: Obst. & Gyn. Socs: BMA; MRCOG; RSM. Prev: Research Fell. St. Mary's Hosp. Med. Sch. Lond.; Regist. (O & G) Chelsea & Westm. Hosp. Riverside HA & Northwick Pk. Hosp. Harrow; Sen. Regist. & Lect. (O & G) Char. Cross & Westm. Hosp. Lond.

STAFFORD, Moyra Patricia Claridge (retired) Uplands, 9 Mill Hill, Shoreham-by-Sea BN43 5TG Tel: 01273 452545 — MRCS Eng. LRCP Lond. 1945 (King's Coll. Hosp.)

STAFFORD, Mr Nicholas David 10 New Walk, Beverley HU17 7AD — MB ChB Leeds 1977; FRCS (Orl.) Eng. 1983. Cons. ENT & Head & Neck Surg. Hull Roy. Infirm.; Prof. ENT Head & Neck Surg. Univ. Hull. Specialty: Otolaryngol. Prev: Cons. ENT Surg. St. Mary's Hosp. & Char. Cross Hosp. Lond.; Sen. Regist. (ENT) St. Mary's & Roy. Marsden Hosps. Lond.; Resid. Etranger Inst. Gustave Roussy, Paris.

STAFFORD, Peter James 27 Burton Street, Loughborough LE11 2DT — MB BS Lond. 1984 (Lond Hosp. Med. Coll.) BSc (1st cl. Hons.) Lond. 1981; MRCP (UK) 1987; MD Lond. 1995. Lect. & Locum Hon. Cons. Cardiol. Glenfield Hosp. Leicester. Specialty: Cardiol. Socs: Brit. Cardiac Soc. Prev: Hon. Sen. Regist. (Cardiol.) Glenfield Gen. Hosp. Leicester; Research Fell. (Cardiol.) Groby Rd. Hosp. Leicester; Regist. (Cardiol.) Roy. Sussex Co. Hosp. Brighton & King's Coll. Hosp. Lond.

STAFFORD, Sarah Jill 22 Ballykennedy Road, Gracehill, Ballymena BT42 2NP — MB BCh BAO Belf. 1996.

STAFFORD, Selma 14 Shirlock Road, London NW3 2HS — MB ChB Manch. 1996.

STAFFURTH, Jean Forbes (retired) Rosedene, 30 Mays Hill Road, Bromley BR2 0HT Tel: 020 8460 3538 — MB BS Lond. 1953 (Char. Cross) DMRT Eng. 1960. Prev: Hon. Cons. Radiother. Chelsea Hosp. for Wom. Lond.

STAFFURTH, John Nicholas Oncology Department, St. Thomas' Hospital, Lambeth Park Road, London SE1 7EH; 1E Westgrove Lane, Greenwich, London SE10 8QP Tel: 020 7928 9292 Fax: 020 7928 9968 Email: lidstonev@staffurthj.freeserve.co.uk — MB BS Lond. 1992 (United Medical and Dental Schools) MRCP (UK) 1995. Regist. Clin.Oncol.St. Thomas' Hosp. Lond. Specialty: Oncol.

STAFFURTH, John Samuel 30 Mays Hill Road, Bromley BR2 0HT Tel: 020 8460 3538 — MRCS Eng. LRCP Lond. 1942 (St. Thos.) MD (Distinc.) Lond. 1948, MB BS 1942; FRCP Lond. 1967, M 1947. Hon. Cons. Phys. Guy's & Lewisham Hosps. Specialty: Gen. Med. Socs: Assn. Phys. Gt. Brit. & Irel.; Fell. Roy. Soc. Med. Prev: Censor R.C.P. Lond.; Res. Asst. Phys. St. Thos. Hosp.; Med. Regist. P. of Wales' Hosp. Plymouth.

STAGG, Caroline Elizabeth Pulteney Practice, 35 Great Pulteney Street, Bath BA2 4BY Tel: 01225 464187 Fax: 01225 485305 — MB BS Lond. 1979 (Char. Cross) DRCOG 1981; MRCGP 1983. Prev: Trainee GP Weymouth VTS.

STAGG, Martin James Albion Medical Practice, 1 Albion Street, Ashton-under-Lyne OL6 6HF Tel: 0161 339 9161 Fax: 0161 343 5131; 41 Moorlands Drive, Mossley, Ashton-under-Lyne OL5 9DB — MB ChB Manch. 1985; MRCGP 1989. Prev: Trainee GP Oldham HA VTS.

STAGKOU, Argyri Institute of Liver Studies, Kings College Hospital, Denmark Hill, London SE5 9RS — Ptychio Iatrikes Thessalonika 1988.

STAGLES, Mr Martin John Crossroads Surgery, 478 Cricklade Rd, Swindon SN2 7BG; 28 Turner St, Swindon SN1 4NJ — MB BS Newc. 1974; FRCS Ed. 1994. Specialty: Ophth.

STAHL, Mr Timothy James 217 Carmel Road N., Darlington DL3 9TF Tel: 01325 483268 — MB ChB Manch. 1967; FRCS Eng. 1974. Specialty: Orthop. Prev: Leverhulme Research Fell. (Orthop. & BioMech.) Leeds Univ.; Sen. Regist. Robt. Jones & Agnes Hunt Orthop. Hosp. Oswestry; Regist. (Accid. & Orthop. Surg.) N. Staffs. Roy. Infirm. Stoke-on-Trent.

STAHLSCHMIDT, Jens Dept. of Histopathology, St James University Hospital, Leeds LS9 7TF Tel: 0113 206 5432 — State Exam Med Hamburg 1993 (Univ. Hambury) MD Hamburg 1994. Specialist Regist. (Histopath.) Leeds Gen. Infirm. Specialty: Histopath. Socs: Internat. Acad. of Path. (Brit. Div.). Prev: SHO (Histopath.) Manch. Roy. Infirm.

STAIANO, Jonathan James 13 Devonshire Place, Handbridge, Chester CH4 7BY Email: JJStaiano@doctors.org.uk — MB BS Lond. 1994 (Guy's Hosp.) MSc (Surgic. Sci.) Univ. Coll. Lond. 2000. Specialty: Plastic Surg.

STAIG, David (retired) St. Kilda, Fairfield Road, Goring-on-Thames, Reading RG8 0EX — MRCS Eng. LRCP Lond. 1955 (Oxf. & Westm.) MA, BM BCh Oxf. 1955; DO Eng. 1959. Prev: Med. Off. Contact Lens Dept. Moorfields Eye Hosp. Lond.

STAIGHT, Guy Barrington 2 Pelham Street, London SW7 2NG Tel: 020 7581 4222 Fax: 020 7581 4676 — MB BS Lond. 1980 (Char. Cross Hosp.) MRCS Eng. LRCP Lond. 1980; MRCP (UK) 1984. Indep. GP Lond.; Dep. Chief Med. Off. Jockey Club. Prev: SHO (Gen. Med.) & Ho. Phys. Northampton Gen. Hosp; Ho. Surg. Char. Cross Hosp. Lond.

STAINER, Gordon Cowes Health Centre, 8 Consort Road, Cowes PO31 7SH Tel: 01983 295251 Fax: 01983 280461; Hillis House, Hillis Gate Road, Northwood, Cowes PO31 8NA Tel: 01983 295088 — MB ChB Birm. 1980; BSc (Psychol.) Birm. 1974; DRCOG 1982; MRCGP 1984. Socs: BMA. Prev: Trainee GP Hereford VTS.

STAINER, Karl John Fallodon Way Medical Centre, 13 Fallodon Way, Henleaze, Bristol BS9 4HT Tel: 0117 962 0652 Fax: 0117 962 0839 — MB ChB Bristol 1988; DRCOG 1990.

STAINER, Mary Ruth Cowes Health Centre, 8 Consort Road, Cowes PO31 7SH Tel: 01983 295251 Fax: 01983 280461; Hillis House, Hillis Gate Road, Northwood, Cowes PO31 8NA Tel: 01983 295088 — MB BCh Wales 1980; DRCOG 1983; MRCGP (Distinc.) 1984. Prev: Trainee GP Hereford VTS; SHO (A & E) Kingston Hosp.

STAINER-SMITH, Andrew Martin East Street Medical Centre, East Street, Okehampton EX20 1AY Tel: 01837 52233; Waterside, Sticklepath, Okehampton EX20 2NH — MB Camb. 1976; MA; BChir 1975; MRCP (UK) 1978; MRCGP 1980. Specialty: Gen. Pract.; Psychosexual Med. Socs: Inst. Psychosexual Med.

STAINES, Frederick Howard (retired) Woolston, Guildford Road, Cranleigh GU6 8PR — (Guy's) MRCS Eng. LRCP Lond. 1942. Prev: GP Group Practice NHS 1948-60.

STAINES, James Edward Health Centre, Bishops Close, Spennymoor DL16 6ED Tel: 01388 811455 Fax: 01388 812034; Hull's Close, 1 Foxes Row, Brancepeth, Durham DH7 8DH Fax: 01388 812034 Email: edward.staines@btinternet.com/ tlaundy@zoom.co.uk — MB BS Newc. 1974; MRCGP 1978. Company Med. Off. Electrolux Home Products. Socs: BMA. Prev: Trainee GP Newc. VTS.

STAINES, Jillian Anne Nottingham Psychotherapy Unit, St. Ann's House, 114 Thorneywood Mount, Nottingham NG3 2PZ Tel: 0115 962 7891; 50 St. Albans Road, Leicester LE2 1GE — MB ChB Leeds 1981; MRCPsych 1987. Sen. Regist. (Psychother.) Nottm. & Trent Region. Specialty: Gen. Psychiat. Prev: Sen. Regist. Rotat. (Psychiat.) Leicester & S. Lincs HA.

STAINES, Jonathan David Crosshouse Hospital, Kilmarnock KA2 0BE Tel: 01563 521133; St. Judes, 3 Ladeside Lane, Kilmaurs, Kilmarnock KA3 2TJ Tel: 01563 538221 — MB BS Lond. 1983; MRCP (UK) 1991. Cons. Paediat. Ayrsh. Centr. Hosp. Irvine & Ayr Hosp. Specialty: Paediat. Prev: Sen. Regist. & Career Regist. (Paediat.) Roy. Hosp. Sick Childr. Glas.; Regist. (Paediat.) Kettering Gen. Hosp.

STAINFORTH, John Nicholas Croft Hall Medical Practice, 19 Croft Road, Torquay TQ2 5UA Tel: 01803 298441 Fax: 01803 296104 — BM (Hons.) Soton. 1976; MRCP (UK) 1979; MRCGP 1985; DRCOG 1985. Specialty: Cardiol. Prev: Research Fell. (Med.) Univ. Soton.; Regist. Rotat. (Med.) N. Staffs. Hosp. Med. Centre Stoke on Trent.

STAINFORTH, Julia Margaret York Hospital, Department of Dermatology, Wiggington Road, York YO31 8HE Tel: 01904 631313 — MB ChB Leeds 1986; MRCP (UK) 1989. Cons. Dermat. York Dist. Hosp. Specialty: Dermat. Socs: Brit. Assn. Dermat.; BMA; Brit. Soc. Dermatological Surg. Prev: Sen. Regist. (Dermat.) Qu. Med. Centre Nottm.; Regist. (Dermat.) Leeds Gen. Infirm.; SHO (Gen. Med.) Leeds East. HA.

STAINSBY, Dorothy National Blood Service, Newcastle Centre, Holland Dr., Barrack Road, Newcastle upon Tyne NE2 4NQ Tel: 0191 219 4436 Fax: 0191 219 4505 Email: dorothy.stainsby@nbs.nhs.uk; 9 Meadow Court, Ponteland, Newcastle upon Tyne NE20 9RB Tel: 01661 824389 — MB BS Newc. 1970; MRCP (UK) 1973; FRCPath 1996, M 1984; FRCP Lond. 1993. Cons. Transfus. Med. Nat. Blood Serv. Newc. u. Tyne.; Hon. Lect. (Med.) Univ. Newc. Specialty: Blood Transfus. Socs: Assn. Clin. Path.; Brit. Soc. Haematol.; Brit. Blood Transfus. Soc. Prev: Cons. Haemat. Shotley Bridge Hosp.; Sen. Regist. (Haemat.) Newc. Hosps.

STAINSBY, Mr George David (retired) 9 Meadow Court, Darras Hall, Ponteland, Newcastle upon Tyne NE20 9RB Tel: 01661 824389 — MB Camb. 1958 (St. Bart.) BChir 1957; FRCS Eng. 1962. Prev: Cons. Orthop. Surg. Newc. Univ. Hosps.

STAINTHORP, David Henry 96 Kennersdene, Tynemouth, North Shields NE30 2NW — BM Soton. 1983.

STAINTON, Richard Timothy The Surgery, Decima St., Bermondsey, London SE1; Broom Cottage, 19 Gilpin Road, Ware SG12 9LZ — MB BS Lond. 1993 (Lond. Hosp. Med. Coll.) DGM RCP Lond. 1995; DRCOG 1996. GP Regist. Lond. Specialty: Gen. Pract.

STAINTON-ELLIS, David Michael (retired) Roke House, 15 Clarefield Drive, Pinkneys Green, Maidenhead SL6 5DW — MB BS Lond. 1956 (St Bart.) DObst RCOG 1961; DIH Eng. 1963; MFOM RCP Lond. 1978. Prev: Sen. Med. Off. Roy. Fleet Auxil. Serv.

STAIRMAND, Rosemary Agnes 18 Valentine Way, Hessett, Bury St Edmunds IP30 9BP — MB ChB Leic. 1985; DCH RCP Lond. 1992.

STAITE, Michael Edward 41 Station Road, Codsall, Wolverhampton WV8 1BY Tel: 01902 843764 — MB ChB Birm. 1990; ChB Birm. 1990. Trainee GP Wolverhampton VTS. Prev: Ho. Off. (Surg.) Dudley Rd. Hosp.; Ho. Off. (Med.) New Cross Hosp. Wolverhampton.

STAITE, Patrick Edward The Grange, Llanon SY23 5LR — MB ChB Birm. 1996.

STAKER, Paul 70 East Street, Sittingbourne ME10 4RU Tel: 01795 428197 — MB BS Lond. 1987; DRCOG 1990; JCPTGP 1991; MRCGP 1991; Dip Sports Med 1996. Socs: Mem. Soc. of Orthopedic Med.
STAKES, Annette Frances Department of Anaesthesia, St James's University Hospital, Beckett St., Leeds LS9 7TF Tel: 0113 206 5580 Email: annette.stakes@leedsth.nhs.uk — MB BS Lond. 1972 (St. Bart.) MRCS Eng. LRCP Lond. 1972; DA Eng. 1975; FFA RCS Eng. 1979. Cons. Anaesth. St. Jas. Univ. Hosp. Leeds. Specialty: Anaesth. Prev: Cons. Anaesth. Calderdale HA; Sen. Regist. (Anaesth.) Yorks. RHA; Regist. (Anaesth.) St. Jas. Hosp. Leeds.
STALDER, Gillian Patricia Mary (retired) Glencairn, Austenwood Common, Gerrards Cross SL9 8NL Tel: 01753 882390 — MB BS Lond. 1960 (St. Bart.) DA Eng. 1969. Assoc. Specialist Anaesth. Oxf. Regional Hosp. Bd. Prev: Ho. Phys. St. And. Hosp. Bow.
STALEY, Christopher John St. Andrews Hospital, Billing Road, Northampton NN1 5DG Tel: 01604 616000 Fax: 01604 232325 — BM BS Nottm. 1977; BMedSci (Hons.) Nottm. 1975, BM BS 1977; MRCPsych 1983. Cons. Psychiat. St Andrews Hosp. Specialty: Gen. Psychiat.
STALEY, Frances Marilyn 39 Sunnyside, Newhall, Burton-on-Trent DE13 8 — MB ChB Sheff. 1965; DObst. RCOG 1967.
STALEY, Margaret Glebelands Avenue Surgery, 2 Glebelands Avenue, London E18 2AB Tel: 020 8989 6272 Fax: 020 8518 8783; 17 Glebe Avenue, Woodford Green IG8 9HB Tel: 020 8504 7906 — MB BS Lond. 1976 (Univ. Coll. Hosp.) DCH Eng. 1978; MRCP (UK) 1979; DRCOG 1982; MRCGP 1983.
STALEY, Petra Katherina The Hollow, Penn Lane, Melbourne, Derby DE73 1EP Tel: 01332 865252 — MB BS Lond. 1988.
STALKER, Malcolm John The Surgery, 24 Eaton Place, Brighton BN2 1EH Tel: 01273 686863 Fax: 01273 623402; 45 Crescent Drive N., Woodingdean, Brighton BN2 6SL — MB BS Lond. 1979 (Middlx.) DRCOG 1982; MRCGP 1985.
STALKER, Robert (retired) 27A Ingham Road, Bawtry, Doncaster DN10 6NN Tel: 01302 710772 — MB ChB Aberd. 1951; DPH Leeds 1961; FFPHM RCP (UK) 1991. Prev: Dir. Pub. Health Doncaster HA.
STALLABRASS, Mr Peter (retired) The Manor House, Peppard Common, Henley-on-Thames RG9 5JE — MB BS Lond. 1955 (St. Thos.) BSc (Hons.) Lond. 1951, MB BS 1955; FRCOG 1975, M 1962, DObst 1957; FRCS Eng. 1959. Cons. Obstetr. & Gynaecol. Roy. Berks. Hosp. Reading; Assoc. Teach. in Obst. St. Mary's Hosp. Med. Sch. Prev: Sen. Regist. Dept. O & G St. Thos. Hosp. & Lambeth Hosp. Lond.
STALLARD, Mr Matthew Charles Tewin Lodge, Tewin Water, Welwyn AL6 0AB Tel: 0143 871 7500 — MB Camb. 1968 (Camb. & St. Bart.) BChir. 1967; FRCS Eng. 1973. Cons. Orthop. Surg. Qu. Eliz. Hosp. Welwyn Garden City & Hertford Co. Specialty: Orthop. Socs: Fell. Brit. Orthop. Assn. Mem. Roy. Soc. Med. Prev: Sen. Regist. (Orthop.) Char. Cross Hosp., St. Mary's Hosp. & Roy.; Nat. Orthop. Hosp. Lond.; Regist. Windsor Gp. Hosps.
STALLARD, Nicholas James 16 Maes Cadwgan, Creigiau, Cardiff CF15 9TQ — MB BCh Wales 1989; FRCA 1995. Cons. (Intens. Care Med.) Univ. Hosp. Wales Cardiff.
STALLARD, Noelle Christine Tewin Lodge, Tewin Water, Tewin, Welwyn AL6 0AB Tel: 01438 717500 — MB BS Lond. 1972 (St. Mary's) FFA RCS Eng. 1976. Specialty: Anaesth. Prev: Sen. Regist. (Anaesth.) Char. Cross Hosp. Lond.; Regist. (Anaesth.) Char. Cross Hosp. Lond.; SHO (Cardiothoracic Surg.) Harefield Hosp.
STALLARD, Sheila 84 Springkell Avenue, Glasgow G41 4EH — MB ChB Aberd. 1981; FRCS Glas. 1986; MD 1997. SpR (Gen. Surg.) Vict. Infirm. Glas. Specialty: Gen. Surg. Special Interest: Breast & Indocrine Surg. Prev: Staff Surg. West. Infirm. Glas.
STALLEY, Linda Fay Springfield House, New Lane, Eccles, Manchester M30 7JE Tel: 0161 789 5858 — BM BS Nottm. 1983; BMedSci (Hons.) 1981; MRCP (UK) 1986; DRCOG 1989.
STALLEY, Nicholas James Preston Road Surgery, 102 Preston Road, Weymouth DT3 6BB Tel: 01305 774466 Fax: 01305 760538 — MB BS Lond. 1974.
STALLWOOD, Mark Ian 12 Barnaby Rudge, Chelmsford CM1 4YG — MB ChB Liverp. 1993; Prim. FRCA Lond. 1998. SHO (Anaesth.) Fazukerley Hosp. Liverp. Specialty: Anaesth. Prev: SHO (Med.) Wrexham Maelor Hosp.; SHO (Anaesth.) Wrexham Maelor Hosp.
STALLWORTHY, Elizabeth Gay Locality Health Centre, Coniston Crescent, Weston Super Mare BS23 3RX Tel: 01934 624942 — MB BS Lond. 1984 (Middlesex Hospital Medical School) DRCOG 1988; MRCGP 1988. Gen. Practitioner.
STALLYBRASS, Frank Clifford (retired) Tregarthen, Shrubberies Hill, Porthleven, Helston TR13 9BH Tel: 01326 564291 — MB BChir Camb. 1947 (Camb. & St. Bart.) MA Camb. 1948, MD 1963.
STAMATAKIS, Mr Jeffrey Demetre Princess of Wales Hospital, Bridgend CF31 1RQ — (King's Coll. Hosp.) BSc (Pharm.) Lond. 1966; MB BS Lond. 1969; FRCS Eng. 1974; MS 1979. Cons. Surg. Princess of Wales Hosp. Bridgend. Specialty: Gen. Surg. Socs: Fell. Roy. Soc. Med. (Pres.); Assn. Coloproctol. Prev: Sen. Regist. (Surg.) King's Coll. Hosp. Lond.; Ho. Off. Hosp. Sick Childr. Gt. Ormond St. Lond.; Ho. Off. St. Jas. Hosp. Lond.
STAMBACH, Thomas Aubrey Gristhouse Farm, Water End, Hemel Hempstead HP1 3BD Tel: 0207 017 4328 — MB BS Lond. 1989.
STAMBOULTZIS, Naoum Flat 8, 37 Croxteth Road, Liverpool L8 3SF — Ptychio Iatrikes Thessalonika 1988.
STAMBULI, Mr Pius Moshi Mangotsfield Surgery, 26 Stockwell Drive, Mangotsfield, Bristol BS16 9DN — MB ChB University of East Africa 1967.
STAMENKOVIC, Steven Aleksandar 14 Frederick Sq, London SE16 5XR — MB ChB Manch. 1992.
STAMER, Jurgen 1 Orchard Dere, Cuddington, Northwich CW8 2UZ Tel: 01606 889044 — State Exam Med Hamburg 1989. Specialist Regist. (Orthop. Surg.) Mersey Region. Specialty: Trauma & Orthop. Surg.
STAMFORD, John Anthony (retired) 32 Rook Wood Park, Horsham RH12 1UB — MB BChir Camb. 1954.
STAMM, Reinhard Gustav Wolfgang 416 Russell Court Complex, Lisburn Road, Belfast BT9 6AA — State Exam Med Marburg 1992.
STAMMERS, Trevor Gordon The Surgery, 2 Church Lane, Merton Park, London SW19 3NY Tel: 020 8542 1174 Fax: 020 8544 1583 — MB BS Lond. 1980; BSc Lond. 1977; DRCOG 1982; MRCGP 1985. 2001, Sen. Tutor (Gen. Pract.) St. Geo. Hosp. Med. Sch., Lond.; Tutor (Gen. Pract.) St. Geo. Hosp. Med. Sch. Lond. Prev: Hon. Regist. St. Geo. Hosp. Lond.; Research Fell. (Gen. Pract.) St. Geo. Hosp. Lond.
STAMP, Elizabeth Jane River Brook Medical Centre, 3 River Brook Drive, Stirchley, Birmingham B30 2SH — BM BS Nottm. 1985; DRCOG 1988; MRCGP 1989.
STAMP, Michael Paul 1 The Meadows, Wilberfoss, York YO41 5PY — MB ChB Manch. 1995. SHO (A & E) Bury Gen. Hosp. Specialty: Accid. & Emerg.
STAMP, Philip Jonathan 65 Malcolm Street, Newcastle upon Tyne NE6 5PL — MB BS Newc. 1991.
STAMP, Robert Albert (retired) Darwin House, Darwing Lane, Fulwood, Sheffield S10 5RG Tel: 0113 230 1414 — MB ChB Leeds 1940; DPM Eng. 1957. Prev: Cons. Psychiat. High Royds Hosp. Ilkley & St. Jas. Hosp. Leeds.
STAMP, Stephen Andrew Wellington House Practice, New Surgery, Station Road, Chinnor OX9 4PL Tel: 01844 351230 — BM BCh Oxf. 1990. Specialty: Gen. Pract.
STAMP, Lord Trevor Charles Bosworth (Private rooms), Royal National Orthop. Hospital Trust, 45-51 Bolsover St., London W1W 5AQ Tel: 020 7387 5070; 15 Ceylon Road, London W14 0PY Tel: 020 7603 0487 Fax: 020 7603 5874 — BChir Camb. 1961; MRCS Eng. LRCP Lond. 1960; MRCP Ed. 1967; FRCP Lond. 1978, M 1967; MD Camb. 1972. Emerit. Cons.UCL Hosp, lond. Hon.Cons.Roy.Nat.Orthop.Hosp.Lond; Cons. Phys. Roy. Nat. Orthopaedic Hosp. Specialty: Endocrinol. Socs: Bone & Tooth Soc. (Hon. Life Mem.); Internat. Skeleton Soc. (Hon. Life Mem.); Nat. Orteopowesis (Mem., Scientif. and Advis. Comm.). Prev: Hon. Sen. Lect. (Hum. Metab.) Univ. Coll. Hosp. & Med. Sch. Lond.; Regist. (Med.) St. Mary's Hosp. Lond.
STAMPFLI, Sarah Louise — MB BS Lond. 1990 (St. Mary's) BSc Lond. 1986; DRCOG 1995. GP Princip. Prev: SHO (Ophth.) N. Devon Dist. Hosp.
STAMPS, Victoria Rebekah John Howard Centre, 2 Crozier Terrace, London E9 6AT — MB BS Lond. 1993.
STANAWAY, Stephen Eric 16 Brompton Avenue, Sefton Park, Liverpool L17 3BU — MB ChB Liverp. 1993.
STANBRIDGE, Andrea Joy — MB BS Lond. 1998.

STANBRIDGE, Judith Elizabeth 51 Redmoss Road, Aberdeen AB12 3JJ Email: jstanbridge@hotmail.com — MB ChB Glas. 1997. Specialty: Accid. & Emerg.

STANBRIDGE, Mr Rex De Lisle St. Mary's Hospital, Praed St., Paddington, London W2 1NY Tel: 020 7886 6038 Fax: 020 7706 7302; Campions, Loudwater Lane, Croxley Green, Rickmansworth WD3 3JD Tel: 01923 774499 Fax: 01923 777567 Email: rex.stanbridge@btinternet.com — MB BS Lond. 1971 (St. Mary's) BSc (Hons.) Lond. 1968; MRCS Eng. LRCP Lond. 1971; FRCS Eng. 1976; MRCP (UK) 1977; FRCP Lond. 1994. Cons. Cardiothoracic Surg. St. Mary's Hosp. Lond.; Cons. Thoracic Surg. Centr. Middlx. Hosp. Lond. Specialty: Cardiothoracic Surg. Socs: Fell. Roy. Soc. Med.; Soc. Thoracic & Cardiovasc. Surg. GB & Irel.; Brit. Thorac. Soc. Prev: Cons. Cardiothoracic Surg. Hammersmith Hosp. Lond.; Sen. Regist. (Cardiothoracic Surg.) Hosp. Sick Childr. Gt. Ormond St., Harefield, Hammersmith & Middlx. Hosps. Lond.; Specialist Research Fell. Cardiac. Surg. Univ. Alabama Birm.

STANBRIDGE, Thomas Nigel Department of Microbiology, Wythenshawe Hospital, Southmoor Road, Manchester M23 9LT Tel: 0161 291 2884/85 Fax: 0161 291 2125 — MRCS Eng. LRCP Lond. 1961 (Guy's) MD Lond. 1973, MB BS 1961; Dip. Bact. (Distinc.) Manch. 1967; FRCPath 1980, M 1968. Cons. Microbiol. Wythenshawe Hosp.; Hon. Lect. in Bact. Univ. Manch. Specialty: Med. Microbiol. Socs: Assn. Clin. Pathols.; BMA. Prev: Sen. Bact. Pub. Health Laborat. Serv.; Lect. in Bact. Univ. Manch.; Sen. Lect. in Med. Microbiol. Welsh Nat. Sch. Med.

STANBURY, Peter Norman (retired) 51 Buxton Avenue, Caversham, Reading RG4 7BT — MRCS Eng. LRCP Lond. 1939 (Camb. & St. Bart.) MA Camb. 1940.

STANBURY, Rosalyn May Toad Hall, 21 Sandown Road, Esher KT10 9TT — MB ChB Bristol 1980; MRCP (UK) 1984; FRCS Eng. 1986; DO RCS Eng. 1986. Specialty: Ophth. Socs: FRCOphth; Sen. Regist. (Med. Ophth.) St. Thos. Hosp. Lond.

STANCLIFFE, James Bennett West Farm Cottages, Seaton, Seaham SR7 0NA Tel: 0191 581 0107 — MB BS Durh. 1964.

STANDAGE, Kevin Francis Bennett Centre, Richmond Terrace, Shelton, Stoke-on-Trent ST1 4ND Tel: 01782 425182 Fax: 01782 425174; 16 Nantwich Road, Woore, Crewe CW3 9SB Tel: 01630 647810 — (Guys) MB BS Lond. 1964; MRCS Eng. LRCP Lond. 1964; MRCPsych 1972; PhD Canada 1977. Cons. Psychiat. Combined Healthcare NHS Trust Stoke-on-Trent; Sen. Clin. Lect. Keele Univ. Specialty: Gen. Psychiat. Socs: Fell. Roy. Soc. Med.; Fell. Roy. Coll. Psychiat.; Fell. RCP Canada. Prev: Head Dept. Psychiat. Vict. Gen. Hosp. Halifax, Nova Scotia, Canada.

STANDART, Sally Collingwood Clinic, St. Nicholas Hospital, Gosforth, Newcastle upon Tyne NE3 3XT Tel: 0191 223 2206 Fax: 0191 223 2206; 2A Holly Avenue, Jesmond, Newcastle upon Tyne NE2 2PY Tel: 0191 281 9497 Fax: 0191 281 9497 — MB ChB Manch. 1982 (Manchester) DRCOG 1987; MRCGP 1988; UKCP 1994. SHO (Psychiat.). Specialty: Gen. Psychiat. Prev: Lect. Primary Health Care Univ. Newc.

STANDEN, Graham Richard Department of Haematology, Bristol Royal Infirmary, Bristol BS2 8HW Tel: 0117 928 2555 Email: g.r.standen@bristol.ac.uk — BM BS Nottm. 1979; MRCP 1983; MRCPath 1990. Cons. in Haemat., Bristol Roy. Infirm.; Sen. Lect. in Haemat., Univ. of Bristol. Specialty: Haematology. Socs: Brit. Soc. of Haemat. Prev: Lect. in Haemat., Univ. of Wales Coll. of Med., Cardiff; HO Posts Nottm. City Hosp.

STANDEVEN, Patricia Anne Howard 3 Gordon Grove, Thanet, Westgate-on-Sea CT8 8NS Tel: 01843 831699 — MB BS Lond. 1975.

STANDFIELD, Mr Nigel John 80 The Avenue, West Wickham BR4 0DZ — MB BS Lond. 1975 (King's Coll. Hosp.) MRCS Eng. LRCP Lond. 1975; FRCS Ed. 1978; FRCS Eng. 1979. Moynihan Medal Assn. Surgs. Gt. Brit. & Irel. 1983; Sen. Regist. (Gen. Surg.) KCH Lond. Specialty: Gen. Surg. Prev: Pfizer Research Fell. Thrombosis Unit King's Coll. Hosp. Lond.; Regist. (Gen. Surg.) King's Coll. Hosp. Lond.; SHO (Gen. Surg.) St. Jas. Hosp. Lond.

STANDING, Beth Louise Pulteney Practice, 35 Great Pulteney Street, Bath BA2 4BY Tel: 01225 464187 Fax: 01225 485305 — BM BCh Oxf. 1988; DCH RCP Lond. 1990; DRCOG 1992; MRCGP 1992. Specialty: Gen. Pract.

STANDING, P A Minden Medical Centre, 2 Barlow Street, Bury BL9 0QP Tel: 0161 764 2652 Fax: 0161 761 5967 — MB ChB Bristol 1970; MB ChB Bristol 1970.

STANDLEY, Carole Derwendeg Medical Centre, Heol Llanelli, Trimsaran, Kidwelly SA17 4AG Tel: 01554 810223; Bronyn Farm, Ferryside SA17 5TW Tel: 01267 267591 — MB ChB Liverp. 1968. Clin. Med. Off. Community/Family Plann. Dyfed HA; Clin. Asst. (Geriat.) Brytnic Hosp. Dyfed HA.

STANDLEY, Thomas David Auger Woodton House, Leiston Road, Aldeburgh IP15 5QD Tel: 01728 454738 — MB ChB Birm. 1996; ChB Birm. 1996; FRCA 2002. SPR Aneasth. East Anglia. Specialty: Anaesth. Prev: SHO Anaesth.Ipswich hosp.

STANDRING, Alexandra Fisher St. Davids, The Sands, Farnham GU10 1JW Tel: 01258 782112 — MB ChB Bristol 1990; DRCOG 1995; MRCGP 1996; DFFP 1997. GP Locum. Socs: MDU.

STANDRING, John Nixon Kingston, 8 Far Dene, Kirkburton, Huddersfield HD8 0QZ Tel: 01484 602450 — MB ChB Manch. 1953; DCH Eng. 1958. Prev: Ho. Phys. Paediat. Bolton Dist. Gen. Hosp.; Ho. Surg. Manch. Roy. Infirm.; RAF Med. Br.

STANDRING, Peter Dr P Standring, Alexandra House, Le Freteanux, St Martin, Jersey JE2 7WG Tel: 01481 725241 Email: p.standring@doctors.org.uk — MB ChB Cape Town 1987 (University of Cape Town) MRCP (UK) 1991; DCH RCP Lond. 1991; PHD,Southampton University 1998. Cons. Paediat., Med. Specialist Gp., Guernsey. Specialty: Paediat. Prev: Regist. (Paediat.) Leeds Gen. Infirm.; Clin. Res. Fell. (Soton. Gen. Hosp.); Regist. Paediat. Respirat. Med. (Adelaide), Australia.

STANEK, Mr Jan Jîri 60 Wimpole Street, London W1G 8AG Tel: 020 7487 4457 Fax: 020 7487 4090 Email: janstanek@aol.com — BM BCh Oxf. 1975; MA Oxf. 1976, BM BCh 1975; FRCS Eng. 1981. Indep. Pract. Lond.; Vis. Prof Plastic Surg Brno Univ Czech RePub. Specialty: Gen. Surg.; Plastic Surg. Socs: Amer. Acad. Cosmetic Surg.; Roy. Soc. of Med.; Ctech Soc. of Aesthetic plastic Surg.s. Prev: Sen. Regist. & Regist. (Gen. Surg.) Westm. Hosp. Lond.; Regist. (Gen. Surg.) Qu. Mary's Hosp. Lond.

STANFIELD, Alan Campbell Lodgehill Road Clinic, Lodgehill Road, Nairn IV12 4RF Tel: 01667 452096 Fax: 01667 456785 — MB ChB Glas. 1977 (University of Glasgow) DRCOG 1982; Cert FPA. 1982; MRCGP 1983. Med. Off. Nairn Town & Couny Hosp.; Dep. Police Surg. Nairn; Med. Off. Brit. Red Cross Soc.; Sen. Lect. (Clin.) Gen. Pract. Univ. of Aberd. Specialty: Gen. Pract. Socs: Highland Med. Soc. Prev: Ho. Off. (Surg.) Stirling Roy. Infirm.; Ho. Off. (Med.) Glas. Roy. Infirm.

STANFIELD, Susan Margaret Lisburn Health Centre, Linenhall St., Lisburn BT28 1LU Tel: 01846 665181; 282A Ballynahinch Road, Hillsborough BT26 6BP Tel: 01846 638847 — MB BCh BAO Belf. 1973; DCH Dub. 1982. SCMO Lisburn. Specialty: Community Child Health.

STANFORD, Andrew James Posterngate Surgery, Portholme Road, Selby YO8 4QH Tel: 01757 700561 Fax: 01757 213295; 10 Silver Street, Riccall, York YO19 6PB Tel: 01757 248442 — MB BS Lond. 1967 (King's Coll. Hosp. Lond.) MRCS Eng. LRCP Lond. 1967; DA Eng. 1970. Specialty: Gen. Pract. Prev: Ho. Phys. & Ho. Surg. King's Coll. Hosp. Lond.; Med. Off. i/c Magila Hosp., Tanzania.

STANFORD, Barbara Jane 144 Castlenau, London SW13 9ET — BM BCh Oxf. 1971; FFA RCS Eng. 1976. Cons. Anaesth. St. Geo. Hosp. Lond. Specialty: Anaesth.

STANFORD, Claire Nicola — MB ChB Leic. 1984; BA Oxf. 1981; DRCOG 1988. Asst. Gp Shrewsbury.

STANFORD, Colin Andrew Callow Fold, Middlehope, Craven Arms SY7 9JT — MB ChB Birm. 1981; DRCOG 1984; MRCGP 1987. Prev: Trainee GP Walsall VTS & BridgN.; SHO (Psychiat.) W. Midl. RHA; Resid. Anaesth. Kingston, Jamaica.

STANFORD, Hermione Mary 11 Gertrude Street, London SW10 0JN — MB BS Lond. 1981.

STANFORD, Margaret Elspeth Anaesthetic Department, Ealing Trust Hospital, Uxbridge Road, Southall UB1 3HW Tel: 020 8574 2444 Fax: 020 8967 5797 Email: stanfordmargie@hotmail.com — MB ChB Cape Town 1973; DA Eng. 1977; FFA RCS Eng. 1979. Assoc. Specialist (Anaesth.) Ealing Trust Hosp. Middlx. Specialty: Anaesth. Prev: Sen. Regist. & Regist. (Anaesth.) Hammersmith Hosp. Lond.; Regist. (Anaesth.) Hillingdon Hosp. Uxbridge.

STANFORD, Michael Francis Ashby Turn Primary Care Centre, The Link, Scunthorpe DN16 2UT Tel: 01724 842051 Fax: 01724 280346 — MB BCh BAO NUI 1973.

STANFORD, Mr Miles Richard 11 Gertrude Street, London SW10 0JN — MB BChir Camb. 1979; MB Camb. 1979, BChir 1978; DO RCS Eng. 1984; FRCS (Ophth.) Eng. 1985; MSc Med. Immunol. Lond. 1986; FCOphth. 1989; MA Camb. 1979, MD 1994. Sen. Lect. (Ophth.) UMDS St. Thos. Hosp. Lond. Specialty: Ophth.

STANG, Fanny (retired) 1 Falmer House, 35 Belsize Park, London NW3 4DY Tel: 020 7431 1554 — MD Vienna 1938; LRCP LRCS Ed. LRFPS Glas. 1944; DPH Manch. 1954; MFCM 1971. Prev: SCM Bromley AHA.

STANGER, Elizabeth The Three Swans Surgery, Rollestone Street, Salisbury SP1 1DX Tel: 01722 333548 Fax: 01722 503626; Brindle Lodge, Nunton, Salisbury SP5 4HZ Tel: 01722 324380 — MB BChir Camb. 1981; BA Camb. 1978; DRCOG 1985; Cert. Family Plann. JCC 1985; Dip. Occ. Med. 1998. GP Princip. (Wom.'s Health Occupat. Med.). Prev: Trainee GP Salisbury VTS.

STANGER, Miles Justin Bay Tree Cottage, Church End, Standlake, Witney OX29 7SG — MB BS Lond. 1988; MSc Manch. 1992; MRCGP 1993; AFOM 2002. GP Med. Off. Specialty: Gen. Pract. Socs: MDDUs; BMA; Soc. of Occupat.al Med. S.O.M. Prev: CMP - UK; Sen. Med. Off. - Lond.

STANGER, Nicholas Robert Yorke St Ann Street Surgery, 82 St. Ann Street, Salisbury SP1 2PT Tel: 01722 322624 Fax: 01722 410624; Brindle Lodge, Nunton Drove, Nunton, Salisbury SP5 4HZ — MB BS Lond. 1982 (St. Thos.) DCH RCP Lond. 1987; MRCGP 1987; Cert. Family Plann. JCC 1987. Prev: Trainee GP Salisbury VTS.

STANGER, Robert Arthur (retired) 71 Peters Road, Locks Heath, Southampton SO31 6EL Tel: 01489 581452 — (St. Thos.) BA, MB BChir Camb. 1948; MRCS Eng. LRCP Lond. 1948. Prev: Ho. Phys. (Obst.) St. Thos. Hosp.

STANGER, Robin John Roe Charles Hicks Centre, 75 Ermine Street, Huntingdon PE29 3EZ Tel: 01480 453038 Fax: 01480 434104 Email: john.stanger@gp-d81050.nhs.uk — MB BS Lond. 1977 (St. Thos.) MRCGP 1986. Socs: GP Asthma Gp. Prev: Trainee GP Ramsbury Wilts.; SHO Balclotha Hosp., NZ.

STANGROOM, Craig Dennis c/o 134 Barkham Ride, Wokingham RG40 4EL; UMN, PO Box 126, Kathmandu, Nepal — BM BS Nottm. 1989; DRCOG 1992; DFFP 1993; MRCGP 1994.

STANHILL, Vivian 88 Dukes Avenue, Theydon Bois, Epping CM16 7HF — MB BS Lond. 1950 (Middlx.) DA Eng. 1955; FFA RCS Eng. 1959. Cons. Anaesth. Redbridge HA. Specialty: Anaesth. Prev: Sen. Regist. Anaesth. United Sheff. Hosps.; Jun. Res. Anaesth. Middlx. Hosp. Lond.; Capt. RAMC.

STANHOPE, Richard Graham Department of Endocrinology, Great Ormond Street Hospital for Children, Great Ormond St., London WC1N 3JH Tel: 020 7905 2139 Fax: 020 7404 6191 Email: r.stanhope@ich.ucl.ac.uk; Department of Paediatric Endocrinology, The Middlesex Hospital, Mortimer St, London W1T 3AA Tel: 020 7380 9221 Fax: 020 7636 2144 — MB BS Lond. 1974 (St. Bartholomews) MRCP (UK) 1977; DRCOG 1980; DCH RCP Lond. 1981; AMRAeS 1982; BSc Lond. 1971, MD 1989; FRCP Lond. 1994; FRCPCH, 1996. p/t Cons. (Paediat. Endocrinol.) Gt. Ormond St. Hosp. for Sick Childr. & Middlx. Hosp. Lond.; Edr. In Chief to Jl. of Paediatric Endocrinol. and Diabetes; Med. Adviser to Contact A Family UK; Cons. (Paediat. Endocrin.) Portland Hosp. For Wom. & Childr. Lond.; Med. Adviser to the Child Growth Assn. UK; Med. Adviser to Congeital Adrenal Hyperplasia Gp. UK; Med. Adviser to Androgen Insensitivity Gp.; Med. Adviser to Families with Pituitary Childr. Specialty: Endocrinol.; Paediat.; Aviat. Med. Socs: Fell. Roy. Soc. Med. (Mem. Sect. Endocrinol. & Progr. Sect.); Eur. Soc Paediat. Endocrinol.; Soc. Endocrinol. (Jt. Progr. Sect.). Prev: Research Fell. (Paediat.) Middlx. Hosp. Lond.; Regist. (Paediat.) Middlx. & Centr. Middlx. Hosps.; SHO St. Bart., Guy's, Brompton, Gt. Ormond St. & Kings Coll. Hosps. Lond.

STANIFORTH, Andrew Denis — MB ChB Birm. 1991; BSc (Class I) Birm. 1988; MRCP UK 1994; DM Nottm. 2000. Specialist Regist. (Cardiol.) Roy. Lond. Hosp. NHS Trust. Specialty: Cardiol. Prev: Research Regist. (Cardiovasc. Med.) Qu. Med. Centre Nottm.; SHO (Med.) Sheff. HA.; SHO (Med.) Leics. HA.

STANIFORTH, Arabella Sophie Caroline — MB BS Lond. 1994 (St. Mary's Hosp. Lond.) BSc (Hons.) Lond. 1991. GP Princip. Bromley. Specialty: Anaesth. Prev: SHO (Anaesth.) Eastbourne Dist. Gen. Hosp.; SHO (Cas.) Kingston Hosp. Surrey; Ho. Off. (Surg.) Northwick Pk. Hosp.

STANIFORTH, Christopher The Health Centre, Beeches Green, Stroud GL5 4BH Tel: 01453 764696 Fax: 01453 756548 Email: chris.staniforth@gp-l84077.nhs.uk; Woodlands, Culver Hill, Amberley, Stroud GL5 5BB — MB BS Lond. 1985 (King's Coll. Hosp. Lond.) MA Oxf. 1986; MRCGP 1989; DCH RCP Lond. 1990; Cert. Family Plann. JCC 1990. Gen. Pract. Trainer; Clin. Asst., Phys. Weavers Croft, PsychoGeriat. Hosp., Stroud, Glos. Socs: BMA; RCGP. Prev: Trainee GP Tunbridge Wells VTS.

STANIFORTH, John The Rugby Surgery, 1-5 Kelvedon Street, Newport NP19 0DW Tel: 01633 261900 — MB BCh Wales 1993; DRCOG 1997; MRCGP 1997. GP Gwent.

STANIFORTH, Mr Paul Royal Sussex Co. Hospital, Eastern Road, Brighton BN2 5BE — MB ChB Birm. 1970; BSc (Anat.) Birm. 1967; BSc (Anat.) Birm. 1967; FRCS Eng. 1975; FRCS Eng. 1975; FRCS Ed. (Orth.) 1981; FRCS Ed. (Orth.) 1981. Cons. Orthop. Surg. Roy. Sussex Co. Hosp. Brighton; Dep. Edr. & Exec. Bd. Mem. Injury. Specialty: Orthop. Socs: Fell. BOA; Brit. Soc. Surg. Hand. Prev: Sen. Regist. (Orthop.) Bristol Roy. Infirm.; Orthop. Fell. Roy. Childr. Hosp. Melbourne; Regist. (Orthop.) Robt. Jones & Agnes Hunt Hosp. OsW.ry.

STANILAND, John Robert Department of Health Care for the Elderly, Ladywell Building, Hope Hospital, Salford M6 8HD Tel: 0161 206 4042 Fax: 0161 206 4031 Email: john.staniland@srht.nhs.uk — MB BChir Camb. 1978 (Univ. of Camb.) MB Camb. 1978, BChir 1977; MA Camb. 1978; MRCP (UK) 1985; FRCP 1998. Cons. Phys. Med. for the Elderly Salford Roy. Hosps. Trust. Specialty: Care of the Elderly. Special Interest: Acute Stroke Med.; Syncope. Prev: Cons. Phys. Med. for the Elderly Wigan & Leigh NHS Trust; Sen. Regist. Rotat. (Med. for the Elderly) N. West. RHA; Regist. (Gen. Med. & Nephrol.) Leeds Gen. Infirm.

STANLEY, Adrian George Department of Cardiovascular Sciences, Clinical Sciences Building, Leicester Royal Infirmary, PO Box 65, Leicester LE2 7LX — BM Soton. 1992 (University of Southampton) BSc Soton. 1991; MRCP (UK) 1996. Clin. Lect. in Med. univ. Leci.; Hon. specialist Regist. in Med. univ. hosp. Leci. NHS Trust. Specialty: Gen. Med.

STANLEY, Adrian John Glasgow Royal Infirmary, Dept. of Gastroenterology, 84 Castle Street, Glasgow G4 0SF Tel: 0141 211 4073 — MB ChB Ed. 1988; MRCP (UK) 1991; MD Edin. 1998; FRCP Edin. 2003; FRCP Glas. 2003. Cons. (Gastro.) Glas. Roy. Infirm. Specialty: Gastroenterol.; Gen. Med. Socs: Brit. Soc. Of Gastroenterol.; Scott. Soc. Of Phys.s; British Association of the Study of the Liver. Prev: Lect. (Med.) Univ. Edin. Roy. Infirm.; Regist. Rotat. (Med.) Edin. Roy. Infirm.; SHO (Med.) William Harvey Hosp. Ashford.

STANLEY, Adrian Michael Charles Street Surgery, Charles Street, Otley LS21 1BJ Tel: 01943 466124; Avalon, 30 Farnley Lane, Otley LS21 2BH Tel: 01943 466868 Fax: 01943 468373 — MB ChB Leeds 1979.

STANLEY, Ann Katharine The Norvic Clinic, St Andrew's Business Park, Thorpe St Andrews, Norwich NR7 0HT Tel: 01603 439614 Fax: 01603 701954 — MB BS Lond. 1986; BSc Lond. 1983; MRCPsych 1992; MMedSc (Psychiat.) Birm. 1993. Cons. (Forens. Psychiat.) Norwich. Specialty: Forens. Psychiat. Prev: Sen. Regist. (Psychiat.) W. Midl. RHA.; Regist. Rotat. (Psychiat.) Birm. HA.; SHO (Med.) United Norwich Hosp.

STANLEY, Barry Park Street Surgery, Park Street, Bootle L20 3DF — MB BChir Camb. 1987; BA Oxf. 1984; T(GP) 1993. Trainee GP York VTS. Prev: SHO (ENT & O & G) York Dist,. Gen. Hosp.; SHO (Geriat.) Halton Gen. Hosp. Runcorn.

STANLEY, Belinda Louise Grant Westbank Practice, The Surgery, Church Street, Starcross, Exeter EX5 1DH Tel: 01626 890368 — MB BS Lond. 1990 (St Thomas's (UMDS)) DFFP 1995. Specialty: Gen. Pract.

STANLEY, Belinda Susan Cumberland Infirmary, Newtown Road, Carlisle CA2 7HY Tel: 01228 814814; The Old Vicarage, Dacre, Penrith CA11 0HH — BM Soton. 1982; MRCP (UK) 1987; FRCP (UK) 1998. Cons. Genitourin. Med. Carlisle Hosps. Trust. Specialty: Genitourinary Medicine. Prev: Lect. & Hon. Sen. Regist. (Genitourin. Med.) Middlx. Hosp. Lond.; Regist. (Genitourin. Med.) St. Mary's Hosp. Lond.; SHO Rotat. (Med.) Soton. HA.

STANLEY, Catherine Anne Mary Rose Heath, The Mount, Heswall, Wirral CH60 4RE — MB BS Lond. 1997.

STANLEY, Charles Kincaid Cross House, 1 Ranmoor Crescent, Ranmoor, Sheffield S10 3GU — MB BS Lond. 1982.

STANLEY, Christopher Paul Larwood Health Centre, 56 Larwood, Worksop S81 0HH Tel: 01909 500233 Fax: 01909 479722 — MB BS Newc. 1982; MRCGP 1989. Prev: Regist. (Respirat. & Gen. Med.) St. Jas. Univ. Hosp. Leeds.

STANLEY, Clare Alexandra 2 Wildwood Terrace, London NW3 7HT Tel: 020 8455 5109 — MB ChB Cape Town 1992. Specialty: Paediat.

STANLEY, Clare Hazel Priorslegh Medical Centre, Civic Centre, Park Lane, Stockport SK12 1GP — MB ChB Manch. 1983; DRCOG 1986; DRCOG 1986; MRCGP 1988; MRCGP 1988.

STANLEY, Mr David The Orthopaedic Department, Northen General Hospital, Sheffield S5 7AU Tel: 0114 243 4343 Fax: 0114 226 6796 Email: claire.faulkner@northngh-tr.trent.nhs.uk; Ranworth, 1 Chorley Road, Fulwood, Sheffield S10 3RJ Tel: 0114 230 4808 — MB BS Lond. 1977 (St George's London) BSc (Physiol., 1st cl. Hons.) Lond. 1974; FRCS Eng. 1985. Cons. (Shoulder & Elbow Surg.) N. Gen. Hosp. Sheff. Specialty: Orthop. Special Interest: Elbow Reconstruction. Socs: Brit. Elbow & Shoulder Soc. (Sec.); Eur. Rheum. Arthrit. Surg. Soc.; Eur. Soc. Surg. of Shoulder & Elbow. Prev: Sen. Regist. (Orthop.) Sheff. Teach. Hosps.

STANLEY, David Peter 67 Middle Park Road, Selly Oak, Birmingham B29 4BH — MB ChB Birm. 1996.

STANLEY, Derek John Peter The Stokes Medical Centre, Braydon Avenue, Little Stoke, Bristol BS34 6BQ Tel: 01454 616767; 26 Russell Grove, Westbury Park, Bristol BS6 7UE Tel: 0117 924 8685 — MB BCh BAO Dub. 1971 (TC Dub.) BA Dub. 1969; DObst RCOG 1973; MRCGP 1980. Specialty: Psychother.; Respirat. Med. Prev: SHO (Obst.) St. Mary's Matern. Hosp. Portsmouth; SHO (Gen. Med. & Paediat.) Glos. Roy. Hosp.

STANLEY, Elizabeth Margaret Gordon (retired) Staples Farm, Datchworth, Knebworth SG3 6RN Tel: 01438 813001 Fax: 01438 814388 Email: stanley@ashwell.com — MRCS Eng. LRCP Lond. 1962 (Roy. Free) Hon. Sen. Lect. (Human Sexuality) St. Geo. Hosp. Med. Sch. Prev: Dir. Human Sexuality Unit St. Geo. Hosp. Med. Sch. Lond.

STANLEY, George Edward Flat 2, 18 Nairn Road, Poole BH13 7NQ — BM Soton. 1988.

STANLEY, Harold Wheldale Plantation House, Salcombe TQ8 8JJ Tel: 01548 842538 — MB BS Lond. 1951 (St. Bart.) MRCS Eng. LRCP Lond. 1949; DA Eng. 1954. Socs: Founder Assoc. MRCGP; Plymouth Med. Soc. & Brit. Med. Acupunc. Soc. Prev: Anaesth. S. Hams Hosp. Kingsbridge; GP Salcombe, Devon; Ho. Surg. & Ho. Surg. Thoracic Unit St. Bart. Hosp. Lond.

STANLEY, Ian Roger 3 Provence Avenue, Brockhall Village, Old Langho, Blackburn BB6 8DF — MB BChir Camb. 1992.

STANLEY, James Charles Rydal Mount, Ruff Lane, Ormskirk L39 4QZ — MB BS Lond. 1998.

STANLEY, James Clive 18 Plantation Road, Lisburn BT27 5BP Tel: 028 92676386 Email: clivestanley@ireland.com — MB BCh BAO Belf. 1978; FRCA; FFA RCSI 1983. Cons. Anaesth. Roy. Gp. Hosps. Belf. Specialty: Anaesth. Socs: BMA; Assn Anaesth. GB & Irel.; Affil. Mem. Amer. Soc. Anesthesiol.

STANLEY, James Derek 46 Brook Lane, Chester CH2 2ED Tel: 01244 40532; 46 Brook Lane, Chester CH2 2ED Tel: 01244 40532 — MB BCh BAO Dub. 1969; BA Dub. 1967, MB BCh BAO 1969. Mem. Med. Bd. DHSS. Prev: Cas. Off. Roy. City of Dub. Hosp.; Ho. Off. Roy. City of Dub. Hosp.

STANLEY, Joanna Ruth 1 Steps End Cottages, Rydal, Ambleside LA22 9LP — MB ChB Manch. 1990. SHO (Cas.) Roy. Lancaster Infirm. Prev: SHO (O & G) Lancaster Infirm.; SHO (Med.) Westmorland Gen. Hosp.; SHO (Paediat.) Roy. Lancaster Infirm.

STANLEY, Joanne Kay The Medical Centre, Pinkham, Cleobury Mortimer, Kidderminster DY14 8QE Tel: 01299 270209 Fax: 01299 270482; 15 Grove Meadow, Cleobury Mortimer, Kidderminster DY14 8AG — MB ChB Birm. 1989; MRCGP 1992. Prev: Trainee GP/SHO Kidderminster Gen. Hosp. VTS; Ho. Off. (Med.) Goodhope Hosp. Sutton Coldfield; Ho. Off. (Surg.) Kidderminster Gen. Hosp.

STANLEY, Professor John Knowles 20 Derby Street West, Ormskirk L39 3NH Tel: 01695 575210 Fax: 01695 575210 — MB ChB Liverp. 1968; FRCS Ed. 1973; FRCS Eng. 1974; MCh Orth Liverp. 1975. p/t Cons. Hand Surg., Wrightington, Wigan and Leigh NHS Trust; Hon. Cons. Hope Hosp., Glan Clwyd Hosp., Alexandra Hosp., Fairfield Hosp., Manch. Childr. Hosp., Roy. Glam. Hosp.; Prof. (Hand Surg.). Orthop. Univ. Manch. Specialty: Orthop. Special Interest: Hand, Wrist, Elbow. Socs: Founder Mem. Brit. Shoulder & Elbow Soc.; (Ex-Pres.) Brit. Assn. Hand Therapists; (Ex-Pres.) NW Physiother. Soc. Prev: Sen. Regist. Roy. Liverp. Hosp., Roy. South. Hosp. Liverp. & Wrightington Hosp. Centre Hip Surg.; Cons. Ormskirk & Dist. Gen. Hosp. 1979-84.

STANLEY, John Steven Dr J. Stanley, Department of Anaesthesia, Newcastle General Hospital, West Road, Newcastle upon Tyne NE4 6BE Tel: 0191 256 3198 Fax: 0191 256 3154 Email: john@stanley.freeserve.co.uk; 13 Moresby Road, Cramlington NE23 3XP Tel: 01670 739499 Email: john@stanleyne.freeserve.co.uk — MB BS Newc. 1987; FRCA 1996. Cons. Anaesth., Newc. Hosp. NHS Trust. Specialty: Anaesth. Socs: Assn. Anaesth.; N. E. Soc. of Anaesth.

STANLEY, Katharine Paula Norfolk & Northwich University Hospital NHS Trust, Colney, Norwich NR4 7UY Tel: 01603 287975 — MB ChB Liverp. 1982; MRCOG 1987. Cons. Obst. & Gyn. Norf. & Norwich Univ. Hosp. NHS Trust. Specialty: Obst. & Gyn.

STANLEY, Mairi Christine 43 Marchmont Road, Edinburgh EH9 1HU Tel: 0131 229 8118 — MB ChB Ed. 1992; DRCOG 1995; MRCGP 1997.

STANLEY, Nigel Noel — MD Camb. 1976 (Camb. & St. Thos.) MB 1964, BChir 1963; FRCP Lond. 1981, M 1967. Cons. Phys. Lister Hosp. Stevenage. Specialty: Gen. Med.; Respirat. Med. Socs: Med. Res. Soc. & Brit. Thoracic Soc. Prev: Regist. (Med.) Roy. Free Hosp. Lond.; Lect. (Med.) Middlx. Hosp. Lond.; Asst. Prof. Med. Univ. Penna. Sch. Med. Philadelphia, USA.

STANLEY, Nigel Noel Staples Farm, Datchworth SG3 6RN Tel: 01438 813 001 — MB BCh Camb. 1963 (Univ. of Camb.) MRCP 1967; MD 1975; FRCP 1981. Cons. in Gen. & Respirat. Med., E. N. Herts. NHS Trust, Stevenage. Specialty: Gen. Med. Special Interest: Respirat. Med. Socs: Brit. Thoracic Soc.; Roy. Soc. of Med. Prev: Lect., Middlx. Hosp. (Lond.); Asst. Prof., Univ. Sch. of Med., Pennsylvania.

STANLEY, Oliver Hugh Southmead Hospital, Bristol BS10 5NB — MB BChir Camb. 1979; DCH Eng. 1980; MRCP (UK) 1981; BA Camb. 1973, MD 1988; FRCP Lond. 1994. Cons. Paediat. (Community) Southmead Hosp. Bristol; Sen. Lect. (Child Disabil.) Univ. Bristol. Specialty: Community Child Health.

STANLEY, Paula Bernadette 131 Rendlesham Road, London E5 8PA — MB BCh BAO NUI 1990.

STANLEY, Peter Hugh Riverside Surgery, Le Molay Littry Way, Bovey Tacey, Newton Abbot TQ13 9QP Tel: 01626 832666 — MB ChB Manch. 1969; BSc (Hons. Physiol.) Manch. 1966; MRCGP 1976.

STANLEY, Philip John Seacroft Hospital, York Road, Leeds LS14 6UH Tel: 0113 264 8164 Fax: 0113 206 2132 Email: p.j.stanley@leeds.ac.uk; 3 Avondale Villas, Thorner, Leeds LS14 3DQ Tel: 0113 289 2846 — MB BS Lond. 1976 (Westm.) MRCS Eng. LRCP Lond. 1976; MRCP (UK) 1978; DTM & H RCP Lond. 1987; MD Lond. 1988; FRCP Lond. 1994. Cons. Phys. (Infec. Dis.) Seacroft Hosp. Leeds; Clin. Sen. Lect. Univ. Leeds. Specialty: Infec. Dis. Prev: Sen. Regist. (Communicable & Trop. Dis.) E. Birm. Hosp.; Regist. (Med.) St. Stephen's Hosp. Chelsea; Clin. Lect. Cardiothoracic Inst. Lond.

STANLEY, Mr Richard Adrian, Wing Cdr. Retd. Caithness General Hospital, Wick KW1 5NS Tel: 01955 605050; Lealands, Bilbster, Wick KW1 5TA Tel: 01955 621237 — (Roy. Free) MB BS Lond. 1970; MRCS Eng. LRCP Lond. 1970; FRCS Eng. 1977. Cons. Surg. Caithness Gen. Hosp. Wick. Specialty: Gen. Surg.; Accid. & Emerg. Socs: Brit. Med. Assn.; Sec. Local Negotiating Comm. Prev: Wing. Cdr. RAF Med. Br.

STANLEY, Richard Sheridan Clerklands, Vicarage Lane, Horley RH6 8AR — MB BS Lond. 1971; MRCS Eng. LRCP Lond. 1971; DObst RCOG 1976.

STANLEY, Richard Stephen Grant — MB BS Lond. 1989 (Roy. Free Hosp. Sch. Med.) BSc (Hons.) Lond. 1986; DRCOG 1993; DCH RCP Lond. 1994; DFFP 1994; MRCGP 1995. GP Princip., Drs Thomas, Cockburn, Georgiou, Stanley, Golding, Hayward & Withers. Specialty: Gen. Pract. Socs: Brit. Med. Acupunct. Soc. Prev:

Clin. Med. Off. (Comunity Paediat.) SW Herts. HA; Resid. Med. Off. (Psychiat.) P. Henry Hosp. Sydney, Austral.

STANLEY, Roger Keith (retired) Lane End, Shore Road, Bosham, Chichester PO18 8QL Tel: 01243 573542 — MRCS Eng. LRCP Lond. 1968 (Char. Cross) MFOM RCP Lond. 1985; AFOM RCP Lond. 1981; Specialist Accredit (Occupat. Med.) JCHMT 1985.

STANLEY, Sally Elizabeth Ann Charles Street Surgery, Charles Street, Otley LS21 1BJ Tel: 01943 466124; Avalon, 30 Farnley Lane, Otley LS21 2BH Tel: 01943 466868 Fax: 01943 468373 — MB ChB Manch. 1980; MRCGP 1984.

STANLEY, Stephen Department of Child Health, Dorset Children's Centre, Damers Road, Dorchester DT1 2LB Tel: 01305 251150; Dairy Cottage, 10 Shitterton, Bere Regis, Wareham BH20 7HU Tel: 01929 471588 — MB ChB Dundee 1973 (St Andrews and Dundee) BSc St. And. 1970; MRCPsych 1982; MCPCH 1996; FRCPCH 1997. Cons. Child & Adolesc. Psychiat. W. Dorset Gen. Hosp. & Dorset Health Care NHS Trust.; Vis. Cons. Purbeck View Sch. for Autism Disorders & Milton Abbey Sch. Specialty: Child & Adolesc. Psychiat. Socs: Assn Family Ther.; Assn. Psychiat. Study Adolesc. Prev: Vis. Cons. Child & Adolesc. Psychiat. Ment. Health Serv. States of Jersey; Cons. Child & Adolesc. Psychiat. W & E Dorset Health Dists.; Sen. Regist. (Child Psychiat.) S. West. HA.

STANLEY, Susan Patricia The Surgery, 223 London Road, Waterlooville PO8 8DA Tel: 02392 263491 Fax: 02392 340504; 110B The Causeway, Petersfield GU31 4LL — BM BS Nottm. 1986; MRCGP 1990. Specialty: Paediat.; Family Plann. & Reproduc. Health.

STANLEY, Trevor Mark New Hayesbank Surgery, Cemetery Lane, Kennington, Ashford TN24 9JZ Tel: 01233 624642 Fax: 01233 637304 — MB BS Lond. 1990 (St. George's Hosp. Med. Sch. Lond.) Dip. Geriat. Med. 1993; DCH 1994; MRCGP 1994; DRCOG 1995; DFFP 1997. Specialty: Gen. Pract.

STANLEY, Wayne Edgar 73 Manor Road, Scarborough YO12 7RT — MB ChB Pretoria 1991.

STANLEY, William John (retired) 8 Crossfield Grove, Marple Bridge, Stockport SK6 5EQ — MB ChB Liverp. 1951; MRCS Eng. LRCP Lond. 1951; DPM Eng. 1959; MD Liverp. 1961; FRCPsych. 1981, M 1972. Prev: Cons. Psychiat. N. West. RHA.

STANLEY-JONES, Jillian Katherine Vivien (Mrs J Aarvold), Foxbury, Westhumble, Dorking RH5 6BQ Tel: 01306 884955 Fax: 01306 884955 — BM BCh Oxf. 1970; MA Oxf. 1970; DObst RCOG 1972; DCH Eng. 1973.

STANLEY-SMITH, Stephen Peter Osmaston Road Medical Centre, 212 Osmaston Road, Derby DE23 8JX Tel: 01332 346433 Fax: 01332 345854; 42 Broadway, Duffield, Belper DE56 4BU Tel: 01332 841424 — MB BS Lond. 1984; BSc Lond. 1981; DRCOG 1988; MRCGP 1989. GP Derby. Specialty: Community Child Health. Socs: Derby Med. Soc.

STANLEY-WHYTE, Elinor Mary (retired) 10 Clatto Place, St Andrews KY16 8SD Tel: 01334 475294 — (St. And.) MB ChB St. And. 1957. Prev: SCMO Lothian HB.

STANNARD, Catherine Faith Jubbs Court, Failand Lane, Failand, Bristol BS8 3SS — MB ChB Liverp. 1984; FCAnaesth. 1989. Sen. Regist. (Anaesth.) E. Anglian RHA. Specialty: Anaesth. Prev: Regist. (Anaesth.) Arrowe Pk. Hosp. Wirral; Regist. (Anaesth.) Nuffield Dept. Anaesth. Oxf.

STANNARD, Clare Louise Brixton Hill Group Practice, 22 Raleigh Gardens, Brixton Hill, London SW2 1AE Tel: 020 86746376 — MB BS Lond. 1996.

STANNARD, Edward John The Surgery, Queens Road, Earls Colne, Colchester CO6 2RR Tel: 01787 222641 Fax: 01787 224634 — MB BS Lond. 1977.

STANNARD, Mr Kevin Peter Dept of Ophthalmology, Royal Victoria Infirmary, Queen Victoria Road, Newcastle upon Tyne NE1 4LP Tel: 0191 232 5131 — MB BS Lond. 1978 (Kings College Hospital Medical School) DO Eng. 1982; FRCS Eng. 1984; FRCOphth 1988. Cons. Ophth. Surg. Roy. Vict. Infirm. Newc. Specialty: Ophth. Prev: Sen. Regist. Kings Coll. Hosp., Moorfields Eye Hosp. & Nat. Hosp. for Nerv. Dis.

STANNARD, Paul John Torbay Hospital, Lawes Bridge, Torquay TQ2 7AA Tel: 01803 654608 Fax: 01803 654651 Email: paul.stannard@nhs.net — MB BS Lond. 1972; FRCOG 1991, M 1978. Cons. (O & G) Torbay Hosp. Torquay. Specialty: Obst. & Gyn. Prev: Lect. (Hon. Sen. Regist.) Char. Cross & W. Lond. Hosps.

STANNARD, Philip Anthony Doncaster Royal Infirmary, Armthorpe Road, Doncaster DN2 5LT; 8 Grange Close, Doncaster DN4 6SE Tel: 01302 532391 — MB BS Lond. 1985; BA Camb. 1981; FRCR 1992. Cons. Radiol. Doncaster Roy. Infirm. & Montagu Hosp. NHS Trust. Specialty: Radiol. Prev: Sen. Regist. (Radiol.) Leeds Gen. Infirm.

STANNARD, Timothy John Friarsgate Practice, Friarsgate Medical Centre, Friarsgate, Winchester SO23 8EF Tel: 01962 853599 Fax: 01962 849982 — BM BS Nottm. 1983.

STANNARD, Wendy Anne 10 Queens Avenue, Heathfield Road, Kings Heath, Birmingham B14 7BU — MB ChB Birm. 1996; ChB Birm. 1996.

STANNERS, Andrew John Pinderfields Hospital, Aberford Road, Wakefield WF1 4DG Tel: 01924 201688 — BM Soton. 1983; MRCP (UK) 1988. Cons. Phys. (c/o Elderly) Pinderfields Hosp. Wakefield. Specialty: Care of the Elderly.

STANNING, Alison Margaret — MB BS Lond. 1985; DRCOG 1988; MRCGP 1989.

STANOWSKI, Maria 10 Campden Hill Square, London W8 7LB Tel: 020 7727 6877 Fax: 020 7727 6877 Email: mstanowski@aol.com — State Exam Rome 1994 (Univ. Rome La Sapienza, Italy) State Exam. Rome 1994. SHO (Psychiat. St Thos. Hosp. Lond. of Old Age); Guys Hosp. Learn. Disabil. Specialty: Ment. Health. Socs: BMA Med. Defence Union & Roy. Coll. Psychiat (Inceptor). Prev: Pre-reg Ho. Off. (Med.) N. Tees Hosp. Stockton on Tees; Pre-reg HO (ENT/Surg.) Freeman Hosp. Newc.; SHO (Psychiat.) Maidstone Kent Greenwich Hosp. Lond.

STANOWSKI, Robert Tollgate Health Centre, 220 Tollgate Road, London E6 5JS Tel: 020 7474 7709 Fax: 020 7445 7715 — MB BS Lond. 1984.

STANSBIE, David Leslie Bristol Royal Infirmary, Department of Chemical Pathology, Bristol BS2 8HW; 6 Charlotte St. S., Bristol BS1 5QB — MB ChB Leeds 1968; PhD Bristol 1977, BSc 1973; MRCPath 1977; FRCPath 1989; MRCP 2002. Cons. Chem. Path. Bristol Roy. Infirm. Specialty: Chem. Path. Prev: Sen. Lect. (Med. Biochem.) Welsh Nat. Sch. Med. Cardiff.

STANSBIE, Mr John Michael (retired) Walsgrave Hospital, Clifford Bridge Road, Coventry CV2 2DX Tel: 024 76 538966; 76 Bransford Avenue, Cannon Park, Coventry CV4 7EB Tel: 024 76 416755 — (Middlx.) BM BCh Oxf. 1966; MA Oxf. 1966; FRCS Eng. 1972. Prev: Cons. ENT Surg. Walsgrave Hosps. NHS Trust.

STANSBY, Mr Gerard Patrick Freeman Hospital, Freeman Road, High Heaton, Newcastle upon Tyne NE7 7DN — MB BChir Camb. 1982; BA Camb. 1982; FRCS Eng. 1987. Specialty: Gen. Surg.

STANSFELD, Professor Stephen Alfred Barts and the London, Queen Marys School of Medicine and Dentistry, Centre for Psychiatry, Medical Sciences Building, Mile End Road, London E1 4NS Tel: 0207 8827727 Fax: 0207 8827924 Email: s.a.stansfeld@qmul.ac.uk; 10 Woodberry Crescent, London N10 1PH Tel: 020 8883 6524 — MB BS Lond. 1975; PhD Lond. 1989, MB BS 1975; MRCP (UK) 1978; MRCPsych. 1982. Hons cons. Psychiat. E. Lond. & the city Health NHS Trust; Prof. of Psychiatry, Barts and the Lond. Qu. Mary Sch. of Med. and Dentistry. Specialty: Gen. Psychiat. Socs: Roy. Soc. Med. (Vice Pres. Psychiat. Sect.). Prev: Reader (Social & Environm. Psychiat. Univ coll.med.Sch.; Vis. Prof. Preven. Med. Univ. Toronto, Canada; Sen. Regist. Maudsley Hosp. Lond.

STANSFIELD, Damian Anthony 7 Hassness Close, Hawkley Hall, Wigan WN3 5RL — MB BS Lond. 1996.

STANSFIELD, David Phillip 2 Cresta House, 12 Ireton St., London E3 4XP Tel: 020 8983 3852 — MB BS Lond. 1989; BSc (Physiol.) Lond. 1988. Regist. (Anaesth.) St. Bart. Hosp. Lond. Specialty: Anaesth. Prev: Regist. (Anaesth.) Moorfields NHS Trust Lond.; SHO (Anaesth.) Milton Keynes NHS Trust & Watford Gen. Hosp.

STANSFIELD, Janet Mary 89 Recreation Road, Reading RG30 4UB — MB BS Lond. 1994 (UMDS) BSc Lond. 1991; MRCP (Lond.) 1997. SHO (Anaesth.) Roy. Berks. Hosp. Reading. Specialty: Anaesth.

STANSFIELD, Margaret Helen West End Medical Practice, 21 Chester Street, Edinburgh EH3 7RF Tel: 0131 225 5220 Fax: 0131 226 1910; 42 Comiston Drive, Edinburgh EH10 5QR Tel: 0131 447 6826 — MB BS Lond. 1969 (St. Thos.) MRCS Eng. LRCP Lond. 1969. Prev: Regist. (Path.) Groote Schuur Hosp. Univ. Cape Town,

S. Africa; Ho. Surg. St. Nicholas Hosp. Lond.; Ho. Phys. Lewisham Hosp. Lond.

STANSFIELD, Rosamund Eileen North Tyneside General Hospital, Newcastle upon Tyne NE29 8NH Tel: 0191 259 6660 Ext: 2386 Fax: 0191 293 2796 — MB BS Newc. 1983 (Newcastle uon Tyne) FCRpath 1998. Cons. Microbiologist N. Tyneside Gen. Hosp. Northumbria Healthcare NHS Trust NE29 8NH. Specialty: Med. Microbiol. Socs: Assn. of Med. Microbiologists; Hospsital Infec. Soc.; Brit. Infec. Soc. Prev: Regist. (Microbiol.) West. Gen. Hosp. Edin.; SHO (Path.) North. Gen. Hosp. Sheff.; Sen. Regist. (Microbiol.) West. Gen. Hosp. Edin.

STANTON, Alan Spencer Solihull Healthcare, 20 Union Road, Solihull B91 3EF Tel: 0121 711 7171 Fax: 0121 711 7212; 45 Goodby Road, Moseley, Birmingham B13 8RH — MB BS Lond. 1981; MSc Lond. 1994, BSc 1979; DCH RCP Lond. 1985; MRCP (UK) 1987. Cons. Community Paediat. Solihull Healthcare; Hon. Sen. Vis. Clin. Lect. Univ. Warwick 1997; Hon. Sen. Clin. Lect. Univ. Birm. 1997. Specialty: Community Child Health. Prev: Regist. (Paediat.) S. Birm. HA.

STANTON, Alice Veronica Department of Clinical & Cardiovascular Pharmacology, Imperial College School of Medicine, St Mary's Hospital, London W2 1NY Tel: 020 7594 3448 Fax: 020 7594 3411 — MB BCh BAO NUI 1984; BSc NUI 1986; MRCPI 1987; PhD NUI 1993. Sen. Lect. Hon. Cons. Clin. Pharm. & Therap. Dept. Clin. & Cardiovasc. Pharm. Nat. Heart Lung Inst. Imperial Coll. Sci. Technol. & Med. Specialty: Pharmacology. Prev: Lect. (Clin. Pharmacol.) Imperial Coll. Sch. Med. Lond.; Lect. (Therap.) Roy. Coll. Surg. Irel. Dub.

STANTON, Anthony John, OBE Secretariat for Londonwide LMCs, BMA House, Tavistock Square, London WC1H 9HT Tel: 020 7387 7418 Fax: 020 7388 2080; 4 Southbank Gardens, Lambourn, Hungerford RG17 7LW — MB BS Lond. 1964 (Westm.) MRCS Eng. LRCP Lond. 1964; DObst RCOG 1971. Sec. Lond. Local Med. Comms. Prev: SHO (O & G) Roy. Hants. Co. Hosp. Winchester; Ho. Phys. Westm. Childr. Hosp.; Surg. Lt. RN.

STANTON, Anthony Walter Burgin Dermatology Unit, Department of Cardiac & Vascular Sciences, St George's Hospital Medical School, London SW17 0RE Tel: 020 8725 5439 Fax: 020 8725 5955 Email: astanton@sghms.ac.uk — MB BCh Wales 1980; BSc (Hons.) Wales 1977; PhD Lond. 1989. Research Fell. (Physiol.) St. Geo. Hosp. Med. Sch. Lond. Socs: Brit. Microcirculat. Soc.

STANTON, Arthur Peter Flat 49, Ivy Lane, Headington, Oxford OX3 9DT — MB BS Sydney 1986.

STANTON, Eleanor Frances Marshfield Road Surgery, 4647 Marshfield Road, Chippenham SN15 1JU Tel: 01249 654466 Fax: 01249 462320 — MB ChB Manch. 1991. Trainee GP Stockport.

STANTON, Elinor Claire Ruth 234 Stoney Lane, Balsall Heath, Birmingham B12 8AW; 45 Goodby Road, Moseley, Birmingham B13 8RH — BM Soton. 1988; DFFP. GP. Prev: SHO (Paediat.) New Cross Hosp. Wolverhampton.

STANTON, Ian David Paul 38 Mayfield Road, Hasbury, Halesowen B63 1BQ — MB BS Lond. 1994.

STANTON, Jean Rosina Dunstable Road Surgery, 163 Dunstable Road, Luton LU1 1BW Tel: 01582 23553 — MB BS Lond. 1983.

STANTON, Jennifer Anne Yeadon Health Centre, 17 South View Road, Yeadon, Leeds LS19 7PS Tel: 0113 295 4040 Fax: 0113 295 4044; 10 Netherfield Road, Guisley, Leeds LS20 9HE Tel: 01943 873284 Fax: 01943 870627 — MB ChB Sheff. 1976.

STANTON, John Albert 143 Derwen Fawr Road, Swansea SA2 8ED Tel: 01792 207935 — MB BCh Wales 1949 (Cardiff) BSc 1946, MB BCh Wales 1949. Col. RAMC T & AVR. Prev: Ho. Phys. Child Health, Dermatol. & Neurol. Depts Roy. Infirm.; Cardiff; Capt. RAMC.

STANTON, Josephine Anne (retired) 13 Canons Drive, Edgware HA8 7RB Tel: 020 8952 1503 Email: susman12000@hotmail.com — MB BS Lond. 1962 (Middlx.) MRCS Eng. LRCP Lond. 1962; BA Open Univ. 1995. Med. Adviser Benefits Agency DSS & The Appeals Service. Prev: Princip. GP.

STANTON, Joy Margaret Airedale General Hospital, Skipton Road, Steeton, Keighley BD20 6TD Tel: 01535 292185 Fax: 01535 655129 — MB ChB Leeds 1975; DA Eng. 1977; FFA RCS Eng. 1984; Dip. Health Serv. Mngmt. York 1994. Cons. Anaesth. Airedale NHS Trust. Specialty: Anaesth. Prev: Sen. Regist. (Anaesth.) Yorks. RHA.

STANTON, Judith Rose 28 Braemar Court, Ashburnham Road, Bedford MK40 1DZ — MB BS Lond. 1989; DRCOG 1991; Cert. Family Plann. JCC 1992; MRCGP 1993; DGM RCP Lond. 1993; T(GP) 1993.

STANTON, Linda Marian (retired) 16 The Callanders, Heathbourne Road, Bushey, Watford WD23 1PU Tel: 020 8950 7760 — (Middlx.) MB BS (Univ. Medal Hons. Path., Obst. & Gyn. & Therap.) Lond. 1961; MRCGP 1974; MA Lond. 1990. Chairp. Barnet LMC; Chairp. Barnet GP Commissioning Gp. Prev: GP Barnet.

STANTON, Mr Martin Barry North London Nuffield Hospital, Calvell Drive, Uplands Park Road, Enfield EN2 7NR Tel: 020 8366 2122 Fax: 020 8367 8032 — MB BS Lond. 1955 (Middlx.) MRCS Eng. LRCP Lond. 1955; DLO Eng. 1958; FRCS Eng. 1963; BA Open 1991. Specialty: Otorhinolaryngol. Socs: Fell. Roy. Soc. Med. (Mem. Sects. Otol. & Laryng.); Brit. Assn. Otol. Prev: Cons. Surg. (ENT) Enfield Hosp. Gp.; Sen. Regist. Roy. Ear & Univ. Coll. Hosps. Lond. & (ENT) Roy. Berks. Hosp. Reading; Regist. Roy. Nat. Throat, Nose & Ear Hosp. Lond.

STANTON, Morris Burmantofts Health Centre, Lincoln Green Road, Leeds LS9 7ST Tel: 0113 248 0321 — MB ChB Leeds 1943; MB ChB (Hons.) Leeds 1943. Prev: Capt. RAMC, Asst. Med. Off. S. Wales Sanat.; Ho. Phys. Lincoln Co. Hosp.

STANTON, Richard Alan Hillview Lodge, Royal United Hospital Bath, Combe Down, Bath BA1 3NG Tel: 01225 324208 — MB BS Lond. 1988; MRCPsych 1993. Cons. (Psychiat. Gen. Adult & Rehabil.) Roy. United Hosp. Bath. Specialty: Gen. Psychiat. Prev: Sen. Regist. (Psychiat.) Univ. Coll. Hosp. Lond.; Clin. Research Fell. & Regist. (Psychiat.) Roy. Lond. Hosp.

STANTON, Robert John The Surgery, High Street, Cheslyn Hay, Walsall WS6 7AB Tel: 01922 701280; Slack Terrace Farm, Dick Edge Lane, Cumberworth, Huddersfield HD8 8YE Tel: 01484 681029 — MB ChB Sheff. 1979.

STANTON, Professor Stuart Lawrence Richard Flat 10, 43 Wimpole St., London W1G 8AE Tel: 020 7486 0677 Fax: 020 7486 6792 Email: sstantonwimpole@yahoo.com; 1 Church Hill, Wimbledon, London SW19 7BN Tel: 020 8879 1678 Fax: 020 8944 5177 — MB BS Lond. 1961 (Univ. Lond. & Lond. Hosp.) MRCS Eng. LRCP Lond. 1961; DObst RCOG 1963; FRCS Eng. 1967; FRCS Ed. 1967; FRCOG 1987, M 1969; FRANZCOG 2001. Cons. Gyn. & Emerit. Prof.St. Geo. Hosp. Lond.; Asst. Edr. Internat. Urogyn. Jl; Examr. RCOG. Specialty: Obst. & Gyn. Socs: Assoc. Mem. BAUS; Blair Bell Res. Soc.; Fell. Roy. Soc.Med. Prev: Prof. Pelvic Reconstruc. & Urogyn. St. Geo. Hosp. Lond.; Research Fell. Inst. Urol. Lond.; Sen. Regist. St. Geo. Hosp. Lond.

STANTON, Susan Margaret Warden Lodge Surgery, Albury Ride, Cheshunt, Waltham Cross EN8 8XE Tel: 01992 622324 Fax: 01992 636900 — MB ChB Bristol 1978; DCH RCP Lond. 1985.

STANTON, Timothy James (retired) 5 North Mill Place, Halstead CO9 2FA Tel: 01787 479003 — MB BS Lond. 1952 (St. Bart.) LMSSA Lond. 1952; DObst RCOG 1954; DA Eng. 1955; FFA RCS Eng. 1958. Prev: Cons. Anaesth. Crawley and Horsham Hosp.s.

STANTON, Tony 2R 3 Trefoil Avenue, Glasgow G41 3PD — MB ChB Glas. 1996. SHO (Gen. Med.) CrossHo. Hosp. Kilmarnock. Specialty: Gen. Med.

STANTON-KING, Kevin David Nene Valley Medical Centre, Clayton, Orton Goldhay, Peterborough PE2 5GP Tel: 01733 366600 Fax: 01733 370711 — MB ChB Leic. 1984.

STANWAY, Andrew Tadeusz 22 Portland Square, London E1W 2QR Tel: 020 7481 3500 Fax: 020 7481 3502 — MB BS Lond. 1968 (King's Coll. Hosp.) MRCS Eng. LRCP Lond. 1968; MRCP (UK) 1971. Psychosexual & Marital Phys. Surrey. Specialty: Psychosexual Med. Socs: Fell. Roy. Soc. Med. Prev: Med. Edr. Update Pub.ations Ltd.; Regist. (Med.) King's Coll. Hosp. Lond.

STANWAY, Penelope Ann 8 Woodhyrst Gardens, Kenley CR8 5LX — MB BS Lond. 1969 (King's Coll. Hosp.) MRCS Eng. LRCP Lond. 1969. Socs: Assoc. Mem. BPA. Prev: Sen. Med. Off. Croydon AHA.

STANWAY, Susannah Jane — MB ChB Bristol 1998.

STANWAY, Tania Lea 29 Kingsway, Frodsham, Warrington WA6 6RU — MB ChB Liverp. 1988; MRCPsych 1992.

STANWELL SMITH, Rosalind Elaine PHLS - Communicable Diseases, Surveillance Centre, 61 Colindale Avenue, London NW9 5EQ Tel: 020 8200 6868 Fax: 020 8200 7868; 60 Agamemnon Road, London NW6 1EH Tel: 020 7794 1063 Mob: 077 7960 8249 Fax: 020 7794 1063 Email:

rstanwellsmith@aol.com — MB BCh Wales 1974; MRCOG 1980; FFCHM 1994. Cons. Epidemiol. PHLS Communicable Dis. Surveillance Centr.; Edr. (Health & Hyg.); Hon. Sen. Lect. Lond.; Sch. of Hyg. & Trop. Med. Specialty: Epidemiol. Prev: Med. Off. Environmen. Health, Bristol; Sen. Regist. (Epidemiol.) PHLS Communicable Dis. Surveillance Centr.; Mem. Scientif. Staff MRC Epidemiol. & Med. Care Unit Northwick Pk. Hosp. Harrow.

STANWORTH, Andrew Ward Kings Road Surgery, 67 Kings Road, Harrogate HG1 5HJ Tel: 01423 875875 Fax: 01423 875885 — MB ChB Leeds 1978. GP Harrogate.

STANWORTH, Mr Peter Antony, TD Walsgrave Hospital, Clifford Bridge Road, Coventry CV2 2DX Tel: 024 7660 2020; Long Meadow Farm, Hob Lane, Burton Green, Kenilworth CV8 1QB Tel: 024 7646 6524 Fax: 024 7646 6524 — BM BCh Oxf. 1968; MA (Physics) Oxf. 1967, BA (Physics) 1962, BM BCh 1968; DCH Eng. 1971; FRCS Eng. 1973. Cons. Neurosurg. Walsgrave Hosp. Coventry; Lt. Col. RAMC (V). Specialty: Neurosurg.; Rehabil. Med. Prev: Cons. Neurosurg. Inst. Neurol. Sc. Glas.; Sen. Regist. (Neurosurg.) Manch. Roy. Infirm. & Radcliffe Infirm Oxf.

STANWORTH, Shirley Elizabeth (retired) Rockcliffe, Castle Road, Wemyss Bay PA18 6AN Tel: 01475 520488 Fax: 0145 522566 — MB ChB Manch. 1959. Assoc. Specialist (Cytol.) Inverclyde Roy. Hosp. Greenock. Prev: Assoc,. Specialist (Cytol.) Inverclyde Roy. Hosp. Greenock.

STANWORTH, Simon Jonathan 15 Ledborough Wood, Beaconsfield HP9 2DJ — BM BCh Oxf. 1987; BA Oxf. 1984; MRCP (UK) 1990; MRCPath 2001. Specialist Regist. (Haemat.) Lond. Specialty: Haematology. Prev: Wellcome Fell. Inst. Molecular Med. Univ. Oxf.; SHo Rotat. Bristol & Stoke on Trent.; Specialist Regist. (Haemat.) Manch.

STAPLE, Gordon 14 Ffordd Dryden, Killay, Swansea SA2 7PA — MB ChB Manch. 1994.

STAPLES, Brian North Cheshire Health, Lister Road, Astmoor West Est, Runcorn WA7 1TW — MB ChB Liverp. 1988; BSc (1st. cl. Hons. Phys.) Lancaster 1981; MPH Liverp. 1991; MFPHM RCP (UK) 1996; DRCOG 1997; DFFP 1998. Cons. (Pub. Health Med.). Specialty: Pub. Health Med.; Gen. Pract. Prev: GP Princip.; GP Regist.; Sen. Regist. (Pub. Health) N. Chesh.

STAPLES, Derrick (retired) 80 Sorby Way, Wickersley, Rotherham S66 1DR — (Sheff.) MB ChB Sheff. 1960. Prev: Asst. Cas. Off. & Ho. Surg. (ENT) Roy. Infirm. Sheff.

STAPLES, Emma Jane 45 Millbeck Green, Collingham, Wetherby LS22 5AG — MB BS Lond. 1996.

STAPLES, Vincent John Water's Edge, Mill Lane, Govilon, Abergavenny NP7 9SA — MB BCh Wales 1985.

STAPLETON, Andrew James — MB BS Lond. 1998.

STAPLETON, Clare Wexham Park Hospital, Wexham Street, Wexham, Slough SL2 4HL Tel: 01753 633185 — MB BS Lond. 1988 (The London Hospital Medical College) MRCP (UK) 1993; FRCA 1995. Cons. in Anaesthetics and Intens. Care, Wexham Pk. Hosp., Slough. Specialty: Anaesth. Socs: BMA; Assn. of Anaesth.s; Soc. of Anaesthetists of South-West Region. Prev: SPR Anaesth., S.-W. Region; Fell. in Anaesth., St Michaels Hosp., Toronto, Canada; Clin. Research Fell., Univ. of Bristol.

STAPLETON, Edward Mark Claremont Bank Surgery, Claremont Bank, Shrewsbury SY1 1RL Tel: 01743 357355; River House, 43 Berwick Road, Shrewsbury SY1 2LS — MB BS Lond. 1985; BSc Immunol. Lond. 1982; MRCGP 1989; DCH RCP Lond. 1989.

STAPLETON, Geoffrey Arthur Gillard The Surgery, The Coppice, Herne Lane, Littlehampton BN16 3BE Tel: 01903 783178 Fax: 01903 859027; 24 The Drive, East Preston, Littlehampton BN16 1QL Tel: 01903 785040 — MB BS Lond. 1964 (Lond. Hosp.) MRCS Eng. LRCP Lond. 1964; DObst RCOG 1966; DA Univ. W. Indies 1968; FFA RCS Eng. 1972. Specialty: Gen. Pract. Prev: Regist. Lond. Hosp. (Whitechapel) & Chase Farm Hosp. Enfield; Princess argt. Hosp. Nassau, Bahamas.

STAPLETON, Mr Simon Robert St John Department of Neurosurgery, Atkinson Morley's Hospital, Wimbledon, London SW20 0NE Tel: 020 8725 4179 Fax: 020 8947 8389; Rosevine, Ockham Road N., Ockham, Woking GU23 6NW — MB BS Lond. 1985; FRCS Eng. 1989; BSc Lond. 1982, MD 1994; FRCS (SN) 1994. Cons. Neurosurg. Atkinson Morley's Hosp. Lond. Specialty: Neurosurg.

STAPLETON, Siobhan 212 Greenford Avenue, London W7 3QT — MB BCh BAO Dub. 1992.

STAPLETON, Thomas The Foundry Cottage, Lane End, High Wycombe HP14 3JS Tel: 01494 881257 — (Oxf.) BM BCh Oxf. 1943; DCH Eng. 1944; FRCP Lond. 1970, M 1947; MA Oxf. 1945, DM 1953; FRACP 1975. Emerit. Prof. Child Health Univ. Sydney & Overseas Fell. Churchill Coll. Camb. Specialty: Paediat. Socs: Hon. FRCPCH; FRCPCH (Hon.); Hon Mem. Paediat. Sect.. Roy.Soc.Med. Prev: Sec-Gen. Internat. Pediat. Assn.; Asst. Dir. Paediat. Unit St. Mary's Hosp. Med. Sch. Lond.; Tutor (Child Health) Univ. Sheff.

STAPLEY, Alison Mary East Surrey Hospital, Canada Drive, Redhill RH1 5RH Tel: 01737 768511; 16 Lavender Close, Redhill RH1 5LP — MB BS Lond. 1996. SHO GP VTS E. Surrey Hosp. Redhill. Specialty: Gen. Pract.

STAPLEY, Margaret Lawson The Health Centre, 114 High Road, South Woodford, London E18 2QS Tel: 020 8491 3310 Fax: 020 8491 3307 — MB ChB Liverp. 1966; DObst RCOG 1968; DCH Eng. 1970. Prev: Regist. (Anaesth.) Lond. Hosp.; Regist. (Paediat.) Windsor Gp. Hosps.; SHO (O & G) Broadgreen Hosp. Liverp.

STAPLEY, Miss Sarah Ann, Surg. Lt.-Cdr. RN 25 Rosedale Close, Crawley RH11 8NQ — MB ChB Glas. 1989; FRCS Eng. 1996. Specialist Regist. (Orthop.) P'boro Dist. NHS Trust. Specialty: Orthop. Prev: Specialist Regist. (Orthop.) Roy. Hosp. Haslar, Gosport.; Dep. Princip. M.O. HMS Illustrious.

STARBUCK, Daniel Augustus — MB ChB Sheff. 1998.

STARBUCK, David Paul New Pond Row Surgery, 35 South Street, Lancing BN15 8AN Tel: 01903 752265 Fax: 01903 851634 — MB ChB Leeds 1979; MRCGP 1983.

STARBUCK, Martin John Shiregreen Medical Centre, 492 Bellhouse Road, Sheffield S5 0RG Tel: 0114 245 6123 Fax: 0114 257 0964; 53 Ranmoor Crescent, Ranmoor, Sheffield S10 3GW — MB ChB Sheff. 1982; DRCOG 1987; MRCGP 1995.

STARCK, Alan Lee 5 Watson Close, Bury St Edmunds IP33 2PG — MB BS Lond. 1996.

STARCK, Gordon Philip St Chad (retired) 74 Hempstead Road, Watford WD17 4ER — (Lond. Hosp.) MA, MB BChir Camb. 1954; MRCS Eng. LRCP Lond. 1954; DObst RCOG 1959. Prev: Regist. (Paediat.) Salisbury Gen. Hosp.

STARCZEWSKA, Mrs Maria (retired) 90 Iveagh House, Loughborough Road, London SW9 7SF Tel: 020 7326 4830 — MB ChB Polish Sch. of Med. 1949.

STARCZEWSKI, Anthony Roman Glan Aber, Red Wharf Bay, Pentraeth LL75 8PZ — MB ChB Manch. 1976; BSc (Hons.) (Med. Biochem.) Manch. 1973, MB ChB (Hons.) 1976; MRCP (UK) 1982. Cons. Phys. (Geriat. Med.) Ysbyty Gwynedd, Bangor. Specialty: Gen. Med. Prev: Sen. Regist. (Geriat. Med.) The Maelor Gen. Hosp. Wrexham; Regist. (Gen. Med.) War Memor. Hosp. Wrexham; SHO (Gen. Med.) Univ. Manch. Hope Hosp. Salford.

STARER, Fritz Lawnswood, 8 Green Lane, Oxhey, Watford WD19 4NJ Tel: 01923 23420 — LRCP LRCS Ed. 1949; LRCP LRCS Ed. LRFPS Glas. 1949; FRCP Ed. 1971, M 1954; FFR 1960; FRCR 1975. Cons. Radiol. Westm. Hosp. Lond. Specialty: Radiol.

STARER, Rachel Didcot Health Centre, Britwell Road, Didcot OX11 7JH — MB ChB Manch. 1986. GP Princip. Didcot Health Centre Didcot Oxon.

STAREY, Nigel Harvey Leonard Prestwood House Surgery, Midway Road, Midway, Swadlincote DE11 7PG Tel: 01283 212373 Email: n.starey@derby.ac.uk; Brook Farm, Snelston, Ashbourne DE6 2GP — MRCS Eng. LRCP Lond. 1977 (Char. Cross) BSc (Hons.) Lond. 1972, MB BS 1977; MRCGP 1983. GP Princip.; Dir. Centre for Primary Care Univ. Derby. Special Interest: Genetics. Prev: GP Burnham on Crouch.; Med. Adviser, N. W. Anglia Health Auth.

STARFORD, Helen 2 Farley Drive, Middlesbrough TS5 8QT — MB ChB Leeds 1994.

STARK, Agnes Macfarlane (retired) 7 Thorp Avenue, Morpeth NE61 1JT Tel: 01670 512737 — MB ChB Glas. 1945 (Univ. Glas.) FRCOG 1981, M 1951, DObst 1948; MD (Commend.) Glas. 1972. Prev: Dir. (Breast Diag.) & Asst. (Gyn. Oncol.) Qu. Eliz. Hosp. Gateshead.

STARK, Allistair Neil Department of Haematology, Dumfries & Galloway Royal Infirmary, Bankend Road, Dumfries DG1 4AP Tel: 01387 241441 Fax: 01387 241344 — MB ChB Glas. 1980 (Glasgow) MRC (UK) 1983; MRCPath 1989. Cons. Haemat. Dumfries & Galloway Roy. Infirm. NHS Trust. Specialty:

Haematology. Socs: Brit. Soc. Haematol. & Assn. Clin. Path.; Fell. Roy. Coll. Pathologists; Fell. Roy. Coll. ??? (Glas.). Prev: Sen. Regist. (Haemat.) North. RHA.

STARK, Cameron Ross Assynt House, Beechwood Business Park, Inverness IV2 3HG — MB ChB Glas. 1985; MRCPsych 1990; MPH Glas. 1991; MFPHM RCP (UK) 1994; FFPHM 1999; MSc Leicester 2000. Cons. Pub. Health NHS Highland; Hon. Sen. Lect. Univ. Aberd.; Hon. Sen. Clin. Lect. Univ. Glas. Specialty: Pub. Health Med. Special Interest: Ment. health; Rural health and health care. Prev: Cons. Pub. Health Ayrsh. & Arran HB.; Regist. (Psychiat.) South. Gen. & Levendale Hosps.

STARK, Daniel Peter Harry Dept of Med.Oncology, Bradford Royal Infirmary, Duchwall Lane, Bradford BD9 6RJ Tel: 01274 364246 Fax: 01274 366745 Email: d.stark@cancermed.leeds.ac.uk — MB BChir Camb. 1993 (Cambridge) MRCP 1995; PhD 2002. Sen. Lect. Med. Oncol., Leeds / Bradford Med. Sch. Specialty: Oncol. Socs: Assoc.Cancer.Phys.

STARK, Edmund George 11 Wycome Road, Hall Green, Birmingham B28 9EN — MB ChB Leeds 1988; MRCGP 1995.

STARK, Gail Lisa — BM BS Nottm. 1994; BMedSci (Hons.) Nottm. 1992; MRCP (Lond.) 1997; DipRCPath 2001. Regist. (Haemat.) Roy. Vict. Infirm. Newc. u. Tyne. Specialty: Haematology. Prev: SHO (Med.) Newc.

STARK, Gavin Peter Victoria Street Medical Group, 7 Victoria Street, Aberdeen AB10 1QW Tel: 01224 641930 Fax: 01224 644081; 6 Ferryhill Place, Aberdeen AB11 7SE — MB ChB Aberd. 1978; MRCGP 1990. Specialty: Gen. Pract.; Plastic Surg. Prev: Facilitator (Gen. Med. Pract.) Grampian HB.

STARK, Gordon David (retired) Craigard, Aberfeldy PH15 2LB Tel: 01887 830529 — MB ChB Ed. 1960; DObst RCOG 1963; FRCP Ed. 1972, M 1964; DCH RCP Lond. 1964; FRCPCH 1997. Cons. Paediat. Roy. Hosp. for Sick Childr. Edin. & St. John's Hosp. Livingston; Hon. Sen. Lect. (Child Life & Health) Univ. Edin. Prev: Cons. Paediat. (Neurol.) King Faisal Specialist Hosp. & Research Centre Riyadh, Saudi Arabia.

STARK, Isobel Mary Webster (retired) 22 Drumlin Drive, Milngavie, Glasgow G62 6LN Tel: 0141 956 2288 — MB ChB Glas. 1947; DObst RCOG 1951.

STARK, Professor James Marshall (retired) 179 Adventurers Quay, Cardiff Bay, Cardiff CF10 4NS Tel: 029 20 492581 Fax: 029 20 492621 — (Univ. Glasgow) MB ChB Glas. 1953; DPath Eng. 1960; FRCPath 1977, M 1965; MD (Commend.) Glas. 1969. Prev: Prof. & Hon. Cons. Med. Microbiol. Univ. Wales Coll. Med. Cardiff.

STARK, Mr Jaroslav Great Ormond Street Hospital for Children NHS Trust, London WC1N 3JH Tel: 020 7831 7593 Fax: 020 7430 1281 — MD Prague 1958 (Charles Univ. Prague) CSc Prague 1968; LAH Dub. 1970; FACS 1978; FACC 1978; FRCS Eng. 1980. Cons. Cardiothoracic Surg. Hosp. Sick Childr. Gt. Ormond St. Lond. Specialty: Cardiothoracic Surg. Socs: Eur. Assn. Cardiothoracic Surg.; Hon. Mem. Amer. Assn. Thoracic Surg. Prev: Asst. (Paediat. Surg.) Chas. Univ. Prague; Sen. Regist. (Surg.) Hosp. Sick Childr. Gt. Ormond St. Lond.; Research Fell. (Cardiol.) Harvard Med. Sch. Boston, USA.

STARK, Jeremy Paul 40 Weigall Road, London SE12 8HE — MB BChir Camb. 1975; MA Camb. 1974. Sen. Regist. (Pub. Health Med.) SE Thames RHA. Prev: GP Ryde I. of Wight; SCMO (Community Child Health) Lewisham & N. Southwark HA.

STARK, John Emanuel (retired) The Old School, Llanigon, Hereford HR3 5QA — MB BChir Camb. 1959 (St. Bart.) FRCP Lond. 1975, M 1961; MD Camb. 1967. Prev: Sen. Lect. & Hon. Cons. Phys. St. Bart. Hosp. Lond.

STARK, Margaret Mary The Forensic Medicine Unit, St George's Hospital Medical School, Cranmer Terrace, Tooting, London SW17 0RE Tel: 020 8725 0015 Fax: 020 8725 0017 — MB BS Lond. 1981 (Westminster) DAB Lond. 1982; DGM RCP 1989; DMJ (Clin.) Soc. of Apothecaries 1992; LLM Wales 1996. Hon. Sen. Lect., Clin. Research Fell., The Forens. Med. Unit, St Geo.'s Hosp. Medicial Sch.

STARK, Michael John (2F1) 15 Bernard Terrace, Edinburgh EH8 9NU — MB ChB Ed. 1996.

STARK, Philip John 11 Wycombe Road, Hall Green, Birmingham B28 9EN — MB ChB Leeds 1982.

STARK, Robert Alexander (retired) Twelve Trees, Bare Lane, Ockbrook, Derby DE72 3RG — MB ChB Glas. 1952; DObst RCOG 1954.

STARK, Ronald David Hill of Park House, Drumoak, Banchory AB31 5HJ Tel: 01330 811400 Fax: 01330 811409 — MB ChB Aberd. 1965; PhD Aberd. 1969; MD Birm. 1973; MRCP (UK) 1973; FRCP Lond. 1985; FFPM RCP (UK) 1989. Indep.Cons. Pharm.Med.; Hon. Sen. Lect. Med. & Therap. Univ. Aberd. Specialty: Pharmaceutical Medicine; Pharmacology. Prev: Clin. Research Fell. (Med.) Univ. Birm.; Canad. MRC Research Fell. & Lect. (Pharmacol.) Univ. Manitoba, Winnipeg, Canada; Chief.Phys.ZenecaPharmaceuts.Alderley PK.

STARKE, Ian Douglas University Hospital Lewisham, Lewisham High St., London SE13 6LH Tel: 020 8333 3379 Fax: 020 8333 3381; Flat 11, Queen's Court, 25/27 Earl's Court Square, London SW5 9DA — MB BS (Hons.) Lond. (Guy's) 1972 (Guy's) MSc (1st Cl. Hons.) 1969; MRCP (UK) 1974; MD Lond. 1985; FRCP Lond. 1993; FRCP Edin. 2003. Cons. Phys. & Sen. Lect. (Med. for Elderly) Univ. Hosp. Lewisham & Guys, Kings & St. Thomas' Med. Sch.s Lond. Specialty: Gen. Med. Socs: Brit. Geriat. Soc.; Brit. Assn. Stroke Physicians. Prev: Sen. Regist. (Gen. & Geriat. Med.) Guy's Hosp. Lond.

STARKEY, Caroline Nicola Department of General Practice and Primary Care, St George's Hospital Medical School, Cranmer Terrace, London SW17 0RE Tel: 020 8725 0056 Fax: 020 8767 7697 Email: cstarkey@sghms.ac.uk; 7 Lattimer Place, London W4 2UD — MB BS Lond. 1985 (Guys Hospital Medical School) MSc Lond. 1994, BSc (Hons.) 1982; DRCOG 1987; DCH RCP Lond. 1989; MRCGP 1990. Clin. Lect., Dept. of Gen. Pract., St Geo.'s Hosp. Med. Sch.; Non-Princip. GP. Specialty: Gen. Pract.

STARKEY, Colin Airedale General Hospital, Skipton Road, Steeton, Keighley BD20 6TD — MB ChB Ed. 1971; FFA RCS Eng. 1976. Specialty: Anaesth.

STARKEY, Graham Bedlingtonshire Medical Group, The Health Centre, Glebe Road, Bedlington NE22 6JX Tel: 01670 822695 — MB BS Newc. 1989 (Newc. u. Tyne) MRCGP 1996; DRCOG 1996. Clin. Asst. Gen. Surg. Wansbeck Gen. Hosp. Ashington. Specialty: Gen. Pract. Prev: PCG Prescribing Lead Centr. PCG, N.D.; Vice Chair, Wawsbeck and Community Prescribing Sub-Comm.

STARKEY, Ian Richard Department of Cardiology, Western General Hospital, Crewe Road S., Edinburgh EH4 2XU Tel: 0131 537 1844 Fax: 0131 537 1844 Email: ian.starkey@luht.scot.nhs.uk; 17 Braekirk Gardens, Kirknewton EH27 8BP Tel: 01506 881231 Fax: 01506 880293 Email: ianstarkey1@compuserve.com — MB ChB Ed. 1975; MRCP (UK) 1977; FRCP Ed. 1989. Cons. Cardiol. West. Gen. Hosp. Edin. Specialty: Cardiol. Socs: Brit. Cardiac Soc.; Scott. Cardiac Soc.; Brit. Cardiovasc. Interven. Soc. Prev: Sen. Regist. (Cardiol.) North. Gen. Hosp. Sheff.

STARKIE, Carol Margaret (retired) Huntroyd, 27 Manor Road N., Edgbaston, Birmingham B16 9JS Tel: 0121 242 2497 — MB ChB Birm. 1963; BSc (Hons. Anat.) Birm. 1960; MRCS Eng. LRCP Lond. 1963; DCH Eng. 1967; FRCPath 1991, M 1979. Prev: Cons. Histopath. Selly Oak Hosp. Birm.

STARKIE, Colin (retired) 142 Sutton Park Road, Kidderminster DY11 6JQ Tel: 01562 823338 — MB ChB Manch. 1932; MD Manch. 1938, BSc Manch. (Anat. & Physiol.) 1928; MRCS Eng. LRCP Lond. 1931; DPH 1933. Prev: MOH Boro. Kidderminster.

STARKIE, David William Health Centre Practice, Bromsgrove Street, Kidderminster DY10 1PG Tel: 01562 822077 Fax: 01562 823733; 47 Staite Drive, Cookley, Kidderminster DY10 3UA Tel: 01562 850132 — BM BS Nottm. 1985; BMedSci Nottm. 1983; MRCGP 1989. Clin. Asst. (Rheum.) Kidderminster Gen. Hosp.; Tutor (Gen. Pract.) Kidderminster. Specialty: Rehabil. Med.; Gen. Pract.; Rheumatol.

STARLING, Andrew James Meridian Surgery, Meridian Way, Peacehaven BN10 8NF Tel: 01273 581999 Fax: 01273 589025 — MB BS Lond. 1985; MRCGP 1991. Gen. Pract. Princip.; GP Trainer. Socs: CICP; CMF.

STARR, David Ralph Plume 11 Frank Dixon Way, Dulwich, London SE21 7ET Tel: 020 8693 6696 Email: david.starr@ukgateway.net — MRCS Eng. LRCP Lond. 1956 (Middlx.) DCH Eng. 1962; MB BS Lond. 1956, DPH 1966. Socs: BMA. Prev: Ho. Phys. Middlx. Hosp. Lond.; Asst. Pathol. Bland-Sutton Inst. Middlx. Hosp. Med. Sch. Lond.; Capt. RAMC.

STARR, Dolores Ramona (retired) 71 Queens Reach, Hampton Court, East Molesey KT8 9DE — (Sheff.) MB ChB Sheff. 1962. JP. Prev: Ho. Surg. & Ho. Phys. City Gen. Hosp. Sheff.

STARR, Mr Donald Gordon Oral and Facial Surgery, Hull Royal Infirmary, Hull HU3 2JZ Tel: 01482 675774 Fax: 01482 675064 Email: don.starr@hey.nhs.uk — MB ChB Glas. 1988; BDS Manch. 1979; FDS RCS Eng. 1983; FRCS Ed. 1993; FRCS (Max-Fac.) 1996. Cons. (Oral & Maxillofacial Surg.)Hull & E.Yorks. Hosps. Specialty: Oral & Maxillofacial Surg. Socs: Fell. Brit. Assn. Oral & Maxillofacial Surg.; Eur. Assn. Cranio-Maxillo. Surg.; Chair Yorks. Regional Comm. Hosp. Dent. Servs. Prev: Sen. Regist. (Maxillofacial Surg.) Leeds Dent. Inst. & Gen. Infirm. Leeds; Sen. Regist. Rotat. (Maxillofacial Surg.) North. Region; Regist. (Maxillofacial Surg.) Middlesbrough Gen. Hosp. & Newc. Gen. Hosp.

STARR, Harry (retired) — MB ChB Sheff. 1962; DObst RCOG 1964. Prev: GP Hornchurch Essex.

STARR, John Michael Royal Victoria Hospital, Craigleith Road, Edinburgh EH4 2DN Tel: 0131 537 5023 Fax: 0131 537 5140 Email: john.starr@ed.ac.uk — MB BS Lond. 1984 (Kings Coll. Lond.) FRCP Edin. Cons. Phys. (Gen. & Geriat. Med.); Reader (Geriat. Med.) Edin. Univ.; Cons. Phys. Lothian Memory Treatm. Centre; Health Foundat. Research Fell. Special Interest: Dementia & Learning Disabil. Prev: Sen. Regist. Hammersmith Hosp. Lond.; Research Fell. Edin. Univ.

STARR, Kathryn Janet Royal Cornhill Hospital, Cornhill Road, Aberdeen AB25 2ZH Tel: 01224 557268; 29 Broadhaven Road, Old Portlethen Village, Aberdeen AB12 4NR Tel: 01224 780556 — MB ChB Aberd. 1972; DObst RCOG 1974; DA 1978; MRCGP 1980; MRCPsych 1983. Locum Cons. Specialty: Child & Adolesc. Psychiat. Prev: Sen. Regist. (Psychiat.) Roy. Cornhill Hosp. Aberd.

STARR, Lesley Margaret Porch Surgery, Beechfield Road, Corsham SN13 9DL Tel: 01249 712232 Fax: 01249 701389 — BM BCh Oxf. 1979 (Cambridge & Oxford) MA 1978; DRCOG 1982; MRCGP 1983. Prev: Asst. GP Corsham & St. Jas. Surg. Bath; Trainee GP Bristol VTS.; Clin. Asst. (Endoscopy) Roy. United Hosp. Bath.

STARR, Matthew Jonathan 63 Harley Street, London W1N 1DD — MB BChir Camb. 1993; MA Camb. 1993.

STARR, Perry Louise 612 Stannington Road, Stannington, Sheffield S6 6AE Email: perry.starr@ukonline.co.uk — MB BS Lond. 1994 (Univ. Coll. & Middlx. Sch. Med.) BSc (Hons.) Lond. 1991. Clin. Research Fell., Centre for Reproductive Med. Walsgrave Hosp. Coventry. Specialty: Obst. & Gyn. Prev: Specialist Regist. (O & G) Solihull Hosp.; SHO (O & G) St. James Hosp. Leeds; SHO (O & G) John Radcliffe Hosp. Oxf.

STARR, Rebecca Louise 17 Grand Avenue, Camberley GU15 3QJ Tel: 01276 61981 — MB ChB Leic. 1989. SHO (O & G) Geo. Eliot Hosp. Nuneaton. Specialty: Obst. & Gyn.

STARRITT, David Raynor The Surgery, Ailsa Muir, The Market Stance, Tarland, Aboyne AB34 4UB Tel: 01339 881281 Fax: 01339 881077; Bonnington, Melgum Road, Tarland, Aboyne AB34 4ZL Tel: 0133 98 81489 — MB BS Lond. 1980; BSc (Hons.) Lond. 1976; DRCOG 1982; MRCGP 2002.

STARRITT, Nicola Elizabeth Flat 1F1, 51 Marchmont Road, Edinburgh EH9 1HT — MB ChB Ed. 1996.

START, Neil John Sett Valley Medical Centre, Hyde Bank Road, New Mills, Stockport SK22 4BP Tel: 01663 743483; 133 Buxton Old Road, Higher Disley, Stockport SK12 2BX Tel: 01663 762889 Email: njstart@gpiag-asthma.org — MB ChB Liverp. 1985; DRCOG 1987; DGM RCP Lond. 1987; MRCGP 1989; AFOM RCP Lond. 1994. GP Princip.; HSE Lead Apptd. Doctor. Specialty: Occupat. Health. Socs: Soc. of Occupat. Med. Prev: Trainee GP Walton & Fazakerley Hosps. Liverp. VTS.

START, Roger David Department of Histopathology, Chesterfield & North Derbyshire Royal Hospital, Calow, Chesterfield S44 5BL Tel: 01246 277271 Ext. 2277 — MB ChB Sheff. 1988; BMedSci Sheff. 1987; MRCPath 1995, D 1992; MD Sheff. 1996. Cons. Histopath. Chesterfield & N. Derbysh. Roy. Hosp. NHS Trust. Specialty: Histopath. Prev: Lect. (Path.) Sheff. Univ. Med. Sch.; Regist. Rotat. (Histopath.) Sheff.; SHO (Histopath.) North. Gen. Hosp. Sheff.

START, Susan Ann 6 Silver Birch Avenue, Sheffield S10 3TA — MB ChB Sheff. 1988; MRCGP.

STASTNY, Dusan (retired) Community Drug Service, Paget House, 2 West St., Leicester LE1 6XP Tel: 0116 247 0200 — MUDr Charles Univ. Prague 1967; MRCPsych 1972. Cons. Psychiat. Leicester HA. Prev: Sen. Regist. (Psychiat.) St. Thos. Hosp. Lond.

STATEN, Paul The Red House Surgery, 241 Queensway, Bletchley, Milton Keynes MK2 2EH Tel: 01908 375111 — MB BS Lond. 1979; MA Camb. 1976; MRCGP 1984; DRCOG 1984.

STATHAM, Alison Mary Latham House Surgery, Latham House Surgery, 31 Lord Street, Ormskirk L40 4BZ; 25 Emmanuel Road, Churchtown, Southport PR9 9RP Tel: 01704 231814 — MB ChB Liverp. 1987; DCH RCP Lond. 1989; DGM RCP Lond. 1990; DRCOG 1991; DFFP 1992; MRCGP 1993. Clin. Asst. - G.U. Med. Prev: Trainee GP S.port.

STATHAM, Barry Nigel Singleton Hospital, Skelly Lane, Swansea SA2 8QA Tel: 01792 285038 Email: barry.statham@swansea-tr.wales.nhs.uk — MB BCh Wales 1975; MRCP (UK) 1977; FRCP Lond 1997. Cons. Dermat. Specialty: Dermat. Special Interest: Contact Dermatitis; Latex Allergy. Prev: Sen. Regist. (Dermat.) Leeds Gen. Infirm.; Regist. (Dermat.) Univ. Hosp. Wales Cardiff; Rotating Regist. (Med.) Univ. Hosp. Wales.

STATHAM, Helen Claire 10 The Pantiles, Bickley, Bromley BR1 2BX — MB BS Lond. 1990; BSc Lond. 1987. SHO (Anaesth.) Bromley Hosp.

STATHAM, John Anthony 6 Hurstwood, Waverton, Chester CH3 7QJ Tel: 01244 336498 Email: JASTAT@aol.com — MB BS Newc. 1975. Specialty: Disabil. Med.; Gen. Pract.

STATHAM, Neil Anthony Beechwood Surgery, 371 Chepstow Road, Newport NP19 8HL Tel: 01633 277771 Fax: 01633 290631 — MB BCh Wales 1981; MRCGP 1985; DRCOG 1985. Prev: Trainee GP Newport VTS.; Ho. Off. (Med.) Neath Gen. Hosp.; Ho. Off. (Surg.) Llandough Hosp. Cardiff.

STATHAM, Mr Patrick Francis Xavier Western General Hospital, Crewe Road, Edinburgh EH4 2XU Tel: 0131 5372101/6 Fax: 0131 537 1133 Email: patrick.statham@ed.ac.uk; 76 Belgrave Road, Edinburgh EH12 6NQ Tel: 0131 476 9209 Email: pfxstatham@netscape.net — MB BS Lond. 1980 (St Bartholomews London) FRCS Ed. 1985; FRCS Eng. 1986; FRCS Surg. Neurol. 1991. Cons. Neurosurg. (Clin. Neurosci.) W. Gen. Hosp. Edin.; Sen. Lect. Dept. Clin. Neurosci.s Univ. of Edin. Specialty: Neurosurg. Socs: Soc. Brit. Neurosurg. (Counc. Mem.); Cervical Spine Soc.; Europ. Skull Base Soc. Prev: Sen. Regist. (Neurosurg.) Dept. Clin. Neurosci. West. Gen. Hosp. Edin.; Regist. (Neurosurg.) Inst. Neurol. Sci. Glas.

STATHAM, Rita (retired) 11 Platt Court, Deganwy Road, Conwy LL31 9DG — (Manch.) MB ChB Manch. 1956; MRCOG 1963; MFFP 1993. Prev: SCMO & Instruc. Doctor (Family Plann.) Nottm. HA.

STATHAM, Roy 24 Victoria Crescent, Nottingham NG5 4DA Tel: 01159 607338 — MB ChB Manch. 1958. Emerit. Cons. Genitourin. Med. Trent RHA. Specialty: Genitourinary Medicine. Socs: Fell. Manch. Med. Soc.; (Ex-Chairm.) Reg. Adv. Sub-Comm. Genitourin. Med. Prev: Med. Off. Trent Regional Blood Trans. Serv.m.; Cons. Genitourin. Trent RHA; Med. Asst. (Venereol.) Sheff. RHB.

STATHER-DUNN, Brenda Lois Seaview, Wisemans Bridge, Saundersfoot SA69 9AU Tel: 01834 812918 — (Oxf. & St. Bart.) BM BCh Oxf. 1953; DLO Eng. 1958. Specialty: Gen. Psychiat. Prev: Assoc. Specialist (Psychiat.) St. David's Hosp. Carmarthen.

STATTER, Neil Richard The Park Surgery, 4 Alexandra Road, Great Yarmouth NR30 2HW Tel: 01493 855672 — MB ChB Sheff. 1973; DObst RCOG 1976; FRCGP 1997, MRCGP 1977. Course Organiser Gt. Yarmouth VTS. Prev: Ho. Phys. Roy. Hosp. Sheff.; Ho. Surg. Roy. Infirm. Sheff.; Trainee Gen. Pract. Doncaster Vocational Train. Scheme.

STAUFENBERG, Ekkehart F A Broadland Clinic Forensic Services - East Anglia & Norwich Epilepsy Clinic, C/o Mrs Julie Allen, Hospital Road, Little Plumstead, Norwich NR13 5EW Tel: 01603 711258 — MD; MRCPsych; MSc. Cons. (Foresic Neuropsychiatry) Norwich; Cons. (Epileptology & Neuropsychiatry) Norwich; Sen. Lect. Sch. of Med. Univ. of E. Anglia. Specialty: Forens. Psychiat.

STAUGHTON, Richard Charles David Chelsea and Westminster Hospital, Fulham Road, London SW10 9NH Tel: 020 8746 8170 Fax: 020 8746 8578; Lister Hospital, Chelsea Bridge Road, London SW1W 8RH Tel: 020 7730 8308 Fax: 020 7823 5541 Email: rstaughton@lineone.net — (Camb. & St. Bart.) MB BChir Camb. 1970; BA Camb. 1967, MA 1970; MRCP (UK) 1973; FRCP Lond. 1986. Cons. Dermat. Chelsea & Westm. Hosp. Lond.; Hon. Cons. Dermat. Roy. Hosp. Chelsea, Brompton Hosp. Lond. & King Edwd. VII Hosp. Lond. Specialty: Dermat. Socs: (Ex-Pres.) St. Johns Dermat.

Soc.; (Ex-Pres.) Derm. Sec. RSM Roy. Soc. Med.; (Ex-Pres.) Dowling Club. Prev: Cons. Dermat. Addenbrooke's Hosp. Camb.; Regist. Skin Dept. St. Thos. Hosp. Lond.; Ho. Phys. St. Bart. Hosp. Lond.

STAUNTON, Avril Felicity Classical Homeopath and Complementary Medicine, British Embassy, USMR 5, BFPO 2; 4115 N. Ridgeview Road, McLean VA 22101, USA Email: dravrilus@aol.com — MRCS Eng. LRCP Lond. 1978 (Liverpool) MB ChB (Hons.) Liverp. 1978; MD Munich 1984. Accreditation procedures for cl.ical Homeopath and Complementary Med., Virginia, USA. Specialty: Obst. & Gyn.; Homeop. Med.; Med. Publishing. Prev: Capt. RAMC GMO Hameln, Acting SMO Detmold; Sen. Regist. Equivalent Obst. and Gyn., Univ. of Munich, Grosshadern; Lect. in Obst. and Gyn., Univ. of Munich, II Frauenklinik, Grosshadern, Univ. of Munich.

STAUNTON, Carmel Rose (retired) 204 Kennington Lane, London SE11 5DN Tel: 020 7735 1770 — MB BCh BAO NUI 1952 (Univ. Coll. Dub.) Prev: GP Lond.

STAUNTON, Donal The Kidgate Surgery, 32 Queen Street, Louth LN11 9AU Tel: 01507 602421 Fax: 01507 601700 Email: staunton-oegpc83006.nhs.uk; 54 Westgate, Louth LN11 9YD Tel: 01507 602421 Fax: 01507 601700 — MB BS Lond. 1980; DRCOG 1982; MA (Physiol. Sci.) Oxf. 1983. Prev: SHO (Paediat.) W. Chesh. Hosp.; SHO (O & G) Norf. & Norwich Hosp.; Ho. Surg. Amersham Gen. Hosp.

STAUNTON, Eamon Bernard Fordingbridge Surgery, Bartons Road, Fordingbridge SP6 1RS Tel: 01425 652123 Fax: 01425 654393 — MB BS Lond. 1979; MRCGP 1986; DCH RCP Lond. 1986.

STAUNTON, Michael Anthony, Col. late RAMC British Liason Officer, Office of the Surgeon General, 5109 Leesburg Pike, Suite 684, Falls Church VA 22041 325, USA Tel: 001 703 681 3161 Fax: 001 703 681 3163 Email: michael.staunton@otsg.amedd.army.mil; 14 Priory Court, Bridgwater TA6 3NR Tel: 001 703 533 1784 Email: stauntonma@aol.com — MB BS Lond. 1979 (St. Bart.) MRCS Eng. LRCP Lond. 1978; MRCGP 1986; MSc (Community Med.) Lond. 1989. Brit. Liason Off. (Med.), Office of the Surg. Gen., 5109 Leesburg Pike, Falls Ch., VA,USA; ATLS Provider 1995; Dep. Preceptor Family Phys. Program for Residents Dewitt Army Hosp. VA USA. Specialty: Gen. Pract.; Pub. Health Med. Socs: Fell. Roy. Soc. Med.; Fell. Roy. Geogr. Soc.; BMA. Prev: Col. Army Med. Servs. Manning & Career Managem. Div.; United Nations Sen. Med. Off. HQ SSW Bosnia Hercogovina Command; Hon. Lect. (Gen. Pract.) Med. Coll. St. Bart. Hosp. Lond.

STAUNTON, Mr Michael Douglas Mary (retired) 25 Regent's Park Road, London NW1 7TL Tel: 020 7267 6171 — (T.C. Dub.) MB BCh BAO Dub. 1949; FRCS Ed. 1957; FRCS Eng. 1957; MA, BA Dub. 1948, LLD 1993, MCh 1962. Mem. Med. Appeal Tribunal. Prev: Cons. Surg. St. Bart. & Homerton Hosps. Lond.

STAUNTON, Neville John Crouch Oak Family Practice, Station Road, Addlestone, Weybridge KT13 2BH Tel: 01932 840123; The Beeches, Guildford Road, Effingham, Leatherhead KT24 5QL Tel: 01372 459236 — MB Camb. 1979 (St.Geo.) BChir 1978. Prev: Asst. Diabetes St. Peter's Hosp. Ottershaw.

STAUNTON, Ruth Mary (retired) 29 Porson Road, Cambridge CB2 2ET — MB ChB Liverp. 1960; DPH 1964 Liverp; DPM Eng. 1973; MA Camb. 1977.

STAUNTON, Thomas Henry Francis Aldersbrook House, 88 Aldersbrook Road, Manor Park, London E12 5DH — MB BS Lond. 1957; MRCS Eng. LRCP Lond. 1957.

STAVELEY, Catharine Diana Tawstock Medical Centre, 7 High Street, Chard TA20 1QF Tel: 01460 67763 Fax: 01460 66044; Knapp House, Waterlake Road, Tatworth, Chard TA20 2SZ Tel: 01460 220460 — MB BS Lond. 1986 (Roy. Free) Specialty: Gen. Pract.

STAVERT-DOBSON, Adrian John 68 Lound Side, Chapeltown, Sheffield S35 2UR — MB ChB Leic. 1997.

STAVRI, Mr George Theodore Dept. Cardiothoracic Surgery, Hammersmith Hospital, Du Cane Road, London W12 0HS; 34, Linton House, 11, Holland Park Avenue, London W11 3RL — MB BS Lond. 1986; FRCS Eng. 1991; MS Lond. 1996. Specialist Regist., Cardiothoracic Surg., Hammersmith Hosp., Lond. Specialty: Cardiothoracic Surg. Prev: Regist. (Rotat.) (Gen. Surg.) Univ. Wales Coll. Med.; Vasc. Research Fell., King's Coll. Hosp.

STAVRON, Karim John 21 Blenkarne Road, London SW11 6HZ — MB ChB Liverp. 1993.

STAVROU, Margaret (retired) 31 Merton Hall Road, London SW19 3PR Tel: 020 8540 7082 — MB BS Lond. 1965 (Roy. Free) MRCS Eng. LRCP Lond. 1963; FRCPath 1984, M 1972. Prev: Cons. (Histopath.) Qu. Mary's Hosp. Roehampton. 1978-96.

STAWARZ, Marek Jerzy Cedars Surgery, 8 Cookham Road, Maidenhead SL6 8AJ Tel: 01628 620458 Fax: 01628 633270 — MB BS Lond. 1987. Trainee GP/SHO Ealing Hosp. VTS. Prev: Regist. (Child Psychiat.) Northwick Pk. Hosp. Harrow.

STAYTE, Wendy Mary Erme House, Mr Gould Hospital, Plymouth PL4 7QD Tel: 01752 272317 Fax: 01752 272361; Port Meadow, 2 Seymour Villas, Totnes TQ9 5QR Tel: 01803 868305 Email: wendysayte@mailcity.com — MB Camb. 1966; BA Camb. 1962, MB 1966, BChir 1965; DCH Eng. 1967; DPM Eng. 1969; MRCPsych 1972. Cons. Child. Psychiat. Plymouth Hosps. Trust. Specialty: Child & Adolesc. Psychiat. Socs: ACPP Scientif. & Med. Network; Roy. Soc. Med. Prev: Cons. Child Psychiat. Parkside Clinic Lond.; Sen. Regist. (Child Psychiat.) Tavistock Clinic Lond.

STAZIKER, Ann Christine 50 Menzieshill Road, Dundee DD2 1PU Tel: 01382 642612 — MB ChB St. And. 1968; FFA RCS Eng. 1973. Cons. Anaesth. Ninewells Hosp. Dundee. Specialty: Anaesth.

STEAD, Alan Lawrence (retired) Bryn Awel, Holyhead LL65 2TF Tel: 01407 2073 — MB ChB St. And. 1948; MD St. And. 1954, MB ChB 1948; DA Eng. 1952; FFA RCS Eng. 1954. Prev: Cons. Anaesth. United Liverp. Hosps. & Liverp. Regional Hosp. Bd.

STEAD, Barbara Elizabeth 5 Springfield Close, Burton on the Wolds, Loughborough LE12 5AN — MRCS Eng. LRCP Lond. 1957 (Leeds) DLO Eng. 1960; FRCS Eng. 1971. Associate Specialist, Leceister Royal Infirmary. Specialty: Otorhinolaryngol. Prev: Supernum. Sen. Regist. (ENT) Nottm. Gen. Hosp.; Regist. Metrop. ENT Hosp. Lond.; Otol. Jt. MRC/NPL Working Gp. on Indust. Noise & Hearing.

STEAD, Brian Roy, TD (retired) 3 Hamilton Road, Newmarket CB8 0NQ Tel: 01638 662454 — MB ChB Ed. 1956; DA Eng. 1958; FFA RCS Eng. 1963. Prev: Cons. Anaesth. Gen. Hosp. Newmarket, W. Suff. Hosp. Bury St. Edmunds &Addenbrooke's Hosp. Camb.

STEAD, Catherine Anne 35 Rugby Road, Brighton BN1 6EB — MB ChB Sheff. 1986.

STEAD, Charlotte Helen Tennyson House Surgery, 20 Merlin Place, Chelmsford CM1 4HW Tel: 01245 260459 Fax: 01245 344287 — MB BS Lond. 1990.

STEAD, Graham William 8 Oakleigh View, West Lane, Baildon, Shipley BD17 5TP — MB ChB Dundee 1975.

STEAD, Harry West Grove, Bramley, Leeds LS13 1HD — MB ChB Leeds 1942. Prev: RAMC; Med. Regist. Halifax Roy. Infirm.

STEAD, Jonathan William Wyndham House Surgery, Fore Street, Silverton, Exeter EX5 4HZ Tel: 01392 860034 Fax: 01392 861165; 17 Cranford Avenue, Exmouth EX8 2HT Tel: 01395 225654 — MB BS Lond. 1974; MPhil Lond. 1993, MB BS 1974; DRCOG 1978; MRCGP 1979.

STEAD, Matthew Sumner Carnewater Practice, Dennison Road, Bodmin PL31 2LB Tel: 01208 72321 Fax: 01208 78478; Kingberry, 38 Rhind St, Bodmin PL31 2EL — BM BCh Oxf. 1981; MA Oxf. 1987, BM BCh 1981; MRCGP 1986; Dip. IMC RCS Ed. 1991.

STEAD, Robert John Macclesfield District General Hospital, Victoria Road, Macclesfield SK10 3BL Tel: 01625 661350 Fax: 01625 663150 — MB ChB Birm. 1977; MRCP (UK) 1980; FRCP Lond. 1994. Cons. Phys. Macclesfield Dist. Gen. Hosp. Specialty: Gen. Med.; Respirat. Med. Socs: Brit. Thorac. Soc.; NW Thoracic Soc. Prev: Postgrad. Clin. Tutor; Sen. Regist. (Gen. & Respirat. Med.) Yorks. RHA; Regist. (Gen. Med. Endocrinol.) Soton. Gen. Hosp.

STEAD, Tanya Louisa 10 Whyteleafe Road, Caterham CR3 5EE — MB ChB Bristol 1998.

STEADMAN, Alison Fay 26 Vitre Gardens, Lymington SO41 3NA — MB ChB Leic. 1992.

STEADMAN, Karen Elaine 8 Crispin Close, Locks Heath, Southampton SO31 6TD — MB ChB Leic. 1989; DCH RCP Lond. 1993; DRCOG 1993; MRCGP 1994. Sen. Regist. (Palliat. Med.) Countess Mt.batten Hse. Soton. Specialty: Palliat. Med. Prev: Trainee GP Kettering VTS.

STEADMAN, Philip William Melvyn St Nicholas Centre, 79b Tewson Road, London SE18 1BB — MB BS Lond. 1989; MSc

Managem. Sci. Lond. 1984, BSc (Hons.) 1974; MRCPsych 1994. Cons. Psychiat. Specialty: Gen. Psychiat. Socs: BMA; Roy. Soc. Med.

STEAN, Martin Leslie Priory Road Surgery, Priory Road, Park South, Swindon SN3 2EZ Tel: 01793 521154 Fax: 01793 512562; Wellview Cottage, Broad Hinton, Swindon SN4 9PA Tel: 01793 731071 — MB BS Lond. 1985 (King's Coll.) DCH RCP Lond. 1988; DRCOG 1988; Cert. Family Plann. JCC 1988; MRCGP 1996. Tutor (Gen. Pract.) Swindon; Lect. (Gen. Pract.) Bath Univ.

STEANE, Patricia Ann, OBE, Deputy Lt. (retired) White Lodge, 279 Gower Road, Sketty, Swansea SA2 7AA Tel: 01792 205396 — MB BS Lond. 1962 (Roy. Free) MRCS Eng. LRCP Lond. 1962; DA Eng. 1964; FFA RCS Eng. 1971. Chairm. Swansea & SW Wales Cancer Inst. Bd. Prev: Med. Dir. & Cons. Anaesth. Swansea NHS Trust.

STEARE, Alison Louise 15 Wellmans Meadow, Kingsclere, Newbury RG20 5HJ — MB BS Lond. 1984 (Char. Cross) DRCOG 1987; MRCGP 1989.

STEARE, Stephen Eric Bayer plc, Stoke Court, Stoke Poges, Slough SL2 4LY Tel: 01635 563052 — MB BS Lond. 1985; MRCP Eng. LRCP (UK) 1988; MD Lond. 1994; Dip Pharm Med 1999. Head Clin. Developm. Bayer plc Newbury. Specialty: Pharmaceutical Medicine. Prev: Clin. Lect. Univ. Coll. Lond.; Regist. (Clin. Cardiol.) Hammersmith Hosp. Lond.

STEARMAN, Andrew Steven Lee 322 Old Shoreham Road, Hove BN3 7HA — MB BS Lond. 1992.

STEARN, Alison Claire 19 Aubrey Road, London E17 4SL — BM Soton. 1995.

STEARN, Margaret Ruth 5 Leckford Place, Oxford OX2 6JB — BM BCh Oxf. 1972; MRCP (U.K.) 1976; FRCP 1998.

STEARNES, Graham Nigel Touchwood, Hill Farm Road, Taplow Village, Maidenhead SL6 0EY Tel: 01628 666173; 60 West Drayton Road, Hillingdon, Uxbridge UB8 3LA Tel: 020 8573 7674 — MB BS Lond. 1975. Specialty: Gen. Pract.

STEARNS, Elizabeth Jane Elford Coroner's Court, Queens Road, Walthamstow, London E17 8QP Tel: 020 8520 7247; Hill Farm, Watling St, Radlett WD7 7HP Tel: 01923 856354 — MRCS Eng. LRCP Lond. 1974 (Guy's) LDS RCS Eng. 1969; MB BS Lond. 1974, BDS (Hons.) 1970; Barrister 1997. HM Coroner for the Eastern Dist. of Greater Lond. Prev: Dep. Coroner Northern Dist. Greater Lond.

STEARNS, Mr Michael Patrick Suite 14, 30 Harley St., London W1G 9PN Tel: 020 7631 4448 Fax: 0207 637 7606; Hill Farm, Watling St, Radlett WD7 7HP Tel: 01923 856354 — MRCS Eng. LRCP Lond. 1974 (Guy's) MB BS Lond. 1974, BDS (Hons.) 1970; FRCS Eng. 1978. Cons. ENT Surg. Roy. Free Hosp. & Barnet Hosp. Lond.; Roy. Nat. Ear, Nose and Throat Hosp., Lond. Specialty: Otolaryngol. Prev: Fellowship Facial Plast. Surg. Portland Oregon, USA.; Sec. Europ. Acad. of Facial Plastic Surg. 1989-94.

STEARS, Anna Jane 11 Cherry Close, Dinas Powys CF64 4RG — MB BS Lond. 1992.

STEBBING, Birgit Middlefield, Hinton Way, Great Shelford, Cambridge CB2 5AN — MB BS Lond. 1968.

STEBBING, Jane Elizabeth The Alresford Surgery, Station Road, Alresford SO24 9JL Tel: 01962 732345; 11 Fair View, Alresford SO24 9PR Tel: 01962 735384 — MB BS Lond. 1984 (Guy's) MA Camb. 1985, BA 1981; DRCOG 1988; DCH RCP Lond. 1989. Prev: Trainee GP/SHO Hants. Co. Hosp. Winchester VTS; SHO (Med.) Ipswich Hosp.; SHO (A & E) Lewisham Hosp. Lond.

STEBBING, Mr John French Royal Surrey County Hospital, Egerton Road, Guildford GU2 7XX Tel: 01483 571122 Ext: 4196 Fax: 01483 464195 Email: jstebbing@uk-consultants.co.uk — MB BS Lond. 1987 (U.M.D.S. (Guy's)) MA Camb. 1988; FRCS Eng. 1991; MS Lond. 1997; FRCS (Gen.) 1998. Cons. (Surg.) Roy. Surrey Co. Hosp. Guild. Specialty: Gen. Surg. Special Interest: Colonoscopy; Colorectal Disease; Inflammatory bowel Dis., including pouch Surg. Socs: Assn. of Coloproctology of Gt. Britain and Irel.; Assn. of Surgeons of Gt. Britain and Irel.; Roy. Soc. of Med. Prev: Sen. Regist. (Gen. Surg.) S. W. Region; MRC Clin. Research Fell. Univ. Oxf.; Regist. Rotat. (Surg.) SW Thames.

STEBBING, Miss Margaret Anne North Hampshire Hospital, Aldermaston Road, Basingstoke RG24 9NA Tel: 01256 313332 Ext: 4310 Fax: 01256 313512 Email: Anne.Stebbing@nhht.nhs.uk — MB BS Lond. 1981 (Guy's) MA Camb. 1982; FRCS Ed. 1986; FRCS Eng. 1986; MD Lond. 1993; T(S) 1993. Cons. Surg. N. Hants. Hosp. Basingstoke. Specialty: Gen. Surg. Socs: Hon Sec Surg. Sect. RSM; BASO; Fell. ASGBI. Prev: Sen. Regist. (Surg.) St. Geo. Hosp. Lond.; Regist. (Surg.) Frimley Pk. Hosp.; SHO (Surg.) Roy. Surrey Co. Hosp. Guildford.

STEBBINGS, Neville Eric The Nottingham Nuffield Hospital, Mansfield Road, Woodthorpe, Nottingham NG5 3FZ Tel: 0115 993 2015 Fax: 0115 967 3005; Munden House, 2 Fairlawn Place, Private Road, Sherwood, Nottingham NG5 4DD Tel: 0115 960 5638 Fax: 0115 960 5638 — (St. Bart.) MB BS Lond. 1950; MRCS Eng. LRCP Lond. 1950. Med. Dir. Center Parcs UK Ltd.; Company Doctor Carlton Television Studios E. Midl.; Theatre Doctor Roy. Centre Nottm. Specialty: Occupat. Health. Socs: Fell. Roy. Soc. Med. Prev: Clin. Asst. City Hosp. Nottm.; Capt. RAMC.

STEBBINGS, Simon Marcus Weston General Hospital, Department of Rheumatology, Grange Road, Uphill, Weston Super Mare NG5 4DD Tel: 01934 636363 — MB BS Lond. 1988; MRCP (UK) 1992; MMed Sc Otago 2001. Cons. (Rheum.) West. Gen. & Southmead Hosp. Bristol. Prev: Regist. (Rheum.) St. Thos. Hosp. Lond.; SHO (HIV & Genitourin. Med.) St. Stephen's & Westm. Hosp. Lond.

STEBBINGS, Mr William Stanley Lewis Norfolk & Norwich University Hospital NHS Trust, Colney Lane, Norwich NR4 7UY Tel: 01603 286423 Fax: 01603 286423 Email: denise.batchelor@nnuh.nhs.uk — MB BChir Camb. 1977 (Camb. & St. Bart.) FRCS Eng. 1981; MChir Camb. (Distinc.) 1988. Cons. Gen. Surg. (Coloproctol.) Norf. & Norwich Hosp.; Hon. Sen. Lect. Univ. E. Anglia; Progr. co-ordinator for Higher Surgic. Train., E. Anglia Region. Specialty: Gastroenterol. Special Interest: Coloproctology. Socs: Fell. Roy. Soc. Med. Prev: Resid. Surg. Off. St. Mark's Hosp. Lond.; Sen. Regist. (Gen. Surg.) St. Bart. Hosp. Lond.; Regist. (Surg.) N. Middlx. Hosp. Lond.

STECHMAN, Michael James 45 Oakwood Avenue, Purley CR8 1AR — MB ChB Birm. 1994.

STECKLER, Thomas Horst Wolfgang 53 Eland Edge, Ponteland, Newcastle upon Tyne NE20 9AY — State Exam Med Berlin 1990.

STEDDON, Simon John Ashdown, 48 Rayleigh Road, Hutton, Brentwood CM13 1AD — MB BS Lond. 1993.

STEDEFORD, Averil (retired) 71 Sandfield Road, Headington, Oxford OX3 7RW Tel: 01865 762383 — MB BS Lond. 1955 (Univ. Coll. Hosp.) DCH Eng. 1958; DObst RCOG 1958; DPM Eng. 1975; MRCPsych 1976. Prev: Cons. Psychol. Med. Sir Michael Sobell Hse. Oxf.

STEDEFORD, Judith Clare Flat 5, Chelholm, Lansdown Road, Cheltenham GL51 6PU — MB BS Lond. 1993 (St. Bart. Med. Coll. Lond.) MRCP (UK) 1996; FRCA 2001. Specialty: Anaesth.

STEDEFORD, Mr Roland David (retired) 23 High Street, Ascott-under-Wychwood, Chipping Norton OX7 6AW — BM BCh Oxf. 1956; MA 1956; PhD Lond. 1960; FRCS Eng. 1961. Prev: Cons. Surg. Havering Hosps. Trust.

STEDMAN, Alan Ernest Weybridge Health Centre, 22 Church Street, Weybridge KT13 8DW Tel: 01932 853366 Fax: 01932 844902 — MB BS Lond. 1967 (St. Geo.) MRCS Eng. LRCP Lond. 1967; DObst RCOG 1970; MRCGP 1984. Prev: Ho. Off. Gen. Med. St. Chas. Hosp. Lond.; Res. Obst. Asst. & Ho Surg. St. Geo. Hosp. Lond.

STEDMAN, Alan Jeffrey 60 Victoria Road, Clacton-on-Sea CO15 6BJ — BM Soton. 1994.

STEDMAN, Brian 82 Canon Street, Winchester SO23 9JQ — MB BS Lond. 1994.

STEDMAN, Caroline Jane Sophia 82 Canon Street, Winchester SO23 9JQ — MB BS Lond. 1994; BSc (Hons.) Lond. 1993. SHO (Med.) Northwick Pk. Hosp. Lond. Specialty: Gen. Med. Prev: Ho. Phys. (Med.) Roy. Free Hosp. Sch. Med.; Ho. Surg. N. Staffs. Roy. Infirm.

STEDMAN, Hamish Gordon Blair Manchester Road Surgery, 63 Manchester Road, Swinton, Manchester M27 5FX Tel: 0161 794 4343 Fax: 0161 736 0669 — MB ChB Manch. 1978; BSc St. And. 1975. Clin. Asst. (O & G) Salford HA; Med. Off. St. Ann's Hospice.

STEDMAN, Juliet Kate The Park Medical Centre, 691 Coventry Road, Small Heath, Birmingham B10 0JL; 36 Clarence Road, Harbone, Birmingham B17 9LG Tel: 01214 261018 — MB ChB Birm. 1993 (Birmingham) DCH 1996. GP Retainer The Pk. Med. Centre, Small Heath. Specialty: Gen. Pract. Socs: Med. Protec. Soc.; BMA; MSS. Prev: GP/Regist. Worcs VTS; SHO Worcester Roy. Infirm.

VTS; Ho. Off. (Gen. Med.) Alexandra Hosp. Redditch & Qu. Eliz. Hosp. Birm.

STEDMAN, Sarah Anne Whitelands, Hyde Road, Long Sutton, Hook RG29 1SP — MB BS Lond. 1978 (Lond. Hosp.) DCH RCP Lond. 1982; DRCOG 1983. Gen. Practitioner Crondall Surrey.

STEDMAN, Stephen Roger 36 Clerence Road, Birmingham B17 9LG — MB ChB Birm. 1993 (Birmingham) FRCA; ChB Birm. 1993. Specialist Regist. (Anaest) Birm Univ Hosp. Specialty: Anaesth.

STEDMAN, Susan Lynda Layer Road Surgery, Layer Road, Colchester CO2 9LA Tel: 01206 546494 Fax: 01206 369912 — MB ChB Sheff. 1974.

STEDMAN, Vanessa Ruth — MB BS Lond. 1991; MRCP (UK) 1995. GP. Specialty: Gen. Pract. Socs: Med. Defence Union. Prev: Regist. (ITU & Med.) Sydney, Austral.

STEDMAN, Yvonne Florence Dingle Barn, Dingle Road, Leigh, Worcester WR6 5JX Tel: 01886 833039 — MB BS Newc. 1975 (Newcastle upon Tyne) DRCOG 1978; MRCGP 1979; DGM RCP Lond. 1992; MFFP 1993. Cons. Family Plann. & Reproduc. Health Care S. Worcs. Community NHS Trust; Hon. Sen. Clin. Lect. (Obst. & Gyn.) Univ. Birm. Specialty: Family Plann. & Reproduc. Health; Genitourinary Medicine. Socs: Chairm. W. Midl. Assn. Family Plann. Doctors. Prev: SCMO Mancunian Community Health Care.

STEED, Andrew John Pathology Laboratory, Calderdale Royal Hospital, Salterhebble, Halifax HX3 0PW Tel: 01422 57171 — MB ChB Manch. 1973; FRCP (1997); FRCPath (1997); BSc (Hons.) Manch. 1969, MSc 1971. Cons. Haemat. Calderdale HA. Specialty: Haematology.

STEED, Andrew John 27 Thornleigh, Newry Road, Armagh BT60 1HT — MB ChB Manch. 1986; BSc (Med. Sci.) St. And. 1983. Med. Off. (Occupat. Health Serv.) Belf.; Clin. Asst. (Cas.) Armagh Community Hosp. Specialty: Occupat. Health. Socs: Soc. Occupat. Med. Prev: Partner Boness Rd. Pract. Grangemouth; Trainee GP Alness; SHO (Psychiat.) St. Lukes Hosp. Armagh.

STEED, Elizabeth Ann Pontcae Surgery, Georgetown, Merthyr Tydfil CF48 1YE; 55 Chester Close, Heolgerrig, Merthyr Tydfil CF48 1SW — MB ChB Liverp. 1983; DRCOG 1985; MRCGP 1987. Prev: Trainee GP Merthyr Tydfil VTS; Ho. Off. (Surg. & Med.) Mid Glam. HA.

STEED, Joan Margaret Dr Martys and Partners, Darley Dale Medical Centre, Two Dales, Matlock DE4 2SA Tel: 01629 733205; Falkland House, 10 New Road, Youlgreave, Bakewell DE45 1WP Tel: 01629 636195 — MB BS Lond. 1978 (Kings Coll. Hosp. Med. Sch. Lond.) DRCOG 1982. Retainer GP. Prev: Retainer GP Drs Dave and Craven, Allen St., Cheadle, Staffs.; Partner at Dr Middleton & Partners Storer Rd Surg. LoughBoro. Leics.

STEEDEN, Andrew Louis Honicknowle Green Medical Centre, Honicknowle Green, Plymouth PL5 3PY Tel: 01752 704364 Fax: 01752 789130; 6 Park Road, Lower Compton, Plymouth PL3 5DR — MB ChB Glas. 1987.

STEEDMAN, Gail Great Barr Group Practice, 912 Walsall Road, Great Barr, Birmingham B42 1TG Tel: 0121 357 1250 Fax: 0121 358 4857 — MB BS Lond. 1974; DCH Eng. 1977; DTM & H Eng. 1978; MRCP (UK) 1979; DRCOG 1987.

STEEDS, Charlotte Emma 21 Canynge Square, Clifton, Bristol BS8 3LA — MB BS Lond. 1996.

STEEDS, John Harold, MBE (retired) Orchard End, Whitehouse Lane, West Bergholt, Colchester CO6 3ET — MRCS Eng. LRCP Lond. 1942 (Univ. Camb. & Middlx.) MB BChir Camb. 1946; MA Camb. 1946; DCH Eng. 1946; FRCGP 1981. Med. Off. Univ. Essex. Prev: Regist. (Paediat.) & Ho. Surg. (Midw. & Gyn.) & Regist. Middlx. Hosp.

STEEDS, Richard Paul 93 Peveril Road, Endcliffe, Sheffield S11 7AQ Tel: 0114 266 4619 — MB BS Lond. 1991; MA Camb. Univ. 1984, BA (Hons.) 1985; MRCP (UK) 1994. Research Regist. (Cardiol.) Roy. Hallamsh. Hosp. Sheff. Specialty: Cardiol.

STEEL, Andrew 189 Arundel Drive, Poulton-Le-Fylde, Blackpool — MB BS Newc. 1981; MRCP (UK) 1984; FRCP Lond 1997. Cons. Integrated Med. Kettering Gen Hosp NHS Trust. Specialty: Gen. Med.; Gastroenterol.; Care of the Elderly. Prev: Sen. Regist. (Geriat. & Gen. Med.) W. Midl. Regional Train. Scheme; Oesoph. Cancer Research Appeal Fell.; Regist. (Gen. Med.) Good Hope Gen. Hosp. Sutton Coldfield.

STEEL, Andrew Christopher 49C Dartmouth Park Road, Dartmouth Park, London NW5 1SU — MB BS Lond. 1996 (St. Bartholomew's Hospital Medical College) BSc Lond. 1993; MRCP London 2001. Specialist Regist. Anaesth. & ICU Imperial Sch. of Anaesth. Lond. Specialty: Gen. Med. Prev: Ho. Phys. St. Bart. Hosp.; Ho. Surg. Bristol Roy. Infirm.; SHO Rotat. (Gen. Med.) Roy. Free Hosp. Hampstead Lond.

STEEL, Andrew Michael Drs GLASS, EL MEKKAWY and STEEL, Springwell Road, Sunderland SR3 4HG Tel: 0191 522 9908 Fax: 0191 528 8294 — MB BS Newc. 1985; MRCGP 1989. Prev: SHO (Paediat.) S. Shields Gen. Hosp.; SHO (Cas.) Ingham Infirm. S. Shields; SHO (Geriat. Med.) Shotley Bridge Gen. Hosp.

STEEL, Mr Anthony Edgar London Otological Centre, 66 New Cavendish St., London W1G 8TD Tel: 020 7637 5111 Email: otolone@btinternet.com; Studland Cottage, Belvedere Road, Burnham-on-Crouch CM0 8AJ Tel: 01621 784093 — MRCS Eng. LRCP Lond. 1949 (St. Mary's) FRCS Eng. 1961. Hon. Cons. ENT Surg. Southend Health Dist.; ENT Adviser (RCS) NE Thames RHA. Specialty: Otorhinolaryngol. Socs: Fell Roy. Soc. Med. (Mem. Sects. Otol. & Laryng.). Prev: Cons. ENT Surg. Southend Health Dist.; Regist. St. Mary's Hosp. Lond. & Hammersmith Hosp.; Lt.-Col. RAMC, TA.

STEEL, Anthony Macpherson (retired) West Street Surgery, 12 West St., Chipping Norton OX7 5AA Tel: 01608 642529 Fax: 01608 645066; 20 Pearce Drive, Chipping Norton OX7 5HY Tel: 01608 643122 — (Ed.) MB ChB Ed. 1963; FRCGP 1982, M 1969. Prev: Med. Off. Nat. Childr. Homes Chipping Norton.

STEEL, Professor Christopher Michael School of Biological & Medical Science, University of St Andrews, Bute Medical Building, St Andrews KY16 9TS Tel: 01334 463558 Fax: 01334 463482 Email: cms4@st-and.ac.uk; 3A The Scores, St Andrews KY16 9AR Tel: 01334 472877 — MB ChB (Hons.) Ed. 1965; FRCP Ed. 1990, M 1968; FRCPath 1992, M 1982; PhD Ed. 1972, BSc (Hons. Physiol.) 1962, DSc 1988; FRSE 1994; FRCS Ed. 1994; F Med Sci 1998. Emerit. Chair Univ. St And.; Hon. Cons. Phys. Lothian HB. Specialty: Genetics. Special Interest: Ethical issues in genetics; Molecular Oncol. Socs: Fell. Roy. Soc. Med.; BMA. Prev: Prof. Med. Sci. Univ. St And.; MRC Trav. Research Fell. (Path.) Kenyatta Nat. Hosp. Nairobi, Kenya; Research Fell. (Med.) West. Gen. Hosp. Edin.

STEEL, Claire Suzanne 1 The Orchard, Hepscott, Morpeth NE61 6HT — MB BS Newc. 1989 (Newcastle) DRCOG 1992; MRCGP 1993. Prev: GP Bristol.

STEEL, Mr David Henry William Sunderland Eye Infirmary, Queen Alexandra Road, Sunderland SR2 9HP Email: dhwsteel@hotmail.com — MB BS Newc. 1989 (Newcastle Upon Tyne) FRCOphth 1993. Cons. Ophthhalmologist, Sunderland eye Infirm. Specialty: Ophth.

STEEL, Dennis Eightlands Road, Dewsbury WF13 2PG Tel: 01924 465929 — MB BS Lond. 1961 (King's Coll. Hosp.) MRCS Eng. LRCP Lond. 1961. Prev: Ho. Surg. & Ho. Phys. Dulwich Hosp.; Ho. Surg. Obst. St. Lukes' Hosp. Bradford.

STEEL, Elizabeth Anne Cumberhead Farm, Lesmahagow, Lanark ML11 0HN — MB ChB Glas. 1994.

STEEL, Elizabeth Anne 21 Berkeley Precinct, Hunters Bar Ecclesall Rd, Sheffield S11 8PN — MB ChB Sheff. 1997.

STEEL, George Mark Ann Burrow Thomas Health Centre, South William Street, Workington CA14 2ED Tel: 01900 603985 Fax: 01900 871131 — MB BS Newc. 1987; MRCGP 1992. Specialty: Gen. Med.

STEEL, Graham 17 Warren Road, Orpington BR6 6JF — MB BCh Wales 1992.

STEEL, Graham Fulton 11- Corsebar Road, Paisley PA2 9PY — MB ChB Glas. 1996.

STEEL, Helen Clare North Oxford Medical Centre, 96 Woodstock Road, Oxford OX2 7NE Tel: 01865 311005 Fax: 01865 311257 — MB BS Lond. 1982 (Oxf. & Univ. Coll. Hosp.) MA Oxf. 1983; MRCGP 1986; DRCOG 1986.

STEEL, Helen Mary HIV Clinical Development, GlaxoSmithKline, Greenford Road, Greenford UB6 0HE Tel: 020 8966 3673 Fax: 020 8966 4529; 31 New Cross Road, London SE14 5DS — MB BS Lond. 1982 (St. Geo. Hosp.) MRCPath 1990; BSc Lond. 1979, MD 1994; FRCPath 1998. Sen. Clin. Research Phys. Glaxo Wellcome plc & Hon. Lect. (Virol.) St. Geo. Hosp. Med. Sch. Lond. Specialty: Pharmaceutical Medicine. Prev: Sen. Regist. (Virol.) St. Geo. Hosp. Lond. & Kingston Hosp. Surrey.

STEEL, James Roger Derriford Hospital, The Primrose Breast Care Centre, Level 7, Plymouth PL6 8DH Tel: 01752 517 563 Fax: 01752 517 562 Email: jim.steel@phnt.swest.nhs.uk — MB BS Lond. 1990 (Guy's Hosp.) BSc Lond. 1989; MRCP 1995; FRCR 1998. Cons. Breat Radiologist, NHS & Nuffied Hosp., Plymouth. Specialty: Radiol.

STEEL, Jonathan Andrew Paul The Street Surgery, 42 The Street, Uley, Dursley GL11 5SY; Cotswold House, Pitt Court, North Nitley, Dursley GL11 6EH — MB ChB Bristol 1985; MRCP (UK) 1988; T (GP) 1991. Prev: Trainee GP/SHO (Paediat.) Cheltenham HA VTS.

STEEL, Judith Margaret, MBE Department of Diabetes, Victoria Hospital, Kirkcaldy KY2 5AN Tel: 01592 643355 Fax: 01592 647090; 3A The Scores, St Andrews KY16 9AR Tel: 01334 472877 Fax: 01334 472877 Email: mandjsteel@aol.com — MB ChB (Hons.) Ed. 1965; FRCP Ed. 1981, M 1968; Cert. JCC Lond. 1976. Assoc. Specialist (Diabetes) Vict. Hosp. Kirkcaldy; Hon. Sen. Lec. Univ. St. Andrews. Specialty: Endocrinol. Socs: BMA; Brit. Diabetic Assn. Prev: Sen. Regist. & Regist. Diabetic Dept. Roy. Infirm. Edin.; SHO (Endocrin.) & Ho. Phys. West. Gen. Hosp. Edin.

STEEL, Kiki Carolyn Mary James Street Surgery, 2 James Street, Boston PE21 8RD Tel: 01205 362556 Fax: 01205 359050; 2 St Andrews, Grantham NG31 9AE Tel: 01476 590522 Fax: 01476 590522 — MB ChB Glas. 1989; DRCOG 1993. Co. Surg. of St John Ambul. Lincs.; Mem. of Lincs. Integrated Volun. Emerg. Serv.; Mem. of Brit. Assn. of Immediate Care. Prev: Trainee GP Grantham.

STEEL, Margaret Rachel (retired) — MB BS Lond. 1953 (Roy. Free) MRCS Eng. LRCP Lond. 1953; DPH Eng. 1965; T(OM) 1991. Prev: Med. Adviser Surrey CC.

STEEL, Mark Dominic Freeman Hospital, Department of Respiratory Medicine, High Heaton, Newcastle upon Tyne NE7 7DN Tel: 0191 2336161 Ext: 27364 Email: mdsteel@doctors.org.uk — MB BS Lond. 1993 (Char. Cross and Westm.) MA Oxf. 1996, BA 1990; MRCP (UK) 1996. Specialty: Respirat. Med.; Gen. Med. Socs: Brit. Thorac. Soc. Prev: Regist. (LAT in Respirat. & Gen. Med.) Mayday Hosp. Croydon; Clin. Res. Fell. (Respir. Med.) Soton. Gen. Hosp.; Regist. (LAT in Respirat. & Gen. Med.) Medway Hosp. Gillingham, Kent.

STEEL, Martin Robert 288 Queens Promenade, Blackpool FY2 9AZ Email: martinsteel@doctors.net.uk — MB BS Lond. 1982; BA Oxf. 1979; MRCGP 1986; MA Oxon 1987; MObstG Liverp. 1991; FRCOG 2002. Cons. O & G Blackpool Vict. Hosp. Specialty: Obst. & Gyn. Special Interest: Minimally Invasive Surg.; Polycystic Ovarian Syndrome. Socs: Brit. Soc. Gyn. Endoscopy. Prev: Sen. Regist. SE Thames Region; Regist. (O & G) St. Davids Hosp. Cardiff & Liverp. Matern. Hosp.; Trainee GP Cleveland VTS.

STEEL, Maxwell — MB BS Newc. 1983.

STEEL, Nicholas Trinity Street Surgery, 1 Trinity Street, Norwich NR2 2BG Tel: 01603 624844 Fax: 01603 766829; 189 Earlham Road, Norwich NR2 3RG — MB ChB Bristol 1988 (Univ. Bristol) DRCOG 1993; MRCGP 1993; T(GP) 1993. GP; Research Fell. Health Policy & Pract. Unit Univ. of Anglia Norwich. Specialty: Gen. Pract. Socs: BMA.

STEEL, Nigel Richard Department of Medicine for the Elderly, Hull Royal Infirmary, Anlaby Road, Hull HU3 2JZ Tel: 01482 674739 Fax: 01482 674026 Email: nigel.steel@hey.nhs.uk — BM BCh Oxf. 1977 (Oxford) MRCP (UK) 1979; FRCP Lond. 1995. Cons. Geriat. (Med. for Elderly) Hull Roy. Infirm., Hull. Specialty: Care of the Elderly. Special Interest: Diabetes. Socs: Brit. Geriat. Soc.; Diabetics UK. Prev: Sen. Regist. (Med. & Geriat.) Hull Roy. Infirm.; MRC Train. Fell. Endocrine Unit (Med.) Roy. Vict. Infirm. Newc.; Regist. (Med.) N. Tees Gen. Hosp. Stockton-on-Tees.

STEEL, Peter Cecil, MBE (retired) The Nook, Withyham Road, Groombridge, Tunbridge Wells TN3 9QP Tel: 01892 863326; Haddiscoe, Withyam Road, Groombridge, Tunbridge Wells TN3 9QS Tel: 01892 864496 — (Camb. & St. Bart.) MB BChir Camb. 1951; MA Camb. 1951. Prev: Ho. Surg. St. Bart. Hosp.

STEEL, Robby Michael OPD 5, St John's Hospital, Livingston Tel: 01506 419666; 12 Ross Gardens, Newington, Edinburgh EH9 3BS — MB ChB Glas. 1993; MA Camb. 1990; MRCPsych. 1997. Cons. in Gen. Adult and Liaison Psychaitry; Hon. Specialist Regist. Roy. Edin. Hosp. Specialty: Gen. Psychiat. Prev: SHO Rotat. (Psychiat.) South. Gen. Hosp. Glas.; Lect. in Psychiat., Univ. of Edin.

STEEL, Robin Easton, MBE (retired) St Johns House Surgery, 28 Bromyard Road, St. Johns, Worcester WR2 5BU Tel: 01905 423612 Fax: 01905 740003; 125 Laugherne Road, Worcester WR2 5LT Tel: 01905 422021 Fax: 01905 748563 — MB BS Lond. 1956 (Univ. Coll. Hosp.) MRCS Eng. LRCP Lond. 1956; DPM Eng 1959; DObst RCOG 1964; FRCGP 1973, M 1968; FRCPsych 1996, M 1994. Treas. W. Midl. LMC. Prev: Chairm. RCGP Ethics Comm. 1989-1992.

STEEL, Sarah Frances Mary Child Development Unit, 40 Upton Road, Norwich NR4 Tel: 01603 508937 Email: sarah.steel@doctors.org.uk — MB ChB Bristol 1988; BSc Bristol 1985; MRCP (UK) 1993; MSc UEA 2000. Cons. Paediat. Norwich Primary Care Trust Childrs. Sevices Norwich; Med. Adviser Adoption and Family Finding Unit. Specialty: Community Child Health. Prev: Sen. Regist. Norwich Community Health Partnership.

STEEL, Shirley Ann Peterborough Hospitals NHS Trust, Peterborough PE3 6DA Tel: 01733 874000; 15 Pingle Lane, Northborough, Peterborough PE6 9BW Tel: 01733 253114 Fax: 01733 252203 — MB BS Lond. 1980 (St Bartholomews Hospital Medical College) FRCOG 1998. Cons. O & G PeterBoro. Hosps. NHS Trust. Specialty: Obst. & Gyn.

STEEL, Stanley Joseph (retired) 23 Grove Road, Bournemouth BH1 3AS Tel: 01202 552785 — (St. Mary's) MB BS Lond. 1944; MRCS Eng. LRCP Lond. 1944; MD Lond. 1949; FRCP Lond. 1974, M 1950. Hon. Cons. Phys. Lond. Chest Hosp.; Hon. Sen. Lect. Nat. Heart & Lung Inst. Prev: Cons. Phys. Barking, Havering & Brentwood Dist. Hosps.

STEEL, Mr William Matthew (retired) Grove House, 11 King St., Newcastle ST5 1EH Tel: 01782 614174 Fax: 01782 714957; Broomrigg Jubilee Path, Kippford, Dalbeattie DG5 4LW Tel: 01556 620630 Fax: 01556 620348 — MB ChB Ed. 1957; FRCS Ed. 1962; FRCS Eng. 1992. Prev: Cons. Orthop. Surg. N. Staffs. Hosp. Centre Stoke-on-Trent.

STEELE, Adrian Paul Hawthorn 29 Mount Ephraim Lane, London SW16 1JE — MB BChir Camb. 1988; BA Camb. 1985, MB BChir 1988; MRCP (UK) 1991. SHO (Anaesth.) St. Bart. Hosp. Lond. Prev: Regist. (Med.) St. And. Hosp. Lond.; SHO (Med.) Roy. Lond. Hosp.; Lect. (Physiol.) Lond. Hosp. Med. Coll.

STEELE, Alison Mary Queen Elizabeth Hospital, Paediatric Department, Sheriff Hill, Gateshead NE9 6SX Tel: 0191 445 2813 — BM Soton. 1985; MRCP (UK) 1990. Cons. (Paediat.) Gateshead Health Trust. Specialty: Paediat.

STEELE, Angela Jane 31 High Street, Milton, Cambridge CB4 6DF Tel: 01223 362804 Mob: 07711 285165 — MB BS Lond. 1985 (St. Thos. Hosp.) DCH RCP Lond. 1987; T(GP) 1990; MRCGP 1997. GP (Palliat. Med.) N. Hants.; Hosp. Practitioner Palliat. Med. Socs: APM. Prev: Trainee GP, Ashford VTS.

STEELE, Ann Helen Cowdenbeath Medical Practice, 173 Stenhouse Street, Cowdenbeath KY4 9DH — MB ChB Ed. 1980; BSc (Med. Sci.) Ed. 1977; DRCOG 1983; MRCGP 1984; DCCH RCP Ed. 1985.

STEELE, Annette Christa Portobello Medical Centre, 14 Codrington Mews, London W11 2EH Tel: 020 7727 5800/2326 Fax: 020 7792 9044 — MB BS Lond. 1986 (St. Mary's Hosp.) BSc Lond. (1st cl. Hons.) 1983, MB BS 1986; Cert. Family Plann. JCC 1988; DRCOG 1988; Dip. Ther. 1997. GP; Tutor (Gen. Pract.) & Clin. Asst. (A & E) St. Mary's Hosp. Lond.; Hon. Med. Ref. Brit. Sub Aqua Club.

STEELE, Anthony Simon Vanpraagh (retired) 145 Bannings Vale, Saltdean, Brighton BN2 8RL Email: steeletonelen@onetel.net.uk — MB BS Lond. 1956 (Univ. Coll. Hosp.) PhD Camb. 1964; MRCGP 1971; DTM & H RCP Lond. 1976. Prev: Med. Off. Usutu Pulp Co. Swaziland.

STEELE, Mr Arthur David McGowan 22 Seymour Walk, London SW10 9NF Tel: 020 7351 3064 Fax: 020 7351 5429 — MB BS Melbourne 1960; DO Eng. 1970; FRCS Eng. 1971; FRACO 1979, M 1977; FRCOphth 1988 Hon 2000. Consg. Ophth. Moorfields Eye Hosp. Lond. Specialty: Ophth. Socs: Fell. Roy. Soc. Med. Prev: Cons. Ophth. Moorfields Eye Hosp. Lond.; Lect. Dept. Clin. Ophth. Moorfields Eye Hosp. & Inst. Ophth. Lond.; SHO Croydon Eye Unit.

STEELE, Caroline Anne 1 Broom Grove, Watford WD17 4RY — MB ChB Leeds 1979; FRCS Ed. 1984.

STEELE, Christopher 29 Parkmount Gardens, Larne BT40 1QN — MB BCh BAO Belf. 1993.

STEELE, Christopher Bodey Medical Centre, 363 Wilmslow Road, Fallowfield, Manchester M14 6XU Tel: 0161 248 6644 Fax: 0161 224 4228; 14 Belfield Road, Didsbury, Manchester M20 6BH Tel:

0161 445 3410 Fax: 0161 445 3423 — MB ChB Manch. 1968. Med. Dir. Stop Smoking Clinic Univ. Hosp. S. Manch.; Med. Presenter 'This Morning Progr.' ITV; Managing Dir. Smokequitters Manch. Socs: Manch. Med. Soc. & Brit. Med. & Dent. Hypn. Soc. Prev: Cons. Smoking Cessation for DERBY FHSA.

STEELE, Elizabeth Sandra Maybole Health Centre and Day Hospital, 6 High Street, Maybole KA19 7BY Tel: 01655 882278 Fax: 01655 889616; Silver Birches, Tarbolton Road, Dundonald, Kilmarnock KA2 9AR Tel: 01563 830902 — MB ChB Ed. 1973. GP Maybole CMO Family Plann. Ayrsh. & Arran HB. Specialty: Family Plann. & Reproduc. Health. Prev: GP Troon.

STEELE, Emma Kristine Royal Jubilee Maternity Service, Grosvenor Road, Belfast BT12 6BJ Tel: 02890 894633 — MB BCh BAO Belf. 1992 (Queen's University) MRCOG 1997; MD 2000. SPR (O & G) Roy. Jubilee Matern. Serv., Belf. Specialty: Obst. & Gyn. Socs: BMA; Roy. Coll. Obst. & Gyn.; Ulster Obst. & Gyn. Soc. Prev: SPR (O & G) Craigavon Area Hosp.; SPR, (O & G) Altnagelvin Hosp. - L'derry; SPR (O & G) Roy. Matern. Hosp. Belf.

STEELE, Gavin John 35C Ommaney Road, New Cross, London SE14 5NS Tel: 020 7358 1384 — MB BS Lond. 1997 (Guy's & St Thos.) GP VTS Lewisham Hosp. Specialty: Gen. Pract. Socs: BMA MPS. Prev: Ho. Surg. Guy's Hosp.; Ho. Phys. Sidcup Kent.

STEELE, George Alfred, TD (retired) 29 Ashleigh Court, Station Road, Arnside, Carnforth LA5 0JH Tel: 01524 761079 — MB ChB Manch. 1948; MRCS Eng. LRCP Lond. 1948; DPH Lond. 1951; BA Open. 1984. Prev: Fact. Med. Off. H. J. Heinz Co. Ltd.

STEELE, Graham Arthur Parkfields, 220 Duffield Road, Derby DE22 1BL Tel: 01332 342263 Fax: 01332 342263 — MB ChB Manch. 1957; DMRD Eng. 1962; FRCR 1995. Cons. Radiol. Derbysh. Roy. Infirm. Specialty: Radiol. Socs: Brit. Soc. Interven. Radiol.; Brit. Inst. Radiol. & Fac. Radiol. Prev: Sen. Regist. (X-Ray) Manch. Roy. Infirm.

STEELE, Herbert Desmond Loughview Surgery, 2 Main Street, Kircubbin, Newtownards BT22 2SP Tel: 028 4273 8532 Fax: 028 4273 8070 Email: d.steele@p283.gp.n-i.nhs.uk; Shore Cottage, Portaferry Road, Greyabbey, Newtownards BT22 2RU Email: dsteele@doctors.org.uk — MB BCh BAO Belf. 1975.

STEELE, Ian Conrad Department of Healthcare for the Elderly, Royal Victoria Hospital, Grosvenor Road, Belfast BT12 6BA Tel: 01232 263320 Fax: 01232 263159; 3 Campbell Chase, Hawthornden Way, Belfast BT4 3LA Tel: 01232 654061 — MB BCh BAO Belf. 1988; MRCP (UK) 1991; MD 1996. Cons. Phys. (Geriat. Med.) Roy. Vict. Hosp. Belf. Specialty: Care of the Elderly.

STEELE, Mr James Alexander Accident & Emergency dept, Altnagelvin Area Hospital, Glenshane Road, Londonderry BT47 6SB Tel: 028 71345171 Fax: 028 71611245 Email: jsteele@alt.n-i.nhs.uk — MB BCh BAO Belf. 1987; FRCS Ed. 1991. Cons., A&E Dept., Altnagelin Area Hosp., Londonderry. Specialty: Accid. & Emerg.

STEELE, James Wallace Birtley Medical Group Practice, Birtley Medical Group, Durham Road, Birtley, Chester-le-Street DH3 2QT Tel: 0191 410 3421 Fax: 0191 410 9672; 16 Larchwood, Harraton, Washington NE38 9BT Tel: 0191 417 4865 — MB ChB Ed. 1972; BSc (Med. Sci. & Bact., Hons.) Ed. 1972, MB ChB 1975. GP Birtley. Prev: Trainee Gen. Pract. Bournemouth & Poole Vocational Train Scheme; Ho. Off. (Gen. Med.) & Ho. Off. (Gen. Surg.) Bangour Gen. Hosp.; Broxburn.

STEELE, Jan Mairi Boyd 58 Hollingbourne Road, London SE24 9ND — MB BS Lond. 1992.

STEELE, Jeremy Peter Charles St. Bartholomew's Hospital, Department of Medical Oncology, West Smithfield, London EC1A 7BE Tel: 020 7601 7900 Fax: 020 7601 7577; 54 New Cavendish Street, London W1G 8TQ Tel: 0207 935 0913 Fax: 0207 486 3248 — MB BS Lond. 1989 (St. Geo. Hosp. Lond.) DA (UK) 1992; MRCP (UK) 1994; MD Lond. 1999. Cons. (Med. Oncol.) St Bartholomew's Hosp., The Roy. Lond. Hosp. and The Lond. Chest Hosp. Specialty: Oncol.; Medico Legal. Special Interest: Mesothelioma. Socs: Assn. Cancer Phys.; Amer. Soc. Clin. Oncol.; Mem., Bd. of Directors, Internat. Mesothelioma Interest Gp. Prev: Specialist Regist. (Med. Oncol.) St. Barts. Hosp. Lond.; Research Fell. (Med.) Roy. Marsden Hosp. & Inst. Cancer Research Sutton; Vis. Fell. Harvard Med. Sch. Boston USA.

STEELE, Katrine 27 Send Road, Send, Woking GU23 7ET — BM Soton. 1993.

STEELE, Mary Christine — MB BS Lond. 1969 (Roy. Free) MRCS Eng. LRCP Lond. 1969. Assoc. Specialist (Dermat.) N. Durh. Acute Hosps. Trust. Specialty: Dermat.

STEELE, Michael (retired) 9 Broadwood, Bolton BL6 4PD Tel: 01204 843317 — MB ChB St. And. 1952; DObst RCOG 1954.

STEELE, Michael Alan Ballywalter Health Centre, Fowler Way, Ballywalter, Newtownards BT22 2PY Tel: 02842 758292 Fax: 02842 758540; 156 Groomsprot Road, Bangor BT20 5PF Tel: 02891 274559 Fax: 02842 758540 — MB ChB Ed. 1982; DRCOG 1984; MRCGP 1986; MRCP (UK) 1994. GP Princip. Ballywalter Health Clinic. Specialty: Gen. Med. Socs: Roy. Coll. Phys.

STEELE, Nicholas Anthony 29 Murvagh Close, Cheltenham GL53 7QX — MB BS Lond. 1994; BSc (Hons.) Lond. 1989. SHO (A & E) Roy. Lond. Hosp. & Homerton Hosp. Lond. Socs: BMA (N. Thames JDC); MDU. Prev: Ho. Off. (Med.) Homerton Hosp. Lond.; Ho. Off. (Renal) St. Bart. Hosp. Lond.; Ho. Off. (Surg.) Whipps Cross Hosp. Lond.

STEELE, Nicholas James The Health Clinic, Weeping Cross, Bodmin Avenue, Stafford ST17 0EG Tel: 01785 662505 Fax: 01785 661064 — MB ChB Birm. 1990; ChB Birm. 1990; MRCGP 1994.

STEELE, Peter Raynor Macdonald 52 Earlsway, Curzon Park, Chester CH4 8AZ Tel: 01244 676932 — MB BChir Camb. 1973 (Middlx.) PhD Camb. 1970, MA 1969; FRCPath 1991, M 1979. Cons. Path. Countess of Chester Hosp. Specialty: Histopath. Prev: Lect. (Path.) Univ. Camb.; Fell. Qu.'s Coll. Camb.

STEELE, Phyllis Sharon — MB BCh BAO Belf. 1991; MRCP (UK) 1994.

STEELE, Raymond Geoffrey 1B Glebe Road, Norwich NR2 3JG — MB BS Melbourne 1991.

STEELE, Richard Thompson Wythall Health Centre, May Lane, Hollywood, Birmingham B47 5PD Tel: 01564 822642 — MB ChB Ed. 1959; MRCGP 1989.

STEELE, Professor Robert James Campbell Department of Surgery and Molecular Oncology, Ninewells Hospital & Medical School, Dundee DD1 9SY Tel: 01382 660111 Fax: 01382 641795 Email: r.j.c.steele@dundee.ac.uk; Redgarth, 11 Rockfield Crescent, Dundee DD2 1JE Tel: 01382 667411 — MB ChB Ed. 1977; BSc (Hons.) Ed. 1974, MD 1983; FRCS Ed. 1984; FRCS Eng. 1996. Prof. Surgic. Oncol. Univ. Dundee; Chairm. Scott. Cancer Trials Colorectal Gp.; Chairm.Sign Colorectal Cancer Focus Gp.; Charim. Colorectal Caner Gp.. Critical Standards for Scotl. Specialty: Gen. Surg. Socs: Assn. Coloproctol.; Assn. Surg.; Brit. Soc. Gastroenterol. Prev: Convenor Educat. Comm. RCS Ed.

STEELE, Russell John Frederick South Western Deanery Office, Directorate of Workforce & Learning, Dean Clarke House, Southernhay East, Exeter EX1 1PQ Tel: 01392 678122 Fax: 01392 671624 Email: russell.steele@dcwdc.nhs.uk; 4 Doriam Close, Exeter EX4 4RS — MB ChB Birm. 1971; DObst RCOG 1973; FRCGP 1991, M 1975; MPhil Exeter 2000. p/t Assoc. Director Postgrad. Gen. Pract. Educat., S. West. Deanery. Specialty: Gen. Pract. Prev: Lect., Sch. Health & Sports Sci., Univ. Exeter; Med. Panel Examrs., RCGP; General Pract., Exeter.

STEELE, Mr Simon Craig Dept of Obstetrics & Gynaecology, Sunderland Royal Hospital, Kayll Road, Sunderland SR4 7TP Tel: 0191 569 9781 Fax: 0191 569 9218 Email: craig.steele@chs.northy.nhs.uk; 32 Fern Avenue, Jesmond, Newcastle upon Tyne NE2 2QX Tel: 0191 281 1995 Email: sc.steele@btinternet.co.uk — MB ChB Leeds 1981 (Leeds University Medical School) MRCOG 1989. cons. O & G Sunderland Roy. Hosp. Sunderland. Specialty: Obst. & Gyn.

STEELE, Sinclair (Joseph Ekow) 18 Girton Avenue, London NW9 9SX — BM BCh Oxf. 1998.

STEELE, Sine 17 Muirden Road, Maryburgh, Dingwall IV7 8EJ — MB ChB Glas. 1997.

STEELE, Mr Stuart James (retired) 10 Harley Street, London W1G 9PF Tel: 0207 467 8312; 35 Tring Avenue, London W5 3QD Tel: 020 8992 2113 Fax: 020 8992 2113 — (Camb. & Middlx.) MB Camb. 1957, BChir 1956; MRCS Eng. LRCP Lond. 1956; MA Camb. 1957; DObst RCOG 1958; FRCS Eng. 1962; FRCOG 1975, M 1964; MFFP 1993. Prev: Emerit. Reader (O & G) Univ. Coll. Lond. Med. Sch.

STEELE, Susan Margaret Accident & Emergency Department, Ninewells hospital & medical school, Dundee DD1 9SY Tel: 01382 660111; Redgarth, 11 Rockfield Cresent, Dundee DD2 1JE Tel:

01382 667411 — MB ChB Ed. 1978. Tayside Univ. Hosp. NHS trust. Specialty: Accid. & Emerg. Prev: Staff Grade Pract. Qu. Med. Centre (NHS Trust) Univ. Hosp. Nottm.

STEELE, Tony 8 Fraser Street, Bristol BS3 4LY — MB ChB Sheff. 1983.

STEELE, William Keith Dunluce Avenue Surgery, 1-3 Dunluce Avenue, Belfast BT9 7AW Tel: 028 9024 0884; 19 Lougherne Road, Hillsborough BT26 6NL Tel: 01846 638660 — MB BCh BAO Belf. 1978 (Qu. Univ. Belf.) FRCGP 1996, M 1983; DCH NUI 1983; MICGP 1987; MD Belf. 1987. Sen. Lect. (Gen. Pract.) Qu. Univ. Belf. Specialty: Dermat. Socs: Assn. Univ. Teach. Gen. Pract. Prev: Janet Nash Trav. Fellowship RSM 1989; Princip. Tutor (Gen. Pract.) (RCGP) Qu. Univ. Belf.

STEELE, William Murray Saltoun Surgery, Fraserburgh AB43 9NH Tel: 01346 514154 Fax: 01346 585228 — MB ChB Aberd. 1971; DObst RCOG 1974. Clin. Asst. (Diabetes) Fraserburgh Hosp.; Hosp. Med. Dir. Fraserburgh Hosp. Specialty: Diabetes. Socs: Aberd. M-C Soc.; (Chairm. & Sec.) Fraserburgh Postgrad. Med. Soc. Prev: Trainee GP Aberd. VTS; Ho. Off. Roy. North. Infirm. Inverness.

STEELE, Yvette Elizabeth Grosvenor Road Surgery, 17 Grosvenor Road, Paignton TQ4 5AZ Tel: 01803 559308 Fax: 01803_ 526702; Chy-Ang-Wheal, Bridgetown Hill, Totnes TQ9 5BA — MB ChB Aberd. 1987; MRCGP 1992; DRCOG 1992. Specialty: Gen. Pract. Prev: Asst. GP Trawden, Lancs.; SHO (Paediat.) Burnley Gen. Hosp.; Trainee GP Guide Post Health Centre N.d.

STEELE-PERKINS, Anthony Peter, Surg. Capt. RN Retd. Brincil Cottage, Kingsdon, Somerton TA11 7LA — (St. Thos.) MB BS Lond. 1968; MRCS Eng. LRCP Lond. 1968; DAvMed Eng. 1976; MSc Lond. 1979; FFOM RCP Lond. 1994, MFOM 1983. Occupat. Phys. Health Servs. BMI. Specialty: Occupat. Health. Socs: Fell. Roy. Soc. Med.; Soc. Occupat. Med. Prev: Dir. Med. Personnel (Navy); Chief Staff Off. (Health & Safety) to Flag Off. Naval Aviat.; MoD Staff of Surg. Gen.

STEEN, Benjamin Meyer 19 Bishopsgate, Wellknowle Place, Glasgow G74 5AX — LRCP LRCS Ed. 1945; LRCP LRCS Ed. LRFPS Glas. 1945; FRFPS Glas. 1947; MRCP Glas. 1962.

STEEN, Caryle Ann (retired) 35 Cholmeley Park, London N6 5EL Tel: 020 8340 1122 Fax: 020 8340 9879 — MB BS Lond. 1958 (Lond. Hosp.) MRCS Eng. LRCP Lond. 1958; FRCGP 1992, M 1972. Hon. Clin. Asst. (Obst.) & Hon. Sen. Clin. Lect. (Gen. Pract.) Univ. Coll. Hosp. Lond. Prev: GP Lond.

STEEN, Heather Jean Cupar Street Clinic, Falls Road, Belfast BT13 2LJ Tel: 01232 327613; Killyloob, 85 Old Kilmore Road, Moira, Craigavon BT67 0NA — MB BCh BAO Belf. 1978; DCH RCP Glas. 1981; MRCP (UK) (Paediat.) 1984. Cons. Paediat. Roy. Belf. Hosp. Sick Childr. N. & W. Belf. H & SS Trust. Specialty: Paediat. Socs: BMA & Brit. Paediat. Soc.; Irish Thoracic Soc.

STEEN, Jillian Sara Muriel Medicines Control Agency, Market Towers, 1 Nine Elms Road, London SW8 5NQ Tel: 020 7273 0260 Fax: 020 7273 0134 — MB BS Lond. 1967 (Lond. Hosp.) MB BS (Hons.) Surg. Lond. 1967; Dip Pharm Med RCP (UK) 1979; MBA Lond. 1986; FFPM 1990. Sen. Med. Assessor Med. Control Agency. Specialty: Pharmaceutical Medicine. Socs: Fell. Fac. Pharmaceut. Phys. Prev: Regist. (Anaesth.) & Ho. Surg. Surgic. Unit. Lond. Hosp.; Med. Adviser Ciba-Geigy UK Ltd.; Commercial Affairs Manager IMS Clin. Servs.

STEEN, Leslie (retired) 7 St Mary's Road, Prestwich, Manchester M25 1AQ — LRCP LRCS Ed. LRFPS Glas. 1950; DPM Eng. 1959; MRCPsych 1971. Prev: Cons. Psychiat. Stockport Dist. HA & Prestwich Hosp.

STEENE, Laura St Helen's Medical Centre, 151 St. Helens Road, Swansea SA1 4DF Tel: 01792 476576 Fax: 01792 301136 — MB BCh Wales 1985.

STEEP, Elke Doctors Residence, Macclesfield District General Hospital, Victoria Road, Macclesfield SK10 3BL — State Exam Med. Berlin 1990.

STEER, Brian Oldways End, 28 Upper Carlisle Road, Eastbourne BN20 7TN Tel: 01323 722314 Email: dbsteer@aol.com — MB BS Lond. 1967 (Univ. Coll. Hosp.) MRCS Eng. LRCP Lond. 1967; FFA RCS Eng. 1972. Cons. Anaesth. Eastbourne Health Dist. Specialty: Anaesth. Socs: BMA & E.bourne Med. Soc. Prev: Sen. Regist. Char. Cross Hosp. Lond.; Regist. Nat. Hosp. Nerv. Dis. & Char. Cross Hosp. Lond.

STEER, Charles (retired) Ballacreg, Dreemskerry, Ramsey IM7 1BA Tel: 01624 815148 Fax: 01624 815148 — (Guy's) MB BS Lond. 1950; MRCGP 1957. Prev: Sen. Ho. Phys. (O & G) Cornelia Gen. Hosp. Poole.

STEER, Charles Gabriel The Surgery, 15 Brackendale, 25 Gloucester Road, Kingston upon Thames KT1 3RL Tel: 020 8546 8864 Fax: 020 8541 0217; 26 Cranes Park, Surbiton KT5 8AD Tel: 020 8399 8008 — MB BS Lond. 1978 (Univ. Coll. Hosp.) BA (2nd cl. Hons. Eng. Sci.) Oxf. 1970, MA 1980; DRCOG 1980; MLCOM 1992.

STEER, Christopher Richard Paediatric Department, Victoria Hospital, Hayfield Road, Kirkcaldy KY2 5AH Tel: 01592 261155; 14 Bellhouse Road, Aberdour, Burntisland KY3 0TL Tel: 01383 860738 — (Ed.) BSc (Hons. Physiol.) Ed. 1969, MB ChB 1971; DCH RCPS Glas. 1974; MRCP (UK) 1976; FRCP Ed. 1986; FRCPCH 1997. Cons. (Paediat.) Vict. Hosp. Kirkcaldy Fife; Clin. Dir. (Obst. & Gyn. & Paediat.) Acute Unit Fife HB; Hon. Clin. Tutor Dept. Child Life & Health Edin. Univ.; Hon. Sen. Lect. Child Life & Health Aberd. Univ.; Hon. Sen. Lect. Preclin. Studies St. And. Univ. Specialty: Paediat. Socs: Brit. Paediat. Assn.; Scott. Paediat. Soc.; Roy.Soc. of Med. Prev: Sen. Regist. (Paediat. Neurol.) & Regist. (Paediat.) Roy. Hosp. Sick; Childr. Edin.; SHO Infec. Dis. Unit City Hosp. Edin.

STEER, Christopher Victor Orpington Hospital, Quebec Ward, Cararod Wing, Sevenoaks Road, Orpington BR6 9JU Tel: 01689 815277 Fax: 01689 815279; Oakenhill, Hosey Hill, Westerham TN16 1TB — MB ChB Birm. 1982 (Birm) MRCOG 1985; MD Birm. 1993. Cons. O & G FarnBoro. Hosp. Specialty: Obst. & Gyn.

STEER, Graham Lansley 20 Primrose Hill, Brentwood CM14 4LT — MB ChB Bristol 1969; DA Eng. 1971; FFA RCSI 1976. Cons. Anaesth. Havering Hosp. Trust; Hon. Cons. Anaesth. Italian Hosp. Lond. & St. Luke's Hosp. for Clergy Lond. Specialty: Anaesth. Prev: Sen. Regist. St. Mary's Hosp. Lond.

STEER, Mr Howard William Bush House, Romsey Road, East Wellow, Romsey SO51 6BG — MB BS Lond. 1970 (St. Thos. Hosp.) PhD Lond. 1968, BSc 1965; MRCS Eng. LRCP Lond. 1970; FRCS Eng. 1975. Cons. Surg. Soton. Gen. Hosp. Specialty: Gen. Surg. Prev: Reader (Surg.) Oxf. Univ.

STEER, Jane Anne Royal Free Hampstead NHS Trust, Pond St, London WC1E 6BD Tel: 020 7794 0500 — MB BS Lond. 1990; MSc Lond. 1994; MRCPath 1999. Cons. Roy. Free Hosp. Specialty: Med. Microbiol. Prev: Sen Regist (Clin Medicol) Univ Coll. Lond Hosp; Research Fell. (Clin. Microbiol.) Univ. Coll. Hosp. Lond.; Regist. (Clin. Microbiol.) Univ. Coll. Lond. Hosps.

STEER, Janet Mary Blackthorn Surgery, 73 Station Road, Netley Abbey, Southampton SO31 5AE Tel: 023 8045 3110 Fax: 023 8045 2747 — BM BCh Oxf. 1980 (St Thomas's and Oxford) BSc Lond. 1966, MSc 1969; Cert. Family Plann. JCC 1982; DRCOG 1984; MFFP 1994. Sen. Clin. Med. Off. (Family Plann.) Soton. Family Plann. Serv.

STEER, Keith Alistair 132 Weston Park, Hornsey Vale, London N8 9PN Tel: 01563 574237 Email: jeremystirling@aol.com — MB BS Lond. 1987 (Middlx.) BSc (Hons.) Leeds 1978; MSc Soton. 1979; PhD Lond. 1982; MRCP (UK) 1991; FRCP 2000. Cons. Metabol. Med. Northwick Pk. Hosp. Harrow. Specialty: Diabetes; Gen. Med.; Endocrinol. Socs: Brit. Diabetic Assn. (Med. & Scientif. Sect.); Soc. for Endocrinol. Brit. Thyroid Assoc. Prev: Lect. (Med., Diabetes & Endocrinol.) Univ. Bristol; Regist. (Med., Diabetes & Endocrinol.) Northwick Pk., Edgware Gen. & St. Mary's Hosps. Lond.; Regist. (Chem. Path.) Univ. Coll. & Middlx. Sch. Med.

STEER, Professor Philip James Academic Department Obstetrics & Gynaecology, Chelsea & Westminster Hospital, 369 Fulham Road, London SW10 9NH Tel: 020 8846 7892 Fax: 020 8846 7880 Email: p.steer@ic.ac.uk; 48 Langley Avenue, Surbiton KT6 6QR Tel: 020 8390 3913 — MB BS Lond. 1971 (Guy's & King's Coll. Hosps.) MRCS Eng. LRCP Lond. 1971; FRCOG 1989, M 1977; BSc (1st cl. Hons.) Lond. 1968, MD 1986; T(OG) 1991. Prof. (Obst.) Fac. of Med. Imperial Coll. Lond.; Director of Perinatal Servs. Chelsea & Westm. Hosp. Lond. Specialty: Obst. & Gyn. Socs: Blair Bell Res. Soc.; (Pres.) Brit. Assn. Perinatal Med.; Fell. Roy. Soc. Med. Prev: Head Dept Matern. Fetal Med. Imp. Coll. Sch. Med. Lond.; Ch.ill Fell. 1981; Prof. & Head Dept. Char. Cross & Westm. Med. Sch. Lond.

STEER, Sophia Elizabeth Dept. of Rheumatology, Guy's Hospital, St Thomas' St, London SE1 9RS — MB BS Lond. 1993 (Guy's)

MRCP (UK) 1996. ARC Clin. Lect., Dept. of Rheum., Guy's Hosp., Lond. Specialty: Rheumatol.; Research.

STEERE, Christopher Edwin Neston Medical Centre, 14-20 Liverpool Road, Neston, South Wirral CH64 3RA; Delsany, 286 Telegraph Road, Heswall, Wirral CH60 7SQ — MB ChB Liverp. 1980.

STEERS, Mr Alfred James Wanklyn 16 Cammo Crescent, Edinburgh EH4 8DZ — MB BS Lond. 1967 (Middlx.) FRCS Eng. 1972. Specialty: Neurosurg.

STEFAN, Martin David 41 Telford House, Tiverton St., London SE1 6NY — MB BS Lond. 1989.

STEFANI, Terence Antony Whitstable Health Centre, Harbour Street, Whitstable CT5 1BZ Tel: 01227 594400 Fax: 01227 771474; Brookfield, 127 South St, Whitstable CT5 3EL Tel: 263949 — MB ChB Sheff. 1970; DCH Eng. 1972; MRCP (UK) 1973; DObst RCOG 1973. Hosp. Pract. (Paediat.) Kent & Canterbury Hosp. Socs: Chairm. 1st aid Train. panel Roy. Nat. Life Boat Inst.; BMA & Mem. Brit. Paediat. Assn. Prev: SHO (Gen. Med./Gen. Paediat./ Neonat.) Dudley Rd. Hosp.; SHO (Anaesth.) Cheltenham Hosp.

STEFANUTI, Eric (retired) 4 Silverdale Close, Sheffield S11 9JN Tel: 0114 236 9219 — MB ChB Sheff. 1959.

STEFANUTTO, Tiscia Bernadette 21 Park Avenue, The Mumbles, Swansea SA3 4DU — MB ChB Cape Town 1993.

STEFFEN, Gundula Margarete 12 St Vincent Road, Wallasey CH44 8BJ — State Exam Med Munster 1991. SHO (Anaesth.) Roy. L'pool Univ. Hosp. Specialty: Anaesth.

STEGER, Mr Adrian Churchill 74 Croxted Road, London SE21 8NP — MB BS Lond. 1977 (St Thomas's) MS Lond. 1990, MB BS 1977; FRCS Glas. 1982; FRCS Eng. 1998. Cons. Surg. Univ. Hosp. Lewisham; Hon. Sen. Lect. (Surg.) United Med. & Dent. Schs. of Guys & St Thos. Specialty: Gen. Surg. Socs: Fell. Roy. Soc. Med.; Brit. Soc. Gastroenterol.; Surg. Research Soc. Prev: Sen. Regist. (Surg.) King's Coll. Hosp. Lond.; Clin. Lect. Univ. Coll. Hosp.; Regist. (Surg.) Roy. Postgrad. Med. Sch. & Hammersmith Hosp. Lond.

STEGGALL, Emily Anne 11 Woodland Road, Weston Super Mare BS23 4HF — MB BS Lond. 1998.

***STEGGALL, Margaret Anne** 266 Heeley Road, Selly Oak, Birmingham B29 6EN — MB ChB Birm. 1998; ChB Birm. 1998. Ho. Off. Rotat. (Med. Surg. Paediat.) Birm. Heartlands Hosp.

STEGGLES, Mr Brian George Higher Newton, Metherell, Callington PL17 8DF Tel: 01579 350154 — MB BS Lond. 1970 (King's Coll. Hosp.) LDS RCS Eng. 1962; BDS Lond. 1962; MRCS Eng. LRCP Lond. 1970; FRCS Ed. 1994; Dip. IMC RCS Ed. 1995; FIMC RCS Ed. 2001. Gen. Pract. Locum; Hon. Lect. Plymouth Postgrad. Med. Sch.; Chairm. Fac. Pre-Hosp. Care RCS Edin. Specialty: Accid. & Emerg. Socs: Resusc. Counc.; Examr. Advis. Bd. Immediate Med. Care Roy. Coll. Surg. Edin.; Plymouth Med. Soc. Prev: Regist. (Oral Surg.) Roy. Free Hosp.; Lect. (Oral Surg.) King's Coll. Hosp.

STEIGER, Christine Ann Alder Hey Royal Liverpool Childrens Hospital, Eaton Road, Liverpool L12 2AP Tel: 0151 252 5195 — MB BS Newc. 1983; MRCP (UK) 1986. Cons. Paediat. (Community Child Health) Alder Hey Hosp. Liverp. Specialty: Community Child Health. Prev: Sen. Regist. (Community Child Health) Alder Hey Hosp. Liverp.; Sen. Regist. (Community Child Health) Northwick Pk. Hosp. & Nottm.

STEIGER, Malcolm Jonathan Walton Centre for Neurology & Neurosurgery, Liverpool L9 7LJ Tel: 0151 525 3611 Fax: 0151 529 5512 Email: malcolm.steiger@thewaltoncentre.nhs.uk — MB BS Newc. 1983 (Newcastle-upon-Tyne) MRCP (UK) 1986; MD Newc. 1995; FRCP 1999. Cons. Neurol. Walton Hosp. Neurol. & Neurosurg. Liverp. Specialty: Neurol. Special Interest: Movement Disorders. Prev: Research Fell. Inst. Neurol. Nat. Hospial Nerv. Disorders Lond.; Sen. Regist. (Neurol.) Nat. Hosp. Neurosurg. & Neurosurg. Lond.; Regist. (Med.) Nottm. AHA.

STEIN, Professor Alan Leslie University of Oxford, Warneford Hospital, Department of Psychiatry, Oxford OX3 7JX Tel: 01865 223911 Fax: 01865 226384 Email: alan.stein@psych.ox.ac.uk — MB BCh Witwatersrand 1979; FRCPsych 1996, M 1984. Prof. of Child Health & Adolesc. Psychiat. Specialty: Child & Adolesc. Psychiat. Prev: Prof. of Child Family Ment. Health, Roy. Free Univ. Coll. Med. Sch., UCL, Tavistock Clinic; Leopold Muller Prof. Child & Family Ment. Health.

STEIN, Alexander Geoffrey 65 Marlborough Mansions, Cannon Hill, London NW6 1JS — MB BS Lond. 1973; MRCS Eng. LRCP Lond. 1973.

STEIN, Andrew George Walsgrave Hospital, Clifford Bridge Road, Coventry CV2 2DX Tel: 02476 535135 Fax: 02476 535160 Email: andy.stein@uhcw.nhs.uk — BMedSci Nottm. 1984; MD Leicester; BM BS Nottm. 1984; MRCP (UK) 1988. Cons. Nephrologist/General Phys. Specialty: Gen. Med. Socs: Renal Association; BMA.

STEIN, Claudia Elisabeth World Health Organisation, GPE/EBD, 20 Avenue Appice, Geneva CH-1211, Switzerland Tel: 00 41 22 791 3234 Fax: 00 41 22 791 4328 Email: pheath@dorset.swest.nhs.uk; 4 Blencowe Drive, Chandlers Ford, Eastleigh SO53 4LZ Tel: 01703 275571 — State Exam Med Essen 1989 (Univ. Essen, Germany) MSc (Pub. Health) Lond. 1997; PhD (Epidemiol.) Soton. 1997; DLSHTM (Pub Health) Lond 1998; MFPHM London 2000. Med. Office Epidemiologist; Consulant to WHO, Geneva. Specialty: Epidemiol.; Pub. Health Med. Socs: Fell. Roy. Soc.Med.; BMA; Chamber Phys. (Germany). Prev: MRC Research Fell. (Environm. Epidemiol.) Soton. Univ.; Sen. Regist. in Pub. Health, Wessex Roation; SHO Rotat. (Med.) Soton. Univ. Hosps.

STEIN, David Dawson (retired) 15 Stamford Avenue, Hayling Island PO11 0BJ Tel: 02392 468296 — (Ed.) MB ChB Ed. 1945. Surg. Lt. RNVR. Prev: Ho. Phys. Roy. Hants. Co. Hosp. Winchester & Perth Roy. Infirm.

STEIN, Emma Leonore (retired) 16 The Paddocks, Wembley HA9 9HH Tel: 020 8904 3872 — MB BS Lond. 1947 (Roy. Free) Deans Medal Clin.Med 1946; MB BS Lond. 1947; DMRD Eng. 1951. Prev: GP S. Harrow.

STEIN, Fiona Caroline Glendaruel, Picklers Hill, Abingdon OX14 2B — MB BS Nottm. 1982; MRCGP 1987; DRCOG 1987.

STEIN, Gaby Flat 2, Peace Court, 8 Swynford Gardens, London NW4 4XL — MB ChB Cape Town 1989.

STEIN, George Willowbrook Medical Practice, Brook St., Sutton-in-Ashfield NG17 1ES — MRCS Eng.; LRCP Lond. 1962; MRCS Eng. LRCP Lond. 1962. Chairm. Mem. Dep. Coop.; JMC Mem. Socs: BMA. Prev: Clin. Asst. (Psychiat.) King's Mill Hosp. Sutton-in-Ashfield.

STEIN, George Stanley 25 Beadon Road, Bromley BR2 9AS — (UCH) MB BS Lond. 1968; MRCP (UK) 1972; DCH Eng. 1973; MRCPsych 1976; M Phil 1979; FRCPsych 1995. Cons. Psychiat. Cane Hill & FarnBoro. Hosp. Orpington Kent; Hon. Sen. Lect. KCH Lond.; Asst. Edr. Brit. Jl. Psychiat. Specialty: Gen. Psychiat. Prev: Regist. Maudsley Hosp. Lond.; Regist. (Med.) Hackney Hosp. Lond.

STEIN, Jennifer Ann 18A Buttermarket, Thame, Oxford OX9 3EP Tel: 01865 260150 Fax: 01865 260150 — MB BCh BAO NUI 1987 (Univ. Coll. Cork, N.U.I.) BSc Lond. 1974; PhD Newc. 1978; MRCPsych 1992. Cons. Psychiat. Psychoth. The Univ. of Oxf. Counselling Serv. for Stud.s Oxf.; Cons. Psychiatric Psychotherapist Aylesbury Vale Ment. Health Care Trust Aylesbury; Cons. Psychiatric Psychotherapist and Jungian Analyst in Private Pract. Oxf. Specialty: Psychother. Socs: Exec. Comm. for Psychother. Fac. Roy. Coll. of Psychiat.s; Soc. of Analyt. Psychol. Prev: Cons. Psychiat. Psychoth.Rockingham Forest NHS Trust Kettering.

STEIN, Professor John Frederick Magdalen College, Oxford OX1 4AU Email: john.stein@physiol.ox.ac.uk — BM BCh Oxf. 1966 (St Thomas's Hosp.) MSc, MA Oxf. 1965; MRCP Lond. 1968; FRCP Lond. 1999. Lect. (Neurophysiol.) Oxf. Univ.; Fell. & Tutor (Med.) Magdalen Coll. Specialty: Ophth.; Neurosurg.; Clin. Neurophysiol. Socs: Physiol. Soc.; Assn. Brit. Neurol.; Brit. Dyslexia Assn. (Scientif. Adv.).

STEIN, Kenneth William Thomas 7 Esplanade Terrace, Joppa, Edinburgh EH15 2ES — MB ChB Bristol 1987.

STEIN, Linda (retired) Careston Manse, Brechin DD9 6SA Tel: 01356 630366 — MB ChB Manch. 1973; DCH Eng. 1975; DObst RCOG 1975; MRCP (UK) 1978.

STEIN, Penelope Effie Department of Haematology, Cambridge Institute for Medical Research, University of Cambridge, Cambridge CB2 2XY Tel: 01223 762660 Fax: 01223 336788; 27 Hinton Avenue, Cambridge CB1 7AR Tel: 01223 520646 — MB BChir Camb. 1983; BMedSci Nottm. 1980; MSc Lond. 1987; PhD Camb. 1990. Wellcome Sen. Fell. (Clin. Sci.) Univ. of Camb. Specialty:

Chem. Path. Prev: Research Assoc. Univ. Alberta; Lister Fell. (Haemat.) Univ. Camb.

STEIN, Robert Colin Ludwig Institute for Cancer Research, 91 Riding House St., London W1W 7BS Tel: 020 7878 4060 Fax: 020 7878 4040 Email: rstein@ludwig.ucl.ac.uk; 20 Walcot Square, Kennington, London SE11 4TZ — PhD Camb. 1978, MA 1978; MB BChir Camb. 1982; MRCP (UK) 1986. Clin. Scientif. Fell. & Sen. Lect. & Hon. Cons. Med. Oncol. Ludwig Inst. for Cancer Research & Dept. Oncol. Univ. Coll. Lond. Med. Sch. Specialty: Oncol. Prev: Lect. & Hon. Sen. Regist. (Med. Oncol.) St. Geo. Hosp. Med. Sch. Lond.; Sen. Regist. (Med. Oncol.) Middlx. & Univ. Coll. Hosps. Lond.; Regist. (Gen. Med.) Whipps Cross Hosp. Lond.

STEIN, Samuel Mark Family Consultation Clinic, Dunstable Health Centre, Priory Gardens', Dunstable LU6 3SU Tel: 01582 707660 Fax: 01582 707659 Email: sbcht1@business.ntl.com — MB BCh Witwatersrand 1986; MRCPsych.; BA (Criminol.) 1994. Cons. (Child, Adolesc. & Family Psychiat.) S. Beds. Comm. Health Care Trust. Specialty: Child & Adolesc. Psychiat. Prev: SHO & Regist. Train. Oxf.; Specialist Regist. Train. St Mary's Hosp. Imperial Coll. Lond.

STEIN, Tarrant Robert Dr Robson and Partners, Manzil Way, Cowley Road, Oxford OX4 1XD Tel: 01865 242109; 19 Abberbury Road, Iffley, Oxford OX4 4ET Tel: 01865 777989 — MB BS Lond. 1966 (King's Coll. Hosp.) MRCS Eng. LRCP Lond. 1966; DObst RCOG 1968; MRCGP 1974.

STEINBERG, Benjamin (retired) 7 Saxholm Dale, Bassett, Southampton SO16 7GZ Tel: 023 8076 0177 — MB ChB BAO Belf. 1946; DPM Lond. 1951; MD Belf. 1955; FRCPsych 1974, M 1971. Emerit. Cons. Psychiat. Soton. & SW Hants. Health Dist. Prev: Cons. & Clin. Asst. (Psychiat.) Knowle Hosp. Fareham.

STEINBERG, Derek (retired) Princess Elizabeth Hospital, Bell House Clinic, Le Vauquiedor, Guernsey GY1 2SB — MB BS Lond. 1965 (Lond. Hosp.) MRCS Eng. LRCP Lond. 1965; DPM Eng. 1968; FRCPsych 1979, M 1972; MPhil Lond. 1972. p/t Vis. Cons. Psychiat. States of Guernsey Health Bd.; Trustee Bethlem Roy. & Maudsley Hosp. Art & Hist. Collections Trust. Prev: Cons. Psychiat. & Vis. Sen. Tutor Ticehurst Hse. Hosp. Sussex.

STEINBERG, Mark Westbury Medical Centre Tel: 020 8346 6919 Fax: 020 8346 6919 — MB ChB Manch. 1995; DRCOG 1997. SHO (Acc. & Emerg.). Prev: SHO (Obstet & Gyn. & Paediat.).

STEINBERG, Myer (retired) — (Dub.) MB BCh BAO Dub. 1941.

STEINBERG, Stanley Westbury Medical Centre, 205 Westbury Avenue, Wood Green, London N22 6RX Tel: 020 8888 3021 Fax: 020 8888 6898 — MB BCh BAO Dub. 1960 (TC Dub.) BA Dub. 1959. Prev: Ho. Phys. & Ho. Surg. Dr. Steevens' Hosp. Dub.; SHO (Cas. & Orthop.) Roy. Vict. Hosp. Bournemouth; Resid. Med. Off. Bearsted Memor. Hosp. Hampton.

STEINBERG, Stanley Victor Castlemilk Health Centre, 71 Dougrie Drive, Glasgow G45 9AW Tel: 0141 531 8585 Fax: 0141 531 8596; 6 Berryhill Drive, Giffnock, Glasgow G46 7AS Tel: 0141 638 7828 Fax: 0141 638 7828 — MB ChB Glas. 1970; BSc (Hons.) Glas. 1968. Prev: Ho. Surg. South. Gen. Hosp. Glas.; Ho. Phys. Raigmore Hosp. Inverness.

STEINBERG, Stephen David 13 Howard Walk, London N2 0HB Tel: 020 8455 1587 — MB BS Lond. 1983. Socs: Fell. Roy. Soc. Med.; Brit. Acupunc. Soc. Prev: Clin. Asst. (Rheum.) Chase Farm Hosp. Hosp. Enfield; SHO Char. Cross Hosp. Lond.; SHO (Rheum.) Princess Alexandra Hosp. Harlow.

STEINBERG, Victor Leonard (retired) 22 Holne Chase, London N2 0QN Tel: 020 8458 2764 — MB BS Lond. 1951 (St. Bart.) FRCP Ed. 1971, M 1957; DPhysMed. Eng. 1958; FRCP Lond. 1988. Prev: Cons. Rheum. Wembley Hosp.

STEINBERGS, Gerardo Gustavs Fullwell Cross Health Centre, 1 Tomswood Hill, Barkingside, Ilford IG6 2HG Tel: 020 8500 0231 Fax: 020 8491 1598; 95 Queens Road, Buckhurst Hill IG9 5BW — MB BS Lond. 1982; DRCOG 1984; Cert. Family Plann. JCC 1985; MRCGP 1987. Princip. GP Fullwell Cross Health Centre Barkinside Essex; Club Med. Off. W. Ham United Football Club. Specialty: Cardiol. Socs: Sec. of Ilford Med. Soc. Prev: Assoc. Course Organiser Redbridge VTS. 1990-1993; Sec. of Ilford Med. Soc. 1986-1996.

STEINBRECHER, Mr Henrik Alex Department of Paediatric Surgery, Southampton University NHS Trust, Southampton General Hospital, Tremona Road, Southampton SO16 6YD Tel: 023 8079 8464 Fax: 023 8079 4750 — MB BS Lond. 1986; FRCS Eng. 1990; MS Soton. 1995; FRCS Paediat. 1997. Cons. (Paediat. Surg.) Soton. Univ. NHS Trust Soton Gen Hosp. Specialty: Paediat. Surg.

STEINER, David Arthur Ridgeway, Mitchel Troy Common, Monmouth NP25 4JB Tel: 01600 775433 Fax: 01600 712020 — MB ChB Liverp. 1972; T(GP) 1993. Prev: GP Jersey, CI; Med. Off. St. Francis Hosp., Zambia; Ho. Off. Ormskirk & Dist. Gen. Hosp. Ormskirk.

STEINER, Eduard Samuel Roundwood Surgery, Wood Street, Mansfield NG18 1QQ Tel: 01623 648880 Fax: 01623 631761; La Corbiere, Cauldwell Drive, Mansfield NG18 4SL Tel: 01623 653615 Fax: 01623 653615 Email: edsteiner1@aol.com — MB ChB Liverp. 1974; DCH RCPS Glas. 1976; Dip Thpc Nottm. 1996. GP Princip.; PCT Exec. Comm. Chairm. Prev: Regist. (Paediat.) Nottm. City Hosp.; Regist. & SHO (Paediat.) King's Mill Hosp. Mansfield.

STEINER, Eleanor Margaret (retired) Atlantic House, Ellenabeich, Isle of Seil, Oban PA34 4RF Tel: 01852 300593 — (Aberd.) MB ChB Aberd. 1961; DPH Aberd. 1966; MFCM 1972; MRCGP 1976; MICGP 1984; FRSH 1997. Prev: Mem. Indep. Tribunal Serv.

STEINER, Gerhard Martin (retired) Sheffield Childrens Hospital, Western Bank, Sheffield S10 2TH Tel: 0114 271 7000 Fax: 0114 271 7514 Email: martin@fulwoody@EMON.co.uk; The Dormers, 584 Fulwood Road, Sheffield S10 3QE Tel: 0114 230 4943 Fax: 0114 230 4943 Email: MARTIN@fulwood1.demon.co.uk — (St. Mary's) MB BS Lond. 1956; MRCS Eng. LRCP Lond. 1956; DCH Eng. 1959; DObst RCOG 1960; FRCP Lond. 1980, M 1962; DMRD 1965; FFR 1967; FRCR 1980. Hon. Clin. Lect. Sheff. Univ.; Cons. Radiol. Sheff. Childr. Hosp. Prev: Instruc. (Radiol.) Yale Univ. Med. Sch., USA.

STEINER, Hans 30 Elm Grove, Killingworth, Newcastle upon Tyne NE12 7AN — MB ChB Bristol 1959; MD Bristol 1974.

STEINER, Helen Rebecca 584 Fulwood Road, Sheffield S10 3QE Tel: 0114 230 4943 — MB BS Lond. 1990; MRCGP; BSc Lond. 1987; DObst Auckland 1992. GP non-principal.

STEINER, Jane 155 Risca Road, Newport NP20 3PP — MB BCh Wales 1977.

STEINER, Janice Ann Oxford Therapeutics Consulting Ltd., Magdalen Centre, Oxford Science Park, Oxford OX4 4GA Tel: 01865 784874 Fax: 01865 784874 Email: jansteiner@oxrx.com — (Sydney) MB BS Sydney 1969; FRACP 1975; DPhil Oxf. 1980; FRCP 2003. Dir. Oxf. Therap. Cons. Ltd. Specialty: Pharmaceutical Medicine; Pharmacology. Special Interest: Tumour Vaccines; Clin. Trials; Gene. Ther. Socs: Brit. Pharm. Soc; Fell. Fac. of Pharmaceut. Med.; Brit. Assn. of Pharmaceut. Phys. Prev: Europ. Med. Dir. Gensia Europe Ltd; Head of Clin. Support, Roche Products Ltd; Dir. of Clin. Pharmacol. Searle Research & Developm. UK.

STEINER, John 28 Park Drive, London NW11 7SP Tel: 020 8458 8303 — MB ChB New Zealand 1958 (Otago) PhD Camb. 1964; DPM Lond. 1967; FRCPsych. 1981, M 1971. Specialty: Psychother. Socs: Brit. Psychoanal. Soc. Prev: Cons. Psychother. Tavistock Clinic Lond.; Cons. Psychiat. Maudsley Hosp. Lond.

STEINER, Marion Ruth Southmead Health Centre, Ullswater Road, Bristol BS10 6DF; 57 Ravenswood Road, Redland, Bristol BS6 6BP — MB BS Lond. 1985 (London) MRCGP 1989; DRCOG 1989; MFFP 1995; LFHom 1997. GP Bristol. Prev: Princip. GP Newc.

STEINER, Michael Charles 28 Park Drive, London NW11 7SP — MB BS Lond. 1990.

STEINER, Nicholas Brian Michael The Hollies Surgery, The Green, Great Bentley, Colchester CO7 8PJ Tel: 01206 250691 Fax: 01206 252496; Rectory Lodge, Rectory Road, Weeley Heath, Clacton-on-Sea CO16 9BH Tel: 01255 830379 — MB ChB Bristol 1972.

STEINER, Mr Robert Emil, CBE 12 Stonehill Road, London SW14 8RW Tel: 020 8876 4038 — MD NUI 1957 (Univ. Coll. Dub.) MB BCh BAO 1941; DMR Eng. 1945; FFR 1952; FRCP Lond. 1965, M 1959; Hon. FACR 1965; Hon. FRACR 1971; Hon. FFR RCSI 1972; FRCR 1975; FRCS Eng. 1982. Emerit. Prof. Radiol. Univ. Lond. At Postgrad. Med. Sch. Hammersmith Hosp. Specialty: Radiol. Socs: FRCR (Ex-Pres. & Warden); Brit. Inst. Radiol. (Ex-Pres. & Edr. Brit. Jl. Radiol.). Prev: Civil Cons. Radiol. to Med. Dir. Gen. (Naval); Cons. Adviser (Radiol.) DHSS; Pres. & Warden Roy. Coll. Radiols.

STEINER, Roy Raymond Woodbridge Road Surgery, 165-167 Woodbridge Road, Ipswich IP4 2PE Tel: 01473 256251; 59 Linksfield, Rushmere St. Andrew, Ipswich IP5 1BA — MB BS Lond. 1983 (Westm.) DRCOG 1987; DCH RCP Lond. 1987; MRCGP 1988;

DFFP 1993. Specialty: Gen. Pract. Prev: Trainee GP Harold Hill Essex; Trainee Community Paediat. HornCh.; Clin. Med. Off. (Family Plann. & Child Health) HornCh.

STEINER, Timothy John Imperial College London, Division of Neuroscience & Mental Health, St Dunstan's Road, London W6 8RP Tel: 020 8846 1191 Fax: 020 8846 1183 Email: t.steiner@imperial.ac.uk — MB BS Lond. 1976 (Char. Cross) BSc (Hons.) Lond. 1969, PhD 1975; LLM Wales 1991; MFPM RCP (UK) 1994; MA Wales 1997; FFPM RCP (UK) 1998; MRCP Lond. 2002; MSc London 2002. Reader (Clin. Physiol.) Imperial Coll. Lond.; Hon. Cons. Clin. Physiol. Char. Cross Hosp. Lond. Specialty: Clin. Physiol.; Pharmaceutical Medicine. Socs: Internat. Headache Soc. Mem. Council. (Chairm. Ethics Comm., Mem. Clin.Trials Comm.); Brit. Assn. for the Study of Headache; World Headache Alliance Hon. Secretary (Counc. Mem.). Prev: Sen. Lect. (Clin. Physiol.) Char. Cross & Westm. Med. Sch. Lond.; Lect. (Experiment. Neurol.) Char. Cross & Westm. Med. Sch. Lond.

STEINERT, Jack 30 Vicarage Road, East Sheen, London SW14 8RU Tel: 020 8876 9505 — MB ChB Birm. 1956; DPM Eng. 1965; FRCPsych 1977, M 1971. Vis. Cons. Psychiat. Roehampton Priory Hosp. Lond.; Hon. Sen. Clin. Lect. Imperial Coll Lond. Specialty: Gen. Psychiat. Socs: BMA. Prev: W. Lond. Healthcare Trust Ealing; Cons. Psychiat. Springfield Hosp. Lond.; Sen. Regist. St. Geo. Hosp. Lond. & Springfield Hosp. Lond.

STEINGOLD, Harry Castlemilk Health Centre, 71 Douglas Drive, Cadtlemilk, Glasgow G45 9AW Tel: 0141 531 8500; 5 Humbie Gate, Newton Mearns, Glasgow G77 5NH Tel: 0141 639 8321 — MB ChB Glas. 1950.

STEINGOLD, Mr Raymond Frank George Eliot NHS Trust, Nuneaton CV10 7DJ Tel: 024 768 65119 Email: raymond.steingold@geh.nhs.uk — MB ChB Manch. 1971 (Manchester) FRCS Eng. 1978. Cons. Orthop. Surg. Nuneaton. Specialty: Orthop. Socs: Fell. Brit. Orthop. Assn. Prev: Sen. Regist. (Orthop.) Harlow Wood Hosp. & Leic. Roy. Infirm.; Tutor & Hon. Regist. (Orthop.) Univ. Dept. Orthop. Hope Hosp. Manch.; Orthop. Regist. Preston Roy. Infirm.

STEINHARDT, Stephen Ian Steinhardt and Partners, The Surgery, 5A Brookfield Road, Gloucester GL3 3HB Tel: 01452 617295 Fax: 01452 617296; Springfield House, Little Witcombe, Gloucester GL3 4TU — MB ChB Bristol 1973; DObst RCOG 1976; MRCGP 1978; D.Occ.Med. RCP Lond. 1995. Prev: SHO (Cas. & Orthop.) Cheltenham Gen. Hosp.; SHO (Obst.) Southmead Hosp. Bristol; SHO (Paediat.) Cheltenham Childr. Hosp.

STEINLECHNER, Mr Colin Wolfgang Brett North Devon District Hospital, Raleigh Park, Barnstaple EX31 4JB Tel: 01271 322577 Email: colin.steinlechner@ndevon.swest.nhs.uk — MB BS Lond. 1992 (St Thomas's) BSc (Hons) Lond. 1989; FRCS Eng 1996; FRCS (Tr & Orth) 2003. Cons. N. Devon Dist. Hosp. Specialty: Trauma & Orthop. Surg.; Orthop.

STEKELMAN, Sharon 237 Alexandra Park Road, London N22 7BJ Tel: 020 8888 9428 Fax: 020 8888 9428 Email: sharonos@hotmail.com — MB BS Lond. 1962 (King's Coll. Lond. & St. Geo.) MRCS Eng. LRCP Lond. 1962; DPM Eng. 1971. Specialty: Psychother. Socs: Brit. Psychoanal. Soc. Prev: Clin. Asst. Portman Clinic & Centre Psychother. Lond.; Sen. Regist. Earls Ct. Child Guid. Unit; Regist. (Psychiat.) Halliwick Hosp. Lond.

STELFOX, Dora Elizabeth Church Street Surgery, 1 Church Street, Newtownards BT23 4FH Tel: 028 9181 6333 Fax: 028 9181 8805; 3 Old Belfast Road, Newtownards BT23 4SG Tel: 01247 819647 — MB BCh BAO Belf. 1979; DCH 1981; DRCOG 1983; MRCGP 1984. Socs: BMA & Ulster Med. Soc.

STELL, Ian Michael Princess Royal University Hospital, Farnborough Common, Orpington BR6 8ND Tel: 01689 863526 Fax: 01689 863542 Email: ian.stell@bromleyhospitals.nhs.uk — MB BS Lond. 1984; DRCOG 1987; DCH RCP Lond. 1987; MRCP (UK) 1988; MRCGP 1989; DTM & H RCP Lond. 1990; Dip. Epid. FPHM RCP (UK) 1994; FRCS Ed. 1995. Cons. (A & E Med.) Bromley NHS Trust. Specialty: Accid. & Emerg. Prev: Lect. (A & E) Guy's Hosp. Lond.

STELLER, Philip Harold 23 Marle Croft, Whitefield, Manchester M45 7NB — MB ChB Manch. 1972; FFA RCS Eng. 1978. Cons. Anaesth. N. Manch. Gen. Hosp. Specialty: Anaesth.

STELLMAN, Rose Margaret Fraser (retired) 7 Finch Court, 10 Lansdown Road, Sidcup DA14 4EN Tel: 020 8309 9522 — (Aberd.) MB ChB Aberd. 1939. Prev: PMO (Child Health) Bexley Health Dist.

STELLON, Anthony John Abbey Practice, 107 London Road, Temple Ewell, Dover CT16 3BY Tel: 01304 821182 Fax: 01304 827673; 125 Whitstable Road, Canterbury CT2 8EQ Tel: 01227 453086 Email: stellon@btinternet.com — MB BS Lond. 1977 (Roy. Free Hosp. Lond.) MRCS Eng. LRCP Lond. 1977; MRCP (UK) 1980; Dip. Med. Acupunc. 1995; Dip. Occ Med. 1999. Hosp. Pract. (Gastroenterol.) Buckland Hosp. Dover. Specialty: Gastroenterol. Socs: Brit. Med. Acupunct. Soc. Prev: Regist. (Med.) Liver Unit King's Coll. Hosp. Lond.; SHO Rotat. (Gen. Med.) North. Gen. Hosp. Sheff.; Ho. Surg. Barnet Gen. Hosp.

STENHOUSE, Craig William St. Werburghs House, Wood Lane, Hanbury, Burton-on-Trent DE13 8TG — MB ChB Leic. 1986.

STENHOUSE, Emily Jane Whinfell House, 5 Claremont Drive, Bridge of Allan, Stirling FK9 4EE — MB ChB Glas. 1996. SHO (O & G) Glas. Specialty: Obst. & Gyn.

STENHOUSE, George (retired) 166 Southbrae Drive, Jordanhill, Glasgow G13 1TX Tel: 0141 954 9594 — MB ChB Glas. 1966; PhD Glas. 1973, BSc (Hons.) 1963; FRCR 1980. Prev: Lect. (Physiol.) Univ. Glas.

STENHOUSE, Jeremy Nicol Health Centre, Faringdon SN7 7EZ Tel: 01367 242388 — MB BChir Camb. 1958 (Camb. & Oxf.) MA, MB Camb. 1958, BChir 1957; DObst RCOG 1961. Prev: Anaesth. Regist. Launceston Gen. Hosp. Tasmania; Ho. Surg. & Ho. Phys. Radcliffe Infirm. Oxf.; Obst. Ho. Surg. Churchill Hosp. Oxf.

STENHOUSE, Peter Granger 7 Beech Avenue, Bearsden, Glasgow G61 3EU — MB ChB Glas. 1998.

STENHOUSE, Philip Daniel 91A Friern Road, London SE22 0AZ — MB BS Lond. 1993; BDS Lond. 1985.

STENHOUSE, Robin Balfour (retired) Karoo, 10 Sandybed Lane, Scarborough YO12 5LH — (St. Geo.) MB BChir Camb. 1960; DObst RCOG 1965; DPM Eng. 1968. Clin. Asst. (Psychiat.) Ellis Centre, Scarboro. Prev: Surg. Lt. RN.

STENHOUSE, Shirley McLean Gretna Surgery, Central Avenue, Gretna DG16 5NA — MB ChB Glas. 1987; MRCGP 1991. Prev: Trainee GP Crieff Health Centre; SHO (O & G & Med.) Stirling Roy. Infirm.; SHO (Psychiat.) Bellsdyke Hosp. Larbert.

STENHOUSE, Thomas Grove Road Surgery, 3 Grove Road, Solihull B91 2AG Tel: 0121 705 1105 Fax: 0121 711 4098; 6 The Crescent, Solihull B91 1JP Tel: 0121 705 1821 — MB ChB Birm. 1976; DRCOG 1980; MRCGP 1984.

STENNER, Jonathan Maurice Crathorne 77 High Street, Buckden, St Neots, Huntingdon PE19 5TA — BChir Camb. 1990.

STENSON, Benjamin James Consultant Neonatologist, Simspon Memorial Maternity Pavilion, Edinburgh — MB ChB Ed. 1986; MRCP (UK) 1990; MD Ed. 1997; FRCPCH 1998. Cons. Neonatologist. Specialty: Neonat. Prev: Research Fell. & Hon. Regist. (Neonat. Paediat.) Univ. Edin.

STENSON, Keith, TD The Surgery, Torton Hill Road, Arundel BN18 9HG Tel: 01903 882517/882191 Fax: 01903 884326 — MB BS Lond. 1965 (Westm.) MRCS Eng. LRCP Lond. 1965; DObst RCOG 1971; MRCGP 1975. Hosp. Pract. (Geriat.) Worthing & Southlands NHS Trust; Col. RAMC(V). Socs: Hon. Progr.. Sec. Med. Off. Sch.Assn. Prev: Ho. Phys. Roy. Vict. Hosp. Bournemouth; Ho. Surg. Westm. Hosp. Lond.

STENSON, Susan Laura Sandygate, Church St., East Markham, Newark NG22 0SA Tel: 01777 871036 — MB BS Lond. 1998 (King's Coll.) Ho. Off. (Gen. Med.& Endocrin.) Glouc. Roy. Hosp. Specialty: Gen. Med. Prev: PRHO (Surg.) Worc Roy. Infirm.

STENT, Venetia Mary 50 Fir Road, Hanworth, Feltham TW13 6UJ Tel: 020 8898 0253 Fax: 020 8893 3864 — MB BS Lond. 1980 (St Bartholomews) MRCGP 1985.

STENTIFORD, Norman Henry (retired) The Oaks, Strawmoor Lane, Oaken, Codsall, Wolverhampton WV8 2HY Tel: 01902 761557 Email: bim@stent.eu.org — MB ChB Bristol 1960; FRCP Lond. 1980, M 1963. Cons. Phys. Russells Hall Hosp. Dudley. Prev: Cons. Phys. Burton Rd. Hosp. Dudley.

STENTON, Kay Jeanette 9 Bishopdale Rise, Mosborough, Sheffield S20 5PE — MB ChB Sheff. 1995.

STENTON, Samuel Christopher Department of Respiratory Medicine, Royal Victoria Infirmary, Newcastle upon Tyne NE1 4LP Tel: 0191 232 5131 Fax: 0191 227 5224 — MB BCh BAO Belf.

1981; BSc Belf. 1978; MFOM RCP Lond. 1995; FRCP (UK) 1999. Cons. Phys. Roy. Vict. Infirm. & Assoc. Hosps. NHS Trust; Sen. Lect. (Med.) Univ. Newc. Specialty: Respirat. Med.; Occupat. Health. Prev: Lect. (Med.) Univ. Newc.; Regist. (Med.) Newc. HA.

STEPHAN, Talal Fouad Mansfield Community Hospital, Stockwell Gate, Mansfield NG18 5QJ Tel: 01623 785151 Fax: 01623 785180; Cornerstone Lodge, 72 Main St, Papplewick, Nottingham NG15 8FE Tel: 0115 964 0099 — MB ChB Baghdad 1971; FRCP Glas.; FRCPI; Dip. Cardiol. Lond 1983. Cons. Rehabil. Med. Mansfield Community Hosp.; Exec. Comm. Mem. - Mansfield Primary Care Trust. Specialty: Rehabil. Med. Socs: BMA; Brit. Soc. Rehabil. Med. Prev: Sen. Regist. (Rehabil. Med.) Derbysh. Roy. Infirm.; SCMO (Rehabil. Med.) Haywood Hosp. Stoke-on-Trent; Career Regist. (Gen. & Geriat. Med.) W. Midl. RHA.

STEPHEN, Alan James Lower Ericstane, 7A West Montrose St., Helensburgh G84 9NF — MB ChB Glas. 1974.

STEPHEN, Alexander Kynoch (retired) Ivycroft, 153 Redcar Lane, Redcar TS10 2DZ — MB ChB Aberd. 1951.

STEPHEN, Andrew Alexander Linden Medical Group, Linden Medical Centre, Linden Avenue, Kettering NN15 7NX Tel: 01536 512104 Fax: 01536 415930; The Spinney, 16B Harrington Road, Loddington, Kettering NN14 1JZ Tel: 01536 711993 — (Sheff.) MB ChB Sheff. 1969; DObst RCOG 1971; DCH Eng. 1973; MRCGP 1980. Gen. Med. Practitioner; Med. Off. SATRA (Shoe & Allied Trades Research Assoc.) Kettering. Socs: BMA. Prev: SHO (Paediat.) Sheff. Childr. Hosp.; SHO (Obst.) Jessop Hosp. Sheff.; Ho. Off. (Med.) North. Gen. Hosp. Sheff.

STEPHEN, Annie Margaret (retired) Broad Reach, Inchberry Road, Fochabers IV32 7QA Tel: 01343 821637 — (Aberd.) MB ChB Aberd. 1940.

STEPHEN, Mr Arthur Buchan Orthopaedic Department, Queens Medical Centre, Clifton Boulevard, Nottingham NG7 2UH Tel: 0115 924 9924 — MB BS Lond. 1993 (Univ. Coll. & Middx. Hosp. Med. Sch.) BSc Lond. 1990, MB BS 1993; FRCS (Eng) 1997. Specialty: Trauma & Orthop. Surg.

STEPHEN, Catherine Margaret 99 Rannoch Drive, Bearsden, Glasgow G61 2ER — MB ChB Aberd. 1986 (Univ. Aberd.) Clin. Assis. Care of Elderly,Gartnavel Gen. Hosp. Glas. Specialty: Care of the Elderly. Prev: Liaison Phys. (c/o Elderly) Newc. City Trust; Trainee GP Dumfries & Galloway HB; SHO Rotat. (Med.) Newc. Gen. Hosp.

STEPHEN, Doris Leonora (retired) 40 Denhill Park, Newcastle upon Tyne NE15 6QH — MB ChB Aberd. 1949.

STEPHEN, Elizabeth Daphne Storey (retired) Royal Oak House, Royal Oak Mews, Mayfield TN20 6AL Tel: 01435 872632 — MB ChB St. And. 1942; DA Eng. 1945; FFA RCS Eng. 1954. Hon. Cons. Anaesth. Maidstone & Tunbridge Wells Health Dist. & Kent HA. Prev: Cons. Anaesth. Maidstone & Tunbridge Wells Health Dist.

STEPHEN, George Portlethen Group Practice, Portlethen Medical Centre, Bruntland Road, Aberdeen AB12 4QP Tel: 01224 780223 Fax: 01224 781317; 53 Crollshillock Place, Newtonhill, Stonehaven AB39 3RF Tel: 01569 30511 — MB ChB Aberd. 1970; MRCGP 1976. Prev: Resid. Ho. Off. (Med. & Surg.) Aberd. Roy. Infirm.; Trainee GP Aberd. VTS.

STEPHEN, George Willson The Health Centre, Trenchard Avenue, Thornaby, Stockton-on-Tees TS17 0DD Tel: 01642 762636 Fax: 01642 766464; Lewins, Fieldhouse Lane, Kirklevington, Yarm TS15 9LS Tel: 01642 781110 — MB ChB Aberd. 1961; DObst RCOG 1964; DA Eng. 1972; MRCGP 1982. Socs: BMA. Prev: Anaesth. S. Teesside Hosp. Gp.; Ship's Surg. Roy. Fleet Auxil. Serv.

STEPHEN, George Wilson 30 Flanchford Road, London W12 9ND — MB ChB Aberd. 1956; FFA RCSI 1962; FFA RCS Eng. 1963. Specialty: Anaesth.

STEPHEN, Helen Janet The Old School Surgery, The Old School, The Square, Ellon AB41 7GX Tel: 01651 851777 Fax: 01651 852090 — MB ChB Aberd. 1969; DCH Glas. 1972; MRCP (UK) 1979.

STEPHEN, Mr Ian Bruce Murray New Barn, 39A Grange Road, Broadstairs CT10 3ER Tel: 01843 867848 Fax: 01843 868536 Email: ibms@btinternet.com — (Camb. & St. Bart.) MB BChir Camb. 1968; MRCS Eng. LRCP Lond. 1968; FRCS Eng. 1973. Ind. Cons. Orthrop. Foot & Ankle Surg.; Cases Comm. Mem. Med. Protec. Soc. Specialty: Orthop.; Trauma & Orthop. Surg. Socs: Fell. BOA & Roy. Soc. Med.; Pres. 2000/2001 Brit. Orthop. Foot Surg. Soc.; Expert Witness Inst. Prev: Sen. Regist. (Orthop.) Princess Eliz. Orthop. Hosp. Exeter; Regist. (Orthop.) Bristol Roy. Infirm.; Research Fell. (Orthop.) McGill Univ. Montreal, Canada.

STEPHEN, John Francis (retired) 25 Vivian Terrace, Davidsons Mains, Edinburgh EH4 5AW — (Ed.) MB ChB Ed. 1950; DObst RCOG 1954.

STEPHEN, Mr John Gordon 12 The Willows, Bishop Auckland DL14 7HH — MB BChir Camb. 1970; FRCS Eng. 1973; MA Camb. 1970, MChir 1984. Cons. Surg. Bishop Auckland Gen. Hosp. & Darlington Mem. Hosp.; Hon. Clin. Lect. (Surg.) Univ. Newc. Specialty: Gen. Surg. Socs: Brit. Soc. Gastroenterol.; Assn. Surg.; Assn. Up. GI Surgeons (AUGIS).

STEPHEN, Linda Jane Epilepsy Unit, Western Infirmary, Dumbarton Road, Glasgow G11 6NT — MB ChB Glas. 1989; DRCOG 1992; DCH 1993; T(GP) 1994; MRCGP 1994; DFFP 1997. Dep. Dir. & Epilepsy Unit West. Infirm. Glas. Specialty: Pharmacology.

STEPHEN, Margaret Elizabeth (retired) Parkside, 124B South Street, Armadale, Bathgate EH48 3JU Tel: 01501 730700 — MB ChB Aberd. 1967. Prev: Res. Ho. Surg. Woodend Gen. Hosp. Aberd.

STEPHEN, Mark James By The Way, Mingoose Vale, Mount Hawk, Truro TR4 8RY — MB ChB Manch. 1994.

STEPHEN, Mary Ross Royal Infirmary, Department of Pathology, 84 Castle St., Glasgow G4 0SF Tel: 0141 211 4264 Fax: 0141 211 4884 — MB ChB Glas. 1971 (Glasgow) MRCPath 1994. Cons. Cytopath. Roy. Infirm. Glas. Specialty: Histopath.

STEPHEN, Robert Strachan Aultoun Croft, Ardallie, Peterhead AB42 5BN — MB ChB Aberd. 1977.

STEPHEN, Stewart Anderson (retired) 1 East Campbell Court, Longniddry EH32 0NW Tel: 01875 853470 — MB ChB St. And. 1950 (Dundee) FRCP Ed. 1973, M 1956. Prev: Cons. Phys. (Geriat.) Sanderson Hosp. Galashiels.

STEPHEN, Walter Taylor Woodside Medical Group A, 80 Western Road, Woodside, Aberdeen AB24 4SU Tel: 01224 492631 Fax: 01224 276173 — MB ChB Aberd. 1973; MRCGP 1977.

STEPHEN, William John (retired) 27 New Street, Wells BA5 2LE Tel: 01749 672642 — MB ChB Bristol 1956; DObst RCOG 1960; Tr. Fell Nuff. Found. 1972; Tr. Fell. RCGP 1980; MRCGP 1996. Prev: Nuffield Trav. Fell. 1972.

STEPHEN, William Simpson Younie Albyn Medical Practice, 30 Albyn Place, Aberdeen AB10 1NW Tel: 01224 586829 Fax: 01224 213238; 172 Deeside Gardens, Aberdeen AB15 7PX Tel: 01224 325024 — MB ChB Aberd. 1973; MRCGP 1979. Hon. Clin Tutor Dept. Gen. Pract. Univ. Aberd.

STEPHENS, Adrian David Kings College Hospital, Demark Hill, London SE5 9RS Tel: 020 7346 4152 Fax: 020 7346 3514; 54 Telfords Yard, Wapping, London E1W 2BQ Tel: 020 7680 1474 — MRCS Eng. LRCP Lond. 1963 (St. Bart.) MD Lond. 1980, MB BS 1963; FRCPath 1988, M 1976. Cons. Haemat. Kings Coll. Hosp. Lond. Specialty: Haematology. Socs: Brit. Soc. Haematol. Prev: Cons. Haemat. St. Bart. Hosp. Lond.; Lect. (Med.) St. Bart. Hosp. Med. Coll. Lond.; Sen. Regist. (Haemat.) & Ho. Surg. St. Bart. Hosp. Lond.

STEPHENS, Alison Rhona (retired) 28 High Street, Eynsham, Witney OX29 4HB — (Edinburgh) MB ChB Ed. 1958; DObst RCOG 1960; DCH RCPS Glas. 1961; MFFP 1993. Prev: Asst. GP Oxf.

STEPHENS, Andrew David Elm Hayes Surgery, High Street, Paulton, Bristol BS39 7QJ Tel: 01761 413155 Fax: 01761 410573 — MB BS Lond. 1990 (Middlx. Hosp. Med. Sch. Lond.) BSc Lond. 1987; DRCOG 1996; DFFP 1997; MRCGP 1998. GP Princip., Dr. Roy and Partners, Elm Hayes Surg., High St., Paulton. Specialty: Dermat.; Pharmacology; Gen. Psychiat. Socs: BMA; RCGP. Prev: GP Princip., Dr. Slade and Partners, Irnham Lodge Surg., Minehead, Som. TA24 5RG.

STEPHENS, Brian Alexis Fenwick (retired) Tollgate House, Wing, Leighton Buzzard LU7 0PW — MRCS Eng. LRCP Lond. 1942 (St. Mary's) MRCGP 1962. Med. Off. StockGr. Pk. Sch. Prev: Clin. Asst. Med. Roy. Bucks. Hosp. Aylesbury.

STEPHENS, Caroline Jane Bridge Street Surgery, 67 Bridge Street, Cambridge CB2 1UU Tel: 01223 355060 Fax: 01223 460812; 43 Herbert Street, Cambridge CB4 1AG Tel: 01223 321320 — BM Soton. 1981. Dep. Police Surg. Camb. Socs: LMC.

STEPHENS, Caroline Susan 12 Kirkintilloch Road, Bishopbriggs, Glasgow G64 2AX — MB ChB Glas. 1986.

STEPHENS, Carys Llywella Brynawel, 10 Parc-yr-Afon, Carmarthen SA31 1RL — MB BS Lond. 1962 (Cardiff) DA Eng.

1967. Regist. (Anaesth.) Merthyr & Aberdare Hosp. Gp. Specialty: Anaesth.

STEPHENS, Catherine Joan Myfanwy Poole Hospital NHS Trust, Longfleet Road, Poole BH15 2JB Tel: 01202 665511; Sancroft House, Canford Magna, Wimborne BH21 3AF — MB BS Lond. 1981; MRCP (UK) 1984; FRCP (UK) 1998. Cons. Dermat. Poole Hosp. Specialty: Dermat. Prev: Sen. Regist. (Dermat.) St. John's Dermat. Centre Lond.; Regist. (Dermat.) St. Thos. Hosp. Lond.

STEPHENS, Catriona Alison Blackthorne House, Queen Street, Farthinghot, Brackley NN13 5NY — MB BS Lond. 1993.

STEPHENS, Charles Philip — MB BS Lond. 1992; MRCP Lond. 1999; MRCGP 2000. GP Cornw.

STEPHENS, Christine — MB ChB Sheff. 1986. GP Retainer Micklover, Derby. Specialty: Gen. Pract.

STEPHENS, Christopher Roman Victor Street Surgery, Victor Street, Shirley, Southampton SO15 5SY Tel: 023 8077 4781 Fax: 023 8039 0680 — MB BS Lond. 1979 (Guy's) MRCGP 1983; DCH RCP Lond. 1984; DRCOG 1985. Sen. Lect. (Primary Med. Care) Sch. Med. Soton. Univ. Specialty: Gen. Pract.

STEPHENS, Clare Alice Torrington Park Health Centre, Torrington Park, North Finchley, London N12 9SS Tel: 020 8343 9122 Email: clare.stephens@barnet-pct.nhs.uk; 16 The Ridgeway, London N3 2PH — MB BS Lond. 1990; DRCOG 1994; MRCGP 1995. GP; Clinica Adviser Educat. & Train. Barnet PCT. Prev: Regist. (Gen. Pract.) Lond.; SHO Rotat. (Obst.) Univ. Coll. Hosp. Lond.; Clin. Lect. (Primary Care) Univ. Coll. Lond.

STEPHENS, Cyril Joakim (retired) Whitefriars, Carmel St., Great Chesterford, Saffron Walden CB10 1PH Tel: 01799 530612 Fax: 01799 531584 — MRCS Eng. LRCP Lond. 1953 (Westm.) BA Camb. 1949; DA Eng. 1955; FFA RCS Eng. 1962. Prev: Cons. Anaesth. W. Essex Dist.

STEPHENS, David Elm Lodge Surgery, 2 Burbage Road, London SE24 9HJ Tel: 020 7733 3073 Fax: 020 7924 0710 — MB BS Lond. 1977; MRCS Eng. LRCP Lond. 1977; DRCOG 1982; MRCGP 1982. Trainer (Gen. Pract.) SE Thames Region; Tutor (Gen. Pract.) KCH Lond.; GP Cons. Lambeth, Southwark & Lewisham Health Commiss. Socs: Socialist Med. Assn. Prev: SHO (O & G) Greenwich Dist. Hosp. Lond.; SHO (Med. & Paediat.) Guy's Hosp. Lond.; Ho. Phys. Addenbrooke's Hosp. Camb.

STEPHENS, David Edward Orchard Lea, 23 Mount St, Bishops Lydeard, Taunton TA4 3AN — Dip. Med. Acupunc; LMSSA Lond. 1962.

STEPHENS, David Francis Fisk (retired) Mary Potter Health Centre, Gregory Blvd, Hyson Green, Nottingham NG5 4DB Tel: 0115 960 8882 — LRCP LRCS Ed. 1948 (Roy. Colls. Ed.) Cert Contracep. & Family Plann. RCOG & RCGP; LRCP LRCS Ed. LRFPS Glas. 1948; MRCGP 1966. JP City of Nottm. Prev: Ho. Phys. Roy. Edin. Hosp. Ment. Disorders.

STEPHENS, David John (retired) Downham Cottage, Lechlade GL7 3DL Tel: 01367 252075 — MB ChB Leeds 1949; DObst RCOG 1953; MRCGP 1959. Prev: GP Lechlade.

STEPHENS, Derek Dillwyn Ty Heulog, Love Lane, Brightlingsea, Colchester CO7 0QQ Tel: 01206 302711 — BM BCh Oxf. 1949; BM BCh Oxon. 1949.

STEPHENS, Douglas Alan (retired) 43 Greystoke Park, Gosforth, Newcastle upon Tyne NE3 2DZ Tel: 0191 217 0409 Fax: 0191 217 0409 Email: alapat@ukonline.co.uk — MB ChB Birm. 1956; DPM Eng. 1961; FRCPsych 1977, M 1971. Med. Mem. North. Ment. Health Review Tribunal Nottm. Prev: Direct. Clin. Serv. (Psychiat.) N. Tyneside Gen. Hosp.

***STEPHENS, Elizabeth Angela** 16 Ravenscar terrace, Leeds LS8 4AU — MB BS Newc. 1998; MRCP 2001. Specialist Regist. (Haemat.) Leeds. Specialty: Gen. Med. Prev: PRHO Sunderland Roy. Hosp.; PRHO N. Tyneside Hosp; SHO (Med.) Sunderland Roy. Hosp.

STEPHENS, Elizabeth Ann 28 Enfield Avenue, Liverpool L23 0SZ Tel: 0151 476 9174 — MB BS Lond. 1993; BSc Lond. 1990; DRCOG 1995; DFFP 1995. Specialty: Family Plann. & Reproduc. Health.

STEPHENS, Emily Christdasi Peters 73 Pollard Lane, Bradford BD2 4RW Tel: 01274 636273 — LMS Punjab 1951; LMS Ludhiana Punjab India 1951; LAH Dub. 1968. Hosp. Pract. (Genitourin. Med.) St. Lukes Hosp. Bradford. Specialty: Genitourinary Medicine.

STEPHENS, Enid Winifred Brett (retired) 5 Sherrardspark Road, Welwyn Garden City AL8 7JW Tel: 01707 324069 — LRCP LRCS Ed. 1944 (Anderson Coll. Glas.) LRCP LRCS Ed. LRFPS Glas. 1944. Prev: GP Hertford.

STEPHENS, Fraser Renfree 97 Firgrove Road, Southampton SO15 3ET Email: firstepheus@hotmail.com — MB ChB Aberd. 1991; FRCA.

STEPHENS, Frederick Graham (retired) 15 Forth-an-Nance, Portreath, Redruth TR16 4NQ — MB BS Lond. 1965; MRCS Eng. LRCP Lond. 1965.

STEPHENS, Geoffrey Paul Holmes Chapel Health Centre, London Road, Holmes Chapel, Crewe CW4 7BB — MB ChB Otago 1971.

STEPHENS, Helen Elizabeth 17 Kestrel Avenue, Staines TW18 4RU — MB BS Lond. 1988.

STEPHENS, Henry Michael Alcwyn Thomson and Partners, The Medical Centre, Oak Street, Lechlade GL7 3RY Tel: 01367 252264 — MB BS Lond. 1983; MRCP (UK) 1986; MRCGP 1989; DRCOG 1989; Dip. Pract. Dermat. Wales 1991.

STEPHENS, Imogen Freya Dawn Western Sussex PCT, Bramber Building, 9 College Lane, Chichester PO19 6FX Tel: 01243 770770 Fax: 01243 815300 — MB ChB Ed. 1983 (Edin.) MRCOG 1988; MFFP 1994; BSc (Hons.) Ed. 1980, MD 1994; MPH Glas. 1995; MFPHM 1998. Dir. Public Health, Western Sussex PCT. Specialty: Pub. Health Med. Prev: Sen. Regist. (Pub. Health Med.) Argyll & Clyde HB; Specialist Wom. Health Glas.; CRC Research Fell. Gyn. Oncol.

STEPHENS, Janice Mary City Walls Medical Centre, St. Martin's Way, Chester CH1 2NR Tel: 01244 357800; Flaxyards Cottage, Rhuddal Heath, Tarporley CW6 9HJ — MB ChB Leic. 1987; DCH RCP Lond. 1990; DRCOG 1991; MRCGP 1992.

STEPHENS, Jeffrey Wayne Dept of Endocrinology, Middlesex Hospital, UCL Hospitals, London W1T 3AA — MB BS Lond. 1994 (St. Mary's Hosp. Med. Sch. Lond.) BSc (Hons.) Lond. 1993; Dip. ALS 1996; MRCP (UK) 1997. Specialist Regist. (Endocrinol. Diabetes/Gen. Med.) Middlx. Hosp. Lond. Specialty: Endocrinol.; Diabetes; Gen. Med. Socs: Soc. of Endocrinol.; Diabetes UK. Prev: SHO Rotat. (Med.) Northwick Pk. Hosp. Harrow; Ho. Off. St. Mary's Hosp. & Ealing Hosp.; Specialist Regist. (Endocrine / Diabetes) Roy. Free Hosp. Lond, UCL Hosp. Lond., Chase Farm Hosp. Enfield.

STEPHENS, Jessica Northfield House, Turweston, Brackley NN13 5JX Tel: 01280 705378 — MB BS Lond. 1984; DRCOG 1987.

STEPHENS, Joan (retired) 1 The Glebe, Cumnor, Oxford OX2 9QA Tel: 01865 864660 — MB BS Durh. 1948 (Newc.) MFFP 1993. Prev: Div. Surg. St. John Ambul. Brig.

STEPHENS, John 44 Beech Way, Blackmore End, Wheathampstead, St Albans AL4 8LY Tel: 01438 833333 Fax: 01438 833536; 44 Beech Way, Blackmore End, Wheathampstead, St Albans AL4 8LY Tel: 01438 833333 Fax: 01438 833536 Email: john@thestephens.org.uk — MB BS Lond. 1973; MRCS Eng. LRCP Lond. 1973; DRCOG 1976.

STEPHENS, John David 29 Crossways, Shenfield, Brentwood CM15 8QY; 93 Harley Street, London W1N 1DF — MB BS Lond. 1967 (Guy's) MRCS Eng. LRCP Lond. 1967; MRCP (UK) 1970; MD Lond. 1979; FRCP Lond. 1993. Cons. Cardiol. Barking Havering & Riedbridge NHS Trust; Hon. Cons. Cardiol. Barts & the Lond. Hosps. NHS Trust. Specialty: Cardiol. Socs: Brit. Cardiac Soc. Prev: Sen. Regist. (Cardiol.) St. Bart. Hosp. Lond.; Regist. (Cardiol.) Brompton Hosp. Lond.; Med Research Fell. (Cardiol.) Harvard Univ. Med. Sch. & Peter Bent Brigham Hosp. Boston, USA.

STEPHENS, John Patrick Bournemouth West Community Mental Health Team, Hahnemann House, Hahnemann Road, Westcliff, Bournemouth BH2 5JW Tel: 01202 584440 Fax: 01202 584444 — MB BS Lond. 1990 (St. Mary's Hosp. Lond.) MRCPsych 1995. Cons. Psychiat. St Ann's Hosp. Poole Dorset; ASM Lond. 1990. Specialty: Gen. Psychiat.; Geriat. Psychiat. Socs: Roy. Coll. of Psychiat.s. Prev: Sen. Regist. (Liaison Psychiat.) St. Geo. Hosp. Tooting; Sen. Regist. (Gen. Ad. Psychiat.) Grayling Well Hosp. Chichester; Regist. (Forens. Psychiat.) Shaftsbury Clinic & (Liaison Psychiat.) St. Geo. Hosp. Lond.

STEPHENS, John Richard Dynevor The Harvey Practice, Magna House, 81 Merley Lane, Wimborne BH21 3BB Tel: 01202 841288 Fax: 01202 840877; Stour Cottage, High St, Spetisbury, Blandford Forum DT11 9DW Email: jrdstephens@lineone.net — BM Soton. 1986 (Univ. Soton.) MRCP (UK) 1990; DCH 1991; DRCOG 1992;

DFFP 1993; MRCGP 1993. Hosp. Practitioner G.U. Med., Roy. Bournemouth Hosp. Specialty: Gen. Pract.

STEPHENS, Katharine 27 Commondale, Putney, London SW15 1HS — MB ChB Bristol 1997. PRHO (Med.) Torbay Hosp.; PRHO (Surg.) NDDH. Specialty: Gen. Surg. Socs: BMA; MPS.

STEPHENS, Mr Keith MacGregor, Brigadier (retired) Palmer House, Moulton, Richmond DL10 6QG Tel: 01325 377937 Email: brigkim@aol.com — MB BS Lond. 1964 (St Bartholomews MS Lond.) FRCS Ed. 1974. Prev: Commanding Off. Duchess of Kent Hosp.

STEPHENS, Laura Catherine Rebecca The Laurels, 12 Venn Gardens, Hartley, Plymouth PL3 5PW — MB BCh Wales 1996. SHO (Psychiat. of the Elderly) Mt.gould Hosp. Plymouth. Specialty: Gen. Psychiat.; Geriat. Psychiat. Prev: SHO (Gen. Adult Psychiat.) Glenbourne Unit, Derriford Plymouth; SHO (Rehabil. Psychiat.) Scott Hosp. Plymouth.

STEPHENS, Marjory Stevenson Kilsyth Medical Partnership, Kilsyth Health Centre, Burngreen Park, Glasgow G65 0HU Tel: 01236 822081 Fax: 01236 826231 — MB ChB Dundee 1975.

STEPHENS, Mark Department of Histopathology, Central Pathology Laboratory, Hartshill Road, Hartshill, Stoke-on-Trent ST4 7PA Tel: 01782 716662 — MB BCh Wales 1982; MRCPath 1988. Cons. Histopath. Centr. Path. Laborat. Stoke-on-Trent. Specialty: Histopath. Prev: Sen. Regist. (Histopath.) Univ. & City Hosps. Nottm.; Regist. (Histopath.) Univ. Hosp. Wales Cardiff; SHO (Path.) Univ. Hosp. Wales Cardiff.

STEPHENS, Matthew Francis Tamour Flat 1, 1 Malvern Road, Stoneygate, Leicester LE2 2BH — MB ChB Leic. 1994.

STEPHENS, Michael Redford 13 Windmill Close, Llantwit Major, Vale of Glamorgan, Cardiff CF14 9BL Tel: 01446 792465 Email: redfordstephens@aol.com — MD Bristol 1975; MB ChB 1963; FRCP Ed. M 1969. Cons. Cardiol. Univ. Hosp. Wales Cardiff; Lect. (Cardiol.) Welsh Nat. Sch. Med. Cardiff. Specialty: Cardiol.

STEPHENS, Myles David Buckingham (retired) 49 Kings Court, Bishop's Stortford CM23 2AB Tel: 01279 652719 Fax: 01279 466572 Email: stephmdb@onetel.net.uk — MRCS Eng. LRCP Lond. 1956 (King's Coll. Hosp.) MB BS 1956; Dobst RCOG 1958; DMJ (Clin.) Soc. Apoth. Lond. 1970; MRCGP 1971; Dip Pharm Med RCP (UK) 1978; MD Lond. 1985; FFPM RCP (UK) 1990. Cons. WHO Uppsala Mt.ing Centre (UMC); Pharmaceut. Cons. Bishop's Stortford. Prev: GP Minehead.

STEPHENS, Mr Neville Aubrey (retired) 19 Bakehouse Hill, Dullingham, Newmarket CB8 9XJ Tel: 01638 508221 — (King's Coll. Hosp.) MB BS Lond. 1948; FRCS Eng. 1953. Cons. Surg. Dartford & Gravesham Health Dist. Prev: Regist. (Urol.) & Sen. Regist. (Surg.) King's Coll. Hosp. Lond.

STEPHENS, Nicola Gay Maesycoed, Gwbert Road, Cardigan SA43 1PH — MB BCh Wales 1990.

STEPHENS, Nicola Jane — MB ChB Liverp. 1998.

STEPHENS, Nigel Graham Dept. of Cardiology, Northwich Park Hospital, Harrow HA1 3UJ Tel: 020 8869 3182 Fax: 020 8869 3176 — MB BS Lond. 1988; PhD Lond. 1985; MRCP (UK) 1991. Cons. Cardiol. & Dir. Cardiol. Northwich Pk. Hosp. Harrow. Specialty: Cardiol. Socs: Brit. Cardiac Soc.; Brit. Cardiovasc. Interven. Soc. Prev: Sen. Regist. (Cardiol.) Addenbrooke's & Papworth Hosps. Camb.; Lect. (Med.) Camb. Univ.; Regist. (Cardiol.) Hammersmith Hosp. Lond.

***STEPHENS, Paul Charles** 1 Brae Grove, Ballygowan, Newtownards BT23 5TP — MB ChB Glas. 1998 (Glasgow) BSc (Hons) Glas. 1996; MB ChB Glas 1998.

STEPHENS, Peter John The Warren Medical Practice, The Warren, Uxbridge Road, Hayes UB4 0SF — MB ChB Liverp. 1978.

STEPHENS, Robert Charles Meredith 7 Archer Road, Penarth CF64 3HW — MB BS Lond. 1993; BA Oxf. 1990; FRCA 2000. Research Fell. (Aneas & Critcal Care)Institute of Child Health UCL Lond. Specialty: Anaesth. Prev: SHO (Anaesth.) Kingston Hosp. Surrey.

STEPHENS, Sheila Joan (retired) Downham Cottage, Lechlade GL7 3DL Tel: 01367 252075 — MB ChB Leeds 1951; DObst RCOG 1953. Assoc. Specialist (Path.) Princess Margt. Hosp. Swindon. Prev: Med. Asst. (Cytol.) Swindon & Cirencester Hosp. Gp.

STEPHENS, Professor Simon Dafydd Glyn University Hospital of Wales, Welsh Hearing Institute, Cardiff CF14 4XW Tel: 029 2074 3474 Fax: 029 2073 3563 Email: stephensd@cardiff.ac.uk; Pen y Bryn, Llan-maes, Llanilltud Fawr, Llantwit Major CF61 2XR Tel: 01446 792403 Email: dafydda/glyn@lineone.net — (Char. Cross) MPhil Lond. 1973, BSc (Special Physiol.) 1962; MB BS Lond. 1965; MRCS Eng. LRCP Lond. 1965; DHMSA 1980; MRCP (UK) 1984; FRCP Lond. 1994. Dir. Welsh Hearing Inst.; Hon. Prof. Univ. Wales Coll. Med.; Audiol. Phys. Univ. Hosp. of Wales, Cardiff. Specialty: Audiol. Med. Socs: (Pres.) Internat. Assn. Phys. Audiol.; (Pres.) Internat. Collegium of Rehabil. Audiol.; (Exec. Comm.) Internat. Soc. Audiol. Prev: Cons. Audiol. Med. Roy. Nat. ENT Hosp. Lond.; Clin. Research Fell. Inst. Sound & Vibration Research Univ. Soton.; Psychoacousticist MRC Applied Psychol. Unit Camb. & Nat. Physical Laborat.

STEPHENS, Virginia Joan The Bell Surgery, York Road, Henley-on-Thames RG9 2DR Tel: 01491 843250 Fax: 01491 411295; Mole End, Crowsley Road, Lower Shiplake, Henley-on-Thames RG9 3LD Tel: 0118 940 4058 — MB BS Lond. 1978 (St. Bart.) MRCS Eng. LRCP Lond. 1978; DRCOG 1996. Specialty: Gen. Pract.

STEPHENS, Wendy Jean 57 Hartopp Road, Leicester LE2 1WG — MB ChB Leic. 1997.

STEPHENS, William Philip — MB BS Lond. 1972 (Westm.) AKC; MRCS Eng. LRCP Lond. 1972; DCH Eng. 1975; DObst RCOG 1975; MRCP (UK) 1976; MD Lond. 1982; FRCP Lond. 1991. Cons. Phys. Trafford Gen. Hosp. Davyhulme Manch. & Alexandra Hosp. Cheadle; Chief Med. Off. Friends Provident Life Off. Specialty: Gen. Med.; Diabetes. Socs: Fell. Manch. Med. Soc.; Brit. Diabetic Assn.; BMA. Prev: Sen. Regist. (Med.) Manch. Roy. Infirm.; Lect. (Med.) Univ. Manch.; Ho. Off. Westm. Hosp. Lond.

STEPHENSON, Mr Brian Mark Woodsdale, St. Brides Netherwent, Penhow, Newport NP26 3AS Tel: 01633 400850 Fax: 01633 234252 — MB BS Lond. 1983 (St. Barth.) BSc (Hons.) Lond. 1980, MB BS 1983; FRCS 1987; MSc Lond. 1992, MS 1992. Cons. Gen. & Colorect. Surg. Roy. Gwent Hosp. Newport. Specialty: Gen. Surg. Prev: Sen. Regist. (Surg.) Univ. Hosp. Wales Cardiff Roy. Infirm. & Newport Hosp.; Clin. Research Fell. (Surg.) Leeds Gen Infirm.; Regist. Rotat. (Surg.) Univ. Hosp. Wales.

STEPHENSON, Caroline Mary Elizabeth 22 The Fairway, Bar Hill, Cambridge CB3 8SR; 205 Hills Road, Cambridge CB2 2RN Tel: 01223 214925 — MB BChir Camb. 1990; BSc (Experim. Psychol.) Sussex 1980; PhD Camb. 1984; DRCOG 1993; MRCGP 1994; MRCPsych 1997. Specialty: Gen. Psychiat.; Gen. Pract.

STEPHENSON, Catherine Jane The Great Barn, Howsham, York YO60 7PH — MB ChB Ed. 1994; Dip. Of Child Health, Univ. of Otago, 1997; Dip. Of Obst, Otago, 1998.

STEPHENSON, Charles Roger Brooklea Clinic, Wick Road, Bristol BS4 4HU; Mill House, Woollard, Pensford, Bristol BS39 4HX Tel: 01761 490352 — MB ChB Ed. 1973; MRCP (UK) 1976; DRCOG 1977; MRCGP 1977.

STEPHENSON, Charmian Louise Paula 38 Lebanon Park, Twickenham TW1 3DG Email: rnorth@globalnet.co.uk — BM BCh Oxf. 1992; MA Camb. 1993; DFFP 1996; MRCGP 1996. Specialty: Gen. Pract. Socs: BMA; Mem. of RCGP. Prev: Regist. (Gen. Pract.) St. John's Health Centre Woking; Trainee GP/SHO St. Peter's Hosp. NHS Trust; Asst. GP Chiswick Health Centre ('97-'98).

STEPHENSON, Christopher John 11 Cragside, Sedgfield, Stockton-on-Tees TS21 2DU — MB ChB Sheff. 1989.

STEPHENSON, Clare 29 Parry Street, Ton Pentre, Pentre CF41 7AQ Tel: 01443 434791 — BM BS Nottm. 1995; BMedSci Nottm. 1993, BM BS 1995. SHO (Anaest.) Roy. Gwent Newport. Socs: MPS. Prev: (Anat. Demonst., Newc. Med. Sch.).; HO (Surg.) Newc.Gen.; HO (Med.) Ayr.

STEPHENSON, Clare Anne The Surgery, 1 Troy Close, Tadworth Farm, Tadworth KT20 5JE — MB BS Lond. 1980; MRCP (UK) 1983; MRCGP 1993.

STEPHENSON, Clare Judith Oxford Natural Health Centre, 3 Church Cowley Road, Oxford OX4 3JR Tel: 01865 715615 — BM BCh Oxf. 1988 (Camb. & Oxf.) MA Camb. 1982; MRCP (UK) 1991; MSc (Pub. Health Med.) Lond. 1997; (Licentiate in Acupunc.) 1998. p/t Acupunc. in Private Pract.; Lect. in Clin. Med., Coll. of Integrated Chinese Med., Reading. Specialty: Gen. Pract.; Acupunc.; Pub. Health Med. Special Interest: Acupunc. Socs: Brit. Med. Acupunc. Soc.; Brit. Acupunc. Counc.; BMA. Prev: Specialist Regist. (Pub. Health Med.) Oxf.; Trainee GP Oxf.; SHO (Psychiat.) Tindal Centre, Aylesbury.

STEPHENSON, Daniel Timothy 193 Popes Lane, London W5 4NH Tel: 020 8579 0592 — MB ChB Manch. 1995; BSc (Hons.) Manch. 1992. SHO (Med.) Northern Gen. Hosp. Sheff. Specialty: Accid. & Emerg. Prev: SHO (A & E) Hope Hosp. Salford.

STEPHENSON, David Kenneth Department of Anaesthesia, Derbyshire Royal Infirmary NHS Trust, London Road, Derby DE1 2QY Tel: 01332 347141 — MB ChB Manch. 1971; FFA RCS Eng. 1977. Staff Grade Anaesth. Derbysh. Roy. Infirm.; Emerit. Cons. Anaesth. N. Notts. HA. Specialty: Anaesth. Socs: Assn. Anaesth. GB & Irel.; PANG; BSOA. Prev: Cons. Anaesth. & Pain Control. Centr. Notts. HA; Lect. (Anaesth.) Manch. Univ.; Sen. Regist. (Anaesth.) Manch. AHA (T).

STEPHENSON, Deborah Angela Lilly House, Priestley Road, Basingstoke RG24 9NL Tel: 01256 315000 Fax: 01256 775719 Email: debs@lilly.com — MB BS Lond. 1985 (St Geo.) MRCPsych 1990; MFPM RCP Lond. 2002; FFPM RCP Lond. 2004. Sen. Clin. Research Phys., Eli Lilly & Co., Basingstoke; Head HTA Strategy. Specialty: Pharmaceutical Medicine. Prev: Clin. Research Phys. Eli Lilly & Co., Basingstoke.; Hon. Assoc. Psychiat. Chelsea & Westm. Hosp.; Europ. Clin. Research Phys. Lilly Research Centre Windlesham Surrey.

STEPHENSON, Geoffrey Victoria Road Health Centre, Victoria Road, Washington NE37 2PU Tel: 0191 416 2578 Fax: 0191 416 6091 Email: geoff.stephenson@gp-a89617.nhs.uk; Whyteleafe, 10 Underhill Road, Cleadon Village, Sunderland SR6 7RS — MB BS Newc. 1974 (Newc. u. Tyne) MRCGP 1978. Bd. Mem. Sunderland Teachg. PCT; Clin. Governance Lead, PEC Mem., Sunderland Teachg. PCT. Specialty: Gen. Pract.

STEPHENSON, Iain 6 Granby Croft, Bakewell DE45 1ET; 4 Langton House Cottages, Main St, Tur Langton, Leicester LE8 0PJ Email: istephen@globalnet.co.uk — MB BChir Camb. 1993 (Addenbrookes) BA (Hons.) Camb. 1991; MRCP Ed. 1997. Specialist Regist. (Infec. Dis.s) Leicester Roy. Infirm. Specialty: Infec. Dis.; HIV Med.; Gen. Med. Socs: Brit. Infect. Soc. Prev: Regist. (Infec. Dis.s) N. Staffs. Hosp. Stoke on Trent.

STEPHENSON, James Reginald 4 Highlands, Ashtead KT21 2SD — MB BS Lond. 1980; MSc Lond. 1986, MB BS 1980; MA Oxf. 1985; MRCPath 1986. Cons. Med. Microbiol. St Helier NHS Trust Carshalton. Specialty: Med. Microbiol.

STEPHENSON, Jane Tracy Church View Surgery, Market Hill, Hedon, Hull HU12 8JE Tel: 01482 899348 — MB ChB Birm. 1993; MRCGP (distinchin); MRCGP 1993. GP Regist. Ch. View Surg. E. Yorks. GP Princip.-. Specialty: Gen. Pract. Socs: MRCGP.

STEPHENSON, Jennifer Ann Walkley House Medical Centre, 23 Greenhow Street, Sheffield S6 3TN Tel: 0114 234 3716; Stannington Medical Centre, Uppergate Road, Stannington, Sheffield S6 6BX Tel: 0114 234 5303 Fax: 0114 234 3113 — MB ChB Sheff. 1981; DCH RCP Lond. 1984; Cert. Family Plann. JCC 1984; DRCOG 1985; MRCGP 1985. Trainer (Gen. Pract.) Sheff. VTS specialising in flexible train.; Mem. Sheff. LMC; GP Represen. Cervical Cytol. Working Party; GP Represen. Local Diabetes Servs. Advis. Gp. Specialty: Gen. Pract. Socs: BMA; RCGP. Prev: Trainee GP/SHO Barnsley VTS; Ho. Off. (Med. & Dermat.) Roy. Hallamsh. Hosp. Sheff.; Ho. Off. (Orthop.) North. Gen. Hosp. Sheff.

STEPHENSON, Jeremy David Fairfield Medical Centre, Lower Road, Bookham, Leatherhead KT23 4DH Tel: 01372 378166 Fax: 01372 374734 — BM BS Nottm. 1989.

STEPHENSON, Professor John Burdett Primmer Fraser of Allander Neurosciences Unit, Royal Hospital Sick Children, Yorkhill, Glasgow G3 8SJ Tel: 0141 201 0141 Fax: 0141 201 9270; 27 Charles Crescent, Lenzie, Glasgow G66 5HH Tel: 0141 776 5589 Email: john@jbpstephenson.com — (Oxf. & St. Thos.) BM BCh Oxf. 1960; MA Oxf. 1960; DCH Eng. 1965; FRCP Lond. 1979, M 1965; FRCP Glas. 1984, M 1982; DM Oxf. 1991; FRCPCH 1996; HonFRCPCH 2000. Hon. Sen. Research Fell., Div. of Developm. Med., Univ. of Glas.; Hon. Prof. Med. Paediat. Neurol. Univ. Glas. Not Retd. Specialty: Paediat. Neurol. Socs: Assn. Brit. Neurol.; Brit. Paediat. Neurol. Assn.; Internat. Child Neurol. Assn. Prev: Retd. Cons. Paediat. Neurol. Roy. Hosp. Sick Childr. Glas.; Sen. Regist. (Med. Paediat. & Neurol.) Roy. Hosp. Sick Childr. Glas.; Fell. (Neurol.) Hosp. Sick Childr. Toronto, Canada.

STEPHENSON, John David Green Lane Surgery, 2 Green Lane, Belper DE56 1BZ Tel: 01773 823521 Fax: 01773 821954 — MB ChB Leeds 1986; DCH RCP Lond. 1991; DRCOG 1992. Prev: SHO (Paediat.) York Dist. Hosp.

STEPHENSON, Judith Mary UCL Medical School, Dept STD, Mortimer Market Centre, Off Capper Street, London WC1E 6AU Email: jstephen@gum.ucl.ac.uk; 66 Trinity Church Square, London SE1 4HT — MD Lond. 1994; MSc 1991, MB BS 1985; MRCP (UK) 1988; MA Oxf. 1993; FFPHM RCP (UK) 1998. Sen. Lect. (Epidemiol.) UCL Med. Sch. Lond. Specialty: Epidemiol.

STEPHENSON, Kay Ann 26 Tansy Close, Guildford GU4 7XN — MB ChB Liverp. 1996.

STEPHENSON, Kenneth Dowson (retired) 185 Coniscliffe Road, Darlington DL3 8DE Tel: 01325 468247 — MB BS Durh. 1952; DA Eng. 1957. Hosp. Pract. (Anaesth.) Darlington Memor. Hosp. Prev: Ho. Phys. & Ho. Surg. Roy. Vict. Infirm. Newc.

STEPHENSON, Kevin Silksworth Health Centre, Silksworth, Sunderland SR3 2AN Tel: 0191 521 0252 — MB ChB Leeds 1986.

STEPHENSON, Lauren Kristina Oak Lodge Medical Centre, 234 Burnt Oak Broadway, Edgware HA8 0AP Tel: 020 8952 1202 Fax: 020 8381 1156; 70 Friern Barnet Lane, Friern Barnet, London N11 3NB — MB BChir Camb. 1988 (Cambridge) MA Camb. 1990; DRCOG 1992; MRCGP 1992. Prev: Trainee GP/SHO Edgware Gen. Hosp. VTS; Ho. Off. (Med.) QE II Hosp. Welwyn Garden City; Ho. Off. (Surg.) Newmarket Gen. Hosp.

STEPHENSON, Margaret Anne (retired) 185 Coniscliffe Road, Darlington DL3 8DE Tel: 01325 468247 — MB BS Durh. 1954 (Newc.) Clin. Asst. (Venereol.) Darlington Memor. Hosp.; Clin. Asst. in ENT Darlington Memor. Hosp. Prev: Sen. Surgic. Ho. Off. & Ho. Phys. Darlington Memor. Hosp.

STEPHENSON, Matthew Thomas 1 Blackheath Park, London SE3 9RN — MB BS Lond. 1987.

STEPHENSON, Patricia Mary Central Health Clinic, Mulberry St., Sheffield S1 Tel: 0114 271 6790; 33 Dore Road, Sheffield S17 3NA Tel: 0114 235 2508 — MB ChB Leeds 1975; DCH RCP Lond. 1977; DFFP 1994. Clin. Med. Off. (Family Plann. & Reproduc. Health) Sheff. Specialty: Family Plann. & Reproduc. Health.

STEPHENSON, Paul Seamus Christmas Maltings Surgery, Camps Road, Haverhill CB9 8HF Tel: 01440 702203 Fax: 01440 712198; Wheel Cottage, The St, Great Wratting, Haverhill CB9 7HQ — BM BCh Oxf. 1987; MA Oxf. 1984; DRCOG 1989; DGM RCP Lond. 1990; MRCGP 1991. Editorial Bd. Mem. Primary Care Resp. Jl. Specialty: Gen. Pract. Prev: Trustee, Nat. Asthma Campaign.

STEPHENSON, Peter (retired) Flat One, Dockendale Hall, Whickham, Newcastle upon Tyne NE16 4EN — MB BCh Witwatersrand 1952; FRCP Lond. 1974, M 1960. Cons. Phys. Gateshead & Dist. Hosp. Gp. Prev: Research Asst. Cardiol. Roy. Vict. Infirm. Newc.

STEPHENSON, Philip Bernard Ommanney Eynsham Medical Group, Eynsham Medical Centre, Conduit Lane, Witney OX29 4QB Tel: 01865 881206 Fax: 01865 881342 — MB BChir Camb. 1984 (Cambridge and St Thomas') MA Camb. 1985; DCH RCP Lond. 1987; DRCOG 1987; MRCGP 1988. Specialty: Gen. Pract. Prev: Ho. Surg. St. Thos. Hosp. Lond.; Cas. Off. Poole Gen. Hosp.; Trainee GP Reading VTS.

STEPHENSON, Ralph Harry, TD Rowcroft Medical Centre, Rowcroft Retreat, Stroud GL5 3BE Tel: 01453 764471 Fax: 01453 755247 — MB BS Lond. 1967 (King's Coll. Hosp.) MRCS Eng. LRCP Lond. 1967; DObst RCOG 1969; DA Eng. 1973. Anaesth. Stroud Gen. Hosp. Prev: SHO (Anaesth.) Gloucester Roy. Hosp.; SHO (Obst.) Redhill Gen. Hosp.; Ho. Surg. & Ho. Phys. King's Coll. Hosp.

STEPHENSON, Richard Hudson Bicester Health Centre, Coker Close, Bicester OX26 6AT Tel: 01869 249333 Fax: 01869 320314; Upper Aynho Grounds, Aynho, Banbury OX17 3AY Tel: 01869 810607 Fax: 01869 320314 — MB BChir Camb. 1967 (St. Thos.) MA, MB Camb. 1967, BChir 1966; DMRD Eng. 1969; DObst RCOG 1969; FRCGP 1997. Socs: Brit. Inst. Radiol.; RCGP. Prev: Regist. (Radiol.) St. Thos. Hosp. Lond.; Ho. Off. St. Peter's Hosp. Chertsey; Ho. Off. (Surg.) Lambeth Hosp.

STEPHENSON, Mr Richard Neal Department of Urology, Western General Hospital, Crewe Road S., Edinburgh EH4 2XU Tel: 0131 537 1581; 79 Orchard Brae Avenue, Edinburgh EH4 2UR — MB ChB Bristol 1982; FRCS Eng. 1988; FRCS (Urol.) 1994. Sen. Regist. (Urol.) Lothian HB. Specialty: Urol. Socs: Assoc. Mem. BAUS. Prev: Lect. (Urol.) Univ. Edin.; Research Regist. (Renal Transpl.) Univ. Sheff.; Regist. (Urol.) Princess Roy. Hosp. Hull.

STEPHENSON, Robert John Toft Road Surgery, Toft Road, Knutsford WA16 9DX Tel: 01565 632681 — MB BS Lond. 1983 (Roy. Free (Clinical) Camb. Univ. (Pre-clinical)) BA Camb. 1980; MRCGP 1988; DRCOG 1988; D.Occ Med. RCP Lond. 1995. GP Partner Toft Rd. Surg. Knutsford Chesh.; Company Doct. Ilford Mobberley. Prev: Trainee GP Macclesfield VTS.

STEPHENSON, Robert Vivian (retired) Pentland House, Bradford Road, Sherborne DT9 6BP Tel: 01935 814173 — (Camb. & St. Thos.) MB BChir Camb. 1957; BA Camb. 1957; FRCOG 1974, M 1961; MA Camb 1997. Prev: Cons. O & G Yeovil Dist. Hosp. & Yeatman Hosp. Sherborne.

STEPHENSON, Roger Edwin Fair Park Surgery, Fair Park, Bow, Crediton EX17 6EY Tel: 01363 82333 Fax: 01363 82841 — MB BS Lond. 1980; MA Camb. 1981; MRCGP 1987.

STEPHENSON, Rosalind The Gables, Rodridge Lane, Station Town, Wingate TS28 5HB Tel: 01429 837648 — MB ChB Glas. 1996. SHO (Psychiat.). Specialty: Gen. Psychiat.

STEPHENSON, Ruth Nicole Anaesthetics Department, Aberdeen Royal Infirmary, Aberdeen AB25 2ZN Tel: 01224 681818; 83 Fountainhall Road, Aberdeen AB15 4EA — MB ChB Ed. 1987; FFA RCSI 1992; FRCA 1993. Sen. Regist. (Anaesth.) Aberd. Roy. Infirm. Specialty: Anaesth.

STEPHENSON, Sarah Jane Stanley Road Surgery, 204 Stanley Road, Bootle L20 3EW Tel: 01676 41557 — MB BS Lond. 1983; DRCOG 1986; MRCGP 1988. GP Liverp. Specialty: Paediat.

STEPHENSON, Professor Terence John Dean's Office, Faculty of Medicine & Health Sciences, The Medical School, Queens Medical Centre, Nottingham NG7 2UH Tel: 0115 970 9380 Fax: 0115 970 9974 Email: terence.stephenson@nottingham.ac.uk — BM BCh Oxf. 1983; BSc (1st cl. Hons.) Bristol 1979; MRCP (UK) 1986; DM Nottm. 1992; FRCP Lond. 1995; FRCPCH Lond. 1997. Dean of Fac. of Med. & Health Sci., Nottm.; Prof. of Child Health, Univ. of Nottm.; Hon. Cons. Paediat., Queens Hosp. Centre, Nottm. Specialty: Paediat. Socs: Neonat. Soc.; Paediat. Research Soc.; Roy. Coll. of Paediat. and Child Health. Prev: Sen. Lect. & Lect. (Child Health) Univ. Nottm.; SHO Nat. Hosp. Nerv. Dis. Lond.; Ho. Phys. Profess. Med. Unit Oxf.

STEPHENSON, Timothy John Royal Hallamshire Hospital, Department of Histopathology, Glossop Road, Sheffield S10 2JF Tel: 0114 271 2213 Fax: 0114 271 2200 Email: tim.stephenson@sth.nhs.uk — MB ChB Sheff. 1981; MA Camb. 1982, BA (1st cl. Hons.) 1978; MB ChB (Hons.) Sheff. 1981; FRCPath 1996, M 1988; MD Sheff. 1995; Dip. Health Serv. Mgt. Open 1996; MBA Open 1999. Cons. Sheff.Teachg.. Hosps. NHS Foundat. Trust & Hon. Clin. Sen. Lect. Sheff. Univ.; Clin. Director Laborat. Med. Diectorate Sheff. Teachg. Hosps.; Edr. Bull. Roy. Coll. Patholgoists Lond. Specialty: Histopath. Socs: Fell. Roy. Soc. Med.; Assn. Clin. Path.; Internat. Acad. Path. Prev: Sen. Lect. (Path.) Univ. Sheff.; Ho. Off. Profess. Med. & Profess. Surg. Units Roy. Hallamsh. Hosp. Sheff.

STEPHENSON, Mr Timothy Patrick Department of Urology, University Hospital of Wales, Heath Park, Cardiff CF14 4XW — MB BS Lond. 1963; FRCS Eng. 1970; MS Lond. 1977.

STEPHENSON, Tony 12 The Cloisters, Newcastle upon Tyne NE7 7LS — MB BS Lond. 1986; MRCGP 1990.

STEPHENSON, Trevor Buteland Terrace Health Centre, Buteland Terrace, Newbiggin-by-the-Sea NE64 6NS Tel: 01670 816796 Fax: 01670 818797; 15 Southgate Wood, Southgate, Morpeth NE61 2EN — MB BS Durh. 1965 (Newc.) DCH RCPS Glas. 1969. Socs: BMA. Prev: SHO (O & G) & (Paediat.) W. Cumbld. Hosp.

STEPHENSON, Victoria Jane Doghurst Cottage, Doghurst Lane, Chipstead, Coulsdon CR5 3PL Tel: 01737 556548; Doghurst Cottage, Doghurst Lane, Chipstead, Coulsdon CR5 3PL — MB ChB Leeds 1998.

STEPP-SCHUH, Kerstin Kirchroder, Tremorvah Crescent, Truro TR1 1NL Tel: 01872 271014 Email: steppschuh@compuserve.com — State Exam Med. Bonn 1991. Specialty: Gen. Surg.

STEPTOE, Adele Marjorie Ashington House, Ashington Way, Westlea, Swindon SN5 7XY Tel: 01793 614840 Fax: 01793 491191 — MB BCh Wales 1987 (Univ. Wales Coll. Med.) DRCOG 1992; DGM Lond. 1992; MRCGP 1993. GP Princip. Socs: BMA. Prev: Trainee GP Trowbridge; Trainee GP/SHO Roy. United Hosp. Bath; GP Princip. Cheltenham.

STERA, Hanna 131 Eastcote Road, Ruislip HA4 8BJ — LMSSA Lond. 1993.

STERGIDES, Anthimos Char Scartho Medical Centre, 26 Waltham Road, Grimsby DN33 2QA Tel: 01472 871747 Fax: 01472 276050; 7 Scartho Road, Grimsby DN33 2AB Tel: 01472 878651 — Ptychio Iatrikes Athens, Greece 1973; Ptychio Iatrikis Athens, Greece 1973. Clin. Asst. (Gastroenterol.), Grimsby Dist. Gen. Hosp. Prev: Regist. & SHO (Gen. Med.) Grimsby Dist. Gen. Hosp.; SHO (Med. & ITU.) Staffs. Gen. Infirm.

STERLAND, John Helmerow 23 Juniper Gardens, Shenley, Radlett WD7 9LA — MB BS Lond. 1982 (Roy. Free) Docc Med 2001. Occupational Physician IBC Motors, Luton; SpR, Kings Coll. Hosp. Specialty: Dentistry/Orthodontics. Prev: GP London Colney; Forensic Medical Examiner; SHO (Geriat., Orthop. & Cas.) Maidstone Hosp.

STERLAND, Mairi Elizabeth (retired) Amberside, Pentrich, Ripley, Derby DE5 3RH Tel: 01773 743216 — MB ChB Aberd. 1949. Prev: Ho. Surg. O & G St. Martin's Hosp. Bath.

STERLING, Graham Murray (retired) General Hospital, Tremona Road, Southampton SO16 6YD Tel: 023 8077 7222; Vermont House, Withers Lane, East Boldre, Brockenhurst SO42 7WX Tel: 01590 612378 — MRCS Eng. LRCP Lond. 1960 (St. Geo.) MD Camb. 1969, MB 1961, BChir 1960; FRCP Lond. 1977, M 1964. Cons. Phys. Soton. Univ. Hosps. Trust; Hon. Clin. Sen. Lect. (Med.) Univ. Soton. Prev: Sen. Lect. (Med.) Univ. Soton.

STERLING, (IJ) Nuala, CBE Southampton General Hospital, Southampton SO16 6YD Tel: 023 8079 4656 Fax: 023 8079 6965; Vermont House, Withers Lane, East Boldre, Brockenhurst SO42 7WX Tel: 01590 612378 — MB BS Lond. 1960 (St. Geo.) MRCS Eng. LRCP Lond. 1960; FRCP Lond. 1982, M 1971. Cons. Phys. Emerit. Geriat. Med. Soton. Univ. Hosp. Trust; Mem. Independant review pannel for advertising of Med.s 2000; Vice Chairm. S. RAC (Distinc. Awards) 2000-03. Specialty: Gen. Med. Socs: Med. Wom. Federat. (Pres. 1989-90) & Brit. Geriat. Soc. (Counc. Mem. 1987-89). Prev: Mem. (Ex-Chairm.) Standing Med. Advisory Comm.; Lect. (Geriat. Med.) Univ. Soton.; Lect. (Med.) Univ. Calif. San Francisco, USA.

STERLING, Jane Carolyn Department of Dermatology, Box 46, Addenbrooke's Hospital, Hills Road, Cambridge CB2 2QQ Tel: 01223 216501 Fax: 01223 216863 Email: jane.sterling@addenbrookes.nhs.uk; Downing College, Cambridge CB2 1DQ — MB BChir Camb. 1978; PhD Camb. 1991, MA 1980; FRCP Lond. 1997, M 1981. Lect. (Dermat.) Camb. Univ. & Hon. Cons. Dermat. Addenbrooke's Hosp. Camb. Specialty: Dermat. Special Interest: Viral Skin Disease; Vulval Skin Disease. Socs: Brit. Assn. Dermat.; Soc. Gen. Microbiol.; Brit. Soc. Investig. Dermat. Prev: Hon. Sen. Lect. St. John's Inst. Dermat. Lond.; Hon. Cons. Dermat. St. John's Dermat. Centre St. Thos. Hosp. Lond.; MRC Clin. Scientist Fell. Camb.

STERLING, Victor James (retired) Dromore, 23 Larchfield Park, Newcastle BT33 0BB Tel: 028437 23668 — (Belf.) MB BCh BAO Belf. 1942.

STERN, Adam Bernard The Wapping Health Centre, 22 Wapping Lane, London Tel: 0207 481 9376 — MB BS Lond. 1988 (King' Coll. Lond.) MRCGP 1996. Prev: Trainee GP Lond.; SHO (Paediat., O & G & Geriat. Med.) Newham Gen. Hosp.

STERN, Colin Michael Macleod St. Thomas's Hospital, London SE1 7EH Tel: 020 7928 9292 Fax: 020 7960 5631 Email: colin.stern@gstt.sthames.nhs.uk; 24 Clearwater Place, Long Ditton, Surbiton KT6 4ET Tel: 020 8398 2676 — (St. Thos.) MA, MB Camb. 1967, BChir 1966; FRCP Lond. 1983, M 1969; DCH Eng. 1970; PhD Lond. 1978; FRCPCH 1997. Cons. Paediat. St. Thos. Hosp. Lond.; Assoc. Regional Dean of Postgrad. Med., Lond. Specialty: Paediat. Special Interest: Fatigue Syndrome; Paediatric Immunol. Socs: Roy. Soc. of Med. Lond., Chairman Acad. Bd. Prev: Sen. Lect. (Immunol.) Roy. Postgrad. Med. Sch. Lond.; Hon. Cons. (Paediat.) Hammersmith Hosp. Lond.; Postgrad. Subdean UMDS Guy's & St. Thos. Hosp. Lond.

STERN, David Michael Manor Surgery, Osler Road, Headington, Oxford OX3 9BP Tel: 01865 762535 — MRCS Eng. LRCP Lond. 1969 (Lond. Hosp.) BSc Lond. 1966, MB BS 1969; MRCGP 1984; FRCGP 1999. GP Headington; Clin. Tutor (Gen. Pract.) Univ. Oxf.

STERN, Mr David Michael, CBE (retired) 32 Thames Point, Fairways, Teddington TW11 9PP — MB BChir Camb. 1929; MRCS

Eng. LRCP Lond. 1928; FRCS Eng. 1932; FRCOG 1942. Prev: Prof. (Obst.) Univ. Khartoum.

STERN, Gerald Malcolm Woolavington Wing, The Middlesex Hospital, Mortimer St., London W1T 3AA Tel: 020 7376 0627 Fax: 020 7937 0438 — MB BS Lond. 1954 (Lond. Hosp.) FRCP Lond. 1970, M 1958; MD Lond. 1965. Emerit. Cons. Neurol. Univ. Coll. Lond. Hosp. & Nat. Hosp. for Neurol. & Neurosurg. Qu. Sq. Lond. Specialty: Neurol. Socs: Assn. Brit. Neurols. & Assn. Phys. GB & Irel. Prev: 1st Asst. Dept. Neurol. Univ. Newc.; Sen. Regist. (Neurol.) Lond. Hosp.; Research Assoc. (Neurol.) Columbia Univ., New York.

STERN, Gillian 42 Southwood Avenue, London N6 5RZ Tel: 020 8348 1351 Fax: 020 8348 1357 — MB ChB Witwatersrand 1971; BSc (Med.) Witwatersrand 1967; MRCPsych 1989. Cons. Child & Adolesc. Psychiat. Haringey Health Care, Lond. Specialty: Child & Adolesc. Psychiat. Socs: BMA; Roy. Coll. Psychiat.; Assoc. Brit. Assn. Psychotherapists.

STERN, Glenn Marvin The Surgery, 939 Green Lanes, Winchmore Hill, London N21 2PB Tel: 020 8360 2228 Fax: 020 8360 5702 — MB BS Lond. 1969 (Univ. Coll. Hosp.) BSc Lond. 1966; DCH Eng. 1971; MRCP (UK) 1973; MRCP (UK) 1973; DObst RCOG 1973. GP Princip. Stern, Patel & Noor Lond.; Treasury Med. Off. Specialty: Gen. Med. Socs: Roy. Soc. Med. Prev: Ho. Phys. Evelina Childr. Hosp. (Guy's Hosp.) Lond.; SHO (Med.) Poole Gen. Hosp.; SHO (O & G) Whittington Hosp. Lond.

STERN, Professor Harold (retired) 16 Hill Rise, Hampstead Garden Suburb, London NW11 6NA Tel: 020 8458 3966 — MB ChB Glas. 1946; PhD Glas. 1953; FRCPath 1971, M 1964. Emerit. Prof. Virol. Univ. Lond. & St. Geo. Hosp. Med. Sch. Prev: Cons. Virol. St. Geo. Hosp. Lond.

STERN, Jeremy Samuel St George's Hospital, Department of Neurology, Ground Floor, Atkinson Morley's Wing, Blackshaw Road, London SW17 0QT Tel: 020 8725 4631 Email: jeremy.stern@stgeorges.nhs.uk — MB BChir Camb. 1991 (Camb. & Univ. Coll. Lond.) MA Camb. 1992; MRCP (UK) 1994; DHMSA 1995. Cons. Neurol. Frimley Pk. Hosp. Surrey; Cons. Neurol. St Geo. Hosp. Lond. Specialty: Neurol. Special Interest: Movement Disorders.

STERN, Julian Michael St Marks Hospital, Watford Rd, Harrow HA1 3UJ Tel: 020 8235 4089 Fax: 020 8235 4001 Email: julian.stern@nwlh.nhs.uk — MB ChB Cape Town 1985 (Univ. of Cape Town) MRCPsych 1991; (Full Mem., Lincoln centre for Psychother.) Lond. 2004. Cons. (Psychother.) St. Marks Hosp. Lond. Specialty: Psychother. Prev: Cons. (Psychother.) Roy. Lond. Hosp.; Sen. Regist. Maudsley Hosp.

STERN, Morag Campbell 23 Stoughton Drive S., Oadby, Leicester LE2 2RJ Tel: 0116 270 7978 — MB ChB St. And. 1966 (Dundee) MD (Hons.) Dundee 1971; MRCP (UK) 1973; MFPHM RCP (UK) 1992. Cons. Pub. Health Med. & Med. Adviser Coventry HA. Specialty: Pub. Health Med. Prev: Sen. Regist. (Pub. Health Med.) Trent RHA.; Asst. Phys. Midl. Asthma & Allergy Treatm. Centre Derby; GP Leicester.

STERN, Myra 10 Beaufort Drive, London NW11 6BU — MB ChB Cape Town 1985; MRCP (UK) 1992; PhD Cape Town 1992. Sen. Regist. & Research Fell. Roy. Brompton Hosp. Nat. Heart & Lung Inst. Specialty: Respirat. Med.

STERN, Peter Max 16 High Street, Great Baddow, Chelmsford CM2 7HQ; 14 Lister Tye, Chelmsford CM2 9LS — MB BS Lond. 1984; MRCGP 1990.

STERN, Richard Stephen St. Anthony's Hospital, London Road, North Cheam, Sutton SM3 9DW Tel: 020 8337 6691 Fax: 020 8337 0816; Springfield Hospital, 61 Glenburnie Road, London SW17 7DJ — MB BS Lond. 1967 (Char. Cross) MRCS Eng. LRCP Lond. 1967; DPM Eng. 1970; FRCPsych 1986, M 1972; MD Lond. 1972. Cons. Psychiatrist, Priory Hosp., Roehampton, London. Specialty: Gen. Psychiat. Prev: Cons. Psychiatrist, South West Lond. & St. George's Mental Health Trust, Lond.; Sen. Lect., Institute of Psychiatry, Lond.

STERN, Sidney The Chalthorpe Clinic, 4 Arthur Road, Edgbaston, Birmingham B15 2UL Tel: 021 455 7585; 3 Oakwood Avenue, Borehamwood WD6 1SP Tel: 020 8953 9140 — MB ChB Glas. 1957; FRCOG 1981, M 1966. Specialty: Obst. & Gyn. Socs: Brit. Menopause Soc. Prev: Vis. Cons. Dept. Gyn. Manor Ho. Hosp. Golders Green; Sen. Cons. O & G Murtala Mohammed Hosp. Kano, Nigeria; Regist. (O & G) Solihull & E. Birm. Hosp.

STERN, Simon Carl Maxim East Surrey Hospital, Deparment of Haematology, Canada Avenue, Redhill RH1 5RH Tel: 01737 768511 Ext: 6473 Fax: 01737 231694 Email: simon.stern@sash.nhs.uk — MB BS Lond. 1987 (St Geo.) MRCP (UK) 1992; MRCPath 1998. Cons. Haematologist, Surrey and Sussex Healthcare NHS Trust, E. Surrey Hosp., Redhill Surrey, RH1 5RH; Cons. Haematologist, BUPA Gatwick Pk. Hosp., Horley, Surrey. Specialty: Haematology. Special Interest: Blood Transfusion; Haemato-Oncology. Socs: Brit. Soc. for Haemat.; UK Myeloma Forum; Brit. Blood Transfus. Soc. Prev: Sen. Regist. (Haemat.) Chelsea & Westminster Hosp. Lond.; Sen. Regist. (Haemat.) Hammersmith Hosp. Lond.; Lect. & Hon. Sen. Regist. (Haemat.) Char. Cross Hosp. Lond.

STERN, Steven Richard The Surgery, Brede Lane, Sedlescombe, Battle TN33 0PW Tel: 01424 870225 — MB ChB Bristol 1978; BSc (Hons.) Bristol 1975, MB ChB 1978; MRCP (UK) Paediat. 1982; DRCOG 1988; Cert. Family Plann. JCC 1988. Specialty: Paediat. Prev: Trainee GP Hastings VTS; SHO (O & G) Buchanan Hosp. Hastings; Sen. Regist./Regist. (Paediat.) Roy. Hosp. Sick Childr. Edin.

STERNBERG, Alexander Justin — MB ChB Bristol 1991 (Bristol University) BSc Bristol 1988; MRCP (UK) 1996; MRCPath 2001. MRC Clin. Research Fell. Weatherall Inst. Molecular Med. Oxf. Specialty: Haematology. Prev: Specialist Regist. (Haemat.) John Radcliffe Hosp. Oxf.; SHO (Haemato-Oncol.) Roy. Marsden Hosp. Fulham Rd.; SHO (Gen. Med.) Taunton.

STERNBERG, Simon 187 Mendip House, Market Square, Edmonton, London N9 0TD Tel: 020 8803 9638 — MB BS Lond. 1948 (Lond. Hosp.) MRCS Eng. LRCP Lond. 1948. Assoc. Specialist St. Michael's Hosp. Enfield. Prev: Med. Asst. St. Michael's Hosp. Enfield; SHO Infec. Dis. & Chest Units Plaistow Hosp.; Capt. RAMC.

STERNDALE BENNETT, (Winifred) Anne (retired) E12 Tower Lane, Bearstead, Maidstone ME14 4JJ Tel: 01622 737921 Fax: 01622 737921 — MB BS Lond. 1947 (King's Coll. Hosp.) MRCS Eng. LRCP Lond. 1947; DO Eng. 1953. Prev: Ophth. Kent CC.

STERNE, Adrian Patrick The Country Medical Centre, 122 Ballinlea Road, Armoy, Ballymoney BT53 8TY Tel: 028 2075 1266 Fax: 028 2075 1122; 4 Semicock Road, Ballymoney BT53 6PX Tel: 01265 665604 — MB BCh BAO Belf. 1984; DRCOG 1987; MRCGP Ed. 1988; DCH RCPSI 1989.

STERNE, Austin John 127 Swanshurst Lane, Birmingham B13 0AS — MB ChB Birm. 1991; ChB Birm. 1991.

STERRY, Mark Julian Gwyn Grove Road Surgery, 3 Grove Road, Solihull B91 2AG Tel: 0121 705 1105 Fax: 0121 711 4098 — MB BCh Wales 1990 (UWCM) DFFP 1993; T(GP) 1994; MRCGP 1994; DRCOG 1995; Dip. Palliat. Med. 1997. Med. Off. Marie Curie Centre, Warren Pearl, Solihull. Specialty: Palliat. Med. Prev: Trainee GP/SHO Wolverhampton VTS.

STEUER, Alan Department of Rheumatology, Charing Cross Hospital, Fulham Palace Road, London W6 8RF; 49 Foscote Road, London NW4 3SE — MB BS Lond. 1991; BSc Lond. 1988; MRCP (UK) 1994. Specialist Regist. (Rheum. & Gen. Med.) Char. Cross Hosp. Specialty: Rheumatol.; Gen. Med.

STEUER, Lara Rachelle 49 Foscote Road, London NW4 3SE — MB BChir Camb. 1992.

STEVEN, Mr Alastair Matthew 6 Beaton Lane, Dundonald, Kilmarnock KA2 9JS Email: alastair.steven@virgin.net — MB ChB Glas. 1992.

STEVEN, Carolyn Margaret 7 Dora Road, London SW19 7EZ Tel: 020 8947 6314 Fax: 020 8947 6314 — (Glas.) MB ChB Glas. 1968; DA Eng. 1971; FFA RCS Eng. 1976. Cons. (Anaesth.) St. Helier Hosp. Carshalton; Hon. Sen. Lect. St. Geo. Hosp. Med. Sch. Lond. Specialty: Anaesth. Socs: Obst. Anaesth. Assn.; Brit. Assn. Day Surg.; BMA & Assn. Anaesth. Gt. Brit. & Irel. Prev: Sen. Regist. (Anaesth.) St. Thos. Hosp. Lond.; Regist. (Anaesth.) Glas. Roy. Infirm. & St. Thos. Hosp. Lond.

STEVEN, Colin Alexander 9 Ainslie Close, Aylestone Hill, Hereford HR1 1JH — MB BS Lond. 1968. Specialty: Occupat. Health. Prev: Med. Off. Brit. Petroleum Abu Dhabi Marine Areas, V.A.E.; Med. Off. Lockheed Aircraft Internat. Riyadh, Saudi Arabia.

STEVEN, Grace Campbell (retired) 29 Strathview Terrace, Balfron, Glasgow G63 0PU — MB ChB Glas. 1949.

STEVEN, Jenny The Spa Medical Practice, Ombersley Sweet East, Droitwich Spa GL9 8RD — MB ChB Liverp. 1992.

STEVEN, John Douglas Stirling Royal Infirmary, Stirling FK8 2AU Tel: 01786 434000 Email: john.steven@fvah.scot.nhs.uk; 10 Dargai

Terrace, Dunblane FK15 0AU Tel: 01786 823664 Email: john.steven@fvah.scot.nhs.uk — MB ChB Ed. 1970; FRCOG 1989, M 1976. Cons. (O & G) Stirling Roy. Infirm. Specialty: Obst. & Gyn. Prev: Sen. Regist. (O & G) Ninewells Hosp. Dundee; Regist. (O & G) West. Gen. Hosp. Edin.

STEVEN, John Mark 47A Roman Road, Bearsden, Glasgow G61 2QP — MB ChB Glas. 1992.

STEVEN, Karen 2 Brora Road, Bishopbriggs, Glasgow G64 1HX — MB ChB Glas. 1990.

STEVEN, Malcolm Monteith Raigmore Hospital, Inverness IV2 3UJ Tel: 01463 704000 Fax: 01463 705640 — MB ChB Aberd. 1974; MRCP (UK) 1977; MD Aberd. 1985; FRCP Glas. 1988; FRCP Ed. 1995. Cons. Phys. (Med. & Rheum.) Highland Acute Hosps. Trust; Hon. Clin. Sen. Lect. Univ. Aberd. Specialty: Rheumatol. Socs: (Counc.) Brit. Soc. of Rheum.; Brit. Soc. of Rheum.; Scott. Soc. Phys. Prev: Sen. Regist. Centre for Rheum. Dis. Glas.; Regist. (Gen. Med.) Aberd. Teach. Hosps.; Regist. (Gen. Med.) Clin. Research Unit Walter & Eliza Hall Inst. Med. Research Melbourne.

STEVEN, Neil Matthew Institute for Cancer Studies, University of Birmingham, Edgbaston, Birmingham B15 2TA Tel: 0961 199219 Fax: 0121 414 3263 Email: n.m.steven@bham.ac.uk; 12 Elmcroft Road, Birmingham B26 1PJ Tel: 0121 784 8677 — MB BS Lond. 1986; BA (Hons.) Camb. 1983; MRCP (UK) 1990; DTM & H RCP Lond. 1993; PhD 1998; PhD Birm. 1998. MRC Clin. Scientist. Inst. Of Cancer Studies, Univ. of Birm. Specialty: Oncol. Socs: Assn. Cancer Phys. Prev: CRC Lect. (Med. Oncol.) Univ. Birm.; MRC Train. Fell. (Infect. & Cancer Studies) Univ. Birm.; Regist. (Infect. & Trop. Med.) Birm. Heartlands Hosp.

STEVEN, Robert Edward 35 Osmaston Road, Stourbridge DY8 2AL — MB ChB Liverp. 1993.

STEVEN, Rukshana Ramzan 16 Kyle Drive, Giffnock, Glasgow G46 6ES — MB ChB Glas. 1993.

STEVENS, Andrea Mary — MB BS Lond. 1991; MRCP (UK) 1994; FRCR 1999. Regist. (Clin. Oncol.) Birm. Oncol. Centre. Specialty: Oncol. Prev: SHO Rotat. (Med.) Glos. Roy. Hosp.; SpR W. Midl.s Clin. Oncol. Train. Progr.

STEVENS, Professor Andrew John Henrik Department of Public Health and Epidemiology, The University of Birmingham, Edgbaston, Birmingham B15 2TT Tel: 0121 414 6768 Fax: 0121 414 7878 — MB BS Lond. 1983; BA Camb. 1975; MSc Lond. 1986; MFCM RCP (UK) 1989; FFPHM RCP (UK) 1995. Prof. Pub. Health Med. Univ. Birm. Specialty: Pub. Health Med. Prev: Sen. Lect. (Pub. Health Med.) Wessex Inst. Pub. Health Med.; Cons. Pub. Health Med. Lewisham & N. Southwark HA.

STEVENS, Angela Felicity The Maudsley Hospital, Denmark Hill, London SE5 — MB BS Lond. 1992; BSc (Hons.) Microbiol. & Virol. Warwick Univ 1981; PhD Microbiol. Leics. 1985; MRCPsych 2001. Specialty: Gen. Psychiat.

STEVENS, Mrs Ann Wyn (retired) Sunset, Old Carnon Hill, Carnon Downs, Truro TR3 6LF Tel: 01872 862975 — MB ChB Liverp. 1962. Med. Off. (Occupat. Health) Roy. Cornw. Hosp. Trust. Truro. Prev: Ho. Surg. & Ho. Phys. David Lewis North. Hosp. Liverp.

STEVENS, Anna Miranda Hamlyn 4 Roman Grove, Leeds LS8 2DT — MB BChir Camb. 1993.

STEVENS, Anthony Baxter Occupational Health Unit, Royal Hospitals Trust, Grosvenor Road, Belfast BT12 6BB Tel: 02890 894611 Fax: 02890 263163 — MB BCh BAO Belf. 1982 (Qu. Univ. Belf.) MRCP (UK) 1985; MFOM RCP Lond. 1991, AFOM 1989; MD Belf. 1991; FRCP 1997; FFOM 1997. Cons. Occupat. Med. Roy. Hosps. Trust Belf.; Sen. Hon. Lect. (Occupat. Med.) Qu. Univ. Belf.; Director Risk and Occupat. Health Serv.s Roy. Hosp. Belf. Specialty: Occupat. Health. Socs: Fell. Ulster Med. Soc.; Soc. Occupat. Med.; Brit. Occupat. Hyg. Soc. Prev: Cons. Occupat. Med. EHSSB; Sen. Regist. (Occupat. Med.) EHSSB; Research Fell. (Med.) Qu. Univ. Belf.

STEVENS, Anthony Edward (retired) The Somerfield Hospital, London Road, Maidstone ME16 0DU Tel: 01622 831542 Fax: 01622 832200; The Old Vicarage, Marden, Tonbridge TN12 9AG Tel: 01622 832200 — MB BS Lond. 1952 (Char. Cross) FRCP Lond. 1975, M 1958. Prev: Cons. Phys. The Maidstone Hosp.

STEVENS, Anthony George (private rooms), 5 The Orchard, North Petherwin, Launceston PL15 8LW Tel: 01566 785546 — BM BCh Oxf. 1963 (Oxf. & Char. Cross) BA (Hons.) Reading 1955; BA (Hons.) Oxf. 1959; DPM Eng. 1969; MA Oxf. 1965, DM 1975; MRCPsych 1996. Specialty: Psychother. Socs: Fell. Roy. Soc. Med. Prev: Sen. Regist. Horton Hosp. Epsom; Ho. Surg. Roy. Surrey Co. Hosp. Guildford; Research Fell. Qu. Anna Maria Inst. Child Health Athens.

STEVENS, Anthony John (retired) 42 Chiswick Quay, London W4 3UR Tel: 020 8995 1222 Fax: 020 8995 1222 Email: anaes@johnstevens.co.uk — (Charing Cross) MB BS Lond. 1963; MRCS Eng. LRCP Lond. 1963; DA (UK) 1965; FFARACS 1970; FANZCA 1992. Private Pract. Prev: Cons. Anaesth. Hammersmith Hosp. Trust.

STEVENS, Arabella Paula Latchetts, Wellgreen Lane, Kingston, Lewes BN7 3NS — MB ChB Manch. 1998.

STEVENS, Claire Elizabeth Appletree Medical Practice, 47a Town Street, Duffield, Belper DE56 4GG Tel: 01332 841219/01332 844200 — BM BS Nottm. 1984; DRCOG 1987; MRCGP 1990. GP Duffield Derby.

STEVENS, Clare Valentine Bramble Cottage, 99 Horsham Road, Cranleigh GU6 8DZ Email: clarestevens@lineone.net — MB BS Lond. 1997.

STEVENS, David Brook, MBE Nobles Hospital, Douglas IM4 4RJ Tel: 07624 493403 Fax: 01624 651277 Email: dbs@mms.org.im; Ashley, Eleanora Drive, Douglas IM2 3NN Tel: 01624 675063 Fax: 01624 675063 Email: dbs@mms.org.im — MB ChB Ed. 1969; BSc Ed. 1966; DMRD Ed. 1974. Dir. I. of Man Motorsport Med. Servs.; Med. Delegate to ACU & FIM; Chairm. Isle of Man Paramedic Steering Comm. Specialty: Radiol.; Accid. & Emerg. Socs: Roy. Coll. Radiol. & BASICS; Mem. Fac. of Pre-Hosp. Immediate Care Roy. Coll. Surg. Edin. Prev: Cons. Radiol. Noble's Hosp. I. of Man.

STEVENS, David George, Wing Cdr. RAF Med. Br. Retd. Green Lane Hospital, Devizes SN10 9DS Tel: 01380 731325 — MB BS Lond. 1978 (St. Bartholomews) BSc Lond. 1972; Cert. Family Plann. JCC 1982; MRCGP 1983; MRCPsych. 1989. Cons. Psychiat. Wilts. Ment.. Health Care Trust. Specialty: Gen. Psychiat. Prev: Cons. Psychiat. Princess Alexandra RAF Wroughton; Regist. Highfield Adolesc. Unit Warneford Hosp. Oxf.; Regist. Felix Post Unit Maudsley Hosp. Lond.

STEVENS, David Laurence Department of Neurology, Gloucestershire Royal Hospital, Gloucester GL1 3NN; Springfield Lawn, The Park, Cheltenham GL50 2SD Tel: 01242 237921 Fax: 01242 522424 — MB BS Lond. 1961 (Guy's) MRCS Eng. LRCP Lond. 1961; FRCP Lond. 1980, M 1966; MD Lond. 1977; FRCP Ed. 1997. Cons. NeUrol. in Private Pract.; Trustee, Variant Crentzfeld & Jakob Dis. Trust, UK; Cons. NeUrol. Gloucestershire Roy. Hosp., Cheltenham Gen. Hosp., Bristol. Specialty: Neurol.; Medico Legal. Socs: World Federat. Neurol. Research Comm. Huntington's Chorea (Sec.Gen.); World Federate. Neurol Finance Comm. (Mem.); Assn. of Brit. Neurol. Topics. Prev: Cons. Neurol. Glos. Roy. Hosp., Cheltenham Gen. Hosp. & Frenchay Hosp. Bristol; Ho. Surg. & Ho. Phys. St. Olave's Hosp. Lond.; Sen. Regist. (Neurol.) Gen. Infirm. Leeds.

STEVENS, Mr David Michael (retired) 36 The Empire, Grand Parade, Bath BA2 4DF — MB BS Lond. 1944 (King's Coll. Hosp.) MRCS Eng. LRCP Lond. 1943; DLO Eng. 1948; FRCS Ed. 1952. Cons. ENT Surg. Bath Clin. Area. Prev: Sen. ENT Regist. United Cardiff Hosps.

STEVENS, David William Paediatric Department, Gloucestershire Royal Hospital, Gloucester GH 3NW Email: david.stevens@bristol.ac.uk — MB BS Lond. 1963 (Westm.) MRCS Eng. LRCP Lond. 1964; MRCP (UK) 1970; DCH Eng. 1971; FRCP Lond. 1989; FRCPCH 1997. Cons. Paediat. Glos. Roy. Hosp.; Sen. Lect., Univ. of Bristol Dept of Child Health. Specialty: Paediat. Special Interest: Gen. Paediat.; Nutrit.; Nutritional anaemics. Prev: Sen. Regist. Roy. Hosp. for Sick Childr. Bristol; Wellcome Fellowsh. Hist. of Med.

STEVENS, Deborah St. Julia's Hospice, Trelissick Road, Hayle TR27 4JA Tel: 01736 751216 Fax: 01736 751355; Elm Cottage, Relubbus, Penzance TR20 9EP Tel: 01736 763417 — MB BS Lond. 1982. Med. Direct. St. Julia's Hospice St. Michael's Hosp. Cornw.; Hon. Cons. (Palliat. Med.) Roy. Cornw. Hosps Trust. Specialty: Palliat. Med.

STEVENS, Diana Claire The New Surgery, Lindo Close, Chesham HP5 2JN Tel: 01494 782262; Stavacre, Bellingdon, Chesham HP5 2XW — MB BS Lond. 1979; DCH RCP Lond. 1984; Cert. Family Plann. RCOG & RCGP 1984; MRCGP 1986. GP Chesham.

Socs: BMA & Med. Protec. Soc. Prev: Clin. Med. Off. W. Lambeth HA; SHO (Paediat.) Char. Cross Hosp. Lond.

STEVENS, Dominic John Charles 86 Numa Court, Brentford Dock, Brentford TW8 8QF — MB ChB Bristol 1964; MRCGP 1977; MSc (Clin. Trop. Med.) Lond. 1983. GP Bolton. Prev: Dist. Med. Off. Luapula Province, Zambia; SHO (Ment. Health) Bristol Roy. Infirm.; Ho. Surg. & Ho. Phys. King's Lynn Gen. Hosp.

STEVENS, Eileen Denise Trafford General Hospital, Moorside Road, Davyhulme, Manchester M41 5SL; 90 Bollington Road, Stockport SK4 5ES — MB ChB Manch. 1985; MRCP (UK) 1988. Clin. Asst. (Med. & Geriat.) Trafford Gen. Hosp. Manch. Specialty: Gen. Med. Socs: Brit. Geriat. Soc.; Roy. Soc. Med; Mem. Med. Soc. Prev: Regist. (Geriat.) Salford HA; Regist. (Med.) Trafford Dist. Gen. Hosp.; SHO (Gen. Med.) N. Manch. Gen. Hosp.

STEVENS, Fiona Maureen Department of Medicine, University College Hospital, Galway, Republic of Ireland Tel: 00 353 91 524222 Fax: 00 353 91 750540; 36 Manton Hollow, Marlborough SN8 1RR Tel: 01672 53219 — MB BS Lond. 1965 (St. Geo.) MRCS Eng. LRCP Lond. 1965; MRCP (UK) 1970; FRCP Lond. 1988; MD NUI 1993. Lect. (Med.) Galway Regional Hosp.

STEVENS, Graham Colin 42 High Street, Harrington, Northampton NN6 9NU — MB ChB Leic. 1994; BSc (Hons.) Leic. 1992. SHO (A & E) Kettering Gen. Hosp. Specialty: Accid. & Emerg.

STEVENS, Gwyneth Mary (retired) 3 Rodney Close, Rodney Road, New Malden KT3 5AA — MRCS Eng. LRCP Lond. 1950 (Sheff.) DCH Eng. 1955.

STEVENS, Howard Martin Kennoway Medical Group, Jordan Lane, Kennoway, Leven KY8 5JZ Tel: 01333 350241 Fax: 01333 352884; 4 Lundin View, Leven KY8 5TL Tel: 01333 421 589 Email: howard@hms60.freeserve.co.uk — MB ChB Aberd. 1983 (Aberdeen) Clin. Asst. (Geriat.) Glenrothes. Specialty: Gen. Pract. Socs: Roy. Coll. Gen. Pract.; BMA; Brit. Med. Accupuncture Soc. Prev: SHO (ENT) Aberd. Roy. Infirm.; SHO (O & G) Princess of Wales Hosp. Bridgend; Trainee GP Bridgend M. Glam.

STEVENS, Howard Peter 52 The Chase, Clapham Old Town, London SW4 0NH Tel: 020 7738 8423 — MB BS Lond. 1988; MA (Oxon) 1983; MRCP (UK) 1991; PhD (Lond) 1998. Cons. Dermatolgist (F/T) - Barnet & Chase Farm Gen. Hosp. Specialty: Dermat. Prev: Wellcome Research Train. Fellowship & Hon. Sen. Regist. Roy. Lond. Hosp. Lond.; Regist. (Dermat.) Roy. Free Hosp. Lond.; Regist. (Gen. Med.) Watford Gen. Hosp.

STEVENS, Ian Ipswich Hospital NHS Trust, Heath Road, Ipswich IP4 5PD — Artsexamen Utreacht 1988. Cons. (Anaesth.) Ipswich Hosp. NHS Trust. Specialty: Anaesth. Special Interest: Acute Pain; Depth of Anaesth.; Difficult Airway.

STEVENS, Isobel Mary (retired) 29 Woolsington Park South, Woolsington, Newcastle upon Tyne NE13 8BJ Tel: 0191 286 3001 — MB ChB Glas. 1950. Prev: Clin. Asst. (Med.) Newc. AHA (T).

STEVENS, Jacqueline Ann John Tasker House Surgery, 56 New Street, Dunmow CM6 1BH — MB BS Lond. 1992 (St. Georges) Gen. Practitioner, Asst. Gt. Dunmold. Specialty: Gen. Pract. Prev: SHO Rotat. N. Hants. Hosp. Basingstoke; GP Regist. Alton Health Centre, Hants. Locum GP - N. Essex.

STEVENS, James Clement — MB BS Lond. 1998; MRCP 2001. Locum Reg. (Neurol.) West. Gen. Hosp. Edin. Specialty: Gen. Med.

STEVENS, Jane Frances 3 Clarendon Street, Cambridge CB1 1JU Tel: 01223 316046 Fax: 01223 500248 — MB BS Lond. 1976 (Univ. Coll. Lond.) MRCP (UK) 1979; DIH Eng. 1983; MFOM 1990. Cons. Occupat. Health. Specialty: Occupat. Health. Socs: Soc. Occupat. Med. & Roy. Soc. Med. Prev: Head of Occupat. Health Glaxo Research & Developm. Greenford; Regist. (Gen. Med.) St. Stephen's Hosp. Lond.; SHO (Thoracic Med.) Brompton Hosp. Lond.

STEVENS, Jeremy David Anaesthetic Department, Royal Hospital Trust, Calow, Chesterfield S44 5BL Tel: 01246 277271; Sparrow Busk Cottage, Clowne Road, Barlborough, Chesterfield S43 4EN Tel: 01246 570358 Fax: 01246 570229 — MB BS Lond. 1982 (St. Bart.) FFA RCSI 1989. Cons. Anaesth. Roy. Hosp. Trust. Chesterfield. Specialty: Anaesth. Socs: Med. Protec. Soc.; HCSA; Pain Soc. Prev: Sen. Regist. & Regist. Roy. Hallamsh. Hosp. Sheff.; Regist. (Anaesth.) & Research Regist. (Acute Pain) York Dist. Hosp.

STEVENS, John Edwin 13 All Saints Road, Headington, Oxford OX3 7AU — MB BS Lond. 1974; FFA RCS Eng. 1979. Cons. Anaesth. & Direct. of Paediat. IC, John Radcliffe Hosp., Headington, Oxf.. Specialty: Anaesth.

STEVENS, John Robert David South West London & St George's Mental Health Trust, Department of Psychotherapy, Harewood House, Springfield Hospital, London SW17 7DJ Tel: 020 8682 6682 Fax: 020 8682 6476 Email: john.stevens@swlstg-tr.nhs.uk; 'Earnsdale', 2 Whitepost Hill, Redhill RH1 6BD Tel: 01737 277706 Fax: 01737 277709 Email: john.stevens@surreyoaklands.nhs.uk — MB BS Lond. 1976 (Char. Cross) MRCPsych 1980; T(Psych) 1991. Cons. Psychiat. in Psychother. Specialty: Psychother. Socs: Assn. Psychoanalyt. Psychother. NHS. Prev: Cons. Psychother. Springfield Hosp. S. W. Lond. & St Geo.'s Ment. Health. NHS Trust; Cons. Psychother. Surrey Oaklands NHS Trust; Cons. Psychiat. Gender Identity Clinic (Psychiat.) Char. Cross Hosp. Lond.

STEVENS, Jonathan Paul 8B Carleton Gardens, Brecknock Road, London N19 5AQ — MB ChB Manch. 1989; BSc Hons. Manch. 1986. Research Fell. & Hon. Regist. Roy. Postgrad. Med. Sch. Lond.; RMO Portland Hosp. for Wom. & Childr. Lond. Specialty: Infec. Dis. Socs: Fell. Roy. Soc. Med. Prev: Interne (Neonatol.) Clinique Port Roy,. Paris.; SHO (Paediat.) Hammersmith Hosp. & Hosp. Sick Childr. Lond.

STEVENS, Judith Mary Queen Alexandra Hospital, Wessex Renal & Transplant Unit, Southwick Hill Road, Portsmouth PO6 3LY Tel: 023 9228 6000 Ext: 1003 Fax: 023 9228 6461 — MB BS Newc. 1981; MD Newc. 1991; FRCP Lon. 2000. Cons. Nephrologist. Qu. Alexandra Hosp., Portsmouth. Specialty: Nephrol. Prev: Sen. Regist. (Nephrol.) St. Mary's Hosp. Portsmouth; Regist. (Renal) Qu. Eliz. Hosp. Adelaide.; Research Fell. Roy. Postgrad. Med. Sch. Lond.

STEVENS, Mr Julian Douglas Moorfields Eye Hospital, City Road, London EC1V 2PD Tel: 020 7253 3411 Fax: 020 7253 4696 Email: 100437.663@compuserve.com; John Saunders Suite, Bath St, London EC1V 9EL Tel: 020 7566 2699 Fax: 020 7566 2608 Email: julianstevens@compuserve.com — MB Camb. 1983 (Univ. Camb.) MA Oxf. 1985, BA 1980; BChir 1982; MRCP (UK) 1986; FRCOphth 1988; DO RCS Eng. 1988; FRCS Eng. 1988. Cons. Ophth. Moorfields Eye Hosp. Lond. Specialty: Ophth. Socs: Eur. Soc. Cataract & Refractive Surgs.; Soc. Cataract & Refractive Surgs. UK & Irel.; Amer. Soc. Cataract & Refractive Surgs. Prev: Corneal & Refractive Fell. Moorfields Eye Hosp. Lond.; Sen. Regist. (Ophth.) Moorfields Eye Hosp. Lond.; Regist. (Ophth.) Oxf. Eye Hosp.

STEVENS, Katharine Lindsey Haughton Accident & Emergency Department, St. Helier's Hospital, Wrythe Lane, Carshalton SM5 1AA Tel: 020 8296 2276 Fax: 020 8288 1837 — MB BChir Camb. 1979 (Univ. Camb. & Middlx. Hosp.) MA Camb. 1978; MRCP (UK) 1983; FFAEM 1993; FRCP Lond. 1994. Clin. Dir. A & E Servs. St Helier's Hosp. Carshalton; Examr. FRCS (A & E); Hon. Sen. Lect. St. Geo. Hosp. Med. Sch. Univ. Lond.; Advanced Trauma Life Support Instruc. & Course Director; Paediat. Advanced Life Support Instruc.; Dep. Dist. Surg. St. Johns Ambul. Specialty: Accid. & Emerg. Socs: Fell. Roy. Soc. Med.; Brit. Assn. Accid. & Emerg. Med.; Fell. Roy. Soc. of Arts. Prev: Cons. Manager A & E St. Geo. Hosp. Lond.

STEVENS, Kathleen Mary (retired) 19 Moore Avenue, Harton, South Shields NE34 6AA Tel: 0191 456 0539 — (Durh.) MB BS Durh. 1945, CPH 1947. Prev: Princip. Community Clinician Durh. AHA.

STEVENS, Keith Douglas Department of Anaesthesia, Arrowe Park Hospital, Arrowe Park Road, Upton, Wirral CH49 5PE Tel: 0151 604 7056 Fax: 0151 604 7126 Email: stevenskds@btinternet.com — MB ChB Cape Town (Univ. of Cape Town) FFA South Africa. Cons. Anaesth., Wirral Hosps. NHS Trust. Specialty: Anaesth. Special Interest: Acute Pain.

STEVENS, Lesley Carol Connaught House, Royal Hampshire County Hospital, Romsey Road, Winchester SO22 5DG Tel: 01962 825128 — MB BS Lond. 1986 (St. Bart. Hosp. Lond.) MRCPsych 1991. Cons. (Psychiat.). Specialty: Gen. Psychiat.

STEVENS, Liam Francis Newtown Surgery, 147 Lawn Avenue, Great Yarmouth NR30 1QP Tel: 01493 853191 Fax: 01493 331861; 147 Lawn Avenue, Great Yarmouth NR30 1QP — MB BS Lond. 1982 (St. Mary's) DRCOG 1985; MRCGP 1986. Prev: Ho. Surg. King Edwd. VII Hosp. Windsor; Ho. Phys. St. Chas. Hosp. Lond.

STEVENS, Linda Eileen Whetstone Lane Health Centre, 44 Whetstone Lane, Birkenhead CH41 2TF Tel: 0151 647 9613 Fax: 0151 650 0875 — MB ChB Liverp. 1974; DObst RCOG 1976; DCH Eng. 1978; MRCGP 1979. Prev: GP Nottm.

STEVENS, Lydia Mary 62 Dukes Avenue, London W4 2AF — BM Soton. 1995.

STEVENS, Mark 46 Yarningale Road, Coventry CV3 3EL — MB BS Lond. 1997.

STEVENS, Mark Andrew John Malvern House, 41 Mapperley Road, Nottingham NG3 5AQ Tel: 0115 841 2006 Fax: 0115 841 2006 — BChir Camb. 1981; DRCOG 1985; MRCGP 1987. Prev: Trainee GP Aylesbury VTS; SHO (Paediat.) St. Thos. Hosp. Lond.

STEVENS, Mark Norton Frambury Lane Surgery, Frambury Lane, Newport, Saffron Walden CB11 3PY; 15 Hurdles Way, Heathfield, Duxford CB2 4PA Tel: 01223 835525 — MB BS Lond. 1972 (St. Thomas') Specialty: Gen. Pract.

STEVENS, Martin John Minsmere House, The Ipswich Hospital, Heath Road, Ipswich IP4 5PD Tel: 01473 704221 — MRCS Eng. LRCP Lond. 1967 (St. Thos.) MRCP (UK) 1972; FRCPsych 1986, M 1975; FRCP Lond. 1995. p/t Cons. Psychiat. (Geriat. Psychiat.) Ipswich Hosp. Specialty: Geriat. Psychiat.; Gen. Psychiat. Special Interest: Electroconvulsive Therapy. Socs: Brit. Geriat. Soc. Prev: Sen. Regist. (Psychol. Med.) Newc. Univ. Hosp.; Regist. (Gen. Med.) Gen. Hosp. Burton on Trent; Serv. Director, Old Age Psychiat., E. Suff. Local Health Servs. NHS Trust.

STEVENS, Matthew James 170 Mayals Road, Mayals, Swansea SA3 1HF — MB BCh Wales 1995. SHO (O & G) GPVTS Scheme. Socs: BMA cl.ic; MDU. Prev: SHO Elderley Med. 6 mths. Australia (Orthop. Anaesth.); SHO A&E; Ho. Off. Gen. Surg.

STEVENS, Matthew Thomas 9 Strangeways, Larkhill, Salisbury SP4 8LN — BM Soton. 1996.

STEVENS, Maxine (retired) 4 Walworth Gate, Darlington DL2 2UB Tel: 01325 312440 — MB ChB Manch. 1959; DPH Lond. 1962.

STEVENS, Michael Charles Garston Birmingham Children's Hospital, NHS Trust, Birmingham B4 6NH Tel: 0121 333 8412 Fax: 0121 333 8241 — MD Lond. 1983 (St. Mary's) MB BS (Hons.) 1974; MRCP (UK) 1976; FRCP Lond. 1992; FRCPCH 1997. Cons. Paediatric Oncologist Birm. Childr.'s Hosp. NHS Trust. Specialty: Paediat. Socs: Internat. Soc. of Paediat. Oncol.; UK Childr.'s Cancer Study Gp. Prev: Med. Dir. Birm. Childr.'s Hosp. NHS Trust; Chairm. UK Childr.s Cancer Study GP.

STEVENS, Michele Ann 16 Wyndham Road, London W13 9TE Tel: 0208 840 4595 — MB BS Lond. 1990 (St. Bartholow's Hospital, London) FRCA 1997. Spr (Anaest) Green Charlottes & Chelsea. Hosp. Lond. Specialty: Anaesth. Prev: SHO (Anaesth.) Chelsea & Westm. Hosp. Lond.; SHO (Cardiothoracic Surg.) St. Bart. Hosp. Lond.; Regist. (Anaesth.) Chelsea & Westm. Hosp. Lond.

STEVENS, Monica Rosemary Clare Northgate Practice, Northgate, Canterbury CT1 1WL — MB BS Lond. 1988 (St. Mary's Medical School) DFFP. Trainee GP Medway VTS., GP Retainer; CMO Family Plann., Canterbury. Prev: Ho. Surg. Bucklands Hosp. Dover; Ho. Phys. Kent & Canterbury Hosp.; Med.s VTS.

STEVENS, Nigel Bradley, Surg. Lt.-Cdr. RN Windsor Crescent Surgery, 6 Windsor Crescent, Val Plaisant, St Helier JE2 4TB Tel: 01534 32341 Fax: 01534 870635; 12 Le Feugerel, Le Mont de la Pulente, St Brelade, Jersey JE3 8HB — MB BCh Wales 1982; MRCGP 1987.

STEVENS, Paul Edward, Squadron Ldr. RAF Med. Br. Retd. Department of Renal Medicine, Kent & Canterbury Hospital, Ethelbert Road, Canterbury CT1 3NE Tel: 01227 766877 Fax: 01227 783073; Milestone Barn, Hode Lane, Bridge, Canterbury CT4 5DL — MB BS Lond. 1980 (London Hospital Medical College) BSc (Hons.) Lond. 1977, MB BS 1980; MRCP (UK) 1985; FRCP 1996. Cons. Nephrol. & Dir. Renal Servs. Kent & Canterbury Hosp. Specialty: Nephrol. Socs: Eur. Dialysis & Transpl. Assn.; Renal Assn. Prev: Cons. Phys. & Nephrol. Princess Mary's RAF Hosp. Halton; Lect. & Hon. Sen. Regist. (Gen. Med. & Nephrol.) Char. Cross Hosp. Lond.; Sen. Regist. (Renal Med.) Princess Mary's Hosp. Halton.

STEVENS, Paul George Cathcart Practice, 8 Cathcart Street, Ayr KA7 1BJ Tel: 01292 264051 Fax: 01292 293803; 3 Ewenfield Park, Ayr KA7 2QG Tel: 01292 265442 — MB ChB Glas. 1976 (Glasgow) DRCOG 1977. Specialist (Genito-Urin. Med.) Heathfield Clinic Ayr. Specialty: Genitourinary Medicine.

STEVENS, Peter John Newbold Surgery, 3 Windermere Road, Newbold, Chesterfield S41 8DU Tel: 01246 277381 Fax: 01246 239828 — MB ChB Ed. 1969; DObst RCOG 1972; FRCGP 1994, M 1977. Prev: SHO (Obst.) West. Gen. Hosp. Edin.; Med. Off. St. Kitts, W. Indies.

STEVENS, Peter John, OBE (retired) South Orchard, College Lane, East Grinstead RH19 3JR Tel: 01342 325963 Fax: 01342 325963 Email: stevens.pj@doctors.org.uk — MB ChB Birm. 1949; DCP Lond 1955; DTM & H Eng. 1960; FRCPath 1972, M 1964; MD Birm. 1968. Prev: Cons. Path. Qu. Vict. Hosp. E. Grinstead.

STEVENS, Philip Harold (retired) The Surgery, Bissoe Road, Carnon Downs, Truro TR3 6JD Tel: 01872 863221; Sunset, Old Carnon Hill, Carnon Downs, Truro TR3 6LF Tel: 01872 863221 — MB ChB Liverp. 1961; MRCS Eng. LRCP Lond. 1961; BSc (Hons. Anat.) Liverp. 1958. Prev: GP Cornw.

STEVENS, Philip John Washington House Surgery, 77 Halse Road, Brackley NN13 6EQ Tel: 01280 702436; 5 Broad Lane, Evenley, Brackley NN13 5SF Tel: 01280 702879 — MB BCh Wales 1978; DRCOG 1983; MRCGP 1984.

STEVENS, Richard Charles Harrisson Orchard Court Surgery, Orchard Court, Orchard Road, Darlington DL3 6HZ Tel: 01325 465285 Fax: 01325 284034; The Surgery, Orchard Court, Darlington DL3 6HZ Tel: 01325 465285 Fax: 01325 284034 — MB BS Newc. 1987 (Newc. u. Tyne) MRCGP 1993; DRCOG 1993; DFFP 1993. Clin. Asst. (Asthma) Darlington Memor. Hosp. Prev: Stud. Health Off. Hawkes Bay Polytechnic, NZ; Trainee GP Cleveland VTS.

STEVENS, Richard Jeffrey The Heberden Unit, Amersham Hospital, Amersham HP7 0JD Tel: 01494 734079 Fax: 01494 734504 — MB BS Lond. 1984 (St. Mary's Hosp. Med. Sch. Lond.) BSc Lond. 1981; MRCP (UK) 1988; FRCP (UK) 2001. Cons. Rheum. S. Bucks. NHS Trust. Specialty: Rheumatol.; Gen. Med. Prev: Sen. Regist. St. Thos. Hosp. Lond.

STEVENS, Richard Murray East Oxford Health Centre, Manzil Way, Cowley Road, Oxford OX4 1XD Tel: 01865 791850 Fax: 01865 727358 — BM BCh Oxf. 1980; MA 1980; DRCOG 1983; MRCGP 1984; FRCGP 1998. Hosp. Pract. (Gastroenterol.) John Radcliffe Hosp. Oxf. Socs: Chairm. Primary Care Soc. For Gastroenterol.

STEVENS, Robert Hartley 23 Egerton Road, Whitefield, Manchester M45 7FU Tel: 0161 796 6773 — MB BCh BAO Belf. 1987; BSc Belf. 1984; MSc Manch. 1993. Sen. Regist. (Pub. Health Med.) NW RHA. Specialty: Pub. Health Med. Socs: Fac. Pub. Health Med. Prev: SHO (Path.) N. Manch. Gen. Hosp.; Ho. Off. (Med. & Surg.) Roy. Lancaster Infirm.

STEVENS, Robert William Arrowe Park Hospital, Arrowe Park Road, Upton, Wirral CH49 5PE Tel: 0151 678 5111 — MB ChB (Hons.) Liverp. 1974; BSc (Hons. Biochem.) Liverp. 1971; FFA RCS Eng. 1979. Cons. Anaesth. Wirral Hosp. NHS Trust. Specialty: Anaesth. Prev: Sen. Regist. (Anaesth) Notts. AHA (T); Regist. (Anaesth.) Liverp. AHA (T).

STEVENS, Roger John Roborough Surgery, 1 Eastcote Close, Southway, Plymouth PL6 6PH Tel: 01752 701659 Fax: 01752 773181; Gaillac, Yelverton PL20 6DW Tel: 01822 855560 — MB BS Lond. 1966 (King's Coll. Hosp.) MRCS Eng. LRCP Lond. 1965. Prev: SHO (Psychol. Med.) St. Pancras Hosp. Lond.; Resid. Med. Off. King Edw. VII Memor. Hosp. Bermuda; Ho. Phys. & Ho. Surg. King's Coll. Hosp. Lond.

STEVENS, Roger Julian Geoffrey Frenchay Hospital, Department of Surgery, Bristol BS16 1LE Tel: 0117 970 1212 — MB ChB (Commend.) Aberd. 2002; BSc (Hons. Physiol. & Pharmacol.) Lond. 1995; MSc (Vasc. Technol. & Med. Distinc.) Lond. 1996. SHO Surgic. Rotat. Frenchay Hosp. Bristol; RAFT Research Fell. (RAFT Inst.) Mt. Vernon Hosp. Middlx. Specialty: Plastic Surg. Special Interest: Skin Cancer. Socs: RSM; BMA. Prev: SHO (A & E) Countess of Chester Hosp.; Vis. Med. Stud., Dept. of Plastic & Reconstruc. Surg., Mayo Clinic, Rochester, Minnesota, USA; Hon. Research Fell. (Acad. Surg. Unit) St Mary's Hosp. Lond.

STEVENS, Rosemary Frances 35 Princess Gardens, Holywood BT18 0PN — MB BCh BAO Belf. 1980.

STEVENS, Rosemary Jane 27 Ford Park Road, Mutley Plain, Plymouth PL4 6RD — MB BS Lond. 1965 (King's Coll. Hosp.) AKC; MRCS Eng. LRCP Lond. 1965; MB BS Lond. 1966. Prev: Clin. Asst. (Child Psychiat.) Nuffield Clinic Plymouth; Ho. Surg. King's Coll. Hosp. Lond.

STEVENS, Roy 13 Balmoral Road, Lytham St Annes FY8 1ER — MB ChB Liverp. 1976; MRCP (UK) 1980; FRCP Lond. 1995; FRCPCH 1996. Cons. Paediat. Vict. Hosp. Blackpool. Specialty: Paediat.

STEVENS, Sarah Anne 20 Catherines Close, Great Leights, Chelmsford CM3 1RX — MB BS Lond. 1990.

STEVENS, Thomas Guy Lambeth Hospital, 108 Landor Road, London SW9 9NT — MB BChir Camb. 1991; MRCPsych. Cons. Psychiat. Lambeth Hosp. Lond. Specialty: Psychiatry.

STEVENS, Vivian John Rodier The Avenue Surgery Partnership, 14 The Avenue, Warminster BA12 9AA Tel: 01985 846224 Fax: 01985 847059 Email: vjrs@wanadoo.co.uk — MB BS Lond. 1980 (Char. Cross) BSc Lond. 1976; MRCS Eng. LRCP Lond. 1980; DRCOG 1987; MRCGP 1988; BA (Open) 1998. Specialty: Gen. Pract.; Acupunc. Socs: Clin. Soc. of Bath. Prev: Clin. Asst. (Psychogeriat.) Warminster.

STEVENS-KING, Angela 31 Kenton Park Road, Harrow HA3 8UB — MB ChB Sheff. 1994.

STEVENSON, Alan David St James Medical Centre, 9 Herbert Street, Pontardawe, Swansea SA8 4EB Tel: 01792 830089 Fax: 01792 830089; 281 Clasemont, Morriston, Swansea SA6 6BT — MB BS Lond. 1988.

STEVENSON, Alastair Gordon Moffat 11 Netherhouse Avenue, Lenzie, Kirkintilloch, Glasgow G66 5NF — MB ChB Glas. 1997 (Glasgow University)

STEVENSON, Alison Wendy New Craigs Hospital, 6-16 Leachkin Road, Inverness IV3 8NP Tel: 01463 242860 ext3615; Hollybank, Station Road, Evanton, Dingwall IV16 9YW — MB ChB Glas. 1986. Specialty: Alcohol & Substance Misuse.

STEVENSON, Allan John Murray Department of Radiology, Western General Hospital, Crewe Road, Edinburgh EH4 2XU — MB ChB Ed. 1979; MRCP (UK) 1982; DMRD Ed. 1986; FRCR 1988; FRCPE 1999. Cons. Radiol. Western Gen. Hosps. NHS Trust Edin.; Head of Dept., Radiol., West. Gen. Hosp., Edin. Specialty: Radiol. Special Interest: Oncol. Imaging. Socs: Roy. Coll. of Radiologists; Roy. Coll. of Physicians; Scott. Radiological Soc. Prev: Cons. Radiol. E. & West. Gen. Hosps. Edin.; Sen. Regist. (Radiol.) Roy. Infirm. Edin.; Regist. (Radiol.) Roy. Infirm. Edin.

STEVENSON, Angela Margery (retired) 270 Merville Garden Village, Newtownabbey BT37 9TT — MB BCh BAO Belf. 1969.

STEVENSON, Ann Iwan North Cardiff Medical Centre, Excalibur Drive, Thornhill, Cardiff CF14 9BB Tel: 029 2075 0322 Fax: 029 2075 7705 — MB BCh Wales 1966; MRCGP 1983. GP Llanishen.

STEVENSON, Anne Grant Bangholm Medical Centre, 21-25 Bangholm Loan, Edinburgh EH5 3AH Tel: 0131 552 7676 Fax: 0131 552 8145; 18A Merchiston Park, Edinburgh EH10 4PN — MB ChB Aberd. 1980; DRCOG 1982; MRCGP 1984. Hosp. Practitioner (Genitourin. Med.) Roy. Infirm. Edin.

STEVENSON, Anthony John Maxwell, OBE (retired) 6 Ingleside Crescent, Lancing BN15 8EN — MRCS Eng. LRCP Lond. 1941.

STEVENSON, Beryll Janette (retired) Alt Tigh, Rosemount, Tain IV19 1ND Tel: 01862 893996 — MB ChB Glas. 1959. Prev: Assoc. Specialist Yorks Reg. Blood Transfus. Serv. Leeds.

STEVENSON, Brian John (retired) The Surgery, Highwood Road, Brockenhurst SO42 7RY Tel: 01590 622272 Fax: 01590 624009; The Surgery, Station Road, Sway, Lymington SO41 6BA Tel: 01590 682617 Fax: 01590 682226 — (Lond. Hosp.) BSc (Physiol.) Lond. 1956; MB BS Lond. 1958; DObst RCOG 1960; DCH Eng. 1962; FRCGP 1981, M 1975. Prev: SHO Qu. Eliz. Hosp. Childr. Lond.

STEVENSON, Brian John Psychopharmacology Unit, School of Medical Sciences, University Walk, Bristol BS8 1TD; 14 Cornwallis Avenue, Bristol BS8 4PP Email: brian_j.stevenson@virgin.net — MA Hons (II) in Physics Oxford; MSc in Digial Electronics, Lond.; MB ChB Leic. 1992. Research Fell.; Hon. Regist. Avon Alcohol Serv. Specialty: Gen. Psychiat.

STEVENSON, Christopher James (retired) 16 Kingsland, Jesmond, Newcastle upon Tyne NE2 3AL Tel: 0191 281 2959 — MB BS Lond. 1945 (Lond. Hosp.) MRCS Eng. LRCP Lond. 1945; FRCP Lond. 1971, M 1947; MD Lond. 1952; MFOM RCP Lond. 1981. Hon. Cons. Dermat. Newc. HA. Prev: Cons. Dermat. Roy. Vict. Infirm. Newc.

STEVENSON, Christopher John Infirmary Drive Medical Group, Consulting Rooms, Infirmary Drive, Alnwick NE66 2NR Tel: 01665 602388 Fax: 01665 604712 — MB BS Newc. 1978; DCH RCPS Glas. 1982; MRCGP 1983.

STEVENSON, Claire Elizabeth 56 Broadwells Crescent, Westwood Heath, Coventry CV4 8JD — MB ChB Manch. 1982; DRCOG 1986. Prev: Trainee GP Warks. & Coventry VTS.

STEVENSON, Claire Winchester Flat 4 Lawley House, 37 Clevedon Road, Twickenham TW1 2TW — MB ChB Glas. 1972.

STEVENSON, David Castlehill Health Centre, Castlehill, Forres IV36 1QF Tel: 01309 672707; West Park House, Forres IV36 1HB Tel: 01309 672883 — MB ChB Glas. 1982; DRCOG (Birmingham) 1986; MRCGP Edin. 1999. GP Princip. Socs: Highland Med. Soc.; Hon. Life Mem. Glas. Univ. MC Soc.; Moray Med. Soc. Prev: SHO (O & G) Raigmore Unit Highland Health Bd.; SHO (ENT & Ophth.) Raigmore Unit.; GP Trainee, Foyers Invernesshire.

STEVENSON, David James 92 Hillview Drive, Clarkston, Glasgow G76 7JD — MB ChB Glas. 1994.

STEVENSON, David John Douglas Public Health Sciences, University of Edinburgh Medical School, Teviot Place, Edinburgh EH8 9AG Tel: 0131 667 3748 Fax: 0131 650 6909 Email: david.stevenson@ed.ac.uk — MB ChB Glas. 1957; MA Camb. 1958; DTM & H Liverp. 1961; DPH Glas. 1964; MD Glas. 1965; FFPH 1993. Hon. Fell. Pub. Health Sci. Univ. Edin. Specialty: Trop. Med. Socs: Life Mem. Freshwater Biol. Assn.; Soc. Scientif. Exploration; Roy. Soc. Trop. Med. & Hyg. (Comm. Mem. Scott. Br.). Prev: Sen. Lect. (Internat. Community Health) Liverp. Sch. Trop. Med.; Govt. Med. Off. Malawi; Research Adviser Tribhuwan Univ., Nepal.

STEVENSON, Ede (retired) Brynmoor House, Harpers Lane, Bolton BL1 6HR Tel: 01204 41052 Fax: 01204 841052 — MB ChB Manch. 1961; DObst RCOG 1963; DCH Eng. 1964.

STEVENSON, Gary Ferryhill Medical Practice, Durham Road, Ferryhill DL17 8JJ Tel: 01740 651238 Fax: 01740 656291; 2 Walkworth Lane, Spennymoor DL16 6UY Tel: 01388 812455 — BM Soton. 1984.

STEVENSON, Gary Scot — MB ChB Glas. 1990; BSc (Hons.) Glas. 1987; MRCPsych 1996; M.Phil (Ed.) 1997; Dip. FMSA 1999. Cons. Psychiat. (Old Age). Specialty: Gen. Psychiat. Socs: Med. & Dent. Defence Union Scotl. Prev: Specialist Regist. (Psychiat.); Regist./SHO (Psychiat.) SE Scotl. Train. Scheme; SHO Dunedin Pub. Hosp., NZ.

STEVENSON, Geoffrey Roy East Quay Medical Centre, East Quay, Bridgwater TA6 5AZ Tel: 01278 423474 — MB BS Lond. 1953; MRCS Eng. LRCP Lond. 1953; DObst RCOG 1957.

STEVENSON, George Telford (retired) Southampton General Hospital, Tremona Road, Southampton SO16 6YD Tel: 023 8079 6639 Fax: 023 8070 4061 Email: G.T.Stevenson@soton.ac.uk; 9 Meadowhead Road, Bassett, Southampton SO16 7AD Tel: 023 8076 9092 — MB BS Sydney 1955; MD Sydney 1962; DPhil Oxf. 1965; FRCPath 1993. Vis. Prof. Sch. Med. Univ. Soton. Prev: Resid Med. Off. Sydney Hosp.

STEVENSON, Guy Cuthbert House, All Saints, City Road, Newcastle upon Tyne NE1 2DA Tel: 0191 209 5591; 10 Otterburn Terrace, Jesmond, Newcastle upon Tyne NE2 3AP Tel: 0191 281 7437 — MB BS Newc. 1977; MLCOM 1987; MSc (Sports Med) 1997; Reg. Osteopath GOsC 2000. Specialist (Orthop. Med.) Newc. u. Tyne. Specialty: Sports Med. Socs: Brit. Assn. Sport & Med.; Brit. Inst. Manip. Med. Prev: Surg. Lt. Cdr. RN.

STEVENSON, Helen Lenore 4 Willow Way, Crosby, Liverpool L23 2TP — MB ChB Liverp. 1997.

STEVENSON, Mr Ian Michael 34 St Michaels Road, Crosby, Liverpool L23 7UN — MB ChB Liverp. 1966; FRCS Ed. 1971 (Liverp.); FRCS Eng. 1971. Cons. Surg. Walton Hosp. Liverp. & Fazakerley Hosp. Liverp.; Surg. Tutor RCS Eng. Specialty: Gen. Surg. Socs: Liverp. Med. Inst. & Vasc. Soc. Gt. Brit. & Irel. Prev: Sen. Surgic. Regist. Walton Hosp. Liverp. & David Lewis. North. Hosp.; Liverp.

STEVENSON, Ilbury Hugh The Poplars Surgery, 17 Holly Lane, Erdington, Birmingham B24 9JN Tel: 0121 373 4216 Fax: 0121 382 9576 — MB BS Lond. 1959 (St. Mary's) DObst RCOG 1964. Prev: Govt. Med. Off. Gibraltar; Ho. Surg. (Obst.) Cheltenham Matern. Hosp.; Clin. Asst. & Hosp. Pract. Jaffray Hosp. Birm.

STEVENSON, Mr James 3 Hillside Cottages, Dalry KA24 4DP — MB ChB Glas. 1983; FRCS Ed. 1987; DA (UK) 1989.

STEVENSON, James Duncan Cedar Lodge, 36 Lakeside Road, Branksome Park, Poole BH13 6LS Tel: 01202 761464 — MB BS Lond. 1971; BSc Lond. 1968, MB BS 1971; FRCR 1980. Cons. Radiol. E. Dorset Health Care Dist. Specialty: Radiol. Prev: Sen. Regist. (Radiol.) St. Geo. Hosp. Lond.; Ho. Phys. (Neurol.) St. Thos. Hosp. Lond.; Med. Regist. Kingston Hosp.

STEVENSON, James Gordon 21 Kilmahew Avenue, Cardoss, Dumbarton G82 5NG — MB ChB Glas. 1971; MRCP (UK) 1973.

STEVENSON, Janet Audrey Margaret Morris (retired) Causewell Cottage, The Street, Darsham, Saxmundham IP17 3QA Tel: 017228 668369 — MRCS Eng. LRCP Lond. 1943 (W. Lond.) DPH Lond. 1947. Prev: Train. Med. Off. FPA.

STEVENSON, Janet Elaine 27 Rankin Road, Edinburgh EH9 3AW — MB BS Lond. 1988. Sen. Regist. (Pub. Health Med.) N. RHA. Specialty: Radiol. Prev: SHO (Pub. Health Med.) Centr. Birm. HA.

STEVENSON, Jean Grange Road Surgery, Grange Road, Bishopsworth, Bristol BS13 8LD Tel: 0117 964 4343 Fax: 0117 935 8422 — MB BS Newc. 1969.

STEVENSON, Jean Frances 9 Briant's Close, Pinner HA5 4SY — MB ChB Leeds 1975; BSc (Pharmacol.) St. And. 1970.

STEVENSON, John (retired) 1 Bramble Edge, Broadmayne, Dorchester DT2 8HE — MRCS Eng. LRCP Lond. 1945 (King's Coll. Hosp.) Prev: Ho. Surg. King's Coll. Hosp.

STEVENSON, John Curtis Royal Brompton Hospital, Faculty of Medicine, Imperial College London, Metabolic Medicine, Sydney Street, London SW3 6NP Tel: 020 7351 8112 Fax: 020 7351 8771 Email: j.stevenson@imperial.ac.uk; Holyrood, Police Station Road, Hersham Village, Walton-on-Thames KT12 4JQ — MB BS Lond. 1972 (Kings Coll. Hosp.) MRCP (UK) 1979; FRCP Lond. 1993; FESC 1997. Reader Fac. of Med. Imperial Coll. Lond.; Cons. Phys., Roy. Brompton Hosp.; Hon. Med. Off., Esher RFC. Specialty: Endocrinol. Special Interest: coronary heart Dis. Preven.; menopause and HRT; osteoporosis. Socs: Endocrine Soc. USA; Fell. Europ. Soc. Cardiol.; Internat. Menopause Soc. Prev: Hon. Cons. Phys. St Mary's Hosp. Lond.; Dir. Wynn Inst.. Imperial Coll. Lond.; Cons. Endocrinol. Wynn Inst. for Metab. Research Lond.

STEVENSON, John Erskine David — MB Camb. 1977; BA Camb. 1973, MB 1977, BChir 1976; DRCOG 1978; MRCGP 1980. Prescribing Lead N. Herts & Stevenage PCT Exec Bd. Prev: Clin. Governance Lead, Stevenage PCG; Clin. Asst. (Diabetes), Lister Hosp., Stevenage.

STEVENSON, Mr John Howard 38 Ruskin Park, Hillsborough Old Road, Lisburn BT27 Tel: 0184 62 70458 — MB BCh BAO Belf. 1973; DObst RCOG 1976; FRCS Ed. 1977.

STEVENSON, John James (retired) The Spinney, Ottery St Mary EX11 1LE Tel: 01404 822525 Email: john@exrays.freeserve.co.uk — MB ChB Ed. 1941; DMR Lond 1945; MD Ed. 1950; FFR RCSI 1962. Prev: Dir. Diag. X-Ray Roy. Marsden Hosp. & St. Peter's Hosp. Gp. (Inst. Urol.).

STEVENSON, John Laing Stotfold Bury, Stotfold, Hitchin SG5 4NU Tel: 01462 730966 — MB BS Lond. 1952 (St. Mary's) MRCS Eng. LRCP Lond. 1952; DObst RCOG 1957. Prev: O & G Ho. Surg. Geo. Eliot Hosp. Nuneaton; Capt. RAMC; Ho. Phys. & Ho. Surg. Harold Wood Hosp.

STEVENSON, John Samuel (retired) 20 Belbrough Lane, Huton Rudby, Yarm TS15 0HY Tel: 01642 700603 — (Roy. Colls. Ed.) LRCP LRCS Ed. LRFPS Glas. 1944. Prev: SHO Ballochmyle Hosp. Mauchline.

STEVENSON, John Stevenson Kennedy (retired) — (Glas.) MB ChB Glas. 1955; DObst RCOG 1957; FRCGP 1972, M 1964. Prev: Sen. Lect. Dept. Gen. Pract. Univ. Edin.

STEVENSON, Miss Katherine Elizabeth DBCG, PO Box 12650, London SE3 9ZZ Tel: 020 8852 8522 Fax: 020 8852 8522 Email: eyes@dbcg.co.uk — BM Soton. 1979; DO RCS Eng. 1983; FRCS Eng. (Ophth.) 1984. Specialty: Ophth. Prev: Sen. Regist. Moorfields Eye Hosp. Lond.; Regist. (Ophth.) Oxf. Eye Hosp.; SHO (Ophth.) Soton. Eye Hosp.

STEVENSON, Kirsteen Morag Child & Family Therapy Service, Battenburg Avenue Clinic, Battenburg Avenue, North End, Portsmouth PO2 0TA Tel: 023 92 653433 — MB BS Lond. 1981; MRCPsych 1987. Cons. Child & Adolesc. Psychiat. Portsmouth City Primary Care Trust. Specialty: Child & Adolesc. Psychiat. Prev: Sen. Regist. (Child Psychiat.) Lond. Hosp.

STEVENSON, Laura Vyvian 1 Drummond Place, Edinburgh EH3 6PH — MB ChB Ed. 1992.

STEVENSON, Lee 181 Langley Hall Road, Solihull B92 7HB — MB ChB Sheff. 1989.

STEVENSON, Madeline Claire — MB ChB Glas. 1998.

STEVENSON, Margarita Carmeno 14 First Street, Chelsea, London SW3 2LD Tel: 020 7584 0658 Fax: 020 7225 0518; 14 First Street, Chelsea, London SW3 2LD Tel: 020 7584 0658 Fax: 020 7225 0518 — MB BS Lond. 1962 (St. Bart. & Char. Cross) FRCOG; MRCS Eng. LRCP Lond. 1962; MBBS 1962; MRCS Eng LRCP Lond. 1962; DOBT 1965; MRCOG 1968, DObst 1965; MRCOG 1968; FRCOG 1978. State Nures Gyn. Lond. Specialty: Obst. & Gyn. Socs: Roy. Soc. Med.; Fell.Med. Soc. Lond.; Worshipful Soc. Apoth. Lond. Prev: Sen. Med. Off. Home Office; Resid. Obst. Providence Hosp. Seattle America; Hon. Cons. Gyn. Southgate Hosp. Lond.

STEVENSON, Marian Pearl 77 Athlestan Way, Stretton, Burton-on-Trent DE13 0XT — MB BS Lond. 1969.

STEVENSON, Mary Elizabeth Cedar Lodge, 36 Lakeside Road, Branksome Park, Poole BH13 6LS Tel: 01202 761464 — MB BS Lond. 1972 (St. Thos.) DObst RCOG 1974. Clin. Asst. (Anaesth.) Roy. Bournemouth Hosp. & Poole Gen. Hosp. Specialty: Anaesth. Socs: Assn. Anaesth.; BMA; Roy. Soc. Med. Prev: Regist. (Anaesth.) Poole Gen. Hosp. & Kingston Gen. Hosp.; SHO & Regist. (Anaesth.) St. Thos. Hosp. Lond.

STEVENSON, Mary J Ardinning, Moor Road, Strathblane, Glasgow G63 9EX Tel: 01360 770308 — MB ChB Glas. 1967; FRCR 1985. Cons. Radiol. Roy. Alexandra Hosp. Paisley. Specialty: Radiol.

STEVENSON, Mary Margaret Department of Genitourinary Medicine, Guest Hospital, Tipton Road, Dudley DY1 4SE Tel: 01384 244856 Fax: 01384 244826 — MB ChB Glas. 1987; DTM & H RCP Lond. 1991; MRCP (UK) 1992. Cons. (Genitourin. Med.) Guest Hosp. Dudley. Specialty: Genitourinary Medicine. Prev: Sen. Regist. (Genitourin. Med.) Gen. Hosp. Birm.; Regist. (Genitourin. Med.) Gen. Hosp. Birm.

STEVENSON, Maureen Michaela Maghera Health Centre, 3 Church Street, Maghera BT46 5EA Tel: 028 7964 2579 Fax: 028 7964 3002; 11 Ardmoneen Court, Magherafelt BT45 5NX Tel: 01648 301179 — MB BCh BAO Belf. 1988; DCH RCPSI 1991; DRCOG 1991; MRCGP 1992. Prev: Ho. Off. Ipswich Gen. Hosp. Queensland, Austral.

STEVENSON, Michael Denis Seascale Health Centre, Seascale CA20 1PU Tel: 01946 728101; The Old Rectory, Bootle, Millom LA19 5TH Email: mdstevenson@doctors.net.uk — MB BS London 1982 (Royal Free Hosp. School of Medicine) MRCGP London; BDS Univ. Birmingham 1974. GP; Scheme Organiser, W. Cumbria V.T.S. Specialty: Gen. Pract. Socs: BMA.

STEVENSON, Nicola Jane 69 Quarry Street, Liverpool L25 6HA — MB ChB Liverp. 1994.

STEVENSON, Nicola Jane Lowther Medical Centre, 1 Castle Meadows, Whitehaven CA28 7RG Tel: 01946 692241 Fax: 01946 590617; 1 Victoria Villa, Moor Row, Wigton CA24 3JX Tel: 01946 813112 — MB ChB Birm. 1985; DRCOG 1991; MRCGP 1992. Prev: Trainee GP W. Cumbld. Hosp. Whitehaven VTS; SHO (Ophth.) Birm. Eye Hosp.; Temp. Lect. (Anat.) Univ. Birm.

STEVENSON, Pamela 5 Drummond Avenue, Auchterarder PH3 1NX — MB ChB Ed. 1967.

STEVENSON, Pamela Susan Old Age Psychiatry, Bensham Hospital, Gateshead NE8 4YL Tel: 0191 445 6681; 8 Alverstone Avenue, Low Fell, Gateshead NE9 6EU Tel: 0191 482 2138 — MB BS Newc. 1979; Cert. JCPTGP 1984; MRCPsych 1986. Specialist Regist. Old Age Psychiat. Newc. Gen. Hosp. Newc. Specialty: Geriat. Psychiat.

STEVENSON, Paul Anthony 8 Lyndhurst Road, Wallasey CH45 6XA — MB ChB Bristol 1963; FRCPath 1990. Cons. Haemat. Walton Hosp. Liverp. Specialty: Haematology. Prev: Research Regist. (Leukaemia) Bristol Childr. Hosp.

STEVENSON, Pauline Frances (retired) Swallowfield, Wheeler's Lane, Linton, Maidstone ME17 4BN Tel: 01622 743392 Email: tpwaters@freenetname.co.uk — MB ChB Bristol 1956; DCH Eng. 1959; DTM & H Liverp. 1962; MRCPsych 1976; DPM Eng. 1977. Cons. Child & Adolesc. Psychiat. Maidstone, Kent; Mem. Inst. Gp. Anal. 1982. Prev: Cons. Child & Adolesc. Psychiat. N. Wilts.

STEVENSON, Peter Robert 37 Coed y fron, Holywell CH8 7UJ Tel: 01352 716886 — MB ChB Liverp. 1979; DRCOG 1985; MRCGP 1987; MFPHM 1997. Cons. (Pub. Health Med.) N. Wales Health Auth. Specialty: Pub. Health Med.

STEVENSON, Philip George 9 Meadowhead Road, Southampton SO16 7AD — BChir Camb. 1990; MRCP 1993.

STEVENSON, Robert (retired) 270 Melville Garden Village, Whitehouse, Newtownabbey BT37 9TT — MB BCh BAO Belf. 1966; DObst RCOG 1968.

STEVENSON, Robert Duncan Ardinning, Moor Road, Strathblane, Glasgow G63 9EX Tel: 014170308 — MD Glas. 1978; MB ChB (Commend) 1967; MRCP (U.K.) 1971. Cons. Gen. & Respirat. Med. Glas. Roy. Infirm. & Stobhill Gen. Hosp. Glas. Specialty: Respirat. Med. Prev: Sen. Regist. (Med. & Respirat. Dis.) West. Infirm. Glas. & Glas. Roy. Infirm.; Lect. (Med.) West. Infirm. Glas.

STEVENSON, Robert Newton Department of Cardiology, Huddersfield Royal Infirmary, Huddersfield HD3 3EA Tel: 01484 22191; 104 Main Gate, Hepworth, Huddersfield HD9 1TJ — MB BS Lond. 1983 (London Hospital) MRCP (UK) 1986; BSc Lond. 1980, MD 1993; FRCP Lond. 1998. Cons. Phys. (Cardiol & Med.) Huddersfield Roy. Infirm. Specialty: Cardiol. Socs: Brit. Cardiac Soc. Prev: Research Fell. Regist. (Cardiol.) Lond. Chest Hosp.; Regist. (Med.) Univ. Coll. Hosp. Lond.

STEVENSON, Robert Rowan (retired) 60 Northwold Avenue, West Bridgford, Nottingham NG2 7JD Tel: 0115 981 9053 — MB ChB St. And. 1945; BSc. 1942, MB ChB St. And. 1945; MRCGP 1960. Prev: Ho. Surg. & Regist. (Med.) Roy. Infirm. Dundee.

STEVENSON, Thomas (retired) 4 Lonsdale Road, Newton Abbot TQ12 1DT — MB ChB Glas. 1942.

STEVENSON, Thomas Charles (retired) Brymoor House, Harpers Lane, Smithills, Bolton BL1 Tel: 01204 841052 — MB ChB Manch. 1957; FRCOG 1977, M 1963.

STEVENSON, Thomas Henry 59 Strangford Road, Downpatrick BT30 6SL — MB BCh BAO Dub. 1974.

STEVENSON, Timothy Richard Thomas Northbourne Medical Centre, Eastern Avenue, Shoreham-by-Sea BN43 6PE Tel: 01273 464640; 67 The Green, Southwick, Brighton BN42 4FX — MB BCh BAO NUI 1984; DRCOG 1987; MRCGP 1988. Prev: SHO (Paediat.) Edgware Gen. Hosp.; Trainee GP Lond.; SHO Edgware Gen. Hosp. VTS.

STEVENSON, Valerie Lynne The National Hospital for Neurology & Neurosurgery, Queen Square, London WC1N 3BG Tel: 020 7837 3611 — MB BS Newc. 1991 (Newc. u. Tyne) MRCP (UK) 1994; CCST (Neurol.) 2004. Cons. Neuro. The Nat. Hosp. for Neurol. & Neurosurg. Lond. Specialty: Neurol. Prev: Research Fell. Inst. Neurol. Lond.

STEVENSON, William (retired) 1 Vivian Park Drive, Aberavon, Port Talbot SA12 6RT — MB BCh Wales 1944 (Cardiff) BSc Wales 1941, MB BCh 1944. Prev: Surg. Regist. Morriston Gen. Hosp. Swansea.

STEVENSON, William John Consett Medical Centre, Station Yard, Consett DH8 5YA Tel: 01207 216116 Fax: 01207 216119 — MB BCh BAO Belf. 1977 (Queens)

STEVENSON, William Thomas John 6 Flowerfields, Catterall, Preston PR3 1YU Tel: 01995 600593 Email: wtjs@compuserve.com — MRCS Eng. LRCP Lond. 1980; BM Bch Oxf 1981. Cons. (Radiol.) Vict. Hosp. Blackpool. Specialty: Radiol. Prev: Cons. Radiol. W. Wales Hosp. Carmarthen.; Cons. Radiol. Princess Roy. Hosp. Telford.

STEVENTON, David Michael Hawthorn House, 2 Walton Lane, Brocton, Stafford ST17 0TT — MB BS Lond. 1986.

STEVENTON, Nicholas Barrie 2 Railway Cottages, Itchen Abbas, Winchester SO21 1BA — MB BChir Camb. 1991.

STEVENTON, Paul Nigel Integrated Care Partnership, Fitznell Manor Surgery, Chessington Road, Ewell, Epsom KT17 1TF Tel: 020 8394 1471 Fax: 020 8393 9753 — MB BS Lond. 1977; DCH RCP Lond. 1981; DRCOG 1983; MRCGP 1983. GP Princip., IT Specialist, Integrated Care Partnership, Ewell, Epsom, Surrey; Chairm. Doctors Indep. Network. Specialty: Gen. Pract. Socs: Roy. Soc. of Med. (Fell.). Prev: Sen. Med. Off. (RDF) North. Irel.

STEWARD, Colin Graham Oncology Day Beds, Bristol Royal Hospital for Children, Upper Maudlin St., Bristol BS2 8BJ Tel: 0117 342 8523 Fax: 0117 342 8628 — BM BCh Oxf. 1984; MA Camb. 1985; MRCP (UK) 1987; PhD Bristol 1994. Cons. Reader Bone Marrow Transpl. Roy. Hosp. Sick Childr. Bristol. Specialty: Paediat.; Haematology; Genetics. Socs: Fell. Roy. Coll. Paediat. & Child Health; Roy. Coll. Phys. Prev: Regist. (Oncol.) Bristol Childr. Hosp.; Regist. (Paeadiat.) Addenbrooke's Hosp. Camb.; Regist. Hosp. Sick Childr. Gt. Ormond St. Lond.

STEWARD, John Aubrey Welsh Cancer Intelligence and Surveillance Unit, 14 Cathedral Road, Cardiff CF11 9LJ Tel: 029 2037 3500 Fax: 029 2037 3511; 21 Augustan Close, Caerleon, Newport NP18 3DJ Tel: 01633 421240 — MB BCh Wales 1970 (Cardiff) BA (Hons.) Open 1982; MSc Math. Statistics & Computing Wales 1984; MFPHM 1986; PhD Wales 1995. Dir. Welsh Cancer Intelligence & Surveillance Unit (Velinde NHS Trust). Specialty: Epidemiol. Prev: Cons. (PHM) Gwent 1990; Asst. Dir. Welsh Breast Screening Serv.; Sen. Lect. (Pub. Health Med.) UWCM 1989.

STEWARD, Kathleen Anne Hillfoot Surgery, 126 Owlcotes Road, Pudsey LS28 7QR Tel: 0113 257 4169 Fax: 0113 236 3380 — MB BS Newc. 1984; BA (Hons.) Camb. 1981; DRCOG 1987; MRCGP 1989.

STEWARD, Mr Mark Arnold 157 Hartshead Lane, Hartsead, Liversedge WF15 8AJ — MB ChB Leeds 1988; FRCS Ed. 1996. Specialist Regist. (Gen. Surg.) N. Western Deanery. Specialty: Gen. Surg. Prev: Clin. Surgic. Research Fell. (Breast Cancer) Leeds Gen. Infirm.; SHO (O & G) St. Jas. Univ. Hosp. Leeds; SHO Rotat. (Surg.) Leeds Gen. Infirm.

STEWARD, Mark Rider Potterells Medical Centre, Station Road, North Mymms, Hatfield AL9 7SN Tel: 01707 273338 Fax: 01707 263564; 28 The Shaws, Welwyn Garden City AL7 2HR Tel: 01707 884552 — MB BS Lond. 1991. Princip. GP N. mymms Herts.

STEWARD, Ronald Edgar (retired) Adams, Wrotham Road, Meopham, Gravesend DA13 0JH Tel: 01474 813586 Email: ronsteward@lineone.net — MB ChB Ed. 1959. Prev: Regist. (Cas.) & SHO (Gen. Surg.) W. Hill Hosp. Dartford.

STEWARD, Sarah Elizabeth The Cottage, Wilmington, Polegate BN26 5SJ — MB BS Lond. 1985; MRCGP 1991.

STEWARD, Professor William Patrick Department of Oncology, Leicester Royal Infirmary, Leicester LE1 5WW Tel: 0116 258 7597 Fax: 0116 258 7599 — MB ChB Manch. 1977; MRCP (UK) 1979; PhD Manch. 1988; FRCP Glas. 1992; FRCPC 1995. Prof. Med. Oncol. Univ. Leicester. Specialty: Oncol. Special Interest: GI Cancer; Sarcoma. Socs: Roy. Coll. of Physicians, Lond.; Assn. of Cancer Physicians. Prev: Prof. Oncol. Qu. Univ. Kingston Ont., Canada; Sen. Lect. (Med. Oncol.) Beatson Oncol. Centre Glas.

STEWART, Adrian John 49 St Margarets Street, Rochester ME1 1UG — MB BCh BAO Belf. 1985; MRCP (UK) 1988.

STEWART, Adrian Johnston 12 Rosevale Avenue, Lisburn BT17 9LG Email: johnston-stewart@tiscali.co.uk — MB BCh BAO Belf. 1983; MFPM; MRCGP.

STEWART, Adriel Lyndthorpe, 3 Waringmore, Moira, Craigavon BT67 0LG — MB BS Lond. 1992.

STEWART, Agnes Campbell (retired) Woodlands, Inverdruie, Aviemore PH22 1QH Tel: 01479 811765 — MB ChB Ed. 1961; Dip. Clin Hyp. Sheffield; BSc. OU 1998. Staff Grade (Dermat.) Barnsley Dist. Gen. Trust Hosp. Prev: GP Barnsley.

STEWART, Aileen Joy Masterton Health Centre, 74 Somerville Street, Burntisland KY3 9DF — MB ChB Aberd. 1990; DRCOG 1992; MRCGP 1994; DFFP 1994; DCCH RCGP 1996. Staff Grade (Community Paediatrics) Masterton Health Centre, Fife. Specialty: Community Child Health. Prev: SHO (Community Paediat.) Dumfries & Galloway Community NHS Trust; SHO (Paediat. & Cas.) Dumfries & Galloway Roy. Infirm.; SHO (Psychiat.) Crichton Roy. Hosp. Dumfries.

STEWART, Alaisdair Garnett Chest Clinic, Medway Hospital, Gillingham ME7 5NY Tel: 01634 830000 Fax: 01634 833837; Cooling House, Main Road, Cooling, Rochester ME3 8DH — MB BChir Camb. 1982; MRCP (UK) 1986; MA Camb. 1983, MD 1993. Cons. Phys. (Thoracic Med. & Allergy) Medway Hosp. Gillingham. Specialty: Respirat. Med.; Intens. Care; Gen. Med. Socs: Brit. Thorac. Soc.; Eur. Soc. Clin. Respirat. Physiol.; Brit. Soc. Allergy & Clin. Immunol. Prev: Sen. Regist. (Med.) Addenbrooke's Hosp. Camb.; Lect. (Med.) Univ. Sheff.; Regist. (Med.) Roy. Hallamsh. Hosp. Sheff. & Lincoln Co. Hosp.

STEWART, Alan Charles (cons. rooms), Biolab Medical Unit, 9 Weymouth Street, London W1W 6DB; 30 The Drive, Hove BN3 3JD Tel: 01273 487003 Fax: 01273 488641 — MB BS Lond. (Guy's) 1976 (Guy's) MRCS Eng. LRCP Lond. 1976; MRCP (UK) 1979. Indep. Cons. Pract. Nutrit. & Homoeop.; Med. Adviser Wom. Nutrit. Advis. Serv. Lewes. Specialty: Homeop. Med. Prev: Informat. Off. Brit. Soc. Nutrit Med.

STEWART, Alan Douglas Wayside House, Clare, Sudbury CO10 8NP Tel: 01787 277638 — MB ChB Bristol 1946; DObst RCOG 1950. Prev: Ho. Surg. Bristol Roy. Infirm.; O & G Ho. Surg. Wom. Hosp. Wolverhampton; Ho. Phys. Worcester Roy. Infirm.

STEWART, Alan John Church Street Surgery, 30 Church Street, Dunoon AB15 5NB — MB ChB Ed. 1990; MRCGP 2001. GP Princip. Specialty: Paediat.
STEWART, Alan Keith (retired) 33 Station Road, Cambridge CB1 5ER Tel: 01223 880607 — MB ChB Manch. 1966 (Univ. Manch.) MSc Manch. 1963; MRCP Lond. 1969.
STEWART, Alan Leslie Department of Clinical Oncology, Christie Hospital, Wilmslow road, Withington, Manchester M20 4BX Tel: 0161 446 3000 Fax: 0161 446 3414 Email: alan.stewart@christie-tr.nwest.nhs.uk — MD Aberd. 1981; MB ChB 1975; FRCR 1985. Cons. Clin. Oncol. Christie Hosp. & Holt Radium Inst. Manch. Specialty: Oncol.; Radiother. Prev: Sen. Regist. (Radiother.) Christie Hosp. & Holt Radium Inst. Manch.; Research Fell. & Regist. (Clin. Pharmacol.) Christie Hosp. & Holt Radium Inst. Manch.
STEWART, Alastair Fulton Struthers 51 St Patricks Road N., St. Annes on Sea, Lytham St Annes FY8 2HB Tel: 01253 712185 — MB BS Lond. 1960 (St. Bart.) DObst RCOG 1965. Prev: Cas. Off. Paddington Gen. Hosp.; Ho. Surg. Sutton & Cheam Hosp.; Ho. Phys. Bethnal Green Hosp. Lond.
STEWART, Alastair Ian 23 Blardenon Drive, Cumbernauld, Glasgow G68 9BE — MB ChB Ed. 1984.
STEWART, Alexander Ullapool Medical Practice, The Health Centre, Market Street, Ullapool IV26 2XE Tel: 01854 612015/612595 Fax: 01854 613025 — MB ChB Glas. 1974; MRCGP 1979.
STEWART, Alexander George Cheshire &Merseyside Health ProtectionTeam, Microbiology Laboratory, Countess of Chester Health Park, Liverpool Road, Chester CH2 1UL Tel: 01244 366766 Fax: 01244 366782 Email: astewart@nwhpa.nhs.uk — MB ChB Glas. 1974; DTM & H RCP Lond. 1976; DRCOG 1976; MPH Liverpool 2000; MFPHI Dub. 2004; MFPHM 2004. Cons. in Health Protec. Specialty: Pub. Health Med. Special Interest: Environm. Pub. Health. Socs: Soc. for Environm. GeoChem. & Health, Bd. Mem.; Brit. Thyroid Assn., Mem.; Europ. Assn. for Cancer Educat., Bd Mem. Prev: Specialist Regist. Pub. Health, Merseyside; Problem based learning Tutor, Med. Fac., Liverp. Univ.; Research Fell., Dept of Health care Educat., Univ. of Liverp.
STEWART, Alexander Ian, TD Worston Hall, Great Bridgeford, Stafford ST18 9QA Tel: 01785 282203 — MB ChB Birm. 1971; BSc (Physiol. Hons.) Birm. 1968; FFA RCS Eng. 1976. Cons. Anaesth. N. Staffs. Hosp. Specialty: Anaesth. Prev: Sen. Regist. (Anaesth.) W. Midl. RHA.
STEWART, Alexander Macrae (retired) Fair Oak, 5 Woodlands Drive, Thelwall, Warrington WA4 2EU Tel: 01925 261968 Fax: 01925 261968 — (Liverp.) MB ChB Liverp. 1953; DIH Soc. Apoth. Lond. 1963; MFOM RCP Lond. 1978. Prev: Gp. Med. Off. Simon Engin. Ltd. Cheadle Heath.
STEWART, Alexander Rae 35 Morningside Park, Edinburgh EH10 5HD — MB ChB Glas. 1958.
STEWART, Alisdair George (retired) 4 Margaret Road, Harrogate HG2 0JZ Tel: 01423 569480 — MB ChB St. And. 1960; LMCC 1962; FRCP Ed. 1976, M 1965; FRCP Lond. 1980, M 1966. Cons. Phys. Harrogate HA. Prev: Research Fell. (Med.) McGill Univ.
STEWART, Alison Jane — MB ChB Ed. 1998.
STEWART, Alison Jill Hospiscare, Dryden Road, Exeter EX2 5JJ — MB BS (Hons.) Lond. 1991 (Roy. Free) BSc (Hons.) Lond. 1988; DCH RCP Lond. 1995; DFFP 1998; MRCGP 1998. Clin. Asst. (Palliat. Med) Hospiscare Exeter. Specialty: Gen. Pract.; Palliat. Med. Prev: SHO (Palliat. Med.) Marie Currie Centre, Fairmile Edin.; Trainee GP Roy. Devon & Exeter Hosp.; SHO (Paediat.) Glos. Roy. Hosp.
STEWART, Alison Lesley Stonehaven Medical Group, Stonehaven Medical Centre, 32 Robert Street, Stonehaven AB39 2EL Tel: 01569 762945 Fax: 01569 766552; 84 Arduthie Road, Stonehaven AB39 2EH Tel: 01569 65533 — MB ChB Dundee 1979; DCH Glas. 1981; DRCOG 1983.
STEWART, Alison Margaret Western Infirmary, Dumbarton Road, Glasgow G11 6NT Tel: 0141 211 2000 Ext: 3389; 27 Rosemont, Westerwood, Cumbernauld, Glasgow G68 0HL — MB ChB Glas. 1991; MRCP (UK) 1994. Specialist Regist. (Endocrin.) Western Infirm. Gals. Specialty: Gen. Med.; Diabetes; Endocrinol. Socs: Brit. Diabetic Assn.; Caledonian Soc. Endocrinol.; Soc. For Endocrin. Prev: Specialist Regist. (Gen. Med., Diabetes & Endocrinol.) South. Gen. Hosp. NHS Trust Glas.; Specialist Regist. Stirling Roy. Infirm.
STEWART, Alison Martin 1500 Warwick Road, Knowle, Solihull B93 9LE Tel: 01564 772010 Fax: 01564 771224; 10 Diddington Lane, Hampton-in-Arden, Solihull B92 0BZ Tel: 01675 442832 — BM Soton. 1976; MRCP (UK) 1980; MRCGP 1983.
STEWART, Alistair Bryce 7 Church Mews, 17 Church Road, Parkstone, Poole BH14 8VF — BM Soton. 1998; MRCS Lond. 2001. Research Fell., Urol., Soton.
STEWART, Amanda Grace Elizabeth Mary Frinton Road Surgery, 68 Frinton Road, Holland-on-Sea, Clacton-on-Sea CO15 5UW — MB ChB Glas. 1983. GP; SHO (A & E) Colchester Gen. Hosp. Prev: SHO (Accid. & Orthop.) South. Gen. Hosp. Glas.; Ho. Off. (Med.) South. Gen. Hosp. Glas.; Ho. Off. (Surg.) Hairmyres Hosp. E. Kilbride.
STEWART, Amy Alexander — MB ChB Glas. 1997.
STEWART, Andrea Diane 58 Waddington Avenue, Coulsdon CR5 1QF — MB ChB Birm. 1992.
STEWART, Mr Andrew 1 Derwent Close, Claygate, Esher KT10 0RF — MB BS Lond. 1986 (King's College Hospital London) BDS Lond. 1979; FDS RCS Eng. 1985; FRCS Glas. 1990. Cons. Oral & Maxillofacial Surg. Qu. Mary's Hosp. Lond. & St. Helier Hosp. Carshalton. Specialty: Oral & Maxillofacial Surg. Prev: Sen. Regist. (Oral & Maxillofacial Surg.) Qu. Vict. Hosp. E. Grinstead; Sen. Regist. (Oral & Maxillofacial Surg.) Univ. Coll. Hosp. Lond.; Regist. (Oral & Maxillofacial Surg.) Qu. Mary's Hosp. Lond.
STEWART, Andrew David 12 Burnside Gardens, Stonehaven AB39 2FA — MB ChB Aberd. 1998.
STEWART, Andrew Draycott Flat 2, Trident House, 14 West St., Portsmouth PO1 2JW — MB ChB Manch. 1978; BSc (Psychol.) Manch. 1975, MB ChB 1978; DObst 1981; MRCP (UK) 1982; DCH RCP Lond. 1982; FRACP 1988. Cons. Paediat. Gisborne Hosp. New Zealand. Specialty: Paediat.
STEWART, Andrew Hugh Robert 742 Saintfield Road, Carryduff, Belfast BT8 8AT — BChir Camb. 1995.
STEWART, Andrew James Department of Haematology, Royal Infirmary, Lauriston Place, Edinburgh EH3 9YW Tel: 0131 536 1000; 1 Cramond Glebe Terrace, Cramond, Edinburgh EH4 6NR Tel: 0131 312 8891 — MB ChB Ed. 1988 (Oxford and Edinburgh) BA Oxf. 1985; MRCP (UK) 1991; Dip. RCPath. 1995. Lect. in Haemat. Edin. Univ. Specialty: Haematology. Prev: Regist. (Nephrol.) Leeds Gen. Infirm.; Regist. (Haemat.) Roy. Infirm. Edin.
STEWART, Andrew Norman The Surgery, 6 College Road, Eastbourne BN21 4HY Tel: 01323 735044 Fax: 01323 417705 — MB ChB Aberd. 1986; DCH RCPS Glas. 1989; MRCGP 1990. GP Princip. Socs: E.bourne Med. Soc. Prev: Trainee GP Eastbourne HA VTS.
STEWART, Andrew Peter Gunnislake Health Centre, The Orchard, Gunnislake PL18 9JZ Tel: 01822 836241 Fax: 01822 833757; Barnwell, Bealbury Farm, St. Mellion, Saltash PL12 6RX — MB BS Lond. 1974 (Char. Cross) DRCOG 1976; MRCGP 1980. Ment. Health Lead E. Cornw. PCG; Mem. Cornw. & Isles of Scilly LMC. Specialty: Gen. Pract. Socs: BMA; Assn. BRd.casting Doctors; Roy. Coll. Gen. Pract. Prev: Regist. (Geriat. Med.) Barncoose Hosp. Redruth; SHO (Obst.) W. Lond. Hosp.; Ho. Phys. (Gen. Med.) Char. Cross Hosp. Lond.
STEWART, Andrew Peter 5 Lambert Drive, Sale M33 5WP — MB ChB Aberd. 1998.
STEWART, Andrew Peter Owen (retired) 22 Pennine Grove, Huntroyde, Burnley BB12 9AB Tel: 01282 772389 — MB BS Lond. 1953 (Guy's) Prev: Ho. Phys. Guy's Hosp.
STEWART, Angela Jane 15 Park Road, Winchester SO22 6AA Tel: 01962 852172 Fax: 01962 852172 — MB BS Lond. 1966 (Roy. Free) MFFP; MB BS (Hons.) Obst. Lond. 1966; MRCS Eng. LRCP Lond. 1966; DObst RCOG 1969; MFFP 1993. SCMO Soton. Community Health Trust; Sen. Clin. Med. Off. Loddon N. Hants. Community Trust. Specialty: Pub. Health Med. Socs: Assoc. Mem. Inst. Psychosexual Med. Prev: Med. Off. Brit. Rail; GP Eltham; SHO FarnBoro. Hosp. Kent.
STEWART, Angus John Trumpington Street Medical Practice, 56 Trumpington Street, Cambridge CB2 1RG Tel: 01223 361611 Fax: 01223 356837; 80 Holbrook Road, Cambridge CB1 7ST Tel: 01223 704713 — MA Camb. 1983, MB BChir 1982; DRCOG 1985; MRCGP 1986; DCH RCP Lond. 1986; AFOM 1990. Med. Off. John Lewis Partership; Sch. Med. Off. Leys Sch.; Med. Off. Hexcel Composites.

STEWART, Ann-Marie 37A Westbourne Road, Sheffield S10 2QT — MB ChB Sheff. 1994.

STEWART, Anne Highfield Family & Adolescent Unit, Warneford Hospital, Warneford Lane, Oxford OX3 7JX Tel: 01865 226280 Fax: 01865 226381 — MB BS Lond. 1978 (St. Bart.) BSc Lond. 1975; DCH RCP Lond. 1985; MRCPsych 1985. Cons. Child & Adolesc. Psychiat. Highfield Family & Adolesc. Unit Oxf. Specialty: Child & Adolesc. Psychiat. Prev: Sen. Lect. Wellington Sch. Med., NZ.

STEWART, Anne Briar 284 Telegraph Road, Heswall, Wirral CH60 7SG — MB ChB Ed. 1978; MRCP (UK) 1983. Cons. Emerg. & Ambulatory Paediat. Alder Hey Childr. Hosp. Liverp. Specialty: Accid. & Emerg.

STEWART, Anne Elizabeth St Lukes Hospice, Turnchapel, Plymouth PL9 9XA; North Beneknowle, Diptford, Totnes TQ9 7LU — MB BS Lond. 1983; BSc Lond. 1981, MB BS 1983; MRCGP 1987. Staff Grade (Palliat. Care) St Lukes Hospice Turnchapel Plymouth. Prev: Trainee GP Plymouth VTS.

STEWART, Anne Linn (retired) 9 Abbotsford Avenue, Rutherglen, Glasgow G73 3NX Tel: 0141 647 3422 — MB ChB Glas. 1960.

STEWART, Audrey Elizabeth (retired) 55 Broad Street, Portsmouth PO1 2JD Tel: 023 9282 3045 Fax: 023 9229 5961 — (Manch.) MB ChB. Manch. 1949; DObst. RCOG 1951. Prev: Sen. Dept. Med. Off. City Portsmouth Health Dept.

STEWART, Barbara Jane Armstrong Deer Park Medical Centre, 6 Edington Square, Witney OX28 5YT Tel: 0118 986 2277 ext 2288 Fax: 0118 975 0297 — MB BS Lond. 1985; BA Camb. 1982; MRCP (UK) 1989; Dip. Epidemiol. RCP (UK) 1993. Cons. Paediat. (Community Child Health). Specialty: Paediat. Prev: Sen. Regist. (Paediat. & Community Child Health) Churchill Hosp. Oxf.; Research Fell. (Community Paediat.) Radcliffe Infirm. Oxf.

STEWART, Barbara Janet Clare Firhill Medical Practice, 167 Colinton Mains Drive, Edinburgh EH13 9AF — MB ChB Ed. 1992.

STEWART, Belinda Rosemary Tyjarrett, Brunant Rd, Clydach, Abergavenny NP7 0NG Tel: 01873 832272 — MB BCh Wales 1990; MRCGP 1995. GP Trainee Brecon; Locum GP Mon. Prev: Trainee GP Abergavenny; Vocat. Train. Abergavenny.

STEWART, Bruce Alexander Dept. of Microbiology, East Surrey Hospital, Canada Avenue, Redhill RH1 5RH Tel: 01737 768511 Email: bruce@doctors.org.uk — MB ChB Birm. 1989 (Birmingham) MRCP UK 1993; MSC, Lond, 1996; MRCPath, 1999. Cons. Microbiologist Surrey & Sussex Healthcare Trust. Specialty: Med. Microbiol. Socs: BMA; Brit. Soc. For Antimicrobial Chemo.; Assn of Med. Microbiologists.

STEWART, Carol Calsayseat Medical Group, 44 Powis Place, Aberdeen AB25 3TS Tel: 01224 634345 Fax: 01224 562220 — MB ChB Dundee 1988.

STEWART, Carol Margaret Bathgate Health Centre, Mid St, Bathgate EH48 1PT; 25 Saltcoats Gardens, Bellsquarry S., Livingston EH54 9JD Tel: 01506 419439 — MB ChB Ed. 1990; BSc Ed. 1988, MB ChB 1990; MRCP (UK) 1994; DRCOG 1995; MRCGP 1997. Retainee GP. Bathgate Heath Centre. Bathgate. Prev: SHO Marie Curie Centre Fairmile Edin.; SHO (Med.) North. & West. Gen. Hosps. Edin.

STEWART, Charles Glyndwr 29 Sandy La, Caldicot, Newport NP26 4NA — MB BCh Wales 1997; BSc (Med. Sci.) 1994.

STEWART, Charles Malcolm Edge of Beyond, Sene Park, Hythe CT21 5XD — MB BS Lond. 1970; MRCOG 1981; T(OG) 1991. Cons. (Gynaecol. & Dep. Med. Dir.) E. Kent Hosps. NHS Trust. Specialty: Obst. & Gyn. Prev: Clin. Research Fell. Hon. Sen. Regist. Dept. O & G St.; Med. Sch. Lond.

STEWART, Charles Peter (retired) 35 Woodside Walk, Hamilton ML3 7JD Tel: 01698 281590 — MB ChB Glas. 1951.

STEWART, Charles Rodger University Hospitals of Leicester NHS Trust, Leicester General Hospital, Gwendolem Road, Leicester LE5 4PW Tel: 0116 258 4833; Bardon Croft, 4 Knighton Rise, Oadby, Leicester LE2 2RE Tel: 0116 270 6230 — MB ChB Glas. 1965; FRCOG 1982, M 1970; T(OG) 1991. Cons. - Obstretics and Gyn. Leicester Gen. Hosp.; Hon. Clin. Lect. Univ. Leicester. Specialty: Obst. & Gyn. Socs: BMA (Sec. Leics. & Rutland Div.); N. Eng. Obst. Soc.; Birm. and Midl.s Obsterical Soc. Prev: Sen. Lect. Univ. Leicester Med. Sch.; Sen. Lect. Univ. Otago & Hon. Cons. (Gyn.) N. Canterbury Hosp. Bd., NZ.

STEWART, Charles Teasdale Trades Lane Health Centre, Causewayend, Coupar Angus, Blairgowrie PH13 9DP Tel: 01828 627318 — MB ChB Glas. 1984.

STEWART, Christopher David The Taymount Surgery, 1 Taymount Terrace, Perth PH1 1NU Tel: 01738 627117 Fax: 01738 444713 — MB BCh BAO Belf. 1988; MB BCh Belf. 1988.

STEWART, Clare Isobel Louise Glaxo Day Hospital, Ashludie Hospital, Monifieth, Dundee DD5 4HQ Tel: 01382 527831 Fax: 01382 527852; 22 Cedar Road, Broughty Ferry, Dundee DD5 3BB — MB ChB Dundee 1988; DGM RCPS Glas. 1994. Staff Grade Phys. (Med. for Elderly) Glaxo Day Hosp. Monifieth. Specialty: Care of the Elderly.

STEWART, Clyne Robert Bruce (retired) 18 Sandringham Court, Porthill, Shrewsbury SY3 8LL Tel: 01743 355743 — (Aberd.) MB ChB Aberd. 1947.

STEWART, Colin John Reid Strathwood, Milndavie Road, Strathblane, Glasgow G63 9EN — MB ChB Glas. 1983.

STEWART, Colin Peter Urquhart The Pines, 38 Seafield Road, Broughty Ferry, Dundee DD5 3AN Tel: 01382 779513 Fax: 01382 480194 — MB ChB Dundee 1973; DMedRehab Eng. 1979; MD Dundee 1986. Specialty: Rehabil. Med. Socs: BMA (Ex-Chairm. NCCG Sub Comm. SCHMS); Fell. Internat. Soc. Prosth. & Orthotics. Prev: Assoc. Specialist (Prosth. & Orthotics) Tort Centre, Ninewells Hosp, Dundee; Regist. (Prosth. & Orthotics) Dundee Limb Fitting Centre Broughty Ferry; Regist. (Geriat. Rehabil.) Ashludie Hosp. Monifieth.

STEWART, Dan (retired) 16 Eversley Crescent, London N21 1EJ Tel: 020 8360 1512 — MB BS Lond. 1951 (St. Mary's) DObst RCOG 1955; MRCGP 1977. Prev: GP Staff Wood Green & Southgate Hosps. & Enfield War Memor. Hosp.

STEWART, David Manchester Childrens Hospitals NHS Trust, Royal Manchester Childrens Hospital, Department Intens. Care Med., Hospital Road, Pendlesbury, Manchester M27 4HA Tel: 0161 727 2468 Fax: 0161 727 2198 Email: david.stewart@man.ac.uk; Children's Hospital Los Angeles, 4650 Sunset Boulevard, Los Angeles, California 90068, USA Tel: 323 664 0728/323 669 2557 Email: dstewart@chla.scu.edu — MB ChB Leic. 1986; FRCPCH; BSc (Hons.) Manch. 1981; MRCP (UK) 1991. Cons. Paediat. Intens. Care Manch. Childr. Hosps. NHS Trust; Lead Clinician Train. & Clin. Pract. Developm.; Lead Clinician High Dependency Unit. Specialty: Paediat. Socs: Paediat. Intens. Care Soc.; Soc. Critical Care Med. Prev: Clin. Fell. (Paediat. Critical Care) Toronto Hosp. for Sick Childr.; Sen. Regist. Rotat. W. Midl. RHA; Regist. Rotat. (Paediat.) W. Middlx. Univ. Hosp. & Westm. Childr. Hosp.

STEWART, David Armour 9 Dornoch Avenue, Griffnock, Glasgow G46 6QH — MB ChB Glas. 1981; MRCP (UK) 1985.

STEWART, David George Telford 37 Main Street, Castlerock, Coleraine BT51 4RA — MB BCh BAO Belf. 1979; MSc (Community Med.) Ed. 1983; MFCM RCP 1984; FFPHM RCP (UK) 1994. Dir. (Pub. Health) EHSSB Belf. Specialty: Pub. Health Med.

STEWART, David Graeme Wordsley Hospital, Department of Dermatology, Stream Road, Dudley DY8 5QX Tel: 01384 244 55 Fax: 01384 244 51 — MB ChB Aberd. 1985; MRCP (UK) 1991; FRCP 2001. Cons. (Dermatol.) Univ. Hosp. Birm. Specialty: Dermat. Prev: Sen. Regist. (Dermatol.) Univ. Hosp. Birm.; Regist. The Birm. Skin Hosp.

STEWART, David Hamilton 7 Glenwater Close, Axmouth, Seaton EX12 4BT — MB ChB Cape Town 1952; FRCOG 1973, M 1959.

STEWART, David John (retired) Wayside, South Stoke, Bath BA2 7DJ Tel: 01225 832031 — (Univ. Glas.) MB ChB Glas. 1944; LM Rotunda 1957. Prev: Clin. Med. Off. Bath Health Dist.

STEWART, David Patrick Edward 12 Meenaleck Walk, Londonderry BT48 8HL — MB BCh BAO Belf. 1990.

STEWART, David Patterson Dr MacLean and Partners, Monifieth Health Centre, Victoria Street, Dundee DD5 4LX Tel: 01382 534301 Fax: 01382 535959 — MB ChB Dundee 1988; DRCOG 1990; MRCGP 1992.

STEWART, David Winterburn Wishaw Health Centre, Kenilworth Avenue, Wishaw ML2 7BQ Tel: 01698 373341 — MB ChB Glas. 1973; DObst RCOG 1976.

STEWART, Denis John Alexander The Health Centre, Station Road, Bawtry, Doncaster DN10 6RQ Tel: 01302 710210 Fax: 01302 710261; 9 Arundel Drive, Ranskill, Retford DN22 8PG Tel: 01302

710210 — MB ChB Dundee 1980; BSc St. And. 1976; DRCOG 1982.

STEWART, Donald Norman, OStJ, TD (retired) High Down, Mount Pleasant, Bishop's Tawton, Barnstaple EX32 0BS Tel: 01271 374548 — MRCS Eng. LRCP Lond. 1942 (Char. Cross) DLO Eng. 1963. Prev: Asst. ENT Surg. Croydon Gp. Hosps.

STEWART, Mr Douglas James Royal Preston Hospital, Sharoe Green Lane, Preston PR2 9HT; 14 Uplands Chase, Fulwood, Preston PR2 7AW Tel: 01772 865009 — MB ChB Aberd. 1969; FRCS Ed. 1973; ChM Aberd. 1979. Cons. Gen. Surg. Roy. Preston Hosp. Specialty: Gen. Surg. Socs: Assn. of Surg. of GB & Irel.; Assn. of Coloproctol. of GB & Irel.

STEWART, Duncan Bernard The Surgery, 28 Wilbury Road, Hove BN3 3JP Tel: 01273 733830 Fax: 01273 207424 — MB BS Lond. 1967 (Guy's) MRCS Eng. LRCP Lond. 1967; DObst RCOG 1969. Med. Off. Roedean Sch. Brighton & Harewood Ct. RMBI Home. Socs: Brighton & Sussex M-C Soc.

STEWART, Edmund Central Health Centre, North Carbrain Road, Cumbernauld, Glasgow G67 1BJ Tel: 01236 737214 Fax: 01236 781699; Craigmarloch Medical Centre, 17 Auchinsee Way, Craigmarloch, Cumbernauld G68 0EZ Tel: 01236 780700 Fax: 01236 780344 — MB ChB Glas. 1991.

STEWART, Eleanor Janet 295 Merville Garden Village, Newtownabbey BT37 9TY — MB BCh BAO Belf. 1981; FRCS Ed. 1986.

STEWART, Elizabeth Jane Colhoun Leigh Infirmary, The Prosser White Dermatology Centre, The Avenue, Leigh WN7 1HS Tel: 01942 264061 Fax: 01942 264016 Email: elizabeth.stewart@wwl.nhs.uk — MB ChB Glas. 1980; MRCP (UK) 1983; FRCP Glas. 1996. Cons. Dermatol. Wrightington, Wigan & Leigh NHS Trust; Hon. Cons. Dermatol. Hope Hosp. Salford. Specialty: Dermat. Special Interest: Atopic Eczema; Leg Ulcers; Skin Cancer. Socs: Brit. Assn. Dermatol.

STEWART, Elizabeth Mary (retired) 4 Margaret Road, Harrogate HG2 0JZ Tel: 01423 569480 — MB ChB St. And. 1960 (Dundee) Prev: SCMO (Community Child Health) Harrogate Health Care Trust.

STEWART, Elspeth Jane 24 Durbin Park Road, Clevedon BS21 7EU — MB ChB Glas. 1977.

STEWART, Esther Caroline Ann Antrim Hospital, Bush Road, Antrim BT41 2RL Tel: 028 9442 4000 Ext: 4869 Email: caroline.stewart@uh.n-i.nhs.uk — MB BCh BAO Belf. 1990 (Qu. Univ. Belf.) DCH RCPS Glas. 1992; MRCPI 1995; MRCPCH 1996. Cons. Paediat. Antrim Hosp. Belf. Specialty: Paediat. Special Interest: Paediatric diabetes.

STEWART, Ewen Andrew Rose Garden Medical Centre, 4 Mill Lane, Edinburgh EH6 6TL Tel: 0131 554 1274 Fax: 0131 555 2159 — MB ChB Ed. 1991; BSc MedSci (Bacteriol.) Ed. 1989; MRCGP 1995; DFFP 1995. Asst. Primary Care Facilitator (HIV/AIDS) Lothian Health. Specialty: Gen. Pract. Prev: Regist. Kobler Centre Chelsea & Westm. Hosp. Lond.; Hosp. Pract. (Diabetes) EGH.

STEWART, Fiona Jane Department of Medical Genetics, Level A, Belfast City Hospital, Lisburn Road, Belfast BT9 7AB Tel: 02890 263874 Fax: 02890 236911 — MB BS Lond. 1985; MRCP (UK) 1989; MA Belf. 1997. Cons. Med. Genetics Belf. City Hosp. Specialty: Genetics. Socs: Brit. Paediat. Assn. & Clin. Genetics Soc. Prev: Sen. Regist. (Med. Genetics) Belf. City Hosp.

STEWART, Fiona Karen Orchard House Psychogeriatric Day Hospital, Union St., Stirling FK8 1NY Tel: 01786 474161; 92 Thriepland Wynd, Perth PH1 1RH Tel: 01738 630643 — MB ChB Dundee 1986. Clin. Asst. (Old Age Psychiat.) Orchard Hse. Psychogeriat. Day Hosp. Stirling. Specialty: Geriat. Psychiat.

STEWART, Frances Ellen 5 Archery Road, Leamington Spa CV31 3PT — MB ChB Glas. 1979.

STEWART, Frances Maria Apartment 2/L, 107 Crown Road North, Glasgow G12 9HS — MB BCh BAO Belf. 1995.

STEWART, Frank Ian — MB ChB Ed. 1965; DCH RCPS Glas. 1969; FRCGP 1995, M 1971. Gen. Practitioner; Hosp. Pract. (Paediat.) W. Lothian NHS Trust.

STEWART, Gavin Davidson Fair Oak, 5 Woodlands Drive, Thelwall, Warrington WA4 2EU Tel: 01925 261968 Fax: 01925 261968; 7 Lapworth Oaks, Station Lane, Lapworth, Solihull B94 6L6 Tel: 01564 785091 Fax: 01564 785093 Email: stewartgd@aol.com — MB BS Newc. 1985; BA (Ist cl. Hons.) Lond. 1979; MB BS (Hons.) Newc. 1985; MRCP Lond. 1988; FRCR 1991. Cons. Radiol. (Diagn. Radiol.) Warwick Dist. Gen. Hosp. Specialty: Radiol. Prev: Sen. Regist. & Regist. Rotat. (Diagn. Radiol.) Manch. Roy. Infirm.; SHO Rotat. (Med.) Leicester Roy. Infirm.

STEWART, George MacLeod (retired) 4 Ashview Close, Ashford TW15 3RF Tel: 01784 255162 — (Aberd.) MB ChB Aberd. 1959; DTM & H Eng. 1964; DPH Aberd. 1969; DIH Eng. 1970; MFCM RCP (UK) 1972; FFPHM RCP (UK) 1994. Prev: Cons. Communicable Dis. Control & Princip. Med. Off. Control Unit Lond. (Heathrow) Airport.

STEWART, Georgina Houston (retired) 3 Lexden Terrace, Tenby SA70 7BJ Tel: 01834 844772 — MB ChB Glas. 1962 (Glas.) DTM & H Liverp. 1975; Dip. Community. Med. Ed. 1977; FFCM 1988, M 1980; DIH Soc. Apoth. Lond. 1986; FRCP 1996.

STEWART, Gillian Elizabeth Glencree, 68 Old Mountfield Road, Omagh BT79 1EH — MB ChB Aberd. 1992.

STEWART, Mr Gordon Ayr Hospital, Ayr KA6 6DX Tel: 01292 610555; 'Alyth', 63 Monument Road, Ayr KA7 2UE Tel: 01292 880610 — MB ChB Glas. 1973; BSc (Hons. Physiol.) Glas. 1971, MD 1985, MB ChB 1973; FRCS Glas. 1978. Cons. Gen. Surg. & Vasc. Surg. Ayrsh. & Arran Acute Hosps. NHS Trust. Specialty: Gen. Surg. Socs: Vasc. Soc. GB & Irel. & Assn. Surgs. GB & Irel.; Eur. Vasc. Soc.; Venous Forum RSM. Prev: Lect. (Surg.) & Sen. Regist. St. Thos. Hosp. Lond.; Sen. Specialist Surg. Cade Unit PM RAF Hosp. Halton.

STEWART, Gordon Duff (retired) Lammasfield, Baring Road, Cowes PO31 8DW — LRCP LRCS Ed. 1955; LRCP LRCS Ed. LRFPS Glas. 1955; DPM Eng. 1965; FRCPsych 1990, M 1971. Prev: Sen. Med. Off. HM Prison Pk.hurst.

STEWART, Professor Gordon Thallon 29/8 Inverleith Place, Edinburgh EH3 5QD Tel: 0131 5522648 Fax: 0131 552 7987 Email: epishoe@gifford.co.uk; 3 Lexdon Terrace, Tenby SA70 7BJ Tel: 0131 552 2648 Fax: 0131 552 7987 — (Glas.) BSc Glas. 1939; MB ChB Glas. 1942; DTM & H Liverp. 1947; MD (High Commend.) 1949; FRCPath 1963; FRCP Glas. 1975, M 1972; FFPHM 1972. Emerit. Prof. Pub. Health Univ. Glas. Specialty: Pub. Health Med.; Infec. Dis. Special Interest: Behaviour in relation to health; Preven. Med. Socs: Emerit. Fell. Infec. Dis. Soc., USA; Fell. Med. Soc. Lond.; Fell. Roy. Statistical Soc. Prev: Cons. Phys. Gtr. Glas. HB; Vis. Prof. Dow Med. Coll. Karachi, Pakistan 1953-54 & Cornell Univ. Med. Coll. New York City, USA 1970-72; Cons. (Epidemiol.) WHO (1953 onward).

STEWART, Gordon Walker Rayne Institute, University College & Middlesex Med. School, University St., London WC1E 6JJ Tel: 020 7679 6193 Fax: 020 7679 0967 Email: g.stewart@ucl.ac.uk — (Edin.) BSc Sussex 1971; MB ChB Ed. 1976; MRCP (UK) 1978; MD Ed. 1984; MSc Lond. 1989; FRCP 1996. Sen. Lect. & Hon. Cons. Phys. Univer. Coll. & Middlx. Hosps. Specialty: Gen. Med.; Haematology. Prev: Wellcome Sen. Fell. (Clin. Sci.) Rayne Inst. Univ. Coll. Lond.; Lect. (Med.) St. Marys Hosp. Med. Sch. Lond.

STEWART, Graham Royal Alexandra Hospital NHS Trust, Paisley PA2 9PN Tel: 0141 887 9111 Fax: 0141 580 4364 — MB ChB Ed. 1982; FRCPCH; MRCP (UK) 1988; FRCP Glasgow 2000. Cons. Paediat. Argyll & Clyde Acute Hosp.s NHS Trust. Specialty: Paediat. Socs: Neantol. Soc.; Brit. Assn. Permatal Med.

STEWART, Graham Alexander — MB ChB Glas. 1991; MRCP (UK) 1995. SpR Nephrology, Ninewells Hospital, Dundee. Specialty: Nephrol. Prev: SHO (Med.) & Ho. Off. (Surg.) Dumfries & Galloway Roy. Infirm.; Ho. Off. (Med.) Glas. Roy. Infirm.; SHO (Renal Med.) West. Infirm. Glas.

STEWART, Gregor St John Angus 49 Lynn Grove, Gorleston, Great Yarmouth NR31 8AR — MB ChB Glas. 1962; DObst RCOG 1965; DA Eng. 1965. Prev: GP Gt. Yarmouth.

STEWART, Gregory (retired) — MB Camb. 1963 (Guy's) FRCPsych 1986, M; MA Camb. 1972, MB 1963, BChir 1962; MRCP Lond. 1966. Sen. Lect. (Developm. Psychiat.) Univ. Coll. & Middlx. Hosp. Lond.; Cons. Horizon Trust & Bloomsbury Community Trust Lond.

STEWART, Grizel D'Rastricke Springhall Farm, Sheriff Mountain, Londonderry BT47 — MB BCh BAO Belf. 1946. Med. Asst. N.W. Special Care Serv. N. Irel. Prev: Regist. (Psychiat.) Lancaster Moor Hosp.

STEWART, Harold Markinch Medical Practice, Markinch Health Centre, 19 High Street, Glenrothes KY7 6ER Tel: 01592 610640 Fax: 01592 612089 — MB BCh BAO Belf. 1979.

STEWART, Harold 16 Ferncroft Avenue, Hampstead, London NW3 7PH Tel: 020 7435 8696 — MB BS Lond. 1947 (Univ. Coll.

Hosp.) MRCS Eng. LRCP Lond. 1947; FRCPsych 1978, M 1971. Specialty: Psychother. Socs: Brit. Psychoanal. Soc. Prev: Cons. Psychother. Adult Dept. Tavistock Clin.; Cons. Phys. & Cons. Psychiat. Paddington Centre for Psychotherap.; Clin. Asst. (Psychol. Med.) Univ. Coll. Hosp. Lond.

STEWART, Harold Charles, CBE, KStJ 41 The Glen, Green Lane, Northwood HA6 2UR Tel: 01923 824893 — MB BChir Camb. 1931 (Univ. Coll. Hosp.) FRSE; MA Camb. 1934, MD 1936; PhD Lond. 1942; FRCP Lond. 1968, M 1949; FFA RCS Eng. 1969. Emerit. Prof. Pharmacol. Univ. Lond.; DL; Chairm. Buttle Trust for Childr.; Pres. Sir Halley Stewart Trust for Research; Patron Med. Counc. on Alcoholism; Vice-Pres. St. Christophers Hosp. Terminal Cases. Specialty: Pharmacology. Socs: Physiol. & Pharmacol. Socs.; Hon. Vice-Pres. Stewart Soc. Prev: Head Pharmacol. St. Mary's Hosp. Med. Sch.; Dir.-Gen. St. John Ambul. Assn.; Hon. Med. Adviser & Mem. Commonw. Counc., Brit. Commonw. Ex-Servs. League.

STEWART, Hazel Elizabeth Coleraine Health Centre, Castlerock Road, Coleraine BT51 3HP Tel: 028 7034 4834 Fax: 028 7035 8914; 10 Rectory Road, Ballyrashane, Coleraine BT52 2LR — MB BCh BAO Belf. 1976; MRCGP 1983.

STEWART, Helen Susan Churchill Hospital, Old Road, Headington, Oxford OX3 7LJ Tel: 01865 226 026 Fax: 01865 226 011 — MB BCh Wales 1988; MRCP (UK) 1991. Cons. Clin. Specialist, Churchill Hosp., Oxf. Specialty: Genetics.

STEWART, Helen Valerie Ann Mursdale Surgery, Mursdale, Tarbert PA29 6XG Tel: 01583 421206; Glenralloch Cottage, Tarbert PA29 6XX Tel: 01330 820052 — MB ChB Glas. 1985; MRCP (UK) 1988; MRCGP 1990; DCCH RCP Ed. 1992. Assoc. GP. Specialty: Gen. Pract.

STEWART, Herbert James 4 Royal Oaks, Kesh Road, Maze, Lisburn BT27 5RP Tel: 01846 622732 — MB BCh BAO Belf. 1986 (Queens University, Belfast) DRCOG 1991; DFFM 1997. Locum GP; Primary Care Pract. A & E Dept. Master Infirmorum Host, Belf. Specialty: Gen. Pract. Socs: Ulster Med. Soc.; BMA.

STEWART, Mr Hugh Donald Royal Lancaster Infirmary, Orthopaedic Department, Ashton Road, Lancaster LA1 4RP — MB BS Lond. 1974 (Lond. Hosp.) FRCS Eng. 1979. Cons. Traum. & Orthop. Surg. Lancaster & Kendal. Specialty: Orthop. Prev: Cons. Orthop. St. Vincents Hosp. Melbourne, Austral.; Sen. Regist. (Orthop.) Derbysh. Roy. Infirm. & Harlow Wood Orthop. Hosp. Mansfield; Regist. (Orthop.) Derbysh. Roy. Infirm.

STEWART, Hugh Harkness Archiebald — (Univ. Glas.) MB ChB Glas. 1985; MRCGP 1989; LLB Glas. 1994; Dip. LP Glas. 1995; MPhil Glas. 1996. Medico Legal Adviser Glas. Specialty: Medico Legal. Socs: BMA. Prev: GP Glas.; SHO (Psychiat.) Gartnavel Roy. Hosp. Glas.; SHO (O & G) Qu. Mother's Hosp. Glas.

STEWART, Hugh Vaughan University Hospital of North Durham, North Road, Durham DH1 5TW Tel: 0191 333 2295; 9 Larches Road, Durham DH1 4NL Tel: 0191 383 1301 — MB ChB Univ. Zimbabwe 1984 (Zimbabwe) MRCPCH; MRCP (UK) 1992; MSc Trop. Med. Liverp. 1995. Cons. (Paediat.) UHND Durh. Specialty: Paediat. Socs: N. of Eng. Paediatric Soc.

STEWART, Mr Iain 220 Moss Heights Avenue, Cardsnald, Glasgow G52 2UB; 17 Mertylfarm View, Braunton EX33 1QH — MB ChB Glas. 1990; FRCS Ed. 1994; DRCOG 1997; MRCGP 1998. GP Locum; GP Regist. Warwick Pract. Specialty: Gen. Pract. Prev: SHO Anaesth., N. Devon Dist. Hosp.; GP Regist. N.am Pract.

STEWART, Iain Douglas 240 Bennett Street, Long Eaton, Nottingham NG10 4HH — MB ChB Glas. 1981.

STEWART, Iain Macphail (retired) 25 Boclair Road, Bearsden, Glasgow G61 2AF Tel: 0141 942 1615 — MB ChB St. And. 1958; DPH St. And. 1964; DIH Dund 1968; MFCM 1973. Prev: Community Med. Specialist (Gt.er Glas. Health Bd.).

STEWART, Ian MacDonald — MB ChB St. And. 1968; MRCP (UK) 1972; FRCP 1991; FRCP Ed. 1991. Cons. Rheum. Vict. Hosp. Blackpool. Specialty: Rheumatol. Prev: Cons. Rheum. Wrightington Hosp.; Sen. Regist. (Rheum.) Manch. AHA (T).

STEWART, Ian McLennan (retired) Manor Farm House, Sessay, Thirsk YO7 3BE Tel: 01845 501521; Lloyds Bank, 49 London Road N., Lowestoft NR32 1BL Tel: 01502 569316 — LMSSA Lond. 1952 (St. Mary's) DPM Eng. 1962; MRCPsych 1971. Med. Sch. St. Mary's Lond. Prev: Cons. Forens. Psychiat. Stockton Hall Psychiat. Hosp.

STEWART, Mr Ian Park Derriford Hospital, Derriford, Plymouth PL6 8DH — MB ChB Bristol 1962; BSc Bristol 1959, MB ChB 1962; FRCS Eng. 1969. Cons. A & E Dept. Plymouth Gen. Hosp. (Freedom Fields Br.). Specialty: Accid. & Emerg. Socs: BMA. Prev: Surgic. Regist. United Sheff. Hosps.; Surg. Regist. Plymouth Gen. Hosp.; Surg. Regist. Birm. Accid. Hosp.

STEWART, Ian Smith Flat 12, Beechgrove, 149 Crown Road S., Glasgow G12 9DP — MB ChB Glas. 1974; DMRD Eng. 1979; FRCR 1981.

STEWART, Iris Dorothy Margaret 69 Brookfield Avenue, Poynton, Stockport SK12 1JE — MB ChB Manch. 1963; MSc Manch. 1980, MB ChB 1963; DO Eng. 1973; Cert JCC Lond. 1977; MFCM RCP Lond. 1982. Socs: Manch. Med. Soc.; Fell. Roy. Inst. Pub. Health & Hyg.

STEWART, Isabella (retired) 74 The Common, Parbold, Wigan WN8 7EA Tel: 01257 462173 — MB ChB Glas. 1957.

STEWART, Isaiah Casey Combined Assessment Unit, Royal Infirmary of Edinburgh, 51 Little France Crescent, Edinburgh EH16 4SA Tel: 0131 242 1410 Fax: 0131 242 1410 Email: casey.stewart@luht.scot.nhs.uk; Lyndhurst, 5 Brae Park, Edinburgh EH4 6DJ — MB ChB Ed. 1978; BSc (Med. Sci.) Ed. 1975; MRCP (UK) 1980; MD 1987; FRCP Ed. 1994. Clin. Director for Acute Med. Roy. Infirm. of Edin. & West. Gen. Hosp. Specialty: Gen. Med. Prev: Cons. Phys. Roy. Infirm. Edin.

STEWART, James Alexander David Leicester General Hospital, Gwendolen Road, Leicester LE5 4PW Tel: 0116 258 4787 Email: james.stewart@uhl-tr.nhs.uk; The Paddocks, The Old Stables, Rolleston LE7 9EN Tel: 0116 259 6430 Email: james.stewart@uhl-tr.nhs.uk — MB ChB Leic. 1991 (Leicester) MRCP (UK) 1994; LLM Cardiff 2000. Cons. Phys. & Gastroenterologists, Univ. Hosps. of Leicester. Specialty: Gastroenterol.; Gen. Med.; Medico Legal. Socs: Brit. Soc. of Gastroenterologists; Soc. of Acute Med.; Brit. Assn. of Parenteral & Enternal Nutrit. Prev: SHO Rotat. (Med.) Leicester & P'boro.; Specialist Regist. (Med. & Gastroenterol.) Leicester Roy. Infirm.

STEWART, James Douglas Meeks Road Surgery, 10 Meeks Road, Falkirk FK2 7ES Tel: 01324 619930 Fax: 01324 627266; The Stable House, Braco, Dunblane FK15 9RA Tel: 01786 880204 — MB ChB Dundee 1968; FRCPath 1986, M 1974; MRCGP 1979. Prev: Regist. Path. Stirlingsh. Area Laborat. Serv.; Jun. Ho. Off. (Med. & Surg.) Stirling Roy. Infirm.; Sen. Regist. (Path.) Glas. Roy. Infirm.

STEWART, James Francis Norman Health Centre, 14 Market Place, Carluke ML8 4AZ Tel: 01555 752150 Fax: 01555 751703; 27 Quarry Road, Lawhill, Carluke ML8 5HB — MB ChB Glas. 1980; MRCGP 1984; DRCOG 1984; DFFP 1993.

STEWART, James Frederick Garfield c/o Department of Ophthalmology, Western Infirmary, Dumbarton Road, Glasgow G11 6NT — MB ChB Otago 1982. Specialty: Ophth.

STEWART, James Ian McKay Department of Anaesthetics, University Hospital of Wales, Heath Park, Cardiff CF14 4XN — MB BS Newc. 1989 (Newc. upon Tyne) FRCA 1995. Cons. Anaesth. Univ. Hosp. of Wales, Cardiff. Specialty: Anaesth. Special Interest: Paediatric Anaesth. and Analgesia. Socs: APA; AAGBI. Prev: Cons. Anaesth. Queens Med. Centre, Univ. Hosp. Nottm.

STEWART, James Martin (retired) 13A Davenant Road, Oxford OX2 8BT Tel: 01865 553067 — (T.C. Dub.) MB BCh BAO Dub. 1944.

STEWART, James Sinclair (retired) 2 Calderwood Court, Montpellier Parade, Cheltenham GL50 1UA Tel: 01242 578070 — MB BS Lond. 1955 (Middlx.) FRCP Lond. 1975, M 1960; MD Lond. 1970. Hon. Sen. Lect. Char. Cross & Westm. Med. Sch. Lond.; Hon. Cons. Phys. (Gastroenterol.) W. Middlx. Univ. Hosp. Isleworth & Teddington Memor. Hosp.; Edx-Examr. RCP Lond. Prev: Tutor & Sen. Regist. (Med.) Roy. Postgrad. Med. Sch. Lond. & Hammersmith Hosp.

STEWART, James Wallace (retired) Hatherleigh, Tower Road, Hindhead GU26 6SP Tel: 01428 604770 — MB BS Lond. 1944 (Middlx.) MRCS Eng. LRCP Lond. 1944; FRCPath 1963; FRCP Lond. 1980, M 1973. Prev: Cons. Haemat. Lond. Clinic.

STEWART, Jane Alison Reproductive Medicine, Bioscience Centre, International Centre for Life, Times Square, Newcastle upon Tyne NE1 4EP; Department of Gynaecology, Royal Victoria Infirmary, Queen Victoria Road, Newcastle Upon Tyne NE1 4LP — MB ChB Ed. 1988; BSc (Hons) (Ed) 1986; MRCOG 1994; MD Ed. 2001. Cons. (Reproductive Med. & Gyn.); Hon. Clin. Lect., Univ. of

Newcastle-Upon-Tyne Med. Sch. Special Interest: Fertil. Preservation; Infertil.

STEWART, Jennie Patterson (retired) 1/30 Claycot Park, Ladywell Avenue, Corstorphine, Edinburgh EH12 7LG Tel: 0131 334 4768 — MB ChB St. And. 1930. Prev: Ho. Surg. & Obstetr. Redlands Hosp. Wom. Glas.

STEWART, Jill Amanda Northamptonshire Centre For Oncology, Northampton Gen NHS Trust, Northampton NN1 5BD Tel: 01604 545238 Email: jill.stewart@ngh.nhs.uk — MB BS Lond. 1973 (Middlx.) FRCR 1979. Clin. Oncologist, Northamptonshire Centre For Oncol. Northampton Gen NHS Trust Northampton NN1 5BD. Specialty: Oncol. Prev: Sen. Regist. & Regist. (Radiother.) Churchill Hosp. Oxf.

STEWART, Mrs Joan Elizabeth 13 Howard Place, St Andrews KY16 9HL — MB ChB St. And. 1946. Prev: Med. Off. W. Scotl. Blood Transfus. Serv.; Ho. Surg. Dundee Roy. Infirm. & Roy. Hosp. Sick Childr. Edin.; Jun. Hosp. Med. Off. King's Cross Hosp. Dundee.

STEWART, John (retired) Bentink Crescent, Troon Tel: 01292 314110 — MB ChB Glas. 1945 (Univ. Glas.) MB ChB (Commend.) Glas. 1945; FRCPath 1971, M 1964. Prev: Cons. Pathol. Ayrsh. Hosp. Gp.

STEWART, John Alexander Bannatyne Plandons, Long Melford, Sudbury CO10 9ET — MB BS Lond. 1949 (St. Thos.) MRCS Eng. LRCP Lond. 1949; DObst RCOG 1954. Prev: Ho. Phys. Salisbury Gen. Infirm.; Ho. Phys. & Cas. Off. Lambeth Hosp.; Obst. Ho. Surg. Roy. Berks. Hosp. Reading.

STEWART, John Alexander Mackenzie (retired) Sunnylaw, 42 Bonhard Road, Scone, Perth PH2 6QB Tel: 01738 552454 — MB ChB Glas. 1949; MRCGP 1960. Prev: Ho. Surg. Glas. Roy. Infirm.

STEWART, John Angus 89 Wyke Road, Weymouth DT4 9QN Tel: 0130 575681 — MB BS Lond. 1948 (Guy's) LMSSA Lond. 1947. Prev: Ho. Surg. Torbay Hosp. Torquay; Capt. RAMC.

STEWART, John Barrie (retired) 20 The Gables, Oxshott, Leatherhead KT22 0SD Tel: 01372 843378 Fax: 01372 844497 — MB ChB Ed. 1957; DTM & H Lond 1961; DRCPath 1967; FRCPath 1981, M 1969. Prev: Cons. Histopath. Epsom Gen. Hosp.

STEWART, John Charles Marshall Marshallstown, Downpatrick BT30 8AL; Efamol Ltd., Woodbridge Meadows, Guildford GU1 1BA — MB ChB Dundee 1978; BSc Belf. 1966; PhD (Chem.) Camb. 1969; MFPM 1990. Med. Dir. Scotia Pharmaceut. Guildford.

STEWART, John Gordon (retired) 1 Wallings Lane, Silverdale, Carnforth LA5 0SA Tel: 01524 701325 Email: doc@gordon3.freeserve.co.uk — MB ChB Glas. 1951. Prev: GP Atherstone.

STEWART, John Gordon Hume Argyll Street Surgery, 246 Argyll Street, Dunoon PA23 7HW Tel: 01369 702067 Fax: 01369 706680 — MB ChB Glas. 1973; MRCGP 1977.

STEWART, John Hatrick Stoneyburn Health Centre, 73 Main Street, Stoneyburn, Bathgate EH47 8BY — MB BCh Dublin 1983 (Trinity College, Dublin) MRCGP Edin. 1988. Specialty: Gen. Pract.

STEWART, John Hirst (retired) Dorter House, Buccleuch St., Melrose TD6 9LD — MB ChB Glas. 1950; MRCGP 1980. Prev: GP Milngavie.

STEWART, John Hubert Hall, OBE (retired) 43 Coolsythe Road, Randalstown, Antrim BT41 3HF Tel: 01849 472801 — (Belf.) MB BCh (Hons.) BAO Belf. 1952. Additional Dep. Forens. Med. Off. Antrim Sub-Div. Roy. Ulster Constab; JP. Prev: Resid. Ho. Off. Roy. Vict. Hosp. Belf. & Roy. Belf. Hosp. Sick Childr.

STEWART, John Lumsdaine (retired) Apartment 36, Hometay House, 2 High St., Monifieth, Dundee DD5 4BN Tel: 01382 533555 — MD Ed. 1955; MB ChB 1945; MFCM 1974. Prev: SCMO Norf. AHA.

STEWART, John Malcolm The Anchorage, Green Road, Thorpe, Egham TW20 8QN Tel: 01344 843185 Fax: 01344 843185 — MB ChB St. And. 1956; DTM & H Eng. 1964. Cons. Adviser in Travel Med. to Boots Health and Beauty. Prev: Sen. Med. Off. Brit. Airways Health Serv.; Regtl. Med. Off. Life Guards; GP Portsmouth.

STEWART, John Matthew Archibald Craig (retired) 1 Villiers Crescent, Eccleston, St Helens WA10 5HP Tel: 01744 23810 — MB ChB Birm. 1950; BSc Birm. 1947; DPM Eng. 1955; MRCPsych 1971. Prev: Cons. Psychiat., Sen. Hosp. Med. Off. & Sen. Regist. (Psychiat.) Rainhill Hosp.

STEWART, Mr John Oscar Reginald (retired) 2 Northgate, Lincoln LN2 1QS Tel: 01522 523231 — MB BCh BAO Belf. 1945 (Qu. Univ. Belf.) MB BCh BAO (Hons.) Belf. 1945; FRCS Eng. 1951; DHMSA 1990. Prev: Cons. Surg. Co. Hosp. Lincoln & Horncastle War Memor. Hosp.

STEWART, John Owen (retired) 26 Conway Mews, Brompton, Gillingham ME7 5BD Tel: 01634 403880 Fax: 01634 403880 — MRCS Eng. LRCP Lond. 1965 (Univ. Coll. Hosp.) BSc (Anat.) Lond. 1960, MB BS 1965; DObst. RCOG 1967; FRCPath 1986, M 1974. Prev: Cons. Path. Dist. Laborat. Severalls Hosp. Colchester.

STEWART, John Simon Watson, Bt Dept of Radiotherapy, Charing Cross Hospital, London W6 8AF — MB BS Lond. 1980; BSc Lond. 1977, MB BS 1980; MRCP (UK) 1983; FRCR 1986; FRCP Lond. 1994. Cons. Radiother. & Oncol. St. Mary's Hosp. Lond. & Sen. Lect. (Radiother. & Oncol.) Imperial Sch. of Med. Specialty: Oncol. Socs: ASCO; ESTRO; RAD Soc. Prev: Clin. Research Fell. Imperial Cancer Research Fund.

STEWART, John Stewart Simpson 74 The Common, Parbold, Wigan WN8 7EA — MB ChB Glas. 1951.

STEWART, John Tytler (retired) 4 Larch Road, Glasgow G41 5DA Tel: 0141 427 2832 — MB ChB Glas. 1955; FRCOG 1978, M 1964. Prev: Cons. O & G Stobhill Gen. Hosp. Glas.

STEWART, Mr Jonathan Department of General Surgery, Manor Hospital, Moat Road, Walsall WS2 9PS Tel: 01922 656649 Fax: 01922 656958 Email: dianne.jones@walsallhospitals.nhs.uk — MD Leeds 1986; MB ChB 1978; FRCS Eng. 1982; FRCS Ed. 1982; T(S) 1991. Cons. Surg.; Clin. Sub Dean, Walsall Manor Hosp. / Birm. Univ. Specialty: Gen. Surg. Special Interest: Colorectal and laparoscopic Surg. Socs: Roy. Coll. of Surgeons of Eng.; Roy. Coll. of Surgeons of Edin. Prev: Cancer Research Campaign Fell. MRC Camb.

STEWART, Jonathan 269 Craigie Drive, Dundee DD4 7UE — MB ChB Dundee 1992.

STEWART, Joseph Gordon The Highlands, 4 Highlands Gardens, St Leonards-on-Sea TN38 0HT Tel: 01424 433234 — MB ChB Glas. 1952.

STEWART, Karen Rosalind 2 Queensway, Grantham NG31 9QD — MB ChB Leic. 1991.

STEWART, Kathleen Heyland (retired) 9 Prior Bolton Street, London N1 2NX Tel: 020 7359 1862 — MB BCh BAO Belf. 1943; DObst RCOG 1947.

STEWART, Kay 17 Vicar Lane, Woodhouse, Sheffield S13 7JH — MB ChB Glas. 1994; BSc (Hons.) Glas. 1992. SHO (Med.) N. Gen. Hosp. Sheff. Specialty: Gen. Med. Prev: SHO (Med.) Airedale Gen. Hosp. Keighley.

STEWART, Keith Ramsay St Martin's Hospital , East Kent Children's Hearing Service, Temple Ward, Canterbury CT1 1TD Tel: 01227 812278; 3 Park House, 41 East Street, Faversham ME13 8AU Tel: 01795 534559 Fax: 01795 534559 Email: keith.kpas@lineone.net — MRCS Eng. LRCP Lond. 1969 (Guy's) DObst RCOG 1971; MSc Manch. 1993. Assoc. Special. community Paediat. Audiol. Specialty: Audiol. Med. Socs: Fell. Roy. Soc. Med.; Brit. Soc. Audiol.; Brit. Assoc. Communtiy DRS in Audiol. Prev: Ho. Surg. (ENT) Guy's Hosp. Lond.; Ho. Phys. Guy's Hosp. Gp.; Gen. Practitioner Huntingdon 1974-1999.

STEWART, Mr Kenneth John — MB ChB Aberd. 1990 (Aberdeen) BMedBiol Aberd. 1989; FRCS Ed. 1995; MD 1999; FRCS Ed. Plast. 2001. SpR Plastic Surg., Edin. Specialty: Plastic Surg. Socs: Fell. Roy. Coll. Surgs. Ed.; Brit. Assoc. Plastic Surg. Trainee Assoc.; Brit. Assoc. Head & neck Oncologists. Assoc. Prev: Research Regist. (Plastic & Reconstruc. Surg.) St. Geo. Hosp. Sydney, Austral.; SpR Plastic Surg., Aberd. Roy. Infirm.; Cranicracial Fell. Chelsea & W. Minster Hosp.

STEWART, Kenneth Macbeth (retired) 4 Holt Drive, Kirby Muxloe, Leicester LE9 2EX Tel: 0116 239 3542 — MB ChB Ed. 1953; DTM & H Liverp. 1957. Prev: Ho. Phys. & Ho. Surg. (Obst.) Bangour Hosp.

STEWART, Kenneth McLauchlan Woodlands, Inverdrive, Aviemore PH22 1QH — MB ChB Ed. 1958.

STEWART, Mr Kenneth Sloan Four Winds, Loftbrae, Gargunnock, Stirling FK8 3DH Tel: 01786 73776 — (Ed.) MD Ed. 1977, MB ChB 1962; FRCOG 1983, M 1969, DFM 1988, DObst. 1966; FRCS Ed. 1969. Cons. Obst. Stirling Roy. Infirm. Specialty: Obst. & Gyn. Prev: Sen Research Fell. Univ. Rhodesia & Cons. Harari Hosp. Salisbury; Sen. Regist. & Clin. Tutor Qu. Eliz. Med. Centre Birm.; Regist. Aberd. Roy. Infirm.

STEWART, Mr Kenneth Sutherland (retired) 5 Gainsborough Drive, Gunton Park, Lowestoft NR32 4LX Tel: 01502 584934 Fax: 01502 584934 — LRCP LRCS Ed. LRFPS Glas. 1944; FRCS Ed. 1952. Prev: Cons. Orthop. Surg. Gt. Yarmouth & Waveney HA.

STEWART, Kevin Owen Royal Hampshire County Hospital, Romsey Road, Winchester SO22 5DG Tel: 01962 825569 Fax: 01962 825570 — MB BCh BAO Belf. 1982; FRCP 1997, MRCP (UK) 1985. Cons. Phys. Roy. Hants. Co. Hosp. Winchester. Specialty: Care of the Elderly. Prev: Cons. Phys. Newham HA; Sen. Regist. (Geriat. Med.) Whittington & Roy. North. Hosps. Lond.; Sen. Regist. (Geriat.) Islington & Bloomsbury HA.

STEWART, Laura 26 Scotstoun Park, South Queensferry EH30 9PQ — MB ChB Ed. 1991 (Univ. Edin.) MRCP (UK) 1994. Specialist Regist. Paediat. Roy. Hosp. for Sick Childr. Yorkhill Glas. Specialty: Paediat. Prev: Regist. (Paediat.) Ninewells Hosp. Dundee.

STEWART, Mr Laurence Herbert The Western General Hospital, Crewe Road South, Edinburgh EH4 2XU Tel: 0131 537 1586; BUPA Murrayfield Hospital, 122 Corstorphine Road, Edinburgh EH12 6UD Tel: 0131 334 0363 — MB ChB Aberd. 1982; FRCS Ed. 1986; MD Aberd. 1994; FRCS (Urol) 1996. Cons. Urol. West. Gen. Hosp. Edin.; Cons. Urol. BUPA Murrayfield Hosp., Edin. Specialty: Urol. Special Interest: Female Urology; Lower Urinary Tract Dysfunction. Socs: Internat. Continence Soc.; Bristish Assn. Urological Surgeons; FRCS. Prev: Sen. Regist. (Urol.) Cardiff Roy. Infirm. Wales & Aberd. Roy. Infirm.; Sen. Regist. (Urol.) ChristCh. Pub. Hosp., NZ.

STEWART, Lawrence Guthrie (retired) 39 Kings Road, Elderslie, Johnstone PA5 9LY Tel: 01505 22060 — MB ChB Glas. 1958.

STEWART, Lesley Jane Benview, off Culterhouse Road, Peterculter AB14 0NT — MB ChB Aberd. 1968; DCH RCPS Glas. 1979. Specialty: Gen. Pract.

STEWART, Linda Bryson Department of Neuroanaesthesia, Institute of Neurological Sciences, Southern General Hospital, 1345 Govan Road, Glasgow G51 4TF — MB ChB Glas. 1987 (Univ. Glas.) FRCA 1991. Cons. Neuroanaesth. South. Gen. Hosp. Glas. Specialty: Anaesth. Prev: Sen. Regist. (Anaesth.) Roy. Infirm. Ed.; Research Fell. (Neuroanaesth. & Neurosurg.) Glas. Univ.

STEWART, Margaret Pathology Department, Royal Lancaster Infirmary, Ashton Road, Lancaster LA1 4RB Tel: 01524 583793 — MB BS Lond. 1975 (Lond. Hosp.) BSc Lond. 1972; MRCPath 1986. Cons. Histopath. Morecambe Bay Acute Hosps. NHS Trust. Specialty: Histopath. Prev: Sen. Regist. (Histopath.) Derby Roy. Infirm., City Hosp., Univ. Hosps. Nottm. & Lancaster Moor Hosp.; Regist. (Path.) Leeds Gen. Infirm.

STEWART, Margaret Elizabeth Hairmyres Hospital, East Kilbride, Glasgow G75 8RG Tel: 01355 572640 — MB ChB Aberd. 1974; BMedBiol Aberd. 1971; MRCP (UK) 1978; FRCP Glas. 1989. Cons. Phys. (Geriat. Med.) Hairmyres Hosp. Specialty: Care of the Elderly; Rehabil. Med. Socs: Brit. Soc. for Rehabil. Med.; Brit. Geriat. Soc.; Pk.inson's Dis. Soc. Prev: Cons. Phys. (Geriat. Med.) Law Hosp. Carluke; Sen. Regist. (Geriat. Med.) Gtr. Glas. Health Bd. West. Dist.; Regist. (Med. & Haemophilia) Glas. Roy. Infirm.

STEWART, Margaret Helen Department of Community Health, Udston Hospital, Hamilton ML3 9LA — MB ChB Glas. 1974.

STEWART, Margaret Jean Winter (retired) The Anchorage, Green Road, Thorpe, Egham TW20 8QN Tel: 01344 843185 Email: zen.genie@zen.co.uk — (St. And.) MB ChB St. And. 1956; DPH Eng. 1971; MFCM 1974; FFPHM RCP (UK) 1990. Prev: Dir. Health Purchasing & Pub. Health SW Surrey HA Guildford.

STEWART, Margaret McGregor (retired) 9 Bartholomew Terrace, Exeter EX4 3BW Tel: 01392 431732 — MB ChB Glas. 1945. Prev: Clin. Med. Off. (Community Health) SW Surrey & NE Hants. HAs.

STEWART, Margaret Roberta (retired) 13A Davenant Road, Oxford OX2 8BT Tel: 01865 553067 — MB BCh BAO Belf. 1943.

STEWART, Margaret Sheila Wayside, South Stoke, Bath BA2 7DJ — MB ChB Manch. 1989. SHO (Ophth.) Ayr. Hosp.

STEWART, Mr Mark — MB BS Lond. 1970; MRCS Eng. LRCP Lond. 1970; FRCS Eng. 1977; MS Lond. 1984. Cons. Surg., Darent Valley Hosp. Dartford Kent. Specialty: Gen. Surg. Special Interest: Colorectal Surg. Socs: Assoc. Mem. Brit. Assn. Urol. Surg.; Assn. Surg.; Assn. of Colo-rectal Surg. (ACPGBI). Prev: Cons. Surg. & Sen. Lect. Baragwanath Hosp. & Univ. Witwatersra Johannesburg, S. Afr.

STEWART, Mary Dickson Cameron Greater Glasgow Primary Care Trust, Great Western Road, Glasgow G12 0XH — MB ChB Aberd. 1991. p/t Clin. Assist. (Psychiat.) Alcohol & Drug Servs.; Clin. Assist. Breast Screening Progr.

STEWART, Mary Elizabeth Fife Primary Care NHS Trust, Whyteman's Brae Hospital, Whyteman's Brae, Kirkcaldy KY1 2ND Tel: 01592 643355 Fax: 01592 643790 — MB ChB Aberd. 1981; MRCPsych 1986; T(Psychiat.) 1992. Cons. Gen. Adult Psychiat. Fife Primary Care NHS Trust Whyteman's Brae Hosp. Kirkcaldy. Specialty: Gen. Psychiat. Prev: Sen. Regist. (Psychiat.) Roy. Edin. Hosp.; Research Regist. Crichton Roy. Hosp. Dumfries; Regist. (Psychiat.) Glas. HB.

STEWART, Mrs Mary Felicity Department of Clinical Biochemistry, Salford Royal Hospitals NHS Trust, Stott Lane, Salford M6 8HD Tel: 0161 206 4971 Fax: 0161 788 7443 Email: felicity.stewart@srht.nhs.uk — MB BS Lond. 1980 (Univ. Coll. Hosp.) BSc (Biochem.) Lond. 1977, MD 1992; MRCPath 1993; FRCPath 2002. p/t Cons. Chem. Path. Salford Roy. Hosp.s NHS Trust Salford. Specialty: Chem. Path. Special Interest: Endocrine Biochemistry; Hyperlipidaemia; Porphyria. Socs: Assn. Clin. Biochem.; Soc. Endocrinol.; Heart UK. Prev: Sen. Regist. (Chem. Path.) Manch. Roy. Infirm. & Salford Roy. Hosp.s NHS Trust Salford; Regist. (Chem. Path.) Wythenshawe Hosp. Manch.

STEWART, Mary Patricia Dunlop 10 Meeks Road, Falkirk FK2 7ES Tel: 01324 619930; The Stable House, Feddal, Braco, Dunblane FK15 9RA Tel: 01786 880204 — MB ChB Glas. 1968. Prev: Jun. Ho. Off. (Med. & Surg.) Stirling Roy. Infirm.

STEWART, Mary Wendover St James Road Surgery, 22 St. James Road, Torpoint PL11 2BH Tel: 01752 812404 Fax: 01752 816436 — MB ChB Cape Town 1970; MB ChB Cape Town 1970.

STEWART, Michael John James Cook University Hospital, Middlesbrough TS4 3BW Tel: 01642 854623 Fax: 01642 854190 — MB ChB Ed. 1986; MRCP (UK) 1989; MD Ed. 1997; FCRP Ed. 2000; FRCP Lond. 2003. Cons. Cardiol. James Cook Univ. Hosp. Middlesbrough. Specialty: Cardiol. Socs: Brit. Hypertens. Soc. Brit. Cardiac. Soc. Prev: Sen. Regist. Cardiovasc. Med. South. Gen. Hosp. Glas.; Career Regist. (Cardiol.) Glas. Roy. Infirm.; Brit. Heart Fondat. Jun. Research Fell. Dept. Cardiol. W. Gen. Hosp. Edin.

STEWART, 0 Michael Peter MacGregor, QHS, Col. L/RAMC Cliffords Farm, Ovington, Richmond DL11 7DD Fax: 01833 627850 — MB ChB Aberd. 1979; FRCS Glas. 1988; FRCS (Orth.) 1994. Cons. Orthopaedic & Trauma Surg. Sir James Cook Univ. Hosp. Middlesbrough; Defence Cons. Adviser. Specialty: Trauma & Orthop. Surg.; Medico Legal. Socs: Fell. BOA; Brit. Shoulder & Elbow Soc.; Combined Serv.s Orthopeadic Soc. Prev: Cons. Orthop. & Trauma Surg. S. Durham NHS Trust; Cons. Adviser (Orthops. & Trauma) DGAMS.

STEWART, Moira Connell Department of Child Health, Institute of Clinical Science, Grosvenor Road, Belfast BT12 6BJ; 5 The Point, Groomsport, Bangor BT19 6JN Tel: 028 9146 4701 — MB BCh BAO Belf. 1977; DCH Dub. 1981; MRCP (UK) 1982; MD Belf. 1986; FRCP Lond. 1994. Cons. Paediat. & Sen. Lect. Inst. Clin. Sci. Belf. Specialty: Paediat. Socs: RCPCH Ulster Paediatric Soc.; Fac. of Paediat., Roy. Coll. of Physicians of Irel.

STEWART, Morag Elmbank Group, Foresterhill Health Centre, Westburn Road, Aberdeen AB25 2AY Tel: 01224 696949 Fax: 01224 691650 — MB ChB Aberd. 1994 (Univ. Aberd.) DFFP; MRCGP. Specialty: Gen. Pract. Socs: BMA.

STEWART, Mr Murray 5 King Edward Road, Jordanhill, Glasgow G13 1QW — MB ChB Aberd. 1986; FRCS Glas. 1990; FRCS Ed. 1994. Career Regist. (ENT) Roy. Alexandra Hosp. Paisley; Clin. Asst. (A & E) West. Infirm. Glas. Specialty: Otolaryngol. Socs: Assoc. Mem. Brit. Assn. Otolaryngol. Head & Neck Surgs.; Otolaryngol. Research Soc. Prev: SHO Rotat. (Surg.) W. Scotl. Train. Scheme.

STEWART, Murray Willis 6 Woodlands Grange, Forest Hall, Newcastle upon Tyne NE12 9DF — BM Soton. 1984; MRCP (UK) 1989; DM Soton. 1995. Cons. Phys. (Diabetes & Endocrinol.) Newc.; Hon. Sen. Lect. Newc. Univ. Specialty: Diabetes; Gen. Med. Prev: MRC Lect. & Sen. Regist. (Diabetes & Endocrinol.) Newc. Univ.; Regist. (Med., Diabetes & Endocrinol.) Roy. Vict. Infirm. Newc. u. Tyne; Regist. (Med.) CrossHo. Hosp. Kilmarnock.

STEWART, Myra Judith 47 Brackendale, Potters Bar EN6 2LP — MB ChB Birm. 1996.

STEWART, Neil Grant 12d St Saviours Road, London SW2 5HD — MB ChB Ed. 1993.

STEWART, Nicholas Church Lane Medical Centre, Orchid Rise, Off Church Lane, Scunthorpe DN15 7AN Tel: 01724 864341 Fax: 01724 876441 — MB ChB Sheff. 1986. Trainee GP Lancaster VTS. Prev: Ho. Off. (Gen. Med.) York Dist. Hosp.; Ho. Off. (Gen. Surg.) Pontefract Gen. Infirm.

STEWART, Mr Owen Gavin Department of Ophthalmology, Hull & East Yorkshire Eye Hospital, Fountain Street, Hull HU3 2JS Tel: 01482 328541 Ext: 605332 Email: owenstewart@fsmail.net; Bearders Barn, North Raod, Lund, Driffield YO25 9TF — MB BS Newc. 1993; FRCOphth 1997. Cons. (Ophthalmologist) Hull & E. Yorks. Eye Hosp. Hull. Specialty: Ophth. Special Interest: Cornea & Anterior Segment Surg. Socs: MDU; UK & Irel. Cataract & Refractive Surgeons (UKIERS). Prev: SHO (Ophth.) St. Jas. Univ. Hosp. Leeds; SHO (Ophth.) Bradford Roy. Infirm.; SHO (Ophth.) N. Riding Infirm. Middlesbrough.

STEWART, Pamela Doris Beckwath, Romaldkirk, Barnard Castle DL12 9EE — MB ChB Cape Town 1985 (Univ. Cape Town)

STEWART, Patricia Antonia East Aquhorthies Farmhouse, Inverurie AB51 5JL — BM Soton. 1982; DIP Clin Micro, Lond. Hosp. Med. Coll 1987; MRCPath 1998. Specialty: Med. Microbiol. Prev: Sen. Regist. In Med. MicroBiol. P/T, Soton. Gen. Hosp.

STEWART, Patricia Jean Martin, Barr and Stewart, Eastwick Park Avenue, Great Bookham, Leatherhead KT23 3ND Tel: 01372 452081 Fax: 01372 451680; 4 Sayers Close, Fetcham, Leatherhead KT22 9PE Tel: 01372 450485 — MB ChB St. And. 1968; DObst RCOG 1971.

STEWART, Patrick Carlin 23 Eastleigh Drive, Belfast BT4 3DX — MB BCh BAO Belf. 1992.

STEWART, Paul Alexander Forest Glades Medical Centre, Bromsgrove Street, Kidderminster DY10 1PG — MB ChB Birm. 1978. GP Medico-Legal Advisor Independ. Med.; Hon. Med. Adviser Wyre Forest Athletics Assn.; Med. Off. Brit. Sugar Kidderminster. Specialty: Gen. Pract. Prev: Regist. (Radiother. & Oncol.) Velindre Hosp. WhitCh. Cardiff; Regist. (Med.) New Cross Hosp. Wednesfield Wolverhampton; SHO (O & G) Wordsley Hosp. Stourbridge.

STEWART, Professor Paul Michael Department of Medicine, Queen Elizabeth Hospital, Edgbaston, Birmingham B15 2TH Tel: 0121 627 2380 Fax: 0121 627 2384 Email: p.m.stewart@bham.ac.uk; Broadlands, Salter Street, Hockley Heath, Solihull B94 6BY — MB ChB Ed. 1982 (Edinburgh) MRCP (UK) 1985; MD Ed. 1989; FRCP Lond. 1995; F Med Sci 1999. Prof. of Med. & Hon. Cons. Phys. Birm.; Prof. Med. Specialty: Endocrinol.; Gen. Med. Socs: Endocrine Soc.; Soc. for Endocrinol.; Acad. of Med. Sci. Prev: Lect. & Hon. Sen. Regist. (Med.) Qu. Eliz. Hosp. Birm.; Sir Stanley Davidson Lect. (Med.) Univ. Edin.; MRC Train. Fell.

STEWART, Pauline Mary Drymen Road Surgery, 96 Drymen Road, Bearsden, Glasgow G61 2SY Tel: 0141 942 9494; 24 Station Road, Bearsden, Glasgow G61 4AL — MB ChB Glas. 1978; MRCGP 1987. Prev: Trainee GP Guildford VTS.

STEWART, Peter 20 Whiteley Wood Road, Sheffield S11 7FE — BM BCh Oxf. 1971; MRCOG 1979. Cons. O & G Sheff. Health Auth. Specialty: Obst. & Gyn.

STEWART, Mr Peter Alexander Hamilton The Yorkshire Clinic, Bingley BD16 1TW Tel: 01274 550856 Fax: 01274 550803; 15 Prospect Place, Harrogate HG1 1LB Tel: 01423 523357 Fax: 01423 523357 — (St. Thos.) MB BS Lond. 1964; FRCS Ed. 1970; FRCS Eng. 1971. Cons. Urol Surg. The Yorks. Clinic. Binley. Specialty: Urol. Socs: Brit. Assn. Urol. Surgs.; Fell. Roy. Soc. Med. (Ex Hon. ; Sec. ; Vice-Pres. & Pres.). Prev: Sen. Regist. (Urol.) Leeds; Transpl. Research Fell. & Hon. Sen. Regist. (Surg.) St. Thos. Hosp. Lond.; Cons. Urol. Surg. Bradford Hosps. NHS Trust.

STEWART, Philippa Jane 1 Borrowdale Close, Gamston, Nottingham NG2 6PD — MB BCh Wales 1993.

STEWART, Rebekah Angela Louise 66 The Causeway, Edinburgh EH15 3PZ — MB BChir Camb. 1990; FRCS 1994; FRCR 1997. Specialty: Radiol.

STEWART, Rhona Margaret Royal Hospital, Calow, Chesterfield S44 5BL Tel: 01246 277271 — MB BS Lond. 1973 (Middlx.) MRCP (UK) 1978; FRCPath 1992, M 1981; FRCP Lond. 1992. Cons. Haemat. Roy. Hosp. Chesterfield. Specialty: Haematology. Prev: Cons. Haemat. Scunthorpe & Goole Hosps.

STEWART, Robert Charles (4F2) 9 Warrender Park Terrace, Edinburgh EH9 1JA — MB ChB Ed. 1996.

STEWART, Robert Clifford, Lt.-Col. RAMC c/o Ulster Bank, Shaftesbury Square, Belfast BT2 — MB BCh BAO Belf. 1949; DTM & H Eng. 1961; FRCPath 1976, M 1964. Asst. Prof. Path. RAM Coll. Millbank. Socs: Assn. Clin. Pathols. & Path. Soc. Gt. Brit.

STEWART, Robert Curle Park Medical Centre, Shavington Avenue, Newton Lane, Chester CH2 3RD Tel: 01244 324136 Fax: 01244 317257; Rock House, Village Road, Christleton, Chester CH3 7AS Tel: 01244 332657 — MB ChB Manch. 1979; DRCOG 1981; MRCGP 1991. Clin. Asst. (Coloscopy) Chester. Specialty: Obst. & Gyn. Prev: Trainee GP Cheadle Hulme Health Centre Manch.; SHO (Paediat.) Booth Hall Childr. Hosp. Manch.; SHO (O & G) St. Mary's Hosp. Manch.

STEWART, Mr Robert D Kettering General Hospital, Rothwell Road, Kettering NN16 8UZ — MB BS Lond. 1973; MRCS Eng. LRCP Lond 1973; FRCS Lond. 1977; MS Lond. 1984. Cons. (Surg.) Kettering General Hospital. Specialty: Gen. Surg. Special Interest: Breast Dis. Socs: Brit. Assn. of Surgic. Oncologists.

STEWART, Robert Evan (retired) 9C/1 Merchiston Park, Edinburgh EH10 4PW Tel: 0131 229 7717 — MB ChB Glas. 1949; DObst RCOG 1953; FRCGP 1981, M 1963. Prev: Med. Off. & Princip. Lect. (Health Educat.) Moray Ho. Coll. Edin.

STEWART, Robert Gregor 26 Westfield Grove, Wakefield WF1 3RS Tel: 01924 2344 — MB ChB Glas. 1946 (Univ. Glas.) Prev: Capt. RAMC; Cas. Off. Manor Hosp. Walsall; Ho. Surg. Whiston Co. Hosp. Whiston.

STEWART, Robert Ian Friarsgate Medical Centre, Winchester Child Guidance, Winchester SO23 8EF Tel: 01962 855477; Morecroft, Muss Lane, King's Somborne, Stockbridge SO20 6PE — MB ChB Glas. 1977; BA (Hons.) N. Carolina 1972; MRCPsych. 1981. Cons. Child & Family Psychiat. Roy. Hants. Co. Hosp. Winchester. Specialty: Child & Adolesc. Psychiat.

STEWART, Robert James Section of Epidemiology, Institute of Psychiatry, De Crespigny Park, Denmark Hill, London SE5 8AF — MB ChB Leeds 1991; MSc London 2000. Specialty: Geriat. Psychiat. Socs: Roy. Coll. Psychiat.

STEWART, Robert More The Surgery, Old Road, Elham, Canterbury CT4 6UH Tel: 01303 840213 Fax: 01303 893817; White Gate House, Acrise, Folkestone CT18 8JU — MB BS Lond. 1978; MRCS Eng. LRCP Lond. 1978; DRCOG 1980. GP Princip.; Chairm. Shepway PCG. Socs: Local Med. Comm. (Kent.). Prev: Regist. (Psychiat.) Hammersmith & St. Bernards Hosp.; SHO (Obst.) W. Lond. & Char. Cross Hosp. Lond.; SHO (Paediat.) Whipps Cross Hosp. Lond.

STEWART, Roberta Aitchison (retired) 17 Framingham Road, Sale M33 3ST Tel: 0161 973 2876 — (Victoria University Manchester) MB ChB Manch. 1946. Prev: Gen. Practitioner,Wythen Shawe Manch.

STEWART, Roderick James Ballenmuir, Newbold, Forres IV36 — MB ChB St. And. 1963; DObst RCOG 1966.

STEWART, Ronald Dawson Miller Maryhill Practice, Elgin Health Centre, Maryhill, Elgin IV30 1AT Tel: 01343 543788 Fax: 01343 551604 — MB ChB Aberd. 1978; MRCP (UK) 1981; DRCOG 1983; MRCGP 1984. Prev: Regist. (Med.) S. Grampian Health Dist.; Research Fell. (Med.) Univ. Aberd.; SHO (Obst.) Bellshill Matern. Hosp.

STEWART, Rorie John Gordon Old Machar Medical Practice, 526 King Street, Aberdeen AB24 5RS Tel: 01224 480324 Fax: 01224 276121; 25 Tarvit Avenue, Cupar KY15 5BN — MB ChB Dundee 1987; BMSc (Hons.) Dund 1984; MRCGP 1991. Specialty: Dermat.

STEWART, Rosamund Chad Hanwell Health Centre, 20 Church Road, Hanwell, London W7 1DR Tel: 020 8579 7337 Fax: 020 8579 7337; 5 Park Avenue, London SW14 8AT Tel: 020 8878 7114 — MB BS Lond. 1978 (Char. Cross) DRCOG 1981.

STEWART, Rosemary Anne 98A Galgorm Road, Ballymena BT42 1AA — MB BCh BAO Belf. 1992; FRCS (Orl) 1996 (Edin).

STEWART, Rosemary Jean 4390 Comanche Drive, Boulder CO 80303, USA Tel: 00 1 303 4942903 Fax: 00 1 303 4923674; 8 Dean Terrace, Edinburgh EH4 1ND — MB ChB Ed. 1988; DRCOG 1991; MRCGP 1995. Consultancy Research Assoc. Univ. Colarado, Boulder, USA. Specialty: Gen. Pract. Prev: GP/Regist. Links Med. Centre Edin.

STEWART, Sheila Christine (retired) Cormorants, Channel Way, Fairlight, Hastings TN35 4BP Tel: 01424 813676 — (Royal Free

Hospital) MRCS Eng. LRCP Lond. 1961; MB BS Lond. 1962; DObst RCOG 1965; DPM Eng. 1974; MRCPsych 1978.

STEWART, Sheila Louise Elvang, Queenshaugh, Riverside, Stirling FK8 1XH — MB ChB Glas. 1987; FRCR 1993. Specialty: Radiol. Prev: Cons. (Radiol.) Southern Gen. Hosp. Glas.; Cons. (Radiol.) Falkirk & Dist. Roy. Infirm.; Regist. (Radiodiag.) South. Gen. Hosp. Glas.

STEWART, Susan Department of Pathology, Papworth Hospital, Papworth Everard, Cambridge CB3 8RE Tel: 01480 830541 Fax: 01480 831192 — MB BChir Camb. 1979; MB BChir Camb. 1978; MA Camb. 1979; FRCPath 1996, M 1984. Cons. Histopath. Papworth Hosp. Camb.; Assoc. Lect. (Path.) Univ. Camb. Specialty: Histopath.

STEWART, Suzanne Dorothy Liskey House, 12 Myrtle Road, Victoria Bridge, Strabane BT82 8QB — MB BS Lond. 1993. Specialty: Gen. Pract.

STEWART, Sylvia (retired) Orchard Wall, Earleswood, Cobham KT11 2BZ Tel: 01932 864233 — MB BS Lond. 1947 (Roy. Free) MRCS Eng. LRCP Lond. 1947; DA Eng. 1950; FFA RCS Eng. 1954. Prev: Cons. Anaesth. Reading Gp. Hosps.

STEWART, Mr Terence James Lake House, Holly Park Road, Killinchy, Newtownards BT23 6SN Tel: 02897 542662 Fax: 02897 542662 — MB BCh BAO Belf. 1964 (Qu. Univ. Belf.) FRCS Eng. 1971. Cons. Otolaryngol. Ulster Independent Clinic. Specialty: Otolaryngol.; Paediat. Socs: Mem. Of Brit. Assoc. of Otorhinolaryngologists - Head & Neck Surg.s; Mem. Of Irish otoLaryngol. Soc. Prev: Sen. Regist. Eye & Ear Clinic Roy. Vict. Hosp. Belf.; Research & Clin. Fell. Mass. Eye & Ear Infirm. Boston, USA; on Staff Mass. Eye & Ear Infirm. & Instruc. Harvard Med. Sch.

STEWART, Thomas Wilfred (retired) 3 Aughton Road, Southport PR8 2AF Tel: 01704 566088 Fax: 01704 566088 — MB ChB Manch. 1955; FRCP Ed. 1973, M 1963. Prev: Cons. Dermat. Roy. Liverp. Hosp., Southport & Formby DGH & Ormskirk & Dist Gen. Hosp.

STEWART, Timothy Dennis Stanley 44 Wyke Avenue, Ash, Aldershot GU12 6EA — MB ChB Cape Town 1986.

STEWART, Victoria Rosalind 2 Montpelier Villas, Brighton BN1 3DH — BM BS Nottm. 1998.

STEWART, Wendy Adele Dept of Biomollecular sciences, University of Manchester Institute of science and Technology, Sackville St., Manchester M60 1QD Email: wendy.stewart@stud.umist.ac.uk; 15 Elm Grove, Manchester M20 6PQ — MB ChB Manch. 1995; MRCP (LOND) 1998. Haemat. Research Assoc., U.M.I.S.T, Manch. Specialty: Haematology. Prev: SHO in Med., Manch. Roy. Infirm. AUG 1997-Oct 1998; SHO in Med. Roy. Bolton Hosp. AUG 1996- AUG 1997.

STEWART, Wilfred Ewart (retired) Garvary Rectory, Killyuilly, Enniskillen — MB BCh BAO Belf. 1961; MRCOG 1967, DObst 1963. Cons. (O & G) Erne Hosp. Enniskillen. Prev: Med. Off. Jubilee Matern. Hosp. Belf.

STEWART, William The Stables, Craigie Village, Kilmarnock KA1 5LY — MB ChB Glas. 1993.

STEWART, William Bryce (retired) Ringans Well, Raitloan, Nairn IV12 5SA Tel: 01667 453211 — MB ChB Glas. 1958; DObst RCOG 1960. Med. Adviser, Benefits Agency, Inverness. Prev: Ho. Phys. South. Gen. Hosp. Glas. & Lennox Castle Matern. Hosp.

STEWART, William Gordon Argyle House, 3 Lady Lawson St., Edinburgh EH3 0QH Tel: 0131 222 5301 — MB ChB Dundee 1983. Med. Adviser Benefits Agency Edin.; Med. Off. Glenrothes RFC. Specialty: Disabil. Med. Prev: SHO (Psychiat.) Stratheden Hosp. Cupar.; SHO (Paediat.) Vict. Hosp. Kirkealdy; Princip. GP, Possil Pk. Glas.

STEWART, William Kinnear (retired) Stanmore, 18 Station Crescent, Invergowrie, Dundee DD2 5DT Tel: 01382 562755 — MB ChB (Distinc.) St. And. 1948; FRCP Lond. 1974, M 1953; FRCP Ed. 1970, M. 1966; MD (Hons.) St. And. 1972; PhD Dundee 1980.

STEWART, William Muir, OBE, Brigadier late RAMC Retd. Bell Rotary House, Abbeyfield Society, 10-12 King's Road, Belfast BT5 6JJ Tel: 028 9065 5587 — MB BCh BAO Belf. 1935; MB BCh BAO, QUB 1935; DPH Eng. 1950.

STEWART-BROWN, Professor Sarah Lynette The Medical School, University of Warwick, Coventry CV4 7AL Email: sarah.stewart-brown@warwick.ac.uk — BA Oxon 1971 (Westm.) BM BCh Oxf. 1974; MA Oxon. 1975; MRCP (UK) 1979; MFCM 1986; PhD Bristol 1989; FFPHM RCP (UK) 1995; FRCP Lond. 1995; FRCPCH 1997. Prof. (Public Health) The Med. Sch. Univ. Warwick; Hon. Cons. (Public Health Med.) Coventry PCT. Specialty: Pub. Health Med. Special Interest: Acad. Pub. Health; Emotional & Social Developm. & Impact on Health in Adulthood; Parenting & Parent-child relationship. Socs: Fell. Fac. of Pub. Health of RCP; Fell. Roy. Coll. of Phys.; Fell. Roy. Coll. Of Paediat. & Child Health. Prev: Dir. Health Servs. Research Unit Dept. Pub. Health & Primary Care Univ. Oxf.; Hon. Cons. Oxon. DHA; Reader in Health Servs. Research Univ., of Oxf.

STEWART-JONES, John Halkett Place Surgery, 84 Halkett Place, St Helier, Jersey JE1 4XL Tel: 01534 36301 Fax: 01534 887793; L'Arc en Ciel, 4 Clos du Parcq, Richmond Road, St Helier, Jersey JE2 3GL Tel: 01534 737119 Fax: 01534 504987 — MB BS Lond. 1974 (Lond. Hosp. Med. Coll.) DRCOG 1977; MRCGP 1978. Prev: SHO (Chest & Gen. Med. & Paediat.) St. Woolos Hosp. Newport; SHO (O & G) Roy. Gwent Hosp. Newport.

STEYN, Anne Marjory Meltham Road Surgery, 9 Meltham Road, Lockwood, Huddersfield HD1 3UP Tel: 01484 432940 Fax: 01484 451423; 33 Deanhouse, Holmfirth HD9 3UG Tel: 01484 689266 — MB ChB Aberd. 1987 (Aberdeen) GP Huddersfield. Specialty: Paediat.; Obst. & Gyn.; Palliat. Med. Socs: BMA. Prev: Trainee GP Port Glas. VTS; SHO Aberd. Matern. Hosp.; SHO (Geriat.) Bridge of Weir Hosp.

STEYN, Mr John Hofmeyr, CStJ Albyn Hospital, 21-24 Albyn Place, Aberdeen AB10 1RW Tel: 01224 595993 Fax: 01224 584797; 3 Louisville Avenue, Aberdeen AB15 4TT Tel: 01224 318450 — (Cape Town) MB ChB Cape Town 1952; FRCS Eng. 1957; PhD Aberd. 1967; FRCS Ed. 1973. Chairm. Albyn Hosp. Aberd.; Emerit. Cons. Urol. Aberd. Roy. Infirm. Specialty: Urol. Socs: Brit. Assn. Urol. Surgs.; Hon. Mem. S. Afr. Urol. Assn. Prev: Cons. i/c Dept. Urol. Aberd. Roy. Infirm.

STEYN, John Peter Blackhall Medical Centre, 51 Hillhouse Road, Edinburgh EH4 3TH Tel: 0131 332 7696 Fax: 0131 315 2884 — MB ChB Aberd. 1979; FRCGP 1996, M 1984.

STEYN, Michael Paul 118C Moulsham Street, Chelmsford CM2 0JW Email: sunways@ukgateway.net — MB ChB Aberd. 1984; DRCOG 1986; MRCGP 1988; FFA RCSI 1991; MSc Aberd. 1995. Cons. Anaesth. Specialty: Anaesth. Socs: Assoication of Burns & Reconstruc. Anaesth.s; Brit. Burns Assn. Prev: Trainee GP Dumfries & Galloway Health Bd. VTS.; Sen. Regist. (Anaesth.) Grampian HB.; Const. Anaesth. Mid Essex Hosps. Trust.

STEYN, Mr Richard Stephen The Cardiothoracic Centre, Thomas Drive, Liverpool L14 3PE Tel: 0151 228 1616; 8 Harrison Hey, Liverpool L36 5YR — MB ChB Aberd. 1984 (Aberdeen) DRCOG 1990; MRCGP 1991; T(GP) 1991; FRCS Ed. 1991; Dip. IMC RCS Ed. 1996. Specialist Regist. (Cardiothoracic Surg.) Cardiothoracic Centre Liverp. Specialty: Cardiothoracic Surg. Socs: Soc. Cardiothoracic Surg. GB & Irel.; BASICS.

STHYR, Leslie Valdemar c/o Midland Bank, 39 Tottenham Court Road, London W1 — MRCS Eng. LRCP Lond. 1942 (Middlx.) MD Lond. 1950, MB BS 1948; FRCP Lond. 1973, M 1953. Socs: Brit. Geriat. Soc. Prev: Phys. Supt. & Cons. Geriat. St. John's Hosp. Battersea; Asst. Phys. (Geriat.) Buckinghamsh. Area; Sen. Regist. Qu. Mary's Roehampton Hosp.

STIBE, Catharina Magdalene Helen 23 Meadowbrook, Oxted RH8 9LT — MRCS Eng. LRCP Lond. 1983 (Sheff.) Specialty: Ophth.; Neurol.

STIBE, Eva 161A Southgate Road, Islington, London N1 3LE — MB BCh Wales 1987; FRCS Ed. 1993.

STIBY, Emma Katherine The Red House, Sanderstead Road, South Croydon CR2 0AG — MB ChB Leic. 1989. SHO (A & E) Belf. City Cas.

STICKLAND, Jane Katherine Duchess of kent House, Dellwood Hospital, Liebenraod Road, Reading Tel: 0118 958 8952 — BM Soton. 1987; DRCOG 1992; MRCGP 1995. Clin. Asst. (Palliat. Med.) Duchess of Kent Hse. Reading. Specialty: Palliat. Med.

STICKLEY, Eileen Angela 3 Blenheim Road, Wakefield WF1 3JZ — MB BCh BAO Dub. 1973.

STIDOLPH, Mr Neville Edsell, Wing Cdr. (retired) 15 Tretawn Park, Mill Hill, London NW7 4PS — BM BCh Oxf. 1937 (Oxf. & St Mary's) BA Cape Town 1932; BA Oxf. 1937; FRCS Eng. 1947. Med. Chairm. War Pens. Appeal Tribunals Eng. & Wales; Mem. Ct.

Examrs. & Penrose May Tutor in Clin. Surg. RCS Eng. Prev: Surg. & Urol. Whittington Hosp.

STIDOLPH, Paul Neville IIAC Secretariat (CMG), 6th Floor, The Adelphi, 1-11 John Adam St., London WC2N 6HT Tel: 020 7962 8412 Fax: 020 7712 2330 — MRCS Eng. LRCP Lond. 1979 (Addenbrooke's, Cambridge) LDS RCS Eng. 1974; MA Camb. 1981, BA Med. Scs. 1976; DRCOG 1983; MSc (Occupat. Med.) Lond. 1990. Med. Sec. to the Indust. Injuries Advisery Counc. (IIAC), Dept. for Work & revisions, Lond., WC2N 6HT. Specialty: Civil Serv. Socs: Fell.Amer. Acad. of Disabil. Evaluating Phys.s; Europ. Union of Med. Ass. & Social Sec. (EUMASS); Coun. Mem. Assur. Med. Soc. (AMS). Prev: CMO's Represen. to the Appeals Serv.; Med. Policy Manager, Med. Policy Gp. DSS Lond.; Sen. Med. Off. BAMS DSS Lond. (N.) Region.

STIER, Susan The Surgery, Parkwood Drive, Warners End, Hemel Hempstead HP1 2LD Tel: 01442 250117 Fax: 01442 256185 — MB ChB Leeds 1991.

STIERLE, Cornelia 45 Sydney Road, Sheffield S6 3GG Tel: 0114 268 0112 — State Exam Med. Heidelberg 1988.

STIFF, Graham Howard St Marys Road Surgery, St. Marys Road, Newbury RG14 1EQ Tel: 01635 31444 Fax: 01635 551316 — MB BS Lond. 1988 (St. Mary's) BSc Physiol. Lond. 1983; MRCGP 1996; (Dist) Cert Med Education 2000. GP Princip. St Marys Rd. Newbury; Clin. Asst. (A & E) Newbury Dist. Hosp.; Vocational Trainer. Specialty: Gen. Pract. Socs: Fell. Roy. Soc. Med.; Brit. Assn. Accid. & Emerg. Med. Prev: GP/Regist. Manor Surg. Oxf.; Regist. (Med.) & SHO (Anaesth.) Roy. Berks. Hosp. Reading; SHO (Paediat.) Radcliffe Hosp. Oxf.

STIFF, James Howard The Surgery, 382 Upminster Road North, Rainham RM13 9RZ Tel: 01708 553120 Fax: 01708 553120 — MRCS Eng. LRCP Lond. 1959 (St. Mary's) FRCGP 1981, M 1968; Cert. Family Plann. JCC 1975; DFFP 1993. Socs: Barking & Havering Med. Audit Advis. Gp. & LMC; (Ex-Provost) NE Lond. Fac. Roy. Coll. Gen. Practs.; BMA (Ex-Chairm. NE Thames Regional Counc.).

STIGGELBOUT, Hendrik Jan Shotton Lane Surgery, 38 Shotton Lane, Shotton, Deeside CH5 1QT Tel: 01244 812094 Fax: 01244 811728 — Artsexamen Amsterdam 1984; MRCGP 1989.

STILES, Mark Andrew Speedwell Surgery, 1 Speedwell Street, Paddock, Huddersfield HD1 4TS Tel: 01484 531786 Fax: 01484 424249; Croft Cottage, 36 Greenhill Bank Road, New Mill, Holmfirth HD9 1ER Tel: 01484 681360 — MB ChB Leeds 1985; MRCGP 1989; DRCOG 1990; DCH RCP Lond. 1990. Prev: Trainee GP Clitheroe Health Centre.

STILES, Mr Peter James Hawks View, 5 Fairway, Merrow, Guildford GU1 2XG Tel: 01483 562296 Fax: 01483 562296 — MB BS Lond. 1956 (Guy's) MRCS Eng. LRCP Lond. 1956; FRCS Eng. 1961. Emerit. Orthop. Surg. Roy. Surrey Co. Hosp. Guildford; Orthopaedic Adviser, various aid organisations. Specialty: Orthop.; Medico Legal. Socs: Fell. Roy. Soc. Med.; Fell. BOA; World Orthopaedic Concern. Prev: Cons. Orthop. Surg. SW Surrey Dist.; Chief Asst. & Sen. Regist. (Orthop. Surg.) St. Bart. Hosp. Lond.; Cons. Orthop. Surg. Rowley Bristow Orthop. Hosp.

STILGOE, Jemima Rya 47 Dryburgh Road, London SW15 1BN; 6 East Shrubbery, Redland, Bristol BS6 6SX — MB BS Lond. 1993 (St mary Hosp.) DRCOG 1995; DCH 1997; MRCGP 1999.

STILL, Mabel Alexandra 10 Abbey Water, Romsey SO51 8EJ — MB BCh Wales 1966; DA Eng. 1969; MRCGP 1981. GP Southampton.

STILL, Ronald McKinnon (retired) 9/5 Whistlefield Court, 2 Canniesburn Road, Bearsden, Glasgow G61 1PX Tel: 0141 942 3097 — MB ChB Glas. 1956; FRCOG 1976, M 1963. Cons. Gyn. Glas. Nuffield Hosp. & Ross Hall Hosp. Glas.; Health Care Internat. Med. Centre Beardmore St. Glas. Clydebank. Prev: Cons. Gyn. Stobhill Gen. Hosp. Glas. & Cons. Obst. Roy. Matern. Hosp.

STILL, Sarah 15 East Hill, Oxted RH8 9AF — BM Soton. 1995 (Soton) DRCOG 1998; DCH 1999. GP Regist. Riverside Pract., Winch. Specialty: Gen. Pract. Prev: SHO GP VTS Roy. Hants Co. Hosp. Winch.

STILLEY, Dores (retired) 5 Ainslie Place, Edinburgh EH3 6AR — MB ChB Ed. 1948. Prev: Med. Adviser Derby Diocesan Adoption Comm.

STILLMAN, Kim Canterbury Health Centre, 26 Old Dover Road, Canterbury CT1 3JB — MB ChB Liverp. 1982. Trainer GP Canterbury; Police Surg. Hosp. Pract. (Venereol.) Canterbury.; Course organiser, Canterbury VTS.

STILLMAN, Paul Leacroft Medical Practice, Ifield Road, Ifield, Crawley RH11 7BS Tel: 01293 526441 Fax: 01293 619970; Claybrooke Haywards, Pound Hill, Crawley RH10 3TR Tel: 01293 882100 — MB ChB Bristol 1969; DObst RCOG 1974. Course Organiser Crawley & Horsham VTS. Prev: Trainee GP Cirencester VTS; Chairm. SW Thames Regional Audio Visual Gp & Crawley & Horsham Med. Soc.; Ho. Surg. & Cas. Off. Southmead Hosp. Bristol.

STILLMAN, Richard Huntley (retired) Caldy Manor, Caldy Wood, Wirral CH48 2HY — MRCS Eng. LRCP Lond. 1943. Prev: Squadron Ldr. RAF Div. Surg. St. Johns Ambul.

STILLWELL, Jennifer Margaret Swan House, 12A Cuxham Road, Watlington OX49 5JW — MRCS Eng. LRCP Lond. 1962; MRCS Eng LRCP Lond. 1962; MFCH 1989. SCMO Wycombe HA.

STILLWELL, Mark Douglas The Surgery, Welbeck Street, Creswell, Worksop S80 4HA Tel: 01909 721206; Manor Lodge, Worksop Road, Whitwell, Worksop S80 4ST — MB ChB Sheff. 1987; DCH RCP Lond. 1990; DRCOG 1991. GP Princip. Specialty: Sports Med. Prev: Trainee GP Worksop VTS.

STILLWELL, Susan — MB ChB Sheff. 1987; DCH RCP Lond. 1990; DRCOG 1991; MRCOG 1992. Clin. Asst. (Gyn.) & Clin. Med. Off. (Family Plann.) Notts. Specialty: Obst. & Gyn.

***STILWELL, Claire Helen** 40 Corvedale Road, Selly Oak, Birmingham B29 4LQ — MB ChB Leeds 1998.

STILWELL, Mr John Harry 81 Longmeadow Road, Knowsley Village, Prescot L34 0HW Tel: 0151 548 6094 Fax: 0151 545 0975 — BM BCh Oxf. 1972; BSc (Biochem., Hons.) Liverp. 1967; LMSSA Lond. 1972; FRCS Eng. 1977. Cons. Hand Surg. Wrightington Hosp., Wigan & Alder Hey Childr. Hosp. Liverp. Specialty: Plastic Surg. Special Interest: Hand & Wrist, including Dupuytrens & Congenital. Socs: Brit. Assn. Plastic Surg.; Brit. Soc. Surg. Hand. Prev: Cons. Plastic Surg. Whiston Hosp. Prescot; Fell. Hand Surg. Univ. Louisville, Kentucky, USA; Sen. Regist. (Plastic Surg.) Whiston Hosp. Prescot.

STILWELL, Ray (retired) Two Gates, Fore St., Wylye, Warminster BA12 0RQ Tel: 01985 248363 — MB BS Lond. 1961 (Guy's) MRCS Eng. LRCP Lond. 1961; DObst RCOG 1963; DA Eng. 1963; MRCGP 1973.

STIMMLER, Anthony 6A North Western Avenue, Watford WD25 9GP Tel: 01923 672086; 68 Flower Lane, Mill Hill, London NW7 2JL Tel: 020 8959 2269 — MB BS Lond. 1982 (Lond. Hosp.) Cert. Family Plann. JCC 1984; DRCOG 1984; D.Occ.Med. RCP Lond. 1995. Occupat. Health Phys. Lewisham & N. Southwark HA. Specialty: Gen. Pract. Socs: Soc. Occupat. Med. Prev: SHO (Psychiat.) Goodmayes; SHO (Obst.) Newham Matern. Hosp.; SHO (Paediat.) Newham Gen. Hosp.

STIMMLER, Leo 11 Landscape Road, Warlingham CR6 9JB — MRCS Eng. LRCP Lond. 1954 (Guy's) MD Lond. 1966, MB BS 1954; FRCP Lond. 1974, M 1960. Cons. Paediat. Guy's Hosp. Lond. Specialty: Paediat. Socs: Brit. Paediat. Assn. Prev: Sen. Research Fell. Inst. Child Health Birm.; Lect. in Paediat. Univ. Birm.; Research Fell. Univ. Colo. Denver, USA.

STIMPSON, Graham George Blackberry Hill Hospital, Fishponds, Bristol BS16 2EW Tel: 0117 965 6061; 12 Challoner Court, Bristol BS1 4RG — MB BS Lond. 1965 (Guy's) MRCS Eng. LRCP Lond. 1965; DPM Eng. 1969; MRCPsych 1972. Cons. Psychother. Blackberry Hill Hosp. Bristol; Clin. Lect. (Ment. Health) Bristol Univ. Specialty: Psychother.

STIMPSON, Victor Barry (retired) 265 Chells Way, Stevenage SG2 0HN Tel: 01438 313001 Fax: 01438 362322 — MB ChB Ed. 1958.

STINCHCOMBE, Claire Elizabeth 5 Cherry Close, Shillingford, Wallingford OX10 7HG — MB ChB Birm. 1993.

STINSON, Deborah Mary S. W. London & St Georges Mental Health NHS Trust, St. Helier, Sutton Hospital, Cotswold Road, Sutton SM2 5NF Tel: 020 8296 4342 Fax: 020 8296 4342; 5 Palace Road, East Molesey KT8 9DJ — MB BCh BAO Belf. 1981; MRCPsych 1986. Cons. Psychiat. Sutton Hosp. Surrey. Specialty: Geriat. Psychiat.

STINSON, Ian Rodney The Parklands Medical Practice, Park Road, Bradford BD5 0SG Tel: 01274 227575 Fax: 01274 693558; The Medical Centre, 30 Buttershaw Lane, Bradford BD6 2DD Tel: 01274 678464 Fax: 01274 693558 — DCH RCP Lond. 1982; BSc (Hons.)

Leeds 1985, MB ChB (Distinc. Path.) 1988; Cert Family Plann JCC 1992; T(GP) 1993; MRCGP 1993. Specialty: Gen. Pract. Socs: BMA; MRCGP.

STINSON, Pauline Gladys 82 Derryfubble Road, Dungannon BT71 7PW — MB BCh BAO Belf. 1996.

STINSON, Mr Robert (retired) Cloghmore, 8 Greystone Road, Antrim BT41 1HD Tel: 028 9442 8367 Fax: 028 9442 8367 — (Qu. Univ. Belf.) MB BCh BAO Belf. 1947; FRCS Ed. 1962. Hon. Cons. Surg. Antrim Area Hosp. N. Health & Social Servs. Bd. Ballymena. Prev: Cons. Surg. Massereene Hosp. Antrim & Waveney Hosp. Ballymena.

STINSON, Sara Isabel (retired) 2 Lavenham Road, Grimsby DN33 3EX — (Leeds) MB ChB Leeds 1946; DObst RCOG 1950; DCH Eng. 1953. Prev: GP Humberside FPC.

STIRLAND, Alison Margaret Womens Community Health Services, CELFACS, St Leonard's Hospital, Nutall St., London N1 5LZ Tel: 020 7601 7100 Fax: 020 7601 7903 — MB ChB Ed. 1987; MRCGP 1991; DRCOG 1991; MFFP 1995. Clin. Asst. Archway Sexual Health Clinic Whittington Hosp. Lond. Specialty: Genitourinary Medicine. Socs: Scientif. Study of VD. Prev: CMO (Family Plann. & Genitourin. Med. in Community) Open Doors Sexual Health Project; SCMO St. Bart. Hosp. & CMO City & Hackney Community Servs. NHS Trust.

STIRLAND, Emma Prospect House, Bulls Cross, Sheepscombe, Stroud GL6 7HU — MB BS Lond. 1980.

STIRLAND, Hilary (retired) Swithland, Hazelwood Lane, Chipstead, Coulsdon CR5 3QZ Email: hilary.eggington@virgin.net — (St. Thos.) MB BS Lond. 1960; DObst RCOG 1961; MFCM RCP (UK) 1983; FFPH 1988; FRCPCH 1997. Prev: Hon. Sen. Lect. St. Geo. Hosp. Med. Sch. Lond.

STIRLAND, John David 56 Holymoor Road, Holymoorside, Chesterfield S42 7DX Tel: 01246 566723 — MRCS Eng. LRCP Lond. 1956 (St. Mary's) BA Camb. 1953, MB 1957, BChir. 1956; DPM Eng. 1960; FRCPsych 1985, M 1971. Cons. Psychiat. Chesterfield Hosp. Specialty: Gen. Psychiat. Prev: Regist. Shenley Hosp. St. Albans; Sen. Regist. Dept. Psychiat. United Sheff. Hosps.

STIRLING, Mr Alistair John 7 Chad Road, Edgbaston, Birmingham B15 3EN Tel: 0121 454 2991 Fax: 0121 454 9008; 119 Gough Road, Edgbaston, Birmingham B15 2JG Tel: 0121 440 3157 — MB ChB Birm. 1977; FRCS Ed. 1981. Cons. Orthop. Surg. Roy. Orthop. Hosp.; Hon. Sen. Lect. Univ. Birm. Specialty: Trauma & Orthop. Surg. Socs: Brit. Scoliosis Soc. Exec. Comm.; Brit. Assn. of Spinal Surg.; Soc. for Back Pain Research. Prev: MRC Research Fell. Univ. Leeds; Lect. (Orthop.) Univ. Leeds.

STIRLING, Amanda Jane Dr McElhone and Partners, Townhead Surgery, 6-8 High St., Irvine KA12 0AY Tel: 01294 273131 Fax: 01294 312832; 3 Old Hillfoot Road, Ayr KA7 3LW — MB ChB Ed. 1989; BSc Ed. 1988, MB ChB 1989; DRCOG 1992; MRCGP 1994.

STIRLING, Andrew Mark 46 Findhorn Place, Grange, Edinburgh EH9 2NS — MB ChB Glas. 1991.

STIRLING, Anne Whitehead Cumberland House, Jordangate, Macclesfield SK10 1EG Tel: 01625 428081 Fax: 01625 503128 Email: anne.stirling@gp-n81062.nhs.uk — MB ChB Glas. 1968; DCH RCPS Glas. 1970; MRCP (UK) 1975; Dip. Prescri Sci. Liverpool 2000. Princip. Gen. Pract. Cumbld. Ho. Macclesfield; Prescribing Lead. Eastern Chesh. P.C.G. Socs: BMA; BMS (Brit. Menopause Soc.); AFMS (Anglo-French Med. Soc.). Prev: Regist. (Paediat. Med.) Roy. Hosp. Sick Childr. Glas.; SHO (Gen. Med.) South. Gen. Hosp. Glas.; Ho. Off. Roy. Infirm. Glas.

STIRLING, Carol Ann — MB ChB Glas. 1989; MRCP (UK) 1993; MRCPath 2003. Specialty: Haematology.

STIRLING, Christina Fionna Margaret Whiteoak, 3 West Common Close, Harpenden AL5 2LJ Tel: 01582 764166 — MB BS Lond. 1984 (Guy's) MA Camb. 1985; MRCP (UK) 1989. Prev: SHO (O & G) Mayday Hosp. Croydon; SHO (Paediat.) City Gen. Hosp. Stoke on Trent; SHO (Paediat.) Qu. Eliz. Hosp. Childr. Lond.

STIRLING, Gavin Mair (retired) 1 Inch Avenue, Dovecot Park, Aberdour, Burntisland KY3 0TF Tel: 01383 860295 — MB ChB Glas. 1928.

STIRLING, George Anthony (retired) 50 Cyprus Road, Mapperley Park, Nottingham NG3 5EB — MB BS Durh. 1952; MD Durh. 1958; FRCPath 1974.

STIRLING, George Scott (retired) The Beeches, Burnhead of Auld Girth, Dumfries DG1 1JN — MB ChB Aberd. 1949; DPM Eng. 1954; FRCPsych 1977, M 1971; FRCP Glas. 1986, M 1984. Prev: Cons. Psychiat. & Med. Admin. Crichton Roy. Hosp. Dumfries.

STIRLING, Heather Fiona Department of Paediatrics, Walsgrave Hospital NHS Trust, Clifford Bridge Road, Walsgrave, Coventry CV2 2DX Tel: 024 76 602020 Fax: 024 76 622197; 101 Ullenhall Road, Knowle, Solihull B93 9JH Tel: 01564 773468 — MB ChB Liverp. 1981 (Liverpool University) BSc (Hons.) Liverp. 1978; MRCP (UK) 1985; DCCH RCP Ed. 1986; MD Liverp. 1995; FRCP Lond. 1997. Cons. Paediat. Walsgrave Hosp. Coventry. Specialty: Paediat.

STIRLING, James Beattie Murcar, 56 Bailie Drive, Bearsden, Glasgow G61 3AH Tel: 0141 942 2120 — MB ChB Glas. 1945; DA Eng. 1953. Socs: Scott. Soc. Anaesths. & Assn. Anaesth. Gt. Brit. & Irel. Prev: Cons. Anaesth. Stobhill Gen. Hosp. & Roy. Hosp. Sick Childr. Glas.; Flight Lt. RAFVR; Sen. Regist. Anaesth. West. Infirm. Glas.

STIRLING, Jennifer Stewart The Balfron Practice, Skimped Hill Health Centre, Skimped Hill Lane, Bracknell RG12 1LH Tel: 01344 306613 Fax: 01344 306614; Courthope, Longhill Road, Chavey Down, Bracknell RG12 9UB — MB ChB Glas. 1977.

STIRLING, Jeremy Mowat — MB ChB Leeds 1987; MRCPsych 1992. Cons. (Addic. & Gen. Psychiat.) Ayrsh. & Arran. Specialty: Gen. Psychiat.

STIRLING, Joanne Louise 14 Croy Avenue, Newton Mearns, Glasgow G77 5SG Tel: 0141 639 7295 — MB ChB Manch. 1994; BSc St. And. 1991; MRCPCH 2001. SpR (Paediatrics) RHSC Glasg. Specialty: Paediat. Prev: SHO (A & E) Vict. Hosp. Blackpool; Ho. Surg. Glas. Roy. Infirm.; Ho. Off. (Med.) Vict. Hosp. Blackpool.

STIRLING, John Grime 7 Nursery Gardens, Beverley HU17 8NS — MB BCh BAO Dub. 1980.

STIRLING, Jonathan Agnew Templepatrick Surgery, 80 Castleton, Templepatrick, Ballyclare BT39 0AZ Tel: 028 9443 2202 Fax: 028 9443 3707; 56A Ballybentragh Road, Dunadry, Antrim BT41 2HJ Tel: 01849 433348 — MB BCh BAO Dub. 1982; BSc (1st cl. Hons.) Belf. 1979; MB BCh BAO Belf. 1982; DCH Dub. 1985; DRCOG 1985; MRCGP 1986.

STIRLING, Julie Allison Violet Bank, Duke Street, Belhaven, Dunbar EH42 1NT — MB ChB Ed. 1990. GP E. Linton.

STIRLING, Kenneth Whyte Alloa Health Centre, Marshill, Alloa FK10 1AB Tel: 01259 216476; 27 Benview Terrace, Devon Village, Fishcross, Alloa FK10 3AR — MB ChB Glas. 1981; MRCP (UK) 1984; MRCGP 1987; DRCOG 1988; FRCP Glas. 1994. Prev: Regist. (Cardiac Med.) West. Infirm. Glas.

STIRLING, Lucy Caroline Medawar Building, Molecular Nociception Group, Department of Biology, University College London, London WC1E 6BT Tel: 020 7679 7943; Flat 23, 1 Prince of Wales Road, London NW5 3LW Tel: 020 7284 0917 — MB BS Lond. 1987 (St Barts.) MRCGP 1993; MSc 1999. Clin. Train. Fell. Molecular Nociception Univ. Coll. Lond.; Hon. Cons. (Palliat. Med.) Univ. Coll. Hosp. NHS Trust. Specialty: Palliat. Med. Socs: Assn. Palliat. Med. Prev: Research Fell., Molecular Nociception, Univ. Coll. Lond.; Sen. Registar, Palliat. Med., Roy. Marsden Hosp. Fulham Rd. Lond. SW4; Sen. Regist. (Palliat. Med.) Roy. Free Hosp. & Edenhall Marie Curie Centre Lond.

STIRLING, Pauline Williamina Margaret Catherine (retired) 15 Willowbed Avenue, Chichester PO19 2JE Tel: 01243 785300 — MB ChB Ed. 1932; DPM Eng. 1937. Prev: Cons. Psychiat. Friern & Halliwick Hosps. Lond.

STIRLING, Mr Richard John 64 Park Road, Buxton SK17 6SN — MB ChB Leic. 1986; BSc (Hons.) Leic. 1984, MB ChB 1986; FCOphth 1991, M 1990. Cons. Ophth. Darlington Memor. Hosp. Specialty: Ophth.

STIRLING, Robert Wilson — MB ChB Glas. 1977; FRCPath 1996, M 1986. Wansbeck Gen. Hosp., Ashington, Northumberland (Changing Jan 2002 to here). Specialty: Histopath. Prev: Cons. Histopath. W. Middlx. Univ. Hosp. Isleworth.

STIRLING, Sarah Louise 9 Stamperland Drive, Clarkston, Glasgow G76 8HD — MB ChB Glas. 1994. Specialty: Gen. Med.

STIRLING, Susanna Clare 33 Endcliffe Rise Road, Sheffield S11 8RU — MB ChB Sheff. 1992; DCH Coll Paeds, S Afr 1995; MSC (MCH) UCL 1997; MPH 2000; DFPHM 2000. Specialist Regist. Pub. Health Med., Trent Deanery. Specialty: Pub. Health Med.

STIRLING, Thomas Boyd (retired) 25 Longwood Road, Aldridge, Walsall WS9 0TA Tel: 01922 452470 Fax: 01922 452551 — MB ChB Birm. 1946.

STIRLING, Valda Anne 7 Nursery Gardens, Beverley HU17 8NS — MB BS Adelaide 1976; MFCM 1987; DFFP 2003. Specialty: Pub. Health Med.

STIRLING, Mr William John Craigavon Area, Hospital Group Trust, 68 Lurgan Road, Craigavon BT63 5QQ; 71 Drumnacanvy Road, Portadown, Craigavon BT63 5LY — MB BCh BAO Belf. 1970; FRCS Ed. 1975. Cons. Surg. Craigavon Area Hosp. Specialty: Gen. Surg.

STIRLING, William Neil (retired) Westmead, 24 Ladygates, Betley, Crewe CW3 9AN — MB ChB Glas. 1950 (Glasgow) MRCGP 1959. Prev: Police Surg., City of Stoke on Trent.

STIRRAT, Mr Allan Norman Department of Orthopaedics, Sunderland District General Hospital, Kayll Road, Sunderland SR4 7TP Tel: 0191 565 6256 — MB ChB Dundee 1979; FRCS Ed. 1984. Cons. Orthop. Surg. Sunderland HA. Specialty: Orthop. Socs: Brit. Orthop. Assn. & Brit. Soc. Surg. Hand.; Brit. Elbow & Shoulder Soc. Prev: Sen. Regist. (Orthop.) St. Mary's Hosp. Paddington & Roy. Nat. Orthop.Hosp. Stanmore; Regist. (Orthop.) Northwick Pk. Hosp. Harrow; Sen. Resid. (Orthop.) Mass. Gen. Hosp. Boston, USA.

STIRRAT, Fiona Wallace 48 Ashburnham Gardens, South Queensferry EH30 9LB Fax: 0131 319 2361 Email: istirrat@aol.com — MB ChB Glas. 1981 (Glasgow University) DRCOG 1985; MRCGP 1986. Asst. GP.

STIRTON, Rosalind Fiona (retired) Westcotes House, Westcotes Drive, Leicester LE3 0QU; 5 Lindisfarne Road, Syston, Leicester LE7 1QJ — BM BS Nottm. 1981; BMedSci Nottm. 1979, BM BS 1981; MRCPsych 1986. Locum Cons. Child & Adolesc. Psychiat. Leics. NHS Trust. Prev: Cons. Child & Adolesc. Psychiat. Leic. NHS Trust.

STIRZAKER, Ljuba Oxfordshire Health Authority, Richards Building, Old Road, Headington, Oxford OX3 7LG Tel: 01865 227186 Fax: 01865 226894 Email: ljuba.stirzaker@oxon-ha.anglox.nhs.uk; 4 Wellington Place, Oxford OX1 2LD — BM BCh Oxf. 1981; MA 1989; MSc Community Med. Lond. 1990; MFPHM RCP (UK) 1993. Cons. Pub. Health Med. Oxf.shire Health Auth.. Specialty: Pub. Health Med. Prev: Cons. Pub. Health Med. Glos. Health Auth.; Sen. Regist. PHM Oxf. RHA.

STITSON, Mr David James, Squadron Ldr. RAF Med. Br. Derriford Hospital, Level 11, Plymouth PL6 8DH Tel: 01752 777111 — MB BS Lond. 1991 (St. Bart. Hosp. Lond.) FRCS Eng. 1996. Cons. Surg. (Orthop. & Trauma) Derriford Hosp. Plymouth. Specialty: Trauma & Orthop. Surg. Socs: Brit. Orthop. Train. Assn. Prev: Specialist Regist. (Orthop. & Trauma) Derriford Hosp. Plymouth.

STITSON, Richard Norman Michael 25 Swift Way, Thurlby, Bourne PE10 0QA — MB ChB Aberd. 1992; BMedBiol. (Hons.) 1990. SHO (Histopath.) QMC, Nottm. Specialty: Histopath. Prev: SHO3 (Haemat.) WGH, Edin.; MRC Clin. Train. Fell. (Genetics) Univ. Camb.

STITT, Geoffrey Woodford Grosvenor House Surgery, 6 Warwick Square, Carlisle CA1 1LB Tel: 01228 525041 Fax: 01228 515786; Woodend, Heads Nook, Carlisle CA8 9AE Tel: 01228 560426 — MB BS Durh. 1965; DObst RCOG 1969; MRCGP 1972. Socs: BMA.

STIVAROS, Stavros Michael Woodfield House, Hill Rd, Penwortham, Preston PR1 9XH — MB ChB Manch. 1997.

STOATE, Howard Geoffrey Alvan Albion Surgery, Pincott Road, Bexleyheath DA6 7LP Tel: 020 8304 8334 Fax: 020 8298 0408; 36 Heathclose Road, Dartford DA1 2PU — MB BS Lond. 1977; DRCOG 1979; FRCGP 1993, M 1981; MSc Gen. Pract. Lond. 1989. Tutor (Gen. Pract.) Qu. Mary's Hosp. Sidcup. Specialty: Gen. Pract. Prev: Clin. Asst. (Respirat. Med.) Brook Gen. Hosp. Lond.; Trainer (Gen. Pract.) Kent; Chair Research Ethics Comm. Bexley HA.

STOBART, James Andrew Harley Huddersfield Road Surgery, 6 Huddersfield Road, Barnsley S70 2LT — MB ChB Sheff. 1989; BMedSci 1986; DRCOG 1993; MRCGP 1994.

STOBBS, Ian Peter The Health Centre, Testwood Lane, Totton, Southampton SO40 3ZN Tel: 023 8086 5051 Fax: 023 8086 5050 — MB ChB Manch. 1968.

STOBIE, Fiona Jane 24 Dronachy Road, Kirkcaldy KY2 5QL — MB ChB Glas. 1992.

STOCK, David — MB ChB Liverp. 1979; MRCPath 1986. Cons. Histopath. E. Glam. Gen. Hosp. Specialty: Histopath. Socs: Roy. Coll. Path. & Internat. Acad. Path. Prev: Sen. Regist. (Histopath.) Middlesbrough Gen. Hosp. & Roy. Vict. Infirm. Newc.; Regist. (Path.) Broadgreen Hosp. & Alder Hey Childr. Hosp. Liverp.

STOCK, David James 13C Weston Park, London N8 9SY Tel: 020 8342 9957 — MB BS Lond. 1990; BSc Lond. 1989.

STOCK, Mr Douglas Graham, Brigadier RAMC Guy's Nuffield House, Newcomen St., London SE1 1YR Tel: 0207 955 5000 Ext: 5978 Fax: 0207 955 4754; Greenshaw House, Wrotham Road, Meopham Green, Gravesend DA13 0AU Tel: 01474 815859 Fax: 01474 815889 — MB BS Lond. 1962 (Char. Cross) MRCS Eng. LRCP Lond. 1963; FRCS Eng. 1967; T(S) 1991. Cons. Orthop. Surg. Defence Secondary Care Agency. Specialty: Orthop. Socs: Fell. BOA; BMA. Prev: Ho. Surg. & Ho. Phys. & Cas. Off. Mt. Vernon Hosp.; Cons. Advisor Orthop. Surg. D.G.A.M.S.

STOCK, Jeremy Guy Louis Conquest Hospital, The Ridge, St Leonards-on-Sea TN37 7RD Tel: 01424 755255; Blackthorne House, The Thorns, Guestling, Hastings TN35 4LR Tel: 01424 814851 — MB ChB Sheff. 1977; FFA RCS Eng. 1981. Cons. Anaesth. Hastings & Rother NHS Trust. Specialty: Anaesth. Socs: Assn. Anaesth. & BMA. Prev: Cons. Anaesth. Sheff. HA; Sen. Regist. (Anaesth.) Wessex RHA; Lect. (Anaesth.) Univ. Calgary Alberta, Canada.

STOCK, Peter Royston (retired) 3 Kellaway Crescent, Westbury-on-Trym, Bristol BS9 4TE Tel: 0117 924 3131 — MB ChB Bristol 1957.

STOCK, Richard David Crouch End Health Centre, 45 Middle Lane, Crouch End, London N8 8PH; 5 Horse Shoe Lane, London N20 8NJ Tel: 020 8446 0401 — MB BS Lond. 1980; Cert. Family Plann. JCC 1984; MRCGP 1984. Prev: Trainee GP Northwick Pk. Hosp. Harrow VTS; Ho. Phys. & Ho. Surg. St. Mary's Hosp. Lond.

STOCK, Sarah Jane Elizabeth — MB ChB Manch. 1998.

STOCK, Mr Simon Everitt Bishop Auckland General Hospital, Bishop Auckland DL14 6AD Tel: 01388 454000 Fax: 01388 454135; Spence House, Hamsterley, Bishop Auckland DL13 3QF Tel: 01388 488468 — MD Newc. 1988; MB BS 1980; FRCS Ed. 1985; FRCS Eng. 1985. Cons. Surg. Bishop Auckland Gen. Hosp. Specialty: Gen. Surg. Socs: Christ. Med. Fellowsh.; Assn. Surg.; Brit. Soc. of Gastroenterol. Prev: Sen. Regist. (Surg.) North. RHA.

STOCKDALE, Andrew David Walsgrave Hospital, Coventry Radiotherapy & Oncology Centre, Clifford Bridge Road, Coventry CV2 2DX Tel: 024 7660 2020 Fax: 024 7653 8900 — MB BS Lond. 1979 (Westm.) BSc Lond. 1976; MRCP (UK) 1982; FRCR 1985. Cons. Clin. Oncol. Walsgrave Hosp. Coventry; Vis. Cons. Clin. Oncol. Solihull Hosp., W. Midl. Specialty: Oncol. Prev: Sen. Regist. (Radiother.) St Luke's Hosp. Guildford; Sen. Regist. & Regist. (Radiother.) Westm. Hosp. Lond.

STOCKDALE, Anna Victoria Kate 21 Vale Road, Wilmslow SK9 5QA — MB ChB Manch. 1997.

STOCKDALE, Elizabeth Joan Noel Department of Diagnostic Radiology, Royal Aberdeen Childrens Hospital, Westburn Road, Aberdeen AB25 2ZG Tel: 01224 681818 Fax: 01224 840659; 1 Grant Road, Banchory AB31 5UW Tel: 01330 823096 — MB ChB Aberd. 1971 (University of Aberdeen) DMRD Eng. 1977; FRCR 1979; MBA Strathclyde 1995; FRCPCH 1997. Cons. Aberd. Roy. Hosps. Trust; Clin. Sen. Lect. Univ. Aberd. Specialty: Radiol.; Paediat. Socs: Eur. Soc. Paediat. Radiol.; Brit. Med. Ultrasound Soc.; Brit. Soc. Paediat. Radiol. Prev: Sen. Regist. St. Geo. Hosp. Lond.; Regist. Roy. Nat. Orthop. Hosp. Lond.; SHO (Surg.) Profess. Surg. Unit. Hosp. Sick Childr. Gt. Ormond St. Lond.

STOCKDALE, Helen Elizabeth 318 Tadcaster Road, York YO24 1HF — MB ChB Birm. 1996.

STOCKDALE, Robert Christopher Arden Cottage, The Common, Earlswood, Solihull B94 5SQ Tel: 01564 702506 — MB ChB Birm. 1967. Specialty: Gen. Med. Prev: Regist. (Gen. Surg. & Thoracic Surg.) Qu. Eliz. Hosp. Birm.; Regist. (Cas.) Gen. Hosp. Birm.

STOCKDALE, Walter Trevor 6 Peckitt Street, York YO1 1SF Tel: 01904 639171 Fax: 01904 633881; 318 Tadcaster Road, York YO24 1HF Tel: 01904 705217 — MB ChB Leeds 1966; DObst RCOG 1968. Prev: Ho. Off. (Surg. & Med.) York Co. Hosp.; Ho. Off. (Obst.) Matern. Hosp. York.

STOCKER, Catherine Anne Rhynern, Station Road, Bere Ferrers, Yelverton PL20 7JS — MB BS Lond. 1989; MRCGP 1994.

STOCKER, David Ian Department of Genitourinary Medicine, Central Outpatients Department, Hartshill Road, Stoke-on-Trent ST4 7PA — MB ChB Birm. 1975.

STOCKER, John Charles 30 Sundial House, Les Rocquettes, Alderney, Guernsey GY9 3TF Tel: 01481 822077 Fax: 01481 823900 — MB BS Lond. 1978 (Lond. Hosp. Med. Coll.) Socs:

Alderney Med. Assn. Prev: Resid. Med. Off. K. Edwd. VII Hosp. for Offs.
STOCKER, Judith — MB ChB Leeds 1998.
STOCKER, Mary Elizabeth The Coach House, Bickleigh, Plymouth PL6 7AL — MB ChB Bristol 1995.
STOCKILL, Ruth Antonia Fieldhead Hospital, Ouchthorpe Lane, Wakefield WF1 3SP — MB ChB Liverp. 1988.
STOCKING, Anthony John Hubert The Coatham Surgery, 18 Coatham Road, Redcar TS10 1RJ Tel: 01642 483495 Fax: 01642 487520 — MB BS Lond. 1975; DRCOG 1980.
STOCKLEY, Andre George Ings (retired) 27 Campden Road, South Croydon CR2 7ER Tel: 020 8688 3089; 27 Campden Road, South Croydon CR2 7ER — MB BS Lond. 1945 (Guy's) LMSSA Lond. 1944. Prev: Ho. Surg. Guy's Hosp.
STOCKLEY, Andrew Thomas Whitefields Surgery, Hunsbury Hill Road, Camp Hill, Northampton NN4 9UW Tel: 01604 760171 Fax: 01604 708528; 16 Beech Close, Bugbrooke, Northampton NN7 3RB Tel: 01604 831370 — BM BCh Oxf. 1979 (Oxford) MA Oxf. 1979; MRCGP 1984. Specialty: Gen. Pract.
STOCKLEY, Mr Ian Connaghyn, 239 Graham Road, Ranmoor, Sheffield S10 3GS Tel: 0114 263 0646 Fax: 0114 263 0686 Email: i.stockley@sheffield.ac.uk — MD Sheff. 1994; MB ChB 1979; FRCS Eng. 1983. Cons. Orthop. Surg. N. Gen. Hosp. Sheff. Specialty: Orthop. Socs: Brit. Orthop. Research Soc. & Brit. Orthop. Foot Surg. Soc.; Brit. Hip. Soc.; Europ. Hip Soc. Prev: Sen. Regist. (Orthop.) North. Gen. Hosp. Sheff.; Clin. Fell. Mt. Sinai Hosp. Toronto, Canada; Sir Harry Platt Research Fell. Hope Hosp. Salford.
STOCKLEY, Jane Manuela Worcestershire Royal Hospital, Charles Hastings Way, Worcester WR5 1DD Tel: 01905 760177 Fax: 01905 760863; Ryall Hill, Ryall Lane, Upton Upon Severn, Worcester WR8 0PN — MB ChB Birm. 1981; FRCPath 1997, M 1989. Cons. Microbiol. Worcester Roy. Infirm. Worcester Roy. Hosp. Specialty: Med. Microbiol.
STOCKLEY, Richard Arthur 6 Tennyson Street, Leicester LE2 1HS — MB ChB Leic. 1995.
STOCKLEY, Robert Andrew 10 Swarthmore Road, Selly Oak, Birmingham B29 4JR — MD Birm. 1978; DSc Birm. 1986, MD 1978, MB ChB 1971; MRCP (UK) 1973; FRCP Lond. 1984. Prof. Med. Qu. Eliz. Hosp. Birm.; Edit. Bd. Europ. Respirat. Jl. & Internat. Jl. Biochem.; Wolfson Research Fell. RCP. Specialty: Gen. Med. Socs: Brit. Lung Foundat. Research Comm.; (Chairm. Chest Research Comm.) Chest, Heart & Stroke Assn.; Assn. Phys. Prev: Lect. (Med.) Univ. Birm.; Chairm. Nat. Asthma Campaign Reseach Comm. 1995.
STOCKLEY, Simon Nicholas The Health Centre, Sunningdale Drive, Eaglescliffe, Stockton-on-Tees TS16 9EA Tel: 01642 780113 Fax: 01642 791020; 189 Durham Road, Stockton-on-Tees TS19 0PX — MB ChB Birm. 1985 (Birmingham) Dip. IMC RCS Ed. 1991; MRCGP 1992. Specialty: Paediat. Dent.
STOCKLEY, William David Kenmore Medical Centre, 60-62 Alderley Road, Wilmslow SK9 1PA Tel: 01625 532244 Fax: 01625 549024 — MB BS Lond. 1963 (King's Coll. Hosp.) DObst RCOG 1965; DCH RCPS Glas. 1966; MRCGP 1976. Hosp. Pract. (Paediat.) Wythenshawe Gen. Hosp. Manch.
STOCKMAN, Alan 27 Fenaghy Road, Galgorm, Ballymena BT42 1HW — MB BCh Belf. 1998.
STOCKMAN, Neil Joseph Thomas 46 Cotswold Avenue, Belfast BT8 6NA — MB BCh BAO Belf. 1995.
STOCKPORT, John Christopher 5 Glen View, Rhyd-y-Foel, Abergele LL22 8EB — MB ChB Manch. 1996. Surg. SHO Glan Clwyd Hosp. Denbighsh. Specialty: Gen. Surg.
STOCKS, David Allen 4 Garth Avenue, Collingham, Wetherby LS22 5BJ — MB BS Lond. 1975; DIH Eng. 1980; AFOM RCP Lond. 1981; DRCOG 1983; MA Health Care Ethics, Leeds 2001. General Practioner.
STOCKS, Philippa Jane Department of Pathology, Kettering General Hospital, Rothwell Road, Kettering NN16 8UZ Fax: 01623 26575 — MB BS Lond. 1974 (St. Bart.) MRCS Eng. LRCP Lond. 1974; FRCPath 1996, M 1985. Cons. (Histopath.) Kettering Gen. Hosp. NHS Trust. Specialty: Histopath. Socs: Assn. Clin. Pathologists. Prev: Cons. (Histopath.) King's Mill Centre; Sen. Regist. (Histopath.) Soton. Gen. Hosp. & Leicester Roy. Infirm.
STOCKTON, Emma Fiona Department of Anaesthetics, Northampton General Hospital, Cliftonville, Northampton NN1 5BD — MB BS Lond. 1997. Specialty: Anaesth.
STOCKTON, Glyn 13 Hazel Street, Leicester LE2 7JN — MB ChB Leic. 1997 (Leicester) SHO (Surg.) PeterBoro. Hosps. NHS Trust PeterBoro. Specialty: Gen. Surg. Prev: Ho. Off. (Med.) Geo. Eliot Hosp. Nuneaton; Ho. Off. (Surg.) Geo. Eliot Hosp.; SHO (Urol.) PeterBoro. Hosp. NHS Trust.
STOCKTON, Martyn Graham Princes Park Health Centre, Wartling Road, Eastbourne BN22 7PF Tel: 01323 744644 Fax: 01323 736094; 19A Upland Road, Eastbourne BN20 8EN Tel: 01323 735361 — MB ChB Birm. 1976.
STOCKTON, Michael Ronald St. Gemma's Hospice, Harrogate Road, Moortown, Leeds LS17 6QD Tel: 0113 269 3231; The Lodge, Cookridge Lane, Cookridge, Leeds LS16 7LG — MB ChB Leeds 1988; MRCGP 1992. Cons. (Palliat. Med.) St. Gemma's Hospice Leeds. Specialty: Palliat. Med.
STOCKTON, Paul Anthony 4 Prestwick Close, Upton Locus, Widnes WA8 9DY — MB ChB Liverp. 1993. Cons. Phys. Whiston Hosp. Merseyside. Prev: SHO (Med.) Whiston Hosp. Merseyside.; Ho. Off. Whiston Hosp. Merseyside.
STOCKWELL, Angela Jane Royal Cornwall Hospital, Treliske, Truro TR1 3LJ; Chyverton Castle, Zelam, Truro TR1 3LJ — MB BS Lond. 1974; MRCS Eng. LRCP Lond. 1974; FRCS (Ophth.) Ed. 1985; FCOphth. Lond. 1988. Cons. Ophth. Roy. Cornw. Hosp. Trust Treliske Hosp. Truro. Specialty: Ophth.
STOCKWELL, Margaret Caldwell 41 Abercrombie Drive, Bearsden, Glasgow G61 4RR Tel: 0141 942 5755 Email: maggie.stockwell@btinternet.com — MB ChB Glas. 1969; DObst RCOG 1971; DA Eng. 1972; FFA RCS Eng. 1975. Cons. Anaesth Glas. Roy. Infirm. Specialty: Anaesth. Prev: Cons. Anaesth. South. Gen. Hosp. Glas.; Sen. Regist. & Regist. (Anaesth.) Glas. Roy. Infirm.
STOCKWELL, Martin Andrew Department of Anaesthesia, St Helier Hospital, Wrythe Lane, Carshalton SM5 1AA Tel: 020 8644 4343 Fax: 020 8296 2951; 45 Chatsworth Avenue, Wimbledon Chase, London SW20 8JZ — MB BS Lond. 1981; FFA RCS Eng. 1986. Cons. ANaesth. & ITU St. Helier NHS Trust Lond. Specialty: Intens. Care. Socs: Assn. Anaesth & Intens. Care Soc.
STOCKWELL, Robert Charles Radiology Department, Chorley & South Ribble District General Hospital, Chorley PR7 1PP Tel: 01257 245878; The Old Barn, Pickup Bank, Hoddlesden, Darwen BB3 3QQ — MB ChB Manch. 1987 (St. And. & Manch.) FRCR 1994. Cons. Radiol. Chorley & S. Ribble Dist. Gen. Hosp. Specialty: Radiol. Prev: Sen. Regist. & Regist. (Radiol.) North. Region; SHO (Gen. Surg.) Halton Dist. Hosp.
STOCKWELL, William Stephen (retired) 13 Cardean Way, Balgeddie, Glenrothes KY6 3PW Tel: 01592 743733 — MB ChB Glas. 1969 (Glasgow) MRCPath 1976; FRCPath 1988.
STODDARD, Mr Christopher James 12 Slayleigh Lane, Fulwood, Sheffield S10 3RF Tel: 0114 230 9284 Fax: 0114 230 7107 — MD Sheff. 1977; MB ChB Sheff. 1971; FRCS Eng. 1976. Cons. Gastrointestional Surg., Sheff. Teachg. Hosps. NHS Trust; Regional Speciality Advsior, Gen. Surg., Trent Region; Sec., Assn. of Upper GI Surg. Specialty: Gen. Surg. Special Interest: Oesophago Gastric Surg. Socs: Brit. Soc. Gastroenterol.; Assn. Coloproctol.; (Sec.) Assn. Upper G.I. Surg. Prev: Clin. Fell. in Surg. McMaster Medica Centre, Hamilton; Sen. Lect. in Surg., Univ. of Liverp.
STODDARD, David Royston 10 Chestnut Close, Duffield, Derby DE56 4HD — MB BS Lond. 1968 (Roy. Free) MRCS Eng. LRCP Lond. 1968.
STODDARD, Emma Louise 6 Mistletoe Road, Jesmond, Newcastle upon Tyne NE2 2DX — MB BS Newc. 1999; DCROG 2003; MRCGP (Distinc.) 2004. Salaried GP, Chester-le-St.
STODDART, Bethan Ceri 20 Corisande Road, Birmingham B29 6RH — BM BS Nottm. 1996.
STODDART, Mr David 65 Powdermill Brae, Gorebridge EH23 4HY; 33 Marywood Square, Strathbungo, Glasgow G41 2BN — MB ChB Manch. 1992; FRCS Ed. 1996; FFAEM 2000. Locum Cons. A&E CrossHo. Hosp. Specialty: Accid. & Emerg. Prev: SHO (A & E & Orthop.) Addenbrooke's Hosp. Camb.; SHO (A & E) Roy. Lancaster Infirm.; SHO (Med.) Westmorland Gen. Hosp.
STODDART, Donald George Shettleston Health Centre, 420 Old Shettleston Road, Glasgow G32 7JZ Tel: 0141 531 6220 Fax: 0141 531 6206; The Hollies, 16 Richmond Drive, Cambuslang, Glasgow G72 8BH Tel: 0141 641 1183 — MB ChB Glas. 1980; BSc Glas. 1979; DRCOG 1984.

STODDART, Helen Alma Road Surgery, Alma Road, Kingswood, Bristol BS15 4EJ Tel: 0117 961 1774 — BSc Lond. 1981, MB BS 1984; DRCOG 1987; DCH RCP Lond. 1987; MFPHM 1994; MRCGP 1998. p/t GP Principal Bristol. Specialty: Gen. Pract.; Pub. Health Med. Socs: Mem. Roy. Coll. of Gen. Practitioners.; Brit. Med. Assn. Prev: Clin. Lect. Primary Health Care, Univ. of Bristol; Trainee GP Portslade Health Centre; Trainee GP Univ. Coll. Hosp. Lond. VTS.

STODDART, James William Anderson 18 Dee Place, Dundee DD2 4JH — BM BCh Oxf. 1998.

STODDART, Joseph Charles 3 Kingsland, Newcastle upon Tyne NE2 3AL Tel: 0191 232 5131 — MD Newc. 1965; MB BS Durh. 1956; FRCA 1993; FRCP Lond. 1994. Cons. Anaesth. Roy. Vict. Infirm. Newc. u. Tyne; Cons. i/c Intens. Ther. Unit Roy. Vict. Infirm. Newc. u.Tyne; Civil Cons. Anaesth. RAF; Cons. Intens. Ther. North. RHA. Specialty: Anaesth. Socs: Anaesth. Research Gp. & Intens. Care Soc.; (Counc.) Roy. Coll. Anaesth. Prev: Regist. (Anaesth.) Roy. Vict. Infirm. Newc.; Med. Off (Research) RAF Inst. Aviat. Med. FarnBoro. Hants.; 1st Asst. (Anaesth.) Univ. Newc.

STODDART, Mark Grainger Dumfries & Galloway Royal Infirmary, Bankend Road, Dumfries DG1 4AP Tel: 01387 241091/01387 246246 — MB ChB Aberd. 1985; BMedBiol. 1985; FRCOphth 1993. Cons. (Ophth.) Dumfries & Galloway Roy. Infirm. Specialty: Ophth. Special Interest: Oculoplastic and Lacrimal Surg. Socs: BMA & N. Eng. Ophth. Soc.; Brit. Oculoplastic Surg. Soc. Prev: Regist. Rotat. (Ophth.) Roy. Vict. Infirm. Newc. u. Tyne; SHO (Ophth.) Roy. Vict. Infirm. Newc.; SHO (Ophth.) Cheltenham Gen. Hosp.

STODDART, Norman (retired) Mayfield Farm, Wilsill, Harrogate HG3 5EB Tel: 01423 711778 — MB BS Lond. 1961 (Guy's) MRCS Eng. LRCP Lond. 1961; FRCGP 1997. Prev: ICI Computer Fell. RCGP.

STODDART, Patricia Elizabeth Burns Watling Street Surgery, 162 Watling Street East, Towcester NN12 6DB — MB ChB Aberd. 1974; DObst RCOG 1976; MRCGP 1980.

STODDART, Peter Anthony Anaesthetic Department, The Royal Hospital for Sick Children, St Michaels Hill, Bristol BS2 8ET Tel: 0117 928 5203 — MB BS Lond. 1984; BSc Lond. 1981; DA (UK) 1987; MRCP (UK) 1989; FCAnaesth 1991. Cons. Paediat. Anaesth. The Roy. Hosp. for Sick Childr. Bristol. Specialty: Anaesth. Prev: Regist. (Anaesth.) Gt. Ormond St. Hosp. Lond.; Asst. Prof. Univ. Virgina, USA.

STODDART, Peter Gavin Pilditch Tableland, Burton Row, Brent Knoll, Highbridge TA9 4BW — MD Bristol 1987; BA Oxf. 1974; MB BS Lond. 1977; DMRD Eng. 1982; FRCR 1983. Cons. Diag. Radiol. Weston Health Trust. Specialty: Radiol.

STODDART, Peter Ronald 108 Queens Road, Leicester LE2 3FL Tel: 0116 707067 — MB BCh Wales 1968 (Cardiff) Socs: BMA.

STODELL, Malcolm Anthony Luton and Dunstable Hospital, Luton LU4 0DZ Tel: 01582 497233; Chestnut Tree Farm, Ampthill Rd, Maulden, Bedford MK45 2DP — MB BS Lond. 1972 (Guy's) MRCS Eng. LRCP Lond. 1972; MRCP (UK) 1976; FRCP Lond. 1994. Cons. Phys. Rheum. & Gen. Med. Luton & Dunstable Hosp. Luton. Specialty: Gen. Med. Socs: Brit. Soc. Rheum. Mem. Prev: Sen. Regist. Rotat. (Rheum.) Westm., Char. Cross & St. Stephen's Hosps. Lond.; Regist. (Gen. Med.) St. Helier Hosp. Carshalton.

STOECKER, Holger Rhynern, Station Road, Bere Ferrers, Yelverton PL20 7JS — State Exam Med Munster 1992.

STOKELL, Richard Alexander Victoria Park Health Centre, Bedford Avenue, Birkenhead CH42 4QJ Tel: 0151 922 1600; 45 Waterpark Road, Birkenhead CH42 8PN — MB ChB Manch. 1984; DRCOG 1986; MRCGP 1988. Prev: Trainee GP Ormskirk & Dist. Gen. Hosp. VTS.

STOKER, Alex Patrick 6A Blackheath Park, London SE3 9RR — MB BS Lond. 1998.

STOKER, Catherine Jane War Memorial Health Centre, Crickhowell NP8 1AG Tel: 01873 810255 — MB BS Lond. 1982; DRCOG 1985; MRCGP 1986.

STOKER, Mr David Lawson Department of Surgery, North Middlesex University Hospital, Sterling Way, London N18 1QX Tel: 020 8887 2461 Fax: 020 8887 2369 Email: dls@dr.com — MB ChB Ed. 1979 (Edinburgh University Medical School) FRCS Ed. 1983; FRCS Eng. 1984; BSc (Med. Sci.) Ed. 1976, MD 1990. Cons. Gen. Surg. N. Middlx. Hosp. Lond.; Clin. Assoc. Prof. St. Geo. Sch. of Med. Grenada; Divisional Director for Anaesthetics & Surg. Specialty: Gen. Surg. Special Interest: Endoscopy and ERCP; Laparoscopic Hernia Surg.; Upper GI Cancer Surg. Socs: Assn. Endoscopic Surgs.; Brit. Soc. Gastroenterol.; Fell. Assn. Surgs. Prev: Assoc. Med. Dir. N. Middlx. Hosp. Lond; Lead Clinician - Surg.; Sen. Regist. (Gen. Surg.) St. Bart. Hosp. Lond. & N. Middlx. Hosp. Lond.

STOKER, Dennis James Royal National Orthopaedic Hospital, 45-51 Bolsover St., London W1P 8AQ; 3 Pearces Orchard, Henley-on-Thames RG9 2LF Tel: 01491 575756 Fax: 01491 575756 Email: stoker@aj3.demon.co.uk — MB BS Lond. 1951 (Guy's) MRCS Eng. LRCP Lond. 1951; FRCP Lond. 1976, M 1958; DMRD Eng. 1969; FFR 1971; FRCR 1975; FRCS Eng. 1992. Cons Radiol Roy Nat Hosp; Orthop.Cons. Radiol Frimley Pk. Hosp. (frimley sy.). Specialty: Radiol. Socs: Fell. (Ex-Dean & Vice-Pres.) Roy. Coll. Radiol.; Fell. Roy. Soc. Med.; Founder Mem. Internat. Skeletal Soc. Prev: Dean Inst. Orthop. Univ. Lond.; Cons. Phys. RAF.

STOKER, Jeffrey Alan 41 Settrington Road, Scarborough YO12 5DL — MB ChB Leeds 1994.

STOKER, John Brandon (retired) Sowood, 13A Culduthel Road, Inverness IV2 4AG Tel: 01463 232141 — MB ChB Leeds 1961; BSc; FRCP Lond. and Edin. Prev: Cardiol. St. James Hosp. Leeds.

STOKER, Nigel Richard Brandon — MB ChB Leeds 1992.

STOKER, Mr Thomas Alan Mayfield 6A Blackheath Park, London SE3 9RR Tel: 020 8852 2669 — MB BChir Camb 1962 (Guy's) MD Camb. 1969, MA; MRCS Eng. LRCP Lond. 1962; FRCS Eng. 1967. Cons. Surg. Qu. Eliz. NHS Trust Lond. SE18; Cons. Surg. Greenwich Dist. Hosp. Specialty: Gen. Surg. Socs: Fell. Assn. of Surg.s; Ex-Pres. W. Kent M-C Soc.; Brit. Soc. Surg. Oncols. Prev: Lect. (Surg.) Westm. Hosp. Lond.; Res. Surg. Off. Roy. Marsden Hosp Lond.; Ho. Surg. Guy's Hosp. Lond.

STOKES, Cathryn Elizabeth Saxonbury House Surgery, Croft Road, Crowborough TN6 1DL Tel: 01892 652266 Fax: 01892 668607 — BM BS Nottm. 1986; MPhil Nottm. 1984, BMed Sci 1983; DGM RCP Lond. 1989; DRCOG 1990; MRCGP 1991; DFFP 1997; D.Occ.Med 2000.

STOKES, Christopher Simon Dashwood, Station Road, Staveley, Kendal LA8 9NB — MB ChB Bristol 1986; BSc Bristol 1983; MRCP (UK) 1990; DRCOG 1992.

STOKES, E. Joan (retired) Ossicles, Newnham Hill, Henley-on-Thames RG9 5TL Tel: 01491 641526 — MB BS Lond. 1937 (Univ. Coll. Hosp.) MB BS (Hons.) Lond. 1937; MRCS Eng. LRCP Lond. 1937; FRCP Lond. 1958, M 1939; FRCPath 1963. Cons. Clin. Bacteriol. Univ. Coll. Hosp. Lond. Prev: Pub. Health Bacteriol. Sector IV Watford.

STOKES, Elizabeth Louise Monkspath Surgery, 27 Farmhouse Way, Monkspath, Solihull B90 4EH Tel: 0121 711 1414 — MB BS Lond. 1989.

STOKES, Iain Michael Nevill Hall Hospital, Brecon Road, Abergavenny NP7 7EG Tel: 01873 732146 Fax: 01873 732147 Email: iain.stokes@gwent.wales.nhs.uk — MB BCh Wales 1971; MRCOG 1977; FRCOG 1989. Cons. O & G Nevill Hall Hosp. Abergavenny. Specialty: Obst. & Gyn. Prev: Sen. Regist. (O & G) Univ. Hosp. of Wales, +St Davids Hosp. Cardiff & Roy. Gwent Hosp. Newport.

STOKES, Jacqueline Margaret The Firs, Crapstone, Yelverton PL20 7PJ Tel: 01822 853068 Fax: 01822 859340 — (Bristol) MB ChB Bristol 1983; DRCOG 1987; DA (UK) 1989. Sessional GP Tavistock; Clin. Asst. (Anaesth.) Plymouth. Prev: Clin. Asst. (Anaesthetics) Tavistock & Plymouth; Princip. Stannary Surg. Tavistock Devon; SHO (Anaesth.) Roy. Devon & Exeter Hosp.

STOKES, John Fisher (retired) Ossicles, Newnham Hill, Henley-on-Thames RG9 5TL Tel: 01491 641526 — MB BChir Camb. 1937 (Camb. & Univ. Coll. Hosp.) MRCS Eng. LRCP Lond. 1937; FRCP Lond. 1947, M 1939; MD Camb. (Prox. Acc. Raymond Horton-Smith Prize) 1947; FRCP Ed. 1975. Consg. Phys. Univ. Coll. Hosp. Prev: Lt.-Col. RAMC.

STOKES, Judith Mary 5 Finney Bank Road, Sale M33 6LR — MB ChB Manch. 1989; BSc (Hons.) 1984. SHO (Prosth.s) Manch. Roy. Infirm.

STOKES, Mathew James The Shamba, Wotton Crescent, Wotton-under-Edge GL12 7JZ; 7 High Street, Wotton-under-Edge GL12 7DE — MB ChB Pretoria 1990; BSc Witwatersrand 1985.

STOKES, Mr Maurice Anthony Department of Surgery, Daisy Hill Hospital, 5 Hospital Road, Newry BT35 8DR Tel: 01693 65511 Fax: 01693 68869; Lisnegar, 23 Well Road, Warrenpoint, Newry BT34 3RS Tel: 016937 52998 — MB BCh BAO NUI 1980 (Univ.

Coll. Dub.) BSc (Anat.) NUI 1982; FRCSI 1986; MCh NUI 1991. Cons. Surg. (Gen. Surg.) Daisy Hill Hosp. Newry. Specialty: Gen. Surg. Socs: Fell. Surg. GB & Irel.; RAMI; BASO. Prev: Sen. Regist. (Gen. Surg.) Irish Train. Scheme; Lect. (Surg.) Univ. Auckland, NZ; Regist. (Surg.) Hosp. Hosp. Salford & Roy. Hosp. Wolverhampton.

STOKES, Michael John Horsefair Practice, Horse Fair, Rugeley WS15 2EL Tel: 01889 582244 Fax: 01899 582244 — MB ChB Birm. 1988 (Birmingham) DRCOG Brim.; DFFP Birm. GP Horsefair, Rugeley, Staffs.; Family Plann. Med. Off., 1st Community Health, Stafford.

STOKES, Michael John 39 The Green, Barton under Needwood, Burton-on-Trent DE13 8JD — MB ChB Birm. 1962; DCH Eng. 1966; MRCP (UK) 1973. Cons. (Paediat.) S.E. Staffs. Health Dist. Specialty: Paediat. Prev: Sen. Regist. (Paediat.) King's Coll. Hosp. Lond.; Regist. (Paediat.) Copthorne Hosp. Shrewsbury; Regist. (Paediat.) United Newc. Hosps.

STOKES, Monica Anne Department of Anaesthesia, University of Birmingham, Edgbaston, Birmingham B15 2TH — BM BS Nottm. 1981; BMedSci Nottm. 1979; FFA RCS Eng. 1986. Sen. Lect. (Anaesth.) Univ. Birm.; Hon. Cons. Birm. Childr. Hosp. NHS Trust. Specialty: Anaesth. Prev: Lect. (Anaesth.) Univ. Birm.

STOKES, Paul Robert Alexander 18 Meadowhead Road, Southampton SO16 7AD Tel: 023 8076 7902 — MB ChB Birm. 1997 (Birmingham University) BSc (Hons) Birm. SHO in A&E, John Radcliffe Hosp., Oxf. Specialty: Accid. & Emerg. Prev: Ho. Off. Surg., Alexandra Hosp., Redditch; Ho. Off. Med./ Cardology, Qu. Eliz. Hosp., Birm.

STOKES, Peter John Alresford Surgery, Station Road, Alresford SO24 9JL Tel: 01962 732345 Fax: 01962 736034 — MB BS Lond. 1984 (Westm.) BSc (Basic Med. Sci. & Physiol.) Lond. 1981, MB BS 1984; MRCGP 1991. Prev: Regist. & SHO (Med.) Roy. Devon & Exeter Hosp. Exeter; SHO (Obst.) Freedom Fields Hosp. Plymouth; SHO (A & E) St. Helier Hosp. Surrey.

STOKES, Robert Andrew Tottington Health Centre, 16 Market Street, Tottington, Bury BL8 4AD Tel: 01204 885106 Fax: 01204 887717 — MB ChB Manch. 1986; MRCGP 1990; DRCOG 1990.

STOKES, Thomas Christopher 87 Kidbrooke Grove, Blackheath, London SE3 0LQ — MD NUI 1981; MB BCh BAO NUI 1971; MRCP (UK) 1974; MRCPI 1976; MSc Lond. 1979; FRCP Lond. 1989. Cons. Phys. Qu. Eliz. Hosp. Woolwich; Hon. Cons. Phys. St. Thos. Hosp. Lond. Specialty: Gen. Med.; Respirat. Med.; Allergy. Prev: Sen. Regist. (Respirat. Med.) Addenbrookes Hosp. Camb. & Papworth; Hosp.; Clin. Lect. Cardiothoracic Inst. & Brompton Hosp.

STOKES, Timothy Newman Department of General Practice & Primary Health Care, University of Leicester, Leicester General Hospital, Gwendolen Road, Leicester LE5 4PW Tel: 0116 258 4873 Fax: 0116 258 4982 Email: tns2@le.ac.uk — MB ChB Ed. 1989; BA Oxf. 1985; MPhil Camb. 1987; MA Oxf. 1989; MRCGP 1993; MPH Notts. 1997; PhD Leicester 2002. p/t Sen. Lect. Gen. Pract. Univ. of Leicester; GP E. Leics. Med. Pract., Leics. Specialty: Gen. Pract.; Research. Prev: Trainee GP Airedale HA.; Ho. Off. (Surg.) York Dist. Hosp.; Ho. Off. (Med.) City Hosp. Edin.

STOKES, Victoria Valerie Lyndhurst Surgery, 2 Church Lane, Lyndhurst SO43 7EW Tel: 023 8028 2689 Fax: 023 8028 2918; 63A Southampton Road, Lymington SO41 9GH Tel: 01590 670401 — MB ChB Leeds 1993. GP Regist, Lyndhurst Surg. Hants. Specialty: Gen. Pract. Prev: SHO Rotat. (Med.) Huddersfield Roy. Infirm. Huddersfield, W. Yorks.

STOKES-LAMPARD, Helen Jayne Department of Primary Care & General Practice, The Medical School, University of Birmingham, Birmingham B15 2TT Email: h.j.stokeslampard@bham.ac.uk; The Cloisters Medical Practice, Greenhill Health Centre, Church Street, Lichfield WS13 6JL; 14 Holte Drive, Four Oaks, Sutton Coldfield B75 6PR — MB BS Lond. 1996 (St. Geo.) DFFP 1998; DRCOG 2000; MRCGP 2002; MSc 2003. GP Princip. The Cloisters Med. Pract., Lichfield; Clin. Research Fell. Univ. of Birm. Specialty: Obst. & Gyn.; Gen. Pract. Special Interest: Women's Health; Cancer Screening. Socs: BMA; RCGP.

STOKKEREIT, Colin Redlands, Mount Tavy Road, Tavistock PL19 9JL; 50 Benson Road, Grays RM17 6DL — MB BS Lond. 1994; BSc (Biochem.) Lond. 1991. Prev: SHO (A & E) Lister Hosp. Stevenage; Ho. Off. (Surg.) Lister Hosp. Stevenage; Ho. Off. (Gen. Med.) King Geo. Hosp. Goodmayes.

STOKOE, David 9 Linkside, Higher Bebington, Wirral CH63 5PE — MB ChB Liverp. 1987.

STOKOE, Eric (retired) 9 Hall Farm, Shincliffe, Durham DH1 2UE Tel: 0191 386 4807 — (Camb. & Durh.) MRCS Eng. LRCP Lond. 1950; MA Camb. 1952, MB BChir 1951; DIH Soc. Apoth. Lond. 1961. Prev: GP Durh. City.

STOKOE, Margaret Ann — MB ChB Dundee 1983; DCH RCP Lond. 1986; Cert. Prescribed Equiv. Exp. JCPTGP 1989; Cert. Family Plann. JCC 1990; DRCOG 1990.

STOKOE, Norman Leslie (retired) 26 Morningside Place, Edinburgh EH10 5EY Tel: 0131 447 8966 — MB ChB Ed. 1945; DO Eng. 1951; FRCS Ed. 1953; FRACS 1958; FRCOphth Lond. 1988. Prev: Cons. Ophth. Surg. E. Fife Hosp. & Edin. Roy. Infirm.

STOLAR, Mark 91 Palmerston Road, Walthamstow, London E17 6PU Tel: 020 8520 7115; 27 Nevin Drive, Chingford, London E4 7LL Tel: 020 8529 1271 — MRCS Eng. LRCP Lond. 1959; DM Cairo 1954, MB BCh 1950. Prev: Med. Regist. Wanstead Hosp. Lond.; Clin. Asst. (Gen. Med.) Battersea Gen. Hosp.; Clin. Asst. (Neurol.) Qu. Mary's Hosp. for E. End. Lond.

STOLKIN, Colin 30 Talfourd Road, London SE15 5NY Tel: 020 7701 1321 — BM BCh Oxf. 1969; MA. Lect. Dept. Anat. King's Coll. Lond. Prev: Sen. Research Fell. (Ment. Health Foundat. & Research Trust) MRC; Neuro-immunol. Project Dept. Zool. Univ. Coll. Lond.; MRC Jun. Research Fell. Dept. Neuropath. Inst. Psychiat. Lond.

STOLL, Basil Arnold 5 Milton Court, Highfield Road, London NW11 9LY — MRCS Eng. LRCP Lond. 1939 (Westm.) DTM & H Eng. 1946; DMRT Eng. 1947; DMRD Eng. 1948; DMR Lond 1948; FFR 1951; FRCR 1975. Hon. Cons. Dept. Radiother. St. Thos. Hosp. & Roy. Free Hosp. Lond.; Vis. Prof. Univ. Witwatersand S. Afr.; Edr. Revs. on Endocrine-Related Cancer; Dep. Edr. Clin. Oncol.; Clin. Edr. BioTher. Specialty: Oncol.; Radiother. Socs: Brit. Breast Gp. Prev: Cons. Radiotherap. Cancer Inst. Melb. & Lect. in Radiother. Monash & Melb. Univs.; Hon. Radiotherap. P. Henry's Hosp. Melb.

STOLL, Henry (retired) 2 Spencer Close, Regents Park Road, Finchley, London N3 3TX Tel: 020 8346 1848 — (Guy's) MRCS Eng. LRCP Lond. 1937. Prev: Chairm. Hampstead Div. BMA.

STOLL, Lionel Julian 27 Hollycroft Avenue, Hampstead, London NW3 7QJ Tel: 020 7435 2656 — MRCS Eng. LRCP Lond. 1933 (Guy's) FRCGP 1971. Socs: Fell. BMA (Ex-Pres. & Chairm. Metrop. Cos. Br.); Fell. Hunt. Soc.; Osler Club. Prev: Clin. Asst. Metrop. ENT Hosp. Lond.; Squadron Ldr. RAF; Phys. CharterHo. Rheum. Clinic.

STOLLARD, Mr Gordon Edmund, RD (retired) Falaise, Appartment 6, 14 West Overcliff Drive, Bournemouth BH4 8AA Tel: 01202 763564 Email: stollge@aol.com; Randabel, 6 Throstle Nest Drive, Harrogate HG2 9PB Tel: 01423 872249 Email: stollge@aol.com — (Univ. Coll. Hosp.) MB BS Lond. 1965; MRCS Eng. LRCP Lond. 1965; FRCS Eng. 1972. Prev: Sen. Regist. (Orthop.) Princess Eliz. Orthop. Hosp. Exeter.

STOLLERY, Nigel Alexander Smeeton Road Health Centre, Smeeton Road, Kibworth, Leicester LE8 0LG Tel: 0116 279 3308 Fax: 0116 279 3320 — MB BS Lond. 1989. Specialty: Accid. & Emerg.

STONE, Adam Francis Minto 5 Deepdene Mansions, Rostrevor Road, Fulham, London SW6 5AQ Tel: 020 7731 5395 — MB BChir Camb. 1991; MA Camb. 1992; MRCP (UK) 1994. Regist. SW Thames RHA. Specialty: Gastroenterol.

STONE, Alan Kenneth Laxey Medical Centre, New Road, Laxey IM4 7BF Tel: 01624 676212; 43 Cronk Avenue, Birchill, Onchan, Douglas IM3 3DE Tel: 01624 623557 — MB ChB Aberd. 1979; MRCGP 1986. Gen. Med. Pract.

STONE, Alan Martin Meddygfa Canna Surgery, 27 Wyndham Cresent, Canton, Cardiff CF11 9EE Tel: 029 2034 1547 Fax: 029 2064 0499 — MB BS Lond. 1984; DCH RCP Lond. 1987; DRCOG 1988; MRCGP 1988.

STONE, Alexander, SBStJ Cranford, Hillside Drive, Woolton, Liverpool L25 5NS Tel: 0151 428 2155 Fax: 0151 421 1070 — (Liverp.) MRCS Eng. LRCP Lond. 1943; MB ChB Liverp. 1944; FRCGP 1969, M 1952. Hon. Lect. (Gen. Pract.) Univ. Liverp. Prev: Dir. Studies (Gen. Pract.) Univ. Liverp.; Corps Surg. St. John Ambul. Brig.

STONE, Alexander George Henry 1 Regents Place, Loughton IG10 4PP — MB BS Lond. 1994; FRCA Lond. 1998. SpR St. Bart. & Lond. Sch. of Anaesth. Specialty: Anaesth. Prev: SHO (Anaesth.)

Whipps Cross Hosp. Lond.; SHO (A & E) Roy. Lond. & Homerton Hosps.; Ho. Off. (Gen. Med.) St. Bart. & Homerton Hosps. Lond.

STONE, Alison Louise Rosemount, 31 Main Road, Portskewett, Newport NP26 5SA — MB BS Lond. 1984.

STONE, Andrew Brian 30 Eton Rise, Eton College Road, London NW3 2DF — MB BS Lond. 1996; BSc (Hons) Lond. 1993 (Physiol).

STONE, Andrew David Royston Church Street Surgery, Church Street, Spalding PE11 2PB Tel: 01775 722189 Fax: 01775 712164 — MB BS Lond. 1984 (Kings Coll. Hosp. Med. Sch.) AKC 1984; DGM RCP Lond. 1987; DRCOG 1988. Specialty: Gen. Pract. Prev: Ho. Off. (Surg.) King's Coll. Hosp. Lond; SHO (Paediat. & O & G) All St.s Hosp. Chatham Kent.; SHO (Obst & Gyn.) Chatham Kent & Trainee GP Canterbury.

STONE, Anna Mary 15 Rodbourne Road, Harborne, Birmingham B17 0PN — MB ChB Birm. 1995.

STONE, Anthony Royston 23 Cross Street, Ystrad, Pentre CF41 7RF — MB ChB Manch. 1993.

STONE, Anthony William 23 The Close, Cleadon, Sunderland SR6 7RG — MB ChB Leeds 1987; DRCOG 1992; MRCGP 1994.

STONE, Audrey Mary (retired) The Manor House, Tollerton, York YO61 1QQ Tel: 01347 838454 Fax: 01347 838454 — (Middlx.) MRCS Eng. LRCP Lond. 1957; DA Eng. 1960. Clin. Asst. (Anaesth.) York Dist. Hosp. Prev: Instruc. in Anaesth. Johns Hopkins Hosp. Baltimore, U.S.A.

STONE, Barnet (retired) Stoneacre, Paris Farm, Common Road, Lingfield RH7 6BZ Tel: 01342 833816 — MB ChB Manch. 1931.

STONE, Beryl Cynthia Keymer House, West Hill, Ottery St Mary EX11 1UW — MB BS Lond. 1951 (King's Coll. Hosp.)

STONE, Brian Edwin Shanklin Medical Centre, 1 Carter Road, Shanklin PO37 7HR Tel: 01983 862245 Fax: 01983 862310 — MRCS Eng. LRCP Lond. 1961 (St. Bart.) DObst RCOG 1964. Prev: Asst. Co. Med. Off. I. of Wight; Ho. Surg. Redhill Gen. Hosp.; Ho. Phys. & Ho. Surg. (O & G) St. Mary's Hosp. Newport.

STONE, Carol Anne — MB ChB Glas. 1997.

STONE, Christine Janet Health Promotion Unit, Beckenham Hospital, 379 Croydon Road, Beckenham BR3 3QL Tel: 020 8289 6658 Fax: 020 8282 3242 — MRCS Eng. LRCP Lond. 1965 (St. Mary's) Primary Care Ment. Health Facilitator Bromley Health. Prev: Ho. Phys. Prospect Pk. Hosp. Reading; Ho. Surg. Roy. Berks. Hosp. Reading.; Partner W. Wickham.

STONE, Mr Christopher Anthony Royal Devon & Exeter Healthcare Trust, Barrack Road, Exeter EX2 5DW Tel: 01392 402633 — MB ChB Manch. 1990; FRCS Eng. 1994; FRCS Ed. 1994; MSc Lond. 1996. Cons. in Plastic and Reconstruc. Surg.; Instruc. in Emerg. Managem. of Severe Burns. Specialty: Plastic Surg. Socs: Brit. Burns Assn.; Assoc. Mem. Brit. Assn. Plastic Surgs. Prev: SHO (Gen. Surg.) Wythenshawe Hosp.; SHO (Plastic Surg.) Radcliffe Infirm.; SHO (Orthop.) Mt. Vernon Hosp.

STONE, Christopher Michael 87A St Georges Drive, Pimlico, London SW1 4DB — MB BS Lond. 1983.

STONE, Mr Colin David Payne Crawley Hospital, West Green Drive, Crawley RH11 7DH Tel: 01293 600325 Fax: 01293 600341 — MB ChB Ed. 1971; BSc (Hons.) Ed. 1968; FRCS Ed. 1976. Cons. Orthop. Surg. Crawley Hosp. New E. Surrey Hosp. Redhill. Specialty: Orthop. Socs: Brit. Orthop. Assn.; Brit. Soc. Surg. Hand. Prev: Sen. Regist. (Orthop.) W. Midl. RHA; Regist. (Orthop.) Lothian HB.

STONE, David Gordon Harvey (retired) Flowers Court Coach House, Pangbourne, Reading RG8 8ES Tel: 0118 984 1510 — (St. Thos.) MB BS Lond. 1943; MRCS Eng. LRCP Lond. 1943; FRCP Lond. 1972, M 1948. Prev: Cons. Paediat. W. Berks. HA.

STONE, Professor David Hope Yorkhill Hospital, Paediatric Epidemiology and Community Health (PEACH) Unit, Glasgow G3 8SJ Tel: 0141 201 0178 Fax: 0141 201 6943 Email: d.h.stone@clinmed.gla.ac.uk — MB ChB Ed. 1972 (Ed. & Glas.) MRCP (UK) 1974; FFCM 1987, MFCM 1979; MD Ed. 1982; FRCP Glas. 1990; FRCPCH 1997. Prof. (Paediat. Epidemiol. & Community Health) Univ. Glas.; Sen. Lect. (Paediat. Epidemiol.) Univ. Glas.; Hon. Cons. Paediat. Epidemiol. Yorkhill NHS Trust. Specialty: Pub. Health Med. Prev: Lect. (Community Med.) St. Thos. Hosp. Med. Sch. Lond.; Sen. Lect. (Epidemiol.) B.G. Univ. Negev, Israel.; Hon. Cons. Pub. Health Med. Gtr. Glas. HB.

STONE, David Lewis Papworth Hospital, Papworth Everard, Cambridge CB3 8RE Tel: 01480 364361 Fax: 01480 364799 — MB BS Lond. 1971 (Charing Cross Hosp.) BSc Lond. 1968; MRCS Eng. LRCP Lond. 1971; MD Lond. 1985; FRCP Lond. 1992; FRCP Ed 1997. Cons. Cardiol. Papworth & W. Suff. Hosp. Trusts; Medical Director, Papworth NHS Trust. Specialty: Cardiol. Special Interest: Cardiac imaging; Med. Educat. Prev: Assoc. Dean Camb. Sch. Clin. Med.

STONE, Diana Rachel Glynn House, Probus, Truro TR2 4JS — BM BS Nottm. 1992; MRCP (UL) 1999.

STONE, Elizabeth Jeanne Pine Paddock, Whitchurch Hill, Reading RG8 7PB Tel: 0118 984 4345 — MB BS Lond. 1967 (King's Coll. Hosp.) DRCOG 1993. Socs: BMA. Prev: Trainee GP West. Elms Surg. Reading; SHO (O & G) Roy. Berks. Hosp. Reading; CMO E. Berks. Health Auth.

STONE, Frances 719 Walmersley Road, Bury BL9 5JN — MB ChB Manch. 1975.

STONE, Gordon Victor The Carn, Flichity, Inverness IV2 6XD Tel: 01808 521401 — MB ChB Aberd. 1969; Dip. Community. Med. Ed. 1976; FFCM 1987, M 1977. Dir. Of Informat. & Clin. Effectiveness Highland NHS Bd.; Hon. Sen. Lect. (Community Med.) Univ. Aberd. Socs: Fac. Community Health (Irel.). Prev: Gen. Manager. Highland HB; Chief Med. Off. & Dir. Pub. Health Highland HB; Flight Lt. RAF Med. Br.

STONE, Ian Mitchell Falmouth Road Surgery, 78 Falmouth Road, London SE1 4JW Tel: 020 7407 4101/0945 Fax: 020 7357 6170 — MB Camb. 1980; BChir 1979.

STONE, James Ciaran Waterside Health Centre, Glendermot Road, Londonderry BT47 6AU Tel: 028 7132 0100 Fax: 028 7134 9323; 8 Glenaden Hill, Altnagelvin, Londonderry BT47 2LJ — MB BCh BAO Belf. 1972; MRCGP 1977; FRCGP 1996.

STONE, James Michael 425 Seaside, Eastbourne BN22 7RT — MB BS Lond. 1997 (Roy. Free Hosp. Sch. of Med., Lond.) BSc; MRCPsych. SpR (Psychiatry) Maudsley Hosp.

STONE, Jennifer Ann Stracey Castle Street Surgery, 67 Castle Street, Salisbury SP1 3SP Tel: 01722 322726 Fax: 01722 410315; 7 Queensberry Road, Salisbury SP1 3PH Tel: 01722 326220 — MB BS Lond. 1968 (King's Coll. Hosp.) MRCS Eng. LRCP Lond. 1968; DObst RCOG 1971. Socs: BMA. Prev: GP with Newton, Dunn & Partners; Med. Off. Quarriers Homes; Clin. Asst. (Psychiat.) Dykebar Hosp. Paisley.

STONE, John Peter William Sheet Street Surgery, 21 Sheet Street, Windsor SL4 1BZ Tel: 01753 860334 Fax: 01753 833696; 12 Ruston Way, Ascot SL5 8TG Tel: 01344 873720 — MB BS Lond. 1986 (Roy. Free Hosp. Sch. Med.) Mem. Berks. LMC. Socs: Windsor Med. Soc.

STONE, Jonathan Western General Hospital, Department of Clinical Neurosciences, Crewe Road, Edinburgh EH4 2XU Tel: 0131 537 1000 Email: Jon.Stone@ed.ac.uk — MB ChB Ed. 1992 (Edinburgh University) MRCP (UK) 1995. Specialist Regist. (Neurol) W. Gen. Hosp. Specialty: Neurol. Special Interest: Functional Neurol. Symptoms/Conversion disorder. Socs: Brit. Neuropsychiat. Assn.; Assoc. of Brit. Neurols. Prev: SHO (Psych.) Roy. Vict. Infirm. Newc.; Regist. (Gen. Med.) Walkato Hosp., Hamilton, NZ; Regist. (Neurol.) Newc. Gen. Hosp.

STONE, Julian Philip 1 Park Street, Maidenhead SL6 1SN — MB BS Lond. 1994.

STONE, Karen Elizabeth Ponfefract General Infirmary, Friarwood Lane, Pontefract WF8 1PU — MB ChB Birm. 1990; MRCP (UK) 1995. Specialist Regist. (Paediat.) Yorks. Region. Specialty: Paediat. Prev: Regist. (Paediat.).

STONE, Katherine Peta 37 Napoleon Avenue, Farnborough GU14 8LZ — BM BCh Oxf. 1998.

STONE, Kenneth Arrowsmith, TD, OStJ (retired) 2 School Close, Cottingwood Lane, Morpeth NE61 1DY Tel: 01670 517411 — MB BS Durh. 1950 (Newc.) MRCGP 1974. Clin. Asst. (Psychiat.) St. Geo. Hosp. Morpeth.

STONE, Mr Kenneth Harold (retired) North London Nuffield Hospital, Cavell Drive, Enfield EN2 7PR Tel: 020 8440 0157; Ridings, 84 Copse Wood Way, Northwood HA6 2UB Tel: 01923 824255 — MB BS Lond. 1950 (St. Mary's) MRCS Eng. LRCP Lond. 1950; FRCS Eng. 1956. Indep. Cons. Surg. (Orthop.) N. Lond. Nuffield Hosp.; Hon. Lect. Inst. Orthop. Prev: Cons. Surg. (Orthop.) Barnet, Enfield & Haringey HAs.

STONE, Mr Laurence Donald 1 Almacs Close, Blundellsands, Liverpool L23 6XT Tel: 0151 924 3752 — MB BS Lond. 1980 (Westm.) MRCS Eng. LRCP Lond. 1980; FRCS Eng. 1984; DRCOG

1987; DCH RCP Lond. 1987. Research Assoc. Dept. Gen. Pract. Univ. Liverp. Prev: Profess. Regist. (Surg.) Roy. Marsden Hosp. Lond.; Profess. Regist. (Surg.) Roy. Liverp. Hosp.

STONE, M J Pedmore Road Surgery, 22 Pedmore Road, Lye, Stourbridge DY9 8DJ Tel: 01384 422591 — MB ChB Bristol 1997; DRCOG; MRCGP. GP; Clin. Assisitant, Dudley H.A. Gastroenterol.

STONE, Malcolm St Mary's Surgery, Church Close, Andover SP10 1DP Tel: 01264 341424 Fax: 01264 336792; 9 Cottage Green, Goodworth Clatford, Andover SP11 7RZ — MB BS Lond. 1984; DRCOG 1987; MRCGP 1988. Princip. GP Andover Hants.

STONE, Mr Martin Ye Olde Forge, Llanmartin, Newport NP18 2EB Tel: 01633 413073 Fax: 01633 411148 Email: marjan@globalnet.co.uk — (Liverp.) MB ChB Liverp. 1968; FRCOG 1986, M 1973; MD Liverp. 1979. Cons. O & G Roy. Gwent Hosp. Newport. Specialty: Obst. & Gyn. Socs: BMA; (Pres.) Welsh Obst. & Gyn. Soc.; (Ex Chairm.) Lond. Obstetric & Gyn. Soc. Prev: Sen. Regist. (O & G) St. Geo. Hosp. Lond. & Soton. Gen. Hosp.; Regist. (O & G) Char. Cross Hosp. Lond.; Ho. Surg. (O & G) United Liverp. Hosps.

STONE, Mr Martin Hope Department of Orthopaedic Surgery, The General Infirmary, Leeds LS1 3EX Tel: 0113 392 6902 Fax: 0113 392 3770; Glenroyd, 1 West Park Grove, Roundhay, Leeds LS8 2HQ Tel: 0113 266 0481 — MB ChB Glas. 1979; FRCS Ed. 1983; MPhil Strathclyde 1987; FRCS Eng. 1997. Cons. Orthop. & Trauma Surg. Gen. Infirm. Leeds. Specialty: Orthop. Socs: Fell. BOA; Brit. Hip Soc. (Exec. Comm.). Prev: Sen. Regist. (Orthop.) Soton. Gen. Hosp.; Regist. (Orthop. Surg.) Glas. Roy. Infirm.

STONE, Michael Christopher Cuffley Village Surgery, Maynards Place, Cuffley, Potters Bar EN6 4JA Tel: 01707 875201 Fax: 01707 876756 — MB BS Lond. 1987; MRCGP 1991. Prev: Trainee GP Pilgrim Gen. Hosp. VTS.

STONE, Michael David 7 Headlands Road, Bramhall, Stockport SK7 3AN — MB ChB Dundee 1994.

STONE, Michael Derek Bone Research Unit, Llandough Hospital, Academic Centre, Penlan Road, Penarth CF64 2XX Tel: 029 2071 6957 Fax: 029 2070 7628 Email: stonemd@cardiff.ac.uk; 78 TreeTops, Portskewett, Newport NP26 5RT Tel: 01291 421988 Email: mikestone6@compuserve.com — MB BS Lond. 1984 (Oxford University and London Hospital) BA Oxf. 1981; MRCP (UK) 1987; DM Nottm. 1997; FRCP (UK) 1998. Cons. Phys. Med. (c/o the Elderly) Llandough Hosp. Penarch; Dir. of Bone Research. Specialty: Care of the Elderly; Gen. Med. Socs: Med. Adviser Nat. Osteoporosis Soc.; Bone & Tooth Soc.; Brit. Geriat. Soc.

STONE, Michael John Trafford Training Centre, Birch Road, Off Isherwood Road, Carrington, Manchester M30 4BH Tel: 0161 868 8750 Fax: 0161 868 8853 Email: mike.stone@manutd.co.uk; 11 Chiltern Close, Hazel Grove, Stockport SK7 5BQ Tel: 0161 285 9328 — MB ChB Manch. 1974; DRCOG 1976; MRCP (UK) 1980; Dip Sports Med 1998. Club doctor, Manch. United. Specialty: Sports Med. Socs: Brit. Assn. of Sport and Exercise Med.; Roy. Soc. of Med.; UKADIS. Prev: Gen. Practitioner, Beech Ho.. Hazel Gr.

STONE, Michele Patricia Whitehead Health Centre, 17B Edward Road, Whitehead, Carrickfergus BT38 9RU Tel: 028 9335 3454 Fax: 028 9337 2625; 19 Old Shore Road, Trooperstone, Greenisland, Carrickfergus BT38 8PF Tel: 01960 369951 — MB BCh BAO Belf. 1986; DRCOG 1989; MRCGP 1990; Cert. Family Plann. JCC 1991.

STONE, Natalie Marie Royal Gwent Hospital, Cardiff Road, Newport NP20 2UB — MB BS Lond. 1992; MRCP (UK) 1995. Specialty: Dermat.

STONE, Nicola Doctors' Mess, Kent and Sussex Hospital, Mount Ephraim, Tunbridge Wells TN4 8AT — BM BS Nottm. 1995.

STONE, Patricia Ann Department of Respiratory Physiology, North West Lung Centre, Wythenshawe Hospital, Southmoor Road, Manchester M23 9LT Tel: 0161 291 2493 Fax: 0161 291 5020 — MB ChB Manch. 1975 (Manchester) Assoc. Specialist (Sleep Laborat.) Wythenshawe Hosp. Manch. Specialty: Respirat. Med. Socs: Fell. Manch. Med. Soc.; Brit. Thorac. Soc.; Brit. Sleep Soc. Prev: Research Fell. (Respirat. Physiol.) Wythenshawe Hosp. Manch.; Med. Off. Nat. Blood Transfus. Serv.; Research Asst. (Respirat. Med.) Manch. Roy. Infirm.

STONE, Patrick Charles 74 Lambton Road, London SW20 0LP — MB BChir Camb. 1991; MA Camb. 1990, MB BChir 1991; MRCP (UK) 1993. MacMillan Lect. (Palliat. Med.) Roy. Lond. Hosp. Specialty: Palliat. Med. Socs: Assn. Palliat. Med.

STONE, Pauline Ann The Western Infirmary, Dumbarton Road, Glasgow G11 6NT Tel: 0141 211 2069; 6 Turnberry Avenue, Glasgow G11 5AQ — MB ChB Leeds 1981; FRCS Ed. 1985; FFARCS 1988. Cons. Anaesth. West. Infirm. Glas.; Hon. Clin. Sen. Lect. Specialty: Anaesth. Prev: Sen. Regist. (Anaesth.) Cardiff; Regist. (Surg.) & SHO (Anaesth.) Roy. Infirm. Edin.

STONE, Peter Gordon Department of Anaesthesia, York Hospital, Wigginton Road, York YO31 8HE Tel: 01904 725399 Fax: 01904 726896 Email: peter.stone@york.nhs.uk — MB BS Lond. 1985 (Christ's Coll., Camb. & Middlx. Hosp. Med. Sch.) MA Camb. 1986, BA 1982; MRCP (UK) 1988; FRCA 1992. Cons. in Anaesth. & Intens. Care Med. York Hosps. NHS Trust. Specialty: Anaesth. Socs: Intens. Care Soc.; BMA; AAGBI. Prev: Sen. Regist. (Anaesth.) Oxf. & S. Bucks.; Fell. Critical Care Med. Harvard Med. Sch. Boston, USA; Regist. & SHO Rotat. (Gen. Med.) Roy. Lond. Hosp.

STONE, Philip Thomas Medway Maritime Hospital, Gillingham ME7 5NY Tel: 01634 830000 Email: ptstone@btinternet.com; 8, Mansell Drive, Borstal, Rochester ME1 3HX Email: ptstone@btinternet.com — MB BS Lond. 1972 (Westm.) AKC; DMRD 1980. Assoc. Spec. In Radiology; Cons. Radiol. To HM Prison Serv. Specialty: Radiol. Prev: Sen. Regist. & Regist. (Radiol.) Lond. Hosp. Whitechapel; Regist. (Radiol.) Qu. Mary's Hosp. Roehampton.

STONE, Richard Malcolm Ellis Forth Floor, Barkat House, 117 - 118 Finshley Road, London NW3 5HT Tel: 020 7472 6060 — BM BCh 1970; MA (Jurisprudence) Oxf. 1963, BM BCh 1970; DObst RCOG 1972; MRCGP 1975. Medico-Legal Practitioner. Prev: Panel Mem. of Stephen Lawrence Inquiry (1997-99); Panel Mem. David Bennett Inquiry (2002-04) into death of black psychiatric Pat.

STONE, Richard Vernon (retired) Boundary Cottage, Boundary Lane, Over Peover, Knutsford WA16 8UJ Tel: 01625 861204 — MB BChir Camb. 1943 (Camb. & Manch.) FRCP Lond. 1972, M 1945; MA Camb. 1943, MD 1950. Prev: Hon. Cons. Phys. Trafford AHA.

STONE, Robert Hellesdon Medical Practice, 343 Reepham Road, Hellesdon, Norwich NR6 5QJ Tel: 01603 486602 Fax: 01603 401389 — MB ChB Sheff. 1977; Dip Health Science UEA 2000.

STONE, Robert Anthony Taunton & Somerset Hospital, Musgrove Park, Taunton TA1 5DA Tel: 01823 333444 Fax: 01823 336877 Email: robert.stone@tauntonsom-tr.swest.nhs.uk — MB BS Lond. 1983 (St. Thos.) BSc Lond. 1980, MB BS 1983; MRCP (UK) 1986; PhD Lond. 1993; FRCP 1999. Cons. Phys. Gen. & Respirat. Med. Taunton & Som. Hosp. Taunton. Specialty: Gen. Med. Prev: Sen. Regist. (Gen. & Respirat. Med.) St. Bart. & Whipps Cross Hosps. Lond.

STONE, Ruth Lloyd 5 Church Road, Whitchurch, Cardiff CF14 2DX — MB BS Lond. 1985; MRCGP 1994.

STONE, Sally Ann Orchard Court Surgery, Orchard Court, Orchard Road, Darlington DL3 6HS Tel: 01325 465285 Fax: 01325 284034 — MB BS Newc. 1987 (Newcastle) MRCP 1990; MRCGP 1993. GP; Primary Care Bd. Mem. Specialty: Gen. Pract.

STONE, Sheldon Paul Department of Medicine for Elderly People, Royal Free Hospital, Pond St., London NW3 2QG — MB BS Lond. 1980; BSc (Hons.) Lond. 1977, MB BS 1980; MRCP (UK) 1984. Lect. (Gen. & Geriat. Med.) Hackney, Homerton, Whipps Cross & St. Bart. Hosps. Lond. Specialty: Care of the Elderly. Socs: Brit. Geriat. Soc. & Med. Disabil. Soc. Prev: Regist. (Neurol.) Char. Cross Hosp. Lond.; Regist. (Med.) Mt. Vernon Hosp. N.wood.

STONE, Timothy David 12 Paxhill La, Twyning, Tewkesbury GL20 6DU — MB ChB Birm. 1997.

STONE, Weland Dinnis (retired) The Manor House, Tollerton, York YO61 1QQ Tel: 01347 838454 Fax: 01347 838454 — (St. Thos.) DM Oxf. 1968, BM BCh 1956; FRCP Lond. 1977, M 1960. Cons. Phys. York Health Dist. Prev: Sen. Regist. Dudley Rd. Hosp. Birm.

STONEBRIDGE, Mr Peter Arno Vascular Diseases Research Unit, Ninewells Hospital & Medical School, Dundee DD1 9SY — MB ChB Manch. 1980; FRCS Ed. 1986; ChM Manch. 1991. Cons. Surg. Ninewells Hosp. Dundee.; Professor of Vascular Surg. Specialty: Surgery, Vascular.

STONEHAM, John Russell Ewhurst Lodge, Windfall Wood Common, Blackdown, Haslemere GU27 3BX Tel: 01428 708066 Fax: 01428 707350 Email: jrs@hive.demon.co.uk; Roundals Farm, Roundals Lane, Hambledon, Godalming GU8 4EA Tel: 01428 682708 Fax: 01428 683575 — (Guy's) MB BS Lond. 1969; MRCS Eng. LRCP Lond. 1969; DA Eng. 1971; FFA RCS Eng. 1973. Cons. Anaesth. S.W. Surrey (Guildford) Health Dist. Specialty: Anaesth.

Prev: Res. (Anaesth.) Vancouver Gen. Hosp.; Sen. Regist. (Anaesth.) Guy's Hosp. Lond.; Regist. (Anaesth.) St. Lukes Hosp. Guildford & Farnham Hosp.

STONEHAM, Mark David, Surg. Lt. RN Retd. Nuffield Department of Anaesthesia, Oxford Radcliff NHS Hospital, Oxford OX3 9DU Tel: 01865 221590 Fax: 01865 220027 — MB BChir Camb. 1987; MA Camb. 1987; FRCA 1994; Dip. Med. Care Catastrophies Soc. Apoth. Lond. 1995. Cons. (Anaesth.) Oxf. Specialty: Anaesth. Prev: Vis. Instruc. Univ. Michigan Med. Center, USA; Anaesth. Regist. Bristol, Exeter.

STONEHAM, Michael David Millbarn Medical Centre, 34 London End, Beaconsfield HP9 2JH Tel: 01494 675303 Fax: 01494 680214; 113 Brands Hill Avenue, High Wycombe HP13 5PX — MB BS Lond. 1971 (Roy. Free) BSc Lond. 1968; MRCS Eng. LRCP Lond. 1971; MRCGP 1976. Research GP Unit of Healthcare Clin. Epidemiol. Oxf. Socs: Chiltern Med. Soc. Prev: Trainee GP High Wycombe VTS; Ho. Surg. New End Hosp. Lond. (Roy. Free); Ho. Phys. Stoke Mandeville Hosp. Aylesbury.

STONEHILL, Edward 138 Harley Street, London W1N 1AH Tel: 020 7935 0554; Hornbeams, The Bishops Avenue, London N2 0BJ Tel: 020 8458 2237 Fax: 020 8455 1996 — MRCS Eng. LRCP Lond. 1961 (Middlx.) MD Lond. 1972, MB BS 1961; DPM Eng. 1965; FRCPsych 1978, M 1971. Emerit. Med. Director, Florence Nightingale Hosps., Lond.; Emerit. Cons. Psychiat. Centr. Middlx. Hosp. Lond. Specialty: Gen. Psychiat. Socs: (Ex-Pres.) Soc. Psychosomatic Res.; Fell. RSM; BMA. Prev: Cons. Psychiat. Centr. Middlx. Hosp. Lond. & Shenley Hosp.; Cons. Psychiat. Imperial Coll. Sc. & Tech. Lond; Research Fell., Hon. Lect. & Hon. Sen. Regist. Acad. Dept. Psychiat. St. Geo. Hosp. Lond.

STONEHOUSE, Walter Patrick Bowman (retired) 82 Mossley Road, Grasscroft, Oldham OL4 4HA Tel: 0145 77 874951 — MRCS Eng. LRCP Lond. 1938 (Camb. & Guy's) DPH Leeds 1950. Prev: Sen. Ho. Surg. & Cas. Off. N. Riding Infirm.

STONELAKE, Angela Virginia Lindisfarne, Gubeon Wood, Tranwell Woods, Morpeth NE61 6BH — BM BS Nottm. 1993; DTM & H Liverp. 1996; MRCPCH Lond. 1999. GP Retainer Leeds 2003; Leeds VTS. Specialty: Paediat. Prev: Medical Officer, Nepal 2000; SHO (Paediat.) City Hosp. Nottm.; SHO (Obst.) City Hosp. Nottm.

STONELAKE, Paul Anthony 85 Belmont Road, Uxbridge UB8 1QU Tel: 01895 255472 — BM BS Nottm. 1993; BMedSci Nottm. 1991. SHO (Anaesth.) Derbysh. Roy. Infirm. NHS Trust. Specialty: Anaesth.

STONELAKE, Mr Paul Simeon Russells Hall Hospital, Department of Surgery, Dudley DY1 2HQ Tel: 01384 456 111 Email: paul.stonelake@dgoh.nhs.uk — BM BS Nottm. 1985 (Nottingham) BMedSci (Hon.) 1983; FRCS Ed. 1990; FRCS Eng. 1990; DM Nottm. 1996. Cons. Surg. Dudley Gp. Hosps.NHS Trust, Dudley, West Midlands; Hon. Sen. Lect. Univ. Birm. Specialty: Gen. Surg. Socs: Brit. Assn. Surgic. Oncol.; ACPGBI; BBG. Prev: Cons. Surg. City Hosp. Birm.; Lect. (Surg.) Univ. Birm. & Hon. Sen. Regist. W. Mild. RHA.

STONEMAN, Margaret Elizabeth Riley (retired) 9 Trapfield Close, Bearsted, Maidstone ME14 4HT Tel: 01622 737039 — (Manch.) MB ChB Manch. 1947; DCH Eng. 1950; MD Manch. 1959; FRCP Lond. 1977, M 1963; FRCPCH 1997. Prev: Cons. Paediat. Maidstone & Medway Health Dists.

STONER, Bryan Anthony (retired) Combe Water, Periton Road, Minehead TA24 8DU Tel: 01643 705330 Email: bstone@btinternet — MB BS Lond. 1967 (Roy. Free) MRCS Eng. LRCP Lond. 1967; MRCGP 1976. Prev: GP Minehead.

STONER, Edward Alexander Princess Alexandra Hospital, Hamstel Road, Harlow Tel: 01279 827821 Email: ed.stoner@btinternet.com — MB ChB Manch. 1990 (Manchester) MRCP (UK) 1993; MD Lond. 2000. Regist. Rotat. (Gastroenteol.) Newham Gen. Hosp. & Lond. Hosp.; Specialist Regist. Roy. Lond. Hosp.; Clin. Developm. Director for Emerg. Care. Specialty: Gen. Med.; Gastroenterol. Socs: Bristish Soc. of Gastroenterol.; Roy. Soc. of Med.; Roy. Coll. of Physicians, Lond. Prev: Res. Fell. Roy. Lond. Hosp.

STONER, Jill Mary 475 Manchester Road, Bury BL9 9SH — MB BS Lond. 1985; DRCOG 1988; MRCGP 1989.

STONER, Katherine Barbara Jarvis Breast Screening Centre, Stoughton Road, Guildford GU1 1LJ Tel: 01483 783200 — MB ChB Cape Town 1982; BSc (Med.) 1978; FFRAD (D) (SA) 1989; FRCR 1993. Cons. Radiol. Jarvis Breast Screening Centre Guildford; Cons. Radiol. Epsom Gen. Hosp. Specialty: Radiol.

STONER, Sarah Jane Dr Fishtal & Partners, 113 Anerley Road, Anerley, London SE20 8AJ Tel: 020 8778 8027 — MB BS Lond. 1994; DRCOG; MRCGP.

STONER, Sarah Jane 5 Watlington Road, Harlow CM17 0DX — MB BS Lond. 1992.

STONES, Nigel Anthony Priorslegh Medical Centre, Civic Centre, Park Lane, Stockport SK12 1GP Tel: 01625 872299 — MB ChB Manch. 1980; MRCP (UK) 1983; DRCOG 1985; MRCGP 1986. Hosp. Pract. (Endocrinol.) Univ. Hosp. S. Manch. Specialty: Dermat.

STONES, Robert William University Department of Obstetrics & Gynaecology, Princess Anne Hospital, Coxford Road, Southampton SO16 5YA Tel: 023 8079 6033 Fax: 023 8078 6933 — MB BS Lond. 1979; DTM & H RCP Lond. 1981; MRCOG 1988; MD Lond. 1994. Sen. Lect. (O & G) Univ. Soton. Specialty: Obst. & Gyn. Prev: Lect. (O & G) Univ. Soton. & St. Mary's Hosp. Med. Sch. Lond.; Research Fell. (Anat.) Univ. Coll. Lond.

STONES, Robin Nicholas, SBStJ Manchester Road Medical Centre, 27-31 Manchester Road, Knutsford WA16 0LY Tel: 01565 633101 Fax: 01565 750135; 20 Rockford Lodge, Knutsford WA16 8AH — MB ChB Manch. 1983 (Manchester) DRCOG 1986; Cert. Family Plann. JCC 1986; MRCGP 1987. GP Princip.; Hosp. Pract. (Dermat.) Trafford Gen. Hosp. Manch. Specialty: Dermat. Socs: BMA. Prev: Trainee GP Lancaster VTS; SHO (ENT) Beaumont Hosp. Lancaster; Ho. Off. (Orthop. & Gen. Surg.) Roy. Preston Hosp.

STONEY, Mr Philip John Furness General Hospital, Dalton Lane, Barrow-in-Furness LA14 4LF Tel: 01229 870870 — MB ChB Glas. 1978; BSc (Hons.) Glas. 1975; FRCS Ed. (Gen.) 1983; FRCS Ed. (ENT) 1986. Cons. Otolaryngol. Furness Gen. Hosp. Barrow-in-Furness. Specialty: Otolaryngol.

STONHAM, Joseph Lincoln County Hospital, Department of Anaesthetics , Greenwell Road, Lincoln LN2 5QY Tel: 01522 512512 — MB BS Lond. 1973; FFA RCS Eng. 1979. Cons. Anaesth., Lincoln Co. Hosp. Specialty: Anaesth. Prev: Regist. (Anaesth.) Soton. Gen. Hosp. Vis. Asst. Prof. Anaesth. Univ.; Texas S. West. Med. Sch. Dallas Texas, U.S.A.; Regist. (Anaesth.) Soton. Gen. Hosp.

STOODLEY, Mr Brian John 21 Lushington Road, Eastbourne BN21 4LG Tel: 01323 410441 Fax: 01323 410978 Email: lushington_clinic@lineone.net; Tuckvar, West St, Alfriston, Polegate BN26 5UX Tel: 01323 870443 — (St. Bart.) MRCS Eng. LRCP Lond. 1962; MB BChir Camb. 1963; MChir Camb. 1973, MA 1963; FRCS Eng. 1967. p/t Hon. Cons. Surg. Dist. Gen. Hosp. Eastbourne & Uckfield Hosp. Specialty: Gen. Surg. Special Interest: Irritable Bowel: Anal Incontinence. Socs: Fell. Roy. Soc. Med.; Fell. Assn. Surgs.; Fell Assn. Coloprctol. Prev: Sen. Regist. (Surg.) St. Bart. Hosp. Lond.; RSO (Surg.) St. Mark's Hosp. Lond.; Const. Surg., Dist. Gen. Hosp., Eastbourne and Uckfield Hosp.

STOODLEY, Katharine Joanna 83 Pickmere Road, Sheffield S10 1GZ — MB ChB Sheff. 1993.

STOODLEY, Neil Gordon North Bristol NHS Trust, Department of Neuroradiology, Frenchay Hospital, Bristol BS16 1LE — BM BCh Oxf. 1985; FRCS Eng. 1989; FRCR 1997. Cons. (Neuroradiol.) Frenchay Hosp. Bristol. Specialty: Radiol. Socs: Brit. Soc. Neuroradiologists; Europ. Soc. Neuroradiol. Prev: Cons. (Neuroradiol.) Univ. Hosp. Wales; Sen. Regist. (Diagnostic Radiol.) John Radcliffe Hosp. Oxf.; Sen. Regist. (Neuroradiol.) Radcliffe Infirm. Oxf.

STOPPARD, Elizabeth Rosemary Royal Berkshire & Battle Hospitals NHS Trust, Reading — MB ChB Manch. 1997; BSc (Hons) St And 1994.

STOPPARD, Miriam 207 Maidenhead Road, Windsor SL4 5HF — MD Newc. 1966; MB BS Durh. 1961; FRCP 1998. Socs: Fell. Roy. Soc. Med.; Assoc. Mem. Heberden Soc. Prev: Managing Dir. Syntex Pharmaceut. Ltd. Maidenhead; Med. Dir. Syntex Pharmaceut. Ltd. Maidenhead; Sen. Regist. (Dermat.) Bristol Roy. Hosp.

STORAH, Peter Kenneth (retired) Yew Tree Cottage, Stafford Avenue, Halifax HX3 0BH Tel: 01422 356513 Fax: 01422 356513 — MB BCh BAO Dub. 1948 (TC Dub.) DObst RCOG 1950; DA RCPSI 1952; FFA RCSI 1962; MD Dub. 1965. Prev: Cons. Anaesth. Roy. Halifax Infirm. & Halifax Gen. Hosp.

STORER, David The General Infirmary, Great George St., Leeds LS1 3EX Tel: 0113 292 3204 Fax: 0113 292 6771 — (Sheff.) MB

ChB Sheff. 1967; DPM Eng. 1970; FRCPsych 1988, M 1972. Cons. Psychiat. Leeds Gen. Infirm.; Sen. Clin. Lect. Univ. Leeds. Specialty: Gen. Psychiat.

STORER, James Ivan 10 Heathland Crescent, Boldmere, Sutton Coldfield B73 5EP — MB ChB Birm. 1970; DRCOG 1972; MRCGP 1975. GP Sutton Coldfield.

STORER, John Richard (retired) Westfield House, Westbrook St, Blewbury, Didcot OX11 9QA Tel: 01235 850651 Email: jgstorer@care4free.net — MB ChB Birm. 1960; DObst RCOG 1963. Prev: Princip., GP.

STORER, Nigel Raymond Bewbush Medical Centre, Bewbush Place, Bewbush, Crawley RH11 8XT Tel: 01293 519420 — BM Soton. 1982; DRCOG 1985; MRCGP 1986.

STORES, Professor Gregory University of Oxford, Park Hospital for Children, Old Road Headington, Oxford OX3 7LQ Tel: 01865 226515 Fax: 01865 762358 Email: gregory.stores@psych.ox.ac.uk; North Gate House, 55 High St, Dorchester-on-Thames, Wallingford OX10 7HN Tel: 01865 34115 — MB ChB Manch. 1967; BA (Hons. Psychol.) Manch. 1960; MRCP (UK) 1970; DPM Eng. 1971; FRCPsych 1981, M 1972; MD 1977; BA (Hons.) (Psychol.) Manch. 1960, MD 1977; FRCP Lond. 1983; MA Oxon 1988. Prof. of Developm. NeuroPsychiat., Univ. of Oxf.; Hon. Cons. Oxf. HA; Fell. of Linacre Coll., Univ. of Oxf. Specialty: Child & Adolesc. Psychiat. Socs: Roy. Coll. Psychiat. (Child Psychiat. Sec.); Brit. Paediat. Neurol. Assn.; Fell.Roy.Coll.Phys. Prev: Cons. Neuropsychiat. & EEG Pk. Hosp. Childr. Oxf.; Lect. (Developm. Med.) Univ. Dept. Psychiat. & Pk. Hosp. Childr. Oxf.; Clin.Reader.Child & Adult Psychiat.Univ.Oxf.

STORES, Olga Patricia Rahma 445 Streetsbrook Road, Solihull B91 1QZ — MB ChB Manch. 1967. Prev: Research Fell. Dept. Regius Prof. Med. Radcliffe Infirm. Oxf.; Clin. Asst. Oxf. Univ. Dept. Psychiat. Warneford Hosp. Oxf.; Regist. (Psychiat.) Bootham Pk. & Naburn Hosps. York.

STOREY, Alan Brett Valentine House, 1079 Rochdale Road, Manchester M9 8AJ Tel: 01254 771315; 5 Spinningfield Way, Heywood OL10 2LF — MB BS Lond. 1985; DRCOG 1989. Prev: Trainee GP Manch.; SHO (A & E & Gen. Med.) Goldcoast Hosp., Austral.; SHO (Psychiat.) Fairfield Gen. Hosp. Bury.

STOREY, Dawn Edinburgh Cancer Centre, Crewe Road, Edinburgh EH4 Tel: 0131 537 1000 — BM BS Nottm. 1995; BMedSci Nottm. 1993; DRCOG 1997. SpR Med. Oncol. Ed. Specialty: Gen. Pract. Prev: SHO (Med.) Stirling Roy. Infirm.; SHO (Palliat. Med.) Marie Curie Centre Edin.; SHO (Clin. Oncol.) West. Gen. Hosp. Edin.

STOREY, Elizabeth Clare — MB ChB Leic. 1998.

STOREY, Geoffrey Oldroyd (retired) Pine Grove, Kentsford Rd, Grange-over-Sands LA11 7BB Tel: 015395 34483 — MD Camb. 1956 (Camb. & Lond. Hosp.) MB BChir 1942; FRCP Lond. 1971, M 1948; DPhysMed Eng. 1953. Prev: Cons. Rheumat. Hackney & Roy. Lond. Hosp.

STOREY, Imogen Clare — MB ChB Birm. 1998.

STOREY, John Loftus 21 Michel Grove, East Preston, Littlehampton BN16 2SX Tel: 01903 783687 — MB BS Lond. 1957; MRCS Eng. LRCP Lond. 1957; LDS RCS Eng. 1964; BDS Lond. 1964.

STOREY, Mark Edward The Surgery, Kirk Road, Houston, Johnstone PA6 7AR Tel: 01505 613240 Email: mark.storey@nhs.net — MB ChB Glas. 1993 (Glasgow) BSc (Hons) Physiol. 1990. Specialty: Gen. Pract.

STOREY, Neil David The Coach House, 3 Kennedy Drive, Helensburgh G84 9AP — MB ChB Glas. 1991.

STOREY, Peter Brett (retired) 2 Brunswick Square, Penrith CA11 7LL Tel: 01768 865006 — MB BS Lond. 1953 (St. Mary's) FRCP Lond. 1973, M 1959; DPM Lond. 1963; MD Lond. 1970; FRCPsych 1975, M 1971. Hon. Cons. Psychiat. St. Geo. & Springfield Hosps. Lond. Prev: Med. Administr. Springfield Hosp. Lond.

STOREY, Robert George Nixon 20 Ballyclander Road, Downpatrick BT30 7DZ — MB BCh BAO Belf. 1970; FRCOG 1991. Cons. O & G Downe Hosp. Downpatrick Matern. Hosp. & Belf. City Hosp. Specialty: Obst. & Gyn. Socs: Ulster Obst. & Gyn. Soc.; BSCCP. Prev: Sen. Regist. (O & G) Belf. City Hosp.; Regist. (O & G) Roy. Matern. Hosp. Belf.; Lect. (O & G) Univ. Nairobi, Kenya.

STOREY, Susan Mary Islington Child & Family Consultation Service (CFCS), Northern Health Centre, 594 Holloway Road, London N7 6LB Tel: 0207 445 8150 Email: sue.story@nhs.net — MB ChB Bristol 1988; BSc Bristol 1985; MRCPsych 1993. Cons. In Child & Adolesc. Psychiat. Islington CFCS, Lond. Specialty: Child & Adolesc. Psychiat. Prev: Sen. Regist. (Child & Adolesc. Psychiat.) Tavistock Clinic Lond.

STOREY, Victor Charles Marks Gate Health Centre, Lawn Farm Grove, Chadwell Heath, Romford RM6 5LL Tel: 020 8590 7066; 130 Harley Street, London W1N 1AH — MB BS Lond. 1953 (St. Bart.) LMSSA Lond. 1952.

STORK, Ann Frances 52 The Sanctuary, Cardiff CF5 4RX — BM BS Nottm. 1990.

STORK, Sheila — DAvMed. Fac. Occupat Med.; MB BS Lond. 1985; MFOM for Occupational Medicine 1998; Accredit Specialist Aviat & Occupat Med 1998. Chief Med. Off., Nat. Air Traffic Serv.s; Med. Examr. CAA; Med. Examr. JOA; Med. Examr. FOA. Specialty: Occupat. Health; Aviat. Med.; Gen. Pract. Socs: Fac. Occupat. Med.; Roy. Agronautical Soc. Prev: Head of Aeromed. Centre and Ocupational Health Serv.s for the Civil Aviat. Auth.; Head of Aeromed. Sect. CAA.

STORM, Marion Croft House, Maynestone Road, Chinley, High Peak SK23 6AH — MB ChB Ed. 1983. Socs: Roy. Coll. Psychiat.

STORMONT, Fiona Claire Flat 5, 27 Warrington Crescent, London W9 1ED — MB BS Lond. 1989.

STORR, Bernard Stanley Harold (retired) Copse End, Chart Road, Chart Sutton, Maidstone ME17 3RB Tel: 01622 843881 — MRCS Eng. LRCP Lond. 1944 (Westm.) BA Camb. 1941; DMRD Eng. 1949. Prev: Cons. Radiol. Brighton & Mid-Downs HAs.

STORR, Emma Faithfull Harehills Corner Surgery, 209 Roundhay Road, Leeds LS8 4HQ — MB BS Lond. 1983 (Guy's Hosp. Lond.) BA (Social Anthropol.) Sussex 1976; DRCOG 1986; MRCGP 1987; PGCLTHE Leeds 1999. Sen. Teachg. Fell. in Primary Care; Salaried GP. Special Interest: Med. Humanities. Prev: GP Tower Hamlets.

STORR, John Nicholas Paul Cumberland Infirmary, Department of Paediatrics, Carlisle CA2 7HY Tel: 01228 523444 — MD Cape Town 1989; MB ChB 1976; FRCP 1997; FRCPCH 1997. Cons. Paediat. Carlisle. N. Cumbria Acute NHS Trust. Specialty: Paediat. Prev: Sen. Regist. (Paediat.) Selly Oak Hosp. Birm.

STORR, Teresa Mary Swallows Waite, Seaville, Silloth, Carlisle CA7 4PT Tel: 016973 61156 — MB BS Newc. 1982; DRCOG 1984; MRCGP 1986. Clin. Asst. (Haemat. & Oncol.) Cumbld. Infirm. Carlisle. Specialty: Oncol.; Radiother.

STORRAR, David Allan Helsby Street Medical Centre, 2 Helsby Street, Warrington WA1 3AW Tel: 01925 637304 Fax: 01925 570430; 4 Marlborough Crescent, Grappenhall, Warrington WA4 2EE — MB ChB Manch. 1984; BSc Hons. (Biochem.) St. And. 1977. Princip. GP Warrington.

STORRIE, Marion Pettigrew Newbyres Medical Group, Gorebridge Health Centre, 15 Hunterfield Road, Gorebridge EH23 4TP Tel: 01875 820405 Fax: 01875 820269 — MB ChB Edinburgh 1977; MB ChB Edin 1977. GP Edin.

STORRING, Roderick Alexander 42 Felstead Road, Wanstead, London E11 2QJ Tel: 020 8989 5853 Fax: 020 8989 1942 — MB BS Lond. 1966; FRCP Lond. 1986. p/t Cons. Phys. (Thoracic & Gen. Med.) King Geo. Hosp. Ilford & Roding Hosp. Ilford. Specialty: Gen. Med. Special Interest: Asbestos related Dis. & other Indust. chest diseases.

STORROW, Kim Johanna Peverell Park Surgery, 162 Outlands Road, Peverell, Plymouth PL2 3PR Tel: 01752 791438 Fax: 01752 783623 — MB BCh Wales 1982; DCH RCP Lond. 1987. GP Peverell Pk. Surg. Plymouth. Socs: Local Med. Comm. Represent. Prev: GP Plympton Health Centre Plymouth.

STORRS, Charles Nicholas (retired) Warwick Hospital, Lakin Road, Warwick CV34 5BW Tel: 01926 495321; Brook Farm, Hanley Swan, Worcester WR8 0EQ Tel: 01684 310796 — MB BChir Camb. 1964 (St. Thos.) MB Camb. 1964, BChir 1963; DCH Eng. 1967; FRCP Lond. 1985, M 1969. Cons. Paediat. Warwick Hosp. Prev: Sen. Regist. (Paediat.) Churchill Hosp. Oxf.

STORRS, Mr Thomas John Chequers, Nackington Park, Nackington Road, Canterbury CT4 7AX Tel: 01227 454441 Fax: 01277 454150 Email: storrs@netlineuk.net — (Guy's) FDS RCS Eng. 1972, L 1966; BDS (Hons.) 1966; MB BS Lond. 1970; MRCS Eng. LRCP Lond. 1970. Cons. Maxillofacial Surg. Kent & Canterbury Hosp. Specialty: Oral & Maxillofacial Surg. Socs: Fell. Brit. Assn. Maxillofacial Surg.; BMA; Centr. Cons. & Specialists Comm.

STORY, Clive Alwyn Bentham Medical Practice, Grasmere Drive, High Bentham, Lancaster LA2 7JP Tel: 01524 261202 Fax: 01524 262905 — MB BS Newc. 1966.
STORY, Doris (retired) 14 Ferndene Court, Moor Road S., Newcastle upon Tyne NE3 1NN — MB BS Durh. 1953; DPH Durh. 1958; MFCM 1972. Prev: SCM (Child Health) N. Tyneside HA.
STORY, Peter 7 Dene Road, Northwood HA6 2AE Tel: 01923 823928 — MRCS Eng. LRCP Lond. 1942 (St. Bart.) MD Lond. 1950, MB BS 1947; FRCPath 1969, M 1963. Consg. Haemat. St. Bart. Hosp. Lond. Specialty: Haematology. Prev: Lt.-Col. RAMC; Brit. Postgrad. Med. Federat. Trav. Fell. (Haematol.) Washington Univ.St. Louis, USA; Cons. Haemat. Inst. Orthop. Roy. Nat. Orthop. Hosps. Stanmore.
STORY, Peter Sean The Medical Centre, Gun Lane, Strood, Rochester ME2 4UW Tel: 01634 290655 — MB BS Newc. 1971; DObst RCOG 1975; MRCGP 1980.
STORY, Thomas William 29 Parker Street, Barrow-in-Furness LA14 5RN — MB BS Lond. 1980.
STORY, Timothy Simon Chard Road Surgery, Chard Road, St. Budeaux, Plymouth PL12 5AL Tel: 01752 363111 — MB BS Lond. 1992 (St. Geo. Hosp. Lond.) DRCOG; DCH RCP Lond.; BSc (Clin. Pharmacol.) Lond. 1989; MRCGP 2002. GP Regist. Portview Surg. Higher Portview Saltash Cornw. Specialty: Paediat. Prev: SHO (O & G) Derriford Hosp. Plymouth; SHO (Paediat.) St. Richards Hosp. Chichester; SHO (A & E) St. Geo. Hosp. NHS Trust Lond.
STOSSEL, Mr Clifford Alain Flagstones, Millbank, Headcorn, Ashford TN27 8JG Tel: 01622 890702 Fax: 01622 891636 — MB BS Lond. 1961 (St. Mary's) MRCS Eng. LRCP Lond. 1962; FRCS Ed. 1968; FRCS Eng. 1970. Cons. Orthop. Surg. Maidstone Health Dist. Specialty: Orthop. Socs: Fell. BOA; BMA. Prev: Sen. Regist. (Orthop.) St. Mary's & Roy. Nat. Orthop. Hosps. Lond.; Regist. (Surg.) W. Herts. Hosp. Hemel Hempstead.
STOTESBURY, Stanley Neville (retired) 40 Malmains Drive, Frenchay, Bristol BS16 1PJ Tel: 0117 956 7984 — (Bristol & Westm.) MRCS Eng. LRCP Lond. 1948. Prev: Ho. Surg. (Orthop.) Westm. Hosp.
STOTHARD, Mr John Consultant Hand & Orthopaedic Surg., James Cook University Hospital, Marton Road, Middlesbrough TS4 3BW Tel: 01642 854214 Fax: 01642 854375 — MB ChB Ed. 1971; FRCS Ed. 1976; MD Ed. 1980; FRCS Ed. (Orth.) 1981. Cons. Hand Surg. S. Tees Acute Unit NHS Trust; Vis. Prof. Sch. Health Univ. Teesside; Hon. Clin. Lect. Fac. of Med. Univ. Newc. Specialty: Trauma & Orthop. Surg. Prev: Cons. Orthop. Surg. N. Tees Health NHS Trust; Sen. Regist. (Orthop. Surg.) N. RHA; Research Assoc. MRC Decompression Sickness Research Team.
STOTHER, Mr Ian George Glasgow Nuffield Hospital, Beaconsfield Road, Glasgow G12 0PJ Tel: 0141 334 9441 Fax: 0141 339 1352; 13 Moncrieff Avenue, Lenzie, Glasgow G66 4NL Tel: 0141 776 5330 — MB BChir Camb. 1970 (St. Geo.) MA Camb. 1970; FRCS Ed. 1974; FRCS Glas. 1981. Cons. Orthopaedic Surg. & Clin. Director Trauma & Orthapaedics N. Glas. Univ. Hosp. NHS Trust; Cons. Orthop. Surg. Glas. Roy. Infirm.; Hon. Sen. Clin. Lect. Univ. Glas. Specialty: Orthop.
STOTHERS, James 14 Darvel Crescent, Ralston, Paisley PA1 3EF — MB ChB Glas. 1956.
STOTT, Caroline Jayne Emperor's Gate Centre for Health, First Floor, 49 Emperors Gate, London SW7 4HJ Tel: 020 8237 5333 Fax: 020 8237 5344; 28 Stamford Brook Avenue, Stamford Brook, London W6 0YD Tel: 020 8563 2026 — BM BS Nottm. 1989 (Univ. Nottm.) BMedSci Nottm. 1987; DRCOG 1993; MRCGP 1994. GP. Socs: Brit. Med. Acupunc. Soc. Prev: Trainee GP/SHO (Psychiat.) Lond.
STOTT, Mrs Catherine Mary Ware Road Surgery, 77 Ware Road, Hertford SG13 7EE Tel: 01992 587961; 20 Harwood Close, Tewin, Welwyn AL6 0LF — MB BCh BAO NUI 1965 (Cork) Clin. Asst. (Paediat.) Hertford Co. Hosp. Prev: Intern Regional Gen. Hosp. Limerick; Clin. Asst. (Psychiat.) & SHO (Paediat.) Qu. Eliz. II Hosp. Welwyn Gdn. City.
STOTT, Christopher Simon — MB BS Lond. 1982 (Charing Cross) DRCOG 1984; DMJ 2001. GP Princip.; Princip. Forens. Med. Examr. (Police Surg.) Lond. Metrop. Police. Specialty: Gen. Pract. Socs: Assn. Police Surg.; BMA.
STOTT, David Brian (retired) Thatched Cottage, Kerry Lane, Eccleshall, Stafford ST21 6EJ Tel: 01785 850271 — (Manch.) MB ChB Manch. 1947; MRCS Eng. LRCP Lond. 1947. Prev: Ho. Surg. Manch. Roy. Infirm.
STOTT, Professor David James Academic Section of Geriatric Medicine, Royal Infirmary, Glasgow G4 0SF Tel: 0141 211 4976 Fax: 0141 211 4944 — MB ChB Glas. 1981; MRCP (UK) 1984; MD Glas. 1988; FRCP Glas. 1994; FRCP (Ed.) 1997. David Cargill Prof. Geriat. Med. Univ. Glas. (1994-); Hon. Cons. Geriat. Med. Glas. Roy. Infirm. (1994-). Specialty: Care of the Elderly. Socs: Med. Res. Soc. & Brit. Geriat. Soc.; Brit. Assn. of Stroke Physicians. Prev: Sen. Lect. & Hon. Cons. Geriat. Med. Univ. Glas.; Sen. Regist. (Geriat. & Gen. Med.) Gtr. Glas. HB.
STOTT, David Rowland Patel and Partners, Broom Lane Medical Centre, 70 Broom Lane, Rotherham S60 3EW Tel: 01709 364470 Fax: 01709 820009; Kimberworth Park Medical Centre, Laydon Road, Rotherham SG1 3QH — MB ChB Sheff. 1980; BSc. Sheff. 1976, MB ChB 1980. Hosp. Pract. (A & E) N. Gen. Hosp., Sheff.
STOTT, Denise Gaye Department of Anaesthetics, Stoke Mandeville Hospital, Mandeville Road, Aylesbury HP21 8AL Tel: 01296 315262; Keepers Cottage, 5 Burts Lane, Long Crendon, Aylesbury HP18 9AJ — MB ChB Sheff. 1982 (Univ. Sheff. Med. Sch.) FRCA 1988. Cons. Anaesth. Stoke Mandeville Hosp. Specialty: Anaesth. Prev: Cons. Anaesth. Withington Hosp. Manch.; Regist. (Anaesth.) Withington Hosp. Manch. & Stepping Hill Hosp. Stockport; Sen. Regist. (Anaesth.) NW RHA.
STOTT, Donald Verney (retired) 35 Tavistock Road, Crownhill, Plymouth PL5 3AF — MB BS Lond. 1940 (King's Coll. Hosp.) MRCS Eng. LRCP Lond. 1940. Prev: GP Plymouth 1951-82.
STOTT, Ian Mark — BM BS Nottm. 1998. Regist. HO.(Gen Med.) Qu Med Centre. Nottm. Specialty: Gen. Med. Prev: Pre Regist. HO. (Gen Surg & Urol.) City Hosp. Nottm.
STOTT, Janet Elizabeth Stockton Heath Medical Centre, The Forge, London Road, Warrington WA4 6HJ Tel: 01925 604427 Fax: 01925 210501; 15 Edenbridge Gardens, Appleton, Warrington WA4 5FH — BM BS Nottm. 1983; BMedSci Nottm. 1981. Prev: SHO (Med., O & G & Paediat.) Warrington Dist. Gen. Hosp.
STOTT, Jenefer Anne Vaughan Parklands Surgery, 4 Parklands Road, Chichester PO19 3DT Tel: 01243 786827; 25 Lyndhurst Road, Chichester PO19 2LE Tel: 01243 784157 — MB BS Lond. 1989; DRCOG 1993. Prev: SHO (Geriat.) St. Richard's Hosp. Chichester; SHO (Psychiat.) Southlands Hosp. Worthing.
STOTT, John Richard Rollin Well Lane House, Well Lane, Lower Froyle, Alton GU34 4LP Tel: 01420 23783 — MRCS Eng. LRCP Lond. 1963 (Middlx.) MB Camb. 1964, BChir 1963; MA Camb. 1964; DCH Eng. 1965; MRCP Lond. 1969; DIC 1974; DAvMed FOM RCP Lond. 1985. Princip. Med.Off.DERA Centre for Human Sci.s. Specialty: Aviat. Med. Socs: Aerospace Med. Assn. & Biol. Engin. Soc. Prev: Sen. Regist. (Clin. Measurem.) Westm. Hosp. Lond.; Ho. Phys. & Cas. Med. Off. Middlx. Hosp. Lond.
STOTT, Mr Mark Anthony Department of Urology, Royal Devon & Exeter Hospital (Wonford), Barrack Road, Exeter EX2 5DW — MD Bristol 1990; MB ChB 1980; FRCS Eng. 1985. Cons. Urol. Exeter HA. Specialty: Urol. Prev: Sen. Regist. (Urol.) E. Anglian RHA; Research Regist. (Urol.) Ham Green Hosp. Bristol.
STOTT, Professor Nigel Clement Halley, CBE Coastguard Cottage, Oxwhich, Swansea SA3 1LS Tel: 01792 390 0746 Fax: 02920 626608 Email: stottoxwich@aol.com — MB ChB Ed. 1966 (Univ. Ed.) BSc (Hons.) Ed. 1964; FRCP Ed. 1980 M 1969; FRCGP 1987, M 1979; T(GP) 1991; FMedSci 1998. Emerit. Prof. of Gen. Pract., Univ. of Wales, Coll. of Med. Specialty: Gen. Pract. Socs: Acad. of Med. Sci.; BMA; Cardiff Med. Soc. (Mem.).
STOTT, Peter Charles The Surgery, 1 Troy Close, Tadworth Farm, Tadworth KT20 5JE Tel: 01737 362327 Fax: 01737 373469 — MB Camb. 1975; BChir 1974; Cert JCC Lond. 1976; DRCOG 1976; DCH Eng. 1977; FRCGP 1989, M 1979.
STOTT, Richard Anthony Philip Old Cottage Hospital Surgery, Alexandra Road, Epsom KT17 4BL Tel: 01372 724434 Fax: 01372 748171; 52 Manor Green Road, Epsom KT19 8RN Tel: 01372 728692 — MB BS Lond. 1972 (St. Thos. Hosp. Lond.) DCH Eng. 1975; MRCP (UK) 1979; FRCP Ed. 1992.
STOTT, Robin Bradley 15 Egerton Drive, Greenwich, London SE10 8JS Tel: 020 8692 4667 Email: stott@dircon.co.uk — MB BChir Camb. 1967; MA Camb. 1967; MRCS Eng. LRCP Lond. 1967; FRCP Lond. 1981, M 1969. Cons. Phys. Lewisham Trust.; Sub-Dean, Guys, Kings & St Thos. Sch. of Med. & Dent. Specialty: Gen. Med.

Prev: Cons. Phys. Lewisham Hosp. Lond.; Sen. Lect. (Med.) Univ. Zimbabwe.

STOTT, Shiona Margaret Department of Anaesthetics, Stobhill Hospital, Balornock Road, Glasgow G21 3UW Tel: 0141 201 3005; 15 South Erskine Park, Bearsden, Glasgow G61 4NA Tel: 0141 942 7341 — MB ChB Glas. 1984; FRCA 1989. Cons. Anaesth. Stobhill Hosp. Glas. Specialty: Anaesth. Prev: Sen. Regist. (Anaesth.) West. Infirm. Glas.; Regist. (Anaesth.) Roy. Infirm. Glas.

STOTT, Stephen Alexander Aberdeen Royal Infirmary, Department of Anaesthetics, Foresterhill, Aberdeen AB25 2ZN — MB ChB Bristol 1985; FRCA.

STOTT, William Bethune (retired) 43 Kingsway Court, Hove BN3 2LQ — LRCP LRCS Ed. 1921 (Univs. Aberd., Ed. & Camb.) LRCP LRCS Ed. LRFPS Glas. 1921; DPH Camb. 1925. Prev: MOH Cuckfield RD & Cuckfield & Burgess Hill UDs.

STOTTER, Miss Anne Department of General Surgery, Glenfield General Hospital, Groby Road, Leicester LE3 9QP Tel: 0116 287 1471 Fax: 0116 258 3950 — MB BS Lond. 1978; MA Camb. 1974, PhD 1975; FRCS Eng. 1982; FRCS Ed. 1982. Cons. Gen. Surg. Glenfield Gen. Hosp. Leics. Specialty: Gen. Surg. Special Interest: Breast Cancer. Socs: Brit. Assn. of Surgic. Oncol.; Assn. of Surgeons of Eng. Prev: Sen. Lect. in Gen. Surg., St Marys' Hosp., Praed St., Lond.

STOUT, Alan William 22a Bridge Road, Helens Bay, Bangor BT19 1TH — MB BCh BAO Belf. 1995.

STOUT, David Brian — MB ChB Leeds 1997.

STOUT, Edward Laverick (retired) 49 Hesligton Lane, York YO10 4HN Tel: 01904 623050 — BA Camb. 1948; MRCS Eng. LRCP Lond. 1953. Prev: GP York.

STOUT, Ian Hugh Department of Psychiatry of Later Life, Meadowbrook, Stott Lane, Salford M6 8DD Tel: 0161 772 3766 Fax: 0161 772 3772; 25 Warwick Drive, Hale, Altrincham WA15 9EA — MB ChB Manch. 1974; MB ChB (Hons.) Manch. 1974; FRCPsych 1995, M 1978; MSc (Psychiat.) Manch. 1981. Cons. Psychogeriat. Ment. Health Servs. Salford NHS Trust; Hon. Clin. Lect. (Psychiat.) Manch. Univ. Specialty: Geriat. Psychiat. Prev: Sen. Regist. (Psychiat.) Tameside Gen. Hosp.; Clin. Research Fell. (Psychiat.) Univ. Manch.; Sen. Regist. (Psychiat.) Univ. Hosp. S. Manch.

STOUT, John Clark Peterhead Group Practice, The Health Centre, Peterhead AB42 2XA Tel: 01774 474841 Fax: 01774 474848; Kirkton House, Markethill, Longside, Peterhead AB42 4TD — MB ChB Dundee 1983; DRCOG 1985; MRCGP 1987.

STOUT, Robert James (retired) 113 Imperial Road, Gillingham ME7 5PH Tel: 01634 307793 — MB BS Lond. 1943 (Lond. Hosp.) MRCS Eng. LRCP Lond. 1941; DA Eng. 1942; FFA RCS Eng. 1954. Prev: Cons. Anaesth. Medway Health Dist.

STOUT, Professor Robert William Department of Geriatric Medicine, Whitla Medical Building, 97 Lisburn Road, Belfast BT9 7BL Tel: 01232 335777 Fax: 01232 325839 Email: r.stout@qub.ac.uk; 3 Larch Hill Drive, Craigavad, Holywood BT18 0JS Tel: 01232 422253 Fax: 01232 428478 — MB BCh BAO Belf. 1965; FRCP Lond. 1979, M 1967; DSc Belf. 1989, MD Belf. 1970; FRCP Ed. 1988; FRCPI 1989; FRCPS Glas. 1995; FMedSci Belf 1998. p/t Director Research & Developm. North. Irel. Health & Social Servs.; Cons. Phys. Belf. City Hosp. Specialty: Care of the Elderly. Socs: Pres. Ulster Med. Soc.; Assn. Phys; Pres. Brit. Geriat. Soc. Prev: Dean Fac. Med. & Health Sci. Qu. Univ. Belf.; Prof. Geriat. Med. Qu. Univ. Belf.; Eli Lilly MRC Trav. Fell. & Vis. Scientist Dept. Med. Univ. Washington, Seattle, USA.

STOUT, Ronald Christie Hospital NHS Trust, Withington, Manchester M20 4BX Tel: 0161 446 3000 Fax: 0161 446 3352; 9 Fairfax Avenue, Didsbury, Manchester M20 6AJ Tel: 0161 434 6596 — MB ChB Liverp. 1973 (Liverpool) FRCR 1980; FRCP 1996. Cons. Radiother. & Oncol. Christie Hosp. & Holt Radium Inst.; Hon. Lect. Univ. Manch. Inst. Cancer Studies. Specialty: Oncol.; Radiother. Socs: BMA; Fell. Roy. coll. Phys. Eng.; Fell. Roy. Coll. Radiol.

STOUT, Thomas Vincent Caerphilly District Miners' Hospital, St. Martin's Road, Caerphilly CF83 2WW Tel: 029 2085 1811 — MB BS Lond. 1963 (Univ. Coll. Hosp.) DCMT Lond. 1966; MRCOG 1971, DObst 1967. Cons., Caerphilly Miners Hosp. Specialty: Genitourinary Medicine. Prev: Sen. Regist. (O & G) St. David's Hosp. Bangor; Regist. (O & G) Torbay Hosp. Torquay; Regist. (O & G) North. Gen. Hosp. Sheff.

STOVES, Catherine 16 Hillston Close, Naisberry Park, Hartlepool TS26 0PE Tel: 01429 260755 — MB BS Newc. 1968; DA Eng. 1970.

STOVES, John 29 Rutland Road, Wallsend NE28 8QL — MB ChB Ed. 1991.

STOVES, Robert The Health Centre, Alfred Squire Road, Wednesfield, Wolverhampton WV11 1XU Tel: 01902 575033 Fax: 01902 575013 — BM BS Nottm. 1991. Trainee GP/SHO (Obst.) Sandwell Dist. Gen. Hosp. Socs: MDU.

STOVIN, Oliver John The Surgery, Glpathorne Road, Oundle, Peterborough PE8 4JA Tel: 01832 273408; 135 Glapthorne Road, Oundle, Peterborough PE8 5BA Tel: 01832 274493 — MB BS Lond. 1983; BA Oxf. 1980; DRCOG 1986; MRCGP 1988. Prev: Trainee GP Camb. VTS; SHO (Med.) Jas. Paget Hosp. Gt. Yarmouth.

STOVIN, Patricia Helen Kidgate Surgery, 32 Queen Street, Louth LN11 9AU Tel: 01507 602421 Fax: 01507 601700; Grove House, 54 Westgate, Louth LN11 9YD Tel: 01507 602421 — MB BS Lond. 1980 (St. Mary's Hosp. Lond.) DRCOG 1982. Specialty: Gen. Pract.

STOVIN, Peter George Ingle (retired) 307 Hills Road, Cambridge CB2 2QS — MB BChir Camb. 1950 (Lond. Hosp.) MRCP Lond. 1952; FRCPath 1973, M 1963. Prev: Cons. Pathol. Papworth & Hinchingbrooke Hosps.

STOVIN, Sybille Elizabeth (retired) 307 Hills Road, Cambridge CB2 2QS — MB BS Lond. 1950; MRCS Eng. LRCP Lond. 1950. Prev: SCMO (Family Plann.) Camb. HA.

STOW, Pamela Jean (retired) 6 Harrow Road, Knockholt, Sevenoaks TN14 7JT — MB BS Lond. 1957 (Univ. Coll. Hosp.) DA Eng. 1959; FFA RCS Eng. 1967. Cons. Anaesth. Croydon & Warlingham Pk. Hosp. Gp. Prev: Ho. Phys. Univ. Coll. Hosp.

STOW, Rachael Elizabeth 32 Moorcroft Dr, Sheffield S10 4GW — MB ChB Dundee 1997.

STOW, Sophia Luise Low Farm, Wilden Road, Colmworth, Bedford MK44 2NN — MB BS Lond. 1993.

STOWE, Helen Elizabeth Rose Cottage,, 4, Alexandra Terrace,, Kelsall, Tarporley CW6 0RW Tel: 01829 751396 — MB BS Newc. 1993 (Newc. u. Tyne) DRCOG 1997; Dip Fam. Plan. 2001. Specialty: Gen. Pract.; Family Planning. Socs: BMA. Prev: SHO QEQM Hosp. Margate, c/o the Elderly.

STOWE, Roy (retired) 1 Pilgrims Way, Canterbury CT1 1XS Tel: 01227 471441 — MB BS Lond. 1953 (Univ. Coll. Hosp.) JP. Prev: Ho. Phys. Univ. Coll. Hosp.

STOWELL, Gillian Margaret Ide Lane Surgery, Ide Lane, Alphinton, Exeter EX2 8UP Tel: 01392 439868 Fax: 01392 493513; 14 Marlborough Road, Exeter EX2 4TJ Tel: 01392 437364 — MB ChB Bristol 1976 (Univ. Bristol) MRCGP 1981.

STOWER, Mr Michael John York District Hospital, Wigginton Road, York YO31 8HE Tel: 01904 725972 Fax: 01904 726886 Email: michael.j.stower@york.nhs.uk; Bramble End, Derwent Lane, Dunnington, York YO19 5RR Tel: 01904 489312 Email: mjstower@aol.com — MB ChB Bristol 1975; FRCS Eng. 1979; DM Nottm. 1983. Cons. Urol. York. Specialty: Urol.; Oncol. Special Interest: Prostate and Bladder Cancer. Socs: Brit. Assn. Urol. Surg.; BMA; Brit. Prostate Gp. Prev: Sen. Regist. S W. RHA; Regist. (Surg.) Nottm. & Derby.

STOYLE, Mr Thomas Frederick 15 Roundhill Close, Syston, Leicester LE7 1PP Tel: 0116 260 2729 Fax: 0116 246 1076; Broadmead, 12 Southernhay Road, Leicester LE2 3TJ Tel: 0116 270 8654 — MB BS Lond. 1953 (St. Geo.) LMSSA Lond. 1953; DObst RCOG 1955; FRCS Eng. 1961. Emerit. Cons. Orthop. Surg. Leicester Roy. Infirm. & Glenfield Gen. Hosp. Leicester. Specialty: Orthop. Socs: Fell. BOA; Brit. HIV Soc.; Brit. Soc. Childr. Orthop. Surg. Prev: Sen. Regist. (Orthop.) Sheff. Roy. Infirm.; Regist. (Orthop.) St. Bart. Hosp. Lond.; Ho. Off. (Orthop.) & Cas. St. Geo. Hosp. Lond.

STRACEY, Doreen Mary Josephine (retired) 15 Mortlake House, 512 High Road, Chiswick, London W4 5RH Tel: 020 8995 2880 — MB BS Punjab 1930; MRCOG 1949. Prev: GP Lond.

STRACEY, Pamela Mary (retired) 34 The Fairway, Braunton EX33 1DZ Tel: 01271 816170 — MB BS Lond. 1958 (Roy. Free) MRCS Eng. LRCP Lond. 1958; DA Eng. 1960; FFA RCS Eng. 1963; T(Anaesth) 1991. Cons. Anaesth. Eliz. G. Anderson Hosp. Lond. & Moorfields Eye Hosp. Lond. Prev: Specialist Anaesth. Univ. NSW, Austral.

STRACH, Mr Eric Hugo (retired) 7 Tower Way, Woolton Park, Liverpool L25 6EB Tel: 0151 428 3806 Email:

eric.strach@btopenworld.com — MD Prague 1938; FRCS Eng. 1951; MChOrth. Liverp. 1952. Prev: Cons. Orthop. Surg. St. Helens Hosp. & Whiston Hosp.

STRACHAN, Alasdair Neil 194 Queensway, Cheadle SK8 3HH — MB ChB Sheff. 1989; DRCOG 1991; DTM & H Lond. 1993; MRCGP 1993. Specialty: Anaesth.

STRACHAN, Alexander Gregory 23 Cherry Orchard Road, Lisvane, Cardiff CF14 0UD Tel: 0114 763072 — MB ChB Sheff. 1996 (Sheffield) Specialty: Gen. Pract. Socs: BMA; MDU.

STRACHAN, Alexandra Mary Jane 28 Chalcot Square, London NW1 8YA — MB BS Lond. 1994.

STRACHAN, Bruce Taylor 6 Glendale Road, Peterhead AB42 1AE — MB ChB Aberd. 1993.

STRACHAN, Charles Douglas Scott Low Moor House, 167 Netherlands Avenue, Low Moor, Bradford BD12 0TB Tel: 01274 606818 Fax: 01274 691684; Lime House, Simm Carr Lane, Shibden, Halifax HX3 7UL — MB ChB Aberd. 1986; DCH RCP Lond. 1990; MRCGP 1994. GP Bradford. Specialty: Gen. Pract.

STRACHAN, Mr Colin John Logan (cons. rooms), Sussex Nuffield Hospital, Warren Road, Woodingdean, Brighton BN2 6DX Tel: 01273 627 064 Fax: 01273 627040 Email: penny.thomas@lineone.net; Braidlea, Beacon Road, Ditchling, Hassocks BN6 8UL Tel: 01273 842984 Fax: 01273 846864 Email: colin.strachan@btinternet.com — MB ChB Glas. 1966; FRCS Ed. 1970; MD Birm. 1979; FRCS Glas. 1987; FRCS Eng. 1996. Cons. Vasc. & Gen. Surg.; Arris & Gale Lect. RCS. Specialty: Gen. Surg. Special Interest: Anti-doping drug policy for golf; Golf injuries. Socs: Assn. Surg.; Vasc. Surg. Soc. Prev: Hon. Cons. Surg. Brighton Acute Health Care Trust; Sen. Lect. (Surg.) Qu. Eliz. Hosp. Birm.; MRC Research Fell. (Vasc. Surg.) King's Coll. Hosp. Lond.

STRACHAN, David Andrew Shebburn Surgery, Main Street, New Abbey, Dumfries DG2 8BY Tel: 01387 850263 Fax: 01387 850468; Gillfoot Farm, New Abbey, Dumfries DG2 8HD Tel: 01387 850225 Email: daveandsue@medix-uk.com — MB ChB Aberd. 1985. Prev: Trainee GP/SHO Dumfries & Galloway VTS; Ho. Off. (Med.) Aberd. Roy. Infirm.; Ho. Off. (Surg.) Dumfries & Galloway Roy. Infirm.

STRACHAN, David Buchan (retired) Southville, Stanningley, Pudsey, Leeds Tel: 0113 270361 — MB ChB Aberd. 1948. Prev: Ho. Surg. N. Ormesby Hosp. Middlesbrough.

STRACHAN, David Grant (retired) 20 Denham Green Terrace, Edinburgh EH5 3PD Tel: 0131 552 3178 — MB ChB Ed. 1957; DObst RCOG 1961. Prev: Ho. Surg. (ENT) Roy. Infirm. Edin.

STRACHAN, Professor David Peter Department of Public Health Sciences, St. George's Hospital Medical School, Cranmer Terrace, London SW17 0RE Tel: 020 8725 5429 Fax: 020 8725 3584 Email: d.strachan@sghms.ac.uk; 157 Hayes Chase, West Wickham BR4 0JD — MB ChB Ed. 1981; MRCP (UK) 1985; MRCGP 1985; MSc (Dist.) (Epidemiol.) Lond. 1986; FFPHM RCP (UK) 1995, M 1989; MD (Dist.) Ed. 1990; FRCP Lond. 1996. Prof. (Epidemiol.) St. Geo. Hosp. Med. Sch. Lond.; Hon. Cons. Pub. Health Med. Wandsworth HA. Specialty: Epidemiol. Prev: Sen. Lect. (Epidemiol.) St. Geo. Hosp. Med. Sch. Lond.; Lect. (Epidemiol.) Lond. Sch. Hyg. & Trop. Med.; Wellcome Research Train. Fell. (Clin. Epidemiol.) Dept. Community Med. Univ. Edin.

STRACHAN, Mr David Richard ENT Department, Bradford Royal Infirmary, Duckworth Lane, Bradford BD9 6RJ Tel: 01274 364439 Fax: 01274 366549 Email: david.strachon@ bradfordhospitals.nhs.uk — MB ChB Leeds 1986; FRCS Eng. 1992; FRCS Ed. 1992; FRCS (ORL.) 1997; Dip. HSM York 1997. Cons. Ear Nose & Throat Surg. The Yorks. Clinic Bradford Rd. Bingley BD16 1TW; Hon. Sen. Lect., Middlx. Univ., Lond.; H.M. Anat. Demonst., Dept. of Health; Cons. Ear Nose & Throat Surg., The Yorks. Clinic, Bradford Rd., Bingley. Specialty: Otorhinolaryngol. Socs: Assoc. Mem. Brit. Assn. Otorhinol. Head & Neck Surgs.; Eur. Acad. Facial Plastic Surg.; Roy. Soc. Med. Prev: Regist. (Otolaryngol.) Leeds, Yorks. & Hull; Trainee Geo. Portmann Foundat. Bordeaux, France; Sen. Regist. (Leeds, Bradford, Hull).

STRACHAN, David Selby (retired) 75 Marwood Drive, Great Ayton, Middlesbrough TS9 6PD Tel: 01642 723800 Email: davidzena@doctors.org.uk — MB ChB Glas. 1949; DObst RCOG 1958; FRCGP 1979, M 1960. Prev: GP MiddlesBoro.

STRACHAN, Fiona Margaret Flat 10, Howburn Court, 173 Hardgate, Aberdeen AB11 6YA Tel: 01224 573065 — MB ChB Aberd. 1991; MRCP (UK) 1994. Career Regist. (Diabetes & Endocrinol.) Aberd. Roy. Infirm. Specialty: Diabetes.

STRACHAN, Mr George Mathieson 4 Frederick Street, Inverallochy, Fraserburgh AB43 8XU — MB ChB Aberd. 1976; FRCS Glas. 1993; FRCS Ed. 1994. Staff Grade (A & E) Roy. Vict. Infirm. Newc. u. Tyne. Specialty: Accid. & Emerg.

STRACHAN, Gordon Robert Henrietta Street Health Centre, 109A Henrietta Street, Girvan KA26 9AN Tel: 01465 713343 Fax: 01465 714591 — MB ChB Manch. 1993.

STRACHAN, Hilary Margaret Christine Crown Avenue Surgery, 12 Crown Avenue, Inverness IV2 3NF Tel: 01463 710777 Fax: 01463 714511 — MB ChB Aberd. 1984.

STRACHAN, Mr Ian MacDonald (retired) 1 Beech Hill Road, Sheffield S10 2SA Tel: 0114 268 4242 — MB ChB St. And. 1959; DO Eng. 1963; FRCS Ed. 1965; FCOphth 1990. Cons. Ophth. Centr. Sheff. Childr. Hosp. Trust. Prev: Sen. Regist. Dundee Roy. Infirm.

STRACHAN, James (retired) Lower Lime House, Simm Carr Lane, Shibden, Halifax HX3 7UL — MB ChB Aberd. 1950. Prev: Clin. Asst. (Rheum.) Halifax Gen. Hosp.

STRACHAN, James Christopher Marnan Harwich Hospital, 419 Main Road, Harwich CO12 4EX Tel: 01255 201200; 7 Queens Road, Dovercourt, Harwich CO12 3TH Tel: 01255 506420 — MB BS Lond. 1964 (Westm.) FRCS Ed. 1971. Specialty: Gen. Surg. Socs: Colchester Med. Soc.; BMA & Colchester Med. Soc. Prev: GP; Clin. Asst. (Surg.) Colchester Gp. Hosps.; Rotating Regist. (Surg.) United Sheff. Hosps.

STRACHAN, James Gerrit — MB ChB Ed. 1973 (University of Edinburgh) MPhil Ed. 1979, BSc (Med. Sci.) 1970; FRCPysch 1993, M 1977. Cons. Psychiat. Roy. Edin. Hosp.; Hon. Sen. Lect. Univ. Edin. Specialty: Gen. Psychiat. Socs: Chairm. Scott. Sec.Gen. Psych. RCPsych. 1996 - 2000; Union Europeénne des médesins Spécialistes - Sect. of Psychol. 2001. Prev: Lect. Univ. Utrecht, Netherlands; Cons. Psychiat. Min. Justice Pieter Baan Centre Utrecht.

STRACHAN, James Wallace (retired) 40 The Avenue, Girvan KA26 9DS Tel: 01465 713513 — MB ChB Glas. 1962; DObst RCOG 1964. Prev: Ho. Off. (Med. & Surg.) Glas. Roy. Infirm.

STRACHAN, Mr John Charles Haggart (retired) 126 Harley Street, London W1N 1AH Tel: 020 7935 0142; 28 Chalcot Square, London NW1 8YA — MB BS Lond. 1961 (St. Mary's) MRCS Eng. LRCP Lond. 1961; FRCS Eng. 1966; FRCS Ed. 1966. Prev: Cons. Orthop. Surg. Roy. Ballet Co.

STRACHAN, Mr John Robert South Warwickshire General Hospitals NHS Trust, Lakin Road, Warwick CV34 5BW Tel: 01926 495321 Fax: 01926 482602; Oak Farm House, Ufton Fields, Ufton, Leamington Spa CV33 9NZ Tel: 01926 612237 — MB BS Lond. 1977 (University of London) FRCS Eng. 1982; MS Lond. 1990; T(S) 1991. Cons. Urol. S. Warks. Gen. Hosp.s NHS Trust. Specialty: Urol. Prev: Sen. Regist. St. Mary's Hosp. Lond.; Sen. Regist. Roy. Marsden Hosp. Lond.; Research Regist. Inst. Urol. & King's Coll. Hosp. Lond.

STRACHAN, Katherine Anne 28 Beacon Road, Ditchling, Hassocks BN6 8UL — MB ChB Glas. 1996.

STRACHAN, Kenneth Alexander Boyd Peterhead Group Practice, The Health Centre, Peterhead AB42 2XA Tel: 01774 474841 Fax: 01774 474848; Ravenscraig Cottage, Inverugie, Peterhead AB42 3DS — MB ChB Aberd. 1979.

STRACHAN, Kenneth Flory (retired) The Village Farm, Offchurch, Leamington Spa CV33 9AP Tel: 01926 435239 — (St. Mary's) MB BS Lond. 1941. Prev: RAMC 1942-47.

STRACHAN, Kerry Jane 41 Ratcliffe Road, Sheffield S11 8YA Tel: 0114 268 1938 — MB ChB Sheff. 1992; BSc Sheff. 1987; DRCOG 1995; MRCGP 1997. Specialty: Gen. Pract. Prev: Trainee GP/SHO (Psychiat.) N.lands Day Hosp. Sheff.

STRACHAN, Lesley May Aberdeen Royal Infirmary, Foresterhill, Aberdeen AB25 2ZN Tel: 01224 681818 — MB ChB Aberd. 1993; DA (UK) 1995; FRCA 1997. Cons. Anaesth. Aderd. Roy. Infirm. Specialty: Anaesth. Special Interest: Plastic & Emerg. Surg. Prev: Specialist Regist. (Anaesth.) Aberd. Roy. Infirm.; SHO (Anaesth.) Aberd. Roy. Infirm.

STRACHAN, Michael Charles — MB BS Lond. 1980; DRCOG 1984; MRCGP 1985. GP Trainer Maidstone. Specialty: Educat.

STRACHAN, Pauline Anne Cedar Lodge, 64 Springfield Avenue, Aberdeen AB15 8JB — MB ChB Aberd. 1984; MRCGP 1988.

STRACHAN, Robert Alexander Hawthorns Surgery, 331 Birmingham Road, Sutton Coldfield B72 1DL Tel: 0121 373 2211

Fax: 0121 382 1274; 57 Somerville Road, Sutton Coldfield B73 6HJ — MB ChB Aberd. 1966; DObst RCOG 1970; FRCGP 1986, M 1972. Partner GP; Assoc. Adviser (Gen. Pract.) W. Midl. RHA. Specialty: Gen. Pract. Prev: GP Course Organiser W. Midl. RHA.

STRACHAN, Mr Roger David The James Cook University Hospital, Department of Neurosurgery, Marton Road, Middlesbrough TS4 3BW Tel: 01642 854413 Fax: 01642 854118 Email: roger.strachan@stees.nhs,uk — MB ChB Ed. 1979; FRCS Ed. 1986; FRCS (SN) 1994; BSc (Med. Sci.) Ed. 1976, MD 1995. Cons. Neurosurg., Dept. of Neurosurg. The James Cook University Hospital. Specialty: Neurosurg. Socs: Soc. Brit. Neurol. Surg.; Soc. Research into Hydrocephalus and Spina Bifida (SRHSB); Internat. Neuromodulation Soc. Prev: Sen. Regist. (Neurosurg.) Manch. Roy. Infirm. & Hope Hosp. Salford; Regist. (Neurosurg.) Middlesbrough Gen. Hosp.; Research Regist. (Surg.) Univ. Newc.

STRACHAN, Stephanie Ruth 9 Glen Hazel, Wyatts Green, Brentwood CM15 0PE — BM BS Nottm. 1996. SHO (Med.) Qu.'s Med. Centre Nottm. Specialty: Gen. Med.

STRACHAN, Mr William Ellis (retired) — MB ChB Aberd. 1954; FRCS Ed. 1962. Prev: Sen. Regist. (Surgic Neurol.) Roy. Infirm. Edin.

STRADLING, Andrew James c/o 31 Field Barn Drive, Weymouth DT4 0EE — MB BS Lond. 1996 (University College London) SHO (Neurosurg.) Addenbrooke's Hosp. Camb.; SHO (A & E) UCL. Specialty: Accid. & Emerg.

STRADLING, Angele Mabel Peggy (retired) Apple Acre, Sampford Brett, Taunton TA4 4LB Tel: 01984 632545 — MB BS Lond. 1944 (Univ. Coll. Hosp.) MRCS Eng. LRCP Lond. 1942; DCH Eng. 1947; DPH Eng. 1967; FFPHM 1979, M 1973. Prev: SCM. (Child Health) Brent & Harrow AHA.

STRADLING, Hugh Alan The Health Centre, Banks Road, Haddenham, Aylesbury HP17 8EE Tel: 01844 291874 Fax: 01844 292344 — MB BS Lond. 1973; BSc Lond. 1970, MB BS 1973; MRCP (UK) 1976; MRCGP 1978; DRCOG 1979; Dip. Palliat. Med. Wales 1994.

STRADLING, Professor John Reginald Oxford Centre for Respiratory Medicine, Churchill Hospital, Oxford OX3 7LJ Tel: 01865 225236 Fax: 01865 225221 Email: john.stradling@orh.nhs.uk — MB BS Lond. 1976 (Middlx.) MRCP (UK) 1978; BSc Lond. 1973, MD Lond. 1981; FRCP Lond. 1992. Cons. Respirat. & Sleep Med. Churchill Hosp. Oxf.; Prof. for Respirat. Med., univ Oxf. Specialty: Respirat. Med. Socs: Brit. Thorac. Soc. & Sleep Res. Soc. Prev: MRC Trav. Fell. (Med.) Univ. Toronto, Canada; Sen. Regist. Oxf. Hosps.; Regist. Hammersmith Hosp. Lond.

STRADLING, Patricia Ann Walnut Corner, 27B The Gables, Haddenham, Aylesbury HP17 8AD — MB BS Lond. 1973; BSc Lond. 1970, MB BS 1973; DA Eng. 1976.

STRADLING, Peter (retired) Apple Acre, Sampford Brett, Taunton TA4 4LB Tel: 01984 632545 — MB BS Lond. 1942 (Univ. Coll. Hosp.) MRCS Eng. LRCP Lond. 1942; MD Lond. 1947; FRCP Lond. 1966, M 1947. Prev: Dir. Chest Clinic & Sen. Lect. (Respirat. Dis.) Roy. Postgrad. Med. Sch. Hammersmith Hosp. Lond.

STRAFFEN, Anne Mary — MB BS Lond. 1983 (St mary's Hosp. Med. Sch., Lond.) FRCPath; BSc 1980; MRCPath 1991. Cons. Chem. Pathologist, Barnsley DGM, Barnsley. Specialty: Chem. Path.

STRAHAN, Mr Jack (retired) Skerry, Drumgay, Enniskillen BT74 4GH Tel: 02866 323498 — MB BCh BAO Belf. 1956; MCh Belf. 1971, MB BCh BAO 1956; DObst RCOG 1958; FRCS Ed. 1962. Prev: Cons. Surg. Erne Hosp. Enniskillen.

STRAIN, Anne Geraldine 9 Tudor Grove, Omagh BT78 1HJ Tel: 01662 245713; 44 Derrybard Road, Fintona, Omagh BT78 2JH — MB BCh BAO Belf. 1989; DMH Belf. 1991; T(GP) 1993. SHO St. Luke's Hosp., Armagh. Specialty: Gen. Med.; Gen. Psychiat.; Ment. Health. Prev: Trainee GP/SHO S. Tyrone Hosp. Dungannon.

STRAIN, Ethel Olivia (retired) 12 South Drive, Hartlepool TS26 8NQ Tel: 01429 272650 — (T.C. Dub.) MB BCh BAO Dub. 1946. Prev: Clin. Med. Off. (Hartlepool) Retd.

STRAIN, George Andrew (retired) 12 South Drive, Hartlepool TS26 8NQ Tel: 01429 272650 — MB ChB St And. 1933. Prev: Flight Lt. RAFVR.

STRAIN, Graham Barbour Cumbernauld Road Surgery, 804 Cumbernauld Road, Glasgow G33 2EH Tel: 0141 770 5234 Fax: 0141 770 0850 — MB ChB Glas. 1981. Prev: Trainee GP New Galloway VTS; GP Cascais, Portugal.

STRAIN, Gregory John 36 Pencombe Drive, Wolverhampton WV4 5EW — MB BS Lond. 1986.

STRAIN, Harriet Anne 1 Downes Road, Marshalswick, St Albans AL4 9NS — MB BS Lond. 1986; MRCGP 1990.

STRAIN, John William, DFM (retired) 1 Castle View, Egremont CA22 2NA — (Lond. Hosp.) MRCS Eng. LRCP Lond. 1952. Prev: SBStJ.

STRAIN, William David 10 St Johns Avenue, Walton, Liverpool L9 2BS — MB ChB Liverp. 1996.

STRAITON, John Alexander Department of Neuroradiology, Leeds General Infirmary, Leeds LS1 3EX Tel: 0113 392 3683 Fax: 0113 392 5196 Email: john@bsnr.co.uk — MB ChB Glas. 1981; MRCP (UK) 1984; FRCR 1988; T(R) (CR) 1991; FRCP Glas. 1995. Cons. Neuroradiol. Leeds Gen. Infirm. Specialty: Radiol.

STRAITON, John Michael Culver Farm, Old Compton Lane, Farnham GU9 8EJ Tel: 01252 724924 Fax: 01252 724924 — MB BS Lond. 1955 (Char. Cross) MRCS Eng. LRCP Lond. 1955; DA (UK) 1957; DO Eng. 1959; MRCOphth 1992. Assoc. Specialist Moorfields Eye Hosp. Specialty: Ophth. Socs: Fac. Ophth. RCS Eng.; Fac. Anaesth. RCS Eng. Prev: Chief Clin. Asst. Moorfields Eye Hosp.; Asst. Med. Off. Moorfields Eye Hosp.; Resid. Anaesth. Char. Cross Hosp.

STRAITON, Nicholas 6 Colin Road, Paignton TQ3 2NR — MB BS Lond. 1979.

STRAKER, Diana Mary Norden House Surgery, Avenue Road, Winslow, Buckingham MK18 3DW Tel: 01296 713434; Homefield, Oving, Aylesbury HP22 4HN Tel: 01296 641737 — MB ChB Manch. 1985; DRCOG 1988; MRCGP 1990. Socs: Buckingham & Dist. Med. Soc. Prev: Trainee GP/SHO Aylesbury VTS; Ho. Off. (Gen. Surg.) Oldham Dist. Hosp.; Ho. Off. (Gen. Med.) Altrincham Gen. Hosp.

STRANDERS, Alan Patrick O'Connell Davenport House Surgery, Bowers Way, Harpenden AL5 4HX Tel: 01582 767821 Fax: 01582 769285; 34 Park Hill, Harpenden AL5 3AT Tel: 01582 713159 — MB BS Lond. 1972 (Middlx.) MRCS Eng. LRCP Lond. 1972; DObst RCOG 1975. Specialty: Haematology.

STRANEX, Stephen Belvior Park Hospital, Northern Ireland Radiotherapy Centre, Hospital Road, Belfast BT8 8JR Tel: 01232 491942; 10 Hampton Court, Holywood BT18 0HU Tel: 01232 425992 — MB BCh BAO Belf. 1977; FFR RCSI 1984. Cons. N. Irel. Radiother. Centre Belf. Specialty: Oncol.

STRANG, Cecil Duncan (retired) Strathlyn, Kilmahog, Callander FK17 8HD Tel: 01877 330074 Email: duncan@istrang.freeserve.co.uk — (Glas.) MB ChB Glas. 1957; DObst RCOG 1959; MRCGP 1970. Prev: GP Strathclyde.

STRANG, Christopher James Ballantyne Mortimer Surgery, Victoria Road, Mortimer Common, Reading RG7 1HG Tel: 0118 933 2436 Fax: 0118 933 3801; Wisteria House, Mortimer Lane, Mortimer, Reading RG7 3AJ Tel: 01734 332572 — MB BS Lond. 1981; DRCOG 1986; MRCGP 1987. Socs: BMA & Reading Med. Soc. Prev: Med. Off. Save The Childr. Sudan; Trainee GP Windsor VTS; SHO Roy. Cornw. Hosp. Truro.

STRANG, Mr Francis Alexander — MB Camb. 1960 (Camb. & St. Bart.) BA Camb. 1956; BChir Camb. 1959; FRCS Eng. 1964. Retd. Cons. Neurosurg. Manch. Roy. Infirm.; Expert Witness Neurosurg. Manch. Specialty: Neurosurg. Prev: Lect. Neurosurg. Univ. Manch. & Hon. Cons. Manch. Roy. Infirm.; Sen. Regist. Dept Neurosurg. Qu. Eliz. Hosp. Birm.; Regist. Dept. Neurol. Surg. St. Bart. Hosp. Lond.

STRANG, Gladys Elsa McArthur (retired) 26 Malcolmson Close, Edgbaston, Birmingham B15 3LS Tel: 0121 454 8335 — MB ChB St. And. 1937; DPM Eng. 1964; MRCPsych 1973. Hon. Cons. Highcroft Hosp. Birm. Prev: Retited.

STRANG, Graham Duncan Macgregor The Medical Centre, 4 Bracklinn Road, Callander FK17 8EJ Tel: 01877 331001 Fax: 01877 331720; The Orchard, Kilmahog, Callander FK17 8HD Tel: 01877 331669 — MB ChB Glas. 1983; DRCOG 1992. Med. Mem. Nursing Home Inspection Team for Forth Valley HB; Exec. Mem. NW Forth Valley Locality. Prev: SHO (Cardiothoracic) West. Infirm. Glas.; SHO (Thoracic Med.) Hairmyres Hosp. E. Kilbride; Trainee GP Argyll.

STRANG, Ian Guthrie (retired) 29 Moorside Road, Eccleshill, Bradford BD2 2HB Tel: 01274 636433 — (Leeds) LMSSA Lond. 1960.

STRANG, Isabella 4 Dunchurch Road, Paisley PA1 3JW — MB ChB Glas. 1972; DObst RCOG 1974; FFA RCSI 1978.

STRANG, James Ian George Deate Medical Unit, Royal Glamorgan Hospital, Llantrisant CF72 8XR — MB BS Lond. 1969; MRCS Eng. LRCP Lond. 1969; MRCP (UK) 1972.

STRANG, Jeffrie Ritchard Midnight Lodge, Scawton, Thirsk YO7 2HG Tel: 01845 597454 Email: strangjrs@aol.com — MB ChB Glas. 1972; MPH Harvard 1977; MFPHM 1992; FFPHM 2000. Director of Pub. Health/Medical Director. Specialty: Pub. Health Med. Prev: Acting Director of Pub. Health N. Yorks HA; Cons. Pub. Health Med. N. Yorks. HA.

STRANG, Professor John Stanley National Addiction Centre, 4 Windsor Walk, Denmark Hill, London SE5 8AF — MB BS Lond. 1973 (Guy's Hosp.) MRCS Eng. LRCP Lond. 1973; MRCPsych 1977; FRCP 1993; MD 1995. Prof. Psychiat. of Addic. & Dir. Addic. Research Unit Nat. Addic. Centre Lond. Specialty: Gen. Psychiat.; Alcohol & Substance Misuse. Prev: Cons. Psychiat. Drug Depend. Manch.; Regist. & Sen. Regist. Maudsley & Bethlem Roy. Hosps.

STRANG, Louis 87 Bidston Road, Birkenhead CH43 6TS — (Glas.) M.B., Ch.B. Glas. 1944. Prev: Paisley.

STRANG, Robert Archibald 69 Elms Lane, Wembley HA0 2NS — MB ChB Glas. 1933; DPH 1937.

STRANG, Timothy Iain — MB ChB Manch. 1986; DCH RCP Lond. 1988; FCAnaesth 1991. Cons. Anaesth. Univ. Hosp. of S. Manch. Specialty: Anaesth. Socs: Difficult Airway Soc.; ACTA. Prev: Sen. Regist. (Anaesth.) NW RHA; Attend. Phys. Univ. Calif., Irvine, USA; SHO (Paediat. & Anaesth.) Booth Hall Hosp. Manch.

STRANG WOOD, Susi Sundial House, 29 High St., Skelton-in-Cleveland, Saltburn-by-the-Sea TS12 2EF Tel: 01287 654175 Fax: 01287 654075 — MB ChB Glas. 1973; Cert. Master Tr NLP; MRCGP 1979. Managem. Cons.; Psychother. Cleveland. Specialty: Psychother. Socs: UKCP. Prev: Princip. Gen. Pract.s Redcar; Occupat. Health Physics.

STRANGE, Julian William Nevill 26 Kingsgate Road, Winchester SO23 9PG — MB ChB Bristol 1994.

STRANGE, Stephen William Sarehole Surgery, 60 Colebank Road, Hall Green, Birmingham B28 8EY Tel: 0121 777 1315 Fax: 0121 777 0865 — MB ChB Birm. 1983; Dip Occ. Med. Roy. Coll. Phys.; DGM RCP.; Dip. Ther. (Wales); BSc (Hons) Birm. 1980; MRCGP 1995. Socs: Birm. Local Med. Comm.; Small Pract.s Assn. (SPA).

STRANGEWAYS, Janet Edna Margaret Merton, Sutton & Wandsworth Health Authority, The Wilson, Cranmer Road, Mitcham CR4 4TP Tel: 020 8687 4529 Fax: 020 8687 4565; 22 Hamilton Way, Finchley, London N3 1AN Tel: 020 8346 0196 — (Roy. Free) MB BS Lond. 1966; MRCS Eng. LRCP Lond. 1966; FRCPath 1986, M 1973. Cons. Communicable Dis. Control Merton, Sutton & Wandsworth HA; Hon. Sen. Lect. (Microbiol.) St. Geo. Hosp. Med. Sch. Lond. Specialty: Pub. Health Med.; Med. Microbiol. Socs: Brit. Infec. Soc.; Hosp. Infec. Soc.; BMA. Prev: Cons. Med. Microbiol. St. Geo. Healthcare NHS Trust Lond.; Regist. (Path.) Radcliffe Infirm. Oxf.; Trainee Bact. Pub. Health Laborat. Portsmouth.

STRANGEWAYS, Peter Robert (retired) Furrows, 101 Sutton Veny, Warminster BA12 7AW Tel: 01985 840403 Fax: 01985 840403 Email: pstrangeways@doctors.org.uk — (St. Thos.) MB BChir Camb. 1963; MA Camb. 1964. Hon. Med. Adviser, Wessex MS Ther. Centre Warminster, Wilts. Prev: Med. Advisor Glos. FHSA.

STRANKS, Mr Geoffrey John The North Hampshire Hospital, Aldermaston Road, Basingstoke RG24 9NA Tel: 01256 473202 Ext: 3147; Mulberry Corner, Ibworth Road, Hannington, Tadley RG26 5TL Tel: 01256 782820 — MB BS Lond. 1983 (St. Geo.) BSc Lond. 1980; FRCS Ed. 1988; FRCS (Orth.) 1995. Cons. in Trauma and Orthopaedic Surg.; Private Pract. and Medico-legal. Specialty: Trauma & Orthop. Surg. Special Interest: Jt. Replacement (Hip & Knee) Trauma. Socs: BOA.

STRANKS, Sarah Jane 7 Watlow Gardens, Buckingham MK18 1GQ — MB ChB Dundee 1990; DRCOG 1993. Clin. Asst. (A & E) Wycombe Gen. Hosp.

STRANTZALIS, George Department of Neurosurgery, Walsgrave Hospital, Clifford Bridge Road, Walsgrave, Coventry CV2 2DX — Ptychio Iatrikes Athens 1981.

STRATFORD, Andrew John The Health Centre, Elm Grove, Mengham, Hayling Island PO11 9AP Tel: 023 9246 6216 — MB BS Lond. 1970 (Char. Cross) MRCS Eng. LRCP Lond. 1969; DObst RCOG 1971. Clin. Asst. (Ment. Subn.) Hants. AHA (T).

STRATFORD, Karen Anne Llynfi Surgery, Llynfi Road, Maesteg CF34 9DT Tel: 01656 732115 Fax: 01656 864451 — MB BCh Wales 1988; BSc Wales 1983, MB BCh 1988; DGM RCP Lond. 1991; MRCGP 1992.

STRATFORD, Maria 56 Pondcroft Road, Knebworth SG3 6DE Tel: 01438 811040 — Lic Med. New U. Lisbon 1978.

STRATH, Iain Douglas The Health Centre, 2 The Tanyard, Cumnock KA18 1BF Tel: 01290 422723 Fax: 01290 425444 — MB ChB Aberd. 1985; DCH RCPS Glas. 1989; DRCOG 1991; MRCGP 1992.

STRATHDEE, Geraldine Mary 113 Hayes Chase, West Wickham BR4 0HY Email: geraldine.strathdee@oxleas.nhs.uk — MB BCh BAO Belf. 1977. Regist. Maudsley Hosp. Beckenham.

STRATHERN, Colin Holmes Coats 99 Fenwick Road, Griffnock, Glasgow G46 6JA — MB ChB Glas. 1995.

STRATHERN, Hugh Murray Altnabreac, Kilmacolm PA13 4AZ — MB ChB Glas. 1950; DObst RCOG 1954; DMRD Eng. 1957; FFR 1964; FRCR 1975. Cons. Radiol. i/c Inverclyde Roy. Hosp. Greenock, Dunoon Gen. Hosp. & Vict. Hosp. Rothesay. Specialty: Radiol. Socs: Brit. Inst. Radiol. & BMA. Prev: Cons. Radiol. i/c Hairmyres & Assoc. Hosps. E. Kilbride.

STRATON, Rae Hervey (retired) The Paddocks, 1 Provost St., Fordingbridge SP6 1AY Tel: 01425 652391 — (Bristol) M.B., Ch.B. Bristol 1945.

STRATON, Thomas (retired) The Paddocks, 1 Provost St., Fordingbridge SP6 1AY Tel: 01425 652391 — MB ChB Bristol 1945. Prev: Ho. Phys. Bristol Roy. Infirm.

STRATTON, David Salisbury District Hospital, Dept of Child Health, Salisbury SP2 8BJ Tel: 01722 425272 Fax: 01722 425284 Email: dr.d.stratton@shc-tr.swest.nhs.uk; Matrimony Farmhouse, Charlton-All-Saints, Salisbury SP5 4HA Tel: 01722 329720 Email: davidstratton100@hotmail.com — MB BS Lond. 1967 (Guy's) MRCS Eng. LRCP Lond. 1967; DCH Eng. 1971; DObst RCOG 1971; MRCP (UK) 1972; FRCPCH 1998. Cons. Paediat. Salisbury Dist. Hosp. Specialty: Paediat. Socs: BMA Royl coll. Paed. & Child Health. Prev: Regist. (Paediat.) Lond. Hosp.; Lect. Child Health Lond. Hosp. Med. Sch. & Univ. Bristol; Sen. Regist. (Paediat.) Ahmadu Bello Univ. Hosp. Zaria, Nigeria.

STRATTON, Frederick Justin Department of Pathology, Birch Hill Hospital, Rochdale OL12 9QB Tel: 01706 377777 — MB ChB Manch. 1974; FRCPath 1992, M 1980; MBA Manch. 1993; MHSM 1994. Cons. Chem. Path. Rochdale Healthcare NHS Trust & Bury Health Care NHS Trust; Clin. Teach. (Med.) Univ. Manch. Specialty: Chem. Path. Prev: Med. Dir. Rochdale Healthcare NHS Trust; Sen. Regist. (Chem. Path.) Manch. AHA (T).

STRATTON, Jonathan David Hillingdon Hospital, Hillingdon, Uxbridge UB8 3NN — MB BS Lond. 1992; MRCP (UK) 1995. Regist. (GIM) Hillingdon Hosp. Specialty: Nephrol.; Gen. Med. Prev: SHO (Med.) St. Mary's Hosp. Portsmouth; Renal Regist. Lister Hosp. Stevenage; Renal Regist. St. Mary's London.

STRATTON, Michael Rudolf 6 Creighton Road, London NW6 6ED Tel: 020 8918 4087 — MB BS Lond. 1982; BA Oxf. 1979; PhD 1989; MRCPath 1991. Prof. Cancer Genetics; Hon. Cons. Roy. Marsden Hosp. Lond. Specialty: Genetics. Prev: Sen. Regist. (Neuropath.) Inst. Psychiat. Lond.; MRC Research Fell. Inst. Cancer Research Lond.; Regist. (Histopath.) Hammersmith Hosp. Lond.

STRATTON, Paul Newark Road Surgery, 501a Newark Road, South Hykeham, Lincoln LN6 8RT Tel: 01522 537944 Fax: 01522 510932 — MB BS Lond. 1971 (Lond. Hosp.) DObst RCOG 1973; DCH Eng. 1974; Cert JCC Lond. 1974; MRCGP 1977; DCCH RCP Ed. 1984; FRCGP 1997. Prev: Ho. Phys. St. Helen's Hosp. Hastings; Ho. Off. (Obst.) W. Chesh. Matern. Hosp.; SHO (Paediat.) Chester City Hosp.

STRATTON, Richard John Rheumatology Department, The Royal Free Hospital, London NW3 2QG Tel: 020 7794 0500 — MB BS Lond. 1988; MA Oxf. 1985; MRCP Lond. 1991; MD Lond. 1999. Sen. Regist. (Rheumatol.) Roy. Free Hosp. Lond.; PhD Stud. (Vasc. Biol.) King's Coll. Lond.; Regist. (Rheumatol. & Gen. Med.) Guy's Hosp. Lond. Specialty: Gen. Med.; Rheumatol. Prev: Research Regist. Roy. Free Hosp. Lond.

STRAUGHAN, Donald William, OBE (retired) 9 Beaufort West, Bath BA1 6QB Tel: 01225 789926 Fax: 01225 789926 Email: donald@straughan.co.uk — (Westm.) PhD Lond. 1959, BSc (Hons.)

1956; MB BS (Hons.) Lond. 1961; MRCS Eng. LRCP Lond. 1961. Prev: Wellcome Prof. Pharmacol. Sch. Pharmacy Univ. Lond.

STRAUGHAN, Stephen James Bramblehaies Surgery, College Road, Cullompton EX15 1TZ Tel: 01884 33536 Fax: 01884 35401; Manor Farmhouse, Bradninch, Exeter EX5 4NW Tel: 01392 881904 — MB ChB Leeds 1980; DA (UK) 1985; MRCGP 1987. Hosp. Practioner (Anaesth.) Roy. Devon & Exeter Trust. Socs: Soc. Orthop. Med.

STRAUSS, Julian Paul Penny's Hill Practice, St Mary's Road, Ferndown BH22 9HB Tel: 01202 897200 — BM Soton. 1980; DCH RCP Lond. 1984; DRCOG 1984; MRCGP 1984; MRCPsych 1988. GP Ferndown Health Centre Dorset.

STRAW, Robert George Flat 12, Janeleigh Court, 193 Fosse Rd S., Leicester LE3 0FY — MB ChB Leic. 1996.

STRAWBRIDGE, Ms Louise Catherine Barnet General Hospital, Wellhouse Lane, Barnet EN5 3DJ Tel: 020 8216 4000 — MB ChB Ed. 1993. Specialist Reg. In Obst. and Gyn. Specialty: Obst. & Gyn.

STRAWBRIDGE, Walter Glyndwr Caradoc (retired) 1 Tyfica Road, Pontypridd CF37 2DA Tel: 01443 3273 — MB BCh Wales 1958 (Cardiff) MD Wales 1958, BSc, MB BCh 1953; Dip. Bact. Lond 1961; FRCPath 1974, M 1963. Prev: Dep. Dir. Pub. Health Laborat. Birm.

STRAWFORD, Ian David Glastonbury Surgery, Feversham Lane, Glastonbury BA6 9LP Tel: 01458 833666 Fax: 01458 834536; 66 Barton House, Butleigh, Glastonbury BA6 8TH — MB ChB Birm. 1985; DCH RCP Lond. 1989; MRCGP 1990.

STRAWFORD, Julie Upton Medical Partnership, 18 Sussex Place, Slough SL1 1NS Tel: 01753 522713 Fax: 01753 552790 — MB ChB Bristol 1976.

STRAY, Colin Michael 20 Guildford Road, Stoneygate, Leicester LE2 2RB Tel: 0116 270 6106 — MB BS Lond. 1967 (Westm.) FFA RCS Eng. 1972. Cons. Anaesth. Leicester Univ. Hosp.s Trust. Specialty: Anaesth. Socs: BMA. Prev: Sen. Regist. (Anaesth.) Birm. AHA (T); Regist. (Anaesth.) Bristol Roy. Infirm.; SHO (Anaesth.) Soton. Hosp. Gp.

STREAHORN, David 23 Bush Road, Bushvale, Dungannon BT71 6QE — MB BCh BAO Belf. 1971.

STREATHER, Christopher Paul 60 Burbage Road, London SE24 9HE Tel: 020 8725 1673 Fax: 020 8725 7068 Email: chris.streather@stgeorges.nhs.uk — MB BS Lond. 1987; MRCP (UK) 1990; MA Oxf. 1994; FRCP UK 2002. Cons. Renal Phys., St Georges Hosp., Lond.; Clin. Director Med., St Georges Hosp., Lond. Specialty: Gen. Med. Special Interest: Cardiovascular Disease in Renal Medicine. Socs: Renal Assn. Prev: Regist. (Renal Med.) King's Coll. Hosp., Roy. Sussex Co. Hosp. & St Thos. Hosp. Lond.; Sen. Research Fell. & Hon. Clin. Lect. (Renal Med.) King's Coll. Hosp. Lond.

STREDDER, David Hugh 2 Maddison Street, Southampton SO14 2BN — MB ChB Leeds 1978; MRCP (UK) 1983; Dip. Pharm. Med. RCP (UK) 1986; MFPM RCP (UK) 1989; MRCGP 1996; DRCOG 1997; DFFP (RCOG) 1997.

STREET, David Frank (retired) 6 Oast Court, Yalding, Maidstone ME18 6JY Tel: 01622 814495 — (St. Bart.) MB BS Lond. 1943; MRCS Eng. LRCP Lond. 1943; DMRD Eng. 1957. Prev: Cons. Radiol. Orsett, Basildon & St. And. Hosps.

STREET, Karen Nicola 71 Woodcote Avenue, Kenilworth CV8 1BG — BM BCh Oxf. 1994.

STREET, Mark Nicholas 39 Peartree Avenue, Newhall, Burton-on-Trent — MB BS Lond. 1985.

STREET, Martin Kinman Coorparoo, Bridgelands Barcombe, Lewes BN8 5BW — MB ChB Birm. 1978; FFA RCS Eng. 1983; FFA RCSI 1983. Specialty: Intens. Care.

STREET, Murray John The Surgery, 21 Queens Road, Brighton BN1 3XA Tel: 01273 328080 Fax: 01273 725209; 20 East Drive, Queens Park, Brighton BN2 2BQ Tel: 01273 603538 — MB BCh Wales 1980 (University Wales) BSc Wales 1975; DRCOG 1982; MRCGP 1985. Specialty: Gen. Pract.

STREET, Miss Patricia Department of Obstetrics, Royal Berkshire Hospital, Cravon Road, Reading RG1 5AN Tel: 01189 878117; Halsinger Farm, Halsinger, Braunton EX33 2NL Tel: 01271 814504 Fax: 01271 816139 — MRCS Eng. LRCP Lond. 1974 (Roy. Free Sch. Med. Lond.) MRCOG 1982; FRCOG 1997. Cons. Obst. Roy. Berks. Hosp. Reading; Dep. Police Surg. Thames Valley Police Reading. Specialty: Obst. & Gyn. Socs: Cert. Mem. BSCCP; Soc. Police Surg. Prev: Assoc. Specialist (O & G) Roy. Berks. Hosp. Reading; Regist. (O & G) Roy. Berks. Hosp. Reading; Regist. (O & G) N. Manch. Gen. Hosp.

STREET, Roger Geoffrey (retired) Tilford, Yealm Road, Newton Ferrers, Plymouth PL8 1BQ Tel: 01752 872073 — (St. Thos.) MB BChir Camb. 1964; MA Camb. 1964; DObst RCOG 1970. Prev: Principle in Gen. Pract.,Warminster, Wilts.

STREET, Simon Haswell Exeter Surgery, Kidlington Health Centre, Exeter Close, Oxford Road, Kidlington OX5 1AP Tel: 01865 375 215 — MB ChB Birm. 1974; DRCOG 1977; MRCGP 1978; MCl Sc 1991. Assoc. Director Oxf. PGMDE. Specialty: Gen. Pract. Prev: Tutor (Pub. Health & Primary Care) Univ. Oxf.; Trainee GP Oxf. VTS; Ho. Phys. Gen. Hosp. Birm.

STREET, Simon Quentin Ingarfield 6 St Mary's Road, Poole BH15 2LH — MB ChB Birm. 1988; ChB Birm. 1988; DCH RCP Lond. 1995; DRCOG 1995; MRCGP 1995. Staff Paediat. (Community Child Health) Poole. Specialty: Community Child Health.

STREETEN, Naomi Clare 30 York Road, Tunbridge Wells TN1 1JY — MB BS Lond. 1997; FRCA 2001.

STREETER, Graham Stuart — MB BS Lond. 1982 (Charing Cross Hospital) DCH RCP Lond. 1985; MRCGP 1986; DRCOG 1986. GP Trainer Maidstone VTS.

STREETER, Helen Louise Cransley Hospice, St. Mary's Hospital, London Road, Kettering NN15 7PW; Eddonelea, Church Lane, East Haddon, Northampton NN6 8DB — MB BS Lond. 1989 (Roy. Free Hosp. Sch. Med.) MRCGP 1993; DCH RCP Lond. 1993; DRCOG 1994. Staff Grade (Palliat. Med.) Cransley Hospice Kettering. Specialty: Palliat. Med. Prev: Clin. Asst. (Palliat. Med.) Cransley Hospice Kettering.

STREETLY, Allison Bexley and Greenwich Health Authority, 221 Erith Road, Bexleyheath DA7 6HZ Tel: 020 8298 6171 Fax: 020 8298 6183 Email: allisonstreetly@ics.bexgreen-ha.sthames.nhs.uk; Department of Public Health Medicine, UMDS, Capital House, 42 Weston St, London SE1 Tel: 020 7955 4945 Email: allison.streetly@kcl.ac.uk — MB BChir Camb. 1985; BA (Hons.) Camb. 1981; MSc Lond. 1989; MFPHM RCP Lond. 1992. Acting Dir. Pub. Health Bexley & Greenwich; Sen. Lect. (Pub. Health Med.) UMDS. Specialty: Pub. Health Med. Prev: Sen. Regist. (Pub. Health Med.) SE Thames RHA.

STREETLY, Matthew James 99 Glyndebourne Gardens, Corby NN18 0QA — BM BS Nottm. 1994.

STREETS, Carole Ann Derriford Hospital, Plymouth PL6 8PH Tel: 01752 777111 Email: carole.streets@phnt.swest.nhs.uk; 2 Bradford Cottages, Buckland Monachorum, Yelverton PL20 6ES Tel: 01822 853473 Email: 2cstreets@2bradroh.freeserve.co.uk — MB ChB Bristol 1992 (Univ. Bristol) BSc (Hons.) Bristol 1989; MRCP (UK) 1996. SHO (Anaesth.) Derriford Hosp. Plymouth. Specialty: Anaesth. Socs: BMA; Assoc. of Anaesth. Of GB & Ire.; Roy. Coll. Phys. Prev: SHO (Med.) Derriford Hosp. Plymouth; SHO (A & E) & Ho. Off. (Med.) Roy. United Hosp. Bath; Ho. Off. (Surg.) Frenchay Hosp. Bristol.

STREFFORD, Teresa Isabel 24 Carlton Road, Northwich CW9 5PN — MB ChB Leeds 1997.

STREHLE, Eugen-Matthias 5 Trotwood, Limes Farm, Chigwell IG7 5JN — State Exam Med Munich 1990; MD Munich 1993. SHO (Paediat., Paediat. Neurol. & Neonatol.) Roy. Preston Hosp. & Sharoe Green Hosp. Prev: SHO (Hosp. & Community Paediat.) Birch Hill Hosp. Rochdale; SHO (Paediat. & Neonatol.) City & Heartlands Hosp. Birm. & Solihull Hosp.

STREIT, Catherine Elizabeth Longrigg Medical Centre, Leam Lane Estate, Felling, Gateshead NE10 8PH Tel: 0191 469 2173 Fax: 0191 495 0893 — Dip Fed 1981 Switzerland. GP Gateshead, Tyne & Wear.

STRELAU-SOWINSKA, Jadwiga 31 Thornway, Bramhall, Stockport SK7 2AQ — MB BCh BAO NUI 1958; MRCPsych 1971. Cons. (Child Psychiat.) Stockport AHA.

STRELITZ, Norma Sylvia White House, Slateway, Pitton, Salisbury SP5 1ED Tel: 01722 712236 — (Liverp.) MB ChB Liverp. 1955; DMRT Liverp. 1961.

STRELLING, Malcolm Keith (retired) Sarnia, Westella Road, Yelverton PL20 6AS Tel: 01822 853219 — MB BS Lond. 1953 (Guy's) DRCOG 1958; DCH RCP Lond. 1958; FRCP Ed. 1975; FRCP Lond. 1976; FRCPCH 1996. Prev: Cons. Paediat. Plymouth.

STRENS, Lucy Henrietta Alban Manor House, Betsham, Southfleet, Gravesend DA13 9LZ — BChir Camb. 1996; BA Camb. 1994; MB Camb. 1997; MA Camb. 1998; MRCP 1998. MRC Clin. Research Fell. Inst. of Neurol. Lond. Specialty: Gen. Med. Prev: Med. SHO Rotat. Roy. Lond. Hosps. Trust.

STRETTON, Christopher Martin (retired) The Little House, Wallsworth Hall, Sandhurst GL2 9PA Tel: 01452 730232 — MB ChB Birm. 1964; MRCS Eng. LRCP Lond. 1964; DObst RCOG 1966; MRCGP 1980; MMedSc Leeds 1985. Prev: GP & Med. Ref. Gloucester Crem.

STRETTON, Trevor Bannister (retired) 12 Hill Top Avenue, Cheadle Hulme, Cheadle SK8 7HN Tel: 0161 485 1361 — MB ChB Manch. 1955; FRCP Lond. 1972, M 1957. Prev: Cons. Phys. Manch. Roy. Infirm. & Sen. Lect. (Med.) Univ. Manch.

STREULE, Michael John (retired) Broomfield Cottage, Broomfield Hill, Great Missenden HP16 9PD Tel: 01494 863940 — (St. Mary's) MB BS Lond. 1959; LMSSA Lond. 1959; DObst RCOG 1961. Prev: GP, Bucks.

STREVENS, Maurice John 187 Upton Road, Bexleyheath DA6 8LY — MB BCh Wales 1969; MRCP (U.K.) 1973.

STRICH, Sabina Jeannette (retired) 1 Folly Bridge Court, Oxford OX1 1SW Tel: 01865 251741 — BM BCh Oxf. 1949; DM Oxf. 1956; MRCPath 1963; MRCP Lond. 1967; FRCPsych 1980, M 1973. Prev: Cons. Child Psychiat. Croydon.

STRICK, Miss Margaret Joy Royal Victoria Infirmary, Queen Victoria Road, Newcastle upon Tyne NE1 4LP Tel: 0191 232 5131 — MB BCh Witwatersrand 1989; FRCS Glas. 1995. Specialist Regist. (Plastic Surg.) Roy. Vict. Infirm. Newc. Specialty: Plastic Surg. Prev: Ho. Phys. Perth Roy. Infirm; SHO (Plastic Surg.); W. Norwich Hosp.

STRICKLAND, Andrew David Springfield, Yarm Way, Leatherhead KT22 8RQ — BM BS Nottm. 1995.

STRICKLAND, Ian David Kingston Hospital, Kingston upon Thames KT2 7QB Tel: 020 8546 7711 Fax: 020 8547 1786; Court Cottage, 23 Catherine Road, Surbiton KT6 4HA Tel: 020 8399 7995 Fax: 020 8287 0885 Email: i_d_strickland@compuserve.com — (Lond. Hosp.) MB Camb. 1967, BChir 1966; FRCP Lond. 1984, M 1968. Cons. Phys. Kingston Hosp. Surrey. Specialty: Gen. Med.; Gastroenterol. Socs: Brit. Soc. Gastroenterol. Prev: Sen. Regist. & Lect. (Med.) Lond. Hosp.; Ho. Off. (Surg.) & Ho. Phys. Lond. Hosp.

STRICKLAND, John Esse Talbot (retired) Sizergh, Le Pont Vaillant Lane, Vale, Guernsey GY6 8BN Tel: 01481 55771 — MB BS Lond. 1946 (Lond. Hosp.) MRCS Eng. LRCP Lond. 1939. Prev: Venereol., Special Treatm. Clinic Bd. of Health Guernsey.

STRICKLAND, Nicola Hilary Department of Imaging, Hammersmith Hospital, Imperial College School of Medicine, Du Cane Road, London W12 0HS Tel: 020 8383 4956 Fax: 020 8383 3121 Email: nstrickland@hhnt.nhs.uk — BM BCh Oxf. 1984; MA (Hons.) Oxf. 1985; MRCP (UK) 1987; FRCR 1991; FRCP UK 2000. Cons. & Sen. Lect. (Radiol.), Hammersmith Hosp., Imperial Coll. Sch. Med. Lond. Specialty: Radiol. Socs: Pres. Anglo-French Med. Soc.; Ex-Pres. EuroPACS Soc. & Radiol. Sect. RSM. Prev: Sen. Regist. (Radiol.) Hammersmith Hosp. Lond.; SHO (Cardiol. & Thoracic Med.) Brompton Hosp. Lond.; SHO (Med. ITU) St. Thos. Hosp. Lond.

STRICKLAND, Paul, OBE 2 Stonehill Road, E. Sheen, London SW14 8RW Tel: 020 8876 0568 Fax: 020 8876 7842; Northwood Consulting Rooms, 25B Green Lane, Northwood HA6 2XJ Tel: 0192 74 26948 — (King's Coll. Lond.) MB BS Lond. 1943; MRCS Eng. LRCP Lond. 1943; DMR Lond 1947; FRCP Lond. 1975, M 1952; FFR 1952; FRCR 1975. Med. Manager (Imaging) Mt. Vernon Hosp. N.wood. Specialty: Oncol.; Radiother. Socs: Fell. Linnean Soc. Prev: Cons. Radiother. Mt. Vernon Hosp. & Radium Inst. Northwood; Vis. Radiother. Hillingdon Hosp., Hertford Co. Hosp., Herts. & Essex Gen. Hosp. & Wexham Pk. Hosp. Slough.

STRICKLAND, Paul John Elmham Surgery, Holt Road, Elmham, Dereham NR20 5JS — MB ChB Bristol 1982; DRCOG 1984; DCH RCP Lond. 1985; MRCGP 1986.

STRICKLAND, Paul Laurence Department of Psychiatry, Meadowbrook, Stott Lane, Salford M6 8DD Tel: 0161 772 3730 Fax: 0161 772 3715 Email: p.strickland@man.ac.uk — MB ChB Manch. 1986; BSc (Hons.) (Physiol.) Manch. 1983, MB ChB 1986; MRCPsych 1990; MMedSc. Leeds 1992. Lect. Hon. Cons. Psychiat. Univ. Manch. & Salford Ment. Health Trust. Specialty: Gen. Psychiat. Socs: Manch. Med. Soc.; Soc. Psychosomatic Research. Prev: Clin. Research Fell. (Psychiat.) Univ. Manch. Withington Hosp. Manch.; Sen. Regist. (Gen. Psychiat.) Univ. Hosp. S. Manch. & Withington Hosp.Manch.; Regist. (Gen. Psychiat.) St. Jas. Hosp. Leeds.

STRIDE, Amanda 5 Bowring Mead, Moretonhampstead, Newton Abbot TQ13 8NP Tel: 01647 440278 — MB ChB Birm. 1995 (Univ. Birm.) MB ChB (Hons.) Birm. 1995. SHO (Gen. Med.) Roy. Devon & Exeter Hosp. (Wonford). Specialty: Gen. Med. Prev: HO. (Gen. Med.) Manor Hosps. Walsall; Ho. Off. (Orthop. & Gen. Surg.) MusGr. Pk. Hosp. Taunton.

STRIDE, Jean Gray (retired) 123 Sussex Road, Petersfield GU31 4LB Tel: 01730 264314 — (St. Mary's) MB BS Lond. 1954; DCH Eng. 1958. Prev: GP Petersfield.

STRIDE, John Stanley Charles Portobello Medical Centre, 14 Codrington Mews, London W11 2EH Tel: 020 7727 5800/2326 Fax: 020 7792 9044; 7 Stonehill Close, London SW14 8RP — MB BS Lond. 1976 (Char. Cross) MRCS Eng. LRCP Lond. 1974; Cert. Family Plann. JCC 1980; LFHom Lond. 1996. Prev: Regist. (Psychiat. & Community Med.) P. of Wales Hosp. Sydney, Austral.; SHO (Paediat.) Wexham Pk. Hosp. Slough; Ho. Phys. Char. Cross Hosp. Lond.

STRIDE, Jonathan David 74 Lower Northam Road, Hedge End, Southampton SO30 4FT — MB ChB Birm. 1995.

STRIDE, Peter Charles Department of Anaesthetics, Cumberland Infirmary, Carlisle CA2 7HY — MB ChB Birm. 1980; FFA RCS Eng. 1986. Cons. Anaesth. Cumbld. Infirm. Carlisle. Specialty: Anaesth.

STRIESOW, Mrs Hannah Hedwig (retired) 138 Claremont Road, Forest Gate, London E7 0PX Tel: 020 8472 5873 — (Halle & Freib.) Staatsexamen, Halle 1932. Prev: Ho. Surg. Lond. Jewish Hosp.

STRIGNER, Andrew Ernest 17 Harley Street, London W1G 9QH Tel: 020 7935 4543 Fax: 020 7436 8819 — MB BS Lond. 1952 (Guy's) MFHom 1954. Specialty: Gen. Med.; Psychother. Socs: Vice-Pres. McCarrison Soc.; Fell. Roy. Soc. Med.; Med. Soc. Lond. Prev: Mem. Counc. Inst. Study & Treatm. Delinq.; Honeyman Gillespie Lect. (Mat. Med.) Roy. Lond. Homoeop. Hosp.; Asst. Phys. Paediat. & Cardiol. Out-pat. Depts. Roy. Lond. Homoeop. Hosp.

STRIGNER, Peter Bernard Kirkwood House, Biggar ML12 6PP Tel: 01899 220164 — MB BS Lond. 1975 (Guy's) MRCS Eng. LRCP Lond. 1975; DRCOG 1978; MRCP (UK) 1982. GP Princip./Partner Biggar Med. Pract. Socs: Regional Fell., Roy. Soc. of Med.; Scott. McCarrison Soc. Prev: Full-time Dep., Healthcall, Edin.; GP Princip./Partner Llangollen Health Centre; GP Trainer Wrexham VTS.

STRIKE, Philip Christopher 3 Woodland Grove, Pontefract WF7 7EP — MB BS Lond. 1991; MRCP (UK) 1995. Specialty: Cardiol.

STRINATI, Mair — MB BS Lond. 1997.

STRINGER, Bevyl Margaret Mid Anglia Community Health Trust, Child Health Centre, Hospital Road, Bury St Edmunds IP33 3ND Tel: 01284 775071; Twin Cottage, Twin Cottage, North Street, Great Dunham, King's Lynn PE32 2LR — (Roy. Free) MB BS Lond. 1967; MRCS Eng. LRCP Lond. 1967; DObst RCOG 1969; DCH Eng. 1971. SCMO Mid Anglia Community Health Trust. Specialty: Community Child Health. Socs: Brit. Paediat. Assn. Prev: SCMO Blackburn Hyndburn & Ribble Valley HA; Deptm. Med. Off. W. Riding CC; Clin. Med. Off. Wilts. AHA.

STRINGER, Jane The Health Centre, Greenside, Cleckheaton BD19 5AN Tel: 01274 872200; Toothill Cottage, Tooothill Lane, Rastrick, Brighouse HD6 2SE — MB ChB Leeds 1980; DRCOG 1983; MRCGP 1984.

STRINGER, Joan Karen Breidden, Calcott Lane, Bicton, Shrewsbury SY3 8EX — MB BCh Wales 1987 (Welsh Nat. Sch. Med.) Cert. Family Plann. JCC 1990; DRCOG 1990; MRCGP 1991. Prev: SHO (ENT) Shrewsbury; SHO (Psychiat.) NW Hosp. Denbigh; SHO (Cas.) Shrewsbury.

STRINGER, Jonathan Whitby Group Practice, Chester Road, Whitby, Ellesmere Port CH65 6TG Tel: 0151 355 6144 Fax: 0151 355 6843 Email: jon.@stringer16.fsnet.co.uk; 16 Liverpool Road, Chester CH2 1AE — MB ChB Liverp. 1981; MRCS Eng. LRCP Lond. 1981. GP Princip. Specialty: Gen. Pract.

STRINGER, Julian Roy Riverside Medical Practice, Roushill, Shrewsbury SY1 1PQ Tel: 01743 352371 Fax: 01743 340269 — MB BCh Wales 1987; DRCOG 1989; Cert. Family Plann. JCC 1990; MRCGP 1991. Specialty: Gen. Pract. Prev: Trainee GP Rossett

Chesh. & Welshpool Powys; SHO (Psychiat.) NWH Denbigh; SHO (ENT) Shrewsbury.

STRINGER, Kathryn Rachael Flat 8, 130-132 Talbot Road, London W11 1JA Tel: 020 7792 9501 — BM BS Nottm. 1992; BMedSci Nottm. 1990; MRCP (UK) 1995. Specialist Regist. (Anaesth.) N. W. Thames Region. Specialty: Anaesth.

STRINGER, Mr Mark David St James's University Hospital, Children's Liver & G.I. Unit, Gledhow Wing, Leeds LS9 7TF Tel: 0113 206 6689 Fax: 0113 206 6691 — MB BS Lond. 1980 (Guy's Hosp.) MRCP (UK) 1984; FRCS Eng. 1985; BSc Lond. 1977, MS 1990; FRCS (Paediat.) 1993; FRCP Lond. 1996; FRCPCH 1998. Cons. Paediatric Hepatobiliary/Transpl. Surg. Leeds Teachg. Hosp. NHS Trust. Specialty: Paediat. Surg.; Transpl. Surg. Socs: Fell. Roy. Soc. Med.; Int. Pediatr. Transpl. Assn.; Brit. Soc. Paediat. Gastroenterol., Hepatol. & Nutrit. Prev: Lect. (Paediat. Surg.) King's Coll. Hosp. Lond.; Sen. Regist. (Paediat. Surg.) Hosp. Sick Childr. Lond.

STRINGER, Rhona (retired) — MRCS Eng. LRCP Lond. 1955; DObst RCOG 1956; FRCOG 1975, M 1962. Hon. Cons. O & G Scunthorpe & Goole NHS Trust. Prev: Hon. Cons. Colposcopy & Laser North. Gen. Hosp. Sheff.

STRINGER, Romola Mary Sprint Mill, Burneside, Kendal LA8 9AQ Tel: 01539 725168 — MB BChir Camb. 1975; DRCOG 1979.

STRINGFELLOW, Helen Frances Dept. of Hisopathology, Royal Preston Hospital, Sharoe Green Lane, Preston PR2 9HT Tel: 01772 710149 — MB ChB Manch. 1991; BSc (Hons) 1989; MRCPath 1998. Cons. (Pathol.) Roy. Preston Hosp. Specialty: Histopath. Socs: Int. Acad. Of Pathol.; BMA; Assoc. Clin. Pathologists.

STRINGFELLOW, Michael John Shirley Avenue Surgery, 1 Shirley Avenue, Shirley, Southampton SO15 5RP Tel: 023 8077 3258/1356 Fax: 023 8070 3078; 29 Shirley Avenue, Southampton SO15 5NF Tel: 02380 704109 — BM Soton. 1982 (Southampton University) MRCP (UK) 1986; MRCGP 1990. GP Shirley Avenue Surg. Soton. Specialty: Gen. Med.

STRITCH, William Alan (retired) 12 Netherbank, Galashiels TD1 3DH Tel: 01896 664730 — MB ChB Ed. 1962. Prev: Med. Off. DHSS Norcross Blackpool.

STRIVENS, Edward Chapel Farm, Dilham, North Walsham NR28 9PZ Tel: 01692 536483 Fax: 01692 535318 — MB BS Lond. 1993 (Char. Cross) BSc Jordan 1992. Prev: SHO Roy. Lond. Hosp.; Ho. Surg. Norf. & Norwich Hosp.; Ho. Phys. Chelsea & Westm. Hosp. Lond.

STRIVENS, Thomas Edward Alan (retired) Chapel Farm, Dilham, North Walsham NR28 9PZ Tel: 01692 536483 Fax: 01692 535318 — MB BS Lond. 1955 (Char. Cross) DObst RCOG 1964; DA Eng. 1974. Prev: GP Norf.

STROBEL, Professor Stephan Peninsulat Medical School, ITTC Building, Tamar Science Park, Davy Road, Plymouth PL6 8BX — MD Frankfurt 1972; PhD Ed. 1984; MRCP (UK) 1990; FRCP Lond. 1994; FRCPCH 1996. Director of Clin. Educat., Peninsular Med. Sch., Plymouth; Chair of Peninsula Postgraduate Health Institute. Specialty: Paediat. Prev: Prof. Paediat. Univ. Frankfurt, Germany.; Vice Dean for Educat. - Train. Inst. Child Health Lond.; Prof. Paediat. & Clin. Immunol. UCL.

STRODE, Christopher Edmund (retired) 96 Kennington Road, Kennington, Oxford OX1 5PE Tel: 01865 735594 — BM BCh Oxf. 1953; DObst RCOG 1958. Prev: Ho. Surg. Cas. & Orthop. Depts. Battle Hosp. Reading.

STRODE, Michael (retired) Flat 6, The Red House, Warrs Hill Road, North Chailey, Lewes BN8 4JE — MB BS Lond. 1946 (St. Thos.) MRCS Eng. LRCP Lond. 1946. Prev: Assoc. Specialist (Paediat.) Chailey Heritage Craft Sch. & Hosp. Chailey.

STRODE, Patricia Ann 148 Baslow Road, Sheffield S17 4DR; Anselm, White Edge Drive, Baslow, Bakewell DE45 1SJ — MB ChB Sheff. 1980; DRCOG 1983.

STROMBERG, Peter 21 Woodside, Craigends, Houston, Johnstone PA6 7DD — MB ChB Glas. 1973; BSc (Pharmacy) (1st cl. Hons.) Strathclyde 1969; MRSC, CChem 1977; MCB 1980; MRCPath 1981. Cons. Clin. Biochem. Argyll & Clyde Health Bd. Specialty: Biochem. Prev: Regist. & Sen. Regist. (Clin. Biochem.) Glas. Roy. Infirm.

STROMMER, Thomas Rochus Staunton Group Practice, 3-5 Bounds Green Road, Wood Green, London N22 8HE Tel: 020 8889 4311 Fax: 020 8826 9100; 30 Braydon Road, Stamford Hill, London N16 6QB Tel: 020 8802 9577 — State Exam Med. Heildelberg 1989.

STRONACH, Anita Jane 23 Brooke Avenue, Chester CH2 1HQ — MB ChB Birm. 1990; ChB Birm. 1990.

STRONACH-HARDY, Sally 43 King's Road, Sherborne DT9 4HX — MB BS Lond. 1967. Specialty: Occupat. Health.

STRONG, Alastair Martin Priory Road Surgery, Priory Road, Park South, Swindon SN3 2EZ Tel: 01793 521154 Fax: 01793 512562; 8 Magdalen Road, Wanborough, Swindon SN4 0BG Tel: 01793 790934 — MB ChB Sheff. 1988; MRCGP 1994. Prev: Trainee GP Swindon VTS.

STRONG, Alexandra McMillan Millar Department of Dermatology, Monklands Hospital, Monkscourt Avenue, Airdrie ML6 0JS Fax: 01236 713156 — MB ChB Glas. 1972; MRCP (UK) 1976; FRCP Glas. 1989. Cons. Dermatolgist Monklands Hosp. Airdrie. Specialty: Dermat. Prev: Sen. Regist. (Dermat.) Roy. Infirm. Glas.

STRONG, Professor Anthony John King's College Hospital, Denmark Hill, London SE5 9RS — MB ChB Ed. 1966 (Edinburgh) FRCS Ed. 1970; MA Oxf. 1979, BA 1963, DM 1995. Cons. Neurosurg. Guy's, King's Coll. & Maudsley Hosps.; Prof. of Neurosurg., King's Coll. Lond. Specialty: Neurosurg. Prev: Reader (Neurosurg.) Univ. Newc.; MRC Fell. Inst. Neurol. Lond.; Sen. Regist. (Neurosurg.) Nat. Hosp. Nerv. Dis. Lond.

STRONG, Clare Karola — MB ChB Bristol 1979; MRCP (UK) 1985.

STRONG, Daniel Peter 5 Nursery Barns, Woodborough, Pewsey SN9 5PF — MB ChB Birm. 1995.

STRONG, David Alan The Deanery, 19 The Front, Middleton One Row, Darlington DL2 1AS Tel: 01325 332241 — MB BChir Camb. 1956 (Univ. Coll. Hosp.) MA, MB Camb. 1956, BChir 1955. Prev: Med. Asst. A & E Dept. Watford Gen. Hosp.

STRONG, Emma Patricia Wellforce, 28 Wilkinson St., Sheffield S10 2GB Tel: 0114 276 9500 — MB BS Calcutta 1966 (Calcutta Med. Coll.) MFHom 1997. Clin. Asst. Gen. Pract. Bilsthrope, Nottm; Private Homoeop. Pract. Specialty: Homeop. Med. Socs: Fac. Homoeopath. Prev: GP Sheff.; Med. Adviser For Benefits Agency Nottm.

STRONG, Professor John Anderson, CBE (retired) 12 Lomond Road, Edinburgh EH5 3JR Tel: 0131 552 2865 — (T.C. Dub.) FRSE; Hon. FRCP Ed. 1994; MB BCH BAO DUB. 1937; MA, MD Dub. 1967, BA 1937; FRCP Lond. 1962, M 1946; FRCP Ed. 1957, M 1954; Hon. FRCPI 1980; Hon. FACP 1980; Hon. FCPP 1981; FRCGP ad eundem 1982. Hon. Lt.-Col. RAMC; Hon. Fell. Trinity Coll. Dub. 1982; Fell. Roy. Soc. of Edin., FRSE. Prev: Pres. Roy. Coll. Phys. Edin.

STRONG, Mr John David Eugene (retired) Golwg-y-Mynydd, Llangorse, Brecon LD3 7UG Tel: 01874 658292 — MB BChir Camb. 1951 (St. Bart.) MB BChir Cambl. 1951; MA Camb. 1951; DO Eng. 1956; FRCS Eng. 1971. Cons. Ophth. Princess Margt. Hosp. Swindon & Savernake Hosp. MarlBoro. Prev: Sen. Regist. (Ophth.) Roy. Vict. Infirm. Newc.

STRONG, John Edward 4 Riverside, Church Road, Holywood BT18 9DB Tel: 028 9042 3568 — MB BCh BAO Belf. 1970; DObst RCOG 1974; FFA RCSI 1976. Cons. Anaesth. Belf. City Hosp. Specialty: Anaesth. Prev: Regist. (Anaesth.) Ulster Hosp. Dundonald; Ho. Off. Roy. Vict. Hosp. Belf.; Regist. Lagan Valley Hosp. Lisburn.

STRONG, Mr Nicholas Patrick Department of Ophthalmology, Royal Victoria Infirmary, Newcastle upon Tyne NE1 4LP Tel: 0191 282 4736 Fax: 0191 282 5525; Deneholme, Allendale Road, Hexham NE46 2DH Tel: 01434 606511 Email: n.p.strong@ncl.ac.uk — MB Camb. 1984; PhD (Physiol.) Calif. 1981; BChir 1983; FRCS Glas. 1987; FCROphth. 1989. Cons. Roy. Vict. Infirm. Newc. u. Tyne. Specialty: Ophth. Prev: Sen. Regist. (Ophth.) Leicester Roy. Infirm.; Regist. (Ophth.) Moorfields Eye Hosp.; SHO (Ophth.) King Edwd. VII Hosp. Windsor.

STRONG, Patrick Martin Bolton Radiology, 57 Chorley New Road, Bolton BL1 4QR Tel: 01204 23270; Sandford, 8 Carlton Road, Heaton, Bolton BL1 5HU Tel: 01204 43591 — MB BCh Wales 1977; DMRD Eng. 1981; FRCR 1985. Cons. Radiol. Bolton HA. Specialty: Radiol. Socs: Manch. Med. Soc. & Bolton Med. Soc. Prev: Sen. Regist. (Diag. Radiol.) Manch. Hosps.; Regist. (Diag. Radiol.) Manch. Hosps.; SHO (Neurosurg.) Plymouth Gen. Hosps.

STRONGE, Kenneth Alfred Newtownards Health Centre, Frederick Street, Newtownards BT23 4LS — MB BCh BAO Belf. 1978; DRCOG Lond. 1980. GP Newtownards Health Centre.

STRONKHORST, Carolina Heleentje The Flat, Perridge House, Pilton, Shepton Mallet BA4 4EN — Artsexamen Amsterdam 1991.

STROOBANT, John University Hospital Lewisham, High St., Lewisham, London SE13 6LH Tel: 020 8333 3136 Fax: 020 8690 1963 — MB BS Sydney 1973; DCH Eng. 1976; DRCOG 1978; MRCGP 1979; FRCP Lond. 1993; FRCPCH 1997. Cons. Paediat. With an Interest in Respirat. Med., Univ. Hosp. Lewisham; Hon. Sen. Lect., Clin. Tutor. Specialty: Paediat.; Respirat. Med.; HIV Med. Socs: BMA. Prev: Staff Neonat. Roy. Hosp. for Wom., Sydney; Cons. Paediat. Whipps Cross Hosp. Lond.; Research Fell. Hosp. Sick Childr. Lond.

STROSS, William Paul St Richard's Hospital, Department of Haematology, Chichester PO19 6SE Tel: 01243 831651 Fax: 01243 831413 Email: paul.stross@rws-tr.nhs.uk; 12 The Avenue, Chichester PO19 5PU Tel: 01243 530245 Email: wps@stross.net — MB ChB Bristol 1981; MRCP (UK) 1984; MRCPath 1992; FRCP 1999. Cons. Haemat. St Richard's Hosp. Chichester; Cons. Haemat. King Edwd. VII Hosp. Midhurst. Specialty: Haematology. Prev: Sen. Regist. (Haemat.) John Radcliffe Hosp. Oxf.; Regist. (Haemat.) Sheff. HA; SHO (Med.) S. West. RHA.

STROUD, Catherine Rachel 5 Holmewood Drive, Rowlands Gill NE39 1EL — MB ChB Sheff. 1996.

STROUD, Sir Charles Eric 84 Copse Hill, Wimbledon, London SW20 0EF — MB BCh Wales 1945 (Cardiff) BSc Wales 1945, MB BCh (Distinc. Pub. Health &; For. Med., Path. & Bact., Surg, Obst. & Gyn.) 1948; FRCP Lond. 1968, M 1955; DCH Eng. 1955. Hon. Med. Dir. Childr. NAtionwide Med. Research Fund; Hans Sloane Fell. Overseas Off. RCP; Emerit. Prof. Child Health King's Coll. Univ. Lond. Specialty: Paediat. Socs: Brit. Paediat. Assn.; (ex-Pres.) Club de Pediatrie Sociale d'Europe. Prev: Prof. Child Health King's Coll. Sch. Med. & Dent.; Asst. to Dir., Dept. Paediat. Guy's Hosp. Lond.; Hon. Lect. Univ. E. Africa, Kampala & Med. Off. Uganda Govt.

STROUD, David Stuart 12 Walnut Grove, Worlington, Bury St Edmunds IP28 8SF — MB ChB Sheff. 1995.

STROUD, Joanna Elizabeth — MB BCh Wales 1997.

STROUD, Michael Adrian, OBE Institute of Human Nutrition, Southampton General Hospital, Tremona Road, Southampton SO16 6YD Tel: 023 8079 6317 Fax: 023 8079 6317; Mole House, Langley, Liss GU33 7JP — MB BS Lond. 1979; MRCP (UK) 1984; FRCP Lond. 1994; FRCP (Ed) 1994; MD 1996; BSc Lond. 1976, MD 1996. Sen. Lect. (Med. Gastro. Nutrit.); Hon. Cons. Phys. Specialty: Gastroenterol.; Gen. Med. Socs: BSG. Prev: Chief Scientist (Physiol.) DRA Centre for Human Sci.s FarnBoro. Hants.; Sen. Regist. (Gastroenterol.) & Research Fell. (Nutrit.) Soton. Gen. Hosp.

STROUD, Ronald Alan (retired) Easter Barn, Worthing Road, Swanton Morely, Dereham NR20 4QD Tel: 01362 637008 — MB BS (Hons. Midw. & Gyn., & Applied Pharmacol. & Therap.) Lond. 1955 (St. Bart.) DObst RCOG 1961. Prev: GP Pangbourne.

STROUDLEY, Jessica Lisa 95 Langthorne Street, Fulham, London SW6 6JU — MB BCh Wales 1982; FRCR 1994. Cons. Radiol., Ealing Hosp. Lond. Specialty: Radiol.

STROUTHIDIS, Nicholas Gabriel — MB BS Lond. 1997.

STROUTHIDIS, Theodore Department of Medicine for the Elderly, Conquest Hospital, St Leonards-on-Sea TN37 7RD Tel: 01424 755255 Fax: 01424 846183 — MB ChB Alexandria 1962; FRCP Lond. 1982, M 1969; LMSSA Lond. 1970. Cons. Phys. (Geriat.) Hastings & Rother NHS Trust; Cons. Med. Adviser Internat. Med. Rescue Lond. Specialty: Gen. Med. Socs: BMA; Brit. Geriat. Soc. Prev: Sen. Regist. (Geriat.) Guy's Hosp. Lond.; Ho. Phys. St. Helier Hosp. Carshalton.

STROUTHOS, Marios 42 Cissbury Ring N., Woodside Park, London N12 7AH Tel: 020 8445 4824 — MB BS Lond. 1987 (University of London & St Mary's Hospital Medical School) MRCPsych 1992; MSC (Ment. Health Sc.) 1994. Specialty: Child & Adolesc. Psychiat. Socs: RCPsych.

STROVER, Alister Roger Matthew Cumberland Infirmary, Newton Road, Carlisle CA2 7HY Tel: 01228 523444; Bank House, Kirkoswald, Penrith CA10 1DQ Tel: 01768 898658 — MB BS Lond. 1994. SHO (Paediat.). Specialty: Geriat. Psychiat. Socs: Med. Protec. Soc.; BMA; Protec. Soc. Prev: GP Regist. St Pauls Sq. Carlisle; SHO (Psychiat.) Argyll & Bute Hosp.; 1st Year Ho. Surg. Wellington Hosp., New Zealand.

STROVER, Mr Angus Everett Droitwich Knee Clinic, St. Andrews Road, Droitwich WR9 8YX Tel: 01905 794858 Fax: 01905 795916; 10 Hengrave Road, Honor Oak, London SE23 3NW Tel: 020 8699 5778 Fax: 020 8291 5139 — MB ChB Cape Town 1962; FRCS Ed. 1979. Cons. Knee Clinic Droitwich Private Hosp.; Edr. Isokinetics & Exercise Sci. Specialty: Orthop.; Sports Med. Socs: Brit. Assn. Surg. Knee; Internat. Soc. Arthroscopy, Knee Surg. & Orthop. Med. (ISAKOS). Prev: Cons. Trauma & Orthop. Surg. Alexandra Hosp. Redditch.

STROWBRIDGE, Nicholas Foster, Col. L/RAMC Medical Reception Station, Ypres Road, Colchester CO7 7NL Tel: 01206 782947 Email: mrscolchester@army.mod.uk.net; Weeping Ash Cottage, Ardleigh Road, Great Bromley, Colchester CO7 7TL Email: nstrow@aol.com — MB BS Lond. 1977 (St. Thos.) DA (UK) 1980; DFFP 1995; MSc (Sport & Exercise Med.) 2003. Sen. Med. Off. M.R.S. Colchester. Specialty: Gen. Pract. Prev: SHO (Anaesth.) Guy's Hosp. Lond.

STROWGER, Timothy Benjamin Clive 16 Westholme, Letchworth SG6 4JB — MB BS Lond. 1994.

STRUBBE, Patricia Anna Maria Josepha St. Elizabeth Hospice, 565 Foxhall Road, Ipswich IP3 8LX Tel: 01473 727776 Fax: 01473 274717; Regency House, Lower St, Great Bealings, Woodbridge IP13 6NL Tel: 01473 735325 Email: patricia.wyard@btinternet.com — MD Ghent 1983 (State University Ghent Belgium) MRCGP 1994; Dip. Palliat. Med. Wales 1995. Dep. Med. Dir. St. Eliz. Hospice Ipswich; Hon. Cons. Palliat. Med. Ipswich Hosp. NHS Trust. Specialty: Palliat. Med. Prev: GP Suff.

STRUBE, Allen George (retired) 33 Goffs Park Road, Crawley RH11 8AX Tel: 01293 612900 — MB Camb. 1956 (Lond. Hosp.) BChir 1955; DObst RCOG 1961; MRCP Lond. 1968. Prev: GP Audit Facilitator W. Sussex.

STRUBE, Gillian (retired) 33 Goffs Park Road, Crawley RH11 8AX Tel: 01293 612900 — (Guy's) MB BS Lond. 1958; MRCS Eng. LRCP Lond. 1958; DCH Eng. 1960. Asst. GP Burgess Hill W. Sussex; Med. Expert Witness. Prev: Med. Adviser W. Sussex Family Health Servs. Auth. Chichester.

STRUBE, Patrick John South Bucks Trust, Wycombe Hospital, Queen Alexandra Rd, High Wycombe HP11 2TT — MB ChB Leeds 1975; DRCOG 1978; FRCA. 1982. Cons. Anaesth. & Intens. Care S. Bucks. NHS Trust Hosps. Specialty: Anaesth.; Intens. Care. Prev: Sen. Regist. Middlx. Hosp., Brompton Hosp. & Northwick Pk. Hosp.; Sen. Med. Off. King Edwd. VIII Hosp. Durban S. Africa.

STRUDLEY, Martin Robert Upper Gordon Road Surgery, 37 Upper Gordon Road, Camberley GU15 2HJ Tel: 01276 26424 Fax: 01276 63486 — MB BS Lond. 1980; MRCP (UK) 1984; DCH RCP Lond. 1984.

STRUDWICK, Richard Harold (retired) Kingston Lodge, 18 Avenue Road, Leamington Spa CV31 3PQ Tel: 01926 831139 — MB ChB Birm. 1944; DTM & H (Medal Trop. Med.) Liverp. 1946; DPH Lond. 1958; MFCM 1973; MFPHM RCP (UK) 1989. Chief Med. Off. Div. of Family Health WHO Geneva, Switz. Prev: Asst. Dir. Health Servs. S.E. Asia Region WHO.

STRUGNELL, Madeline Jane 4 The Orchard, Badswell Lane, Appleton, Abingdon OX13 5LF — BM Soton. 1995.

STRUIK, Siske Sybrich 94 Avondale Road, Liverpool L15 3HF — Artsexamen Utrecht 1993; Artsexamen Utrect 1993.

STRUNIN, Professor Leo Anaesthetics Unit, The Royal London Hospital, Whitechapel, London E1 1BB Tel: 020 7377 7725 Fax: 020 7377 7126 — MB BS Durh. 1960; FFA RCS Eng. 1964; MD Newc. 1974; FRCPC 1980. BOC Prof. Anaesth. Bart's and The Lond., Qu. Mary Sch. Med. & Dent. Specialty: Anaesth. Socs: Pres AAGBI. Prev: Prof. & Head Dept. Anaesth. Univ. Calgary, Canada; Pres. Roy. Coll. Anaesth.

STRUTHERS, Agnes Dykes Southside Road Surgery, 43 Southside Road, Inverness IV2 4XA Tel: 01463 710222 Fax: 01463 714072 — MB ChB Glas. 1980; DRCOG 1982; MRCGP 1984.

STRUTHERS, Professor Allan David Department Clinical Pharmacology and Therapeutics, Ninewells Hospital, Dundee DD1 9SY; Bech na Mara, 5 Riverview, Newport-on-Tay DD6 8QX — MB ChB Glas. 1977; MB ChB (Hons.) Glas. 1977; DCH Glas. 1979; MRCP (UK) 1980; BSc (Hons.) Glas. 1973, MD 1984; FCRP Ed. 1990; FRCP Glas. 1990; FRCP Lond. 1992; FESC 1994. Prof. Of

Cardiovasc. Med. & Theraputics & Cons. Phys. Ninewells Hosp. Med. Sch. Dundee. Specialty: Gen. Med. Prev: Sen. Regist. (Med.) Roy. Postgrad. Med. Sch. & Qu. Charlotte's Matern. Hosp. Lond.; Regist. (Med.) Stobhill Hosp. Glas.; SHO (Child Health) Roy. Hosp. Sick Childr. Glas.

STRUTHERS, Charles Alexander Clouds Hill House, St. George, Bristol BS6 7LD — MB ChB Bristol 1977.

STRUTHERS, Gavin Douglas North Ormesby Health Centre, Elizabeth Terrace, North Ormesby, Middlesbrough TS3 6EN Tel: 01642 247196; 33 Fearnhead, Marton, Middlesbrough TS8 9XN — MB ChB Glas. 1978; BSc Glas. 1975; DRCOG 1981; MRCGP 1983. Specialty: Occupat. Health. Socs: Soc. Occupat. Med.

STRUTHERS, George Robert Bromson Hall, Ashorne, Warwick CV35 9AD Tel: 01926 651046 Email: gstruthers@doctors.org.uk; 5 Davenport Road, Earlsdon, Coventry CV5 6QA Tel: 02476 672997 — MB Camb. 1974 (King's Coll. Hosp.) MRCP (UK) 1977; FRCP Lond. 1994. Cons. Rheum. Univ. Hosps. of Coventry and Warks. NHS Trust. Specialty: Rheumatol. Socs: Fell. Roy. Soc. Med.; Midl. Rheum. Soc.; Brit. Soc. Rheum. Mem. of Counc. 2000. Prev: ARC Michael Mason Research Fell. & Hon. Lect. St. Geo. Hosp. Kogarah & Univ. New S. Wales Sydney; Sen. Regist. (Med. Rheum.) Qu. Eliz. Hosp. Birm.; Regist. (Med.) Musgr. Pk. Hosp. Taunton.

STRUTHERS, Ian Robertson Struthers and Partners, 436 Mosspark Boulevard, Glasgow G52 1HX Tel: 0141 882 5494 Fax: 0141 883 1015; 14 Falkland Street, Glasgow G12 9PR — MB ChB Glas. 1976; BSc Glas. 1974; MRCP (UK) 1979; DRCOG 1982; MRCGP 1983.

STRUTHERS, James Keith 2 Campden Way, Handforth, Wilmslow SK9 3JA — MB ChB Witwatersrand 1988; MRCPath 1993.

STRUTHERS, Jean Orr (retired) 17 Douglas Avenue, Langbank, Port Glasgow PA14 6PE Tel: 01475 540661 — (Glas.) MB ChB Glas. 1954; FRCOG 1973, M 1958; MD Glas. 1967. Prev: Cons. O & G Roy. Alexandra Hosp. Paisley.

STRUTHERS, John Langford (retired) 27 Kellett Road, Southampton SO15 7PS Tel: 023 8077 2226 — MB BChir Camb. 1955 (Camb. & St. Bart.) Prev: GP Soton.

STRUTHERS, Linda Jane 97 Nethercraigs Road, Paisley PA2 8SG — MB ChB Dundee 1990 (Univ. Dundee) Specialist Regist. (Paediat.) Whipps Cross Hosp. Lond. Specialty: Paediat. Prev: SHO (Paediat.) Qu. Eliz. Hosp. Childr. Lond.; SHO (Paediat.) St. Mary's Hosp. Lond. & Qu. Med. Centre Nottm.

STRUTHERS, Richard Alexander 20 Gamekeepers Park, Edinburgh EH4 6PA — MB ChB Bristol 1992.

STRUTHERS, Simon Langford 2 Seamans Cottage, Seamans Lane, Minstead, Lyndhurst SO43 7FU — MB ChB Leic. 1992.

STRUTT, Kristina Leila 10 Buxton Old Road, Macclesfield SK11 7EL — MB BS Lond. 1984 (The Middlesex Hospital Medical School) MA Camb. 1985; MRCP (UK) 1988; Dip. Pharm. Med. 1991; MFPHM 1993. Med. Adviser (Oncol.) Zeneca Pharmaceut. Specialty: Pharmaceutical Medicine. Prev: Regist. (Med.) Roy. Berks. Hosp. Reading.

STRUTT, Matthew David 73 Pier Avenue, Herne Bay CT6 8PG Tel: 01227 367206 — MB BS Lond. 1994 (St. Bartholomew's) MSc Lond. 1991, BSc 1989. Regist. Virol./Microbiol. Dulwich/Kings Coll. Hosp. Specialty: Med. Microbiol. Prev: Regist. Med. Microbiol. Greenwich Dist. Hosp.

STRUTTE, Lesley Janet Fraser Brookside Farmhouse, Pitney, Langport TA10 9AQ Tel: 01458 250126 Fax: 01458 250126 — (St. Geo.) MB BS Lond. 1970; DObst RCOG 1973; MFHom 1989.

STRYCHARCZYK, Kazimierz Julian Crouch End Health Centre, 45 Middle Lane, Crouch End, London N8 8PH — MB BS Lond. 1986; BSc Lond. 1983, MB BS 1986; DRCOG 1990; MRCGP 1991.

STRYJAKIEWICZ, Eugene Glenn 4 Colston Crescent, Wilford Hill, West Bridgford, Nottingham NG2 7FT — MB ChB Sheff. 1980.

STRYMOWICZ, Christine Green Woods, 3 Essenden Road, Sanderstead, South Croydon CR2 0BW Tel: 020 8657 0141 — LRCP LRCS Ed. LRCPS Glas. 1971 (Med. Acad. Wroclaw) MB Wroclaw 1963. Regist. St. Thos. Hosp. Lond. Socs: BMA.

STRZELECKA, Maria Jozefa (retired) 107 Coombe Lane, London SW20 0BD — MB BCh BAO Dub. 1961; MA Dub. 1961.

STUART, Alan Graham Childrens Heart Unit, Bristol Children's Hospital, St Michaels Hill, Bristol BS2 8BJ Tel: 0117 928 3324 Fax: 0117 928 3341 — MB ChB Dundee 1982 (Univ. Dundee) MRCP (UK) 1985; FRCPCH 1997; FRCP Lond. 1998. Cons. Cardiol. (Congen. Heart Dis.) United Bristol Combined Hosp. Trust; Hon. Sen. Lect. (Med.) Bristol Univ. Specialty: Paediat. Cardiol. Socs: Brit. Paediat. Assn.; Brit. Paediat. Cardiac Assn.; Brit. Cardiac. Soc. Prev: Cons. (Congen. Heart Dis.) Univ. Hosp. of Wales; Sen. Regist. (Cardiol. & Paediat.) W. Midl. RHA; Hon. Sen. Regist. & Research Fell. (Child Health) Univ. Newc. u. Tyne.

STUART, Alexander Barclay Bridge of Allan Health Centre, Fountain Road, Bridge of Allan, Stirling FK9 4EU Tel: 01786 833210; 1 Allanwaterr Gardens, Bridge of Allan, Stirling FK9 4DW Tel: 01786 833210 — MB BChir Camb. 1980; BSc (Hons.) St. And. 1974; DRCOG 1983. Med. Off. i/c H.M. Inst. Cornton Vale Stirling. Specialty: Accid. & Emerg.

STUART, Andrew Brian Douglas The Park End Surgery, 3 Park End, South Hill Park, London NW3 2SE Tel: 020 7435 7282 — MB BS Lond. 1991 (Univ. Coll. Middlx. Hosps.) DRCOG 1994; MRCGP 1995. GP. Specialty: Gen. Pract. Prev: Hon. Sen. Lect. Acad. Fell. GP Regist.

STUART, Angus Erskine (retired) Ardshiel, Isle Ornsay, Isle of Skye IV43 8QS — MB ChB Glas. 1948; FRS Ed. 1970, PhD 1959; FRCP Ed. 1970, M 1959. Prev: Prof. (Path.) Univ. Newc.

STUART, Anthony Leslie Gordon 2 Regents Court, Balcombe Road, Poole BH13 6DY — (St. Mary's) MRCS Eng. LRCP Lond. 1943. Prev: Med. Off. Lond. Airport (Heathrow).

STUART, Brenda Margaret Brighton and Sussex University Hospital Trust, The Princess Royal Hospital, Lewes Road, Haywards Heath RH16 4EX Tel: 01444 441881 — MB BS Lond. 1988 (St Georges Hospital Medical School) FRCP 1992. Cons. (Rheum.) Mid Sussex NHS Trust, Princess Roy. Hosp., Haywards Heath. Specialty: Rheumatol. Prev: Sen. Regist. (Rheum.) Poole, Bournemouth & ChristCh. Hosps.; Regist. Soton. Gen. Hosp.; Regist. (Med.) Roy. S. Hants. Hosp. & Salisbury Dist. Gen. Hosp.

STUART, Brian Sansom Victoria Infirmary, Department of Anaesthesia, Glasgow G42 9TY Tel: 0141 201 5320 Fax: 0141 201 5318; Craigievar, Ford Road, Newton Mearns, Glasgow G77 5AB Tel: 0141 639 5300 — MB ChB Aberd. 1969; FFA RCS Eng. 1974; MPhil (Law & Ethiss in Med.) Glas. 1998. Cons. (Anaesth.) Vict. Infirm. Glas. Specialty: Anaesth. Special Interest: Intens. Care; Law/Ethics. Prev: Sen. Regist. (Anaesth.) West. Infirm. Glas.; Research Fell. (Surg.) West. Infirm. Glas.; Regist. (Anaesth.) Vict. Infirm. Glas.

STUART, Catriona Anne The White House, 11 Claremont Drive, Bridge of Allan, Stirling FK9 4EE — MB BS Lond. 1977.

STUART, Mr David Wallington (retired) St. Mary's, 1 Poolfield Avenue, Keele Road, Newcastle ST5 Tel: 01782 619260 — MB BS Lond. 1945 (St. Mary's) DLO Eng. 1953; FRCS Eng. 1959; FRCS Ed. 1959. Cons. ENT Surg. N. Staffs. Roy. Infirm. Stoke-on-Trent; Mem. Midl. Inst. Otol.; Mem. N. Staffs. Med. Inst. Prev: Wing Cdr. RAF Med. Br., ENT Specialist.

STUART, Douglas (retired) 491 Nuthall Road, Nottingham NG8 5DD Tel: 0115 978 3156 — MB ChB Aberd. 1954 (Aberdeen) Prev: Gen. Practitioner Nottm.

STUART, Elsa Anita 61 Hazel Crescent, Kidlington OX5 1EJ — MB ChB Bristol 1998.

STUART, Fiona Elizabeth Oak Cottage, London Road, Woore, Crewe CW3 9RQ — MB ChB Birm. 1996.

STUART, Fiona Margaret Ottershaw Surgery, 3 Bousley Rise, Ottershaw, Chertsey KT16 0JX Tel: 01932 875001 Fax: 01932 873855; 12 Wilson Drive, Ottershaw, Chertsey KT16 0NT — MB BS Lond. 1987; DRCOG 1991. Specialty: Gen. Med.

STUART, Forbes MacKenzie 23 Keirsbearth Court, Kingseat, Dunfermline — MB ChB Aberd. 1974; DRCOG 1977; MRCGP 1978.

STUART, Gillian (retired) 34 West Stonebridge, Orton Malborne, Peterborough PE2 5LU; 34 West Stonebridge, Orton Malborne, Peterborough PE2 5LU — MB ChB Birm. 1964; BSc. Birm. 1961, MB ChB 1964; MRCP Lond. 1968; DFFP 1993.

STUART, Gordon William Rosemary, Royal Esplanade, Ramsgate CT11 0 Tel: 01843 591450 — (Aberd.) M.B., Ch.B. Aberd. 1944. Mem. (Ex. Chairm.) Kent Family Pract. Comm. (FCP) & Kent Local Med. Prev: R.A.M.C.; Ho. Surg. & Res. Anaesth. King Geo. Hosp. Ilford.

STUART, Ian (retired) Lagavaigh, 14 Brothock Meadows, Letham Grange, Arbroath DD11 4QN Tel: 01241 890488 — MB ChB Aberd. 1955; DObst RCOG 1957.

STUART, Ian Michael Giffard Doctors Surgery, 68 Giffard Drive, Cove, Farnborough GU14 8QB Tel: 01252 541282 Fax: 01252 372159 — MB ChB Leeds 1981; DRCOG 1984; MRCGP 1987. Chair., Black Water Valley Doctors CoOperat.; Bd. Mem., Blackwater Valley PCG.

STUART, Ian Mitchell (retired) Snushalls, 135 Old London Road, Hastings TN35 5LY Tel: 01424 420768 — MB BS Lond. 1957; DObst RCOG 1963.

STUART, Irvine Renfrew Blythe Practice, 1500 Warwick Road, Knowle, Solihull B93 9LE Tel: 01564 779280 Fax: 01564 772010 Email: irvinestuart@blythepractice.co.uk — MB BS Newc. 1974; BDS Newc. 1969; DRCOG 1976; MRCGP 1978; FRCGP 2004. Course Organiser Solihull VTS. Specialty: Gen. Pract.; Educat.; Acupunc. Special Interest: Cardiovasc. Dis.

STUART, Jack Macfarlane (retired) Blythways, Coleshill B46 1AH Tel: 01675 463301 — MB ChB Birm. 1942; DCH Eng. 1947; DObst RCOG 1950; MRCGP 1952; MBE 2002. Prev: GP Coleshill.

STUART, Jacqueline Mary Elizabeth Queens Road Surgery, Queens Road, Blackmill, Consett DH8 0BN — MB BS Newc. 1986; MRCGP 1990.

STUART, James Douglas South Queensferry Medical Practice, The Health Centre, 41 The Loan, South Queensferry EH30 9HA Tel: 0131 331 1396 Fax: 0131 537 4433; 1 Essex Road, Edinburgh EH4 6LF Tel: 0131 339 0894 — MB ChB Ed. 1971; BSc (Med. Sci.) Ed. 1968; MRCGP 1975; DObst RCOG 1975; Dip. Occ. Med. 1996. Prev: Ho. Phys. Roy. Infirm. Edin.; Ho. Surg. Roy. Hosp. Sick Childr. Edin.; SHO (Neurol.) North. Gen. Hosp. Edin.

STUART, James MacNaughton (retired) The Health Protection Agency (SW), The Wheelhouse, Bonds Mill, Bristol Road, Stonehouse GL10 3RF Tel: 01453 829740 Fax: 01453 829741 Email: james.stuart@hpa.org.uk; Tankard Spring House, High Street, Chalford, Stroud GL6 8DW — MB Cantab. 1975 (Camb. Middlx. Hosp.) MA Cantab BChir 1974; DCH RCP Lond. 1979; DRCOG 1979; MFCM 1988; T(PHM) 1991. Prev: Director, Health Protec. Agency S. W.

STUART, Professor John (retired) 12 Brueton Avenue, Solihull B91 3EN Tel: 0121 705 1443 — MD Ed. 1971; MB ChB 1960; FRCP Ed. 1972, M 1965; FRCPath 1979, M 1972. Prof. Haemat. Univ. Birm. Prev: Cons. Haemat. Qu. Eliz. Hosp. Birm.

STUART, John Paton (retired) 3 Clifton House, Queen Parade, Harrogate HG1 5PW Tel: 01423 521025 — (Leeds) MB ChB Leeds 1946, DPH 1967; MFCM 1972. Prev: Div. Med. Off. W. Riding CC.

STUART, Joyce Cameron Department of Anaesthetics, Western General Hospital, Edinburgh Tel: 0131 537 1666 — MB ChB Aberd. 1986; FRCA 1990; MPhil Medical Law & Ethics, University of Glasgow 2000. Cons. Critical Care & Anaesth. West. Gen. Hosp. Edin. Specialty: Anaesth.; Intens. Care; Medico Legal. Prev: Cons. (Anaesth.) Vict. Hosp. Kirkcaldy; Sen. Regist. (Anaesth.) Edin. Roy. Infirm.; SHO (Anaesth.) Ninewells Hosp. Dundee.

STUART, Kenneth Crichton (retired) 2 Waterside Close, Darley Abbey, Derby DE22 1JT Tel: 01332 550206 Fax: 01332 550206 — MB ChB Ed. 1956; DObst RCOG 1962; MRCGP 1966.

STUART, Sir Kenneth Lamonte (retired) The Barbados High Commission, 1 Great Russell St., London WC1B 3JY Tel: 020 7631 4975 Fax: 020 7323 6872; 3 The Garth, Cobham KT11 2DZ Tel: 01932 863826 Fax: 01932 860427 — MB BCh BAO Belf. 1948; DSc (Hon.) Belf. 1986, MD 1952; FRCP Lond. 1965, M 1952; FRCP Ed. 1960, M 1952; FACP 1977; FFPM RCP (UK) 1991; FFPHM RCP (UK) 1995. Hon. Med. & Scientif. Adviser Barbados High Commiss. Lond.; Gresham Prof. Physic Gresham Coll. Lond.; Mem. Counc. King's Coll. Lond. Prev: Prof. & Head, Dept. Med. & Dean Med. Fac. Univ. W. Indies, Jamaica.

STUART, Lynda Maria 3 The Garth, Cobham KT11 2DZ — MB BS Lond. 1993.

STUART, Margaret Anne Evelyn (retired) Lych Gate, Bakeham Lane, Englefield Green, Egham TW20 9TZ Tel: 01784 432724 — (Lond. Hosp.) MRCS Eng. LRCP Lond. 1952; DCH Eng. 1971. Prev: Clin. Asst. (Paediat.) Ashford Hosp. Middlx.

STUART, Mary Helen The Surgery, 18 Hove Park Villas, Hove BN3 6HG Tel: 01273 776245 Fax: 01273 324202 — MB ChB Aberd. 1976; BSc Aberd. 1971, MB ChB 1976; DRCOG 1979; DCH Eng. 1980. GP Princip. Hove. Specialty: Gen. Pract.

STUART, Michael Hillier Queensway Surgery, 75 Queensway, Southend-on-Sea SS1 2AB Tel: 01702 463333 Fax: 01702 603026; Fair Havens Hospice, 126 Chalkwell Avenue, Westcliff on Sea SS0 8HN Tel: 01702 344879 — MB ChB Leeds 1962. Hon. Med. Dir. Fair Havens Hospice Westcliff on Sea. Specialty: Otorhinolaryngol. Socs: Founder Mem. Assn. Palliat. Med.; Assur. Med. Soc. Prev: Regist. (ENT) Southend Gen. Hosp.; Resid. Aural Off. Gen. Infirm. Leeds; SHO (Accid. & Orthop.) Roy. Halifax Infirm.

STUART, Mr Michael James 22 Marle Croft, Whitefield, Manchester M45 7NB — MB BS Lond. 1985 (St. Thomas' Hosp. Med. School) FRCS Ed. 1992; FFAEM 1997. Cons./Hon. Lect. In A & E Clin. Dir., Manch. Roy. Infirmary. Specialty: Accid. & Emerg. Prev: Sen. Regist. Rotat. (A & E) Manch.; Regist. (A & E) Manch.; Regist. (Emerg. Med.) Brisbane, Austral.

STUART, Nancy (retired) 15 Oak Tree Lodge, Harlow Manor Park, Harrogate HG2 0QH — MB ChB Manch. 1950. Prev: Clin. Med. Off. (Community Child Health) Leeds E. Dist. HA (T).

STUART, Nicholas Simon Andrew Department of Oncology, Ysbyty Gwynedd, Penrhosgarnedd, Bangor LL57 2PW Tel: 01248 384150 Fax: 01248 384505 — BM Soton. 1979; MRCP (UK) 1983; T(M) 1991; DM Soton. 1991; FRCP 1998. Prof. of Cancer Studies Univ. Bangor; Hon. Cons. Oncol. Gwynedd Hospital Bangor; Hon. Cons. Oncol. N. Wales Cancer Centre, Rhyl. Specialty: Oncol. Socs: ACP; BACR; ASCO.

STUART, Olivia Mary Christmas Cottage, Little Longstone, Bakewell DE45 1NN — MB ChB Birm. 1993.

STUART, Patricia Joy — MB ChB Leeds 1955; MRCGP 1968.

STUART, Mr Paul Robert Freeman Hospital, Freeman Road, Newcastle upon Tyne NE7 7DN Tel: 0191 233 6161 Fax: 0191 251 1927 Email: prs@stuart-orthopaedics.co.uk — MB BS Newc. 1983; FRCS Eng. 1987; FRCS Ed. 1987. Cons. Orthop. (Hand & Upper Limb Surg.) Freeman Hosp. Newc. u. Tyne. Specialty: Orthop. Special Interest: Rheumatoid UL Surgery; Wrist Injury / Disease. Socs: Brit. Soc. Surg. Hand; Brit. Orthop. Assn.; Brit. Orthopaedic Research Soc. Prev: Hand Fell. Trent RHA; Research Fell. Mayo Clinic Rochester, Minnesota, USA; Sen. Regist. (Orthop.) North. RHA.

STUART, Peter, ERD Pejong, 74 Longlands Road, Carlisle CA3 9AE Tel: 01228 525718 — MB ChB Glas. 1949 (Glas.) DA Eng. 1954; FFA RCS Eng. 1955. Cons. Anaesth. Carlisle & E. Cumbld. Hosp. GP.; Lt.-Col. RAMC, T & AVR, Cons. in Anaesth. Specialty: Anaesth. Socs: BMA & Assn. Anaesths. Gt. Brit. & Irel. Prev: Sen. Regist. Anaesth. Glas. Roy. Infirm.; Vis. Instruc. in Anaesth. Univ. Rochester & Vis. Fell. in Anaesth.; Strong Memor. Hosp. Rochester, New York.

STUART, Ranald McKenzie Department of Radiology, Royal Perth Hospital, Wellington Street, Perth 6008, Western Australia, Perth, Australia; 35 Honister Avenue, High West Jesmond, Newcastle upon Tyne NE2 3PA — MB ChB Ed. 1991; BSc Ed. 1989; FRCS 1999. Radiol. Fell., Roy. Perth Hosp., Perth, Australia. Specialty: Radiol. Prev: SpR in Radiol., Newc. upon Tyne Hosps. Trust; SHO (Med.) Roy. Infirm., West. Gen. Hosp. Edin. & New Cross Hosp. Wolverhampton; Ho. Off. West. Gen. Hosp. & Roy. Infirm. Edin.

STUART, Richard Alexander Oakwood, Bushell Road, Neston, South Wirral CH64 9QB — MB ChB Liverp. 1993; BSc (Hons) 1984; DROGG 1998. Specialty: Paediat. Dent.

STUART, Mr Robert Cornelius 5 Kylepark Crescent, Uddingston, Glasgow G71 7DQ — MB BCh BAO NUI 1982; FRCSI 1987; MCh NUI 1993; FRCSI (Gen.) 1995. Sen. Lect. & Hon. Cons. (Upper Gastrointestinal Surg.) Glas. Roy. Infirm. Specialty: Gen. Surg. Prev: Sen. Regist. (Surg.) St. Jas. Hosp. Dub.; Vis. Lect. (Surg.) P. Wales Hosp. Shatin, Hong Kong.

STUART, Robert Darrell 4 Kings Court, Kings Avenue, Buckhurst Hill IG9 5LU — MB ChB Leeds 1994.

STUART, Ruth (retired) 2 Waterside Close, Darley Abbey, Derby DE22 1JT Tel: 01332 550206 Fax: 01332 550206 — MB ChB Ed. 1956.

STUART, Susan Heaton Road Surgery, 41 Heaton Road, Heaton, Newcastle upon Tyne NE6 1TP Tel: 0191 265 5509 Fax: 0191 224 1824; 21 Northumberland Avenue, Forest Hall, Newcastle upon Tyne NE12 9NR — MB BS Newc. 1969.

STUART, Terence Michael Old Hall Grounds Health Centre, Old Hall Grounds, Cowbridge CF71 7AH Tel: 01446 772237 Fax: 01446 775883 — MB BCh Wales 1979; DRCOG 1982; MRCGP 1983.

STUART, Wendy Hazel 4 Marine Crescent, Great Yarmouth NR30 4ER — MB BS Lond. 1987; DRCOG 1989; FRCA 1995. Specialty: Anaesth.

STUART, Wesley Paul 12 Balgreen Avenue, Edinburgh EH12 5ST — MB ChB Ed. 1991.

STUART, William Edgar (retired) 5 Crossways, Craigends, Houston, Johnstone PA6 7DG Tel: 01505 614765 — MB BS Durh. 1944.

STUART-BUTTLE, Charles Derek George Dunorlan Medical Group, 64 Pembury Road, Tonbridge TN9 2JG Tel: 01732 352907 Fax: 01732 367408 Email: charles.stuart-buttle@gp-g82042.nhs.uk; 9 Holden Road, Tunbridge Wells TN4 0QG — MB BS Lond. 1980 (St. Bartholemews) DRCOG 1983. Partner. Prev: Dir. of Read Code Developm. NHS Centre for Coding & cl.ification, GP Tadworth.

STUART MORROW, Carol 10A Nutley Terrace, London NW3 5SB Tel: 020 7935 9366 Fax: 020 7935 9366; 9 Blandford Close, Hampstead Garden Suburb, London N2 0DH Tel: 020 8455 6544 — MB ChB Liverp. 1964; Dip Forens Pyschother Lond. 1996. Psychoanalytic Psychotherapist and Specialist in Psychosexual Medicines. Specialty: Psychosexual Med.; Psychother. Socs: Brit. Confederation of Psychother.; Inst. of Psychosexual Medicines. Prev: Instruct. Sen. Med. Off. Margt. Pyke Centre Study & Train.; Ho. Phys. Poole Gen. Hosp.; Ho. Surg. King Edwd. VII Hosp. Windsor.

STUART-SMITH, Karen Dept. of Anaesthesia, Glan Clwyd Hospital, Rhyl LL18 5UJ Tel: 01745 583910 — MD Glas. 1990 (University of Glasgow) BSc (Hons.) Glas. 1982, MB ChB 1985; FRCA 1991. Cons. Anaesth. Specialty: Anaesth.; Pharmacology. Prev: Post-Doctoral Research Fell. (Physiol.) Mayo Clinic Rochester, USA; SHO (Anaesth.) Vict. Infirm Glas.; Attend. Anaesthesiol. John Hopkins Hosp. Baltimore, Maryland, USA.

STUART-SMITH, Sara Elizabeth Department of Haematology, St Mary's Hospital, Praed Street, London W12 Tel: 020 8383 0000 — MB BS Lond. 1996 (Royal Free Hospital School of Medicine) BSc 1995 Lond; MRCP 1999 Lond. Haemat. Specialist Regist., Hammersmith Hosp., Lond. Specialty: Haematology. Socs: Roy. Coll. of Phys.s, Lond.

STUART-SMITH, Susan Jane The Tavistock Clinic, 120 Belsize Lane, London NW3 5BA; The Barn, Serge Hill, Abbots Langley WD5 0RY — MB BS Lond. 1989 (Univ. Coll. Hosp. Lond.) MA Camb. 1982; MRC Psych 1997. Specialist Regist. Tavistock Clinic. Specialty: Psychother. Prev: Regist. Rotat. Oxf.

STUART TAYLOR, Malvena Elizabeth Southampton General Hospital, Department of Anasethetics, Tremonia Road, Southampton SO16 6YD Tel: 023 8079 6135 Fax: 023 8079 4348 Email: malvena.stuart-taylor@suht.swest.nhs.uk — MB BS Lond. 1978 (Roy. Free) BSc Lond. 1975; FRCA 1985. p/t Cons. Anaesth. Soton. Gen. Hosp.; Assoc. Dean for PRHO's Wessex Deanery Winchester. Specialty: Anaesth. Special Interest: Undergraduate & Postgrad. Educat. Socs: Soc. Computing & Technol. in Anaesth.; Pain Soc.; Royal College of Anaethetists.

STUBBENS, Gillian Church Street Practice, 8 Church Street, Southport PR9 0QT Tel: 01704 538414 Fax: 01704 539239 — MB ChB Bristol 1982; DRCOG 1984; Cert. Family Plann. JCC 1984. GP Southport. Prev: GP Barnsley; Clin. Med. Off. Barnsley HA; Trainee GP St Ives, Camb. VTS.

STUBBING, John Frederick Dept. of Anaestaetics, Southampton General Hospital SO16 6YD Tel: 02380 796720 Fax: 02380 794348 — MB BS Lond. 1976; MRCS Eng. LRCP Lond. 1976 (Charing Cross Hospital) Cons. Anaesth., Soton. Gen. Hosp. Specialty: Anaesth. Special Interest: Pain Med.; Post Grad. Med. Educat. Socs: Pain Soc.; Assn. of Anaesth.

STUBBINGS, Clive Alan Exmouth Health Centre, Claremont Grove, Exmouth EX8 2JF Tel: 01395 273001 Fax: 01395 273771; Tolpedn, 23 Cranford Avenue, Exmouth EX8 2HU Tel: 01395 274473 — MB BChir Camb. 1974 (Univ. Coll. Hosp.) MB Camb. 1974, BChir 1973; MA Camb. 1974; MRCP (UK) 1975; MRCGP 1977. GP Princip. Prev: Course Organiser (Gen. Pract.) Exeter Postgrad. Med. Sch. Exeter VTS; Research Fell. (Gen. Pract.) Univ. Exeter.

STUBBINGS, Martin Andrew Gosford Hill Medical Centre, 167 Oxford Road, Kidlington OX5 2NS Tel: 01865 374242 Fax: 01865 377826; 63 Bicester Road, Kidlington OX5 2LD Tel: 01865 376185 — MB BS Lond. 1977.

STUBBINGS, Ronald (retired) 85 Dovercourt Road, Dulwich, London SE22 8UW — MB BS Lond. 1959 (St. Bart.) AFOM RCP Lond. 1979; DHMSA 1979. Prev: Med. Off. BP Co. Ltd. Lond.

STUBBINGS, Susan Margaret Exmouth Health Centre, Claremont Grove, Exmouth EX8 2JF Tel: 01395 273001 Fax: 01395 273771; Tolpedn, 23 Cranford Avenue, Exmouth EX8 2HU Tel: 01395 274473 Email: clivestubb@eclipse.co.uk — MB BS Lond. 1973 (Univ. Coll. Hosp.) BSc Lond. 1970, MB BS 1973; MRCGP 1978. Specialty: Haematology.

STUBBINGTON, Hayley Louise Trinity Hill, Bungalown, Trinity Hill, Medstead, Alton GU34 5LT — MB BS Lond. 1992.

STUBBINS, John Haydn (retired) Hathaway, 4 Dynevor Avenue, Neath SA10 7AG Tel: 01639 644671 — MB ChB Ed. 1962; DPH Wales 1966; MFCM 1973. Prev: Cons. Pub. Health Med. M. Glam. HA.

STUBBS, Arthur (retired) Myrtle Cottage, The Street, Kirkby-Le-Soken, Frinton-on-Sea CO13 0EG — MB ChB Sheff. 1959; DObst RCOG 1962.

STUBBS, Benjamin Herbert Rex — MB BS Lond. 1994; MSc Lond. 1986; BSc Birm. 1995; MRCGP 2000.

STUBBS, Emma Jane Darenth Dene, Shoreham Road, Otford, Sevenoaks TN14 5RP — MB BS Lond. 1993.

STUBBS, John Richard Campion (retired) 13 Victoria Road, Dumfries DG2 7NU Tel: 01387 255343 Email: john@stubbs343.fsnet.co.uk — MB BS Durh. 1958; FFA RCS Eng. 1967. Prev: Cons. Anaesth. Dumfries & Galloway Roy. Infirm.

STUBBS, Lesley Anne 2 Cathedral Drive, Fairfield, Stockton-on-Tees TS19 7JT — MB BS Newc. 1981. Clin. Med. Off. (Child Health) S. Tees HA.

STUBBS, Martin Campbell 11 Broadlands, Carnoustie DD7 6JY — MB ChB Dundee 1994.

STUBBS, Paul Gerard Pontardawe Health Centre, Pontardawe, Swansea SA8 4JU Tel: 01792 863103 Fax: 01792 865400 — MB BCh Wales 1979; MRCGP 1984; DRCOG 1985.

STUBBS, Peter Damian Hartcliffe Health Centre, Hareclive Road, Bristol BS13 0JP Tel: 0117 964 2839 Fax: 0117 964 9628 — MB ChB Bristol 1971; DObst RCOG 1973; MRCGP 1975. Specialty: Gen. Pract.

STUBBS, Peter John 22 St Georges Road, Richmond TW9 2LE — MB BS Lond. 1982; MRCPI 1986; MRCP (UK) 1987. Med. Regist. W. Middlx. Univ. Hosp. Isleworth. Prev: SHO (Nephrol.) St. Peter's Gp. of Hosps. Lond.; Ho. Off. (Cardiol.) Roy. Free Hosp. Lond.

STUBBS, Robert Paul Tickle and Stubbs, 28 West Street, Earls Barton, Northampton NN6 0EW Tel: 01604 810219 Fax: 01604 810401; 48 Northampton Road, Earls Barton, Northampton NN6 0HE — MB ChB Sheff. 1986; DRCOG 1989; MRCGP 1990.

STUBBS, Valerie Margaret Myrtle Cottage, 80 The Street, Kirby-le-Soken, Frinton-on-Sea CO13 0EG Tel: 01255 677954; Myrtle Cottage, 80 The St, Kirby-le -Soken, Frinton-on-Sea CO13 0EG Tel: 01255 677954 — MB ChB Sheff. 1961.

STUBGEN, S O The Coach House Surgery, 27 Canterbury Road, Herne Bay CT6 5DQ Tel: 01227 374040 — MB ChB Pretoria 1985; MB ChB Pretoria 1985. Gen. Med. Practitioner.

STUBINGTON, Mr Simon Richard The Michael Heal Department of Urology, Mid Cheshire Hospitals NHS Trust, Leighton Hospital, Middlewich Road, Leighton, Crewe CW1 4QJ Tel: 01270 612010 Fax: 01270 250168 Email: simon.stubington@mcht.nhs.uk; Private Medical Practice, The South Cheshire Private Hospital, Leighton, Crewe CW1 4QP Tel: 01270 612310 (Sec.) — MB BS Lond. 1987 (St Thos.) BSc Lond. 1984; FRCS Ed. 1992; FRCS Eng. 1992; FRCS (Urol) 1999; DM Nottm 1999. Cons. Urological Surg., Mid Chesh. Hosps. NHS Trust, Leighton, Crewe; Cons. Urological Surg., The S. Chesh. Private Hosp., Leighton, Crewe. Specialty: Urological Surgery. Special Interest: Laparoscopic renal Surg.; Holmium LASER Prostate Surg. Socs: Fell. Roy. Soc. Med.; Brit. Assoc. Urol. Surg.; BAUS Sect. EndoUrol. Prev: Transpl. Research Fell. (Surg.) Nottm. City Hosp.; Regist. (Surg.) Nottm. City Hosp.; SHO (Surg.) Leeds Gen. Infirm.

STUBLEY, Michael Walter Aughton Surgery, 19 Town Green Lane, Aughton, Ormskirk L39 6SE Tel: 01695 422384 — MB BS Lond. 1976; MRCS Eng. LRCP Lond. 1976. Specialty: Dermat.

STUCKE, Sally Kathleen Nevill Hall Hospital, Brecon Road, Abergavenny NP7 7EG Tel: 01873 732485; Lower Pant-y-Goida, Talycoed Lane, Llantilio Crossenny, Abergavenny NP7 8TH — MA Camb. 1983; MB BS Lond. 1987; MRCP Lond. (UK) 1993; FRCPCH

Lond. 1997. Cons. Paediat. (Community Child Health) Gwent Healthcare Trust. Specialty: Community Child Health. Socs: Fell. Roy. Coll. Paediat. & Child Health; Brit. Assn. Community Child Health; Welsh Paediat. Soc. Prev: Regist. (Paediat.) Bristol; Regist. (Neonat.) Bristol; Regist. (Community Child Health) Bristol.

STUDD, Clive Department of Anaesthetics, Royal Sussex County Hospital, Brighton — MB ChB Leeds 1969; FFA RCS Eng. 1975. Cons. Anaesth. Roy. Sussex Co. Hosp. Brighton. Specialty: Anaesth. Prev: Sen. Regist. (Anaesth.) Bristol Roy. Infirm.; Specialist in Anaesth. Princess Alexandra's RAF Hosp. Wroughton; SHO Anaesth. Leeds Gen. Infirm.

STUDD, Professor John William Winston Lister Hospital, Chelsea Bridge Road, London SW1W 8RH Tel: 020 7730 5433 Fax: 020 7823 6108; 120 Harley Street, London W1G 7JW Tel: 020 7486 0497 Fax: 020 7224 4190 Email: harley @studd.co.uk — (Birm.) MB ChB Birm. 1962; FRCOG 1986, M 1967; DSc Birm. 1994, MD 1971. Prof. Of Gynaecol. Chelsea & Westm. Hosp. Lond.; Dir. Fertil. & Endocrinol. Centre Lister Hosp. Lond.; Examr. Univs. Lond., Birm., Nottm. & Camb. & RCOG; Chairm. Menopause & PMS Trust; Pub.ats. Off. RCOG; Vice Pres. - Nat. Osteoporosis Soc. Specialty: Obst. & Gyn. Socs: Fell. Roy. Soc. Med. (Pres. Sect. Obst. & Gyn.); (Pres.) Internat. Soc. Reproduc. Med.; (Chairm.) Nat. Osteoporosis Soc. Prev: Cons. O & G King's Coll. & Dulwich Hosp.; Sen. Lect. & Cons. (O & G) Univ. Nottm.; Lect. & Sen. Regist. (O & G) Univ. Birm.

STUDDS, Christopher John 47 Ecton Avenue, Macclesfield SK10 1RD — MB BS Lond. 1986.

STUDDY, John Denman (retired) 86 Braiswick, Colchester CO4 5AY Tel: 01206 853487 — MB BS Lond. 1950 (St. Bart.) MRCPsych 1971. Prev: Cons. Psychiat. Bridge Hosp. Witham.

STUDDY, Peter Robert Harefield Hospital, Harefield, Uxbridge UB9 6JH Tel: 01895 823737 — MD Lond. 1983 (Roy. Free) FRCP Lond. 1989. Cons. Phys. Roy. Brompton & Harefield NHS Trust & W. Herts NHS Trust. Specialty: Gen. Med.; Respirat. Med.

STUDHOLME, Katrine Madge 10 Park Road, Abingdon OX14 1DS Tel: 01235 530722 — MRCS Eng. LRCP Lond. 1955 (Lond. Hosp.) MB Camb. 1956, BChir 1955; MRCGP 1979. Indep. Psychotherapist Abingdon. Specialty: Psychother. Prev: GP 1960-1990.

STUDHOLME, Thomas James 432 Springvale Road, Crookes, Sheffield S10 1LQ — MB ChB Otago 1993.

STUDLEY, Mr John George Noel James Paget Hospital NHS Trust, Lowestoft Road, Gorleston, Great Yarmouth NR31 6LA Tel: 01493 452452 — MB BS Lond. 1973 (Middlx.) FRCS Eng. 1978; MS Lond. 1986. Cons. Gen. Surg. Jas. Paget Hosp. Gt. Yarmouth. Specialty: Gen. Surg. Prev: Sen. Regist. (Gen. Surg.) Northampton Gen. Hosp., Hammersmith Hosp. & Roy. Postgrad. Med. Sch.; Regist. Rotat. (Gen. Surg.) Bloomsbury HA; Research Fell. (Surg.) State Univ. N.Y., Buffalo.

STUMPER, Oliver Friedrich Wilhelm The Heart Unit, Children's Hospital, Steelhouse Lane, Birmingham B4 6NH Tel: 0121 333 9442 Fax: 0121 333 9441 Email: oliver.stumper@bhamchildrens.wmids.nhs.uk — (Bonn, Germany) PhD Rotterdam 1991 University Rotterdam, NL; MD Bonn 1988 University Bonn; State Exam Med. Bonn 1988. Cons. Paediat. Cardiol.; Hon. Sen. Lect. Univ. Birm.; Hon. Cons. Cardiol. Qu. Eliz. Hosp. Birm. Specialty: Paediat. Cardiol. Socs: Brit. Paediat. Cardiol. Assn.; Eur. Soc. Cardiol. Prev: Sen. Regist. (Paediat. Cardiol.) Birm. Childrs. Hosp.; Sen. Research Fell. Hosp. Necker, Paris.

STUMPFLE, Richard 29 Clockhouse Place, London SW15 2EL Email: rstumpfle@doctors.net.uk — MB ChB Ed. 1997; BSc Ed. 1995; MRCP 2001.

STUPPLE, Jeremy Mark Gifford The Medical Centre, 15 Cawley Road, Chichester PO19 1XT Tel: 01243 786666/781833 Fax: 01243 530042; Kilindi, Itchenor, Chichester PO20 7DH Tel: 01243 511304 Fax: 01243 514780 — MB BS Lond. 1983; MRCGP 1986; DCH RCP Lond. 1986; DRCOG 1986.

STURDEE, David William Solihull Hospital, Department of Obstetrics & Gynaecology, Solihull B91 2JL Tel: 0121 424 5390 Fax: 0121 424 5389 Email: david.sturdee@heartsol.wmids.nhs.uk; 44 Mirfield Road, Solihull B91 1JD Tel: 0121 705 1759 — (St. Thos.) MB BS Lond. 1969; DObst 1971; DA Eng. 1972; FRCOG 1988, M 1975; MD Birm. 1979. Cons. O & G Solihull & Birm. Heartlands Hosp.; Sen. Clin. Lect. Univ. Birm.; Co-Edr. in Chief Jl. Internat. Menopause Soc. - The Climacteric 1997-. Specialty: Obst. & Gyn. Socs: BMA (Ex. Chairm. Solihull Div.); (Ex-Chairm.) Brit. Menopause Soc.; Brit. Soc. Colpos. & Cerv. Path. Prev: Edr. Diplomate 1993-9; Sen. Regist. (O & G) Walsgrave Hosp. Coventry & Birm. Matern. Hosp.; Research Fell. (O & G) Univ. Birm.

STURDY, Mr David Eric Rothesay, 22 Stow Park Circle, Newport NP20 4HF Tel: 01633 264646 — MB BS Lond. 1950 (Guy's) FRCS Eng. 1956; MS Lond. 1960. Surg. Roy. Gwent Hosp.; Urol. St. Woolos Hosp. Newport. Socs: Brit. Assn. Urol. Surgs.; Assn. Surg. Prev: Sen. Regist. (Surg.) Roy. Infirm. Preston & Hosp. Sick Childr. Gt. Ormond St.; Regist. Roy. Marsden Hosp. Lond.; Auth. Essentials and Outline of Urology.

STURDY, John Laurence (retired) 91 Gledhow Lane, Leeds LS8 1NE — MB ChB Liverp. 1978. Prev: Staff Grade Geriat. Psychiat. Leeds Comm & Ment. Health Trust.

STURDY, Roger Elston High Noon, Ladock, Truro TR2 4PW Tel: 01726 882386 — MB Camb. 1973; MA Camb. 1976, MB 1973, BChir 1972; MRCPsych 1979. Specialty: Child & Adolesc. Psychiat. Prev: Sen. Regist. (Child Psychiat.) Lond. Hosp.; Asst. Dir. Lond. Med. Gp. & Soc. Study Med. Ethics; Regist. (Psychol. Med.) Hosp. Sick Childr. Lond.

STURGE, Joan Claire — MB BS 1965 (Middlx.) MPhil Lond. 1972, MB BS 1965; DCH RCPS Glas. 1967; DPM Eng. 1970; MRCPsych 1971; FRCPCH 1995. Cons. Child Psychiat. Northwick Pk. Hosp. Harrow Middlx. HA1 3UJ; Serv. Harrow. Specialty: Child & Adolesc. Psychiat. Socs: Fellow 1991.

STURGE, Richard Arthur 45 Eaton Rise, London W5 2HE Tel: 020 8997 8972 Fax: 020 8997 4427 Email: sturgera@aol.com — (Guy's) MB BS Lond. 1965; MRCP (UK) 1971; FRCP Lond. 1986. Cons. Rheum. Barnet & Chase Farm Hosp.s NHS Trust. Specialty: Rheumatol. Socs: BMA & Brit. Soc. Rheum. Prev: SHO MRC Rheum. Unit Taplow; Med. Regist. Guy's Hosp. Lond.; Sen. Regist. (Gen. Med. & Rheum.) Char. Cross & St. Stephens Hosps.

STURGEON, David Alexander Department Psychological Medicine, University College Hospital, Gower St., London WC1E Tel: 020 7387 9300 Ext: 8585 Fax: 020 7387 1710 — BM BCh Oxf. 1971; MA Oxf. 1971; FRCPsych 1986, M 1976. Cons. Liason. Psychiat. & Hon. Sen. Lect. (Fac. Clin. Sci.) Univ. Coll. Lond. Specialty: Gen. Psychiat. Socs: Fell. Internat. Coll. Psychosomatic Med. (Treas.). Prev: Sen. Lect. (Ment. Health) Univ. Coll. Lond.; Hon. Cons. (Psychiat.) Univ. Coll. Hosp. Lond.; Leverhulme Research Fell. Univ. Coll. Hosp. Med. Sch. Lond.

STURGEON, James Liddell Motherwell Health Centre, 138-144 Windmill Street, Motherwell ML1 1TA Tel: 01698 265193 Fax: 01698 253324 — MB ChB Glas. 1968.

STURGESS, Mr Dale Anthony 7 Bowerfield Avenue, Hazel Grove, Stockport SK7 6HZ — MB ChB Manch. 1981; FRCOphth 1991; FRCS Ed. 1991. Specialty: Ophth. Socs: Fell. Roy. Coll. Surg. Edin.; Fell. Roy. Coll. Ophth.; BMA. Prev: SHO (Ophth.) Stepping Hill Hosp. Stockport; SHO (Neurol. & Neurosurg.) Midl. Centre for Neurol. & Neurosurg.; SHO (Ophth.) Wolverhampton Eye Infirm.

STURGESS, Hugh Hopwood House, The Vineyard, Lees Road, Oldham OL4 1JN Tel: 0161 682 6297; 8 North Nook, Austerlands, Saddleworth, Oldham OL4 3QR — MB ChB Manch. 1981; DRCOG 1986; MRCGP 1986. Local Med. Off. Civil Serv.; Dep. Police Surg.

STURGESS, Ian 24 Ethelbert Road, Canterbury CT1 3NE — MB ChB Leeds 1982.

STURGESS, Lucy Bethan — MB BS Lond. 1998.

STURGESS, Michael John Hayes Court, 50 Hayes Lane, Kenley CR8 5LA — MB BCh Wales 1971.

STURGESS, Richard Patrick 47 Rose Mount, Oxton, Birkenhead CH43 5SQ — MB BS Lond. 1984 (Middlx.) BSc Lond. 1981; MRCP (UK) 1987; MD Lond. 1996. Cons. Phys. (Gen. Med. & Gastroenterol.) Aintree Hosps. Liverp. Specialty: Gastroenterol. Socs: Brit. Soc. Gastroenterol. Prev: Sen. Regist. Roy. Liverp. Univ. Hosps.; Research Fell. St. Thos. Hosp. Lond.; Regist. Inst. Liver Studies King's Coll. Hosp.

STURGISS, Stephen Noel Department of Obstetrics & Gynaecology, Royal Victoria Infirmary, Newcastle upon Tyne NE1 4LP Tel: 0191 232 5131; 61 Whinfell Road, Darras Hall, Newcastle upon Tyne NE20 9EW — MB ChB Manch. 1982; MRCOG 1988; MD Newc. 1993. Cons. Obst. & Fetal Med. RUI Newc. Specialty: Obst. & Gyn.

STURLEY, Rachel Helen Royal Devon & Exeter Hospital (Heavitree), Gladstone Road, Exeter EX1 2ED Tel: 01392 405049 Fax: 01392 405061 — MB ChB Sheff. 1980; MRCOG 1985; MD Sheff. 1994. Cons. O & G Roy. Devon & Exeter Hosp. Specialty: Obst. & Gyn. Socs: Brit. Diabetic Assn.; BSCCP. Prev: Sen. Regist. (O & G) Roy. Devon & Exeter Hosp.; Regist. (O & G) Southmead Hosp. Bristol; Research Regist. (Obst. & Diabetes) Roy. United Hosp. Bath.

STURMAN, Daniel Robert — MB ChB Sheff. 1998. Ho. Off. Surg.Urol.Stepping Hill Hosps.tockport. Specialty: Gen. Surg.; Urol. Prev: Ho. Off. Med. Stepping Hill Hosp. Stockport.

STURMAN, Janette May 23 Brompton Walk, Darlington DL3 8RT Tel: 01325 488541 — MB ChB Glas. 1984; MRCGP; Cert AvMed (Gen.); DRCOG 1988. Specialty: Family Plann. & Reproduc. Health. Socs: BMA. Prev: Trainee GP Stokesley VTS & GuisBoro.

STURMER, Heidi Louise 2 Mansfield Avenue, Quorn, Leicester LE12 8BD; 2 Mansfield Avenue, Quorn, Leicester LE12 8BD — MB BS Lond. 1993 (Charing Cross and Westminster) DRCOG; DFFP; BSc (Intercalated) Lond. 1990; DCH RCP Lond. 1995; MRCGP 1997. Specialty: Gen. Pract.

STURRIDGE, Bernadette Frances 72 Margaret Road, Barnet EN4 9NX — MB BS Lond. 1988.

STURRIDGE, Mr Marvin Francis (retired) The Middlesex Hospital, Mortimer St., London W1T 3AA Tel: 020 7636 8333; Crendon, 23 Minton Road, Felpham, Bognor Regis PO22 7JN Tel: 01243 822377 — MB BS Lond. 1952 (Middlx.) FRCS Eng. 1958; MS Lond. 1965. Archiv. Middlx. Hosp. Prev: Cons. Thoracic Surg. Middlx. Hosp.

STURROCK, Angela Mary Blackwoods Medical Centre, 8 Station Road, Muirhead, Glasgow G69 9EE Tel: 0141 779 2228 Fax: 0141 779 3225 — MB ChB Glas. 1993; MRCGP 1997. GP Partner. Prev: SHO (Gyn.) West. Univ. NHS Trust Glas.

STURROCK, David (retired) Lanemead, Common Road, Corston, Malmesbury SN16 0HL Tel: 01666 823429 Fax: 01666 826484 — MB ChB Glas. 1950; MSc Lond. 1965. Prev: Home Off. Insp. Animals (Scientif. Procedures) Act 1986.

STURROCK, Maureen Margaret Douglas Inch Centre, 2 Woodside Terrace, Glasgow G3 7UY Tel: 0141 211 8000 Fax: 0141 211 8005 — MB ChB Aberd. 1974; DObst RCOG 1976; MRCPsych 1979; T(Psych) 1991. Cons. Forens. Psychiat. Gtr. Glas. Community & Ment. Health Servs. Trust. Specialty: Forens. Psychiat. Prev: Cons. Forens. Psychiat. Mersey RHA.

STURROCK, Nigel David Crighton Nottingham City Hospital NHS Trust, Hucknall Road, Nottingham NG5 1PB Tel: 0115 969 1169 Fax: 0115 962 7959 — MD Dundee 1994; MB ChB 1988, BMSc (Hons.) 1985; MRCP (UK) 1991; FRCP (UK) 2001. Cons. (Diabetes & Endocrinol.) City Hosp. Nottm.; Clin. Director, acute Med., city Hosp., Nottm. Specialty: Diabetes; Endocrinol. Socs: Soc. for Endocrinol.; Nottm. M-C Soc.; Diabetes UK. Prev: Sen. Regist. (Diabetes Mellitus & Endocrinol.) City Hosp. Nottm.; Regist. (Med.) QMC Nottm.; Research Fell. (Clin. Pharmacol.) Univ. Dundee.

STURROCK, Professor Roger Davidson Centre for Rheumatic Diseases, University Department of Medicine, Royal Infirmary, 10 Alexandra Parade, Glasgow G31 2ER Tel: 0141 211 4687/8 Fax: 0141 211 4878 — MRCS Eng. LRCP Lond. 1969 (Westm.) MD Lond. 1977, MB BS 1969; MRCP (UK) 1971; FRCP Glas. 1983; FRCP Lond. 1985. McLeod/ARC Chairm. Rheum. Univ. Glas. Specialty: Gen. Med.; Rheumatol. Socs: Fell. Roy. Soc. Med.; Brit. Soc. Rheum.; Brit Soc Rheumatol. (Ex-Pres.). Prev: Sen. Lect. & Cons. Phys. Centre Rheum. Dis. Roy. Infirm. Glas.; Lect. (Rheum. & Med.) Centre for Rheum. Dis. & Univ. Dept. Med. Glas. Roy. Infirm.; Research Asst. (Rheum.) Westm. Hosp. Lond.

STURROCK, Susan Marjory 11 Craster Drive, Arnold, Nottingham NG5 8SL — MB ChB Dundee 1988; DRCOG 1997; DFFP 1998. GP. Specialty: Gen. Pract. Prev: SHO (O & G) City Hosp. Nottm.; GP/Regist. Bakersfield Med. Centre Nottm.; SHO (Psychiat.) Qu.s Med. Centre. Nottm.

STURT, Tessa Mary Albion Health Centre, 333 Whitechapel Road, London E1 1BU Tel: 020 7247 1730 Fax: 020 7247 2589 — MB BS Lond. 1984; DRCOG 1990; MRCGP 1992. Specialty: Obst. & Gyn.

STURTON, Edwin William (retired) 32A Skinner Street, Creswell, Worksop S80 4JH Tel: 01909 721535 — BM BCh Oxf. 1956; DObst RCOG 1958; MRCGP 1978. Prev: Ho. Phys. & Ho. Surg. (ENT) Radcliffe Infirm. Oxf.

STURTON, Peter Richard Abbey Medical Practice, 95 Monks Road, Lincoln LN2 5HR Tel: 01522 530334 Fax: 01522 569442; The Coach House, Weir St, Lincoln LN5 8DU Tel: 01522 529763 — MB ChB Dundee 1983. Prev: Trainee GP Chesterfield VTS; Ho. Off. (Med.) King's Cross Hosp. Dundee; Ho. Off. (Orthop.) Dundee Roy. Infirm.

STURZAKER, Mr Hugh Gerard Coastal Clinic, 4 Park Road, Gorleston, Great Yarmouth NR31 6EJ Tel: 01493 601770 Fax: 01493 442430 Email: hsturzaker@aol.com; Hobland House, Hobland, Great Yarmouth NR31 9AR Tel: 01493 665287 Email: hsturzaker@aol.com — BM BCh Oxf. 1966 (Oxf. & Guy's) MRCS Eng. LRCP Lond. 1966; MA Oxf. 1966; BM BCh. Oxf. 1966; FRCS Ed. 1971; FRCS Eng. 1972. p/t Cons. Surg. Jas. Paget Hosp. Gorleston, Gt. Yarmouth. Specialty: Gen. Surg. Socs: Fell. Roy. Soc. Med.; BMA; Assn. of Coloproctolgy of Gt. Britain & N Irel. Prev: Sen. Regist. (Surg.) Guy's Hosp. Lond.; Ho. Surg. Guy's Hosp.; Research Fell. (Surg.) St. Mark's Hosp. Lond.

STUTCHFIELD, Peter Roy Glan Clwyd District General Hospital, Rhyl LL18 5UJ Tel: 01745 583910; Glas Coed, Pen-yr-Allt, Whitford, Holywell CH8 9DD — MB BS Lond. 1977 (Univ. Coll. Hosp.) BSc (Hons. Genetics) Lond. 1974; MRCP (UK) 1981; FRCP Lond. 1995. Cons. Paediat. Glan Clwyd Hosp. Rhyl; Clin. Teach. Child Health Univ. of Wales Coll. of Med. Specialty: Paediat.; Neonat.; Endocrinol. Socs: Brit. Soc. Paediat. Endocrinol.; Brit. Assn. Perinatal Med.; Roy. Coll. Paediat. and Child Health. Prev: Sen. Regist. (Paediat.) Roy. Liverp. Hosp. Alder Hey; Regist. (Paediat.) Birm. Childr. Hosp.; SHO (Paediat. Respirat. & Intens. Care) Hosp. Sick Childr. Gt. Ormond St. Lond.

STUTTAFORD, Irving Thomas 8 Devonshire Place, London W1N 1PB Tel: 020 7486 7166 Fax: 020 7935 1063; 36 Elm Hill, Norwich NR3 1HG Tel: 01603 615133 — (Oxf. & W. Lond) MRCS Eng LRCP Lond 1959. Med. Columnist 'The Times', Oldie. Specialty: Genitourinary Medicine; Occupat. Health; Med. Publishing. Socs: Roy. Soc. Med.; Chelsea Clin.; BMA. Prev: Med. Correspondant to The Times, Options, Elle; Sen. Med. Adviser to Barclays Bank, The Rank Org. The Hunting Gp., C.E. Andersons & Sons Ltd., & other Cos.; Primary Care Phys. (UK).

STUTTARD, Ana Maria 37A Burghley Road, London N8 — Lic Med. Lisbon 1977.

STUTTARD, Carl Albert Reepham Surgery, Smugglers Lane, Reepham, Norwich NR10 4QT Tel: 01603 870271 Fax: 01603 872995 — MB ChB Liverp. 1977; MRCGP 1982.

STUTTARD, Gareth Lincoln 41 Clive Road, Pattingham, Wolverhampton WV6 7DJ — MB ChB Birm. 1998.

STUTTARD, Susan South Milford Surgery, High St., South Milford, Leeds LS25 5AA Tel: 01977 682202 Fax: 01977 681628; Prebendal House, Church Lane, Monk Fryston, Leeds LS25 5ES Tel: 01977 681207 — BM BS Nottm. 1987 (Nottingham) BMedSci Nottm. 1985; MRCGP 1992. Socs: BMA; POWAR. Prev: Trainee GP Nottm.; SHO (Psychiat.) Leics.

STUTZ, Joanna Alexandra — MB BChir Camb. 1989; MA 1989; FRCR 1997.

STYLE, Anne Marion (retired) Muncaster House, Loweswater, Cockermouth CA13 0RU Tel: 01900 85318 — MB BS Lond. 1950 (W. Lond. & Univ. Coll. Lond.) MRCS Eng. LRCP Lond. 1950. SCMO W. Cumbria DHA. Prev: Ho. Surg. Fulham Hosp.

STYLES, Caroline Jane 40 Crockerton Road, London SW17 7HG — MB BChir Camb. 1993.

STYLES, Caroline Louise Bristol Royal Infirmary, Marlborough St., Bristol BS2 8HW Tel: 0117 923 0000; Flat 3, 15 Victoria Square, Clifton, Bristol BS8 4ES Tel: 0117 973 3711 — MB BChir Camb. 1990; MA Camb. 1991; MRCP (UK) 1993; FRCR 1997. Specialist Regist. Bristol Roy. Infirm. Specialty: Radiol. Prev: Regist. (Radiol.) Qu. Med. Centre Nottm.; SHO (Med.) City Hosp. Nottm. & Newham Gen. Hosp. Lond.

STYLES, Hilary Frances (retired) Lower Mitton Farm, Mitton, Penkridge, Stafford ST19 5QW Tel: 01785 780507 — MB ChB Manch. 1964; DObst RCOG 1967. Prev: Ho. Surg. Univ. Dept. Orthop. Manch. Roy. Infirm.

STYLES, John Trevor (retired) Lower Mitton Farm, Mitton, Penkridge, Stafford ST19 5QW Tel: 01785 780507 — MB BS Lond. 1964 (Univ. Coll. Hosp.) BSc (Hons. Anat.) Lond. 1961; MB BS (Hons., Distinc. Obst. & Gyn.) Lond. 1964; MRCS Eng. LRCP Lond.

1964; FFA RCS Eng. 1968. Cons. Anaesth. Roy. Wolverhampton Hosps. NHS Trust. Prev: Sen. Regist. (Anaesth.) United Birm. Hosps.

STYLES, Richard John Whitchurch Surgery, Bell Street, Whitchurch RG28 7AE Tel: 01256 892113 Fax: 01256 895610 — MB ChB Bristol 1974; DRCOG 1976; FRCGP 1995, M 1978. Course Organiser Mid Wessex VTS Examr. RCGP; RCGP Convenor of Jt. Hosp. Vis. Wessex Region. Prev: Trainee GP Univ. Bristol VTS; SHO (O & G) Southmead Hosp. Bristol.

STYLIANIDES, Labrini The Old Rectory, Rectory Rd, Tolleshunt Knights, Maldon CM9 8EZ — MB BS Lond. 1990.

SU, Mr Archibald Paul Ching Chung Rivermead, Creekview Road, South Woodham Ferrers, Chelmsford CM3 5YL — MB BS Lond. 1964 (Univ. Coll. Hosp.) FRCS Eng. 1973. Cons. ORL & Head & Neck Surg. Basildon & Thurrock Gen. Hosp.s NHS Trust. Specialty: Otorhinolaryngol. Socs: Fell. Roy. Soc. Med.; Mem. BMA; Brit. Assoc. of Otorhinolaryngologists Head & Neck Surg.s. Prev: Sen. Regist. (Otolaryng.) Nottm. Univ. Hosp.; Regist. (Otolaryng.) Southend Gen. Hosp.; Ho. Surg. Roy. Ear Hosp. (Univ. Coll. Hosp.) Lond.

SU, Robin Chee Wei 87 Colwith Road, Hammersmith, London W6 9EZ — MB BS Lond. 1985.

SUARES, Mark Woodlands Surgery, Pilch Lane, Huyton, Liverpool L14 0JE Tel: 0151 489 1806 Fax: 0151 489 0920.

SUAREZ, Valerie Histopathology Department, Staffordshire General Hospital, Weston Road, Stafford ST16 3SA — MB BS Lond. 1979 (Lond. Hosp.) BSc Lond. 1976; MRCPath 1986; FRCPath 1997. Cons. Histopath. Mid. Staffs Gen. Hosps. Trust. Specialty: Histopath.

SUBAK-SHARPE, Robert John County Hospital, Hereford HR1 2ER Tel: 01432 355444; The Poppies, Shelwick, Hereford HR1 3AL Tel: 01432 356054 — MB ChB Glas. 1979; MRCOG 1986; FRCOG 1998. Cons. O & G Co. Hosp. Hereford. Specialty: Obst. & Gyn. Prev: Sen. Regist. Rotat. (O & G) Wales; In Vitro Fertilisation Co-ordinator & Research Regist. Roy. Postgrad. Med. Sch. Hammersmith Hosp. Lond.; Regist. (O & G) Walton & Fazakerley Hosps. Liverp.

SUBANANDAN, P Green Street Surgery, 48 Green Street, Enfield EN3 7HW Tel: 020 8804 3200 Fax: 020 8443 2615 — MB BS Sri Lanka 1973; MB BS Sri Lanka 1973.

SUBASH CHANDRAN, Rajagopalan 34 Belmont Road, Bangor LL57 2LL Tel: 01248 364251 Email: subash@hotmail.com — MB BS Madras 1973; MD Madras 1976; MRCP (UK) 1990. Trust Specialist Phys. (Med. & c/o Elderly) Ysbyty Gwynedd Bangor. Specialty: Gen. Med. Prev: Clin. Asst. (c/o Elderly) & Regist. (Geriat. Med.) Ysbyty Gwynedd Bangor; SHO (Gen. Med.) Watford Gen. Hosp.; SHO (Geriat. Med.) Doncaster.

SUBASH CHANDRAN, Srinivasan Sandling House, Sandling Lane, Sandling, Maidstone ME14 3AH — MB BS Madras 1974.

SUBASINGHE, Suranganie Zita Augusta Southend General Hospital, Eye Unit, Prittlewell Chase, Westcliff on Sea SS0 0RY Tel: 01702 435555; 20 Cranley Avenue, Westcliff on Sea SS0 8AH Tel: 01702 390359 — MB BS Ceylon 1967; DO Eng. 1970; FRCS Ed. 1976; MS (Ophth.) Colombo 1988; FRCOphth 1989. p/t Cons. Ophth. Southend Gen. Hosp. Specialty: Ophth. Socs: BMA; RSM; (Counc.) Coll. Ophth. Sri Lanka. Prev: Cons. Ophth. Southend Gen. Hosp.; Cons. Ophth. Sri Jayewardena Pura Gen. Hosp., Sri Lanka; Cons. Ophth. MoH, Kuwait.

SUBBERWAL, Kamini Windermere Gardens Surgery, 49 Windermere Gardens, Redbridge, Ilford IG4 5BZ Tel: 020 8550 9195 Fax: 020 8550 3746 — MB BS Rayishankar U 1971; MB BS Rayishankar U 1971.

SUBBIAH, Shanmugam Ribblesdale House Medical Centre, Market Street, Bury BL9 0BU Tel: 0161 764 7241 Fax: 0161 763 3557; 74 Rudgwick Drive, Bury BL8 1YE — LRCP LRCS Ed. 1979; LRCP LRCS Ed. LRCPS Glas. 1979; DRCOG 1982; MRCGP 1983.

SUBBU, Venkata Subramanyam Morrison Road Surgery, Morrison Road, Port Talbot SA12 6TH Tel: 01639 887790 Fax: 01639 888093; The Croft, 99 Penycae Road, Port Talbot SA13 2EG — MB BS Andhra 1967 (Andhra Med. Coll. Visakhapatnam) DA Eng. 1971. Prev: Regist. (Anaesth.) Neath Gen. Hosp.

SUBESINGHE, Nyanissara 52 Traps Lane, New Malden KT3 4SA Tel: 020 8942 8812 — MB BS Ceylon 1971; MRCP (UK) 1981.

SUBHANI, Moinuddin Wyken Medical Centre, Brixham Drive, Coventry CV2 3LB Tel: 024 7668 9149 Fax: 024 7666 5151; The Garden House, Lower Road, Barnacle, Coventry CV7 9LD Tel: 024 76 604793 — MB BS Karachi 1962 (Dow Med. Coll.) MRCGP 1977. Princip. GP. Specialty: Dermat. Socs: BMA; MBMAS. Prev: SHO, Ho. Surg. & Ho. Phys. I. of Thanet Hosp. Gp.; Resid. Med. Off. Holywell Hosp. Watford.

SUBHEDAR, Nimish Vasant NICU Liverpool Womens Hospital, Crown St., Liverpool L8 7SS Tel: 0151 708 9988 Email: nvsubhedar_lwh@yahoo.com; 40 Village Road, Oxton, Birkenhead CH43 6TY — MB ChB Bristol 1988; MRCP (UK) 1991; MD (liverpool) 1998. Cons. Neonat. Paediat., Liverp. Wom.s Hosp. Specialty: Neonat. Socs: RCPCH.

SUBOTSKY, Fiona Eleanor Department of Child & Family Psychiatry, King's Collge Hospital, Denmark Hill, London SE5 9RS Tel: 020 7346 3219 Fax: 020 7346 3221 — MB BS Lond. 1966 (St. Bart.) BSc (Psychol.) Lond. 1971; MRCPsych 1975. Cons. Child & Adolesc. Psychiat. S. Lond. & Maudsley Trust Lond. Specialty: Child & Adolesc. Psychiat. Socs: Fell. Roy. Coll. Psychiats.; Fell. Med. Woms. Federat. (Past Treas. Lond. Assn. of MWF); BMA. Prev: Med. Dir. Bethlem & Maudsley Trust; Cons. Child Psychiat. King's Coll. Hosp. Lond. & Brixton Child Guid. Unit; Sen. Regist. (Psychol. Med.) Hosp. Sick Childr. Gt. Ormond St. Lond.

SUBRAHMANYAM, Pasapula Chinna Ordnance Road Surgery, 171 Ordnance Road, Enfield Lock, Enfield EN3 6AD Tel: 01992 761185 Fax: 01992 760938; 4 Foxes Lane, Cuffley, Potters Bar EN6 4JB — MB BS Sri Venkateswara 1969 (Kurnool Med. Coll.) GP Enfield. Prev: Regist. & SHO St. Geo. Hosp. Lincoln; SHO (Surg.) Co. Hosp. Louth; SHO W. Kent Gen. Hosp. Maidstone & Kent & Canterbury Hosp.

SUBRAMANIAM, Kumari Pushpa 22 North Drive, Stoke Mandeville Hospital, Aylesbury HP21 9AN — MB BS Rani Durgavati 1985; MRCP (UK) 1993.

SUBRAMANIAM, Muruga Kumar Parklands, Wymington Road, Rushden NN10 9EB Tel: 01933 396000 — MB BS (Hons.) Sri Lanka 1976 (University of Ceylon) LMSSA Lond. 1989; T(GP) 1994. Clin. Asst. (Ophth.) Kettering Gen. Hosp. Specialty: Ophth.

SUBRAMANIAM, Sickan 358 Marfleet Lane, Hull HU9 5AD — MB BS Madras 1975.

SUBRAMANIAM, Mr Srinivasan Kings Mill Hospital, Mansfield Road, Sutton-in-Ashfield NG17 4JL; 15, 53 Stoney Street, Nottingham NG1 1LX — MB BS Mysore 1984; FRCS Glas. 1990; FRCOphth 1990. Cons. Ophthalm. Kings Mill hosp. Specialty: Ophth. Socs: BMA. Prev: Fell.Med.Retinal.Serv.Moofields Eye.Hosp; Fell.anteria segmentServ.moorfields Eye hosp.; Specialist Regist. N Thames Rotat.

SUBRAMANIAN, Geeta c/o Old Church Hospital, Oldchurch Road, Romford RM7 0BE; 53 Great Cullings, Romford RM7 0YJ — MB BS Madras 1980 (Jipmer, Pondicherry, India) DCH RCP Lond. 1980; MRCP (UK) 1981. Cons. Paediat. Havering Hosp. Trust Romford. Specialty: Neonat. Socs: Brit. Paediat. Assn. Prev: Cons. Neonat. King Abdulaziz Hosp. Jeddah, Saudi Arabia.

SUBRAMANIAN, Mr Kodaganallur Ananthakrishnier 1 Harlow Road, Rainham RM13 7UP Tel: 01708 552072 Fax: 01708 524408 — MB BS Madras 1969 (Madras University) DFFP; MS; FRCS Glas.; FRCS Ed. Socs: BMA.

SUBRAMANIAN, Pallipuram Bharathan Hurst Road Health Centre, Hurst Road, Walthamstow, London E17 3BL Tel: 020 8503 6710 Fax: 020 8521 8293 — MB BS Madras 1958 (Stanley Med. Coll.) Prev: Regist. (Cas.) & Regist. (Orthop.) Whipps Cross Hosp. Lond.; SHO W. Cumbld. Gp. Hosps.

SUBRAMANIAN, Shobha Consultant Paediatrician, Castleford and Normanton District Hospital, Lumley Street, Hightown, Castleford WF10 5LT Tel: 01924 201688 — MB BS Bombay 1986 (Grant Medical College, Bombay) MD Bombay 1989; MRCP 1993. Sen. Regist. (Paediat.) Pinderfields Hosp., Aberford Rd., Wakefield; Cons. Community Paediat., Princess Roy. Hosp. Hudderfield. Specialty: Paediat. Socs: BMA. Prev: Sen. Regist. (Paediat.) S. Tyneside NHS Trust.

SUBRAMANIAN, Thiruppathy 15 Maple House, King's Mill Hospital, Mansfield Road, Sutton-in-Ashfield NG17 4NY — MB BS Madras 1984.

SUBRAMANYAM, M Cranbury Surgery, 16 Cranbury Avenue, Southampton SO14 0LQ Tel: 023 8022 2660 Fax: 023 8022 2660 — MB BS Mysore 1963; MB BS Mysore 1963.

SUBRAMANYAM, Pisipati Varsha Gemini Vale, 3 Birchwood Grove, Hampton TW12 3DU Tel: 020 8941 5882 — MB BS Madras

1965; MRCOG 1973, DObst 1968. Asst. Prof. (O & G) King Abdul Aziz Hosp. Univ. Riyadh, Saudi. Prev: SHO Ashford Hosp. Middlx.; Ho. Surg. Edgware Gen. Hosp.; Ho. Off. Watford Gen. Hosp.

SUBZPOSH, Mr Syed Yafis Ali 59 Wheeleys Road, Edgbaston, Birmingham B15 2LL Tel: 0121 242 3698 — MB BS Aligarh 1979; MCh (Orth.) Liverp. 1989.

SUCHAK, Kirtikumar Kalyanji Centre Point Surgery, Centre Point, Fairstead, King's Lynn PE30 4SR Tel: 01553 772063 Fax: 01553 771463 — MB BS Sambalpur 1971 (S.S. Med. Coll. Burla) LRCP LRCS Ed. LRCPS Glas. 1975. Socs: BMA. Prev: SHO Accid., Emerg. & Orthop. Dept. Ashington Gen. Hosp.; SHO (Gen. Med.) Dunston Hill Hosp. Gateshead; SHO (Chest Dis.) Kelling Hosp. Holt.

SUCHAK, Vinesh Mansukh — MB BCh Wales 1993 (Univ. Wales Coll. Med.) BSc (Physiol.) Wales 1990. GP Partner. Specialty: Gen. Pract. Prev: GP Trainee.

SUCHDEV, Mr Manjit Singh 7-8 Croxdale Terrace, Pelaw, Gateshead NE10 0RR Tel: 0191 469 2337; 43 Callander, Ouston, Chester-le-Street DH2 1LG Tel: 0191 410 9446 — MB BS Punjab 1975; MS Punjab 1978, MB BS 1975; FRCS Ed. 1983; DRCOG 1985; MRCGP 1989. GP Gateshead.

SUCHY, Katja Christina 6 Londrina Terrace, Berkhamsted HP4 2NA — State Exam Med. Munich 1991.

SUCKLE, Norman Edward Blantyre Health Centre, 64 Victoria Street, Blantyre, Glasgow G72 0BS Tel: 01698 823260; Gleniffer House, Braehead Road, Thorntonhall, Glasgow G74 5AQ Tel: 0141 644 3833 — MB ChB Glas. 1962; DObst RCOG 1964. Specialty: Gen. Pract.

SUCKLING, Heather Cullenbel (retired) 93 Ribblesdale Avenue, London N11 3AQ Tel: 020 8368 6130 Email: heathers@doctors.org.uk; 93 Ribblesdale Avenue, London N11 3AQ Tel: 020 8368 6130 Email: heathers@doctors.org.uk — (Roy. Free) MB BS Lond. 1963; DObst RCOG 1965; FRCGP 2001. p/t Prof. Developm. Spine Tutor Roy. Free & Univ. Coll. Sch. of Med.; Hon. Clin. Asst. in Psychother., Camden and Islington Ment. health and Social care NHS Trust. Prev: Cons. to BIS Healthcare, advising on Educat. for Primary Care in Macedonia.

SUCKLING, Ian Gerard Sandsend Surgery, East Row, Sandsend, Whitby YO21 3SU Tel: 01947 895356 Fax: 01947 895581; (branch Surgery) Hazeldene, 9 Coach Road, Sleights, Whitby YO22 5AA Tel: 01947 810775 Fax: 01947 810667 — MB ChB Liverp. 1983; MRCGP 1990; DGM RCP Lond. 1993. Specialty: Occupat. Health. Prev: Cas. Off. RN Hosp. StoneHo..; Sen. Med. Off. RM Poole Dorset.

SUCKLING, Rebecca Jo 75 Festing Road, London SW15 1LW — MB BS Lond. 1996.

SUCKLING, Rupert John Rotherham Health Authority, Rotherham SG5 2QU — MB ChB Ed. 1992. Specialist Regist. Pub. Health, Rotherham HA.

SUD, Suman Kumar 711 Alum Rock Road, Alum Rock, Birmingham B8 3JA Tel: 0121 328 1746 — MB ChB Leeds 1975; LDS RCS Eng. 1983; BChD Leeds 1983. Prev: Trainee GP Coventry & Birm. VTSs.

SUDAN, Sandeep 81 Park Road, Hendon Central, London NW4 3PA — MB BS Lond. 1993 (Kings College London) BSc 1990. Specialist Regist (Anaesth.) William Harvey Hosp. Ashford Kent. Specialty: Anaesth.

SUDARSANAM, Padhmavathi 1 Duchess Grove, Knighton Lane, Buckhurst Hill IG9 5HA Tel: 020 8498 9766 Fax: 020 8498 9766 — LRCP LRCS Ed. 1986; LRCP LRCS Ed. LRCPS Glas. 1986; MFFP 1994. SCMO Wom.'s Health Servs., THHT, Mile End. Specialty: Family Plann. & Reproduc. Health.

SUDARSHAN, Catherine Dushyanthy 9 Alverton Drive, Newton Aycliffe DL5 7PP — BM Soton. 1991. SHO (A & E) Tameside Gen. Hosp. Ashton-under-Lyne. Specialty: Cardiothoracic Surg. Prev: Ho. Off. (Cardiol. & Gen. Med.) Hull Roy. Infirm.; Ho. Off. (Cardiothoracic Med.) North. Gen. Hosp. Sheff.

SUDARSHAN, Gururau 6 Sheldon Grove, Newcastle upon Tyne NE3 4JP — MB BS New Delhi, India 1981; FFA RCSI 1989; FCAnaesth. 1990.

SUDARSHI, Sonali — MB BS Lond. 1998.

SUDBURY, John Roger (retired) Malvern, Cameron Close, Ingatestone CM4 9HA Tel: 01277 356006 — BM BCh Oxf. 1948 (Lond. Hosp.) MA Oxf. 1950, BM BCh 1948; DObst RCOG 1950; MRCP Lond. 1952. Prev: Jun. Med. Regist. & Res. Accouch. Lond. Hosp.

SUDBURY, Peter Russell Wexham Park Hospital, Slough SL2 4HL Tel: 01753 633000 — BM BCh Oxf. 1986; MA Camb. 1985, BA (Natural Sci.) 1982; MRCPsych 1990; MBA Oxf. Brookes 1996. Cons. (Psychiat. & Addic.s) Wexham Pk. Hosp. Slough. Specialty: Gen. Psychiat.; Alcohol & Substance Misuse. Socs: BMA; Soc. Study Addic.

SUDDER, Jennifer Ailsa 9 Battock Terrace, Torphins, Banchory AB31 4JD — MB ChB Aberd. 1997.

SUDDERICK, Mr Robert Malcolm Mount Alvernia Hospital, Harvey Road, Guildford GU1 3LX Tel: 01483 451460 Fax: 01483 451459; Amberley, Grantley Avenue, Wonersh, Guildford GU5 0QN Tel: 01483 898622 — MB BS Lond. 1983; BDS Liverp. 1974; FDS RCS Eng. 1978; FRCS Eng. 1988; FRCS Ed. 1988. Cons. Otolaryngol. Roy. Surrey Co. Hosp. Guildford. Specialty: Otolaryngol. Socs: Brit. Assn. Otol.; BMA; Roy. Soc. Med. Prev: Sen. Regist. (Otolaryngol.) Char. Cross Hosp. Lond. & Mayday Hosp. Croydon; Regist. (Otolaryngol.) Char. Coss Hosp. Lond.; SHO (Otolaryngol.) Univ. Hosp. Qu. Med. Centre Nottm.

SUDDERUDDIN, Ameena Pretoria Road Surgery, 1 Pretoria Road, Leytonstone, London E11 4BB Tel: 020 8539 3232 — MB BS 1972.

SUDDES, Kevin Paul The Coach House, Boycott Manor, Dadford Road, Buckingham MK18 5JZ — MB ChB Leeds 1982.

SUDDICK, Evelyn Mabel (retired) 25 South Drive, Fulwood, Preston PR2 9SR Tel: 01772 862674 — MB ChB Liverp. 1962; DObst RCOG 1964; DTM & H Liverp. 1964. Prev: Community Child Health Doc. Blackpool Wyre, rfylde Community NHS Trust.

SUDDLE, Abid Raza 59 Clarendon Rise, London SE13 5EX — MB BS Lond. 1993.

SUDDLE, Asim Nadeem 75 Old Ford End Road, Bedford MK40 4LY — MB ChB Glas. 1992.

SUDELL, Anthony John Cumbria and Lancashire Strategic Health Authority Tel: 01772 647092 Email: anthony.sudell@clha.nhs.uk — MB BS Lond. 1981 (St. Mary's) MA Oxf. 1983; MSc Manch. 1988; MFPHM 1989. Cons. Pub. Health Med. NW Lancs. HA. Specialty: Pub. Health Med. Prev: Sen. Regist. (Community Med.) N. West. RHA.

SUDELL, Christopher Joseph Meden Vale Medical Centre, Egmanton Road, Meden Vale, Mansfield NG20 9QN Tel: 01623 845694 Fax: 01623 844550; 24 St. Peter's Avenue, Church Warsop, Mansfield NG20 0RZ — MB ChB Sheff. 1986; BSc Lond. 1981. Prev: SHO (O & G) Doncaster Roy. Infirm.; Trainee GP Sheff.; SHO (Paediat.) Childr. Hosp. Sheff.

SUDELL, Joanna Mary The Nightingale Practice, 10 Kennighall Road, London E5 8BY — MB BS Lond. 1985; DRCOG 1988; DCH RCP Lond. 1988; MRCGP 1989.

SUDELL, Raymond Paul Meden Vale Medical Centre, Egmanton Road, Meden Vale, Warsop, Mansfield NG20 9QN Tel: 01623 845694 Fax: 01623 844550 — MB ChB Sheff. 1988; MRCGP 1992.

SUDELL, William Alexander Hamilton Road Surgery, 201 Hamilton Road, Felixstowe IP11 7DT Tel: 01394 283197 — MB BS Lond. 1978 (Guy's) BSc (Hons.) Lond. 1975; MRCS Eng. LRCP Lond. 1978; DRCOG 1982; MSc Glasgow 1991; AFOM RCP Lond. 1992; DFFP 1993; OFFP 1993. Med. Advisor Cranes Fluid Systems. Specialty: Occupat. Health. Socs: BMA; Soc. Occupat. Med. Prev: Trainee GP Brighton VTS; Ho. Phys., Ho. Surg. & SHO (Med. & Cardiol.) Guy's Hosp. Lond.

SUDHA, Immaneni Kanaka Cranham Health Centre, 117 Marlborough Gardens, Upminster RM14 1SR Tel: 01708 222722 Fax: 01708 640961; 45 Viking Way, Brentwood CM15 9HY Tel: 01277 219963 — MB BS Sri Venkateswara 1975 (Sri Venkateswara Univ.) DCH 1986; MRCP (UK) 1987; DRCOG 1987; MRCGP 1990. GP Trainer Upminster; B & H MAAG Co-Chairm.

SUDHAKAR, Chundarathil 27 Norman Avenue, South Croydon CR2 0QH Tel: 020 8660 5393 Fax: 020 8239 92450 — MB BS Andhra 1967 (Andhra Med. Coll. Vizag) GP Tutor S. Croydon; Sen. Tutor (Gen. Pract.) St. Geo. Hosp. Med. Sch. Lond. Prev: SHO (Surg.) St. Chas. Hosp. Lond. & Vict. Hosp. Worksop; SHO (Surg. & Urol.) Kent & Canterbury Hosp.

SUDHAKAR, Mr Joseph Ebenezer Norht Tees General Hosptial, Dept. of Orthopaedics, Hardwick, Stockton-on-Tees TS19 8PE Tel:

01642 617617 Fax: 01642 624902; 2 School Lane, Barbon, Carnforth LA6 2LP Tel: 015242 76388 Fax: 015242 76316 Email: joesudhakar@btinternet.com — MB BS Kerala 1987; FRCS Eng. 1993. Specialist Regist. In Orphopaedic Suregy. Specialty: Orthop. Socs: BMA; BOA; MDU.

SUDHAKAR, K St John's Surgery, 2 Greenfield Walk, Huyton, Liverpool L36 0XP Tel: 0151 489 9067.

SUDHAKAR, Madhwapathi c/o Department of Anaesthetics, Prince Charles Hospital, Merthyr Tydfil CF47 9DT — MD BS Sri Venkateswara 1986.

SUDHAKAR RAO, Settipalli 17 Applewood Close, St Leonards-on-Sea TN37 7JS — MB BS Osmania 1980.

SUDHAKARAN, Nadarajan 21 Westbourne Gardens, Hove BN3 5PL — MB BCh Wales 1995.

SUDHEER, Kondaveeti 4 Thompson Close, Folkestone CT19 5UA — MB BS Sri Venkateswara 1973.

SUDLOW, Catherine Lucy Moore Department of Clinical Neurosciences, University of Edinburgh, Western General Hospital, Edinburgh EH4 2XU — BM BCh Oxf. 1991; BA (Hons.) Med. Sci. Camb. 1988; MRCP (UK) 1994; MSc (Epidemiol.) Lond. 1997. Wellcome Clin. Scientist. Specialty: Neurol.; Epidemiol. Socs: Steering Comm. - Antithrombotic Ther. Trialists Collaboration; Assn. Brit. Neurols.; Cochrane Stroke Gp. Prev: Hon. Regist. (Neurol.) Radcliffe Infirm. NHS Trust, Oxf.; Regist. (Med. Neurol.) West. Gen. Hosp. Edin.; Regist. (Gen. Med.) Worthing Hosp. W. Sussex.

SUDLOW, Elizabeth Mary 58 Craigleith View, Edinburgh EH4 3JY Tel: 0131 337 2022 — MB BS Lond. 1964 (St. Thos.) SCMO Lothian Region Family Plann. Serv.; Clin. Asst. Colposcopy Unit Roy. Infirm. Edin. Prev: Ho. Surg. St. Thos. Hosp. Lond.; Ho. Phys. N. Staffs. Roy. Infirm. Stoke-on-Trent.

SUDLOW, Michael Frederick 58 Craigleith View, Edinburgh EH4 3JY Tel: 0131 337 2022 — MB BS Lond. 1964 (St. Thos.) FRCP Lond. 1983, M 1967; FRCP Ed. 1982. Cons. Phys. & Hon. Sen. Lect. (Med.) Roy. Infirm. Edin. Specialty: Gen. Med.; Respirat. Med. Prev: Ho. Phys. St. Thos. Hosp. Lond.; Ho. Surg. Qu. Eliz. Hosp. Birm.

SUDLOW, Mr Robin Andrew 82 Burnham Road, Leigh-on-Sea SS9 2JS — MB BS Lond. 1972 (Lond. Hosp.) FRCS Eng. 1979. Cons. Orthop. Surg. Southend Gen. Hosp. Specialty: Orthop. Socs: Fell. Brit. Orthop. Assn.; Fell. Roy. Soc. of Med. Prev: Lect. The Lond. Hosp.; Sen. Regist. (Orthop.) Notley Hosp.; Sen. Regist. Roy. Nat. Orthop. Hosp. Lond.

SUDLOW, Sheila Ludham Surgery, Staithe Road, Ludham, Great Yarmouth NR29 5AB Tel: 01692 678611 Fax: 01692 678295; Rosecroft, Church Road, Catfield, Great Yarmouth NR29 5AX Tel: 01692 580646 — MB ChB Manch. 1977; DRCOG 1979; MRCGP 1981. Prev: GP Stalham.

SUE-LING, Mr Henry Michael Leeds General Infirmary, Great George St., Leeds LS1 3EX Tel: 01132 923467 Fax: 01132 923635; St Catherine's, College Farm Lane, Linton, Wetherby LS22 4HR — MB ChB Leeds 1980; MD Leeds 1986; FRCS Glas. 1986; FRCS Eng. 1987. Cons. Surg. Leeds Gen. Infirmay. Specialty: Gen. Surg. Socs: BMA; Assn. Surg.; Brit. Soc. Gastroenterol.

SUEKE, Henri Morris St George's Hospital, Blackshaw Road, London SW17 0QT Email: hsueke@hotmail.com — MB ChB Liverp. 2002; BSc (Hons.) Liverp. 2001; MRCOphth (Part 1) Lond. 2004. SHO (Neurosurg.) St Geo. Hosp. Lond.

SUETT, Mark James Crantock, Westgate, Bridgnorth WV16 5BL — MB ChB Birm. 1997.

SUFFERN, Margaret Alison (retired) 6 Cundall Way, Harrogate HG2 0DY Tel: 01423 503142 — MB ChB Leeds 1943. Prev: Matern. & Child Welf. Off. Leeds.

SUFFERN, Walter Sefton (retired) 6 Cundall Way, Harrogate HG2 0DY Tel: 01423 503142 — MB ChB Leeds 1942; MRCS Eng. LRCP Lond. 1942; MD Leeds 1947; FRCP Lond. 1970, M 1948. Prev: Cons. Phys. Harrogate Gen. Hosp. & Ripon Hosp.

SUFFIELD, Mervyn John Trinity Care, 15 Musters Road, West Bridgeford, Nottingham NG2 7PP Tel: 01159 455485; The Cottage, Winchester Road, Waltham Chase, Southampton SO32 2LG — MB BS Newc. 1975. Dir. of Care. Specialty: Gen. Pract.; Occupat. Health. Socs: Coll. Occup. Health. Prev: Princip. Gen. Pract. Occupat. Health Specialty.

***SUFFLING, Hannah** — MB ChB Bristol 1998. HO. (Gen Med & Neuro) Roy Devon & Exeter Hosp. Specialty: Gen. Surg.

SUFFLING, Norford John (retired) 20 Spur Hill Avenue, Parkstone, Poole BH14 9PH — (St. Thos.) MB BS Lond. 1963; DPM Eng. 1973; MRCPsych 1975; FRCPsych 1998. Prev: Cons. Psychiat. E. Dorset Health Dist.

SUFRAZ, Reshad Bowden House Clinic, London Road, Harrow HA1 3JL Tel: 020 8966 7000 Fax: 020 8864 6092 — MB BS Lond. 1988 (Univ. Coll. Hosp.) BSc Lond. 1985; MRCPsych 1994; MA (Clin. Psychol.) Pepperdine 1996. Assoc. Specialist (Psychiat.) Bowden Ho. Clinic Harrow; Resid. Med. Off. Bowden Ho. Clinic. Specialty: Gen. Psychiat. Socs: BMA; MPS; Roy. Coll. Psychiats.

SUGANTHI, Damal Pathangi London Road Medical Centre, Cavendish House, 515 London Road, Thornton Heath CR7 6AR Tel: 0208 2399002 Fax: 0208 2399003; 8 Sprucedale Gardens, Shirley, Croydon CR0 5HU Tel: 0208 654 5049 — MB BS Madras 1964; MRCOG 1974, DObst 1967. Clin. Asst. (Obst.) Mayday Hosp. Thornton Heath Surrey. Socs: Fell. Roy. Soc. Med.; BMA. Prev: SHO (O & G) Beckenham Matern. Hosp., Greenwich Dist. Hosp. & Lewisham Gp. Hosps.

SUGARMAN, Philip Ashley St Andrew's Group of Hospitals, Billing Road, Northampton NN1 5DG — MB ChB Liverp. 1983; MRCPsych 1987; MSc Manch. 1990. Med. Dir. St Andrew's Gp. Hosps. Specialty: Forens. Psychiat. Prev: Cons. Forens. Psychiat. Invicta Community Care NHS Trust; Regional Adviser Forens. Psychiat. S. E. Region NHS Exec.; Sen. Regist. Reaside Clinic Birm.

SUGARMAN, Mr Philip Morris 3 Leamington Avenue, Manchester M20 2WQ — MB BS Lond. 1988; BSc Lond. 1985, MB BS 1988; FRCS Ed. 1994. Specialist Regist. (A&E) Mersey Deanery. Specialty: Accid. & Emerg.

SUGARS, Kenneth Hugh, Surg. Capt. RN Retd. 11 Waudby Close, Walkington, Beverley HU17 8SA Tel: 01482 861056 — MB ChB Ed. 1965; MRCGP 1971. Company Med. Off. BAE Systems Brough and Clariant UK Beverley. Specialty: Occupat. Health. Socs: Soc. Occupat. Med. Prev: Dir. Med. Personnel Med. Directorate Gen. (Naval); Adviser Gen. Pract. to Med. Dir. Gen. (Navy).

SUGDEN, Mr Brian Anthony 8 Balcomie Crescent, Troon KA10 7AR Tel: 01292 311009 — MB BS Newc. 1970; FRCS Glas. 1976. Cons. Surg. CrossHo. Hosp. Kilmarnock. Specialty: Gen. Surg.

SUGDEN, Brian David Sugden and Ndirika, The Health Centre, Curtis Street, Hucknall, Nottingham NG15 7JE Tel: 0115 963 3580 Fax: 0115 963 3733 — MB BS Lond. 1973; MRCGP 1977. GP Hucknall; Clin. Tutor Gen. Pract. Univ. Nottm.

SUGDEN, Christopher John St Andrew's Hospice, Henderson Street, Airdrie ML6 6DJ Tel: 01236 766957 Fax: 01236 748786; 59 Lubnaig Road, Newlands, Glasgow G43 2RX — MB ChB Aberd. 1976; FFA RCS Eng. 1980. Med. Dir. St. And.Hospice Airdrie Lanarksh.; Cons. Anaesth. Lanarksh. Acute Hosp.s NHS Trust. Specialty: Palliat. Med.; Anaesth. Prev: Cons. Anaesth. S. Gen. Hosp. NHS Trust.

SUGDEN, Elaine Margaret Department of Clinical Oncology, Churchill Hospital, Oxford OX3 7LJ Tel: 01865 225659; 36 North Hinksey Village, Oxford OX2 0NA Tel: 01865 728128 — BM BCh Oxf. 1972; MA Oxf. 1972; DCH Eng. 1975; FCR Eng 1975; FRCR England 1990. Cons in Clin. Onocol. Specialty: Oncol.; Radiother.

SUGDEN, Jacqueline Janet Chenies, Lakeview Road, Furnace Wood, Felbridge, East Grinstead RH19 2QB — BM Soton. 1995.

SUGDEN, Joanna Helen Rosedale, Bluntisham Rd, Colne, Huntingdon PE28 3LY — BChir Camb. 1996; MB BChir Camb. 1996; DTM & H Liverp 1998. GP Regist. Foundry La. Surg. Leeds. Specialty: Gen. Pract. Prev: SHO (Rheumat.) Leeds United Teachg. Hosps.; SHO (A&E) S. Manch. Univ. Hosps. Trust; Ho. Off. (Gen. Surg.) Ipswich Hosp.

SUGDEN, John Christopher Hawthorne Farm, Little Fenton, South Milford, Leeds LS25 6HF Tel: 0193781 7462 — MB ChB Leeds 1968; BSc (Hons.) Leeds 1965; MB ChB (Hons.) Leeds 1968; FFA RCS Eng. 1972. Cons. Anaesth. Leeds Gen. Infirm. & Sen. Clin. Lect. Univ. Leeds. Specialty: Anaesth.

SUGDEN, John Harrison (retired) Hingabank Farm, Deepdale Dent, Sedbergh LA10 5RD — MB ChB St. And. 1963; DPM Leeds 1974. Prev: Regist. (Psychiat.) Lynfield Mt. Hosp. Bradford.

SUGDEN, John Samuel 50 Totley Brook Road, Dore, Sheffield S17 3QT — MRCS Eng. LRCP Lond. 1954; DObst RCOG 1957; MRCGP 1965.

SUGDEN, Kenneth Heaver (retired) Holly Bank, Rogues Hill, Penshurst, Tonbridge TN11 8BQ — MRCS Eng. LRCP Lond. 1936 (St. Bart.) MRCS Eng., LRCP Lond. 1936. Prev: Asst. Co. Med. Off.

SUGDEN, Kenneth John (retired) Cruckend Cottage, 15 The Island, Upper Tean, Stoke-on-Trent ST10 4JE Tel: 01538 723962 Email: jsbrbkbuff@aol.com — (St. Bart.) MB BS Lond. 1959; MRCS Eng. LRCP Lond. 1959; DObst RCOG 1963; Cert FPA 1974. Prev: Managing Dir. On Call Ltd.

SUGDEN, Paul Elliot 52 Pirie Road, Congleton CW12 2EF — MB ChB Manch. 1994.

SUGG, David James Berriedale, Mayfield Lane, Wadhurst TN5 6JE Tel: 01892 782959 — MB ChB Manch. 1988; DRCOG 1991; MRCGP 1996. Prev: GP/Regist. HildenBoro. Med. Gp. Tonbridge; GP Kawana Waters 7 Day Med. Centre Minyama Queensland, Austral.; SHO (A & E & ENT) Roy. Preston Hosp.

SUGGETT, Nigel Ross 2 Fernwoods, Bartley Green, Birmingham B32 3RL — BM BCh Oxf. 1994; FRCS (Eng.) 1998. Specialist Regist. (Gen. Surg.) W. Midl. Rotat. Specialty: Gen. Surg. Prev: SHO Rotat. (Surg.) Birm. Heartlands Hosp.; SHO (Gen. Surg.) Sandwell Gen. Hosp.; SHO (Gen. Surg.) Qu.'s Hosp., Burton-on-Trent.

SUGHRA, Ghulam 19 Surig Road, Canvey Island SS8 9EP Tel: 01268 695331 — MB BS Punjab 1971.

SUGRUE, Mr Denis Lambert (retired) 2 Fieldway, Trentham, Stoke-on-Trent ST4 8AQ Tel: 01782 657953 — (Univ. Coll. Dub.) MCh NUI 1953, MB BCh BAO 1950; DLO Eng. 1953. Prev: Cons. Phys. Genitourin. Med. N. Staffs Hosp. Centre & Dist. Gen. Hosps.Stafford.

SUGUMAR, Kanagalingam 27 Hamond Close, South Croydon CR2 6BZ — LRCP LRCS Ed. LRCPS Glas. 1995.

SUGUNAKARA RAO, Mr Yalamanchili Venkata Krishna 8 Bronte Close, Kettering NN16 9XN — FRCSI 1984; FRCS Glas. 1984.

SUHAIL, Mohammed 6 Reaper Crescent, Highgreen, Sheffield S35 3FH — MB ChB Dundee 1993.

SUHARWARDY, John Mohammed Ally Eye Department, Royal Oldham Hospital, Rochdale Road, Oldham OL1 2JM Tel: 0161 627 8192 Fax: 0161 627 8478 — MB ChB Manch. 1986 (Univ. of Manch.) FRCOphth 1990; MD 2001. Cons. Ophth. Pennine Acute Trust (Oldham). Specialty: Ophth. Special Interest: Gloucoma; Small Incision Cataract Surg. Prev: Sen. Regist., Birm. & Midl. (W. Midlands) Eye Centre.

SUKHIA, Viraf Dara 6 Fulmer Way, London W13 9XQ Tel: 020 8840 4259 — MB BS Poona 1966 (B.J. Med. Coll.) DObst RCOG 1968; DCH Eng. 1969. Prev: Regist. (Paediat.) King Edwd. Hosp. Ealing & Perivale Matern. Hosp.; SHO Paediat. Soton. Childr. Hosp.; SHO Neonat. Paediat. Whittington Hosp. Lond.

SUKUMAR, Pathmajani Dove Dale, 22 Over Hill Road, Wilmslow Park, Wilmslow SK9 2BE Tel: 01625 539659 — LMSSA Lond. 1993. SHO (c/o the Elderly) Univ. Hosp. S. Manch.; GP Regist. Specialty: Gen. Pract. Prev: SHO (Paediat.) Macclesfield D.G.H.

SUKUMARAN, Suparna 149 Saltram Crescent, London W9 3JT Tel: 020 8960 6771 — MB ChB Liverp. 1989; DCCH RCGP 1993; MRCPsych 1996. Cons. Child & Adolesc. Psyhiatrist W. Lond. Ment. Health Trust. Specialty: Child & Adolesc. Psychiat. Socs: BMA; Roy. Soc. of Med. Prev: SHO & Regist. Rotat. (Psychiat.) UMDS Lond.; SHO Rotat. (Paediat.) Char. Cross & Westm. Hosps. Lond.; SHO Rotat. (Med.) Roy. Liverp. Hosp.

SUKUMARAN, Suryagopal Obulisamy The Frank Swire Health Centre, Nursery Lane, Ovenden, Halifax HX3 5TE Tel: 01422 355535 — MB BS Madras 1970; DCH RCPSI 1977; JCPTGP Lond. 1982; MFCH Lond. 1989. GP. Specialty: Gen. Pract.; Paediat. Socs: Med. Protec. Soc.; Fac. Community Health.

SUKUMARAN NAIR, Cheripadi Lakshmi, Park Farm Villas, South Newsham, Blyth NE24 4HA — MB BS Mysore 1974 (Kasturba Med. Coll.) BSc, MB BS Mysore 1974. SHO Wharfedale Gen. Hosp. Otley. Prev: SHO (Med.) Gen. Hosp. Chester-le-St.; SHO (Geriat.) Wharfedale Gen. Hosp. Otley.

SUKUMARAN NAIR, Parameswara Kurup Frimley Park Hospital NHS Trust, Portsmouth Road, Frimley, Camberley GU15 5UJ Tel: 01276 604604; 13 Falmouth Close, Camberley GU15 1EA — MB BS Kerala 1974; DCH RCPSI 1985; Dip. Thoracic Med. Lond 1988; Dip. Respirat. Med. RCPSI 1989. Staff Grade (Paediat. Med.) Frimley Pk. Hosp. NHS Trust. Specialty: Paediat.; Respirat. Med.

SUKUMARAN NAIR, Sethulekshmy Frimley Park Hospital NHS Trust, Portsmouth Road, Frimley, Camberley GU16 7UJ; 13 Falmouth Close, Camberley GU15 1EA — MB BS Kerala 1974; MD Kerala 1979; MRCOG 1991; FRCOG 2003. Staff Gyn. & Obst. Frimley Pk. Hosp. NHS Trust.

SULAIMAN, H M Riverside Centre for Health, Park Street, Liverpool L8 6QP Tel: 0151 706 8306.

SULAIMAN, Mohamed Zubayr Careem Gloucestershire Royal Hospital, Department of Genitourinary Medicine, Great Western Road, Gloucester GL1 3NL Tel: 01452 394462 Fax: 01452 394466; 3 Ellesmere Grove, Cheltenham GL50 2QQ Tel: 01242 252576 — MB ChB St And. 1972; FRCOG 1996, M 1981. Cons. Phys. (Genitourin. Med. & HIV Med.) Glos.; Cons. Phys. (Genitourin. Med. & HIV Med.) Cheltenham. Specialty: Genitourinary Medicine. Socs: Brit. Soc. Colpos. & Cerv. Path.; Brit. Assn. of Sexual Health & HIV. Prev: Cons. Phys. (Genitourin. Med.) Gt. Yarmouth & Waveney HA; Sen. Regist. (Genitourin. Med.) Roy. Hallamsh. Hosp. Sheff. & Gen. Hosp. Nottm.

SULAIMAN, Mr Shah Khalid Dept of Orthopaedic, Walsall Manor Hospital NHS Trust, Moat Rd, Walsall WS2 9PS; 160 The Mall, Fendon, Pinner HA5 9TH — MB BS Karachi 1977; FRCS (Orth); MRCS Eng. LRCP Lond. 1979; FRCS Ed. 1982. Cons (Orthop) Surg. Specialty: Orthop. Socs: BFO; BMA.

SULAIMAN, Syed Ayaz Lutfi 49 Castle Road, Colne BB8 7AR — MB ChB Liverp. 1997.

SULAIMAN, Syed Mahmood Urfi 49 Castle Road, Colne BB8 7AR — MB ChB Leeds 1992.

SULAIVANY, Taha-Ismail Abbo Ground Floor Flat, 123 Hamilton Place, Aberdeen AB15 5BD — MB ChB Mosul 1978; MRCP (UK) 1989; MRCPI 1989.

SULCH, David Antony 1 Winston Drive, Isham, Kettering NN14 1HS — MB BS Lond. 1986.

SULE, Bamidele Adebola 129 Mowbray Road, Cambridge CB1 7SP — MB ChB Obafemi Awolowu U, Nigeria 1984.

SULE, Hem Dattatray Moss Side Medical Centre, 16 Moss Side Way, Leyland, Preston PR26 7XL Tel: 01772 466004 Fax: 01772 622897 — MB BS Jiwaji 1968.

SULE, Kuldip Kaur 163 Dunstable Road, Luton LU1 1BW — MB BS Lond. 1986; MRCGP 1992.

SULE, Sulabha Hem Moss Side Medical Centre, 16 Moss Side Way, Leyland, Preston PR26 7XL Tel: 01772 466004 Fax: 01772 622897 — MB BS Jiwaji 1970; MRCOG 1984.

SULE SUSO, Josep Staffordshire Oncology Centre, North Staffs Hospital Trust, Princes Road, Stoke-on-Trent ST4 7LN; 80 Dartmouth Avenue, Westlands, Newcastle ST5 3PA — LMS Autonoma Barcelona 1988. Clin. Asst. (Oncol.) Staffs. Oncol. Centre N. Staffs. Hosp. Trust. Specialty: Oncol.; Radiother. Prev: Research Fell. (Experim. Oncol.) Nat. Cancer Inst. Milan, Italy; SHO (Oncol. Radiolther.) N. Staffs Roy. Infirm. Stoke-on-Trent.

SULEMAN, Abdulrahim Eaglestone Health Centre, Standing Way, Eaglestone, Milton Keynes MK6 5AZ Tel: 01908 679111 Fax: 01908 230601 — MB BCh Wales 1972; DObst RCOG 1974.

SULEMAN, Adil Shabaz — MB ChB Dundee 1994; MRCGP 1999. Specialty: Gen. Pract.

SULEMAN, Mohammad Ishaque Manor Park Medical Centre, High St., Polegate BN26 5DJ Tel: 01323 482301 Fax: 01323 484848; 7 Weatherby Close, Park Lane, Eastbourne BN21 2XB Tel: 01323 502041 — MB BS Karachi 1961 (Dow. Med. Coll.) Hosp. Pract. Diabetic & Cardiac Clinics Dist. Gen. Hosp. Eastbourne. Specialty: Cardiol.; Diabetes. Socs: BMA; E.bourne Med. Soc. Prev: Regist. (Med.) Eastbourne Hosp. Gp.; SHO (Med. & Paediat.) St. Helen's Hosp. Hastings; Ho. Off. (Paediat.) Evelina Childr. Hosp. Guy's Hosp. Lond.

SULEMAN, Mohammed Hanif Jamal 10 Poole Street, Blackburn BB1 3JS — MB ChB Sheff. 1998.

SULEMAN, Mr Shamshudeen Karmali Epsom General Hospital, Epsom KT8 7EG Tel: 01372 735735 Fax: 01372 745351 — LRCPI & LM, LRSCI & LM 1958; FRCS Ed. 1965; FFAEM 1996. Cons. A & E Med. Epsom Gen. Hosp. Specialty: Accid. & Emerg. Socs: RSM Fell.; BAEM Fell. Prev: Sen. Orthop. Specialist MoH Kenya; Assoc. Prof. Orthop. Univ. Agakhan Karachi, Pakistan.

SULEMAN, Subeena Tubussum 99 Thornbury Road, Birmingham B20 3DE — MB ChB Glas. 1997.

SULEMAN, Zora 78 Third Avenue, Bordesley Green, Birmingham B9 5RL — MB ChB Leeds 1994.

SULH, Jaswinder Singh 18 Sussex Place, Slough SL1 1NR — MB ChB Manch. 1987; DCH RCP Lond. 1991; DRCOG 1992; MRCGP 1993.

SULIMAN, Abdel Moneim Hussein Cardiology Department, Newham General Hospital, Glen Road, Plaistow, London E13 8SL Tel: 020 7476 4000 Fax: 020 7363 8350; 239 Prince Regent Lane, Plaistow, London E13 8SD Tel: 020 7474 7307 — MB BS Khartoum 1976; MB BS Khartoum Sudan 1976; DTCD Wales 1984; MSc Cardiovasc. Studies Leeds 1988; MRCPI 1989.

SULIMAN, Mohamed El Ghazali Rahmtalla The Endocrine Unit, Q Floor, Royal Hallamshire Hospital, Glossop Road, Sheffield S10 2JF — MB BS Khartoum 1985; MRCP (UK) 1993.

SULKE, Alfred Neil Eastbourne General Hospital, Department of Cardiology, Kings Drive, Eastbourne BN21 2UB Tel: 01323 423747 — BM Soton. 1983; BSc (Hons. Biochem.) Sussex 1977; MRCP (UK) 1986; DM Soton. 1991; FACC 1995; UMDS 1995; FRCP 2000; FESC 2004. Cons. (Cardiol.) Eastbourne Gen. Hosp. & St. Thos. Hosp. Lond. Specialty: Cardiol. Socs: Brit. Pacing & Electrophysiol. Gp.; N. Amer. Soc. Pacing & Electrophys.; Fell. Amer. Coll. Cardiol. Prev: Hon. Sen Lect. (Teacher) Univ of Lond.; Sen. Regist. (Cardiol.) Guy's Hosp. Lond.; Research Regist. & Regist. (Cardiol.) Guy's Hosp. Lond.

SULLIVAN, Angela Jane Northcroft Surgery, Northcroft Lane, Newbury RG14 1BU Tel: 01635 31575 Fax: 01635 551857; Frogmill, Pound Lane, Burghclere, Newbury RG20 9JR Tel: 01635 278541 — MB ChB Leeds 1975; DRCOG 1977; DCH Eng. 1978; MRCP (UK) 1980; MRCGP 1983. Prev: Regist. (Gen. Med.) Roy. Berks. Hosp. Reading; SHO (Med.) Radcliffe Infirm. Oxf.; SHO (O & G) & (Paediat.) Soton. Gen. Hosp.

SULLIVAN, Anita Louise Lung Investigation Unit, 1st Floor Nuffield House, Queen Elizabeth Hospital, Edgbaston, Birmingham B15 2TH — MB ChB Manch. 1994.

SULLIVAN, Ann Kathleen 264 Trinity Road, London SW18 3RQ — MB BS Tasmania 1988; MRCP (UK) 1995; Dip GU Med 2001.

SULLIVAN, Anne Cestria Health Centre, Whitehill Way, Chester-le-Street DH2 3DJ Tel: 0191 388 7771 Fax: 0191 387 1803; 173 Gilesgate, Durham DH1 1QH — MB BS Lond. 1971; MRCS Eng. LRCP Lond. 1971; DObst RCOG 1973.

SULLIVAN, Brendan Anthony St. Georges Lodge, 123 Fronks Road, Dovercourt, Harwich CO12 4EF Tel: 01255 502909 — MB Camb. 1978; MA Camb. 1978, MB 1978, BChir 1977; MLCOM 1989.

SULLIVAN, Brian Anthony Pantysgawen Farm, Thornhill Road, Cardiff CF14 9UA Tel: 029 2062 3054 — MB BCh Wales 1974; FRCR 1979. Cons. Radiol. Roy. Gwent Hosp. Newport. Specialty: Radiol. Socs: Brit. Soc. Skeletal Radiol.; Eur. Soc. Skeletal Radiol.; Brit. Soc. Interven. Radiol.

SULLIVAN, Carol Linda Singleton Hospital, Sketty, Swansea SA2 8QA Tel: 01792 205666 Fax: 01792 285244; 15 Roger Beck Way, Sketty, Swansea SA2 0JF — BM BCh Oxf. 1987; BA (Hons.) Oxf. 1984; MRCP (UK) 1991; FRCPCH 1997. Cons. Paediat. Singleton Hosp. Swansea. Specialty: Paediat. Prev: Sen. Regist. (Paediat.) Nottm. & Derby Hosps.; Regist. (Paediat.) Bristol & Exeter; SHO (Paediat. Cardiol.) Childr. Hosp. Birm.

SULLIVAN, Caroline Frances 18 Midland Avenue, Nottingham NG7 2FD — MB ChB Liverp. 1982; MRCPsych 1987.

SULLIVAN, Caroline Mary 481C Hulloway Road, London N19 4DD Tel: 020 7272 8004 — MB ChB Manch. 1996. SHO (A & E) UCLH Lond.

SULLIVAN, Charles Anthony (retired) 35 Urney Road, Strabane BT82 9DA — LAH Dub. 1951.

SULLIVAN, Charlotte Anne Flat 3 Balmoral Court, 1 Scotland Street, Birmingham B1 2RU — MB BS Lond. 1992 (St. George's Hosp. Med. Sch. Lond.) BSc (Hons.) Lond. 1991; FRCOphth 1996. Specialist Regist. (Ophth.). Specialty: Ophth. Socs: Fell. Roy. Coll. Of Ophthal.

SULLIVAN, Christine June The Health Centre, 80 Knaresborough Road, Harrogate HG2 7LU Tel: 01423 883212; 6 Stone Rings Close, Harrogate HG2 9HZ Tel: 01423 872737 — MB ChB Bristol 1978; DRCOG 1981.

SULLIVAN, Christobel Jean 5 Elston Hall, Elston, Newark NG23 5NP Tel: 01636 525657 — MB BS Lond. 1965; MRCS Eng. LRCP Lond. 1965; MB BS (Hons. Surg.) Lond. 1965. Asst. Specialist Dermat. Grantham Hosp. & INCS. Specialty: Dermat. Socs: Lincoln Med. Soc. Prev: GP Newark; Hon. Surg. Newmarket Gen. Hosp.; Hon. Phys. Brit. Milit. Hosp. Singapore.

SULLIVAN, Dorothy Beatrice House 4, Cauedside Farm, Steading, St Andrews KY16 9TY — MB ChB Glas. 1980; DRCOG 1985; MRCGP 1987; MSc (Med. Sci.) Glas. 1997. GP Princip.

SULLIVAN, Francis Michael Blantyre Health Centre, Victoria St., Blantyre, Glasgow G72 0BS Tel: 0141826331; 124 Kylepark Drive, Uddingston, Glasgow G71 7DE — MB ChB Glas. 1980; MB ChB (Hons.) Glas. 1980; MRCP (UK) 1983; MRCGP 1984; PhD (Clin. Epidemiol.) Glas. 1991; FRCP Glas. 1994. Sen. Lect. (Gen. Pract.) Glas. Prev: Lect. (Gen. Pract.) Univ. Glas.; Cons. Phys. Seychelles.

SULLIVAN, Frederick Donald The Fountain Medical Centre, Sherwood Avenue, Newark NG24 1QH; 5 Elston Hall, Top St., Elston, Newark NG23 5NP — MB BS Lond. 1964 (Westm.) MRCS Eng. LRCP Lond. 1964; DA Eng. 1966; FFA RCS Eng. 1971. Specialty: Anaesth. Socs: Assn. Anaesths. Prev: Sen. Regist. (Anaesth.) N. Staffs. Gp. Hosps.; Specialist in Anaesth. RAF; Ho. Phys. Westm. Hosp. Lond.

SULLIVAN, Gary St. Tydfil's Hospital, Merthyr Tydfil CF47 0SJ Tel: 01685 723244 — MB BCh Wales 1982 (Univ. Wales Coll. Med.) MRCGP 1987; MRCPsych 1993; MSc (Psychiat.) Wales 1996; MD Wales 2003. Cons. Psychiat., N. Glam. NHS Trust, St. Tydfil's Hosp., Merthyr Tydfil; Clin. Director, Ment. Health, N. Glam. NHS Trust. Specialty: Gen. Psychiat. Socs: Brit. Assn. of Med. Managers; BHSM.

SULLIVAN, Geoffrey (retired) 16 Kingsway, Penwortham, Preston PR1 0AP Tel: 01772 742365 — MB ChB Manch. 1950. Prev: Cons. Radiol. Preston & Chorley.

SULLIVAN, Graham Howell (retired) 2 Freemantle Road, Leicester LE2 2EL Tel: 0116 270 5276 — (St. Mary's) MB BS Lond. 1952. Prev: Jun. Specialist Dermat. RAMC.

SULLIVAN, Jillian Valerie Health Clinic, 407 Main Road, Dovercourt, Harwich CO12 4ET Tel: 01255 201299 Fax: 01255 201270; St. Georges Lodge, 123 Fronks Road, Dovercourt, Harwich CO12 4EF — MB BS Lond. 1976; MRCS Eng. LRCP Lond. 1976; DRCOG 1979.

SULLIVAN, John Marcus Moorside Surgery, 1 Thornbridge Mews, Bradford BD2 3BL Tel: 01274 626691 — MB ChB Leeds 1987; DRCOG 1991; MRCGP 1992; T(GP) 1992. Prev: Trainee GP Bradford VTS.

SULLIVAN, Mr Jonathan Gerald Bristol Urological Institute, Southmead Hospital, Bristol BS10 5NB; 9 Julian Road, Sneyd Park, Bristol BS9 1NQ Tel: 0117 962 6130 — MB BS Lond. 1989 (Kings Coll. Hosp. Lond.) FRCS Eng. 1995. Specialist Regist. (Urol.) Southmead Hosp. Bristol. Specialty: Urol. Prev: SHO (Gen. Surg./Urol.) Cheltenham Gen. Hosp.; SHO (Urol.) Inst. of Urol. Middlx. Hosp. Lond.

SULLIVAN, Marianne Antoinette Louise The Practice Of Health, 31 Barry Road, Barry CF63 1BA Tel: 01446 700350 Fax: 01446 420795; Home Farm, Sully, Penarth CF64 5UF Tel: 01222 530263 — MB BCh Wales 1975; Cert. Family Plann. JCC 1977. Socs: Barry Med. Soc.

SULLIVAN, Mark Lemon Street Surgery, 18 Lemon Street, Truro TR1 2LZ Tel: 01872 73133 Fax: 01872 260900; 2 Creekside View, Tresiscllan, Truro TR2 4BS Tel: 01326 240123 — MB ChB Birm. 1976; MRCGP 1987; MFHom 1991. GP; Homoeop. Phys. Cornw. Specialty: Gen. Pract. Socs: BMA. Prev: GP Mullion Cornw.; SHO (Med.) Walsgrave Hosp. Coventry; SHO (Obst.) Roy. Cornw. Hosp. Truro.

SULLIVAN, Mr Mark Edward 40 The Avenue, Worminghall, Aylesbury HP18 9LE — MB BS Lond. 1989; FRCS Ed. 1993.

SULLIVAN, Martin James Kingsway Surgery, 37 The Kingsway, Swansea SA1 5LP Tel: 01792 650716 Fax: 01792 456902 — BM Soton. 1994; DRCOG 1997; MRCGP 1998. GP Princip. Kingsway Surg. Swansea. Specialty: Gen. Pract. Socs: Chairm. Gt.er Swansea GP Co-op. Prev: GP Regist. Kingsway Surg. Swansea.

SULLIVAN, Mr Michael Francis Consulting Rooms, The Princess Grace Hospital, 42-52 Nottingham Place, London W1U 5NY Tel: 020 7486 4970 Fax: 020 7935 5467; 12 Gloucester Crescent, London NW1 7DS Tel: 020 7485 4473 Email: mfsullivan@aol.com — (Camb. & St. Mary's) MB Camb. 1962, BChir 1961; MRCS Eng. LRCP Lond. 1961; FRCS Eng. 1967. Cons. Orthop. Surg. Roy. Nat.

Orthop. Hosp. Lond. Specialty: Orthop. Socs: Fell. (Counc.) BOA; BMA; (Pres.) Europ. Spine Soc.

SULLIVAN, Michael John Llwyn Brwydrau Surgery, 3 Frederick Place, Llansamlet, Swansea SA7 9RY Tel: 01792 771465 Email: michael.j.sullivan@gp.w98005.wales.nhs.uk — MB BCh Wales 1979; DRCOG 1983. Exam. Med. Off. & Exam. Med. Phys. DHSS. Socs: BMA.

SULLIVAN, Navina 2A Jennings Road, St Albans AL1 4NT — MB ChB Natal 1989; MSc (Mother & Child Health) Lond. 1992; DCH RCPI 1994. Socs: BMA. Prev: Trainee GP/SHO (Gen. Med.) Princess Alexandra Hosp. Harlow; Regist. (O & G) S. Afr.

SULLIVAN, Paul Andrew Sullivan, Jones, Evans and Deignan, Ringland Health Centre, Ringland Circle, Newport NP19 9PS Tel: 01633 277011 Fax: 01633 290706 — MB BS Lond. 1982 (St. Mary's Hosp. Lond.) MRCGP 1987; Dip Ther 1999. Specialty: Gen. Pract.

SULLIVAN, Paul Major Patrick Moorfield Eye Hospital, London EC1V 2PD; 5 Tolmers Ave, Cuffley, Potters Bar EN6 4QE — MB BS Lond. 1984; MD Lond. 1991; FCOphth 1992. Cons. Moorfields Eye Hosp. Lond. Specialty: Ophth. Socs: Brit. Diabetic Assn.; Brit. Ophth. Photogr. Assn. Prev: Sen. Regist. & Fell. Moorfields Eye Hosp. Lond.; Regist. Soton. Eye Hosp.; Research Fell. Hammersmith Hosp. Lond.

SULLIVAN, Peter Bernard Department of Paediatrics, John Radcliffe Hospital, Oxford OX3 9DU Tel: 01865 220934 Fax: 01865 220479 — MB ChB Manch. 1980; DRCOG 1984; FRCP Lond. 1997, M (UK) 1985; BSc Manch. 1975, MD 1991; MA Oxf. 1994; FRCPCH 1997. Univ. Lect. & Hon. Cons. Paediat. John Radcliffe Hosp. Oxf. Specialty: Paediat.; Gastroenterol. Socs: Brit. Soc. Paediat. Gastroenterol. & Paediat. Research Soc.; Eur. Soc. Paediat. Gastroenterol. & Nutrit.; Pres. Commonw. Assn. Paediat. Gastroenterol. & Nutrit. Prev: Sen. Lect. (Paediat.) Chinese Univ., Hong Kong; Lect. (Child Health) Char. Cross & Westm. Med. Sch. Lond.; Clin. Research Fell. Dunn Nutrit. Laborat. Univ. Camb.

SULLIVAN, Peter Michael (retired) Ballyferriter, 81 Compton Road, Wolverhampton WV3 9QH Tel: 01902 423047 — MB ChB Birm. 1953. Prev: GP Bilston W. Midl.s.

SULLIVAN, Ralph Bentham Medical Practice, Grasmere Drive, High Bentham, Lancaster LA2 7JP Tel: 01524 261202 Fax: 01524 262222905; 2 Richmond House, Hawes Road, Ingleton, Carnforth LA6 3AN Tel: 015242 41885 Fax: 015242 41825 Email: ralph@giffard.demon.co.uk — MB ChB Manch. 1977; DRCOG 1983; MRCGP 1984; Dip Ther. Newc. 1996.

SULLIVAN, Raymond Patrick Glebefields Health Centre, St Mark's Road, Tipton DY4 0UB; 63 Clifton Road, Sutton Coldfield B73 6EN — MB BCh BAO NUI 1987; DCH 1990. GP. Specialty: Medico Legal; Occupat. Health; Gen. Pract. Socs: PgDL UCE 2000.

SULLIVAN, Shona Clare Royal Glamorgan Hospital, Llantrisant CF72 8XR Tel: 01443 443591 Email: shona.sullivan@pr-tr.wales.nhs.uk — MB BCh Wales 1974 (Welsh Nat. Sch. of Med.) FRCS Eng. 1979; FCOphth 1984. Cons. Ophth. Roy. Glam. Hosp. Llantrisant. Specialty: Ophth. Special Interest: Ophthalmic Plastic and Reconstructive Surgery. Socs: Eur. Soc. Oculoplastic & Reconstruc. Surg. Prev: Sen. Regist. Univ. Hosp. Wales Cardiff.

SULLIVAN, Stephen Kevan Brackenwray Farm, Kinniside, Cleator CA23 3AG Tel: 01946 862604 Email: brackenwray@aol.com — MB BS Lond. 1969; DObst RCOG 1972. Locum GP.

SULLIVAN, Terence James PO Box 760, Morden SM4 6QS Tel: 020 8640 8640 Fax: 020 8640 8640 — MB BS Lond. 1975 (St. Mary's Lond.) MRCS Eng. LRCP Lond. 1975; DA (UK) 1982; MRCA 2001. Medicolegal Reporting. Specialty: Medico Legal. Socs: Assn. Anaesth. - Elected; Soc. Advancem. Anaesth. in Dent.; Dent. Sedation Teach.s Gp. Prev: Cons. Anaesth. Dudley Gp. of Hosps.; Indep. Anaesth. (Day Care Dent.) Surrey; Cons. Anaesth., Libya.

SULLIVAN, Thomas James (retired) 69 Corinium Gate, Cirencester GL7 2PX — MB BChir Camb. 1949 (Westm.) MA Camb. 1950, MB BChir 1949; PhD Lond. 1960. Prev: Sen. Lect. Pharmacol. & Therap. St. Thos. Hosp. Med. Sch. Lond.

SULLIVAN, Valerie Joan Flatt Walks Health Centre, 3 Castle Meadows, Catherine Street, Whitehaven CA28 7QE Tel: 01946 692173 Fax: 01946 590406; Brackenwray Farm, Kinniside, Cleator CA22 2TB Tel: 01946 862604 — MB BS Lond. 1971 (St. Geo. Hosp.) BSc Lond. 1966.

SULLIVAN, Vera Alma (retired) Rus-in-Urbe, 6 Beechcote Avenue, Portadown, Craigavon BT63 5DG Tel: 028 3833 3709 — (Belf.) MD Belf. 1955, MB BCh BAO 1946; DPM Dub. 1949; MRCPsych 1971. Cons. Psychiat. Learning Disabilty South. Health & Social Servs. Bd.

SULLIVAN, William Roy The Surgery, Abbey End, Kenilworth, Coventry CV8 1LF Tel: 01926 52576 — MB ChB Ed. 1959.

SULLIVAN STANDEN, Anne Kingsbury Court Surgery, Church Street, Dunstable LU5 4RS Tel: 01582 663218 Fax: 01582 476488 — MB BCh NUI 1961.

SULLMAN, Barry 118 Second Avenue, Manor Park, London E12 6EL — MB ChB Dundee 1988.

SULLY, Mr Lance Department Plastic Surgery, City Hospital, Nottingham NG5 1PB Tel: 0115 969 1169 Ext: 46790 Fax: 0115 962 7939; 11Regent Street, Nottingham NG1 5BS Tel: 0115 947 5475 Fax: 0115 924 1606 — MB Camb. 1966 (St. Geo.) BChir 1965; FRCS Eng. 1973. Cons. Plastic Surg. Nottm. HA. Specialty: Plastic Surg.

SULTAN, Mr Abdul Hameed Mayday University Hospital, London Road, Croydon CR7 &YE Tel: 0208 401 3161 Fax: 0208 401 3681 Email: abdul.sultan@mayday.nhs.uk — MB ChB S. Africa 1979 (Univ. of Natal) MD (Natal) 1995; FRCOG (RCOG.) 2004. Cons. Obst. & Gyn., Croydon; Hon. Sen. Lect., St. George's Hosp. Med. Sch. Specialty: Obst. & Gyn. Special Interest: Obstetric Perineal Trauma; Urogynaecology. Socs: Brit. Med. Soc.; Internat. continence Soc.; Brit. Soc. of Urogynaecology. Prev: Sen. Regist., St. Geo. Hosp., Lond.

SULTAN, Helen Yasmin 22 St Ronan's Road, Harrogate HG2 8LE — BChir Camb. 1996.

SULTAN, M S The Surgery, 226 Mitcham Road, Tooting, London SW17 9NN Tel: 020 8672 7868 Fax: 020 8672 8630 — MB BS Madras 1973; MB BS Madras 1973.

SULTAN, Mahmoud Gamal El-Din Riyadh Military Hospital, D161, PO Box 7897, Riyadh 11159, Saudi Arabia Tel: 00 966 1 4625209 Fax: 009661 462509; 98 Redgrove Park, Cheltenham GL51 6QZ Tel: 01242 512451 — MB BCh Ain Shams 1969; FRCOG 1997, MRCOG 1982. Cons. Obst. & Gyn. Riyadh Milit. Hosp., Saudi Arabia.; Asst. Director of Obst. Riyadh Milit. Hosp. Saudi Arabia. Specialty: Obst. & Gyn.

SULTAN, Mohammad Lower Broughton Health Centre, Great Clowes Street, Salford M7 1RD; 20 Sefton Drive, Worsley, Manchester M28 2NQ — MB BS Punjab 1967 (King Edwd. Med. Coll. Lahore) BSc Punjab (Pakistan) 1966, MB BS 1967; DCH RCPSI 1972. Specialty: Paediat. Socs: Fell. Manch. Med. Soc.; BMA. Prev: SHO (Gen. Surg.) Mayo Hosp. Lahore, Pakistan; SHO (Paediat. Infec. & Chest Dis.) Castle Hill Hosp. Cottingham; SHO (Paediat.) Bradford Gp. Hosps.

SULTAN, Muhammad Khaled Care Principles, Linden House, Market Weighton, York YO43 4LA — MD Damascus 1983; MRCPsych; CCST (LD). Cons. Psychiat. (Learning Disabil.). Specialty: Gen. Psychiat.

SULTAN, Vimala 21 West Way, Carshalton SM5 4EN — MB BS Madras 1975.

SULTANA, Afzal Mohi Uddin Woodside Lodge, 12 Victoria Avenue, Sunderland SR2 9PZ — MB BS Karachi 1985; MRCOG 1993.

SULTANA, Ayesha Ashma The Surgery, 1 Boundary Court, Snells Park, Edmonton, London N18 2TB — MB BS Calcutta 1971; DGO 1973; DRCOG 1979. GP Lond.; Clin. Asst. Diabetic Centre, N. Middlx. Hosp., Sterling Way, Edmonton.

SULTANA, Khurshid 39 Braemar Avenue, Wood Green, London N22 7BY Tel: 020 8889 3790 — MB BS Karachi 1958; DObst RCOG 1966. CMO City & Hackney Health Dist.

SULTANA, Kishwar 19 Romilly Crescent, Canton, Cardiff CF11 9NP — MB BCh Wales 1991.

SULTANA, Razia 2 Llanddennis Road, Roath Park, Cardiff CF23 6EF Tel: 029 2075 5555 — MB BS Dacca 1969.

SUMANASURIYA, Rudrani Champa Wexham Park Hospital, Slough SL2 4HL Tel: 01753 633166 Fax: 01753 691343; 152 Old Woking Road, Woking GU22 8LE — MB BS Colombo 1980; MRCP (UK) 1986; MRCS Eng. LRCP Lond. 1987.

SUMARIA, Mahendra Kumar Mulchand Brierley Hill Health Centre, Albion Street, Brierley Hill DY5 3EE Tel: 01384 77382 Fax: 01384 483931 — MB BS Saurashtra 1972 (M. P. Shah Med. Coll.)

MRCGP 1977. Prev: Trainee Gen. Pract. Dudley Vocational Train. Scheme; Ho. Off. (Gen. Med.) & Ho. Off. (Gen. Surg.) Dudley AHA.

SUMATHIPALA, Sanjeewa 2 West Green Close, Edgbaston, Birmingham B15 2LA — MB ChB Birm. 1995.

SUMBWANYAMBE, Nawa Wilfred X-Ray Department, Diana, Princess of Wales Hospital, Scartho Road, Grimsby DN33 2BA Tel: 01472 874111 Ext.7758 Fax: 01472 875450; Mundawanga, 218A Station Road, New Waltham, Grimsby DN36 4PH Tel: 01472 828907 — MB ChB Zambia 1982; DMRD Ed. 1988; FRCR 1990; T(R)(CR) 1991. Cons. Radiol. Dist. & Gen. Hosp. Grimsby. Specialty: Radiol. Socs: Fell. Roy. Coll. Radiol.; Brit. Med. Ultrasound Soc.; Brit. Inst. Radiol. Prev: Sen. Regist. (Radiol.) Hull Roy. Infirm.; Regist. (Radiol.) Roy. Infirm. Edin.

SUMERAY, Mark Stephen Ethicon Ltd, PO BOX 408, Bankhead Ave, Edinburgh E11 4HE Tel: 0131 442 5563 — MS Lond. 1998 (University College and Middlesex School of Medicine) BSc (1st cl. Hons.) Lond. 1987; MB BS Lond. 1990; FRCS Eng. 1994; FRCS Ed. 1994. Vice Pres. Clin. Trials, Ethicon. Specialty: Research. Socs: Roy. Soc. Med. Prev: Brit. Heart Foundat. Jun. Research; Fell. (Cardiothoracic Surg.) Middlx. Hosp. Lond.; Specialist Regist. (Cardiothorac Surg.) E. Lond. Rotat.

SUMIRA, Roman Peter Studfall Medical Centre, Studfall Avenue, Corby NN17 1LG Tel: 01536 401371 Fax: 01536 401300 — MB ChB Leic. 1985. Specialty: Gen. Pract.

SUMITRA, John Vijayakumar Department of Community Paediatrics, Royal Berkshire Hospital NHS Trust, 3 Craven Road, Reading RG1 5LF Tel: 0118 931 5878 Fax: 0118 975 0297; 11 Longworth Avenue, Tilehurst, Reading RG31 5JU Tel: 0118 941 0525 — MB BS Bangalore 1969; M.D. (Paediat.); DCCH RCP Ed. 1983; MSc Community Paediat. Lond. 1991; MRCPCH 1997. SCMO (Child Health) Roy. Berks. Hosp. NHS Trust. Specialty: Community Child Health. Socs: Fac. Comm. Health. Prev: Clin. Med. Off. Norwich HA; Regist. (Paediat.) Brown Memor. Hosp. Ludhiana, India; Asst. Paediat. ETCM Hosp. Kolar, India.

SUMMER, Mick 14 Croyde Close, Leicester LE5 4WG — MB ChB Leic. 1995.

SUMMERELL, Joan Mary (retired) 7 Hill Crest, Langland, Swansea SA3 4PW — MB BCh Wales 1956; DCP Lond 1968; FRCPath 1982, M 1970. Cons. Morbid Anatomist W. Glam. AHA.

SUMMERFIELD, Brian John The Surgery, The Limes Medical Centre, Trinity Square, Margate CT9 1QY Tel: 01843 227567 Fax: 01843 222720 Email: Brian.Summerfield@gp-G92052.nhs.uk; Balcombe House, 11A Avenue Gardens, Cliftonville, Margate CT9 3BD Fax: 01843 292407 Email: bjsummerfield@doctors.org.uk — (Sheff. Univ.) MB ChB Sheff. 1972; DRCOG 1976. Prev: Regist. (Med.) North. Gen. Hosp. Sheff.; SHO (Obst.) St. John's Hosp. Chelmsford.

SUMMERFIELD, Derek Anton Medical Foundation for Care of Victims of Torture, 96 Grafton Road, London NW5 3EJ Tel: 020 7813 7777 Fax: 020 7813 0011; 55 Denman Road, London SE15 5NS — MB BS Lond. 1977; BSc (Hons.) Cape Town 1970; MRCPsych 1985. Psychiat. Med. Found. For c/o Victims of Torture.; Hon. Sen. Lect. (Psychiat.) St. Geo. Hosp. Med. Sch. Lond.; Research Assoc. Refugee Studies Progr., Oxf. Univ. Specialty: Gen. Psychiat. Prev: Sen. Regist. (Psychiat.) St. Geo. Hosp. Lond.

SUMMERFIELD, Hilary Ann (retired) Meadowside, Piddletrenthide, Dorchester DT2 7QX Tel: 07300 348284 — MB BCh Oxf. 1970; MRCP (UK) 1972. Family Plann. and Well Wom. Serv. N. Dorset PCT. Prev: CMO Family Plann. & Well Wom. Serv. Barnet Community Healthcare Trust.

SUMMERFIELD, Professor John Arthur Department of Medicine, Imperial College School of Medicine at St Mary's, London W2 1PG Tel: 020 7886 6365 Fax: 020 7724 9369 — MB BS Lond. 1979 (Lond. Hosp.) MB BS Lond. 1970; MRCP (UK) 1972; MD Lond. 1976; FRCP Lond. 1985. Prof. Med. Imperial Coll. Sch. Med. Lond.; Clin. Dir. Of Med. St Mary's NHS Trust. Specialty: Gastroenterol. Socs: Assn. Phys.; Brit. Soc. Gastroenterol.; Eur. Assn. Study Liver. Prev: Wellcome Trust Sen. Fell. & Hon. Cons. Phys. Roy. Free Hosp. Lond.; MRC Clin. Research Fell. Roy. Free Hosp. Lond.; Lect. (Med.) Roy. Free Hosp.

SUMMERFIELD, Karen Elizabeth St Peters Street Medical Practice, 16 St Peters Street, London N1 8JG Tel: 020 7226 7131 Fax: 020 7354 9120 — MB BChir Camb. 1990; MA Camb. 1990, MB BChir 1990; DCH RCP Lond. 1991; DRCOG 1992; MRCGP 1993. GP.

SUMMERFIELD, Oliver John 25 Kildare Terrace, London W2 5JT — MB BS Lond. 1998.

SUMMERFIELD, Richard John West Wood House, Church Lane, Sparsholt, Winchester SO21 2NJ — MB BChir Camb. 1974; MA Camb. 1973; FRCA 1981. Specialty: Anaesth.

SUMMERHAYES, John Lionel Vickery (retired) Brocklands Cottage, Ridgeway Lane, Lymington SO41 8AA Tel: 01590 674060 — MB BS Lond. 1949 (King's Coll. Hosp.) MRCS Eng. LRCP Lond. 1948; MRCP Lond. 1952; DObst RCOG 1956; MRCGP 1968. Prev: Regist. (Med.) King's Coll. Hosp. Lond.

SUMMERHAYES, Peter James Sandown Medical Centre, Melville Street, Sandown PO36 8LD Tel: 01983 402464 Fax: 01983 405781 — MB BS Lond. 1973.

SUMMERHAYS, Beatrice Gabrielle Community Child Health Department, Dunsbury Way, Leigh Park, Havant PO9 5BG Tel: 023 9248 2154 Fax: 023 9247 1892 — MB BS Lond. 1979 (Westm.) BSc Lond. 1976. SCMO (Community Child Health) Portsmouth CIM Primary Care Trust; Sen. Doctor (Child Protec.) Portsmouth & SE Hants. HA. Specialty: Community Child Health. Socs: Roy. Coll. Paediat. & Child Health. Prev: GP W. Bromwich W. Midl.; Trainee GP Braintree; Clin. Med. Off. (Community Child Health) Havant.

SUMMERLY, Myrtle Enid (retired) 6 Airdall Spinney, Stone ST15 8AZ Tel: 01785 615938 — MB ChB Birm. 1955; DCH Eng. 1960; FFCM 1985, M 1980. Prev: Dir. Pub. Health N. Staffs. HA.

SUMMERS, Alison Rael Kidderminster Health Centre, Worcestershire Specialist Children's Services, Bromsgrove Street, Kidderminster DY10 1PG Tel: 01562 820091; Lineholt Grange, Lyth Lane, Lineholt, Ombersley, Droitwich WR9 0LG Tel: 01905 621670 — MB ChB Birm. 1972. Community Paediat. Wyre Forest PCT; Clin. Asst. (Ear, Nose & Throat). Specialty: Community Child Health; Otolaryngol.

SUMMERS, Andrew Hendford Lodge Medical Centre, 74 Hendford, Yeovil BA20 1UJ Tel: 01935 470200 Fax: 01935 470202; Sheepslake House, Longlands Lane, East Coker, Yeovil BA22 9HN — MB BS Lond. 1977; DRCOG 1983; MRCGP 1985.

SUMMERS, Beatrice Anne Department of Neurology, Staffordshire General Hospital, Weston Road, Stafford ST16 3SA Tel: 01785 230238 Fax: 01785 230237 — (Univ. Coll. Hosp.) BChir Camb. 1974; MA Camb. 1975; MB 1975; FRCP 1997 M (UK) 1977. Cons. Neurol. M. Staffs. Gen. Hosp. NHS Trust. Specialty: Neurol. Socs: Brit. Pharm. Soc. Prev: Sen. Regist. (Neurol.) Inst. Psychiat. Lond.; Regist. Nuffield Dept. Clin. Med. John Radcliffe Hosp. Oxf.; SHO (Neurol.) Nat. Hosp. Nerv. Dis. Qu. Sq.

SUMMERS, Mr Bruce Neville Department of Orthopaedics, The Princess Royal Hospital, Telford TF1 6TF Tel: 01952 641222; Cheswell House, Cheswell, Newport TF10 9AD — MB BS Lond. 1976 (Middlx.) FRCS Eng. 1981; T(S) 1991. Cons. Orthop. Surg. Princess Roy. Hosp. Telford. Specialty: Orthop. Prev: Sen. Regist. (Orthop.) Middlx. Hosp. Lond.; Regist. (Orthop.) Robt. Jones & Agnes Hunt Orthop. Hosp. OsW.ry.

SUMMERS, Miss Claire Lucy 9 Dalton Gardens, Davyhulme, Manchester M41 5TH Tel: 0161 747 6376 — MB ChB Manch. 1983; FRCS Glas. 1988; DCH RCP Lond. 1990; FFAEM 1994. Cons. A & E Med. Trafford Gen. Hosp. Manch. Specialty: Accid. & Emerg. Prev: Sen. Regist. (A & E Med.) Addenbrooke's Hosp. Camb. & Norf. & Norwich Hosp.

SUMMERS, Donald William Bates Health Centre, Llanfairfechan LL33 0NH Tel: 01428 680021; Hafod y Bryn, Mount Road, Llanfairfechan LL33 0HD Tel: 01428 680500 — MRCS Eng. LRCP Lond. 1958 (Char. Cross)

SUMMERS, Douglas Joseph The Gables Health Centre, 26 St Johns Road, Bedlington NE22 7DU Tel: 01670 829889 Fax: 01670 820841 — MB ChB Sheff. 1988. GP Bedlington, N.d.

SUMMERS, Edward James The Coatham Surgery, 18 Coatham Road, Redcar TS10 1RJ Tel: 01642 483495 Fax: 01642 487520; 26 Saltscar, Redcar TS10 2PH — MB ChB Leeds 1984; DRCOG 1988; MRCGP 1988. Prev: Trainee GP Boston VTS.

SUMMERS, Elizabeth Mary (retired) 8 Alderwood Grove, Edenfield, Ramsbottom, Bury BL0 0HQ Tel: 01706 826655 — MB ChB Liverp. 1959; MB ChB (Hons. cl. 2, Distinc. Surg.) Liverp; DObst RCOG 1961. Prev: SCMO Salford HA.

SUMMERS, Geoffrey David Kidderminster General Hospital, Bewdley Road, Kidderminster DY11 6RJ Tel: 01562 823424; The Little Oak, Far Forest, Kidderminster DY14 9EA — MB BChir Camb. 1974; MA Camb. 1974; MRCP (UK) 1976; T(M) 1991; FRCP Lond. 1992. Cons. Phys.Worchestershire Acute Hosps. NHS Trust. Specialty: Gen. Med.; Respirat. Med. Socs: Midl. Thoracic Soc. & Brit. Thoracic Soc. Prev: Lect. (Med.) St. Thos. Hosp. Med. Sch. Lond.; Regist. (Med.) Centr. Middlx. Hosp. Lond.; SHO (Med.) Walton Hosp. Liverp.

SUMMERS, Gillian Denise Sandy Health Centre Medical Practice, Northcroft, Sandy SG19 1JQ; Alwyn House, 17 St Neots Road, Sandy SG19 1LE Tel: 01767 681171 Fax: 01767 681171 — MB BCh Wales 1977; DRCOG 1983; MRCGP 1984. Prev: Dep. Police Surg. N. Beds.

SUMMERS, Graham Taybank Medical Centre, 10 Robertson Street, Dundee DD4 6EL Tel: 01382 461588 Fax: 01382 452121 — MB ChB Dundee 1987. Specialty: Gen. Pract. Socs: Forfarshire Med. Assn. Prev: Trainee GP Tayside HB VTS; Ho. Off. (Med.) Ninewells Hosp. Dundee; Ho. Off. (Surg.) Stracathro Hosp. Angus.

SUMMERS, Gregory Dominic Department of Rheumatology, Derbyshire Royal Infirmary, London Road, Derby DE1 2QY Tel: 01332 347141 Fax: 01332 254989 Email: greg.summers@sdah-tr.trent.nhs.uk — MB ChB Manch. 1976; MRCP (UK) 1979; BSc Manch. 1973, MD 1987; FRCP Lond. 1995. Cons. (Rheum.) Derbysh. Roy. Infirm. Derby. Specialty: Rheumatol. Special Interest: Osteoporosis.

SUMMERS, Henry Arthur Hamilton (retired) 8 Princes Avenue, Walsall WS1 2PH Tel: 01922 627047 — MB BCh BAO Belf. 1942; DPH Belf. 1948. Prev: SCM (Environment Health) Walsall AHA.

SUMMERS, Isobel Margaret Rosemary 9 Adams Road, Cambridge CB3 9AD Tel: 01223 61805 — MB Camb. 1974; BChir 1973.

SUMMERS, Jeffrey, Squadron Ldr. RAF Med. Br. Retd. Maidstone Hospital , Kent Oncology Centre, Hermitage Lane, Maidstone Tel: 01622 225111 Fax: 01622 225252 Email: jsummers@koc.mtw-tr.nhs.uk — MB BCh Wales 1983 (WELSH Nat. Sch. OF Med., CARDIFF Univ.) MRCP (UK) 1989; FRCR 1994. Cons. Clin. Oncologist, Kent Oncol. Centre. Specialty: Oncol. Prev: Regist. (Clin. Oncol.) Addenbrooke's Hosp. Camb.

SUMMERS, Judith Alison East Lancashire Health Authority, 31-33 Kenyon Road, Lomeshaye Estate, Nelson BB9 5SZ Tel: 01282 610215 — MB ChB Leeds 1979; DTM & H Liverp. 1981; MFPHM 1990; MRCPsych 1998. Specialty: Pub. Health Med.; Gen. Psychiat. Socs: Fac. Pub. Health Med.

SUMMERS, Judith Ann The Pasque Hospice, Head of Medical Services, Great Bramingham Lane, Streatley, Luton LU3 3NT — MB BS Lond. 1977; MRCS Eng. LRCP Lond. 1977.

SUMMERS, Lesley Ann Haleacre Unit, Amersham Hospital, Whileden St., Amersham HP7 0JD — MB BS Lond. 1981. Clin. Asst. (Psychiat.) Amersham Hosp. Specialty: Gen. Psychiat. Prev: Clin. Asst. (Psychiat.) Drug Dependency Clinic Amersham Hosp. Bucks.; Regist. (Psychiat.) The Lond. Hosp.

SUMMERS, Lucinda Kate Mary Department of Endocrinology, Diabetes & Metabolic Medicine, St Thomas' Hospital, Lambeth Palace Road, London SE1 7EH Tel: 020 7928 9292 Fax: 020 7928 4458; 24 Lee Road, London SE3 9RT Tel: 020 8852 8214 — MB BS Lond. 1990 (University Hospital London & King's College Sch. Med. & Dent) BSc Lond. 1987; MRCP (UK) 1993; Dphil Oxford, 1998. Lect. (Med.) Dept. of Endocrinol., Diabetes & Metab. Med. St Thos. Hosp. Lond.; Hon. Regist. St Thos. Hosp. Lond. Specialty: Diabetes; Endocrinol.; Gen. Med. Socs: Endocrine Soc.; Brit. Diabetic Assn. (Med. & Scientif. Sect.); Eur. Assn. for Study Diabetes. Prev: Research Regist./Hon. Regist. Oxf. Radcliffe Infirm.; Regist. (Med.) Middlx. Hosp., Regist. (Med.) Basildon Hosp. Essex.

SUMMERS, Lucy Jane Gillies and Overbridge Medical Partnership, Brighton Hill, Sullivan Road, Basingstoke RG22 4EH — MB BChir Camb. 1969 (Guy's) DCH Eng. 1971; MRCP (UK) 1981; DRCOG 1987.

SUMMERS, Lynne Worthen Sentry Hill, Henley Road, Marlow SL7 2DQ Tel: 01628 486444 Fax: 01628 476560; 12 Dartmouth Court, South Embankment, Dartmouth TQ6 9DG Tel: 01803 834238 — MB BS Lond. 1976; MRCS Eng. LRCP Lond. 1976. Socs: Chiltern Med. Soc. & BMA.

SUMMERS, Margaret Windsor 128 Coventry Road, Nuneaton CV10 7AD — MB ChB Sheff. 1965.

SUMMERS, Maria (retired) 1 St Margaret's Drive, Leire, Lutterworth LE17 5HW — DPM 1961 Manch; MB BCh BAO NUI 1952; MD NUI 1967. Prev: Cons. Child Psychiat. Clatterbridge Hosp. Bebington & Dir. Child Guid. Clin. Ellesmere Port.

SUMMERS, Philip David 10 Ravensdon Street, London SE11 4AR — MB BS Lond. 1993.

SUMMERS, Richard Thomas Fern House Surgery, 125-129 Newland Street, Witham CM8 1BH Tel: 01376 502108 Fax: 01376 502281; Schills Barn, Lanham Green Road, Cressing, Braintree CM7 8DR — MB BS Lond. 1989 (St. Bart. Lond.) Specialty: Gen. Pract.

SUMMERS, Roderick Olaf Cheney 27 Barnetts Lane, Kidderminster DY10 3HJ — MB BChir Camb. 1962; DObst RCOG 1964; MA Camb. 1965; MRCP Lond. 1967; MRCGP 1978. Socs: BMA. Prev: Ho. Phys. Gen. Hosp. Birm.; Ho. Surg. Gen. Hosp. Hereford; Med. Regist. Gen. Hosp. Birm.

SUMMERS, Ronald (retired) 353 Arbroath Road, Dundee DD4 7SQ Tel: 01382 456682 — (St. And.) MB ChB St. And. 1943; DTM & H Liverp. 1949. Prev: Squadron Ldr. R. Aux. AF.

SUMMERS, Sarah Helen Sheepslake House, Longlands Lane, East Coker, Yeovil BA22 9HN — MB BS Lond. 1978; BSc (Hons.) Biochem. Lond. 1975, MB BS 1978; DRCOG 1982.

SUMMERS, Stephen Paul The Park Medical Group, Fawdon Park Road, Newcastle upon Tyne NE3 2PE Tel: 0191 285 1763 Fax: 0191 284 2374; 10 Belle Grove W., Spital Tongues, Newcastle upon Tyne NE2 4LT — MB ChB Manch. 1984; MRCGP 1988; DRCOG 1988.

SUMMERS, Stephen Robert Gayton Road Health and Surgical Centre, Gayton Road, King's Lynn PE30 4DY Tel: 01553 762726 Fax: 01553 696819; 323 Wootton Road, King's Lynn PE30 3AX — MB BS Lond. 1979; Cert. Family Plann. RCOG & RCGP 1983; DRCOG 1983; FRCGP 1997, M 1986; MRCGP 1986; MFHom 1995; Dip. Med. Acupunct. 1997. GP King's Lynn. Specialty: Homeop. Med. Prev: Med. Off. Providenciales Health Centre Turks & Caicos Is.; SHO (A & E) & (Paediat.) Qu. Eliz. Hosp. King's Lynn.

SUMMERS, Susan Katharine Mount Chambers Surgery, 92 Coggeshall Road, Braintree CM7 9BY Tel: 01376 553415 Fax: 01376 552451; Schills Barn, Lanham Green Road, Cressing, Braintree CM7 8DR — MB BS Lond. 1989 (St. Bart. Lond.) Specialty: Gen. Pract.

SUMMERS, William Brown 27 Ashfield Road, Clarkston, Glasgow G76 7TX Tel: 0141 644 1599 — MB ChB Glas. 1938; DPH Glas. 1946. Chest Phys. Belvedere Hosp.

SUMMERS, Yvonne Jane Christie Hospital NHS Trust, Department of Medical Oncology, Wilmslow Road, Withington, Manchester M20 2BX Tel: 0161 446 3000; Ettrick, Lock 7, Crinan Canal, Cairnbaan, Lochgilphead PA31 8SQ — MB ChB Manch. 1993 (St. Andrews and Manchester) BSc 1990; MRCP (UK) 1996. Clin. Lect. (Med. Oncol.) Christie Hosp. Manch. Specialty: Gen. Med.; Oncol.

SUMMERSCALES, Adrian Alvaston Medical Centre, 14 Boulton Lane, Alvaston, Derby DE24 0GE Tel: 01332 571322; 16 Main Street, Ambaston, Derby DE72 3ES — BM BS Nottm. 1987. Socs: Derby Med. Soc.; Brit. Assn. Sport & Med.

SUMMERSKILL, Shirley Catherine Wynne (retired) 58 Compayne Gardens, London NW6 3RY Tel: 020 7328 4774 — BM BCh Oxf. 1958 (St. Thos.) MA Oxf. 1958. Prev: Med. Off. Blood Transfus. Serv.

SUMMERSKILL, William Storith Markham EBS Teaching Coordinator, NHS South Region, Department of Medical Education, University of Bristol, Bristol; Pincott Farm, Coopers Hill, Upton St Leonards, Gloucester GL3 4RX — MB BS Lond. 1986 (St. Mary's) DRCOG 1988; MRCGP 1990; DCH RCP Lond. 1990; DFFP 1996; MSc (Oxon.) 2000. Prev: Trainee GP/SHO Portsmouth VTS; Ho. Surg. Qu. Alexandra Hosp. Portsmouth; Ho. Phys. Roy. United Hosp. Bath.

SUMMERTON, Ailie Mary 7 Hall Walk, Welton, Brough HU15 1PN — BM BCh Oxf. 1984; MA Camb. 1985. Sen. Regist. (Chem. Path.) Sheff. HA. Specialty: Chem. Path. Prev: Regist. (Chem. Path.) Roy. Hallamsh. Hosp. Sheff.; SHO Rotat. (Path.) N. Staffs. HA; SHO & Ho. Off. (Med.) N. Staffs. HA.

SUMMERTON, Christopher Barry Trafford General Hospital, Moorside Road, Davyhulme, Manchester M41 5SL Tel: 0161 746 2846 Fax: 0161 746 2761; 24 Parsonage Road, Heaton Moor,

Stockport SK4 4JR Tel: 0161 291 9047 Fax: 0161 291 9048 — MB BChir Camb. 1983 (Camb. Univ.) MRCS Eng. LRCP Lond. 1982; BA Camb. 1979, MA 1983; MRCP (UK) 1986; MD Camb. 1992; FRCP Ed 1999; FRCP (Lond.) 2000. Cons. (Gastro. & Gen. Med.) Trafford Gen. Hosp.; Hon. Cons. (Phys.) Hope Hosp. Salford; Hon. Lect. in Med., Uni. Of Manch. Specialty: Gen. Med.; Gastroenterol. Socs: Brit. Soc. Gastroenterol.; Brit. Assn. Study Liver; Brit. Assn. Paren. & Ente. Nutrit. Prev: Sen. Regist. (Gastroenterol. & Gen. Med.) N. Manch. Gen. Hosp.; Sen. Regist. (Gastroenterol. & Gen. Med.) Manch. Roy. Infirm.; Research Regist. & Regist. (Med.) Addenbrooke's Hosp. Camb.

SUMMERTON, Mr Duncan John, Surg. Cdr. RN Solent Department of Urology, St. Mary's Hospital, Portsmouth PO3 6AD Tel: 023 9228 6000 Ext: 2305 Email: djsummerton@clara.net — MB ChB Leic. 1987; BSc Leic. 1984; FRCS Eng. 1994; FRCS Ed. 1994; FRCS (Urol.) 2000. Cons. Urol., Solent Dept. of Urol., Portsmouth; Cons. Adviser in Urol. to Med. Director Gen. (Navy). Specialty: Urol. Special Interest: Urethral reconstruction; Urethral stricture Dis.; Urological Oncol. Socs: Brit. Assn. of Urological Surg.s (BAUS); Ex-Hon. Sec. of the Specialist Urological Regist.s Gp. (Surg); Roy. Naval Med. Soc. Prev: Specialist Regist. (Urol.) RN Hosp. Haslar; Sen. Regist., Inst. of Urol., Lond.; Specialist Regist. (Wessex Rotat.).

SUMMERTON, Nicholas The Surgery, Manlake Avenue, Winterton, Scunthorpe DN15 9TA Tel: 01724 732202 Fax: 01724 734992 — BM BCh Oxf. 1984 (Oxford) MA Oxf. 1986, BA 1981; DRCOG 1987; MRCGP 1988; MPH Leeds 1994; MFPHM RCP (UK) 1995; DM Oxf. 2002. Clin. Sen. Lect. (Primary Care Med.) Univ. Hull. Specialty: Gen. Pract. Prev: Sen. Regist. (Pub. Health) Huddersfield; Regist. (Pub. Health) Bradford HA; GP Skelman Thorpe Huddersfield.

SUMMORS, Andrew Charles Anaesthetics Department, Norfolk & Norwich Hospital, Brunswick Road, Norwich NR1 3SR — MB BS Queensland 1990.

SUMMORS, Rachel Emma Fonmon Cottage, Station Road, Llantwit Major CF61 1ST Tel: 01446 794251 — MB BS Lond. 1989; DRCOG 1995; MRCGP 1997. GP Longterm Locum at present. Specialty: Gen. Pract.

SUMNALL, Andrew Gordon Dyneley House Surgery, Newmarket Street, Skipton BD23 2HZ Tel: 01756 799311 Fax: 01756 707203; 21 Gainsborough Court, Skipton BD23 1QG Tel: 01756 791510 — BM BCh Oxf. 1986 (Oxford) BA Camb. 1983; DRCOG 1988; MRCGP 1990. Clin. Asst. (Geriat.) Skipton Gen. Hosp. Prev: Trainee GP Cambs. VTS.

SUMNER, Alexander Harold 15 Market Street, Ramsbottom, Bury BL0 0JQ; 61 Cromwell Avenue, Highgate, London N6 5HP — MB ChB Liverp. 1988. SHO (A & E)St. Bart. Hosp. Lond. Prev: SHO Regional Thoracic Unit Fazakerley Hosp. Liverp.

SUMNER, David James Old Road West Surgery, 30 Old Road West, Gravesend DA11 0LL Tel: 01474 352075/567799 Fax: 01474 333952 — MB ChB Sheff. 1980; DCH RCP Lond. 1984.

SUMNER, David William, TD (retired) Flat 2, Gledhow Manor, 350 Gledhow Lane, Leeds LS7 4NH Tel: 0113 266 4024 — MB ChB Manch. 1950 (manchester) BSc Manch. 1947; FRCP Lond. 1974, M 1958; FRCP Ed. 1982. Mem. Med. Appeal Tribunal. Prev: Cons. Neurol. & Hon. Clin. Lect. (Neurol.) Univ. Leeds.

SUMNER, Deborah Wycombe General Hospital, High Wycombe HP11 2TT Tel: 01494 526161; Barracks House, Barracks Hill, Coleshill, Amersham HP7 0LN — MB BS Lond. 1980; FRCS Eng. 1985; MRCOG 1988. Cons. O & G Wycombe Gen. Hosp. Specialty: Obst. & Gyn. Prev: Sen. Regist. (O & G) Pembury Hosp. & St. Thos. Hosp. Lond.; SHO (Gen. Surg.) Reading Hosps.; SHO (O & G) Qu. Charlotte's & Chelsea Hosps. Lond.

SUMNER, Deborah Jane The Hollies, 10 Elbow Lane, Formby, Liverpool L37 4AF Tel: 01704 877600 Fax: 01704 833811 — MB ChB Liverp. 1984; MRCGP 1992.

SUMNER, Edward 49 Gordon Mansions, Torrington Place, London WC1E 7HG Tel: 020 7637 0968 Fax: 020 7829 8866 — BM BCh Oxf. 1966 (Univ. Coll. Hosp.) MA Oxf. 1966; FRCA 1971. Cons. Anaesth. Hosp. Sick Childr. Gt. Ormond St. Lond.; Edr.-in-Chief Paediat. Anaesth. Specialty: Anaesth. Prev: Sen. Regist. (Anaesth.) St. Thos. Hosp. Lond.; Regist. (Anaesth.), Ho. Surg. & Ho. Phys. Univ. Coll. Hosp. Lond.

SUMNER, Helen Mary 3 Laurel Bank, Foxhouses Road, Whitehaven CA28 8AD Tel: 01946 692750 — MB ChB Aberd. 1962.

SUMNER, Keith Robert (Surgery), 53 Borough St., Castle Donington, Derby DE74 2LB Tel: 01332 810241 Fax: 01332 811748; 35 Towles Pastures, Castle Donington, Derby DE74 2RX Tel: 01332 810241 — MB ChB Birm. 1975; DCH Eng. 1978; MRCGP 1980; DRCOG 1981. Trainer (Gen. Pract.) Nottm. VTS.

SUMNER, Margaret Anne Ellen (retired) Flat 2, Gledhow Manor, 350 Gledhow Lane, Leeds LS7 4NH Tel: 0113 266 4024 — MB ChB Manch. 1954 (Manch) DA Eng. 1957. Prev: Clin. Med. Off. (Vaccination & Immunisation) Leeds E. HA.

SUMNER, Mary Clare (retired) Kemp Lodge Nursing Home, Park Road, Waterloo, Liverpool L22 3XG — MB ChB Liverp. 1955; MRCS Eng. LRCP Lond. 1955; DMRD Liverp. 1961.

SUMNER, Michael 50 Parson Street, Congleton CW12 4ED — MB ChB Birm. 1980; DRCOG 1985; MRCGP 1985; MSc (Occ. Health) Birm. 2002. Civil. Med. Pract. M.O.D. Prev: GP Cent. Birm. VTS; Trainee GP Centr. Birm. VTS.

SUMNER, Michael John Centeon Limited, Centeon House, Market Place, Haywards Heath RH16 1DB Tel: 01444 447424; Myrtle Cottage, The Common, Dunsfold, Godalming GU8 4LE Tel: 01483 200570 — MB BS Lond. 1990; MRCP (UK) 1993; Dip Pharm. Med. 1996. Clin. & Med. Affairs Manager Centeon Ltd. Specialty: Pharmaceutical Medicine.

SUMNER, Tina Louise Heywood and Partners, 119 Wren Way, Farnborough GU14 8TA Tel: 01252 541884 Fax: 01252 511410 — MB BS Lond. 1995.

SUMNERS, David George Albany Lodge, Church Crescent, St Albans AL3 5JB Tel: 01727 834330 Fax: 01727 834182 — MB BS Lond. 1978 (Univ. Coll. Hosp.) BSc (Hons.) Lond. 1974; MRCPsych 1983; FRCPsych 2001. Cons. Psychiat. W. Herts. Community Trust; Cons. Psychiat. The Brain Injury Rehabil. Trust. Specialty: Gen. Psychiat. Socs: BMA & Brit. Soc. Rehabil. Med. Prev: Cons. Psychiat. & Med. Dir. Barnet Healthcare NHS Trust; Sen. Regist. (Psychiat.) Middlx. Hosp. Lond.; Regist. (Psychiat.) Guy's Hosp. Lond.

SUMNERS, Susan Mary Watling Medical Centre, 42 London Road, Stanmore HA7 4NU Tel: 020 8958 4237 Fax: 020 8905 4809 — MB BS Lond. 1976 (Roy. Free) MRCS Eng. LRCP Lond. 1976; MRCGP 1981.

SUMPTER, Katherine Anne Royal Marsden Hospital, Sutton SM2 5PT Email: kate.sumpter@rmh.nthames.nhs.uk; Garden Flat, 30 Barclay Road, London SW6 1EH — MB BS Lond. 1992 (St. Bartholomew's) MRCP 1995. SpR (Med. Oncol.) Roy. Marsden Hosp. Fulham Rd. Lond. Specialty: Oncol. Prev: Research Fell.

SUMPTION, Catherine Anne 16 Creighton Road, London NW6 6ED — MB BS Lond. 1986.

SUMPTION, John Carlyon 3 Windsor Avenue, Radyr, Cardiff CF1 8BW Tel: 02920 842291 — MB BS Lond. 1950 (St. Mary's) MRCS Eng. LRCP Lond. 1949; DA Eng. 1951; FFA RCS Eng. 1954. Cons. Anaesth. E. Glam. Gen. Hosp. Pontypridd. Specialty: Anaesth. Prev: Sen. Regist. Anaesth. United Birm. Hosps.; Regist. Anaesth. United Cardiff Hosps.; Specialist Anaesth. RAMC.

SUMPTION, Nanno Joyce Corris House, Radyr, Cardiff Tel: 029 2084 2291 — MB BCh Wales 1949 (Cardiff) BSc, MB BCh Wales 1949. Clin. Med. Off. S. Glam. AHA (T).

SUMPTON, John Roy (retired) One Hundred, Austin Fields, King's Lynn PE30 1RS — MB BS Lond. 1958 (Univ. Coll. Hosp.)

SUMRA, Rupinder 19 Campion Road, Leamington Spa CV32 5XF — MB ChB Manch. 1990; DCH RCP (UK) 1993; DRCOG 1995; MRCGP 1995; DFFP 1995.

SUN WAI, Wong Yen Seng 16A Vicarage Road, London E10 5EA Tel: 0208 925 7433; 18 Cook Street, Port Louis, Mauritius Tel: 00 230 21 22027 — MB BCh BAO NUI 1988; FRCA 1995. Clin. Research Phys. Internat. Clin. Trials Lond. Prev: Acting Sen. Regist. & Regist. Rotat. Roy. Lond. Hosp. & Whipps Cross Hosp. Lond.

SUNAK, Yashvir Raymond Road Surgery, 34 Raymond Road, Upper Shirley, Southampton SO15 5AL Tel: 023 8022 7559 Fax: 023 8033 4028; 21 Spindlewood Close, Glenwood Avenue, Bassett, Southampton SO16 3QD Tel: 02380 767002 — MB ChB Liverp. 1974; DRCOG 1976. GP Soton.; Clin. Asst. (Learning Disabil.) Soton. Community NHS Trust; Med. Mem. of Indep. Tribunal Serv.; Occupat. Health Phys. John Lewis partnership. Specialty: Occupat. Health. Socs: Soc. Occupat. Med.; Soton. Med. Soc. Prev: Trainee

GP Aldermoor Health Centre & Victor St. Surg.; SHO (O & G) Soton. Gen. Hosp.; SHO (Paediat.) Alder Hey Childr. Hosp. Liverp.

SUNDAR, Mr Manthravadi Sivakama 5 Broadhalgh, Rochdale OL11 5LX — MB BS Andhra 1976; FRCS Ed. 1985; MCh (Orthop.) Liverp. 1991.

SUNDAR ESWAR, Dr 185 Machon Bank Road, Netheredge, Sheffield S7 1PH — MB BS Madras 1989; MRCOG 1994.

SUNDAR RAO, Mr Praveen 40 Magdalen Road, Thornton-Cleveleys FY5 3EF — MB BS Madras 1988; FRCS Glas. 1992.

***SUNDARALINGAM, Janaki** 56 Compton Road, London SW19 7QD — MB BS Lond. 1998 (Charing Cross & Westm. Med. Sch.) MB BS Lond 1998. Ho. Off. (Surg.) W. Middx Hosp. Isleworth. Prev: Ho. Off. (Med.) Chelsea & Westm. Hosp. Lond.

SUNDARALINGAM, Jeyanthi 43 Alwyne Road, London SW19 7AE — MB BS Lond. 1994; BA (Hons.) Camb. 1991. SHO (Gyn. & Oncol.) Hammersmith Hosp. Lond. Prev: Ho. Off. (Surg.) Chelsea & Westm. Hosp. Lond.; Ho. Off. (Med.) Mayday Hosp. Lond.

SUNDARALINGAM, Sinnappu 19 Fareham Close, Fulwood, Preston PR2 8FH — MB BS Sri Lanka 1972; FFA RCSI 1983. Specialty: Anaesth.

SUNDARALINGAM, Visvalingam 34 Millwell Crescent, Chigwell IG7 5HY Tel: 020 8500 3050 — MB BS Ceylon 1963. GP.

SUNDARARAJAN, Prabhavati Thursby Surgery, 2 Browhead Road, Burnley BB10 3BF Tel: 01282 422447 Fax: 01282 832575 — MB BS Bombay 1973; MB BS Bombay 1973.

SUNDARESAN, Maryse Lakshmi Department of Histopathology, North Middlesex Hospital, Sterling Way, London N18 1QX — MB BS Lond. 1982 (Guy's Hospital Medical School) MRCPath 1994. Cons. Histopath. N. Middlx. Hosp. Specialty: Histopath. Prev: Sen. Regist. (Histopath.) King's Coll. Hosp. Lond.; Regist. (Histopath.) Hammersmith Hosp. Lond.

SUNDARESAN, Rathiranie Fairfield, Oxhey Lane, Pinner HA5 4AN Tel: 020 8421 2109 — MB BS Ceylon 1955 (Colombo) DPH Lond. 1967. SCMO Harrow HA. Socs: BMA. Prev: MOH Dehiwela, Ceylon.

SUNDARESAN, Thirunavukkarasu The Health Centre, London Road, Tilbury RM18 8EB Tel: 01375 842504; Fairfield, Oxhey Lane, Pinner HA5 4AN Tel: 020 8421 2109 — MB BS Ceylon 1954; DCH RCPS Glas. 1968. Socs: BMA. Prev: SHO (O & G) PeterBoro. Hosp.; SHO (Psychiat.) Hillingdon Hosp.; GP Badula, Ceylon.

SUNDARESAN, Vasiharen MRC Centre for Developmental Neurobiology, 4th Floor, New Hunts House, Guy's Hospital Campus, King's College, London Bridge, London SE1 1UL Tel: 020 7848 6807 Mob: 07711 250841 Fax: 020 7848 6816 Email: vasi.sundaresan@kcl.ac.uk; Department of Histopathology, St. Thomas' Hospital, Lambeth Palace Road, London SE1 7EH Tel: 020 7928 9292 — MB BS Lond. 1981; MRCP (UK) 1985; MRCPath 1989; PhD Lond. 1993; FRCPath 1999; FRCP 2003. Sen. Lect. (Histopath.. Path.) Hon. Cons. Guys St Thomas Hosp. Kings Coll. Lond. Specialty: Histopath. Prev: MRC Clin. Scientist Fell., MRC, Camb.; Clin. Research Fell. Cancer Research Campaign Univ. & MRC Clin. Oncol. Radiother. Units Camb.; Regist. (Histopath.) Addenbrooke's Hosp. Camb. & Char. Cross Hosp. Lond.

SUNDERLAND, Anne Renfrew Health Centre, 103 Paisley Road, Renfrew PA4 8LL Tel: 0141 886 3535 Fax: 0141 885 0098; Kirkton Lodge, Northview Road, Bridge of Weir PA11 3EX Tel: 01505 612876 — MB ChB Glas. 1979; DRCOG 1982. Prev: Trainee GP Paisley VTS.

SUNDERLAND, Mr Graham Thomas Department of Surgery, Southern General Hospital NHS Trust, 1345 Govan Road, Glasgow G51 4TF Tel: 0141 201 1655 Fax: 0141 201 1674 Email: gtsunderland@compuserve.com — MB ChB Glas. 1980; BSc (1st cl. Hons. Physiol.) Glas 1977; FRCS Glas. 1984; MD Glas. 1988. Cons. Surg. South. Glas. Hosps. NHS Trust. Specialty: Gen. Surg. Prev: Sen. Regist. Rotat. (Gen. Surg.) Glas.; Research Fell. Univ. Dept. Surg. Glas. Roy. Infirm.; Lect. Univ. Surg. Chinese Univ. Hong Kong.

SUNDERLAND, Mr Henry (retired) 1 Rose Hill Court, Bessacarr, Doncaster DN4 5LY — MB BChir Camb. 1951 (King's Coll. Hosp.) MChir Camb. 1961, MB BChir 1951; FRCS Eng. 1957. Prev: Cons. Gen. Surg. Doncaster Roy. Infirm.

SUNDERLAND, John Robert Towcester Medical Centre, Link Way, Towcester NN12 6HH Tel: 01327 359953 Fax: 01327 358929 — MB ChB Leeds 1975; DRCOG 1979; MRCGP 1981.

SUNDERLAND, Lesley Anne (retired) The Street Lane Practice, 12 Devonshire Avenue, Leeds LS8 1AY Tel: 0113 295 3838 Fax: 0113 295 3842; 10 Hillcrest Rise, Cookridge, Leeds LS16 7DL Tel: 0113 285 7719 Email: lesleys@doctors.org.uk — MB ChB Sheff. 1987; DRCOG 1989; Cert. Family Plann. JCC 1990.

SUNDERLAND, Robert Birmingham Childrens Hospital, Steelhouse Lane, Birmingham B4 6NH Tel: 0121 333 8168 — MB ChB Ed. 1974 (Edinburgh) MRCP (UK) 1977; MD Ed. 1982; FRCP (L) 1996; FRCPCH 1997. Cons. Paediat. Birm. Childr. Hosp.; Hon. Sen. Clin. Lect. (Child Health) Birm. Univ. Specialty: Paediat. Prev: Sen. Regist. (Paediat.) W. Midl. RHA; Regist. (Paediat. Path.) Childr. Hosp. Sheff.; Regist. Childr. Hosp. Sheff. & St. Finbarr's Hosp. Cork.

SUNDERLAND, Robin Woodlands, Penn St., Amersham HP7 0PX — MB BS Lond. 1998.

SUNGUM-PALIWAL, Sobharani Park View Clinic, 60 Queensbridge Road, Moseley, Birmingham B13 8QE — MD Marseilles 1980 (Faculty of Medicine, Marseille) DTM & H Marseilles 1980; MRCPsych 1985. Cons. Child & Adolesc. Psychiat. & Hon. Sen. Clin. Lect. (Paediat. & Child Health) Birm. Childr.s Hosp. Specialty: Child & Adolesc. Psychiat. Special Interest: Autistic Spectrum Studies. Socs: BMA; Assn. Child Psychol. & Psychiat.; Brit. Psychol. Soc. Prev: Sen. Regist. (Child & Adolesc. Psychiat.) W. Midl. RHA; Regist. (Psychiat.) Nottm. Train. Scheme.

SUNIL BABU, Velikkakathu Springfield University Hospital, London SW17 7DJ Tel: 020 8682 6325 Fax: 020 8682 6868; 2 Southwood Avenue, Coulsdon CR5 2DT — MB BS Kerala 1985; MRCPsych 1993. Cons. (Psychiat.) S. Merton Elderly Team Springfield Hosp. Lond.; Hon. Sen. Lect. (Psychiat.) St. Geo. Hosp. Med. Sch. Lond. Specialty: Geriat. Psychiat.; Gen. Psychiat. Socs: Brit. Neuropsychiat. Assn. Prev: Sen. Regist. Sutton Hosp. Sutton.

SUNMAN, Wayne Department of Care of the Elderly, City Hospital, Hucknall Road, Nottingham NG5 1PB Tel: 0115 969 1169 Fax: 0115 960 8409 Email: wsunman@ncht.org.uk — MB ChB Ed. 1983; BSc Ed. 1981; MRCP (UK) 1986; MD Liverp. 1998; FRCP Lond. 2002. Cons. (Geriat. & Gen. Med.) Nottm. Specialty: Care of the Elderly; Gen. Med. Socs: Med. Res. Soc.; Brit. Geriat. Soc. Prev: Sen. Regist. (Geriat. & Gen.) Oxf.; Hon. Sen. Regist. (Therap.) Liverp. Univ.; Clin. Research Fell. (Therap.) St. Mary's Hosp. Lond.

SUNTER, James Peter Causey Bridge End Farm, Marley Hill, Newcastle upon Tyne NE16 5EG — MD Newc. 1981; MB BS 1971; FRCPath 1992, M 1980; DMJ Path.) Soc. Apoth. Lond. 1985. Home Off. Path.; Hon. Cons. Histopath Gateshead Hosp. NHS Trust; Hon. Lect. Univ. Newc.; Assn. Clin. Path. & Brit. Assn. Forens. Med. Specialty: Forens. Path. Socs: Path. Soc.

SUNTHA, Sinnathurai Orrell Road Practice, Bradshaw Street, Orrell, Wigan WN5 0AB Tel: 01942 222321 Fax: 01942 620327 — MD Moscow 1971; MD Peoples Friendship Univ. Moscow 1971; LRCP LRCS Ed. LRCPS Glas. 1977; DRCOG 1977; DCH RCPSI 1978. Prev: Regist. (Chest & Infec. Dis.) Ayrsh. & Arran Health Bd.; SHO (Paediat.) Seafield Childr. Hosp. Ayr; SHO (A & E) Kilmarnock Infirm.

SUNTHANKAR, Gita Clapham Park Surgery, 72 Clarence Avenue, Clapham, London SW4 8JQ — MB BCh Wales 1989 (Univ. Hosp. Wales) BSc (Hons) Wales 1985; DTM & H Liverp. 1992; DRCOG (Bristol) 1992; MSc (Publ. Health) 1996. GP Princip.

SUNTHARALINGAM, Ganeshalingam 69 Hillside Ave, Worthing BN14 9QT — MB BChir Camb. 1990; BA Camb. 1988, MB BChir 1990.

SUNTHARALINGAM, Murugasu (retired) 69 Hillside Avenue, Worthing BN14 9QT — MB BS Ceylon 1964 (Colombo) MRCP Lond. 1973; FRCP Lond. 1988. Cons. Phys. (Geriat. Med.) Worthing Health Dist. Prev: Sen Regist. (Geriat. Med.) Ipswich Hosp.

SUNTHARALINGAM, Shiamala 7 Brangwyn Crescent, London SW19 2UA — MB BS Lond. 1997.

SUNTHARANATHAN, Ariamalar 10 Marvell Close, Pound Hill, Crawley RH10 3AL Tel: 01293 512273 — MB BS Sri Lanka 1977; MB BS Sri Lanka Ceylon 1977.

SUPER, Maurice 120 Fog Lane, Didsbury, Manchester M20 6SP Tel: 0161 445 4927 Fax: 0161 445 4927 Email: maurice.super@man.ac.uk/maurice.super@manchester.ac.uk; 120 Fog Lane, Didsbury, Manchester M20 6SP Tel: 0161 445 4927 Fax: 0161 445 4927 Email: maurice.super@man.ac.uk — MB BCh Witwatersrand 1959; DCH RCPS Glas. 1965; FRCP Ed. 1977, M 1965; MD Cape Town 1978; MSc Ed. 1979; FRCP Lond. 1992; FRCPCH 1997. Hon. Cons. Paediat. Geneticist & Hon. Lect. Roy.

Manch. Childr. Hosp. Specialty: Genetics; Paediat. Special Interest: Cystic fibrosis heterozygote effects, cystic fibrosis All aspects. Socs: (Counc.) Manch. Med. Soc.; Brit. Hum. Genetic Soc.; Roy. Coll. Paediat. & Child Health. Prev: Cons. Paediat. S. West. Afr. Admin.

SUPER, Patricia Abbey Medical Centre, 87-89 Abbey Road, London NW8 0AG; Flat 1, 91 Cranfield Gardens, London NW6 3EA — MB ChB Stellenbosch 1992; DFFP 1997; DRCOG 1997. GP Regist. Abbey Med. Centre. Specialty: Gen. Pract. Socs: BMA. Prev: SHO (O & G) Roy. Free Hosp. Lond.; SHO (Anaesth.) Guy's Hosp. Lond.

SUPER, Mr Paul Anthony Birmingham Heartlands & Solihull NHS Trust, Bardesley Green E., Birmingham B9 5SS Tel: 0121 766 6611; 109 Old Station Road, Hampton in Arden, Solihull B92 0HE Email: sup3r@aol.com — MB BS Lond. 1987 (Royal Free. Hosp.) BSc Glas. 1982; FRCS Eng. 1991; FRCS (Gen.) 1998. Cons. (Surg.) Upper GI & Gen. Surg. Birm. Heartlands & Solihull NHS Trust. Specialty: Gen. Surg. Prev: Sen. Regist. Northern Gen. Hosp. Sheff.; Sen. Regist. Roy. Hallamshire Hosp. Sheff.; Lect. (Surg.) St. Mary's Hosp. Med. Sch. Lond.

SUPPLE, David Lincoln Preston Park Surgery, 2a Florence Road, Brighton BN1 6DP Tel: 01273 559601/566033 Fax: 01273 507746; 35 Rugby Road, Brighton BN1 6EB — MB BS Lond. 1983; MRCGP 1989.

SUPPLE, Mohammed Arif Towcester Medical Centre, Link Way, Towcester NN12 6HH; 73 West End, Silverstone, Towcester NN12 8UY Tel: 01327 858147 — MB BS Lond. 1982; DRCOG 1987; MRCGP 1989.

SUPPLE, Neelam Tahseen 11 Hathaway Green Lane, Stratford-upon-Avon CV37 9HX — MB BS Lond. 1984; BSc (Hons.) Lond. 1981, MB BS 1984; MRCP (Paeds) UK 1994; MRCGP 2001.

SUPPREE, David Alastair Hampstead Medical Practice, 91 Heath Street, London NW3 6SS Tel: 020 7435 5055 Fax: 020 8458 5100; 73 Hodford Road, London NW11 8NH Tel: 020 8935 5234 — MB ChB Liverp. 1975. p/t Asst. GP; Medicolegal expert. Specialty: Acupunc.; Medico Legal. Special Interest: Medicolegal; Diabetes; Psychiat. Socs: ADA; Expert Witness Inst.; Assoc. RCGP.

SUPRAMANIAM, Ganesan Watford General Hospital, Vicarage Road, Watford WD18 0HB Tel: 01923 217695 Fax: 01923 217841; 11 Macdonald Close, Chesham Bois, Amersham HP6 5LZ Tel: 01494 728523 Fax: 01494 434458 — MB BS Ceylon 1971 (Colombo) DCH Eng. 1975; MRCP (UK) 1977; MSc (Nutrit.) Lond. 1978; FRCP Lond. 1992; FRCPCH 1996. Cons. Paediat. Watford Gen. Hosp. Specialty: Paediat. Socs: BMA; Roy. Coll. of Paediat. & Child Health; Sec. Gen. Commonw. Assoc. for Ment. Handicap & Developm.al Disabilities (CAMHADD). Prev: Sen. Regist. (Paediat.) St. Mary's Hosp. Lond.; Regist. (Paediat.) Dept. Child Health St. Geo. Hosp. Lond.; SHO (Paediat.) N. Middlx. Hosp. & St. Mary's Hosp. Lond.

SUR, Sujit Kumar Birleywood Health Centre, Birleywood, Skelmersdale WN8 9BW Tel: 01695 723333 Fax: 01695 556193; 56 Elmers Green, Skelmersdale WN8 6SB — MB BS Calcutta 1967.

SURALIWALA, Mr Khushroo Homi Ormskirk & District General Hospital, Surgical Directorate, Wigan Road, Ormskirk L39 2AZ Tel: 01695 656164 Fax: 01695 656261 Email: helen.fynn@southportandormskirk.nhs.uk — MB BS Gujarat 1980 (B. J. Med. Coll. Ahmedabad, India & Univ. Liverp.) MS (Orthop.) Gujarat 1983; MChOrth Liverp. 1990; FRCS 2003. Cons. Orthop. Surg. Southport & Ormskirk NHS Trust; Hon. Sen. Lect. (Sports Rehabil.) Univ. of Salford. Specialty: Orthop. Special Interest: Knee Surg.; Sports Injury. Socs: Brit. Assn. Surg. Knee; Brit. Orthop. Assn.; Brit. Orthop. Foot Surg. Soc. Prev: Regist. Wrightington Hosp. UK; Regist. Robt. Jones Orthop Hosp. Oswestry; Assitant Prof. (Orthop.) BI Med. Coll. Ahmedabad India.

SURAWY, Andrzej Jerzy The Surgery, 17 Battersea Rise, London SW11 1HG Tel: 020 7228 0195 Fax: 020 7978 5119 — MB BS Lond. 1971 (Westm.) MRCS Eng. LRCP Lond. 1977; MRCGP 1984.

SURAWY, Jerzy (retired) Dromquinna, Birchall Close, Leek ST13 5RQ — MB BCh BAO NUI 1952; DPM Eng. 1963; MRCPsych 1971. Prev: Cons. Psychiat. Stallington Hosp. Blythe Bridge.

SURDHAR, Harminderjeet Singh 10 Grafton Road, Birmingham B21 8PL — MB BS Lond. 1996.

SURENDRA KUMAR, Dhushyanthan 46 Kelburn Close, Northampton NN4 0RA — MB ChB Bristol 1993. SHO (Med.) Bristol Roy. Infirm.; Chairm. SW Jun. Doctors' Comm. Specialty: Gen. Med.

SURENDRA KUMAR, Rajasundram Meadow View, Roman Park, Little Aston Park, Sutton Coldfield B74 3AF Tel: 0121 360 7360 Fax: 0121 366 6977 — MB BS Ceylon 1967 (Peradeniya) Hosp. Pract. St. Margt. Hosp. Gt. Barr & N.croft Hosp. Birm.; Police Surg. Birm. Prev: Clin. Asst. (Rheum.) Selly Oak Hosp. Birm.

SURENDRAKUMAR, Sylvia Mathiraratnam Meadow View, 1 Roman Park, Roman Lane, Sutton Coldfield B74 3AF — MB BS Ceylon 1967; Dip. Community Paediat. Warwick 1983. SCMO (Child Health) Walsall AHA. Prev: Clin. Med. Off. (Child Health) Walsall AHA.

SURENTHIRAN, Sabaratnam 19 Pickhurst Park, Bromley BR2 0UE — MB BS Colombo 1982; MB BS Colombo Sri Lanka 1982; MRCP (UK) 1989.

SURENTHIRAN, Sangaralingam Shanmuga 68 Westmount Road, London SE9 1JE — MB BS Lond. 1985.

SURESH-BABU, Mirajkar Vithal Lincoln County Hospital, Greetwell Road, Lincoln LN2 5QY Tel: 01522 573 176 Fax: 01522 573 176 Email: suresh.babu@ulh.nhs.uk — MRCP Irel. 1993; DCH Madras 1989; MB BS India 1986 (Univ. of Madras, India) Cons. Paediat. Specialty: Paediat. Special Interest: Paediatric Gastroenterol. Socs: Brit. Soc. of Paediatric Gastroenterol. & Nutrit.; Roy. Coll. of Paediat. and Child Health. Prev: Sen. Regist. in Paediatric Gastroenterol., Booth Hall Childr. Hosp., Manch.

SURESH, Cheriyil Gangadhara Kurup Department of Cardiology, Royal Oldham Hospital, Rochdale Road, Oldham OL1 2JH Tel: 0161 627 8492 Fax: 0161 627 8474 Email: britmed@aol.com — MD Kerala 1987; MB BS Kerala 1983; MRCP (UK) 1990. Assoc. Specialist (Cardiol.). Specialty: Cardiol.

SURESH, Krishnmurthy c/o Drive P. P. Jana, 9 Tamarind Close, Hempstead, Gillingham ME7 3ST — MB BS Madras 1988; MRCP (UK) 1992.

SURESH, Tharayil Royal Scottish National Hospital, Forth Valley Primary Care NHS Trust, Larbert FK5 4SD Tel: 01324 570700; 2 Skelmorlie Place, Stenhousemuir, Larbert FK5 4UU Tel: 01324 562484 — MB BS Kerala 1969; DPM Leeds 1980. Cons. Psychiat. (locum) Loch View, Forth Valley PCT Larbert. Specialty: Ment. Health. Socs: Affil. Mem. Roy. Coll. Psychiat; BMA; Hosp. Cons. & Specialist Assn. Prev: Cons. Psychiat. Govt. Ment. Hosp. Calicut, India; Regist. (Psychiat.) Stanley Royd Hosp. Wakefield & St. Luke's Hosp. Huddersfield.

SURESH BABU, Mr Gokarakonda Department of Urology, James Paget Hospital, Great Yarmouth NR31 6LA Tel: 01493 452452; 15 Winstanley Road, Thorpe St. Andrew, Norwich NR7 0YH Tel: 01603 439212 — MB BS Nargarjuna 1978 (Guntur Medical College A.P. India) MB BS Nagarjuna 1978; MS (Gen. Surg.) Chandigarh 1982; FRCS Ed. 1986. Cons. Urol. James Paget Hosp. Gt. Yarmouth. Specialty: Urol. Socs: Med. Defence Union; BAUS; RCS Edin. Prev: Regist. (Urol.) N. Manch. Gen. Hosp.

SURESH BABU, Pillanna White Lodge, 15 St Giles Avenue, Scartho, Grimsby DN33 2HA — MB BS Mysore 1981.

SURESH SHETTY, Vorvady 1 Eastacombe Rise, Heanton, Barnstaple EX31 4DG — MB BS Mysore 1974.

SURESHKUMAR, Thambipillai 23 Milton Road, London E17 4SP — MB BS Colombo 1982.

SURI, Anil Kumar Ferndale Unit, Fazakerley Hospital, Longmoor Lane, Liverpool L9 7AL Tel: 0151 529 3206 — MD Panjab 1977 (Govt. Med. Coll. Patiala) MB BS 1970; MRCPsych 1974. Cons. Psychiat. Fazakerley Hosp. Liverp.; Hon. Clin. Lect. (Psychiat.) Univ. Liverp. Specialty: Gen. Psychiat. Prev: Lect. (Psychiat.) Univ. Liverp.

SURI, Avinash Chander New North Road Surgery, 563 New North Road, Hainault, Ilford IG6 3TF Tel: 020 8500 3054 Fax: 020 8501 3025 — MB BS Aligarh Muslim 1971; MB BS Aligarh Muslim 1971; MRCS Eng. LRCP Lond. London 1981.

SURI, Avtar Singh Birchills Health Centre, 23-27 Old Birchills, Walsall WS2 8QH Tel: 01922 614896 Fax: 01922 35073 — MB BS All India Inst. Med. Sci. 1972; MB BS All India Inst. Med.Sci. 1972.

SURI, Deepak Whittington Hospital, London N19 5NP Tel: 820 7288 5490 — MB BS Lond. 1992 (Middlesex) MRCP Lond. 1989; BSc Lond. 1989. Cons. Gastroenterologist, Whittington Hosp., Lond. Specialty: Gastroenterol. Prev: SHO St. Geo.'s Hosp. Lond.; SpR Gastroenterology/Hepatology, Roy. Free Hosp.; SpR Gastroenteroloy, The Middlx. Hosp.

SURI, Harminder Singh, Air Commodore RAF Med. Br. The Surgery, 25 Greenwood Avenue, Beverley HU17 0HB Tel: 01482 881517 Fax: 01482 887022 — MB BS Lond. 1977; BSc Guru Nanak Dev 1972; LMSSA Lond. 1985. Police Surg. Specialty: Gen. Med.

SURI, Ranjan 118 Canterbury Road, Harrow HA1 4PB Tel: 020 8723 6412 — MB ChB Manch. 1994 (Manchester) MRCPaed. 1997. Paediat. Regist. Northwick Pk. Hosp. Harrow. Specialty: Paediat. Socs: RCPCH.

SURI, Shailesh 118 Canterbury Road, Harrow HA1 4PB — MB ChB Birm. 1992.

SURI, Shobha Burscough Health Centre, Stanley Court, Lord Street, Burscough, Ormskirk L40 4LA Tel: 01704 894997 — MB BS Gauhati 1972.

SURI, Shubhada Sanjay Rotherham District General Hospital, Moorgate Road, Oakwood, Rotherham S60 2UD Tel: 01709 820000; 11 Woolgreaves Avenue, Sandal, Wakefield WF2 6DX Tel: 01924 259648 — MB BS Univ. Poona 1986 (Byramjee Jeejeebhoy) MRCP (UK) 1995. Staff Grade (c/o Elderly). Specialty: Care of the Elderly. Socs: BMA.

SURI, Sushil Burscough Health Centre, Stanley Court, Lord Street, Burscough, Ormskirk L40 4LA Tel: 01704 894997; 3 Backmoss Lane, Burscough, Ormskirk L40 4BD — MB BS Delhi 1968.

SURI, Yash Pal Memorial Hospital, Holyhurst Road, Darlington DL3 6HX Tel: 01325 380100 Fax: 01325 743622 — MB BS Agra 1958; BSc Agra 1953; ECFMG 1965; DTM & H Liverp. 1969; MRCP (UK) 1973; FRCP Glas. 1988; FRCP Ed. 1991. Cons. Phys. Geriat. Med. Memor. Hosp. Darlington & Richardson Hosp. Bernard Castle; Vis. Prof. Czechoslovakia Fac. of Med. Univ. Bratislava. Specialty: Gen. Med. Socs: Nat. Exec. Comm. & Div. Chairm. UK Overseas Doctors Assn.; Eur. Tissue Repair Soc. Prev: Sen. Regist. (Geriat. Med.) S. Cleveland HA; Regist. (Gen. Med.) Leigh Infirm.

SURIYA, Anar 6 Thornhill Close, Blackpool FY4 5BR — MB ChB Dundee 1991.

SURRIDGE, John Giles c/o Department of Endoscopy, The Royal Bournemouth Hospital, Castle Lowe E., Bournemouth BHT 1DW Tel: 01202 303626; Koyana, 224 Sanbanks Road, Poole BH14 8HA Tel: 01202 700688 Fax: 01202 706544 — BM BCh Oxf. 1960 (St. Thos.) MA Oxf. 1960; DObst RCOG 1965. Assoc. Specialist (Med.) Roy. Vict. Hosp. Bournemouth. Specialty: Gastroenterol. Socs: BMA. Prev: GP Bournemouth; Sen. Med. Off. (Cas.) St. Thos. Hosp. Lond.

SURRIDGE, Julia Mary 224 Sandbanks Road, Poole BH14 8HA — MB BS Lond. 1990 (St. Bartholomew's London) DRCOG 1994; DCH 1997. Community Paediat. SHO Brighton. Specialty: Paediat. Socs: MPS. Prev: Trainee GP Chichester VTS; Paediat. SHO Brighton; Paediat. SHO Portsmouth.

SURRIDGE, Nicholas John Bellingham Green Surgery, 24 Bellingham Green, London SE6 3JB Tel: 020 8697 7285 Fax: 020 8695 6094; 87 Bromley Road, London SE6 2UF — MB BS Lond. 1980 (King's Coll. Hosp.) BSc (1st cl. Hons.) Lond. 1977; LMSSA 1980.

SURTEES, Ann Curliss House, Corby Glen, Grantham Tel: 0147 684251 — MB ChB Leeds 1953. Prev: Ho. Surg. O & G Hosp. Wom. & Matern. Hosp. Leeds.

SURTEES, Helen Frances Anne Studholme Medical Centre, 50 Church Road, Ashford TW15 2TU; 143 Church Street, Staines TW18 4XZ — MB BS Lond. 1987.

SURTEES, Mr Peter Sunderland Royal Hospital, Kayll Road, Sunderland SR4 7TP — MB BS Newc. 1975; FRCS Ed. 1983. Specialty: Gen. Surg. Prev: Cons. Gen. Surg. Roy. Halifax Infirm.

SURTEES, Ridley Alexander (retired) Curliss House, Corby Glen, Grantham — MB ChB Leeds 1954; MRCGP 1968.

SURTEES, Robert Alexander Harrison Institute of Child Health, 30 Guilford St., London WC1N 1EH; 134 Victoria Road, London N22 7XQ — BM BCh Oxf. 1980; MA, 1980; PhD Lond. 1992; FRCP Lond. 1995; FRCPCH 1997. Sen. Lect. (Paediat. Neurol.) Inst. Child Health Univ. Lond.; Hon. Cons. Neurol. Hosp. Sick Childr. Gt. Ormond St. Lond. Specialty: Paediat. Neurol.; Neurol.

SURTEES, Stanley John Postgraduate Medical Centre, District General Hospital, Eastbourne BN21 2UD Tel: 01323 414967 Fax: 01323 414932 — MB ChB Liverp. 1952; FRCP Ed. 1982, M 1960; DTM & H Liverp. 1960; FRCPath 1976, M 1964; DHMSA 1992. Hon. Cons. Path. Clin. Chem., Med. Archiv. Eastbourne Hosp. Trust. Specialty: Chem. Path. Socs: Assn. Clin. Biochem.; Path. Soc.; Assn. Clin. Path. Prev: Sen. Lect. (Path.) & Erasmus Wilson Demonst. RCS Eng.; Regist. (Path.) St. Jas. Hosp. Lond. & Walton Hosp. Liverp.

SURY, Michael Roy Joseph Great Ormond Street Hospital for Children, Great Ormond St., London WC1A 7AS Tel: 020 7829 8865 Fax: 020 7829 8866 — MB BS Lond. 1980; DA Eng. 1982; FFA RCS Eng. 1985. Cons. Anaesth. Gt. Ormond St. Hosp. for Child. NHS Trust.; Clin. Dir. & Med. & Urol. Directorate, Gt. Ormond St. Specialty: Anaesth.

SURYANARAYAN SETTY, Raja Seetharamaiah, MBE The Royal Oldham Hospital, Rochdale Road, Oldham OL1 2JH Tel: 0161 624 0420 Fax: 0161 627 8694; 34 Epping Close, Chadderton, Oldham OL9 9ST Tel: 0161 678 6002 Fax: 0161 345 6704 — (Bangalore Med. Coll.) BSc Mysore 1958; MB BS Bangalore 1970; DTM & H Liverp. 1973; Cert. Family Plann. JCC 1996. Assoc. Specialist Oldham AHA. Specialty: Care of the Elderly. Prev: SHO Sheff. & Bradford HA.

SURYAVANSHI, Vijay Singh c/o Weybridge Medical (UK) Ltd., Freepost KT4605, Weybridge KT13 8BR — MB BS Jiwaji 1974.

SUSHILA, Sivathanu 11 Arthur Road, Farnham GU9 8PB Tel: 01252 710490 — MB BS Madras 1954 (Madras Med. Coll.) DCH Eng. 1957; MRCP Ed. 1959; FRCP Ed. 1994. Specialty: Paediat. Socs: BMA. Prev: Reader (Paediat.) Madras Med. Coll.; Regist. Liverp. RHB.

SUSMAN, Maurice Daniel (retired) 13 Canons Drive, Edgware HA8 7RB Tel: 020 8952 1503 — MB ChB Manch. 1951; DPH Eng. 1965; FFPHM 1991. Med. Ref. W. Herts Crematorium Watford Herts. Prev: Cons. Communicable Dis. Control Barnet HA.

SUSMAN, Rachel Davida 13 Canons Drive, Edgware HA8 7RB Tel: 020 8952 1503 Fax: 020 8952 1503 — MB BS Lond. 1994. Research Fell. Roy.Hosp.For Wom. Sydney Australia. Specialty: Paediat.

SUSNERWALA, Shabbir Saifuddin Rosemere Cancer Centre, Royal Preston Hospital, Sharoe Green Lane, Fulwood, Preston PR2 9HT Tel: 01772 522909 Fax: 01772 522955 — MB BS Bombay 1983; DMRT Lond. 1994; FRCR 1995. Cons. Clin. Oncol. Specialty: Oncol.; Radiother.

SUSSAMS, Roger William (retired) 349 Wrotham Road, Istead Rise, Gravesend DA13 9EF Tel: 0147 483 2494 — MB BS Lond. 1962 (Westm.) MFOM RCP Lond. 1980; DIH Eng. 1981. Prev: Occupat. Phys. Wellcome Foundat. Ltd. Gp. Occupat. Health Serv.

SUSSEX, Janet Elisabeth North Street House Surgery, 6 North Street, Emsworth PO10 7DD Tel: 01243 373538 — MB BS Lond. 1972 (St. Mary's Hosp. Lond.) DObst RCOG 1975; DCH Eng. 1976.

SUSSKIND, Werner (retired) 1B Ramsay Court, Eaglesham Road, Newton Mearns, Glasgow G77 5DJ Tel: 0141 639 3265 Fax: 0141 639 3265 Email: wsusskind@hotmail.com — (Glas.) MB ChB Glas. 1956; FRCP Glas. 1972, M 1962; FRCP Ed. 1976, M 1963; T(M) 1991. Prev: Cons. Dermat. Vict. Infirm. Glas.

SUSSMAN, Helen Sarah Greenmantle, 3 Washington Close, Reigate RH2 9LT — MB BS Lond. 1975; BSc (Hons.) Lond. 1971; FFPM RCP (UK) 1994. Specialty: Pharmaceutical Medicine. Prev: Med. Manager Ciba-Geigy Ltd Horsham; Med. Adviser Farmitalia Carlo Erba Ltd Barnet.

SUSSMAN, Jonathan David Greater Manchaster Neuroscience Centre, Hope Hospital, Stott Lane, Salford M6 8HD Tel: 0161 206 4591 Fax: 0161 206 2933 — MB ChB Leeds 1986; MRCP (UK) 1989; PhD (Cantab.) 1998; FRCP 2001. Cons. Neurol. Specialty: Neurol. Prev: Research Asst. MRC Centre for Brain Repair Camb.; Lect. (Neurol.) Univ. of Sheff.; Regist. (Med.) Univ. Hosp. of Wales Cardiff.

SUTARIA, Nilesh 2 Akehurst Close, Copthorne, Crawley RH10 3QQ — MB ChB Leeds 1990.

SUTARIA, Mr Praful Dahyabhai Blackheath Hospital, Lee Terrace, Blackheath, London SE3 9UD Tel: 020 8318 7722 Fax: 020 8318 2542; 106 St. Georges Road, London SE1 Tel: 020 7261 9165 — MB BS Nagpur 1965; FRCS Ed. 1968. Cons. Surg. Orthop. Greenwich Dist. Hosp. Specialty: Orthop. Socs: Fell. Brit. Soc. Surg. Hand.; Fell. BOA. Prev: Sen. Regist. (Orthop.) Char. Cross Hosp. Lond., Northwick Pk. Hosp. Harrow & Roy. Nat. Orthop. Hosps.

SUTCLIFF, John Robert Harvey (retired) Melroyd End, Bicknacre, Chelmsford CM3 4HA — MB BS Lond. 1966 (St. Bart.) MRCP (UK) 1973; DObst RCOG 1974; FRCGP 1994, M 1977. Trainer (Gen. Pract.) Essex FPC; Med. Off. Hosp. & Homes St. Giles. Prev: Regist. (Med.) United Norwich Hosps.

SUTCLIFFE, Alastair Gordon Royal Free & University College Medical School, University College London, London NW3 5QG Tel: 020 7830 2049 Fax: 020 7830 2049; 17 Eastholm, London NW11 6LR Tel: 020 8201 9244 — MB ChB Manch. 1987; MD; FRCPCH; MRCP (UK) 1992. Sen. Lect. (Paediat.) Roy. Free & Univ. Coll. Med. Sch. Lond.; Hon. Cons. Paediat. Specialty: Paediat. Socs: Brit. Paediat. Assn.; BMA; Assn. Research Infant & Child Developm. Prev: Lect. (Child Health) Roy. Free Hosp. Lond.; Sen. Regist. (Paediat.) Roy. Free Hosp. & Moorfields Eye Hosp. Lond.; Lect. (Child Health) Univ. Manch.

SUTCLIFFE, Alistair Paul Moor Lodge, Brackenhill Lane, Eskdaleside, Whitby YO22 5ER — MB ChB Aberd. 1993; BSc (1st cl. Hons.) Lond. 1987; MB ChB (Hons.) Aberd. 1993; DFFP 1996; DRCOG 1997; MRCGP 1998. Specialty: Gen. Pract. Prev: SHO (Med.) John Radcliffe Hosp. Oxf.; SHO (O & G) Raigmore, Abred.; SHO (Paediat.) Aberd.

SUTCLIFFE, Anne Josephine Queen Elizabeth Hospital, Egbaston, Birmingham B15 2TH Tel: 0121 472 1311 Email: anne.sutcliffe@uhb.nhs.uk — MB ChB Birm. 1974; BSc (Hons.) Birm. 1971; FFA RCSI 1978; FFA RCS Eng. 1979. Cons. in Anaesth. & Critical Care, Qu. Eliz. Hosp., Birm.; Med. Lead Heart of Eng. Critical Care Network. Specialty: Intens. Care; Anaesth. Special Interest: Neuro and Trauma. Socs: Assn. Anaesth. (Ex-Mem. Counc.); (Ex-Brit. Rep.) Internat. Trauma Anaesth. & Critical Care Soc. (Chairm., Finance Comm.); ESA. Prev: Lead Clinician Neuroscis. Critical Care Area; Ruscoe Clark Memor. Lect.; Cons. Anaesth. Birm. Accid. Hosp.

SUTCLIFFE, Gordon Edward (retired) Heathfield, Sandy Way, Maybury, Woking GU22 8BB Tel: 01483 773178 — MB BS Lond. 1943 (St. Thos.) MRCS Eng. LRCP Lond. 1942.

SUTCLIFFE, Ian Michael Dewsbury & District Hospital, Halifax Road, Dewsbury WF13 4HS Tel: 01924 816141 Fax: 01924 512059 Email: ian.sutcliffe@midyorks.nhs.uk; 179 Leeds Road, Lofthouse, Wakefield WF3 3NE Tel: 01924 824110 — MB BS Lond. 1991 (St Geo.) BSc (Psychol. as applied to Med. 2.1) Lond. 1989; MRCP (UK) 1996. Cons. Phys. with an interest in Respirat. Med., Mid-Yorks, Newsbury. Specialty: Respirat. Med. Socs: BMA; Brit. Thorac. Soc.

SUTCLIFFE, James Edward Lawrence (retired) Seskinore, 49 Shore Road, Carrickfergus BT38 8UA Tel: 01232 862241 — MB BCh BAO Belf. 1950; DObst RCOG 1952; MRCGP 1968. Prev: Ho. Off. Roy. Vict. Hosp. Belf.

SUTCLIFFE, Mr John Christopher The London Spine Clinic, 119 Harley Street, London W1G 6AU Tel: 020 7616 7200 Fax: 020 7486 4601 — MB ChB Ed. 1983; FRCS Ed. 1988; FRCS (SN) 1992. Cons. Neurosurg. Roy. Lond. Hosp. & Harley St. Lond. Specialty: Neurosurg. Socs: Brit. Neurol. Surg. Soc. Prev: Sen. Regist. (Neurosurg.) Roy. Lond. Hosp.; Regist. (Neurosurg.) Roy. Hallamsh. Hosp. Sheff.

SUTCLIFFE, Mr Jonathan Richard 102 Waterloo Road, Southport PR8 3AY Tel: 01704 575615 — MB ChB Leeds 1991; FRCS 1998. SHO Postgrad. Surgic. Train. Scheme St. Jas. Univ. Hosp. Leeds. Specialty: Paediat. Surg.

SUTCLIFFE, Kim Caroline The Corners, 11 West End, Guisborough, Redcar TS14 6NN — MB BCh BAO Belf. 1985 (Qu. Belf.) DGM RCP Lond. 1988; DRCOG 1989; DCH RCPS Glas. 1989; MRCGP 1990; DFFP 1993. Specialty: Community Child Health.

SUTCLIFFE, Lesley Kathleen Glenfields, Blind Lane, Isle Abbotts, Taunton TA3 6RH Tel: 01460 281205 — MB BS Lond. 1976 (Lond. Hosp.) DRCOG 1978; T(GP) 1991; MFFP 1993; Registered Coloscopist - 2000. Staff grade - Gyn., Contraceptive & Sexual Health, Taunton & Som. Hosp.; Clin. Asst. - Genito-urinary Med., Yeovil Hosp. Specialty: Family Plann. & Reproduc. Health.

SUTCLIFFE, Mr Martin Logan Rockleigh, 51 Roman Bank, Stamford PE9 2ST Tel: 01780 63728 — MB ChB Sheff. 1969; FRCS Eng. 1974. Cons. Orthop. Surg. P'boro. Dist. Hosp., Edith Cavell Hosp., Co. Hosp. Doddington, Fitzwilliam Hosp. P'boro. & Stamford & Rutland Memor. Hosp.; Recognised Clin. Teach. Univ. Camb.; Hon. Clin. Tutor Univ. Leicester. Specialty: Orthop. Socs: Fell. BOA; BMA. Prev: Sen. Regist. Sheff. AHA (T); Regist. Rotat. (Surg.) Roy. Hosp. Sheff.; Regist. (Orthop.) King Edwd. VII Orthop. Hosp. Sheff.

SUTCLIFFE, Melanie Kate Sheffield Children's Hospital, Western Bank, Sheffield S10 2TH Tel: 0114 271 7000; 33 Wyston Brook, Hilton, Derby DE65 5JB Tel: 730448 Email: msutcliffe@doctorsnet.org.uk — MB BS Lond. 1997 (St. George's Hosp. Med. Sch.) BSc (Ost.) 1992 CNNA. Specialty: Paediat.

SUTCLIFFE, Mr Michael Matthew Lister (retired) Underwood, Waterhouse Lane, Kingswood, Tadworth KT20 6HT Tel: 01737 832532 Email: MLSutcl@aol.com — MB BS Lond. 1954 (Univ. Coll. Hosp.) FRCS Eng. 1963. Prev: Cons. Surg. Mayday Healthcare Croydon.

SUTCLIFFE, Moira Caroline Fishponds Health Centre, Beechwood Road, Fishponds, Bristol BS16 3TD Tel: 0117 908 2365 Fax: 0117 908 2377 — MB ChB Bristol 1985. Trainee GP Bristol VTS. Prev: SHO (ENT) MusGr. Pk. Hosp. Taunton.

SUTCLIFFE, Nicholas Peter Health Care International, Beardmore St., Clydebank G81 4HX Tel: 0141 951 5611 Fax: 0141 951 5603 — MB ChB Manch. 1982; BSc Manch. 1979; MRCP (UK) 1985; FCAnaesth 1989. Sen. Regist. (Anaesth.) Roy. Liverp. Hosp. Specialty: Intens. Care. Prev: Regist. (Anaesth.) Glas. Roy. Infirm.; Regist. (Renal Med.) Glas. Roy. Infirm.

SUTCLIFFE, Norman Howard (retired) 16 Burnham Road, Leigh-on-Sea SS9 2JU Tel: 01702 474724; 91 Rushbottom Lane, Benfleet SS7 4EA Tel: 013745 754311 — MB BS Lond. 1960 (Westm.) MRCS Eng. LRCP Lond. 1959. Prev: SHO (Obst.) & Ho. Phys. City Hosp. Derby.

SUTCLIFFE, Nurhan (retired) Bloomsbury Rheumatology Unit, 4th Floor, Arthur Stanley House, 40-50 Tottenham St., London W1T 4NJ Tel: 020 7380 9230 Fax: 020 7380 9278; 17 Eastholm, London NW11 6LR Tel: 020 8201 9244 — Tip Doktoru Istanbul 1987; MRCP (UK) 1993; MD 2001. Specialist Regist. (Rheum.) Middlx. Hosp. Lond. Prev: Regist. Hope Hosp. Manch.

SUTCLIFFE, Penelope Jane 42 Petworth Road, Haslemere GU27 2HX — MB BS Lond. 1992.

SUTCLIFFE, Rachel Christine The Mount House Surgery, Beech Close, Warboys, Huntingdon PE28 2RQ — BChir Camb. 1992.

SUTCLIFFE, Richard Lawrence Guy, DFC (retired) 5 Berkeley Close, Green Park, Northampton NN1 5BJ Tel: 01604 638501 — (St. Thos.) MB BS Lond. 1953; MRCS Eng. LRCP Lond. 1953; FRCP Ed. 1975, M 1967. Prev: Cons. Phys. (Geriat. Med.) Northampton HA & St. And. Hosp. Northampton.

SUTCLIFFE, Roderick Ian Academic Unit of Primary Care, 20 Hyde Terrace, University of Leeds, Leeds LS2 9LN Tel: 0113 343 4193 Fax: 0113 343 4181 Email: r.i.sutcliffe@leeds.ac.uk; 109 Cragg Road, Mytholmroyd, Hebden Bridge HX7 5FB Tel: 01422 882082 — MB ChB Liverp. 1976; FRCGP 1994, M 1980; DRCOG 1980; MMedSci Sheff. 1995. Sen. Lect. in Primary Care Teachg. Leeds; GP Princip. Leeds. Specialty: Gen. Pract.; Educat. Prev: Cons. Primary Med. Care Sheff. Health; Course Organiser Calderdale VTS; GP Sheff. Halifax & Hebden Gp. Pract.

SUTCLIFFE, Vanessa Jane 42 Englands Way, Chard TA20 1EF — BM BS Nottm. 1998.

SUTCLIFFE, Veronica Anne Ardingly Court Surgery, Ardingly Court, 1 Ardingly Street, Brighton BN2 1SS Tel: 01273 688333 Fax: 01273 671128 — MB BS Lond. 1990 (UCL) BSc Lond. 1987; DTM & H RCP Lond. 1992; DRCOG 1994; DCH RCP Lond. 1995; MRCGP 1995. GP Brighton. Specialty: Gen. Pract. Prev: Trainee GP/SHO Brighton VTS; Ho. Surg. Roy. Sussex Co. Hosp. Brighton; Ho. Phys. W. Norwich Hosp.

SUTER, Catherine Mary Willingham Medical Practice, 52 Long Lane, Willingham, Cambridge CB4 5LB Tel: 01954 260230 Fax: 01954 206204; 71 Cottenham Road, Histon, Cambridge CB4 9ET Tel: 01223 565326 — MB BS Lond. 1980 (Univ. Coll. Hosp.) BSc (Hons.) Lond. 1975; DRCOG 1982.

SUTERIA, Yasmin 1 Bentham Close, Bury BL8 3DL — BM Soton. 1995.

SUTHERBY, Elizabeth Kim Maudsley Hospital, Denmark Hill, London SE5 8AZ Tel: 020 7703 6333 — MB BS Lond. 1986; MRCPsych 1992. Sen. Regist. (Psychiat.) Maudsley Hosp. Lond. Specialty: Gen. Psychiat. Socs: BMA.

SUTHERLAND, Aeneas Rose (retired) 8 Grange Road, St Andrews KY16 8LF Tel: 01334 73747 — MB ChB Ed. 1943; DA Eng. 1954. Prev: Cons. Anaesth. Law Hosp. Carluke.

SUTHERLAND, Mr Alasdair George Dept. Orthopaedics, Polwarth Building, Foresterhill, Aberdeen AB25 2ZD Email: ort025@abdn.ac.uk — MB ChB Aberd. 1990; FRCS Ed. 1994; FRCS Ed (Tr&Orth) 1999; MD (Hons) Aberd. 2003. Sen. Lect. & Cons. (Orthop.) Aberd. Specialty: Orthop. Socs: Socute Inst. Orthopeche et de Traumatol. (SICOT); Fell. BOA. Prev: SHO Rotat. (Surg.) Aberd. Hosps.; Regist (Orthop.) Roy. Infirm.; Lect. (Orthop.) Univ. Aberd.

SUTHERLAND, Alastair Mackie 12 Newtonlea Avenue, Newton Mearns, Glasgow G77 5QA Tel: 0141 639 1434 — MB ChB Glas. 1959.

SUTHERLAND, Andrew Sharp Kelso Medical Group Practice, Health Centre, Inch Road, Kelso TD5 7LF Tel: 01573 224424 Fax: 01573 226388; Goshen Bank, Edenside Road, Kelso TD5 7BS — MB ChB Ed. 1979; DRCOG 1981; MRCGP 1993.

SUTHERLAND, Anne Bryson (retired) 48 Ravelston Gardens, 48 Ravelston Gardens, Edinburgh EH4 3LF Tel: 0131 337 3921 — MB ChB Ed. 1951; MD Ed. 1958; FRCS Ed. 1963. Prev: Cons. Plastic Surg. Plastic & Maxillofacial Unit SE Region Scotl.

SUTHERLAND, Anthony Michael Leemont, Le Bequet Road, Village de Putron, St Peter Port, Guernsey — MB BS Newc. 1993. SHO (A & E) Guernsey. Socs: BMA.

SUTHERLAND, Bruce 35 Springfield Gardens, Aberdeen AB15 7RX — MB ChB Aberd. 1976.

SUTHERLAND, Cassandra Jane The Old Vicarage, Mabe, Penryn TR10 9JG — MB ChB Liverp. 1987; FRCA 1994. Cons. (anaesth.) Roy. Cornw. Hosp. Truro. Specialty: Anaesth. Prev: Clin. Research Fell. (Anaesth.) Derriford Hosp. Plymouth.; Specialist Regist. SW Sch. Anaesth.

SUTHERLAND, Ceri Jane 68A Downhham Road, London N1 5BG — MB ChB Ed. 1992.

SUTHERLAND, Charles George Grant Department of Pathology, Royal Alexandra Hospital, Paisley PA2 9PN Tel: 0141 580 4162 Fax: 0141 580 4164 Email: charles.sutherland@rah.scot.nhs.uk — MB ChB Dundee 1979; MRCPath 1987. Cons. Histopath. Roy. Alexandra Hosp. Paisley. Specialty: Pathology, General.

SUTHERLAND, Christine Annette Hastings 23 Norwood Drive, Giffnock, Glasgow G46 7LS — MB ChB Glas. 1991 (Glasgow) MRCPsych 1995. Staff Grade Psychiat. Greater Glas. Primary Care Trust. Specialty: Gen. Psychiat. Prev: SHO S. Sector Psychiat. Serv. Community & Ment. Health Unit Greater Glas.

SUTHERLAND, Claire — MB ChB Glas. 1998.

SUTHERLAND, David Findlay Woodside Health Centre, Barr Street, Glasgow G20 7LR Tel: 0141 531 9556 Fax: 0141 531 9555; 46A Dalziel Drive, Glasgow G41 4HY — MB ChB Aberd. 1982; DRCOG 1984; MRCGP 1986. Prev: Trainee GP West. Infirm. Glas. VTS.

SUTHERLAND, David Thompson (retired) 26 Dallam Drive, Sandside, Milnthorpe LA7 7LL; 30 Ashleugh Court, Station Road, Arnside, Carnforth LA5 0JH Tel: 01524 761140 — MB ChB Aberd. 1947.

SUTHERLAND, Derek James 10 Woodside Drive, Sanquhar, Forres IV36 2UF — MB ChB Aberd. 1994.

SUTHERLAND, Donald Hall, DFC (retired) 5 Kinnaber Road, Hillside, Montrose DD10 9HE Tel: 01674 830285 — MB ChB Glas. 1951; DMRD Eng. 1959. Cons. Radiol. Stracathro Hosp. Brechin; Hon. Sen. Lect. Univ. Dundee. Prev: Sen. Regist. Dept. Radiodiag. Roy. Infirm. Aberd.

SUTHERLAND, Dorothy Anne (retired) 13 Clayton Drive, Prestatyn LL19 9RW — MB ChB Aberd. 1950; DCH Eng. 1955. Assoc. Specialist Paediat. Glan Clwyd Hosp.

SUTHERLAND, Edmond McIntosh (retired) 12 Runcorn Close, Greenlands, Redditch B98 7PU — BM BCh Oxf. 1964; BA Oxf. 1960, BM BCh 1964; DPM Eng. 1968; MRCPsych 1972. Prev: Research Sen. Regist. Oxf. RHB.

SUTHERLAND, Elisabeth (retired) Mill House, Grinton, Richmond DL11 6HL Tel: 01748 884279 — MB ChB Sheff. 1951; MRCGP 1974.

SUTHERLAND, Eric Lynton (retired) Mill House, Grinton, Richmond DL11 6HL Tel: 01748 884279 — MB ChB Sheff. 1951 (Sheff) DPM Eng. 1958; FRCPsych 1980. Prev: Cons. Psychiat. Winterton Hosp.

SUTHERLAND, Fraser Tullis 14 Atholl Gardens, Kilwinning KA13 7DQ; 270 Queen's Road, Aberdeen AB15 8DR Tel: 01224 318157 — MB ChB Aberd. 1989. Specialty: Gen. Pract.

SUTHERLAND, George Roberton (retired) 22 Montrose Drive, Bearsden, Glasgow G61 3LG Tel: 0141 942 7802 — (Ed.) MB ChB (Distinc.) Ed. 1955; FRCP Ed. 1971, M 1959; DMRD Ed. 1965; FFR 1967; FRCR 1975; MRCP (Glas.) 1984; FRCP Glas. 1986. Prev: Cons. Nuffield Hosp. & Bon Ssecour Hosp. Glas.

SUTHERLAND, George Ross 25 Howard Place, Edinburgh EH3 5JY — MB ChB Ed. 1972; MRCP (UK) 1975. Head of Cardiac Ultrasound Thorax Center Ziekenhuis Dijrzegt, Rotterdam, The Netherlands. Prev: Cons. Paediat. Cardiol. Soton. Gen. Hosp.

SUTHERLAND, Glenys Ann The Harlequin Surgery, 160 Shard End Crescent, Shard End, Birmingham B34 7BP — MB ChB Leeds 1974; MRCGP 1981.

SUTHERLAND, Gordon Archibald Directorate of Anaesthesia, Royal Infirmary, Alexandra Parade, Glasgow G31 3ER; 45 Laxton Drive, Lenzie, Glasgow G66 5LX — MB ChB Glas. 1974; FRCA 1980. Cons. (Anaesth.) Glas. Roy. Infirm. Specialty: Anaesth. Prev: Clin. Fell. (Anaesth.) McGill Univ. Montreal Canada.

SUTHERLAND, Graeme Munro Abbey Health Centre, East Abbey Street, Arbroath DD11 1EN Tel: 01241 870307 Fax: 01241 431414 — MB ChB Glas. 1978.

SUTHERLAND, Graham Crieff Health Centre, King Street, Crieff PH7 3SA Tel: 01764 652456 Fax: 01764 655756; Schiehallion, 27 Strathearn Terrace, Crieff PH7 3BZ Tel: 01764 655459 — MB ChB Ed. 1990; MRCGP 1995. Specialty: Gen. Pract.

SUTHERLAND, Hamish Watson (retired) Redstones, 9 Marchbank Road, Bieldside, Aberdeen AB15 9DJ Tel: 01224 867017 — MB ChB St. And. 1957; DObst RCOG 1960; FRCOG 1976, M 1964. Hon. Clin. Reader (Obst. & Gyn.) Univ. Aberd.; Hon. Cons. O & G Aberd. Roy. Hosps. Trust. Prev: Reader & Cons. O & G Aberd. Roy. Hosps. Trust.

SUTHERLAND, Helen Bruce (retired) Park Towers, 30 Marlborough Road, Ryde PO33 1AB Tel: 01983 611644 — MB ChB Glas. 1920; DPH Lond. 1930. Prev: Anaesth. Roy. I. of Wight Co. Hosp. Ryde.

SUTHERLAND, Helen Claire 2 Park Lane, Hale, Altrincham WA15 9JS — BM BS Nottm. 1993.

SUTHERLAND, Iain Alasdair Keith Chastleton, Newton Drive, Framwellgate Moor, Durham DH1 5BH Tel: 01385 46171 — MB Camb. 1972; BChir 1971; DCH Eng. 1973; DObst RCOG 1976.

SUTHERLAND, Iain Alexander Pembroke House, 32 Albert Road, N.E. Lincolnshire, Cleethorpes DN35 8LU Tel: 01472 691033 Fax: 01472 291516 — MB ChB Aberd. 1967; DRCOG 1972.

SUTHERLAND, Ian Alexander — MB ChB Ed. 1978. GP Princip. Pathhead Midlothian EH37 5PP. Socs: MRCGP.

SUTHERLAND, Ian Alexander 10 Waverley Road, Farnborough GU14 7EY — MB BS Lond. 1965 (Guy's) MRCS Eng. LRCP Lond. 1965; DA Eng. 1967; FFA RCS Eng. 1970. Cons. Anaesth. Frimley Pk. Hosp. Specialty: Anaesth. Prev: Sen. Regist. (Anaesth.) Char. Cross Hosp. Lond.; Staff Anaesth. St. Radboud Ziekenhuis Nijmegen Univ., Netherlands; Regist. (Anaesth.) Guy's Hosp. Lond.

SUTHERLAND, Ian Boyd (retired) Flat 1, 8 Chesterfield Road, Eastbourne BN20 7NU Tel: 01323 739777 — (Ed.) MB ChB Ed. 1949, DPH 1953; FFCM 1972; FRCP Ed. 1983, M 1982. Prev: Regional Med. Off. S. West. RHA.

SUTHERLAND, Ian Crawford (retired) Green Meadows, Prinsted, Emsworth PO10 8HS Tel: 01243 372504 Email: sutherland.i@virgin.net — MRCS Eng. LRCP Lond. 1957 (St. Mary's) DObst RCOG 1962; DA Eng. 1964; FFA RCS Eng. 1968. Cons. Anaesth. Portsmouth & S.E. Hants. HA. Prev: Cons. Anaesth. Portsmouth & S.E. Hants. HA.

SUTHERLAND, Ian Ross Sturry Surgery, 53 Island Road, Sturry, Canterbury CT2 0EF — MB ChB Aberd. 1988; MRCGP 1996. GP Princip., Dr Molony & Partners, Sturry Surg., Sturry, Kent. Specialty: Gen. Pract. Prev: Locum GP Queensland, Australia; Locum GP Montpellier Health Care, Cheltenham; GP Trainee, Shipston-on-Stour.

SUTHERLAND, James Andrew The New Surgery, 209 Sheffield Road, Killamarch, Sheffield S21 8DZ Tel: 01909 770347 — MB BS Newc. 1981; MRCGP 1986.

SUTHERLAND, Jamie 26 Furze Hill Drive, Poole BH14 8QL — BM Soton. 1990.

SUTHERLAND, Jane Katriona Royal Edinburgh Hospital, Morningside Park, Edinburgh EH10 5HF — MB ChB Ed. 1993; MRCPsych.

SUTHERLAND, Janet Shirley (retired) 8 Grange Road, St Andrews KY16 8LF Tel: 01334 73747 — MB ChB Glas. 1958. Prev: Clin. Med. Off. (Family Plann.) Ninewells Hosp. Dundee.

SUTHERLAND, Joanne (retired) Strathard, Drumnadrochit, Inverness IV63 6XP Tel: 01456 450230 — MB ChB Ed. 1957; DCH

RFPS Glas. 1962; MRCPsych 1984. Prev: Clin. Asst. (Psychiat. Research) Highland Psychiat. Research Gp. Craig Dunain Hosp. Inverness.

SUTHERLAND, John (retired) Fernbank, Miller Avenue, Wick KW1 4DF Tel: 01955 5326 — MB ChB Glas. 1952. Prev: Ho. Surg. Law Hosp. Carluke & Overtoun Matern. Hosp. Dumbarton.

SUTHERLAND, John Douglas (retired) Craig Ben Cottage, Kinlochspelve, Isle of Mull PA62 6AA Tel: 0168 04 224 — MB ChB Ed. 1956.

SUTHERLAND, John Forbes Wilson, MBE (retired) 25 MacDonald Drive, Knockothie, Ellon AB41 8BD Tel: 01358 723801 — MB ChB Glas. 1955; DObst RCOG 1957. Prev: GP Peterhead.

SUTHERLAND, John Graham 107 Sunnyside Road, Aberdeen AB24 3LT — MB ChB Aberd. 1994. Specialty: Accid. & Emerg.

SUTHERLAND, John Hugh (retired) Glan y Mor Surgery, Poles, Dornoch IV25 3HZ — MB ChB Ed. 1951; MRCGP 1969.

SUTHERLAND, Karen Elizabeth — MB ChB Glas. 1998.

SUTHERLAND, Mrs Kathryn Anne 25 Bangholm Loan, Edinburgh EH5 3AH Tel: 0131 552 7676 Fax: 0131 552 8145; 25 Howard Place, Edinburgh EH3 5JY — MB ChB Ed. 1974 (Edinburgh) MRCP (UK) 1977. Gen. Practitoner. 25 Bangholm Loan, Edin.; Hosp. Practitioner, Lipid Clinic (Cardiol.) Roy. Infirm. Edin. Specialty: Cardiol. Socs: Brit. Hyperlipid. Assn.; SHARP.

SUTHERLAND, Linda Mary Jasmine Park (ward 6), City Hospital, Aberdeen Tel: 01224 663131; 77 Fountainhall Road, Aberdeen AB15 4EA Tel: 01224 644170 — MB ChB Aberd. 1979. Clin. Asst. (Med. for Elderly) City Hosp. Aberd. Specialty: Care of the Elderly. Prev: Sessional Med. Off. Aberd. & NE Scotl. Blood Transfus. Serv.; Clin. Asst. (Psychogeriat.) Farnham Rd. Hosp. Guildford; Regist. Rotat. (Psychiat.) Aberd.

SUTHERLAND, M Shona McPhail Department of Opthalmology, Queen Margaret Hospital, Dunfermline KY12 9SU — MB ChB Glas. 1988; FRCOphth 1997. Cons. Opthalmology, Qu. Margt. Hosp. Dunfermline. Specialty: Ophth. Prev: Specialist Regist. (Ophth.) Ninewells Hosp. Dundee.

SUTHERLAND, MacKenzie Stewart 70 Chestnut Drive, Marton, Middlesbrough TS7 8BX Tel: 01642 273332 — MB ChB Aberd. 1962; DPM Ed. & Glas. 1967; Dip. Psychother. Aberd. 1970; MRCPsych 1973. Indep. Cons. Psychiat.; Hon. Cons. N. Tees Gen. Hosp. Stockton. Specialty: Gen. Psychiat. Socs: Fell. Roy. Soc. Med. Prev: Sen. Regist. NE (Scotl.) RHB; Regist. Profess. Unit Ross Clinic Aberd.; Exchange Regist. (Psychiat.) Univ. W. Indies.

SUTHERLAND, Mary Veronica (retired) 18 Cantley Manor Avenue, Cantley, Doncaster DN4 6TN — (St. And.) MB ChB St. And. 1956. Prev: GP Tickhill.

SUTHERLAND, Paul Dudley Southampton General Hospital, Tremona Road, Southampton SO16 6YD; 43 Beech Grange, Landford, Salisbury SP5 2AL Email: paulsutherland@hotmail.com — BM BCh Oxf. 1991 (Oxford) FRCA 1996. Cons. Anaesth. Specialty: Anaesth.

SUTHERLAND, Rachel Jane 1 The Drive, Adel, Leeds LS16 6BG — MB ChB Leeds 1990. Trainee GP N. Worcs. HA VTS.

SUTHERLAND, Robert William 35 Dalhousie Terrace, Edinburgh EH10 5PD — MB ChB Ed. 1986; DA (UK) 1990; FRCA 1992. Cons. Anaesth. West. Gen. Hosp. NHS Trust Edin. Specialty: Anaesth.

SUTHERLAND, Sandra Jane The Surgery, St Couan Crescent, Kirkcowan, Newton Stewart DG8 0HH Tel: 01671 830206 Fax: 01671 404163 — MB ChB Aberd. 1984; DRCOG 1986; DCCH RCP Ed. 1989; MRCGP 1989.

SUTHERLAND, Lady Sheena (retired) Houndwood House, Eyemouth, Edinburgh TD 14 5TW Tel: 01890 761 200 Email: s.sutherland@bushinternet.com — MB ChB Aberd. 1963; MRCPath 1982. Hon. Cons. Roy. Infirm. Edin. NHS Trust. Prev: Cons. Virol. Dulwich PHL King's Coll. Hosp. & Hon. Sen. Lect. King's Coll. Sch. Med. & Dent.

SUTHERLAND, Sheilah Dorothy 7 Rupert Close, Henley-on-Thames RG9 2JD Tel: 01491 575577 — (Manch.) MD Manch. 1963, MB ChB 1957. Socs: Fell. Manch. Med. Soc.; Hon. Fell. Soc. Chiropodists. Prev: Sen. Lect. Anat. Univ. Manch; Ho. Surg. & Ho. Phys. Manch. Roy. Infirm.; JP.

SUTHERLAND, Stephanie Claire Claro House, Stratton Chase Drive, Chalfont St Giles HP8 4NS Tel: 01494 874647 Fax: 01494 874605 — MB BS Newc. 1991. SHO (Paediat.). Specialty: Paediat.

SUTHERLAND, Thomas Worsley (retired) 70 Batley Road, Alverthorpe, Wakefield WF2 0AD Tel: 01924 372857 — MD Leeds 1953; MB ChB 1940; FCPath 1966. Reader & Sen. Lect. (Path.) Univ. Leeds. Prev: Hon. Cons. Pathol. Gen. Infirm. Leeds.

SUTHERST, John Richard 20 Bath Street, Waterloo, Liverpool L22 5PS Tel: 0151 920 0791 Fax: 0151 928 7821 Email: jrs.bathst@blueyonder.co.uk — MB ChB Sheff. 1963; FRCOG 1980, M 1967; MD Sheff. 1980. p/t Cons. (Gyn.) Liverp. Wom. Hosp. Specialty: Obst. & Gyn. Socs: Internat. Continence Soc.; Assoc. Mem. BAUS; Internat. Urogyn. Assn. Prev: Reader (Clin. O & G) Univ. Liverp. & Hons. Cons. (Obst. & Gyn.) Liverp. HA; Sen. Lect. (O & G) Univ. Liverp.; Cons. (O & G) Arrowe Park Hospital, Wirral.

SUTLIEFF, Patricia Ann Foster House Surgery, 23 Cockett Road, Langley, Slough SL3 7TQ Tel: 01753 580484 Fax: 01753 580501 — MB BS Lond. 1973 (St. Geo.) BSc Lond. 1970; DRCOG 1976; DA Eng. 1976; Cert. Family Plann. JCC 1977. GP Langley Berks. Prev: GP Hayes & Slough; SHO (Obst. & Anaesth.) Northwick Pk. Hosp. Harrow.

SUTTIE, Gillian Mary (retired) Ferniehirst, 13 Lockhart Place, Hawick TD9 9JR Tel: 01450 372979 — MB ChB Aberd. 1962.

SUTTIE, Keith Young 3 Kilspindie Road, Dundee DD2 3JP Tel: 01382 611472 — MB ChB Dundee 1991. Regist. (O & G) Walsgrave Hosp. Coventry.

SUTTON, Adrian Graham Lyndale, 90 Woodford Road, Bramhall, Stockport SK7 1PB — MB BS Lond. 1977 (Univ. Coll. Hosp.) BSc (Hons.) (Psychol.) Lond. 1974, MB BS 1977; FRCPsych 1994, M 1981. Cons. Child & Family Psychiat. Winnicott Centre Centr. Manch. Health Care Trust; Hon. Assoc. Lect. Vict. Univ. Manch. Specialty: Child & Adolesc. Psychiat. Prev: Sen. Regist. Child Guid. Train. Centre & Whitting Hosp. Lond.; Sen. Regist. (Child & Family) Tavistock Clin. Lond.; Regist. (Psychol. Med.) Univ. Coll. Hosp. Lond.

SUTTON, Alan Roade Medical Centre, 16 London Road, Roade, Northampton NN7 2NN Tel: 01604 862218 Fax: 01604 862129; 9 Lodge Avenue, Collingtree, Northampton NN4 0NQ Tel: 01604 766804 — MB ChB Sheff. 1967; DObst RCOG 1970. Clin. Asst. Grafton Manor Brain Injury Unit. Prev: Lect. (Health Educat.) Northampton Boro.; Ho. Off. (Surg. & Paediat.) & SHO (O & G) Northampton Gen. Hosp.

SUTTON, Amanda — MB ChB Bristol 1986; DRCOG 1989; Cert. Family Plann. JCC 1989; MRCGP 1990. Partner in Gen. Pract., Dukes Avenue Pract., Lond. N10. Prev: Trainee GP St. Johns Way Lond.

SUTTON, Andrew Gordon Charles 45 Algarth Road, Pocklington, York YO42 2HL — MB BChir Camb. 1993 (Addenbrooke's Clin. Sch. Camb.) MA Camb. 1994; MRCP (UK) 1996. Research Regist. (Cardiol.) S. Cleveland Hosp. Middlesbrough. Specialty: Cardiol.

SUTTON, Andrew Nicholas Sullivan Way Surgery, Sullivan Way, Scholes, Wigan WN1 3TB Tel: 01942 243649 Fax: 01942 826476; The Old School House, 254 Withington Lane, Aspull, Wigan WN2 1JA Tel: 01942 492904 — MB ChB Manch. 1982.

SUTTON, Ann Mary Yorkhill NHS Trust, Glasgow G3 8SJ Tel: 0141 201 0557 Fax: 0141 201 9352 — MB BS Lond. 1974 (King's Coll.) DCH Eng. 1976; MRCP (UK) 1980; FRCP Glas. 1988; FRCPCH 1997. Cons. Paediat. Yorkhill NHS Trust Glas.; Hon. Sen. Lect. Glas. Univ. Specialty: Paediat.

SUTTON, Anthony John (retired) Hazel Cottage, Whinburgh, Dereham NR19 1QR — MB BS Lond. 1956 (Lond. Hosp.) Prev: Ho. Surg. Lond. Hosp.

SUTTON, Caroline Judith 1 The Avenue, South Moulescoomb, Brighton BN2 4GF; 26 St. Leonards Gardens, Hove BN3 4QB — MB BS Lond. 1979; DCH RCP Lond. 1983; MRCP (UK) 1986.

SUTTON, Christopher Derek 8 Acorn Way, Wigston LE18 3YA — MB BCh Wales 1993.

SUTTON, Professor Christopher James Gabert Guildford Nuffield Hospital, Stirling Road, Guildford GU2 7RF Tel: 01483 555833 Fax: 01483 555835 Email: csutton@uk-consultants.co.uk; Gunner's Farm, Stringers Common, Guildford GU4 7PR — (St. Mary's) MB BChir Camb. 1967; MA Trinity College, Cambridge 1967; FRCOG 1987. Cons. Gyn. Roy. Surrey Co. Hosp. Guildford; Prof. Of Gynaecol. Surg. Uni. Of Surrey, Guildford; Hon. Lect. Roy. Lond. Hosp. Univ. Lond.; Clin. Tutor Imperial Coll. Sch., Uni. Lond. Specialty: Obst. & Gyn. Socs: Brit. Soc. Of Gynaecol. Endoscopy; Euro. Soc. Of Gynaecol. Endoscopy; Gynaecol. Club of GB & Ire.

Prev: Cons. O & G St. Luke's Hosp. Guildford; Sen. Regist. Addenbrooke's Hosp. Camb. & St. Mary's Hosp. Lond.; Cons. Lautoka Hosp., Fiji.

SUTTON, Claire Louise — MB ChB Birm. 1998; MRCP.

SUTTON, David Alfred Owen Department of Medicine for the Elderly, Llandough Hospital, Penarth CF64 2XX Tel: 029 2071 1711 Fax: 029 2070 0877 — MB ChB Bristol 1962; MRCP (UK) 1973; FRCP Lond. 1991; MA Wales 1993. Cons. Phys. Llandough Hosp. NHS Trust. Specialty: Care of the Elderly. Prev: Sen. Regist. (Geriat. Med.) Bournemouth & E. Dorset & Char. Cross Hosps.; Regist. (Gen. Med.) Roy. Gwent Hosp. Newport.

SUTTON, David Nicholas 2A Ashleigh Grove, West Jesmond, Newcastle upon Tyne NE2 3DL — MB ChB Liverp. 1995. Specialty: Oral & Maxillofacial Surg.

SUTTON, David Nigel Shackleton Department of Anaesthetics, Southampton General Hospital, Tremona Road, Southampton SO16 6YD Tel: 023 8079 6135 Fax: 023 8079 4348 Email: david.sutton@suht.swest.nhs.uk — BM Soton. 1978; DA Eng. 1983; FFA RCS Eng. 1985. Cons. Anaesth. Soton. Univ. Hosps. NHS Trust. Specialty: Anaesth. Socs: Assn. Anaesth. of GB & Irel.; BASICS; Roy. Coll. Anaesth. Prev: Clin. Servs. Director, Critical Care; Sen. Regist. (Anaesth. & IC) Soton. Gen. Hosp.; Resid. Anaesth. King Edwd. VII Memor. Hosp., Bermuda.

SUTTON, Derek Richard (retired) 17 Kirk Lane, Walkington, Beverley HU17 8SN — MB BS Lond. 1964 (St. Bart.) MRCS Eng. LRCP Lond. 1964; FRCP Lond. 1982, M 1968; MD Lond. 1972. Prev: Phys. & Gastroenterol. Hull Roy. Infirm.

SUTTON, Dorothy Everett Carnforth Clinic, Market St, Carnforth LA5 9JU Tel: 01524 732259; Walker Lane Barn, Snape Raike Lane, Goosnargh, Preston PR3 2EU Tel: 01995 640655 — MB ChB St. And. 1967; MSc Audiol. Med. Manch. Univ. 1990. SCMO (Audiol.) Preston HA. Specialty: Audiol. Med.

SUTTON, Elizabeth Joan (retired) 29 Halsall Lane, Formby, Liverpool L37 3NN — (Roy. Free) MRCS Eng. LRCP Lond. 1949; DCH . Lond. 1953; DPH Liverp. 1961; FFCM RCP (UK) 1984, M 1972. Prev: Community Phys. (Child Health) Sefton HA.

SUTTON, Emma Jane 2B Crossland Road, Chorlton, Manchester M21 9DG — BM BS Nottm. 1991.

SUTTON, Emma Michelle 31 Burghley Road, St. Andrews, Bristol BS6 5BL — MB ChB Bristol 1994.

SUTTON, Fay Julie Castle Mead Medical Centre, Hill Street, Hinckley LE10 1DS Tel: 01455 637659 Fax: 01455 238754; The Old Rectory, Church St, Sapcote, Leicester LE9 4FG Tel: 0116 23451 — MB ChB Bristol 1974; DRCOG 1976. Lect. (Gen. Pract.) Leicester Univ.

SUTTON, Mr Frederick Raymond (retired) 2 Blunts Hall Drive, Witham CM8 1LZ Tel: 01376 513614 — MB BS Lond. 1943 (King's Coll, Hosp.) MRCS Eng. LRCP Lond. 1943; FRCS Eng. 1949. Prev: Sen. Surg. Rush Green Hosp. Romford.

SUTTON, Gaius Backholer (retired) Kirkiboll House, Tongue, Lairg IV27 4XL Tel: 01847 611255 — MB ChB Bristol 1957; DObst RCOG 1959; DCH RCP Lond. 1961; DA (UK) 1961. Prev: GP Highland HB.

SUTTON, Mr George Augustine 38 Harborne Road, Edgbaston, Birmingham B15 3HE Tel: 0121 452 1083 Fax: 0121 455 8485 — MB BCh BAO NUI 1967 (Univ. Coll. Dub.) DCH NUI 1969; FRCS Ed. 1977; FRCOphth 1989. Ophth. Birm. & Midl. Eye Hosp. & Good Hope Hosp.; Cons. Ophth. Birm. HA; Clin Tutor Birm. Univ. Specialty: Ophth. Socs: Fell. Roy. Soc. Med.; UK IOL Soc.; Europ. Soc. (Oculoplastic) Surg.s.

SUTTON, George Christopher 6 The Ridings, Cobham KT11 2PT Tel: 01372 843335 — (Univ. Coll. Hosp.) MA, MD Camb. 1971, MB BChir 1958; FRCP Lond. 1977, M 1962. Sen. Lect. Nat. Heart & Lung Inst. Imp. Coll. Sch. Med. Lond.; Hon. Cons. Roy. Brompton & Nat. Heart Hosp. Lond. & Harefield Hosp. Middlx. Specialty: Cardiol. Socs: Fell. Amer. Coll. Cardiol.; Brit. Cardiac Soc. Prev: Sen. Regist. (Cardiol.) Brompton Hosp. Lond.; Ho. Phys. & Ho. Surg. Univ. Coll. Hosp. Lond.; Regist. (Med.) Addenbrooke's Hosp. Camb.

SUTTON, Graham Cunningham Health Protection Agency, White Rose House, Wakefield WF1 1LT Tel: 01924 213035 Fax: 01924 21370 — MB ChB Ed. 1975; MSc (Human Genetics) Ed. 1977; PhD Ed. 1981; FFPH RCP (UK) 1996, M 1986. Cons. Pub. Health, Health Protection Agency. Specialty: Pub. Health Med.

SUTTON, Mr Graham Leslie James The Anchorage, Lands End Road, Old Burlesdon, Southampton SO31 8DN Tel: 023 8040 2385 — BM Soton. 1978; FRCS Ed. 1982; FRCS Eng. 1982; MS Soton. 1989. Cons. Vasc. Surg. Qu. Alexandra Hosp. Portsmouth. Specialty: Gen. Surg. Socs: BMA. Prev: Sen. Clin. Vasc. Fell. St. Mary's Hosp. Lond.; Sen. Regist. (Surg.) Wessex RHA.

SUTTON, Helen Ersy (retired) Manderley, 34 Bower Gardens, Shady Bower, Salisbury SP1 2RL Tel: 01722 323902 — MB BS Lond. 1956 (Univ. Coll. Hosp.) MSc Nuclear Med. Lond. 1983; BA Winchester 2000. Prev: Sen. Med. Off. DHSS.

SUTTON, Helen Joan (retired) 119 Moor End Road, Mellor, Stockport SK6 5PT Tel: 0161 427 2550 — MRCS Eng. LRCP Lond. 1954 (Camb. & Oxf.) BA Camb. 1951, MB BChir 1956. Prev: Assoc. Specialist (Geriat.) Barnes Hosp. & Manch. Roy. Infirm.

SUTTON, Ian John 33 St Helena Way, Horsford, Norwich NR10 3EA — MB ChB Birm. 1992.

SUTTON, Jacqueline Frances 14A Finney Drive, Chorlton, Manchester M21 9DS — MB BS Lond. 1993.

SUTTON, James Francis 120 Poplar Road, Dorridge, Solihull B93 8DQ — MB ChB Leic. 1994.

SUTTON, Jane Cecilia (retired) The Health Centre, Whyteman's Brae, Kirkcaldy KY1 2NA Tel: 01592 641203; Westhall, 31 Links Road, Lundin Links, Leven KY8 6AT Tel: 01333 320323 — MB ChB Liverp. 1959. Prev: Ho. Off. Childr. Hosp. Liverp.

SUTTON, Jean Margaret Park Road Surgery, 25 Park Road, St Helens WA9 1DG Tel: 01744 738735 Fax: 01744 454624; Lonsdale, 14 Laurel Road, West Park, St Helens WA10 4AX Tel: 01744 24285 — MB ChB Liverp. 1989 (Univ. Liverp. Med. Sch.) DRCOG 1992. Princip. GP. Specialty: Obst. & Gyn. Socs: Med. Defence Union; BMA; Christians in Caring Professions. Prev: Trainee GP/SHO (Psychiat.) Fazakerley Hosp. & (Paediat. & Cas.) Alder Hey Hosp. Liverp.

SUTTON, John Andrew Clinical Pharmacology Unit, Royal Surrey County Hospital, Egerton Road, Guildford GU2 7XX Tel: 01483 51122 Fax: 01483 455375; The Cedars, Vanzell Road, Easebourne, Midhurst GU29 9BA Tel: 01730 817150 — MB BS Lond. 1966; DObst RCOG 1968; FFA RCSI 1976; MD Lond. 1989. Dir. Clin. Pharmacol. Unit Guildford. Specialty: Pharmaceutical Medicine. Socs: Brit. Pharm. Soc.; Brit. Assn. Pharmaceut. Phys. Prev: Head Clin. Pharmacol. Units Roussel Beecham.

SUTTON, John Baden The Surgery, 141 Long Causeway, Adel, Leeds LS16 8EX Tel: 0113 293444 Fax: 0113 295 3440 — MB ChB Leeds 1975; BSc (Pharmacol.) Leeds 1973; DRCOG 1977; Cert. JCC Lond. 1977. Gen. Practitioner Princip. Leeds. Socs: GP Airways Gp. Prev: SHO (A & E) Gen. Infirm. Pontefract; SHO (O & G) & Ho. Surg. St. Jas. Hosp. Leeds; Ho. Phys. Leeds Gen. Infirm.

SUTTON, Jonathan Department of Pathology, The General Infirmary, Leeds LS1 3EX Tel: 0113 392 7836 Fax: 0113 392 7839 — MB BS Lond. 1977; BA CANTAB 1971; MRCPath 1985. Specialty: Histopath.

SUTTON, Julian Kingsley 30 Hill Top Avenue, Cheadle Hulme, Cheadle SK8 7HY Tel: 0161 485 3668 — BM BCh Oxf. 1994 (Oxford University Medical School) BA (Hons. Physiol. Sci.) Oxf. 1991. Specialty: Infec. Dis.

SUTTON, Juliet Clare Poplar Grove Surgery, Meadow Way, Aylesbury HP20 1XB Tel: 01296 482554 Fax: 01296 398771 — BSc (Hons.) Lond. 1985, MB BS 1988; DCH RCP Lond. 1990; MRCGP 1992. Prev: Trainee GP Hemel Hempstead; SHO (Psychiat.) Hill End Hosp. St. Albans; Ho. Off. (Surg.)& (Med.) Hemel Hempstead.

SUTTON, Katherine Jane Meadway Health Centre, Meadway, Sale M33 4PS Tel: 0161 905 2880 — MB ChB Ed. 1985; DRCOG 1988; Cert. Family Plann. JCC 1990; T(GP) 1991; MRCGP 1991. Prescribing & Coronary Heart Dis. Lead, Trafford S. PCT. Socs: Roy. Med. Soc. Edin.

SUTTON, Keith Henry (retired) Foxgloves, Holt Forest, Wimborne BH21 7DU Tel: 01258 840832 — MB BS Lond. 1954 (Univ. Coll. Hosp.) DObst RCOG 1964; MRCGP 1976. Prev: GP Lond. & Bournemouth.

SUTTON, Laurence Neil Main X-Ray, The Calderdale Royal Hospital, Salterhebble, Halifax HX3 0PW Tel: 01422 357171; Century House, 2 Heath Avenue, Manor Heath Road, Halifax HX3 0EA Tel: 01422 360253 — MB ChB Leeds 1979; BSc (Hons.) (Pharmacol.) Leeds 1976, MB ChB 1979; FRCR 1988; FRCP 2001.

Cons. Diag. Radiol. Halifax Hosps.; Clin. Director Diagnostic Imaging Calderdale & Huddersfield NHS Trust. Specialty: Radiol. Socs: Roy. Coll. Phys. Lond. Prev: Sen. Regist. (Radiol.) Leeds.

SUTTON, Lisa Jayne 18 Minster Close, Off Churchfields, Barry CF63 1FL Tel: 01446 700731 — MB BS Lond. 1986. Clin. Med. Off. Welsh Blood Transfus. Serv. Prev: SHO A & E Colchester Gen. Hosp.; Trainee GP Colchester.

SUTTON, Lynne Joanne 7 Thorney Close, Lower Earley, Reading RG6 3AF — BMedSci Nottm. 1993; BM BS Nottm. 1995. Locum Staff Grade (A & E). Specialty: Gen. Med. Socs: BMA; MPS. Prev: SHO (Med.) St. Richards Hosp. Chichester.

SUTTON, Margaret Amelia Winifred (retired) Foxgloves, Holt Forest, Wimborne BH21 7DU Tel: 01258 840832 — MB ChB Liverp. 1956. Prev: SCMO (Adult Health) Newham Health Dist.

SUTTON, Mary Elizabeth (retired) North Ridge, Edinburgh Road, Kings Worthy, Winchester SO23 7NY Tel: 01962 883649 Email: marytayl@aol.com — MB BS Lond. 1973; DCH Eng. 1976; FRCPCH 1997. Prev: Cons. Paediat. (Community Child Health) Soton. Community Serv. NHS Trust.

SUTTON, Mr Michael Cheltenham General Hospital, Cheltenham GL53 7AN Tel: 01242 272361 Fax: 01242 272403; Lansdown Lodge, Lansdown Road, Cheltenham GL51 6QL Tel: 01242 520900 Fax: 01242 253816 — BM BCh Oxf. 1967 (Oxf. & Guy's) MA Oxf. 1967; FRCS Eng. 1973; FRCOG 1990, M 1977. Cons. O & G Cheltenham Hosps. Specialty: Obst. & Gyn. Prev: Sen. Regist. & Regist. (O & G) Westm. Hosp. Lond.; Maj. RAMC.

SUTTON, Paul Adrian Riverside Surgery, Barnard Avenue, Brigg DN20 8AS Tel: 01652 650131 Fax: 01652 651551; Beechwood Lodge, 10 Scawby Lodge, Broughton, Brigg DN20 0AF Tel: 01652 658857 — MB ChB Leeds 1978; MRCGP 1988. GP Brigg N. Lincs.; Bd. Mem. & Clin. Governance Lead N. Lincs PCG. Prev: Clin. Research Fell. (Pub. Health Med.) Univ. Hull.; Med. Adviser E. Riding HA; GP Winteron Scunthorpe.

SUTTON, Mr Paul Mark Northern General Hospital, Herries Road, Sheffield S5 7AU Tel: 014 226 6251 — MB ChB Sheff. 1990; FRCS Ed. 1994; FRCS Eng. 1994; FRCS 1999. Cons. Orthopeadic Sugeon. Specialty: Orthop. Socs: Fell. Brit. Orth. Assn.; Mem. Internat. Soc. Arllronary, Knee Surg. & Spnts Orthop. Med. (ISAKOM). Prev: SHO Rotat. (Gen. Surg.) Leeds Gen. Infirm.; Regist. (Orthop.) Yorks. Regional Train. Scheme.

SUTTON, Peter Douglas (retired) Lamont, Southdown Road, Seaford BN25 4HU Tel: 01323 898560 — MB BS Lond. 1945 (Middlx.) DMRD Eng. 1954; FFR 1962; FRCR 1975. Hon. Civil Cons. (Radiol.) RAF. Prev: Cons. Advisor Radiol. RAF.

SUTTON, Peter Morgan (retired) Manderley, 34 Bower Gardens, Shady Bower, Salisbury SP1 2RL Tel: 01722 323902 — MB BS Lond. 1956 (Univ. Coll. Hosp.) BSc (Hons. Anat.) Lond. 1953; FRCPath 1976, M 1964. Prev: Dir. Pub. Health Laborat. Serv. Centre Applied Microbiol. & Research Porton Down.

SUTTON, Peter Robert Beverley Road Surgery, 840 Beverley Road, Hull HU6 7HP Tel: 01482 853270; 12 Hallwalk, Snuffmill Lane, Cottingham HU16 4RL Tel: 01482 848162 — MB ChB Leeds 1968. Clin. Asst. (Dermat.) Princess Roy. Hosp. Hull. Specialty: Dermat. Prev: SHO (Paediat. & Obst.) & Ho. Off. Wakefield Hosp. Gp.

SUTTON, Philip Henry 7 Clover Road, Aylsham, Norwich NR11 6JW Tel: 01263 733972 — MB BS Lond. 1940 (Westm.) BSc Lond. 1937; MRCS Eng. LRCP Lond. 1940; FRCP Lond. 1973, M 1947; MD Lond. 1947. Prev: Cons. Chest Phys. Norwich Health Dist.; Ho. Phys. Radcliffe Infirm. Oxf.; R.A.F. Med. Br. 1941-46.

SUTTON, Philip Percy University Hospital of Hartlepool, The General Hospital, Hartlepool TS24 9AH Tel: 01429 266654 Fax: 01429 235389; West View House, West Park Lane, Sedgefield, Stockton-on-Tees TS21 2BX Tel: 01740 620140 — MB BS Newc. 1975; BSc Newc. 1973, MD 1984; FRCP Ed. 1991; FRCP Lond. 1993. Cons. Phys., N.Tees & Hartlepool NHS Trust; Hon. Clin. Lect., Univ. of Newc. Specialty: Respirat. Med. Socs: Brit. Thorac. Soc. Prev: Sen. Regist. Aberd. Roy. Infirm.; Lect. Roy. Free Hosp. Sch. Med. Lond.; Regist. Ninewells Hosp. Dundee.

SUTTON, Pylotis Gan Stuart (retired) 11 Bexley Lane, Sidcup DA14 4JW Tel: 020 8300 8548 — (Middlx.) MRCS Eng. LRCP Lond. 1948. Prev: Ho. Surg. Co. Hosp. Hereford.

SUTTON, Rebecca Sian 4 Whalley Avenue, Chorlton, Manchester M21 8TU — MB ChB Manch. 1997.

SUTTON, Professor Richard 149 Harley Street, London W1G 6DE Tel: 020 7935 4444 Fax: 020 7935 6718 — (King's Coll. Hosp.) MRCS Eng. LRCP Lond. 1964; MB BS Lond. 1964; FRCP Lond. 1983, M 1967; FACC 1975; DSc (Med.) Lond. 1988; FESC 1989; FAHA 2000. Prof. Clin. Cardio. & Cons. Cardiol. Roy. Brompton Hosp. Lond. & Chelsea & Westm. Hosp.; Hon. Cons. Cardiol. St. Luke's Hosp. Lond.; Edr.-in-Chief EUROPACE 1998-. Specialty: Cardiol. Socs: BMA; Brit. Cardiac Soc.; (Sub. Comms.) Europ. Heart Rhythum Assn. Prev: Chairm. Europ. Working Gp. Cardiac Pacing of the Europ. Soc. Cardiol.; Cons. Cardiol. Westm. Hosp. Lond.; Sen. Regist. & Dir. Cardiac Catheterisat. Laborat. Nat. Heart Hosp. Lond.

SUTTON, Richard James 17 Kirk Lane, Beverley HU17 8SN — MB BS Lond. 1990; FRCS (Eng) 1996; FRCS (Gen. Surg.) 2002. BASO Clinical Fellow in Oncoplastic Surgery.

SUTTON, Professor Robert University of Liverpool, Division of Surgery & Oncology, Royal Liverpool University Hospital, Daulby Street, Liverpool L69 3GA Tel: 0151 706 4170 Fax: 0151 706 5826 Email: r.sutton@liverpool.ac.uk — MB BS Lond. 1980 (King's Coll. Hosp.) BA (Anthropol. & Psychol.) (Hons.) Durh. 1974; FRCS Eng. 1984; DPhil Oxf. 1989; FRCS (Gen.) 1992. Hunt. Prof. RCS Eng. (1990-1). Specialty: Gen. Surg. Special Interest: Pancreatitis; Hepatopancreatobiliary disorders. Socs: Pancreatic Soc. of GB and Irel.; Assoc. Surg. GB and Irel.; Soc. Acad. Res. Surg. Prev: Reader (Surg.) Univ. Liverp., Hon. Cons. Surg., Roy. Liverp. Univ. Hosp.; Sen. Lect. (Surg.) Univ. Liverp.; Lect. (Surg.) Univ. Liverp.

SUTTON, Roger Barrie Owen 212 Anerley Road, Penge, London SE20 8TJ — MB BS Lond. 1972; FDS RCS Eng. 1974, L 1966; BDS Lond. 1966, MB BS 1972.

SUTTON, Roger Malcolm Havant Health Centre Suite C, PO Box 44, Civic Centre Road, Havant PO9 2AT Tel: 023 9247 4351 Fax: 023 9249 2524; 2 Taswell Road, Southsea PO5 2RG Tel: 01705 756926 — BM Soton. 1983 (Southampton) DRCOG 1988; MRCGP 1989. Socs: Christian Med. Soc. Prev: SHO (O & G) St. Mary's Hosp. Portsmouth; SHO (ENT/Geriat./Cas.) Qu. Alexandra Hosp. Portsmouth.

SUTTON, Mr Ronald Arthur Beechfield, 11 Beech Hill, Hexham NE46 3AG Tel: 01434 602021 Fax: 01434 602021 — MB BS Durh. 1963; FRCS Ed. 1969. Cons. Orthop. Surg. Hexham Gen. Hosp. Specialty: Orthop. Socs: Inter. Med. Soc. Paraplegia. Prev: Sen. Regist. & Regist. (Orthop. Surg.) Roy. Vict. Infirm. Newc.; Sen. Regist. (Orthop. Surg.) Univ. Dept. Orthop. Nuffield Orthop. Hosp.

SUTTON, Ruth Helen Harvey House Surgery, 13-15 Russell Avenue, St Albans AL3 5HB Tel: 01727 831888 Fax: 01727 845520; 31 Alma Road, St Albans AL1 3AT — MB ChB Leic. 1991; MRCGP 1995; DFFP 1995.

SUTTON, Stanley Edward (retired) 9 Richard Road, Crosby, Liverpool L23 8TD — (Manch.) MB ChB Manch. 1950. Prev: Capt. RAMC.

SUTTON, Stanley Grahame 35 Montagu Gardens, Wallington SM6 8EP Tel: 020 8647 1135 — MB BChir Camb. 1957; MRCS Eng. LRCP Lond. 1954; DObst RCOG 1959; DCH Eng. 1959; DA (UK) 1961. Specialty: Genitourinary Medicine. Socs: Sutton Med. Soc.; Internat. Organisat. Mycoplasmol.; Brit. Med. Laser Assn. Prev: SHO (Anaesth.) Ronkswood Hosp. Worcester; SHO (Paediat.) W. Pk. Hosp. Macclesfield; SHO (Infec. Dis.) Cherry Tree Hosp. Stockport.

SUTTON, Timothy Mark 13 Holmfield Way, Weston Favell, Northampton NN3 3BJ Tel: 01604 240831 Email: tsutton@middlemore.co.nz — MB ChB Bristol 1992; BSc Bristol 1989; MRCP (UK) 1996. Cons. (Cardiol.) Auckland, New Zealand. Specialty: Cardiol. Prev: SHO (Med.) Northampton Gen. Hosp.; Ho. Off. (Med.) Bristol Roy. Infirm.; Ho. Off. (Surg.) Bristol Roy. Infirm.

SUTTON, Vera Estelle 40 Holne Chase, Hamstead Garden Suburb, London N2 0QQ Tel: 020 8455 0825 Fax: 020 8458 7188; 40 Holne Chase, Hampstead Garden Suburb, London N2 0QQ Tel: 020 8455 0825 Fax: 020 8458 7188 — (Leeds) MB ChB Leeds 1957. Med. Off. to Various Life Insur. Companies. Specialty: Gen. Psychiat. Socs: Affil. RCPsych; Fell. Roy. Soc. Med. & Med. Soc. Lond.; Assur. Med. Soc. & Roy. Coll. Psychiat. Prev: Hon. Clin. Asst. Friern & Halliwick Hosps. Lond.; Med. Off. Marie Stopes Clinic Lond.; Ho. Phys. & Ho. Surg. (O & G) St. Jas. Hosp. Leeds.

SUTTON, Wendy Elizabeth 25 Dewberry, Coulby Newham, Middlesbrough T58 0XH — MB BChir Camb. 1994; DRCOG 1996; MRCGP 1997. Specialty: Gen. Pract.

SUTTON COULSON, Thomas (retired) Graylings, Bascombe Road, Churston Ferrers, Brixham TQ5 0JX Tel: 01803 842703 — (Oxf. & Middlx.) MA, BM BCh Oxf. 1939; MRCS Eng. LRCP Lond. 1939. Prev: RAMC 1939-45.

SUVARNA, Jeremy Rafe, Squadron Ldr. RAF Med. Br. Retd. Medicines & Healthcare Products Regulatory Agency, 1 Nine Elms Lane, London SW8 5NQ — MB BS Lond. 1988 (Roy. Free Hosp.) BSc (Hons.) Lond. 1985; DAvMed FOM RCP Lond. 1992; Dip. IMC RCS Ed. 1995; Dip Pharm Med 2000; MFPM 2000. Sen. Med. Assessor, Medicines & Healthcare Products Regulatory Agency. Specialty: Pharmaceutical Medicine. Prev: Med. Adviser Boehringer Ingelheim Ltd. Bracknell Berks; Team Ldr. Medicines Control Agency.

SUVARNA, Simon Kim Northern General Hospital (Sheffield Teaching Hospitals), Department of Histopathology, Herries Road, Sheffield S5 7AU Tel: 0114 271 4942 Fax: 0114 271 4006 — MB BS Lond. 1984 (Middlx.) BSc (Hons.) Lond. 1981; MRCP (UK) 1987; FRCPath 1993. Cons. Histopath. & Cytopath. Sheff. Teaching Hosp. Specialty: Histopath. Prev: Sen. Regist. (Histopath.) Sheff.; Regist. (Histopath.) St. Mary's Hosp. Lond.; SHO (Histopath.) Univ. Coll. Hosp. Lond.

SUXENA, Shesh Raj Audley Health Centre, Church St., Audley, Stoke-on-Trent ST7 8EW Tel: 01782 721345 Fax: 01782 723808 — MB BS Osmania 1955; MRCP (UK) 1965.

SUZUKI, Iris Ingeborg 13 Wicker Street, London E1 1QF — MB BS Lond. 1993.

SVASTI-SALEE, Derek 9 Bruges Place, London NW1 0TE — MB BS Lond. 1998.

SVENNE, Mr Dzintars 15 Downhills Way, London N17 6AN Tel: 020 8888 4269; 62 Woodland Drive, Berry Hill, Mansfield NG18 4JL — MB BS Lond. 1963 (RCSI) LRCPI & LM, LRCSI & LM 1958; FRCSI 1966; DMRD Eng. 1969. Cons. Radiol. Centr. Notts. Health Dist. Specialty: Radiol. Socs: Fell. Roy. Soc. Med.; Assn. Surgs. E. Afr. Prev: Sen. Regist. (Radiol.) & Clin. Tutor Nottm. Univ. Hosp. Gp.; Sen. Regist. (Neurosurg.) & Hon. Clin. Lect. Dept. Surg. Mulago Hosp.; (Makerere Univ.) Kampala, Uganda.

SVENSSON, William Edward Nuclear Medicine, Imaging Department, Charing Cross Hospital, Fulham Palace Road, Hammersmith, London W6 8RF Tel: 020 8383 0129 Fax: 020 8846 1426 Email: wsvensson@hhnt.nhs.uk; 1 High Park Road, Richmond TW9 4BL Tel: 020 8876 0997 — LRCPI & LM, LRSCI & LM 1974 (Ireland) LRCPI & LM, LRCSI & LM 1974; FRCSI 1979; FRCR 1988. Cons. Radiol. Char. Cross Hosp.; Hon. Sen. Lect. Hammersmith Hosp. Specialty: Radiol.; Nuclear Med. Socs: Fell. Roy. Soc. Med.; Brit. Inst. Radiol. Prev: Sen. Regist. (Nuclear Med. & Ultrasound) Roy. Marsden Hosp. Lond.; Regist. (Diag. Radiol.) Roy. Free Hosp. Lond.; Cons. Radiol. Ealing Hosp.

SVERRISDOTTIR, Anna Wisteria Cottage, 74 Park Road, Alrewas, Burton-on-Trent DE13 7AJ — Cand Med et Chir Reykjavik 1984; FRCS Ed. 1993; FRCS (Gen. Surg.) 1999.

SVOBODA, Daniel 17 Cherry Tree Avenue, Scarborough YO12 5DX — MB ChB Otago 1990.

SVOBODA, Vladimir Henry John (retired) 92 Heath Road, Petersfield GU31 4EL Tel: 01730 264884 Fax: 01730 264884 Email: v.h.j.svoboda@btinternet.com — (Chas. Univ. Prague) MUDr Prague 1955; DMRT Eng. 1969; FFR 1970; LMSSA Lond. 1972. Prev: Cons. Radiother. St. Mary's Gen. Hosp. Portsmouth.

SWABY, Martin John Manston Surgery, 72-76 Austhorpe Road, Leeds LS15 8DZ Tel: 0113 264 5455 Fax: 0113 232 6181; Carlton House, 149 Primrose Lane, Leeds LS15 7QZ — MB ChB Leeds 1974; DRCOG 1977.

SWADDLE, Margaret Brooklyn, Corchester Terrace, Corbridge NE45 5NS — (Roy. Free) MRCS Eng. LRCP Lond. 1968; MB BS Lond. 1968; DObst RCOG 1970.

SWADE, Shelley Naomi St Quintins Health Centre, St. Quintin Avenue, London W10 6NX Tel: 020 8960 5677 Fax: 020 8968 5933 — MB ChB Cape Town 1975; Dip. Ven. Soc. Apoth. Lond. 1981; Dip. Ther. Lond. 1997; MSc Lond. 1999.

SWAEBE, Clare Isobel 1 Cotswold Way, Ashby-de-la-Zouch LE65 1ET — MB ChB Leeds 1992.

SWAGE, Thoreya Hananne 20 Edward Road, Farnham GU9 8NP Tel: 01252 726432 Fax: 01252 726432 Email: t.swage@btinternet.com — MB BS Lond. 1985; MA Oxf. 1993. Cons. in Healthcare Managem. Prev: Dir. Primary Care Developm. W Surrey HA; Locality Manager Ealing, Hammersmith & Hounslow HA; Area Manager Ealing, Hammersmith & Hounslow FHSA.

SWAI, Elishita Andrews c/o Department of Anaesthesia, South Tyneside District Hospital, Harton Lane, South Shields NE33 Tel: 0191 202 4046 Fax: 0191 202 4046; 62 Murrayfields, West Allotment, Newcastle upon Tyne NE27 0RF Tel: 0191 270 9007 Fax: 0191 270 9007 — MB ChB E. Afr. 1970 (Unvi. Of Makerere. Uganda) FRCA 1974. S. Tyneside NHS Trust; Assoc. Specialist. Specialty: Anaesth. Socs: BMA; NE Soc. Anaesth. Prev: Cons. Anaesth.Al-Amiri Hosp. Kuwait.

SWAIN, Alison Jane Hockley Medical Practice, 247 South Road, Hockley, Birmingham B18 5JS Tel: 0121 554 1757 Fax: 0121 554 1757; 133 Wentworth Road, Harborne, Birmingham B17 9SU — MB ChB Birm. 1986; DRCOG 1990. Prev: Trainee GP Birm. VTS; SHO Dudley Rd. Hosp. VTS; SHO (Med.) Selly Oak Hosp. Birm.

SWAIN, Anna Victoria 201 Sandyford Road, Sandyford, Newcastle upon Tyne NE2 1NP — MB BS Newc. 1998; MB BS Newc 1998.

SWAIN, Anne Frances 41 Willow Road, London NW3 1TN — MB BS Lond. 1973 (Roy. Free) MRCS Eng. LRCP Lond. 1973; MRCP (UK) 1976; FRCP Lond. 1993. Cons. Dermat. Luton & Dunstable Hosp. Luton. Specialty: Dermat.

SWAIN, Archana 16 Royal Lodge Road, Belfast BT8 7UL — MB BS Urkal 1970.

SWAIN, Catherine Mary 25 Brookside Way, Wall Heath, Kingswinford DY6 9AW — MB ChB Birm. 1985; MRCGP 1995.

SWAIN, Christopher Paul 41 Willow Road, Hampstead, London NW3 1TN — MRCS Eng. LRCP Lond. 1971 (St. Bart.) BA Oxf. 1964; MD Lond. 1986, BSc 1968, MB BS 1972; MRCP (UK) 1974; FRCP Lond. 1990. Cons. & Sen. Lect. (Gastroenterol.) Lond. Hosp. Specialty: Gastroenterol. Prev: Sen. Regist. St. Geo. Hosp. Lond.

SWAIN, David Geoffrey Department of Elderly Medicine, Arden Lodge Annexe, Yardley Green Hospital, Yardley Green Road, Birmingham B5 9PX Tel: 0121 766 6611 Fax: 0121 753 0653; 133 Wentworth Road, Birmingham B17 9SU — MB BS Lond. 1981 (Roy. Free) BSc Lond. 1978, MB BS Lond. 1981; MRCP (UK) 1984; FRCP 1998. Cons. Phys. Elderly Med. - Birm. Heartlands. Hosp. Specialty: Care of the Elderly. Prev: Sen. Regist. (Geriat.) Sandwell Hosp. Birm.

SWAIN, David Leslie, LVO, QHP, Surg. Capt. RN The Royal Naval Hospital, Haslar, Gosport PO12 2AA Tel: 023 9258 4255 — MB ChB Bristol 1964; DObst RCOG 1971; DA Eng. 1972; FRCA Eng. 1975. Cons. Adviser Anaesth. RN Hosp. Haslar. Specialty: Anaesth. Prev: Med. Off. i/c RN Hosp. Plymouth; Dir. Naval Offs. Appointing (Med.); Cons. Adviser (Anaesth.) Med. Directorate Gen. (Naval).

SWAIN, Mr Debadutta Rabinandan 75 Carnleigh Drive, Brooklands, Sale M33 3PT — MB BS Patna 1974; FRCS Ed. 1982; FRCS Glas. 1983.

SWAIN, Elizabeth Doctors Surgery, 18 Union Street, Kirkintilloch, Glasgow G66 1DH Tel: 0141 776 1238 Fax: 0141 775 2786; 7 Woodilee Cottages, Lenzie, Glasgow G66 3UA Tel: 0141 776 3879 — MB ChB Dundee 1973; DObst RCOG 1975; MRCGP 1981; DTM & H Liverp. 1981. Prev: Med. Supt. Ch. of Christ Centr. Nigeria Alushi Med. Centre Plateau State, Nigeria.

SWAIN, Kiran Behari Oldpark Road Surgery, 460 Oldpark Road, Belfast BT14 6QG Tel: 028 9074 6535 Fax: 028 9074 7768; 16 Royal Lodge Road, Belfast BT8 7UL Tel: 01232 746535 — MB BS Utkal 1971; MICGP 1985; PhD Qu. Univ. Belf. 1996. Research Fell. (Cardiac) Ulster Hosp. Specialty: Cardiol.

SWAIN, Rosemary Anne Hamilton St Pauls Medical Centre, St Pauls Square, Carlisle CA1 1DG Tel: 01228 524354 Fax: 01228 616660; 12 Portland Square, Carlisle CA1 1PY Tel: 01228 24354 — MB BS Lond. 1980; MRCGP 1984; DRCOG 1985.

SWAIN, Mr William David Department of Orthopaedics, Royal Victoria Hospital, Grovuenor Road, Belfast BT12 6BA Tel: 028 9089 4762 — MB BCh BAO Belf. 1986 (Queen's University Belfast) BSc Belf. 1983; FRCSI 1990; FRCS (Orth.) 1997. Cons. Orthop. Surg. Specialty: Orthop. Prev: SHO Rotat. (Gen. Surg.) Lisburn Co. Antrim.

SWAINE, Christina Anne 5 Mushroom Field, Kingston, Lewes BN7 3LE — MB BS Lond. 1993; BSc (Hons.) Physiol. Lond. 1988.

SWAINE, Christopher Norman Anaesthetic Department, Royal Sussex County Hospital, Eastern Road, Brighton BN2 5BE — MB BS Lond. 1979; MA, MB BS Lond. 1979.

SWAINE, David John The Surgery, School Hill House, 33 High Street, Lewes BN7 2LU — BSc Lond. 1988, MB BS 1991; DRCOG 1992; DFFP 1993; MA MRCGP 1994; DCH RCP Lond. 1994.

SWAINE, Josephine Mary (retired) 15 Loom Lane, Radlett WD7 8AA — MB BCh Wales 1963 (Cardiff) DObst RCOG 1965. Prev: SCMO (Family Plann. & Reproduc. Health Care) W. Herts.Community Health (NHS) Trust St. Albans.

SWAINSBURY, Joanna Shaw Nuffield House Surgery, The Stow, Harlow CM20 3AX Tel: 01279 425661 Fax: 01279 427116 — MB BS Lond. 1978. GP Harlow.

SWAINSON, Catherine Jane 6 Connor Way, Gatley, Cheadle SK8 4HF — MB BS Newc. 1986; FRCS Ed. 1990; FRCR 1994. Cons. Radiol. The Roy. Oldham Hosp. Oldham. Specialty: Radiol. Prev: Sen. Regist. (Diag. Radiol.) Manch. RHA.

SWAINSON, Charles Patrick NHS Lothian, Royal Infirmary of Edinburgh, 52 Little france crescent, Edinburgh EH16 4SA Tel: 0131 242 3306 Fax: 0131 242 3302 Email: charles.swainson@luht.scot.nhs.uk — MB ChB Ed. 1971 (Edinburgh) MRCP (UK) 1974; FRCP Ed. 1985; FFPHM 2002. Med. Director NHS Lothian, Edin.; Cons. Renal Phys., Roy. Infirm. of Edin. Specialty: Nephrol. Special Interest: Cardiovascular Disease; Transplant. Socs: Internat. Soc. Nephrol.; Renal Assn.; Brit. Assn. of Med. Managers. Prev: Sen. Lect. (Med.) Univ. Otago ChristCh., NZ.

SWAINSON, Susanna Monica Arbory Street Surgery, Arbory Street, Castletown IM9 1LN; 23 Victoria Road, Castletown IM9 1EN Tel: 01624 823686 Fax: 01624 823686 — MB BCh BAO Belf. 1977.

SWAINSTON, David George (retired) — MB BS Durh. 1965; DA Eng. 1970. Prev: Med. Off. Drug Concern Clinic.

SWALE, Jim 3 Cranmore Way, London N10 3TP — MB BS Lond. 1945.

SWALE, Nicholas Frederick Holyoake The Smithy, 2 Lower South Wraxall, Bradford-on-Avon BA15 2RR; Box Surgery, London Road, Box, Corsham SN13 8NA — BM Soton. 1995; MRCGP (Merit); DFFP. GP Assist. Box Surgery, Wiltshire. Specialty: Gen. Med. Prev: SHO (Med.) Roy. Hants. Co. Hosp. Winchester.

SWALE, Victoria Jane Royal London Hospital, Department of Dermatology, London E1 1BB Tel: 020 7377 7383 — BM Soton. 1992; MRCP (UK) 1995. SPR Barts & the Lond. NHS Trust. Specialty: Dermat. Prev: Research Fell. (Dermatol.) Roy. Lond. & St. Bart. Sch. of Med. & Dent.; SPR (Dermat.) Roy. Free Hosp.; SHO (Dermat.) Guy's & St. Thos. Hosp. Trust Lond.

SWALES, Brendan Joseph The Briers, 28 Victoria Road, Sheffield S10 2DL Tel: 0114 266 8090 — MB ChB Sheff. 1982 (Sheffield) DRCOG 1986; MRCGP 1989. Hosp. Pract. (Geriat. Med. & Assessm. & Rehabil.) Sheff. Specialty: Gen. Pract. Socs: LMC; DMC.

SWALES, Brian Geoffrey (retired) 6 Palmaston Close, Haverbreaks, Lancaster LA1 5BS Tel: 01524 69682 — MRCS Eng. LRCP Lond. 1961 (Leeds) DObst RCOG 1963; DA Eng. 1965; FFA RCS Eng. 1972. Prev: Cons. Anaesth. Lancaster Acute Hosps. NHS Trust & Westmorland Hosps. NHS Trust.

SWALES, Caroline Louise Lever Faberge Ltd, PO Box 69, Port Sunlight, Wirral CH62 42D — MB ChB Leeds 1988. Cons. (Occup. Phys.) Unilever Port Sunlight Wirral. Specialty: Occupat. Health. Prev: Trainee Phys. (Occupat. Health) ICI Runcorn.

SWALES, Hilary Anne Southampton General Hospital, Tremora Rd, Southampton SO16 6YD — MB ChB Leeds 1986; FRCA 1993. Cons. (Anaesth.) Soton. Gen. Hosp. Specialty: Anaesth. Prev: SHO (Anaesth.) York Dist. Hosp. & Leeds Gen. Infirm.; Ho. Off. Profess. Med. Unit St. Jas. Hosp. Leeds; SHO (A & E) Leeds Gen. Infirm.

SWALES, Mr John Saunders — MB ChB Sheff. 1979; FRCS Eng. 1983; DRCOG 1986. Prev: Regist. (Gen. Surg.) Leicester Roy. Infirm.

SWALES, Miss Nola Vanessa Flat 2, 18 Vernon Road, Edgbaston, Birmingham B16 9SH Tel: 0121 454 9128; XX, The Common, Goathland, Whitby YO22 5AN Tel: 01947 896257 — MB ChB Dundee 1992; FRCS Ed. 1996. Regist. (Gen. Surg.) Hereford Co. Hosp. Specialty: Gen. Surg. Socs: BMA. Prev: Sen. SHO Birm.; SHO Rotat. Heartlands & Solihull.

SWALES, Philip Patrick Richard 21 Morland Avenue, Leicester LE2 2PF; 6 Orlando Road, Clarenton Park, Leicester LE2 1WN Tel: 0116 270 6104 — MB BS Lond. 1997 (St Barthemews Hospital Med. College) BSc Lond. 1994. SHO, Gen. Med. Rotat., Leicester. Specialty: Gen. Med. Prev: SHO, Coronary Care Unit, Leicester Roy. Infirm., Leicester; Sen. Ho. Off., Gastroenterol., Glenfield Gen. Hosp., Leicester.

SWALES, Valerie Susan Elm Lane Surgery, 104 Elm Lane, Sheffield S5 7TW Tel: 0114 245 6994 Fax: 0114 257 1260; The Briers, 28 Victoria Road, Sheffield S10 2DL Tel: 0114 266 8090 — MB ChB Sheff. 1982; MRCGP 1989.

SWALLOW, Elizabeth Bryony Chestnut Tree Cottage, Willows Green, Chelmsford CM3 1QH — MB BS Lond. 1997.

SWALLOW, Hugh Malcolm Streatley Hall, Sharpenhoe Road, Streatley, Luton LU3 3PS Tel: 01582 881680; 19 Cardiff Road, Luton LU1 1PP Tel: 01582 31831 Fax: 01582 454142 — MB BS Lond. 1955 (St. Geo.) MRCS Eng. LRCP Lond. 1955; DObst RCOG 1959. Hosp. Pract. (ENT) Luton & Dunstable Hosp.; Med. Off. S. Beds. Hospice.

SWALLOW, James Howard (retired) Chestnut Tree Cottage, Willows Green, Chelmsford CM3 1QH Tel: 01245 361472 — MB BChir Camb. 1952 (Lond. Hosp.) MRCS Eng. LRCP Lond. 1952; FRCP Lond. 1974, M 1959. Prev: Cons. Phys. Mid-Essex HA.

SWALLOW, James William Wellington Health Centre, Chapel Lane, Wellington, Telford TF1 1PZ Tel: 01952 226000; The Grange, Upton Magna, Shrewsbury SY4 4TZ Tel: 01743 709386 — MB ChB Birm. 1989.

SWALLOW, Julia (retired) The Cedars, Cholesbury Road, Wigginton, Tring HP23 6JQ — (Leeds) BSc (Hons. Physiol.) Leeds 1959, MB ChB 1961. SCMO S.W. Herts. Dist. Prev: Clin. Med. Off. Derbysh. AHA & Leics AHA(T).

SWALLOW, Malcolm Bryan Market Surgery, Warehouse Lane, Wath-On-Dearne, Rotherham S63 7RA Tel: 01709 877524 Fax: 01709 875089 Email: malcolm.swallow@gp-c87029.nhs.uk; 89 Rockingham Road, Swinton, Mexborough S648EE — MB BS Lond. 1982; DCH RCP Lond. 1986; DRCOG 1987; MRCGP 1988.

SWALLOW, Michael David Northgate Village Surgery, Northgate Avenue, Chester CH2 2DX Tel: 01244 390396; 58 Greenfield Crescent, Waverton, Chester CH3 7NH Tel: 01244 332250 — MB ChB Sheff. 1961. Prev: Regist. (Med.) North. Gen. Hosp. Sheff.; Sen. Ho. Phys. Chesterfield Roy. Hosp.; Ho. Phys. & Ho. Surg. Roy. Infirm. Sheff.

SWALLOW, Michael William, OBE (retired) 15 Deramore Drive, Belfast BT9 5JQ Tel: 028 9066 9042 Fax: 028 9066 9042 Email: swallow.mw@tesco.net — MB BS Lond. 1952 (Westm.) FRCP Lond. 1972, M 1958. Neurol. Roy. Vict. Hosp. Prev: Sen. Regist. (Neurol.) Univ. Coll. Hosp.

SWALLOW, Patricia Diana Margaret Rose (retired) Chestnut Tree Cottage, Willows Green, Chelmsford CM3 1QH Tel: 01245 361472 Fax: 0243 360774 Email: di.swallow@btinternet.com — (Middlx.) MB BS Lond. 1962; MRCS Eng. LRCP Lond. 1962; FRCA 1969. Prev: Cons. Anaesth. St. And. Centre Broomfield Hosp. Chelmsford.

SWALLOW, Peter Nigel 100 High Street, Olney MK46 4BE — MB BS Lond. 1998.

SWALLOW, Rodney Alan 1 Holbeche Crescent, Fillongley, Coventry CV7 8ES Tel: 01676 541261 Email: rodney@swallowpcg.freeserve.co.uk — MB BChir Camb. 1972; MA Camb. 1972. Chairm. Coventry N. PCG; Co-Chariman of Professional Exec. Comm. of Coventry PCT. Specialty: Diabetes.

SWALLOW, Rosemary Alexandra Chestnut Tree Cottage, Willows Green, Chelmsford CM3 1QH Tel: 01245 361472 Fax: 01245 361472 — MB BS Lond. 1994; MRCP UK 1997. LAT Gen. Med. Regist. & Endocrinol. Bristol Roy. Infirm. Bristol. Prev: SHO Rotat. John Radcliffe NHS Trust Oxf.

SWAMI, Atul Bhai Addenbrooke's Hospital, Box 93, Hills Road, Cambridge CB2 2QQ Tel: 01223 245151 Fax: 01223 216066; 96 Cotelands, Chichester Road, Croydon CR0 5UF — MB BCh Wales 1984; MRCP (UK) 1987; FRCA 1990. Cons. Neurosci. Critical Care Unit Addenbrookes Hosp. Camb. Specialty: Intens. Care. Prev: Cons. Anaesth. & Ex-Dir. Neuroanaesth. Servs. Addenbrooke's Hosp. Camb.; Sen. Regist. (Anaesth.) Roy. Free Hosp. Lond. & Nat. Hosp. Neurol.; SHO (Anaesth.) Univ. Coll. & Middlx. Hosps. Lond.

SWAMI, Mr Kuchibhotla Satyanarayana Aberdeen Royal Infirmary, Ward 44, Aberdeen AB25 2ZN Tel: 01224 554629 Fax: 01224 840726; 2 Primrose Bank Drive, Cults, Aberdeen AB15 9PF — MB BS Andhra 1977 (Andhra Med. Coll., India) FRCS Ed. 1987; Dip. Urol. Lond 1990; FRCS (Urol.) 1994. Cons. Urol. Surg. Aberd. Roy. Infirm.; Cons. Urol. Surg. Albyn Hosp., Aberd. Specialty: Urol.

Socs: Brit. Assn. Urol. Surg.; Eur. Assn. Urol.; Sociéte Internat. D'Urologie. Prev: Sen. Regist. (Urol.) Aberd. Roy. Infirm.; Clin. Research Fell. Bristol Urol. Inst.; Regist. (Urol.) Southmead Hosp. Bristol.

SWAMI, Manohar Lal Russell Street Surgery, 79 Russell Street, Reading RG1 7XG Tel: 0118 959 2131 Fax: 0118 959 3112; 5 Goodwin Close, Calcot, Reading RG31 7ZW — MB BS Rajasthan 1970; MRCPI 1981. Thames Valley Police Surg. (Newbury & Didcot.). Prev: Med. Off. Univ. Leeds; SHO & Regist. (Gen. Med.) N.gate Hosp. Gt. Yarmouth; SHO (Gen. Med.) Cromer & Dist. Hosp. Norf.

SWAMI, Pinakiprasad Maganbhai Oak Road Surgery, 1 Oak Road, Canvey Island SS8 7AX Tel: 01268 692211 — MB BS Baroda 1960.

SWAMI, Sadhana Russell Street Surgery, 79 Russell Street, Reading RG1 7XG Tel: 0118 959 2131 Fax: 0118 959 3112 — MB BS Rajasthan 1973.

SWAMPILLAI, Janice Suhanthi The Steps, Boxford, Sudbury CO10 5HP — MB BS Lond. 1997 (Char. Cross & Westm.)

SWAMY, Gowri Narayana The Medical Centre, The Strand, Kirkholt, Rochdale OL11 2JG — MB BS Madras 1975.

SWAMY, Master Shivalingappa Associate Specialist, Department Health & Care of the Elderl, 1 Lpapford Close, Mapperley, Nottingham NG3 5SQ Tel: 0115 920 9419 — MB BS Mysore 1955 (Mysore Med. Coll.) Assoc. Specialist Nottm. HA.

SWAN, Alexander Julian Newton Medical Practice, Park St., Newtown SY16 1EF Tel: 01686 626221; Pinefields, Pines Gardens, Llanidloes Road, Newtown SY16 1EY Tel: 01686 629733 — MB BS Lond. 1988; DRCOG 1991; MRCGP 1992. Prev: Trainee GP/SHO (Psychiat.) Northampton Gen. Hosp. VTS; Ho. Off. (Gen. Med.) Burton on Trent Gen. Hosp.; Ho. Off. (Gen. Surg.) St. Thos. Hosp.

SWAN, Charles Henry James Mencom House, 2 Gower St, Newcastle-under-Lyme ST5 1EH — (Birm.) MB ChB Birm. 1961; FRCP Lond. 1979, M 1967; MD Birm. 1969; FRCP Ed. 1994. Specialty: Gastroenterol. Socs: Brit. Soc. Gastroenterol. (Mem. Comm. Endoscopy Sect.- Mem. Counc. & Vice-Pres. Endoscopy); Assn. Phys. Prev: Cons. Phys. (Gastroenterol.) N. Staffs. Hosp. Centre Stoke-on-Trent; Sen. Regist. Gen. Hosp. Birm.; US Pub. Health Serv. Research Fell. New York Med. Coll., USA.

SWAN, Elspeth Anne Street House, Westward, Wigton CA7 8AF — MB BS Newc. 1988; MA Camb. 1989; MRCGP 1992.

SWAN, Ethne (retired) 6 Rosedene Close, Birchill, Onchan, Douglas IM3 3HU Tel: 01624 76218 — MB ChB Glas. 1963; MFFP 1993. Prev: Family Plann. Clin. Med. Off.

SWAN, Frances Ann Arran Surgery, 40 Admiral Street, Glasgow G41 1HU Tel: 0141 429 2626 Fax: 0141 429 2331 — MB ChB Glas. 1986; DRCOG 1988; MRCGP 1990.

SWAN, Harold Thomas (retired) 4 Albert Terrace, Edinburgh EH10 5EA Tel: 0131 447 1167 — MB ChB Ed. 1944; FRCP Lond. 1974, M 1949; DCH Eng. 1951; MD Ed. 1961; FRCPath 1973, M 1963; FRCP Ed. 1985; DLitt Sheff. 1992. Hon. Lect. (Hist. of Med.) Univ. Sheff. Prev: Clin. Dean Fac. Med. Univ. Sheff.

SWAN, Mr Iain Ruairidh Cameron Royal Infirmary, Department of Otolaryngology, Glasgow G31 2ER Tel: 0141 211 4695 Fax: 0141 552 8411 Email: iain@ihr.gla.ac.uk; 3 Manor Road, Jordanhill, Glasgow G14 9LG Tel: 0141 959 5586 — MB ChB Glas. 1976 (University of Glasgow) FRCS Ed. 1980; MD Glas. 1985. Sen. Lect. (Otolaryngol.) Univ. Glas.; Cons. Otol. MRC Inst. Hearing Research (Scott. Sect.) Roy. Infirm. Glas; Hon. Cons. Otolaryngol. Roy. Infirm. Glas. Specialty: Otolaryngol.

SWAN, Ian Robert Bradford Road Medical Centre, 60 Bradford Road, Trowbridge BA14 9AR Tel: 01225 754255; Little Priory, Bathwick Hill, Bath BA2 6LA — MB ChB Glas. 1974 (Glasgow) Dobst RCOG 1976 1976; MRCGP 1981; Dip. Astmma 1997; DFFP 1997. GP; GP Trainee.

SWAN, Ingrid Louise Hamilton Blackhouse, Eyemouth TD14 5LR — MB ChB Glas. 1980; DRCOG 1982; MRCGP 1985; MRCPsych 1988. Assoc. Specialist Dingleton Hosp. Melrose. Specialty: Geriat. Psychiat.

SWAN, John David (retired) 42 Linkswood, Compton Place Road, Eastbourne BN21 1EF Tel: 01323 731397 — LRCP LRCS Ed. 1938 (Univ. & Roy. Colls. Ed.) LRCP LRCS Ed. LRFPS Glas. 1938; MRCGP 1952. Prev: Capt. RAMC 1940-46.

SWAN, Jonathan William Cardiology Department, North Manchester General Hospital, Manchester M8 6RL Tel: 0161 795 4567; Barwood House, Grants Lane, Ramsbottom BL0 9DB — MB ChB Manch. 1983; DRCOG 1985; MRCP (UK) 1988; MD Manch. 1994. Cons. Cardiol. N. Manch. Gen. Hosp. Specialty: Cardiol. Prev: Sen. Regist. (Cardiol.) Manch. Roy. Infirm.; BMS Cardiovasc. Research Fell. Brompton Hosp. Lond.; Regist. (Cardiol.) Harefield Hosp. & Kings Coll. Hosp. Lond.

SWAN, Joseph (retired) 12 Snaefell Crescent, Onchan, Douglas IM3 4NJ Tel: 01624 626209 — MB ChB Glas. 1963; DPH 1966.

SWAN, Katharine Olive 99 Rosses Lane, Ballymena BT42 2SQ — MB BCh BAO Belf. 1990; MB BCh Belf. 1990.

SWAN, Kathleen Mary Sundon Medical Centre, 142-144 Sundon Park Road, Sundon Park, Luton LU3 3AH Tel: 01582 571130 Fax: 01582 564452; 44 Kingsdown Avenue, Luton LU2 7BU — MB ChB Sheff. 1977.

SWAN, Lorna Level 4 Cardiology, Western Infirmary, Glasgow G11 6NT Tel: 0141 211 2987 Fax: 0141 339 2800 Email: ls11n@clinmed.gla.ac.uk; 82 Micklehouse Road, Springhill, Baillieston, Glasgow G69 6TG — MB ChB Glas. 1992; MRCP (UK) 1995. Clin. Research Fell. (Med. & Therap.) West. Infirm. Glas. Specialty: Cardiol.

SWAN, Mr Marc Christopher Radcliffe Infirmary, Department of Plastic & Reconstructive Surgery, Oxford OX2 6HE; Trinity College, Oxford OX1 3BH — MB BS Lond. 1996 (St Mary's) BSc (Neurosci.) Lond. 1993; MRCS Eng. 2000. Clin. Research Fell. Radcliffe Infirm. Oxf. Prev: Regist. (Plastic & Reconstruc. Surg.) Groote Schuur Hosp. Cape Town; SHO (Vasc. Surg.) St Mary's Hosp. Lond.; SHO (Orthop.) St Mary's Hosp. Lond.

SWAN, Marion PO Box 43, Windermere LA22 0GR Tel: 015394 31025 — MB BS Newc. 1972; MRCPsych 1977; FRCPsych 1997. Indep. Forens. Psychiat. Cumbria. Specialty: Forens. Psychiat. Prev: Cons. Forens. Psychiat. North. RHA; Sen. Regist. (Forens. Psychiat.) North. RHA; Sen. Regist. (Psychiat.) St. Luke's Hosp. Middlesbrough.

SWAN, Melanie Jane 14 Larch Way, Ferndown, Wimborne BH21 9SS — MB BS Lond. 1987; MRCP (UK) 1991.

SWAN, Philippa Ann (retired) The River House, Tarrant Rushton, Blandford Forum DT11 8SD Tel: 01258 452403 — MB ChB Ed. 1946; DObst RCOG 1949. Prev: Ho. Phys. & Ho. Surg. Deaconess Hosp. Edin.

SWAN, Sandra Elizabeth Wargrave Surgery, Victoria Road, Wargrave, Reading RG10 8BP Tel: 0118 940 3939 Fax: 0118 940 1357; 4 Holly Cross, Crazies Hill, Wargrave, Reading RG10 8QB Tel: 01734 403483 — MB ChB St. And. 1968; DObst RCOG 1970.

SWAN, Timothy Fraser Wesleyan Chapel, Barningham, Richmond DL11 7DU — MB ChB Liverp. 1991; BSc (Hons) Biochem. Liverp. 1986. HM Forces Doctor.

SWAN, William Gordon Dunblane Medical Practice, Heatlh Centre, Well Place, Dunblane FK15 9BQ Tel: 01786 822595 Fax: 01786 825298 — MB ChB Aberd. 1972; DObst RCOG 1975.

SWANA, Albert Siampisani Lancashire Care NHS Trust, EMI Unit, The Mount, Whalley Road, Accrington BB5 6AS Tel: 01254 294706 Email: albert.swana@mail.bhrv.nwest.nhs.uk — MB ChB Zambia 1985. Cons., Old Age Psychiat., Lancs. Care NHS Trust, Blackburn, Lancs. Specialty: Gen. Psychiat. Special Interest: Old Age Psychiat.

SWANI, Mohan Singh 265 Baldwins Lane, Hall Green, Birmingham B28 0RF Tel: 0121 744 1290; 37 Brueton Avenue, Solihull B91 3EN Tel: 0121 704 2321 Fax: 0121 704 2321 — MB ChB Sheff. 1958; DObst RCOG 1962.

SWANN, Alan Bedford Imperial College Health Centre, Watts Way, London SW7 1LU Tel: 020 7594 9401 Fax: 020 7594 9407 Email: a.swann@ic.ac.uk — BM Soton. 1978 (Southampton) AFOM RCP Lond. 1988. Dir. Occupat. Health Imperial Coll. of Sci. Technol. & Med. Lond. Specialty: Occupat. Health. Prev: GP Princip. Imperial Coll. Med. Partnership Lond.; Trainee GP Willesden; SHO Cent. Middlx. Hosp. Lond.

SWANN, Alan George Castleside Unit, Newcastle General Hospital, Westgate Road, Newcastle upon Tyne NE4 6BE Tel: 0191 273 6666; 1 Bridge End Cottage, Warden, Hexham NE46 4SH — MB BCh BAO Dub. 1983; MRCPI 1986; MRCGP 1987; MRCPsych 1990. Cons. Old Age Psychiat. Castleside Unit Newc. Gen. Hosp.; Clin. Director. Specialty: Geriat. Psychiat.

SWANN, Alison Rosehill Surgery, 189 Manchester Road, Burnley BB11 4HP Tel: 01282 428200 Fax: 01282 838492; Witton Lodge,

School Lane, Simonstone, Burnley BB12 7HR Tel: 01282 771711 — MB ChB Dundee 1973 (St Andrews) DObst RCOG 1975; MRCGP 1977; Dip. Pract. Dermat. Wales 1991. Prev: Clin. Med. Off. Burnley HA; SHO (Anaesth.) Roy. Hosp. Sick Childr. Edin.; SHO (Obst.) Elsie Inglis Matern. Hosp. Edin.

SWANN, Cynthia Mary 32 Abbotts Way, Highfield, Southampton SO17 1NS — MB ChB Leeds 1972; MRCGP 1976. Prev: Univ. Phys. Univ. Health Serv. Univ. Soton.; Lect. (Primary Med. Care) Univ. Soton.

SWANN, David Graham — MB BCh Bristol 1980; BSc Bristol 1977; FRCA 1989. Cons. Anaesth. Roy. Infirm. Edin.; Sen. Lect., Univ. of Edin. Specialty: Anaesth.; Intens. Care. Socs: BMA; SICS; ICS.

SWANN, Debra Elizabeth — MB BS Lond. 1990 (Charing Cross & Westminster) MRCGP Lond. 1997; MA (The Ethics of Cancer and Palliative Care) Keele 2003. Cons. Palliat. Med. Lond.; Cons. in Palliat. Med., St. Christopher's Hospice, Sydenham, Lond. Specialty: Palliat. Med. Socs: BMA; RSM; Assn. of Palliat. Med. Prev: SHO (A & E) Yorks.; SpR rotation in Palliative Medicine, Jan. 98-May 2002.

SWANN, Mr Ian James Kirklea, 7 Campsie Road, Strathblane, Glasgow G63 9AB — MB BS Newc. 1971 (Newc. u. Tyne) FRCS Eng. 1976; FRCS Eng. 1976; DFM Glas. 1989; DFM Glas. 1989; FFAEM 1993; FFAEM 1993. Cons. Admin. Charge of A & E Glas. Roy. Infirm.; Hon. Clin. Sen. Lect. Glas. Univ. Specialty: Accid. & Emerg. Prev: Clin. Dir. (A & E Med.) Glas.; Sen. Regist. (A & E) Glas. Roy. Infirm.; Regist. Rotat. (Gen. Surg.) Newc. AHA (T).

SWANN, Ian Lonsdale Burnley General Hospital, Casterton Avenue, Burnley BB10 2PQ Tel: 01282 474167 Fax: 01282 474156; Witton Lodge, School Lane, Simonstone, Burnley BB12 7HR Tel: 01282 71711 — MB ChB St. And. 1970; DCH Eng. 1976; FRCP Ed. 1985; FRCP (UK) 1997; FRCPCH 1997. Cons. Paediat. N. West. RHA; Clin. Dir. Burnley Health Care Trust; Hon. Lect. Univ. Liverp. Med. Sch; Prin. Regional Examr. NW. Region RCPCH. Specialty: Paediat. Socs: Fell. Manch. Med. Soc.; FRCPCh.; Roy. Coll. Paedia. & Child Health. Prev: Sen. Regist. (Paediat.) Univ. Hosp. Wales Cardiff; Regist. (Neonat. Paediat.) Simpson Memor. Matern. Pavil. Edin.; Regist. (Paediat. Med.) Roy. Hosp. Sick Childr. Edin.

SWANN, James Cyprian (retired) 104 Hayes Way, Beckenham BR3 6RT Tel: 020 8650 3673 — MB BS Lond. 1959 (Lond. Hosp.) DObst RCOG 1961; DMRD Eng. 1963; FFR 1965; FRCR 1975. Prev: Cons. Radiol. BMI Sloane Hosp. Beckenham & Chelsfield Pk. Hosp. The Lond. Hosp. and Bromley Hosps. NHS Trust.

SWANN, John David Grosvenor Street Surgery, 4 Grosvenor Street, St Helier, Jersey JE1 4HB Tel: 01534 30541 Fax: 01534 887948 — MB BCh BAO Belf. 1964; DObst RCOG 1967.

SWANN, Kenneth John Whitley Road Health Centre, Whitley Road, Whitley Bay NE26 2ND Tel: 0191 253 1113; 36 Arden Court, Hadrian Park, Wallsend NE28 9YB Tel: 0191 280 7545 — MB BS Newc. 1983; MRCGP 1987.

SWANN, Mr Malcolm (cons. rooms), 9 Beaumont Road, Windsor SL4 1HY Tel: 01753 863063 Fax: 01753 850128; 3 Chantry Place, Kingstable St., Eton, Windsor SL4 6RH Tel: 01753 840328 — MB BS Lond. 1955 (Westm.) MRCS Eng. LRCP Lond. 1955; FRCS Eng. 1960. Cons. Orthop. Surg. Heatherwood & Wexham Pk. Hosp. Trust. Specialty: Orthop. Socs: Fell. Roy. Soc. Med. (Ex-Pres. Orthop. Sect.); Fell. BOA. Prev: Sen. Regist. Roy. Nat. Orthop. Hosp. Lond.; Hon. Sec. Brit. Orthop. Assn.; Ho. Surg. Roy. Marsden Hosp.

SWANN, Margaret Alice 27 Hawthornden Road, Belfast BT4 3JU Tel: 01232 651825 Fax: 01232 651825 — MB BCh BAO Belf. 1968; DCH RCPSI 1970; MD Belf. 1989; LLM Cardiff 2000. Indep. Med. Pract. Belf. Prev: SCMO S. & E. Belf. Community Trust.

SWANN, Richard Ivan Adair West Kent HA, Preston Hall, Aylesford ME20 7NJ — (Camb. & St. Thos.) MA, MB Camb. 1968, BChir 1967; DObst RCOG 1970; MRCGP 1976; MFPHM 1990. Cons. Pub. Health Med. W. Kent. HA. Specialty: Pub. Health Med. Prev: Cons. Pub. Health Med. SE Thames RHA; Sen. Regist. (Community Med.) SE Thames RHA; GP Sutton Valence.

SWANN, Roy Andrew Clinical Microbiology and Public Health Laboratory, Level 5 Sandringham Building, Leicester Royal Infirmary, Leicester LE1 5WW Tel: 0116 258 6505; 15 Chapel Close, Houghton on the Hill, Leicester LE7 9HT — BM BCh Oxf. 1976; MA Camb. 1976; FRCPath 1994, M 1982. Cons. Med. Microbiol. Roy. Infirm. Leic. NHS Trust. Specialty: Med. Microbiol.

SWANNACK, Robert Yorkley Health Centre, Bailey Hill, Yorkley, Lydney GL15 4RS Tel: 01594 562437 — MB BS Lond. 1974.

SWANNELL, Anthony John (retired) The City Hospital, Hucknall Road, Nottingham NG5 1PJ Tel: 0115 969 1169 Fax: 0115 962 7709; 32 Wollaton Vale, Nottingham NG8 2NR — MB Camb. 1963 (Westm.) MB Camb. 1962, BChir 1963; FRCP Lond. 1979, M 1967. Cons. Rheum. Nottm. City Hosp. Trust (T); Clin. Teach. Univ. Nottm. Prev: Sen. Regist. (Rheum.) Canad. Red Cross Memor. Hosp. Taplow & Hammersmith Hosp. Lond.

SWANSON, Mr Alexander James Grenville (retired) Fernbrae Hospital, 329 Perth Road, Dundee DD2 1LJ Tel: 01382 667203; 9 Roxburgh Terrace, Dundee DD2 1NZ Tel: 01382 566022 — MB ChB St. And. 1966; FRCS Ed. 1974. Hon. Sen. Lect. Univ. of Dundee. Prev: Sen. Lect. (Orthop. & Trauma Surg.) Univ. Dundee.

SWANSON, Fiona Margaret 3 Arnprior Place, Alloway, Ayr KA7 4PT — MB ChB Manch. 1987; BSc (Med. Sci.) St. And. 1984. Breast hys. / Screening Ayrsh. Centr. Hosp, Irvine; Staff Grade (Comm. Paediat.) Ayrsh. Centr. Hosp, Irvine. Prev: SHO (Psychiat.) St. Mary's Hosp. N.d.; SHO (Child Psychiat.) Qu. Eliz. Hosp. Gateshead; SHO (Paediat. & Comm. Paediat.) Qu.s Pk. Hosp. Blackburn.

SWANSON, Gilbert Herbert (retired) Tigh na Creige, Crarae, By Minard, Inveraray PA32 8YA — MB ChB Glas. 1949. Prev: Clin. Asst. (ENT) Hull Roy. Infirm.

SWANSON, Lynn 17 Honister Avenue, Jesmond, Newcastle upon Tyne NE2 3PA — MB BS Newc. 1988; DA (UK) 1992. Specialty: Anaesth.

SWANSON, Maureen Ann Cheshire West PCT, 1829 Building, Countess of Chester Health Park, Liverpool Road, Chester CH2 1UL Tel: 01244 650330 Fax: 01244 650396 — MB ChB Liverp. 1976; DRCOG 1979. Med. Dir. (Primary Care) Cheshire West PCT. Specialty: Gen. Pract.

SWANSON, Noel Christopher Paul Child & Family Therapy, 2nd Floor, Osborn Clinic, Osborn Road, Fareham PO16 7ES Tel: 01329 822220 Fax: 01329 282136 — BM Soton. 1982 (Southampton) MRCPsych 1987. Cons. Child & Adolesc. Psych. Child & Fam. Ther. Clinic, Hants. Specialty: Child & Adolesc. Psychiat. Prev: Fell. Psychiat. Dalhousie Univ. Halifax Nova Scotia, Canada; Psychiat. Belize City Hosp., Belize; SHO (Psychiat.) Middlx. Hosp. Lond.

SWANSTON, Alice Catherine Nelson (retired) Flat 14 Yewdale, 196 Harborne Park Road, Harborne, Birmingham B17 0BP — (Roy. Free) MRCS Eng. LRCP Lond. 1933; DPH Lond. 1946; DIH Soc. Apoth. Lond. 1946. Prev: Sen. Med. Off. DHSS.

SWANSTON, James Kelly (retired) Tillypronie, Helmsley, York YO62 5DQ Tel: 01439 770670 — LRCP LRCS Ed. LRFPS Glas. 1934; MRCGP 1962.

SWANSTON, John Stephen Kelly, OStJ, Col. late RAMC Royal Hospital Chelsea, London SW3 4SR Tel: 020 7370 0161 — MB ChB Liverp. 1966 (Liverpool) Asst. Phys. (Gen. Pract.) Roy. Hosp. Chelsea. Specialty: Gen. Pract.; Care of the Elderly; Sports Med. Socs: BMA; Roy. Soc. Med. Prev: Cdr. (Med.) HQ Lond. Dist.; Med. Adviser NATO Forces, Norway; Sen. Med. Off. Episcopi Garrison Cyprus.

SWANTON, Alexander Graham — MB BS Lond. 1998.

SWANTON, Angus Richard (retired) 20 Marsham Lodge, Marsham Lane, Gerrards Cross SL9 7AB Tel: 01753 886302 — (St. Geo.) MRCS Eng. LRCP Lond. 1947. Prev: Med. Off. Civil Aviat. Auth.

SWANTON, Robert Howard 42 Wimpole Street, London W1G 8YF Tel: 020 7486 7416 Fax: 020 7487 2569; 10 Dover Park Drive, Roehampton, London SW15 5BG Email: rhswanton@easynet.co.uk — MB BChir Camb. 1970 (St. Thos.) MRCP (UK) 1971; MA, MD Camb. 1980; FRCP Lond. 1984. Cons. Cardiol. Univ. Coll. Lond. Hosps. Heart Hosp. Lond. Specialty: Cardiol. Socs: BMA; Pres. Brit. Cardiac Soc. (1998-2001); Fell. Europ. Soc. Cardiol. Prev: Sen. Regist. (Cardiol.) Nat. Heart Hosp. Lond.; Regist. (Cardiac) & Ho. Phys. St. Thos. Hosp. Lond.

SWANWICK, Maelie Victoria 34 Leeds Road, Rawdon, Leeds LS19 6HA — MB ChB Leeds 1991; BSc (Hons.) Leeds 1988, MB ChB 1991.

SWANWICK, Timothy London Deanery, 20 Guilford Street, London WC1N 1DZ Tel: 020 7692 3082 Email: tswanwick@londondeanery.ac.uk — MB BS Lond. 1986; MA Camb. 1983; DRCOG 1989; DCH RCP Lond. 1990; FRCGP 2004. Examr.

RCGP; Director of Postgrad. Gen. Pract. Educat., Lond. Specialty: Gen. Pract.

SWAPP, Helen Garden Sunnybank House Medical Centre, Towngate, Wyke, Bradford BD12 9NG Tel: 01274 424111 Fax: 01274 691256 — MB ChB Aberd. 1987 (Aberdeen) MRCGP 1993. Specialty: Acupunc. Prev: Trainee GP Leeds West. HA; SHO (Anaesth.) Roy. Hallamsh. Hosp. Sheff.; SHO Gold Coast Hosp. Queensland, Austral.

SWARBRICK, Edwin Thornton New Cross Hospital, Wolverhampton WV10 0QP Tel: 01902 643027 — MB BS Lond. 1968 (St. Geo., Lond.) MB BS (Hons.) Lond. 1968; MRCP (UK) 1971; MD Lond. 1980; FRCP Lond. 1985. Cons. Phys. & Gastroenterol. New Cross & Roy. Hosps. Wolverhampton; Director of Research & Developm.. Roy. Wolverhampton Hosp. Trust. Specialty: Gen. Med.; Gastroenterol. Special Interest: Endoscopy Train.; Inflammatory Bowel Dis. Socs: Brit. Soc. Gastroenterol.; Roy. Soc. Med.; Midl. Gastroenterol. Soc. Prev: Sen. Regist., St Barthoelmews Hosp., St Marks Hosp. & Gt. Ormond St., Lond.

SWARBRICK, John Gerard Stanley Road Surgery, 204 Stanley Road, Bootle L20 3EW Tel: 0151 922 5719; 37 Prescot Road, Ormskirk L39 4TG Tel: 01695 572882 — MB ChB Dundee 1985; MRCGP 1989. Socs: Guild Catholic Doctors. Prev: GP Poulton-le-Fylde.

SWARBRICK, Mr Michael John Department of Radiology, Royal Hallamshire Hospital, Glossop Road, Sheffield S10 2JF Tel: 0114 276 6222 Fax: 0114 271 3766; 4 Bishopdale Drive, Ridgeway, Sheffield S20 5PH Tel: 0114 248 7811 — BM BCh Oxf. 1986; MA Oxf. 1988, BA 1983; FRCS Eng. 1991; FRCR 1994. Sen. Regist. (Radiol.) Roy. Hallamsh. Hosp. Sheff. Specialty: Radiol. Prev: Regist. (Radiol.) Roy. Hallamsh. Hosp. Sheff.; SHO (Gen. Surg.) Roy. Infirm & Gen. Hosp. Leicester; SHO (Cardiothoracic Surg.) Glenfield Gen. Hosp. Leics.

SWARBRICK, Peter John Benefits Agency, Medical Services, Argyle House, Lady Lawson St., Edinburgh EH3 0QL Tel: 0131 222 5775; 32 West Werberside, Crewe Road S., Edinburgh EH4 1SZ Tel: 0131 332 1931 — (Ed.) MB ChB Ed. 1962; FRCGP 1993, M 1969. Med. Adviser Benefits Agency Edin.; Hon. Fell. Rehabil. Studies Unit Univ. Edin. Specialty: Rehabil. Med.; Disabil. Med. Socs: Fell. Roy. Soc. Med. Edin.; Scott. Soc. Rehabil. Prev: Princip. GP Livinston; SHO Princess Margt. Rose Orthop. Hosp. & West. Gen. Hosp. Edin.; Ho. Surg. Roy. Infirm. Edin.

SWARBRICK, Philomena Mary The Old Vicarage, Colton, Ulverston LA12 8HF — MB ChB Manch. 1984 (Manchester) BSc (Hons. Anat.) Manch. 1981; MRCP (UK) 1993; DRCOG 1994; DFFP 1994; MRCGP (Distinc.) 1995. Specialty: Gen. Pract. Socs: BMA. Prev: Trainee GP Milnthorpe, Cumbria.; Partner GP Cumbria; Macmillan GP Facilitator.

SWARBRICK, Ruth Hanna Homestead, Rew St., Cowes PO31 8NP — MB BS Lond. 1991; E; BSc (Hons.) Lond. 1986, MB BS 1991.

SWAROOP, Mukul Brook Medical Centre, Ecton Brook Road, Northampton NN3 5EN Tel: 01604 401185 Fax: 01604 403268; Wendover, 512 Wellingborough Road, Northampton NN3 3HX Tel: 01604 402787 — MB BS Agra 1969 (S.N. Med. Coll. Agra) DCH Delhi 1972. Hosp. Pract. (Paediat.) Northampton Gen. Hosp. Specialty: Paediat.

SWART, Michael Leslie Department of Anaesthesia, Torbay Hospital, Newton Road, Torquay TQ2 7AA — MB BS Lond. 1987.

SWART, Sonia Sylvia Northampton General Hospital, Cliftonville, Northampton NN1 5BD Tel: 01604 545839 Fax: 01604 545933; Northampton General Hospital, Cliftonville, Northampton NN1 5BD Tel: 01858 545465 Email: sonia.swart@btinternet.com — MB BChir Camb. 1977; MD Camb. 1986, MA, MB 1977, BChir 1976; MRCP (UK) 1979; MRCPath 1986; FRCPath 1992; FRCP 1993. Cons. Haemat. Northampton Gen. Hosp. NHS Trust. Specialty: Haematology. Prev: Lect. Haemat. Dept. of Pharmacol. & Therap. Univ. Leicester.; Cons. Haemat. N. Warks. HA & Rugby HA.

SWARUP, Namita Department of Paediatrics, John Radcliffe NHS Trust, Oxford OX3 9DU — MB BS Ibadan 1989; MRCP (UK) 1995.

SWASH, Professor Michael The Royal London Hospital , Barts and The London NHS Trust and Queen Mary University of London, Neurological Department, London E1 1BB Tel: 020 7377 7472 Fax: 020 7377 7318 Email: mswash@bartsandthelondon.co.uk; Queen Mary University of London, London — MB BS Lond. 1962 (Lond. Hosp.) FRCP Lond. 1977, M 1969; MD Lond. 1973; FRCPath 1991, M 1982. Prof. Neurol. Qu. Mary Coll. of Med. and Dent., Quenn Mary Univ. of Lond.; Chief Med. Off. Swiss Relnsur. (UK) Ltd. Specialty: Neurol. Socs: (Ex-Sec.) Assn. Brit. Neurol.; Hon. Mem. Austral. Assn. Neurols.; Amer. Neuro. Assn. Prev: Chairm. Research Ethics Comm. of E. Lond. City HA; Neurol. (Adjunct Staff) Cleveland Clinic Foundat. Ohio, USA; Prev. Chairman Motor Neurone Dis. Assn.

SWATKINS, Sandra Substance Misuse Team, 27/29 Hallchurch Road, Holly Hall, Dudley DY2 0TQ Tel: 01384 457373 Fax: 01384 244903 Email: sandra.swatkins@dudleyph-tr.wmids.nhs.uk — MB ChB Birm. 1980; MRCPsych 1984. Cons. Psychiat. (Drug & Alcohol Misuse) Dudley Priority Health NHS Trust. Specialty: Alcohol & Substance Misuse.

SWAYNE, Jeremy Michael Deneys Grove House Surgery, Ditcheat West Shepton, Shepton Mallet BA4 5UH Tel: 01749 342314 Fax: 01749 344016 Email: jem.swayne@btinternet.com — (Oxf. & St. Geo.) BA Oxf. 1963; MRCS Eng. LRCP Lond. 1966; BM BCh Oxf. 1967; DObst RCOG 1969; MRCGP 1974; FFHom 1991, M 1983. p/t Dean, Fac. Homeop. Lond.; Homeop. Phys. SW Region. Specialty: Homeop. Med. Special Interest: Christian Healing Min. Prev: Sen. Med. Coding Cons. NHS Centre for Coding & cl.ification; GP Yeovil & Coleford.; Homeop. Phys. Bristol Homoeop. Hosp.

SWAYNE, Philippa Salisbury District Hospital, Salisbury SP2 8BJ Tel: 01722 336262 Fax: 01722 414143 Email: philippa.swayne@salisbury.nhs.uk; Lower Nunton Farm House, Nunton, Salisbury SP5 4HP — MB ChB Bristol 1982 (University of Bristol) DRCOG 1986; FFA RCS Eng. 1988; MRCGP 1989. Cons. Anaesth. Salisbury Dist. Hosp. Specialty: Anaesth. Socs: Assn. Anaesth.; Obst. Anaesth. Assn.

SWEATMAN, Catherine Mary The Surgery, 134 Baffins Road, Portsmouth PO3 6BH Tel: 023 9282 7132 Fax: 023 9282 7025; 7 Hamilton Close, Langstone, Havant PO9 1RP — BM Soton. 1985; DRCOG 1988; MRCGP 1990. Prev: Trainee GP Portsmouth VTS.

SWEATMAN, Martin Charles Michael The Hillingdon Hospital NHS Trust, Pied heath Road, Uxbridge UB8 3NN Tel: 01895 279663 — MB BS Lond. 1976 (St. Bart.) BSc (Hons.) Lond. 1973; MRCS Eng. LRCP Lond. 1976; MRCP (UK) 1980; FRCP Lond. 1995. Cons. Phys., Care of the Elderly; Clin. Director, Care of the Elderly; Coll. Tutor (Medicine). Specialty: Gen. Med.; Care of the Elderly; Respirat. Med. Socs: Assoc. Mem. Brit. Thoracic Soc.; Brit. Geriat. Soc.; Roy. Soc. of Med. Prev: Sen. Regist. St. Thos. & Kent & Canterbury Hosp.; Clin. Research Fell. Cardiothoracic Inst. Brompton Hosp. Lond.; Cons. Phys. Mt. Vernon Hosp. Northwood.

SWEDAN, Hisham Ibrahim Claremont Medical Centre, 29 Claremont Road, London E17 5RJ Tel: 0208 527 1888; 8 Felstead Road, Wanstead, London E11 2QJ — MB BCh Cairo 1972; DGM RCP Lond. 1985.

SWEDAN, Sawsan Kamel Selim Lord Lister Health Centre, 121 Woodgrange Road, Forest Gate, London E7 0EP Tel: 020 8250 7530 Fax: 020 8250 7535; 8 Felstead Road, Wanstead, London E11 2QJ — MB BCh Cairo 1974; DObst. RCPSI 1980; MRCS Eng. LRCP Lond. 1982. GP City & E. Lond. FPC.

SWEENEY, Anthony Martin Tang Hall Surgery, 190 Tang Hall Lane, York YO10 3RL Tel: 01904 411139 Fax: 01904 431224 — MB ChB Liverp. 1981.

SWEENEY, Anthony Niall The Grange, Highfield Road, Hemsworth, Pontefract WF9 4DP Tel: 01977 610009 Fax: 01977 617182 — MB ChB Liverp. 1981; MRCGP 1989. GP Hemsworth.

SWEENEY, Bernard John Gerard 108 Ifield Road, London SW10 9AD — MB BCh BAO NUI 1986; MRCPI 1988.

SWEENEY, Brendan The Crescent Medical Practice, 12 Walmer Crescent, Glasgow G51 1AT Tel: 0141 427 0191 Fax: 0141 427 1581 — MB ChB Glas. 1972; MA Glas. 1966, MB ChB 1972; DObst RCOG 1974; FRCGP 1986, M 1976.

SWEENEY, Brian Edward Fintona Medical Centre, 33 Dromore Road, Fintona, Omagh BT78 2BB Tel: 028 8284 1203 Fax: 028 8284 0545 — MB BCh BAO NUI 1987; LRCPSI 1987.

SWEENEY, Catherine Marie 1 Ridgeway, Epsom KT19 8LD — MB BS Lond. 1997.

SWEENEY, Clare Mary Clanrye Surgery, Newry Health Village, Monaghan Street, Newry BT35 6BW Tel: 028 3026 7639 Fax: 028 3025 7414 — MB BCh BAO Belf. 1990; MB BCh Belf. 1990.

SWEENEY, Cormac James Erne Health Centre, Erne Hospital, Cornagrade Road, Enniskillen BT74 6AY Tel: 028 6632 5638;

Health Centre, Cornagrade Road, Enniskillen BT74 Tel: 01365 325638 Fax: 01365 329446 — MB BCh BAO NUI 1973 (University College Dublin) MICGP 1986. GP Enniskillen. Prev: Regist. (Med.) Altnagelvin Hosp. Londonderry; SHO (Paediat.) St. Anthony, Newfld.; Ho. Phys. & Ho. Surg. Altnagelvin Hosp. Lond.derry.

SWEENEY, David The Grange Clinic, Westfield Avenue, Malpas, Newport NP20 6EY Tel: 01633 855521 Fax: 01633 859490 — BM BS Nottm. 1981; BMedSci Nottm. 1979; DRCOG 1983; MRCGP 1985.

SWEENEY, Denis Oldpark Road Surgery, 460 Oldpark Road, Belfast BT14 6QG Tel: 028 9074 6535 Fax: 028 9074 7768 — MB BCh BAO Belf. 1979.

SWEENEY, Desmond 20 Buchanan Drive, Rutherglen, Glasgow G73 3PE Tel: 0141 647 1824 — LRCP LRCS Ed. 1973 (Anderson Coll. Glas.) Dip. Amer. Bd. Anesth. 1968; LRCP LRCS Ed. LRFPS Glas. 1944 FACA 1973. Cons. Anesth. Auburn Gen. Hosp. Washington USA; Sen. Instruct. Dept. Anaesth. Univ. Hosp. Seattle, Washington. Specialty: Anaesth.; Alcohol & Substance Misuse. Socs: Fell. Roy. Soc. Med.; King Co. Med. Soc.; Fell. Internat. Anesth. Research Soc. Prev: Chief Resid. (Anesth.) King Co. Hosp. Seattle, U.S.A.; Resid. (Anesth.) Washington Hosp. Center, U.S.A.; Capt. RAMC.

SWEENEY, Elizabeth 49 Covertside, Wirral CH48 9UH — MB ChB Bristol 1993.

SWEENEY, Gary Alan Ranworth Surgery, 103 Pier Avenue, Clacton-on-Sea CO15 1NJ Tel: 01255 421344 Fax: 01255 473581; 22 Holland Road, Clacton-on-Sea CO15 6EQ Tel: 01255 429041 Fax: 01255 473581 — MRCS Eng. LRCP Lond. 1978 (St. Bart.) FFA RCSI 1985; MRCGP 1987. GP Princip.; Hosp. Pract. (Anaesth.) Colchester Hosp.; Med. Adviser N. Essex HA. Specialty: Gen. Pract.; Anaesth. Socs: Brit. Assoc. of Med. Managers; Colchester Med. Soc. Prev: Regist. (Anaesth.) Coventry HA; SHO (Anaesth.) Southend Hosp. NE Thames HA; SHO (Paediat. & O & G) St. John's Hosp. Chelmsford.

SWEENEY, Helen Ruth The Surgery, 2 Great Wood Road, Small Heath, Birmingham B10 9QE Tel: 0121 766 8828 Fax: 0121 773 0091 — MB BS Newc. 1989.

SWEENEY, Jennifer Margaret 209 Glasgow Road, Dumbarton G82 1DP — MB ChB Glas. 1993.

SWEENEY, John Nicholas 168 Almond Brook Road, Standish, Wigan WN6 0SS — MB ChB Sheff. 1983; Dip. Gum. (Dist.) 1994 Soc. of Apoth. Lond.; MRCP (UK) 1988; FRCP 1999. Cons. Phys. (G U Med.) Blackpool Vict. & Roy. Preston Hosps. Specialty: Genitourinary Medicine. Prev: Cons. Phys. (G U Med.) Roy. Lond. Hosp.; Sen. Regist. (G U Med.) Roy. Lond. Hosp.; Hon. Sen. Regist. (Immunol.) St. Bart. Med. Coll. Lond.

SWEENEY, Jonathan Edmon 484 West Road, Newcastle upon Tyne NE5 2ET — MB ChB Liverp. 1978.

SWEENEY, Kathleen Mary Majella The Surgery, 1 Marble Arch Terrace, Florence Court, Enniskillen BT92 1EF; Moybrone, Letterbreen, Enniskillen BT74 9EP — MB BCh BAO NUI 1985 (Univ. Coll. Galway) MRCGP 1989; DRCOG 1992. SHO (Dermat.) Roy. Alexandra Hosp. Paisley. Socs: Sligo GP Soc.; Fermanagh GP Assn. Prev: Trainee GP Cumnock Ayrsh.; SHO (O & G) Southmead Gen. Hosp. Glas.; SHO (Paediat.) Booth Hall Manch.

SWEENEY, Kevin Thomas 1016 Great Western Road, Glasgow G12 0NP — LRCP LRCS Ed. 1942; LRCP LRCS Ed. LRFPS Glas. 1942. Socs: Roy. M-C Soc. Glas. & BMA.

SWEENEY, Kieran Gerard St. Leonard's Medical Practice, 34 Denmark Road, Exeter EX1 1SF Tel: 01392 201790 Fax: 01392 201796; 1 Robins Court, Upton Pyne, Exeter EX5 5HZ Tel: 01392 841639 — MB ChB Glas. 1978 (Glasgow) MA Glas. 1971, MB ChB 1978; MRCGP 1982; MPhil Exeter 1996. GP Exeter; Lect. Health Serv. Research RDSU Roy. Devon Exeter NHS Trust; Lect. (Gen. Pract.) Univ. of Exeter. Specialty: Gen. Pract. Socs: Fell. Roy. Soc. Of Arts. Prev: Harkness Fell. Commonw. Fund New York 1991; Vis. Fell. Univ. Washington, Seattle, USA.

SWEENEY, Louise Evelyn X-Ray Department, Royal Belfast Hospital for Sick Children, 180 Falls Road, Belfast BT12 6BE — MB BCh BAO Belf. 1976; DCH RCPS Glas. 1978; DMRD Eng. 1980; FRCR 1983. Cons. Radiol. Roy. Belf. Hosp. Sick Childr. & Roy. Vict. Hosp. Belf. Specialty: Radiol.

SWEENEY, Margaret Mary (retired) 20 Parkway, Ilford IG3 9HU Tel: 020 8599 0776 — (W. Lond.) MRCS Eng. LRCP Lond. 1945.

SWEENEY, Mark Gerard Knightsbridge Medical Centre, 71-75 Pavilion Road, London SW1X 0ET Tel: 020 8237 2600; 4 Gunnersbury Avenue, Ealing Common, London W5 3NH Tel: 020 8752 1994 — MB BS Lond. 1984; MRCGP Lond. 1988; DFFP 1989; DRCOG 1989; Dip Clin Hypn 1997; MSc (Hons.) Lond. 1998. GP Princip. Specialty: Gen. Pract.; Gen. Psychiat.; Paediat.; Obst. & Gyn. Prev: GP Tutor Chelsea & Westm. Hosp.; Chairm. K.C.W. Clin. Audit Advis. Gp.

SWEENEY, Mary Elizabeth 5 Linden Avenue, Liverpool L23 8UL — MB ChB Liverp. 1990.

SWEENEY, Michael Thomas 8 Harbern Close, West Derby, Liverpool L12 8SR — MB ChB Liverp. 1984.

SWEENEY, Patrick Laurie (retired) Fintona Medical Centre, 33 Dromore Road, Fintona, Omagh BT78 2BB Tel: 028 8284 1203 Fax: 028 8284 0545 — LRCPI & LM, LRSCI & LM 1962.

SWEENEY, Peter Martin Red House Surgery, 124 Watling Street, Radlett WD7 7JQ Tel: 01923 855606 Fax: 01923 853577; 9 King Harry Lane, St Albans AL3 4AS Tel: 01727 848072 — MB BS Lond. 1986; DA (UK) 1988; DRCOG 1990; MRCGP 1991.

SWEENEY, Richard Charles Dr Moss and Partners, 28-38 Kings Road, Harrogate HG1 5JP Tel: 01423 560261 Fax: 01423 501099 — MB ChB Leeds 1979; Cert. Family Plann. RCOG 1982; DRCOG 1982; FRCGP 1995, M 1984.

SWEENEY, Thomas Kevin, QHP (retired) Tresanton, Wych Hill Way, Woking GU22 0AE Tel: 01483 828199 — (National Univ. of Irel.; Univ. Coll. Dub.) MB BCh BAO Univ. Coll. Dub. 1949; DTM & H Eng. 1954; TDD Wales 1959; FFCM 1983, M 1972; FFPHM RCP (UK) 1989. Prev: Sen. Med. Off. DHSS.

SWEENIE, Alan Christopher 1/R, 1 Cathkin Road, Langside, Glasgow G42 9UB Tel: 0141 636 6129 — MB ChB Glas. 1993. SHO (Anaesth.) Victor A. Infirm. Glas. Specialty: Anaesth. Prev: SHO (Anaesth.) Hairmyres Hosp. E. Kubride; SHO (A & E) Roy. Alexandra Hosp. Paisley.; SHO (A & E & Orthop.) South. Gen. Hosp. Glas.

SWEENIE, John Fraser Crown Avenue Surgery, 12 Crown Avenue, Inverness IV2 3NF Tel: 01463 710777 Fax: 01463 714511; Tendore Farm, North Kessock, Inverness IV1 3XD — MB ChB Glas. 1981; FRCP 2000 Edin.; MRCP (UK) 1988; MRCGP 1990; Dip Pract. Dermat. Wales 1993. Hon. Lect. (Gen. Pract.) Dundee Univ.

SWEERTS, Michele Irene Edith c/o Watercress Cottage, 1 Oldbury Lane, Wick, Bristol BS15 5QG — MB ChB Cape Town 1975.

SWEET, Amanda Jane 55 Whittington Road, Cheltenham GL51 6BT — MB BCh Wales 1998.

SWEET, David Gordon The Gables, 15 Ormiston Park, Belfast BT4 3JT Tel: 02890 580373; The Gables, 15 Ormiston Park, Belfast BT4 4JT Email: dsweet@ntworld.com — MB BCh BAO Belf. 1990 (Qu. Univ. Belf.) MRCPI 1995; MRCPCH 1996. Specialist Regist. (Train. Paediat.) Belf.; Maj. RAMC (Territorial Army). Specialty: Paediat.

SWEET, David John Stratton Medical Centre, Hospital Road, Stratton, Bude EX23 9BP Tel: 01288 352133 — MB Camb. 1974; BChir 1973; DRCOG 1979; DA 1981. GP Bude; Hon. Doctor Bude Surf Club.

SWEET, Elizabeth Mary (retired) Dunwhillan, 3 Fullarton Crescent, Troon KA10 6LL Tel: 01292 314325 — MB ChB Ed. 1950 (Edinburgh Univ) DCH Eng. 1953; FRCP Ed. 1968, M 1954; DMRD 1959; FFR 1962; FRCR 1975; FRCP Glas. 1983, M 1981. Prev: Cons. Radiol. Roy. Hosp. Sick Childr. & Qu. Mother's Hosp. Glas.

SWEET, Hector Struthers (retired) Gothic Cottage, Lamb Corner, Dedham, Colchester CO7 6DX Tel: 01206 322391 — MB ChB Glas. 1939 (Univ. Glas.) DOMS Eng. 1950.

SWEET, Peter Thomas Maes Mawr, 61 First Avenue, Charmandean, Worthing BN14 9NP Tel: 01903 209192 — MB BS Lond. 1975; MRCS Eng. LRCP Lond. 1975; FFA RCS Eng. 1979. Cons. Anaesth. Worthing HA. Specialty: Anaesth. Prev: Sen. Regist. St. Mary's Hosp. Lond. W2; Regist. St. Bart. Hosp. Lond.

SWEET, Pia Rebecca St Marys Hospital Sidcup NHS Trust, Frognal Avenue, Sidcup DA14 6LT — MB ChB Leic. 1985; FRCA 1994. Cons. in Anaesth. & Pain Managem. Specialty: Anaesth. Special Interest: Pain Management. Socs: Brit. Med. Assn.; Internat. Assn. for the Study of Pain; Roy. Coll. of Anaesth.

SWEET, Stephen Charles Mayne (retired) La Ferme du Pignon, Route des Sages, Torteval, Guernsey GY8 0LB Tel: 01481 263273

Fax: 01481 263905 Email: s.sweet@lineone.net — MB ChB Bristol 1973; DA Eng. 1976; DObst RCOG 1976. Prev: GP Guernsey.

SWEET-ESCOTT, Michael William (retired) Moor Cottage, Guiting Power, Cheltenham GL54 5UE Tel: 01451 850357 — BM BCh Oxf. 1951 (Oxf. & St. Bart.) MA Oxf. 1951; MRCGP 1962. Prev: GP Skipton; .

SWEETEN-SMITH, Beverley Ann Adelaide Medical Centre, 111 Adelaide Road, London NW3 7RY Tel: 020 7722 4135 — MB BS Lond. 1985 (Univ. Coll. Lond.) BSc Nottm. 1980; MRCGP 1990; DRCOG 1990; DTM & H RCP Lond. 1996. GP Princip. Prev: GP Wantage Oxon.; Trainee GP John Radcliffe Hosp. VTS; Flt. Lt. RAF.

SWEETENHAM, Dileas Mary Combe House, Lynbrook Lane, Entry Hill, Bath BA2 5NB Tel: 01225 427110 Fax: 01225 423110 — MB BS Lond. 1956 (Roy. Free) DCH Eng. 1958. Specialty: Gen. Pract. Socs: Hon. Life Mem. Med. Off. Sch. Assn.; Clin. Soc. Bath. Prev: Med. Off. The Roy. Sch. Bath; Resid. Med. Off. Roy. Free Hosp.

SWEETENHAM, Ian Arthur Charles Hicks Centre, 75 Ermine Street, Huntingdon PE29 3EZ Tel: 01480 453038; 12 Church Road, Brampton, Huntingdon PE28 4PW Tel: 01480 355454 — MB BChir Camb. 1988; MA Camb. 1989; MRCGP 1992. GP Tutor Huntingdon; Clin. Asst. (Med. for Elderly) Huntingdon.

SWEETING, Audrey Evelyn (retired) Low Banks, Banks Lane, Riddlesden, Keighley BD20 5BD Tel: 01535 607972 — MB ChB Leeds 1957; BSc (Gen. & Hons.) Lond. 1952 & 1953; DPM Leeds 1978. Prev: Assoc. Specialist (Psychogeriat. & Psychiat.) Airedale Gen. Hosp. Keighley.

SWEETING, Keith William (retired) Low Banks, Banks Lane, Riddlesden, Keighley BD20 5BD — MRCS Eng. LRCP Lond. 1957 (Leeds) Prev: GP Keighley.

SWEETLAND, Helen Margaret Department of Surgery, University of Wales College of Medicine, Heath Park, Cardiff CF14 4XN Tel: 029 2074 2896 Fax: 029 2076 1623; 4 Gateside Close, Cardiff CF23 8PB Tel: 029 2073 3697 — MB ChB Sheff. 1983; FRCS Ed. 1988; MD Sheff. 1992. Reader (Surg.) Univ. Wales Coll. Med. Specialty: Gen. Surg. Prev: Sen. Lect. (Surg.) Univ. Wales Coll. Med.; Sen. Regist. Rotat. (Gen. Surg.) N. Trent Region; Lect. (Surg.) Univ. Sheff. & N. Gen. Hosp. Sheff.

SWEETMAN, Anne Cecilia Portugal Place Health Centre, Portugal Place, Wallsend NE28 6RZ Tel: 0191 262 5252 Fax: 0191 262 0241 Email: anne.sweetman@nhs.net; 26 Rosebery Crescent, Jesmond, Newcastle upon Tyne NE2 1EU Tel: 0191 281 6808 — MB BS Newc. 1975; DRCOG 1978; MRCGP 1979.

SWEETMAN, Bernard Stewart (retired) 9 Westpoint, 49 Putney Hill, London SW15 6RU Tel: 020 8788 7088 — MB BS Lond. 1944 (Middlx.) MRCS Eng. LRCP Lond. 1944. Prev: Local Treasury Med. Off. Med. Adviser Thresher & Co.

SWEETMAN, Brian John Morriston Hospital, Swansea SA6 6NL Tel: 01792 703103 Fax: 01792 703632 — MD Lond. 1986 (St. Thos.) PhD Lond. 1981, MB BS 1968; MRCP (UK) 1972; FRCP Lond. 1994. Cons. Phys. Rheum. Morriston, Singleton, Neath & Llanelli Hosps. Specialty: Rheumatol. Socs: Brit. Soc. Rheum.; Soc. Back Pain Research. Prev: Research Assoc. & Sen. Regist. Guy's Hosp. Lond.

SWEETMAN, Julian Andrew Pontllandffraith Health Centre, Blackwood Road, Blackwood NP12 2YU Tel: 01495 227156 Fax: 01495 220311 — MB ChB Bristol 1991; BSc (Hons.) Bristol 1988.

SWEETMAN, Stella Muriel (retired) 9 Westpoint, 49 Putney Hill, London SW15 6RU — LRCPI & LM, LRSCI & LM 1941 (Lond. Sch. Med. Wom. & Dub.) LRCPI & LM, LRCSI & LM 1941. Prev: Capt. RAMC.

SWEETNAM, Anthony Thomas (retired) 9 Redesdale Gardens, Adel, Leeds LS16 6AT Tel: 0113 267 8591 — MRCS Eng. LRCP Lond. 1963 (Leeds) DA Eng. 1970. Clin. Asst. (Anaesth.) Harrogate Gen. Hosp.

SWEETNAM, Mr David Ian Staveley 6 Dunstable Mews, Devonshire St., London W1G 6BT Tel: 020 7935 5004 Fax: 020 7935 5004 Email: aandcsweetnam@aol.com — MB BS Lond. 1987 (The Middlesex Hospital Medical School) Dip. Sports Med. RCS Ed.; FRCS Eng. 1991; FRCS(Orth) 1996. Sen. Regist. The Roy. Nat. Orthop. Hosp. Trust Stanmore. Specialty: Orthop. Socs: Brit. Orthop. Assn.; Roy. Soc. Med.; Brit. Hip Soc.

SWEETNAM, Sir (David) Rodney, KCVO, CBE 25 Woodlands Road, Bushey WD23 2LS Tel: 01923 223161 Fax: 01923 223161 — (Camb. & Middlx.) MA Camb. 1951, BA 1947; MB BChir Camb. 1950; FRCS Eng. 1955; Hon. FRCS (Glas.) 1997; Hon. FRCS (Irel.) 1997; Hon. FACS 1998; Hon. FCM (SA) 1998; Hon. FDS RCS 1998. Cons. Orthop. Surg. Emerit. The Middlx. Hosp. Lond., UCH (University College Hospital) & Kings Edwd. VII Hosp. Lond.; Fell. UCL. Specialty: Orthop. Socs: Hon. Fell. BOA; Fell. Roy. Soc. Med.; Fell. Roy. Coll. Surg. Eng. Prev: Orthop. Surg. to the Qu.; Pres. Roy. Coll. of Surgs. Eng.; Pres. Brit. Orthop. Assn.

SWENY, Paul Renal Transplant Unit, Royal Free Hospital, London NW3 2QG — MB BChir Camb. 1970; MA, MD Camb. 1979, MB 1970, BChir 1969; MRCP (UK) 1972; FRCP Lond. 1986. Cons. Nephrol. Roy. Free Hosp. Lond. Specialty: Nephrol. Socs: Internat. Soc. of Nephrol.; Amer. Transplantation Soc.; Brit. Transplantation Soc.

SWERDLOW, Anthony John Section of Epidemiology, Institute of Cancer Research, Sutton SM2 5NG Tel: 020 8722 4012 — BM BCh Oxf. 1975; MA Camb. 1976; MFCM 1980; PhD Glas. 1985; FFPHM RCP (UK) 1994, M 1989; MA Oxf. 1990, DM 1990; T(PHM) 1991. Prof. of Epidemiol. Inst. of Cancer Research; Director, Dept. of Health Cancer Screening Eval. Unit, Inst. of Cancer Research; Hon. Cons. in Epidemiol., Roy. Marsden. Prev: Prof. of Epidemiol., Lond. Sch. of Hyg. and Trop. Med.

SWIERCZYNSKI, Stanislaw 9 White Court, 200 West Hill, London SW15 3JB — Lekarz Lublin 1955; Clin. Dip. Paediat. Warsaw 1963; Clin. Dip. Endocrinol. Warsaw 1968. Clin. Asst. (Ment. Handicap) Botleys Pk. Hosp. Chertsey Surrey. Prev: Regist. (Psychiat.) FarnBoro. Hosp. Kent; Clin. Asst. Ment. Handicap Area, Cornw.

SWIESTOWSKI, Ignacy The Black County Family Practice, Health Centre, Queens Road, Tipton DY4 8PH Tel: 0121 557 6397 Fax: 0121 557 1662; 36 Woodcroft Avenue, Tipton DY4 8AE Tel: 0121 557 2446 — LRCPI & LM, LRSCI & LM 1957 (RCSI) LRCPI & LM, LRCSI & LM 1957; DObst RCOG 1959.

SWIETOCHOWSKI, John Patrick Gerard The Doctors House, Victoria Road, Marlow SL7 1DN Tel: 01628 484666 Fax: 01628 891206 — MB ChB Dundee 1977.

SWIFT, Mr Andrew Cree Department of Otolarynology, Head & Neck Surgery, University Hospital Aintree, Aintree NHS Trust, Fazakerley, Liverpool L9 7AL Tel: 0151 529 5258 Fax: 0151 529 5263; 64 Knowsley Road, Cressington Park, Grassendale, Liverpool L19 0PG Tel: 0151 427 6377 Fax: 0151 427 1118 — MB ChB Sheff. 1977 (Sheffield) FRCS Eng. 1981; FRCS Ed. 1984; ChM Sheff. 1989. Cons. ENT Surg. Univ. Hosp. Aintree Liverp.; Clin. Lect. Univ. Liverp. Specialty: Otorhinolaryngol. Socs: BAOL - HNS Full Mem.; RSM Full Mem.; N. Eng. Otoloaryngol. Soc. Prev: Lect. & Sen. Regist. (ENT) Mersey RHA; MRC Research Fell. Univ. Liverp.; Regist. (ENT) Liverp. HA.

SWIFT, Benjamin — MB ChB Leic. 1998.

SWIFT, Professor Cameron Graham Department of Health Care of the Elderly, Kings College School of Medicine & Dentistry, Kings College Hospital (Dulwich), London SE22 8PT Tel: 020 7346 6076 Fax: 020 7346 6476; 8 Spencer Road, Bromley BR1 3SU — MB BS Lond. 1969 (St. Bart.) MRCS Eng. LRCP Lond. 1969; MRCP (UK) 1974; PhD Dundee 1984; FRCP Lond. 1988. Prof. Health c/o Elderly & Cons. Phys. King's Coll. Hosp. Lond.; Prof. Health c/o Elderly Univ. Kent. Specialty: Care of the Elderly. Socs: Brit. Pharm. Soc.; Brit. Geriat. Soc. (Chairm. Scientif. Comm.). Prev: Sen. Lect. & Cons. Phys. (Geriat. Med.) Univ. Wales Coll. of Med. Cardiff; Cons. Phys. (Med. for the Elderly) & Postgrad. Clin. Tutor Hull HA; Trustbank Vis. Prof. ChristCh. Sch. Med. NZ 1994.

SWIFT, Ephraim Frank Flat 24, The Willows, Beechfield Gardens, Southport PR8 2SW — MRCS Eng. LRCP Lond. 1948 (Liverp.)

SWIFT, Gillian Lesley Llandough Hospital, Penlan Road, Penarth CF64 2XX Tel: 029 2071 1711 — MB BCh Wales 1986 (UWCM) BSc Wales 1983; MRCP (UK) 1989; MD Wales 1992; FRCP 1999. Cons. Phys. (Gastroenterol. & Gen. Med.) Llandough Hosp. Cardiff. Specialty: Gastroenterol. Socs: Brit. Soc. Gastroenterol.; Nutrit. Soc.; Eur. Assn. Gastroenterol. & Endoscopy. Prev: Sen. Regist. (Gastroenterol.) Llandough Hosp. Cardiff; Regist. (Med.) Cardiff Roy. Infirm.; Research Regist. (Gastroenterol.) Univ. Hosp. Wales Cardiff.

SWIFT, Graham Roger (retired) The Surgery, Park Lane, Woodstock, Oxford OX20 1UB Tel: 01993 811452 — MB BS Lond. 1956 (Univ. Coll. Hosp.) MRCS Eng. LRCP Lond. 1956; DObst RCOG 1959; Family Plann. Cert RCOG 1981. Apptd. Fact. Doctor. Prev: Ho. Surg. & Ho. Phys. Whittington Hosp. Lond.

SWIFT, Joseph Louis 35 Thorndon Hall, Thorndon Park, Ingrave, Brentwood CM13 3RJ Tel: 01277 811 299 Fax: 01277 811 299 — MB BS Lond. 1951 (Middlx.) MRCS Eng. LRCP Lond. 1951; DPM Eng. 1954; FRCPsych 1979, M 1971. Child & Family Consultation Serv. Specialty: Child & Adolesc. Psychiat.; Medico Legal. Socs: Fell. Roy. Soc. Med.; Assoc. Mem. Brit. Psychoanalyt. Soc. Prev: Med. Dir. Romford Child Guid. Clinic; Cons. Psychiat. Community Ment. Health & Child Guid. Lond. Boro. Newham; Psychiat. Portman Clinic Lond.

SWIFT, Margaret Rosemary Brook Lane Surgery, 27 Brook Lane, Bromley BR1 4PX Tel: 020 8461 3333 Fax: 020 8695 5567; 8 Spencer Road, Bromley BR1 3SU Tel: 020 8460 3215 — MB BS Lond. 1969. GP Bromley.

SWIFT, Michael Andrew The Surgery, Branksomewood Road, Fleet GU51 4JX Tel: 01252 613624 Fax: 01252 816489; Little Orchard, School Lane, Ewshot, Farnham GU10 5BN — MB ChB Bristol 1976; DA Eng. 1979.

SWIFT, Nicholas David 50 Wallasey Village, Wallasey CH45 3NL Tel: 0151 691 2088 Fax: 0151 637 0146; 42 Mount Road, Upton, Wirral CH49 6JB Tel: 0151 604 1934 — MB ChB Manch. 1986; DRCOG 1990. Forens. Med. Examr. Merseyside Police A (Wirral) Div. Specialty: Gen. Pract. Socs: Assn. Police Surg.

SWIFT, Pauline Anne Stravithie Mill, St Andrews KY16 8LT — MB BS Lond. 1994.

SWIFT, Peter George Furmston Leicester Royal Infirmary Children's Hospital, Leicester LE1 5WW Tel: 0116 254 1414 Fax: 0116 258 7637 Email: peter.swift@uhl-tr.nhs.uk; 21 Westminster Road, Leicester LE2 2EH Tel: 0116 221 7376 Email: peterswift@webleicester.co.uk — (Camb. & Guy's) MB Camb. 1969, BChir 1968; MRCS Eng. LRCP Lond. 1968; MA Camb. 1969; MRCP (UK) 1971; DCH Eng. 1972; FRCP Lond. 1984; FRCPCH 1996. Cons. Paediat. & Endocrinol. Leicester Roy. Infirm. Specialty: Paediat.; Diabetes; Endocrinol. Socs: Roy. Coll. Paediat. & Child Health; (Sec-General) Internat. Soc. Paediat. & Adolesc. Diabetes; (Ex-Sec.) Brit. Soc. Paediat. Endocrinol. & Diabetes. Prev: Sen. Regist. (Paediat.) Bristol Hosp. Sick Childr.; Regist. (Paediat.) Sheff. Childr. Hosp.; SHO (Neonat. Paediat.) Univ. Coll. Hosp. Lond.

SWIFT, Mr Robert Ian Mayday Univ. Hosp., Lond. Rd., Croydon Tel: 0208 4013 000 — MB BS Lond. 1983 (King's Coll.) BSc (Hons.) Lond. 1981; FRCS Lond. 1985; FICS 1995; MS Lond. 1995. Cons. Surg. (Colorectal) Mayday Univ. Hosp. Croydon. Socs: Assn. Surg.; AESGBT; RSM.

SWIFT, Sarah Elizabeth St Jame's University Hospital, Beckett St, Leeds LS9 7TF Tel: 0113 206 5231; 127 East Parade, Henworth, York YO31 7YD Tel: 01904 431524 — MB BChir Camb. 1991 (Emmanuel College, Camb./ St. Bartholomew's Hospital Medical Sch, Lond.) MA, MB BChir (Hons.) Camb. 1991; MRCP (UK) 1993; FRCR 1996. Cons. Radiol., St Jame's Uni. Hosp. & Cookridge Hosp., Leeds. Specialty: Pharmacology. Prev: Specialist Regist., Leeds/Bradford, Radiol. Train. Scheme; SHO (Med.) Northwick Pk. Hosp.; Ho. Phys. St. Bart. Hosp. Lond.

SWIFT, Timothy David Speedwell Surgery, 1 Speedwell Street, Paddock, Huddersfield HD1 4TS Tel: 01484 531786 Fax: 01484 424249; Surat Cottage, 2 Meal Hill, Slaithwaite, Huddersfield HD7 5UR Tel: 01484 842983 — MB BS Lond. 1978; MA Camb. 1979, BA 1975; DRCOG 1980; MRCGP (Distinc.) 1982; Dip. Pract. Dermat. Wales 1991. GP Huddersfield; Clin. Asst. (Dermat.) Huddersfield; VTS Course Organiser (Yorkshire Deanery). Specialty: Dermat. Socs: BMA; RCGP.

SWINBURN, Christopher Ralph Taunton And Somerset NHS Trust, Taunton TA1 5DA Tel: 01823 342146 Fax: 01823 343709 Email: chris.swinburn@tst.nhs.uk — MB BChir Camb. 1978 (St. Thos.) MRCP (UK) 1980; MD Camb. 1985; FRCP 1994. Cons. Phys. Thoracic & Gen. Med. Taunton & Som. Hosp. (MusGr. Pk. Br..). Specialty: Respirat. Med. Socs: Fell. Roy. Coll. Phys. (Lond.); Brit. Thorac. Soc. Prev: Sen. Regist. (Thoracic Med.) Freeman Hosp. Newc.; Sir Jules Thorn Research Fell. & Regist. (Med.) Middlx. Hosp. Med. Sch.; SHO (Cardiol. & Neurol.) St. Geo. & Atkinson Morley's Hosp.

SWINBURN, Helen Mary 40 The Pavillions, 140 Cambridge Road, Southend-on-Sea SS1 1HP — BM Soton. 1984. Regist. (Haemat.) Southend Hosp. Essex. Specialty: Haematology.

SWINBURN, Jonathan Murray Amyatt Department of Cardial Research, Northwick Park Hospital, Watford Road, Harrow HA1 3UJ Tel: 020 8869 2547 Fax: 020 8864 0075 — MB BS Lond. 1994 (Char. Cross & Westm.) MA Camb. 1995, BA 1991; MRCP 1997. Clin. Research Fell. (Cardiol.) Northwick Pk. Hosp. Specialty: Cardiol. Prev: Research Regist. (Cardiol.) Northwick Pk. Hosp.; SHO (ITU) Birm. City Hosp.; SHO (Med.) Northwick Pk. Hosp.

SWINBURN, Ralph Teasdale (retired) 45 Woodcroft Road, Wylam NE41 8DH Tel: 01661 852113 — MB BS Durh. 1948; DObst RCOG 1952.

SWINBURNE, Anita Priory Lane Surgery, Priory Lane, Prestatyn LL19 9DH Tel: 01745 854496; 18 Bryneithin Avenue, Prestatyn LL19 9LS Tel: 01745 853219 Email: aswinburne@aol.com — MB ChB Liverp. 1987; MRCGP 1992. Socs: Assn. Police Surg. Prev: Trainee GP Abergele VTS.

SWINBURNE, Kenneth Arthur McLeod Cairns Owen (retired) 16 Foxhill Crescent, Leeds LS16 5PD — MB BChir Camb. 1956 (Camb. & St. Bart.) DMRD Eng. 1966; CBiol,Mbiol 2001. Cons. (Diag. Radiol.) St. Jas. Univ. Hosp. Leeds & Wharfedale Gen.; Hosp. Sen. Clin. Lect. in Diag. Radiol. Univ. Leeds. Prev: Sen. Regist. Diag. Radiol. Gen. Infirm. Leeds.

SWINBURNE, Margaret Layinka 16 Foxhill Crescent, Leeds LS16 5PD — MB ChB Leeds 1951; BSc Leeds 1948; DCH Eng. 1954; FRCP Lond. 1976, M 1957; FRCPath 1975, M 1964; GI Biol. 1995. Prev: Cons. Path. St. Jas. Hosp. Leeds.; Sen. Regist. (Path.) St. Jas. Hosp. Leeds; Jun. Asst. (Path.) Univ. Camb.

SWINBURNE, Paul — MB ChB Ed. 1997.

SWINBURNE, Robert Miles Audley Mills Surgery, 57 Eastwood Road, Rayleigh SS6 7JF Tel: 01268 774981; Wades, Creeksea Ferry Road, Canewdon, Rochford SS4 2EX — MB BS Lond. 1959 (Lond. Hosp.) MRCS Eng. LRCP Lond. 1959; DObst RCOG 1961. Prev: Receiv. Room Off. Lond. Hosp.; Ho. Surg. Gen. Hosp. Rochford.

SWINDALE, Flora Elisabeth 22 Cooper Road, Guildford GU1 3LY Tel: 01483 32306 — MD Basle 1938 (Bonn, Berlin & Basle) Socs: BMA.

SWINDALL, Hilary Jane East Quay Medical Centre, East Quay, Bridgwater TA6 5YB Tel: 01278 444666 Fax: 01278 445448 — MB ChB Sheff. 1977; DRCOG 1979; MRCGP 1999.

SWINDELL, Pamela Joy The Health Centre, Beeches Green, Stroud GL5 4BH Tel: 01453 763980 — MB BS Newc. 1975; MB BS (Hons.) Newc. 1975; MRCP (UK) 1978. Prev: Research Regist. (Microbiol.) Southmead Hosp. Bristol; SHO (Med. & Path.) Southmead Hosp. Bristol.

SWINDELLS, Ann Craigard, Evening Hill, Thursby, Carlisle CA5 6PU Tel: 01228 710944 — MB ChB Bristol 1971. Clin. Med. Off. E. Cumbria HA.; Staff Grade Paediat. (Audiol.) - N. I. Healthcare Trust. Specialty: Audiol. Med.

SWINDELLS, Robin Fraser Cawley Doctors Surgery, Half Moon Lane, Wigton CA7 9NQ Tel: 016973 42254 Fax: 016973 45464; Craigard, Evening Hill, Thursby, Carlisle CA5 6PU Tel: 01228 710944 — MB ChB Bristol 1971; DObst RCOG 1974; MRCGP 1975.

SWINDEN, Josephine Anne — MB BS Lond. 1996; DRCOG 1999; DFFP 2000; MRCGP 2000.

SWINDEN, Stephen John Darnall Health Centre, 2 York Road, Sheffield S9 5DH Tel: 0114 244 1681 Fax: 0114 242 1160 — MB ChB Manch. 1975.

SWINDLEHURST, Amanda Louise The Riverside Surgery, Waterside, Evesham WR11 1JP Tel: 01386 40121 Fax: 01386 442615; Little Orchard, Kersoe, Pershore WR10 3JD Tel: 01386 710607 — MB BS Lond. 1988; DA (UK) 1992; DCH RCP Lond. 1993; MRCGP 1994. Prev: Trainee GP Cheltenham.

SWINDLEHURST, Ruth Alys 20 Woodland Avenue, Lymm WA13 0BJ — MB ChB Leic. 1998.

SWINGLEHURST, Deborah Anne — MB BS Lond. 1993 (Univ. Camb. Jesus Coll. & St. Mary's Hosp. Lond.) MA Camb. 1994; DGM RCP Lond. 1995; DCH RCP Lond. 1996; DRCOG Lond. 1997; MRCGP Lond. 1998; MSc 2003. GP Princip. Norwich Rd. Surg. Ipswich; Teachg. Fell. Dept. of Primary Care UCL. Prev: GP Regist. Lattice Barn Surg. Ipswich; SHO (Med.) Ipswich Gen. Hosp. VTS; SHO (A & E & c/o Elderly) Northampton Gen. Hosp.

SWINGLEHURST, Paul Anthony 18 Windsor Street, Barrow-in-Furness LA14 5JR — MB ChB Liverp. 1997.

SWINGLEHURST, Peter John (retired) 11 Thorpe Road, Staines TW18 3EA Tel: 01784 490786 Fax: 01784 441244 — MB BChir

Camb. 1960 (Camb. & St. Thos.) DObst RCOG 1963. Princip. in Gen. Med. Pract. Prev: Ho. Off. (O & G) Farnham Hosp.

SWINGLER, Rebecca 30 Birch Road, Southville, Bristol BS3 1PF Tel: 0117 966 8360 Email: rebeccaswingler@hotmail.com — MB ChB Ed. 1994. SSHO O & G. Specialty: Obst. & Gyn.

SWINGLER, Robert James Department of Neurology, Ninewells Hospital, Dundee DD1 9SY Tel: 01382 660111 Fax: 01382 425739 — MB BS Lond. 1980 (Guy's) MRCP (UK) 1983; BSc (Hons.) Lond. 1977, MD 1990; T(M) 1991; FRCP Ed. 1998; FRCP 1999. Cons. Neurol. Dundee Teachg. Hosps. NHS Trust; Hon. Sen. Lect. Dundee Univ. Specialty: Neurol. Socs: Ord. Mem. BMA; Ord. Mem. ABN; Corr. Assoc. AAN. Prev: Sen. Regist. (Neurol.) Dundee Gen. Hosps.; MRC Trav. Fellowship CB Day Laborat. Mass. Gen. Hosp. E. Charle Mass., USA; Lect. (Med. Neurol.) Univ. Edin.

SWINHOE, Alexandra Louise Anaesthetic Department, Barnsley District General Hospital NHS Trust, Barnsley S75 2EP Tel: 01226 777976; Deershaw Barn, Deershaw Lane, Cumberworth, Huddersfield HD8 8YB Tel: 01484 682695 — MB ChB Birm. 1991 (Birm. Univ.) ChB Birm. 1991; FRCA 1997. Specialist Regist. Rotat. (Anaesth.) N. Trent Sheff. Specialty: Anaesth. Prev: SHO (Anaesth.) Halifax; SHO (Paediat.) Wordsley; Ho. Off. (Surg.) Russell Hall Hosp. Dudley.

SWINHOE, Crispin Francis Anaesthetic Department, Barnsley District General Hospital, Barnsley S75 2EP Tel: 01226 777 976 Fax: 01226 320375; Deershaw Barn, Cumberworth, Huddersfield HD8 8YB Tel: 01484 682695 — MB BS Lond. 1979 (St. Mary's) MRCGP 1985; DA (UK) 1988; FRCA 1993. Cons. Anaesth. Barnsley Dist. Gen. Hosp.; Clin. Head of Serv. Critical Care. Specialty: Anaesth. Socs: Intens. Care Soc.; Anaesth. Res. Soc. Prev: Sen. Regist. (Anaesth.) Roy. Hallamsh. Hosp. Sheff.; Clin. Research Fell. (Anaesth.) Sheff. Univ.; Ho. Phys. (Med.) RNH Haslar.

SWINHOE, David John Elmwood Medical Centre, 7 Burlington Road, Buxton SK17 9AY Tel: 01298 23019; Crossview Cottage, 147 Green Lane, Buxton SK17 9DG — MB ChB Manch. 1980; MRCOG 1985; MRCGP 1990. Specialty: Obst. & Gyn. Prev: Regist. (O & G) Qu. Mothers Hosp. Glas.

SWINHOE, June Rose 59 Twyford Avenue, London N2 9NR Tel: 020 8883 1591 Email: swinhoe@pasher.demon.co.uk — MRCS Eng. LRCP Lond. 1971 (Roy. Free) MD Lond. 1985, MB BS 1971; FRCOG 1989, M 1975. Cons. O & G King Geo. Hosp. Goodmayes. Specialty: Obst. & Gyn. Socs: Fell. Roy. Soc. Med. Prev: Sen. Regist. Roy. Free Hosp. Lond.; Regist. (O & G) United Liverp. Hosp.; SHO (O & G) Qu. Charlottes & Chelsea Hosps.

SWINHOE, Peter Harrison, OBE, CStJ, Brigadier late RAMC Retd. (retired) The Retreat, Bonchurch Shute, Bonchurch, Ventnor PO38 1NX — (St. Mary's) MRCS Eng. LRCP Lond. 1951; MB Chir Camb. 1952; MA Camb. 1952; DObst RCOG 1954; DTM & H Eng. 1968; MFCM 1973. Prev: Hon. Phys. to HM Qu.

SWINN, Mr Michael James 35 Gresley Road, London N19 3LA — MB BS Lond. 1991; BSc Lond. 1988; FRCS Eng. 1996; MSc 1999; FRCS (Urol) 2002. Specialty: Urol. Prev: SpR St Mary's Hosp., Lond.

SWINSCOE, Anthony William Cedar House Surgery, 14 Huntingdon Street, St. Neots, Huntingdon PE19 1BQ Tel: 01480 406677 Fax: 01480 475167; Stilton Cottage, 18 Alberman St, Eaton Socon St Neots, Huntingdon Tel: 01480 212596 — MB ChB Sheff. 1979; DRCOG 1983; MRCGP 1983.

SWINSCOE, Brian David The Surgery, Bottesford, Nottingham NG13 0AN Tel: 01949 842325 — BM BS Nottm. 1981; BSc (Hons.) Cranwell 1971; BMedSci (Hons.) Nottm. 1979, BM BS 1981.

SWINSON, Brian David 131 Mountsawdel Road, Coleraine — MB BCh Belf. 1998.

SWINSON, Daniel Edmund Bryan 11 Tullis Close, Castlefield, Stafford ST16 1AX — MB BS Lond. 1996; MRCP; BSc Lond. 1993.

SWINSON, David Robert — (King's Coll. Hosp.) MRCS Eng. LRCP Lond. 1965; MB BS Lond. 1965; MRCP (UK) 1970; DPhysMed Eng. 1974; FRCP Lond. 1984. Specialty: Rheumatol. Special Interest: Osteoporosis; Pagets Dis. Socs: Fell. Roy. Soc. Med.; Brit. Soc. Rheum. Prev: Cons. Rheum. & Rehabil. Wrightington Hosp. NHS Trust & Wigan & Leigh NHS Trust.

***SWINSON, Sophie Elizabeth** 11 Tullis Close, Castlefields, Stafford ST16 1AX — MB BS Lond. 1998 (Camb. & St. Mary's) BA (Hons) Cantab 1995; MB BS Lond 1998; MRCPCH 2001. Ho. Off. (Med.) Ealing Hosp. Socs: BMA; MPS; MSS. Prev: Ho. Off. (Surg.) Ealing Hosp.; Ho. Off. (Paediat.) Ealing Hosp.

SWINTON, Susan McLean — MB ChB Aberd. 1997; MRCA 2001. GP Regist. Socs: Med. & Dent. Defence Union of Scotl. (MDDUS). Prev: SHO (Psychiat) Murray Roy. Infirm. Perth; SHO (O & G) Dunedin New Zealand; Regist. (Anaesth.) Lower Hutt New Zealand.

SWINYARD, Peter William Phoenix Surgery, Dunwich Drive, Toothill, Swindon SN5 8SX Tel: 01793 600440 Fax: 01793 600410 Email: peter.swinyard@gp-j83645.nhs.uk — MB BS Lond. 1979 (St. Thos.) Specialty: Gen. Pract. Socs: GPC Represen. for Wilts. and Dorset, GPC Premises subcommittee Chairm. Prev: Trainee GP Colchester VTS.

SWIRE, Herbert Churchfields Surgery, Recreation Road, Bromsgrove B61 8DT Tel: 01527 872163 — MB ChB Birm. 1968; MA Camb. 1964. Indep. Clin. Asst. BromsGr. Socs: BromsGr. & Redditch Med. Soc. Prev: GP BromsGr..

SWIRE, Nina Palliative Care Team, 26 Nassau St., London W1N 7RF Tel: 020 7380 9236; 37 Ninehams Road, Caterham-on-the-Hill, Caterham CR3 5LN Tel: 020 8660 9264 — MB ChB Leeds 1984; MRCP (UK) 1992. Sen. Regist. (Palliat. Med.) Camden & Islington NHS Community Trust. Specialty: Palliat. Med.

SWIRSKY, David Michael Leeds General Infirmary, Great George St., Leeds LS1 3EX Tel: 0113 392 6285 Fax: 0113 392 6286 — MB BS Lond. 1975 (Univ. Coll. Hosp. Med. Sch. Lond.) MRCPath 1987; FRCP Lond. 1993. Cons. Haematologist Leeds Gen. Infirm. Specialty: Haematology. Socs: Brit. Soc. Haematol. Prev: Sen. Lect. & Hon. Cons. Haemat. Hammersmith Hosp. Lond.; Leukaemia Research Fund Train. Fell. (Haemat. Med.) Camb.; Sen. Regist. Hammersmith Hosp. Lond.

SWITALSKI, Boleslaw Jan Dingley Dell, 443 Barnsley Road, Sandel, Wakefield WF2 6BJ Tel: 01924 250988 — MB ChB Polish Sch. of Med. 1942 (Poznan & Polish Sch. of Med.) Prev: Ho. Surg. Roy. Infirm. Edin.; Cas. Off. & Ho. Phys. Chesterfield Roy. Hosp.; Capt. Polish Army Med. Corps. 1942-8.

SWITHINBANK, David Winthrop Stokes Medical Centre, Braydon Avenue, Little Stoke, Bristol BS34 6BQ Tel: 01454 616767 Fax: 01454 616189; 20 Woodland Grove, Stoke Bishop, Bristol BS9 2BB Tel: 0117 968 4400 — MB BS Lond. 1976; DRCOG 1981; MRCGP 1983. Occupat. Phys. Hewlett Packard Ltd. Bristol.

SWITHINBANK, Ian Milne Camborne/Redruth Community Hospital, Barncoose Terrace, Redruth TR15 3ER Tel: 01209 881645 — MB BChir Camb. 1975; MRCP (UK) 1977. Cons. Phys. (s/i in Elderly) Camborne/Redruth Community Hosp. Cornw. Specialty: Care of the Elderly. Prev: Sen. Regist. (Geriat. & Gen. Med.) Dudley Rd., Gen. & Selly Oak Hosps.; Regist. (Neurol.) Frenchay Hosp. Bristol.; Ho. Phys. St. Thos. Hosp. Lond.

SWITHINBANK, Lucy Victoria 20 Woodland Grove, Stoke Bishop, Bristol BS9 2BB — MB BS Lond. 1977; MD Brist. 2000. Assoc. Specialist (Urodynamics) Southmead Hosp. Bristol. Specialty: Rehabil. Med.; Rheumatol.

SWOFFER, Steven John Oak Hall Surgery, 41-43 High Street, New Romney TN28 8BW Tel: 01797 362106 Fax: 01797 366495 — MB BS Lond. 1982; DRCOG 1986. Hon. Med. Off. Littlestone-on-Sea Lifeboat.

SWORD, Andrew James Alton Health Centre, Anstey Road, Alton GU34 2QX Tel: 01420 84676 Fax: 01420 542975; Oakbank, East Worldham, Alton GU34 3AT — MB ChB Manch. 1982; MRCGP 1987. Prev: SHO (O & G) St. Mary's Hosp. Manch.; SHO (A & E) Stockport Infirm.; SHO (Paediat.) N. Manch. Gen. Hosp.

SWORD, Annie Carmichael (retired) Stourvale, 2 Bridge Place, Northbourne, Bournemouth BH10 7EA — MB ChB Ed. 1926 (Univ. Ed.) DPH Lond. 1930. Prev: Asst. Co. Med. Off. Lindsey (Lincs.) CC.

SWORD, Lindsay Jean Watercress Medical Group, Dean Surgery, Ropley, Alresford SO24 0BQ Tel: 01962 772340 Fax: 01962 772551; Oakbank, East Worldham, Alton GU34 3AT — MB ChB Manch. 1982; DRCOG 1986.

SWORDS, Jacqueline Greenford Road Medical Centre, 591 Greenford Road, Greenford UB6 8QH Tel: 020 8578 1764 Fax: 020 8578 8347; 16 Altenburg Avenue, Ealing, London W13 9RN — MB ChB Dundee 1989; DCH RCP Lond. 1991; DRCOG 1992; MRCGP 1993. Specialty: Gen. Med. Prev: Trainee GP Lond. VTS.

SWORDS, Patrick Joseph Kevin Winterton Hospital, Sedgefield, Stockton-on-Tees TS21 3EJ — LRCP LRCS Ed. 1963 (Galway) LAH

Dub. 1958; LRCP LRCS Ed. LRCPS Glas. 1963; LM Coombe 1965; DObst RCOG 1966; DCH NUI 1970; DPM RCPSI 1972; MRCPsych 1974.

SWORN, Michael John (retired) — MRCS Eng. LRCP Lond. 1965 (Lond. Hosp.) LLB Lond. 1985, MB BS 1965; FRCPath 1983, M 1971; Cert BA 1992. Prev: Cons. Histopath & Cytopath. Roy. Hants. Co. Hosp. Winchester.

SYADA, Mr Mounir 152 Harley Street, London W1G 7LH Tel: 020 7935 8868 Fax: 020 7224 2574; Romany, 414 Fulham Palace Road, London SW6 6HX Tel: 020 7385 1184 Fax: 020 7385 1184 — MD Damascus 1971; FRCS Glas. 1982. Cons. Gen. Surg. Cromwell Hosp. & Lond. Bridge Hosp. Lond.; Sec. W. Lond. M-C Soc., Postgrad. Centre Char. Cross Hosp. Lond. Specialty: Gen. Surg. Socs: Fell. Roy. Soc. Med.; Sec. W. Lond. Medico-Chirurgical Soc. Prev: Cons. Gen. Surg. Whittington & Roy. North. Hosp. Lond.; Regist. (Gen. Surg.) St. Stephen's & Roy. Masonic Hosps. Lond.; SHO (Gen. Surg., Urol., Orthop. & Cardiovasc.) Char. Cross, St. Mary's & Hammersmith Hosps.

SYAM, Velayudham Stuart Road Surgery, Stuart Road, Pontefract WF8 4PQ Tel: 01977 703437 Fax: 01977 602334; 46 Dulverton Rise, Pontefract WF8 2PY — MB BS Kerala 1980; MRCP (UK) 1989; DRCOG 1991; MRCGP 1992. GP Pontefract W. Yorks. Specialty: Gen. Med.

SYDENHAM, David John Taylor and Partners, The Surgery, Hexton Road, Barton-le-Clay, Bedford MK45 4TA Tel: 01582 882050 — MB BS Lond. 1970 (Char. Cross) MRCS Eng. LRCP Lond. 1970; DObst RCOG 1973. Specialty: Gen. Pract.

SYDNEY, John Paul Martin Sydney and Partners, St Mary's Medical Centre, Rock St, Oldham OL1 3UL Tel: 0161 620 6667 Fax: 0161 626 2499 — MB ChB Manch. 1975; DCH Eng. 1979; MRCGP Lond. 1981. GP Oldham.

SYDNEY, Margaret Mary (retired) 11 Barnfield Close, Thornton-Cleveleys FY5 2AF — MB BCh BAO Dub. 1969 (Trinity Coll. Dub.) MA Dub. 1968. Med. Policy Adviser DSS HQ's Lancs. Prev: Med. Adviser War Pens. Agency & Med. Off. Benefits Agency Blackpool.

SYDNEY, Michael Aidan Flatt Walks Health Centre, 3 Castle Meadows, Catherine Street, Whitehaven CA28 7QE Tel: 01946 692173 Fax: 01946 590406 — MB ChB Manch. 1967; BSc (Hons. Physiol.) Manch. 1967; MB ChB (Hons.) Manch. 1970; MRCP (UK) 1973; MRCGP 1977.

SYDNEY, Ronald Meadowbank Health Centre, 3 Salmon Inn Road, Polmont, Falkirk FK2 0XF — MB ChB Manch. 1994; BSc (Med. Sci.) St. And. 1991. GP Falkirk. Specialty: Gen. Pract. Prev: Regist. (Gen. Pract.) Denny Health Stirlingsh.; SHO (Psychiat. Geriat. Med. & O & G).

SYED, A A Kingsdowne Surgery, 34 Kingsdowne Road, Surbiton KT6 6LA Tel: 020 8399 9032 Fax: 020 8390 2122.

SYED, Aamir Bakhtiar Fox Hollies Surgery, 511 Fox Hollies Road, Hall Green, Birmingham B28 8RJ Tel: 0121 777 1180 Fax: 0121 777 6265; 157 Swanshurst Lane, Moseley, Birmingham B13 0AS — MB BS Lond. 1984; DRCOG 1988; MRCGP 1991.

SYED, Attiya 192 Lavender Hill, Enfield EN2 8NP Tel: 020 8367 3815 — MB BS Punjab 1965 (Fatima Jinnah Med. Coll.) Clin. Asst. (Accid.) Chase Farm Hosp. Enfield.

SYED, Ghufran Mahmood 38 Gainsborough Road, New Malden KT3 5NU — BM Soton. 1995.

SYED, Iftikhar Ali Manchester Road Surgery, 187 Manchester Road, Burnley BB11 4HP Tel: 01282 420680 Fax: 01282 832031; Oaklands, 332 Burnley Road, Holme in Cliviger, Burnley BB10 4ST — MB BS Karachi 1958; DPH Manch. 1966; MFFP 1991.

SYED, Imran Anwaar 55 Hamilton Avenue, Romford RM1 4RP — MB BS Lond. 1994.

SYED, Junaid Ali Kingsdowne Surgery, 34 Kingsdowne Road, Surbiton KT6 6LA Tel: 020 8399 9032 Fax: 020 8390 2122 — MB BS Lond. 1991 (Char. Cross & Westm.) MRCGP 1996; MBA Lond. 2001. Specialty: Gen. Pract. Socs: BMA. Prev: Trainee GP Roehampton VTS.

SYED, Mubeen Fatima Prenton Medical Centre, 516 Woodchurch Road, Prenton, Birkenhead CH43 0TS Tel: 0151 608 7666 — MB BS Osmania 1978; MRCOG Lond.; MFFP Lond. 1996. Specialty: Gen. Pract.; Family Planning; Womens Health. Socs: BMA; MDU; Roy. Coll. of AP.

SYED, Naila Yasmin Northwood Medical Centre, 10/12 Middleton Hall Road, Kings Norton, Birmingham B30 1BY Tel: 0121 458 5507 — MB ChB Bristol 1990 (Univ. Bristol) MRCGP 1994; DRCOG 1996; DFFP 1996. Specialty: Gen. Pract.

SYED, Naveed Akhtar Leeds North East Primary Care Trust, Beech House, 7A Woodhouse Cliff, Leeds LS6 2HF Tel: 0113 305 9820 Fax: 0113 305 9873; 25 Cowley Crescent, Heaton, Bradford BD9 6LX Tel: 01274 495021 — MB ChB Manch. 1993. Specialist Regist. (Pub. Health Med.) Leeds NE. PCT, Leeds HA, Glos. HA & Avon HA Bristol. Specialty: Pub. Health Med. Prev: SHO (Oncol.) St. Jas. Univ. Hosp. Leeds; SHO (Dermat.) Hope Hosp. Univ. of Manch. Salford; SHO (Gen. Med.) Blackburn Roy. Infimary.

SYED, Onn Abbas 14 Greenford Road, Manchester M8 0NW — MB BCh Wales 1993.

SYED, Rakshan 68 Basing Hill, Wembley HA9 9QR — MB BS Lond. 1996.

SYED, Rizwan Ul Hoda 33 Norborough Road, Wheatley, Doncaster DN2 4AT — BM Soton. 1996.

SYED, Samira Batul 33 Derwent Crescent, Stanmore HA7 2NE — MB BS Lond. 1982 (Univ. Coll. Hosp.) DCCH RCP Ed. RCGP & FCM 1987; DCH RCP Lond. 1990. Assoc. Specialist (Paediatric Dermatology), Gt Orand St Hosp. Specialty: Paediat. Socs: Univ. Coll. Hosp. Old Stud.'s Assn.; BMA. Prev: Staff Grade Paediat. Gt Ormond St. Hosp. Lond.; SHO (O & G) Princess Margt. Hosp. Swindon; Regist. & SHO (Paediat.) Princess Margt. Hosp. Swindon.

SYED, Shahid Hussain Oldham Health Authority, Department Public Health Medicine, Westhulme Avenue, Oldham OL1 2PN Tel: 0161 624 0420; 1 Dunlin Close, Bamford, Rochdale OL11 5PZ Tel: 01706 523005 — MB BS Punjab 1965; FRIPHH 1983. SCMO (Adult Health) Dept. Pub. Health Oldham; Non-Exec. Bd. Mem. Rochdale HA. Specialty: Pub. Health Med. Socs: BMA (Exec. Mem. Oldham Div.); Fac. Comm. Health.; Assn. Local Auth. Med. Advisers. Prev: Med. Off. Provin. Health Servs. Punjab, Pakistan.

SYED, Shamshad Ullah 30 Compton Ave, Sudbury, Wembley HA0 3FD Tel: 020 8903 2737 — MB BS Calcutta 1968.

SYED, Shamsun Nahar 13 Fern Bank Close, Stalybridge SK15 2RZ; 13 Fernbank Close, Stalybridge SK15 2RZ — MB BS Dacca 1966 (Dacca Med. Coll.) Assoc. Specialist in Anaesth. N. West. RHA.

SYED, Shamsuzzoha Babar 39 Park Avenue, Mitcham CR4 2ER — MB BS Lond. 1996; DPH Contab.; DFPHM; MD USA. SpR Pub. Health Med. East. Region.

SYEDAH, Najam Anwar 55 Hamilton Av, Romford RM1 4RP — MB BS Lond. 1997.

SYKES, Alan John The Surgery, 29 High Stile, Leven, Beverley HU17 5NL — MB ChB Dundee 1978; DA Eng. 1982; DRCOG 1984; MRCGP 1986.

SYKES, Andrew 41 Hill Drive, High Ackworth, Pontefract WF7 7LQ — MB ChB Sheff. 1989; BSc Sheff. 1984, MB ChB 1989.

SYKES, Andrew Sykes and Menzies, Littlebury Medical Centre, Fishpond Lane, Spalding PE12 7DE Tel: 01406 22231 Fax: 01406 425008 — BM BCh Oxf. 1977.

SYKES, Andrew John Christie Hospital, Wilmslow Road, Manchester M20 4BX Tel: 0161 446 3354 Fax: 0161 446 3352 Email: andrew.sykes@christie-tr.nwest.nhs.uk — MB ChB Birm. 1989; MRCP (UK) 1992; FRCR 1996. Cons. (Clin. Oncol.) Christie Hosp. Manch. Specialty: Oncol.; Radiother.

SYKES, Anne Charlotte Jenner Health Centre, 201 Stanstead Road, Forest Hill, London SE23 1HU Tel: 020 8690 2231; 32 Manor Way, Beckenham BR3 3LJ — BM BCh Oxf. 1980; MA Camb. 1981; MRCGP 1984; Cert. Family Plann. JCC 1984. Socs: BMA. Prev: GP Leeds & Sydenham Green Lond.; Trainee GP Airedale Health Dist.

SYKES, Annemarie Barnwell House, Skirmett Road, Fingest, Henley-on-Thames RG9 6TH — MB BS Lond. 1998; MRCP Lond. 2002.

SYKES, Catherine Joanne Ladywell medical centre, Edinburgh EH12 7TB — MB ChB Ed. 1988; DRCOG 1992; MRCGP 1993; DCCH RCP Ed. 1994. Specialty: Gen. Pract. Prev: Trainee GP York VTS.

SYKES, Catherine Margaret 58 Kirby Road, Dunstable LU6 3JH Tel: 01582 602927; 41 Seamons Close, Dunstable LU6 3EQ Tel: 01582 603359 — MB BS Lond. 1979 (Char. Cross) MRCS Eng. LRCP Lond. 1979; DRCOG 1981. Gen. Practitioner, Dunstable, Beds; Occupat. Phys. Marks & Spencer (& other companies); Family Plann. Clin. Sector. Specialty: Occupat. Health; Paediat.; Gen. Psychiat. Socs: BMA. Prev: Univ. Luton Stud. Health Doctor.

SYKES, Colin Alexander Abbey Park Hospital, Dalton Lane, Barrow-in-Furness LA14 4TP Tel: 01229 491310/01229 813388; The Villa, Mount Pleasant, Greenodd, Ulverston LA12 7RG Tel: 01229 861459 Email: scolinsykes@aol.com — MB BS Lond. 1967 (St Bart.) MRCS Eng. LRCP Lond. 1967; DObst RCOG 1969; DA Eng. 1970; DCH Eng. 1971; MRCP UK 1972; FRCP Lond. 1985. Cons. Phys. & Cardiol. Specialty: Cardiol. Socs: Brit. Cardiac Soc. Prev: Sen. Regist. (Med.) Clatterbridge Hosp. Bebington, Roy. Liverp. Hosp. & Liverp. Roy. Infirm.; Cons. Gen. Phys. Morecambe Bay NHS Trust.

SYKES, David 27 Longford Road, Bradway, Sheffield S17 4LP — MB BS Newc. 1996.

SYKES, David Paul 2 Second Avenue, Dalton, Huddersfield HD5 9SJ — MB ChB Leeds 1984.

SYKES, David William (retired) Eastcliff, 14 Marine Parade, Budleigh Salterton EX9 6NS — MB ChB Bristol 1959; DObst. 1964; FRCOG 1982, M 1969. Cons. O & G Roy. Devon. & Exeter Hosp. Prev: Lect. (O & G) & Hon. Sen. Regist. Roy. Free Hosp. Lond.

SYKES, Eliot 39 Rectory Park, Morpeth NE61 2SZ — MB BS Newc. 1996.

SYKES, Elizabeth Mary 24 Bury Road, Alverstoke, Gosport PO12 3UD — MB ChB Dundee 1974. Community Paediat. Portsmouth City PCT. Prev: Clin. Med. Off. Portsmouth & SE Hants. HA.

SYKES, George William 7 Avenue Road, Stratford-upon-Avon CV37 6UW — MB BChir Camb. 1947 (Camb. & Manch.) MA Camb. 1947; MRCGP 1962.

SYKES, Hannah Ruth Southport NHS Trust, Town Lane, Kew, Southport PR8 6PN Tel: 01704 704205 — MB BS Lond. 1986; BSc Lond. 1983, MB BS 1986; MRCP (UK) 1989; FRCP 1998. Cons. Phys. & Rheumatol. Southport Hosp. Specialty: Rheumatol. Socs: BSR. Prev: Sen. Regist. (Med. & Rheum.) Mersey RHA; Regist. Rotat. (Rheum. & Med.) North. RHA; SHO (Med.) Newc. HA.

SYKES, Helen Department of Haematology, Kingston Hospital, Galsworthy Road, Kingston upon Thames KT2 7QB Tel: 020 8547 0887 — MB BS Lond. 1970; FRCPath 1989, M 1977. Cons. (Haemat.) Kingston Hosp. Surrey. Specialty: Haematology. Prev: Sen. Research Assoc. (Leukaemia Research Fund Fell.) Dept. Haemat., Med. Univ. Camb.; Lect. (Haemat.) St. Geo. Hosp. Med. Sch. Lond.; Regist. (Clin. Path.) Roy. Marsden Hosp. Lond.

SYKES, Helen Elaine 18 Tynybedw Street, Treorchy, Cardiff CF42 6RA Tel: 01443 774484 — MB BCh Wales 1994. SHO (A & E) E. Glam. Hosp. Specialty: Accid. & Emerg. Prev: Ho. Off. (Gen. Med.) P. Chas. Hosp. Merthyr Tydfil; Ho. Off. (Gen. Surg.) W. Wales Gen. Hosp. Carmarthen.

SYKES, Ian Richard Oakham Surgery, 213 Regent Road, Tividale, Oldbury B69 1RZ Tel: 01384 252274 Fax: 01384 240088 — MB ChB Birm. 1987 (Birmingham) BSc (Hons.) Birm. 1984; DCH RCP Lond. 1990; DRCOG 1991; T(GP) 1992; MRCGP 1992. Gen. Practitioner. Specialty: Gastroenterol. Prev: SHO (Psychiat.) Rubery Hill Hosp. Birm.; SHO (Paediat., Geriat. & A & E) Selly Oak Hosp. Birm.

SYKES, Jennifer Anne Greenford Road, Greenford UB6 0HE Tel: 020 8966 5222 Fax: 020 8966 8383 — MB ChB Manch. 1983 (Univ. Manch.) MRCP (UK) 1988; Cert. Av. Med. 1991. VP Oncol., Muscularskeletal & Inflammatory Clin. Developm., GSK; Hon. Clin. Asst. Hammersmith Hosp. Lond. Specialty: Pharmaceutical Medicine. Socs: Brit. Assn. Pharmaceut. Phys.; Brit. Assn. Sport & Med.; Brit. Assn. Lung Res. Prev: Med. Strategy Head (Internat. Respirat. Med.) Glaxo Wellcome Research & Developm. Uxbridge; Sen. Med. Adviser Allen & Hanbury's Ltd.; Med. Off. (Aero Med. Evacuations) Mondial Asst. (UK) Ltd.

SYKES, Jeremy James William, OStJ Defence Postgraduate Medical Deanery, ICT Centre, Birmingham Research Park, Edgbaston, Birmingham B15 2SQ Tel: 0121 415 8152; 24 Bury Road, Gosport PO12 3UD — MB ChB Dundee 1973; MSc Lond. 1980; FFOM RCP Lond. 1992, M 1985; FRCP RCP Lond. 1996. Defence Postgrad. Med. Dean. Specialty: Occupat. Health. Socs: Soc. Occupat. Med.; Eur. Undersea Biomed. Soc. Prev: Dir. of Health (Navy); Pres. Fac. Occupat. Med.; Head Undersea Med. Inst. of Naval Med.

SYKES, John Edmondson GSK House, Smithkline Beecham International, 980 Great West Road, Brentford TW8 9GS Tel: 020 8047 4825 Fax: 020 8047 6935 Email: john.e.sykes@gsk.com; 11 Long Reach Close, Whitstable CT5 4PA Tel: 01227 277506 Email: jes4771@aol.com — MB BS Lond. 1976 (St Thomas Medical Hospital) BSc Lond. 1973, MB BS 1976; FFA RCS Eng. 1983; FFPM 1994. Vice Pres. Internat. Clin. Developm. & Med. Affairs Middle E. N. Africa/Sub Saharan Africa GlaxoSmithKline Pharmaceut. Specialty: Anaesth.; Pharmaceutical Medicine. Socs: Fell. Fac. of Pharmaceutical Phys.; Fell. Roy. Fac. Anaesthetists. Prev: Dir. & Vice Pres. Smithkline Beecham Internat. London; Med. Dir. SmithKline Beecham Melbourne Australia; Regional Med. Dir. S. E. Asia Beecham Internat. Hong Kong.

SYKES, John Reginald 243 Wilmslow Road, Heald Green, Cheadle SK8 3BQ — MB ChB Sheff. 1981; MRCPsych 1985. Cons. Psychiat. for the Elderly Walton Hosp. Chesterfield.; Med. Director Community Health Care Serv. (N. Derbysh.) HNS Trust. Specialty: Geriat. Psychiat.; Gen. Psychiat. Prev: Lect. North. Gen. Psychiat. Unit Sheff.

SYKES, Kenneth Bryan Sandringham Practice, Sandringham Road Health Centre, Sandringham Road, Doncaster DN2 5JH Tel: 01302 321521 Fax: 01302 761792; 106 Stoops Lane, West Bessacarr, Doncaster DN4 7RY Tel: 01302 370759 — MB ChB Birm. 1974 (University of Birmingham) MRCGP 1980 DRCOG 1979; Dip. Therapeut UWCH 1997. Specialty: Gen. Pract.; Gastroenterol. Prev: Trainee GP Doncaster VTS; SHO (Gen. Med.) Good Hope Hosp. Sutton Coldfield & Coventry AHA; Ho. Phys. Gen. Hosp. Birm.

SYKES, Linda Worsbrough Health Centre, Oakdale, Worsbrough Dale, Barnsley S70 5EG Tel: 01226 204090 Fax: 01226 771966; 29 Mount Vernon Road, Barnsley S70 4DH Tel: 01226 207237 — MB ChB Ed. 1978; DA Eng. 1981; DRCOG 1983; MRCGP 1995. Tutor (Gen. Pract.) Barnsley. Socs: Fac. Anaesth. RCS.

SYKES, Professor Sir Malcolm Keith Treyarnon, Cricket Field Lane, Budleigh Salterton EX9 6PB Tel: 01395 445884 Email: mk.sykes@virgin.net — MB BChir Camb. 1949 (Univ. Coll. Hosp.) MA Camb. 1951; DA Eng. 1953; FFA RCS Eng. 1955; Hon. FANZA 1978; Hon. FCA (SA) 1989. Emerit. Nuffield Prof. Anaesth. Univ. Oxf. Specialty: Anaesth. Prev: Prof. Clin. Anaesth. Roy. Postgrad. Med. Sch. Lond.; Fell. (Anaesth.) Mass. Gen. Hosp. Boston, USA; Rickman Godlee Trav. Fell. Univ. Coll. Hosp. Med. Sch. 1954.

SYKES, Michael Hugh (retired) Hazelwood, 5 Hawksdown, Walmer, Deal CT14 7PH Tel: 01304 372866 — MB BS Lond. 1958 (Westm.) MRCS Eng. LRCP Lond. 1958. Prev: Ho. Surg. Westm. Hosp. Lond.

SYKES, Muriel Grace (retired) 85 Mainway, Alkrington, Middleton, Manchester M24 1LL — MB ChB Liverp. 1955.

SYKES, Nicholas Fenton 23 Thornville Street, Leeds LS6 1RP — MB ChB Leeds 1994.

SYKES, Nigel Philip St. Christopher's Hospice, Lawrie Park Road, London SE26 6DZ — BM BCh Oxf. 1980; MA Oxf. 1981; FRCGP 1995, M 1984; FRSA 2000; ILTM 2002. Cons. Palliat. Med. St. Christopher's Hospice Lond.; Hon. Cons. Palliat. Med. Guy's, St. Thos. & Lewisham Hosps.; Hon. Sen. Lect. Palliat. Med. King's Coll. Lond. Specialty: Palliat. Med. Socs: Assn. Palliat. Med.; Europ. Assn. Palliat. Care. Prev: Macmillan Lect. (Palliat. Med.) Univ. Leeds; Sen. Regist. St. Christopher's Hospice Lond.

SYKES, Oliver Mark Westgate Surgery, Westgate, Otley LS21 3HD — MB BS Newc. 1987; DCH RCPS Glas. 1992; MRCGP 1993; DRCOG 1993.

SYKES, Peter (retired) Brook Farmhouse, Brinkhill, Louth LN11 8QX Tel: 01507 253 — (Sheff.) MB ChB Sheff. 1953; LMSSA Lond. 1953; DPM Eng. 1958; FRCPsych 1976, M 1971. Prev: Mem. Ment. Health Review Tribunal Nottm.

SYKES, Mr Peter Antony Trafford General Hospital, Department of Surgery, Moorside Road, Davyhulme, Urmston, Manchester M41 5SL; 40 Carrwood Avenue, Bramhall, Stockport SK7 2PY Tel: 0161 440 9644 — MB ChB Manch. 1966; FRCS Ed. 1971; FRCS Eng. 1972; MD Manch. 1975. Cons. Surg.; Reviewer for Commiss. of Health Improvement. Specialty: Gen. Surg. Socs: Fell. Manch. Med. Soc.; Assn. Surg. Prev: Sen. Regist. (Surg.) Univ. Hosp. S. Manch.; Regist. (Surg.) Manch. Roy. Infirm.

SYKES, Peter Hugh Wowham, Lansdown Road, Bath BA1 5RB — MB ChB Bristol 1985.

SYKES, Peter Hugh The Surgery, The Corn Stores, 12 Nargate Street, Littlebourne, Canterbury CT3 1UH Tel: 01227 721515; 5 Park Cottages, Park Lane, Preston, Canterbury CT3 1DS — MB BS Lond. 1984; DRCOG 1988.

SYKES, Mr Philip John, OBE St Joseph's Hospital, Harding Avenue, Malpas, Newport NP20 6ZE Tel: 01633 820357 Email: l.bellamy.plas.surg@talk21.com; Applecote, Applethwaite, Keswick CA12 4PP Tel: 017687 75027 Email: sykes.keswick@virgin.net — BA Camb. 1961 (Middlx.) MB Bchir Camb. 1964 1964; MA Camb. 1964; FRCS Eng. 1970; T(S) 1991; FRCS Edin. AdHominem 2001. Cons. Expert Priv. Medico-legal Pratice Plast. & Hand Surg. St Joseph's Hosp. Newport. Specialty: Plastic Surg. Socs: Brit. Soc. Surg. Hand; Brit. Assn. Plastic Surg. Prev: cons.plastic surg.Morrison Hosp.Swansea; Sen. Regist. (Plastic Surg.) Stoke Mandeville Hosp.; Regist. (Surg.) Northampton Gen. Hosp.

SYKES, Phyllis May (retired) 50 Buckingham Place, Downend, Bristol BS16 5TN; 50 Buckingham Place, Downend, Bristol BS16 5TN — (Leeds) MB ChB Leeds 1938.

SYKES, Rachel Anne Plas Meddgy Surgery, 40 Parkhill Road, Bexley DA5 1HU Tel: 01322 522056 Fax: 01322 521345; 7 Walton Road, Sidcup DA14 4LJ — BM BS Nottm. 1977; MRCGP 1981; DRCOG 1981.

SYKES, Rachel Sarah The Surgery, Field Road, Stainforth, Doncaster DN7 5AF Tel: 01302 841202; The Firs, Hay Green, Fishlake, Doncaster DN7 5JY Tel: 01302 844905 — MB ChB Liverp. 1987; DRCOG 1991; MRCGP 1992. GP; Med. Off. Youth Clinic; Hon. Clin. Tutor Sheff. Univ.; GP Trainer. Specialty: Family Plann. & Reproduc. Health. Prev: Trainee GP Doncaster VTS.

SYKES, Richard Vernon (retired) Carrantuohill, Bare Lane, Ockbrook, Derby DE72 3RG Tel: 0332 280852 — MB ChB Manch. 1948.

SYKES, Robert Andrew Sunrise Cottage, Barrack Hill, Kingsthorne, Hereford HR2 8AY — MB BS Lond. 1995 (Roy. Lond. Hosp.) DRCOG 1997. GP Regist. - Much Birch Surg. Heref. Specialty: Gen. Pract.

SYKES, Robin Alastair Morecambe Health Centre, Hanover Street, Morecambe LA4 5LY Tel: 01524 418418 Fax: 01524 832584 — MB ChB Manch. 1985; DRCOG 1988; MRCGP 1991. Socs: Assoc. Mem. Brit. Acupunc. Soc. Prev: Trainee GP Bolton VTS; Ho. Off. (Surg.) Vict. Hosp. Blackpool; Ho. Off. (Med.) Bolton Gen. Hosp.

SYKES, Robin George, TD (retired) Low Bridges, Stocksfield NE43 7SF Tel: 01661 842319 — BM BCh Oxf. 1942; MA Oxf. 1942; DA Eng. 1949; FFA RCS Eng. 1953. Cons. Anaesth. N. Regional Thoracic Surg. Centre, Freeman Hosp. Newc. Prev: Hon. Surg. to H.M. The Qu.

SYKES, Roger Andrew David Ravenscraig Hospital, Inverness Road, Greenock PA16 9HA Tel: 01475 633777 — MB ChB Glas. 1978; MRCPsych 1984; FRCPsych 1999. Cons. Psychiat. Ravenscraig Hosp. Greenock. Specialty: Gen. Psychiat.

SYKES, Rupert 52 Broadway, Bramhall, Stockport SK7 3BU Tel: 0161 439 1823 — MB BS Lond. 1932 (Manch.) MRCS Eng., LRCP Lond. 1932; FRCP Lond. 1969, M 1934; BSc Lond. 1926, MD 1935. Fell. Manch. Med. Soc. Prev: Cons. Phys. Stepping Hill Hosp. Stockport; Cons. Phys. Manch. North. Hosp.; Res. Med. Off. Manch. Roy. Infirm.

SYKES, Seth Alexander Greer The Surgery, Wainfleet Road, Burgh Le Marsh, Skegness PE24 5ED Tel: 01754 810205; 66 Station Road, Burgh Le Marsh, Skegness PE24 5EL Tel: 01754 810275 — MB ChB Edin. 1965.

SYKES, Sheila Grace (retired) Carrantuohill, Bare Lane, Ockbrook, Derby DE72 3RG Tel: 01332 280852 — MB ChB Manch. 1955; DObst RCOG 1958; DPH Ed. 1959; DCH Eng. 1960. Prev: Retd. GP.

SYKES, Steven John Danks, Smith, Sykes and Farrell, 134 Beeston Road, Beeston Hill, Leeds LS11 8BS Tel: 0113 276 0717 Fax: 0113 270 3727 — MB ChB Leeds 1980; DRCOG 1983; MRCGP 1984. Prev: SHO & Ho. Off. Airedale Gen. Hosp. Steeton.

SYKES, Mr Timothy Charles Freeman Pembroke House, Old Mill Lane, Oldbury, Bridgnorth WV16 5EE Tel: 01746 764 3060 Email: sykes@mac.com — MB BCh Wales 1991 (Univ. Wales Coll. Med.) BSc (Physiol.) Wales 1988; FRCS Eng. 1995; FRCS (Gen.) 2003. Regist. (Gen. Surg.) Royal Shrewsbury Hospital. Specialty: Gen. Surg. Prev: Regist. (Gen. Surg.) Heartlands Hosp. Birm.; SHO Rotat. (Surg.) S. Birm.; SHO (Urol.) Roy. Marsden Hosp.

SYLVESTER, Anna Rachel 45 Reddings Road, Birmingham B13 8LW — MB ChB Leeds 1994.

SYLVESTER, Mr Bernard Simon 15 Bruntwood Lane, Cheadle SK8 1HS Tel: 0161 832 7780 — MB BS Lond. 1969 (Lond. Hosp.) FRCS Eng. 1974. Cons. Orthop. Surg. N. Manch. Health Dist. Specialty: Orthop. Socs: Orthop. Research Soc.; Brit. Orthop. Assn. Prev: Regist. (Orthop.) Hammersmith Hosp. Lond.; Regist. (Orthop.) St. Mary's Hosp. Lond.; Lect. Orthop. Surg. Hope Hosp. Salford.

SYLVESTER, Gillian Mary Doctors Surgery, 2 Danson Crescent, Welling DA16 2AT Tel: 020 8303 4204 Fax: 020 8298 1192; 12 Mottingham Gardens, London SE9 4RL Tel: 020 8857 4019 — MB BS Lond. 1961 (Roy. Free) MRCS Eng. LRCP Lond. 1961; DObst RCOG 1966.

SYLVESTER, Nigel Charles Friarsgate Practice, Friarsgate Medical Centre, Friarsgate, Winchester SO23 8EF Tel: 01962 853599 Fax: 01962 849982; Windy Ridge, Cliff Way, Compton Down, Winchester SO21 2AP — MB BS Newc. 1977; MRCGP; DRCOG 1979.

SYLVESTER, Mr Paul Andrew 12 Cothale Vale, Cotham, Bristol BS6 6HR — MB ChB Bristol 1990; FRCS Lond. 1994. Specialty: Gen. Surg.

SYLVESTER, Peter Kirwan (retired) The Cedars, Makeney Road, Duffield, Belper DE56 4BD Tel: 01332 840448 — MB BS Lond. 1950 (Westm.) FFPH, 2003; MRCS Eng. LRCP Lond. 1948; DCH Eng. 1951; DObst RCOG 1952; DPH Lond. 1957; FFCM RCP (UK) 1978, M 1974; FFPHM RCP (UK) 1989. Emerit. Cons. Southern Derbysh. HA. Prev: Dist. Med. Off. South. Derbysh. HA.

SYLVESTER, Stephen Houghton Henry The Surgery, Tennant Street, Stockton-on-Tees TS18 2AT Tel: 01642 613331 Fax: 01642 675612; Greenways, 9 Teesbank Avenue, Eaglescliffe, Stockton-on-Tees TS16 9AY — MB ChB Cape Town 1981; MRCP (UK) 1985; DRCOG 1986; Dip. Med. Educat. Dund 1994; FRCGP 1998. GP Princip. Stockton on Tees; GP Tutor.

SYLVESTER, Susan Elizabeth Westbourne Medical Centre, Milburn Road, Bournemouth BH4 9HJ Tel: 01202 752550 Fax: 01202 769700 — MB BCh Wales 1974.

SYM, Ruth Audrey 8 Beaumont Avenue, Southwell NG25 0BB — MB ChB Glas. 1990.

SYMCOX, Helen Ann Shay Lane Medical Centre, Shay Lane, Hale, Altrincham WA15 8NZ Tel: 0161 980 3835 Fax: 0161 903 9848 — MB ChB Liverp. 1988; BSc Liverp. 1988; DRCOG 1991; MRCGP 1992.

SYME, Adam Iain Cameron Riverside Medical Practice, Ballifeary Lane, Ness Walk, Inverness IV3 5PW Tel: 01463 715999 Fax: 01463 718763 — MB ChB Ed. 1982; FRCGP; MRCP (UK) 1985; DRCOG 1987; MRCGP 1988. GP Princip.

SYME, Mr Brian Allan Crosshouse Hospital, Kilmarnock KA2 0BE; 9 Dunskey Road, Kilmarnock KA3 6FJ — MB ChB Glas. 1991; FRCS Ed. 1996; FRCSEd (Tr & Orth) 2002. Cons. Orthopaedic Surg. Crosshouse Hosp. Kilmarnock. Specialty: Orthop. Prev: Specialist Regist. Orthop. Vict. Infirm.

SYME, David McBride Killin Medical Practice, Laggan Leigheas, Ballechroisk, Killin FK21 8TQ Tel: 01567 820213 Fax: 01567 820805 — DCH RCPS Glas. 1981; MRCGP 1982. GP Killin.

SYME, Mr Ian George 19 Beech Crescent, Newton Mearns, Glasgow G77 5BN — MB ChB Glas. 1975; FRCS Ed. 1979. Cons. Ophth. Surg. StoneHo. Gen. Hosp. Lanarksh. Specialty: Ophth.

SYME, Paul David Borders General Hospital, Melrose, Roxburghshire, Melrose TD6 9BS; Ashtrees, Gattonside, Melrose TD6 9LZ — MB ChB Ed. 1981; BSc Hons 1979, MBCNB 1981; FRCP Ed 1997. Cons. Phys.; Sen. Lect., Edin. Univ. Specialty: Gen. Med.

SYME, Mr William Smith (retired) North Carthat, Collin, Dumfries DG1 3SA — (Glas.) MB ChB Glas. 1957; LMCC 1960; FRCS Glas. 1964; FRCS Ed. 1965. Prev: Cons. Orthop. Surg. Dumfries & Galloway Roy. Infirm.

SYMERS, Dorothy Annie (retired) La Meule, Rue Du Moulin, St Martin, Jersey JE3 6AH Tel: 01534 851582 — (Roy. Free) MB BS Lond. 1945. Prev: Med. Off. J. Lyons & Co. Ltd.

SYMES, Clare (retired) Tudor Cottage, The Street, Brent Eleigh, Sudbury CO10 9NU Tel: 01787 247354 — MB ChB Manch. 1974; MRCGP 1978. Prev: GP Sudbury.

SYMES, David Millman Camster House, 7 Beechdene, Tadworth KT20 5EA Tel: 01737 814714 Fax: 01737 819807 — MB BS Lond. 1955 (St. Mary's) MRCS Eng. LRCP Lond. 1955; Dip. Dermat. Wales 1992. Hon. Clin. Tutor (Dermat.) St. Geo. Hosp. Med. Sch.; Med. Adviser Disablem. Tribunal & Examg. Med. Pract. DSS; Cons. Dermatol. Kingston Hosp. Specialty: Dermat. Socs: Fell. Roy. Soc. Med.; Soc. Occupat. Med.; BMA. Prev: Hon. Hosp. Pract. (Dermat.)

St. Geo. Hosp. Lond.; Sen. Med. Cons. Whittaker Life Scs. Ltd.; Med. Cons. John Brown Engin. & Construc. Ltd.

SYMES, Janet Elizabeth Woodside Barn, Back Lane, Heath Charnock, Chorley PR6 9DJ — MB ChB Manch. 1983; DRCOG 1986; Cert. Family Plann. JCC 1987.

SYMES, John Bernard Lloyd Horsman's Place Surgery, Instone Road, Dartford DA1 2JP Tel: 01322 228363 — MD Malta 1973; MRCOG 1979; M.A. (Med. Ethics and Law) Lond. 1997. Prev: Regist. (O & G) Westm. & St. Stephens Hosps. Lond.; Regist. (O & G) Edgware Gen. Hosp.; SHO (Obst.) Univ. Coll. Hosp. Lond.

SYMES, Mr John Mayland Crossways, Church Road, Binstead, Ryde PO33 3TA — MB BS Lond. 1964 (Char. Cross) MRCS Eng. LRCP Lond. 1964; FRCS Eng. 1970; MS Lond. 1978. Cons. Surg. St Mary's Hosp. Newport I. of Wight. Specialty: Gen. Surg. Prev: Ho. Surg. St. Jas. Hosp. Balham; Lect. in Surg. Lond. Hosp. Med. Coll.; Sen. Regist. Vasc. Surg. Lond. Hosp.

SYMES, Michael Harvey (retired) 21 Priors Court, Back of Avon, Tewkesbury GL20 5US Tel: 01684 290081 Email: mharvey.symes@virgin.net — MB BS Lond. 1949 (St. Mary's) LMSSA Lond. 1948; DPM Eng. 1963; MRCPsych 1971.

SYMES, Michael Herbert Archibald Cromer Group Practice, 48 Overstrand Road, Cromer NR27 0AJ Tel: 01263 513148 — MB BS Lond. 1968 (Westm.) MRCS Eng. LRCP Lond. 1968; DA Eng. 1971; DObst RCOG 1976.

SYMES, Michael Oliver 242 Shirehampton Road, Bristol BS9 2EH — MD Bristol 1963; MB ChB 1959. Cons. Sen. Lect. (Surg.) Univ. Bristol; Hon. Cons. Immunol. Avon AHA (T).

SYMES, Steven Roy Woodside Barn, Back Lane, Heath Charnock, Chorley PR6 9DJ — MB ChB Manch. 1983; Cert. Family Plann. JCC 1987.

SYMINGTON, Alan John Forsyth ThE Elizabeth Courtauld Surgery, Factory Lane West, Halstead CO9 1EX Tel: 01787 475944 Fax: 01787 474506 — (Cambridge) MB Camb. 1977, BChir 1976; DRCOG 1978; MRCGP 1981; DCH RCP Lond. 1981; FRCGP 1998. GP Princip.; GP Tutor Braintree PCG.

SYMINGTON, Lady (Esther Margaret) (retired) Green Briar, 2 Lady Margaret Drive, Troon KA10 7AL Tel: 01292 3157 — MB ChB Glas. 1942. Clin. Asst. (Geriat.) Ayrsh. Centr. Hosp. Irvine. Prev: Clin. Asst. (Geriat.) Cuddington Hosp. Sutton.

SYMINGTON, Ian Stevenson Glasgow Occupational Health, Glasgow Royal Infirmary, 4th Floor Cuthbertson Building, 91 Wishart Street, Glasgow G31 2HT Tel: 0141 211 0427 Fax: 0141 211 0423 Email: Ian.Symington@northglasgow.scot.nhs.uk — (Glas.) MB ChB Glas. 1969; DObst RCOG 1971; FRCP Glas. 1983, M 1973; DIH Soc. Apoth. Lond. 1977; FFOM RCP Lond. 1985, MFOM 1983; FRCP Lond. 1994. Dir. Glasgow Occupational Health & Cons. Occupat. Physician, NHS Greater Glasg.; Hon. Sen. Clin. Lect. Univ. Glas.; Hon. Cons. Univ. Strathclyde. Socs: (Ex-Pres.) Soc. Occupat. Med. Prev: Sen. Employm. Med. Adviser EMAS Lond.; Employm. Med. Adviser EMAS Dundee; Regist. (Respirat. Med.) West. Infirm. Glas.

SYMINGTON, James Joseph Mark Coleraine Hospital, 28A Mountsandal Road, Coleraine BT52 1JA Tel: 01265 44177; 21 Old Coleraine Road, Portstewart, Londonderry BT55 7PZ Tel: 01265 835298 Email: msymington@aol.com — MB BCh BAO Belf. 1985; FFA RCSI 1990. Cons. (Anaesth.) Coleraine Hosp. Specialty: Anaesth. Prev: Sen. Regist. (Anaesth.) Craigavon Area Hosp.

SYMINGTON, Stuart Kevin 248 Coalisland Road, Dungannon BT71 6EP — MB BCh BAO Belf. 1991.

SYMINGTON, Sir Thomas (retired) Green Briar, 2 Lady Margaret Drive, Troon KA10 7AL Tel: 01292 315707 — MB ChB 1941 (Glas.) FRS Ed.; BSc (Hons.) Glas. 1936; MD (Hons.) 1950; FRFPS Glas. 1958; FRCP Glas. 1962; FRCPath 1964. Vis. Prof. Path., Stamford Univ. 1965. Prev: Dir. Inst. Cancer Research Roy. Cancer Hosp. Chester Beatty.

SYMMERS, Eleanor 81 St Albans Road, Edinburgh EH9 2PQ Tel: 0131 667 1716 — MB ChB Glas. 1965. Indep. Counselling Psychother. Edin.; Med. Mem. Appeals. Serv; Hosp. Pract. Med. Rehab. Specialty: Psychother.; Disabil. Med.; Rehabil. Med. Prev: Research Fell. Breast Unit Dept. Clin. Surg. Roy. Infirm. Edin.; Regist. (Psychiat.) Roy. Edin. Hosp.; Regist. Psychiat. Univ. Coll. Hosp. Lond.

SYMMERS, William St Clair Howdenhall Surgery, 57 Howden Hall Road, Edinburgh EH16 6PL Tel: 0131 664 3766 Fax: 0131 672 2114; 81 St Alban's Road, Edinburgh EH9 2PQ Tel: 0131 667 1716 — MB BS (Hons. Obst. & Gyn.) Lond. 1967 (Univ. Coll. Hosp.) BSc (Hons.) Physiol. Lond. 1964; MRCS Eng. LRCP Lond. 1967; MSc (Med. Sci.) Glas. 1983; MRCGP 1984. GP Adviser Roy. Infirm. Edin. NHS Trust. Specialty: Gen. Pract. Prev: Head of WHO MONICA Proj. Univ. Edin. & Hon. Research Fell. (Cardiovasc. Epidemiol. Unit) Univ. Dundee.

SYMMONS, Professor Deborah Pauline Mary ARC Epidemiology Research Unit, University of Manchester Medical School, Oxford Road, Manchester M13 9PT Tel: 0161 275 5044 Fax: 0161 275 5043 — MB ChB 1977; MD Birm. 1987, MB ChB 1977; MRCP (UK) 1980; MD Birm. 1987; FRCP Lond. 1994; MFPHM 1999. Dep. Dir. ARC Epidemiol. Unit Univ. Manch. Med. Sch.; Cons. Rheum. Macclesfield Dist. Gen. Hosp.; Prof. of Rheum. and Musculoskeletal Epidermiology, Univ. of Manch. Specialty: Rheumatol. Prev: Lect. (Rheum.) Univ. Birm.; Regist. (Rheum. & Med.) Guy's Hosp. Lond.

SYMON, David Nicholas Kidd University Hospital of Hartlepool, Holdforth Road, Hartlepool TS24 9AH Tel: 01429 522802 Fax: 01429 522738 Email: david.symon@nth.nhs.uk — MB ChB Glas. 1973; BSc Glas. 1971; FRCP Glas. 1989; FRCP Ed. 1991; FRCP Lond. 1995; FRCPCH 1997. Cons. Paediat. Univ. Hosp. of Hartlepool; Director of R & D, N. Tess & Hartlepool NHS Trust. Specialty: Paediat. Special Interest: Headache, migraine, migraine equivalent syndromes in Childr. and adolescents. Socs: Internat. Headache Soc. (Mem. of Paediatric Sub Comm.); Anglo-Dutch Migraine Assn.; Brit. Assn. for the Study of Headache. Prev: Lect. (Child Health) Univ. Aberd.; Regist. (Med. Paediat.) Roy. Hosp. Sick Childr. Glas.; Regist. Rotat. (Med.) West. Infirm. Glas.

SYMON, Professor Lindsay, TD, CBE (retired) Maple Lodge, Rivar Road, Shalbourne, Marlborough SN8 3QE Tel: 01672 870501 Fax: 01672 870501 — (Aberd.) MB ChB (1st cl. Hons.) Aberd. 1951; FRCS Ed. 1957; FRCS Eng. 1959; Hon. FACS 1994. Prev: Prof. Neurol. Surg. Univ. Lond. Inst. Neurol. Lond. 1978-95.

SYMON, Margaret Allison South Cleveland Hospital, Marton Road, Middlesbrough TS4 3BW Tel: 01642 850850; Tigh an Achadh, Stockton Road, Castle Eden, Hartlepool TS27 4SD Tel: 01429 836612 — MB ChB Aberd. 1982; MRCP (UK) 1985; DA (UK) 1988; FRCA 1989; FRCP Glas. 1995. Cons. Anaesth. S. Tees Acute Hosps. NHS Trust. Specialty: Anaesth. Prev: Sen. Regist. (Anaesth.) Newc. Teach. Hosps.; Regist. (Gen. Med.) Aberd. Teach. Hosps.; Clin. Tutor Univ. Aberd.

SYMON, Michaela Anne Invergowire House, Dundee DD2 1UA — MB ChB Dundee 1994.

SYMON, Rosemary Buckland House, Oxford St., Eddington, Hungerford RG17 0ET Tel: 01488 682658; High Street, Ramsbury, Marlborough SN8 2QT Tel: 01672 20366 — MB BS Lond. 1980 (St. Thos. Hosp. Med. Sch. Lond.) DRCOG 1982; Cert. Family Plann. JCC 1982; MRCGP 1985. GP Principal. Prev: Trainee GP Reading VTS; Clin. Asst. (Ophth.) Princess Margt. Hosp. Swindon; SHO (Anaesth.) St. Thos. Hosp. Lond.

SYMON, Thomas, Lt.-Col. RAMC Medical Centre, Army Foundation College, Harrogate H63 0SE Email: tomsymon@madasafish.com; Medical Centre, Infantry Training Centre, Catterick Garrison DL9 3PS Email: tomsymon@madasafish.com; Parkwood, Lartington, Barnard Castle DL12 9BP Email: tomsymon@madasafish.com — MB ChB Glas. 1966; DFFP 1995. Civil. Med. Practitioner, ITC Catterick. Specialty: Sports Med.; Gen. Pract. Socs: Assoc. RCGP; BMA. Prev: Chief Med. Off. UN Peacekeeping Force Cyprus; Chief Med. Off. Rotyal Brunei Armed Forces SMO ITC Catterick; Sen. Med. Off.,Army Foundat. Coll., Harrogate.

SYMONDS, Professor Edwin Malcolm Scchool of Human Development & Midwifery, Floor D, East Block, University Hospital, Queen's Medical Centre, Nottingham NG7 2UH Tel: 0115 970 9240 Fax: 0115 970 9234; Nursery Cottage, The Green, Car Colston, Nottingham NG13 8JE — MB BS Adelaide 1957; FACOG; FRANZOG; FRCOG 1971, M 1962; MD Adelaide 1970; FFPHM (Distinc.) RCP (UK) 1996. Foundat. Prof. O & G Univ. Nottm.; Edr-in-Chief Curr. Obst. & Gyn. Specialty: Obst. & Gyn. Socs: Fell. Amer. Gyn. & Obst. Soc.; Fell. Hungarian Gyn. Soc.; (Counc.) Med. Defence Union. Prev: Commiss.er of Commonw. Schol.sh. Commiss.; Sen. Regist. (O & G) Univ. Liverp.; Sen. Lect. & Reader (O & G) Univ. Adelaide.

SYMONDS, Ian Martin Derby City General Hospital, Uttoxeter Road, Derby DE22 3NE Tel: 01332 625633 Fax: 01332 625634 Email: ian.symonds@nottingham.ac.uk; 46 Appledore Avenue, Wollaton, Nottingham NG8 2RW Tel: 0115 916 5732 — BM BS Nottm. 1983; BMedSci. Nottm. 1981; MRCOG 1995; DM Nottm. 1995. Sen. Lect. (O & G) Univ. Nottm. Specialty: Obst. & Gyn. Socs: Eur. Assn. for Cancer Research; Brit. Gyn. Cancer Soc. Prev: Lect. (O & G) Univ. Nottm.; Regist. (Gyn.) Birm. Wom. Hosp.; Regist. (O & G) Birm. Matern. Hosp.

SYMONDS, Miss Katherine Elizabeth Hereford County Hospital, Union Walk, Hereford HR1 2ER Tel: 01432 372900 — MB ChB Liverp. 1975; FRCS Ed. 1981; FFAEM 1996. Cons. (A & E) Hereford County Hosp. Specialty: Accid. & Emerg. Special Interest: Paediatric A & E. Prev: Clin. Asst. (A & E) Hereford Gen. Hosp.; Regist. N. Manch. Gen. Hosp. & Roy. Manch. Childr. Hosp.; Cons. A & E Surg. (Paediat. Trauma) Birm. Childr. Hosp.

SYMONDS, Raymond Paul, TD University of Leicester, Department of Oncology, Leicester Royal Infirmary, Leicester LE1 5WW Tel: 0116 258 6294 Fax: 0116 258 7599 Email: paul.symonds@uhl-tr.nhs.uk; 11 Alvington Way, Market Harborough LE16 7NF Tel: 01858 461018 — MB BS Newc. 1972; MRCP (UK) 1975; MD Newc. 1981; FRCR 1982; FRCP Glas. 1989. Reader in Oncol., Leicester Univ.; Vis. Prof. Hahnemann Med. Coll. Philadelphia, USA 1981; Hon. Cons. Leicester Roy. Infirm. Specialty: Oncol. Prev: Cons. Radiother. & Oncol., Beatson Oncol. Centre, Western Infirm. Glas.; MRC Fell. (RadioBiol.), Regist. & Hosp. Office (Radiol.) Roy. Vict. Infirm. Newc.

SYMONDS, Richard Leonard Medway Hospital, Windmill Road, Gillingham ME7 5NY Tel: 01634 830000 Fax: 01634 830082; 141 Butchers Lane, Mereworth, Maidstone ME18 5QD Tel: 01622 812425 Email: r.symonds@virgin.net — MB ChB Birm. 1967; DPM Eng. 1971; FRCPsych 1989, M 1972. Cons. Psychiat. Thames Gateway NHS Trust, Medway Maritime Hosp.; Recognised Teach. United Med. & Dent. Sch. 1988; Cons. Psychiat. Medway Hosp.; Hon. Sen. Lect. Univ. of Kent at Canterbury. Specialty: Gen. Psychiat. Socs: BMA (Exec. Comm. Local Div.); NHSCA. Prev: Cons. Psychiat. Tunbridge Wells HA & Sen. Lect. Kings Coll. Hosp.; Lect. (Psychol. Med.) Welsh Nat. Sch. Med. Cardiff; Sen. Regist. (Psychiat.) WhitCh. Hosp. Cardiff.

SYMONDSON, Alicia Millicent (retired) Landscape, Kinnerley, Oswestry SY10 8DU Tel: 01691 682577 — MB BChir Camb. 1939 (Camb. & Univ. Coll. Hosp.) MA. GP & House Physician, Luton & Dunstable Hospital. Prev: Ho. Phys. Burslem, Haywood & Tunstall Memor. Hosp.

SYMONS, Audrey Jean Cunningham (retired) 6A Thornly Park Avenue, Paisley PA2 7SB Tel: 0141 884 2034 — MB ChB Glas. 1950; DA Eng. 1959; FFA RCS Eng. 1964. Prev: Cons. Anaesth. Roy. Alexandra Infirm. Paisley.

SYMONS, Gareth Vize Yule House, Kew Gdns. Road, Kew, Richmond Tel: 020 8940 4223 — MB BS Lond. 1964 (St. Mary's) FFA RCSI 1973; FFA RCS Eng. 1973. Cons. Anaesth. St. Mary's Hosp. Teach. Gp. Specialty: Anaesth. Prev: Capt. RAMC.

SYMONS, Hugh Francis Brady (retired) 6 Rockhampton Close, London SE27 0NG Tel: 020 8769 5862 — MRCS Eng. LRCP Lond. 1942 (St. Mary's) MRCS. Eng. LRCP Lond. 1942; DphysMed. Eng. 1950. Prev: Cons. Phys. Rheum. & Rehabil. St. Geo. Hosp. Lond.

SYMONS, Iris Elizabeth Department of Anaesthetics, Barnet General Hospital, Wellhouse Lane, Barnet EN5 3DJ — MB ChB Bristol 1972; BSc (Hons.) Bristol 1968; DObst RCOG 1974; FFA RCS Eng. 1977. Cons. Anaesth. Barnet and Chase Farm Hosp.s Trust Barnet, Herts. Specialty: Anaesth. Socs: BMA & Assn. Anaesth.; Assn. of Paediat. Anaesth. Prev: Underlaker Thoraxanestesi Karolinska Hosp. Stockholm.; Sen. Regist. (Anaesth.) Addenbrooke's Hosp. Camb.; Regist. (Anaesth.) Hosp. Sick Childr. Gt. Ormond St.

SYMONS, John Charles Colchester General Hospital, Turner Road, Colchester CO4 5JL Tel: 01206 853535; Moors Farm, Assington, Colchester CO10 5NE Tel: 01787 227379 — MB BChir Camb. 1962 (St. Thos.) MA Camb. 1962; DObst RCOG 1964; DCH Eng. 1965; FRCP Lond. 1971. Cons. Paediat. Essex Co. Hosp. Colchester; Paediat. Dir. NEE HA. Specialty: Paediat. Socs: Brit. Paediat. Assn.; BMA. Prev: Hon. Clin. Asst. Brompton Hosp. Lond.; Ho. Surg. St. Thos. Hosp.; Sen. Regist. (Paediat.) Jenny Lind Hosp. Norwich & Brompton Hosp. Lond.

SYMONS, Kenneth William, VRD Symons Medical Centre, 25 All Saints Avenue, Maidenhead SL6 8EL Tel: 01628 26131; Oaktree House, Cannon Hill, Bray, Maidenhead SL6 2EW Tel: 01628 624575 Fax: 01628 410051 — (Camb. & St. Geo.) MA Camb. 1944; MRCS Eng. LRCP Lond. 1944; MB BChir Camb. 1944. Med. Ref. & Other Insur. Cos. Specialty: Dermat. Socs: Hon. Mem. (Ex-Pres.) Windsor Med. Soc. Prev: Ho. Phys. St. Geo. Hosp.; Surg. Lt.-Cdr. RNR; Assoc. Specialist (Dermat.) K. Edwd. VII Hosp. (Windsor) & Heatherwood Hosp. Ascot.

SYMONS, Lorraine Claire Warwick House Medical Centre, Holway Green, Upper Holway Road, Taunton TA1 2QA — BM BS Nottm. 1989; BMedSc Nottm. 1987; DGM RCP Lond. 1991; DRCOG 1992; MRCGP 1994. Specialty: Gen. Pract.

SYMONS, Michael (retired) 26 Town Walls, Shrewsbury SY1 1TN Tel: 01743 362173 — MB BChir Camb. 1944 (Camb. & Bristol) MA Camb. 1946, MB BChir 1944; MRCS Eng., LRCP Lond. 1944; FRCP Lond. 1975, M 1946; FRCPath 1964. Prev: Cons. Path. Salop. AHA.

SYMONS, Nicola Jane Howsman Little Broom Ing, Calverley Lane, Calverley, Leeds LS28 5QQ — (Leeds) MBChB 1975; DCH 1985; DCCH 1986; FRCPCH 1997. Cons. Community Paediat. Bradford Hosp. Trust. Specialty: Paediat. Socs: BMA; RCPCH.

SYMONS, Rory Charles Francis The Symons Medical Centre, 25 All Saints Avenue, Maidenhead SL6 6EL Tel: 01628 626131 Fax: 01628 410051 — MB BS Lond. 1982 (St. Mary's) DCH RCS Lond. 1986; MRCGP 1986. Clin. Asst. (Rheum.) Wycombe & Amersham Hosps. Specialty: Occupat. Health. Prev: Trainee GP Kentish Town Health Centre Lond.; SHO (A & E, Paediat. & Psychiat.) Univ. Coll. Hosp. Lond.

SYMONS, Sean Benjamin Vize 192 Portnall Road, London W9 3BJ — MB BS Lond. 1995.

SYMONS, Stephanie Jennifer 17 Hall Road, Rusholme, Manchester M14 5HN — MB ChB Manch. 1995.

SYN, Thant Norton Brook Medical Centre, Kingsbridge TQ7 1AE Tel: 01548 853551 Fax: 01548 857741; 6 Pineview Close, Mansfield NG18 4PQ Tel: 01623 421054 — MB BS Med. Inst. (II) Rangoon 1984; MPH Univ. Mahodol, Bangkok 1990; MRCP Ire Paediatrics 1999. Plymouth GP Vocational Train. Scheme; Cert. Educat. Commiss. for Foreign Med. Grads. (USA); Staff Community Paediat. (Child Health Servs.). Specialty: Paediat. Socs: BMA; Assoc. Mem. RCPCH; Brit. Assn. Community Child Health.

SYN, Wing-Kin — MB ChB Sheff. 1998.

SYNDIKUS, Isabella Maria Clatterbridge Centre for Oncology, Bebington, Wirral CH63 4JY Tel: 0151 334 1155 Fax: 0151 482 7675 — MD Munich 1986; State Exam Med. Munich 1986; MRCP (UK) 1989; FRCP Lond. 1992. Cons. Clin. Oncol. Clatterbridge Hosp. Liverp. Specialty: Oncol.; Radiother. Prev: Sen. Regist. (Clin. Oncol.) Middlx. Hosp. Lond.; Regist. (Radiother.) Roy. Marsden Hosp. Sutton; SHO (Gen. Med.) Addenbrooke's Hosp. Camb.

SYNEK, Miroslav H-Villa, Coldeast Hospital, Southampton SO31 7YJ Tel: 01489 570799 Fax: 01489 578490; 39 Corvette Avenue, Warsash, Southampton SO31 9AN — MUDr Charles Univ. Prague 1982 (Fac. Med.) MUDr Charles U, Prague 1982; MD Soton. 1995; DCH Lond. 2000. Staff Grade (Community Paediat.) Portsmouth Health Care Trust. Specialty: Community Child Health. Prev: Research Fell. Univ. Med. Univ. Soton.

SYNGE, Jessie 24 Merrivale, Oakwood, London N14 4SL — MB Calcutta 1951.

SYNNOTT, Mary Bernadette North & South Stoke Primary Care Trusts, Directorate of Public Health, Heron House, Grove Road, Stoke-on-Trent ST4 4LX Tel: 01782 298123 Fax: 01782 298135 — MB BCh BAO NUI 1974 (Univ. Coll. Dub.) FRCPI 1996, M 1978; MD NUI 1985. SCMO (Pub. Health Med.) N. & S. Stoke PCTs. Specialty: Pub. Health Med. Socs: BMA. Prev: SCMO (Pub. Health Med.) N. Staff. HA; Clin. Lect. (Med. Microbiol.) Univ. Birm.; Intern & SHO (Med.) St. Vincent's Hosp. Dub.

SYNNOTT, Mary Eithna 11 Greenpark Road, Rostrevor, Newry BT34 3EY Tel: 0284 1733 8333 Fax: 0284 1773 9454 — MB BCh BAO NUI 1979. Locum A&E Off. Specialty: Gen. Surg. Prev: Chief Med. Off. Oke-Offa Hosp., Ibadan; Chief Med. Off. St. Brendan's Hosp., Nigeria.

SYRED, John Ralph Brantgarth, Guldrey Lane, Sedbergh LA10 5DS Tel: 01539 620239 Fax: 01593 620158 — MB BS Lond. 1969 (St.

Bart.) DA Eng. 1972; DObst RCOG 1972; MRCS Eng. LRCP Lond. 1972; MRCGP 1978.

SYSON, Anneregine Department of Genitourinary Medicine, Dept. GUM, Cardiff Royal Infirmary, Cardiff — MB ChB Leeds 1968; Dip GUM Soc. Apoth. 1989. Assoc. Specialist (Genitourin. Med.) Cardiff Roy. Infirm. Specialty: Genitourinary Medicine.

SYYED, Raheel 319 Albert Drive, Pollockshields, Glasgow G41 5EA Tel: 0141 423 4977 — MB ChB Glas. 1993; MB ChB Glasgow 1993; MRCP Glasgow 1998. Pulmonry Vasc. Fell. Specialty: Gen. Med. Socs: MRCP (Glas.). Prev: SpR (Med.) Oldchurch Hosp.; SpR (Med.) St. Peter's Hosp.; SHO (Med.) StoneHo. Hosp.

SZABADI, Professor Elemer Division of Psychiatry, B Floor, Medical School University Hospital, Queen's Medical Centre, Nottingham NG7 2UH Tel: 0115 970 9336 Fax: 0115 919 4473 Email: elemer.szabadi@nottingham.ac.uk — MD Budapest 1964; Dip. Neurol. Budapest 1968; FRCPsych 1981, M 1974; PhD Ed. 1978; DSc Manch. 1983. Prof. Psychiat. Univ. Nottm. & Hon. Cons. Psychiat. Qu. Med. Centre Nottm. Specialty: Gen. Psychiat. Socs: (Ex-Comm. & Edit. Bd.) Brit. Pharm. Soc.; Brit. Assn. Psychopharmacol. Prev: Reader (Psychiat.) Univ. Manch.; Sen. Lect. (Psychiat.) Univ. Manch. & Lect. (Neurol.) Univ. Budapest; Lect. (Psychiat.) Univ. Edin.

SZABOLCSI, Anna Eva 21 Hermitage Lane, London NW2 2EY — MD Budapest 1972 (Semmelweiss) MRCS Eng. LRCP Lond. 1982. Licenciate in Acupunc. Socs: Brit. Med. Acupunct. Soc.; Primary Care Rheum. Soc.; BMA. Prev: Trainee GP Hampstead; Regist. (Rheumat.) Roy. Free Hosp. Lond.; Regist. Wexham Pk. Hosp.

SZAFRANSKI, Jan Stanislaw 3 Crescent Road, Rowley Park, Stafford ST17 9AW — BM BS Nottm. 1985.

SZAMOCKI, Mrs Janina Zofia Maria (retired) Brookfields, Green Barns Lane, Little Hay, Lichfield WS14 0QN Tel: 01543 480970 — MB ChB Aberd. 1950. Prev: Indep. Homoeop. Pract. Staffs.

SZANTO, Stephen Francis (retired) 39 Kensington Drive, Woodford Green IG8 8LP — LAH Dub. 1962; FRCPI 1982, M 1964; PhD Lond. 1969. Prev: Cons. Phys. in Geriat. Forest & Thames Gps. Hosps. Lond.

SZAREWSKI, Anne Marie Imperial Cancer Research Fund, PO Box 123, Lincoln Inn Fields, London WC2A 3PX Tel: 020 7269 3160 Fax: 020 7269 3429; 5 Priory Terrace, London NW6 4DG Tel: 020 7624 7170 Fax: 020 7372 7510 — MB BS Lond. 1982 (Middlx. Hosp. Med. Sch. Lond.) PhD 1997 Lond.; DRCOG 1984; Cert. Family Plann. JCC 1984; MFFP 1993. Sen. Clin. Research Fell. Imperial Cancer Research Fund Lond.; Instruc. Doctor (Family Plann.) Margt. Pyke Centre Lond. Specialty: Obst. & Gyn. Prev: Clin. Asst. Lydia Dept. St. Thos. Hosp. Lond.; Clin. Asst. (Colposcopy) Roy. North. Hosp. Lond.

SZCZESNIAK, Leszek Andrzej Sussex Road Surgery, 125 Sussex Road, Southport PR8 6AF Tel: 01704 536778 Fax: 01704 532838 — MB ChB Leeds 1976.

SZEKELY, Gabor River Lodge Surgery, Malling Street, Lewes BN7 2RD Tel: 01273 472233 Fax: 01273 486879; Thorny Croft, Wellgreen Lane, Kingston, Lewes BN7 3NS Email: gab.szekely@virgin.net — MB BS Lond. 1980 (St. Geo.) BSc Lond. 1977; DRCOG 1982; MRCGP 1984; DGM RCP Lond. 1993; DFFP 1998.

SZEKELY, John Michael George Clare Surgery, Swan Drive, New Road, Chatteris PE16 6EX Tel: 01354 695888 Fax: 01354 695415 — MB BS Lond. 1980; BSc Lond. 1977; MRCGP 1984. Prev: Trainee GP Boston VTS.

SZEKI, Iren Katalin 34 Brackenfield Road, Gosforth, Newcastle upon Tyne NE3 4DY — MB BS Lond. 1996.

SZEMIS, Andrzej Hubert The Willows, Cordelia Close, Leicester LE5 0LE Tel: 0116 246 0988 Fax: 0116 246 1368 — Lekarz Warsaw 1961. Assoc. Specialist in Psychiat. Specialty: Gen. Psychiat. Socs: Affil. Roy. Coll. of Psychiat.s. Prev: Staff Grade (Psychiat.) Leicester.

SZLOSAREK, Piotr Wojciech 32 Devonshire Road, London N13 4QX — MB BS Lond. 1994.

SZOFINSKA, Barbara Barlow Medical Centre, 8 Barlow Moor Road, Didsbury, Manchester M20 6TR Tel: 0161 445 2101 Fax: 0161 445 9560 — MB ChB Manch. 1990; DFFP 1993; MRCGP 1994. Specialty: Gen. Pract. Prev: Trainee GP Manch. VTS.

SZOLACH, Mrs Maria Regina The Surgery, 127 Trinity Road, Tooting, London SW17 7HJ Tel: 020 8672 3331 — MRCS Eng. LRCP Lond. 1990. GP Lond. Specialty: Gen. Pract. Socs: BMA; Polish Med. Assn. Prev: Trainee GP/SHO Centr. Middlx. Hosp. NHS Trust VTS; Ho. Off. (Med.) OldCh. Hosp.; Ho. Off. (Surg. & Orthop.) Mayday Univ. Hosp.

SZOLLAR, Judit Havering Hospitals, Romford RM7 0BE Tel: 01708 345 5331 Ext: 3273; 66 Savernake Road, London NW3 2JR Tel: 020 7284 1336 Fax: 020 7284 1336 — MD Budapest 1968 (Simmclwcis University Budapest) Paediatrics & Neonatology 1979; Human Genetics 1979; PhD Tncsis Budapest 1981. Cons. Paediat. with s/i in Paediatric Diabetes and Endocrinol., OldCh. and Harold Wood Hosps. Specialty: Paediat.; Neonat. Socs: Roy. Coll. Paediat. and Child Health; Assoc. Mem. of Roy. Coll. of Pathologists Clincal Genetics Soc. Prev: Sen. Lect. (Paediat. & Neonat.) Univ. Semmelweis Budapest, Hungary.

SZULEC, Zdzislaw Jan (retired) 1 The Meadow, Bryants Farm, Lostock, Bolton BL1 5XN Tel: 01204 493053 — MB ChB Polish Sch. of Med. 1947 (Polish Sch. Med. Ed.) Corps. Surg. St. John Ambul. Brig. N. W. Area.

SZULECKA, Teresa Krystyna St. James University Hospital, Department of Psychiatry, Beckett St., Leeds LS9 7FT Tel: 0113 243 3144 Fax: 0113 234 6856; 7 Oaklea Hall Close, Adel, Leeds LS16 8HB — Lekarz Krakow 1970; MRCPsych 1979; MD Brussels 1986. Cons. Psych.Harrogate clinic, Mid Yorks. Nuffield Hosp. Specialty: Gen. Psychiat. Socs: Brit. Neuropysch. Assn. Prev: Cons. Psychiat. Bassetlaw Dist. Gen. Hosp. Worksop.; Cons. Psychiat. Doncaster Roy. Infirm.; Cons. Psychiat. St. James' Univ. Hosp. Leeds.

SZWEDZIUK, Peter 4 Stanley Road, Chatham ME5 8LN — MB BS Lond. 1985.

SZYPRYT, Mr Edward Paul 34 Regent Street, Nottingham NG1 5BT Tel: 0115 956 1300 Fax: 0115 956 1314 — MB BS Lond. 1978 (Roy. Lond. Hosp.) FRCS Eng. 1983. Cons. (Orthop. & Trauma Surg.) Univ. Hosp. NHS Trust Nottm. Specialty: Orthop. Socs: Brit. Assn. for Surg. of the Knee; Fell. & Counc. Mem. BOA; Brit. Orthop. Research Soc. Prev: Sen. Regist. (Trauma & Orthop.) Univ. Hosp. & Harlow Wood Orthop.Hosp. Nottm.; NCB Spinal Research Fell. Harlow Wood Orthop. Hosp. Nottm.; Regist. (Trauma & Orthop.) P. of Wales & St. Geo. Hosp. Sydney, Australia.

SZYSZKO, Janina Maria Chiswick Family Practice, 89 Southfield Road, Chiswick, London W4 1BB Tel: 0208 995 6707 Fax: 0208 995 0750 — MB BS Lond. 1986; BSc (Basic Med. Scis. with Anat.) Lond. 1983; DRCOG 1988; MRCGP 1990. Prev: Trainee GP Chiswick; SHO (A & E & Psychiat.) Hillingdon Hosp.; SHO (Geriat. & O & G) Qu. Mary's Univ. Hosp. Roehampton.

TA, Thuan Chi 120 Rosebery Street, Swindon SN1 2ES — MB BS Lond. 1992.

TAAFFE, Patrick Islwyn, Glandwr, Barmouth LL42 1TG — LAH Dub. 1955.

TAAMS, Mr Karel Otto Derriford Hospital, Plastic Surgery & Burns Unit, Plymouth PL6 8DH Tel: 01752 777111 — Artsexamen Groningen 1988 (Artsexamen Groningen) MMed (Plastic & Reconstruc. Surg.) Witwatersrand 1994; FCS(SA) 1994. Cons. Plastic Surg. Derriford Hosp. Plymouth. Specialty: Plastic Surg. Socs: BAPS; Craniofacial Soc. Prev: Cons. Plastic Surg. Acad. Hosp. Rotterdam, Netherlands.

TABANDEH, Mr Homayoun 30 Palace Court, London W2 4HZ — MB BS Lond. 1985; DO RCS Glas. 1989; FCOphth 1990; MRCP (UK) 1990; FRCS Glas. 1990; MS Lond. 1996. Sen. Regist. Moorfields Eye Hosp. Lond. Specialty: Ophth.

TABANI, Mr Aslam Rashid Accident & Emergency Department, Goodhope Hospital, Rectory Road, Birmingham B75 7RR Tel: 0121 378 2211 Ext: 2101 Fax: 0121 378 6198 — MB BS Karachi 1983; FFAEM; FRCS. Cons. (Accid. & Emerg.) Good Hope Hosp. Birm. Specialty: Accid. & Emerg. Prev: Sen. Regist., A&E Dept., St Thomas' Hosp. Lond.

TABAQCHALI, Mr Mohamed Amin University Hospital of North Tees, Hardwick, Stockton-on-Tees TS19 8PE Tel: 01642 624078 — MB BCh 1982 (Cairo University) FRCS Ed. 1988; FRCS England 1988; FRCS (Gen. Surg.) 1998. Cons. Gen. Surgeon with interest in Colorectal Surgery, North Tees & Hartlepool NHS Trust; Lead Clinician, Trust Cancer Unit, North Tees & Hartlepool NHS Trust; Lead Clin, Cancer Network for Teeside, South Durham & North

Yorkshire. Specialty: Gen. Surg. Socs: BMA Mem.; Assoc. of Surgeons of GB & I; Assoc. of Coloproctologist of GB & I.

TABAQCHALI, Professor Soad (retired) Department of Medical Microbiology, St. Bartholomew's & Royal London School Med. & Dent., St Bartholomew's Hospital, Smithfield, London EC1A 7BE Tel: 020 7601 8401 Fax: 020 7601 8409; 9 Kent Terrace, Regent's Park, London NW1 4RP Tel: 020 7724 3379 — MB ChB St. And. 1958; FRCPath 1986, M 1974; MRCP (UK) 1990; FRCP Lond. 1993. Prof. & Head Dept. Med. Microbiol. St. Bart. & Roy. Lond. Sch. Med. & Dent.; Hon. Cons. Roy. Hosps. NHS Trust; Clin. Dir. (Med. Microbiol.) & Chairm. Infec. Control Comm. Roy. Hosps. NHS Trust Lond. Prev: Reader & Sen. Lect. (Med. Microbiol.) St. Bart. Hosp. Med. Coll. Lond.

TABB, Peter Asquith Knights, Billingshurst — MB ChB St. And. 1969; DCH RCPS Glas. 1972. Prev: GP Billingshurst; Regist. (Paediat.) Dundee Health Dist.; SHO (Med.) Roy. Salop Infirm. Shrewsbury.

TABERNER, Catherine Ruth Hill House, Rue de la Terre Norgiot, St Saviours, Guernsey GY7 9JR — MB ChB Sheff. 1987; MSc, DCH, DFFP.

TABERNER, David Allan 20 Cogshall Lane, Comberbach, Northwich CW9 6BS — BM BCh Oxf. 1970; MRCP (U.K.) 1973; MRCPath 1978. Cons. (Haemat.) Withington Hosp. Manch. Specialty: Haematology. Socs: Brit. Soc. Haemat.; Fell. Manch. Med. Soc. Prev: Sen. Regist. United Manch. Hosps.; SHO (Cardiol.) Brompton Hosp. Lond.; SHO IC Unit St. Thos. Hosp. Lond.

TABERT, James Edward Keir, MBE Castle Street Surgery, 39 Castle Street, Luton LU1 3AG Tel: 01582 729242 Fax: 01582 725192 — MB BS Lond. 1960 (St. Bart.) DObst RCOG 1962. Prev: Ho. Surg. Swindon Matern. Hosp.; Ho. Surg. & Ho. Phys. Sutton & Cheam Hosp.

TABNER, James Anthony The Grove Surgery, Trinity Medical Centre, Thornhill Street, Wakefield WF1 1PG Tel: 0845 6077740 Fax: 01924 200913; 125 Thornes Road, Wakefield WF2 8QD Tel: 01924 374000 — MB ChB Leic. 1983; MRCGP 1988. Prev: Trainee GP Wakefield VTS; SHO (Community Med.) Stockport HA VTS.

TABNER, Shirley Anne 66 Wrenthorpe Lane, Wrenthorpe, Wakefield WF2 0PT Tel: 01924 290908 — MB BS Lond. 1981; DRCOG 1983. SCMO Contracep. & Sexual Health N. Kirklees PCT. Specialty: Family Plann. & Reproduc. Health. Prev: Clin. Med. Off. (p/t) Family Plann. Wakefield & Ponefract Community Trust; Mem. Wakefield VTS; Ho. Surg. & Ho. Phys. Pinderfields Gen. Hosp. Wakefield.

TABONE-VASSALLO, Mr Mario 10 Harley Street, London W1G 9PF Tel: 020 7467 8300 Fax: 020 7467 8312; Dwejra, 80 Vicarage Terrace, Romford Road, London E15 4EE — MD Malta 1971; FRCS Ed. 1976; FRCS Eng. 1977; FFAEM 1994. Specialty: Accid. & Emerg.; Trauma & Orthop. Surg.; Gen. Surg. Socs: Roy. Soc. Med. (Founder & Ex-Pres. & Sec. Sect. Accid. & Emerg. Med.); Founding Fell. Europ. AERO Med. Inst. (Ex-Vice-Pres.); Liveryman Worshipful Soc. Apoth. Prev: Clin. Dir. (A & E) Med. Servs. Malta; Cons. Surg. i/c A & E Dept. Greenwich Dist. Hosp.; Cons. Surg. i/c A & E Dept. N. Middlx. Hosp.

TABONY, Winifred Mary Mains Medical Centre, Park Mains Post Office, 300 Mains Drive, Erskine PA8 7JQ Tel: 0141 812 3230 Fax: 0141 812 5226; 23 Pendicle Road, Bearsden, Glasgow G61 1PT — MB ChB Glas. 1974; MRCGP 1978.

TABOR, Arthur Shand 5 Woodland Drive, Hove BN3 6DH Tel: 01273 557779 — (St. Bart) MB BS Lond. 1958. Prev: Ho. Phys. & Ho. Surg. St. Bart. Hosp.; Ho. Surg. Mayday Hosp.; Squadron Ldr. RAF Med. Br.

TABOR, John Edward Kildonan House, Ramsbottom Road, Horwich, Bolton BL6 5NW Tel: 01204 468161 Fax: 01204 698186; 2 Manor Road, Horwich, Bolton BL6 6AR Tel: 01204 694503 — MB BS Lond. 1982; MA Oxf. 1982; DRCOG 1987; MRCGP 1987.

TABRIZI, Sarah Joanna 11 Rupert House, 54 Nevern Square, London SW5 9PL — MB ChB Ed. 1992; BSc (Hons) 1986; MRCP (UK) 1995; PhD UCL 2000. DoH Nat. Clin. Scientist; Clin. Sen. Lect.; Hon. Cons. Neurologist & Neurosurg. Specialty: Neurol. Socs: ABN. Prev: Specialist Regist. (Neurol.) Roy Free Hosp. Lond.; Regist. (Med.) St. Thos. Hosp. Lond.; Specialist Regist. Neurol., Nat. Hosp. For Neurol. and Neurosurg., Lond.

TACCHI, Derek, TD (retired) 2 Oakfield Road, Gosforth, Newcastle upon Tyne NE3 4HS Tel: 0191 285 2945 Fax: 0191 285 2945 — MB BS Durh. 1948; FRCOG 1965, M 1954; MD Durh. 1961. Prev: Cons. O & G Roy. Vict. Infirm. & Princess Mary Matern. Hosp. Newc.

TACCHI, Mary Jane Ravenswood Clinic, Ravenswood Road, Heaton, Newcastle upon Tyne NE6 5XT — MB BS Lond. 1986 (Westminster) MRCPsych 1991. Cons. (Adult Psychiat.); Clin. Lect. (Psychiat.) Newc. Univ. Specialty: Gen. Psychiat. Socs: BMA; RCPsych.

TACCONELLI, Franco Flat 23, Fletcher Buildings, Martlett Court, London WC2B 5EU — MB BS Lond. 1996; AKC Lond. 1986; BSc Lond. 1986; PhD Lond. 1992. Trainee GP. Specialty: Gen. Pract.

TACHAKRA, Mr Spitman Savak Central Middlesex Hospital, Accident & Emergency Department, Acton Lane, London NW10 7NS Tel: 020 8453 2250 Fax: 020 8453 2764; 83 Barn Hill, Wembley HA9 9LN Tel: 020 8904 0642 Email: sapal.tachakra@tinyworld.co.uk — MB BS Bombay 1964; MS Bombay 1967; FRCS Ed. 1972; FFAEM 1994. Cons. A & E Med. Nat. W. Lond. Hosp.s NHSTRust; Hon. Clin. Sen. Lect. (A & E Med.) Imperial Coll. Lond.; Hon Cons. A&E Med. St. Mary's Hosp. Lond. Specialty: Accid. & Emerg. Special Interest: Telemedicine. Socs: Roy. Soc. Med. (Sec. Telemed Forum & Mem. Counc. Accid. & Emerg. Med.). Prev: Undergrad. Sub-Dean St Mary's Hosp. Med. Sch. Lond.; Mem. Exec. Comm. Brit. Assn. of A & E Med.

TACKLEY, Roger Malcolm Anaesthetic Department, Torbay General Hospital, Torquay TQ2 7AA Tel: 01803 614567 Fax: 01803 654312; Redmayes, 42 Parkhurst Road, Torquay TQ1 4EP Tel: 01803 316 091 Email: r.tackley@scata.org.uk — MRCS Eng. LRCP Lond. 1977 (St. Bart.) BSc (Pharmacol. Hons.) Lond 1973; MB BS Lond. 1977; FRCA Eng. 1982. Cons. Anaesth. Torbay HA. Specialty: Anaesth. Socs: Past Chairm. of SCATA.

TADROS, Amir 8 Whitegale Close, Hitchin SG4 9LP — MB ChB Leic. 1996.

TADROS, Mr Athanassius Naguib Royal Eye Infirmary, Dorset County Hospital, Williams Avenue, Dorchester DT1 2JY Tel: 01305 251150 Fax: 01305 255374 — MB BCh Ain Shams 1977; DO RCPSI 1987; FRCOphth 1990; FRCS (Ophth.) Glas. 1990. Cons. Ophth. Surg. Roy. Eye. Infirm. Dorset Co. Hosp.; Cons. Ophth. Surg., Yeovil Dist. Hosp., Yeovil; Cons. Ophth. Surg. Winterbourne Hosp., Herringston Rd., Dorchester, DT1 2DR; Cons. Ophth. Surg. Yeatman Hosp. Sherbourne. Specialty: Ophth. Special Interest: Anterior Segment; Refractive Aspect of cataract Surgery. Socs: Mem. of Amer. Acad. of Ophth.; Mem. of Europ. Soc. of Cataract and Refractive Surg.; Mem. of Med. Protec. Soc.

TADROS, Fayez Farid 6 Burnaston Crescent, Shirley, Solihull B90 4LT — MB ChB Alexandria 1970. Specialty: Anaesth.

TADROS, Osama Ibrahim 8 Whitegale Close, Hitchin SG4 9LP Tel: 01462 36686 — MB BCh Cairo 1963; DS Cairo 1966, MB BCh 1963, DGO 1971.

TADROS, Wadie Samaan c/o Lloyds Bank, 407-409 Coventry Road, Birmingham B10 0SP — LMSSA Lond. 1973 (Khartoum) MB BS Khartoum 1969; DCH RCPSI 1973; ECFMG Cert 1973. Supervising Phys. & Sen. Phys. (Intern. Med.) Tapline-Badanah Hosp. Saudi Arabia. Prev: Regist. (Gen. Med.) Bolton Roy. Infirm.

TADROS-ATTALLA, Mr Samir Gorgy (retired) Pengarth, 55 Falmouth Road, Truro TR1 2HL Tel: 01872 2663 — MB ChB Alexandria, Egypt 1958 (Alexandria) FRCS Ed. 1966; LMSSA Lond. 1967. Indep. Med. Pract. Truro. Prev: Assoc. Specialist (A & E) Roy. Cornw. Hosp. Truro.

TADROS-CAUDLE, Maria Ernest Villa Sheradrosa, Nelson Avenue, Minster on Sea, Sheerness ME12 3SF — LRCP LRCS Ed. LRCPS Glas. 1976.

TADROSS, Mr Alphonse Atallah James Paget Hospital, Lowestoft Road, Gorlesdon, Great Yarmouth NR31 6LA Tel: 01493 600611; Lotus Villa, New Road, Fritton, Great Yarmouth NR31 9HP — MB ChB Assiut 1973; FRCS Ed. 1988. Assoc. Specialist (Surg.) Jas. Paget Hosp. Gt. Yarmouth. Prev: Regist. (Surg.) Cheltenham Gen. Hosp.

TADROUS, Paul Jospeh Department of Histopathology, Northwick Park & St Mark's NHS Trust, Northwick Park Hospital, Watford Road, Harrow HA1 3UJ — MB BS Lond. 1992 (Lond. Hosp. Med. Coll.) MSc. Image Anal. in Histol. (Distinct.) Lond. 1994. Specialist Regist. in Histopath. Specialty: Histopath. Socs: Path. Soc.; Train. Mem. Assn. Clin. Path.

TAFFINDER, Adrian Paul Health Centre, Poplar Avenue, Gresford, Wrexham LL12 8EP Tel: 01978 852208; 69 Wynnstay Lane, Marford, Wrexham LL12 8LH Tel: 0197 885 2492 — MB BCh Wales 1976; DRCOG 1978; MRCGP 1980. Course Organiser S. Clwyd VTS. Prev: Trainee GP Wrexham VTS; Ho. Phys. Singleton Hosp. Swansea; Ho. Surg. Roy. Gwent Hosp. Newport.

TAFFINDER, Gaenor Ann Health Centre, Poplar Avenue, Gresford, Wrexham LL12 8EP Tel: 01978 852206; 69 Wynnstay Lane, Marford, Wrexham LL12 8LH Tel: 0197 885 2492 — MB BCh Wales 1976; DRCOG 1979; MRCGP 1980. Prev: SHO (Cas.) War Memor. Hosp. Wrexham; Trainee Gen. Pract. Wrexham Vocational Train. Scheme; Ho. Surg. & Ho. Phys. Roy. Gwent Hosp. Newport.

TAFFINDER, Lawrence David (Surgery), Main Road, Stickney, Boston PE22 8AA Tel: 01205 480237; Pennycress, Chapel Lane, Sibsey, Boston PE22 0SN Tel: 01205 750496 — MB BCh Wales 1971; DObst RCOG 1973; Cert. Family Plann. JCC 1977; MRCGP 1977; Dip. Pract. Dermat. Wales 1992. Trainer GP Boston. Prev: Trainee GP Wolverhampton VTS; Ho. Phys. & Ho. Surg. Nottm. Gen. Hosp.

TAFFINDER, Mr Nicholas James William Harvey Hospital, Colorectal Unit, Kennington Road, Willesborough, Ashford TN24 0LZ — MB BChir Camb. 1990; FRCS Eng. 1993. Cons. (Gen. Surg.) William Harvey Hosp. Ashford. Specialty: Gen. Surg. Prev: Regist. (Gen. Surg.) St Mary's Hosp. Lond.; SHO Jean Verdier Hosp., Paris, St Mary's Hosp. Lond. & Qu. Alexandra Hosp. Portsmouth.

TAGBOTO, Senyo Komla 12 Smore Slade Hills, Oadby, Leicester LE2 4UX — MB ChB Ghana 1987; MRCP (UK) 1994. Regist. (Nephrol.) Leicester Gen. Hosp. Specialty: Gen. Med. Prev: Regist. (Nephrol. & Gen. Med.) P'boro. Dist. Hosp.

TAGELDIN, Mr Mohamed Elhosseini 8 Clifton Court, Royal Terrace, Southend-on-Sea SS1 1DX — FRCS Eng. 1978; MA MS Camb. 1990. Staff Grade Pract. N. Middlx. Hosp. Lond. Prev: Regist. (Gen. Surg.) Bishop Auckland Gen. Hosp.; SHO (Gen. Surg.) & Med. Assoc. (Orthop.) W. Suff. Hosp.

TAGG, Catherine Elizabeth Brill View, Woodperry Road, Beckley, Oxford OX3 9UZ — MB BS Lond. 1996.

TAGG, Gillian Valerie St. James University Hospital, Beckett St., Leeds LS9 7TF Tel: 0113 206 4068 Fax: 0113 206 4085 — MB ChB Leeds 1968; DObst RCOG 1970; DPM Leeds 1977; FRCPsych 1995, M 1978. Cons. Child & Adolesc. Psychiat. Leeds Community Ment. Health Trust; Sen. Lect. (Psychiat.) Univ. Leeds. Specialty: Child & Adolesc. Psychiat. Prev: Sen. Regist. (Child & Adolesc. Psychiat.) Yorks. RHA; Regist. (Psychiat.) St. Jas. Univ. Hosp. Leeds; SHO (Psychiat.) Glenside Hosp. Bristol.

TAGGART, Allister James Department of Rheumatology, Musgrave Park Hospital, Stockman's Lane, Belfast BT9 7JB Tel: 01232 669501 Fax: 01232 683191; 65 Richmond Court, Lisburn BT27 4QX Tel: 01846 664832 — MB BCh BAO Belf. 1975; MD Belf. 1982; FRCP Ed. 1989; FRCP Lond. 1994. Dep. Med. Dir. GreenPk. Healthcare Trust. Specialty: Rehabil. Med.; Rheumatol. Socs: Fell. Ulster Med. Soc.; Brit. Soc. Rheum.; (Hon. Sec.) Irish Soc. Rheum. Prev: Cons. Phys. & Sen. Lect. (Therap. & Pharmacol.) Qu. Univ. Belf.

TAGGART, Catherine Mary 22 Newtonbreda Road, Belfast BT8 6AS — MB BCh BAO Belf. 1995.

TAGGART, Christopher Michael Woodside Medical Centre, Jardine Crescent, Coventry CV4 9PL Tel: 024 7669 4001 Fax: 024 7669 5639; The Mill Barn, Ivy Farm Lane, Coventry CV4 7BW Tel: 024 76 416321 — MB ChB Manch. 1981 (Manchester) DRCOG 1984; MRCGP 1985. Princip. GP; Postgrad. Tutor (Gen. Pract.) Coventry & Warks. Hosp.; GP Bd. Mem. W. Coventry PCG; Mem. Coventry Local Med. Comm. Specialty: Gen. Pract. Socs: BMA; Christ. Med. Fellowsh. Prev: Trainee GP Lancaster VTS; Ho. Off. (Med.) Roy. Lancaster Infirm.; Ho. Off. (Surg.) Macclesfield Infirm.

TAGGART, Curphey Clague Ballasalla Medical Centre, Main road, Ballasalla IM9 2RQ Tel: 01624 823243 Fax: 01624 822947 Email: curpheytaggart@manx.net; Hunters Lodge, Bridge Road, Ballasalla IM9 3DQ Tel: 01624 822815 — MB ChB Liverp. 1976; DRCOG 1979; MRCGP 1984.

TAGGART, Professor David Paul Peter John Radcliffe Hospital, Oxford Heart Centre, Oxford OX3 9DU Tel: 01865 221121 Fax: 01856 220244 Email: david.taggart@orh.nhs.uk; 52 Park Town, Oxford OX2 6SJ — MB ChB Glas. 1981; FRCS Glas. 1985; MD (Hons.) Glas. 1989; PhD Glas 1999. Prof. of Cardiovasc. Surg., Univ. of Oxf.; Cons. Cardiothoracic Surg. John Radcliffe Hosp. Oxf. Specialty: Cardiothoracic Surg. Socs: Brit. Cardiac Soc.; Europ. Soc. of Cardiothoracic Surg.; Soc. of Cardiothoracic Surgeons of Gt. Britain & Irel. Prev: Sen. Regist. Roy. Brompton Nat. Heart & Lung Hosp.

TAGGART, George Edward Crouch Farmhouse, Long Mill Lane, Crouch, Borough Green, Sevenoaks TN15 8QD — MB BS Lond. 1991.

TAGGART, Hugh Francis 37 Newlands Road, Glasgow G43 2JG — MB ChB Glas. 1951.

TAGGART, Hugh McAllister Belfast City Hospital, Department of Health Care for The Elderly, Lisburn Road, Belfast BT9 7AB Tel: 0289 032 9241 Fax: 0289 026 3946 Email: hugh.taggart@bch.n-i.nhs.uk; 1 Crawfordsburn Wood, Crawfordsburn, Bangor BT19 1XB Email: hugh.taggart@nirland.com — MB BCh BAO Belf. 1973; MRCP (UK) 1977; MD Belf. 1979; FRCP Glas. 1997, Lond. 1991. Cons. Phys. (Health Care for Elderly) Belf. City Hosp. Specialty: Care of the Elderly. Socs: Fell. Ulster Med. Soc.; Brit. Geriat. Soc.; Amer. Soc. Bone & Mineral Research. Prev: Sen. Lect. (Geriat. Med.) Qu's. Univ. Belf.; Resid. Fell. (Geriat. Med.) Univ. Washington, Seattle, USA.

TAGGART, Ian 252 Nithsdale Road, Dumbreck, Glasgow G41 5AH — MB ChB Aberd. 1983. Cons. Plastic Surg. Cannisburn Hosp. Specialty: Plastic Surg.

TAGGART, Lucy Petronilla 164 Turney Road, London SE21 7JJ — MB BS Lond. 1985; MRCGP 1991.

TAGGART, Michael Borough Green Medical Practice, 34 Maidstone Road, Borough Green, Sevenoaks TN15 8BD; Crouch Farm House, Long Mill Lane, Borough Green, Sevenoaks TN15 8QD Tel: 01732 3161 — MB BChir Camb. 1958 (Camb. & St. Thos.) BA Camb. 1958; DObst RCOG 1959.

TAGGART, Patrick Campbell Millar 378 Higham Lane, Nuneaton CV11 6AP — MB BS Lond. 1971 (King's Coll. Hosp.) BSc (Hons. Physiol.) Lond. 1968; DObst RCOG 1974; DCH Eng. 1974; FFA RCS Eng. 1978. Cons. Anaesth. Geo. Eliot Hosp. NHS Trust Nuneaton. Specialty: Anaesth.

TAGGART, Peter Irwin 12 Blandford Road, Bedford Park, Chiswick, London W4 1DU Tel: 020 8994 8547 — (St. Bart.) MD Lond. 1976, MB BS 1957; FRCP Lond. 1985, M 1964; MRCP Ed. 1964; DSc 2003. Reader (Cardiol.) The Heart Hosp., Univ. Coll. Lond. Hosps. Specialty: Gen. Med. Socs: Brit. Cardiac Soc. & Physiolog. Soc. Prev: Med. Regist. King's Coll. Hosp. Lond.; Leverhulme Research Schol. & Brit. Heart Foundat. Research Fell. & Hon. Sen. Regist. Dept. Cardiol. Middlx. Hosp. Lond.

TAGGART, Simon James Cook University Hospital, Department of Clinical Neurophysiology, Marton Road, Middlesbrough T54 3BW Tel: 01642 282755 — BMedSc Newc. 1992; MB BS Newc. 1993. Consultant in Clinical Neurophysiology. Specialty: Clin. Neurophysiol. Prev: Specialist Regist. Clin. Neurophysiol. Regional Neurosci. Centre Newc. Gen. Hosp.

TAGGART, Simon Charles Ormandy Robin Hood Cottage, Great Staughton, Huntingdon PE19 4BB — MB ChB Manch. 1989 (St Andrews and Manchester) MRCP (UK) 1992; MD Manchester 1996; (Gen. Med & Thoracic Med) CCST 1999. Cons. Phys. Specialty: Respirat. Med. Socs: Brit. Thoracic Soc.; Brit. Lung Foundat. Prev: Sen. Regist. (Thoracic & Gen. Med.).

TAGGART, Thomas Frederick Ormandy 25 Oxford Street, Liverpool L15 8HX — MB ChB Liverp. 1991.

TAGGART-JEEVA, Sakib 47 Colinmander Gardens, Ormskirk L39 4TE — MB ChB Liverp. 1997.

TAGHIPOUR, Jahangir Royal Berkshire & Battle NHS Trust, London Road, Reading RG1 5AN Tel: 0118 987 7022; 132 Chaplin Road, Wembley HA0 4UT Tel: 020 8900 2977 — MD 1979; Dip. Thorac. Med. Lond. 1987; MRCS Eng. LRCP Lond. 1990; DFFP 1995; DRCOG 1996. Staff Grade Reading. Specialty: Accid. & Emerg. Prev: Regist. (A & E) Good Hope Hosp. N. Birm. HA.

TAGHIZADEH, Abdosamad Department of Pathology, Oldchurch Hospital, Romford RM7 0BE — MD Tehran 1958; PhD Lond. 1965. Cons. Histopath. OldCh. Hosp. Romford. Specialty: Histopath.

TAGHIZADEH, Mr Arash Kusha 27A Cyril Mansions, Prince of Wales Drive, London SW11 4HP — MB BS Lond. 1992; BSc Lond. 1989; FRCS (Eng) 1997. Specialty: Urol.

TAGORE, N K Westminster Medical Centre, Aldams Grove, Liverpool L4 3TT Tel: 0151 922 3510 Fax: 0151 902 6071.

TAHA, Ali Said Assa'd Division of Medicine & Gastroenterology, Eastbourne General Hosptial, Eastbourne BN21 2UD Tel: 01323 417400; 22 Ashburnham Road, Eastbourne BN21 2HX — MRCS Eng. LRCP Lond. 1982 (Bristol) MRCPI 1986; MRCP (UK) 1987; PhD Glas. 1993, MD 1990. Cons. Gastroenterol. Eastbourne Gen. Hosp. Specialty: Gastroenterol. Socs: Internat. Mem. Amer. Gastroenterol. Assn.; Brit. Soc. Gastroenterol. Prev: Sen. Regist. (Gastroenterol. & Gen. Med.) South. Gen. Hosp. Glas.; Regist. (Gastroenterol.) Glas. Roy. Infirm.; Regist. (Med.) Falkirk & Dist. Roy. Infirm.

TAHA, Hassan Mohamed Deal Mental Health Centre, Bowling Green Lane, Deal CT14 9UR; 152 New Dover Road, Canterbury CT1 3EJ — MB BS Khartoum, Sudan 1976 (Fac. Med. Univ. Khartoum) DCP 1996; DPM 1997. Assoc. Spec. Gen. Adult Psychiat. Specialty: Geriat. Psychiat. Socs: BMA; MDU; Sudan Med. Assn. Prev: Act. Cons. Thanet Ment. Health Ramsgate.

TAHA, Riem — MB ChB Leic. 1998.

TAHALANI, R P Whiston Road Surgery, 219 Kingsland Rd, London E2 8AN Tel: 020 7739 8625 — MB BS Patna Med. Coll. India 1973.

TAHBAZ, Arash Flat 3, 25 De Vere Gardens, London W8 5AN — MB ChB Bristol 1992.

TAHERI, Shahrad Department of Endocrinology, Imperial College School of Medicine, The Hammersmith Hospital, Du Cane Road, London W12 0HS Tel: 020 8743 2030; 41 Windermere Avenue, London SW19 3EP Tel: 020 8542 2272 — MB BS Lond. 1994 (Barts, Lond.) BSc (Hons.) Lond. 1987; MSc (Human Biol.) Oxf. 1989; MB BS (Hons.) Lond. 1994; MRCP (Lond.) 1997. Wellcome Research Fell. Hammersmith Hosp. Lond. Specialty: Endocrinol.; Gen. Med. Socs: BMA. Prev: Specialist Regist. (Endocrinol.) Hammersmith Hosp. Lond.; Regist. (Gen. Med. & Cardiol.) Ashford Hosp. Middlx.; Research Regist. Hammersmith Hosp. Lond.

TAHERZADEH, Omeed 66F Blomfield Road, Little Venice, London W9 2PA Tel: 020 7266 4315 — MB BS Lond. 1993 (Univ. Coll. Hosp.) BSc Lond. 1989. SHO (Plastics) Morriston Hosp. Swansea. Specialty: Plastic Surg. Prev: SHO (Gen. Surg.) Qu. Eliz. Qu. Mother's Hosp. Margate; SHO (Urol.) Kent & Canterbury Hosp.; SHO (Orthop.) St. Peter's Hosp. Chertsey.

TAHGHIGHI, Jason Payman 1 Lyne Walk, Hackleton, Northampton NN7 2BW — MB ChB Manch. 1991; DFFP 1995; DRCOG 1995. SHO (A & E Med.) Trafford Gen. Hosp. Manch. Prev: SHO (O & G) Trafford Gen. Hosp.; SHO Intens. Care Unit Roy. Preston Hosp.; SHO (Neurol.) Roy. Preston Hosp.

TAHIR, Hasan Imam Syed Flat 3, Balmoral Court, 39 Wembley Park Drive, Wembley HA9 8HE — MB BS Lond. 1996; MRCP; BSc.

TAHIR, Mohammad Zakariya 58 Vicarage Road, West Bromwich B71 1AQ — MB BS Punjab 1964 (King Edwd. Med. Coll. Lahore) MB BS Punjab (Pakistan) 1964; DA Eng. 1968; DLO Eng. 1976.

TAHIR, Muhammad Forest Edge Practice, Manford Way Health Centre, 53 Foremark Close, Ilford IG6 3HS Tel: 020 8500 9938 Fax: 020 8559 9319 — MB BS Newc. 1988; MRCGP 1992.

TAHIR, Saad Sabeh Radiotherapy Department, St. Lukes Hospital, Warren Road, Guildford GU1 3NT; 7 Gill Avenue, Guildford GU2 7WW Tel: 01483 571122 — MB ChB Baghdad 1974; FRCR 1986. Sen. Regist. (Clin. Oncol.) St Luke's Hosp. Guildford. Specialty: Oncol.

TAHIR, Shahed Mehmood 24 Queens Road, Wheatley, Doncaster DN1 2NQ — MB ChB Leeds 1995.

TAHZIB, Farhang 4 The Spinney, Haywards Heath RH16 1PL — MB ChB Aberd. 1976.

TAI, Cheh-Chin — MB BChir 1996.

TAI, Grace Kee Ling 1 Stroud Park Road, Plymouth PL2 3NL — MB BCh BAO NUI 1987; LRCPSI 1987.

TAI, Yeoman Michael Arthur Heath Lane Consulting Rooms, 7/9 Heath Lane, Oldswinford, Stourbridge DY8 1RF Tel: 01384 396146; The Chaucer Hospital, Nackington Road, Canterbury CT4 7AR Tel: 01227 455466 — LRCPI & LM, LRSCI & LM 1961 (RCSI) LRCPI & LM, LRCSI & LM 1961; LAH Dub. 1961; DA Eng. 1963; DObst RCOG 1963; FFA RCSI 1967. Cons. Pain Relief & Palliat. Care E. Kent Pain Managem. Serv. Margate. Specialty: Palliat. Med.; Anaesth. Socs: Assn. Anaesths.; Intractable Pain Soc. Prev: Cons. Anaesth. & Dir. Pain Relief Unit Dudley HA; Sen. Regist. (Anaesth.) United Birm. Hosps. & Birm. RHB; Ho. Surg. & Ho. Phys. & Regist. (Anaesth.) Adelaide Hosp. Dub.

TAIBJEE, Saleem Mustafa — MB ChB Birm. 1998.

TAIG, Christine Stobswell Medical Centre, 163 Albert Street, Dundee DD4 6PX Tel: 01382 461363 Fax: 01382 453423 — MB ChB St. And. 1967.

TAIG, David Retson Coldside Medical Practice, 129 Strathmartine Road, Dundee DD3 8DB Tel: 01382 826724 Fax: 01382 884129 — MB ChB St. And. 1967.

TAILBY, Christine Helen Bridge Cottage, 120 Bridge Lane, Frodsham, Warrington WA6 7HZ Tel: 01928 739562 — MB ChB Dundee 1988. SHO (Anaesth.) Broadgreen Hosp. NHS Trust Liverp. Specialty: Anaesth. Socs: Christ. Med. Fellowsh. Prev: SHO (Anaesth.) Hull Roy. Infirm.

TAILOR, Anilkumar Jayantilal Royal Surrey County Hospital, Egerton Road, Guildford GU2 7XX Tel: 01483 571122 Ext: 2176 Email: anil@tailoruk.freeserve.co.uk — MB BS Lond. 1991 (Kings Coll Hosp.) BSc (Hons.) Lond. 1988; MRCOG 1998. Cons. Gyn. Oncologist. Specialty: Obst. & Gyn. Special Interest: Ultrasonography to discriminate benign and Malig. ovarian masses. Prev: SHO (O & G) Greenwich Dist. Hosp.; Research Regist. & SHO (O & G) King's Coll. Hosp. Lond.; Specialist Regist. (O & G) Southend Gen. Hosp.

TAILOR, Harshad North Street Health Centre, North Street, Ashby-de-la-Zouch LE65 1HU Tel: 01530 414131 — MB ChB Dundee 1989; DRCOG 1993; MMedSci Birm. 1994; MRCGP 1995. GP Leicester; Occupational Physician.

TAILOR, Manubhai Dahyabhai (retired) Shivam, Worcester Road, Great Witley, Worcester WR6 6HR Tel: 01299 896660 — MB ChB Birm. 1962.

TAILOR, Rajesh 95 Hertford Road, E. Finchley, London N2 9BX — MB ChB Dundee 1984.

TAILOR, Rekha Anil John Tasker House, 56 New St., Great Dunmour, Dunmow CM6 1BH; 24 West Hayes, Hatfield Heath, Bishop's Stortford CM22 7DH — MB ChB Manch. 1989; DFFP 1992; DRCOG 1993; MRCGP 1995. GP Retainee. Prev: GP Princip.

TAILOR, Vijay Gulab Hillcrest Surgery, 337 Uxbridge Road, Acton, Wembley W3 9RA Tel: 0208 993 0982 — MB ChB Leic. 1993; Bsc (Hons.) MBchB DRCOG. Gen. Pract. Prinicpal.

TAINE, Diana Landon Greensands Medical Practice, Brook End Surgery, Potton, Sandy SG19 2QS Tel: 01767 260260 Fax: 01767 261777; 18 Gamlingay Road, Waresley, Sandy SG19 3DB — MB BS Lond. 1984; MRCGP 1988.

TAINSH, John Alexander Department of Radiology, Stracathro Hospital, Brechin DD9 7QA Tel: 0135 666 5132; 'Tanglewood', 1A Viewfield Road, Arbroath DD11 2BS Tel: 01241 876210 — MB ChB Aberd. 1977; BMedBiol (Commend.) Aberd. 1974, MB ChB 1977; DMRD Ed. 1983; FRCR 1985; FRCP 1998. Cons. (Radiol.) Tayside Health Bd. Specialty: Radiol. Prev: Sen. Regist. (Radiol.) Tayside Health Bd.; Regist. (Radiol.) Lothian Health Bd. (Edin.); Regist. (Gen. Med.) Grampian Health Bd. (Aberd.).

TAIT, Alan Christopher 9 Ley Hey Road, Marple, Stockport SK6 6PQ — MB ChB Birm. 1972; MRCPsych 1977. Cons. Psychiat. Tameside AHA, Tameside Gen. Hosp. & Community Ment.; Health Centre Hyde. Specialty: Gen. Psychiat. Socs: Assn. Family Therapists.

TAIT, Allan Christie (retired) 56A Craigmillar Park, Edinburgh EH16 5PT — MB ChB Glas. 1941; DPH 1947; DPM Lond. 1948; FRCP Ed. 1969, M 1965; FRCPsych 1971. Prev: Phys. Supt. & Cons. Psychiat. Crichton Roy., Dumfries.

TAIT, Charles Robert Sabine Loddon Vale Practice, Hurricane Way, Woodley, Reading RG5 4UX Tel: 0118 969 0160 Fax: 0118 969 9103; Woodvale House, Spencers Wood, Reading RG7 1AE Tel: 01734 883296 — MB BS Lond. 1968 (St. Bart.) MRCS Eng. LRCP Lond. 1968; DCH Eng. 1970; DObst RCOG 1970. Clin. Asst. (Paediat.) Roy. Berks. Hosp. Reading. Socs: BMA; Reading Path. Soc. Prev: SHO (Paediat.) Roy. Berks. Hosp. Reading.

TAIT, Clare Penelope c/o Prof. P. Haggett, 5 Tunbridge Close, Bristol BS40 8SU — MB BS Lond. 1985; MB BS (Hons.) Lond. 1985; MRCP (UK) 1988. Prev: SHO (Med.) Whittington Hosp. & Hammersmith Hosp. & Brompton Hosp. Lond.

TAIT, Colin Michael Busby Road Surgery, 75 Busby Road, Clarkston, Glasgow G76 7BW Tel: 0141 644 2666 Fax: 0141 644 5171; 26 Church Road, Giffnock, Glasgow G46 6LT — MB ChB Glas. 1973; DObst RCOG 1976; FRCP Glas. 1991. Prev: Regist. (Gen. Med.) Vict. Infirm. Glas.; SHO (O & G) Paisley Matern. Hosp.; SHO (Paediat. Med.) Roy. Hosp. Sick Childr. Glas.

TAIT, David Hamilton Hay Murray Royal Hospital, Muirhall Road, Perth PH2 7BH Tel: 01738 621151 Fax: 01738 440431 Email:

david.tait@tpct.scot.nhs.uk — MB ChB Ed. 1974; BSc Ed. 1971; MRCPsych 1974; FRCPsych 1993, M 1978; BA Open 1986; MBA Stirling 1998. Cons. Psychiat. NHS Tayside, Perth; Hon. Sen. Lect. Univ. Dundee; Librarian, Roy. Coll. of Psychiat.s, Lond.; Med. Director, Huntercombe Edin. Hosp., Binny Est., Ecclesmachan Rd., Uphall, W. Lothian. Specialty: Psychother.; Gen. Psychiat. Socs: Fell., Roy. Coll. of Psychiat.s; Fell., Roy. Soc. of Med.; Brit. Med. Assn. Prev: Sen. Regist. Aberd. Teach. Hosps.; Regist. Roy. Edin. Hosp.

TAIT, Deborah 15 Byng Road, Barnet EN5 4NW — MB ChB Leeds 1998.

TAIT, Diana Mary Royal Marsden Hospital, Downs Road, Sutton SM2 5PT Fax: 020 8661 3370/020 8661 3610 Email: diana.tait@rmh.nthames.nhs.uk — MB ChB Ed. 1975; MRCP (UK) 1978; FRCR 1984; MD Ed. 1988; FRCP 1998. Cons. Clin. Oncol. Roy. Marsden NHS Trust Sutton & Lond.; Hon. Sen. Lect. Univ. Lond. Specialty: Oncol. Special Interest: Breast; Systemic Treatm. for Neuroendocrine Tumours; Upper & Lower GI.

TAIT, Elizabeth Ann (retired) Ham Glebe, Church Road, Ham, Richmond TW10 5HG Tel: 020 8940 8629 — MB BS Lond. 1960 (Char. Cross) DObst RCOG 1961. Prev: GP Lond.

TAIT, Frank George (retired) Jays Cottage, Tisbury Row, Tisbury, Salisbury SP3 6RZ Tel: 01747 870209 — MB BS Melbourne 1947; DPM Eng. 1954; MRCPsych 1972. Prev: Sen. Med. Off. DHSS.

TAIT, Mr Gavin Robert Crosshouse Hospital, Kilmarnock KA2 0BE Tel: 01563 577333 Fax: 01563 577976 — MB ChB Ed. 1980 (Edinburgh) FRCS Glas. 1984. Cons. Orthop. Surg. CrossHo. Hosp. Kilmarnock. Specialty: Orthop. Socs: Brit. Assn. Surg. Knee; Brit. Elbow & Shoulder Soc. Prev: Wellcome Research Asst. Qu. Univ. Belf.; Sen. Regist. (Orthop. Surg.) Vict. Infirm. Glas.

TAIT, Godfrey Beckwith (retired) 16 Crowlees Road, Mirfield WF14 9PJ Tel: 01924 497867 — MD Ed. 1947 (Univ. Ed.) MB ChB 1939; FRCP Ed. 1958, M 1947. Hon. Cons. Gen. Med. Dewsbury Area Hosps. Prev: Sen. Med. Regist. Huddersfield Roy. Infirm.

TAIT, Graeme William Dumfries & Galloway Royal Infirmary, Bankend Road, Dumfries DG1 4AP Tel: 01387 241353 Fax: 01387 241192 Email: g.tait@dgri.scot.nhs.uk — MB ChB Ed. 1982 (Univ. Ed.) MRCP (UK) 1987; MD Ed. 1996; FRCP Glas. 1997. Cons. Phys. & Cardiol. Dumfries & Galloway Roy. Infirm. Specialty: Cardiol. Special Interest: Coronary Artery Disease; Heart failure; hyperlipidaimia. Prev: Clin. Lect. (Med. Cardiol. & Path. Biochem.) Univ. Glas.

TAIT, Hamish Adie Tait and Partners, 68 Pipeland Road, St Andrews KY16 8JZ Tel: 01334 476840 Fax: 01334 466516; 1 Aikman Place, St Andrews KY16 8XS Tel: 01334 473909 Email: hamish.tait@bigfoot.com — MB ChB Glas. 1971 (Glasgow University) DObst RCOG 1973; DCH RCPS Glas. 1974; MRCGP 1978; FRCGP 2002.

TAIT, Mr Iain Stephen Ninewells Hospital, Dundee DD1 9SY — MB ChB Glas. 1986; FRCS Ed. 1990. Specialty: Gen. Surg.

TAIT, Ian Greville (retired) Westfields, 45 Park Road, Aldeburgh IP15 5EN Tel: 01728 452114 — MB BChir Camb. 1954 (St. Bart.) MA, MB Camb. 1954, BChir 1953; DCH Eng. 1957; FRCGP 1977, M 1960; MD Camb. 1981. Prev: GP Aldeburgh Suff.

TAIT, Ian James Nunwell Surgery, 10 Pump Street, Bromyard HR7 4BZ Tel: 01885 483412 Fax: 01885 488739; Ashfields House, Hereford Road, Bromyard HR7 4ET Tel: 01885 482872 — MB ChB Birm. 1982; DRCOG 1986; MRCGP 1987. Specialty: Gen. Pract.

TAIT, Isobel Anne (retired) 4/4 Advocates Close, 357 High Street, Edinburgh EH11 PS Email: anne.tait@cressington.force9.co.uk — MB ChB 1959 (Edin.) MD Ed. 1982; DObst RCOG 1962; Dip Ven 1980; Dip Palliat Med Cardiff 1999. Prev: Cons. Genitourin. Med. Liverp. & Wirral HAs.

TAIT, Jacqueline 17 Station Road, Mintlaw, Peterhead AB42 5EE — MB ChB Aberd. 1983.

TAIT, James Stephen Smithy Cottage, Lighthorne, Warwick CV35 0AU — MB BS Lond. 1998.

TAIT, Mrs Janet Felicity (retired) Westfields, 45 Park Road, Aldeburgh IP15 5EN Tel: 01728 452114 Fax: 01728 454070 — MB BS Lond. 1954 (St. Bart.) Cert. FPA JCC 1960. Prev: Med. Off. Family Plann. Clinics Local Health Partnerships NHS Trust Ipswich.

TAIT, Janis Lairig, Old Mills, Fochabers IV32 7HJ Tel: 01343 820373 — MB ChB Glas. 1978.

TAIT, Karen Fiona 28 Currock Mount, Carlisle CA2 4RF — MB ChB Leeds 1997.

TAIT, Nicholas Karl 224 Banner Dale Road, Ecclesall, Sheffield S11 9FE — MB ChB Birm. 1995.

TAIT, Nicholas Paul Department of Radiology, Hammersmith Hospital, Du Cane Road, London W12 0HN Tel: 020 8383 4924 — MB BChir 1978 (Westm. Med. Sch.) MA Camb. 1979; FRCR 1985. Cons. Interventional Radiologist, Hammersmith Hosps. NHS Trust, Lond. Specialty: Radiol. Socs: Brit. Soc. of Interventional Radiol.; Cardiovasc. and Interventional Soc. of Europe; Europ. Soc. of Gastrointestinal Radiologists. Prev: Cons. Radiologist, N.Tees and Hartlepool NHS Trust, Stockton on Tees, 1988-2000; Sen. Regist., Diagnostic Radiol., Newc. upon Tyne 1984-1988.

TAIT, Robert Campbell Department of Haematology, MacEwan Building, Royal Infirmary, Glasgow G4 0SF Tel: 0141 211 5168 Fax: 0141 211 4931 Email: campbell.tait@northglasgow.scot.nhs.uk — MB ChB Glas. 1984 (Univ. Glas.) BSc (Hons.) Glas. 1981, MB ChB 1984; MRCP (UK) 1987; MRCPath 1993; FRCP Glas. 1997; FRCPath 2001. Cons. Haemat. Glas. Roy. Infirm. Specialty: Haematology.

TAIT, Sheila Angela Elizabeth 66 Bells Burn Avenue, Linlithgow EH49 7LB Tel: 01506 840181 — MB ChB Aberd. 1992; DRCOG 1995; MRCGP 1996. GP. Specialty: Gen. Pract. Socs: BMA. Prev: Clin. Research Phys. Inveresk Clin. Research Edin.; GP Princip. Kingsgate Med. Centre Bathgate; GP Regist. S. Qu.sberry Health Centre.

TAIT, Sheila Kathleen Springbank Surgery, York Road, Green Hammerton, York YO26 8BN Fax: 01423 331433; Carlton Farm, Nun Monkton, York YO26 8EJ — MB ChB Aberd. 1976; MRCOG 1981; MRCGP 1985.

TAIT, Timothy John Department of Rheumatology, Grimsby Hospital, Scartho Road, Grimsby DN33 2BA Tel: 01472 874111 Fax: 01472 875483; Burwell Manor, Burwell, Louth LN11 8PR — MB BS Lond. 1987; BSc Lond. 1984; MRCP (UK) 1991. Cons. Rheum. Grimsby Hosp. Specialty: Rehabil. Med.; Rheumatol. Prev: Sen. Regist. (Rheum) York Dist. Hosp.

TAIT, Mr William Finlayson North Manchester General Hospital, Crumpsall, Manchester M8 6RL — MB ChB Glas. 1978; FRCS Eng. 1982; MD Glas. 1986. Specialty: Gen. Surg. Prev: Regist. (Surg.) Hope Hosp. Salford; Regist. (Surg.) Stepping Hill Hosp. Stockport & Wythenshawe Hosp. Manch.; Research Fell. Univ. Dept. Surg. Univ. Hosp. S. Manch.

TAIT, William Miller (retired) 79 Shaftesbury Avenue, Blackpool FY2 9TT Tel: 01253 592052 — (Glas.) MB ChB Glas. 1957; DObst RCOG 1961; DA S. Afr. 1978. Prev: Med. Advsr War Pens. Agency Norcross Blackpool.

TAIT, Winifred Beech House, Beech Avenue, Hazel Grove, Stockport SK7 4QR Tel: 0161 483 6222; 54 Ladythorn Road, Bramhall, Stockport SK7 2EY Tel: 0161 439 1343 — MB ChB Aberd. 1959.

TAIT, Winifred Anne Regional Infectious Diseases Unit, Western General Hospital, Crewe Road, Edinburgh EH4 2XU Tel: 0131 537 2855 Fax: 0131 537 2878 — MB BChir Camb. 1979; MRCPsych 1985; Mem., Scott. Assn. of Psychoanalytical Psychotherapists 1993. Cons. Psychiat. Regional Infec. Dis. Unit. West. Gen. Hosp. Edin. Specialty: Gen. Psychiat. Prev: Sen. Regist. (Psychiat.) Roy. Edin. Hosp.

TAIWO, Mr Claudius Bola 4 Chestnut Avenue, Gainsborough DN21 1EU — MB BS Ibadan 1980; MB BS Ibadan, Nigeria 1980; FRCS Ed. 1988; FRCS Eng. 1989. Hosp. Surg. (Gen. Surg.) John Coupland Hosp. GainsBoro. Specialty: Gen. Surg. Socs: FICS; Med. Defence Union. Prev: Tutor (A & E) Univ. Leeds.

TAJUDDIN, Meraj Leicester Frith Hospital, Groby Road, Leicester LE3 9QF Tel: 0116 225 5273 Fax: 0116 225 5272 Email: meraj.tajuddin@leicspart.nhs.uk; 58 Wheatfield Close, Glenfield, Leicester LE3 8JD Tel: 0116 287 5259 — MB BS Lond. 1993 (St Barts) BSc 1986; MRCPsych 2002. Specialist Regist. And Honourary Lecturer (Psychiat. & Learning Disabil.) Leicester Frith Hosp. Specialty: Gen. Psychiat.

TAK, Abdul Momin 24 Sunley Gardens, Perivale, Greenford UB6 7PE — MB BS Kashmir 1987.

TAKEDA, Scott 6 Missenden Close, Bedfont Lane, Feltham TW14 9XN — MB BS Lond. 1992.

TAKES, Hendricka Margaret The Karis Medical Centre, Waterworks Road, Edgbaston, Birmingham B16 9AL Tel: 0121 454 0661 Fax: 0121 454 9104; The Vicarage, Sycamore Road, Aston,

Birmingham B6 5UM — MB ChB Birm. 1985; DRCOG 1988; MRCGP 1989.

TAKEUCHI, Elena Erina Flat4 holly Grange, 66-68 Northenden Road, Sale M33 3HA Tel: 0161 2861064 Email: etakeuchink@yahoo.com — MB ChB Manch. 1998.

TAKHAR, Amrit Pal Singh Wansford Surgery and Kings Cliffe Practice, Yarwell Road, Wansford, Peterborough PE8 6PL Tel: 01780 782342 Fax: 01780 783434; Springfield House, 21 Roman Drive, Stibbington, Peterborough PE8 6LL Tel: 01780 783575 Fax: 01780 784088 Email: amrit@btinternet.com — MB ChB Birm. 1983 (Birmingham) BSc (Hons.) Birm. 1980; DCH RCP Lond. 1986; DRCOG 1986; MRCGP 1987. Specialty: Gen. Pract.

TAKHAR, Baldeep 32 Grovewood Hill, Coulsdon CR5 2EL — MB ChB Manch. 1990; DCH RCP Lond. 1993; DRCOG 1994; DFFP 1994. GP Tutor Nottm. Univ. Specialty: Gen. Pract. Prev: SHO (Psychiat.) Derby City Hosp.; Trainee GP Purley; SHO (Paediat.) N. Middlx. Hosp.

TAKHAR, Gurpreet Singh 130 Princes Gardens, London W3 0LL — MB BS Lond. 1989; BSc (Immunol.) Lond. 1986; MRCGP 1993; MBA (INSEAD) 1994. Director of World-wide Business Developm. GlaxoSmithKline; Ex-Internat. Off. BMA Assoc. Gp. Comm.; Vis. Fac. Imperial Coll. Health; Managem. Progr.. Specialty: Pharmaceutical Medicine. Socs: Roy. Coll. of Gen. Practitioners. Prev: Trainee GP St. Bart. Lond. VTS.

TAKHAR, Kuljeet 7 Parkway, Uxbridge UB10 9JX — MB ChB Dundee 1997.

TAKTAK, Mr Sabah George 7 Broomgrove Gardens, Edgware HA8 5SH Tel: 020 8951 3871 — MB ChB Baghdad 1959; LMSSA Lond. 1969; FRCS Ed. 1979. Regist. (Orthop.) Lister Hosp. Stevenage. Specialty: Orthop. Prev: Regist. (Orthop.) W. Lond. Hosp., Roy. North. Hosp. Lond. & Roy. Free; Hosp. Lond.

TAKYI, Alfred 30 Cadewell Park Road, Torquay TQ2 7JU Tel: 01803 615171; 11Cadewell Park, Clayhall, Ilford IG5 0JL Tel: 020 8550 6354 — MUDr Charles Univ. Prague 1971; MUDr Charles U. Prague 1971; Dip. Postgrad. Cert. Psychiat. Budapest 1985. SCMO (Psychiat.) Newham Health Care Trust Lond. Specialty: Gen. Psychiat. Socs: Fell. Roy. Soc. Med. Prev: Staff Grade (Psychiat.) Newham Healthcare Trust Lond.; Clin. Asst. (Psychiat.) Torquay; Regist. (Psychiat.) Dorchester & Lincoln & Torquay.

TALAT, Mahe The Surgery, 49 Tottenham Lane, Hornsey, London N8 9BD — MB BS Sind 1969 (Liaquat Med. Coll.) Prev: SHO (Gen. Med.) Moyle Hosp. Larne; Trainee GP Whitehead Health Centre.

TALATI, Freni (retired) 392 Southcroft Road, London SW16 6QX Tel: 020 8677 2614 — MB BS Bombay 1950 (Grant Med. Coll.) BSc Bombay 1944.

TALATI, Mr Vrandavan Ratilal Chesterfield Royal Hospital, Chesterfield Tel: 01246 77271 — MB BS Gujarat 1963 (B.J. Med. Coll. Ahmedabad) MS Gujarat 1967, MB BS 1963; DLO Eng. 1973; FRCS Ed. 1977. Cons. ENT Surg. Chesterfield Roy. Hosp. Specialty: Otolaryngol. Prev: Sen. Regist. (ENT) Hallamsh. Hosp. Sheff.; Sen. Regist. (ENT) Leicester Roy. Infirm.; Regist. (ENT) Bradford Roy. Infirm.

TALAVLIKAR, Prakash Hari 59 The Ridgeway, Chatham ME4 6PB Tel: 01634 43466 — MD Bombay 1964 (Grant Med. Coll.) MB BS 1962; FRCP Ed. 1986, M 1968. Cons. Phys. c/o Elderly N. Kent Healthcare NHS Trust. Specialty: Care of the Elderly. Socs: Roy. Soc. Med.; Brit. Geriat. Soc. & Indian Cardiol. Soc. Prev: Regist. (Med.) St. Bart. Hosp. Rochester & (Cardiac) West. Gen. Hosp. Edin.; Sen. Regist. (Geriat. Med.) Univ. Hosp. S. Manch.

TALBERT, Alison Wendy Audrey Mvumi Hospital, PO Box 32, Mvumi, Dodoma, Tanzania; c/o 28 Pine Grove, Eccles, Manchester M30 9JL — MB BS Lond. 1983; BA (Hons.) Physiol. Sci. Oxf. 1980; MRCP (UK) 1986. Miss. Doctor Mvumi Hosp. Tanzania. Specialty: Trop. Med.; Paediat. Prev: SHO Hosp. Trop. Dis. Lond.; Ho. Phys. Lond. Hosp.; Ho. Surg. Amersham Gen. Hosp.

TALBOT, Alison Jane Tilehurst Surgery, Tylers Place, Pottery Road, Tilehurst, Reading RG30 6BW Tel: 0118 942 7528 Fax: 0118 945 2405 — BM Soton. 1986; MRCGP 1990; DCH RCP Lond. 1990; DRCOG 1990. Specialty: Dermat.

TALBOT, Andrew William East House, 38 St John's Avenue, Bridlington YO16 4NG Tel: 01262 401921 Fax: 01262 400161 — MB ChB Leeds 1982 (Univ. Leeds) MRCPsych 1987. Cons. Psychiat. Bridlington & Dist. Hosp. N. Humberside. Specialty: Geriat. Psychiat. Prev: Sen. Regist. (Psychiat.) W. Midl. RHA; Tutor (Psychiat.) Univ. Leeds; Regist. Rotat. Leeds Train. Scheme.

TALBOT, Mr Clifford Heyworth (retired) Moorlands Farm, Moorlands Lane, Froggatt, Calver, Hope Valley S32 3ZH Tel: 01433 631876 — MB BChir Camb. 1948 (Camb. & Guy's) MA Camb. 1950, MChir 1957, MB BChir 1948; FRCS Eng. 1953. Prev: Cons. Surg. Roy. Hallamsh. Hosp. Sheff.

TALBOT, Mr David 84 Woodbine Road, Gosforth, Newcastle upon Tyne NE3 1DE — MB BS Newc. 1982; MD Newc. 1988; FRCS Ed. 1989; PhD Newc. 2000. Cons. Surg. Freeman Hosp. Newc. u. Tyne. Specialty: Transpl. Surg. Socs: Eur. Soc. Organ Transpl.; Eur. Liver Transpl. Assn.; Assoc. Mem. Brit. Assn. Paediat. Surgs. Prev: Hon. Sen. Lect. Surg. Univ. Newc.; Sen. Regist. (Renal Transpl.) Newc. u. Tyne; Vis. Fell. Hepatobiliary Unit Qu. Eliz. Hosp. Birm.

TALBOT, Deborah 48 Chesterfield Road, Lichfield WS13 6QW — MB ChB Birm. 1998.

TALBOT, Denis Charles University of Oxford, ICRF Medical Oncology Unit, Churchill Hospital, Headington, Oxford OX3 7LJ Tel: 01865 226183 Fax: 01865 226179; 33 Butts Road, Horspath, Oxford OX33 1RJ Tel: 01865 87542 — MB BChir Camb. 1981; BSc Liverp. 1974; PhD Lond. 1978; MA Camb. 1983; MRCP (UK) 1985; MA Oxf. 1996; FRCP Lond. 1996. Cons. Med. Oncol. Oxf. HA & Imperial Cancer Research Fund; Sen. Clin. Lect. Univ. Oxf. Specialty: Oncol. Socs: Assn. Cancer Phys.; Amer. Soc. Clin. Oncol.; Amer. Assn. Cancer Research. Prev: Sen. Regist. (Med.) Roy. Marsden Hosp. Lond. & Sutton; Regist. (Med. Oncol.) St. Bart. & Homerton Hosp. Lond.; Regist. (Gen. Med.) Newmarket Gen. Hosp.

TALBOT, Mr Ernest Mark Eye Department, Royal Preston Hospital, Sharoe Green Lane, Preston PR2 9HT; 38 Higher Bank Road, Fulwood, Preston PR2 8PE — MB ChB Dundee 1980; DOphth Dub. 1983; FRCS Ed. 1985; FRCOphth 1988. Cons. Ophth. Roy. Preston Hosp.; Hon. Sen. Lect. Univ. Centr. Lancs. Specialty: Ophth. Prev: Sen. Regist. Tennent Inst. Glas.; Regist. & SHO (Ophth.) St. Paul's Eye Hosp. Liverp.

TALBOT, Heather 94 Ashdell Road, Sheffield S10 3DB Tel: 0114 266 0404 — (Roy. Free) MRCS Eng. LRCP Lond. 1967; MB BS Lond. 1967; DObst RCOG 1969; DA Eng. 1972; FFA RCS Eng. 1977. Assoc. Specialist (Anaesth.) Roy. Hallamsh. Hosp. Sheff. Specialty: Anaesth. Prev: Regist. (Anaesth.) Nottm. City Hosp.

TALBOT, Professor Ian Charles Academic Department of Pathology, St. Mark's Hospital, Northwick Park, Watford Road, Harrow HA1 3UJ Tel: 020 8235 4220 Fax: 020 8235 4277 Email: i.talbot@doctors.org.uk; 34 Belitha Villas, London N1 1PD — MB BS Lond. 1964 (King's Coll. Hosp.) MRCPath 1971; MD Lond. 1979; FRCPath 1983. Cons. Histopath. St. Mark's Hosp.; Prof. Histopath. Imperial Coll. Sch. Med. Specialty: Histopath. Special Interest: Gastroenterol.; Gastro-intestinal and tumour Path. Socs: Brit. Soc. Gastroenterol.; Fell. Roy. Soc. Med.; Path. Soc. of GB & Ireland. Prev: Reader Univ. Leicester & Hon. Cons. Pathol. Leics. HA; Sen. Lect. (Morbid Anat.) King's Coll. Hosp. Med. Sch. Lond.; Regist. (Morbid Anat.) Hammersmith Hosp. Lond.

TALBOT, Joanna Louise Rock House, New Road, Penkridge, Stafford ST19 5DN — MB BCh Wales 1994.

TALBOT, Mr John FitzRoy Eye Department, Royal Hallamshire Hospital, Glossop Rd, Sheffield S10 2JF — MB BS Lond. 1970; MRCS Eng. LRCP Lond. 1970; FRCS Eng. 1978; FRCOphth 1988. Cons. Ophth. Roy. Hallamsh. Hosp. Sheff.; Hon. Sen. Lect. Sheff. Univ. Med. Sch.; Treasurer Roy. Coll. of Ophths. Specialty: Ophth. Prev: Sen. Regist. Moorfields Eye Hosp.; Lect. Inst. Ophth.

TALBOT, John Michael Bicester Health Centre, Coker Close, Bicester OX26 6AT Tel: 01869 249333 Fax: 01869 320314; The Barn House, Souldern, Bicester OX27 7JP Tel: 01869 345555 — BM BCh Oxf. 1968; MA, BM BCh Oxf. 1968; DObst RCOG 1974; FRCGP 1997, M 1977. Prev: Regist. Dept. Paediat. & Child Health Univ. Cape Town Red Cross Hosp.; Cape Town S. Africa; Ho. Phys. & Surg. Radcliffe Infirm. Oxf.; SHO Accid. Serv. United Oxf. Hosps.

TALBOT, John Michael (retired) 3 Whitegates Close, Canns Lane, Hethersett, Norwich NR9 3JG Tel: 01603 811709 — MB BS Lond. 1945 (King's Coll. Hosp.) MD Lond. 1952; Dip. Bact. Lond. 1952; FRCPath 1968, M 1963. Prev: Med. Dir. Priscilla Bacon Lodge (Palliat. Care Unit) Norwich.

TALBOT, John Storey Trehafod, Waurnarlydd Road, Sketty, Swansea SA2 0GB Tel: 01792 582139 Fax: 01792 585220 — MB ChB Liverp. 1978; MRCS Eng. LRCP Lond. 1978; MRCPsych 1983.

Cons. Child & Adolesc. Psychiat. Child & Family Clinic Port Talbot.; Vis. Cons. Psychiat. to Hillside Secure Unit, Neath. Specialty: Child & Adolesc. Psychiat. Socs: Chairm. Div. Psychiat. Swansea; Welsh Regional Represen. Child & Adolesc. Psychiat., Roy. Collgege of Psychiat.s. Prev: Sen. Regist. (Child & Adolesc. Psychiat.) Alder Hey Hosp. Liverp. & Young People's Centre Countess of Chester Hosp.; Regist. (Psychiat.) Roy. Liverp. Hosp.

TALBOT, John Stuart Salford Trafford HA, Peel House, Albert St., Eccles, Manchester M30 0NJ Tel: 0161 787 0128 — MB ChB Manch. 1965; DObst RCOG 1969; MRCGP 1976. Med. Adviser Salford & Trafford HA.

TALBOT, Kevin Andrew Radcliffe Infirmary, University Department of Clinical Neurology, Woodstock Road, Oxford OX2 6HE Tel: 01865 224310 Fax: 01865 790493 Email: kevin.talbot@clneuro.ox.ac.uk — MB BS Lond. 1990 (Char. Cross & Westm.) BSc Lond. 1989; MRCP (UK) 1993; DPhil (Oxon) 1999. MRC/GSK Clin.Sci. Fell, Oxford Uni, Dept Human Anat.& Genet.; Hon. Cons. Neurologist. Specialty: Neurol. Prev: Hon. Regist. (Clin. Neurol.) Radcliffe Infirm. Oxf.; Med. Research Counc. Clin. Train. Fell. (Genetics) Univ. Oxf.; SHO Hammersmith Hosp. & Nat. Hosp. for Neurol. & Neurosurg. Lond.

TALBOT, Mark Shoghi New Cross Hospital, Royal Wolverhampton Hospitals, Wolverhampton WV10 0QP — MB BS Lond. 1990; MRCP (UK) 1995.

TALBOT, Martin David Royal Hallamshire Hospital, Glossop Road, Sheffield S10 2JF — MB ChB (Hons. Distinc. Pharmacol. & Obst. & Gyn.) Liverp. 1972; Liverp. 1972; MRCP (UK) 1976; FRCP Lond. 1989; MEd (Medical Educ.) Sheff. 1999. Cons. Phys. (Genitourin. Med.) Roy. Hallamshire Hosp. Sheff.; Hon. Sen. Clin. Lect. Univ. Sheff. Specialty: Genitourinary Medicine; HIV Med. Socs: Assn. Med. Educat.; Assn. Humanistic Psych.; Brit. Assn. Sexual Health & HIV. Prev: Dir. Undergrad. Med. Educat. Sheff. Teachg. Hosps.; Sub-Dean Fac. Med. Univ. Sheff.; Ho. Phys. Liverp. Roy. Infirm.

TALBOT, Mr Nicholas John The Old Dairy, Fore St., Silverton, Exeter EX5 4HP Tel: 01392 861344 — BM BCh Oxf. 1994; BA (Hons.) Oxf. 1991; FRCS (Eng) 1998. SpR (Orthop. & Trauma) Dorryfaro Hosp., Plymouth. Specialty: Trauma & Orthop. Surg. Prev: Senior SHO (Orthop. & Trauma) Newsgrove Park, Taunton; SpR (Orthop. & Trauma) N. Devon Dist. Hosp., Barnstaple; SHO Rotat. (Surg.) Roy. Devon & Exeter Hosp.

TALBOT, Paul Richard Department of Neurology, Greater Manchester Neuroscience Centre, Hope Hospital, Stott Lane, Salford M6 8HD Email: paul.talbot@srht.nhs.uk; Heath Barn, The Heath, Glossop SK13 7QF Email: paultalbot@doctors.org.uk — MB ChB Manch. 1987 (Manchester) MRCP (UK) 1990; MD 1996; FRCP (UK) 2002. Cons. Neurol. - Greater Manch. Neurosci. Unit, Hope Hosp., Salford. Specialty: Neurol. Special Interest: Multiple Sclerosis. Socs: Assn. Brit. Neurol. Prev: Sen. Regist. (Neurol.) Manch. Roy. Infirm.; Research Fell. (Neurol.) Manch. Roy. Infirm.; Regist. (Neurol.) N. Manch. Gen. Hosp.

TALBOT, Mr Peter Albert James Talbot, Ward, Seery and Ahmad, Gardenia Surgery, 2A Gardenia Avenue, Luton LU3 2NS Tel: 01582 572612 Fax: 01582 494553; 355 Old Bedford Road, Luton LU2 7BL — MB ChB Liverp. 1972; FRCS Ed. 1977; MRCGP 1988. Prev: Regist. (Gen. Surg.) Whiston Hosp. Prescot Merseyside; Regist. (Orthop.) Roy. South. Hosp. Liverp.

TALBOT, Mr Robert William Poole General Hospital, Longfleet Road, Poole BH15 2 Tel: 01202 675100; 1 Beaucroft Road, Wimborne BH21 2QW Tel: 01202 887579 Fax: 01202 442615 — MB BS Lond. 1974 (King's Coll. Hosp.) FRCS Eng. 1978; MS Lond. 1984; T(S) 1991. Cons. Gen. Surg. Poole Gen. Hosp. Specialty: Gen. Surg. Socs: Fell. Roy. Soc. Med.; Assoc. of ColoProctol. Prev: Vis. Scientist Mayo Clinic Rochester, USA; RSO St. Marks Hosp. Lond.

TALBOT, Ruth Mary The Grange, The Street, Waltham St. Lawrence, Reading RG10 0JJ — BA Camb. 1978, MB BChir 1981; DCH RCP Lond. 1983; MRCPsych 1987. Indep. Cons. Child and Adolesc. Psychiat. Specialty: Child & Adolesc. Psychiat. Prev: Cons. Child & Adolesc. Psychiat. Merton Child Guid. Serv. Mitcham.; Sen. Regist. (Child Psychiat.) St. Geo. Hosp. Lond.; SHO & Regist. (Rotat.) (Psychiat.) St. Geo. Hosp. Tooting.

TALBOT, Sarah 22 Newberry Road, Weymouth DT4 8LW — BM BCh Oxf. 1997.

TALBOT, Stephen Laurel Farm, Pitney, Langport TA10 9AF Tel: 01458 252266 — MB BS Lond. 1963 (Guy's) MRCS Eng. LRCP Lond. 1963; DRCOG 1965; MRCP Lond. 1966; BA (Hons.) Open 1993. Indep. Phys. Som. Specialty: Cardiol. Socs: BMA; Med. Protec. Soc. Prev: Sen. Regist. Sheff. HA & Hammersmith Hosp. Lond.; Regist. Qu. Eliz. Hosp. Birm.; Regist. MusGr. Pk. Hosp. Taunton.

TALBOT-SMITH, Alison Jane — MB BS Newc. 1993.

TALEB, Sidi Mohammed Taleb and Partners, The Surgery, Burton Road, Swadlincote DE11 7JG Tel: 01283 217036 Fax: 01283 552308 — MRCS Eng. LRCP Lond. 1976.

TALERMAN, Harold Joseph 152 Harley Street, London W1G 7LH Tel: 020 7935 8868 — MB BCh Witwatersrand 1959; DO RCPSI 1968; DO Eng. 1968. Clin. Asst. Moorfields Eye Hosp. Lond. Specialty: Ophth. Socs: Ophth. Soc. UK. Prev: Cons. Eye Surg. Provin. Hosp. & Livingstone Hosp. Port. Eliz., S. Afr.

TALKHANI, Mr Imtiyaz Suleman 1 Osborne Cottage, Highfield, Wrexham LL11 4US — MB BS Karnatak 1986; FRCS Glas. 1992.

TALLACH, Cameron Rowanlea, 5A Upper Breakish, Breakish, Isle of Skye IV42 8PY — MB ChB Aberd. 1968. Hon. Tutor (Family Medicine) Chinese Univ. of Hong Kong. Socs: Hong Kong Med. Soc. & Hong. Kong Coll. Gen. Pract.

TALLACH, James Ross Free Presbyteriam Manse, Isle of Raasay, Kyle IV40 8PB Tel: 01478 660216 Fax: 01478 660216; Free Presbyteriam Manse, Isle of Raasay, Kyle IV40 8PB Email: jamesross@tallach.fsnet.co.uk — MB ChB Aberd. 1967. GP Raasay. Socs: Brit. Med. Assoc. Prev: Med. Off. Mbuma Mission Hosp. Nkai, Zimbabwe.

TALLACK, Fenella Evelyn Riverside Substance Misuse Service, 69 Warwick Road, London SW5 Tel: 020 8846 7777 — MB Camb. 1983; MA Camb. 1984, MB 1983, BChir 1982; MRCPsych 1990. Staff Grade Team Dir. Subst. Misuse Community Team Riverside HA. Socs: BMA. Prev: Regist. (Psychiat.) Kingston Gen. Hosp.; SHO (Psychiat.) PeterBoro. Dist. Hosp.; SHO (Psychiat.) Roy. Edin. Hosp.

TALLACK, John Aidan Machaon, Swallows Cross, Brentwood CM15 0SS Tel: 01277 353206 Email: atallack@fsmail.net — (Aberd.) MB ChB Aberd. 1949. Disabil. Analyst Chelmsford Med. Examinations Centre. Specialty: Civil Serv.; Gen. Med. Socs: Fell. Med. Soc. Lond.; (Ex-Div. Pres.) BMA. Prev: Assoc. Specialist Phys. OldCh. & Rush Green Hosps. Romford.; Enfield.

TALLANT, Neil Peter Barn Surgery, Christchurch Medical Centre, Purewell Cross Road, Christchurch BH23 3AF Tel: 01202 486456 Fax: 01202 486678; 84 Walcott Avenue, Christchurch BH23 2NG Tel: 01202 479856 — BM Soton. 1983; MRCGP 1987; DRCOG 1987. GP. ChristCh..; Clin. Asst. Thoracic Med. Bournemouth Gen. Hosp. Prev: Trainee GP I. of Wight VTS.

TALLANTYRE, Helen Myfanwy Espley Cottage, Espley, Morpeth NE61 3DJ — MB ChB Sheff. 1997.

TALLANTYRE, Patricia Margaret The Gables Health Centre, 26 St. Johns Road, Bedlington NE22 7DU Tel: 01670 829889 Fax: 01670 820841; Espley Cottage, Espley, Morpeth NE61 3DJ Tel: 01670 513396 — MB BChir Camb. 1967 (Camb. & St. Thos.) BA Camb. 1964. Specialty: Gen. Pract. Socs: BMA. Prev: SHO Essex Co. Hosp. Colchester; SHO (Paediat.) Flemming Memor. Hosp. Newc.; SHO (O & G) Princess Mary Matern. Hosp. Newc.

TALLENT, David Neill The Medical Suite, Renaissance Hotel Gatwick, Gatwick Airport, Horley RH6 0BE Tel: 01293 776996 Fax: 01293 823 6498; 26 Grasslands, Smallfield, Horley RH6 9NU Tel: 01342 844952 Email: david.tallent@btinternet.com — MB ChB Sheff. 1981; MRCGP 1989; DAvMed FOM RCP Lond. 1992; AFOM RCP Lond. 1995. Aviat. Med. Off. Civil Aviat. Auth. Gatwick. Specialty: Aviat. Med.; Occupat. Health. Prev: Company Aeromed. Specialist Dan-Air Serv. Ltd. Horley.

TALLENTS, Mr Christopher John, TD Eye Department, Kidderminster General Hospital, Bewdley Road, Kidderminster DY11 6RJ Tel: 01562 823424 Fax: 01562 513062; The White Cottage, Kinlet, Bewdley DY12 3BD Tel: 01299 841238 Fax: 01299 841482 — MB BS Lond. 1964 (Middlx.) BSc (Hons.) Lond. 1961; DO Eng. 1967; FRCS Eng. 1969; LMCC 1973. Cons. Ophth. Kidderminster Gen. Hosp. Specialty: Ophth. Socs: BMA. Prev: Sen. Regist. (Ophth.) King's Coll. Hosp. Lond.; Regist. (Ophth.) Sussex Eye Hosp.; SHO (Ophth.) Leeds Gen. Infirm.

TALLETT, Paul Ronald Inwoods Farm, Five Ashes, Mayfield TN20 6JA — MB BS Lond. 1976 (King's Coll. Hosp.) DRCOG 1978; FRCR 1982. Cons. (Radiol.) Kent & Sussex Hosp. & Nuffield Hosp. Tunbridge Wells. Specialty: Radiol.

TALLIS, Patricia Mary Child Adolescent Mental Health Service, Bristol Royal Hospital for Children, Paul O'Gorman Building, Upper Maudlia St., Bristol BS2 8BJ — MB ChB Liverp. 1988 (Univ. Liverp.) MRCPsych 1994. Sen. Regist. (Child & Adolesc. Psychiat.) Bristol. Specialty: Child & Adolesc. Psychiat. Prev: Regist. Rotat. (Psychiat.) Liverp. Train. Sch.; SHO Rotat. (Psychiat.) Liverp. VTS.

TALLIS, Professor Raymond Courtenay University of Manchester, Clinical Sciences Building, Hope Hospital, Eccles Old Road, Manchester M6 8HD Tel: 0161 787 7164 Fax: 0161 206 5722; 5 Valley Road, Bramhall, Stockport SK4 2BZ Tel: 0161 439 2548 — BM BCh Oxf. 1970 (Oxf. & St Thos.) FRCP Lond. 1988, M 1976; Dlitt Hull 1997; LittD Manch. 2002. Prof. Geriat. Med. Univ. Manch.; Hon. Cons. Phys. (Geriat. Med.) Salford Roy. Hosps. NHS Trust; Vis. Prof. St Geo. Hosp. Med. Sch. Specialty: Care of the Elderly. Special Interest: Epilepsy; Stroke. Socs: Sec. 1942 Club; Fell. Acad. Med. Sci. Prev: Sen. Lect. (Geriat. Med.) Roy. Liverp. Hosp.; Clin. Research Fell. Wessex Neurol. Centre.

TALLON, Grainne Mary 111 Ballylenaghan Park, Primrose Hill, Belfast BT8 6WR; 111 Ballylenaghan Park, Primrose Hill, Belfast BT8 6WR — MB BCh BAO Belf. 1994; MRCP (Glasgow) 1999.

TALLON, Julian Griffith John Mitchell and Partners, The Park Surgery, Old Tetbury Road, Cirencester GL7 1UX Tel: 01285 654733 Fax: 01285 641408 — MB BCh Wales 1985; DCH RCP Lond. 1991. Community Paediat. E. Wilts. Specialty: Gen. Pract. Socs: BMA. Prev: Trainee GP Stroud, Glos.; SHO (Paediat.) E. Glam. Hosp. Pontypridd; Dep. Doctor Melbourne, Austral.

TALLURI, Satish Chandra c/o Dr P.B. Gopal, Department of Anaesthesia, Darlington Memoral Hospital, Holyhurst Road, Darlington DL3 6HX — MB BS Andhra 1984; MRCPI 1993.

TALMUD, Juli Clair 26 Richborough Road, London NW2 3LX — MB ChB Leeds 1998.

TALPUR, Hyder Ally Hanford Health Clinic, New Inn Lane, Hanford, Stoke-on-Trent ST4 8EX Tel: 01782 658047; 3 Sark Close, Newcastle ST5 3LN — MB BS Sind 1970 (Liaquat Med. Coll. Hyderabad) ECFMG Cert. 1976; MRCP (UK) 1982; Cert. Prescribed Equiv. Exp. JCPTGP 1983; FRCPE 1998. Socs: Local Med. Comm.; N. Staffs Docks Corp. Prev: Regist. & SHO (Geriat. Med.) City Gen. Hosp. Stoke-on-Trent; SHO (Chest Med.) Halifax Gen. Hosp.

TALUKDER, Ranadhir High Street Medical Centre, High St, Winsford CW7 2AS Tel: 01606 862767 Fax: 01606 550876; 3 Partridge Close, Swanlow Park, Over, Winsford CW7 1PY Tel: 01606 861618 — (Chittagong Med. Coll. Dacca) MB BS Univ. Dacca 1967; DTM & H Eng. 1975; LRCP LRCS Ed. LRCPS Glas. 1979. Socs: N.wich Med. Soc.; BMA; Overseas Doctors Assn. Prev: Regist. (Gen. Med.) Leeds Gen. Infirm.; Regist. (Gen. Med.) Scunthorpe Gen. Hosp.; SHO (Gen. Med.) Bishop Auckland Gen. Hosp.

TALUKDER, Mr Shyam Benode c/o Dr S. D. Ghosh, Flat 2, Singleton Hospital, Sketty, Swansea SA2 8QA — MB BS Calcutta 1960; DLO RCS Eng. 1967; FRCS Ed. 1971.

TALWAR, Meenakshi — MB BS Lond. 1994 (Univ. Coll. Lond.) MRCPCH. SpR St. George's Hosp. Paediatric Dept Blackshaw Rd. Lond. Prev: SHO Chelsea & Westm. Hosp. Lond.

TALWAR, Sandeep 8 Yeading Avenue, Harrow HA2 9RN — BM Soton. 1987. Specialty: Cardiol.; Gen. Med.

TALWAR, Suneel Leicester Royal Infirmary, Infirmary Square, Leicester LE1 5WW Tel: 0116 254 1414 — MB BS New Delhi 1991; MRCP Ed. 1996.

TALWATTE, Beatrice Yuletine 7 Highview Gardens, Finchley, London N3 3EX Tel: 020 8346 4574 — MB BS Ceylon 1960 (Colombo) DPH Eng. 1968; DTM & H Eng. 1972; DPM Eng. 1974. Regist. & Assoc. Specialist (Psychiat.) Harperbury Hosp. Shenley. Specialty: Gen. Psychiat. Prev: Med. Off. Outpat. Dept. Gen. Hosp. Colombo, Ceylon; Sch. Med. Off. Ceylon; Med. Off. (Matern. & Child Health) Kandy, Ceylon.

TALWATTE, Dhesa Bandu Bandare 7 High View Gardens, Finchley, London N3 3EX — MB BS Ceylon 1958 (Colombo) DA Eng. 1968; DObst RCOG 1968; FFA RCS Eng. 1972. Cons. Anaesth. N. Middlx. Hosp. Lond. Specialty: Anaesth. Socs: Ceylon Med. Assn. Prev: Cons. Anaesth. St. Albans City Hosp. & Gen. Hosp. Kandy, Ceylon; Sen. Regist. (Anaesth.) Roy. Free Hosp. Lond.

TAM, Barbara Sau Man 61 Alma Court, Bristol BS8 2HJ — MB ChB Bristol 1992.

TAM, Darwin Belmont Health Centre, 516 Kenton Lane, Kenton, Harrow HA3 7LT Tel: 020 8427 1213; 11 Ridgeway Court, 1 The Avenue, Hatch End, Pinner HA5 4UT — MB BCh Wales 1990; DRCOG 1994; DCH RCP Lond. 1994; MRCGP 1995. GP Princip.

TAM, Frederick Wai-Keung Renal Unit, Imperial College School of Medicine, Hammersmith Hospital, Du Cane Road, London W12 0NN Tel: 020 8740 3152 Fax: 020 8383 2062; 43 Cotswold Gardens, London NW2 1QT — MB BChir Camb. 1985; MA Camb. 1986, BA 1982; MRCP (UK) 1987; PhD Lond. 1996. Sen. Research Fell. Nat. Kidney Research Fund. Specialty: Nephrol.; Gen. Med. Prev: MRC Train. Fell.; Regist. Rotat. (Med.) Hammersmith & Hillingdon Hosps. Lond.; SHO (Neurol.) St. Jas. Univ. Hosp. Leeds.

TAM, Nicolette Lai Kay Kewins, Newtons Hill, Hartfield TN7 4DH Tel: 01892 770231; 83 Middle Way, Summertown, Oxford OX2 7LE Tel: 01865 511726 — BM BCh Oxf. 1998. HO. (Gen Med.) Milton Keynes Gen Hosp. Specialty: Immunol.; Endocrinol.; Diabetes. Socs: MDU; BMA; Med. Sickness. Prev: HO.(Gen Surg.) John Radcliffe Hosp. Milton Keynes.

TAM, Philip Gordon Emmanuel 28 Montgomerie Terrace, Skelmorlie PA17 5DT — MB BS Lond. 1996.

TAM, Thomas Chris Flat 11 Straffon Lodge, 1 Belsize Grove, London NW3 4XE — MB ChB Leic. 1993.

TAM, Wing Kwong Majumder, Roy and Tam, Greenock Health Centre, 20 Duncan Street, Greenock PA15 4LY Tel: 01475 724477 Fax: 01475 727140 — MD Shantung Christian U 1947. GP Greenock, Renfrewsh.

TAMALE SSALI, Mr Edward Gasterfson 66 Park Hall Road, London SE21 8BW — MB ChB Makerere 1974 (Makerere Med. Sch. Kampala) MRCS Eng. LRCP Lond. 1977; MRCOG 1982, D 1979; FRCS Ed. 1982. Cons. O & G Kuwait Oil Co. Specialty: Obst. & Gyn. Prev: Regist. (O & G) Scarsdale Hosp. Chesterfield; SHO (Gyn.) Newton Abbot Hosp. Devon; SHO (O & G) Nottm. Hosp. Wom.

TAMBAR, Mr Balvir Krishan Burnley District Hospital, Barnsley — MB BS Delhi 1966 (Maulana Azad Med. Coll. New Delhi) FRCS Eng. 1974. Regist. (Gen. Surg.) Barnsley Dist. Gen. Hosp. Specialty: Gen. Surg. Prev: Regist. (Urol.) Ballochmyle Hosp. Mauchline; SHO (Gen. Surg.) Leicester Gen. Hosp. & W. Wales Gen. Hosp.; Carmarthen.

TAMBIAH, Jeymi 28 Wykeham Hosp, Chaucer Place, Off North Rd, Wimbledon, London SW19 1HU Email: j.tambiah@ic.ac.uk — MB ChB Manch. 1993; BSc (Hons.) St. And. 1990; FRCS 1993; FRCS 1998. SHO (Intens. Care) Qu. Mary's Hosp. Sidcup; Research Regist. (Vasc. Surg.) Char Cross. Lond. Specialty: Intens. Care. Prev: SHO.(Cardio Surg.) St Thomas Hosp. Lond.

TAMBYRAJA, Andrew Laksman 58 Heron Drive, Lenton, Nottingham NG7 2DF — BM BS Nottm. 1998; BM BS Nottm 1998.

TAMIMI, Nihad Asad Mohammad Kent & Canterbury Hospital, Ethelbert Road, Canterbury CT1 3NG Tel: 01227 766877 Fax: 01227 783073; 24 Cowdrey Place, Canterbury CT1 3PD Tel: 01227 785932 — MB BS Punjab 1982; MRCP (UK) 1991; MSc Cantab. 1998. Assoc. Specialist (Renal Med.) Kent & Canterbury Hosp.; Mem. Jordanian Med. Counc. Specialist Regist. Specialty: Nephrol. Socs: Eur. Renal Assn.; Brit. Renal Assn. Prev: Research Regist. (Renal) Canterbury; Regist. (Renal) Canterbury; Regist. (Renal) Kuwait.

TAMIN, Jacques Sin Fat, TD Interact Health Management, Port of Liverpool Building, Pier Head, Liverpool L3 2AN Tel: 0151 224 1400 Fax: 0151 224 1401 Email: Jacques.Tamin@interacthealth.co.uk; 10 Leicester Road, Sale M33 7DU Tel: 0161 905 2024 — MB ChB Manch. 1980; DRCOG 1983; MRCGP 1984; Dip. Pract. Dermat. Wales 1990; MFOM RCP Lond. 1994, AFOM 1991; LLM Univ. Wales 1993; FFOM 2001. Med. Director and Chief Occupational Phys., Interact Health Managem.; Cons. Occupat. Health Ciba Specialty Chem. UK; Gp. Occupational Phys., Ciba Specialty Chemicals UK Ltd. Specialty: Occupat. Health. Special Interest: Work-related stress risk assessments. Socs: Soc. Occupat. Med. & Medichem.; Chairm. Soc. of Occupat. Med., N.W. Gp. Prev: Cons. Occupat. Health Salford Community Healthcare Trust; Cons. Occupat. Health Ashworth Hosp.; Clin. Asst. (Occupat. Health) N. Manch. HA.

TAMIN, Sylvio Kin Fat 8 Fern Avenue, Flixton, Manchester M41 5RZ Tel: 0161 746 9579 — MB ChB Manch. 1983. Med. Adviser Schlumberger-Sema Med. Servs.; Occupational Phys. Interact

Health Managem. Ltd. Specialty: Pharmaceutical Medicine. Prev: Clin. Asst. Antenatal Clinic Tameside.; Clin. Research Phys. Medeval Ltd. Univ. Manch.

TAMIZIAN, Onnig Derby City Hospital, Uttoxter Rd, Derby DE22 3NE Tel: 01332 340131; 27 Balmoral Drive, Bramcote Hills, Nottingham NG9 3FU Tel: 0115 925 8371 — BM BS Nottm. 1993; BMSc (1st cl. Hons.) Nottm. 1991. SHO.(Geriats.) Roy Vic Hosp. Edin. Specialty: Gen. Pract. Prev: Specialist Regist. (O & G) Mid Trent Rotat.; Ho. Off. (Med.) Nottm. City Hosp.; Ho. Off. (Surg. & Gyn.) Qu. Med. Centre Nottm.

TAMKIN, Elaine Jean Springfield House, New Lane, Patricroft, Manchester M30 7JE — MB ChB Manch. 1976.

TAMKIN, William Patrick Borcharot Medical Centre, 62 Whitchurch Road, Withington, Manchester M20 1EB Tel: 0161 445 7475 Fax: 0161 448 0466 — MB ChB Manch. 1976; MRCGP 1983; MMedSc (Gen. Pract.) Leeds 1987.

TAMLYN, Geoffrey William (retired) Lancaster House, Springfield Road, Chelmsford CM2 6BP Tel: 01245 357457 — MB BS Lond. 1954 (St. Bart.) DObst RCOG 1956; DA Eng. 1959; MRCGP 1971; BA Open 1996. Prev: Med. Off. New Hall Sch.

TAMLYN, Gregory John The Witterings Health Centre, Cakeham Road, East Wittering, Chichester PO20 8BH Tel: 01243 673434 Fax: 01243 672563 — MB BS Lond. 1978 (Guy's) DRCOG 1981; MRCGP 1986.

TAMLYN, Roger Stanley Pelham, MBE Warren House, 1 Leven Avenue, Talbot Woods, Bournemouth BH4 9LH Tel: 01202 766493 Mob: 07850 506971 — MB BS Lond. 1966 (King's Coll. Hosp.) FRCA; MRCS Eng. LRCP Lond. 1965; FFA RCS Eng. 1977. On sabbatical. Specialty: Anaesth.; Intens. Care. Socs: BMA; Assn. Anaesth. Prev: Sen. Cons. & Head Dept. Anaesth. Resusc. Qu. Eliz. Hosp. Lond.; QHS (Qu.'s Hon. Surg.) / Cons. Anaesth. Frimley Pk. Hosp. / Head (Anaesth.) Roy. Hosp. Haslar Gosport 1996-99; Head (Anaesth. / Resusc. & Intens. Care) Qu. Eliz. Hosp. Lond.

TAMMA, Mr Suryanarayana Goodhope Hospital, Rectory Road, Sutton Coldfield B75 7RR Tel: 0121 378 2211; 3 Clark Way, Heston, Hounslow TW5 9EG — MB BS Berhampur 1977; FRCS Ed. 1987.

TAMMES, Bruin (retired) 14 Fitzjohn's Avenue, London NW3 Tel: 020 7435 1840 — MB ChB Ed. 1957.

TAMPI, Suresh Chandran 1 Millars Croft, Adlington St., Macclesfield SK10 1BD — MB BS Madras 1973 (Jawaharlal Inst. Postgrad. Med. Pondicherry) Staff Surg. (A & E) Macclesfield Dist. Gen. Hosp. Specialty: Accid. & Emerg.

TAMPIYAPPA, Tennent Nirushan 22 Harwood Avenue, Bromley BR1 3DU — MB BS Lond. 1994.

TAMS, Jonathan Tang Hall Surgery, 190 Tang Hall Lane, York YO10 3RL Tel: 01904 411139 Fax: 01904 431224; Church End House, Cow Catton, York YO41 1EA Tel: 01759 372777 — MB ChB Dundee 1976; MRCGP 1982. Trainer (Gen. Pract.) York VTS.

TAN, Anton Tiauw-Lok 85 Highfield S., Birkenhead CH42 4ND — State Exam Med Dusseldorf 1987.

TAN, Boon Bing University Hospital of North Staffordshire, Department of Dermatology, Central Outpatients, Hantshill Road, Stoke-on-Trent ST4 7PA — MB BS Lond. 1987; FRCP; MRCP (UK) 1991. Cons. Dermatol. Univ. Hosp. of N. Staffs. Stoke-on-Trent. Specialty: Dermat. Special Interest: Occupational Dermatitis. Socs: RCP.

TAN, Carol 3 Vyvyan Ter, Bristol BS8 3DF — MB ChB Bristol 1997.

TAN, Chin Yau The Birmingham Skin Centre, Sheldon Block, City Hospital NHS Trust, Dudley Road, Birmingham B18 7QH Tel: 0121 554 3801 Fax: 0121 507 6644 — MB BS Malaysia 1972; MRCP (UK) 1978; FRCP Lond. 1994. Cons. Dermat. Birm. Skin Centre City Hosp. NHS Trust; Hon. Cons. Dermat. Dent. Hosp. Birm.; Hon. Sen. Clin. Lect. Univ. Birm. Specialty: Dermat. Socs: BMA & Brit. Assn. Dermat. Prev: Sen. Regist. (Dermat.) N. Staffs. Hosp. Centre Stoke-on-Trent; Clin. Research Off. Welsh Nat. Sch. Med. Cardiff; Regist. (Dermat.) Univ. Hosp. Wales Cardiff.

TAN, Garry Daniel 18 Wragby Close, Bury BL8 1XD — MB ChB Manch. 1993; MRCP (UK) 1996; DTM & H Lond. 1997. Specialty: Diabetes; Endocrinol.; Gen. Med.

TAN, Jin Yeow Royal London Hospital, Department of Histopathology, Whitechapel, London E1 1BB Tel: 020 7377 7000 — BSc (Hons.) Lancaster 1990; MMedSci Sheff. 1992; MD AUC, Montserrat 1996; LRCP Lond. 1998; LMSSA Lond. 1998; LRCS Eng. LRCP Lond. 1998. Specialist Regist. (Histopath.) Lond. Deanery N. Thames E. Rotat. Specialty: Histopath. Socs: Fell. RSM; BMA; Trainee Mem. Roy. Coll. Path. Prev: SHO (Histopath.) Leics. Roy. Infirm.; SHO (Ophth.) N. Middlx. Univ. Hosp. Lond.; SHO (Ophth.) Princess Alexandra Hosp. Harlow.

TAN, John Bu Leong Quarter Jack Surgery, Rodways Corner, Wimborne BH21 1AP Tel: 01202 848262 Fax: 01202 882368 — MB ChB Bristol 1985; FRCSI 1992; MRCGP 1993; DRCOG 1994; DFFP 1995. Prev: Trainee GP Bournemouth; SHO (Obst, & Gyn.) Poole; SHO (Paediat.) Yeovil.

TAN, Ju Le 16 Radcliffe Road, Croydon CR0 5QE — MB BS Newc. 1993; MRCP. 1996. SHO (Med.) S. Cleveland Hosp. Specialty: Cardiol. Prev: Adult Congen. Heart Dis. Fell. Roy. Bromton Hosp. (2003-2004); Assoc. Cons. Cardiol., Nat. Heart Centre, Singapore (2003); Cardiol. Regist. Rotat. Nat. Heart Centre, Singapore (1999-2002).

TAN, Kai Lee 4 Clearwater Way, Lakeside, Cardiff CF23 6DJ — MB BCh Wales 1993 (Univ. Wales Coll. of Med.) MBA Wales 1996; MRCP 1999. Regist. (Med.) E. Glam. Gen. Hosp. Specialty: Gen. Med. Prev: SHO (Med.) Princess of Wales Hosp. Bridgend; SHO (Med.) Caerphilly Dist. Miner's Hosp.

TAN, Kathryn Choon Beng 4 Wilde Place, Palmers Green, London N13 6DU — MB BCh Wales 1984; MRCP (UK) 1987.

TAN, Kay-Sin Department of Neurology, Pinderfields General Hospital, Wakefield WF1 4DG — MB BS Melbourne 1994 (Melbourne, Australia) Dip. Med. Lond 1996; MRCP (UK) 1997. Specialist Regist. (Neurol.) Pinderfields Gen. Hosp. Wakefield. Specialty: Neurol. Socs: Roy. Coll. Phys. Edin.; Liverp. Med. Inst.; Univ. Melbourne Med. Soc. Prev: SHO Rotat. (Med.) Roy. Liverp. Univ. Hosp.

TAN, Kee Sun Holywood Arches Health Centre, Westminster Avenue, Belfast BT4 1NS Tel: 028 9056 3354 Fax: 028 9065 3846; 17 Massey Avenue, Belfast BT4 2JT Tel: 01232 760200 — MRCS Eng. LRCP Lond. 1968. Specialty: Gen. Pract.

TAN, Kelvin Hiang-Vee 20 Bruce Street, Cardiff CF24 4PJ — MB BCh Wales 1993.

TAN, Khor Heng 91 Travellers Way, Bath Road, Hounslow TW3 — MB BS Queensland 1965; MRCOG 1973. Prev: Regist. (O & G) Eliz. G. Anderson Hosp. Lond.; Ho. Off. Paediat., Gen. Surg. & O & G Govt. Hosps. Singapore.

TAN, Kia Meng Lister II, Plaistow Hospital, Samson Street, Plaistow, London E13 9EH Tel: 020 8586 6419 Fax: 020 8586 6420 Email: meng.tan@newhampct.nhs.uk — MB ChB Glas. 1982 (Univ. Glas.) FRCPCH; MRCP (UK) 1987; MSc Lond. 1991. Cons. Paediat. (Community Child Health) Newham Primary Care Trust. Specialty: Community Child Health.

TAN, Kim-Heung 309 Cinnamon Wharf, Shad Thames, London SE1 2YJ — MB BS Lond. 1986 (Middlx. Hosp. Med. Sch.) MRCP (UK) 1989; MD Lond. 1995. Sen. Regist. (Cardiol.) Guy's Hosp. Lond. Specialty: Cardiol. Socs: Brit. Cardiac Soc.

TAN, Ko Yih Flat 10, 6 Riverview Place, Glasgow G5 8EB — MB ChB Ed. 1994.

TAN, Kristinn Siew-Wei 11 Grays Lane, Downley, High Wycombe HP13 5TZ — MB ChB Sheff. 1998.

TAN, Kuok Chuin Eddie 5 Hinchin Brook, Lenton, Nottingham NG7 2EF — BM BS Nottm. 1997.

TAN, Mr Lam Chin Queen Elizabeth Hospital, Edgbaston, Birmingham B15 2TH Tel: 0121 472 1311 Email: lamchin.tan@uhb.nhs.uk — MB ChB Ed. 1987; FRCS Ed. 1992; MD 2001; FRCS (Gen. Surg.) 2002. cons. Surg. Renal & Laprascopic Univ. Hosp. Birm. NHS Trust. Specialty: Gen. Surg. Special Interest: Laparoscopic Surg. (Advanced); Renal Transpl. Prev: SpR (Renal Transpl.) Portmouth Hopsitals NHS Trust; SpR (Renal Transpl.) Oxf. Radcliffe NHS Trust; SpR (Gen. Surg.) Wessex Region.

TAN, Lan Aik Rectory Road Surgery, 41 Rectory Road, Hadleigh, Benfleet SS7 2NA Tel: 01702 558147 — MB BS Lond. 1988. Regist. Rotat. (O & G) Whipps Cross Hosp., St. Bart. & Homerton Hosp. Lond. Specialty: Obst. & Gyn. Prev: SHO (O & G) Chelsea & Westm. Hosp. & Univ. Coll. Hosp. Lond.

TAN, Li Tee Oncoloy Centre, Addenbrooke's NHS Trust, Hills Road, Cambridge CB2 2QQ Tel: 01223 216555 Fax: 01223 216589 — MB BS Lond. 1985 (Charing Cross and Westm.) MRCP (UK) 1988; FRCR 1992. Cons. Clin. Oncol. Addenbrooke's NHS Trust Camb.;

Cons. Clin. Oncol. Hinchingbrooke Hospm Huntingdon, Cambs.; Cons. Cli. Oncol. PeterBoro. Dist. Gen. Hosp.. Specialty: Oncol.; Radiother.

TAN, Lip-Bun Leeds General Infirmary, Molecular Vascular Medicine, G-Floor Martin Wing, Leeds LS1 3EX Tel: 0113 392 5401 Fax: 0113 932 5395 — MB BChir Camb. 1980 (Oxf. & Camb.) DPhil Oxf. 1977, BSc (Hons.) 1973; MRCP (UK) 1983; FESC 1994; FRCP Lond. 1995. Brit. Heart Foundat./Mautner Sen. Lect. (Cardiovasc. Med.) Univ. Leeds; Hon. Cons. Cardiol. Gen. Infirm. & St Jas. Univ. Hosp. at Leeds. Specialty: Cardiol.; Research. Special Interest: Assessm. of cardiac reserve; Cardiac myocyte apoptosis; End-stage heart failure. Socs: Past Sec. Brit. Assn. of Cardiac Rehabil. Prev: Lect. (Cardiovasc. Med.) John Radcliffe Hosp. Oxf.; MRC Trav. Fell. Cardiovasc. Inst. Michael Reese Hosp. Chicago, USA; Regist. (Cardiol.) E. Birm. Hosp.

TAN, Michael Chor Soon Flax Centre, Ardoyne Avenue, Belfast BT14 7AD; 7 Avonvale, Circular Road, Belfast BT4 2WA — MB BCh BAO Belf. 1986; DCH Dub. 1989; MRCGP 1990.

TAN, Mr Michael Meng Say 3 Acres Brook Road, Higham, Burnley BB12 9BY — MB ChB Glas. 1982; FRCS Ed. 1994; FFAEM 1999.

***TAN, Nicholas Chien Lee** 10 Chatham Street, London SE17 1NY Email: drnicktan@yahoo.com — MB BS Lond. 1998 (UMDS of Guy's and St. Thomas's) BSc (Hons) Lond. 1995; MB BS Lond 1998. PRHD Surg., Guy's Hosp. Specialty: Gen. Surg.

TAN, Patrick Swee Teong Marcham Road Family Health Centre, Marcham Road, Abingdon OX14 1BT Tel: 01235 522602 Email: patrick.tan@gp-k84041.nhs.uk — BM BCh Oxf. 1992 (Oxford) DCH RCP Lond 1994; DRCOG 1995; MRCGP 1996. Specialty: Gen. Pract.

TAN, Peng Hong Montrose, 3 Hendon Avenue, London N3 1UL Tel: 020 8349 4861 Fax: 020 8343 0694 Email: p.tan@imperial.ac.uk — MB BS Lond. 1995 (St Mary's) MRCS 1999; DIC (Immunol.) Lond. 1999; MSc (Immunol.) Lond. 1999; PhD (Path.) Lond. 2004. SpR in Gen. Surg. (Oxford Deanery). Specialty: Gen. Surg. Socs: Soc. of Acad. and Research Surg.; Europ. Gene Ther. Soc.; Brit. Soc. of Immunol. Prev: Clin. Fell. Surg. Addenbrookes Camb.; Clin. Research Fell. Transpl. Immunol. Hammersmith Hosp.; SHO (Vasc. Surg.) St. Marys Hosp. Lond.

TAN, Mr Peter — BM Soton. 1989; FRCS Eng. 1993. Cons (Surg. Vasc.) Doncaster & Bassetlaw Hosps. NHS Trust Doncester. Specialty: Vasc. Med. Prev: SHO Rotat. (Surg.) York Dist. Hosp.

TAN, Robert Seng-Hoon Orleigh Mount, St. Stephens Road, Lansdown, Bath BA1 5PN Tel: 01225 313488 — MB Camb. 1965 (St. Thos.) BChir 1964; MA Camb. 1969; FRCP Lond. 1983, M 1969. Cons. Dermatol. Roy. United Hosp. Bath. Specialty: Dermat. Prev: Sen. Regist. (Dermat.) Westm. Hosp. Lond.; Regist. (Dermat.) St. Thos. Hosp. Lond.; Regist. (Med.) Poole Gen. Hosp.

TAN, Professor Seang Lin Department of Obstetrics & Gynaecology, McGill University, Royal Victoria Hospital, Women's Pavilion, 687 Pine Avenue West, Montreal H31 1A1, Canada Tel: 00 1 514 8431658 Fax: 00 1 514 8431678; The London Women's Clinic, 113/115 Harley St, London W1G 6AP Tel: 0207 487 5050 Fax: 0207435 5850 — MB BS Singapore 1977; MMed (Obst. & Gyn.) Singapore 1982; FRCOG 1995, M 1983; T(OG) 1991; FRCSC 1995. James Edmund Dodds Prof. & Chairm. Dept. Obst. & Gyn. McGill Univ. & Obst. & Gyn. in Chief Roy. Vict. Hosp. Montreal, Canada. Specialty: Obst. & Gyn. Socs: Fell. Roy. Soc. Med.; Amer. Fertil. Soc.; Eur. Soc. Human Reproduc. & Embryol. Prev: Cons. & Sen. Lect. (Obst. & Gyn.) King's Coll. Sch. Med. & Dent. Lond.; Sen. Research Fell. Dept. Obst. & Gyn. King's Coll. Sch. Med. & Dent. Lond.; Sen. Regist. Kandau Karbau Hosp., Singapore.

TAN, Sen Hean 217 Gammons Lane, Watford WD24 5JJ — MB BCh BAO NUI 1966.

TAN, Shani 37 Mount Pleasant Road, Brondesbury Park, London NW10 3EG Tel: 020 8459 3680; 70 Fernhill Road, Singapore 1025, Singapore — MB BS Singapore 1982; FFA RCS Eng. 1988. Hon. Sen. Regist. Hosp. for Sick Childr. Lond.; Clin. Teach. (Anaesth.) Fac. Med. Nat. Univ. Singapore. Socs: Singapore Soc. Anaesthesiol. Prev: Sen. Regist. (Anaesth.) Singapore Gen. Hosp.; Regist. (Anaesth.) Hammersmith Hosp. Lond.

TAN, Si-Yen 23 Buttermere Drive, London SW15 2HW — MB ChB Ed. 1984; MRCP (UK) 1987; MD Ed. 1996. Cons. Nephrol. King's Coll. Hosp. Lond. Specialty: Nephrol. Socs: Eur. Dialysis & Transpl. Assn.; Internat. Soc. Nephrol.; Renal Assn. Prev: Sen. Regist. & Hon. Lect. (Renal) Hammersmith Hosp. Lond.; Research Fell. & Hon. Sen. Regist. Hammersmith Hosp. Lond.; Regist. (Renal) Roy. Infirm. Edin.

TAN, Sil Yee c/o Dr Peter Godfrey, Charlotte Keel Health Centre, Seymore Road, Easton, Bristol BS5 0UA; PO Box 44, Seri Complex 2600, Brunei Darussalam — MB ChB Bristol 1991.

TAN, Simon 47 Vista Road, Clacton-on-Sea CO15 6DG — MB BS Lond. 1994.

TAN, Stella Veronica Su-Ming Neuromuscular Unit, Department of Neurology, Charing Cross Hospital, London W6 8RF — MB BS Lond. 1986; BSc (Infec. & Immunity, 1st cl. Hons.) Lond. 1983, MB BS 1986; MRCP (UK) 1989. Research Regist. (Neurol.) Char. Cross & Chelsea & Westm. Hosps. Lond. Specialty: Neurol. Prev: Regist. (Neurol.) Atkinson Morley's Hosp. Lond.

TAN, Su-Yen 481C Holloway Road, London N19 4DD — MB ChB Manch. 1996.

TAN, Susern Flat 4, 377 Crookesmoor Road, Sheffield S10 1BD — MB ChB Sheff. 1994.

TAN, Swee Wan Elm Lodge, 64 Elm Grove, London SE15 5DE Tel: 020 8692 2209 — MB BS Lond. 1964 (St. Thos.) DObst RCOG 1969.

TAN, Wee Ming Westgate Practice, Greenhill Health Centre, Church St., Lichfield WS13 6JL; 30 Peak Close, Thirlmere Park, Armitage, Rugeley WS15 4TY — MB ChB Sheff. 1989. Trainee GP Lichfield VTS. Prev: SHO (Gen. Med.) Burton Gen. Hosp.

TAN, Yan Mei Darlington Memorial Hospital, Hollyhurst Road, Darlington DL3 6HX Tel: 01325 380100; 12 Lorong 14/37B, Petaling Jaya, Selangor 46100, Malaysia Tel: 01 06 03 7560096 — MB ChB Glas. 1990; MRCP (UK) 1994. SHO Darlington Memor. Hosp. S. Durh. HA. Prev: SHO Castle Hill Hosp. E. Yorks. HA.

TAN ENG LOOI, Carolyn 22 Downsview Road, London SE19 3XB — MB BS Malaya 1980; FRCS Ed. 1985; FRCS Glas. 1985.

TAN HARK HONG, Kenneth Department of Paediatrics, Rotherham District General Hospital, Moorgate Road, Rotherham S60 2UD — MB BS Melbourne 1991.

TAN PHOAY LAY, Christina The Health Centre, 120 Bedford Hill, Balham, London SW12 9HS Tel: 020 8673 1720 — MB BS Lond. 1985 (Lond. Hosp.) DRCOG 1989; MRCGP 1993. Prev: SHO (O & G) The Lond. Hosp.

TAN TONG KHEE, Dr Ilford Cottage, Clifton St., Laugharne, Carmarthen SA33 4QG — MB BS Singapore 1986; FFA RCSI 1995. Specialty: Anaesth.

TANDAY, Jashpal Singh The Thorndike Centre, Longley Road, Rochester ME1 2TH Tel: 01634 817217 — MB BCh Wales 1975; DRCOG 1978; MRCGP 1980. GP Tutor Medway.

TANDON, Anand Prakash Calderdale Royal Hospital, Salterhebble, Halifax HX3 0PW Tel: 01422 224231 Fax: 01422 224471; Heath Lodge, Heath Lane, Halifax HX3 0BZ Tel: 01422 369960 — MD (Med.) Lucknow 1968, MB BS 1964; MRCP (UK) 1973; FRCP Lond. 1988. Cons. Cardiol., Calderdale Roy. Hosp.; Clin. Dir. Acute Med. Specialty: Cardiol. Socs: Brit. Cardiac Soc. & Brit. Pacing & Electrophys. Gp. Prev: Tutor (Med.) Univ. Leeds; Sen. Regist. (Cardiol.) Leeds Gen. Infirm.; Cons. Phys. & Cardiol. Roy. Halifax Infirm. & Halifax Gen. Hosp.

TANDON, Bhaskar 4 Deene Close, Grimsby DN34 5XB — MB BS Delhi 1969.

TANDON, Dinesh Kumar 19 Locksley Close, Stockport SK4 2LW — MB BS Lucknow 1966 (G.S.V.M. Med. Coll. Kanpur) DA Eng. 1973.

TANDON, H P Penketh Health Centre, Honiton Way, Penketh, Warrington WA5 2EY Tel: 01925 725644 Fax: 01925 791017 — MB BS Vikram 1963; MB BS Vikram 1963.

TANDON, Kopal 4 The Drive, Longton, Preston PR4 5AJ — BM BCh Oxf. 1997.

TANDON, Mr Mahendra Kishore Frimley Park Hospital, Portsmouth Road, Frimley, Camberley GU16 7UJ Tel: 01276 692777; 5 Orchard End, Rowledge, Farnham GU10 4EE Tel: 01252 794452 — DO FRC (Ophth.)(K.G.M. Coll. Lucknow) 1963 (K.G.M. Coll. Lucknow) MB BS Lucknow 1963; FRCS Ed. (Ophth.) 1976. Cons. Ophth. Surg. Frimley Pk. Hosp. & Farnham Hosp. Specialty: Ophth. Prev: Regist. (Ophth.) Centr. Middlx. Hosp. Lond.; Out-Pat. Off. Moorfields Eye Hosp. Lond.; Sen. Regist (Ophth.) Kent Co. Ophth.& E. Grinstead Hosp., Maidston.

TANDON, Naresh Kumar 161 Woodlands Road, Sparkhill, Birmingham B11 4ER — MB ChB Dundee 1993.

TANDON, Pradip Kumar Tandon, 71 Grove Road, Wallasey CH45 3HF Tel: 0151 639 4616 Fax: 0151 637 0182; 18 Woodbank Park, Oxton, Birkenhead CH43 9WN Tel: 0151 652 7659 Fax: 0151 637 0182 — MB BS Lucknow 1969; DTM & H Liverp. 1980. Community Paediat. Merseyside; Med. Adviser, Wirral Unified Housing. Specialty: Gen. Pract. Socs: (Dep. Treas.) Overseas Doctors Assn.; BMA. Prev: SCMO Manch.

TANDON, R Tandon, 71 Grove Road, Wallasey CH45 3HF Tel: 0151 639 4616 Fax: 0151 637 0182 — (Kanpur, India) MB BS 1970; DCH 1971; Dip Ven. Liverpool 1993. Specialty: Genitourinary Medicine; Paediat.

TANDON, Mr Roop Kishore New Cross Hospital, The Royal Wolverhampton Hospitals NHS Trust, Wolverhampton WV10 0QP Tel: 01902 642965; 17 Addisland Court, Holland Villas Road, London W14 8DA Tel: 020 7603 6667 Mob: 07790 825983 — MB BS Andhra Univ. India 1961; FRCS Royal Coll. Of Surgeons, Edin. 1970. Hon. Lect. Dept of Primary Care & Population Sciences, UCL & The Roy. Free Hosp, Lond.; Hon. Lect. In Med. Education, Barts & The Lond. Queen Mary's School of med. & Dentistry, Lond. Specialty: Orthop. Socs: Mem. Of Med. Protection; Mem. Naughton Dunn Orthopaedic Club; Sen. Mem. Brit. Orthop. Assn. Prev: Regist. Heatherwood Hosp. Ascot & Roy. Postgrad. Med. Sch. Hammersmith Hosp. Lond.

TANDON, Sankalap 14 Squirrel Way, Loughborough LE11 3GP — BM BS Nottm. 1998; BM BS Nottm 1998.

TANDON, Sneh Lata Rochester Health Centre, Delce Road, Rochester ME1 2EL Tel: 01634 401111; 127 Wilson Avenue, Rochester ME1 2SL Tel: 01634 812064 — MB BS Lucknow 1966 (G.S.V.M. Med. Coll. Kanpur) BSc, MB BS Lucknow 1966. Family Plann. Assn. & IUCD Instruc. Prev: Trainee GP Brent & Harrow VTS; SHO (Surg.) Ulster Hosp. Belf.; SHO (O & G) P. of Wales Gen. Hosp. Lond.

TANDON, Mr Subash Chander Royal Hospital, Cleveland Road, Wolverhampton Tel: 01902 307999; 6 Rowallane Close, Bangor BT19 7SS Tel: 01247 274508 — MB BCh BAO Belf. 1988; FRCSI 1992. Regist. (Orthop.) Roy. Hosp. Wolverhampton. Specialty: Orthop. Socs: BMA & Brit. Orthop. Assn. Prev: SHO (Cas.) E. HB; Ho. Off. Belf. City Hosp.

TANDON, Urmila Rani 161 Woodlands Road, Sparkhill, Birmingham B11 4ER — MB ChB Leic. 1994.

TANDY, Andrew David Department of Child Health, Musgrove Park Hospital, Taunton TA1 5DA Tel: 01823 342690 Fax: 01823 333 6877 — MB BS Lond. 1981 (Univ. Coll. Hosp.) BSc (Hons.) Lond. 1978; DRCOG 1983; MRCGP 1985; DCH RCP Lond. 1985; MRCP (UK) 1990; T(GP) 1991; T(M) (Paediat.) 1993; FRCPCH 1997. Cons. Paediat. Taunton & Som. Hosp. Specialty: Paediat. Socs: BMA; SW Paediat. Club; Brit. Assn. Community Child Health. Prev: Lect. & Hon. Sen. Regist. (Child Health) Univ. Nottm.; Regist. Roy. United Hosp. Bath; Ho. Phys. Univ. Coll. Hosp. Lond.

TANDY, George Graham Byways, Stockswell Road, Hough Green, Widnes WA8 — MRCS Eng. LRCP Lond. 1952 (Liverp.)

TANDY, Jane Catherine 17 Poyner Close, Prices Lodge, Fareham PO16 7YQ — MB ChB Ed. 1983; MRCP (UK) 1986. Cons. c/o Elderly Qu. Alexandra Hosp. Portsmouth. Specialty: Care of the Elderly.

TANEGA, Kara Rosemary McKenna Ferryview Health Centre, 25 John Wilson Street, Woolwich, London SE18 6PZ Tel: 020 8319 5400 Fax: 020 8319 5404 — MB BS Lond. 1988.

TANEJA, Anil Kumar C/o 30 Aycliffe Road, London W12 DLL Email: a.taneja@rbh.nthames.nhs.uk — MB BS Poona 1986. Clin. Research Fell. (Cardiol.). Specialty: Cardiol.; Gen. Med.; Occupat. Health. Special Interest: Cardiol.

TANEJA, Ashok West End Clinic, West End Lane, Rossington, Doncaster DN11 0PQ Tel: 01302 865865 Fax: 01302 868346 — MB BS Delhi 1981; MRCGP 1991.

TANG, Alan Leong Fai The Florey Unit, Royal Berkshire Hospital, Reading RG1 5AN Tel: 0118 987 7205 Fax: 0118 987 7211 Email: alan.tang@rbbh-tr.nhs.uk — MB BS Lond. 1983 (King's Coll.) Dip. GU Med. Soc. Apoth. Lond. 1988; FRCP 1996; DFFP 1996. Cons. Phys. Genitourin. Med. Roy. Berks. Hosp. Reading; Vis. Cons., HMYOI & RC Reading, Forbury Rd, Reading. Specialty: Genitourinary Medicine; Acupunc.; HIV Med. Socs: BMA (Hon. Sec. W. Berks. Div.).; Brit. HIV Assn. Exec. Comm. Mem. Prev: Cons. Phys. Genitourin. Med. Greenwich Dist. Hosp. Lond.; Sen. Regist. (Gen. & Genitourin. Med.) St. Thos. Hosp. Lond.; SHO (Med.) Whittington Hosp. Lond.

TANG, Mr Augustine Tak-Ming Dept. of Cardiothoracic Surgery, Southampon General Hospital, Tremona Rd, Southampton SO16 6YD Tel: 02380 777222 — BM BS Nottm. 1990; BMedSci (Hons.) Nottm. 1988; FRCS Ed. 1994; DM Nottm. 1998. Specialist Regist. (Cardiol Surg.) Wessex.; Hon Surg Research Fell. Liverp. Univ. Hosps. NHS Trust. Specialty: Cardiothoracic Surg. Socs: Soc. Of Cardiothoracic Surg.s of GB & Irel.; Europ. Assn. For Cardiothoracic Surg.; Cardiac Surgic. Research Club. Prev: Brit. Heart Foundat. Research Fell. (Cardiothoracic Surg.) Manch. & Liverp.

TANG, Bruce Yew Wai Annfield Medical Centre, 16 Annfield Place, Glasgow G31 2XE Tel: 0141 554 2989 Fax: 0141 550 3965; 9 Sandfield Avenue, Milngavie, Glasgow G62 8NR Tel: 0141 956 6270 — MB ChB Dundee 1984; DRCOG 1990; MRCGP 1990.

TANG, Carol Pui-Yi 128 Lauriston Road, London E9 7LH — MB BCh Wales 1998. Specialty: Accid. & Emerg.

TANG, Carol Wei Man 37 High Street, Cricklade, Swindon SN6 6AY — MB BCh Wales 1997 (University of Wales College of Medicine) GP VTS Princess of Wales Hosp. Bridgend. Specialty: Gen. Med.; Diabetes; Endocrinol. Prev: Pre-Regist. Ho. Off. E. Glam. Hosp. Ch. Village & Glan Clwyd Hosp. Bodelwyddan Rhyl.

TANG, Christopher Yeong Kee 97 Waterloo Road, Romford RM7 0AA — MRCS Eng. LRCP Lond. 1971.

TANG, Mr Daniel Tung Shing 9 Browgate, Sawley, Clitheroe BB7 4NB Fax: 01200 440374 Email: dtang007@aol.com — MB ChB Sheff. 1982; FRCS Ed. 1991. Cons. Orthop. Surg. Airedale Gen. Hosp. W. Yorks.; Cons. Orthopaedic Surg., Abbey Gisburne Pk. Hosp., Clitheroe. Specialty: Trauma & Orthop. Surg. Special Interest: Shoulder Surg. Socs: Fell. Brit. Orthop. Assn.; Brit. Trauma Soc.; Brit. Med. Assn.

TANG, Dannis Wing Kuen Suite 5, Egmont House, 116 Shaftesbury Avenue, London W1D 5EW — MB ChB Sheff. 1984 (Sheffield) MRCP Paediat. (UK) 1987; DRCOG 1990; DCH RCPS Glas. 1992; MD Sheffield 1997. Research Fell. Qu. Charlotte's & Chelsea Hosp. Lond. Specialty: Neonat.

TANG, Joseph Gordon 11 Malcolm Drive, Surbiton KT6 6QS — BChir Camb. 1987.

TANG, Kare Hung Colchester General Hospital, Department of Medicine, Turner Road, Colchester CO4 5JL Tel: 01206 742219; 7 Hedgelands, Copford, Colchester CO6 1YT — BM Soton. 1991.

TANG, Kim Man Morrill Street Health Centre, Morrill Street, Holderness Road, Hull HU9 2LJ Tel: 01482 323398 Fax: 01482 217957 — MB ChB Manch. 1980.

TANG, Kwok Hung 172 Balgores Lane, Gidea Park, Romford RM2 6BS — MB ChB Ed. 1991; MRCP (UK) 1995. Specialist Regist. Rotat. (Gastroenterol.) S. Thames Region. Specialty: Gastroenterol.

TANG, Sek Cheung 79 Brim Hill, London N2 0EZ — MB BS Lond. 1978; MRCS Eng. LRCP Lond. 1978.

TANG, Siu Cheung 28A Egerton Road, Hartlepool TS26 0BW — MB BS Hong Kong 1977; T(S) 1991.

TANG, Sui Yuen 2 Foreman Place, Merthyr Tydfil CF47 0EJ — MB BS Lond. 1998.

TANG, Wing Yu 9 Triscombe Drive, Llandaff, Cardiff CF5 2PN — MB BCh Wales 1998.

TANG, Yew Cheen Salcombe Gardens, 8 Salcombe Gardens, Mill Hill, London NW7 2NT Tel: 020 8959 6592 Fax: 020 8959 0112 — BM Soton. 1982.

TANG, Yuen-Tsang Katherine 26 Woodberry Way, London N12 0HG — MB BS Hong Kong 1956.

TANG, Yuet Yee Mary Orchard Surgery, Christchurch Medical Centre, Purewell Cross Road, Christchurch BH23 5ET Tel: 01202 481902 Fax: 01202 486887 — MB ChB Manch. 1991 (Univ. Manch.) MRCGP 1996.

TANGANG, Vivian Ngwu Flat 10, Emmanuel House, Distin St., London SE11 6QL — MB BS Lond. 1997.

TANGNEY, David Joseph High Street Surgery, 1st Floor, 97-101 High Street, Fort William PH33 6DG Tel: 01397 703773 Fax: 01397 701068 — MB BCh BAO NUI 1985.

TANGRI, Arun Kumar Riverlyn Medical Centre, Station Road, Bulwell, Nottingham NG6 9AA Tel: 0115 975 2666 Fax: 0115 927 9555; 37 Gunnersbury Way, Nuthall, Nottingham NG16 1QD Tel:

0115 975 4323 — MB BS Poona 1975 (Armed Forces Med. Coll. Poona, India) MRCS Eng. LRCP Lond. 1989.

TANGRI, Charu Derby Royal Infirmary, London Road, Derby DE1 2QY; 37 Gunnersbury Way, Nuthall, Nottingham NG16 1QD Tel: 0115 975 4323 — MB BS Delhi 1979; DO RCPSI 1985; LRCP LRCS Ed. LRCPS Glas. 1986. Staff Grade (Psychiat.) Derby Roy. Infirm.

TANGYE, Sheila Royse (retired) 89 Lonsdale Road, Barnes, London SW13 9DA Tel: 020 8748 4574 — BM BCh Oxf. 1943 (Oxf. & Bristol) MA Oxf. 1947, DM 1951; DCH Eng. 1947, DPM 1960; MRCPsych 1971. Prev: Cons. Psychiat. Roy. Albert Hosp. Lancaster.

TANKEL, Mr Henry Isidore, OBE (retired) 26 Dalziel Drive, Glasgow G41 4PU Tel: 0141 423 5830 Fax: 0141 424 3648 — (Univ. Glas.) MB ChB (Commend.) Glas. 1948; FRCS Ed. 1954; MD (Commend.) Glas. 1958; FRFPS Glas. 1962. Cons. Surg. Glas. Prev: Cons. Surg. South. Gen. Hosp. Glas.

TANKEL, Jeremy William Lanceburn Health Centre, Clarendon Surgery, Churchill Way, Salford M6 5QX Tel: 0161 736 4529 Fax: 0161 736 2724 — MB ChB Glas. 1979; FRCS Glas. 1983; MRCGP 1986; DMJ 1998. Partner Gen. Pract.; Police Surg.; Hon. Lect. Gen. Pract. Univ. of Manch.

TANN, Carolyn Julie 35 Grange Road, Shrewsbury SY3 9DG Email: callytann@hotmail.com — MB ChB Birm. 1997. SHO Paediat.s, Lewisham Hosp. Specialty: Paediat.

TANN, Oliver Richard Thanet House, High St., Chalford, Stroud GL6 8DH — MB BS Lond. 1998.

TANNA, Amratlal Gokaldas 351 London Road, Stoneygate, Leicester LE2 3JX Tel: 0116 270 7086 — MB BS Baroda 1966; DPM Eng. 1975.

TANNA, Aruna Dhirendra Upton Surgery, Waggon Lane, Upton, Pontefract WF9 1JS Tel: 01977 647521; 3 Rosslyn Close, Ackworth, Pontefract WF7 7QF Tel: 01977 610308 — MB BS Bombay 1969 (Grant Med. Coll.)

TANNA, Dhirendra Ranchhoddas (retired) Upton Surgery, Waggon Lane, Upton, Pontefract WF9 1JS Tel: 01977 647521; Lightcliffe, Pontefract Road, Hemsworth, Pontefract WF9 5LW Tel: 01977 616963 — MB BS Bombay 1972 (Grant Med. Coll.) Clin. Asst. (Psychogeriat.) Pontefract HA.

TANNA, Kirit Harold Hill Centre, Gooshays Drive, Romford RM3 9JP Tel: 01708 343815 Fax: 01708 379790 — MB BS Gujarat 1979; MB BS Gujarat 1979.

TANNA, Meeta 4 Winchester Mews, 12A Winn Road, Southampton SO17 1ET — BM Soton. 1997. SHO (Paediat.) Soton. Gen. Hosp. Specialty: Paediat. Socs: BMA; MPS. Prev: PRHO (Med.) Soton.; PRHO (Surg.) Dorchester.

TANNA, Rajendra 392 Greenlane Road, Leicester LE5 4NE — MB ChB Leic. 1995.

TANNA, Shobhana Amritlal 351 London Road, Stoneygate, Leicester LE2 3JX Tel: 0116 270 7086 — MB BS Baroda 1964; DPM Lond. 1974. SCMO (Community Med.) Leics. HA.

TANNA, Vikram Narandas Morarji Clarendon Medical Practice, Clarendon Street, Hyde SK14 2AQ Tel: 0161 368 5224 Fax: 0161 368 4767 — MB BS Lond. 1978 (Middlx.) MA Oxf. 1974; DRCOG 1981; MRCGP 1983; FRCGP 1997; MSc Univ. of Manchester 1999. Gen. Med. Practitioner; GP Postgrad. Tutor Tameside. Socs: Fell. Manch. Med. Soc. Prev: Trainee GP Bramhall Health Centre; SHO Preston VTS; Ho. Surg. Christie Hosp. Manch.

TANNA, Viral The Barnard Medical Practice, 43 Granville Road, Sidcup DA14 4TA — MB BS Lond. 1989; DRCOG 1993; DFFP 1993.

TANNAHILL, Professor Andrew James Health Education Board for Scotland, Woodburn House, Canaan Lane, Edinburgh EH10 4SG Tel: 0131 536 5500 Fax: 0131 536 5501 — MB ChB Glas. 1977 (Univ. Glas.) MB ChB (Hons.) Glas. 1977; MSc (Community Med.) Ed. 1982; MFCM RCP (UK) 1985; FFPHM RCP (UK) 1992; FRCP Ed. 1996; FRCP (Glas.) 1999. Chief Exec.Health Educat. Bd. Scotl.; Vis. Prof. (Centre for Exercise Sci. & Med.) Univ. Glas.; Hon. Sen. Lect. (Epidemiol. & Pub. Health) Univ. Dundee; Hon. Sen. Lect. (Pub. Health) Univ. Glas.; Hon. Fell. (Pub. Health Scis.) Univ. Edin. Specialty: Pub. Health Med. Prev: Sen. Lect. (Pub. Health Med.) Univ. Glas. & Hon. Cons. Pub. Health Med. Gtr. Glas. HB; Specialist Community Med. E. Anglian RHA & Assoc. Lect. (Community Med.) Univ. Camb.

TANNAHILL, Mary Mabel (retired) 12 The Wigdale, Hawarden, Deeside CH5 3LL Tel: 01244 520321 Email: tanjo@doctors.org.uk — MB ChB Glas. 1957; DPH Lond. 1960; DPM Eng. 1962; FRCPsych 1979, M 1971. Cons. Psychiat. N. Wales Hosp. Denbigh. Prev: Sen. Lect. (Psychol. Med.) St. Thos. Hosp. Lond.

TANNER, Andrew Roger North Tees General Hospital, Hardwick, Stockton-on-Tees TS19 8PE Tel: 01642 617617 Fax: 01642 624089 — MB BChir Camb. 1973 (Camb. & Guy's) BA Camb. 1969, MA, MB BChir 1973; MRCP (UK) 1975; FRACP 1979; DM Soton. 1982; FRCP Ed. 1989; FRCP Lond. 1991. Cons. Phys. N. Tees Gen. Hosp. Specialty: Gen. Med. Socs: Brit. Soc. Gastroenterol. Prev: Lect. (Med.) Soton. Gen. Hosp.; Lect. (Med.) Univ. Queensland & Brisbane, Austral.; Sen. Regist. Roy. Brisbane Hosp. Austral.

TANNER, Carless Paul (retired) Rosegarth, Backcrofts, Rothbury, Morpeth NE65 7XY Tel: 01669 621032 — MB BS Durh. 1945 (Newc.) FRCGP 1976, M 1958. Prev: Course Organiser Regional Postgrad. Inst. Med. Sch. Newc.

TANNER, Colin Cedric Frimley Green Medical Centre, 1 Beech Road, Frimley Green, Camberley GU16 6QQ Tel: 01252 835016 Fax: 01252 837908; 5 Henley Drive, Frimley Green, Camberley GU16 6NE — MB BS Lond. 1981 (St. Geo.) DRCOG 1985.

TANNER, Elizabeth Irene (retired) 3 Netheravon Road, Salisbury SP1 3BJ Tel: 01722 322933 — MB BChir Camb. 1954; Dip. Bact. Lond 1961; FRCPath 1976, M 1964. Prev: Cons. Bacteriol. Pub. Health Laborat. Epsom.

TANNER, Gregory Peter Gerrard Taunton Road Medical Centre, 12-16 Taunton Road, Bridgwater TA6 3LS Tel: 01278 720000 Fax: 01278 423691 — MB BS Lond. 1989; BSc (Chem.) Lond. 1984; DFFP 1994; MRCGP 1994; DGM 2002. Sen. Clin. Lect. Univ. Of Bristol (Dept. Of Oncol. & Palliat. Medicine). Prev: GP. Med Centre. Bridgwater.

TANNER, Helena Taunton Road Medical Centre, 12-16 Taunton Road, Bridgwater TA6 3LS Tel: 01278 720000 Fax: 01278 423691; Crossways Barn, Main Road, Middlezoy, Bridgwater TA7 0PD — MB BS Lond. 1989.

TANNER, James Mourilyan Stentwood Coach house, Dunkeswell, Honiton EX14 4RW Email: jgtanner@aol.com — MB BS Lond. 1944 (St. Mary's & Univ. Penna., Philadelphia) MD Penna. 1944; DPM Lond. 1946; PhD Lond. 1953, DSc 1957; FRCP Lond. 1972, M 1963; FRCPsych 1971. Emerit. Prof. Child. Health & Growth Univ. Lond. Specialty: Paediat. Special Interest: Growth and Developm. of Childr., normal and disordered, including growth as a mirror of the health of populations. Socs: Soc. Study Human Biol.; BMA. Prev: Sen. Lect. (Physiol.) St. Thos. Hosp. Med. Sch.; Ho. Phys. Johns Hopkins Hosp. Baltimore; Demonst. (Human Anat.) Oxf.

TANNER, John Albert Oving Clinic, Church Lane, Oving, Chichester PO20 2DG Tel: 01243 773167 Fax: 01243 530567; Ferriby, Taylors Lane, Busham, Chichester PO18 8QQ — MB BS Lond. 1977 (Lond. Hosp.) BSc (Psychol.) Lond. 1973; Dip. Musculoskell Med. Soc. Apoth. Lond. 1993; Dip. Sports Med. Lond 1993. Indep. Orthop. & Sports Phys.; Chairm. Educat. Comm. BIMM; Course Organiser & Clin. Tutor Modular Course; Examr. for Dip. M.S. Med.; Examr. for MSc Sports & Ex. Med.; Instruc. for Internat. Spinal Interven. Soc. Specialty: Rehabil. Med.; Rheumatol.; Sports Med. Socs: Pain Soc.; Brit. Assn. Sport & Med.; Internat. Intradiscal Ther. Soc. Prev: Author Better Back, Back Pain Hodder & Stoughton, RSM Series.

TANNER, John Gwyn Silverbrook, Rhiwsaeson, Pontyclun CF7 — MB BCh Wales 1970 (Welsh Nat. Sch. Med.)

TANNER, Kirsty Jayne 149 Ship Lane, Farnborough GU14 8BJ — MB BS Newc. 1998; MRCP.

TANNER, Professor Malcolm Stuart Division of Child Health, University of Sheffield, The Children's Hospital, Western Bank, Sheffield S10 2TH Tel: 01142 717228 Fax: 01142 755364 Email: m.s.tanner@sheffield.ac.uk — (King's Coll. Hosp.) MSc (Biochem.) Lond. 1977, BSc (1st cl. Hons.) (Pharmacol.) 1966; MB BS Lond. 1969; MRCS Eng. LRCP Lond. 1969; DCH Eng. 1972; MRCP (UK) 1974; FRCP Lond. 1986. Prof. Paediat. Univ. Sheff.; Non-Exec. Dir. Sheff. Childr. Hosp. NHS Trust. Specialty: Paediat. Socs: Brit. Soc. Gastroenterol.; Roy. Coll. Paediat. & Child Health; Eur. Soc. Paediat. Gastroenterol. & Nutrit. Prev: Sen. Lect. (Child Health) Univ. Leicester.

TANNER, Mark Hertford County Hospital, North Road, Potters Bar SG14 1LP — MB BCh Wales 1983; MRCPsych 1994; LLM 1999.

Cons. (Psychiat.) Herford Co. Hosp.; Barrister 1986 Middle Temple. Specialty: Gen. Psychiat. Prev: Regist. (Psychiat.) St. Bernard's Hosp. Ealing; Clin. Research Fell. St. Mary's Hosp. Lond.; Sen. Regist., St Clements Hosp., Lond.

TANNER, Mark Antony 45a Hampstead High Street, Hampstead, London NW3 1QG — MB BS Lond. 1997.

TANNER, Michael Thomas Greystead, High St., Kinver, Stourbridge DY7 6HG Tel: 01384 872200 — MB ChB Birm. 1961.

TANNER, Mr Norman Stuart Brent BUPA Hospital Tunbridge, Fordcombe Road, Fordcombe, Tunbridge Wells TN3 0RD Tel: 01892 740044 Fax: 01892 740085 Email: brenttanner@brenttanner.co.uk; The Oasts, Broadreed Farm, Criers Lane, Five Ashes, Mayfield TN20 6LG Tel: 01825 830409 Fax: 01825 830367 — MB BChir Camb. 1969 (Camb. & St Thos.) MRCS Eng. LRCP Lond. 1969; MA Camb. 1970; FRCS Eng. 1974. Hon. Cons. Plastic Surg. Qu. Vict. Hosp. E. Grinstead; Bupa Hopital Tunbridge Wells, Kent; The Sussex Nuffield Hosp.; The N. Downs Hosp., Surrey; Cons. Plastic and Reconstruc. Surg., Gatwick Pk. Hosp., Horley, Surrey. Specialty: Plastic Surg. Socs: Brit. Assn. Plastic Surg.; Brit. Assn. Aesthetic Plastic Surgs.; Roy. Coll. of Surg.s. Prev: Sen Regist. (Plastic Surg.) Canniesburn Hosp. Glas.; Research Fell. (Head & Neck Unit) Roy. Marsden Hosp. Lond.; Ho. Off. Surg. St. Thos. Hosp. Lond.

TANNER, Patricia Mary (retired) Ashmount, 13 Woodlands Rise, Ilkley LS29 9BU Tel: 01943 608064 — (Univ. Ed.) MB ChB Ed. 1947. Prev: Ho. Phys. Lond. Chest Hosp. & Radcliffe Infirm.

TANNER, Peter Archibald Stuart Witchings, Bakers Hill, Barnet EN5 5QL Tel: 020 8447 0817 — MB BS Lond. 1979; MRCPath 1987. Cons. Histopath. King Geo. & Barking Hosps. Specialty: Histopath. Socs: Brit. Div. Internat. Acad. Path.; Assn. Clin. Path. Prev: Sen. Regist. (Histopath.) Westm. & St. Stephens Hosp. Lond.; Regist. (Histopath.) Barnet Gen. Hosp.; Med. Adviser 'The Human Body' published 1986.

TANNER, Robert Michael Llangollen Health Centre, Regent Street, Llangollen LL20 8HL Tel: 01978 860625 Fax: 01978 860174; Pendraw Garth Isa, Garth, Glyn Ceiriog, Llangollen LL20 7LY — BM BCh Oxf. 1992; BA (Hons.) Oxf. 1989; MRCGP 1996. Specialty: Gen. Pract. Prev: GP/Regist. Aylesbury VTS; SHO (Obst.) Hammersmith Hosp. Lond.; Ho. Surg. John Radcliffe Hosp. Oxf.

TANNER, Simon John 5 Ullswater Grove, Alresford SO24 9NP — BM Soton. 1981; DRCOG 1984; DCH RCP Lond. 1985; MRCGP 1986; MSc Lond. 1994; MFPHM 1996. Cons. (Pub. Health Med.) N. & Mid Hants. Health Auth. Specialty: Pub. Health Med. Prev: GP Alresford, Hants.

TANNER, Stephanie Peta 107 Camberwell Grove, London SE5 8JH — MB BS Lond. 1993.

TANNER, Mr Vaughan Oputhalmic Department, Royal Berkshire Hospital, London Road, Reading RG1 5AN Tel: 0118 987 7158 Fax: 0118 987 8939 — MB BS Lond. 1990 (St. George's Hosp. Lond.) BSc (Hons. Med. Sci.) Lond. 1987; FRCOphth 1994. Cons. Ophthalmic Surg., Roy. Berks. Hosp., Reading; Cons. Ophthalmic Surg., Wing Edwd. VII Hosp., Windsor, BUPA Dunedin Hosp., Reading, Princess Margt. Hosp., Windsor. Specialty: Ophth. Socs: MDU; RCOphth; Amer. Acad. Of Ophth. Prev: Regist. (Ophth.) P. Chas. Eye Unit King Edwd. VII Hosp. Windsor; Specialist Regist (Ophth.) Oxf. Eye Hosp.; Vitreo- retinal Fell. St. Thomas's Hosp. Lond.

TANNETT, Peter Geoffrey 5 Lilac Oval, Hillam, Leeds LS25 5HQ — MB ChB Leeds 1958; DA Eng. 1964; DObst RCOG 1965; FRCA Eng. 1975. Specialty: Anaesth. Socs: Yorks. Soc. Anaesth.; BMA; Assn. Anaesth. Prev: Cons. (Anaesth.) Pinderfields Pontefract Hosp. NHS Trust; Sen. Regist. (Anaesth.) Yorks. RHA; Cas. Off. Gen. Infirm. Leeds.

TANNOCK, Timothy Charles Ayrton (retired) Conservative Central Office, 32 Smith Square, London SW1P 3HH Tel: 0207 984 8235 Fax: 0207 984 8292 — MB BS Lond. 1983; MA Oxf. 1993, BA (Hons.) 1980; MRCPsych 1988; T(Psych) 1994. Mem. of the Europ. Parliament (Lond. Region - Conserv.). Prev: Cons. (Psychiat.) Univ. Coll. Hosp. & Middlx. Hosp. Lond.

TANQUERAY, Andrew Baron 46 West Street, Rochford SS4 1AJ — MB Camb. 1978; BChir 1977; MRCP (UK) 1980; FRCR 1986. Cons. Radiol. Southend Hosp. Specialty: Radiol. Prev: Sen. Regist. St. Thos. Hosp.

TANQUERAY, John Frederic Harlestone Road Surgery, 117 Harlestone Road, Northampton NN5 7AQ Tel: 01604 751832 Fax: 01604 586065; Mulberry House, The Green, Hardingstone, Northampton NN4 7BU Tel: 01604 761876 — MB BChir Camb. 1985 (Cambridge) DRCOG 1987; DCH RCP Lond. 1988; MRCGP 1989; D Med 2002. Gen. Practitioner, Northampton. Specialty: Medico Legal. Socs: Soc. of Expert Witnesses. Prev: GP Ipswich.

TANSER, Susan Jane, Surg. Lt.-Cdr. RN 1 Garfield Road, Southampton SO19 4DA Email: sjtanser@yahoo.com — MB BS Lond. 1990 (St. Bartholomew's) DA; FRCA 1997. Specialty: Anaesth.; Intens. Care.

TANSEY, Alexandra Katherine Philomena (retired) Daventry Road Surgery, 281 Daventry Road, Coventry CV3 5HJ Tel: 024 7650 3485 Fax: 024 7650 5730; Manor Farm, Old Milverton, Leamington Spa CV32 6SA Tel: 01926 339495 — LRCPI & LM, LRSCI & LM 1960 (RCSI) DObst RCOG 1963. Prev: Ho. Off. (Obst.) & Ho. Phys. Paediat. Northampton Gen. Hosp. & Ho.

TANSEY, Bernard John Low Waters Medical Centre, 11 Mill Road, Hamilton ML3 8AA Tel: 01698 283626 Fax: 01698 282839; 4 Carnoustic Court, Bothwell, Glasgow G71 8UB Tel: 01698 853351 — MB ChB Glas. 1966. Med. Off. Philips Elec., Safeway (W. of Scotl.), & Lawrence Scott, Hamilton. Prev: Ho. Phys. Falkirk & Dist. Roy. Infirm.; Ho. Surg. Hairmyres Hosp. E. Kilbride; Ho. Surg. (Obst.) Falkirk Roy. Infirm.

TANSEY, David James 2A Oaklea Road, Wirral CH61 3US — BM BS Nottm. 1989.

TANSEY, John Michael Trent Meadows Medical Centre, 87 Wood Street, Burton-on-Trent DE14 3AA Tel: 01283 845555 Fax: 01283 845222 Email: johntansey@btinternet.com — MB ChB Leic. 1983; DPMC Keele 1991. Prev: Trainee GP Leic. VTS.; Regist. & SHO (Psychiat.) Carlton Hayes Hosp. Leics.

TANSEY, Margaret Therese Low Waters Medical Centre, 11 Mill Road, Hamilton ML3 8AA Tel: 01698 283626 Fax: 01698 282839; 4 Carnoustie Court, Bothwell, Glasgow G71 8UB Tel: 01698 853351 — MB ChB Glas. 1965; DObst RCOG 1967. Med. Off. (Obst.) Bellshill Matern. Hosp. Socs: E. Kilbride Med. Soc. Prev: Ho. Surg. Glas. Roy. Infirm. & Glas. Roy. Matern. Hosp.; Ho. Phys. Belvedere Hosp. Glas.

TANSEY, Mr Michael Alfred Lambert (retired) Manor Farm, Old Milverton, Leamington Spa CV32 6SA Tel: 01926 39495 — LRCPI & LM, LRSCI & LM 1960 (RCSI) FRCS Ed. 1969. Cons. Orthop. Surg. S. Warks. Gp. Hosps. Prev: Res. Surg. Off. Hallam Hosp. W. Bromwich.

TANSEY, Michael James Byron Cromwell Cottage, 9-11 Mill St., Gamlingay, Sandy SG19 3JW Tel: 01767 50719 — MD Cape Town 1981; BSc. St. And. 1970; MB ChB Manch. 1973.

TANSEY, Mr Patrick Alfred Harbison 10 Norwood Avenue, Heaton, Newcastle upon Tyne NE6 5RA — MB BCh BAO NUI 1990; LRCPSI 1990; FRCS Ed. 1994.

TANSEY, Patrick Joseph Victoria Infirmary, Department of Haematology, Langside, Glasgow G42 9TT Fax: 0141 201 5652 — MB ChB Glas. 1973; MRCP (UK) 1976; FRCPath. 1992,M 1980; FRCP Glas. 1989. Cons. Haemat. S. Glas. Univ. NHS Trust. Specialty: Haematology. Special Interest: Lymphomas.

TANSEY, Susan Patricia Servier Research & Deveolpment Unit, Fulmer Hall, Windmill Hill, Slough SL3 6HH Tel: 01753 666345 Fax: 01753 664408 — MB ChB Manch. 1988; DCH RCP Lond. 1992; MRCP (UK) 1994; DPM 2000. Clin. Research Manager Servier R & D. Specialty: Pharmaceutical Medicine; Paediat. Socs: MRCPCH. Prev: SP Reg.Paediat.Roy.Liverp.Childr.s.Hosp; Research Fell.Antenatal TRH Trial Wom..Hosp.Liverp.

TANSLEY, Miss Anne Patricia Cairn Cottage, Montgomery Hill, Frankby, Wirral CH48 1NF — MB ChB Liverp. 1992 (Liverpool) FRCS Ed. 1997. Specialist Regist. (Gen. Surg.) Mersey Region. Specialty: Gen. Surg. Socs: WIST; BMA; ASIT.

TANSLEY, Mr Anthony Gerard The Marches Medical Practice, Mill Lane, Buckley CH7 3HB — MB ChB Liverp. 1986; FRCS Ed. 1992. Specialty: Plastic Surg. Prev: SHO (Plastic SUrg.) Qu. Mary's Hosp. Roehampton & Whiston Hosp.

TANSLEY, Elizabeth Jane Tansley and Partners, Chalkhill Health Centre, Chalkhill Road, Wembley HA9 9BQ Tel: 020 8904 0911 — (St. Mary's) MB BS Lond. 1966; MRCS Eng. LRCP Lond. 1966. Trainer (Gen. Pract.) Middlx. Specialty: Paediat. Socs: BMA. Prev:

Clin. Tutor (Gen. Pract.) Middlx. Hosp. Lond.; Ho. Surg. Paddington Green Childr. Hosp.; Ho. Phys. Chase Farm Hosp. Enfield.

TANSLEY, Margaret Catherine Parkside Family Practice, Eastleigh Health Centre, Newtown Road, Eastleigh SO50 9AG Tel: 023 8061 2032 Fax: 023 8062 9623 — MB BS Lond. 1970 (St. Geo.) DObst RCOG 1972; MRCGP 1976. Prev: Civil. Med. Pract. to Army Tidworth Garrison; Ho. Phys. St. Geo. Hosp. Lond.; Ho. Surg. Salisbury Gen. Infirm.

TANSLEY, Patrick David Thomas 1 Gullet Lane, Kirby Muxloe, Leicester LE9 2BL Tel: 0116 238 6315 — MB BChir Camb. 1994; BSc Lond. 1992; MB BChir Camb. 1995. Socs: Brit. Assn. Clin. Anat.; Roy. Soc. Med.

TANSLEY, Robert Giles 9 South Hill, Guildford GU1 3SY — MB BS Lond. 1989; MPhil Camb. 1994; MRCOG 1995. Med. Assessor MCA. Specialty: Pharmaceutical Medicine. Prev: Med. Affairs Sanofi Winthrop Guildford; Regist. Rotat. Camb. & P'boro.

TANT, Darryl Roderic The Surgery, 37 Castle Street, Luton LU1 3AG Tel: 01582 726123 Fax: 01582 731150; Algonquin, 30 Roundwood Park, Harpenden AL5 3AF Tel: 01582 763362 — MB BChir Camb. 1967 (Camb. & Middlx.) MRCS Eng. LRCP Lond. 1967; MA Camb. 1967; FRCGP 1982, M 1975. GP; Examr. MRCGP Exam. Prev: Course Organiser Luton & Dunstable Hosp. VTS; Tutor (Gen. Pract.) Luton & Dunstable Hosp. Postgrad. Med. Centre; Resid. (Internal Med.) Sunnybrook Hosp. Univ. Toronto, Canada.

TANTAM, Professor Digby John Howard Centre for Psychotherapeutic Studies, University Sheffield, 16 Claremont Crescent, Sheffield S10 2TA Tel: 0114 222 2979 Fax: 0114 275 0226 — BM BCh Oxf. 1972; MA, BA Oxf. 1966; FRCPsych 1991, M 1977; MPH Harvard 1977; BA Open 1985; PhD Lond. 1986. Clin. Prof. Psychother. Univ. Sheff. & Hon. Cons. Psychotherapist (Community Health) Sheff.; Sen. Lect. (Psychiat.) & Hon. Cons. Psychiat. UHSM.; Prof. Psychother. Univ. Warwick & Hon. Cons. Psychotherapist Coventry 1990-95; Vis. Prof. Univ. Zambia; Lect. Inst. Psychiat. Specialty: Psychother. Prev: MRC Train. Fell. Inst. Psychiat. Lond.; Sen. Regist. (Psychiat.) Maudsley Hosp. Lond.; Clin. Fell. (Psychiat.) Harvard Med. Sch., USA.

TANTI, Geoffrey John Llwyn Ygroes Psychiatric Unit, Wrexham Maelor Hospital, Wrexham Technology Park, Wrexham LL13 7TD — MD Malta 1986; MRCPsych 1994; MSc 1999. Cons. Psychiat., Wrexham; Cons. Psychiat. in Learning Disabilities. Specialty: Gen. Psychiat.; Ment. Health.

TANWEER, Kishwer (retired) 36 Woodbourne Avenue, London SW16 1UU Tel: 020 8677 4618 — (Dow Med. Coll. Karachi) MB BS Karachi 1963. Prev: Clin. Med. Off. (Child Health) Sutton Community NHS Trust.

TAO, Miriam Third Floor, 60 Cadogan Square, London SW1X 0EE — MB BS Lond. 1984 (Char. Cross Hosp.) SHO (Med.) Princess Margt. Hosp. Swindon. Socs: BMA. Prev: SHO (Cas.) Hillingdon Hosp. Lond.; SHO (Oncol.) St. Geo. Hosp. Lond.; Ho. Phys. Char. Cross Hosp. Lond.

TAOR, Lesley Patricia Muriel The Beeches, Packhorse Road, Bessels Green, Sevenoaks TN13 2QP — MRCS Eng. LRCP Lond. 1973 (Char. Cross) DRCOG 1977. Prev: Trainee GP Medway VTS; Ho. Surg. (Orthop.) & Ho. Phys. (Geriat. Psychiat. & Dermat.) Char. Cross Hosp. Lond.

TAOR, Pamela Jane (Surgery), 7A Welbeck Road, West Harrow, Harrow HA2 0RQ Tel: 020 8422 3021; Highlands, London Road, Harrow-on-the Hill, Harrow HA1 3JJ Tel: 020 8422 3260 — MB BS Lond. 1963 (Char. Cross) BA (Phil.) Lond. 1986, MB BS 1963. Hosp. Pract. Edgware Gen. Hosp. Specialty: Gen. Psychiat. Prev: Regist. (Psychiat.) Edgware Gen. Hosp.

TAOR, Mr William Stewart Flat 19, Harmont House, 20 Harley St., London W1G 9PH; Highlands, London Road, Harrow HA1 3JJ Tel: 020 8422 3260 Fax: 020 8422 7979 — (Char. Cross) BSc Lond. 1960, MB BS 1962; FRCS Eng. 1967; LLB 2000. Medico-Legal Cons.; Hon. Med. Adviser & Orthop. Surg. Badminton Assn. of Eng. & Internat. Badminton Federat. Specialty: Orthop. Socs: Fell. BOA. Prev: Cons. Orthop. Surg. Parkside Health Dist.; Sen. Regist. Roy. Nat. Orthop. Hosp. & Char. Cross Hosp. Lond.; Cons. Orthop. Surg. Manor Ho. Hosp.

TAPLEY, Michael Philip 7 Mottram Old Road, Stalybridge SK15 2TG — MB BS Lond. 1985. Sen. Hospice Dr. (Palliat. Care Med.) Willow Wood Hospice Ashton-under-Lyne; Family Plann. & Sexual Health CMO Tameside & Manch. PCTs; Assoc. Specialist Stockport PCT. Specialty: Genitourinary Medicine; Gen. Pract.; HIV Med. Socs: BMA. Prev: Clin. Asst. (Genitourin. Med.) Roy. Oldham Hosp.; SHO (Anaesth.) Tameside Gen. Hosp. Ashton-under-Lyne Lancs. & Westm. Hosp. Lond.; SHO (A & E) Qu. Mary's Hosp. Lond.

TAPP, Andrew John Singleton Royal Shrewsbury Hospital, Mytton Oak Road, Shrewsbury SY3 8XQ Tel: 01743 261141 — MB BS Lond. 1982; MRCOG 1989. Cons. O & G Roy. Shrewsbury Hosp. Specialty: Obst. & Gyn. Prev: Sen. Regist. St. Geo. & Mayday Hosp. Lond.

TAPP, Edmund Foxdenton House, Sytchampton, Stourport-on-Severn DY13 9TA Tel: 0190 562 1657 Fax: 0190 562 1657 — (Liverp.) MRCS Eng. LRCP Lond. 1959; MB ChB (Hons.) Liverp. 1959; MD Liverp. 1964; FRCPath 1978, M 1968. Indep. Forens. Pathologist to the Home Office. Specialty: Forens. Path. Socs: Liverp. Med. Inst.; Palaeopath. Assn. Prev: Cons. Path. (Morbid Anat. & Histopath.) Roy. Preston Hosp.; Cons. Path. (Morbid Anat. & Histol.) Withington Hosp. Manch.; Lect. (Path.) & Hon. Lect. (Orthop. Path.) Liverp. Univ.

TAPP, Gwendolyn Rosemary (retired) Mallards, 36 Sea Drive, Felpham, Bognor Regis PO22 7NB Tel: 0124 369 582252 — MB BS Lond. 1950 (Roy. Free) FRC Paed & CH (Hon.); MRCS Eng. LRCP Lond. 1950; DCH Eng. 1952, DPH 1956; MFCM 1974. Prev: Sen. Med. Off. (Child Heath) E. Surrey Health Dist.

TAPP, Martin James Franklin 129 New Road, Brixham TQ5 8DB — MB ChB Bristol 1998.

TAPPER, Geoffrey William The Mount, Salisbury Road, Shaftesbury SP7 8NL Tel: 01747 852872 Fax: 01747 851463 — MB BS Lond. 1955 (Middlx.) DObst RCOG 1961. Examg. Med. Practitioner, Benefit Agency. Prev: Ldr. Dorset Co. Counc.

TAPPER, Roger John Frogmill, Pound Lane, Burghclere, Newbury RG20 9JR — MB BS Lond. 1968 (St. Thos.) DObst RCOG 1970.

TAPPER-JONES, Lorna Maureen Penylan Road Surgery, 100 Penylan Road, Roath Park, Cardiff CF23 5RH Tel: 029 2046 1100 Fax: 029 2045 1623; Maes-y-Coed, 59 Heath Pk Avenue, Cardiff CF14 3RG Tel: 029 2075 1306 — MB BCh Wales 1977; MD Wales 1986, BDS 1972; DRCOG 1980; DCH (UK) 1981; FRCGP 1992, M 1982; MFFP 1993; ILTM 2001. GP Princip.; Sen. Lect. (Gen. Pract.) Univ. Wales Coll. Med. Cardiff; GP Trainer S. Glam. VTS; Examr. Roy. Coll. Gen. Practs. Specialty: Gen. Pract. Socs: Cardiff Med. Soc.; Primary Care Dermat. Soc.; Primary Care Rheum. Soc. Prev: Trainee GP S. Glam. VTS; Lect. (Oral Med.) Welsh Nat. Sch. Med.; Clin. Med. Off. S. Glam. HA.

TAPPIN, Alan Robert (retired) Knapwood House, Littlewick Road, Knaphill, Woking GU21 2JU Tel: 01483 474122 — MB BS Lond. 1959 (St. Mary's) DObst RCOG 1961; DA Eng. 1962; FFA RCS Eng. 1966. Prev: ons. Anaesth. N.W. Surrey Gp. Hosp.

TAPPIN, David Michael Yorkhill NHS Trust, Royal Hospital for Sick Children, Glasgow G3 8SJ Tel: 0141 201 0176 Fax: 0141 201 0837 Email: goda11@udcf.gla.ac.uk; 31 Shawhill Road, Glasgow G41 3RW — MB BS Lond. 1981 (Middlesex Hospital) MRCP (UK) 1986; MD Lond. 1996; MPH (Glas) 1998. Sen. Lect. (Community Child Health) Glas. Univ.; Cons. Paediatrican (Hon.) Roy. Hosp. For Sick Childr., Glasg. Specialty: Community Child Health; Paediat.; Pub. Health Med. Socs: MRCPCH; Fell. Roy. Coll. Phys. & Surg. Glas. Prev: Canterbury Cot Death research fell. ChristCh. New Zealand; Sen lect. Scott Cot Death Trust.

TAPPIN, Michael James — MB BS Lond. 1990; FRCOphth. Cons. (Ophthal. Surg.) Ashford St. Peter's & Roy. Surrey Hosps. Special Interest: Corneal Cataract and Refractive Surg.

TAPPING, Peter John Vine Medical Centre, 69 Pemberton Road, East Molesey KT8 9LJ Tel: 020 8979 4200 Fax: 020 8941 9827; Tandrup, Hill View Road, Claygate, Esher KT10 0TU — MB BS Lond. 1983; MRCGP 1988. GP E. Molesey. Prev: Trainee GP Frimley Pk. Hosp.; Ho. Off. (Med.) Newham Gen. Hosp.; Ho. Off. (Surg.) Lond. Hosp.

TAPPOUNI, Faiz Raphael The Eye Academy, 114A Harley St., London W1G 7EL Tel: 020 7722 6638 Fax: 020 7722 6638; 114A Harley Street, London W1N 1DG Tel: 020 7935 0052 Fax: 020 7935 0072 — MB ChB Baghdad 1963; MD Baghdad 1973; FRCOphth 1989. Cons. Ophth. Eye Acad. Lond.; Mem. Amer. Acad. Ophth.; Mem. Pan Arab Congr. Ophth.; Co-Edr. Afro-Asian Jl. Ophth. Specialty: Ophth. Socs: Eur. Soc. Cataract & Refractive Surgs. Prev: Cons. Ophth. Surg. Al Haitham Hosp.

TAPSELL, Sam Henry John High Noon, 11 Middle St., Nether Heyford, Northampton NN7 3LL — MB BS Newc. 1998.

TAPSFIELD, William George Collingwood Surgery, Hawkeys Lane, North Shields NE29 0SF Tel: 0191 257 1779 Fax: 0191 226 9909 — MB ChB Ed. 1978.

TAPSON, John Stephen Freeman Hospital, Newcastle upon Tyne NE7 7DN Tel: 0191 233 6161 Fax: 0191 213 0370 Email: john.tapson@tfh.nuth.northy.nhs.uk; Hollybush House, Robsheugh, Newcastle upon Tyne NE20 0JQ Tel: 01661 886443 — MB BS Lond. 1976 (Guy's) BSc (Hons.) Lond. 1973; MRCS Eng. LRCP Lond. 1976; MRCP (UK) 1980; MD Newc. 1988; FRCP (UK) 1994. Cons. Nephrol. Freeman Hosp. Newc. u. Tyne. Specialty: Nephrol. Prev: Sen. Regist. (Nephrol.) Roy. Vict. Infirm. Newc.

TARABA, Pam The Surgery, 118 Old Oak Road, London W3 7HG Tel: 020 8740 7328 Fax: 020 8743 2235 — (Charles Univ. Prague) MUDr Prague 1960; MRCS Eng. LRCP Lond. 1973; DPM Eng. 1975. Clin. Asst. in Psychiat. W. Middlx. Hosp.

TARALA, Mrs Christine Thelma Maltings Green Road Surgery, 64 Maltings Green Road, Layer de la Haye, Colchester CO2 0JJ — MB ChB Glas. 1975 (Glasgow) DRCOG 1978. Specialty: Gen. Pract.

TARAPHDAR, S East Street Surgery, 1 East Street, Rochdale OL16 2EG — MB BS Calcutta 1970; MB BS Calcutta 1970.

TARBUCK, Andrew Frederick The Julian Hospital, Bowthorpe Road, Norwich NR2 3TD Tel: 01603 421772 Fax: 01603 421831 Email: andrew.tarbuck@norfmhc-tr.anglox.nhs.uk — BM BCh Oxf. 1986; BA Camb. 1983; MA Camb. 1987; MRCPsych 1990. Cons. in Old Age Psychiat. Norf. Ment. Healthcare NHS Trust. Specialty: Gen. Psychiat. Socs: Inst. Learning & Teachg. in Higher Educat.; Roy. Coll. Psychiat. (East. Region. Represen.) Fac. Old Age Psychiat. Prev: Sen. Regist. (Old Age Psychiat.) Fulbourn Hosp. Camb.; SHO (Psychiat.) Fulbourn Hosp. Camb.

TARBUCK, Mr David Thomas Henrich (retired) Tanglewood, 11 South Lynn Drive, Eastbourne BN21 2JF — MB BS Lond. 1967 (Roy. Free) MRCS Eng. LRCP Lond. 1967; DO Eng. 1971; FRCS Eng. 1975; FRCOphth 1988. Prev: Cons. Opth. Surg. Eastbourne NHS Trust.

TARELLI, Stephen Vincent 4 Greencroft Close, Darlington DL3 8HW — MB ChB Ed. 1968.

TARGETT, Mr John Peter Geoffrey Basildon & Thurrock Univ. Hosps. NHS Trust, Basildon Hospital, Basildon Hospital, Nethermayne, Basildon SS16 5NL Tel: 01268 593611 Email: johntargett@btuh.nhs.uk; Hartswood House, Hartswood Road, Great Warley, Brentwood CM14 5AG — MB BS Lond. 1983 (St. Mary's Hosp. Med. Sch. Lond.) FRCS Eng. 1988; FRCS (Orth.) 1995. Cons. Trauma & Orthop. Basildon Hosp. Essex. Specialty: Trauma & Orthop. Surg. Special Interest: Knee Surgery; Spine Surgery. Socs: Brit. Orthopaedic Assn. Prev: Sen. Regist. & Regist. Rotat. (Orthop.) St. Geo. Hosp. Lond.; Regist. (Gen. Surg. & Orthop.) Basildon Hosp. Essex.

TARGETT, Katherine Lesley 19 Tofts Close, Low Worsall, Yarm TS15 9QA — BM BCh Oxf. 1993.

TARGOSZ, Sarah Alexandra Woodlands, 53 Strathblane Road, Milngavie, Glasgow G62 8HA — MB ChB Manch. 1998.

TARIN, Mr Mohammad Kamran c/o Abdul Quyum, 36 Cemetry Road, Oldbury, Oldbury B68 8SP — MB BS Peshawar 1986; FRCS Ed. 1993.

TARJUMAN, Mr Muhammad 83 Nickleby Road, Chelmsford CM1 4XG — MD Damascus 1971; FRCS Glas. 1986. Regist. (Gen. Surg.) Broomfield Hosp. Chelmsford. Specialty: Gen. Surg. Prev: Regist. (Gen. Surg.) Walsgrave Hosp. Coventry.

TARLETON, David Edward Balliol Ridingleaze Medical Centre, Ridingleaze, Bristol BS11 0QE Tel: 0117 982 2693 Fax: 0117 938 1707; 43A Nore Road, Portishead, Bristol BS20 6JY — MB ChB Birm. 1972.

TARLO, Leonard 28 Lyttelton Road, Droitwich WR9 7AA Tel: 01905 773315 — MB BCh BAO Dub. 1951 (T.C. Dub.) BA Dub. 1948, MB BCh BAO 1951; DPM Eng. 1954; FRCPsych. 1981, M 1971. Hon. Cons. St. Luke's Hosp. for the Clergy Lond. Specialty: Gen. Psychiat. Prev: Cons. Psychiat. Mid. Worcs. Gp. Hosps.; Hon. Clin. Tutor Univ. Birm.; Asst. Psychiat. W. Pk. Hosp. Epsom.

TARLOW, Jonathan Holloway Road Surgery, 94 Holloway Road, London N7 8JG Tel: 020 7607 2323; 16 Greenhalgh Walk, London N2 0DJ Tel: 020 8455 8680 Fax: 020 8458 0182 — MB BS Lond. 1965 (Lond. Hosp.) MRCS Eng. LRCP Lond. 1965; DObst RCOG 1967. Prev: Ho. Phys. & Obst. Ho. Surg. Qu. Eliz. II Hosp. Welwyn Gdn. City; Ho. Surg. Whittington Hosp. Lond.

TARLOW, Michael Jacob (retired) 43 Silhill Hall Road, Solihull B91 1JX Tel: 0121 681 9656 Email: michaeltarlow@blueyonder.co.uk — MB BS Lond 1962 (Guy's) L.L.M. 2000 Univ. of Wales; MB BS Lond. 1962; MSc (Biochem.) Lond. 1965; FRCP Lond. 1982, M 1968; FRCPCH 1997. Prev: Sen. Lect. (Paediat. & Child Health) Univ. Birm.

TARLOW, Samuel Holloway Road Surgery, 94 Holloway Road, London N7 8JG Tel: 020 7607 2323 — MRCS Eng. LRCP Lond. 1937 (Univ. Coll. Hosp.)

TARN, Anne Carolyn Department Chemical Pathology, Mayday University Hospital, London Road, Croydon CR7 7YE; 15 Church Way, Hurst Green, Oxted RH8 9EA Tel: 01883 722953 — MB BS Lond. 1978 (St. Bart.) MD Lond. 1996, MB BS 1978; MRCS Eng. LRCP Lond. 1978; MRCP Lond. 1982; MSc (Clin. Biochem.) Univ. Surrey 1990; MRCPath 1996. Specialty: Chem. Path.

TARN, Mark, Maj. RAMC 28 Swanstead, Basildon SS16 4PE Tel: 01268 474268 — BM Soton. 1990 (Southampton) Specialty: Gen. Psychiat.

TARNESBY, Georgia Miriam Susannah 68 Ossulton Way, London N2 0LB Tel: 020 8883 0224 — MB BChir Camb. 1988 (St. Thomas. Hosp., UMDS) BA 1989; MA Camb. 1989; MRCP (UK) 1991; MBA 1994. Specialty: Cardiol. Prev: Regist. (Cardiol.) Northwick Pk. Hosp. Lond.; SHO (Neurol.) Roy. Free Hosp. Lond.; SHO (Renal & Transpl.) Guy's Hosp. Lond.

TARNOKY, Joan Maureen (retired) 12 Whitby Drive, Reading RG1 5HW Tel: 0118 986 0299 Fax: 0118 986 0299 — (Durh.) FRCPCH; MB BS Durh. 1950; DCH Eng. 1953. Prev: Assoc. Specialist & Regist. (Paediat.) Roy. Berks. Hosp. Reading.

TARNOW-MORDI, William Odita Department of Child Health, University of Dundee, Dundee DD1 9SY Tel: 01382 660111 Fax: 01382 645783; 11 West Park Road, Dundee DD2 1NU — MB Camb. 1976; MB BChir Camb. 1976; MRCP (UK) 1977; DCH Eng. 1978. Reader (Neonat. Med. & Perinatal Epidemiol.) & Hon. Cons. Paediat. Ninewells Hosp. & Med. Sch. Dundee. Specialty: Epidemiol. Socs: Roy. Coll. Paediat. & Child Health; Neonat. Soc.; Brit. Assn. Perinatal Med. Prev: Research Fell. & Hon. Sen. Regist. John Radcliffe Hosp. Oxf.; SHO (Paediat.) Univ. Coll. Hosp. Lond.; SHO Hosp. Sick Childr. Gt. Ormond St.

TARPEY, Joseph Jarlath Department of Anesthestics, Warwick Hospital, Lakin Road, Warwick CV34 5BW Tel: 01926 495321 Fax: 01926 403715 — MB BCh BAO NUI 1985; FFA RCSI 1991. Cons. Anaesth. Warwick Hosp. Specialty: Anaesth. Prev: Vis. Asst. Prof. Oregon Health Sci.s Univ.

TARR, Gillian 25 Penygraig Road, Ystradowen, Cwmllynfell, Swansea SA9 2YP — MB BCh Wales 1984.

TARR, Katherine Elizabeth 25 Hampden Road, Malvern WR14 1NB — MB BS Lond. 1992.

TARR, Terence John Ashlea, 37 Thurstaston Road, Heswall, Wirral CH60 6SB Tel: 0151 342 7087 — MB BS Lond. 1980 (Guy's) FRCA. 1986. Cons. Anaesth. Arrowe Pk. Hosp. Wirral. Specialty: Anaesth. Prev: Lect. & Hon. Sen. Regist. (Anaesth.) Univ. Liverp.; Regist. (Anaesth.) Qu. Vict. Hosp. E. Grinstead; Regist. (Anaesth.) Guy's Hosp. Lond.

TARRANT, Catharine Jane 18 Gertrude Road, West Bridgford, Nottingham NG2 5BY; Department of Psychiatry, Duncan MacMillan House, Porchester Road, Nottingham NG3 6AA Tel: 0115 969300 Ext: 40766 — BM BS Nottm. 1992 (Nottingham) MRCPsych 1996. Clin. Research Worker/Research Fell. Univ. of Nottm. Specialty: Gen. Psychiat.

TARRANT, Mrs Deborah Anne Wellington House Surgery, Henrietta Street, Batley WF17 5DN Tel: 0845 607 7740 — MB BChir Camb. 1985; MA Camb. 1987, MB BChir 1985; DRCOG 1990; MRCGP 1990. Dep. Man. Kirkgate Surg., Wakefield. Socs: BMA. Prev: Trainee GP Wakefield VTS.

TARRANT, Kevin Nigel Brigstock Medical Centre, 141 Brigstock Road, Thornton Heath CR7 7JN Tel: 020 8684 1128 Fax: 020 8689 3647; Hawthorns, 26 Burcott Road, Purley CR8 4AA — MB BS Nottm. 1982; BMedSci (Hons.) Nottm. 1980, MB BS 1982; DRCOG 1985; MRCGP 1986; Dip Occ Health & Safety 1999. Clin. Asst. (Rheum.) Mayday Hosp. Croydon.; Hosp. Practitioner (Rheun). Specialty: Rheumatol. Prev: Clin. Asst. (Diabetes) Mayday Hosp. Croydon.

TARRANT, Paul Douglas 129 Mains Drive, Erskine PA8 7JJ Tel: 0141 812 6033 Fax: 0141 561 3033; 129 Mains Drive, Erskine PA8 7JJ Fax: 0141 561 3033 Email: drptarrant@aol.com — MB ChB Glas. 1976; DRCOG 1979; MRCGP 1979. Director Nazarene Compassionate Ministries - Europe; Adviser Care Counselling for Scotl.; Regist. Nazarene Health Care Fellowship; Mem. Med. Advis. Comm. Ch. of the Nazarene Internat. Specialty: Gen. Pract.; Obst. & Gyn. Socs: Christian Med. Fellowsh. Prev: Mem. Renfrew Dist. Med. Comm.; Mem. GP Sub. Comm. Argyll & Clyde Area Med. Comm.

TARRY, Jennifer Elizabeth Edward House, Timberdine Close, Worcester WR5 2DD — MB ChB Birm. 1973; FRCPsych 2005. Cons. Psychiat. Worcs. Ment. Health Partnership Trust. Specialty: Geriat. Psychiat. Prev: Cons. Psychiat. i/c Elderly Co. Hosp. Durh.

TARSH, Evelyn June (retired) 15 Hillcrest Avenue, London NW11 0EP Tel: 020 8458 7783 — (Liverp.) MB ChB Liverp. 1958; MRCS Eng. LRCP Lond. 1958. Prev: Asst. GP. Ruislip.

TART, Christopher John — MB BS Lond. 1973 (Univ. Coll. Lond. & Westm.) BSc Lond. 1970; FFA RCS Eng. 1979. EMP in Med. Servs.; SEMA Disabil. Med. Prev: Med. Off. Gosport War Memor Hosp.; Trainee GP Wessex VTS.; Regist. (Anaesth.) Magill Dept. Anaesth. Westm. Hosp. Lond.

TARUVINGA, Margaret Gravesend & North Kent Hospital, Bath St., Gravesend DA11 0DG — MB BS W. Indies 1985.

TARVER, David Stephen Dept. of Radiology, Poole Hospital, Longfleet Road, Poole BH15 2JB Tel: 01202 442313 Email: dtarver@email.com — MB BS Lond. 1982; MRCP (UK) 1985; MRCGP 1988; FRCR 1993. Cons. Radiologist, Pool Hosp., Poole, Dorset. Specialty: Radiol.

TARVET, Faye The Cooperage, Mid Shore, Pittenweem, Anstruther KY10 2NW — MB ChB Ed. 1997.

TARZI, Michael David 39 Charlock Way, Guildford GU1 1XY — MB BS Lond. 1997.

TARZI, Naji 5 Belle Vue Close, Staines TW18 2HY — LMSSA Lond. 1962.

TARZI, Ruth Margaret Flat 21 Corfton Lodge, Corfton Rd, Ealing, London W5 2HU — BM BCh Oxf. 1994; MA 1995; MRCP 1997; PhD Univ. London 2003. Spec. Reg. Nephrol & General Med. London Deanery. Specialty: Nephrol.; Gen. Med. Prev: SHO (Haemat.) Kings Coll. Hosp.; SHO (Neurol.) Radcliffe Infirm. Oxf.; SHO (Renal Med.) Hammersmith Hosp. Lond.

TASKER, Angela Doreen Papworth Hospital, Department of Radiology, Papworth Everard, Cambridge CB3 8RE — MB BChir Camb. 1984; MA Camb. 1985, BA (Hons.) 1981; MRCP (UK) 1986; FRCR 1992. Cons. (Radiol.) Papworth Hosp. Camb. Specialty: Radiol. Prev: Sen. Regist. (Radiol.) John Radcliffe Hosp. Oxf.; Regist. (Radiol.) John Radcliffe Hosp. Oxf.; Regist. Rotat. (Med.) St. Thos. Hosp. Lond. & Medway Hosp. Kent.

TASKER, Bronwyn Elizabeth Glenpark Medical Centre, Ravensorth Road, Dunston, Gateshead NE11 9AD — MB BS Newc. 1988 (Newcastle upon Tyne) DCH RCP Lond. 1991; MRCGP 1992; Dip. Therap. 1998. Prev: Trainee GP N.d. VTS.

TASKER, Claire Mary (retired) Grey House, High St., Beckley, Oxford OX3 9UU — MB ChB Birm. 1969.

TASKER, Mr David Gordon Ravenscourt Surgery, 36-38 Tynewydd Road, Barry CF62 8AZ Tel: 01446 733515 Fax: 01446 701326; 8 Minehead Avenue, Sully, Penarth CF64 5TH — MB BCh Wales 1972; FRCS Eng. 1978; MRCGP 1990. Prev: Regist. (Surg.) Addenbrookes Hosp. Camb. & Llandough Hosp.; SHO Profess. Surg. Unit Univ. Hosp. Wales Cardiff.

TASKER, Gillian Dallas Magnolia House Practice, Magnolia House, Station Road, Ascot SL5 0QJ Tel: 01344 637800 Fax: 01344 637823; Tall Trees House, Winchfield Road, Ascot SL5 7EX Tel: 01344 876648 — MB BS Lond. 1982 (Char. Cross) DRCOG 1985; MRCGP 1986; DCH RCP Lond. 1987. Clin. Asst. Breast Clinic King Edwd. VII Hosp. Windsor. Socs: Windsor Med. Soc. Prev: Clin. Med. Off. St. Thos. Hosp. Lond.; Trainee GP Windsor VTS; SHO (Med., Paediat., A & E & O & G) Heatherwood Hosp. Ascot.

TASKER, Heather Yvonne — BM BS Nottm. 1997; DRCOG; DFFP.

TASKER, Ian Thomas Springfield House, 110 New Lane, Eccles, Manchester M30 7JE — MB ChB Sheff. 1991; DRCOG Lond. 1996; MRCGP Lond. 1997. GP Partnership Swinton Manch. Specialty: Gen. Pract.

TASKER, John Anthony West Bar Surgery, 1 West Bar Street, Banbury OX16 9SF Tel: 01295 256261 Fax: 01295 756848; Saddlers Cottage, Main St, North Newington, Banbury OX15 6AJ Tel: 01295 730531 — BM BCh Oxf. 1977; MA, DPhil Oxf. 1978; DCH RCP Lond. 1980; MRCP (UK) 1980; DRCOG 1981; FRCGP 1996, M 1982. Chair Exec. Comm. Cherwell Vale PCT; Tutor (Gen. Pract.) Banbury.

TASKER, John Rendel (retired) 6 Milton Court, Milton Malsor, Northampton NN7 3AX Tel: 01604 858545 — MD Camb. 1951 (Lond. Hosp.) MB BChir 1940; FRCP Lond. 1963, M 1943. Prev: Cons. Phys. Gen. Hosp. & Cynthia Spencer Hospice Northampton.

TASKER, Margaret Silver Birches, 110 Rawlinson Lane, Heath Charnock, Chorley PR7 4DE — MB ChB Ed. 1976; MRCOG 1981, D 1978. Specialty: Obst. & Gyn.

TASKER, Mr Paul Richard Siebert 157 Worsley Road, Worsley, Manchester M28 2SJ — MB BS Lond. 1973 (St. Geo.) FRCS Eng. 1981. Sen. Regist. (Surg.) Morriston & Singleton Hosps. Swansea. Socs: Fell. Manch. Med. Soc.; BMA. Prev: Hon. Surg. Regist. & Markland Research Fell. Dept. Gastroenterol.; Manch. Roy. Infirm; Regist. Rotat. (Surg.) Whittington & Roy. Free; Hosp. Lond.; SHO Rotat. (Surg.) St. Geo. & Roy. Marsden Hosps. Lond.

TASKER, Peter Roy William St James House Surgery, County Court Road, King's Lynn PE30 5SY Tel: 01553 774221 Fax: 01553 692181; Doomsday House, Hall Lane, South Wootton, King's Lynn PE30 3LQ Tel: 01553 673260 — MB BS Lond. 1971; MRCS Eng. LRCP Lond. 1971; DCH Eng. 1977; DRCOG 1978; FRCGP 1989, M 1979. Prev: SHO & Ho. Phys. Profess. Dept. Med. & Ho. Surg. Char. Cross Hosp. Lond.

TASKER, Robert Charles Department of Paediatrics, University of Cambridge, School of Clinical Medicine, Addenbrookes Hospital, Hills Building, Cambridge CB2 2QQ — MB BS Lond. 1983; MA Camb. 1983; DCH RCP Lond. 1985; MRCP (UK) 1986; FRCP (UK) 1996; FRCPCH (UK) 1997; MD Camb. 1999; ILTM (UK) 2002. Univ. Lect. (Paediat. IC) Camb. Univ.; Hon Cons. Phys. (IC) Addenbrooke's Hosp. Camb. Specialty: Paediat.; Intens. Care; Respirat. Med. Prev: Cons. Phys. (IC) Hosp. for Sick Childr. Gt. Ormond St. Lond.; Fell. (Critical Care & Anaesth.) John Hopkins Hosp. USA; Research Regist. Respirat. Unit Hosp. Sick Childr. Gt. Ormond St.Lond.

TASKER, Robert Lucian Hewitt (retired) 21 Willow drive, Clench Warton, King's Lynn PE34 4EN — MRCS Eng. LRCP Lond. 1948 (St. Mary's Medical School, London) Prev: Flight Lt. RAF Med. Br.

TASKER, Timothy Charles Gadsden — MB BS Lond. 1978 (Univ. Coll. Hosp.) BA Oxf. 1974; MRCP (UK) 1981; FFPM RCP (UK) 1994, M 1990; DCPSA (HC) 1999. Clin. Pharmacologist.

TASKER, Mr Timothy Patrick Beaumont Winfield Hospital, Tewkesbury Road, Longford, Gloucester GL2 9WH Tel: 01452 331111; Gloucestershire Royal Hospital, Great Western Road, Gloucester GL1 3P — MB ChB Cape Town 1972; FRCS Ed. 1977. Cons. Orthop. Surg. Gloucester Roy. Infirm. Specialty: Orthop. Socs: Fell. BOA; Fell. Brit. Assn. for Study of Knee Surg.

TASKER, William John Angel Hill Surgery, 1 Angel Hill, Bury St Edmunds IP33 1LU Tel: 01284 753008 Fax: 01284 724744 — MB BS Lond. 1986. GP. Prev: SHO (A & E) Hinchingbrooke Hosp. Huntingdon; SHO (A & E) Qu. Mary's Hosp. Sidcup Kent.; SHO (Health Care for Elderly) Dulwich Hosp. Lond.

TASLIMUDDIN, Abu Siddique Mohammad 43 Barley Lane, Goodmayes, Ilford IG3 8XE — MB BS Dacca 1958; MB BS Dacaca 1958. Prev: GP Dagenham.

TASOU, Anthony London Road Surgery, 49 London Road, Canterbury CT2 8SG Tel: 01227 463128 Fax: 01227 786308 — MB BS Lond. 1984 (St. Bart.) DRCOG 1990. GP Canterbury.

TASSADAQ, Mr Tariq 123 Murray Road, Rugby CV21 3JR — MB BS Punjab 1985; FRCS Ed. 1989.

TASSONE, Peter 22 Manor Road, London Colney, St Albans AL2 1PL — MB ChB Birm. 1995; MRCS Glas. 2002.

TATAM, Margaret Elizabeth Kingsway Surgery, 20 Kingsway, Waterloo, Liverpool L22 4RQ Tel: 0151 920 9000 Fax: 0151 928 2411; 17 Eshe Road N., Blundellsands, Liverpool L23 8UE Tel: 0151 924 3286 — MB ChB Ed. 1973 (Edin.) BSc (Med. Sci.) Ed. 1970; DCH Eng. 1976. Socs: SPA Comm. Mem. Prev: Trainee GP Sighthill Health Centre Edin.; SHO (Anaesth.) Leicester Roy. Infirm.; SHO (Paediat.) West. Gen. Hosp. Edin.

TATE, Alexandra Rowena Flat 2, 38 Sackville Gdns., Hove BN3 4GH — MB BS Lond. 1994; DFFP; MRCGP.

TATE, Andrew Lawson Kilburn Park Medical Centre, 12 Cambridge Gardens, London NW6 5AY Tel: 020 7624 2414 Fax: 020 7624 2489 — MB BS Lond. 1990; MRCGP 1995.

TATE, Ann de Carteret Horsenden House, Little Bealings, Woodbridge IP13 6LX — MB BS Lond. 1967 (Guy's) MRCS Eng. LRCP Lond. 1967; DMRD Eng. 1972; FRCS Ed. 1972; FFR 1974; FRCR 1975. Cons. Radiol. Ipswich Hosp. Specialty: Radiol. Prev: Sen. Regist. (Radiol.) Ipswich Hosp. & Univ. Coll. Hosp. Lond.; Regist. (Radiol.) Univ. Coll. Hosp. Lond.

TATE, Anne Teresa Marie Curie Cancer Care, 89 Albert Embankment, London SE1 7TP Tel: 020 7599 7252 Fax: 020 7599 7260 Email: teresa.tate@mariecurie.org.uk; 15 Park Avenue N., London N8 7RU — MB BS Lond. 1974 (Roy. Free Hosp.) MRCS Eng. LRCP Lond. 1974; FRCR 1981; FRCP Lond. 1997. Med. Adviser Marie Curie Cancer Care, Lond.; Cons. Palliat. Med. & Hon. Sen. Lect. St. Bart. Hosp. Lond. Specialty: Palliat. Med. Socs: Assn. for Palliat. Med.; Roy. Soc. of Med. (Palliat.); Brit. Oncol. Assn. Prev: Clin. Instruc. (Radiat. Oncol.) Univ. Calif. San Diego, USA; Hon. Cons. Palliat. Med. Homerton Hosp. Lond.; Regist. (Radiother.) St. Bart. & Roy. Free Hosps. Lond.

TATE, David William 70 Southfield Road, Nailsea, Bristol BS48 1SE — MB ChB Leeds 1995.

TATE, Mr Geoffrey Thompson (retired) 65 Kent Road, Harrogate HG1 2NH — MB ChB Leeds 1952; FRCS Ed. 1959; FRCS Eng. 1963. Surg. Harrogate Health Dist.

TATE, Graham Harry Austin The Priory Hospital Marchwood, Hythe Road, Marchwood, Southampton SO40 4WU Tel: 023 8084 0044 Fax: 023 8020 7554 Email: austintate@.prioryhealthcare.co.uk; 9 Warwick Road, Southampton SO15 7PF Tel: 023 8077 3785 Fax: 023 8090 6819 Email: tate@zoo.co.uk — MB ChB Birm. 1964 (Birm. Univ.) MRCS Eng. LRCP Lond. 1964; DPM Eng. 1971; FRCPsych 1994, M 1972. Cons. Psychiat. & Med. Dir. Marchwood Priory Hosp.; Gp. Med. Dir., Priory Healthcare.; Chairm. UK Alcohol Forum. Specialty: Gen. Psychiat.; Alcohol & Substance Misuse. Prev: Cons. Psychiat. King Khalid Nat. Guard Hosp. Jeddah, Saudi Arabia; Cons. Psychiat. Roy. S. Hants., Hosp. Soton; Maj. RAMC.

TATE, Janice — BM Soton. 1990.

TATE, Mr Jeremy James Thompson Department of Surgery, Royal United Hospital, Bath BA1 3NG Tel: 01225 824543 Email: jeremy.tate@ruh-bath.swest.nhs.uk — MB BS Lond. 1980; FRCS Ed. 1984; FRCS Eng. 1985; MS Soton. 1989. Cons. Gen. Surg. Roy. United Hosp. Bath. Specialty: Gen. Surg. Socs: Assn. Endoscopic Surg. (Counc. Mem. 1998-1999). Prev: Sen. Regist. (Gen. Surg.) Roy. Free Hosp. Lond.; Lect. Chinese Univ. Hong Kong, Shatin.

TATE, Judith 3 Torquay Gardens, Gateshead NE9 6XB — MB BS Lond. 1987; BSc (Physiol.) Lond. 1984, MB BS 1987; DA (UK) 1990; MRCGP 1992.

TATE, Mary Elsbeth (retired) 91 Hartswood Road, Brentwood CM14 5AG Tel: 01277 226086 — (Roy. Free) MB BS Lond. 1961; MRCS Eng. LRCP Lond. 1961. Prev: Med. Off. Barking, Havering & Brentwood DHA.

TATE, Michael John Middlewich Road Surgery, 6 Middlewich Road, Sandbach CW11 1DL Tel: 01270 767411 Fax: 01270 759305; Townend Barn, Marsh Green Farm, Vicarage Lane, Sandbach CW11 3BU Tel: 01270 764320 — MB ChB Liverp. 1980 (Liverpool) MRCGP 1984. GP; GP Trainer.

TATE, Patricia Ann Christmas Maltings Surgery, Haverhill; 109 Grantchester Meadows, Cambridge CB3 9JN — MB BChir Camb. 1982 (Addenbrookes Cambridge) MA Camb. 1983; DRCOG 1984; DGM RCP Lond. 1985; DCH RCP Lond. 1985; FRCGP 2003. Examr MRCGP; Hon. Clin. Asst. Psychother. Specialty: Psychother. Socs: (Mem. Counc.) Balint Soc.

TATE, Paul Andrew Oldchurch Hospital, Waterloo Road, Romford RM7 0BE — MB BS Lond. 1993.

TATE, Peter Howard Lovel Marcham Health Centre, Marcham Road, Abingdon OX14 1BT Tel: 01235 522602; The Clock House, High St, Culham, Abingdon OX14 4NA Tel: 01235 528052 Fax: 01235 539291 — MB BS Newc. 1968; FRCGP 1983, M 1974. Trainer (Gen. Pract.) Abingdon; VIDEO Convenor MRCGP Exam. Socs: BMA & Oxf. Med. Soc. Prev: Surg. P & O Lines.

TATE, Rachel Mary (retired) 18 Beaulieu Close, Champion Hill, London SE5 8BA — MB ChB Birm. 1945; DObst RCOG 1948; DCH Eng. 1950. Prev: Sen. PMO DHSS.

TATE, MR Robert James The Ipswich Hospital, Heath Road, Ipswich IP4 5PD Tel: 01473 703205 Fax: 01473 703158; Horsenden House, Little Bealings, Woodbridge IP13 6LX Tel: 01473 622995 Fax: 01473 622995 — MB BS Lond. 1968 (Guy's) BDS Lond. 1964; MRCS Eng. LRCP Lond. 1968; LDS RCS Eng. 1963, F 1970. Cons. Oral & Maxillofacial Surg. Ipswich & W. Suff. Hosps. Specialty: Oral & Maxillofacial Surg. Socs: Brit. Assn. Oral Surgs. & BMA; HCSA; Brit. Dent. Assn. Prev: Sen. Regist. (Oral Surg.) Westm. Gp. Hosps.; Lect. (Oral Surg.) Univ. Coll. Hosp. Lond.; Ho. Surg. (ENT) Guy's Hosp. Lond.

TATE, Rodney Temple The Surgery, 4 Old Steine, Brighton BN1 1EJ Tel: 01273 501542 — MB BS Lond. 1962 (St. Mary's) DObst RCOG 1964. Socs: BMA.

TATE, Stephen 5 Strandview Street, Stranmillis, Belfast BT9 5FF — MB BCh BAO Belf. 1995.

TATE, Stephen Richard Holmes Chapel Health Centre, London Road, Holmes Chapel, Crewe CW4 7BB — MB BS Newc. 1983; MRCP (UK) 1986; MRCGP 1989; Dip. Occ. Med. 1996.

TATEK, Josef 17 St Andrews Drive, Bridge of Weir PA11 3HS Tel: 01505 614168 — MD Prague 1962 (Chas. Univ. Prague) LRCP LRCS Ed. LRCPS Glas. 1971. Assoc. Specialist (Orthop.) Roy. Alexandra Infirm. Paisley. Prev: Regist. (Orthop.) Roy. Alexandra Infirm. Paisley. SHO (Surg.) Gen.; Hosp. Tabor, Czechoslovakia; Regist. (Orthop.) 1st Orthop. Clinic Prague, Czechoslovakia.

TATEOSSIAN, Miss Jasmine Krikor Hammersmith Hospital (Cytology Department), 150 Du Cane Road, London W12 0HS Tel: 020 8383 3931; 24 Langside Avenue, Roehampton, London SW15 5QT Tel: 020 8876 5974 — MB BS Lond. 1965 (Roy. Free) MRCS Eng. LRCP Lond. 1963. Assoc. Specialist (Histopath.) Hammersmith & Qu. Charlotte's & Chelsea Hosps. Specialty: Histopath. Prev: Regist. Chelsea Hosp. Wom.; SHO Gyn. Guy's Hosp. Gp. Obst. Off. Roy. Free Hosp. Lond.

TATFORD, Edgar Patrick Wylie, MBE, TD 38 Stone Road, Bromley BR2 9AU Tel: 020 8460 1061 — MB BS Lond. 1951 (Guy's) MRCS Eng. LRCP Lond. 1951; DObst 1957; FRCOG 1973, M 1960; DCH Eng. 1961. Cons. O & G Bromley Hosp. Gp.; Col. late RAMC (V), OC 217 (L) Gen. Hosp. RAMC (V). Specialty: Obst. & Gyn. Socs: Fell. Roy. Soc. Med. Prev: Sen. Regist. (O & G) Guy's Hosp. Lond.; Jun. Lect. (Anat.) St. Bart. Hosp. Lond.; Resid. Med. Off. Chelsea Hosp. Wom. & Qu. Charlotte's Hosp. Lond.

TATHAM, Margaret Elizabeth Goodinge Health Centre, Goodinge Close, North Road, London N7 9EW Tel: 020 7530 4940 — MB BS Lond. 1981; BA (Hons.) (Hist.) Toronto 1970; BA (Hons.) (Physiol.) Oxf. 1978; MRCP (UK) 1984.

TATHAM, Pamela Charity The Garth, 79 Hallgarth St., Durham DH1 3AY Tel: 0191 384 6242; 52 Mitchell Avenue, Jesmond, Newcastle upon Tyne NE2 3LA Tel: 0191 281 0193 — MB BS Lond. 1949 (Univ. Coll. Hosp.) Specialty: Homeop. Med. Socs: Brit. Assn. Allergy & Environm. Med.; (Comm.) Inst. Psionic Med.; Assoc. Mem. Fac. Homoeop. Prev: Clin. Med. Off. Sunderland HA; Med. Off. Colon. Med. Serv. Malaya & N. Borneo.

TATHAM, Peter Frank Baxter Farm, Willoughby-on-the-Wolds, Loughborough LE12 6SY Tel: 01509 880975 — MB BS Lond. 1966 (St. Bart.) MRCS Eng. LRCP Lond. 1966; FFA RCS Eng. 1970. Cons. Anaesth. Nottm. City Hosp. Specialty: Anaesth. Prev: Sen. Regist. (Anaesth.) St. Bart. Hosp. Lond.; Dir. of Anaesth. Papua New Guinea; Regist. (Anaesth.) Hosp. Sick Childr. Gt. Ormond St.

TATHAM, Peter Heathcote Maynards, Cornworthy, Totnes TQ9 7HB Tel: 01803 732733 — MB BChir Camb. 1959 (St. Thos.) MA Camb. 1959; DObst RCOG 1966; Dip. Analyt. Psychol. C.G. Jung Inst. Zürich 1978. Specialty: Psychother.

TATHAM, Richard Hugh Benjamin 4 Elim Terrace, Peverell, Plymouth PL3 4PA Tel: 01752 260202; The Old Hall, Harberton, Totnes TQ9 7SQ — MB BS Lond. 1987; BSc (Hons.) Biochem. Lond. 1984. SHO (Med.) Derriford Hosp. Plymouth. Prev: Trainee GP Saltash Cornw.; SHO (Special Care Baby Unit) & Med. Rotat. Derriford Hosp.

TATLA, Taranjit 52 Portland Street, Derby DE23 8QB — MB BS Lond. 1996.

TATMAN, Maybelle Alice Epidemiology and Biostatistics Unit, Institute of Child Health, 30 Guilford St., London WC1N 1EH Tel: 020 7242 9789; 34 Cobden Road, Brighton BN2 2TJ Tel: 01273 684381 — MB BS Lond. 1984; MRCP (UK) 1987; MSC (Community Paediat.) Lond. 1990. Research Fell. Inst. Child Health Lond.

Specialty: Community Child Health. Socs: Brit. Paediat. Assn. Prev: Regist. (Paediat.) Roy. Lond. Hosp.

TATMAN, Peter John Goldington Avenue Surgery, 85 Goldington Avenue, Bedford MK40 3DB; 107 Warwick Avenue, Bedford MK40 2DH — MB BS Lond. 1980 (Middlx.) DRCOG 1982; MRCGP 1983. Gen. Med. Practitioner.

TATNALL, Frances Melanie — MB BS Lond. 1978 (Roy. Free Hosp.) MRCS Eng. LRCP Lond. 1978; FRCP 1996, MRCP (UK) 1980; MD Lond. 1991. Cons. Dermat. Watford Gen. Hosp. Specialty: Dermat.

TATNALL, Sarah Kate Royal Manchester Children's Hospital, Manchester M27 4HA; 125 Swinton Park Road, Salford M6 7PB — BM BS Nottm. 1995. SHO (Paediat.) Roy. Manch. Childr. Hosp.

TATTAN, Theresa Maria Goretti Cossham Hospital, Lodge Road, Kingswood, Bristol BS15 1LQ — MB BS Lond. 1988 (Royal Free Hospital School of Medicine) MRCPsych 1994; MSc Manch. 1996. Sen. Regist. (Psychiat.). Specialty: Gen. Psychiat.

TATTARI, Ms Christalleni 10 Harley street, London W1G 9PF Tel: 0207 467 8540 Email: ctattari@hotmail.com; 13 Bancroft Avenue, London N2 0AR Tel: 0208 340 0777 — Ptychio Iatrikes Athens 1970 (Univ. Athens) MRCS Eng. LRCP Lond. 1975; FRCS Lond. 1979; T(S) 1994. Indep. Pract. (Plastic Surg.) Nuffield Hosp. Lond.; InDepend. Cosmetic and Aesthetic Surg., King's Oak Hosp. Chase Farm (N.side). Specialty: Plastic Surg. Socs: Europ. Acad. Facial Surg.; BMA. Prev: Cons. Plastic Surg. & Head of Plastic Surg. Unit Tembisa Hosp. Olifansfontein, S. Afr.

TATTERSALL, Anne Elizabeth Meltham Group Practice, 1 The Cobbles, Meltham, Huddersfield HD9 4AH Tel: 01484 347 620 Fax: 01484 347 621 — MB BS Lond. 1970 (Roy. Free) MRCS Eng. LRCP Lond. 1970; DCH Eng. 1972.

TATTERSALL, Christopher William 121 Clifton Drive S., Lytham St Annes FY8 1DX — MB BS Lond. 1970. GP Blackpool.

TATTERSALL, Deborah Jane 123 Anderton Park Road, Moseley, Birmingham B13 9DQ Email: dtattersall@blueyonder.co.uk; 16 Silver St, Chacombe, Banbury OX17 2JR Tel: 01295 710612 — MB ChB Manch. 1991; BSc (Hons.) Manch. 1988; MRCP (UK) 1994; FRCR (UK) 1998. Cons. Radiol. Univ. Hosp. Birm. NHS Trust. Specialty: Radiol. Prev: SHO (Med.) Southmead Hosp. Bristol; Regist. (Radiol.) John Radcliffe Hosp. Oxf.

TATTERSALL, Edward Paul Dove River Practice, Gibb Lane, Sudbury, Ashbourne DE6 5HY Tel: 01283 812455 Fax: 01283 815187 Email: paul.tattersall@sshawebmail.nhs.uk; Threeways, Rolleston on Dove, Burton-on-Trent DE13 9BD Tel: 01283 813532 Email: thetats@inrolleston.fsnet.co.uk — MB BS Lond. 1983 (Roy. Free) DRCOG 1986; Cert. Family Plann. JCC 1986; MRCGP 1987. Socs: BMA; Dispensing Doctors Assn. Prev: Trainee GP Burton on Trent VTS.

TATTERSALL, Hilary Jane Pen y Maes Health Centre, Beech Street, Summerhill, Wrexham LL11 4UF Tel: 01978 756370 Fax: 01978 751870 — MB BCh Wales 1977 (WNSM) DRCOG 1981; Cert. Family Plann. JCC 1981; MRCGP 1981; DFFP 1994.

TATTERSALL, James Erskine 45 Langtons Wharf, Leeds LS2 7EF Tel: 0113 247 0955 Email: jamestattersall@compuserve.com — MB BS Lond. 1980 (Char. Cross) MRCP Lond. 1985; MD Lond. 1995. Staff Grade Nephrol, St.James's Univ. Hosp, Leeds; Med. Director Software Developm. Mediqal Ltd Stevenage. Specialty: Nephrol. Prev: Hon. Cons. Basildon Hosp.; Staff Grade Nephrol. North. Gen. Hosp. Sheff.; Clin. Scientist, Lister Hosp. Stevenage.

TATTERSALL, Jill Marjorie (retired) 1 Brackenbarrow Cottages, Smithy Hill, Lindale, Grange-over-Sands LA11 6LT Tel: 015395 34872 — MB ChB Sheff. 1956; DRCOG; DObst RCOG 1959; DCH Eng. 1959; FFFP RCOG 1997. Prev: Head Family Plann. & Well Wom. Servs. Community & Ment. Health Trust S. Cumbria HA.

TATTERSALL, Joan Mary (retired) 10 North Grange Mews, North Grange Road, Leeds LS6 — MB Leeds 1936; MB, ChB Leeds 1936. Prev: Asst. Med. Off. Dept. Stud. Health Univ. Leeds.

TATTERSALL, Joseph Pen y Maes Health Centre, Beech Street, Summerhill, Wrexham LL11 4UF Tel: 01978 756370 Fax: 01978 751870 — MB BCh Wales 1976 (WNSM) Cert Family Plann 1980; DRCOG 1980; MRCGP 1981; D.Occ.Med. 1995; AFOM 1999. Specialty: Gen. Pract.; Occupat. Health.

TATTERSALL, Mark Lincoln Huntercombe Maidenhead Hospital, Huntercombe Lane S., Taplow, Maidenhead SL6 0PQ Tel: 01628 667881 Fax: 01628 603398 — MB BS Lond. 1981 (Westm. Hosp. Med. Sch.) MRCPsych 1989. Cons. Adolec. & Adult Eating Disorders Huntercombe Manor Hosp. Taplow; Hon. Cons. Eating Disorders St. Geo. Hosp. Lond. Specialty: Gen. Psychiat. Prev: Hon. Cons. Eating Disorders Gt. Ormond St. Childr Hosp. Lond.; Cons. Kingston Hosp. Kingston-upon-Thames; Sen. Regist. St. Geo. Hosp. Lond.

TATTERSALL, Michael Paul Swindon & Marlborough NHS Trust, Great Western Hospital, Swindon SN3 6BB Tel: 01793 604020 — MB BS Lond. 1975 (St Thomas's Hospital London) FFA RCS Eng. 1980. Cons. Anaesth. Swindon & MarlBoro. NHS Trust.; McMillan Cons., Prospect Hospice, Swindon. Specialty: Anaesth.; Palliat. Med. Prev: Sen. Regist. (Anaesth.) Nuffield Dept. Anaesth. Oxf.; Regist. (Anaesth.) Bristol Roy. Infirm.; SHO (Clin. Measurem.) Westm. Hosp. Lond.

TATTERSALL, Nigel Manchester Road Surgery, 187 Manchester Road, Burnley BB11 4HP Tel: 01282 420680 Fax: 01282 832031; Kiddrow Lane Health Centre, Kiddrow Lane, Burnley BB12 6LH Tel: 01282 427979; Shepherds Clough Farm, Dean Lane, Bacup OL13 8RG — MB ChB Aberd. 1985; BSc (Hons.) Aberd. 1980. Prev: Clin. Asst. (Genitourin.) Burnley Health Care NHS Trust.

TATTERSALL, Philip Heap (retired) 8 Ravensworth Terrace, Durham DH1 1QP Tel: 0191 384 3699 — MB ChB Leeds 1955; MRCGP 1963. Prev: GP Durh. City.

TATTERSALL, Rachel Scarlett 4 Oakwood Mount, Leeds LS8 2JG — MB ChB Sheff. 1995; BMedSci Sheff. 1992. SHO (Gen. Med.) St. Jas. Univ. Hosp. Leeds.

TATTERSALL, Professor Robert Booth Curzon House, Curzon St, Gotham, Nottingham NG11 0HQ Email: robert.tattersall@virgin.net — MD Camb. 1975, MB 1968, BChir 1967; MRCP (U.K.) 1970; FRCP Lond. 1980. Specialist Prof. Human Metab. Nottm. 1998; Prof. Clin. Diabetes Nottm. Specialty: Endocrinol. Prev: Prof. Clin. Diabetes Nottm.; Sen. Lect. St. Bart. Hosp. Lond.; Sen. Regist. Diabetic Dept. King's Coll. Hosp. Lond.

TATTERSALL, Sally Jane 350 Upper Richmond Road, London SW15 6TL Tel: 020 8788 0686 — MB BS Lond. 1984 (Westm.) MRCGP 1991. Prev: Trainee GP/SHO Rotat. Qu. Marys Hosp. Roehampton VTS.

TATTERSALL, Toby Spa Road Surgery, Spa Road East, Llandrindod Wells LD1 5ES Tel: 01597 824291 / 842292 Fax: 01597 824503 — MB BS Lond. 1988; DRCOG 1991; MRCGP 1993.

TATTERSFIELD, Professor Anne Elizabeth Division of Respiratory Medicine, Clinical Sciences Building, City Hospital, Hucknall Road, Nottingham NG5 1PB Tel: 0115 840 4772 Fax: 0115 840 4771 Email: anne.tattersfield@nottingham.ac.uk; Priory Barn, The Hollows, Thurgarton, Nottingham NG14 7GY Tel: 01636 830378 — (Newc.) MB BS Durh. 1963; FRCP Lond. 1979, M 1966; MD Newc. 1970. Prof. Respirat. Med. City Hosp. Nottm. Specialty: Respirat. Med. Socs: Brit. Thoracic Soc. (Past Pres.); Acad. of Med. Sci.; Assn. of Physicians. Prev: Sen. Lect. & Reader (Med.) Soton.; Sen. Regist. Lond. Hosp.; Regist. Hammersmith Hosp.

TATTERSFIELD, Helen Grace Oakview Family Practice, 190 Shroffold Road, Downham, Bromley BR1 5NJ Tel: 020 8695 6485 Fax: 020 8695 0830; 29 Stone Road, Bromley BR2 9AX Tel: 0208 460 9993 — MB BS Lond. 1984 (King's Coll. Lond.) MA Oxf. 1984; DRCOG 1989; DCH RCP Lond. 1989; MRCGP 1990; DFFP 1996. Primary Care Phys., Lewisham Hosp.; Bd. Mem., S. lewisham PCG. Specialty: Gen. Pract.

TATTERSFIELD, Mr James Frederick 30 Sauncey Avenue, Harpenden AL5 4QJ Tel: 01582 762919 — (Middlx.) MB BS Lond. 1957; DO Eng. 1964; FRCS Ed. 1967. Cons. Ophth. Surg. Luton & Dunstable Hosp. & St. Albans City Hosp. Specialty: Ophth. Socs: FRCOphth. Prev: Sen. Regist. (Ophth.) Nat. Hosp. Nerv. Dis. Maida Vale & Roy. Free Hosp.; Clin. Asst. Moorfields Eye Hosp.; Regist. St. Mary's Hosp. & W. Ophth. Hosp. Lond. & Addenbrooke's Hosp.

TATTON, Pamela Upholme, Blackamoor Crescent, Dore, Sheffield S17 3GL Tel: 0114 236 0339 — MB ChB Sheff. 1977.

TATTUM, Christine Mary The Tardis Surgery, 9 Queen Street, Cheadle, Stoke-on-Trent ST10 1BH Tel: 01538 753771 Fax: 01538 752557 — MB ChB Manch. 1980; DRCOG 1984; MRCGP 1986. Asst. Occupat. Phys. Stoke-on-Trent. Specialty: Occupat. Health. Prev: Trainee GP/SHO N. Staffs. HA VTS.

TATTUM, Keith Thomas Baddeley Green Surgery, 988 Leek New Road, Stoke-on-Trent ST9 9PB Tel: 01782 533777 Fax: 01782 533333 Email: keith.tattum@nshawebmail.nhs.uk; 988 Leek New Road, Stockton Brook, Stoke-on-Trent ST9 9PB — MB ChB Manch.

1980; BA (Hons.) Hull 1974; DRCOG 1984; FRCGP 1993, M 1986; DFFP 1994. Clin. Lect. Keele Univ.; Clin. Tutor, Univ. Coll. Lond., and Roy. Free Hosps., 1999; Mental Health Lead, North Stoke PCT, 1999. Special Interest: Alternative Models of Primary Care; Arts for Health; Ment. Health in Primary Care. Prev: Lect. (Med.) Sch. Univ. Manch.; SHO (A & E) Wythenshawe Hosp. Univ. Manch. Sch. Med.; Trainee GP N. Staffs. VTS.

TAUB, Pierre-Stanislas Antoine 209 Harrow Road, London W2 5EG Tel: 020 7266 6000 — MB BCh Wales 1990 (University of Wales, College of Medicine) T (GP) 1994; MRC Psych 1997. Cons. Psychiat., Paterson Centre for Ment. Health, Lond. Specialty: Gen. Psychiat.

TAUBE, Mr Martin West Wales General Hospital, Carmarthen SA31 2AF Tel: 01267 227514 Fax: 01267 227514; 21 Swiss Valley, Llanelli SA14 8BS Tel: 01554 774096 Fax: 01554 774096 — MRCS Eng. LRCP Lond. 1975 (Westm.) BSc Lond. 1972, MS 1988, MB BS (Hons.) 1975; FRCS Eng. 1979. Cons. (Urol.) W. Wales Gen Hosp. Carmathen. Specialty: Urol.; Gen. Surg. Prev: Ho. Surg., Regist., Sen. Regist. & Lect. Westm. Hosp. Lond.; Cons. Surg. & Urol. P. Philip Hosp. Llanelli; Marks & Spencer Fell. RCS 1980.

TAUBEL, Jorg Richmond Pharmacology, Atkinson Morley's Hospital, Lopse Hill, London SW20 0NE Tel: 020 8879 7111 Fax: 020 8879 6237 Email: j.taubel@RichmondPharmacology.com — MD Frankfurt 1989; State Exam Med. Frankfurt 1987; Dip Pharm Med Lond. 1999. MD CharterHo. Clin. Research Unit Lond. Specialty: Pharmacology; Pharmaceutical Medicine. Prev: Head Med. Dept. Clin. Pharmacol. Parexel Berlin.

TAUBMAN, Rachel Lucy 101 Westfield Lane, St Leonards-on-Sea TN37 7NF — MB BS Lond. 1993.

TAUDEVIN, Elizabeth Jeanne Elm Grove Surgery, Silver St., Calne SN11 0JD Tel: 01249 812305; 60 Trinity Park, Calne SN11 0QD — MB BChir Camb. 1993; DRCOG 1995; MRCGP 1996. GP Calne. Specialty: Gen. Pract. Prev: Trainee GP/SHO (Psychiat.) Roy. United Hosp. Bath VTS.

TAULKE-JOHNSON, Timothy Desmond c/o Newlands Medical Clinic, Chorley New Road, Bolton BL1 5BP — MB BS Lond. 1977; MRCS Eng. LRCP Lond. 1977.

TAUSSIG, David Christopher 52 Arthur Road, Wimbledon, London SW19 7DS Tel: 020 8946 0316; 20 Mina Road, Old Merton Park, London SW19 3AU — MB BS Lond. 1993 (Char. Cross & Westm. Med. Sch.) BSc (Basic Med. Scis. & Pharmacol.) Lond. 1990; MRCP (UK) 1996; MRCPath 2001. Specialist Regist. (Haemat.) Roy. Lond. Hosp.; ICRF Translational Research Fell., Stem ceil Laborat. Room 504, ICRF, 44 Lincoln's Inn Fields, Lond. Specialty: Haematology. Prev: SHO (Intens. Care) St. Geo. Hosp. Lond.; SHO (Infec. Dis.) St. Geo. Hosp. Lond.; SHO (Gen. Med. with Cardiol.) E. Surrey Hosp. Redhill.

TAUSSIG, Jo-Ann 57 Vainor Road, Wadsley, Hillsborough, Sheffield S6 4AP — MB BS Lond. 1998; MB BS Lond 1998.

TAUZEEH, Shah Mohammad Finchley Memorial Hospital, Granville Road, London N12 0JE — MB BS Calcutta 1981.

TAVABIE, Abdolah The Surgery, 108 Chislehurst Road, Orpington BR6 0DW Tel: 01689 826664 Fax: 01689 890795 — MD Jondishapour 1975 (Jondishapour Univ.) MRCGP; FRCGP 1993. GP; Dean of Postgrad. GP Educat. S. Thames (E.). Specialty: Diabetes.

TAVABIE, Jacqueline Ann The Surgery, 108 Chislehurst Road, Orpington BR6 0DW — MB BS Lond. 1981 (Guy's) BSc (Biochem.) Lond. 1978; DRCOG 1994; MRCGP 1995. GP Orpington.

TAVADIA, Hosie Byram (retired) Stirling Royal Infirmary, Department of Pathology, Stirling FK8 2AU Tel: 01786 434000 — MB ChB Aberd. 1964; DObst RCOG 1966; FRCPath 1982, M 1971. Prev: Lect. (Path.) Roy. Infirm. Glas.

TAVADIA, Sherine Menzies Byram 3F1, 7 Hovelock St., Glasgow G11 5JB — MB ChB Glas. 1993; MRCP(UK) 1996. Specialty: Dermat.

TAVARE, Stephen Myles Sawston Health Centre, Link Road, Sawston, Cambridge CB2 4LB Tel: 01223 832711 Fax: 01223 836096 — MB Camb. 1977; BChir 1976; DRCOG 1979; MRCGP 1981.

TAVARES-MOTT, Nicola Esseuvolon 138 Selwyn Road, Birmingham B16 0HN — MB BS Lond. 1994; BSc Lond. 1991.

TAVERNER, John Patrick (retired) 96 Dorridge Road, Dorridge, Solihull B93 8BS Tel: 01564 775575 — MB BCh Wales 1970; DObst RCOG 1974; MRCGP 1975. Prev: SHO (Allergy & Asthma) St. Davids Hosp. Cardiff.

TAVERNOR, Rosalyn Mary Elizabeth Department of Forensic Psychiatry, Nottingham Healthcare NHS Trust, Duncan Macmillan House, Nottingham NG3 6AA — MB ChB Leeds 1988; MRCPsych 1994. Lect. (Forens. Psychiat.) Liverp. Univ. & Hon. Sen. Regist. Ashworth Hosp. Specialty: Forens. Psychiat.

TAVERNOR, Simon James Department of Psychiatry, B Floor South Block, Queens Medical Centre, Derby Road, Nottingham NG7 2UH Tel: 0115 924 9924 — MB ChB Ed. 1987; BSc (Hons.) Ed. 1985; MRCPsych 1993. Cons. (Psychiat.) Univ. Hosp. Nottm.; Clin. Teach., Nottm. Univ. Specialty: Gen. Psychiat. Socs: Brit. Neuropsychiat. Assn.; Brit. Assn. for PsychoPharmacol. Prev: Clin. Lect. (Psychiat.) Nottm. Univ.; Sen. Regist. Rotat. (Gen. Adult Psychiat.) Mid Trent; Regist. Rotat. (Psychiat.) Gtr. Manch.

TAW, Harry 6 Hillside Road, Southall UB1 2PD — MB BS Med. Inst. (I) Rangoon 1975.

TAWFIK, Rihab Fathi Pinderfields General Hospital, Wakefield WF1 4DG Tel: 01924 201688 Fax: 01924 814864 — (Baghdad, Iraq) MB ChB Baghdad 1969; DCH Baghdad 1976; MRCP (UK) 1979; FRCPCH 1996; FRCP 1999. Cons. Paediat. Pinderfields Hosp. Wakefield. Specialty: Paediat. Socs: Brit. Soc. Paediat. Gastroenterol. & Nutrit.; Yorks. Regional Paediat. Soc. Prev: Sen. Regist. (Paediat. Gastroenterol.) Booth Hall Hosp. Manch.

TAWIA, Anmor 46 Strand Park, Cloughmills, Ballymena BT44 9LL — LRCPI & LM, LRSCI & LM 1963; LRCPI & LM, LRCSI & LM 1963.

TAWN, David Julian Department Diagnostic Radiology, Royal Bournemouth Hospital, Castle Lane E., Bournemouth BH7 7DW Tel: 01202 303626; Elgam House, 32 Arnewood Road, Southbourne, Bournemouth BH6 5DH Tel: 01202 428776 — MB ChB Bristol 1980; FRCR 1988. Cons. Radiol. Roy. Bournemouth & ChristCh. Hosps. NHS Trust. Specialty: Radiol. Prev: Sen. Regist. (Radiodiag.) Bristol Roy. Infirm. & Plymouth Hosp.

TAWODZERA, Percy Bobo-Changadeya Peter c/o Professor Middlemiss, Department of Radiodiagnosis, Bristol Royal Infirmary, Bristol BS2 8HW Tel: 0117 922041 — MB ChB Birm. 1974 (Rhodesia) DMRD Eng. 1981; FRCR 1982.

TAWSE, Bernadette Marie Pudsey Health Centre, 18 Mulberry Street, Pudsey LS28 7XP Tel: 0113 257 0711 Fax: 0113 236 3928; 101 Holt Lane, Leeds LS16 7PJ — MB ChB Aberd. 1972. Specialty: Gen. Pract.

TAWSE, Stephen Barclay The Health Centre, North Road, Stokesley, Middlesbrough TS9 5DY Tel: 01642 710748 Fax: 01642 713037; 12 The Avenue, Stokesley, Middlesbrough TS9 5ET Tel: 01642 711365 — MB BS Lond. 1987; BSc Lond. 1984; DA (UK) 1991; DRCOG 1992; MRCGP 1993. Prev: Trainee GP Leyburn; SHO (Psychiat.) Darlington; SHO (Paediat.) Northallerton.

TAY, Clement Chong Kheng Simpson Centre for Reproductive Health, Royal Infirmary of Edinburgh, Little France, Edinburgh EH16 4SA — MB ChB Glas. 1980; MSc (Med. Sci.) Glas. 1984; FRCS Glas. 1988; MRCOG 1988; FRCOG London 2000. Cons. O & G Simpson Centre for Reproductive Health, Royal Infirmary of Edinburgh, Little France, Edinburgh. Specialty: Obst. & Gyn. Special Interest: Infertil.; Minimal Access Surg.; Polycystic Ovary Syndrome. Prev: Subspeciality Train. Fell. (Reproduc. Med.) & Sen. Regist. (O & G) Roy. Infirm. Edin.; WHO Clin. Research Fell. (Reproduc. Med.) Centre for Reproduc. Biol. Univ. Edin.; Regist. Qu. Mother's Hosp. & West. Infirm. Glas.

TAY, Eugene Sheng Wei Flat 167, Defoe House, Barbican, London EC2Y 8ND — MB BS Lond. 1997.

TAY, Hua Hui 156 Bensham Lane, Thornton Heath, Croydon CR7 7EN — MB BS Lond. 1981; MRCP (UK) 1984.

TAY, Mr Huey Ling ENT Department, Freeman Hospital, High Heaton, Newcastle upon Tyne NE7 7DN; 203 Elmwood House, Melville Grove, Newcastle upon Tyne NE7 7AZ — BM BCh Oxf. 1985; FRCS Ed. 1989; FRCS Eng. 1993.

TAY, Jacqueline I-Yen Clarendon Wing, Leeds General Infirmary, Belmont Grove, Leeds LS2 9NS Tel: 0113 2432799 — MB ChB Leic. 1986 (University of Leicester) MRCOG Leic. 1992; MD Leic. 2003. Cons. (O & G) Leeds Teachg. Hosps. NHS Trust, Leeds. Specialty: Obst. & Gyn.; Gen. Med. Socs: BMA; BFS (British Fertil. Society); BSGE (British Soc. of Gyn. Endoscopists). Prev: Locum Cons., Obstetrics/Gynaecology, Leeds Gen. Infirm., Leeds; Clin. Lect., Obstetrics/Gynaecology, Univ. of Leeds, Leeds.

TAY, Kem Sing The Evergreen Practice, Skimped Hill Health Centre, Skimped Hill Lane, Bracknell RG12 1LH Tel: 01344 306936 Fax: 01344 306966 — LRCP LRCS Ed. 1982; LRCP LRCS Ed. LRCPS Glas. 1982. Socs: BMA & Brit. Med. Acupunc. Soc.

TAY, Paul Yee Siang Flat 6, Eden Court, 79 Clarkehouse Road, Sheffield S10 2LG Tel: 0114 267 0665 — MB BCh BAO Belf. 1992; MRCOG. 1996. SHO (O & G) Roy. Vict. Hosp. Belf.; Clin. Fell. Sheff. Fertil.. Sheff. Specialty: Obst. & Gyn. Prev: SHO (O & G) Ulster Hosp. Dundonald & Roy. Vict. Hosp.; SHO (O & G) Roy Vict Hosp. Belf.; SHO (O & G) Belf. City Hosp. Belf.

TAY, Teck Wah 18 Kensington Manor, Dollingstown, Craigavon BT66 7HR — MB BCh BAO Belf. 1992.

TAY MCGARRY, Guek Siang 9 The Plateau, Piney Hills, Belfast BT9 5QP — MB BCh BAO Belf. 1969.

TAY ZA AUNG, Dr New Health Centre, Third Avenue, Canvey Island SS8 9SU Tel: 01268 683758 Fax: 01268 684057; 85 Long Road, Canvey Island SS8 0JB — MB BS Rangoon 1957; DPH Bristol 1961; DObst RCOG 1967; MRCGP 1974. Prev: SHO Southend & Rochford Gen. Hosps. & Co. Hosp. Griffithstown; Med. Off. Sea & Airport Rangoon, Burma.

TAYABALI, Mujtaba 14 Hauxton Road, Little Shelford, Cambridge CB2 5HJ — MB ChB St. And. 1962.

TAYAL, Mr Nilema 5 East Court, Wembley HA0 3QJ Tel: 020 8904 3590 — FRCS Ed. 1986.

TAYAL, Surupchand Aminchand 21 Angram Drive, Sunderland SR2 7RD — MB BS Gujarat 1977; MD Gujarat 1980; MRCPI 1990. Cons.(Genitourin Med.) Middlesbourough Gen Hosp. Specialty: Genitourinary Medicine; HIV Med. Socs: Soc. Study VD. Prev: Sen. Regist. (Genitourin. Med.) Newc. Gen. Hosp.

TAYAR, René Radiology Department, St Helier Hospital, Wrythe Lane, Carshalton SM5 1AA Tel: 0208 644 4343; 45 Epsom Lane S., Tadworth KT20 5TA Tel: 01737 813582 — MD Malta 1980; MD Malta 1969; FRCR 1980. Cons. Radiol. St. Helier NHS Trust Carshalton Surrey; Hon. Sen. Lect. St. Geo. Hosp. Med. Sch. Lond. Socs: MRAA (UK); Educat. Sec., previously Hon. Sec. Prev: Hon. Sec. MRAA (UK) 1998-2003; Sen. Regist. & Regist. United Bristol Hosps.

TAYLER, David Holroyd Royal Sussex County Hospital, Eastern Road, Brighton BN2 3EW — MB BS Lond. 1981; FFA RCS Eng. 1986. Cons. Anaesth. Roy. Sussex Co. Hosp. Brighton. Specialty: Anaesth. Prev: Sen. Regist. (Anaesth.) King's Coll. Hosp. Lond.

TAYLER, David Ian Lawson Road Surgery, 5 Lawson Road, Broomhill, Sheffield S10 5BU Tel: 0114 266 2860; 225 Ringinglow Road, Bents Green, Sheffield S11 7PT Email: d.tayler@shef.ac.uk — BM (Hons) Soton. 1977; BSc (Engin) (1st cl. Hons.) 1972; MRCP (UK) 1979; DRCOG 1986; MRCGP 1986; FRCP 2002. Hosp. Pract. (Cardiol.) North. Gen. Hosp. Sheff. Specialty: Cardiol. Prev: Research Fell. Cardiol. North. Gen. Hosp. Sheff.; Regist. (Cardiol. & Gen. Med.) King's Coll. Hosp. Lond. & Roy. Sussex.Co. Hosp.

TAYLER, Deborah Jayne Southway Surgery, 2 Bampfylde Way, Southway, Plymouth PL6 6TA — MB BCh Wales 1985; BSc (Physiol.) Wales 1980; DRCOG 1987; MRCGP 1989.

TAYLER, Elizabeth Mary DFID, 1 Palace Street, London SW1E 5HE Email: l-tayler@dfid.gov.uk; The Cottage, The Cottage, Quality Street, Redhill RH1 3BB — BM BCh Oxf. 1988 (Oxford) MRCP (UK) 1991; MSc Fac of Med 1994; MFPHM 1999. Policy Team Leader DFID. Specialty: Pub. Health Med. Prev: ODA Fell. Tuberc. Unit WHO Geneva; Sen. Regist., Pub. health, Oxf. health Auth.; Health Adviser/Deputy Head DFID, Nigeria.

TAYLER, Michael John The Surgery, Margaret Street, Thaxted, Dunmow CM6 2QN Tel: 01371 830213 Fax: 01371 831278; Oakhurst, Park St, Thaxted, Dunmow CM6 2NE Tel: 01371 831059 — MB Camb. 1980; BChir 1979; DRCOG 1983; MRCGP 1985; Dip. IMC RCS Ed. 1993. Prev: Trainee GP Addenbrooke's Hosp. VTS Camb.; Ho. Surg. Addenbrooke's Hosp. Camb.; Ho. Phys. W. Suff. Hosp. Bury St. Edmunds.

TAYLER, Peter James Fairfield Centre, 12 Portland Square, Carlisle CA1 1PY; 24 Woodcroft Road, Wylam NE41 8DH Tel: 01661 852464 Fax: 01661 854044 — BM BCh Oxf. 1976; MA Camb. 1977; MRCP (UK) 1978; MRCPsych 1985; FRCPsych 1997. Cons. Adolesc. Psychiat. Fairfield Centre Carlisle; Cons. Adolesc. Psychiat. Lindisfarne Suite Nuffield Private Hosp. Clayton Rd. Jesmond, Newc.-u-Tyne. Specialty: Child & Adolesc. Psychiat.; Medico Legal. Prev: Sen. Regist. (Child Adolesc. Psychiat.) Nuffield Child Psychiat. Unit Newc.; Regist. (Paediat.) Westm. Childr. Hosp.; Cons. Adolesc. Psychiat. Sir Martin Roth. Young People's Unit Newc. Gen. Hosp.

TAYLER, Robert George Opie (retired) Merlebank, Church Hill, Merstham, Redhill RH1 3BJ Tel: 01737 643178 — MB BChir Camb. 1948 (Guy's) MA Camb. 1946, MB BChir 1948; DObst RCOG 1951. Prev: Clin. Asst. (Surg.) Redhill E. Surrey Hosp.

TAYLER, Timothy Martin Brook Lane Surgery, 233a Brook Lane, Sarisbury Green, Southampton SO31 7DQ Tel: 01489 575191 Fax: 01489 570033; 60 Brook Lane, Warsash, Southampton SO31 9FG Tel: 01489 584297 — MB ChB Bristol 1981; MRCP (UK) 1984. Prev: SHO (Neurol., Cardiol. & Gastroenterol.) Soton. Gen. Hosp.; SHO (Chest Med.) Hall Green Hosp. Bristol.

TAYLOR, Adam David 1 Meadow Close, Hove BN3 6QQ — MB ChB Aberd. 1993.

TAYLOR, Adrian Howard 50 Kewstoke Road, Stoke Bishop, Bristol BS9 1HF — MB BS Lond. 1992; FRCS 1997; FRCS (Trauma & Orth.) 2003. Specialty: Trauma & Orthop. Surg.

TAYLOR, Adrienne Laurel Farm, 20 St Andrew's Road, Old Headington, Oxford OX3 9DL — BM BCh Oxf. 1967; MA, BM BCh Oxf. 1967.

TAYLOR, Aileen Euphemia Macdonald Department of Dermatology, Royal Victoria Infirmary, Queen Victoria Road, Newcastle upon Tyne NE1 4LP Tel: 0191 232 5131; 40 Reid Park Road, Jesmond, Newcastle upon Tyne NE2 2ES — MB ChB Ed. 1976 (Edin.) MRCP (UK) 1980; FRCP 1998. Cons. Dermat. Newc. Hosps. NHS Trust. Specialty: Dermat.

TAYLOR, Alan Furness General Hospital, Pathology Laboratory, Barrow-in-Furness LA14 4LF Tel: 01229 491257 Fax: 01229 491044 Email: alan.taylor@fgh.mbht.nhs.uk — MB ChB Liverp. 1977 (Liverpool) BA (Hons.) Oxf. 1970; FRCPath 1996, M 1984; MA Oxon 1990. Cons. (Chem. Path.) Morecambe Bay Hospitals: Lancaster, Barrow-In-Furness, Kendal; Hon. Lect. Biochem. Dept. Univ. Lancaster. Specialty: Chem. Path. Special Interest: Lipidology. Socs: Assn. Clin. Biochems.; Heart UK. Prev: Ho. Off. Liverp. Roy. Infirm.; Sen. Regist. (Clin. Chem.) Univ. Hosp. Nottm.; Regist. (Clin. Biochem.) Addenbrookes Hosp. Camb.

TAYLOR, Alan David North Devon District Hospital, Raleigh Park, Barnstaple EX31 45B Tel: 01271 322577 Fax: 01271 311541 — MB BS Lond. 1991 (St. Bart. Hosp. Med. Sch.) DPhil (Chem.) Sussex 1986, BSc (Chem.) 1983; MRCP (UK) 1995. Cons. (Cardiol. & Gen. Internal Med.) N. Devon Dist. Hosp. Specialty: Gen. Med.; Cardiol. Socs: MDU. Prev: Specialist Regist. (Cardiol.) Derriford Hosp. Plymouth.; Regist. (Cardiol.) Roy. Devon & Exeter Hosp.; SHO (Med.) Singleton Hosp. Swansea.

TAYLOR, Alan Richard, BEM (retired) 12 Culloden Road, Enfield EN2 8QB — (Lond. Hosp.) MB BS Lond. 1950; DObst RCOG 1952; DTM & H Eng. 1959; MRCGP 1964. Prev: Med. Supt. Med. Serv. & Clinic Chittagong, E. Pakistan.

TAYLOR, Mr Alan Robert Stoke Mandeville Hospital NHS Trust, Mandeville Road, Aylesbury HP01 8AL Tel: 01296 315197 Fax: 01296 315199; Elmhurst, 23 School Lane, Weston Turville, Aylesbury HP22 5SG Tel: 01296 613201 Fax: 01296 615401 — MB BS Newc. 1969; FRCS Ed. 1975; FRCS Eng. 1975. Cons. Gen. Surg. Stoke Mandeville Hosp. Specialty: Gen. Surg. Socs: Brit. Assn Of Research Surg.; Assoc. Of Surg.s GB + Irel.; Soc. Of Acad. and Research surg. Prev: Lect. (Surg.) Univ. Liverp.; Sen. Regist. (Surg.) Roy. Liverp. Hosp. & Broadgreen Hosp. Liverp.; Wellcome Research Fell. & Tutor (Surg.) Roy. Postgrad. Med. Sch.

TAYLOR, Alasdair Royal Lancaster Infirmary, Department of Radiology, Lancaster LA1 4RP — MB ChB Aberd. 1983. Cons.(Radiol.) Morecambe Bay Hosps. Trust & Lancaster & Lakeland Nuffield Hosp. Specialty: Radiol. Special Interest: Magnetic resonance imaging; Gastrointestinal Radiol.; Cancer imaging. Socs: Brit. Soc. of Gastroenterol. (Special Interest Gp. in Gastrointestinal & Abdom. Radiol.).

TAYLOR, Alastair Douglas Kessington Medical Centre, 85 Milngavie Road, Bearsden, Glasgow G61 2DN Tel: 0141 211 5621 — MB ChB Glas. 1992 (Glasgow) DFFP 1994; DRCOG 1995; MRCGP 1996. GP Principle, Kessington Med. Centre, Bearsden. Specialty: Anaesth.; Gen. Pract. Socs: BMA. Prev: SHO Anaesth. Monklands DGH Lanarksh.; GP/Regist. Argyll VTS - Taynvilt Med. Pract.; SHO Med. Lorn & Is.s DGH Oban.

TAYLOR, Alexander James, OBE Grampian Healthcare NHS Trust, Westholme, Woodend Hospital, Aberdeen AB15 6LS Tel: 01224 663131 Fax: 01224 840790; Beechwood, Fyvie, Turriff AB53 8PB Tel: 01651 891349 Fax: 01651 891706 — MB ChB Aberd. 1950; FRCGP 1978, M 1963. Chairm. Grampian Healthcare NHS Trust Woodend Hosp. Aberd.; Hon. Sen. Lect. Univ. Aberd.; Med. Examr. Civil Aviat. Auth. Specialty: Aviat. Med. Prev: Lect. (Gen. Pract.) Univ. Aberd.; GP Fyvie, Turriff; Med. Off. Shapinsay, Orkney.

TAYLOR, Alexandra 30 Bonchurch Road, Southsea PO4 8RZ — MB BS Lond. 1993.

TAYLOR, Alexandra Jayne 12 Haileybury Road, West Bridgford, Nottingham NG2 7BJ — MB BS Lond. 1993.

TAYLOR, Mr Alfred Roy (retired) 4 Watchcroft Drive, Buckingham MK18 1GH Tel: 01280 823551 — MB BS Lond. 1957 (St. Mary's) MRCS Eng. LRCP Lond. 1957; FRCS Eng. 1964. Assoc. Surg. Nuffield Orthop. Centre Oxf. Prev: Cons. Orthop. Surg. Aylesbury Gp. Hosps. & Oxf. Regional Rheum Research Centre Stoke Mandeville Hosp. Aylesbury.

TAYLOR, Aliki Joanna The University of Birmingham, Public Health and Epidemiology, Edgbaston, Birmingham B15 2TT Email: a.j.taylor@bham.ac.uk — MB BS Lond. 1994; MPH Birm. 1999; MFPHM 2001. p/t Cancer Research UK Train. Fell. Specialty: Pub. Health Med.

TAYLOR, Alison Elizabeth 10 St Georges Avenue, Timperley, Altrincham WA15 6HE — MB ChB Manch. 1994.

TAYLOR, Alison Mary Cameron 30 The Drive, Hove BN3 3JD Tel: 01273 778123 — MB BS Lond. 1989 (St. Barts. Hosp. Lond.) DRCOG 1991; MRCGP 1994; MFHom 2003. GP Centr. Ho. Surg. Hove; Homeopathic Phys. Specialty: Obst. & Gyn.; Gen. Pract. Prev: Trainee GP Hove.

TAYLOR, Alison Patricia QEDH, Mindelsohn Way, Edgbaston, Birmingham B15 2QZ — MB ChB Manch. 1988; BA Liverp. 1978; MRCPsych 1992; MMedSci (Psychiat.) Birm. 1996. Cons. (Old Age Psychiat.) S. Birm. Ment. Health Trust. Specialty: Geriat. Psychiat. Prev: Sen. Regist. (Psychiat.) W. Midl. RHA; Regist. Rotat. (Psychiat.) S. Birm. DHA; SHO (Psychiat.) Lancaster Moor Hosp. & Midl. Nerve Hosp. Birm.

TAYLOR, Alistair John The Health Centre, Bank St., Faversham ME13 8QR Tel: 01795 533296 — MB ChB Bristol 1981; DRCOG 1984; MRCGP 1985.

TAYLOR, Amanda Jane Whetstone Lane Health Centre, 44 Whetstone Lane, Birkenhead CH41 2TF Tel: 0151 647 9613 Fax: 0151 650 0875; Beacon Cottage, Moorland Close, Heswall, Wirral CH60 0EL — MB ChB Liverp. 1986; DRCOG 1988.

TAYLOR, Amanda Jane Biggleswade Health Centre, Saffron Road, Biggleswade SG18 8DJ — MB BS Lond. 1992.

TAYLOR, Amanda Victoria Wessex Regional Forensic Psychiatric Services, Ravenswood House, The Knowle Hospital, Fareham PO17 5NA Tel: 01329 836198 Fax: 01329 834780 — MB BS Lond. 1985 (Middlesex) BSc Lond. 1982, MB BS 1985; MRCPsych 1991. Specialty: Forens. Psychiat.

TAYLOR, Andrea Jane Town Medical Centre, 25 London Road, Sevenoaks TN13 1AR Tel: 01732 454545/458844 Fax: 01732 462181; 22 Annetts Hall, Borough Green, Sevenoaks TN15 8DY — MB ChB Leeds 1982; BSc (Chem. Path.) Leeds 1979, MB ChB 1982; DRCOG 1985; MRCGP 1986.

TAYLOR, Andrew Alexander Department of Obstertrics & Gynaecology, Royal Free Hospital, Pond Street, London NW3 2QW — MB BS Newc. 1993.

TAYLOR, Mr Andrew Barrie Wilson Easter Cornhill, South Creake, Fakenham NR21 9LX Tel: 01328 560 — MB ChB Ed. 1964; FRCOG 1983, M 1970, DObst 1967; FRCS Ed. 1971. Cons. O & G Qu. Eliz. Hosp. King's Lynn Norf. Specialty: Obst. & Gyn. Socs: Brit. Soc. Colposcopy; Fell. Edin. Obst. Soc.; Fell. Roy. Soc. Med. Prev: Sen. Regist. & Clin. Tutor Hammersmith Hosp. Lond.; Regist. (Gen. Surg.) Peel Hosp. Galashiels; SHO Simpson Memor. Matern. Pavil., Roy. Infirm. Edin.

TAYLOR, Andrew Damian Hull Royal Infirmary, X-Ray Department, Anlaby Road, Hull HU3 2JZ Tel: 01482 28541 — MB ChB Bristol 1977; FRCR 1986. Cons. Diag. Radiol. Hull & E. Yorks. HA. Specialty: Radiol.; Medico Legal. Socs: Brit. Med. Ultrasound Soc.; Brit. Soc. Of Skeletal Radiologists. Prev: Sen. Regist. (Diag. Radiol.) Char. Cross Hosp. Lond.

TAYLOR, Andrew Frederick 38 Ashden Walk, Tonbridge TN10 3RL — MB BS Lond. 1996; BSc (Lond.) 1993, MB BS 1996; FRCA 2000. SpR (Anaesth.) Kent and Sussex Hosp. Specialty: Anaesth. Prev: SHO (Anaesth.) Redhill & St. Hellier Hosps. Surrey.

TAYLOR, Mr Andrew John Nigel Royal Liverpool Hospital, Prescot Street, Liverpool L7 8XP — MB BS Lond. 1991; BSc Lond. 1988; FRCS Eng. 1995; FRCS (Tr. & Orth.) 2000. Specialty: Orthop.

TAYLOR, Andrew Lionel Johnson St James Medical Centre, 11 Carlton Road, Tunbridge Wells TN1 2HW Tel: 01892 541634 Fax: 01892 545170 — MB BS Lond. 1975 (St. Bartholomews Hosp., Lond.) DRCOG 1977; DCH RCP Lond. 1979; MRCGP 1981. Socs: Christian Med. Fellowsh. Prev: Med. Off. Africa Inland Ch. Kapsowar Hosp., Kenya.

TAYLOR, Andrew Mark Maudsley Hospital, London SE5 8AF — MB BS Lond. 1988.

TAYLOR, Andrew Michael 160 The Dashes, Harlow CM20 3RU — BM Soton. 1992; BSc Sheff. 1988. Specialty: Gen. Med.

TAYLOR, Mr Andrew Michael Uplands, 11 College Street, East Bridgford, Nottingham NG13 8LE — MB BS Lond. 1990; FRCS Eng. 1994; DMed Nottm. 1999; FRCS (Trauma & Orthopaedics) 2000. Socs: Brit. Orthop. Train. Assn.; Brit. Orthopaedic Foot Surg. Soc.

TAYLOR, Andrew Philip 71 Flixborough Road, Burton-upon-Stather, Scunthorpe DN15 9HB — MB ChB Leeds 1990.

TAYLOR, Andrew Richard Beech Tree Surgery, 68 Doncaster Road, Selby YO8 9AJ Tel: 01757 703933 Fax: 01757 213473 — MB ChB Birm. 1988. Clin. Asst. (A & E) Selby War Memor. Hosp. N. Yorks. Specialty: Gen. Pract.

TAYLOR, Andrew Spencer Taylor, Parsons, Donnelly, Kuruvilla and Mulrine, Woolton House Medical Centre, 4/6 Woolton Street, Woolton, Liverpool L25 5JA Tel: 0151 428 4184 Fax: 0151 428 4598; 5 Sunnygate Road, Liverpool L19 9BS — MB ChB Liverp. 1977; MRCGP 1988. Med. Off. Liverp. Marie Curie Centre. Socs: Liverp. LMC.

TAYLOR, Andrew William Leesbrook Surgery, Mellor Street, Lees, Oldham OL4 3DG Tel: 0161 621 4800 Fax: 0161 628 6717; 38 Summershades Lane, Grasscroft, Saddleworth, Oldham OL4 4ED Tel: 01457 878570 Fax: 01457 874894 — MB ChB Manch. 1970. Clin. Asst. (Urodynamics) Oldham HA. Prev: Regist. (Surg.) Preston Roy. Infirm.; SHO Rotat. (Surg.) Manch. Roy. Infirm.; SHO (Urol.) Crumpsall Hosp. Manch.

TAYLOR, Angela Valerie (retired) 30 Trafalgar Road, Birkdale, Southport PR8 2HE Tel: 01704 568800; 30 Trafalgar Road, Birkdale, Southport PR8 2HE — MB ChB Liverp. 1960. Med. Mem. of APPEALS Serv. Prev: Princip. in Gen. Pract.

TAYLOR, Anita Jane Central Health Clinic, 1 Mulberry St., Sheffield S1 2PJ Tel: 0114 271 6815 Fax: 0114 271 6791; 74 Townend Street, Sheffield S10 1NN — MRCS Eng. LRCP Lond. 1971; MFFP 1993. SCMO S.E. Sheff. NHS Primary Care Trust. Specialty: Psychosexual Med. Socs: Fac. Community Health; Inst. Psychosexual Med. Prev: SCMO Community Health Sheff. NHS Trust.

TAYLOR, Anne Kathryn 8 Swann Grove, Cheadle Hulme, Cheadle SK8 7HW — MB ChB Manch. 1991.

TAYLOR, Anthony Department of Physiology, Charing Cross & Westminster Medical School, Fulham Palace Road, London W6 8RF Tel: 020 8846 7593 Fax: 020 8846 7338 — MB BS Lond. 1954 (Lond. Hosp.) BSc Lond. 1951. Prof. Emerit. & Sen. Research Fell. (Physiol.) Char. Cross & Westm. Med. Sch. Lond. Specialty: Gen. Med. Prev: Hon. Cons. & Prof. of Physiol. United Med. Dent. Sch. Guy's & St. Thos. Hosps. Head Div. Phys.

TAYLOR, Anthony James 9 Bowers Croft, Cambridge CB1 8RP — MB BS Lond. 1993.

TAYLOR, Anthony John, CBE (retired) Tir-an-Og, Brooklands, Sarisbury Green, Southampton SO31 7EE Tel: 01489 583199 — (Camb. & Guy's) MA Camb. 1981, BA 1955; MB BChir Camb. 1958. Prev: Co. Med. Off. Cyanamid GB Ltd.

TAYLOR, Anthony John 67 Cleveland Road, North Shields NE29 0NW — MB ChB Leic. 1985; FRCA 1994. Sen. Regist. Rotat. (Anaesth.) Newc. u. Tyne. Specialty: Anaesth.

TAYLOR, Anthony Martin — MB ChB Leeds 1993; FFAEM; MRCP.

TAYLOR, Anthony St John Willow Street Medical Centre, 81-83 Willow Street, Oswestry SY11 1AJ Tel: 01691 653143 Fax: 01691 679130; Hamilton House, Trefonen, Oswestry SY10 9DG Tel: 01691 653417 — MB ChB Birm. 1975; DRCOG 1985. Socs: BMA. Prev:

Regist. (Surg.) Centr. Birm. Dist. HA; Regist. (Orthop.) E. Birm. Hosp.; Regist. (Surg.) Co. Hosp. Hereford.

TAYLOR, Antonia Jane Farnham Health Centre, Hale Road, Farnham GU9 9QS — BM BS Nottm. 1991; DRCOG 1996; DCH 1998; MRCGP 2000.

TAYLOR, Arthur William Outram (retired) Saltoun Hall, Pencaitland, Tranent EH34 5DS Tel: 01875 340262 — (Univ. Ed.) MB ChB Ed. 1939; FRCP Ed. 1972, M 1947. Prev: Ho. Phys. Leith Hosp.

TAYLOR, Mr Barry Anthony Warrington Hospital NHS Trust, Lovely Lane, Warrington WA5 1QG Tel: 01925 662076 Fax: 01925 662042; Lilac Cottage, Pickerings Lock, Crewood Common, Crowton, Northwich CW8 2TX Tel: 01928 788503 — BM BCh Oxf. 1978 (Oxford) MA Camb. 1979; FRCS Eng. 1982; MCh Oxf. 1986. Cons. Gen. Surg. Warrington Dist. Gen. Hosp.; Moynihan Trav. Fell. Assn. Surgs. GB & Irel. Specialty: Gen. Surg. Socs: Ord. Mem. Surg. Research Soc.; Brit. Soc. Gastroenterol.; Assn. Coloproctol. (Counc. Mem.). Prev: Sen. Lect. (Surg.) & Hon. Cons. Surg. Broadgreen & Roy. Liverp. Univ. Hosps.; Lect. & Hon. Sen. Regist. (Surg.) Univ. Wales Coll. Med. Cardiff; Fell. (Colon & Rectal Surg.) Mayo Clinic Rochester, USA.

TAYLOR, Mr Benjamin Anthony Spinal Surgery Unit, Royal National Orthopaedic Hospital Trust, Brockley Hill, Stanmore HA7 4LP Tel: 020 8909 5525 — MB BS Lond. 1980 (Univ. Coll. Hosp.) FRCS Ed. 1985; FRCS Eng. 1986; MCh (Orthop.) Liverp. 1990. Cons. Orthop. Surg. Roy. Nat. Orthop. Hosp. Trust Stanmore; Hon. Cons. Orthopaedic Spinal Surg., Nat. Hosp. for Neurol. and Neurosurg., Lond. Specialty: Trauma & Orthop. Surg. Socs: Founder Mem. Brit. Cervical Spine Soc.; Brit. Scoliosis Soc. Prev: Sen. Regist. (Orthop.) Middlx. Hosp. Lond.; Regist. (Orthop.) Univ. Coll. Hosp. Lond.; Demonst. St. Thos. Hosp. Med. Sch.

TAYLOR, Berenice Penelope 43 Ridgeway Gardens, Hornsey Lane, Highgate, London N6 5NH — MB ChB Sheff. 1968; DObst RCOG 1970. Med. Assessor with the Indep. Tribunal Serv. Specialty: Care of the Elderly. Prev: Clin. Asst. (Geriat. Rehabil.) Roy. Free Hosp. Lond.; GP Bournemouth & Chandler's Ford; Sen. Med. Off. Family Plann. Clinic Liverp.

TAYLOR, Bernard 3/5 Merchant Street, London E3 4LJ Tel: 020 8980 3676; (private), 7 Sharon Gardens, London E9 7RX Tel: 020 8985 1657 — MB BS Lond. 1949 (Guy's) FRCGP 1979, M 1957. Socs: Lond. Jewish Hosp. Med. Soc. & Israel Med. Assn. Brit. Fellowsh. Prev: Capt. RAMC; Ho. Phys. Dudley Rd. Hosp. Birm. & Connaught Hosp. Walthamstow.

TAYLOR, Miss Brenda Anita (retired) 12 Park View, Wootton Bridge, Ryde PO33 4RJ — MRCS Eng. LRCP Lond. 1949; M.B., B.S. Lond. 1949; FRCOG 1976, M 1959. Prev: Cons. O & G I. of Wight Hosp. Gp.

TAYLOR, Brenda Esther (retired) 4 Gray's Orchaid, Thurlaston, Rugby CV23 9LB Tel: 01788 521848 — (Roy. Free) BSc (Hons., Special Anat.) Lond. 1956, MD 1969, MB; BS (Hons. Surg.) 1959; MRCS Eng. LRCP Lond. 1959; FRCP Lond. 1979, M 1963. Prev: Cons. Phys. Preston Health Dist.

TAYLOR, Professor Brent Royal Free & University College Medical School, Department of Paediatrics & Child Health, Royal Free Campus, University College London, London NW3 2PF Tel: 0207 830 2288 Fax: 0207 830 2003 Email: b.taylor@rfc.ucl.ac.uk — MB ChB Otago 1966; FRACP 1977; PhD Bristol 1986; FRCPCH 1998. Prof. of Community Child Health UCL Lond.; Hon. Cons. Paediat. & Director (Child Health) Roy. Free Hampstead NHS Trust Lond. Specialty: Paediat. Special Interest: Use of Routine Data for Research. Prev: Sen. Lect. (Child Health) St Mary's Hosp. Med. Sch. Lond.; Sen. Lect. (Social Paediat. & Epidemiol.) Bristol Univ.; Sen. Lect. (Paediat.) Christchurch Clin. Sch. of Med. New Zealand.

TAYLOR, Brian Oscar Treweek Burches, 4 The Green, Colne Engaine, Colchester CO6 2EZ Tel: 01787 224876 Fax: 01787 224897 Email: ptaylor762@aol.com; 19 Hamilton Road, Cambridge CB4 1BP Tel: 01223 312020 — MRCS Eng. LRCP Lond. 1945 (St. Thos.) MRCGP 1964; MFHom 1971. Hon. Med. Off. Halstead Hosp. Specialty: Homeop. Med. Socs: Colchester Med. Soc. Prev: Asst. Med. Off. Essex Co. Hosp. Black Notley; Ho. Phys. Roy. Surrey Co. Hosp. Guildford; Resid. Med. Off. High Wycombe & Dist. War Memor. Hosp.

TAYLOR, Bruce Lindsay Department of Critical Care Medicine, Portsmouth Hospitals NHS Trust, Queen Alexandra Hospital Cosham PO6 3LY Tel: 02392 286844 Fax: 02392 286844 Email: bruce.taylor@porthosp.nhs.uk; Puriton Lodge, Scant Road E., Hambrook, Chichester PO18 8UG Tel: 01243 573675 — MB ChB Manch. 1979 (St. Andr./Manch.) BSc St. And. 1976; FFARCS Eng. 1984; FANZCA 1990, FFICANZCA 1990; FJFICM 2002. Cons. (Critical. Care Med.) Cons. Anaesth. Qu. Alexandra Hosp. Cosham Hants. Specialty: Intens. Care. Socs: Paediat. Intens. Care Soc.; Assn. Anaesth.; Fell. FICANZCA 1990. Prev: Regist. (Paediat. Intens. Care) Roy. Childrs. Hosps. Melbourne Austral.; Sen . Regist. (Anaesth.) S.W. Rec. Rotat.; Regist. (Anaesth.) Addenbrooke's Hosp. Camb.

TAYLOR, Bruce Weir Claughton Medical Centre, 161 Park Road North, Birkenhead CH41 0DD Tel: 0151 652 1688 Fax: 0151 670 0565; Heathfield, Telegraph Road, Caldy, Wirral CH48 1NZ Tel: 0151 625 6337 — MB BS Nottm. 1982; DRCOG 1985; MRCGP 1986.

TAYLOR, Bryce Leighton Road Surgery, 1 Leighton Road, Linslade, Leighton Buzzard LU7 1LB Tel: 01525 372571 Fax: 01525 850414; 36 Creslow Way, Stone, Aylesbury HP17 8YW Tel: 01296 747980 — MB ChB Manch. 1978; DCH RCP Lond. 1981; DRCOG 1981; MRCGP 1984; Dip. Pract. Dermat. Wales 1991.

TAYLOR, Caecilia Jane Anne Forensic Personality Disorder Service, John Howard Centre, 2 Crozier Terrace, Hackney, London E9 6AT Tel: 020 8510 2120 Fax: 020 8919 8421 — MB BS Lond. 1982 (Roy. Free) BSc Med. Sociol. Lond. 1979; MRCPsych 1986; Dip. Forens. Psychiat. Lond. 1995. Cons. Forens. Psychiat. John Howard Centre, 2 Crozier Terrace, Hackney, London E9 6AT. Specialty: Forens. Psychiat. Special Interest: Personality disorder. Socs: Roy. Coll. Psychiat.; Brit. Med. Assn.; Internat. Assn. of Forens. Psychother. Prev: Sen. Lect. Dept. Forens. Psychiat. Inst. of Psychiat. & Broadmoor Hosp.; Research Psychiat. Genetics Sect. Inst. Psychiat. Lond.; SHO Rotat. (Psychiat.) Roy. Free Hosp. Lond.

TAYLOR, Carl Lucien 33 High Street, Ivinghoe, Leighton Buzzard LU7 9EP — MB BS Lond. 1979 (Roy. Free) MRCPsych 1984. Cons. Psychiat.Milton Keynes Hosp.s. Specialty: Gen. Psychiat. Prev: Cons. Psychiat. W. Cumbld. Hopital Whitehaven; Sen. Regist. (Psychiat.) Fulbourn Hosp. Camb.; Sen. Regist. St. Clements Hosp. Ipswich.

TAYLOR, Caroline Anita The Health Centre, Manor Way, Lee-on-the-Solent PO13 9JG Tel: 02392 550220; 70 Woodrush Crescent, Locks Heath, Southampton SO31 6UP Tel: 01489 602263 — BM Soton. 1994; DRCOG 1996; DFFP 1997; MRCGP 1998. GP Princip.; CMO Family Plann. & Reproductive Health, Southampton & Portsmouth. Specialty: Gen. Pract.; Family Plann. & Reproduc. Health.

TAYLOR, Caroline Grace 16 Tabor Grove, Wimbledon, London SW19 4EB — MB BS Lond. 1989 (St. Thos. Hosp. Med. Sch. (UMDS)) MRCP (UK) 1993; FRCR 1997. Cons. Radiol. Jarvis Breast Scr. Centre, Guildf. Specialty: Radiol. Prev: Regist. (Med.) St. Mary's Hosp. Lond.; SHO (Med.) Medway Hosp. Kent; SHO (A & E) St. Geo. Hosp. Lond.

TAYLOR, Caroline Louise Crown Dale Medical Centre, 61 Crown Dale, London SE19 3NY Tel: 020 8670 2414 Fax: 020 8670 0277; Fairmount, 2A Mount Ephraim Lane, Streatham, London SW16 1JG Tel: 020 8769 5631 — MB BS Lond. 1983 (St. Geo.) DRCOG 1987. Prev: Trainee GP Lond. VTS.

TAYLOR, Caroline Louise 38 Heath Crescent, Halifax HX1 2PR — MB ChB Leeds 1992. Trainee GP York VTS.

TAYLOR, Caroline Margaret Lawton House Surgery, Bromley Road, Congleton CW12 1QG Tel: 01260 275454 Fax: 01260 298412; Brackenrigg, Crouch Lane, Timbersbrook, Congleton CW12 3PT Tel: 01260 276898 — MB ChB Manch. 1986; DRCOG 1988; MRCGP 1990. Socs: BMA; RCGPs & Anglo-German Soc. Prev: SHO/Trainee GP Hope Hosp. Salford VTS; Ho. Surg. & Ho. Phys. Manch. Roy. Infirm.

TAYLOR, Caryl 51 Kimberley Road, Penylan, Cardiff CF23 5DL — MB BS Lond. 1987.

TAYLOR, Catherine Elizabeth Taff Vale Practice, Duffryn Road, Rhydyfelin, Pontypridd CF37 5RW Tel: 01443 406591 Fax: 01443 492900 Email: catherine.e.taylor@care4free.net; 43 Parc-y-Bryn, Creigiau, Cardiff CF15 9SE Tel: 029 2089 2396 — MB ChB Birm. 1981 (Birmingham) MRCGP 1986. GP; Clin. Asst. (Ophth.) Pontypridd & Rhondda NHS Trust. Prev: Sen. Med. Off. (Ophth.) Centr. Hosp. Honiara.

TAYLOR, Catherine Jane 144 Stannington View Road, Sheffield S10 1SS — MB ChB Sheff. 1997.

TAYLOR, Catherine Mary Ferndale, New Road, Henley-in-Arden, Solihull B95 5HY — MB ChB Birm. 1993 (Birmingham) DRCOG. 1997; DFFP. 1997; MRCEP. 1998. GP. Locum. Specialty: Gen. Pract. Prev: SHO (A & E) Worcester Roy. Infirm.; SHO (Ophth.) Worcester Roy. Infirm. VTS; Ho. Off. (Surg.) Qu. Eliz. Hosp. Birm.

TAYLOR, Cecil Frederick (retired) Medical Department, British Steel, Port Talbot Works, Port Talbot SA13 2NG Tel: 01637 872000 Fax: 01639 872560; Brynawelon, 67 Heol Cennen, Ffairfach, Llandeilo SA19 6UW — (Birm.) MB ChB Birm. 1965; DIH Soc. Apoth. Lond. 1977; FFOM RCP Lond. 1991, MFOM 1981. Occupat. Phys. Prev: Chief Med. Off. Brit. Steel plc. (Tinplate).

TAYLOR, Cecilia (retired) Health Centre, Walesmoor Avenue, Kiveton Park, Sheffield S26 5RF Tel: 01909 770213; 41 Dawcarr Lane, Woodall, Harthill, Sheffield S26 7XN Tel: 01909 770070 — MB ChB Leeds 1943; DCH Eng. 1943.

TAYLOR, Chadwick Richard 5 Morninton Road, Sale M33 2DA — MB ChB Manch. 1990.

TAYLOR, Charles Edmunds Darby (retired) Alnwick House, High St., Little Shelford, Cambridge CB2 5ES Tel: 01223 842115 — (Camb. & Middlx.) MB BChir Camb. 1946; Dip. Bact. Lond 1955; MA Camb. 1948, BA 1944, MD 1956; FRCPath 1970. Prev: Dir. Regional Pub. Health Laborat. Camb., Hon. Cons. Microbiol. Camb. HA & Assoc. Lect. Univ. Camb.

TAYLOR, Charles Matheson (retired) Barnards, Redricks Lane, Sawbridgeworth CM21 0RL — MB ChB Aberd. 1945; Dip. Psychol. Lond. 1990. Prev: Ho. Phys. (Paediat.) Whipps Cross Hosp.

TAYLOR, Charles Murray (retired) Moss Cottage, Ledaig, North Connel, Oban PA37 1RX — MB ChB Ed. 1954; BSc (Hons.) Glas. 1942, MB ChB Ed. 1954; DObst RCOG 1956. Prev: Ho. Phys. & Ho. Surg. Roy. Infirm. Edin.

TAYLOR, Charles Peter Brannams Medical Centre, Brannams Square, Kiln Lane, Barnstaple EX32 8GP Tel: 01271 329004 Fax: 01271 346785 — MB BS Lond. 1986.

TAYLOR, Charlotte Jane 15 Birch Tree Court, West St., Hoole, Chester CH2 3PH — MB BS Newc. 1992.

TAYLOR, Miss Christine Jean Accident & Emergency Department, Queen Mary's Hospital, Frognal Avenue, Sidcup DA14 6LT Tel: 020 8302 2678 Email: chris@cjt.co.uk — State Exam Med Bonn 1982; FRCS Ed. 1987. Dir. Emerg. Care Qu. Mary Hosp. Sidcup. Specialty: Accid. & Emerg.

TAYLOR, Christopher Bryan Directorate of Sexual Health, King's Healthcare, 15-22 Caldecot Road, London SE5 9RS Tel: 020 7346 3478 Fax: 020 7346 3486 — MB BS Lond. 1986; FRCP (UK) 1992. Cons. Phys. (HIV & Genitourin. Med.) King's Healthcare Lond. Specialty: Genitourinary Medicine.

TAYLOR, Professor Christopher John Sheffield Children's Hospital, Academic Unit of Child Health, Sheffield S10 2TH Tel: 0114 276 1111 Fax: 0114 275 5364; 153 Dobcroft Road, Sheffield S7 2LT Tel: 0114 235 1015 — MB ChB Liverp. 1973; DCH RCPS Glas. 1975; FRCP (UK) 1978; MD Liverp. 1986. Prof. (Paediat. Gastroenterol.) Univ. Sheff.; Hon. Cons. Paediat. Sheff. Childr. Hosp. Specialty: Paediat.; Gastroenterol. Socs: Brit. Paediat. Assn.; Brit. Soc. Gastroenterol. Prev: Sen. Lect. (Paediat.) Alder Hey Childr. Hosp.

TAYLOR, Christopher John 29 William Court, 6 Hall Road, St Johns Wood, London NW8 9PA — MB BS Lond. 1996 (UCL) FRCA (Part 1); MRCP (Lon). Specialist Regist. in Anaesthetics N. Thames Rotat. Specialty: Paediat. Prev: Princip. Ho. Off (Surg.) Broomfield Hosp. Chelmsford; Princip. Ho. Off (Med.) Mayday Univ. Hosp. Thornton Health; SHO (Gen. Paediat.) Whittington Hosp. Lond.

TAYLOR, Christopher Mark Birmingham Children's Hospital, Birmingham B4 6NH Tel: 0121 333 9227 Fax: 0121 333 9231 Email: cm.taylor@bch.nhs.uk — MB ChB Birm. 1971; FRCPCH; DCH Eng. 1973; MRCP (UK) 1975; FRCP Lond. 1991. Cons. Paediat. & Nephrol. Birm. Childr. Hosp. Socs: International Peadiatric Nephrology Association; International Society for Nephrology; European Renal Association. Prev: Lect. (Paediat. & Nephrol.) Birm. Childr. Hosp. & E. Birm. Hosp.; Research Asst. (Renal Unit) Birm. Childr. Hosp.; Sen. Regist. Univ. Hosp. W. Indies Jamaica.

TAYLOR, Christopher Michael St. James's University Hospital, Roundhay Wing, Beckett St., Leeds LS9 7TF Tel: 0113 243 3144 Fax: 0113 234 6856; 42 The Drive, Adel, Leeds LS16 6BQ Tel: 0113 226 4463 Fax: 0113 226 4463 Email: chris.taylor@cwcom.net — MB BChir Camb. 1977; MA (Hons.) Camb. 1973; MRCPsych 1982. Hon. Clin. Lect. Univ. Leeds; Cons. Psychiat. St. Jas. Univ. Hosp. Leeds. Specialty: Gen. Psychiat.

TAYLOR, Christopher Paul Haslemere Health Centre, Church Lane, Haslemere GU27 2BQ Tel: 01483 783023 Fax: 01428 645065; Fridays Hill House, Fernhurst, Haslemere GU27 3DX Tel: 01428 643480 — MB BS Lond. 1974 (St. Thos.) DRCOG 1977; DA Eng. 1977. GP. Socs: Chairm. Haslemere Med. Soc. Prev: Clin. Asst. in Rehabil. Young Severely Disabled Unit Godwin Unit Haslemere Hosp.; SHO (Anaesth.) St. Thos. Hosp. Lond.; SHO (O & G & Paediat.) Ashford Hosp. Middlx.

TAYLOR, Claire Louise 7 Taironen, Cowbridge CF71 7UA — MS BS Lond. 1991.

TAYLOR, Claire Margaret 56 Lindale Mount, Wakefield WF2 0BH — MB ChB Leeds 1991.

TAYLOR, Clare 65 Sommerville Road, Bristol BS7 9AD — MB ChB Bristol 1990.

TAYLOR, Clare Helen — MB ChB Bristol 1989; BSc (Hons.) Cell Path. Bristol 1989; DRCOG 1995; MRCGP 1996. Specialty: Gen. Pract. Prev: GP Retainee Firs Ho. Surg. Histon Camb.

TAYLOR, Clare Louise 36 Habberley Road, Kidderminster DY11 5PE — MB ChB Manch. 1998. SHO (Infectious Diseases) Roy. Free Hosp., Hampstead. Specialty: Gen. Med. Prev: HO. (Surg.) Roy Lanc Infirm. Lanc.; HO. (Med.) Roy Lanc Infirm. Lanc.; SHO.(Gen Med.) Roy Lanc Infirm. Lanc.

TAYLOR, Clare Petronella Florence Dept of Haematology, The Royal Free Hospital, Pond St, Hampstead, London NW3 2QG Tel: 020 7794 0500 Ext: 8462 Fax: 0207 830 2092 — MB BS Lond. 1985 (Medical College of St Bartholemews Hospital) MRCP (UK) 1988; PhD Lond. 1995; MRCPath 1998. p/t Cons & Hon Sen Lect. (Haemat. & Transfus Med.) Roy Free Hampstead NHS Trust. Lond.; Cons., Nat. Blood Serv., N. Lond.. Specialty: Haematology. Socs: Brit. Soc. of Haemat.; Brit. Blood Transfus. Soc. Prev: Sen. Regist. (Clin. Haemat.) Roy. Free Hosp. Lond.; Clin. Research Fell. Imperial Cancer Research Fund Lond.; Regist. (Haemat.) St. Mary's Hosp. Lond.

TAYLOR, Colette 24 Foxlands Drive, Penn, Wolverhampton WV4 5NA Tel: 01902 339107 — MB ChB Liverp. 1959; DObst RCOG 1961. SCMO Wolverhampton HA. Specialty: Community Child Health.

TAYLOR, Colette Lydie (retired) Barn Cottage, Back Road, Apperknowle, Dronfield S18 4AR Tel: 01246 412259 — (Roy. Free) MB BS Lond. 1949; DA Eng. 1952; FFA RCS Eng. 1954. Prev: Anaesth. Sheff. Sch. Dent. Serv.

TAYLOR, Colin George (retired) 11 Bumbles, 3 Station Road, Little Houghton, Northampton NN7 1AJ Tel: 01604 891452 — MB BS Lond. 1956 (St. Bart.)

TAYLOR, Colin George Department of Haematology, Pembury Hospital, Pembury, Tunbridge Wells TN2 4QJ Tel: 01892 823535; 5 Waverley Drive, Sandown Park, Tunbridge Wells TN2 4RX — MB BS Lond. 1965; MRCS Eng. LRCP Lond. 1965; FRCPath 1984, M 1974; FRCP 1999. Cons. Haemat. Pembury Hosp. Tunbridge Wells. Specialty: Haematology. Socs: Assn. Clin. Path.; Brit. Soc. Haemat. Prev: Regist. & Lect. Kings Coll. Hosp. Lond.

TAYLOR, Craig James Charles 69 Vicarage Road, Harborne, Birmingham B17 0SR — MB ChB Ed. 1993.

TAYLOR, Cynthia Pauline Janet — MB ChB Liverp. 1980; DRCOG 1983; DCH RCP Lond. 1984; MRCGP 1985; MFFP 1994. Gen. Practitioner, Cuffley; Clin. Med. Off. (Family Plann.) Elms Clinic Potters Bar & Garston Clinic, Watford. Prev: Community Med. Off. W. Lambeth HA.

TAYLOR, Daniel John Evelina Childrens Hospital, Guys Hospital, St Thomas St, London SE1; Flat 1, 12 Christchurch Rd, London N8 9QL — MB ChB Liverp. 1996; MRCPCH. 1999. Regist. (Paediat IC.) Guys Hosp. Lond. Specialty: Paediat.

TAYLOR, David 27 Heath Huost Road, London NW3 2RU — (UCHMS) MB BS Lond. 1970; MRCP (UK) 1972; FRCPsych 1989, M 1976. Cons. Psychother. Tavistock Clin. Lond. Specialty: Gen. Psychiat.; Psychother. Socs: Brit. Psychoanal. Soc.; Fell. Roy. Coll. Psychiat. Prev: Hon. Sen. Regist. Maudsley Hosp. Lond.; Research Worker Inst. Psychiat. Lond.; Sen. Regist. Nat. Hosp. Nerv. Dis. Qu. Sq. Lond.

TAYLOR, David Alexander Wycombe Hospital, Department of Thoracic Medicine, Queen Alexandra Road, High Wycombe HP11 2TT Tel: 01494 425453 Email: david.taylor@sbucks.nhs.uk; The Boot, Watts Green, Chearsley, Aylesbury HP18 0DD Tel: 01844 201986 — MB BS Lond. 1990; BSc (Hons.) Lond. 1987; MRCP (UK) 1994; MD Lond. Univ. 2000. Cons. Respirat. Med. Wycombe Hosp. Specialty: Respirat. Med.; Gen. Med. Special Interest: Asthma; COPD; Lung Cancer. Socs: Brit. Thoracic Soc. Prev: Clin. Research Fell. Nat. Heart & Lung Inst.; Clin. Research Phys. (Clin. Pharmacol.) Wellcome Research Laborat. Beckenham; SHO (Gen. Med.) Northwick Pk. Hosp. Lond.

TAYLOR, David Anthony Rosegarth Surgery, Rothwell Mount, Halifax HX1 2XB Tel: 01422 353450/350420 — MB ChB Leeds 1992.

TAYLOR, David Bryan Stuart, TD, CStJ (retired) Easingwold, 498 Chorley New Road, Bolton BL1 5DR Tel: 01204 843406 — MB ChB Manch. 1948; MRCS Eng. LRCP Lond. 1949; DObst RCOG 1964; MRCGP 1978. Prev: Ho. Surg. Ancoats Hosp. Manch. & Matern. Hosp. Hull.

TAYLOR, Professor David Charles Pentre Grange, Llanover, Abergavenny NP7 9EW — MD Lond. 1969 (Char. Cross) MB BS 1960, DPM 1965; FRCPsych 1973, M 1971; FRCP Lond. 1982, M 1976; T(Psych) 1991; FRCPCH (Hon.) 1997. Vis. Prof. Paediat. Neuropsychiat. Hosp. Sick Childr. Gt. Ormond St. Lond. Specialty: Child & Adolesc. Psychiat. Prev: Cons. Pysch. Epilepsy Surg. Program Beaumont Hosp. Dub.; Vis. Psychiat. David Lewis Centre for Epilepsy & St. Piers Lingfield.; Prof. Child & Adolesc. Psychiat. Univ. Manch.

TAYLOR, David Donaldson George Street Surgery, 99 George Street, Dumfries DG1 1DS Tel: 01387 253333 Fax: 01387 253301; Oakfield, Newbridge, Dumfries DG2 0QX Tel: 01387 720122 — MB ChB Aberd. 1976; DRCOG 1979; MRCGP 1980.

TAYLOR, David Geoffrey Barrie Woodlands Road Surgery, 57 Woodlands Road, Northfield, Birmingham B31 2HZ Tel: 0121 475 1065 Fax: 0121 475 6179 — MB ChB Bristol 1978; MRCP Ed. 1982; DRCOG 1984. Princip. GP N.field.

TAYLOR, David George 21 Phoenix Lodge Mansions, Brook Green, London W6 7BG — MB BCh BAO Belf. 1986; MRCPsych, London 1990. Cons. Psychiat. W. Lond. Ment. Health NHS Trust. Specialty: Geriat. Psychiat. Prev: Sen. Regist. (Psychiat.) Char. Cross & Westm. Higher Train. Scheme.; Research Train. Fell. (Psychiat. Neuropath.) Ment. Health Foundat. Roy. Free Hosp. Lond.; Regist. (Psychiat.) Roy. Free Hosp. Lond.

TAYLOR, David John Lochmaben Medical Group, The Surgery, 42-44 High Street, Lockerbie DG11 1NH Tel: 01387 810252 Fax: 01387 811595; Merrick, 2 Rankine Heights, Marjoriebanks, Lochmaben, Lockerbie DG11 1LJ Tel: 01387 811376 — MB ChB Aberd. 1977; DRCOG 1980; MRCGP 1982. Specialty: Gen. Pract. Prev: Trainee GP VTS Dumfries & Galloway Roy. Infirm.; Research Fellowship Univ. Aberd.

TAYLOR, Professor David John Leicester Royal Infirmary, Reproductive Sciences Section, Department of Cancer Studies & Molecular Medicine, Robert Kilpatrick Building, Leicester LE1 6HB Tel: 0116 252 3161 Fax: 0116 252 5846; 28 The Pick Building, Leicester LE1 6HB — MB BS Newc. 1970; FRCOG 1988, M 1975; MD Newc. 1983. Prof. O&G & Vice Dean Univ. Leicester Sch. Med.; Clin. Dir. & Hon Cons. (Women's, Perinatal and Sexual Health Services) Univ. Hosps of Leicester NHS. Specialty: Obst. & Gyn. Prev: Reader (O & G) Univ. Dundee; Scientif. Staff, MRC Reproduc. & Growth Unit Princess Mary Matern. Hosp. Newc.; Ho. Surg. & Ho. Phys. Roy. Vict. Infirm. Newc.

TAYLOR, David Lynton Siam Surgery, Sudbury CO10 1JH Tel: 01787 370444 Fax: 01787 880322 — LMSSA Lond. 1981; MA Camb. 1982, MB ChB 1982; MRCGP 1987; DRCOG 1987.

TAYLOR, David McIntyre Inverkeithing Medical Group, 5 Friary Court, Inverkeithing KY11 1NU Tel: 01383 413234 Fax: 01383 410098 — MB ChB Glas. 1971; MRCGP 1975.

TAYLOR, David Robert Queen Camel Health Centre, Queen Camel, Yeovil BA22 7NG Tel: 01935 850225 Fax: 01935 851247 — MB BS Lond. 1984; DRCOG 1988; DCH RCP Lond. 1988; MRCGP 1990.

TAYLOR, David Russell Department of Dermatology, New Cross Hospital, Wolverhampton WV10 0QD — MB BChir Camb. 1971 (St. Bart.) MB Camb. 1971, BChir 1970; DObst RCOG 1972; MRCP (UK) 1974. Cons. Dermat. Roy. Wolverhampton Hosps. Specialty: Dermat. Socs: Fell. Roy. Soc. Med. Prev: Sen. Regist. (Dermat.) St. Helier Hosp. Carshalton; Regist. (Dermat.) Univ. Coll. Hosp. Lond.; SHO (Gen. Med.) Brook Gen. Hosp. Lond.

TAYLOR, Mr David Samuel Bethany, 14 Leadhall Way, Harrogate HG2 9PG — MB ChB Manch. 1964; DCH Eng. 1966; FRCOG 1983, M 1970, DObst 1967; FRCS Ed. 1973. Cons. O & G Harrogate Health Dist. Specialty: Obst. & Gyn. Prev: Tutor (O & G) Manch. Univ.; Sen. Regist. (O & G) & Regist. (Gyn. Path. & Cytol.) St. Mary'sHosp. Manch.

TAYLOR, Mr David Samuel Irving Consulting Rooms, 234 Great Portland Street, London W1W 5QT Tel: 020 7935 7916 Fax: 020 7323 5430 Email: eyeclinic.234@btconnect.com/ eyeclinic.234gps@btinternet.com; 23 Church Road, Barnes, London SW13 9HE Tel: 020 8878 0305 Fax: 020 8878 1125 — MB ChB Liverp. 1967; DO RCS Eng. 1970; MRCP (UK) 1972; FRCS Eng. 1973; FRCP Lond. 1984; FCOphth 1990; FRCPCH 1998; DSc 2001. Cons. Ophth. Hosp. Sick Childr. Gt. Ormond St. Lond. & Hon. Sen. Lect. Inst. Child Health Lond. Specialty: Ophth. Socs: Internat. Mem. Amer. Assn. Paediat. Ophth. & Strabismus; Counc. Mem. Roy. Lond. Soc. Blind; Roy. Soc. Med. & Brit. Orthoptic Bd. Prev: Fell. Neuroophthol. Univ. Calif. Med. Centre San Francisco, USA; Research Fell. Hosp. Sick Childr. Gt. Ormond St. Lond.; Cons. Ophth. Nat. Hosp. Nerv. Dis. Lond.

TAYLOR, David Stephen Honeysuckers, 36 White Hart Lane, Hockley SS5 4DW Tel: 01302 203083 — MB BS Lond. 1986; MRCGP 1991.

TAYLOR, David William Oakswood, Wingfield Road, Oakerthorpe, Alfreton DE55 7LH — MB ChB Liverp. 1980.

TAYLOR, Dawn Anne 22 Alloway Drive, Newton Mearns, Glasgow G77 5TG — MB ChB Glas. 1992.

TAYLOR, Dawn Margaret Southern Medical Group, 322 Gilmerton Road, Edinburgh EH17 7PR Tel: 0131 664 2148 Fax: 0131 664 8303 — MB ChB Dundee 1980; DRCOG 1982; MRCGP 1984. GP Edin.

TAYLOR, Deborah Anne 141 Dewhirst Road, Syke, Rochdale OL12 9TX — BM BS Nottm. 1993. Specialty: Obst. & Gyn.

TAYLOR, Deborah Hannah College Road Surgery, 50/52 College Road, Maidstone ME15 6SB Tel: 01622 752345 Fax: 01622 758133; The Grange, Maidstone Road, Marden, Tonbridge TN12 9AG Tel: 01622 831264 — MB BS Lond. 1986 (Lond. Hosp.) MRCGP 1989; DRCOG 1991. Specialty: Gen. Pract.

TAYLOR, Derek 8 Clochranhill Road, Alloway, Ayr KA7 4PZ — MB ChB Glas. 1975; BSc (Hons.) Glas. 1971, MB ChB 1975; DCH Eng. 1977; MRCP (UK) 1978.

TAYLOR, Mr Desmond Gerard (retired) Barn Cottage, Back Road, Apperknowle, Dronfield S18 4AR Tel: 01246 412259 Fax: 01246 292213 — MB BCh BAO Belf. 1948 (Qu. Univ. Belf.) FRCS Eng. 1952. Hon. Lect. (Thoracic Surg.) Univ. Sheff. Prev: Thoracic Surg. United Sheff. Hosps. & City Gen. Hosp. Sheff.

TAYLOR, Diane Michele 19 Sutton Hall Drive, Little Sutton, South Wirral CH66 4UQ — MB ChB Liverp. 1981; DRCOG 1984. Gen. Practitionor Princip.; Family Plann. Clinic Medical Off. Specialty: Community Child Health; Family Planning.

TAYLOR, Dorothy Linda Playfield House, Stratheden Hospital, Cupar KY15 5RR — MB BS Lond. 1975; DCH Eng. 1978; MRCPsych 1983. Cons. Child & Family Psychiat. Stratheden Hosp. Cupar. Specialty: Child & Adolesc. Psychiat. Prev: Sen. Regist. Dept. Child & Family Psychiat. Roy. Hosp. Sick Childr.; Glas.

TAYLOR, Edith (retired) Dolcrwm, Roe Wen, Conwy LL32 8TE Tel: 01492 650311 — (King's Coll. Hosp.) MRCS Eng., LRCP Lond. 1939; DObst RCOG 1943; MB BS Lond. 1946. Prev: Ho. Phys. King's Coll. Hosp. & Qu.'s Hosp. Childr.

TAYLOR, Edward Ian Russell 378 Chester Road, Birmingham B36 0LE Tel: 0121 770 3035 — MB ChB Ed. 1958. Socs: BMA. Prev: Ho. Surg. (Orthop.) & Ho. Phys. Stracathro Hosp. Brechin; Squadron Ldr. RAF Med. Br.

TAYLOR, Eithne Gayle Dewsbury Hospital, Department of Dermatology, Halifax Road, Dewsbury WF13 4HS Tel: 01924 816137 — MB ChB Bristol 1987 (Univ. Bristol) BSc Bristol 1984; MRCP (UK) 1990; FRCP 1999. Cons. Dermat. Dewsbury Hosp.; Hon. Sen. Clin. Lect. Univ. of Leeds. Specialty: Dermat. Socs: Brit. Assn. Dermat.; Brit. Soc. of Paediat. Dermatol.; Brit. Soc. for the Study of Vuval Diseases. Prev: Sen. Regist. (Dermat.) Leeds Gen.

Infirm.; Regist. (Dermat.) Roy. Berks. Hosp. Reading; Regist. (Dermat. & Gen. Med.) Wycombe Gen. Hosp.

TAYLOR, Professor Elizabeth 1-2-4 Cameron House, White Cross, South Road, Lancaster LA1 4XJ — MB ChB Aberd. 1972 (Aber.) MRCPsych. Cons. Psychiat. Morecambe Bay Primary Care Trust.

TAYLOR, Elizabeth Ann Saul Rotherham General Hospital, Moorgate Road, Rotherham S60 2UD Tel: 01709 304 550 — MB ChB Dundee 1977; FFA RCSI 1983. Cons. Anaesth. Rotherham Dist. Gen. Hosp. S. Yorks. Specialty: Anaesth.

TAYLOR, Elizabeth Jane Elm Farm, Horpit, Lower Wanborough, Swindon SN4 0AT — MB BS Lond. 1977; DRCOG 1980; Dip Occ Med 1996.

TAYLOR, Elizabeth Patricia 45 Pasture Hill Road, Haywards Heath RH16 1LY — MB ChB Cape Town 1988.

TAYLOR, Elizabeth Rutherford (retired) — (Univ. Coll. Hosp.) MB BChir Camb. 1950. Prev: Cas. Off. N. Lonsdale Hosp. Barrow-in-Furness.

TAYLOR, Ella Storey Cottage, Kirkby Overblow, Harrogate HG3 1HD Tel: 01423 871607 — (Aberd.) MB ChB Aberd. 1946; DPH Glas. 1952.

TAYLOR, Elsie Gladys (retired) 8 Milton Road, Mill Hill, London NW7 4AX Tel: 020 8959 8820 — MB BCh BAO Belf. 1951; DCH Eng. 1953; DObst RCOG 1954.

TAYLOR, Emily Clare 56 Woolwich Road, Belvedere DA17 5EN — MB BS Lond. 1996.

TAYLOR, Miss Emma Jane South Malling Cottage, Lewes Road, Lindfield RH16 2LF Tel: 01273 891286 — MB BS Lond. 1994 (UMDS) FRCS Eng. 1998; FRCS (TR & ONU) Eng 2003. Specialist Regist. (Orthop.) S. E. Thames Rotat. Specialty: Orthop. Prev: SHO (Surg.) Roy. Sussex Co. Hosp. Brighton.

TAYLOR, Emma Jane Stewart Longreach, Crampshaw Lane, Ashtead KT21 2UF Tel: 01372 273506 — MB BS Lond. 1992; DA (UK) 1996. SHO (Anaesth.) Epsom Gen. Hosp. Specialty: Anaesth. Prev: SHO (Neonates) St. Geo. Hosp. Lond.; SHO (Anaesth.) Roy. Hants. Co. Hosp. Winchester.

TAYLOR, Mrs Enid (retired) 60 Wood Vale, London N10 3DN Tel: 020 8883 6146 Email: ttcl00431@blueyonder.co.uk — (Lond. Hosp.) MA Camb. 1969, BA 1954; MB BChir Camb. 1957; FRCS Eng. 1965; FRCOphth 1993. Prev: Cons. Ophth. Surg. N. Middlx. Hosp. Lond.

TAYLOR, Professor Eric Andrew Department of Child & Adolescent Psychiatry, Institute of Psychiatry, De Crespigny Park, London SE5 8AF Tel: 020 7848 0488 Fax: 020 7708 5800 — (Middlx.) MA, MB Camb. 1968, BChir 1968; MRCP (UK) 1973; FRCPsych 1988, M 1975; FRCP Lond. 1986; FMedSci 2000. Prof. Child & Adolesc. Psychiat. Inst. of Psychiat. Lond.; Hon. Cons. (Child & Adolesc. Psychiat.) Bethlem Roy. & Maudsley Hosp. & KCH. Specialty: Child & Adolesc. Psychiat. Prev: Prof. Developm. Neuropsychiat. Inst. Psychiat. King's Coll. Lond.; Sen. Regist. (Child & Adolesc. Psychiat.) Bethlem Roy. & Maudsley Hosps. Lond.; Clin. & Research Fell. (Psychiat.) Mass. Gen. Hosp.

TAYLOR, Eric Hilton (retired) Crab Cottage, Ridley Hill, Kingswear, Dartmouth TQ6 0BY Tel: 01803 752349 — MB BS Lond. 1946 (St. Mary's) MRCS Eng. LRCP Lond. 1944; DTM & H Liverp. 1963. Prev: Med. Off. North. Territory Austral.

TAYLOR, Mr Eric William Inverclyde Royal Hospital, Larkfield Road, Greenock PA16 0XN Tel: 01475 633777 Mob: 0783 169 4953 Fax: 01475 656139 Email: eric.taylor@irh.scot.nhs.uk; 5 Langbank Rise, Kilmacolm PA13 4LF Tel: 01505 872722 Email: e-w-taylor@yahoo.co.uk — MB BS Lond. 1967 (St. Mary's) MRCS Eng. LRCP Lond. 1967; FRCS Eng. 1974; FRCS Glas. 1986. Cons. Surg. Inverclyde Roy. Hosp., Greenock, Argyll and Clyde Acute NHS Trust; Hon. Clin. Sen. Lect. Univ. Glas.; Cons. Gen. Surg. RN Scotl.; Edr. Surgic. Infec. Specialty: Gen. Surg. Socs: Fell. Assn. Surgs.; Surg. Infec. Soc.; Hosp. Infec. Soc. Prev: Surg. Cdr. RN & Cons. Surg. RN Hosp. Haslar; Sen. Regist. (Surg.) Profess. Surg. Unit S. Grampian (Aberd.) Health Dist.

TAYLOR, Evelyn Anne (retired) The Old Farm, 26 Meriden Road, Hampton-in-Ardon, Solihull B92 0BT Tel: 01675 442765 Fax: 01675 443901; Anaesthetic Department, Walsgrave NHS Trust, Clifford Bridge Road, Walsgrave, Coventry CV2 2DX Tel: 01203 602020 — MB ChB Birm. 1970; DA Eng. 1972; FFA RCS Eng. 1975; FFA RACS (Intens. Care) 1982. Cons. Anaesth. & IC Walsgrave Hosp. Coventry. Prev: Regist. Roy. Perth. ICU W. Australia.

TAYLOR, Evelyn June Wycombe General Hospital, High Wycombe HP11 2TT — MB BS Lond. 1972 (Roy. Free) MRCS Eng. LRCP Lond. 1972; DObst RCOG 1974; FFA RCS Eng. 1977; T(Anaesth) 1991. Cons. Anaesth. Wycombe Gen. Hosp. Specialty: Anaesth. Socs: Assn. Anaesth.; BMA. Prev: Sen. Regist. (Anaesth.) W. Midl. & Oxf. HAs; Regist. (Anaesth.) Northwick Pk. Hosp. Harrow; SHO (Anaesth.) Roy. Sussex Co. Hosp. Brighton.

TAYLOR, Fiona Ann Dept of Community Child Health, Grampian University Hosp, Berry Den Rd, Aberdeen AB25 3; 29 Binghill Road, Milltimber, Aberdeen AB13 0JA — MB ChB Aberd. 1989. Staff Grade Community Paediat. Grampian Univ Hosp NHS Trust. Specialty: Community Child Health.

TAYLOR, Fiona Clare 57A Loom Lane, Radlett WD7 8NX — MB BS Lond. 1994. SHO (O & G) St. Johns of Howden Hosp. Livingston. Specialty: Obst. & Gyn.

TAYLOR, Miss Fiona Gillian Mary Apt. 123, 21-33 Worple Road, London SW19 4BG Tel: 020 8946 8860 Email: fgmtaylor@doctors.org.uk — MB BS Lond. 1996 (Roy. Lond. Hosp.) MRCS Ed. 2000. SpR (Surgical) Flinders Med. Centre, Adelaide. Specialty: Gen. Surg. Socs: Roy. Soc. of Med.; Assn. of Surgeons in Train. Prev: SpR (Surgical) Ashford & St. Peters; SHO (A & E); SpR (Surgic.) Worthing & Southlands Hosp.

TAYLOR, Fiona Janet 31A Queens Crescent, Edinburgh EH9 2BA — MB ChB Aberd. 1982. SHO (Psychiat.) Dingleton Hosp. Melrose. Prev: SHO (Psychiat.) Bilbohall Hosp. Elgin.

TAYLOR, Frank (retired) 98 Sudbury Court Drive, Harrow HA1 3TF Tel: 020 8908 1177 — (Middlx.) MB BS Lond. 1948; MD Lond. 1952; DObst RCOG 1952; DCH Eng. 1952. Hosp. Pract. (Infec. Dis.) St. John's Hosp. Uxbridge. Prev: Regist. (Paediat.) Hillingdon Hosp.

TAYLOR, Frank John Barron (retired) Hartford Bridge House, Bedlington NE22 6AQ Tel: 01670 823260 — MB BChir Camb. 1961 (Camb. & Durh.) MRCS Eng. LRCP Lond. 1960. Clin. Asst. N.d. Ment. Health NHS Trust. Prev: GP Blyth.

TAYLOR, Frank Richard Taylor and Partners, The Surgery, Hexton Road, Barton-le-Clay, Bedford MK45 4TA Tel: 01582 528700 Fax: 01582 528714; Taymer House, Luton Road, Silsoe, Bedford MK45 4QP Tel: 01525 860245 Fax: 01525 861889 — LRCPI & LM, LRSCI & LM 1962 (RCSI) Specialty: Gen. Pract.

TAYLOR, Frank Thomas Barnt Green Surgery, 82 Hewell Road, Barnt Green, Birmingham B45 8NF Tel: 0121 445 1704 Fax: 0121 447 8253 — MB ChB Birm. 1981 (Birmingham) DRCOG 1984; MRCGP 1986. GP Barnt Green.

TAYLOR, Frederick Gerard Invergare, Glenarn Road, Helensburgh G84 8LL Tel: 01436 821432 Fax: 01436 821452 — MB ChB Glas. 1961; DObst RCOG 1963; MRCGP 1974; DIH Eng. 1976; MSc (Occupat. Med.) Lond. 1976; FFOM RCP Lond. 1987, MFOM 1981; FRCP Lond. 1993. Cons. Occupat. Phys. Lond.; Corporate Health Adviser Citibank NA. Specialty: Occupat. Health. Socs: Fell. Roy. Soc. Med. (Ex-Pres. Occupat. Med. Sect.); (Ex-Pres. & Treas.) Soc. Occupat. Med. Prev: Chief Med. Off. & Head of Health & Welf. Servs. Marks & Spencer plc.

TAYLOR, Gareth Henry Fisher Little St John Street Surgery, 7 Little St. John Street, Woodbridge IP12 1EE Tel: 01384 382046 — MB BCh Witwatersrand 1986.

TAYLOR, Gavin Beddie (retired) 26 Blackhouse Terrace, Peterhead AB42 1LQ Tel: 01779 472345 — MB ChB Aberd. 1954; MRCGP 1965. Prev: GP Aberd.sh.

TAYLOR, Geoffrey Arnold Northfield Road Surgery, Northfield Road, Blaby, Leicester LE8 4GU Tel: 0116 277 1705; 13 Willoughby Road, Countesthorpe, Leicester LE8 5UA Tel: 0116 277 1428 — MB BChir Camb. 1951 (Guy's) MA, MB BChir Camb. 1951; DObst RCOG 1957. Prev: Asst. Ho. Surg. & Ho. Phys. Guy's Hosp. Lond.; Ho. Surg. (Gyn. & Obst.) Roy. United Hosp. Bath.

TAYLOR, Mr Geoffrey James Wycombe General Hospital, Queen Alexandra Road, High Wycombe HP11 2TT Tel: 01494 426421; Sladmore Farm House, Cryers Hill Road, Cryers Hill, High Wycombe HP15 6LL — MB ChB Birm. 1977 (Brimingham) FRCS Ed. 1982; FRCS Eng. 1982; FRCS (Orthop.) Ed. 1988. Cons. Orthop. & Trauma Surg. Wycombe HA. Specialty: Orthop. Socs: Fell. BOA; BMA; Brit. Elbow & Shoulder Soc. Prev: Sen. Regist. (Orthop.) Guy's & St. Thos. Hosp. Lond.; Regist. (Orthop.) Northwick Pk. Hosp. Harrow; Regist. Rotat. (Orthop.) Roy. Free Hosp. & Windsor HA.

TAYLOR, George (retired) Redbrook, Brookledge Lane, Adlington, Macclesfield SK10 4JU Tel: 01625 829834 — MRCS Eng. LRCP Lond. 1930 (Manch.) DIH Eng. 1949. Cons. Med. Adviser Hawker Siddeley Aviat. Ltd.

TAYLOR, George Abel (retired) 5 Campsie Place, Aberdeen AB15 6HL Tel: 01224 319602 — MB ChB Aberd. 1958; FRCGP 1991, M 1972.

TAYLOR, George Benjamin 18 Palmerston Road, Buckhurst Hill IG9 5LT Tel: 020 8504 1552 — MB BS Lond. 1950 (St. Bart.) MRCS Eng. LRCP Lond. 1949; DObst RCOG 1954; DCH Eng. 1955. Mem. Staff Forest Hosp. Buckhurst Hill.

TAYLOR, George Browne Department of Postgrad Medical Education, Willow Terrace Road, University of Leeds, Leeds LS2 9JT Tel: 0113 343 1501 Fax: 0113 343 1530 Email: g.b.taylor@doctors.org.uk; Buckeye Barn, 8 The Fold, Hessay, York YO26 8LF Email: g.b.taylor@doctors.org.uk — MB BS Newc. 1972 (Newcastle) DObst RCOG 1975; FRCGP 1986, M 1976; MICGP 1987; Ed. D. (Newc.) 2000. Director of Postgrad. GP Educat. Yorks. Deanery Leeds. Prev: Course Organiser Northumbria VTS; Trainee GP Newc. VTS; Ho. Phys. Child Health & Ho. Surg. Roy. Vict. Infirm. Newc.

TAYLOR, George Swan (retired) Eden Holme, Haltwhistle NE49 0AF Tel: 01434 320376 — MB ChB Ed. 1945 (Univ. Ed.) Prev: Ho. Surg. Orthop. Hosp. Larbert.

TAYLOR, Gerald Gershom 53 Gervis Road, Bournemouth BH1 3DQ Tel: 01202 25154 — MRCS Eng. LRCP Lond. 1941 (King's Coll. & Char. Cross)

TAYLOR, Gordon James 12 Old Vicarage Lane, Quarndon, Derby DE22 5JB — MB ChB Sheff. 1956; MRCS Eng. LRCP Lond. 1956; DA Eng. 1958; FFA RCS Eng. 1960. Cons. Anaesth. Nottm. HA. Specialty: Anaesth. Socs: Intrac. Pain Soc. GB & Irel. (Ex-Hon. Sec.). Prev: Sen. Regist. Anaesth. West. Infirm. Glas.; Sen. Ho. Off. Anaesth. Roy. Hosp. Sheff.; Regist. Anaesth. United Sheff. Hosps.

TAYLOR, Graeme Roy 47 Crowtree Lane, Louth LN11 9LL — MB ChB Sheff. 1986.

TAYLOR, Graham Albert William Snakes Lane East Surgery, 178 Snakes Lane East, Woodford Green IG8 7JQ Tel: 020 8539 2077 Fax: 020 8556 1723; 8 Ashfields, Loughton IG10 1SB — MB BS Lond. 1966 (Guy's) MRCS Eng. LRCP Lond. 1966.

TAYLOR, Graham David Heathcroft, Back Lane, Letchmore Heath, Watford WD25 8EF — MB BS Lond. 1980 (Char. Cross Hosp.) BSc (Hons.) Lond. 1977; MRCGP 1988; MBA 1999. Specialty: Pharmaceutical Medicine.

TAYLOR, Graham Errington Budleigh Salterton Medical Centre, 1 The Lawn, Budleigh Salterton EX9 6LS Tel: 01395 441212 Fax: 01395 441244; Greyfriars, Westfield Road, Budleigh Salterton EX9 6SS Tel: 01395 442498 — MB ChB St. And. 1971. Prev: SHO (O & G) Roy. Devon & Exter Hosp. (Heavitree); Ho. Off. (Med.) Maryfield Hosp. Dundee; Ho. Off. (Surg.) Roy. Infirm. Dundee.

TAYLOR, Graham Malcolm St James University Hospital, Beckett St, Leeds LS9 7TF; 19 The Village, Thorp Arch, Wetherby LS23 7AR — MB ChB Manch. 1993. Lect. (Obst & Gyn.) St James Univ Hosp. Leeds. Specialty: Obst. & Gyn. Prev: Specialist Regist. (O & G) Ninewells Hosp. Dundee.

TAYLOR, Graham Paul Royal Cornwall Hospital (Treliske), Gloweth, Truro TR1 3LJ Tel: 01872 252716 Fax: 01872 252017 Email: graham.taylor@rcht.swest.nhs.uk — MB BS Lond. 1972 (St. Geo.) DCH Eng. 1976; DObst RCOG 1976; MRCP (UK) 1977; MSc (Immunol.) Lond. 1988; FRCP Lond. 1994; FRCPCH 1997. Cons. Paediat. Roy. Cornw. Hosp. Truro. Specialty: Paediat. Socs: BMA. Prev: Sen. Regist. (Paediat.) Westm. & W.m. Childr. Hosps. Lond.; Research Fell. & Hon. Sen. Regist. Roy. Postgrad. Med. Sch. Hammersmith Hosp. Lond.; Regist. (Paediat.) St. Mary's Hosp. Lond.

TAYLOR, Graham Philip Wright Fleming Institute, Department of Genitourinary Medicine & Communicable Diseases, Imperial College, Norfolk Place, London W2 1PG Tel: 020 75943910 Fax: 020 75943910 Email: g.p.taylor@ic.ac.uk; Jefferus Wing, St Mary's Hospital, Praed St, London W2 1NY Tel: 020 7886 6790 — MB ChB Birm. 1981 (University of Birmingham Medical School) MRCP (UK) 1987. Sen. Lect./Hon. Cons., Genitourin. Med. Communicable Dis.s, Imperial Coll./St Mary's Hosp. Lond. Specialty: Genitourinary Medicine; HIV Med. Socs: Brit. Infec. Soc.; BHIVA; Roy. Soc. Trop. Med. & Hyg. Prev: Hon. Sen. Regist. (Genitourin. Med. Communicable Dis.) St. Mary's Hosp. Lond.; Chief Med. Off. Centr. Hosp. Honiara, Solomon Is.; Regist. (Med.) Mid. Glam. HA.

TAYLOR, Graham Roy Maryhill Practice, Elgin Health Centre, Maryhill, Elgin IV30 1AT Tel: 01343 543788 Fax: 01343 551604 — MB ChB Aberd. 1985; DRCOG 1988; MRCGP 1989.

TAYLOR, Mr Grahame John Saint Clair Department of Orthopaedics, The Glenfield Hospital, Groby Road, Leicester LE3 9QP Tel: 0116 287 1471 Ext: 3448 — MB ChB Ed. 1981 (Univ. Ed.) FRCS Ed. 1987; FRCS (Orth.) 1995. Cons. Orthop. Surg. Glenfield Hosp. Leicester. Specialty: Orthop. Socs: Brit. Orthopaedic Assn.; Brit. Orthopaedic Research Soc. Prev: Lect. (Orthop.) Surg. Leicester Univ.

TAYLOR, Guinevere Sarah Emily 490 Manchester Road, Rochdale OL11 3EL — MB ChB Leeds 1997.

TAYLOR, Heath Philip 171 St Ann's Hill, London SW18 2RX — MB BS Lond. 1994; BSc (Physiol.) Lond. 1991.

TAYLOR, Helen The Graeme Medical Centre, 1 Western Avenue, Falkirk FK2 7HR — MB ChB Leeds 1994. Specialty: Gen. Pract.

TAYLOR, Helen Denise Clifton Medical Centre, 571 Farnborough Road, Clifton, Nottingham NG11 9DN Tel: 0115 921 1288 — MB ChB Liverp. 1986; DRCOG 1991. GP Principle.

TAYLOR, Helen Elizabeth Anne 4 Vane Road, Thame OX9 3WG — MB ChB Birm. 1984.

TAYLOR, Helen Frances (retired) 7 Hampole Balk, Skellow, Doncaster DN6 8LF — MB ChB Sheff. 1953; MRCS Eng. LRCP Lond. 1954.

TAYLOR, Helen Margaret Ebenezer Cottage, Hollington, Ashbourne DE6 3GB — MB ChB Sheff. 1985; MA Oxf. 1987. Locum Cons. N. Staffs. Specialty: Ment. Health. Prev: Assoc. Specialist (Learning Disabilities) Aston Hall Hosp. Derby.; Clin. Asst. & GP Asst. Aston Hall Hosp. Derby.; Regist. (Psychiat.) Kingsway & Pastures Hosps. Derby.

TAYLOR, Helen Murray Hawkhill, Lunan Bay, Arbroath DD11 4UX — MB ChB Glas. 1990.

TAYLOR, Helen Patricia Derwent Practice, Norton Road, Malton YO17 9RF Tel: 01653 600069 Fax: 01653 698014; Maris Otter House, West St, Swinton, Malton YO17 6SP — MB ChB Sheff. 1986. Clin. Asst. Ophth.

TAYLOR, Henry John Hunter 27 Clarendon Way, Tunbridge Wells TN2 5LD — MB BS Lond. 1993; BSc Lond. 1990; MRCP 1997; FRCR 2001. Cons. (Clin. Oncol.) Kent Oncol. Centre Maidstone. Specialty: Oncol. Prev: SpR (Clin. Oncol.) Roy. Marsden Hosp. Lond.; Specialist Regist. (Clin. Oncol.) St Bartholomews Hosp. Lond.; SHO (Med.) Whipps Cross Hosp. Lond.

TAYLOR, Hilary Elizabeth Park Road Medical Centre, 44 Park Road, Guiseley, Leeds LS20 8AR; 3 Kingfield, Guiseley, Leeds LS20 9DZ — MB ChB Leic. 1984. Prev: Trainee GP Stockport VTS.

TAYLOR, Hilary Jane 5 Wynbreck Dr, Keyworth, Nottingham NG12 5FY — MB BS Newc. 1997. SHO (Med.) Lister Hosp. Stevenage. Specialty: Gen. Med.

TAYLOR, Hugh Fraser Great Bansons Surgery, Bansons Lane, Ongar CM5 9AR Tel: 01277 363028 Fax: 01277 365264 Email: hugh.taylor@gp-f81049.nhs.uk — MB BS Lond. 1976 (Lond. Hosp.) BSc (Psychol.) Lond. 1973; MRCP (UK) 1981; DRCOG 1983. Clin. Asst. (Gastroenterol.) Princess Alexandra Hosp. Harlow; Hosp. Pract. Princess Alexandra Hosp. Harlow. Specialty: Gen. Pract.; Gastroenterol.; Diabetes. Prev: Regist. (Med.) St. Margt.s Hosp. Epping; Regist. (Med.) Lond. Hosp. Whitechapel.

TAYLOR, Hugh William Granby Place Surgery, Granby Place, 1 High Street, Northfleet, Gravesend DA11 9EY Tel: 01474 352447/362252; 3 Old Road W., Gravesend DA11 0LH Tel: 01474 333228 — MB BS Lond. 1982; DRCOG 1985; MRCGP 1987.

TAYLOR, Mr Hugo Wheldon Rowntree Basildon Hospital, Nether Mayne, Basildon SS16 5NL Tel: 01268 533911; Little Styles Cottage, MargarettingTye, Ingatestone CM4 9JX Tel: 01277 840618 Fax: 01277 841339 — MB BS Lond. 1983; FRCS Eng. 1989; FRCS (Gen.) 1997. Cons. (Gen. Surg. Coloproctol. & Breast Surg.) Basildon Hosp. Specialty: Gen. Surg. Special Interest: Colorectal Cancer; Faecal Incontinence; Pelvic Floor. Socs: Worshipful Soc. Apoth.; Brit. Assn. Surg. Oncol. Prev: Sen. Regist. (Gen. Surg.) Roy. Free Hosp. Lond.; Regist. (Gen. Surg.) The Lond. Hosp., Basildon & Roy. Free Hosp.; SHO Pre-Fellowsh. Rotat. (Surg.) St. Bartholomews Hosp. Lond.

TAYLOR, Iain Neil Rowan Cottage, Monktonhill Road, Prestwick KA9 1UJ — MB ChB Aberd. 1982; FFA RCSI 1989. Sen. Regist. (Anaesth.) Vict. Infirm. Glas. Specialty: Anaesth. Prev: Regist. (Anaesth.) Glas. Roy. Infirm.; SHO (Anaesth.) Falkirk & Dist. Roy. Infirm.

TAYLOR, Ian Arthur Mansion House Surgery, Abbey Street, Stone ST15 8YE Tel: 01785 815555 Fax: 01785 815541; 87 Lichfield Road, Stone ST15 8QD Tel: 01785 815060 — (Birm.) MB ChB Birm. 1968; DObst RCOG 1970; DCH Eng. 1971. Prev: SHO (Psychiat.) Bristol Roy. Infirm.; SHO (Obst.) Birm. Matern. Hosp.; Ho. Phys. Qu. Eliz. Hosp. Birm.

TAYLOR, Ian Christie Department Health Care for Elderly People, Ulster Hospital, Dundonald, Belfast BT16 1RH Tel: 01232 484511 Fax: 01232 550415 — MB BCh BAO Belf. 1975; MRCP (UK) 1979; BSc (Hons.) Belf. 1972, MD 1980; FRCP Glas. 1993; FRCP Ed. 1994; FRCP Lond. 1995. Cons. Phys. (Geriat. Med.) Ulster Hosp. Dundonald. Specialty: Care of the Elderly. Socs: Brit. Geriat. Soc. & Ulster Med. Soc. Prev: Cons. Phys. (Geriat. Med.) Roy. Vict. Hosp. Belf.

TAYLOR, Professor Ian Galbraith, CBE (retired) Croft Cottage, Cinder Hill, Whitegate, Northwich CW8 2BH Tel: 01606 882119 — (Manch.) FRCPCH; MB ChB Manch. 1948; DPH Manch. 1954; MD (Gold Medal) Manch. 1962; FRCP Lond. 1977, M 1973. Prev: Ellis Llwyd Jones Prof. of Audiol. & Educat. of Deaf Univ. Manch.

TAYLOR, Ian Keith Sunderland Royal Hospital, Kayll Road, Sunderland SR4 7TP Tel: 0191 565 6256 ext 47348 Fax: 0191 569 9292; 36 Runnymede Road, Ponteland, Newcastle upon Tyne NE20 9HG — MB BS Lond. 1983 (St. Mary's) BSc (Upper 2nd cl. Hons.) Lond. 1979, MB BS 1983; MRCP (UK) 1986; FRCP 1997. Cons. Phys. (Gen. & Respirat. Med.) Sunderland Roy. Hosp. Kayll Rd. Sunderland. Specialty: Gen. Med. Socs: Brit. Thorac. Soc.; Eur. Respirat. Soc.; Amer. Thoracic Soc. Prev: Sen. Lect. (Hon. Cons. Phys.); Nat. Heart & Lung Inst. & Roy. Postgrad. Med. Sch.

TAYLOR, Ian Robert Southampton General Hospital, Tremona Road, Southampton SO16 6YD Tel: 02380 796720 — MB ChB Bristol 1992; DA (UK) 1995; FRCA 1998. Specialist Regist. Rotat. (Anaesth.) Wessex. Specialty: Anaesth. Socs: Obstetric Anaesth.s Assn. Prev: SHO (Anaesth.) Qu. Alexandra Hosp. Portsmouth; SHO (Med.) St. Mary's Hosp. Portsmouth; SHO (Anaesth.) Barnstaple.

TAYLOR, Ian William — MB ChB Manch. 1991; BSc Manch. 1977; PhD Surrey 1981. Head (Clin. Pharm. Unit) Glaxo-Wellcome. Specialty: Pharmaceutical Medicine.

TAYLOR, Professor Irving Department of Surgery, Royal Free and University College Medical School, Charles Bell House, 67-73 Riding House St., London W1W 7EJ Tel: 020 7679 9312 Fax: 020 7636 5176 Email: irving.taylor@ucl.ac.uk; 43 Ridgeway Gardens, Hornsey Lane, Highgate, London N6 5NH Tel: 020 7263 8086 Fax: 020 7263 8085 — (Sheff.) MB ChB Sheff. 1968; FRCS Eng. 1972; ChM Sheff. 1978, MD (Distinc.) 1975; F.MedSci 2000; FRCPS (Hon.) Glas. 2001. Prof. Surg. Univ. Coll. Lond.; Hon. Cons. Univ. Coll. Lond. Hosps. NHS Trust; Vice Dean & Director (Clinical Studies) Roy. Free & Univ. Coll. Med. Sch. Univ. Coll. Lond. Specialty: Gen. Surg.; Oncol. Special Interest: Colorectal cancer; Colorectal liver metastases. Socs: Pres. Soc. Acad. & Research Surg; Assn. Surg. (Ex-Educat. Sec.); (Ex-Sec.) Surgic. Research Soc. Prev: Prof. Surg. Univ. Soton.; Sen. Lect. & Cons. Surg. Broadgreen Hosp. Liverp. & Roy. Liverp. Hosp.; Sen. Regist. (Surg.) Roy. Hosp. Sheff.

TAYLOR, J D M Charlotte Keel Health Centre, Seymour Road, Easton, Bristol BS5 0UA — MB ChB Bristol 1973; MB ChB Bristol 1973.

TAYLOR, Jack Lorimer Aboyne Health Centre, Bellwood Road, Aboyne AB34 5HQ Tel: 01339 886345; Craigston, Birsemore, Aboyne AB34 5EP Tel: 013398 86297 — MB ChB Aberd. 1975 (Aberdeen) DRCOG 1977; MRCGP 1979; FRCGP 1998. Princip. Gen. Pract.; Cas. Off. Aboyne Hosp.; Med. Dir. Aboyne Hosp.; Clin. Tuor Aberd. Univ.; Trainer Gen. Pract. Specialty: Gen. Pract.

TAYLOR, Jacqueline 120E Brondesbury Park, London NW2 5JR — MB BS Newc. 1987.

TAYLOR, James York District Hospital, Departmentof Oral & Maxillofacial Surgery, Wigginton Road, York YO31 8HE — MB BS Lond. 1993; FRCS (Oral & Maxillofacial Surg.); BDS Glas. 1983; FDS RCS Eng. 1988. Special Interest: Facial Deformity; Head & Neck Surg.; Skin Cancer. Socs: Char. Cross Dent. Soc. Prev: Regist. (Oral & Maxillofacial Surg.) St. Margt. Epping & Roy. Lond. Hosp.

TAYLOR, James Aitken Vennel Street Health Centre, 50 Vennel Street, Dalry KA24 4AG Tel: 01294 832523 Fax: 01294 835771; 8 Saint Palladius Terrace, Dalry KA24 5AX Tel: 01294 833621 — MB ChB Dundee 1976; DRCOG 1978; MRCGP 1980. Company Med. Adviser Roche Products Ayrsh. Specialty: Gen. Pract. Socs: (Treas.) Anglo-French Med. Soc.

TAYLOR, James Calbeck (retired) 52 Cleveley Road, Meols, Wirral CH47 8XR Tel: 0151 632 4332 — MB ChB Liverp. 1949 (Liverpool) MD Liverp. 1962, DPH 1955. Prev: SCMO (Community Child Health Serv.) Liverp. HA.

TAYLOR, James Christopher Department of Rheumatology, Nothampton General Hospital, Cliftonville, Northampton NN1 5BD; 50 George Lane, Lewisham, London SE13 6HL Tel: 020 8697 4072 — MB BS Lond. 1990 (Guys Med. Sch.) MRCP Lond. 1993. Cons. Rheumatologist; Specialist Regist. (Rheum & Gen Med.). Specialty: Gen. Med.; Rheumatol.; Sports Med. Special Interest: Metab. Bone Dis. Socs: BMA; BSR; Brit. Soc. for Sport and Exercise Med. Prev: Specialist Regist. (Research Fell.) Osteoperosis.

TAYLOR, James Francis Nuttall Cardiac Wing, Great Ormond Street Hospital for Children, NHS Trust, Great Ormond St., London WC1N 3JH Tel: 020 7430 2987 Fax: 020 7430 2995; 10 Arragon Court, 62 The Avenue, Beckenham BR3 5LA Tel: 020 8650 884 Fax: 020 8663 3309 — (St. Thos.) MRCS Eng. LRCP Lond. 1962; MB BChir Camb. 1962; DCH Eng. 1964; FRCP Lond. 1978, M 1966; MA Camb. 1962, MD Camb. 1976; FRCPCH 1996. Cons. Paediat. Cardiol. Gt. Ormond St. Hosp. Childr. Lond.; Sen Lect. Inst. of Child Health UCL. Specialty: Paediat. Cardiol. Socs: Brit. Cardiac Soc.; Brit. Paediat. Cardiol. Assn.; Assn. Europ. Paediat. Cardiol. Prev: Sen. Regist. (Med.) & Ho. Phys. Thoracic Unit Hosp. Sick Childr. Gt. Ormond St. Lond.; Regist. (Med.) St. Thos. Hosp. Lond.

TAYLOR, James Fraser (retired) Rosehaugh, Rhynie, Huntly AB54 4LJ Tel: 01464 861325 — MB ChB Aberd. 1954; DPH Ed. 1965; DIH Eng. 1965; FFOM RCP Lond. 1990. Prev: Sen. Med. Off. Chloride GP plc.

TAYLOR, James Graham (retired) Karassy, Westwood Road, Windlesham GU20 6LS Tel: 01344 22437; Karassy, Westwood Road, Windlesham GU20 6LS Tel: 01344 22437 — (Birm.) MB ChB Birm. 1940; FFOM RCPI 1977; FFOM RCP Lond. 1979. Cons. in Aviat. & Occupat. Med. to Brit. Airways; Health Screening Phys. Princess Margt. Hosp. Windsor. Prev: Dir. Med. & Safety Serv. Brit. Airways.

TAYLOR, James Michael 2 North Road, Peterhead AB42 1BL — MB ChB Aberd. 1955.

TAYLOR, James Patrick Thursby Surgery, 2 Browhead Road, Burnley BB10 3BF Tel: 01282 422447 Fax: 01282 832575 — MB ChB Manchester 1978; MB ChB Manchester 1978.

TAYLOR, James William 5 Wentworth Drive, Messingham, Scunthorpe DN17 3TZ — MB BS Lond. 1981. Sen. Med. Off. Roy. Fleet Aux.

TAYLOR, Jane Ann Claremont Surgery, 56-60 Castle Road, Scarborough YO11 1XE Tel: 01723 375050 Fax: 01723 378241; 11 Holbeck Hill, Scarborough YO11 2XE Tel: 01723 373557 — MB BS Lond. 1981 (Guy's Hospital) Dip. Therap. Newc. 1998; Dip Occ Med London 1999. GP; Clin. Asst. (Cardiol.); O.H.P. Prev: Clin. Asst. (Diabetes).

TAYLOR, Jane Charmian Gordon Wilson 28 Craigmount Park, Corstorphine, Edinburgh EH12 8EE — MB ChB Glas. 1987. Med. Off. Scott. Nat. Blood Transfus. Serv. Glas.

TAYLOR, Jane Hunt Wallacetown Health Centre, 3 Lyon Street, Dundee DD4 6RF Tel: 01382 459519 Fax: 01382 453110 — MB ChB Aberd. 1982; MRCGP Ed. 1987.

TAYLOR, Jane Rosemary Chrisp Street Health Centre, 100 Chrisp St., Poplar, London E14 6PG Tel: 020 7515 4860; 5 Alloway Road, Bow, London E3 5AS — MB ChB Manch. 1976; MRCGP 1981. GP Lond.

TAYLOR, Janet Irene Hobcroft House, Hobcroft Lane, Mobberley, Knutsford WA16 7QS — MB BCh BAO Dub. 1958 (T.C. Dub.) Prev: Asst. Psychiat. Regist. Hope Hosp. Eccles, Salford Roy. Hosp. & Bridgewater Hosp. Eccles.

TAYLOR, Janet Margaret Old Hall Grounds Health Centre, Old Hall Grounds, Cowbridge CF71 7AH Tel: 01446 772383 Fax: 01446 774022; Crud-y-Gwynt, Love Lane, Llanbleddian, Cowbridge CF71 7JQ Tel: 01446 772295 — MB BCh Wales 1975; Dip Counselling Swansea; Dip Clin Hypn Lond. 2001. Gen. Practitioner,

Dr. R. D. Jones & Partners, The Health Centre, Cowbridge Vale of Glam. CF31 1RQ; Counsellor and Med. Hypnotherapist, The Bridgend Clinic, Princess of Wales Hosp., City Rd., Bridgend, Mid Glam. CF31 1RQ. Specialty: Hypnother. Socs: Brit. Soc. of Med. and Dent. Hypn.; Brit. Soc. of Experim. and Clin. Hypn. Prev: Trainee GP M. Glam. VTS; SHO (O & G) S. Glam. HA (T); SHO (Psychiat.) Morgannwg Hosp. Bridgend.

TAYLOR, Jason Leslie Mascalls Park, Mascalls Lane, Brentwood CM14 5HQ Tel: 01277 302 712 — MB BS Lond. 1977 (Roy. Free Hosp.) MRCS Eng. LRCP Lond. 1977; MRCPsych 1982; MSc (Econ.) 1997. Cons. Psychiat. Warley Hosp. Brentwood. Specialty: Gen. Psychiat. Prev: Sen. Regist. (Psychiat.) Friern, Whittington & Roy Free Hosps. Lond.; Clin. Asst. & Regist. (Psychiat.) Roy. Free Hosp. Lond.

TAYLOR, Jean Elizabeth Culduthel Road Surgery, Ardlarich, 15 Culduthel Road, Inverness IV2 4AG Tel: 01463 712233 Fax: 01463 715479 — MB ChB Aberd. 1965; DObst RCOG 1967.

TAYLOR, Jeffrey Panteg Health Centre, Kemys Street, Griffithstown, Pontypool NP4 5DJ Tel: 01495 763608 Fax: 01495 753925 — MB BCh Wales 1984.

TAYLOR, Jennifer Geraldine 17 Littleworth Grove, Walmley, Sutton Coldfield B76 2XF — MB BCh Wales 1988. SHO (Cas.) Roy. Hosp. Wolverhampton. Prev: Ho. Off. (Med.) W. Wales Gen. Hosp.; Ho. Off. (Surg.) Neath Gen. Hosp.

TAYLOR, Jennifer Louise 32 Busby Road, Carmunnock, Clarkston, Glasgow G76 9BN — MB ChB Aberd. 1998.

TAYLOR, Jeremy David The Old Farm House, Epsom Road, Guildford GU4 7AB — MB BS Lond. 1998.

TAYLOR, Joanna Karen Elizabeth Tir-Na-Og, Brooklands, Sarisbury Green, Southampton SO31 7EE — BM BS Nottm. 1986.

TAYLOR, Joanne Denyse 3 Beeches Walk, Carshalton SM5 4JS — MB BS Lond. 1994.

TAYLOR, Joanne Elizabeth Renal Unit, Dorset County Hospital, Williams Avenue, Dorchester DT1 2JY Tel: 01305 255269 Fax: 01305 254756 — MB BChir Camb. 1985; BSc St. And. 1982; MRCP (UK) 1987; MD Camb. 1992. Dir. (Renal Servs.) Dorset. Specialty: Nephrol. Prev: Sen. Regist. Nottm. City Hosp.; Regist. Qu. Eliz. Hosp. Birm.

TAYLOR, Joby 38 Thirlestane Road, Edinburgh EH9 1AW — MB ChB Ed. 1998.

TAYLOR, John (retired) Ardgowan Medical Practice, 2 Finnart Street, Greenock PA16 8HW Tel: 01475 888155 Fax: 01475 785060 — MB ChB Aberd. 1958; MRCGP 1972.

TAYLOR, John St Giles Road Surgery, St Giles Road, Watton, Thetford IP25 6XG Tel: 01953 889134/881247 Fax: 01953 885167 — MB ChB Liverp. 1969; DObst RCOG 1972; DA Eng. 1972.

TAYLOR, John Rockhaven, 30 Georges Lane, Horwich, Bolton BL6 6RT — MB ChB Ed. 1968.

TAYLOR, John Arnold 20 Downesway, Alderley Edge SK9 7XB — MB ChB Manch. 1966.

TAYLOR, John Brian (retired) Greenbank, Riverside Road, Dittisham, Dartmouth TQ6 0HS Tel: 01803 722380 — MB BCh BAO Belf. 1948; DObst RCOG 1951; DCH Eng. 1952; FRCGP 1970. Prev: Ho. Phys. & Sen. Extern. Surg. Roy. Vict. Hosp. Belf.

TAYLOR, John Christopher, Lt.-Col. RAMC Glencairn, Reidhaven St., Elgin IV30 1QH — MB ChB Aberd. 1981; FFA RCS Eng. 1988. Cons. Anaesth. Dr Gray's Hosp. Elgin. Specialty: Anaesth. Prev: Cons. Anaesth. Brit. Army; Sen. Regist. (Anaesth.) Brit. Army; Regist. (Anaesth.) Aberd. Roy. Infirm.

TAYLOR, John Christopher Kneesworth House Hospital, Bassingbourn-cum-Kneesworth, Royston SG8 5JP Tel: 01763 255600 Fax: 01763 246115 — MRCS Eng. LRCP Lond. 1972 (Guy's) DObst. RCOG 1975; FRCPsych 1993, M 1981. Med. Dir. Partnerships In Care Ltd. Specialty: Forens. Psychiat. Prev: Cons. Forens. Psychiat. Roy. Free, Friern Hosps. Lond. & Wessex RHA; Sen. Regist. (Forens. Psychiat.) Roy. Free Hosp. & HM Prison Holloway.

TAYLOR, Mr John Desmond Renal Unit, Guy's Hospital, Guy's Tower, St Thomas St., London SE1 9RT Tel: 020 7955 4818 Fax: 020 7407 6370 Email: john.d.taylor@kcl.ac.uk; 182 Shakespeare Tower, Barbican, London EC2Y 8DR Tel: 020 7382 9048 Email: johnatguys@aol.com — MB BChir Camb. 1978 (Camb. & Guy's) MRCS Eng. LRCP Lond. 1977; MA Camb. 1978; FRCS Ed. 1982; MD Leicester 1989. Cons. Transpl. Surg. Guy's Hosp. Lond.; Hon. Cons. Transpl. Surg., Kent and Canterbury Hosp.; Hon. Cons. Transpl. Surg. - King's Healthcare, Lond.; Hon. Cons. Transpl. Surg., Gt. Ormond St Hosp. Lond. Specialty: Transpl. Surg. Socs: Roy. Soc. Med.; Brit. Transpl. Soc.; Assn. Surg. Prev: Sen. Regist. (Gen. Surg.) & Regist. Roy. Liverp. Hosp.; Research Fell. (Surg.) Univ. Leics.

TAYLOR, John Edward (retired) 9 Pine Meadows, Kirkella, Hull HU10 7NS Tel: 01482 656366 Email: john@jetaylor11.fsnet.co.uk — MRCS Eng. LRCP Lond. 1953; LDS Leeds 1960. Prev: Ho. Phys. Pinderfields Hosp. Wakefield.

TAYLOR, Mr John Frederic (retired) 34 South Road, Grassendale Park, Liverpool L19 0LT Tel: 0151 427 1148 Fax: 0151 427 1148 Email: johnftaylor@compuserve.com — MB ChB Liverp 1958; DTM & H Liverp. 1963; FRCS Eng. 1966; MD Liverp. 1965, MChOrth 1971. Prev: Cons. Orthop. Surg. Alder Hey Childr. Hosp. Liverp.

TAYLOR, John Frederick, CBE 45 Canonbury Road, London N1 2DG Tel: 020 7359 2548; Burthallan House, Burthallan Lane, St Ives TR26 3AB Tel: 01736 796577 — MB BS Lond. 1957 (St. Geo.) DObst RCOG 1959; DIH Soc. Apoth. Lond. 1960; FFOM RCP Lond. 1985, MFOM 1978; FRCP Lond. 1992. Med. Adviser, Pub. Carriage Office, Lond. Specialty: Occupat. Health. Socs: Fell. Roy. Soc. Med. Prev: Chairm. Transport Comm. Med. Commiss on Accid. Preven.; Chief Med. Off. Dept. of Transport; Sen. Med. Off. Driver & Vehicule Licensing Centre (DVLC).

TAYLOR, Mr John Gibson, VRD (retired) Hill Farm, Downham, Wymondham NR18 0SD Tel: 01603 810462 — FRCS Eng. 1947 (St. Mary's); MRCS Eng. LRCP Lond. 1941; MB BS Lond. 1941. Prev: Cons. Orthop. Surg. Norf. & Norwich Hosp. & Rheum. Unit St. Michael's Hosp. Aylsham; 1st Asst. Accid. Serv. Radcliffe Infirm. Oxf.

TAYLOR, John Henry Keevil (retired) Talisker, Moor Court, Amberley, Stroud GL5 5DA Tel: 01453 873151 — MB BS Lond. 1955 (St. Bart.) DObst RCOG 1959. Prev: GP Middlx.

TAYLOR, John Jarvis States Laboratory, St Helier, Jersey Tel: 01534 59000 — MB BS Lond. 1955 (Char. Cross) FRCPath 1978, M 1966; DMJ Soc. Apoth. Lond. 1982. Dir. States Laborat. Jersey. Specialty: Pathology, General. Prev: Ho. Phys. & Ho. Surg. Char. Cross Hosp.; Res. Clin. Pathol. Qu. Eliz. Hosp. Birm.

TAYLOR, John Langton (retired) 3 Linnet Hill, Rochdale OL11 4DA Tel: 01706 524242 — (Manch.) BSc Manch. 1940, MB ChB 1943; MRCS Eng. LRCP Lond. 1943; FRCP Lond. 1970, M 1948. Prev: Cons. Phys. Rochdale & Dist. Gp. Hosps.

TAYLOR, John Leahy (retired) 18 Thameside, Riverfield Road, Staines TW18 2HA Tel: 01784 452331 Fax: 01784 452331 — MB BS Lond. 1957 (St. Mary's) MRCS Eng. LRCP Lond. 1944; MRCGP 1953; DMJ Soc. Apoth. Lond. 1964. Prev: Sec. Med. Protec. Soc.

TAYLOR, John Mark Stuart Road Surgery, Stuart Road, Pontefract WF8 4PQ Tel: 01977 703437 — MB ChB Sheff. 1984.

TAYLOR, John Nicholas Perth-y-Terfyn, 51 Mount Road, St Asaph LL17 0DH Tel: 01745 583734 — MB ChB Liverp. 1971. Prev: Med. Regist. Mersey RHA; SHO Roy. Liverp. Childr. Hosp.

TAYLOR, John Robert Florence Street Resource Centre, 20-60 Florence St., Glasgow G5 0YZ Tel: 0141 429 2878 — MB ChB Ed. 1987; MPhil Ed. 1996, MB ChB Ed. 1987; MRCPsych 1992. Cons. Psychiat. Levendale Hosp. Glas. Specialty: Gen. Psychiat. Prev: Regist. (Psychiat.) Dingleton Hosp. Melrose.; Sen. Regist. N. Mersey Community Trust Liverp.

TAYLOR, John Stephen Garratt Palmerston Road Surgery, 18 Palmerston Road, Buckhurst Hill IG9 5LT Tel: 020 8504 1552 — MB BS Lond. 1978.

TAYLOR, John Stewart (retired) Oakroyd, Moray Place, Elgin IV30 1NN Tel: 01343 543595 — MB ChB Aberd. 1951. Prev: Ho. Phys. Roy. Infirm. & City Hosp. Aberd.

TAYLOR, John Victor King Cross Surgery, 199 King Cross Road, Halifax HX1 3LW Tel: 01422 330612 Fax: 01422 323740; 41 Savile Park, Halifax HX1 3EX — BM BS Nottm. 1984; BMedSci (Hons.) 1982; MRCGP 1988. Princip GP Halifax.

TAYLOR, Mr John Vincent 62 Warwick Road, Upton CH49 6NF Tel: 0151 641 0628 Email: johnvtaylor@hotmail.com — MB ChB Liverp. 1993; FRSC; BSc (Hons.) Liverp. 1990; FRCS Ed. 1997; ChM Liverp. 2004. SpR Merseyside. Specialty: Gen. Surg.; Surgery, Vascular. Prev: Price Surgic. Research Fell. Univ. of Louisville Kentucky, USA.

TAYLOR, Jonathan Breck Park Slope Surgery, 32 Stoke Road, Blisworth, Northampton NN7 3BT Tel: 01604 858237 Fax: 01604 859437; Grey House, 5 Baker St, Gayton, Northampton NN7 3EZ — MB BS Lond. 1986 (Westm.) DRCOG 1991.

TAYLOR, Jonathan Michael 3 Apple Tree Close, Church St., Boston Spa, Wetherby LS23 6DG — MB ChB Leeds 1982; DRCOG 1986.

TAYLOR, Josephine 29 Merton Hall, Wimbledon, London SW19 3PR — MB BS Lond. 1985.

TAYLOR, Judith O'Mara 106 Harley Street, London W1N 1AF; 8 Prince Albert Road, London NW1 7SR — BM Soton. 1979; MRCP (UK) 1985. Locum Cons. Paediatric Nephrologist Guys Hosp. Lond. Specialty: Paediat.

TAYLOR, Julia Christine 131 Leys Lane, Frome BA11 2JS — MB BS Lond. 1990.

TAYLOR, Julia Marion Ward End Medical Centre, 794A Washwood Heath Road, Ward End, Birmingham B8 2JN Tel: 0121 327 1049 Fax: 0121 327 0964 — MB ChB Manch. 1978; MRCGP 1983; DRCOG 1983.

TAYLOR, Julia Mary National Blood Service Leeds Blood centre, Bridle Path, Leeds LS15 7TW Tel: 0113 2148646 Email: julia.taylor@nbs.nhs.uk — MB ChB Sheff. 1980; MRCP 1983; FRCPath 1998. Cons. in Transfus. Med. Nat. Blood Serv. Leeds. Specialty: Haematology. Prev: Sen. Regist. Char. Cross & Westminster Hosps. Lond.; Regist. Leicester Roy. Infirm.

TAYLOR, Julie Ann Newbold Verdon Medical Practice, St. George's Close, Newbold Verdon, Leicester LE9 9PZ Tel: 01445 822171 Fax: 01445 824968 — BM BS Nottm. 1986; BMedSci Nottm. 1984; DRCOG 1989. Gen. Practitioner Leics. Specialty: Gen. Pract. Prev: Trainee GP Warks.

TAYLOR, Karen Margaret 5 Westerham Close, Trentham, Stoke-on-Trent ST4 8JW — MB ChB Birm. 1993.

TAYLOR, Karey Anne Psychotherapy Department, Warneford Hospital, Headington, Oxford OX3 7JX — BM BCh Oxf. 1985.

TAYLOR, Kathleen Anne Benoran, Torr Road, Bridge of Weir PA11 3BE — MB ChB Glas. 1985; DRCOG 1988; DCCH RCP Ed. 1989; MRCGP 1990. Trainee GP Edin. VTS.; GP Retainer Scheme. Prev: Clin. Asst. Merchiston Hosp. Johnstone; GP Princip. Battersea Lond.; SHO (Psychiat.) Warlingham Pk. Hosp.

TAYLOR, Kay Vivienne Park Road Health Centre, Park Road, Tarporley CW6 0BE Tel: 01829 732401 Fax: 01829 732404 — MB ChB Manch. 1977.

TAYLOR, Keith John 15 Northdene Drive, Rochdale OL11 5NH — MD Manch. 1990; MB ChB 1977; MRCP (UK) 1983. Cons. Phys. Respirat. Med. Glan Clwyd Dist. Gen. Hosp. Rhyl Denbish. Specialty: Respirat. Med.

TAYLOR, Keith William Department of Medicine, Royal London Hospital, Whitechapel, London E1 1BB; 18 Lion Street, Rye TN31 7LB Tel: 01797 222512 — MB BChir Camb. 1955 (King's Coll. Hosp.) PhD Camb. 1960, MA 1955; FRCP Lond. 1994. Emerit. Prof. Biochem. Lond. Specialty: Diabetes. Prev: Hon. Cons. Diabetic Med. King's Coll. Hosp. Lond.; Prof. Biochem. Lond. Hosp. Med. Coll.; Prof. Biochem. & Cons. Chem. Path. Univ. Sydney, Austral.

TAYLOR, Kenneth George The Diabetes & Endocrinology Unit, City Hospital, Dudley Road, Birmingham B18 7QH Tel: 0121 507 4592 Fax: 0121 507 4988; Redstacks, 1 Priory Road, Halesowen B62 0BZ Tel: 0121 602 2142 Fax: 0121 602 2142 Email: kandgtaylor@blueyonder.co.uk — MB BS Lond. 1970 (St. Bartholomew's Hospital Medical School) MRCS Eng. LRCP Lond. 1970; MRCP (UK) 1973; MD Lond. 1978; FRCP Lond. 1987. p/t Cons. Phys. City Hosp. Birm. Specialty: Gen. Med.; Diabetes; Endocrinol. Special Interest: Lipid Disorders. Socs: Diabetes UK; Heart UK. Prev: Sen. Regist. (Med.) Birm. Gen. Hosp.; Hon. Sen. Regist. & Research Fell. St. Bart. Hosp. Lond.

TAYLOR, Professor Kenneth MacDonald Cardiothoracic Surgical Unit, Imperial College School of Medicine, Hammersmith Hospital, Ducane Road, London W12 0NN Tel: 020 8383 3214 Fax: 020 8740 7019 Email: scarroll@ic.ac.uk; 129 Argyle Road, Ealing, London W13 0DB — MD Glas. 1979, MB ChB 1970; FRCS Glas. 1974; FRCS Eng. 1984. Brit. Heart Foundat. Prof. Cardiac Surg. Univ. Lond.; Prof. Cardiac Surg. Imperial Coll. Sch. of Med. at Hammersmith Hosp. Lond. Specialty: Cardiothoracic Surg. Socs: Surg. Research Soc. & Soc. Thoracic & Cardiovasc. Surgs.; FSA 1977; FESC 1995. Prev: Sen. Lect. (Cardiac Surg.) Univ. Glas.; Hall Tutorial Fell. in Surg. Univ. Glas.

TAYLOR, Kobina Arba 47 Linchmere Road, Lee, London SE12 0NB — MB BChir Camb. 1952 (Univ. Coll. Hosp.) MA, MB BChir Camb. 1952. Prev: SHMO S. Wing Bedford Gen. Hosp.; Res. Surg. Off. Roy. Hosp. Chesterfield; Surg. Regist. PeterBoro. Gen. Hosp.

TAYLOR, Lakhbir Kaur Boxworth End Surgery, 58 Boxworth End, Swavesey, Cambridge CB4 5RA Tel: 01954 230202 Fax: 01954 206035 — MB BS Lond. 1982 (St. Bart.) BSc. (Hons.) Lond. 1979. Specialty: Gen. Pract.

TAYLOR, Laura Bradley 122 The Ridgeway, Enfield EN2 8JN — MB BS Lond. 1998.

TAYLOR, Mr Lee James Runcton Manor, Runcton, Chichester PO20 1PS Tel: 01243 528933 Fax: 01243 538214 — MB BS Lond. 1977 (Middlx.) FRCS Eng. 1981. Cons. Orthop. Surg. Roy. W. Sussex NHS Trust. Specialty: Orthop. Special Interest: Arthroscopic Surgery of Knee & Ligament Reconstruction; Decompressive Surgery of Lumbar Spine; Primary/Revision Hip & Knee Arthrosplasty. Prev: Cons. Orthop. Surg. St Richard's Hosp. Chichester; Sen. Regist. Middlx. Hosp. & Roy. Nat Orthop. Hosps. Lond.; Regist. (Orthop.) St Geo. Hosp. Lond.

TAYLOR, Liam Paul Gerard The Grange Clinic, Westfield Avenue, Malpas, Newport NP20 6EY Tel: 01633 855521 Fax: 01633 859490 Email: liam.taylor@gp-w93045.wales.nhs.uk; Newport Locha Health Board, Wentwood Suite, St Cadoc's Hospital, Newport NP18 3XQ Tel: 01633 436200 — MB BCh BAO Belf. 1990; DGM RCPS Glas. 1993; DCH Dub. 1993; DRCOG 1994; MRCGP 1995; Dip Ther, Wales 1998. GP Princip.; Med. Dir. Newport LHB. Specialty: Gen. Pract. Prev: Regist. (Pub. Health Med.) & Cornw. Isles of Scilly Health Auth.; SHO Altnagelvin Hosp. Londonderry; Ho. Off. Mater Hosp. Belf.

TAYLOR, Lilian (retired) — MB ChB Manch. 1959. Prev: Clin. Asst. Dept. Path. High Wycombe Gen. Hosp.

TAYLOR, Lillious McLellan (retired) c/o Purvis, 2 Dalmellington Court, Kittoch Field, East Kilbride, Glasgow G74 4XD Tel: 01355 263602 — MA Glas. 1949, MB ChB 1960; DObst RCOG 1962; DCH RCPS Glas. 1967. Prev: Assoc. Specialist (Dermat.) Vict. Infirm. Glas.

TAYLOR, Linda Elizabeth 4 Beech Close, Highnam, Gloucester GL2 8EG — MB BCh BAO Belf. 1979; DCH Dub. 1982; MRCGP 1988; DCCH Ed. 1989. Clin. Med. Off. (Child Health) Glos. Specialty: Community Child Health.

TAYLOR, Lorna Anne 63-65 Garstang Road, Preston PR1 1LJ Tel: 01772 253554; Moor Hall Cottage, Lower Bartle, Preston PR4 0RU Tel: 01772 723274 — MB BCh Wales 1979; BSc (Hons.) St. And. 1976. GP Preston.

TAYLOR, Lorna Margaret Mayfield Road Surgery, 125 Mayfield Road, Edinburgh EH9 3AJ Tel: 0131 668 1095 Fax: 0131 662 1734; 33 Kingsknowe Drive, Edinburgh EH14 2JY Tel: 0141 443 5590 — MB ChB Ed. 1978; DRCOG 1980; MRCGP 1982.

TAYLOR, Magnus John Avecia Ltd, PO Box 521, Leeds Road, Huddersfield HD1 9GA Tel: 01484 433946 Email: magnus.taylor@avecia.com; 112 Huddersfield Road, Brighouse HD6 3RH — MB ChB Manch. 1976 (Manchester) MRCP (UK) 1981; FFOM RCP Lond. 1993, M 1986; FRCP Lond. 1999. Cons. Occupational Health Phys. Avecia Ltd Manchester; Regional Specialty Adviser Occupat. Med. Specialty: Occupat. Health. Socs: Mem. Soc. of Occupat.al Med. Prev: Sen. Occupat. Health Phys. ICI BioSci.s Huddersfield; Chairm. Soc. Occupat. Med. (Yorksh. Br.); Lect. (Occupat. Med.) Manch. Univ.

TAYLOR, Malcolm Bernard Oakeswell Health Centre, Brunswick Park Road, Wednesbury WS10 9HP Tel: 0121 556 2114; 53 Broadway, Walsall WS1 3EZ — MB ChB Birm. 1969; DObst RCOG 1973. Prev: SHO (O & G) Marston Green Matern. Hosp. Birm.; Ho. Phys. Qu. Eliz. Hosp. Birm.; Ho. Surg. Gen. Hosp. Birm.

TAYLOR, Malcolm Peter (retired) 20 Saxton Avenue, Doncaster DN4 7AX Tel: 01302 370927 — MB ChB Birm. 1955; FRCGP 1974. Prev: GP Doncaster.

TAYLOR, Marcus Ben Depart. Of Diagnostic Radiology, Christie Hospital NHS Trust, Wilmslow Road, Withington, Manchester M20 4BX Tel: 0161 446 3980 — MB ChB Sheff. 1991 (Sheffield) MRCP (UK) 1994; FRCR 1999. Cons. Radiologist, Christie Hosp. NHS Trust, Manch. Specialty: Radiol. Prev: SHO Rotat. (Med.) City Hosp. Birm.; Specialist Regist. Rotat. (Diagn. Radiol.) Manch.

TAYLOR, Margaret (retired) 7 Marina Drive, South Shields NE33 2NH — MB ChB Bristol 1957; FRCPCH; DCH Eng. 1960; DObst RCOG 1961; FRCP Ed. 1980, M 1965. Cons. Paediat. S. Shields Hosp. Gp.

TAYLOR, Margaret Elizabeth Ty Nant, 13 Hermitage Meadow, Snow Hill, Clare, Sudbury CO10 8QQ — MB BS Lond. 1961 (Roy. Free) MRCS Eng. LRCP Lond. 1961. Socs: BMA. Prev: Gyn. Ho. Surg. Roy. Free Hosp. Lond.; Ho. Phys. Qu. Mary's Hosp. Sidcup.

TAYLOR, Margaret Elspeth Jubilee Surgery, Barry's Meadow, High St., Titchfield, Fareham PO14 4EH Tel: 01329 844220; 56A West Street, Titchfield, Fareham PO14 4DF Tel: 01329 847209 — MB ChB Liverp. 1965.

TAYLOR, Margaret Jean (retired) 16 Broadmead, Broadmayne, Dorchester DT2 8EE — LRCP LRCS Ed. 1953; LRCP LRCS Ed. LRFPS Glas. 1953. Asst. (Path.) W. Dorset Gp. Hosps.

TAYLOR, Margaret Joan (retired) 86 Rennets Wood Road, Eltham, London SE9 2NH Tel: 020 8850 0990 — MB ChB Sheff. 1962; MRCPsych 1978.

TAYLOR, Marian Ann (retired) The Birches, Huntington Lane, Ashford Carbonel, Ludlow SY8 4DG — MRCS Eng. LRCP Lond. 1955 (Roy. Free) DCH Eng. 1960; DO Eng. 1982.

TAYLOR, Marion Haddo Medical Group, The Old School, The Square, Tarves, Ellon AB41 7GX Tel: 01651 851777 — MB ChB Aberd. 1992; MRCGP 1996. Gen. Practitioner Haddo Med. Gp. Specialty: Gen. Pract. Prev: Locum Gen. Practioner Aberd.; Locum Gen. Practioner Hereford; Med. Off. St. Michael's Hospice Hereford.

TAYLOR, Marjory Frances Shettleston Health Centre, Shettleston Health Centre, 420 Old Shettleston Road, Glasgow G32 7JZ Tel: 0141 531 6250 Fax: 0141 531 6216; 187 Sandy Hills Road, Mount Vernon, Glasgow G32 9NB — MB ChB Glas. 1988. Prev: SHO (Geriat.) Roy. Alexandra Hosp. Glas.; SHO (A & E) West. Infirm. Glas.; SHO (Med.) Glas. Roy. Infirm.

TAYLOR, Mark Alexander 21 Seventree Road, Londonderry BT47 5QH — MB BCh BAO Belf. 1994.

TAYLOR, Mark Andrew Honley Surgery, Marsh Gardens, Honley, Huddersfield HD9 6AG Tel: 01484 303366 Fax: 01484 303365; Mollicar House, Lumb Lane, Almondbury, Huddersfield HD4 6SZ — MB ChB Leeds 1981; MRCGP 1985. Specialty: Gen. Pract. Socs: Huddersfield Med. Soc. Prev: Trainee GP Huddersfield VTS; Ho. Phys. Chapel Allerton Hosp. Leeds.; Ho. Surg. Leeds Gen. Infirm.

TAYLOR, Mark Bartholomew Longacre House, Crapstone, Yelverton PL20 7PF — MB BS Lond. 1978 (St. Bart.) FFA RCS Eng. 1983. Cons. Dept. Anaesth. & Pain Relief Clinic, Derriford Hosp. Plymouth. Specialty: Anaesth. Prev: Sen. Regist. (Anaesth.) Hammersmith & Char. Cross Hosps. Lond.; Regist. (Anaesth.) Hosp. Sick Childr. Lond.; Fell. Toronto Gen. Hosp.

TAYLOR, Mark Buchanan 131 Brewery Road, Plumstead, London SE18 1NE — MB BS Lond. 1979; MA Camb. 1977; PhD Kent 1984; MRCPath 1993. Lect. (Med. Microbiol.) Lond. Hosp. Med. Coll. Specialty: Med. Microbiol. Prev: Wellcome Train. Fell. St. Mary's Hosp. Lond.; Ho. Surg. Roy. Ear Hosp. Lond.

TAYLOR, Mark Conroy Hill House Surgery, Aspatria, Carlisle CA7 3NG Tel: 016973 20209 Fax: 016973 22333; Teesdale House, High Scales, Aspatria, Carlisle CA7 3NG — MB BS Newc. 1980; Dip Audiol Dip Sports Psychol. 2002 (Newc.); MRCGP 1984; DRCOG 1984. Specialty: Obst. & Gyn.

TAYLOR, Mark Lees 75 The Balk, Walton, Wakefield WF2 6JX; 2 The Cottage, Manse Brae, Croy, Inverness IV2 5PU Tel: 01967 43332 — MB ChB Birm. 1991. Specialty: Gen. Pract. Socs: MRCGP.

TAYLOR, Mark Stuart Magna House Medical Centre, 81 Merley Lane, Merley, Wimborne BH21 3BB Tel: 01202 841288 Fax: 01202 840877; Greenholm, Arrowsmith Road, Canford Magna, Wimborne BH21 3BD Tel: 01202 693366 Email: marktaylor@doctors.org.uk — MB BS Lond. 1975 (Guy's) MRCGP 1989. GP Princip. Magna Ho. Med. Centre; GP Trainer Dorset; Course Organiser Dorset VTS. Prev: Examr. RCGP; RNLI Med. Off.; Clin. Asst. Opht.

TAYLOR, Mr Mark Travers Coventry and Warwickshire Hospital, Stoney Stanton Lane, Coventry CV1 4RH Tel: 02476 246503; Flat 24, Hollymount, 29 Hagley Road, Birmingham B16 9LS Tel: 0121 455 6381 — (Birmingham) MB ChB Birm. 1985; Dip. Sports Med. Lond 1987; MRCP (UK) 1989; FRCS (A&E) Ed. 1991; FRCS Eng. 1992; FRCS (Orth.) 1997. Orthopaedic and Trauma Cons., Coventry and Warks. Hosp. Specialty: Trauma & Orthop. Surg. Socs: BOA; BMA; BASEM. Prev: Regist. (Orthop. & Trauma) Birm. Gen. Hosp.; Specialist Regist. (Orthop. & Trauma) Roy. Orthop. Hosp. Birm.; Orthopaedic and Trauma Cons., Sandwell Hosp. 2000-2002.

TAYLOR, Martin, Capt. 38 Summershades Lane, Grasscroft, Oldham OL4 4ED Email: martintaylor999@hotmail.com — MB ChB Leeds 1998. SHO. (A&E.) PeterBoro. Gen Hosp. Specialty: Accid. & Emerg. Socs: RAMC - Capt. Prev: PRHO. Derriford Hosp Plymouth.; PRHO. Leeds Gen Infirm.

TAYLOR, Martin Charles 7 Westfield Road, Lymington SO41 3PZ — MB BS Lond. 1985; MRCP (UK) 1994. Regist. (Diabetes & Endocrinol.) Soton. Gen. Hosp. Specialty: Endocrinol. Prev: Regist. (Diabetes & Endocrinol.) Roy. Bournemouth Hosp.; Regist. Gen. Hosp. Jersey.

TAYLOR, Mr Martin Christopher King's Mill Centre for Healthcare Services, Mansfield Road, Sutton-in-Ashfield NG17 4JL Tel: 01623 622515; 38 Main Street, Woodborough, Nottingham NG14 6EA Tel: 0115 965 5654 — MB ChB Sheff. 1971; FRCS Ed. 1977. Cons. Urol. King's Mill Hosp. Mansfield; Clin. Director of Surg. King's Mill Hosp. Mansfield. Specialty: Urol. Prev: Clin. Dir. (Urol.) City Hosp. Nottm.; Cons. Urol. Dist. Gen. Hosp. Rotherham; Sen. Regist. City Hosp. Nottm.

TAYLOR, Martin John The Cornerstone Practice, 26 Clwyn Road, March PE15 9BT Tel: 01354 606300 Fax: 01354 656033; Willow Farm, 129 Knight's End Road, March PE15 8QD Tel: 01354 652611 — MB ChB Sheff. 1985; MRCGP 1989.

TAYLOR, Mary (retired) Elm Cottage, Mill Road, Shiplate, Henley-on-Thames RG9 3LW Tel: 0118 940 3046 — (Belf.) MB ChB BAO Belf. 1961; DObst RCOG 1963. Prev: Assoc. Specialist (Anaesth. & IC) Roy. Berks. Hosp. Reading.

TAYLOR, Mary Buchanan Aboyne Health Centre, Bellwood Road, Aboyne AB34 5HQ Tel: 01339 886345; Aboyne Medical Practice, The Health Centre, Aboyne AB34 5HQ Tel: 013398 86345 — MB ChB Aberd. 1974; DCH RCPS Glas. 1976; DRCOG 1978; MRCGP 1979. Partner in Gen. Pract. Socs: Country Mem. Liverp. Med. Inst.; Co-organiser Upper Deeside Med. Gp.

TAYLOR, Mary Helen Department of Anaesthetics, Birmingham Heartlands Hospital, Bordesley Green E., Birmingham B9 5SS Tel: 0121 766 6611; 65 Salisbury Road, Moseley, Birmingham B13 8LB Tel: 0121 449 4838 — MB ChB Birm. 1971; DObst RCOG 1973; DA Eng. 1974; FFA RCS Eng. 1975. Cons. Anaesth. Birm. Heartlands Hosp. Specialty: Anaesth. Prev: Sen. Regist. (Anaesth.) W. Midl. RHA; Sen. Regist. (Anaesth.) Univ. Hosp. Kingston, Jamaica; Regist. (Anaesth.) Walsgrave Hosp. Coventry.

TAYLOR, Matthew Adam 3 Archery Close, Wickersley, Rotherham S66 1DT — MB ChB Manch. 1998; MB ChB Manch 1998.

TAYLOR, Matthew James The Rectory, Well Meadow, Church Road, Newbury RG14 2DR — MB BS Lond. 1991.

TAYLOR, Mavis Gloria Spencer (retired) 78 Kimberley Road, Little Wakering, Southend-on-Sea SS3 0JP Tel: 01702 219279 — (Char. Cross) MB BS (Hons. Surg.) Lond. 1958. Prev: Ho. Surg. Char. Cross Hosp.

TAYLOR, Melvyn Roy Lakeside Practice, The Health Centre, Off Station Road, Doncaster DN6 0JB Tel: 01302 700212 Fax: 01302 707370 — MB ChB Sheff. 1970. Prev: SHO (ENT) Sheff. Roy. Hosp.; Ho. Off. (Gen. Med.) Doncaster Roy. Infirm.; Ho. Off. (Orthop.) Sheff. Roy. Infirm.

TAYLOR, Michael Leverndale Hospital, 510 Crookston Rd, Glasgow G53 7TU Tel: 0141 211 6531 — MB ChB Glas. 1991; MRCPsych 1996; MPhil (Glas) 2000. Cons. Psychiat., Leverndale Hosp. Glas. Specialty: Forens. Psychiat.; Gen. Psychiat. Prev: Specialist Regist. (Psychiat.) Douglas Inch Centre Glas.

TAYLOR, Michael Park Road West Surgery, 11 Park Road West, Crosland Moor, Huddersfield HD4 5RX Tel: 01484 642020/642044 Fax: 01484 460774 — MB ChB Leeds 1978.

TAYLOR, Michael Anthony 1 Windle Grove, Windle, St Helens WA10 6HN — MB BChir Camb. 1991.

TAYLOR, Michael Antony Rollin 5 Drumblefield, Chelford, Macclesfield SK11 9BT — MB BS Lond. 1966; MRCS Eng. LRCP Lond. 1966; MRCP (U.K.) 1971; FRCP Lond. 1986. Cons. Phys. Macclesfield Hosp. Specialty: Gen. Med. Prev: Sen. Med. Regist. St. Jas. Univ. Hosp. Leeds & Univ. Hosp. W. Indies; Kingston Jamaica.

TAYLOR, Michael Arkwright (retired) Eskdale, 112 Sutton Park Road, Kidderminster DY11 6JG — MRCS Eng. LRCP Lond. 1961 (Manch.) DObst RCOG 1964.

TAYLOR, Michael Eric The White House, Llangenny, Crickhowell NP8 1HA — MB BS Lond. 1960; BSc Lond. 1957, MB BS 1960; MRCP Lond. 1965; DMRD Eng. 1967; FFR 1969; FRCR 1975. Cons. Phys. St. Geo. Hosp. Lond. Specialty: Radiol. Socs: Fell. Roy. Soc. Med. Lond.; Brit. Soc. Allergy & Environm. Med. Prev: Sen. Regist.

(Radiol.) Univ. Coll. & Middlx. Hosp. Lond. & Hosp. Sick Childr. Gt.Ormond St. Lond.; Regist. (Med.) Roy. Brompton Nat. Heart & Lung Hosp. Lond.; Ho. Surg. Middlx. Hosp. Lond.

TAYLOR, Mr Michael Francis Scott Department of Orthopaedics, Broomfield Hospital, Court Road, Chelmsford CM1 7ET Tel: 01245 514604 Email: michael.taylor@meht.nhs.uk — MB ChB Bristol 1983; FRCS Ed. 1987; FRCS (Orth.) 1992. Cons. in Trauma & Orthopaedic Surg., Mid Essex Hosps. NHS Trust, Chelmsford (Broomfield Hospital). Specialty: Orthop. Socs: Brit. Orthopaedic Assn.; Brit. Soc. for Surg. of the Hand; Brit. Orthopaedic Foot Surg. Soc.

TAYLOR, Michael James Yatton Family Practice, 155 Mendip Road, Yatton, Bristol BS49 4ER Tel: 01934 832277 Fax: 01934 876085; Stablegrove, West Hay Road, Wrington, Bristol BS40 5NR Tel: 01934 863504 Fax: 01934 863599 — MB BS Lond. 1985; MA Camb. 1982; DRCOG 1988; MRCGP 1989. Socs: BMA.

TAYLOR, Michael John Clayton Health Centre, 89 North Road, Clayton, Manchester M11 4EJ Tel: 0161 223 9229 Fax: 0161 223 1116 — MB ChB Manch. 1961; DObst RCOG 1962.

TAYLOR, Michael Stuart 34 Bramwith Road, Nethergreen, Sheffield S11 7EZ Tel: 0114 230 8352 — MB ChB Manch. 1994. SHO (Med.) N. Derbysh. Roy. Hosp. Chesterfield. Specialty: Gen. Med.

TAYLOR, Michael William 46 Newlands Crescent, Aberdeen AB10 6LH Tel: 01224 315202 — MB ChB Aberd. 1975; BSc Aberd. 1970; MRCP (UK) 1977; FRCGP 1992, M 1980; FRCP Ed. 1993. Dir. of Post Grad. Gen. Pract. Educat. Post Grad. Centre Aberd. Roy. Infirm.; Sen. Lect. Dept. Gen. Pract. & Primary Care Foresterhill Health Centre Westburn Rd. Aberd.

TAYLOR, Moira Elizabeth Stockport NHS Trust, Department of Microbiology, Department of Laboratory Medicine, Stepping Hill Hospital, Poplar Grove, Stockport SK2 7JE — MB ChB Manch. 1985 (Manchester) MSc (Molecular Microbiol) Manch. 1993; MRCPath 1994. Cons. (Microbiologist) Stockport NHS Trust Stockport. Specialty: Med. Microbiol.

TAYLOR, Murray George (retired) Beaconscroft, Peak Lane, Compton Dundon, Somerton TA11 6NZ Tel: 01458 274284 — (St. Bart.) MB BS Lond. 1952; DObst RCOG 1957. Prev: Regist. (Med.) Weymouth & Dist. Hosp.

TAYLOR, Myles James Overton 18 Quarry Hollow, Headington, Oxford OX3 8JR — BM BCh Oxf. 1989.

TAYLOR, Neil Malcolm Frimley Park Hospital, Department of Anaesthesia, Portsmouth Road, Frimley, Camberley GU21 4JQ — MB BS West. Australia 1985; FRCA 1993. Cons. Anaesth. Frimley Pk. Hosp. Camberley. Specialty: Anaesth. Special Interest: Obstetric Anaesth.

TAYLOR, Nia Jane 3 Beddoes Drive, Bayston Hill, Shrewsbury SY3 0BU — BM BCh Oxf. 1998.

TAYLOR, Nicholas Charles Gwion Castle, Llandysul SA44 4LE — MB ChB St. And. 1971; DCH Eng. 1973; MRCP (UK) 1976. Cons. Phys. & Cardiol. W. Wales Hosp. Carmarthen. Specialty: Cardiol. Socs: Brit. Cardiac Soc. Prev: Hon. Sen. Regist. Papworth Hosp. Camb.; Regist. Nat. Heart Hosp. Lond.

TAYLOR, Nicholas Howard 97 London Road, Gloucester GL1 3HH Tel: 01452 522079 Fax: 01452 387884; 12 Claremont Road, Bishopston, Bristol BS7 8DQ — MB BS Lond. 1978 (St. Geo.) DRCOG 1982; MRCGP 1983.

TAYLOR, Nicholas John, Maj. RAMC Almond Road Surgery, Almond Road, St. Neots, Huntingdon PE19 1DZ Tel: 01480 473413 Fax: 01480 406906; The Priory, 26 West St, Godmanchester, Huntingdon PE29 2HG — MB BChir Camb. 1983; MA Camb. 1983; DRCOG 1987; MRCGP 1988. Prev: Regtl. Med. Off. 1st Bn. Green Howards Osnabruck BAOR; SHO (Med.) Camb. Milit. Hosp. Aldershot; Ho. Phys. (Neurol.) St. Bart. Hosp. Lond.

TAYLOR, Nicholas Mark 246 Meadow Head, Sheffield S8 7UH — MB ChB Leeds 1985.

TAYLOR, Nicholas Patrick, Maj. RAMC Dr Moss and Partners, 28-38 Kings Road, Harrogate HG1 5JP Tel: 01423 560261 Fax: 01423 501099; 14 St. James Drive, Harrogate HG2 8HT — MB BS Newc. 1985; MRCGP 1991; DCH RCP Lond. 1991. Specialty: Paediat. Prev: Ho. Off. (Gen. Med.) Dryburn Gen. Hosp. Durh.; Ho. Off. (Gen. Surg.) Cumbld. Infirm. Carlisle.; Unit Med. Off. 35RE.

TAYLOR, Nicholas Robert 20 Lightborne Road, Sale M33 5EA — MB ChB Bristol 1998.

TAYLOR, Nigel Geoffrey Mytholmroyd Health Centre, Thrush Hill Raod, Mytholmroyd, Hebden Bridge HX7 5AQ Tel: 01422 882291 — MB BS Lond. 1991 (King's Coll. Sch. Med. & Dent.) DFFP 1996.

TAYLOR, Nigel William Gervase Bradgate Surgery, Ardenton Walk, Brentry, Bristol BS10 6SP Tel: 0117 959 1920 Fax: 0117 983 9332 — MB BS Lond. 1978 (Westm.) BA Camb. 1973; DRCOG 1981; MRCGP 1982.

TAYLOR, Nora Louise (retired) 6 London Road, Uppingham, Oakham LE15 9TJ — LRCP LRCS Ed. LRFPS Glas. 1951 (Ed.) DFFP 1993.

TAYLOR, Norman Henry Lancaster (retired) Northside, 15 Eastfield, Westbury-on-Trym, Bristol BS9 4BH Tel: 0117 962 2163 — (St. Geo.) MB BS Lond. 1959; DObst RCOG 1963. Prev: Ho. Surg. (Orthop.) St. Geo. Hosp. Lond.

TAYLOR, Norval Richard William (retired) 258 Staines Road, Twickenham TW2 5AR Tel: 020 8894 2342 — (Univ. Ed.) MB ChB Ed. 1947; MRCP Ed. 1956; MFPHM RCP (UK) 1974; FRCP Ed. 1997. Prev: Sen. Med. Off. Dept. Health & Social Security.

TAYLOR, Ormond Hargreaves (retired) 47 Crowtree Lane, Louth LN11 9LL Tel: 01507 603685; 47 Crowtree Lane, Louth LN11 9LL Tel: 01507 603685 — MB ChB St. And. 1947 (Dundee) DObst RCOG 1951. Prev: Ho. Surg. Vict. Hosp. Burnley & Hull Matern. Hosp.

TAYLOR, Mr Ormond Mark Kettering General Hosptial NHS Trust, Rothwell Road, Kettering NN16 8UZ — MB ChB Sheff. 1983; FRCS Ed. 1990; MD Sheff. 1995; FRCS (Gen.) 1996. Cons. Gen. Surg. Kettering Gen. Hosp. NHS Trust. Specialty: Gen. Surg. Prev: Sen. Regist. (Gen. Surg.) Yorks.; Research Fell. Univ. Dept. Surg. Leeds Gen. Infirm.

TAYLOR, Professor Pamela Jane Broadmoor Hospital, Crowthorne RG45 7EG Tel: 01344 754398 Fax: 01344 754385 — MB BS Lond. 1971; MRCS Eng. LRCP Lond. 1971; MRCP (UK) 1974; FRCPsych 1989, M 1976. Prof. of Forens. Psychiat.; Chairm. Roy. Coll. of Psychiat.s Working Gp. on Treatm. in Security. Specialty: Forens. Psychiat. Socs: Amer. Psychiat. Assn.; RSM. Prev: Prof. Special Hosp. Psychiat. Dept. Forens. Psychiat. Inst. Psychiat. Univ. Lond.; Hon. Cons. (Psychiat.) Bethlem & Maudsley Hosps. & Broadmoor Hosp.; Head of Med. Servs. Special Hosps. Serv. Auth. Lond.

TAYLOR, Patricia Anne Summerleaze House, Kilmington, Axminster EX13 7RA — MB BS Lond. 1986 (King's College Hospital London) DA (UK) 1989. SCMO (Anaesth.) Exeter Community Trust. Specialty: Anaesth. Prev: Regist. (Anaesth.) Yeovil Dist. Hosp.; SHO (Anaesth.) Roy. Devon & Exeter Hosp.; SHO (Neonat. Paediat.) Southmead & Bristol Matern. Hosps.

TAYLOR, Patrick Keith (retired) 35 Glebe Road, Long Ashton, Bristol BS41 9LJ — MRCS Eng. LRCP Lond. 1966; MRCOG 1971, DObst 1969; FRCOG 1989. Prev: Cons. (GU Med.) Bristol Roy. Infirm.

TAYLOR, Paul Alexander Colville 2 St Werburghs Road, Chorlton-cum-Hardy, Manchester M21 0TN Tel: 0161 881 6721; 11 Hilary Road, Taunton TA1 5BH Tel: 01823 333915 — MB ChB Manch. 1987; BSc (Hons.) Manch. 1985; DRCOG 1991; MRCGP 1992.

TAYLOR, Paul Anthony Hanham Surgery, 33 Whittucks Road, Hanham, Bristol BS15 3HY Tel: 0117 967 5201 Fax: 0117 947 7749; 17 Sunnyvale Drive, Longwell Green, Bristol BS30 9YH — MB BS Lond. 1987; DRCOG 1991; MRCGP 1991; DCH RCP Lond. 1992. GP Bristol.

TAYLOR, Paul Francis The Croft & Tinshill Medical Practice, 8 Tinshill Lane, Leeds LS16 7AP Tel: 0113 267 3462 Fax: 0113 230 0402; 4 Highfield Drive, Rawdon, Leeds LS19 6EY Tel: 0113 250 7664 — MB ChB Leeds 1969; DObst RCOG 1975.

TAYLOR, Paul Martin Department of Clinical Radiology, Manchester Royal Infirmary, Manchester M13 9WL; Bell in The Thorn, 111 Belthorn Road, Belthorn, Blackburn BB1 2NY — MB ChB Manch. 1977; MRCP (UK) 1981; FRCR 1985; FRCP 2000. Cons. Radiol. Centr. Manch. Healthcare Trust; Hon. Clin. Sen. Lect. Univ. Manch. Specialty: Radiol. Prev: Sen. Lect. (Diagn. Radiol.) Univ. Manch.

TAYLOR, Paul Richard Philip 5a Thornsett Road, Sheffield S7 1NA — MB ChB Sheff. 1992.

TAYLOR, Pauline Felicity (retired) 4 Vicarage Close, Vicarage Way, Ringmer, Lewes BN8 5LF Tel: 01273 813660 — MB ChB St.

And. 1950. Prev: Med. Off. I/c St. Luke's Hosp. Chabua, India & St. Luke's Hosp. Ummedpur India.

TAYLOR, Penelope Rose Anne Royal Victoria Infirmary, Newcastle upon Tyne NE1 4LP Tel: 0191 232 5131 Fax: 0191 230 0651; Buckeye Barn, 8 The Fold, Hessay, York YO26 8LF Tel: 01904 737223 Email: penny.taylor@doctors.org.uk — MB BS Newc. 1972. Assoc. Specialist (Haemat.) Roy. Vict. Infirm. Newc. u. Tyne. Specialty: Haematology. Prev: Regist. (Haemat.) Roy. Vict. Infirm. Newc.; Ho. Phys. & Profess. Ho. Surg. Roy. Vict. Infirm. Newc. u. Tyne.

TAYLOR, Peter Anthony Airlea, Crapstone, Yelverton, Plymouth — MB BS Lond. 1965 (Lond. Hosp.) MRCS Eng. LRCP Lond. 1964; FFA RCS Eng. 1968. Cons. (Anaesth.) Plymouth Gen. Hosp. Specialty: Anaesth. Socs: BMA & Assn. Anaesths. Prev: SHO (Anaesth.) St. Margt.'s Hosp. Epping; Regist. (Anaesth.) Char. Cross Hosp Lond.; Sen. Regist. (Anaesth.) St. Thos. Hosp. Lond.

TAYLOR, Peter Bruce (retired) 14 Dunearn Street, Broughty Ferry, Dundee DD5 3NP Tel: 01382 738978 Email: peter.taylor1@tinyworld.co.uk — MB ChB Aberd. 1967; FFA RCS Eng. 1975. Examr. to St. And.Ambul. Brig. Prev: Cons. Anaesth. Ninewells Hosp.

TAYLOR, Peter Charles Kennedy Institute of Rheumatology, Imperial College, 1 Aspenlea Road, Hammersmith, London W6 8RF — BM BCh Oxf. 1985; BA Camb. 1982; MA Camb. 1986; PhD Lond. 1996; FRCP 2000. Reader in Experim. Rheum.; Hon. Cons. Phys., Imperial Coll. Lond.; Hon. Cons. Phys., Char. Cross Hosp., Lond. Specialty: Rheumatol. Special Interest: Rheumatiod Arthritis. Prev: Lect. (Rheum.) Char. Cross Hosp. Lond.; Research Fell. (Arthritis & Rheum.) Kennedy Inst. Rheum. Lond.; Regist. & SHO Rotat. (Gen. Med.) N. Staffs. HA.

TAYLOR, Mr Peter Charles Andrew North West London Hospitals NHS Trust, Central Middlesex Hospital, Acton Lane, London NW10 7NS Tel: 020 8965 5733 Fax: 020 8453 2100 — MRCS Eng. LRCP Lond. 1975 (St Mary's) FRCSI (Otol.) 1984; FICS 1990. Cons. ENT Surg. N. W. Lond. NHS Trust; Hon.Cons. ENT Surg. Char. Cross Hosp. Lond. Specialty: Otolaryngol. Socs: Hunt. Soc.; RSM; BADS. Prev: Regist. (ENT Surg.) United Bristol Hosps. & Southmead Hosp.; SHO (ENT Surg.) St. Mary's Hosp. Lond.; Cas. Off. St. Mary's Hosp. Lond.

TAYLOR, Peter Christopher Department of Haematology, Rotherham District General, Rotherham S60 2UD Tel: 01709 820000 Fax: 01709 830694; Mootings, Sitwell Grove, Rotherham S60 3AY — MB ChB Sheff. 1977; MRCP (UK) 1982; MRCPath 1986. Cons. Haemat., Rotherham Dist. Gen. Hosp. Specialty: Haematology. Socs: Assn. Clin. Paths.; Brit. Soc. Haemat. Prev: Sen. Regist. (Haemat.) Roy. United Hosp. Bath; Regist. (Haemat.) Roy. Hallamsh. Hosp. Sheff.; Regist. (Med.) Rotherham Dist. Gen. Hosp.

TAYLOR, Mr Peter David The Sycamores, Longden, Shrewsbury SY5 8EX — MB ChB Glas. 1984; FRCS Ed. 1989; DRCOG 1996. GP. Specialty: Gen. Surg. Prev: Regist. (Gen. Surg.) Newc. HA.

TAYLOR, Peter John 5 Royal Chase, Dringhouses, York YO24 1LN — MB ChB Leeds 1987; DRCOG 1991; MRCGP 1992. Med. Adviser for Civil Serv. Leeds. Specialty: Civil Serv. Prev: SHO (O & G) Princess Roy. & Hull Matern. Hosps.; SHO (ENT Surg. & Infec. Dis.) Seacroft Hosp. Leeds; SHO (Med. for Elderly) St. Jas. Hosp. Leeds.

TAYLOR, Mr Peter John, Surg. Cdr. RN Dept. Vascular Surgery, Level 1, Peterborough District Hospital, Thorpe Road PE3 6DA Tel: 01733 878709 — MB BS Lond. 1987 (Lond. Hosp. Med. Coll.) DA (UK) 1990; FRCS Eng. 1992; DTMH, Liverpool. 1996; FRCS 2003. Cons. Gen. & Vasc. Surg., MDHU. P'boro.; Cons. Gen. Surg., Roy Navy, Full Time. Specialty: Gen. Surg. Socs: Affil. Mem., Vasc. Surg. Soc. Of Brit. And N. Ire.; Affil. Mem., Europ. Soc. Of Vasc. + EndoVasc. Surg.; Mem., Milit. Surgic. Soc. Prev: Regist. (Gen. Surg.) Raigmore Hosp. NHS Trust; Cons.Surg. Kisiizi Hosp. Uganda; Specialist Regist. (Gen. Surg), Roy. Utd Hosptial. Bath.

TAYLOR, Peter Leon 514 Scott Hall Road, Leeds LS7 3RA Tel: 0113 620780 — MB ChB Leeds 1953.

TAYLOR, Peter Neil The Dairy House, Stratton, Dorchester DT2 9RU — MB BS Lond. 1983; MRCP (UK) 1986; FRCR 1991. Cons. Radiol. W. Dorset Gen. Hosps. NHS Trust. Specialty: Radiol. Prev: Sen. Regist. (Radiol.) Leeds.

TAYLOR, Mr Peter Richard Guy's & St. Thomas' NHS Foundation Trust, Department of Surgery, Lambeth Palace Road, London SE1 7EH Tel: 020 7403 3893 Fax: 020 7403 2323 Email: taylorvasc@aol.com — MB BChir Camb. 1979; MA 1980; FRCS Eng. 1983; MChir Camb. 1990. Cons. (Vasc. Surg.) Guy's St. Thos. Hosp. Trust; Hon. Cons. Vasc. Surg. KCH; Hon. Cons. Vasc. Surg. Univ. Hosp. Lewisham. Specialty: Gen. Surg.; Surgery, Vascular. Special Interest: Carotoid Dis.; Endoluminal Treatm.; Thoracic & Abdom. Aortic Path. Socs: Vasc. Surg. Soc. & Europ. Vasc. Surg. Soc.; Assn. Surg.; Internat. Soc. for Cardiovasc. Surg. Prev: Sen. Lect. & Hon. Cons. Surg. (Vasc. Surg.) Guy's & Lewisham Hosps.; Sen. Regist. (Gen. Surg.) Guy's Hosp. Lond.; Sen. Fell. (Vasc.) St. Mary's Hosp. Lond.

TAYLOR, Philip James Ralph Axminster Medical Practice, St Thomas Court, Church Street, Axminster EX13 5AG Tel: 01297 32126 Fax: 01297 35759 — MB BS Lond. 1984; MA Oxf. 1981; MRCGP 1989; T(GP) 1991. Med. Audit Advis. Gp. Coordinator Exeter Dist.

TAYLOR, Philip James Steevens Denton Turret Medical Centre, 10 Kenley Road, Slatyford, Newcastle upon Tyne NE5 2UY Tel: 0191 274 1840; 14 Highlaws, South Gosforth, Newcastle upon Tyne NE3 1RQ Tel: 0191 284 7775 — MB BS Newc. 1984; DRCOG 1987; MRCGP 1988; Cert. Family Plann. JCC 1988.

TAYLOR, Philip John Hanscombe House Surgery, 52A St Andrew Street, Hertford SG14 1JA — MB BCh BAO Dub. 1971; FRCA 1980. Prev: Ho. Off. Meath Hosp. Dub.

TAYLOR, Mr Philip John The James Cook University Hospital, Marton Road, Middlesbrough TS4 3BW Tel: 01642 854891 Fax: 01642 282733 Email: philip.taylor@stees.nhs.uk; Spring House, Great Broughton, Stokesley, Middlesbrough TS9 7HX Tel: 01642 778389 — MB ChB Sheff. 1970; FRACGP 1979; MRACOG 1983; MRCOG 1985; FRCOG 2000. Cons O & G The James Cook Univ. Hosp. Specialty: Obst. & Gyn. Prev: Lect. (O & G) Univ. Aberd.; Regist. Roy. Infirm. Ed.; Regist. (O & G) Newc., Austral.

TAYLOR, Phillip West House, 30 Southlands Mount, Riddlesden, Keighley BD20 5HH — BM BCh Oxf. 1988; BA Oxf. 1986, BM BCh 1988. SHO (Anaesth.) Norf. & Norwich Hosp.

TAYLOR, Phillipa Anne London Lane Clinic, Kinnaird House, 37 London Lane, Bromley BR1 4HB Tel: 020 8460 2661 Fax: 020 8464 5041 — MRCGP; MB BCh Witwatersrand 1983.

TAYLOR, Phyllis 53 Gervis Road, Bournemouth BH1 3DQ Tel: 01202 555154 Fax: 01202 555154 — MB BS Lond. 1947 (Roy. Free) DCH Eng. 1949. Gen. Practitioner (Private).

TAYLOR, Rachel Ann Close Farm Surgery, 47 Victoria Road, North Common, Bristol BS30 5JZ — MB BCh Wales 1992 (Univ. Wales Coll. Med.) DRCOG 1994; DCH RCP Lond. 1995; DFFP 1995; MRCGP 1996; T(GP) 1996. GP N. Common Bristol. Prev: SHO Gwent HA.

TAYLOR, Rachel Sarah 31 Thirlmere Road, Hinckley LE10 0PE; 111 Mayola Road, Clapton, London E5 0RG — MB BS Lond. 1994. Specialty: Gen. Med.

TAYLOR, Rachel Sophie 43 Newport Road, Edgmond, Newport TF10 8HQ Tel: 01952 812511 — MB ChB Sheff. 1993 (Sheffield) DFFP. 1997; MRCGP. 1997. Specialty: Gen. Pract.; Family Plann. & Reproduc. Health. Prev: GP. Worcester.

TAYLOR, Ralph Lionel 86 Rennets Wood Road, Eltham, London SE9 2NH Tel: 020 8850 0990 — MB ChB Sheff. 1960; DObst. RCOG 1962; DMRD Eng. 1971; FFR 1973; FRCR 1975. Cons. Radiologist, Blackheath Hosp., Lond. SE3 9UD; Hon. Cons. Radiol. Qu. Eliz. Hosp. (NHS Trust) Lond. SE18 4QH. Specialty: Radiol. Prev: Sen. Regist. (Radiol.) St. Bart. Hosp. Lond.; Regist. (Radiol.) Lond. Hosp.; Asst. Cas. Off. & ENT Ho. Surg. Roy. Infirm. Sheff.

TAYLOR, Reginald David (retired) — MB BCh Dublin 1958 (Dub.) DDbsb RCOG 1967. Prev: GP E.leigh, Hants.

TAYLOR, Richard 2 Haigh Head, Hoylandswaine, Sheffield S30 6JJ Tel: 01226 765827; Walderslade, Elsecar, Barnsley S74 9LJ Tel: 01226 743221 — MB ChB Liverp. 1975; MRCGP 1981. Clin. Asst. (Genito-Urin. Med.) Barnsley Dist. Gen. Hosp. Prev: Trainee Gen. Pract. Barnsley Vocational Train. Scheme; SHO (Endocrine Path.) Jessop Hosp. Wom. Sheff.; SHO (O & G) St. Catherine's Hosp. Birkenhead.

TAYLOR, Richard Andrew Stephen The Surgery, High Street, Fenny Compton, Leamington Spa CV47 2YG Tel: 01295 770855 Fax: 01295 770858; 1 Brook Street, Fenny Compton, Leamington Spa CV47 2YH — BM BCh Oxf. 1981; MA Camb. 1982; DRCOG 1984; DCH RCP Lond. 1985; MRCGP 1985.

TAYLOR, Richard Charles Henry The Surgery, Sandy Lane, Brewood, Stafford ST19 9ES Tel: 01902 850206 Fax: 01902 851360; Westgate, Dean Street, Brewood, Stafford ST19 9BU Tel: 01902 850594 — MB BS Lond. 1968 (Guy's) MRCS Eng. LRCP Lond. 1968; DObst RCOG 1973. Prev: Ho. Surg. Guy's Hosp.; Ho. Phys. St. Olave's Hosp. Lond.; SHO Harari Gen. Hosp. Salisbury, Rhodesia.

TAYLOR, Richard Geoffrey Taylor and Partners, Shirehampton Health Centre, Pembroke Road, Shirehampton, Bristol BS11 9SB Tel: 0117 916 2226 Fax: 0117 916 2206 Email: richard.taylor@gp-L81008.nhs.uk; 5 Cotham Grove, Cotham, Bristol BS6 6AL — MB ChB Birm. 1976; DRCOG 1979; MRCGP 1981; D.Occ.Med. RCP Lond. 1995; AFOM 1999. GP Bristol; Occupat. Phys. SITA Contract Serv. Specialty: Occupat. Health.

TAYLOR, Richard John Alexander 17 Hallfield, Ulverston LA12 9TA Tel: 01229 587611 — BSc (Hons.) Newc. 1969, MB BS 1972; DObst RCOG 1974; DCH RCPS Glas. 1975; MRCGP 1976. Socs: Hon. Treas. Local BMA Div.. Prev: GP Chelmsford Essex; Trainee GP E. Cumbria VTS.

TAYLOR, Richard Matthew 703 Shadwell Lane, Leeds LS17 8ET — BM BCh Oxf. 1989; BA (Hons.) Oxf. 1986, BM BCh 1989.

TAYLOR, Richard Thomas (retired) 11 Church Walk, Kidderminster DY11 6XY Tel: 01562 60010 Fax: 01562 748371 — (Westm.) MB Camb. 1960, BChir 1959; FRCP Lond. 1979, M 1965. Prev: Cons. Phys. Kidderminster Gen. Hosp.

TAYLOR, Richard Waring (retired) White House Farm, Main Street, Keyham, Leicester LE7 9JQ Tel: 0116 259 5415 — MB BChir Camb. 1964 (Westm.) DObst RCOG 1965; MRCGP 1973. Prev: GP Leicester.

TAYLOR, Richard Winston Martin 107 Weavers Way, London NW1 0XG — MB BS Lond. 1990 (Univ. Coll. Lond.) BSc (Hons.) Lond. 1987; MRCPsych 1996. Regist. (Psychiat.) Maudsley Hosp. Lond. Specialty: Forens. Psychiat.

TAYLOR, Robert Bryce 11 Eccleston Gardens, St Helens WA10 3BN — MRCS Eng. LRCP Lond. 1937 (Lond. Hosp.) DPM Eng. 1948; MRCPsych 1972.

TAYLOR, Robert Capel (retired) Westerton, Balloch, Alexandria G83 8NA Tel: 01389 753064 — (Glas.) MB ChB Glas. 1952; DA Eng. 1956. Prev: Cons. Anaesth. Vict. Infirm. Glas.

TAYLOR, Robert Henry Paediatric Intensive Care Unit, Royal Belfast Hospital for Sick Children, 180 Falls Road, Belfast BT12 6BE Tel: 01232 263056; 57 Ballyhanwood Road, Belfast BT5 7SW Tel: 01232 487303 — MB BCh BAO Belf. 1982; FFA RCS Dub. 1986; MA (Med. Ethics and Law) Belf. 1997. Cons. Paediat. Anaesth. & Paediat. Intens. Care Roy. Belf. Hosp. for Sick Childr. Specialty: Anaesth. Prev: Clin. Fell. (Paediat. Anaesth.) Hosp. for sick Child. Toronto.

TAYLOR, Mr Robert Horace Eye Department, York District Hospital, Wigginton Road, York YO31 8HE Tel: 01904 725612 Fax: 01904 726343 Email: rtaylor@yorkeyes.demon.co.uk — MB BS Lond. 1985 (Guy's) MRCS Eng. LRCP Lond. 1984; DO RCS Eng. 1989; FRCS Glas. 1990; FRCOphth 1993. Cons. Ophth. York Dist. Hosp. Specialty: Ophth. Socs: Int. Mem. Amer. Assoc. Paediat. Ophthl. & Strabismus Surg.s; UK & Irel. Soc. Cataract & Refractive Surg.s; Oxf. Ophth. Congr. Prev: Fell. Paediat. Ophth. Toronto Canada; Sen. Regist. Roy. Hallamsh. Hosp. Sheff.; Regist. (Ophth.) Birm. & Midl. Eye Hosp.

TAYLOR, Mr Robert Stewart Ashtead Hospital, The Warren, Ashtead KT21 2SB Tel: 01372 276874 Fax: 01372 276874; 10 Catherine Court, Lake Road, Wimbledon, London SW19 7EW — MS Lond. 1973, MB BS 1957; MRCS Eng. LRCP Lond. 1957; FRCS Eng. 1962; FRCS Ed. 1962. Cons. Vasc. Surg. & Hon. Sen. Lect. St. Geo. Hosp. Lond.; Hon. Cons. Surg., Epsom.; Gen. Hosp., Epsom, Surrey. Specialty: Vasc. Med. Socs: Fell. Assn. Surgs.; Internat. Cardiovasc. Soc. & Vasc. Surg. Soc. GB & Irel.; GP & Ire. Vasc. Surg. Soc. - Counc. Mem. Prev: Sen. Regist. (Surg.) Lond. Hosp.; Cons. Gen. & Vasc. Surg. Epsom Gen.; Cons. Gen. & Vasc. Surg. St Geo.'s.

TAYLOR, Roderick Gordon Calderdale Royal Hospital, Halifax HX3 0PW — MB BS Lond. 1975 (Roy. Free) MRCP (UK) 1978; BSc (1st cl. Hons.) Lond. 1972, MD 1986; FRCP Lond. 1994. Cons. (Gen. & Respirat. Med.) Calderdale & Huddersfield NHS Trust. Specialty: Respirat. Med. Socs: Brit. Thorac. Soc. Prev: Lect. (Thoracic Med. & Physiol.) Roy. Free Hosp. Sch. Med. Lond.; Research Regist. (Respirat. Unit) Roy. Postgrad. Med. Sch.; SHO (Thoracic Med.) Brompton Hosp.

TAYLOR, Professor Rodney Hemingfield Ealing Hospital NHS Trust, Uxbridge Road, Southall UB1 3HW Tel: 020 8967 5375 Fax: 020 8967 5771 Email: Rodney.Taylor@eht.nhs.uk — MB BS Lond. 1972 (Univ. Coll. Hosp.) BSc Bristol 1965; MRCS Eng. LRCP Lond. 1972; MRCP (UK) 1976; MD Lond. 1984; FRCP Lond. 1987; DHMSA 1992; DPhilMed 1994; MBA OUBS 1996; FRIPH 2001. Med. Dir. & Cons. Phys. & Gastroenterol. Ealing Hosp.; Pres., Fac. Hist. Phil. Med, Soc. Apoth. Lond.; Examr. Hist. Med. Soc. Apoth. Lond. Specialty: Gastroenterol. Socs: Med. Res. Soc.; Brit. Soc. Gastroenterol.; Fell. Med. Soc. Lond. Prev: Wellcome Sen. Research Fell. Clin. Sc. & Sen. Lect. (Gastroenterol.) Centr. Middlx. Hosp. & Middlx. Hosp. Med. Sch. Lond.; RCP/RN Prof. Med & Assoc. Postgrad. Dean RDMC; Research Assoc. Univ. Laborat. Physiol. Oxf.

TAYLOR, Roger Edward Cookridge Hospital, Leeds LS16 6QB Tel: 0113 267 3411; 26 Firs Drive, Harrogate HG2 9HB Tel: 01423 815360 — MB BS Lond. 1976 (St. Bart.) MA Oxf. 1973; MRCP (UK) 1979; FRCR 1984; FRCP Ed. 1992; FRCP 1998. Cons. Clin. Oncol. Cookridge Hosp. Leeds. Specialty: Oncol. Socs: UK Childr. Cancer Study Gp. & Internat. Soc. Paediat. Oncol. Prev: Sen. Lect. & Hon. Cons. Radiat. Oncol. Univ. Edin. & West. Gen. Hosp. Edin.; I.C.R.F. Research Fell. & Hon. Sen. Regist. (Clin. Oncol.) W., Gen. Hosp. Edin.; Regist. (Radiother. & Oncol.) Lond. Hosp. Whitechapel.

TAYLOR, Roger George (retired) Fairways, Dudley Avenue, Westgate-on-Sea CT8 8PT Tel: 01843 831675 Email: rogertaylor999@aol.com — MB BS Lond. 1958; DObst RCOG 1959.

TAYLOR, Rosalind Ann Hospice of St Francis, 27 Shrublands Road, Berkhamsted HP4 3HX Tel: 01442 862960 Fax: 01442 877685; Low House, 33 High St, Ivinghoe, Leighton Buzzard LU7 9EP Tel: 01296 668266 Fax: 01296 668266 — MB BChir Camb. 1980 (Westm.) MA Camb. 1981; DRCOG 1984; MRCGP 1986. Med. Dir. Hospice of St. Frances, Berkhamsted. Specialty: Palliat. Med. Prev: Asst. Phys. (Palliat. Med.) W. Cumbld. Hosp.; GP Cockermouth.; GP St. Neots Cambs.

TAYLOR, Ross Jenkins University of Aberdeen, Dept. U General Practice, Foresterhill Health Centre, Westburn Road, Aberdeen AB25 2AY Tel: 01224 553972; Westburn Medical Group, Foresterhill Health Centre, Westburn Road, Aberdeen AB25 2AY Tel: 01224 559595 — MB ChB Aberd. 1966 (Aberdeen 1966) DCH Lond. 1970; FRCGP 1982, M 1972; MD Aberd. 1981; FRCP Edin 2001. Sen. Lect. (Gen. Pract.) Univ. Aberd. Specialty: Gen. Pract. Socs: Assn. Study Med. Educat. & Nutrit Soc.

TAYLOR, Rowena Frances Halstead The Chest Clinic, Whipps Cross Hospital, Whipps Cross Road, London E11 1NR Tel: 020 8539 5522 — MB BS Lond. 1981; FRCP (UK) 1984; MD Lond. 1996. Cons. Phys. (Thoracic & Gen. Med.) Whipps Cross Hosp. Lond. Specialty: Respirat. Med. Prev: Sen. Regist. Whipps Cross Hosp. Lond.; Clin. Tutor & Research Regist. (Cystic Fibrosis) Roy. Brompton Hosp. Lond.; Regist. (Med.) Lond. Chest Hosp. & Whittington Hosp.

TAYLOR, Professor Roy University of Newcastle upon Tyne, Medical School, Department of Medicine, Framlington Place, Newcastle upon Tyne NE2 4HH Tel: 0191 232 5131 Fax: 0191 222 0723; 40 Reid Park Road, Jesmond, Newcastle upon Tyne NE2 2ES — MB ChB Ed. 1976; BSc (Hons. Bacteriol.) Ed. 1973; MD Ed. 1985; FRCP Lond. 1989; FRCP Ed. 1991. Prof. Med. & Metab. & Hon. Cons. Phys. Roy. Vict. Infirm. Newc. Specialty: Diabetes. Socs: Soc. Magnetic Resonance; Brit. Diabetic Assn.; Assn. Phys. Prev: 1st Asst. (Med.) Freeman Hosp. Newc.; Vis. Prof. Med. Yale Univ. 1990-91; Regist. (Med.) Newc. AHA.

TAYLOR, Roy Charles (retired) Hill House, Cheney Hill, Rodmersham, Sittingbourne ME9 0AH — MB BS Lond. 1954 (St. Bart.) MRCS Eng. LRCP Lond. 1954; DObst RCOG 1956. Prev: O & G Ho. Surg. Lewisham Hosp.

TAYLOR, Russell John (retired) 17 Outwoods Road, Loughborough LE11 3LX Tel: 01509 267456 Email: russell.j.taylor@cwcom.net — (Leeds) MB ChB Leeds 1957. Prev: GP Princip., Bridge St. Med. Pract. LoughBoro.

TAYLOR, Ruth Diana 21 Cunningham Hill Road, St Albans AL1 5BX — MB BS Lond. 1992.

TAYLOR, Ruth Elizabeth Dept. of Psychiatry, Institute of Psychiatry, De Crepigny Park, London SE5 8AF Tel: 020 7848 0757 Fax: 020 7848 0757 — MB ChB Manch. 1985; BSc (1st. cl. Hons.)

Psych. Manch. 1985; MB ChB Manch. 1988; MRCPsych 1993. Res. Fell. Inst. Of Psych.; Hon. Clin. Asst. (Neuropsychiat.) Nat. Hosp. Neurol. & Neurosurg. Qu. Sq. Lond. Specialty: Gen. Psychiat. Prev: Regist. (Psychiat.) Manch. Roy. Infirm.; SHO (A & E Med.) St. Bart. Hosp. Lond.; Ho. Off. (Gen. Med.) Salford Roy. & Hosp. Hosps. Salford.

TAYLOR, Ruth Louise Arden Cottage, King Street, Silverton, Exeter EX5 4JG — MB BS Lond. 1996.

TAYLOR, Sally Margaret — MB ChB Manch. 1982; DRCOG 1986; Cert Family Planning JCC 1987; MRCGP 1989. Specialty: Gen. Pract. Special Interest: Gen. Pract. Educat. Prev: GP Princip. Paddington Green Health Centre Lond. Aug. 1990-July 2003; GP Trainer 1993-2003; Trainee GP Kentish Town Health Centre Lond. VTS.

TAYLOR, Samuel Geoffrey (retired) 23 Rusham Park Avenue, Egham TW20 9LZ Tel: 01784 432448 — MB BChir Camb. 1957 (Camb. & St. Mary's) MRCS Eng. LRCP Lond. 1956; BA Camb. 1957; DObst RCOG 1958. Prev: Ho. Surg. (Obst.) King Edwd. VII Hosp. Windsor.

TAYLOR, Sandra Jane Theatre Royal Surgery, 27 Theatre Street, Dereham NR19 2EN Tel: 01362 852800 Fax: 01362 852819; Sunset View, Fakenham Road, Horningtoft, Dereham NR20 5DP — MB ChB Ed. 1979 (Edinburgh) DCH Lond. 1982; MRCGP 1983. GP; Clin. Asst. GU Med. Norf. & Norwich Hosp. Specialty: Gen. Pract.; Genitourinary Medicine.

TAYLOR, Sandra Jean Mawbey Brough Health Centre, 39 Wilcox Close, London SW8 2UD Tel: 020 7622 3827 Fax: 020 7498 1069 — MB ChB Bristol 1989; T(GP) 1994; DFFP 1994; (Dist.) MRCCeP 1999. GP. Specialty: Gen. Pract. Prev: Dist. Med. Off. Luapula Province, Zambia.

TAYLOR, Sara Dillwyn 68 Hammersmith Grove, London W6 7HA — LRCPI & LM, LRSCI & LM 1976; LRCPI & LM, LRCSI & LM 1976.

TAYLOR, Sarah Anissa 27 Crosbie Road, Birmingham B17 9BG — MB ChB Liverp. 1998.

TAYLOR, Sarah Catryn 14 High Laws, Newcastle upon Tyne NE3 1RQ — MB BS Newc. 1984.

TAYLOR, Sarah Jane X Ray Department, The Great Western Hospital, Marlborough Road, Swindon SN3 6BB Tel: 01793 604020 — MB BS Lond. 1981 (St. Bart.) BSc Lond. 1978; FRCR 1987. Cons. Radiol. The Great Western Hospital Swindon. Specialty: Radiol. Prev: Clin. Fell. (Radiol.) McMaster Univ. Hamilton Ontario, Canada; Sen. Regist. (Radiol.) Stoke City Gen. Hosp. & N. Staffs. Infirm.; Regist. Birm. Hosps.

TAYLOR, Sarah Jane 17 Whitfield Park, Ringwood BH24 2DX — MB BS Lond. 1990; MRCGP 1994; Dip. Occ. Med. Lond. 1998. Specialist Regist., Occupat. Med. Soton. Univ. Hosp. NHS Trust. Specialty: Occupat. Health. Socs: SOM.

TAYLOR, Sarah Jane Chesterfield Drive Surgery, Ipswich IP1 6DW — MB ChB Dundee 1996.

TAYLOR, Sarah Katherine St Georges Medical Centre, Field Rd, Wallasey CH45 5LN Tel: 0151 630 2080; 55 Brimstage Road, Heswall, Wirral CH60 1XE Tel: 0151 342 3599 — MB BS Lond. 1992 (St Georges Hospital, London) DRCOG 1998.

TAYLOR, Sarah Lucy 18 Kings Drive, Heaton Moor, Stockport SK4 4DZ — MB ChB Birm. 1991 (Birmingham) DCH RCP Lond. 1994; MRCGP 1995; DFFP 1995. GP Princip. Specialty: Gen. Pract.

TAYLOR, Mr Scott Garry Flat 31, 22 Cleveland St, Glasgow G3 7AE — MB ChB Glas. 1993; FRCS RCPS (Glas.) 1997. Research Fell. Univ. Dept. of Surg. Western Infirm. Glas. Specialty: Gen. Surg. Prev: SHO Rotat. (Surg.) Monkland Dist. Gen. Hosp. Airdrie.

TAYLOR, Sharon Elisa — MB BS Lond. 1992; MRCPsych; MRCP; BSc. SpR (Child Psychiat.) St. Mary's Hosp. Lond.; Hon. Lect. (Child & Adolesc. Psychiat.) Imperial Coll./St. Mary's Higher Train. Scheme St. Mary's Hosp.

TAYLOR, Sian Margaret 33 Russet Gardens, Emsworth PO10 8DG — MB ChB Bristol 1990. GP Non Princip. Specialty: Gen. Psychiat. Prev: SHO (Psychiat.) St. Jas. Hosp. Portsmouth.

TAYLOR, Simon Christopher PO Box 140, Richmond Delivery Offices, Richmond Tel: 01748 833441 — MB BCh Wales 1997 (University of Wales) DMCC (Soc. Of Apothacaries, Lond.) 2000. GP. Brit. Army; SHO Orthop. Socs: Haywood Club; BASICS; BAEM. Prev: SHO Orthop., Frimley Pk. Hosp.; SHO A&E, Lewisham Hosp.

TAYLOR, Simon Wheldon 1 Pump Court, Temple, London EC4Y 7AA Tel: 020 7827 4000 Fax: 020 7827 4100; September Cottage, Monks Lane, Wadhurst TN5 6EN — MB BChir Camb. 1987; MA Camb. 1987. Barrister-at-Law. Socs: BMA; Liveryman Worshipful Soc. Apoth. Prev: Ho. Off. Lond. Hosp.

TAYLOR, Stephanie Jane Caroline Dept of General Practice and Primary Care, St Barts Royal London School of Med. & Dentistry, University of London, London E1 4NS; 15 Courtnell Street, London W2 5BU — MB BS Lond. 1984 (Roy. Free) DCH RCP Lond. 1986; DRCOG 1989; MRCGP 1989; MSc Lond. Sch. Hyg. & Trop. Med. Lond. 1993; MFPHM RCP (UK) 1996; MD Lond. 2002. Sen. Clin. Lect. in Health Serv.s Research & Developm., St Barts.; Hon. Cons. Pub. Health Med. Barking Havering and Redbridge NHS Trust, Essex. Specialty: Pub. Health Med.; Gen. Pract.

TAYLOR, Stephen 37 Villiers Street, Leamington Spa CV32 5YH Tel: 01926 833188 Fax: 01926 833265 — MB ChB Leic. 1992 (Leicester) DTM & H RCP Lond. 1994; MRCP (UK) 1996. Specialist Regist. (Genitourin. Med.) Birm. Heartlands Hosp. Specialty: Genitourinary Medicine. Socs: BMA, MSSVD & BHIVA. Prev: SHO (Infec. Dis. & Trop. Med.) Birm. Heartlands Hosp.; SHO (Infec. Dis. & Trop. Med.) Birm. Heartlands Hosp.

TAYLOR, Stephen Anselm Willis (retired) 25 Boscobel Road, Walsall WS1 2PL Tel: 01922 628366 Fax: 01922 627 607 Email: dsawtaylor@aol.com — MB BS Lond. 1957.

TAYLOR, Stephen Charles (retired) 11 Ironbridge Path, Fordham, Ely CB7 5LJ — MB Camb. 1971; BChir 1970; DObst RCOG 1974. Prev: Ho. Surg. King's Coll. Hosp. Lond.

TAYLOR, Stephen Gordon The Long House, 73 East Trinity Road, Edinburgh EH5 3EL Tel: 0131 552 4919; 16 West Ferryfield, Edinburgh EH5 2PU Tel: 0131 551 2620 — MB ChB Ed. 1984 (Edinburgh) DRCOG 1986; DCH RCP Glas. 1987; MRCGP 1989.

TAYLOR, Stephen James 3 Mosswook Park, Manchester M20 5QW — MB ChB Manch. 1989 (Manchester) Socs: MRCGP.

TAYLOR, Mr Stuart Alexander Netley House, Gravel Hill, Wombourne, Wolverhampton WV5 9HA Tel: 01902 892135 — (King's Coll. Hosp.) MRCS Eng. LRCP Lond. 1966; MS Lond. 1980, MB BS 1968; FRCS Eng. 1972. Cons. Surg. The Roy. Wolverhampton Hosps. NHS Trust. Specialty: Gen. Surg. Prev: Sen. Surg. Regist. King's Coll. Hosp. Lond.; Ho. Surg. & Ho. Phys. Kings Coll. Hosp. Lond.

TAYLOR, Stuart Andrew 8 Chapel Drive, Balsall Common, Coventry CV7 7EQ — MB BS Lond. 1994.

TAYLOR, Susan Aline Park Surgery, Aline Park, Lochaline, Morvern, Oban PA34 5XT Tel: 01967 421252 Fax: 01967 421303 — MB ChB Glas. 1985.

TAYLOR, Susan Glenfield Hospital, Groby Road, Leicester LE3 9QP Tel: 0116 287 1471; 9 Swithland Court, Brand Hill, Woodhouse Eaves, Loughborough LE12 8SS Tel: 01509 890971 — MB BS Lond. 1971 (Roy. Free) MRCS Eng. LRCP Lond. 1971; DA Eng. 1974; FFA RCS Eng. 1980. Cons. Anaesth. Glenfield Hosp. Leicester. Specialty: Anaesth. Prev: Sen. Regist. (Anaesth.) Leicester AHA; Regist. (Anaesth.) Roy. Nat. Throat, Nose & Ear Hosp. Lond.; Regist. (Anaesth.) Roy. Free Hosp. Lond.

TAYLOR, Susan Barrie George Street Surgery, 99 George Street, Dumfries DG1 1DS Tel: 01387 253333 Fax: 01387 253301 — MB ChB Aberd. 1976; DRCOG 1978; MRCGP 1980.

TAYLOR, Susan Diane Holly Tree House, 278 Church Road, Frampton Cotterell, Bristol BS36 2BH — MB ChB Sheff. 1971; FFA RCS Eng. 1976. Specialty: Anaesth.

TAYLOR, Susan Doris Dickson (retired) 86 Heathcote Grove, Chingford, London E4 6SF Tel: 020 8529 2527 — (Qu. Univ. Belf.) MB BCh BAO Belf. 1941. Prev: Med. Off. Cytol. Clinics Redbridge & Waltham Forest AHA. Late Med.

TAYLOR, Susan Elizabeth 9 Turf Lane, Cullingworth, Bradford BD13 5EJ — BM Soton. 1989. SHO (O & G) Roy. United Hosp. Bath. Specialty: Obst. & Gyn. Prev: Regist. (Psychiat.) Roy. S. Hants. Hosp. Soton.

TAYLOR, Susan Jane Rotherfield Surgery, Rotherfield, Crowborough TN6 3QW Tel: 01892 852415/853288 Fax: 01892 853499; Brook Health Centre, Crowborough Hill, Crowborough TN6 2ED Tel: 01892 652850 — MB BS Lond. 1980; DRCOG 1983; Dip. Pract. Dermat. Wales 1994. Specialty: Gen. Med. Prev: Clin. Asst. (Dermat.) Kent & Sussex Hosp. Tunbridge Wells; GP Sittingbourne; Trainee GP Crawley VTS.

TAYLOR, Susan Mary Rudrashetty and Partners, Mary Potter Health Centre, Gregory Boulevard, Hyson Green, Nottingham

NG7 5HY — BM BS Nottm. 1987; DCH RCP Lond. 1990; MRCGP 1991; DRCOG 1991. Trainee GP/SHO Nottm. HA & Qu. Med. Centre Nottm.

TAYLOR, Terence Anthony Health Centre, Pier Road, Tywyn LL36 0AT Tel: 01654 710238 Fax: 01654 712143 — MB BCh BAO NUI 1985; MRCGP 1989. GP Tywyn.

TAYLOR, Thomas Cochrane, KStJ (retired) 19 Redcar Road, Marske-by-the-Sea, Redcar TS11 6BS Tel: 01642 485138 — MB BS Durh. 1945; DLO Eng. 1952. Chair. BMA S. Tees Div.

TAYLOR, Thomas Gilchrist 39 Midmills Road, Inverness IV2 3NZ — MB ChB Aberd. 1965; MRCPath 1974.

TAYLOR, Thomas Henry (retired) 60 Wood Vale, London N10 3DN Tel: 020 8883 6146 Email: ttcl00431@blueyonder.co.uk — (Lond. Hosp.) MB BS Lond. 1954; FFA RCS Eng. 1960; FRCA 1992. Prev: Cons. Anaesth. Roy. Lond. Trust.

TAYLOR, Thomas Lauder Outram Wellington Health Centre, Chapel Lane, Wellington, Telford TF1 1PZ Tel: 01952 226000 — MB ChB Ed. 1968; MRCOG 1977; Cert JCC Lond. 1979. Prev: Regist. (O & G) Wythenshawe Hosp. Manch.; Ho. Phys. & Ho. Surg. Roy. Infirm. Edin.; Surg. Lt. RN (Gen. Serv. Medal).

TAYLOR, Thomas William Department of Clinical Radiology, Ninewells Hospital, Dundee DD1 9SY Tel: 01382 660111 — MB ChB Ed. 1984; BSc (Hons.) Ed. 1982; DMRD Ed. 1990; FRCR 1991. Cons. Radiol. Tayside Univ. Hosps. NHS Trust. Specialty: Radiol. Prev: Sen. Regist. (Radiol.) Roy. Infirm. & West. Gen. Hosp. Edin.

TAYLOR, Timothy Chadwick (retired) The Spinney, Brooklands, Hammerwood, East Grinstead RH19 3QA Tel: 01342 322494 — MB BChir Camb. 1960 (Westm.) MA, MB Camb. 1960, BChir 1959; DObst RCOG 1964. Prev: GP Lingfield, Surrey.

TAYLOR, Timothy Mackford St Richards Hospital, Spitalfield Lane, Chichester PO19 6SE Tel: 01243 788122; Three Anchor Bay, 2 Downview Road, Barnham, Bognor Regis PO22 0EE — MB BS Lond. 1984; BSc Lond. 1981, MB BS 1984; MRCP (UK) 1989. Cons. Paediat. St. Richards Hosp. Chichester. Specialty: Paediat. Prev: Sen. Regist. St. Geo. Hosp. Lond.

TAYLOR, Timothy Michael Winn Taunton Road Medical Centre, 12-16 Taunton Road, Bridgwater TA6 3LS Tel: 01278 444400 Fax: 01278 423691 — MB Camb. 1987; BChir 1986; MA Oxf. 1988. Specialty: Gen. Med.

TAYLOR, Tom Horsfield (retired) 211 Brodie Avenue, Liverpool L19 7NB Tel: 0151 427 1494 — MRCS Eng. LRCP Lond. 1926 (Leeds) MRCS Eng., LRCP Lond. 1926. Prev: Hon. Surg. Out-pats. Beckett Hosp. Barnsley.

TAYLOR, Mr Trevor Childs Royal Belfast Hospital for Sick Children, Falls Road, Belfast BT12 6BE Tel: 028 9063 2835 Email: trevor.taylor@royalhospitals.n-i.nhs.uk; 27 Hawthornden Road, Belfast BT4 3JU Tel: 028 9065 6302 Fax: 028 9065 1825 Email: tctaylor@dnet.co.uk — MB BCh BAO Belf. 1968; FRCS Ed. 1972; FRCS Eng. 1995. Cons. Orthop. Surg. Roy. Hosps. Trust Belf. Specialty: Orthop. Socs: Fell. BOA; Ulster Med. Soc. Prev: Tutor (Surg.) Qu. Univ. Belf.; Clin. Orthop. Study Fell. Hosp. Sick Childr. Toronto, Canada; Cons. Bloorview Childr. Hosp. Willowdale, Canada.

TAYLOR, Valerie Eileen 27 Orchard Street, Aberdeen AB24 3DA — MB ChB Aberd. 1995; BSc Med. Sci. (Hons.) Aberd. 1993; FRCA 2003. Specialist Regist. Aberd. Roy. Hosps. NHS Trust. Specialty: Anaesth.

TAYLOR, Valerie Margaret 24 West Drive, Harrow Weald, Harrow HA3 6TS — MB ChB Glas. 1978; FFA RCS Eng. 1982. Cons. Anaesth. Roy. Nat. Orthop. Hosp. Stanmore. Specialty: Anaesth.

TAYLOR, Vernon Rostron The Surgery, 74A Worcester Road, Hagley, Stourbridge DY9 0NH Tel: 01562 882474; Windover Cottage, Field Lane, Clent, Stourbridge DY9 0JA Tel: 01562 884529 — MB ChB Liverp. 1958.

TAYLOR, Victor Norman (retired) 86 Heathcote Grove, Chingford, London E4 6SF — (Qu. Univ. Belf.) MB BCh BAO Belf. 1941. Prev: Orthop. Ho. Surg. & Cas. Off. Kent & Sussex Hosp.

TAYLOR, Vivien Mary 31 Wimbolt Street, London E2 7BX — BM Soton. 1977; DRCOG 1980; MRCGP 1982; MSc Lond. 1989.

TAYLOR, Walter Noel Alexander (retired) 6 London Road, Uppingham, Oakham LE15 9TJ Tel: 01572 822802 — (St. Bart.) MB BS Lond. 1951; MRCS Eng. LRCP Lond. 1951; DObst RCOG 1959. Prev: Surg. Lt. RN.

TAYLOR, Walter Robert John 26 Pitchford Road, Heath Farm, Shrewsbury SY1 3HS — MB BS Lond. 1981; MRCP (UK) 1988.

TAYLOR, Wendy Barbara Newcastle General Hospital, NCCT, Westgate Road, Newcastle upon Tyne NE4 6BE Tel: 0191 256 3579; 12 Boundary Gardens, High Heaton, Newcastle upon Tyne NE7 7AA — MB BS Newc. 1979; MRCP (UK) 1982; BMedSc Newc. 1976, MD 1987; FRCR 1990. Cons. Clin. Oncol. Newc. Gen. Hosp. Specialty: Oncol.; Radiother. Socs: Brit. Gyn. Cancer Soc. Prev: Sen. Regist. & Regist. (Radiother. & Oncol.) Newc. Gen. Hosp.; Research Regist. (Clin. Pharmacol.) Univ. Newc.

TAYLOR, Wendy Jane Taybank Medical Centre, 10 Robertson Street, Dundee DD4 6EL Tel: 01382 461588 Fax: 01382 452121; Windrush Cottage, 13 Bonfield Road, Strathkinners KY16 0DA Tel: 01334 850710 — MB ChB Dundee 1989; MRCGP 1995.

TAYLOR, Wendy Jane 17 Lawford Road, London W4 3HS — MB ChB Bristol 1981; MRCP (UK) 1984; MSc Lond. 1988; FRCR 1989. Sen. Regist. Neuroradiol. Hosp. Sick Childr. & Nat. Hosp. Neurol. & Neurosurg. Specialty: Radiol. Prev: Sen. Regist. (Radiol.) Roy. Free Hosp. Lond.

TAYLOR, William Flat 10, 48 Handsworth Wood Road, Birmingham B20 2DT — MB ChB Birm. 1964; BSc (Physiol.) Birm. 1961, MB ChB 1964; MRCP Lond. 1969.

TAYLOR, William 2 Hollytree Road, Liverpool L25 5PA — MB ChB Liverp. 1969; DObst RCOG 1971; MRCPath 1978. Cons. Histopath. & Gastrointest. Endoscopist Univ. Hosp. Aintree, Liverp. Specialty: Histopath.

TAYLOR, William (retired) 5 Priory Gardens, St Andrews KY16 8XX Tel: 01334 478522 — MB ChB Glas. 1951; DObst RCOG 1960; MRCGP 1974. Med. Ref. Dundee Benefits Agency. Prev: GP Ardrie.

TAYLOR, Mr William Arthur Stewart — MB ChB Glas. 1984; FRCS Glas. 1988. Cons. Neurosurg., Southern Gneral Hopitsl, Glas. Specialty: Neurosurg. Prev: Regist. Rotat. (Surg.) W. of Scot.; Sen. Regist. (Neurosurg.) Atkinson Morley's Hosp. Wimbledon.

TAYLOR, William Douglas White Lodge Practices, 21 Grosvenor Street, St Helier, Jersey JE1 4HA Tel: 01534 873786; Clairfield, Maufant, St Saviour, Jersey JE2 7HQ Tel: 01534 861441 — MB ChB Glas. 1960. Prev: Ho. Phys. & Ho. Surg. Ballochmyle Hosp. Mauchline; Ho. Surg. Matern. Hosp. Swindon.

TAYLOR, William Edwin Elmbank Group, Foresterhill Health Centre, Westburn Road, Aberdeen AB25 2AY Tel: 01224 696949 Fax: 01224 691650; 63 Cairnlee Avenue E., Cults, Aberdeen AB15 9NU Tel: 01224 861642 — MB ChB Aberd. 1979; FRCGP 1994, M 1983; DCH RCP Lond. 1983; DRCOG 1983. Dir. Quality Assur. Initiatives RCGP Scotl.; Med. Off. Liberty Aberd. Socs: Soc. Occupat. Med.; Aberd. M-C Soc. Prev: Trainee GP Dumfries & Galloway; Ho. Phys. Aberd. City Hosp.; Ho. Surg. Aberd. Roy. Infirm.

TAYLOR, William Gledhill (retired) 7 Bridge Close, Burniston, Scarborough YO13 0HS Tel: 01723 870547 — MB ChB Leeds 1953; DIH Soc. Apoth. Lond. 1973; MFOM RCP Lond. 1978. Prev: Sen. Med. Off. Imperial Chem. Industries plc.

TAYLOR, Mr William Gordon Bywell, Chester Road, Rossett, Wrexham LL12 0HN — MB ChB Leeds 1980; MRCOG 1988; MObstG Liverp. 1990; Dip. Obst. Ultrasound RCOG 1992; FRCOG 2000. Cons. Obst. Gyn. Wrexham Maelor Hosp. Specialty: Obst. & Gyn. Socs: Brit. Med. Ultrasound Soc. Prev: Sen. Regist. Liverp. Matern. Hosp.; Regist. Newc. u. Tyne Gen. Hosp. & Roy. Liverp. Hosp.

TAYLOR, William Halstead (retired) Department of Medical Microbiology, Duncan Building, Royal Liverpool Hospital, Prescot St., Liverpool L7 8XW Tel: 0151 706 2000; Clare House, 16 Salisbury Road, Cressington Park, Liverpool L19 0PJ Tel: 0151 427 1042 Email: drwhtaylor@hotmail.com — (Oxf.) BA (1st cl. Hons. Animal Physiol.) 1946; BM BCh Oxf. 1948; MA Oxf. 1949; FRCP Lond. 1971, M 1950; DM 1957. Emerit. Cons. Liverp. HA & Emerit. Cons. Metabol. Med. Halton Gen. Hosp. Runcorn. Prev: Cons. Chem. Path. & Head of Dept. Liverp. HA.

TAYLOR, William Ian McMath Upper Kirkstone, La Route De La Haule, St Lawrence, Jersey JE3 1BA Tel: 01534 601124 Fax: 01534 68482 — MRCS Eng. LRCP Lond. 1964; MA Camb. 1965, BA 1961, MB BChir 1964. Specialty: Paediat. Socs: Jersey Med. Soc.

TAYLOR, William Nigel 182 Church Road, Litherland, Liverpool L21 5HE Tel: 0151 949 0281 Fax: 0151 949 0271 — MB ChB Liverp. 1983 (Univ. Liverp.) BSc (Hons.) Liverp. 1978; T(GP) 1991;

DFFP 1993. Salaried PMS GP, Bootle and Litherland PCT. Specialty: Gen. Med.; Accid. & Emerg.; Sports Med. Socs: N. W. Soc. of Family Plann. Prev: Trainee GP Bridge of Allan VTS; SHO (O & G) Ninewells Hosp. Dundee; SHO (Gen. Surg.) Hexham Gen. Hosp. N.d.

TAYLOR, William Reginald (retired) 61 Efflinch Lane, Barton-under-Needwood, Burton-on-Trent DE13 8EU Tel: 01283 712356 — MB ChB Sheff. 1956. Prev: GP Burton-on-Trent.

TAYLOR, Willson Davidson Glaxo Department of Dermatology, James Cook University hospital, Marton Road, Middlesbrough TS4 3BW Tel: 01642 854701 Fax: 01642 854763 Email: willson.taylor@stee.nhs.uk — MB ChB Aberd. 1969; MRCP (UK) 1974; FRCP Ed. 1985; FRCP Lond. 1989. Cons. Dermatol. S. Tees Acute Hosp. Specialty: Dermat. Special Interest: Deptm. Managem.; Paediatric Dermat. Socs: Brit. Assn. of Dermat.; Roy. Soc. of Med.; Roy. Coll. of Phys.

TAYLOR, Yvonne Thornliebank Health Centre, 20 Kennishead Road, Thornliebank, Glasgow G46 8NY Tel: 0141 531 6901 Fax: 0141 638 7554 — MB ChB Glas. 1963; FRCP Glas. Prev: Regist. Inst. Radiotherap. Glas.

TAYLOR, Zoe Leigh — MB ChB Aberd. 1998.

TAYLOR-BARNES, Kathryn Shere Surgery, Gomshall Lane, Shere, Guildford GU5 9DR Tel: 01483 202066 — MB BCh BAO NUI 1996; LRCPI; DCH 2001. Gen. Pract. Regist., Shere Surg., Shere. Specialty: Gen. Pract.

TAYLOR-HELPS, Douglas Frederick Derwent Practice, Norton Road, Malton YO17 9RF Tel: 01653 600069 Fax: 01653 698014 — MB ChB Manch. 1980; MRCGP 1985.

TAYLOR-ROBERTS, Matthew Giles William Westcourt, 12 The Street, Rustington, Littlehampton BN16 3NX Tel: 01903 784311 Fax: 01903 850907; Yew Tree Cottage, Warningcamp, Arundel BN18 9QJ — MB BS Lond. 1980; DRCOG 1985; Cert. Family Plann. JCC 1985.

TAYLOR-ROBERTS, Timothy David The Surgery, 35A High Street, Wimbledon, London SW19 5BY Tel: 020 8946 4820 Fax: 020 8944 9794 — MB BS Lond. 1971; BSc Lond. 1967; DObst RCOG 1975. Prev: Ho. Phys. St. Mary's Hosp. Lond.

TAYLOR-ROBINSON, Professor David Division of Medicine, Imperial College, London W2 1NY; 6 Vache Mews, Vache Lane, Chalfont St Giles HP8 4UT Tel: 01494 580324 Fax: 01494 580324 — MB ChB Liverp. 1954; MD (NE Roberts Prize) Liverp. 1958; FRCPath 1977, M 1965; MRCP (UK) 1996. Emerit. Prof. Genitourin. Microbiol. & Med. Imperial Coll. Sch. Lond. Specialty: Med. Microbiol.; Genitourinary Medicine. Socs: Soc. Gen. Microbiol.; Med. Soc. Study VD; Path. Soc. Prev: Head Div. Sexually Transm. Dis. MRC Clin. Research Centre Harrow; Mem. Scientif. Staff MRC Common Cold Unit Salisbury; Christiana Hartley Fell. (Bact.) Univ. Liverp.

TAYLOR-ROBINSON, David Carlton 1 Courtland Road, Liverpool L18 2EG — MB ChB Leeds 1998.

TAYLOR-ROBINSON, John Winston Belle Vale Health Centre, Hedgefield Road, Liverpool L25 2XE Tel: 0151 487 0514 Fax: 0151 488 6601; 97 Menlove Avenue, Calderstones, Liverpool L18 3HP Tel: 0151 722 1681 — MRCS Eng. LRCP Lond. 1971 (Liverp.) Prev: Ho. Surg. & Ho. Phys. St. Helens Gen. Hosp.; Ho. Off. (Obst.) Liverp. Matern. Hosp.

TAYLOR-ROBINSON, Katharine 32 Dacre Road, Hitchin SG5 1QJ — MB ChB Leeds 1998.

TAYLOR-ROBINSON, Simon David Hammersmith Hospital, Gastroenterology Unit, Imperial College School of Medicine, Du Cane Road, London W12 0HS Tel: 020 8383 3266 Fax: 020 8749 3436 — MB BS Lond. 1984; MRCP (UK) 1989; MD Lond 1996; FRCP UK 2001. Reader in Med. (Hepat. & Gastroenterology) Imperial Coll. Lond. Specialty: Gastroenterol. Special Interest: Hepatitis; Liver Cancer. Prev: Research Fell. (Gastroenterol.) NMR Unit, Roy. Postgrad. Med. Sch., Hammersmith Hosp., Lond.; Regist. (Gastroenterol.) Roy. Free Hosp. Lond.

TAYLOR-SHEWRING, Mrs Dorothy A (retired) 37 Fox Hill, Selly Oak, Birmingham B29 4AG Tel: 0121 472 2857 — (Liverp.) M.B., Ch.B. Liverp. 1923.

TAYLOR-SMITH, Robert George The Gables, 12 Albany House, 85 Manor Drive, Wembley HA9 8DJ — MB BS Lond. 1992.

TAYLOR-SMITH, Sarah Rachael — BM Soton. 1997.

TAYOB, Yunus St. Albans & Hemel Hempstead Trust Hospitals, St. Albans City Hospital, Waverley Road, St Albans AL3 5PN Tel: 01727 866122 Fax: 01727 841390; 4 Douglas Road, Harpenden AL5 2EW Fax: 01442 219251 — MB BCh BAO Dub. 1977; MFFP; MA 1979, MB BCh BAO Dub. 1977; MRCOG 1983. Cons. O & G St. Albans City & Hemel Hempstead Hosps.; Examr. RCOG & PLAB & United Examg. Bd. Specialty: Obst. & Gyn. Socs: Inst. Obst. & Gyn. Irel.; Blair Bell Res. Soc.; Nat. Assn. Family Plann. Doctors. Prev: Lect. & Hon. Sen. Regist. Roy. Free Hosp. Lond.; Regist. Middlx. Hosp. Lond.; Research Fell. Margt. Pyke Centre Lond.

TAYTON, Mr Keith John Jeremy Stoneycroft House, Shirenewton, Chepstow NP16 6RQ Tel: 01291 641747 Fax: 01291 641747 — (Roy. Free) MB BS Lond. 1968; MRCS Eng. LRCP Lond. 1968; FRCS Eng. 1973. Cons. Orthop. Surg. Roy. Gwent Hosp., Newport. Specialty: Trauma & Orthop. Surg. Socs: Fell. BOA.; BMA. Prev: Sen. Lect. (Traum. & Orthop. Surg.) Welsh Nat. Sch. Med. Cardiff; Sen. Regist. (Orthop.) S. Glam. AHA (T); Regist. (Orthop.) Nuffield Orthop. Centre Oxf.

TAYTON, Robert Geoffrey Thatcham Medical Practice, Bath Road, Thatcham RG18 3HD Tel: 01635 867171 Fax: 01635 876395 — MB BS Lond. 1970 (King's Coll. Hosp.) AKC; MRCS Eng. LRCP Lond. 1970; DObst RCOG 1973; DCH Eng. 1974; MRCGP 1975. Prev: Trainee GP Tunbridge Wells VTS; Ho. Phys. King's Coll. Hosp. Lond.; Ho. Surg. Kent & Sussex Hosp. Tunbridge Wells.

TAYYAB, Mohammad 17 New Haeth Close, Wednesfield, Wolverhampton WV11 1XX — MB BS Bahauddin Zakariya U Pakistan 1984; MRCPI 1994; MRCOG 1994.

TAYYEBI, Gulam Ali Russell Medical Centre, Upper Russell Street, Wednesbury WS10 7AR Tel: 0121 556 5470 Fax: 0121 505 1157 — MB BS Vikram 1969.

TCHAMOUROFF, Stephan Elias (retired) 18 Palmeira Avenue, Hove BN3 3GB Tel: 01273 736285 — LMSSA Lond. 1961 (St. Bart.) DObst 1967; FRCOG 1987, M 1970. Cons. Genitourin. Med. Brighton HA. Prev: Sen. Regist. (Genitourin. Med.) Univ. Coll. Hosp. Lond.

TCHIKHIAEVA, Tatiana University Hospital of Hartlepool, Woldforth Road, Hartlepool TS29 9AH — Vrach Kubanskij Med Inst 1993. (Accid. & Emerg.) Univ. Hosptial Hartlepool.

TEAGO, Philippa Jane Health Centre, Purbeck, Stentonbury, Milton Keynes MK14 2LB Tel: 01908 318989 — MB ChB Manch. 1984.

TEAGUE, Gillian Department of Paediatrics, Vowden Hall, Torbay Hospital, Totnes TQ2 7AA Tel: 01803 614567; Rydon House, Stoke Gabriel, Totnes TQ9 6SP Tel: 01803 782547 — MB ChB Bristol 1968; DCH Eng. 1972. Clin. Asst. (Paediat.) Torbay Hosp. Torquay.

TEAGUE, Isabel The Surgery, Worcester Road, Great Witley, Worcester WR6 6HR Tel: 01299 896370 Fax: 01299 896873; 43 Eardiston, Tenbury Wells WR15 8JJ Tel: 01584 881240 Fax: 01584 881353 — MB BS Lond. 1991 (Univ. Coll. and Middl. Sch. of Med.) BSc Lond. 1988; DFFP 1994; MRCGP 1995. Clin. Med. Off. Family Plann. (p/t). Specialty: Gen. Pract.; Family Plann. & Reproduc. Health. Socs: BMA; RCGP. Prev: Trainee GP Worcs.; SHO (Paediat.) Worcester Roy. Infirm.; Bd. Mem. Malvern Hills PCG.

TEAGUE, Robin Harry, OBE Torbay Hospital, Lawes Bridge, Torquay TQ2 7AA Tel: 01803 614567 Fax: 01803 654896; Rydon House, Stoke Gabriel, Totnes TQ9 6SP Tel: 01803 782547 Fax: 01803 782955 — MB ChB Bristol 1968; MRCS Eng. LRCP Lond. 1968; MRCP (UK) 1974; MD Bristol 1976; FRCP Lond. 1986. Cons. Phys. Torbay Hosp. Torquay. Specialty: Gastroenterol. Socs: Brit. Soc. Gastroenterol. Prev: Cons. Sen. Lect. Univ. Liverp.

TEAHON, Catherine Department of Gastroenterology, Nottingham City Hospital Trust, Hucknall Road, Nottingham NG5 1PB — MB BCh BAO NUI 1981; MRCPI 1984; MD NUI 1991, MMedSci 1985. Specialty: Gastroenterol.; Pharmacology; Gen. Med.

TEALE, Charles Department of Medicine for the Elderly, Seacroft Hospital, York Road, Leeds LS14 6UH Tel: 0113 264 8164; 3 Lidgett Park Road, Leeds LS8 1EE Tel: 0113 266 1123 — BM Soton. 1983; MRCP (UK) 1986; MD Leeds 1992; FRCP 1998. Cons. Phys. (Elderly) Seacroft aand St James Hosp. Leeds; Sen. Clin. Lect. Fac. Med. Leeds Univ. Specialty: Care of the Elderly. Socs: Brit. Geriat. Soc. Prev: Sen. Regist. Leeds Hosps.; Regist. Leeds Hosps.

TEALE, Glyn Robert Birmingham Women's NHS Trust, Edgbaston, Birmingham B15 2TG; 6 Swiss Farm Road, Copthorne, Shrewsbury SY3 8XB — MB BS Lond. 1989; BSc Biochem. Lond. 1986, MB BS (Hons.) 1989; MRCP (UK) 1993. Research Fell., Birm. Wom.'s NHS Trust.

TEALE, Katherine Frances Helen Department of Anaesthetics, Manchester Royal Infirmary, Oxford Road, Manchester M13 9WL — MB ChB Ed. 1987; DA (UK) 1989; FRCA. 1992. Specialty: Anaesth. Prev: SHO (Anaesth.) Stobhill Hosp. Glas.

TEALE, Stephen James Insch Health Centre, Rannes Street, Insch AB52 6JJ Tel: 01464 821500 Fax: 01464 821527 — MB ChB Dundee 1988.

TEALE, Teresa Elizabeth The Surgery, 4 Station Road, Frimley, Camberley GU16 7HF Tel: 01276 62622 Fax: 01276 683908; 1 Chestnut Avenue, Camberley GU15 1LT Tel: 01276 24693 — MB ChB Glas. 1967; DObst RCOG 1970. Prev: SHO (O & G) Roy. Matern. Hosp. Belf.

TEALL, Angela Jane Microbiology Department, Queen Elizabeth Hospital, Stadium Road, Woolwich SE18 4QH Tel: 020 8836 5699; 12 Garlies Road, Forest Hill, London SE23 2RT Tel: 020 8699 0386 — MB BS Lond. 1977; MA (Univ. of Surrey) 2001 (Wimbledon School of AA); MRCP Lond. 1981; MRCPath 1984; MSc Lond. 1984; BA Fine Art Lond. Inst. 1998. Cons. Microbiologist Qu. Eliz. NHS Trust. Specialty: Med. Microbiol. Socs: BMA. Prev: Sen. Regist. (Microbiol.) Univ. Coll. & Middlx. Hosp.; Cons. Microbiol. Greenwich Healthcare NHS Trust.

TEALL, John Graham Church Grange, Bramblys Drive, Basingstoke RG21 8QN Tel: 01256 29021 — MRCS Eng. LRCP Lond. 1957 (Birm.) LMSSA Lond. 1955; DObst RCOG 1957; DA Eng. 1959. Clin. Asst. (Dermat.) Basingstoke & N. Hants. Health Dist.; Med. Cons. Automobile Assn., Lancia SpA (Competitions) Turin & Fed. Internat. de l'Automobiliste. Specialty: Dermat. Socs: BMA. Prev: Clin. Research Asst. St. John's Hosp. Lond. Ho. Surg. & Ho. Phys.; Manor Hosp. Walsall; Obst. Ho. Phys. & Ho. Anaesth. Roy. Hants. Co. Hosp. Winchester.

TEANBY, Mr David Nigel Whiston Hospital, Prescot L35 5DR Tel: 0151 426 1600 Fax: 0151 430 1094 — MB ChB Liverp. 1980; FRCS Eng. 1988; FRCS (Orth.) 1995. Cons. Orthop. Surg. Whiston Hosp. Merseyside. Specialty: Orthop. Socs: Hon. Fell. BOA; Brit. Trauma Soc.; Brit. Assn. Surg. Knee. Prev: Sen. Regist. Hope Hosp. Salford.

TEARE, Celia Margaret Lila Wantage Health Centre, Church Street Practice, Wantage OX12 7AY Tel: 01235 770245 Fax: 01235 770727; 60 Newbury Street, Wantage OX12 8DF — MB BS Lond. 1971; MRCGP 1976.

TEARE, Erica Louise Department of Microbiology, New Writtle St., Chelmsford CM2 0YX Tel: 07767 886521 Fax: 01245 492496; Smallfields, Mill Road, Stock, Ingatestone CM4 9LL Tel: 01277 840524 — MB BS Lond. 1977 (St. Geo.) MSc Lond. 1982, BSc (Hons.) 1974; MRCS Eng. LRCP Lond. 1977; FRCPath 1996, M 1983. Cons. Med. Microbiol. Mid-Esses Hospitals NHS Trust. Specialty: Med. Microbiol. Socs: (Counc.) Roy. Soc. Med.; (Counc.) Hosp. Infec. Soc.; Assn. Med. Microbiol. Prev: Asst. Med. Microbiol. Pub. Health Laborat. Dulwich; Lect. (Med. Microbiol.) Westm. Hosp. Lond.; Regist. (Med. Microbiol.) & SHO (Path.) Westm. Hosp. Lond.

TEARE, Helen Caroline Woodlands, Lezayre Road, Ramsey IM8 2LN — MB BS Lond. 1989. Specialty: Obst. & Gyn.

TEARE, Julian Paul GI Unit, St Mary's Hospital, Paddington, London W2 1NY Tel: 0207 886 1072 Fax: 0207 886 6871 — MB BS Lond. 1984; MRCP (UK) 1988; MD Lond. 1995; FRCP 2000. Cons. Gastroenterol. St. Mary's Hosp. Lond.; Mem. Med. Counc. on Alcoholism. Specialty: Gastroenterol. Socs: Brit. Soc. Gastroenterol.; Amer. Gastoenterol. Assn. Prev: Sen. Regist. (Gen. Med. & Gastroenterol.) St. Mary's Hosp. Lond.; Regist. (Gen. Med. & Gastroenterol.) St. Thos. Hosp. Lond.; Regist. (Med.) Canterbury Hosp.

TEARE, Lara Jane 26 Temple Road, Dorridge, Solihull B93 8LF — MB ChB Bristol 1998.

TEASDALE, Andrew Richard Department of Anaesthetics, Royal Devon & Exeter Hospital, Barrack Road, Exeter EX2 5DW Tel: 01392 402474 Fax: 01392 402473 Email: andrew.teasdale@rdehc-tr.swest.nhs.uk — MB ChB Zimbabwe 1984; LRCP LRCS Ed. LRCPS Glas. 1986; FCAnaesth. 1989. Cons. in Anaesth. Roy. Devon & Exeter Healthcare Trust Exeter. Specialty: Anaesth. Prev: Regist. (Anaesth.) Soton. Gen. Hosp.; Asst. Prof. (Anaesth.) UWMC Seattle; Sen. Regist. (Anaesth.) Leeds Gen. Infirm.

TEASDALE, Mr Colin (retired) Derriford Hospital, Derriford Road, Plymouth PL6 8DH Tel: 01752 777111 Fax: 01752 763436; Nuffield Hospital, Derriford Road, Plymouth PL6 8BG Tel: 01752 775861 Fax: 01752 768969 — MB BS Lond. 1969 (Lond. Hosp.) BSc Lond. 1966, MS 1983, MB BS 1969; FRCS Eng. 1974. Cons. Gen. Surg. Plymouth HA. Prev: Sen. Regist. (Surg.) Bristol Health Dist. (T).

TEASDALE, Mr Derek Hall (retired) 8 Mytchett Heath, Mytchett, Camberley GU16 6DP Tel: 01252 546859 — MB BS Lond. 1942 (King's Coll. Hosp.) MRCS Eng. LRCP Lond. 1942; FRCS Eng. 1949. Hon. Cons. Surg. Rochdale Infirm. & Birch Hill Hosp. Rochdale; Penrose May Teach. RCS. Prev: Surg. Adviser RCS Eng. NW RHA.

TEASDALE, Diane Elizabeth Larwood Health Centre, 56 Larwood, Worksop S81 0HH Tel: 01909 500233 Fax: 01909 479722 — MB ChB Sheff. 1992 (Sheffield) Dip Palliat Care 1999. GP; Med Off. Hospice of Good Shephard.Retfold. Specialty: Gen. Pract.; Palliat. Med.

TEASDALE, Eric Leslie AstraZeneca, Global Safety, Health and Environment, 15 Stanhope Gate, London W1K 1LN Tel: 01625 512510 Fax: 01625 517824 Email: eric.teasdale@astrazeneca.com; Badgers Bend, 5 Eaton Drive, Alderley Edge SK9 7RA Tel: 01625 585854 Email: eric.teasdale@astrazeneca.com — MB ChB Aberd. 1972; Cert Family Planning JCC 1975; M 1976; AFOM 1979; DIH Soc. Apoth. Lond. 1979; CIH Dund. 1979; MFOM 1983; FRCGP 1993; FFOM RCP Lond. 1993; MIEMA 1998; FIOSH.RSP 1999; FRCP 1999; FACOEM 2000; FIEMA 2003. Gp. Chief Med. Off. AstraZeneca; Dir. Global SH & E Strategy; Mem. Internat. Commiss. Occupat. Health. Specialty: Occupat. Health. Socs: Soc. Occup. Med. Prev: Chief Med. Off. Zeneca; Trainee GP Aberd. VTS; Div. Med. Off. ICI.

TEASDALE, Professor Graham Michael University Department Neurosurgery, Institute of Neurological Sciences, Southern General Hospital, Glasgow G51 4TF Tel: 0141 201 2019 — MB BS Durh. 1963 (Durham) MRCP Lond. 1966; FRCS Ed. 1971; FRCS Glas. 1981; T(S) 1991; F Med Sci 1999; FRSE 2001; FRCS (Eng.) 2001. Prof. Neurosurg. Univ. Glas.; Hon. Cons. Neurosurg. S. Gen. Hosp. Glas.; Chairm. Europ. Brain Injury Consortium. Specialty: Neurosurg. Socs: Soc. Brit. Neurol. Surg.; Internat. Neurotrauma Soc. Prev: Pres.Soc. of Breast Neurol. Surg.

TEASDALE, Katherine Childrens Hospital, Western Bank, Sheffield S10 2TH — MB ChB Sheff. 1989; MRCP (UK) 1993; DTM & H Liverp. 1994.

TEASDALE, Kathryn Jane 28 Granville Road, Oxted RH8 0DA — MB BS Lond. 1991 (St. Geo. Hosp. Med. Sch.) DRCOG 1995; DFFP 1995; MRCGP 1996. Specialty: Gen. Pract. Prev: Trainee GP Epsom, Surrey.

TEATHER, Stephen John Richmond House Surgery, Richmond Terrace, Station Road, Whitchurch SY13 1RH Tel: 01948 662870; 52 Pear Tree Lane, Whitchurch SY13 1NQ — MB ChB Birm. 1975; DRCOG 1977; DCH Eng. 1978.

TEBB, James Barry Tunstall Washway Road Medical Centre, 63-65 Washway Road, Sale M33 7SU Tel: 0161 962 4354 Fax: 0161 962 0046 — MB ChB Manch. 1968. Prev: SHO (Cardiac Surg.) Manch. Roy. Infirm.; SHO (Orthop. & Cas.) Pk. Hosp. Davyhulme; Ho. Off. (Surg.) Unit. Manch. Roy. Infirm.

TEBBETT, John Ernest (retired) 122 Urmston Lane, Stretford, Manchester M32 9BQ — MB ChB Birm. 1949. Ex-Officio Mem. Trafford LMC Chairm.; Mem. Trafford Family Pract. Comm. Prev: Ho. Surg. Gen. Hosp. Birm.

TEBBIT, Anne 19 Pennine Rise, Scissett, Huddersfield HD8 9JE — MB BS Lond. 1991.

TEBBOTH, Louise Ina Joan 24 Cleveland Way, London E1 4UF — MB ChB Sheff. 1998 (Sheffield) MB ChB Sheff 1998. GP (VTS: Guy's & St Thomas's).

TEBBS, Veronica Margaret — MB BS Newc. 1980; MRCGP 1984; FFPHM 2001. Assoc. Med. Dir. 3M Health Care Ltd & Europ. Clin. Developm. Manager, Basal Cell Carcinoma Project; Clin. Asst., Dept. of Dermat., Qu.s Med. Centre, Nottm. Specialty: Dermat.; Immunol.; Oncol. Prev: Head Drug Safety Copenhagen; Head (Med.) Milton Keynes; Head (Rheum. & Consumer Med.) Nottm.

TEBBUTT, Isabel Helen Walletts, Great Warley St, Great Warley, Brentwood CM13 3JE Tel: 01277 227557 Email: sbwg@wallets.fsnet.co.uk — MB BS Lond. 1977 (St. Geo.) MFFP; DCH Eng. 1980; FRCOG 1995, M 1982. Cons. O & G Harold Wood Hosp. Romford. Specialty: Obst. & Gyn. Prev: Cons. O & G Stoke Mandeville Hosp. Aylesbury; Sen. Regist. (O & G) Hammersmith Hosp. Lond.; Hon. Clin. Tutor (O & G) W. Chesh. Hosp.

TEBBUTT, Niall Christopher 15 Wimbledon Drive, Stourbridge DY8 2PQ — BM BCh Oxf. 1989.

TEBBY, Susan Jane Norwood, 57 Elworth St., Sandbach CW11 1HA Tel: 01270 763454 — MB ChB Manch. 1986; BSc (Hons.) Pharm. Med. Manch. 1983; MRCP (UK) 1990; FRCR 1997. Specialist Regist. (Diag. Radio.) N. Staffs. Hosp. Specialty: Radiol. Prev: Regist. Rotat. (Med.) N. Staffs. Roy. Infirm. & City Gen. Hosp Stoke-on-Trent.; Regist. Rotat. (Diag. Radiol.) N. W. RHA.

TECKHAM, Paul Ng Soon Harold Wood Hospital, 14 Hospital Crescent, Gubbins Lane, Romford RM3 0BJ — MB ChB Leeds 1982.

TEDBURY, Michael John St Johns Medical Centre, 62 London Road, Grantham NG31 6HR Tel: 01476 590055 Fax: 01476 400042 — MB BS Newc. 1976 (Lond.) MRCGP 1980.

TEDD, Clive Barron Saltaire Medical Centre, Richmond Road, Shipley BD18 4RX Tel: 01274 593101 Fax: 01274 772588 — MRCS Eng. LRCP Lond. 1970; DA Eng. 1973.

TEDD, Rachael Jane 7 Craven Cl, Fulwood, Preston PR2 9PU — MB ChB Glas. 1997.

TEDDERS, Brian Claudy Health Centre, Irwin Crescent, Claudy, Londonderry BT47 4AB Tel: 028 7133 8371 — MB BCh BAO NUI 1978; LRCPI & LM, LRCSI & LM 1978.

TEDDERS, Raphael Andrew The Health Centre, Cemmaes Road, Machynlleth SY20 8LB; Brickfield House, Brickfield St, Machynlleth SY20 — MB BCh BAO NUI 1979; LRCPI & LM, LRCSI & LM BAO 1979.

TEDDY, Mr Peter Julian Department of Neurological Surgery, The Radcliffe Infirmary, Oxford OX2 6HE Tel: 01865 224941 Fax: 01865 224898; St. Peters College, Oxford OX1 2DL Tel: 01865 278900 — BM BCh Oxf. 1972; MA, DPhil, BSc 1972; FRCS Eng. 1977. Cons. Neurosurg. Radcliffe Infrim. Oxf. & Nat. Spinal Injuries Centre Stoke Mandeville Hosp. Aylesbury; Sen. Research Fell. St. Peter's Coll. Oxf.; Clin. Lect. Univ. Oxf. Med. Sch. Specialty: Neurosurg. Socs: Soc. Brit. Neurol. Surg. & Internat. Assn. Study of Pain; Internat. Med. Soc. Paraplegia; Brit. Cervical Spine Soc. Prev: Dir. Clin. Studies Univ. Oxf. Med. Sch.; Asst. Edr. Brit. J. Neurosurg.; Clin. Director (Neurosci.), Radcliffe Infirm., Oxf..

TEDSTONE, Ian Keith Newthorpe Medical Practice, Eastwood Clinic, Nottingham Road, Nottingham NG16 3HB Tel: 01773 760202 — BM BS Nottm. 1994.

TEE, Dudley Edward Handbury (retired) 1 St Aubyns Mead, Rottingdean, Brighton BN2 7HY Tel: 01273 302635 — MB BS Lond. 1954 (King's Coll. Hosp.) FRCPath 1976, M 1965. Prev: Head of Immunol. King's Coll. Sch. Med. & Dent.

TEE, Michael Kevin John Tasker House Surgery, 56 New Street, Great Dunmow, Dunmow CM6 1BH Tel: 01371 873774 Fax: 01371 873793 Email: miketee@jth.demon.co.uk; Meadow Cottage, High St, Widdington, Saffron Walden CB11 3SG Tel: 01799 542626 — MB BChir Camb. 1985; BSc (Hons.) St. And. 1980; DLO RCS Eng. 1988; DRCOG 1989; MRCGP 1990. Clin. Asst. (Ear, Nose & Throat). Socs: LMC; Vice-chair. PCT.

TEEBAY, Peter French (retired) 17 Hale Road, Hale Village, Liverpool L24 5RB Tel: 0151 425 3742 Fax: 0151 425 3742 — MB ChB Liverp. 1956; MRCS Eng. LRCP Lond. 1956; MRCGP 1971; Dip Ad Educat Liverp. 1971. Lect. (Gen. Pract.) Liverp. Univ. Prev: Clin. Asst. (Psychiat.) Rainhill Hosp. Prescot.

TEECE, Stewart Conway 40 Beverley Road, Nunthorpe, Middlesbrough TS7 0HN — MB ChB Glas. 1995.

TEED, Alison Rhona Wellspring Surgery, St. Anns Health Centre, St. Anns, Well Road, Nottingham NG3 3PX Tel: 0115 9505907/8 Fax: 0115 988 1582 — MB BCh Wales 1985; DRCOG 1990. Specialty: Obst. & Gyn. Prev: GP Newport, Gwent; SHO (Urol. & A & E) Cardiff Roy. Infirm.; SHO (Geriat. & O & G) Llandough Hosp. Cardiff.

TEED, Henry (retired) 466 Loose Road, Maidstone ME15 9UA Tel: 01622 743948 — MB BS Lond. 1957 (St. Geo.) DObst RCOG 1960; DCH Eng. 1961. Prev: Ho. Surg. (O & G) St. Mary Abbot's Hosp. Kensington.

TEELOCK, Boodhun 49 Newlands Court, Forty Avenue, Wembley HA9 9LZ — MB ChB Ed. 1950.

TEENAN, David William NHS Ayrshire & Arran General Hospitals Division, Ophthalmology Department, Ayr Hospital, Dalmellington Road, Ayr KA6 6DX — MB ChB Dundee 1993; FRCS Ed.; FRCOphth. Cons. Ophth. NHS Ayrsh. & Arran. Specialty: Ophth. Prev: Acting Cons. Ophth. Univ. Hosp. Wales Cardiff.

TEENAN, Mr Robert Paul 1 Erskine Avenue, Glasgow G41 5AL — MB ChB Glas. 1981; FRCS Glas. 1985; MD Glas. 1990; FRCS (Gen.) 1995. Cons. Surg. Glas. Roy. Infirm. Specialty: Gen. Surg.

TEES, Ernest Carroll (retired) 6 Templars Place, St. Peter St., Marlow SL7 1NU Tel: 016284 71113 — MB BCh BAO Dub. 1953 (T.C. Dub.) MA Dub. 1939, MB BCh BAO 1953. Prev: Ho. Off. City & Co. Hosp. Londonderry.

TEGNER, Henry The Surgery, 1 Forest Hill Road, London SE22 0SQ Tel: 020 8693 2264 Fax: 020 8299 0200 — MB BS Lond. 1969 (Lond. Hosp.) DObst RCOG 1973; MSc Lond. 1993; FRCGP 2000. Course Organiser Lewisham VTS. Prev: Ho. Phys. Mile End. Hosp.; Ho. Surg. Lond. Hosp.; Squadron Ldr. RAF Med. Br.

TEH, Corina Poh Ling 1 Foxes Close, Hermitage Walk, The Park, Nottingham NG7 1PG; Flat 3, Tower Mansions, 86/87 Grange Road, London SE1 — BM BS Nottm. 1987; BMedSci. (Hons.) 1985; MRCP (UK) 1992; DRCOG 1993; MRCGP 1993; DFFP 1994. Specialty: Paediat.

TEH, Hui-Pin (retired) St. John's Hospital, Livingston EH54 6PP Tel: 01506 419666; 3 Morningside Place, Edinburgh EH10 5ES Tel: 0131 447 4507 — MB BCh BAO Dub. 1964; FFA RCS Eng. 1968. Cons. Anaesth. St. John's Hosp. Livingston W. Lothian. Prev: Cons. Anaesth. Bangour Gen. & City Hosps. Edin.

TEH, James Lip Ze Nuffield Orthopaedic Centre NHS Trust, Windmill Road, Headington, Oxford OX3 7LD Tel: 01865 227337 — MB BS Lond. 1991; BSc (Hons.) Psychol. Lond. 1987; MRCP (UK) 1994; FRCR 1997. Cons. Musculoskeletal Radiologist Nuffield Orthopaedic Centre, Oxf. Specialty: Radiol. Socs: Roy. Coll. of Physicians; Roy. Coll. of Radiologists; Brit. Soc. of Skeletal Radiologists. Prev: Specialist Regist. (Radiol.) Lond.

TEH, Lee Gek Whitevale Medical Group, 30 Whitevale Street, Glasgow G31 1QS — MB ChB Aberd. 1978.

TEH, Lee-Suan Blackburn Royal Infirmary, Department of Rheumatology, Ward 13, Level 5, Bolton Road, Blackburn BB2 3LR Tel: 01254 294484 Fax: 01254 294423 Email: lee-suan.teh@mail.bhrv.nwest.nhs.uk; 28 Cholmondeley Road, Salford M6 8NH Tel: 0161 7430392 Email: lsteh@btinternet.com — MB ChB (Commend.) Aberd. 1984; MRCP (UK) 1987; MD Aberd. 1994; FRCP Glas. 1997; FRCP Lond. 2000. Cons. Rheum. Blackburn Roy. Infirm. Specialty: Rheumatol. Special Interest: Systemic Lupus Erythematosis. Socs: Brit. Soc. of Rheum.; Brit. Soc. of Immunol.; Brit. Isles Lupus Assessm. Gp. Prev: Sen. Regist. (Rheum.) Manch.; Research Fell. Arthritis & Rheum. Counc.; Regist. (Rheum.) Univ. Hosp. Wales.

TEHAN, Brian Edwin Department of Anaesthesia, Glan Clwyd Hospital, Bodelwyddan, Rhyl LL18 5UJ Tel: 01745 583910 Fax: 01745 583143 Email: drbrian.tehan@cd-tr.wales.nhs.uk; Ty Canol, Copthorn Road, Upper Colwyn Bay, Colwyn Bay LL28 5YP Tel: 01492 531284 — MB BCh BAO NUI 1986; FFA RCSI 1992; Spec. Accredit. Anaesth. RCSI (Fac. Anaesth.) 1995. Cons. Anaesth. & Intens. Care Glan Clwyd Hosp.; Clin. Director Anaerthesia; Treas. Welsh Intens. Care Soc. Specialty: Anaesth.; Intens. Care. Socs: Welsh Soc. Anaesth.; Sec. Welsh Intens. Care Soc.; Intens. Care Soc. Prev: Sen. Regist. (Anaesth.) & Fell. Cardiothoracic Anaesth. Leeds Gen. Infirm.; SHO (Anaesth.) St. Jas. Univ. Hosp. Leeds.

TEIMORY, Masoud Worthing Hospital, Park Avenue, Worthing BN11 2DH — MB ChB Bristol 1986; FRCOphth 1991. Clin. Director of Head & Neck Surg. Special Interest: Cataract & Refraction Surg.; Squint & Neuro-ophthalmol.

TEJANI, Sakkar (retired) 107 Cadogan Gardens, South Woodford, London E18 1LY Tel: 020 8989 7974 — MB BS Bombay 1956 (Grant Med. Coll.) MRCGP 1966.

TEJURA, Bindu Albert Einstein Medical Centre, 5501 Old York Road, Philadelphia PA 19141, USA Tel: 215 456 7890 Fax: 215 473 7566 Email: btejura@aol.com; 88 Trinity View, Caerleon, Newport NP18 3SW — MB BCh Wales 1992; BSc (Hons) Pharmacology. Specialty: Gen. Med.

TEJURA, Harsit 88 Trinity View, Caerleon, Newport NP18 3SW — MB BCh Wales 1993.

TEK, Vinod 95 Grosvenor Road, Ilford IG1 1LB — LMSSA Lond. 1997.

TEKLE, Iyassu Ashurst Health Centre, Lulworth, Ashurst, Skelmersdale WN8 6QS Tel: 01695 732468 Fax: 01695 555365 — MB BCh N U Ireland 1979; MB BCh N U Ireland 1979.

TEKRIWAL, Alok Kumar Department of Ophthalmology, County Hospital, Lincoln LN2 5QY — MB BS Patna 1988; FRCOphth 1994.

TELANG, Shammohan Maharudra Gray Hill Surgery, Woodstock Way, Caldicot, Newport NP26 5AB; Momon's Folly, Wedgwood Drive, Portskewett, Newport NP6 4TL Tel: 01291 420252 — MB BS Poona 1955 (B. J. Med. Coll. Poona) Apptd. Fact. Doctor. Prev: Regist. (Orthop.) Cardiff Roy. Infirm.; SHO (Cas.) Sassoon Hosp. Poona; Ho. Surg. St. Woolos Hosp. Newport.

TELESZ, Ann Marysia Health Centre, Handsworth Avenue, Highams Park, London E4 9PD Tel: 020 8527 0913 Fax: 020 8527 6597 — MB BS Lond. 1980 (Univ. Coll. Hosp.) MA Oxf. 1978, BA (Biochem.) 1975; DRCOG 1984; MRCGP 1985. Trainer; Course Organiser Whipps Cross Hosp. VTS.

TELFER, Aileen Hazel 34 Grange Terrace, Edinburgh EH9 2LE — MB ChB Ed. 1990. SHO (Gen. Med. & Infec. Dis.) Castle Hill Hosp. Hull. Specialty: Gastroenterol.

TELFER, Alexander Borland Meikle (retired) Kinmuir, 167 Mugdock Road, Milngavie, Glasgow G62 8NB Tel: 0141 956 1371 — MB ChB Glas. 1956; FFA RCS Eng. 1963; FRCP Glas. 1984, M 1982. Cons. Anaesth. Glas. Roy. Infirm.; Hon. Clin. Lect. Anaesth. Univ. Glas. Prev: Sen. Regist. Univ. Dept. Anaesth. & Ho. Off. (Anaesth.) Glas. Roy.Infirm.

TELFER, Carol Ann Linda 14 Sorbie Drive, Stonehouse, Larkhall ML9 3NL — MB ChB Glas. 1987.

TELFER, Ian Dept of Psychiatry, Tameside Central Hosp, Fountain St, Ashton-under-Lyne OL6 9RW Tel: 0161 331 5094 — MB ChB Liverp. 1979; MRCPsych 1985. Cons.(Psychiat.) W. Pennine Health Auth.. Specialty: Alcohol & Substance Misuse. Socs: MDU.

TELFER, James Robert Mill Road Surgery, Mill Road, Market Rasen LN8 3BP Tel: 01673 843556 Fax: 01673 844388 — MB BS Lond. 1984; MRCGP 1988; MA Camb. 1992.

TELFER, Mr John Robert Currie 78 Hainburn Park, Fairmilehead, Edinburgh EH10 7HJ — MB ChB Ed. 1985; FRCS Glas. 1991. Specialist Regist. (Plastic Surg.) St. John's Hosp. at Howden Livingstone. Specialty: Plastic Surg. Prev: SHO (Plastic Surg.) Char. Cross Hosp., St. Geo. Hosp. & Qu. Mary's Univ. Hosp. Lond.

TELFER, John Robin (retired) Ellenthorpe, Church Road, Lympstone, Exmouth EX8 5JT — MB BS Lond. 1965 (King's Coll. Hosp.) DCH Eng. 1967; DObst RCOG 1968. Prev: SHO (O & G & Paediat.) Freedom Fields Hosp. Plymouth.

TELFER, June Mary 10 Woodburn Gardens, Aberdeen AB15 8JA — MB ChB Ed. 1994.

TELFER, Mr Martin Ronaldson — MB BS Lond. 1985; BDS 1977; FDS RCS Eng. 1985; FRCS Ed. 1988. Cons. Oral & Maxillofacial Surg. York Dist. Hosp.; Dep. Lead Cancer Clinician - York Trust. Specialty: Oral & Maxillofacial Surg.

TELFER, Nicholas Roland Dermatology Centre, Hope Hospital, Stott Lane, Salford M6 8HD Tel: 0161 787 1010 Fax: 0161 962 2054 Email: nrtelfer@aol.com — MB ChB Manch. 1981; MRCP (UK) 1984; FRCP Lond. 1998. Cons. Dermat. & Dermat. Surg. Dermat. Centre Manch. Specialty: Dermat. Socs: Brit. Assn. Dermat.; Fell. Amer. Coll. of MOHS Micrographic Surg. & Cutaneous Oncol.; Fell. Amer. Soc. Dermatologic Surg. Prev: Asst. Prof. & Fell. MOHS & Dermat. Surg. Div. Dermat. Univ. Calif. Los Angeles, USA; Sen. Regist. (Dermat.) Skin Hosp. Manch.

TELFER, Trevor Percival (retired) Cob End, Oast Court, Yalding, Maidstone ME18 6JY — MB BS Melbourne 1948 (Melb.) DPath. Eng. 1955; FRCP Lond. 1988, M 1957; FRCP Ed. 1983, M 1957; MCPA 1958; FRCPath 1972, M 1964. Cons. Path. St. Bart. Hosp. Rochester. Prev: Regist. (Clin. Path.) Univ. Coll. Hosp.

TELFER BRUNTON, William Andrew Truro Public Health Laboratory, Penventinnie Lane, Treliske, Truro TR1 3LQ Tel: 01872 254900 Fax: 01872 222198 — MB ChB Ed. 1973; BSc (Hons.) (Bact.) Ed. 1970; FRCPath 1982, M 1980; FRCP Ed. 1998. Cons. Microbiol., Dir. Pub. Health Laborat. Truro; JP. Specialty: Med. Microbiol. Socs: Assn. Clin. Path.; Brit. Soc. Study of Infec.; Assn. Med. Microbiol. Prev: Lect. (Bact.) & (Clin. Chem.) Univ. Edin.

TELFORD, Anne Marie Tower Hill, Armagh BT61 9DR Tel: 01861 410041 Fax: 01861 414551; 107 Old Kilmore Road, Moira, Craigavon BT67 0NA — MB BCh BAO Belf. 1975 (Queens University Belfast.) MRCP (UK) 1980; MD Belf. 1982; FFPHM RCP (UK) 1994, M 1988; FRCP (UK) 1999. Dir. Pub. Health SHSSB. Specialty: Pub. Health Med. Prev: Cons. Pub. Health Med. NHSSB; Sen. Regist. (Community Med.) NHSSB Ballymena.

TELFORD, David Ronald Department of Microbiology, Royal Lancaster Infirmary, Ashton Road, Lancaster LA1 4RP Tel: 01524 583770 Fax: 01524 583798; Aldcliffe, Carr Bank, Milnthorpe LA7 7LB Tel: 01524 761529 — MB ChB Manch. 1971 (Manchester) Dip. Bact. Manch. 1978; FRCPath. 1990, M 1978. Cons. Microbiol. Morecambe Bay Hosps. NHS Trust; Cons. Communicable Dis. Control Morecambe Bay HA; Hon. Reader (Biol. Sci.) Lancaster Univ.; Dep. Med. Dir. Morcambe Bay Hosps. NHS Trust. Specialty: Med. Microbiol.; Infec. Dis. Prev: Cons. Microbiol. Leeds Pub. Health Lab.; Sen. Regist. (Microbiol.) Manch. AHA; Tutor (Communicable Dis.) Manch. Univ.

TELFORD, Karen Jane 4 Friars Court, Coleraine BT51 3JH — MB ChB Bristol 1991.

TELFORD, Michael Edwin Fournier Pharmaceuticals Ltd, 19-20 Progress Business Centre, Whittle Parkway, Slough SL1 6DQ Tel: 01753 740400 Fax: 01753 740444 Email: m.telford@fournier.fr — MB BS Lond. 1983 (St Mary's) T(GP) 1987; Dip. Pharm. Med. RCP (UK) 1997; AFPM RCP Lond. 1998; MFPM RCP Lond. 2002. Med. Dir. Fournier Pharmaceuticals Ltd. Slough. Specialty: Pharmaceutical Medicine; Gen. Med.; Gen. Pract. Socs: (Dep. Chairm. Exec. Comm 2002) Brit. Assn. Pharmaceut. Phys.; Fell. Roy. Soc. Med. Prev: Sen. Med. Affairs Phys., Bayer plc, Newbury; Med. Adviser Yamanouchi Pharma Ltd. W. Byleet; GP Hampton.

TELFORD, Richard Jonathan Dept. of Anaesthetics, Royal Devon & Exeter NHS Trust, Barback Road, Exeter EX2 5DW Tel: 01392 402474 Fax: 01392 402472 Email: richard.telford@rdehc-tr.swest.nhs.uk — MB BS Lond. 1981 (St. Bart.) BSc (Hons.) Lond. 1978, MB BS 1981; FFA RCS Eng. 1985. Cons. Anaesth. Roy. Devon & Exeter Hosps. Specialty: Anaesth. Socs: Brit. Med. Assn.; Coll. of Anaesth.; Vasc. Anaesth. Soc. Prev: Sen. Regist. (Anaesth.) St. Geo. Hosp. Lond.; Regist. (Paediat. Anaesth.) Roy. Liverp. Childr. Hosps.; Regist. (Anaesth.) Guy's Hosp.

TELFORD, Rosemary Margaret The Robert Darbishire Practice, Rusholme Health Centre, Walmer Street, Manchester M14 5NP Tel: 0161 225 6699 Fax: 0161 248 4580 — MB ChB Manch. 1983; DRCOG 1986; DCH RCP Lond. 1987; MRCGP 1988. Hon. Lect. (Gen. Pract.) GP Tutor. Prev: Dist. Med. Off. Katherine North. Terr., Austral.; GP Chippenham; Trainee GP Northwick Pk. Hosp. Harrow VTS.

TELFORD, Sydney Bruce (retired) Channel Farm, Oakridge, Winscombe BS25 1NJ Tel: 01934 843247 Email: btel682804@aol.com — MB BCh BAO Dub. 1949 (T.C. Dub.) DTM & H Eng. 1960; FFCM 1986, MFCM 1974. Prev: SCM S. West. RHA & Avon HA.

TELLECHEA ELORRIAGA, Francisco Javier 11 Simpson Street, Crosshouse, Kilmarnock KA2 0BD — LMS Basque Provinces 1989.

TELLER, Richard Henry Marshall Finchley Road Surgery, 682 Finchley Road, Golders Green, London NW11 7NP Tel: 020 8455 9994 — MB BS Lond. 1988; MA Oxf. 1982; MRCGP 1992.

TELLING, Jeremy Philip The Priory Surgery, 326 Wells Road, Bristol BS4 2QJ Tel: 0117 949 3988 Fax: 0117 778250 — MB ChB Bristol 1956; DObst RCOG 1961. Prev: Act. Maj. RAMC.

TELLWRIGHT, Joseph Michael (retired) Manor Farm, Hunsterson, Nantwich CW5 7RB Tel: 01270 520353 — MB Camb. 1956; BChir 1955.

TEMPERLEY, Christine The Medical Centre, 4 Craven Avenue, Thornton, Bradford BD13 3LG Tel: 01274 832110/834387 Fax: 01274 831694; 32 Lidget, Oakworth, Keighley BD22 7HH Tel: 01535 642008 — MB ChB Leeds 1989. GP. Specialty: Gen. Pract. Prev: Trainee GP York VTS; SHO (Psychiat.) Lynfield Mt. Hosp. Bradford.

TEMPERLEY, David Edward Royal Albert Edward Infirmary, Wigan Lane, Wigan WN1 2NN Tel: 01942 244000; 67 Framingham Road, Sale, Manchester M33 3RH Tel: 0161 972 0004 — MB BCh BAO Dub. 1984; MB BCh BAO (Dub.) 1984; MRCPI 1986; FRCR 1991. Cons. Radiol.Wrightington, Wigan & Leigh NHS Trust. Specialty: Radiol. Prev: Regist. (Radiol.) N. West. RHA.

TEMPERTON, Helen Clair 6 Clifton House, 131 Cleveland St., London W1T 6QE — MB BCh Wales 1995.

TEMPEST, Heidi Victoria 19 Langham Road, Cambridge CB1 3SD — BChir Camb. 1996.

TEMPEST, Janet Elizabeth The Surgery, 14 Manor Road, Beckenham BR3 5LE Tel: 020 8650 0957 Fax: 020 8663 6070 — MB BS Lond. 1982; MRCGP 1986. GP Beckenham.

TEMPEST, Lynda Carole Hamilton Road Surgery, 201 Hamilton Road, Felixstowe IP11 7DT Tel: 01394 283197 Fax: 01394 270304; 31 Foxgrove Lane, Felixstowe IP11 7JU — MB ChB Sheff. 1975 (Sheffield) DRCOG 1977. Prev: Trainee Gen. Pract. Sheff. Vocational Train. Scheme; Ho. Phys. & Ho. Surg. Doncaster Roy. Infirm.

TEMPEST, Pernell Kate 34 Chyandor Close, St. Blazey, Par PL24 2LP — MB BS Lond. 1992.

TEMPLE, Adrian James 1a Marsh Road, Weymouth DT4 8JD Tel: 01305 773243 — MB BS Lond. 1968 (St. Geo.) MRCS Eng. LRCP Lond. 1968; FRCS Eng. 1975. Private practitioner, Weymouth, Dorset & Hosp. Practitioner (Rheumat.). Specialty: Gen. Med.; Rheumatol. Prev: GP, Weymouth, Dorset.

TEMPLE, Mr Andrew John Lovington Grange, Lovington Lane, Lower Broadheth, Worcester WR2 6QQ Tel: 01905 640992 — MB BS Lond. 1994; BSc Lond. 1991; FRCS Lond. 1998. Specialist Rotat. (Orthop.) W. Midl. Specialty: Orthop. Prev: SHO Rotat. (Surg.) Roy. Berks. Hosp.

TEMPLE, Andrew Richard 19 Welland Vale Road, Leicester LE5 6PX — MB ChB Leeds 1994. Ho. Off. (Surg.) Leeds Gen. Infirm. Prev: Ho. Off. (Respirat. Med.) St. Jas. Univ. Hosp. Leeds.

TEMPLE, Celia Margaret Rose Garden Medical Centre, 4 Mill Lane, Edinburgh EH6 6TL Tel: 0131 554 1274 Fax: 0131 555 2159 — MB ChB Sheff. 1984; MRCGP 1988.

TEMPLE, Dean Russell Orchard Medical Practice, Innisdoon, Crow Hill Drive, Mansfield NG19 7AE Tel: 01623 400100 Fax: 01623 400101; Ashworth, 2 St. Chads Close, Mansfield NG18 4DS Tel: 01623 654177 — MB ChB Leic. 1987. Prev: SHO (Geriat. & A & E) Kings Mill Hosp. Sutton-in-Ashfield; Trainee GP/SHO Mansfield VTS.

TEMPLE, Isabel Karen Wessex Clinical Genetic Service, Department of Child Health, Princess Anne Hospital, Coxford Road, Southampton SO16 5YA Tel: 023 8079 6625 Fax: 023 8079 4346; South Ploverfield, Long Lane, Bursledon, Southampton SO31 8DA — MB ChB Birm. 1981; MRCP (UK) 1984; FRCP Lond. 1995. Cons. Clin. Genetics Soton. Gen. Hosp.; R & D Soton. Univ. Hosps. Trust; Hon. Sen. Lect. Univ. of Soton. Specialty: Genetics. Socs: (Comm.) Clin. Genetics Soc. Prev: Sen. Regist. (Genetics) Hosp. for Sick Childr. Gt. Ormond St.

TEMPLE, John Darcus Derby Road Health Centre, 292 Derby Road, Lenton, Nottingham NG7 1QG Tel: 0115 947 4002 Fax: 0115 924 0783 — MB Camb. 1970 (Middlx.) BChir Camb 1969; MA Camb. 1970; DObst RCOG 1973; MRCGP 1976; Dip. Med. Educat. Dund 1995. GP Nottm.; Lect. (Gen. Pract.) Univ. Nottm. since 1981. Prev: Trainee GP Teeside VTS; SHO (Psychiat.) Lond. Hosp.; Ho. Phys. W. Middlx. Hosp.

TEMPLE, Professor Sir John Graham Wharncliffe, 24 Westfield Road, Edgbaston, Birmingham B15 3QG Tel: 0121 454 2445 Fax: 0121 454 2445 Email: jgtemple@rcsed.ac.uk — MB ChB (Hons.) Liverp. 1965; MRCS Eng. LRCP Lond. 1966; FRCS Ed. 1969; FRCS Eng. 1970; ChM Liverp. 1977; F med Sci 1998; FRCP 1999; FHKCS 2001; FRACS 2002. President Royal College of Surgeons of Edinburgh; Chair, Specialist Training Authority; Examr. RCS Edin.; Prof. Surg. Birm. Univ.; Special Adviser to CMO (Postgrad. Educat.); Chairm. COPMED. Specialty: Gastroenterol.; Educat. Socs: BMA & Surgic. Res. Soc.; Roy. Soc. Med.; (Counc.) Roy. Coll. Surgs. Edin. Prev: Postgrad Dean Birm. Univ. & W. Midl. Region (1991-2000); Sen. Lect. (Surg.) Univ. Manch.; Hon. Cons. Surg. Salford AHA (T).

TEMPLE, Jonathan Mark Fraser Gwent Health Authority, Mamhilad, Pontypool NP4 0QN Email: mtemple@pha2.demon.co.uk — MB BChir Camb. 1980; DRCOG 1981; Cert. Family Plann. JCC 1982; MRCGP 1983. Regist. (Pub. Health) Gwent HA. Specialty: Pub. Health Med. Prev: GP Glynneath W. Glam.

TEMPLE, Louis Norman Department of Cellular Pathology, Epsom General Hospital, Dorking Road, Epsom KT18 7EG Tel: 01372 735735 Ext: 6085 Fax: 01372 735274 Email: louis.temple@epsomsthelier.nhs.uk — MB BS Lond. 1972 (St. Bart.) MRCS Eng. LRCP Lond. 1972; MRCPath 1985; FRCPath 1996. Cons. Cellular Pathologist, Epsom and St Helier Univ. Hosp. NHS Trust. Specialty: Histopath. Special Interest: Cervical Cytol.; Gastrointestinal Path.; Urological Path. Socs: IAP; ACP; BSCC.

TEMPLE, Margaret Eleanor (retired) Sandleford, 33 Mount Sandel Road, Coleraine BT52 1JE — MB BCh BAO Dub. 1953; DA Eng. 1956.

TEMPLE, Lady Margaret Jillian Leighton (retired) Wharncliffe, 24 Westfield Road, Edgbaston, Birmingham B15 3QG Tel: 0121 454 2445 Fax: 0121 454 2445 Email: jgtemple@rcsed.ac.uk — MB ChB Liverp. 1965 (Liverp.) FFPHM; SCMO, HOB, PCT; MRCS Eng. LRCP Lond. 1966; MFFP 1993. Prev: Med. Off. (Family Plann.) Sefton AHA.

TEMPLE, Melanie Jayne, Squadron Ldr. RAF Pierremont Unit, Department of Liaison Psychiatry, Hollyhurst Road, Darlington DL3 6HX — MB ChB Glas. 1994; MRCPsych 1999. p/t Cons. (Liaison Psychiat.) Darlington Memor. Hosp.; Cons. (Militar. Psychiat.) DCMH Catterick. Specialty: Gen. Psychiat. Prev: SpR (Gen. Psychiat.) Dept. Liaison Psychiat., Leeds Gen. Infirm.; SHO (Gen. Psychiat.) Duchess of Kent Hosp. Catterick.

TEMPLE, Nicholas Owen Thomas Tavistock and Portman NHS Trust, Tavistock Centre, 120 Belsize Lane, London NW3 5BA Tel: 020 7435 7111 Fax: 020 7447 3709 Email: ntemple@tavi-port.nhs.uk; Stanfield House, 86 Hampstead High St, London NW3 1RE Tel: 020 7794 1259 — MB ChB Bristol 1969; BSc (Hons. Anat.) Bristol 1966, MB ChB 1969; DPM Scot. 1972; FRCPsych 1991, M 1973. p/t Cons. Psychiat. Pychother.Tavistock Clin.; Chief Exec., Tavistock and Portman NHS Trust. Specialty: Psychother. Special Interest: Psychosomatic Illness. Socs: Brit. Psychoanal. Soc. Prev: Cons. Psychother. Maudsley Hosp. Lond., King's Coll. Hosp. 4 Portman Clinic Lond.

TEMPLE, Paul Ian Accident & Emergency Department, Kings Mill Centre for Health Care Services NHS Trust, Sutton-in-Ashfield NG17 4JL Tel: 01623 622515; 14 Charnwood Lane, Arnold, Nottingham NG5 6PE Tel: 0115 926 4332 — MB ChB Sheff. 1987; BSc Sheff. 1984; MRCGP 1995; DFFP 1995; Dip. IMC RCS Ed. 1995. Staff Grade (A & E) Kings Mill Centre Notts. Specialty: Accid. & Emerg. Prev: Trainee GP Mansfield VTS.

TEMPLE, Mr Robert Hartley Department of Otolaryngology, Countness of Chester Hospital, Liverpool Road, Chester CH2 1UL Tel: 01244 366374 — MB ChB Sheff. 1991; FRCS Ed. (Orl.) 1995; FRCS Ed. ORL-HNS 2000. Specialist Regist. (OtoLaryngol.) Manch.; 2003 Cons. Otolaryngolist, Countess of Chester. Specialty: Otolaryngol. Socs: Forum Mem. Roy. Soc. Med.; BAO - HNS. Prev: SHO Rotat. (Otolarnyngol.) Roy. Liverp. Hosp.

TEMPLE, Robert Mark Department of Renal Medicine, Birmingham Heartlands Hospital, Bordesley Green E., Birmingham B9 5SS Tel: 0121 424 2157 — MB ChB Birm. 1982; FRCP Ireland; MRCP (UK) 1986; MD Birm. 1992. Cons. Nephrol. Birm. Heartlands Hosp. Specialty: Nephrol.; Gen. Med. Socs: FRCP Edin.; FRCP Lond. Prev: Sen. Regist. (Nephrol.) Portsmouth; Wellcome Lect. (Med.) Univ. Edin.; Regist. (Nephrol.) Edin.

TEMPLE, Rosemary Christine Norfolk and Norwich Hospital, Brunswick Road, Norwich NR1 3SR Tel: 01603 286771 Fax: 01603 287320; 8 Montague Road, Cambridge CB4 1BX Tel: 01223 311360 — MB BS Lond. 1977; MA Camb. 1977; MRCP (UK) 1980; FRCP (UK) 1999. Cons. Endocrinol. & Diabetes Norf. & Norwich Hosp. Specialty: Gen. Med. Socs: Eur. Assn. for Study Diabetes; Brit. Diabetic Assn. Prev: SCMO (Endocrinol. & Diabetes) Norf. & Norwich Hosp.; Sen. Regist. (Endocrinol.) Addenbrooke's Hosp. Camb.; Lect. (Endocrinol. & Metab.) Lond. Hosp.

TEMPLE, Sarah Elizabeth Basement Flat, 86 Disraeli Road, London SW15 2DX — MB BChir Camb. 1986.

TEMPLE-MURRAY, Anne Pauline Upton Village Surgery, Wealstone Lane, Upton, Chester CH2 1HD Tel: 01244 382238 — BM BS Nottm. 1984; BMedSci Nottm. 1982. GP Chester Retainer Scheme. Specialty: Gen. Pract. Prev: GP Beeston, Nottm.

TEMPLETON, Professor Allan Department of Obstetrics & Gynaecology, University of Aberdeen, Foresterhill, Aberdeen AB25 2ZD Tel: 01224 550590 Fax: 01224 684880 Email: allan.templeton@abdn.ac.uk; Templeton, Knapperna House, Udny, Ellon AB41 6SA Tel: 01651 842481 — MB ChB Aberd. 1969; MRCOG 1974; FRCOG 1987, M 1974; MD (Hons.) Aberd. 1982; FMedSci 2002. Prof. O & G Univ. Aberd.; Pres., Roy. Coll. of Obst. & Gyn. Specialty: Obst. & Gyn. Socs: Brit. Fertil. Soc.; Soc. for Study of Fertil.; ESHRE. Prev: Hon. Sec. Roy. Coll. of Obst. & Gyn.; Sen. Lect. (O & G) Univ. Edin.

TEMPLETON, Andrew Martin (Surgery), 90 Emscote Road, Warwick CV34 5QJ Tel: 01926 492311; 1 Farm Road, Lillington, Leamington Spa CV32 7RP — MB BS Lond. 1967 (Univ. Coll. Hosp.) MRCS Eng. LRCP Lond. 1967; DObst RCOG 1973. Prev: Resid. Obst. Brit. Milit. Hosp. Rinteln; Garrison Med. Off. Hemer.

TEMPLETON, David James 5 Brownside Avenue, Cambuslang, Glasgow G72 8BL — MB ChB Aberd. 1995.

TEMPLETON, Hilary Margaret (retired) 73 Newberries Avenue, Radlett WD7 7EL — MB BCh Wales 1973. Prev: GP Watford.

TEMPLETON, James Douglas (retired) 72 Castlebay Court, Largs KA30 8DP Tel: 01475 673815 — MB ChB Glas. 1954 (Glasgow) FRCPsych 1982, M 1971. Prev: Cons. Psychiat. & Psychotherap. Dept. South. Gen. Hosp. Glas.

TEMPLETON, Professor John The Beeches, 170 Oulton Road, Stone ST15 8DR — (Belfast) MB BCh BAO Belf. 1961; FRCSC 1970; FRCS Eng. 1991; FRCS Glas. 1993. Emerit. Prof. Traum. Orthop. Surg. Keele Univ.; Hon. Cons. Surg. (Ortho.) Nuffield Orthopaedic Centre Oxf.; Med. Dir. Nuffield Orthopaedic Centre Oxf. Specialty: Orthop. Socs: Fell. BOA; Girdlestone Orthop. Soc. Prev: Cons. Orthop. Surg. N. Staffs. Roy. Infirm., Stoke on Trent; Dean Fac. of Health, Keele Univ.; Asst. Prof. Surg. McGill Univ. Montreal, Canada.

TEMPLETON, John Stewart (retired) 62a South St, Perth PH2 8PD — MB ChB Glas. 1957. Prev: Europ. Regional Med. Dir. A.H. Robins Co.

TEMPLETON, Lynn Margaret Clydebank Health Centre, Kilbowie Road, Clydebank G81 2TQ Tel: 0141 952 2080; 9 Sandfield Avenue, Milngavie, Glasgow G62 8NR — MB ChB Glas. 1985; MRCGP 1989.

TEMPLETON, Mr Peter Alexander Leeds General Infirmary, Great George St, Leeds LS1 3EX; 5 Lammas Court, Scarcroft, Leeds LS14 3JS — MB BCh BAO Belf. 1987 (Queen's Univeristy Belfast) FRCS (Eng) 1991; FRCS (Orth) 1996. Cons. (Trauma & Orthop.) Leeds Gen Infirm. Leeds; Sen Clin Lect. Univ. Leeds. Specialty: Trauma & Orthop. Surg.; Medico Legal.

TENANT-FLOWERS, Melinda Directorate of Sexual Health, The Caldecot Centre, King's Healthcare NHS Trust, 15-22 Caldecot Road, London SE5 9RS Tel: 020 7346 4535 Fax: 020 7346 3486 Email: melinda.tenant-flowers@kingsch.nhs.uk; 13 Hillsborough Road, London SE22 8QE Tel: 020 7735 1732 — MB BChir Camb. 1982 (Newc. u. Tyne & Camb.) BSc (Hons.) Durham. 1976; MRCPI 1987. Cons. Sexual Health Kings Healthcare Lond. Specialty: Pharmaceutical Medicine. Socs: BMA; Assn. Sexual Health Med.; Soc. Study VD. Prev: Sen. Lect. (Sexual Health Med.) Sydney Hosp., Austral.; Clin. Lect. (Genitourin. Med.) Middlx. Hosp. Lond.; Sen. Regist. (Genitourin. Med.) Westm. & St. Stephens Hosps. Lond.

TENCH, David William Park House, Manchester Mental Health Partnership, Gen. Hospital, Delaunays Road,, Manchester M8 5RL Tel: 0161 720 2421; 59 Moorfield Road, Salford, Manchester M6 7EY Tel: 0161 737 1086 — MB ChB Manch. 1984; MSc Manch. 1993, MB ChB 1984; MRCPsych. 1989. Cons. Psychiat. For The Elderly, Manch. Ment. Health Partnership. Specialty: Geriat. Psychiat. Socs: Fell. Of Manch. Med. Soc. Psychiat. Sec.; Of the Fac. of Old Age Psychiat., Roy. Coll. Of Psychiat. Prev: Sen. Regist. (Psychiat.) Withington Hosp. Manch.; Research Fell. (Psychiat.) Hope Hosp. Salford.; Cons. Psychiat. The Roy. Oldham Hosp.

TENDALL, John David 1 Hillside, London NW5 1QT — MB BS Lond. 1973.

TENG, Judy Min Hsien 28 Holne Chase, London N2 0QN — MB BS Lond. 1984; MRCP (UK) 1988. Regist. (Paediat.) St. Mary's Hosp. Lond. Specialty: Paediat. Prev: Regist. (Paediat. Neonat.) Univ. Coll. Hosp. Lond.

TENGKU ISMAIL, Tengku Saifudin Flat 1/2, 18 Cornwall St., Glasgow G41 1AQ — MB ChB Glas. 1995.

TENNANT, Allan William The Firs, Cadney Road, Howsham, Market Rasen LN7 6LA — BM Soton. 1985.

TENNANT, Barry Desmond Gloucester House Medical Center, 17 Station Road, Urmston, Manchester M41 9JS Tel: 0161 748 7115; 62 Lock Lane, Partington, Manchester M31 4PP — MB ChB Manch. 1961.

TENNANT, David North Tyneside General Hospital, Rake Lane, North Shields NE29 8NH; 6 Beechways, Durham DH1 4LG — MB ChB Ed. 1978 (Edinburgh) BSc Ed. 1975; DCH RCP Lond. 1983; MRCP (UK) 1983; FRCR 1991; Cert Med Educat 2002. Cons. Radiol. N. Tyneside Hosp. N. Shields. Specialty: Radiol. Socs: Fell. Roy. Coll. Radiol.; Brit. Inst. Radiol.; BMA. Prev: Cons. Radiol. Dryburn Hosp. Durh.

TENNANT, Francesca Dorothy Bournewood Community NHS Trust, Trust HQ, Goldsworth Park Centre, Woking GU21 3LQ Tel: 01483 728201; 16 Well Close, Horsell, Woking GU21 4PT Tel: 01483 765613 — MB ChB Liverp. 1980; DCH RCP Lond. 1988; Dip. Community Paediat. Warwick 1993. Community Med. Off. (Child Health) Bournewood Community NHS Trust; Assoc. Specialist (Paediat. Audiol.) Woking. Specialty: Community Child Health. Socs: Brit. Assn. Community Child Health; Brit. Assn. Community Drs in Audiol.

TENNANT, Nicola Jayne Tamara, 3A Duff Avenue, Elgin IV30 1QS — MB ChB Aberd. 1997.

TENNANT, Rachel Caroline Flat 2, 10 Henfield Road, London SW19 3HU — MB BS Lond. 1996.

TENNANT, Sally Jane 40 Ashmore Road, Maida Vale, London W9 3DF; 40C Ashmore Road, Maida Vale, London W9 3DF — MB BS Lond. 1993 (St Marys Hospital Medical School) FRCS 1997. Specialty: Orthop.

TENNANT, Mr William George E Floor, West Block, University Hospital, Queens Medical Centre, Nottingham NG7 2UH Fax: 0115 970 9150 Email: billt@qmcvascular.demon.co.uk — (Edinburgh) MB ChB Ed. 1982; FRCS Ed. 1987; BSc (Med. Sci.) Ed. 1979, MD 1993; FRCS (Gen.) 1994. Cons. Vasc. & Gen. Surg. Qu. Med. Centre Nottm. Specialty: Gen. Surg.; Vasc. Med.

TENNEKOON, Mahinda Forest Road Medical Centre, 354-358 Forest Road, Walthamstow, London E17 5JL Tel: 020 8520 6060 Fax: 020 8521 6505; 12B Sinnot Road, London E17 Tel: 020 8527 2512 — MB BS Ceylon 1962; DCH Eng. 1966. GP Redbridge & Waltham Forest FPC. Socs: Med. Protect. Soc. Prev: Regist. (Paediat.) Whipps Cross Hosp. Lond.; SHO (Med.) Barking Hosp.; SHO (Paediat., Neurol. & Rheumat.) Princess Alex. Hosp. Harlow.

TENNEKOON, Milinda Satyajith South Street Surgery, 83 South Street, Bishop's Stortford CM23 3AP — MB BS Lond. 1991; MRCGP 1995.

TENNENT, Thomas Duncan St George's Hospital, Orthopaedic Department, Blackshaw Road, London SE17 0QT Tel: 020 8725 2032 — MB BS Lond. 1992 (St. Bart's Hosp.) BSc (Hons) Essex 1987; FRCS (Eng) 1996; FRCS (Tr. & Orth.) 2001. Cons. St Geo. Hosp. Lond. Specialty: Trauma & Orthop. Surg. Socs: Brit. Orthopaedic Assn.; Brit. Elbow & Shoulder Soc.; RCS (Eng.).

TENNENT, Thomas Gavin Church Farm, Church Lane, Harwell, Didcot OX11 0EZ — BM BCh Oxf. 1961; DPM Eng. 1967; DM Oxf. 1970; FRCPsych 1979, M 1971.

TENNET, Hilary Mary 39A Malone Park, Belfast BT9 6NL — MB BCh BAO NUI 1973.

TENTERS, Michael Teodors The Surgery, Park Lane, Stubbington, Fareham PO14 2JP Tel: 01329 664231 Fax: 01329 664958 — MB BS Lond. 1983; BSc (Hons.) (Physiol.) Lond. 1980, MB BS 1983; MRCOG 1986; MRCGP 1988. Specialty: Gen. Pract.

TEO, Andrew Chien Wei 11 Celandine Court, Yateley GU46 6LP — MB BS Lond. 1992.

TEO, Cuthbert Eng-Swee Department of Forensic Medicine, Guy's Hospital, London SE1 9RT Tel: 020 7407 0378 Fax: 020 7403 7292 — MB BS Singapore 1988; MB BC Singapore 1988; DMJ (Path.) Soc. Apoth. Lond. 1993. Hon. Clin. & Research Assoc. (Forens. Med.) UMDS Lond. Specialty: Forens. Path. Socs: Brit. Acad. Forens. Sci.; Assn. Police Surg.

TEO, Ho Teck Ho Tit Christopher 73 Brynland Avenue, Bishopston, Bristol BS7 9DZ — MB ChB Glas. 1979.

TEO, Hong-Giap Trafford General Hospital, Moorside Road, Manchester M41 5SL Tel: 0161 748 4022; Apartment 24, Whitworth House, 53 Whitworth St, Manchester M1 3WS Tel: 0161 236 7523 — MB ChB Sheff. 1995 (Sheffield University) SHO (Gen. Med.) Trafford Gen. Hosp. Moorside Rd. Manch. Specialty: Gen. Med. Socs: Med. Protec. Soc.

TEO, Hoon Seong Department of Anaesthetics, West Suffolk Hospital, Hardwick Lane, Bury St Edmunds IP33 2QZ; 107 Dudley Road, Manchester M16 8BW — MB ChB Bristol 1991.

TEO, Nee Beng Flat 23, Forrestburn Court, Monkscourt Avenue, Airdrie ML6 0JS — MB ChB Glas. 1994.

TEO, Swee Guan 79 Burgoyne Road, London N4 1AB — MB BS New South Wales 1996 (The University of New South Wales,

Australia) MB BS (1st Cl. Hons) New South Wales 1996; BSc Med. 1996. SHO (Med.) The Whittington Hosp. Lond. Specialty: Gen. Med.

TEO, Mr Tiew-Chong The Queen Victoria Hospital, Holtye Road, East Grinstead RH19 3DZ Tel: 01342 410210 Fax: 01342 315512; 3 Meridian Way, East Grinstead RH19 3GB Tel: 01342 410210 — MB ChB Aberd. 1982; FRCS Ed. 1987; MD (Hons.) Aberd. 1991; FRCS (Plast) 1995. Sen. Regist. (Plastic Surg.) Qu. Vict. Hosp. E. Grinstead. Specialty: Plastic Surg. Socs: Med. Protec. Soc. Prev: Sen. Regist. St. Thos. Hosp. Lond.; Regist. Wexham Pk. Hosp. Slough; Research Fell. Harvard Univ. Boston, USA.

TEODORCZUK, Andrew Michael 72 Mallard Pl, Twickenham TW1 4SR — MB ChB Ed. 1997.

TEOH, Chia-Meng Flat 10, 6 Riverview Place, Glasgow G5 8EB — MB ChB Ed. 1994.

TEOH, Leok-Kheng Kristine — MB BChir Camb. 1991; BA Camb. 1988; FRCS Eng. 1996. Specialist Regist. (Cardiothoracic Surg.) W. Lond. Rotat.

TEOH, Robin Elizabeth Araburn, 29 Cranwells Park, Bath BA1 2YD — MB ChB Bristol 1980; DA Eng. 1984; MRCGP 1986; DRCOG 1986. Prev: Lect. (Primary Care Med.) Malaysia; Med. Off. Leics. Hospice.; GP in Singapore.

TEOH, Siew Koon 44 Clarence Terrace, Regents Park, London NW1 4RD — MB BS Lond. 1982. SHO (Med.) (Rotat.) Camb. HA.

TEOH, Tiong Ghee St Marys Hospital, Dept of Obstetrics & Gynaecology, Praed St, London W2 1NY Tel: 020 7886 6691 Fax: 020 7886 2169; 3A Victoria Grove Mews, Notting Hill, London W2 4LN — MB BCh BAO NUI 1987; LRCPSI 1987; MRCOG 1992; MRCPI 1993; MD 1996. Cons. (Obst & Gyn.) St Marys Hosp. Lond. Specialty: Obst. & Gyn. Socs: RSM; Soc. for Matern. and Foetal Med. Prev: Serv. Dir. Obst.

TEOH, Yee Ping Trust Office, Law Hospital NHS Trust, Carluke ML8 5ER — MB BS Melbourne 1996.

TEOH, Yin Yin 76 Hawthorn Avenue, Glasgow G61 3NQ — MB BCh BAO Belf. 1993.

TEOTIA, Narendra Pal Singh Mill Lane Surgery, 135 Mill Lane, Chadwell Heath, Romford RM6 6RS Tel: 020 8599 6835 Fax: 020 8983 8063 — MB BS Lucknow 1969.

TEPER, Emma Lucy — MB BS Lond. 1998.

TEPPER, Rachel (retired) 1a Hanover Gardens, Salford, Manchester M7 4FQ Tel: 0161 795 6668 — MB ChB Manch. 1940. Prev: Clin. Med. Off. N. Manch. HA.

TERIBA, Aderemi Hakeem Health Services Department, University of Lagos, Lagos, Nigeria; 3 Wareham House, Fentiman Road, London SW8 1AZ — MB BS Ibadan 1972; MMedSci (Gen. Pract.) Leeds 1988; MRCGP 1989. Director (Health Serv.) Univ. Lagos. Prev: SHO (Paediat.) E. Birm. Hosp.; SHO (Geriat.) Newc. Gen. Hosp.

TERLESKI, Michelle Jane Tywyu, Yr Ala, Pwllheli LL53 5BN — MB BS Lond. 1981; BSc Lond. 1978, MB BS Lond. 1981; MRCGP 1986. Freelance GP. Prev: GP BasCh. Shewsbury; Trainee GP Shrewsbury VTS; Ho. Surg. Char. Cross Hosp.

TERLEVICH, Ana 1 Bradrushe Fields, Cambridge CB3 0DW — MB ChB Bristol 1997.

TERNENT, Thomas Culcheth Surgery, Thompson Avenue, Culcheth, Warrington WA3 4EB Tel: 01925 765101 Fax: 01925 765102 — MB ChB Manch. 1966; DObst RCOG 1968; DIH Eng. 1978.

TERRELL, Clare (retired) Manor House, Alderton, Woodbridge IP12 3BL Tel: 01394 411334 — (Univ. Coll. Hosp.) MB BS Lond. 1960; DCH Eng. 1966; DMRT Eng. 1968; FFR 1972. Cons. Palliat. Med. Guy's Hosp. Lond. Prev: Med. Dir. St. Eliz. Hospice Ipswich.

TERRELL, Emily Sarah 19 Springfield, Kegworth, Derby DE74 2DP — BM Soton. 1997.

TERRELL, Helen Mary 52 Midsummer Road, Snodland ME6 5RP — MB ChB Birm. 1994.

TERRELL, John Davidson (retired) 47 Longlands Road, Carlisle CA3 9AE Tel: 01228 525986 Fax: 01228 525986 — (Univ of Glas) DCH Eng. 1956; MB ChB Glas. 1951, DPH 1957; FFCM 1981, M 1973. Prev: DMO W. Cumbria Health Auth.

TERREROS BERRUETE, Orlando 47 Vicarage Gardens, Scunthorpe DN15 7BA — LMS Basque Provinces 1988.

TERRILL, Lisa Maria Stone Cottage, 12 High Road, Manthorpe, Grantham NG31 8NG — MB BS Lond. 1991.

TERRIS, Alexander James McDonnell Dr Terris and Partners, The Hart Surgery, York Road, Henley-on-Thames RG9 2DR Tel: 01491 843200 Fax: 01491 411296; Harpsden Gate, Harpsden Way, Henley-on-Thames RG9 1NS Tel: 0149157 574691 — MB BS Lond. 1968 (St. Mary's) MRCP (UK) 1971. GP Princip. Hart Pract. Henley Oxon.; Med. Off. Shiplake Coll. Prev: Med. Off. Shiplake Coll.; Regist. (Med.) Amersham Hosp.; SHO (Neurol.) Soton. Gp. Hosps.

TERRIS, Mark Grampian University Hospital Trust, Aberdeen Royal Infirmary, Foresthill, Aberdeen AB25 2YA; 63 Clifton Road, Aberdeen AB24 4RN — MB ChB Aberd. 1998; MB ChB Aberd 1998. SHO.(Med Paediat.) Roy Aberd Childr Hosp. Specialty: Paediat. Prev: HO. (Gen Surg & Orthop.); HO. (Rheum & Cardio.).

TERRY, Anne Elizabeth Ashurst, 5 Appold St, London EC2A 2HA — MB BS Lond. 1991; DRCOG 1995. Specialty: Gen. Pract.

TERRY, Catherine Margaret Twin Oaks Medical Centre, Ringwood Road, Bransgore, Christchurch BH23 8AD Tel: 01425 672741 Fax: 01425 674333 — BM Soton. 1984; BSc Soton. 1968; MSc Surrey 1971; DGM RCP Lond. 1987; DRCOG 1988; Cert. Family Plann. JCC 1988; DFFP 1993. Specialty: Gen. Pract. Socs: Brit. Med. Acupunct. Soc.; BMA. Prev: SHO (A & E) Roy. Hants. Co. Hosp. Winchester.

TERRY, Dennis Arthur 41 High Street, Colney Heath, St Albans AL4 0NS Tel: 01727 565 — MB BS Lond. 1964 (Univ. Coll. Hosp.) MRCS Eng. LRCP Lond. 1964; DPM Eng. 1974; MRCPsych 1976.

TERRY, Diana Margaret Susan Sir Humphry Davy Department Anaesthesia, Bristol Royal Infirmary, Bristol BS2 8HW Tel: 0117 928 2163 Fax: 0117 928 2098 Email: diana.terry@ubht.swest.nhs.uk — MB BS Lond. 1975 (King's Coll. Hosp.) FFA RCSI 1979; FFA RCS Eng. 1980. p/t Cons. Anaesth. Bristol Roy. Infirm. Specialty: Anaesth. Special Interest: Dent. Anaesth.; Orthopaedic Anaesth.; Resusitation Train. Socs: (Counc.) Assn. Dent. Anaesth.; (Counc.) Soc. Analgesia and Anxiety Control in Dent. (SAAD); Resusc. Counc. UK. Prev: Sen. Regist. (Anaesth.) Middlx. Hosp. Lond.

TERRY, Elizabeth Juliet Lawnside, Ridgeway Moor, Ridgeway, Sheffield S12 3XW — MB ChB Manch. 1985; DRCOG 1988; MRCGP 1990. GP Retainer Sothall Med. Centre Sheff. Prev: Trainee GP Linton Cambs. VTS.; SHO (Paediat.) Hinchingbrooke Hosp. Huntingdon; SHO (O & G) Rosie Matern. Hosp. Camb.

TERRY, Gordon 'Westaways', Lowes Barn Bank, Durham DH1 3QP — MB BS Durh. 1966; FRCP Lond. 1982, M 1970; FRCP Ed. 1985. Cons. Phys. Bishop Auckland Gen. Hosp.; Hon. Clin. Lect. Univ. Newc. Specialty: Gen. Med. Socs: Brit. Cardiac Soc. Prev: Cons. Phys. Dryburn Hosp. Durh.; Sen. Regist. (Med.) Newc. Univ. Gp. Hosps.; Regist. (Med. & Cardiol.) Aberd. Roy. Infirm.

TERRY, Helen Jane Department of Elderly Medicine, St. Luke's Hospital, Bradford — BM BCh Oxf. 1986; MA Camb. 1987; MRCP (UK) 1989. Cons. Geritrician, Bradford Hosp.s NHS Trust, Bradford. Specialty: Care of the Elderly; Gen. Med. Prev: Sen. Regist. (Geriat. & Gen. Med.) & Regist. (Gen. Med.) Univ. Hosp. Nottm.; SHO (Gen. Med.) Univ. Hosp. Nottm.; Sen. Regist. (Geriat. & Gen. Med.) St. Jas. Hosp., Leeds.

TERRY, Jack 4 Bennett's Copse, Wood Drive, Chislehurst BR7 5SG Tel: 020 8467 7271 — MB BS Lond. 1951 (King's Coll. Hosp.) MRCS Eng. LRCP Lond. 1951.

TERRY, Julia Marion Park Surgery, Hursley Road, Chandlers Ford, Eastleigh SO53 2ZH — MB BS Lond. 1991 (The Royal Lond. Hosp.) BSc (Hons.) (Path.) 1988; FRCS Eng. 1995; MRCGP 1999; DFFP 1999. GP, Chandlers Ford, Hants. Prev: GP Locum, W.Sussex; GP Regist. The Med. Centre, Cawley Rd., Chichester.

TERRY, Kathryn Jane 1 Complins, Holybourne, Alton GU34 4EH — MB BS Lond. 1994.

TERRY, Patrick Michael St Quintin Aldermoor Surgery, Aldermoor Close, Southampton SO16 5ST Tel: 02380 241000 Fax: 02380 241010 — MB BS Lond. 1980; MRCOG 1986; MRCOG 1986; T (M) 1991; T(M) 1991; T(GP) 1994; MFFP 1994; MFFP 1994; MRCGP 1994; T (GP) 1994; MRCGP 1994. Princip. Gen. Pract. Specialty: Gen. Pract.

TERRY, Paula Miriam — MB ChB Manch. 1991; DA (UK) 1995; DIMC-RCS Edin. 1999; FRCS (A&E) Edin. 1999. Specialist Regist., Emerg. Med., Hope Hosp.; Med. Director, Gtr. Manch. Co. Fire Serv. Specialty: Accid. & Emerg.; Gen. Med.; Intens. Care.

TERRY, Mr Peter Brian 60 Forest Road, Aberdeen AB15 4BP Tel: 01224 317560 — MD Ed. 1987; MB ChB 1976; FRCS Ed. 1981. Cons. & Hon. Sen. Lect. (O & G) Aberd. Matern. Hosp. Specialty:

Obst. & Gyn. Prev: Sen. Lect. & Hon. Cons. (O & G) Aberd. Matern. Hosp.; Sen. Regist. (O & G) Aberd. Matern. Hosp.; Regist. (O & G) Dudley Rd. Hosp. Birm.

TERRY, Robert Sidney (retired) Mill Cottage, Gladestry, Kington HR5 3NY — MB BS Lond. 1960 (Guy's) Asst. Gen. Practitioner Prev: Paediat. Ho. Phys. Worcester Roy. Infirm.

TERRY, Robin Eric Richmond House Surgery, Richmond Terrace, Station Road, Whitchurch SY13 1RH Tel: 01948 662870 — MB ChB Birm. 1975; DRCOG 1979; MPhil 2000.

TERRY, Roger Walter Patrick (retired) The Ledges, Redbrook Road, Monmouth NP25 3LZ Tel: 01600 715725 — MB ChB Birm. 1967. Prev: Regist. (Orthop.) S. Warks. Hosp. Gp.

TERRY, Mr Roland Mark Princess Royal University Hospital, ENT Department, Farnborough Common, Orpington BR6 8ND — MB BS Lond. 1978; FRCS Eng. 1982. Cons. ENT. Surg. Specialty: Otorhinolaryngol. Special Interest: Head & Neck Cancer; Thyroid & Salivary Gland Surg. Socs: Fell. Roy. Soc. Med.; Brit. Assn. Otol. Head & Neck Surg. Prev: Sen. Regist. Yorks RHA; Research Fell. Univ. Leeds.

TERRY, Roland Mervyn Stanley (retired) 7 Tower Close, Orpington BR6 0SP — MB Calcutta 1944; DMRD Eng. 1950.

TERRY, Susan Hazel (retired) 47 Mill Lane, Dorridge, Solihull B93 8NN — MRCS Eng. LRCP Lond. 1965 (St. Mary's) MRCOG 1971, DObst 1966; DPM Eng. 1975. Prev: Cons. Adult Ment. Handicap Coventry, N. Warks. & S. Warks. HAs.

TERRY, Sydney Walter Wellington (retired) 67 Minster Way, Bath BA2 6RJ Tel: 01225 466430 — MB BS Madras 1941; DTM & H Eng. 1947; DPH Lond. 1948; MFCM 1972. Prev: SCM Wilts. AHA.

TERRY, Mr Timothy Robin Leicester General Hospital, Gwendolen Road, Leicester LE5 4450 Tel: 0116 258 4450 — MRCS Eng. LRCP Lond. 1975 (King's Coll. Lond. & St. Geo.) BSc (Hons.) Lond. 1972, MS 1987, MB BS 1975; FRCS Eng. 1980. Cons. Urol. & Hon. Clin. Tutor Leicester Univ. Hosps. Specialty: Urol. Socs: Brit. Assn. Urol. Surgs.; Corres. Mem. Amer. Urol. Assn. Prev: Sen. Regist. Leeds Univ. Hosps.; Regist. Rotat. (Urol.) Char. Cross Hosp. Lond. & Eastbourne Hosp.; Wellcome Surg. Research Regist. Profess. Surg. Unit St. Geo. Hosp. Lond.

TERVIT, Nicola Margaret — MB ChB Glas. 1994. Specialty: Obst. & Gyn.

TESCHKE, Caroline Jean 20 Manor Farm Road, Dorchester-on-Thames, Oxford OX10 7HX — MB BS Newc. 1979; BA (Hons.) Lond. 1968; MRCP (UK) 1985.

TESFAYE, Solomon Royal Hallamshire Hospital, Floor P, Glossop Road, Sheffield S10 2JF Tel: 0114 271 2709 Fax: 0114 271 3708; 4 Cherry Tree Road, Sheffield S11 9AA Tel: 0114 250 7696 — MB ChB Bristol 1984 (Bristol University Medical School) MRCP (UK) 1988; MD Bristol 1994; FRCP 2001. Hon. Sen. Clin. Lect. Univ. of Sheff. Specialty: Diabetes; Gen. Med. Socs: Brit. Diabetic Assn.; BMA; Internat. Diabetes Federat. Prev: Cons. Phys. & Diabetol. Roy. Hallamsh. Hosp. Sheff./ Hon. Sen. Clin. Lect. (Univ. of Sheff.); Sen. Regist. (Diabetes & Endocrinol.) Roy. Liverp. Hosp.; Research Regist. (Diabetes) Roy. Hallamsh. Hosp. Sheff.

TESFAYOHANNES, Mr Biniam Northern General Hospital NHS Trust, Herries Road, Sheffield S5 7AU Tel: 0114 243 4343 Fax: 0114 256 0472 — MB ChB Sheff. 1982; FRCS Ed. 1988; FFAEM 1994. Cons. A & E N. Gen. Hosp. NHS Trust Sheff. Specialty: Accid. & Emerg.

TESH, Anne Elizabeth Christina Bridge Farm, Sweffling, Saxmundham IP17 2BA — MB ChB Sheff. 1995.

TESH, Dorothy Eileen (retired) 20 Hillgrove Crescent, Kidderminster DY10 3AP — MB ChB Birm. 1965; MRCPsych 1984. Prev: Cons. (Ment. Handicap) Lea Castle Hosp. Kidderminster.

TESTA, Professor Humberto Juan The Alexandra Hospital, Mill Lane, Cheadle SK8 2PX Tel: 0161 428 3656 Fax: 0161 491 3867; 27 Barcheston Road, Cheadle SK8 1LJ Tel: 0161 428 6873 — MD Buenos Aires 1979; Medico 1962; PhD Manch. 1972; FRCP Lond. 1986; FRCR 1988. Cons. (Nuclear Med.) Priv. Pract. The Alexandra Hosp. Cheadle. Specialty: Nuclear Med.

TETLEY, Giles Holdenhurst Road Surgery, 199 Holdenhurst Road, Bournemouth BH8 8DF Tel: 01202 558337 — MB BS Lond. 1972 (Univ. Coll. Hosp.) DObst RCOG 1974; DA Eng. 1975; FFA RCS Eng. 1977. Specialty: Anaesth. Prev: Regist. (Anaesth.) Roy. Berks. Hosp. Reading; SHO (Paediat.) Northampton Gen. Hosp.

TETLOW, Stanley 3 Highbury Close, Springwell, Gateshead NE9 7PU Tel: 0191462532 — MB BS Durh. 1958. Prev: Ho. Phys. & Ho. Surg. Roy. Vict. Infirm. Newc.

TETSTALL, Ann Philippa Rivermead Gate Medical Centre, 123 Rectory Lane, Chelmsford CM1 1TR Tel: 01245 348688 Fax: 01245 458800 — MB BS Lond. 1978; MRCP (UK) 1981.

TETTENBORN, Michael Adrian Frimley Children's Centre, Church Road, Frimley, Camberley GU16 7AD Tel: 01483 782861 Fax: 01483 782999 Email: mike.tettenborn@shb-tr.nhs.uk — MB ChB Bristol 1971; DCH Eng. 1973; DRCOG 1976; FRCP Lond. 1994; FRCPCH 1996. Cons. Child Health Blackwater Valley and Hants PCT and Frimley Pk. Hosp. NHS Trust. Specialty: Paediat. Prev: Cons. (Child Health) Eastbourne & Co. NHS Trust; Sen. Regist. (Paediat.) Guy's Hosp. Lond.; Regist. (Paediat.) John Radcliffe Hosp. Oxf.

TETTMAR, Richard Eden (retired) Chelmsford Public Health Laboratory, New Writtle St., Chelmsford CM2 0YX — MB BS Lond. 1972 (Lond. Hosp.) MRCS Eng. LRCP Lond. 1972; DPath Eng. 1977; FRCPath 1991, M 1979.

TEUNISSE, Frank Surgery Gord, Levenwick, Shetland ZE2 9HX Tel: 01950 422240; Glenlea, Southpunds, Levenwick, Shetland ZE2 9HX Tel: 01950 422427 — Artsexamen Amsterdam 1988; Artsexamen Free Univ Amsterdam 1988; MRCGP 1993; T(GP) 1993. Prev: Trainee GP Inverness.

TEUTEN, Anthony Robert (retired) 5 Beaufort Road, Ealing, London W5 3EB Tel: 020 8997 2884 — (St. Mary's) MB BS Lond. 1949. Prev: GP Lond.

TEVERSON, Eric Fern House Surgery, 125-129 Newland Street, Witham CM8 1BH Tel: 01376 502108 Fax: 01376 502281; Barnardiston House, 35 Chipping Hill, Witham CM8 2DE Tel: 01376 502266 — MB BS Lond. 1978; DRCOG 1982. Prev: GP Kings Lynn VTS; Ho. Phys. Kingston Hosp.; Ho. Surg. Lond. Hosp.

TEW, Christopher John Lister Hospital, Coreys Mill Lane, Stevenage SG1 4AB Tel: 01438 314333 Fax: 01438 781147 — MB BS Lond. 1976; BSc Lond. 1973, MB BS 1976; MRCP (UK) 1982; MRCPath 1985; FRCP (London) 2000. Cons. Haemat. Lister Hosp. Stevenage. Specialty: Haematology. Prev: Lect. (Haemat.) Char. Cross & Westm. Med. Sch. Lond.; Sen. Regist. (Haemat.) W.m. Hosp. Lond.; Regist. (Gen. Med.) Redhill Gen. Hosp.; Regist. (Haemat.) St. Bart. Hosp. Lond. Regist. (Haemat.) St. Bart. Hosp. Lond.

TEW, David Neil Princess Margaret Hospital, Okus Road, Swindon SN1 4JU — MB BS Lond. 1984; FRCA. 1989.

TEW, Elizabeth The Windsor Road Surgery, Windsor Road, Garstang, Preston PR3 1ED Tel: 01995 603350 Fax: 01995 601301; Blencathra, Cabus Nook Lane, Cabus, Preston PR3 1AA Tel: 01524 791146 — MB BS Newc. 1972; DCCH RCP Ed. 1984. GP Garstang. Socs: Fac. Fam. Plann. & Reproduc. Health Care. Prev: Ho. Surg. & Ho. Phys. Newc. Gen. Hosp.; Trainee GP Newc. VTS.

TEW, Jeremy Simon Touraj Westminster And Pimlico General Practice, 15 Denbigh Street, London SW1V 2HF Tel: 020 7834 6969 Fax: 020 7931 7747 — MB BS Lond. 1992.

TEW, John Anthony The Windsor Road Surgery, Windsor Road, Garstang, Preston PR3 1ED Tel: 01995 603888 Fax: 01995 601301; Blencathra, Cabus Nook Lane, Cabus, Preston PR3 1AA Tel: 01524 791146 — MB BS Newc. 1972; MRCGP 1976. Hosp. Pract. (Psychiat.) Roy. Preston Hosp. Specialty: Gen. Pract. Prev: Trainee Gen. Pract. Newc. Vocational Train. Scheme; Ho. Surg. & Ho. Phys. Newc. Gen. Hosp.

TEW, Josephine Hewgill 94 Inkerman Street, Luton LU1 1JD Tel: 01582 415381; Ansley House, Woburn, Milton Keynes MK17 9PU Tel: 01525 290656 — BM BCh Oxf. 1952 (St. Bart.) DCH Eng. 1958. Specialty: Paediat. Socs: Brit. Paediat. Assn. & Soc. Pub. Health. Prev: SCMO Beds. HA; Ho. Phys. St. Martin's Hosp. Bath & SHO Roy. United Hosp. Bath; Ho. Surg. (Obst.) City of Lond. Matern. Hosp.

TEW, Robert Patrick Limeleigh Medical Group, 434 Narborough Road, Leicester LE3 2FS Tel: 0116 282 7070 Fax: 0116 289 3805 — MB ChB Leic. 1988.

TEWARI, Rohini Mira 19 Station Road, Cippenham, Slough SL1 6JJ — MB BS Lond. 1993.

TEWARI, Sidhartha Lea Castle, Wolverley, Kidderminster DY10 3PP Tel: 01562 850461 — MB BS Ranchi 1982; Dip. Psychiat. Ed. 1991; MRCPsych 1992. Cons. Psychiat. Worcs. Specialty: Ment. Health.

TEWARI, Sushil Kumar 87 St Albans Avenue, Hartshead, Ashton-under-Lyne OL6 8XN Tel: 0161 339 9547 — MB BS Jiwaji 1970. Specialty: Orthop.

TEWARI, Vinod Kumar Trentham Road Surgery, 37 Trentham Road, Kirkby, Liverpool L32 4UB Tel: 0151 546 3711 Fax: 0151 548 4265 — MB BS Banaras Hindu 1971; MD (Dip. Clinic Hypnosia) Sheff. Gen. Practitioner with Cardiol. interest; Private for Acupunc. and Hypn. in Kirkby, Liverp. L32 4UB. Socs: BMA; IMA UK; Brit. Med. and Dent. Hypnotic Soc.

TEWARY, Mr Ashok Kumar Walsall Hospital Trust, Moat Road, Walsall WS2 9PS — FRCS; MS Panjab; MB BS Panjab 1978; FRCS Ed. 1988; FRCS Eng. 1990. Specialty: Otolaryngol.

TEWSON, Edward Timothy Cayley, GM (retired) The Manor, Ickford, Aylesbury HP18 9HS Tel: 01844 339255 — BM BCh Oxf. 1951; DObst RCOG 1953. Prev: Ho. Phys. Radcliffe Infirm. Oxf.

TEWSON, Gillian Rosemary The Surgery, Norwich Road, Saxlingham Nethergate, Norwich NR15 1TP Tel: 01508 499208; Skeets Hill Farm House, Shotesham St Mary, Norwich NR15 1UR — MB BS Lond. 1980; DRCOG 1983; MRCGP 1985.

TEWSON, Jocelyn Manor, Ickford, Aylesbury HP18 9HS Tel: 01844 339255 — MB BS Lond. 1949; DCH Eng. 1954; MRCGP 1975. Prev: Sen. Ho. Phys. Churchill Hosp. Oxf.; Paediat. Ho. Phys. & Surgic. Ho. Surg. Radcliffe Infirm. Oxf.

TEWSON, Penelope Jane Hall Farm House, High St., Great Abington, Cambridge CB1 6AE — MB BS Lond. 1968 (Roy. Free) DObst RCOG 1970; DCH Eng. 1971. GP Linton Cambs. Prev: Regist. (Paediat.) P.s Margt. Hosp. Swindon; SHO (Paediat.) Radcliffe Infirm. Oxf.; Ho. Phys. Roy. Free Hosp.

THA, Zan Crabbs Cross Surgery, 38 Kenilworth Close, Crabbs Cross, Redditch B97 5JX Tel: 01527 544610 Fax: 01527 540286 — MB BS Med. Inst. (I) Rangoon 1973 (Rangoon, Burma) ECFMG (USA) 1979; DRCOG 1981; MRCGP 1981; DCCH RCP Ed. 1984; MICGP 1985. Princip. GP Crabbs Cross Surg. Redditch. Socs: BMA; Burmese Doctors Assn.

THACKER, Andrew Jonathan 168 Causeway Green Road, Oldbury, Oldbury B68 8LJ — MB ChB Birm. 1988; ChB Birm. 1988. SHO (A & E) Dudley Rd. Hosp. Birm. Prev: Ho. Off. Sandwell Dist. Gen. Hosp.; Ho. Off. Gen. Hosp. Birm.

THACKER, Betty Victoria 24 Rugby Close, Newcastle ST5 3JN — MB ChB Birm. 1955; MRCS Eng.; LRCP Lond. 1955; DObst. RCOG 1957; DA Eng. 1958; FFA RCS Eng. 1961. Cons. Anaesth. Stoke-on-Trent Gp. Hosps. Specialty: Anaesth. Socs: BMA. Prev: Regist. (Anaesth.) United Birm. Hosps.; Sen. Regist. (Anaesth.) Roy. Hosp. Wolverhampton; Cons. Anaesth. Dudley Rd. Hosp. Birm.

THACKER, Bharat Gunvantray The Consulting Rooms, Oxhey Drive, South Oxhey, Watford WD19 7RU Tel: 020 8459 5550; 59 Morley Crescent E., Stanmore HA7 2LG — MB ChB Glas. 1989; DRCOG 1991; Cert. Family Plann. JCC 1992; MRCGP 1993. Clin. Asst. Willesden Gen. Hosp. Specialty: Cardiol. Socs: BMA. Prev: Trainee GP Paisley; Trainee GP Rendrewsh. VTS; Ho. Off. (Surg.) Dumfries & Galloway Hosp. Ho. Off. (Med.) Roy. Aberd. Hosp.

THACKER, Mr Charles Robert 15 Bincleaves Road, Weymouth DT4 8RS Tel: 01305 785891 — MB BS Lond. 1974 (St. Mary's) MRCS Eng. LRCP Lond. 1974; FRCS Eng. 1979. Cons. Orthop. Surg. W. Dorset Gen. Hosps. NHS Trust. Specialty: Orthop. Socs: Fell. BOA; BMA. Prev: Sen. Regist. (Orthop. & Trauma) Soton. & Portsmouth HAs; Regist. (Surg.) St. Mary's & Qu. Alexandra Hosp. Portsmouth; SHO (Orthop. & Trauma) Roy. United Hosp. Bath.

THACKER, Elizabeth Julie Royal Cornwall Hospital, Treliske, Truro TR1 3LJ; Helnoweth Farm, Gulval, Penzance TR20 8YP — MB BS Lond. 1985. Staff Grade (Nephrol.) Renal Unit. Roy. Cornw. Hosp. Truro. Specialty: Nephrol.

THACKER, Justin Gray McDougall 15 Rowcroft, Hemel Hempstead HP1 2JF — MB ChB Ed. 1992; MRCOG 1994; MRCP (UK) 1996; DTM & H 1998. SHO (Paediat. Surg.) Edin. Specialty: Paediat. Socs: Med. & Dent. Defence Union Scotl. Prev: SHO (Med. Paediat.) Edin.

THACKER, Michael Puttrell Arnewood Practice, Milton Medical Centre, Avenue Road, New Milton BH25 5JP Tel: 01425 620393 Fax: 01425 624219; Far Forest, South Drive, Ossemsley, New Milton BH25 5TN — MB BS Lond. 1972 (Westm.) MRCS Eng. LRCP Lond. 1972; MRCGP 1977; FRCGS 2002. Prev: Trainee GP Bournemouth & Poole VTS; Ho. Surg. Westm. Hosp. Lond.; Ho. Phys. Gen. Hosp. Nottm.

THACKER, Richard Henry Lister House Surgery, 35 The Parade, St Helier JE2 3QQ Tel: 01534 36336 Fax: 01534 35304; Melrose, St. Clement Inner Road, St Helier, Jersey JE2 6QP Tel: 01534 35285 Fax: 01534 25659 — MRCS Eng. LRCP Lond. 1965; LMCC Canada 1970; DObst 1970. Prev: GP Squamish BC, Canada; Flight Lt. RAF Med. Br.

THACKER, Sarah Lucia 225 Broad Lane, Coventry CV5 7AQ — MB BS Lond. 1990.

THACKER, Simon John Marazion Surgery, Gwallon Lane, Marazion TR17 0HW Tel: 01736 710505 Fax: 01736 711205 Email: simon.thacker@marazion.cornwall.nhs.uk; Helnoweth Farm, Gulval, Penzance TR20 8YP — MB BS Lond. 1985; DCH RCP Lond. 1988.

THACKER, Simon Philip Derby City General Hospital, Uttoxeter Road, Derby DE22 3NE Tel: 01332 625553; 5 Hardy Close, Barton under Needwood, Burton-on-Trent DE13 8HG — MB ChB Birm. 1988; BSc (Hons.) Birm. 1987; MB ChB (Hons.) Birm. 1988; MRCPsych 1993; CCST 1997. Cons. (Old Age Psychiat.) Derby City Gen. Hosp. Specialty: Geriat. Psychiat. Socs: BMA; RCPsych. Prev: Sen. Regist. Rotat. (Old Age Psychiat.) Nottm.; Regist. Rotat. (Psychiat.) Birm.; SHO (Med.) Dudley Rd. Hosp. Birm.

THACKRAY, Colin Peter Rhoslan Surgery, 4 Pwllycrochan Avenue, Colwyn Bay LL29 7DA Tel: 01492 532125 Fax: 01492 530662 — MB ChB Liverp. 1982; DRCOG 1984; DGM RCP Lond. 1986; MRCGP 1987. Specialty: Gen. Pract.

THACKRAY, Jennifer Erdmuthe 24 Vincent Gardens, London NW2 7RP — MB BS Lond. 1994.

THACKRAY, Peter Oak Tree Lodge, 157 West Ella Road, Kirk Ella, Hull HU10 7RN Tel: 01482 658161 Email: 106515.1144@compuserve.com — MB BS Durh. 1962; DObst RCOG 1966; FFPM RCP (UK) 1989. Specialty: Pharmaceutical Medicine. Socs: Brit. Assn. Pharmaceut. Phys. Prev: Dir. Med. Research Europe/Africa Div. Vick Internat. Egham; Med. Supt. Wenchi Methodist Hosp., Ghana; Flight Lt. RAF Med. Br.

THACKRAY, Simon Dominic Rhodes, Maj. RAMC Castle Hill Hospital , Department of Cardiology, Cottingham Email: simonthackray@hotmail.com — MB BS Lond. 1993 (St Geos.) MRCP Lond. 1998. Specialist Regist. Yorks. Cardiol. Train. Rotat.; Lect. in Clinical Cardiol. Specialty: Cardiol. Socs: Roy. Army Med. Corps. Prev: Research Regist. (Cardio.) Univ of Hull.; Specialist Regist. PeterBoro. & Papworth Hosp.; Med. Regist. Rotat. Roy. P. Alfred Hosp. Sydney, Australia.

THACKSTONE, Stanley Irvine (retired) Cremorne, Roughcote Lane, Cookshill, Caverswall, Stoke-on-Trent ST11 9EG Tel: 01782 392561 — MB ChB Leeds 1956; MRCGP 1965. Prev: Ho. Phys. Seacroft Gen. Hosp. Leeds.

THADANI, Helen Dept of Chemical Pathology and Endocrinology, St Thomas Hospital, Lambeth Palace Rd, London SE1 7EH Tel: 020 7928 9292 Ext: 3542; 34 South Lodge Drive, Oakwood, London N14 4XP — MB BChir Camb. 1995; BSc (Hons.) Camb. 1990. Specilaist Regist. Guys & St Thomas's Hosp NHS Trust. Lond. Prev: Specialist Regist. Oxf. Deanery John Radcliffe Hosp. Oxf.; Hon. Research Regist. King's Coll. Sch. Med. & Dent. Lond.; SHO (Clin. Chem., Endocrinol. & Metab. Med.) King's Coll. Hosp. Lond.

THAIN, Alexander Buchan (retired) Castle Coach House, Inverugie, Peterhead AB42 3DN Tel: 01779 838274 — MB ChB Aberd. 1959; DObst RCOG 1966; CIH Dund 1974; MFOM RCP Lond. 1984. Prev: Head Occupat. Health ADCO Abu Dhabi, UAE.

THAIN, Annie (retired) Minfield, Pipegate, Market Drayton TF9 Tel: 0163 081418 — MB ChB Aberd. 1921; MB ChB (1st Cl. Hnrs.) Aberd. 1921. Prev: Ho. Phys. Westm. Hosp.

THAKAR, Bharati Ranee Mayday University Hospital, 530 London Road, Thornton Heath, Croydon Tel: 020 8401 3154 Fax: 020 8401 3651 Email: ranee.thakar@mayday.nhs.uk — MB BS Karnatak, India 1988; MRCOG 1994. Cons. Urogynaecologist. Socs: Fac. Fam. Plann.; Med. Protec. Soc. Prev: Clin. Research Fell. Middlx.; Regist. Mayday Univ. Hosp.; Regist. Worcester Roy. Infirm.

THAKE, Ann Isobel Smith The Laurie Pike Health Centre, 95 Birchfield Road, Handsworth, Birmingham B19 1LH Tel: 0121 554 0621 Fax: 0121 554 6163; 47 Somerville Road, Sutton Coldfield B73 6HH — MD Sheff. 1987; MB ChB 1969; DObst RCOG 1971. Lect. Dept. Gen. Pract. Birm. Univ. Prev: Clin. Asst. Genetics W. Midl. RHA.

THAKER, Chandrakant Shankerlal Burgess Road Surgery, 357a Burgess Road, Southampton SO16 3BD; 10 Spindlewood Close,

Bassett, Southampton SO16 3QD Tel: 02380 767645 — MB BS Bombay 1974 (Grant Med. Coll.) GP; Clin. Asst. (ENT) Roy. Soton. Hopsital.

THAKER, Dilesh Arrowe Park Hospital, Arrowe Park Road, Wirral CH49 5PE — MB ChB Liverp. 1998.

THAKER, Kantilal Kalidas Knowsley Medical Centre, 9-11 Knowsley St., Bury BL9 0ST Tel: 0161 764 1217 Fax: 0161 764 6155; 9 Rothbury Close, Bury BL8 2TT — MB BS Gujarat 1971.

THAKER, Pinakin Kumarbhai The Surgery, 65 Church Street, Cannock WS11 1DS — MB BS Gujarat 1971 (B.J. Med. Coll. Ahmedabad)

THAKERAR, Jayendra Gordhandas The Surgery, 192 Tudor Drive, Kingston upon Thames KT2 5QH Tel: 0208 549 9030 Fax: 0208 974 9020; Ham Clinic, Ashburnham Road, Ham, Richmond TW10 7NF Tel: 020 8940 9442 — MB BS Bombay 1971. Med. Off. Family Plann. Clinic W. Molesey. Specialty: Gen. Pract. Socs: Roy. Soc. Med.; Overseas Doctors Assn.; BMA. Prev: Clin. Asst. (Rheum.) Croydon Gen. Hosp.; Sessional Med. Off. Family Plann. Clinic Richmond.

THAKKAR, Bhalchandra Chhaganlal The Clinic, Barbers Avenue, Rawmarsh, Rotherham S62 6AD Tel: 01709 526277; 8 Broom Lane, Rotherham S60 3EL Tel: 01709 305309 Fax: 01709 305309 Email: bhal1wk@yahoo.co.uk — MB BS Calcutta 1960 (National Medical College) BSC Baroda India. B.O.C. Med. Adviser.

THAKKAR, Chandrashekhar Hirjibhai The London Hospital , Barts and the London NHS Trust, Neuro X-Ray Department, Whitechapel Road, London E1 1BB Tel: 020 7377 7000 Ext: 2434/2435 Mob: 07956 420 298 Fax: 020 7377 7165 Email: mrctuk@yahoo.co.uk; St. Bartholomew's Hospital , Barts and the London NHS Trust, Neuro X-Ray Department, Q.E. Block, Ground Floor, West Smithfield, London EC1A 7BE Tel: 020 7601 8301 Mob: 07956 420298 Fax: 020 7601 8323 — MB BS Bombay 1972; MD Bombay 1975; DMRD Lond. 1977; FRCR 1979. Cons. Radiol. The Roy. Lond. Hosp. Whitechapel,Lond.; Cons. Neuroradiol. St. Barts. Hosp. Lond.; Cons. Neuroradiol. The Lond. Imaging Centre., Lond.; Cons. Neuroradiol., The Lond. Clinic. Lond.; Cons. Neuroradiol. King Edwd. VII Hosp. Lond. Specialty: Radiol. Socs: Fell. Roy. Coll. Radiol. Prev: Cons. Neuroradiol. Bombay Hosp. India; Sen. Regist. The Lond. Hosp. Whitechapel. Lond.

THAKKAR, Mr Dushyant Hirjibai 53 Russell Road, Moor Park, Northwood HA6 2LP Tel: 01923 835638 Fax: 01923 835638 — MB BS Bombay 1972; MS (Orth.) Bombay 1974; DOrth Bombay 1974; FCPS (Orth.) Bombay 1975; MChOrth Liverp. 1978; FRCS (Trauma & Orth.) UK 2000. Cons. Orthopaedic Surg. Medway Maritime Hosp. Gillingham Kent; Staff Orthopaedic Surg., Old Ch., Essex. Socs: Overseas Fell. Brit. Orthop. Assn.; Mem. Indian Orthop. Assn. Prev: Hon. Asst. Prof. (Orthop.) Topiwala Nat. Med. Coll. Univ., Bombay; Lect. (Orthop) Univ. Sheff.; Regist. (Orthop.) Roy. Liverp. Hosp.

THAKKAR, Ila Dushyant 53 Russell Road, Northwood HA6 2LP Tel: 01923 835638 Fax: 01923 835638 — MB BS Gujarat 1976; DGO TC Dub. 1979; DA Eng. 1981; DA (UK) 1987. Gen. Practitioner, Barnet Health Auth. Specialty: Gen. Pract. Prev: Regist. (Anaesth.) Morriston Hosp. Swansea.; Regist. (Anaesth.) Northwick Pk. Hosp., Harrow & Harefiled Hosp.

THAKKER, Bishan Department of Bacteriology, Lister Building, Royal Infirmary, Castle Street, Glasgow G12 0SF Tel: 0141 211 4640 — MB ChB Ed. 1985; MRCPath 1993. Cons. Bacteriol. Roy. Infirm. Glas. Specialty: Med. Microbiol.

THAKKER, Pradumal 18 Westmorland Gardens, Peterborough PE1 5HU — MB BS Newc. 1989.

THAKKER, Professor Rajesh Vasantlal University of Oxford, Nuffield Orthopaedic Centre, Nuffield Department of Clinical Medicine, Botnar Research Centre, Headington, Oxford OX3 7LD Tel: 01865 227971 Fax: 01865 227972 Email: rajesh.thakker@ndm.ox.ac.uk — MB BChir Camb. 1981; BA 1977; MA 1981; MRCP UK 1983; FRCP Lond. 1993; MD Camb. 1994; FRCP (Ed) 1997; FRCPath 1998; FMedSci 1999. May Prof. of Med., Univ. of Oxf., Oxf., and Consulatant Phys. and Endocrinologist at John Radcliffe Hosp., Oxf.. Specialty: Endocrinol. Socs: Assn. Phys.; (Ex-Chairm.) N. Amer. Paediat. Bone & Mineral Working Gp.; Amer. Soc. of Bone & Mineral Research. Prev: Prof. Med & Cons Phy/ Endocrin & MRC Clin. Scientist ImperialColl. Sch. of Med., Lond.; Hon. Cons. Phys. (Endocrinol.) Northwick Pk. Hosp. Harrow; MRC Train. Fell. & Hon. Sen. Regist. Middlx. Hosp. Med. Sch. Lond.

THAKKER, Yogini Department of Child Health, Milton Keynes PCT, Standing Way, Eaglestone, Milton Keynes MK6 5LD — MB ChB Manch. 1982; DRCOG 1985; DCH RCP Lond. 1986; MRCP (UK) 1989. Cons. Community Paediat. Milton Keynes PCT. Specialty: Paediat.

THAKOR, Ranjit Sinh The Surgery, 2-6 Halsbury Street, Leicester LE2 1QA Tel: 0116 273 0044 Fax: 0116 249 0810; 30/32 Loughborough Road, Leicester LE4 5LD Tel: 01162 268 2727 Fax: 01162 261 1223 — MB ChB Birm. 1974 (Birmingham) DRCOG 1977; MRCGP 1978. Prev: Trainee GP Kettering Vocations Train. Scheme; Ho. Surg. Dudley Rd. Hosp. Birm.; Ho. Phys. Gen. Hosp. Birm.

THAKOR, Surendra Balwantray 8 Starfield Avenue, Littleborough OL15 0NG Tel: 01706 41409 — MB BS Gujarat 1962 (B.J. Med. Coll. Ahmedabad) DA Gujarat 1963. Hosp. Pract. (Anaesth.) Burnley, Pendle, Rossendale AHA. Prev: Clin. Asst. (Anaesth.) Burnley, Pendle, Rossendale AHA; Regist. (Anaesth.) Burnley Health Dist.

THAKORE, Jogin Hemant Academic Department of Psychological Medicine, 3rd Floor, Alexandra Wing,, The Royal London Hospital, London E1 1BB Tel: 020 7377 7344 Fax: 020 7377 7343 — MB BCh BAO Dub. 1986; MRCPsych 1993; PhD Lond. 1995. Sen. Lect. (Psychol. Med.) St. Barth. & The Roy. Lond. Sch. of Med. & Dent. Specialty: Gen. Psychiat. Socs: Inst. Soc. Psychoneuroendocrinol.; Brit. Neuroendocrine Gp.; Brit. Assn. Psychopharmacol. Prev: Lect. (Psychol. Med.) St. Bart. Hosp. Lond.

THAKORE, Mr Shobhan Bansidhar 9 Clovis Duveau Drive, Dundee DD2 5JA — MB ChB Dundee 1992; BMSc (Hons.) Dund 1989; DRCOG 1994; FRCS Ed. 1996. Specialist Regist. (A&E.) Ninewells Hosp. Dundee. Specialty: Accid. & Emerg. Prev: SHO (Intens. Care) Qu. Margt. Hosp. Dunfermline.

THAKRAR, Diviash Narendra Northwood Health Centre, Neal Close, Acre Way, Northwood HA6 1TH Tel: 01923 820844 Fax: 01923 820648 — MB BS Lond. 1993.

THAKRAR, Jayshree Prabhudas 42 Christchurch Avenue, Kenton, Harrow HA3 8NJ Tel: 020 8907 0936 — Artsexamen Utrecht 1991.

THAKRAR, Navinchandra Amarshi Holly Road Medical Centre, 2A Holly Road, Chiswick, London W4 1NU Tel: 020 8994 0976 Fax: 020 8994 3685; 34 Lea Gardens, Wembley HA9 7SE Fax: 020 8994 3685 — MB BS Bombay 1972 (Grant Med. Coll.) GP Lond.; Mem. Ealing, Hammersmith & Hounslow LMC; Sec. Overseas Doctor's Assn.

THAKRAR, Pankaj Mohanlal Havant Health Centre Suite C, PO Box 44, Civic Centre Road, Havant PO9 2AT Tel: 023 9247 4351 Fax: 023 9249 2524 — BM Soton. 1987; DCH RCP Lond. 1990; DRCOG 1991; MRCGP 1993. Prev: Trainee GP Leicester & Market HarBoro..

THAKUR, Baleshwar Plungington Road Surgery, 100 Plungington Road, Preston PR1 7UE Tel: 01772 250574 — MB BS Patna 1962. Clin. Asst. Sharoe Green Hosp. Fulwood.

THAKUR, Indra Mohan Department of Paediatrics, Darlington Memorial Hospital, Hollyhurst Road, Darlington DL3 6HX Tel: 01325 380100; 100 Cleveland Avenue, Darlington DL3 7BE Tel: 01325 281427 — MB BS Patna 1979; FRCPI 1992. Cons. Paediat. Darlington Memor. Hosp. Co. Durh. Specialty: Paediat.

THAKUR, Makhan Chandra Thakur & Partners, Silver Lane Surgery, 1 Suffolk Court, Leeds LS19 7JN Tel: 0113 250 5988 Fax: 0113 250 3298; 62 West End Lane, Horsforth, Leeds LS18 5EP Tel: 0113 258 4664 Fax: 0113 250 3298 — MB BS Gauhati 1963 (Assam Med. Coll. Dibrugarh) DPM Leeds 1972. Specialty: Geriat. Psychiat. Socs: BMA.

THAKUR, Meenakshi 498 Uxbridge Road, Pinner HA5 4SL — MB BS Lond. 1988; DCH RCP Lond. 1992; MRCGP 1993.

THAKUR, S C Speke Health Centre, North Parade, Speke, Liverpool L24 2XP Tel: 0151 486 1695.

THAKUR, Miss Shakti Birmingham & Midland Eye Centre City Hospital, Dudley Road, Birmingham — MB BS Lond. 1990 (University of London, St. George's Hospital Medical School) FRCS Ed. 1995; FRCOphth 1996. Specialist Regist. (Ophth.) W. Midl.s. Specialty: Ophth. Prev: SHO (Cas.) St. Geo. Hosp. Lond.; SHO (Ophth.) N. Middlx. Hosp. Lond. & Edgware Gen. Hosp.; SHO (Ophth.) Centr. Middx Hosp.

THALAKOTTUR, Joy Mathew Purbeck Health Centre, Purbeck, Stantonbury, Milton Keynes MK14 6BL Tel: 01908 318989 Fax: 01908 319493 — (Bangalore Medical College) MB BS Bangalore 1972; DORCP&S (Dublin) 1985; DORCS (Lond.) 1985. Gen. Med. Practitioner; Ophth. Med. Practitioner. Specialty: Ophth. Prev: Clin. Asst. Ophth.

THALANGE, Nandu Kumar Sidramappa Norfolk & Norwich University Hospital, Jenny Lind Children's Department, Colney Lane, Norwich NR4 7UY Tel: 01603 286349 Email: nandu.thalange@nnuh.nhs.uk — MB BS Lond. 1988; MRCP (UK) 1992. Cons. (Paed./Paed. Endocrin.) Norf. & Norwich Univ. Hosp. Norwich. Prev: Cons. (Paed./Paed. Endocrin.) Surrey & Sussex NHS Trust; SpR (Paed.) Addenbrooke's Hosp. Camb.; SHO (Paediat.) King's Coll. Hosp. Lond. & Southend Hosp.

THALAYASINGAM, Balasingam 16 Middlewood Road, Lanchester, Durham DH7 0HL Tel: 01207 520693; 16 Middlewood Road, Lanchester, Durham DH7 0HL — (Newc.) MB BS Durh. 1960; MRCS Eng. LRCP Lond. 1961; DObst RCOG 1964; DCH Eng. 1964; MRCP (U.K.) 1970; FRCP Ed. 1987; FRCP Lond. 1988; FRCPCH 1997. Hon. Cons., N. Durh. Univ. Hosp.; Examr. MRCP (UK) RCP of Edin. & Lond.; Examr. PLAB; Examr. R.C.P.C.H; Locum Cons. Paediat., S. Tyneside health NHS Trust, Palmers Community Hosp. Specialty: Paediat. Socs: BMA; Fell. Roy. Soc. Med. Prev: Sen. Regist. (Rheum. & Med.) City Hosp. Nottm.; Fell. (Gastroenterol.) St. Christopher's Hosp. Childr. (Temple Univ.) Philadelphia, USA; Fell. (Neonatol.) Wayne State Univ. Michigan, USA.

THALAYASINGAM, Marie Edna Laleeni Westbourne Surgery, Kelso Grove, Shiney Row, Houghton-le-Spring DH4 4RW Tel: 0191 385 2512 Fax: 0191 385 6922 — MB BS Ceylon 1971 (Peradeniya) DCH RCPS Glas. 1982; DFFP 1993. GP Princip.; W.bookne Surg. Kelso Gr. Shiney Row Tyne & Wear. Socs: BMA; MDU; DFFP. Prev: SHO (Paediat.) S. (Manch.) Health Dist. (T); Ho. Off. (Paediat.) & Ho. Off. (O & G) Gen. Hosp. Kandy, Sri Lanka.; N.ernbia Vocational Train. for Gen. Pract.

THALLER, Mr Vladimir Theodor — BM BS Nottm. 1976 (Nottingham University) FRCOphth; BMedSci 1973; FRCS Eng. 1984. Cons. Ophth. Surg. Plymouth HA. Specialty: Ophth. Socs: Fell. Roy. Coll. Ophth.; Eur. Soc. Oculoplastic & Reconstruc. Surg. Prev: Resid. & Oculoplastic Fell. Moorfields Eye Hosp.

THALLON, David Frank Edmonstone (Surgery), Rothschild House, Chapel St., Tring HP23 6PU Tel: 01442 822468 Fax: 01442 825889; The Laurels, 14 Station Road, Tring HP23 5NG Tel: 01442 823172 — MB BChir Camb. 1961 (St. Thos.) MA, MB Camb. 1961, BChir 1960; DObst RCOG 1961. Socs: BMA; Roy. Soc. Med. Prev: Ho. Surg. St. Thos. Hosp. Hydestile; Ho. Phys. (O & G) St. Thos. Hosp. Lond.; Resid. Med. Off. Burton Gen. Hosp.

THAM, Lawrence Chiew Hong Homerton University Hospital, Homerton Row, London E9 6SR Tel: 020 8510 7302 Fax: 020 8510 7668 — MB BS Newc. 1988. Cons. Anaesth. Homerton Univ. Hosp. Lond.; Cons. in Intens. Care Med. St Bart. Hosp. Lond. Specialty: Anaesth.

THAM, Nirangalie Cockfosters Medical Centre, Heddon Court Avenue, Cockfosters, Barnet EN4 9NB Tel: 020 8441 7008 — MB BS Lond. 1983; DRCOG 1986.

THAM, Siew Wan Division of Disability, Department of Mental Health Services, St. Georges Hospital, Jenner Wing, Cranmer Terrace, London SW17 0RE; 9 Barnes Avenue, Barnes, London SW13 9AA Tel: 020 8741 7631 — MB BChir Camb. 1990; BA Camb. 1987, MB BChir 1990; MA Camb. 1991. Regist. (Psychiat.) St. Geo. Hosp. Lond.; Regist. (Disabil.) Dept. Ment. Health Sci. St. Geo. Hosp. Lond. Prev: SHO (Psychiat.) Roy. Lond. Hosp.

THAM, Tony Chiew Keong Ulster Hospital, Dundonald, Belfast BT16 1RH Tel: 028 9056 1344 Fax: 028 9056 1396 Email: ttham@utvinternet.com; 43 New Forge Lane, Belfast BT9 5NW Tel: 028 9028 0620 — MB BCh BAO Belf. 1985; MRCP (UK) 1988; MD Belf. 1990; FRCP 2000; FRCPI 2000. Cons. Phys. & Gastroenterol. Ulster Hosp. Dundonald Belf. Specialty: Gastroenterol.; Gen. Med. Socs: Brit. Soc. Gastroenterol.; Ulster Soc. Gastroenterol.; Ulster Soc. Internal Med. Prev: Gastroenterol. Fell. Brigham & Wom.s Hosp. Harvard Med. Sch. Boston, Mass., USA; Sen. Regist. & Sen. Tutor (Gastroenterol.) Inst. Clin. Sci. Qu.s Univ. & Roy. Vict. Hosp. Belf.; Regist. (Gen. Internal Med.) & Sen. Home Off., Belf. Teachg.. Hosp.

THAMAN, Rajesh 91 Princes Avenue, Surbiton KT6 7JW — MB BS Lond. 1994.

THAMBAPILLAI, Mr Augustus Jayaseelan Dept. of Audiological Medicine, St Ann's Hospital, St Ann's Road, London N15 3TH Tel: 0208 462 6523 Fax: 0208 442 6769 — MB BS Ceylon 1972; DLO (RCS) Eng. 1986; FRCS Edin. 1987; MSc UCL 1994. Cons. (Audiological Med.). Specialty: Audiol. Med. Socs: BMA; BAAP; IAAP. Prev: Sen. Regist. in Audiogical Med., Roy. Nat. Throat Nose & Ear Hospiatl; Staff Surg. ENT, N. Riding Infirm., MiddlesBoro.

THAMBAPILLAI, Ravindraseelan St. Elmo, 201 Church Hill Road, Barnet EN4 8PQ — MB BS Sri Lanka 1973 (Colombo) DCH RCP Lond. 1983; MRCP (UK) 1984.

THAMBAR, Isaac Vanniasingham (retired) Department of Genitourinary Medicine, Royal Infirmary, Blackburn BB2 3LR Tel: 01254 687304; 11A Somerset Avenue, Wilpshire, Blackburn BB1 9JD — MB BS Ceylon 1960; MRCP (UK) 1976; FRCP Ed. 1991; FRCP Lond. 1994. Prev: Cons. Genitourin. Med. Roy. Infirm. Blackburn Gen. Hosp. Burnley & Gen. Hosp. Bury.

THAMBIRAJAH, Gladstone Ravindraraj Chesterfield & North Derbyshire Royal Hospital, Chesterfield S44 5BL Tel: 01246 277271 — MB BS Peredeniya 1979; LRCP LRCS Ed. LRCPS Glas. 1987; MRCOG 1995. Staff Grade (O & G) Chesterfield Roy. Hosp. NHS Trust. Specialty: Obst. & Gyn.

THAMBIRAJAH, Muthusamy Subramaniam Child & Family Consultation Centre, 161 Eccleshall Road, Stafford ST16 1PD Tel: 01785 222708; 8 Thelsford Way, Solihull B92 9NR Tel: 0121 705 8388 — MB BS Ceylon 1967; LMSSA Lond. 1985; MRCPsych 1987. Cons. Child & Adolesc. Psychiat. Child & Family Consult. Centre Stafford. Specialty: Community Child Health.

THAMBIRAJAH, Sharmini Anaesthetics Department, Rotherham District General Hospital, Moorgate Road, Rotherham S60 2UD — MB BS Peradeniya 1979; MB BS Peradeniya, Sri Lanka 1979.

THAMIZHAVELL, Mr Ramasamy Chakravarthy Accident & Emergency Department, Kettering General Hospital, Kettering NN16 8UZ — MB BS Madras 1975; FRCS Glas. 1990. Cons. A & E Kettering Gen. Hosp. Specialty: Accid. & Emerg. Prev: Staff Grade (A & E) Bedford Hosp.

THAMMANNA, Dr 60 Keward Avenue, Wells BA5 1TS Tel: 01749 675036 — MB BS Mysore 1970. Clin. Asst. (Psychiat.) Barrow Hosp. Bristol; Med. Off. Barleywood Treatm. Centre Wrington W. Som.

THAMPI, Annette Adult Mental Health Services, Claydon Community Mental Health Service, Claydon, Melbourne Vic. 3168, Australia; 3 Coolsara Park, Lisburn BT28 3BG Tel: 01846 679066 — MB ChB Bristol 1991 (Univ. Bristol) MRCPsych 1995. Sen. Regist. (Psychiat.) Melbourne. Austral. Specialty: Gen. Psychiat. Socs: BMA; Ulster Med. Soc.; Roy. Coll. Psychiat. Prev: Sen. Regist. (Psychiat.) Holywell Hosp. Antrim; Sen. Regist. Jt. Research Holywell Hosp. Antrim.; SHO (Psychiat.) Windsor Hse. Belf. City Hosp.

THAMPY, Reshma Sreekumaran 9 Lorne Crescent, Bishopbriggs, Glasgow G64 1XU — MB ChB Glas. 1998.

THAN, Min The Surgery, 62/64 Church St., Bilston WV14 0AX Tel: 01902 496065 Fax: 01902 496384; Tinacre Top, 40 Tinacre Hill, Wightwick, Wolverhampton WV6 8DA Tel: 01902 579279 — MB BS Rangoon 1981; DTCD Wales 1987; DGM RCP Lond. 1992. Specialty: Care of the Elderly. Prev: Regist. (Gerontol.) Medway Hosp. Gillingham.

THAN, Nilar Flat 4, 23 Bainbrigge Road, Leeds LS6 3AD Tel: 0113 274 7285; 24 Buttermere Drive, Kendal LA9 7PA Tel: 01539 733807 — MB ChB Leeds 1993; MRCP UK; BSc (Hons.) Leeds 1990; MB ChB (Hons.) Leeds 1993. Specialist Regist. (Renal Med.) Leeds Gen. Infirm. Specialty: Nephrol. Socs: BMA; MDU; Eur. Dialysis & Transpl. Assn.

THAN, Soe Paediatircs Dept, Chesterfield & North Derbyshire, Royal Hospital, Calew, Chesterfield S42 7HY Tel: 01246 277271 Ext: 3023 Fax: 01246 552620 Email: than_soe@doctors.org.uk — MB BS Med. Inst. (I) Rangoon 1987; MRCPCH; MRCP (UK) 1995. Specialty: Paediat. Special Interest: Neonatology.

THAN HTAY, Dr 11 Love Lane, Halifax HX1 2BQ Tel: 01422 356609 — MB BS Med. Inst. (I) Rangoon 1973; DA (UK) 1983. Assoc. Specialist (Anaesth.) Halifax Roy. Infirm. Specialty: Anaesth. Prev: Clin. Asst. & Regist. (Anaesth.) Halifax Roy. Infirm.; SHO (Anaesth.) Eastbourne Gen. Hosp.

THAN KYAW, Dr 155 Manchester Road, Swinton, Manchester M27 4FH Tel: 0161 794 6901 Fax: 0161 728 4877; 37 Granary Lane, Worsley, Manchester M28 7PH Tel: 0161 794 7363 — MB BS Burma 1972; MSc; MFCH.

THAN NYUNT, Martin Paul Accident Emergency Department, Royal Infirmary of Edinburgh, Lauriston Place, Edinburgh EH3 9YW Tel: 0131 229 2477; Middle House, High St, Harby, Newark NG23 7EB Tel: 01522 703456 — MB BS Lond. 1991. SHO (A & E Med.) Roy. Infirm. Edin. Socs: Brit. Assn. Accid. & Emerg. Med.

THAN THAN SWE, Dr 283 Queslett Road, Birmingham B43 7HB — MB BS Rangoon 1971; MB BS Med Inst (I) Rangoon 1971.

THANABALASINGHAM, Sri Thalayasingham Health Control Unit, Terminal 3 Arrivals, Heathrow Airport, Hounslow TW6 1NB Tel: 020 8745 7208 Fax: 020 8745 6181 Email: st.hcu@virgin.net; Jesmin, 18 Sheridan Gardens, Kenton, Harrow HA3 0JT Tel: 020 8907 3814 — (Univ. Ceylon, Peradeniya, Sri Lanka) MB BS Ceylon 1972; DTM & H RCP Lond. 1986; MRCPI 1986; FRCP (Ireland) March 2000. Clin. Director/Senior Port Med. Off., Health Control Unit, Terminal 3 Arrivals, Heathrow Airport, Hounslow, Middlx.; Associate Specialist (General Medicine) Cardiology, Gastroenterology and Inf. Disease (Gen. Med. & Infec. Dis.) W. Middlx. Univ. Hosp. Isleworth; Assoc. Specialist (Chest Med.) Hillingdon Hosp. Hillingdon. Specialty: Gen. Med. Special Interest: Infec. Dis. & Trop. Med.; Ischaemic Heart Dis., Hypertens. & Congestive Cardiac Failure Dysrhythmias; Trop. Cardiol. Socs: Fell. of Roy. Soc. of Trop. Med. and Hyg.; British Thoracic Society; Brit. Med. Assn. Prev: Regist. (Infec. Dis. & Trop. Med.) W. Middlx. Univ. Hosp. Isleworth; SHO (Gen. Med.) N. Tyneside Gen. Hosp.; Ho. Off. (Gen. Med.) Gen. Hosp. Colombo, Sri Lanka.

THANABALASINGHAM, Yasothara Department of ENT, Northwick Park Hospital, Harrow HA1 3UJ Tel: 020 8864 3232; Jesmin, 18 Sheridan Gardens, Kenton, Harrow HA3 0JT Tel: 020 8907 3814 — MB BS Sri Lanka 1976; MB BS Univ. Sri Lanka 1976; DLO RCS Eng. 1984; LMSSA Lond. 1990. Clin. Asst. (ENT) Northwick Pk. Hosp. Harrow Hillingdon Hosp Uxbridge; Clin. Asst. (ENT) Ealing Hosp Uxbridge Rd. Southall. Specialty: Otolaryngol. Prev: SHO (ENT) W. Middlx. Unit. Hosp. Isleworth & N. Tyneside Gen. Hosp.; Ho. Off. (Gen. Med.) Gen. Hosp. Kurunegala, Sri Lanka.

THANDA, Khin Myo — (Institute of Medicine (I) Rangoon, Burma) DRCOG Lond.; MB BS Med Inst (I) Rangoon 1975; MB BS Med Inst (I) Rangoon 1975. Specialty: Obst. & Gyn.; Paediat.

THANDI, Himat Singh Parklands Medical Practice, The Medical Centre, 30 Buttershaw Lane, Bradford BD6 2DD — MB ChB Ed. 1997.

THANDI, Karamvir Singh 46 Wadhurst Road, Birmingham B17 8JE — MB ChB Birm. 1992.

THANDI, Rajvir Singh — MB ChB Birm. 1994 (Birmingham) DRCOG 1997; MRCGP 1998. Princip. Gen. Practitioner, N.brook Gp. Pract., 93 N.brook Rd, Olton, Solihull B90 3LX, W. Midl.s. Specialty: Gen. Pract.

THANGA, Vakees 30 Shelton Road, Merton Park, London SW19 3AT — MB BS Lond. 1986; DCH RCP Lond. 1989. Trainee GP Lond. VTS. Socs: MDU. Prev: SHO (Paediat.) Hammersmith Hosp. Lond.; SHO (A & E) Lewisham Hosp.; SHO (Geriat.) St. Geo. & Rushgreen Hosps.

THANGARAJ, Irene Latha 38 Redbourne Avenue, Finchley, London N3 2BS — MB BS Madras 1986; MRCP (UK) 1996. Sen. Regist. (Gen. & Geriat. Med.) Watford Gen. Hosp. Specialty: Care of the Elderly. Prev: Regist. (c/o Elderly) Barnet Gen. Hosp.; SHO (c/o Elderly & Gen. Med.) Barnet Gen. Hosp.

THANGARAJASINGAM, Vythialingam (retired) 328 Pickhurst Rise, West Wickham BR4 0AY; 73 Kingston Road, Wimbledon, London SW19 1JN — MB BS Ceylon 1956; DCH RCP Lond. 1962; DTM & H Liverp. 1962. Prev: Clin. Asst. (Family Plann.) FarnBoro. Hosp. Orpington.

THANGKHIEW, Irene (retired) — MB BS Gauhati 1966; Dip. Bact. Lond 1968; MSc (Bact.) Manch. 1970; MRCPath 1994. Prev: Assoc. Specialist Med. Microbiol.

THANKEY, Kishorchandra Lalji The Surgery, Riversley Road, Nuneaton CV11 5QT Tel: 024 7638 2239/7664 2409 Fax: 024 7632 5623 — MB BS Rajasthan 1973.

THANT, Moe 5 Chaffinch Close, Skippingdale, Scunthorpe DN15 8EL; Anaesthetic Department, Scunthorpe General Hospital, Scunthorpe DN16 — MB BS Med. Inst (I) Rangoon 1985; DA Lond. 1994. Staff Grade Anaesth. Specialty: Anaesth.

THAPA, Shailendra 31 Golding Throughfare, Chelmsford CM2 6TU Tel: 01245 608854 — MB BS Bahauddin Zakariya Univ. 1988. Clin. Research. Instit of Psychiat. Specialty: Gen. Psychiat. Socs: MRCPsych.

THAPA, Than Bahadur The Machylilleth Health Centre, Forge Road, Machynlleth SY20 8EQ Tel: 01654 702601 Fax: 01654 3688; Maes-y-Gynesh, Garth Road, Machynlleth SY20 8HQ Tel: 01650 702601 Fax: 01654 3688 — MB BS Gauhati 1959; DPH Calcutta 1963; DTM & H Ed. 1967; MRCP (UK) 1970; FRCP Ed 1998. GP; Clin. Asst. Bro Ddyfi Community Hosp. Specialty: Accid. & Emerg. Prev: Regist. (Med.) Princess Margt. Hosp. Swindon.

THAPAR, Ajay Kumar Department of General Practice, Rusholme Health Centre, Walmer St., Rusholme, Manchester M14 — MB ChB Dundee 1984; BSc (Hons.) Physiol. Dund 1980; DCH RCP Lond. 1988; DRCOG 1989; MRCGP 1990. Lect. (Gen. Pract.) Univ. Manch. Specialty: Gen. Pract. Prev: Lect. (Gen. Pract.) Univ. Wales Coll. Med.; GP Aberbargoed, M. Glam.

THAPAR, Professor Anita Child and Adolescent Psychiatry Section, Dept of Psychological Medicine, University of Wales College of Medicine, Heath Park, Cardiff CF14 4XN Tel: 029 2074 3241 Fax: 029 2074 7839 — MB BCh Wales 1985; MRCPsych 1989; PhD Wales 1995. Prof. (Child & Adolesc. Psychiat.) Univ of Wales Coll of Med. Specialty: Child & Adolesc. Psychiat. Prev: Sen. Lect. (Child & Adolesc. Psychiat.) Univ. Manch.; MRC Research Fell. Univ. Wales Coll. Med. Cardiff; Sen. Regist. Rotat. (Child & Adolesc. Psychiat.) S. Wales.

THAPAR, Nikhil — BM (Hons.) Soton. 1993; BSc (Hons) 1992; MRCP (UK) 1997; MRCPCH 1997; PhD Lond. 2005. Clinician Scientist and Lect. in Paediatric Gastroenterol.; Specialist Regist. in Paediat. Gastroenterol., Gt. Ormond St. Hosp., Lond. Specialty: Neonat.; Paediat. Socs: Brit. Soc. of Developm. Biol.; Brit. Soc. of Paediatric Gastroenterol., Hepat. and Nutrit. Prev: Specialist Regist. in Paediatric Gastroenterol., St Bartholemew's and the Roy. Lond. Hosp.; Specialist Regist. in Paediat., St Marys Hosp. Portsmouth.

THAPAR, Rama Silver Street Medical Centre, 159 Silver Street, London N18 1PY Tel: 020 8807 1057 Fax: 020 8345 5259 — MB BS Delhi 1970; Cert. Family Plann. JCC 1972. Specialty: Obst. & Gyn.

THAPAR, Vineet Knowle Green Surgery, Staines Health Centre, Knowle Green, Staines TW18 1XD Tel: 020 8399 6622 Fax: 020 8390 4470 — BM Soton. 1986; DRCOG 1989; MRCGP 1991. Specialty: Gen. Med. Socs: BMA; Brit. Med. Acupunct. Soc. Prev: Regist. (Med.) Qu. Eliz. II Hosp. Brisbane, Austral.; SHO (Paediat.) Wexham Pk. Hosp. Slough; SHO (O & G) Heatherwood Hosp. Ascot.

THARAKAN, Joseph Princess Alexandra Hospital, Hamstel Road, Harlow CM20 2QX Tel: 01279 444455 — MB BS 1990 (Grant) MRCP 1990; MD 1990. Consultant Physician/Medicine; Hon. Gastroenterolgist, St. Mary's Hosp., Isle of Wight. Specialty: Gen. Med.

THARAKAN, Parayil Mohan Brenkley Avenue Health Centre, Brenkley Avenue, Shiremoor, Newcastle upon Tyne NE27 0PR Tel: 0191 219 5708 — MB BS Kerala 1974. GP Newc.

THARAKARAM, Sriramulu Pembury Hospital, Department of Dermatology, Tonbridge Road, Pembury, Tunbridge Wells TN2 4QJ — MB BS Madras 1979. Cons. Dermat. Maidstone & Tunbr. Wells NHS Trust.

THARMARAJAH, Pritam 42 Lucerne Road, Thornton Heath, Croydon CR7 7BA — MB BS Lond. 1996.

THARMARATNAM, Anand Kumaresh 21 Iverna Court, Wrights Lane, London W8 6TY Email: 106056.2037@compuserve.com — MB BS Lond. 1992 (University College London) Res. Phys. Quintiles Transnat. Lond. Specialty: Pharmaceutical Medicine. Prev: SHO (Anaesth.).

THARMARATNAM, Dushen 243 High Kingsdown, Bristol BS2 8DG — MB ChB Bristol 1998.

THARMARATNAM, Suresh — MB BS Lond. 1987 (Char. Cross & Westm. Med. Sch.) MRCOG 1992; DAdv Obst. Ultrasound 1998. Cons. (O & G) Belf. City Hosp. Belf.; Cons. (O&G) Roy. Jubilee Matern. Hosp. Belf. Specialty: Obst. & Gyn. Socs: Ulster Obst. & Gyn. Soc.; Brit. Med. Ultrasound Soc.; BMA. Prev: Sen. Regist. (O & G) Ant. Area Hosp. Antrim; Lect./Sen. Regist. (O & G) Roy. Matern. Hosp. Belf.; Regist. (O & G) St. Bart. & King Geo. Hosps. Lond.

THARMASEELAN, Kanagasingam 19 Cheriton Avenue, Bromley BR2 9DL Tel: 020 8464 1577 — MB BS Sri Lanka 1974; MRCS Eng. LRCP Lond. 1986; DO RCS Glas. 1987; FCOphth 1990. Staff Grade Ophalmologist, Essex Co. Hosp., Colchester. Specialty: Ophth. Socs: FRCO. Prev: Clin. Med. Off., Roy. Eye Infirm., Plymouth.

THARUMARATNAM, Devika Bosede 23 Gainsborough Gardens, Edgware HA8 5TA — MB BS Lond. 1994.

THATCHER, Mr Matthew James Medicines Control Agency, Market Towers, 1 Nine Elms Lane, London SW8 5NQ — MB BS Lond. 1977; MB BS (Hons.) Lond. 1977; FRCS Ed. 1982; FRCS Eng. 1982; DMRD 1984; DRCOG 1988. Sen. Med. Off. Med. Control Agency. Specialty: Pharmaceutical Medicine.

THATCHER, Professor Nicholas Department Medical Oncology, Christie Hospital, Manchester M20 4BX Tel: 0161 446 3745 Fax: 0161 446 3299 — MB BChir Camb. 1971; MRCP (UK) 1972; DCH Eng. 1973; DMRT Eng. 1974; PhD Manch. 1980; FRCP Lond. 1984. Prof. & Cons. Med. Oncol. Christie Hosp. Manch. Specialty: Oncol. Prev: Chairm. MRC Lung Cancer Working Party; Chairm. UK Coordinating Comm. on Cancer Research (Trials).

THATCHER, Peter Graham 46 Cornflower Lane, Shirley Oaks, Croydon CR0 8XJ — MB BS Lond. 1993.

THAVA, Vallipuram Raj Department of Radiology, Lincoln County Hospital, Greetwell Road, Lincoln LN2 5QY Tel: 01522 573457/573266 Fax: 01522 573241 Email: raj.thava@ulh.nhs.uk — MB BS Sri Lanka 1974; MRCS Eng. LRCP Lond. 1985; FRCR 1990; T(R) (CR) 1992. Cons. Radiol. Lincoln Hosps. NHS Trust. Specialty: Radiol. Special Interest: Hepatobiliary Imaging; Interventional Radiol. Prev: Cons. Radiol. Grimsby Hosp. NHS Trust; Sen. Regist. (Radiol.) W. Midl. RHA.

THAVABALAN, Ponnappa Bobby Essex County Hospital, Essex Rivers Healthcare Trust, Lexden Road, Colchester CO3 3NB Tel: 01206 834558 — MB BS Ceylon 1962; Dip. Dermat. Lond. 1968; FRCP Ed. 1989; FRCP Lond. 1994. Cons. Genitourin. Med. Colchester. Specialty: Genitourinary Medicine. Socs: BMA; Assn. GU Med. Prev: Sen. Regist. (Venereol.) Westm. Hosp. Lond.; Regist. (Dermat. & Venereol.) Univ. Coll. Hosp. Lond.

THAVAPALAN, Muruganandan Thavapalan and Partners, 55 Little Heath Road, Bexleyheath DA7 5HL Tel: 01322 430129 Fax: 01322 440949 — MB BS Sri Lanka 1974; MRCS Eng. LRCP Lond. 1982; MRCGP 1992. Specialty: Dermat. Prev: Clin. Asst. (Thoracic Med.) Brook Hosp. Lond.; Clin. Asst. (Dermat.) Brook Hosp. Lond.

THAVAPALAN, Nandani Dora 18 Heathwood Walk, Bexley DA5 2BP Tel: 01322 559942 — MB BS Sri Lanka 1973; MRCPsych 1986. Assoc. Specialist (Psychiat.) Greenwich Dist. Hosp. Lond. Specialty: Gen. Psychiat.

THAVARAJ, Manchulaa 23 Lyndhurst Crescent, Swindon SN3 2RW — MB ChB Dund. 1998.

THAVARAJAH, Vaithilingam Muthusamy Nobles Hospital, Westmoreland Road, Douglas — MB BS Sri Lanka 1974; LRCP LRCS Ed. LRCPS Glas. 1987.

THAVASOTHY, Murali 31 Stivichall Croft, Coventry CV3 6GP — MB BS Lond. 1990.

THAVASOTHY, Rajaratnam Coventry Mental Health Unit, Walsgrave Hospital, Clifford Bridge Road, Coventry CV2 2TE Tel: 02476 602020; 31 Stivichall Croft, Coventry CV3 6GP Tel: 02476 414275 Fax: 02476 538920 — MB BS Ceylon 1959; DPM Eng. 1969; MRCP (UK) 1971; MRCPsych 1972. Cons. Psychiat. Coventry Ment. Health Unit; Hon. Sen. Clin. Lect. (Clin. Psychiat.) Univ Birm. Specialty: Gen. Psychiat. Prev: Sen. Regist. Fulbourn Hosp. & United Camb. Hosps.; Vis. Cons. Psychiat., Univ. of Warwick.

THAWDA WIN, Dr 10 Mapledale Avenue, Croydon CR0 5TA — MB BS Med. Inst. (I) Rangoon 1976.

THAYALAN, Aingarapillai Samuel Occupational Health Department, Kingston Hospital, Galsworthy Road, Kingston upon Thames KT2 7Q13 Tel: 020 8546 7711 Ext: 2615 Email: samual.thayalan@kingstonhospital.nhs.uk; 45 High Drive, New Malden KT3 3UD Tel: 020 8546 7711 — MB BS Peradeniya, Sri Lanka 1982 (Univ. of Peradeniya, Sri Lanka) MRCS Eng. LRCP Lond. 1987; MRCP (UK) 1990; AFOM RCP (UK) 1993. Cons. Occupational Physician, Occ. Health Dept, Kingston Hospital; Cons. Occ. Health Physician, St. Helier Hosp.,. Specialty: Occupat. Health. Socs: Soc. Occupat. Med.; BMA; Assoc. of NHS Occ. Physicians. Prev: Sen. Registrar in Occ. Med., Newcastle Health Authority.

THAYALAN, Sumathy 45 High Drive, New Malden KT3 3UD Tel: 020 8408 0368 — LRCP LRCS Ed. 1993; MBBS LRCP LRCS Ed. LRCPS Glas. 1993; DCH 1997. GP Regist. Epsom.

THÉ, Ing Thay (retired) 7 Queen Elizabeth Street, London SE1 2LP Tel: 020 7407 1069 — MB BS Lond. 1944 (Guy's) DTM & H Eng. 1948. Prev: Ho. Phys. Postgrad. Med. Sch. Lond. & Guy's Hosp. FarnBoro.

THEAKER, Jeffrey Michael Southampton General Hospital, Southampton Tel: 02380 796980 Email: jtheaker@doctors.net.uk — MB BS Lond. 1980; MA Oxf. 1982; MRCPath 1986; MD 1987; FRCPath 1993. Cons. Histopath. Soton. Univ. Hosp.; BUPA Soton, Wessex Nuffield & Sarum Rd. Hosp. Specialty: Histopath.; Dermatopathology. Special Interest: Urological, Breast, Head and Neck Path.. Oncological Path.. Prev: Clin. Lect. Nuffield Dept. Path. & Bacteriol. John Radcliffe Hosp. Oxf.

THEAN, See Yin Lennard Harold No 03-55 Mayer Mansion, 55 Devonshire Road, Singapore 239855, Singapore Email: ithean@mbox4.singnet.com.sg; 22 Holybank Court, 193 London Road, Leicester LE2 1ZF — MB ChB Leic. 1990; FRCS Ed. 1997. Specialist Regist. Singapore Nat. Eye Centre. Specialty: Ophth.

THEANO, Ginette South London and Maudsley NHS Trust, The Crescent Res. Centre, Salcot Crescent, New Addington,, Croydon CR0 0JJ — LMS Madrid 1965; Licenciatura in Medicina (Madrid) 1966; Dip. Psychiat. Madrid 1967; DPM Eng. 1970; MRCPsych 1972; FRCPsych 1989. Cons. Psychiat. S. Lond. and Maudsley NHS Trust. Specialty: Gen. Psychiat.; Womens Health. Socs: Brit. Assn. Psychopharmacol.; Croydon Medico-Legal Soc.; Roy. Coll. of Psychiat.s. Prev: Sen. Regist. (Psychol. Med.) Guy's Hosp. Lond.; Regist. Croydon AHA; SHO Runwell Hosp. Essex.

THEAR-GRAHAM, Michael Robert Parc-y-Bont, Newport Road, Llantarnam, Cwmbran NP44 3AF Tel: 01633 433166 Fax: 01633 433166 Email: drgraham@glam.ac.uk; 14 Longhouse Grove, Henllys, Cwmbran NP44 6HQ Tel: 01633 864919 Fax: 01633 864919 — MB ChB Ed. 1985; JCPTGP Wales 1992. Indep. Dispensing GP Gwent. Specialty: Audiol. Med.

THEBE, Phaudaraj Raj Department of Pathology, Dartford & Gravesham NHS Trust, Joyce Green Hospital, Dartford DA1 5PL Tel: 01322 227242 Fax: 01322 283532; 40 Lamorbey Close, Sidcup DA15 8BA Tel: 020 8302 3814 — MB BS Jiwaji 1979; DCP Lond 1988; MRCPath 1993. Cons. Histopath. & Cytopath. Dartford & Gravesham NHS Trust. Specialty: Histopath. Socs: IAP (Brit. Div.); BSCC.

THEBRIDGE, Peter Jonathan Yardley Green Medical Centre, 73 Yardley Green Road, Bordesley Green, Birmingham B9 5PU Tel: 0121 773 3838 Fax: 0121 506 2005; 45 Kingslea Road, Solihull B91 1TQ Tel: 0121 704 9608 — MB ChB Manch. 1981; DRCOG 1984; MRCGP 1985.

THEIN, Michael 647 Great West Road, Osterley, Isleworth TW7 4PZ — MB BS Lond. 1998.

THEIN, Myint Parnwell Medical Centre, Peterborough PE1 4YL Tel: 01733 896112 Fax: 01733 892286 — MB BS Rangoon 1975; DTM UK Liverp.; MB BS Med. Inst. (I) Rangoon 1975.

THEIN, Professor Swee Lay Dept. of Haematological Medicine, GKT School of Medicine, King's Denmark Hill Campus, Bessemer Road, London SE5 9PJ Tel: 020 7346 1682/020 7346 1689 Fax: 020 7346 5178 — MB BS Malaya 1975; MRCP (UK) 1977; MRCPath (Haemat.) 1981; FRCPath 1993; FRCPA 1998; DSc 1999. Prof. in Heamatology & Hon. Cons. King's Healthcare Trust, Lond. Specialty: Haematology; Genetics. Prev: Wellcome Sen. Research Fell. & Hon. Cons. Oxf. RHA.

THEIN THEIN WYNN, Dr Freeman Hospital, Care of the Elderly Department, Newcastle upon Tyne NE7 7DN — MB BS Med. Inst. (I) Rangoon 1965; FRCP; MRCP (UK) 1971. Cons. Phys. (Care of Elderly), Freeman Hosp., Newc. Upon Tyne. Specialty: Care of the Elderly. Socs: Fac. Community Health; Brit. Geriat. Soc. Prev: SCMO (Elderly) Newc. City Health Trust.

THEIVENDRA, Muttiah Town Surgery, 37 Cecil Road, Enfield EN2 6TJ Tel: 020 8342 0330 Fax: 020 8342 0330 — MB BS Sri Lanka 1975; LRCP LRCS Ed. LRCPS Glas. 1984.

THELWALL-JONES, Hugh (retired) 89 Harley Close, Telford TF1 3LF Tel: 01952 247182 Fax: 01952 247183 Email: hugh.t@virgin.net — MRCS Eng. LRCP Lond. 1965 (Camb. & Middlx.) MA Camb. 1966; MB BChir Camb. 1966; DObst 1968;

FRCOG 1983, M 1970; T(OG) 1991. Prev: Gp. Med. Dir. Brit. United Provident Assn.

THELWELL, Christine Margaret 49 Wolds Drive, Keyworth, Nottingham NG12 5FT — MB ChB Glas. 1990.

THELWELL, John Reginald (retired) 49 Eaton Mews, Handbridge, Chester CH4 7EJ — (Manch.) MB ChB Manch. 1959. Prev: Ho. Off. (Obst.) Withington Hosp. Manch.

THEMEN, Mr Arthur Edward George Department of Orthopaedics, Royal Berkshire Hospital, Reading RG1 5AN Tel: 01189 875111; Berkshire Independent Hospital, Wensley Road, Coley Park, Reading RG1 6UZ Tel: 01189 902 8000; Whitley Glebe, 11 Glebe Road, Reading RG2 7AG Tel: 01734 752097 — MB Camb. 1965; MA Camb. 1968; FRCS Eng. 1969; FRCS Ed. 1969. Cons. Orthop. Surg. Roy. Berks. Hosp. Reading. Specialty: Orthop. Socs: Fell. BOA. Prev: SHO Postgrad. Med. Sch.; Sen. Regist. (Orthop.) Roy. Nat. Orthop. Hosp. Stanmore; Regist. (Orthop.) St. Mary's Hosp. Lond.

THEN, Kong Yong 20 Regent Close, Edgbaston, Birmingham B5 7PL Tel: 020 7231 1502 — MB BS Lond. 1995 (St. Geo. Hosp. Med. Sch. Lond.) MSc Lond. 1999; FRCS Ed. 1999. SpR Birm. & Midl. Eye Centre. Specialty: Ophth. Socs: Med. Defense Union; BMA. Prev: SHO (Ophth.) Roy. Eye Infirm. Plymouth; Ho. Off. (ENT & Surg.) Manor Hosp. Walsall; Ho. Off. (Med.) Yeovil Hosp. Som.

THENABADU, Asoka Lakshman 29 Longdown Lane North, Epsom KT17 3HY Tel: 020 8393 7819 Fax: 020 8786 7826 Email: statlocums@aol.com — MB BS Ceylon 1968; DCH; MRCPCH. Locum Cons. (Paediat.). Specialty: Paediat.

THENUWARA, Charitha 14 Blendon Road, Bexley DA5 1BW — MB BS Lond. 1998.

THENUWARA, Clarence Dayasiri The Surgery, 118 Restons Crescent, Eltham, London SE9 2JJ Tel: 020 8859 7941 Fax: 020 8859 2382 — MB BS Ceylon 1967. Socs: Mem. Brit. Acupunture Counc.; Mem. Brit Med. Acupunture Soc.

THEOBALD, Andrew John Bedgrove Surgery, Brentwood Way, Aylesbury HP21 7TL Tel: 01296 330330 Fax: 01296 399179; Hundred Acre Wood, Ashendon Farm Barns, Ashendon, Aylesbury HP18 0HB Tel: 01296 651869 Email: theo@bucksnet.co.uk — MB ChB Dundee 1987; DRCOG 1989; DCCH RCP Ed. 1990; MRCGP 1991; T(GP) 1991. Clin. Asst. Cancer Care & Chemother. Unit Stoke Mandeville Hosp. NHS Trust Aylesbury. Prev: Trainee GP Aylesbury VTS; Ho. Off. (Med.) Stoke Mandeville Hosp.; Ho. Surg. Amersham Gen. Hosp.

THEOBALD, Janet Louisa Mary — MB ChB Aberd. 1993; MB ChB (Hons) Aberd. 1993 (Aberdeen) BSc Leeds 1981. Specialty: Gen. Psychiat. Socs: Austral. Med. Assn.; BMA. Prev: Regist. (Psychiat.) Alfred Gp. Hosps. Melbourne, Austral.

THEOBALD, John Arthur (retired) 2A Retreat Road, Topsham, Exeter EX3 0LF Tel: 01392 875498 — (Guy's) MRCS Eng. LRCP Lond. 1956; MB BS Lond. 1957; DPH Lond. 1961; MFCM 1974. Prev: Sen. Med. Off. (Pub. Health Med.) Exeter & N. Devon HA.

THEOBALD, Nicholas John Anthony Chelsea & Westminster Hospital, 369 Fulham Road, London SW10 9NH Tel: 020 8846 6149 Email: nick.theobald@chelwest.nhs.uk — MB BS Lond. 1983 (Guy's) DRCOG 1985; MRCGP 1987; Dip GU Med. 1997; MSc (STI/HIV) UCL/LSHTM 2004. Assoc. Specialist GUM/ HIV Chelsea & Westm. Hosp. Lond. Specialty: Genitourinary Medicine; HIV Med. Prev: GP Swindon; Trainee GP Rotat. Swindon VTS; Ho. Surg. Roy. Devon & Exeter Hosp.

THEODORE, Cecelia Maria 27 Methley Street, Kennington, London SE11 4AL Tel: 020 7582 2448 — MB BCh BAO Dub. 1985; BA Dub. 1985; MRCP (UK) 1991; Dip. GU Med. Soc. Apoth. Lond. 1992; DFFM 1995. Cons. GU & HIV Med. Mayday Univ. Hosp. Croydon. Specialty: Genitourinary Medicine. Socs: Med. Soc. Study VD; Assn. GU Med.; Brit. Soc. Colposc. & Cervic. Pathol. Prev: Sen. Regist. (Genitourin. Med. & HIV) Char. Cross Hosp. Lond.; MRC Research Fell. Roy. Lond. Hosp.

THEODOROU, Maria 124 Woodside Road, London N22 5HS — MB BS Lond. 1998.

THEODOROU, Mr Nikitas Alfred — MRCS Eng. LRCP Lond. 1972 (Char. Cross) MS Lond. 1985, MB BS 1972; FRCS Ed. 1977; FRCS Eng. 1977. Cons. Surgeon, Hammersmith Hosp.s NHS Trust, Dept. of Gastrointestinal Surgey.; Honorary Senior Lecturer Imperial College School of Medicine. Specialty: Gen. Surg. Prev: Sen. Regist. Char. Cross Hosp.; Cons. Surg. W. Middlx. Univ. Hosp.; Regist. (Surg.) Mt. Vernon Hosp. Northwood.

THEODOROU, Stanley 14 Acre End Street, Eynsham, Witney OX29 4PA — MB BS New South Wales 1985; MRCPsych 1994.

THEODOSIOU, Catherine Anne 5 Morningside Park, Edinburgh EH10 5HD — MB ChB Ed. 1997.

THEODOSIOU, Louise Joyce Stepping Hill Hospital, Poplar Grove, Stockport SK2 7JE Tel: 0161 419 2063 — MB ChB Manch. 1997; BSc (Hons.) St. And.; MRCPsych. Socs: MDU; BMA.

THEODOSSI, Andrew 26 Roedean Crescent, London SW15 5JU Tel: 020 8876 6346 Fax: 020 8401 3495 — MB BS Lond. 1971; MRCP (UK) 1974; MD Lond. 1985; FRCP Lond. 1986. Cons. Phys. (Gastroenterol.) Mayday Hosp. Lond. Specialty: Gastroenterol. Socs: Fell. Roy. Soc. Med.; Brit. Soc. Gastroenterol. Prev: Sen. Regist. (Gen. Med. & Gastroenterol.) Westm. Hosp. Lond.; Clin. Research Fell. Liver Unit King's Coll. Hosp. Lond.

THEODOSSIADIS, Alexander North Manchester General Hospital, Crumpsall, Manchester M8 5RB Tel: 0161 720 2037 Fax: 0161 720 2073 — Ptychion Iatrikis Athens 1968; MRCS Eng. LRCP Lond. 1971; DPM Eng. 1972; FRCPsych 1996, M 1973. Cons. Psychiat. N. Manch. Gen. Hosp. Specialty: Gen. Psychiat. Socs: Fell. Manch. Med. Soc. Prev: Sen. Regist. (Psychiat.) Manch. AHA (T); Regist. (Psychiat.) Bristol Health Dist. (T); SHO (Psychiat.) Profess. Unit Glenside Hosp. Stapleton.

THEODOULOU, Megan Tara 24 Aston Street, Oxford OX4 1EP — MB BS Lond. 1989.

THEOLOGIS, Tim Nuffield Orthopaedic Centre, Windmill Road, Headington, Oxford OX3 7LD Tel: 01865 227475 Fax: 01865 227250; 117 Kingston Road, Oxford OX2 6RW — MD Athens 1985; FRCS England; MSc Oxford 1991; PhD Athens 1994. Cons. Orthopaedic Surg., Nuffield Orthopaedic Centre, Oxf.; Hon. Sen. Clin. Lect., Univ. of Oxf. Specialty: Paediat. Surg. Socs: Brit. Orthopaedic Assn.; Brit. Soc. of Childrens Orthopaedic Surg.; European Society of Motion Analysis. Prev: Fell., Hosp. for sick Childr., Toronto, Canada.

THEOPHANOUS, Markos 17 Erylmore Road, Liverpool L18 4QS — MB ChB Liverp. 1991.

THEOPHILOPOULOS, Nicky Tameside General Hospital, Fountain Street, Ashton-u-lyne, Ashton-under-Lyne OL6 9RW Tel: 0161 3315289; 4 Congleton Close, Alderley Edge SK9 7AJ — Ptychio Iatrikes Athens 1968; MD 1985; Ph D 1992. Cons. in Adult Psychiat., Pennine Care NHS Trust, Ashton-Upon-Lyne, Lancs. Specialty: Gen. Psychiat. Special Interest: Psychopharmacology. Socs: Roy. Coll. of Psychiat.

THEOPHILUS, Mary Neelamala 121 Rosemallion House, Treliske Hospital, Treliske, Truro TR1 3LJ — MB ChB Ed. 1998.

THEOPHILUS, Samuel Wilfred Jyotichandra (retired) 9 Southernhay Close, Leicester LE2 3TW — MB BS Madras 1956 (Christian Med. Coll. Vellore) DA Eng. 1967; FFA RCSI 1974. Prev: Cons. Anaesth. Leicester Roy. Infirm.

THERAPONDOS, Georgios Panayiotis 3/5 Gilmour's Entry, Edinburgh EH8 9XL — MB ChB Ed. 1992; BSc Med. Sci. (Hons.) Ed. 1991; MRCP (UK) 1996. Clin. Research Fell. (Med.) Roy. Infirm. Edin. Specialty: Gastroenterol.

THERON, Johanna Susanna 8 Harefield Close, Enfield EN2 8NQ — MB ChB Stellenbosch 1987.

THET TUN, Dr The Surgery, Elm Lodge, The Cricket Green, Mitcham CR4 4LB Tel: 020 8648 5030 — MB BS Rangoon 1955. Prev: Hosp. Pract. (Obst.) St. Helier Hosp. Carshalton; Sen. Med. Off. Burma Rlys.; Cas. Off. Hertford Co. Hosp.

THET WIN, Dr 22 Tyrley Close, Compton, Wolverhampton WV6 8AP — MB BS Med. Inst. Mandalay 1973; DO RCPSI 1983.

THETHRAVUSAMY, Mr Joseph Aloysius 43 Stayton Road, Sutton SM1 1QY — MB BS Madras 1949; FRCS Eng. 1960.

THETHY, Ragbir Singh 629 Kings Road, Birmingham B44 9HW — MB ChB Manch. 1990.

THEVA, Rajalakshmi 5 Silver Lane, Purley CR8 3HJ — MB BS Ceylon 1969; DPM Eng. 1984; MRCPsych 1985. Cons. Psychiat. Surrey Oaklands NHS Trust. Specialty: Ment. Health. Prev: Cons. Psychiat. Croydon Ment. Handicap Unit.

THEVATHASAN, Mr Lionel Jeyakumar 41 Bushey Road, London SW20 8TE Email: lionelthe@hotmail.com — MB BS Lond. 1994 (St. Bartholomew's London) FRCS (Eng.) 1998. Research Fell. (Neurosurg.) Addenbrooke's Hosp. Camb. Specialty: Neurosurg.

THEVATHASAN, Muthuveloe Court House Practice, Tonyfelin Surgery, Bedwas Road, Caerphilly CF83 1XN Tel: 029 2088 7316 — MB BS Ceylon 1954; DTCD Wales 1961; DPH Eng. 1962.
THEVATHASAN, Pravin Asrajit 5 Mayfield Park, Shrewsbury SY2 6PD — MB BS Lond. 1988; MRCPsych.
THEVENDRA, Sabaratnam Forum Health Centre, 1A Farren Road, Wyken, Coventry CV2 5EP Tel: 024 7626 6370 Fax: 024 7663 6518 — MB BS Ceylon; MRCOG 1977.
THEW, Melanie Elizabeth Barn 1 Hall Farm, Westhorpe, Southwell, Nottingham NG2 0NG Tel: 01636 815102 — BM BS Nottm. 1994; BMedSci Nottm. 1992. SHO (Anaesth.) Roy. Devon & Exeter Hosp. Specialty: Anaesth. Prev: SHO (Med.) Torbay Hosp. Torquay; SHO (A & E) Roy. United Hosp. Bath.
THEW, Ronald James Latham House Medical Practice, Sage Cross Street, Melton Mowbray LE13 1NX Tel: 01664 854949 Fax: 01664 501825; 16 Asfordby Place, Asfordby, Melton Mowbray LE14 3TG Tel: 01664 813771 Fax: 01664 501825 Email: rjthew@aol.com — MB BS Lond. 1968 (St. Bart.) MRCS Eng. LRCP Lond. 1968; DCH Eng. 1970; DObst RCOG 1970; DA Eng. 1971; FRCGP 1987, M 1979. Chair Melton PCG. Socs: Leic. Med. Soc. Prev: SHO (Anaesth.) Poole Gen. Hosp.; SHO (Paediat.) Redhill Gen. Hosp.; Ho. Off. (Obst.) Redhill Gen. Hosp.
THEWLES, Michael John Manchester Road Surgery, 484 Manchester Road, Sheffield S10 5PN Tel: 0114 266 8411 — MB ChB Sheff. 1977; MRCGP 1981.
THEXTON, Penelope Jane St Bartholomew's Sexual Health Centre, St Bartholomew's Hospital, West Smithfield, London EC1A 7BE Tel: 020 7601 8092 Fax: 020 7601 8601; 36 Albert Street, London NW1 7NU Tel: 020 7387 7370 Email: penny.thexton@dial.pipex.com — MB BS Lond. 1986; BA Camb. 1976; DCH RCP Lond. 1989; MRCGP 1990. Clin. Asst. Dgum St. Bart. Hosp. & Med. Off. Med. Express Clinic. Lond. Specialty: Gen. Pract.
THEXTON, Robina 42 St Mary's Avenue Central, Norwood Green, Southall UB2 4LT Tel: 020 8574 4195 — MB BS Lond. 1951 (Roy. Free) MRCS Eng. LRCP Lond. 1950. Socs: Inst. Psychosexual Med. Prev: Instruc. Med. Off. (Family Plann.) Ealing Health Dist.; Ho. Phys. Roy. Free Hosp.; Ho. Surg. Roy. Lond. Homoep. Hosp.
THIAGALINGAM, Namasivayam Mayday University Hospital, London Road, Croydon CR7 7YE Tel: 020 8401 3000; 7 Clarice Way, Wallington SM6 9LD Tel: 020 6695375 Fax: 020 7732359 — MB BS Colombo 1985. Associate Specialist. Specialty: Accid. & Emerg.
THIAGARAJAH, Mr Kadampamoorthy Amaranath North Middlesex University Hospital, Stirling Way, London N18 1QX Tel: 020 8887 2466 Fax: 020 8887 2256; 23 Houndsden Road, London N21 1LU Tel: 020 8360 9532 Fax: 020 8360 9532 Email: k.a.t.hound@btinternet.com — (Peradeniya) MB BS Ceylon 1970; FRCS Ed. 1982; FRCOpth 1989. Cons. Ophth. N. Middlx. Hosp. Lond. Specialty: Ophth. Socs: Oxf. Ophth. Congr.; Internat. Mem. Amer. Acad. Ophth.; Fell. RSM. Prev: Cons. Ophth. King Khalid Hosp., Saudi Arabia; Sen. Regist. (Ophth.) Roy. Hallamsh. Hosp. Sheff.; Regist. (Ophth.) Derbysh. Roy. Infirm. Derby.
THIAGARAJAH, Karthigesu (retired) 92 Windmill Hill Drive, Bletchley, Milton Keynes MK3 7RR — MB BS Ceylon 1956. Prev: GP.
THIAGARAJAH, Sivakkolunthar Greenacres, Homefield Road, Worthing BN11 2HS Tel: 01903 843888 Fax: 01903 843889 — MB BS Ceylon 1971 (Faculty of Medicine University of Ceylon) BCPsych Lond. 1992. Assoc. Specialist (Psychiat.) Worthing Priority Care NHS Trust. Specialty: Gen. Psychiat.
THIAGARAJAN, Jayaraman Lister hospital, East and North Herts NHS Trust, Coreys Mill Lane, Stevenage SN1 4AB Tel: 01438 781086 Fax: 01438 781302 Email: dr.rajan@nhs.net — MB BS Madras 1985; DA (UK) 1988; FCAnaesth 1991. Cons. in Anaesth. and Critical Care; Lead Clinician, Herts and Beds Critical Care Delivery Gp. Specialty: Anaesth.; Intens. Care. Socs: Intens. Care Soc.; Assn. of Anaesthetists.
THIAGARAJAN, Manickam 31 Shore Green, Thornton-Cleveleys FY5 2LT Tel: 01253 822649 — MB BS Lond. 1992 (Kasturba Med. Coll.) MB BS Karnatak 1966.
THIAGARAJAN, Prakash Department of Paediatrics, Jersey General Hospital, Gloucester Street, St. Helien JE1 3QS Tel: 01534 622062 Fax: 01534 622895 Email: p.thiagarajan@gov.je — MB BS Madras 1991; MRCP (UK) 1991; MRCPCH 2002; FRCP, Edin. 2003. Cons. Paediat., Jersey Gen. Hosp., St. Helien, Jersey. Specialty: Paediat. Special Interest: Neonatology. Socs: Brit. Assn. of Perinatal Med.; Roy. Coll. of Phys. of Edin.; Roy. Coll. of Paediat. & Child Health. Prev: Cons. Paediat. & Neonatology, Duneoin Hosp, New Zealand; Clin. Sen. Lect. in Paediat., Univ. of Itago, Duneoin, New Zealand.
THIBAUT, R E Parsons Heath Medical Practice, 35A Parsons Heath, Colchester CO4 3HS Tel: 01206 864395 Fax: 01206 869047 — MB BS London 1977; MB BS London 1977.
THICK, Anthony Patrick Broadway Medical Centre, 164 Great North Road, Gosforth, Newcastle upon Tyne NE3 5JP Tel: 0191 285 2460 — MB BS Lond. 1976 (Royal London) GP Princip. Newc. & N. Tyneside Health Auth. Specialty: Gen. Pract. Socs: Soc. Occupat. Med. Prev: Div. Med. Off. Thames Water Plc.
THICKETT, Charles Roy (retired) 6 Ladderbanks Lane, Baildon, Shipley BD17 6RX Tel: 01274 598490 — MB ChB Sheff. 1950; MRCGP 1960. Prev: Capt. RAMC.
THICKETT, David Richard 26 Hall Drive, London SE26 6XB — MB BS Lond. 1992.
THICKETT, Kathleen Mary 15 West View, Chesterfield S44 6LJ — MB ChB Leeds 1991.
THICKNES, Philip John Lyon (retired) 8 Woodside Avenue, Corbridge NE45 5EL Tel: 01434 632082 Fax: 01434 634416 Email: philipthick@doctors.org.uk — (St. Thos.) MB BChir Camb. 1964; MA Camb. 1964; DObst RCOG 1966; MRCGP 1975. Prev: Princip., Riversdale Surg., Wylam N.umberland.
THIEDE, Mrs Brenda (retired) Great Ghyll, West Scrafton, Leyburn DL8 4RT — MB ChB Leeds 1957.
THILAGARAJAH, Mr Kanagasabai, TD 5 Regents Place, Blackheath, London SE3 0LX Tel: 020 8853 1392 — MB BS Ceylon 1959 (Colombo, Univ. Ceylon) FRCS Ed. 1969; FRCS Eng. 1972; MRCS Eng. LRCP Lond. 1974. Clin. Dir. (A & E) Qu. Mary's Hosp. Sidcup. Specialty: Accid. & Emerg. Socs: Milit. Surg. Soc.; W Kent. M-C Soc.; Roy. Soc. Med. Prev: Cons. A & E N. Middlx. Univ. Hosp.; Regist. (Thoracic Surg.) Preston Hall Hosp. Maidstone; Regist. (A & E, Orthop. & Gen. Surg.) Croydon Gp. Hosps.
THILAGARAJAH, Mr Michael 5 Regents Place, Blackheath, London SE3 0LX — MB BS Lond. 1992 (Char. Cross & Westm.) FRCS Eng. 1997; MSc Lond. 1998. Specialist Regist. In Orthop., SE Thames Region; Specialist Regist. in Orthop. & Trauma - Guy's & St. Thomas' Hosp., Lond. Socs: Brit. Orthop. Assn. Prev: S. E. Thames Spr Rotat.; MSc Research fell. (Surgic. Sci.), Hammersmith.
THILAGARAJAH, Mr Ranjan Broomfield Hospital, Chelmsford CM1 Tel: 01376 562676 Fax: 01376 562676 Email: ranjan@dhet.netkonect.co.uk/springfieldurology@yahoo.co.uk; 37 Deanhill Court, Upper Richmond St W., East Sheen, London SW14 7DJ — MB BS Lond. 1990; FRCS Eng. 1995. Cons. Urol. Broomfield Hosp. Chelmsford. Specialty: Urol. Socs: Fell. Roy. Soc. Med. Prev: Specialist Regist. (Urol.) Cen Middlx. Hosp; Specialist Regist. (Urol.) Colchester Hosp.; Clin. Fell. (Urol)Princess Alexandra Hosp, Bris.AUS.
THILAKAWARDHANA, Wellala Don Punyasena Princess Margaret Hospital, Okus Road, Swindon SN1 4JU Tel: 01793 36231 — MB BS Sri Lanka 1973; DA Eng. 1982.
THILLAIAMBALAM, Navathevi 16 Queens Way, Frimley Green, Camberley GU16 6QB — MB ChB Sheff. 1998.
THILLAINATHAN, Sinnadurai Brownlow Medical Centre, 140 Brownlow Road, Southgate, London N11 2BD Tel: 020 8888 7775 Fax: 020 8888 3450 — MB BS Sri Lanka 1972; LMSSA Lond. 1986.
THILLAINAYAGAM, Andrew V. Gastroenterology Unit, Hammersmith Hospital, Du Cane Road, London W12 0NN Tel: 020 8383 3266 (Academic)/0208 846 1945 (NHS) Fax: 0208 749 3436/ 0208 846 1975 — MB ChB Manch. 1984; MRCP (UK) 1987; MD 1995; FRCP Lond. 2001. Cons. (Gastroenterol.) Hammersmith Hosps. NHS Trust; Hon. Sen. Lect. Imperial Coll. Sch. of Med. Lond.; Hon. Cons., John Radcliffe Hosp., Oxf. Specialty: Gastroenterol.; Gen. Med. Socs: Fell. Roy. Soc. Med.; Brit. Soc. Gastroenterol.; Amer. Gastroenterological Assn. Prev: Sen. Regist. John Radcliffe Hosp. Oxf.; RMO St. Marks Hosp. Lond.; Regist. & Hon. Lect. Med. Coll. St. Bart. Hosp. Lond.
THILLAIVASAN, Kathiravelpillai Department of Anaesthesia, The Edith Cavell Hospital, Bretton Gate, Peterborough PE3 6QR Tel:

01733 874000; 47 Walkers Way, Bretton, Peterborough PE3 9AX Tel: 01733 332449 — MB BS Ceylon 1971 (Colombo) MRCA Lond.; DA (UK). Prev: Clin. Med. Off. (Anaesth.) Edith Cavell Hosp. PeterBoro..; Clin. Asst. (Anaesth.) Pboro. Dist. Hosp.; Regist. (Anaesth.) PeterBoro. Dist. Hosp.

THILO, Julia Belinda Parkside Family Practice, Green Road Surgery, 224 Wokingham Road, Reading RG6 1JT Tel: 0118 966 3366 Fax: 0118 926 3269 — MB BS Lond. 1990; DRCOG 1994; DFFP 1994; MRCGP 1995. Clin. Asst. Genitourin. Clinic Roy. Berks. Hosp. Prev: Trainee GP Reading Scheme; SHO Frimley Pk. Hosp.

THIMMEGOWDA, Hanume Mountain Road Medical Centre, Thornhill, Dewsbury WF12 0BS Tel: 01924 522100 Fax: 01924 522102 — (Karnatak Med. Coll. Hubli) MB BS Karnatak 1967. GP Dewsbury. Prev: Regist. (Geriat. Med.) St. Luke's Hosp. Huddersfield.

THIN, Mairead Jane Blackwood, North Kessock, Inverness IV1 3XD — MB ChB Aberd. 1998.

THIN, Robert Nicol Traquair, OBE 13 Park Avenue, Bromley BR1 4EF Tel: 020 8464 9278 — MB ChB Ed. 1959; FRCP Ed. 1973, M 1964; MD Ed. 1968; FRCP 1988. Clin. Asst., Dept. of Genitourin. Med., Beckham Hosp., Beckham, Kent. Specialty: Genitourinary Medicine. Socs: Fell. Roy. Soc. Med.; (Ex-Pres.) Med. Soc. Study VD; (Ex-Chairm.) Assn. for Genitourin. Med. Prev: Phys. (Genitourin. Med.) St. Thos. Hosp. Lond.; Cons. (Venerol.) St. Peter's Hosps. Lond.; Phys. (Genital Med.) St. Bart. Hosp. Lond.

THIN KYU, Dr 177 Cheltenham Road, Bristol BS6 5RH — MB BS Rangoon 1968.

THIN THIN AYE, Dr Radiology Department, Walsgrave Hospital, Coventry CV2 2DX — MB BS Med. Inst. (I) Rangoon 1965 (Inst. Med. (I) Rangoon) BSc Univ. Rangoon 1958; DMRD Eng. 1970; FRCR 1975. Cons. Radiol. Walsgrave Hosp. Coventry, Coventry & Warks. Hosp. &; Geo. Eliot Hosp. Nuneaton. Specialty: Radiol. Socs: Brit. Inst. Radiol. Prev: Civil Asst. Surg. Rangoon Gen. Hosp., Burma; Civil Asst. Surg. Mandalay Gen. Hosp., Burma; Head Dept. Radiol. Magwe Div. Hosp., Burma.

THIN THIN SAING, Dr 6 Smitham Bottom Lane, Purley CR8 3DA — MB BS Med. Inst. Rangoon 1982; MRCP (UK) 1994. Staff Grade (Paediat.) Law Hosp. Carluke. Specialty: Paediat. Prev: SHO (Paediat.) Plymouth; SHO (Paediat.) Oxf.

THIND, Indra 40 Brookside, Great Barr, Birmingham B43 5DB — MB ChB Leic. 1995.

THIND, Jaishree Castle Hill Hospital, Castle Road, Cottingham HU16 5JQ — MB BS Madras 1983; FRCA 1992. Cons. Anaesth. Castle Hill Hosp. Cottingham. Specialty: Anaesth. Socs: Assn. Anaesth. of Gt. Britain & N.ern Irelans; Brit. Assn of Day Surg.; Intens Care Soc. Prev: Specialist Regist. (Anaesth.) Oxf. Redcliffe Hosp.; Locum Cons., Hillingdon Hosp., Uxbridge, Middlx.; Clin. Fell., Obstetric Anaesth., W.chester Co. Med. Center, Valhalla, New York, USA.

THING, John Rhodes 1 Cambridge Road, Owlsmoor, Sandhurst GU47 0UB Tel: 01344 777015 Fax: 01344 777226 — MB ChB Cape Town 1972 (Univ. Cape Town) BSc S. Afr. 1968; Cert. Family Plann. JCC 1977; MRCGP 1978. GP; Clin. Asst. (Sports Med.) Frimley Pk. Hosp.

THINN, Kyaw Care Principles, Ashley House, Ashley, Market Drayton TF9 4LX Tel: 01630 673800 Fax: 01630 673805 Email: kyaw.thinn@ashleyhouse.careprinciples.com — MB BS Burma 1973; MRCPsych 1985. Cons. Psychiat. (Learning Disabil.) Care Principles, Ashley Ho.; Hon. Sen. Lect. (Psychiat.) Univ. Birm.; Hon. Lect. Fac. Health & Community Care Univ. Centr. Eng. Birm. Specialty: Gen. Psychiat.

THIRKELL, Claire Elizabeth Heathgate Surgery, The Street, Poringland, Norwich NR14 7JT Tel: 01508 494343; 11A The St, Brooke, Norwich NR15 1JW Tel: 01508 550264 — MB BChir Camb. 1984; BSc (Hons.) St. And. 1981; MRCGP 1990. GP Princip. Heathgate Surg. Poringland.

THIRKETTLE, James Leslie (retired) 1 Old Horsham Road, Crawley RH11 8PD — (Char. Cross) MB BS Lond. 1955; FRCP Lond. 1978, M 1961. Prev: Cons. Phys. Crawley Hosp.

THIRLAWAY, Barbara May (retired) Ziarat, 18 Speen Lane, Newbury RG14 1RW — MB BS Punjab 1941 (Lady Hardinge Med. Coll. New Delhi) Prev: Clin. Med. Off. Hants.

THIRLWALL, Miss Andrea Simone, Level 1 11 Holiday St, Berkhamsted HP4 2EE Tel: 01442 864079 — BM BS Nottm. 1993; FRCS CSIG. 1998; FRCS OUT. 1998. Specialist Regist. (ENT.) Oxf. Region. Specialty: Otorhinolaryngol. Socs: MPS; FRS; BAOHNS.

THIRLWALL, Michael Meadowcroft Surgery, Jackson Road, Aylesbury HP19 9EX Tel: 01296 425775 Fax: 01296 330324 Email: drmike.thirlwall@gp-k82018.nhs.uk — MB BS Lond. 1971 (Char. Cross) MRCS Eng. LRCP Lond. 1971; DObst RCOG 1973; FRCGP 1987, M 1975. Examr. (RCGP) 1991-2004. Prev: Course Organiser Aylesbury Health Dist. VTS.

THIRLWALL, Pamela Jane 11 Ripon Road, Killinghall, Harrogate HG3 2DG — MB ChB Leeds 1969.

THIRLWELL, Christina The Mallards, The Causeway, Occold, Eye IP23 7PP — MB BS Lond. 1997.

THIRU, Mr Chittampalam Naranapillai (retired) 158 Anson Road, London NW2 6BH Tel: 020 8452 0170 — MB BS Ceylon 1962; FRCS Ed. 1974. Examg. MO. Prev: GP.

THIRU, Nallasivam 95 Parkhall Road, Walsall WS5 3HS — MB BS Kerala 1969.

THIRU, Yamuna Department Paediatrics, Level 7, QEQM, St Mary's Hospital, South Wharf Road, London W2 1NY Tel: 020 7886 6377 Fax: 020 7886 6284; Mews Flat, Milne House, 3 Norfolk Square, London W2 1RU — MB ChB Leeds 1990 (Leeds University) BSc (Hons.) Leeds 1987, MB ChB 1990; MRCP (UK) 1993; DCH (UK) 1994. Specialty: Paediat.; Intens. Care.

THIRUCHELVAM, Angeeta Conway Medical Centre, Westbourne Road, Luton LU4 8JD Tel: 01582 429953 Fax: 01582 487500 — MB ChB Leeds 1991.

THIRUCHELVAM, Nikesh 90 Cliff Lane, Ipswich IP3 0PJ — MB BS Lond. 1996.

THIRUCHELVAM, Timonthy Rajiv 113 Worple Way, Rayners Lane, Harrow HA2 9SW — MB ChB Liverp. 1996.

THIRUMALA KRISHNA, Mamidipudi c/o Dr A. H. Deshpande, 24 Midgley Drive, Four Oaks, Sutton Coldfield B74 2TW; University Medicine, Level D, Centre Block, Southampton General Hospital, Tremona Road, Southampton SO16 6YD Tel: 01703 794155 Fax: 01703 701771 — MB BS Madras 1989; PhD Soton.; MRCP (UK) 1992; Dip Nat. Bd. Med. Examiners (Gen. Med.) New Delhi 1997. Postdoctoral Clin. Research Fell. Dept. of Med. Univ. of Soton.; Hon. Regist. (Med./Respirat. Med.) Soton. Univ. Hosps. NHS Trust. Specialty: Gen. Med.; Respirat. Med. Socs: Roy. Coll. Phys.; Brit. Assn. Lung Res. Prev: Sen. Resid. (Med. & Cardiol.) Vijaya Health Centre, Madras.

THIRUMAMANIVANNAN, Mr Govindan 3 Shelley Avenue, Manor Park, London E12 6SP — MB BS Madras 1982; FRCS Glas. 1994.

THIRUMAVALAVAN, Mr Vallur Sivaprakasam 20 Milford Gardens, Wembley HA0 2AR Tel: 020 8903 2402 — MB BS Madras 1977; MS (Gen. Surg.) Madras 1983; FRCS Ed. 1985; FRCS Glas. 1985; Dip. Urol. Lond 1989.

THIRUNATHAN, Jegathesvary 18 Laurel Park, Harrow HA3 6AU — MB BS Ceylon 1968.

THIRUNAVUKARASU, Ratnasabapathy (retired) 30 Ennerdale Avenue, Stanmore HA7 2LD Tel: 020 8907 8942 — MB BS Ceylon 1955 (Sri lanka)

THIRUNAVUKKARASU, Sathiamalar Department of Pathology, Cambridge University, Tennis Court Road, Cambridge CB2 1QP Tel: 01223 217163; Department of Pathology, Addenbrookes Hospital, Cambridge CB2 2QQ — MB ChB Leeds 1964; MRCP (UK) 1970; FRCPath 1988, M 1974; Dip. Amer. Bd. Clin. Anat. Path. 1976; MA Camb. 1977; FRCP Lond. 1990. Sen. Lect. Dept. of Path., Univ. of Camb.; Hon. Cons. Path. Addenbrookes Hosp. Camb. Specialty: Pathology, General. Socs: Fell. Roy. Coll. Phys.; Fell., Roy. Coll. of Path. Prev: Cons. Path. Beth Israel Hosp. Boston, USA; Clin. Fell. Harvard Med. Sch. Boston, U.S.A.; Clin. Lect. Sch. of Clin. Med. Univ. Camb.

THIRUNAWARKARISU, Kankanamalage Susitha St. Davids Hospital, Carmarthen SA31 3HB Tel: 01267 237481 — Vrach Moscow 1970; Vrach Peoples Friendship U, Moscow 1970.

THIRUVUDAIYAN, Ponnampalam 326 Philip Lane, London N15 4AB — MB BS Sri Lanka 1972; MRCP (UK) 1986.

THISTLETHWAITE, Jill Elizabeth Medical Education Unit, The Medical School, University of Leeds, Leeds LS2 9LN Tel: 0113 233 4179 — MB BS Lond. 1981; BSc (Hons.) Lond. 1978; DRCOG 1984; MRCGP (Distinc.) 1985. Sen. Lect. (Community-Based Teachg.) Med. Sch. Univ. Leeds.

THIT THIT, Dr 93 Shakespeare Road, Luton LU4 0HT Tel: 01582 580946 — MB BS Med. Inst. (I) Rangoon 1982; MRCP (UK) 1995. Staff Grade (Med. for Elderly) Luton & Dunstable Hosp. Specialty: Care of the Elderly. Socs: BMA; Brit. Geriat. Soc.

THIYAGARAJAN, Chinnaya Asari 2 Marlborough Road, Aylesbury HP21 8AU — MB BS Madras 1975.

THO, Jia Haur St Bartholomew's Hospital, Department of Clinical Neurosciences, 38 Little Britain, London EC1A 7BE Email: jhtho@doctors.org.uk — MB BCh BAO NUI 1999. Specialist Regist. (Clin. Neurophysiol.) Lond. Deanery Rotat. Specialty: Neurol. Socs: MRCP; MDDUS; Assoc. Mem. Brit. Stroke Phys. Prev: SHO (Gen. Med.) Staffs. Gen. Hosp.; SHO (Gen. Med.) Roy. Liverp. Hosps.; PRHO (Gen. Surg.) Glas. Roy. Infirm.

THOBURN, Charles Royston Flat 76, Boss House, Boss St., London SE1 2PT — MB BS Lond. 1994.

THOM, Alexander Anderson Parkhead Hospital, 81 Salamanka Street, Glasgow G31 5ES Tel: 0141 211 8300 — MB ChB Glas. 1991; BSc (Hons) Glas. 1988; MRCPsych. 1997. Cons. (Gen. Psychiat.) Glas. Specialty: Gen. Psychiat.

THOM, Alexander William Rose (retired) 24 Marina Court, Alfred St., Bow, London E3 2BH Tel: 020 8981 1508 — (Univ. Ed.) LRCP LRCS Ed. LRFPS Glas. 1947.

THOM, Barry Thornton (retired) 6 Glen Rise, Brighton BN1 5LP Tel: 01273 558177 — (St. Bart.) MB BS Lond. 1956; Dip. Bact. 1965; FRCPath 1978, M 1966. Prev: Dir. Pub. Health Laborat. Roy. Sussex Co. Hosp. Brighton.

THOM, Carolyn Margaret Harrison 82 Warren Road, Blundellsands, Liverpool L23 6UG — MB ChB Ed. 1971; MRCOG 1979. Cons. (O & G) Mill Rd. Matern. Hosp. & Roy. Liverp. Hosp. Specialty: Obst. & Gyn.

THOM, Christopher Henry The Maidstone Hospital, Hermitage Lane, Maidstone ME16 9QQ Tel: 01622 224819 Fax: 01622 224018 Email: chris_thom@lineone.net; Old Hill House, Old Loose Hill, Loose, Maidstone ME15 0BN — MB Camb. 1982; BChir Camb. 1981; MRCP (UK) 1985; FRCP (Lond) 1999. Cons. Phys. Special Responsibilty The Elderly Maidstone & Tunbridge Wells NHS Trust. Specialty: Care of the Elderly; Gen. Med. Special Interest: Parkinson's Dis.; Stroke. Socs: BMA; Brit. Geriat. Soc. Prev: Sen. Regist. (Geriat. & Gen. Med.) St. Thoms. Hosp Lond.; Sen. Regist. (Geriat. & Gen. Med.) Kent & Canterbury Hosp.; Lect. (Med.) Univ. Maiduguri Nigeria.

THOM, Duncan Edward 115 Seedhill Road, Paisley PA1 1RD — MB ChB Glas. 1994.

THOM, Margaret Helen Charnwood, Duke Street, Belhaven, Dunbar EH42 1NT Tel: 01368 863668 — MB BS Lond. 1973 (King's Coll. Hosp.) FRCOG 1990, M 1978. Specialty: Obst. & Gyn. Socs: Fell. Roy. Soc. Med.; Blair Bell Res. Soc. Prev: Cons. O & G., Gt. Portland St. Lond.; Cons. O & G Guy's Hosp. Lond.; Sen. Regist. (O & G) Qu. Charlotte's Matern. Hosp. & Chelsea Hosp. for Wom.

THOM, Margaret Vivien Martin House Hospice for Children, Grove Rd, Clifford, Wetherby LS23 6TX Tel: 01937 844836 — MB BCh BAO Belf. 1984; DGM RCP Lond. 1986; DCH Dub. 1987; DRCOG 1987; MRCGP 1988; Dip. Palliat. Med. Cardiff 1994. Clin. Asst. Amrtin Ho. Hospice for Childr. Specialty: Palliat. Med. Prev: Cons. Palliat. Med. P. if Wales Hospice & Pontefract Hosp NHS Trust; Med. Director P. of Wales Hospice Pontefract.

THOM, Maria Helene National Hospital For Neurology & Neruosurgery, Division of Neuropathology, Queens Street, London WC1N 3BG Tel: 0207 837 3611 Fax: 0207 916 9546 Email: m.thom@ion.ucl.ac.uk — MB BS Lond. 1988; BSc Lond. 1985, MB BS 1988; FRCPath 1995. Sen. Lect. / Hon. Cons. (Neuropath.). Specialty: Neuropath. Special Interest: Epilepsy. Socs: Mem. Roy. Coll. Of Pathologists; Mem. BNS.

THOM, Martin George — MB ChB Dund. 1998.

THOM, Peter McGregor Van Den Bergh Foods Ltd., Brooke House, Manor Royal, Crawley RH10 9RQ Tel: 01293 648299 Fax: 01293 648900; Conifers, 3 Birdhaven, Wrecclesham, Farnham GU10 4PB Tel: 01252 725667 — MB ChB Aberd. 1970; Assoc. Fac. Occupat. Med. RCP Lond. 1980. Foods Med. Adviser Unilever (UK) Crawley. Specialty: Occupat. Health. Socs: Soc. Occupat. Med. Prev: Med. Off. Brit. Steel Corp. Motherwell.

THOM, Ruth Balami Old Hill House, Old Loose Hill, Loose, Maidstone ME15 0BN Tel: 01622 744833 — LMSSA 1997; MBBS. 1988; MSC Lond. 1993; LMSSA LRCP LRCS Lond. 1997. Specialty: Gen. Pract.

THOM, Simon Alasdair McGillivray The Peart-Rose Clinic, St. Mary's Hospital, London W2 1NY Tel: 020 7886 1172 Fax: 020 7886 6145 Email: s.thom@ic.ac.uk; 26 Kingswood Avenue, Queens Park, London NW6 6LL — MB BS Lond. 1976 (St. Mary's) MRCP (UK) 1979; MD Lond. 1992; FRCP Lond. 1996. Sen. Lect. & Hon. Cons. Phys. (Clin. Pharmacol. & Therap.) St. Mary's Hosp. & Med. Sch. Lond. Specialty: Pharmacology. Socs: Brit. Hypertens. Soc.; Brit. Pharm. Soc. Prev: Regist. (Med.) St. Mary's Hosp. Lond.; SHO Rotat. (Med.) Newc. AHA (T).

THOM, William Flockhart Yealm Medical Centre, Yealmpton, Plymouth PL8 2EA — MB BChir Camb. 1985 (Camb. Univ. Westm. Hosp.) MA Camb. 1985; MRCGP 1988. Princip. Gen. Pract.; GP Trainer. Specialty: Gen. Pract. Socs: BMA; Plymouth Med. Soc.; RCGP. Prev: Course Organiser Plymouth GPVTS; GP Southwold; Trainee GP Plymouth VTS.

THOM, William Francis John Maxwell (retired) 51 Gunters Mead, 37 Copsem Lane, Esher KT10 9HJ Tel: 01372 849588 — LRCP LRCS Ed. LRFPS Glas. 1940; DTM & H Eng. 1947; DCH Eng. 1947; DPH Ed. 1948. Prev: Hon. Lt.-Col. IMS, IAMC (Mentioned in Dispatches).

THOM, William Reid 9 Kitchener Street, Wishaw ML2 7JQ — MB ChB Aberd. 1981.

THOM, William Tod, OBE (retired) Wanda Cottage, Station Road, Eddleston, Peebles EH45 8QN Tel: 01721 730277 — MB ChB Ed. 1940; DTM & H Ed. 1950; FFCM 1979, M 1974. Prev: Dir. Med. Servs. Somaliland, Protectorate.

THOMAS, A G St Laurence's Medical Centre, 32 Leeside Avenue, Kirkby, Liverpool L32 9QU Tel: 0151 549 0000 Fax: 0151 547 4747.

THOMAS, Abraham 2 Fairholme Close, Saughall, Chester CH1 6AH — MB BS Nigeria 1979; MRCPI 1990.

THOMAS, Adrian Graham Booth Hall Childrens Hospital, Charlestown Road, Blackley, Manchester M9 7AA Tel: 0161 795 7000 Fax: 0161 220 5072 Email: agthomas@manu.demon.co.uk — MB ChB Manch. 1981; BSc (Physiol.) (Hons.) Manch. 1978, MD 1991, MB ChB 1981; MRCP (UK) 1984; FRCP (Ed.) 1997. Cons. Paediat. Gastroenterol. Booth Hall Childr. Hosp. Manch. Specialty: Paediat. Socs: Eur. Soc. Paediat. Gastroenterol. & Nutrit.; Co-Chairm. Quality of Life Working Gp.; Europ. Soc. Paediatric Gastroenterol. & Nutrit. Prev: Hon. Sen. Regist. Hosp. Sick Childr. Lond.; Tutor (Child Health) Univ. of Manch.

THOMAS, Adrian Mark Kynaston Department of Nuclear Medicine, Princess Royal University Hospital, Farnborough Common, Orpington BR6 8ND Email: adrian.thomas@btinternet.com; 3 Cedar Copse, Bickley, Bromley BR1 2NY Tel: 0208 467 6808 Email: adrian.thomas@btinternet.com — MB BS Lond. 1978 (Univ. Coll. Lond. & Univ. Coll. Hosp.) BSc (Hons.) Lond. 1975; MRCP (UK) 1981; FRCR 1984; FRCP Lond. 1996. Cons. Radiol. Bromley Hosps. NHS Trust; Honorary Senior Lecturer, Faculty of Health and Sciences, Canterbury Christ Church University College, Canterbury, Kent. Specialty: Radiol.; Nuclear Med. Special Interest: Hist. of Radiol.; Chest Radiol.; Head & Neck Radiol. Socs: Fell. Roy. Soc. Med. (Mem. Counc. Sect. Radiol.); Hon Sec. Brit. Inst. of Radiol.; Chairm., Radiol. Hist. and Heritage Charitable Trust. Prev: Sen. Regist. (Radiol. & Diagn. Imaging) Hammersmith Hosp. & Hillingdon Hosp. Uxbridge; Regist. (Radiol. & Diagn. Imaging) Hammersmith Hosp.

THOMAS, Alan Donald NHS Grampian, Aberdeen Royal Infirmary, Anaesthetic Department, Aberdeen AB25 2ZN Tel: 01224 681818 — MB ChB Bristol 1981; FFA RCSI 1989; MSc Robert Gordon Uni. Aberdeen 2000. Cons Anaesth, NHS Grampian, Aberd. Specialty: Anaesth.; Hyperbaric Medicine. Socs: N. E. of Scotl. Soc. Anaesth. Prev: Cons. Anaesth. Tayside Hosps. NHS Trust (Stracathro & Dundee); Sen. Regist. (Anaesth.) Aberd. Roy. Hosp. NHS Trust; Med. Off. Brit. Antarctic Survey Aberd.

THOMAS, Alan John Crud Yr Awel, Penrhyndeudraeth LL48 6NG — MB ChB Sheff. 1992.

THOMAS, Alastair Lloyd 52 Long Copse Lane, Emsworth PO10 7UR Tel: 01243 373434 — MB BS Lond. 1967 (Guy's) MRCS Eng. LRCP Lond. 1967; MRCP (UK) 1972; FRCP Lond. 1990. Cons. Rheum. Portsmouth & S.E. Hants. HA. Specialty: Rheumatol. Socs: BMA. Prev: Sen. Regist. (Rheum.) Univ. Hosp. Wales, Cardiff;

Research Fell. Univ. Michigan Hosp. Ann Arbor, USA; Regist. (Med.) Cardiff. Roy. Infirm.

THOMAS, Alec Jeremy 34 Church Street, Oswestry SY11 2SP Tel: 01691 652929; Croeswylan Way, Croeswylan Lane, Oswestry SY10 9PT Tel: 01691 670181 — MB BS Lond. 1959 (St. Mary's) MRCS Eng. LRCP Lond. 1959; DObst RCOG 1961; Cert. Family Plann. JCC 1976. Specialty: Obst. & Gyn. Socs: BMA. Prev: Resid. Med. Off. Qu. Charlotte's Hosp. Lond.; Cas. Off. & Resid. Off. (O & G) St. Mary's Hosp. Lond.; Hosp. Pract. (O & G) Shrewsbury Gp.

THOMAS, Alexandra Jane 32 Mountfield Gardens, Kenton, Newcastle upon Tyne NE3 3DB Tel: 01642 471952 — MB ChB Dundee 1994; FRCSEd (A+E); DRCOG 1996. Specialist Regist. Accid. and Emerg., North. Region. Specialty: Accid. & Emerg. Socs: BMA. Prev: SHO (Gen. Med.) Middlesbrough Gen. Hosp.; SHO (ENT & Ophth. & Dermat.) N. Riding Infirm.; SHO (A & E) Middlesbrough Gen. Hosp.

THOMAS, Aleyamma Lalita Department of Histopathology, Greenwich District Hospital, Vanburgh Hill, London SE10 9HE Tel: 020 8312 6023; 10 Eastlands Crescent, London SE21 7EG Tel: 020 8693 2424 Fax: 020 8693 2424 — MB BS Panjab 1970 (Christian Med. Coll.) MD 1975; FRCPath 1990. Cons. Histo/cytopath. Greenwich Dist. Hosp. Lond. Specialty: Histopath. Prev: Lect./Sen. Regist. Path. Qus. Med. Centre Nottm.; Regist. Path. Qu. Mary's Univ. Hosp. Roehampton.

THOMAS, Alfred Arthur Llewellyn Haslemere Health Centre, Church Lane, Haslemere GU27 2BQ Tel: 01428 653881 Fax: 01428 645065; High Garth, High Lane, Haslemere GU27 1BD Tel: 01428 644418 Email: alfred.thomas@btinternet.com — (St. Thos.) MB BS Lond. 1956; DObst RCOG 1958. Hosp. Pract. (Med.) Haslemere Hosp. Socs: BMA.

THOMAS, Alfred Evan 18 Villiers Road, Woodthorpe, Nottingham NG5 4FB Tel: 0115 960 9264 — MB ChB Manch. 1944; BSc Manch. 1941, MB ChB (Hons.) 1944; FRCP Lond. 1972, M 1949. Cons. Phys. City Hosp. Nottm. Specialty: Gen. Med. Prev: Surg. Lt. RNVR; Med. Regist. Manch. Roy. Infirm.; Sen. Med. Regist. Sheff. Roy. Infirm.

THOMAS, Alfred Theophilous 41 Garden Avenue, Mitcham CR4 2EE Tel: 020 8648 9371 — Vrach Odessa 1974; DTM & H Liverp. 1978; MRCP (UK) 1983.

THOMAS, Alison Jane Holly Lodge, London Road, Addington, Maidstone ME16 0LP — MB BS Lond. 1991 (Char. Cross & Westm.) MRCGP 1995. Specialty: Gen. Pract.

THOMAS, Alison Jane 47 Coleraine Road, London SE3 7PF Tel: 020 8852 9975 — MB ChB Birm. 1992. Cas. Off. Gosford Hosp. NSW, Austral. Prev: SHO Qu. Eliz. Hosp. Birm.; Ho. Off. (Med.) Good Hope Hosp.

THOMAS, Alison Michaela 23 Insole Grove West, Llandaff, Cardiff CF5 2HH — MB ChB Bristol 1993.

THOMAS, Allan Eric (retired) 67 Thornhill Road, Plymouth PL3 5NG Tel: 01752 672412 — (Cardiff) MRCS Eng. LRCP Lond. 1945.

THOMAS, Alun Hugh William Brown Centre, Manor Way, Peterlee SR8 5TW Tel: 0191 554 4544 Fax: 0191 554 4552 Email: hugh.thomas@gp-a83012.nhs.uk — MB BChir Camb. 1978; MA Camb. 1978; MRCGP 1982.

THOMAS, Amanda Jane Hart Community Paediatrics, St James's University Hospital, Beckitt St., Leeds LS9 7TF Tel: 0113 206 5923 Fax: 0113 206 4877 Email: amanda.thomas@leedsth.nhs.uk — MB BS Lond. 1982; DCH RCP Lond. 1985; MMed. Sci. Leeds 1998; MA Univ. of York 2003. Cons. Community Paediat., St James Univ. Hosp., Leeds; Full Time (Child Protect.) E. Leeds PCT. Specialty: Community Child Health. Socs: BMA; RCPCH; BACCH. Prev: SCMO (Child Protec. & Audiol.) LCMHT; Clin. Med. Off. (Child Health & Family Plann.) York HA & E. Surrey HA; Trainee GP Carshalton Surrey.

THOMAS, Andrew 3 Shelsley Close, Penkridge, Stafford ST19 5EF — MB ChB Liverp. 1982; MRCOG 1988. Princip. GP. Prev: Regist. (O & G) St. Mary's Hosp. Portsmouth.

THOMAS, Mr Andrew Martin Charles The Royal Orthopaedic Hospital, Woodlands, Northfield, Birmingham B31 2AP Tel: 0121 685 4005 Fax: 0121 685 4100 — MB BS Lond. 1977 (London Hospital Medical College) FRCS Ed. 1982; FRCS Eng. 1983. Cons. Orthop. Surg. Roy. Orthop. Hosp. Birm. & Univ. Hosp. Birm.; Med. Dir. Roy. Orthop. Hosp. Birm.; Hon. Sen. Lect. Univ. Birm. Specialty: Orthop. Socs: Brit. Orthop. Research Soc.; Internat. Soc. Study Lumbar Spine; Rheumatoid Arthritis Surg. Soc. Prev: Hon. Research Fell. Physiol. Univ. Birm.; Sen. Regist. Roy. Orthop. Hosp. Birm.; Regist. (Neurosurg.) Qu. Eliz. Hosp. Birm.

THOMAS, Mr Andrew Philip Wolverhampton Nuffield Hospital, Wood Road, Tettenhall, Wolverhampton WV6 8LE Tel: 01527 835166 Fax: 01527 835166 Email: apt@apthomas51.pressure.co.uk — MB BChir Camb. 1976; FRCS Eng. 1980; FRCS Ed. (Orth.) 1986. Specialty: Orthop.

THOMAS, Angela Eleine Royal Hospital for Sick Children, Department of Haematology, Sciennes Road, Edinburgh EH9 1LF Tel: 0131 536 0433 Fax: 0131 536 0430 Email: angela.thomas@luht.scot.nhs.uk — MB BS Lond. 1980 (St Bart.) MRCP (UK) 1983; FRCP Ed. 1994; PhD Lond. 1995; FRCPath 1996; FRCPCH 1997. Cons. Haemat. (Paediat.) Roy. Hosp. Sick Childr. Edin.; Hon. Sen. Lect. Edin. Specialty: Haematology. Prev: Hon. Sen. Regist. (Haemat.) Char. Cross Hosp. Lond.; Clin. Research Fell. Centre for the Genetics of Cardiovasc. Disorders Rayne Inst. Lond.; Sen. Regist. (Haemat.) St. Bart. Hosp. Lond.

THOMAS, Anita Jane Derriford Hospital, Plymouth PL6 8DH — MB ChB Bristol 1975; MB ChB (Distinc. Clin. Path.) Bristol 1975; MRCP (UK) 1978; PhD Soton. 1991; FRCP Lond. 1992. Cons. Phys. in Gen. & Geriat. Med. & Assoc. Med. Dir. (Med. Educat.); Clin. Subdean (Plymouth) Peninsula Med. Sch.; Lead Assessor GMC Professional Perform. Procedures; Mem. DH Expert Gp. on Vit.s & Minerals; Examr. RCP; Mem. DH/FSA Scientif. Advis. Commitee Nutrit. Specialty: Gen. Med. Socs: Nutrit. Soc.; Assn Study Med. Educat.; Roy. Soc. Med. Prev: Mem. (Counc.) Roy. Coll. Phys. (Hon. Sec. Comm. Med. Educat., Train. & Staffing) Gen. Internal Med. Comm.; Sen. Lect. (Geriat. Med.) & Hon. Cons. Phys. Univ. Soton.; MRC/AFRC Special Train. Fell. Nutrit. 1985-1987.

THOMAS, Ann (retired) — MB BCh Wales 1954; BSc Wales 1951, MB BCh 1954; DObst RCOG 1957; MSc Manch. 1978; FCMI 1988, M 1979; MFCM 1982. Prev: Cons. Pub. Health Med. S. Glam.

THOMAS, Ann Elizabeth Isca General Practice Unit, Cadoc House, High Street, Caerleon, Newport NP18 1AZ Tel: 01633 423886 Fax: 01633 430153 — MB BCh Wales 1977; BSc (Hons.) Wales 1972. Princip. GP Gwent. Specialty: Obst. & Gyn.

THOMAS, Anna-Jane Bargoed Hall Family Health Centre, Cardiff Road, Bargoed CF81 8NY Tel: 01443 831211 — MB BCh Wales 1996 (University of Wales College of Medicine) Specialty: Gen. Pract.

THOMAS, Anna Kathryn Llys Ifor, Crescent Road, Caerphilly CF83 1XY Tel: 029 2088 1994 — MB BCh Wales 1975; DRCOG 1977; DCH Eng. 1980; MRCPsych 1987; LLM Wales 1997. Cons. Forens. Psychiat. for People for People with Learning Disabilities. Specialty: Forens. Psychiat.; Gen. Psychiat. Socs: Wales Medico-Legal Soc. Prev: Cons. Forens. Psychiat. Caswell Clinic Bridgend; Sen. Regist. Psychiat. of Learning Disabil., Forens. Psychiat.; Sen. Med. Off. Welsh Off. Cardiff.

THOMAS, Anna Margaret The Groes, Hope Mountain, Caergwrle, Wrexham LL12 9HF — MB BCh Wales 1995.

THOMAS, Anna May 4 Kings Court, Kings Avenue, Buckhurst Hill IG9 5LU — MB BS Lond. 1996.

THOMAS, Anne Gwendolen Glenview, Glasllwch Lane, Newport NP20 3PS Tel: 01633 62517 — MB BCh Wales 1950 (Cardiff) BSc Wales 1947, MB BCh 1950; DObst RCOG 1952. Sen. Med. Off. Gwent Health Auth. Prev: Res. Pathol. Mass. Gen. Hosp. Boston; Asst. Clin. Pathol. Univ. Wales; Res. Clin. Pathol. Radcliffe Infirm. Oxf.

THOMAS, Anne Louise Department of Oncology, Leicester Royal Infirmary, Leicester LE1 5WW Tel: 0116 258 7597 Fax: 0116 258 7599; 3 The Barns Wold Farm, Kinoulton Lane, Nottingham NG12 3EQ — BM Soton. 1991 (Univ. Soton.) MRCP (UK) 1994; Phd. 1999. Cons. (Med. Oncol.) Leicester Roy. Infirm. Specialty: Oncol. Prev: Clin. Research Fell. (Med. Oncol.) City Hosp. Nottm.; Med. Regist. QMC Nottm.; Specialist Regist. (Med. Oncol.) Leicester Roy. Infirm.

THOMAS, Anne Margaret The Surgery, White Cliff Mill Street, Blandford Forum DT11 7DQ Tel: 01258 452501 Fax: 01258 455675; Tilhayes, Church Hill, Iwerne Minster, Blandford Forum DT11 8LS Tel: 01747 811658 — MB BS Lond. 1978 (St. Bart.) MB BS (Hons. Med.) Lond. 1978; MRCP (UK) 1981; DCH 1981; MRCGP 1983; DRCOG 1984. Specialty: Gen. Med. Prev: Trainee GP

Islington VTS Lond.; SHO Hosp. Sick Childr. Gt. Ormond St.; SHO (Obst.) Mothers Hosp. Lond.

THOMAS, Anne Myfanwy (retired) Institute of Neurological Sciences, Glasgow G51 4TF Tel: 0141 201 2490 Fax: 0141 201 2510 Email: myfanwy.thomas@sgh.scot.nhs.uk; 27 Rowallan Gardens, Broomhill, Glasgow G11 7LH Tel: 0141 339 7988 Fax: 0141 339 7988 — (Roy. Free) MD Lond. 1985, MB BS 1968; DCH RCPS Glas. 1971; FRCP Glas. 1989; FRCP 1998. Cons. Neurol. Inst. Neurol. Sci. Glas.; Hon. Sen. Clin. Lect. Univ. Glas.

THOMAS, Anne Stella Mary (retired) Cardiff Road Medical Centre, Cardiff Road, Taffs Well, Cardiff CF15 7YG Tel: 029 2081 0260 Fax: 029 2081 3002 — MRCS Eng. LRCP Lond. 1965.

THOMAS, Anthony (retired) Radiology Department, Norfolk & Norwich Hospital, St. Stephen's Road, Norwich NR1 3SR Tel: 01603 286094 — MB BS Lond. 1963 (Guy's) MB BS (Hons.) Lond. 1963; MRCS Eng. LRCP Lond. 1963; DObst RCOG 1965; DMRD Eng. 1969; FRCR 1975, FFR 1972. Cons. Radiol. Norf. & Norwich Health Care NHS Trust. Prev: Sen. Regist. (Radiol.) St. Mary's Hosp. & Nat. Hosp. Nerv. Dis. Lond.

THOMAS, Anthony Bainbridge The Wynd Surgery, 9 The Wynd, Marske-by-the-Sea, Redcar TS11 7LD Tel: 01642 477133 Fax: 01642 475150; Sundon, 2 Windsor Road, Saltburn-by-the-Sea TS12 1BQ Tel: 01287 622393 — MB BS Durh. 1966; DObst RCOG 1969. Prev: SHO (O & G) Preston Hosp. N. Shields; SHO (Paediat.) Qu. Eliz. Hosp. Gateshead; Ho. Phys. & Ho. Surg. Middlesbrough Gen. Hosp.

THOMAS, Anthony Leonard 14 Linkway Avenue, Ashton-in-Makerfield, Wigan WN4 8XE — MB ChB Sheff. 1989.

THOMAS, Antony 60 Walmesley Road, Leigh WN7 1XN — MB BS Madras 1988; MRCP (UK) 1994.

THOMAS, Antony Noel Department Anaesthesia, Hope Hospital, Eccles Old Road, Salford M6 8HD; 38 Hillington Road, Sale M33 6GP — MB BS Lond. 1982; FFA RCS Eng. 1987. Cons. Anaesth. Hope Hosp. Salford. Specialty: Anaesth.

THOMAS, Antony Russell 5 Stepney Rise, Scarborough YO12 5BP Email: antony.thomas1@btopenworld.com — MB ChB Leeds 1990.

THOMAS, Archibald Lloyd (retired) 149 Stoddens Road, Burnham-on-Sea TA8 2DE Tel: 01278 4172 — LMSSA Lond. 1930 (Guy's) MRCS Eng. LRCP Lond. 1931; DIH Eng. 1947. Prev: Med. Off. Roy. Arsenal Woolwich.

THOMAS, Arnallt Ty-Gwyn, 382 Pentregethin Road, Gendros, Swansea SA5 8AH — LMSSA Lond. 1960.

THOMAS, Arnold Owen West House, Westgate, Cowbridge CF7 — MB BCh Wales 1952.

THOMAS, Arthur Glannrafon Surgery, Glannrafon, Amlwch LL68 9AG Tel: 01407 830878 Fax: 01407 832512 — MB ChB Liverp. 1967. Socs: BMA.

THOMAS, Arthur Richard Pinfold Health Centre, Field Road, Bloxwich, Walsall WS3 3JP Fax: 01922 775132; Oakwood, Roman Road, Little Aston Park, Sutton Coldfield B74 3AQ — MB ChB Birm. 1962; DA Eng. 1965; DObst RCOG 1965. Socs: BMA. Prev: SHO Anaesth. Dudley Rd. Hosp. Birm.; Sen. Ho. Surg. ENT Dept. Qu. Eliz. Hosp. Birm.; Ho. Surg. Heathfield Rd. Matern. Hosp. Birm.

THOMAS, Arthur Robinson, MBE, VRD (retired) Upper Gulmswell, Combe-in-Teignhead, Newton Abbot TQ12 4RE Tel: 01626 873420 — MB BChir Camb. 1958 (Paris, Camb. & St. Geo.) MRCS Eng. LRCP Lond. 1928; MA Camb. 1931; DMRE 1933. Prev: Hon. Radiol. Newton Abbot Hosp.

THOMAS, Barbara Ann, OBE (retired) Jarvis Screening Centre, Stoughton Road, Guildford GU1 1LJ Tel: 01483 783200 Fax: 01483 783299; Copsen, Knoll Road, Frith Hill, Godalming GU7 2EL Tel: 01483 422949 — MB BChir Camb. 1960 (Camb. & Middlx.) MA Camb. 1960; DObst RCOG 1960; MRCR 1988. Mem. - Margt. Gp. - Breast Cancer Screening - Age Trial. Prev: Director - Jarvis Breast Cancer, Screening, Diagnostic and Nat. Train. Centre, Guildford.

THOMAS, Barbara Elizabeth (retired) 116 Newmarket Road, Norwich NR4 6SA Tel: 01603 452394 — BM BCh Oxf. 1948; BM BCh Oxf.; MA Oxf. 1950; FFA RCS Eng. 1954. Prev: Assoc. Specialist (Anaesth.) Norf. & Norwich Hosp.

THOMAS, Barbara Elsie Clark Avenue Surgery, Clark Avenue, Pontnewydd, Cwmbran NP44 1RY Tel: 01633 482733 Fax: 01633 867758 — MB BCh Wales 1966 (Cardiff) Prev: Ho. Surg. & Ho. Phys. E. Glam. Hosp. Pontypridd.

THOMAS, Benny 53 Chaucer Avenue, Cranford, Hounslow TW4 6NA — MB BS Lond. 1987 (Royal Free Hospital London) DRCOG Lond.; MRCP Lond. 1995. Regist. (Neurol.) Morriston Hosp. Swansea. Specialty: Neurol.; Gen. Pract.

THOMAS, Bernard 70 Everton Road, Liverpool L6 2EW — MB ChB Manch. 1988; DRCOG 1991; MRCGP 1992. GP Liverp. Prev: Assoc. GP. NWRHA.

THOMAS, Beryl Irene Evans Church Surgery, Portland St., Aberystwyth SY23 2DX Tel: 01970 4855; Orlandon, 31 North Parade, Aberystwyth SY23 2JN Tel: 01970 623808 — MB BCh Wales 1959 (Cardiff) DCH Eng. 1961; DPH Lond. 1964; MFCM 1972. Prev: Dep. MOH Cards. CC; Ho. Phys. Maelor Hosp. Wrexham; SHO (Paediat.) Neath Gen. Hosp.

THOMAS, Brett Morgan Grosvenor Avenue Surgery, 20 Grosvenor Avenue, Hayes UB4 8NL Tel: 020 8845 7100 Fax: 020 8842 4401; 34 Rickmansworth Road, Harefield, Uxbridge UB9 6JX — MB BS Lond. 1980 (Char. Cross) Clin. Asst. (Gastroenterol.) Mt. Vernon Hosp. Specialty: Gastroenterol. Prev: SHO (Thoracic Surg.) Harefield Hosp.; SHO (ENT) Mt. Vernon & Hillingdon Hosps. N.wood.

THOMAS, Brian Michael (retired) 35 Alderney Ave, Hounslow TW5 0QN Tel: 020 8570 2926 — MB BS Lond. 1958 (St. Mary's) MRCS Eng. LRCP Lond. 1958; FRCP Lond. 1981, M 1962; DMRD Eng. 1965; FFR 1967; FRCR 1975. Prev: Cons. Radiol. Univ. Coll. Hosp. & St. Marks Hosp.

THOMAS, Bronwen Ellen 27 Strange Road, Garswood, Ashton-in-Makerfield, Wigan WN4 0RX — MB ChB Liverp. 1972.

THOMAS, Bronwen Neilson (retired) Fay Cottage, 37 Penyfai Lane, Llanelli SA15 4EN — MB BCh Wales 1951 (Cardiff) BSc, MB BCh Wales 1951. JP. Prev: Sen. Hosp. Med. Off. Llanelli Chest Centr.

THOMAS, Carol Adelaide Portswood Road Surgery, 186-188 Portswood Road, Portswood, Southampton SO17 2NJ Tel: 023 8055 5181 Fax: 023 8036 6416 — MB BS Lond. 1979 (Middlesex Hospital University of London) T (GP) 1992; DFFP 1995. GP Soton.; Clin. Asst. (Breast Surg.) Soton. Univ. Hosp. Trust. Roy. S. Hants. Hosp. Specialty: Family Plann. & Reproduc. Health. Prev: Regist. (Haemat.) Guy's Hosp. Lond.

THOMAS, Caroline Frances Louise Barons Farm, Plantation Rd, Turton, Bolton BL7 0BZ — MB ChB Dundee 1993.

THOMAS, Caroline Lucy 12C Bernard Island House, Royal United Hospital, Bath BA1 3NG; 59 Western Road, Hagley, Stourbridge DY9 0JX — BM Soton. 1992. Ho. Off. Roy. United Hosp. Bath.

THOMAS, Caroline Margaret Jean Lletymaelog, Llandeilo SA19 7HY Tel: 01558 823541 Email: carolthomas@doctors.org.uk — MB BS Lond. 1969 (Roy. Free Hosp.) MRCS Eng. LRCP Lond. 1969; DObst RCOG 1972; DCH Eng. 1975; FRCP (UK) 1997, MRCP 1979. Cons. Community Paediat. (child Developm.) MSc Dept. UHW Cardiff. Specialty: Paediat. Socs: Fell. Roy. Soc. Med.; Brit. Paediat. Assn.; Welsh Paediat. Soc. Prev: Cons. Community Paediat. P. Philip Hosp. Llanelli; Sen. Regist. Llaudough Hosp. Cardiff.

THOMAS, Carys Wyn Merrywood, 31 Deepdene Wood, Dorking RH5 4BE Tel: 01306 882482; Merrywood, 31 Deepdene Wood, Dorking RH5 4BE Tel: 01306 882482 — MB BS Lond. 1998 (Univ Coll + Middlesex School of Med.) BA Camb 1995; MA Camb 1999. Specialty: Gen. Surg. Socs: BMA; MS; MDU.

THOMAS, Catherina Myfanwy Wickenwood, 49 Hinton Way, Great Shelford, Cambridge CB2 5AZ — MB BS Lond. 1980 (Royal Free Hospital School of Medicine) DRCOG 1984; DCH RCP Lond. 1984; MRCGP 1985; DOH 1998; Dip GU Med 2001. Prev: GP Camb.

THOMAS, Cathryn Patricia Ley Hill Surgery, 228 Lichfield Road, Sutton Coldfield B74 2UE Tel: 0121 308 0359 Fax: 0121 323 2682 — MB ChB Birm. 1984 (Birmingham) FRCGP 1995, M 1989. Sen. Lect. (Gen. Pract.) Univ. of Birm. Prev: Lect. (Gen. Pract.) Univ. Birm.

THOMAS, Cecilia Elizabeth Brynderwen Surgery, Crickhowell Road, St. Mellons, Cardiff CF3 0EF Tel: 029 2079 9921 Fax: 029 2077 7740; 14 Lake Road E., Roath Park, Cardiff CF23 5NN — MB BCh Wales 1978; MRCGP 1982; Dip. Palliat. Med. Wales 1992; DFFP 1995; PCR - Univ. Of Bath 1999. Hon. Lect. Gen. Pract. Univ. of Wales Coll. of Med.; Trainer in Family Plann.

THOMAS, Cenydd William Gorwel, Pendine, Carmarthen SA33 4PQ — MB BS Lond. 1998.

THOMAS, Charles Ernest Allen (retired) Trefusis, Buttermilk Lane, Pembroke SA71 4TL Tel: 01646 682912 — (Lond. Hosp.) LMSSA Lond. 1950; MRCS Eng. LRCP Lond. 1954. Prev: SHO (Anaesth.) Chelmsford Hosp. Gp.

THOMAS, Christine Margaret St Hilary Brow Group Practice, 204 Wallasey Road, Wallasey CH44 2AG Tel: 01695 574170 — MB ChB Liverp. 1983. Specialty: Dermat.

THOMAS, Christine Suzanne 110 Elthorne Park Road, London W7 2JJ — MB BS Lond. 1989; FRCA 1996. Cons. Anaesth. The W. Middx. Univ. Hosp. Trust, Isleworth. Specialty: Anaesth. Prev: Specialist Regist. (Anaesth.) Middlx. Hosp.

THOMAS, Mr Christopher David 24 Briarsmount, Heaton Mersey, Stockport SK4 2EB Tel: 0161 442 1421 Fax: 0161 442 1421 Email: christhomas1@compuserve.com — MB ChB Manch. 1992; FRCS Eng. 1997. Specialist Regist. (Orthop.) N. W. Region. Specialty: Trauma & Orthop. Surg. Socs: Manch. Med. Soc.; BMA. Prev: Research Fell. Orthop. Surg. Manch. Roy. Infirm.

THOMAS, Christopher Elwyn 12 Brickmarkers Lane, Colchester CO4 5WP — MB ChB Ed. 1993.

THOMAS, Christopher James County Hospital, Hereford HR1 2ER Tel: 01432 355444; Paradise House, Lower Paradise Frm., Marden, Hereford HR1 3EN — MB BS Lond. 1972; MRCS Eng. LRCP Lond. 1972; MRCP (UK) 1976; MRCPsych 1977. Cons. Psychiat. Hereford Co. Hosp. Specialty: Gen. Psychiat. Prev: Cons. Liaison Psychiat. Leicester Roy. Infirm.

THOMAS, Christopher Peter Alma Road Surgery, Alma Road, Romsey SO51 8ED Tel: 01794 513422 Fax: 01794 518668; Brackenwood Cottage, Rudd Lane, Michelmersh, Romsey SO51 0NG — MB BS Lond. 1984; DRCOG 1987; MRCGP 1988.

THOMAS, Christopher Stuart Department of Psychiatry, Laurente House, Wythenshawe Hospital, Manchester M23 9LT Tel: 0161 291 6925 Fax: 0161 291 6907 — MD Wales 1992; MRCPsych 1984; T(Psych) 1991. Cons. Psychiat. & Hon. Lect. Univ. Hosp. S. Manch. Specialty: Gen. Psychiat. Prev: Sen. Lect. (Psychiat. Med.) Univ. Otago, NZ.

THOMAS, Christopher William (retired) Garian, 4 Dinglewood Close, Westbury-on-Trym, Bristol BS9 2LL Tel: 0117 968 3726 Fax: 0117 968 3726 Email: chris@dinglewood.freeserve.co.uk — (Ed.) MB ChB Ed. 1957. Prev: Ho. Phys., Ho. Surg. & SHO (Cas.) Roy. Gwent Hosp. Newport.

THOMAS, Claire 84 Brookfield Road, Grimsby DN33 3JL — BM BS Nottm. 1994. Specialty: Anaesth.

THOMAS, Claire Daphne Royal Shrewbury Hospital, Mytton Oak Road, Mytton Oak, Shrewsbury SY3 8XQ Tel: 01743 261000 Email: cdthomas@doctors.org.uk; 25 Bull St, Harborne, Birmingham B17 0HH Tel: 0121 426 2018 — MB ChB Birm. 1993 (Birmingham) MRCPCH 1998. Ho. Off. (Paediat.) Mackay Base Hosp. Mackay, Austral. Specialty: Paediat. Prev: Ho. Off. & Resid. Med. Off. (O & G) Mt. Isa Base Hosp., Austral.; Ho. Off. (Med.) Birm. Heartlands Hosp.

THOMAS, Claire Philippa Flat 6, Ulverdale Road, Chelsea, London SW10 0SN — MB BS Lond. 1994; MRCP; MRCPath; BSc Lond. 1987; Dphil (Oxon.) 1991; MSc Lond. 2003. Specialty: Med. Microbiol.; Infec. Dis.

THOMAS, Colin Charles 11 Woodbank Avenue, Gerrards Cross SL9 7PY — MB BChir Camb. 1983; MA Camb. 1983; MFOM RCP Lond. 1994, A 1990. Sen. Med. Off. BBC TV. Specialty: Occupat. Health. Prev: Cons. Occupat. Phys. Southend Hosp.; Med. Off. Ford Motor Co. Dagenham; Ho. Phys. New Addenbrooke's Hosp. Camb.

THOMAS, Colin Hugh — MB ChB Birm. 1968; FFA RCS Eng. 1972. Cons. Anaesth. Birm. InDepend. Pract. Specialty: Anaesth. Prev: Cons. Anaesth. Birm. Accid. Hosp.; Cons. Anaesth. Roy. Orthop Hosp. Birm.

THOMAS, Cyril Geoffrey Arthur (retired) 116 Newmarket Road, Norwich NR4 6SA Tel: 01603 452394 — BM BCh Oxf. 1948 (Oxf. & St. Thos.) MA Oxf. 1949; FRCP Lond. 1987, M 1952; FRCPath 1970. Prev: Cons. Microbiol. Norf. & Norwich Hosp.

THOMAS, Dafydd Huw Vaughan The Health Centre, Hermitage Road, St John's, Woking GU21 8TD Tel: 01483 723451 Fax: 01483 751879 — MB BCh Wales 1980; DRCOG 1985; MRCGP 1986.

THOMAS, Dafydd Wyn Department of Anaesthesia and Intensive Care, Morriston Hospital, Swansea SA6 6NL Tel: 01792 703468 Fax: 01792 703470; Cynghordy, Salem, Abertawe, Swansea SA6 6PD Tel: 01792 842598 — MB BCh Wales 1978; FFA RCS Eng. 1984. Cons. (Anaesth. & IC) Swansea. Specialty: Anaesth.; Intens. Care. Socs: Soc. Anaesth. of Wales; Counc. Mem. Autologous Transfus. s/i Gp.; Dep. Regional Advisor for Anaesth. Wales.

THOMAS, Damion Block 9 Southampton General Hospital, Tremona Road, Southampton SO16 6YD — BM Soton. 1998.

THOMAS, Daniel Ashley Gorwel, Welsh Hook Road, Hayscastlecross, Haverfordwest SA62 5NY — MB ChB Liverp. 1968; DObst RCOG 1970; FFA RCS Eng. 1975. Cons. (Anaesth.) Withybush Hosp. HaverfordW.. Specialty: Anaesth.

THOMAS, Daniel Lewis Charles Hereford House, 51 Westerfield Road, Ipswich IP4 2UU Tel: 01473 254555 — MB BS Lond. 1945 (Lond. Hosp.) MD Lond. 1953 MB BS 1945, DPM 1950; MRCPsych 1971. Socs: BMA. Prev: Cons. Psychiat. Suff. Ment. Hosps.; Sen. Hosp. Med. Off. Runwell Hosp.; Sen. Regist. Dept. Psychiat. St. Geo. Hosp. Lond.

THOMAS, Daniel Phillip Pennant, Rhosmaen, Llandeilo SA19 6NP — MB BS Lond. 1990.

THOMAS, David 31 Lizban Street, Blackheath, London SE3 8SS — MB BS Lond. 1975; FFA RCS Eng. 1980. Sen. Regist. (Anaesth.) Lond. Hosp. Specialty: Anaesth.

THOMAS, David Adrian QMCUH, Nottingham NG7 2UH Tel: 0115 924 9924 Fax: 0115 849 3294 Email: david.thomas@mail.qmcuh-tr.trent.nhs.uk — MB ChB Birm. 1981; MRCPCH; DCH RCP Lond. 1986; MRCP (UK) 1987. Cons. Paediat. & Intensivist Qu.s Med. Centre Nottm. Specialty: Paediat.; Intens. Care; Respirat. Med. Socs: Paediat. Intens. Care Soc. Prev: Sen. Regist. (Paediat.) City Hosp. & Qu. Med. Centre Nottm.

THOMAS, David Arthur Long Lane Surgery, 15 Long Lane, Liverpool L19 6PE Tel: 0151 494 1445; 121 Alder Road, Liverpool L12 2BA — MB ChB Liverp. 1954; BSc (Hons. Physiol.) Liverp. 1951. Specialty: Gen. Pract. Socs: Liverp. Med. Inst.

THOMAS, David Brynmor Bute Medical Buildings, Queens Terrace, St Andrews KY16 9TS Tel: 01334 76161 — MB BS Lond. 1956 (Univ. Coll. Lond. & Univ. Coll. Hosp.) FRS Ed.; BSc (Special) Lond. 1952, MB BS 1956; FRCPath 1977, M 1974; DSc Birm. 1976; FIBiol. 1976; FRCP Ed. 1984. Bute Prof. Anat. & Experim. Path. Univ. St. And. Socs: Fell. Roy. Soc. Med. Prev: Master, United Coll. St. Salvator & St. Leonard St. Andrews; Sen. Lect. Histol. & Cellular Biol. Univ. Birm.; Nuffield Lect. Path. Univ. Oxf.

THOMAS, David Charles 36 Granville Road, Oxted RH8 0DA Tel: 01883 712423 — MB ChB Sheff. 1983; DA 1986; DRCOG 1991. Specialty: Anaesth.; Otolaryngol.

THOMAS, David Colwyn West Winds, Caswell Road, Newton, Swansea SA3 — MB BS Lond. 1947 (St. Bart.) MRCS Eng. LRCP Lond. 1942. Mem. Min. of Pens. & Nat. Insur. Med. Bds. Socs: BMA. Prev: Phys. & Anaesth. EMS Hosp. Morriston; Ho. Surg. Swansea Gen. & Eye Hosp.; Capt. RAMC.

THOMAS, David Derek Maendy Place Medical Centre, 1 Maendy Place, Weatherall Street, Aberdare CF44 7AY Tel: 01685 872146 Fax: 01685 884767 — MB BCh Wales 1976; DRCOG 1978.

THOMAS, Professor David Fraser Morgan St James's University Hospital, Department of Paediatric Urology, Clinical Sciences Building, Leeds LS9 7TF Tel: 0113 206 5114 Fax: 0113 206 4140 Email: d.f.m.thomas@leeds.ac.uk — MB BChir Camb. 1971 (Camb./Guys) MA Camb. 1971; MB Camb. 1971; MRCP (UK) 1973; FRCS Eng. 1976; FRCPCH 1997; FRCP Lond. 1997; FRCP Ed. 1997. Cons. Paediat. Urol. Leeds Teachg. Hosps. NHS Trust; Associate Editor British Journal of Urology; Prof. Paed. Surg. Leeds Uni. Specialty: Paediat. Surg. Socs: Eur. Soc. Paediat. Urol.; Exec. Brit. Assn. Paediat. Surg.; Counc. Brit. Assn. Urol. Surg. (1995-1998). Prev: Sen. Clin. Lect. Univ. Leeds; Sen. Regist. Hosp. Sick Childr. Gt. Ormond St. Lond.; Wellcome Research Fell. Inst. Child Health Lond.

THOMAS, David Gareth Green Close Surgery, Green Close, Kirkby Lonsdale, Carnforth LA6 2BS Tel: 015242 71210 Fax: 015242 72713 — (Bombay) MA Cantab; MB BS London 1980. GP Carnforth, Lancs.

THOMAS, David Gareth 2 Lambourn Avenue, Eastbourne BN24 5PQ — BM Soton. 1998.

THOMAS, David Gareth Hughes Iet Wen, Morfa Nefyn, Pwllheli LL53 6AR — MB BCh Wales 1949 (Cardiff) BSc MB BCh Wales 1949. Sen. Med. Off. Roy. Fleet Auxil. Prev: Ho. Surg. Llandough Hosp. Cardiff; RN; Res. Med. Off. H.M. Stanley Hosp. St. Asaph.

THOMAS, David Gary 4 Brookfield Park Road, Cowbridge CF71 7HJ — MB BCh Wales 1981; FFA RCS Lond. 1985. Cons. Anaesth. Princess of Wales Hosp. Bridgend. Specialty: Anaesth. Prev: Sen. Regist. (Anaesth.) Cardiff & Swansea; Regist. (Anaesth.) St. Mary's Hosp. Lond.; SHO (Anaesth.) Swansea.

THOMAS, David George Chastleton, Newton Drive, Framwellgate Moor, Durham DH1 5BH Tel: 0191 384 6171; 5 Goodwell Lea, Brancepeth, Durham DH7 8EN Tel: 0191 378 4465 — MB BCh Wales 1993 (Univ of Wales.)

THOMAS, David Geraint BUPA Occupational Health, PO Box 15, Gresty Road, Crewe CW2 6BT Tel: 01270 453100 Fax: 01270 453101 Email: thomasda@bupa.com; 14 Nevis Drive, Crewe CW2 8UH Tel: 01270 214241 Email: thomcrewe@aol.com — MRCS Eng. LRCP Lond. 1974; AFOM RCP Lond. 1995. Med. Off. Brit. Railways Crewe. Specialty: Occupat. Health. Socs: Fell. Roy. Soc. Med.; Soc. Occupat. Med. Prev: SHO (Surg.) Manch. Roy. Infirm. & Sharoe Green Hosp. Preston.

THOMAS, David Gerard Department of Anaesthesia, Dryburn Hospital, North Road, Durham DH1 5TW Tel: 0191 386 4911; 10 Richmond Crescent, Vicars Cross, Chester CH3 5PB — MB BS Newc. 1980; Dip. Obst. Auckland 1988; FFA RCSI 1990. Cons. Anaesth. Dryburn Hosp. Durh. Specialty: Anaesth. Socs: Assn. Anaesth.; Obst. Anaesth. Assn.

THOMAS, Professor David Glyndor Treharne The National Hospital for Neurology & Neurosurgery, Queen Square, London WC1N 3BG Tel: 020 7837 3611 Fax: 020 7278 7894 Email: neurological.surgery@ion.ucl.ac.uk; 14 Montagu Square, London W1H 2LD Tel: 020 7486 8566 — (St. Mary's) MRCS Eng. LRCP Lond. 1966; MA Camb. 1968, BA 1963, MB 1967, BChir 1966; MRCP (UK) 1970; FRCS Ed. 1972; FRCP Glas. 1985; FRCS Eng 1998. Prof. Neurosurg. Nat. Hosp. Neurol. & Neurosurg. Lond.; Sen. Lect. Inst. Neurol. Lond.; Cons. Neurosurg. Nat. Hosps. Nerv. Dis. Lond. & Northwick Pk. Hosp. Specialty: Neurosurg. Socs: Fell. Roy. Soc. Med.; Soc. Brit. Neurol. Surgs.; Pres. Europ. Soc. Stereotactic & Func.al Neurosurg. Prev: Sen. Regist. (Neurosurg.) Inst. Neurol. Scs. South. Gen. Hosp. Glas.; SHO (Neurol.) St. Mary's Hosp. Lond.; Asst. Lect. (Anat.) St. Mary's Hosp. Med. Sch. Lond.

THOMAS, David Gordon Borough Green Medical Practice, Quarry Hill Road, Borough Green, Sevenoaks TN15 8RQ Tel: 01732 883161 Fax: 01732 886319 — MB BChir Camb. 1969 (Camb. & Guy's) DCH Eng. 1971; MRCGP 1989. Prev: Regist. (Paediat.) Pembury Hosp. Tunbridge Wells; Ho. Phys. Roy. Devon & Exeter Hosp.; Ho. Surg. Guys Hosp. Lond.

THOMAS, Mr David Gwyn 3 Haugh Lane, Sheffield S11 9SA — MB BS Lond. 1962 (Middlx.) FRCS Eng. 1967; FRCP 1999. Cons. Urol. Surg. Spinal Injuries Unit Northern Gen. Hosp., Sheff.; Hon. Clin. Lect. Urol. Univ. Sheff. Specialty: Urol. Prev: Hon. Clin. Lect. Spinal Injuries Univ. Sheff.; Sen. Regist. Dept. Urol. Sheff.

THOMAS, David Hugh (retired) 61 Stakesby Road, Whitby YO21 1JF — MB ChB Leeds 1956; DObst RCOG 1961. Local Treasury Med. Off. Prev: GP Whitby.

THOMAS, David Hywel Llwyn-y-Piod, Peniel, Carmarthen SA32 7AA — BM BS Nottm. 1997.

THOMAS, David Ian 18 Pilkington Avenue, Sutton Coldfield B72 1LA — MB ChB Birm. 1981; DA (UK) 1985; FCAnaesth. 1990.

THOMAS, David Iorwerth (retired) 34 Widewell Road, Roborough, Plymouth PL6 7DW — (Guy's) MRCS Eng. LRCP Lond. 1941. Prev: Ho. Surg. Northampton Gen. Hosp. & Selly Oak Hosp. Birm.

THOMAS, Mr David James Department Urology, Freeman Hospital, Newcastle upon Tyne; 2 Cadaway House, Greenside, Ryton NE40 4SH — MB BS Lond. 1985; FRCS Ed. 1989; FRCS Eng. 1990. Research Regist. (Urol.) Freeman Hosp. Newc. u. Tyne. Specialty: Urol. Prev: Regist. (Surg.) St. Mary's Hosp. Portsmouth; Regist. (Surg.) Qu. Alexandra Hosp. Cosham Portsmouth; SHO Rotat. (Surg.) Bristol Roy. Infirm.

THOMAS, David James 31 Smith Street, Chelsea, London SW3 4ER Tel: 020 7352 5899 — MB BS Lond. 1943 (St. Mary's) MRCS Eng. LRCP Lond. 1942; LRCP Lond. 1942; DCH Eng. 1944; MRCP Lond. 1946; MD Lond. 1947; MRCGP 1960. Specialty: Gen. Pract. Socs: BMA (Late Chairm. Local Br.). Prev: Clin. Asst. Vict. Hosp. Childr. Tite St.; Ho. Phys. King Edwd. Memor. Hosp. Ealing.

THOMAS, Mr David Jeffrey Glan Clwyd Hospital, Rhyl LL18 5UJ Tel: 01745 583910 Fax: 01745 583143; Plas Ffordd Ddwr, Llandyrnog, Denbigh LL16 4ET Tel: 01824 790316 — MB BS Lond. 1965 (St. Mary's) MRCS Eng. LRCP Lond. 1964; FRCS Ed. 1970; FRCOG 1983, M 1970. Cons. O & G Clwyd N. Health Dist. Specialty: Obst. & Gyn. Socs: Fell. N. Eng. Obst. & Gyn. Soc.; Welsh Obst. & Gyn. Soc. Prev: Sen. Regist. (O & G) Westm. Hosp. Lond.; Ho. Surg. (Gyn.) Samarit. Hosp. Lond.; Ho. Surg. (Obst.) St. Mary's Hosp. Lond.

THOMAS, David John (retired) Wooletts, Cherry Tree Lane, Fulmer, Slough SL3 6JE Tel: 01753 662147 Fax: 01753 664023 — (Camb. & Birm.) MB BChir Camb. 1970; MA Camb. 1970; MRCP (UK) 1972; MD Birm. 1977; FRCP Lond. 1985. Cons. Neurol. St. Marys Hosp. Lond.; Sen. Lect. Inst. Neurol. & Hon. Cons. (Neurol.) Nat. Hosp. Neurol. & Neurosurg. & Chalfont Centre for Epilepsy. Prev: Research Fell. St. Thos. Hosp. Lond. & Nat. Hosp. Nerv. Dis. Qu. Sq. Lond.

THOMAS, David John Bowen 4 Chandos Close, Buckhurst Hill IG9 5HS Tel: 020 8505 0421 — MD Lond. 1978 (St. Thos.) MB BS 1971; MRCP (UK) 1974; FRCP Lond. 1993. Cons. Phys. Mt. Vernon & Hillingdon Hosps.; Sen. Regist. Med. Unit St. Bart. Hosp. Lond. Specialty: Gen. Med. Socs: Brit. Diabetic Assn.; Med. Res. Soc. Prev: Sen. Regist. Whipps Cross Hosp. Lond.; Regist. Basingstoke Dist. & Soton. Univ. Hosp.; Wessex Research Fell.

THOMAS, David Kermac Macmeikan (retired) The White Cottage, Braywood, Oakley Green, Windsor SL4 4QF Tel: 01628 621250 — MB BS Lond. 1953 (Univ. Coll. Hosp.) DObst RCOG 1957; MRCGP 1963. Prev: Ho. Surg. Univ. Coll. Hosp.

THOMAS, David Lewis Royal Gwent Hospital, Cardiff Road, Newport NP20 2UB — MB BCh Wales 1976; FFA RCS Eng. 1980. Cons. Anaesth. Roy. Gwent Hosp. Newport. Specialty: Anaesth.

THOMAS, David Malcolm University Hospital of Wales, Heath Park, Cardiff CF14 4WZ Tel: 029 2074 6645 Fax: 029 2074 6661 — MB BChir Camb. 1984; MD Camb. 1994; FRCP 2000. Clin. Director of Med., Cardiff & the Vale NHSTrust; Cons. Phys. (Nephrol.) Univ. Hosp. Wales. Specialty: Gen. Med.; Nephrol.

THOMAS, David Michael Marlow and Partners, The Surgery, Bell Lane, Stroud GL6 9JF Tel: 01453 883793 Fax: 01453 731670 — MB BS Lond. 1983; MRCP Lond. 1986; DA (UK) 1988; FRCP Lond. 2002. Clin. Research Fell., Dept. of Gen. Pract. & Primary Care,University of Aberdeen>; Primary Care Advisor, Gloucestershire Research & Development Support Unit.

THOMAS, Mr David Michael Gloucester Royal Hospital, Department of ENT, Gloucester GL1 3NN Tel: 0845 422 6186; Tottmoor, Shipton Oliffe, Cheltenham GL54 4JQ Fax: 0845 422 6432 — MB BS Lond. 1987 (Char. Cross & Westm.) BSc Cardiff 1982; FRCS Eng. 1991; FRCS (Otol.) 1993; FRCS (Orl.) 1997. Cons. (Otolaryngol.) Cheltenham Gen Gloucester Hosp.& Clin. Dir. For Otolaryngol. Specialty: Otolaryngol.; Otorhinolaryngol.; Oncol. Socs: BAO; H+NS; BAHNO. Prev: Sen. Regist. (ENT) Southmead Hosp. Bristol; Regist. (ENT) St. Mary's Hosp. Lond.; Sen. Regist. (ENT) Roy. Devon & Exeter Hosp.

THOMAS, Mr David Michael Department of Urology, Queen's Hospital NHS Trust, Belvedere Road, Burton-on-Trent DE13 0RB Tel: 01283 566333 Ext: 4011 Fax: 01283 593087; (cons. rooms), 181 Rolleston Road, Burton-on-Trent DE13 0LD Tel: 01283 563045 — MB BChir Camb. 1971 (Middlesex Hospital) MA Camb. 1971; FRCS Eng. 1975. Cons. Urol. Burton Hosp. NHS Trust. Specialty: Urol. Socs: BAUS. Prev: Sen. Regist. (Urol.) Middlx. Hosp. & St. Peters Hosp.

THOMAS, David Michael Spa Medical Centre, Snowberry Lane — MB BS Lond. 1990; DRCOG 1994; MRCGP 1995. GP Princip. Melksham Wiltsh. Specialty: Gen. Pract. Socs: MDU & BMA. Prev: GPUTS, St Albans.

THOMAS, David Michael Marryat, Kippington Road, Sevenoaks TN13 2LH — MB BS Lond. 1975 (Guy's) BSc (Hons.) Lond. 1972; MRCS Eng. LRCP Lond. 1975.

THOMAS, David Owen Goldacre Farm, Farway, Colyton EX24 6DH — MB ChB Sheff. 1991.

THOMAS, David Rhys Lowfield Road, 5 Lowfield Road, Shaw Heath, Stockport SK2 6RW Tel: 0161 480 8249 Fax: 0161 474 0290; 27 Heath Road, Stockport SK2 6JJ Tel: 0161 419 9001 — MB BS Lond. 1964; MRCS Eng. LRCP Lond. 1964; MRCP Lond. 1967.

THOMAS, Mr David Rhys Good Hope Hospital, Rectory Road, Sutton Coldfield B75 7RR Tel: 0121 378 2211 Ext: 2386 Fax: 0121

311 1074; The Dell, 33 Hartopp Road, Sutton Coldfield B74 2QR Tel: 0121 308 6344 — MB BCh Wales 1965 (Welsh) FRCS Eng. 1971. p/t Cons. Surg. N. Birm. HA.; Hon. Lect., Birm. Univ. Specialty: Urol. Socs: BAMS.

THOMAS, David Richard Bryn Villa, Gorslas, Llanelli SA15 5AT — MB BS Lond. 1978; MA Camb. 1978; MRCS Eng. LRCP Lond. 1978.

THOMAS, Mr David Richard (retired) 6 North Avenue, Ashbourne DE6 1EZ Tel: 01335 345800 Email: d.thomas@pobox.com — MB BS Lond. 1961 (St. Geo.) MRCS Eng. LRCP Lond. 1961; FRCS Eng. 1967. Cons. Surg. Derbysh. Roy. Infirm. & Derbysh. Childr. Hosp.; Clin. Teach. Univ. Nottm.; DL Derbysh. Prev: Ho. Phys. (Med.) & Ho. Surg. (Surg.) St. Geo. Hosp. Lond.

THOMAS, David Richard Brynmor (retired) Messers Herbert Smith, Exchange House, Primrose St., London EC2A 2HS Tel: 020 7374 8000 Fax: 020 7374 0888; Old Orchard, The St, Plaxtol, Sevenoaks TN15 0QG Tel: 01732 811070 — MB ChB Ed. 1987 (Univ. of Edin.) Partner Messers Herbert Smith Lond. Prev: Ho. Surg. Vasc. Surg. Unit. Glas. Roy. Infirm.

THOMAS, David Roger 14 Lake Road E., Roath Park, Cardiff CF23 5NN — MB BCh Wales 1978; MRCPsych 1984. Cons. Forens. Psychiat., Bro Morgannwg Trust, Glanrhyd Hosp., Bridgend. Specialty: Forens. Psychiat.

THOMAS, David Vaughan Philipps (Surgery), 83 Grove Road, Sutton SM1 2DB Tel: 020 8642 1721; 51 Southway, Carshalton Beeches, Carshalton SM5 4HP Tel: 020 8642 8973 — MRCS Eng. LRCP Lond. 1971 (Guy's) DFFP 1994. Socs: Brit. Assn. Sport & Med. Prev: Regist. Accid. & Orthop. Dept. St. Peter's Hosp. Chertsey; Cas. Off. Guy's Hosp.; Asst. Med. Off. Brookfield Cott. Hosp. Newfoundld., Canada.

THOMAS, Debbie Bevan Ty-Elli Group Practice, Ty Elli, Llanelli SA15 3BD Tel: 01554 772678 / 773747 Fax: 01554 774476; 10 Squirrel Walk, Fforest, Pontarddulais, Swansea SA4 1UH — MB BCh Wales 1988; DRCOG 1991; MRCGP 1992. Clin. Asst. GU Med.

THOMAS, Deborah Jane 5 Clovelly Road, Emsworth PO10 7HL — MB BS Lond. 1987.

THOMAS, Deborah Jane — MB ChB Ed. 1993. Locum GP Deopham Norf. Specialty: Obst. & Gyn. Prev: SHO (O & G) Colchester.

THOMAS, Deborah Karen 18 Fosse Way, London W13 0BZ — MB BS Lond. 1993.

THOMAS, Dhanesvari Northampton General Hospital, The Eye Department - Singlehurst Ward, Cliftonville, Northampton NN1 5BD — MB ChB Natal 1991.

THOMAS, Donald Alexander (retired) 64 Hutton Village, Hutton, Brentwood CM13 1RU — MRCS Eng. LRCP Lond. 1956 (Camb. & St. Mary's) DA Eng. 1961; FFA RCS Eng. 1967. Cons. Anaesth. Havering Health Dist. Prev: Sen. Regist. (Anaesth.) Barnet Gen. Hosp.

THOMAS, Donald Glynne Department of Occupational medicine, Royal Liverpool University NHS Trust, Liverpool L14 Tel: 0151 282 6765 Fax: 0151 282 6815; 5 Church Farm Court, Neston Road, Willaston, South Wirral CH64 2XP — (Liverp.) MB ChB Liverp. 1968; Assoc. Fac. Occupat. Med. RCP Lond. 1979. Clin. Dir. (Occupat. Med.) Liverp. Trusts, Univ. Hosps., Mersey Regional Bd. & Nat. Blood Transfus. Serv.; Cons. Anaesth. Mersey RHA. Specialty: Occupat. Health. Socs: Liverp. Soc. Anaesth. & Soc. Occupat. Med.; Fell. Roy. Soc. Med. Prev: Med. Asst. (A & E) Chester Roy. Infirm.; Regist. (Radiol.) Robt. Jones & Agnes Hunt Orthop. Hosp. Oswestry; Regist. (Anaesth.) Clatterbridge Hosp. Bebington.

THOMAS, Donald John, MBE, KStJ 22 Bowham Avenue, Bridgend CF31 3PA Tel: 01656 653130 — MB BCh Wales 1954 (Cardiff) BSc Wales 1951; FFOM RCP Lond. 1985, MFOM 1978; Specialist Accredit. (Occupat. Med.) RCP Lond. 1978. Specialty: Occupat. Health. Socs: Soc. Occupat. Med.; BMA (Exec. Mem. Mid-Glam. Div.); Cardiff PG Fed.Chest Dis. Prev: Company. Assoc. Brit. Ports. Swansea & Cardiff; Med. Off. i/c Radiol. Servs. S. Wales Area Nat. Coal Bd. & Nat. Smokeless Fuels Ltd.; SHO Miners' Chest. Dis. Treatm. Centre Llandough Hosp.

THOMAS, Dorothy Spencer Windyridge, Swaines Road, Bembridge PO35 5XS — MB BS Lond. 1921 (King's Coll.) MRCS Eng. LRCP Lond. 1921. Prev: Med. Off. Knowle Hosp. Fareham; Clin. Asst. Neurol. Dept. & Obst. Ho. Surg. King's Coll. Hosp.

THOMAS, Douglas Gordon 388 Westdale La, Mapperley, Nottingham NG3 6ES — MB ChB Birm. 1997.

THOMAS, Mr Douglas Wilfred Glyder, Gwaelodygarth Close, Merthyr Tydfil CF47 8DX — MRCS Eng. LRCP Lond. 1943 (Camb. & Westm.) BA Camb. 1940; FRCS Eng. 1949.

THOMAS, Duncan Porter (retired) The Old Barn, North Green, Kirtlington, Kidlington OX5 3JZ Tel: 01869 350930 Email: dpt@patrol.i-way.co.uk — (Oxf. & St. Bart.) MB BS Lond. 1954; MSc Oxf. 1952, DPhil 1958; MD Lond. 1964; FRCPath 1980, M 1973. Prev: Head Div. Haemat. Nat. Inst. Biol. Standards & Control Potters Bar.

THOMAS, Edna June (retired) (Surgery), 5 Strawberry Place, Glyn Mefus, Morriston, Swansea SA6 7AQ Tel: 01792 771072; Cefn Eithin, School Lane, Middleton, Rhossili, Swansea SA3 1PJ Tel: 01792 390563 — MB ChB Birm. 1958. Prev: Ho. Surg. & Ho. Phys. Morriston Hosp. Swansea.

THOMAS, Edward Gwyn 32 Cedar Avenue, Hazlemere, High Wycombe HP15 7DW Tel: 01494 712065 — MB BCh Wales 1974; FFPM RCP (UK) 1995. Specialty: Pharmaceutical Medicine.

THOMAS, Edward Hartley (retired) 2 Cranford Gardens, Marple, Stockport SK6 6QQ Tel: 0161 427 3500 Email: thomcran@btinternet.com — MB ChB Manch. 1960; DObst RCOG 1961; DA Eng. 1962; MRCGP 1968. Prev: GP Stockport.

THOMAS, Elaine 2 Melbourne Crescent, Beaconside, Stafford ST16 3JU — MB ChB Leeds 1985; DRCOG 1989; Dip. Community Paediat. Warwick 1993. Staff Grade Doctor Premier Health NHS Trust. Specialty: Community Child Health.

THOMAS, Eleanor Elizabeth 13 Southernhay Road, Stoneygate, Leicester LE2 3TN Tel: 0116 270 8058 — MB BS Lond. 1993 (St Marys Hosp. NHS Sch.) BSc Hons 1990; MRCP 1998. SHO (Community Paediat.) Frencham Hosp. Bristol. Specialty: Paediat. Prev: SHO (Neonat.) St Michaels Hosp. Bristol; SHO (Paediat.) Australia; SHO (Paediat.) Lewisham Hosp. Lond.

THOMAS, Eleri Wyn 57 Porset Close, Caerphilly CF83 1PQ — MB BCh Wales 1998.

THOMAS, Elfyn Owen Heulfryn, Ty Mawr, Lon Pentraeth, Menai Bridge LL59 5HR — MB BS Lond. 1990.

THOMAS, Elizabeth Ann Irnham Lodge Surgery, Townsend Road, Minehead TA24 5RG Tel: 01643 703289 Fax: 01643 707921 — MB BCh Wales 1982.

THOMAS, Elizabeth Ann Chilcoate Surgery Practice, Hampton Avenue, St Marychurch, Torquay TQ1 3LA Tel: 01803 323123/314240 Fax: 01803 322001; Iona, 27 Shiphay Avenue, Torquay TQ2 7ED Tel: 01803 605359 — MB BS Lond. 1983; DRCOG 1990; MRCGP 1991. Specialty: Gen. Med. Prev: Trainee GP Ivybridge Health Centre Devon; Regist. (Gen. Med.) Plymouth Gen. Hosp.; SHO (O & G & A & E) Plymouth Gen. Hosp.

THOMAS, Elizabeth Margaret 10 Airbles Drive, Motherwell ML1 3AS — MB ChB Glas. 1976; DRCOG 1979; DCH Eng. 1980; MRCGP 1980.

THOMAS, Emily Jane Bridge Ways, Little Bookham St., Bookham, Leatherhead KT23 3HR — BM BCh Oxf. 1998; BM BCh Oxf 1998.

THOMAS, Emma Elizabeth 26 Brentford Avenue, Crosby, Liverpool L23 2UZ — MB ChB Birm. 1993.

THOMAS, Mr Emrys Maelor 117 Burbage Road, Dulwich, London SE21 7AF Tel: 020 7274 8703 — MB BS Lond. 1957 (King's Coll. Hosp.) MRCS Eng. LRCP Lond. 1957; FRCS Eng. 1967. Cons. Orthop. Surg. King's Coll. Hosp. Lond. & Roy. Masonic Hosp. Specialty: Orthop. Socs: Fell. Roy. Soc. Med. & Brit. Orthop. Assn. Lond. Prev: Ho. Phys. & Ho. Surg. King's Coll. Hosp. Lond.; Surg. Regist. Roy. Postgrad. Med. Sch. & Hammersmith Hosp. Lond.; Sen. Orthop. Regist. King's Coll. Hosp. Rotat. Train. Scheme.

THOMAS, Eric Jackson 23 Westbourne Terrace, Shiney Row, Houghton-le-Spring DH4 4QT Tel: 0191 852512; 7 High Friarside, Burnopfield, Newcastle upon Tyne NE16 6AN Tel: 01207 71624 — MB BS Durh. 1949. Mem. Med. Bd. Min. of Social Security; Div. Med. Off. St. John Ambul. Brig. Socs: BMA. Prev: Ho. Surg. Roy. Vict. Infirm. Newc.; Ho. Phys. Stobhill Hosp. Glas.

THOMAS, Eryl Ann James Paget Hospital NHS Trust, Lowestoft Road, Gorleston, Great Yarmouth NR31 6LA Tel: 01493 452400 Fax: 01493 453387 Email: eryl.thomas@jpaget.nhs.uk — MB ChB Bristol 1982; MRCP (UK) 1985; FRCR 1989. Cons. Radiol. Jas. Paget NHS Trust Gt. Yarmouth. Specialty: Radiol. Socs: Roy. Coll. of Radiologists; Roy. Coll. of Phys.s; JPH Ethics Advis. Gp. Prev: Cons.

Radiol. Broadgreen Hosp. NHS Trust Liverp.; Sen. Regist. (Radiol.) Bristol Roy. Infirm. & Plymouth Gen. Hosp.

THOMAS, Essillt Balgay, Grange Lane, Alvechurch, Birmingham B48 7DJ — MB ChB Liverp. 1959.

THOMAS, Ewan Llywelyn Gerafon Surgery, Benllech, Llandudno — MB ChB Manch. 1982.

THOMAS, Ewart Royston (retired) Four Winds, Bynea, Llanelli SA14 9PR Tel: 01554 59597 — MRCS Eng. LRCP Lond. 1955 (Lond. Hosp.) Prev: Ho. Surg. & Ho. Phys. St. And. Hosp. Bow.

THOMAS, Ffion Jones Bryn-y-Mor Farm, Pembrey Mountain, Burry Port SA16 0BX — MB BCh Wales 1989.

THOMAS, Frank Melville York Medical Practice, St John's Health Centre, Oak Lane, Twickenham TW1 3PA Tel: 020 8744 0220 Fax: 020 8892 6855; Lansdowne, 187 Percy Road, Twickenham TW2 6JS — MB BS Lond. 1978 (Char. Cross University of Wales) BDS Wales 1972; LDS RCS Eng. 1973; Cert. Family Plann. JCC 1984. Specialty: Urol.; Otorhinolaryngol.; Sports Med. Socs: Fell. Roy. Soc. Med.; BMA. Prev: Trainee GP W. Middlx. Hosp. VTS; SHO & Demonst. (Anat.) Char. Cross. Hosp. Lond.; Ho. Surg. (Urol., ENT & Oral Surg.) Char. Cross Hosp. Lond.

THOMAS, Gail Golygfa Hardd, Caerbryn Square, Penygroes Road, Ammanford SA18 — MB BCh Wales 1989; MRCGP 1993.

THOMAS, Gail Elizabeth Darent Valley Hospital, Darenth Wood Road, Dartford DA2 8DA Tel: 01322 428628 Fax: 01322 428635 Email: gthomasmdphd@yahoo.com — MD South Illinois 1986 (Chicago) BA South. Illinois 1977; PhD 1982; Surgic. Oncol. Fellowsh. 1993. Cons. Surg. (Gen. & Breast); Cons. to Lymphatic Filiarsis Program, The Carter Centre, Atlanta, GA USA; Dir. Carter Centre UK. Specialty: Oncol. Special Interest: Breast Cancer. Socs: Soc. of Surgic. Oncol.; Brit. Assn. of Surgic. Oncologists; Assn. of Wom. Surgeons. Prev: Cons. Surgic. Oncologist, Long Br., NJ USA.

THOMAS, Gareth Boxbush, 243 Rushmere Road, Ipswich IP4 3LU Tel: 01473 712088 Fax: 01473 712088 — MB BS Lond. 1969 (St. Mary's) MRCS Eng. LRCP Lond. 1969; FRCOG 1987, M 1974; MD Lond. 1979; LLM Wales 1996. p/t Cons. (O & G) Ipswich Hosp.; Dep. Med. Dir. Ipswich Hosp. NHS Trust. Specialty: Obst. & Gyn.; Medico Legal. Socs: Eur. Assn. Gyn. & Obst.; RSM; E. Anglian Obst. and Gynacology Soc. Prev: Sen. Regist. John Radcliffe Hosp. Oxf.; Lect. (O & G) Univ. Coll. Hosp. Lond.; Resid. Med. Off. Qu. Charlotte's Matern. Hosp. Lond.

THOMAS, Gareth Andrew Osbert Department of Gastroenterology, University Hospital of Wales, Heath Park, Cardiff CF4 4QW Tel: 029 2074 3291 Email: gareth.thomas@uhw-tr.wales.nhs.uk — MB BS Lond. 1988 (St. Bart.) FRCP; FRCP (UK) 1991; BSc (1st cl. Hons.) Lond. 1985, MD 1995. Cons. Phys. & Gastroenterol. Univ. Hosp. Wales Cardiff. Specialty: Gastroenterol. Socs: Brit. Soc. Gastroenterol.; Roy. Coll. of Physicians. Prev: Sen. Regist. (Gastroenterol.) & Regist. (Med.) Univ. Hosp. Wales Cardiff.

THOMAS, Mr Gareth Edward Melbourne (retired) 9 Forest Road, Branksome Park, Poole BH13 6DQ — MB BS Lond. 1952 (St. Bart.) MRCS Eng. LRCP Lond. 1951; FRCS Ed. 1959. Hon. Cons. ENT Surg. Bournemouth & E. Dorset Hosp. Gp. Prev: Sen. Regist. (ENT) Cardiff Roy. Infirm.

THOMAS, Gareth Lewis 50 The Coverdales, Gascoigne Estate, Barking IG11 7JY — BM BS Nottm. 1994.

THOMAS, Gareth Lewis — MB BS Newc. 1994 (Newcastle) BMedSc (Hons.) Newc. 1993; MRCP (UK) 1998; FRCA 2001. SHO Rotat. (Anaesth./IC) S. Manch. Sch. Anaesth.; Specialist Regist. Anaesth. NW Rotat. (2000 - 2005); Sen. Regist. Intens. Care, Westmead Hosp., Sydney, Aus. Specialty: Anaesth.; Intens. Care. Prev: Ho. Phys. Roy. Vict. Infirm. Newc.; Ho. Surg. Newc. Gen. Hosp.; SHO Rotat. (Med.) Roy. Vict. Infirm. & Freeman Hosp. Newc. u. Tyne.

THOMAS, Gareth Owen 9 Tocil Croft, Cannon Park, Coventry CV4 7DZ — MB ChB Birm. 1996.

THOMAS, Gareth Rees Victoria Gardens Surgery, Victoria Gardens, Neath SA11 1HW Tel: 01639 643786 Fax: 01639 640018 — MRCS Eng. LRCP Lond. 1975.

THOMAS, Gavin David Peggottys, Little Cheney, Dorchester DT2 9AN — MB BS Lond. 1996.

THOMAS, Gaynor (retired) 24 St John's Road, Hazel Grove, Stockport SK7 5HG Tel: 0161 483 2724 — MB ChB Manch. 1957; DA Eng. 1960. Prev: Assoc. Specialist Stepping Hill Hosp. Stockport & Stockport Infirm.

THOMAS, Gaynor Caroline Cherrytree Cottage, Broadfield, Saundersfoot SA69 9DG — MB BCh Wales 1998.

THOMAS, George Douglas Hylton Department of Pathology, Calderdale Royal Hospital, Salterhebble, Halifax HX3 0PW Tel: 01422 224885 — MB ChB Liverp. 1973; MRCPath 1981; FRCPath 1994. Cons. Histopath. & Morbid Anat. Yorks. RHA. Specialty: Histopath. Prev: Sen. Regist. (Histopath.) Yorks, RHA.

THOMAS, George Martin (retired) — MB ChB Ed. 1957; DObst RCOG 1962; FRCGP 1984, M 1969.

THOMAS, Geraint Huw Saxonbrook Medical, Maidenbower Square, Crawley RH10 7QH Tel: 01293 547315 Fax: 01293 613439; Long Acre, Effingham Road, Crawley RH10 3HY Tel: 01342 713893 — MB BCh Wales 1987.

THOMAS, Gillian Dawn Department of Clinical Oncology, Leicester Royal Infirmary, Leicester LE1 5WW — MB BS Lond. 1980 (Char. Cross Hosp.) MRCS Eng. LRCP Lond. 1980; FRCR 1987; T(R) (CO) 1992; MD 1996. Cons. (Clin Oncol.) Derbysh. Roy Infirm. Derby. Specialty: Oncol.; Radiother. Prev: Clin. Research Fell. (Immunol.) Univ. Birm.; SHO/Regist. (Radiother.) Velindre Hosp. Cardiff VTS.; Sen. Regist. (Radiother./Oncol.) Clin. Acad. Unit. Roy. Marsden Hosp. Sutton.

THOMAS, Glenna (retired) Swn-y-Mor, Overton, Gower, Swansea SA3 1NR Tel: 01792 391244 — MB BCh Wales 1952; DObst RCOG 1956.

THOMAS, Gordon Oswald (retired) 30 Western Road, Abergavenny NP7 7AD Tel: 01873 857711 Fax: 01873 857711 — MB BS Lond. 1961 (Univ. Coll. Hosp.) MRCS Eng. LRCP Lond. 1961; FRCP Lond. 1981, M 1965; FCCP 1995. Prev: Cons. Phys. (Gen. & Thoracic Med.) Nevill Hall Hosp. Abergavenny.

THOMAS, Gordon Robert Williams The Surgery, Trentham Mews, New Inn Lane, Stoke-on-Trent ST4 8PX Tel: 01782 657159 — MB ChB Birm. 1980.

THOMAS, Graham David Meddygfa Star Surgery, Gaerwen, Anglesey LL60 6AH Tel: 01248 714533 — MB ChB Aberd. 1993; MRCGP 1997. Dr. Ben Alofs, examen Amsterdam. Specialty: Gen. Pract. Prev: Trainee GP Gwynedd; GP Castellfryn Surg., Star.

THOMAS, Graham Edgar (retired) 243 Forest Road, Tunbridge Wells TN2 5HT Tel: 01892 526503 — (St. Thos.) MB BS Lond. 1965; MRCS Eng. LRCP Lond. 1965; MRCP (UK) 1970; MD Lond. 1977; FRCP Lond. 1992.

THOMAS, Gregory Patrick Lorne Flat 21, 43 Bartholomew Close, London EC1A 7HN — BM BCh Oxf. 1998; MA Camb. 1995; MRCS 2002. Surg. John Radcliff Hosp. Oxf. Specialty: Gen. Surg. Prev: Phys. Milton Keynes Gen Hosp.

THOMAS, Gruffydd John The Queen Edith Medical Practice, 59 Queen Ediths Way, Cambridge CB1 8PJ Tel: 01223 247288 Fax: 01223 213459; 6 Stanley Road — MB ChB Bristol 1992; MRCGP 1996; DRCOG 1996. GP Qu. Edith Med. Pract. Specialty: Gen. Pract. Prev: Trainee GP/SHO Roy. Devon & Exeter NHS Trust.

THOMAS, Gwenyth Adfer Medical Group, Llanelli Town Centre, Thomas Street, Llanelli SA15 3JH Tel: 01554 775555 Fax: 01554 778868 — MB BCh Wales 1984 (Univ. Wales Sch. of Med. Cardiff) DRCOG 1987. Prev: Trainee GP W. Wales Gen. Hosp. Carmarthen.

THOMAS, Gwyn David (retired) 22 Court Crescent, Bassaleg, Newport NP10 8NH Tel: 01633 895045 — MB BS Lond. 1956 (Guy's) MRCS Eng. LRCP Lond. 1956; DA Eng. 1964; FFA RCS Eng. 1965. Prev: Cons. Anaesth. Glan Hafren NHS Trust.

THOMAS, Gwynallt Watkins (retired) Meadow Cottage, Alpington, Norwich NR14 7NG — MB BS Lond. 1960 (Univ. Coll. Hosp.) MRCS Eng. LRCP Lond. 1960; DObst RCOG 1962; DA Eng. 1965; FFA RCS Eng. 1968. Prev: Cons. Anaesth. Norwich Health Dist.

THOMAS, Hannah Mari (retired) Ystrad Isa, Denbigh LL16 4RL Tel: 01745 812550 Fax: 01745 813345 — MB BCh Wales 1956. GP Denbigh. Prev: Med. Ref. Welsh Office.

THOMAS, Hawys Olwen Wordsworth Surgery, 97 Newport Road, Roath, Cardiff CF14 0XA — MB BCh Wales 1993; DRCOG; MRCGP. Specialty: Gen. Med.

THOMAS, Hayley Rebecca 8 Eardley Road, Heysham, Morecambe LA3 2PH — MB ChB Manch. 1997.

THOMAS, Helen Catherine Lisson Grove Medical Centre, 3-5 Lisson Grove, Mutley, Plymouth PL4 7DL Tel: 01752 205555 Fax: 01752 205558; 24 Thorn Park, Mannamead, Plymouth PL3 4TD

Tel: 01752 666133 — MB ChB Birm. 1986; ChB Birm. 1986; DRCOG 1989.

THOMAS, Helen Joan Roycroft, Madden and Thomas, Chelford Surgery, Elmstead Road, Macclesfield SK11 9BS Tel: 01625 861316 Fax: 01625 860075 — MB ChB Liverp. 1989 (Liverpool) MRCGP 1993. Clin. Asst. (Gen. Med.) E. Chesh. Trust.

THOMAS, Helen Joanna 15 Wayland Close, Adel, Leeds LS16 8LT Tel: 0113 267 0388 — MB ChB Leic. 1987; DRCOG 1989; DGM RCP Lond. 1991; MRCGP 1992; DCCH 1996; DCCH 1997. Specialty: Community Child Health.

THOMAS, Helen Lucy 34 Poplar Avenue, Putnoe, Bedford MK41 8BL Tel: 01234 346551 — BM Soton. 1990; MSc (Med. Anthropol.) Brunel Univ. 1998. Prev: Locum CMO Community Paediat. Richmond Twickenham & Roehampton; Researcher Centre for Social Research & Educat. Bogota Colombia; Grade 8 Dr Dept. of Epidemiol. Colombian Nat. Inst. of Health Bogota Colombia.

THOMAS, Helen Mair 57 Milton Road, London SW14 8JP — MB BS Lond. 1986; DRCOG 1993. Prev: Trainee GP Lond.; SHO (O & G) Bristol; SHO (A & E) Lond.

THOMAS, Helen Ruth 68 St Guthiac St, Hereford HR1 2EX — MB ChB Manch. 1998. SHO. Hereford Hosp. Prev: PRHO. (Med & Surg.) City Gen Hosp. Stoke-On-Trent.

THOMAS, Professor Howard Christopher Department of Medicine, St. Mary's Hospital, London W2 1PG Tel: 020 7886 6454 Fax: 020 7724 9369 Email: h.thomas@ic.ac.uk — MB BS (Hons.) Newc. 1969; BSc (Hons.) Newc. 1966; PhD Glas. 1975; FRCPS Glas. 1978; FRCP Lond. 1979; MRCPath 1981; FRCPath 1986. Prof. Med. Imp. Coll. Sch. Med. St. Mary's Hosp. Lond.; Dean (Clin.) Imp. Coll. Fac. Med.; Cons. Phys. & Hepatol. St Mary's Hosp. Lond. Specialty: Gastroenterol. Socs: Fell. Roy. Soc. Med.; Counc. Europ. Assn. Study of Liver; (Trustee) Brit. Liver Trust. Prev: Prof. Med. Roy. Free Hosp. Med. Sch. Lond.

THOMAS, Howard Glyn North Swindon Practice, Home Ground Surgery, Thames Avenue, Haydon Wick, Swindon SN25 1QQ Tel: 01793 705777 — MB ChB Ed. 1972; MRCGP 1980.

THOMAS, Mr Howard James Watkins (retired) Station Road Surgery, 46 Station Road, New Barnet, Barnet EN5 1QH Tel: 020 8441 4425 Fax: 020 8441 4957; 15 Hasluck Gardens, Barnet EN5 1HS — MB BS Lond. 1965 (Univ. Coll. Hosp.) MRCS Eng. LRCP Lond. 1964; FRCS Ed. 1971; FRCS Eng. 1974. Prev: Resid. Surg. Off. Barnet Gen. Hosp.

THOMAS, Hugh Alistair Barton, Horn Lane, Plymstock, Plymouth PL9 9BR Tel: 01752 407129; Bridge Park Cottage, 117 Goutsford, Ermington, Ivybridge PL21 0NY Tel: 01548 830192 — MB BS Lond. 1975; MRCS Eng. LRCP Lond. 1975. GP Plymstock, Devon.

THOMAS, Hugh Falcon College Road Surgery, 6 College Road, Eastbourne BN1 4HY Tel: 01323 735044 — MB ChB Leic. 1986; BSc (Hons.) (Environm. Sci.) Salford 1973; MSc Aston 1978; Cert. Av. Med. 1988; MFPHM RCP (UK) 1994. Gen. Practitioner. Specialty: Gen. Pract.; Epidemiol. Prev: Epidemiologist MRC Epidemiol. Unit Llandough Hosp. Penarth; Sen. Regist. (Pub. Health Med.) Wessex RHA; Regist. (Community Med.) Canterbury & Thanet HA.

THOMAS, Mr Hugh James McKim 9 Lucknow Avenue, Mapperley Park, Nottingham NG3 5AZ Tel: 0115 960 7823; 34 Regent Street, Nottingham NG1 5BT Tel: 0115 956 1304 Fax: 0115 956 1314 — (Cardiff) MB BCh Wales 1955; FRCS Eng. 1963. Cons. Orthop. Surg. Univ. Hosp. Nottm. & Nottm. City Hosp. Specialty: Orthop. Socs: Fell. Brit. Orthop. Assn.; Brit. Soc. Childr. Orthop. Surg.; Brit. Cervical Spine Soc. Prev: Lect. in Orthop. Surg. Univ. & Roy. Infirm. Manch.; Hon. Cons. Orthop. Surg. Robt. Jones & Agnes Hunt Hosp. Oswestry; Orthop. Regist. Roy. Nat. Orthop. Hosp. Lond.

THOMAS, Hugh Williams (retired) 31 Fairway, Trentham, Stoke-on-Trent ST4 8AS Tel: 01782 657539 — MB ChB Glas. 1949; FRCGP 1978, M 1960.

THOMAS, Huw Daniel 50 Victoria Road, Penarth CF64 3HZ — MB BCh Wales 1998.

THOMAS, Huw Gerwyn Irnham Lodge Surgery, Townsend Road, Minehead TA24 5RG Tel: 01643 703289 Fax: 01643 707921; Woodcombe Farm House, Woodcombe, Minehead TA24 8SB — MB BCh Wales 1983; DRCOG 1989; MRCGP 1990.

THOMAS, Huw Glyn Claremont Surgery, The Wilderness Medical Centre, Cookham Road, Maidenhead SL6 8AN — MB BS Lond. 1996; BSc; DRCOG; MRCGP; DFFP.

THOMAS, Huw Jeremy Wyndham Department of Gastroenterology, St. Mary's Hospital, Praed St., London W2 1NY Tel: 020 7886 1208 Fax: 020 7886 1138; 66 Harley Street, London W1G 7HO Tel: 020 7631 0966 Fax: 020 7631 5341 — MB BS Lond. 1982 (Camb. & Lond. Hosp.) MA Camb. 1982; PhD Lond. 1991; FRCP (M 1985) 1997. Cons. Phys. & Gastroenterol. St. Mary's Hosp. Lond.; Hon. Cons. (Phys. & Gastroenterol.) King Edwd. VII Hosp. Lond.; Sen. Lect. & Hon. Cons. Phys. CR-UK Colorectal Unit St. Mark's Hosp. Harrow. Specialty: Gastroenterol.

THOMAS, Huw Morgan Department of General Paediatrics, Southmead Hospital, Westbury-on-Trym, Bristol BS10 5NB Tel: 0117 959 5582 Fax: 0117 959 5282 Email: Thomas_H@southmead.swest.nhs.uk — MB BS Lond. 1983 (Univ. Coll. Hosp. Lond.) BSc Lond. 1980; MRCP (UK) 1989; FRCPCH 1997. Cons. Paediat. Southmead Hosp. Bristol; Cons. Respirat. Paediat.Bristol Roy. Hosp. for Childr. Specialty: Paediat.; Respirat. Med.; Allergy. Socs: Roy. Coll. of Paediat. and Child Health; Brit. Thoracic Soc. Prev: Sen. Regist. (Paediat.) Roy. Hosp. for Sick. Childr. Bristol.

THOMAS, Mr Huw Owen 31 Rodney Street, Liverpool L1 9EH Tel: 0151 703 2900; Pinwydden, 18 Pine Walks, Prenton, Prenton CH42 8NE Fax: 01515132494 Email: verstapp@aol.com — MB BCh Wales 1966 (Welsh National School of Medicine) ECFMG 1966; FRCS (Ed) 1971; FRCS Eng. 1972; MChOrth Liverp. 1973. Medico-Legal Cons. Specialty: Orthop. Socs: Low Friction Soc.; Med. Appeal Tribunal; Liverp. Med. Inst. Prev: Late Capt. TAVR; Sen. Cons. Orthop. Surg. Arrowe Pk., Clatterbridge Hosps. Wirral & BUPA Murrayfield Hosp. Wirral; Sen. Regist. (Orthop.) Liverp. Roy. Infirm. & Wrightington Hosp. Appley Bridge.

THOMAS, Hywel Gwyn X Ray Department, Musgrave Park Hospital, Taunton TA1 5DA Tel: 01823 342406 Email: hywel.thomas@tst.nhs.uk — MB ChB Birm. 1983 (Birmingham) MRCP (UK) 1987; FRCR 1990. Cons. Diag. Radiol. MusGr. Pk. Hosp. Taunton. Specialty: Radiol. Socs: Assoc. Mem. Med. Defence Union; Inst. Radiol.; Brit. Soc. Interven. Radiol. Prev: Sen. Regist. & Regist. (Diag. Radiol.) John Radcliffe Hosp. Oxf.; SHO (Neurosurg.) Walsgrave Hosp. Coventry.

THOMAS, Hywel Lloyd Profiad Ltd., 20-24 Vachel Road, Reading RG1 1NY Tel: 0118 951 0707 Fax: 0118 951 0606; Goodwood, Boulston, Haverfordwest SA62 4AG Tel: 01437 768794 Fax: 01437 763517 — MB BS Lond. 1981 (St. Bart.) DRCOG 1984; MRCGP 1985; DCH RCP Lond. 1987. Managing Dir. Profiad Ltd.; Comp. Sec. Rifleman Research Ltd. Specialty: Gen. Pract. Prev: GP HaverfordW.

THOMAS, Ian McDougall Llynyfran Surgery, Llynyfran Road, Llandysul SA44 4JX Tel: 01559 363306 Fax: 01559 362896; Glancwerchyr, Maesllyn, Llandysul SA44 5LD Tel: 01239 851505 — MB BCh Wales 1976 (Cardiff) DRCOG 1980. Specialty: Community Child Health.

THOMAS, Illtyd Richard John 43 New Road, Cockett, Swansea SA2 0GA — MB BChir Camb. 1992; BA (Hons.) 1989, MB BChir Camb. 1992. Specialty: Gen. Med.

THOMAS, Mr Iowerth Huw (retired) 17 Holmfield Road, Leicester LE2 1SD — MD Newc. 1983; MB BS 1974; FRCS Ed. 1980.

THOMAS, Ivor Gareth Queen Margaret Hospital, Whitefield Road, Dunfermline KY12 0SU Tel: 01383 623623 Fax: 01383 627044; 50 The Muirs, Kinross KY13 8AU — MB ChB Ed. 1984; MRCPsych 1989. Cons. Old Age Psychiat. Fife HB Dunfermline. Specialty: Geriat. Psychiat. Prev: Sen. Regist. (Psychait.) N. Region; Regist. (Psychiat.) Aberd.

THOMAS, Iwan Richard, TD Crinnis House, Les Bois, Layer de la Haye, Colchester CO2 0EX Tel: 01206 738273 Email: ir.thomas@virgin.net — (Middlx.) MB BS Lond. 1965; MSc Surrey 1971; AFOM RCP Lond. 1995. Indep. p/t. Occupat. Phys. Specialty: Occupat. Health. Socs: Fell. Roy. Soc. Med.; Soc. Occupat. Med. Prev: Area.Med.Advis,Post Office EHS; RMO 22nd Special Air Serv. Regt.; Ho. Surg. & Ho. Phys. St. And. Hosp. Billericay.

THOMAS, Jacob Department of Psychiatry, Pilgrim Hospital, Sibsey Road, Boston PE21 9QS Tel: 01205 364801 Ext: 3506; Karimparampil, Tiruvalla 5, PO Kerala State, India — MB BS Mysore 1973 (Kasturba Med. Coll. Mangalore) BSc (Chem.) Kerala 1963;

DPM Eng. 1977; FRCPsych 1993, M 1978; Dip. Health Serv. Managem. York 1992. Cons. Psychiat. Pilgrim Hosp. Boston. Specialty: Gen. Psychiat. Prev: Sen. Regist. St. Bart. & N. Middlx. Hosps. Lond. & Goodamyes Hosp. Ilford.

THOMAS, Jacqueline Anne Overdale Medical Practice, 207 Victoria Avenue, Borrowash, Derby DE72 3HG Email: jackie.hull@gp-c81066.nhs.uk — MB ChB Manch. 1993; BSc (Hons.) Manch. 1991; Dip. Child Health 1996; MRCGP 1997; MPH Nott. 2002.

THOMAS, James Alexander 53 Main Street, Embsay, Skipton BD23 6RD — MB BS Lond. 1994.

THOMAS, Mr James Andrew 70 St Ambrose Road, Heath, Cardiff CF14 4BH Tel: 029 2061 2919 — MB BCh Wales 1987; FRCS Eng. 1992. Cons. (Urol.) Bridgend & Dist. NHS Trust. Specialty: Urol. Socs: Assoc. Mem. BAUS; BMA; MDU. Prev: Specialist Regist. (Urol.) S Wales Train. Scheme; Regist. Rotat. (Surg.) Cardiff.

THOMAS, James Clannie 19 Somersham Road, Bexleyheath DA7 4SA — MB BCh BAO NUI 1971.

THOMAS, Mr James Nigel ENT Department, King's College Hospital, Denmark Hill, London SE5 9RS Tel: 020 7346 5338 Fax: 020 7346 5337; ENT Department, Bromley Health Trust, Farnborough Hospital, Farnborough Common, Orpington BR6 8ND Tel: 01689 814285 — MA Oxf. 1968; BM BCh Oxf. 1968; FRCS Eng. 1974. Cons. Surg. ENT Dept. King's Coll. Hosp. Lond. Specialty: Otolaryngol. Prev: Cons. Surg. ENT Dept. Groote Schuur Hosp. Capetown; 1st Asst. ENT Dept. Radcliffe Infirm. Oxf.

THOMAS, James Picton Douglas (retired) Ty Cornel, Rudry, Caerphilly CF83 3DD Tel: 029 2075 4765 — MD Camb. 1956 (St. Bart.) BA Camb. 1944, MD 1956, MB BChir 1948; FRCP Lond. 1970, M 1953. Hon. Cons. Phys. Univ. Hosp. Wales Cardiff. Prev: Sen. Lect. (Med.) Welsh Nat. Sch. Med.

THOMAS, James Roger Leighton 28 Maresfield Gardens, London NW3 5SX Tel: 020 7435 4737 Fax: 020 7433 1334 — MB BS Lond. 1966 (St Thos.) AFOM; DRCOG; MRCS Eng. LRCP Lond. 1965; DObst RCOG 1968. Med. Advis. Ernst & Young & Morgan Crucible Co. Ltd.; Examg. Phys. United Nations Lond. Socs: Assoc. Fac. Occupat. Med. Prev: Ho. Surg. St. Thos. Hosp. Lond.; Ho. Phys. Lewisham Hosp. & Princess Louise Kensington Hosp. Childr. Lond.

THOMAS, James Stephen Idris Bryn-Villa, Gorslas, Llanelli SA14 7LP — MB BS Lond. 1981.

THOMAS, Jane Elizabeth Goodwood, Boulston, Haverfordwest SA62 4AG Tel: 01437 765297 — MB ChB Bristol 1982; DCH RCP Lond. 1987; DA (UK) 1988.

THOMAS, Jane Margaret 12 Ardwick Road, London NW2 2BX — MB ChB Liverp. 1987.

THOMAS, Jane Mary 84 Wyresdale Road, Lancaster LA1 3DY Tel: 01524 382682; 34 Bury Old Road, Whitefield, Manchester M45 6TF — MB ChB Manch. 1987. Primary Health Care Adviser for Develop. Countries Working with Non-Govt.al Aid Organisations. Socs: Fell. Roy. Soc. of Trop. Med. & Hyg.

THOMAS, Janet Department of Clinical Haematology, Royal United Hospital, Combe Park, Bath BA1 3NG; 15 Park Hill, Shirehampton, Bristol BS11 0UH — MB BS Lond. 1966 (Roy. Free) MRCS Eng. LRCP Lond. 1966; FRCPath 1972. Assoc. Specialist (Haemat.) Roy. United Hosp. Bath. Specialty: Haematology. Prev: Sen. Regist. (Haemat.) Kingston Hosp. Kingston-upon-Thames & St. Thos.Hosp. Lond.

THOMAS, Janet Rhondda NHS Trust, Albert Road, Pontypridd CF37 1LA Tel: 01443443789 Fax: 01443 443791; Bedford Falls, 24 Danygraig Drive, Talbot Green, Pontyclun CF72 8AQ Tel: 01443 223385 Fax: 01443 223385 — MB BCh Wales 1969 (Cardiff) MFFP 1993. Cons. (Family Plann. & Reproduct. Health Care); Progr. Co-ordinator for Gwent; Treas. Welsh Family Plann. Doctors Gp.; Cervical Screening Wales. Specialty: Family Plann. & Reproduc. Health. Socs: Treas. Welsh Family Plann. Doctors Gp.; Fac. Community Health; Fac. Fam. Plann. Prev: GP Pontyclun & Kenilworth; SHO (O & G) Walsgrave Hosp. Coventry; Ho. Off. (Paediat.) Gulson Rd. Hosp. Coventry.

THOMAS, Janet Beynon Ty Maen Cottage, South Cornelly, Bridgend CF33 4RE Tel: 01656 746404 — MRCS Eng. LRCP Lond. 1965; MB BS Lond. 1965; DTM & H RCP Lond. 1986.

THOMAS, Janet Mary 92 Ulleswater Road, Southgate, London N14 7BT — MB ChB Bristol 1978; DRCOG 1980; DCH Eng. 1982.

THOMAS, Jean Alero Department of Infectious & Tropical Diseases, London School of Hygiene & Tropical Medicine, Keppel St., London WC1E 7HT Tel: 020 7927 2289 Fax: 020 7927 2303 — (St Mary's Hospital London) MB BS Lond. 1970; MSc Oxf. 1976; MRCPath 1991. Sen. Clin. Lect. Specialty: Histopath.; Virology.

THOMAS, Jeffery Llewellyn Edward Watson (retired) Rectory Lodge, Cosheston, Pembroke Dock SA72 4UJ — MB BS Lond. 1958 (Westm.) MRCS Eng. LRCP Lond. 1958; DA Eng. 1962, DTM & H 1961; FFA RCS Eng. 1963. Prev: Cons. Anaesth. W. Glam. HA.

THOMAS, Jenkyn Powell 36 Clos Brenin, Pontyclun CF72 9GA — MB BS Lond. 1955.

THOMAS, Jennifer 19 Y Teras, Creigiau, Cardiff CF15 9NG — MB BCh Wales 1993.

THOMAS, Jennifer Anne Tudor Lea, Sutton Close, Cookham, Maidenhead SL6 9QU Tel: 01628 524859 — MB BS Lond. 1996 (Charing Cross and Westminster Medical School) MRCP (UK) 2001. SpR (Histopathology) St James' Hosp., Leeds. Specialty: Gen. Med. Prev: SHO (Med.) Soton. Gen. Hosp.

THOMAS, Jeremy Simon 14 Cleeve Lawns, Bristol BS16 6HJ — MB BCh Wales 1992.

THOMAS, Jeremy St John Western General Hospital, Department of Pathology (LUHD), Crewe Road, Edinburgh EH4 2XU Tel: 0131 537 1961 Fax: 0131 537 1013 Email: jeremy.thomas@luht.scot.nhs.uk — MB BS Lond. 1978 (St. Thos.) MA Oxf. 1980, BA 1975; MRCS Eng. LRCP Lond. 1978; MRCP (UK) 1981; MRCPath 1986; T(Path) 1991; FRCP Ed. 1992; FRCP Glas. 1994; FRCPath 1997. Cons. Histopath. & Cytol. W. Gen. Hosp. Edin. Specialty: Histopath. Prev: Sen. Regist. (Path.) West. Infirm. Glas.; SHO (Gen. Med.) West. Infirm. Glas.; Ho. Surg. St. Thos. Hosp. Lond.

THOMAS, Joan (retired) 76 Wimmerfield Avenue, Killay, Swansea SA2 7DA — MB BCh Wales 1944 (Cardiff) BSc, MB BCh Wales 1944; DObst RCOG 1946. Prev: GP Swansea.

THOMAS, Joan Margaret 1 The Courtway, Bone Mill Lane, Enborne, Newbury RG20 0EU — MB BS Lond. 1973 (Univ. Coll. Hosp.) MRCP (UK) 1977; FRCP 1995. Consultant in Respiratory Medicine, Royal Berkshire & Battle Hospitals NHS Trust.

THOMAS, Joanna Clare Plas Ffordd Ddwr, Llandyrnog, Denbigh LL16 4ET — MB ChB Liverp. 1998.

THOMAS, John The Vale of Neath Practice, Bodfeddyg, 102 High Street, Neath SA11 5AL Tel: 01639 722431 — MB BCh Wales 1963 (Cardiff) Prev: SHO (Gen. Med.) St. David's Hosp. Cardiff; Regist. (Chest & Gen. Med.) Llangwyfan Hosp.; SHO (O & G) H. M. Stanley Hosp. St. Asaph.

THOMAS, Mr John Alun Beynon (retired) West Hill, 26 Fairwater Road, Llandaff, Cardiff CF5 2LE Tel: 029 2056 2763 — MB BCh Wales 1937 (Cardiff) BSc, MB BCh Wales 1937; DLO Eng. 1943; FRCS (Orl.) Eng. 1949. Prev: Cons. Otol. MRC Inst. Hearing Research (Welsh Sect.) Univ. Hosp. Wales.

THOMAS, John Berian (retired) Tan-y-Castell, Llanmill, Narberth SA67 8UE Tel: 01834 860435 — MRCS Eng. LRCP Lond. 1943 (Middlx.) Cons. Accid. Surg. Pembroke Co. War Memor. Hosp. HaverfordW.. Prev: Clin. Asst. Orthop. Surg. PeterBoro. & Dist. Memor. Hosp.

THOMAS, John Berwyn (retired) The Cottage, Buttons Farm, Wadhurst TN5 6NW Tel: 01892 782848 — MB BCh Wales 1955 (Cardiff) DA Eng. 1961; FFA RCS Eng. 1965. Cons. Anaesth. Tunbridge Wells Health Dist. Prev: Sen. Regist. Westm. & Brompton Hosps. Lond.

THOMAS, John Delwyn (retired) 33 Edyvean Close, Bilton, Rugby CV22 6LD Tel: 01788 817236 — BSc Wales 1945; MB BCh Wales 1949.

THOMAS, John Geraint Penarth Health Centre, Stanwell Road, Penarth CF64 3XE Tel: 029 2070 3039 — MB BCh Wales 1971; DObst RCOG 1974.

THOMAS, John Gethin Marsham Street Surgery, 1 Marsham Street, Maidstone ME14 1EW Tel: 01622 752615/756129 — MB BS Lond. 1977; DRCOG 1981.

THOMAS, John Glyn 12 Beresford Road, Birkenhead CH43 1XG — MB BS Liverp. 1968; MRCS Eng. LRCP Lond. 1967.

THOMAS, John Gwyn (retired) Ystrad Isa, Denbigh LL16 4RL Tel: 01745 812550 Fax: 01745 813345 — MB BCh Wales 1956 (Cardiff) BSc Wales 1952; DObst RCOG 1960; DCH Eng. 1961;

FRCGP 1974, M 1965. Approved Med. Off. Ment. Health Act EMP Wales. Prev: Mem. Advis. Body (Gen. Pract.) Welsh Med. Comm.

THOMAS, John Hirwain (retired) 134 Victoria Avenue, Porthcawl CF36 3HA — MRCS Eng. LRCP Lond. 1940 (Cardiff) FRCP Lond. 1975, M 1950; DCH Eng. 1950. Prev: Cons. Phys. Geriat. Bridgend Gen. Hosp. & Morgannwg Ment. Hosps.

THOMAS, John Lumley (retired) 5 Meridian Way, Newcastle upon Tyne NE7 7RU Tel: 0191 266 2504 — MB BS Durh. 1955; DPH Newc. 1968. Prev: GP Wallsend.

THOMAS, John Samuel Bryn-Coed, 114 Sketty Road, Swansea SA2 0JX Tel: 01792 208626; Arosfa, Llangoedmôr, Cardigan SA43 2LT — (Welsh National School of Medicine) MB BCh Wales 1966; DObst RCOG 1969; DA Eng. 1971; FFA RCS Eng. 1971. Cons. Anaesth. W. Glam. HA Swansea. Specialty: Anaesth. Socs: BMA & Assn. of Anaesth. Gt. Brit. & Irel.; BMA. Prev: Ho. Phys. & Ho. Surg. Morriston Hosp. Swansea; SHO (Anaesth.) Nuffield Dept. Anaesth. Radcliffe Infirm. Oxf.; Sen. Regist. (Anaesth.) Univ. Hosp. of Wales Cardiff.

THOMAS, Jonathan Mark Greenbank Road Surgery, 29 Greenbank Road, Liverpool L18 1HG Tel: 0151 733 3224 Fax: 0151 734 5147; 4 Penhale Close, Aigburth, Liverpool L17 5BT Tel: 0151 726 0915 — MB ChB Liverp. 1987.

THOMAS, Jonathan Martin 47 Old Road, Llanelli SA15 3HR — MB ChB Manch. 1993.

THOMAS, Jose Nevill Hall Hospital, Brecon Road, Abergavenny NP7 7EG Tel: 01873 732991 Fax: 01873 732913 — MB BS Kerala 1977; MD Inst. Med. Sci. India 1981; MRCP (UK) 1987; FRCP 2001. Cons. Phys. (Gen. & Resp. Med.) Nevill Hall Hosp.; Hon. Cons. Phys. Llandough Hosp. Penarth. Specialty: Respirat. Med. Socs: Brit. Thorac. Soc.; Welsh Thoracic Soc.; Soc. Phys. in Wales. Prev: Cons. Phys. (Thoracic Med.) Caerphilly Dist. Miner's Hosp.; Lect. Univ. Wales Coll. Med.; Regist. (Thoracic Med.) Llandough Hosp. S. Glam. HA.

THOMAS, Mr Joseph Meirion The Lister Hospital, Chelsea Bridge Road, London SW1W 8RH Tel: 020 7631 4498 Fax: 020 7259 9552 — MB BS Lond. 1969 (wESTM.) FRCS Eng. 1975; MS Lond. 1979; FRCP 1998. Cons. Surg. Oncol. Roy. Marsden Hosp. Lond. Specialty: Gen. Surg. Prev: Resid. Surgic. Off. St. Mark's Hosp. Lond.; Sen. Regist. (Surg.) St. Geo. Hosp. St. Jas. Hosp. Lond. & Roy. Marsden Hosp. Sutton.

THOMAS, Joyce Lilian, OBE (retired) 72 East Dulwich Grove, Dulwich, London SE22 8PS — MD Liverp. 1978, MB ChB 1948; DCH Eng. 1970; FFCM 1982, M 1978; FFPHM RCP (UK) 1988. Hon. Cons. Pub. Health Med. W. Glam. DHA; Sen. Lect. Sch. Postgrad. Studies Med. & Health Care Swansea.

THOMAS, Judith Clatterbridge Hospital, Bebington CH63 4JY Tel: 0151 334 4000; Pinwydden, 18 Pine Walks, Prenton, Birkenhead CH42 8NE Tel: 0151 608 3909 Fax: 0151 513 2494 Email: verstapp@aol.com — MB ChB Liverp. 1975 (Liverpool) BSc (Hons.) Liverp. 1972, MB ChB 1975; Cert Family Planning JCC 1986; BA (Hons) Open 2001. p/t Clin. Asst. (Diag. Ultrasound) Clatterbridge Hosp., Bebington & Arrowe Pk. Hosp. Upton Wirral. Specialty: Radiol. Prev: SHO (Med.) & Ho. Off. Broadgreen Hosp. Liverp.; Sessional Screening BUPA Murrayfield Med. Centre.

THOMAS, Judith Anne The Deepings Practice, Godsey Lane, Market Deeping, Peterborough PE6 8DD Tel: 01778 579000 Fax: 01778 579009; 194 Eastgate, Deeping St. Jas., Peterborough PE6 8RD Tel: 01778 346098 — MB ChB Leic. 1982; DRCOG 1986; MRCGP 1986.

THOMAS, Judith Barbara Department of Public Health, Sunderland Teaching Primary Care Trust, The Childrens Centre, Durham Road, Sunderland Tel: 0191 565 6256 — MB BChir Camb. 1978; FFPHM RCP (UK); MA Camb. 1978; MSc Newc. 1989; MFPHM RCP (UK) 1990. Dir. (Pub. Health) Sunderland Health Auth. Specialty: Pub. Health Med.

THOMAS, Judith Mary Longwater Lane Medical Centre, Longwater Lane, Old Costessey, Norwich NR8 5AH Tel: 01603 742021 Fax: 01603 740271; Talisker, Tuttles Lane W., Wymondham NR18 0DZ Tel: 01953 606532 — MB BS Newc. 1974 (Newcastle-upon-Tyne) GP Princip.; Clin. Med. Off. Well Wom. Clinic Norwich.; Specialist Police Surg. Norf. Constab.

THOMAS, Julia Elizabeth Trevithick Surgery, Basset Road, Camborne TR14 8TT Tel: 01209 716721 Fax: 01209 612488 — MB BS Lond. 1994.

THOMAS, Julia Susanne 12 Dalebury Road, London SW17 7HH Tel: 020 8682 9742 — MB ChB Manch. 1990 (Manchester) Specialty: Gen. Pract. Prev: Trainee GP/SHO Ealing Hosp. VTS.

THOMAS, Julian Edward Royal Victoria Infirmary, Institute of Child Health, Queen Victoria Road, Newcastle upon Tyne NE1 4LP Tel: 0191 202 3033 Fax: 0191 202 3022 Email: j.e.thomas@ncl.ac.uk — MB BS Newc. 1982; MRCP (UK) 1985; MD Newcastle 1998. Ann Coleman Sen. Lect. in Paediatric Gastroenterol. and Nutrit., Univ. of Newc. Specialty: Paediat. Prev: Clin. Research Fell. Dunn Nutrit. Laborat. Camb.

THOMAS, Julie Greenmount, Bradford Road, Sherborne DT9 6BP Tel: 01935 813977 — MB BS Lond. 1998; MB BS Lond 1998. PRHO. (Gen Surg.) Colchester Gen Hosp.) Colchester. Essex. Prev: PRHO. (Med.) Dorset Co. Hosp. Dorchester.

THOMAS, Kannankara Mathew Harraton Surgery, 3 Swiss Cottages, Vigo Lane, Washington NE38 9AB Tel: 0191 416 1641 — MB BS Kerala 1974. GP Washington Tyne & Wear.

THOMAS, Karen Elizabeth 4 Grove Road, Speen, Newbury RG14 1UH — MB BS Lond. 1986.

THOMAS, Karen Elizabeth Copsen, Knoll Road, Frith Hill, Godalming GU7 2EL Email: karenthomas5@yahoo.com — BM BCh Oxf. 1990; MA Camb. 1991, B 1987; MRCP (UK) 1993. Cons. Radiologist, Hosp. for sick Childr., Toronto, Ontario. Specialty: Radiol. Prev: Cons. Radiologist, St Mary's Hosp. and Gt. Ormond St. Hosp., Lond.

THOMAS, Karen Jane Dunorlan Medical Group, 64 Pembury Road, Tonbridge TN9 2JG Tel: 01732 352907 Fax: 01732 367408; Rosenlaui, 3 Higham Gardens, Tonbridge TN10 4HZ — MB BS Lond. 1985 (St. Thos.) DRCOG 1989; DFFP 1994. Prev: Trainee GP Redhill VTS.

THOMAS, Katherine Eleanor 53 Main Street, Embsay, Skipton BD23 6RD — MB BS Lond. 1994.

THOMAS, Kathleen Anne The Laser Centre, Frenchay Hospital, Frenchay, Bristol BS16 1LE Tel: 0117 975 3807; 7 Collingwood Road, Redland, Bristol BS6 6PB — MB ChB Bristol 1983; DRCOG 1987; MRCGP 1989. Staff Grade, Laser Centre, Frenchay Hosp., Bristol. Specialty: Plastic Surg. Prev: Gen. Pract., Asst., Bristol.

THOMAS, Kathleen Mary (retired) 18 Kings Avenue, Woodford Green IG8 0JA — MB BS Queensland 1963 (Queensld.) MRCPath 1972. Cons. Histopath. Whipps Cross Hosp. Lond.

THOMAS, Kathleen Mary (retired) Sails, West Street, Seaview PO34 5ER Tel: 01983 612679 — MB BCh BAO Dub. 1947 (T.C. Dub.) BA Dub. 1947; DO Eng. 1961. Prev: Med. Off. Oji River Settlem. Nigeria Leprosy Serv.

THOMAS, Kathrin Jane Margaret Thompson Medical Centre, 105 East Millwood Road, Speke, Liverpool L24 6TH Tel: 0151 425 3331 Fax: 0151 425 2272 — MB ChB Leic. 1986; DRCOG 1994; MRCGP 1994. Specialty: Gen. Pract.

THOMAS, Kathryn Mary Jane St. Thomas Medical Group, Cowick St., Exeter EX4 1HJ Tel: 01392 676606 Fax: 01392 264424 Email: k.m.thomas@exeter.ac.uk; 14 Bagshot Avenue, Exeter EX2 4RN — MB BS Lond. 1981 (Royal Free Hospital School of Medicine, London) DA Eng. 1984; DRCOG 1985; MRCGP 1986. GP St Thomas Med. Gp.; Princip. Med. Off. Univ. Exeter. Specialty: Gen. Pract. Prev: Trainee GP Tiverton VTS; SHO (Paediat. & Anaesth.) Roy. Devon & Exeter Hosp.

THOMAS, Kathryn Patricia Abbotswood Medical Centre, Defford Road, Pershore WR10 1HZ Tel: 01386 552424 — MB ChB Leeds 1983 (Leeds University Medical School) DCH RCP, Lond 1986; DRCOG 1986; MRCGP 1987. GP.

THOMAS, Kathryn Samantha 18 The Whimbrels, Rest Bay, Porthcawl CF36 3TR — MB BS Lond. 1989.

THOMAS, Kay 27 Kenyon Street, London SW6 6JZ — MB BS Lond. 1994.

THOMAS, Keith Microbiology Department, Chesterfield & North Derbyshire Royal Hospital, Calow, Chesterfield S44 5BL Tel: 01246 552270 — MB BCh Wales 1974; FRCPath 1993, M 1981. Cons. Microbiol. Roy. Hosp. Chesterfield. Specialty: Med. Microbiol.

THOMAS, Keith Heathbridge House, The Old Bridge, Kenfig Hill, Bridgend CF33 6BY Tel: 01656 740359 Fax: 01656 745400; Gwalia House, 4 Oaklands Drive, Bridgend CF31 4SH Tel: 01656 668433 — MRCS Eng. LRCP Lond. 1955 (Lond. Hosp.) Prev: Ho. Surg. Orthop. & Accid. Dept. Lond. Hosp.; Ho. Phys. Anaesth. Div.

RAF Hosp. Ely; JHMO Paediat. & Obst. Dept. Northampton Gen. Hosp.

THOMAS, Keith David 30 Howecroft Croft, Eastmead Lane, Bristol BS9 1HJ — BM BCh Oxf. 1993.

THOMAS, Keith Lewis Salop House Surgery, Salop House, Chapel Street, Tregaron SY23 6HA Tel: 01974 298218 Fax: 01974 298207; Rhandir, Lampeter Road, Tregaron SY25 6HG — MB BS Lond. 1983; DGM RCP Lond. 1985; DCH RCP Lond. 1986; DRCOG 1987; MRCGP 1987. Clin. Asst. Geriat. Med. Dyfed.

THOMAS, Mr Kelvin Einstein Brook Cottage, Rodsley, nr. Brailsford, Ashbourne DE6 3AL Tel: 01335 330471 — MB BS Lond. 1955 (Guy's) BA Johns Hopkins Univ. 1950; DLO Eng. 1960; FRCS Eng. 1962. Emerit. Cons. ENT Surg. Univ. Hosp. Nottm. Socs: Fell. Roy. Soc. Med. (Mem. Sect. Otol. & Laryngol.); Fell. Roy. Soc. Arts; Med. Art Soc. Prev: Sen. Regist. (ENT) & Asst. Ho. Phys. & Ho. Surg. Guy's Hosp. Lond.; Sen. Regist. (ENT) Addenbrooke's Hosp. Camb.

THOMAS, Kenneth Bruce (retired) 4 Glen Eyre Road, Southampton SO16 3FZ Tel: 023 8058 6701 — MRCS Eng. LRCP Lond. 1943 (Liverp.) MD Liverp. 1972, MB ChB 1943. Prev: GP Waterlooville.

THOMAS, Kerry Wynn Bron-y-Garn Surgery, Station St., Maesteg CF34 9AL Tel: 01656 733262; Sisial-y-Nant, 18B Yr-Ysfa, Maesteg CF34 9AG — MB BCh Wales 1983.

THOMAS, Mr Kevin Southport & Ormskirk Hospital NHS Trust, Town Lane, Kew, Southport PR8 6PN Tel: 01704 547471; 10 Breeze Road, Birkdale, Southport PR8 2HG — MB ChB Liverp. 1991; MRCOG 1997; MD 2003. Specialty: Obst. & Gyn.

THOMAS, Mr Kevin James Trefynys, Llangristiolus, Bodorgan LL62 5DN — MB BS Lond. 1985 (St. Bart. Hosp. Lond.) FRCS Ed. 1993. Cons. (Urulogist) Ysbbyty Gwynedd. Specialty: Urol. Prev: Sen. Regist. (Urol.) Univ. Hosp. Wales.

THOMAS, Kevin Ross Pontcae Surgery, Dynevor Street, Georgetown, Merthyr Tydfil CF48 1YE Tel: 01685 723931 Fax: 01685 377048; 7 Lon y Brynnau, Brynna Farm, Cwmdare, Aberdare CF44 8PU — MB ChB Manch. 1989 (Manchester) MB ChB (Hons.) Manch. 1989; Dip. IMC RCS Ed. 1992; DRCOG 1993; MRCGP 1993. Chairman Methyr Tydfil LHG. Specialty: Gen. Pract. Prev: SHO (A & E Med. & O & G) P. Chas. Hosp. Merthyr Tydfil.

THOMAS, Kizhakkekara Thomas 36 Norford Way, Rochdale OL11 5QS Tel: 01706 344454 — MB BS Kerala 1968; MRCPsych 1976. Cons. Psychiat. (Learning Disabil.) Lancs.; Mem. Med. Specialists Comm.; Mem. Clin. Care Team & Head Learning Disabil. Servs. Specialty: Ment. Health.

THOMAS, Lee Spencer 13 Eshelby Close, Liverpool L22 3XT — MB ChB Dund. 1998.

THOMAS, Mr Lewis Philip (retired) Glenview, Glasllwch Lane, Newport NP20 3PS Tel: 01633 243001 — MB BCh Wales 1944 (Cardiff) BSc Wales 1941, MCh 1959, MB BCh 1944; FRCS Eng. 1947. Prev: Cons. Surg. Roy. Gwent Hosp. Newport.

THOMAS, Linzi Ann Singleton Hospital, Swansea SA2 8QA Tel: 01792 205666 Fax: 01792 285033 Email: drlinzit@yahoo.co.uk — MB BCh Wales 1988; MD; MRCP (UK) 1991. Cons. Gastroenterologist. Specialty: Gen. Med. Prev: Research Fell., Guys and St. Thomas' Hosps.; SHO (Med.) W. Glam. HA.; Regist. (Med.) S. West. RHA.

THOMAS, Lynda Joan Cottage Hospital, 27a Birmingham Road, Sutton Coldfield B72 1QH Tel: 0121 255 4032 Fax: 0121 321 1299; The Dell, 33 Hartopp Road, Four Oaks, Sutton Coldfield B74 2QR Tel: 0121 308 6344 — MB ChB Birm. 1973; Dip. Community Paediat. Warwick 1985; MRCPCH 1996; MSc Comm. Child Health Warwick 1999. Assoc. Specialist S. Birm. Primary Care Trust. Specialty: Community Child Health. Socs: Fac. Community Health. Prev: SCMO NBC Community Health Trust & Good Hope Hosp.

THOMAS, Mair Croesawdy, Llandre, Bow St., Aberystwyth SY23 5BZ Tel: 01970 828726 — MB BCh Wales 1997 (University of Wales College of Medicine Cardiff) SHO GP VTS Bridgend. Specialty: Gen. Pract. Socs: BMA; MSS; MDU. Prev: Ho. Off. (Surg.) W. Wales Gen. Hosp. Carmarthen; Ho. Off. (Med.) Singleton Hosp. Swansea.

THOMAS, Mair Eleri Morgan 21 Park Avenue, London NW11 7SL Tel: 020 8455 7600 — (Univ. Ed.) BSc Ed. 1941; MB ChB (Ed) 1942; DPH Eng. 1947; FRCPath 1963; MFCM RCP (UK) 1972; MFPHM RCP (UK) 1989; MRI (UK) 2001. Emerit. Cons. Microbiol. Univ. Coll. Lond. Hosp. NHS Trust. Specialty: Med. Microbiol.; Epidemiol. Socs: Fell. Path. Soc.; Fell. Roy. Soc. Med.; Internat. Organisat. Mycoplasmol. Prev: Cons. Epidemiol. Centr. Publ. Health Laborat. Colindale; Cons. Microbiol. & Hon. Sen. Lect. Univ. Coll. Hosp.; Cons. Path. Eliz. G. Anderson Hosp. Lond.

THOMAS, Malcolm David 51 Laws Street, Pembroke Dock, Pembroke Tel: 01646 683113 — MB BCh Wales 1969 (Cardiff) DObst RCOG 1971.

THOMAS, Maliakal Cherian 9 Tranby Lane, Analby, Hull HU10 7DR — MB BS Kerala 1965.

THOMAS, Maliampurackal Sebastian (retired) 38 Hutton Close, Westbury-on-Trym, Bristol BS9 3PT Tel: 0117 968 5486 Fax: 0117 968 5486; Jusmax, 38 Hutton Close, Westbury on Trym, Bristol BS9 3PT Tel: 0117 968 5456 — MB BS Kerala 1968 (Med. Coll. Trivandrum) BSc Kerala 1963. Clin. Asst. Rehabil. Unit Ham Green Hosp. Bristol; Clin. Asst. (Genitourin. Med.) Princess Margt. Hosp. Swindon. Prev: Clin. Asst. (A & E) Bristol Roy. Infirm.

THOMAS, Margaret David (retired) 39 Heathpark Avenue, Cardiff CF14 3RF Tel: 029 2075 6524 Email: gethyn@tinyworld.co.uk — MB BCh Wales 1956. Prev: Clin. Asst. Dept. Child Health S. Glam. HA (T).

THOMAS, Margaret Louise The Surgery, St. Mary's Road, Newbury RG14 1ES Tel: 01189 883134; 23 Cheviot Close, Newbury RG14 6SQ Tel: 01635 40246 Fax: 01635 35069 Email: m.l.thomas@lineone.net — MB ChB Sheff. 1977; Mem. Inst. Psychosexual Medicine; DRCOG 1985; MFFP 1995; MRCGP 2002. GP. Specialty: Family Plann. & Reproduc. Health; Gen. Pract.; Psychosexual Med. Socs: Fac. Fam. Plann. & Reproduc. Health Care; IPM. Prev: Cons. in Family Plann. & Reproductive Health Care.

THOMAS, Margaret Marsh The Surgery, Astonia House, High Street, Baldock SG7 6BP Tel: 01462 892458 Fax: 01462 490821; Newstead, Oaks Close, Hitchin SG4 9BN Tel: 01462 433258 Fax: 01462 433258 — MB BS Lond. 1968 (Roy. Free) MRCS Eng. LRCP Lond. 1968; DObst RCOG 1970. Socs: RSM.

THOMAS, Margaret Susan Bradgate Surgery, Ardenton Walk, Brentry, Bristol BS10 6SP Tel: 0117 959 1920 Fax: 0117 983 9332 — MB ChB Bristol 1970; DObst RCOG 1971; DPM Eng. 1974. GP Bristol. Prev: Sen. Regist. (Child Psychiat.) Bristol Roy. Hosp. Sick Childr.

THOMAS, Margot Ross Flat 2, 101 St Johns Way, Archway, London N19 3RG — MB BS Lond. 1984.

THOMAS, Margot Vivienne (retired) Gelli, Idole, Carmarthen SA32 8DG — MB BCh BAO Dub. 1960 (TC Dub.) MA Dub. 1960. Clin. Asst. (Adult Psychiat.) W. Wales. Prev: Med. Off. Serv. Childr. Schs. JHQ Rhinedahlen, BAOR BFPO 40.

THOMAS, Marian (retired) Berwyn, Pentraeth Road, Menai Bridge LL59 5RR Tel: 01248 712794 — (Manch.) MB ChB Manch. 1965; SR 1998. Prev: Cons. Community Paediat.

THOMAS, Marjorie Mitchell Seafield, Cardross, Dumbarton G82 5LD Tel: 01389 841342 — MB ChB Ed. 1965; DObst RCOG 1967. Assoc. Specialist (A & E) Vale of Leven Hosp. Alexandria. Prev: Asst. & Assoc. Specialist (Surg.) Vale of Leven Hosp. Alexandria.

THOMAS, Mark Countisbury Avenue Surgery, 152 Countisbury Avenue, Llanrumney, Cardiff CF3 5YS Tel: 029 2079 2661 Fax: 029 2079 4537 — MB BCh Wales 1980.

THOMAS, Mark Edward Renal Unit, Leicester General Hospital, Gwendolyn Road, Leicester LE5 4PW Tel: 0116 249 0490; 23 Wimborne Road, South Knighton, Leicester LE2 3RQ — MB BS Lond. 1983 (Westm. Med. Sch. Univ. Lond.) BSc Lond. 1980; MRCP (UK) 1988. Sen. Regist. (Nephrol.) Leicester Gen. Hosp. Specialty: Nephrol. Prev: Sen. Regist. (Med.) Leicester Roy. Infirm.; Research Fell. Washington Univ. St. Louis USA; Research Fell. (Nephrol.) Roy. Free Hosp. Lond.

THOMAS, Mark Greenslade 54 Southmoor Road, Walton Manor, Oxford OX2 6RD — MB ChB Auckland 1977.

THOMAS, Mark Lloyd Dept. Anaesthesia, Great Ormond St. Hospital, London WC1N 3JH Tel: 023 8077 7222; Dept of Anaesthesia, Great Ormond St Hospital, London WC1 — MB BChir Camb. 1989; BSc Lond. 1987; FRCA 1994. Regist. Rotata. (Anaesth.) Char. Cross Hosp. Lond. Specialty: Anaesth.; Paediat. Prev: SHO (Anaesth.) Hinchingbrooke Hosp. & Roy. Lond. Hosp.;

SHO (Cardiol. & Cas.) Roy. Adelaide Hosp., Austral.; Regist. Rotat. (Anaesth.) Char. Cross Hosp. Lond.

THOMAS, Mark Richard 11 Frederick Square, London SE16 5XR — MB BS Lond. 1993 (Lond. Hosp. Med. Coll.) BSc (Hons.) Sociol. Applied to Med. Lond. 1991; MRCP (UK) 1997. Specialist Regist. (Neonatology) St. Geo.'s Hosp. Lond. Specialty: Paediat. Prev: SHO (Paediat. Oncol.) Roy. Marsden Hosp.; SHO (Paediat.) St. Geo. Hosp. Lond.; SHO (Paediat.) Whittington NHS Trust.

THOMAS, Mark Stephen Llynyfran Surgery, Llynyfran Road, Llandysul SA44 4JX Tel: 01559 364000 Fax: 01559 364001 — MB BS Lond. 1987 (St. Geos. Lond.) DFFP 1996; MRCGP 2003.

THOMAS, Martin Murmur-Y-Coed, Bethesda Bach, Llanwnda, Caernarfon LL54 5SG — MB ChB Liverp. 1996 (Liverpl.) BSc (Hons.) Liverp. 1991. GP Regist. Gwynedd VTS. Prev: Ho. Off. Med. & Surg. Southport & Forming NHS Trust.

THOMAS, Mr Martin Harford St Peter's Hospital, Guildford Road, Chertsey KT16 0PZ; The Holme, Clay Lane, Headley, Epsom KT18 6JS — MB BS Lond. 1969 (St Thos.) MRCS Eng. LRCP Lond. 1969; FRCS Eng. 1974; MS Lond. 1980. Cons. Surg. St. Peter's Hosp. Chertsey. Specialty: Gen. Surg.; Surgery, Vascular. Socs: Fell. Roy. Soc. Med.; Vasc. Surg. Soc.; Assn. Surg. GB & Irel. Prev: Sen. Regist. (Surg.) St. Thos. Hosp. Lond.; Clin. Research Fell. Scripps Clinic, Calif. USA; Research Fell. (Surg.) King's Coll. Hosp. Med. Sch. Lond.

THOMAS, Martin John Llwynbedw Medical Centre, 82/86 Caerphilly Road, Birchgrove, Cardiff CF14 4AG Tel: 029 2052 1222 Fax: 029 2052 2873; The Nook, 22 Westbourne Crescent, Cardiff CF14 2BL Tel: 029 2069 2227 — MB BCh Wales 1975 (Cardiff) BSc (Med. Biochem.) (Hons.) Wales 1972; MRCGP 1980.

THOMAS, Martin Paul 17 Marsdale Drive, Nuneaton CV10 7DE — MB ChB Leic. 1992.

THOMAS, Martin Peter Thomas and Partners, Churchwood Surgery, Pontypool Meidical Centre, Pontypool NP4 6Dh Tel: 01495 752444 Fax: 01495 767820 — MB BS Lond. 1983; MRCGP 1990. Specialty: Gen. Med.

THOMAS, Martyn Geoffry The Riverside Practice, The Health Centre, Marylebone Road, March PE15 8BG Tel: 01354 661922 Email: martyn.thomas@gp-d81603.nhs.uk — MB BS Lond. 1983 (Roy. Free) BSc Lond. 1980; DRCOG 1986; MRCGP 1988; DGM RCP Lond. 1991; DFFP 2003. Specialty: Gen. Pract. Prev: SHO (Paediat.) Whipps Cross Hosp. Lond.; Ho. Surg. Basildon Gen. Hosp.; Ho. Phys. Whipps Cross Hosp.

THOMAS, Martyn Rhys c/o Dept of Cardiology, Kings College Hospital, Denmark Hill, London SE6 9RS Tel: 020 8346 3748 Fax: 020 7346 3489; 43 Canadian Avenue, Catford, London SE6 3AU Tel: 020 8690 3003 Email: mttwins@aol.com — MD Lond. 1993; MB BS 1982; MRCP (UK) 1985; FRCP 1999. Cons. Cardiol. King's Coll. Hosp. Lond. Specialty: Cardiol. Prev: Research Regist. (Cardiol.) Kings Coll. Hosp. Lond.; Sen. Regist. (Med. & Cardiol.) Kings Coll. Hosp. Lond.; Regist. Med. Unit. St. Mary's Hosp. Lond.

THOMAS, Mary Bowie (retired) Chorad, Little Bay, Kingarth, Rothesay PA20 9NP Tel: 01700 831228 — (Univ. Glas.) MB ChB Glas. 1944. Prev: Regist. Bellshill Matern. Hosp. & William Smellie Matern. Hosp. Lanark.

THOMAS, Mary Frances 27 Cornes Close, Winchester SO22 5DS — MB BS Lond. 1968 (St. Mary's) MRCS Eng. LRCP Lond. 1968; MRCOG 1976, DObst. 1970. SCMO (Adult Servs.) Winchester Health Auth. Prev: Regist. (O & G) Roy. Hants. Co. Hosp. Winchester; Paediat. Regist. St. Mary's Hosp. Portsmouth.

THOMAS, Mary Parker Smith, MBE 31 Fairway, Trentham, Stoke-on-Trent ST4 8AS Tel: 01782 657539 — MB ChB Glas. 1949. Prev: Med. Off. Matern. Sect. Ayrsh. Centr. Hosp. Irvine; Med. Off. Stobhill Hosp. Glas. & Ballochmyle Hosp.

THOMAS, Mary Patricia Thurleigh Road Practice, 88A Thurleigh Road, London SW12 8TT Tel: 020 8675 3521 Fax: 020 8675 3800 — MB ChB Sheff. 1990. Sports Phys.GP Notts Forest FC & FA; Clin. Asst. (Rheum.). Specialty: Gen. Pract.; Sports Med. Socs: BASM; BMA; MRCGP.

THOMAS, Mathew Koduvathrail Birmingham Heartlands Surgery, Gray Street, Bordesley Village, Birmingham B9 4LS Tel: 0121 772 2020 — MB BS Panjab 1965 (Christian Med. Coll. Ludhiana) DCH Eng. 1968. Prev: Clin. Med. Off. (Child Health) Birm. AHA; Regist. (Geriat. & Med.) St. Luke's Hosp. Huddersfield; SHO (Gen. Med. & Paediat.) Horton Gen. Hosp. Banbury.

THOMAS, Matthew Poole Hospital, Department of Medicine for the Elderly, Longfleet Road, Poole BH15 2JB Tel: 01202 448160 Fax: 01202 442993 — MB BS Lond. 1988 (London Hospital Medical College) MRCP (UK) 1991; FRCP 1999; FRCP Edin 2003. Cons.(community/) Geriatrician. Specialty: Care of the Elderly. Socs: Brit. Geriat. Soc. Prev: Research Fell. & Hon. Sen. Regist. Roy. Bournemouth Hosp.; Sen. Regist. Rotat. (Geriat. Med.) Wessex; Regist. Rotat. Jersey & Soton.

THOMAS, Matthew James Colman 15 (1F2) Spottiswoode Street, Edinburgh EH9 1EP — MB ChB Ed. 1996.

THOMAS, Miss Medi Angharad West Wales General Hospital, Carmarthen SA31 2AF Tel: 01267 227585 — MB BS Lond. 1985; FRCS (ORL-HNS). Cons. ENT Surg. W. Wales Gen. Hosp. Carmarthen. Specialty: Otorhinolaryngol.

THOMAS, Megan Ruth Blenheim House Child Development Centre, 145-147 Newton Drive, Blackpool FY3 8LZ Tel: 01253 651615 Fax: 01253 397008 Email: Dr.Thomas@bfwhospitals.nhs.uk; 52 Albany Road, Lytham St Annes FY8 4AS Tel: 01253 738371 Fax: 01253 738371 — MB ChB Manch. 1988 (St Andrews and Manchester) BSc St. And. 1985; DRCOG 1991; MRCP Paediat. Glas. 1992. p/t Cons. (Community Paediat.) Blenheim Hse. Child Developm. Centre Blackpool. Specialty: Paediat. Socs: FRCPCH. Prev: Sen. Regist. (Paediat.) Blackpool Vict. Hosp.; Sen. Regist. (Paediat.) Ninewells Hosp. & Med. Sch. Dundee; Regist. (Paediat.) Mater Misercordiae Hosp. Brisbane, Australia.

THOMAS, Michael Copsen, Knoll Road, Frith Hill, Godalming GU7 2EL Tel: 01483 422949 — MB BChir Camb. 1966 (St. Mary's) FRCP Lond. 1977, M 1962; MA Camb. 1960, MD 1966. Cons. Cardiol. King Edwd. VII Hosp. Midhurst; Hon. Phys. Roy. Brompton Hosp. Lond. Specialty: Gen. Med. Socs: Brit. Cardiac Soc. Prev: Mem. Scientif. Staff & Cons. Phys. MRC Cardiovasc. Research Unit Roy.; Postgrad. Med. Sch. Hammersmith Hosp. Lond.; Ho. Phys. (Med.) St. Mary's Hosp.

THOMAS, Michael Albert 85 Pentre Road, Pontardulais, Swansea SA4 8HR — MB BCh Wales 1992.

THOMAS, Michael David Guardian Medical Centre, Guardian Street, Warrington WA5 1UD Tel: 01925 650226 Email: mike.thomas@gp-n81012.nhs.uk; 25 Woodbridge Close, Appleton, Warrington Tel: 01925 601518 Email: mike.thomas@onetel.net — MB ChB Manch. 1961; BSc (Anat. Hons.) Manch. 1959; DA Eng. 1965; DObst RCOG 1966; FRCGP 1995, M 1974. GP Partner.

THOMAS, Mr Michael Graham Bristol Royal Infirmary, Department of Surgery, 4th Floor, Marlborough Street, Bristol BS2 8NW Tel: 0117 928 3066 Fax: 0117 925 2786; 45 Sydenham Hill, Cothons, Bristol BS6 5SL — MB BS Lond. 1984 (Middlx.) MS Lond. 1994, BSc (1st cl. Hons.) 1981; FRCS Eng. 1989; FRCS Ed. 1989; FRCS (Gen.) 1996. Cons. Colorectal Surg. United Bristol Healthcare NHS Trust. Specialty: Gen. Surg. Socs: Brit. Soc. Gastroenterol.; Assn. Coloproctol.; Surgic. Rese. Soc. Prev: Lect. (Surg.) Univ. Liverp.

THOMAS, Michael Harford (retired) Coppice House, Bradford-on-Avon — MB ChB Bristol 1942. Prev: Ho. Surg. & Cas. Off. Bristol Roy. Infirm.

THOMAS, Michael John Evan 219 Inverness Place, Cardiff CF24 4RY — MB BCh Wales 1993.

THOMAS, Michael John Glyn, Col. late RAMC Retd. The Bloodcare Foundation, 3 Cholseley Drive, Fleet GU51 1HG Tel: 01252 622060 Fax: 01252 622331 Email: michaeljb.thomas2@virgin.net; The Bloodcare Foundation, P.O.Box 558, Horsham RH12 5WJ Tel: 01403 262652 Fax: 01403 262657 Email: clinical@bloodcare.org.uk; 3 Cholseley Drive, Fleet GU51 1HG Tel: 01252 622060 Fax: 01252 622331 Email: michaeljg.thomas2@virgin.net — MB BChir Camb. 1963 (St. Bart.) LMSSA Lond. 1962; MA Camb. 1963; DTM & H RCP Lond. 1964; FRCP Ed 1997. Clin. Dir. Blood Care Foundat.; Chairm. Data & Satety Monitoring Bd. HemclinicIntern. Clin. Trials; Med. Cons. to Dideco - Blood Managem. & Zeal Med.; Indep. Cons. Transfus. Med. Hook. Specialty: Blood Transfus.; Trop. Med. Socs: Fell. BMA; Brit. Blood Transfus. Soc.; Internat. Soc. Blood Transfus. Prev: Dir. Army Blood Transfus. Serv. Aldershot.

THOMAS, Miles Alexander 28 Harnwood Road, Salisbury SP2 8DB Tel: 01722 320893 — MB BS Lond. 1983. GP Shrewton, Wilts.

THOMAS, Millicent Anne Department of Patholopgy, Inverclyde Royal Hospital, Larkfield Road, Greenock PA16 0XN; 12 Mosspark Road, Milngavie, Glasgow G62 8NJ — MB ChB Ed. 1978; MRCPath 1987. Cons. Path. Inverclyde Roy. Hosp. Greenock. Specialty: Histopath. Prev: Cons. Cytopath. Glas. Roy. Infirm.

THOMAS, Miranda Rebecca — MB ChB Bristol 1997; DRCOG 1999; DCH 2000; MRCGP 2001; DFFP 2002. Specialty: Gen. Pract.

THOMAS, Mivart Gwynrudd West 121 Harley Street, London W1G 6AX Tel: 020 7224 0402 Fax: 020 7224 0403; 30 Red Post Hill, Dulwich, London SE24 9JQ Tel: 020 7274 6599 — MRCS Eng. LRCP Lond. 1965 (Camb. & St. Bart.) MA Camb. 1965; MRCPsych 1971. Dep. Med. Director (Psychol. Med.) Cromwell Hosp. Lond. Specialty: Gen. Psychiat. Socs: Fell. Med. Soc. Lond.; Amer. Psychiat. Assn.; Indep. Doctors Forum. Prev: Asst. Prof. Clin. Psychiat. New Jersey Med. Sch. USA; Dir. Dept. Psychiat. Jersey City Med. Center, USA; Asst. Prof. Psychiat. Rutgers Univ. New Jersey, USA.

THOMAS, Moira Jean Department of Immunology, Western Infirmary, Glasgow — MB ChB Glas. 1987; MRCPath Glas.; MRCP (UK).

THOMAS, Nancy Elizabeth The Surgery, 612 Saffron Lane, Leicester LE2 6TD Tel: 01162 911212 Fax: 01162 910300 — MB BS Newc. 1977; MRCGP 1982.

THOMAS, Neil Howard Mailpoint 021, Department of Child Health, Southampton General Hospital, Tremona Road, Southampton SO16 6YD Tel: 023 8079 4457 Fax: 023 8079 4962 Email: neil.thomas@suht.swest.nhs.uk; Denbigh, Shepherds Lane, Compton, Winchester SO21 2AD — MB BChir Camb. 1983 (King's Coll. Hosp.) MA Camb. 1983; DCH RCP Lond. 1987; MRCP (UK) 1987; FRCPCH 1997; FRCP 1999. Cons. Paediat. Neurol. Soton. Gen. Hosp. Specialty: Paediat. Neurol. Prev: Sen. Regist. (Paediat.) Guy's Hosp. Lond.; Research Fell. (Paediat.) Roy. Postgrad. Med. Sch. Lond.; Regist. (Paediat.) Hammersmith Hosp.

THOMAS, Neil Martin 34 Cheriton Grove, Tonteg, Pontypridd CF38 1PF — MB ChB Liverp. 1992.

THOMAS, Mr Neil Philip The Hampshire Clinic, Basing Road, Basingstoke RG24 7AL Tel: 01256 819222 Fax: 01962 761152 — MB BS Lond. 1974; BSc (Hons.) Lond. 1971; FRCS Eng. 1978. Cons. Orthop. Surg. N. Hants. Hosp., The Hants. Clinic & Wessex Nuffield Hosp. Specialty: Orthop. Socs: Fell. Roy. Soc. Med.; (Pres.) BRT. Assn. Surg. Of Knee (BASK) 2002-2004; Ass. Ed. Journal of Bone & Joint Surg. - Ed. Board Mem.1997 -2001. Prev: Sen. Regist. Rotat. (Orthop.) Univ. Coll. Hosp. & Westm. Hosp. Lond.; Regist. (Gen. Surg.) Univ. Coll. Hosp. Lond.; SHO Rotat. (Surg.) Northwick Pk. Hosp. Harrow.

THOMAS, Neil Rhys Launceston Close Surgery, 9-10 Launceton Close, Winsford CW7 1LY Tel: 01606 861200 — MB BCh Wales 1983; MRCGP 1988; DRCOG 1990.

THOMAS, Mr Nicholas Wake Macmeikan King's College Hospital, Denmark Hill, London SE5 9RS Tel: 020 7346 3288 Fax: 020 7346 3280; 3 Radlet Avenue, Forest Hill, London SE26 4BZ Tel: 020 8291 7739 Email: nwm.thomas@virgin.net — MB BS Lond. 1988 (Lond. Hosp.) FRCS Glas. 1992; FRCS Eng. 1992; FRCS (SN) 1997. Specialty: Neurosurg. Socs: Fell. Roy. Soc. Med.; BMA; Soc. of Brit. Neurosurgeons. Prev: Spinal Fell. (Neurosurg.) Ohio State Univ. Ohio, USA; Regist. (Neurosurg.) Atkinson Morley Hosp.; Sen. Regist. (Neurosurg.) Gt. Ormond St. Hosp. & Nat. Hosp. for Neurol & Neurosurg. Qu. Sq. Lond. & Atkinson Morley's Hosp. Lond.

THOMAS, Nicola Frances 48 Villiers Crescent, Eccleston, St Helens WA10 5HR — MB ChB Manch. 1997.

THOMAS, Professor Nigel Brett North Manchester General Hospital, Delaunays Road, Crumpsall, Manchester M8 5RB Tel: 0161 795 4567; 10 Juniper Close, Sale M33 6JT — MRCS Eng. LRCP Lond. 1981 (St. Bart.) BSc (Hons.) Lond. 1978, MB BS 1981; FRCR 1987. Cons. (Radiol.) N. Manch. Gen. Hosp.; Hon. Vis. Prof., Univ. of Salford. Specialty: Radiol.

THOMAS, Nigel Eugene (retired) Cottage View, Stonewalls, Burton, Rossett, Wrexham LL12 0LG Tel: 01244 571436 — (Liverp.) MB ChB Liverp. 1958; DCH Eng. 1961; DPH Eng. 1962.

THOMAS, Noel Bell Bron-y-Garn Surgery, Station Street, Maesteg CF34 9AL Tel: 01656 733262 Fax: 01656 735239; Bron-y-Garn, Maesteg CF34 9AL — MB ChB Ed. 1968 (Camb. & Ed.) MA Camb. 1965; DObst RCOG 1970; DCH Eng. 1972; MFHom 2000. GP (NHS). Prev: Ho. Phys. Edin. Roy. Infirm.; SHO Paediat. Amersham Gen. Hosp.

THOMAS, Norman Armsden The Surgery, Caerffynnon, Dolgellau LL40 1LY Tel: 01341 422431 — MB ChB Birm. 1945; DObst RCOG 1950. Med. Off. Dolgellau & Barmouth Dist. Hosp. Prev: Ho. Surg. Dudley Rd. Hosp. Birm.; Ho. Surg. MRC Burns Unit Birm. Accid. Hosp.; Hon. Maj. RAMC.

THOMAS, Norman Spencer (retired) 25 Alvechurch Highway, Lydiate Ash, Bromsgrove B60 1NZ — (King's Coll. Hosp.) MB BS Lond. 1951; MRCS Eng. LRCP Lond. 1951; DA Eng. 1957; FFA RCS Eng. 1962. Prev: Cons. Anaesth. Selly Oak Hosp. Birm.

THOMAS, Olive Mary (retired) Perivale, Higher Metherell, Callington PL17 8DD Tel: 01579 350737 Email: oandg@ukgateway.net — (Manchester) MB ChB Manch. 1950; DPH Manch. 1954. Prev: Med. Off. (Family Plann.) Wigan HA.

THOMAS, Osmond Leopold 110 Westcotes Drive, Leicester LE3 0QS — MB BS West Indies 1985.

THOMAS, Owain Rhys 41 Dol-Y-Llan, Miskin, Pontyclun CF72 8RY — MB BCh Wales 1997.

THOMAS, Owen Gethin (retired) Maesgwyn, 75 Pengam Road, Ystrad Mynach, Hengoed CF82 8AB Tel: 01443 813248 — MB BS Lond. 1948 (St. Bart.) Prev: Lt. RAMC.

THOMAS, Owen Maelgwyn (retired) 65 Sandringham Road, Swindon SN3 1HT — MB ChB Leeds 1956. Prev: Ho. Phys. & Ho. Surg. Swansea Gen. Hosp.

THOMAS, Mr Palakuzhyil Thomas 6 Sunningdale Close, Kirkham, Preston PR4 2TG Tel: 01772 672722 — MB BS Aligarh Muslim, India 1968; FRCSI 1986. Assoc. Specialist (Gen. Surg.) Blackpool Vict. Hosp. Specialty: Gen. Surg.

THOMAS, Pamela Jill Everton Road General Practice, 70 Everton Road, Liverpool L6 2EW Tel: 0151 260 5050 — MB ChB Manch. 1986; MRCGP 1991; DFFP 1993; Dip. Ther. 1997. GP (p/t). Specialty: Gen. Pract. Prev: Trainee GP Harpenden; Trainee GP Rugby VTS.

THOMAS, Pamela Wayne (retired) The Old Manse, 46 Westgate, Cowbridge CF71 7AR Tel: 01446 773322 — MB BCh Wales 1962 (Cardiff) DObst RCOG 1964; DPH Wales 1966. Prev: SCMO (Genetics) M. Glam. AHA.

THOMAS, Patricia Anne (retired) 43 Monument Lane, Rednal, Birmingham B45 9QQ Tel: 0121 453 2964 — MB ChB St. And. 1957; DO Eng. 1965; MCOphth 1990. Prev: Assoc. Specialist (Ophth.) BromsGr. & Redditch Health Dist.

THOMAS, Patricia Catherine Garburn House, Westmorland General Hospital, Burton Road, Kendal LA9 7RG Tel: 01539 795253 Fax: 01539 795361; Verandah Cottage, Nether Burrow, Kirby Lonsdale, Carnforth LA6 2RJ Tel: 015242 74223 — MB ChB Birm. 1974; MRCPsych 1978. Cons. Psychiat. Bay Community Trust. Specialty: Gen. Psychiat. Prev: Sen. Regist. (Psychiat.) Univ. Coll. Hosp. Lond.; Research Fell. (Psychiat.) Univ. Coll. Hosp. Med. Sch. Lond.; Regist. (Psychiat.) Shelton Hosp. Shrewsbury.

THOMAS, Paul 9 Victoria Avenue, Forest Hall, Newcastle upon Tyne NE12 8AX — MB BS Newc. 1988; MRCP (UK) 1994. SpR (Anaesth.) North. Deanery. Specialty: Anaesth. Prev: SHO (Anaesth.) Dryburn Hosp.

THOMAS, Mr Paul Anthony Department of Surgery, Whipps Cross University Hospital, London E11 1NR Tel: 020 8535 6606; 22 King's Avenue, Buckhurst Hill IG9 5LP Tel: 020 8505 3203 — MB BS Lond. 1968 (Lond. Hosp.) FRCS Eng. 1973; BSc Lond. 1965, MS 1977; MCI Arb 1999. Med. Director, Whipps Cross Univ. Hosp.; Undergrad. Tutor Whipps Cross Hosp. Lond.; Mem. of Intercolleges Exam. Bd. in Gen. Surg.; CME Tutor RCS Eng.; Regional Adviser Surg. NE Thames; Edr. Brit. Jl. Hosp. Med.; Chairm. Higher Surg. Train. Comm. NE Thames; Mem. Exam. Comm. RCS Eng.; Mem. Edit. Bd. FRCS Supplm.; Cons. Gen. & Gastrointestinal Surg. Whipps Cross Univ. Hosp. Lond. Specialty: Gen. Surg. Socs: Surg. Research Soc.; Brit. Soc. Gastroenterol.; Assn. Endoscopic Surgs. Prev: Organiser Whipps Cross Hosp. Advanced Surgic. Course Lond.; Tutor (Surg.) RCS; Chairm. Physiol. Sect. Appl. Basic Sci Exam. RCS.

THOMAS, Paul David Taunton and Somerset NHS Trust, Musgrove Park, Taunton TA1 5DA Tel: 01823 333444 — MB BChir Camb. 1988; MRCP (UK) 1992; DTM & H Liverp. 1993; MD (Lond.) 2001. Cons. Phys./Gastroenterologist, Taunton & Som. Hosp. Specialty: Gastroenterol.; Gen. Med. Prev: Research Fell. St. Mark's & St. Thos. Hosps.; Regist. Chelsea & Westm. Hosp. Lond.

THOMAS, Paul David Gipping Valley Practice, Kirby Rise, Barham, Ipswich IP6 0AS Tel: 01473 832832 Fax: 01473 830200 — (Roy. Free) BSc (Hons. Physiol.) Dund 1974; MSc (Ergonomics) Loughborough 1975; MB BS Lond. 1984; MRCGP 1988. Specialty: Accid. & Emerg.; Gen. Pract.; Obst. & Gyn. Socs: BASICS; Disp. Doctors Assn. (Mem. Nat. Comm.). Prev: Trainee GP Ipswich VTS; Research Off. MRC Div. Bioeng. Harrow.

THOMAS, Professor Paul Rhodri — MB ChB Bristol 1979; DCH Lond. 1983; MRCGP 1986; MD Liverp. 2003; FRCGP 2004. p/t General Practitioner; Prof. Primary Care Research Educat. & Developm. Thames Valley Univ. & Brent Primary Care Trust. Specialty: Gen. Pract. Socs: BMA; MRCGP. Prev: Sen. Lect. Imperial College; Director W. Lond. Research Network; R&D Cons. Brent Primary Care Trust.

THOMAS, Mr Paul Roderick Spensley St. Helier Hospital, Carshalton SM5 1AA Tel: 020 8644 4343 — MB BS Lond. 1978 (Bart.) FRCS Eng. 1982; MS Lond. 1991. Cons. Surg. (Gen. & Vasc. Surg.) St. Helier Hosp. Carshalton. Specialty: Gen. Surg. Socs: (Ex-Counc.) Vasc. Surgic. Soc.; Surgic. Research Sc.

THOMAS, Mrs Pauline Julia (retired) 6 Hunter Place, Louth LN11 9LG Tel: 01507 603473 — MB ChB St. And. 1959. Prev: Clin. Med. Off. N. Lincs. DHA.

THOMAS, Pauline Mary Ann 16 Frankland Terrace, Emsworth PO10 7BA Tel: 01243 378870 — (Roy. Free) MB BS Lond. 1954. SCMO Portsmouth Healthcare Trust. Specialty: Family Plann. & Reproduc. Health.

THOMAS, Peter Bowden Flat 3, 57 Arlingford Road, London SW2 2ST — MB BS Lond. 1992.

THOMAS, Mr Peter Brian Macfarlane University Hospital of North Staffordshire, Princes Road, Stoke-on-Trent ST4 7NL Tel: 01782 554857 Email: p.b.m.thomas@keele.ac.uk — MB BS Lond. 1975 (St. Thos.) FRCS Eng. 1981; FRCS Ed. 1981. Cons. & Sen. Lect. (Orthop. Surg.) Keele; Cons. Orthop. Surg. N. Staffs. Roy. Infirm. Specialty: Orthop. Special Interest: Hands; Limb Reconstruction; Problem Fractures. Socs: Brit. Hand Soc.; Brit. Orthopaedic Assn.; Brit. Trauma Soc. Prev: Sen. Regist. Robt. Jones & Agnes Hunt Orthop. Hosp. Oswestry; Research Fell. (Orthop.) St. Luke's Episcopal Hosp. & Methodist Hosp. Houston, Texas; Regist. (Surg.) Univ. Hosp. Wales Cardiff.

THOMAS, Peter Cadwalladr A&E Department, Milton Keynes General Hospital, Standing Way, Eaglestone, Milton Keynes MK6 5LD Tel: 01908 243931 Email: peter.thomas@mkgeneral.nhs.uk — MB ChB Liverp. 1981; FRCS Glas. 1989; FFAEM 1998. Cons. A&E Med. . Milton Keynes Hosp.; Clin. Director A&E; Assoc. Tutor, Oxf.

THOMAS, Peter Daniel Spence (retired) The Hill, Baldersby, Thirsk YO7 4PH Tel: 01765 640332 — MB BChir Camb. 1950 (Camb. & Lond. Hosp.) MA Camb. 1950; MRCS Eng. LRCP Lond. 1950; DCH Eng. 1973. Prev: Gen. Practitoner, Bedale, N. Yorks.

THOMAS, Peter Howard Lower Farm House, Llysworney, Cowbridge CF71 7NQ Tel: 01446 772450 — MB BCh Wales 1944 (Cardiff) MD Wales 1955; FRCGP 1969; Pres. Medal RCGP 1998. Morgan E. Williams Award 1955; Hon. Curator, Museum RCGP. Specialty: Homeop. Med. Socs: Counc. (Ex-Pres.) Hist. Med. Soc. Wales; Fac. Hom. (Bristol & SW Br.). Prev: Ho. Phys. Welsh Nat. Sch. Med.

THOMAS, Professor Peter Kynaston, CBE Inst. Of Neurology, Queen Square, London WC1N 3BG Tel: 020 7837 3611; 33 West Hill Park, Merton Lane, London N6 6ND Tel: 020 8340 3365 Email: pkt.hotline@virgin.net — (Univ. Coll. Lond. & Univ. Coll. Hosp.) MB BS Lond. 1950; MRCS Eng. LRCP Lond. 1950; FRCP Lond. 1967, M 1956; DSc Lond. 1971, BSc (1st cl. Hons.) 1947, MD 1957; FRCPath 1990. Emerit. Prof. Roy. Free Hosp. Sch. Med. & Inst. Neurol. Lond.; Hon. Cons. Neurol. Roy. Free Hosp., Nat. Hosp. Neurol. Neurosurg. Qu. Sq. & Roy. Nat. Orthop. Hosp. Lond. Specialty: Neurol. Socs: Assn. Brit. Neurols.; Assn. Phys.; Hon. Mem. Amer. Neurol. Assn. Prev: Asst. Prof. Neurol. McGill Univ. Montreal; Sen. Regist. Acad. Unit, Nat. Hosp. Qu. Sq.; Regist. (Neurol.) Middlx. Hosp. Lond.

THOMAS, Peter Leslie Portswood Road Surgery, 186-188 Portswood Road, Portswood, Southampton SO17 2NJ Tel: 023 8055 5181 Fax: 023 8036 6416 — MB BS Lond. 1980 (Middlx.) BSc Lond. 1980; FRCS (Orl.) Eng. 1987; T(GP) 1990. GP Soton.; Occupat. Phys. GPSI ENT Soton City PCT, GEC Marconi Infrared Ltd, Phillips Electronics. Specialty: Occupat. Health; Otolaryngol. Socs: Small Pract.s Assoc.; Primary Care Spec. Gp. of Brit. Computer Soc.; GP Asthma Gp. Prev: Regist. (ENT Surg.) Roy. Gwent Hosp.

THOMAS, Peter Leslie Bupa Wellness Centre, Centurian Court, 64 London Road, Reading RG1 5AS Tel: 01189 062800 Fax: 01889 062801 Email: thomaspe@bupa.com — MB BS Lond. 1969 (St. Thos.) DObst RCOG 1972; Dip. Sports Med. Scott. Roy. Coll. 1997. Sen. Orthopaedic and Sports Phys.; Med. Commiss. Mem. FISA; Med. Off. Olympic Med. Inst.; Fell. Inst. of Sports Med. Specialty: Sports Med. Prev: Team Doctor GB Rowing Team; Maj. RAMC.

THOMAS, Peter Walter Vaughan Red Bank Group Practice, Red Bank Health Centre, Unsworth Street, Manchester M26 3GH Tel: 0161 724 0777 Fax: 0161 724 8288; Woodthorpe, 28 South Downs Road, Hale, Altrincham WA14 3HW Tel: 0161 928 0668 — MB ChB Manch. 1980 (Manchester) DRCOG 1985; DCH RCP Lond. 1986; MRCGP 1987. Occupat. Health Phys. Rochdale Hosp. NHS Trust & Salford Univ. Sch. of Nursing; Vice-Chairm. & Commissioning Lead Bury S. PCG; Med. Off. Bury Hospice. Specialty: Gen. Pract.; Occupat. Health; Palliat. Med. Prev: Paediat. Dubai-Lond. Clinic, Dubai, UAE; Trainee GP Barlow Med. Centre Manch.; SHO & Ho. Off. S. Manch. Hosps.

THOMAS, Philip Andrew Heath Lane Surgery, Earl Shilton, Leicester LE9 7PB Tel: 01455 844431 Fax: 01455 442297; The Lodge, Station Road, Earl Shilton, Leicester LE9 4LU — MB ChB Manch. 1974.

THOMAS, Philip David St. Davids, Lower Road, Hockley SS5 5JU — MB BCh BAO Dub. 1972; BA; BSc (Hons.) Wales 1968.

THOMAS, Philip Fredric Lane Head Farm Cottage, Heptonstall, Hebden Bridge HX7 7PB — MB ChB Manch. 1972; DPM Eng. 1978; FRCPsych 1995, M 1980; MPhil. Ed. 1984; MD Manch 2000. Cons. Psychiat. Bradford Outreach Team; Sen. Research Fell., Centre for Citizenship and Community, Ment. Health, Univ. of Bradford. Specialty: Gen. Psychiat. Prev: Cons. Psychiat. Ysbyty Gwynedd & Manch. Roy. Infirm.; Lect. & Hon. Sen. Regist. (Psychiat.) Roy. Edin. Hosp.

THOMAS, Mr Philip James Dept. of Urology, Sussex House, 1 Abbey Road, Brighton BN2 1H Tel: 01273 696955; The Gables, 56 Southover High St., Lewes BN7 1JA — MB BS Lond. 1981; FRCS Lond. 1986; FRCS (Urol.) 1992. Cons. (Urol.) Brighton Health Care Trust; Cons. Urol. (Urol.) Char. Cross Hosp. Lond. Specialty: Urol. Prev: Sen. Regist. (Urol.) Guy's Hosp. Lond.

THOMAS, Phillip Morriston Hospital, Morriston, Swansea SA6 6NL Tel: 01792 703889; The Coach House, Penmaen, Swansea SA3 2HA — MB BCh Wales 1979; MRCP (UK) 1982; FRCP Lond. 1996. Cons. Cardiol. Morriston Hosp. Swansea. Specialty: Cardiol. Prev: Cons. Cardiol. Singleton Hosp. Swansea; Lect. & Hon. Sen. Regist. St. Mary's Hosp. Lond. & Northwick Pk. Hosp. Harrow.

THOMAS, Phyllis Marion (retired) 49 Cilddewi Park, Johnstown, Carmarthen SA31 3HP — MB BCh Wales 1957. Prev: Assoc. Specialist St. Davids Hosp. Carmarthen.

THOMAS, Phyllis Menna 45 Westbury Road, Northwood HA6 3DB Tel: 01923 823712 — MB BCh Wales 1952 (Cardiff) BSc (Chem.) Wales 1944, MB BCh 1952. Clin. Asst. (Dermat.) Mt. Vernon Hosp. & Edgware Gen. Hosp. Prev: Ho. Phys. Roy. Infirm. Cardiff; SHO (Psychiat.) Fulbourn Hosp. Camb.; Beal Research Fell. Stanford Med. Sch. San Francisco, USA.

THOMAS, Mr Puthenparampil George Parkgate Medical Centre, Netherfield Lane, Parkgate, Rotherham S62 6AW Tel: 01709 514500 Fax: 01709 514490 — MB BS Panjab 1980; FRCS Ed. 1987. GP. Specialty: Orthop. Prev: Regist. (Orthop.) Qu. Eliz. Hosp. Gateshead.

THOMAS, Rachel Gillian 190 Jarrom Street, Leicester LE2 7DF — MB ChB Leic. 1997.

THOMAS, Rachel Hannah — MB BS Lond. 1993 (St. Mary's Paddington) MRCGP 1998. GP Locum Cardiff Area.

THOMAS, Mr Ravi Department of Rehabilitation, Raigmore Hospital, Inverness IV2 3UJ Tel: 01463 70400; 2 Inshes View, Westhill, Inverness IV2 5DS Tel: 01463 793458 — MB BS Kerala 1970 (Med. Coll. Trivandrum) MS (Orthop.) Panjab 1974. Med. Off. (Rheum. & Rehabil.) Raigmore Hosp. Inverness. Prev: Regist. (Orthop.) Raigmore Hosp. Inverness.

THOMAS, Rebecca Elizabeth 177 Kingshayes Road, Walsall WS9 8RZ — MB BS Lond. 1997.

THOMAS, Rhian Princess Street Surgery, Princess Street, Gorseinon, Swansea SA4 4US Tel: 01792 895681 Fax: 01792 893051; The Gnoll, 2 Bryntywod, Llangyfelach, Swansea SA5 7LE Tel: 01792 792343 — MB BS Lond. 1985 (St Bartholomew's Hospital) DCH RCP Lond. 1990; MRCGP 1993. GP.

THOMAS, Mr Rhidian de Winton Melbourne Charing Cross Hospital, Department of Orthopaedics, Fulham Palace Road, London SW8 Tel: 020 8846 1475 Fax: 020 8967 5625 Email: rhidian.thomas@ic.ac.uk — MB BS Lond. 1986 (St Bart. Hosp. Med. Sch.) BSc 1983; FRCS Ed. 1991; FRCS (Orth) 1997; MS 1998. Cons., Orthop., Char. Cross Hosp. Lond.; Hon. Sen. Lect., Imperial Coll. Sch. of Med., Lond. Specialty: Orthop.; Trauma & Orthop. Surg. Special Interest: lower limb sports injuries, knee and ankle arthroscopic and ligament repair. Socs: BOA; BOSTA; BMA.

THOMAS, Mr Rhys Hywel 5 Archer Road, Penarth CF64 3HW — MB BS Lond. 1990 (Univ. Coll. Hosp.) FRCS Glas. 1995; FRCS (Orth) 2000. Specialty: Orthop.

THOMAS, Richard Charles Royal Hampshire County Hospital, Romsey Road, Winchester SO22 5DG; 14 West Street, Titchfield, Fareham PO14 4DH — MB BS Lond. 1991 (St Mary's) DA (UK) 1996; FRCA 1996; FRCA 1998. Cons. (Anaesth. & Intens. Care Med.). Specialty: Anaesth.

THOMAS, Richard Cherian 9 Tranby Lane, Anlaby, Hull HU10 7DR — MB BS Newc. 1996.

THOMAS, Richard David Radiology Department, Royal Devon & Exeter Hospital (Wonford), Barrack Road, Exeter EX2 5DW — MB ChB Liverp. 1985; MRCP (UK) 1988; FRCR 1991. Cons. Radiol. Roy. Devon & Exeter Hosp. Wonford. Specialty: Radiol. Prev: Sen. Regist. (Radiol.) Soton. Univ. Hosps.; Regist. (Radiol.) Soton. Gen. Hosp.; SHO (Med.) Truro Hosps.

THOMAS, Richard Gerwyn Tanyfron Surgery, 7-9 Market Street, Aberaeron SA46 0AS Tel: 01545 570271 Fax: 01545 570136; Brynhyfryd, Crossways, Ffosyffin, Aberaeron SA46 0HD — MB BS Lond. 1982; MRCGP 1986.

THOMAS, Richard Huw 19 Smithies Avenue, Sully, Penarth CF64 5SS — MB ChB Manch. 1985.

THOMAS, Richard John Hayling Island Health Centre, Elm Grove, Hayling Island PO11 9AP — BM Soton. 1993; MRCGP; DGM RCP Lond. 1995. SHO (O & G) Portsmouth NHS Trust; GP Princip., E. Hants. PCT. Specialty: Gen. Pract.

THOMAS, Richard John 9 Beckett Road, Worcester WR3 7NH Tel: 01905 451034 — MB BS Lond. 1973; MRCS Eng. LRCP Lond. 1973. Clin. Asst. (Thoracic Med.) Worcestershire Royal Hosp. Prev: GP Droitwich, Worcs.

THOMAS, Mr Richard Stephen Alban BUPA Hospital, Leicester LE2 2FF Tel: 01162 653650 Fax: 01162 653651; The Oaks, 6 Main Street, Queiniborough, Leicester LE7 3DA — (St Bart.) MA, MB BChir Camb. 1964; FRCS Eng. 1970. Cons. Otolaryngol. Leicester AHA (T). Specialty: Otolaryngol. Socs: Sect. Roy. Soc. Med. & Examr. Otolaryngol. RCS Eng.; BMA; FRCS. Prev: Sen. Regist. (ENT) St. Bart. Hosp. & Roy. Marsden Hosp. Lond.; Sen. Regist. Roy. Nat. Throat, Nose & Ear Hosp. Lond.; Ho. Phys. & Ho. Surg. (ENT) St. Bart. Hosp. Lond.

THOMAS, Richard Stephen Lloyd Heath Hill Practice, Heath Hill Road South, Crowthorne RG45 7BN Tel: 01344 777915 — MB BS Lond. 1974 (Char. Cross) DRCOG 1979; Cert JCC Lond. 1980; DCH Eng. 1980; MRCGP 1981.

THOMAS, Robert James 12 Philadelphia Road, Porthcawl CF36 3DP — MB ChB Leic. 1984; MRCP (UK) 1988. Regist. (Oncol. & Radiother.) Middlx. Hosp. Lond. Specialty: Oncol.; Radiother.

THOMAS, Robert Stephen Rainbow Medical Centre, 333 Robins Lane, St Helens WA9 3PN Tel: 01744 811211 — MB ChB Liverp. 1978; DRCOG 1982; BA Open 1989; MSc Aberystwyth 1998. Specialty: Gen. Pract.

THOMAS, Roderic David The Cardiac Centre, Royal United Hospital, Combe Park, Bath BA1 3NG Tel: 01225 428331 Fax: 01225 825441; Rowley House, Combe Hay, Bath BA2 7EF Tel: 01225 832188 — MB BChir Camb. 1968 (St. Thos.) MD Camb. 1978, MA 1969; MRCP (UK) 1970; FRCP Lond. 1986. Cons. Phys. & Cardiol. Roy. United Hosp. Bath. Specialty: Cardiol. Socs: Brit. Cardiac Soc. Prev: Sen. Regist. (Med. & Cardiol.) Leeds Gen. Infirm. & Killingbeck Hosp.; Regist. (Med.) St. Thos. Hosp. Lond.

THOMAS, Roderick Lister Barn Surgery, Christchurch Medical Centre, Purewell Cross Road, Christchurch BH23 3AF Tel: 01202 486456 Fax: 01202 486678 — MB BS Lond. 1976 (Westm.) MRCS Eng. LRCP Lond. 1976; D.Occ.Med. RCP Lond. 1995. Med. Off. (Occupat. Health) Roy. Bournemouth Hosp.; Chairm. ChristCh. PCG. Specialty: Occupat. Health. Prev: SHO (Med.) Kent & Canterbury Hosp.; SHO (Med.) Roy. Vict. Hosp. Bournemouth; Ho. Phys. (Radiother.) Westm. Hosp. Lond.

THOMAS, Roger David Corporate Medical Group Office of the Chief Medical Adviser, Department of Work & Pensions, 1-11 John Adam Street, London WC2N 6HT Tel: 020 7712 2003; Allambi, Long Hill, Seale, Farnham GU10 1NQ — MB BS Lond. 1973 (St. Mary's Hosp.) DRCOG 1977. Med. Policy Adviser DSS Lond. Specialty: Civil Serv.

THOMAS, Roger Walwyn Old Road Surgery, Old Road, Llanelli SA15 3HR Tel: 01554 775555 Fax: 01554 778868; Y Graig, Caswell St, Llanelli SA15 1BS Tel: 01554 759500 Fax: 01554 759500 — MB BCh BAO Dub. 1970. Exam. Med. Off. Attendance Allowance Bd. & Co-op. Insur. Company; Company Doctor S. Wales Region Thysseu GB Ltd.

THOMAS, Rosemary Ann Natalie Torrington Health Centre, New Road, Torrington EX38 8EL Tel: 01805 622247 Fax: 01805 625083 — MB ChB Bristol 1984; DRCOG Lond. 1988; Cert. Family Plann. JCC 1989; MRCGP Lond. 1989. Prev: Trainee GP Taunton VTS; SHO (Geriat. Med., A & E & O & G) Som. HA.

THOMAS, Roslyn Margaret Northwick Park and St Mark's Hospital, Watford Road, Harrow HA1 3UJ Tel: 020 8869 3941 Fax: 020 8869 2927 — MB BS Queensland 1970 (Univ. of Queensland) FRCPCH; FRCPCH; MRCP (UK) 1975; FRCP Lond. 1993. Cons. Neonat. Paediat. Northwick Pk. & St. Marks Hosp. with s/i Neonatol. Specialty: Paediat.; Neonat. Socs: Neonat. Soc.; Brit. Assn. Perinatal Med.; Roy. Coll. of Paediat. and Child Health. Prev: Sen. Regist. (Paediat.) Univ. Coll. Hosp. Lond.

THOMAS, Rosser Ian Heol Fach Surgery, Heol Fach, North Cornelly, Bridgend CF33 4LD Tel: 01656 740345 Fax: 01656 740872; 5 Church View, Laleston, Bridgend CF32 0HF Tel: 01656 654077 — MB BCh Wales 1978; MRCGP 1981; DRCOG 1981.

THOMAS, Ruth Cameron (retired) Meadow Cottage, Alpington, Norwich NR14 7NG — BM BCh Oxf. 1965 (Oxf. & St. Bart.) MA Oxf. 1966, BM BCh 1965; FFA RCS Eng. 1969. Prev: Cons. Anaesth. Norwich Health Dist.

THOMAS, Ruth Ellen 19 Nightingale Road, Rickmansworth WD3 7DE — MB BS Lond. 1988.

THOMAS, Mr Ryland James Department of Orthopaedic Surgery, New Cross Hospital, Wolverhampton WV10 0QP Tel: 01902 642961 — (Lond. Hosp.) MB BS Lond. 1966; MRCS Eng. LRCP Lond. 1966; DObst RCOG 1968; FRCS Eng. 1971. Cons. Orthop. Surg. Roy. Wolverhampton NHS Hosps. Trust. Specialty: Orthop. Socs: BMA; BOA.

THOMAS, Samuel Jeffrey Isca General Practice Unit, Cadoc House, High Street, Caerleon, Newport NP18 1AZ Tel: 01633 423886 Fax: 01633 430153 — MB BCh Wales 1981; BSc Wales 1972; PhD Wales 1976; DRCOG 1985. GP Caerleon.; Med. Dir. Cadoc Health Care. Specialty: Occupat. Health; Gen. Pract.; Gen. Med.

THOMAS, Sarah Family Doctor Unit Surgery, 92 Bath Road, Hounslow TW3 3LN Tel: 020 8577 9666 Fax: 020 8577 0692; 20 St. Pauls Close, Hounslow TW3 3DE Tel: 020 8572 0158 Fax: 020 8572 0158 — MB BS Lond. 1985; DRCOG 1988; DCH RCP Lond. 1992.

THOMAS, Sarah Elizabeth Don Valley House, Saville Street East, Sheffield S4 7UQ; Tapton Heights, 29 Taptonville Road, Broomhill, Sheffield S10 5BQ — MB ChB Sheff. 1975; DipMed; MB ChB (Hons.) Sheff. 1975; MRCP (UK) 1978; DTM & H Liverp. 1979. Cons. Dermat. Barnsley Dist. Gen. Hosp.; Postgrad. Dean Med. Specialty: Dermat.

THOMAS, Sarah Emma Maesymeillion, Crundale, Haverfordwest SA62 4DG — MB BCh Wales 1993.

THOMAS, Shan Elizabeth Mary Ashleigh Surgery, Napier Street, Cardigan SA43 1ED Tel: 01239 621227 — MB BCh Wales 1981; DRCOG 1983; DCH RCP Lond. 1985. Specialty: Community Child Health; Family Planning.

THOMAS, Shanthi Eucharista Antonita Princess Alexandra Hospital, Hamstel Road, Harlow CM20 1QX Tel: 01279 444455

Fax: 01279 416846; The Orchard, Much Hadham SG10 6BS Tel: 01279 827036 Email: shanthi@dr-thomas.com — MB BS Ceylon 1971 (Univ. of Sri Lanka) FRCPath 1995, M 1983; MSc Lond. 1984, MD 1990; MBA 1998. Cons. Chem. Path. Princess Alexandra Hosp., Harlow, Essex. Specialty: Chem. Path. Socs: Fell. Roy. Soc. Med. Prev: Sen. Regist. St. Mary's Hosp. Lond.; Sen. Regist. Northwick Pk. Hosp. Harrow; Med. Reviewer, Commiss. for Health Improvement.

THOMAS, Sheena Dawn 'Islwyn', 9 Plas Cadwgan Road, Ynystawe, Swansea SA6 5AG — MB BCh Wales 1997.

THOMAS, Sheena Diane Department of Palliative Care, Salisbury District Hospital, Salisbury SP2 8BJ Tel: 01722 336262; The Briars, 78 Campbell Road, Salisbury SP1 3BG Tel: 01722 332322 — MB BCh Wales 1976. Sessional Clin. Asst. (Palliat. Care) Salisbury Dist. Hosp. Prev: SHO Univ. Hosp. Wales & E. Glam. Hosp.; Clin. Med. Off. S. Glam. & Leicester HA.

THOMAS, Shona Alison 13 Stamfordham Close, Rudchester Park, Wallsend NE28 8ER — MB ChB Manch. 1989; MRCGP 1994; T(GP) 1994. Trainee GP Blackburn. Specialty: Gen. Pract.

THOMAS, Sian Beaumont Villa Surgery, 23 Beaumont Road, St Judes, Plymouth PL4 9BL Tel: 01752 663776; The Forge, Dorsley Barns, Old Plymouth Road, Totnes TQ9 6DN Tel: 01803 863892 — MB BS Lond. 1988 (Royal Free Hospital School of Medicine) DRCOG 1991; MRCGP 1992. GP Princip.

THOMAS, Sian Elizabeth Sydenham Green Group Practice, 26 Holmshaw Close, London SE26 4TH Tel: 020 8676 8836 Fax: 020 7771 4710; 90 Barn Mead Road, Beckenham BR3 1JD Tel: 020 8676 8836 Fax: 020 7771 4710 — MB BS Lond. 1981; DRCOG 1984; MRCGP 1986.

THOMAS, Sian Rachel 43 Patrickhill Road, Glasgow G11 5BY Tel: 0141 339 0585 — BM Soton. 1991; MRCP (UK) 1995. Lect. Neurol. Southern Gen. Hosp. Glas. Specialty: Neurol.

THOMAS, Simon Hugh Lynton Wolfson Unit of Clinical Pharmacology, University of Newcastle upon Tyne, Claremont Place, Newcastle upon Tyne NE1 4LP Tel: 0191 222 5644 Fax: 0191 261 5733 Email: simon.thomas@ncl.ac.uk; 28 Elmfield Road, Gosforth, Newcastle upon Tyne NE3 4BA — MB BS Lond. 1981; MRCP (UK) 1984; BSc (Hons.) Lond. 1978, MD 1991; FRCP 2000. Cons. Phys. & Sen. Lect. Freeman Hosp. & Univ. Newc. Specialty: Pharmacology; Gen. Med. Socs: Brit. Pharm. Soc.; Amer. Soc. Clin. Pharmacol. & Therap.; Brit. Toxicology Soc. Prev: Sen. Regist. (Med. & Clin. Pharmacol.) Freeman Hosp. Newc.; Regist. (Med.) & Lect. St. Thos. Hosp. Lond.; SHO Lond. Chest Hosp., Brompton Hosp. & Roy. Free Hosp. Lond.

THOMAS, Simone Yvette Anne Cheddar Medical Centre, Roynon Way, Cheddar BS27 3NZ Tel: 01934 742061 Fax: 01934 744374 — MB BS Lond. 1987 (Roy. Free Hosp. Lond.)

THOMAS, Stanley Long Byre, Hay Hedge Lane, Bisley, Stroud GL6 7AN — MD Wales 1956 (Cardiff) MB ChB 1949. Emerit. Prof. Physiol. Manch. Univ.

THOMAS, Stephen David Dept Of Anaesthesia, The Cardiothoracic Centre, Thomas Drive, Liverpool L14 3PE Tel: 0151 228 1616; Pinelodge, 1 Hanson Park, Oxton, Prenton CH43 9JN Tel: 0151 652 7656 — MB ChB Liverp. 1984 (Liverp) DA (UK) 1990; FCAnaesth. 1991. Cons.(Anaesth.) The Cardio Centre. Liverp. Specialty: Anaesth. Socs: Jun. Mem. Liverp. Soc. Anaesth.; Train. Mem. Assn. AnE.h. Prev: Sen. Regist. Rotat. (Anaesth.) Merseyside; Clin. Lect. (Anaesth.) Univ. Liverp.; Regist. Rotat. Merseyside.

THOMAS, Stephen Mark Diabetes & Endocrine Day Centre, Guys & St. Thomas' Trust, St thomas' Hospital, Lambeth Palace Road, London Email: stephen.m.thomas@gstt.nhs.uk; 56 Selkirk Road, Twickenham TW2 6PX — BM Soton. 1986; MRCP (UK) 1989. Specialty: Nephrol.; Diabetes; Endocrinol.

THOMAS, Stephen Michael James Fisher Medical Centre, 4 Tolpuddle Gardens, Bournemouth BH9 3GQ Tel: 01202 522622 — MB BS Lond. 1972 (St. Thos.) DObst RCOG 1976. Prev: SHO (Paediat.) Poole Gen. Hosp.; SHO (Med.) Roy. Nat. Hosp. Bournemouth; Ho. Phys. & Ho. Surg. Salisbury Gen. Hosp.

THOMAS, Stephen Rhys Department of Cystic Fibrosis, Royal Brompton Hospital, London SW3 6NP; 53 Chatsworth Avenue, Merton Park, London SW20 8JZ Tel: 020 8543 2507 — MB BS Newc. 1988; MRCP Ed. 1991. Research Fell. & Hon. Regist. (Cystic Fibrosis) Roy. Brompton Hosp. Lond. Specialty: Respirat. Med. Socs: Brit. Thorac. Soc. Prev: Regist. Rotat. (Respirat. & Gen. Med.) SE Scotl.; SHO (Med.) City Hosp. Edin. & Christie Hosp. Manch.

THOMAS, Steven Guy Dolhaul, Llangoedmor, Cardigan SA43 2LH — MB ChB Leeds 1991.

THOMAS, Steven John 79 St Albans Road, Bristol BS6 7SQ — MB BCh Wales 1996.

THOMAS, Steven Mark Department of Radiology, Northern General Hospital, Herries Road, Sheffield S5 7AU Tel: 0114 243 4343 Fax: 0114 271 4747 Email: s.m.thomas@sheffield.ac.uk — MB BS Lond. 1988; MRCP UK 1991; FRCR 1995; MSc Sheffield 2000. Clin. Sen. Lect. and Hon. Cons. Radiologist, Univ. of Sheff. Specialty: Radiol. Socs: Brit. Soc. Interven. Radiol.; Cardiovasc. & Interven. Radiol. Soc. Europe; Soc.Cardiovasc & Interven.al Radiol. Prev: Sen. Regist. Rotat. (Diagn. Radiol.) St. Geo. Hosp. Lond.; Regist. Rotat. (Diagn. Radiol.) St. Geo. Hosp. Lond.; EndoVasc. Fell., Northern Gen. Hosp. Sheff.

THOMAS, Steven Noel 61 Walkley Road, Sheffield S6 2XL — MB ChB Sheff. 1993; MRCGP 1997. SHO (Med.) Sheff. Specialty: Gen. Med.

THOMAS, Stuart Alan Readesmoor Medical Group Practice, 29-29A West Street, Congleton CW12 1JP — MB ChB Birm. 1989; MRCGP 1993; DFFP 1993; DCH RCP Lond. 1993. Specialty: Gen. Pract.

THOMAS, Stuart Ian Merlins, 63 Shepherds Lane, Beaconsfield HP9 2DU — BM Soton. 1998.

THOMAS, Stuart Kynaston (Surgery), 7 South Parade, Llandudno LL30 2LN; Dursley, 9A Whitehall Road, Rhos-on-Sea, Colwyn Bay LL28 4HW Tel: 01492 540775 — MB ChB (Hons.) Liverp. 1970; DObst RCOG 1972. Specialty: Dermat.

THOMAS, Stuart Winston Wellspring Medical Centre, Park Road, Risca, Newport NP11 6BJ Tel: 01633 612438 Fax: 01633 615958; Ffynon Oer Farm, Panylan Road, Bassaleg, Newport NP1 9RW — MB BCh Wales 1981 (University Hospital Wales) DRCOG 1985; MRCGP 1987.

THOMAS, Mr Sunil Soloman West Midlands Regional Plastic Surgery Unit, Wordsley Hospital, Stourbridge DY8 5QX Tel: 01384 401401 Fax: 01384 244436; 9 Crookham Close, Harborne, Birmingham B17 8RR Tel: 01384 244322 — MB BS Panjab 1981 (Christian Med. Coll. Ludhiana, Punjab) MS Punjab 1985; FRCSI 1996. Staff (Plastic Surg.) Good Hope & Wordsley Hosps. W. Midl. Specialty: Plastic Surg. Socs: BMA; Eur. Wound Managem. Soc.; Assn. Surgs. India.

THOMAS, Susan Dinas Powys Health Centre, 75 Cardiff Road, Dinas Powys CF64 4JT Tel: 029 2051 2293 Fax: 029 2051 5318 — MB BCh Wales 1979 (Welsh Nat. Sch. Med.) DRCOG 1982. Socs: Cardiff Med. Soc.

THOMAS, Susan Joan Regional Child Development Centre, St James's University Hospital, Leeds LS9 7TF Tel: 0113 206 5870 — MB BS Newc. 1975; MRCP (Paediat.) (UK) 1982. Cons. Paediat. St Jas. Univ. Hosp. Leeds. Specialty: Paediat.

THOMAS, Susan Marguerite Lilliput Surgery, Elms Avenue, Lindisfarne, Poole BH14 8EE Tel: 01202 741310 Fax: 01202 739122 — MB BS Lond. 1981 (St. Thos.) MRCGP 1985; DRCOG 1985.

THOMAS, Susan Mary Tindal Centre, Bierton Road, Aylesbury HP20 1HU Tel: 01296 393363 Fax: 01296 399332; The Chiltern Hospital, London Road, Great Missenden HP16 0EN Tel: 01494 890890 Fax: 01494 890250 — MB BS Lond. 1982 (Roy. Free) MRCPsych 1988. p/t Cons. Psychiat. Buckinghamshire Mental Health Trust. Specialty: Gen. Psychiat. Prev: Sen. Regist. (Psychiat.) Maudsley Hosp. Lond.; Regist. (Psychiat.) Fulbourn Hosp. Camb.

THOMAS, Susanna Jane 11 Fane Road, Oxford OX3 0RZ — BM BCh Oxf. 1990.

THOMAS, Syamala Mary Mayday Healthcare NHS Trust, Mayday University Hospital, 530 London Road, Croydon CR7 7YE Tel: 020 8401 3452 Fax: 020 8401 3458 Email: syamala.thomas@mayday.nhs.uk — MB BS India 1971 (Christian Med. Coll., Vellen, India) MRCPath 1981; FRCPath 1993. Cons. Histopath. / Cytopathologist, Mayday Healthcare NHS Trust, Croydon; Med. Director, Mayday Healthcare NHS Trust, Croydon. Socs: Roy. Coll. of Pathologists; Assn. of Clin. Pathologists; Brit. Soc. of Clin. Oncol.

THOMAS, Tabitha Sophie Low Birks, Sedbergh LA10 5HQ — BChir Camb. 1996.

THOMAS, Thekanady Mathew Cedar House Surgery, 14 Huntingdon Street, St. Neots, Huntingdon PE19 1BQ Tel: 01480 406677 Fax: 01480 475167 — MB BS Lond. 1986.

THOMAS, Thelma Margaret 3 Montpelier Road, London W5 2QS Tel: 020 8998 3567 — MB BS Lond. 1969 (St. Mary's) MRCP (UK) 1972; MFCM 1979; MRCGP 1983. GP. Prev: Mem. Clin. Scientif. Staff MRC Epidemiol. & Med. Care Unit.

THOMAS, Thomas 4 Carlton Close, Rushden NN10 9EL — MB BS Nagpur, India 1975.

THOMAS, Mr Thomas Glyn 4 Redditch Close, Wirral CH49 2QJ — MB ChB Liverp. 1990; FRCS Eng. 1994.

THOMAS, Mr Thomas Glyn (retired) Manyara, Bushy Ruff, Ewell Minnis, Dover CT16 3EE Tel: 01304 822321 Fax: 01304 367036 — MB BS Lond. 1951 (Guy's) FRCS Eng. 1959. Prev: Cons. Orthop. Surg. S.E. Kent and Canterbury Hosp.

THOMAS, Thomas Peter Lloyd Llys-y-Coed, Llanddarog, Carmarthen SA32 8NU — MB BS Lond. 1973 (St. Mary's) MRCS Eng. LRCP Lond. 1973; FRCP 1992, M 1976; T (M) 1991. Cons. Phys. P. Philip Hosp. Dyfed. Specialty: Gen. Med.

THOMAS, Thomas Richard Suite D, Havant Health Centre, Civic Centre Road, Havant PO9 2AP Tel: 023 9247 5010 Fax: 023 9249 2392; Pentwyn, Ferry Road, Hayling Island PO11 0BY — MB BCh Wales 1972; BSc (Hons. Anat.) Wales 1969. Med. Off. (Family Plann., Vasectomies) St. Mary's Hosp. Family Plann. Clinic Porstmouth.

THOMAS, Tina Elisabeth Robin Hill, Welsh St. Donats, Cowbridge CF71 7SS — MB BCh Wales 1989.

THOMAS, Tom Dulyn Llewelyn (retired) Plas-y-Wern, New Quay SA45 9ST Tel: 01545 580230 — MB ChB Liverp. 1952; DPH Liverp. 1956; MD Liverp. 1966; MFCM 1973.

THOMAS, Trevor Anthony 14 Cleeve Lawns, Downend, Bristol BS16 6HJ — MB ChB St. And. 1964; FFA RCS Eng. 1969. Cons. Anaesth. United Bristol Healthcare Trust; Hon. Clin. Lect. Univ. Bristol. Specialty: Anaesth. Socs: Obst. Anaesth. Assn. (Ex. Pres., Ex Hon. Sec.); Soc. of Anaesth.s of the S. West. Region (Ex. Pres., Ex Hon. Sec. and Ex-Edr. Anaesth. Points W.; Roy. Soc. of Med. Sect. of Anaesth. (Ex Monorary Sec.). Prev: Chairm. Div. Anaesth. Brist. Health Dist.; Chairm. Hosp. Med. Comm. Bristol & W. HA; Research Asst. Univ. Toronto, Canada.

THOMAS, Tudor Huw 10 Bryn Castell, Radyr, Cardiff CF15 8RA — MB BS Lond. 1989.

THOMAS, Mr Tudor Lloyd Turner Rise Consulting Rooms, 55 Turner Road, Colchester CO4 5JY Tel: 01206 752888 Fax: 01206 752223 — MRCS Eng. LRCP Lond. 1971 (Middlx.) MB BS Lond. 1971, BDS 1966; FRCS Eng. 1976. Cons. Orthop. Surg. Colchester & Roy. Lond. Hosps.; Regional Speciality Adviser; Trauma and Orthop.; Regional Adviser, Essex and Hertfordshire. Specialty: Orthop. Socs: Quality Assurance Comm. Royal College of Surgeons of England; Past Pres. Orthopaedic Section of Royal Society of Med. Prev: Reg. Spec. Adv. N. Thames East 1997-2002.

THOMAS, Valerie Anne Department of Cellular Pathology, St Georges Hospital, Blackshaw Road, Tooting, London SW17 0RE Tel: 020 8725 2448 Fax: 020 8767 2984 — MB BS Lond. 1986 (St. George's HMS) PhD Lond. 1984, BSc 1980; MRCPath 1991. Cons. Cytopath. and Histiopath St. Geo. Hosp. Lond.; Hon. Sen. Lect. St. Geo. Hosp. Lond. Specialty: Histopath. Prev: Lect. & Hon. Sen. Regist. (Histopath.) Roy. Free Hosp. Lond.

THOMAS, Vaughn Llewellyn Farne House, Armstrong Road, Brockenhurst SO42 7TA — LRCP LRCS Ed. 1978 (Univ. Rhodesia) MB ChB 1978; LRCP LRCS Ed. LRCPS Glas. 1978; FFARCS Eng. 1983; DCH RCP Lond. 1984.

THOMAS, Vivian, Group Capt. RAF Med. Br. Health Consultancy, Preston Lodge Court, Preston Deanery, Northampton NN7 2DS — MB BCh Wales 1970 (Cardiff) DObst RCOG 1972; MRCGP 1976; DAvMed Eng. 1978; AFOM RCP Lond. 1980. Sen. Occupat. Phys. Sedgwick Noble Lowndes Health Consult. Northampton; Med Dir medigold Health Consultancy. Specialty: Occupat. Health. Prev: PMAN 5 (RAF); Pres. Med. Bd. OASc; Oc Med. Wing RAF Wegberg.

THOMAS, Vivien Joy Ensom Magill Department of Anaesthetics, Chelsea & Westminster Hospital, Fulham Road, London SW10 9NH Tel: 020 8746 8026 Fax: 020 8746 8801; The Holme, Clay Lane, Headley, Epsom KT18 6JS — (St. Mary's) MB BS Lond. 1969; FFA RCS Eng. 1974. Cons. Anaesth. Chelsea & Westm. Hosp. Lond. Specialty: Anaesth. Socs: Assn. Anaesth.; Assn. Paediatric Anaesth. Prev: Sen. Regist. (Anaesth.) Westm. Hosp. Lond. & St. Geo. Hosp. Lond.; SHO (Anaesth.) St. Thos. Hosp. Lond.

THOMAS, Walter Hugh Muriau Cadarn, Llan-Talyllyn, Brecon LD3 7TG Tel: 01874 658344 — MB BS Lond. 1960 (St. Mary's) MRCS Eng. LRCP Lond. 1960; FRCS 1963; MD Connecticut 1967; FRCSC 1968. Cons. Surg. P. Chas. Gen. Hosp. Merthyr Tydfil; Hon. Surgic. Teach. Welsh Nat. Sch. Med. Specialty: Gen. Surg. Prev: Cons. Surg. St. Catherines Canada; Cons. Surg. RAMC; Research Assoc. (Surg.) Yale Univ. USA.

THOMAS, William Alfred 18 Villiers Road, Woodthorpe, Nottingham NG5 4FB; South Woodville, St. Margaret's Road, Bowdon, Altrincham WA14 2AW — MB ChB Sheff. 1973; FFA RCS Eng. 1979. Cons. Anaesth. Wythenshawe Hosp. Manch. Specialty: Anaesth. Prev: Sen. Regist. (Anaesth.) St. Bart. Hosp. Lond.; Regist. (Anaesth.) Hosp. Sick Childr. Gt. Ormond St. Lond.

THOMAS, William Cledwyn Teilo, MBE, KStJ, TD Fay Cottage, 37 Penyfai Lane, Llanelli SA15 4EN Tel: 01554 2678; 6 Brynfield Court, Swansea SA3 4TF Tel: 01792 369753 — MRCS Eng. LRCP Lond. 1950 (St. Bart.) DL Dyfed; Police Surg. (A Div.) Dyfed Powys Police; Occupat. Health Phys. & Clin. Asst. (Haemat.) P. Phillip Hosp. Llanelli. Specialty: Occupat. Health. Prev: Venereologist W. Wales Hosp. Carmarthen; Regtl. Med. Off. 4th Bn. RRW TAVR Lt. Col.; Surg. Lt. RNVR.

THOMAS, Mr William Ernest Ghinn Royal Hallamshire Hospital, Glossop Road, Sheffield S10 2JF Tel: 0114 271 3142 Fax: 0114 271 3512; Ash Lodge, 65 Whirlow Pk Road, Whirlow, Sheffield S11 9NN Tel: 0114 262 0852 Fax: 0114 236 3695 Email: thomas@wegt.freeserve.co.uk — MB BS Lond. 1972 (St. Geo.) AKC 1969; MRCS Eng. LRCP Lond. 1972; FRCS Eng. 1977; BSc Lond. 1969, MS 1980. Hon. Sen. Lect. Sheff. Univ.; Cons. Surg. & Clin. Dir. Surg. Roy Hallam Sh. Hosp. Sheff.; Surgic. Skills Tutor RCS Eng.; Gen. Med. Counc. Phase 2 Assessor. Specialty: Gen. Surg.; Gastroenterol.; Endocrinol. Socs: Fell. Assn. Surg.; Brit. Soc. Gastroenterol.; Surg. Research Soc. Prev: Sen. Regist. (Surg.) United Bristol Hosps.; Cons. Surg. & Clin. Dir. Surg. Roy. Hallamsh. Hosp. Sheff.; Regist. (Surg.) Addenbrooke's Hosp. Camb.

THOMAS, Mr William Gareth Morvah Farmhouse, Saltash PL12 5AB — MB BS Lond. 1973 (Lond. Hosp.) BSc (Biochem.) Lond. 1970; MRCS Eng. LRCP Lond. 1973; FRCS Ed. 1979; FRCS Eng. 1980. Cons. Orthop. Surg. Plymouth HA. Specialty: Orthop. Socs: Brit. Scoliosis Soc.; Brit. Assn. Surg. Knee; Brit. Elbow & Shoulder Soc. Prev: Sen. Regist. (Orthop.) Soton. Gen. Hosp.; Regist. (Surg.) St. Thos. Hosp. Lond.; SHO (Surg.) Bristol Roy. Infirm.

THOMAS, William Gethyn (retired) 39 Heath Park Avenue, Cardiff CF14 3RF Tel: 029 2075 6524 Email: gethyn@tinyworld.co.uk — MB BCh Wales 1956. Prev: Phys. i/c Res. Staff. & Stud.s Univ. Hosp. Wales & Univ. Wales Coll. Med.

THOMAS, William Ioan 16 Heol Gwys, Upper Cwmtwrch, Swansea SA9 2XQ — MB BCh Wales 1997.

THOMAS, William Kenneth Aylesbury Partnership, Aylesbury Medical Centre, Taplow House, Thurlow Street, London SE17 2XE Tel: 020 7703 2205 — MB BS Lond. 1959 (King's Coll. Hosp.) MRCS Eng. LRCP Lond. 1959. Socs: S. Lond. Obst. Soc. Prev: Ho. Phys. St. And. Hosp. Bow; Ho. Surg. Obst. St. Giles' Hosp. Lond.; Outpat. Off. Roy. Nat. Throat, Nose & Ear Hosp. Lond.

THOMAS, Mr William Michael Leicester General Hospital, Gwendolen Road, Leicester LE5 4PW Tel: 0116 249 0490; The Willows, Wartnaby Road, AB Kettleby, Melton Mowbray LE14 3JJ — MB BCh Wales 1982; FRCS Ed. 1987; DM Nottm. 1991. Cons. Gen. Surg. Leicester Gen. Hosp. Specialty: Gen. Surg. Prev: Sen. Regist. (Gen. Surg.) Leicester Hosps.; MRC Research Fell. (Surg.) Nottm. Univ.

THOMAS, Mr William Robert Griffith 5 Dyffryn Road, Gorseinon, Swansea SA8 3BX — MB BCh Wales 1957; FRCS Ed. 1965; FRCS Eng. 1965. Cons. Surg. W. Wales Gen. Hosp. Carmarthen.

THOMAS, Wilson Royal Oldham Hospital, Rochdale Road, Oldham OL1 2JH — MB BS Punjab 1981; MD (Gen. Med.) Punjab 1985; FRCP 2002. Chest Clinic Roy. Oldham Hosp. Rochdale Rd. Oldham.

THOMASON, Frederic William Lower Crows Nest Farm, Kiln Lane, Milnrow, Rochdale OL16 3TR — MB ChB Manch. 1976; DRCOG 1978.

THOMASON, Janie Keith Medical Group, Health Centre, Turner St, Keith AB55 5DJ Tel: 01542 882244 Fax: 01542 881002; Cockmuir

House, Longmorn, Elgin IV30 8SL — MB ChB Aberd. 1980; DCH RCP Glas. 1983; MRCGP 1984. Clin. Asst. (Diabetes) Dr. Gray's Hosp. Elgin.

THOMASSON, David Ian 34 Coope Road, Bollington, Macclesfield SK10 5AE — MB ChB Manch. 1990.

THOMASSON, Jane Elizabeth Rachel The Dairy House, Stratton, Dorchester DT2 9RU — MB ChB Bristol 1986; FRCA 1992. Clin. Asst. (Anaesth.) W. Dorset Gen. Hosps. NHS Trust. Specialty: Anaesth. Prev: Regist. (Anaesth.) Yorks. Region Train Scheme; Regist. (Anaesth.) Plymouth Gen. Hosps.

THOMERSON, Derek George (retired) 55 Mountfield, Hythe, Southampton SO45 5AQ Tel: 023 8084 4088 — (St. Mary's) LMSSA Lond. 1956; MB BS Lond. 1959. Prev: Port Health Med. Off. Soton.

THOMERSON, Myfanwy Celia Rosalind 55 Mountfield, Hythe, Southampton SO45 5AQ — (Manch.) MB ChB Manch. 1952; DRCOG 1958; Dip. Med. Acupunc. 1997. Socs: Brit. Med. Acupunct. Soc.

THOMPSELL, Amanda Ann Bence 41 Vine Street, London EC3N 2AA — MB BS Lond. 1982 (Char. Cross) DRCOG 1985; DGM RCP Lond. 1986; MRCPsych 1997. Regist. (Psychiat.) Roy. Free Hosp. Lond. Specialty: Geriat. Psychiat. Prev: Clin. Asst. (Med. for Elderly) Roy. Free Hosp. Lond. & Diagn. Unit Eliz. Garrett Anderson.

THOMPSETT, Caroline 40 Tavistock Court, Tavistock Square, London WC1H 9HG — MB BS Lond. 1985 (Roy. Free) FRCA 1991. Sen. Regist. (Anaesth.) St. Mary's Hosp. Lond. Specialty: Anaesth.

THOMPSON, Mr Adrian Charles ENT Department, Queen's Hospital, Burton-on-Trent DE13 0RB Tel: 01283 566333 Ext: 4543 Fax: 01283 593004 — MB ChB Leeds 1982; FRCS Ed. 1986; FRCS Eng. 1988; FRCS (Orl.) 1993. Cons. ENT Surg. Burton Hosps. NHS Trust. Specialty: Otolaryngol. Socs: Brit. Assn. Otol. Head & Neck Surg.; Brit. Assn. Head & Neck Oncol.; Brit. Assn. of Endocrine Surgs. Prev: Sen. Regist. Rotat. (ENT) Nottm. & Derby Train. Scheme; Regist. (ENT) Univ. Hosp. Nottm. & Vict. Infirm. Glas.; SHO (Plastic Surg.) St. Luke's Hosp. Bradford.

THOMPSON, Aidan William 18 Corrina Park, Dunmurray, Belfast BT17 0HA — MB BCh BAO Belf. 1995.

THOMPSON, Alan Brian Robert The Surgery, 20 Lee Road, Blackheath, London SE3 9RT Tel: 020 8852 1235 Fax: 020 8297 2193 — MB BS Lond. 1979 (St. Mary's) MRCS Eng. LRCP Lond. 1979; MRCP (UK) 1983; DCH RCP Lond. 1985; MRCGP 1988.

THOMPSON, Mr Alan Clive 14 Osborne Close, Harrogate HG1 2EF — MB BS Lond. 1985; BSc (Hons.) Lond. 1982, MB BS 1985; FRCS Eng. 1991. Regist. (Surg.) Roy. Lond. Hosp. Specialty: Gen. Surg.

THOMPSON, Professor Alan James National Hospital for Neurology & Neurosurgery, Queen Square, London WC1N 3BG Tel: 020 7837 3611 Fax: 020 7813 6505 Email: a.thompson@ion.ucl.ac.uk — MD Dub. 1985; MB BCh BAO 1979; FRCP Lond. 1994; FRCPI 1995. Prof. (Clin. Neurol. & Neurorehabilitation) Inst. of Neurol. Lond.; Clin. Director (Clin. Neurosciences) Univ. Coll. Lond. Hosps.; Cons. Neurol. Nat. Hosp. for Neurol. & Neurosug. Specialty: Neurol.; Rehabil. Med. Special Interest: Multiple Sclerosis; Neurorehabilitation. Socs: Assn. Brit. Neurol; Amer. Neurol. Assn.; Europ. Neurol. Soc. Prev: Sen. Lect. Inst. of Neurol.; Reader (Clin. Neurol.) Univ. Dept. Clin. Neurol. Inst. of Neurol.; Cons. Neurol. Whittington Hosp.

THOMPSON, Alan James 189 Cooden Sea Road, Bexhill-on-Sea TN39 4TH — BM Soton. 1998.

THOMPSON, Alan Richard 189 Cooden Sea Road, Cooden, Bexhill-on-Sea TN39 4TH — MB BS Lond. 1969 (Univ. Coll. Hosp.) DA Eng. 1973; FFA RCS Eng. 1975. Cons. (Anaesth.) Hastings Health Dist. Specialty: Anaesth. Prev: Sen. Regist. (Anaesth.) Soton. & S.W. Hants. Health Dist. (T); Regist. (Anaesth.) Univ. Coll. Hosp. Lond.; Ho. Surg. & Ho. Phys. Metrop. Hosp. Lond.

THOMPSON, Professor Alastair Mark Ninewells Hospital, Department of Surgery & Molecular Oncology, Dundee DD1 9SY Tel: 01382 633936 Email: a.m.thompson@dundee.ac.uk — MB ChB Ed. 1984; BSc (Hons) 1982; MD. 1991; FRCS Ed. 1991; FRCS (Gen.) 1995. Professor of Surgical Oncology, Univ. Dundee; Hon Cons. Surg. Specialty: Gen. Surg. Special Interest: Breast Cancer. Socs: Assn. of Surg.s of Gt. Britain & Irel.; Brit. Oncological Assn.; Brit. Assn. for Cancer Research. Prev: Hon. Regist. Univ. Dept. Surg. Roy. Infirm. Ed. Lothian HB; Regist. (Surg.) Raigmore Hosp. Inverness; SHO West. Infirm. Glas.

THOMPSON, Mr Albert Edward The Consulting Rooms, York House, 199 Westminster Bridge Road, London SE1 7UT Tel: 020 7928 3019 Fax: 020 7928 3019 — MB BS Lond. 1955 (St. Mary's) FRCS Eng. 1959; MS Lond. 1966. Specialty: Gen. Surg. Prev: Cons. Surg. St. Thos. Hosp. & Roy. Marsden Hosp. Lond.; Asst. Dir. Surgic. Unit St. Mary's Hosp. Lond.; Sen. Regist. (Surg.) St. Mary's Hosp. Lond.

THOMPSON, Alexander John 61 St Clares Court, Lower Bullingham, Hereford HR2 6PY Tel: 01432 343062 — MB BS Lond. 1994 (Roy. Lond. Hosp. Med. Coll.) DRCOG 1996. GP Non-Princip.; Health Promotion Off. Heref. HA. Specialty: Gen. Pract. Prev: SHO Hereford Hosps. NHS Trust VTS; Ho. Off. (Med.) King Geo. Hosp. Ilford; Ho. Off. (Surg.) Epsom.

THOMPSON, Alice Mary Susan Park Lane Cottages, Hawstead, Bury St Edmunds IP29 5NX Tel: 01284 753296 — MB BS Lond. 1966 (St. Bart.) MRCS Eng. LRCP Lond. 1966; DCH Eng. 1971; DObst RCOG 1975; MRCP (UK) (Paediat.) 1984. Cons. Paediat. W. Suff. Gen. Hosp. Bury St Edmunds. Specialty: Paediat. Prev: Assoc. Specialist (Paediat.) W. Suff. Gen. Hosp. Bury St Edmunds.; Dep. Police Surg. Suff.

THOMPSON, Mr Alistair Graham 81 Harborne Road, Edgbaston, Birmingham B15 3HG Tel: 0121 455 9496 Fax: 0121 455 9496 — (Univ. of Birm.) MB ChB Birm. 1965; FRCS Ed. 1972; T(S) 1991; FRCS Eng. 1995. Cons. Orthop. Surg. Roy. Orthop. Hosp. NHS Trust, Birm. Specialty: Orthop. Special Interest: Spinal Diformity; Spinal Surg. Socs: Pres. Brit. Scoliosis Res. Soc.; Internat. Fell. Scoliosis Research Soc. USA; Fell. Brit. Orthopaedic Assn.

THOMPSON, Alistair Robin Tytler Seven Brooks Medical Centre, 21 Church Street, Atherton, Manchester M46 9DE Tel: 01942 882799 Fax: 01942 873859 — (Glas.) MB ChB Glas. 1970; FRCGP 1996. GP Assoc. Dir. Salford & Trafford HA. Specialty: Gen. Pract. Socs: BMA; RCGP. Prev: SHO (Obst.) Paisley Matern. Hosp.; SHO (Anaesth.) Glas. Roy. Infirm.

THOMPSON, Allan Christopher Division of Psychiatry, North Tees General Hospital, Hardwick, Stockton-on-Tees TS19 8PE — BM Soton. 1979.

THOMPSON, Mr Andrew Royal Albert Edward Infirmary, Wigan Tel: 01942 773051; 84 Bucklow Gardens, Lymm WA13 9RQ Tel: 01925 756940 — MB ChB Manch. 1991; FRCS Eng. 1995; FRCS (Urol.) 2001. Cons. Urol. Roy. Albert Edwd. Infirm., Wigan. Specialty: Urol. Socs: BAUS; RCS. Prev: Specialist Regist. (Urol.) NW Region; Demonst. (Anat.) Univ. Leeds.

THOMPSON, Andrew 121 Humber Road S., Beeston, Nottingham NG9 2EX — MB BS Lond. 1996.

THOMPSON, Andrew Leech Meadow Cottage, Sheinton, Cressage, Shrewsbury SY5 6 — MB BS Lond. 1998.

THOMPSON, Andrew Christopher 22 Southfield Drive, Hazlemere, High Wycombe HP15 7HB — MB ChB Bristol 1998.

THOMPSON, Andrew James 2 Berkeley Hall, Saintfield Road, Lisburn BT27 5QZ — MB BCh BAO Belf. 1989 (Queens University Belfast) MRCP; MB BCh Belf. 1989. Specialty: Paediat. Socs: MRCPCH.

THOMPSON, Andrew Jeffrey Stafford Road Surgery, 60 Stafford Road, Cannock WS11 2AQ Tel: 01543 503332 Fax: 01543 503010; Squirrel's Leap, Denefield, Penkridge, Stafford ST19 5JF Email: ajtho@lineone.net — MB ChB Liverp. 1979; DRCOG 1982. GP Cannock. Socs: Cannock & Mid Staffs. Med. Socs.; BMA.

THOMPSON, Andrew John Park Road Medical Centre, 44 Park Road, Guiseley, Leeds LS20 8AR Tel: 01943 872113; 152 Bradford Road, Menston, Ilkley LS29 6ED Tel: 01943 872583 — MB ChB Leeds 1980; MRCGP 1984.

THOMPSON, Andrew Joseph Department of Radiology, Kettering General Hospital, Kettering NN16 8UZ Tel: 01536 492000 Fax: 01586 492473; 6 Captains Court, Horton, Northampton NN7 2AX Tel: 01604 870211 — MB ChB Liverp. 1971 (Liverpool) DMRD Liverp. 1975; FRCR 1977. Cons. Radiol. Kettering Gen. Hosp. Specialty: Radiol.

THOMPSON, Andrew Keith Dept of Histopathology, The Medical School, University of Birmingham, Birmingham B15 2TT Tel: 0121 414 4016; 7 Cornfield Croft, Sutton Coldfield B76 1SN Tel: 0121 378 2342 — MB ChB Leeds 1988. Specialist Regist. Histopath. W. Midl. Regional Traning Scheme. Specialty: Histopath. Prev: Ho. Off.

(Gen. Surg.) Bradford Roy. Infirm.; Ho. Off. (Gen. Med.) Huddersfield Roy. Infirm.

THOMPSON, Andrew Maurice The Strand Practice, 2 The Strand, Goring-by-Sea, Worthing BN12 6DN Tel: 01903 243351 Fax: 01903 705804; Whiteridge, 12 Longlands, Charmandean, Worthing BN14 9NT Tel: 01903 231568 — MB BS Lond. 1990 (Guy's Hospital) DRCOG 1993; DFFP 1993; MRCGP 1994.

THOMPSON, Andrew Paul The Surgery, 174 Rookery Road, Handsworth, Birmingham B21 9NN Tel: 0121 554 0921; 114 West Avenue, Handsworth Wood, Birmingham B20 2LY Tel: 0121 686 5461 Fax: 07000 329362 — MB ChB Birm. 1989 (Birmingham) DGM RCP Lond. 1991; MRCGP 1993; DFFP 1993. Specialty: Gen. Pract. Socs: Fell. Roy. Soc. Med. Prev: Trainee GP Birm.; SHO (O & G) Dist. Gen. Hosp. W. Bromwich; SHO (Geriat. & A & E) & Ho. Off. (Med.) Russells Hall Hosp. Dudley.

THOMPSON, Andrew Philip Westerhope Medical Group, 377 Stamfordham Road, Westerhope, Newcastle upon Tyne NE5 2LH Tel: 0191 243 7000 Fax: 0191 243 7006 — MB BS Newc. 1987 (Newcastle upon Tyne) DA (UK) 1989; MRCGP 1994. GP Princip. W.erhope Med. Gp. Specialty: Gen. Pract. Prev: Trainee GP N.d. VTS; SHO (Paediat. & Med.) Qu. Eliz. Hosp. Gateshead; SHO (Anaesth.) Newc. u. Tyne.

THOMPSON, Angela North Warwickshire PCT, Child Health Services, Riversley Park Centre, Coton Road, Nuneaton CV11 5TY Tel: 02476 378611; 17 Hargrave Close, Coventry CV3 2XS Tel: 01203 448351 — MB ChB Liverp. 1980; DCH RCP Lond. 1983; DCCH RCP Ed. 1984; MRCPH 1992; MSc Warwick 2002. Assoc. Specialist (Palliative Care/Child Health) N. Warks. PCT. Specialty: Community Child Health; Paediat.; Palliat. Med. Socs: Brit. Assn. Community Child Health; RCPCH; ACT Counc. Mem. Prev: SCMO (Child Health) Warks. HA; Clin. Med. Off. (Child Health) Coventry HA.

THOMPSON, Angela Claire 36 Sherwood Drive, Marske, Redcar TS11 6DR — MB ChB Liverp. 1996 (Liverpool) DGH - RCPCH 1999. Specialty: Gen. Pract.

THOMPSON, Angela Mary Stewart 6 Highgate Road, Altrincham WA14 4QZ Tel: 0161 928 4862 — (Liverp.) MB ChB Liverp. 1960; DObst RCOG 1962. Clin. Med. Off. Trafford AHA. Socs: Fac. Community Health; Assoc. Mem. Brit. Paediat. Soc. Prev: Ho. Surg. & Ho. Phys. Broadgreen Hosp. Liverp.; Ho. Surg. Mill Rd. Matern. Hosp. Liverp.

THOMPSON, Angus James Radiology Department, Woodend Hospital, Aberdeen AB15 6XS Tel: 01224 663131; 48 Camperdown Road, Aberdeen AB15 5NU Tel: 01224 633804 — MB ChB Aberd. 1980; DMRD Aberd. 1984; FRCR 1986. Head Radiol. Woodend Hosp., Aberd. Specialty: Radiol. Prev: Cons. Radiol. Dundee Hosps. & Carlisle Hosps.; Vis. Prof. Kwong Wah Hosp. Kowloon Hong Kong 1991; Sen. Regist. (Diagn. Radiol.) Roy. Surrey Co. Hosp. Guildford.

THOMPSON, Ann Veronica 30 Cleveland Road, South Woodford, London E18 2AL Tel: 020 8530 4917 Fax: 020 8530 4917 — MB BChir Camb. 1974 (Cambridge and St. Thomas' Hospital) MA Camb. 1974; MA Camb. 1974; DObst RCOG 1975; Dobst RCOG 1975. p/t Hosp. Practitioner Chingford Osteoporosis Clinic Lond. Specialty: Rheumatol.; Gen. Pract. Prev: GP Oxf.; Research Regist. (Community Med. & Gen. Pract.) Univ. Oxf.

THOMPSON, Anne Elizabeth Child, Adolescent & Family Services, Moore House, 10/11 Lindum Terrace, Lincoln LN2 5RS — MB BS Newc. 1985; MRCP (UK) 1988; MRCPsych 1991. Cons. (Child & Adolesc. Psychiat.) Lincoln. Specialty: Child & Adolesc. Psychiat. Prev: Lect. (Child & Adolesc. Psychiat.) Univ. Nottm.; Sen. Regist. North. RHA; Regist. Rotat. (Psychiat.) Newc.

THOMPSON, Anne Mary The Surgery, 48 Mulgrave Road, Belmont, Sutton SM2 6LX Tel: 020 8642 2050 — BM Soton. 1978; DFFP 1995. Specialty: Gen. Pract.

THOMPSON, Anne Rosemary Robinson, Ashton, Leung, Solari and Thompson, James Preston Health Centre, 61 Holland Road, Sutton Coldfield B72 1RL Tel: 0121 355 5150 — MB ChB Birm. 1980; MRCGP 1984.

THOMPSON, Anne Tait Avon Medical Centre, Academy Street, Larkhall ML9 2BJ Tel: 01698 882547 Fax: 01698 888138; Garngour, 22 Hill Road, Stonehouse, Larkhall ML9 3EA — MB ChB Glas. 1983; DRCOG 1986; MRCGP 1987. GP StoneHo. Socs: BMA.

THOMPSON, Anthony Baird Tamarisk, Frogspool, Truro TR4 8RU — MB ChB Liverp. 1989.

THOMPSON, Anthony Michael 30 Myrtlefield Park, Belfast BT9 6NF Tel: 01232 665094 Email: amt@myrtlfld.dnet.co.uk; 6 Heathmount, Portstewart BT55 7AP Tel: 01265 833845 — MB BCh BAO Belf. 1976; DRCOG 1978; FFR RCSI 1985. Cons. Radiol. Downe Hosp. Downpatrick & Roy. Vict. Hosp. Belf. Specialty: Radiol. Socs: Roy. Coll. Radiol. & Fell. Ulster Med. Soc.; Brit. Med. Ultrasound Soc.; Amer. Röentgen Ray Soc. Prev: Sen. Regist. Univ. Hosp. Nottm.; Regist. (Radiol.) Roy. Vict. Hosp. Belf.; SHO & Ho. Off. Craigavon Area Hosp.

THOMPSON, Ashley George Gyton (retired) c/o Westminster Bank, 62 Victoria St., London SW1 — MB BCh Camb. 1914 (St. Geo.) MA (Nat. Sc. Trip.) Camb. 1911, MD 1924, MB BC DPH. Prev: MOH Boro. Lambeth.

THOMPSON, Barbara (retired) Heathcliffe, 14 Green Head Road, Utley, Keighley BD20 6EA Tel: 01535 602875 — MB ChB Sheff. 1963; DObst RCOG 1966. Prev: SCMO Airedale HA.

THOMPSON, Barbara Clare (retired) Newlands, Whitchurch Hill, Reading RG8 7PN — MB BS Lond. 1962; MRCS Eng. LRCP Lond. 1962. Prev: Community Paediat. (Presch. Audiol.) Roy. Berks. & Battle Hosp. NHS Trust Reading.

THOMPSON, Basil Ainsworth (retired) Northgate House, 1 Upper Northgate Street, Chester CH1 4EE Tel: 01244 342977 — MB ChB Sheff. 1952; MRCS Eng. LRCP Lond. 1953; MRCGP 1961; DIH Soc. Apoth. Lond. 1963; AFOM RCP Lond. 1990.

THOMPSON, Brenda Mildred (retired) 705 Aylestone Road, Leicester LE2 8TG Tel: 0116 283 2325; 94 Stoughton Road, Oadby, Leicester LE2 4FN Tel: 0116 271 6400 — MB BS Lond. 1961 (Roy. Free) MRCS Eng. LRCP Lond. 1961. Prev: Ho. Surg. & Ho. Phys. Gt. Yarmouth & Gorleston Hosp.

THOMPSON, Bryan Eykyn Lombe, MBE (retired) 60A London Road, Kilmarnock KA3 7DD — MB BChir Camb. 1951; LMSSA Lond. 1949. Prev: Med. Supt. St. Luke's Hosp. PO Hiranpur, Dist. Pakur, Bihar, India.

THOMPSON, Caroline Creed Taunton & Somerset Hospital, Musgrove Park, Taunton TA1 5DA Tel: 01823 333444 Fax: 01823 342411; Welham Rise, Charlton Mackrell, Somerton TA11 7AJ Fax: 01458 224219 — MB ChB Birm. 1983; DA (UK) 1985; DRCOG 1989; MRCGP 1992; DLO 2000. Staff Grade Surg. ENT Dept., Taunton & Som. Hosp. Specialty: Otorhinolaryngol. Socs: BMA; MDU. Prev: GP Principle, Glastonbury.

THOMPSON, Carolyn Irene Royal Infirmary of Edinburgh, Lauriston Place, Edinburgh — MB ChB Ed. 1980; FRCRP (Ed.); MRCP (UK) 1983. Cons. in Gum, NHS Lothian, Edin. Specialty: Genitourinary Medicine. Prev: Cons. in Gum, Fife Acute Hosp.s NHS Trust.

THOMPSON, Catherine Susannah Department of Medicine, Salisbury District Hospital, Salisbury SP2 8BL — MB BS Lond. 1990; BSc Lond. 1987, MB BS 1990; MRCP 1994. Cons. in Respirat. and Gen. Med.

THOMPSON, Catriona (retired) 101/2 Greenbank Drive, Edinburgh EH10 5GB — MB ChB Ed. 1960; DA (Eng.) 1963; FFA RCS Eng. 1970. Prev: Cons. Anaesth. Ayrsh. & Arran HB.

THOMPSON, Catriona Jane Kwinchens, Old High Road, Brightwell-cum-Sotwell, Wallingford OX10 0QF — BM Soton. 1995.

THOMPSON, Cecilia Mary Hill Lane Surgery, 162 Hill Lane, Southampton SO15 5DD Tel: 023 8022 3086 Fax: 023 8023 5487 — MB BS London 1976; MRCGP Lond. 1980. GP Soton. Socs: RCGP; BMA.

THOMPSON, Cedric Francis Derek High Street Surgery, 46 High Street, Kelvedon, Colchester CO5 9AG Tel: 01376 572906 Fax: 01376 572484 Email: cedric.thompson@gp-f81011.nhs.uk; 6 Brockwell Lane, Kelvedon, Colchester C05 9BB Tel: 01376 570660 — MB BS Lond. 1975 (Westminster) DRCOG 1979; MRCGP 1981.

THOMPSON, Mr Charles Edward Rosslyn (retired) 138 Spilsby Road, Boston PE21 9PE Tel: 01205 364387 — MB BChir Camb. 1958 (Middlx.) MA Camb. 1958; FRCS Ed. 1964. Prev: Cons. Surg. S. Lincs. Health Dist.

THOMPSON, Christine Louise Chipping Surgery, 1 Symn Lane, Wotton-under-Edge GL12 7BD Tel: 01453 842214; 23 Hawkesbury Road, Hillesley, Gloucester GL2 7RE Email: christine.gordon@btinternet.com — MB ChB Bristol 1986; DRCOG 1991. GP. Prev: Trainee GP Bath VTS; SHO (Infec. Dis. & Respirat. Med.) Ham Green Hosp. Bristol.

THOMPSON, Christine Mary 52 Boston Place, London NW1 6ER Tel: 020 7402 3550 Fax: 020 7402 3550; 11 Blackwell Scar, Darlington DL3 8DL Tel: 01325 464914 Fax: 01325 464914 — (St. Bart.) MB BS Lond. 1955; DPH Lond. 1967; DIH Eng. 1968; Spec. Accredit. (Occupat. Med.) RCP Lond 1979; MFOM RCP Lond. 1979. Med Adviser Penguin Books Ltd. Harmondsworth Middlx. Specialty: Occupat. Health. Socs: Fell. Roy. Soc. Med.; BMA.

THOMPSON, Professor Christopher Priory House, Randall's Way, Leatherhead KT22 Tel: 01372 860400 Fax: 01372 860401 — MB BS 1977 (Univ. Coll. Lond.) MPhil Lond. 1984, BSc 1974; FRCPsych. 1991, M 1982; MD Lond. 1987; FRCP 1995; MRCGP 2000. Director Healthcare Servs., Priory Gp.; Vis. Prof. of Psychiat. Univ. of Soton. Specialty: Gen. Psychiat. Socs: Fell. Collegium Internat.e Neuropsychopharmacologicum (CINP); Founder Int. Soc. Affective Disorders; Brit. Assn. Psychopharmacol. Prev: Prof. Psychiat. Univ. Soton. & Head of Sch. of Med.; Sen. Lect. Char. Cross & Westm. Med. Sch. Lond.

THOMPSON, Claire Lorraine 6 Castle Street, Inner Avenue, Southampton SO14 6HA — MB ChB Sheff. 1990.

THOMPSON, Claire Louise Ravenstone, The Park, Cheltenham GL50 2RP Tel: 01242 234504 — MB ChB Birm. 1995. Specialty: Gen. Pract.

THOMPSON, Craig Antony Pavilion Flat, University Road, Aberdeen AB24 3DR — MB ChB Aberd. 1986; BMedBiol. Aberd. 1985. SHO (Accid. Emerg. & Gen. Surg.) Hairmyres Hosp. E. Kilbride Glas. Prev: SHO (Thoracic Surg.) Hairmyres Hosp. E. Kilbride Glas.; SHO (Orthop. A & E) StoneHo. Hosp. StoneHo.; SHO (A & E) Roy. Sussex Co. Hosp. Brighton.

THOMPSON, Craig Stephen County Hospital, North Road, Durham DH1 4ST Tel: 0191 333 3434 — MB BS Newc. 1991. Staff Grade (Gen. Psychiat.) Gen. Hosp. Durh. Specialty: Gen. Psychiat. Prev: Regist. (Gen. Psychiat.) St. Luke's Hosp. Middlesbrough.

THOMPSON, Damien Harold Michael 13 Rectory Square, London E1 3NQ — MB BS Lond. 1994.

THOMPSON, Daniel Owl End, Newfield Lane, Sheffield S17 3DB — MB BS Lond. 1998.

THOMPSON, Daniel Stenhouse Luton & Dunstable Hospital, Luton LU4 0DZ Tel: 01582 497214 Fax: 01582 497214 Email: dan.thompson@ldh-tr.anglox.nhs.uk; 16 Hollybush Lane, Harpenden AL5 4AT Tel: 01582 460739 — MB BS Lond. 1965 (Univ. Coll. Hosp.) BSc (Physiol.) Lond. 1962; MRCS Eng. LRCP Lond. 1965; FRCPath 1984, M 1972. Cons. Haemat. Luton & Dunstable Hosp. Specialty: Haematology. Socs: Brit. Soc. Haematol.; Assn. Clin. Path. Prev: Sen. Regist. (Haemat.) Univ. Coll. Hosp. Lond.; Sen. Regist. (Haemat.) Roy. Perth Hosp., W. Austral.; Ho. Phys. Univ. Coll. Hosp.

THOMPSON, Mr David Hope Hospital, Stott Lane, Salford, Manchester M6 8HD; Squirrel Chase, Heighley Castle Way, Madeley, Crewe CW3 9HF Tel: 01782 750778 — MB BS Lond. 1991 (Guy's Hosp. Lond.) FRCS Eng. 1996. Specialist Regist. In Radiol., N. W. Rotat., Hope Hosp. Manch. Specialty: Radiol. Prev: SHO Rotat. (Surg.) Kent & Canterbury Hosp.; SHO (Urol.) Harold Wood Hosp. Romford; SHO(Surg)Roy. Hants. Co. Hosp.

THOMPSON, David Frederick John Westby House Farm, Rawcliffe Road, St Michaels, Garstang, Preston PR3 0UE — MRCS Eng. LRCP Lond. 1957 (St. Mary's) DObst RCOG 1959. Dir. BUPA Manch. Med. Centre. Socs: Fell. Manch. Med. Soc.; Soc. Occupat. Health. Prev: Med. Dir. BUPA Manch. Med. Centre; Regist. (O & G) Sharoe Green Hosp. Preston.

THOMPSON, David George Department of Medicine, Hope Hospital, Salford M6 8HD Tel: 0161 787 4363 Fax: 0161 787 4364 — MB BS Lond. 1972; MRCP (UK) 1974; BSc Lond. 1969, MD 1980; FRCP Lond. 1992; FMedSci 2000. Prof. & Hon. Cons. Med. & Gastroenterol. Hope Hosp. Specialty: Gastroenterol. Socs: Amer. Gastroenterol. Assn.; (Sec.) Brit. Soc. Gastronterol.; Physiol. Soc. Prev: Wellcome Trust Sen. Lect. (Med.) Lond. Hosp. Med. Coll.; Lect. (Med.) Lond. Hosp.; SHO Hammersmith Hosp.

THOMPSON, David John Headquarters, The Masion, Mansion Park, Tongue Lane, Leeds LS6 4QT Tel: 0113 231 6716 Fax: 0113 231 6718 — MB BS Lond. 1970 (Middlx.) MSc Manch. 1980; FRCPsych 1991. Cons. Psychiat. Malham Hse. Day Hosp. Leeds; Sen. Clin. Lect. Univ. Leeds. Specialty: Gen. Psychiat. Prev: Cons. Psychiat. Airedale Gen. Hosp. Keighley; Sen. Regist. (Psychiat.) Withington Hosp. Manch.

THOMPSON, David Robert Peter Newtownstewart Medical Centre, 5 Millbrook Street, Newtownstewart, Omagh BT78 4BW Tel: 028 8166 1333 Fax: 028 8166 1883; Brandon House, Newtownstewart, Omagh — MB BCh BAO Belf. 1974.

THOMPSON, Denys Ridley Southview, Lower St., Whiteshill, Stroud GL6 6AR Tel: 01453 751581 — (Leeds & Oxf.) BSc Leeds 1963; BM BCh Oxf. 1965; DObst RCOG 1972; MRCGP 1978. Specialty: Blood Transfus. Prev: SHO Accid. Serv., Ho. Surg. & Ho. Phys. Radcliffe Infirm. Oxf.; Ho. Off. (Obst.) Churchill Hosp. Oxf.

THOMPSON, Desmond George The Surgery, 20 Lee Road, Blackheath, London SE3 9RT Tel: 020 8852 1235 Fax: 020 8297 2193; 83 Guibal Road, Lee, London SE12 9HF — MB BS Lond. 1983 (St. Bart.) DRCOG 1986; MRCGP 1989; Dip Sports Med Bath Univ. 2001. GP Princip. Prev: GP Lewisham & Southwark VTS; Ho. Surg. Hackney Hosp. Lond.; Ho. Phys. St. Bart. Hosp. Lond.

THOMPSON, Dinah Deborah (retired) Saunders, Church St., Coggeshall, Colchester CO6 1TX Tel: 01376 561245 — MB BChir Camb. 1949 (Camb. & King's Coll. Hosp.) MA Camb. 1950; DPM Eng. 1968. Prev: Cons. Psychiat. Severalls Hosp. Colchester.

THOMPSON, Mr Dominic Nolan Paul Department of Neurosurgery, Great Ormond Street Hospital for Children, NHS Trust, London WC1N 3TH Email: thompd@gosh.nhs.uk — MB BS Lond. 1986 (Char. Cross & Westm. Med. Sch.) BSc (Anat.) Lond. 1983, MB BS 1986; FRCS 1990; FRCS Eng. 1990; FRCS (SN) 1997. Cons. Paediat. Neurosurg. Gt. Ormond St. Hosp. For Childr. NHS Trust; Hon. Cons. Neurosurg.; Nat. Hosp. for Neurol. and Neurosurg., Qu. Sq. Lond.. Specialty: Neurosurg. Prev: Sen. Regist. (Neurosurg.) Atkinson Morley's Hosp. & Nat. Hosp. Qu. Sq.; Research Fell. (Neurosurg. & Craniofacial) Hosp. Sick Childr. Gt. Ormond St. Lond.; Regist. (Neurosurg.) Nat. Hosp. Qu. Sq. Lond.

THOMPSON, Edward Eustace Michael (retired) Tregenna, Brooks Drive, Hale Barns, Altrincham WA15 8TR Tel: 0161 980 4113 — MB ChB Liverp. 1959; DObst RCOG 1964; FFA RCS Eng. 1967. Cons. Anaesth. S. Manch. Health Dist. (T). Prev: Sen. Regist. (Anaesth.) United Manch. Hosps.

THOMPSON, Professor Edward John National Hospital, Institute of Neurology, Queen Square, London WC1N 3BG Tel: 020 7837 3611 Fax: 020 7837 8553 Email: e.thompson@ion.ucl.ac.uk — MD Rochester 1968 (Univ. Rochester, USA) FRCPath 1989, M 1979; PhD Lond. 1966, DSc 1992; FRCP Lond. 1996; MRCP Lond. 1999. Prof. & Hon. Cons. Chem. Path. Inst. Neurol. Nat. Hosp. for Neurol. & Neurosurg. Lond. Specialty: Chem. Path. Prev: on Staff Zool. Dept. Univ. Coll. Lond., Nat. Inst. Health Bethesda, USA.

THOMPSON, Elinor Mary South and West Devon Health Authority, The Lescaze Offices, Dartington, Totnes TQ9 6JE — MB ChB Bristol 1983; MFCM 1989. Cons. Pub. Health Med. S. & W. Devon HA. Specialty: Pub. Health Med.

THOMPSON, Elizabeth Anita Bristol Homeopathic Hospital, Cotham Hill, Bristol BS6 6JU Tel: 0117 973 1231 Fax: 0117 923 8759 — MB BS Lond. 1987; MRCP (UK) 1991; MFHom 1995. Cons. Homeopathic Phys. & Hon. Sen. Lect. (Palliat. Care). Specialty: Homeop. Med.; Palliat. Med.

THOMPSON, Elizabeth Ann 27 Moor Park Road, Northwood HA6 2DL Tel: 01923 827361 — MB BChir Camb. 1966 (Camb. & St. Mary's) MA Camb. 1966. Prev: SHO (Anaesth.) & Ho. Surg. Hillingdon Hosp. Uxbridge; Ho. Phys. St. Mary's Hosp. Lond.

THOMPSON, Elizabeth Claire 69 Valley Drive, Kirk Ella, Hull HU10 7PW — MB ChB Liverp. 1991. Specialty: Gen. Pract.

THOMPSON, Elizabeth Georgina Emily 1 Hackwood Park, Hexham NE46 1AX — MB ChB Manch. 1998.

THOMPSON, Elizabeth Hildred St Margaret's Somerset Hospice, Heron Drive, Bishops Hull, Taunton TA1 5HA Tel: 01823 259394 Fax: 01283 345900; Green End, Rowford, Cheddon Fitzpaine, Taunton TA2 8JY Tel: 01823 451529 — MB ChB Manch. 1971; Dip. Pallial. Med. 1995. Sen. Med. Off. (Palliat. Med.) St. Margt. Som. Hospice Taunton. Specialty: Palliat. Med.

THOMPSON, Elizabeth Jacqueline 36 Park Road, Ipswich IP1 3SU — MB ChB Ed. 1964; FFA RCS Eng. 1972. Specialty: Anaesth.

THOMPSON, Elizabeth Mary Department of Histopathology, St. Mary's Hospital, London W2 1NY Tel: 020 7886 1770 Fax: 020 7886 6068 Email: m.thompson@ic.ac.uk; 88 Grange Road, London W5 3PJ — MB BChir Camb. 1977 (Camb. & Middlx.) MA Camb. 1977; MRCP (UK) 1980; FRCPath 1995, MRCPath 1983; MD Camb.

1993. Cons. Histopath. St. Mary's Hosp. Lond. Specialty: Histopath. Socs: Assn. Clin. Path.; Renal Assn.; Internat. Acad. Path. Prev: Sen. Lect. (Histopath.) Roy. Postgrad. Med. Sch. Lond.; MRC Train. Fell. Roy. Postgrad. Med. Sch. Lond.; Sen. Regist. (Histopath.) Hammersmith Hosp. Lond. & Northwick Pk. Hosp. Harrow.

THOMPSON, Elizabeth Mary Mater Informorum Hospital, Crumlin Road, Belfast BT14 6AB Tel: 028 9074 1211 — MB BCh BAO Belf. 1976; FFA (I) RCS; FRCA Eng. 1981. Cons. Anaesth. Mater Informorum Hosp. Belf. Specialty: Anaesth.

THOMPSON, Emma Carol Margaret Frenchay Healthcare Trust, Blackberry Hill Hospital, Manor Road, Fishponds, Bristol BS16 2EW; 91 Richmond Road, Montpelier, Bristol BS6 5EP — MB ChB Bristol 1983; Dip. Psychoan Observat. Studies East. Lond.; DRCOG 1986; MRCGP 1988; MRCPsych 1991. Clin. Asst. in Psychoth. 1 session per week Frenchay Healthcare Trust. Specialty: Psychother. Prev: Staff Grade, Regist. & SHO (Psychiat.) United Bristol Healthcare NHS Trust; Trainee GP Avon VTS.

THOMPSON, Eric John Bertha House, 71 Malone Road, Belfast BT9 6SB — MB BCh BAO Belf. 1947. Prev: Ho. Surg. & Ho. Phys. W. Norf. & King's Lynn Gen. Hosp.

THOMPSON, Euan James 70/4 St Leonard's Street, Edinburgh EH8 9RA — MB ChB Ed. 1996.

THOMPSON, Fiona Charlotte 10 Old Downs, Hartley, Longfield DA3 7AA — BM BS Nottm. 1996.

THOMPSON, Fiona Jane Department of Pediatrics, Northampton General Hospital, Cliftonville, Northampton NN1 5BD Tel: 01604 545522 Fax: 01604 545640 Email: fionathompson@ngh.nhs.uk; Meadowbrook, 12/13 Lower Harlestone, Northampton NN7 4EW Tel: 01604 820840 Email: kennetjthompson@ol.com — MB BS Lond. 1987 (Med. Coll. St. Bart. Hosp. Univ. Lond.) FRCPCH; MRCP (UK) 1991; DCH RCP Lond. 1991. Cons. Paediat. Northampton Gen. Hosp. Specialty: Paediat. Socs: Neonat. Soc. Prev: Research Fell. (Paediat.) King's Coll. Hosp. Lond.; Sen. Regist. (Paediat.) Northampton Gen. Hosp. & John Radcliffe Hosp. Oxf.

THOMPSON, Fiona Jane — MB ChB Leeds 1997.

THOMPSON, Frank Derek 27 Moor Park Road, Northwood HA6 2DL — MB Camb. 1965 (Camb. & St. Mary's) BChir 1964; MRCP (U.K.) 1971; FRCP Eng. 1983. Cons. (Nephrol.) St. Peter's Hosp. Lond. Harefield & Mt. Vernon Hosp.; Hon. Cons. (Nephrol.) Nat. Heart Hosp. Lond. Northwood; Hon. Sen. Lect. Inst. Urol Lond. Specialty: Urol. Prev: Renal Regist. St. Philip's Gp. Hosps.; Lect. in Nephrol. Inst. Urol. Lond.; Ho. Surg. St. Mary's Hosp.

THOMPSON, Gaynor Louise 24 Woods Grove, Burniston, Scarborough YO13 0JD — MB BS Newc. 1991.

THOMPSON, Geoffrey Robert Royal Shrewsbury Hospital, North Mytton Oak Road, Copthorne, Shrewsbury SY3 8BR Tel: 01743 231122; The Old Barn, Great Ness, Shrewsbury SY4 2LE — MB ChB Manch. 1966; FFA RCS Eng. 1972. Cons. Anaesth. Salop AHA. Specialty: Anaesth. Socs: Fell. Manch. Med. Soc. Prev: Sen. Regist. & Regist. (Anaesth.) Manch. Roy. Infirm.; Regist. (Anaesth.) Ashton-under-Lyne Gen. Hosp.

THOMPSON, Geoffrey Stuart (retired) 6 Highgate Road, Altrincham WA14 4QZ Tel: 0161 928 4862 — (Camb. & Univ. Coll. Hosp.) MB BChir Camb. 1951; FRCP Lond. 1974, M 1960; MA Camb. 1954, MD 1965. Prev: Cons. Phys. Wythenshawe Hosp. Manch.

THOMPSON, Professor Gilbert Richard Imperial College Faculty of Medicine, Metabolic Medicine, Hammersmith Hospital, Du Cane Road, London W12 0NN Tel: 020 8994 6143 Fax: 020 8994 6143 Email: g.thompson@imperial.ac.uk — (St. Thos.) MB BS Lond. 1956; FRCP Lond. 1973, M 1959; MD Lond. 1963. Emerit. Prof. Clin. Lipidol. Imperial Coll. 1998; Hon. Con. Phys. Hamersmith Hopital Lond. 1998; Cons. Clin. Lipidology Cromwell Hosp. 2002. Specialty: Gen. Med. Special Interest: Lipidology. Socs: (Ex-Chairm.) Brit. Hyperlipidaemia Assn.; (Ex- Chairm.) Brit. Atherosclerosis Soc.; (Ex-Chairm.) RSM Forum on Lipids in Clin. Med. Prev: Research Fell. Harvard Med. Sch. & Mass. Gen. Hosp. Boston, USA; Asst. Prof. Baylor Coll. Med. & Methodist Hosp. Houston, USA; Vis. Prof. McGill Univ. & Roy. Vict. Hosp. Montreal, Canada.

THOMPSON, Gillian 48A Loanends Road, Nutts Corner, Crumlin BT29 4YW — MB BCh. Belf. 1998.

THOMPSON, Gillian Mary The Health Centre, Main Road, Radcliffe-on-Trent, Nottingham NG12 2GD Tel: 0115 933 3737; 360 Musters Road, West Bridgford, Nottingham NG2 7DA — MB ChB Manch. 1977; MRCGP 1981.

THOMPSON, Gordon (retired) 157 Reads Avenue, Blackpool FY1 4HZ Tel: 01253 627061 Fax: 01253 627061 — MB ChB Sheff. 1959; DIH Soc. Apoth. Lond. 1966. Prev: Med. Off. DHSS Blackpool.

THOMPSON, Gordon Henry Health Centre, Forum Way, Cramlington NE23 6QN Tel: 01670 712821 Fax: 01670 730837; 28 Easedale Avenue, Melton Park, Gosforth, Newcastle upon Tyne NE3 5TB Tel: 01632 2182 — MB BS Durh. 1965; DObst RCOG 1971.

THOMPSON, Graham David Donnington Medical Practice, Wrekin Drive, Donnington, Telford TF2 8EA Tel: 01952 605252 Fax: 01952 677010; The Lees, Potters Bank, Red Lake, Telford TF1 5EP — MB BS Lond. 1968 (St. Bart.) MRCS Eng. LRCP Lond. 1968; DObst RCOG 1970; DCH Eng. 1972. Prev: Regist. (Paediat.) Wolverhampton AHA; Regist. (Med.) Cheltenham.

THOMPSON, Mr Graham Michael Moorfields Duke Elder Department, Department of Ophthalmology, St. George's Hospital, Tooting, London SW17 0QT Tel: 020 8725 2062 Fax: 020 8725 3026 — MB BS Lond. 1973; DO Eng. 1976; FRCS Eng. 1979; FRCOphth 1989. Cons. Ophth. St. Geo. Hosp. Lond.; Hon. Sen. Lect. St. Geo. Hosp. Med. Sch. Lond. Specialty: Ophth. Prev: Sen. Regist. (Ophth.) St. Barts. Hosp. Lond.; Sen. Regist. & Regist. Moorfields Eye Hosp. Lond.

THOMPSON, Harold Wellesley Karl (retired) 307 London Road, Appleton, Warrington WA4 5JB Tel: 01925 264211 — MB BCh BAO Belf. 1953. Med. Off. Laporte Chem.s & other Cos. Prev: Sen. Extern. Ho. Surg. Roy. Vict. Hosp. Belf.

THOMPSON, Harry Edwin George Street Surgery, 16 George Street, Alderley Edge SK9 7EP Tel: 01625 584545/6; Davenport House Farm, Upcast Lane, Wilmslow SK9 6EH Tel: 01625 590337 — MB ChB Dundee 1983; BSc Dund 1979; DRCOG 1985; MRCGP 1987.

THOMPSON, Helen Macfarlane, MBE (retired) 60A London Road, Kilmarnock KA3 7DD — MB ChB Glas. 1947; DObst. 1951.

THOMPSON, Henry (retired) 7 Clarry Drive, Four Oaks Est., Sutton Coldfield B74 2RA Tel: 0121 323 2549 — MD Glas. 1954; MB ChB 1948; FRCPath 1975. Reader (Path.) Univ. Birm.; Cons. Pathol. Gen. Hosp. Birm. Prev: Ho. Surg. Glas. Roy. Infirm.

THOMPSON, Hilary Frances Brooklands Medical Practice, 594 Altrincham Road, Brooklands, Manchester M23 9JH Tel: 0161 998 3818 Fax: 0161 946 0716; Woodlawn, Belmont Road, Hale, Altrincham WA15 9PT Tel: 0161 928 2535 — MB BS Lond. 1972; BSc Lond. 1969, MB BS (Hons. Med.) 1972; DCH Eng. 1975; MRCP (UK) 1975; DRCOG 1976; MRCGP 1992. Princip. Gen. Pract. Prev: Trainee Gen. Pract. Lond. (Whittington Hosp.) Vocational Train.; Scheme; Ho. Phys. & Ho. Surg. Lond. Hosp.

THOMPSON, Howard Michael Fern Bank, Water Lane, St Agnes TR5 0QZ Tel: 01872 552040 Email: hthompson@doctors.org.uk — MB ChB Birm. 1988; FRCA 1994. Cons. (Anaesth. & Pain Managem.) Roy. Cornw. Hosp. Truro. Specialty: Anaesth. Socs: Assn. Anaesth.; Brit. Pain Soc. Prev: Cons. (Anaesth. & Pain Managem.) Pilgrim Hosp. Boston; Sen. Regist. Leicester; Regist. (Anaesth.) Leicester.

THOMPSON, Hudson Taylor, MBE (retired) 9 Cotswold Way, Trenewydd Park Est., Risca, Newport NP11 6QT Tel: 612797 — MRCS Eng. LRCP Lond. 1950.

THOMPSON, Mr Hugh Hilary Lister Hospital, Coreys Mill Lane, Stevenage SG1 4AB Tel: 01438 781103 Fax: 01438 781154 Email: hilary.thompson@nhs.net; Priory Cottage, Charlton, Hitchin SG5 2AA Tel: 01462 431409 — MB BS Lond. 1971 (Lond. Hosp.) MS Lond. 1982, BSc (1st cl. Hons. Anat.) 1968; MB BS (Hons. Distinc. Med.) Lond. 1971; FRCS Eng. 1977. Cons. Surg. Lister Hosp. Stevenage. Specialty: Gen. Surg. Socs: Assn. Surg.; Assn. Coloproctol.; Assn. Endoscopic Surgs. Prev: Sen. Lect. Surg. Lond. Hosp. Med. Coll.; Fell. Dept. Surg. UCLA Los Angeles, USA; Ho. Off. Birm. Accid. Hosp.

THOMPSON, Ian (retired) Mill Street Medical Centre, Mill Street, St Helens WA10 2BD Tel: 01744 23641 Fax: 01744 28398; 47 Eccleston Gardens, St Helens WA10 3BJ Tel: 01744 602162 — MRCS Eng. LRCP Lond. 1968.

THOMPSON, Ian Davenport (retired) 63 St Martin's Road, Finham, Coventry CV3 6FD Tel: 024 7641 1522 — (Birm.) MB ChB

Birm. 1956; DA Eng. 1959; FFA RCS Eng. 1962. Prev: Cons. Anaesth. Coventry Hosp. Gp.

THOMPSON, Ian George Chestnuts Surgery, 70 East Street, Sittingbourne ME10 4RU Tel: 01795 423197 Fax: 01795 430179; 205 Borden Lane, Sittingbourne ME9 8HR — MB BS Durh. 1966 (Newc.) DObst RCOG 1968; MRCGP 1973.

THOMPSON, Ian McKim 36 Harborne Road, Birmingham B15 3AJ Tel: 0121 456 1402 — MB ChB Birm. 1961. Indep. Medico (Vice President), legal Pract.. BMA. Socs: Hon. Mem. Med. Colls. of Spain. Prev: Mem. GMC.

THOMPSON, Ian Philip Cousley 11 Lennys Road, Derryadd, Craigavon BT66 6QS — MB BCh BAO Belf. 1988; DRCOG 1992; MRCGP 1995; DLO 2002. Stafff Surg. ENT Antrim Area Hosp. Specialty: Otorhinolaryngol. Prev: SHO (ENT) Ulster Hosp.; Clin. Asst. (ENT) Downe Hosp. Belf.

THOMPSON, Ian Richard — MB BS Lond. 1998 (King's Coll. Hosp.) BA (Hons.) Oxf. 1995. SHO (GUM/HIV) St Bart. & The Lond. Hosps.

THOMPSON, Ian Wallace 29 Brownlow Lane, Cheddington, Leighton Buzzard LU7 0SS — MB ChB Ed. 1978.

THOMPSON, Irene Margaret (retired) 2 Cedar Park, Bleary, Portadown, Craigavon BT63 5LL — (Belf.) MB BCh BAO Belf. 1947; DPH Belf. 1949; MD Belf. 1952; MFCM 1972. Prev: Asst. Chief Admin. Med. Off. East. Health & Social Servs. Bd.

THOMPSON, Ivan Horden Group Practice, The Health Centre, Peterlee SR8 1AD Tel: 0191 587 0808 Fax: 0191 587 0700; 3 Woodfield, Peterlee SR8 1DB Tel: 0191 586 8218 Fax: 0191 586 8218 — (Bristol) MB ChB Bristol 1957; MRCGP 1968. Co. Surg. St. John Ambul. Brig. Socs: Fell. Roy. Soc. Med.

THOMPSON, Jacqueline 35 Ross Avenue, Inverness IV3 5QJ — MB ChB Leeds 1996; BSc (Hons.) Leeds 1994.

THOMPSON, Jacqueline Mary Holmgarth House, Carthorpe, Bedale DL8 2LF — MB ChB Leic. 1985; DRCOG 1989; MRCGP 1994.

THOMPSON, Jacqueline Russell Daudsons Mains Medical Centre, 5 Quality St, Edinburgh EH4 5BP Tel: 0131 336 2291 Fax: 0131 336 1886 Email: jacquelinethompson@orange.net; 615 Gosford Place, Edinburgh EH6 4BJ Tel: 0131 530 1185 — MB ChB Ed. 1993; MRCGP; DRCOG. 1998; DFFP. 1999. GP Princip., Daudsons Mains Med. Centre, Edin..; SHO (O&G), Southmead, Bristol. Specialty: Gen. Pract. Prev: SHO. (A & E.) Frenehay Hosp. Bristol.; SHO. (Psychiat.) Cornw..; SHO. (Med.) Cornw..

THOMPSON, Jacqueline Susan Park Medical Centre, 164 Park Road, Peterborough PE1 2UF Tel: 01733 552801 Fax: 01733 425015 — MB BS Lond. 1980; LMSSA Lond. 1980; DRCOG 1985.

THOMPSON, James 73 Kiltaire Crescent, Ivertowers Grange, Airdrie ML6 8JG — MB ChB Glas. 1974; DObst RCOG 1976; DFFP 1997.

THOMPSON, James Francis Webster The Old Vicarage, South St., Roxby, Scunthorpe DN15 0BJ — MB BS Lond. 1975; BA (Physics) Oxf. 1970; FFA RCS Eng. 1979. Cons. Anaesth. Scunthorpe Gen. Hosp. Specialty: Anaesth.

THOMPSON, James Reid The Surgery, 5 Kensington Place, London W8 7PT Tel: 020 7229 7111 Fax: 020 7221 3069 — MB BCh BAO Belf. 1988 (Qu. Univ. Belf.) MRCGP 1996. GP. Specialty: Gen. Pract. Prev: Trainee GP Char. Cross Hosp. Lond. VTS; SHO (Genitourin. Med.) Chelsea & Wesm. Hosp. Lond.; SHO (Med.) Hammersmith Hosp. Lond. & Harefield Hosp.

THOMPSON, Jane Louise 2 Gar Street SO23 8GQ Tel: 01962 843040 Email: fleet.thompsons@virgin.net — MB BS Lond. 1968 (Middlx.) DFFP 1993. Specialty: Obst. & Gyn. Socs: Christ. Med. Fellowsh. Prev: Clin. Med. Off. W. Surrey & NE Hants. HAs; Ho. Surg. (Gyn. & Obst.) & Ho. Phys. (Paediat.) Middlx. Hosp. Lond.; Ho. Phys. Mayday Hosp. Thornton Heath.

THOMPSON, Jane Maureen (retired) 6 Albion Place, Lower Upnor, Rochester ME2 4XD — MB BCh BAO Dub. 1964; BA Dub. 1962, MB BCh BAO 1964; DCH RCPSI 1966.

THOMPSON, Jane Sarah Chatham House, Doncaster Gate, Rotherham S65 1DW Tel: 01709 304808 Fax: 01709 304886 — MB ChB Sheff. 1987. Staff Grade Doctor (Child & Adolesc. Psychiat.) Chatham Hse. Rotherham. Specialty: Gen. Pract.; Child & Adolesc. Psychiat.; Trop. Med. Prev: Clin. Asst. (Adolesc. Unit) North. Gen. Hosp. Sheff.

THOMPSON, Jeremy Charles St Martins Practice, 319 Chapeltown Road, Leeds LS7 3JT Tel: 0113 262 1013 Fax: 0113 237 4747 — MB ChB Leeds 1983; DRCOG 1987; MRCGP 1990. Specialty: Gen. Pract. Socs: Nat. Inst. Med. Herbalists.

THOMPSON, Jeremy Neil Trelawney Avenue Surgery, 425 Trelawney Avenue, Langley, Slough SL3 7TT Tel: 01753 775545 Fax: 01753 775545; 39 Burroway Road, Langley, Slough SL3 8EH Tel: 01753 541047 — MB BS Newc. 1975; MRCP (UK) 1978; MRCGP 1983. Specialty: Gen. Pract.

THOMPSON, Mr Jeremy Nowell Chelsea & Westminster Hospital, Department of Surgery, 369 Fulham Road, London SW10 9NH Tel: 020 8746 8463 Fax: 020 8746 8282 Email: gisurg@chelwest.nhs.uk; 88 Grange Road, London W5 3PJ — MB BChir Camb. 1977; MChir Camb. 1988, BA 1974; FRCS Eng. 1980. Cons. Surg. Chelsea & Westm. Hosp. & Roy. Marsden Hosp. Lond.; Clin. Director of Surg., Chelsea and Westm. Hosp. Specialty: Gen. Surg. Socs: Fell. Assn. Surgs.; Brit. Soc. Gastroenterol.; Pancreatic Soc. Prev: Cons. Surg. Ealing & Hammersmith Hosp. Lond.; Sen. Lect. (Surg.) Roy. Postgrad. Med. Sch. Lond.; Lect. Acad. Surg. Unit St. Mary's Hosp. Lond.

THOMPSON, Joanna Jane The Surgery, Bellingham, Hexham NE48 2HE — MB BS Newc. 1987; MRCGP.

THOMPSON, Joanne 9 Westerdale Road, Seaton Carew, Hartlepool TS25 2AE — MB BChir Camb. 1988.

THOMPSON, Joanne Helen The Surgery, Vicarage Lane, Walton on the Naze CO14 8PA Tel: 01255 674373 Fax: 01255 851005 — MB BS Lond. 1988; DRCOG 1993.

THOMPSON, John (retired) PO Box 1428, Glasgow G52 3QS — MD Glas. 1964; MB ChB 1943; DPH 1948.

THOMPSON, John (retired) Crossways, Frodesley, Shrewsbury SY5 7HA Tel: 01694 731262 — MB ChB Liverp. 1950; DObst RCOG 1955. Prev: GP Wirral.

THOMPSON, John 1 Lichfield Close, Denshaw, Oldham OL3 5SF — MB ChB Manch. 1991.

THOMPSON, John Andrew Spring Gardens Health Centre, Providence Street, Worcester WR1 2BS Tel: 01905 681681 Fax: 01905 681699; 15 Yew Tree Close, London Road, Worcester WR5 2LH — MB ChB Bristol 1972; DA Eng. 1975; DObst RCOG 1976. Prev: Ho. Surg. Bristol Roy. Infirm.; SHO (Paediat.) Bristol Childr. Hosp.; SHO (Anaesth.) Roy. Devon & Exeter Hosp. (Wonford) Exeter.

THOMPSON, John Brian The Health Centre, 20 Duncan Street, Greenock PA15 4LY Tel: 01475 724477 Fax: 01475 727140; Suilven, 7 Hilltop Crescent, Gourock PA19 1YW — MB ChB Glas. 1975; DRCOG 1977; DA Eng. 1979.

THOMPSON, John Bruce Mount Farm Surgery, Lawson Place, Bury St Edmunds IP32 7EW Tel: 01284 769643 Fax: 01284 700833; Park Lane Cottages, Hawstead, Bury St Edmunds IP29 5NX — MB BChir Camb. 1968 (St. Bart.) BA Camb. 1964; MRCP (UK) 1970.

THOMPSON, John Charles Barnshaw Bodnant, Water St., Penygroes, Caernarfon LL54 6LU Tel: 01286 880203 Fax: 01286 880629 Email: john.thompson@gp-W94042.wales.nhs.uk — MB ChB St And. 1969; DObst 1971; MRCGP (Distinc.) 1974. GP & Clin. Asst. (Psychiat.) Gwynedd HA. Socs: BMA; Welsh Psychiat. Soc. Prev: SHO (O & G) Robroyston Hosp. Glas.; Ho. Surg. Dunfermline & W. Fife Hosp.; Ho. Phys. Bangour Gen. Hosp. Broxburn.

THOMPSON, John Clifford Seven Brooks Medical Centre, 21 Church Street, Atherton, Manchester M46 9DE Tel: 01942 882799 Fax: 01942 873859 — MB ChB Liverp. 1979; DRCOG 1980; MRCGP 1995.

THOMPSON, Mr John Frederick Royal Devon & Exeter Hospitals, Barrack Road, Exeter EX2 5DW Tel: 01392 402739 Email: john.thompson@rdehc-tr.nhs.uk — MB BS Lond. 1982; FRCS Ed. 1986; FRCS Eng. 1986; MS Soton. 1990. Cons. (Gen. & Vasc.) Surg. Roy. Devon & Exeter Hosps. Specialty: Gen. Surg. Special Interest: Vasc. Socs: Jt. Vasc. Research Gp. (Treas.); Brit. Blood. Transfus. Soc. (Counc.); Assn. Surg. GB & Irel. Prev: Wessex Research Fell. Soton. Univ. Hosps.; SHO & Demonst. (Anat.) Char. Cross & Westm. Med. Sch. Lond.; Lect. (Surg.) & Sen. Regist. Univ. Bristol & Bristol Roy. Infirm.

THOMPSON, John Mark 121 Dalkeith Road, Edinburgh EH16 5AJ — MB BS Newc. 1998.

THOMPSON, John Michael Hazel Cottage, School Lane, Pirbright, Woking GU24 0JW — MB BS Lond. 1982; MRCS Eng. LRCP Lond. 1981.

THOMPSON, John Paul University of Wales College of Medicine, University Hospital of Wales, Heath Park, Cardiff CF14 4XN — MB ChB Sheff. 1985 (Sheff. Univ.) BMedSci (1st. cl. Hons.) 1984; MRCP (UK) 1990. Sen. Lect. in Clin. Pharmacol., Univ. of Wales Coll. of Med., Cardiff. Specialty: Pharmacology. Special Interest: Clinical Toxicology. Socs: Eur. Assn. Poisons Control Centres & Clin. Toxicol.; Amer. Acad. of Clin. Toxicology; Brit. Toxicol. Soc.

THOMPSON, Professor John Warburton 1 Hackwood Park, Hexham NE46 1AX Tel: 01434 608552 Fax: 01434 608552; 1 Hackwood Park, Hexham NE46 1AX Tel: 01434 608552 Fax: 01434 608552 — MB BS Lond. 1948 (Lond. Hosp.) MB BS (Hons.) Surg., Hyg. & Forens. Med. Lond. 1948; PhD Lond. 1960; FRCP Lond. 1981, M 1977; Dip. Med. Acupunc. 1995. Hon. Phys. & Hon. Cons. in Med. Studies, St. Oswald's Hospice, Newcatle upon Tyne (Palliat. Med., especially the control of Chronic Pain).; Emerit. Prof. Pharmacol. Univ. Newc. u. Tyne; Emerit. Cons. Clin. Pharm. Newc. HA; Cons. in Pain Managem. with special Refer. to mechanisms and Managem. of chronic pain problems (Private Pract.). Specialty: Pharmacology; Palliat. Med.; Acupunc. Socs: Brit. Pharm. Soc.; Internat. Assn. Study of Pain; The Pain Society. Prev: Prof. Pharmacol. Univ. Newc.; Sen. Lect. (Pharmacol.) Inst. Basic Med. Scs. RCS Eng. & St. Geo. Hosp. Med. Sch. Lond.; Research Asst. (Applied Pharmacol.) Univ. Coll. & Univ. Coll. Hosp. Med. Sch.

THOMPSON, Jonathan Andrew Richard West Kirby Health Centre, Grange Road, Wirral CH48 4HZ Tel: 0151 625 9171 Fax: 0151 625 9171; Millyea, 47 Farr Hall Drive, Lower Heswall, Wirral CH60 4SE — MB ChB Liverp. 1985 (Liverpool) Dip Primary Care Therapeutics 1999. Specialty: Gen. Pract.

THOMPSON, Jonathan Lee 33 Old Lansdowne Road, Manchester M20 2PA — BM BS Nottm. 1986; BMedSci (Hons.) Nottm. 1984.

THOMPSON, Jonathan Paul Whytecote Cottage, 21 Station Road, Littlethorpe, Leicester LE9 5HS — MB ChB Leic. 1988; BSc (Med. Sci.) Leic. 1986; FRCA 1994; MD Leic. 2002. Sen. Lect. & Hon. Cons. (Anaesth.& Crit. Care) Leicester Univ. Dept. Anaesth.

THOMPSON, Josephine Amanda Temple Sowerby Medical Practice, Temple Sowerby, Penrith CA10 1RZ Tel: 017683 61232 Fax: 017683 61980; Nunwick Hall, Great Salkeld, Penrith CA11 9LN — MB BCh Wales 1989; DCH RCP Lond. 1993; DFFP 1993; DRCOG 1994. Off. (Family Plann.) Penrith Dist.; Trainee GP Penrith Retainer Scheme. Prev: SHO (Cas.) Greenwich Lond. VTS; Ho. Off. (Gen. Med.) E. Glam. Gen. Hosp. Pontypridd; Ho. Off. (Neurosurg. & Gen. Surg.) Univ. Hosp. Wales Cardiff.

THOMPSON, Judith Ann Sunnyside Doctors Surgery, 150 Fratton Road, Portsmouth PO1 5DH Tel: 023 9282 4725 Fax: 023 9286 1014; St. Andrews, 9 Eastern Parade, Southsea PO4 9RA Tel: 023 9275 6938 Fax: 023 9275 6438 — MB ChB Bristol 1970; DObst RCOG 1972. Specialty: Family Plann. & Reproduc. Health. Socs: Nat. Assn. Family Plann. Doctors; BMA (Mem. Sec. Portsmouth & SE Hants. Div.). Prev: Trainee GP Portsmouth & SE Hants. HA; SCMO (Family Plann.) Portsmouth & SE Hants. HA; Clin. Asst. Breast Clinic Qu. Alexandra Hosp. Portsmouth.

THOMPSON, Julie Ann Croft Cottage, 98 Leeds Road, Liversedge WF15 6AA — MB ChB Leeds 1998.

THOMPSON, Juliet Anne St. Paul's Surgery, Oram's Mount, Winchester SO22 5DD Tel: 01962 853599 — BM BS Nottm. 1990 (Nottingham) DRCOG 1993; MRCGP 1994.

THOMPSON, Justin Rhys North Holmwood Surgery, 1 Bentsbrook Close, North Holmwood, Dorking RH5 4HY Tel: 01306 885802 — BMedSci Nottm. 1983, BM BS 1985; DCH RCP Lond. 1990; MRCGP 1990. GP Dorking.

THOMPSON, Karen Jill Wellway Medical Group, Wellway, Morpeth NE61 1BJ Tel: 01670 517300; The Cottage, Threeways, Tranwell Woods, Morpeth NE61 6AQ Tel: 01670 511286 — MB BS Lond. 1990; DRCOG 1993; MRCGP 1994. Prev: SHO (Gen. Med. & Geriat.) Qu. Eliz. Hosp. Gateshead; SHO (O & G) Hexham Gen. Hosp.; SHO (Paediat.) N. Tyneside Hosp.

THOMPSON, Katherine Mary 28 Holmwood Gardens, Westbury-on-Trym, Bristol BS9 3EB — MB BS Newc. 1979.

THOMPSON, Kenneth John The Surgery, The Cannons, Fisher Street, Leven KY8 3HD Tel: 028 2565 2854; 58 Donibristle Gardens, Dalgety Bay, Dunfermline KY11 9NQ Tel: 01383 820354 — MB ChB Dundee 1988. Princip. Gen. Pract. Specialty: Gen. Pract. Prev: SHO (O & G) Forth Pk. Matern. Hosp. Kirkcaldy.; SHO (Cardiothoracic Surg.) Roy. Infirm. Edin.

THOMPSON, Kenneth Robin Bangor Health Centre, Newtownards Road, Bangor BT20 4LD Tel: 028 9146 9111 — MB BCh BAO Belf. 1971.

THOMPSON, Kenneth Whitton Newlands Medical Centre, Borough Road, Middlesbrough TS1 3RX Tel: 01642 247401 Fax: 01642 223803 Email: K.thompson@lineone.net; 11 Southwood, Coulby Newham, Middlesbrough TS8 0UE Tel: 01642 593554 Fax: 0870 130 9903 Email: k.thompson@lineone.net — (Edinburgh) MB ChB Ed. 1960. p/t Indust. Med. Off.; Locum GP.

THOMPSON, Kerry Coral Old Dairy Cottage, Clay Lane, Crossbush, Arundel BN18 9RS — BM (Clin. & Hons.) Soton. 1987 (Southampton) BSc (1st cl. Hons.) Psych. & Physiol. Soton. 1983; MRCP (UK) 1991; PhD 1998. Cons. Phys./Gastroenterlogist, Worthing and Southlands NHS Trust, Worthing Hosp., Worthing. Specialty: Gastroenterol.; Gen. Med. Prev: SpR Gastroenterol., Roy. Hants. Co. Hosp., Winchester.

THOMPSON, Kevin Orion Thorpewood Medical Group, 140 Woodside Road, Thorpe St. Andrew, Norwich NR7 9QL Tel: 01603 701477 Fax: 01603 701512; The Paddock, 2 Meadows Lane, Thorpe St. Andrew, Norwich NR7 0QX Tel: 01603 701220 Fax: 01603 701512 — MB BChir Camb. 1973 (Camb. & Guys) MRCS Eng. LRCP Lond. 1971; MB Camb. 1973, MA, BChir 1972. Socs: BMA. Prev: Med. Regist. Norf. & Norwich Hosp.; SHO (O & G) Norf. & Norwich Hosp.

THOMPSON, Lawrence Edward Crumlin Medical Practice, 5 Glenavy Road, Crumlin BT29 4LA Tel: 028 9442 2209 Fax: 028 9442 2233 — MB BCh BAO Belf. 1973; DObst RCOG 1975; MRCGP 1981.

THOMPSON, Lucy Victoria Lovemead Group Practice, Roundstone Surgery, Polebarn Circus, Trowbridge BA14 7EH — MB BS Lond. 1989; MRCP (UK) 1993. Prev: Trainee GP/SHO Bath VTS.; SHO Rotat. (Med.) Bournemouth & Poole Hosps.

THOMPSON, Mabel Mary Helen (retired) 8 Manor Way, Blackheath, London SE3 9EF Tel: 020 8852 4938; 8 Manor Way, Blackheath, London SE3 9EF Tel: 020 852 4938 — MB BCh BAO Dub. 1950 (Dub.Trinity College) BA Dub. 1947, MB BCh BAO 1950. Prev: GP Lond.

THOMPSON, Malcolm Charles 18 Greenhill Main Road, Greenhill, Sheffield S8 7RD — MB ChB Manch. 1977; MRCOG 1983, D 1980; MRCGP 1985; MRNZCOG 1985; DGM RCP Lond. 1989; MLCOM 1993; DCH (RCP Lond.) 1994; DCH RCP Lond. 1994; DA (UK) 1995; FRCA 1997. Specialty: Anaesth. Socs: Brit. Med. Acupunct. Soc.; Pain. Soc. Prev: Specialist Regist. Rotat. (Anaesth.) SE Thames; GP Buller, NZ.

THOMPSON, Malcolm Charles Friarage Hospital, Northallerton DL6 1JG Tel: 01607 779911 — MB ChB Manch. 1973; DCH Eng. 1976; DRCOG 1977; FFA RCS Eng. 1981. Cons. Anaesth. Friarage Hosp. Northallerton. Specialty: Anaesth. Socs: Assn. Anaesth. Gt. Brit. & Irel.; Intens. Care Soc. Prev: Sen. Lect. (Milit. Anaesth.) Brit. Army; Sen. Regist. (Anaesth.) Guy's Hosp. Lond.; Trainee GP King's Lynn VTS.

THOMPSON, Malcolm George (retired) Rotherhurst, 3 The Avenue, Orpington BR6 9AS Tel: 01689 824240 — MB BS Lond. 1950 (Guy's) MRCS Eng. LRCP Lond. 1950. Prev: Hosp. Pract. (Surg.) Orpington Hosp.

THOMPSON, Margaret Jane Johnston Ashurst Hospital, Lyndhurst Rd, Southampton SO40 7AR Tel: 023 8074 3030 Fax: 023 8074 3033; 3 Sandy Lane, Titchfield, Fareham PO14 4ER Tel: 01329 847234 Fax: 01329 847236 — MB ChB Glas. 1970; DCH RCPS Glas. 1972; DObst RCOG 1973; MRCP (UK) 1975; FRCPsych 1994, M 1979; FRCP Glas. 1988; FRCHCP 1999. Child Psychiat.; Reader / Cons. Child Pyschiat. Specialty: Child & Adolesc. Psychiat. Socs: Assn. Child Psychol. & Psychiat.; Brit. Paediat. Assn.; Maru Soc. Prev: Sen. Regist. Wessex RHA; Lect. (Child & Adolesc. Psychiat.) Univ. Glas.; Hon. Sen. Regist. (Child & Family Psychiat.) Roy. Hosp. Sick Childr. Glas.

THOMPSON, Mark Graham The Old Farm Surgery, 67 Foxhole Road, Paignton TQ4 3TB Email: thompson@wanderers70.freeserve.co.uk — MB ChB Bristol 1994; DRCOG 1999. GP VTS Bath. Specialty: Gen. Pract. Socs: BMA. Prev: SHO (Anaesth.); SHO (Acc. & Emerg.); SHO (O & G).

THOMPSON, Mark John Thornbury Health Centre, Eastland Road, Thornbury, Bristol BS35 1DP Tel: 01454 412167 Fax: 01454 419522 — MB ChB Bristol 1991.

THOMPSON, Mark Wakefield Handbridge Medical Centre, Greenway Street, Handbridge, Chester CH4 7JS Tel: 01244 680169 Fax: 01244 680162; 7 Hoole Park, Hoole, Chester CH2 3AN Tel: 01244 313103 — MB BS Lond. 1983; MRCGP; MA Camb. 1984. Prev: Trainee GP Chester VTS; Trainee GP East. Suburbs VTS Melbourne; Family Plann. ChristCh. N.Z.

THOMPSON, Mary Adela (retired) Shankill Health Centre, 135 Shankill Parade, Belfast BT13 1SD Tel: 01232 247181 — MB BCh BAO Belf. 1960.

THOMPSON, Mary Dymock 84 Moorside N., Newcastle upon Tyne NE4 9DU Tel: 0191 273 8637 — MD Durh. 1947; MB BS 1940, DPH 1960. Prev: Childh. Tuberc. Phys. Newc.; Paediat. Regist. Qu. Charlotte's Hosp.; Res. Med. Off. Babies Hosp. Newc.

THOMPSON, Matthew Graham Park Lane Cottages, Hawstead, Bury St Edmunds IP29 5NX — BM Soton. 1993 (Southampton) Specialty: Gen. Psychiat.

THOMPSON, Matthew James Central Microbiologial Laboratories, Western General Hospital, Crewe Road, Edinburgh EH4 2XU — MB ChB Glas. 1989.

THOMPSON, Professor Matthew Merfyn St Georges Hospital Medical School, Department of Vascular Surgery, Blackshaw Road, London SW17 0QT; 120 St Leonard's Road, East Sheen, London SW14 7NJ Tel: 020 8725 3205 Fax: 020 8725 3495 — MB BS Lond. 1987 (St Bart.) MA Camb. 1988; MD (Distinc.) Leic. 1994; FRCS Eng. 1994; FRCS 1998. Cons. (Vascular & Enolovascular Surgery) St Georges Hosp.; Lect. (Surg.) Univ. Leicester.; Prof Surg. St Georges Hosp. Med. Sch. Specialty: Gen. Surg. Prev: Cons.(Vascul EndoVasc. Surg.) Leics Roy Infirm.

THOMPSON, Maureen Kerry Judith 39 Mountsandel Road, Coleraine BT52 1JE Tel: 01265 51151 — MB ChB Manch. 1994 (Manchester) Specialty: Gen. Pract.

THOMPSON, Michael Alan St Peter & St James Hospice, North Common Road, North Chailey, Lewes BN8 4ED Tel: 01444 471598 — MB BS Lond. 1987; DCH RCP Lond. 1992; DRCOG 1992; MFHom 2004.

THOMPSON, Michael Alexander Gateways, Church Lane, Stanway, Colchester CO3 8LR — MB BS Lond. 1970 (Guy's) MRCS Eng. LRCP Lond. 1970; MRCP (U.K.) 1975; FFA RCS Eng. 1976. Cons. Dept. Anaesth. Guy's Hosp.; Fell. Roy. Soc. Med. & Med. Soc. Lond. Specialty: Anaesth. Prev: Regtl. Med. Off. 3rd Bn. Roy. Regt. of Fusiliers; Trainee (Anaesth.) Brit. Milit. Hosp. Rinteln; Specialist in Anaesth. Roy. Herbert Hosp. Woolwich.

THOMPSON, Michael Ernest 21 Gardenfield, Skellingthorpe, Lincoln LN6 5SP Tel: 01522 684084 — MB ChB Sheff. 1968; DObst RCOG 1970; MRCGP 1975; FFOM RCP Lond. 1994, MFOM 1982, AFOM 1980; DIH Eng. 1982. Cons. Occupat. Phys. Specialty: Occupat. Health. Socs: Soc. Occupat. Med. Prev: Cons. Occupat. Med. Lincoln Hosps. NHS Trust; Area Med. Off. Brit. Rail Doncaster; Clin. Asst. (Diabetes) Doncaster Roy. Infirm.

THOMPSON, Mr Michael Harrison Southmead Hospital, Department of Surgery, Southmead, Bristol BS10 5NB Tel: 0117 959 5163 Fax: 0117 959 5168 — MB BS Newc. 1968; FRCS Eng. 1973; MD Newc. 1979. Cons. Surg. Southmead Hosp. Bristol. Specialty: Gen. Surg. Special Interest: Biliary Dis. Socs: Assn. Endoscopic Surgs. Prev: Lect. (Surg.) Univ. Bristol.

THOMPSON, Michael Hugh Luton & Dunstable Hospital, Dunstable Road, Luton LU4 0DZ Tel: 01582 491122 Fax: 01582 497280; 8 Green Close, Stanbridge, Leighton Buzzard LU7 9JL Tel: 01525 210478 — BM BCh Oxf. 1973; FRCP; FRCPCH; DCH Eng. 1977; MRCP (UK) 1977. Cons. Paediat. Luton & Dunstable Hosp. Specialty: Paediat. Prev: Sen. Regist. (Paediat.) Roy. Alexandra Childr. Hosp. Brighton; Sen. Regist. (Paediat.) King's Coll. Hosp. Lond.

THOMPSON, Michael Joseph Glebe House Surgery, 19 Firby Road, Bedale DL8 2AT Tel: 01677 422616 Fax: 01677 424596 — MB ChB Leic. 1985; MRCGP 1989; DRCOG 1989; Cert. Family Plann. JCC 1989. Specialty: Gen. Pract.

THOMPSON, Mr Michael Reginald Queen Alexandra, Cosham Hospital, Portsmouth Tel: 023 92 286710 Fax: 02392 286710; 5 Teapot Row, Clocktower Drive, Southsea PO4 9YA Tel: 023 92 756938 Fax: 01705 838170 — (Sheff.) MB ChB Sheff. 1966; FRCS Eng. 1971; MD Sheff. 1980. Cons. Surg. Qu. Alexandra Hosp. Portsmouth. Specialty: Gen. Surg.; Gastroenterol. Socs: Fell. (Counc. Mem.) Roy. Soc. Med. (Sec. Sect. Coloproctol.); Brit. Soc. Gastroenterol. (Sec); Assn of ColoProctol. GB+I (Sec). Prev: Sen. Regist. (Gen. Surg.) Bristol Roy. Infirm.; Regist. (Surg.) Roy. Infirm. Sheff.; Lect. (Surg.) Univ. Manch.

THOMPSON, Michael Robert Northland Surgery, 79 Cunninghams Lane, Dungannon BT71 6BX Tel: 028 8772 752 Fax: 028 8772 7696; 7 Riverdale, Tamnamore, Dungannon BT71 6PZ Tel: 01868 723126 Email: mthom80931@aol.com — MB BCh BAO Belf. 1984; MB BCh Belf. BAO 1984; MRCGP 1991.

THOMPSON, Michael William Benedict Portslade Health Centre, Church Road, Portslade, Brighton BN41 1LX Tel: 01273 422525 Fax: 01273 413510 — MB BS Lond. 1987 (Char. Cross & Westm. Med. Sch. Lond.) DCH 1990; DRCOG 1991; MRCGP 1992; T(GP) 1993; DTM & H 1993.

THOMPSON, Mr Neill Stuart 8 Greystown Avenue, Belfast BT9 6UJ — MB BCh BAO Belf. 1990; FRCS Ed. 1994.

THOMPSON, Nichola Jane Magrathea, 51 Woodham Waye, Woking GU21 5SJ — MB ChB Bristol 1974; DCH Eng. 1980.

THOMPSON, Nicholas Montgomery House Surgery, Piggy Lane, Bicester OX26 6HT Tel: 01869 249222; 22 West End, Launton, Bicester OX26 5DF Tel: 01869 321366 Fax: 01869 249888 Email: nickthompson@pgec-horton.demon.co.uk — MB BS Lond. 1972 (Middlx.) DObst RCOG 1974; DCH Eng. 1975; MRCGP 1978; FRCGP 1999. Course Organiser Banbury VTS Oxf. Region.

THOMPSON, Nicholas Paul Dept. of Medicine, Freeman Hospital, Newcastle upon Tyne NE7 7DN Tel: 0191 284 3111 Fax: 0191 223 1249 Email: nick.thompson@tfh.nuth.northy.nhs.uk — MB BS Lond. 1987 (St. Bart.) MRCP (UK) 1990; MD Lond. 1996; FRCP 2001. Cons. (Gastroenterol. & Gen. Phys.) Newc. Upon Tyne. Specialty: Gastroenterol. Socs: Brit. Soc. Gastroenterol. Prev: Clin. Research Fell. Roy. Free Hosp. Med. Sch.; Sen. Regist. (Gastroenterol.) Newc.

THOMPSON, Norris Ferguson Doctors Surgery, 18 Union Street, Kirkintilloch, Glasgow G66 1DH Tel: 0141 776 1238 Fax: 0141 775 2786; Glengyle, 4 Douglas Avenue, Lenzie, Kirkintilloch, Glasgow G66 4NU Tel: 0141 776 2778 — MB ChB Glas. 1965; FRCGP 1994, M 1974. Assoc. Adviser (Gen. Pract.) Glas.; Hon. Clin. Sen. Lect. Univ. Glas. Prev: Ho. Phys. & Ho. Surg. West. Infirm. Glas.

THOMPSON, Patricia Diane (retired) 218 Christchurch Road, Newport NP19 8BJ — MRCS Eng. LRCP Lond. 1964 (Sheff.) Prev: GP Caerphilly M. GLam.

THOMPSON, Patricia Mary (retired) 1 Embankment Gardens, London SW3 — MRCS Eng. LRCP Lond. 1952 (Roy. Free) MRCS Eng. LRCP Lond. (Feb.) 1952.

THOMPSON, Paul Consultant Psychiatrist, Argyll and Bute Hospital, Lochgilphead PA31 8LD Tel: 01546 602323 — MB Camb. 1987; PhD Leeds 1982, BSc (Hons.) 1978; BChir 1986; MRCPsych 1993. Cons. Psychiat. Specialty: Gen. Psychiat. Special Interest: Old Age Psychiat.

THOMPSON, Paul Northumberland House, 4337 Stourport Rd, Kidderminster DY11 7BL; 12 Imperial Avenue, Kidderminster DY10 2RA — MB BS Lond. 1994 (London Hospital) DRCOG; MRCCGP.

THOMPSON, Paul Warren Department of Rheumatology, Poole General Hospital, Poole BH15 2JB Tel: 01202 442123 Fax: 01202 660147 Email: xad90@dial.pipex.com — MD Lond. 1990; MB BS 1977; MRCP (UK) 1982; FRCP 1996. Cons. Rheum. & Rehabil. Poole Gen. Hosp.; Hon. Sen. Lect. Roy. Lond. Hosp. Med. Coll. Specialty: Rehabil. Med.; Rheumatol. Socs: Brit. Soc. Rheum.; Amer. Coll. Rheum.; Roy. Soc. Med. Prev: Sen. Lect. (Rheum.) Lond. Hosp. Med. Coll. Lond.; Sen. Regist. (Rheum.) Lond. Hosp. Whitechapel.; ARC Research Fell. (Lond. Hosp.).

THOMPSON, Penelope Jane Bell House, Grand Bouet, St Peter Port, Guernsey GY1 2SB; St Leonards, Les Eturs, Castel, Guernsey GY5 7DT — MB ChB Sheff. 1980; MRCP (UK) 1984; MRCPsych 1989. Cons. Child & Adolesc. Psychiat. States of Guernsey. Specialty: Child & Adolesc. Psychiat. Prev: Cons. Child & Adolesc. Psychiat. Pk. Hosp. Oxf.

THOMPSON, Peter c/o Ellison Unit, Bensham Hospital, Bensham, Gateshead NE8 4YL Tel: 0191 402 6680 — MB BS Newc. 1980; FRCPsych 1995, M 1984. Cons. Psychiat. (Psychogeriat.) N. RHA; Hon. Clin. Lect. Univ. Newc. Specialty: Geriat. Psychiat. Socs: BMA.

Prev: Sen. Regist. (Psychiat.) North. RHA; Regist. & SHO (Psychiat.) Newc. HA.

THOMPSON, Peter David 7 Park View, Kingsmark, Chepstow NP16 5NA Tel: 01291 623643 Email: thomopd@aol.com — MB ChB Bristol 1966; DObst RCOG 1968; MRCGP 1976. Prev: SHO (Thoracic Surg.) Frenchay Hosp. Bristol; Ho. Phys. Bristol Roy. Infirm.

THOMPSON, Peter John 154 Grand Drive, Raynes Park, London SW20 9LZ — MB BS Lond. 1985; MRCOG 1993. Sen. Regist. (O & G) Roy. Free Hosp. Lond. Specialty: Obst. & Gyn. Prev: MRC Research Fell. (Pennatol.) Kings Coll. Hosp. Lond.

THOMPSON, Peter John St Melor Surgery, St Melor House, Edwards Road, Amesbury, Salisbury SP4 7LT Tel: 01980 622474 Fax: 01980 622475 — MB BS Lond. 1976 (Univ. Coll. Hosp.) BDS Lond. 1968; FDS RCS Eng. 1972; MRCS Eng. LRCP Lond. 1976; DRCOG 1980. Socs: BMA. Prev: SHO (O & G) Plymouth Gen. Hosp.; Ho. Phys. Bromley Hosp.; Ho. Surg. FarnBoro. Hosp. Kent.

THOMPSON, Mr Peter John McKim Wier Cottage, Millbank, Fladbury, Pershore WR10 2QA — MB ChB Birm. 1992; FRCS 1997. Specialist Regist. (Orthop.) NW Thames Rotat. Specialty: Orthop. Prev: SHO Northwick Pk. Hosp. Harrow; Neurosurg. SHO Qu. Sq. Lond.; Gen. Surg. SHO Chase Farm Hosp. Enfield.

THOMPSON, Mr Peter Kenneth 50 Gloucester Terrace, London W2 3HH Tel: 020 7723 0517 Email: peter.k.thompson@kingsch.nhs.uk; Pitt Cottage, Bowling Green Close, Putney Heath, London SW15 3TE Tel: 020 8788 7815 — MB BS Lond. 1990 (Lond. Hosp. Med. Coll.) BSc (Hons.) Lond. 1987; FRCS Ed. 1994. Clin. Fell. (Intrathoracic Transpl.) St. Geo. Hosp. Lond. Specialty: Cardiothoracic Surg. Socs: Med. Protec. Soc.; Roy. Soc. Med. Prev: SHO (Cardiothoracic) Middlx. Hosp. Lond.; SHO (Vasc. Surg.) St. Mary's Hosp. Lond.; Ho. Phys. (Cardiol. & Gen. Med.) Roy. Lond. Hosp. Whitechapel.

THOMPSON, Mr Peter Melville, RD Department of Urology, Kings College Hospital, Denmark Hill, London SE5 9RS Tel: 0207 737 4000; 7 Crescent Place, London SW3 2EA Tel: 020 7352 1301 Fax: 020 7352 1310 Email: pmturology@aol.com — MB BS Lond. 1970 (Kings Coll. Hosp.) MRCS Eng. LRCP Lond. 1970; FRCS Eng. 1975. Cons. Urol. Surg. Kings Health Care Trust Hosps. Specialty: Urol. Socs: Fell. Roy. Soc. Med.; Brit. Assn. Urol. Surgs.; Brit. Med. Assn. Prev: Sen. Regist. (Urol.) King's Coll. Hosp. Lond.; Sen. Regist. (Surgic.) Baragwanath Hosp. Johannesburg, S. Afr; Regist. (Surg.) King's Coll. Hosp. Lond.

THOMPSON, Peter Wentworth, MBE (retired) 58 John Batchelor Way, Penarth CF64 1SD Tel: 029 2070 3418 — MB BChir Camb. 1949 (Camb. & St. Geo.) MRCS Eng. LRCP Lond. 1949; FRCA. 1953; DA Eng. 1953. Prev: Cons. (Anaesth.) Univ. Hosp. Wales Cardiff.

THOMPSON, Petrie Bourne 119 Haberdasher Street, London N1 6EH Tel: 020 7608 2965; 71 Oldfield Road, London N16 0RR Tel: 020 7249 3725 — MB BS Lond. 1976 (Univ. Coll. Hosp.) MRCPsych 1983. Psychiat. Adviser Inner City Centre Lond. Specialty: Psychother. Prev: Sen. Regist. Cassel Hosp.; Regist. Maudsley Hosp.

THOMPSON, Philip Michael 3 Queen Anne's Gardens, London W4 1TU — MB BS Lond. 1996; MRCP. 1999; MA. 1999. Specialist Regist. (Radiol.). Specialty: Radiol.

THOMPSON, Rachel Elizabeth (retired) Northgate House, 1 Upper Northgate St, Chester CH1 4EE Tel: 01244 342977 — MRCS Eng. LRCP Lond. 1952. Prev: GP Chester.

THOMPSON, Ralph Cecil William (retired) 37 Marine Parade, Dovercourt, Harwich CO12 3RG Tel: 01255 502791 — (Guy's) MB BS Lond. 1944; DA Eng. 1952; FFA RCS Eng. 1954. Hon. Cons. Char. Cross Hosp. Lond. Prev: Cons. (Anaesth.) Roy. Masonic Hosp. Lond.

THOMPSON, Richard Charles Fernyhough Priory Medical Group, Cornlands Road, Acomb, York YO24 3WX Tel: 01904 781423 Fax: 01904 784886 — BM BS Nottm. 1989.

THOMPSON, Richard Damian Queen Elizabeth Hospital, Birmingham B15 2TH — MB BS Lond. 1992; BSc (Physiol.) Lond. 1989; MRCP (UK) 1995; PhD Lond. 2002. Cons. Phys. Qu. Eliz. Hosp. Birm. Specialty: Respirat. Med.; Gen. Med.

THOMPSON, Richard James The Old Rectory, Stapleford Tawney, Romford RM4 1TD — BM BS Nottm. 1993; BMedSci 1991; FRCS Eng. 1997. Specialty: Paediat. Surg.

THOMPSON, Richard John Glenview, 341 Crystal Palace Road, E. Dulwich, London SE22 9JL — BM BCh Oxf. 1987; MRCP (UK) 1994. Research Fell. (Paediat.) Univ. Coll. Lond. Med. Sch. Specialty: Paediat. Socs: Brit. Paediat. Assn. Prev: Lect. (Paediat.) UCL Med. Sch. 1994-1995.

THOMPSON, Richard John Bridgewater Family Medical Practice, Drumcarrig, Bridgwater St., Whitchurch SY13 1QH Tel: 01948 662128 Fax: 01948 666550; Heatherfield House, Hollins Lane, Tilstock, Whitchurch SY13 3NT Tel: 01948 880480 Email: r.thompson@freeuk.com — MB ChB Birm. 1979; DRCOG 1982; Cert. Family Plann. JCC 1982; MRCGP 1984. Hosp. Pract. Shrops. HA; Med. Adviser WhitCh. Community Hosp.; Dep. Police Surg. W. Mercia Police. Specialty: Gen. Pract.

THOMPSON, Richard Norman John Bradbury Medical Practice, 10-12 Lisburn Road, Belfast BT9 6AA Tel: 028 9032 3035 — MB BCh BAO Belf. 1985.

THOMPSON, Sir Richard Paul Hepworth St Thomas' Hospital, London SE1 7EH Tel: 020 7188 2504 Fax: 020 7188 2510 Email: richard.thompson@kcl.ac.uk; 36 Dealtry Road, London SW15 6NL Tel: 020 8789 3839 Fax: 020 8788 3492 — (Oxf. & St. Thos.) BA Oxford 1962; BM BCh Oxf. 1964; FRCP Lond. 1979, M 1966; MA, DM Oxf. 1971. Cons. Phys. St. Thos. Hosp. Lond.; Phys. to HM the Qu.; Hon. Phys. King Edwd. VII Hosp. Offs.; Treas. Roy. Coll. Physicians, Lond. Specialty: Gastroenterol.; Gen. Med. Prev: Phys. to HM Household; MRC Clin. Research Fell. & Hon. Lect. Med. Liver Unit Kings Coll. Hosp. Lond.; Research Asst. Gastroenterol. Unit Mayo Clinc Rochester, USA.

THOMPSON, Richard Stewart The Old Laundry, Neatishead, Norwich NR12 8AD — MRCS Eng. LRCP Lond. 1969.

THOMPSON, Richard William Graham St Thomas Surgery, Rifleman Lane, St. Thomas Green, Haverfordwest SA61 1QX Tel: 01437 762162 Fax: 01437 776811; Fox Hollow, RHOS, Haverfordwest SA62 4AU — ChB Birm. 1986; DCH RCP Lond. 1989; Cert. Family Plann. JCC 1992; DRCOG 1992; MRCGP 1993. Specialty: Gen. Pract. Socs: Roy. Coll. Gen. Practitioners.

THOMPSON, Robert John (retired) The Plough, The Street, Guston, Dover CT15 5ET — MRCS Eng. LRCP Lond. 1971; FFA RCS Eng. 1975. Sen. Regist. (Anaesth.) St. Bart. Hosp. Lond.; Specialist (Anaesth.) Academisch Ziekenhuis Groningen Netherlands; Cons. (Anaesth.) East Kent Hospitals Trust. Prev: Regist. (Anaesth.) Salisbury Health Dist.

THOMPSON, Robert Martin The Kennels, Middle Lane, Hutton Buscel, Scarborough YO13 9LS Tel: 01723 863594 — MB BS Lond. 1980; DRCOG 1982.

THOMPSON, Robert Miles Hawthorn, New Road, Old Snydale, Pontefract WF7 6HE — MB BS Lond. 1977.

THOMPSON, Robert Noel Department of Rheumatology, Aintree Hospitals NHS Trust, Liverpool L9 7AL Tel: 0151 529 3341; 12 Riverbank Road, Heswall, Wirral CH60 4SG Tel: 0151 342 8457 — MB BCh BAO NUI 1973; MRCP (UK) 1980; FRCP Lond. 1992. Cons. Rheum. Univ. Hosp. Aintree Liverp.; Clin. Dir. (Rheum.) Univ. Hosp. Aintree Liverp. Specialty: Rheumatol.; Gen. Med. Socs: Brit. Soc. Rheum. Prev: Fell. Rheum. Univ. Alberta, Canada; Sen. Regist. (Rheum. & Rehabil.) Manch. Univ. Rheum. Dis. Centre, Hope, Withington & Roy. Infirm. Manch.

THOMPSON, Robert Tester The Surgery, 59 Sevenoaks Road, Orpington BR6 9JN Tel: 01689 820159; 59 Sevenoaks Road, Orpington BR6 9JN Tel: 01689 20159 — MB BS Lond. 1978 (Guy's) DRCOG 1982; MRCGP 1983.

THOMPSON, Rodney Julian Wesley The Grange, 7 The Orchards, Four Oaks, Sutton Coldfield B74 2PP — MB ChB Birm. 1976; MRCGP 1983.

THOMPSON, Roger Woodseats Medical Centre, 4 Cobnar Road, Woodseats, Sheffield S8 8QB Tel: 0114 274 0202 Fax: 0114 274 6835; Owl End, Dore Moor Est., Newfield Lane, Sheffield S17 3DB — MB ChB Sheff. 1971.

THOMPSON, Roger Humphrey Leech Meadow Cottage, Sheinton, Cressage, Shrewsbury SY5 6DN — MB BS Lond. 1967 (Lond. Hosp.)

THOMPSON, Roger Martin The Marches Surgery, Drs Thompson, Knight, Knight, Fisher, Edwards & Wall, Westfield Walk, Leominster HR6 8HD Tel: 01568 614141; Pound House, Brockmanton, Leominster HR6 0QU Tel: 01568 760606 — MB BS Lond. 1973 (Lond. Hosp.) DObst RCOG 1975; MRCGP 1977. Specialty: Gen. Pract. Prev: Trainee GP Preston VTS; Ho. Phys. Bethnal Green Hosp.; Ho. Surg. (Cardiothoracic Surg.) Lond. Hosp.

THOMPSON, Professor Ronald Augustine, MBE, TD (retired) 37 Grange Hill Road, Kings Norton, Birmingham B38 8RE Tel: 0121 458 3549 — MB BS Lond. 1958 (Univ. Coll. Hosp.) BSc (Anat.) Lond. 1955; MRCS Eng. LRCP Lond. 1958; FRCP Lond. 1979, M 1963; FRCPath 1981, M 1971. Prev: Cons. Immunol. E. Birm. Hosp.

THOMPSON, Ronald Leslie Ernest Altnagelvin Hospital, Glenshane Road, Londonderry BT47 6SB; North West Independent Hospital, Church Hill House, Ballykelly, Londonderry BT49 9HS — MB BCh BAO Belf. 1981. Cons. Surg. Altnagelvin Area Hosp. Londonderry. Specialty: Gen. Surg. Special Interest: Breast Surg.; Laparoscopic Surg. Socs: Brit. Assn. Surgic. Oncol.

THOMPSON, Ruth Elizabeth — MB ChB Dundee 1997.

THOMPSON, Sara Anne Station Road Surgery, 24 Station Road, Long Buckby, Northampton NN6 7QB Tel: 01327 842360 Fax: 01327 842302; Bridge House, Murcott, Long Buckby, Northampton NN6 7QR Tel: 01327 842850 — MB BS Newc. 1982; MRCGP 1986; DRCOG 1986. Trainer GP Northampton. Specialty: Gen. Pract.

THOMPSON, Sharon Elizabeth 38 Kilnford Drive, Dundonald, Kilmarnock KA2 9ET — MB ChB Aberd. 1995.

THOMPSON, Shirley Margaret Creighton (retired) Cherry Cottage, 5 The Square, Kenilworth CV8 1EF Tel: 01926 59996 — MB BS Durh. 1950. Prev: Clin. Asst. (Psychiat.) S. Warks. Hosp. Gp.

THOMPSON, Simon Abington Health Complex, Doctors Surgery, 51A Beech Avenue, Northampton NN3 2JG Tel: 01604 791999 Fax: 01604 450155 — MB ChB Aberd. 1982; MRCGP 1986; DRCOG 1986. Socs: BMA.

THOMPSON, Simon David Risca Surgery, St. Mary Street, Risca, Newport NP11 6YS Tel: 01633 612666 — MB BS Lond. 1979; MRCGP 1984.

THOMPSON, Simon Gower Amersham Health Centre, Chiltern Avenue, Amersham HP6 5AY Tel: 01494 434344; 54 Hogg Lane, Holmer Green, High Wycombe HP15 6PZ — MRCS Eng. LRCP Lond. 1972 (Guy's) MRCGP 1979.

THOMPSON, Simon Patrick Ringwood Health Centre, The Close, Ringwood BH24 1JY Tel: 01425 478901 Fax: 01425 478239; 24 Gravel Lane, Ringwood BH24 1LN — MB BS Lond. 1981 (St Thomas') DRCOG 1986. Prev: Trainee GP Salisbury; SHO (Cas. Orthop.) Derby Roy. Infirm.; Ho. Phys. Salisbury Gen. Infirm.

THOMPSON, Mr Stanley Graham, RD (retired) Abbey House, Great Massingham, King's Lynn PE32 2JG Fax: 01485 520254 — MB BS Lond. 1953 (St. Bart.) FRCS Eng. 1961. Prev: Cons. Surg. W. Norf. & Wisbech HA.

THOMPSON, Stephen John 2 St Nicholas Drive, Whitesmocks, Durham DH1 4HH — MB BS Newc. 1985. Regist. (Histopath.) Newc. Gen. Hosp. Specialty: Histopath.

THOMPSON, Mr Stephen Keith Fairfield Cottage, Croft Drive E., Caldy, Wirral CH48 1LS Tel: 0151 625 9081 — MB ChB Liverp. 1968; FRCS Ed. 1973; MChOrth Liverp. 1976. Cons. Orthop. Surg. Roy. Liverp. Hosp. & Warrington Dist. Gen.; Regist. (Orthop. Surg.) Liverp. AHA (T). Specialty: Orthop.

THOMPSON, Stephen William Waterloo Medical Centre, 178 Waterloo Road, Blackpool FY4 3AD — MB ChB Manch. 1991.

THOMPSON, Mr Stuart David 35 Bridle Road, Wollaston, Stourbridge DY8 4QE — MB BS Lond. 1989; FRCS Ed. 1994. Clin. Research Fell. (Surg.) Univ. Hosp. Edgbaston. Specialty: Otolaryngol.

THOMPSON, Susan Mary 16 Meadow Brook Road, Birmingham B31 1NE — MB ChB Birm. 1972; FRCS Eng. 1981; FRCOphth 1992. Cons. Ophth. Dudley & Sandwell HAs. Specialty: Ophth.

THOMPSON, Susan Mary 144-150 High Road, Willesden, London NW10 2PT Tel: 020 8459 5550; 27 Asmuns Hill, London NW11 6ES Tel: 020 8455 1731 — MB BS Lond. 1980; MRCGP 1985.

THOMPSON, Sylvia Ann Sussex Place Surgery, 63 Sussex Place, Bristol BS2 9QR Tel: 0117 955 6275 Fax: 0117 955 8666 — MB BCh BAO Belf. 1984; MB BCh Belf. 1984; MRCGP 1990.

THOMPSON, Terence Joseph 2 Shelley Grove, Southport PR8 6HA — MB BCh BAO NUI 1984.

THOMPSON, Thomas Roy (retired) East House, Shoreston Hall, Seahouses NE68 7SX Tel: 01665 720052 — MB BS Durh. 1952. Prev: Mentioned in Despatches 1955.

THOMPSON, Timothy Mark Thatcham Medical Practice, Bath Road, Thatcham RG18 3HD Tel: 01635 67171 — MB BS Lond. 1973; DObst RCOG 1975; MRCGP 1977.

THOMPSON, Trevor David Barnes 20 Milner Road, Glasgow G13 1QL Tel: 0141 954 9326 Email: doctortrev@bigfoot.com — MB BS Lond. 1990 (Oxford and St. Mary's) BA Oxf. 1986; DRCOG 1992; MRCGP 1995; MFHom 1996. Higher Professional Train. Fell. Univ. of Glas.; Dir. MIRTH! Internet Consultancy Phys. (Homoeopathy). Specialty: Homeop. Med.; Gen. Pract. Prev: Clin. Researcher Glas. Homoeop. Hosp.; SHO (Homoeop.) Glas. Homoeop. Hosp.

THOMPSON, Trevor Henry Raymond Ely Bridge Surgery, 23 Mill Road, Ely, Cardiff CF5 4AD Tel: 029 2056 1808 Fax: 029 2057 8871 — MB BCh Wales 1981; DRCOG 1984; MRCGP 1986.

THOMPSON, Trevor Joseph 30 Rathmena Avenue, Ballyclare BT39 9HX — MB BCh BAO Belf. 1990; MB BCh Belf. 1990.

THOMPSON, Valerie The Barn, Church Walks, Christleton, Chester CH3 7AF — LLB Southampton 1975 (Liverpool) MB ChB Liverp. 1996. GP Regist. Bunbury Med. Pract. Specialty: Pathology, General. Prev: SHO Rotat. (Surg.) Liverp. & Chester.

THOMPSON, Valerie Mary (retired) The Fieldings, Papermill Lane, South Moreton, Didcot OX11 9AH — (Roy. Free) MB BS Lond. 1948; MRCS Eng. LRCP Lond. 1948; FRCOG 1969, M 1953; FRCS Eng. 1958. Prev: Cons. Gyn. Roy. Free Hosp.

THOMPSON, Wendy Christine Ruby 31 Girdlers Road, London W14 0PS — MB BS Lond. 1986.

THOMPSON, William 14 Avon Close, The Bryn Estate, Pontllanfraith, Blackwood NP12 2GB — MB BCh Wales 1983.

THOMPSON, William Department Obstetrics & Gynaecology, Institute of Clinical Science, Grosvenor Road, Belfast BT12 6BJ Tel: 01232 894600 Fax: 01232 328247 Email: w.thompson@qub.ac.uk — (Qus. Univ. Belf.) MB BCh BAO (Hons.) 1961; DObst RCPI 1963; FRCOG 1980, M 1967; BSc (Hons.) Belf. 1958, MD 1975. Prof. O & G Qu. Univ. Belf.; Cons. Obst. Roy. Matern. Hosp. Belf.; Cons. Gyn. Roy. Vict. Hosp. Belf.; Cons. Obst. & Gyn. Belf. City Hosp. Specialty: Obst. & Gyn. Socs: Treas. Internat. Federat. Fertil. Soc.; Brit. Fertil. Soc.; Brit. Menopause Soc. Prev: Lect. (O & G) Kandang Kerbau Hosp., Univ. Singapore.

THOMPSON, Mr William Arthur Lisle, TD (retired) 22 Fford Llechi, Rhosneigr LL64 5JY Tel: 01407 810505 — (Liverp.) MChOrth Liverp. 1956, MB ChB 1947; FRCS Ed. 1955. Prev: Cons. Orthop. Surg. Walton & Fazakerley Hosps. Liverp.

THOMPSON, William Bruce Church Walk Surgery, 28 Church Walk, Lurgan, Craigavon BT67 9AA Tel: 028 3832 7834 Fax: 028 3834 9331 — MB BS Lond. 1985 (St Bart.) DCH Dub. 1989; MRCGP 1990; DRCOG 1990; Dip. Sports Med. Scotl. 1993; FFSEM (RSI) 2002. General Practitioner; Lect. Univ. of Ulster; Clin. Asst. Orthops. & Sports Med. Craigavon Area Hosp. Portadown. Specialty: Orthop.; Sports Med.; Gen. Pract.; Orthopaedic Medicine. Special Interest: Orthopaedic & Sports Medicine. Socs: Amer. Coll. Sports Med.; Soc. Orthopaedic Med. Lond. 1997 (Fellow); Brit. Assn. Sport & Exercise Med.

THOMPSON, William David North Tees General Hospital, Stockton-on-Tees TS19 8PE Tel: 01642 617617 — MB BS Newc. 1980 (Newc. u. Tyne) MRCP (UK) 1983; FRCR 1987; FRCP Ed. 1995. Cons. Radiol. Cleveland. Specialty: Radiol. Socs: Brit. Med. Ultrasound Soc. Prev: Sen. Regist. & Regist. (Radiol.) Newc.

THOMPSON, William Douglas Department of Pathology, Medical School, Aberdeen Royal Infirmary, Aberdeen AB25 2ZD Tel: 01224 681818 Fax: 01224 663002; East Law, Durno, Pitcaple, Inverurie AB51 5EU Tel: 0146 76 681401 — MB ChB Glas. 1970; FRCPath 1990, M 1978; PhD Glas. 1981; DSc Aberd. 1996. Sen. Lect. (Path.) Aberd. Roy. Infirm. Specialty: Histopath. Socs: Path. Soc.; Brit. Atherosclerosis Soc.; Internat. Fibrinogen Research Soc. Prev: Lect. (Path.) Glas. Roy. Infirm.

THOMPSON, William Joseph (retired) The Margaret Thompson Medical Centre, 105 East Millwood Road, Speke, Liverpool L24 6TH Tel: 0151 425 3339 Fax: 0151 425 2272; 43 Danford Lane, Solihull B91 1QD Tel: 0121 704 1645 — (Liverp.) MB ChB Liverp. 1961; DTM & H Liverpool 2000. Prev: Ho. Surg. & Ho. Phys. & SHO (O & G) Walton Hosp. Liverp.

THOMPSON, William Michael Cardiff Community Healthcare Trust, Ely Hospital, Cowbridge Road W., Cardiff CF2 5DW Tel: 029 2056 2323 Fax: 029 2055 5047 — MB BCh Wales 1989. Sen. Regist. (Learning Disabilities) Cardiff Community Healthcare Trust. Specialty: Ment. Health.

THOMPSON, William Stanley (retired) 395 Sandyfields Road, Lower Gornal, Dudley DY3 3DJ Tel: 01902 882938 — LRCP LRCS Ed. LRFPS Glas. 1951.

THOMS, Gavin Malcolm Macthomas Department of Anaesthesia, Manchester Royal Infirmary, Oxford Road, Manchester M13 9WL Tel: 0161 276 4551 Fax: 0161 273 5685 Email: gavin.thoms@man.ac.uk; 1 Hungry Lane, Bradwell, Hope Valley S33 9JD — MB ChB Ed. 1971; DCH Eng. 1973; FRCA 1976; MSc Manch. 1985; MFPHM 1985; FFPHM 1998. Cons. Anaesth. Manch. Roy. Infirm.; Hon. Sen. Research Fell. (Anaesth.) Manch. Univ. Specialty: Anaesth.; Epidemiol. Socs: Assn. of Anaesth.s; Soc. Computing & Technol. in Anaesth.; Assn. Anesth. Clin. Directors. Prev: Sen. Research Fell. Manch. Univ.; Director of Pub. Health Manch. Health Auth.; Sen. Med. Off. Dept. of Health Leeds.

THOMSITT, Mr John (retired) (cons. rooms), 4 Manston Terrace, Exeter EX2 4NP Tel: 01392 435053 Fax: 01392 435301 — MB BS Lond. 1960; FRCS Eng. 1969; FRCOphth 1988. Cons. Ophth. Eng. W. of Eng. Eye Unit Roy. Devon & Exeter Hosp. Wonford. Prev: Sen. Lect. (Clin. Ophth.) Univ. Lond. Moorfields Eye Hosp. Lond.

THOMSON, Mr Adrian Alexander Gordon Underbank House, Charlestown, Hebden Bridge HX7 6PE Tel: 01422 844355 — MB BChir Camb. 1969; MA Camb. 1967; FRCS Eng. 1975. Cons. (Health Managem.) Medico-Legal Ltd. Specialty: Gen. Surg. Prev: Cons. (Gen. Surg.) Rochdale.

THOMSON, Alan Robert The Maltings Family Practice, 10 Victoria Street, St Albans AL1 3JB Tel: 01727 853296 Fax: 01727 862498 — MB BChir Camb. 1986; MA Camb. 1989, BA 1984, MB BChir 1986. Specialty: Gen. Med.

THOMSON, Alan Roderick 41 Braeside Avenue, Aberdeen AB15 7ST — MB ChB Aberd. 1990.

THOMSON, Alan Sinclair Castlehill Health Centre, Castlehill, Forres IV36 1QF Tel: 01309 672221 Fax: 01309 673445; Montana, Nelson Road, Forres IV36 1DR Tel: 01309 673023 — MB ChB Aberd. 1984; BSc Aberd. 1978; MRCGP 1988.

THOMSON, Alan Walter Dr Campbell and Partners, 246 Argyll Street, Dunoon PA23 7HW Tel: 01369 703279 Fax: 01369 704430 — MB ChB Ed. 1976; FFARCSI 1985; MRCGP 1986.

THOMSON, Alasdair James 34 Riversdale, Gravesend DA11 8SR — MB ChB Aberd. 1979.

THOMSON, Alastair Grant Old Town Surgery, 13 De la Warr Road, Bexhill-on-Sea TN40 2HG Tel: 01424 219323 Fax: 01424 733940; The Tall House, Heatherdune Road, Bexhill-on-Sea TN39 4HB Tel: 01424 214385 — MB ChB Bristol 1979; DCH RCP Lond. 1983; MRCGP 1984; DRCOG 1984.

THOMSON, Alastair James Western General Hospital, Crewe Road South, Edinburgh EH4 2XU — MB ChB Ed. 1993 (Edinburgh) MRCP (UK) 1996; FRCA 1999. Specialist Regist. (Anaesth.) Edin.; Research Fell. Dept. of Med. Sci. Univ. of Edin. Specialty: Anaesth. Prev: SHO (Anaesth.) Glas.; SHO (Med.) Edin.

THOMSON, Alexander McFarlane 53 New Abbey Road, Dumfries DG2 7LZ — MB ChB Manch. 1998.

THOMSON, Alison Jean Abbotswood, Gattonside, Melrose TD6 9NS Tel: 0189 682 2754 — MB ChB Ed. 1966 (Edin.) DObst RCOG 1968; MRCP (UK) 1972; FRCP Ed. 1984. Specialty: Paediat. Socs: Scott. Paediat. Soc. & Brit. Paediat. Soc. Prev: Sen. Regist. (Paediat.) Roy. Aberd. Childr. Hosp.; Regist. (Paediat.) Edin. North. Hosp. Gp.; Resid. Hosp. Sick Childr. Toronto, Canada.

THOMSON, Alison Jean Marin Ancrum Medical Centre, 12-14 Ancrum Road, Dundee DD2 2HZ Tel: 01382 669316 Fax: 01382 660787; Beach Cottage, 71 Beach Crescent, Broughty Ferry, Dundee DD5 2BG Tel: 01382 730321 Email: alison.thompson@blueyonder.co.uk — MB ChB Dundee 1981; DRCOG 1984. GP Tayside. Prev: Med. Off. E. Scotl. Blood Transfus. Serv. Dundee.

THOMSON, Alison Joyce Midlock Medical Centre, 7 Midlock Street, Glasgow G51 1SL Tel: 0141 427 4271 Fax: 0141 427 1405 — MB ChB Glas. 1984; MRCGP 1989. Gen. Practitioner - Princip.

THOMSON, Alistair David — MB ChB Glas. 1981; MRCGP 1984; Cert. Prescribed Equiv. Exp. JCPTGP 1986; Cert. Family Plann. JCC 1988; DFFP 1993. Socs: Assn. Course Organisers.

THOMSON, Alistair Park (retired) 1 Albion Terrace, Saltburn-by-the-Sea TS12 1JW — MB ChB Glas. 1959; CIH Dund 1978; DIH Soc. Apoth. Lond. 1979; MFOM RCP Lond. 1980. Prev: Wilton Area Med. Off. Teeside Operat. ICI, C & P plc Cleveland.

THOMSON, Alistair Peter James Leighton Hospital, Crewe CW1 4QJ Tel: 01270 612289; 2 The Avenue, Alsager, Stoke-on-Trent ST7 2AN Tel: 01270 873569 — MB BChir Camb. 1977 (King's Coll. Hosp.) DRCOG 1979; DCH Eng. 1980; MRCP (UK) 1981; MD Camb. 1991; FRCP Lond. 1994; FRCPCH 1997. Cons. Paediat. Mid Chesh. Hosps. NHS Trust, Leighton Hosp. Crewe; Hon. Cons. Paediat. Roy. Liverp. Childr. Hosp.; Hon. Clin. Lect. Univ. Liverp.; PostGrad. Clin. Tutor and Director of Med. Educat., Mid Chesh. Hosps & NHS Trust, Crewe.; Hon. Lect. Dept. Med. Micro.Univ. Liverp. Specialty: Paediat. Socs: Nat. Assn. Clin. Tutors (Chair). Prev: Sen. Regist. Rotat. (Paediat.) Mersey RHA; Research Fell. & Hon. Regist. St. Thos. Hosp. Lond.; Regist. St. Thos. Hosp. Lond. & Pembury Hosp.

THOMSON, Andrew (retired) High Corrie, Stanley, Perth PH1 4PG Tel: 01738 828540 — (Edinburgh University) MB ChB Ed. 1950; DObst RCOG 1960; MRCGP 1967. Prev: GP Stanley.

THOMSON, Andrew John Department of Obstetrics & Gynaecology, Royal Alexandra Hospital, Coriebar Road, Paisley PA2 9PN Tel: 0141 580 4275 Fax: 0141 580 4364 Email: andrew.thomson@rah.scot.nhs.uk — MB ChB Glas. 1989 (Glasgow) BSc (Hons) (Pharmacology) 1986; MRCOG 1994; MD (Hons) Glas. 1999. Cons. O & G. Specialty: Obst. & Gyn. Prev: Clin. Lect. in O & G; Specialist Regist.

THOMSON, Andrew McLean MRC Molecular Haematology Unit, Institute of Molecular Medicine, John Radcliffe Hospital, Oxford OX3 9DS Tel: 01865 222395 Fax: 01865 222500 Email: athomson@worf.molbiol.ox.ac.uk; September Cottage, 69B North St, Middle Bacon, Chipping Norton OX7 7BZ Tel: 01869 347649 — MB ChB Glas. 1990; BSc (Hons.) Glas. 1987; DPhil Oxf. 1997. MRC Post Doctoral Research Fell. MRC Molecular Haemat. Unit Inst. Molecular Med. Univ. Oxf. Specialty: Haematology. Prev: Specialist Regist. (Virol.) St. Mary's Hosp. Lond.; SHO (Path.) Stirling Roy. Infirm.; Ho. Off. (Surg.) Stirling Roy. Infirm.

THOMSON, Andrew McMurray Paterson 7 Rannoch Avenue, Bishopbriggs, Glasgow G64 1BU — MB ChB Glas. 1947. Asst. Phys. Stobhill Gen. Hosp. Glas. Specialty: Care of the Elderly.

THOMSON, Andrew Scott The Atherstone Surgery, 1 Ratcliffe Road, Atherstone CV9 1EU Tel: 01827 713664 Fax: 01827 713666; The Firs, Shadows Lane, Congerstone, Nuneaton CV13 6NF — MB ChB Ed. 1987; MRCGP 1993. Prev: SHO (Gen. Pract.) Nuneaton VTS; SHO (Gen. Med.) Geo. Eliot Hosp. Nuneaton.

THOMSON, Angus John Malcolm Arrowe Park Hospital, Upton, Wirral CH49 5PE Tel: 0151 678 5111; 1 Quarry Road West, Heswall, Wirral CH60 6RE Tel: 0151 342 6493 Email: gus@doctors.org.uk — MB ChB Liverp. 1993; DFFP 1997; MRCOG 1999. Specialist Regist. O & G, Mersey Region. Specialty: Obst. & Gyn. Socs: Brit. Fertil. Soc. Prev: Specialist Regist. (O & G) Mersey Deanery N. W. Region.

THOMSON, Anne Helen Department of Paediatics, John Radcliffe Hospital, Headington, Oxford OX3 9DU Tel: 01865 221496 — MD Aberd. 1987; MB ChB 1976; FRCP Lond. 1994. Cons. Paediat. Respirat. Dis. John Radcliffe Hosp. Oxf. Specialty: Paediat. Prev: Lect. (Child Health) Univ. Leic.; Research Fell. (Neonat. Respirat.) Hammersmith Hosp. Lond.

THOMSON, Brian James 22 Lymington Road, London NW6 1HY — MB ChB Ed. 1980; MRCP (UK) 1983; PhD CNAA 1992. MRC Train. Fell. Nat. Inst. for Med. Research Lond.; MRC Clin. Sci. Fell. Addenbrooke's Hosp. Camb. Specialty: Gen. Med. Prev: Regist. (Med.) Roy. Infirm. Edin.

THOMSON, Bruce Ewan (retired) Knoweside, Ferntower Road, Crieff PH7 3DH Tel: 01764 653048 Fax: 01764 653048 — MB BS Lond. 1962 (Lond. Hosp.) MRCS Eng. LRCP Lond. 1962; DObst RCOG 1965; MRCGP 1977; MA Oxf. 1980.

THOMSON, Bruce Forsyth Morrison Lincluden Surgery, 53 Bellshill Road, Uddingston, Glasgow G71 7PA Tel: 01698 813873; 10 Gleneagles Park, Bothwell, Glasgow G71 8UT Tel: 01698 852856 — MB ChB Glas. 1981; DRCOG 1984; MRCGP 1985.

THOMSON, Carl Craggs Farm House, Little Broughton, Cockermouth CA13 0YG Tel: 01900 825244 Fax: 01900 829354 Email: carlthomson@doctors.org.uk — MB ChB Ed. 1967; MRCP (UK) 1970. Specialty: Gen. Med. Prev: Cons. Phys. W. Cumbld. Hosp. Hensingham 1997-1998.

THOMSON, Carolyn Margaret 9 Milton Crescent, Edinburgh EH15 3PF — MB ChB Aberd. 1985.

THOMSON, Catherine Robertson Health Centre, Park Drive, Stenhousemuir, Larbert FK5 3BB Tel: 01324 570570 Fax: 01324 553632 — MB ChB Glasgow 1977. GP Larbert.

THOMSON, Catriona Woodside, Copperas Lane, Haigh, Wigan WN2 1PB — MB ChB Manch. 1989.

THOMSON, Charles Wilson (retired) The Pound, 32 Brookfield Road, East Budleigh, Budleigh Salterton EX9 7EL Tel: 01395 446008 — MB BS Durh. 1953; FFA RCS Eng. 1961.

THOMSON, Christopher Bruce (retired) 584 Bath Road, Bristol BS4 3LE Tel: 0117 971 2132 — MRCS Eng. LRCP Lond. 1956 (Guy's) DIH Dund 1970; FFOM RCP Lond. 1982, MFOM 1979. Prev: Sen. Employm. Med. Adviser Health & Safety Exec.

THOMSON, Clare Mary Meadowside Medical Centre, Meadowside, Mountbatten Way, Congleton CW12 1DY Tel: 01260 272331 Fax: 01260 277964 — MB ChB Manch. 1979; BSc St. And. 1976. Specialty: Diabetes.

THOMSON, Colin Charles Buchanan 24 Longdean Park, Hemel Hempstead HP3 8BZ — BM BCh Oxf. 1998.

THOMSON, Colin Hugh (retired) Troisdorf, Hereford Road, Weobley, Hereford HR4 8SW — MB ChB Ed. 1952. Prev: Ho. Surg. & Ho. Phys. Cumbld. Infirm. Carlisle.

THOMSON, Daniel Ferguson 1 Ledcameroch Crescent, Bearsden, Glasgow G61 4AD Tel: 0141 942 7513 — MB ChB Glas. 1964; FFA RCS Eng. 1968. Cons. (Anaesth.) Vict. Infirm. Glas. Specialty: Anaesth. Prev: Sen. Regist. Glas. Roy. Infirm.; Sen. Specialist Natal Provin. Hosp. Admin. S. Africa.

THOMSON, David Alexander, OBE (retired) Evendine House, Colwall, Malvern WR13 6DT Tel: 01684 540948 — (Glas.) MB ChB Glas. 1938; MRCOG 1948; MRCGP 1958.

THOMSON, David James Ramsay Gibb No. 1 Serjeants Inn, London EC4 Tel: 020 7387 5798 Email: dthomson@no1serjeantsinn.com; 52 Rawstorne Street, London EC1V 7NQ Tel: 020 7278 9251 Email: clerks@barnards_inn_chambers.co.uk — MB ChB Sheff. 1985; LLB (Hons.) 1992; LLM (Hons.) 1993. Barrister at Law; GP Retainer Scheme; Regt. Surg. Inns of Ct. & City of Lond. Yeomanry. Socs: Fell. Roy. Soc. Med.; Med. Pract. Union.; Soc. Doctors in Law. Prev: GP Lond.; SHO (Surg.) Brompton & Roy. Marsden Hosps.; Demonst. & Lect. Leeds Med. & Dent. Sch.

THOMSON, Mr David Stewart 35 Champion Hill, London SE5 8BS — MB ChB Manch. 1977; BSc St. And. 1974; FRCS Eng. 1981. Head Clin. Research Lorex Synthelabo (UK). Specialty: Pharmaceutical Medicine.

THOMSON, Derek Adam Haltwhistle Medical Group, Haltwhistle Health Centre, Greencroft Avenue, Haltwhistle NE49 9AP Tel: 01434 320077 Fax: 01434 320674; Sholl, Fairholme, Comb Hill, Haltwhistle NE49 9EX Tel: 01434 321182 — MB BS Newc. 1983; MRCGP 1988. PEC GP Northd. Care Trust; Med. Director Northumbria Healthcare Trust.

THOMSON, Donald Mark Melven (retired) Pinkacre, Leigh on Mendip, Bath BA3 5LX Tel: 01373 812230 — MB ChB Bristol 1954. Prev: Med. Off. Uganda Med. Dept.

THOMSON, Donald McDonald McKenzie Medical Centre, 20 West Richmond Street, Edinburgh EH8 9DX Tel: 0131 667 2955; 72 Craighall Road, Edinburgh EH6 4RG Tel: 0131 552 5069 — MB ChB Ed. 1971; BSc Ed. 1968; MRCP (UK) 1973; FRCGP 1990, M 1975; FRCP Ed. 1990. Sen. Lect. (Gen. Pract.) Univ. Edin.; Assoc. Dean (Admissions) Fac. Med. Univ. Edin. Specialty: Gen. Pract. Prev: Lect. (Gen. Pract.) Univ. Edin.

THOMSON, Douglas John The Park Medical Practice, Maine Drive Clinic, Maine Drive, Derby DE21 6LA Tel: 01332 665522 Fax: 01332 678210 — MB ChB Glas. 1975.

THOMSON, Mr Douglas Stormonth (retired) 38 Christ Church Road, Cheltenham GL50 2PW Tel: 01242 515932 — (Durh.) MB BS Durh. 1945; DOMS Eng. 1950; FRCS Ed. 1960. Prev: Cons. Ophth. Surg. N. Glos. Clin. Area.

THOMSON, Duncan George c/o 15 Spylaw Bank Road, Colinton, Edinburgh EH13 0JW — MB ChB Aberd. 1987.

THOMSON, Elaine Sheila Wallacetown Health Centre, 3 Lyon Street, Dundee DD4 6RF Tel: 01382 459519 Fax: 01382 453110; Bellfield, 3 Bank Street, Newport-on-Tay DD6 8AU — MB ChB Dundee 1992; DRCOG 1995; DFFP 1995; MRCGP 1996.

THOMSON, Elizabeth Jean (retired) 114 West King Street, Helensburgh G84 8DQ Tel: 01436 672673 — MB ChB Glas. 1963; DObst RCOG 1964; FRCPath 1982, M 1969. Cons. Microbiol. Monklands Hosp. Airdrie. Prev: Cons. Bact. Belvidere Hosp. Glas.

THOMSON, Emma Cassandra 11 Kelvin Dr, Glasgow G20 8QG — MB ChB Glas. 1997.

THOMSON, Fiona Jane Dept. Of Medicine for the Elderly, Hull Royal Infirmary, Anlaby Road, Hull HU3 2JZ — MB ChB Manch. 1984; BSc St. And. 1981; MD Manch. 1992; FRCP 1998. p/t Cons. Phys. (Geriat. Med.) Hull and E. Yorks. Hosps. Trust. Prev: Sen. Regist. (Gen. & Geriat. Med.) Roy. Oldham, Hope & Ladywell Hosps. Salford; Tutor (Gen. & Geriat. Med.) Manch. Roy. Infirm.; SHO (Gen. Med.) Hope Hosp. Salford.

THOMSON, Gail Lindsay Brownlee Centre, Gartnavel General Hospital, Glasgow; 11/5 Queenshill, South Groathill Avenue, Edinburgh EH4 2LL — MB ChB Ed. 1994. SHO (Infect. Dis.) Gartnavel Hosp. Glas. Specialty: Infec. Dis.

THOMSON, Mr Gary George John Bonnyrigg Health Centre, High Street, Bonnyrigg EH19 2DA Tel: 0131 663 7272 — MB ChB Ed. 1977 (Edinburgh) FRCS Ed. 1983. Specialty: Gen. Surg.; Paediat. Surg.

THOMSON, George Alexander Diabetes Unit, The Kings Mill Centre for Health Care Services, Mansfield Road, Sutton-in-Ashfield NG17 4JL Tel: 01623 622515 Ext: 3272 Fax: 01623 672332; 50B Roland Avenue, Nuthall, Nottingham NG16 1BB Tel: 0115 975 7266 — MB ChB Glas. 1988; MB ChB (Commend.) Glas. 1988; MRCP (UK) 1991; FRCS (Edinburgh) 1999. Cons. Phys. (Diabetes & Endocrinol.) The Kings Mill Centre for Health Care Servs. Nottm. Specialty: Gen. Med.; Diabetes; Endocrinol. Socs: Collegiate Mem. Roy. Coll. Phys & Surg. Glas.; FRCP Edin.; Diabetes UK. Prev: Sen. Regist. (Med., Diabetes & Endocrinol.) Univ. Hosp. Nottm.; Sen. Regist. (Med., Diabetes & Endocrinol.) Derbysh. Roy. Infirm.; Career Regist. (Diabetes & Endocrinol.) South. Gen. Hosp. Glas.

THOMSON, George Douthwaite Moore House Lodge, Whalton, Morpeth NE61 3UX — MB BS Durh. 1962.

THOMSON, George Edward Brookside Health Centre, Brookside Road, Freshwater PO40 9DT Tel: 01983 753433 Fax: 01983 753662 — MB BS Lond. 1976. Clin. Asst. (Rheum.) St. Mary's Hosp. Newport, IOW.

THOMSON, George Jeremy (retired) Ravenswood, Tighnabruaich PA21 2EE Tel: 01700 811603 — MB ChB Glas. 1957. Prev: Ho. Phys. Roy. Infirm. Glas.

THOMSON, Mr George John Lyle Royal Preston Hospital, Sharoe Green Lane, Fulwood, Preston PR2 9HT Tel: 01772 716565 Fax: 01772 710315; 16 Oakley Park, Heaton, Bolton BL1 5XL Tel: 01204 843693 Email: geo_thomson@hotmail.com — MB ChB Glas. 1977 (Glasgow) FRCS Glas. 1982; MD Glas. 1989. Cons. Surg. Roy. Preston Hosp. Specialty: Gen. Surg.; Vasc. Med. Socs: Manch. Med. Soc.; Vasc. Surg. Soc. GB & Irel.; Assn. Surg.

THOMSON, Graeme Arthur Department of Haematology, Chelsea & Westminster Hospital, 369 Fulham Road, London SW10 9NH Tel: 0208 746 8201 Fax: 0208 746 8202 Email: Graeme.Thompson@chelwest.nhs.uk — Artsexamen Amsterdam 1990; BSc (Hons.) Immunol. Glas. 1981. Lect. & Assoc. Specialist (Haematology), Chelsea and Westm. Hosp.; Sen. Regist. (On Call Rota) Char. Cross Hosp. Lond. & Chelsea Westminster Hosp. Specialty: Haematology. Socs: Fell. Roy. Soc. Med.; Brit. Soc. Haematol.; Brit. Soc. Immunol. Prev: Regist. (Haemat.) Roy. Devon & Exeter Hosp. (Wonford); Regist. (Blood Transfus.) NE Scotl. Blood Transfus. Centre Roy. Infirm. Aberd.; Lect. Hon Sen. Regist (Haemat.) Roy. PostGrad. Med. Sch. Hammersmith Lond..

THOMSON, Mr Hamish Gray The Chiltern Hospital, London Road, Great Missenden HP16 0EN Tel: 01494 890890; Alscot Cottage, Alscot Lane, Longwick, Princes Risborough HP27 9RU Tel: 01844 343382 — MB BS Lond. 1981 (St. Bart.) FRCS Ed. 1985; FRCS Eng. 1987; T(S) 1991. Cons. Otolaryngol. Wycombe Gen. Hosp. High Wycombe & Amersham Hosp. Specialty: Otolaryngol. Socs: BMA & BAOL. Prev: Sen. Regist. (ENT) W. Midl. Train. Scheme; Regist. (ENT) Roy. Nat. Hosp. Lond.; SHO Rotat. (Gen. Surg.) Bristol.

THOMSON, Harry Robbins (retired) The Warren, Rhosneigr, Anglesey LL64 5QT Tel: 01407 811282 — MB BS Lond. 1941 (Middlx.) FRCP Lond. 1975, M 1948; MD Lond. 1949. Prev: Cons. Phys. (Geriat.) Coventry & N. Warks.

THOMSON, Helen W (retired) 24 Rowan Road, Dumbreck, Glasgow G41 5BZ Tel: 0141 427 0771 — MB ChB Glas. 1964. Prev: SCMO Community Child Health Servs. Gtr. Glas. Health Bd.

THOMSON, Hilary Ann Burnham Health Centre, Minniecroft Road, Burnham, Slough SL1 7DE Tel: 01628 605333 — MB BS Lond. 1981; MRCGP 1986; DRCOG 1986.

THOMSON, Horace Norman Michaelson (retired) Denville, Coulardbank Road, Lossiemouth IV31 6ED Tel: 01343 813865 Fax: 01343 813865 — MB ChB Aberd. 1944; DPH Aberd. 1965. Prev: Med. Off. & Lect. (Health Educat.) Aberd. Coll. of Educat.

THOMSON, Hugh Eric Gordon (retired) 24 Woodlands Grove, Stockton Lane, York YO31 1DL Tel: 01904 424530 — MB ChB St. And. 1957. Prev: GP York.

THOMSON, Mr Hugh James Department of Surgery, Heartlands Hospital, Birmingham B9 5SS Tel: 0121 766 6611 Fax: 0121 773 6897; 18 Hampshire Drive, Birmingham B15 3NZ Tel: 0121 455 7327 — MB ChB Aberd. 1977; FRCS Ed. 1981; FRCS Eng. 1981; ChM Aberd. 1984. Cons. Surg. Heartlands Hosp. Birm.; Hon. Clin. Lect. (Surg.) Univ. Birm. Specialty: Gen. Surg. Socs: Christ. Med. Fellowsh.; Brit. Soc. Gastroenterol.; BMA. Prev: Sen. Regist. (Surg.) Addenbrooke's Hosp. Camb.; Regist. (Surg.) West. Gen. Hosp. Edin.; Regist. (Surg.) Aberd. Roy. Infirm.

THOMSON, Ian Andrew Thomson and Partners, The Medical Centre, Oak Street, Lechlade GL7 3RY Tel: 01367 252264 — MB BS Lond. 1979; DRCOG.

THOMSON, Ian Bruce Clackmannan and Kincardine Medical Practice, Health Centre, Main Street, Clackmannan FK10 4QX Tel: 01259 723725 Fax: 01259 724791; 3 Linnmill Cottage, Clackmannan, Alloa FK10 3PY Tel: 01259 723975 — MB ChB Dundee 1980. Prev: Trainee GP Greenock & Gourock VTS; SHO (Surg.) Perth Roy. Infirm.; SHO (Med.) Stracathro Hosp.

THOMSON, Ian Copland (retired) Tanera House, Riccall, York YO19 6PT Tel: 01757 248319 — MB ChB Ed. 1959; DObst RCOG 1961. Prev: Princip., Gen. Pract., Beech Tree Surg., Selby, N. Yorks.

THOMSON, Ian George Torr Farm, Areton Gifford, Kingsbridge TQ7 4EP Tel: 01548 559172 Fax: 01548 559172 Email: wruthomson@aol.com — BM BCh Oxf. 1955 (Oxf. & Middlx.) MA, BM BCh Oxf. 1955; DPM Eng. 1966; FRCPsych 1984, M 1971. Medicolegal work. Specialty: Gen. Psychiat. Special Interest: Personality Disorders. Prev: Cons. Psychiat. I. of Wight Hosp. DHA; Dist. Surg. S. Africa.

THOMSON, Ian Howie, OStJ (retired) 51 Heatherwood, Seafield, Bathgate EH47 7BX Tel: 01506651070 — MB ChB Ed. 1947 (Univ. Ed.) AFOM RCP Lond. 1982. Prev: Sen. Med. Off. Brit. Steel Corpn. Scotl.

THOMSON, James Burt Department of Anaesthesia, Wishaw General Hospital, Wishaw ML21 0DP — MB ChB Ed. 1973 (Edinburgh) BSc (Med. Sci.) Ed. 1970; FFA RCS Eng. 1977. Cons. Anaesth. Wishaw Gen. Hosp. Specialty: Anaesth. Socs: Europ. Soc. of Regional Anaesth.-Life Mem.; Brit. Soc. of Orthopaedic Anaesth.s.

THOMSON, James Ewing Inverclyde Royal Hospital, Greenock PA16 0XN Tel: 01475 633777; Raasay, 14 Douglas Avenue, Langbank, Port Glasgow PA14 6PE — MB ChB Glas. 1970; MRCP (UK) 1973; FRCP Glas. 1983; FRCP Ed. 1988. Cons. Phys. Inverclyde Roy. Hosp. Greenock. Specialty: Gen. Med.

THOMSON, James Laing Gordon (retired) Little Begbrook, Begbrok Park, Frenchay, Bristol BS16 1NF Tel: 0117 957 0161 — (St. Bart.) MD Lond. 1950, MB BS 1945; DMRD Eng. 1948; FRCP Lond. 1971, M 1952; FRCR 1975. Prev: Cons. Radiol. Frenchay Hosp. & Roy. Infirm. Bristol.

THOMSON, James Morris Dott 9 Morgan Street, Dundee DD4 6QE — MB ChB St. And. 1969; BSc St. And. 1966; DObst RCOG 1974.

THOMSON, James Phillips Spalding (retired) Master's Lodge, Charterhouse, Chaterhouse Square, London EC1M 6AN Tel: 020 7253 0272 Email: jamespsthomson@aol.com — (Middlx.) MB BS Lond. 1962; MRCS Eng. LRCP Lond. 1962; DObst RCOG 1964; FRCS Eng. 1969; MS Lond. 1974; DM Lambeth 1987. Prev: Emerit. Cons. Surg. St. Marks Hosp. for Intestinal & Colorectal Disorders NW Lond. NHS Trust.

THOMSON, Janet McMurray Glen 8 Bath Street, Stonehaven AB39 2DH — MB ChB Glas. 1978; MRCGP 1984. GP Glas.

THOMSON, Janette Kennedy 1 Ledcameroch Crescent, Bearsden, Glasgow G61 4AD Tel: 0141 942 7513 — MB ChB Glas. 1966. GP Clydebank Health Centre.

THOMSON, Janice The Old Station Surgery, Heanor Road, Ilkeston DE7 8ES Tel: 0115 930 1055; 50B Roland Avenue, Nuthall, Nottingham NG16 1BB Tel: 0115 854 7628 — MB ChB Dundee 1990; DFFP 1993; DRCOG 1993; MRCGP 1994. Prev: Trainee GP Vict. Infirm. VTS.

THOMSON, Jean The Anaesthetic Department, Calderdale Royal Hospital, Salterhebble, Halifax HX3 0PW — MB ChB Birm. 1973; FRC Anaes. Eng. 1977; DRCOG 1979. Specialty: Anaesth.

THOMSON, Jennifer Clair 7 Naworth Drive, Carlisle CA3 0DD — MB ChB Manch. 1998.

THOMSON, Joan Hairmyres Hospital, Eaglesham Road, East Kilbride, Glasgow G75 8RG — MB ChB Ed. 1970; DPM Ed. 1973; FRCPsych 1992, M 1974; BSc (Med. Sci.) (Hons. Bact.) Ed. 1968, MD 1980. Cons. Gen. Psychiat. Hairmyres Hosp. E. Kilbride. Specialty: Gen. Psychiat.

THOMSON, Joan Elizabeth Dykebar Hospital, Grahamston Road, Paisley PA2 7DE Tel: 0141 884 5122 Fax: 0141 884 7162 — MB ChB Glas. 1983; MRCPsych. 1988. Cons. Psychiat., NHS Argylle & Clyde, Paisley. Specialty: Gen. Psychiat.

THOMSON, Joan Elizabeth Govan Health Centre, 5 Drumoyne Road, Glasgow G51 4BJ Tel: 0141 440 1212; 21 Russell Drive, Bearsden, Glasgow G61 3BB — MB ChB Glas. 1968; DA Eng. 1970.

THOMSON, John Kintore, 24 Rowan Road, Dumbreck, Glasgow G41 5BZ Tel: 0141 427 0771 Fax: 0141 427 0771 — MB ChB 1960; DObst RCOG 1962; FRCP Glas. 1973, M 1965; MD Glas. 1973; FRCP Ed. 1992; FChs Soc. Chirop & Podiat Lond. 1996. Cons. (Dermat.) Glas. Roy. Infirm. (Retd.). Specialty: Dermat.

THOMSON, John Alexander (retired) 13 Russell Drive, Bearsden, Glasgow G61 3BB Tel: 0141 942 6302 — (Glasgow University) FRCP Edin. 2003; MB ChB Glas. 1956; MRCP Lond. 1961; FRFPS Glas. 1961; FRCP Glas. 1968; MD Glas. 1970; PhD Glas. 1974; FRCP Lond. 1975. Prev: Reader (Med.) & Cons. Phys. Univ. Dept. Med. Roy. Infirm. Glas.

THOMSON, John Blackwood (retired) 10 Carnoustie Gardens, Glenrothes KY6 2QB Tel: 01592 755268 — (Manch.) MB ChB Manch. 1959.

THOMSON, John Duncan Ross The Barn, High St., Waddington, Lincoln LN5 9RF — BM BS Nottm. 1993; MRCP (UK) 1996.

THOMSON, John Richard (retired) No. 11, John Murray Court, Motherwell ML1 2QW Tel: 01968 252798 — (Glas.) MB ChB Glas. 1950. Prev: Med. Off. RAAMC.

THOMSON, John Stewart St. Clair House, 34 Hutcheon St., Aberdeen AB25 3TB — MB ChB Aberd. 1995. Specialty: Cardiol.

THOMSON, Joseph Howard Crumlin Medical Practice, 5 Glenavy Road, Crumlin BT29 4LA Tel: 028 9442 2209 Fax: 028 9442 2233; Park House, Crumlin BT29 4BW Tel: 0184 94 52209 — MB BCh BAO Belf. 1973; DObst RCOG 1975; MRCGP 1980. Prev: Sen. Med. Off. Harbour Breton Newfld..

THOMSON, Julia 3a Alexandra Grove, Finsbury Park, London N4 2LG — BM Soton. 1997. SHO (Paediat.) Roy Free. Specialty: Paediat.

THOMSON, Julie Simpson Medical Group, Bathgate Primary Centre, Whitburn Road, Bathgate EH48 2SS Tel: 01506 655155; Annacht, 1 Simpson Crescent, Bathgate EH48 1BL Tel: 01506 654688 — MB ChB Ed. 1982 (Edinburgh) MRCGP 1987.

THOMSON, Keith Derek North Hampshire Hospital, Department of Anaesthesia, Aldermaston Road, Basingstoke RG24 9NA Tel: 01256 313461 Fax: 01256 354224; Brookside Farm, Winkfield Road, Ascot SL5 7LT Tel: 01344 886147 Email: keith.t2@ukonline.co.uk — MB BS Lond. 1976 (University College Hospital London) BSc Ed. 1969; DA Eng. 1979; FFA RCS Eng. 1981; DRCOG 1982. Cons. Anaesth. N. Hants. Hosp. Basingstoke Hants. Specialty: Anaesth.

THOMSON, Keith Thomas Engleton House Surgery, 2 Villa Road, Radford, Coventry CV6 3HZ Tel: 024 7659 2012 Fax: 024 7660 1913 Email: keith.thomsom@nhs.net — MB ChB Leeds 1975.

THOMSON, Kenneth Fletcher Malcolm, TD, OStJ (retired) 41 Heslington Lane, York YO10 4HN Tel: 01904 622159 — BM BCh Oxf. 1951 (Oxf. & St. Thos.) DLO Eng. 1954. Prev: Area Surg. St. John Ambul. Brig. (Off. Brother).

THOMSON, Kevin James 26 Seaforth Road, Golspie KW10 6TJ — MB ChB Glas. 1997.

THOMSON, Kirsty Jane 15 Spylaw Bank Road, Edinburgh EH13 0JW — MB ChB Aberd. 1989.

THOMSON, Lawrence Mackinnon (retired) 49 Westland, Martlesham Heath, Ipswich IP5 3SU Tel: 01473 612188 — MB BS Lond. 1962 (Middlx.) Prev: GP Ipswich.

THOMSON, Lesley Fiona 21 Hunts Mead, Billericay CM12 9JA — MB ChB Leeds 1986.

THOMSON, Lindsay Dorothy Greig Department of Psychiatry, The University of Edinburgh, Kennedy Tower, Morningside Park, Edinburgh EH10 5HF Tel: 0131 537 6509 Fax: 0131 537 6508 Email: l.d.g.thomson@ed.ac.uk/ldgt@staffmail.ed.ac.uk — MB ChB Ed. 1987; MRCPsych 1991; MPhil Ed. 1994; MD Ed. 2000. Sen. Lect. (Forens. Psychiat.) Univ. Edin.; Hon. Cons. Forens. Psychiat. The State Hosp. Carstairs Lanark. Specialty: Forens. Psychiat. Prev: Sen. Regist. (Adult Psychiat. & Forens. Psychiat.) Roy. Edin. Hosp.; Research Fell. (Psychiat.) Univ. Edin.; Regist. Rotat. (Psychiat.) Roy. Edin. Hosp. Lothian HB.

THOMSON, Lucy Anne Baronscourt Surgery, 89 Northfield Broadway, Edinburgh EH8 7RX Tel: 0131 657 5444 Fax: 0131 669 8116; Kilfinan, 19 Glenesk Crescent, Eskbank, Dalkeith EH22 3BW — MB BS Lond. 1990 (Univ. Coll. Hosp. Middlx.) DRCOG 1994; MRCGP (Distinc.) 1995; DFFP 1995. Specialty: Gen. Pract.

THOMSON, Lucy Elizabeth Victoria Park Health Centre, Bedford Avenue, Birkenhead; 11 Harringay Avenue, Mossley Hill, Liverpool L18 1JE Tel: 0151 734 0432 — MB ChB Liverp. 1993; DRCOG 1996; DFFP 1997. GP Retainer. Specialty: Gen. Pract. Prev: GP Regist.

THOMSON, Margaret Shah and Thomson, Bute House Medical Centre, Ground Floor, Luton LU1 1QJ Tel: 01582 729428 Fax: 01582 417762 Email: margaretthompson@gp-e81048.nhs.uk — MB ChB Ed. 1971. Specialty: Gen. Pract.

THOMSON, Mrs Margaret Ann Sonning Common Health Centre, Wood Lane, Sonning Common, Reading RG4 9SW Tel: 01734 722188 Fax: 01734 724633; The Strip, Shepherds Green, Rotherfield Greys, Henley-on-Thames RG9 4QW — BM BCh Oxf. 1964; MA Oxf. 1964, BM BCh 1964; DCH RCP Eng. 1967; MRCP (UK) 1970. Prev: Med. Off. (Paediat.) Radcliffe Infirm. Oxf.; Sen. Regist. (Haemat.) Roy. Postgrad. Med. Sch. Hammersmith Hosp. Lond.

THOMSON, Margaret Anne Rees 1 Whitefauld Road, Dundee DD2 1RH Tel: 01382 566622 Email: robert.smith3@which.net — MB ChB Dundee 1974; FRCOG 1995; MFFP 1996; MRCOG 1999. Cons. O & G & Hon. Sen. Lect. Ninewells Hosp. & Med. Sch. Dundee.; Director Scott. Hydaticliform Mole Follow-up Serv. Specialty: Obst. & Gyn.; Family Plann. & Reproduc. Health.

THOMSON, Marion Taylor (retired) 4 Grove House, The Grove, Epsom KT17 4DJ Tel: 01372 742743 — MB ChB Glas. 1939; DPH 1943; MFCM 1972. Prev: SCMO Som. HA.

THOMSON, Mary Forsyth (retired) 19 Stokesley Road, Marton, Middlesbrough TS7 8DT Tel: 01642 275691 — (Glas.) MB ChB Glas. 1952.

THOMSON, Mary Janette (retired) 35 Newland Park Drive, York YO10 3HR Tel: 01904 423992 — (Edinburgh) MB ChB Ed. 1963; DObst RCOG 1965. Prev: GP York & Bromley.

THOMSON, Matilda Kennedy (retired) 11 Orchard Toll, Edinburgh EH4 3JF Tel: 0131 315 2747 — (Glas.) MB ChB Glas. 1939.

THOMSON, Mr Matthew Perekkatt (retired) 10 Levaghery Close, Portadown, Craigavon BT63 5HL Tel: 028 3833 6579 — MB BS Kerala 1958; DLO Eng. 1967; FRCS Ed. 1977. Cons. ENT Surg. Craigavon Area Hosp. Gp. Trust. Prev: Cons. ENT Surg. Craigavon Area Hosp. Gp. Trust.

THOMSON, Melvyn Fyffe Denmuir Farm, Newburgh, Cupar KY14 6JQ — MB ChB Glas. 1970; FFA RCSI 1977. Cons. Anaesth. & Hon. Sen. Lect. Univ. Dundee. Specialty: Anaesth.

THOMSON, Merran Ann Hammersmith Hospital, Department of Paediatrics & Neonatal Medicine, Du Cane Road, London W12 0NN Tel: 020 8383 3270 Fax: 020 8740 8281 Email: merran.thomson@imperial.ac.uk — MB ChB Manch. 1982 (Manch. & St Andrews) MRCP (UK) 1988. Cons. (Perinatology) Neonat. Units Hammersmith & Qu. Charlotte Hosps. Lond. Specialty: Neonat. Socs: Eur. Soc. Paediat. Research; Fell. Roy. Coll. Paediat. and Child Health; Neonat. Soc. Prev: Cons. & Hon. Clin. Lect. (Perinatol.) Neonat. Unit Hope Hosp. Salford; Sen. Regist. & Hon. Clin. Lect. (Paediat.) Neonat. Unit Birm. Matern. Hosp.

THOMSON, Michael Little Shannon, 87 Crock Lane, Bridport DT6 4DH Tel: 01308 458133 Email: michael.thomson2@virgin.net; PO Box 20, Murambinda Mission Hospital, Muranbinda, Zimbabwe Tel: 01308 458133 Fax: 01308 458133 Email: michael.thomson2@virgin.net — (Guy's) MB BS Lond. 1965; DObst RCOG 1967; FRCGP 1993, M 1975. p/t Locum GP. Prev: Ho. Surg. & Ho. Phys. Orpington Hosp.; Ho. Surg. (Obst.) Boscombe Hosp.

THOMSON, Michael Andrew University Department of Paediatric Gastroenterology, Royal Free Hospital, Pond St., London NW3 2QG Tel: 020 7830 2781 Fax: 020 7830 2146 Email: mthomson@rfhsm.ac.uk; Tanera House, Riccall, York YO19 6PT — MB ChB Aberd. 1985; DCH Lond. 1987; MRCP (Paediat.) UK 1990; FRCPCH 1997. Cons. Paediat. (Gastroenterol. & Nutrit.) Roy. Free Hosp. Lond.; Hon. Sen. Lect. (Paediat. Gastroenterol.) Roy. Free Hosp. Sch. Med. Lond. Specialty: Paediat. Socs: Brit. Paediat. Assn.; Brit. Soc. Paediat. Gastroenterol. & Nutrit.; BMA. Prev: Lect. Liver Transpl. Birm. Childr. Hosp.

THOMSON, Michael David (retired) Little Pednavounder, Coverack, Helston TR12 6SE Tel: 01326 280140 — MB ChB St. And. 1944.

THOMSON, Michael Roy Burnham Medical Centre, Love Lane, Burnham-on-Sea TA8 1EU Tel: 01278 795445 Fax: 01278 793024; Burnham Medical Centre, Love Lane, Burnham-on-Sea TA8 1EU Tel: 01278 782283 — MB ChB Bristol 1972; BSc Bristol 1969, MB ChB 1972; MRCP (U.K.) 1975; DRCOG 1977; MRCGP 1980.

THOMSON, Morven Elizabeth (retired) 30 Roehampton Close, London SW15 5LU Tel: 020 8876 3979 — MB ChB Glas. 1950; MRCPsych 1978; DPM Eng. 1978. Prev: Vis. Cons. Psychiat. Priory Hosp. Lond.

THOMSON, Professor Neil Campbell Department of Respiratory Medicine, Division of Immunology, Infection and Inflamation, University of Glasgow and Western Infirmary, Glasgow G11 6NT Tel: 0141 211 3241 Fax: 0141 211 3464 Email: n.c.thomson@clinmed.gla.ac.uk; Gryffe Lodge, Florence Drive, Kilmacolm PA13 4JN — MB ChB 1972 (University of Glasgow) MRCP (UK) 1975; MD Glas. 1980; FRCP Glas. 1986; FRCP Lond. 1990. Prof. of Respirat. Med. Univ. Glas.; Hon. Cons. Western Infirm. Glas. Specialty: Respirat. Med. Special Interest: Asthma. Socs: Brit. Thorac. Soc.; Amer. Thoracic Soc.; Assoc. of Phys. Prev: Research Fell. McMaster Univ. Hamilton Canada; Jun. Doctor Glas. Teach. Hosps.; Hon. Prof. Univ. Glas.

THOMSON, Nigel Stuart, TD Folly Farm, Bressingham, Diss IP22 2AS — MB ChB Manch. 1976 (Manchester) MRCP (UK) 1980; FRCP 2001. Prev: Tutor (Child Health) Univ. Manch.

***THOMSON, Noah Dominic** — MB BS Lond. 1997; DCH, DRCOG, DFFP; BSc (Hons.) Lond. 1994. Ho. Off. King Edwd. VII Hosp. Midhurst.

THOMSON, Patricia Helen Gibb 14 Crosbie Court, Craigend Road, Troon KA10 6ES — MB ChB Glas. 1967; DCH RCPS Glas. 1974. MPH Glas. Prev: SCMO (Child Health) Ayrsh. & Arran.

THOMSON, Penelope Jane Foxmoor Nurseries, Wellington TA21 9PH — MB BS Lond. 1982.

THOMSON, Penelope Jane 49 Wroxham Gardens, Potters Bar EN6 3DJ — MB BS Lond. 1983. Staff Grade in Dermat., Barnet Hosp., Barnet. Specialty: Dermat.

THOMSON, Peter Gifford Greyswood Practice, 238 Mitcham Lane, London SW16 6NT Tel: 020 8769 0845/8363 Fax: 020 8677 2960 Email: doctortee@tiscali.co.uk — (Westminster) BSc Lond. 1982, MB BS 1985; DCH RCP Lond. 1988; MRCGP 1990; MSc (Sports Medicine) Lond. 2002.

THOMSON, Peter Gordon 8 Galachlaw Shot, Edinburgh EH10 7JF Tel: 0131 445 1001 — MB ChB Ed. 1970; MRCOG 1976. Cons. O & G St. John's Hosp. Livingston. Specialty: Obst. & Gyn.

THOMSON, Professor Peter James Oral & Maxillofacial Surgery, School of Dental Sciences, University of Newcastle, Framlington Place, Newcastle upon Tyne NE2 4BW Tel: 0191 222 8290 Email: peter.thomson@nd.ac.uk — MB BS Newc. 1988 (Newcastle) MSc Manch. 1993, BDS 1982; BDS 1982; FDS RCS Eng. 1990; FRCS Ed. 1992; MSc 1993; PhD Manch. 1997. Prof. Oral & Maxillofacial Surg. Univ. Newc. u. Tyne. Specialty: Gen. Surg. Socs: Fell. of the Brit. Assn. of Oral & Maxillofacial Surg.; Brit. Assn. of Head & Neck Oncol.; Brit. Assn. of Day Surg.

THOMSON, Rachel Wildway, Clarendon Drive, Dundee DD2 1JU — MB ChB Aberd. 1998.

THOMSON, Professor Richard Geoffrey School of Population and Health Science, (Epidemiology and Public Health), Medical School, Newcastle upon Tyne NE2 4HH Tel: 0191 222 8760 Fax: 0191 222 8211 Email: richard.thomson@ncl.ac.uk — BA Oxf. 1979; BM BCh Oxf. 1982; MRCP (UK) 1985; MD Newc. 1990; FFPHM RCP (UK) 1996, M 1990; FRCP Lond. 1996. Prof. of Epidemiol. and Pub. Health, Newc. Univ. Med. Sch.; Director, UK Quality Indicator Poject, Newc. Specialty: Pub. Health Med. Prev: Sen. Lect. in Pub. Health Med., Newc. Univ. Med. Sch.; Dir. Health Strategy North. RHA; Sen. Regist. (Community Med.) N. RHA.

THOMSON, Richard Simon Greenheart, Highfields, East Horsley, Leatherhead KT24 5AA — MB ChB Ed. 1996.

THOMSON, Robert Cunningham Glen Meadowbank Health Centre, 3 Salmon Inn Road, Falkirk FK2 0XF Tel: 01324 715446 Fax: 01324 717986; 37 St. Ninians Road, Linlithgow EH49 7BN Tel: 01506 842679 — MB ChB Ed. 1978.

THOMSON, Mr Robert George Nighy (retired) Friarscroft, 31 Highgate Avenue, Fulwood, Preston PR2 8LN Tel: 01772 719515 — MB BS Lond. 1960 (St. Bart.) MRCS Eng. LRCP Lond. 1960; FRCS Eng. 1966. Cons. Urol. Preston & Chorley Hosp. Gp. Prev: Research Fell. To Merseyside Assn. Kidney Research.

THOMSON, Robert John Tanera House, Riccall, York YO19 6PT — MB BS Newc. 1989. Regist. (Community Psychiat.) Wiakato HB Hamilton, NZ. Specialty: Gen. Psychiat.

THOMSON, Robert McNeill Woodside, Copperas Lane, Haigh, Wigan WN2 1PB Tel: 01942 831047 — MB ChB Manch. 1949; FRCOG 1971, M 1955, DObst 1951; DCH Eng. 1952. Cons. O & G Wigan & Leigh Hosp. Gp.; Chairm. Med. Exec. Comm. & Cons. Staff Comm.; Cons. Mem. DMT Wigan DHA. Specialty: Obst. & Gyn. Socs: Fell. Manch. Med. Soc.; N. Eng. Obst. & Gyn. Soc. Prev: Lect. (O & G) Univ. Manch.; 1st Asst. O & G St. Mary's Hosps. Manch.; Sen. Ho. Surg. (Obst.) Qu. Charlotte's Matern. Hosp. Lond.

THOMSON, Robert Scott (retired) Cathcart Practice, 8 Cathcart Street, Ayr KA7 1BJ Tel: 01292 264051 Fax: 01292 293803; 8 Blackburn Road, Ayr KA7 2XQ Tel: 01292 266407 Fax: 01292 280824 — MB ChB Glas. 1963; DObst RCOG 1965. Prev: Clin. Asst. (Psychiat.) Ayrsh. & Arran HB.

THOMSON, Roderick David Anthony Baird Health Centre, St Thomas' Hospital, Lambeth Palace Road, London SE1 7EH — MB BS W. Indies 1989; DCH RCP Lond. 1996; DFFP 1998. CMP MoD.

THOMSON, Rodney Gordon 4 Redthorne Way, Cheltenham GL51 3NW Tel: 01242 251310 — MRCS Eng. LRCP Lond. 1971. Prev: Regist. (O & G) Riyadh; GP Austral.

THOMSON, Roger Geoffrey Trumpington House, 56 High Street, Dulverton TA22 9DW Tel: 01398 323333 Fax: 01398 324030 — MB BS Lond. 1983 (Char. Cross Hosp. Lond.) MRCGP 1989; DCH RCP Lond. 1990. Socs: RSM. Prev: Sen. Med. Off. N.ants.

THOMSON, Ruth Ballantine Rowena, 53 Glebe St., Dumfries DG1 2LZ — MB ChB Ed. 1968; DCH Eng. 1971; DObst RCOG 1972; MRCP (UK) 1975; FRCP Glas. 1985. Cons. (Paediat.) Dumfries & Galloway Roy. Infirm. Dumfries. Specialty: Paediat. Socs: Brit. Soc. Study Infec.; Brit. Paediat. Assn. Prev: Sen. Regist. & Regist. (Paediat.) Roy. Hosp. Sick Childr. Glas.; Regist. (Infec. Dis.) Belvidere Hosp. Glas.

THOMSON, Samuel Alastair Braids Medical Practice, 6 Camus Avenue, Edinburgh EH10 6QT Tel: 0131 445 5999; Braids Medical Practice, 6 Camus Avenue, Edinburgh EH10 6QT Tel: 0131 445 5999 — MB ChB Aberd. 1978; MRCP (UK) 1980; MRCGP 1985.

THOMSON, Samuel Wood (retired) Mansfield, Easter St., Duns TD11 3DW Tel: 01361 882963 — MB BS Lond. 1945 (St. Bart.) MRCS Eng. LRCP Lond. 1945; DOMS Eng. 1948; DObst RCOG 1948; DTM & H Liverp. 1949; MRCGP 1968. Prev: Mem. Nigerian Med. Counc.

THOMSON, Sarah Renata Sitwell and Partners, Little Common Surgery, 82 Cooden Sea Road, Bexhill-on-Sea TN39 4SP Tel: 01424 845477 Fax: 01424 848225; The Tall House, Heatherdune Road, Bexhill-on-Sea TN39 4HB Tel: 01424 214385 — MB ChB Bristol 1980; MB ChB (Hons.) Bristol 1980; DRCOG 1983; MRCGP 1984.

THOMSON, Sean Douglas 12 Cedar Close, Borehamwood WD6 2ED — MB ChB Otago 1992.

THOMSON, Sheila Evelyn Gordon (retired) 24 Woodlands Grove, Stockton Lane, York YO31 1DL Tel: 01904 424530 — MB ChB St. And. 1956. Clin. Asst. Special Centre Epilepsy Neuro-Psychiat. Unit Bootham Pk. Hosp. York. Prev: Med. Adviser to Macmillan Nurses York.

THOMSON, Sheila Mairi Jean (retired) 62 Countesswells Road, Aberdeen AB15 7YE Tel: 01224 316387 — (Aberd.) MB ChB Aberd. 1946. Prev: Community Phys. Grampian HB.

THOMSON, Sheila Margaret Paisley Road West Surgery, 1808 Paisley Road West, Glasgow G52 3TS Tel: 0141 211 6660 Fax: 0141 211 6662 — MB ChB Glas. 1970.

THOMSON, Simon James Tanners, Highfields Lane, Kelvedon, Colchester CO5 9BE — MB BS Lond. 1983; FFA RCS Eng. 1988. Cons. Anaesth. Basildon & Thurrock Hosp. Trust. Specialty: Anaesth. Socs: Pres. of Internat. Neuromodulation Soc. (UK and Ireland); Sec. of Internat. Neuromodulation Soc. (World).

THOMSON, Stanley Andrew (retired) 46 Love Lane, Stourbridge DY8 2LD Tel: 01384 394333 — (Glas.) M.B., Ch.B. Glas. 1945. Med. Off. Swinford Old Hall, Stourbridge; Chairm. Dudley Local Med. Comm.; Mem. Dudley FPC. Prev: Ho. Surg. Roy. Infirm. Glas.

THOMSON, Sir Thomas James, KBE, CBE, OBE (retired) 1 Varna Road, Jordanhill, Glasgow G14 9NE Tel: 0141 959 5930 — MB ChB Glas. 1945; FRFPS Glas. 1949; FRCP Lond. 1969, M 1950; FRCP Glas. 1964, M 1962; FRCP Ed. 1981; FRCPI 1983; Hon. FACP 1983; Hon. LLD Glas. 1988. Prev: Chairm. Gtr. Glas. HB.

THOMSON, William Tawelfan, Llanegwad, Nantgaredig, Carmarthen SA32 7NJ Tel: 01267 290578 — MB ChB Liverp. 1975; FFA RCS Eng. 1982. Cons. Anaesth. Carmarthen & Dist. NHS Trust. Specialty: Anaesth. Prev: Sen. Regist. (Anaesth.) N. West. RHA; Regist. (Anaesth.) Cardiff Hosps.; SHO (Anaesth.) Nottm. Hosps.

THOMSON, William Black Govan Health Centre, 5 Drumoyne Road, Glasgow G51 4BJ Tel: 0141 531 8400 Fax: 0141 531 8404; Westfield Health Centre, 71 Hillington Road S., Glasgow G52 2AE Tel: 0141 882 2222 Fax: 0141 882 4321 — MB ChB Glas. 1975; DRCOG 1977; MRCGP 1979. Specialty: Dermat.

THOMSON, William Bruce (retired) Chantry House, Vicarage Close, Cookham, Maidenhead SL6 9SE Tel: 01628 528022 — MB BS Lond. 1951 (St. Mary's) BSc Lond. 1948, MD (Med.) 1952; FRCP Lond. 1972, M 1954. Prev: Cons. Phys. Chiltern AMI Hosp. Gt. Missenden Bucks.

THOMSON, William George (retired) 19 Chinthurst Park, Shalford, Guildford GU4 8JH Tel: 0114 222 0482 Email: bill@wgthomson.freeserve.co.uk/s.goodacre@sheffield.ac.uk — MB ChB Aberd. 1947; DMJ (Clin.) Soc. Apoth. Lond. 1969, DIH 1967; MFOM RCP Lond. 1978; Specialist Accredit. (Occupat. Med.) RCP Lond. 1978; Cert. Av Med. RCP Lond. & CAA 1978. Med. Adviser Legal & Gen. Assur. in Pre-Retirement Educat.; Med. Adviser Retirement Counselling Serv. Prev: Cons. Phys. H. Shepherd & Co. Ltd. (Engin.).

THOMSON, Mr William Hamish Fearon Gloucester Royal Hospital, Great Western Road, Gloucester GL1 3NN Tel: 01452 528555 Fax: 01452 394813 — (St. Bart.) MB BS Lond. 1961; FRCS Eng. 1967; MS Lond. 1975. Cons. Surg. Gloucester AHA. Specialty: Gen. Surg. Socs: Assn. Surg.; Assn. Coloproctol. Prev: Sen. Regist. (Surg.) Soton. Univ. Hosp.

THOMSON, William John (retired) Nelson, Little Court, Elie, Leven KY9 1AU — MB ChB St. And. 1955. Prev: GP Fife.

THOMSON, Mr William Old 1 Brownside Avenue, Cambuslang, Glasgow G72 8BL Tel: 0141 583 1997 — MB ChB Glas. 1971; FRCS Glas. 1976. Cons. Surg. Hairmyres Hosp. E. Kilbride. Specialty: Gen. Surg.

THOMSON, William Oliver (retired) 7 Silverwells Court, Bothwell, Glasgow G71 8LT — MB ChB Glas. 1947 (Univ. Glas.) DPH Glas. 1951, DPA 1956; DIH Soc. Apoth. Lond. 1958; MD (Commend.) Glas. 1958; FFCM 1977, M 1974; Dip. Scott. Counc. Health Educat. 1979; MRCP (UK) 1986; FRCP Glas. 1988. Prev: Chief Admin. Med. Off. Lanarksh. HB.

THOMSON, William Stenhouse Taylor (retired) Ar Dachaidh, Mid-Letters, Strachur, Cairndow PA27 8DP — MB ChB Glas. 1945; BSc (Hons. Biochem.) 1951; PhD Glas. 1954; M 1970; FRCP Glas. 1972; FRCPath 1973. Prev: Cons. Biochem. South. Gen. Hosp. Glas.

THOMSON, Winifred Isobel (retired) Colinton Surgery, 296B Colinton Road, Edinburgh EH13 0LB Tel: 0131 441 4555 Fax: 0131 441 3963; 15 Spylaw Bank Road, Edinburgh EH13 0JW Tel: 0131 441 2337 — MB ChB Ed. 1961.

THOMSSEN, Henrike Kennedy Institute of Rheumatology, Sunley Division, 1 Lurgan Avenue, London W6 8LW Tel: 020 8741 8966 Fax: 020 8563 0399 — State Exam Med Munich 1988; State Exam Med. Munich 1988; MD Munich 1989.

THONET, Mr Robert Gustave Nicholas Kingston and Queen Mary's Hospitals, Galsworthy Road, Kingston upon Thames KT2 7QB Tel: 020 8355 2027 Fax: 020 8355 2871; Devon Lodge, 17 Portsmouth Avenue, Thames Ditton KT7 0RU Tel: 020 8398 0046 Fax: 020 8398 0046 — MB BS Lond. 1971 (Westm.) MRCS Eng. LRCP Lond. 1971; FRCS Ed. 1977; FRCS Eng. 1977; MRCOG 1979; FRCOG 1991. Cons. O & G Qu. Mary's Univ. Hosp. Lond. Specialty: Obst. & Gyn. Socs: N. Eng. Obst. & Gyn. Soc.; Brit. Menopause Soc.; Brit. Fertil. Soc. Prev: Sen. Regist. (O & G) Univ. Hosp. S. Manch.; Regist. (O & G) Camb. HA; Resid. Med. & Surg. Off. Qu. Charlotte's & Chelsea Hosp. for Wom. Lond.

THONG, Kok Foon MacMillan Surgery, 10 Dulas Road, Kirkby, Liverpool L32 8TL Tel: 0151 546 2908 Fax: 0151 548 0704; 13 Stanley Avenue, Birkdale, Southport PR8 4RU Tel: 01704 66205 — MB BS Newc. 1980; MRCPI 1987. Specialty: Cardiol. Socs: Roy. Coll. Phys. Irel.; Roy. Soc. Med. Lond. Prev: Regist. (Cardiol.) Centr. Middlx. Hosp. Lond.; Med. Rotat. Univ. Aberd.

THOO, Chee Kong 62 Queens Drive, Mossley Hill, Liverpool L18 0HF — MB ChB Liverp. 1988; DTM & H Liverp. 1991. Specialty: Cardiol.

THOPPIL, Joseph Philip 106 Ancrum Street, Spital Tongues, Newcastle upon Tyne NE2 4LR — MB BS Newc. 1998.

THORBURN, Douglas Queen Elizabeth Hospital, Liver Unit, Birmingham B15 2TF Tel: 0121 472 1311 Ext: 2393 Email: douglas.thorburn@uhb.nhs.uk — MB ChB Glas. 1990; MRCP (UK) 1993; MD Glas. 2002; FRCP Glas. 2004. Specialty: Gastroenterol.; Gen. Med.

THORBURN, John Stuart 548 Meanwood Road, Leeds LS6 4JN Tel: 0113 741313 — MD Leeds 1949; MB ChB 1943. Med. Off. T. Walls & Son Leeds Area. Prev: Regist. Dermat. Dept. Leeds Gen. Infirm.; Capt. RAMC.

THORBURN, Pamela Joyce 38 Pendicle Road, Bearsden, Glasgow G61 1EE — MB ChB Glas. 1990; MRCGP 1994.

THORBURN, Robert Anthony Frederick Holmes Chapel Health Centre, London Road, Holmes Chapel, Crewe CW4 7BB Tel: 01477 533100 Fax: 01477 532563; 87 Portree Drive, Holmes Chapel, Crewe CW4 7JF — BM BCh Oxf. 1990; MA Camb 1992; MRCP (UK) 1994. Gen. Practitioner, Holmes Chapel Health Centre. Specialty: Gen. Pract. Prev: SHO Rotat. (Med.) N. Staffs. Hosp.; Trainee GP N. Staffs. VTS.

THORBURN, Rosalind Jane Community Child Heatlh, Guardian House, Warrington WA5 1TP Tel: 01925 405713 Fax: 01925 405725; 15 Portland Road, Bowdon, Altrincham WA14 2PA Tel: 0161 928 1748 Fax: 0161 926 8436 — MB BS Lond. 1971; MRCS Eng. LRCP Lond. 1971; MRCP (UK) 1975; FRCPCH 1997. Cons. Paediat. (Community Child Health) Warrington Community NHS Trust. Specialty: Community Child Health. Socs: FMRCPCH. Prev: Cons. Paediat. Community Child Health Addenbrooke's Hosp. Camb.; Sen. Regist. (Paediat.) Addenbrooke's Hosp. Camb.; Lect. (Paediat.) Univ. Coll. Hosp. Lond.

THORBURN, Terence Guy Tilhurst, Thursley, Godalming GU8 6QD — BM BS Nottm. 1997.

THORBURN, William (retired) 5 Craigton Cottages, Craigton, Milngavie, Glasgow G62 7HQ Tel: 0141 956 5813 — (Glas.) MB ChB Glas. 1943. Prev: Ho. Phys. West. Infirm. Glas.

THORBURN, William Stuart Farfield Group Practice, St Andrew's Surgeries, West Lane, Keighley BD21 2LD Tel: 01535 607333 Fax: 01535 611818 — MB ChB Leeds 1975; BSc (Hons. Physiol.) Leeds 1972, MB ChB 1975.

THORES, Orison Alistair 5 Haven's Edge, Old Golf Course, Limekilns, Dunfermline KY11 3LJ — MB ChB Aberd. 1960; DObst RCOG 1963; DCH RCPS Glas. 1963; FRCP Canada 1972; FFCM 1979; AFOM RCP Lond. 1983. Sen. Med. Off. Scott. Home & Health Dept. Prev: Community Med. Specialist Fife Health Bd.; Research Fell. Univ. Brit. Columbia; Sen. Med. Cons. Min. Health Ontario.

THORIS, Sigrid 1 Doune Gardens, Glasgow G20 6DJ — Cand Med et Chir Reykjavik 1989.

THORLEY, Anthony Philip Bath Addictions Service, Camden House, Bath Mental Health Care Trust, Bath NHS House, Combe Park, Bath BA1 3QE — MRCS Eng. LRCP Lond. 1970 (Univ. Coll. Hosp.) MA, MB BChir Camb. 1970; FRCPsych 1984, M 1974. Cons. Psychiat. Newc. Healthcare Trust Newc. u. Tyne; Sen. Med. Off. (Addic.) DoH; Hon. Cons. Psychiat. Bethlem Roy. & Maudsley Hosps. Lond. Specialty: Alcohol & Substance Misuse. Prev: Dir. Centre for Alcohol & Drug Studies St. Nicholas Hosp. Newc. u.Tyne; Research Psychiat. Addic. Research Unit Inst. Psychiat. Lond.; Sen. Regist. & Regist. Bethlem Roy. & Maudsley Hosps. Lond.

THORLEY, Claire Hamilton 1 Parkfield Close, Hartlebury, Kidderminster DY11 7TW — MB ChB Birm. 1987; BSc (Hons. Anat.) Birm. 1984; DRCOG 1991; T(GP) 1992; MRCGP 1992. GP Asst. Ombersley Med. Pract. Specialty: Family Plann. & Reproduc. Health. Prev: GP Asst. Davenal Ho. Surg. BromsGr.; GP Asst. The Med. Centre Chaddesley Corbett.

THORLEY, Clive Graham — MB ChB Birm. 1987; BSc (Hons. Anat.) Birm. 1984; MRCGP 1992; T(GP) 1992. GP Princ. Kidderm. Prev: Trainee GP Hay-on-Wye; SHO (Med., Psychiat., Paediat. & O & G) Worcester Roy. Infirm.; Ho. Off. (Surg.) Qu. Eliz. Hosp. Birm.

THORLEY, Helen Black Firs, Birks Drive, Ashley heath, Market Drayton TF9 4PQ — MB BS Lond. 1977; MRCPsych. 1983; Dip. Psychother. Univ. Liverp. 1994. Cons. Psychiat. City Gen. Hosp. Stoke-on-Trent. Specialty: Gen. Psychiat. Prev: Cons. Psychiat. St. Geo. Hosp. Stafford.

THORLEY, John Newlyn Treleaver, Mithian Downs, St Agnes TR5 0PY — MB BS Lond. 1970 (St. Mary's) MRCS Eng. LRCP Lond. 1970; DA Eng. 1976.

THORLEY, Kevan John Higherland Surgery, 3 Orme Road, Poolfields, Newcastle ST5 2UE Tel: 01782 717044 Fax: 01782 715447 — MB BChir Camb. 1977 (Camb./Middlx. Hosp.) MB Camb. 1977, BChir 1976; MA Camb. 1976; DRCOG 1978; MRCGP 1985; Dip. Occ. Med. 1995. GP Trainer, Higherland Surg. Newc.-u-Tyne. Socs: Internat. Soc. Perinatal Med. & Psychol.; Brit. Holistic Med. Assn. (Chairm. N. Midl. Div.).

THORLEY, Nicola Jane Manor House Surgery, Manor Street, Glossop SK13 8PS — BM BCh Oxf. 1994; MA Cantab. 1991; DRCOG 1997; DFFP 1998. GP. Specialty: Gen. Pract.

THORLEY, Rosemary Ann Windrush Health Centre, Welch Way, Witney OX28 6JS Tel: 01993 702911 Fax: 01993 700931 — MB BS Lond. 1985.

THORMAN, Christopher Andrew Laird Wymondham Medical Partnership, Postmill Close, Wymondham NR18 0RF Tel: 01953 602118 Fax: 01953 605313; Greenfields, Dykebeck, Wymondham NR18 9PL Tel: 01953 607211 — (Nottingham) BMedSci. Nottm. 1978, BM BS 1980; DCH RCP Lond. 1983; DRCOG 1984; MRCGP 1985.

THORMAN, Neil Anthony 80A Leader Road, Sheffield S6 4GH — MB ChB Sheff. 1994.

THORMOD, Clare Elisabeth 20 Alberta House, Blackwall Way, London E14 9QH — MB BS Lond. 1987; MRCGP 1991. Occupat. Health Phys., Marks and Spencer.

THORN, Christopher Charles Flat 14, The Merchant's House, 66 North St., Leeds LS2 7PN — MB BS Lond. 1998.

THORN, David Roger Lakenham Surgery, 1 Ninham Street, Norwich NR1 3JJ Tel: 01603 765559 Fax: 01603 766790 — MB ChB Leeds 1970; T(GP) 1991. Prev: SHO (Obst.) Norf. & Norwich Hosp.; Ho. Phys. & Ho. Surg. St. Jas. Hosp. Leeds.

THORN, Jennifer Beatrice 1 Burnbrae, Maybury Drive, Edinburgh EH12 8UB — MB BS Lond. 1970; MRCS Eng. LRCP Lond. 1970. Chief Med. Off. (Family Plann. & Psychosexual Counselling) Lothian Health Bd. Family Plann. & Well Wom. Servs.

THORN, Vivienne Mary Barton Surgery, Lymington House, Barton Hill Way, Torquay TQ2 8JG Tel: 01803 323761 Fax: 01803 316920; Inchcolme, 5 St Margarets Road, St Marychurch, Torquay TQ1 4NW Tel: 01803 311325 Fax: 01803 326691 — MB ChB Ed. 1979; BSc (Med. Sci.) Ed. 1976, MB ChB 1979; MRCGP 1988.

THORNBER, Andrew John 14 Greystoke Close, Berkhamsted HP4 3JJ; 5 Hawsley Road, Beesonend, Harpenden AL5 2BL — MB ChB Liverp. 1991; BSc (Hons.) Microbiol. 1986. Trainee GP Qu. Eliz. II Hosp. Welwyn Gdn. City VTS.

THORNBER, Doreen Rosemary St. James Hospital, Portsmouth; Child & Family Therapy Service, Havant Health Centre, Petersfield Road, Havant PO9 2AG — MB BS Lond. 1956 (St. Mary's) DMP Eng. 1965; MRCPsych 1972. Cons. Child Psychiat. Wessex Unit for Parents & Childr. & Hants. Child Guid. Serv. Prev: Ho. Surg. Hertford Co. Hosp.; Ho. Phys. Cuckfield Hosp.

THORNBER, Mark Merryhills, Rumbling Bridge, Kinross KY13 0PX — MB ChB Glas. 1990.

THORNBER, Stephen Heath House Surgery, Free School Lane, Halifax HX1 2PS Tel: 01422 365533 Fax: 01422 345851; 19 Rocks Road, Halifax HX3 0HR Tel: 01422 352923 — MB ChB St. And. 1967.

THORNBERRY, Mr David John Disablement Services Centre, 1 Brest Way, Off Morlaix Drive, Derriford, Plymouth PL6 5XW Tel: 01752 792777; Leeward, Church Hill, Whitchurch, Tavistock PL19 9EL Tel: 01822 614848 — MB BChir Camb. 1974 (Camb. & St. Thos.) MRCS Eng. LRCP Lond. 1974; MA Camb. 1974; FRCS Eng. 1980. Cons. Rehabil. Med. Derriford Hosp. Plymouth. Specialty: Rehabil. Med. Socs: Brit. Soc. Rehabil. Med.; Internat. Soc. Prosth.s & Orthotics; Posture & Mobility Gp. of Eng. & Wales. Prev: Med. Off. & Hon. Cons. Prosth. Rehabil. Disablem. Servs. Centre Princess Eliz. Orthop. Hosp. Exeter; Med. Off. Artific. Limb Centre Qu. Mary's Hosp. Roehampton; Regist. Wolverhampton Hosps.

THORNBERRY, Elizabeth Anne Gloucestershire Royal Hospital, Department of Anaesthetics, Great Western Road, Gloucester GL1 3NN Tel: 01452 394812 Fax: 01452 394485 — MB BS Lond. 1977 (King's Coll. Hosp.) FFA RCS Eng. 1982. Cons. Anaesth. Glos. Roy. NHS Trust. Specialty: Anaesth. Socs: Obst. Anaesth. Assn.; Soc. for Educat. in Anaesth. UK; Brit. Soc.y of Orthopaedic Anaesth. Prev: Cons. Anaesth. Portsmouth Hosps. NHS Trust; Sen. Regist. Soton. HA; Regist. Bristol Roy. Infirm.

THORNBURGH, Imogen Lucy Forge Cottage, 2 Linton Rd, Loose, Maidstone ME15 0AE — BM BS Nottm. 1997; MRCPCH; BMedSci Nottm. 1995. SpR (Paed.) Oxf. Specialty: Paediat. Prev: SHO (Paediat.) Qu.s Med. Centre. Nottm.

THORNBURY, Gail Donna 274 Saintfield Road, Belfast BT8 6PD — MB BCh BAO Belf. 1985; MRCP (UK) 1989; FRCR 1990. Sen. Regist. (Radiol.) Roy. Vict. Hosp. Belf. Specialty: Radiol.

THORNBURY, Keith Douglas 2 Riverview Street, Belfast BT9 5FD — MB BCh BAO Belf. 1982; MB BCh Belf. 1982.

THORNE, Alison Alice Cottage, 2 The Green, Culham, Abingdon OX14 4LZ — MB ChB Manch. 1993.

THORNE, Mrs Anne Kathryn Churton House, Church Pulverbatch, Shrewsbury SY5 8BZ Tel: 0174 373270 — MB BCh Wales 1969 (Lond.) DObst RCOG 1971. GP Westbury Salop Wom.'s Retainer Scheme. Prev: Govt. Med. Off. Dominica, W. Indies; Govt. Med. Off. Solomon Is.

THORNE, Bernadette Mary Harcourt Medical Centre, Crane Bridge Road, Salisbury SP2 7TD Tel: 01722 333214 Fax: 01722 421643; 3 Wrenscroft, Salisbury SP2 8ET — MB BS Lond. 1981 (Char. Cross) MRCS Eng. LRCP Lond. 1981; MRCGP 1985; DRCOG 1985. GP Princip.

THORNE, Christopher Paul Mount Pleasant Health Centre, Mount Pleasant Road, Exeter EX4 7BW Tel: 01392 55262 Fax: 01392 270497 — BM BS Nottm. 1984; MRCGP 1988.

THORNE, Mrs Dorothy Helen (retired) The Gin Case, Castle Hill, Hayton, Brampton CA8 9JA Tel: 01228 670749 — (Camb. & Bristol) BA Camb. 1937; MRCS Eng. LRCP Lond. 1943.

THORNE, Mr John Anthony 11 Ashfield Road, Cheadle SK8 1BB — MB BS Lond. 1990; BSc Lond. 1987; FRCS Eng. 1994. Specialist Regist. (Neurosurg.) Manch. Roy. Infirm. & Hope Hosp. Salford. Specialty: Neurosurg.

THORNE, Martin Geoffrey (retired) The Old Bell House, Market Place, Somerton TA11 4NJ Tel: 01458 270038 — MD Camb. 1953 (Guy's) MB BChir 1945; FRCP Lond. 1969, M 1949. Prev: Cons. Phys. Torbay Hosp. Torquay.

THORNE, Napier Arnold (retired) 3 Rosewood, 11 Park Road, Haslemere GU27 2NJ Tel: 01428 644224 — MB BS Lond. 1945 (St Bart.) MRCS Eng. LRCP Lond. 1945; FRCP Lond. 1972, M 1949; MD Lond. 1949. Prev: Cons. Dermat. Roy. Lond. Hosp.

THORNE, Pamela Mary Tarr Steps, 21 Back Lane, Bilbrough, York YO23 3PL Tel: 01937 531819 — MRCS Eng. LRCP Lond. 1956 (Leeds) DObst RCOG 1958; DO Eng. 1961; MCOphth 1989. Clin. Asst. (Ophth.) Co. Hosp. York. Specialty: Ophth. Socs: NOTB Assn.; York Med. Soc. Prev: Regist. (Ophth.) K. Edwd. VII Hosp. Windsor; SHMO (Ophth.) Sheff. RHB.; Resid. Surg. Off. Roy. Eye Hosp. Lond.

THORNE, Richard John Thorne Farend, Faringdon Rd, Abingdon OX14 1BB — MB BChir Camb. 1965 (Oxf.) Socs: BMA. Prev: Demonst. (Human Anat.) Oxf. Univ.; SHO (Accid. Serv.), Ho. Phys. & Ho. Surg. Radcliffe Infirm. Oxf.

THORNE, Rosemary Jane Rother House Medical Centre, Alcester Road, Stratford-upon-Avon CV37 6PP Tel: 01789 269386 Fax: 01789 298742; Aldeen House, Lighthorne Road, Kineton, Warwick CV35 0JL Tel: 01926 640767 — MB BS Lond. 1974 (Middlx.)

THORNE, Sara Angela Queen Elizabeth Hopsital, Edgbaston, Birmingham B15 2TH Tel: 0121 627 2959 Fax: 0121 627 2862 — MB BS Lond. 1986 (Royal Free) MD Lond. 1993; FRCP (UK) 2003. Cons. Cardiol. & Hon. Sen. Lect. Qu. Elzabeth Hosp. Birm.. Specialty: Cardiol. Prev: Cons (Cardio.) Roy Brompton Hosp. Lond.; Lect. (Cardiol.) Roy. Brompton Hosp. Lond.; Regist. (Cardiol.) Gt. Ormond St. Hosp. Lond.

THORNE, Simon James 21 Woodfield Park, Amersham HP6 5QH — MB ChB Leeds 1996.

THORNE, Theophilus Crowhurst, MC (retired) 2 St Andrews Road, Rochford SS4 1NP Tel: 01702 544181 — MRCS Eng. LRCP Lond. 1940 (Guy's) DA Eng. 1947; FFA RCS Eng. 1954; FRCA Eng. 1992. Prev: Cons. Anaesth. Rochford & Southend Gen. Hosps.

THORNE, William Ivor John Churton House, Church Pulverbatch, Shrewsbury SY5 8BZ; Churton House, Church Pulverbatch, Shrewsbury SY5 8BZ Tel: 0174 373270 — MB ChB Ed. 1969; MA Oxf. 1966; BSc Ed. 1966, MB ChB 1969; DTM & H Liverp. 1972; MRCGP 1982. Clin. Asst. Roy. Shrewsbury Hosp. Prev: Dist. Med. Off., Dominica W. Indies; Chief Med. Off., Solomon Is.s.

THORNELEY, Christopher William The Old Stables, Swanton Morley Road, Worthing, Dereham NR20 5HS — MB BS Lond. 1997.

THORNELOE, Mr Michael Hugh Woodburn, Wood Lane, Parkgate, South Wirral CH64 6QZ — MB BCh BAO Dub. 1970; FRCS Eng. 1975.

THORNETT, Andrew Martyn Dept. of Psychiatry, University of Southampton, Royal South Hants Hospital, Southampton SO14 0YG — MB BCh Wales 1993. Clin. Research Fell. Dept. Psychiat., Univ. Southampton. Specialty: Gen. Psychiat. Prev: SHO Rotat. (Psychiat.) Chichester.

THORNETT, Judith Ann Well Lane Surgery, Well Lane, Stow on the Wold, Cheltenham GL54 1EQ Tel: 01451 830625 Fax: 01451 830693; Chestnut Court, College Farm, Wyck Rissington, Cheltenham GL54 2PN Tel: 01451 810991 Fax: 01451 810991 Email: thornett@wyckrissington.freeserve.co.uk — MB ChB Birm. 1984; DCH RCP Lond. 1989; DRCOG 1989; MRCGP 1990. Partner Gen. Pract. Stow-on-the-Wold, Glos. Prev: GP Kidderminster.

THORNHAM, John Rodger Norton Medical Centre, Billingham Road, Norton, Stockton-on-Tees TS20 2UZ Tel: 01642 360111 Fax: 01642 558672; Morton Grange Cottage, Church Lane, Nunthorpe, Middlesbrough TS7 0PE Tel: 01642 320092 — MB BS Newc. 1971; FRCGP 1986, M 1976; DObst RCOG 1976. Assoc. Adviser (Gen. Pract.) Univ. Newc. u. Tyne.; Chairm. PCG.

THORNHILL, John David Stenhouse Medical Centre, Furlong Street, Arnold, Nottingham NG5 7BP Tel: 0115 967 3877 Fax: 0115 967 3838; 51 Burlington Road, Sherwood, Nottingham NG5 2GR — MB ChB Sheff. 1980; MRCGP 1986. Trainer (Gen. Pract.) Nottm.

***THORNHILL, Professor Martin Hope** St Barts. and The Royal London Oral Disease Research Centre, Clinical Sciences Building, 2 Newark St., London E1 2AD Tel: 020 7295 7154/020 7882 7154 Fax: 020 7295 7159/020 7882 7159 Email: m.h.thornhill@mds.qmw.ac.uk — MB BS Lond. 1978 (Kings) BDS Lond. 1982, PhD 1990, MSc 1986; FDS RCS Ed. 1988; FFD RCSI 1992; T(S) 1992. Prof. Clin. Oral Sci. Univ. of Lond. & Cons. in Oral Med. Specialty: Oral & Maxillofacial Surg. Socs: BDA; Internat. Assn. Dent. Research; Brit. Soc. Oral Med. Prev: Prof. Med. in Dent. Univ. of Manch.; Sen. Lect. (Oral Med.) Dept. Oral Med. & Periodont. Lond. Hosp. Med. Coll.; Lect. (Oral Med.) Lond. Hosp. Med. Coll.

THORNHILL, Robert John University Hospitals Coventry NHS Trust, Walsgrave Hospital, Clifford Bridge Road, Coventry CV2 2DX Tel: 024 7660 2020; Well Cottage, Newcastle Road South, Brereton, Sandbach CW11 1SA — MB ChB Birm. 1995; Dip IMC RCS Ed. 2003. Specialist Regist. (Anaesth.) W. Midl. Deanery. Specialty: Anaesth.; Intens. Care; Pre Hospital Care. Socs: Assn. Anaesth.; Intens. Care Soc.; BMA. Prev: Clin. Fell. Emerg. Med. - Birm. Heartlands Hosp.; Clin. Fell. PICU: Birm. Childr.s Hosp.; SHO (Anaesth. & ITU) Univ. Hosp. Birm.

THORNICROFT, Professor Graham John Section of Community Psychiatry (PRiSM), Health Services Department, Institute of Psychiatry, De Crespigny Park, London SE5 8AF — MB BS Lond.

1984; MA Camb. 1980; MA Camb. 1980; MRCPsych 1988; MRCPsych 1988; MSc Lond. 1989; MSc (Epidemiol.) Lond. 1989; Phd Lond. 1995; PhD Lond. 1995; MFPM 1999; FRCPsych 2000. Cons. Psychiat. S. Lond. Maudsley NHS Trust (SL&M); Prof. & Dir. Sect. of Community Psychiat.; Head, Helath Serv.s Research Dept, Inst. of Psychiat.; Director of R&D (SL&M); (PRiSM). Specialty: Gen. Psychiat.

THORNICROFT, Sylvia Gill (retired) 8 Caversfield Close, Littleover, Derby DE23 7SR Tel: 01332 510090 — MB ChB Sheff. 1958; DCH Eng. 1961; MRCP Ed. 1968.

THORNILEY-WALKER, Edward George Anthony Aitken, Thorniley-Walker, Lombard and Booth, Medical Centre, Gibson Court, Boldon Colliery NE35 9AN Tel: 0191 519 3000 Fax: 0191 519 2020; 34 Hawthorn Road, South Gosforth, Newcastle upon Tyne NE3 4DE Tel: 0191 284 7136 — MB BS Newc. 1985; DRCOG 1990; MRCGP 1994. Prev: GP Kirkbymoorside; Trainee GP Gr. Med. Gp. Gosforth; SHO (Paediat.) S. Shields Gen. Hosp.

THORNING, Geoffrey Phillip 58 Elderfield Road, London E5 0LF; 58A Granby Road, Eltham, London SE9 1EN Tel: 020 8319 0317 — MB BS Lond. 1996 (Kings College London) BA Camb. 1991. SHO (Med.) Qu. Marys Hosp. Sidcup. Specialty: Gen. Med. Prev: Ho. Off. (Surg.) Greenwich Dist. Hosp.; Ho. Off. (Med.) Kings Coll. Hosp. Lond.

THORNINGTON, Roger Edgar Department of Anaesthesia, Royal Liverpool Childrens Hospital, Alder Hey, Eaton Road, Liverpool L12 2AP Tel: 0151 228 4811/0151 252 5223 Fax: 0151 252 5460 Email: ret@liv.ac.uk; Quarrystones, 166 Quarry St, Liverpool L25 6DZ Tel: 0151 428 4518 Fax: 0151 252 5460 — MB BS Lond. 1968; FFA S. Afr. 1976; FRCA 1991. Cons. Paediat. Anaesth. Liverp. HA. Specialty: Anaesth. Socs: Liverp. Soc. Anaesth.; Assn. Paediat. Anaesth. Prev: Cons. Anaesth. Red Cross War Memor. Childr. Hosp. Cape Town.

THORNLEY, Andrew Peter Lambgates Surgery, 1-5 Lambgates, Hadfield, Glossop SK13 1AW Tel: 01457 869090 — MB ChB Leeds 1996. GP Princip.

THORNLEY, Barbara Ann Holly Tree House, 48A Main Road, Middleton Cheney, Banbury OX17 2LT — MB BS Lond. 1966 (Roy. Free) MRCS Eng. LRCP Lond. 1966; DA Eng. 1969; FFA RCS Eng. 1972. Cons. Anaesth. Horton Hosp. Banbury; Assoc. Dir. of Postgrad. Med. Educat. Oxf. Deanery. Specialty: Anaesth. Socs: BMA; Assn. Anaesth.; R.S.M. Prev: Sen. Regist. (Anaesth.) Roy. Berks. Hosp. Reading; Sen. Regist. & Regist. (Anaesth.) Radcliffe Infirm. Oxf.

THORNLEY, Craig Norman — MB ChB Otago 1992.

THORNLEY, Philip Courtside Surgery, Kennedy Way, Yate, Bristol BS37 4DQ — MB ChB Sheff. 1982; DRCOG 1985. Socs: Doctors Accid. Rescue Team; S. Yorks. Medico-Legal Soc. Prev: SHO (A & E) Rotherham Dist. Gen. Hosp.

THORNLEY, Sarah Kate Maryport Group Practice, Alneburgh House, Ewanrigg Road, Maryport CA15 8EL Tel: 01900 815544 Fax: 01900 816626; Bridge End, Deanscales, Cockermouth CA13 0SL Tel: 01900 827378 — MB ChB Leeds 1989; MRCGP 1994; DCCH RCP Ed. 1994. GP Princip. Specialty: Gen. Pract. Prev: Trainee GP W. Cumbld. Hosp. Cumbria VTS.

THORNS, Andrew Roger 59 Vale Road, Claygate, Esher KT10 0NL — MB BS Lond. 1989; DCH RCP Lond. 1992; MRCGP 1995. Specialty: Palliat. Med.

THORNS, Rosemary Feldon Lane Surgery, Feldon Lane, Halesowen B62 9DR Tel: 0121 422 4703; Locksley Cottage, Belbroughton, Stourbridge DY9 0DG — MB BS Newc. 1985; Cert. Family Plann. JCC 1988; DGM RCP Lond. 1988; DRCOG 1990.

THORNTON, Albert John The Glen, Summerhill, Kingswinford, Brierley Hill — MB ChB Birm. 1963; MRCS Eng. LRCP Lond. 1963.

THORNTON, Andrew Moor End, Irton, Holmrook CA19 1YQ — MB ChB Manch. 1967; MRCS Eng. LRCP Lond. 1967; DA Eng. 1972.

THORNTON, Andrew Chalbury Unit, Weymouth Community Hospital, Melcombe Avenue, Weymouth DT4 7TB Tel: 01305 762522 Fax: 01305 762526 — MB ChB Leeds 1986; MRCPsych 1992. Cons. Psychiat. for the Elderly, Weymouth Community Hosp. Weymouth. Specialty: Gen. Psychiat.; Geriat. Psychiat. Prev: Regist. Rotat. (Psychiat.) Camb. VTS.; Sen. Regist. in Gerontology & Old age Psychiat., N. W. TS.

THORNTON, Andrew Joseph The Bridge Street Centre, Foundry Bridge, Abertillery NP13 1BQ Tel: 01495 322682 — MB ChB Birm. 1985.

THORNTON, Andrew Shepherd Northlands Surgery, North Street, Calne SN11 0HH Tel: 01249 812091 Fax: 01249 815343 — MB BS Lond. 1977 (Lond. Hosp.) MA Camb. 1975; DCH RCP Lond. 1981; MRCGP 1983.

THORNTON, Anna Sara Constance 5 Sloane Street, London SW1 — MB BS Lond. 1975 (Middlx.) DMRD Eng. 1980; FRCR 1983. Cons. Radiol. Newham Gen. Hosp. Lond. Specialty: Radiol. Socs: FRCR. Prev: Sen. Regist. Univ. Coll., Gt. Ormond St., Maida Vale & Lond. Hosps.; Regist. Westm. Hosp. Lond.

THORNTON, Barbara Ann Four Winds, Glenmore Rd E., Crowborough TN6 1RE — MB ChB Manch. 1976.

THORNTON, Catherine Walker (retired) Fasgadh, Kilmichael, Glassary, Lochgilphead PA31 8QJ Tel: 0154 65 226 — MB ChB Glas. 1945 (St. And. & Univ. Glas.) Prev: Anaesth. Walsall Gp. Hosps.

THORNTON, Claire Maureen Histopathology Department, Institute of Clinical Science, Royal Group of Hospitals Trust, Grosvenor Road, Belfast BT12 6BA Tel: 02890 240503 Fax: 02890 233643; 38 Ranfurly Avenue, Bangor BT20 3SJ Tel: 02891 467049 — MB BCh BAO Belf. 1983; MRCPath 1990. Cons. Perinatal/Paediat. Path. Roy. Vict. Hosp. Belf. Specialty: Histopath.

THORNTON, Daniele Alexandra Allesley Park Medical Centre, Whitaker Road No.2, Coventry CV5 9JE Tel: 024 7667 4123 Fax: 024 7671 8166; Orchard House, Banbury Road, Kineton, Warwick CV35 0JY Tel: 01926 642515 — (Leeds) MB ChB Leeds 1988; DFFP 1992; T(GP) 1992; MRCGP 1993.

THORNTON, Daphne Parkway Medical Centre, 2 Frenton Close, Chapel House Estate, Newcastle upon Tyne NE5 1EH Tel: 0191 267 1313 Fax: 0191 229 0630 — MB BS Newc. 1986; MRCGP 1992; DRCOG 1992.

THORNTON, David John Queensview Medical Centre, Thornton Road, Northampton NN2 6LS Tel: 01604 713315 Fax: 01604 714378 — MB ChB Bristol 1968.

THORNTON, David Mark 13 Avondale Road, Chesterfield S40 4TF Tel: 01246 277879 — MB ChB Birm. 1987. Staff Grade (A & E) Chesterfield Roy. Hosp. Calow Chesterfield. Specialty: Accid. & Emerg.; Gen. Pract. Socs: Ordinary Mem. Roy. Soc. Med. Prev: SHO (A & E) Kings Mill Hosp. Mansfield Notts.; GP/Regist. CNDRH VTS.

THORNTON, David Michael Grange Practice, Allerton Health Centre, Bell Dew Road, Bradford BD15 7NJ — MB ChB Sheff. 1982; BSc Sheff. 1979, MB ChB 1982.

THORNTON, Eric John, Air Commodore RAF Med. Br. c/o DDMed Pers, DGMS (RAF), HQPTC, RAF Innsworth, Gloucester GL3 1EZ — MB ChB Dundee 1972; DAvMed. Eng. 1981; MFOM RCP Lond. 1989. Specialty: Occupat. Health.

THORNTON, Helen Louise 22 Bloomfield Drive, East Rainton, Houghton-le-Spring DH5 9SF — MB BS Newc. 1993.

THORNTON, John Andrew (retired) 8 Beaumond Green, Winchester SO23 8GF Tel: 01962 851574 — MB BS Lond. 1951 (Guy's) MRCS Eng. LRCP Lond. 1951; DA Eng. 1953; FFA RCS Eng. 1954; MD Lond. 1969; FFA RACS 1983. Prev: Prof. & Head Dept. Anaesth. & Intens. Care Chinese Univ. of Hong Kong Shatin NT, Hong Kong.

THORNTON, John Douglas (retired) 2 Green Hill Road, Leeds LS12 3QA Tel: 0113 263 9099 — MB ChB Leeds 1947.

THORNTON, John Noel Dickson Copnor Road Surgery, 111 Copnor Road, Portsmouth PO3 5AF Tel: 023 9266 3368 Fax: 023 9278 3203; 18 Craneswater Park, Southsea PO4 0NT — MB ChB Birm. 1985; DRCOG 1988; MRCGP 1989. GP Portsmouth. Prev: SHO BromsGr. & Redditch VTS; Ho. Surg. Birm. Accid. Hosp.; Ho. Phys. Good Hope Hosp. Sutton Coldfield.

THORNTON, John Richard St Peter's Hospital, Guildford Road, Chertsey KT16 0PZ Tel: 01932 872000 Fax: 01932 722229; The Runnymede Hospital, Guildford Road, Chertsey KT16 0RQ Tel: 01932 877833 Fax: 01932 877834 — MD Bristol 1982; MB ChB (Hons.) 1974; FRCP 1997. Cons. Phys. Ashford Hosp. Middlx. & St Peter's Hosp. Surrey. Specialty: Gastroenterol. Socs: Brit. Soc. Gastroenterol. Prev: Lect (Med.) St. Jas. Hosp. & Gen. Infirm. Leeds; Clin. Regist. & MRC Research Fell. (Med.) Bristol Roy. Infirm.

THORNTON, Leonard Countess of Chester Hospital, Liverpool Road, Chester CH2 1UL — MB ChB Glas. 1980; MRCPsych 1984. Cons. Child & Adolesc. Psychiat. Countess of Chester Hosp. Specialty: Child & Adolesc. Psychiat. Prev: Cons. Adolesc. Psychiat. Preswich Hosp. Manch.

THORNTON, Leslie Stuart Hugh (retired) Fairoak, Taplow Common Road, Burnham, Slough SL1 8LP — MB ChB Glas. 1940.

THORNTON, Margaret Elizabeth (retired) 23 Shelsley Drive, Moseley, Birmingham B13 9JU Tel: 0121 449 0531 — (Birm.) MB ChB Birm. 1951; DCH Eng. 1954, DA 1955; FFA RCS Eng. 1961. Prev: Cons. Anaesth. & Pain Relief W. Birm. HA.

THORNTON, Mark Julian Radiology Dept, Southmead Hosp, Westbury, Bristol BS10 5NB; 10 Royal Park, Clifton, Bristol BS8 3AW Tel: 0117 946 7885 — MB ChB Bristol 1987; MRCP (UK) 1991; FRCR 1995. Cons.(Radiol.). Specialty: Radiol. Socs: Fell. Roy. Soc. Med. Prev: Sen. Regist. Rotat. (Clin. Radiol.) SW Region; Regist. (Clin. Radiol.) Bristol; SHO (Neurosurg., Neurol. & Med.) Frenchay Hosp.

THORNTON, Maureen (retired) 54 Deramore Park S., Belfast BT9 5JY Tel: 01232 660186 — MB BCh BAO Belf. 1955.

THORNTON, Michael Campion (retired) Turnstones, 36 Salford, Audlem, Crewe CW3 0BJ Tel: 01270 811621 — (St. Geo.) MB BChir Camb. 1952; DObst RCOG 1957. Prev: Cas. Off. St. Geo. Hosp. Lond.

THORNTON, Patrick Dominic 6 North Link, Glen Road, Belfast BT11 8HW — MB BCh BAO Belf. 1991; MB BCh Belf. 1991.

THORNTON, Paul Elmwood Health Centre, Huddersfield Road, Holmfirth, Huddersfield HD9 3TR Tel: 01484 683138 Fax: 01484 689711; Wood Farm, Wood Lane, Holmfirth, Huddersfield HD9 3JB Tel: 01484 688614 — MB BS Lond. 1985; DCCH RCP Ed. 1989. Prev: Trainee GP Huddersfield.

THORNTON, Paul George Newsome 43 Granby Hill, Bristol BS8 4LS Tel: 0117 929 9113 Email: paul.thornton@which.net — MB ChB Bristol 1970; DA Eng. 1972; FFA RCS Eng. 1975. Cons. (Anaesth.) united Britol Healthcare Trust. Specialty: Anaesth. Prev: Sen. Regist. (Anaesth.) Avon AHA (T); Regist. (Anaesth.) Bristol Health Dist. (T); SHO (Anaesth.) Alder Hey Childr. Hosp. Liverp.

THORNTON, Peter John The Surgery, 20-22 Westdale Lane, Carlton, Nottingham NG4 3JA Tel: 0115 961 9401 — MB ChB Leeds 1970.

THORNTON, Peter William Carnoustie Medical Group, Dundee Street, Carnoustie DD7 7RB Tel: 01241 859888 Fax: 01241 852080; Rimuhau, 49 Carlogie Road, Carnoustie DD7 6EW — MB ChB Ed. 1972 (Edinburgh) BSc Ed. 1969; DA Eng. 1975; DObst RCOG 1975; FRCGP 1995, M 1978; MFFP 1994. GP Princip. Carnoustie Med. Gp.; Mem. GP Clin. Advis. Panel Med. & Dent. Defence Union of Scotl. Specialty: Gen. Pract. Socs: BMA. Prev: SHO (Paediat. & Plastic Surg.) Perth Roy. Infirm.; Ho. Surg. Roy. North. Infirm. Inverness; Ho. Phys. Deaconess Hosp. Edin.

THORNTON, Rebecca Jane The Lodge, Manor Farm, Shropham, Attleborough NR17 1DX — MB ChB Leeds 1991.

THORNTON, Richard John 45 Steep Hill, Lincoln LN2 1LU — MB BS Lond. 1971; FFA RCS Eng. 1976. Specialty: Anaesth.

THORNTON, Robert, Col. late RAMC — MD Ed. 1988; MB ChB 1974; DAvMed FOM RCP Lond. 1979; MFOM 1985, A 1981; DIH Soc. Apoth. Lond. 1984; MSc (Occupat. Med.) Lond. 1984; FFOM 1999. Asst. Dir. Med. Plans MOD. Specialty: Occupat. Health. Socs: Fell. Aerospace Med. Assoc. Prev: Assit Dir Med Policy MOD; Cons. Adviser Aviat. Med. HQ DAAC; Research Med. Off. Inst. Aviat. Med. FarnBoro.

THORNTON, Robert David Bewicke Medical Centre, 51 Tynemouth Road, Wallsend NE28 0AD Tel: 0191 262 3036 Fax: 0191 295 1663 — MB BS Newc. 1978; MRCGP 1982.

THORNTON, Robert John 26 Arran Hill, Thrybergh, Rotherham S65 4BH — BM BS Nottm. 1998.

THORNTON, Sandra Joy Engleton House Surgery, 2 Villa Road, Coventry CV6 3HZ Tel: 01484 688614 Fax: 01484 689711; Wood Farm, Wood Lane, Holmfirth, Huddersfield HD9 3JB Tel: 01484 688614 — MB BS Lond. 1984; DCH RCP Lond. 1986. Prev: Trainee GP Huddersfield.

THORNTON, Sarah Jane 24 Mount Pleasant, Nangreaves, Bury BL9 6SP — MB ChB Leeds 1991. Regist. (Anaesth.) Hope Hosp. Salford. Specialty: Anaesth. Socs: BMA; Train. Mem. Assn. Anaesth.; Manch. Med. Soc. Prev: SHO (ICU & Neurosurg.) N. Manch. Gen. Hosp.; SHO (Anaesth.) Huddersfield Roy. Infirm.; SHO (Anaesth.) Stepping Hill Hosp. Stockport.

THORNTON, Sarah Jane 22 Mitton Avenue, Barrowford, Nelson BB9 6BD — MB BS Lond. 1998.

THORNTON, Simon John CARE Nottingham, The Park Hospital, Sherwood Lodge Drive, Nottingham NG5 8RX Tel: 0115 967 1670 Fax: 0115 967 3542 Email: info@care-ivf.com — MB BChir Camb. 1981 (Cambridge University) MA Camb. 1983; MRCOG 1986; MD Melbourne 1990; FRCOG 1999. Med. Dir. CARE, The Pk. Hosp. Nottm. Specialty: Obst. & Gyn. Special Interest: Egg Donation; Infertil.; IVF. Socs: Brit. Fertil. Soc.; Amer. Soc. Reproduc. Med. Prev: Med. Dir. NURTURE Qu.s Med. Centre Nottm.; Sen. Regist. (Reproduc. Med.) Jessop Hosp. Sheff.; IVF Co-ordinator Roy. Wom. Hosp. Carlton, Vict., Austral.

THORNTON, Professor Steven Department Biological Sciences, University of Warwick, Coventry CV4 7AL Tel: 024 76 572747 Fax: 024 76 523568 Email: Sthornton@bio.warwick.ac.uk — BM Soton. 1983; DM Soton. 1989; MRCOG 1989. Prof. (O & G) Univ. Warwick; Hon. Cons. Obst., Univ. Hosps. of Coventry and Warks. Specialty: Obst. & Gyn. Special Interest: Labour; Preterm labour. Socs: Soc. Endocrinol.; Physiol. Soc.; Society for Gynaecologic Investigator. Prev: Lect. Hon. Cons. (Materno-fetal Med.) Rosie Matern. Hosp. Camb.; MRC Clin. Sci. Camb.; Birthright Train. Fell.

THORNTON, Susan Mary Brook House, Dam Lane, Leavening, Malton YO17 9SF Tel: 01653 658249 — BM BS Nottm. 1985 (Nottingham) BMedSci Nottm. 1983; DCH RCP Lond. 1989; DRCOG 1989; MRCGP 1990. p/t Princip. GP Sherburn & Rillington Pract., Malton, N. Yorks. Specialty: Gen. Pract. Prev: Asst. GP Derwent Surg. Malton Retainer Scheme.

THORNTON, Timothy James Pickering Surgery, Southgate, Pickering YO18 8BL; Middleton Hall, Middleton, Pickering YO18 8NX Tel: 01751 472283 — MB BChir Camb. 1977.

THORNTON, Timothy John Health Centre, 80 Knaresborough Road, Harrogate HG2 7LU Tel: 01423 883212 — MB BS Lond. 1974 (Guy's) MRCS Eng. LRCP Lond. 1974; DRCOG 1979; MRCGP 1980. Princip. in Gen. Pract. Harrogate. Prev: Squadron Ldr. Med. Off. RAF.

THORNTON, Vyvian Granville Four Winds, Glenmore Road E., Crowborough TN6 1RE — MB BS Lond. 1977; MRCS Eng. LRCP Lond. 1977.

THORNTON, William Dickson, CB, QHP (retired) 54 Deramore Park South, Belfast BT9 5JY — MB BCh BAO Dub. 1954; MD Dub. 1968; FFCM RCP (UK) 1979, M 1974; FFPHM RCP (UK) 1989. Prev: Dep. Chief Med. Off. DHSS N. Irel.

THORNTON-CHAN, Eddie Wing Cheong Clarendon Medical Practice, Clarendon Street, Hyde SK14 2AQ Tel: 0161 368 5224 Fax: 0161 368 4767; Grove End Farm, Blossoms Lane, Woodford, Stockport SK7 1RF — MB ChB Dundee 1983. Specialty: Cardiol. Prev: SHO (Paediat.) Bury Gen. Hosp.; SHO (Gen. Med.) Salford HA.

THORNTON-SMITH, Alexander Nathan 101 Roseberry Road, Epsom Downs, Epsom KT18 6AB — MB BS Lond. 1996 (King's College School Medicine and Dentistry) BSc Lond. 1993. Specialty: Accid. & Emerg.

THOROGOOD, Alan 71 Endsleigh Court, Colchester CO3 3QW Tel: 01206 575915 — (Westm.) MRCS Eng. LRCP Lond. 1951; DA Eng. 1955; FFA RCS Eng. 1957. Cons. Anaesth. Colchester Hosp. Gp. Specialty: Anaesth. Socs: Assn. Anaesths. & Intractable Pain Soc.; BMA. Prev: Sen. Regist. (Anaesth.) Qu. Vict. Hosp. E. Grinstead; Instruc. (Anaesth.) Univ. Wash. & Staff Anaesth. Veteran's Admin. Hosp. Seattle, USA.

THOROGOOD, Christopher The Medical Centre, Badgers Crescent, Shipston-on-Stour CV36 4BD Tel: 01608 661845 Fax: 01608 663614; Walnut Cottage, Upper Brailes, Banbury OX15 5AZ Tel: 01608 685581 Fax: 01608 685191 — MB BS Lond. 1975 (Roy. Free) MRCS Eng. LRCP Lond. 1975; DCH Eng. 1977; DRCOG 1978; FRCGP 1997, M 1979. GP Warks. HA; Course Organiser Banbury Dist. Oxf. Region; Examr. Roy. Coll. Gen. Pract.

THOROGOOD, Simon Vernon Department of Radiology, Royal Cornwall Hospitals Trust, Truro TR1 3LT Tel: 01872 250000 Fax: 01872 225314 Email: simon.thorogood@rcht.swest.nhs.uk; Greenacre, St. Clement, Truro TR1 1SZ Tel: 01872 278023 Email: simon@sthorogood.freeserve.co.uk — MB BS Lond. 1987. Cons. Radiol. Roy. Cornw. Hosps. Trust. Specialty: Radiol. Socs: FRCR;

RCP. Prev: Sen. Regist. (Radiol.) Bristol Roy. Infirm.; Regist. (Radiol.) Plymouth Gen. Hosp.; Regist. (Gen. Med.) Poole Hosp.

THORP, Jennifer Susan Audley Mills Surgery, 57 Eastwood Road, Rayleigh SS6 7JF Tel: 01268 774981; 14 Hall Park Avenue, Westcliff on Sea SS0 8NR Tel: 01702 77330 Fax: 01268 770176 — MB ChB Sheff. 1967; DObst RCOG 1969. Prev: Ho. Surg. (O & G) & Ho. Phys. OldCh. Hosp.; Romford.

THORP, Josephine Mary 32 Middleton Drive, Milngavie, Glasgow G62 8HT — MB ChB (Hons.) Leeds 1970; MRCP (UK) 1973; FRCA 1976. Cons. Anaesth.Lanarksh. Seute Hosp.s NHS Trust. Specialty: Anaesth.

THORP, Julie Kathryn Pine Lodge, The Green, Carleton, Pontefract WF8 3NJ — MB ChB Leeds 1998.

THORP, Nicola Jayne Maria Louise Clatterbridge Centre for Oncology, Bebington, Wirral CH63 4JY Tel: 0151 334 4000 Fax: 0151 482 7675 Email: nicky.thorp@ccotrust.nhs.uk; 33 Cheltenham Avenue, Liverpool L17 2AR Tel: 0151 733 5272 — MB ChB Leic. 1990; MRCP (UK) 1994; FRCR 1998. Cons. (Clin. Oncol.) Clatterbridge Centre Oncol. Wirral. Specialty: Oncol.; Radiother. Prev: Regist. (Clin. Oncol.) Clatterbridge Centre Oncol. Wirral.

THORP, Suzanne Louise 50 Danford Lane, Solihull B91 1QG Tel: 0121 711 3422 — MB ChB Birm. 1995. SHO (Paediat.) Sheff.. Childr. Hosp. Specialty: Accid. & Emerg. Prev: SHO (Paediat.) Liver Unit Birm. Childr. Hosp.; Ho. Off. (Gen. Surg.) Sandwell Dist. Gen. Hosp. Birm.

THORP, Tom Anthony John (retired) Harcombe House, Harcombe, Sidmouth EX10 0PR Tel: 01395 597480 — (Manch.) MB ChB Manch. 1949; DPH Liverp. 1952; DO Eng. 1960; MRCOphth 1990. Prev: Ophth. Med. Pract. Chesh. FPC.

THORP, Tom Anthony Simon Royal Sussex County Hospital, Eastern Road, Brighton BN2 5BE Tel: 01273 609060 Fax: 01273 609060; 11 Crown Hill, Seaford BN25 2XJ Fax: 01323 873416 Email: devereux@ukonline.co.uk — MB ChB Liverp. 1980; DA (UK) 1985; FFA RCSI 1988; MRCA 2001. Cons. Anaesth. & Pain Relief Brighton and Sussex University Hospitals. Specialty: Anaesth.; Chronic Pain. Socs: Assn. Anaesth.; Pain Soc.; Roy. Soc. Med. Lond. Prev: Hon. Cons. Pain Relief Guy's Hosp. Lond.; Sen. Regist. (Anaesth.) Qu. Med. Centre Nottm.

THORP-JONES, Daryl John 4 Northmead, Ledbury HR8 1BE — MB BS Lond. 1998; MB BS Lond 1998.

THORPE, Mr Andrew Christopher Department of Urology, City Hospitals, Sunderland SR4 7TP Tel: 0191 565 6256; 4 Ivy Road, Gosforth, Newcastle upon Tyne NE3 1DB — MB BCh Wales 1981; FRCS Ed. 1985; MS Wales 1993; FRCS (Urol) 1994. Cons. Urol. City Hosps. Sunderland. Specialty: Urol. Prev: Sen. Regist. (Urol.) Freeman Hosp. Newc.; Regist. (Paediat. Surg.) Lond. Hosp.; Regist. (Urol.) & Research Fell. Roy. Lond. Hosp.

THORPE, Mr Anthony Peter Department of Radiology, Royal Aberdeen Hospital, Westburn Road, Aberdeen AB25 2ZG; Foresters Croft, McGray Hill, Stonehaven AB39 3QA — MB ChB Birm. 1984; BSc (Hons.) Birm. 1981, MB ChB 1984; FRCS Eng. 1989; FRCR 1994; MRad (D) 1996. Cons. Radiol. Specialty: Radiol. Prev: Fell. in Interview. Radiol. Glas.; Regist. (Emerg. Med.) Fremantle, West. Austral; SHO (Orthop.) Nottm. HA.

THORPE, Anthony Wilfred (retired) 53 Church Street, Emley, Huddersfield HD8 9RP Tel: 01924 840127 — (Leeds) MB ChB Leeds 1957. Prev: GP Wakefield.

THORPE, Christopher Michael 28 Beaufort Avenue, Langland, Swansea SA3 4NU — MB BS Lond. 1985; FRCA 1992. Sen. Regist. (Anaesth.) Edin.

THORPE, Elizabeth Jane 56 St Christopher Mews, Wallington SM6 — MB BS Lond. 1997; DRCOG; DFFP.

THORPE, Frederick Graham (retired) Haslams Cottage, High Lane Farm, 71 Falkland Road, Ecclesall, Sheffield S11 7PN Tel: 0114 266 6692 — MB ChB Sheff. 1952; DPM Eng. 1957; FRCPsych 1978, M 1971. Prev: Cons. Childr. Psychiat. Sheff. HA (T).

THORPE, George William (retired) 10 Parkfields, Arden Drive, Dorridge, Solihull B93 8LL Tel: 01564 772768 — MB ChB (Hons) Birm. 1950; MRCS Eng. LRCP Lond. 1950; MRCP Lond. 1952; FRCGP 1983, M 1972. Prev: Regional Adviser (Gen. Pract.) W. Midl. RHA & Univ. Birm.

THORPE, Gerald William The Shambles, Moxons Lane, Waddington, Lincoln LN5 9QF — MB BS Lond. 1977; DCH RCP Lond. 1980; FRCR 1983. Cons. Radiol. Lincoln Hosps NHS Trust. Specialty: Radiol. Prev: Sen. Regist. (Radiol.) Manch. HA; SHO (Med.) Doncaster Roy. Infirm.; SHO (Paediat.) Leic. Gen. Hosp. & P'boro. Dist. Hosp.

THORPE, Graham John (retired) 36 Barnbrook Road, Sarisbury Green, Southampton SO31 7BQ Tel: 01489 480181 Email: thorpepatgraham@yahoo.co.uk — MB BS Lond. 1956 (Char. Cross) DTM & H (Warrington Yorke Medal) Liverp. 1961; FRCP Lond. 1977, M 1962. Prev: Cons. Phys. (Palliat. Med.) Countess Mt.batten Hse. Moorgreen Hosp. Soton.

THORPE, Jacqueline 289 Thorpe Road, Longthorpe, Peterborough PE3 6LU — BM BS Nottm. 1996.

THORPE, Mr James Andrew Charles Department of Cardiothoracic Surgery, Leeds General Infirmary, St George St., Leeds Tel: 0113 392 5897 Fax: 0113 392 5092; The Poplars, 22 Fink Mill, Morsforth, Leeds LS18 4DH Tel: 0113 281 9349 — MB ChB Leeds 1972; FRCS Ed. 1976; FRCS Eng. 1977; FECTS 1998. Cons. Thoracic Surg. Leeds Gen. Infirm. Specialty: Cardiothoracic Surg. Socs: Soc. of Thoracic & Cardiovasc. Surg.; Eur. Soc. Pneumonol.; Eur. Assn. Cardioth. Surg. Prev: Cons. Cardiothoracic Surg. Roy. Hallamsh. Hosp. & North. Gen. Hosp. Sheff.; Sen. Regist. (Cardiothoracic Surg.) Birm. Hosps.; Regist. (Surg.) Papworth Hosp. Camb.

THORPE, John Wainwright Edith Cavell Hospital, Department of Neurology, Bretton Gate, Peterborough PE3 9GZ Tel: 01733 875272 Email: john.thorpe@pbh-tr.nhs.uk; 12 Pepys Road, London SE14 5SB Email: thorpeje@aol.com — MB BS Lond. 1988; BA (Hons.) Oxf. 1985; MRCP (UK) 1991; MD 1999. Cons. Neurologist P'boro. Hosps. NHS Trust; Cons. Neurologist Addenbrookes Hosp. Camb. Specialty: Neurol. Special Interest: Multiple Sclerosis. Socs: Assoc. Mem. Assn. Brit. Neurol. Prev: Locum Cons. Neurologist Roy. Free Hosp.; SpR Neurol. Roy. Free Hosp.; SpR Neurol. Nat. Hosp. Qu. Sq.

THORPE, Margaret Oatway (retired) Flat 2, 49 Westbourne Villas, Hove BN3 4GG Tel: 01273 722055 — (Toronto) MD Toronto 1932; MCPS Alta. 1937; DObst RCOG 1944. Prev: Asst. Venereol. H.M. Prison Holloway.

THORPE, Maric John Langridge 32 Steventon, Daresbury Park, Sandymoor, Runcorn WA7 1UB — MB ChB Liverp. 1993.

THORPE, Mark Adrian, Maj. RAMC Retd. Smallbrook Surgery, 48 Boreham Road, Warminster BA12 9JR Tel: 01985 846700 Fax: 01985 846700 — MB BS Lond. 1983; MRCGP 1987.

THORPE, Michael Hamilton (retired) 28 Beaufort Avenue, Langland, Swansea SA3 4NU Tel: 01792 368780 — MB ChB Sheff. 1958; FFA RCS Eng. 1963. Prev: Cons. Anaesth. Singleton Hosp. Swansea.

THORPE, Mr Nigel Christopher Hillcrest, 11 Church Farm Road, Heacham, King's Lynn PE31 7JB — MB BS Lond. 1981; FRCS Ed. 1988; FRCS Eng. 1988.

THORPE, Mr Paul Lawrence Patrick John Taunton & Somerset NHS Trust, Somerset Spinal Surgery Service, Musgrove Park Hospital, Taunton TA1 5DA Tel: 01823 344825 Mob: 07768 386154 Fax: 01823 343444 Email: Paul.Thorpe@tst.nhs.uk; Somerset Nuffield Hospital, Staplegrove, Taunton TA2 6AN Tel: 01823 443232; Forde House, 9 Upper High Street, Taunton TA1 3PX Tel: 01823 462870 Fax: 01823 462870 Email: plpjt@doctors.org.uk/plpjt@hotmail.com — MB ChB Leic. 1991; FRCS Ed. 1996; FRCS (Trauma & Orthop.) Ed. 2001. Cons. Orthopaedic & Spinal Surg. Specialty: Orthop.; Deformity, Cervical, ThoracoLumbar surgery. Special Interest: Spinal Surg. including deformity,cervical & thoracolumbar Surg.; Medico-legal. Socs: Brit. Assn. of Spinal Surgeons; Brit. Cervical Spine Soc.; AO Alumni Assn. Prev: Specialist Regist. (Orthop.) S. W. Rotat.; SHO Rotat. (Surg.) Frenchay Hosp. Bristol; SHO (Orthop. & A & E) Roy. Hallamsh. Hosp. Sheff.

THORPE, Penelope Anne Department of Histopathology, West Middlesex University Hospital, Twickenham Road, Isleworth TW7 6AF Tel: 020 8321 5860 Email: anne.thorpe@whuh-tr.nthames.nhs.uk — MB BS Lond. 1980 (Royal Free) BSc (Hons.) Ed. 1971; PhD Camb. 1975; MRCPath 1986; FRCpath 1997. Cons. Histopath. W. Middlx. Univ. Hosp. Specialty: Histopath.

THORPE, Richard William Thorpe, Burgess and Menzies, Moulton Medical Centre, High St, Spalding PE12 6QB Tel: 01406 370265 Fax: 01406 373219 — MB ChB Sheff. 1985; MMedSci Nottm. 1996. Clin. Asst. (Geriat.) Welland Hosp. Spalding; Med. Off. Holbeach Hosp. Socs: BMA; Roy. Soc. Med.

THORPE, Ronald Stanley Gostelyns, Stoke Holy Cross, Norwich NR14 8LW Tel: 01508 2288 — MB ChB Birm. 1942; DMRD Eng. 1947; FRCR 1975. Specialty: Radiol. Socs: Norwich M-C Soc. Prev: Ho. Surg. Burntwood EMS Hosp; Capt. RAMC 1943-47.; Regist. (Radiol.) Birm. United Hosp.

THORPE, Russell John The Old Links Surgery, 104 Highbury Road East, Lytham St Annes FY8 2LY Tel: 01253 713621; Haymon, 150 St Annes Road E., Lytham St Annes FY8 23HW Tel: 01253 712481 — MB ChB Liverp. 1982. Prev: Trainee GP Wirral HA VTS; Ho. Off. Southport Gen. Infirm.

THORPE, Sheila Christine (retired) Meadowside, Ropley, Alresford SO24 0DS Tel: 01962 773202 — MB ChB Glas. 1952; DObst RCOG 1962; MRCGP 1974. Prev: Regist. (O & G) Fulham Hosp. & Fulham Matern. Hosp.

THORPE, Susan Sheila Standerton, Seymour Road, Mannamead, Plymouth PL3 5AT — MB BS Lond. 1984. Regist. (O & G) Lewisham & Guy's. Hosps. Lond. Specialty: Obst. & Gyn. Prev: SHO (O & G) St. Mary's Hosp. Portsmouth; SHO (O & G) King's Coll. & Dulwich Hosps. Lond.

THORPE-BEESTON, John Guy Chelsea and Westminster Hopspital, Fulham Road, London SW10 9NH — MB BChir Camb. 1984; MRCOG 1989; MA Camb 1985, MD 1991; FRCOG 2001. Cons. O & G Chelsea & Westm. Hosp. Lond. Specialty: Obst. & Gyn. Prev: Sen. Regist. (O & G) St. Mary's Hosp. Lond.; SHO (O & G) Kings Coll. Hosp. Lond.; SHO (Surg.) Hammersmith Hosp. Lond.

THOULD, Anthony Keith (retired) Idless Mill, Idless, Truro TR4 9QS Tel: 01872 272593 — (St. Bart.) MD Lond. 1960, MB BS (Hnrs.) 1954; FRCP Lond. 1974, M 1958. Cons. Rheum. Roy. Cornw. Hosp. (City) Truro; Surg. Lt. Cdr. RNR. Prev: Sen. Regist. (Med.) & Ho. Surg. St. Bart. Hosp. Lond.

THOULD, Geoffrey Robert Devon Health Protection Unit, The Lescaze Offices, Shinner's Bridge, Dartington, Totnes TQ9 6JE Tel: 01803 866665 — MB BS Lond. 1986; BSc (Hons.) Durham. 1981; MB BS (Distinc.) Lond. 1986; MSc (Pub. Health) Lond. 1995; MFPHM 1998. Cons., Communicable Dis. Control (Pub. Health Med.),Devon Health Protec. Unit. Specialty: Pub. Health Med. Prev: Sen. Regist. (Pub. Health Med.) S. & W. RHA; Regist. (Pub. Health Med.) SE Thames RHA; Regist. (Microbiol.) Bristol Roy. Infirm.

THOUNG, Mehm Tin 8 Church Green, Roxwell, Chelmsford CM1 4NZ — MB BS Western Australia 1985; FRCA 1993.

THOW, Jonathan Charles York Hospital, Wiggington Road, York YO31 8HE Tel: 01904 725624 — MD Newc. 1991; MB BS Newcastle 1982 (Newcastle upon Tyne) MRCP (UK) 1985; FRCP Lond. 1998. Cons. Phys. Diabetes & Endocrinol. York Dist. Hosp.; Hon. Clin. Reader, Hull York Med. Sch. Specialty: Endocrinol.; Diabetes. Prev: Sen. Regist. (Med.) Manch. Roy. Infirm.; Regist. (Gen. Med.) Newc. Gen. Hosp.

THOW, Mary Elizabeth (retired) Sighthill Health Centre, Calder Road, Edinburgh EH11 4AU Tel: 0131 453 5335; The Old Manse, 45 Lanark Road, Edinburgh EH14 1TL Tel: 0131 443 4685 — MB BS Lond. 1957 (Roy. Free) Prev: GP Princip. Sighthill Health Centre Edin. EH11 4AU.

THRASHER, Adrian James Molecular Immunology Unit, Institute of Child Health, 30 Guilford St., London WC1N 1EH Tel: 020 7813 8490; Manor Farm Barns, Little Staughton, Bedford MK44 2BH — MB BS Lond. 1986; MRCP (UK) 1989; PhD Lond. 1995. Wellcome Trust Sen. Fell. in Clin. Sci. & Hon. Cons. Immunol. Gt. Ormond St. Hosp.for Childr. NHS Trust.; Hon. Sen. Regist. UCL Sch. Med. & Gt. Ormond St. Hosp. Lond. Prev: Clin. Lect. & Hon. Regist. Rayne Inst. Univ. Coll. Hosp. Lond.; Lect. (Molecular Med.) & Regist. (Gen. Med.) Univ. Coll. Hosp.

THREEPURANENI, Gopichand 22 Holder Drive, Cannock WS11 1TL — MB ChB Leic. 1995.

THRELFALL, Alexandra Katherine Walnut Tree House, Oxford Road, Old Marston, Oxford OX3 0PH Tel: 01865 242071 — BM Soton. 1977; DRCOG 1979; DCH RCP Lond. 1981; MRCGP 1984.

THRELFALL, Alison Louise Testvale Surgery, 12 Salisbury Road, Totton, Southampton SO40 3PY Tel: 023 8086 6999/6990 Fax: 023 8066 3992; 3 Blackwater House, Emery Down, Lyndhurst SO43 7FJ Tel: 02380 283022 — MB ChB Birm. 1981 (Birmingham) FPA 1985; DRCOG 1985; MRCGP 1985; Diploma in Healthcare Ethics (Kings Coll. Lond.) 2003.

THRELFALL, Ann Elizabeth Edenfield Road Surgery, Cutgate Shopping Precinct, Edenfield Road, Rochdale OL11 5AQ Tel: 01706 344044 Fax: 01706 526882; 110 Bury Road, Edenfield, Ramsbottom, Bury BL0 0ET — MB ChB Manch. 1981.

THRELFALL, James Anthony — BM BS Nottm. 1997.

THRES, Grace Veronica The Hazard, Widemouth Bay, Bude EX23 0AQ — MB ChB Bristol 1945 (Bristol & Univ. Tulane) DPH Eng. 1958.

THRIPPLETON, Lucy Kate 25 Grove Street, Wantage OX12 7AB — MB BS Lond. 1997.

THRIPPLETON, Sean Arthur The Surgery, Worsley Road, Immingham, Grimsby DN40 1BE — MB BS Lond. 1987; DRCOG 1991; MRCGP 1992.

THROSSELL, Jane Ann Lynfield Mount Hospital, Heights Lane, Bradford BD9 6DP Tel: 01274 494194 Fax: 01274 483494 — MB BS Newc. 1974; DPM Leeds 1977; MRCPsych 1978. Cons. Psychiat. Bradford Community Health Trust. Specialty: Gen. Psychiat.

THROWER, Andrew James 14 Cliffside Gardens, Leeds LS6 2HA — MB ChB Leeds 1998.

THROWER, Dorothy Frances (retired) 2 Highfields, Warsash Road, Warsash, Southampton SO31 9JE Tel: 01489 579168 — MB ChB Bristol 1955; DObst RCOG 1958; DCH Eng. 1957, DPH 1966. Prev: Clin. Med. Off. (Community Health) Portmouth & SE Hants. HA.

THROWER, Michelle Mary 33 The Kyles, Ravenscraig, Kirkcaldy KY1 2QG Tel: 01592 205699 — MB ChB Dundee 1990; MRCGP 1994. Prev: Trainee GP Fife.

THROWER, Patricia Ann St Georges Medical Centre, 7 Sunningfields Road, Hendon, London NW4 4QR Tel: 020 8202 6232 Fax: 020 8202 3906; Links Cottage, Holders Hill Crescent, London NW4 1NE Tel: 020 8203 2217 — MB BS Lond. 1974 (St. Bart.) FRCP 2001. GP Princip.; Clin. Director Barnet PCT. Prev: Sen. Regist. (Gen. Med. & Rheum.) St. Bart. Hosp. Lond.

THROWER, Stephanie Mary (Surgery), Wadeslea, Elie, Leven KY9 1EA Tel: 01333 330302; The Manse, Pittenweem, Anstruther KY10 2LR Tel: 01333 311255 — MB ChB St. And. 1963. Prev: Clin. Asst. Playfield Ho. Cupar & PDU Vict. Hosp. Kirkcaldy; Asst. Med. Off. Falmouth Hosp. Trelawny Jamaica.

THRUSH, David Cyril Little Beacon, Court Road, Newton Ferrers, Plymouth PL8 1DA Tel: 01752 872503 — (Camb. & St. Geo.) MD Camb. 1973, MB 1966, BChir 1965; FRCP Lond. 1982, M 1968. Cons. Neurol. Devon AHA. Specialty: Neurol. Socs: Assn. Brit. Neurol. & W. Country Phys. Assn.

THRUSH, Roger (retired) Pinfold Health Centre, Field Road, Bloxwich, Walsall WS3 3JP Fax: 01922 775132; 9 St. Margaret's, Streetly, Sutton Coldfield B74 4HU Tel: 0121 353 8858 — MB BS Lond. 1968 (St. Bart.) DObst RCOG 1970; DCH RCP Lond. 1971; MRCGP 1972. Prev: Trainee GP Newc. VTS.

THRUSH, Steven 9 St Margarets, Sutton Coldfield B74 4HU — MB BS Lond. 1992.

THULBOURNE, Mr Terence (retired) Rivendell, Auchterhouse, Dundee DD3 0RF — (Sheff.) MB ChB (Hnrs.) Sheff. 1960; FRCS Eng. 1969. Prev: Retd. Cons. Orthop. Dundee Roy. Infirm.

THUM, Annabel Maxine Elizabeth Highgate Group Practice, 4 Notrh Hill, Highgate, London N6 4QH Tel: 0208 340 6628; 14 Denewood Road, Highgate, London N6 4AJ Tel: 0208 341 2558 — MB ChB Bristol 1987; DRCOG 1990; MRCGP 1991. Prev: Trainee GP Capelfield Surg. Claygate; SHO (A & E) Kingston Hosp. Kingston u. Thames; SHO (Psychiat.) The Priory Roehampton.

THURAIRAJ, Thillairaj 6 The Pastures, Bixley Farm, Ipswich IP4 5UQ Tel: 01473 715108 — MB BS Sri Lanka 1980. SCMO (Psychiat. for Elderly) Minsmere Hse., St. Clements & Gen. Hosp. Ipswich. Specialty: Geriat. Psychiat. Prev: Staff Grade (Psychiat. for Elderly) Barnet Gen. & Napsbury Hosp. Herts.

THURAIRAJA, Ramesh 24 Malcolm Drive, Surbiton KT6 6QS — BM Soton. 1998.

THURAIRAJAH, Adrian 32 St John's Road, Wembley Central, Wembley HA9 7JQ Tel: 020 8902 0118 — MB BS Ceylon 1954.

THURAIRAJAH, Guhaeni York Road Surgery, 55 York Road, Ilford IG1 3AF Tel: 020 8514 0906 Fax: 020 8553 3323 — MB BS Ceylon 1971.

THURAIRAJAH, Krishni 92 Helmsdale Avenue, Dundee DD3 0NW — MB ChB Dundee 1993; DRCOG 1996; MRCGP 1998. GP.

THURAIRAJASINGAM, Sornaghandimalar (retired) 8 Fir Tree Avenue, Worsley, Manchester M28 1LP — MB BS Ceylon 1953;

DMRD Eng. 1962; FFR 1969; FRCR 1975. Cons. Radiol. Salford AHA (T).

THURAISINGAM, Adrian Ivo 24 Castle Bank, Stafford ST16 1DJ — MB ChB Manch. 1995.

THURAISINGAM, Chelliah Paul (retired) 24 Castle Bank, Stafford ST16 1DJ Tel: 01785 241040 — MB BS Ceylon 1950; DTM & H Ceylon 1953. Prev: GP Stafford.

THURGOOD, Michael Clive Fairwater Medical Centre, Fairwater Square, Fairwater, Cwmbran NP44 4TA Tel: 01633 869544 — MB BCh Wales 1992; MRCGP 1996; DRCOG 1997. GP. Specialty: Gen. Pract. Socs: Roy. Coll. Gen. Pract.; BMA. Prev: Trainee GP Cardiff; SHO (O & G) Cardiff.

THURKETTLE, Alison Jayne City Medical Practice, 60, Portland St, Lincoln LN5 7LB Tel: 01522 876800 Fax: 01522 876803 — MB ChB Leeds 1984 (University of Leeds) DRCOG 1987. Asst. GP Lincoln. Specialty: Gen. Pract.

THURLBECK, Sarah Margaret St. George's Hospital, Blackshaw Road, London SW17 0QT Tel: 020 8725 3648 Fax: 020 8725 3938 — MB BS Lond. 1980; MRCP (UK) 1983; FRCPC 1990. Cons. Paediat. St. Geo. Hosp. Lond. Specialty: Paediat.

THURLEY, Patricia Ann (Surgery), 3 Cape Road, Warwick CV34 4JP Tel: 01926 499988; 33 Blacklow Road, Warwick CV34 5SX Tel: 01926 491673 — MRCS Eng. LRCP Lond. 1967 (Liverp. & Birm.) Prev: Ho. Surg. & Ho. Phys. Warneford Gen. Hosp. Leamington Spa.

THURLEY, Patricia Elizabeth X-Ray Department, Whipps Cross Hospital, Leytonstone, London E11 Tel: 020 8539 5522; 16 Grove Hill, South Woodford, London E18 2JG Tel: 020 8989 0623 Email: pethurley@aol.com — MB BS Lond. 1970 (Westm.) BSc (Special) Lond. 1967; MRCS Eng. LRCP Lond. 1970; DCH Eng. 1972; DMRD Eng. 1974; FRCR 1981. Cons. Radiol. Whipps Cross Hosp. Lond. Specialty: Radiol. Prev: Clin. Asst. (Radiol. & Ultrasound) Whipps Cross Hosp. Lond.; Regist. (Radiol.) Westm. Hosp. Lond.

THURLOW, Alexander Cresswell Department of Anaesthesia, St. George's Hospital, Blackshaw Road, London SW17 0QT Tel: 020 8672 1255; 17 Belvedere Drive, London SW19 7BU Tel: 020 8946 0240 — MB BS Lond. 1964 (St. Mary's) MRCS Eng. LRCP Lond. 1964; FFA RCS Eng. 1968. Cons. Anaesth. St. Geo. Hosp. Lond. Specialty: Anaesth. Socs: BMA; Assn. Anaesths. Prev: Sen. Regist. (Anaesth.) St. Thos. Hosp. Lond. & Hosp. Sick Childr. Gt. Ormond St.; Regist. (Anaesth.) St. Geo. Hosp. Lond.

THURLOW, Beverley Anne Beatrice (retired) 214 Moss Delph Lane, Aughton, Ormskirk L39 5BJ Tel: 01695 422067 — MB ChB Liverp. 1963; DObst 1965; MRCOG 1970. Assoc. Specialist - Child Health Alder Hey Childrs. Hosp. NHS Trust. Prev: Clin. Med. Off. S. Sefton HA.

THURLOW, John Horning Road Surgery, Horning Road West, Hoveton, Norwich NR12 8QH Tel: 01603 782155 Fax: 01603 782189; Church Farm, Upper St, Horning, Norwich NR12 8NL — MB BS Lond. 1969 (St. Bart.) MRCS Eng. LRCP Lond. 1969; DCH Eng. 1971. Prev: SHO Ipswich & E. Suff. Hosps.; SHO (Obst.) Roy. Berks. Hosp. Reading; Ho. Surg. St. Bart. Hosp. Lond.

THURLOW, Susan Kristina Grosvenor Avenue Surgery, 20 Grosvenor Avenue, Hayes UB4 8NL Tel: 020 8845 7100 Fax: 020 8842 4401 — MB BS Lond. 1989; DRCOG 1993; MRCGP 1994.

THURNELL, Mr Christopher Alain Flat 4, 21 Fog Lane, Didsbury, Manchester M20 0AR Email: christhurnell@hotmail.com — MB ChB Manch. 1990 (Manchester) BSc (Hons.) Manch. 1984, MB ChB 1990; MRNZCOG 1998; MRCOG 1999; FRANZCOG 2001. Cons. (O & G) Rotorua Hosp. Rotorua, New Zealand. Specialty: Obst. & Gyn. Prev: Regist. (O & G), Countess of Chester, Chester; Regist. (O & G) Cheltenham Hosp. Cheltenham; Demonst. (Anat.) Univ. Manch.

THURRELL, Wendy Pamela Consultant Cellular Pathology, Cellular Pathology, Kennington Road, Willesborough, Ashford TN24 0LZ — MB BS Lond. 1983; MRCPath 1992; FRCPath 2002.

THURSBY-PELHAM, Anna Katherine 2 Woodlands Avenue, New Malden KT3 3UN — MB ChB Dundee 1996.

THURSBY-PELHAM, Fergus William Vaughan 2 Woodlands Avenue, New Malden KT3 3UN — MB BS Lond. 1998.

THURSFIELD, Sian Rhiannon 40A Lichfield Road, London NW2 2RG — MB BS Lond. 1993.

THURSFIELD, William Reginald Ritchie (retired) Red Cross Cottage, Salterns, Seaview PO34 5AG Tel: 01983 613115 — MB BS Lond. 1946 (St. Thos.) MRCS Eng. LRCP Lond. 1945; DMRD Eng. & Lond 1950; LMCC 1954. Prev: Cons. Radiol. I. of Wight & Portsmouth Hosp. Gp.

THURSTAN, John Whieldon Holywell House Surgery, Holywell Street, Chesterfield S41 7SD Tel: 01246 273075 Fax: 01246 555711; Wych Cottage, Common Lane, Cutthorpe, Chesterfield S42 7AN — MB ChB Sheff. 1979; DRCOG 1983. Socs: MRCGP.

THURSTAN, Nigel David Antony Chard Road Surgery, Chard Road, Plymouth PL5 2UE Tel: 01752 363111; 62 Windemere Crescent, Plymouth PL6 5HX — MB ChB Manch. 1971.

THURSTON, Mr Andrew Vernon Consultant Urologist, St Albans City Hospital, St Albans AL3 5PN Tel: 01721 897116 — MB BChir Camb. 1978; MA Camb. 1978; FRCS Eng. 1982. Cons. Urol. W. Herts Hosp.s. Specialty: Urol. Socs: Brit. Assn. Urol. Surgs. & Brit. Prostate Gp.; Amer. Urological Assn. Prev: Regist. (Urol.) Portsmouth HA; Demonst. (Anat.) Camb. Univ.; Cons. (Urol.) Doncaster.

THURSTON, Anne Marguerite J M Waters and Partners, 21 Beaufort Road, Southbourne, Bournemouth BH6 5AJ Tel: 01202 433081 Fax: 01202 430527; The Glen, Beckley, Christchurch BH23 7ED — MB BS Lond. 1981 (Guy's) DRCOG 1984; MRCGP 1985; DCH RCP Lond. 1986. Specialty: Gen. Pract. Socs: BMA. Prev: Trainee GP Guy's Hosp. VTS; Clin. Med. Off. & Ho. Phys. Guy's Hosp. Lond.

THURSTON, Brian John Lisson Grove Medical Centre, 3-5 Lisson Grove, Mutley, Plymouth PL4 7DL Tel: 01752 205555 Fax: 01752 205558; Clinkland Farm House, Ermingston, Ivybridge PL21 9JY Email: brianthur@aol.com — MB BChir Camb. 1979 (Cambridge & Westminster) DRCOG 1986; DCH RCP Lond. 1986. Prev: SHO (A & E) Torbay Hosp. Torquay; SHO (Paediat.) Roy. Devon & Exeter Hosp. Exeter; SHO (O & G) Camb. HA.

THURSTON, Caroline (retired) Corner House, Plump Rd, Tharston, Norwich NR15 2YR — MB ChB Sheff. 1989; BSc (Hons.) Soton. 1983; FRCA (Pt. I) 1993; FFARCSI (Pt. II) 1994.

THURSTON, Eric Wistan, OStJ (retired) 11 Ryder Seed Mews, Pageant Road, St Albans AL1 1NL Tel: 01727 856112 — (Char. Cross Hosp.) MB BS Lond. 1948. Prev: Capt. RAMC.

THURSTON, Professor Herbert University of Leicester, Leicester Warwick Med. Sch., School of Medicine, Robert Kilpatrick Clinical Sciences Building, Leicester Royal Infirmary, PO Box 65, Leicester LE2 7LX Tel: 0116 252 3183 Fax: 0116 252 3188; Linden House, Loddington Road, Tilton-on-the Hill, Leicester LE7 9DE — MB ChB (Hons.) Manch. 1966; MRCP (UK) 1970; BSc (Hons.) Manch. 1964, MD 1980; FRCP Lond. 1981. Prof. Med. & Cons. Phys. Univ. Leicester & Leicester Roy. Infirm. Specialty: Gen. Med. Socs: Assn. Phys. & Med. Research Soc.; Internat. Soc. of Hypertens.; Cardiac Soc. Research Assn. Prev: SHO Profess. Med. Unit & Ho. Phys. & Ho. Surg. Manch. Roy. Infirm.; Lect. (Med.) Univ. Manch.

THURSTON, Hilary Ann Sefton Health Authorities, Burlington House, Crosby Road N., Waterloo, Liverpool L22 0QB Tel: 0151 920 5056 Fax: 0151 920 1035 — MB ChB Liverp. 1983; DRCOG 1986; MRCGP 1989; MPH Liverp. 1991; MFPHM 1998. Specialty: Pub. Health Med.; Gen. Pract. Socs: BMA. Prev: Sp. Regist. (Pub. Health Med.) Mersey RHA; Trainee GP Merseyside VTS; RMO (Psychiat.) Vict., Austral.

THURSTON, John Gavin Bourdas Vessels, Bessels Green Road, Sevenoaks TN13 2PT Tel: 01732 458367 — MRCS Eng. LRCP Lond. 1961 (Guy's) MB BS Lond. 1961; BS 1967; MRCP Lond. 1967; FRCP 1992; FFAEM 1993; FIFEM 2004. Cons. Emerg. Phys. A/E Darent Valley Hosp., Dartford; Phys. Grand Order Water Rats; Maj. Incident Doctor, RFU Twickenham. Specialty: Accid. & Emerg.; Cardiol. Socs: BMA; BAEM; RCP. Prev: Cons. Phys. i/c A & E Dept. Qu. Mary's Hosp. Roehampton; Sen. Regist. (Gen. Med. & Cardiol.) Westm. Hosp. Lond.

THURSTON, John Vernon (retired) Actons Cottage, Buckholt La, Bexhill-on-Sea TN39 5AX Tel: 01424 830415 — MB BS Lond. 1948 (St. Mary's) MRCS Eng. LRCP Lond. 1945; DObst RCOG 1950.

THURSTON, Julia Sarah Wargrave Surgery, Victoria Road, Wargrave, Reading RG10 8BP Tel: 0118 940 3939 Fax: 0118 940 1357 — MB BS Lond. 1981 (Guy's) DRCOG 1984; MRCGP 1985. Socs: BMA. Prev: Trainee GP Guy's Hosp. VTS Lond.

THURSTON, Kenneth The Surgery, Lydford Mews, 23 High Street, East Hoathly, Lewes BN8 6DR Tel: 01865 840943 Fax: 01865 841309; Hollyhocks Thomas Turner Drive, East Hoathly, Lewes BN8 6QF — MRCS Eng. LRCP Lond. 1974 (Sheff.) Specialty: Gen.

Pract. Prev: SHO (A & E Orthop. & Gen. Surg.) Leicester Roy. Infirm.; Demonst. (Anat.) Univ. Leicester; Ho. Phys. (Cardiol. & Gen. Med.) North. Gen. Hosp. Sheff.

THURSTON, Nicola Garden Cottages, Trewsbury House, Coates, Cirencester GL7 6NY — MB BS Lond. 1994.

THURSTON, Stephen Charles Wymondham Medical Partnership, Postmill Close, Wymondham NR18 0RF — MB ChB Leic. 1985; DRCOG 1989. Prev: Trainee GP Leicester VTS.

THURSTON, Timothy John New Milton Health Centre, Spencer Road, New Milton BH25 6EN Tel: 01425 621188 Fax: 01425 620646; The Glen, Beckley, Christchurch BH23 7ED — (Guy's) BSc Lond. 1979, MB BS 1982; DRCOG 1985; DCH RCP Lond. 1986; MRCGP 1986. Prev: Ho. Phys. Guy's Hosp. Lond.; Older Person's Lead New Forest PCT.

THURSZ, Mr Anthony David Standing Stones, Kinniside, Cleator CA23 3AQ Tel: 01946 861415 Fax: 01946 861415; Standing Stones, Kinniside, Cleator CA23 3AQ Tel: 01946 861415 Fax: 01946 861415 — (King's Coll. Hosp.) MA, MB BChir Camb. 1953; MRCS Eng. LRCP Lond. 1953; FRCOG 1976, M 1963, DObst 1956; FRCS Ed. 1963. Specialty: Obst. & Gyn. Socs: Fell. Manch. Med. Soc. & N. Eng. Obst. & Gyn. Soc. Prev: Cons. O & G Vale of Leven Hosp. Alexandria; Cons. O & G W. Cumbld. Hosp. Gp.; Sen. Regist. (O & G) Newc. Gen. Hosp.

THURSZ, Mark Richard Imperial College School of Medicine, Department of Medicine, St Mary's Hospital, Praed St., London W2 1PG Tel: 020 7594 3641 Fax: 020 7724 9369 Email: m.thursz@ic.ac.uk — MB BS Lond. 1986; MRCP (UK) 1989; MD Lond. 1997. Sen. Lect. & Hon. Cons. (Med. & Gastroenterol.) St. Mary's Hosp. Med. Sch. Imperial Coll. Lond. Specialty: Gastroenterol. Socs: Brit. Soc. Gastroenterol.; Eur. Assn. Study Liver; Assn. of Phys.s. Prev: Regist. (Med. & Gastroenterol.) Northwick Pk. Hosp.

THURTLE, Owen Anthony Woodbridge Road Surgery, 165-167 Woodbridge Road, Ipswich IP4 2PE Tel: 01473 256251; 43 Cowper Street, Ipswich IP4 5JA Tel: 01473 278022 — MB BS Newc. 1973; MRCP (UK) 1977; DRCOG 1984; MRCGP 1985; T (M) 1991; T (GP) 1991. Specialty: Rheumatol. Prev: Sen. Regist. (Rheum & Rehabil.) Soton. & Portsmouth; Regist. (Med.) York Health Dist.

THUSE, Mr Makarand Ganesh Manor Hospital, Moat Road, Walsall WS2 9PS Tel: 01922 721172; 29 Carlton Croft, Streetly, Sutton Coldfield B74 3JT — MB BS Bombay 1969 (Seth G.S. Med. Coll.) Dip. Orthop. CPS Bombay 1972; MS (Gen. Surg.) Bombay 1972; FRCS Ed. 1975; FRCS Eng. 1975; DMRD Eng. 1981; FRCR 1983. Cons. Radiol. Walsall Heath Dist. Manor, Little Aston Hosps. Specialty: Radiol. Prev: Sen. Regist. (Radiol.) W. Midl. RHA; Regist. (Surg.) Gravesend & N. Kent Hosp. & Dartford & Gravesham Health Dist.; Regist. (Surg.) Qu. Mary's Hosp. Sidcup.

THWAITE, Dawn Sarah Trem-Y-Bryn, Carreghofa Lane, Llanymynech SY22 6LA; Trem-Y-Bryn, Carreghofa Lane, Llanymynech SY22 6LA Tel: 01691 830083 — MB BS Lond. 1994; BSc Basic Med. Scs. & Physiol. (1st cl. Hons.) Lond. 1991; MRCP Pt. I 1996; DFFP. 1998; DRCOG. 1998. GP Regist. Montgomery Med Pract. Powys. Prev: SHO (GUM & HIV) Chelsea & Westminster Hosp.; SHO (O & G) FarnBoro. Hosp. Kent; SHO Rotat. (Med.) Kings Coll. Hosp. Lond.

THWAITE, Erica Louise 95 Avon Road, Billinge, Wigan WN5 7SF — MB BS Lond. 1991 (King's College London) MRCP 1994; FRCRI 1996; DMRD 1997. Specialist Regist. (Radiol.) Mersey Region. Specialty: Radiol.

THWAITE, Linda Jane 364 Hale Road, Halebarns, Altrincham WA15 8SY — MB ChB Sheff. 1989 (Sheffield) DRCOG 1992; MRCGP 1995. Specialty: Gen. Pract.

THWAITES, Alison Jane 47 Lonsdale Road, Birmingham B17 9QX — MB ChB Birm. 1988; ChB Birm. 1988.

THWAITES, Barnaby Christopher — MB BS Lond. 1979 (Roy. Free) FRCP; BSc (Genetics & Biol.) Manch. 1974. Cons. Cardiologist Royal Hampshire County Hospital; Hon. Cons. Cardiol. N. Hants. Hosp. & Soton. Gen. Hosp. Specialty: Cardiol. Socs: Brit. Pacing & Electrophysiol. Gp.; Brit. Cardiac Soc. Prev: Cons. Phys. & Cardiol. Holberton Hosp. Antigua, W. Indies.; Regist. Nat. Heart Hosp. Lond.; Hon. Cons. Cardiol. Freeman Hosp. Newc.

THWAITES, Ian Guy Marlhurst, Southwater, Horsham RH13 9BY Tel: 01403 730153 — MB BChir Camb. 1967 (St. Thomas' Hospital Lond.) DCH Eng. 1970; MLCOM 1991; DMS Med. 1993. Indep. Phys. (Musculoskeletal Med.) Horsham. Specialty: Orthop. Socs: Brit. Inst. Musculoskeletal Med. Prev: GP Horsham, Sussex.

THWAITES, Richard John Department of Paediatrics, St. Mary's Hospital, Portsmouth PO3 6AD Tel: 023 92 286000 Fax: 023 92 866101 — MB BS Lond. 1985; BA Camb. 1982; BA Camb. 1982; MRCP (UK) 1991; MRCP UK 1991. Cons. Paediat. St. Mary's Hosp. Portsmouth. Specialty: Paediat. Prev: Lect. (Neonatol.) United Med. Sch. Guy's & Thos. Hosp. Lond.; Lect. (Child Health) Med. Coll. St. Bart. Hosp. Lond.

THWAITES, Rosemary North View, Copt Hewick, Ripon HG4 5BY — MB ChB Manch. 1994.

THWAITES, Sheila Margaret (retired) 5 Arlington Close, Goring-by-Sea, Worthing BN12 4ST Tel: 01903 244265 — MB BS Lond. 1960; MRCS Eng. LRCP Lond. 1960; DObst RCOG 1964.

THWAITES, Susan Valerie Millway Medical Practice, Hartley Avenue, Mill Hill, London NW7 2HX Tel: 020 8959 0888 Fax: 020 8959 7050 — MB BS Lond. 1971 (Char. Cross) MRCS Eng. LRCP Lond. 1971; DObst RCOG 1973; MRCGP 1984.

THWAY, Yi Histopathology Department, Chelmsford & Essex Centre, New Writtle St., Chelmsford CM2 0PT Tel: 01245 513468 Fax: 01245 513464 — MB BS Inst. Med. Rangoon 1972; MRCPath 1983; FRCPath 1995. Cons. Pathol. Chelmsford & Essex Hosp. Specialty: Pathology, General. Socs: Internat. Acad. Path. & BMA. Prev: Regist. Shrodells Hosp. Watford; Lect. & Hon. Sen. Regist. Westm. Med. Sch. Lond.

THYNE, Douglas Hamish Scott 2nd Flat, 17 Comely Bank St, Edinburgh EH4 1AP — MB ChB Ed. 1996; DFFP; MRCGP. Gen. Pract. Locum Edin. Specialty: Gen. Pract. Socs: BMA; RCGP; FFP. Prev: Surg. Ho. Off. Dumfries & Galloway Roy. Infirm. Dumfries; Med. Ho. Off. Cumbld. Infirm. Carlisle; Paediat. SHO Perth Roy. Infirm. Perth.

THYVEETIL, Mable Das Department of Histopathology, Wexham Park Hospital, Slough SL2 4HL Tel: 01753 633457; 3 Edenham Close, Lower Earley, Reading RG6 3TH Tel: 0118 966 9678 — MB BS Kerala 1983; BSc (Zool.) Lond. 1975; MB BS Kerala 1981; MRCPath 1993. Assoc. Specialist (Histopath.) Wexham Pk. Hosp. Slough; Mem. Internat. Acad. Path. (Brit. Div.). Specialty: Histopath. Socs: Med. Defence Union. Prev: Staff Grade & Regist. (Histopath.) Wexham Pk. Hosp.

TIAH, Howard Anthony 7 Benson Street, Linthorpe, Middlesbrough TS5 6JQ — MB BCh BAO NUI 1983.

TIBBALLS, Jonathan Mark Radiology Department, Royal Free Hospital, Pond St., Hampstead, London NW3 2QG Tel: 020 7830 2170 Fax: 020 7830 2316 Email: jonathan.tibballs@royalfree.nhs.uk — MB BS Lond. 1987; MRCP (UK) 1990; FRCR 1994; FRANZCR 1998; FRACR 1998. Cons.(Radiol & Hon Sen Lect.). Specialty: Radiol. Special Interest: Hepatobiliary-Pancreatic Imaging & Interven.; Liver Transplantation; Vasc. Interven. Prev: SHO (Gen. Med., Neurol. & Gasteroenterol.) OldCh. Hosp. Romford.

TIBBATTS, Lucy Margaret 240 Longmore Road, Shirley, Solihull B90 3ES — BChir Camb. 1996; MB BChir Camb. 1996; MA Camb. 1998. SHO (Gen. Med.) Norwich. Specialty: Gen. Med.

TIBBITTS, Adrian Richard Haytons Bent, Nett Road, Shrewton, Salisbury SP3 4HB — MB Camb. 1969 (St. Thos.) BChir 1968. Barrister-at-Law Middle Temple. Socs: BMA. Prev: Ophth. Ho. Surg. St. Thos. Hosp.; Ho. Phys. Chapel Allerton Hosp. Leeds.

TIBBLE, Helen Clare 7 Nicholas Crescent, Fareham PO15 5AQ — MB ChB Leic. 1990.

TIBBLE, Jeremy Alexander 96 Hamlets Way, Mile End, Bow, London E3 4SY; Department of Gastroenterology, King's College Hospital, Denmark Hill, London SE5 Tel: 020 7346 6044 — MB BS Lond. 1990; MRCP (UK) 1993; MSc (Distinction) Lond. 1999. Research Fell. (Gastroenterol.) King's Coll. Hosp. Lond. Specialty: Gen. Med. Prev: Regist. Rotat. (Gastroenterol.) King's Coll. Hosp. Lond.; SHO Rotat. (Med.) Newham Gen. Hosp.

TIBBLE, Michael John Kenneth St Peters Street Medical Practice, 16 St Peters Street, London N1 8JG Tel: 020 7226 7131 Fax: 020 7354 9120 — MB BS Lond. 1965 (Westminster) MRCS Eng. LRCP Lond. 1965. Specialty: Gen. Pract. Socs: MDU.

TIBBLE, Rachel Katherine The Quest, Bendarroch Road, West Hill, Ottery St Mary EX11 1TS — MB ChB Leic. 1992.

TIBBOTT, Christopher William Downing Street Surgery, 4 Downing Street, Farnham GU9 7PA Tel: 01252 716226 Fax: 01252 322338; Millington, 37 Echo Barn Lane, Farnham GU10 4NG Tel:

01252 716075 — MB BS Lond. 1973 (King's Coll. Hosp.) AKC; BSc (Hons.) Lond. 1970; DRCOG 1977; MRCGP 1980.

TIBBS, Christopher Joceyln St George's Hospital, Blackshaw Road, London SW17 0QT Tel: 020 8675 1255 Fax: 020 8780 2338 Email: christopher.tibbs@stgeorges.nhs.uk; Bunchfield, Lynchmere Ridge, Haslemere GU27 3PP — MB BS Lond. 1984 (Univ. Oxf. & St. Thos. Hosp. Med. Sch.) MA Oxf. 1979; FRCP 1999. Cons. Gastroenterol. St. Geo.'s Hosp. Lond.; Cons. Gastoenterology Qu. Mary's Roehampton. Specialty: Gastroenterol.; Gen. Med. Special Interest: Therapeutic Endoscopy; Viral Hepatitis. Socs: Brit. Soc. Gastroenterol.; Brit. Assn. Study Liver (Comm. Mem.); Eur. Assn. Study Liver Dis. Prev: Lect. Inst. Liver Studies King's Coll. Hosp. Lond.; Regist. (Med.) St. Richard's Hosp. Chichester & St. Thos. Hosp. Lond.

TIBBS, Mr David John, MC (retired) 31 Davenant Road, Oxford OX2 8BU Tel: 01865 515259 Email: david.tibbs1@ntlworld.com — (Guy's) MRCS Eng. LRCP Lond. 1942; MB BS Lond. 1943; FRCS Eng. 1948; MS Lond. 1959; MA Oxf. 1965. Hon. Cons. Surg. John Radcliffe Hosp. Oxf. Prev: Reader (Surg.) Univ. Durh.

TIBBS, Philip Graydon North Street House Surgery, 6 North Street, Emsworth PO10 7DD Tel: 0143 373538; Mays Coppice Farm House, Rowlands Castle, Havant PO9 5NE Tel: 01705 413239 — BM BCh Oxf. 1980; MA Oxf. 1982, BA 1977, BM Bch 1980; DRCOG 1982; MRCGP 1984. Prev: Trainee GP Portsmouth VTS; Ho. Phys. John Radcliffe Hosp. Oxf.; Ho. Surg. Roy. United Hosp. Bath.

TIBBUTT, David Arthur Perry Point, 4 Whittington Road, Worcester WR5 2JU Tel: 01905 355451 Email: david@tibbutt.co.uk — BM BCh Oxf. 1967; MRCP (UK) 1971; MA Oxf. 1967, DM 1977; FRCP Lond. 1983. Adviser for CPD in Uganda (Honorary). Specialty: Cardiol.; Trop. Med. Socs: Brit. Cardiac Soc.; BMA; W Midl. Region Phys. Assn. Prev: Cons. Phys. Worcester Roy. Infirm.; Clin. Director (Med.) Worcester Roy. Infirm; Sen. Regist. (Gen. Med.) Radcliffe Infirm. Oxf.

TIBBY, Shane Martin Paediatric Intensive Care, Guy's Hospital, London SE1 9RT; 69 Cornhill Avenue, Hockley SS5 5BY — MB ChB Otago 1987; MRCP (UK) 1994.

TIBREWAL, Mr Sheo Bhagwan Greenwich District Hospital, London SE10 9HE Tel: 020 8312 6099 Fax: 020 8312 6152; The Blackheath Hospital, Lee Terrace, London SE3 9UD Tel: 020 8295 5795 Fax: 020 8295 5795 — MB BS 1973; FRCS Eng. 1980; FICS 1990; T(S) 1991. Cons. Orthop. Surg. Greenwich HA. Specialty: Trauma & Orthop. Surg. Socs: Fell. Roy. Soc. Med.; Fell. BOA; Hunt. Soc. Prev: Lect. (Orthop. Surg.) Univ. Newc.; Sen. Regist. (Orthop. Surg.) St. Bart. Hosp. Lond.; Regist. (Orthop. Surg.) Nuffield Orthop. Centre Oxf.

TIBREWAL, Suresh Prasad The Surgery, 136 Richmond Road, London E8 3HN Tel: 020 7254 2298 — MB BS Ranchi 1978; LMSSA 1984; DCH RCPS Glas. 1985; DRCOG 1989. Prev: SHO (O & G) N. Middlx. Hosp. Lond.; SHO (A & E) Chase Farm Hosp. Enfield; SHO (Paediat.) Roy. Berks. Hosp. Reading.

TICE, Mr John William Sunley Trauma & Orthopaedic Directorate, Southampton General Hospital, Tremona Road, Southampton SO16 6YD Tel: 02380 796249; The Old Rectory, Southampton SO32 1JH Tel: 01489 860866 — MB BS Lond. 1988; FRCS (Tr & Orth); MA (Engin. Sci.) Oxf. 1983; FRCS Eng. 1993. Cons. Orthopaedic Surg., Southampton gen.Hosp.; Regist.Rotat (Orthop) St Geo.Hosp.Lond. Specialty: Orthop.; Trauma & Orthop. Surg. Socs: Brit. Orthop. Assn.; Roy. Soc. Med.; Brit. Trauma Soc. Prev: SHO Rotat. (Surg.) St. Mary's Hosp. Lond.; Asst. Lect. (Anat.) Med. Coll. St. Bart. Hosp. Lond.; Ho. Surg. Homerton Hosp. Lond.

TICEHURST, Peter Rowland Ampleforth Surgery, Back Lane, Ampleforth, York YO62 4EF Tel: 01439 788215 Fax: 01439 788002; 50 Bondgate, Helmsley, York YO62 5EZ Tel: 01439 770098 — (Guy's) MB BS Lond. 1969; MRCS Eng. LRCP Lond. 1969. Med. Off. Thos. The Baker Helmsley; Med. Off. Ampleforth Coll. & Jun. Sch. Socs: Med. Off. Sch. Assn. Prev: Ho. Surg. Qu. Mary's Hosp. Sidcup; Ho. Phys. Pembury Hosp.

TICEHURST, Mr Richard Norman (retired) Kingswood, Starvecrow Lane, Peasmarsh, Rye TN31 6XN Tel: 01424 882575 — MB BChir Camb. 1943 (Guy's) MRCS Eng. LRCP Lond. 1942; MChir Camb. 1952, MA, MB BChir 1943; FRCS Eng. 1948. Prev: Cons. Gen. Surg. & Urol. Hastings Gp. Hosps.

TICKLE, Caroline 22 Dunholme Road, Newcastle upon Tyne NE4 6XE — MB BS Newc. 1998.

TICKLE, Elaine Kirsty Tyn Gadlas, Waynfawr, Caernarfon LL55 4BZ Tel: 01286 650031 — MB ChB Liverp. 1996 (Liverpool) BSc (Hons.) Liverp.1993, MB ChB 1996. SHO. (GP UTS.). Specialty: Gen. Pract.; Gen. Med.; Accid. & Emerg. Prev: MO (Gen. Duty).

TICKLE, Simon Andrew Tickle and Stubbs, 28 West Street, Earls Barton, Northampton NN6 0EW Tel: 01604 810219 Fax: 01604 810401; 142 Ardington Road, Northampton NN1 5LT Tel: 01604 635258 — MB ChB Manch. 1982; BSc St. And. 1979; MRCGP 1987. Specialty: Gen. Pract. Socs: BMA; Med. Protec. Soc. Prev: Trainee GP Chester VTS; Ho. Phys. Tameside Gen. Hosp.; Ho. Surg. Salford Roy. Hosp.

TICKTIN, Stephen Jan Flat 29 Church Garth, Pemberton Gardens, London N19 5RN — MD Toronto 1973; MA Toronto 1969; MRCPsych 1982. Indep. Psychiat. Lond.; Vis. Lect. Sch. Psychother. & Counselling Regent's Coll. Lond. Specialty: Gen. Psychiat. Prev: Clin. Asst. (Child & Adolesc. Psychiat.) Centr. Middlx. Hosp. Lond.; Regist. N.gate Clinic Lond.; SHO Roy. Free & Friern Hosps. Lond.

TIDBURY, Penelope Jane — MB BS Lond. 1980; MRCPath 1997. Cons. Cyto and Histiopathologist. Great West Hosp., Swindon. Specialty: Histopath. Prev: Sen. Regist. (Histopath.) Bloomsbury & Islington DHA; Lect. Chinese Univ. Hong Kong, Shatin.

TIDESWELL, David James Hillside, High St., Bloxham, Banbury OX15 4LT — MB BS Newc. 1998.

TIDLEY, Michael Gwyn Department of Occupational Health, Princess of Wales Hospital, Cotty Road, Bridgend CF31 1RG Tel: 01656 752 158 Fax: 01656 752 153 — MB ChB Bristol 1989; AFOM 1997; MFOM 1999. Cons. in Ocupational Med., Bro Borgannwg NHS Trust, Bridgend; Mem. of Welsh Affairs Forum, Fac. of Occupational Med.; Dep. Regional Speciailty Adviser, Wales; Chairm. of Welsh Regional Gp., (ANHOPS). Specialty: Occupat. Health. Special Interest: Fitness for work; Ill Health Reitrement. Socs: Soc. of Occupat.al Med.; Assn. of NHS Occupational Physcians (ANHOPS). Prev: Specialist in Ocupational Med. - BMI Health Servs.; Specialist Regist. in Ocupational Med. - Civil Serv./BMI Health Servs.

TIDMAN, Jill Sheelagh Maureen Slateford Road Surgery, 79 Slateford Road, Edinburgh EH11 1QW Tel: 0131 313 2211; 30 Greenhill Gardens, Edinburgh EH10 4BP Tel: 0131 447 1102 — MB BS Lond. 1978 (Guy's) MRCS Eng. LRCP Lond. 1977; DRCOG 1980; MRCGP 1982; T(GP) 1991. Prev: GP Carshalton; Trainee GP Guy's Hosp. Lond. VTS.

TIDMAN, Michael John Department of Dermatology, The Royal Infirmary, Lauriston Place, Edinburgh EH3 9YW Tel: 0131 536 2051; 30 Greenhill Gardens, Edinburgh EH10 4BP Tel: 0131 447 1102 — (Guy's) MRCS Eng. LRCP Lond. 1977; BSc (Hons.) Lond. 1974, MD 1986, MB BS 1977; MRCP (UK) 1979; FRCP Ed. 1991. Cons. Dermat. Roy. Infirm. Edin. Specialty: Dermat. Prev: Sen. Regist. Dermat. Guy's Hosp. Lond.; MRC Train. Fell. Inst. Dermat. Lond.; Hon. Regist. St. John's Hosp. Dis. Skin Lond.

TIDMARSH, David (retired) Pine House, Quarry Lane, Yateley GU46 6XW Email: dtid@globalnet.co.uk — (St. Bart.) MB BChir Camb. 1958; DPM Eng. 1964; MD Camb. 1977; FRCPsych 1992. Prev: Cons. Psychiat. Broadmoor Hosp. Crowthorne.

TIDMARSH, Mark Douglas Cumberland Infirmary, Carlisle CA2 7HY — MB ChB Leic. 1988; BSc (Biochem.) Liverp. 1982; MB ChB (Hons.) Leic. 1988; FRCA 1994. Regist. Rotat. (Anaesth.) Leicester & Derby; Cons. Anaesth. Carlisle. Specialty: Anaesth. Prev: SHO Rotat. (A & E Gen. Med. & Endocrinol.) Leicester Roy. Infirm.; Ho. Off. (Surg.) P'boro. Dist. Gen. Hosp.

TIDNAM, Peter Frederick (retired) Brougham House, 7 Scotton St., Wye, Ashford TN25 5BU Tel: 01233 813582 — MB BS Lond. 1963 (St. Geo.) MRCS Eng. LRCP Lond. 1963; DA Eng. 1966; FFA RCS Eng. 1971. Prev: Cons. Anaesth. Westm. Hosp. Lond. & Qu. Mary's Hosp. Roehampton.

TIDSWELL, Alexander Thomas 7 Plumian Way, Balsham, Cambridge CB1 6EG — MB BChir Camb. 1992.

TIDSWELL, Andrew Thomas Harrison Herbert Avenue Surgery, 268 Herbert Avenue, Poole BH12 4HY Tel: 01202 743333 Fax: 01202 738998 — MRCS Eng. LRCP Lond. 1975; DRCOG 1981. Med. Direct. (Occupat. Health) Employm. Med. Servs. Poole. Specialty: Occupat. Health. Socs: Soc. Occupat Med.

TIDSWELL, Philip Royal Preston Hospital, Sharoe Green Lane N., Fulwood, Preston PR2 9HT Tel: 01772 522558 Fax: 01772 523643; 56 Stubbins Street, Ramsbottom, Bury BL0 0NL Tel: 01706 828001 Fax: 01706 828001 — MB BS Lond. 1984 (Cambridge; London)

MA Camb. 1984; MRCP (UK) 1987; FRCP 1999. Cons. Neurol. Roy. Preston Hosp. & Blackburn Roy. Infirm. Specialty: Neurol. Socs: Assn. Brit. Neurol.; N. Eng. Neurol. Assn. Prev: Sen. Regist. & Regist. Rotat. (Neurol.) Leeds Gen. Infirm. & St Jas. Univ. Hosp. Leeds; Research Regist. (Neurol.) Roy. Hallamsh. Hosp. Sheff.

TIDY, Gerald The Portmill Surgery, 114 Queen Street, Hitchin SG4 9TH Tel: 01462 434246 — MRCS Eng. LRCP Lond. 1969 (St. Mary's) Prev: SHO (Med.) Cheltenham Gen. Hosp.; Psychiat. Resid. St. Brendan's Hosp. Bermuda; SHO (O & G) Qu. Eliz. II Hosp. Welwyn Gdn. City.

TIERNAN, Diarmuid Gerard Mary The Granary, Manor House, 58 Churchgate Way, Terrington St. Clement, King's Lynn PE34 4LZ — MB BCh BAO NUI 1982; DRCOG 1988. GP Terrington St. Clement (Rheumatology). Specialty: Care of the Elderly. Prev: Clin. Asst. (c/o Elderly & Rheum.) Qu. Eliz. Hosp. King's Lynn, Norf.; GP Birtley, Tyne & Wear & Hunstanton, Norf.

TIERNEY, Christopher John Appleton Village Surgery, 2-6 Appleton Village, Widnes WA8 6DZ Tel: 0151 423 2990 Fax: 0151 424 1032; 28 Knowsley Road, Liverpool L19 0PG — MB ChB Manch. 1977 (Manchester) DRCOG 1979; MRCGP 1983. Med. Adviser Liverp. FHSA.

TIERNEY, Dawn Maria 71 Ely Road, Littleport, Ely CB6 1HJ — MB BS Lond. 1994.

TIERNEY, Edward The Medical Centre, Market St., Whitworth, Rochdale OL12 8QS Tel: 01706 852238 Fax: 01706 853877 — LRCPI & LM, LRSCI & LM 1964 (RCSI) LRCPI & LM, LRCSI & LM 1964; MRCGP 1975. Med. Off. Buckley Hall Prison. Socs: BMA; IMA; Assn. Police Surg. Prev: Police Surgs. Rochdale; Ho. Surg. Richmond Hosp. Dub.; SHO (Anaesth.) Rochdale Hosp. Gp.

TIERNEY, Francis Benbecula Medical Practice, Griminish Surgery, Griminish, Isle of Benbecula HS7 5QA Tel: 01870 602215 Fax: 01870 602630 — MB ChB Sheff. 1984 (Sheffield) DRCOG 1987; MRCGP 1990; DA (UK) 1991; DFFP 1996. Ltd. Specialist (Anaesth.) Uist and Barra Hosp., Isle of Benbecwa. Specialty: Gen. Pract.; Anaesth. Prev: SHO (Anaesth.) Trent RHA; Trainee GP Portree I. of Skye VTS; SHO (Paediat., Gen. Med. & O & G) Highland HB.

TIERNEY, Gillian Maria 12 Stanhope St, Stanton-By-Dale, Ilkeston DE7 4QA — BM BS Nottm. 1991; BMedSci (Hons.) Nottm. 1989; FRCS Eng. 1995; DM 1999. Specialty: Gen. Surg.

TIERNEY, Jacqueline Naomi 70 The Crest, Birmingham B31 3QA — MB ChB Liverp. 1993.

TIERNEY, Mr John Department of Surgery, Hammersmith Hospital, Du Cane Road, London W12 0NN — MB BCh BAO NUI 1987; FRCSI 1991.

TIERNEY, John Patrick 28 Regents Court, Coalisland, Dungannon BT71 4SB — MB BCh BAO Belf. 1993.

TIERNEY, Nicholas Mark 1 Wentworth Drive, Sale M33 6PW — MB ChB Manch. 1982.

TIERNEY, Patrick Brendan Clontiloret, Shawforth, Rochdale — LRCPI & LM, LRSCI & LM 1969; LRCPI & LM, LRCSI & LM 1969.

TIERNEY, Patrick Thomas Francis New Pond Row, 35 South St., Lancing BN15 8AN Tel: 01903 752265 Fax: 01903 851634 — MB BS Lond. 1975 (Univ. Coll. Hosp.) Cert. Prescribed Equiv. Exp. JCPTGP 1981. Specialty: Cardiol. Prev: Ho. Phys. Stoke Mandeville Hosp. Aylesbury; Ho. Surg. Univ. Coll. Hosp. Lond.

TIERNEY, Mr Paul Alexander Southmead Hospital, Department of ENT Surgery, Westbury-on-Trym, Bristol BS10 5NB Tel: 0117 959 6221 Fax: 0117 959 5850 — BM BCh Oxf. 1989; BA (Physiol.) Oxf. 1986; FRCS Eng. 1993; FRCS (Orl. Hons.) Eng. 1999. Specialty: Otorhinolaryngol. Socs: BAO.

TIFFIN, Emma Jane 7Walden Road, Huntingdon PE29 3AZ — MB BS Lond. 1992; BSc (Hons) 1991; MRCGP 1998.

TIFFIN, Nicholas John 3 Arthur Street, Penrith CA11 7TT — MB BCh Wales 1995.

TIFFIN, Paul Alexander University Dept of Psychiatry, Royal Victoria Infirmary, Newcastle upon Tyne NE1 — MB BS Newc. 1997; B.Med.Sci (Hons). Newc. 1994. SHO (Psychiat. Rotat.) North. Deanery. Specialty: Gen. Psychiat.

TIFFIN, Peter Arnold Crawford 28 Lethnot Street, Broughty Ferry, Dundee DD5 2QS — MB BS Newc. 1987.

TIGCHELAAR, Eibert Frank St James House Surgery, County Court Road, King's Lynn PE30 5SY Tel: 01553 774221 Fax: 01553 692181 — Artsexamen Rotterdam 1988. Specialty: Alcohol & Substance Misuse.

TIGG, Alison 25 Grummock Avenue, Ramsgate CT11 0RP — MB BS Lond. 1989; MRCP (UK) 1995. Specialty: Gen. Med.

TIGHE, Brian Stanley 8 Westfield Road, Basingstoke RG21 3BW — MB BS Lond. 1996 (Char. Cross & Westm.) BSc (Hons.) Lond. 1991; DCH Lond. 1998; DRCOG Lond. 2003. Specialty: Gen. Pract. Socs: MRCGP.

TIGHE, Jane Elizabeth Tertowie Grange, Kinellar, Aberdeen AB21 0TP Fax: 01224 790557 — MB BS Lond. 1985 (St. Thomas's Hosp. Med. Sch.) PhD Lond. 1995, BSc 1982; MRCP (UK) 1988; FRCP Ed 2000; FRCPath 2003. Cons. Haemat. Aberd. Roy. Infirm. Specialty: Haematology. Socs: Brit. Soc. Haematol. Prev: Sen. Regist. (Haemat.) Univ. Coll. Hosp. Lond.; MRC Research Fell. (Haemat.) RPMS Lond.; Regist. (Haemat.) Hammersmith Hosp. Lond.

TIGHE, Professor John Richard (retired) 9 Eden Park Close, Batheaston, Bath BA1 7JB — MD Wales 1962 (Cardiff) BSc Wales 1950, MD 1962, MB BCh 1953; FRCP Lond. 1974, M 1958; FRCP Ed. 1971, M 1958; FRCPath 1975, M 1963. Emerit. Prof. Histopath. Univ. Lond. Guy's and St Thomas's Hosp. Med. Sch. Prev: Prof. Histopath. UMDS Lond.

TIGHE, Karen Elaine Dept. of Anaesthetics, Leicester Royal Infirmary, Infirmary Road, Leicester LE1 5WW — MB ChB Manch. 1986; DA (UK) 1989; MRCP (UK) 1990; FRCA 1993; CCST 1994. Cons. Anaesth. Leicester Roy. Infirm. Specialty: Anaesth. Prev: Sen. Regist. Rotat. Nottm. & E. Midl.; Regist. Derby City Hosp. & Nottm. Univ. Hosp.; Regist. (Anaesth.) Qu.s Med. Centre Univ. Hosp. Nottm.

TIGHE, Mr Mark Joseph Warrington Hospital, Lovely Lane, Warrington WA5 1QG — MB ChB Liverp. 1989; FRCS Ed. 1993. Specialty: Gen. Surg.

TIGHE, Mary Department of Haematology, Musgrove Park Hospital, Taunton TA1 5DA Tel: 01823 271049; 22 Holway Avenue, Taunton TA1 3AR Tel: 01823 271049 — MB ChB Ed. 1973; DRCOG 1976; MRCP (UK) 1978. Assoc. Specialist (Haemat. & Oncol.) Taunton & Som. NHS Trust. Specialty: Haematology. Prev: Med. Off. Taunton & Som. Hosp. MusGr. Pk. Br. Married Wom. Doctors Retainer Scheme; SHO Taunton & Som. Hosp. (MusGr. Pk. Br.); Ho. Off. Norf. & Norwich Hosp. & W. Norwich Hosp.

TIGHE, Michael Richard Woodlands House, West Norwich Hospital, Bowthorpe Road, Norwich — MB BS Lond. 1984; MRCP (UK) 1987; MD Lond. 1994.

TIGHE, Nicola Jane The Coach House, South Woodville, St Margarets Rd, Altrincham WA14 2AW — MB ChB Liverp. 1997.

TIGHE, Robert John (retired) 1 Law Court, Wygate Park, Spalding PE11 3FG Tel: 01775 761097 — (Birm.) MRCS Eng. LRCP Lond. 1946. Prev: Ho. Surg. Gen. Hosp. Birm.

TIGHE, Sean Quentin Miles, Surg. Cdr. RN Retd. Anaesthetic Department, Countess of Chester Hospital NHS Trust, Chester CH2 1UL Tel: 01244 365461 Fax: 01244 365435; 38 Glan Aber Park, Chester CH4 8LF Tel: 01244 683086 — MB BS Lond. 1978 (Guy's) MRCS Eng. LRCP Lond. 1978; FFA RCS Eng. 1984. Cons. Anaesth. Countess of Chester Hosp. NHS Trust. Specialty: Anaesth.; Intens. Care. Socs: Intens. Care Soc.; Assn. Anaesth.; BMA. Prev: Cons. Anaesth. & Head Dept. RNH Plymouth; Cons. Anaesth. & Sen. Lect. RNH Haslar; Hon. Sen. Regist. Glas. Roy. Infirm.

TIGHE, Shelagh Maureen (retired) 9 Eden Park Close, Batheaston, Bath BA1 7JB — (Sheff.) MD Sheff. 1963, MB ChB 1952; MRCS Eng. LRCP Lond. 1952; DCH Eng. 1954; FRCP Lond. 1977, M 1958. Prev: Cons. Dermat. Ashford Hosp. Middlx. & Teddington Memor.

TIJSSELING, Andreas Charles Ferryhill Medical Practice, Durham Road, Ferryhill DL17 8JJ Tel: 01740 651238 — Artsexamen Amsterdam 1986. GP Ferryhill, Co. Durh.; Clin. Asst. Dermat. BAG Hosp. (p/t).

TILAK-SINGH, Deepa C-7 Maryfield Terrace, Dumfries DG1 4UG — MB BS Poona 1987.

TILBURY, Jonathan Gregory 104 Strathmore Avenue, Coventry CV1 2AF — MB ChB Birm. 1975.

TILDESLEY, Geoffrey (retired) Cadzowbank, 19 Coniscliffe Road, Hartlepool TS26 0BT — MB ChB Birm. 1962; MRCP Lond. 1966; FRCP Lond. 1982, M 1966. Cons. Phys. Hartlepool Gp. Hosps. Prev: Sen. Regist. (Gen. Med.) Welsh Hosp. Bd. & United Cardiff Hosps.

TILDSLEY, Gemma Jane Department of Histopathology, Princess Royal Hospital, Lewes Road, Haywards Heath RH16 — MB BS

Lond. 1984 (Westm.) MRCPath 1991. Cons. Histopath. Princess Roy. Hosp. Haywards Health Sussex. Specialty: Histopath.

TILEY, Christopher George Westchester, Huntingdon Road, Cambridge CB3 0LG Tel: 01223 276331 — MB BS Lond. 1992; BSc Lond. 1989; MRCP (UK) 1996.

TILEY, Michael John Harperhall, Elsrickle, Biggar ML12 6QZ — MB ChB Aberd. 1973; DObst RCOG 1976.

TILEY, Sarah Josephine Prescott Surgery, Prescott Road, Baschurch, Shrewsbury SY4 2DR Tel: 01939 260210 Fax: 01939 260752 — BM BCh Oxf. 1988; DCH RCP Lond. 1992; DFFP 1994; MRCGP 1994. GP Partner Prescott Surg. Basch. Specialty: Gen. Pract. Prev: Assoc. GP Tarrington & Leintwardine; Trainee GP Mansfield VTS; SHO Roy. Shrewsbury Hosp. VTS.

TILFORD, Maureen Patricia Tilford, Rash and Burrell, Health Centre, Lawson Road, Norwich NR3 4LE Tel: 01603 427096 Fax: 01603 403704; Mulberry House, 3 Newmarket Road, Cringleford, Norwich NR4 6UE Tel: 01603 504710 — MB ChB Glas. 1972; Cert. Family Plann. JCC 1988. Socs: Doctor-Healer Network; Brit. Soc. for Med. & Dent. Hypn. Prev: Trainee GP Twickenham; SHO (Cas.) W. Middlx. Hosp.; SHO (Paediat.) Hillingdon Hosp. Middlx.

TILFORD, Trevor John (retired) 32 Greenacres, Little melton, Norwich NR9 3QU Tel: 01603 814180 — MB BS Lond. 1965 (St. Geo.) MRCS Eng. LRCP Lond. 1964; DObst RCOG 1968. Prev: GP Norwich.

TILL, Arthur Michael Yew Trees, 12 Larkspear Close, Gloucester GL1 5LN Tel: 01452 525141 — MB BS Lond. 1962 (Middlx.) DObst RCOG 1964. Specialty: Obst. & Gyn. Prev: Ho. Surg. (ENT) Middlx. Hosp. Lond.; Ho. Off. (O & G) Roy. Lancaster Infirm.; Maj. RAMC (Specialist O & G).

TILL, Christopher Brian Wright The Chase, Highknott Road, Arnside, Carnforth LA5 0AW — BM Soton. 1987; FRCA 1993. Cons. Anaesth. Lancaster Acute NHS Trust. Specialty: Anaesth. Socs: Manch. Med. Soc.; Intens. Care Soc.

TILL, Janice Anne Department of Paediatrics, Royal Brompton Hospital, Sydney St., London SW3 6NP Tel: 020 7351 8546 Fax: 020 7351 8622; 179 Engadine Street, Southfields, London SW18 5DU — MB BS Lond. 1982 (St Bart. Hosp. Med. Sch.) BSc (Immunity & Infec.) Lond. 1979; MD Lond. 1994. Cons. Paediat. Electrophysiol. Roy. Brompton & Harefield NHS Trust; Hon. Sen. Lect. Nat. Heart & Lung Inst. Specialty: Cardiol.; Paediat. Cardiol. Socs: BMA; Paediat. Electrophysiol. Gp.; N. Amer. Pacing & Electrophysiol. Gp. Prev: Research Regist. (Paediat. Cardiol.) Brompton Hosp. Lond.; Lect. (Paediat. Electrophysiol.) Roy. Brompton Hosp.

TILL, Mr Kenneth Reed's Court, Lydeard St Lawrence, Taunton TA4 3RX Tel: 01984 667388 Fax: 01984 667388 Email: 106036.3500@compuserve.com — (St. Geo.) Hon. FRCPCH; MRCS Eng. LRCP Lond. 1944; MA Camb. 1945; MB BChir Camb. 1946; FRCS Eng. 1953. Hon. Cons. Neurol. Surg. Hosp. Sick Childr. Gt. Ormond St. & Univ. Coll. Hosp. Lond.; Hon. Civil Cons. RAF. Specialty: Neurosurg. Socs: Internat. Soc. Paediat. Neurosurg.; Soc. Brit. Neurol. Surgs.; Internat. Assoc. Mem. Amer. Assn. of Neurol. Surg. Prev: Neurol. Surg. Univ. Coll. Hosp. Lond.; Sen. Regist. (Neurosurg.), Cas. Off. & Res. Anaesth. St. Geo. Hosp.

TILL, Morwenna Margaret (retired) Reed's Court, Lydeard St Lawrence, Taunton TA4 3RX Tel: 01984 667388 Fax: 01984 667388 Email: 106036.3500@compuserve.com — (Camb. & Roy. Free) BA Camb. 1941; MB BChir Camb. 1944; DCH Eng. 1946. Prev: Sen. Research Fell. (Haemat.) Inst. Child Health Lond. Clin. Research.

TILL, Noorjahan (retired) 26A Campbell Road, Southsea PO5 1RN Tel: 023 9281 7732 — MB BS Bihar 1966 (Darbhanga Med. Coll.) DPM Eng. 1979; MB AcC Brit. Coll. Acupunc. Lond. 1995. Prev: Assoc. Specialist St. Jas. Hosp. Portsmouth.

TILL, Richard James Ashley (retired) Roundhay Road Surgery, 209 Roundhay Road, Leeds LS8 4HQ Tel: 0113 249 0504 Fax: 0113 248 0330 — MB ChB Leeds 1965; DObst RCOG 1967.

TILL, Richard John Wright 17 Upper Pines, Banstead SM7 3PU — MB ChB Birm. 1981.

TILL, Simon Harold Royal Hallamshire Hospital, Department of Rheumatology, Beech Hill Road, Sheffield S10 2JF Tel: 0114 271 1941 Fax: 0114 271 1844; 7 Grove Road, Dore, Sheffield S17 4DJ — MB ChB Sheff. 1989; MRCP (UK) 1992. Cons. (Rheum & Sport Med.). Specialty: Rheumatol.; Sports Med. Prev: Sen Regist. (Gen. Med. & Rheum.) Chesterfield Roy. Hosp.

TILLEARD-COLE, Professor Richard Reginald Rupert, OBE, Col. (cons. rooms), 5 Walton Street, Oxford OX1 2HG Tel: 01865 554754; Roubartelle Abbas, Clifton Hampden, Abingdon OX14 3EQ Tel: 01865 407722 — BM BCh Oxf. 1954 (Oxf. & St Bart.) BA Oxf. 1950; MA Oxf. 1954; DPM Lond. 1960; MRCPsych 1971; FRCPsych 1976. Cons. Psychiat. & Dir. Oxf. Inst. Psychiat.; Hon. Cons. St. And. Hosp. Northampton; May & Baker Prof. Psychiat. & Hon. Fell. Worcester Coll. Oxf. (Oxf.); Pres. Oxf. Postgrad. Fellowship of Psychiat.; Dep. Hon. Col. & Master Oxf. Univ. Off's Train. Corps.; Pres.; Tilleard-Cole Med. Soc. Worcester Coll. Oxf. Specialty: Gen. Psychiat.; Hypnother.; Med. Publishing. Socs: Liveryman Soc. of Apoth. Lond.; Fell. Brit. Soc. Med. & Dent. Hypn.; Oxf. Soc. Of Med. Prev: Tutor (Neuro-Anat.) Univ. Oxf. (Worcester Coll.); Psychiat. Warneford Hosp. Oxf.; Col. Wilts. Regt.

TILLER, Gillian 79 Grayswood Drive, Mytchett, Camberley GU16 6AS — MB BS Lond. 1981.

TILLER, Jane Margaret South London & Mandsley NHS Trust, Denmak House, London SE5 8AZ — MB ChB Glas. 1986; MRCPsych. Cons. Adult Psychiat. & Clin. Direct. S.rah. Specialty: Gen. Psychiat. Prev: Researcher & Hon. Sen. Regist. (Psychiat.) Inst. Psychiat. Lond.

TILLETT, Angela Jane 17 St Bernard Road, Colchester CO4 0LE Tel: 01206 845103 — MB BS Lond. 1987; DRCOG 1991; DCH RCP Lond. 1992; MRCP (UK) 1994; MRCGP 1994. Specialty: Paediat. Prev: Regist. (Paediat.) Ipswich Hosp.

TILLETT, David Robin Fraser (retired) Bennett House, Coombe Park, Kingston upon Thames KT2 7JB Tel: 020 8546 5983 Fax: 020 8547 3603 — MRCS Eng. LRCP Lond. 1962 (St. Geo.) DA Eng. 1969; FFA RCS Eng. 1971. United Kingdom Amer. Univeristy of The Caribbean, St Maarten Netherland Antilles. Prev: Sen. Regist. (Anaesth.) St. Thos. Hosp. Lond.

TILLETT, Richard Ian Laccohee Wonford House Hospital, Exeter EX2 5AF Tel: 01392 403446 — MB BS Lond. 1969; MRCPsych 1977; FRCPsych 1998. Cons. Psychiat. & Psychother. Exeter & Dist. Community NHS Trust. Specialty: Gen. Psychiat.; Psychother. Prev: Sen. Regist. (Psychiat.) Glenside Hosp. Bristol.

TILLEY, Alison Jane Dept. of Occupational Health, Whitefriars, Leurins Nead, Bristol BS1 2NT Tel: 01179 282223 — MB BS Lond. 1988 (Middlx. Hosp. Med. Sch.) DRCOG 1993; MRCGP 1994; DOM 1999. Clin. Asst. in Ocupational Health. Specialty: Occupat. Health. Prev: Locum GP Bristol.

TILLEY, Elisabeth Ann Turret Lodge, 29 Slipper Road, Emsworth PO10 8BS; Turret Lodge, 32 Havant Road, Emsworth PO10 7JG — (St. Mary's) BSc (2nd cl. Hons. Physiol.) Lond. 1977, MB BS 1980; MRCP (UK) 1983; FRCR 1986. Cons. Radiol. Qu. Alexandra Hosp. Portsmouth. Specialty: Radiol. Prev: Sen. Regist. (Radiol.) St. Geo. Hosp. Lond.

TILLEY, Emma Jane Westcourt, 12 The Street, Rustington, Littlehampton BN16 3NX Tel: 01903 777000 Fax: 01903 850907 — MB BS Lond. 1988 (St. Bart. Hosp. Med. Coll.) DCH RCP Lond. 1993; DRCOG 1994. GP. Specialty: Gen. Pract. Socs: BMA. Prev: Regist. (Med. Diabetes & Endocrinol.) Worcester Roy. Infirm.; SHO (Paediat.) Cheltenham Gen. Hosp.

TILLEY, James Howey MacDonald (retired) 7 The Avenue, Nunthorpe, Middlesbrough TS7 0AA Tel: 01642 316412 — (The London Hospital) MA (Hons. Chem.) Camb. 1938; MB BChir Camb. 1944; DPH Liverp. 1946; MFCM 1973. Prev: Area Specialist (Pub. Health Med.) Cleveland HA.

TILLEY, Jane Anne Appleby House, Kingston Bagpuize, Abingdon OX13 5AP — MB BCh Wales 1995.

TILLEY, Jane Marie Flat B, 3 Manstone Road, Cricklewood, London NW2 3XH — MB BS Lond. 1994. Specialty: Anaesth. Socs: Med. Defence Union; BMA.

TILLEY, John Stewart Pulteney Practice, 35 Great Pulteney Street, Bath BA2 4BY Tel: 01225 464187 Fax: 01225 485305 — MB BS Lond. 1975; MRCS Eng. LRCP Lond. 1974; MRCGP 1990.

TILLEY, Marelle Margaret Ellen Motherwell Health Centre, 138-144 Windmill Street, Motherwell ML1 1TB Tel: 01698 266688 Fax: 01698 253230; 1 Thanes Gate, Bothwell, Glasgow G71 7HS — MB ChB Glas. 1986; DRCOG 1991; MRCGP 1992. Socs: BMA.

TILLEY, Nicola Jane 226 Barton Road, Kettering NN15 6RZ — MB ChB Birm. 1992.

TILLEY, Peter John Boston The James Cook University Hospital, Neurology Department, Middlesbrough TS4 3BW Tel: 01642 854308 — MB BS Newc. 1967; MRCP (U.K.) 1971; FRCP Lond. 1984. Cons. Neurol. N. RHA. Specialty: Neurol. Socs: BMA & Assn. Brit. Neurol. Prev: Sen. Regist. (Neurol.) Newc. Gen. Hosp.; Fell. (Neurol.) Mayo Clinic Rochester USA; Regist. (Neurol.) Roy. Vict. Infirm. Newc.

TILLEY, Rebecca Elizabeth Cambridge Microbiology & Public Health Laboratory, Addenbrookes Hospital, Hills Road, Cambridge CB2 2QW Tel: 01223 257035; 59 Laceys Lane, Exring, Newmarket CB8 7HN — MB BS Lond. 1996 (Univ. Coll. Lond.) BSc (Hons.) Hist. Med. Lond. 1993; MSc (Clin. Microbiol.) 1998; DTM & H Lond. 2000.

TILLEY, Rosalinde Caron 15 Bellew Street, Tooting, London SW17 0AD Tel: 020 8946 6053 Fax: 0870 054 8423 Email: ros@bellew.demon.co.uk — BSc (Sociol. Appl. Med. & Basic Med. Sci.) Lond. 1989; MB BS (Hons.) Lond. 1992; FRCA 1998. Specialist Regist. (Anaesth.) S. W. Thames Rotat. Specialty: Anaesth. Socs: Intens. Care Soc.; Anaesth. Assn.; Obst. Anaesth. Assn. Prev: Regist. & SHO (ITU) Roy. Brompton Hosp. Lond.; SHO (Respirat. Med.) Roy. Brompton Hosp. Lond.; SHO (Anaesth.) Whittington Hosp. Lond.

TILLING, Keith John (retired) Tregate, West End, Cholsey, Wallingford OX10 9LW — MB BS Lond. 1955 (Lond. Hosp.) DPM Eng. 1959; MRCPsych 1971. Prev: Cons. Psychiat. Fair Mile Hosp. Wallingford & Roy. Berks. Hosp. Reading & Eldon Day Hosp. Reading.

TILLMAN, David McGill Department of Dermatology, Western Infirmary, Dumbarton Road, Glasgow G11 6NT — MB ChB Glas. 1981; PhD (Biochem.) Glas. 1976; MRCP (UK) 1984; FRCP Glas. 1994. Sen. Lect. (Dermat.) Univ. Glas.; Hon. Cons. (Dermat.) Gtr. Glas. HB. Specialty: Dermat. Prev: Regist. (Dermat.) W. Infirm. Glas.; Clin. Scientist/Hon. Med. Regist. MRC Blood Pressure Unit. West. Infirm. Glas.

TILLMAN, Mr Roger Michael Royal Orthopaedic Hospital, Bristol Road S., Northfield, Birmingham B31 2AP Tel: 0121 685 4145 Fax: 0121 685 4102 — MB ChB Manch. 1984 (Manch. Univ.) FRCS Ed. 1988; FRCS (Orth.) 1993. Cons. Orthop. Surg. Roy. Orthop. Hosp. Birm.; Hon. Sen. Clin. Lect. in Surg. Univ. of Birm. Specialty: Orthop. Special Interest: Bone and Soft Tissue Tumours. Socs: Brit. Orthop. Oncol. Soc.; Brit. Assn. Surg. Knee; Brit. Orthop. Assoc. Prev: Sen. Regist. Wrightington Hosp., Roy. Preston Hosp. & Manch. Roy. Infirm.; Demonst. (Anat.) Univ. Bristol.

TILLOTT, Rebecca Claire 63 Illingworth, Windsor SL4 4UP — MB ChB Manch. 1998.

TILLSON, Christopher Bodnant Surgery, Menai Avenue, Bangor LL57 2HH Tel: 01248 364567 Fax: 01248 370654 — MB BS Lond. 1976 (St. Thos.) DRCOG Lond. 1981; MRCGP Lond. 1981 FP Cert. 1981.

TILLY, Adam 72 Northumberland Avenue, Gidea Park, Hornchurch RM11 2HP — MB BS Lond. 1986 (St. Bart. Hosp. Med. Sch.) DCH RCP Lond. 1992. Staff Grade (Community Child Health) City & Hackney HA. Specialty: Community Child Health. Socs: Brit. Assn. of Community Doctors in Audiol.; Brit. Soc. of Audiol. Prev: SHO (Paediat.) OldCh. Hosp.; SHO (Paediat.) Riverside H.A.; SHO (Paediat.) Char. Cross Hosp. Lond.

TILLY, Helen Victoria Saffrons, Gables Road, Church Crookham, Fleet GU52 6QZ Tel: 01252 621430 — MB BS Lond. 1988.

TILSED, Mr Jonathan Victor Thomas Castle Hill Hospital, Castle Road, Cottingham HU16 5JQ Email: jonathan.tilsed@hey.nhs.uk — MB BS Lond. 1988 (St Mary's) FRCS Eng. 1993; FRCS (Gen. Surg.) 1999. Specialty: Gen. Surg. Socs: Mem. Assn. Coloproctology GB & Irel.; Mem. Amer. Soc. Colon & Rectal Surgeons; Fell. Assn. Surg. GB & Irel. Prev: Clin. Lect. (Surg.) St Bart. & The Roy. Lond. Sch. Med. & Dent.; RCS Research Fell. Inst. Cancer Research; Specialist Regist. (Gen. Surg.) SE Thames Regional Higher Train. Scheme.

TILSEN, Elizabeth Mary (retired) Priors Gate, 92B Tettenhall Road, Wolverhampton WV6 0BX — MB ChB Birm. 1954; DObst RCOG 1956; DCH Eng. 1958; MRCP Lond. 1966. Prev: Sen. Regist. & Cons. Phys. (Geriat. Med.) New Cross Hosp. Wolverhampton.

TILSLEY, David William Owen 15 Greenways, Beckenham BR3 3NG — MB BS Lond. 1983.

TILSLEY, George Nigel Wykeham (retired) Dodington House, Dodington, Nether Stowey, Bridgwater TA5 1LF Tel: 01278 741238 — MB ChB Sheff. 1952; MRCS Eng. LRCP Lond. 1952. Prev: GP Sheff.

TILSLEY, Timothy Mark Mill Street Surgery, Mill Street, North Petherton, Bridgwater TA6 6LX Tel: 01278 662223 Fax: 01278 663727; Dodington House, Dodington, Nether Stowey, Bridgwater TA5 1LF — MB ChB Sheff. 1982. Clin. Forens. Phys. Som. Prev: Trainee GP Milnthorpe VTS; SHO (Geriat.) Lancaster Roy. Infirm.; SHO (Orthop. & Cas.) Roy. Hallamsh. Hosp. Sheff.

TILSTON, Mr Michael Paul Grimsby Health NHS Trust, Scartho Road, Grimsby DN33 2BA Tel: 01472 874111; Brinkhill House, Main St, Fulstow, Louth LN11 0XF — MB BS Lond. 1980; FRCS Ed. 1984. Cons. Surg. Grimsby Gen. Hosp. Specialty: Gen. Surg.

TILSTON, Simon Iain Graham Hooklaw Farm, Lethame, Strathaven ML10 6RW Tel: 01357 522019 — MB ChB Dundee 1992; DRCOG 1995; MRCGP 1997; DIP DERM 2002. Specialty: Gen. Pract.; Dermat.

TILSTON, Stephanie Jane The Coach House, Braeside Gardens, York YO24 4EZ — MB ChB Dund. 1998.

TILZEY, Anthea Jane Department of Virology, St Thomas' Hospital, London SE1 7EH Tel: 020 7922 8167 Fax: 020 7922 8387 Email: anthea.tilzey@kcl.ac.uk — MB BS Lond. 1978; MA Oxf. 1980; MRCP (UK) 1983. Cons. (Virol.) Guys & St. Thos. Trust Lond.; Hon. Sen. Lect. United Med. & Dent. Schs. Guy's & St Thos. Hosp. Specialty: Virology. Socs: Eur. Soc. Clin. Virol.; Soc. Gen. Microbiol. Prev: Assoc. Specialist (virol.) Guys & St. Thos. Trust. Lond.; Sen. Regist. (Virol.) St. Thos. Hosp. Lond.; Regist. (Med. & Genitourin Med.) St. Thos. Hosp. Lond.

TILZEY, Susan Elizabeth 42 Corrance Road, London SW2 5RH — MB Camb. 1985; BChir 1984.

TIMANS, Anita Rita Psycological Therapies Service, Leonard Lodge, Leonard Road, Croydon CR0 2UL Tel: 020 8700 8832; 129 Auckland Rise, London SE19 2DY Tel: 020 8653 7958 — MB BS Lond. 1984; MRCPsych 1990. Cons. Psychotherapist S. Lond. & Muadsley NHS trust. Specialty: Psychother.; Gen. Psychiat. Socs: Hon. Mem. Latvian Psychiat. Assn. Prev: Sen. Regist. (Psychother.) Pathfinder Trust Springfield Hosp. Tooting Bec; Sen. Regist. (Psychiat.) St. Geo.'s Hosp. Lond.; Regist. & SHO Rotat. (Psychiat.) St. Geo. Hosp. Lond.

TIMBERLAKE, Anthony Herbert 13 Shrubbery Avenue, Worcester WR1 1QN — MB ChB Birm. 1962.

TIMBERLAKE, Carolyne Marie Princess Royal University Hospital, Farnborough Common, Orpington BR6 8ND Email: carolyne.timberlake@bromleyhospitals.nhs.uk — MB BS Lond. 1989; FRCA Lond. 1994. Cons. (Anaesthetics & Pain Management) Bromley Hosps. NHS Trust. Specialty: Anaesth. Socs: Pain Society; Roy. Coll. of Anaesthetists; Brit. Med. Acupunc. Soc.

TIMBERLAKE, Timothy 51 Keswick Road, Bournemouth BH5 1LR Tel: 01202 303535 Fax: 01202 469936 Email: timothytimberlak@aol.com; Orchard Farm, Leigh Common, Wincanton BA9 8LF Tel: 01747 841207 Fax: 01747 840088 — (Westm.) MB BS Lond. 1966; MRCS Eng. LRCP Lond. 1966; DObst RCOG 1968. Sen. Med. Assoc. Eurodoc Ltd.; Lect. Sclerother. E. Midl.s Coll.; Lect. Sclerother. The Grace Sch. Specialty: Gen. Med. Socs: GP Writers Assn. Prev: Sen. Partner, Tumberlake. Blackurore, Ladd, Jenkins, W. Moors, Dorest.; Med. Off. i/c Troops Petroleum Centre W. Moors; Resid. Obst. Asst. Kingston Hosp.

TIMBURY, Morag Crichton (retired) 22 Monckton Court, Strangways Terrace, Holland Park Road, London W14 8NF Tel: 020 7602 3345 — MB ChB Glas. 1953; PhD Glas. 1966, MD 1960; FRCPath 1976, M 1964; FRCP Glas. 1974, M 1972; FRSE 1979; FRCP Lond. 1994. Prev: Dir. Centr. Pub. Health Laborat. Lond.

TIMLIN, Clive Edward Underwood Surgery, 139 St. Georges Road, Cheltenham GL50 3EQ Tel: 01242 580644 Fax: 01242 253519; 2 Yew Tree Close, Shipton Oliffe, Cheltenham GL54 4JT — MB BS Lond. 1972 (St. Mary's)

TIMLIN, Mark Andrew 35 Northwick Avenue, Kenton, Harrow HA3 0AA — BM Soton. 1995.

TIMMINS, Alan James H.M. Young Offenders Centre, Glen Parva, Tigers Road, Wigston, Leicester LE18 4TN — MB ChB Birm. 1974. Sen. Med. Off. Health Care Serv. for Prisoners Wigston. Prev: Regist. & SHO (Psychiat.) Highcroft Hosp. Birm.; Ho. Phys. Birm. Gen. Hosp.

TIMMINS, Andrew Clive 18 Willoughby Road, Chelmsford CM2 6UT — MB ChB Birm. 1981.

TIMMINS, Bryan Christopher Kemsley Division, National Centre for Brain Injury Rehabilitation, St Andrews Hospital, Billing Road, Northampton NN1 5DG Tel: 01604 629696 — MB ChB Leeds 1986; MRCPsych 1992; MRCP (UK) 1996. Cons. (Brain Injury Rehabil.) Kemsley Unit, Northampton. Specialty: Disabil. Med.; Gen. Psychiat. Prev: Cons. DKMH Catterick, N. Yorks.; Regist. Posts Cardiol. QEMH Lond.; Sen. Specialist (Psychiat.) QEMH Lond. & Maudsley Hosp. Lond.

TIMMINS, David John Grant Southwell House Surgery, Southwell House, Back Lane, Rochford SS4 1AY Tel: 01702 545241 Fax: 01702 546390; Botelers, Hall Road, Rochford SS4 1NN Tel: 01702 545241 — MB BS Lond. 1970 (Middlx.) DObst RCOG 1974; Cert. Family Plann. RCOG & RCGP 1974; FRCGP 1985, M 1975; DFFP 1993. Specialty: Gen. Pract.

TIMMINS, Derek John 8 Douglas Road, West Kirby, Wirral CH48 6EB; Royal Liverpool and Broadgreen University Hospital, Prescot St, Liverpool L7 8XP Tel: 0151 706 2630 Fax: 0151 706 5821 — MB ChB Liverp. 1977; Cert. Family Plann. JCC 1982; DRCOG 1982; MRCGP 1982; MRCP (UK) 1985; Dip. Ven. Liverp. 1986; FRCP Lond. 1995; MFFP 1996; Dip. Psychosexual Med. 1997; Dip. Occ. Med. 1998; LLM Cardiff 1999; FRCP Ed 1999; MBA Open 2000. Cons. Phys. Liverp. HA; Hon. Lect. (Genito-urin Med.) Univ. Liverp. Specialty: Genitourinary Medicine; Family Plann. & Reproduc. Health; HIV Med. Socs: Med. Soc. Study VD; Brit. Soc. of Colposcopists. Prev: Sen. Regist. (Genito-urin. Med.) Middlx. Hosp. Lond.

TIMMINS, S F Newington Road Surgery, 100 Newington Road, Ramsgate CT12 6EW Tel: 01843 595951 Fax: 01843 853387 — Artsexamen Utrecht 1991; Artsexamen Utrecht 1991.

TIMMINS, William Leonard (retired) Roswen, 22 Western Terrace, Falmouth TR11 4QP Tel: 01326 314922 — MB BS Lond. 1950 (St. Bart.) MRCS Eng. LRCP Lond. 1949; DObst RCOG 1951; MRCGP 1968. Prev: Ho. Surg. St. Bart. Hosp.

TIMMIS, Adam David London Chest Hospital, Department of Cardiology, Bonner Road, London E2 9JX Tel: 020 8983 2413 Fax: 020 8983 2279 — MB BChir Camb. 1974; MA Camb. 1975; MRCP (UK) 1976; MD Camb. 1983; FRCP Lond. 1993; FESC 1994. Prof. of Clin. Cardiol., Barts & The Lond. NHS Trust. Specialty: Cardiol. Special Interest: Acute Coronary Syndromes; Intens. Cardiol. Socs: Brit. Cardiac Soc. Prev: Sen. Regist. (Cardiol.) Guy's Hosp. Lond.; Research Fell. Massachusett's Gen. Hosp. Boston, USA; Regist. (Cardiol.) King's Coll. Hosp. Lond.

TIMMIS, Christopher Grant Eastcote Health Centre, Abbotsbury Gardens, Eastcote, Ruislip HA5 1TG Tel: 020 8866 0121 Fax: 020 8866 8382; 54 Waxwell Lane, Pinner HA5 3EN — MB Camb. 1977; MA Camb. 1976; BChir 1976; DRCOG 1981; MRCGP 1983. GP Trainer Pinner. Socs: Roy. Coll. Gen. Pract.

TIMMIS, John Benjamin 12 Ringwood Avenue, London N2 9NS — MB BS Lond. 1975; FRCR 1982; DMRD Eng. 1982. Cons. (Radiol.) Whittington & Roy. N. Hosps. Lond. Specialty: Radiol.

TIMMIS, Paul Kenneth 54A Victoria Park Road, London E9 7NB Tel: 020 8533 5986 — MB ChB Sheff. 1986; DA (UK) 1992; FRCA 1994. Cons. Anaesth. Whipps Cross Hosp. Lond. Specialty: Anaesth.; Intens. Care. Prev: Regist. Rotat. (Anaesth.) St. Bartholomews Hosp. Lond.; SHO (Med.) Hereford Co. Hosp.; SHO (Anaesth.) Colchester.

TIMMIS, Mr Peter (retired) Cherry Trees, Shootersway Lane, Berkhamsted HP4 3NP Tel: 01442 863727 — MB BS Lond. 1948 (St Bart.) MRCS Eng. LRCP Lond. 1946; FRCS Eng. 1954. Prev: Cons. ENT Surg. Luton & Dunstable Hosp. & W. Herts. Hosp. Hemel Hempstead.

TIMMIS, Robert Gerald The Hadleigh Practice, Hadleigh House, 20 Kirkway, Broadstone BH18 8EE Tel: 01202 692269; 24 Lower Golf Links Road, Broadstone BH18 8BH — MB BS Lond. 1988 (Univ. Coll. & Middlx. Sch. Med.) DRCOG 1991; MRCGP 1992. Specialty: Gen. Pract. Prev: Trainee GP Brighton HA VTS; Ho. Off. (Med.) Mt. Vernon Hosp.; Ho. Off. (Surg.) Stoke Mandeville Hosp.

TIMMONS, James Anthony 76 Caledonia Road, Saltcoats KA21 5AP — MB ChB Glas. 1974; DRCOG 1976.

TIMMONS, Maria Therese Grace No.8 Dovecote Farm, Waldridge Lane, Chester-le-Street DH2 2NQ — MB BCh BAO NUI 1983.

TIMMONS, Mr Michael John Department of Plastic Surgery, Bradford Royal Infirmary, Bradford BD9 6RJ — MB BChir Camb. 1974 (Camb. & Guy's) MB Camb. 1974, BChir (Distinc. Obst. & Gyn.) 1973; MChir Camb. 1988, MA 1974; FRCS Eng. 1978. Cons. Plastic Surg. Bradford & Airedale NHS Trusts. Specialty: Plastic Surg. Socs: Brit. Soc. Surg. Hand; Brit. Assn. Plastic Surg. Prev: Regist. (Surg.) Addenbrooke's Hosp. Camb.; Regist. (Plastic Surg.) Mt. Vernon Hosp. Northwood; Sen. Regist. (Plastic Surg.) Leeds & Bradford HAs.

TIMMONS, Michael Joseph London Road Medical Practice, 12 London Road, Kilmarnock KA3 7AE Tel: 01563 523593 Fax: 01563 573552 — MB ChB Ed. 1981; MSc Glas. 1973, BSc 1969; BSc (Med. Sci.) St. And. 1978; DRCOG 1983. Lect. (Aviat. Med.) Brit. Aerospace Flying Coll. Prestwick; Clin. Asst. (Cardiol.) CrossHo. Hosp. Kilmarnock. Specialty: Aviat. Med. Socs: Assoc. Mem. RCGP.; BMA. Prev: Regist. (Geriat. Med.) N. Ayrsh. Dist. Gen. Hosp.; SHO (Orthop., A & E) N. Ayrsh. Dist. Gen. Hosp.; SHO (Paediat.) N. Ayrsh. Dist. Gen. Hosp.

TIMMS, Celia Mary Joyce West Pikefish Farmhouse, Pike Fish La, Laddingford, Maidstone ME18 6BH — MB ChB Bristol 1997.

TIMMS, Damian Patrick Havant Health Centre Suite E, PO Box 40, Havant PO9 2AG — MB ChB Bristol 1976; DA Eng. 1981; DRCOG 1982; MRCGP 1984. Regist. (Anaesth.) RN. Hosp. Haslar. Specialty: Anaesth. Prev: Regist. (Anaesth.) Qu. Alexandra's Hosp. Cosham; SHO (Cas.) RN Hosp. Haslar Gosport.

TIMMS, Matthew Adam John Lingmel, Thurstaton Rd, Heswall, Wirral L60 6RY — MB ChB Bristol 1997.

TIMMS, Mr Michael Steven Royal Infirmary, Blackburn BB2 3LR Tel: 01254 294409 Fax: 01254 294060; Great Mitton Hall, Great Mitton, Clitheroe BB7 9PQ Tel: 01254 826150 — MB ChB Leeds 1980; FRCS Ed. 1986; FRCS Eng. 1987; T(S) 1992. Cons. Otolaryngol. Blackburn Roy. Infirm. & Burnley Gen. Hosp. Specialty: Otorhinolaryngol. Socs: Brit. Assn. of Otorhinolatyngologists / Head and Neck Surg.s; Europ. Acad. of Facial Plastic Surg. (Joseh Soc.).; Roy. Soc. of Med. Prev: Sen. Regist. Lect. (Otorhinolaryng.) N.W. Regional Train. Scheme, Manch. Roy. Infirm.

TIMMS, Philip Wingrave Guy's, King's and St thomas's School of Medicine, Start Team, Master's House, London SE11 4TH Tel: 020 840 0653 Fax: 020 840 0657 — MRCS Eng. LRCP Lond. 1976 (Guy's) MRCPsych 1985. Sen. Lect. (Community Psychiat.) Guy's, King's & St Thomas's Sch. of Med.; Hon. Cons.; S. Lond. & Maudsley Trust. Specialty: Gen. Psychiat. Prev: Sen. Regist. (UMDS Psychiat.) Guy's Hosp. Lond.

TIMMS, Roger Francis Acle Medical Centre, Bridewell Lane, Acle, Norwich NR13 3RA Tel: 01493 750888 Fax: 01493 751652; Rose Farmhouse, Broad Road, Fleggburgh, Great Yarmouth NR29 3DD Tel: 01493 368273 — MB BS Lond. 1980 (King's Coll. Med. Sch.) Hosp. Practitioner (Dermat.) Jas. Paget Hosp. Norf. Specialty: Dermat. Socs: BMA; Norf. & Norwich Medico-Chirurgical Soc. Prev: Trainee GP Leicester VTS; Ho. Surg. King's Coll. Hosp. Lond.; Ho. Phys. St. Helen's Hosp. Hastings.

TIMMS, Ronald Lionel Thundersley Hall, 192 Church Road, Thundersley, Benfleet SS7 4PL Tel: 01268 792583 — MRCS Eng. LRCP Lond. 1948 (Guy's)

TIMNEY, Aidan Patrick Trinity House Surgery, 17 Irish Street, Whitehaven CA28 7BU Tel: 01946 693412 Fax: 01946 592046; Elvet, Low Moresby, Whitehaven CA28 6RX Tel: 01946 694257 Fax: 01946 694257 — MB BS Durh. 1964; DIH Eng. 1979.

TIMONEY, Mr Anthony Gerard Mary Bristol Urological Institute, Southmead Hospital, Bristol BS37 9XE Tel: 0117 959 5154 Fax: 0117 950 2229 Email: anthony-timoney@bui.ac.uk — MB BCh BAO NUI 1981 (Dub.) FRCS Ed. 1985; FRCSI 1985; MCh 1995. p/t Cons. Urol. N. Bristol NHS Trust Bristol; Hon. Sen. Lect. in Surg., Univ. of Bristol. Specialty: Urol. Special Interest: Interstitial Cystitis; Laparoscopy; Stone and Prostate Dis. Socs: BAUS; BMA; Europ. Assn. of Urol.

TIMONEY, Norma 150 Park Hill Road, Birmingham B17 9HD — MB ChB Bristol 1992; BA (BDen Sc) Dub. 1981; FDS RCS Eng. 1986; FRCS Eng. 1995. Regist. Rotat. (Plastic Surg.) Higher Specialist Train. W. Midl. Specialty: Plastic Surg. Socs: Brit. Craniofacial Soc. Prev: Regist. & SHO (Plastic Surg.) Roy. Devon & Exeter Hosp.; SHO (Plastic Surg.) Frenchay Hosp.; SHO Rotat. (Gen. Surg.) MusGr. Pk. Hosp. Taunton.

TIMOTHY, Adrian Robert Guy's and St. Thomas' NHS Trust, Department Clinical Oncology, c/o Cancar Management Offices, 4th Floor, Thomas Guy House, Guy's Hospital, St. Thomas' Street,

London SE1 9RT Tel: 0207 955 4547 Fax: 0207 955 8857 — MB BS Lond. 1969 (Westm.) MRCS Eng. LRCP Lond. 1969; DMRT Eng. 1974; FRCR 1976; FRCP Lond. 1988. Cons. Clin. Oncologist, Guy's & St. Thomas' Hosp. Specialty: Oncol. Special Interest: Radiat. Prev: Cons. Radiother. & Oncol. St. Thos. Hosp. Lond.; Gordon Hamilton Fairley Fell. St. Bart. Hosp. Lond.; Fell. Radiat. Therap. Harvard Med. Sch. Boston USA.

TIMOTHY, Elizabeth Molly (retired) 22 Parkwood Avenue, Roundhay, Leeds LS8 1JW — MB BS Madras 1959 (Christian Med. Coll. Vellore) MFPHM; DObst RCOG 1963; DCH Eng. 1964; DPH Leeds 1970; MFCM 1986. Specialist in Community Med. Child Health Plann. & Informat. Dewsbury Dist. HA. Prev: Sen. Regist. (Community Med.) Leeds Gen. Infirm.

TIMOTHY, Irene (retired) 6 Millrace Drive, Fullers Drive, Wistaston, Crewe CW2 6XG Tel: 01270 665242 — (Christian Med. Coll. Vellore, India) MB BS Madras 1957; DObst RCOG 1966; MRCOG 1980; MFFP 1994. Prev: Assoc. Specialist Mid Chesh. Hosps. Trust.

TIMOTHY, Mr Jacob Department of Neurosurgery, Leeds General Infirmary, Leeds LS1 — MB BS Lond. 1991; FRCS Eng. 1996; FRCS (SN) 2002. Cons. Neurosurg. Specialty: Neurosurg. Prev: SHO (Gen. Surg.) Kent & Canterbury Hosp.; SHO (Orthop.) Greenwich Hosp.; SHO (Cardiothoracic) Roy. Brompton Hosp.

TIMPANY, Margaret Mary (retired) Home Breeze House, Beach St, Bare, Morecambe LA4 6BT Tel: 0180 420772 — MB ChB Ed. 1943; DPH Birm. 1947. Prev: Clin. Med. Off. Lancaster Health Dist.

TIMPERLEY, Andrew Colin 8 Middleton Way, Leasingham, Sleaford NG34 8LN — MB ChB Leeds 1990.

TIMPERLEY, Mr Andrew John 2 The Quadrant, Wonford Road, Exeter EX2 4LE Tel: 01392 437070 Email: jtimperley@bigfoot.com — MB ChB Manch. 1981; FRCS Ed. 1986. Cons. Orthop. & Trauma Exeter. Specialty: Orthop.

TIMPERLEY, Jane Clare Anaesthetic Dept., Ninewells Hospital, Dundee Tel: 01382 660 111 — MB ChB Dundee 1987; DA (UK) 1989; MRCGP 1993; FRCA (UK) 1998. Specialist Regist. Anaesth. Ninewells Hosp. Dundee. Specialty: Anaesth. Prev: Staff Doctor in Anaesth. Dumfries & Galloway Roy. Infirm. Dumfries; Specialist Regist. Anasthesia W.Yorks.

TIMPERLEY, Jonathan 9 Welton Mount, Leeds LS6 1ET — MB ChB Leeds 1994.

TIMPERLEY, Lorretta Rose Holly Tree Cottage, Ashiestiel, Galashiels TD1 3LJ; Borders Community Health Services, Dingleton Hospital, Melrose TD6 9HN Tel: 01896 822727 Fax: 01896 823807 — MB ChB Dundee 1991; MA (Hons.) Ed. 1969; PhD Ed. 1977. Staff Grade (Psychiat.). Specialty: Gen. Psychiat. Prev: SHO (Psychiat.) Crichton Roy. Hosp. Dumfries.

TIMPERLEY, Malcolm Richard — MB ChB Liverp. 1980; MRCPsych 1987. Cons. Psychiat. Tees & NE Yorks. NHS Trust. Specialty: Gen. Psychiat.

TIMPERLEY, Walter Richard (retired) — (Oxf.) DM Oxford 1970; BM BCh Oxf. 1961; FRCPath 1981, M 1969; MA Oxf. 1961, DM 1970. Prev: Cons. Neuropath. & Hon. Clin. Lect. (Path.) United Sheff. Hosps. & Univ. Sheff.

TIMSON, Ian Roe Lee Surgery, 367 Whalley New Road, Blackburn BB1 9SR Tel: 01254 680075 Fax: 01254 695477 — MB ChB Manch. 1985; MRCGP 1989; T(GP) 1991. Prev: Trainee GP Clitheroe VTS.

TIN, Nyan Kyaw Leacroft Medical Practice, Ifield Road, Ifield, Crawley RH11 7BS Tel: 01293 526441 Fax: 01293 619970 — MB BS Rangoon 1976; MB BS Med Inst (I) Rangoon 1976; MRCGP 1988. GP Gambrill & partners.

TIN LOI, Shay Fho 34A Little Norsey Road, Billericay CM11 1BL — MB BS Lond. 1976; MRCS Eng. LRCP Lond. 1976; MRCP (UK) 1979; FFA RCS Eng. 1983. Specialty: Anaesth.

TINCELLO, Douglas Gordon University of Leicester, PO Box 65, Leicester LE2 7LX Tel: 0116 258 8391 Fax: 0116 273 1620 Email: dgt4@le.ac.uk — MB ChB Ed. 1989; MRCOG 1995; BSc (Med. Sci.) Ed. 1987, MD 1995. Sen. Lecturer/Honorary Cons. Urogynaecologist. Specialty: Obst. & Gyn. Socs: Internat. Continence Soc.; Internat. Urogynaecology Assn.; Editor, B,J Obstet Gynaecol. Prev: Clin. Lect. Univ of Liverp.; Research Regist. Liverp. Wom.'s Hosp.; Specialist Regist. (O & G) Mersey Deanery.

TINCKLER, Mr Laurence Francis, TD Maelor General Hospital, Wrexham Tel: 01978 291100; Priddbwll Bonc, Farm Llansilen, Oswestry SY10 7QB Tel: 0169 791455 Fax: 01691 791455 — (Liverp.) MB ChB (Hons.) Liverp. 1945; MRCS Eng. LRCP Lond. 1946; FRCS Eng. 1950; MD Liverp. 1962, ChM 1955; DTM & H Liverp. 1959; FACS 1966. Cons. Gen. & Urol. Surg. Maelor Gen. Hosp. Wrexham; Head of Dept. Surg. Riyadh Al-Kharj Milit. Hosp. Saudi Arabia; Chief of Urol. K. Fahad Hosp. Al Baha, Saudi Arabia; Hon. Research Assoc. Dept. Surg. Univ. Liverp.; Lt. Col. RAMC(V) O.C. Surgic. Div. 203 (Welsh) Gen. Hosp.; Med. Dir. Curnow Shipping Ltd. Specialty: Gen. Surg. Socs: Fell. Roy. Soc. Med.; Brit. Assn. Urol. Surgs.; BMA. Prev: Cons. Surg. K. Edwd. Memor. Hosp. Falkland Is.s; Prof. Surg. Univ. Singapore & Hon. Cons. Surg. Brit. Milit. Hosp. Singapore; Vis. Prof. Surg. Univ. Calif. Los Angeles.

TINCOMBE, Michael Robert Park Surgery, 278 Stratford Road, Shirley, Solihull B90 3AF Tel: 0121 241 1700 Fax: 0121 241 1821 — MRCS Eng. LRCP Lond. London 1975; MRCS Eng. LRCP Lond. London 1975.

TINDAL, Margaret Taylor 30 Newlands Road, Glasgow G43 2JD Tel: 0141 632 1583 — MB ChB Glas. 1926; FRFPS Glas. 1931; MD (Commend.) 1933; FRCP Glas. 1983, M 1962. Prev: Muirhead Research Schol. Roy. Hosp. Sick Childr. Glas.; Extra Disp. Phys. Glas. Roy. Infirm.; Hon. Disp. Phys. Roy. Hosp. Sick Childr. Glas.

TINDALL, Hilary Department of Diabetes, North Middlesex Hospital, Sterling Way, London N18 1QX — MD Leeds 1983; MB ChB 1972; MRCP (UK) 1977; FRCP Lond. 1994; FRCP Ed. 1997. Specialty: Endocrinol.; Diabetes.

TINDALL, Mark Julian 26 Swanmore Road, Littleover, Derby DE23 3SD — MB ChB Sheff. 1997.

TINDALL, Nicholas John Wellington Road Surgery, Wellington Road, Newport TF10 7HG Tel: 01952 811677 Fax: 01952 825981 Email: tindalls@medix-uk.com; 22 Newport Road, Edgmond, Newport TF10 8HQ Tel: 01952 814668 — MB ChB Birm. 1980 (Birmingham) DRCOG 1983. Med. Off. Lilleshall Sports Injury Centre Newport. Prev: Trainee GP N. Staffs. HA VTS.

TINDALL, Mr Stuart Frederick Scunthorpe General Hospital, Cliff Gardens, Scunthorpe Tel: 01724 290114 — MB ChB Sheff. 1969; FRCS Eng. 1974; MCh Sheff. 1985. Cons. Urol. Scunthorpe & Grimsby Hosps.; Div.al Director Surg., North. Lincs. & Goole Hosps., NHS Trust. Specialty: Urol.; Gen. Surg. Special Interest: Laparoscopic and Endoscopic Surg. Socs: BMA; Assoc. Mem. BAUS; Brit. Assn. of Med. Managers. Prev: Sen. Regist. (Gen. Surg.) Hallamsh. Hosp. Sheff.; Research Asst. Dept. Surg. Sheff. Univ.; Rotating Surg. Regist. Sheff. Roy. Infirm.

TINDALL, Professor Victor Ronald, CBE 4 Planetree Road, Hale, Altrincham WA15 9JJ Tel: 0161 904 8222 Fax: 0161 904 8333 — (Liverp.) MB ChB Liverp. 1951; DObst RCOG 1955; FRCS Ed. 1961; FRCOG 1974, M 1961; MD Liverp. 1962; MSc Manch. 1976; FRCS Eng. 1991. Emerit. Prof. O & G Univ. Manch. Socs: Fell Roy. Soc. Med. Prev: Cons. O & G Univ. Hosp. Wales Cardiff & Welsh Hosp. Bd.; Sen. Lect. Welsh Nat. Sch. Med. Cardiff; Wellcome Vis. Prof. S. Afr. 1986.

TINDLE, John Edward (retired) Gwernant, Tanygroes, Cardigan SA43 2JS Email: john_tindle@whsmithnet.co.uk/ jtindle@compuserve.com — (Roy. Free) MB BS Lond. 1956; MRCS Eng. LRCP Lond. 1956. Designated Examr. Austral. High Commiss. Prev: Med. Adviser Old Ct. Hosp. Lond.

TINEGATE, Hazel Nancy Todridge Farm, Middleton, Morpeth NE61 4RE — MB BS Lond. 1975; MRCP (UK) 1979; MRCPath 1983; T(Path) 1991. Cons. Haemat. N. Tyneside Gen. Hosp. Specialty: Haematology. Prev: Sen. Regist. (Haemat.) Freeman Hosp. Newc.

TINER, Richard Stephen Association of the British Pharmaceutical Industry, 12 Whitehall, London SW1A 2DY Tel: 020 7747 1404 Fax: 020 7747 1400 Email: rtiner@abpi.org.uk/scosshall@abpi.org.uk — MB BS Lond. 1974 (Middlx. Hosp.) DRCOG 1977; MFPM 1999. Med. Dir. Assn. Brit. Pharmaceut. Industry Lond. Specialty: Pharmaceutical Medicine. Socs: Roy. Soc. Med.; BMA; Brit. Assn. of Pharmaceutical Phys.s. Prev: GP French Weir Health Centre Taunton & Trainee GP Taunton VTS; SHO Kettering Gen. Hosp. N.ants.

TING, Alison Yih-Hua 14/8 East Parkside, Edinburgh EH16 5XL — MB ChB Ed. 1997; MRCPCH (UK).

TING, Mr Philip Yuen Cho First/Floor, 19 Gerrard Street, London W1D 6JG — MB BS Lond. 1989; FRCS Ed. 1994. Specialty: Gen. Pract.

TING, Simon Chow Hwa 300 Bellhouse Road, Shiregreen, Sheffield S5 0RE — MB ChB Sheff. 1996.

TINGEY, Mr William Robert The Chiltern Hospital, London Road, Great Missenden HP16 0EN Tel: 01494 890890; Flat 4, Teal House, The Millstream, London Road, High Wycombe HP11 1AE Tel: 01494 539939 Fax: 01494 539939 Email: wrtinge@uk-consultants.co.uk — MB BS Lond. 1969 (St. Bart.) MRCS Eng. LRCP Lond. 1969; FRCS Eng. 1975; FRCOG 1992, M 1977. Cons. Gyn., Private Pract.; Examr. DRCOG Course Guys & Thomas's; Examr. Univeristy of Lond. MBBS Guy's and Thomas's; Examr. FRCOG Course Guys & Thomas's. Specialty: Obst. & Gyn. Socs: Hysteroscopy Soc.; Europ. Endoscopy Soc.; Pelvic Floor Soc. Prev: S. Bucks NHS Trust; Cons. Obsterician & Gynaecologist; Sen. Regist. (O & G) Oxf. & Northampton.

TINKER, Andrew BHF Laboratories and Department of Medicine, Room 420, The Rayne Institute, 5 University Street, University College London, London WC1E 6JJ Tel: 020 7679 6391 Fax: 020 7691 2838 Email: a.tinker@ucl.ac.uk; 34 Green End Dell, Green End Road, Boxmoor, Hemel Hempstead HP1 Tel: 01442 216902 Fax: 01442 216902 — MB BS Lond. 1987 (Roy. Free) BA Oxf. 1984; MRCP (UK) 1990; PhD Lond. 1993; FRCP UK 2004. Prof. of Molecular Med. Specialty: Pharmacology. Prev: Reader; Wellcome Sen. Research Fell. (Clin. Sci.), Sen. Lect. & Hon. Cons. (Clin. Pharmacol.) Univ. Coll. Lond.; Postdoctoral Research Fell. Univ. Calif., San. Francisco.

TINKER, Andrew James 9 Greystone Close, Burley in Wharfedale, Ilkley LS29 7RS Tel: 01943 865587 — MB ChB Leic. 1987 (Leics.) MB ChB Leics. 1987; MRCP (UK) 1990. Staff Grade, Palliat. Med. Marie Curie Hospice Bradford. Specialty: Gastroenterol.; Haematology. Prev: Regist. (Med.) Southland Hosp., New Zealand; Regist. (Med.) Whiston Hosp.; SHO (Med.) E. Birm. Hosp.

TINKER, Gladys Mary Llandough Hospital NHS Trust, Llandough Hospital, Penlan Road, Penarth CF64 2XX Tel: 029 2071 1711 Fax: 029 2070 8973; 7 Cae Garn, Heol-y-Cyw, Bridgend CF35 6LD — MB ChB Ed. 1969; BSc (Med. Sci.) Ed. 1966; MRCP (UK) 1976; Dip. Palliat. Med. Wales 1992; FRCP Ed. 1993; MSc Wales 1994. Cons. Phys. (Geriat. Med.) Llandough Hosp. NHS Trust. Specialty: Care of the Elderly. Prev: Sen. Regist. W. Wales Hosp. Carmarthen; Regist. St. David's Hosp. Cardiff; SHO (Geriat. Unit) Univ. Hosp. of Wales Cardiff.

TINKER, Jack The Royal Society of Medicine, 1 Wimpole St., London W1G 0AE Fax: 020 290 2977 Email: jack.tinker@roysocmed.ac.uk; 1 Rectory Road, Barnes, London SW13 0DU — (Manch.) BSc, MB ChB Manch. 1960; FRCS Glas. 1966; FRCP Lond. 1980, M 1969; DIC 1971; FRSA 1998. p/t Emerit. Dean The Roy. Soc. of Med.; Governor Expert Witness Inst.; Emerit. Cons. Phys. Univ. Coll. Hosps.; Edr. in Chief Hosp. Med.; Med. Adviser Rio Tinto plc. Specialty: Gen. Med. Socs: Fell. Roy. Soc. Med.; Fell. Roy. Soc. of Arts. Prev: Dean The Roy. Soc. of Med.; Dean & Postgrad. Med. Univ. Lond. & NW Thames; Postgrad. Sub-Dean Middlx. Hosp. Med. Sch.

TINKER, Michael David The Surgery, Bowholm, Canonbie DG14 0UX Tel: 01387 371313 Fax: 01387 371244; Hillside, 1 Hillside Crescent, Langholm DG13 0EE — MB ChB Ed. 1969; DObst RCOG 1971; FRCP 2002. Course Organiser E. Cumbria VTS; N. Region Summative Assessm. Coordinator. Specialty: Gen. Pract.; Educat.

TINKER, Noel Richard 2 Northfield Close, South Lane, Brough HU15 2EW — MB ChB Liverp. 1993.

TINKER, Rachel Mary Moss Valley Medical Practice, Gosber Road, Eckington, Sheffield S21 4BZ — MB BS Lond. 1987 (Char. Cross & Westm. Med. Sch.) DRCOG 1993; MRCGP 1995; M Ed 2003.

TINKLER, Anne Marie Brockley House, Pilgrims Way, Guildford GU4 8AD — MB ChB Manch. 1983; DRCOG 1986; MRCGP 1987.

TINKLER, George Geoffrey Portway Surgery, 1 The Portway, Porthcawl CF36 3XB Tel: 01656 304204 Fax: 01656 772605; 128 West Road, Nottage, Porthcawl CF36 3RY — MB BCh Wales 1972; DObst RCOG 1974; MRCGP 1976; Cert. Family Plann. JCC 1977. Clin. Asst. (Behaviour Ther.) Morganwg Hosp. Bridgend; GP Trainer Porthcawl; Local health Group Board Member Bridgend.

TINKLER, Joanna Mary Hope Cove, Cuddington Way, Sutton SM2 7HY Tel: 020 8661 1996; First Floor Flat, 52 Hamilton Rd, Wimbledon, London SW19 1JF — MB BS Lond. 1993; DCH RCP Lond. 1996; DRCOG 1996; MRCPCH Lond. 1999. SHO (Paediat.) Qu. Marys Childr Hosp. Surrey. Specialty: Paediat. Prev: SHO (Neonates.) St Helier Hosp. Surrey.; SHO (Paediat.) Roy Surrey Co. Hosp. Guildford.; Med Regist. ChristCh.. NZ.

TINKLER, Richard Frederick William The Surgery, 34 Teme Street, Tenbury Wells WR15 8AA Tel: 01584 810343 Fax: 01584 819734; Kitchen Hill, Orleton, Ludlow SY8 4HP Tel: 01568 780369 — MB BS Lond. 1973 (St. Geo.) BSc West. Austral. 1968; DCH Eng. 1975; DA Eng. 1977. Hosp. Pract. (Anaesth.) & Clin. Asst. (Cas.) Tenbury & Dist. Hosp. Specialty: Anaesth. Socs: Assn. Anaesth. Prev: SHO (Paediat., O & G & Anaesth.) N. Staffs. Hosp. Centre Stoke-on-Trent.

TINKLER, Robert 713 Yardley Wood Road, Birmingham B13 0PT Tel: 0121 444 3597; 95 Hither Green Lane, Abbey Park, Redditch B98 9BN — MB ChB Birm 1955 (Birm.)

TINKLER, Sandra Dawn 70 Broomfield Avenue, Battlehill Estate, Wallsend NE28 9AE — MB ChB Dundee 1984; MRCP (UK) 1988; MSc (Clin. Oncol.) Ed. 1991; FRCR 1992. Cons. Clin. Oncol. Wessex Radiother. Centre Roy. S. Hants. Hosp. Specialty: Oncol.; Radiother. Prev: Sen. Regist. (Radiat. Oncol.) Newc. Gen. Hosp.; Regist. (Radiat. Oncol.) West. Gen. Hosp. Edin.

TINKLIN, Tracy Susan Derbyshire Childrens Hospital, Uttoxeter Rd, Derby DE22 3NE — BM Soton. 1988; MRCP (UK) 1993.

TINLINE, Colin Carmichael — MB ChB Ed. 1971; FRCPsych 1993, M 1977; DPM Eng. 1977. Cons. & Adolesc. Psychiat., PearTree Centre, Redditch. Specialty: Child & Adolesc. Psychiat. Prev: Sen. Regist. Nuffield Child Psychiat. Unit Newc.; Regist. (Psychiat.) Newc. HA; SHO Centr. Hosp. Warwick.

TINNION, Shirley Anne Meadowcroft Surgery, Jackson Road, Aylesbury HP19 9EX Tel: 01296 425775 Fax: 01296 330324 — BSc (Hons.) Lond. 1984, MB BS 1987; DRCOG 1990; DCH RCP Lond. 1990; MRCGP 1991; FRCGP 2000; DIC DipENT 2002. GP Princip. Prev: Ho. Phys. Stoke Mandeville Hosp. Aylesbury; Ho. Surg. Amersham Hosp.; Trainee GP Stoke Mandeville Hosp. Aylesbury.

TINSA, Jazwinder Singh 7 Elwells Close, Bilston WV14 9YH — MB ChB Aberd. 1992.

TINSLAY, Pamela Ivy 4 Romney Chase, Emerson Park, Hornchurch RM11 3BJ — MB BS Lond. 1959 (Roy. Free) MRCS Eng. LRCP Lond. 1959; DPH Glas. 1967; MFCM 1972. Hon. Cons. Pub. Health Med. Barking & Havering HA. Specialty: Pub. Health Med. Prev: Cons. Communicable Dis. Control Barking & Havering HA; Dist. Community Phys. Havering Health Dist.

TINSLEY, Ellis George Frederick (retired) Brooklands, Carleton Road, Skipton BD23 2BE Tel: 01756 792338 — (Camb. & St. Mary's) MB Camb. 1957, BChir 1956; FRCPath 1976, M 1964. Prev: Cons. Path. Airedale Gen. Hosp. Keighley.

TINSLEY, Helen Margaret Meyer Street Surgery, 20 Meyer Street, Cale Green, Stockport SK3 8JE Tel: 0161 480 2882 Fax: 0161 480 0583; 20 Harrisons Drive, Woodley, Stockport SK6 1JY — MB ChB Manch. 1974 (Manchester) ECFMG Cert 1975; MFFP 1994. Specialty: Gen. Pract. Socs: Fac. Fam. Plann. & Reproduc. Health; Brit. Menopause Soc.; BDA.

TINSLEY, Michael John, Col. late RAMC Clifton, 76 Main St., Keyworth, Nottingham NG12 5AD — MB ChB Manch. 1966; BSc Manch. 1963; DObst RCOG 1970; MRCGP 1976. Cdr. Med. 2 (UK) Div. E Dist. Specialty: Pub. Health Med. Prev: IFOR Theatre Surg.; Med. Advis. Allied Forces NW Europ.; Cdr. Med. BMH Iserlohn.

TINSON, Ruth Elizabeth 30 Links Way, Eden Park, Beckenham BR3 3DQ — MB BS Lond. 1998.

TINT, Aung Khine 81 Heaton Road, Withington, Manchester M20 4GW Email: atint@btinternet.com — MB BS Med Inst (I) Rangoon 1996. Specialist Regist. (Psychiat.) Macclesfield Gen. Hosp. Specialty: Gen. Psychiat.

TINTO, Barbara Anne Oakbank, Lamlash, Brodick KA27 8LH — MB ChB Glas. 1976; DRCOG 1978.

TINTO, Elizabeth Isabella London Street Practice, 72 London Street, Reading RG1 4SJ Tel: 0118 957 4640 Fax: 0118 959 7613; 5 Fallowfield Close, Cavesham, Reading RG4 8NQ Tel: 01734 470253 — MB ChB Aberd. 1977; DRCOG 1982.

TINTO, Richard Graham Lamlash Medical Centre, Lamlash, Brodick KA27 8NS Tel: 01770 600516 Fax: 01770 600132; Oakbank, Lamlash, Brodick KA27 8LH Tel: 0177 06 00517 — MB ChB Glas. 1971; MRCP (UK) 1978; MRCGP 1981. Prev: Regist. (Med.) Hairmyres Hosp. E. Kilbride; Med. Off. All St.s' Hosp. Transkei, S. Afr.

TINTO, Sujaee Asoka Samarasekara (retired) 5 Carnoustie Court, Bothwell, Glasgow G71 8UB — MB BS Ceylon 1965 (Colombo) DSM Ed. 1969; MRCGP 1977.

TINTON, Marilyn Margaret Longcroft Clinic, 5 Woodmansterne Lane, Banstead SM7 3HH Tel: 01737 359332 Fax: 01737 370835; 37 Ewell Downs Road, Ewell, Epsom KT17 3BT — MB BS Lond. 1973; DRCOG 1976; DCH Eng. 1977.

TIONG, Ho Yee 27 Lower Road, Beeston, Nottingham NG9 2GT — BM BS Nottm. 1997.

TIPLADY, Peter North Cumbria Health Authority, 4 Wavell Drive, Rosehill, Carlisle CA1 2SE Tel: 01228 603500 Fax: 01228 603612; The Arches, The Green, Wetheral, Carlisle CA4 8ET Tel: 01228 561611 Email: petertiplady@ncha.demon.co.uk — MB BS Durh. 1965; MRCGP 1972; FFPHM RCP (UK) 1986. Dir. (Pub. Health) N. Cumbria HA. Specialty: Pub. Health Med. Socs: BMA.

TIPLADY, Trevor John (retired) Evelyn House, Ramsbury, Marlborough SN8 2PA Tel: 01672 520288 — MB BS Lond. 1955 (King's Coll. Hosp.) MRCS Eng. LRCP Lond. 1955; DObst RCOG 1959. Prev: Clin. Asst. (Obst.) & Stroke Rehabil. Unit Savernake Hosp. MarlBoro.

TIPPER, Rebecca Jane — MB ChB Ed. 1988; MRCGP 1996; MRCPsych 1999; MPhil Ed. 2000. SHO (Psychiat.) Dingleton Hosp. Melrose; Specialist Regist. in Gen. Adult Psychiat., Roy. Edin. Hosp. Specialty: Gen. Psychiat. Prev: GP/Regist. Edin.; SHO (Geriat. & Gen. Med.) Haddington.

TIPPETT, Richard Jonathan Downside House, St. Boniface Rd, Ventnor PO38 1PJ — MB BS Lond. 1997.

TIPPETT, Susan Anne Nightingale Surgery, Greatwell Drive, Cupernham Lane, Romsey SO51 7QN Tel: 01794 517878 Fax: 01794 514236; 22 The Thicket, Whitenap, Romsey SO51 5SZ Tel: 01794 516028 — MB ChB Leeds 1975; DRCOG 1977; MRCGP 1980.

TIPPETTS, Alice Elizabeth Ekams, PO 216, Kununurra WA 6743, Australia Tel: 08 91 681288; 8 Oakfield Street, Heavitree, Exeter EX1 2QT Tel: 01392 424704 — BM Soton. 1988; DRCOG 1992; MRCGP 1994; Austral Med Counc 1999. Med. Off. (GP) in Aboriginal Health in rural Australia. Specialty: Gen. Pract. Prev: Sen. Med. Off. Carnarvon Aboriginal Med. Serv. Austral.; Long Term GPO Locum Exeter; Trainee GP Exeter VTS.

TIPPETTS, Ranette 22 Sitwell Villas, Morton, Alfreton DE55 6GX Tel: 01246 864602; 12 Deighton Close, St Ives, Huntingdon PE27 3JJ Tel: 01480 463704 — MB ChB Birm. 1995; ChB Birm. 1995. SHO Neonatology, Addenbrookes Hosp. Specialty: Paediat. Prev: SHO (Paediat.) Birm. Heartlands; SHO (A & E) Bristol Roy. Infirm.; PRHO (Surg.) City Hosp. Birm.

TIPPING, Conal Gerard 1 Inglewood, Lurgan, Craigavon BT67 9LS — MB BCh Belf. 1998.

TIPPING, Jonathan Peter Musgrove Park Hospital, Accident & Emergency Department, Taunton TA1 5DA — MB BCh Wales 1988; MRCGP 1993.

TIPPING, Kathryn Elizabeth 31 Bramley Road, Bramhall, Stockport SK7 2DW — MB BS Lond. 1993.

TIPPING, Philip James 24 Penine Avenue, Riddings, Alfreton DE55 4AE Tel: 01773 602707; Crofters Barn, Knowts Hall Farm, Golden Valley, Riddings, Alfreton DE55 4ES Tel: 01773 749058 — MB ChB Liverp. 1988; Cert. Family Plann. JCC 1991. Prev: SHO (Paediat.) Chester; SHO (O & G) Whiston; SHO (Geriat.) Chester.

TIPPING, Thelma Ruth Royal Glamorgan Hospital, Ynysmaerdy, Llantrisant, Pontypridd CF72 8XR Tel: 01443 443443 Fax: 01443 443248; 10 Clinton Road, Penarth CF64 3JB Tel: 02920 712673 — MB BCh Wales 1979 (Welsh National School of Medicine) BSc (Hons.) (Maths) Wales 1973, MB BCh 1979; FFA RCSI 1985. Roy. Glamprgan Hosp. Lllantrisant. Specialty: Anaesth. Prev: Cons. Anaesth. Manor Hosp. Walsall.

TIPPLE, Berndine Gesiene Everest House Surgery, Everest Way, Hemel Hempstead HP2 4HY Tel: 01442 240422 Fax: 01442 235045 — BM Soton. 1983; DRCOG 1986; Cert. Family Plann. JCC 1986. Socs: BMA. Prev: Trainee GP Harpenden VTS; SHO (O & G & Gen. Med.) Luton & Dunstable Hosp.

TIPPLE, Ronald Whitaker, Surg. Capt. RN Cree, Crapstone, Yelverton PL20 7PG — MB BCh Wales 1938 (Cardiff) BSc, MB BCh Wales 1938; DLO Eng. 1947.

TIPPLES, Melanie Kate 20 Nella Road, London W6 9PB — MB BS Lond. 1992; MBBS FRCSED MRCOG. SPR OBS and Gynae, N. W. Thames, year 5. Specialty: Obst. & Gyn. Prev: SHO (O & G) St. Thos. Hosp. Lond.

TIPPU, Naveed Iqbal Park Avenue Surgery, 27 Park Avenue, Dover CT16 1ES Tel: 01304 206463 Fax: 01304 216066; 74 Archers Court Road, Whitfield, Dover CT16 3HU Tel: 01304 826766 Email: tippu@lineone.net — MB BS Oshanir 1980; LRCP LRCS Ed. LRCPS Glas. 1983; MRCP (UK) 1988; Dip. Addict Behaviour St. George's Med. Sch. 1995; LFHOM (Licenciete Fellow in Homeopathy) Royal London Homoeopathic Hospital 1998. Princip. Gen. Pract. Socs: Roy. Coll. Phys.; Fac. Homoeop. Prev: Regist. (Gen. Med.) Basildon Hosp.; SHO Rotat. (Gen. Med.) Gen. Hosp. & Ingham Infirm. S. Shields.

TIPTAFT, Mr Richard Charles Emblem House, 27 Tooley Street, London SE1 2PR Tel: 020 7403 4303 Fax: 020 7403 5303; 42 Gloucester Circus, Greenwich, London SE10 8RY — MB BS Lond. 1972; BSc (Hons. Physiol.) Lond. 1969 1969; FRCS Eng. 1976. Cons. Urol.Guy's & St. Thomas' Hosps. Trust Lond. Specialty: Urol. Prev: Sen. Lect. Urol. & Hon. Cons. Surg. Urol. Lond. Hosp.; Hon. Cons. Urol. Newham HA; Resid. (Urol.) Yale New Haven Med. Centre USA.

TIPTON, Carolyn Mary Newra House, 63 Willoughby St, Crieff PH5 2AE — MB BS Lond. 1988; DRCOG 1991; MRCGP 1992. Prev: GP Crieff Retainer Scheme.; GP Princip.

TIPTON, Richard Henson (retired) Gyfres Farm, Bucks Hill, Chipperfield, Kings Langley WD4 9BR Tel: 01923 267664 Email: rht1@ndirect.co.uk — MB BS Lond. 1960 (Univ. Coll. Hosp.) DObst RCOG 1963; FRCOG 1978, M 1965; MD Sheff. 1971. Prev: Cons. O & G Watford Gen. Hosp.

TIRUNAWARKARISU, Kanawadi Pillai St. David's Hospital, Carmarthen SA31 3HB Tel: 01267 237481; Brynawelon, 2 Alltycnap Road, Johnstown, Carmarthen SA31 3QY — MB BS Ceylon 1971; MRCPsych 1984. Regist. (Psychiat.) St. David's Hosp. Carmarthen. Specialty: Gen. Psychiat. Prev: Regist. (Child Psychiat.) Bod Difyr Clinic Colwyn Bay; Regist. & SHO Winwick Hosp. Warrington.

TIRUPATHI-RAO, Marada Tonypandy Health Centre, Winton Field, Tonypandy CF40 2LE Tel: 01443 433284 Fax: 01443 436848 — MB BS Andhra 1972. GP Tonypandy, M. Glam.

TISCHKOWITZ, Mark Derek Karl-Eugen White's Farmhouse, Upp End, Manuden, Bishop's Stortford CM23 1BT — MB ChB Liverp. 1993.

TISDALE, John Bartholomew Tregony Road Surgery, Tregony Road, Probus, Truro TR2 4JZ; The Surgery, Mill Lane, Grampound, Truro TR2 4RU — MB ChB Liverp. 1976.

TISDALL, Jennifer Mary (retired) The Red House, 23 Furzehatt Road, Plymstock, Plymouth PL9 8QX Tel: 01752 402356 Fax: 01752 402366 Email: jentisdl@netcomuk.co.uk — (King's Coll. Hosp.) MB BS Lond. 1956. Prev: SCMO (Family Plann.) Devon AHA.

TISDALL, Michael Walter (retired) The Red House, 23 Furzehatt Road, Plymstock, Plymouth PL9 8QX Tel: 01752 402356 — (Middlesex Hospital) MB Camb. 1956, BChir 1955; BA Middlesex Hospital 1955; DCH Eng. 1958; DObst RCOG 1959.

TISI, Mr Paul Vincent Bedford Hospital, Department of Vascular Surgery, Kempston Road, Bedford MK42 9DJ Tel: 01234 792186 Fax: 01234 792187 — MB BS Lond. 1988; FRCS Ed. 1992; MS Soton. 1999; FRCS Gen. Surg. 1999. Cons. Vasc. & Gen. Surg. Bedford Hosp.; Cons. Vasc. Surg. Luton & Dunstable Hosp. Specialty: Surgery, Vascular. Special Interest: Aortic Aneurysms; Carotid Artery Surg.; Peripheral Vasc. Dis. Socs: Eur. Soc. Vasc. Surg.; Association of Surgeons of GB & Ireland; Vascular Surgical Society of GB & Ireland. Prev: Specialist Regist. (Vasc. Surg.) Soton. Gen. Hosp.; Specialist Regist. (Surg.) St Richard's Hosp. Chichester; Research Fell. (Vasc. Surg.) Roy. S. Hants. Hosp. Soton.

TISSAINAYAGAM, Melwyn Balendra Jeganathan (retired) 15 Meadowvale, Darras Hall, Ponteland, Newcastle upon Tyne NE20 9NF; No 8, Chelsea Gardens, Colombo 3, Sri Lanka — MB BS Ceylon 1964; MRCOG 1976. Prev: Med. Off. DSS Newc.

TITCHMARSH, Michael Reid (retired) 24 Castlegate, York YO62 5AB Tel: 01439 770620/01439 771860 — MB ChB Liverp. 1965; DObst RCOG 1967.

TITCOMB, Daniel Robert 27 Woodland Gr, Bristol BS9 2BD — MB ChB Bristol 1997; BSc (Hons) UCL 1993; MRCS (Eng) 2000. Specialty: Gen. Surg.

TITCOMB, Margaret Louise The Falkland Surgery, Monks Lane, Newbury RG14 7DF — MB BS Lond. 1982; MRCGP 1988. GP.

TITCOMBE, Donald Hereward Macalister (retired) 9 Harefield Drive, Wilmslow SK9 1NJ Tel: 01625 27396 — MB ChB Manch 1940 (Manch.) Prev: Ho. Surg. & Clin. Asst. Aural Dept. Manch. Roy. Infirm.

TITCOMBE, Jane Louisa Mary Ware Road Surgery, 77 Ware Road, Hertford SG13 7EE Tel: 01992 587961 — MB ChB Dundee 1977; MRCGP 1984. Clin. Asst. (Dermat.) Qu. Eliz. II Hosp. Welwyn Gdn. City. Specialty: Dermat. Socs: Scott. Dermat. Soc.; Dowling Club. Prev: Regist. (Gen. Med.) Perth Roy. Infirm.; Regist. (Dermat.) Tayside HB; SHO (Dermat.) Ninewells Hosp. Dundee.

TITE, Lorraine Jean 20 Chanctonbury Chase, Redhill RH1 4BB — MB BS Lond. 1998.

TITFORD, Joan Elvira (retired) 1 Tollers Lane, Coulsdon CR5 1BE — (Univ. Coll. Hosp.) MRCS Eng. LRCP Lond. 1943. Prev: Regist. (O & G) New End Hosp. Hampstead.

TITHERIDGE, Katherine Louise Gold Street Medical Centre, 106 Gold Street, Wellingborough NN8 4ES Tel: 01933 223429 Fax: 01933 229240 — BM BS Nottm. 1997.

TITHERIDGE, Ruth Elsie 3 Chapman Lane, Flackwell Heath, High Wycombe HP10 9AZ Tel: 01628 523972 — MB BS Lond. 1983 (Char. Cross Hosp. Med. Sch.) DRCOG 1987; MRCGP Lond. 1987; DCH RCP Lond. 1987. Prev: GP Bedford.

TITLEY, Jeremy Victor East Hill Farm, West Knoyle, Warminster BA12 6AN — MB BS Lond. 1968.

TITLEY, Mr Oliver Garth Sellyoak Hospital, University Hospital Birmingham NHS Trust, Raddlebarn Road, Sellyoak, Birmingham B29 6JD Tel: 021 627 8602; 43 Woodville Road, Harborne, Birmingham B17 9AR Tel: 0121 427 1432 — MB ChB Birm. 1986; MSc Birm. 1992; FRCS Eng. 1992; FRCS (Plast) 1998; CCST 1999. Cons. Plastic Surg., Unversity Hosp., Birm.; Cons. Plastic Surg., Good Hope Hosp., Sutton Coldfield. Specialty: Plastic Surg. Socs: Full BAPS; Assoc. BSSH. Prev: SHO (Plastic Surg.) Wexham Pk. Hosp. Slough; SHO (Plastic Surg.) W. Midl. Regional Plastic & Jaw Surg. Unit; SHO Rotat. (Gen. Surg.) Leicester.

TITLEY, Roger George The Surgery, 20 Southwick Street, Southwick, Brighton BN42 4TB Tel: 01273 592723/596077; 7 Mill Hill, Shoreham-by-Sea BN43 5TG Tel: 01273 455247 — MB BS Lond. 1965 (St. Mary's) MRCS Eng. LRCP Lond. 1964; DObst RCOG 1967. Police Surg. Shoreham by Sea; Port Med. Off. HMA Shoreham by Sea Lifeboat. Prev: Ho. Surg. (O & G) Odstock Hosp. Salisbury; Ho. Surg. & Ho. Phys. Salisbury Infirm; Ho. Surg. (Orthop.) Paddington Gen. Hosp.

TITMAS, Gordon John (retired) 7 The Bull Meadow, Streatley-on-Thames, Reading RG8 9QD Tel: 01491 874057 — (Newc. u. Tyne) MB BS Newc. 1968; DObst RCOG 1972; MRCGP 1975; Dip. Palliat. Med. Wales 1991.

TITMAS, John Michael (retired) 706 Finchley Road, London NW11 7ND Tel: 020 8458 7371 — (Middlx.) MRCS Eng. LRCP Lond. 1947; MB BS Lond. 1949; DPH Lond. 1963. Prev: Civil. Ophth. Specialist RAF Centr. Med. Estab. Lond.

TITMUSS, Sarah Jane The Old Rectory, Madresfield, Malvern WR13 5AB Tel: 01425 403413/01684 572495 Fax: 01425 402032 — MB BS Lond. 1982 (University College Hospital London) BSc (Hons.) Lond. 1977; DRCOG 1985; DCH RCP Lond. 1988.

TITORIA, Manoj Wrightington Hospital, Hall Lane, Appley Bridge, Wigan WN6 9EP Email: manoj.titoria@ntlworld.com — BSc 1960; MB BS Lucknow 1967; DA 1972; FFARCSI 1975. Consultant Anaesthetist. Specialty: Anaesth. Socs: Fell. Assoc. Anaesth. GB & Irel.; Internat. Anaesthesis Research Soc., USA. Prev: Cons. Anaesth. Ormskirk & Dist. Gen. Hosp.

TITTERINGTON, Mary Barbara 7 Horseshoe Lane, Brackagh, Portadown, Craigavon BT62 3RS Tel: 01762 840415 — MB BCh BAO Dub. 1974. Clin. Med. Off. Health Centre Portadown.

TIVY-JONES, Mr Peter North West Wales Hospitals Trust, Bangor LL57 2PW — MB BS Lond. 1970 (Westm.) MRCS Eng. LRCP Lond. 1970; FRCS Ed. 1975; MRCOG 1976. Cons. N. W. Wales Hosp.sTrust. Specialty: Obst. & Gyn. Socs: BMA; HCSA. Prev: Sen. Regist. St. David's Hosp. Bangor; Regist. (O & G) St. Mary's & Samarit. Hosps. Lond.; Resid. Med. Off. Qu. Charlotte's Hosp. Wom. Lond.

TIWARI, Alok 42 Pollards Green, Chelmsford CM2 6UH — MB BS Lond. 1996.

TIWARI, Indrajit Department of Gatroenterology, Broomfield Hospiral, Chelmsford CM1 7ET Tel: 01245 514097 Fax: 01245 514864 Email: itiwari@hotmail.com — MB BS Allahabad 1971 (MLN Med. Coll., Allahabad, India) MD India 1975; MRCPI 1980; FRCPI 1990. Assoc. Specialist Gatroentrlogy, Broomfield Hosp. Chelmsford. Specialty: Gen. Med. Socs: Mem. Brit. Soc. of Gastroenterol.; Fell. Roy. Soc. of Med. (1993); Mem. Saudi Gastroenterol. Assn. Prev: Cons. Gastroenterologist Milit. Hosp. South. Region, Saudi Arabia; Regist. Med. Cumbld. Infirm. Carlisle; Regist. Med. Univ. Hosp. NHS, Cardiff.

TIWARI, Mr Indu Bhushan, Group Capt. RAF Med. Br. Retd. (retired) 66 A Arundell, Ely CB6 1BQ — MB BS Nagpur 1961; FRCS Ed. 1969. Prev: Regist. (Surg.) W. Cumbld. Hosp. Hensingham.

TIWARI, Kala 87 St Alban's Avenue, Hartshead, Ashton-under-Lyne OL6 8XN Tel: 0161 339 9547 Fax: 0161 223 7282 — MB BS Banaras Hindu 1968; BSc (Hons.) Banaras Hindu 1962. GP Manch. PCT. Prev: Clin. Med. Off. (Family Plann.) Stockport HA.

TIWARI, Ninawatie Vimal Wrafton House Surgery, Wrafton House, 9-11 Wellfield Road, Hatfield AL10 0BS Tel: 01707 265454 Fax: 01707361286 — MB ChB Aberd. 1975 (Aberdeen) Cert. Family Plann. JCC 1978; DRCOG 1979; DCH RCP Lond. 1986; MRCGP 1987. Sstaft Screde Community Prediatrician, W. Herts Trust. Specialty: Community Child Health; Gen. Pract.; Community Child Health. Prev: Clin. Med. Off. Dacorum & St. Albans Community NHS Trust.; Trainee GP St. Mary's Hosp. Lond. VTS; Hosp. Med. Off. Shenley Hosp.

TIWARI, Prem Prakash The Surgery, Deep Croft, 21 Croft Road, Edwalton, Nottingham NG12 4BW.

TIWARI, Ram Krishna Nelson Health Centre, Cecil Street, North Shields NE29 0DZ Tel: 0191 257 1191 Fax: 0191 258 4961 — MB BS Lucknow 1972. GP N. Shields Tyne & Wear.

TIWARI, Ravindra Butetown Health Centre, Loudown Square, Docks, Cardiff CF10 5UZ Tel: 029 2046 2347 Fax: 029 2045 3080.

TIWARI, Shobhi Rani The Surgery, Deep Croft, 21 Croft Road, Edwalton, Nottingham NG12 4BW.

TIWARY, Ram Nain 504 New Cross Road, London SE14 6TJ — MRCS Eng. LRCP Lond. 1968; MSc (Med. Sci.) Glas. 1985.

TIZARD, Eleanor Jane Childrens Renal Unit, Bristol Royal Hospital for Children, Upper Maudlinst, Bristol BS2 8BJ Tel: 0117 342 8881 — MB BS Lond. 1979 (Middlesex) FRCP; MRCP (UK) 1981. Cons. Paediatric Nephrologist, Royal Hosp. for Children, Bristol. Specialty: Paediat. Socs: Liveryman Soc. Apoth. Lond.; Fell. Roy. Coll. Paediat. & Child Health; Brit. Assn. Paediat. Nephrol.

TIZZARD, Simon Peter Lamport, Stowe, Buckingham MK18 5AB — MB BS Lond. 1996; BA Cantab 1993.

TJANDRA, Mr Janwar Joe Department of Surgery, University Hospital of Wales, Heath Park, Cardiff CF4 4XN Tel: 029 2074 2756 — MB BS Melbourne 1981; FRCS Glas. 1985; FRCS Eng. 1986; FRACS 1989. Sen. Lect. & Cons. Surg. Univ. Hosp. Wales. Socs: Amer. Soc. Colon & Rectal Surg. Prev: Clin. Assoc. Cleveland Clinic Foundat., USA; Sen. Regist. Roy. Melbourne Hosp. Austral.

TLUSTY, Peter John The Belgravia Surgery, 24-26 Eccleston Street, London SW1W 9PY Tel: 020 7590 8000 Fax: 020 7590 8010 — MB BS Lond. 1980 (Char. Cross Hosp.) BSc Lond. 1977; MRCS Eng. LRCP Lond. 1980; FRCS Ed. 1986. Sen. Partner Gen. Pract. Specialty: Gen. Pract.; Gen. Surg.; Obst. & Gyn. Prev: SHO (Obst.) Westm. Hosp. Lond.; SHO (Surg.) St. Jas. Hosp. Lond.; Resid. Med. Off. (Obst.) Qu. Charlottes Hosp. Lond.

TO, Meekai Stephanie 45 Farnes Drive, Romford RM2 6NT Tel: 01708 760043 — BM BS Nottm. 1994; BMedSci 1992. Research Fell. Harris Birthright Centre Kings Coll. Hosp. Lond. Specialty: Obst. & Gyn. Socs: RSM. Prev: SHO Qu. Charlottes & Chelsea Hosp.

TO, Mr Shun Suen Princess Margaret Hospital, Okus Road, Swindon SN1 4JU — MB ChB Ed. 1974; FRCS Ed. 1979; DLO Eng. 1981; FRCS Eng. 1982. Cons. ENT Surg. Princess Margt. Hosp. Swindon. Specialty: Otolaryngol. Prev: Sen. Regist. (ENT) W. Midl. RHA; Regist. (Gen. Surg.) Burton-on-Trent Gen. Hosp.; Regist. (Gen. Surg.) Nazareth Hosp. (EMMS), Israel.

TO, Ting Hoi Cross Deep Surgery, 4 Cross Deep, Twickenham TW1 4QP Tel: 020 8892 8124 Fax: 020 8744 9801; 30 Ravensbourne Road, Twickenham TW1 2DQ Tel: 020 8892 2805 — MB BS Lond. 1978 (Roy. Free) DRCOG 1979.

TOAL, Brendan Jude Donegall Road Surgery, 293 Donegall Road, Belfast BT12 5NB Tel: 028 9032 3973 — MB BCh BAO Belf. 1982; MB BCh Belf. 1982.

TOAL, Martin John Biogen Ltd, 5D Roxborough Way, Foudation Park, Maidenhead SL6 3UD Tel: 01628 501000; 10 Larchmoor Park, Gerrards Cross Rd, Stoke Poges, Slough SL2 4EY Tel: 01753 662198 — MB BCh BAO Belf. 1988; DMH Belf. 1992; DPH Belf. 1995; MSc (Pub. Health) Newc. 1997; MFPHMI. 1998; MFPHM 1999. Med. Dir., Biogen Ltd. Specialty: Pharmaceutical Medicine. Socs: (Counc.) BMA (Ex-Chairm. N. Irel. Jun. Doctors Comm.) (Chairm. Pub. Health; BMA Counc. Mem. Prev: Regional Med. Adviser, Bristol- Myers Lauss Pharaceutics Lts; SHO (Psychiat.) Tyrone & Fermanagh Hosp. Omagh; SHO Rotat. (Psychiat.) N. Irel.

TOAL, Patrick Anthony Tattykeel House, 126 Doogary Road, Omagh BT79 0BN — MB BCh BAO Belf. 1993; DGM RCPS Glas. 1995; DRCOG 1996; DCH Dub. 1996. GP/Regist. Foyleside Med. Pract. Derry. Prev: SHO (O & G Paediat. & Med.) Altnagelvin Hosp. Derry.

TOAL, Surgeon Captain Patrick Francis, SBStJ, Surg. Capt. RN Retd. (retired) Willow End, 1B Glebe Park Avenue, Bedhampton, Havant PO9 3JR Tel: 02392 479363 — MB BCh BAO NUI 1949; Specialist Accredit. (Occupat. & Community Med.); DPH (Hnrs.) 1965; DIH Dund 1969; FFCM 1979, M 1974; MFOM RCP 1980. Prev: Dir. Health & Research (Navy).

TOALE, Eamon 15B Windsor Road, London W5 3UL — MB BCh BAO NUI 1991.

TOASE, Peter David Huntingdon Road Surgery, 1 Huntingdon Road, Cambridge CB3 0DB Tel: 01223 364127 Fax: 01223 322541 — MB BS Lond. 1972 (St. Thos.) DCH Eng. 1975; DObst RCOG 1975; MRCGP 1977. Prev: Trainee GP Wessex VTS; Ho. Phys. St. Peter's Hosp. Chertsey; Ho. Surg. Brook Gen. Hosp. Lond.

TÖRÖK, Robert Zoltàn — MB BS Lond. 1995 (Guys - UMDS) Dip. IMC RCS Ed. 1997; FRCA (Primary) London 1998; MRCS (Ed. A & E) 2000. SpR, A&E Kings. Coll. Hosp. Specialty: Accid. & Emerg. Socs: Ass. Mem. Brit. Ass. A&E Med.; Fac. of A & E Med.; Brit. Ass Immediate Care Doctor.

TOBEY, Ilona West Street Surgery, 16 West Street, Newport PO30 1PR Tel: 01983 522198 Fax: 01983 524258 — MB ChB Bristol 1970; DCH Eng. 1973.

TOBIANSKY, Robert Ian Colindale Hospital, Silkstream Unit, Colindale Avenue, London NW9 5HG Tel: 020 8952 2381 Fax: 020 8205 8911 — MB BCh Witwatersrand 1986; MRCPsych 1992. Cons. Old Age Psychiat. Colindale Hosp. Lond. Specialty: Geriat. Psychiat.

TOBIAS, Andrew John 11 Browning Road, Lancing BN15 0PY Tel: 01903 761088 Fax: 01903 761088 Email: andy@andytobias.freeserve.co.uk — BM BS Nottm. 1980; BMedSci Nottm. 1978; MRCGP 1984; DRCOG 1984; Cert. Av. Med. 1993; (Advanced Course in Aviat. Med.) Kings Coll. 2000. Authorised Aviat. Med. Examr. for UK CAA; Freelance GP. Prev: Full Time NHS GP. Lancing, W. Sussex; Hosp. Practitioner, Urol., Worthing & Southlands, NHS Trust, S.

TOBIAS, Anthony Richard 3 Sefton Avenue, Mill Hill, London NW7 3QB Tel: 020 8959 0369 — MB ChB Manch. 1991; DFFP; BSc St. And. 1988; DRCOG 1994; MRCGP 1996. NHS GP Princip., Barnet HA, Mill Hill, N. Lond. Prev: GP Regist. E. Kilbride; SHO (Gen. Med.) Ayr Hosp.; SHO (Paediat.) CrossHo. Hosp.

TOBIAS, Catherine Mary Royal Manchester Childrens Hospital, Pendlebury, Manchester M27 4HA — MB BS Newc. 1987; MRCGP 1991; MRCPsych 1995. Specialty: Child & Adolesc. Psychiat. Prev: Trainee GP Northumbria VTS; Research Regist. Univ. Manch.; Sen. Regist. Rotat. (Child & Adult Psychiat.) Manch.

TOBIAS, Edward Spencer Institute of Medical Genetics, Yorkhill NHS Trust, Glasgow G3 8SJ Tel: 0141 201 0365 — MB ChB (Commend) Glas. 1990 (Univ. Glas.) BSc (Hons.) Molecular Biol. Glas. 1987; MRCP (UK) 1993; PhD Glas. 1997; CCST (Med. Genetics) 2001. Hon. Cons. (Med. Genetics) Inst. Med. Genet., Yorkhill Hosp. Glas.; Glaxo-Wellcome Senior Clinical Research Fellow, Beason Institute for Cancer Research, Glasgow. Specialty: Genetics. Special Interest: Molecular Genetics of Cancer. Socs: RCPS Glas.; Brit. Soc. Human Genetics; Brit. Assn. for Cancer Research. Prev: Clin. Research Sci. Beatson Inst. for Cancer Research Glas.1996-7; MRC Train. Fell. (Biochem. & Molec. Biol.) Univ. Glas.1993-1996; SHO Rotat. (Med.) West. Infirm. Glas.1991-1993.

TOBIAS, Gabriela Jill The Surgery, 52B Well Street, London E9 7PX Tel: 020 8985 2050 Fax: 020 8985 5780; 48 Northchurch Road, London N1 4EJ Tel: 020 7249 2326 — MB BS Lond. 1973; DCH Eng. 1977; MRCGP 1978. Cochair Exec., City & Hackney PCT. Prev: Clin. Fell. in Med. Mass. Gen. Hosp. Boston, U.S.A.; Regist. (Geriat.) St. Thos. Hosp. Lond.; Ho. Phys. Univ. Coll. Hosp. Lond.

TOBIAS, Professor Jeffrey Stewart Meyerstein Institute of Oncology, Middlesex Hospital, London W1 Tel: 020 7637 1214 Fax: 020 7637 1201 Email: j.tobias@uclh.org; 48 Northchurch Road, London N1 4EJ Tel: 020 7249 2326 — MB BChir Camb. 1972 (St. Bart.) BA Camb. 1968, MD 1977, MA, MB 1972, BChir 1971; MRCP (UK) 1973; FRCR 1979; FRCP Lond. 1990. Cons. Radiother. & Oncol. Univ. Coll. Hosp. & Middlx. Hosp. Lond.; Prof. Cancer Med. Univ. Coll. & Middlx. Sch. Med. Specialty: Oncol. Socs: Founder Mem. (Ex-Hon. Sec.) Brit. Oncol. Assn.; Counc. RCRadiol. Prev: Clin. Dir. Meyerstein Inst. Oncol. Middlx. Hosp. Lond.; Lect. (Radiother. & Oncol.) Roy. Marsden Hosps. Lond.; Fell. (Med. Oncol.) Harvard Med. Sch. Boston, USA.

TOBIAS, John Avrom Elmwood Avenue Surgery, 3 Elmwood Avenue, Newton Mearns, Glasgow G77 6EH Tel: 0141 639 2478 Fax: 0141 639 6708 — MB ChB Glas. 1986 (Glasgow) Cert. Family Plann. JCC 1989; MRCGP 1990. Hon. Clin. Sen. Lect. Dept. Gen. Pract. Univ. Glas. Specialty: Gen. Pract. Socs: RCGP. Prev: GP Aberd. VTS.

TOBIAS, Jonathan Harold Rheumatology Unit, Bristol Royal Infirmary, Bristol BS2 8HW Tel: 0117 928 2907 — MB BS Lond. 1984; MA Camb. 1985; MRCP (UK) 1987; PhD Lond. 1994, MD 1991; FRCP (UK) 1999. Reader (Rheum.) Univ. Bristol & United Bristol Hosp. Trust. Specialty: Rheumatol. Socs: Amer. Soc. Bone & Mineral Research; Bone & Tooth Soc. (Treas.); Brit. Soc. Rheum. (Comm. Mem.). Prev: ARC Clin. Research Fell. & Hon. Sen. Regist. (Rheum.) St. Geo. Hosp. Med. Sch. Lond.; MRC Research Train. Fell. St. Geo. Hosp. Med. Sch. Lond.; Regist. (Med.) St. Richard's Hosp. Chichester & St. Geo. Hosp. Lond.

TOBIAS, Lazarus (retired) 1 Hough Lane, Wilmslow SK9 2LG Tel: 01625 530851 — (Glas.) MB ChB Glas. 1938. Prev: Sen. Res. Med. Off. Manor Ho. Hosp. Golders Green.

TOBIAS, Martin PO Box 30412, Kilburn, London NW6 42Q Mob: 0771 433 5820; 18 Marston Close, Swiss Cottage, London NW6 4EU Tel: 020 7328 2092 — MB ChB Manch. 1954; DObst RCOG 1957. Indep. GP Lond. Prev: Med. Off. Esso Petroleum Co. Ltd. Lond.; SHO (Surg.) Ashton-under-Lyne Gen. Hosp.; Flight Lt. RAF Med. Br.

TOBIAS, Michael Avalon, Swiss Hill, Alderley Edge SK9 7DP Tel: 01625 583815 Fax: 01625 583815 Email: mike_tobias@hotmail.com — (Manch.) MB ChB Manch. 1963; DA Eng. 1965; DObst RCOG 1965; FRCA. Eng. 1968. Specialty: Anaesth. Socs: Fell. Manch. Med. Soc.; BMA; N. W. Regional Pain Gp. Prev: Cons. Anaesth. Wythenshawe Hosp. Manch.; Instruc. (Anaesth.) Mass. Gen. Hosp. Boston, USA; Sen. Regist. (Anaesth.) Univ. Hosp. W. Indies, Jamaica.

TOBIAS, Myer (Surgery) 49 Belle Vale Road, Liverpool L25 Tel: 0151 487 8660; 157 Menlove Avenue, Calderstones, Liverpool L18 3EE Tel: 0151 722 2384 — LRCP LRCS Ed. 1954 (Glas.) LRCP LRCS Ed. LRFPS Glas. 1954. SCMO Liverp. AHA (T); Instruc. Doctor Jt. Comm. Contracept. Lond. Prev: Ho. Phys., Ho. Surg. & Ho. Off. (O & G) Sharoe Green Hosp. Preston.

TOBIAS, Naomi Frances Bradleys Practice, Buckley Health Centre, Padeswood Road, Buckley CH7 2JL Tel: 01244 549628 — MB ChB Manch. 1979; DRCOG 1982; MRCGP 1983.

TOBIN, Caoimhin Padraig The White Rose Surgery, Exchange Street, South Elmsall, Pontefract WF9 2RD — MB BCh BAO NUI 1990; DObst RCPI 1993; DCH RCPSI 1993; Diploma in Practical Dermat., Cardiff 2000. GP Trainer. Prev: Trainee GP Som.

TOBIN, David Edward The Grayshott Surgery, Boundary Road, Grayshott, Hindhead GU26 6TY Tel: 01428 604343 — MB BS Lond. 1979; MRCS Eng. LRCP Lond. 1979; DA (UK) 1982; DRCOG 1984. Prev: Trainee GP Windsor VTS.

TOBIN, Francis Anthony Law Street Surgery, 49-51 Laws Street, Pembroke Dock SA72 6DJ Tel: 01646 683113 / 682002 Fax: 01646 622273 — MB BCh BAO NUI 1987.

TOBIN, Geoffrey Brian The Surgery, 25 Alms Hill, Bourn, Cambridge CB3 7SH Tel: 01954 719313 Fax: 01954 718012; Ave. House, High St, Madingley, Cambridge CB3 8AB — MRCS Eng. LRCP Lond. 1974 (Guy's) BSc Lond. 1971, MB BS 1974; MRCP (UK) 1977. Specialty: Gastroenterol. Prev: Regist. (Med.) Addenbrookes

Hosp. Camb.; SHO Brompton Hosp. Lond.; Resid. Med. Off. Nat. Heart Hosp. Lond.

TOBIN, Gerald William 7 Manor Park, Redland, Bristol BS6 7HJ Tel: 0117 907 1720; United Bristol Healthcare NHS Trust, Bristol BS1 3NU Tel: 0117 928 6314 — MD Dub. 1987; MB BCh BAO 1977; FRCPI 1992, M 1980; FRCP Lond. 1998. Cons. Phys. c/o Elderly United Bristol Health Care NHS Trust. Specialty: Care of the Elderly.

TOBIN, Jean Margaret Department of GU Medicine, St. Mary's Hospital, Milton Road, Portsmouth PO3 6AD — MB BS Lond. 1968 (Roy. Free) MRCS Eng. LRCP Lond. 1968; MRCOG 1973; FRCOG 1989, M 1973; MFFP 1995. Cons. Phys., GU Med., St. Mary's Hosp., Portsmouth; Cons. Civil. Adviser in GU Med. to the Roy. Navy. Specialty: Genitourinary Medicine; HIV Med. Socs: Sec. Brit. Federat. against Sexually Transm. Dis.s; Chairm. BMA Dermato-Venerology sub-comm.

TOBIN, John O'Hara (retired) 4 Gladstone Road, Headington, Oxford OX3 8LJ Tel: 01865 750926 — BM BCh Oxf. 1942; MA, DM Oxf. 1991, BM BCh 1942; Dip. Bact. Manch. 1948; FRCPath 1970, M 1963; FRCP Lond. 1979, M 1971. Prev: Dir. Pub. Health Laborat. Oxf.

TOBIN, Judith Ann Heathfield Medical Centre, Lyttelton Road, Hampstead Garden Suburb, London N2 0EE Tel: 020 8458 9262 Fax: 020 8458 0300; 39 Southway, London NW11 6RX Tel: 020 8458 4617 — MB BCh Wales 1978; DRCOG 1980; DCH Eng. 1981; MRCGP 1984.

TOBIN, Martin Damian c/o Mr M. J. Rogers, 46 Wilga Road, Welwyn AL6 9PS — MB ChB Leic. 1988.

TOBIN, Michael John William Ringmead Medical Practice, Great Hollands Health Centre, Great Hollands Square, Bracknell RG12 8WY Tel: 01344 454338 Fax: 01344 861050; Lynton House, Lower Wokingham Road, Crowthorne RG45 6BT Tel: 01344 774080 — MRCS Eng. LRCP Lond. 1973 (Leeds) DObst RCOG 1975. Specialty: Gen. Pract.

TOBIN, Michael Vincent Pinderfields Hospital, Aberford Road, Wakefield WF1 4DG Tel: 01924 212519; 5 Fennel Court, Carr Lane, Sandal, Wakefield WF2 6TS Email: carmelo.aquilina@ntlworld.com — MB BCh BAO NUI 1979; MRCP (UK) 1983; MD NUI 1991; FRCP 1998. Cons. Phys. Gastroenterol. Pinderfields Hosp. Wakefield. Specialty: Gastroenterol.; Gen. Med. Prev: Sen. Regist. (Med. & Gastroenterol.) Walton Hosp. Liverp.; Research Fell. (Med.) Hope Hosp. Salford; Sen. Regist. Broadgreen & Walton Hosps. Liverp.

TOBIN, Simon David Manning Norwood Avenue Practice, 11 Norwood Avenue, Southport PR9 7EG Tel: 01704 226973 Fax: 01704 505758 — MB BS Lond. 1989; BSc (Hons.) Lond. 1986; DCH RCP Lond. 1992; DRCOG 1993; MRCGP 1994. Specialty: Gen. Pract.

TOBIN, Tracy Ann c/o Mr M. J. Rogers, 46 Wilga Road, Welwyn AL6 9PS — MB ChB Leic. 1989.

TOBY, John Paxton, CBE Chinkwell House, Great Brington, Northampton NN7 4HY Tel: 01604 770292 Email: johntobyuk@aol.com — (St. Bart.) MB Camb. 1965, BChir 1964; MRCP (U.K.) 1969; FRCGP 1980, M 1972; FRCP 1995; FFPHM 1998. Assoc. Regional Adviser GPVTS Oxf. HA. Socs: Chairm. of Counc. Roy. Coll. of GPs. Prev: Hosp. Pract. (Gen. Med.) Northampton Gen. Hosp.; Course Organiser Gen. Pract. Train. Northampton Health Dist.; Regist. (Med.) Northampton Gen. Hosp.

TOD, Edward David Macrae, OBE APCET Tel: 020 8665 1138 Fax: 020 8665 1118; The Firs, Budiam Road, Sandhurst TN18 5JY — MB ChB Ed. 1952; FRCGP 1993, M 1971; Dip. Criminol. Lond. 1984. Ed. PCG NHS; Cons. Scorpio Ltd.; JP; Chief Exec. APCET. Socs: Fell. Med. Soc. Lond.; Liveryman Soc. Apoth.; Med. Jl.ists Assn. Prev: Dir. Forum for Indep. Research in Health Keele Univ.; Hon. Research Fell. (Clin. Epidemiol. & Social Med.) St. Geo. Hosp. Med. Sch.

TOD, Ian Alexander Arthur Upper Eden Medical Practice, The Medical Centre, Brough CA17 4AY Tel: 017683 41294 Fax: 017683 41068 — MB BS Newc. 1977; DRCOG 1980; MRCGP 1981. Specialty: Physiother.; Psychother.; Rehabil. Med.

TODD, Alastair Stewart (retired) 10 Gillies Terrace, Broughty Ferry, Dundee DD5 3LF Tel: 01382 477758 — (Durh.) MB BS Durh. 1949; MD Durh. 1961; FRCPath 1976, M 1964. Prev: Cons. Haemat. Ninewells Hosp. Dundee.

TODD, Alison Agnes Jean Flat 11, Magnolia Lodge, 73 Chingford Avenue, London E4 6SX — MB ChB Aberd. 1988; BA Durham. 1993.

TODD, Alistair William Hill House, Braehead, Avoch IV9 8QL — MB ChB Dundee 1981; MRCP (UK) 1984; FRCR 1987. Cons. Radiol. Raigmore Hosp. Inverness. Specialty: Radiol. Prev: Regist. (Radiol.) Newc. HA.

TODD, Alwyn Edward Brooklands, 303 Belstead Road, Ipswich IP2 9EH — MB ChB Leeds 1960.

TODD, Andrew James The Old Rectory, St. Mary Church, Cowbridge CF71 7LT — MRCS Eng. LRCP Lond. 1961 (W. Lond.) Sen. Med. Off. Home Office; Hon. Clin. Asst. (Psychiat.) Univ. Wales.

TODD, Andrew Martin 9 Colquhoun Drive, Bearsden, Glasgow G61 4NQ — MB ChB Aberd. 1995.

TODD, Barras James (retired) 12 Gravel Hill, Croydon CR0 5BB Tel: 020 8654 6406 Email: barras.todd@virgin.net — MB BS Lond. 1952 (Char. Cross)

TODD, Mr Brian David Stepping Hill Hospital, Poplar Grove, Stockport SK2 7JE Tel: 0161 483 1010; Croft House, Maynestone Road, Chinley, High Peak SK23 6AH Tel: 01663 750568 — MB ChB Ed. 1980 (Edinburgh) FRCS Ed. 1984; FRCS Ed. (Orth.) 1991. Cons. Trauma & Orthop. Surg. Stockport HA; T&O Surgeon at Stockport NHS Trust (Acute). Specialty: Orthop.; Trauma & Orthop. Surg. Socs: Brit. Orthop. Assn.; NW Spine Gp.; Manch. Med. Soc. Fell. Prev: Sen. Regist. (Orthop.) Sheff. Hosps.; Regist. (Orthop.) Roy. Sussex Co. Hosp. Brighton & St. Thos. Hosp. Lond.; Surg. Tutor RCS Eng.

TODD, Mr Bryan Seymour Accident Department, John Radcliffe Hospital, Headington, Oxford OX3 9DU — MB BChir Camb. 1979; DPhil Oxf. 1989, MA 1982; FRCS Eng. 1984. Clin. Asst. (A & E Med.) John Radcliffe Hosp.; Research Off. (Neonat. Telemonitoring) Oxf. Univ. Specialty: Accid. & Emerg. Prev: Research Fell. Progr. Research Gp. Oxf. Univ.; Regist. (Gen. Surg.) Princess Margt. Hosp. Swindon.

TODD, Catherine Louise Mowbray House, Malpas Road, Northallerton DL7 8FW Tel: 01609 775281 Fax: 01609 778029; Harewood House, 28 Harewood Lane, Northallerton DL7 8BQ Tel: 01609 773198 — MB ChB Leeds 1982; DO RCS Eng. 1986; MRCGP 1988. Specialty: Ophth.

TODD, Ceri 4 The Bryn, Derwen Fawr, Swansea SA2 8DD — MB BCh Wales 1992; MRCGP 1996.

TODD, Charles (retired) 5 Richmond Crescent, Bangor BT20 5QD Tel: 028 9147 2758 — MB BCh BAO Belf. 1964.

TODD, Colin Eric Campbell Radiology Department, Kingston Hospital NHS Trust, Galsworthy Road, Kingston upon Thames KT2 7QB Tel: 0208 546 7711 Ext: 2130 Fax: 0208 934 3559 Email: colin.todd@kingstonhospital.nhs.uk; 15 Elm Road, Chessington KT9 1AF — MB BS Lond. 1979 (Roy. Free) FRCS Ed. 1984; FRCR 1990. Cons. Radiol. Kingston Hosp. Trust, Kingston Upon Thames; Cons. Radiologist, Parkside Hosp., Wimbledon; Cons. Radiologist, New Vict. Hosp. Specialty: Radiol.; Nuclear Med. Socs: BSIR; RSNA; CIRSE. Prev: Sen. Regist. (Radiol.) Guy's Hosp. Lond.; Regist. (Radiol.) Westm. Hosp. Lond.; SHO (Cardiothoracic Surg.) Soton. Gen. Hosp.

TODD, David 1 Riverside Gardens, Barrow-in-Furness LA13 0DD Tel: 01229 821032 Fax: 01229 824689 — MB BS Lond. 1967 (Char. Cross) Med. Dir. Morecambe Bay Occupat. Health Serv. Barrow-in-Furness; Med. Adviser Brit. Gas. HRL, Tronic, Colony Gift Corporation. Specialty: Occupat. Health. Socs: Soc. Occupat. Med.; Roy. Soc. Med.; Mem. of Expert Witness Inst. Prev: Ho. Surg. W. Hill Hosp. Dartford; Ho. Phys. Joyce Green Hosp. Dartford.

TODD, David Anthony 156 Everton Road, Hordle, Lymington SO41 0HB — MB BS Sydney 1998.

TODD, David Bryan 17 Orford Gardens, Strawberry Hill, Twickenham TW1 4PL Email: mpmdbt@bath.ac.uk — MB BChir Camb. 1984; MA Oxf. 1982; DRCOG 1988; DCH RCP Lond. 1989; MRCGP 1990; DA (UK) 1992; FRCA 1994. GP; Sports Med. Course. Socs: BMA; Frenchay Hosp. Triathlon Club. Prev: Regist. Rotat. (Anaesth.) S. Western RHA.

TODD, Mr Denis Oliver University Health Service, 5 Lennoxvale, Belfast BT9 5BY Tel: 028 9033 5520 Fax: 028 9033 5661 — MB BCh BAO Belf. 1977; DObst 1980; FRCS Ed. 1981; MRCGP 1983; MFOM RCP Lond. 1987, A 1985; MFOM RCPI 1986; Cert AvMed

1987; FFOM RCPI 1997; FFOM RCP Lond. 1998; FRCP Lond. 1999. Sen. Med. Off. Qu. Univ. Belf. Specialty: Occupat. Health. Socs: Pres. Soc. Occupat. Med. (UK); (Ex Gp. Chairm.) Occupat. Med.; BMA. Prev: GP Cherryvalley & Med. Off. DHSS (N.. Irel.).

TODD, Derick Morris Cardiothoracic Centre, Thomas Drive, Liverpool L14 3PE Tel: 0151 293 2394 Email: derick.todd@ctc.nhs.uk — MB ChB Ed. 1991; BMedSci (Hons.) Ed. 1989; MRCP Ed. 1994. Cons. (Cardiol.). Specialty: Cardiol. Prev: Regist. Rotat. (Cardiol.) Trent Region; Research Regist. Manch. Heart Centre; SHO Rotat. (Med.) Lothian HB Edin.

TODD, Elizabeth Anne 7 Cathedral Rise, Lichfield WS13 7LP — MB ChB Manch. 1984.

TODD, Elizabeth Jane Bradley Stoke Surgery, Brook Way, Bradley Stoke North, Bristol BS32 9DS Tel: 01454 616262 Fax: 01454 619161 — MB ChB Bristol 1979; BSc (Hons.) Lond. 1968, PhD 1974; Cert. Family Plann. JCC 1985; Cert Prescribed Equiv. Exp. JCPTGP 1987. GP Bristol. Specialty: Ophth.; Occupat. Health; Sports Med. Socs: Soc. Occupat. Med.

TODD, Miss Felicity Nicola A&E Dept, Bradford Royal Infirmary, Duckworth Lane, Bradford BD9 6RJ Tel: 01274 364457 Email: felicity.todd@bradfordhospitals.nhs.uk — MB ChB Liverp. 1987; FRCS Ed. 1994; FFAEM 1998. Cons.(A&E.) Brad Roy Infim. Specialty: Accid. & Emerg. Socs: Brit. Assn. Accid. & Emerg. Med.; Assn. Study Med. Educat.; Eur. Resusc. Counc. Prev: Regist. (A & E) N. Trent Doncaster; Sen. Regist.. Yorks. Deanery 1996-1998.

TODD, Geoffrey Robert George Antrim Area Hospital, Antrim BT41 2RL — MB BCh BAO Belf. 1975; MRCP (UK) 1979. Cons. Chest Phys. Antrim Area Hosp. Specialty: Gen. Med. Prev: Cons. Phys. Moyle Hosp. Larne.

TODD, Mr George Buchanan Coniston Broad Chalke, Salisbury SP5 5DH Tel: 01722 780595 — MB BChir Camb. 1966 (Univ. Coll. Hosp.) MRCS Eng. LRCP Lond. 1965; FRCS Eng. 1970. Cons. Surg. (ENT) Salisbury NHS Health Care Trust. Specialty: Otorhinolaryngol. Socs: Roy. Soc. Med. (Mem. Otol. & Laryngol. Sects.). Prev: Sen. Regist. (ENT) St. Thos. Hosp. Lond.; Sen. Surg. Off. Roy. Nat. Throat, Nose & Ear Hosp. Lond.; Sen. Lect. W. Indies Jamaica.

TODD, Gillian Bees 6th Floor, Churchill House, Churchill Way, Cardiff CF10 2TW Tel: 029 2022 6216 Fax: 029 2023 0106; 20 High Fields, Cardiff CF5 2QA Tel: 029 2057 8244 — MB BCh Wales 1966; FFPHM 1987. Chief Exec. Bro Taf HA. Specialty: Pub. Health Med. Prev: Chief. Exec. S. Glam. DHA; Chief Exec. S. Birm. Acute Unit; Dist. Gen. Manager Centr. Notts. HA.

TODD, Graham Philip Anthony 1 Alexandra Road, Brookvale, Basingstoke RG21 7RG — BMedSci Sheff. 1993; MB ChB Sheff. 1994. HO (Psych./Surg./Med.) NGH Sheff. Prev: SHO (Geriat.) Bradford; Ho. Surg. (Emerg.) Middlemore Hosp. Auckland, NZ; SHO (Orthop.) Auckland.

TODD, Iain Charles Astley Ainslie Hospital, 133 Grange Loan, Edinburgh EH9 2HL Tel: 0131 537 9087 Fax: 0131 537 9087; 48 The Green, Pencaitland, Tranent EH34 5HE Tel: 01875 340832 Fax: 0131 537 9080 — MD Ed. 1991; BSc Ed. 1976, MD 1991, MB ChB 1979; MRCP (UK) 1982. Cons. (Rehabil. Med.) Astley Ainslie Hosp. Edin. Specialty: Rehabil. Med.; Rheumatol. Socs: Brit. Cardiac Soc.; Brit. Soc. For Rehab. Med.; Brit. Assoc. of Stroke Phys.s. Prev: Sen Regist. (Rehabil. Med.) Astley Ainslie Hosp. Edin.; Regist. (Gen. Med.) Vict. Infirm. Glas.; Regist. & SHO (Gen. Med. Rotat.) Hull.

TODD, Iain Mathieson (retired) 2 Gartness Court, Drymen, Glasgow G63 0AX — MB ChB Glas. 1948 (Univ. Glas.) MRCGP 1973. Prev: Ho. Surg. West. Infirm. Glas.

TODD, Ian Douglas Hutchinson (retired) 455 Parrs Wood Road, Didsbury, Manchester M20 5NE Tel: 0161 445 9497; Lanton Hill Farm, Jedburgh TD8 6SY Tel: 01835 63275 — MB ChB Aberd. 1950; FRCP Lond. 1975, M 1958; DMRT Eng. 1960; FFR 1962; FRCR 1975. Prev: Dep. Dir. (Radiother.) & Cons. (Radiother. & Oncol.) Christie Hosp. & Holt Radium Inst. Manch.

TODD, Ian Michael 14 St Peters Avenue, Weston Super Mare BS23 2JU — BM BCh Oxf. 1983.

TODD, Sir Ian Pelham, KBE (retired) 4 Longmead Close, Farleigh Road, Norton St Philip, Bath BA2 7NS Tel: 01373 834081 — (St. Bart. & Univ. Toronto) Hon. FRCS Glas.; Hon. FRCSC; Hon. FACS; Hon. FRACS; Hon. FCS (SA); MRCS Eng. LRCP Lond. 1944; DCH Eng. 1947; FRCS Eng. 1949; MD Toronto 1945, MS 1956. President RCS Eng., 86-89. Prev: Dir. Overseas Doctors Higher Train. Scheme RCS Eng.

TODD, James Andrew 1 Crag View, Sutton-in-Craven, Keighley BD20 7QE Tel: 01535 631852 — MB ChB Manch. 1993 (Manchester) SHO. (Psychiat.) Leeds. Specialty: Gen. Psychiat.; Forens. Psychiat.; Geriat. Psychiat. Prev: SHO. (Psychiat.); GP Regist. Springfield Med Cen. Bingley.; SHO. (Psychiat.) Airedale Gen Hosp. Keighley/.

TODD, James Gordon Eastfield, Tandlehill Road, Kilbarchan, Johnstone PA10 2DQ — MB ChB Glas. 1975; FRCA Eng. 1979. Cons. Anaesth, N. Glas. Hosps. Univ. NHS Trust. Specialty: Anaesth. Socs: Assn. Anaesth. Gt. Brit. & Irel.; Anaesth. Research Soc. Gt. Brit. Prev: Cons. Anaesth. W. Infirm. Glas. & Inst. Neurol. Sci. Glas.; Sen. Regist. (Anaesth.) West. Infirm. Glas.; Regist. (Anaesth.) Roy. Infirm. Glas.

TODD, James Peter (retired) The Red House, 47 Clayton Road, Jesmond, Newcastle upon Tyne NE2 4RQ Tel: 0191 281 5425 — MB BS Durh. 1960; DObst RCOG 1964.

TODD, Jennifer Ann Trinity Hospice, 30 Clapham Common Northside, London SW4 0RN Tel: 020 7787 1000 — MB ChB Manch. 1990 (St Andrews) BSc St. And. 1987; DRCOG 1993; MRCGP 1994; MA (ethics) 2000. Cons. (Palliat. Med.) Trinity Hospice. Specialty: Palliat. Med. Socs: APM; RCGP. Prev: Specialist Regist. (Palliat. Med.) S. Thames Rotat.

TODD, John Bedlington Medical Group, Glebe Road, Bedlington NE22 6JX Tel: 01670 822695 Fax: 01670 531860; 13 Sweethope Dene, Morpeth NE61 2DZ — MB ChB Leeds 1985; BSc (Hons.) Physiol. Leeds 1982; MRCGP 1989. Specialty: Gen. Pract.

TODD, Mr John Kirkland (retired) 9 Colquhorn Drive, Bearsden, Glasgow Tel: 0141 942 0908 — MD Glas. 1962; BSc Glas. 1955, MD (Hons.) 1962, MB ChB 1958; FRCS Ed. 1963; FRCS Glas. 1963. Prev: Cons. Surg. Roy. Infirm. Glas.

TODD, John Neild (retired) Meadow Breeze, Llanddew, Brecon LD3 9ST Tel: 01874 610 902 — MB BS Lond. 1952 (St. Bart.) FFCM 1985, MFCM 1982. Prev: Dir. Pub. Health Sheff. HA.

TODD, John Ovenstone, Wing Cdr. RAF Med. Br. Retd. Moray Health Services, Doctor Gray's Hospital, Elgin IV30 1SN Tel: 01343 543131; Kyle Lodge, Lochiepots Road, Miltonduff, Elgin IV30 8WL Email: 106731.3026@compuserve.com — MB ChB Aberd. 1979; MRCPsych 1985; MRCGP 1990; T(Psych) 1991; T(GP) 1991; DAvMed 1991; AFOM RCP Lond. 1992. Cons. Psychiat. Doctor Gray's Hosp. Elgin. Specialty: Gen. Psychiat. Prev: Sen. Med. Off. RAF St. Athan; Hon. Regist. Warneford Hosp. Oxf.; Clin. Assoc. Psychogeriat. Maudsley Hosp. Lond.

TODD, John Reynard Comrie 1 Barnton Park Dell, Edinburgh EH4 6HW Tel: 0131 476 0024 — MB ChB St. And. 1966; DObst RCOG 1968. Prev: SHO (O & G) Dundee Roy. Infirm.; Anaesth. Centr.lasarett Uddevalla, Sweden; Research Fell. (Ophth.) Univ. Toronto, Canada.

TODD, June Lorraine Red Reap Surgery, 31 Coton Road, Nuneaton CV11; 29 Seneschal Road, Chelesmore, Coventry CV3 5LF — MB ChB Sheff. 1972; DObst RCOG 1974; MRCGP 1977.

TODD, Katharine Hilda Lesley (retired) Spindle Tree, Pant Lane, Austwick, Lancaster LA2 8BH — MRCS Eng. LRCP Lond. 1961 (Leeds) MA Oxf. 1939; DObst RCOG 1965. Prev: Clin. Asst. Cas. & Accid. Dept. Bradford Roy. Infirm.

TODD, Kathryn Helen Collum House, 214 Leckhampton Road, Cheltenham GL53 0AW — MB BS Lond. 1992.

TODD, Killingworth Richard (retired) 18 Bshop Road, Nether Stowey, Bridgwater TA5 1NP — (Univ. Coll. Hosp.) MB BS Lond. 1942. Prev: Cas. Surg. Regist. Edgware Gen. Hosp.

TODD, Kim Paula Knight, Todd, Jackson and Mather, Hawthorn House Medical Centre, 28-30 Heaton Road, Newcastle upon Tyne NE6 1SD Tel: 0191 265 5543/6246 Fax: 0191 276 2985; 41 Manor Fields, Benton, Newcastle upon Tyne NE12 8AG — BM BS Nottm. 1981; MRCGP 1986.

TODD, Mairi Jane Alleyn — MB BS Lond. 1984 (St. Bartholomews) MRCGP 1989. p/t Sessional GP; GP Locum 2003. Socs: BMA; MRCGP; MDDUS. Prev: GP Trainer; Partner Queensbridge GP Practice 1992-2003; GP Halesworth.

TODD, Margaret Mary (retired) The Gables, 3 Main Road, Biddenham, Bedford MK40 4BB Tel: 01234 353357 — MB BCh BAO NUI 1951 (Univ. Coll. Dub.) LM Coombe 1953. Prev: GP Bedford.

TODD, Marie Colette Springburn Health Centre, 200 Springburn Way, Glasgow G21 1TR Tel: 0141 531 9681 Fax: 0141 531 6705; 9 Colquhoun Drive, Bearsden, Glasgow G61 4NQ Tel: 0141 942 0908 — MB ChB Glas. 1965; DA Eng. 1969. GP Glas. Prev: Late Anaesth. Krankenhaus Wattwil, Switz..

TODD, Neil James Department of Microbiology, St. James' University Hospital, Beckett St., Leeds LS9 7TF Tel: 01532 433144 Fax: 01532 837085; Lynn Dene, Back Lane, Barkston Ash, Tadcaster LS24 9PL — MB ChB Bristol 1984; BA Oxf. 1981; MRCPath 1991. Cons. Microbiol. St. Jas. Univ. Trust Hosp.; Hon. Sen. Lect. (Microbiol.) Univ. Leeds. Specialty: Med. Microbiol. Prev: Sen. Regist. (Microbiol.) Yorks. RHA.

TODD, Neville Barras Totnes Hospital, Coronation Road, Totnes TQ9 5GH Tel: 01803 862622 — MB BS Lond. 1978; DRCOG 1980; MRCGP 1982; MRCPsych 1988. Cons. (Old Age Psychiat.) S. Devon Healthcare Trust Torbay. Specialty: Geriat. Psychiat. Prev: Sen. Regist. (Psychiat.) St. Lawrences Hosp. Bodmin; Sen. Regist. (Psychiat.) Moorhaven Hosp. Plymouth.

TODD, Mr Nicholas Vyner Department of Neurosurgery, Regional Neurosciences Centre, Newcastle General Hospital, Newcastle upon Tyne NE4 6BE Tel: 0191 273 8811 Fax: 0191 273 0117; Foulmartlaw, Gallowmill, Morpeth NE61 3TZ Tel: 01661 881694 — MD Lond. 1987 (Guy's) MB BS 1978; FRCS Eng. 1982. Cons. Neurosurg. Regional Neurosci. Centre Newc. u. Tyne. Specialty: Neurosurg. Prev: Sen. Regist. (Neurosurg.) Inst. Neurosci. Glas.; MRC Research Fell.

TODD, Norman Alexander (retired) 16 Ormonde Drive, Glasgow G44 3SJ — MB ChB Glas. 1951; DPM Eng. 1959; FRCP Ed. 1976, M 1961; FRCPsych 1979, M 1972. Cons. Psychiat., Levendale Hosp., Glas. Prev: Regist. Psychiat. Unit, Stobhill Hosp. Glas.

TODD, Olive Isobel (retired) 18 Bishop Road, Nether Stowey, Bridgwater TA5 1NP — (W. Lond.) MRCS Eng., LRCP Lond. 1947. Prev: Ho. Surg. Roy. Salop. Infirm. Shrewsbury.

TODD, Oliver Rowland The Gables, 3 Main Road, Biddenham, Bedford MK40 4BB Tel: 01234 353357 — MRCS Eng. LRCP Lond. 1952 (King's Coll. Hosp.) Prev: GP Bedford; Ho. Phys. Brook Hosp. Woolwich; Ho. Surg. (Obst.) St. And. Hosp. Billericay.

TODD, Pamela Margaret Box 46 Department of Dermatology, Addenbrookes NHS Trust, Hills Road, Cambridge CB2 2QQ — MB BS Lond. 1984; BSc Lond. 1981; MRCP (UK) 1987; FRCP 2000. Cons. Dermatol., Addenbrooke Hosp., Camb.; Assoc. Lect. Univ. of Camb. Med. Sch. Specialty: Dermat. Socs: Brit. Med. Assoc.; Melanoma study Gp.; Brit. Soc for Study of Vulval Dis. Prev: Regist. (Dermat.) Glas. Roy. Infirm.; Dermat. Sen. Regist. Roy. Hosps., Lond.; Dermat. Regist. Kings Coll. Hosp., Lond.

TODD, Peter Graham (retired) Redbourn, The Spinney, Bassett, Southampton SO16 7FW Tel: 023 8076 8763 — (St. Thos.) MD Lond. 1941, MB BS (Hons. Surg. & Path.) 1939; MRCS Eng. LRCP Lond. 1939; FRCP Lond. 1964, M 1940; DCH Eng. 1944. Prev: Phys. Roy. S. Hants. Hosp., Soton. Gen. Hosp. & Hythe Hosp.

TODD, Peter James Sunnymount, 10 Oldfield Way, Heswall, Wirral CH60 6RG — MB BS Lond. 1973 (Middlx.) MRCP (UK) 1975; DCH Eng. 1978; FRCP Lond. 1990. Cons. (Paediat.) Arrowe Pk. Hosp. Merseyside. Specialty: Paediat. Prev: Sen. Regist. (Paediat.) Roy. Liverp. Childr. Hosp. & Alder Hey Childr.; Hosp.

TODD, Richard George The Shrubbery, 65A Perry Street, Northfleet, Gravesend DA11 8RD Tel: 01474 356661 Fax: 01474 534542; 84 Whitehill Road, Gravesend DA12 5PH — MB BS Newc. 1981; DRCOG 1984; MRCGP 1985.

TODD, Mr Robert Marshall 9 Oaklands Drive, Bishop's Stortford CM23 2BZ Tel: 01279 53166 — MB ChB Glas. 1956; FRCS Ed. 1971. Cons. Ophth. Herts. & Essex Gen. Hosp. Bishop's Stortford. Specialty: Ophth. Prev: Cons. in Ophth. RAF Hosp. Cosford.

TODD, Robert McLaren (retired) 17 Beauclair Drive, Liverpool L15 6XG Tel: 0151 722 2218 — (Camb. St. Bart. & Harvard) MA Camb. 1941, MD 1946, MB BChir 1940; MRCS Eng. LRCP Lond. 1940; DCH Eng. 1943; FRCP Lond. 1965, M 1945. Prev: Reader in Child Health. Univeristy of Liverp..

TODD, Mr Ronald Stanley 29 Boundary Drive, Moseley, Birmingham B13 8NY Tel: 0121 442 2672 — MB ChB Liverp. 1954; DObst RCOG 1956; FRCS Ed. 1960; FRCS Eng. 1961. Mem. Ct.. Examrs. RCS Eng. Socs: Liverp. Med. Inst. Prev: Cons. Surg. Clwyd HA; Hon. Sen. Surg. Regist. Liverp. Roy. Infirm. & Broadgreen Hosp.; Demonst. (Anat.) & Lect. (Surg.) Univ. Liverp.

TODD, Rose Miriam (retired) The Red House, 47 Clayton Road, Jesmond, Newcastle upon Tyne NE2 4RQ Tel: 0191 281 5425 — MB BS Durh. 1960.

TODD, Ruth Louise 1 Lealholm Way, Guisborough TS14 8LN — MB BS Newc. 1993 (Newcastle) DRCOG 1996; MRCGP 2001. Hospice Phys. Teesside Hospice Middlesborough; Clin. Asst. in Diabetes. Specialty: Gen. Pract. Prev: SHO (Palliat. Med.) Teesside Hospice Middlesbrough.

TODD, Sarah Elizabeth 87 Allensbank Road, Cardiff CF14 3PP — MB BCh Wales 1990.

TODD, Stephen Andrew 30 Rutherglen Park, Bangor BT19 1DD — MB BCh BAO Belf. 1997.

TODD, Virginia Ann Lakeside Health Centre, Tavy Bridge, Thamesmead, London SE2 9UQ Tel: 020 8310 3281 — MB BS Lond. 1966; DObst RCOG 1971; DCH Eng. 1971; FRCP Canada 1974.

TODD, William Health Centre, Linwood, Johnstone PA5 7DG Tel: 01505 21051; 9 Crossways, Houston, Johnstone PA6 7DG Tel: 01505 613729 — MB ChB Glas. 1947. Socs: BMA. Prev: Chief Med. Off. Nchanga Consolidated Copper Mines Ltd. (Broken Hill; Div.) Kabwe, Zambia; Med. Supt. Miss. Hosp. Jalna, India.

TODD, William George 4 Merchiston Crescent, Edinburgh EH10 5AN Tel: 0131 229 5400 — MB ChB Aberd. 1943.

TODD, William Taylor Andrew Monklands Hospital, Infectious Diseases Unit, Monkscourt Avenue, Airdrie ML6 0JS Tel: 01236 712134 Fax: 01236 712449; 17 Crosshill Drive, Rutherglen, Glasgow G73 3QT Tel: 0141 647 7288 Email: wtat@ntlworld.com — MB ChB Ed. 1977; BSc (Hons.) Ed. 1974. MB ChB 1977; FRCP Ed. 1988; FRCP Glas. 1990; T(M) 1991. Cons. Phys. Gen. Med. & Communicable Dis. Monklands Dist. Gen. Hosp.; Speciality Adviser Infec. to Chief Med. Off. (Scotl.). Specialty: Infec. Dis. Socs: Roy. Medicochirurgical Soc. Glas.; Scott. Soc. Phys.; Coun. Mem. Brit. Infec. Soc. Prev: Sen. Regist. (Communicable Dis.) City Hosp. Edin.; Lect. (Med.) Harare, Zimbabwe; Regist. (Gen. Med. Endocrinol.) Roy. Infirm. Edin.

TODD-POKROPEK, Cecilia Jane 18 Stone Mill Way, Leeds LS6 4RG — MB ChB Liverp. 1997.

TODES, Cecil Jacob (retired) 38 Clifton Hill, London NW8 0QG Tel: 020 7624 4533 — MRCS Eng. LRCP Lond. 1960 (W. Lond.) BDS Witwatersrand 1953; FDS RCS Eng. 1956; DPM Eng. 1965; FRCPsych 1985, M 1971. Prev: Cons. Child Psychiat. Paddington Centre for Psychother.

TODMAN, Elaine Ferndean, 4 Falkland Road, Montpelier, Bristol BS6 5JT — MB ChB Bristol 1996.

TODMAN, Rodney Claud Frederick (retired) 14 Dovehouse Court, Grange Road, Olton, Solihull B91 1EW Tel: 0121 705 8685 — MB ChB Ed. 1944. Prev: GP Druids Heath Birm.

TODMAN, Roger Herbert Department of Child Health, Willows Child Development Centre, Pedders Lane, Ashton, Preston PR2 2TR Tel: 01772 401472 Fax: 01772 768122; 6 Ascot Road, Thornton-Cleveleys FY5 5HN Tel: 01253 866150 — MB ChB Liverp. 1976; DCCH RCP Ed. 1991. SCMO (Child Health) Guild Community Health Care Preston. Specialty: Community Child Health. Socs: Fac. Community Health.

TOEG, Daniel Caversham Practice, 4 Peckwater Street, London NW5 2UP Tel: 020 7530 6500 Fax: 020 7530 6530 — MB ChB Manch. 1985 (Manchester University) BSc (Hons.) Manch. 1982; MRCP (UK) 1988; MRCGP 1992; T(GP) 1992; DFFP 1998.

TOELLNER, Christoph Barthold Weavers Lane Surgery, 1 Weavers Lane, Whitburn, Bathgate EH47 0SD Tel: 01501 740297 Fax: 01501 744302 — State Exam Med Bonn 1986; MD Bonn 1988. GP Whitburn. Specialty: Gen. Pract.; Gastroenterol.; Respirat. Med. Socs: BMA; Roy. Coll. Gen. Pract.; Med. Protec. Soc.

TOES, Norman Antony (retired) 56 Mayfield Road, Writtle, Chelmsford CM1 3EL Tel: 01245 421729 — MB BS Lond. 1949 (Lond. Hosp.) MRCS Eng. LRCP Lond. 1949; DObst RCOG 1954. Prev: Sen. Med. Off. Prison Med. Serv. Home Office.

TOFAZZAL, Nasima Singleton Hospital, Histopathology Department, Swansea NHS Trust, Sketty, Swansea Tel: 01792 285546 Fax: 01792 285537 Email: nasima.tofazzal@swansea-tr.wales.nhs.uk — MB BS Dhaka 1987 (Dhaka Med. Coll. Bangladesh) MPhil Dhaka Bangladesh 1992; Diploma (Cytol.) Roy. Coll. of Pathologist 2000; MRCPath Roy. Coll. of Pathologist UK 2000. Cons. Histo & Pathologist Swansea NHS Trust. Specialty:

Histopath. Special Interest: Cytopathology. Socs: Association of Clinical Pathologists; BSCC; MPS. Prev: Specialist Regist. (Histopath.) S. W. Region Lond. 1997 - 2000.

TOFF, Nicholas James 12 St Annes Close, Winchester SO22 4LQ — MB BS Lond. 1981 (Charing Cross) BSc (Hons.) Lond. 1977; DRCOG 1983; Cert. Av. Med. 1987; FRCA 1988. Specialty: Anaesth.; Aviat. Med. Prev: Regist. (Anaesth.) Bristol Extended Train. Scheme; SHO (Anaesth.) Southmead Hosp. Bristol; SHO (Anaesth.) Roy. Hants. Co. Hosp.

TOFF, Penelope Rebecca 20 Chatham Road, Oxford OX1 4UY Tel: 01865 721495 — MB BS Lond. 1986; BSc Basic Med. Scs. & Psychol. Lond. 1983. SHO (Paediat.) Oxf. Radcliffe Hosp. Trust. Prev: SHO (A & E) Oxf. Radcliffe Hosp. Trust; SHO (Genitourin. Med.) St. Mary's Hosp. Trust Lond.; SHO & Clin. Med. Off. (Family Plann. & Wom. Health) Lothian HB.

TOFF, William Daniel Tilcocks, 4 West Hill, Aspley Guise, Milton Keynes MK17 8DN — MB BS Lond. 1981 (Univ. Coll. Hosp.) BSc (Hons.) Lond. 1978.

TOFT, Anthony Douglas, CBE Endocine Clinic (OPD2), Royal Infirmary, Edinburgh EH16 5QA Tel: 0131 242 1480 Fax: 0131 242 1485/0131 536 2091 — BSc Ed. 1966, MD 1976, MB ChB 1969; MRCP (UK) 1971; FRCP Ed. 1980; FRCP Lond. 1992; Hon. FACP 1993; Hon. FRACP 1993; FRCPI 1993; FRCP Glas. 1993; FRCS Ed. 1993; Hon. FFPharm Med. 1994; Hon. FRCGP 1994; Hon. FRCPC 1994. Cons. Phys. Roy. Infirm. Edin. Specialty: Endocrinol. Socs: Assn. Phys. Prev: Ho. Surg. & Ho. Phys. Roy. Infirm. Edin.

TOFT, Kristan Celia 36 Paddock Close, Radcliffe-on-Trent, Nottingham NG12 2BX — MB ChB Leeds 1989.

TOFT, Neil John 20 Craighouse Terrace, Edinburgh EH10 5LJ — MB ChB Ed. 1994. Specialty: Pathology, General.

TOFTS, Louise Jane The Bays, West Edge, Marsh Gibbon, Bicester OX27 0HA — MB BS Lond. 1998.

TOGHILL, Peter James (retired) 119 Lambley Lane, Burton Joyce, Nottingham NG14 5BL Tel: 0115 931 2446 Fax: 0115 931 2446 Email: ptoghill@dialstart.net — (Univ. Coll. Hosp.) MB BS Lond. 1955; MRCS Eng. LRCP Lond. 1955; DObst RCOG 1959; FRCP Ed. 1973, M 1961; MRCP (UK) 1962; MD Lond. 1966; FRCP Lond. 1975. Prev: Emerit. Cons. Phys. Univ. Hosp. Nottm.

TOGOBO, Ambrose Kofi Whipps Cross Hospital, Whipps Cross Road, Leytonstone, London E11 1NR Tel: 020 8539 5522; 59 King's Road, Leytonstone, London E11 1AU Tel: 020 8558 4171 Fax: 020 8539 5552 — Vrach Lvov Med Inst. USSR 1971; DTM & H Liverp. 1973; DA (UK) 1981; Cert. Family Plann. JCC 1986; MRCA 2002. Assoc. Specialist & Clin. Asst. (Anaesth.) Whipps Cross Hosp. Lond. Specialty: Anaesth. Socs: BMA; Med. Protec. Soc. Prev: SHO (Anaesth.) Basildon Hosp.; SHO (Anaesth. & O & G) King's Mill Hosp.; SHO (Obst.) Firs Matern. Hosp. Nottm.

TOH, Chee Tse Accident & Emergency Department, Central Middlesex Hospital NHS Trust, Acton Lane, Park Royal, London NW10 7NS — MB BS Lond. 1990; BSc (Hons.) (Pharm. with Basic Med. Sc.) 1987.

TOH, Cheng Hock Department of Haematology, Royal Liverpool University Hospital, Prescot St., Liverpool L7 8XP Tel: 0151 706 4322 Fax: 0151 706 5810 Email: toh@liv.ac.uk — MB ChB (Hons.) Sheff. 1985 (Univ. Sheff.) MRCP (UK) 1988; MRCPath 1994; MD Sheff. 1995; FRCP (UK) 1999; FRCPath (UK) 2002. Reader / Hon. Cons. in Haemat., Univ. of Liverp.; Director, Roald Dahl Haemostasis and Thrombosis Centre, Roy. Liverp. Univ. Hosp. Specialty: Haematology. Socs: Brit. Soc. Haematol. & Thrombosis; Internat. Soc. of Thrombosis and Haemostasis. Prev: Sen. Regist. (Haemat.) Sheff. Hosps.; Post-Doctoral Fell. (Haemat.) Qu. Univ. Kingston, Canada; Regist. (Haemat.) Roy. Hallamsh. Hosp. Sheff.

TOH, Khay-Wee 38 Burr Close, London E1W 1NB — MB BS Lond. 1994.

TOHANI, Vinod Kumar Southern Health and Social Services Board, Tower Hill, Armagh BT61 9DR Tel: 028 3741 0041 Fax: 028 3741 4551 — MB BCh BAO Dub. 1976; BA Dub. 1974, MA 1977; MSc (Community Med.) Univ. Lond. 1982; MICGP 1984; MFCM RCP (UK) 1986; MFPHM RCPI 1992; FFPHM 2001. Cons. Communicable Dis. Control SHSSB Craigavon; Chairm. Pub. Health Med. & Community Health N. Irel.; Mem. of NI Food Standard Advisery Comm. 2000-2003. Specialty: Pub. Health Med. Socs: BMA; Soc. for Social Med.; Travel Assn. Prev: SCM WHSSB; Specialist (Community Med.) Burnley, Pendle & Rossendale HA.

TOHILL, Martin 47 Derramore Heights, Magherafelt BT45 5RX Tel: 02879 301575 Email: martintohill@occupationalhealth.fsnet.co.uk — MB BCh BAO Belf. 1989; DRCOG 1992; DFFP 1993; MRCGP 1994; DOccMed 2000. Occupational Health Phys.; Med. Ref.; GP Locum. Specialty: Occupat. Health; Gen. Pract. Socs: BMA; BMAS; SOM. Prev: Trainee GP/SHO (Paediat.) Ulster Hosp. Dundonald; SHO (Psychiat.) Tyrone & Fermanagh; SHO (Med.) & Ho. Off. Mid Ulster Hosp.

TOHILL, Mel Patrick 5 Dorchester Park, Belfast BT9 6RH — MB BCh BAO Belf. 1997.

TOKE, Eric (Surgery), 2 Radnor Place, Liverpool L6 4BD Tel: 0151 263 3100; (home), 5 Dudlow Gardens, Liverpool L18 2HA Tel: 0151 722 1871 — MB ChB Liverp. 1950; FRCGP 1987. JP; Clin. Asst. (Psychiat.) & Clin. Med. Off. Liverp. DHA; Local Med. Off. Civil Serv. Socs: Liverp. Med. Inst.; Merseyside Med.-Legal Soc.

TOLAN, Damian John Michael St James Univ. Hospital, Leeds LS9 7TF — MB ChB Leeds 1997. Sen Ho. Off., St James' Univ. Hosp. Leeds.

TOLAN, Emma Louise 13 Euxton Cl, Bury BL8 2HY — MB ChB Leeds 1997.

TOLAN, Shaun Paul 58 Albion Street, St Helens WA10 2HD — MB BCh Wales 1997.

TOLAND, Jane Mary Paula 8 Stockmans Drive, Belfast BT11 9AU — MB BCh BAO Belf. 1988; MB BCh Belf. 1988.

TOLAND, Mary Waterside Health Centre, Glendermot Road, Londonderry BT47 6AU Tel: 028 7132 0100 Fax: 028 7134 9323; 110 Caw Hill Park, Londonderry BT47 6XX — MB BCh BAO NUI 1986; MRCP (UK) 1989; DCH NUI 1990; DRCOG 1991; MRCGP 1992. Specialty: Gen. Pract.

TOLAND, William James Whiteabbey Health Centre, 95 Doagh Road, Newtownabbey BT37 9QN Tel: 028 9086 4341 Fax: 028 9086 0443 — MB BCh BAO Belf. 1971; DObst 1973.

TOLBA, Mr Mahmoud Abd-Allah Orchard House, High Halden, Ashford TN26 3BS Tel: 01580 240333 — MB BCh Cairo 1972; MSc Cairo 1980; MRCOG 1993. Assoc. Specialist (Gyn.) Benenden Hosp. Cranbrook. Specialty: Obst. & Gyn. Socs: Exec. Comm. Brit. Soc. (Psychosomatics in Obst. & Gyn.); Eur. Assn. Obst. & Gyn.

TOLCHER, Rosamond Anne Family Planning Service, Central Health Clinic, East Park Terrace, Southampton SO14 0YL Tel: 023 8090 2506 Fax: 023 8090 2600; Beech House, 123B Newton Road, Warsash, Southampton SO31 9GY Tel: 01489 578324 — BM (Hons. Distinc. Clin. Med. & Med. Sci.) Soton. 1985; DRCOG 1987; MFFP 1994. Cons. (Family Plann. & ReProduc. Health). Specialty: Family Plann. & Reproduc. Health. Prev: SHO (A & E & Paediat.) Soton. Gen. Hosp.; SHO (O & G) Princess Anne Hosp. Soton.

TOLE, Mr Derek Michael Bristol Eye Hospital, Lower Maudlin Street, Bristol BS1 2LX Tel: 0117 928 4697 Email: derek.tole@bristol.ac.uk — MB ChB Manch. 1982; FRCOphth; DGM 1987; MRCGP 1988. Cons. (Ophth.) Bristol Eye Hosp. Specialty: Ophth. Special Interest: Corneal & External Eye Disease. Prev: GP Belford.; Trainee GP S.W. Cumbria VTS.

TOLEMAN, Susan Elizabeth Portchester Health Centre, West Street, Portchester, Fareham PO16 9TU Tel: 023 9237 6913 Fax: 023 9237 4265 — BM Soton. 1977.

TOLHURST, Professor David Erskine Guy's Nuffield House, Newcomen St.,, London SE1 1YR Tel: 020 7955 4761; 47 Aylesford Street, London SW1V 3RY — (Otago University, New Zealand) MB ChB New Zealand 1959; FRCS Lond. 1966; PhD Rotterdam 1988. Cons. Plastic Surg. Guy's Nuffield Ho. Lond.; Co-Edr. Europ. Jl. of Plastic Surg. Specialty: Plastic Surg. Socs: Brit. Assn. Plastic Surg.; Historian Europ. Assn. of Plastic Surg. Prev: Marks Fell. & Sen. Regist. Qu. Vict. Hosp. E. Grinstead; Cons. Plastic Surg. Wellington Hosp. New Zealand; Prof. (Plastic Surg.) Leiden Univ. Netherlands.

TOLHURST, Jacqueline Crook Log Surgery, 19 Crook Log, Bexleyheath DA6 8DZ Tel: 020 8304 3025 Fax: 020 8298 7739; 27 Spring Vale, Bexleyheath DA7 6AR Tel: 01322 523918 — MB ChB Ed. 1986; DCH RCP Lond. 1989; MRCGP Lond. 1996. GP Princip. Bexleyheath; Community Med. Off. Greenwich Healthcare Trust & Oxleas NHS Trust. Specialty: Gen. Pract. Prev: GP/Regist. Eltham; SHO (Paediat.) Borders Gen. Hosp. Melrose; SHO (O & G) Simpsons Matern. Memor. Hosp. Edin.

TOLHURST, Jennifer Elizabeth Dept. Pathology, Glasgow Royal Infirmary, 84 Caslte St, Glasgow G4 0SF — MB ChB Glas. 1992. Specialty: Histopath.

TOLHURST-CLEAVER, Christopher Lewis 17 West Road, Bowdon, Altrincham WA14 2LD Tel: 0161 928 6803 Fax: 0161 927 7036 Email: t.cleaver@virgin.net — MB ChB Sheff. 1971; DObst RCOG 1976; FRCA Eng. 1977. Cons. (Anaesth.) S. Manch. Univ. Hosp.; Hon. Clin. Lect. Vict. Univ. Manch.; Hon. Sec. Anaes Sect. Manch. Med. Soc. Specialty: Anaesth. Special Interest: Paediatrics; Plastics; Regional. Socs: Europ. Soc. Regional Anaesth.; Assn. Anaesth. GB & Irel.; APA. Prev: Sen. Regist. (Anaesth.) Brompton & Westm. Hosps. Lond.; Vis. Asst. Prof. (Anaesth.) Univ. Texas, Dallas; Regist. (Anaesth.) Sheff. AHA (T).

TOLIA, Mr Jitendra Jayantilal Luton and Dunstable Hospital, Lewsey Road, Luton LU4 0DZ Tel: 01582 497329 — MB ChB Glas. 1975 (Univ. Glas.) FRCS Ed. (Ophth.) 1980; FRCOphth 1992. Cons. Ophth. Luton & Dunstable Hosp.; Cons. Ophth. St Albans City Hosp. Specialty: Ophth. Special Interest: Cararacts; LASIK; Macular Degeneration. Socs: FRCOphth. Prev: Cons. Ophth. Ysbyty Gwynedd Bangor; Sen. Regist. Qu. Med. Centre Nottm.; Hon. Lect. Nottm. Univ.

TOLIA, Kusum Jagdish Barking Medical Group Practice, 130 Upney Lane, Barking IG11 9LT Tel: 020 8594 4353/5709 Fax: 020 8591 4686 — (Royal College of Surgeons Dublin, Ireland) MB BCh N U Ireland 1979; MB BCh N U Ireland 1979; MRCGP RCGP 1987.

TOLIAS, Mr Christos 46 Weymoor Road, Harbourne, Birmingham B17 0RY — Ptychio Iatrikes Greece 1988; FRCS Eng. 1994. Specialist Regist. (Neurosurg.). Specialty: Neurosurg. Prev: Specialist Regist. (Neurosurg.) Liverp.; Research Regist (Neurosurg.) Walsgrave Hosp. Coventry.

TOLLAND, Elizabeth Mary West Suffolk Drug Advisory Service, Blomfield House Health Centre, Looms Lane, Bury St Edmunds IP33 1HE Tel: 01284 775275; Spencers Farm, Polstead Heath, Colchester CO6 5BD Tel: 01787 210503 Email: tollwick@aol.com — MB BS Newc. 1974 (Newcastle upon Tyne) SCMO Substance Misuse; DFFP RCOG 1993; MSc Addictive Behaviour 2000. Med Off. (Paediat) Suufolk.; Family Plann. Doctor. Specialty: Community Child Health; Alcohol & Substance Misuse; Family Plann. & Reproduc. Health. Socs: MRCPCH; Brit. Assn. Community Child Health. Prev: Community Med. Off. W. Suff. HA.

TOLLAND, John (retired) 10 Skottowe Crescent, Great Ayton, Middlesbrough TS9 6DS Tel: 01642 723513 — (Roy. Colls. Ed. & Qu. Univ. Belf.) LRCP LRCS Ed. LRFPS Glas. 1938; DPH Belf. 1947; MFCM 1973. Prev: Dist. Community Phys. S. Tees Health Dist.

TOLLAND, Julia Patricia Flat 4, 64 Osborne Park, Belfast BT9 6JP Tel: 07759 659824 — MB BCh Belf. 1998 (Queens University Belfast) MRCP Ed.; BSc (Med. Gen.). Regist. (Gen Med.) Belf. City Hosp. Specialty: Gen. Med.

TOLLAST, Anthony Richard Sunnyside Doctors Surgery, 150 Fratton Road, Portsmouth PO1 5DH Tel: 023 9282 4725 Fax: 023 9286 1014 — BM Soton. 1983; Cert. Family Plann. JCC 1985; DRCOG 1986; MRCGP 1987; Dip. Pract. Dermat. Wales 1993. Clin. Asst. (Dermat.) St. Mary's Hosp. Portsmouth. Prev: Trainee GP Portsmouth VTS; Ho. Surg. & Ho. Phys. St. Mary's Hosp. Portsmouth.

TOLLER, Ruth Anne Royal Victoria Hospital, Jedburgh Road, Dundee DD2 1SP Tel: 01382 423181; 3 Duffus Court, Dundee DD4 9BU — MB BS Newc. 1976; MRCGP 1980. Clin. Med. Off. (Department of Medicine for the Elderly) Tayside Health Bd. Specialty: Care of the Elderly.

TOLLETT, Barbara Joan Fleet Medical Centre, Church Road, Fleet GU51 4PE Tel: 01252 613327 Fax: 01252 815156 — MB ChB Birm. 1981.

TOLLEY, Mr David Anthony Murrayfield Hospital, Corstorphine Road, Edinburgh EH12 6UD Tel: 0131 334 0363 Fax: 0131 334 7338; Loquhariot Farm, Gorebridge EH23 4PB Tel: 01875 820860 — MB BS Lond. 1970 (Kings Coll. Hosp.) MRCS Eng. LRCP Lond. 1970; FRCS Eng. 1975; FRCS Ed. 1983; FRCP Edin. 2003. Cons. Urol. Surg. West. Gen. Hosp. Edin.; Dir. Scott. Lithotriptor Centre West. Gen. Hosp.; Hon. Sen. Lect. Univ. Edin. Specialty: Urol. Socs: Counc. Roy. Coll. of Surg.s Edin.; (Counc.) Brit. Assn. Urol. Surgs.; Soc. Internat.e d'Urologie, Europ. Prev: Sen. Regist. (Urol.) Gen. Infirm. Leeds; Sen. Regist. (Urol.) Kings Coll. Hosp. Lond.; Regist. (Urol. & Transpl.) Hammersmith Hosp. Lond.

TOLLEY, Ian Philip Hellesdon Medical Practice, 343 Reepham Road, Hellesdon, Norwich NR6 5QJ Tel: 01603 486602 Fax: 01603 401389 Email: ian.tolley@nhs.net — MB ChB Leic. 1985; MRCGP 1989; DRCOG 1989. GP Norwich.

TOLLEY, Jennifer Mary Manor Park Surgery, Bell Mount Close, Leeds LS13 2UP Tel: 0113 295 4302 Fax: 0113 295 4321 — MB BS Newc. 1974; DRCOG 1976. GP Leeds. Prev: SHO (O & G) Airedale Gen. Hosp.; SHO (Gen. Med.) Darlington Memor. Hosp.; SHO (O & G) Roy. Berks. Hosp. Reading.

TOLLEY, Martin Stephen Bellevue Medical Centre, 26 Huntingdon Place, Edinburgh EH7 4AT Tel: 0131 556 2642 Fax: 0131 557 4430 — MB BS Lond. 1982; MA Camb. 1978, BA 1974; DCH RCP Lond. 1985; MRCGP 1988. Clin. Asst. Princess Alexandra Eye Pavil. Roy. Infirm. Edin. Specialty: Ophth. Prev: Trainee GP Sheff. VTS; Ho. Phys. St. Bart. Hosp. Lond.; Ho. Surg. Whipps Cross Hosp. Lond.

TOLLEY, Michael Edward Carlton House, 17 High Green, Great Shelford, Cambridge CB2 5EG — MRCS Eng. LRCP Lond. 1964 (Univ. Coll. Hosp.) BSc Lond. 1961, MB BS 1964; DA Eng. 1967; FFA RCS Eng. 1969. Cons. Anaesth. Addenbrookes Hosp. Camb. Specialty: Anaesth. Prev: Sen. Regist. (Anaesth.) Addenbrooke's Hosp. Camb.; Regist. (Anaesth.) United Camb. Hosps.; SHO (Anaesth.) Soton. Hosps. Gp.

TOLLEY, Mr Neil Samuel St Mary's Hospital, Praed Street, Paddington, London W2 1NY Tel: 020 7886 1091 Fax: 020 7886 1847 — MB BCh Wales 1982 (Cardiff) DLO RCS Eng. 1987; FRCS Ed. 1988; MD Wales 1988; FRCS Eng. 1989. Cons. ENT & Head & Neck Surg. St. Mary's & Ealing NHS Trust; Regional Adviser in Otolaryngol., Roy. Coll. of Surg.s (Eng.); Program Director Specialist Train. Comm. N. Thames. Specialty: Otolaryngol. Special Interest: Paediatric Airway; Thyroid. Socs: Eur. Acad. Facial Surg.; Brit. Assn. Otorhinol.; Brit. Assn. Paediatric Otolaryngologists. Prev: Sen. Regist. Roy. Nat. Throat, Nose & Ear Hosp.; Jun. Cons. Groote Schuur Hosp. Cape Town, S. Afr.; Sen. Regist. Sir Chas. Gairdner Hosp. Perth, West. Austral.

TOLLEY, Peter Frederick Richmond 23 Beechcroft Drive, Ellesmere Port, South Wirral CH65 6PD — MB ChB St. And. 1973.

TOLLIDAY, John Douglas Lyngford Park Surgery, Fletcher Close, Taunton TA2 8SQ Tel: 01823 333355 Fax: 01823 257022 — MB ChB Manch. 1978; MRCGP 1986. Prev: Ho. Phys. & Ho. Surg. Stepping Hill Hosp. Stockport; Trainee GP Exeter VTS.

TOLLINS, Alan Peter Elsdale Street Surgery, 28 Elsdale Street, London E9 6QY Tel: 020 8985 2719 — MB BS Lond. 1983.

TOLMAC, Jovanka West London Mental Health NHS Trust, Adolescent Community Team, Windmill Lodge, Uxbridge Road, Southall UB1 3EU Tel: 020 8354 8800 Email: j.tolmac@ic.ac.uk — MD Belgrade 1989; MRCPsych. Specialist Regist. (Psychiat. Child & Adolesc.) Ealing Hosp. Lodon. Specialty: Child & Adolesc. Psychiat. Special Interest: Adolesc. Psychiat.

TOLMAN, Cae Jonathan 11 Holtdale Drive, Leeds LS16 7RT — MB ChB Leeds 1997.

TOLMIE, John Lorimer Duncan Guthrie Institute of Medical Genetics, Yorkhill Hospitals, Yorkhill, Glasgow G3 8SJ Tel: 0141 339 8888; 85 Hughenden Lane, Hyndland, Glasgow G12 9XN — MB ChB Glas. 1980; BSc (Hons.) Glas. 1977; MRCP (UK) 1983; FRCP Glas. 1994. Cons. Clin. Genetics Yorkhill Hosp. Glas. Specialty: Genetics. Socs: Clin. Genetics Soc.

TOLUFASHE, Ezekiel Ajibola — MB BS Lagos 1977; MRCP (UK) 1987. Specialty: Care of the Elderly.

TOMA, Mr Abbad St George's Hospital, Blackshaw Road, London SW17 0QT Tel: 020 8725 2054 — MB BCh BAO NUI 1986; LRCSI 1986; LRCPI 1986; FRCS Ed. 1994; FRCS (ORL) 1997. Cons. ENT Surg. St Geo. & Kingston NHS Trusts Lond. Specialty: Otolaryngol. Special Interest: Rhinology & Facial Plastic Surg.

TOMAR, Surendra Singh College Street Health Centre, College Street, Leigh WN7 2RD Tel: 01942 671085 Fax: 01942 680477 — MB BS Indore 1971.

TOMB, Joseph John (retired) 96 Crwafordsburn Road, Newtownards BT23 4UH — MB BCh BAO Belf. 1947.

TOMBLESON, Philip Michael John, MBE Health Centre, Lewes Road, Ditchling, Hassocks BN6 8TT Tel: 01273 842570; Little Ash, 30 Lewes Road, Ditchling, Hassocks BN6 8TU Tel: 01273 844099 Fax: 01273 845747 — MB BS Lond. 1960 (Guy's) MRCS Eng. LRCP Lond. 1960; DObst RCOG 1962; DA Eng. 1962; FRCGP 1989,

M 1968. Chairm. OSCE Panel, PLAB Exam., GMC Lead Assessor, GMC Performance Procedure. Prev: Course Organiser Mid-Sussex Vocational Train. Scheme; Convenor of Panel Examnrs. MRCGP Exam.

TOMBLIN, Maeve Philomena Mary Worle Health Centre, 125 High St, Worle, Weston Super Mare BS22 6HB Tel: 01934 510510 Fax: 01934 522088 — MB BCh BAO NUI 1981; DObst RCPI 1985.

TOMBOLINE, David Spencer The Health Centre, Milman Road, Reading RG2 0AY Tel: 01734 862285; 5 Hartsbourne Road, Earley, Reading RG6 5PX — MB BS Lond. 1986; DRCOG 1989; DCH RCP Lond. 1990; T (GP) 1991.

TOMBS, David George 3 The Paddock, Winshill, Burton-on-Trent DE15 0BB — MB ChB Birm. 1982; MRCPsych 1987; MMedSci Leeds 1989. Cons. Psychiat. Pastures Hosp. Derby. Specialty: Gen. Psychiat. Socs: Derby Med. Soc. Prev: Lect. Univ. Leeds.

TOMEI, Louise Dawn Quercus, Parkwood Road, Nutfield, Redhill RH1 4HD — MB ChB Leic. 1991; BSc (Hons.) Lond. 1986; DRCOG. 1995; DFFP. 1996; MRCGP. 1996.

TOMES, Doris Helen (retired) c/o National Westminster Bank, 18 Cromwell Place, London SW7 — MRCS Eng. LRCP Lond. 1927 (Westm.) Prev: Asst. Co. Med. Off. Devon C.C.

TOMES, Joanna Susan Boundary Road, Grayshott, Hindhead GU26 6TY — MB BS Lond. 1987.

TOMETZKI, Andrew John Peter Bristol Royal Hospital For Children, Upper Maudlin Street, Bristol BS2 8BJ Tel: 0117 342 8853 Fax: 0117 342 8857 Email: andrew.tometzki@ubht.swest.nhs.uk — MB ChB Sheff. 1985 (Sheffield Medical School) MRCP (UK) 1991; FRCP 1999. Cons. Paediatric Cardiol., UBHT Bristol. Specialty: Cardiol. Socs: Brit. Cardiac Soc.; Brit. Paediat. Cardiac Assn. Prev: Regist. (Paediat. Cardiol.) Roy. Liverp. Childr. Hosp. & Roy. Hosp. Sick Childr. Glas.; ECMO Research Fell.; Sen. Regist. (Paediat. Cardiol.) Roy. Hosp. Sick Childr. Edin.

TOMIAK, Richard Henry Herbert Merck, Sharpe & Dohme, Hertford Road, Hoddesdon EN11 9BU Tel: 01992 467272 Fax: 01992 451066; 12 Hartington Road, Chiswick, London W4 Tel: 020 8995 5629 — MB BChir Camb. 1981; MA Camb. 1982, MB BChir 1981; Dip. Pharm. Med. RCP UK. 1987; MFPM 1989; FFPM 1998. Dir. Med. Affairs Merck, Sharpe & Dohme Hoddesdon. Specialty: Pharmaceutical Medicine. Prev: Sen. Med. Adviser Syntex Pharmaceut.

TOMIC, Damian Anton Fyffe, Northfield Avenue, Pinner HA5 1AR — MB BS Lond. 1990.

TOMINEY, Damian Paul Tominey, 17 Upper Lattimore Road, St Albans AL1 3UD Tel: 07831 399852 — MB BS Lond. 1971 (Univ. Coll. Hosp.) BSc (Hons.) Lond.; DObst RCOG 1974; T(GP) 1991. Private Practitioner. Specialty: Gen. Pract. Special Interest: Nursing Home Developm. Socs: Soc. Apoth.; BMA. Prev: Indep. Med. Pract. St. Albans; Exec. Med. Off. DHSS.

TOMISON, Arden Randall Fromeside Clinic, Blackberry Hill Hospital, Stapleton, Bristol BS16 1ED Tel: 0117 958 3678 — MB ChB Dundee 1979; M 1984; FRCPsych 1997. Cons. Forens. Psychiat. & Head Forens. Psychiat. Avon & Wilts. Ment. Health NHS Trust; Hon. Sen. Lect., Ment. Health Univ., Bristol. Specialty: Forens. Psychiat. Prev: Sen. Regist. (Forens. Psychiat.) Langdon Hosp.; Clin. Dir. (Ment. Health) Frenchay Healthcare NHS Trust.

TOMKINS, Professor Andrew Mervyn Centre for International Child Health, Institute of Child Health, University College London, 30 Guildford Street, London WC1N 1EH Tel: 0207 905 2123 Fax: 0207 404 2062 Email: a.tomkins@ich.ucl.ac.uk; 9, Haddon Court, Shakespeare Road, Harpenden AL5 5NB Tel: 01582 768121 — MB BS Lond. 1966 (Middlx.) MRCS Eng. LRCP Lond. 1966; MRCP Lond. 1969; FRCP 1981; FFPHM 1996; FRCPCH 1997; FAcadMS 2001. Hon. Cons. Paediat. Hosp. for Childr. Gt. Ormond St. Lond.; Hon. Cons. Phys. Hosp. Trop. Dis. & UCH. Specialty: Trop. Med. Prev: Sen. Lect. (Clin. Nutrit.) Lond. Sch. Hyg. & Trop. Med. Lond.; Sen. Regist. (Med.) Ahmadu Bello Univ. Zaria, Nigeria; Clin. Sci. MRC Fajara, The Gambia, W. Afr.

TOMKINS, Christine Margaret Paris House, The Rocks Road, E. Malling, West Malling ME19 6AU — MB BCh Manch. 1980; BSc Manch. 1977; MB BCh (Hons.) Manch. 1980; DO RCS Eng. 1983; FRCS Eng. 1984; FCOphth 1989; MBA Lond. 1997. Professional Servs. Dir. Med. Defence Union. Prev: Regist. (Ophth.) & SHO (Ophth.) St. Thos. Hosp. Lond.; Hon. Lect. (Anat.) Univ. Manch.; SHO (Ophth.) Char. Cross Lond.

TOMKINS, Michael James 9 Hawkesbury Road, Shirley, Solihull B90 2QR — MB BS Lond. 1988; MRCP (UK) 1993.

TOMKINS, Susan Elizabeth Department of Clinical Genetics, St Michaels Hospital, Southwell Street, Bristol BS2 8EG Tel: 0117 928 5107 — MB ChB Leic. 1988; MRCP (Paediat.) (UK) 1994. Specialty: Genetics.

TOMKINSON, Alun Kenbrook, Upper Canning Street, Ton Pentre, Pentre CF41 7HG — MB BCh Wales 1987.

TOMKINSON, John Spencer County Hospital, North Road, Durham DH1 4ST Tel: 0191 333 3477 Fax: 0191 333 3400 Email: john.tomkinson@cddps.northy.nhs.uk — BM BS Nottm. 1978 (Nottingham) BMedSci (Hons.) Nottm. 1975; MRCPsych 1982. Cons. Psychiat., Co. Durh. and Darlington Priority Servs. NHS Trust, Durh. Specialty: Gen. Psychiat.; Psychother. Prev: Sen. Regist. (Psychiat.) Yorks. RHA; Regist. (Psychiat.) Nottm. HA; Hon. Clin. Lect. Univ. Leeds.

TOMKINSON, Julian Stuart The Barn, 17 Oaks Lane, Bradshaw, Bolton BL2 3BR — MB ChB Manch. 1995.

TOMLIN, Pamela Irene Royal Preston Hospital, Sharoe Green Lane, Preston PR2 9HT; 13 Billinge Avenue, Blackburn BB2 6SD — MB Camb. 1972; BChir 1971; DCH RCP Lond. 1973; MRCP (UK) 1977; FRCP Lond. 1992; FRCPCH 1997. Cons. Paediat. Neurol. Roy. Preston Hosp. N. West. RHA. Specialty: Paediat. Neurol.

TOMLIN, Peter James (retired) Radnor House, The Headlands, Downton, Salisbury SP5 3HJ — MB BS Lond. 1957 (Lond. Hosp.) FFA RCS Eng. 1962. Prev: Sen. Regist. Hammersmith Hosp. Lond.

TOMLINS, Christopher David Corbett Royal Berkshire and Battle Hospitals NHS Trust, Royal Berkshire Hospital, Reading RG1 5AN Tel: 0118 987 7668 Fax: 0118 987 7675 Email: christopher.tomlins@rbbh.tr.nhs.uk — (Guy's) FDS RCS Eng. 1973, LDS 1963; BDS Lond. 1964; MRCS Eng. LRCP Lond. 1969; MB BS Lond. 1969. Cons. Oral Surg. Roy. Berks. Hosp. Reading; Cons. Oral and Maxillofacial Surg., W. Berks. Community Hosp., Newbury; Cons. Oral and Maxillofacial Surg., BUPA Dunedin Hosp. Reading; Cons. Oral and Maxillofacial Surg., Berks. Independant (Capio Reading) Hosp. Reading. Specialty: Oral & Maxillofacial Surg. Socs: Fell. RCS Eng.; Fell. Brit. Assn. Oral & Maxillofacial Surg.; BMA. Prev: Sen. Regist. (Oral Surg.) Westm. Hosp. Gp.; Regist. (Oral Surg.) Eastman Dent. Hosp. Lond.; Ho. Surg. (Orthop.) Guy's Hosp.

TOMLINS, Frank Geoffrey 14 Alderton Hill, Loughton IG10 3JB — MB BChir Camb. 1948 (Univ. Coll. Hosp.) MA MB BChir Camb. 1948. Prev: Ho. Surg. Obst. Unit Univ. Coll. Hosp.; Ho. Phys. W. Kent Gen. Hosp. Maidstone; Asst. Med. Off. Brit. Rlys. West. Region.

TOMLINSON, Andrew Alan Directorate of Anesthesia, City General, North Staffs Hospital, Newcastle Road, Stoke-on-Trent ST4 6QG Tel: 01782 715444; 2 Granville Avenue, Newcastle ST5 1JH — MB BS Lond. 1975 (Roy. Free) MRCS Eng. LRCP Lond. 1975; FRCA 1980. Cons. Anaesth. N. Staffs. Hosp. Specialty: Anaesth. Prev: Sen. Regist. (Anaesth.) Soton. HA; Staff Anaesth. Shanta Bhawan Hosp. Kathmandu, Nepal; Regist. (Anaesth.) Sheff. HA.

TOMLINSON, Anne Patricia The Orchard Surgery, Bromborough Village Road, Bromborough, Wirral CH62 7EU Tel: 0151 343 2084 Fax: 0151 343 9437; 15 West Drive, Upton, Wirral CH49 6JX Tel: 0151 677 1605 — MB BCh Wales 1977; DCH Eng. 1979; DRCOG 1980; MRCGP 1981. Prev: Clin. Med. Off. Wirral HA. NHS Trust; Trainee GP Clatterbridge VTS.

TOMLINSON, Sir Bernard Evans, CBE (retired) — MB BS Lond. 1943 (Univ. Coll. Hosp.) MRCS Eng. LRCP Lond. 1943; FRCP Lond. 1965, M 1944; MD Lond. 1962; FCPath 1964; Hon. MD Newc. 1993. Prev: Hon. Emerit. Prof. Path. Univ. Newc.

TOMLINSON, Brian (retired) 7 Clwyd Avenue, Prestatyn LL19 9NG Tel: 01745 857040 — MB ChB Leeds 1952. Prev: GP Prestatyn.

TOMLINSON, Christopher James 31 Yorton Cottage, Shrewsbury SY4 3EU — BM BS Nottm. 1993; BMedSci Nottm. 1991.

TOMLINSON, Clare Jacqueline 26 Willow Drive, Droitwich WR9 7QE Tel: 01905 796461 — BM Soton. 1985. GP Regist., Worcs. Specialty: Civil Serv. Prev: GP Regist., Pershore; SHO (O & G) Worcester Roy. Infirm. VTS; Ref. & Adjudicating Med. Pract. for Benefits Agency Med. Servs.

TOMLINSON, David Robert 21 Holmsdale Avenue, London SW14 7BQ — MB BS Lond. 1985.

TOMLINSON, David Robert — BM (Hons.) Soton. 1995; BSc (Hons.) Soton. 1994.

TOMLINSON, Diane Church Farm House, Arminghall, Norwich NR14 8SG — MB BS Lond. 1981; MRCGP 1986; DRCOG 1987; MRCPsych 2004.

TOMLINSON, Ellen Oi-Lun High Gable, 62 Banks Road, Pound Hill, Crawley RH10 7BP Tel: 01293 526509 — BSc (Hons.) St. And. 1982; MB BChir Camb. 1984; MRCPI 1986; DRCOG 1990; MRCGP 1993. Prev: Trainee GP Lewisham VTS; SHO Rotat. (Med.) St. Jas. Hosp. Leeds.

TOMLINSON, Frank Edwin (retired) 89 Westgate, Tranmere Park, Guiseley, Leeds LS20 8HH Tel: 01943 872927 — MB ChB Leeds 1957; DObst RCOG 1961. Prev: GP Shipley, W. Yorks.

TOMLINSON, Garry Nelson The Health Centre, Bridge Street, Thorne, Doncaster DN8 5QH Tel: 01405 812121 Fax: 01405 741059; Wrancarr Mill, Wrancarr Lane, Moss, Doncaster DN6 0DP — MB ChB Auckland 1974; DRCOG 1979; DPM Eng. 1981. GP Doncaster AHA. Prev: Regist. (Psychiat.) Fair Mile Hosp. Wallingford; SHO (O & G) Odstock Hosp. Salisbury; Trainee GP Liphook.

TOMLINSON, Geoffrey Charles Glenbourne, Momaix Drive, Dernford, Plymouth PL6 5AF Tel: 01752 761 3120; Rose Wollas, Rose, Truro TR4 9PH Tel: 01872 573583 Email: gtomlinson@doctors.org.uk — MB BCh Wales 1974; DPM Leeds 1977; MRCPsych 1979. Cons. Psychiat. Glenbourne Community Trust 1999; Psychiat. Adviser to Centre for Ment. Health Servs. Developm. Specialty: Gen. Psychiat. Socs: Brit. Assn. Behavioural & Cognitive Psychother.; Roy. Coll. Psychiats. Prev: Cons. Psychiat. North. Birm. Ment. Health Trust; Cons. Psychiat. Trengweath Ment. Health Unit Redruth; Sen. Regist. (Psychiat.) Mapperley Hosp.

TOMLINSON, Ian Philip Mark London Research Institute, Cancer Research UK, 44, Lincoln's Inn Fields, London WC2A 3PX — BM BCh Oxf. 1992; PhD Camb. 1988, MA 1989, BA 1985; MRC Path 1999. Head, Molecular & Populat. Genetics Laborat., ICRF, Lond.; Prof. of Clin. Genetics, Imperial Coll., Colorectal Cancer Unit,St Mark's Hosp. Harrow; Hon. Cons. in Clin. Genetics, Churchill Hosp., Oxf. Specialty: Genetics. Special Interest: Cancer Genetics; Clinical Cytogenetics; Molecular Genetics. Prev: Sen. Clin. Res. Fell., Oxf.; Sen. Clinician Research Fell. Inst. Cancer Research Sutton; Research Fell. Cancer Genetics Laborat. Imperial Cancer Research Fund Lond.

TOMLINSON, Ian Walter Castle Hill Hospital, Castle Road, Cottingham HU16 5JQ Tel: 01482 875875; 7 Allanhall Way, Kirkella, Hull HU10 7QU Tel: 01482 654291 — MD Lond. 1982 (Kings London) MB BS 1971; MRCP (UK) 1977; FRCP Lond. 1993. Cons. Rheum.Hull & E. Yorks. Hosp. NHS Trust. Specialty: Rheumatol.; Gen. Med. Prev: Cons. Rheum. E. Yorks. & ScarBoro. Hosp. Trusts.; Regist. (Gen. Med.) Leicester Gen. Hosp.; Lect. (Rheum.) Univ. Manch.

TOMLINSON, Isobel Mary Moorcroft Medical Centre, Butteslon Street, Hanley, Stoke-on-Trent ST1 3NJ — MB BS Lond. 1975 (Roy. Free) MRCS Eng. LRCP Lond. 1975; DRCOG 1977; MRCGP 1984. GP Princip. Prev: GP Newc. Staffs.; Trainee GP Wessex VTS; Clin. Asst. Shanta Bhawan Hosp. Kathmandu, Nepal.

TOMLINSON, Jean Mowat 3 Long Acres Close, Coombe Dingle, Bristol BS9 2RF Tel: 0117 968 2079 — MRCS Eng. LRCP Lond. 1948 (Univ. Coll. Lond. & W. Lond. Hosp.) Prev: Lady Med. Off. Seremban & Penang, Malaya.

TOMLINSON, John David Director of Public Health, Broxtowe & Hucknall PCT, Headquarters, Priory Court, Derby Rd, Nottingham NG9 2TN Tel: 0115 875 4913 Fax: 0115 875 4910 — MB ChB Liverp. 1980; DRCOG 1985; MRCGP 1986; MFPHM RCP (UK) 1994; FFPHM RCP (UK) 2000. Director of Pub. Health, Broxtowe & Hucknall PCT; Clin. Tutor Leicester Univ. Med. Sch., Nottm. Univ. Med. Sch. & Nottm. Sch. Pub. Health. Specialty: Pub. Health Med. Prev: Cons. Pub. Health Med. Leics. Health.

TOMLINSON, John Fielding Fartown Health Centre, Huddersfield HD2 2QA Tel: 01484 544318 — MB ChB Manch. 1952. Socs: Huddersfield Med. Soc.

TOMLINSON, John Howard Rosegarth House, Clifton Road, Tettenhall, Wolverhampton WV6 9AP — MB ChB Manch. 1974; FFA RACS 1982. Cons. (Anaesth.) Wolverhampton DHA. Specialty: Anaesth.

TOMLINSON, John Montgomery Royal Hampshire County Hospital, Romsey Road, Winchester SO22 5DG Tel: 01962 824443; Clays Farm, East Worldham, Alton GU34 3AD Tel: 01420 82210 Fax: 01420 543060 — MB BS Lond. 1959 (Middlx.) DObst RCOG 1962; FRCGP 1984, M 1965. Clinician (Men's Sexual Health) Roy. Hants. Co. Hosp. Winchester; Cons. (Men's Sexual Health) Sarum Rd. Hosp. Winchester SO22 5HA. Socs: BMA; Int. Soc. Study Adult Male (ISSAM); Euro. Soc. Sex. Med. (ESSM). Prev: Hon. Sen. Lect. (Primary Med. Care) Univ. Soton. Med. Sch.; Sen. Partner, Tomlinson & Partners Alton; Assoc. Adviser Profess. Developm. Wessex Region.

TOMLINSON, Joy Elizabeth Mary 83 Milton Road, Kirkcaldy KY1 1TP — MB ChB Glas. 1993.

TOMLINSON, Kenneth Mills (retired) 4 Cook's Place, Newent GL18 1TR Tel: 01531 821129 — MB BS Lond. 1949 (St. Thos.) MRCS Eng. LRCP Lond. 1940. Prev: JP.

TOMLINSON, Marjorie Jane Weston General Hospital, Grange Road, Uphill, Weston Super Mare BS23 4TQ — MB ChB Liverp. 1977; MRCP (UK) 1981; FRCR 1995. p/t Cons. (Clin. Oncol.) Weston Gen. Hosp., Weston-Super-Mare and Bristol Oncol. centre. Specialty: Oncol. Special Interest: Breast and Colorectal Cancer. Prev: Sen. Regist. in Clin. Oncol., Haemat. and Oncol. Centre, Bristol.

TOMLINSON, Mr Mark Antony Clinical Research Unit, Ingleby House, St. George's Hospital, Blackshaw Road, Tooting, London SW17 0QT Tel: 020 8725 0177 — MB BS Lond. 1990 (St. Geo. Hosp.) FRCS Eng. 1995. Research Regist. (Vasc. Surg.) St. Geo. Hosp. Lond. Specialty: Gen. Surg. Prev: SHO (Colorectal Surg. & Cardiothoracic Surg.) St. Geo. Hosp. Lond.; SHO (Plastic Surg.) Salisbury Dist. Hosp.; SHO (Gen. Surg.) St. Helier Hosp. Carshalton.

TOMLINSON, Mark John Vine House, New Street, Ledbury HR8 2DX — MB BCh Wales 1985; DRCOG 1988; MRCGP 1989; Dip. Pharm. Med. RCP (UK) 1996; AFPM 2001; MFPM 2002. Med. Dir. Sequani Clin. Ledbury. Specialty: Pharmaceutical Medicine; Gen. Pract. Prev: Med. Manager Sanofi Winthrop Ltd. Guildford; Director (Cardiovasc. + Metab.s), Bristol - Myers Squibb, P.ton, New Jersey.; Asst. GP Cohuna Vict., Austral.

TOMLINSON, Patricia Outram (retired) Clay's Farm, East Worldham, Alton GU34 3AD Tel: 01420 82210 Fax: 01420 543060 — MB BS Lond. 1957 (Guy's) MRCS Eng. LRCP Lond. 1957; DCH Eng. 1961. Prev: Sch. Med. Off. Lord Mayor Treloar Coll. for Disabled Boys & Girls.

TOMLINSON, Paul Alexander Department of Anaesthesia, City Hospital, Hucknall Road, Nottingham NG5 1PB — MB ChB Bristol 1973; FFA RCS Eng. 1981. Specialty: Anaesth.

TOMLINSON, Piers Sunnymead, Tring Road, Long Marston, Tring HP23 4QL — BM Soton. 1994.

TOMLINSON, Rachel Jane The Health Centre, Victoria Street, Marsden, Huddersfield HD7 6DF Tel: 01484 844332 Fax: 01484 845779 — MB ChB Leeds 1988.

TOMLINSON, Mr Richard John Rostron 8 Church Street, Southport PR9 0QT Tel: 01704 533666 — MB ChB Manch. 1970; FRCS Eng. 1974.

TOMLINSON, Robert Cyril Green Cottage, Moor Lane, Kirk Ireton, Ashbourne DE6 3JE — MB ChB Liverp. 1995.

TOMLINSON, Robert James (retired) Brackley, 15 Crooklands Drive, Garstang, Preston PR3 1JH Tel: 01995 603752 — MB BS Lond. 1962 (St. Bart.) MRCS Eng. LRCP Lond. 1962; DObst RCOG 1964. Prev: SHO (O & G) St. Mary's Hosp. Kettering.

TOMLINSON, Simon David 9 Glendale Grove, Spital, Wirral CH63 9FP — MB ChB Birm. 1991; ChB Birm. 1991.

TOMLINSON, Professor Stephen University of Wales College of Medicine, Cardigan House, Heath Park, Cardiff CF14 4XN Tel: 029 2074 2029 Fax: 029 2074 5306 Email: tomlinsons@cardiff.ac.uk — MB ChB (Hons.) Sheff. 1968; MRCP (UK) 1971; MD Sheff. 1976; FRCP Lond. 1982; FMedSci 1998. Vice-Chancellor Univ. Wales Coll. Med. Cardiff; Hon. Cons. Phys., Cardiff & Vale NHS Trust. Specialty: Diabetes. Socs: Pres. Assn. Physicians Gt. Britain & Irel. 2002-2003 (Hon. Sec. & Treas. 1988-1998); GMC Team Ldr., Peninsula Med. Sch.; Vice-Chairm. UUK Health Comm. Prev: Prof. (Med.) & Dean (Fac. Med. Dent. & Nursing) Univ. Manch.; Hon. Cons. Phys. Manch. Roy. Infirm.; Reader (Med.) & Wellcome Trust.

TOMLINSON, Stewart John Medwyn Surgery, Moores Road, Dorking RH4 2BG Tel: 01306 882422 Fax: 01306 742280 — MB BS Lond. 1994; DFFP 1997 Lond.; MRCGP (Distinc.) 1998 Lond.; DRCOG 1997 Lond.; BSc. (Hons.) Lond. 1991, MB BS 1994. GP Princip. Dorking Surrey. Specialty: Gen. Pract. Socs: RCGP; RCOG.

TOMLINSON, Sydney Brian (retired) 10 Tetley Court, Hollins Hall, Hampsthwaite, Harrogate HG3 2GP — MB ChB Leeds 1944; MRCGP 1953. Prev: Regist. Dept. Paediat. & Child Health Gen. Infirm. Leeds.

TOMMEY, Martin Frederick Miller Street Surgery, Miller Street, Off Kings Street, Newcastle ST5 1JD Tel: 01782 711618 Fax: 01782 713940 — MB BS Lond. 1971; MRCS Eng. LRCP Lond. 1971.

TOMMINS, Kathryn Sarah Morrill Street Health Centre, Holderness Road, Hull HU9 2LJ Tel: 01482 320046; 18 Hambling Drive, Beverley HU17 9GD — MB ChB Manch. 1978; MRCGP 1982. GP Hull.

TOMNAY, Joyce 16 Mansion House Road, Glasgow G41 3DN — MB ChB Aberd. 1973.

TOMOS, Hywel Wynn New Cross Surgery, 48 Sway Road, Morriston, Swansea SA6 6HR Tel: 01792 771419; Port Reath, Balaclava Road, Glais, Swansea SA7 9HH — MB BCh Wales 1991; MRCGP 1995. Specialty: Gen. Pract.

TOMPKIN, David Michael Bankes Woodlands Surgery, 5 Woodlands Road, Redhill RH1 6EY Tel: 01737 761343 Fax: 01737 770804; 5 Cronks Hill Road, Redhill RH1 6LY Tel: 01737 247659 — MB BS Lond. 1974 (St. Thos.) MRCS Eng. LRCP Lond. 1974. Prev: Med. Off. Port Saunders Hosp. Newfld.; Ho. Off. (Orthop.) & SHO (O & G) St. Thos. Hosp. Lond.

TOMPKINS, David Stewart Leeds Public Health Laboratory, Bridle Path, York Road, Leeds LS15 7TR Tel: 0113 264 5011 Fax: 011320 603655 — MB ChB Birm. 1976; FRCPath 1994, M 1982. Cons. Microbiol. Pub. Health Laborat. Leeds.; Hon. Cons. Leeds Teachg. Hosp.s NHS Trust. Specialty: Med. Microbiol. Socs: Assn. Med. Microbiol.; Hon. Sec. Assn. of Med. Microbiologists 1995-1997; Vice-Pres. Acd. Clin. Microbiologists (India). Prev: Cons. Microbiol. Bradford; Lect. Univ. Leeds.

TOMPKINS, Geoffrey David (retired) The Thatched Cottage, Chignal Smealy, Chelmsford CM1 4SZ Tel: 01245 441034 Fax: 01245 441034 Email: tompkins@tinyworld.co.uk — MB BS Lond. 1955 (Lond. Hosp.) JP.; Dep. Coronor E. Dist. Gt Lond. Area. Prev: Ho. Surg. Hillingdon Hosp.

TOMPKINSON, John Michael Park Surgery, 60 Ilkeston Road, Heanor DE75 7DX Tel: 01773 531011 Fax: 01773 534440 — BM BS Nottm. 1988; BMedSci (Hons.) Nottm. 1995. Specialty: Gen. Pract.

TOMS, Mr Andoni Paul The Old Rectory, 6 Church Road, Swainsthorpe, Norwich NR14 8PH — MB BS Lond. 1991; FRCS Eng. 1995; FRCR 2000. Cons. Radiologist, Norf. & Norwich Univ. Hosp. NHS Trust Norwich. Specialty: Radiol. Prev: Regist. (Radiol.) Addenbrooke's NHS Trust Camb.

TOMS, Andrew David Royal Shrewsbury Hospital, Shrewsbury SY3 8XQ; 26 Acton Burnell, Shrewsbury SY5 7PQ — MB ChB Birm. 1992. Specialty: Orthop.

TOMS, David Anthony 2 Regent Street, Nottingham NG1 5QB Tel: 0115 947 4755 Fax: 0115 950 8174; The Manor House, Main St, Aslockton, Nottingham NG13 9AL Tel: 01949 850374 — MB BS Lond. 1960 (Univ. Coll. Hosp. Lond.) MRCS Eng. LRCP Lond. 1960; DObst RCOG 1962; DCH Eng. 1963; MRCP Lond. 1967; DPM 1968; FRCPsych. 1982, M 1972. Indep. Psychiat. Notts.; Emerit. Cons. Psychiat. N. HA. Specialty: Gen. Psychiat. Socs: Soc. Psychosomatic Research. Soc.; Nottm. M-C Soc. Prev: Sen. Regist. (Psychiat.) St. Geo. Hosp. Lond.; Regist. (Psychiat.) Claybury Hosp. Woodford Bridge, Essex; Ho. Phys. Univ. Coll. Hosp. Lond.

TOMS, Elaine Stella Greenwood and Sneinton Family Medical Centre, 249 Sneinton Dale, Sneinton, Nottingham NG3 7DQ Tel: 0115 950 1854 Fax: 0115 958 0044; 12 Nuthall Grove, Glen Parva, Leicester LE2 9HU — MB ChB Birm. 1982; MB ChB (Hons.) Birm. 1982; MRCP (UK) 1985; MRCGP 1989. Prev: Regist. Rotat. (Med.) Kettering & Leicester Hosps.; SHO (Rotat.) City Hosp. Nottm.

TOMS, Graham Christopher Oldchurch Hospital, Romford RM7 0BE Tel: 01708 746090; 47 Beacontree Road, Leytonstone, London E11 3AX — MD Manch. 1989; MB ChB 1979; MRCP (UK) 1982. Lect. (Metab. & Endocrinol.) Lond. Hosp. Med. Coll.

TOMS, Graham Ralph Parade Surgery, The Parade, Liskeard PL14 6AF Tel: 01579 342667 Fax: 01579 340650; Tremellick Cottage, St. Cleer, Liskeard PL14 6RP Tel: 01579 343306 — MB BS Lond. 1984; DRCOG 1987; MRCGP 1988; DA (UK) 1990. Prev: Trainee GP Chertsey VTS; Ho. Surg. Univ. Coll. Hosp. Lond.; Ho. Phys. Roy. Devon & Exeter Hosp.

TOMS, Julian Stanley Martyn Portree Medical Centre, Portree, Isle of Skye IV51 9BZ Tel: 01478 612013 Fax: 01478 612340; Creag-a-Charran, Staffin Road, Portree IV51 9HP Tel: 01478 612961 — (Camb. & St. Bart.) MA Camb. 1971, MB BChir 1970; DCH Eng. 1972; DObst RCOG 1973; MRCGP 1974; MRCP (UK) 1984; DFFP 1996; FRCP Ed. 1997. GP Portree, Isle of Syke; Clin. Asst. Portree Hosp.; GP Trainer, Portree Med. Centre. Specialty: Neurol. Prev: SHO (Psychiat.) Craig Dunain Hosp. Inverness; SHO (Paediat.) Roy. Cornw. Hosp. Truro; SHO (Neurol.) Dundee Roy. Infirm.

TOMS, Mark Edwin 43 Woburn Av, Farnborough GU14 7HQ — MB ChB Sheff. 1997.

TOMS, Rhinedd Margaret The Lakes Mental Health Centre, Turner Road, Colchester CO4 5JL Tel: 01206 228740 Fax: 01206 844182; 45 Oaks Drive, Colchester CO3 3PS Tel: 01206 549547 — MB BChir Camb. 1967 (Camb. & Westm.) BChir 1967; MRCS Eng. LRCP Lond. 1967; MA Camb. 1968; FRCPsych 1993, M 1981. Cons. Psychiat. N. Essex Ment. Health Partnership NHS Trust; Hon. Cons. Psychiat. St. Luke's Hosp. for Clergy Lond. Specialty: Gen. Psychiat. Socs: BMA. Prev: Sen. Regist. (Psychiat.) Severalls Hosp. Colchester; Supernum. Regist. (Psychiat.) Severalls Hosp. Colchester; Med. Off. (Staff Health) Lambeth Lewisham & Southwark AHA.

TOMSON, Charles Richard Vernon Department of Renal Medicine, Southmead Hospital, Bristol BS10 5NB Tel: 0117 959 5225 Fax: 0117 950 8677 Email: tomson_c@southmead.swest.nhs.uk; 40 Caledonia Place, Bristol BS8 4DN — MB BCh Oxf. 1981 (Oxford) FRCP (UK); MRCP (UK) 1984; DM Oxf. 1990. Cons. Nephrol. Southmead Hosp. Bristol. Specialty: Nephrol. Socs: Educ. Sec. Renal Assn.; Mem., Renal Assn. Train. Educat. & Research Subcomm.; Mem., Roy. Coll. Phys.s (Lond.) CPD Advisery Gp. Prev: Cons. Nephrol. St. Bart. Hosp. Lond.; Lect. (Med.) Leicester Univ.; MRC Train. Fell. RVI Newc. u. Tyne.

TOMSON, Christopher Mark Calder Blackthorn Surgery, 73 Station Road, Netley Abbey, Southampton SO31 5AE Tel: 023 8045 3110 Fax: 023 8045 2747; 33 Old Priory Close, Hamble, Southampton SO31 4QP Tel: 02380 457950 Fax: 01703 457950 Email: marktomson@compuserve.com — MB BS Lond. 1985; MRCGP 1993. GP Trainer.

TOMSON, David Peter Carey Collingwood Surgery, Hawkeys Lane, North Shields NE29 0SF Tel: 0191 257 1779 Fax: 0191 226 9909; 20 Rothbury Terrace, Heaton, Newcastle upon Tyne NE6 5XH — BM BCh Oxf. 1985; BA (Hons.) Camb. 1982; MRCGP 1990. GP Partner; Hon. Lect. Newc. Med. Sch.; Vice-Chairm. Riveside PCG.

TOMSON, Michael John Francis 72 Southgrove Road, Sheffield S10 2NQ — MB BS Lond. 1982 (Univ. Camb. & Lond. Hosp.) BA Camb. 1979; DCH RCP Lond. 1986; Cert. Family Plann. JCC 1987; DRCOG 1987; MRCGP 1989. GP; CME Tutor; VTS Tutor. Specialty: Gen. Pract. Prev: Regist. (Child Psychiat.) Tavistock Clinic Lond.; SHO (Paediat. & Community Paediat.) Paddington & N. Kensington HA; SHO Rotat. (Med.) Romford.

TOMSON, Peter Riley Vernon (retired) The Abbots House, Abbots Langley WD5 0AR Tel: 01923 264946 Email: peter.tomson@btinternet.com — MB BChir Camb. 1950 (Camb. & Univ. Coll. Hosp.) DObst RCOG 1954; FRCGP 1973, M 1961. Prev: Capt. RAMC.

TONER, Christopher Charles 3 Ridgeway Crescent Gardens, Orpington BR6 9QH — BM Soton. 1986.

TONER, Geraldine Gertrude 3 Laurel Park, Randalstown, Antrim BT41 3HJ — MB BCh BAO Belf. 1975; DCH Eng. 1979. Prev: GP. Antrim Health Centre Antrim.

TONER, Mr Joseph Gerard The Ulster Hospital, Paediatric Department, Belfast BT16 0RH Tel: 028 9056 4812 Fax: 028 9026 3594 — MB BCh BAO Belf. 1979; FRCS Ed. 1983. Cons. (Otolaryngol.) Ulster Hosp. Dundonald, Belf. City Hosp.; Hon. Sen. Lect., Queens Univ., Belf.; Director N. Irel. Cochlear Implant Centre. Specialty: Otolaryngol. Socs: Politer Soc.; Collegieum. Prev: Sen. Regist. (Otolaryngol.) Belf. City Hosp.

TONER, Joseph Michael St Woolos Hospital, Newport NP20 4SZ Tel: 01633 238317; 13 Dorallt Close, Henllys, Cwmbran NP44 6EY Tel: 01633 480256 — MB BS Lond. 1977; BSc (Hons.) Lond. 1974; FRCP (UK) 1997, M 1980. Cons. Phys. Roy. Gwent & St. Woolos Hosp. Newport. Specialty: Gen. Med.; Care of the Elderly; Rehabil. Med. Prev: Cons. Geriat. Med. St. Woolos Hosp. Newport.

TONER, Professor Peter Gilmour Department of Histopathology, Cheltenham General Hospital, Sandford Road, Cheltenham GL53 7AN — MB ChB Glas. 1965; FRCPath 1984, M 1971; DSc Glas. 1972; FRCP Glas. 1984, M 1982. Cons. Histopath., Gloucestershire Hosps. NHS Trust; Prof. Emerit., The Queens Univ. of Belf. Specialty: Histopath. Socs: Path. Soc. GB & Irel.; Assn. of Clin. Pathologists; Internat. Acad. of Pathologists. Prev: Musgrave Prof. Path. Qu. Univ. Belf.; Prof. (Path.) Univ. Glas.; Vis. Prof. (Path.) Univ. Colorado Med. Centre Denver USA.

TONES, Brian John Silsden Health Centre, Elliott Street, Silsden, Keighley BD20 0DG Tel: 01535 652447 Fax: 01535 657296; Low Shann Farm, High Spring Gardens Lane, Keighley BD20 6LN Tel: 01535 600001 — MB ChB Birm. 1973 (Birmingham) MRCGP 1978. GP; Course Organiser Airedale VTS; Clin. Asst. (Cardiol.).

TONG, David (retired) 18 Selborne Road, Sidcup DA14 4QY Tel: 020 8300 1032 — MRCS Eng. LRCP Lond. 1966 (Guy's) BSc (Hons.) Anat. 1963, MB BS Lond. 1966; MRCP (UK) 1972; DMRT Eng. 1974; FRCR 1976; FRCP Lond. 1992. Prev: Cons. (Radiother. & Oncol.) Guy's & St Thomas' Hosp. NHS Trust.

TONG, Grant Ying Kit Consultant Anaesthetist, Inverclyde Royal Hospital, Larkfield Road, Greenock PA16 0XN — MB ChB Glas. 1989; FRCS Glas. 1995; FRCS Glas. 1995; FRCA 1997; FRCA 1997. Specialist Regist. (Anaesth.) Glas. Specialty: Anaesth. Prev: SHO (Anaesth.) Glas.; SHO (Surg.) Monklands Hosp. Airdrie; SHO (A & E) West. Infirm. Glas.

TONG, Jeffrey Leighton, Maj. RAMC Frimley Park Hospital, Portsmouth Rd, Camberley GU16 7UJ Tel: 01276 604604; 2 Elton House, Rodney Place, Clifton, Bristol BS8 4HZ Tel: 0117 923 8691 — MB ChB Birm. 1991; DA (UK) 1996; FRCA (UK) 1998. Specialist Regist. (Anaest.) Frimley Pk. Hosp. Surrey. Specialty: Anaesth. Socs: Med. Defence Union; Train. Mem. Assn. AnE.h.; BPAS. Prev: Specialist Regist. (Anaesth.) John Radcliffe Hosp. Oxf.; Specialist Regist. (Anaesth.) Bristol Roy. Infirm.; SHO (Anaesth.) Frimley Pk. Hosp. Camberley.

TONG, Nigel Anthony The Barn, Back Lane, Aughton, Ormskirk L39 6SX — MB ChB Liverp. 1986.

TONG, Terence 4 Neville Drive, London N2 0QR Tel: 020 8455 4488 — MB BCh BAO NUI 1983; LRCPI & LM, LRCSI & LM 1983. Socs: BMA. Prev: Ho. Off. (Urol. & Surg.) Oldham Roy. Infirm.; Ho. Off. (Med.) Oldham & Dist. Gen. Hosp. & Oldham Roy. Infirm.

TONG, Timothy 4 Neville Drive, London N2 0QR — MB BS Lond. 1992.

TONG, William The Binfield Practice, Binfield Health Centre, Terrace Road North, Bracknell RG42 5JG Tel: 01344 425434 Fax: 01344 301843; 7 Caswall Close, Binfield, Bracknell RG42 4EF Tel: 01344 422734 Email: willtong@mcmail.com — MB BS Lond. 1982 (Westm. Hosp.) BSc (Hons.) Biochem. Lond. 1977. Company Occupat. Health Phys. Bracknell. Specialty: Gen. Pract. Socs: Brit. Assn. Sport & Med.; Brit. Med. Acupunct. Soc.; Assoc. Mem. Soc. Occupat. Med.

TONGE, Ann Elizabeth 118 Banstead Road S., Sutton SM2 5LJ — MB ChB Bristol 1981.

TONGE, Anne Rogerson 8 Dartford Road, Sevenoaks TN13 3TQ Tel: 01732 452046 — MB ChB Birm. 1959. Indep. Analyt. Psychother. Kent.

TONGE, Barbara Lesley (retired) Heathfield, Tarvin Road, Littleton, Chester CH3 7DF Tel: 01244 335059 — MB BS Lond. 1955 (Roy. Free) MRCS Eng. LRCP Lond. 1955; DCH Eng. 1963. Prev: GP Chester.

TONGE, Gillian Margaret Peterloo Medical Centre, 133 Manchester Old Road, Middleton, Manchester M24 4DZ Tel: 0161 643 5005 Fax: 0161 643 7264 — MB ChB Manch. 1992; DCH RCP Lond. 1995; DRCOG 1995; MRCGP 1996. Trainee GP Birch Hill Hosp. Rochdale VTS. Specialty: Gen. Pract.

TONGE, Helen Wilson (retired) 32 Eslington Terrace, Newcastle upon Tyne NE2 4RN Tel: 0191 281 1816 — (Edin.) MB ChB Ed. 1943. Prev: Clin. Med. Off. S. Tyneside HA.

TONGE, Hilda Margaret Royal United Hospital, Combe Park, Bath BA1 3NG Tel: 01225 428331; 2 Widcombe Crescent, Bath BA2 6AH — MB BS Lond. 1978; PhD Rotterdam 1987; MRCOG 1988; FRCOG 2000. Cons. O & G Roy. United. Hosp. Bath. Specialty: Obst. & Gyn. Socs: BMA & Brit. Med. Ultrasound Soc. Prev: Sen. Regist. (O & G) Roy. United Hosp. Bath & Bristol; Research Regist. Qu. Charlotte's Matern. Hosp. Lond.; Regist. (O & G) Bristol Matern. Hosp.

TONGE, Jennifer Louise (retired) House of Commons, Westminster, London SW1A 0AA Tel: 020 7219 4596 Fax: 020 7219 4596 Email: tonge@cix.co.uk; 5 Bush Road, Kew Green, Richmond TW9 3AN Tel: 020 8948 1649 Email: j.tonge@cix.co.uk — (Univ. Coll. Hosp.) MB BS Lond. 1964; MFFP 1993; FFFP (Hon.) 2002. MP. Prev: Sen. Managem. Community Health Servs. W. Lond. Healthcare Trust.

TONGE, Jeremy Marcus Adrian Elm Hayes Surgery, Paulton, Bristol BS39 7QJ Tel: 01761 413155 Email: jeremy@tonge.co.uk — MB BS Lond. 1993 (St Mary's) DRCOG 1995; DFFP 1995; MRCOG 1998. SHO (Obst. & Gyn.) Basingstoke.; SHO (Obst. & Gyn.) Winchester NHS Trust; Sen. SHO. (Obst & Gyn.) Chichester; GP Paulton / Chippenham; GP Regist. Bath. Specialty: Obst. & Gyn. Prev: SHO (Paediat. & Neonates) Poole NHS Trust; SHO Capital Coast Health, NZ; SHO (O & G) Soton. NHS Trust.

TONGE, John Riverside Health Surgery, Riverside Walk, Retford DN22 6AA Tel: 01777 706661; Longacre, 69 Town St, Lound, Retford DN22 8RT Tel: 01777 817982 — MB ChB Sheff. 1973; MRCP (UK) 1978. GP Princip.; GP Adviser to Doncaster & Bassetlaw Acute Hosps. NHS Trust. Socs: Exec. Comm., Bassetlaw PCT. Prev: Regist. (Med.) Roy. Infirm. Sheff.; Non-Exec. Dir. Bassetlaw Hosp. & Community Serv. Trust.

TONGE, Kathryn Anne The Hillingdon Hospital, Pield Heath Rd, Uxbridge UB8 3NN Tel: 01895 238282 Fax: 01895 279215 — MB BS Lond. 1988 (Univ. Oxf. & St. Mary's Hosp. Med. Sch.) MA (Hons.) Oxf. 1989, BA (Hons.) 1985; MRCP (UK) 1991. Cons. (Gastoenterol.) The Hillingdon Hosp. Uxbridge. Specialty: Gastroenterol.; Gen. Med. Prev: Sen Regist. Chelsea & Westminster & St Marks Hosp.

TONGE, Keith Angus Dept. Radiology, St Thomas' Hospital, London SE1 7EH Tel: 020 7928 9292 Ext: 2436 Fax: 020 7261 0405 Email: keith.tonge@gstt.sthames.nhs.uk; 5 Bush Road, Kew, Richmond TW9 3AN Tel: 0208 948 1649 Fax: 0208 948 1649 — MB BS Lond. 1965 (Univ. Coll. Hosp.) BSc Lond. 1962; MRCS Eng. LRCP Lond. 1965; DMRD Eng. 1970; FFR 1973; FRCR 1975. Cons. Radiol. Guy's & St. Thos. Hosp. Trust. Specialty: Radiol. Socs: RSM Sect. Radiol. Counc.lor. Prev: Research Fell. Roy. Marsden Hosp. Lond.; Sen. Regist. (Radiol.) United Birm. Hosps.

TONGE, Mary Francella Rebecca 85 Yvonne Road, Redditch B97 5HT — MB ChB Birm. 1978.

TONI, Eric Edward The Surgery, 106 Cowper Road, Rainham RM13 9TS Tel: 01708 550276 Fax: 01708 552620 — MB BS London 1977; MB BS London 1977.

TONKIN, Lisa Vivyan Minster Cottage, Highmoor Hill, Caldicot, Newport NP26 5PF — MB BCh Wales 1998.

TONKIN, Ralph William (retired) 11 Muirton, Aviemore PH22 1SF — MB ChB Ed. 1945; FRCPath 1974, M 1963; FRCP Ed. 1979, M 1976. Prev: Sen. Lect., Dept. Bacteriol. Univ. Edin. Roy. Infirm. Edin.

TONKIN, Richard Douglas (retired) 66 Noel Road, Islington, London N1 8HB Tel: 020 7359 1279 — MB BS Lond. 1939 (St. Geo.) MRCS Eng. LRCP Lond. 1939; FRCP Lond. 1955, M 1945; MD Lond. 1946. Pres. Research Counc. for Complementary Med. Prev: Dir. Diagn. Unit Lond. Clinic.

TONKS, Alison Mary BMJ Editorial, BMA House, Tavistock Square, London WC1H 9JR Email: atonks@bmj.com — MB ChB Bristol 1985; FRCA 1990. Freelance Edr. and writer, BMJ Lond.

TONKS, Clive Malcolm (retired) 10 Anselm Road, Pinner HA5 4LJ Tel: 020 8428 3894 Fax: 020 8621 4764 — MB ChB Leeds 1955; FRCP Lond. 1980, M 1959; DPM Lond. 1962; FRCPsych 1974, M 1971. Prev: Cons. Psychiat. St. Mary's Hosp. & Med. Sch. Lond.

TONKS, Joyce Margaret (retired) 10 Anselm Road, Pinner HA5 4LJ Tel: 020 8428 3894 Fax: 020 8621 4764 — MB ChB Leeds 1957. Prev: SCMO Harrow DHA.

TONKS, Wendy Stella Saltaire Medical Centre, Richmond Road, Shipley BD18 4RX Tel: 01274 593101 Fax: 01274 772588 — MB BS Newc. 1981; DRCOG 1986; MRCGP 1996. Specialty: Gen. Pract.

TONNESMANN, Margarete Elisabeth Hedwig Pauline 41A Aberdare Gardens, London NW6 3AL Tel: 020 7624 5688 — MD Kiel 1958 (Gottingen, Bonn, Dusseldorf & Hamburg) State Exam. Med. Hamburg 1951. Hon. Cons. Psychother. & Med. Sociologist King's Coll. Hosp. Lond. Specialty: Psychother. Socs: Assoc. Mem. Brit. Psychoanal. Soc.

TONUCCI, Daniela Francesca Maria 26 Windsor Road, London N3 3SS — MB ChB Bristol 1995.

TOOBY, David John 34 The Ridgeway, Chatham ME4 6PD Tel: 01634 45979 — MRCS Eng. LRCP Lond. 1959 (St. Bart.) BSc Lond. 1956, MB BS 1959; DObst RCOG 1962.

TOOGOOD, Andrew Alan 10 Finbury Close, Olton, Solihull B92 8DH — MB ChB Manch. 1987; MRCP (UK) 1991. Clin. Research Fell. (Hon. Regist.) Christie Hosp. NHS Trust Manch. Specialty: Endocrinol. Socs: Soc. Endocrinol. & Growth Hormone Research Soc.

TOOGOOD, Mr Giles John St James University Hospital, Leeds LS9 7TF; 81 North Lane, Roundhay, Leeds LS8 2QJ — BM BCh Oxf. 1986; FRCS Ed. 1990; DM 1995; FRCS (Gen) 1996. Cons. (Surg.). Specialty: Gen. Surg.; Transpl. Surg.

TOOGOOD, Shirley Joyce (retired) 31 Kendal End Road, Barnt Green, Rednal, Birmingham B45 8PY Tel: 0121 445 2627 — MB BS Lond. 1956 (King's Coll. Hosp.) Dist. Med. Off. W. Birm. HA. Prev: SCM Birm. HA.

TOOKE, Professor John Edward Peninsula Medical School, ITTC Building, Tamar Science Park, Davy Road, Plymouth PL6 8BX Tel: 01752 764263 Fax: 01752 764226 Email: john.tooke@pms.ac.uk — BM BCh Oxf. 1974 (Oxford) MRCS Eng. LRCP Lond. 1974; DM Oxf. 1982, MA, MSc 1974; MRCP (UK) 1977; FRCP Eng. 1993; DSC Oxon. 1998. Dean Pennisula Med. Sch.; Hon. Cons. Phys. Roy. Devon & Exeter Hosp.; Prof. (Vasc. Med.) Univ. Exeter. Specialty: Diabetes; Vasc. Med. Socs: Pres. Brit. MicroCirc. Soc.; Acad. of Med. Sci.; Vice-Pres., Europ. Soc. for Microcirculation. Prev: Wellcome Sen. Lect. Char. Cross & Westm. Med. Sch. Lond.; Hon. Cons. Phys. Endocrine Unit Char. Cross Hosp. Lond.; Lect. (Med.) Leeds Gen. Infirm.

TOOKMAN, Adrian Jeffrey Marie Curie Hospice Hampstead, 11 Lyndhurst Gardens NW3 5NS Tel: 020 7830 2905 Email: adrian.tookman@mariecurie.org.uk — MB BS Lond. 1976 (Char. Cross) MRCS Eng. LRCP Lond. 1976; FRCP 1982. Med. Director Marie Curie Hospice Hampstead; Cons. Palliat. Med. Roy. Free Hosp. NHS Trust Lond. Specialty: Palliat. Med. Prev: Regist. (Rheum.) Whittington Hosp. Lond.; Resid. Med. Off. Roy. North. Hosp. Lond.; SHO (Med. Ophth.) St. Thos. Hosp. Lond.

TOOLEY, Mr Alan Hunter (retired) 26 The Avenue, Linthorpe, Middlesbrough TS5 6PD Tel: 01642 818750 Fax: 01642 822949 — MB BS Lond. 1953 (King's Coll. Hosp.) MRCS Eng. LRCP Lond. 1953; FRCS Eng. 1957. Prev: Cons. Surg. S. Tees Acute Trust Hosps.

TOOLEY, Deborah Ann Department of Anaesthetics, St. James University Hospital, Beckett St., Leeds LS9 7TF; The Lodge, Potterton, Barwick in Elmet, Leeds LS15 4NN Tel: 0113 281 1186 Fax: 0113 281 1186 — MB ChB Auckland 1990; MB ChB Auckland 1989; Dip. Obs. Auckland 1993; DA (Eng.) 1996. Specialist Regist. (Anaesth.) St. James Univ. Hosp. Leeds. Specialty: Anaesth.; Intens. Care. Socs: Assn. Anaesth.; Intens. Care Soc. Prev: SHO (Anaesth.) W. Yorks.; Regist. (A & E) UK & New Zealand; SHO (O & G) New Zealand.

TOOLEY, Ian Russell Littlewick Medical Centre, 42 Nottingham Road, Ilkeston DE7 5PR Tel: 0115 932 5229 Fax: 0115 932 5413 — MB BS Newc. 1983; DRCOG 1986; MRCGP 1987. Trainee GP Northumbria VTS.

TOOLEY, James Ross — MB BS Lond. 1993; MRCPCH; MRCP (UK) 1996. Cons. (Neonatal Med.). Specialty: Paediat. Prev: Clin. Research Fell. Univ. of Bristol; Specialist Regist. (Paediat.) Addenbrookes Hosp. Camb.; Regist. (Paediat.) Norf. & Norwich Hosp.

TOOLEY, Peter John Hocart PT Pharma Consultancy (Gernsey) Ltd., Les Miellies, L'Ancresse, Vale, Guernsey GY3 5AZ Tel: 01481 242607 Fax: 01481 242505 Email: tooleyp@aol.com; Les Mielles, L'Ancresse, Vale, Guernsey GY3 5AZ Tel: 01481 244543 Email: tooleyp@aol.com — MB BS Lond. 1964 (Lond. Hosp.) MRCS Eng. LRCP Lond. 1963; DObst 1965; MRCGP 1971; DMJ Soc. Apoth. Lond. 1981; DFFP RCOG 1993; LLM (Wales) 1994. Cons. Pharmaceut. Med.; Contract Med. Dir. Sankyo Pharma (UK); Contract Med. Dir. Alliance Pharmaceut.; Contract Med. Dir. Mayne plc. Specialty: Pharmaceutical Medicine. Socs: Fell. Roy. Soc. Med.; BMA; Brit. Acad. Forens. Sci. Prev: Head of Med. Affairs Janssen-Cilag Ltd (UK); GP Twyford.

TOOLIS, Francis Haematology Department, Dumfries & Galloway Royal Infirmary, Bankend Road, Dumfries DG1 4AP Tel: 01387 246246 Fax: 01387 241344 Email: f.toolis@dgri.scot.nhs.uk — MB ChB Ed. 1972; FRCP (E,G,L), FRCPath, MBA. Cons. Haemat. Dumfries & Galloway Roy. Infirm. Specialty: Haematology. Socs: Coll. of Amer. Pathologists; Amer. Soc. of Hematology; Europ. Soc. of Haemat.

TOOMEY, Peter John York District Hospital, Wiggington Road, York YO31 8HE Tel: 01904 631313 Email: peter.j.toomey@excha.yhs-tr.northy.nhs.uk — MB BS Lond. 1983; FFA RCSI 1989. Cons. Anaesth. York Health Servs. NHS Trust. Specialty: Anaesth. Prev: Cons. Anaesth. Stoke Mandeville Hosp. Aylesbury; Sen. Regist. (Anaesth.) Yorks. RHA.

TOOMEY, Mr William Francis (retired) 23 Allander Drive, Torrance, Glasgow G64 4LA Tel: 01360 620410 — MB ChB Glas. 1946 (Univ. Glas.) FRFPS Glas. 1949; FRCS Glas. 1962. Prev: Cons. Surg. Roy. Alexandra Hosp. Paisley.

TOON, Christiane Gertrud Erika 51 Gorsebank Road, Hale Barns, Altrincham WA15 0BB — MD Hamburg 1962; State Exam. Med. Hamburg 1961; Dip. Anaesth. Hamburg 1969. Assoc. Specialist (Anaesth.) Wythenshawe Hosp. Manch. Specialty: Anaesth.

TOON, Peter Dennis Canterbury Health Centre, 26 Old Dover Road, Canterbury CT1 2LS Tel: 01227 452444 Email: petertoon@aol.com — MRCS Eng. LRCP Lond. 1977 (King's Coll. Hosp.) AKC 1974; BSc (1st cl. Hons.) Lond. 1974, MB BS 1977; DPMSA (Distinc.) 1982; MSc Oxf. 1983; DCH RCP Lond. 1983; MRCGP 1984; Cert Med Educat (Distinc. Distance Learning) OU 1999. GP Asst. Specialty: Gen. Pract. Special Interest: ethics, primary care Developm. outside UK, IT in Gen. Pract. Socs: Grad. Mem. Brit. Psychol. Soc.; Balint Soc.; Inst. of Teachg. and Learning. Prev: GP Princip. Hackney Lond. E8; Edr. RCGP Pub.ations; Educat. Facilitator LIZEI Progr. N. Thames.

TOON, Philip Gerald Mulberry House, Cox Lane, Rossett, Wrexham LL12 0BH — MB ChB Manch. 1974; MRCOG 1982; T(OG) 1991.

TOONE, Brian Kenneth 4 Grove Park, Camberwell, London SE5 8LT Tel: 020 7733 3499 Email: brian.toone@btinternet.com — (St. Geo.) MB BS Lond. 1962; MRCP (UK) 1967; MPhil Lond. 1973; FRCPsych 1988, M 1973; FRCP Lond. 1988. Hon. Cons. Psychiat. Maudsley & Bethlem Roy. Hosps.; Hon. Sen. Lect. Inst. Psychiat. Specialty: Gen. Psychiat. Socs: Brit. Neuropsychiat. Assn.; Brit. Assn. Psychopharmacol. Prev: Sen. Regist. & Regist. Maudsley & Bethlem Roy. Hosps. Lond; Lect. & Sen. Lect. Inst. Psychiat.; Cons. Psychiat. Maudsley & Bethlem Roy. Hosps. & King's Coll. Hosp. Lond.

TOONE, Peter Charles St Clements Surgery, Tanner Street, Winchester SO23 8AD Tel: 01962 852211 Fax: 01962 856010 — MB BS Lond. 1970 (King's Coll. Hosp.) MRCS Eng. LRCP Lond. 1971; DCH Eng. 1973; DObst RCOG 1974; MRCGP 1981.

TOONE, Robin Philip Donovan Old Mill Surgery, Marlborough Road, Nuneaton CV11 5PQ Tel: 024 7638 2554 Fax: 024 7635 0047; 97 Milby Drive, Nuneaton CV11 6GD Tel: 01203 385771 — MRCS Eng. LRCP Lond. 1965 (Guy's) DObst RCOG 1967. Prev: Ho. Surg. Putney Hosp.; Cas. Off. Padd. Gen. Hosp.; Obst. Ho. Off. Bromley Hosp.

TOOP, Dorothy Margaret (retired) Auchochan House Flat 79, New Trows Road, Lesmahagow, Lanark ML11 0JS Tel: 01555 890035 Email: bdtoop@compuserve.com — (Univ. Ed.) MB ChB Ed. 1944; DObst RCOG 1967. Prev: Med. Off. Saiburi Christian Hosp. S. Thailand.

TOOP, Kenneth Monro The James Cook University Hospital, Marton Road, Middlesbrough TS4 3BW Tel: 01642 854857 Fax: 01642 854857 Email: ken.toop@stees.nhs.uk; 604 Yarm Road, Eaglescliffe, Stockton-on-Tees TS16 0DQ Tel: 01642 780780 — MB ChB Ed. 1972 (Univ. Ed.) FRCOG 1995, M 1980. Cons. Obst. & Gyn., James Cook Univ. Hosp., Middlesbrough. Specialty: Obst. & Gyn. Special Interest: Endocrinol.; Generaust; Menopause. Socs: Christian Med. Fellowsh. (Exectuive Comm.); N. E. Manopause Gp. (Founder); Brit. Menopause Soc. Prev: Sen. Regist. Manch. & Oldham HAs; Regist. Aberd. Teachg. Hosps.; SHO West. Gen. Hosp. Edin.

TOOP, Michael James Department of Pathology, Harrogate District Hospital, Lancaster Park Road, Harrogate HG2 7SX Tel: 01423 553056 Fax: 01423 553229 Email: miketoop@csi.com —

MB Camb. 1979 (Cambridge) BChir 1978; MRCP (UK) 1983; MRCPath 1986; FRCPath 1996. Cons. Chem. Path. Harrogate HA. Specialty: Chem. Path.; Diabetes; Endocrinol. Prev: Sen. Regist. (Chem. Path.) Birm. HA.

TOOP, Robert Leslie 5 The Elms, Ellington, Morpeth NE61 5LH Tel: 01670 860428 — MB BS Newc. 1970; DObst RCOG 1972; DIH Eng. 1980. Med. Dir. Occupat. Health Med. Servs. Specialty: Occupat. Health. Socs: Assoc. Fac. Occupat. Med. RCP Eng; Soc. Occupat. Med. Newc. Br.. Prev: Phys. Occupat. Health N. Eng. Indust. Health Serv. Newc.

TOOP, William James (retired) 23 Erskine Hill, Polmont, Falkirk FK2 0UH Tel: 01324 715873; Auchlochan House, Flat 79, Lesmahagow, Motherwell ML1 0JS Tel: 01555 890035 Email: bdtoop@compuserve.com — (Univ. Ed.) MB ChB Ed. 1938; DTM & H Ed. 1947. Prev: Med. Off. China Inland Mission Hosp. Dali, Yunnan, China.

TOOR, Mr Karamjit Singh 79a Scotts Road, Southall UB2 5DF Tel: 020 8574 0637 — MB BS Panjab 1966; MB BS Panjab (India) 1966; DO Eng. 1970; FRCS Eng. 1975.

TOORAWA, David Ahmed Lincoln House Surgery, Wolsey Road, Hemel Hempstead HP2 4TU Fax: 01442 244554; The Orchard, 152 St. Johns Road, Hemel Hempstead HP1 1NR Tel: 01442 254366 Fax: 01442 244554 — MB BS Lond. 1967 (Univ. Coll. Hosp.) DObst RCOG 1969; MRCGP 1978. Socs: BMA. Prev: Ho. Surg. (Obst.) Vict. Matern. Hosp. Barnet SHO (Path.) Barnet Gen. Hosp.

TOOSEY, Joyce Brenda Metcalf (retired) Fairways, 8 Wealdhurst Park, Broadstairs CT10 2LD Tel: 0841 860166 — (Lond. Sch. Med. Wom.) MB BS Lond. 1941; MRCS Eng. LRCP Lond. 1941; DPH Eng. 1943. Prev: MOH Blandford Boro. & RD, Wimborne & Cranborne RD & Wimborne UD &.

TOOSY, Ahmed Tahir Coombe Farm, Oaks Road, Croydon CR0 5HL — MB BS Lond. 1994.

TOOSY, Tahir Hafeez The Coppice, West Drive, Carshalton SM5 4EL Tel: 020 8642 2308 — MB BS Punjab 1967 (King Edwd. Med. Coll. Lahore) MB BS Punjab (Pakistan) 1967.

TOOTH, Barbara Park House Medical Centre, 18 Harvist Road, London NW6 6SE Tel: 020 8969 7711 Fax: 020 8969 8880; 37 Arlington Road, Camden, London NW1 7ES — MB BS Lond. 1963 (London Hospital Whitechapel) Socs: Roy. Soc. of Med.

TOOTH, David Roy Kiveton Park Primary Care Centre, Chapel Way, Kiveton Park, Sheffield S26 6QU Tel: 01909 770213 Fax: 01909 772793 — MA (Hons.) Camb. 1989; MB BChir Camb. 1989; DCH RCP Lond. 1992; DFFP 1993; MRCGP 1993.

TOOTH, Elisabeth Ann (retired) 29 Sunningdale Close, Handsworth Wood, Birmingham B20 1LH Tel: 0121 523 8392 — (Univ. Coll. Hosp.) MB BS Lond. 1958; DObst RCOG 1960; FRCOG 1979, M 1965. Prev: Cons. Gyn. & Obst. Sandwell Dist. Gen. Hosp. W. Bromich.

TOOTH, Jacqueline Anne Owlthorpe Medical Centre, Moorthorpe bank, Sheffield S20 6PD Tel: 0114 247 7852 Fax: 0114 248 3691; 53 Ribblesdale Drive, Regency Court, Ridgeway, Sheffield S12 3XE — MB ChB Sheff. 1978; DRCOG 1980.

TOOTH, John Anthony (retired) 17 Chesham Road, Wilmslow SK9 6EZ Tel: 01625 582337 — MB ChB Birm. 1955; Dip. Bact. Lond 1964; FRCPath 1977, M 1965; MRCP Lond. 1968. Cons. Bacteriol. United Manch. Hosps.; Hon. Lect. in Bact. Univ. Manch. Prev: Sen. Bacteriol. Pub. Health Laborat., Soton. Gen. Hosp.

TOOTH, Julie Suzanne 1 Birch Grove, Meir Heath, Stoke-on-Trent ST3 7JN — MB ChB Leeds 1991.

TOOTHILL, Susan Valerie St John's Hill Surgery, 39 St. John's Hill, Sevenoaks TN13 3NT Tel: 01322 663111/663237 Fax: 01322 614867; 73 Pollyhaugh, Eynsford, Dartford DA4 0HE — MB BS Lond. 1980.

TOOVEY, Angela Joy 2 Goldington Road, Bedford MK40 3NG Tel: 01234 351341 Fax: 01234 341464 — MB ChB Manch. 1978; DRCOG 1980; DCH RCP Lond. 1981; MRCGP 1983. Specialty: Community Child Health; Obst. & Gyn.

TOOVEY, Anthony Rupert Goldington Road Surgery, 2 Goldington Road, Bedford MK40 3NG Tel: 01234 351341 — MB ChB Manch. 1978; MRCP (UK) 1981; DRCOG 1986; MRCGP 1987.

TOOZE, Reuben Matthew Dept of Histopathology, Adden Brookes Hospital, Box 235, Hills Rd, Cambridge CB2 2QQ Tel: 01223 217163 Email: tmt22@cam.ac.uk; 11 Milford St, Cambridge CB1 2LP — MB BS Lond. 1992 (St Barts.) PhD Lond. 1998. Specialist Regist. Specialty: Histopath. Prev: Clin Research Fell. Camb Univ.

TOOZS-HOBSON, Mr Philip Milton Brimingham Womens Hosp, Metchley Park, Edgbaston, Birmingham B15 2TG — MB BS Lond. 1989 (St Marys Hosp. Med. Sch.) MRCOG 1994; MFFP 1996. Cons. O&G Brimingham Wom.'s Hosp. Birm. Specialty: Obst. & Gyn. Socs: ICS. Prev: Research Regist. (Urodynamics) King's Coll. Hosp. Lond.; Regist. (O & G) Chelsea & Westm. Hosp. Lond.; SHO (A & E) St. Mary's Hosp. Lond.

TOPA, Giuseppe Nicola Francesco 7 Castle Street, Tunbridge Wells TN1 1XJ — State Exam Perugia 1989.

TOPHAM, Clare Ann Royal Surrey County Hospital, St Luke's Cancer Centre, Egerton Road, Guildford GU2 7XX; Rudgwick Grange, Tismans Common, Horsham RH12 3BS — MB BS Lond. 1967 (Guy's) MRCS Eng. LRCP Lond. 1967; DMRT Eng. 1974; FRCR 1975. Cons. Radiotherap. & Oncol. St Luke's Hosp. Guildford & Crawley. Specialty: Oncol. Socs: BMA. Prev: Regist. & Sen. Regist. (Radiother. & Oncol.) Westm. Hosp. Lond.

TOPHAM, Emma Jane Wild Harrys, Hayes La, Slinfold, Horsham RH13 0SL — BM BCh Oxf. 1997.

TOPHAM, Mr John Harcourt (cons. rooms), Goring Hall Hospital, Bodiam Avenue, Goring-By-Sea, Worthing BN11 4PN Tel: 01903 506699 Fax: 01903 242348 — MRCS Eng. LRCP Lond. 1967 (Guy's) BDS 1963; MB BS Lond. 1967; FRCS Eng. 1972. Cons. ENT Surg. Roy. Sussex Co. Hosp. Brighton, Worthing Hosp. & Roy. Alexandra Childr. Hosp. Brighton. Specialty: Otolaryngol. Socs: Brighton & Sussex M-C Soc.; Fell. Roy. Soc. Med. Prev: Regist. & Sen. Regist. (ENT) Lond. Hosp.; Ho. Surg. & Ho. Phys. Guy's Hosp. Lond.

TOPHAM, Katherine Mary HQ LWCTG(G), Normandy Barracks BFPO 16 — BM Soton. 1985; DFFP 1993.

TOPHAM, Lawrence Garth, OStJ, Surg. Capt. RN Retd. (retired) Tilings, Holt Close, Wickham, Fareham PO17 5EY Tel: 01329 832072 — MB ChB Leeds 1937; MD Leeds 1946; FRCP Ed. 1967, M 1957; MRCP Lond. 1969. Prev: Hon. Phys to HM the Qu./Prof. Med. Roy. Navy & RCP Lond.

TOPHAM, Liam Arthur Top Flat, 9 Sherwood Rise, Nottingham NG7 6JG — BM BS Nottm. 1993.

TOPHAM, Peter Stewart 10 St Agnes Way, Horeston Grange, Nuneaton CV11 6TN — MB ChB Birm. 1988; ChB Birm. 1988.

TOPHAM, Simon Paul James Street Family Practice, 49 James Street, Louth LN11 0JN Tel: 01507 611122 Fax: 01507 610435; 132 Newmarket, Louth LN11 9EN Tel: 01507 610561 Email: simon.topham@virgin.net — MB BS Newc. 1987. GP Partner. Specialty: Sports Med.; Family Plann. & Reproduc. Health.

TOPHILL, Mr Paul Robert Northern General Hospital, Princess Royal Spinal Injuries Unit, Herries Road, Sheffield S5 7AU Tel: 0114 271 5645 Fax: 0114 271 5649 Email: paul.tophill@sth.nhs.uk — MB ChB Leic. 1981 (Leicester) FRCS Eng. 1987; FRCS (Urol.) 1995; MD Sheff. 1997. Cons. Urol. Surg.; Cons. Urol. Surg., Claremount Hosp., Sheff. Specialty: Urol.; Neurol.

TOPIWALA, Nimisha Prakash 7A Station Road, London N21 3SB — MB BS Lond. 1998.

TOPLEY, Elizabeth (retired) 1 Wickens Place, High St, West Malling ME19 6NB Tel: 01732 849442 — MB BS Lond. 1939 (University College) MD Lond. 1952. Prev: Prof. Ibarapa Project Univ. Coll. Hosp. Ibadan, Nigeria.

TOPLEY, Elizabeth Mary Childhealth Service, Mansfield Community Hospital, Stockwellgate, Mansfield NG18 5QJ; 21 Greendale Ave, Edwinstone, Mansfield NG21 9NA Tel: 01623 785198 — MB ChB Sheff. 1978. Specialty: Community Child Health. Socs: MRCGP.

TOPLIS, Mr Philip John Dept. Obstetrics & Gynaecology, Frimley Park Hopital Trust, Camberley GU16 5UJ; Wyck Farm House, Wyck Lane, Wyck, Alton GU34 3AL — MB ChB Bristol 1973 (Bristol University) FRCS Glas. 1979; FRCS Ed. 1979; FRCOG 1993, M 1980. Cons. O & G W. Surrey & NE Hants. HA. Specialty: Obst. & Gyn. Socs: Fell. Roy. Soc. Med.; Brit. Soc. Colpos. & Cerv. Path.; Brit. Soc. Gyn. Endoscopy. Prev: Sen. Regist. John Radcliffe Hosp. Oxf.; Regist. (O & G) Guy's Hosp. & Char. Cross Hosp. Lond.; Resid. Qu. Charlottes & Chelsea Hosp. for Wom. Lond.

TOPP, Dudleigh Oscar, Capt. RAMC Retd. (retired) 21 Old Bincombe Lane, Sutton Poyntz, Weymouth DT3 6NB — MB BS Lond. 1949 (Char. Cross) DMJ Soc. Apoth. Lond. 1962; DPM Eng.

1965; FRCPsych 1980, M 1971; MFCM 1972. Prev: PMO Home Office, Prison Dept.

TOPP, Judith Mary Oak Hill Health Centre, Oak Hill Road, Surbiton KT6 6EN Tel: 020 8399 6622 Fax: 020 8390 4470; 6 King Charles Road, Surbiton KT5 8PY Tel: 020 8399 1004 — MB BS Lond. 1975 (St. Bart.) DCH Eng. 1977; DRCOG 1978; MRCGP 1980. Prev: SHO (Obst.) Northwick Pk. Harrow; SHO (Paediat.) Qu. Mary's Hosp. Childr. Carshalton; Ho. Surg. St. Bart. Hosp. Lond.

TOPPER, Ruth P J Kaye and Partners, Northwick Surgery, 36 Northwick Park Road, Harrow HA1 2NU Tel: 020 8427 1661 Fax: 020 8864 2737 — MB ChB Manch. 1975.

TOPPING, Adam Partington 33 Broughton Way, Rickmansworth WD3 8GW — MB ChB Leic. 1992.

TOPPING, Joanne Liverpool Women's Hospital, Crown Street, Liverpool L8 7SS — MB ChB Liverp. 1984. Specialty: Obst. & Gyn.

TOPPING, Miss Nicola Claire 6 Meadow Walk, Chapel Allerton, Leeds LS7 4RN — MB ChB Leeds 1992; MB ChB (Distinc.) Psychiat. Leeds 1992; DRCOG 1994; MRCOPHTH 1999. Specialist Regist. Yorks. Ophth. Rotat. Prev: SHO (Ophth.) Leeds Gen. Infirm.; SHO (Ophth.) Birm. & Midl. Eye Centre.

TOPPING, Susan 114 Ashtons Green Drive, St Helens WA9 2AT — MB BCh Wales 1980.

TOPPING, Walter Alan Lodge Health, 20 Lodge Manor, Coleraine BT52 1JX Tel: 028 7034 4494 Fax: 028 7032 1759 — MB BCh BAO Belf. 1975; DCH RCPSI 1978; MRCGP 1979. GP Trainer.

TOPPLE, Nicola Anne North Staffordshire Hospital, Newcastle Road, Stoke-on-Trent ST4 6QG — MB ChB Sheff. 1993; FRCS (Royal College of Radiologists) 2001. Specialist Regist. Rotat. (Radiol.) N. Staffs. Specialty: Radiol. Socs: Roy. Coll. Radiol. Prev: SHO (Med.) Roy. Shrewsbury Hosp.

TORABI, Kouros Crownhill Surgery, 103 Crownhill Road, Plymouth PL5 3BN Tel: 01752 771713 — MD Tehran 1967; MD Tehran 1967.

TORBET, Mr Thomas Edgar (retired) 66 Netherblane, Blanefield, Glasgow G63 9JP — MB ChB Glas. 1953; FRCOG 1973, M 1960, DObst 1957; FRCS Ed. 1967. Cons. O & G South. Gen. Hosp. Glas. Prev: Sen. Regist. (O & G) Ayrsh. Centr. Hosp. Irvine.

TORBOHM, Ingo Karl-Heinz Bryn Teg, Gwalchmai, Holyhead LL65 4RB — State Exam Med Lubeck 1990.

TORE, Vidyadhar Baosingh Department of Anaesthesia, Grantham & District Hospital, 101, Manthorpe Road, Grantham NG31 8DW Tel: 01476 565232 Email: anil.tore@ulh.nhs.uk — MB BS Mumbai 1985; DA, MD, University of Mumbia, India; DA, FRCA, Royal College of Anaesthetist; FRCA Lond. 1994. Consultant Anaesthetist. Specialty: Anaesth. Socs: Fell. Roy. Coll. Anaesth.; Assn. of Anaesthetists of Gt. Britain & Irel.

TORKINGTON, Albert Peter James Roseberry Topping, 1 Westgate Drive, Bridgnorth WV16 4QF — MB ChB Ed. 1969.

TORKINGTON, Jared Mill House, Michelham Priory, Upper Dicker, Hailsham BN27 3QN — MB BS Lond. 1991.

TORKINGTON, Mark John 23 Hill Street, Carnforth LA5 9DY — MB ChB Manch. 1987; DCH RCP Lond. 1990. Trainee GP Lancs. VTS. Specialty: Dermat.

TORLESSE, Ruth Mary Treverbyn, Main St., Stillington, York YO61 1LG Tel: 01347 810203 — MB ChB Ed. 1994 (Edinburgh) Specialty: Gen. Pract.

TORLEY, Denis Francis (retired) — MB ChB Glas. 1959; DPM Eng. 1965; MRCPsych 1972. Prev: Cons. Psychiat. Dykebar Hosp. Paisley.

TORLEY, Donna Flat 3/1, 71 Ashley St., Glasgow G3 6HW — MB ChB Glas. 1998.

TORMEY, Vincent Joseph Dept of Immunology, Royal Free Hospital, Pond St, London NW3 2QG Tel: 020 7794 0500 — MB BCh BAO Dub. 1989; BA (Biochemistry) 1991; MRCPI 1992; PhD (Immunology) 1999; MRCPath 2000. Cons. Immunol. Roy. Free Hosp. Lond. Specialty: Immunol.

TORNEY, John James 1 Westland Avenue, Newcastle BT33 0BZ — MB BCh BAO Belf. 1993.

TORODE, Nigel Basil Park Lane Medical Centre, 82 Park Lane, Bedhampton, Havant PO9 3HN; Cambric Cottage, Woodmancote, Emsworth PO10 8RD Tel: 01243 373456 — BM Soton. 1980 (Southampton) DRCOG 1982; MRCGP 1984. Specialty: Gen. Pract.

TORODE, Stewart Arthur, OBE Barnston, Park Close, Fetcham, Leatherhead KT22 9BD — MB ChB Ed. 1966; DPhysMed. Eng. 1971; MRCP (UK) 1976; FRCP Ed. 1990. Cons. Rheumatologist to Hinder Centre, Crowsborough & Royal Sussex County Hospital, Brighton; Cons. Rheumatologist at King Edwd. VIIth Hosp., Midhurst.; Cons. Rheumatologist at Epsom Day Surg. Unit, Epsom, Surrey. Specialty: Rheumatol. Socs: Brit. Soc. Rheum.; Brit. Assn. Rehabil. Med. Prev: Cons. Rheum & Rehabil. DSMRU RAF Headley Ct. Epsom; Cons. Adviser Rheum. & Rehabil. RAF; Med. Dir. & Cons. Rheum. & Rehabil. Horder Centre Arthritis CrowBoro.

TOROK, Zoltan 37A Ladysmith, Gomeldon, Salisbury SP4 6LE — MB ChB Sheff. 1966; MSc Surrey 1968; PhD Lond. 1979; MFOM RCP Lond. 1983. Specialty: Occupat. Health. Socs: Soc. Occupat. Med.; Soc. Clin. Neurophysiol. (EEG).

TOROSSIAN, Feirooz Sinbad Bedros Balham Health Centre, 120 Bedford Hill, London SW12 9HS Tel: 020 8673 1720 Fax: 020 8673 1549; 56 Windermere Avenue, London SW19 3ER — MB ChB Basrah 1980; MRCOG 1991; MRCGP 1994. Specialty: Obst. & Gyn.

TORPEY, Nicholas Peter Addenbrooks Dialysis Centre, Addenbrookes Hospital, Box 118, Hills Rd, Cambridge CB1 1QQ Tel: 01223 245151; 1 Delles ottage, Carmen St, Great Chesterford, Saffron Walden CB10 1NR Tel: 01799 531305 — MB BS Lond. 1994 (St Georges Hospital Medical School London) PhD Camb. 1991; MRCP (UK) 1997. Research Fell. (Nephrol.) Anglia Region, Addenbrookes Hosp. Specialty: Nephrol.; Gen. Med.

TORQUATI, Fabio Roberto Woodlea House Surgery, 1 Crantock Grove, Bournemouth BH8 0HS Tel: 01202 300903 Fax: 01202 304826; 27 Egerton Road, Bournemouth BH8 9AY — MB BS Lond. 1987.

TORR, Mrs Barbara 45 St Werburgh's Road, Chorlton-cum-Hardy, Manchester M21 0UN Tel: 0161 881 6560 — MB ChB Manch. 1951; BDS 1946. Dent. Off. Pk. Hosp. Davyhulme. Prev: Asst. Lect. Dent. Sch. Manch. Univ.; Orthop. Ho. Surg. Manch. Roy. Infirm.; Demonst. Manch. Dent. Hosp.

TORR, James Bernard Doughty 45 St Weyburgh's Road, Chorlton-cum-Hardy, Manchester M21 0UN Tel: 0161 881 6560 — MD Manch. 1957; MB ChB 1948, BDS 1969. Fell. Manch. Med. Soc. Prev: Lect. (Oral Surg.) Manch. Dent. Hosp.; Lect. in Anat. Manch. Univ.; Squadron Ldr. RAF Med. Br.

TORRANCE, Aileen Muriel 7 Fairlight Road, Hythe CT21 4AD Tel: 01303 265787 — MB ChB Ed. 1973; DA Eng. 1977. Clin. Asst. (Anaesth.) William Harvey Hosp. Ashford Kent & St. Martin's Hosp. Canterbury Kent. Specialty: Anaesth.

TORRANCE, Alison Meta Elizabeth Craiglockhart Surgery, 161 Colinton Road, Edinburgh EH14 1BE Tel: 0131 455 8494 Fax: 0131 444 0161 Email: a.torrance@connectfree.co.uk — MB ChB Dundee 1975.

TORRANCE, Caroline Jane Aberdare Hospital, Aberdare CF44 0RF — MB BS Lond. 1982; FRCS Ed. 1986; DRCOG 1989; Dip. GU Med. Soc. Apoth. Lond. 1995; Dip Palliat Med Cardiff 2000. Staff Grade (Palliat. Med.) N. Glam. NHS Trust. Specialty: Palliat. Med. Prev: Clin. Asst. (Genitourin. Med.) Roy. Gwent Hosp. Newport.; Regist. (Radiol.) Manch. AHA; SHO (Gen. Surg.) Northampton Gen. Hosp.

TORRANCE, Ian Leitch 23 Eliot Place, Blackheath, London SE3 0QL — MB ChB Dundee 1980; MRCGP 1986; MFOM RCP (UK) 1993. Cons. Occupat. Phys.; Hon. Sen. Clin. Lect. (Occupat. Med.) Inst. Occupat. Health Univ. Birm. Specialty: Occupat. Health. Socs: Soc. Occupat. Med.; Assoc. of Local Auth. Med. Advisers. Prev: Director of Occcupational Health Roy. Hosp.s NHS Trust Lond.; Gp. Occupat. Health Adviser Nat. Grid Company Lond.; Med. Off. Brit. Coal Gateshead.

TORRANCE, Mr John Daly (retired) 6 St Thomas Road, Lytham St Annes FY8 1JL Tel: 01253 724302 — MB ChB Glas. 1959; FRCS Ed. 1967. Prev: Cons. Orthop. Surg. Vict. Hosp. Blackpool.

TORRANCE, John Malcolm Castle Surgery, 5 Darwin Street, Castle, Northwich CW8 1BU Tel: 01606 74863 Fax: 01606 784847; 5 Darwin Street, Northwich CW8 1BU — MB ChB Manch. 1974; DRCOG 1978; MRCGP 1980.

TORRANCE, Marion Elizabeth 3 Greenbank Crescent, Edinburgh EH10 5TE — MB ChB Manch. 1985; MRCP (UK) 1992; MSc Lond. 1993. Cons. Community Paediat. China. Specialty: Community Child Health. Socs: RCPCH; BACCH. Prev: Cons. Comm. Paed. Nothd.;

Sen. Regist. (Community Child Health) North. & Yorks. Region; SCMO (Paediat.) Camden & Islington.

TORRANCE, Mary Heather (retired) 3 Greenbank Crescent, Edinburgh EH10 5TE Tel: 0131 447 3230 — MB ChB Ed. 1949; MRCP Lond. 1953. Prev: SCMO (Community Med.) Lothian Health Bd.

TORRANCE, Thomas Charles Dover Health Centre, Maison Dieu Road, Dover CT16 1RH Tel: 01304 865544; 51 Crabble Lane, Dover CT17 0NY Tel: 01304 202525 — MB ChB Glas. 1970. Prev: GP Trainer Kirkmuirhill; Med. Regist. StoneHo. Hosp.; Jun. Ho. Off. Glas. Roy. Infirm.

TORRANCE, William Nisbet Spearhead Associates, Spearshill, Tayport DD6 9HT Tel: 01382 552248 — MB ChB St. And. 1963; Dip. Soc. Med. Ed. 1972. Indep. Consultancy (Pub. Health Med.) Spearhead Assocs. Tayport; Hon. Sen. Lect. (Community & Occupat. Med.) Univ. Dundee. Specialty: Pub. Health Med. Socs: BMA & Scott. Soc. Med. Admin.s. Prev: Cons. Pub. Health Med. Tayside HB; Med. Admin. Ninewells Hosp. & Med. Sch. Dundee; Research Fell. (Community Med.) East. RHB (Scotl.).

TORRENS, James Derek Longwater Lane Medical Centre, Longwater Lane, Old Costessey, Norwich NR8 5AH Tel: 01603 742021 Fax: 01603 740271 — MB BCh Belfast 1973; MB BCh Belfast 1973.

TORRENS, Rebecca Louise Lower Mill Cottage, Furnace Lane, Madeley, Crewe CW3 9EU — MB BS Newc. 1996.

TORRES, Maria Do Rosario Carvalho Bellevue Medical Centre, 26 Huntingdon Place, Edinburgh EH7 4AT — Lic Med Coimbra 1980.

TORRIE, Edwin Peter Hodgett X-Ray Department, Royal Berkshire Hospital, London Road, Reading RG1 5AN Tel: 01734 877930; Cranhull Cottage, The Old Orchard, Mill Lane, Calcot, Reading RG31 7RS Tel: 01734 417592 — MB BCh BAO Belf. 1973; DMRD 1981; FRCR 1983. Cons. Radiol. Roy. Berks. Hosp. Reading. Specialty: Radiol.

TORRY, Michael John William Sutton Moors, 1 Overhill Road, Wilmslow SK9 2BE — BM BS Nottm. 1996.

TORRY, Rebecca Bermondsey and Lansdowne Medical Centre, The Surgery, Decima Street, London SE1 4QX Tel: 020 7407 0752 Fax: 020 7378 8209; St. George's Vicarage, 89 Westcombe Pk Road, London SE3 7RZ Tel: 020 8858 3006 — MB Camb. 1980; BChir 1979; DObst RCOG 1982; MRCGP 1983. Gen. Pract. Princip.; Course Organiser, Guys & St. Thomas' GP Vocational Train. Scheme, Lond. SE1.

TOSE, John Melvin Whitley Bay Health Centre, Whitley Road, Whitley Bay NE25 2ND Tel: 0191 253 1113; 13 Ashfield Grove, Whitley Bay NE26 1RT — MB BS Newc. 1972; MRCGP 1976.

TOSE, Jonathan Central Surgery, Stanhope Parade, Heal Gordon St, South Shields NE33 4JP — MB BS Newc. 1994.

TOSELAND, Michael Anthony The Thatched Cottage, 20 Meadow Lane, Little Houghton, Northampton NN7 1AH Tel: 01604 891751 — MB ChB Birm. 1954; MRCS Eng. LRCP Lond. 1954. Med. Adviser KAB seatings Northampton. Prev: Ho. Surg. (O & G) & Ho. Phys. Solihull Hosp.

TOSELAND, Olga Rosemary Stacey House, Hardingstone, Northampton Tel: 01604 61382 — MB ChB Birm. 1954; MRCS Eng. LRCP Lond. 1954; DA Eng. 1961; FFA RCS Eng. 1964. Cons. Anaesth. Kettering Gen. Hosp. Specialty: Anaesth. Socs: BMA. Prev: Ho. Surg. (ENT) & Sen. Regist. Anaesth. Qu. Eliz. Hosp. Birm.; Sen. Regist. Anaesth. N. Staffs. Roy. Infirm. Stoke-on-Trent.

TOSH, Grahame Cameron Southend Hospital, Prittlewell Chase, Westcliff on Sea SS0 0RY Tel: 01702 221401 Fax: 01702 221413 Email: dr.tosh@hospital.southend.nhs.uk; Palliative Care Team Office, Basildon Hospital, Nethermayne, Basildon SS16 5NL Tel: 01268 53088 Fax: 01268 53088 — MB BS Lond. 1985; FCAnaesth. 1990. Cons. Palliat. Med. Southend & Basildon Hosps. Specialty: Palliat. Med. Prev: Cons. Palliat. Med. & Med. Dir. Fair Havens Hospice.

TOSH, Joseph Lupset Surgery, off Norbury Road, Wakefield WF2 8RE Tel: 01924 376828 Fax: 01924 201649; 109 Cumbrian Way, Lupset Park, Wakefield WF2 8LA — MB BCh BAO Dub. 1971; DCH RCPS 1973; DObst RCOG 1974; MRCGP 1975.

TOSHNER, David 5 Douglas Avenue, Giffnock, Glasgow G46 6NX — MB ChB Glas. 1966. Prev: Regist. Dept. Mat. Med. & Therap. Stobhill Gen. Hosp. Glas.; Phys. i/c Asthma Rehabil. Inst. Arad, Israel; Cons. Allergist Hadassah Med. Sch. Jerusalem.

TOSHNIWAL, Mishrilal Hiralal 42 Burnside Gardens, Lodge Road, Walsall WS5 3LB — MB BS Poona 1969.

TOSSON, Safwat Roushdy 9A Coniscliffe Road, Hartlepool TS26 0BS — MB ChB Ain Shams 1976; MRCOG 1983; MObstG Liverp. 1984. Cons. O & G N. Tees & Hartlepool NHS Trust; Co Lead Abnormal Uterine Bleeding Clinic. Specialty: Obst. & Gyn. Prev: Lead Clinician Urogynaecology & Pelvic reconstruction Surg.; Sen. Regist. Roy. Gwent Hosp.; Regist. Taunton, Liverp. & Arrowe Pk. Hosps.

TOSTEVIN, Miss Philippa Mary Jane St Georges Hospital, Blackshaw Road, Tooting, London SW17; Kingwood, Elmgrove Road, Cobham Tel: 01932 860345 — BSc Lond. 1986; FRCS Oto. Lond. 1996; FRCOG 1997. Specialist Regist. (Otolaryngol.) S. W. Thames. Specialty: Otolaryngol. Prev: SHO (Paediat. Surg.) John Radcliffe Oxf.; SHO (OtoLaryngol.) Roy. Nat. ENT Hosp.; SHO (NeoSurg.) Arkinson Morley Hosp.

TOSZEGHI, Anthony de 56 Elsworthy Road, London NW3 3BU Tel: 020 7722 5208 Fax: 020 7586 5704 — (Univs. Vienna & Pecs) MD Pecs 1943; LRCP LRCS Ed. LRFPS Glas. 1959; MBA Durh. 2000. Clin. Asst. Roy. Free Hosp. Lond. Specialty: Otorhinolaryngol. Socs: BMA. Prev: Cons. Clin. Haemat. & Med. Peterfy Hosp. Budapest.

TOTE, Subodh Prabhakar 3 Wilmington Gardens, Barking IG11 9TW — MB BS Lond. 1993.

TOTH, Mathias West Mount, 32 King Edward Avenue, Dartford DA1 2HZ Tel: 01322 220060 Fax: 01322 400428 — State Exam Med Hamburg 1987; MD Hamburg 1991; MRCP (UK) 1997. Specialist Regist. Gen & Geriat. Med. Specialty: Gen. Med. Socs: Roy. Coll. Phys.; Brit. Geriat. Soc.

TOTHAM, April NBS Bristol, Southmead Road, Bristol BS10 5ND — MB BS Lond. 1972 (Middlx.) DObst RCOG 1975; DA Eng. 1979. Assoc. Specialist (Transfus.) NBS Bristol. Specialty: Blood Transfus.; Haematology. Prev: Clin. Asst. (Paediat. Oncol.) United Bristol Healthcare Trust; Clin. Med. Off. (Child Health) Bath Dist. HA; GP Rendcomb.

TOTHILL, Catherine Louise Westfield, Hognaston, Ashbourne DE6 1PU — MB BS Lond. 1992.

TOTHILL, Geoffrey 35 Laburnum Road, Chertsey KT16 8BY Mob: 07973 311796 Email: geoff@medicalescorts.co.uk — MB BS Lond. 1988; Cert AvMed. Chief Med. Off. 1st Assist Ltd (Aviation & Assistance/Travel Medicine). Special Interest: Accid. & Emerg. Med. Socs: Fac. Mem. Clin. Considerations in Aviat. Transfer (CCAT). Prev: SHO (Neurosurg.) Roy. Lond. Hosp. Trust.; SHO (A & E) Lewisham Hosp. Lond.; SHO (Cardiothoracic Surg.) St. Thos. Hosp. Lond.

TOTHILL, Sally Anne Ladywell Medical Centre (West), Ladywell Road, Edinburgh EH12 7TB Tel: 0131 334 3602 Fax: 0131 316 4816; 30 Craigmount Terrace, Edinburgh EH12 8BW — MB ChB Ed. 1982 (Edin.) BSc (Med. Sci.) 1979; DRCOG 1985; MRCGP 1986; LFHOM 1997; MFHom 2001. GP Trainer. Specialty: Gen. Pract. Prev: SHO (Rehabil. Med.) Astley Ainslie Hosp. Edin.; SHO (A & E) Bangour Gen. Hosp. Broxburn; SHO (O & G) Vict. Hosp. Kirkcaldy.

TOTMAN, Marissa Bernadette — BM BCh Oxf. 1997; MA 1994 Cantab; DRCOG; DFFP; MRCGP; DCH.

TOTTEN, Eileen Sycamore House, Tile Barn, Woolton Hill, Newbury RG20 9UZ — MB ChB Glas. 1977.

TOTTEN, Joseph Wilson Sycamore House, Tile Barn, Woolton Hill, Newbury RG20 9UZ Tel: 01635 255584 Fax: 01635 255584 — MB ChB Glas. 1977; DPM Eng. 1984; MFPM 1989. Gp. R & D Dir. Shire Pharmaceut. plc Andover. Specialty: Pharmaceutical Medicine. Socs: Fac. Pharmaceut. Med.; Fell. Roy. Soc. Med. Prev: Vice-Pres. Clin. R & D Astra Charnwood LoughBoro.; Dir. of Developm. Fisons plc.

TOTTLE, Anthony John — MB BCh Wales 1983; MRCP (UK) 1986; FRCR 1990. Cons. Radiol. Glos. Roy. Hosp. Specialty: Radiol. Prev: Sen. Regist. (Radiodiag.) SW RHA; Regist. (Radiodiag.) Bristol & West. HA; SHO (Gastroenterol.) Frenchay Hosp. Bristol.

TOTTLE, John Alan Gothelney Cottage, Charlynch Lane, Charlynch, Bridgwater TA5 2PG Tel: 01278 652493 — MB BS Lond. 1950 (Char. Cross.) MRCS Eng. LRCP Lond. 1950; DPH Eng. 1956. Prev:

Cas. Off. Watford Peace Memor. Hosp.; Ho. Surg. Taunton & Som. Hosp.; Ho. Surg. (Obst.) Musgrave Pk. Hosp. Taunton.

TOTTLE, Sarah 26 North Hill, Fareham PO16 7HP Tel: 01329 513858 — MB ChB Birm. 1993; DCH 1997; DRCOG 1998; MRCGP 1998. GP Regist. Drayton Surg. Drayton Hants. Specialty: Gen. Pract. Prev: SHO (O & G) St Richard's Hosp. Chichester; SHO (Paediat.) St Richard's Hosp. Chichester; SHO (Orthop.) Qu. Alexandra Cosham.

TOTTS, Kaye Susan 252 Croham Valley Road, South Croydon CR2 7RD — MB BS Newc. 1988; FRCS (A&E) Ed 1996. Specialist Regist. (A&E) Sunderland Roy. Infirm. Specialty: Accid. & Emerg.; Gen. Med. Prev: SHO (Orthop.) Hexham; SHO (A & E) Sunderland & S. Shields Hosps.; SHO (Anaesth.)Aberd. Roy. Infirm.

TOU, Samson Iong Heng 1st Floor Flat 16 Craigie Street, Aberdeen AB25 1EL — MB ChB Aberd. 1997.

TOUBIA, Mrs Nahid Farid Rainbo, 59 Bravington Road, London W9 3AA Tel: 020 8968 5573 Fax: 020 8968 5573; 42 Milman Road, London NW6 6EG Email: ntoubia@aol.com — MB ChB Cairo 1974 (QASR AL Aini- Egypt) FRCS Eng. 1980; MSC. ECON. Unitversity of London, 1989. Pres. of Internat. Not-For-Profit-Organisation(Charity); Adjunct Prof. Clin. Pub. Health, Columbia Univ., Sch. of Pub. Health, New York. Specialty: Gen. Surg.; Family Plann. & Reproduc. Health.

TOUGH, Alison Margaret Baillieston Health Centre, 20 Muirside Road, Baillieston, Glasgow G69 7AD Tel: 0141 531 8040; Glencairn, 2 Heather Place, Lenzie, Kirkintilloch, Glasgow G66 4UJ — MB ChB Dundee 1977; MRCGP 1981. Prev: Trainee GP S. Qu.sferry Health Centre; Community Paediat. Train. The Sch. of Community Paediat. Edin.

TOUGH, Harry Gordon 106 Church Way, Weston Favell, Northampton NN3 3BQ — MB ChB Aberd. 1956; DPM Eng. 1963; FRCPsych 1982, M 1972. Cons. Psychiat. Mayfair Centre Community Ment. Health Kettering. Specialty: Gen. Psychiat.

TOUGH, Sandra Livingstone 10 The Firs, Salters Road, Newcastle upon Tyne NE3 4PH — MB ChB Aberd. 1980; MRCPsych 1985.

TOUN, Akumoere Yinkori — MB BS Lond. 1989; MRCP (UK) 1992. Specialty: Gen. Med.

TOUNJER, Isfendiar Ali 48 Eburne Road, London N7 6AU — LMSSA Lond. 1960.

TOUQUET, Mr Robin, RD Accident and Emergency Department, St. Mary's Hospital, Praed St., London W2 1NY Tel: 020 7886 1200 Fax: 020 7886 6366 — MB BS Lond. 1971 (Westm.) DCH Eng. 1973; DObst RCOG 1974; MRCGP 1976; FRCS Eng. 1979; T(S) 1991; FFAEM 1993. Cons. A & E Med. St. Mary's Hosp. Lond.; Fac. Prof. A&E Med.; Hon. Clin. Sen. Lect. Imperial Coll. Lond.; Regional Adviser Med. Counc. on Alcohol. Special Interest: Alcohol misuse. Socs: Med. Counc. on Alcohol; Brit. Assn. A& E Med. Prev: Sen. Regist. (A & E) St. Geo. & Mayday Hosps. Lond.; Regist. (Surg.) Univ. Coll. Hosp. Lond.; GP Faversham, Kent.

TOURISH, Paul Gerard 2 Mill Lane, Houghton Green, Warrington WA2 0SU — MB BCh BAO NUI 1989.

TOURLE, Colin Alfred Brook Cottage, Mill Lane, Hellingly, Hailsham BN27 4HD — MB BS Lond. 1965 (King's Coll. Hosp.) MRCS Eng. LRCP Lond. 1965; DObst RCOG 1967. Socs: BMA. Prev: Ho. Phys. King's Coll. Hosp. Lond.; Ho. Surg. Dulwich Hosp. Lond; Ho. Surg. (Obst.) Cuckfield Hosp. Sussex.

TOVEY, David Ian Herne Hill Group Practice, 74 Herne Hill, London SE24 9QP Tel: 020 7274 3314 Fax: 020 7738 6025; 46 Dalmore Road, London SE21 8HB — MB ChB Bristol 1983; DCH RCP Lond. 1987; MRCGP 1989; FRCGP 2000. Tutor (Gen. Pract.) King's Coll. Hosp. Lond. Prev: Trainee GP Wimbledon VTS; SHO (Paediat.) St. Marys Hosp. Lond.; Trainee GP/SHO GP Middlx. Hosp. Lond. VTS.

TOVEY, Mr Frank Ivor, OBE (retired) 5 Crossborough Hill, Basingstoke RG21 4AG Tel: 01256 461521 Fax: 01256 323696 — (Bristol) MB ChB (Hons.) Bristol 1944; MRCS Eng. LRCP Lond. 1944; FRCS Eng. 1947; ChM Liverp. 1962. Hon. Research Fell. (Surg.) Univ. Coll. Lond. Prev: Cons. Surg. Basingstoke & Dist. Hosp.

TOVEY, Gail Frances 7 Uplands Dr, Wolverhampton WV3 8AB — MB ChB Birm. 1997.

TOVEY, John Ernest (retired) 17 Patricia Avenue, Worthing BN12 4NE Tel: 01903 505163 — MB ChB Bristol 1952; MD Bristol 1960; FRCPath 1973, M 1964.

TOVEY, Lucas Alfred Derrick (retired) Old Charm Cottage, Old Scriven, Knaresborough HG5 9DY — MD Bristol 1957; MB ChB 1950; FRCPath 1973, M 1964; FRCOG 1989. Prev: Cons. Haemat. & Path. Yorks. RHA.

TOVEY, Peter John (retired) 160 St.ly Road, Birmingham B23 7AH Tel: 0121 350 2323 Fax: 0121 382 0169; 41 Greenside Road, Erdington, Birmingham B24 0DJ Tel: 0121 373 2826 — MB ChB Birm. 1960; MRCS Eng. LRCP Lond. 1960. Ho. Off. (Surg.) Dudley Rd. Hosp. Prev: Ho. Phys. Hallam Hosp. W. Bromwich.

TOVEY, Ronald Brian The Stapleford Centre, 25a Eccleston St, Belgravia, London SW1W 9NP Tel: 020 7823 6840 Fax: 020 7730 3409 — MB BS Lond. 1983; BSc Hons. Lond. 1979, MB BS 1983. Specialty: Alcohol & Substance Misuse; Gen. Psychiat.; Ment. Health.

TOWELL, John Douglas Middleway Surgery, Middleway, St. Blazey, Par PL24 2JL Tel: 01726 812019 Fax: 01726 816464; 39 Trevance Park, Tywardreath, Par PL24 2PY Tel: 01726 815959 — MB ChB Leeds 1969; Cert. Counselling Exeter 1989.

TOWER, Julian Edmund Christopher (retired) Grassgarth, Natland, Kendal LA9 7QH — MB BChir Camb. 1953 (St. Thos.) MRCGP 1964. Prev: Resid. Obst. Off. St. Thos. Hosp.

TOWERS, David George Cape Hill Medical Centre, Raglan Road, Smethwick B66 3NR Tel: 0121 558 0871 Fax: 0121 555 6125; 31 Wheatsheaf Road, Birmingham B16 0RZ — MB ChB Birm. 1973 (Birmingham) MRCGP 1977. Prev: SHO (Psychiat.) All St.s Hosp. Birm.; Trainee GP Birm. VTS; Ho. Off. Dudley Rd. Hosp. Birm.

TOWERS, Elizabeth Andrea Burnside, Chelford Road, Prestbury, Macclesfield SK10 4AW — MB ChB Sheff. 1970.

TOWERS, Elizabeth Madge Whitley House Surgery, Moulsham Street, Chelmsford CM2 0JJ Tel: 01245 352194 Fax: 01245 344478 — MB BS Lond. 1982.

TOWERS, Mr John Francis 52 Mount Ephraim Lane, Streatham, London SW16 1JD — MRCS Eng. LRCP Lond. 1967 (Liverp) LDS Liverp. 1961; FFD RCSI 1969; FDS RCPS Glas. 1969; MSc Lond. 1980, MDS 1982; FRCS Ed. 1985. Cons. Oral & Maxillo-facial Surg. St. Geo. Hosp. Lond. & Mayday Hosp. Croydon. Specialty: Oral & Maxillofacial Surg. Socs: Fell. Brit. Assn. Oral Surgs.; BMA. Prev: Sen. Lect. (Oral Surg.) Univ. Lond.; Sen. Regist. (Oral Surg.) St. Geo. Hosp. Gp.; Regist. (Oral Surg.) United Liverp. Hosps.

TOWERS, Jonathan Robert 7 Bossell Road, Buckfastleigh TQ11 0DE Tel: 01364 42534 Fax: 01364 644057 — MB ChB Sheff. 1985; DA 1990; MRCGP 1992.

TOWERS, Judith Sarah Neurology Department, Royal United Hospital, Bath; 277 Bloomfield Road, Bath BA2 2NT — MB BS Lond. 1988; MRCGP 1992. Staff Grade, Acute stroke Care.

TOWERS, Malcolm Kinsey 93 Harley Street, London W1G 6AD Tel: 020 7935 9242 Fax: 020 7487 2831; 44 Dene Road, Northwood HA6 2DE Tel: 01923 821216 — (Lond. Hosp.) MB BChir Camb. 1946; MRCP (UK) 1951; FRCP Lond. 1970. Specialty: Cardiol. Socs: Fell. Roy. Soc. Med.; Brit. Cardiac. Soc. Prev: Cardiol. Harefield Hosp.; Cons. Cardiometrics Hosps. For Dis. of Chest Lond.; 1st Asst. Inst. Cardiol.

TOWERS, Shona Hamilton (retired) 22 Stocks Lane, Chester CH3 5TF Tel: 01244 318528 — MB ChB Liverp. 1956; MD Liverp. 1968, MB ChB 1956; FRCOG 1975. Prev: Consult. (O & G) Chester Health Dist.

TOWERS, Simon John Bridge Street Practice, 21 Bridge Street, Driffield YO25 6DB Tel: 01377 253441 Fax: 01377 241962 — BM BCh Oxf. 1975; MRCGP 1979; DRCOG 1979; M.Med sci 1999. Prev: Trainee GP Bristol VTS; Ho. Phys. King's Coll. Hosp. Lond.; Ho. Surg. FarnBoro. Hosp. Kent.

TOWERS, Stephen 3 Hall Court, Sutton in Craven, Keighley BD20 7NF — MB ChB Sheff. 1982; MD Camb. 1983.

TOWERS, Susan Marie The Ridge Medical Practice, 3 Paternoster Lane, Great Horton, Bradford BD7 3EE Tel: 01274 502905 Fax: 01274 522060 — MB ChB Manch. 1985.

TOWEY, Raymond Martin 8 White House Close, Solihull B91 1SL Email: raytowey@africaonline.co.ug — MB ChB Manch. 1967; FFA RCS Eng. 1972. Miss. Doctor, Tanzania. Specialty: Anaesth. Prev: Cons. Anaesth. Guy's Hosp. Lond.

TOWIE, Hugh Gerald The Abbey Practice, The Family Health Centre, Stepgates, Chertsey KT16 8HZ Tel: 01932 561199 Fax: 01932 571842 — MB ChB Glas. 1977; MRCGP 1984.

TOWLE, Natalie Deborah 24 St.John's Avenue, Churchdown, Gloucester GL3 2DD Tel: 01452 713036; 6 Beeches Road, Charlton Kings, Cheltenham GL53 8NQ Tel: 01242 260497 — MB BS Lond. 1991 (University of London (University College & Middlesex)) DGM RCP Lond. 1993; DFFP 1995; DRCOG 1995; MRCGP Lond. 1996. Retainer Gen. Pract. Specialty: Gen. Pract. Prev: GP Regist. Cheltenham; SHO (O & G) Worcester Roy. Infirm.; SHO (Oncol.) Cheltenham Gen. Hosp.

TOWLER, Adam Hilltop House, Bourton on the Hill, Moreton-in-Marsh GL56 9AL; 11 Holders Lane, Birmingham B13 8NL Tel: 0121 449 3803 Email: adam.towler@virgin.net — BM BCh Oxf. 1992; BA Oxf. 1989, BM BCh 1992; MRCP. 1995. Staff Grade (Dermatol.) New Cross Hosp. Wolverhampton. Specialty: Dermat.; Accid. & Emerg.; Gen. Med. Prev: SHO (Gen. Med.) St. Jas. Univ. Hosp. Leeds.

TOWLER, Gillian Margaret Whitehorse Vale Surgery, Whitehorse Vale, Barton Hills, Luton LU3 4AD Tel: 01582 490087; 8 Barton Avenue, Dunstable LU5 4DF Tel: 01582 662795 — MB ChB Bristol 1971; DObst RCOG 1973; DCH Eng. 1975. Princip. in Gen. Pract. Socs: Assoc. Mem. RCGP.; BMA.

TOWLER, Gillian Mary Haxby Group Practice, Haxby & Wigginton Health Centre, The Village, Wigginton, York YO32 2LL — MB ChB Manch. 1990; DCH RCP Lond. 1995; MRCGP 1996; DRCOG 1996. GP Principle, Haxby Gp. Pract., York. Specialty: Gen. Pract. Socs: York Med. Soc.

TOWLER, Hamish Moray Andrew Whipps Cross University Hospital, Whipps Cross Road, London E11 1NR — MB ChB Aberd. 1979 (University of Aberdeen) BMedBiol Aberd. 1976; MRCP (UK) 1982; FRCS Ed. 1987; FRCOphth 1989; FRCP Ed 2000; MD UNSW 2002. Cons. (Ophth.) Whipps Cross Hosp. Lond. Specialty: Ophth. Special Interest: Retina; Uventis. Prev: Lect. (Ophth.) Moorfields Eye Hosp. Lond.; Lect. (Ophth.) Univ. Aberd.; Sen. Regist. (Ophth.) E. Anglia RHA.

TOWLER, Joan Norma (retired) 7 Belmont Avenue, Baildon, Shipley BD17 5AJ Tel: 01274 592915 — (Leeds) MB ChB Leeds 1946, DPH 1953; MFCM 1972; DCH RCPS Glas. 1972. Prev: SMO Bradford DHA.

TOWLER, Mr Julian Max 3 Penrith Avenue, Dunstable LU6 3AN — BM BCh Oxf. 1967 (St. Thos.) FRCS Eng. 1973. Cons. Urol. Surg. Luton & Dunstable Hosp. Specialty: Urol. Prev: Sen. Regist. (Urol.) Aberd. Roy. Infirm.; SHO (Gen. Surg.) Cheltenham Gen. Hosp.; Regist. (Urol.) Newc. Gen. Hosp.

TOWLERTON, Glyn Richard Magill Dept. of Anaesth., Chelseaa & Westm. Hospital, Fuutam Road, London SW10 Tel: 020 8746 8026 — MB BS (Hons.) Lond. 1990 (St. Bartholomew's London) BSc Lond. 1987; MRCP (UK) 1993; FRCA 1996. Anaesth. Cons. Director Pain Managem. Unit Chelsea & W.minister Lond. Specialty: Anaesth. Socs: BMA; RCA; RCP.

TOWLSON, Katherine Louise Vale of Leven DGH, Alexandria G83 0UA Tel: 01389 603924; Hillend Cottage, Quarry Road, Fintry, Glasgow G63 0XD Tel: 01360 860576 Fax: 01360 860535 — MB BS Lond. 1986; LMSSA Lond. 1985; BA (Hons.) Camb. 1982, MA 1986; DCCH RCP Ed. 1987; MRCPsych 1990. Cons. (Child & Adolesc. Psychiat.) Vale of Leven Dist. Gen. Hosp. Specialty: Child & Adolesc. Psychiat. Prev: Sen. Regist. (Child & Adolesc. Psychiat.) W. Scotl. Train. Scheme; Regist. (Psychiat.) Roy. Edin. Hosp.

TOWN, Valerie Joan Kings Road Surgery, 67 Kings Road, Harrogate HG1 5HJ Tel: 01423 875875 Fax: 01423 875885 — MB ChB Sheff. 1983.

TOWNELL, Mr Nicholas Howard Tayside University Hospitals Trust, Ninewells Hospital & Medical School, Dundee DD1 9SY; Rosebank, Hillside, Montrose DD10 9HZ — MB BS Lond. 1972; FRCS Eng. 1977; FRCS Ed. 1993. Cons. Urol.; Clin. Director for Surg. and Oncol.; Apptd. Tutor (Minimally Invasive Surg.) RCS Edin; Hon. Sen. Lect. (Surg.) Univ. Dundee. Specialty: Urol. Socs: Soc. Minimally Invasive Ther.; Brit. Assn. Urol. Surgs. Prev: Sen. Regist. (Gen. Surg. & Urol.) Roy. Free Hosp. Lond.

TOWNEND, Anne Mary The Health Centre, 20 Cleveland Square, Middlesbrough TS1 2NX Tel: 01642 245069 Fax: 01642 230388; 8 High Green, Great Ayton, Middlesbrough TS9 6BJ Tel: 01642 722695 — MB BS Newc. 1979; MRCGP 1983.

TOWNEND, Mr Ian Ralph Department of Urology, Doncaster Royal Infirmary, Armthorpe Road, Doncaster DN2 5 Tel: 01302 366666 Fax: 01302 320098; 22 Partridge Flatt Road, Bessacarr, Doncaster DN4 6SD Tel: 01302 533293 — MB ChB Ed. 1973; FRCS Eng. 1979; FRCS Ed. 1979; MS Soton. 1986. Cons. Urol. Doncaster Roy. Infirm. Specialty: Urol. Socs: Fell. Roy. Soc. Med.; Brit. Assn. Urol. Surgs.; Brit. Soc. for EndoUrol. Prev: Pharmaceut. Phys. Rhone-Poulenc Rorer; Hon. Sen. Regist. & Research Fell. (Surg.) Soton. Univ.; Regist. (Gen. Surg. & Urol.) Hallamsh. Hosp. Sheff.

TOWNEND, Mr John Richard Leslie St. Helens House, 2 The Drive, Chichester PO19 5RE Tel: 01243 530411 Fax: 01243 530411 Email: jtownend@headandneck.co.uk; St. Helens House, 2 The Drive, Chichester PO19 5RE — MB BS Lond. 1971 (Oxf.) FDS RCS Eng. 1974, L 1966; BDS Lond. 1967; MRCS Eng. LRCP Lond. 1971. Cons. (Maxillofacial Surg.) St Richards Hosp. Chichester; Hon. Cons., King Edwd. VII Hosp., Midhurst; Hon. Clin. Tutor UMDS Lond. Specialty: Oral & Maxillofacial Surg. Special Interest: Dental Implants; facial Skin cancer; salivary Gland disease. Socs: Fell. Brit. Assn. Oral & Maxillofacial Surg.; Eur. Acad. Facial Plast. Surg.; UK Regist. Expert Witnesses. Prev: Sen. Regist. (Oral Surg. & Plastic & Jaw Surg.) Sheff. HA; Regist. (Oral Surg.) & SHO (Plastic Surg.) Oxf. HA.

TOWNEND, Michael Smithy Cottage, Millhouse, Hesket Newmarket, Wigton CA7 8HR Tel: 016974 78477 Fax: 016974 78477; Lorton Park Cottage, High Lorton, Cockermouth CA13 9UG Tel: 016974 78477 Fax: 016974 78477 — (Leeds) MB ChB (Hons.) Leeds 1962; Dip Travel Med Glasg. 1996. Writer & Lect. on Travel Health, Travel Health Adviser; Hon. Clin. Teach., Univ. of Glas.; Tutor in travel Med., St Martins Coll., Lancaster; Medico-legal Examr. Socs: Internat. Soc. Travel Med.; Brit. Travel Health Assn.; BMA.

TOWNEND, Richard Hugh Malcolm (retired) 22 Wingfield Road, Alfreton DE55 7AN — LRCPI & LM, LRSCI & LM 1957; LRCPI & LM, LRCSI & LM 1957. Prev: Ho. Surg., Ho. Phys. & Ho. Surg. (O & G) Vict. Hosp. Keighley.

TOWNEND, William James King 64 Errwood Road, Manchester M19 2QH — MB ChB Leeds 1992.

TOWNER, Christine Hazle 56 Limpsfield Road, Sanderstead, South Croydon CR2 9EB Tel: 020 8657 3067 — MB BS Lond. 1955 (Westm.) FRCP Ed. 1980 M 1964. Cons. Phys. Croydon Health Auth. Specialty: Gen. Med. Socs: BMA & Brit. Geriat Soc. Prev: SHO Geriat. Unit, W. Middlx. Hosp. Isleworth; Regist. Dept. Geriat. Med. United Camb. Hosps; Sen. Regist. Geriat. Unit, Brighton Gen. Hosp.

TOWNER, Helen Denise The New Aylesford Surgery, R. B. L. U., Aylesford, Maidstone Tel: 01622 882384 — MB ChB Bristol 1981; Cert. Family Plann. JCC 1985; DRCOG 1985; MRCGP 1987. Trainee GP Maidstone. Prev: Cas. Off. West. Regional Hosp. Pokhara Nepal; SHO (Paediat. & Med.) Maidstone Gen. Hosp.

TOWNLEY, Adam David 3 North Square, London NW11 7AA — MB ChB Manch. 1998.

TOWNLEY, Alison National Blood Service, Leeds Blood Centre, Bridle Path, Leeds LS15 7TW Tel: 0113 214 8600 Fax: 0113 214 8696 — MB ChB Sheff. 1974. Assoc. Specialist Nat. Blood Serv. Leeds. Specialty: Blood Transfus.

TOWNLEY, Paul Andrew West End Medical Practice, 1 Heysham Road, Heysham, Morecambe LA3 1DA Tel: 01524 831931 Fax: 01524 832516; 379 Heysham Road, Morecambe LA3 2BP Tel: 01524 853509 — MB ChB Manch. 1980; MRCGP 1984; DRCOG 1984.

TOWNLEY, Stephen Anthony 2 Spinney View, Liverpool L33 7XX — MB BCh Wales 1993 (UWCM) BSc (Hons) (Wales) 1990; MRCP (UK) 1997. Specialty: Anaesth.

TOWNSEND, Adrian Philip The Surgery, New Street, Stockbridge SO20 6HG Tel: 01264 810524 Fax: 01264 810591 Email: adrian.townsend@gp-j82016.nhs.uk — MB ChB Manch. 1981; BSc (Med. Sci.) St. And. 1978. GP Stockbridge. Prev: SHO Rotat. Hastings AHA.

TOWNSEND, Alain Robert Michael Institute of Molecular Medicine, John Radcliffe Hospital, Hedington, Oxford OX3 9DU Tel: 01865 752328; 6 Polstead Road, Oxford OX2 6TN Tel: 01865 512714 — MB BS Lond. 1977 (St. Mary's) MB BS (Distinc. Med.) Lond. 1977; MRCP (UK) 1979; PhD Lond. 1984.

TOWNSEND, Alan Swainson, MBE (retired) Wegberg, Cronk Drine, Union Mills, Douglas IM4 4NG Tel: 01624 851525 — (St.

Mary's) MB BS Lond. 1956; MRCS Eng. LRCP Lond. 1956; DObst RCOG 1958; FRCOG 1977, M 1964. Prev: Cons. O & G I. of Man.

TOWNSEND, Angela Joy Woodpecker Cottage, Bailey End Lane, Ross-on-Wye HR9 5TR — MB BS Lond. 1986; BSc Lond. 1983; MRCOG 1990.

TOWNSEND, Mr Arthur Carlisle (retired) Slipper House, Emsworth PO10 8BS — MB BChir Camb. 1950 (Middlx.) FRCS Eng. 1959. Prev: Orthop. Surg. Kent & Sussex Hosp.

TOWNSEND, Mr Calver 114 Harley Street, London W1G 7JJ Tel: 020 7935 1565 Fax: 020 7224 1752 Email: ct.114harleystreet@btopenworld.com; The Northwood Consulting Rooms, 7 Greenhill Court, 25B Green Lane, Northwood HA6 2VZ Tel: 01923 826948 Fax: 01923 778283 Email: marciac@lineone.net — MB BS Lond. 1967 (Middlx.) DO Eng. 1972; FRCS Eng. 1975; FRCOphth 1988. Hon. Cons. (Ophth. Surg.) St. Mary's NHS Trust & W. Eye Hosp. Lond. Specialty: Ophth. Special Interest: Laser Ther. for retinal diseases; Small incision cataract Surg. Socs: Fell. Roy. Soc. Med.; UK & Irel. Soc. Cataract & Implant Surgs.; BMA. Prev: Resid. Surg. Off. Moorfields Eye Hosp. Lond.; Sen. Ho. Off. W. Eye Hosp. Lond.; Ho. Off. (Ophth. & Dermat.) Middlx. Hosp.

TOWNSEND, Mr Calver 114 Harley Street, London W1G 7JJ Tel: 0207 9351 565 Fax: 0207 2241 752 Email: ct.114harleystreet@btopenworld.com — MB BS London 1967 (Middlx. Hosp. Med. Sch.) FRCOphth, DO 1972; FRCS 1974. Cons. Ophth. Surg. in Private Pract. Only. Specialty: Ophth. Special Interest: Laser Treatm. Retinal Vasc. Dis.; Small Incision Cataract & Implant Surg. Socs: Roy. Soc. of Med.; United Kingdom and Irel. Soc. of Cataract & Redfractive Surg.; Europ. Soc. of Cataract & Refractive Surg. Prev: Cons. Ophth. Surg., West. Eye Hosp. & St. Marys, Lond.

TOWNSEND, Carolyn Louise Meadow View, Dean La, Cookham, Maidenhead SL6 9AF — BM BCh Oxf. 1997.

TOWNSEND, Catherine Rose (retired) Silverwood, The Fairway, Weybridge KT13 0RZ Tel: 019323 47648 — MB BS Lond. 1959 (Roy. Free) MRCS Eng. LRCP Lond. 1959; DO Eng. 1966; MRCOphth 1988. Clin. Asst. Roy. Free Hosp. Lond.; Clin. Asst. West. Ophth. Hosp. Lond.; Clin. Asst. St. Peter's Hosp. Chertsey. Prev: Regist. Roy. Eye Hosp. Lond.

TOWNSEND, Christopher John c/o Meadway, Carlton Lane, Wirral CH47 3DB — MB ChB Birm. 1991; BSc Birm. 1991, MB ChB 1991. Short Term Overseas Program. Coordinator Tear Fund Teddington. Prev: Ho. Off. (Med.) Kidderminster; Ho. Off. (Surg.) Newcross & Wolverhampton.

TOWNSEND, Christopher Stephen Salop Road Medical Centre, Salop Road, Welshpool SY21 7ER Tel: 01938 553118 Fax: 01938 553071 — MB BS Newc. 1971; MRCGP 1975.

TOWNSEND, David William Bute House, Grove Medical Centre, Wootton Grove, Sherborne DT9 4DL Tel: 01935 810900 Fax: 01935 810901; Sheeplands, Sheeplands Lane, Sherborne DT9 4BW Tel: 01935 815362 — MB BS Lond. 1973 (Middlx.) DRCOG 1979. GP Sherborne; Clin. Asst. (Ophth.) Sherborne.

TOWNSEND, Mr Edward Richard Lambettis, Horn Hill, Rickmansworth Lane, Gerrards Cross SL9 0QU Tel: 01895 828580 — MB BS Lond. 1970; MRCS Eng. LRCP Lond. 1970; FRCS Eng. 1976. Cons. Thoracic Surg. Harefield, Hillingdon, King Edwd. VII, Wexham Pk. & Northwick Pk. Hosps. Specialty: Cardiothoracic Surg. Prev: Sen. Regist. (Cardiothoracic Surg.) St. Geo. & Soton Hosps.; Regist. (Cardiothoracic Surg.) Kings Coll. Hosp. & Brook Gen. Hosp. Lond.

TOWNSEND, Eric William John (retired) Culmer, 39 Fore St., Shaldon, Teignmouth TQ14 0EA Tel: 01626 873741 — MRCS Eng. LRCP Lond. 1940 (Bristol) Prev: Med. Off. Molesey Hosp.

TOWNSEND, Giles Edward — MB BS Lond. 1995.

TOWNSEND, Helen Angus (retired) St. Edmunds Lodge, Park Road, Haslemere GU27 2NL — (Adelaide) MB BS Adelaide 1949. Prev: Assoc. Med. Director, Revlon Health Care, E.bourne, E. Sussex.

TOWNSEND, Horace Robert Allen (retired) 9 St Blaize Court, Cirencester GL7 1JA Tel: 01285 885263 — MB BCh BAO NUI 1952; FRCP Ed. 1974, M 1971. Prev: Cons. Clin. Neurophysiol. Nat. Hosp. Nerv. Dis. Qu. Sq. Lond.

TOWNSEND, Mr John (retired) Health Control Unit, Terminal 3, Heathrow Airport, Hounslow TW6 1NB Tel: 020 8745 7419 Fax: 020 8745 6181; 89E Victoria Drive, London SW19 6PT Tel: 020 8785 7675 — (St. Bart.) BSc (Hons.) (Physiol.) Lond. 1956; MB BS Lond. 1959; MRCS Eng. LRCP Lond. 1959; DObst RCOG 1962; FRCS Ed. 1969. Prev: Sen. Clin. Med. Off. Health Control Unit Heathrow Airport Lond.

TOWNSEND, John Crispin The Shrubbery, 65A Perry Street, Northfleet, Gravesend DA11 8RD Tel: 01474 356661 Fax: 01474 534542 — MB ChB Sheff. 1980; MRCPath 1987; DRCOG 1992. Prev: Trainee GP Lewisham VTS; Specialist (Chem. Path.) Woden Valley Hosp., Austral.

TOWNSEND, John Stafford The Harrowby Lane Surgery, Grantham NG31 9NS Tel: 01476 79494; 18 New Beacon Road, Grantham NG31 9JR — MB BS Lond. 1974.

TOWNSEND, Judith Margaret Redhill, 85 Wyke Road, Weymouth DT4 9QN — MB ChB Bristol 1977; MRCPsych 1984.

TOWNSEND, Mr Julian Charles Francis (retired) 17 Townsend Drive, St Albans AL3 5RB Tel: 01727 862565 — MB BChir Camb. 1957 (St. Geo.) FRCS Eng. 1964. Prev: Cons. Surg. St. Albans City Hosp.

TOWNSEND, Laura Zoe The Gate Cottage, Reading Road N., Fleet GU51 4AQ — MB BS Lond. 1998.

TOWNSEND, Mark Redhill, 85 Wyke Road, Weymouth DT4 9QN — MB ChB Bristol 1977; DRCOG 1979.

TOWNSEND, Mary (retired) 31 Cromley Road, High Lane, Stockport SK6 8BU — MB BS Lond. 1944 (Roy. Free) DCH Eng. 1946; MRCP Lond. 1948; MFCM 1973. Prev: SCM (Child Health) Stockport AHA.

TOWNSEND, Michael Stephen Arnold (retired) Earle House, 9 High St, Spalding PE11 1TW Tel: 01775 722020 Fax: 01775 714378 Email: msat@d-lweb.net — MB BChir Camb. 1965 (St. Geo.) MA Camb. 1966; DObst RCOG 1967; FRCGP 1988, M 1971. On Lincolnshire Supplementary Locum List; Med. Adviser to S. Holland Dist. Counc. Prev: GP Princip., Ch. St. Surg., Spalding, Lincs.

TOWNSEND, Neal William Hathaway 29 Rutland Avenue, Freckleton, Preston PR4 1HL — MB ChB Manch. 1995.

TOWNSEND, Mr Paul Leslie Gordon Department of Plastic Surgery, Frenchay Hospital, Frenchay, Bristol BS16 1LE — MB BS Lond. 1963 (Univ. Coll. Hosp.) BSc (Hons.) Lond. 1960; FRCS Eng. 1968; FRCS Canada 1972. Cons. Plastic Surg. Frenchay Hosp. Bristol.; Trustee, Skin Cancer Research Fund. Specialty: Plastic Surg. Special Interest: Lower Limb Trauma; Skin Cancer. Socs: Brit. Assn. of Plastic surgeons; Brit. Assn. of Aesthetic Plastic Surgeons; Cossham Med. Assn. Prev: Sen. Regist. (Plastic Surg.) Frenchay Hosp. Bristol; Regist. (Plastic Surg.) Odstock Hosp. Salisbury.

TOWNSEND, Peter 19 Crofton Drive, Baglan, Port Talbot SA12 8UL — MB BS Lond. 1989.

TOWNSEND, Mr Peter Thomas 28 Whitecroft, Horley RH6 9BZ Fax: 01293 822973 Email: peter@gynaesurgeon.com — MB BS Lond. 1975 (Guys Hospital) MRCS Eng. LRCP Lond. 1975; FRCOG 1992, M 1979. Cons. O & G E. Surrey and Sussex NHS Trust. Specialty: Obst. & Gyn.

TOWNSEND, Philip Simon The Health Centre, Gibson Lane, Kippax, Leeds LS25 7JN Tel: 0113 287 0870 Fax: 0113 232 0746 — MB ChB Liverp. 1987.

TOWNSEND, Raymond Francis (retired) Fairacre, The Byeway, West Wittering, Chichester PO20 8LJ Tel: 01243 514481 — MRCS Eng. LRCP Lond. 1936 (Westm.) MRCGP 1968. Prev: Consg. Med. Off. Henry Wiggin & Co. Hereford; Med. Regist. Westm.

TOWNSEND, Roger Maurice 8 Blenheim Gardens, Reading RG1 5QG — MB BS Lond. 1993; BSc Lond. 1990, MB BS 1993.

TOWNSEND, Stephen John Bitterne Park Surgery, 28 Cobden Avenue, Bitterne Park, Southampton SO18 1BW Tel: 023 80585 655/6 Fax: 023 8055 5216 — MB BS Newc. 1976; MRCGP 1989. Prev: Surg. Lt.Cdr. RN.

TOWNSHEND, David Nicholas 225 Osborne Road, Newcastle upon Tyne NE2 3LB — MB BS Newc. 1997.

TOWNSHEND, Jennifer Margaret Parkgate Health Centre, Park Place, Darlington DL1 5LW Tel: 01325 462762; West House, The Lendings, Startforth, Barnard Castle DL12 9AD — MB BS Newc. 1974; MRCGP 1979.

TOWNSHEND, Neil William Norman Barn Close Surgery, 38-40 High Street, Broadway WR12 7DT Tel: 01386 853651 Fax: 01386 853982; Peel House, High St, Broadway WR12 7AJ — MB BS Lond. 1980; DRCOG 1983. Chief Med. Off. Internat. Luge Federat.;

Chairm. Nat. Sports Med. Inst. UK. Prev: Mem. (Vice-Chairm.) Brit. Olympic Assn.

TOWNSLEY, Andrew Easterhouse Health Centre, 9 Auchinlea Road, Glasgow G34 9HQ Tel: 0141 531 8170 Fax: 0141 531 8110 — MB ChB Glas. 1988.

TOWNSLEY, Gerald Stewart (retired) — MRCS Eng. LRCP Lond. 1969 (St. Thos.) Dip. IMC RCS Ed. 1989. Prev: Gp Southwold.

TOWNSLEY, William London IRYO Centre, 234/236 Hendon Way, London NW4 3NE Tel: 020 8202 7272 Fax: 020 8202 6222; 12 Wymondham, Queensmead, St. Johns Wood Park, London NW8 6RD Tel: 020 7722 3866 Fax: 020 7722 3866 — MRCS Eng. LRCP Lond. 1943 (Middlx.) Med. Ref. Various Insur. Cos.; Cons. Lond. Info. Centre (Rash Dematol.). Specialty: Dermat. Socs: Brit. Med. Laser Assn. Prev: Ho. Surg. Qu. Alexandra Hosp. Portsmouth; Capt. RAMC.

TOWNSON, Peter John Hope Farm Medical Centre, Hope Farm Road, Great Sutton, South Wirral CH66 2WW Tel: 0151 357 3777 Fax: 0151 357 1444; Ravenswood, Mill Lane, Willaston, South Wirral CH64 1RW Tel: 0151 327 6324 — MB ChB Liverp. 1979.

TOWRISS, Mark Hamilton Bottisham Medical Practice, Tunbridge Lane, Bottisham, Cambridge CB5 9DU Tel: 01223 811203 Fax: 01223 811853 — MB BS Newc. 1977 (Newcastle-upon-Tyne) DCH RCP Lond. 1984; MRCGP 1985. Princip. GP Bottisham. Prev: Regist. (Med.) Dunedin Pub. Hosp., NZ; Ho. Phys. Newc. Gen. Hosp.; Ho. Surg. Shotley Bridge Hosp. Durh.

TOWSE, Margaret Susan (retired) — MB ChB Manch. 1975; MRCPsych 1979; MSc Manch. 1981. Prev: p/t Cons. Psychiat. (Psychother.) N. Manch. Gen. Hosp.

TOWSON, Nigel Bernard Dene Towson and Partners, Juniper Road, Boreham, Chelmsford CM3 3DX Tel: 01245 467364 Fax: 01245 465584; The Surgery, Strutt Close, Hatfield Peverel, Chelmsford CM3 2HB Tel: 01245 380324 Fax: 01245 381488 — MB BS Lond. 1972 (Roy. Free) MRCS Eng. LRCP Lond. 1972; DRCOG 1973; FRCGP 1996, M 1980. Lect. (Primary Care & Populat. Studies) Roy. Free Hosp. Sch. Med.; Course Organiser Chelmsford VTS. Socs: Chelmsford Med. Soc. Prev: Ho. Phys. (Gen. Med.) Luton & Dunstable Hosp.; Ho. Surg. (Gen. Surg. & Obst.) Roy. Free Hosp. Lond.

TOWUAGHANTSE, Mr Emmanuel Flat 20, Kent Court, North Acre, London NW9 5GF — MB BS Benin 1978; B BS Benin 1978; FRCS Ed. 1985.

TOY, Alison Jane Mechie and Partners, 67 Owen Road, Lancaster LA1 2LG Tel: 01524 846999 Fax: 01524 845174 — MB BS Lond. 1983; MRCGP 1988.

TOY, Elizabeth Winifred Exeter Oncology Centre, Royal Devon & Exeter Hospital, Barrack Road, Exeter EX2 5DW — MB BS Lond. 1993 (St Georges Med. Sch.) MRCP (UK) 1996; FRCR (UK) 2000. Cons. Clin. Oncologist, Exeter Oncol. Centre; Cons. Clin. Oncologist, Torbay Hosp. Specialty: Oncol. Special Interest: Gastro Intestional Malignancy; Thoracic Malignancy. Socs: Brit. Thoracic Oncol. Gp.; Amer. Soc. of Clin. Oncol.; Brit. Oncol. Assn. Prev: SpR Velindre Hosp., Cardiff; Clin. Research Fellow- Brit. Columbia Cancer Agency, Canada; Sen. Ho. Off. Med., Roy. Devon & Exter Hosp.

TOY, John Leslie Cancer Research UK, 61 Lincoln's Inn Fields, London WC2A 3PX; Chalmadale, Troutstream Way, Loudwater, Rickmansworth WD3 4LB — MB ChB Leeds 1968; MRCP (UK) 1973; PhD CNAA 1981; FFPM RCP (UK) 1994, M 1989; FRCP 1993. Med. Dir., CRUK; Hon. Cons. Phys. Hammersmith Hosp. Lond. Specialty: Oncol. Socs: Roy. Soc. Med. (Ex Pres. Counc. Oncol. Sect.). Prev: Sen. Med. Off., Dept. of Health; Vice-Pres. (Clin. Investig.) SmithKline Beecham; Lect. & Hon. Sen. Regist. (Med.) Univ. Leeds & Leeds Gen. Infirm.

TOY, Matthew Jonathan Chalmadale, Troutstream Way, Loudwater, Rickmansworth WD3 4LB — MB ChB Leeds 1998.

TOY, Rosemary Gade House Surgery, 99B Uxbridge Road, Rickmansworth WD3 7DJ Tel: 01923 775291 Fax: 01923 711790; Chalmadale, Troutstream Way, Rickmansworth WD3 4LB — MB ChB Leeds 1970; DCH RCPS Glas. 1972; DFFP RCOG 1998.

TOYE, Rosemary Directorate of Imaging, The Medway NHS Trust, Medway Maritime Hospital, Windmill Road, Gillingham ME7 5NY Tel: 01634 838954 Fax: 01634 813275 Email: rosemary.toye@medway.nhs.uk — MB BS Lond. 1984 (King's Coll. Hosp.) MA Oxon. 1983; AKC 1984; FRCR Eng. 1990. Clin. Director of Breast Screening Medway; Cons. Medway Maritime Hosp. Specialty: Radiol. Special Interest: Breast Imaging; Interventional Radiol. Socs: BSIR; RSNA; BIR. Prev: Cons. Greenwich Dist. Hosp. Lond.; Cons. Univ. Hosp. Lewisham Lond.; Hon. Fell. S. Bank Univ.

TOYN, Caroline Elisabethe Department of Pathology, Dudley Road Hospital, Birmingham Tel: 0121 554 3801; 35 Eastfield Road, Westbury on Trym, Bristol BS9 4AE Tel: 0117 962 9479 — MB ChB Glas. 1985; BSc (Hons) Glas. 1982, MB ChB 1985. Regist. (Path.) Dudley Rd. Hosp. Birm. Specialty: Pathology, General.

TOYN, Joanne Louise 10 Belvedere Drive, Dukinfield SK16 5NW — MB BS Lond. 1998.

TOYNBEE, Jean Constance (retired) Chapel Cottage, Ganthorpe, York YO60 6QD — BM BCh Oxf. 1948; BM BCh Oxon. 1948.

TOYNE, Anushya The Grantham Centre, Beckett House, Grantham Rd, London SW9 90L Email: anushyatoyne@aol.com; 122 Harbut Road, London SW11 2RE Tel: 020 7228 7028 — MB BS Lond. 1991 (Roy. Free Hosp. Lond.) DRCOG 1996; MRCGP 1998. GP Partner, The Grantham Centre, Beckett Ho., Grantham Rd, Stockwell, Lond. Specialty: Gen. Pract. Prev: GP Regist. Lond.; SHO (Paediat.) Watford Gen. Hosp.; SHO Rotat. (O & G & Gen. Med.) Lister Hosp. Stevenage.

TOYNTON, Christopher John (retired) The Medical Specialist Group, Alexandra House, Les Frieteaux, St Martin's, Guernsey GY1 1XE; La Rocque Balan, L'Ancresse, Guernsey GY3 5AL Tel: 01481 245422 Fax: 01481 246685 — MB BS Lond. 1961 (St. Thos.) DObst RCOG 1967; DLO RCS Eng. 1985. Surg. (ENT) Princess Eliz. Hosp. Guernsey. Prev: SHO (Gyn. & Obst.) Buchanan Hosp. St. Leonards-on-Sea.

TOYNTON, Nicola Jane Yealm Medical Centre, Yealmpton, Plymouth PL8 2EA Tel: 01752 880567 Fax: 01752 880582; Lower Marsh Farm, Landulph, Saltash PL12 6NG Tel: 01752 848041 — MB BS Lond. 1983 (St. Thomas Hosp. Med. Sch. Lond. Univ.) DRCOG 1986; MRCGP 1987; DCH RCP Lond. 1987; FRCGP 2004. GP Princip. Yealmpton. Specialty: Gen. Pract. Prev: Trainee GP Tunbridge Wells VTS; Ho. Surg. (Gen. Surg. & ENT) St. Thos. Hosp. Lond.

TOYNTON, Mr Stephen Clement Derriford Hospital, Department of Otorhinolarynogology, Level 7, Plymouth Hospitals NHS Trust, Plymouth SE1 7EH Tel: 01752 763164 Email: steve.toynton@phnt.swest.nhs.uk — MB BS Lond. 1986; FRCS (ORL); FRCS (Otol.) Eng. 1991. Cons. (Otorhinolarynogol.) Derriford Hosp. Plymouth; Advis. (Otol.) Diving Dis. Research Centre Plymouth. Specialty: Otorhinolaryngol. Special Interest: Middle Ear Reconstruc. Surg.; Paediatric ENT. Socs: British Association of Otorhinolarynogology- Head & Neck Surgery; Royal College of Surgeons. Prev: Sen. Regist. (ENT) St Thos. Hosp. Lond.; Sen. Regist. (ENT) Gt. Ormond St. Hosp. Lond.; Tutor Specialist (ENT) Christchurch Pub. Hosp. New Zealand.

TOZER, Amanda Jane 266 Broadway N., Walsall WS1 2PT — MB BCh Wales 1990.

TOZER, Rita Doreen Clarissa (retired) 7A Wendover Lodge, Church St., Welwyn AL6 9LR Tel: 01438 715989 — MB BS Lond. 1949 (Roy. Free) MRCS Eng. LRCP Lond. 1949; DObst RCOG 1950. Prev: Sen. Med. Off. (Family Plann.) Barnet HA.

TOZER, Roger David Worthing Hospital, Lyndhurst Road, Worthing BN11 2DH Tel: 01903 205111 Fax: 01903 285101 — MB BS Lond. 1981; FRCP (UK) 1986. Cons. Phys. (Med. for the Elderly) Worthing Hosp. Specialty: Care of the Elderly. Prev: Sen. Regist. St. Geo. Hosp. Lond.

TRACE, Jonathan Paul Ian Fallon and Partners, 1 Houghton Lane, Shevington, Wigan WN6 8ET Tel: 01257 253311 Fax: 01257 251081 — MB ChB Liverp. 1976.

TRACE, Thomas (retired) 2 Sutton Close, Folkestone CT19 5LL Tel: 277750 — MB ChB Liverp. 1954; DPH Cardiff 1969; FFCM 1979, M 1974. DMO S.E. Kent Health Auth. Prev: DCP Lewisham Dist., Lambeth, & Southwark HA.

TRACEY, Colin Anthony The Orchard Surgery, Commercial Road, Dereham NR19 1AE Tel: 01362 692916 Fax: 01362 698347 — MB BS Lond. 1976.

TRACEY, Dennis Michael NHS Highland, Department of Public Health Medicine, Assynt House, Beechwood Park, Inverness IV2 3HG Tel: 01463 717123 Fax: 01463 717666 Email: Dennis.Tracey@hhb.scot.nhs.uk — MB ChB Sheff. 1976; MRCGP 1982; MFPHM 1989. Cons. in Pub. Health Med.; Hon. Clin. Sen. Lect. (Pub. Health Med.) Univ. Aberd. Specialty: Pub. Health Med.

Socs: World Conf. of Family Doctors (WONCA). Prev: Sen. Health Adviser, DFID; Med Dir. Highland Primary Care NHS Trust.; Tuberc. Advisor Min. Health Lesotho.

TRACEY, Fergal 26 Inishowen Park, Portstewart BT55 7BQ — MB BCh BAO Belf. 1985.

TRACEY, Miriam Ellen 19 Ardmore Park, Finaghy, Belfast BT10 0JJ — MB ChB Dundee 1991.

TRACEY, Noreen Geraldine Teresa 5 Hackett Villas, Omagh BT78 1LU; 73 Greystown Avenue, Belfast BT9 6UH — MB BCh BAO Belf. 1986; MRCP (UK) 1989; FFR RCSI 1992; FRCR 1993. Cons. Radiol. Belf. City Hosp. Specialty: Radiol.

TRACEY, Susan 60 Crown Drive, Inverness IV2 3QG — MB ChB Sheff. 1976; DRCOG 1978; MRCGP 1994. Locum GP Highlands of Scotl. Prev: Hon. Sen. Lect. Dept. Family Med. Univ. Of Pretoria S. Africa; Med. Off. Transkei S. Afr.; Asst. GP Sheff.

TRACEY, Turlough John Coleraine Health Centre, Castlerock Road, Coleraine BT51 3HP Tel: 028 7034 4834 Fax: 028 7035 8914 — MB BS Lond. 1990.

TRACEY, Vivien Vaile (retired) 1 Fountain Court, Ipswich Road, Norwich NR1 2QA Tel: 01603 625359 — (Cardiff) BSc, MB BCh Wales 1944; DCH Eng. 1947; DPH Lond. 1961; FFCM 1976, M 1972. Specialist Community Med. Northampton Dist. HA. Prev: Sen. Med. Off. N.ants. CC.

TRACY, Hilda Joan Dale End Road, Barnston, Wirral CH61 1DD — MB ChB Liverp. 1957; PhD Liverp. 1965, MB ChB 1957.

TRACY, Peter Michael 10 Beech Grove., Porthcawl CF36 5DP — MB BCh Wales 1980.

TRAFFORD, Paul Jeremy Flat D, Shalstone Manor, Shalstone, Buckingham MK18 5LT — MB ChB Liverp. 1983 (Liverpool) BSc (Biochem.) Liverp. 1978, MB ChB 1983. Specialty: Anaesth.; Sports Med. Socs: Liverp. Med. Inst. & Liverp. Soc. Anaesth.; Assn. Anaesth.

TRAFFORD, Penelope Anne Watling Medical Centre, 108 Watling Avenue, Burnt Oak, Edgware HA8 0NR Tel: 020 8906 1711 Fax: 020 8201 1283; 42 London Road, Stanmore HA7 4NU Tel: 020 8958 4237 — MB BS Lond. 1979; MRCGP 1984. GP Princip., Assoc. Dean, The Lond. Deanery.

TRAFFORD, Peter Alan (retired) Timsbury, off Portway, Wells BA5 2BB Tel: 01749 673254 — (St. Thos.) MRCS Eng. LRCP Lond. 1942; MB BS Lond. 1943; DPM Eng. 1972. Prev: Sen. Med. Off. HM Prison Med. Serv.

TRAFFORD, Peter Damian Occupational Health Unit, Jubliee House, Jubliee St., Blackburn BB1 1EP Tel: 01254 587883 Fax: 01253 589630 Email: damian.trafford@capita.co.uk; 45 Dukes Brow, Blackburn BB2 6DH Tel: 01254 56056 Email: drafford@doctors.org.uk — MB BS Lond. 1974 (Lond. Hosp. Med. Coll.) DRCOG 1977; AFOM RCP Lond. 1993; MSc Manch. 1996; MFOM RCP Lond. 1997. Occupational Health Cons., Capita plc and Blackburn with Darwen Boro. Counc. Specialty: Occupat. Health. Socs: Assn. Local Auth. Med. Advisors; Soc. Occupat. Med. Prev: Occupat. Phys. Rochdale Healthcare NHS Trust; GP Glos.; Sen. Med. Adviser Blackburn Boro. Counc.

TRAFFORD, Rachel Margaret James Street Surgery, Workington CA14 2DF Tel: 01900 62241 — MB ChB Ed. 1992; DRCOG 1995. GP Princip. James St., Workington. Specialty: Gen. Pract. Socs: Med. Protec. Soc.; BMA. Prev: GP Trainee St Pauls Sq. Carlisle; SHO (O & G) City Gen. Hosp. Carlisle; GP Princip., Lond. Rd., Carlisle.

TRAGEN, David 5 Kilmalcolm Close, Prenton CH43 9QT Tel: 0151 652 4775/07812 040509 Email: davetragen@hotmail.com — MB ChB Manch. 2000. SHO, Anaesth., King's Mill Hosp., Mansfield. Specialty: Anaesth. Prev: SHO, Anaesth., Queen's Med. Centre, Nottm.; Resid., Anaesth., Roy. Melbourne Hosp., Australia; Resid., Emerg. Dept., Roy. Melbourne Hosp., Australia.

TRAGEN, Dawn Justine 44 Parkstone Avenue, Whitefield, Manchester M45 7QH — MB ChB Manch. 1994 (Manchester) DRCOG 1997. GP Cheadle Hulme, Chesh. Specialty: Gen. Pract. Prev: SHO (Med.) N. Manch. Gen. Hosp.; SHO (O & G) N. Manch. Gen. Hosp.; SHO (Paediat.) Booth Hall Childr.'s Hosp.

TRAGEN, Leslie 5 Kilmalcolm Close, Prenton CH43 9QT Tel: 0151 652 4775 — MB ChB Liverp. 1951; DObst RCOG 1958; MRCGP 1965. Med. Advis. & Examr. Nestor Disabil. Anal. Specialty: Disabil. Med. Socs: Liverp. Med. Inst.; Birkenhead & Wallasey Med. Socs. Prev: Dep. Police Surg. Merseyside Police; GP Wirral FPC; Capt. RAMC Jun. Anaesth. Specialist.

TRAHERNE, John Bernard 48 Brixton Water Lane, London SW2 Tel: 020 7274 1521 — MB BS Lond. 1958 (King's Coll. Hosp.) MRCS Eng. LRCP Lond. 1958. Prev: ENT Clin. Asst. Lond. Hosp. & Roy. Nat. Throat, Nose & Ear Hosp.; Ho. Phys. Belgrave Hosp. Childr.

TRAIL, Mr Ian Alexander Wrightington Hospital, Hall Lane, Appley Bridge, Wigan WN6 9EP — MB ChB Manch. 1978; FRCS Ed. 1982; FRCS Eng. 2002. Cons. Orthop. Surg. Wrightington Hosp. Wigan. Specialty: Orthop. Special Interest: Hand, Wrist, Elbow, Shoulder. Socs: Brit. Soc. Surg. of Hand; Brit. Orthop. Assn.; Brit. Elbow Shoulder Soc. Prev: Sen. Regist. (Orthop.) NW RHA.

TRAILL, Charles Gordon The Surgery, Sydenham House, Mill Court, Ashford TN24 8DN Tel: 01233 645851 Fax: 01233 638281; Leighton House, Church Road, Kennington, Ashford TN24 9DQ — MB BS Lond. 1969; DObst RCOG 1971; MRCGP 1976. Clin. Asst. (Dermat.) Kent & Canterbury Hosp.; CMO Paediatric Audiol. Ashford Kent. Specialty: Dermat.

TRAILL, Erica Ruth Bochruben House, Torness, Inverness IV2 6TZ — MB ChB Ed. 1985.

TRAILL, Lilias McAlpine (retired) Bellevue, 2 Pendreich Road, Bridge-of-Allan, Stirling FK9 4PZ — MB ChB Glas. 1944; DPH 1967; MFCM 1972. Prev: Sen. Med. Off. (Community Med.) Forth Valley HB.

TRAILL, Zoe Christina 10 St Andrews Road, Headington, Oxford OX3 9DL — MB BS Lond. 1986; FRCR; MRCP.

TRAIN, Jean Dick (retired) Cathkin, 4 Nunholm Place, Dumfries DG1 1JR Tel: 01387 53033 — MB ChB Glas. 1951. Prev: SCMO Dumfries & Galloway Health Bd.

TRAIN, Jonathan James Andrew 30 Avenue Road, Doncaster DN2 4AQ Email: jon_train@compuserve.com — MB ChB Bristol 1983; FRCA. 1990; MBA 1995. Cons.(Anaest.) Doncaster Roy Infirm. Doncaster. Specialty: Anaesth.; Intens. Care. Socs: BMA & Assn. Anaesth. Prev: Sen. Regist. Rotat. (Anaesth.) Roy. Free Hosp. Lond.; Fell. Cardiothoracic Anaesth. Acad. Ziekenmuis Groningen, Netherlands.

TRAIN, Mr Thomas Scott Rutherford (retired) Cathkin, 4 Nunholm Place, Dumfries DG1 1JR Tel: 01387 253033 — MD Glas. 1959, MB ChB 1951; FRCOG 1970, M 1956; FRCS Glas. 1981. Prev: Cons. O & G Dumfries & Galloway Hosp. Gp.

TRAINER, Jean Forbes (retired) Westfield Bungalow, Kirkfieldbank, Lanark ML11 9UH Tel: 01555 661285 — MB ChB Ed. 1952. Prev: Cas. Off. & Ho. Off. (Orthop.) Law Hosp. Carluke.

TRAINER, Peter James Department of Endocrinology, Christie Hospital, Wilmslow Road, Manchester M20 4BX Tel: 0161 446 3664/0161 446 3772 — MB ChB Ed. 1983; BSc Ed. 1980; MRCP (UK) 1986; MD 1997; FRCP 1998. Cons. (Endocrinol.) Christie Hosp. Specialty: Endocrinol. Prev: Sen. Lect., Hon. Cons. (Endocrinol.) St. Bart. Hosp. Lond.

TRAN, Ann Dao Shadbolt House, Salisbury Road, Worcester Park KT4 7BX Tel: 0208 3304096 — MB ChB Bristol 1990; MRCGP 1995. Specialty: Accid. & Emerg. Socs: BMA & Med. Defence Union; MDU; RCGP. Prev: Trainee GP/SHO Exeter VTS; Asst. Ship's Doctor P & O Cruises (UK) Ltd. Soton.

TRAN, Anna Thi Huyen 24 The Glade, Coventry CV5 7BU — MB ChB Leic. 1998.

TRAN, Huong Nam Paul 42 Station Road, Bearsden, Glasgow G61 4AL — MB BCh BAO Belf. 1986. Specialty: Oral & Maxillofacial Surg.

TRAN, Minh Ngoc 8 Tasman Cl, Mickleover, Derby DE3 9LF — MB ChB Manch. 1997.

TRAN, Tan Loc 11 Lytton Road, Pinner HA5 4RH — MB BS Lond. 1978.

TRANMER, Christopher Kings Avenue Surgery, 23 Kings Avenue, Buckhurst Hill IG9 5LP Tel: 020 8504 0122 Fax: 020 8559 2984; 17 Queens Avenue, Woodford Green IG8 0JE Tel: 020 8505 5171 — (Roy. Free) MRCS Eng. LRCP Lond. 1967; MB BS Lond. 1967; MRCGP 1975; Dip. Primary Care Rheum. Bath Univ. 1998. Hosp. Pract. (Rheum. & Rehabil.) King Geo. Hosp. Ilford. Socs: BMA; Forest Med Soc; Ilford Med soc. Prev: Regist. (Gen. Med.) King Geo. Hosp. Ilford; SHO (O & G) Ilford Matern. Hosp.; SHO (Paediat.) Qu. Eliz. II Hosp. Welwyn Garden City.

TRANMER, Francoise Marie 17 Queens Avenue, Woodford Green IG8 0JE — MB BS Lond. 1997.

TRANMER, Louise Solange Wanstead Place Surgery, 45 Wanstead Place, Wanstead High Street, London E11 2SW Tel: 020 8989 2019 Fax: 020 8532 1124; 17 Queens Avenue, Woodford Green IG8 0JE Tel: 020 8505 5171 Fax: 020 8559 2812 Email: ctranmer@ndirect.co.uk — MB BS Lond. 1970 (Roy. Free) MRCS Eng. LRCP Lond. 1969. Clin. Asst. in Colposcopy, Whipps Cross Univ. Hosp. Prev: Ho. Surg. King Geo. Hosp. Ilford; Ho. Phys. Barking Hosp.

TRANTER, Alan William (retired) 33 Stanley Avenue, Beckenham BR3 6PU Tel: 020 8658 8986 — MB BS Lond. 1951 (Char. Cross) MB BS (Hons. Surg.) Lond. 1951; MRCS Eng. LRCP Lond. 1951; DPH Eng. 1958, DCH 1954; FFCM 1978, M 1972. Prev: Dist. Med. Off. Bromley AHA.

TRANTER, John Victor (retired) 37 Burland Avenue, Tettenhall, Wolverhampton WV6 9JJ Tel: 01902 753388 — MB ChB Birm. 1957; MRCS Eng. LRCP Lond. 1958. Prev: Gen. Practioner Drs Tranter & Fowler Wolverhampton.

TRANTER, Julie Islip Medical Practice, Bletchingdon Road, Islip, Kidlington OX5 2TQ Tel: 01865 371666 Fax: 01865 842475 — BM BCh Oxf. 1985; MRCGP 1989.

TRANTER, Liam Kevin Flat 4, 8 Cambridge Rd, Kingston upon Thames KT1 3JY — MB ChB Otago 1997.

TRANTER, Richard — MB ChB Manch. 1994; MRCPsych.

TRANTER, Richard Church Street Surgery, 27-28 Church St, Whitehaven CA28 7EB Tel: 01946 693660; 3 Round Close Park, Scilly Banks, Whitehaven CA28 8UH Tel: 01946 67276 — MB ChB Birm. 1987; DCH RCP Lond. 1990; MRCGP 1991.

TRANTER, Mr Robert Martyn David Sussex Nuffield Hospital, Warren Road, Wooding Dean, Brighton BN2 6DX Tel: 01273 627032 Fax: 01273 627033 Email: rtranter@uk-consultants.co.uk; Foxdown, 50 Longhill Road, Ovingdean, Brighton BN2 7BE Email: bren.bob@virgin.net — MB ChB Bristol 1974; BDS Birm. 1967; FDS RCS Eng. 1972; FRCS Eng. 1979. Cons. Otolaryngol. Brighton & Princess Roy. Hosp. Haywards Heath. Specialty: Otolaryngol. Special Interest: Head and Neck Surg.; Skull Base Surg. Socs: Mem. of Exec. HCSA; Co. Chairm. HCSA for Sussex; Treas. Federat. Indep. Pract. Orgs. Prev: Sen. Regist. Qu. Eliz. Hosp. Birm.; SHO (Oral Surg.) Plymouth Gen. Hosp.; SHO (Plastic Surg.) Frenchay Hosp. Bristol.

TRAPIELLA, Beatriz 20 Melrose Close, Southsea PO4 8EZ — LMS Basque Provinces 1992.

TRAPNELL, David Hallam (retired) Dumbles Cottage, Woodend Lane, Awre, Newnham GL14 1EP — (Middlx.) BA (1st cl. Hons. Nat. Sc. Trip. Pt. 1) Camb 1949, MA 1953, MD 1963, MB BChir 1952; FRCP 1975, M 1957; DMRD Eng. 1959; FFR 1961; FRCR 1975. Prev: Cons. Radiol. Westm. Hosp.

TRAPNELL, Mr John Eliot (retired) Ropewind, Snails Lane, Blashford, Ringwood BH24 3PG — MB BChir Camb. 1954 (Middlx.) MD Camb. 1966, MA, MB BChir 1954; FRCS Eng. 1961. Hon. Cons. Surg. Roy. Bournemouth Hosp. Prev: Pres. Pancreatic Soc. Gt. Brit. & Irel. 1980.

TRAQUAIR, Katharine Ann — MB ChB Aberd. 1997.

TRAQUAIR, Katherine Elizabeth Corona (retired) Rothiemay House, Huntly AB54 7ND — MB ChB Ed. 1942. Prev: Surg. Regist. Hairmyres Hosp. E. Kilbride.

TRASK, Colin William Lawson Southend Hospital, Prittlewell Chase, Westcliff on Sea SS0 0RY Tel: 01702 221223 Fax: 01702 221039 Email: colin.trask@southend.nhs.uk — BM BCh Oxf. 1974; BA Oxf. 1972; MA Oxf. 1974; FRCR 1982. Cons. (Radiother. & Oncol.) Southend Hosp.; Hon. Sen. Lect. (Clin. Oncol.) UCL; Clin. Director Oncol., Southend Hosp.; Lead Clinician, S. Essex Cancer Network. Specialty: Oncol.; Radiother. Special Interest: Breast; Lung. Prev: Sen. Regist. (Radiother. & Oncol.) Univ. Coll. Hosp. Lond.

TRASK, Michael Darien 4 Dunham Rise, Altrincham WA14 2BB — MB ChB Manch. 1968; DObst RCOG 1970; FFA RCS Eng. 1975. Cons. Anaesth. Salford AHA (T). Specialty: Anaesth. Socs: Assn. Anaesths.

TRATHEN, Bruce Christopher The Old Plough, 7 The Street, Wallington, Baldock SG7 6SW — MB BS Lond. 1989.

TRATHEN, Duncan Paul 117 Green Dragon Lane, London N21 1HE; 36B Durley Road, London N16 5JS — MB BS Lond. 1994.

TRAUB, Anthony Ivor 6 Broomhill Park Central, Belfast BT9 5JD — MD Belf. 1980; MD (Hons.) Belf. 1980, MB BCh BAO 1972; FRCOG 1989, M 1977. Cons. & Sen. Lect. Midw. & Gyn. Qu. Univ. Belf. Specialty: Obst. & Gyn.

TRAUB, Michael Max 9 De Freville Avenue, Cambridge CB4 1HN — MB BS Lond. 1973; MRCS Eng. LRCP Lond. 1973; MRCP (U.K.) 1976. Sen. Regist. (Neurol.) Lond. Hosp. Specialty: Neurol. Prev: SHO (Med.) King's Coll. Hosp. Lond.; SHO IC St. Thos. Hosp. Lond.

TRAUE, Denise Carolyn 9 Meadow Way, Potters Bar EN6 2NJ — MB BS Lond. 1996. Specialty: Gen. Med.

TRAVELL, Paul David Littlewick Medical Centre, 42 Nottingham Road, Ilkeston DE7 5PR Tel: 0115 932 5229 Fax: 0115 932 5413 — MB ChB Leic. 1983; MRCGP 1988; DRCOG 1988. Prev: SHO (Ophth.) PeterBoro. Gen. Hosp.

TRAVENEN, Michael James Longshut Lane West Surgery, 24 Longshut Lane West, Stockport SK2 6SF Tel: 0161 480 2373 Fax: 0161 480 2660 Email: miketravenen@hotmail.com — MB ChB Manch. 1972.

TRAVERS, Anne Frances South Humber Health Authority, Health Place, Wrawby Road, Brigg DN20 8GS Tel: 01652 659659; 27 Oakwell Mount, Leeds LS8 4AD — MB ChB Leeds 1977; BSc (Hons.) Leeds 1974, MB ChB 1977; MRCP (UK) 1981; MPH 1994; MFPHM 1996. Cons. (Pub. Health Med.) S. Humber Health Auth. Specialty: Pub. Health Med. Socs: Soc. Social Med.; Brit. Geriat. Soc.; Assn. UK Pub. Health. Prev: Sen. Regist. (Geriat.s) Leeds Gen. Infirm.; Assoc. Research Fell. Univ. Coll. Lond.; Med. Off. St. Peter's Mission Hosp. Chisumbanje, Zimbabwe.

TRAVERS, Carolyn Victoria Ashley House, Church Lane, Hampsthwaite, Harrogate HG3 2HB — MB BCh Wales 1982.

TRAVERS, Mr Eric Horsley (retired) 10 Martlets, West Chiltington, Pulborough RH20 2QD Tel: 01798 813127 — MB ChB Ed. 1936; MRCS Eng. LRCP Lond. 1939; FRCS Eng. 1941. Prev: Cons. Surg. N. Teesside Hosp. Gp.

TRAVERS, James (retired) c/o Fisher, 28 Octavia Terrace, Greenock PA16 7SR — MB ChB Glas. 1935 (Univ. Glas.)

TRAVERS, John Francis Croftfoot Road Surgery, 30 Croftfoot Road, Glasgow G44 5JT Tel: 0141 634 0431 Fax: 0131 633 5284 — MB ChB Glas. 1979.

TRAVERS, Peter Rowlstone Covox Centre, The Old Mill, Tudor St., Exeter EX4 3BR Tel: 01392 430997; 38 Winchester Avenue, Exwick, Exeter EX4 2DJ Tel: 01392 277660 — MB BS Lond. 1942 (St. Thos.) MRCS Eng. LRCP Lond. 1942; DPhysMed. Eng. 1954. Indep. Sports Med. & Rehabil. Cons. Covox Centre Exeter; Cons. (Physical & Sports Med.) Broadmeadow Sports Centre, Devon. Specialty: Physiother. Prev: Convenor Med. Advis. Comm. Brit. Amateur Athletic Bd.; Lect. (Physiol. & Sports Med.) Sch. Educat. Univ. Exeter; Wing Cdr. (Ret) RAF Med. Br.

TRAVERS, Raymond Francis Rampton Hospital Authority, Retford DN22 0PD Tel: 01777 247759 Fax: 01777 247221 — MB BCh BAO NUI 1984; LRCPI & LM, LRCSI & LM 1984; MRCPsych 1991. Cons.(Forens Psychait.) Rampton Hosp Auth.; Sen Lect.(Hon) Univ of Sheff. Specialty: Psychother.; Rehabil. Med.; Pub. Health Med. Socs: Liverp. Psychiat. Soc.; Brit. Neuropsychiat. Soc.; Linc Med Soc. Prev: Sen. Regist. (Forens. Psychiat.) Scott Clinic Merseyside.

TRAVERS, William John Elton South Forest Locality, Mental Health Centre, 21 Thorne Close, London E11 4HU Tel: 020 8535 6948 Fax: 020 8535 6822 — MB BS Newc. 1981; DRCOG 1984; MRCGP 1985; MRCPsych. 1988. Cons. Psychiat. N. E. Lond. Ment. Health Trust, Lond. Specialty: Gen. Psychiat. Prev: Sen. Regist. Rotat. (Psychiat.) St. Bart. Hosp. Lond.

TRAVIS, Alison 2 Newlands Road, Cockermouth CA13 0AH Tel: 01900 824084 — BM BS Nottm. 1996; BMedSci Nottm. 1994. SHO (Gen. Med.) York Dist. Hosp. Specialty: Gen. Med. Prev: Jun. Ho. (Gen. Surg. & Med.) Qu. Med. Centre. Nottm.

TRAVIS, Charles David Elms Surgery, 5 Derby Street, Ormskirk L39 2BJ Tel: 01695 571560 Fax: 01695 578300 — MB ChB Liverp. 1970; DObst RCOG 1972; MRCGP 1977.

TRAVIS, Michael John Institute of Psychiatry, De Crespigny Park, Camberwell, London SE5 8AF — MB BS Lond. 1990 (Guy's Hosp.) BSc (Hons.) Lond. 1987; MRCPsych 1994. Lect. & Hon. Cons. IoP & Maudsley Lond. Specialty: Gen. Psychiat. Prev: Lect. & Hon. Sen. Regist. Inst. Psychiat. Lond.; Sen. Regist. (Psychiat.) St. Bart. & Homerton Hosps. Lond.; Hon. Sen. Regist. (Psychiat.) Bethlem & Maudsley Hosps. Lond.

TRAVIS, Paul Polkyth Surgery, 14 Carlyon Road, St Austell PL25 4EG Tel: 01726 75555; 22 Churchtown Road, Gerrans, Truro

TR2 5DZ Tel: 07739 251484 — MB Camb. 1984; BSc St. And. 1980; BChir 1983.

TRAVIS, Peter James Grove Surgery, 3 Grove Road, Solihull B91 2AG Tel: 0121 705 1105 Fax: 0121 711 4098; Woodside, 232 Streetsbrook Road, Solihull B91 1HF Tel: 0121 705 7867 — (Manchester) MB ChB Manch. 1967; DObst RCOG 1969; FRCGP 1987, M 1974. Socs: BMA & Assur. Med. Soc. Prev: Ho. Off. (Surg., Med. & Obst.) Withington Hosp. Manch.

TRAVIS, Phyllida Jane 4 Lyncroft Gardens, London W13 9PU Tel: 020 8579 9000 — MB BS Lond. 1981; MA Oxf. 1981; DCH RCP Lond. 1986; DRCOG 1987; MRCGP 1987; Msc (Health Plann. & Financing) Lond. 1994. Technical Off. WHO.

TRAVIS, Simon Piers Leigh John Radcliffe Hospital, Gastroenterology Unit, Headley Road, Oxford OX3 9DU Tel: 01865 851072 — MB BS Lond. 1981; MRCP (UK) 1987; DPhil Oxf. 1992; FRCP 1998; MA Oxon 2002. Cons. Phys. & Gastroenterol. Oxf. Specialty: Gastroenterol. Socs: Chairm. IBD Sect. Brit. Soc. of Gastroenterol. Prev: Sen. Regist. (Gastroenterol. & Gen. Med.) John Radcliffe Hosp. Oxf.; Jun. Research Fell. Linacre Coll. Oxf.; Regist. St. Thos. Hosp. Lond.

TRAVIS, Susan Elisabeth 291 Oldham Road, Rochdale OL16 5HX; 18 Spencer Lane, Bamford, Rochdale OL11 5PE Tel: 01706 369603 — MB ChB Manch. 1980; BSc St. And. 1977; DCH RCP Lond. 1982; DRCOG 1983.

TRAVLOS, John Staffordshire General Hospital, Weston Road, Stafford ST16 3SA Tel: 01785 257731 Ext: 4547 — MB BCh; FRCS; FCS (SA Orth); Mmed (Orth). Cons. Orthopaedic Surg. Specialty: Trauma & Orthop. Surg.

TRAYNER, Iris Aird McNeil 42 Rivermeads Avenue, Twickenham TW2 5JQ Tel: 020 8898 7144 — MB BS Lond. 1962 (St. Mary's) MRCS Eng. LRCP Lond. 1961. Clin. Asst. Dept. Chem. Path. Hammersmith Hosp. Lond.; Research Fell. MRC Lipoprotein Team Hammersmith Hosp. Lond. Specialty: Chem. Path. Socs: Fell. Roy. Soc. Med.; Brit. Hyperlipidaemia Assn. Prev: Ho. Surg. St. Mary's Hosp. Padd.; Research Asst. Dept. Endocrinol. Hammersmith Hosp. Lond.; Regist. Dept. Chem. Path. Hammersmith Hosp. Lond.

TRAYNER, Justin William Glenfield Surgery, 111 Station Road, Glenfield, Leicester LE3 8GS — MB ChB Leic. 1990. SHO (O & G) Sorrento Matern. Hosp. Moseley Birm. Prev: Ho. Off. (Gen. Surg.) Geo. Eliot Hosp. Nuneaton; Ho. Off. (Gen. Med.) Leicester Gen. Hosp.

TRAYNOR, Christine Patricia 137 Osbaldwick Lane, York YO10 3AY — MB ChB Leic. 1995. Specialty: Gen. Med.

TRAYNOR, David Bernard Pennells and Partners, Gosport Health Centre, Bury Road, Gosport PO12 3PN Tel: 023 9258 3344 Fax: 023 9260 2704 — MB ChB Manch. 1976; MRCGP 1980; DRCOG 1980.

TRAYNOR, James Philip 582 Crow Road, Glasgow G13 1NP Tel: 0141 954 7823 — MB ChB Aberd. 1994; MRCP UK 1997. SHO (Nephrol.) Stobhill Hosp. Glas. Specialty: Nephrol. Prev: SHO (Neph. & Med.) Monklands Dgm Lanarks.

TREACHER, David Floyd Mead Ward, Intensive Care Unit, St. Thomas' Hospital, London SE1 7EH Tel: 020 7928 9292 Fax: 020 7922 8240 Email: david.treacher@gstt.sthames.nhs.uk; 23 Cole Park Road, Twickenham TW1 1HP Tel: 020 8892 0849 — MB BS Lond. 1975 (St. Thos. Lond.) BA (Hons.) Oxf. 1972; MRCP (UK) 1978; FRCP Lond. 1992. Cons. Phys. & Dir. of Intens. Care. Guy's & St. Thos. Hosp. NHS Trust Lond. Specialty: Intens. Care; Respirat. Med.; Gen. Med. Socs: BMA; Brit. Thorac. Soc.; Eur. Soc. Intens. Care.

TREACY, Finbarr Patrick (retired) 108 Monton Road, Eccles, Manchester M30 9HG — LRCPI & LM, LRCSI & LM 1950.

TREACY, Patrick Joseph Knockaraven Garrison, Enniskillen BT74 4AE — MB BCh BAO NUI 1986; LRCPSI 1986.

TREACY, Peter John Department of Surgical & Anaesthetic Sciences, Floor K, Royal Hallamshire Hospital, Sheffield S10 2JF Tel: 0114 282 1290 Fax: 0114 271 3791 — MB BS Adelaide 1984; MD Adelaide 1994; FRACS 1994. Clin. Lect. (Gen. Surg.) Univ. Sheff.; Sen. Regist. Roy. Hallamsh. Hosp. Sheff. Specialty: Gen. Surg. Prev: Sen. Regist. Roy. Adelaide Hosp., Austral.

TREADGOLD, Nicholas John Pollok Health Centre, 21 Cowglen Road, Glasgow G53 6EQ Tel: 0141 531 6860 Fax: 0141 531 6808 — MB ChB Leeds 1985.

TREADGOLD, Ursula Ann Anderby, Gore End, Newbury RG20 0PH — BM Soton. 1991. Specialty: Accid. & Emerg.

TREADWELL, Elizabeth Anne 144 Henwick Road, Worcester WR2 5PB — MB ChB Birm. 1967; DPM Eng. 1974. Clin. Asst. (Psychiat.) Worcester Roy. Infirm. (Newtown Br.). Prev: Clin. Asst. (Psychiat.) Powick Hosp.; Regist. (Psychiat.) Powick Hosp.; Ho. Surg. & Ho. Phys. Worcester Roy. Infirm.

TREAGUST, Janette Denise — MB BS Lond. 1988; BSc (Hons.) Lond. 1985; DRCOG 1991; MRCGP 1992; MFPHM 2000. Sen. Regist. (Pub. Health Med.) Som. Avon Health Auth. Specialty: Gen. Pract.; Pub. Health Med.

TREANOR, Orla Teresa 8 Greenan Road, Newry BT34 2PJ; 15 Cairnshill Park, Belfast BT8 6RG Tel: 01232 729 5918 — MB BCh BAO Belf. 1994; DCH Dublin 1997; DRCOG Lond 1997; MRCOP 1998. Socs: DMA; MPS.

TREASADEN, Ian Henry West London Mental Health NHS Trust, Three Bridges Secure Unit, Uxbridge Road, Southall UB1 3EU — MB BS Lond. 1975 (Lond. Hosp.) MRCS Eng. LRCP Lond. 1975; ECFMG Cert 1975; MRCPsych 1979. Cons. Forens. Psychiat. Three Bridges Secure Unit, Lond.; Hon. Sen. Lect. (Forens. Psychiat.) St Mary's Hosp. Campus, Imperial Coll. Sch. of Med. Lond. Specialty: Forens. Psychiat. Socs: BMA. Prev: Sen. Regist. (Forens. Psychiat.) Maudsley Hosp. Bethlem Roy. Hosp. & Broadmoor Special Hosp. Lond.; Research Fell. & Hon. Sen. Regist. (Forens. Psychiat.) Univ. Soton.

TREASURE, Janet Linda Kings College London, Department of Psychiatry, 5th Floor Thomas Guy House, Guy's Hospital, London SE1 9RT Tel: 0207 9554247 Fax: 0207 9552976 Email: j.treasure@iop.kcl.ac.uk — MB BS Lond. 1978 (St. Thos.) PhD Lond. 1975, BSc 1973; MRCS Eng. LRCP Lond. 1978; MRCP (UK) 1980; FRCPsych 1995, M 1984; FRCP 1999. Cons. Eating Disorder Unit Maudsley Hosp. Lond. Specialty: Gen. Psychiat. Prev: Sen. Lect. Inst. Psychiat. Lond.; Regist. Maudsley Hosp.; SHO St. Helier Hosp.

TREASURE, Joanna Consultant Cellular Pathologist, Southport & Ormskirt NHS Trust, Southport District General Hospital, Southport PR8 6TN Tel: 01695 583651 — MB BS Lond. 1985; MA Camb. 1986, BA 1982; MRCPath 1994. Cons. Cellular Path. S.port& Ormskirk NHS Trust. Specialty: Histopath. Socs: Assn. Clin. Path.; Internat. Acad. Path.; Brit. Soc. for Clin. Cytol. Prev: Cons. Cellular Path. Ormskirk & Dist. Gen. Hosp.; Clin. Lect. (Path.) & Hon. Sen. Regist. Univ. Manch.; Regist. (Histopath.) Soton. Gen. Hosp.

TREASURE, Richard Anthony Robert Plas Ffynnon Medical Centre, Middleton Road, Oswestry SY11 2RB Tel: 01691 655844 Fax: 01691 668030; Bryn Teg, Hengoed, Oswestry SY10 7EH Tel: 01691 653402 Fax: 01691 671864 — MB BS Lond. 1981; MRCP (UK) 1984; MRCGP 1989. Specialty: Gen. Pract. Prev: Trainee GP Brecon VTS; Regist. (Med.) Char. Cross Hosp. Lond.; SHO (Med.) Westm. Hosp. Lond.

TREASURE, Professor Tom Professor Cardiothoracic Surgery, Guy's and St. Thomas's, London SE1 9RT — (Guy's) MD Lond. 1982, MS 1978, MB BS 1970; MRCS Eng. LRCP Lond. 1970; FRCS Eng. 1975. Cons. Cardiothoracic Surg. Guy's Hospital. Socs: EACTS; ESTS; BTS. Prev: Cons. Cardiothoracic Surg St Geo.'s Hosp.; Cons. Cardiothoracic Surg. Middlx. & Univ. Coll. Hosps.; Sen. Regist. Lond. Chest & Brompton Hosp. Lond. & Ho. Surg. Thoracic Unit. Guy's Hosp. Lond.

TREASURE, Wilfrid Muirhouse Medical Group, 1 Muirhouse Avenue, Edinburgh EH4 4PL Tel: 0131 332 2201; 16/1 Broughton Road, Edinburgh EH7 4EB Tel: 0131 556 7650 — MB BS Lond. 1983; MA Camb. 1977; MB BS Camb. 1983; MRCP (UK) 1985; Cert. Family Plann. JCC 1990; DRCOG 1990; MRCGP 1990; DCH RCP Lond. 1991; T(GP) 1991. Specialty: Vasc. Med.

TREBBLE, Timothy — MB BS Lond. 1991.

TREBLE, Mr Nicholas John Department of Orthopaedics, North Devon District Hospital, Raleigh Park, Barnstaple EX31 4JB Tel: 01271 322747; Muddiford House, Muddiford, Barnstaple EX31 4EZ Tel: 01271 850822 — MB ChB Liverpool 1977; MRCS Eng. LRCP Lond. 1977; FRCS Eng. 1983; MChOrth. Liverp. 1985. Cons. Orthop. Surg. S. West. RHA. Specialty: Orthop. Socs: Fell. BOA; Brit. Soc. of Childr.'s Orthopaedic Surg.s; Brit. Assn. of Knee Surgs. Prev: Sen. Regist. Mersey RHA; Clin. Research Fell. Roy. Childr. Hosp., Melbourne.

TREDGET, Janet Mair Priory Medical Practice, 48 Bromham Road, Bedford MK40 2QD Tel: 01234 262040 Fax: 01234 219288 — MB ChB Sheff. 1983; MRCGP 1987; DRCOG 1987.

TREDGETT, Michael William 1 Bagnall Cottages, Cinderhill Road, Nottingham NG6 8SD — MB ChB Ed. 1991.

TREDGOLD, Barnaby 13 Florence Road, Brighton BN1 6DL — MB BS Lond. 1996.

TREDGOLD, Christopher Francis — MB BChir Camb. 1967 (Univ. Coll. Hosp.) MRCS Eng. LRCP Lond. 1967; DObst RCOG 1969; FRCGP 1993, M 1973.

TREE, Andrea Mary Hollies Surgery, Elbow Lane, Liverpool L37 4AF Tel: 01704 877600 Fax: 01704 833811 — MB ChB Liverp. 1981; DRCOG 1985; MRCGP 1990. GP Formby. Prev: Trainee GP Formby VTS.

TREE, Deborah Anne 5 Lyndale Close, Leyland, Preston PR25 3DT — MB ChB Liverp. 1983.

TREE-BOOKER, David Anselm Lupset Surgery, off Norbury Road, Wakefield WF2 8RE Tel: 01924 376828 Fax: 01924 201649 — MRCS Eng. LRCP Lond. 1978; Cert. FPA 1981.

TREFZER, Siegfried 3 Sandwell Crescent, London NW6 1PB — State Exam Med Berlin 1987.

TREGASKES, Sarah Nadine — MB BS Lond. 1998. Specialty: Gen. Pract.

TREGASKIS, Brian Francis Belford Hospital, Fort William PH33 6BS Tel: 01397 702481; St. Clement, Spean Bridge PH34 4EN Tel: 01397 712657 Email: tregaskis@compuserve.com — MB BS Lond. 1981 (Middlx.) MRCP (UK) 1984; FRCP Ed. 1995. Cons. Phys. (Gen. Med. & Gastroenterol.) Belford Hosp. Fort William; Postgrad. Tutor 1994. Specialty: Gastroenterol. Socs: Brit. Soc. Gastroenterol.; (Asst. Sec.) RCP Edin.; Nutrit. Soc. Prev: Sen. Regist. (Med.) Leicester; Regist. (Med.) Dundee & Roy. Cornw. Hosp. Truro; Mem. Soc. Apoth.

TREGASKIS, Moira St. Clement, Lodge Gardens, Spean Bridge PH34 4EN — MB ChB Ed. 1979; BSc Ed. 1976; DRCOG 1982; Cert. Family Plann. JCC 1982. Doctors Highland Retainer Scheme. Prev: GP Truro; CMO Leics.; Trainee GP Bath VTS.

TREGEAR, Cecilia — D Med y Cir Colombia 1977. Med. Dire. Wimpole Med. Centre Lond. Specialty: Gen. Med. Special Interest: Anti-ageing Med. to slow down ageing; Skin Rejuvenation. Socs: Roy. Soc. Med.; Brit. Cosmetic Doct. Assn.; Amer. Soc. Anti-aging Med. Prev: Regist. (Int. Med. & Nuclear Med.) St Thos. Hosp. & Roy. Masonic Hosp. Lond.; Clin. Asst. (Nuclear Med.) St Thos. Hosp. Lond.

TREGER, Aubrey 27 Langdale Court, Kingsway, Hove BN3 4HF — MB BCh Witwatersrand 1971.

TREGILLUS, Eva Victoria (retired) Rockmount, Mill Hill Top, Reeth, Richmond DL11 6SQ Tel: 01748 884710 — MB ChB Liverp. 1942; MD Liverp. 1946. Prev: GP Darlington FPC.

TREGILLUS, John (retired) Rockmount, Mill Hill Top, Reeth, Richmond DL11 6SQ Tel: 01748 884710 — MB ChB Birm. 1943; MRCS Eng. LRCP Lond. 1943; MD Birm. 1951; FRCPath 1963. Prev: Sen. Cons. Pathol. Memor. Hosp. Darlington.

TREHAN, Anubha 62 Carrwood, Halebarns, Altrincham WA15 0EP Tel: 0161 980 2428 — MB ChB Manch. 1995. SHO (Med.) Blackburn.

TREHAN, Mr Ashwini Kumar Department of Obstetrics, Dewsbury & District Hospital, Halifax Road, Dewsbury WF13 4HS Tel: 01924 512000 Fax: 01924 512262 Email: clinic@endometriosis-consultant.co.uk; Oxford House, 436 Oxford Road, Cleckheaton BD19 4LB Tel: 01274 870567 — MB BS Ranchi 1978; MRCOG 1983; DRCOG 1985; FRCS Ed. 1986. Cons. O & G Dewsbury Health Care. Specialty: Obst. & Gyn. Socs: Roy. Coll. of Obstetricians and Gynaecologists; Roy. Coll. of Surgeons of Edin.; Brit. Soc. of Gyn. Endoscopy. Prev: Sen. Regist. (O & G) St. Thos. Hosp. Lond.

TREHAN, Vijay Kumar Brooks Bar Medical Centre, 162-164 Chorlton Road, Old Trafford, Manchester M16 7WW Tel: 0161 226 7777 Fax: 0161 232 9963; 62 Carrwood, Halebarns, Altrincham WA15 0EP Tel: 0161 980 2428 — MB BS Jammu & Kashmir 1969 (Govt. Med. Coll. Srinagar) Med. Off. Lancs. Cricket Club. Prev: SHO (Orthop.) Roy. Cornw. Hosp. (City) Truro; SHO (Orthop.) Winford Orthop. Hosp.; SHO (A & E) Weston-Super-Mare Gen. Hosp.

TREHARNE, Anne Elizabeth East & Gloucestershire NHS Trust, Child Health Services Department, County Offices, St Georges Road, Cheltenham GL50 3ES Tel: 01242 516235; Aballava, 18 Wincel Road, Winchcombe, Cheltenham GL54 5YE — MB ChB Manch. 1955. SCMO (Community Child Health) E. Glos. NHS Trust. Socs: Fac. Comm. Health; SW Paediat. Club. Prev: Clin. Med. Off. Cumbria & Carlisle; Sen. Med. Off. Manch.

TREHARNE, Christopher James Ty-Elli Group Practice, Ty Elli, Llanelli SA15 3BD Tel: 01554 772678 / 773747 Fax: 01554 774476 — MB BCh Wales 1983. Clin. Asst. (Endoscopy) Dyfed.

TREHARNE, Eifion Ty Elli, Vauxhall, Llanelli SA15 Tel: 01554 772678; 19 Swiss Valley, Llanelli SA14 8BS Tel: 01554 774102 — MB ChB Leeds 1957.

TREHARNE, Elizabeth Jayne Riverdale, Old Mill Lane, Cowley, Uxbridge UB8 2JH Tel: 01895 230741 Fax: 01895 230741 — MB BCh Wales 1986; DCH RCP Lond. 1989. GP Retainer.

TREHARNE, Mr Gareth David 29 Burlington Road, Withington, Manchester M20 4QA — MB ChB Leic. 1992; FRCS (Ed.) 1997. Specialist Regist.(Gen Surg.) Manc. Specialty: Gen. Surg. Prev: Research Fell. Dept. Surg. Leic. Univ.

TREHARNE, Ian Alan Lloyd Turner Rise Consulting Rooms, 55 Turner Road, Colchester CO4 5JY Tel: 01206 752228 Fax: 01206 752223; 1 Les Bois, Layer De La Haye, Colchester CO2 0DT Tel: 01206 738258 — MB ChB Aberd. 1972; FRCOG 1994, M 1978. Cons. O & G Essex Rivers Trust Colchester. Specialty: Obst. & Gyn.

TREHARNE, Ian Raymond Willowbrook Health Centre, Cottingham Road, Corby NN17 2UR Tel: 01536 260303 Fax: 01536 406761; Dallington House, Kettering Road, Geddington, Kettering NN14 1AW Tel: 01536 742267 — BM BCh Oxf. 1968; MA, BM BCh Oxf. 1968; DObst RCOG 1971; MRCGP 1975; DIH 1981; AFOM 1981. Specialty: Occupat. Health.

TREHARNE, Miss Linda Jane Dallington House, 6 Kettering Road, Geddington, Kettering NN14 1AW — MB ChB Bristol 1994; BSc (Hons) Anat Sci. (Bris.) 1991; FRCS (Eng) 1998. Specialty: Plastic Surg.

TREHARNE, Philip Gordon 8 Tebourba Drive, Alverstoke, Gosport PO12 2NT Tel: 023 9250 3240 — MRCS Eng. LRCP Lond. 1947 (Camb. & St. Bart.) MA, MB BChir Camb. 1947. Prev: Ho. Surg. St. Bart. Hosp.; Sen. Ho. Surg. Woolwich Memor. Hosp.; Capt. RAMC.

TREHARNE JONES, Robert The Mill Stone, 8 Oxlea Road, Wellswood, Torquay TQ1 2HF Tel: 01803 214864 Email: tjwizard@tiscali.co.uk — MRCS Eng. LRCP Lond. 1979 (St. Bart.) LMSSA Lond. 1978; Cert. Family Plann. JCC 1984; Cert. Prescribed Equiv. Exp. JCPTGP 1985. Health Informatician; Marketing Dir. Sullivan Cuff Med. Computing; Managing Dir. Wizard Wheeze GP Computing Cons.; Med. Edr. Regatta Magazine; Managing Dir. UpFront Med. Communications. Special Interest: Asthma; Pract. Managem.; Primary Care IT. Socs: Brit. Assn. Sport & Med.; Primary Health Care Specialist Gp., Brit. Computer Soc.; UK Counc., Health Informatics Professionals. Prev: SHO (O & G) Princess Roy. Hosp. Hull; SHO (Psychiat.) Roy. Cornw. Hosp. Truro; Demonst. (Human Morphol.) Nottm. Univ.

TREIP, Cecil Stanley (retired) 25 High Street, Waterbeach, Cambridge CB5 9JU — MB BS Lond. 1947 (Lond. Hosp.) PhD Lond. 1962, MD 1952; MA Camb. 1962; FRCPath 1973, M 1963. Univ. Lect. (Path.) Univ. Camb.; Hon. Cons. Neuropath. Addenbrooke's Hosp. Camb. Prev: Univ. Sen. Asst. Path. Addenbrooke's Hosp. Camb.

TRELEAVEN, Jennifer Gillian Royal Marsden Hospital, Downs Road, Sutton SM2 5PT Tel: 020 8661 3200 Fax: 020 8643 7958 — MD Camb. 1987; BA (Psychol.) Leic. 1967; MA Camb. 1976, MD 1987, MB BChir 1974; MRCP (UK) 1977; FRCPath 1994, M 1982; FRCP Lond. 1993. Cons. Haemat. And Hon. Sen. Lect. Roy. Marsden Hosps. Specialty: Haematology.

TRELINSKI, Marek Jerzy Bridge Surgery, St Peters Street, Stapenhill, Burton-on-Trent DE15 9AW Tel: 01283 563451 Fax: 01283 500896; Norwood Cottage, Hall Grounds, Rolleston-on-Dove, Burton-on-Trent DE13 9BS Tel: 01283 813816 — MB BS Lond. 1976 (St. Mary's) BSc (Hons.) Lond. 1972; MRCS Eng. LRCP Lond. 1975; DCH Eng. 1979; DRCOG 1980; MRCGP 1981. Princip. (Gen. Pract.) Burton on Trent. Prev: Trainee GP Sidcup VTS; SHO (Gen. Med.) Ramsgate Wing, Thanet Dist. Hosp.; Ho. Phys. & Ho. Surg. St. Mary's Hosp. Lond.

TRELIVING, Linda Rose Royal Cornhill Hospital, Aberdeen AB25 2ZH — MB ChB Glas. 1981; MRCPsych 1985. Cons. Psychiat. In Psychother., Roy. Cornhill Hosp. Aberd. Specialty: Gen. Psychiat.; Psychother. Prev: Cons. Psychiat. In Psychother.,

Psychother. Dept., Dundee; Cons. Psychiat. Roy. Dundee Liff Hosp. (Special Responsibil. for Psychother.).

TRELOAR, Adrian Joseph Room 19, Memorial Hospital, Shooters Hill, London SE18 Tel: 020 8336 6407 Fax: 020 8836 6384 — MB BS Lond. 1984; BSc Lond. 1981, MB BS 1984; DCH RCP Lond. 1988; DRCOG 1988; MRCP (UK) 1989; MRCGP 1989; MRCPsych 1991. Cons. & Sen. Lect. (Psychiat. in old age) UMDS Guy's & Dxleas Trust. Kent. Specialty: Geriat. Psychiat. Socs: EAGP; IPA. Prev: Sen. Regist. (Psychiat.) Maudsley Hosp. Lond.; Regist. Rotat. (Psychiat.) Guy's Hosp. Lond.; GP Sandwell.

TRELOAR, Emma Jane Southmead Hospital, Westbury on Tryn, Bristol BS10 Tel: 0116 249 0490; 10 The Park, Portishead, Bristol BS20 7LT Tel: 0116 255 8669 — MB ChB Leic. 1997 (University of Leicester) SHO (O & G) Leicester Gen. Hosp.; SHO. (Neonate.) Southmead Hosp.; SHO. (Gyn.) Frenchay Hosp.; SHO. (Obs.) Southmead Hosp. Specialty: Obst. & Gyn. Prev: PRHO (Oncol./Gen. Med.) Leicester Roy. Infirm.; PRHO (Gyn./Gen. Surg.) Leicester Roy. Infirm.

TREMAINE, Kenneth James Benefits Agency Medical Services, Government Buildings, Flowers Hill, Bristol BS4 5LA Tel: 0117 971 8311 Fax: 0117 971 8482; 18 Wiltshire Avenue, Yate, Bristol BS37 7UF — MB ChB Bristol 1976. Med. Off. Benefits Agency. Specialty: Disabil. Med. Socs: Brit. Med. Acupunct. Soc. Prev: GP Bristol.

TREMBALOWICZ, Franciszek Czeslaw (retired) 18 Firwood Close, Hampden Park, Eastbourne BN22 9QL Tel: 01323 504714 — Med. Dipl. Lwow 1937; DMRD Eng. 1958. Cons. Radiol. Pinderfields Gen. Hosp. Wakefield. Prev: Regist. Radiol. Dept. Roy. Infirm. Cardiff.

TREMBATH, Professor Richard Charles Leicester Genetics Centre, Leicester Royal Infirmary NHS Trust, Infirmary Square, Leicester LE1 5WW Tel: 0116 258 5736 Fax: 0116 258 6057 — MB BS Lond. 1981 (Guy's) BSc (Hons.) Lond. 1978; MRCP (UK) 1984; FRCP Lond. 1996. Prof. (Med. Genetics) Univ. of Leicester. Specialty: Genetics. Socs: Brit. Clin. Genetics Soc.; Amer. Soc. Human Genetics. Prev: Lect. (Med. Genetics.) ICH Lond.; SHO Brompton Hosp. & Lond. Chest Hosp.; Jun. Lect. (Med.) Guy's Hosp. Med. Sch. Lond.

TREML, Jonathan Mayday University Hospital, Croydon CR7 7YE Tel: 020 8401 3000; 128 Central Road, Morden SM4 5RL Tel: 020 8640 4456 — MB BS Lond. 1994 (Char. Cross & Westm.) BA (Hons.) Oxf. 1991; MRCP (UK) 1997. Specialist Regist. (Gen. Med. & Geriat. Med.) Mayday Hosp. Specialty: Care of the Elderly; Gen. Med. Prev: Specialist Regist. (Gen. Med. & Geriat. Med.) Crawley Hosp.; SHO (Gen. Med.) Qu. Mary's Univ. Hosp. Lond.

TREMLETT, Catherine Helen West Suffolk Hospital, Harwick Lane, Bury St Edmunds IP33 2QZ — MB ChB Manch. 1991; MRCPath; MSc; BSc (Hons.) St And. 1988. Cons. (Med. Microbiol.) W. Suff. Hosps. NHS Trust. Specialty: Med. Microbiol. Prev: SHO (Med. Microbiol.) Whiston Hosp. Prescot.; Ho. Off. (Surg. & Med.) Withington Hosp. Manch.

TREMLETT, Joanne Catherine 49 London Road, Twyford, Reading RG10 9EJ — MB Camb. 1984; MA Camb. 1985, MB 1984, BChir 1983. Trainee Windsor VTS. Prev: Ho. Off. Addenbrookes Hosp. Camb. & Hinchinbrook Hosp. Huntingdon.

TREMLETT, Michael Richard 60 Langbaurgh Road, Hutton Rudby, Yarm TS15 0HL — BM Soton. 1982; DA (UK) 1985; DCH RCP Lond. 1986; FRCA. 1990. Cons. Anaesth. James Cook Hosp. Middlesbrough. Specialty: Anaesth. Prev: Sen. Regist. (Anaesth.) Newc.; Regist. Rotat. (Anaesth.) Bristol; Vis. Asst. (Anaesth.) Johns Hopkins Hosp. Baltimore, MD, USA.

TREMLETT, Pauline Diane Ballington Manor, Wylye, Warminster BA12 0QF Tel: 01985 483 2345 — MB ChB Liverp. 1968. Prev: Clin. Asst. (Rheum.) W. Hill Hosp. Dartford.; SHO Renal Unit Roy. Devon & Exeter Hosp.; SHO (Obst.) City Hosp. Exeter.

TRENCH, Alistair John Merrylaw, Doune Road, Dunblane FK15 9AR Tel: 01786 823552 — MB ChB Ed. 1968; FFA RCS Eng. 1973. Cons. Anaesth. Roy. Infirm. Stirling & Roy. Inform. Edin.; Regist. (Anaesth.) Bangour Gen. Hosp. Broxburn; Ho. Phys. Milesmark Hosp. Dunfermline. Specialty: Anaesth. Socs: Soc. Anaesths. Gt. Brit. & Irel.

TRENCHARD, Peter John Clement (retired) 25 Park Road, Rushden NN10 0RW Tel: 01933 358009 — MB BS Lond. 1967 (Guy's) MRCS Eng. LRCP Lond. 1967; DObst RCOG 1969; MRCGP 1979. Indep. GP & Hon. Clin. Assis. Northants. Heartlands NHS Trust. Prev: Hon. Asst. Rockingham Forest NHS Trust.

TREND, Patrick St John The Royal Surrey County Hospital, Guildford GU2 7XX — MB BS Lond. 1979 (St. Thos.) PhD Lond. 1987, MB BS 1979; MA Oxf. 1980; FRCP 1997. Cons. Neurol. Roy. Surrey Co. Hosp. Guildford. Specialty: Neurol.

TREND, Ulla Doncaster Gate Hospital, Rotherham S65 1DW Tel: 01709 820000; Bole Hill Cottages, Norton, Sheffield S8 8QE — MB ChB Manch. 1977; BSc St. And. 1974; DCH RCP Lond. 1983; MRCPsych 1989; MSc Nottm. 1994. Cons. Community Paediat. Rotherham Priority Health Trust. Specialty: Paediat.

TRENDELL-SMITH, Nigel Jeremy Department of Histopathology, Charing Cross Hospital, Fulham Palace Road, London W6 8RF Tel: 020 8846 1234; 27 North End Road, Yatton, Bristol BS49 4AW Tel: 01934 833565 — MB BS Lond. 1989; BSc Lond. 1986; DRCPath Lond. 1994. Sen. Regist. (Histopath.) Char. Cross Hosp. Lond. Specialty: Histopath. Prev: Demonst. (Path.) Univ. Bristol.

TRENFIELD, John Dennis Stuart 5 Julian Close, Sneyd Park, Bristol BS9 1JX Tel: 0956 420794 — MB BS Lond. 1996; MRCS Ed. 2001. SpR Accid. & Emerg. Specialty: Gen. Surg. Prev: SHO (Surg.) Kingston Hosp.

TRENFIELD, Sarah Margaret Flat 34, Carrara Wharf, Ranelagh Gardens, Fulham, London SW6 3UJ — (University of Bristol) Primary FRCA 1997 - Roy. Coll. Anaesth.; BDS Bristol 1988; FDS RCS Eng. 1993; MB ChB Bristol 1995. SHO Anaesth. St Mary's Hosp. Paddington Lond.; Specialist Regist. (Anaesth.) Imperial Sch. of Med. Specialty: Anaesth.; Oral & Maxillofacial Surg.

TRENHOLM, Philip William Christie Hospital, 550 Wilmslow Road, Withington, Manchester M20 4BX Tel: 0161 446 3000 — MB ChB Manch. 1992; MRCP (UK) 1997. Specialist Regist. (Clin. Oncol.) Chrisie Hosp. Manch. Specialty: Oncol.; Radiother.

TRENT, Michael Paul The Cobham Health Centre, 168 Portsmouth Road, Cobham KT11 1HT Tel: 01932 867231 Fax: 01932 866874 — MB BS Lond. 1980.

TRENT, Robert Sidney Woodside Medical Centre, Jardine Crescent, Coventry CV4 9PL Tel: 024 7669 4001 Fax: 024 7669 5639; 29 Turnlands Close, Walsgrave, Coventry CV2 2PT Tel: 024 76 611440 — MRCS Eng. LRCP Lond. 1976.

TRENT, Roger John Western Infirmary, Dumbarton Road, Glasgow G11 6NT Tel: 0141 211 2000; 214 Nithsdale Road, Glasgow G41 5HD Tel: 0141 427 5607 — BM Soton. 1985; MRCP (UK) 1989; DA (Roy Coll Anaesths) 1990; MD (Univ of Aberdeen) 1998. Research Fell. Cardiol. Aberd. Specialty: Cardiol.

TRENT, Sally Louise 76 Comeragh Road, London W14 9HR — MB BS Lond. 1993; BSc Lond. 1990; MRCP (UK) 1996; FRCR 2000. Specialty: Oncol.

TRESADERN, Mr John Christopher The Royal Infirmary, Infirmary Road, Blackburn BB2 3LR Tel: 01254 263555 — BM BCh Oxf. 1972; BA (Hons.) Oxf. 1969; FRCS Eng. 1977; ChM Manch. 1984. Cons. Gen. Surg. Blackburn Roy. Infirm. Specialty: Gen. Surg.

TRESEDER, Andrew Stephen Morriston Hospital, Department of Geriatric Medicine, Morriston, Swansea SA6 6NL Tel: 01792 703384 — MB BCh Wales 1974; DCH Eng. 1977; FRCP (UK) 1980. Cons. Phys. (Geriat. Med.) W. Glam. HA. Specialty: Gen. Med.

TRESIDDER, Andrew Philip Tavender Glanvill and Partners, Springmead Surgery, Summerfields Road, Chard TA20 2EW Tel: 01460 63380 Fax: 01460 66483 — MB BS Lond. 1983; DRCOG 1986; MRCGP 1988. Socs: Brit. Holistic Med. Assn.; Brit. Assn. of Flower Essence Producers.

TRESIDDER, Ian Robert Southover Medical Practice, Bronshill Road, Torquay TQ1 3HD Tel: 01803 327100 Fax: 01803 316295 — MB BS Lond. 1986; BSc Lond. 1983, MB BS 1986; MRCP (UK) 1989; DRCOG 1991; MRCGP 1991. Hosp. Pract. (Respirat. Med.) S. Devon Healthcare Torbay Hosp. Prev: SHO (A & E) Torbay Hosp. Torquay.

TRESIDDER, Jane Scott Boulton Clinic, Wyndham St., Alvaston, Derby DE24 0EP Tel: 01332 574823; 61 West End, Wirksworth, Derby DE4 4EG Tel: 01629 823953 — MB BS Lond. 1970 (St. Thos.) DObst RCOG 1972; DTM & H Liverp. 1973; DCH Eng. 1978; MRCP (Paediat.) (UK) 1983; FRCP Lond. 1995. Cons. Community Paediat. South. Derbysh. HA. Specialty: Paediat. Socs: Brit. Paediat. Assn. (Community Paediat. Gp.). Prev: Sen. Regist. (Community Paediat.) Dept. Child Health Nottm. HA; Regist. (Community

Paediat.) Univ. Hosp. Nottm. HA; Regist. (Paediat.) Derbysh. Child. Hosp.

TRESIDDER, Nicholas John Hassengate Medical Centre, Southend Road, Stanford-le-Hope SS17 0PH Tel: 01375 673064 Fax: 01375 675196 — MB BS Lond. 1980; DRCOG 1983; MRCGP 1984.

TRESILIAN, Kathleen Edith (retired) 19 Wyndham Street, Brighton BN2 1AF — MB BS Lond. 1927 (Lond. Hosp. & Vienna) MRCS Eng., L.R.C.P. Lond. 1923. Prev: Clin. Asst. St. John's Skin Hosp. Leicester Sq. & Lond. Hosp.

TRESMAN, Robert Lewis 50 Oakfield Avenue, Hitchin SG4 9JD — MB BS Lond. 1981 (Univ. Coll. Hosp.) PhD Lond. 1971, BSc (Hons. Anat.) 1966, MB BS 1981; MRCPsych 1986. Prev: Regist. (Psychiat.) Lond. Hosp.; Regist. (Psychiat.) Goodmayes Hosp. Ilford.

TRETHOWAN, William Nicholas Department of Occupational Medicine, Royal Shrewsbury Hospital, Mytton Oak Road, Shrewsbury SY3 8XQ Tel: 01743 231122; Shrubbery, Westbury, Shrewsbury SY5 9QX — MB BS Lond. 1974; MRCS Eng. LRCP Lond. 1974; MRCP (UK) 1978; MFOM RCP Lond. 1987. Cons. Occupat. Med. Roy. Shrewsbury Hosp. Specialty: Occupat. Health.

TREVAIL, Philip Roy Pool Health Centre, Station Road, Pool, Redruth TR15 3DU Tel: 01209 717471 Fax: 01209 612160 Email: phil.trevail@pool.cornwall.nhs.uk; Mayfield Whitehall, Scorrier, Redruth TR16 5BB — BM Soton. 1986; DRCOG 1990; MRCGP 1992; DFFP 1995. Gen. Practitioner; Med. Manager Assn. Cornw. Doctors on Call (Kernow Doc). Specialty: Gen. Pract. Prev: Trainee GP/SHO Roy. Cornw. Hosp. Truro; SHO (A & E) Roy. Hants. Co. Hosp. Winchester; Police Surg. Camborne.

TREVAN, Anthony Charles (retired) 27 Cheam Road, Ewell, Epsom KT17 1QX Tel: 020 8393 5445 Fax: 020 8393 5445 — (St. Bart.) MB BS Lond. 1951; DObst RCOG 1953; DCH Eng. 1954; MRCGP 1975.

TREVARTHEN, Franklyn David Aviation Medical Practice, 10 Hertford Road, Digswell, Welwyn AL6 0EB Tel: 01438 714056 Fax: 01438 840617 Email: dtrevar934@aol.com — MB BS Lond. 1960 (Univ. Coll. Hosp.) DObst RCOG 1962; DMJ (Clin.) Soc. Apoth. Lond. 1970; Cert Av Med MoD (Air) & CAA 1973; MFOM RCP Lond. 1983. Med. Examr. CAA (UK), FAA (USA) & CAD (Hong Kong, China); Med. Off. Avia Special Welwyn Garden City; Med. Off. Cedesa Letchworth; Examining Medical Practitioner DSS. Specialty: Occupat. Health; Aviat. Med.; Medico Legal. Socs: Soc. Occupat. Med.; Internat. Soc. Travel Med.; Fell. Roy. Aeronautical Soc. (Aviat. Sect.). Prev: Hon. Cons. Occupat. Health Luton & Dunstable Hosp. NHS Trust; Med. Off. Dunstable & Plant Med. Off. Luton Vauxhall Motors Ltd.; Med. Off. Avdel Ltd. & GKN Lincoln Electric Ltd. Welwyn Gdn. City.

TREVELYAN, Mary Harriet (retired) Sighthill Health Centre, Calder Road, Edinburgh EH11 4AU Tel: 0131 537 7030 Fax: 0131 537 7005 — MB BS Lond. 1963; DObst RCOG 1967. Prev: Lect. (Social Med.) St. Thos. Hosp. Med. Sch. Lond.

TREVELYAN, Nicola Clare 56 Plymouth Place, Leamington Spa CV31 1HN — MB ChB Manch. 1994 (Manchester) BSc St. And. 1991; MRCP 1998. Regist. (Paediat.) Walsgrave Hosp. Coventry.; SHO (Paediat.) Northampton Gen. Hosp. Specialty: Paediat. Prev: Regist. (Paediat.) Auckland Healthcare Ltd., NZ; SHO (Paediat.) Liverp. Woms. Hosp. & Alder Hey Hosp.

TREVELYAN, Thomas Arnold Onion Patch, 8 The Spinney, Itchenor, Chichester PO20 7DF Tel: 01243 511038 Fax: 01243 512489 — (St. Thos.) MB BChir Camb. 1967; MRCGP 1973. Part time GP. Socs: BMA. Prev: GP Princip., Kensington 1970-1999.

TREVELYAN, Thomas Rhys Sconce, Llannefydd, Denbigh LL16 5EY — MB BChir Camb. 1973; MRCPsych 1977.

TREVELYAN THOMAS, Mary Kate Middle Farm House, Long Crichel, Wimborne BH21 5JU — MB BS (Hons. Surg.) Lond. 1978 (Westm.) MA Camb. 1979; MRCGP 1983.

TREVETT, Andrew James Horroquoy, Harray, Orkney KW17 2JT Tel: 01856 761410 — MB ChB Glas. 1987; MA Camb. 1984; DTM & H Liverp. 1990; MRCP Glas. 1990; MD (Hons.) Glas. 1995; DRCOG 1996; MRCGP 1996. GP Stromness Orkney; Wellcome Vis. Lect. Specialty: Infec. Dis. Socs: Fell. Roy. Sch. Trop. Med. & Hyg.; PNG Med. Soc. Prev: SHO (Med.) Vict. Infirm. Glas.

TREVETT, Mr Michael Charles West Meadow, Bell Lane, Lower Broad Heath, Worcester WR2 6RR Tel: 01905 641038 — MB ChB Cape Town 1982; FCS(SA) 1993; M Med (Orthop.) Cape Town Univ. 1994; FRCS (E) 1996. Cons. Orthop. Specialty: Orthop.

TREVOR, Alison Jane Castlefields Health Centre, Chester Close, Castlefields, Runcorn WA7 2HY Tel: 01928 566671 Fax: 01928 581631 — MB BChir Camb. 1986; MA Camb. 1987; DRCOG 1990. Clin. Med. Off. (Family Plann.) Chester & Halton Community NHS Trust. Prev: Trainee GP Warrington Dist. Gen. Hosp. VTS; SHO (A & E) Macclesfield Dist. Gen. Hosp.

TREVOR, Sally Parkfield Medical Centre, The Walk, Potters Bar EN6 1QH Tel: 01707 651234 Fax: 01707 660452; 58 Bradmore Way, Brookmans Park, Hatfield Heath, Hatfield AL9 7QX Tel: 01701 647133 — MB BS Lond. 1990; BSc Lond. 1987; DRCOG 1994; MRCGP 1994.

TREW, Mr David Richard West Kent Eye Centre, Princess Royal University Hospital, Farnborough Common, Orpington BR6 8ND Tel: 01689 865684 — MB BS Lond. 1983 (Westm. Hosp.) MA Camb. 1980; DO RCS Eng. 1987; FRCS Eng. 1988; FRCOphth 1993. Cons. Ophth.West Kent Eye Hosp.; Assoc. Med. Director (Clin. Governance) Bromley Hosp. NHS Trust; Cons. Ophth. Surg., Qu. Mary's Sidcup NHS Trust; Clin. Director for Ophth., Princess Roy. Univ. Hosp. Specialty: Ophth. Socs: S.. Ophth. Soc.; Fell. Roy. Soc. Med.

TREW, Geoffrey Howard Institute of Obstetrics & Gynaecology, Hammersmith Hospital, Du Cane Road, London W12 0NN Tel: 020 8383 2372 Fax: 020 8383 2371; Lodge Hill Farm, Haw Lane, Bledlow Ridge, High Wycombe HP14 4JQ — MB BS Lond. 1984 (St. Geos. Lond.) MRCOG 1991. Cons. Gyn. Hammersmith Hosp. Lond.; Hon. Sen. Lect. Imperial Coll., Lond.. Specialty: Obst. & Gyn. Socs: Brit. Fertil. Soc.; Amer. Soc. Reproduc. Med.; Brit. Soc. Gyn. Endoscopy. Prev: Sen. Regist. (O & G) Hammersmith Hosp. Lond.; Sen. Regist. & Lect. (O & G) Roy. Lond. Hosp.; Regist. (O & G) Guy's Hosp. Lond.

TREW, Judith Mary 10 Jock Inkson's Brae, Elgin IV30 1QE — MB ChB Glas. 1984; DCH Glas. 1988; MRCGP 1990. Specialty: Community Child Health. Prev: Clin. Med. Off. Ayrsh. & Arran HB.; Staffgrade Community Paediat.

TREW, Julie Mildred 47 Landrock Road, London N8 9HR — MB BS Lond. 1977.

TREW, Robert James Blencathra, 1 Fulthorpe Grove, Wynyard, Billingham TS22 5QZ Tel: 01740 644499 — MB ChB Ed. 1962; DObst RCOG 1969. Prev: GP Princip. N. Croydon Med. Centre Thornton Heath Surrey; SHO Accid. Luton & Dunstable Hosp. Luton; SHO (Med. & Surg.) Roy. Manch. Childr. Hosp.

TREWBY, Catherine Scott Clifton Court Medical Practice, Victoria Road, Darlington DL1 5JN; Hurgill House, 24 Hurgill Road, Richmond DL10 4BL — MB BS Lond. 1973; MRCP (UK) 1976; MRCGP 1980; FRCP 2003. Prev: SHO & Ho. Phys. St. Geo. Hosp. Lond.; Paediat. Regist. St. Peter's Hosp. Chertsey.

TREWBY, Peter Nicholas Memorial Hospital, Darlington DL3 6HX — MD Camb. 1980; MB 1972, BChir 1971; MRCP (UK) 1973; FRCP Lond. 1986. Cons. Phys. Darlington Memor. Hosp. Specialty: Gen. Med. Socs: Fell. Roy. Soc. Med.; Brit. Soc. Gastroenterol. Prev: SHO Brompton Hosp. Lond.; Regist. King's Coll. Hosp. Lond.; Sen. Regist. (Med.) St. Mary's Hosp. Lond.

TREWEEKE, Paul Stewart Department Radiology, North Devon District Hospital, Barnstaple EX31 4JB Tel: 01271 322619; Witham, Bydown, Swimbridge, Barnstaple EX32 0QB Tel: 01271 830170 — MB BS Lond. 1979; FRCR 1986. Cons. Radiol. N. Devon Dist. Hosp. Specialty: Radiol. Prev: Sen. Regist. (Radiol.) Char. Cross Hosp. Lond.; Regist. (Radiol.) St. Thos. Hosp. Lond.

TREWHELLA, Mrs Jean Dorothy (retired) The Old Rectory, Stansfield, Sudbury CO10 8LT — MB ChB Bristol 1955. Prev: Assoc. Specialist St. Ebba's Hosp. Epsom.

TREWHELLA, Matthew John The Mill, Killerby, Darlington DL2 3UQ — MB BS Lond. 1981; BA (Hons.) Oxf. 1977; FRCR 1987. Cons. Radiol. N. Tees Gen. Hosp. Stockton-on-Tees. Specialty: Radiol. Prev: Cons. (Radiol.) Princess of Wales RAF Hosp. Ely; Hon. Clin. Asst. (Radiol.) Hosp. for Sick Childr. Gt. Ormond St. Lond.; Hon. Regist. (Radiol.) Middlx. Hosp. Lond.

TREWIN, Peter John Heselton Balance Street Health Centre, Balance Street, Uttoxeter ST14 8JG Tel: 01889 562145 Fax: 01889 568164 Email: petertrewin@doctors.org.uk; Hill House, Denstone, Uttoxeter ST14 5HL Tel: 01889 590767 — MB BS Lond. 1983 (Char. Cross) DRCOG 1986; DCH RCP Lond. 1986. School Medical Officer. Prev: Trainee GP Mid Sussex VTS; Cas. Off. Cuckfield Hosp.

TREWINNARD, Barry Francis White House Surgery, Weston Lane, Weston, Southampton SO19 9HJ Tel: 023 8044 9913 Fax: 023 8044 6617; The White House, Weston Lane, Woolston, Southampton SO19 9HJ Tel: 01703 449913 — MB ChB Manch. 1975.

TREWINNARD, Karen Rosemary 279 Upper Deacon Road, Bitterne, Southampton SO19 5JJ — BM Soton. 1979; Cert. Family Plann. JCC 1982; MFFP 1993. Instruc. Doctor Family Plann. & Well Wom. Serv. Portsmouth; Med. Jl.ist Freelance Columnist Wom. Alive Magazine; Natural Family Plann. Teach. Catholic Marriage Advis. Counc. Specialty: Obst. & Gyn. Socs: Affil. Mem. Med. Jl.ists Assn.; Assn. BRd.casting Doctors.

TREWINNARD, Philip James 1082 Huddersfield Road, Scouthead, Oldham OL4 4AG — MB ChB Manch. 1978.

TREZIES, Allister James Harris 41 Downs Hill, Beckenham BR3 5ET — MB BS Lond. 1991.

TREZISE, Catherine Anne 6 Mill Lane, Hoobrook, Kidderminster DY10 1XP — MB ChB Birm. 1986; BSc (Hons.) Pharmacol. Birm. 1983, MB ChB 1986; DGM RCP Lond. 1992; MRCPsych 1997. SCMO Learning Disabil. Psychiat. Specialty: Ment. Health. Prev: Clin. Med. Off. (Psychiat.) Burton Rd. Hosp. Dudley.; Specialist Regist. W. Midl. Train. Scheme Learning Disabil. Psychiat.

TRIAY, Charles Henry 109 St Georges Square Mews, London SW1V 3RZ; PO Box 207, San Pedro, Alcantara, Malaga 29670, Spain Tel: 34 5278 0540 Fax: 34 5278 6534 Email: triaymedic@mercuryin.es — MB BS Lond. 1982. Prev: SHO (Paediat. & A & E) St. Mary's Teach. Gp.

TRIBE, Elizabeth Mary (retired) 255 Canford Lane, Westbury on Trym, Bristol BS9 3PF — MB BS Lond. 1954 (Middlx.)

TRIBLEY, Anthony Richard Winchcombe Medical Practice, The Surgery, Abbey Terrace, Winchcombe, Cheltenham GL54 5LL Tel: 01242 602307 Fax: 01242 603689 — BM BCh Oxf. 1989; MA Oxf. 1993, BA 1986; DCH RCP Lond. 1992; DRCOG 1993; MRCGP 1994. Specialty: Gen. Pract.

TRICKER, Mr John Antony Lessenden House, Rimpton, Yeovil BA22 8AB Tel: 01935 850922 Fax: 01935 822196 — MB BS Lond. 1966 (St. Bart.) MRCS Eng. LRCP Lond. 1966; FRCS Eng. 1973. Cons. Orthop. & Traum. Surg. Yeovil Dist. Hosp. Specialty: Orthop. Socs: Fell. BOA. Prev: Clin. Lect. (Orthop. Surg.) Univ. Oxf.; Hon. Sen. Regist. Nuffield Orthop. Centre & John Radcliffe Hosp. Oxf.

TRICKETT, Alan Charles Henry (retired) Roe Beech, Beaulieu Road, Lyndhurst SO43 7DA Tel: 023 8028 2732 — MB ChB Ed. 1961; DObst RCOG 1963; MRCGP 1969.

TRICKETT, Anthony Robert, MBE Hoy & Walls Health Centre, Bayview, Longhope, Stromness KW16 3PA Tel: 01856 701209 Fax: 01856 701224; Glebelands, Longhope, Stromness KW16 3PA Tel: 01856 701460 — (Manch.) MRCS Eng. LRCP Lond. 1964; FRSH 1996. GP Is. of Hoy, Orkney; HMA Longhope Lifeboat (RNLI). Socs: Fell. Roy. Soc. Med.; Fell. Roy. Soc. Health. Prev: Asst. Lect. (Anat.) Univ. Manch.; SHO (Path., Surg. & Paediat.) Roy. Manch. Childr. Pendlebury.

TRICKETT, Jonathan Paul Roe Beech, Beaulieu Road, Lyndhurst SO43 7DA — MB BS Lond. 1994.

TRICKEY, Mr Nicholas Robert Allan 4 Albany Road, Windsor SL4 1HL Tel: 01753 866311 Fax: 01753 850817; 4 Priory Close, Sunningdale, Ascot SL5 9SE Tel: 01344 623687 Fax: 01344 872425 — MB BS Lond. 1962 (St. Mary's) MRCS Eng. LRCP Lond. 1962; MB BS (Hons. Obst. & Gyn.) Lond. 1962; FRCS Eng. 1967; FRCOG 1983, M 1970. Specialty: Obst. & Gyn. Prev: Cons. O & G Heatherwood Hosp. Ascot & King Edwd. VII Hosp. Windsor.; Sen. Regist. (O & G) Soton. Gen. Hosp. & St. Geo. Hosp. Lond.; Regist. (O & G) St. Mary's Hosp. Lond.

TRICKLEBANK, Barry The Swan Medical Centre, 4 Willard Road, Yardley, Birmingham B25 8AA Tel: 0121 706 0216 Fax: 0121 707 3105 — MB ChB Birm. 1986.

TRICKS, Charles David Wrington Vale Medical Practice, Station Road, Wrington, Bristol BS40 5NG Tel: 01934 862532 Fax: 01934 863568; The Cottage, Ladymead Lane, Langford, Bristol BS40 5EF Tel: 01934 852652 — BM BCh Oxf. 1978 (Oxford) BA 1975; DRCOG 1980; MRCGP 1982. Specialty: Gen. Pract.

TRICKS, Norman Charles (retired) Templars, Stoford, Halse, Taunton TA4 3JJ Tel: 01823 433466 — MB ChB Bristol 1952; MRCS Eng. LRCP Lond. 1951. Prev: Ho. Phys. & Cas. Off. Bristol Roy. Infirm.

TRIEMAN, Noam Barnet, Enfield & Haringey Mental Health NHS Trust, Mental Health Unit, Chase Farm Hospital Site, The Ridgeway, Enfield EN2 8JL Tel: 0845 111 4000 Ext: 1337 Fax: 020 8364 6711 Email: noam.trieman@beh-mht.nhs.uk; The Priory Hospital North London, Grovelands House, The Bourne, Southgate, London N14 6RA Tel: 020 8882 8191 — MD (Distinc.) The Hebrew Univ., Jerusalem, Israel 1980; MRCPsych. Cons. Psychiat. Barnet, Enfield & Haringey Ment. Health NHS Trust; Privat. Vis. Cons. Psychiat. The Priory Hosp. N. Lond. Specialty: Gen. Psychiat. Special Interest: Depression; Stress & Anxiety Disorders; Dynamic Psycho-therapy. Socs: BMA; Roy. Coll. of Psychiatrists. Prev: Sen. Lect. (Community Psychiat.) Roy. Free & Univ. Coll. Med. Sch. Lond.

TRIFFITT, David James Bramley House, Mill Orchard, E. Hanney, Wantage OX12 0JH Tel: 01235 868314; 74 Sunningwell Road, Oxford OX1 4SX Email: davetriff@hotmail.com — MB BS Lond. 1992 (London Hospital Medical College) MRCGP 1997; DRCOG 1997. GP Clin. Asst. S. Oxf. Health Centre. Specialty: Gen. Pract.; Sports Med. Socs: MDU; BMA. Prev: GP Regist. Eynsham, Oxon.; SHO (O & G) Leicester Gen. Hosp.; Med. Rep. Raleigh Internat. Expedition to Belize.

TRIGG, Cecilia Jane ST Mary's Hospital, Praed Street, Paddington, London W2 1NY Tel: 020 7886 1149; Cage Farm Lodge, 68 The Ridgeway, Tonbridge TN10 4NN — MB BS Lond. 1983; MRCP (UK) 1986; MD Lond. 1992; (CCST) Immunology 1999. Cons. Allergist, St Mary's Hosp., Praed St., Paddington Lond. Specialty: Allergy. Socs: Fell. Roy. Soc. Med.; Brit. Thorac. Soc. (Mem.); Brit. Soc. Allergy Clin. Immunol. (Mem.). Prev: Sen. Regist. In Allergy, Guy's Hosp. Lond.; Research Fell. Dept. Respirat. Med. St. Bart. Hosp. Lond.; SHO & Regist. Rotat. Kings Coll. Hosp. Lond.

TRIGG, Hilary Anne Fairlands Medical Centre, Fairlands Avenue, Worplesdon, Guildford GU3 3NA Tel: 01483 594250 Fax: 01483 598767 Email: hat@doctors.org.uk; 39 Ashenden Road, Guildford GU2 7XE Tel: 01483 573339 — MB BS Lond. 1981 (King's Coll.) DCH RCP Lond. 1984; DRCOG 1985; MRCGP 1986. Prev: Trainee GP Guildford VTS; Ho. Surg. Brook Gen. Hosp. Woolwich; Ho. Phys. Dulwich Hosp. King's Health Dist.

TRIGG, Kenneth Haddon (retired) Middle Fell, Rockshaw Road, Merstham, Redhill RH1 3BZ Tel: 01737 643313 — MB BS Lond. 1954 (King's Coll. Hosp.) DObst RCOG 1958; FRCGP 1976, M 1965. Prev: Provost S.W. Thames Fac. RCGP.

TRIGG, Sarah Louise 98 Upper Cliff Road, Gorleston, Great Yarmouth NR31 6AL — BM Soton. 1998.

TRIGG, Susan Elizabeth Ellis Clifton Surgery, 151-153 Newport Road, Roath, Cardiff CF24 1AG Tel: 029 2049 4539 Fax: 029 2049 4657 — MB BCh Wales 1987; MRCGP 1992.

TRIGGS, Angharad Jane 99 King George V Dr N., Heath, Cardiff CF14 4EH — MB BCh Wales 1998.

TRIGWELL, Peter John Department of Liaison Psychiatry, Leeds General Infirmary, Great George St., Leeds LS1 3EX Tel: 0113 392 5246 Fax: 0113 392 8389 Email: peter.trigwell@leedsth.nhs.uk — MB ChB Leeds 1989; MRCPsych 1993; MMedSc Leeds 1994. Cons. Liaison Psychiat. And Psychosexual Leeds Gen. Infirm.; Hon. Sen. Clin. Lect. Univ. Leeds. Specialty: Gen. Psychiat.; Psychosexual Med. Prev: Research Sen. Regist. (Psychiat.) St James' Univ. Hosp. Leeds; Sen. Regist. (Psychiat.) Leeds Gen. Infirm.; Sen. Regist. (Psychiat.) High Royds Hosp. Leeds.

TRIKAS, Athanasios Hammersmith Hospital, Department of Cardiology, Echocardiography Section, Du Cane Road, London W12 0NN — Ptychio Iatrikes Athens 1984.

TRIKHA, Sanjay Paul 151 Heaton Road, Bradford BD9 4RZ — MB BS Lond. 1997.

TRILL, Andrea Susan 51 Grosvenor Park, London SE5 0NH — MB BS Lond. 1990; BSc, MB BS (Hons.) Lond. 1990.

TRIMBLE, Mr David Keith George 6 Grenroe, Moira, Craigavon BT67 0DT Tel: 01846 613265 — MB BCh BAO Belf. 1995; FRCSI. 1999. SHO. (ENT Surg.) Antrim Area Hosp. N. Irel.. Specialty: Otorhinolaryngol.

TRIMBLE, Professor Elisabeth Ruth, CBE Department of Clinical Biochemostry and Metabolic Medicine, Queen's University of Belfast Fax: 02890 236143 Email: e.trimble@qub.ac.uk — MB BCh BAO Belfast (Queen's Univ., Belfast) MB; MD; FRCP London; DCH; FRCPath. Prof. Clin. Biochemistry & Metabolic Med.; Cons. Chemical

Pathologist. Specialty: Chem. Path.; Endocrinol. Socs: Diabetes UK; Euro. Assoc. for the study of Diabetes; American Diabetes Assoc.

TRIMBLE, Freda Mary 155 Ballyskeagh Road, Drumbeg, Dunmurry, Belfast BT17 9LL — MB BCh BAO Belf. 1982; MB BCh Belf. 1982.

TRIMBLE, Ian Michael Geoffrey Black and Partners, Sherwood Health Centre, Elmswood Gardens, Nottingham NG5 4AD Tel: 0115 985 8822 Fax: 0115 933 9050; 23 Tavistock Avenue, Mapperley Park, Nottingham NG3 5BD Tel: 0115 985 7401 — BM BS Nottm. 1982; MPhil Nottm. 1980, BMedSci 1979; MRCGP 1988. Sen. GP Adviser DoH; GP Adviser NHSE. Prev: GP Princip.

TRIMBLE, Karl Thomas 41 Boden Road, Birmingham B28 9DL — MB ChB Liverp. 1993.

TRIMBLE, Professor Michael Robert Department of Clinical Neurology, Institute of Neurology, National Hospital, Queen Square, London WC1N 3BG Tel: 020 7837 3611 Fax: 020 7837 3611 Email: mtrimble@ion.ucl.ac.uk — MB ChB (Hons) Birm. 1970; BSc (1st Class Hons) Birm. 1967; MRCP 1972; MRCPsych 1975; MPhil Lond 1976; FRCPsych 1982; FRCP Lond. 1986; MD 1993. Prof. Inst. Neurol. Lond.; Cons. Nat. Hosp. Neurol. & Neurosurg. Dis. Qu. Sq. Lond. Specialty: Neurol.; Gen. Psychiat. Socs: Fell. Amer. Psychiat. Assn.; Fell. Roy. Soc. Med.; Brit. Neuropsychiatric Assn. (Chairm.).

TRIMBLE, Peter Henry Chester — MB BCh BAO Belf. 1985.

TRIMBLE, William George Clements Dunluce Health Centre, 1 Dunluce Avenue, Belfast BT9 7HR; 16 Cleaver Park, Malone Road, Belfast BT9 5HX — MB BCh BAO Dub. 1965; FRCGP 1986, M 1971.

TRIMLETT, Richard Henry James Pen-y-Fai Nurseries, Pen-y-Fai, Bridgend CF31 4LX — MB BS Lond. 1992.

TRIMMING, Helen Mary Dr Ayre & Partners, Hartlepool Health Centre, Victori Road, Hartlepool T26 8DB; 25 St Edmunds Green, Sedgefield TS21 3H7 — MB BChir Camb. 1994; DRCOG 1998; DFFP 1998; MRCGP 1999. GP salaried, Hartlepool PCT; GP s/i Palliat. Care Hospice, Hartlepool. Specialty: Gen. Pract. Prev: GP Regist. Cleveland VTS; Salaried GP, McKenzie Ho., Hartlepool; GP Regist., Sedgefield.

TRIMMINGS, Mr Nigel Peter Dept. of Orthopaedics, Royal Hampshire County Hospital, Romsey Road, Winchester SO22 5DG Tel: 01962 824979 — MB BS Lond. 1975 (St. Mary's) MRCS Eng. LRCP Lond. 1975; FRCS Eng. 1980. Cons. Surg. Orthop. Roy. Hants. Co. Hosp. Winchester; Hon. Clin. Prof., St Geo.'s Univ., Grenada, W. Indes. Specialty: Trauma & Orthop. Surg. Socs: Fell. BOA; Brit. Elbow & Shoulder Soc.; Roy. Soc. Med. - Mem. of Counc. Commail Orthopadiesetion. Prev: Sen. Regist. (Orthop.) Roy. Free & Windsor Gp.

TRINDER, Johanna Homefield, Wilkes Farm, Doynton, Bristol BS30 5TJ — MB BS Lond. 1990 (Charing Cross and Westminster) MRCOG 1995. Research Regist. (O & G). Specialty: Obst. & Gyn.

TRINDER, Thomas John 16 Manor Hill, Carnesure Manor, Killinchy Road, Comber, Newtownards BT23 5FN Tel: 01247 870422 — MB BCh BAO Belf. 1986; FFA RCSI 1990; MD Belf. 1995. Cons. (Anaesth. & Intens. Care) Ulster Hosp. Belf.; Dir. Intens. Care. Specialty: Intens. Care. Socs: Assn. Anaesth.; Intens. Care Soc. Irel.; Soc. Critical Care Med. Prev: Chief Regist. (Intens. Care Unit) Roy. Adelaide Hosp., Australia; Research Fell. Regional Intens. Care Unit Roy. Hosps. Belf.

TRING, Frederick Charles (retired) Spring House Farm, Gowland Lane, Cloughton, Scarborough YO13 0DU Tel: 01723 870395 — LDS 1966; MB ChB Sheff. 1967; PhD Sheff. 1982, MA 1972, MD 1973; MRCGP 1976. Prev: Cons. Dermat. Bradford, Airedale & Wharfedale Hosps.

TRING, Ian Charles Department of Anaesthesia, Scarborough Hospital, Woodlands Drive, Scarborough YO12 6QL Tel: 01723 368111; Spring House Farm, Gowland Lane, Cloughton, Scarborough YO13 0DU Tel: 01723 870319 — MB BS Lond. 1981 (St. Bart.) MRCS Eng. LRCP Lond. 1981; DA Eng. 1983; FFA RCSI 1985; FRCA 1997. Cons. Anaesth. ScarBorough. Hosp. Specialty: Anaesth. Socs: Assn. Dent. Anaesth.; Assn. Anaesth.; Yorks. Soc. Anaesth. Prev: Sen. Regist. Rotat. (Anaesth.) Yorks. RHA.

TRING, Jonathan Patrick 28 Leicester Road, Uppingham, Oakham LE15 9SD — MB ChB Leeds 1989; FFA RCSI 1996.

TRINICK, Thomas Richard The Ulster Hospital, Belfast BT16 1RH Tel: 028 9048 4511 Ext: 2600 Fax: 028 9048 7131 Email: tom.trinick@ucht.n-i.nhs.uk; 3 Malone Meadows, Belfast BT9 5BG Tel: 028 9066 7803 Fax: 028 9066 7803 Email: Thomas.Trinick@btinternet.com — MB BCh BAO Belf. 1977 (Qu. Univ Belf.) MRCP (UK) 1981; FRCPath 1995, M 1986; BSc (Hons.) Belf. 1975, MD 1988; FRCP Ed. 1996; FRCP Lond. 1998; FRCPI 2000. Cons. Chem. Path. and General Phys. Ulster Hosp. Belf. And Chairm. of the Regional Med. Audit Comm., N.I.; Hon. Clin. Lect., Clin. Biochemistry, Qu.s Univ. of Belf.; Lect. in BioMed. Sci.s, Univ. of Ulster; Chairman E. Medical Advisory Committee Belfast. Specialty: Chem. Path.; Gen. Med.; Diabetes. Special Interest: Vasc. Dis. and androgen Defic. Socs: Hyperlip. Assn.; Irish Cardiac Soc.; Irish Angiology Soc. Prev: NI Regional Tutor in Clin. Biochem.ry; Sen. Regist. (Chem. Path.) Roy. Vict. Hosp. Belf.; Sen. Regist. Clin. Biochem.ry and Metab. Med. Roy. Vict. Infirm. Newc. upon Tyne.

TRIPATHI, Bharat Prasad Golf Course Road Surgery, 11 Golf Course Road, Livingston EH54 8QF — MB BS Punjab 1967 (Govt. Med. Coll. Patiala) MB BS Punjabi 1967. GP Livingston.

TRIPATHI, Dharam Narain St Nicholas Health Centre, Saunder Bank, Burnley BB11 2EN Tel: 01282 422528 Fax: 01282 832834 — MB BS Lucknow 1958; MB BS Lucknow 1958.

TRIPATHI, Dharmendra Pati The Jersey Practice, Heston Health Centre, Cranford Lane, Hounslow TW5 9ER Tel: 020 8321 3434 Fax: 020 8321 3440 — MB BS Patna 1968 (Patna Med. Coll.) DTD Patna 1971; DTCD Wales 1976. SHO Cefn Mably Hosp. Socs: Fell. Internat. Federat. Sports Med. Athens; Coll. Chest Phys. U.S.A.

TRIPATHI, Dhiraj 4/6 West Savile Gardens, Edinburgh EH9 3AB — MB ChB Ed. 1994; MRCP (UK) 1999. SpR (Gastroenter./Gen. Int. Med.) Edin.

TRIPNEY, Robert Edmiston Scott Delapre Medical Centre, Gloucester Avenue, Northampton NN4 8QF Tel: 01604 761713; 17 Favell Way, Northampton NN3 3BZ Tel: 01604 403396 — MB ChB Ed. 1961; DObst RCOG 1963; DCH Eng. 1965; MRCP Lond. 1969. Hosp. Pract. (Electrocardiog.) Northampton Gen. Hosp. Specialty: Gen. Med. Socs: BMA; CMF. Prev: Pres. N.ants. Med. Soc.

TRIPP, Joanna Claire Scott 20 Inverleith Gardens, Edinburgh EH3 5PS — MB BS Lond. 1987.

TRIPP, John Howard Department of Child Health, Royal Devon & Exeter Hospital (Wonford), Barrack Road, Exeter EX2 5DW Tel: 01392 403148 Fax: 01392 403158 Email: jhtripp@ex.ac.uk; Pixie Cottage, Alphington, Exeter EX2 8TD Tel: 01392 270392 — MB BS Lond. 1968 (Guy's) MRCP (UK) 1971; BSc Lond. 1965, MD 1979; FRCP Lond. 1986; FRCPCH 1997. Sen. Lect. (Child Health) Univ. Exeter Postgrad. Med. Sch.; Cons. Paediat. Roy. Devon & Exeter Hosp. Exeter. Specialty: Paediat. Socs: Brit. Soc. Allergy & Clin. Immunol.; Fell. Coll. Paediat. & Child Health; Fell. RCP. Prev: Sen. Regist. Hosp. Sick Childr. Gt. Ormond St. Lond.; Research Fell. Inst. Child Health Lond.

TRIPP, Sarah Jane Carreg-y-Borth, Telford Road, Menai Bridge LL59 5DT — MB ChB Leeds 1991.

TRIPPE, Helen Ruth West Surrey Health Authority, The Ridgewood Centre, Old Bisley Road, Camberley GU16 9QE Tel: 01276 671718; Summerfield, Park Road, Winchester SO22 6AA — BM Soton. 1985; BA Birm. 1967; MFPHM RCP (UK) 1994. Cons. Pub. Health Med. W. Surrey Health Auth. Camberley Surrey. Specialty: Pub. Health Med. Prev: Sen. Regist. (Pub. Health Med.) Wessex Inst. Pub. Health Med. Winchester; Vis. Fell. Fac. Educat. Univ. Soton.; Regist. (Pub. Health Med.) Salisbury Dist. Health Auth.

TRISCOTT, Ann Patricia (retired) — MB ChB Birm. 1961; DA Eng. 1964; FFA RCS Eng. 1969. Prev: Cons. Anaesth. Harefield Hosp. Middlx.

TRISTRAM, Amanda Jane Renby Fold Farm Cottage, Mossy Lea Rd, Wrightington, Wigan WN6 9SA — MB ChB Sheff. 1991; MRCOG. 1998. SHO (Obst & Gyn.) Manch. Specialty: Obst. & Gyn. Prev: SHO (O & G) Sheff.

TRISTRAM, Stephen John North Hampshire Hospital, Department of Surgery, Aldermaston Road, Basingstoke RG24 9NA Tel: 01256 313569; Walnut Tree House, 5 Paddock Fields, Old Basing, Basingstoke RG24 7DB Tel: 01256 328327 Email: drstristram@aol.com — MB ChB St. And. 1968; DObst RCOG 1971. Sen. Med. Advis. Provensis Ltd S. Harefield Middlx.; Assoc. Specialist (Surg.) N. Hants. Hosp.; Practising rights: The Hants. Clinic, Basingstoke, Parkside Hosp. Wimbledon, Ashtead Hosp. Socs: BMA; Roy. Soc. Med. Prev: Med. Off. Sun Life Financial of Cananda, Basingstoke, Hants.

TRITTON, Barbara Antoinette 62 Windsor Drive, Chelsfield, Orpington BR6 6HD Tel: 01689 852204; Quinneys, The Hillside, Pratts Bottom, Orpington BR6 7SD Tel: 01689 58257 — MB BS Lond. 1966 (Westm.) MRCS Eng. LRCP Lond. 1965. Mem. Bromley LMC. Prev: Ho. Surg. Westm. Childr. Hosp.; Ho. Phys. FarnBoro. Hosp. Kent.

TRIVEDI, Alka Deepak Warrington Road Surgery, 429A Warrington Road, Abram, Wigan WN2 5XB Tel: 01942 866277 Fax: 01942 866198 — MB BS Indore 1973.

TRIVEDI, Deepak Warrington Road Surgery, 429A Warrington Road, Abram, Wigan WN2 5XB Tel: 01942 607627 Fax: 01942 261747 — MB BS Indore 1973.

TRIVEDI, Devyani Vipin Scarisbrick Practice, 13 Scarisbrick New Road, Southport PR8 6PX Tel: 01704 531114 Fax: 01704 533794; 13 Scarisbrick New Road, Southport PR8 6PX — MB BS Gujarat 1966 (B.J. Med. Coll. Ahmedabad) DGO 1968; MFFP 1993. GP Southport; Sen. Clin. Med. Off. St. Helen's & Knowsley HA. Prev: Regist. (O & G) St. Helier Hosp. Carshalton.

TRIVEDI, Hemant Vishvanath Parker Drive Medical Centre, 122 Parker Drive, Leicester LE4 0JF Tel: 0116 235 3148; 16 All Saints Road, Thurcaston, Leicester LE7 7JD Tel: 0116 236 3076 Fax: 0116 236 3076 — MB BS Bombay 1966 (Grant Med. Coll.) Socs: LMS; BMA; LMC. Prev: SHO (Obst.), SHO (Gyn.) & SHO (Surg.) Leicester Roy. Infirm.

TRIVEDI, Janakbala 6 Gaudi Walk, Rogerstone, Newport NP10 0AG — MB BS Calcutta 1964; DObst RCOG 1972.

TRIVEDI, Jitendrakumar Shreeji Medical Centre, 22 Whitby Road, Slough SL1 3DQ Tel: 01753 527988 Fax: 01753 530269 — MB BS Baroda 1974; MB BS Baroda 1974.

TRIVEDI, Kathryn Louise Greenways, Gussage All Saints, Wimborne BH21 5ET — MB ChB Sheff. 1997.

TRIVEDI, Kiran Mayee Great Barr Group Practice, 912 Walsall Road, Great Barr, Birmingham B42 1TG Tel: 0121 357 1250 Fax: 0121 358 4857; 27 Athlone Road, Walsall WS5 3QU — MB BS Vikram 1961; DObst RCOG 1971.

TRIVEDI, Kirit Girijashankar 8 Walnut Drive, Bishop's Stortford CM23 4JT — MB BS Gujarat 1972.

TRIVEDI, Monica 27 Athlone Road, Walsall WS5 3QU — MB BS Lond. 1996; MRCP (Lond.) 1999.

TRIVEDI, Ravi Shanker 51 Stambourne Way, Upper Norwood, London SE19 2PY Tel: 020 8653 6865 — MB BS Lucknow 1942; DTM & H Eng. 1955.

TRIVEDI, Sanjay Hemant 16 All Saints Road, Thurcaston, Leicester LE7 7JD — MB ChB Sheff. 1997.

TRIVEDI, Mr Satish Kumar 83 Woodstock Avenue, Golders Green, London NW11 9RH Tel: 020 8458 8288; 83 Woodstock Avenue, Golders Green, London NW11 9RH — MB BS Jiwaji 1974 (G. R. Med. Coll. Gwalior (MP)) DO RCS Eng. 1976; FRCS Ed. 1983; FRCS Glas. 1984. Specialty: Ophth.

TRIVEDI, Vipin Ambalal Scarisbrick Practice, 13 Scarisbrick New Road, Southport PR8 6PX Tel: 01704 531114 Fax: 01704 533794 — MB BS Gujarat 1966 (B.J. Med. Coll. Ahmedabad) DA Gujarat 1968. Socs: Assoc. Mem. RCGP; Indian Soc. Anaesth.; BMA. Prev: Regist. (Anaesth.) Roy. Infirm. Aberd., Moorfields Eye Hosp. (City Rd. Br.) Lond. & City Hosp. Nottm.

TRIVEDI, Vishnuprasad Jagjivandas 49 Corfton Road, London W5 1AQ — MRCS Eng. LRCP Lond. 1978; LCPS Bombay 1945; LAH Dub. 1957.

TROKO, David Memba 2 Longmeadow Close, Sutton Coldfield B75 7SQ Tel: 0121 240 4165 Email: dtroka@hotmail.com/ memba@lineone.net — MD Liberia 1981; BSc Liberia 1975. Staff Grade (Accid. & Emerg.) Good Hope Hosp. Sutton Coldfield. Specialty: Accid. & Emerg.; Orthop. Special Interest: Hand Trauma.

TROLLEN, Robert Michael Milton Medical Centre, 109 Egilsay Street, Glasgow G22 7JL Tel: 0141 772 1183 Fax: 0141 772 2331; 25 Clevenden Gardens, Kelvinside, Glasgow G12 0PU Tel: 0141 357 5641 — MB ChB Glas. 1972. Mem. LMC. Socs: BMA; Occupational Med. Servs.

TROMANS, Anthony Matthew 13 Russell Street, Wilton, Salisbury SP2 0BG — MB ChB Manch. 1978.

TROMANS, Jonathan Paul National Public Health Service of Wales, Temple of Peace & Health, Cathays Park, Cardiff CF10 3NW Tel: 02920 402479; 3 Vale Court, Cowbridge, Cowbridge CF71 7ES Tel: 01446 773485 — BM BCh Oxf. 1976 (Oxford) BA (1st cl.) Oxf. 1972; MFPHM RCP (UK) 1993. Cons. Pub. Health Med.,Nat. Pub. Health Serv.Wales. & Pub. Health Dir. Rhondda Cynon Taf Local Health Board. Specialty: Pub. Health Med. Prev: Sen. Med. Off., Nat. Assembly for Wales, Cardiff; Sen. Regist. (Pub. Health Med.) Health Promotion Auth. For Wales Cardiff; Princip. GP Cowes I. of Wight.

TROMANS, Philip Marcel Chesterfield Royal Hospital, Calow, Chesterfield S44 5BL Tel: 01246 277271 Email: philip.tromans@chesterfieldroyal.nhs.uk — MB ChB Liverp. 1973; FRCOG 1992, M 1978. Cons. O & G Chesterfield & N. Derbysh. Roy. Hosp. Specialty: Obst. & Gyn. Socs: N. Eng. Obst. & Gyn. Soc.; (Co. Chairm.) Derbysh. Hosp. Cons. & Specialists Assn. Prev: Lect. (O & G) Univ. Liverp.; Hon. Sen. Regist. Liverp. HA.

TROMPETAS, Alexander Selsdon Park Medical Practice, 95 Addington Road, South Croydon CR2 8LG Tel: 020 8657 0067 Fax: 020 8657 0037; Marlowes, Tandridge Road, Warlingham CR6 9LS Tel: 01883 627027 — Ptychio Iatrikes Ioannina 1985 (Med. Sch. Univ. Ioannina, Greece) MBBS Ioannina Greece 1985; MRCGP 1990. Sen. Partner Selsdon Pk. Med. Pract.; Tutor (Gen. Pract.) Croydon; Chairm. Centr. Croydon PCG; Starnet Lead GP (S. Thames Region). Specialty: Gen. Pract. Prev: Clin. Asst. (HIV) Croydon; Chairm. Centr. Croydon Commissioning Gp.

TROMPETER, Richard Simon Great Ormond Street Hospital for Children NHS Trust, London WC1 3JH Tel: 020 7813 8305 Fax: 020 7829 8841 Email: trompr@gosh.nhs.uk — MB BS Lond. 1970 (Guy's) MRCS Eng. LRCP Lond. 1970; MRCP (UK) 1973; FRCP Lond. 1989; FRCPCH 1997. Cons. Paediat. (Nephrol.) Hosp. for Childr. Gt. Ormond St. Lond.; Sen. Clin. Lecturer; Inst. of Nephrol.; UCLH Lond. Specialty: Paediat.; Nephrol. Socs: Internat. Soc. of Nephrol.; Internat. Soc. of Paeditrics & Nephrol.; Brit. Transpl. Soc. Prev: Cons. Paediat. Roy. Free Hosp. & Med. Sch. Lond.; Lect. & Hon. Sen. Regist. (Paediat.) Guy's Hosp. Lond.; Research Fell. Inst. Child Health Lond. & Regist. Hosp Sick Childr. Gt. Ormond St.

TROMPETER, Sara 1 Holt Close, London N10 3HW Tel: 020 8444 8985 — MB ChB Bristol 1997; BSc (Hons) Psychol. 1994. Paediat. SHO UCH Hosp., Lond. Specialty: Paediat. Socs: BMA. Prev: SHO ATE Kings Coll. Hosp., Windsor; Ho. Off. (Surg.) Whipps Cross Hosp. Lond.; Ho. Off. (Med.) Bristol Roy. Infirm.

TROOP, Anne Catherine Long Meadow, Shawes Drive, Anderton, Chorley PR6 9HR Tel: 01257 480604 — MB ChB Liverp. 1980; DMRD Liverp. 1984; FRCR 1986. Cons. Radiol. Roy. Albert Edwd. Infirm. Wigan. Specialty: Radiol.

TROOP, Patricia Ann, CBE Dept of Health, Richmond House, 79 Whitehall, London SW1A 2NS Tel: 020 7210 5591 Fax: 020 7930 4636 Email: pat.troop@doh.gsi.gov.uk — MB ChB Manch. 1971; FRCP 2002 (Elected); MSc Manch. 1979; FFCM 1986, M 1980; MA Cambridge 1988. Dep. Chief Med. Off., Dept. of Health; Vis. Prof. at the Lond. Sch. of Hyg. Specialty: Pub. Health Med. Prev: Regional Director of Pub. Health (E.ern Region, Formerly Anglia & Oxf., formerly E. Anglia Chief Camb. HA & Camb FHSA.

TRORY, Graham Howard Hartlepool Healthcentre, Victoria Road, Hartlepool TS26 8DB Tel: 01429 278139 Fax: 01429 864004 — MB ChB Dundee 1988. Trainee GP Bangor VTS.

TROSS, Samantha Zoisa 23 Kitchener Road, Thornton Heath, Croydon CR7 8QN Email: zoisa1@aol.com — MB BS Lond. 1992; FRCS Eng. 1997. SHO Rotat. (Surg.) Roy. Lond. Hosp.; Specialist Regist. (Orthop.) S.E Thames. Specialty: Orthop. Prev: SHO (Orthop. Surg.) Mayday Univ. Hosp. Thornton Heath.; SHO (A & E) St. Geo. Hosp. Trust; Demonst. (Anat.) Qu. Mary & Westfield Coll. Lond.

TROSSER, Alan Highbury Grange Health Centre, Highbury Grange, London N5 2QB Tel: 020 7226 2462 — MB BS Lond. 1978 (Univ. Coll. Hosp.) BSc Lond. 1973; MRCP (UK) 1980. Prev: Research Fell. & Hon. Regist. (Cardiac) King's Coll Hosp. Lond.

TROTMAN, Ivan Frank 74 Moor Lane, Rickmansworth WD3 1LQ — MB BS Lond. 1971; MRCP (UK) 1975; MD Lond. 1988; FRCP Lond. 1994. Cons. Phys. & Dir. (Palliat. Med.) Mt. Vernon Hosp. Northwood. Specialty: Gastroenterol.; Gen. Med.; Palliat. Med. Socs: Brit. Soc. Gastroenterol. & Assn. Palliat. Med. Prev: Sen. Regist. & Research Fell. Dept. Gastroenterol. Centr. Middlx. Hosp. Lond.; Sen. Regist. (Gen. Med. & Geriat.) United Oxf. Hosps.; Squadron Ldr. (Med. Specialist) RAF Med. Br.

TROTT, Leonard Inglis Bryn Elfed, Pontrhydyfen, Port Talbot SA12 9TN Tel: 01639 896244 — MB BCh Wales 1957.

TROTT, Peter Alan Department of Cytopathology, Royal Marsden Hospital, Fulham Road, London SW3 6JJ Tel: 020 7352 8171; Flat 1, 20-21 Marylebone High St, London W1M 3PE Tel: 020 7224 4617 — MB BChir Camb. 1966 (Guy's) MRCS Eng. LRCP Lond. 1959; FRCPath 1984, M 1972. Cons. Path. (Cytol.) Roy. Marsden Hosp. & Dir. Path. The Lond. Clinic Edr. Cytopath.; Cons. Cytopath. to Army. Specialty: Histopath. Socs: (Pres.) Brit. Soc. Clin. Cytol. Prev: Cons. Path. (Cytol.) St. Stephen's Hosp. Lond.; Research Fell. (Path.) St. Pauls Hosp. Lond.

TROTTER, Barbara Marion (retired) Half Acre, Southfields, Speldhurst, Tunbridge Wells TN3 0PD — (Liverp.) MB ChB Liverp. 1947; DA Eng. 1953. Prev: Asst. Anaesth. Kingston Hosp. Gp.

TROTTER, Carol Agnes 11 Holmesland Lane, Botley, Southampton SO30 2EH — MB ChB Dundee 1973; MRCPsych 1977. Cons. Psychiat. (Psychogeriat.) St. Jas. Hosp. Portsmouth. Mem. BMA. Specialty: Geriat. Psychiat.

TROTTER, Christopher 50 Browmere Drive, Croft, Warrington WA3 7HR — MB ChB Aberd. 1979.

TROTTER, Mr Geoffrey Alan 28 Buckingham Close, Petts Wood, Orpington BR5 1SA Tel: 01689 833441 Fax: 01622 723066 — MB ChB Liverp. 1975; FRCS Eng. 1980; MS Soton. 1986. Cons. Gen. Surg. Maidstone Hosp. Specialty: Gen. Surg. Prev: Sen. Regist. (surg.) Guy's Hosp. Lond.; Regist. (Surg.) Basingstoke Dist. Hosp.; Regist. & Tutor (Surg.) Bristol Teach. Hosps.

TROTTER, Geoffrey Gerald Rushbottom Lane Surgery, 91 Rushbottom Lane, Benfleet SS7 4EA Tel: 01268 754311 — MB BS Lond. 1976.

TROTTER, John King (retired) Spindlewood, Tredrea Gdns, Perran-ar-Worthal, Truro TR3 7QG Tel: 01872 863468 — MRCS Eng. LRCP Lond. 1946 (Lond. Hosp.) DA Eng. 1954; FFA RCS Eng. 1957. Prev: Cons. Anaesth. W. Cornw. Clin. Area.

TROTTER, Matthew Ian Sunset Cottage, Blackpond Lane, Lower Bourne, Farnham GU10 3NW — MB ChB Birm. 1995; MRCS Eng. 1998. Otolaryngol., head and neck Surg., W. Midlands.

TROTTER, Penelope Anne Musgrove Park Hospital, Taunton TA1 5; Church Hill Cottage, Halse, Taunton TA4 3AB Tel: 01823 432815 — MB BS Lond. 1980 (Lond. Hosp.) DCH RCP Lond. 1985; DRCOG 1985; MRCGP 1986. Staff Doctor Gyn. (gynaecology & colposcopy) Som. HA. Specialty: Family Plann. & Reproduc. Health. Prev: Clin. Asst. (Colposcopy) Som. HA; Trainee GP N.umbrian VTS.

TROTTER, Philip Miles 92 Blenheim Place, Aberdeen AB25 2DY — MB ChB Aberd. 1976; MRCPsych 1981; FRCPsych 1998. Cons. Psychiat. Roy. Cornhill Hosp. Aberd. Specialty: Gen. Psychiat. Prev: Cons. Pscyhiat. Stratheden Hosp. Cupar & Kingseat Hosp. Newmachar; Lect. (Psychiat.) Univ. Dundee; Regist. Roy. Cornhill Hosp. Aberd.

TROTTER, Robin Fenwick Goodacre and Partners, Swadlincote Surgery, Darklands Road, Swadlincote DE11 0PP Tel: 01283 551717 Fax: 01283 211905; 4 Home Farm, Geary Lane, Bretby, Burton-on-Trent DE15 0QE Tel: 01283 702221 — MB ChB Birm. 1980; MRCGP 1986. Specialty: Gen. Pract. Prev: Trainee GP Measham; Ho. Phys. & SHO (Med.) Burton on Trent Gen. Hosp.

TROTTER, Simon Edward Dept of Histopathology, Birmingham Heartlands Hospital, Bordesley Green E., Birmingham B9 5SS Tel: 0121 685 5877 Fax: 0121 685 5898 Email: set@doctors.org.uk — MB BS Lond. 1980 (Lond. Hosp.) MRCPath 1992. Cons.(Histopath & Cytopath.) Heartlands & Solihull NHS Trust. Specialty: Histopath. Socs: Fell. Roy. Soc. Med.; Internat. Acad. Path. (Brit. Div.). Prev: Sen. Regist. (Histopath.) Roy. Brompton & Nat. Heart & Lung Inst. Lond.

TROTTER, Simon Hony Links Medical Centre, 4 Hermitage Place, Edinburgh EH6 8BW Tel: 0131 554 1036 Fax: 0131 555 3995; 7 Stirling Road, Edinburgh EH5 3HZ — MB ChB Ed. 1975; BA Camb. 1972; DRCOG 1977; MRCGP 1982.

TROTTER, Timothy Nigel Anaesthetic Department, Glenfield General Hospital, Leicester — MB ChB Manch. 1981; BSc St. And. 1978; MB ChB (Hons.) Manch. 1981; DRCOG 1984; MRCGP (Distinc.) 1985; FCAnaesth 1989. Cons. Anaesth. Glenfield Gen. Hosp. Specialty: Anaesth. Prev: Lect. (Anaesth.) Univ. Leic.

TROUGHTON, Alison Mary Josephine Gray and Troughton, The Health Centre, Tavanagh Avenue, Craigavon BT62 3BU Tel: 028 3835 1393 — MB BCh BAO Belf. 1987; DCH Dub. 1990; Dip. Ment. Health Belf. 1990; MRCGP 1991; DRCOG 1992. GP Partner Job share. Prev: Trainee GP Stranraer; SHO Craigavon Area Hosp.

TROUGHTON, Alvan Harold 45 Victoria Road, Cirencester GL7 1ES; Department of Radiology, Princess Margaret Hospital, Swindon SN1 4JU — MB ChB Bristol 1978; MRCP (UK) 1983; FRCR 1989; FRCP 1998. Cons. (Radiol.) Princess Margt. Hosp. Swindon. Specialty: Radiol.

TROUGHTON, Kimberley Elizabeth Vance 2 Lime Kiln Lane, Aghalee, Craigavon BT67 0EZ; 94 Church Road, Randalstown BT41 3JW — MB BCh BAO Belf. 1990; DCH Dub. 1993; MRCP (UK) 1994. Cons. Community Paediat., Antrim Area Hosp., Antrim, N.I. Specialty: Paediat.

TROUGHTON, Thomas William Eric The Health Centre, High Street, Catterick Village, Richmond DL10 7LD Tel: 01748 811475 Fax: 01748 818284; Oakleigh House, Brompton-on-Swale, Richmond DL10 7HN — MB BCh BAO Belf. 1980; DRCOG 1982.

TROUGHTON, Timothy St John — MB BCh BAO Belf. 1992; DGM RCPS Glas. 1994; DCH Dub. 1995; DRCOG 1995; MRCGP 1996; DFFP 1997. Specialty: Gen. Pract.

TROUGHTON, Victoria Andrea Greenwich & Bexley Cottage Hospice, 185 Bostall Hill, Abbey Wood, London SE2 0QX Tel: 020 8312 2244 Fax: 020 8312 0202; 154 Wricklemarsh Road, Blackheath, London SE3 8DP — BM Soton. 1994; DMH Belf. 1996. Specialty: Palliat. Med.

TROULI, Charikliа Flat 3, Brockley Hill House, Royal National Orthopaedic Hospital, Brockley Hill, Stanmore HA7 4LP — Ptychio Iatrikes Athens 1986.

TROUNCE, Christopher Charles McIntosh, Trounce and Harvey, Health Centre, Orchard Way, Kingsbridge TQ7 2LB Tel: 01548 580214 Fax: 01548 581080 — MB BS Lond. 1978; MRCP (UK) 1982; MRCGP 1984.

TROUNCE, David Quartermaine (retired) 63 Madeira Park, Tunbridge Wells TN2 5SX Tel: 01892 529942 — (Guy's) MB BS Lond. 1944; MRCS Eng. LRCP Lond. 1945; FRCP Lond. 1973, M 1949; DCH Eng. 1949; MD Lond. 1950. Prev: Cons. Paediat. Harlow Hosp. Gp.

TROUNCE, John Quartermaine Royal Alexandra Hospital for Sick Children, Brighton BN1 3JN Tel: 01273 328145 Fax: 01273 736685 — MB BS Lond. 1976 (Guy's) MRCS Eng. LRCP Lond. 1976; DCH RCP Lond. 1980; MRCP (UK) 1981; MD Leic. 1994; FRCP Lond. 1994; FRCPCH 1997. Cons. Paediat. Roy. Alexandra Hosp. for Sick Childr. Brighton. Specialty: Paediat. Socs: Neonat. Soc.; Paediat. Intens. Care Soc. Prev: Sen. Regist. (Paediat.) Qu. Med. Centre Nottm.; Regist. (Paediat.) Leics. Roy. Infirm.; SHO (Paediat.) Qu. Eliz. Hosp. Childr. Lond.

TROUNCE, Professor John Reginald (retired) Farnehill, Ightham, Sevenoaks TN15 9HE Tel: 01732 882556 — (Guy's) MB BS (Hons. Med. & Path.) Lond. 1943; MRCS Eng. LRCP Lond. 1943; FRCP Lond. 1964, M 1944; MD Lond. 1946. Emerit. Prof. Clin. Pharm. & Emerit. Phys. Guy's Hosp. Lond. Prev: Sen. Asst. & Sen. Regist. (Med.) Guy's Hosp. Lond.

TROUNCE, Nicholas David Heene and Goring Practice, 145 Heene Road, Worthing BN11 4NY Tel: 01903 235344 Fax: 01903 247099; 9 Landsdowne Court, Worthing BN11 5HD Tel: 01903 49889 — MB BChir Camb. 1976 (Westm.) BA Camb. 1973; DCH Eng. 1979; DRCOG 1981. Princip. GP Worthing. Prev: SHO (Med.) St. Heliers Carshalton; SHO (Paediat.) St. Richards Hosp. Chichester; SHO (O & G) St. Richards Hosp. Chichester.

TROUNCE, Richard Fleming Lincoln Road Practice, 63 Lincoln Road, Peterborough PE1 2SF Tel: 01733 565511 Fax: 01733 569230 — MB BS Lond. 1983; DCH RCP Lond. 1988.

TROUNSON, William Noy 42 Church End, Biddenham, Bedford MK40 4AR — MB BS Lond. 1977; MRCP (UK) 1981.

TROUP, David Farquharson Arrochar Surgery, Kirkfield Place, Arrochar G83 7AE Tel: 01301 702531 Fax: 01301 702746; 35 George Street, Helensburgh G84 7EU Tel: 01436 674474 — MB ChB Aberd. 1976; MRCGP 1980. Socs: Assoc. Mem. Fac. Homoeop.; Brit. Soc. Experim. & Clin. Hypn.; BASICS. Prev: GP Turriff; Trainee GP Aberd. VTS.

TROUP, Dorothy Iona (retired) 61 Woodside Drive, Forres IV36 2UF Tel: 01309 675724 — MB ChB Ed. 1949; DObst RCOG 1954. Prev: Med. Adviser Dorothy Ho. Foundat. Bath.

TROUP, Douglas (retired) Group Practice Centre, Old Chester Road, Great Sutton, South Wirral — MB ChB Glas. 1951; DObst RCOG 1955.

TROUP, John Duncan Gordon Kirkton House, Cairnie, Huntly AB54 4TR Tel: 01466 760207 Fax: 01466 760300 Email: john.troup@kirkton-house.fsnet.co.uk — MRCS Eng. LRCP Lond. 1949 (St. Thos.) DSc Med. Lond. 1989, PhD 1968; FFOM (Hons.) RCP Lond. 1994, MFOM 1985. Hon. Sen. Research Fell. (Orthop. Surg.) Univ. Aberd. Specialty: Occupat. Health; Research; Medico Legal. Socs: Fell. Ergonomics Soc. Prev: Cons. & Vis. Prof. Inst. Occupat. Health, Helsinki; Hon. Cons. Phys. Roy. Free Hosp. Lond.; Research Fell. Inst. Orthop. & Dir. Dawn Trust Unit for Spinal Research.

TROUTON, Thomas Graham Antrim Hospital, 45 Bush Road, Antrim BT41 2RL Tel: 028 944 24287 Fax: 028 944 24679 Email: tom.trouton@uh.n-i.nhs.uk; 74 Ballinderry Road, Lisburn BT28 2QS — MB BCh BAO Belf. 1983; MRCP (UK) 1986; BSc (Hons.) Belf. 1980, MD 1989; FRCP Ed. 1996; FRCP Lond. 1997. Cons. Cardiol. Antrim Hosp.; Hon. Cons. Roy. Gp. Hosps. Belf. Specialty: Cardiol. Socs: BMA; Coun. Mem. Irish Cardiac Soc.; Brit. Cardiac Soc. Prev: Clin. Research Fell. Cardiol. Mass. Gen. Hosp. & Harvard Med. Sch. Boston, USA; Sen. Regist. (Cardiol.) Roy. Vict. Hosp. Belf.; Research Fell. Roy. Vict. Hosp. Belf.

TROWBRIDGE, Michael David The Veterinary Surgery, Ralphs Ride, Bracknell RG12 9LG; 2 Kingfisher Drive, Barnstaple EX32 8QW — MB BS Lond. 1992.

TROWELL, Geoffrey Mark Highbridge Medical Centre, Pepperall Road, Highbridge TA9 3YA Tel: 01278 783220 Fax: 01278 795486; 50 Rectory Road, Burnham-on-Sea TA8 2BZ Tel: 01278 764230 — MB BS Lond. 1987 (Char. Cross & Westm. Med. Sch.) DRCOG 1991; MRCGP 1993. Police Surg. Som. Specialty: Gen. Pract.

TROWELL, Hugh Miles Sandown Medical Centre, Melville Street, Sandown PO36 8LD Tel: 01983 402464 Fax: 01983 405781 Email: hugh.trowell@gp-j84013.nhs.uk — MB BS Lond. 1988 (St. Thomas' Hospital, London) DRCOG 1992, prize medal; Cert. Family Plann. JCC 1992; T(G) 1992; MRCGP 1992. GP I. of Wight. Specialty: Gen. Pract. Prev: Trainee GP I. of Wight VTS; SHO (Psychiat.) Newcroft Hosp. Newport, I. of Wight.

TROWELL, Jeremy Everard Pathology Laboratory, Ipswich Hospital NHS Trust, Heath Rd, Ipswich IP4 5PD Tel: 01473 703735 — (St. Bart.) BChir 1967; MB Camb. 1968; MRCPath 1974. Cons.Histopath, Ipswich Hosp. NHS Trust. Specialty: Histopath. Socs: Path. Soc.; Assn. of Clin. Pathologists. Prev: Ho. Surg. Roy. Berks. Hosp. Reading; Ho. Phys. Ronkswood Hosp. Worcester; Lect. Path. Univ. Birm.

TROWELL, Joan Mary John Radcliffe Hospital, Oxford OX3 9DU Tel: 01865 220944 Fax: 01865 751100 — MB BS Lond. 1964 (Roy. Free) MRCS Eng. LRCP Lond. 1964; FRCP Lond. 1987, M 1967. Oxf. Regional Fell. in Hepat., Nuffield Dept. of Med., Oxf. Univ.; Med. Mem. of Gen. Med. Counc.; Chairm. GMC Fitness to Pract. Comm.; Mem. of the Informat. Standards Bd. of the NHS Nat. Progr. for IT. Specialty: Gastroenterol. Socs: Med. Wom.'s Federat., Past Pres. 1998-1999; Brit. Soc. of Gastroenterol.; Brit. Assn. for the Study of the Liver. Prev: Regist. (Med.) Hammersmith Hosp. & Addenbrooke's Hosp. Camb.; Ho. Phys. Brompton Hosp. Lond.; Dep. Dir. Clin. Studies Oxf. Univ. Med. Sch.

TROWELL, Joanna Elizabeth 3 St Stephen's Close, Willerby, Hull HU10 6DG — MB BS Lond. 1996.

TROWELL, Judith Ann 45 Heath Drive, Potters Bar EN6 1EJ Tel: 01707 652205 — (Roy. Free) M Br PA Soc.; MRCS Eng. LRCP Lond. 1965; MB BS Lond. 1965; DCH Eng. 1969; DPM Eng. 1976; FRCPsych 1983, M 1976. Cons. Psychiat. Child & Family Dept. Tavistock Clinic Lond.; Hon. Sen. Lect. Roy. Free Hosp. Sch. Med.; Vice Pres. Young Minds. Specialty: Child & Adolesc. Psychiat. Socs: Brit. Psychoanal. Soc.; Internat. Soc. for Preventaion of Child Abuse & Neglect. Prev: Prof. of Child Mental Health, Westmidlands Regional Health Authority, UC Worcester.

TROWER, Christopher Simon Geoffrey, Squadron Ldr. RAF Med. Br. Retd. Poplar Grove Surgery, Meadow Way, Aylesbury HP20 1XB Tel: 01296 482554 Fax: 01296 398771; Speen Lodge, 36 Chiltern Road, Wendover HP22 6DA Tel: 01296 623744 Email: trowerchristopher@hotmail.com — MB BS Lond. 1974 (St. Bart.) MRCS Eng. LRCP Lond. 1973; DRCOG 1976; MRCGP 1979; FRCGP 1999. Princip. Partner Walton Gr. Surg. Aylesbury; Med. Adviser Bucks. HA; Bd. Mem./Clin. Governance Lead Aylesbury Vale PCG; GP Mem. Vale of Aylesbury PCT. Specialty: Gen. Pract. Socs: BMA (Exec. Bucks. Div.); (Chairm.) Assn. Primary Care Med. Advisors; Vice-Chairm. Iain Rennie Hospice at Home. Prev: Chairm. Assn. of Primary Care Med. Advisers; GP Chalfont St. Peter; Sen. Med. Off. RAF Locking.

TROWER, Katharyne Jayne Longacre, 76 Preston Crowmarsh, Wallingford OX10 6SL — BM BS Nottm. 1997.

TROWER, Tyrone Paul Balidon Centre, Summerlands Hosp, Preston Rd, Yeovil BA20 2BX Tel: 01935 424511; Linden Lea, Ryme Road, Yetminster, Sherborne DT9 6JY — BM Soton. 1988; MRCPsych 1993. Cons.(Child & Adoles Psychiat.) Som.. Specialty: Child & Adolesc. Psychiat. Prev: Regist. (Psychiat.) St. Jas. Hosp. Portsmouth & Knowle Hosp. Fareham; Regist. (Psychiat.) Roy. S. Hants. Hosp. Soton.; SHO (Psychiat.) Craylingwell Hosp. Chichester.

TROWER-GREENWOOD, Brian Goodall 48 Firs Road, Houghton on the Hill, Leicester LE7 9GU — MB BS Lond. 1959 (St. Thos.) PhD Lond. 1966, BSc (Hons. Physiol.) 1956; MB BS (Hons. Surg.) Lond. 1959; MRCS Eng. LRCP Lond. 1961. Hon. Lect. (Path.) Univ. Leicester. Socs: Pharmacol. Soc.; Path. Soc.; Brit. Soc. Immunol. Prev: Mem. Scientif. Staff Inst. Animal Physiol. Camb.; Lect. Sherrington Sch. of Physiol. St. Thos. Hosp.; Head Path. R & D Laborats. Fisons Pharmaceuts.

TROWLER, Eric Patrick Brookland House, 501 Crewe Road, Wistaston, Crewe CW2 6QP Tel: 01270 67250 — MB ChB Manch. 1959.

TROYACK, Anthony David East Barnet Health Centre, 149 East Barnet Road, Barnet EN4 8QZ Tel: 020 8440 7417 Fax: 020 8447 0126 — MB ChB Leeds 1968; DObst RCOG 1970. Specialty: Gen. Pract.

TRUCKLE, Simon — MB BS Lond. 1996 (Roy. Lond.) DRCOG Lond. 2000; MRCGP 2002. GP.

TRUDGILL, Michael John Ashley, Squadron Ldr. RAF Med. Br. Station Medical Centre, RAF Linton on Ouse, York YO6 2AD Tel: 01347 848261; Ivy House, High St, Clophill, Bedford MK45 4BE Tel: 01525 860529 Fax: 01525 60529 — MB BCh Wales 1989; Dip. IMC 1995; MRCGP 1996; DAvMed 1997. Sen. Med. Off. Flight Med. Off. GP/Aviat. Med. Linton on Ouse York. Specialty: Aviat. Med. Socs: Roy. Aeronaut. Soc. Prev: Med. Off. RAF Leeming Med. Off. Ascension Is.

TRUDGILL, Nigel John Sandwell General Hospital, Lyndon, West Bromwich B71 4HJ Tel: 0121 553 1831 — MB ChB Sheff. 1988; MRCP (UK) 1991. Cons. Phys. & Gastroenterol., Sandwell Gen. Hosp.; Hon. Clin. Sen. Lect., Univ. of Birm. Specialty: Gastroenterol. Special Interest: Oesophagus. Socs: MRCP.

TRUE, Rodney Charles (retired) 15 Southcrofts, Nantwich CW5 5SG Tel: 01270 610206 — MB ChB Leeds 1967; DPM Eng. 1971; MRCPsych 1972. Cons. Psychiat. Mersey RHA. Prev: Sen. Regist. Birm. AHA (T).

TRUEMAN, Angela Margaret City Hospital, Hucknall Road, Nottingham NG5 1PJ Tel: 0115 969 1169; Pear Tree Cottage, Padleys Lane, Burton Joyce, Nottingham NG14 5EB Tel: 0115 969 1169 — (Roy. Free) MRCS Eng. LRCP Lond. 1967; BSc Lond. 1964, MB BS 1967; MRCP (UK) 1971; FRCP Lond. 1987. Cons. Phys. (Geriat. Med.) City Hosp. Nottm. Specialty: Gen. Med.

TRUEMAN, Christopher John Ashby Turn Primary Care Centre, The Link, Scunthorpe DN16 2UT — MB BCh Wales 1985.

TRUEMAN, Freda Adelaide (retired) 12Llys Llewelyn, Meadow Farm, Llantwit fardre, Pontypridd CF38 2HQ Tel: 01446 732089 Fax: 01443 207889 — (Manch.) MB ChB Manch. 1951. Prev: Assoc. Specialist (Trauma & Orthop. Surg.) S. Glam. AHA (T).

TRUEMAN, Geoffrey Bruce 11 Hanover Drive, Chislehurst BR7 6TA — MB ChB Manch. 1987; DRACOG 1990, M 1995. Regist. (O & G) Roy. Bournemouth Hosp. Specialty: Obst. & Gyn.

TRUEMAN, Mark David The Surgery, 2 Crescent Bakery, St. Georges Place, Cheltenham GL50 3PN Tel: 01242 226336 Fax: 01242 253587; Glenroy, 14 Church Road, St Marks, Cheltenham GL51 7AN Tel: 01242 227852 — (Univ. Coll. Hosp.) BSc (Hons.) (Genetics) Lond. 1976, MB BS 1979; DRCOG 1982; DA (UK) 1985; MFA RCS Eng. 1986; DCH RCP Lond. 1988. Specialty: Anaesth. Prev: Regist. (Anaesth.) Cheltenham & Dist. HA.

TRUEMAN, Richard Simon Church Grange Health Centre, Bramblys Drive, Basingstoke RG21 8QN Tel: 01256 329021 Fax: 01256 817466; 27 Belvedere Gardens, Chineham, Basingstoke RG24 8GB Tel: 01256 332654 — MB ChB Aberd. 1987; MRCGP 1991. Specialty: Gen. Pract. Socs: BMA.

TRUEMAN, Trevor 2 Viewfield, Como Rd, Malvern WR14 2TH Tel: 01684 573722 — MB ChB Birm. 1972; BSc (Hons. Anat.) Birm. 1969; MRCP (UK) 1976; MD Birm. 1982. Socs: (Chairm.) Oromia Support Gp. (Human Rights & Pro-Democracy Organisat.).

TRUESDALE, Peter Jeffrey (retired) Trehill Cottage, Heathfield, Tavistock PL19 0LB Tel: 01822 810716 — (Leeds) MB ChB Leeds 1955; DPH Lond. 1963; DIH Eng. 1970; MFCM 1974; FFOM RCP Lond. 1985, MFOM 1979; MFPHM 1989. Prev: Hon. Phys. to HM the Qu.

TRUMAN, Kirstie Helen Cypher House, 8 Goose Island, Maritime Quarter, Swansea SA1 1UB — MB BCh Wales 1997.

TRUMAN, Lucy Ann 4 Somermead Court, Maltsters Way, Lowestoft NR32 3PQ — BM Soton. 1994 (Univ. Soton.) BSc (Biochem. Physiol.) Lond. 1990. SHO (ENT) Edin. Specialty: Otorhinolaryngol. Prev: SHO (A & E) Dunfermline; Ho. Off. (Med.) Bournemouth; Ho. Off. (Surg.) Aberd.

TRUMP, Professor Dorothy St Mary's Hospital, University of Manchester , Academic Unit of Medical Genetics, Hathersage Road, Manchester M13 0JH Tel: 0161 276 6903 Email: dorothy.trump@manchester.ac.uk — MB BChir Camb. 1988 (Camb. & Roy. Lond. Hosp.) BA Camb. 1985; MRCP UK 1991; MD Camb. 1996. Prof. (Human Molecular Genetics) Univ. Manch. Specialty: Genetics; Research. Special Interest: Genetic Eye Dis. Socs: Brit. Soc. for Human Genetics; Assn. for Research in Vision and Ophth.; Assn. of Physicians. Prev: Sen. Lect. & Hon. Cons. (Clin. Genetics) Addenbrooke's Hosp..; Wellcome Clinician Scientist & Hon. Sen. Regist. (Med. Genetics) Addenbrooke's Hosp. NHS Trust Camb.; MRC Train. Fell. (Molecular Med.) RPMS Hammersmith Hosp. Lond.

TRUMPER, Anne Louise 45 Moor Allerton Crescent, Leeds LS17 6SH — MB ChB Manch. 1986. SHO (Anaesth.) Trafford Gen. Hosp. Manch.

TRUMPER, Michele Josephine 1 Louisa Gardens, London E1 4NG — MB BS Lond. 1996.

TRUSCOTT, Douglas Ellis (retired) Twin View, Higher Carvossa, Ludgvan, Penzance TR20 8AJ — (Lond. Hosp.) MB BS Lond. 1945; DMRD Eng 1951; FRCR 1994. Prev: Cons. Radiol. W. Cornw. Hosp.

TRUSCOTT, Janet Hilary 5 Kent Road, Bishopston, Bristol BS7 9DN — MB ChB Liverp. 1971; MRCPsych 1977. Cons. Psychiat. Southmead Hosp. Bristol. Specialty: Gen. Psychiat. Prev: Sen. Lect. (Ment. Health) Univ. Bristol; Sen. Regist. (Psychiat.) Bristol; Hon. Lect. (Ment. Health) Univ. Bristol.

TRUST, Patrick Martin Bank Street Surgery, 46-62 Bank Street, Alexandria G83 0LS Tel: 01389 752419 Fax: 01389 710521; Beaumaris, Church Avenue, Cardross, Dumbarton G82 5NS Tel: 01389 841387 — MB BS Lond. 1971; FRCGP 1996, M 1982. Hosp. Pract. (Geriat.) Vale of Leven Hosp. & Dumbarton Jt. Hosp.; Chairm. Argyll & Clyde HB (Primary Care Audit Comm.). Prev: Assoc. Adviser (Gen. Pract). Dumbarton Dist. Univ. Glas.; Regist. MRC Blood Pressure Unit West. Infirm. Glas.; SHO (Med.) Hammersmith Hosp. Lond.

TRUTER, Keith William Campbell Langley Corner, Ifield Green, Crawley RH11 0NF Tel: 01293 527114 Fax: 01293 553510; 9 Selbourne Close, Pound Hill, Crawley RH10 3SA Tel: 01293 885303 Email: keithtruter2@aol.com — BM BCh Oxf. 1974; MA Oxf. 1975; MRCGP 1982; DRCOG 1982. Princip. Dr. Royds-Jones & Partners, Crawley. Specialty: Obst. & Gyn. Socs: Roy. Coll. Gen. Practitioners. Prev: SHO (O & G) St. Richards Hosp. Chichester.; Trainee GP Crawley; SHO (Med.) Brit. Milit. Hosp. Hong Kong.

TRY, Jacqueline Louise Faversham Meadows, Mumfords Lane, Chalfont St Peter, Gerrards Cross SL9 8TQ — MB ChB Leic. 1987.

TRYE, Caroline Julia 59 Northumberland Road, Leamington Spa CV32 6HF — MB BCh Wales 1991 (Univ. Wales Coll. Med.) DCH RCP Lond. 1995; DRCOG 1995; MRCGP 1996. Specialty: Gen. Pract.

TRYTHALL, David Arthur Heaton 21 Lossie Drive, Iver SL0 0JR — MRCS Eng. LRCP Lond. 1946; MD Lond. 1950, MB BS 1946; MRCP (UK) 1949.

TRYTHALL, Janet Dr Gray's Hospital, Elgin IV30 1SN Tel: 01343 543131; Seaview, Covesea, Duffus, Elgin IV30 5QS Tel: 01343 814816 — MB BS Newc. 1971 (Univ. New. u. Tyne) DObst RCOG 1973; FFA RCS 1982. Assoc. Specialist (Anaesth.) Doctor Gray's Hosp. Elgin. Specialty: Anaesth. Prev: Trainee GP Blyth N.d. VTS; Regist. (Anaesth.) Newc. AHA (T); Med. Off. Nchanga Consolidated Copper Mines (Broken Hill Div.) Kabwe, Zambia.

TRZCINSKI, Christopher John Markfield Medical Centre, 24 Chitterman Way, Markfield LE67 9WU Tel: 01530 249461 Fax: 01530 245668; 13 Jonathan Close, Groby, Leicester LE6 0DM — BM Soton. 1984; DCH RCP Lond. 1987; DRCOG 1988; MRCGP 1991. Prev: Trainee GP Salisbury HA VTS.

TRZECIAK, Andrzej Wladyslaw The Health Centre, Chapel Street, Thirsk YO7 1LG Tel: 01845 523154 Fax: 01845 526213 — MB BS Lond. 1983.

TSAGURNIS, Ioannis University Hospitals of Coventry & Warwickshire NHS Trust, Clifford Bridge Road, Walsgrave, Coventry CV2 2DX Tel: 024 7653 5230; 11 Welford Road, Sutton Coldfield B73 5DP — State Exam Med. Dusseldorf 1987. Cons. (Intens. Care) Univ. Hosps. Coventry & Warwicksh. NHS Trust.

TSAHALINA, Efthalia 75 Lewsey Road, Luton LU4 0EN — Ptychio Iatrikes Ioannina 1991.

TSAI, Her Hsin Castle Hill Hospital, Castle Road, Cottingham HU16 5JQ — MB ChB Aberd. 1983; MRCP (UK) 1986; MD (Hons.) Aberd. 1991. Cons. (Gastroent.). Prev: Regist. (Med.) Grampian Health Bd.

TSAI-GOODMAN, Beverly Department of Paed. Cardiology, Ward 32, Royal Hospital for Sick Children, Upper Maudlin St., Bristol BS2 8DJ Tel: 0117 921 5411 — BM Soton. 1990; MRCP (UK) 1994. SpR in Paediatric Cardiol. Specialty: Paediat.

TSAKONAS, Dionyssios Room 153 Nurses Home, Royal Orthopaedic Hospital, Woodlands, Northfield, Birmingham B31 2AP — Ptychio Iatrikes Athens 1985.

TSAM, Linda 19 Tangmere, Harrison St., London WC1H 8JG — MB BS Lond. 1992 (UCL) BSc (Hons.) Lond. 1989, MB BS 1992; MRCP (UK) 1997. Specialty: Med. Microbiol.

TSAMIS, Michail Room 14, Floor 1, Parkstone House, Poole Hospital, 35 Parkstone Road, Poole BH15 2NG — State Exam Rome 1993.

TSANG, Bing 19A Tunstall Crescent, Leicester LE4 9DX — MB BS Lond. 1991.

TSANG, David Tze Kwan 44 Ethelbert Gardens, Gants Hill, Ilford IG2 6UN — MB BS Lond. 1994; MRCP; FRCR.

TSANG, Mr Geoffrey Man Kwan 5 Blyth Close, Walton, Chesterfield S40 3LN — MB ChB Birm. 1987; FRCS Ed. 1991.

TSANG, Hoo Kee 10 Old Post Road, Holyhead LL65 2RL — MB BCh Wales 1997.

TSANG, Pierre Bridgeton Health Centre, 201 Abercromby Street, Glasgow G40 2DA Tel: 0141 531 6670 Fax: 0141 531 6505 Email: drpierretsang@hotmail.com — MB ChB Glas. 1978 (Univ. Glas.) Specialty: Gen. Pract. Special Interest: Accupuncture.

TSANG, Said Wan Mandy 85 Mote Hill, Hamilton ML3 6EA — MB ChB Glas. 1998.

TSANG, Mr Thomas Tat Ming Jenny Lind Children's Department, Norfolk & Norwich Hospital, Norwich NR1 3SR Tel: 01603 287171 Fax: 01603 287584 — MB BS Hong Kong 1982; BSc (Hons.) Lond. 1977; FRCS Ed. 1987. Cons. Paediat. Surg. Norf. & Norwich Hosp. Specialty: Paediat. Surg. Socs: Fell. Roy. Coll. Surgs. Edin.; Brit. Assn. Paediat. Surg. Prev: Higher Surgic. Trainee (Paediat. Surg.) Qu. Med. Centre Univ. Hosp. Nottm.; Sen. Regist. (Paediat. Surg.) John Radcliffe Hosp. Oxf.; Regist. Roy. Manch. Childr. Hosp.

TSANG, Wai-Ming 55 Lamplighters Close, Hempstead, Gillingham ME7 3NZ — LRCP LRCS Ed. 1983 (Taiwan) LRCP LRCS Ed. LRCPS Glas. 1983. Ho. Off. Stracathro Hosp. Brechin. Prev: Resid. Radiol. Dept. Nat. Taiwan Univ. Hosp. Taiwan.

TSANG, Woon Chau 11 The Thistles, Westlands, Newcastle ST5 2HL — MB BCh BAO Belf. 1991 (Queen's University Belfast) MB BCh Belf. 1991; FRCS (Ed.) 1997. Specialty: Gen. Surg.

TSANG, Woon Choy 28 Lambert Park, Dundonald, Belfast BT16 1LG — MB BCh BAO Belf. 1988.

TSANG, Woon Kam 28 Lambert Park, Dundonald, Belfast BT16 1LG Tel: 01232 489076 — MB ChB Sheff. 1995 (Univ. Sheff.) SHO (O & G) Sheff. Specialty: Obst. & Gyn. Prev: (SHO) (O & G) Sheff.; SHO (A&E) Sheff.; SHO (Geuito-Urin. med.) Sheff.

TSANG WAN MEI, Mona 11 Abdale Road, London W12 7ER — MB BS Hong Kong 1971.

TSANG WING KEUNG, Dr 11 Abdale Road, London W12 7ER Tel: 020 8743 2031 — MB BS Hong Kong 1969; DObst RCOG 1973; FRCOG 1990, M 1975. Prev: Cons. O & G Tung Wah Gp. Hosps. Hong Kong; SCMO Tower Hamlets HA.

TSANGARIDES, Mr Georgios Andreas County Hospital, Lincoln LN2 5QY, Egypt Tel: 01522 512512 — Ptychio Iatrikes Athens 1969; FRCS Ed. 1991. Staff Grade Orthop. Co. Hosp. Lincoln LN2 5QY. Specialty: Orthop.
TSAVELLAS, Mr George — MB BS Lond. 1990; FRCS Ed. 1996; FRCS Eng. 1996; FRCS (Gen. Surg.) 2003. Gen. Surg. E. Kent Hosp. NHS Trust. Specialty: Gen. Surg.
TSE, Bonnie Si-Wang The Glebe Surgery, Monastery Lane, Storrington, Pulborough RH20 4LR Fax: 01903 740700 — MB BS Lond. 1979; DCH RCP Lond. 1981; MRCGP 1987.
TSE, David Tit Kin 53 Icknield Drive, Ilford IG2 6SE — MB BS Lond. 1978.
TSE, Nan Yuin 7 Ulster Road, Margate CT9 5RZ — MB ChB Leeds 1996.
TSE, Wai Yee Department of Nephrology, Queen Elizabeth Medical Centre, Edgbaston, Birmingham B15 2TH Tel: 0121 472 1311 Fax: 0121 627 2527 Email: w.y.tse.1@bham.ac.uk; 1 Nortune Close, Wychall Lane, King's Norton, Birmingham B38 8AJ Tel: 0121 459 8956 — MB ChB Leeds 1989; BSc (Hons.) Leeds 1986, MB ChB (Hons.) 1989; MRCP (UK) 1992. Regist. Rotat. (Gen. Med. & Nephrol.) Qu. Eliz. Med. Centre Birm. Specialty: Nephrol. Prev: SHO Rotat. (Med.) Newc.; Train. Fell. MRC.
TSE, Yin Ha Anissa 6 Farfield Grove, Beeston, Nottingham NG9 2PW — BM BS Nottm. 1992.
TSE SAK KWUN, Pin Cheong Kwun, 6 Waverley Avenue, Fleetwood FY7 8BN Tel: 01253 778448; 27 Princes Way, Fleetwood FY7 8PG Tel: 01253 875179 — MB ChB Manch. 1985 (St Andrews and Manchester) BSc (Hons) St. And 1980; DRCOG 1987; DCH RCP Lond. 1988; MRCGP 1989.
TSEKOURAS, Anastasios Department of Plastic Surgery, Countess of Chester Hospital, Liverpool Road, Chester CH2 1BQ — Ptychio Iatrikes Athens 1987. Regist. (Plastic Surg.) Countess of Chester Hosp. Specialty: Plastic Surg.
TSENG, Evelin Hing Ying Tanglewood, Hawthorne Road, Bickley, Bromley BR1 2HN Tel: 020 8295 0935 — MB BS Lond. 1975 (Guy's) MRCS Eng. LRCP Lond. 1975; MRCP (UK) 1979; MSc Lond. 1995. Cons. (Community Paediat.s) Ravenshourne NHS Trust Kent. Specialty: Community Child Health. Prev: Sen. Regist. (Optimum Health Servs.) Lond.
TSEUNG, Ka Wai Manor Farm Medical Centre, Manor Farm Road, Huyton, Liverpool L36 0UB Tel: 0151 480 1244 Fax: 0151 480 6047; 271 Menlove Avenue, Woolton, Liverpool L25 7SA — MB ChB Liverp. 1980 (Liverpool) BSc (Hons.) Liverp. 1976, MB ChB 1980.
TSEUNG, Man Hong — MB ChB Liverp. 1987; BSc (Hons) Liverp. 1984; DRCOG 1991; Cert. Family Plann. JCC 1991; MRCGP 1993. GP Princip.; Clin. Lead in Palliat. Med. for Runcorn & Widnes PCG. Specialty: Community Child Health; Palliat. Med. Prev: Trainee GP Ormskirk Dist. Gen. Hosp.; SHO (Paediat.) Alder Hey Hosp. Liverp.; SHO (Cardiothoracic Med.) Broadgreen Hosp. Liverp.
TSIAPRAS, Dimitrios 41 Aldbourne Road, London W12 0LW — Ptychio Iatrikes Athens 1984. Specialty: Cardiol.
TSINTIS, Panayiotis Andrea 14 Peterborough Drive, Lodge Moor, Sheffield S10 4JB — MB ChB Sheff. 1983; MRCP (UK) 1987. Sen. Med. Off. Med. Control Agency DoH. Prev: Regist. (Med.) Glas. Roy. Infirm.; SHO (Gen. & Geriat. Med.) Nether Edge Hosp. Sheff.; SHO (A & E) Roy. Hallamsh. Hosp. Sheff.
TSO, Marie Teresa Bik Yan 28 Meadowbank, Watford WD19 4NP — MB ChB Glas. 1987.
TSOI, Kenney Cham Fai 99 Elmhurst Drive, Hornchurch RM11 1NZ — MB BS Lond. 1997.
TSOKODRYI, Casper Southend Hospital, Prittlewell Chase, Westcliff on Sea SS0 0RY — MB BS Lond. 1984.
TSOLAKIS, Marios Georgiou Flat 59, Viceroy Court, Wilmslow Road, Didsbury, Manchester M20 2RH — MB ChB Manch. 1990 (Univ. Manch.) MRCGP 1995. Specialty: Gen. Pract. Socs: BMA; Med. Protec. Soc. Prev: Trainee GP/SHO Univ. Liverp.
TSUI, Janice Chung Sze 50 Grosvenor Road, Petts Wood, Orpington BR5 1QU Tel: 01689 825528 — BChir Camb. 1996; MB Camb. 1997. SHO (A & E) Whittington Hosp. Lond. Specialty: Accid. & Emerg. Prev: Pre-Registration Ho. Off. (Med.) Addenbrookes; Pre-Registration Ho. Off. (Surg./Urol.) Norf. & Norwich Hosp.
TSUI, Mr Steven Shi Lap Department of Cardiothoracic Surgery, Papworth Hospital, Papworth, Cambridge CB3 8RE Tel: 01480 364297 Fax: 01480 364332 Email: stephen.tsui@papworth.nhs.uk — MB BChir Camb. 1988 (Univ. Camb.) FRCS Eng. 1992; MA Camb. 1989, MD 1996; FRCS (Cth.) 1997. Cons. (Cardiothoracic Surg.) Papworth Hosp. Specialty: Cardiothoracic Surg. Special Interest: Transplantation; Valve Surg.; Ventricular Assist Devices. Prev: Research Fell. Duke Univ. Med. Center, USA.
TUANO, Raquel 1 Cropton Way, Manor Fard, Hindley Green, Wigan WN2 4RT — MB ChB Leic. 1998.
TUBBS, Diana Barbara 48 Ridgmont Road, Seabridge, Newcastle ST5 3LB — MB BS Lond. 1970 (St. Bart.) MRCS Eng. LRCP Lond. 1970; DCH Eng. 1974. Clin. Asst., Community Paediat., Univ. Hosp. of N. Staffs. Prev: Clin. Asst. (Cystic Fibrosis) Newc.; SHO (Paediat.) Hammersmith Hosp. Lond.
TUBBS, Mr Oswald Nigel Nuffield Hospital, 22 Somerset Road, Edgbaston, Birmingham B15 2QQ Tel: 0121 456 2000 Fax: 0121 452 2881; 41 Ellesboro Road, Harborne, Birmingham B17 8PU Tel: 0121 427 3272 Fax: 0121 428 4561 Email: nigel@tubbs.freeserve.co.uk — MB BChir Camb. 1963 (St Thos.) MA Camb. 1962; MRCS Eng. LRCP Lond. 1964; FRCS Eng. 1970; FICS 1977. Cons. Surg. Univ. Hosp. and Roy. Orthopaedic Hosp. Birm.; Hon. Lect. Surg. Univ. Birm.; Edr. Injury Brit. Jl. Accid. Surg. Specialty: Trauma & Orthop. Surg. Socs: Brit. Orthop. Assn.; Fell. Inst. of Sports Med.; Brit. Assn. for Surg. of Knee. Prev: Sen. Surg. Regist. Robt. Jones & Agnes Hunt Orthop. Hosp. Oswestry; SHO (Thoracic Surg.) St. Thos. Hosp.; Ho. Surg. Nat. Hosp. Nerv. Dis. Qu. Sq.
TUBBS, Sophie Clare 34 Rocks Lane, London SW13 0DB — MB BS Lond. 1997.
TUBMAN, Terese Margaret 22 Churchtown Road, Gerrans, Portscatho, Truro TR2 5DZ.
TUCK, Alison Wendy Watledge Surgery, Barton Road, Tewkesbury GL20 5QQ — MB ChB Bristol 1981; DRCOG 1985; MFFP 1994. SCMO/Instruc. Doctor (Family Plann.) Worcester. Specialty: Family Plann. & Reproduc. Health.
TUCK, Barry Austin Avenue Road Surgery, 28A Avenue Road, Malvern WR14 3BG Tel: 01684 561333 Fax: 01684 893664 — MB ChB Birm. 1981; MRCGP 1985; DRCOG 1985.
TUCK, Christine Scott (retired) 9 Bootham Crescent, York YO30 7AJ Tel: 01904 623841 — MB BS Lond. 1963 (Lond. Hosp.) FRCS Ed. 1968; FRCOG 1986, M 1971. Prev: Cons. (O & G) York Health Dist.
TUCK, Edgar Allen Marshall (retired) 5 Monkswood, Silverstone, Towcester NN12 8TG Tel: 01327 857469 — MB BS Lond. 1954 (St. Mary's) MRCS Eng. LRCP Lond. 1953.
TUCK, Gillian Wansford & King's Cliffe Practice, Old Hill Farm, Yarwell Road, Wansford, Peterborough PE8 6PL Tel: 01780 782342 Fax: 01780 783434; Drift End, First Drift, Wothorpe, Stamford PE9 3JL — MB ChB Manch. 1971; DA Eng. 1973.
TUCK, Harry Angell (retired) Grange Cottage, Thorpe Lane, Cawood, Selby YO8 3SG Tel: 01757 268168 — MB BS Lond. 1937 (Westm.) Prev: Regional Med. Off. Regional Med. Serv. (E. Midl. Div.) DHSS.
TUCK, Jeremy John Hobart, Lt.-Col. Commanding Officer, 5 General Support Medical Regt., Fulwood Barracks, Preston PR2 8AA Tel: 01772 260500 — MB BS Lond. 1983 (Lond. Hosp.) MSc (Public Health) Lond.; MRCGP 1993. Specialist Regist. Pub. Health Med. Specialty: Pub. Health Med. Socs: Fell. Roy. Soc. of Med. Yeomen; Worshipful Soc. Apoth. Prev: Staff Off. (Med. Br.) Permanent Jt. HQ, Northwood.
TUCK, Jonathan Stephen Department of Radiology, Wythenshawe Hospital, Southmoor Road, Manchester M23 9LT — MB ChB Glas. 1980 (Glas. Univ.) FRCS Glas. 1984; FRCR 1989. Cons. Radiologist, Wythenshawe Hosp. Specialty: Radiol. Socs: Brit. Soc. Interven. Radiol.; CIRSE. Prev: Sen. Regist. (Diagn. Radiol.) Manch. Roy. Infirm.; Vis. Asst. Prof. Radiol. Univ. Maryland Med. Systems Baltimore, USA; Sen. Regist. (Diagn. Radiol.) Christie Hosp. Manch.
TUCK, Michael Elmitt (retired) Channel View Surgery, 3 Courtenay Place, Teignmouth TQ14 8AY Tel: 01626 774656 — MB BChir Camb. 1959 (Middlx.) MA, MB Camb. 1959, BChir 1958; DObst RCOG 1960. Prev: Ho. Phys. & Ho. Off. Dept. O & G Middlx. Hosp. Lond.
TUCK, Simon Julian Peterborough District Hospital, Thorpe Road, Peterborough PE3 6DA — MB ChB Manch. 1971; MRCP (UK)

1975; DCH Eng. 1977; FRCP Lond. 1995; FRCPCH 1997. Cons. Paediat. P'boro. Dist. Hosp. Specialty: Paediat. Special Interest: Neonatal Paediatrics. Socs: Neonat. Soc.; Roy. Soc. of Med. Prev: Sen. Regist. (Paediat.) Addenbrooke's Hosp. Camb.; Sen. Regist. (Paediat.) Norf. & Norwich Hosp.

TUCK, Stephen Paul 25 Chantry Way E., Swanland, North Ferriby HU14 3QF; 95 Townsgate, Silkstone, Barnsley S75 4SW — MB ChB Leeds 1993; BSc. SHO Rotat. (Med.) The Roy. Hallamshire Hosp., Sheff. Socs: BMA. Prev: SHO (Neurol.) Pinderfield Wakefield; SHO Rotat. (Med.) Barnsley Dist. Gen. Hosp. S. Yorks.; Ho. Off. (Surg.) St. James Univ. Teachg. Hosp.

TUCK, Susan Catherine Channel View Surgery, 3 Courtenay Place, Teignmouth TQ14 8AY Tel: 01626 774656 — MB BS Lond. 1959 (Middlx.) Prev: Ho. Surg. Middlx. Hosp.; Ho. Phys. Princess Alice Hosp. E.bourne.

TUCK, Susan Margaret Department Obst. & Gyn., Royal Free Hospital, Hampstead, London NW3 2QG Tel: 020 7794 0500 — MD Bristol 1984; MB ChB 1974; FRCOG 1992, M 1980, D 1977; DCH Eng. 1977; MRCGP 1978. Cons. O & G Roy. Free Hosp. Lond. Specialty: Obst. & Gyn. Socs: Fell. Roy. Soc. Med. Prev: Sen. Regist. John Radcliffe Hosp. Oxf.; Regist. King's Coll. Hosp. Lond.

TUCKER, Andrew John Kirkham Medical Practice, St Albans Road, Torquay TQ1 3SL Tel: 01803 323541 Fax: 01803 314311; Hill Park Farm, Lower Gabwell, Stokeinteignhead, Newton Abbot TQ12 4QR — MB BS Lond. 1979 (St. Bart.) BSc (Hons.) Lond. 1975, MB BS 1979; DRCOG 1981; MRCGP 1984. Specialty: Obst. & Gyn. Prev: SHO (O & G) St. Bart. Hosp. Lond.; SHO (Geriat. & Paediat.) Crawley Hosp.

TUCKER, Andrew John Westlands Medical Centre, 20B Westlands Grove, Portchester, Fareham PO16 9AD Tel: 023 9237 7514 — BM Soton. 1990; MRCGP 1994; DRCOG 1994. Trainee GP/SHO Portsmouth & SE Hants. VTS. Prev: Ho. Off. (Med.) St. Mary's Hosp. Portsmouth; Ho. Off. (Surg.) Poole Gen. Hosp.

TUCKER, Anna Katherine 37 Barkfield Lane, Liverpool L37 1LY — MB ChB Liverp. 1994; DRCOG 1996. Gen. Practitioner Neston Surg. Mellocu La. Neston S. Wirral. Specialty: Gen. Pract. Prev: GP Regist. Manor Health Centre Liscard Wirral; GP Regist. Villa Med. Centre Prenton Wirral.

TUCKER, Mr Antony Gower Bradford Royal Infirmary, Duckworth Lane, Bradford BD9 6RJ Tel: 01274 364118 — MB ChB Sheff. 1972; FRCS Eng. 1977. Cons. ENT Bradford Roy. Infirm. Specialty: Otolaryngol.; Otorhinolaryngol. Prev: Sen. Regist. (ENT) Liverp. AHA (T); Regist. (ENT) Avon AHA (T); SHO (Plastic Surg.) Nottm. City Hosp.

TUCKER, Audrey Kathleen Princess Grace Hospital, Nottingham Place, London W1M 3FD Tel: 020 7486 1234 Fax: 020 7486 1084; 391 Lauderdale Tower, Barbican, London EC2Y 8NA Tel: 020 7628 0126 Fax: 020 7628 0126 — (St. Bart.) MB BS Lond. 1964; DMRD Eng. 1967; FFR 1970. Cons. Radiol. Princess Grace Hosp. Lond. Specialty: Radiol. Socs: Fell. Roy. Soc. Med.; Fell. Med. Soc. Lond. Prev: Cons. Radiol. St. Bart. Hosp. Lond.; Sen. Regist. (Diag. Radiol.) Middlx. Hosp. Lond.; Ho. Surg. St. Bart. Hosp.

TUCKER, Barbara Rose 13 Letchworth Avenue, Chatham ME4 6NP — MB BS Lond. 1964 (Lond. Hosp.) Prev: Ho. Surg. & Ho. Phys. St. Bart. Hosp. Rochester.

TUCKER, David Stone (retired) 10 West Cliff, Southgate, Gower, Swansea SA3 2AN Tel: 01792 234737 Fax: 01792 234737 Email: dst@southgate71.fsnet.co.uk — MB BS Lond. 1958 (King's Coll. Hosp.) MRCS Eng. LRCP Lond. 1956; MRCGP 1973. Prev: Ho. Surg. Bolingbroke Hosp. Lond.

TUCKER, Dawn Louise 60 St Peters Road, West Mersea, Colchester CO5 8LN — MB BS Lond. 1996.

TUCKER, Graham Paul Nines and Partners, Shoreham Health Centre, Pond Road, Shoreham-by-Sea BN43 5US Tel: 01273 440550 — MB Camb. 1976; BChir 1975; DCH Eng. 1978; DRCOG 1979; MRCGP 1980. Specialty: Community Child Health. Prev: Ho. Phys. OldCh. Hosp. Romford; Trainee GP Windsor VTS.

TUCKER, Helen Holme (retired) 3 Selby Close, Westlands, Newcastle ST5 3JB Tel: 01782 615168 — MB BS Lond. 1967 (Roy. Free) MRCS Eng. LRCP Lond. 1967; MFFP 1993. Prev: SCMO (Community Gyn. & Family Plann.) N. Staffs. Hosp. Centre NHS Trust.

TUCKER, Howard Simon 3 Weaver Ct, Torquay TQ2 7RT — MB BCh Wales 1997.

TUCKER, John Borders General Hospital, Melrose TD6 9BD — MB ChB Ed. 1975; MRCP (UK) 1978; FRCPath 1996, M 1984; FRCP Lond. 1996. Cons. Haemat. Borders Gen. Hosp. Melrose. Specialty: Haematology. Socs: Brit. Soc. Haematol.; Assn. Clin. Path.; BMA. Prev: Cons. Haemat. Good Hope Hosp. Sutton Coldfield; Clin. Research Fell. ICRF (Med. Oncol.) St Bart. Hosp. Lond.; Sen. Regist. & Regist. (Haemat.) Roy. Infirm. Edin.

TUCKER, John Burnard (retired) Netherwayes, 1 Sidmouth Road, Honiton EX14 1BE Tel: 01404 42317 Fax: 01404 42317 — (Bristol) MB ChB Bristol 1941.

TUCKER, Mr John Keith 77 Newmarket Road, Norwich NR2 2HW Tel: 01603 614016 Fax: 01603 766469 Email: ktucker77@aol.com; The Mill House, Mill Road, Barnham Broom, Norwich NR9 4DE Tel: 01603 759470 Fax: 01603 759580 Email: ktucker@aol.com — MB BS Lond. 1968 (Char. Cross) MRCS Eng. LRCP Lond. 1968; FRCS Eng. 1973. Cons. Orthop. Surg. Norf. & Norwich Hosp. Specialty: Orthop. Socs: BMA; Hon. Sec. Brit. Hip Soc.; Brit. Orthop. Assn. Prev: Sen. Regist. (Orthop.) St. Bart. Hosp. Lond.; Regist. (Surg.) Addenbrooke's Hosp. Camb.; Ho. Surg. Char. Cross Hosp. Lond.

TUCKER, John Shackleton St Luke's Hospital, Little Horton Lane, Bradford BD5 0NA Tel: 01274 365213; Spring Head, 436 Haworth Road, Allerton, Bradford BD15 9LL — MB ChB (Hons. Distinc. Med.) Leeds 1966; BSc (cl. II Hons.) Leeds 1966; MRCP (UK) 1972; FRCP Lond. 1987. Cons. Phys. (Geriat. Med.) St. Luke's Hosp. Bradford. Specialty: Care of the Elderly. Socs: Brit. Geriat. Soc. Prev: Ho. Phys. Leeds Gen. Infirm.; Lect. (Med. & Geriat. Med.) Univ. Manch.

TUCKER, Kerry Elizabeth 3 Rosebery Av, Colchester CO1 2UJ — MB ChB Birm. 1997.

TUCKER, Kevan Paul Little Harwood Health Centre, Plane Tree Road, Blackburn BB1 6PH Tel: 01535 600488; 46 James Hall Gardens, Walmer, Deal CT14 7TA Tel: 01304 364077 — MB ChB Leeds 1987. Trainee GP. Airdale VTS. Prev: Pre-Regist. Hse. Jobs (Med.) Roy. Halifax Infirm. & Leeds Gen. Infirm. (Surg. Urol.).

TUCKER, Matthew Harold — MB ChB Birm. 1998.

TUCKER, Peter William, MBE, TD (retired) 31 Julians Acres, Berrow, Burnham-on-Sea TA8 2LX Tel: 01278 780526 — (Lond. Hosp.) MB BChir Camb. 1950; DObst RCOG 1952; MRCGP 1960. Prev: Capt. RAMC.

TUCKER, Philippa Margaret Mill Road Surgery, 61 Mill Road, Mile End, Colchester CO4 5LE Tel: 01206 845900 Fax: 01206 844090 — MB BS Newc. 1980.

TUCKER, Phillip James (retired) Stonecross Surgery, 25 Street End Road, Chatham ME5 0AA; 13 Letchworth Avenue, Chatham ME4 6NP — (Lond. Hosp.) MB BS Lond. 1964. Prev: Ho. Off. (Surg.) Whipps Cross Hosp. Lond.

TUCKER, Roderick John (retired) 3 Selby Close, Westlands, Newcastle ST5 3JB Tel: 01782 615168 — MB BS Lond. 1966 (Roy. Free) FRCGP 1986; MRCGP 1971; DFFP 1993. Prev: GP Wolstanton, Newc., Staffs.

TUCKER, Sam Michael 152 Harley Street, London W1G 7LH Tel: 020 7935 1858 Fax: 020 7224 2574; 65 Uphill Road, Mill Hill, London NW7 4PT Tel: 020 8959 0500 Fax: 020 8906 2406 Email: sammtucker@btinternet.com — (Witwatersrand) MB BCh Witwatersrand 1952; DCH Eng. 1957; FRCP Ed. 1973, M 1961; FRCP Lond. 1990; FRCPCH 1997. p/t Hon. Cons. Paediat. Hillingdon Hosp. & Mt. Vernon Hosp. Northwood; Hon. Dir. Research Hillingdon Hosp. & Brunel Univ.; Hon. Lect. (Paediat. & Cardiol.) Inst. Dis. of Chest Brompton Hosp. Lond; Assoc. Prof. Dept. Mech. Engin. Brunel Univ. W. Lond; Asst. Prof. Brunel Univ. Uxbridge Dept of Mechanical Engin.; Director Newborn Hearing Unit Hillingdon Hosp. Specialty: Paediat. Special Interest: Learning problems in Childr.; Newborn hearing. Socs: Brit. Paediat. Assn. & Brit. Cardiac Soc.; Roy. Soc. Med. (Ex-Pres. Sect. Paediat.); Counc. Mem. Roy. Soc. Med. (Sen Treas.). Prev: Sen. Regist. (Paediat.) St. Geo. Hosp. Lond.; Regist. (Paediat.) Middlx. Hosp. & Qu. Eliz. Hosp. Childr. Lond.

TUCKER, Sarah Catherine 3 Weaver Court, Torquay TQ2 7RT Tel: 01803 400564 — MB ChB Bristol 1992; FRCS Lond. 1998. SHO (Surg.) Torbay Gen. Specialty: Plastic Surg. Prev: SHO (Plastics) Morriston Swansea; SHO (Orthop.) Cardiff Roy. Infirm.; SHO (Gen. Surg.) Gwent.

TUCKER, Sian Elizabeth 32 Millers Meadow, Rainow, Macclesfield SK10 5UE — BM BS Nottm. 1994.

TUCKER, Simon Christopher Department of Dermatology, Dorset County Hospital, Williams Avenue, Dorchester DT1 2JY Tel: 01305 255103 Fax: 01305 255291 Email: simon.tucker@wdgh.nhs.uk — MB ChB Birm. 1992; MRCP UK 1995; FRCP UK 2004. Cons. Dermatol., W. Dorset Gen. Hosps. NHS Trust, Dorchester. Specialty: Dermat. Special Interest: Contact Dermatitis; Skin cancer. Socs: Brit. Assn. of Dermatologists; Roy. Soc. of Med. Prev: Specialist Regist. in Dermat., Salford Roy. Hosps. NHS Trust 1997-2000; SpR Dermat. Burnley Gen. Hosp. 1996-1997.

TUCKER, Stephen Robert Ipswich Hospital , Suffolk Mental Health Partnerships NHS Trust, Minsmere House, Heath Road, Ipswich IP13 0EU — MB BS Lond. 1983; MRCPsych 1991. Specialty: Geriat. Psychiat.

TUCKER, Mr Stewart Kenneth 34A Waterlow Road, London N19 5NH — MB BS Lond. 1988; FRCS Eng. 1992. Regist. (Orthop.) Univ. Coll. & Middlx. Hosps. Specialty: Orthop. Prev: SHO (A & E) Univ. Coll. Hosp. Lond.:; SHO (Orthop. & Gen. Surg.) Watford Gen. Hosp.

TUCKER, Susan Elizabeth 196 Redmayne Drive, Chelmsford CM2 9XE — MB BS Lond. 1989. Specialty: Gen. Pract.

TUCKER, Mrs Valerie Alberta Elsie (retired) La Maison de Haut, Rue Des Messuriers, St Peters, Guernsey GY7 9SL Tel: 01481 265191 — (St. Thos.) MB BS Lond. 1953; DA Eng. 1955. Prev: Ho. Phys. & Resid. Anaesth. St. Thos. Hosp.

TUCKER, William Frank Gordon Alexandra Hospital, Woodrow Drive, Redditch B98 7UB; 2 Inett Way, Manor Oaks, Droitwich WR9 0DN — MB BS Lond. 1976 (St. Geo.) MRCS Eng. LRCP Lond. 1976; MRCP (UK) 1978; FRCP (Lond) 2000. Cons. Dermat. N. Worcs. Health Dist. Specialty: Dermat. Prev: Sen. Regist. & Tutor (Dermat.) Roy. Hallamsh. Hosp. Sheff.; Regist. (Dermat.) St. Mary's Hosp. Lond.

TUCKERMAN, James Gerard Seafield Medical Centre, Barhill Road, Buckie AB56 1FP Tel: 01542 835577 Fax: 01542 835092 — MB ChB Aberd. 1976.

TUCKEY, Jacqui Ellen Ella Gordon Unit, St Marys Hosp, Milton Rd, Portsmouth PO3 6; 12 Myers Close, Swanmore, Southampton SO32 2RN — MB ChB Bristol 1988 (Univ. Bristol) MRCOG 1993. Specialist Regist. Comm Gyn. St Marys Hosp. Portsmouth. Specialty: Obst. & Gyn. Prev: Regist. (O & G) Roy. Gwent Hosp. Newport; Specialist Regist.(Ob + Gyn.) N. Hants Hosp. Basingstoke; Clin. Ass.(Ob + Gyn.) Roy United Hosp. Bath.

TUCKEY, Jennifer Patricia Royal United Hospital, Bath BA1 3NG Tel: 01225 428331; Wier House, Lower Stoke, Limpley Stoke, Bath BA2 7FR Tel: 01225 723103 — MB ChB Bristol 1983; DCH RCPS 1987; FRCA 1989. Cons. Anaesth., Roy. United Hosp. Bath. Specialty: Anaesth. Socs: Obst. Anaesth. Assn.; Assn. Anaesth.; Clin. Soc. Bath. Prev: Staff Grade Anaesth. Bath; Regist. (Anaesth.) Plymouth & Portsmouth; SHO (Paediat.) Poole Bournemouth.

TUCKFIELD, Christopher John 37 Glisson Road, Cambridge CB1 2HA — MB BS Sydney 1984.

TUCKLEY, Catharine Mary (retired) 17 Horwood Avenue, Derby DE23 6NX Tel: 01332 348423 — MB ChB Aberd. 1962.

TUCKLEY, Jonathan Marc Clouds Cottage, Fore Street, Holbeton, Plymouth PL8 1NE — MB BS Lond. 1991; BSc (Hons.) 1988; DA 1993; Dip Obst (Distinc.) New Zealand 1998; MRCGP (Distinc.) 2002. SHO (Anaesth.) Roy. Cornw. Hosp. Treliske Truro.

TUCKMAN, Emanuel (retired) 27 Downside Crescent, London NW3 2AN Tel: 020 7794 5725 — MD Lond. 1963 (Univ. Coll. Hosp.) MB BS 1944; DCH Eng. 1945, DTM & H 1947. Prev: Nuffield Trav. Fell. 1963.

TUCKWELL, Gareth David Hospice In The Weald, Maidstone Road, Pembury, Tunbridge Wells TN2 4TA Tel: 01892 820 503 Email: gareth.tuckwell@hospiceintheweald.org.uk; 2 Sutherland Road, Tunbridge Wells TN1 1SE Tel: 01892 519318 Email: gareth@tuckwell-family.co.uk — MB BS Lond. 1971 (St. Bart.) MRCS Eng. LRCP Lond. 1971; DObst RCOG 1973; MRCGP 1977; Dip. Palliat. Med. Wales 1992. Med. Director Hospice In The Weald; Trustee of St Columba's Fellowsh. (Chair); Trustee Macmillan Cancer Relief. Specialty: Palliat. Med. Special Interest: Holistic Healthcare. Socs: Fell. Roy. Soc. Med.; BMA; Assn. Palliat. Med. Prev: Dir Macmillan Cancer Relief; Med.Dir Burrswood Hosp.Tunbridge Wells.

TUCKWELL, Leonard Arthur Aysgarth, 132 Earnsdale Road, Darwen BB3 1JA — MB BS Sydney 1958; MRCOG 1973; FRCOG 1985; DFFP 1999. InDepend. Cons. Gynaecologist Darwen Lancs; Clin. Med. Off. (Family Plann.) Bolton Hosp. NHS Trust. Specialty: Obst. & Gyn. Prev: Cons. (O & G) Blackburn, Hyndburn & Ribble Valley HA; Lect. O & G Univ. Bristol.

TUCKWELL, Wendy Ann 80 Bank End Lane, Huddersfield HD5 8EN Tel: 01484 311034 — MB ChB Leeds 1969; DObst RCOG 1974; MPH Leds 1999. Specialty: Gen. Pract. Socs: BMA. Prev: GP Hull.

TUDBALL, Patricia 23 Tegfan, Pontyclun CF72 9BP — MB BCh Wales 1986. Staff Grade (Gen. Psychiat.) Gwent Community Health Care Trust. Specialty: Gen. Psychiat.

TUDBERRY, Rachel Alice 31 Percy Road, London N21 2JA — MB BS Lond. 1997.

TUDDENHAM, Alfred David, SBStJ (retired) 24 Seaway Avenue, Friars Cliff, Christchurch BH23 4EX Tel: 01425 275880 — MB BS Lond. 1953 (Guy's) MRCS Eng. LRCP Lond. 1953; MRCGP 1971; Assoc. Fac. Occupat. Med. RCP Lond. 1979. Soton. Approved Med. Examr. Roy. Commercial Union & other insur. cos. Prev: Div. Med. Off. Brit. Rlys. South. Region, Brit. Rail Maintenance Ltd., Brit. Sealink (UK) Ltd. Portsmouth Assoc. Brit. Ports.

TUDDENHAM, Professor Edward George Denley Haemostasis and Thrombosis Research Group, MRC Clinical Sciences Centre, Imperial College School of Medicine, Hammersmith Hospital, Du Cane Road, London W12 0NN Tel: 020 8383 8235 Fax: 020 8383 8273 Email: edward.tuddenham@csc.mrc.ac.uk — (Westm.) MB BS Lond. 1968; FRCP Lond. 1987, M 1974; FRCPath 1987, M 1975; MD Lond. 1985; FRCP Ed 1997. MRC Clin. Sci. Staff, Dir. Haemostasis Research Gp. Clin. Sci. Centre Imperial Coll. Sch. Med. Lond.; Prof. Haemostais Imp. Coll. Sch. of Med. & Hon. Cons. Haemat. Hammersmith Hosp. Lond. Specialty: Haematology. Socs: World Federat. Haemophilia; Internat. Soc. Thrombosis & Hemostasis; Fell. of the Acad. of Med. Sci. Prev: Sen. Lect. (Haemat.) & Co-Dir. Haemophilia Centre Roy. Free Med. Lond.; Lect. (Haemat.) Welsh Nat. Sch. Med. Cardiff; Regist. (Path.) United Liverp. Hosps.

TUDDENHAM, Laurence Marcus Central Scotland Healthcare, Old Denny Road, Larbert FK5 4SD — MB ChB Ed. 1996. SHO (Psychiat.) Centr. Scotl. Healthcare NHS Trust.

TUDOR, Gareth Raymond Princess of Wales Hospital, Department of Radiology, Coity Road, Bridgend CF31 1RQ — MB BCh Wales 1989; MRCP; FRCR; BSc (Hons.) Wales 1986.

TUDOR, Gary John 11 St John Street, Manchester M3 4DW — MB ChB Manch. 1976.

TUDOR, Gary Paul Parkhill Medical Practice, Parkhill Road, Torquay TQ1 2AR Tel: 01803 212459 — MB ChB Manch. 1990; DRCOG; MRCGP; DFFP; BSc (Hons); Dip IMC; MSc Wales 1983. SHO (A & E) Roy. Devon & Exeter Hosp.

TUDOR, John (retired) Mortimer's Farm House, Foxton, Cambridge CB2 6RR Tel: 01223 870352 — (King's Coll. Hosp.) MB BS Lond. 1957; MRCS Eng. LRCP Lond. 1957; DObst RCOG 1960; DMRD Eng. 1971; FFR 1973. Cons. (Diag. Radiol.) Addenbrookes Hosp. Camb. Prev: Sen. Regist. Dept. Radiodiag. Hammersmith Hosp. Lond.

TUDOR, Mr John Colin Winton House, Portsdown Hill Road, Portsmouth PO6 1BE Tel: 023 92 389044 Fax: 01705 793 894 Email: jtudor30@hotmail.com — (St. Bart.) MA, MB Camb. 1967 BChir 1966; DO Eng. 1972; FRCS Ed. 1974; FRCS Eng. 1975; FRCOphth 1993. Cons. Ophth. Qu. Alexandra Hosp. Eye Unit Portsmouth. Specialty: Ophth. Socs: Amer. Acad. Ophth.,; BMA & Hosp. Cons. & Specialist Assn. Prev: Sen. Regist. Soton. Eye Hosp.; Regist. (Ophth.) Bristol Eye Hosp.

TUDOR, John Gowen The Church Street Practice, David Corbet House, 2 Callows Lane, Kidderminster DY10 2JG Tel: 01562 822051 Fax: 01562 827251; The Goddes farm House, The Greenway, Rock, Bewdley DY14 9SN Tel: 01299 832163 — MB ChB Birm. 1984; BSc (Hons.) Birm. 1981.

TUDOR, Mary Maud (retired) 8 South Bourne Close, Selly Park Road, Selly Park, Birmingham B29 7LU Tel: 0121 471 4154 — MB BCh BAO NUI 1942; Sch. Dent. Anaesth. Birm. Prev: Sen. Res. Anaesth. Qu. Eliz. Hosp. Birm.

TUDOR, Nerys Llwyd Trannon, 4 Bryn Eryl, Ruthin LL15 1DT Tel: 01824 23150 — MB BS Lond. 1963 (Roy. Free & Cardiff) Clin. Med. Off. Clwyd HA. Prev: Paediat. Ho. Off. E. Glam. Hosp. Ch. Village, Ho. Surg. Caerphilly; Dist. Miner's Hosp.

TUDOR, Mr Richard Gowen — MB ChB Birm. 1979; FRCS Eng. 1983; FRCS Ed. 1983; BSc (Hons.) (Anat.) Birm. 1976, MD 1987. Cons. Surg. Worcs. NHS Trust; Hon. Sen. Clin. Lect. (Surg.) Univ. Birm. Specialty: Gen. Surg. Prev: Lect. (Surg.) Univ. Birm.; Research Fell. Gen. Hosp. Birm.; Ho. Surg. Profess. Unit Qu. Eliz. Hosp. Birm.

TUDOR, Virginia Sarah Northfield Health Centre, 15 St. Heliers Road, Northfield, Birmingham B31 1QT Tel: 0121 478 1850 Fax: 0121 476 0931 — MB ChB Birm. 1978; DRCOG 1981.

TUDOR DE SILVA, Hewavasam Patuwata Badathuruge 14 Hawkwood, Maidstone ME16 0JQ — MB BS Sri Lanka 1973.

TUDOR-JONES, Thomas 50 Westport Avenue, Ridgewood Park, Mayals, Swansea SA3 5EQ Tel: 01792 402207 Fax: 01792 295952 — (Birm.) MB ChB Birm. 1959; DObst RCOG 1961; DPH Wales 1971. Dir. Occupat. Health Serv. Univ. Coll. Swansea; Clin. Asst. (Dermat.) Singleton Hosp. Swansea. Specialty: Occupat. Health. Prev: MOH Port Talbot Municip. Boro.; SHO (Obst.) Mt. Pleasant Hosp. Swansea; Ho. Phys. & Surg. Swansea Gen. Hosp.

TUDOR MILES, Andrew Peter Tudor (retired) The Surgery, 35A High Street, Wimbledon, London SW19 5BY Tel: 020 8946 4820 Fax: 020 8944 9794; 77 Bolingbroke Grove, London SW11 6HB — MB BS Lond. 1966 (St. Geo.) FRCGP 1991, M 1980. Med. Adviser Youngs Brewery; Hon. Med. Off. All Eng. Lawn Tennis Club; Hon. Med. Off. Kings Coll. Sch. Wimbledon. Prev: Regist. (Med.) St. Thos. Gp. Hosps.

TUDOR-THOMAS, William Richard (retired) Old Orchard, Pardys Hill, Corfe Mullen, Wimborne BH21 3HW Tel: 01929 603940 Fax: 01202 603940 Email: a2wtt@aol.com — MB BS Lond. 1971; DObst RCOG 1976. Vice-Chairm. Poole Hosp. NHS Trust; HMA, Dorset ME Support Gp. Prev: Sen. Partner, Swange Med. Pract.

TUDOR-WILLIAMS, Trevor Gareth — MB BS Lond. 1977 (St. Thos.) MRCP (UK) 1982. Sen. Lect. in Paediatric Infec. Dis.s. Imperial Coll.. Lond. Specialty: Paediat.; Infec. Dis. Socs: Harveian Soc. Lond.

TUDWAY, Andrew John Christie 13 Wykeham Gate, Haddenham, Aylesbury HP17 8DF — MB Camb. 1970; BA Camb. 1966, MB 1970, BChir 1969; FRCPath 1988, M 1976. Cons. (Histopath.) Stoke Mandeville Hosp. Aylesbury. Specialty: Histopath. Prev: Lect. Path. Univ. Bristol.

TUDWAY, David Christie Birmingham Heartlands Hospital, Radiology Department, Bordesley Green East, Birmingham B9 5ST Tel: 0121 424 2000 Ext: 42283 Fax: 0121 766 6919 Email: david.tudway@heartsol.wmids.nhs.uk — MB BS Lond. 1971; MRCP UK 1975; FRCR Lond. 1982. Cons. Radiologist, Birm. Heartlands and Solihull NHS Trust; Practising Radiologist, BUPA Parkway Hosp., Solihull. Specialty: Radiol. Special Interest: Ultrasound; Uroradiology. Socs: Roy. Coll. of Radiologists; Brit. Med. Ultrasound Soc. Prev: Clin. Director Radiol., Birminbgham Heartlands and Solihull NHS Trust.

TUFAIL, Adnan 20 Orchard Castle, Cardiff CF14 9BA; Jules Stein Eye Institute, 100 Stein Plaza, UCLA, Los Angeles 90024, USA — MB BS Lond. 1989; FRCOphth 1994. Fell. Ophth. Jules Stein Eye Inst. UCLA Los Angeles, USA. Prev: SHO Moorfields Eye Hosp.

TUFFILL, Mr Sidney George (retired) 57 Fitzjames Avenue, Croydon CR0 5DN Tel: 020 8654 6333 — (King's Coll. Hosp.) LLB Lond.; MRCS Eng. LRCP Lond. 1942; MB BS (Hons., Distinc. Forens. Med. & Pub. Health) Lond. 1942; FRCS Eng. 1947.

TUFFIN, Mr James Robert Maxillofacial Unit, University Hospital of South Manchester, Wythenshawe, Manchester M23 9LT Tel: 0161 291 4993 Fax: 0161 291 4996 — BM Soton. 1983 (Univ. Soton.) BDS Lond. 1974; FDS RCS Eng. 1978; FRCS Ed. 1989. Cons. Oral & Maxillofacial Surg. S. Manch. Univ. Hosps. Trust; Cons. Oral & Maxillofacial Surg. Stockport Hosps. Trust. Specialty: Oral & Maxillofacial Surg. Socs: Fell. Brit. Assn. Oral & Maxillofacial Surg.; BMA; Eur. Assn. Cranio-Maxillo. Surg. Prev: Sen. Regist. (Oral & Maxillofacial Surg.) NW RHA.

TUFFNELL, Derek John Bradford Teaching Hospitals NHS Trust, Duckworth Lane, Bradford BD9 6RJ Tel: 01274 364520 Fax: 01274 366690 Email: derek.tuffnell@bradfordhospitals.nhs.uk — MB ChB Leeds 1983; MRCOG 1988; FRCOG 2000. Cons. O & G Bradford NHS Trust. Specialty: Obst. & Gyn. Prev: Sen. Regist. (O & G) Yorks. RHA; Regist. (O & G) St. Jas. Hosp. Leeds.

TUFFREY, Catherine 27 Moor Croft Drive, Longwell Green, Bristol BS30 7DB — BM BS Nottm. 1994. SHO (Neonates) Southmead Hosp. Bristol. Specialty: Paediat. Socs: RCP; RCPCH. Prev: SHO Rotat. (Paediat.) Roy. United Hosp. Bath.

TUFFT, Nigel Richard 22 Parker Bowles Drive, Market Drayton TF9 3EU — MB ChB Bristol 1988.

TUFNELL, Guinevere Child & Family Service, The Traumatic Stress Clinic, 73 Charlotte Street, London W1T 4PL Tel: 020 7530 3666 Fax: 020 7530 3677 Email: guinevere.tufnell@nhs.net — MB BS Lond. 1977 (Royal Free) MA Camb. 1967; MRCPsych 1981; FRCPsych 2001. Cons. Child & Adoloescent Psychiat., Camden & Islington PCT d. Specialty: Child & Adolesc. Psychiat. Socs: Roy. Coll. Psychiat.s. Prev: Cons. Psychiat.. Child & Adoloescent Psychiat., Forest Healthcare Trust, Lond..

TUFT, Stephen John Moorfields Eye Hospital, 162 City Road, London EC1V 2PD Tel: 020 7253 3411 Fax: 020 7566 2019 Email: stuft@compuserve.com — MB BChir Camb. 1978 (King's Coll. Hosp.) MRCS Eng. LRCP Lond. 1977; FRACS 1983; FRACO 1983; FRCOphth 1990; MD Camb. 1992. Cons. Ophth. Moorfields Eye Hosp. Lond. Specialty: Ophth. Socs: BMA. Prev: Cons. Ophth. ChristCh., NZ; Lect. (Clin. Ophth.) Moorfields Eye Hosp. Lond.; Research Fell. Inst. Ophth. Lond.

TUGGEY, Justin Mark 23 Rockwood Road, Calverley, Leeds LS28 5AB Email: jtuggey@doctors.org.uk — MB ChB Leeds 1994.

TUITE, Mr Jeremy Dennis Broomfield Hospital, Court Road, Chelmsford CM1 7ET Tel: 01245 514201 Fax: 01245 514644 — MB ChB Leeds 1975; FRCS Eng. 1981. Cons. Orthop. Surg. Mid Essex Hosp. NHS Trust. Chelmsford. Specialty: Orthop. Socs: Brit. Orth. Assn.; Brit. Elbow & Shoulder Soc. Prev: Sen. Regist. Roy. Nat. Orthop. Hosp.

TUKE, John Underwood Bute House, Grove Medical Centre, Wootton Grove, Sherborne DT9 4DL Tel: 01935 812226 Fax: 01935 817055; Frampton Farm, Leigh, Sherborne DT9 6HJ — MB BS Lond. 1963; MRCS Eng. LRCP Lond. 1963; DObst RCOG 1965.

TUKE, John Wilson Millside House, Mill Road, Buxhall, Stowmarket IP14 3DS Tel: 01449 737643 Fax: 01449 737512 Email: jw@tuke.keme.co.uk — (Newcastle) MB BS Durh. 1956; DCH RCPS Glas. 1968; MRCGP 1969; FRCPCH 1998; MFPHM 2000. InDepend. Cons. In Pub. Health Med. Socs: BMA. Prev: Cons. Pub. Health Med. Suff. HA; GP Morpeth.

TULLBERG, Harriet Teresa Wynn Carnewater Practice, Dennison Road, Bodmin PL31 2LB Tel: 01208 72321 Fax: 01208 78478; Kingsberry, 38 Rhind St, Bodmin PL31 2EL Tel: 01208 76867 — MB ChB Bristol 1983; DRCOG 1986; MRCGP 1990. Specialty: Gen. Pract.

TULLETT, David Charles 33B Aldermans Hill, Hockley SS5 4RP — MB BChir Camb. 1988; BA Camb. 1982; MRCPsych 1993.

TULLETT, Mr William Melville Accident & Emergemcy Department, Western Infirmary, Dumbarton Road, Glasgow G11 6NT Tel: 0141 211 2651 Fax: 0141 339 3046; 47 Thomson Drive, Bearsden, Glasgow G61 3PA Tel: 0141 942 0686 — MB ChB Aberd. 1978; MRCP (UK) 1981; FRCS Ed. 1987; Dip. Forens. Med. Glas 1989; FRCPS Glas. 1991; FFAEM 1994; Dip. Sports Med. 1997. Cons. (A & E & Intens. Ther.) West. Infirm. Glas. Specialty: Accid. & Emerg. Socs: Brit. Assn. Accid. & Emerg. Med.; ICS. Prev: Sen. Regist. (A & E) West. Infirm. Glas.; Regist. (Med.) West. Infirm. Glas.

TULLEY, Margaret Mary Brookside Surgery, Brookside Close, Gipsy Lane, Earley, Reading RG6 7HG — MB BS Lond. 1979; DCH RCP Lond. 1982; DRCOG 1982; MRCGP 1983.

TULLEY, Paul Nicholas 10 Ennerdale Road, Formby, Liverpool L37 2EA Tel: 01704 877264 — MB BS Lond. 1993; BSc (Biochem. & Immunol.) Lond. 1990, MB BS 1993. SHO (A & E) Char. Cross Hosp. Lond. Prev: Demonst. (Anat.) Char. Cross & Westm. Med. Sch. Lond.; Ho. Surg. Char. Cross Hosp. Lond.; Ho. Phys. W. Middlx. Hosp. Lond.

TULLO, Mr Andrew Brent Manchester Royal Eye Hospital, Oxford Road, Manchester M13 9WH Tel: 0161 276 5522 Fax: 0161 272 6618 Email: atullo@central.cmht.nwest.nhs.uk — MB ChB Bristol 1974 (Univ. Bristol) MD Bristol 1982; FRCS Glas. 1983; FRCOphth 1992. Cons. Manch. Roy. Eye Hosp.; Hon. Sen. Lect. Univ. Manch.; Vis. Prof. UMIST. Specialty: Ophth. Socs: BMA; (Treas.) Europ. Eye Bank Assn. Prev: Wellcome Trust Research Fell. Univ. Bristol; Sen. Regist. Manch. Roy. Eye Hosp.

TULLOCH, Alexander David 158 Durham Road, London SW20 0DG — MB BS Lond. 1998.

TULLOCH, Alexander Kinnison (retired) 20 Jedburgh Road, Dundee DD2 1SR Tel: 01382 566447 — MB ChB St. And. 1941 (Dundee) DOMS Eng. 1948. Prev: Cons. Ophth. Ninewells Hosp. Dundee, Roy. Infirm. Dundee, King's.

TULLOCH, Alistair John (retired) 36 Church Lane, Wendlebury, Bicester OX25 2PN Tel: 01869 243278 — MB ChB Aberd. 1950; MD Aberd. 1976; DObst RCOG 1956; FRCGP 1975, M 1959. Hon. Research Fell. Unit of Health Care Epidemiol. Univ. Oxf.

TULLOCH, Barrie Charles Mews Close Health Centre, Mews Close, Ramsey, Huntingdon PE26 1BP Tel: 01487 812611 Fax: 01487 711801; 59 Main Street, Great Gidding, Huntingdon PE28 5NU Tel: 01832 293236 Fax: 01487 711801 — MB ChB Leeds 1963. Prev: Ho. Phys. & Ho. Surg. St. Jas. Hosp. Leeds; Ho. Surg. (Obst.) St. Mary's Hosp. Leeds; Ho. Phys. (Paediat. & Dermat.) St. Jas. Hosp. Leeds.

TULLOCH, Mr Christopher John Low Carlbury, Piercebridge, Darlington DL2 3TP — MB ChB Liverp. 1977; MCh Orthop. Liverp. 1984, MB ChB 1977; FRCS Ed. 1982; FRCS Eng. 1982. Cons. Orthop. Surg. N. Tees Gen. Hosp. Stockton-on-Tees. Specialty: Orthop. Socs: Fell. BOA. Prev: Sen. Regist. (Orthop.) Mersey RHA.

TULLOCH, Mr David Neill, Surg. Cdr. RN Retd. Department of Urology, Western General Hospital, Crewe Road, Edinburgh Tel: 0131 537 1582 Email: dnt@doctors.net — MB BS Lond. 1979 (St Bartholomew's) FRCS Ed. 1986. Cons. Urol. Western Gen. Hosp. Edin. Specialty: Urol. Socs: Brit. Assn. Urol. Surgs. Prev: Cons. Urol. RN Hosp. Haslar; Sen. Regist. (Urol.) Inst. Urol. & St. Bart. Hosp. Lond.

TULLOCH, James Stuart 8 North Parade, Bootham, York YO30 7AB — MB BS Newc. 1997.

TULLOCH, Janet Gillespie The Vicarage, 15 St John's Hill, Wimborne BH21 1BX Tel: 01202 883490 — MB ChB Dundee 1977; DO RCS Eng. 1983. Staff Grade (Ophth.) Roy. Bournemouth Hosp. Specialty: Ophth. Prev: Clin. Asst. (Ophth.) Newc. Gen. Hosp.; Regist. (Ophth.) Newc. Gen. Hosp.; SHO (Ophth.) Manch. Roy. Eye Hosp.

TULLOCH, John Alexander, MC (retired) Woodvale, Edzell, Brechin DD9 7TF Tel: 01356 648234 — MB ChB Ed. 1943 (Univ. Ed.) FRCP Ed. 1956, M 1948; MD Ed. 1950; FRCP Lond. 1974, M 1963. Prev: Cons. Phys. Stracathro Hosp. Brechin.

TULLOCH, Lynda Joyce Craiglockhart Surgery, 161 Colinton Road, Edinburgh EH14 1BE Tel: 0131 455 8494 Fax: 0131 444 0161; 21-5 Russell Gardens, Edinburgh EH12 5PP Tel: 0131 538 7484 Email: ljt@doctors.org.uk — MB ChB Ed. 1983; DRCOG 1985; MRCGP 1987. Specialty: Gen. Pract.

TULLOCH, Pamela Mary Buchanan Marlborough Medical Practice, The Surgery, George Lane, Marlborough SN8 4BY Tel: 01672 512187 Fax: 01672 516809; Hillside, Granham Hill, Marlborough SN8 4DG — MB ChB Ed. 1979; DRCOG 1981; MRCGP 1984. Specialty: Gen. Pract.

TULLOH, Robert Michael Rhys Bristol Royal Hospital for Children, Congenital Heart Unit, Paul O'Gorman Building, Upper Maudlin Street, Bristol BS2 8JN Tel: 0117 342 8853 Fax: 0117 342 8857 Email: robert.tulloh@ubht.swest.nhs.uk — BM BCh Oxf. 1984 (Oxford) BA Oxford 1981; MA Oxf. 1985; MRCP (UK) 1987; MRCPCH 1996; FRCPCH 1997; DM Oxford 2003. Cons. Paediat. Cardiol. Roy. Bristol Hosp. for Childr. Specialty: Paediat. Cardiol. Special Interest: Pulm. Hypertens. Socs: Brit. Cardiac Soc.; Fell. Roy. Soc. Med. Prev: Cons. Paediat. Cardiol. Guy's & St. Thomas's Hosp. Lond.; Brit. Heart Foundat. Research Fell. Inst. Child Health; Sen. Regist. (Paediat. Cardiol.) Roy. Brompton Hosp. Lond.

TULLY, Adrian Mark Vale of Leven Dist. Gen. Hospital, Alexandria G83 0UA Tel: 01389 754121 — MB ChB Dundee 1977; FRCA 1984. Cons. Anaesth. Argyll & Clyde Acute Servs. NHS Trust; Hon. Sen. Clin. Lect. Fac. of Med. Glas. Univ. Specialty: Anaesth.

TULLY, Beryl Angela (retired) 6 Falcondale Walk, Westbury-on-Trym, Bristol BS9 3JG — MB ChB Bristol 1962. Prev: SCMO Southmead Health Serv. NHS Trust & United Bristol Hosp. Trust.

TULLY, Elizabeth Margaret Knox 5 Trafalgar Place, Bath Road, Devizes SN10 2AN — MB BCh BAO Belf. 1988; MB BCh Belf. 1988; MRCGP 1992. Trainee GP Doncaster VTS. Prev: Jun. Ho. Off. Tyrone Co. Hosp. Omagh.

TULLY, Kathryn Nicola The Ross Practice, Keats House, Bush Fair, Harlow CM18 6LY Tel: 01279 692747 Fax: 01279 692737; 13 Hampton Gardens, Sawbridgeworth CM21 0AN — MB BS Lond. 1985 (Lond. Hosp. Med. Coll. Univ. Lond.) DRCOG 1990; MRCGP 1994. Specialty: Obst. & Gyn. Prev: Trainee GP Crawley VTS; SHO (O & G & Psychiat.) Crawley.

TULLY, Winifred Margaret Michal Whiteways, 17 Kennedy Road, Shrewsbury SY3 7AB — MRCS Eng. LRCP Lond. 1959 (Guy's) DCH Eng. 1961. Prev: Med. Off. Family Plann Assn.; Med. Off. Brook Advisory Centre for Young People.

TUMA, Tuma Abdul-Karem Hartlepool General Hospital, Holdforth Road, Hartlepool TS24 9AH Tel: 01429 522826 Fax: 01429 863983 — MB ChB Mosul Iraq 1973 (Mosul, IRAQ.) MRCPsych 1982. Cons. (Old Age Psychiat.). Specialty: Geriat. Psychiat.

TUMATH, David Edward Ferguson The Bethesda Medical Centre, Palm Bay Avenue, Cliftonville, Margate CT9 3NR Tel: 01843 209300 Fax: 01843 209301 — MB BCh BAO Belf. 1971. Hosp. Pract. (Diabetes) Qu. Eliz. the Qu. Mother Hosp. Margate. Socs: Fell. Roy. Soc. Med.; Christian Med. Fellowsh. Mem.; BMA Mem.

TUMMALA, Venkateswara Rao 4 Parkwood Avenue, Roundhay, Leeds LS8 1JW — MB BS Andhra 1972. SCMO Barnsley Community & Priority Servs. Trust.

TUMMAN, Jonathan James Wilfred Department of Urology, Manchester Royal Infirmary, Oxford Road, Manchester M13 9WL Email: jtumman@yahoo.co.uk — MB ChB Manch. 1995; MRCSED 1999. Clin. Fell., Urol., Manch. Roy. Infirm. Specialty: Urol. Socs: BMA; Internat. Continence Soc. (UK). Prev: Ho. Off. (Med.) Manch. Roy. Infirm.; Sho Urol.Roy.Lancs.Hosp.; SHO Rotat. Gen. Surg. Roy. Oldham Hosp.

TUN, May Sanyu 2 St Aubyns Avenue, London SW19 7BL — MB BS Lond. 1982.

TUN, Si Thu Vicarage Lane Surgery, 189 Vicarage Lane, Blackpool FY4 4NG Tel: 01253 838997 Fax: 01253 699375 — MB BS Med Inst (I) Rangoon 1973; MB BS Med Inst (I) Rangoon 1973.

TUN, Victor Whyteleafe Surgery, 19 Station Road, Whyteleafe CR3 0EP Tel: 01883 624181 Fax: 01883 622498; 3 Wheat Knoll, Kenley CR8 5JT Tel: 020 8645 0272 — MB BS Lond. 1980 (Guy's Hospital) DRCOG 1983.

TUN MIN, Dr H2 Unit, Bolton General Hospital, Minerva Road, Farnworth, Bolton BL4 0JR Tel: 01204 390390; 9 Renfrew Drive, Beaumont Chase, Off Wigan Road, Bolton BL3 4XX — MB BS Mandalay 1976; DO RCSI 1995. Clin. Asst. (Ophth.) Bolton Gen. Hosp. & Hope Hosp. Salford. Prev: SHO Jas. Paget Hosp. Gt. Yarmouth & Leighton Hosp. Crewe.

TUNBRIDGE, Anne Jacqueline — MB ChB Birm. 1993; DTM & H Liverp. 1995; MRCP Lond. 1999. SHO (Gen. Med.) Poole Hosp. Dorset; Clin. Lect. in Infec. Diseases, Univ. of Sheff. Specialty: Infec. Dis. Prev: Med. Pract. Bethesda Hosp. Ubombo, Kwazulu/Natal S. Afr.; SHO (Paediat.) St. Peter's Hosp. Chertsey; SHO (A & E) N. Middlx. Hosp. Lond.

TUNBRIDGE, Ronald David Gregg Department of Medicine, Manchester Royal Infirmary, Manchester M13 9WL Tel: 0161 276 4156 Fax: 0161 274 4833; 55 Manor Drive, Manchester M21 7QG Tel: 0161 448 9590 — (St. Mary's) MRCS Eng. LRCP Lond. 1968; MB BS Lond. 1968; MRCP (UK) 1970; MD Lond. 1982; FRCP Lond. 1984. Sen. Lect. (Med.) Univ. Manch.; Hon. Cons. Phys. & Hosp. Dean (Clin. Studies) Manch. Roy. Infirm. Specialty: Gen. Med. Socs: Brit. Hypertens. Soc. Prev: Lect. (Med.) St. Mary's Hosp. Med. Sch. Lond.; MRC Jun. Research Fell. St. Mary's Hosp. Steroid Unit Lond.

TUNBRIDGE, William Michael Gregg — BChir Camb 1964 (Univ. Coll. Hosp.) MA Camb 1965; MRCS Eng. LRCP Lond. 1965; MB Camb 1965; DTM & H Liverp. 1967; FRCP Lond. 1979, M 1968; MD Camb 1977. Dir. of Postgrad. Med. Educat. & Train. Univ. Oxf. & Postgrad. Dean (Oxf.); Hon. Cons. Phys. John Radcliffe Hosp. & Radcliffe Infirm. Oxf.; Prof.ial Fell. Wadham Coll. Oxf. 1994-. Specialty: Gen. Med.; Diabetes; Endocrinol. Socs: Soc. Endocrinol.; Thyroid Club (Ex-Pres.); Diabetes UK. Prev: Cons. Phys. Newc. Gen. Hosp.; Sen. Lect. (Med.) Univ. Newc.; Regist. (Med.) Hammersmith Hosp.

TUNE, George Sydney c/o X-Ray Department, Friarage Hospital, Northallerton DL6 1JG — MB ChB Manch. 1974; PhD Bristol 1962, BA 1959; DMRD Eng. 1978. Cons. Radiol. Friarage Hosp. Northallerton, St. John of God Hosp. Specialty: Radiol. Prev: Sen. Regist. (Radiol.) Univ. Hosp. S. Manch.; Ho. Surg. Manch. Roy. Infirm.; Ho. Phys. Vict. Hosp. Blackpool.

TUNG, Kean Tat (Kenneth) Southampton General Hospital, Level B, Southampton Oncology Centre, Tremona Road, Southampton SO16 6YD — BM BCh Oxf. 1982; MRCP (UK) 1985; FRCR 1990; T(R) (CR) 1992; FRCP 1999. Cons. Radiol. Soton. Univ. Hosp. Trust. Specialty: Radiol.

TUNG, Mun-Yee Florence Road, London W5 3UA — MB BS Lond. 1996.

TUNGEKAR, Muhammad Fahim Muhammad Yousuf Department of Histopathology, St. Thomas Hospital, London SE1 7EH Tel: 020 7928 9292; 18 Woodville Road, Leytonstone, London E11 3BH — MB BS Bombay 1973 (Grant Medical College, Bombay) MD Bombay 1975; FRCPath 1991, M 1979. Sen. Lect. & Cons. Histopath. St. Thos. Hosp. Lond. Specialty: Histopath. Socs: Internat. Acad. Path. (Brit. Div.); Assn. Clin. Path.; Nat. Acad. of Med. Sci. (India). Prev: Assoc. Prof. & Cons. Histopath. Univ. Kuwait; Sen. Regist. (Histopath.) St. Geo. Hosp. Med. Sch. Lond.; Lect. Grant Med. Coll. Bombay.

TUNGLAND, Ole Petter The Central Sheffield University Hospitals, North Trent Medical Audiology, Royal Halamshire Hospital, Glossop Road, Sheffield S10 2JF Tel: 0114 271 1853 Fax: 0114 271 1855 — Cand Med Oslo 1973; T(M) 1991. Cons. Audiol. Med. Sheff. Teachg. Hosps. Specialty: Audiol. Med. Prev: Cons. Audiol. Med. Hosp. Sick Childr. Gt. Ormond St. Lond.; Sen. Cons. ENT Audiol. Ring Med. Centre Oslo, Norway; Cons. ENT Skövde Centre Hosp. Sweden Vestfold Centre Hosp. Tønsberg, Norway.

TUNIO, Mr Ali Murad Department of Surgery, University College of London Medical School, 67-73 Riding House St., London W1W 7EJ — MRCS Eng. LRCP Lond. 1987; FRCS Ed. 1991.

TUNIO, Fazal The Surgery, Elm Tree Medical Centre, Elm Tree Avenue, Stockton-on-Tees TS19 0UW Tel: 01642 603330 Fax: 01642 675656 — MB BS Sind 1968 (Liaquat Med. Coll.) Prev: Cas. Med. Off. Middlesbrough Gen. Hosp.; Trainee GP Kingsbury Lond.

TUNKEL, Sarah Alisa 8 Corringham Court, Corringham Road, London NW11 7BY — MB BS Lond. 1989 (Univ. Coll. Lond.) Healthcare Consultancy, Delotte & Touche Lond.; Research Fell. Fetal Med. Kings Coll. Hosp. Sch. of Med. Dent. Specialty: Obst. & Gyn.

TUNN, Edward James Department of Rheumatology, Royal Liverpool Hospital, Liverpool — MD Glas. 1990; BSc (Hons.) Glas. 1976, MD 1990, MB ChB 1978; MRCP (UK) 1981. Cons. Rheum. Roy. Liverp. Hosp. Specialty: Rheumatol.

TUNNADINE, Charles Henry John 6 Lewes Road, Ditchling, Hassocks BN6 8TT — MB BS Lond. 1981.

TUNNADINE, David Edward (retired) Europa House, West St., Bassett Road, Leighton Buzzard LU7 1DD Tel: 01525 851888; 1 Copper Beech Way, Leighton Buzzard LU7 3BD Tel: 01525 372524 Fax: 01525 377298 — (Guy's) BA, MB BChir Camb. 1953; DObst RCOG 1956; FRCGP 1983, MRCGP 1969. Prev: Res. Med. Off. Beckenham Matern. Hosp.

TUNNEY, Patrick James 10 Willow Tree Court, Brooklands Road, Sale M33 3SE — MB BCh BAO NUI 1984; MRCPI 1993.

TUNNICLIFF, Malcolm 1 Turn Furlong, Kingsthorpe, Northampton NN2 8BZ — MB BS Lond. 1997.

TUNNICLIFFE, William Stuart Inglemere, Moseley Road, Hallow, Worcester WR2 6NJ — MB BCh Witwatersrand 1986; MRCP (UK) 1992; MSc (Epidemiol.) Lond. 1994. Research Regist. Chest Research Inst. E. Birm. Hosp.; Research Regist. Heartlands Research Inst. Birm. Specialty: Respirat. Med.

TUNSTALL, Michael Eric (retired) University Medical School, Department of Environmental and Occupational Medicine, Foresterhill, Aberdeen AB25 2ZD Tel: 01224 558189; 9 South Headlands Crescent, Newtonhill, Stonehaven AB39 3TT Tel: 01569 730228 — (Univ. Coll. Hosp.) MB BS Lond. 1952; MRCS Eng. LRCP Lond. 1952; DObst RCOG 1955; DA Eng. 1956; FFA RCS Eng. 1959. Hon. Cons. Anaesth. Aberd. Roy. Hosps. NHS Trust; Hon. Research Fell. (Environm. & Occupat. Med.) Univ. Aberd. Prev: Cons. Anaesth. Aberd. Hosps.

TUNSTALL, Nigel Robert 131 Kinson Road, Bournemouth BH10 4DG — MB BS Lond. 1990.

TUNSTALL, Patricia June St. Helens & Knowsley Health Authority, Cowley Hill Lane, St Helens WA10 2AP Tel: 01744 33722; Brookside Cottage, 1 Fiveways, Springfield Lane, Eccleston, St Helens WA10 5EL Tel: 01744 26588 — DObst RCOG 1968; MB ChB Liverp. 1966, MCommH 1975; MFCM 1986; MFPHM 1990. Cons. Pub. Health Med. St. Helens & Knowsley HA. Specialty: Pub. Health Med. Prev: Regional SCM (Special Servs.) Mersey RHA; Cons. Pub. Health Med. Mersey RHA.

TUNSTALL, Shaun 10 Grenville Avenue, Preston PR5 4UA — MB ChB Leeds 1990.

TUNSTALL, Susan Rebecca Macmillan Unit, Frenchay Hospital, Bristol BS16 1LE — MB BS Newc. 1986. Cons. (Palliat. Med.) Frenchay Hosp. Bristol. Specialty: Palliat. Med.

TUNSTALL PEDOE, Dan Sylvester 29 Meynell Crescent, London E9 7AS Tel: 020 8986 2762 — MB BChir Camb. 1965 (St. Bart.) MA 1965; FRCP Lond. 1979, M 1967; DPhil Oxf. 1970. Sen. Lect. & Cons. (Med. & Cardiol.) St. Bart. & Homerton Hosps. Lond.; Med. Dir. Lond. Marathon. Specialty: Cardiol. Socs: Life Vice-Pres. Brit. Assn. Sports & Med.; Roy. Soc. Med. (Pres. Sports Med. Sect.). Prev: Research Physiol. Cardiovasc. Research Inst. San Francisco, USA; Sen. Regist. Radcliffe Infirm. Oxf.; Ho. Phys. St. Bart. Hosp. Lond.

TUNSTALL-PEDOE, Professor Hugh David Cardiovascular Epidemiology Unit, Ninewells Hospital & Medical School, Dundee DD1 9SY Tel: 01382 644255 Fax: 01382 641095 — MB BChir Camb. 1965 (Camb. & Guy's) MB (Distinc. Surg., Gyn & Obst.) Camb. BChir 1965; FRCP Lond. 1981, M 1967; MA Camb. 1965, BA (1st cl. Hons.) 1961, MD 1977; FFPHM RCP (UK) 1981, M 1978; FRCP Ed. 1986. Prof. & Dir. Cardiovasc. Epidemiol. Unit & Sen. Lect. (Med.) Ninewells Hosp. Univ. Dundee; Hon. Cons. Cardiol. & Pub. Health Med. Dundee Teachg. Hosps. NHS Trust. Specialty: Cardiol. Socs: Fell. Europ. Soc. Cardiol.; Assn. Phys. Prev: Sen. Lect. (Epidemiol.) & Hon. Phys. St. Mary's Hosp. Med. Sch. Lond.; Lect. (Med.) Lond. Hosps.; Mem. Clin. Scientif. Staff. MRC Social Med. Unit.

TUNSTALL-PEDOE, Oliver Daniel 4 Hill Street, Broughty Ferry, Dundee DD5 2JL — MB BChir Camb. 1996.

TUPPEN, Jonathan James Avenue Road Surgery, 2 Avenue Road, Warley, Brentwood CM14 5EL Tel: 01277 212820 Fax: 01277 234169; 42 Junction Road, Brentwood CM14 5JN Email: jtuppen@doctors.org.uk — MB ChB Manch. 1984; DRCOG 1987; MRCGP 1988. Co. Chairm., Exec. Comm., Billericay Brentwood & Wickford PCT, Trust HQ. Prev: Regist. (Med. for Elderly) Qu. Mary's Hosp. Sidcup; Trainee GP Lond. VTS.

TUPPEN, Nicola Michelle 4 Luton Avenue, Broadstairs CT10 2DH — MB ChB Birm. 1995.

TUPPER, Annemarie Dora (retired) 97 Cambridge Road, West Wimbledon, London SW20 0PU Tel: 020 8946 5486 — (Roy. Free) MB BS Lond. 1952; DObst RCOG 1955; DPhysMed. Eng. 1968. Prev: Cons. Rehabil. Univ. Coll. Hosp. Lond.

TUPPER, Catherine Helen Atkinson Health Centre, Market St., Barrow-in-Furness LA14 2LR — BM BS Nottm. 1983; BMedSci (Hons.) Nottm. 1981; MRCGP 1990; MFFP 1993. Cons. (Family Plann. & Reproductive Health Care). Specialty: Family Plann. & Reproduc. Health. Prev: Head Family Plann. S. Cumbria.

TUPPER, David James Luepin Basingstoke District Hospital, Basingstoke RG24 9NA Tel: 01256 817718 — MB ChB Leeds 1973; MRCP (UK) 1978; FRCP Lond. 1995. Cons. Geriat. Basingstoke Dist. Hosp. Specialty: Care of the Elderly. Socs: Internat. Soc. Quality Assur. Health Care. Prev: Sen. Regist. (Geriat. Med.) Soton. Gen. Hosp.; Regist. (Gen. Med.) Co. Hosp. Hereford; SHO (Gen. Med.) WillesBoro. Hosp. Ashford.

TUPPER, Nicholas Adrian 37 Wadbrough Road, Sheffield S11 8RF — MB ChB Sheff. 1995 (University of Sheffield) Med. SHO, Doncaster.

TUPPER, Ruth Carol Anne Holywell Ho. Med. Centre, Chesterfield; 5 Harlech Green, Lodge Moor, Sheffield S10 4NR — MB ChB Sheff. 1997; DRCOG; MRCGP; DCH; DFFP. GP Holywell Ho. Med. Centre Chesterfield. Specialty: Gen. Pract. Socs: Med. Protec. Soc.; BMA; RCGP. Prev: Pre-Regist. Ho. Off. (Gen. Surg.); Pre-Regist. Ho. Off. (Gen. Med.); SHO Med., Palliat. Care, Orthop., Obst. & Gyn., Paediat.

TUPPER-CAREY, Darrell Alexander 13 The Avenue, Colchester CO3 3PA Tel: 01206 575517 — MB ChB Birm. 1987; FCAnaesth. Cons. (Anaesth.) James Paget Hosp. Gt Yarmouth. Specialty: Anaesth.; Intens. Care. Prev: SHO (Anaesth.) Birm. Hosp.; SHO (Med.) Russells Hall Hosp. Dudley W. Midl.; Ho. Off. Dudley Rd. Hosp. Birm. & WalsGr. Hosp. Coventry.

TURA, Jenny Elizabeth Heath Lane Surgery, Earl Shilton, Leicester LE9 7PB Tel: 01455 844431; 8 Browns Close, Sapcote, Leicester

LE9 4FZ — MB ChB Leic. 1984. Prev: Trainee GP Leics. VTS; SHO (Psychiat.) Carlton Hayes Hosp.; SHO (A & E) Leicester Roy. Infirm.

TURBERFIELD, Laura Marion Temple Cowley Health Centre, Templar House, Temple Road, Oxford OX4 2HL Tel: 01865 777024 Fax: 01865 777548 — BM BCh Oxf. 1987; BA Camb. 1984; DRCOG 1990. Prev: Trainee GP Kidlington Health Centre Oxon.; SHO (Gen. Med., O & G & Dermat.) Oxf. HA.

TURBERVILLE, Stephen Matthew 23 Hawthorn Close, Wallingford OX10 0SY Tel: 01903 873739 — MB BS Lond. 1992 (St. Geo. Hosp. Med. Sch.) SpR (Child & Adolesc. Pschiatry) Oxf. Specialty: Geriat. Psychiat. Prev: SHO (Paediat.) St. Mary's Hosp. Lond., Hillingdon Hosp. Uxbridge & Southlands Hosp. Shoreham-by-Sea; SHO (A & E) St. Helier Hosp. Carshalton; SHO (Psychiat.) Fair Mile Hosp. Cholsey.

TURBERVILLE SMITH, Rupert John The Bridges Medical Centre, 26 Commercial Road, Weymouth DT4 7DW Tel: 01305 774411 — MB BS Lond. 1992.

TURBIN, Diana Rose Abbeys Meads Medical Practice, Elstree Way, Swindon SN25 4YX — (Univ. Coll. Hosp.) BSc Lond. 1981, MB BS 1984; MRCP (UK) 1987; DCH RCP Lond. 1987. GP Swindon. Specialty: Gen. Pract.

TURBITT, Deborah Ann 12 Cheverell House, Pritchards Road, London E2 9BN Tel: 020 7739 8971 — MB BS Lond. 1986.

TURCK, Walter Peter George 98-100 Market Street, Edenfield, Ramsbottom, Bury BL0 0JL Tel: 0170682 2435 — MB ChB St. And. 1963; FRCP Ed. 1977, M 1968; FRCP Lond. 1980, M 1968. Cons. Phys. Fairfield Gen. Hosp, Bury. Specialty: Gen. Med. Prev: Cons. Phys. Bury Gen. Hosp. & Rossendale Gen. Hosp.; Cons. Phys. Alice Ho Miu Ling Nethersole Hosp.; Clin. Lect. Univ. Dept. Med. Hong Kong.

TURCZANSKA, Ewa Hillside, Bodfari, Denbigh LL16 4DE — MB BS Lond. 1981.

TUREK, Tamara Anne Hathaway Surgery, 32 New Road, Chippenham SN15 1HR Tel: 01249 447766 Fax: 01249 443948 — MB ChB Dundee 1986.

TURFITT, Edward Neil Petroc Group Practice, The Surgery, St Columb Major, St Columb TR9 6AA Tel: 01637 880359 Fax: 01637 881482; Polwithen, St Columb TR9 6BA Tel: 01637 880511 — (Guy's) MB BS Lond. 1968; MRCS Eng. LRCP Lond. 1968; DObst RCOG 1974; Cert JCC Lond. 1978. Clin. Asst. (Colposcopy) Cornw.. Specialty: Obst. & Gyn. Prev: Ho. Surg. & Ho. Phys. Beckenham Hosp.; Resid. Obst. Brit. Milit. Hosp. Munster; Maj. RAMC.

TURFITT, Mary Elizabeth The Perranporth Surgery, Perranporth TR6 0PS Tel: 01872 572255 — MB BS Lond. 1968 (Guy's) MRCS Eng. LRCP Lond. 1968; Cert JCC Lond. 1978. Prev: Ho. Surg. Orpington Hosp.; Ho. Phys. St. Nicholas' Hosp. Plumstead.

TURFREY, Deborah Jane 30 Station Road, Bearsden, Glasgow G61 4AL — MB BS Lond. 1990 (St. Mary's Hosp. Lond.) FRCA 1995. Specialist Regist. (Anaesth.) Glas. Specialty: Anaesth. Prev: Research Fell. (Anaesth.) Glas. Univ.

TURFREY, Donna Marie Ferrers Cottage, Lullington Road, Edingale, Tamworth B79 9JA — MB BS Lond. 1994.

TURK, Edward Peter (retired) Sunny Meadow Farm, Long Buckby Wharf, Northampton NN6 7PP Tel: 01327 842574 — MB BChir Camb. 1974 (Camb. & St. Bart.) MRCPath 1982.

TURK, Gary Nicholas Antrim Health Centre, Station Road, Antrim BT41 4BS Tel: 028 9441 3940 Fax: 028 9441 3949 — MB BCh BAO Belf. 1982; MRCGP 1987.

TURK, Jeremy Psychiatry Corridor, Jenner Wing, St. Georges Hospital Medical School, Cranmer Terrace, London SW17 0RE Tel: 020 8725 5531/1068 Fax: 020 8725 3592 Email: j.turk@sghms.ac.uk; 10 Rocombe Crescent, London SE23 3BL — MB BS Lond. 1982 (Middlx. Hosp. Med. Sch.) BSc (Hons.) Lond. 1979; DCH RCP Lond. 1984; MRCPsych 1986; MD Lond. 1995; FRCPCH 1997, M 1996. Reader Developm. Psychiat., St. Geo. Hosp. Med. Sch. Lond.; Hon. Cons. Child & Adolesc. Psychiat.; S. W. Lond. & St George's Ment. Health NHS Trust. Specialty: Child & Adolesc. Psychiat. Special Interest: Autism; Behavioural Phenotypes; Childr. & Young People with Learning Disabilities. Socs: Pres., Learning Disabil. Sect., Roy. Soc. Med.; Full Mem. Child Psychiat. Research Soc.; Soc. Study Behavioural Phenotypes. Prev: Wellcome Research Fell. (Psychiat.) Inst. Child Health Lond.; Sen. Regist. (Child Psychiat.) Hosp. for Sick Childr. Gt. Ormond St. Lond.; Regist. (Psychiat.) Bethlem & Maudsley Hosps. Lond.

TURK, Professor John Leslie Flat 21, Lulworth Court, 13 Cannon Hill, London N14 7DJ — (Guy's) DSc Lond. 1967, MD 1959, MB BS (Hnrs.) 1953; MRCS Eng., LRCP Lond. 1953; FRCPath 1974, M 1963; FRCP Lond. 1975, M 1970; FRCS Eng. 1978. Emert. Prof. Path. Univ. Lond. Socs: Path. Soc. & Brit. Soc. Immunol. Prev: Sir William Collins Prof. of Path. Roy. Coll. Surg. & Univ. Lond.; Reader in Immunol. Inst. Dermat. Lond.; Mem. Scientif. Staff, MRC, Nat. Inst. Med. Research.

TURK, Theresa (retired) Flat 21, Lulworth Court, 13 Cannon Hill, London N14 7DJ — MB BS Lond. 1950 (W. Lond.) MB BS (Hnrs Path.) Lond. 1950; MRCS Eng. LRCP Lond. 1950; DCH Eng. 1953. Prev: Paediat. Regist. W. Middlx. Hosp. Isleworth.

TURKIE, Peter Victor High Street Surgery, 15 High Street, Overton, Wrexham LL13 0ED Tel: 01978 710666 Fax: 01978 710494 (Call before faxing); Fairfield, 32 Salop Road, Overton-on-Dee, Wrexham LL13 0EH Tel: 01978 710595 — MB BS Lond. 1969 (St. Geo.) MRCP (UK) 1974. GP; Med. Adviser N. Wales HA. Prev: Regist. (Med.) Liverp. RHB.

TURKINGTON, Douglas Newcastle City Health NHS Trust, Department of Psychiatry, Royal Victoria Infirmary, Newcastle upon Tyne NE1 4CP Tel: 0191 232 5131 Fax: 0191 227 5281; 5 Gerrard Close, Briere Dene, Whitley Bay NE26 4NS Tel: 0191 251 6343 Fax: 0191 223 2206 Email: dougturk@aol.com — MB ChB Glas. 1981; MRCPsych 1986; FRCPsych 1998. Sen. Lect. (Liason Psychiat.) & Cons. Psychiat. at Roy. Vict. Infirm. Newc.-u-Tyne. Specialty: Gen. Psychiat. Prev: Cons. Psychiat. St. Nicholas Hosp. Newc.; Sen. Regist. (Psychiat.) Roy. Hallamsh. Hosp. Sheff.; Sen. Regist. (Psychiat.) Bassetlaw Dist. Gen. Hosp. Worksop.

TURKINGTON, John Ronald Andrew Castle Practice, Carrickfergus Health Centre, Taylors Avenue, Carrickfergus BT38 7HT Tel: 028 9336 4193 Fax: 028 9331 5947 — MB BCh BAO Belf. 1996.

TURKINGTON, Peter Malcolm Hope Hospital , Salford Royal NHS Trust, Department of Respiratory Medicine, Stott Lane, Salford M6 8HD — MB ChB Leeds 1993 (Leeds Univ.) MRCP 1996; MD Leeds Univ. 2003; MD Leeds 2003. Consultant, Respir. & Gen. Med., Salford Royal NHS. Specialty: Gen. Med. Special Interest: Obstructive sleep apnoea; Sleep disorders; Respirat. failure. Socs: Brit. Thoracic Soc.; Europ. Respiratrory Soc.; Amer. Thoracic Soc. Prev: Specialist Regist., Respiratury Med., Yorks.

TURLE, George Charles (retired) 5 Moorfield, Canterbury CT2 7AN Tel: 01227 65448 — MD Lond. 1952 (Char. Cross) MB BS 1948; DPM Eng. 1951; FRCPsych 1987, M 1972. Prev: Cons. Psychiat. In-pat. Adolesc. Unit St. Augustines Hosp. Canterbury.

***TURLEY, Andrew Jones** 156 Blair Athol Road, Banner Cross, Sheffield S11 7GD Tel: 0114 268 5273; 7 Hill Close, Darlington Tel: 01325 461885 — MB ChB Sheff. 1998 (Sheffield) BMedSci (Hons) 1995; MB ChB Sheff 1998. HO. Northern Gen Hosp. Sheff..; Rotat Med. Qu.s Gen Cen. Nottm.

TURLEY, Isabel Mary Area F, X-Ray Department, Wythenshawe Hospital, Southmoor Road, Manchester M23 9LT — MB ChB Manch. 1976; DMRD Eng. 1980; FRCR 1982. Cons. Radiol. Wythenshawe Hosp. Manch. Specialty: Radiol.

TURLEY, James Francis Woodlands Park Health Centre, Canterbury Way, Wideopen, Newcastle upon Tyne NE13 6JL Tel: 0191 236 2366 Fax: 0191 236 7619; 15 Albany Mews, Gosforth, Newcastle upon Tyne NE3 4JW Tel: 0191 284 0026 — MB BS Durham 1966.

TURLEY, Jeanette Marie Windsor House Surgery, Corporation Street, Morley, Leeds LS27 9NB Tel: 0113 252 5223 Fax: 0113 238 1262 — MB ChB Sheff. 1988; MRCGP 1994.

TURLEY, Simon Jack — MB BS Lond. 1977 (Guy's) MRCS Eng. LRCP Lond. 1977.

TURLEY, Stephen Anthony The Avenues Medical Group, 27-29 Roseworth Avenue, Gosforth, Newcastle upon Tyne NE3 1NB Tel: 0191 285 8035; 12 Bloomsbury Court, Newcastle upon Tyne NE3 4LW — MB BCh BAO Belf. 1986; DRCOG 1989; MRCGP 1991; D.Occ.Med. RCP Lond. 1996. Prev: Trainee GP Northumbria; SHO (O & G) Newc. Gen. Hosp.; Ho. Off. Belf. City Hosp.

TURNBERG, Daniel 5 Broadway Avenue, Cheadle SK8 1NN — MB ChB Leeds 1994.

TURNBERG, Lord Leslie Arnold, KBE (retired) House Of Lords, London SW1A Tel: 020 8200 1295 — (Manch.) MB ChB Manch. 1957; FRCP Lond. 1973, M 1961; MD Manch. 1966; FRCP Ed.

1993; FRCPI 1993; FRCPS 1994; DSc Salford 1996; DSc Manch. 1998. Prev: Chairm. Bd. of Pub. Health Laborat. Serv. Lond.

TURNBULL, Adam Lothian (retired) Pippins, North Warren, Aldeburgh IP15 5QF Tel: 01728 452888 — BM BCh Oxf. 1947 (Oxf. & Lond. Hosp.) DM Oxf. 1955, BM BCh 1947; FRCP Lond. 1969, M 1952. Prev: Phys. Lond. Hosp.

TURNBULL, Alastair John — MD Lond. 1985 (St Thomas's Hospital London) BSc Lond. 1979, MB BS 1982; MRCP (UK) 1985; T(M) 1993; FRCP 1998. Cons. Phys. & Gastroenterol. York. Dist. Hosp. Specialty: Gastroenterol. Prev: Sen. Regist. (Gen. Med. & Gastroenterol.) Freeman Hosp. Newc. u Tyne; Research Fell. & Hon. Sen. Regist. Rayne Inst. St. Thos. Hosp. Lond.; Regist. (Med.) & Ho. Phys. St. Thos. Hosp. Lond.

TURNBULL, Alexander David Beech Hill Medical Practice, 278 Gidlow Lane, Wigan WN6 7PD Tel: 01942 821899 Fax: 01942 821752; 102 Whitley Crescent, Wigan WN1 2PU — MB ChB Glas. 1971; MRCGP 1975; Dip. Med. Ethics Keele 1991. Specialty: Gen. Pract. Socs: GP Writers Assn. Prev: Benefits Agency.

TURNBULL, Mr Andrew Robert Rathmullen House, 4A Combe Road, Bath BA2 5HX Tel: 01225 837484 — MB BS Lond. 1967 (St. Thos.) FRCS Eng. 1972; MS Soton. 1977. Hons. Cons. Gen. & Vasc. Surg. Bath Roy. United Hosp. NHS Trust. Specialty: Gen. Surg.; Vasc. Med. Prev: Lect. & Hon. Sen. Regist. (Surg.) Surg. Div. Fac. Med. Soton. Univ.; Regist. (Surg.) Soton. Univ. Hosp.

TURNBULL, Anna Therese Mary Doctors Surgery, Half Moon Lane, Wigton CA7 9NQ Tel: 016973 42254 Fax: 016973 45464; The Ghyll, Carwath Bridge, Rosley, Wigton CA7 8AU — MB ChB Aberd. 1981; MRCGP 1985; DRCOG 1985. GP Wigton.

TURNBULL, Anne 8 Lochview Road, Bearsden, Glasgow G61 1PP — MB ChB Glas. 1992. SHO (A & E) South. Gen. Hosp. Glas. Specialty: Gen. Pract.

TURNBULL, Anne Elizabeth Department of Radiology, Derby City General Hospital, Uttoxeter Road, Derby DE22 3NE Tel: 01332 340131; Springfield House, Moor Lane, Ockbrook, Derby DE72 3SA — BM BCh Oxf. 1983; MA Oxf. 1985; FRCR 1990. Cons. Radiol. Derby City Hosp. & Derby Roy. Infirm. Specialty: Radiol. Prev: Sen. Regist. (Radiol.) Qu. Med. Centre Nottm.

TURNBULL, Christopher James Arrowe Park Hospital, Upton, Wirral CH49 5PE Tel: 0151 678 5111 — MB BChir Camb. 1975 (Westm.) MA Camb. 1971; DObst RCOG 1976; MRCP (UK) 1977; MRCGP 1979; DCH Eng. 1979; FRCP Lond. 1993. Cons. Phys. (Geriat. Med.) Arrowe Pk. Hosp. Upton. Specialty: Care of the Elderly. Special Interest: Community Care; Diabetes; Movement Disorders. Socs: Brit. Med. Assn.; Brit. Geriat. Soc. (Train. & Clin. Pract & Effectiveness Comms.); Roy. Coll. Phys. (Spec. Adv. & Jt. Spec. Comms.). Prev: Chairm. Mersey Specially Train. Comm.; Clin. Dir. (Med. for Elderly) Arrowe Pk. Hosp.; Sen. Regist. (Geriat.) Clatterbridge Hosp. Wirral.

TURNBULL, Colin Michael Main X-Ray Department, Western General Hospital, Crewe Road, Edinburgh EH4 2XU Tel: 0131 537 2042 Fax: 0131 537 1027; 31 Inveralmond Drive, Cramond, Edinburgh EH4 6JX Tel: 0131 312 6765 — MB ChB Ed. 1971; BSc (Med. Sci.) Ed. 1969; MRCP (UK) 1974; DMRD Ed. 1976; FRCR 1978; FRCP Ed. 1988. Cons. Cardioradiol. West. Gen. Hosp. Edin.; Hon. Sen. Lect. (Radiodiag.) Univ. Edin. Specialty: Radiol. Socs: Fell. Roy. Coll. Phys.; BMA; Fell. Roy. Coll. Radiol. (Clin. Dir. For Radiol. LUHT). Prev: Sen. Regist. & Regist. (Radiodiag.) Roy. Infirm. Edin.; SHO (Gen. Med.) East. Gen. Hosp. Edin.

TURNBULL, David Hepburn (retired) 11 Tewkesbury Avenue, Marton, Middlesbrough TS7 8NB — (Newc.) MB BS Durh. 1942; MRCP Lond. 1948; MD Durh. 1953. Prev: Resid. Med. Off. Roy. Vict. Infirm. Newc. u. Tyne.

TURNBULL, Donald Malcolm Westwinds, Redburn Row, Chilton Moor, Houghton-le-Spring DH4 6PX — MB BS Durh. 1950. Prev: Ho. Phys. Dryburn Hosp. Durh.; Ho. Surg. Gyn. Roy. Vict. Infirm. Newc. upon Tyne.

TURNBULL, Douglass Matthew Department of Neurology, The Medical School, University of Newcastle upon Tyne, Framlington Place, Newcastle upon Tyne NE2 4HH — MB BS Newc. 1976; MRCP (UK) 1978; PhD Newc. 1984, MD 1984; FRCP Lond. 1991. Prof. Neurol. Univ. Newc.; Hon. Cons. Neurol. Newc. AHA. Specialty: Dentistry/Orthodontics.

TURNBULL, Edith Barton 15 Carrick Drive, Coatbridge ML5 1JX — MB ChB Glas. 1948.

TURNBULL, Gael Lundin (retired) 12 Strathearn Place, Edinburgh EH9 2AL — MD Pennsylvania USA 1951 (Univ. Pennsylvania) BA Camb. 1948; MCPS 1956; DA Eng. 1957. Prev: Hosp. Pract. (Anaesth.) Kidderminster & Dist. HA & S. Cumbria HA.

TURNBULL, George Anthony (retired) Hawthorn Bank, Silverdale, Carnforth LA5 0SQ Fax: 01524 702210 — MB BS Durh. 1955; FRCOG 1978, M 1965. Cons. O & G N. Lancs. S. Westmorland Hosp. Gp. Prev: Cons. O & G N. Lancs. S. Westmorland Hosp. Gp.

TURNBULL, Georgina Helen Longwitton Hall, Longwitton, Morpeth NE61 4JJ — MB BS Lond. 1996.

TURNBULL, Gordon James, Wing Cdr. RAF Med. Br. Retd. Ticehurst House Hospital, Ticehurst, Wadhurst TN5 7HU Tel: 01580 200391 Fax: 01580 201006; The Brewery House, Broad Town, Swindon SN4 7RE Tel: 01793 731569 Fax: 01793 731569 — MB ChB Ed. 1973 (Edinburgh) BSc (Med. Sci.) Ed. 1970; FRGS 1977; MRCP (UK) 1979; FRCPsych 1995, M 1982; FRCP Ed. 1995; FRSA 1999. Clin. Dir. Traum. Stress Managem. Centre Ticehurst Hse. Hosp. Wadhurst; Cons. Psychiat. Civil Aviat. Auth.; Hon. Sen. Lect. Psychiat.Univ.Kent. Specialty: Gen. Psychiat. Prev: Cons. Psychiat. Princess Alexandra Hosp. RAF Wroughton.

TURNBULL, Helen Elizabeth 4 Hollycross, Crazies Hill, Reading RG10 8QB — MB ChB Ed. 1998.

TURNBULL, Ian William X-Ray Department, Hope Hospital, Eccles, Salford Email: iwturnbull@medleg.freeserve.co.uk; 3 New Hall Avenue, Heald Green, Cheadle SK8 3LQ Tel: 0161 437 5924 — MB ChB Ed. 1971; BSc Ed. 1968; DMRD Ed. 1975; FRCR 1978. Cons(Neuro.) Hope Hosp. Eccles, Salford, Manch.; Lect. Dept. Diagn. Radiol. Univ. Manch.; Vis. Prof. Univ. Hosp. Lond., Ontario, Canada. Specialty: Radiol. Socs: Fell. Roy. Soc. Med.; F. Ch.S; Brit. Soc. Neuroradiol. Prev: Sen. Regist. (Radiol.) Soton. Gen. Hosp.; SHO (Med. Renal Unit) & Regist. (Radiol.) Roy. Infirm. Edin.

TURNBULL, Jane Claire (retired) South Durham Health Care NHS Trust, Archer Street Clinic, Darlington DL3 6LT Tel: 01325 465218; 12 Cleveland Terrace, Darlington DL3 7HA Tel: 01325 482279 — MB BS Newc. 1970; DCH RCP Lond. 1986. Prev: Clin. Med. Off. N.d. HA.

TURNBULL, Lesley Susan Department of Pathology, The Women's Hospital, Catharine St., Liverpool L8 7 Tel: 0151 709 1000; Stable Cottage, Gunley Hall, Marton, Welshpool SY21 8JL — MB ChB Ed. 1979; BSc (Hons.) (Bact.) Ed. 1976, MB ChB 1979; MRCPath 1986. Cons. Cytol. Wom. Hosp. Liverp. & Roy. Liverp. Hosp.; Hon. Lect. Liverp. Med. Sch. Specialty: Histopath. Socs: BMA. Prev: Cons. Histopath. St. Geo. Hosp. Med. Sch. Lond.; Sen. Regist. (Histopath.) N. West. RHA.

TURNBULL, Lindsay Wilson 30 Kaimes Road, Edinburgh EH12 6JT — MB ChB Ed. 1979; BSc (Hons.) (Path.) Ed. 1976, MB ChB 1979. SHO (Gen. Med.) Roy. Infirm. Edin. Socs: BMA. Prev: Ho. Phys. & Ho. Surg. Roy. Infirm. Edin.

TURNBULL, Malcolm John Uxbridge Health Centre, George St., Uxbridge UB8 1UB Tel: 01895 231925 Fax: 01895 813190; The Corner Cottage, 45 Stratton Road, Beaconsfield HP9 1HR — BM BCh Oxf. 1969; MA, BM BCh Oxf. 1969; DObst RCOG 1971.

TURNBULL, Margaret Helen Fleming (retired) 17 Orchard Drive, Bridgnorth WV16 4HY Tel: 01746 763080 — (Ed.) MB ChB Ed. 1945, DPH 1953. Prev: Asst. Co. Med. Off. & Sch. Med. Off. Salop CC.

TURNBULL, Mark King Street Surgery, 22A King Street, Hereford HR4 9DA Tel: 01432 272181 Fax: 01432 344725 — MB BS Lond. 1988; DCH RCP Lond. 1991; DRCOG 1991; MRCGP 1993. Clin. Asst. (Cardiol.) Hereford Co. Hosp.

TURNBULL, Michael Robert (retired) Fellbeck, Rogerfield, Keswick CA12 4BQ Tel: 01768 772442 Email: michael.turnbull@dunelm.org.uk — MB BS Durh. 1966.

TURNBULL, Nigel Bruce Hereward Medical Centre, Exeter Street, Bourne PE10 9XR Tel: 01778 373399 Fax: 01778 391713 — MB ChB Sheff. 1970; DCH RCPS Glas. 1972; MRCGP 1975.

TURNBULL, Penny Jo Top Flat S., 38 Thomson St., Aberdeen AB25 2QP — MB ChB Aberd. 1997.

TURNBULL, Peter Providence Surgery, 12 Walpole Road, Boscombe, Bournemouth BH1 4HA Tel: 01202 395195 Fax: 01202 304293 — MB BCh Wales 1978; BA Nat. Sc. Camb. 1975; MRCP (UK) 1981. GP Princip. Bournemouth. Prev: Regist. Cardiac. Dept. St. Thos. Hosp. Lond.; Regist. (Gen. Med.) Poole Gen. Hosp.; Ho. Phys. Med. Unit Univ. Hosp. Cardiff.

TURNBULL, Susan Mildred Department of Health, Wellington House, 133-155 Waterloo Road, London SE1 8UG Tel: 020 7972 4378 Fax: 020 7972 4559; 18 Pewley Way, Guildford GU1 3PY Tel: 01483 830822 Email: susan.turnbull@virgin.net — MB BS Newc. 1981; MRCGP 1985. Sen. Med. Off. (Communicable Dis.s) Brit. Dept. of Health. Specialty: Civil Serv. Prev: Med. Adviser Driver & Vehicle Licensing Agency; GP Blaydon-on-Tyne; Trainee GP E. Cumbria VTS.

TURNBULL, Mr Timothy John (cons. rooms), 32 The Drive, Hove BN3 3JD Tel: 01273 820082 Fax: 01273 731137 — MB BS Lond. 1974; FRCS Eng. 1978. Cons. Orthop. Surg. Roy. Sussex Co. Hosp. & Roy. Alexandra Hosp. Sick Childr. Brighton. Specialty: Orthop. Socs: Fell. BOA & Roy. Soc. Med.; Brit. Assn. for Surg. of Knee; Brit. Orthopaedic Foot Surg. Soc. Prev: Sen. Regist. (Orthop.) Roy. Lond. Hosp. & Roy. Nat. Orthop. Hosps. Lond.; Clin. Fell. Hosp. for Sick Childr., Toronto.

TURNER, Agnes Jane 13 Upper Malone Crescent, Upper Malone Rd, Belfast BT9 6PR Tel: 01232 201095 — MB BCh BAO Belf. 1996. SHO (Anaesth) Antrim Area Hosp. Antrim. Specialty: Anaesth. Prev: Jun. Ho. Off. Belf. City Hosp. Belf.

TURNER, Mr Alan Gordon, Deputy Lt. Edith Cavell Hospital, Peterborough Hospitals NHS Trust, Bretton Gate, Peterborough PE3 9GZ Tel: 01733 874000 Fax: 01733 875369 Email: alan.turner@pbh-tr.nhs.uk; Millstone, 48 Main Street, Ailsworth, Peterborough PE5 7AF Tel: 01733 380666 Fax: 01733 380666 — (Char. Cross London University) BSc Lond. 1965; MRCS Eng. LRCP Lond. 1968; MB BS Lond. 1968; FRCS Eng. 1973; FRCS Ed. 1973. Cons. Urol. P'boro. & Stamford Hosps. & Med. Dir. P'boro. Hosp. NHS Trust. Specialty: Urol. Socs: Fell. Roy. Soc. Med.; Brit. Assn. Urol. Surgs. Prev: Lect. (Urol. & Renal Transpl.) Char. Cross Hosp. Lond.; Lect. (Urol.) Inst. Cancer Research & Roy. Marsden Hosp. Lond.; Regist. (Urol.) Char. Cross Hosp. Lond.

TURNER, Alan Muir Wessex Nuffield Hospital, Winchester Road, Chandler's Ford, Eastleigh SO50 2DW Tel: 023 8026 0919; 4 Hiltingbury Road, Chandler's Ford, Eastleigh SO53 5SW Tel: 01703 253019 — MB BChir Camb. 1973 (Guy's) MB Camb. 1973, BChir 1972; MRCP (UK) 1975; FRCP Lond. 1991. Cons. Neurol. Wessex Neurol. Centre Soton., Qu. Alexandra Hosp. & St. Mary's Hosp. Portsmouth. Specialty: Neurol. Prev: Regist. (Neurol.) Nat. Hosp. Nerv. Dis. Qu. Sq. Lond.; Regist. (Neuropsychiat.) St. Thos. Hosp. Lond.

TURNER, Alastair Ronald 12 Froghall Road, Aberdeen AB24 3JL — MB ChB Aberd. 1997.

TURNER, Albert (retired) 25 Station Lane, Mickle Trafford, Chester CH2 4EH Tel: 01244 301748 — MB ChB Liverp. 1954; MRCGP 1977. Prev: Ho. Phys. Sefton Gen. Hosp.

TURNER, Alison Jane 28 Jenner House, Restell Close, Vanbrugh Hill, London SE3 7UW — MB BS Lond. 1989.

TURNER, Alison Robertson Church Street Surgery, 30 Church Street, Dunoon PA23 8BG Tel: 01369 703482/702778 Fax: 01369 704502; Westgate, Toward, Dunoon PA23 7UA Tel: 01369 870251 Email: alisonturner@doctors.org.uk — MB ChB Glas. 1970. Socs: BMA; MWF.

TURNER, Mr Alistair 35 Wrottesley Road, Tettenhall, Wolverhampton WV6 8SG — MB BCh Wales 1973 (Welsh National School Medicine) BSc (Hons.) Wales 1970, MB BCh 1973; FRCS Eng. 1978; FRCS Ed. 1978; MChOrth Liverp. 1983. Cons. Orthop. Surg. Roy. Hosp. & New Cross Hosp. Wolverhampton. Specialty: Orthop. Socs: Fell. BOA; Brit. Soc. Childr. Orthop. Surg. Prev: Sen. Lect. (Orthop. Surg.) Univ. Liverp.; Regist. (Orthop. & Trauma) Nuffield Orthop. Centre Oxf.; Regist. Christie Hosp. & Holt Radium Inst. Manch.

TURNER, Mr Allan Roderick Queen Margaret Hospital, Dunfermline KY12 0SU Tel: 01383 623623 Fax: 01383 674004; 34 Couston Street, Dunfermline KY12 7QW — MB ChB Ed. 1965; FRCS Ed. 1971; FRCS Eng. 1972. Cons. Gen. Vasc. Surg. Qu. Margt. Hosp. NHS Trust; Hon. Sen. Lect. Univ. Edin.; Examr. RCS Ed.; Regional Adviser to R. Coll. of Surg.s of Edin. Specialty: Gen. Surg. Socs: BMA; Vasc. Soc. GB; Assn. Surg. Prev: Asst. Prof. Surg. Pahlavi Univ. Shiraz, Iran; Regist. (Surg.) Clatterbridge Hosp. Bebington, Broadgreen Hosp. Liverp. & Glas. Roy. Infirm.

TURNER, Andrea Dept. Of Immunobiology, Kings College London, Guys Hospital, St Thomas Street, London SE1 3UL — MB BChir Camb. 1991; MRCP (UK) 1994. MRC Clin. Research Fell., ImmunoBiol. Dept. Guy's Hosp. Lond. Specialty: Paediat.; Immunol.

TURNER, Andrew Frere Lowesmoor Medical Centre, 93 Lowesmoor, Worcester WR1 2SA Tel: 01905 723441 Fax: 01905 724987; 288 Bath Road, Worcester WR5 3ET Tel: 01905 769153 — MB BS Lond. 1984 (Westminster Medical School) DRCOG 1989. Socs: Primary Care Soc. Gastroenterol.

TURNER, Andrew James Leslie Manchester Royal Infirmary, Department of Clinical Virology, 3rd Floor Clinical Sciences Building 1, Oxford Road, Manchester M13 9WL Tel: 0161 276 5688 Fax: 0161 276 5477 — MB ChB Manch. 1979; Dip. Bact. Manch. 1985; MRCPath 1989; FRCPath 1997. Cons. Virol. Specialty: Virology.

TURNER, Andrew Neil Renal Medicine (MRU, University of Edinburgh, Royal Infirmary, Lauriston Place, Edinburgh EH3 9YW Email: htttp://renux.dmed.ed.ac.uk/edren — BM BCh Oxf. 1980; MA Camb. 1981; MRCP (UK) 1984; PhD Lond. 1992; FRCP Lond. 1996; FRCP Ed. 1997. Prof. Nephrol. Univ. Edin. Specialty: Nephrol. Socs: Renal Assn.; Brit. Soc. Immunol.; Assn. Phys.s. Prev: Sen. Lect. & Hon. Cons. Med. & Therap. Univ. of Aberd.; Research Fell. Renal Unit Roy. Postgrad. Med. Sch. Lond.; Regist. (Med.) York Dist. Hosp.

TURNER, Angus William Mure Flat 6, 192 Bedford Hill, London SW12 9HL — MB BS Lond. 1986.

TURNER, Anita Jacqueline 42 Haddricks Mill Road, Newcastle upon Tyne NE3 1QL — MB BS Newc. 1990.

TURNER, Anne Curtis (retired) The Old Vicarage, Church Road, Combe Down, Bath BA2 5JJ Tel: 01225 833226 Fax: 01225 833226 — MB BS Lond. 1962 (St. Thos.) MFFP 1993. Prev: SCMO (Family Plann.) Bath.

TURNER, Anne Marie 14 Brisbane Grove, Hartburn, Stockton-on-Tees TS18 5BW — BM BS Nottm. 1997.

TURNER, Archibald (retired) 7A Larchlea S., Darras Hall, Ponteland, Newcastle upon Tyne NE20 9LW Tel: 01661 823068 — (Newc.) MB BS Durh. 1952. Prev: Clin. Med. Off. Gateshead HA.

TURNER, Arthur Francis (retired) Meadows Cottage, Radipole Village, Weymouth DT4 9RY Tel: 01305 782763 — MB BCh BAO Belf. 1934; DPH Lond. 1937. Prev: Co. MOH Dorset.

TURNER, Barbara Anne 507 North Drive, Thornton-Cleveleys FY5 2HY — MB BS Lond. 1993. Specialty: Anaesth.

TURNER, Benjamin Charles 3 Bridgelands, Copthorne, Crawley RH10 3QW Fax: 01342 719577; 3 Bridgelands, Copthorne, Crawley RH10 3QW — MB BS Lond. 1992 (St. Bart. Hosp. Lond.) BSc Lond. 1989; MRCP (UK) 1995. Specialist Regist. (Diabetes, Endocrinol. & Gen. Med.); Research Fell. Roy. Bournemouth Hosp. & St. Thos. Hosps. Lond. Specialty: Diabetes; Gen. Med.; Diabetes. Socs: Diabetic Assn. Prev: Specialist Regist. (Diabetes, Endocrinol. & Gen. Med.) Qu. Alex. Hosp. Portsmouth; Specialist Regist. (Diabetes, Endocrinol. & Gen. Med.) Princess Margt. Hosp. Swindon; SHO (Gen. Med.) Roy. Sussex Co. Hosp. Brighton.

TURNER, Benjamin Patrick Flat 1, Lenton Abbey, Derby Road, Beeston, Nottingham NG9 2SN — MB BS Lond. 1991.

TURNER, Beryl Rachel (retired) Sandalwood, 21 Courtyard Gardens, Wrotham, Sevenoaks TN15 7DS — MB ChB Liverp. 1943. Prev: Chest Phys. SE Thames HA.

TURNER, Beverley Anne Dronfield Health Centre, High Street, Dronfield, Sheffield S18 1PY Tel: 01246 419040 Fax: 01246 291780 — MB ChB Leeds 1972; MRCGP 1976; FRCGP 2004.

TURNER, Caroline Mallorie Irwin St Martins Practice, 319 Chapeltown Road, Leeds LS7 3JT Tel: 0113 262 1013 Fax: 0113 237 4747 — BM Soton. 1980; DRCOG 1982; MRCGP 1989. Specialty: Palliat. Med.

TURNER, Carolyn Joan Old School Surgery, Church St., Seaford BN25 1HH Tel: 01323 890072; 25 Blatchington Hill, Seaford BN25 2AJ — MB BS Lond. 1987 (King's Coll. Sch. Med. & Dent.) Princip. GP Seaford. Prev: Princip. GP Crowthorne, Berks.; GP Princip. Newhaven.

TURNER, Charles Godfrey Bodidris, 10 Park Road West, Sutton-on-Sea, Mablethorpe LN12 2NQ Tel: 01507 442296 — MRCS Eng. LRCP Lond. 1959 (Leeds) Prev: Regist. (Anaesth.) Harrogate Gen. Hosp.; SHO (Obst.) ScarBoro. Gen. Hosp.; Ho. Surg. & Ho. Phys. Otley Gen. Hosp.

TURNER, Charlotte Flat 2, 10 Friars Walk, Exeter EX2 4AY — BM BCh Oxf. 1988.

TURNER, Charlotte Elizabeth, Maj. 125 Kings Ride, Camberley GU15 4LJ — MB BS Lond. 1991.

TURNER, Christopher Brian Hodson and Partners, Park Farm Medical Centre, Allestree, Derby DE22 2QN Tel: 01332 559402 Fax: 01332 541001; 39 Burley Lane, Quarndon, Derby DE22 5JR Tel: 01332 840138 — MB BS Lond. 1973 (Roy. Free) MRCS Eng. LRCP Lond. 1973; MRCGP 1978; DCH Eng. 1978; DRCOG 1978. Prev: SHO A & E Dept. Lond. Hosp.; Ho. Surg. Roy. Free Hosp.; Ho. Phys. St. And. Hosp. Lond.

TURNER, Christopher Mitchell 10 Coden Terrace, Haymarket, Edinburgh EH11 2BJ — MB ChB Ed. 1992. Specialty: Gen. Psychiat.

TURNER, Claire Louise Susan 72 Chiltern Drive, Surbiton KT5 8LW — MB ChB Birm. 1996 (Birmingham) ChB Birm. 1996.

TURNER, Clare Elizabeth 16 Vandra Close, Malvern WR14 1EJ Tel: 01684 567209 — MB BCh Wales 1998.

TURNER, Clare Louise Houghton Farmhouse, Ringmore, Kingsbridge TQ7 4HH — MB BS Lond. 1988; DCH RCP Lond. 1991; MRCPCH 2000. Staff Grade Paediat. Derriford Hosp. Plymouth. Specialty: Paediat.

TURNER, Claudia Louise 10 Throwley Drive, Herne Bay CT6 8LP — MB BS Lond. 1997. SHO (Paediat.) The St. Helier NHS Trust Surrey. Specialty: Paediat.

TURNER, Claudia Louise St Richmonds Hospital, Spitalfield Lane, Chichester PO19 6SE — MB BS Lond. 1997 (St George's Hosp. Med. Sch. Lond.) MRCPCH. Specialist Regist. (Paediat.) St Richards Hosp. Chichester. Specialty: Paediat. Prev: Specialist Regist. (Paediat.) St Peter's Hosp. Chertsey.

TURNER, Colin The Health Centre, Elm Grove, Mengham, Hayling Island PO11 9AP Tel: 023 9246 6224 — MB ChB Bristol 1983; MRCGP 1987; DRCOG 1987. GP Hayling Is. Hants. Specialty: Paediat.

TURNER, Colin Mure (retired) Podkin Farm, High Halden, Ashford TN26 3HS — MB ChB Glas. 1944.

TURNER, David Alexander Hatfield Road Surgery, 70 Hatfield Road, Ipswich IP3 9AF — MB BS Lond. 1971; MRCS Eng. LRCP Lond. 1971; DCH Eng. 1975; FRCP (UK) 2002. Hosp. Pract. (Gen. & Chest Med.) Ipswich Hosp. Specialty: Gen. Med.

TURNER, David Charles Turner, Hart, Appleton and Briggs, Woodsend Medical Centre, School Place, Corby NN18 0QP Tel: 01536 407006 Fax: 01536 401711; 16 Church Lane, Dingley, Market Harborough LE16 8PG Tel: 01858 535319 Fax: 01536 401711 Email: dcturner2@aol.com — MB BS Lond. 1969 (St. Geo.) MRCGP 1985; Dip. Med. Educat. Dund 1994. GP Corby; Cons. Weetabix, Golden Wonder, Orchard Ho. Foods. Specialty: Gen. Med. Socs: Brit. Assn. Performing Arts Med.; BMA. Prev: Regist. (Path.) Roy. Hants. Co. Hosp. Winchester & St. Geo. Hosp. Lond.; Ho. Phys. Epsom Dist. Hosp.; Ho. Surg. St. Geo. Hosp. Lond.

TURNER, David John Gosford House, 3 Noel Road, Oulton Broad, Lowestoft NR32 3JS Tel: 01502 564263 Email: caritas@totalise.co.uk — MB ChB Ed. 1960; DA Eng. 1964; FFA RCS Eng. 1967. Cons. Anaesth. Jas. Paget Hosp. Gt. Yarmouth. Specialty: Anaesth. Socs: BMA; E. Anglian Assn. Anaesth. Prev: Sen. Regist. (Anaesth.) Roy. Infirm. Edin.; Regist. (Anaesth.) Ipswich & E. Suff. Hosp.

TURNER, David John Pencester Surgery, 10/12 Pencester Road, Dover CT16 1BW Tel: 01304 240553 Fax: 01304 201773 — MB ChB Ed. 1978.

TURNER, David Patrick James 2 School Lane, Stanton-by-Dale, Ilkeston DE7 4QJ — MB ChB Leic. 1989.

TURNER, David Paul Ventnor Medical Centre, 3 Albert Street, Ventnor PO38 1EZ Tel: 01983 852787 Fax: 01983 855447; Fowlsdown Farm, Whiteley Bank, Ventnor PO38 3AF — MB ChB Birm. 1977.

TURNER, Professor David Robert Department of Histopathology, Taunton and Somerset Hospitals, Musgrove Park, Taunton TA1 5DA Tel: 01823 342267 Fax: 01823 344431 — (Guy's) MB BS Lond. 1962; MRCS Eng. LRCP Lond. 1962; PhD Lond. 1969; FRCPath 1984, M 1972. Cons. Hispopathologist Taunton and Som. Hosp.; Emerit. Prof. Path. Nottm. Univ.; Emerit. Cons. Histopath. Univ. Hosp. Nottm.; Mem. WHO Comm. cl.ificat. & Nomenclature of Renal Dis.; Advis. Edr. Internat. Dictionary of Med. & Biol.; Adviser Edr. Jl. Clin. Path. & Internat. Jl. Experim. Path; CPA Insp. Specialty: Histopath. Socs: BMA; Path. Soc.; Roy. Soc. Med. Prev: Vice-Dean Univ. Nottm. Med. Sch.; Cons. Histopath. MusGr. Pk. Hosp. Taunton; Reader & Prof. Histopath. Guys Hosp. Med. Sch. Lond.

TURNER, Deborah Celia Greenhill Health Centre, 482 Lupton Road, Sheffield S8 7NQ Tel: 0114 237 2961 — MB ChB Sheff. 1978; DRCOG 1980; DCCH RCP Ed. 1983. Socs: BMA. Prev: SHO (Paediat.) Sheff. Childr. Hosp.; SHO (Gyn. & Obst.) Jessop Hosp. Wom. Sheff.

TURNER, Deborah Louise Torbay Hospital, Department of Haematology, Lawes Bridge, Torquay TQ2 7AA — MB BS Lond. 1992 (Roy. Free) BSc (Hons.) 1989; MRCP (UK) 1996; MRCPath 2001. Cons. (Haemat.) Torbay Hosp. Specialty: Haematology.

TURNER, Delphine Ruth 35 Station Road, Felstead, Dunmow CM6 3HD — MB BS Lond. 1976; FRCP.

TURNER, Mr Derek Thomas Leslie 109 Spilsby Road, Boston PE21 9PE Tel: 01205 361913 — MB BS Lond. 1968 (Guy's) FRCS Eng. 1973; MS Soton. 1981. Cons. Urol. Pilgrim Hosp. Boston; Clin. Director (Urol.) United Lincs. Hosps. Specialty: Urol. Socs: BMA; Brit. Assn. Urol. Surgs. Prev: Lect. (Surg.) Soton. Univ.

TURNER, Mr Douglas Patrick Breen (retired) 74 Leicester Road, Uppingham, Oakham LE15 9SD Fax: 01325 464914 — MRCS Eng. LRCP Lond. 1939 (Liverp.) FRCS Eng. 1948. Prev: Cons. Gen. Surg. Broadgreen Hosp. & Mill Rd. Matern Hosp. Liverp.

TURNER, Duncan 6 Traquair Park W., Edinburgh EH12 7AL — MB ChB Aberd. 1997.

TURNER, Edward Charles Shiregreen Medical Centre, 492 Bellhouse Road, Sheffield S5 0RG Tel: 0114 245 6123 Fax: 0114 257 0964 — MB ChB Sheff. 1988; DRCOG 1992. Specialty: Gen. Pract.

TURNER, Elaine Inglis Killin Medical Practice, Laggan Leigheas, Ballechroisk, Killin FK21 8TQ Tel: 01567 820213 Fax: 01567 820805 — MB ChB Ed. 1983; BSc (Hons.) Ed. 1980; DRCOG 1987. Prev: Regist. (Clin. Biochem.) Roy. Infirm. Edin.; Research Regist. (O & G) Roy. Vict. Infirm. Newc. u. Tyne.

TURNER, Mr Eric Anderson (retired) 19B School Road, Moseley, Birmingham B13 9ET Tel: 0121 449 8217 — MB ChB Glas. 1940; FRCS Eng. 1949. Prev: Neurosurg. Qu. Eliz. Hosp. Birm.

TURNER, Erin Sinclair 25 All Saints Road, Kings Heath, Birmingham B14 7LL — MB ChB Birm. 1991; ChB Birm. 1991.

TURNER, Ethel Barbara (retired) 4 Mortain Road, Rotherham S60 3BX Tel: 01709 370169 — MB ChB Sheff. 1962. Prev: Cons. Genitourin. Phys. Rotherham Dist. Gen. Hosp.

TURNER, George Craven (retired) 25 Timms Lane, Formby, Liverpool L37 7DW Tel: 0170 48 31323 — MB ChB Leeds 1947; MD Leeds 1957, MB ChB 1947; FRCPath 1969, M 1963. Prev: Dir. Liverp. Regional Pub. Health Laborat.

TURNER, Mr George Stewart Manchester Royal Eye Hospital, Oxford Road, Manchester M13 9WH Tel: 0161 276 1234 — MB BS Lond. 1977 (St. Geo.) MRCP (UK) 1982; FRCS Eng. 1984. Cons. Ophth. Manch. Roy. Eye Hosp. Specialty: Ophth. Socs: Assn. Research in Vision & Ophth. Prev: Cons. Ophth. Taunton & Som. Hosp.; Lect. (Clin. Ophth.) Inst. Ophth. Lond.; Resid. Surgic. Off. Moorfields Eye Hosp. Lond.

TURNER, Gerald McDonald Ambrose (retired) Dove Cottage, 2 Ragleth View, Ludlow Road, Little Stretton, Church Stretton SY6 6RF — MB ChB Ed. 1949; FRCP Ed. 1971, M 1955. Prev: Cons. Phys. Dunoran Home (Guy's Hosp.) Bromley.

TURNER, Gillian Elrick Norfolk & Norwich University Hospital, Department of Haematology, Norwich NR4 7UY Tel: 01603 286286 Fax: 01603 286918 Email: gill.turner@nnuh.nhs.uk — MB ChB Ed. 1981; BSc (Hons.) Med. Sci. Ed. 1978, MD 1992; FRCPath 2000; FRCP (Edin) 2000. Cons. Haematol. Norf. - Norwich NHS Trust, Norwich. Specialty: Haematology. Prev: Sen. Regist. (Haemat. & Blood Transfus.) North. RHA.; Regist. (Haemat.) West. Gen. Hosp. Edin.; Regist. (Med.) Roy. Infirm. Edin.

TURNER, Gillian Frances Lymington Infirmary, East Hill, Lymington SO41 9ZH Tel: 01590 676085; Arnewood Corner, Arnewood Bridge Road, Sway, Lymington SO41 6ER — MB BS Lond. 1981; MRCS Eng. LRCP Lond. 1981; MRCP (UK) 1983; FRCP Lond. 1994. Cons. Phys. Geriat. Med. Soton. & Lymington. Specialty: Care of the Elderly. Socs: Brit. Geriat. Soc.; Hosp. Cons. & Spec. Assn. Prev: Sen. Regist. W. Midl.

TURNER, Gillian Margaret X-Ray Department, Derby City General Hospital, Uttoxeter, Derby DE22 3NE Tel: 01332 340131 Fax: 01332 625844; The Mount, Yeldersley, Ashbourne DE6 1LS — MB

BS Lond. 1984 (Univ. Coll. Hosp. Med. Sch.) BSc Lond. 1981; FRCR 1992. Cons. Radiol. Derby City Gen. Hosp. Specialty: Radiol. Prev: Sen. Regist. (Radiol.) Nottm. HA.

TURNER, Guy Allan, Surg. Cdr. RN Retd. Anaesthetic Department, Royal West Sussex Hospital, Spitalfield Lane, Chichester PO19 6SE Tel: 01243 788122 Fax: 01243 831600; 72A West Gate, Chichester PO19 3HH Tel: 01243 783923 — MB BS Lond. 1975 (Westminster) MRCS Eng. LRCP Lond. 1975; FFA RCS 1981. Cons. Anaesth. St. Richards Hosp. Chichester. Specialty: Anaesth. Prev: Cons. Anaesth. Intens. Care Unit RN Hosp. Haslar Gosport.

TURNER, Gwendoline Department of Clinical Genetics, Ashley Wing, St James University Hospital, Leeds Tel: 0113 243 3144; 68 Duchy Road, Harrogate HG1 2EZ Tel: 01423 506772 — MB ChB Ed. 1967. Cancer Research UK Cancer Genetics Building St. James Hosp., Leeds. Specialty: Genetics. Prev: ICRF Genetic Epidemiol. St. Jas. Hosp. Leeds; Dep. Clin. Genetics St. Jas. Hosp. Leeds.

TURNER, Harriet Jemima Holcroft, Common Lane, Lower Stretton, Warrington WA4 4PD — MB BS Newc. 1998; MB BS Newc 1998.

TURNER, Helen Mary (retired) Bodnant, Keighley Road, Colne BB8 7HL Tel: 01282 865615 — MRCS Eng. LRCP Lond. 1950 (Roy. Free) DPH Manch. 1966; MFCM 1973; FRCPCH 1997. Prev: SCMO Burnley HA.

TURNER, Henry Richard 10 Armit Place, St Andrews KY16 8RE Tel: 01334 75198 — MB ChB St. And. 1945 (St. Andrews) FFA RCS Eng. 1962, DA Eng. 1960. Specialty: Anaesth.

TURNER, Hugh Dundonald Coxhoe Medical Practice, 1 Lansdowne Road, Cornforth Lane, Coxhoe, Durham DH6 4DH Tel: 0191 377 0340 Fax: 0191 377 0604 — MRCS Eng. LRCP Lond. 1989; MA Oxf. 1984, BA (Hons. Physiol.) 1980. Socs: Fell. Roy. Soc. Health; ARM Represen. N. Durh. Div.; BMA Hon. Sec. North Durham Div. 1998-pres. Prev: Trainee GP Cleveland VTS; SHO (Med.) S. Cleveland Hosp. & Roy. Shrewsbury Hosp.

TURNER, Ian Mark 50 Woodlands Park, Whalley, Clitheroe BB7 9UG — MB ChB Dundee 1997.

TURNER, Ian Maxwell The Surgery, Sandy Lane, Brewood, Stafford ST19 9ES Tel: 01902 850206 Fax: 01902 851360 — MB ChB Liverp. 1972; DCH Eng. 1976; DRCOG 1977.

TURNER, Jacqueline Susan South Parade Surgery, 1 South Parade, Penzance TR18 4DJ Tel: 01736 362082 Fax: 01736 332933 — MB BS Lond. 1968; MRCS Eng. LRCP Lond. 1968.

TURNER, Mr James Andrew (retired) Carey House, Magham Down, Hailsham BN27 1PR Tel: 01323 844646 — MB BS Lond. 1947 (Guy's) FRCS Eng. 1954.

TURNER, Jean (retired) Carey House, Magham Down, Hailsham BN27 1PR Tel: 01323 844646 — MB BS Lond. 1949 (Roy. Free)

TURNER, Mrs Jean Gillean Cameron 34 Couston Street, Dunfermline KY12 7QW Tel: 01383 729689 Email: jmacraeturner@hotmail.com — MB ChB Aberd. 1966; FRCS Ed. 1970; FRCS Eng. 1972; B.Mus (Hons.) Ed. 1999. Peripatetic Locum Cons. Surg., remote and rural Hosps. of Scotl., mainly West. Isles Hosp., Stornoway. Specialty: Gen. Surg. Socs: Assoc. of Surg. Of Gt. Brit. & Irel. (Fell.); Viking Surgic. Club. Prev: Cons. Gen. Surg. (Long Term Locum) Withybush Hosp. Haverfordw.; Cons. Gen. Surg. (Long Term Locum) Dunfermline & W. Fife Hosps; & Noble's Hosp. I. of Man.

TURNER, Mrs Jean McGiven Springburn Health Centre, 200 Springburn Way, Glasgow G21 1TR Tel: 0141 531 9691 Fax: 0141 531 6705; Beechwood, 1 Balmore Road, Milngalvie, Glasgow G62 6ES — MB ChB Aberd. 1965; DA Eng. 1970. GP Glas. Prev: Regist. Anaesth. Aberd. Roy. Infirm.; Regist. Anaesth. South. Gen. Hosp. Glas.

TURNER, Jennifer Jane Le Moaillage, La Route de Rocquaine, St Pierre du Bois, Guernsey GY7 9HU — MB BS Lond. 1990; RCGP.

TURNER, Joanna 12A Grey Point, Helen's Bay, Bangor BT19 1LE — MB BCh BAO Belf. 1992.

TURNER, Joanna Judith Bitterne Park Surgery, 28 Cobden Avenue, Southampton SO18 1BW Tel: 023 8058 5655 Fax: 023 8055 5215; Chase Grove, Waltham Chase, Southampton SO32 2LF Tel: 01489 891416 — MB ChB Bristol 1988; MRCP (UK) 1992; DTM & H RCP Lond. 1993; T(GP) 1996; MRCGP Lond. 1997.

TURNER, Joanna Margaret 17 Summerhill Street, Newcastle upon Tyne NE4 6EJ — MB BS Newc. 1994.

TURNER, Joanna Patricia Rushall Medical Centre, 107 Lichfield Road, Rushall, Walsall WS4 1HB Tel: 01922 622212 Fax: 01922 637015 — MB BS Lond. 1986; DCH RCP Lond. 1990; DRCOG 1991; MRCGP 1992.

TURNER, Joanne Louise — MB BS Lond. 1989; MRCPsych 1994. Specialty: Gen. Psychiat.; Psychother.

TURNER, John Consett Medical Centre, Station Yard, Consett DH8 5YA Tel: 01207 216116 Fax: 01207 216119; 9 Kempton Close, Derwent Braes, Shotley Bridge, Consett DH8 0UB Tel: 01207 501797 — MB BS Newc. 1980; DRCOG 1984; MRCGP 1984. GP Consett.

TURNER, John Chatterton Shipley (retired) Miller's Cottage, Walkern Mill, Walkern, Stevenage SG2 7NP Tel: 01438 861250 — MRCS Eng. LRCP Lond. 1953 (Middlx.) MA Camb. 1955, MB BChir 1954; DObst RCOG 1956.

TURNER, John Edward — (Univ. Coll. Hosp.) MRCS Eng. LRCP Lond. 1969; BSc Lond. 1966, MB BS 1969; DObst RCOG 1972; MRCGP 1975; Dip. Palliat. Med. Wales 1991; MFFP 1993. Clin. Asst. Renal Unit Kent & Canterbury Hosp. Specialty: Gen. Med. Prev: SHO (Med. & O & G) Cuckfield Hosp.; Ho. Surg. Ipswich & E. Suff. Hosp.

TURNER, John Halifax, SBStJ Magnolia House, 27 Carisbrooke Gardens, Knighton, Leicester LE2 3PR Tel: 0116 210 7740 Fax: 0116 210 7741 Email: jht3@le.ac.uk — MB BChir Camb. 1971 (Guy's) MB Camb. 1972 BChir 1971; MA Camb. 1972. Clin. Lect. Dept. of Gen. Pract. & Primary Care Leicester Univ.; Teachg. Assoc. Drs Platts, Drucquer, Sharp, Shaw & Ward; Educat. Coord. Leics. GP. Salaried scheme. Specialty: Gen. Pract. Socs: Leic. Med. Soc.; AUDGP; CMF. Prev: Ho. Surg. & Ho. Phys. (Gen. Med.) St. Nicholas Hosp. Plumstead.; Sen. Partner Gen. Pract. (Retd.) Leics.

TURNER, John Jeffrey University Hospital Aintree, Lower Lane, Liverpool L9 7AL Tel: 0151 529 2392 Fax: 0151 529 2420 Email: johnjturner@aht.nwest.nhs.uk — (St. Mary's) MRCS Eng. LRCP Lond. 1966; MB BS Lond. 1966; MRCP (UK) 1972; FRCP Lond. 1988. Cons. Phys. Univ. Hosp. Alm Tree Liverp.; Clin. Dir. & Head Med. Servs. Aintree Hosps.; Hon. Clin. Lect. Univ. Liverp.; Ex Clin. Director & Head of Med. Servs. Specialty: Gen. Med. Special Interest: Med. in the Elderly. Socs: Liverp. Med. Inst.; Brit. Geriat. Soc.(Former Counc. Mem. & Mersey Regional Chair). Prev: Sen. Regist. (Nuffield Dept. Med.) Radcliffe Infirm. Oxf.; Regist. (Med. & Endocrinol.) St. Vincent's Hosp. Dub.; Ho. Phys. (Med. Unit) St. Mary's Hosp. Lond.

TURNER, John Morris Department of Anaesthesia, Addenbrookes Hospital, Hills Road, Cambridge CB2 2QQ Tel: 01223 217434; 29 Church Street, Little Shelford, Cambridge CB2 5HG Tel: 01223 842344 — MB ChB Bristol 1965; FFA RCS Eng. 1970. Cons. Anaesth. Camb. HA. Specialty: Anaesth. Socs: BMA. Prev: Cons. Anaesth. Midl. Centre Neurosurg. & Neurol. Smethwick; Lect. (Anaesth.) Univ. Leeds; Sen. Regist. (Anaesth.) United Birm. Hosps.

TURNER, John Robert Bentley (retired) Glenturner, 3 Summer Meadow, The Uplands, Mill Hill Lane, Pontefract WF8 4HZ Tel: 01977 704762 Fax: 01977 704762 — MB ChB Leeds 1954; FRCP Lond. 1978, M 1960. Prev: Mem. Med. Appeals Tribunals.

TURNER, John Robinson (retired) Corner House, Cropton, Pickering YO18 8HH Tel: 01751 417586 — MRCS Eng. LRCP Lond. 1952 (Sheff.) Prev: Surg. Cunard SS Company.

TURNER, John Scott Adult Intensive Care Unit, Royal Brompton National Heart & Lung Hospital, Sydney St., London SW3 6NP — MB ChB Cape Town 1980; FCP(SA) 1988; MMed. 1989. Doverdale Fell. Roy. Brompton & Nat. Heart Hosp. Lond. Specialty: Gen. Med. Prev: Cons. Surg. ICU Groote Schuur Hosp. Cape Town S. Africa; Sen. Regist. (Respirat.) Groote Schuur Hosp. Cape Town, S. Africa.

TURNER, John Sydney (retired) 7 Crynfryn Buildings, Aberystwyth SY23 2BD Tel: 01970 612045 — MRCS Eng. LRCP Lond. 1947 (Univ. Coll. Hosp.) Prev: Gen. Pract. Tregaron & Ceredigion.

TURNER, John Victor Cedar House Surgery, 14 Huntingdon Street, St. Neots, Huntingdon PE19 1BQ Tel: 01480 406677 Fax: 01480 475167; 28 Woodlands, St. Neots, Huntingdon PE19 1UE — MB BS Newc. 1968. Socs: BMA.

TURNER, Mr John William (retired) 15 Springkell Drive, Pollokshields, Glasgow G41 4EZ Email: m800jwt@aol.com — MB BS Lond. 1956 (King's Coll. Hosp.) MRCS Eng. LRCP Lond. 1956; FRCS Ed. 1962; FRCS Glas. 1974. Prev: Sen. Regist. Dept. Surg. Neurol. Roy. Infirm. Edin.

TURNER, Jonathan Andrew McMahon, QHP, RD Royal Bournemouth Hospital, Castle Lane E., Bournemouth BH7 7DW Tel: 01202 303626 Fax: 01202 704863 Email: jonathan.turner@rbch-tr.swest.nhs.uk — (Middlx. Hosp. Med. Sch.) MB BS Lond. 1970; MRCP (UK) 1973; FRCP Lond. 1990. Cons. Phys. E. Dorset Health Dist.; Director Roy. Navy Reserves Med. Br. Specialty: Gen. Med.; Respirat. Med. Special Interest: Asbestos Related Lung Dis. Socs: Brit. Thoracic Soc.; Europ. Respirat. Soc.; Amer. Thoracic Soc. Prev: Lect. (Med.) Middlx. Hosp. Med. Sch. Lond.; Regist. (Med.) Centr. Middlx. Hosp. Lond.

TURNER, Joseph Edward 25 Westland Road, Knebworth SG3 6AS — MB BS Lond. 1992.

TURNER, Joseph Greenwood 13 Promenade, Southport PR8 1QY Tel: 01704 536398 — MRCS Eng. LRCP Lond. 1950 (St. Mary's)

TURNER, Julian Geoffrey Litchdon Medical Centre, Landkey Road, Barnstaple EX32 9LL Tel: 01271 23443 Fax: 01271 25979; Higher Westaway, Newton Tracey, Barnstaple EX31 3PL Tel: 01271 858417 — MB BS Lond. 1969 (Middlx.) DObst RCOG 1971; DCH Eng. 1977; FRCGP 1988, M 1978; DFFP 1995. Examr. RCGP. Socs: Fell. Roy. Soc. Med. Prev: Regist. (Med.) Chas. Gardner Hosp. Perth, W. Austral.; Regist. (Med.) Launceston Gen. Hosp. Tasmania, Austral.; SHO (O & G) N. Devon Dist. Hosp. Barnstaple.

TURNER, Julian Paul Marine Medical, Blyth Health Centre, Thoroton Street, Blyth NE24 1DX Tel: 01670 396520 Fax: 01670 396537; 12 Caseton Close, Whitley Bay NE25 9PL Tel: 0191 253 2912 — MB BS Newc. 1982. SHO (Gen. Med.) Freeman Hosp. Newc.

TURNER, Julie Annabel 83 Bushey Wood Road, Sheffield S17 3QD — MB ChB Manch. 1993. Specialist Regist., Med. Microbiol. Specialty: Med. Microbiol. Prev: SHO (Microbiol.) North. Gen. Hosp. Sheff.

TURNER, Justin Andrew 2 Chapel Fold, Leeds LS6 3RG — MB ChB Leeds 1992.

TURNER, Karina Louise The Charter Medical Centre, 88 Davigdor Road, Hove BN3 1RF Tel: 01273 738070/770555 Fax: 01273 220 0883 — MB ChB Manch. 1992.

TURNER, Katherine Jane Drumchapel Health Centre, 80-90 Kinfauns Drive, Glasgow G15 7TS Tel: 0141 211 6120 Fax: 0141 211 6128 — MB ChB Sheff. 1977.

TURNER, Kevin James Punchetts, West Riding, Tewin Wood, Welwyn AL6 0PD — BM BCh Oxf. 1993; FRCS Eng. 1997; DM Oxf. 2002. SpR (Urol.) West. Gen. Hosp. Edin. Specialty: Urol. Prev: SHO (Urol.) Churchill Hosp. Headington, Oxf.; Demonst. (Anat.) Univ. Camb.

TURNER, Linda Margaret Middle House, Solefields Road, Sevenoaks TN13 1PJ — MB ChB Manch. 1991; MRCP (UK) 1994; FRCR 1998. Cons. Radiologist, Bromley Hosps. NHS Trust, S. Lond. Specialty: Radiol.

TURNER, Lisa Maudsley Hospital, Denmark Hill, London SE5 8AZ Tel: 020 7703 6333 — MB ChB Bristol 1989; BSc Bristol 1986, MB ChB 1989; MRCPsych 1994. Regist. (Psychiat.) Maudsley Hosp. Lond. Specialty: Gen. Psychiat. Prev: SHO (Path.) Southmead Hosp. Bristol; Ho. Off. Southmead Hosp. Bristol; Ho. Off. Weston Gen. Hosp. Weston Super Mare.

TURNER, Lynda Anne North Tees Primary Care Trust, Univ. Hosp. of N. Tees, Hardwick, Stockton-on-Tees TS19 8PE — MB BS Newc. 1977; MFFP. 1993; MIPM. 1999. Lead Clinician (Family Plann. & Reproductive Healthcare) N. Tees PCT; Sen. Clinic Med. Off. (Family Plann.) Gateshead HA. Prev: Clinician (Familiy Plann.) N Tees & Hartlepool NHS Trust.

TURNER, Lynda Mary Beechvale, 11 Quarterlands Road, Drumbeg, Lisburn BT27 5TN — MB BCh BAO Dub. 1983; DRCOG 1987.

TURNER, Marc Leighton Royal Infirmary of Edinburgh , Edinburgh and SE Scotland Blood Transfusion Centre, 51 Little France Crescent, Edinburgh EH16 4SA Tel: 0131 242 7520 Fax: 0131 242 7514 Email: marc.turner@ed.ac.uk/ marc.turner@snbts.csa.scot.nhs.uk — MB ChB Manch. 1982; MRCP (UK) 1987; PhD Ed. 1996; MRCPath 1997; FRCP (Ed) 1999; FRCPath 2005. Sen. Lect. Univ. Edin.; Clin. Director, Edin. and SE Scotl. Blood Transfus. Centre; Assoc. Med. Director, Clin. / Non-Clinicial Servs., NHS Lothian; Hon. Cons. Haemat. Lothian Univ. Hosps. Trust; Hon. Cons. Haemat. Scott. Nat. Blood Transfus. Serv. Specialty: Haematology; Blood Transfus. Socs: Brit. Soc. For Haemat.; Brit. Blood Transfus. Soc.; Internat. Soc. for Experim. Haemat. Prev: Sen. Regist. (Transfus. Med.) Edin. & SE Scotl. Blood Transfus. Serv.; Clin. Research Fell. (Haemat.) Edin. Roy. Infirm.; Regist. (Haemat.) Edin. Roy. Infirm.

TURNER, Margaret Anne (retired) 17 Wyedale Crescent, Bakewell DE45 1BE — MB ChB Manch. 1953.

TURNER, Margaret Deborah Occupational Health Department, Centre for Occupational Health, 45 Bush Road, Antrim BT41 2RL Tel: 01849 424407 Fax: 01849 424402; 10 Windsor Heights, Old Glenarm Road, Larne BT40 1UL — MB BCh BAO Belf. 1985 (Qu. Univ. Belf.) DCH Dub. 1987; DRCOG 1988; MRCGP 1990. Clin. Med. Off. (Occupat. Health) N. Health & Social Servs. Bd.; Forens. Med. Off. P.A.N.I. Specialty: Occupat. Health. Socs: BMA; Assn. Police Surg.; Soc. Occupat. Med. Prev: Trainee GP Ballymena; SHO (Gen. Med.) Moyle Hosp. Larne; SHO (O & G) Route Hosp. Ballymoney.

TURNER, Mark Andrew Consultant Psychiatrist, Duchess Kent Psych Hospital, Horne Rd, Catterick Garrison DL9 4; 44 Milbourne Road, Bury BL9 6PX — MB ChB Liverp. 1989; MRCP (UK) 1992; MA 1993; MRCPsych 1995; MSC 1998; Mphil 1999. Gen. Adult Psychiat. Specialty: Gen. Psychiat.; Forens. Psychiat. Prev: Lect. Forens. Psychiat., Inst. Psychiat., Lond.; Sen. Reg. NeuroPsychiat. St. Thomas's Hosp., Lond.

TURNER, Mark Anthony Benjamin 53 Lowther Cr, Leyland, Preston PR26 6QA — MB ChB Manch. 1997.

TURNER, Mark Augustine Timothy 8 Chiffon Way, Salford, Manchester M3 6AB Tel: 0161 834 6135 — MB ChB Manch. 1991; DRCOG 1993; MRCP (UK) 1994. Research Fell. (Child Health) Univ. Manch.; Hon. Regist. Manch. Childr. Hosp.; Clin. Fell. Centr. Manch. NHS Trust. Specialty: Paediat.

TURNER, Mark Stephen Cardiology Department, South West Cardiothoracic Centre, Derriford Hospital, Plymouth PL6 8DH Tel: 01752 792661 Fax: 01752 792666; 5 Dalewood Rise, Laverstock, Salisbury SP1 1SE — MB ChB Bristol 1990; MB ChB (Hons.) Bristol 1990; MRCP (UK) 1996. Specialist Regist. (Cardiol.)'. Specialty: Cardiol.; Gen. Med. Prev: Regist. (Gen. Med. & Cardiol.) Derriford Hosp. Plymouth.

TURNER, Martin Robert Skyways Medical Centre, 2 Shelley Crescent, Hounslow TW5 9BJ Tel: 020 8569 5688 Fax: 020 8577 9952 — MB ChB Sheff. 1977. Specialty: Dermat. Prev: SHO (Psychiat.) Hillingdon Hosp. Middlx.; SHO (A & E) Ashford Hosp. Middlx.; SHO (Dermat. & Geriat.) Highlands Hosp. Lond.

TURNER, Martin St John Larkfield Centre,, Garngaber Avenue, Lenzie, Glasgow G66 3UG Tel: 0141 776 7100 Fax: 0141 776 7462 — MB BS Lond. 1984 (Roy. Free Hosp. Lond.) MA, BA (Hons.) Camb. 1981; MRCPsych 1989; MPhil Ed. 1990; T(Psych) 1994. Cons. Psychiat. Stobhill Hosp. Glas.; Hon. Clin. Sen. Lect. (Psychol. Med.) Univ. Glas. Specialty: Gen. Psychiat. Socs: Roy. Soc. Med.; Roy. Coll. Psychiat. Prev: Sen. Regist. (Psychiat.) W. Scotl. Train. Scheme Gtr. Glas. HB; Sen. Med. Research Fell. Roy. Edin. Hosp.; Regist. Roy. Edin. Hosp.

TURNER, Mary The Malt House, Cuddington, Aylesbury HP18 0AS — MB ChB Ed. 1960; DObst RCOG 1962.

TURNER, Matthew Edward Clay 78 Northwood Road, Whitstable CT5 2EZ — MB BS Lond. 1993 (St. Geo.) MRCP (UK) 1997. Specialty: Paediat.

TURNER, Matthew William Harding 5 Humberstone Road, Cambridge CB4 1JD — MB BChir Camb. 1992.

TURNER, Maurice John The Paddocks, 9 Boxwood Way, Warlingham CR6 9SB — MB Camb. 1955 (Camb. & Bristol) BChir 1954; DMRD Eng. 1959; FRCR 1962; FRCP Ed. 1979, M 1963. Specialty: Radiol. Prev: Cons. Radiol. The Lond. Clinic, Lond. Hosp. Whitechapel & Torbay Hosp. Torquay.

TURNER, Maxwell Herman (retired) 59 Middlefield Lane, Hagley, Stourbridge DY9 0PY Tel: 01562 882228 — MB ChB Liverp. 1947; MRCS Eng. LRCP Lond. 1947; MMSA Lond. 1956.

TURNER, Michael Arthur Scarborough Hospital, Scalby Road, Scarborough YO12 6QJ — MB ChB Ed. 1966; FFA RCS Eng. 1971; FFA RACS 1979. Cons. Anaesth. ScarBoro. Hosp. Specialty: Anaesth. Socs: Assn. Anaesths. & Obst. Anaesth. Assn. Prev: Cons. Anaesth. Dunedin Pub. Hosp. & Lect. (Anaesth.) Univ Otago Dunedin, NZ; Sen. Regist. Dundee Gen. Gp. Hosps.

TURNER, Michael John Dept. of Cellular Pathology, Wycombe Hospital, High Wycombe HP11 2TT Fax: 01494 425674 — MB BS

Lond. 1973 (Westm. & King's Coll.) BSc Lond. 1970; MRCPath 1980; FRCPath 1990. Cons. Histopath. Wycombe Gen. Hosp. High Wycombe Bucks. Specialty: Histopath. Socs: Assn. of Clin. Pathologists; Internat. Acad. of Path. Prev: Sen. Regist. (Histopath.) Westm. Med. Sch. Lond.; Sen. Regist. (Histopath.) St. Stephens Hosp. Lond.

TURNER, Michael Skinner Lawn Tennis Association, Queen's Club, Palliser Road, London W14 9EG Tel: 020 7381 7071 Fax: 020 7381 3001 Email: michael.turner@lta.org.uk; 30 Devonshire Street, London W1G 6PU Fax: 020 7228 7495 — MB BS Lond. 1970 (St Thos.) MRCS Eng. LRCP Lond. 1970; MD Washington 1972. Chief. Med. Adviser Jockey Club & Horse Racing Auth.; Memb. Ind. Sports Rev. Bd.; Chief Med. Adviser Lawn Tennis Assoc. Specialty: Sports Med.; Occupat. Health. Socs: Editorial Bd. Mem. of the Brit. Journal of Sports Med.; Treasurer of Brit. Assoc. of Sport and Exercise. Med.; Europ. Comm. Memb. Soc. for Tennis Med. & Sci. Prev: Dir. Med. Servs. Brit. Olympic Assn.; Chief Med. Adviser Brit Ski & Snow Bd. Fed and Memb. Med. Comm. FIS; Chief Med. Adviser Texaco.

TURNER, Mr Murdo Alexander (retired) The Oaks, Glasson, Carlisle CA7 5DT — MB ChB (Ed.) 1956; FRCS (Ed.) 1959; FRCS (Glas.) 1974. Prev: Cardiothoracic Surg. Greater Glas. Health Bd. 1966-1993, Glas..

TURNER, Naomi (retired) 59 Middlefield Lane, Hagley, Stourbridge DY9 0PY Tel: 01562 882228 — MRCS Eng. LRCP Lond. 1953 (Sheff.) DCH Eng. 1957. Prev: Clin. Asst. (Paediat.) Corbett Hosp. Stourbridge & Wordsley Hosp.

TURNER, Neil 19 Ryecroft Avenue, Whitton, Twickenham TW2 6HH — MB BS Lond. 1980; DRCOG 1983; MRCGP 1984. Specialty: Diabetes.

TURNER, Neville Brindley 18 Appleton Drive, Whitmore, Newcastle ST5 5BT Tel: 01782 680540 — MB ChB Ed. 1990 (Univ. Ed. Med. Soc.) DA Lond. 1994. Staff Anaesth. N. Staff. Hosp. Specialty: Anaesth.

TURNER, Nicholas Arden Medical Centre, Church Road, Tiptree, Colchester CO5 0HB Tel: 01621 816475 Fax: 01621 819902 — MB ChB Leic. 1984; MRCGP 1990.

TURNER, Nicholas Charles 13 Belbroughton Road, Oxford OX2 6UZ — BM BCh Oxf. 1997.

TURNER, Mr Nicholas Owen 9 The Davids, Bournville Copse, Birmingham B31 2EX Tel: 0121 477 9455 Fax: 0121 476 6003 Email: nickclaireturner@aol.com — MB ChB Birm. 1983; FRCS Eng. 1990. Cons. ENT Surg. Walsall Hosps. NHS Trust; Cons. ENT Surg. BUPA Hosp. Little Ashton; Mem ASFGB Med. Comm.; Hon Med Adviser to Englisth Sch.s swimming assoc. Specialty: Otolaryngol. Socs: BMA & Med. Defence Union; Midl. Inst. Otol.; B. A. O.H. N S. Prev: Regist. (ENT) Russells Hall Hosp. Dudley, Qu. Eliz. Hosp., Dudley Rd. Hosp. Birm., Walsgrave Hosp. & Coventry & Warwick Hosp.

TURNER, Nicola Simone The Hall Practice, Hampden Road, Chalfont St. Peter, Gerrards Cross SL9 9SA Tel: 01753 887311 Fax: 01753 890639 — BM Soton. 1992; BSc (Hons.) Psychol. Soton. 1991; DRCOG 1994; MRCGP 1996. Specialty: Gen. Pract.

TURNER, Norman Robert Balfour (retired) (Surgery), 304 Tollcross Road, Glasgow G31 4UR; 18 West Coats Road, Cambuslang, Glasgow G72 8AB — LRCP LRCS Ed. 1943; LRCP LRCS Ed. LRFPS Glas. 1943. Prev: Cas. & Exam. Surg. Colvilles Clyde Iron Works.

TURNER, Patricia Elizabeth May Staffordshire County Council, Occupational Health Unit, 15 Tipping St., Stafford ST16 2LN Tel: 01785 276280 Fax: 01785 224410; 51 Cocknage Road, Dresden, Stoke-on-Trent ST3 4AT Tel: 01782 312541 — MB BCh Wales 1965 (Cardiff) AFOM RCP Lond. 1991. Co. Occupat. Health Phys. Staffs. CC. Specialty: Occupat. Health. Socs: Fell. Roy. Soc. Med.; Soc. Occupat. Med. Prev: GP Stoke-on-Trent; Med. Off. Michelin Tyre Co. Stoke-on-Trent; Sen. Med. Off. Achimota Sch. Hosp. Ghana.

TURNER, Patricia Margaret The Corner Surgery, 180 Cambridge Road, Southport PR9 7LW Tel: 01704 505555 Fax: 01704 505818; 40 Coudray Road, Southport PR9 9PE — MB BS Lond. 1974. Specialty: Gen. Med. Prev: SHO (Cas. & Microbiol.) Roy. Lond. Hosp.

TURNER, Paul The Health Centre, Pond Road, Shoreham-by-Sea BN43 5US Tel: 01273 440550 Fax: 01273 462109; 291 Upper Shoreham Road, Shoreham-by-Sea BN43 5QA Tel: 01273 463755 — MB BS Lond. 1969 (St. Bart.) MRCS Eng. LRCP Lond. 1969; DObst RCOG 1971. Prev: Ho. Phys. & Ho. Surg. Bury Gen. Hosp.; Ho. Off. (O & G) Fairfield Gen Hosp.

TURNER, Paul — MB BS Lond. 1996 (St Geo.) BSc Lond. 1993; MRCPCH 1999; MSc (Med. Microbiol.) Lond. 2004. Specialist Regist. (Med. Microbiol.) Univ. Coll. Hosp. Lond. Specialty: Med. Microbiol. Prev: SHO (Microbiology) Roy Free Hosp. Lond.; Regist. (Paediat.) Roy. Children's Hosp. Melbourne Australia; SHO (Paediat.) Guy's Hosp. Lond.

TURNER, Paul Christopher Thomas 39 Repton Road, West Bridgford, Nottingham NG2 7EP — MB BS Lond. 1985.

TURNER, Paul Jeremy C.T. & Angio Department, Pinderfields Hospital, Aberford Road, Wakefield WF1 4 Tel: 01924 213708 — MB ChB Leeds 1985; MRCP (UK) 1989; FRCR 1994. Cons. International Radiol. Pinderfields Hosp., Mid Yorks Trust. Specialty: Radiol. Socs: Roy. Coll. Radiol.; Brit. Soc. of Interven.al Radiol.; CIRSE. Prev: Sen. Regist. (Radiol.) St. Jas. Univ. Hosp. Leeds, Leeds Gen. Infirm. & Bradford Roy. Infirm.

TURNER, Paul Robert Wilson The Karis Medical Centre, Waterworks Road, Edgbaston, Birmingham B16 9AL Tel: 0121 454 0661 Fax: 0121 454 9104 — MB ChB Birm. 1991; ChB Birm. 1991.

TURNER, Paul Stephen Haverhill Road, Stapleford, Cambridge CB2 5BX Tel: 01223 842429 — MB BS Lond. 1983 (St. Mary's) BSc (Med. Sci.) Lond. 1980, MB BS 1983. SHO (Trop. Dis.) Hosp. Trop. Dis. St. Pancras Lond. Prev: SHO (A & E) Dunfermline & W. Fife Hosp.; Ho. Off. (Orthop.) Dunfermline & W. Fife Hosp.; Ho. Off. Gen. Med. Hosp. St. Cross Rugby.

TURNER, Pauline 22 Springfield Crescent, Uddingston, Glasgow G71 7LN — MB ChB Glas. 1998.

TURNER, Peter 20 High Mill Road, Hamsterley Mill, Rowlands Gill NE39 1HE — MB BS Newc. 1970; BSc (Anat.) Newc. 1967, MB BS 1970; MRCP (U.K.) 1974; FRCP Lond. 1989. Locum Cons. (Palliative Care) St. Bede Unit Gateshead. Specialty: Gen. Med. Prev: Cons. Phys. Qu. Eliz. Hosp. Gateshead.

TURNER, Mr Peter John The Joint Clinic, Orchard House, Victoria Square, Droitwich WR9 8DN Tel: 01905 799116 Fax: 01905 798249 Email: info@joint-clinic.co.uk; Owl Hill Farm, Dunhampton, Stourport-on-Severn DY13 9SS Tel: 01905 621053 Fax: 01905 621458 Email: turnerpj@aol.com — MB ChB Cape Town 1965; FCS Orth (SA) (Cape Town) 1986. Cons. Specialist Knee Surg. Droitwich Spa Hosp.; Cons. Specialist Knee Surg. BUPA Hosp. S. Bank Worcs. Specialty: Trauma & Orthop. Surg.; Orhopaedic Surgery. Special Interest: Cruciate Ligament Reconstruction; High Tibial Osteotomics; Patella Femoral Realignment. Socs: Brit. Assn. of Surg. of the Knee; Internat. Soc. of Arthroscopy Knee Surg. & Orthopaedic Sports Med.; Europ. Soc. of Sports Traumatology Knee Surg. & Arthroscopy. Prev: Cons. Orthop. Surg. Groote Schuur Hosp. Cape Town; Cons. Orthop. Surg. Princess Alice Orthop. Hosp. Cape Town; Cons. Orthop. Surg. Wynberg Hosp. Cape Town, S. Afr.

TURNER, Peter Percival, OBE (retired) Kitwells Lodge, Green Street, Shenley, Radlett WD7 9BD Tel: 020 8953 7229 — MB BS Lond. 1945 (Lond. Hosp.) FRCP Lond. 1971, M 1953; MD Lond. 1950, MB BS 1945, DPH 1959; DIH Eng. 1959. Prev: Cons. Phys. Edgware Gen. Hosp.

TURNER, Mr Philip Gartside Ryley Mount, 432 Buxton Road, Stockport SK2 7JQ Tel: 0161 483 9333 Fax: 0161 419 9913 — MB ChB Manch. 1978; FRCS Eng. 1982; FRCS Ed. 1982. Cons. Orthop. Surg. Stockport HA. Specialty: Orthop. Prev: Sen. Regist. (Orthop.) Withington Hosp. Manch.

TURNER, Philip James Eardley and Partners, Biddulph Medical Centre, Well Street, Biddulph, Stoke-on-Trent ST8 6HD Tel: 01782 512822 Fax: 01782 510331 — BM BS Nottm. 1987 (Nottingham) BMedSci (Hon.) Nottm. 1985; Dip. GU Med. Soc. Apoth. Lond. 1990; Cert. Family Plann. JCC 1990; MRCGP 1991. GP Princip. The Med. Centre, Biddulph Stoke on Trent; GP Research fell. N. Staffs. GP Research Network. Specialty: Gen. Pract. Prev: Staff Grade (Genitourin. Med.) Countess of Chester NHS Trust; Regist. (Emerg.) Waikato Hosp., NZ; Trainee GP Doncaster VTS.

TURNER, Mr Philip John Stanwell Road Surgery, 95 Stanwell Road, Ashford TW15 3EA Tel: 01784 253565 Fax: 01784 244145; 28 Fordbridge Road, Ashford TW15 2SG Tel: 01784 244636 — MB ChB Sheff. 1977; FRCS Ed. 1981; DRCOG 1984.

TURNER, Rachel 3 Bridgelands, Copthorne, Crawley RH10 3QW — MB BS Lond. 1993 (St. Bartholomew's Hospital London) BSc

Lond. 1990; DRCOG 1995. GP. Specialty: Gen. Pract. Prev: SHO (Psychiat.) Seymour Clinic Swindon; SHO (Cas.) Roy. Sussex Co. Hospial Brighton.; SHO (Elderly Care) Poole Gen. Hosp.

TURNER, Richard Duke 68 Duchy Road, Harrogate HG1 2EZ Tel: 01423 506772 — MB ChB Ed. 1967; FFCM RCP (K) 1993, M 1985. Cons. Pub. Health Med. E. Riding HA.; Director of Pub. Health S. Leeds Primary Care Trust. Specialty: Pub. Health Med. Prev: SCM (Informat. & Research) Yorks. RHA; Manager Health Policy Anal. Unit Yorks RHA.

TURNER, Richard George North Hampshire Hospital, Allergy Department , Ground Floor, Aldermaston Road, Basingstoke RG24 7NA Tel: 01256 314972 Fax: 01256 314796 Email: richard.g.turner@btopenworld.com — (Char. Cross Hosp., Univ. of Lond.) MB BS Lond. 1970; MRCS Eng. LRCP Lond. 1970; MRCP (U.K.) 1974. Hon. Clin. Teach. Univ. Soton. Specialty: Allergy. Socs: Brit. Soc. of Allergy & Clin. Immunol.; Brit. Soc. Allergy & Environm. Med.; BMA. Prev: Fell. Internal Med. Ochsner Med. Foundat. New Orleans, USA; Ho. Phys. Nat. Hosp. Nerv. Dis. Lond.; Regist. (Med.) Lambeth & St. Thos. Hosp. Lond.

TURNER, Richard John Duncan Macmillan House, Nottingham Healthcare (NHS) Trust, Dorchester Road, Nottingham NG3 6AA Tel: 01159 249924; Punch Bowl House, 111 Main St, Woodborough, Nottingham NG14 6DA Tel: 0115 965 2539 — MB ChB St. And. 1969; DPM Eng. 1972; FRCPsych 1990, M 1974; MD Dundee 1977. Cons. Psychiat. Nottm. Healthcare Trust, Univ. Hosp.; Med. Dir. Nottm. Healthcare Trust; Clin. Teach. Univ. Nottm. Med. Sch. Specialty: Gen. Psychiat. Prev: Assoc. Postgrad. Dean Nottm. Med. Sch.; Lect. (Ment. Health) Bristol Univ.

TURNER, Richard John Churchill Hospital, Department of Dermatology, Old Road, Oxford OX3 7LS Tel: 01865 228258 Fax: 01865 228260 Email: richard.turner@orh.nhs.uk — MB BCh Wales 1989; MRCP (UK) 1992; FRCP UK 2003. Cons. (Dermatol.) Surg.; Hon. Sen. Clin. Lect. (Oxf.); Clin. Tutor (Trinity Coll.). Specialty: Dermat. Special Interest: Skin Cancer; Surg. Socs: Exec. Comm. Brit. Soc. of Dermat.; Brit. Assn. of Dermat.; Brit. Soc. Dermatologic Surg. Prev: Lect. (Dermat.) Univ. Wales Coll. Med. Cardiff.; Regist. (Gen. Med. & Endocrinol.) Caerphilly Miners Hosp. M. Glam.; Sen. Reg (Dermatol.) RVI.

TURNER, Richard John Newbold (retired) 125 Finchfield Lane, Wolverhampton WV3 8EY Tel: 01902 763108 — (St. Thos.) MB BChir Camb. 1963; MA Camb. 1964; FFA RCS Eng. 1967. Cons. Anaesth. The Roy. Wolverhampton NHS Trust. Prev: Sen. Regist. (Anaesth.) United Birm. Hosps.

TURNER, Robert John The Topsham Surgery, The White House, Holman Way, Exeter EX3 0EN Tel: 01392 874646 Fax: 01392 875261; Walnut Cottage, Oil Mill Lane, Clyst St Mary, Exeter EX5 1AH Tel: 01392 877262 — MB BS Newc. 1978; DA Eng. 1981; MRCGP 1983.

TURNER, Rodney Martin (retired) Flat 2, 59 Mount Ararat Road, Richmond TW10 6PL Tel: 0818 332 2167 — MB BS Durh. 1951 (Newc.) FRCGP 1980, M 1960. Prev: Sen. Lect. (Gen. Pract.) United Dent. & Med. Sch. Lond.

TURNER, Ronald William (retired) 2 Connaught Close, Connaught Gardens, Clacton-on-Sea CO15 6HL Tel: 01255 422282 — MB ChB Leeds 1957; DObst. RCOG 1962; DLO Eng. 1963; MRCGP 1968. Prev: Ho. Surg. (ENT) Leeds Gen. Infirm.

TURNER, Rosalie Jane 29 Rectory Road, Frampton, Cotterell, Bristol BS36 2BN — MB ChB Sheff. 1986; MRCGP 1993.

TURNER, Rosemary Christine 5 Osmund Close, Worth, Crawley RH10 7RG Tel: 01293 884250 — MB BS Lond. 1983; MRCP (UK) 1986; FRCP (UK) 1999. Cons. Palliat. Care Brighton. Specialty: Palliat. Med. Prev: Sen. Regist. Roy. Marsden Hosp. Sutton; Regist. (Gen. Med. & Med. Oncol.) Guy's Hosp. Lond.

TURNER, Roy Sydney Leonard 16 Vicarage Road, Kidlington OX5 2EL — (Oxf.) LMSSA Lond. 1956; MA, BM BCh Oxf. 1957. Socs: Oxf. Med. Soc. Prev: Ho. Phys. Osler Hosp. Oxf.; Ho. Phys. & Paediat. Ho. Off. Roy. Berks. Hosp.

TURNER, Rupert Jonathan Clay 78 Northwood Road, Whitstable CT5 2EZ — MB ChB Birm. 1993; MRCP 1997; DCH 1997. Specialty: Paediat.

TURNER, Ruth Vivien Trenchard Avenue, Thornaby, Stockton-on-Tees TS17 0EE Tel: 01642 762921 — MB BChir Camb. 1985 (Cambridge) DRCOG 1990.

TURNER, Sandra Lynne Christie Hospital NHS Trust, Wilmslow Road, Withington, Manchester M20 4BX Tel: 0161 446 3000; 8 Windermere Close, Choleywood, Rickmansworth WD3 5LF — MB BS Sydney 1987.

TURNER, Sarah Louise 20 Sefton Avenue, Heaton, Newcastle upon Tyne NE6 5QR — MB BS Newc. 1992.

TURNER, Scott David Theatre Royal Surgery, 27 Theatre Street, Dereham NR19 2EN Tel: 01362 852800 Fax: 01362 852819 — MB ChB Ed. 1988; Dip. IMC RCS Ed. 1990. Specialty: Gen. Pract.

TURNER, Sheelagh Maria Cruddas Park Surgery, 178 Westmorland Road, Cruddas Park, Newcastle upon Tyne NE4 7JT — MB BS Newcastle 1974; MB BS Newc. 1974. GP Newc.

TURNER, Simon 88 Rockingham Road, Kettering NN16 9AD — MB ChB Dundee 1997.

TURNER, Simon John Shipley Peartree Lane Surgery, 110 Peartree Lane, Welwyn Garden City AL7 3XW Tel: 01707 329292; 62 Peartree Lane, Welwyn Garden City AL7 3UH Tel: 01707 329292 — MB BS Lond. 1980 (Middlx.)

TURNER, Simon Julian 4 Twyford Close, Manchester M20 2YR — MB ChB Manch. 1993.

TURNER, Stacy Lee Llanberis, Caernarfon LL55 4EL — MB ChB (Hons.) Liverp. 1997; BSc (Hons. Cell Biol.) Liverp. 1994.

TURNER, Stephen Denys The Health Centre, Thame OX9 Tel: 0184 421 2553 — MB Camb. 1959 (Camb. & St. Thos.) BChir 1958; DObst RCOG 1961; FRCGP 1987.

TURNER, Stephen Lindsay 45 Blythswood Crescent, Largs KA30 8HX — MB ChB Glas. 1995.

TURNER, Mr Stephen Michael Department Orthopaedics, Coventry & Warwickshire Hospital, Stoney Stanton Road, Coventry CV1 4FH Tel: 024 76 224055; Earlsdon Consulting Rooms, 15 Palmerston Road, Earlsdon, Coventry CV5 6FH Tel: 024 76 678472 Fax: 01203 678818 — MB ChB Liverp. 1978; ChM Liverp. 1993, MB ChB 1978; FRCS Ed. 1983. Cons. Orthop. Surg. Coventry HA. Specialty: Orthop. Socs: Fell. Brit. Orthop. Soc.; Brit. Soc. Surg. Hand. Prev: Sen. Regist. (Orthop. Surg.) NW RHA; Regist. (Orthop.) Guy's, Lewisham & Brighton Hosp.; Tutor (Orthop.) Univ. Manch.

TURNER, Stephen Richard Doctors Surgery, Newton Way, Baildon, Shipley BD17 5NH Tel: 01274 582506 Fax: 01274 532426; 9 Belmont Rise, Baildon, Shipley BD17 5AN Tel: 01274 587207 — MB ChB Ed. 1973; DObst RCOG 1975; DA Eng. 1978; Cert JCC Lond. 1979. Prev: Ho. Off. (Surg.) Roy. Hosp. Sick Childr. Edin.; Ho. Off. (Med.) Bangour Gen. Hosp. Broxburn; Trainee Gen. Pract. Livingston Vocational Train. Scheme.

TURNER, Stuart William 7 Devonshire Street, London W1W 5DY Tel: 020 7323 9890 Fax: 020 7323 9903 Email: s.turner@traumaclinic.org.uk — MB BChir Camb. 1977 (Univ. Camb. & Middlx.) MD Camb. 1987, MA 1977; MRCP (UK) 1981; FRCPsych 1994, M 1981; FRCP Lond. 1996. Cons. Psychiat.; Hon. Chair of Trustees, Refugee Ther. Centre; Hon. Sen. Lect. (Psychiat.) Roy. Free & Univ. Coll. Med. Sch. Lond.; Trustee, Redress. Specialty: Gen. Psychiat. Special Interest: Emotional Reactions to Adverse and Traum. Experiences. Socs: Fell. RSM; Treas., Internat. Soc. for Traum. Stress Studies. Prev: Campus Dean (Community) Roy. Free & Univ. Coll. Med. Sch.; Med. Dir. Camden & Islington Community Trust; Pres., Europ. Soc. for Traum. Stress Studies.

TURNER, Susan — MB ChB Manch. 1989 (University Manchester) MSc Pharmacol. Manch. 1982, BSc Pharmacy 1980; PhD Med. Biophysics Manch. 1984; MFOM 1997; Cert. Occupat. Med. 1997. Sen. Clin. Fell. In Occ. & Environmental Health, Univ. of Manch; Hon. Cons. In Occ. Med., Central Manch. & Manch. Children's Univ. Hosp. NHS Trust, Manch. Specialty: Occupat. Health. Socs: Roy. Pharmaceut. Soc.; Fac. Occupat. Med.; Soc. Occupat. Med. Prev: Cons. Occ. Med., Pennine Acute Hosp.s NHS Trust, Roy. Bolton Hosp., & Trafford Gen. Hosp. (Locum App.).

TURNER, Susan Eve Heather Grange, Hurst Road, Biddulph, Stoke-on-Trent ST8 7RU — MB ChB Leic. 1991; DFFP 1994; DRCOG 1994; MRCG P 1995. Specialty: Gen. Pract.; Family Plann. & Reproduc. Health.

TURNER, Susan Margaret 67 Greenville Drive, Low Moor, Bradford BD12 0PT — MB ChB Liverp. 1994; MRCP(UK) Edin. 1997. Specialty: Gastroenterol.; Gen. Med.

TURNER, Suzanne Dale Pitt Farm, Ancient Lane, Hatfield Woodhouse, Doncaster DN7 6PJ — MB ChB Sheff. 1986; MRCGP 1990.

TURNER, Thomas Blake Mountsandel Surgery, 4 Mountsandel Road, Coleraine BT52 1JB Tel: 028 7034 2650 Fax: 028 7032 1000; 7 Forrest Park, Coleraine BT52 1JJ — MB BCh BAO Belf. 1972; DCH RCPSI 1975; DObst RCOG 1975; FRCGP 1994, M 1976. Specialty: Paediat. Socs: BMA. Prev: SHO (Gen. Med. & Psychiat.) Craigavon Area Hosp.

TURNER, Thomas Liley Yorkhill NHS Trust, Glasgow G3 8WD Tel: 0141 201 0000; Highlands, Moor Rd, Strathbalne, Glasgow G63 9EY — MB ChB St. And. 1966; FRCPCH; MB ChB (Commend.) St. And. 1966; MRCP (U.K.) 1971; FRCP Ed. 1982; FRCP Glas. 1982. Cons. (Paediat.) Qu. Mother's Hosp. & Roy. Hosp. Sick Childr. Glas. Specialty: Paediat.

TURNER, Trevor Howard Department of Psychological Medicine, St. Bartholomews Hospital, West Smithfield, London EC1A 7BE Tel: 020 7601 7946 Fax: 020 7601 7097 — MB BS Lond. 1976 (St. Bartholomews) BA (Hons. Classics) Bristol; FRCPsych 1994, MRCPsych 1981; MD Lond. 1990. Cons. Psychiat. St. Bartholomews Hosp. & Homerton Hosp. Lond.; Clin. Director, E. Lond. and the City Ment. Health NHS Trust, Lond. Specialty: Gen. Psychiat. Prev: Lect. Inst. Psychiat. Lond.; Lect. & Hon. Sen. Regist. St. Bartholomews Hosp. Lond.; Regist. Maudsley Hosp. Lond.

TURNER, Wayne Mark 74 Leander Avenue, Choppington NE62 5BD Tel: 01670 812443 — MB ChB Leic. 1993.

TURNER, William (retired) 1 Premiere Park, Ilkley LS29 9RQ — (Leeds) MB ChB (2nd cl. Hons.) Leeds 1950; DPH Leeds (Distinc.) 1957; LLB Lond. 1958; FFCM 1972. Prev: Regional Med. Off. Yorks. RHA.

TURNER, William David Watson Mark Street Surgery, 2 Mark St., Rochdale OL12 9BE Tel: 01706 48255 Fax: 01706 526640; 5 Tyrone Drive, Rochdale OL11 4BE Tel: 01706 368424 — MB ChB Glas. 1966. Socs: BMA. Prev: Ho. Phys. & Ho. Surg. & SHO O & G Birch Hill Hosp. Rochdale.

TURNER, William Dundonald (retired) 25 Ashfield Road, Leicester LE2 1LB Tel: 0116 270 8336 — MB ChB Sheff. 1950; DA Eng. 1952; FFA RCS Eng. 1954. Anaesth. Leicester Hosp. Gps. Prev: Sen. Regist. (Anaesth.) United Sheff. Hosps.

TURNER, Mr William Henry Department of Urology, Princess Royal Hospital, Saltshouse Road, Hull HU8 9HE Tel: 01482 701151 Fax: 01482 676635 — BM BCh Oxf. 1983 (Camb. & Oxf.) MD Camb 1997, MA 1984; FRCS Eng. 1987; FRCS (Urol.) 1997. Sen. Regist. (Urol.) Princess Roy. Hosp. Hull. Specialty: Urol. Socs: Internat. Continence Soc.; Assoc. Mem. BAUS; Jun. Mem. Europ. Assn. Urol. Prev: Resid. Urol. Inselspital Bern, Switz.; Research Fell Univ. Dept. Pharmacol. Oxf.; Regist. (Urol.) Churchill Hosp. Oxf.

TURNER, William Joseph (retired) Peel House Medical Centre, Avenue Parade, Accrington BB5 6RD Tel: 01254 237231 Fax: 01254 389525; Aysgarth, The Syke, Grindleton, Clitheroe BB7 6SQ — MB ChB Liverp. 1966. Prev: SHO, Cas. Off., Ho. Surg. & Ho. Phys. Walton Hosp. Liverp.

TURNER, William Wilson 51 Cocknage Road, Dresden, Stoke-on-Trent ST3 4AT; Alma House, 89 Blurton Road, Blurton, Stoke-on-Trent ST3 2BS — MB BCh Wales 1962 (Cardiff) Clin. Asst. (Psychiat.) St. Edwd. Hosp. N. Staffs. HA. Socs: Fell. Roy. Soc. Med. Prev: Sen. Med. Off. i/c Achimota Sch. Hosp., Ghana.

TURNER, Winston Murray Leslie (retired) Bodnant, Keighley Road, Colne BB8 7HL Tel: 01282 865615 — MRCS Eng. LRCP Lond. 1938 (Univ. Coll. Hosp.) MD Lond. 1945, MB BS (Hnrs.) 1938; DLO Eng. 1942; FRCP Lond. 1971, M 1945; DCH Eng. 1949; FRCPCH 1997. Prev: Cons. Paediatr. Burnley Health Dist.

TURNER, Yvonne Jane School Cottage, School Lane, Washington, Pulborough RH20 4AP — MB BS Lond. 1990.

TURNER-PARRY, Alison Joanne 10 Windmill Rise, Poppleton Road, York YO26 4TX — MB ChB Leeds 1998. Specialty: Paediat.

TURNER-STOKES, Professor Lynne Frances Northwick Park Hospital, Regional Rehabilitation Unit, Watford Road, Harrow HA1 3UJ Tel: 020 8869 2800 Fax: 020 8869 2803 Email: lynne.turner-stokes@kcl.ac.uk; 55 Fitzroy Park, Highgate, London N6 6JA Tel: 020 8340 2464 Fax: 020 8340 2227 Email: lynne.turner-stokes@dial.pipex.com — MB BS Lond. 1979; MA (Phys. Sci.) Oxf. 1983, BA 1976; MRCP (UK) 1982; DM Oxf. 1989. Cons. Rehabil. Med. Regional Rehabil. Unit. Northwick Pk. Hosp. Lond.; Herbert Dunhill Chair Rehabil. King's Coll. Lond.; Hon. Prof. Assoc. Reader Brunel Univ.; Vis. Reader Imperial Coll. Lond. Specialty: Rehabil. Med. Socs: Brit. Soc. Rheum.; Soc. Research Rehabil.; (Exec. Counc.) Brit. Soc. Rehabil. Med. Chair: Research & Clin. Standards Subcommittee; Clin. Guidelines Coordinator. Prev: Sen. Regist. (Rheum. & Rehabil.) Northwick Pk. & Middlx. Hosp.; Research Regist. (Rheum.) Middlx. Hosp. Lond.; Regist. Rotat. (Gen. Med.) Univ. Coll. Hosp. Lond.

TURNER-WARWICK, Professor Dame Margaret Elizabeth Harvey, DBE Pynes House, Silver Street, Thorverton, Exeter EX5 5LT Tel: 01392 861173 Fax: 01392 860940 — BM BCh Oxf. 1950; MA, DM Oxf. 1956; PhD Lond. 1961; FRACP 1983; Hon. DSc New York 1985; FACP 1988; FRCP Ed. 1988; FRCPC 1989; FFOM RCP Lond. 1990; FFPHM RCP (UK) 1990; Hon. DSc Lond. 1990; FRCGP 1990; Hon. DSc Exeter 1990; FRCPS Glas. 1991; FRCA 1991; Hon. DSc Camb. 1993, Oxf. 1992, Sussex 1992, Hull 1991; FRCPath 1992; FRCPSI 1992; FRCS Eng. 1993; FRCR 1994; FRCPCH 1996; Hon. DSc Leics. 1998. Hon. Consg. Phys.; Emerit. Prof. Med. Lond. Univ.; Hon. Bencher Middle Temple; Fell. UCL 1991; Hon. Fell. LMH Oxf.; Hon. Fell. Girton Camb.; Hon. Fell. Imperial Coll. 1996; Hon. Fell. Green Coll. Oxf. Specialty: Respirat. Med. Socs: Assn. Phys.; (Ex-Pres.) Brit. Thoracic Soc.; Fell. (Ex-Pres.) RCP Lond. Prev: Pres. Roy. Coll. Phys. Lond.; Dean Cardiothoracic Inst.; Prof. Med. Cardiothoracic Inst.

TURNER-WARWICK, Mr Richard Trevor Pynes House, Thorverton, Exeter EX5 5LT Tel: 01392 860940 — BM BCh Oxf. 1949; MA Oxf., BSc 1946; FRCS Eng. 1954; FRCP Lond. 1980, M 1955; DM Oxf. 1957, MCh 1962; FACS 1970; Hon. FRACS 1981; Hon. DSc New York 1987; FRCOG 1990; Hon. FACS 1997. Emerit. Cons. Surg. Middlx. Hosp., Inst. Urol. & Univ. Coll. Med. Sch. Lond.; Robt. Luff Foundat. Fell. Reconstruc. Urol.; Sen. Lect. Inst. Urol.; Emerit. Cons. Surg. Middlx. Hosp.; Cons. Urol. St. Peter's Hosp.; Hon. Cons. Urol. Surg. Roy. P. Alfred Hosp. Sydney. Specialty: Gen. Surg. Socs: Fell. Urol. Soc. Austral.; Counc. RCS Eng. (Hunt. Prof. 1957 & 77); Assn. Surg. (Moynihan Prize 1958). Prev: Sen. Urol. Cons. K. Edwd. VII Hosp. Offs., Hosp. St. John & St. Eliz. & Roy. Nat. Orthop. Hosp. Lond.; Resid. Columbia Presbyt. Med. Center New York; Res. Surg. Off. St. Paul's Hosp.

TURNEY, John Harry Leeds General Infirmary, Great George St., Leeds LS1 3EX Tel: 0113 392 3757 Fax: 0113 392 6560; 35 The Avenue, Roundhay, Leeds LS8 1JG Tel: 0113 266 5882 — MB BChir Camb. 1975 (King's Coll. Hosp.) MA Camb. 1974; MRCP (UK) 1978; FRCP Lond. 1990; T(M) 1991. Cons. Phys. & Nephrol. Leeds Gen. Infirm.; Mem., Comm. of Safety of Devices. Specialty: Nephrol. Socs: (Pres.) Brit. Renal Symp.; (Exec. Comm.) Renal Assn. Prev: Sen. Regist. Qu. Eliz. Hosp. Birm.

TURNEY, Mr Joseph Pett (retired) Fairwater, Dinham, Ludlow SY8 1EH Tel: 01584 874800 — MB BS Lond. 1941 (Univ. Coll. Hosp.) MB BS (Hnrs. Distinc. in Surg.) Lond. 1941; MRCS Eng. LRCP Lond. 1941; FRCS Eng. 1948. Prev: Maj. RAMC.

TURNEY, Theresa Mary Brown and Partners, 35 Saughton Crescent, Edinburgh EH12 5SS Tel: 0131 337 2166 Fax: 0131 313 5059; 5 Corrennie Gardens, Edinburgh EH10 6DG — MB BS Newc. 1981; DRCOG 1985; DCCH RCP Ed. 1986; MRCGP 1986.

TURNILL, Adelaide 75 Ermine Street, Huntingdon PE29 3EZ Tel: 01480 453038 Fax: 01480 434104 — MB BCh BAO Belf. 1969. GP; Hosp. Practitioner (Old Age Psychiat.) Hinchingbrooke Hosp. Huntingdon. Specialty: Geriat. Psychiat. Prev: Clin. Asst. in Psychogeriat. Med. (Ment. Health for the Elderly) Hinchingbrooke Hosp. Huntingdon.

TURNOCK, Mr Richard Roulston Department Paediatric Surgery, Royal Liverpool Children's NHS Trust, Eaton Road, Liverpool L12 2AP Tel: 0151 252 5477 Fax: 0151 252 5677 Email: mick.turnock@rlch.nwest.nhs.uk — MB ChB Liverp. 1977; FRCS Ed. 1982; FRCS (Paediat.) 1992; FRCS Eng. 2000. Cons. Paediat. Surg. Roy. Liverp. Childr. Hosp.; Hon. Sec. and Treas., Brit. Assn. of Paediatric Surgeons. Specialty: Paediat. Surg. Special Interest: Ano-Rectal Infections. Prev: Medical Director RLC NHS Trust 2000-2003.

TURNPENNY, Peter Douglas Royal Devon & Exeter Hospital, Clinical Genetics Department, Gladstone Road, Exeter EX1 2ED Tel: 01392 405726 Fax: 01392 405739 Email: peter.turnpenny@rdehc-tr.swest.nhs.uk — MB ChB Ed. 1977; BSc Ed. 1974; DRCOG 1980; DCH RCP Lond. 1982; MRCP (UK) 1986; FRCPCH 1997, M 1996; FRCP 1998. Cons. Clin. Geneticist Roy. Devon & Exeter NHS Foundat. Trust; Hon. Sen. Clin. Lect. Peninsula Med. Sch. Exeter. Specialty: Genetics. Special Interest: Dysmorphic Syndromes; Med. Ethics. Socs: Brit. Soc. of Human Genetics; Europ. Soc. of Human

Genetics; Amer. Soc. of Human Genetics. Prev: Sen. Regist. (Clin. Genetics) Aberd.

TURPIN, Claude Dunbar Hillcroft, Buckingham Road, Brackley NN13 7EL Tel: 01280 704340 — (TC Dub.) BA Dub. 1943, MB BCh BAO 1947; LM Rotunda Hosp. 1947.

TURPIN, David Frank 39 Mons Street, Hull HU5 3SZ — MB BS Lond. 1989.

TURPIN, Jean Alexandra (retired) Lingmoor, 160 Queen Alexandra Road, Sunderland SR3 1XL Tel: 0191 522 7489 Email: docturpin@aol.com — MB BS Durh. 1952; DPH Newc. 1968; BA 1999. Prev: Sen. Med. Off. Health Dept. Sunderland Co. Boro.

TURPIN, Philip John Yardley Green Medical Centre, 75 Yardley Green Road, Bordesley Green, Birmingham B9 5PU Tel: 0121 773 3737; 1 Station Road, Hampton in Arden, Solihull B92 0BJ — BM BCh Oxf. 1983; BA Oxf. 1980; DCH RCP Lond. 1986; MRCGP 1988. Prev: SHO (Gen. Med.) Derby Roy. Infirm.; SHO (Paediat., Infec. Dis. & Geriat. Med.) E. Birm. Hosp.; SHO (O & G) Solihull Hosp.

TURRELL, Charlotte Mary Kent & Sussex Hospital, Mount Ephraim, Tunbridge Wells TN4 8AT; April Cottage, Westdown Lane, Burwash Common, Etchingham TN19 7JT Tel: 01435 883398 — MB BS Lond. 1998; MB BS Lond 1998. HO. (Surg.) Kent + Sussex Hosp.

TURTLE, Alan Manson Richhill Clinic, 6 Greenview, Maynooth Road, Richhill, Armagh BT61 9PD; 46 Maynooth Road, Richhill, Armagh BT61 9RG — MB BCh BAO Belf. 1976; DRCOG 1979.

TURTLE, Frances 164 Knockan Road, Rathkenny, Ballymena BT43 7LP; 12 Millburn Mews, Ballyclare BT39 9DP — MB ChB Ed. 1990; MRCP. Gen. Med. Locum Med Off. Antrim. Specialty: Gen. Med. Prev: Staff Grade (Cardiol.) Ballymena.; Research Fell. (Cardiol.) Roy. Gp. of Hosps. Belf.

TURTLE, James Audley Westgate Bay Avenue Surgery, 60 Westgate Bay Avenue, Westgate-on-Sea CT8 8SN Tel: 01843 831335 Fax: 01843 835279 — MB BS Lond. 1973 (Middlx.) DRCOG 1978.

TURTLE, Mark Jonathan Department of Anaesthetics, West Wales General Hospital, Carmarthen SA31 2AF Tel: 01267 235151 Fax: 01267 237181 Email: mark.turtle@carmarthen.nhs.wales.uk — MB BS Lond. 1975 (Guy's) MRCS Eng. LRCP Lond. 1975; FFA RCS 1981. Cons. Anaesth. W. Wales Gen. Hosp. Carmarthen. Specialty: Anaesth. Socs: Internat. Assn. Study of Pain; Intens. Care Soc.; BMA. Prev: Sen. Regist. Bristol & Weston HA; Regist. Salford HA.

TURTON, Catherine Louise Ash House, Main St., Barkston Ash, Tadcaster LS24 9PR — MB ChB Leeds 1994.

TURTON, Charles William Gilmour Bankside, Ditchling Common, Burgess Hill RH15 0SJ Tel: 01444 233307 — MB BS Lond. 1970 (King's Coll. Hosp.) MRCP (UK) 1973; MD Lond. 1980; FRCP 1988. Cons. Phys. (Respirat. Med.) Brighton & Sussex Univ Hosps. NHS Trust. Specialty: Gen. Med.; Respirat. Med. Prev: Sen. Regist. (Med.) Brompton Hosp. Lond.; Sen. Regist. Roy. Free Hosp. Lond.; Regist. (Med.) St. Geo. Hosp. Lond.

TURTON, Edmund Philip Leo Ash House, Main St., Barkston Ash, Tadcaster LS24 9PR — MB ChB Leeds 1992.

TURTON, Jane Llandough Hospital, Penlan Road, Penarth CF64 2XX Tel: 029 2071 6957 Fax: 029 2071 6957 — MB ChB Manch. 1987; DCH RCP Lond. 1992; DGM RCP Lond. 1993; MSc Cardiff 1994; MRCGP 1995. Clin. Asst. (Day Hosp. & Bone Reseach Unit) Llandough Hosp., Cardiff & Valo NHS Trust Penarth. Specialty: Care of the Elderly; Osteop. Prev: Regist. (Gen. Pract.) Cardiff; SHO (c/o Elderly) Llandough Hosp.; SHO (Paediat. & Obst.) Univ. Hosp. of Wales.

TURVEY, Andrew John — MB BS Lond. 1988 (St. Bartholomew's Hospital Medical College) BSc (Hons.) Lond. 1985, MB BS 1988; FRCA 1994. Cons.(Anaest.)Bromley Hosp. Kent. Specialty: Anaesth.; Intens. Care. Socs: Assn. Anaesth.; Obst. Anaesth. Assn.; ICS. Prev: Specialist Regist. (Anaesth.) St. Mary's Hosp. Lond.; Regist. (Anaesth.) Roy. Marsden Hosp. Lond.

TURVEY, Joanne Sarah 51 Waverley Avenue, Twickenham TW2 6DQ — MB BS Lond. 1998.

TURVILL, James Lawrence 15 Pickwick Road, London SE21 7JN — MB ChB Manch. 1988; BSc (Med Sci) St. And. 1985; MB ChB (Hons.) Manch. 1988; MRCP (UK) 1991. Research Fell. (Digestive Dis.) Research Centre Med. Coll. St. Bart. Hosp. Lond. Specialty: Gastroenterol.

TURVILL, Jonathan William, Surg. Cdr. RN Cockenzie & Port Seton Health Centre, Avenue Road, Cockenzie, Prestonpans EH32 0JL Tel: 01875 812998 Fax: 01875 814421 — MB BCh Wales 1977 (Welsh National School of Medicine) MRCGP 1983; DRCOG 1984. Occupat. Phys. BMI Healthcare. Specialty: Gen. Pract. Prev: Princip. Med. Off. HMS Rooke, Gibraltar; Princip. Med. Off. RN SQ Cochrane; Sen. Med. Off. UKSU AfS., Naples.

TURVILL, Phyllis 9 Denning Road, London NW3 1ST Tel: 020 7794 6114 — MB BS Lond. 1966 (St. Bart.) MRCS Eng. LRCP Lond. 1966; DMJ Soc. Apoth. Lond. 1978. Sen. Forens. Med. Examr. Metrop. Police; Med. Adviser Brit. Agencies for Adoption & Fostering. Socs: Assn. Police Surgs. Gt. Brit.; Med. Wom. Federat. Prev: Ho. Phys. & Ho. Surg. St. Margt.'s Hosp. Epping; Paediat. Ho. Phys. Whipps Cross Hosp. Lond.

TURVILL, Shelagh Bernadette 15 Pickwick Road, London SE21 7JN — MB BS Lond. 1992; MB BS (Hons.) Lond. 1992. Specialist Regist. (Anaesth.) N. Thames Rotat. Specialty: Anaesth. Socs: Freeman Worshipful Soc. Apoth. Lond. Prev: SHO (Anaesth.) St. Thomas Hosp. Lond.

TURVILLE, Sheila Anne Broadford Medical Practice, High Road, Broadford, Isle of Skye IV49 9AA Tel: 01599 534257 Fax: 01599 534107 — MB ChB Aberd. 1980; DRCOG 1986.

TURYA, Elitham B Trafford NHS Trust, Moorside Road, Davyhulme, Manchester M41 5SL Tel: 0161 746 2382 Fax: 0161 746 2381 Email: elitham.turya@trafford.nhs.uk — MB ChB Makerere 1975; MSc Lond. 1981; MRCP RCPI 1983; MBA Warwick 2001. Cons. (Child Health). Specialty: Community Child Health. Special Interest: Enuresis; Adoption. Socs: Royal College Paediatric & Child Health (FRCPCH); British Association Medical Managers; BACCH. Prev: SR Community Paediat. NWRHA Manch.

TUSON, Mr Julian Richard Donagh Department of Radiology, John Radcliffe Hospital, Oxford Tel: 01865 220825; 14 Coburg Wharf, Liverpool L3 4EB — MB BChir Camb. 1980; FRCS Eng. 1985; BA Camb. 1976, MA, MChir 1991; FRCR 1995. Sen. Regist. (Radiol.) John Radcliffe Hosp. Oxf. Specialty: Radiol. Prev: Clin. Supervisor Sch. Clin Med. & Hon. Sen. Clin. Research Fell. (Surg.) Univ. Camb.; Regist. Rotat. (Surg.) Addenbrooke's Hosp. Camb. & St. Geo. Hosp. Lond.

TUSON, Mr Kenneth William Rhodes Nuffield Hospital, Consultant Rooms, Kingswood Road, Tunbridge Wells TN2 4UL Tel: 01892 541346 Fax: 01892 515689 Email: k.tuson@nuffield-woc.freeserve.co.uk; Gyll cottage, Vale Road, South St., Mayfield TN20 6DB Tel: 01435 873216 — (Manch.) MB ChB Manch. 1966; FRCS Ed. 1971; FRCS Lon. 1998. Cons. (Orthop. Surg.) Maidstone & Tunbridge Wells NHS Trust; Cons. (Ortho. Surg.) The Horder Centre for Arthritis Crowborough E. Sussex. Specialty: Orthop.; Trauma & Orthop. Surg. Special Interest: Jt. Replacement Surg. Socs: Fell. BOA; World Orthop. Concern (Intern. Pres.); Hosp. Cons. & Special. Assn. Vice Pres. Prev: Sen. Regist. (Orthop.) King's Coll. Hosp. Lond.; Regist. Univ. Dept. Orthop. Manch. Roy. Infirm.; Asst. Resid. (Surg.) Vancouver Gen. Hosp., Canada.

TUT, Thomas Than 9 The Avenue, Mansfield NG18 4PN — MB BS Med. Inst. (I) Rangoon 1975.

TUTHILL, David Paul 21 Weardale Gardens, Enfield EN2 0BA — MB BCh Wales 1990.

TUTIN, Alan Frederick Merrow Park Surgery, Kingfisher Drive, Guildford GU4 7EP Tel: 01483 503331 Fax: 01483 303457; Woodstock, 6 Hillier Road, Guildford GU1 2JQ — MB BS Newc. 1974; BSc.

TUTIN, Angela Myfanwy Merrow Park Surgery, Kingfisher Drive, Guildford GU4 7EP Tel: 01483 503331 Fax: 01483 303457; Woodstock, 6 Hillier Road, Guildford GU1 2JQ — MB BS Newc. 1973; DObst RCOG 1975.

TUTT, Andrew Nicholas James Royal Marsden Hospital, Fulham Road, London SW3 6JJ Tel: 020 7352 8171 Email: andrewt@icr.ac.uk; 15 Allestree Road, London SW6 6AD — MB ChB Bristol 1990 (Bristol Univ.) MRCP (UK) 1993; FRCR 1997. Hon. Specialist Regist. (Clin. Oncol.) Roy. Marsden Hosp. Lond.; Clin. Research Fell. Inst. Cancer Research. Specialty: Oncol.; Radiother. Prev: SHO (Gen. Med.) Hosp. Centre Stoke-on-Trent.

TUTTE, Kevin Philip Somers Town Health Centre, Blackfriars Close, Southsea PO5 4NJ Tel: 023 9285 1199 Fax: 023 9281 4626 — MB ChB Birm. 1980; MRCGP 1985.

TUTTLE, Sheena Gilbert Road Medical Group, 39 Gilbert Road, Bucksburn, Aberdeen AB21 9AN Tel: 01224 712138 Fax: 01224 712239 — MB ChB Aberd. 1965; MB ChB Aberd. 1965; MD Aberd. 1971.

TUTTON, Elizabeth Vanda Mary Castleton Health Centre, 2 Elizabeth Street, Castleton, Rochdale OL11 3HY Tel: 01706 658905 Fax: 01706 343990; 5 Bowling Green Way, Bamford, Rochdale OL11 5QQ — MB ChB Manch. 1979; DRCOG 1981.

TUTTON, Geoffrey Robert Cronehills Health Centre, West Bromwich B70 Tel: 0121 553 6277 — MB ChB Birm. 1970; MRCGP 1978.

TUTTON, Mr Miles Kenneth 17 Blackfriars, Chester CH1 2NU Tel: 01244 342460 Fax: 01244 342460 — MB BS Lond. 1974 (Lond. Hosp.) BSc (Biochem., Hons.) Lond. 1970; MRCS Eng. LRCP Lond. 1974; FRCS Eng. 1978; DO Eng. 1981; FRCS Eng. (Ophth.) 1983. Cons. Ophth. Countess of Chester Hosp. NHS Trust. Specialty: Ophth. Socs: Fell. Roy. Coll. Ophth.; Fell. Roy. Soc. Med.; Counc. Mem. UKISCRS. Prev: Sen. Regist. (Ophth.) Manch. Roy. Eye Hosp.; Regist. (Ophth.) Soton. Eye Hosp.; Clin. Asst. Moorfields Eye Hosp. Lond.

TUTTY, Christopher Leake (retired) 8 Hall Park, Berkhamsted HP4 2NU Tel: 01442 862150 — MB BS Lond. 1950 (St. Thos.) DObst RCOG 1955. Prev: Ho. Surg. St. Thos. Hosp. Lond.

TUXFORD, Ann Félicité (retired) 34 Styal Road, Wilmslow SK9 4AG — MB ChB St. And. 1957; MD (Commend) Dundee 1969. Prev: Lect. (Bact. & Virol.) Univ. Manch.

TUXFORD, Keith (retired) 4 Royds Avenue, Accrington BB5 2LE Tel: 01254 236351 — (Manch.) MB ChB Manch. 1948; MRCS Eng. LRCP Lond. 1948. Prev: GP Accrington.

TWADDLE, Shona Passfoot Cottage, Balmaha, Glasgow G63 0JQ — MB ChB Glas. 1993. Specialist Regist. (Chem Path/ Clin Biochem.) Nothingham City Hosp. Specialty: Chem. Path.

TWAIJ, Mohammed Hussain Abdul Rassol Ali East Surrey Hospital, Redhill RH1 5RH; 5 Mayfield Road, Sutton SM2 5DU — MB ChB Baghdad 1976; DCH RCP Lond. 1983. Staff Paediat. E. Surrey Hosp. Redhill. Specialty: Paediat. Prev: Sen. Regist. (Paediat.) Stoke Mandeville Hosp.

TWAMLEY, Huw William James The Old Rectory, Wolvesnewton, Chepstow NP16 6NY — MB ChB Manch. 1996.

TWARDZICKI, Halina Maria Ludwika (retired) — MB ChB Birm. 1963. Locums (Occasional) only. Prev: GP Havering.

TWEDDEL, Ann Cowan University Hospital of Wales, Department of Cardiology, Heath Park, Cardiff CF14 4XW Tel: 029 2074 7747 Fax: 029 2074 4096 — MB ChB Glas. 1972; FESC,MBA (Open); MD Glas. 1993. Dir. Nuclear Cardiol. Univ. Hosp. Wales Cardiff. Specialty: Cardiol.

TWEDDELL, Alan Leonard Health Protection Agency, Shrub Hill Road, Worcester WR4 9RW Tel: 01905 760000 — MB BS Queensland 1971; MRCOG 1982; MFPHM RCP (UK) 1990; FFPHM RCP (UK) 1998. Cons. Health Protection Agency. Specialty: Pub. Health Med. Prev: Cons. Pub. Health Med. Worcs. HA; Sen. Regist. (Community Med.) W. Midl. RHA.

TWEDDELL, Gillian Anne 36 Riverside Gardens, Busby, Glasgow G76 8EP — MB ChB Glas. 1988; DRCOG 1992.

TWEDDELL, William Hillman 33 Rangeways, Kingswinford DY6 8PN — LRCPI & LM, LRSCI & LM 1958; LRCPI & LM, LRCSI & LM 1958. GP Kingswinford.

TWEDDLE, Deborah Anne Department of Child Health, Royal Victoria Infirmary, Queen Victoria Road, Newcastle upon Tyne NE1 4LP Tel: 0191 202 3033 Fax: 0191 202 3060 Email: d.a.tweddle@ncl.ac.uk; 25 Wolveleigh Terrace, Gosforth, Newcastle upon Tyne NE3 1UP Tel: 0191 213 2405 — MB ChB Manch. 1991; BSc (Hons.) Manch. 1988; MB ChB (Hons.) Manch. 1991; MRCP (UK) 1994; PhD Newc. Univ. 2002. Dept. of Health Clin. Scientist, Lect. & Hon. Specialist Regist. (Paediat. Oncology) Sch. Clin. Med. Sci. & N.Institute Cancer Research Newc.; Research Assoc. & Hon. Regist. (Paediat. Oncol.) Child Health Dept. & Cancer Research Unit Univ. Newc. u. Tyne. Specialty: Paediat. Special Interest: Neuroblastone; Translational Research. Socs: BMA; MDU; Roy. Coll. Paediat. & Child Health. Prev: Clin. Fell. (Paediat. Oncol.) Leukaemia Research Fund; SHO (Paediat.) John Radcliffe Hosp. Oxf.; Sen. Supervisory Resid. Duke Paediat. Hosp. Durh., N. Carolina, USA.

TWEED, Carolyn Susan 459 Whirlowdale Road, Sheffield S11 9NG — MB ChB Sheff. 1980; DRCOG 1983; MRCGP 1984; FRCR 1992. Specialty: Radiol.

TWEED, Charles Robert Carlton Hall, Carlton-on-Trent, Newark NG23 6NW Tel: 01636 821421 — MB BS Lond. 1991.

TWEEDALE, John Lindsay Great Shelford Health Centre, Ashen Green, Great Shelford, Cambridge CB2 5EY Tel: 01223 843661 Fax: 01223 844569; 4 Finch's Close, Stapleford, Cambridge CB2 5BL Tel: 01223 845651 — MB ChB Bristol 1980; MRCGP 1985; DRCOG 1985; DA (UK) 1987.

TWEEDDALE, Martin Department of Critical Care, Queen Alexandra Hospital, Cosham, Portsmouth PO6 3LY Tel: 023 9228 6558 Fax: 023 9228 6967 Email: martin.tweeddale@porthosp.nhs.uk — MB BS Lond. 1967 (Westm.) PhD Lond. 1965; FRCPC (Internal Med.) Montreal, Canada 1972; FRCP Lond. 2000; FRCA 2004. Clin. Director & Cons. (Critical Care) Qu. Alexandra Hosp. Portsmouth. Specialty: Intens. Care. Special Interest: Critical Care Med. Socs: Intens. Care Soc.; Soc. of Critical care Med. Prev: Director, Intens. Care Unit, Vancouver Gen. Hosp., Vancouver, Canada.

TWEEDIE, David Gilbert Castle Hill, Lower Fulbrook, Warwick CV35 8AS Tel: 01926 624686 — MB BS Lond. 1962 (Westm.) FFA RCS Eng. 1966. Cons. Anaesth. S. Warks. HA. Specialty: Anaesth. Socs: Fell. Roy. Soc. Med. Prev: Sen. Regist. (Anaesth.) Liverp. RHB; Regist. (Anaesth.) Broadgreen Hosp. Liverp.; SHO (Anaesth.) Westm. Hosp. Lond.

TWEEDIE, Dawn Mary Finlayson Street Practice, 33 Finlayson Street, Fraserburgh AB43 9JW Tel: 01346 518088 Fax: 01346 510015 — MB ChB Dundee 1986.

TWEEDIE, Ian Edward Department of Anaesthesia, University Hospital Aintree NHS Trust, Lower Lane, Liverpool L9 7AL Tel: 0151 529 5152 Fax: 0151 529 5155 — MB ChB Liverp. 1981 (Liverpool) FFA RCS Eng. 1987; DA (UK) 1987. Cons. Anaesth. Univ. Hosp. Aintree NHS Trust Liverp.; Cons. Neuroanaesthetics The Walton Centre. Specialty: Anaesth. Socs: Treas. of Liverp. Soc. of Anaestuetists; Chairm. of Assn. of Mersey ICU's. Prev: Vis. Asst. Prof. of Anesthesiol. Oregon Health Scs. Univ., USA.

TWEEDIE, Mr James Hamilton Buckingshire Hospitals NHS Trust, Mandeville Road, Aylesbury HP21 8AL Tel: 01296 316559 Fax: 01296 315296; Loosley House, Loosley Row, Princes Risborough HP27 0PF Tel: 01844 346819 — MB BS Lond. 1973 (St. Bart.) MS Lond. 1984, BSc (Hons.) 1970; FRCS Ed. 1978; FRCS Eng. 1979. Cons. Surg. (Gen. Surg.) Stoke Mandeville Hosp. Aylesbury. Specialty: Gen. Surg. Socs: Assn. Endoscopic Surgs.; Fell. Assn. of Coloproctol. GB & Irel.; Assn. Of Surg.s GB & Irel. Prev: Sen. Regist. (Gen. Surg.) Univ. Hosp. Nottm.; Research Fell. Univ. Missouri Colombia, USA; Sen. Regist. St. Mark's Hosp. for Dis. of Colon & Rectum Lond.

TWEEDIE, Roderick John The Deepings Practice, Godsey Lane, Market Deeping, Peterborough PE6 8DD Tel: 01778 579000 Fax: 01778 579009; 66 West End, Langtoft, Peterborough PE6 9LU Tel: 0140 24 345034 — MB ChB Glas. 1973; DObst RCOG 1975; MRCGP 1978. Prev: Chairm. Welland PCG; Chairm. P'boro. GP Forum; Course Organiser P'boro. VTS.

TWEEDIE-STODART, Nancy Marjorie 2 Balfour Place, St Andrews KY16 9RQ Tel: 01334 473223 — (Ed.) MB ChB Ed. 1950; DPM Eng. 1960. Affil. RCPsych. Prev: Cons. Child Psychiat. Preston Health Dist.; Cons. Psychiat. Roy. Cornhill Hosp. Aberd.; SHO Maudsley Hosp. Lond.

TWEEDLE, Mr David Ernest Frederick (retired) The Beeches Consulting Centre, Mill Lane, Cheadle SK8 2PY Tel: 0161 491 2908 Fax: 0161 428 1692 Email: deft@the-beeches.com; 5 Bramway, Bramhall, Stockport SK7 2AP Tel: 0161 440 0273 — MB ChB St. And. 1964; FRCS Ed. 1969; ChM Dund 1974; FRCS Eng. 1988. Prev: Cons. Surg. Univ. Hosp. S. Manch. & The Christie Hosp. Manch.

TWEEDLE, Isabella Simpson 10 Brookdale Road, Bramhall, Stockport SK7 2NW Tel: 0161 440 0588 — MB ChB St. And. 1965; DA Eng. 1968; DCP Sheff. 1993. SCMO (Child Health) N. Manch. Specialty: Community Child Health. Socs: Manch. Med. Soc.; BAACH. Prev: Clin. Med. Off. Manch. Hosp. & Community NHS Trust; Clin. Asst. (Anaesth.) Gateshead Health Dist.; SHO (Anaesth.) W. Cumbld. Hosp. Hensingham.

TWEEDLE, Mr James Richard 23 Victoria Place, Kings Park, Stirling FK8 2QT Email: james.tweedle@ntlworld.com — MB ChB Glas. 1989; FRSC (Urol.) 2000. Cons. (Urol.) Forth Valley.

TWEEDY, Mark Hans 52 Queens Gardens, Bayswater, London W2 3AA — MB BS Lond. 1978.

TWELVES, Nigel Ponteland Medical Group, Thornhill Road, Ponteland, Newcastle upon Tyne NE20 9PZ Tel: 01661 825513 Fax: 01661 860755 — MB BS Newc. 1988.

TWENA, Diane Michelle Baronsmere Road Surgery, 39 Baronsmere Road, East Finchley, London N2 9QD Tel: 020 8883 1458 Fax: 020 883 8854; 62 Kingsley Way, London N2 0EW — MB ChB Manch. 1988; BSc (Hons.) Manch. 1985; MRCGP 1993. SHO (Psychiat.) Chase Farm Hosp. Enfield NE Thames RHA.

TWENEY, Jessica Cornelia St Helier Bluebell Medical Centre, 356 Bluebell Road, Sheffield S5 6BS Tel: 0114 242 1406 Fax: 0114 261 8074 — MB ChB Bristol 1983; BSc (Hons.) Bristol 1980; DRCOG 1989. Gen. Pract. Clin. Asst. (Elderly Psychiat.) Sheff. Prev: Clin. Govern. Lead N. Sheff. PCT.

TWENTYMAN, Llewelyn Ralph (retired) Willoughby, Dale Road, Forest Row RH18 5BP Tel: 01342 822151 — MB BChir Camb. 1943 (Camb. & Univ. Coll. Hosp.) MRCS Eng. LRCP Lond. 1943; FFHom. 1959. Prev: Cons. Phys. Roy. Lond. Homoeop. Hosp.

TWENTYMAN, Orion Peter Department of Respiratory Medicine, Norfolk & Norwich University Hospital, Colney Lane, Norwich NR4 7UY Tel: 01603 289646 Fax: 01603 289640 Email: orion.twentyman@nnuh.nhs.uk — BM Soton. 1979 (Univ. Soton.) MRCP (UK) 1982; PhD Soton. 1994. Cons. Phys. Norf. & Norwich Hosp. Specialty: Respirat. Med.; Gen. Med. Socs: Brit. Thorac. Soc.; Medical Research Society. Prev: Sen. Regist. (Respirat. & Gen. Med.) Papworth & Addenbrooke's Hosps. Camb.; MRC Investigator Univ. Soton.; Regist. (Med.) Manch. Roy. Infirm.

TWIDDY, Peter Jonathan McIntosh, Gourlay and Partners, Stockbridge Health Centre, 1 India Place, Edinburgh EH3 6EH Tel: 0131 225 9191 Fax: 0131 226 6549; 46 Hillpark Avenue, Edinburgh EH4 7AH — MB ChB Ed. 1985; DCCH RCP Ed. 1991; MRCGP 1993. Specialty: Gen. Pract.

TWIDELL, Sara Mary Beckingham Bridgford House, Horninghold, Market Harborough LE16 8DH Tel: 01858 555204 — MB ChB Ed. 1993.

TWIGG, Annette Isobel The Surgery, 16 Watford Road, Crick, Northampton NN6 7TT Tel: 01788 822203 Fax: 01788 824177 — BM BS Nottm. 1984.

TWIGG, Caroline Evelyn — MB ChB Leeds 1987; DRCOG 1990; MRCGP 1991; DCCH RCP Ed. 1993. Socs: Nat. Assn. Non-Princip.s.

TWIGG, Lesley Judith Syston Health Centre, Melton Road, Syston, Leicester LE7 2EQ — MB ChB Leic. 1982; MRCGP 1988. Prev: SHO (Med.) Leicester Roy. Infirm.

TWIGG, Simon Frank Guilsborough Surgery, High Street, Guilsborough, Northampton NN6 8PU Tel: 01604 740210/740142 Fax: 01604 740869; Witherford, 5 Foxhill Road, West Haddon, Northampton NN6 7BQ Tel: 01788 87762 — BMedSci (Hons.) Nottm. 1982, BM BS 1984; DCH RCP Lond. 1986.

TWIGG, Steven James 2 Clifton Park Road, Clifton, Bristol BS8 3HL Email: steve.twigg@blueyonder.co.uk — MB BChir Camb. 1993; BA (Hons.) Camb. 1990; MRCP UK 1997; FRCA 2001. Cons. Gloucestershire Roy. Hosp. Specialty: Anaesth.; Intens. Care.

TWIGLEY, Alison Jane Lewsey Road, Luton LU4 0DZ Tel: 01227 766877 Fax: 01277 783191 — MB BS Lond. 1976 (St. Mary's) MRCS Eng. LRCP Lond. 1976; FFA RCS Eng. 1980. Cons. Anaesth. Luton & Dunstable Hosp. Specialty: Anaesth. Socs: Assn. Anaesth.; Assn. Of Obstetric Anaesth.; Brit. Orthopaedic anaesth. Assn. Prev: Sen. Regist. (Anaesth.) Hammersmith Roy. Postgrad. Hosp.; Regist. (Anaesth.) Char. Cross Hosp. Lond.; SHO (Anaesth.) Edgware Gen. Hosp. Lond.

TWINE, Martin Richard Bounds Green Group Practice, Gordon Road, Bounds Green, London N11 2PF Tel: 020 8889 1961; Home Farm Cottage, Ponsbourne Park, Newgate Street Villiage, Hertford SG13 8QT Tel: 01707 872377 Email: martintwine@csi.com — MB BS Lond. 1983 (Univ. Coll. Hosp.) BA (Physiol. Sc.) Oxf. 1980; DCH RCP Lond. 1986; DRCOG 1986; MRCGP 1987; DGM RCP Lond. 1987; MFHom 1994. GP Tutor UCL. Specialty: Homeop. Med. Prev: Trainee GP Northwick Pk. Hosp. VTS; Ho. Surg. Barnet Gen. Hosp.; Ho. Phys. Northampton Gen. Hosp.

TWINEM, Gillian Shirin 10 Colvil Street, Belfast BT4 1PS — MB BCh BAO Belf. 1989.

TWINER, David Anthony Neil Lansdowne Surgery, Waiblingen Way, Devizes SN10 2BU Tel: 01380 722939 Fax: 01380 723790; Olive House, High St, Rowde, Devizes SN10 2ND — (Westm.) MB BS Lond. 1964; DA Eng. 1971; DObst RCOG 1971. Clin. Asst. Deviles Community Hosp. Specialty: Gen. Pract. Socs: Clin. Soc. Bath & Med. Offs. Sch. Assn. Prev: Regist. (Anaesth.) Roy. Berks. Hosp. Reading; Ho. Surg. (Surg.) & Cas. Off. Westm. Hosp.; Anaesth. Devizes Hosps.

TWINHAM, Douglas John 2 The Paddock, Swanland, North Ferriby HU14 3QW Tel: 01482 633261 Fax: 01482 633258 — MB ChB Leeds 1965. Socs: Hull Med. Soc.

TWINING, Daniel Hugh (retired) Rivendell, Kingsale Road, Salcombe TQ8 8AS Tel: 01548 842757 — (Oxf. & Univ. Coll. Hosp.) BM BCh Oxf. 1940.

TWINING, Peter Department of Radiology, Queens Medical Centre, Nottingham NG7 2UH Tel: 0115 970 1064 Fax: 0115 970 1064 Email: peter.twining@nottingham.ac.uk — MB BS Lond. 1979 (Guys Hospital) MRCS Eng. LRCP Lond. 1979; FRCR 1985. Cons. Radiol. Specialty: Radiol.

TWISLETON-WYKEHAM-FIENNES, Mr Alberic George Consultant Surgeon, St George's Hospital, London SW17 0QT Tel: 0208 725 5584 Fax: 0208 725 3495 Email: fiennes@sghms.ac.uk; 19 Pendarves Road, London SW20 8TS Tel: 020 8946 0597 — MB BS Lond. 1976 (St. Bart.) BSc (Hons.) Lond. 1973, MS 1987, MB BS 1976; FRCS Eng. 1981. Cons. Surg., St. George's Hosp., Lond.; ATLS Instruc. RCS Eng. 1989; AO Foundat. Vis. Prof. & Martin Allgöwer Trauma Schol. 1990, Switz. Specialty: Gen. Surg. Prev: Lect. & Hon. Sen. Regist. (Surg.) St. Geo. Hosp. Med. Sch. Lond.; Wellcome Clin. Research Fell. St. Geo. Hosp. Lond.; Ho. Surg. St. Bart. Hosp. Lond.

TWIST, Andrew Mark 457 Liverpool Road, Ainsdale, Southport PR8 3BN — MB ChB Liverp. 1984. SHO (Infec. Dis.) Fazakerley Hosp. Liverp. Prev: SHO (A & E) Southport Gen. Infirm.

TWIST, Donald Chisnall 42 Briestfield Road, Thornhill, Dewsbury WF12 0PW Tel: 01924 452202 — MB ChB Leeds 1950. Prev: Ho. Phys. Ackton Hosp. Nr. Pontefract; Asst. Cas. Off. Pontefract. Gen. Infirm.; Capt. RAMC.

TWIST, John Stuart (retired) Rosskeen, Crich, Matlock Tel: 0177 385 2466 — MRCS Eng. LRCP Lond. 1942 (Leeds) MRCS Eng., LRCP Lond. 1942. Prev: Ho. Phys. St. Jas. Hosp. Leeds.

TWIST, Joyce Rosalie (retired) Maranatha, 22 Main Road, Littleton, Winchester SO22 6PS Tel: 01962 880475 Email: pat-twist@beeb.net — MB ChB Liverp. 1945; DCH Eng. 1947; DObst RCOG 1948; LMCC 1950. Prev: Clin. Med. Off. Winchester & Mid Hants. Family Plann. Serv.

TWIST, Mr Mark Henry Clinton Felpham and Middleton Health Centre, 109 Flansham Park, Felpham, Bognor Regis PO22 6DH Tel: 01243 582384 Fax: 01243 584933 — MB BS Lond. 1989 (St. Bartholomews) BSc Lond. 1986; FRCS Eng. 1993; DRCOG 1995; MRCGP 1996. Specialty: Gen. Pract.

TWIST, William Andrew 353 Gathurst Road, Orrell, Wigan WN5 8QE — MB ChB Birm. 1988; ChB Birm. 1988.

TWISTON DAVIES, Mr Ceri William The General Hospital, St Helier, Jersey JE1 3QS Tel: 01534 622483 Fax: 01534 621415; Le Hurel Farm, Ruette Pinel, Mont Cochon, St Lawrence, Jersey JE3 1HF Tel: 01534 864072 Fax: 01534 869122 Email: twiston@jerseymail.co.uk — MB BS Lond. 1976 (Middlx.) MRCS Eng. LRCP Lond. 1976; FRCS Ed. 1981. p/t Cons. Orthop. Surg. States of Jersey. Specialty: Orthop. Special Interest: ATLS Instruc. Socs: Fell. BOA; Liveryman Worshipful Soc. Apoth. Prev: Sen. Regist. Wessex Regional Orthop. Train. Scheme; Regist. (Gen. Surg. & Orthop.) Yeovil Dist. Hosp.; Cas. Off. (Surg.) & Demonst. (Anat.) Middlx. Hosp. Lond.

TWITCHEN, Michael John Unit of Medicine in Relation to Oral Disease, Floor 22, Guy's Tower, Guy's Hospital, London SE1 9RT Tel: 020 79555 2323; 27 Lime Grove, The Dell, Angmering, Littlehampton BN16 4HA — MB BS Lond. 1993; BDS Lond. 1986; LDS RCS Eng. 1986; LMSSA Lond. 1993; FFD RCSI 1996. Lect. (Med. in Relation to Oral Dis.) Guy's Hosp. Lond. Prev: SHO (Med.) Worthing Hosp. Sussex.

TWITE, Mark David 24 Elm Grove, Garboldsham, Diss IP22 2RY — MB BChir Camb. 1994; MRCP (Paediat.) 1997. Specialty: Paediat.

TWITE, Simon Jonathan 42 Bridgemere Drive, Framwellgate Moor, Durham DH1 5FG Tel: 0191 386 2429 — MB ChB Ed. 1996 (Edinburgh) BSc. (Hons.) Med. Sci. Ed. 1995. SHO Med. Rotat. Dryburn Hosp. Co. Durh. Specialty: Gen. Med. Prev: PRHO (Surgic.) CrossHo. Hosp. Kilmarnock Scotl.; PRHO (Med.) Borders Gen. Hosp. Melrose Scotl.

TWIVY, Samuel Barstow Willow Cottage, 16 Moor End, Eaton Bray, Dunstable LU6 2HN Tel: 01525 220543 — (Lond. Hosp.) MRCS Eng. LRCP Lond. 1951.

TWOHEY, Linda Caroline Department of Anaesthetics, Kettering General Hospital NHS Trust, Rothwell Road, Kettering NN16 8UZ Tel: 01536 492746 — MB BS Lond. 1982 (Univ. Camb. & Fac. Clin. Scis. Univ. Coll. Lond.) MA Camb. 1983; FFARCS Eng. 1988. Cons. Anaesth. Kettering Gen. Hosp. Specialty: Anaesth. Prev: Sen. Regist. Rotat. (Anaesth.) Northampton & Oxf.; Regist. (Anaesth.) Harefield Hosp. Middlx.; Regist. (Anaesth.) The Lond. Hosp.

TWOHIG, Michael McDermot Royal Sussex County Hospital, Eastern Road, Brighton BN2 5BE Tel: 01273 609060 Fax: 01273 609060 — MB BChir Camb. 1975 (Camb. & King's Coll. Hosp.) MA Camb. 1974; FFA RCS Eng. 1979. Cons. Anaesth. Brighton & Sussex Univ. Hosp. NHS Trust. Specialty: Anaesth. Socs: Hon. Sec. SE Soc. Of Anaesth. Prev: Sen. Regist. (Anaesth. & Intens. Care) Kings Coll. Hosp. Lond.

TWOMEY, Alan Francis John 59 Castleton Avenue, Wembley Park, Wembley HA9 7QE — MB BS Lond. 1996; BSc Lond. 1995.

TWOMEY, Catherine Ann Scartho Medical Centre, 26 Waltham Road, Grimsby DN33 2QA Tel: 01472 871747 Fax: 01472 276050; Fieldgate Lodge, Main Road, Ashby cum Fenby, Grimsby DN37 0QW Tel: 01472 828348 — MB BS Lond. 1986; BSc Lond. 1983, MB BS 1986; MRCGP 1990. GP. Specialty: Genitourinary Medicine. Socs: Roy. Coll. Gen. Pract.

TWOMEY, James Aiden Department of Neurophysiology, Pinderfields General Hospital, Aberford Road, Wakefield WF1 4DG — MD NUI 1986; MB BCh BAO 1973; MRCP (UK) 1977; FRCP Lond. 1994. Cons. Clin. Neurophysiol. Pinderfields Gen. Hosp. Wakefield. Specialty: Clin. Neurophysiol. Prev: Sen. Regist. (Clin. Neurophysiol.) Leeds Gen. Infirm. & St. Jas. Hosp. Leeds; Regist. (Neurol.) Derbysh. Roy. Infirm.; SHO Rotat. Withington Hosp. Manch. & Christie Hosp. Manch.

TWOMEY, Jerome Christopher Medical Centre, Okehampton EX20 1AY Tel: 01837 52233; Elmfield House, Hatherleigh, Okehampton EX20 3JY — MB BChir Camb. 1958 (St. Mary's) MA, MB Camb. 1958, BChir 1957; MRCOG 1967. Specialty: Obst. & Gyn. Prev: Surg. Cdr. RN; Sen. Specialist (O & G) RN Hosp. Malta.

TWOMEY, John (retired) 43 Hillview Road, Banchory, Aberdeen AB31 4EE — MB BCh BAO NUI 1948 (Univ. Coll. Cork) DTM & H Eng. 1955; DPH Lond. 1963; FMCM 1984, M 1972. Prev: SCM. Coventry Health Dist.

TWOMEY, John Lawrence 3 Ealing Village, London W5 2LY — MB BCh BAO NUI 1993.

TWOMEY, Mr John Matthew 4 Haines Hill, Taunton TA1 4HW — MB BS Lond. 1978 (Guy's) BSc Lond. 1975; MRCS Eng. LRCP Lond. 1978; MRCP (UK) 1982; FRCS Eng. 1985. Cons. Ophth. Taunton. Specialty: Ophth.

TWOMEY, John Michael The Mary Potter Health Centre, Gregory Boulevard, Hyson Green, Nottingham NG7 5HY — MB BCh BAO NUI 1955 (Cork)

TWOMEY, Michael James 57 The Common, Parbold, Wigan WN8 7EA — MB BCh BAO NUI 1983.

TWOMEY, Michael Patrick Keiran Keepers Cottage, Barrock Park, Southwaite, Carlisle CA4 0JS Tel: 01697 473461 — (Cork) MB BCh BAO NUI 1960; DPM Eng. 1966; MRCOG 1969; MRCPsych 1977. Cons. Psychiat. Sedgefield Community Hosp. Cons. Psychiat. Specialty: Geriat. Psychiat. Socs: (Hon. Sec.) Soc. Clin. Psychiat.; Roy. Soc. Med. Prev: Cons. Psychiat. Garlands Hosp. Carlisle; Cons. O & G Mullingar Co. Hosp. & Letterkenny Gen. Hosp.; Regist. Dumfries & Galloway Roy. Infirm.

TWOMEY, Patrick Joseph 7 Culverhay, Wotton-under-Edge GL12 7LS Tel: 01453 844830 — MB BCh BAO NUI 1980. Trainee GP Wotton-under-Edge.

TWOMEY, Paul Anthony Scartho Medical Centre, 26 Waltham Road, Grimsby DN33 2QA Tel: 01472 871747 Fax: 01472 276050; 239 Louth Road, Holton Le Clay, Grimsby DN36 5AE Tel: 01472 828348 — MB BS Lond. 1986; MA Camb. 1986; DGM RCP Lond. 1989; MRCGP 1990. Specialty: Care of the Elderly. Socs: BMA. Prev: Trainee GP Grimsby VTS.

TWOMEY, Peter James Golden — MB BS Lond. 1984; DCH RCP Lond. 1987; DRCOG 1988; MRCGP 1991. GP Devon. Specialty: Audiol. Med. Prev: SHO (Paediat.) Kingston Hosp.; SHO (O & G) Centr. Middlx. Hosp.; SHO (A & E) Lewisham & Guy's Hosp.

TWORT, Antony Edward Peter (retired) Bryn Tor, Deanery Road, Godalming GU7 2PQ Tel: 01483 415823 — MB BS Lond. 1948 (St. Thos.) DPH Lond. 1954; MRCP Lond. 1958; MFCM 1972. Prev: Dist. Community Phys. Winchester & Centr. Hants. Health Dist.

TWORT, Charles Hamish Crampton St Thomas Hospital, London SE1 7EH Tel: 020 7188 5185 Fax: 020 7188 5173 Email: charles.twort@kcl.ac.uk — MB BChir Camb. 1976; MRCP (UK) 1978; MA Camb. 1977, MD 1990; FRCP Lond. 1993; FRCP Ed. 1993. Sen. Lect. (Med.) GKT Sch. of Med. Lond.; Postgraduate Dean GKT School of Medicine & Director of PostGrad. Educat. Guy's & St. Thos. Hosps. Trust Lond. Socs: British Thoracic Society.

TWORT, Richard John 200 Ardgowan Road, London SE6 1XA Tel: 020 8698 9662 Fax: 020 8461 2457 Email: dickietwort@compuserve.com — MB BChir Camb. 1979; MA Camb. 1976, MB BChir 1979; MRCGP 1984. Clin. Med. Off. Nat. Blood Auth. Specialty: Blood Transfus. Prev: GP S. Lond.

TWYBLE, Thomas Stewart (retired) 94 Southchurch Boulevard, Southend-on-Sea SS2 4UZ Tel: 01702 465319 — LRCP LRCS Ed. LRFPS Glas. 1960. Prev: SHO Purdysburn Hosp. Belf.

TWYCROSS, Robert Geoffrey (retired) Sir Michael Sobell House, Churchill Hospital, Oxford OX3 7LJ Tel: 01865 225 891 Fax: 01865 741 867; Tewsfield, Netherwoods Road, Headington, Oxford OX3 8HF Tel: 01865 764197 Fax: 01865 742274 Email: robtwy@yahoo.com — (Univ. Oxf.) BM BCh Oxf. 1965; FRCP Lond. 1980, M 1969; DM Oxf. 1977; FRCR 1996. Emerit. Clin. Reader in Palliat. Med., Univ. Oxf; Director, World Health Organisation's Collaborative Centre for Palliat. Care; Accademic Dir., Oxf. Internat. Centre for Palliat. Care. Prev: Research Fell. St. Christopher's Hospice Lond.

TWYDELL, Helen Jane 34 Park Road, Southborough, Tunbridge Wells TN4 0NX Tel: 01892 542700 — MB BS Lond. 1998; MB BS Lond 1998. Specialty: Gen. Med.

TWYMAN, Derek Gould (retired) 9 Queenswood House, Crane Bridge Road, Salisbury SP2 7TW — MB Camb. 1956; BChir 1955; DObst RCOG 1962. Prev: Ho. Surg. & Ho. Phys. Memor. Hosp. Cirencester.

TWYMAN, Mr Roy Sean Epsom General Hospital, Epsom KT18 7EG Tel: 01372 735110 — MB BS Lond. 1982 (Westm.) FRCS Eng. 1986; FRCS (Orth.) 1992. Cons. Orthop. Surg. Epsom Gen. Hosp. Specialty: Orthop. Prev: Sen. Regist. (Orthop.) Middlx. Hosp. & Roy. Nat. Orthop. Hosp. Lond.; Regist. (Orthop.) Westm. Hosp. Lond.

TWYMAN, Victor Ronald (retired) Holme Leys, Burmington, Shipston-on-Stour CV36 5AR Tel: 01608 664215 — MB BS Lond. 1954 (Char. Cross) DObst RCOG 1960. Prev: Princip. GP Newark Notts.

TYAGI, Mr Arun Kumar Willow End, 4 Church Grove, Wexham, Slough SL3 6LF — MB BS Meerut India 1974; BSc Agra India 1967; FRCS (Eng.) 1980. Assoc. Specialist (Gen. Surg.) Wexham Pk. Hosp. Berks. Special Interest: Laparascopic Surg.

TYAGI, Mr Dinesh Chandra 14 Farm Grove, Rugby CV22 5NQ Tel: 01788 71911 — MB BS Lucknow 1962 (G.S.V.M. Med. Coll. Kanpur) BSc Agra 1957; FRCS Ed. 1979.

TYBULEWICZ, Aniela Teresa 31 Queen's Crescent, Newington, Edinburgh EH9 2BA Tel: 0131 667 7842 — MB BS Lond. 1990; MRCP (UK) 1994. Paediat. Specialist Regist. Roy. Hosp. for Sick Childr. Edin. Specialty: Paediat. Socs: Brit. Paediat. Assn.

TYBULEWICZ, Suzanna Maria Eat Calder Medical Practice, 197 Main St, East Calder, Livingston EH53 0EW Email: susanna.tybulewicz@wlt.scot.nhs.uk — MB BS Lond. 1989; DRCOG 1993. Specialty: Gen. Pract.

TYDEMAN, Graham Stephen John Barruchlaw Lodge, Brighouse, Bathgate EH48 3DW — MB BCh Wales 1985; BSc Cardiff 1983.

TYE, Jennifer Christine Dudley Gp. of Hosps. NHS Trust, Russell's Hall Hospital, Dudley DY1 2HQ Tel: 01384 244076 — MB BS Lond. 1991 (Kings Coll., Lond.) FRCA 1998. Cons. Anaesth., Russell Hall Hosp., Dudley. Specialty: Anaesth. Special Interest: Obstetric Anaesth. Socs: Obstetric Anaesth. Assn.; Difficult Airway Soc.

TYERMAN, Gillian Veronica Rotherham Road Medical Centre, 100 Rotherham Road, Barnsley S71 1UT Tel: 01226 282587 — MB ChB Sheff. 1977; MRCGP 1981.

TYERMAN, Kay Sarah North View, Edmundbyers, Consett DH8 9NJ — MB BChir Camb. 1992; MA Camb. 1993; MRCP (UK) 1995. Specialty: Paediat.

TYERMAN, Peter Frank Rotherham Road Medical Centre, 100 Rotherham Road, Barnsley S71 1UT Tel: 01226 282587 Fax: 01226 291900; Swaithe Villa, Low Swaithe, Worsbrough, Barnsley S70 3QF — MB ChB Sheff. 1977; MRCGP 1981.

TYERS, Mr Anthony Gordon Salisbury District Hospital, Salisbury SP2 8BJ Tel: 01722 336262 Fax: 01722 322871; Huckleberry, Bouverie Close, Salisbury SP2 8DY Fax: 01722 339538 — MB BS Lond. 1970 (Char. Cross) MRCS Eng. LRCP Lond. 1970; FRCS Eng. 1975; DO Eng. 1977; FRCS Ed. (Ophth.) 1980; FRCOphth 1989. Cons. Ophth. Surg. Salisbury Dist. Hosp. Specialty: Ophth. Socs: Fell. Roy. Soc. Med.; Comm. Mem. Europ. Soc. Ophth. Plastic & Reconstruc. Surg.; BMA. Prev: Sen. Regist. Middlx. Hosp. & Moorfields Eye Hosp. Lond.; Fell. Mass. Eye & Ear Infirm. Boston, USA; Resid. Surg. Off. Moorfields Eye Hosp. Lond.

TYERS, David John — MB ChB Leic. 1980; DRCOG 1987; MRCGP 1987.

TYERS, Rachael Natalie Sian 38 Caerphilly Road, Bassaleg, Newport NP10 8LF — MB BCh Wales 1995.

TYERS, Renee Constance Barbara New Hall Hospital, Salisbury SP5 4EY Tel: 01722 331021; Salisbury District Hospital, Salisbury SP2 8BJ Tel: 01722 336262 — Artsexamen Utrecht 1980; DO Eng. 1985; MRCOphth 1989. Clin. Asst. (Ophth.) Salisbury Dist. Hosp. Specialty: Ophth. Socs: Fell. Roy. Soc. Med.; BMA. Prev: Clin. Asst. Moorfields Eye Hosp. Lond.; SHO (Ophth.) St. Bart. Hosp. Lond.; Resid. (Ophth.) Acad. Med. Centre Amsterdam.

TYLDEN, Elizabeth 322 South Lambeth Road, London SW8 1UQ Tel: 020 7720 6622 Fax: 020 7498 7248; St. Julians, Sevenoaks TN15 0RX Tel: 01732 458261 Fax: 01732 454005 — MB BChir Camb. 1943 (Camb. & Lond. Sch. Med. Wom. and West Lond. Hosp.) BA (Nat. Sc. Trip.) Camb. 1939 MA 1943; MRCS Eng. LRCP Lond. 1943; MRCPsych 1971. Hon. Cons. Psychiat. Bromley Hosp.; Chairm. Lambeth Drugline; Pres. Stepping Stones Club. Specialty: Alcohol & Substance Misuse; Child & Adolesc. Psychiat.; Gen. Psychiat. Socs: Roy. Soc. Med.; Marcé Soc.; Founder Mem. Expert Witness Inst. Prev: Hon. Research Fell. Acad. Dept. Psychiat. UCH & Middlx. Hosp.; Mem. DHSS Working Party on The Treatm. of Drug Addic.; Mem. Comm. on Health of Hosp. Staff.

TYLDESLEY, David Barry Anaesthetic Department, Ysbyty Gwynedd, Bangor LL57; Castellor, 19 Overlea Avenue, Deganwy, Llandudno Tel: 01492 83646 — MB BCh Wales 1979. Clin. Asst. (Anaesth.) Gwynedd HA. Prev: Regist. (Anaesth.) Gwynedd HA; SHO (Anaesth.) Withington Hosp. Manch. & Gwynedd HA.

TYLDESLEY, Roy Cooke (retired) 9 Woodland Court, Knoll Hill, Bristol BS9 1NR Tel: 0117 968 2399 — MB ChB Ed. 1951; FRCGP 1980, M 1973. Prev: Phys. i/c BUPA Health Screening Bristol.

TYLDESLEY SMITH, Jeanette Thelma Ashbrooke (retired) Beaconsfield, Golf Road, Gourock PA19 1DQ Tel: 01475 633936 — MB ChB Glas. 1963; BSc (Hons.) Glas. 1960; DPM Ed. & Glas. 1968; FRANZCP 1985, M 1974. Prev: Cons. Psychiat. Argyll & Clyde HB.

TYLEE, André Trevor Stonecot Surgery, 115 Epsom Road, Sutton SM3 9EY Tel: 020 8644 5187; 18 Lower Hill Road, Epsom KT19 8LT Tel: 01372 812157 — MB BS Lond. 1978 (Guy's) FRCGP 1994, M 1984; MD Lond. 1994; MRCPsych 1996. Sen. Lect. (Sect. Epidemiol. & Primary Care) Inst. Psychiat. Lond.; Dir. RCGP Unit for Ment. Health Educat. Inst. Psychiat. Lond.; Hon. Sen. Lect. (Gen. Pract.) St. Geo. Hosp. Specialty: Gen. Pract. Socs: Roy. Soc. Med.; Assn. Univ. Depts. Gen. Pract.; Med. Scientif. Network. Prev: Ment. Health Foundat. Research Fell.; SHO Nuffield Ho. Guys Hosp.; Ho. Phys. Guy's Hosp.

TYLER, Arthur Kenneth Fossicks, Sheet, Petersfield Tel: 01730 62494 — BM BCh Oxf. 1942; BA (Hons.) 1939, BM BCh Oxon. 1942; DPhysMed Eng. 1947. Hon. Cons. Phys. (Rheum. & Rehabil.) Portsmouth & S.E. Hants. Health Dist. Specialty: Gen. Med. Socs: Fell. Roy. Soc. Med.; Med. Disabil. Soc. Prev: Med. Dir. Qu. Alexandra Cerebral Palsy Day Unit; Regist. Dept. Physical Med. Hosp. Sick Childr. Gt. Ormond St.; Asst. Med. Off. Dept. Physical Med. St. Thos. Hosp.

TYLER, Christopher Kenneth Graburn County Hospital, Greetwell Road, Lincoln LN2 5QY Tel: 01522 512512 — MB BS Lond. 1980; FFA RCS Eng. 1985. Dir. Intens. Care & Cons. Anaesth. Co. Hosp. Lincoln. Specialty: Intens. Care; Anaesth. Prev: Clin. Tutor Univ. Nottm.

TYLER, Clare Louise Wearne Cottage, Brookland Corner, Somerton Road, Langport TA10 9SN — MB BCh Wales 1992.

TYLER, Geoffrey James Nevells Road Surgery, Letchworth SG6 4TS Tel: 01462 683051; 111 Norton Road, Letchworth SG6 1AG Tel: 686339 — MB ChB Leeds 1966 (Lond.) DObst RCOG 1968. Socs: Primary Care Soc. in Rheum.; Local Med. Comm.; GP Writers Assn. Prev: Ho. Phys. St. James Univ. Hosp. Leeds; Ho. Surg. BromsGr. Gen. Hosp.; Ho. Off. (Obst.) Cuckfield Hosp.

TYLER, Jacqueline Ann 12 Manor Close, Blisland, Bodmin PL20 4JY — MB BS Lond. 1981 (St. George's Hospital Medical School) Private GP Cornw. Specialty: Sports Med.; Forens. Path. Prev: GP Harlow & Ware.

TYLER, Janet Barbara (retired) 31 Brooks Road, Wylde Green, Sutton Coldfield B72 1HP Tel: 0121 686 5869 — MB BS Lond. 1959 (King's Coll. Hosp. Lond.) MRCS Eng. LRCP Lond. 1959. Med. Adviser to Adoption Panel Nch Midl.s. Prev: SCMO (Child Health and Family Plann.) N. Birm. Community Trust.

TYLER, Jean Elizabeth Bristol Disablement Services Centre, Westbury-on-Trym, Bristol BS10 5NB; Mill Cottage, Kinver Grange, Ferney, Dursley GL11 5AB — MB ChB Bristol 1979 (Bristol Univ.) DA Lond. 1981; MSc Lond. 1986. Specialty: Rehabil. Med. Prev: Dist. HIV Preven. Coordinator Pub. Health Med. Glos. Health; Sen. Regist. (Community Med.) NW Thames RHA; SHO (Geriat.) Guy's Hosp. Lond.

TYLER, John Edward Warley Medical Centre, Ambrose House, Kingsway, Oldbury B68 0RT Tel: 0121 421 8400 Fax: 0121 421 8418; 154 Lightwoods Hill, Smethwick B67 5ED Email: john.tyler@btinternet.com — MB ChB Birm. 1975; BSc (Hons., Med. Biochem.) Birm. 1972; DRCOG 1978. Sen. Partner Warley Med. Centre; Med. Off. Lemförder UK, Darlaston & Birwelco Ltd.; PEC Vice Chairman Oldbury & Smethwick PCT. Specialty: Gen. Pract. Socs: BMA. Prev: Trainee GP Kidderminster VTS; GP Member Oldbury & Smethwick PCT; SHO Midl. Centre Neurosurg. & Neurol. Smethwick.

TYLER, Mark Andrew Hamlet House, 2B High St, Benwick, March PE15 0XA Tel: 01354 677373 — MB ChB Manch. 1993; DFFP. Specialty: Gen. Pract.

TYLER, Mark John Cheam Family Practice, The Knoll, Parkside, Cheam, Sutton SM3 8BS Tel: 020 8770 2014 Fax: 020 8770 1864 — MB BS Lond. 1987; DCH RCP Lond. 1991; MRCGP 1992. Specialty: Community Child Health. Prev: Trainee GP Henfield Health Centre; SHO (O & G) Southlands Hosp. Shoreham-by-Sea.

TYLER, Mr Michael Paul Howard Stoke Mandeville NHS Trust Hosp., Aylesbury HP21 8AL — MB ChB Aberd. 1988; FRCS Eng. 1992; ChM Aberd. 1998; FRCS (Plast.) 1999. Plastic Surg. Stoke Mandeville Hosp. Aylesbury. Specialty: Plastic Surg. Prev: Specialist Regist. (Plastic Surg.) Radcliffe Infirm. Oxf.

TYLER, Patricia Valerie St. Paul's Vicarage, Hawkstone Close, Newcastle ST5 1HT — MB ChB Manch. 1963. Specialty: Community Child Health.

TYLER, Philippa Anne Church Orchard, Church Lane, Kingston, Canterbury CT4 6HY — MB BS Lond. 1998; BSc 1995. HO. (Surg / Orthop.) Whillington Hosp. Lond. Prev: Ho. Off. (Med.) N. Middlx. Hosp. Lond.

TYLER, Robert John The Health Centre, Water St., Port Talbot SA12 6HR Tel: 01639 891376 — MB BCh Wales 1957.

TYLER, Roger Medhurst Woodnook Cottage, Woodnook Lane, Old Brampton, Chesterfield S42 7JF; Royal Hospital, Chesterfield S44 5BL Tel: 01246 277271 Fax: 01246 552620 — BM BCh Oxf. 1972; DCH Eng. 1975; MRCP (UK) 1976. Cons. Paediat. Roy. Hosp. Chesterfield. Specialty: Paediat. Prev: Sen. Regist. (Paediat.) Qu. Mary's Hosp. Childr. Carshalton & St.; Geo. Hosp. Lond.; Regist. (Paediat.) Notts. AHA (T).

TYLER, Shantha Stephnie Arumaiammal Brimington Medical Centre, Foljambe Road, Brimington, Chesterfield S43 1DD Tel: 01246 220166 Fax: 01246 208221; 12 Rose Avenue, Calow, Chesterfield S44 5TH — MB BS Lond. 1973 (King's Coll. Hosp.) DCH Eng. 1975; FP Certificate 1984. GP Princip.; Hon. Clin. Tutor Sheff. Med. Sch. Specialty: Gen. Pract. Prev: Clin. Asst. (Psychogeriat.) N. Derbysh. HA; Trainee GP Nottm. VTS; SHO (Paediat.) Sydenham Childr. Hosp.

TYLER, Vera Jean (retired) Herons Lake, St. Giles-in-the-Wood, Torrington EX38 7HZ — MFFP 1993; MIPM 1996; MB ChB Liverp. 1957. Sen. Clin. Med. Off. N. Devon. Healthcare Trust. Prev: Med. Off. Milk Marketing Bd. Dartington Crystal & Savage Industs. Torrington.

TYLER, Xenia Margaret Department of Histopathology and Cytopathology, Norfolk and Norwich Hospital, Brunswick Road, Norwich NR1 3SR Tel: 01603 289897 Fax: 01603 286017; St Mary's House, 10 Crome Road, Norwich NR3 4RQ Tel: 01603 622158 — MB ChB Leic. 1984; MRCPath 1991. Cons. Path. Norf. & Norwich Hosp. Specialty: Histopath. Socs: Assn. Clin. Pathol.; (Brit. Div.) Internat. Acad. Path. Prev: Cons. Path. Roy. Berks. Hosp. Reading; Sen. Regist. (Histopath.) Northampton Gen. Hosp. & John Radcliffe Hosp. Oxf.; Regist. (Histopath.) Leicester Roy. Infirm. & Gen. Hosp.

TYM, Elizabeth Leigh 17 Humberstone Road, Cambridge CB4 1JD Tel: 01223 562610 — MB ChB Sheff. 1955; MRCS Eng. LRCP Lond. 1955; DPM Eng. 1975; MRCPsych 1976; MA Camb. 1988. Cons. (Old Age Psychiat.) P'boro. Dist. Hosp.; Assoc. Lect. Camb. Univ; Cons. Psych. Rochford Hosps. Southend on Sea. Specialty: Geriat. Psychiat. Prev: Research Assoc. (Psychiat.) New Addenbrooke's Hosp. Camb.; Unit Med. Dir. N. Ryde Hosp. Sydney NSW, Austral.

TYMENS, Darren Craig The Surgery, 1 Kew Gardens Road, Richmond TW9 3HN Tel: 020 8940 1048 Fax: 020 8332 7644 — MB BChir Camb. 1993.

TYMMS, David James Royal Albert Edward Infirmary, Wigan Lane, Wigan WN1 2NN Tel: 01942 822341 — MB ChB Leeds 1975; MD Leeds 1986; FRCP Lond. 1994. Cons. Phys. Roy. Albert Edwd. Infirm. Wigan. Specialty: Gen. Med.; Diabetes; Endocrinol. Prev: Sen. Regist. (Gen. Med., Diabetes & Endocrinol.) Bath & Soton.; Lect. (Med.) Gen. Infirm. Leeds; William Hewitt Research Fell. (Med.) Gen. Infirm. Leeds.

TYNAN, Michael John 5 Ravensdon Street, London SE11 4AQ Email: michaeljtynan@aol.com — MD Lond. 1971; MB BS 1958; FRCP Lond. 1983, M 1978. Emerit. Prof. (Paediat. Cardiol.) Kings Coll. Lond. Prev: Joseph Levy Prof. Paediat. Cardiol. Guy's Hosp. Med. Sch. Lond.

TYNAN, Paul Francis King Street Surgery, 38 King Street, Lancaster LA1 1RE Tel: 01524 32294 Fax: 01524 848412 — MB BS Lond. 1984.

TYNE, Hilary Louise 25 Riversmead, Hoddesdon EN11 8DP — MB ChB Liverp. 1998.

TYRE, Nigel William Ferguson Mental Health Service for the Elderly, Hundens Lane, Darlington DL1 1 Tel: 01325 382639 — MB ChB Dundee 1976. Specialty: Geriat. Psychiat.

TYRELL, Martin Scott (retired) Burwood, Burlings Lane, Knockholt, Sevenoaks TN14 7PF — MRCS Eng. LRCP Lond. 1956 (Guy's) LDS RCS Eng. 1952; DObst RCOG 1958; MRCGP 1966.

TYRER, Malcolm Dennis and Partners, The Medical Centre, Folly Lane, Warrington WA5 0LU Tel: 01925 417247 Fax: 01925 444319 Email: malcolm.tyrer@gp-n81056.nhs.uk; 26 Littlecote Gardens, Appleton, Warrington WA4 5DL Tel: 01925 601780 — MB ChB Leeds 1985 (LEEDS) DRCOG 1990; DCCH RCGP 1991; MRCGP 1991; DFFP 1996. Princip., Gen. Pract., Folly La. MC, Warrington; UnderGrad. Tutor, Univ. of Liverp..; GP Trainer; Vocational Train. scheme organiser - Warrington. Specialty: Gen. Pract. Prev: Maj. RAMC.

TYRER, Professor Peter Julian Head of Department of Psychological Medicine, Faculty of Medicine, Imperial College, St Dunstan's Road, London W6 8RP Tel: 020 8846 7390 Fax: 020 8846 7372 — MB BChir Camb. 1966 (St. Thos.) MD Camb. 1975, BA 1966; MRCP Lond. 1968; DPM Eng. 1969; FRCPsych 1979, M 1973; FRCP Lond. 1993; MFPHM RCP (UK) 1993; FFPHM RCP (UK) 1998; FMedSci 1999. Prof. Community Psychiat. St. Mary's Hosp. Med. Sch. & Hon. Cons. Psychiat. NW Lond. Ment. Health NHS Trust. Specialty: Gen. Psychiat. Prev: Cons. Psychiat. Notts. AHA (T); Sen. Lect. (Psychiat.) Univ. Soton.; Clin. Research Fell. MRC.

TYRER, Professor Stephen Patrick Department of Psychiatry, Leazes Wing, Royal Victoria Infirmary, Newcastle upon Tyne NE1 4LP Tel: 0191 281 0886 Fax: 0191 222 6162 Email: s.p.,tyrer@ncl.ac.uk; 3 Brandling Park, Newcastle upon Tyne NE2 4QA Email: sptyrer@yahoo.com — MB BChir Camb. 1966 (Camb. & Middlx.) DPM Eng. 1969; FRCPsych 1987, M 1972; LMCC 1978; MA Camb. 1982. p/t Prof. of Psychiat.; Clin. Sen. Lect. Univ. Newc. Specialty: Ment. Health; Gen. Psychiat. Socs: Roy. Soc. Med.; Fell. Canad. Coll. Neuropsycopharmacol.; Internat. Assn. Study of Pain. Prev: Cons. Psychiat in Neurorehab Roy. Vict Infirm Necastle upon Tyne & Prudhoe Hosp., N.d; Vis. Prof. Dept. Psychiat. McMaster Univ. Hamilton, Ontario, Canada; Sen. Lect. (Psychiat.) Univ. Newc.

TYRIE, Christine Mary Eastlands Clinic, 19 Eastlands, Clifton Road, Newcastle upon Tyne NE4 6XH — MB BS Newc. 1978; DRCOG 1980; MRCPsych 1983; MA Leeds 1993. Specialty: Gen. Psychiat. Special Interest: Factitous Disorder; Stress,Womens Ment. health problems. Socs: BMA; MDU; Expert Witness Inst. Prev: Med. Director Newc. Nuffield Hosp.; Cons. Psychiat. Roy. Vict. Infirm. Newc.; Private Pract.: Lindisfarne Suite, Nuffield Hosp., Clayton Rd., Newc. upon Tyne.

TYRRELL, Betty Moyra (retired) Ash Lodge, Dean Lane, Whiteparish, Salisbury SP5 2RN Tel: 01794 884352 — MB ChB Sheff. 1949. Prev: Clin. Med. Off. Wilts. AHA.

TYRRELL, Christopher Guy 6 The Armoury, London Road, Shrewsbury SY2 6PA Tel: 01743 235606 — MB ChB Manch. 1980.

TYRRELL, Christopher John Department of Radiotherapy & Oncology, Derriford Hospital, Plymouth PL6 8DH Tel: 01752 763995 Fax: 01752 763992 — MB ChB (Hons.) Bristol 1970; MRCP (UK) 1972; FRCR (Ther.) 1975; FRCP Lond. 1991. Cons. Clin. Oncol. Plymouth & Cornw. HA's. Specialty: Oncol.; Radiother. Prev: Hon. Sen. Lect. Univ. Plymouth Postgrad. Med. Sch.; Lect. & Regist. (Radiother.) Roy. Marsden Hosp.; Ho. Phys. & Ho. Surg. Bristol Roy. Infirm.

TYRRELL, David Arthur John, CBE (retired) Ash Lodge, Dean Lane, Whiteparish, Salisbury SP5 2RN Tel: 01794 884352 Fax: 01794 884352 — (Sheff.) MB ChB (Hons.) Sheff. 1948; FRCP Lond. 1965, M 1949; MD (Distinc.) Sheff. 1953; FRCPath 1971, M 1964; FRS 1970; Hon. DSc Sheff. 1979; DM (Hon.) Soton. 1990. Prev: Dir. Common Cold Unit Salisbury.

TYRRELL, Graham Robert Shere Surgery and Dispensary, Gomshall Lane, Shere, Guildford GU5 9DR Tel: 01483 202066 Fax: 01483 202761; Orchard Leigh, Combe Lane, Shere, Guildford GU5 9JD Tel: 01483 203332 — MB BS Lond. 1974 (St George's Medical School London) DObst RCOG 1976.

TYRRELL, Jennifer Clare Children's Centre, Royal United Hospital, Bath BA1 3NG — MB BS Lond. 1977 (Westm.) MA Oxf. 1978; DCH Eng. 1980; MRCP (UK) 1981; DM Nottm. 1991; FRCP Lond. 1996. Cons. Paediat. Roy. United Hosp. Bath. Specialty: Paediat. Socs: Roy. Coll. Paediat. & Child Health. Prev: Sen. Regist. (Paediat.) John Radcliffe Hosp. Oxf.

TYRRELL, Judith Mary Highfield, 1 Chalgrove Road, Sutton SM2 5JT Tel: 020 8643 3844 — MB BCh BAO Dub. 1973; DCH NUI 1975; DObst RCOG 1975; MRCP (UK) 1980. Associate Specialist in Diabeties, St. Helier Hosp. Carshalton; Clinical Champion for Diabetes, Sutton, Merton PCT. Specialty: Diabetes. Prev: Assoc. Specialist in Diabetes, Chelsea, Westm. NHS Trust.

TYRRELL, Malcolm Franklin (retired) — MB BS Lond. 1961 (King's Coll. Lond. & St. Geo.) MRCS Eng. LRCP Lond. 1961; DA Eng. 1963; FRCA 1966. Prev: Cons. Anaesth. Westm. Hosp. Lond. & Qu. Mary's Univ. Hosp. Roehampton.

TYRRELL, Mr Mark Richard c/o Kent & Sussex Hospital, Mount Ephraim, Tunbridge Wells TN4 8AT — MB BChir 1984; FRCS Eng.; FRCS Ed.; DIC; PhD. Cons. Vasc. & Gen. Surg. Specialty: Surgery, Vascular.

TYRRELL, Nicolette Marie St Andrews Medical Centre, 30 Russell Street, Eccles, Manchester M30 0NU Tel: 0161 707 5500 Fax: 0161 787 9159 — MB ChB Manch. 1982; MRCGP 1986; DRCOG 1986. Single handed Gen. Practitioner. Prev: SHO (O & G) Hope Hosp. Salford.

TYRRELL, Philippa Jane Hope Hospital, Clinical Sciences Building, Salford M6 8HD Tel: 0161 206 5586 Fax: 0161 206 5586 Email:

pippa.tyrrell@srht.nhs.uk; 4 Fulshaw Avenue, Wilmslow SK9 5JA — MB BS Lond. 1981; MA Camb. 1982; MRCP (UK) 1985; MD Lond. 1992; FRCP 2000. Sen. Lect. (Stroke Med.) Univ. Manch. & Hon. Cons. Salford Roy. Hosps. NHS Trust. Specialty: Care of the Elderly. Special Interest: Acute Stroke; Inflammation in Stroke; Post Stroke Pain. Socs: Brit. Assn. Stroke Phys. Prev: Sen. Regist. (c/o Elderly) Char. Cross Hosp. Lond.; Research Regist. MRC Cyclotron Unit Hammersmith Hosp. Lond.; Regist. (Med.) St. Mary's Hosp. Lond.

TYRRELL, Prudencia Norah Mary — MB BCh BAO Dub. 1984; MRCPI 1987; FRCR 1991. Cons. Radiol. Robt. Jones & Agnes Hunt Orthop. & Dist. Hosp. NHS Trust Oswestry. Specialty: Radiol. Prev: Sen. Regist. (Radiol.) W. Midl.; Regist. (Radiol.) W. Midl.; Regist. (Med.) Meath Hosp. Dub.

TYRRELL, Richard Francis Eastney Health Centre, Highland Road, Southsea PO4 9HU Fax: 023 9273 4900 — MB BS Lond. 1979 (Charing Cross) MRCS Eng. LRCP Lond. 1978. Hon. Lect. (Gen. Pract.) Univ. Soton.

TYRRELL, Simon Nicholas 4 Redland Drive, Kirk Ella, Hull HU10 7UZ — MD Leeds 1993; MB ChB Manch. 1980; MRCOG 1985; T(OG) 1991. Cons. O & G Hull Matern. Hosp. Specialty: Obst. & Gyn. Socs: N. Eng. Obst. & Gyn. Soc.; Brit. Med. Ultrasound Soc. Prev: Lect. & Regist. (O & G) St. Jas. Hosp. Leeds; SHO (O & G) Wythenshawe Hosp. Manch.

TYRYNIS THOMAS, Sian Angharad Birchwood Surgery, North Walsham NR28 0BQ; Old Manor Farm House, The Hill, Swanton Abbott, Norwich NR10 5EA Tel: 01692 538224 — MB BS Lond. 1987.

TYSON, Anthony John The Surgery, Front Street, Pelton, Chester-le-Street DH2 1DE — MB BS Newc. 1977; MRCGP 1981.

TYSON, Claudine Margaret (retired) Otterford Mill, Otterford, Chard TA20 3QL — MB ChB Birm. 1957; DObst RCOG 1959.

TYSON, Victor Claud Henry (retired) Highfield, Hill Lane, Hathersage, Hope Valley S32 1AY Tel: 01433 650232 — (Sheff.) MB ChB Sheff. 1948. Prev: Adjudicating Med. Auth. DHSS Sheff. & Barnsley.

TYTHERLEIGH, Mr Matthew Grosvenor — MB BS Lond. 1992 (St. Bart. Hosp. Lond.) FRCS Eng. 1996. Specialist Regist. (Gen. Surg.) Oxf. Deanery. Specialty: Gen. Surg.

TYTLER, Jennifer Ann 5 Devisdale Court, Altrincham WA14 2AU — MB ChB Birm. 1977; DRCOG 1980; DCH 1980; FFA RCS Eng. 1983. Specialty: Anaesth.

TZABAR, Yoav Haim Cumberland Infirmary, Newtown Rd, Carlisle CA2 7HY Tel: 01228 523444 — MB ChB Dundee 1984; DA (UK) 1990; FRCA 1993. Cons.(Anaest.) Cumbld. Infirm. Carlisle. Specialty: Anaesth.; Intens. Care. Prev: Sen. Regist. (Anaesth.) Univ. Wales Coll. Med. Cardiff; Med. Off. Brit. Antartic Survey; Regist. (Anaesth.) Aberd. Roy. Hosp.

TZIFA, Constantina Doctor's Residence, Wordsley Hospital, Stream Road, Stourbridge DY8 5QX — Ptychio Iatrikes Thessalonika 1991.

TZOULIADIS, Vissarion (retired) 129A Hadham Road, Bishop's Stortford CM23 2QD Tel: 01279 656895 — Ptychio Iatrikes Athens 1953; DMRD Eng. 1960. Prev: Cons. Radiol. Herts. & Essex Gen. Hosp. Bishop's Stortford & Princess Alexandra Hosp. Harlow.

U-KING-IM, Jean Marie Kim Sin Flat E, Ashtree House, 3 Claremont Road, Newcastle upon Tyne NE2 4AN — MB BS Newc. 1998.

UBEROI, Raman The John Radcliffe, Radiology Department, Level 2, Headley Way, Headington, Oxford OX3 9DU Tel: 01865 220816 Fax: 01865 220801 Email: raman.uberoi@orh.nhs.uk — MB BChir Camb. 1985; BMSc (Path.) Dundee 1983; MRCP (UK) 1988; FRCR 1992. Cons. Interven. Radiol. Specialty: Radiol. Socs: BMA; Brit. Soc. Interven. Radiol. Prev: Cons. Vasc. Radiol. Qu. Eliz. Hosp. Gateshead; SHO (Med., Rheum. & Geriat.) Treliske Hosp. Truro; SHO (A & E) Roy. Vict. Infirm. Newc.

UBEROY, Vijayinder Kumar 30 Dorian Road, Hornchurch RM12 4AN — MB BS Poona 1971 (Armed Forces Med. Coll. Poona) DTCD Delhi 1972. SHO Ipswich Hosp. (Foxhall Wing).

UBHAYAKAR, Gaurang Narayan North Hampshire Hospital, Department of Radiology, Aldermaston Road, Basingstoke RG24 9NA Tel: 01256 313478 Email: gaurang.ubhayakar@nhht.nhs.uk — BM Soton. 1988; MRCP 1993; FRCR 1999. Cons. Radiol. N. Hants. NHS Trust. Specialty: Radiol. Special Interest: Interventional Radiol. Socs: Brit. Soc. Interventional Radiol.

UBHI, Baljinder Singh 95 Heworth Village, York YO31 1AN — MB ChB Leeds 1992; BSc (Hons.) 1987; MRCP 1997. Lect. (Paediat. Child Heath) St. Jas. Univ. Hosp. Leeds. Specialty: Paediat.

UBHI, Mr Charanjeit Singh Nottingham City Hospital, Hucknall Road, Nottingham NG5 1PB Tel: 0115 969 1169 Email: cubhi@ncht.trent.nhs.uk; 27 Melton Gardens, Edwalton, Nottingham NG12 4BJ Tel: 0115 923 4060 — MB ChB Manch. 1977; FRCS Ed. 1982; FRCS Eng. 1983; MD Manch. 1987. Cons. Nottm. City Hosp. Specialty: Gen. Surg. Socs: Brit. Assn. of Endocrine Surgs.; Assn. Surg.s of GB & NI. Prev: Cons. Gen. Surg. Univ. Hosp. Qu. Med. Centre Nottm.; Lect. St Jas. Univ. Hosp. Leeds; Lect., St.James' Univ. Hosp., Leeds.

UBHI, Satpaul Rectory Lodge, Church View, Patrington, Hull HU12 0SQ — MB ChB Sheff. 1990; DCH RCP Lond. 1992; DRCOG 1993.

UBHI, Mr Sukhbir Singh Leicester Royal Infirmary, Infirmary Square, Leicester LE1 5WW Tel: 0116 254 1414 Fax: 0116 258 6083 — MB ChB Leic. 1983 (Leicester) FRCS Ed. 1988; FRCS Eng. 1989; MD Leic. 1994. Cons. Gen. Surg., Leicester Roy. Infirm., Leicester; Cons. Gen. Surg. Leicester Roy. Infirm. Specialty: Gen. Surg. Prev: Research Fell. (Surg.) Univ. Leicester; Regist. (Surg.) Soton. & Salisbury.; Higher Surg. Trainee Leicester Hosps.

UBHI, Verjinderpal Singh 75 Westway, London SW20 9LT Tel: 020 8540 5553 — MB BS Lond. 1980 (St. Bart.) DCH RCP Lond. 1983; MRCGP 1984; DRCOG 1984. Prev: Trainee GP St. Bart./Hackney Hosps. VTS; Ho. Surg. St. Bart. Hosp. Lond.; Ho. Phys. P. of Wales Hosp. Lond.

UBOGAGU, Matthew North Middlesex Hospital, Edmnton-Sterling Way, London N18 1QX — State Exam Higher Med Inst Sofia 1977. Staff Grade (Obst. & Gyn.) N. Middlx. Hosp. Specialty: Obst. & Gyn. Special Interest: Minimal Access Surg.

***UBOGU, Emamoke Eromedoghene** — MB ChB Birm. 1998; DRCOG 2001. GP Sherwood Ho. Med. Pract., Edgbaston, Birm. Specialty: Gen. Pract. Socs: MDU; BMA. Prev: SHO A & E - Dudley (Rysells Hall Hosp.); SHO Pub. Health - Sand Well Gen.; SHO Obs & Gynae - Wolverhampton (new cross).

UDAL, Michael Stannard Gosbury Hill Health Centre, Orchard Gardens, Chessington KT9 1AG Tel: 020 8397 2142 Fax: 020 8974 2717; 85 Common Road, Claygate, Esher KT10 0HU Tel: 01372 62329 — BM BCh Oxf. 1968 (Oxford Univ/Kings Coll Lond) DObst RCOG 1970; DCH Eng. 1971; MRCGP 1982; FRCGP 1996. Prev: Ho. Off. (Med. Surg. & O & G) Kings Coll. Hosp. Lond.; Ho. Off. (Paediat.) FarnBoro. Hosp., Kent.

UDDIN, Farakh Javed 27 New Way Road, Leicester LE5 5UA Email: fjuddin@doctors.org.uk — MB ChB (Hons) Leeds 1998; BSc (Hons) Leeds 1995.

UDDIN, Mr Jimmy Mohamed 59 Rowfant Road, London SW17 7AP — BChir Camb. 1991 (Cambridge University) MA Camb. 1991, BChir 1991; FRCOphth 1995. Specialist Regist. E. Anglia, Norf. & Norwich Hosp. Specialty: Ophth. Socs: AAD (Amer. Acad. of Opthinology). Prev: SHO (Ophth. & Plastics) Gt. Ormond St. Hosp. Lond.

UDDIN, Kutub 21 Rampart Street, London E1 2LA — MB BS Lond. 1998.

UDDIN, Md Mashuk 73 Disraeli Road, London E7 9JU — MRCS Eng. LRCP Lond. 1993.

UDDIN, Shahana 37 Freemantle Road, Barkingside, Ilford IG6 2BD — MB BS Lond. 1996.

UDEJIOFO, Susan Frances 56 Louth Road, Sheffield S11 7AW; 484 Manchester Road, Sheffield S10 5PN — MB ChB Sheff. 1987; MRCGP 1991.

UDEN, John Anthony Bampton Surgery, Landells, Bampton, Oxford OX18 2LJ — MB BS Lond. 1985.

UDENZE, Christopher Chukwuekelua NDU Surgery, St Anns Health Centre, St Anns, Nottingham NG3 3PX Tel: 0115 950 5455 Fax: 0155 958 8493 — MB BS Lond. 1986.

UDESHI, Umesh Laxmidas Kidderminster Hospital, Bewdley Road, Kidderminster DY11 6RJ Tel: 01562 823424 Fax: 01562 513014 — MB BCh Wales 1979; FRCR 1986. Cons. Radiol. Worcs. Acute Hosps. NHS Trust. Specialty: Radiol. Socs: Brit. Inst. Radiol. & Brit. Med. Ultrasound Soc.; Magnetic Resonance Radiologists Assn. Prev: Sen. Regist. & Regist. (Radiol.) W. Midl. RHA; SHO (Med.) Bridgend Gen. Hosp.

UDEZUE, Emmanuel Olisaebuka Saudi Arabian Oil Company, Medical Services Organisation, Aramco Box. 7490, Udhailiyah, near DHAHRAN 31311, Saudi Arabia Tel: 00 966 3 577 8687 Fax: 00 966 3 577 8687 Email: manevans@hotmail.com/ manevans@yahoo.com; 3A Winston Avenue, Branksome, Poole BH12 1PA Tel: 01202 718460 — MB BS Ibadan 1973; (5 DISTINCTIONS IN FINAL MB, BS) IBADAN, NIGERIA 1973 (Univ. of Ibadan Med. Sch., Nigeria) DHMSA Soc. Apoth, Lond. 1978; MSc (Clin. Trop. Med.) Lond. 1982; FACTM 1982; MRCPI 1982, FRCPI 1998. Head of Internal Med., Aramco Al Hasa Med. Center, Saudi Arabia. Specialty: Gen. Med. Special Interest: COST-EFFECTIVE CARE IN DEVELOPING COUNTRIES, DIABETES, MALARIA, AND SICKLE CELL Dis.. ACUTE Med. CARE. PHYSICAL FITNESS AND WHOLESOME WELLNESS. Socs: Fell. Roy. Soc. Trop. Med. & Hyg.; Fell. Fac. Hist. Med. & Pharmacy Soc. Apoth.; Brit. Diabetic Assn. Prev: Cons. Phys. Aramco Med. Serv.s, S. Arabia; Cons. Phys. & Lect. (Pharmacol. & Therap.) Univ. Nigeria & Teachg. Hosp. Enugh, Nigeria; Regist. (Med.) Roy. Lond. Hosp., Luton & Dunstable & St. Mary's Hosps. Luton.

UDO, Ededet Akpan 112 Jubilee Avenue, Romford RM7 9LT — MB BS Lagos 1981; MRCOG 1990.

UDOEYOP, Mr Udoeyop Walter 24 Spring Shaw Road, Orpington BR5 2RH — MB BS Ibadan 1980; FRCS Ed. 1994.

UDOKANG, Mariel Jane Bournbrook Medical Practice, 480 Bristol Road, Selly Oak, Birmingham B29 6BD Tel: 0121 472 0129 — MB ChB Birm. 1974; MRCGP 1978; T(GP) 1991; MRCP (UK) 1993.

UDUKU, Ngozi Ola-Adetokunbo New Surgery, 2 Morley Road, London SE13 6DQ Tel: 020 8297 7999 Fax: 020 8297 7880 — MB ChB Leic. 1984; BSc (Hons.) Leic. 1982; DRCOG 1988; MRCGP 1994. Med. Examr. Metrop. Police; GP Tutor Kings Coll. Sch. Med. & Dent. Specialty: Pub. Health Med.

UDWADIA, Zarir 20 Cranford Lodge, Victoria Drive, London SW19 6HH — MB BS Bombay 1985; MRCP (UK) 1988.

UFF, Jeremy Stephen Department Clinical Pathology, Gloucester Royal Infirmary, Great Western Road, Gloucester GL1 3NN — MB BChir Camb. 1971; MA, MB Camb. 1971, BChir 1970; MRCP (UK) 1972; MRCPath 1976. Cons. Gloucestershire Roy. Hosp. Gloucester. Specialty: Histopath. Prev: Sen. Lect. St. Geo. Hosp. Med. Sch. Lond.; Sen. Regist. (Histopath.) Hammersmith Hosp. Lond.; SHO (Med.) Lond. Hosp.

UFODIAMA, Bertram Enechukwu 20 Meadowcroft Road, Outwood, Wakefield WF1 3TA Tel: 01924 871975 — MB BS Nigeria 1980; MRCP (UK) 1994. Staff Grade Paediat. Pinderfields Gen. Hosp. Wakefield. Specialty: Paediat. Socs: MRCPCH.

UGARGOL, Chandrashekar Prabhakar Prospect House Medical Centre, 84 Orrell Road, Orrell, Wigan WN5 8HA Tel: 01942 222321 Fax: 01942 620327 — MB BS Bombay 1966.

UGBOMA, Ike Anthony Francis 24 Monarch Court, Lyttelton Road, London N2 0RA — MB BS Lond. 1996.

UGBOMA, Koyi James 3 Mount Drive, Wembley Park, Wembley HA9 9ED — BM BCh Nigeria 1976; LMSSA Lond. 1984; MSc (Clin. Nuclear Med.) Lond. 1985. Specialty: Nuclear Med.

UGLOW, Mr Michael George Southampton University Hospital, Tremona Road, Southampton SO16 6YD Tel: 023 8079 4850; Gainsborough House, Winchester, Boorley Green, Southampton SO32 2DH Tel: 01489 788329 — MB BS Lond. 1989 (St. George's Hospital Medical School, London) FRCS Eng. 1993; FRCS (Tr & Orth) 1999. Cons. Orthopaedic Surgeon, Southampton Univ. Hosp.; Ingham Fell., The New Childrs. Hosp. Sydney Australia. Specialty: Trauma & Orthop. Surg. Socs: Brit. Orthopaedic Trainees Assoc., Pres.., 98/99; Brit. Orthopaedic Foot Surg. Soc.; Brit. Soc. Childr.'s Orthopaedic Surg. Prev: Regist. (Orthop.) Portsmouth; Regist. (Orthop.) Soton. Gen. Hosp.; Regist. (Orthop.) Basingstoke.

UGLOW, Paul Andrew 10 Galloway Drive, Kennington, Ashford TN25 4QQ — MB BS Lond. 1998; MB BS Lond 1998.

UGOCHUKWU, Uchechukwu Ogugua 77A Stratford Road, London E13 0JN — LRCP LRCS LRCPS Ed., Glas. 1998; BM BCh Nigeria 1979.

UGOJI, Uchechi Ugochukwu 51 Brookfield Avenue, Loughborough LE11 3LN — MB ChB Glas. 1963; MRCP (UK) 1969; FRCPC 1972; FRCP Glas. 1992. Specialty: Gen. Med.; Dermat.

UGWU, Clement Nwokolo Halton General Hospital, Runcorn WA7 2DA Tel: 01928 714567 Fax: 01928 715666 — MD Kharkov 1971 (Kharkov Med. Inst.) FRCPI; MD (Hons.) Kharkov Med. Inst. 1971; MRCS Eng. LRCP Lond. 1975; MRCPI 1979. Cons. Phys. (Geriat. Med.) Halton Health Dist. Specialty: Gen. Med. Prev: Sen. Regist. (Geriat. Med.) N. Tees Gen. Hosp. Stockton-on-Tees; Regist. (Med.) N. Lonsdale Hosp. Barrow-in-Furness; Ho. Off. (Gen. Surg.) Oldham & Dist. Gen. Hosp.

UGWUMADU, Mr Augustin Nnamdi Department of Obstetrics & Gynaecology, St. Georges Hospital, Blackshaw Road, London SW17 0QT Tel: 020 86721255 Ext: 0506 Fax: 020 8725 0078 Email: augwumad@sghms.ac.uk — MB BS Lagos 1986 (Univ. Lagos Coll. Med., Nigeria) MRCOG 1994. Cons. Obst. & Gynaecoogist & Hon. Sen. Lecturer St. Geo.s Hopsital, Lond. Specialty: Endocrinol.; Obst. & Gyn.; Research; Immunol. Special Interest: Anti-oestrogens; Gen. Gyn.; High-risk Obst. Prev: Regist. (O & G) St Peter's Hosp. Chertsey; Regist. (O & G) St. Helier Hosp. Carshalton & Qu. Mary's Hosp. Roehampton; SNR. Regist. (O&G) St. Geo.s Hosp. 2000-2001.

UHAMA, Joseph Nnajiuba c/o Dr C Ezechukwu, 5 Cobland Road, London SE12 9SD — State DMS Pavia 1994.

UHEBA, Mr Mokhtar Ali 35 Gilbert Road, Camberley GU16 7RD — MB BCh Al Fatah, Libya 1981; FRCS Glas. 1990.

UITENBOSCH, Martin The Surgery, Denmark Street, Darlington DL3 0PD Tel: 01325 460731 Fax: 01325 362183 — Artsexamen Amsterdam 1987. GP Darlington, Co. Durh.

UKACHI-LOIS, Justice Onyemuche 11 Swingate Close, Lordswood, Chatham ME5 8RH — MB BS Lond. 1986.

UKACHUKWU, Ijeoma 80 Tanfield Avenue, Neasden, London NW2 7RT Tel: 020 8452 9051 — MB BS Lond. 1994 (St Mary's Paddington) MRCGP 1998 - RCGP; BSc, Hons, (Lond.) 1992; DRCOG 1996; DFFP 1998. GP Asst., Ealing Pk. Health Centre, Lond. Specialty: Gen. Pract. Socs: BMA.

UKRA, Mr Hani Abdul Hameed Rashid 51 Friars Place Lane, London W3 7AQ Tel: 020 8248 9682 — MB ChB Baghdad 1972 (Univ. Baghdad) FRCS Glas. 1983; LRCP LRCS Ed. LRCPS Glas. 1985. Specialty: Orthop. Prev: Cons. Orthop. & Trauma Surg. Al-Hammadi Hosp. Olaya, Riyadh, Saudi Arabia; Cons. Orthop. Salalah, Oman.

ULAHANNAN, Thomas John Gloucester Royal Hospital, Department of Diabetes & Endocrinology, Gloucester GL1 3NN Tel: 08454 226276 Fax: 08454 226304 Email: thomas.ulahannan@glos.nhs.uk — MB ChB Leeds 1991; BSc (Med. Microbiol.) 1988; MRCP (UK) 1994; CCST 1999; FRCP RCP Lond. 2004. Cons. Phys. (Diabetes, Endocrinol., Gen. Med.) Gloucester Roy. Hosp. Specialty: Gen. Med.; Diabetes; Endocrinol. Special Interest: Insulin Pump Ther. Socs: Soc. For Endocrinol. Prev: Sen. Regist. (Gen. Med.) John Radcliffe Hosp. Oxf.; Sen. Regist. (Diabetes & Endocrinol.) Radcliffe Infirm. Oxf.

ULLAH, Mr Aamer Saeed 2 Cutler Close, Marton-in-Cleveland, Middlesbrough TS7 8QD — MB BS Lond. 1993 (Charing Cross & Westminster) FRCS 1998. Specialty: Orthop.

ULLAH, Habib Plane Trees Group Practice, 51 Sandbeds Road, Pellon, Halifax HX2 0QL Tel: 01422 330860; 18 Gatesgarth Crescent, Lindley, Huddersfield HD3 3LG Tel: 01484 460349 — MB ChB Bristol 1978. Police Surg. Huddersfield (W. Yorks. Police). Socs: Roy. Coll. of Gen. Practitioners (Assoc.); Brit. Soc. for Heart Failure; Primary Care Cardiovasc. Soc.

ULLAH, Hadayat Patel and Partners, 4 Bedford Street, Bletchley, Milton Keynes MK2 2TX Tel: 01908 377101 Fax: 01908 645903 — MB ChB Glas. 1990.

ULLAH, Khan Mohmad Shafi 34 Marquis Road, London N4 3AP — MB BS Dacca 1963.

ULLAH, Mahmood Iqbal 14 Galston Avenue, Newton Mearns, Glasgow G77 5SF — MB ChB Glas. 1972; DObst. RCOG 1974; DCH RCPS Glas. 1976; MRCP (UK) 1977; FRCP Glas. 1988; T(M) 1991. Cons. Phys. Qu.s Pk. Clinic. Specialty: Respirat. Med. Prev: Chairm. Med. Divis. Al Shaty Teachg. Hosp., Jeddah; Cons. Phys. Heathfield Hosp. Ayr; Lect. (Med.) Middlx. Hosp.

ULLAH, Mr Ramzan Mohammed 25 Hampton Manor, Belfast BT7 3EL — MB BCh BAO Belf. 1989; FRCS Ed. 1993.

ULLAH, Saif 49 Cranleigh Gardens, Luton LU3 1LS — MB BS Karachi 1982.

ULLAH, Mr Shakir 29 Broadlands, Shann Park, Keighley BD20 6HX — MB BS Peshawar 1979; FRCS Ed. 1989.

ULLEGADDI, Ashok Fakirappa Royal Shrewsbury Hospital, Shelton, Shrewsbury SY3 8DN Tel: 01743 231122; 58 Primrose

Drive, Sutton Park, Shrewsbury SY3 7TP — MB BS Mysore 1968 (Kasturba Med. Coll. Manipal) DPM RCPSI 1987. Assoc. Specialist (Psychiat.) Shrops. HA. Specialty: Geriat. Psychiat.

ULLEGADDI, Rajesh 58 Primrose Drive, Shrewsbury SY3 7TP Tel: 01743 245826 — MB ChB Aberd. 1994. SHO (Gen. Med.) Walsgrave Hosp. Coventry. Specialty: Gen. Med.

ULLIOTT, Elaine Elizabeth Jane Huthwaite Health Centre, New Street, Huthwaite, Sutton-in-Ashfield NG17 2LR Tel: 01623 513147 Fax: 01623 515574; Homeston Farm, 10 Alfreton Road, Newton, Alfreton DE55 5TP — MB ChB Sheff. 1980; DRCOG 1983; CPDC Warwick 2001.

ULLYATT, Kim Joy O'Grady-Peyton International, Centre Ct., 1301 Stratford Road, Hall Green, Birmingham B28 9HH — MB ChB Orange Free State 1995.

ULYATT, The Hon. Mrs Frances Margaret (retired) 8 Market Place, Tetbury GL8 8DA Tel: 01666 504009; 8 Cambridge Road, London SW11 4RS Tel: 020 7924 5211 — (Lond. Sch. Med. Wom.) MB BS Lond. 1943; DA Eng. 1948; FFA RCS Eng. 1957. Prev: Cons. Anaesth. Croydon & Warlingham Hosp. Gp.

ULYETT, Ian Hartsholme, Main Road, Asby, Workington CA14 4RT — MB ChB Sheff. 1977; FFA RCS Eng. 1982. Cons. (Anaesth.) W. Cumbld. Hosp. Specialty: Anaesth. Socs: Assn. Anaesths. Prev: Sen. Regist. (Anaesth.) N. West. RHA; Regist. (Anaesth.) Sheff. AHA; Regist. (Anaesth.) Oldham AHA.

UMACHANDRAN, Velaitham 10 Nightingale Way, London E6 5JR — MB BS Sri Lanka 1976; MRCP (UK) 1983.

UMAPATHEE, P Bentley Health Centre, Askern Road, Bentley, Doncaster DN5 0JX Tel: 01302 874416 Fax: 01302 875820 — MRCS Eng. LRCP Puvanasundaram; MB BS Sri Lanka 1975; MB BS Sri Lanka 1975.

UMAPATHY, Arumugam Bath Road Surgery, 450 Bath Road, Cippenham, Slough SL1 6BB Tel: 01628 602564 Fax: 01628 660122 — MB BS Ceylon 1972; MB BS Ceylon 1972.

UMAR, Mr Abdulqadir 31 Sneckyeat Court, Hensingham, Whitehaven CA28 8PG; 31 Sneckyeat Court, Hensingham, Whitehaven CA28 8PG — MB BS Ahmadu Bello, Nigeria 1979; FRCS Ed. 1990. Specialist Regist., Roy. Vict. Infirm., Newc. Specialty: Gen. Surg.; Gastroenterol. Socs: Pancreatic Club; Affil. Mem. Assn. of Surgs. of GB & Ire; BMA. Prev: Specialist Regist. Freeman Hosp. Newc.; Specialist Regist. (Surg.) W. Cumbld. Hosp. Whitehaven; Regist. (Surg.) Wansbeck Hosp.

UMARIA, Nina 5A Wynford Road, London N1 9QN — MB BS Lond. 1992.

UMARJI, Shamim Ismail Mohamed 3 Osborne Road, Clifton, Bristol BS8 2HA — BM BCh Oxf. 1996 (Oxford) SHO, Surgic. Rothation, Bristol, Roy. Infirm. Specialty: Orthop.; Gen. Surg. Socs: Oriel Coll. Med. Soc. Oxf. Prev: A & E, St Thomas's Hosp. Lond.

UMBRICH, Paul 4 Heron Way, Langton Road, Norton, Malton YO17 9AX — MB ChB Manch. 1991.

UMEBUANI, Victor Chukwudi Edgworth Medical Centre, 354 Bolton Road, Turton, Bolton BL7 0DU Tel: 01204 852226 — MB ChB Nigeria 1977.

UMEH, Chukwuemeka Frederick 1 Perivale Drive, Strawberry Fields, Oldham OL8 2JJ — MB BS Nigeria 1986; MRCP (UK) 1993.

UMEH, Hilary Ndubueze Royal Berkshire Hospital, London Road, Reading RG1 5AN Tel: 01189 875111 Email: hilary.umeh@rbbh.nhs.uk — MB BS Ibadan 1976; FRCS Eng 1983; FRCS (Gen Surg) 2000. Cons. Surg., Roy. Berks. Hosp.; Cons. Surg., W. Berks. Community Hosp.; Cons. Surg.,BUPA Dunedin Hosp., Reading; Cons. Surg., Capio Hosp. Reading; Cons. Surg., Thames Valley Nuffielfd Hosp., Wexham Pk.; Honoraray Cons. Surg., Wexham Pk. Hosp., Slough. Specialty: Gen. Surg. Socs: Brit. Assn. of Surgic. Oncol.; Assn. of Surgeons of Gt. Britain and Irel.; Assn. of Breast Surgeons. Prev: Locum Cons. Surg., RBH Reading; Specialist Regist., Newham Gen. Hosp., Lond.; Assoc. Specialist, Roy. Berks. and Battle NHS Trust, Reading.

UMERAH, Francis Ngozi The Children's Centre, 70 Walker St., Hull HU3 2HE Tel: 01482 221261 Fax: 01482 617606; 737 Beverley Road, Hull HU6 7ES Tel: 01482 859652 — MB BS Lagos 1983; DCH RCP Lond. 1995; MRCP (UK) 1995. Cons. Paediat. Hull & E. Riding Community Health NHS Trust Hull; Cons. Paediat., Hull Roy. Infirm., Anlaby Rd., Hull. Specialty: Community Child Health; Paediat.; Neurol. Prev: Clin. Med. Off. (Child Health) Community & Priority Servs. NHS Trust Barnsley.

UMESH, Sharan Harrogate District Hospital, Lancaster Park Road, Harrogate HG2 7SX Tel: 01423 555304 Fax: 01423 553367 Email: umesh.sharan@hhc-tr.northy.nhs.uk — MB BS Panta Med. Coll. India 1971; MD Panta Univ. India; MRCP UK. Cons. Phys. (Gen. Med. / Med. for the Elderly). Specialty: Gen. Med. Special Interest: Cardiol.; Geriat. Med. Socs: Brit. Geriat. Soc. Prev: Assoc. Specialist (Med.).

UMESH, Shivanna 15 Cormorant Avenue, Houston, Johnstone PA6 7LG Tel: 01505 613462 — MB BS Mysore 1974; DCH RCPSI 1980; LRCP LRCS Ed. LRCPS Glas. 1983; DCH RCPS Glas. 1983; DCCH RCP Ed. 1984. SCMO (Hearing Impairment) Johnstone Health Centre; Med. Pract. Roy. Hosp. Sick Childr. Glas. Specialty: Paediat. Socs: Brit. Assn. Community Drs in Audiol. Prev: Clin. Med. Off. Linwood Health Centre Renfrewsh.

UMNUS, Lutz 18 Clarence Road, Warrington WA4 2PQ Fax: 01925 486965 — State Exam Med Rostock 1992. GP Warrington. Specialty: Gen. Pract. Socs: MDU.

UMO-ETUK, Joanna Mkpo-Etuk Oldchurch Hospital, Department of Anaesthesia, Waterloo Road, Romford RM7 0BE Tel: 01708 708443 — MB BS Benin 1983; FRCA 1994. Cons. Anaesth.; Anaesth. Represen. (Med. Advis. Comm.) BUPA Roding Hosp. Specialty: Anaesth. Special Interest: Paediatric Anaesthesia. Socs: Assn. Anaesth.

UMOREN, Denis Mbong Ikpe Lodge, Linden Road, Yeovil BA20 2BH — MB BS Lagos 1979 (Coll. Of Med. Univ. of Lagos.) MRCOG 1988. Assoc. Specialist, O & G, Yeovil Dist. Hosp., Yeovil, Som.. Specialty: Obst. & Gyn.; Family Plann. & Reproduc. Health; Trop. Med. Socs: Brit. Soc. for Colposcopy & Cervical Path..

UMPLEBY, Mr Henry Clark Department Surgery, Royal United Hospital, Combe Park, Bath BA1 3NG Tel: 01225 824542 Fax: 01225 824542 — MB ChB Bristol 1975; FRCS Eng. 1980; T(S) 1991. Cons. Gen. Surg. Roy. United Hosp. Bath. Specialty: Gen. Surg. Socs: RCS (Eng.); Assn Surg.; Brit. Assn. Surg. Oncol. Prev: Wellcome Surgic. Research Fell. 1982; Lect. Univ. Soton. 1984-87.

UMPLEBY, Madeline Hilda Jane (retired) Flat 3, 37 Arundell Road, Weston Super Mare BS23 2QH Tel: 01934 412182 — MRCS Eng. LRCP Lond. 1921 (Roy. Free & St. Geo.) DPH Eng. 1928.

UMRANI, Wali Mohummed The Surgery, 152 Plashet Road, Upton Park, London E13 0QT Tel: 020 8472 0473 Fax: 020 8471 2243 — LMSSA London 1969.

UN, Emine Nevin 222 Nithsdale Road, Pollokshields, Glasgow G41 5PZ Email: ekremkizinevin@yahoo.com — Tip Doktoru Istanbul 1968; FFA RCSI 1986. Cons. (Anaesth.) Prin. Chas. Hosp. Merthyr Tydfil. Specialty: Anaesth. Socs: Founder Mem. Internat. Assn. Study Pain; Anaesth. Res. Soc.; Diplomate Europ. Acad. Anaesth. 1985. Prev: Locum Cons. Stoke Mandeville Hosp. Aylesbury; Cons. Neuroanaesth. Inst. Neurol. Sci. Glas.; Lect. (Anaesth.) Vict. Univ. Manch.

UNADKAT, M D Oak Lane Medical Centre, 6 Oak Lane, Twickenham TW1 3PE Tel: 020 8894 1730 Fax: 020 8893 8667.

UNADKAT, M M Oak Lane Medical Centre, 6 Oak Lane, Twickenham TW1 3PA.

UNCLE, Kenneth Albert The Orchards Health Centre, Gascoigne Road, Barking IG11 7RS Tel: 020 8594 1311; 130 Upney Lane, Barking IG11 9LT Tel: 020 8594 4353 — MB BS Lond. 1982 (Westminster Hospital Medical School) BSc (1st cl. Hons.) Birm. 1975.

UNCLES, David Roy Department of Anaesthesia, Worthing Hospital, Lyndhurst Road, Worthing BN11 2DH Tel: 01903 205111; Amballa, Golden Acre, East Preston, Littlehampton BN16 1QP Tel: 01903 786007 Fax: 01903 786007 — MB BS Lond. 1985; FFA RCSI 1991; FRCA 1992. Specialty: Anaesth. Prev: Asst. Prof. Health Scis. Centre Charlottesville Virginia, USA.; Sen. Regist. Nuffield Dept. Anaesth. Oxf.

UNDERHILL, Fiona Eastwood Road Medical Centre, London E18 Tel: 020 8530 4108; 28 Monkhams Avenue, Woodford Green IG8 0EY — MB BS Lond. 1982; DRCOG 1984.

UNDERHILL, Gillian Susan Department of Virology, Public Health Laboratory, St. Mary's General Hospital, Milton Road, Portsmouth PO3 6AQ Tel: 0239 282 4652 Fax: 0239 282 4652 — MRCS Eng. LRCP Lond. 1978 (St. Mary's) BSc Lond. 1975, MB BS 1978; MRCPath 1985; FRCPath 1996. Cons. Virol. Pub. Health Laborat. St. Mary's Gen. Hosp. Portsmouth. Specialty: Virology. Prev: Sen.

Regist. (Virol.) St. Mary's Hosp. Lond.; Trainee Path. St. Mary's Hosp. Lond.; Ho. Off. (Surg.) Vict. Hosp. Blackpool.

UNDERHILL, Helen Clare 14 Foxgrove Avenue, Beckenham BR3 5BA — MB BS Lond. 1988; MRCP (UK) 1991; DCH RCP Lond. 1991.

UNDERHILL, Helen Louise — BM Soton. 1997. Anaesth. Soton. Gen. Hosp. Specialty: Anaesth.

UNDERHILL, Simon Wrexham Maelor Hospital, Croesnewydd Road, Wrexham LL11 7TD Tel: 01978 291100; The Hermitage, Hindford, Oswestry SY11 4NP — MB ChB Leeds 1977; FRCA 1983. Cons. Anaesth. Wrexham Maelor Hosp. Specialty: Anaesth.

UNDERHILL, Mr Timothy John Mill Stream Cottage, Whatlington, Battle TN33 0ND — MB ChB Bristol 1980; FRCS Ed. 1984. Cons. A & E Med. Hastings HA. Specialty: Accid. & Emerg. Prev: Sen. Regist. (A & E Med.) Trent RHA.

UNDERHILL, Yvonne Margaret The Surgery, High Street, Heathfield TN21 8JD Tel: 01435 864999; Millstream Cottage, Whatlington, Battle TN33 0ND — MB BS Lond. 1981; MRCP (UK) 1984. Gen. Practitioner. Specialty: Cardiol. Prev: GP Nottm.; Trainee GP Salisbury VTS; SHO (O & G) Salisbury HA.

UNDERWOOD, Alan David The Health Centre, Manor Road, Beverley HU17 7BZ Tel: 01482 862733 Fax: 01482 864958 — MB ChB Ed. 1988.

UNDERWOOD, Betty Park Gate Surgery, 28 St. Helens Road, Ormskirk L39 4QR Tel: 01695 72561 Fax: 01695 571709; 25 Greetby Hill, Ormskirk L39 2DP — MB ChB Liverp. 1961; DObst RCOG 1964; DFFP 1993.

UNDERWOOD, Caroline Jane Croft House, Lamonby, Penrith CA11 9SS — MB ChB Birm. 1976; DRCOG 1978; Cert JCC Lond. 1978; MRCGP 1981; DCH RCP Lond. 1982. Prev: SHO (Paediat.) Qu.s Pk. Hosp. Blackburn; Ho. Phys. Ronkswood Br. Worcester Roy. Infirm.; Ho. Surg. Castle St. Br. Worcester Roy. Infirm.

UNDERWOOD, Christine Lavinia 6 Mallaig Avenue, Dundee DD2 4TW Tel: 01382 643066 — MB ChB Dundee 1974 (Dundee Univ.) DObst RCOG 1976; MFHom ECP Lond. 1986. Clin. Asst. Homoeop. Clinic Butterburn Clinic Dundee; Research Assoc. Dept of Med. Ninewells Hosp. & Med. Sch. Dundee. Specialty: Vasc. Med.

UNDERWOOD, Elizabeth Marion Lucy Medical Centre, 12 East King Street, Helensburgh G84 7QL Tel: 01436 673366 Fax: 01436 679715; Helensburgh Medical Centre, 12 East King St, Helensburgh G84 7QL Tel: 01436 673366 — MB ChB Liverp. 1987; DRCOG 1992; DFFP 1993; MRCGP 1994. Specialty: Gen. Pract. Prev: Trainee GP Alloa Health Centre.

UNDERWOOD, Felicity Susan Harriet 266 Wollaton Road, Beeston, Nottingham NG9 2PP — MB BS Lond. 1993.

UNDERWOOD, Gayle Henderson 41 Philips Street, Bainsford, Falkirk FK2 7JE — MB ChB Aberd. 1986; DCH RCPS Glas. 1988. SHO (Palliat. Med.) Marie Curie Centre Glas.

UNDERWOOD, Ian Richard Claypath Medical Practice, 26 Gilesgate, Durham DH1 1QW Tel: 0191 333 2830 Fax: 0191 333 2836; 13 The Grove, North End, Durham City, Durham DH1 4LU Tel: 0191 386 3968 — MB ChB Aberd. 1968. GP Durh.; Clin. Asst. (Ophth.) Univ. Hosp. of N. Durh.

UNDERWOOD, Professor Sir James Cressee Elphinstone Department of Pathology, University of Sheffield Medical School, Beech Hill Road, Sheffield S10 2RX Tel: 0114 271 2501 Fax: 0114 226 1464 Email: jceu@shef.ac.uk; 258 Fulwood Road, Sheffield S10 3BL — MB BS Lond. 1965 (St. Bart.) MRCS Eng. LRCP Lond. 1965; FRCPath 1972; MD Lond. 1973. Joseph Hunter Prof. Path. Univ. Sheff. Med. Sch.; Hon. Cons. Centr. Sheff. Univ. Hosps.; Pres. Roy. Coll. of Pathologists. Specialty: Histopath. Socs: Path. Soc.; Internat. Acad. Path. Prev: Edr. Histopathol.; Reader (Path.) Univ. Sheff. Med. Sch.; Regist. (Path.) St. Bart. Hosp. Lond.

UNDERWOOD, Jeremy Robert Argyle House, 3 Lady Lawson St., Edinburgh EH3 0XY; 19 Main Street, Low Valley Field, Dunfermline KY12 8TF — MB ChB Leic. 1980; DRCOG 1988; MRCGP 1989. Specialty: Civil Serv.

UNDERWOOD, Margaret Cramond Cestria Health Centre, Whitehill Way, Chester-le-Street DH2 3DJ Tel: 0191 388 7771 Fax: 0191 387 1803; 13 The Grove, North End, Durham DH1 4LU Tel: 0191 386 3968 — (Univ. Aberd.) MB ChB Aberd. 1968; DObst RCOG 1971. GP Chester-le-St..

UNDERWOOD, Mr Mark Anthony Brincliffe, 7 St Michael Drive, Helensburgh G84 7SF Tel: 01436 674381 Email: mauip@clinmed.gla.ac.uk — MB ChB Liverp. 1987; MB ChB (Hons.) Liverp. 1987; FRCS Ed. 1991; MD Liverp. 1996; FRCS (Urol.) Ed. 1998. Cons. Urol. Glas. Roy. Infirm. Specialty: Urol. Prev: Career Regist. (Urol.) South. Gen. Hosp. Glas.; Clin. Research Fell. Glas. Roy. Infirm.; Lect. (Urol.) Glas. Roy. Infirm.

UNDERWOOD, Paul Martyn 25 Lime Road, Oxford OX2 9EQ — MB ChB Leeds 1994.

UNDERWOOD, Richard (retired) 25 Greetby Hill, Ormskirk L39 2DP Tel: 01695 576229 Email: home@runderwood.worldonline.co.uk — MB ChB Liverp. 1961.

UNDERWOOD, Professor Stephen Richard Royal Brompton Hospital, Sydney St., London SW3 6NP Tel: 020 7351 8811 Fax: 020 7351 8822 Email: r.underwood@ic.ac.uk; 2A Mount Ephraim Lane, Streatham, London SW16 1JG Tel: 020 8769 5631 — BM BCh Oxf. 1977; MA Oxf. 1976; MRCP (UK) 1979; MD Lond. 1994; FRCP Lond. 1996; FRCR 1996. Prof. Cardiac Imaging Imperial Coll. Sch. Med. & Hon. Cons. Roy. Brompton Hosp. Lond.; Hon. Cons. Roy. Marsden Hosp. Lond.; Hon. Sen. Lect. UCL. Specialty: Cardiol.; Nuclear Med.; Radiol. Socs: Brit. Cardiac Soc.; Fell. Europ. Soc. Cardiol.- Co-Chair, Educat. Comm.; Brit. Nuclear Cardiol. Soc- Post Chairm. Prev: Hon. Sen. Regist. (Cardiol.) Middlx. Hosp.; Regist. (Gen. Med.) The Lond. Hosp.; SHO (Gen. Med.) The Radcliffe Infirm. Oxf.

UNDERWOOD, Susan Mary Anaesthetic Department, Bristol Royal Infirmary, Bristol BS2 8HW — MB ChB Bristol 1981 (Univ. Bristol) DA (UK) 1985; FRCA Eng. 1986. Cons. Anaesth. Bristol Roy. Infirm. Specialty: Anaesth. Socs: Assoc. of Cardiothoracic Anaesth.s; Soc. Of Anaesth.s of the S. W. Region; Roy. Coll. of Anaesth.s. Prev: Sen. Regist. (Anaesth.) Roy. Lond. Hosp.

UNDERWOOD, Thomas James 29 Bishop Street, Shrewsbury SY2 5HB Tel: 01743 243776 — MB ChB Liverp. 1996; Dip Trop Med.& Hygiene - Liverp. 1997; DRCOG Birm. 2002.

UNDERWOOD, Trevor Alan Chancellor House Surgery, 6 Shinfield Road, Reading RG2 7BW Tel: 0118 931 0006 Fax: 0118 975 7194 — MRCS Eng. LRCP Lond. Lond. 1978; MB BS Lond. 1980.

UNDERWOOD-WHITNEY, Anthony John (retired) Old Vicarage Cottage, Sutton Maddock, Shifnal TF11 9NG Tel: 01952 730676 — MB BChir Camb. 1945 (Westm.) BA Camb. 1942. Prev: RAF VR Med. Br.

UNGAR, Alexander Moorthwaite Cottage, Wigton CA7 0LZ — BM BCh Oxf. 1962.

UNGAR, Stuart Charles The Ground Floor Consulting Suite, The Princess Grace Hospital, 42/52 Nottingham Place, London W1U 5NY Tel: 020 7580 6789 Fax: 020 7224 3836 Email: stuungar@aol.com; 49 Tottenham Street, London W1T 4RZ — (Roy. Free) MB BS Lond. 1968, Acad. Dip. Gen. Biochem. 1965; MRCS Eng. LRCP Lond. 1968; MRCP (UK) 1971. Med. Off. Nat. Transcommunications & Indep. Television Commiss.; Med. Dir. The Doctors Laborat. Socs: Fell. Roy. Soc. Med. & Med. Soc. Lond.; Counc.Mem.Indep.Doctors.Forum. Prev: Regist. Psychiat. Unit. St. Mary Abbots Hosp. Lond.; Regist. Qu. Charlotte's Hosp. Lond.; SHO (Respirat. Med.) Roy. Postgrad. Med. Sch. Lond.

UNGAR-SARGON, Julian Yehuda The Gainsborough Clinic, 80 Lambeth Road, London SE1 7PW Tel: 020 8346 7019 Fax: 020 8346 7019; Suite 17, Mayflower Lodge, Regents Park Road, London N3 Tel: 020 346 7019 — (The Roy. Lond. Hosp. Med. Coll.) MRCS Eng. LRCP Lond. 1974; MB BS Lond. 1974; MTS (Harvard) 1988; MA Brandeis 1992; PhD (Brandeis Uni) 1999. Indep Pract. Lond., Neurol.; Dir., E.M.G. Laborat. The GainsBoro. Clinic Lond.; Cons. The GainsBoro. Clinic. Lond. Specialty: Neurol. Socs: Amer. Acad. Neurol. (Bd. Eligible); Diplomate, Amer. Acad. Pain Managem. (Bd. Certified); Diplomate, Bd. of Clin. Electrodiagnostic Med. (Bd. Certified). Prev: Asst. Prof. Med. Coll. Pennsylvania, USA; Instruc. Harvard Med. Sch. Boston Mass., USA.; Med. Dir., Lifeline Med. Center, Indiana, USA.

UNGARO, Anna Rita Shakespeare Road Surgery, 17 Shakespeare Road, Bedford MK40 2DZ Tel: 01234 327337 — MB BS Lond. 1991.

UNIA, Catherine The Alec Turnbull Clinic, East Oxford Health Centre, Cowley Road, Oxford OX4 1XD Tel: 01865 456666; 2 Chilswell Road, Oxford OX1 4PJ Tel: 01865 723445 — MB ChB Birm. 1975; MFFP. Mem. of Fac. & Family Plann. & Reproductive Healthcare; Sen. Clin. Med. Off. Specialty: Family Plann. & Reproduc. Health. Socs: British Menopause Society.

UNITT, Helen Margaret 32 Brook Lane, Nanpantan, Loughborough LE11 3RA — MB ChB Leeds 1991; BSc (1st cl. Hons. Biochem.) Leeds 1988; DRCOG 1993; DCH RCP Lond. 1994; DFFP 1994; MRCP (London) 1997. SHO (Paediat.) Leicester Roy. Infirm.; Long Term Locum GP LoughBoro. Specialty: Paediat. Prev: Trainee GP Derby VTS.

UNNI, Ambat Govindan Royal Alexandra Hospital, Care Of The Elderly, Corsebar Road, Paisley PA2 9PN — MB BS Calicut Med. College-Kerala 1967 (Calicut Med. Coll.) MRCPI 1980; FRCPI 1991.

UNNIKRISHNAN, Manghat 32 Hallfield, Ulverston LA12 9TA Tel: 01229 54780 — MB BS Madras 1961 (Stanley Med. Coll. Madras) FRCP Glas. 1982, M 1966. Cons. Phys. in Geriat. Furness Gen. Hosp. Barrow-in-Furness. Specialty: Gen. Med. Socs: BMA; Assoc. Mem. Brit. Geriat. Soc. Prev: Ho. Phys. Pinderfields Gen. Hosp. Wakefield; Med. Regist. N. Lonsdale Hosp. Barrow-in-Furness; Asst. in Geriat. Doncaster Hosp. Gp.

UNSWORTH, Anthony (retired) 4 Upper Linney, Ludlow SY8 1EF Tel: 01584 877314 — MB ChB Liverp. 1951; DObst RCOG 1955.

UNSWORTH, David Joseph Southmead Hospital, Bristol BS10 5ND Tel: 0117 959 5629 Email: joeunsworth@hotmail.com — MB BS Lond. 1987; BSc (Hons.) Biochem. Leeds 1977; PhD (Immunol.) Lond. 1982, MB BS 1987; MRCP (UK) 1991; MRCPath 1993; FRCP 1999. Cons. Clin. Immunol. Southmead Hosp. Bristol. Specialty: Immunol. Prev: Sen. Regist. (Clin. Immunol.) Addenbrooke's Hosp. Camb.; SHO Rotat. (Med.) Hammersmith Hosp. Lond.

UNSWORTH, Francis James Swn-yr-Afon, Abercegir, Machynlleth SY20 8NR Tel: 01650 511821 — MB ChB Manch. 1955.

UNSWORTH, James Oak Tree Lane Centre, 91 Oak Tree Lane, Selly Oak, Birmingham B29 6JA Tel: 0121 627 8221 — MB ChB Sheff. 1980 (Sheffield.) MRCP (UK) 1983; FRCP (UK) 1996. Cons. in Rehabil. Med., Southern Birm. Community Health Trust. Specialty: Rehabil. Med.; Rheumatol.

UNSWORTH, Philip Francis Department of Microbiology, Tameside General Hsopital, Ashton-under-Lyne OL6 9RW Tel: 0161 331 6500 Fax: 0161 331 6496; 1 Pine Road, Didsbury, Manchester M20 6UY Tel: 0161 445 6480 — MB ChB Manch. 1971; BSc (Hons) Manch. 1968, MB ChB 1971; FRCPath 1989, M 1977. Cons. Microbiol. Tameside & Glossop Trusts; Hon. Clin. Lect. in Med. Microbiol., Manch. Univ. Specialty: Med. Microbiol. Socs: Hosp. Infec. Soc. Assn. Clin. Paths. and Assoc. Med. Microbiologists. Prev: Sen. Microbiol. Centr. Pub. Health Laborat. Lond.; Lect (Microbiol.) St. Thos. Hosp. Med. Sch. Lond.; Asst. Lect. (Path.) Middlx. Hosp. Med. Sch. Lond.

UNTER, Charles Ernest Marcell Department of Paediatrics, The Maidstone Hospital, Hermitage Lane, Maidstone ME16 9NN Tel: 01622 224204 Fax: 01622 224495; Silver Fern, Church Road, Offham, West Malling ME19 5NY Tel: 01732 872800 — MB BS Lond. 1975 (Char. Cross) MRCS Eng. LRCP Lond. 1975; DRCOG 1977; FRACP 1986. Cons. Paediat. Maidstone and Tunbridge wellls NHS Trust, Maidstone Hosp., Maidstone; Med. Director Maidstone and Tunbridge Wells NHS Trust; Hon. Cons. Paediat., Kings Coll. Hosp., Lond. Specialty: Paediat. Socs: Fell. Roy. Coll. Paediat. & Child Health; Brit. Paediatric Respirat. Soc.; Brit. Med. Assn. Prev: Cons. Paediat. Taranaki Area HB, NZ; Sen. Regist. P. of Wales Childr. Hosp. Sydney, Austral.; Regist. (Paediat.) ChristCh. Hosp., NZ.

UNWIN, Mr Andrew John Phoenix House, 9 Nightingale Walk, Windsor SL4 3HS Tel: 01753 868622 Fax: 01753 868642 Email: unwinaj@aol.com — MB BS Lond. 1988; BSc (Hons.) 1985; FRCS 1992; FRCS (Orth) 1995. Cons. Orthopaedic Surg. Windsor Orthopaedic Clinic, Windsor; Clin. Lect. in Anat., Imperial Col. Lond. Specialty: Trauma & Orthop. Surg. Socs: Edu. Sec., Rheum. Arth. Surg. Soc.; Brit. Ortho. Assn; Anat. Soc. Prev: Lect. (Anat.) Char. Cross & Westm. Med. Sch. Lond.; Registra Rotat. N. W. Thames; Cons. Orthop. Surg., Wrexham Pk. Hosp., Berks.

UNWIN, Arthur Benson (retired) 112 Cambridge Street, London SW1V 4QF Tel: 020 7235 2333 Fax: 020 7235 2333 — MB BChir Camb. 1941 (St. Thos.) MRCS Eng. LRCP Lond. 1941; BA (Hons.) Camb. 1938, MA 1942. Prev: Ho. Phys. St. Jas. Hosp. Balham & St. Thos. Hosp.

UNWIN, David Edmund John The Surgery, Ravenghyll, Kirkoswald, Penrith CA10 1DQ Tel: 01768 898560 Fax: 01768 898905 — MB BChir Camb. 1976 (Univ. Coll. Hosp.) MA Camb. 1976; DCH Eng. 1980; DRCOG 1981; MRCGP 1983. Prev: Ho. Phys. Whittington Hosp. Lond.; Ho. Surg. Addenbrooke's Hosp. Camb.

UNWIN, David John Shore Farm, Marsh Road, Banks, Southport PR9 8DX — MB ChB Liverp. 1982.

UNWIN, Elizabeth Finola (retired) Lindow House, Londow Lane, Wilmslow SK9 5LH Tel: 01625 531149; 3 Westfield, St Margarets Road, Bowdon, Altrincham WA14 2AW — MB BCh BAO Belf. 1950; DCH Eng. 1954. Prev: Res. Med. Off. Booth Hall Childr. Hosp. Manch.

UNWIN, Helen Margaret Beech Hill Medical Practice, 278 Gidlow Lane, Wigan WN6 7PD Tel: 01942 821899 Fax: 01942 821752 — MB BS Lond. 1985; DRCOG 1988; MRCGP 1990. GP Wigan.

UNWIN, Jonathan Rosebank Surgery, 153B Stroud Road, Gloucester GL1 5JQ Tel: 01452 522767 — MB BS Lond. 1981 (St. Mary's Hosp.) DRCOG 1986; MRCGP 1986. Clin. Asst. (O & G & X-Ray) Glos.

UNWIN, Lesley Gladys Blantyre Health Centre, 64 Victoria Street, Blantyre, Glasgow G72 0BS Tel: 01698 826331 — MB ChB Glas. 1987; MRCGP 1992.

UNWIN, Michael Richard Princess Road Surgery, 471-475 Princess Road, Withington, Manchester M20 1BH Tel: 0161 445 7805 Fax: 0161 448 2419 — MB ChB Manch. 1985; BSc St. And. 1982.

UNWIN, Nigel Christopher Department of Epidemiology & Public Health, University of Newcastle, Newcastle upon Tyne NE2 4HH; 60 Rothbury Terrace, Newcastle upon Tyne NE6 5XJ — BM BCh Oxf. 1984. Specialty: Epidemiol.

UNWIN, Paul William Borough Green Medical Practice, Quarry Hill Road, Borough Green, Sevenoaks TN15 8BE Tel: 01732 883161 Fax: 01732 886319; Wrotham Surgery, St. Mary's Road, Wrotham, Sevenoaks TN15 Tel: 01732 882009 — MB BS Lond. 1986; DRCOG 1989; DGM RCP Lond. 1989; DCH RCP Lond. 1991; MRCGP Lond. 1992; Dip Ent 2002. Prev: Clin. Asst. (ENT) Sevenoaks.

UNWIN, Philip Roger Harpsden Court Farm, Harpsden, Henley-on-Thames RG9 4AT Tel: 01491 578382 — MB BS Lond. 1982 (St Mary's) DRCOG 1986; MRCGP 1988; Dip Occ Med 2000. GP Henley-on-Thames; Med. Off. Microsoft UK Reading. Specialty: Occupat. Health. Socs: Soc Occ Med.

UNWIN, Professor Robert John Centre for Nephrology, Institute of Urology & Nephrology, Royal Free and University College, Medical School, Middlesex Hospital, London W1W 7EY Tel: 020 76799302 Fax: 020 7637 7006 Email: robert.unwin@ucl.ac.uk; Dellwood, 4 Uplands Close, Gerrards Cross SL9 7JH Tel: 01753 885654 — BM (Hons.) Soton. 1976; MRCP (UK) 1978; PhD Lond. 1983; FRCP Lond. 1994. Hon. Cons. Phys. Univ. Coll. Lond. Hosp. Trust; Prof. (Nephrol. & Physiol.) 1997. Specialty: Nephrol.; Gen. Med. Prev: Reader (Nephrol. & Physiol.) Univ. Coll. Lond. Med. Sch.; Hon. Cons. Phys. & Sen. Lect. (Renal Med. & Physiol.) Middlx. Hosp. Lond.; Sen. Lect. (Clin. Pharmacol.) Roy. Postgrad. Med. Sch. Hammersmith Hosp. Lond.

UNWIN, Rosamond Sylvia — MB BS Lond. 1982 (Univ. Coll. Hosp.) LMSSA Lond. 1982; DA (UK) 1984; MRCGP 1990; DTM & H Liverp. 1991. G.P. Specialty: Trop. Med. Socs: Christ. Med. Fellowsh. Prev: Trainee GP Northallerton VTS.; Primary Health Care Facilitator, NE Nigeria.

UNWIN, Thomas Alasdair Edmund 4 Firbank Drive, Woking GU21 7QT; 4 Firbank Drive, Woking GU21 1QT — MB BS Lond. 1986; BSc (Physiol.) Lond. 1981; MRCGP 1990; DTM & H Liverp. 1991; MSc Lond. 1998. TCO Dept. for Internat. Developm. (DFID). Specialty: Trop. Med.; Gen. Pract. Socs: Fell. Roy. Soc. Med.; Christ. Med. Fellowsh.; Roy. Soc. Trop. Med. & Hyg. Prev: Clin. Lect. TeleMed. Roy. Free Hosp. Sch. Med.; Sen. Med. Off. LCCN Med. Progr. Nigeria; Trainee GP W. Cumbria VTS.

UNYOLO, Paul Michael 3 Castledykes Road, Dumfries DG1 4SN Tel: 01387 257716 — MB ChB Manch. 1984. Regist. (Gen. Surg.) Monklands & Bellshill NHS Trust. Specialty: Gen. Surg. Prev: SHO (Orthop.) Dumfries & Galloway Acute & Matern. NHS Trust; SHO (Gen. Surg.) Cornw. & I. of Scilly HA.

UPADHYAY, Mr Ajay Kumar 20 The Glebe, Hawley, Blackwater, Camberley GU17 9BB Tel: 01276 600216 — MB BS Delhi 1980; FRCS Ed. 1984; FRCS Glas. 1985. Regist. Surg. Crawley Hosp. Sussex. Socs: Fell. Roy. Soc. Med. Prev: Regist. (Surg. & Urol.)

Rushgreen & OldCh. Hosp. Romford; SHO (Surg.) St. Mary's Hosp. Newport; SHO (Orthop.) Redhill Gen. Hosp.

UPADHYAY, Bipin Bhaishankar Fieldhead Hospital, Ouchthorpe Lane, Wakefield WF1 3SP Tel: 01924 327467 Fax: 01924 327461 — MB ChB Nairobi 1977 (University of Nairobi Medical School) MRCPsych 1987. Cons. Psychiat. Learning Disabil. Serv.s Fieldhead Hosp. Wakefield. Specialty: Ment. Health; Gen. Psychiat. Socs: Assn. Child Psychol. & Psychiat.; Amer. Assn. Ment. Retardation; Europ. Assn. Ment. Health in Ment. Retardation. Prev: Cons. (Psychiat. & Gen. Psychiat.) Dewsbury Dist. Hosp.; Sen. Regist. (Psychiat.) Fieldhead Hosp. Wakefield; Sen. Regist. (Psychiat.) High Royds Hosp. Ilkley & Meanwood Pk. Hosp. Leeds.

UPADHYAY, Mahendra Hughes and Partners, The Health Centre, Forge Road, Machynlleth SY20 8EQ Tel: 01654 702224 Fax: 01654 703688 — MB BS Gauhati 1971; MB BS Gauhati 1971.

UPADHYAY, Mr Ramesh Narasimhacharya 9 Mold Road Estate, Gwersyllt, Wrexham LL11 4AA Tel: 01978 753566 — MB BS Osmania 1967; MS (ENT) Osmania 1973, MB BS 1967; DLO RCPSI 1983.

UPADHYAY, Sunil Kumar Princess Royal Hospital, Department of Radiotherapy & Oncology, Salthouse Road, Hull HU8 9HE Tel: 01482 676875 Fax: 01482 676545 — MB BS Lucknow 1975; MD (Radiother.) Delhi 1980, DMRT 1978. Cons. (Clin. Oncol.) Princess Roy. Hosp. Hull. Specialty: Oncol.; Radiother.; Oncol.; Palliat. Med. Special Interest: Breast and lung cancer. Prev: Assoc. Specialist (Clin. Oncol.) Princess Roy. Hosp. Hull; Staff Radiat. Oncol. Princess Roy. Hosp.

UPADHYAY, Vipul Amritlal c/o Mr. B. B. Konnur, 38 Sevington Road, Hendon, London NW4 3RX — MB BS Gujarat 1986.

UPADHYAYA, Ajaya Kumar Herts & Essex Hospital, Bishops Stortford Tel: 01279 827509 Fax: 01279 827156 — MB BS Berhampur 1977; DPM Bombay 1980; MD Chandigarh 1983; MRCPsych 1987; FRCPC, Canada 1995; FRCPsych 2004. Cons. Psychiat., Herts. Partnership Trust, Herts & Essex Hosp., Bishops Stortford, Herts; Hon. Sen. Lect. in Psychiat., Univ. Coll., Lond. Specialty: Gen. Psychiat. Special Interest: Old Age Psychiat.

UPADHYAYA, Geetha 29 Deighton Avenue, Sherburn in Elmet, Leeds LS25 6BR Tel: 01977 683715 Fax: 01274 223306 — MB BS Madras 1972 (Mdras University) MD Madras 1984; PhD Madras 1990. Specialty: Chem. Path. Socs: Assn. Clin. Biochem.; BMA.

UPADHYAYA, Linda Mary c/o Grove Cottage, Lowfield Heath, Crawley RH11 0PY Tel: 01293 551129 — MB ChB Sheff. 1984. Specialist Paediat. Karuna Vihar Charity India.

UPADHYAYA, Rachna Rashmi 711 Pointwest, 116A Cromwell Road, Kensington, London SW7 4XH — MB BCh Wales 1994; DFFP 1998; MRCGP 2000; DIC Imp. Coll. Lond. 2000; MBA Imp. Managem. Sch. Lond. 2000.

UPCHURCH, Francis Charles Medeva Pharma Ltd., Regents Park, Kingston Road, Leatherhead KT22 7PQ Tel: 01372 364002 Fax: 01372 364155 — MB ChB Birm. 1977; BSc Birm. 1972; DRCOG 1981; MFPM RCP (UK) 1993. Med. Dir., Europe, Medeva Pharma Ltd. Specialty: Pharmaceutical Medicine. Prev: Assoc. Med. Dir. Allen & Hanburys Glaxo; GP Penzance; Trainee GP Taunton VTS.

UPCHURCH, Susan Marlowe Partnership, Shakespeare House Health Centre, Shakespeare Road, Basingstoke RG24 9DS Tel: 01256 328860 Fax: 01256 351911; Bees Cottage, Easton Greg, Malmesbury SN16 0PL Tel: 01666 840943 — MB ChB Manch. 1969; DObst RCOG 1971. Prev: SHO (Obst.) N. Herts. Hosp. Hitchin; Ho. Surg. W. Herts. Hosp. Hemel Hempstead; Ho. Phys. St. Helier Hosp. Carshalton.

UPILE, Tahwinder 11 Botany Avenue, Bradford BD2 1EU — MB ChB Manch. 1992.

UPJOHN, Adam Carnegie (retired) 15 Ferry Path, Cambridge CB4 1HB — MRCS Eng. LRCP Lond. 1958 (Edin., Sheff.)

UPJOHN, Clive Henry Critchett (retired) 4 Clark Place, Belford NE70 7LT Tel: 01668 213224 — MB BChir Camb. 1940 (Camb. & Middlx.) MRCS Eng. LRCP Lond. 1939; MA, MD Camb. 1951, MB BChir 1940; FRCP Lond. 1972, M 1941; DCH Eng. 1948. Prev: Cons. Paediat. Bromley Health Dist.

UPJOHN, Gillian Margaret (retired) 15 Ferry Path, Cambridge CB4 1HB — MB ChB Sheff. 1958; MRCGP 1977.

UPPAL, Gurjeet Singh White City Health Centre, Australia Road, Shepherds Bush, London W12 7PH Tel: 020 8749 4145 — BM Soton. 1986; Cert. Family Plann. JCC 1988; DRCOG 1989; MRCGP 1992. Specialty: Gen. Med. Prev: SHO (O & G) W. Dorset Hosp. Dorchester; SHO (Orthop.) Weymouth & Dist. Hosp.; SHO (Paediat.) Brisbane, Austral.

UPPAL, Harmandeep Kaur Uppal Villa, Minster Drive, Minster on Sea, Sheerness ME12 2LA — MB BS Lond. 1996.

UPPAL, Harpreet Singh 16 Pinto Close, Birmingham B16 9EP — MB ChB Manch. 1994.

UPPAL, Manjinder Singh Flat 4, 28 Lennox Road S., Southsea PO5 2HU; 26 Park Lane, Slough SL3 7PF — BM Soton. 1989; DRCOG 1992; MRCGP 1993.

UPPAL, Rajanpal Singh 38 Shirland Mews, London W9 3DY — MB BS Lond. 1993.

UPPAL, Mr Rakesh 149 Harley Street, London W1G 6DE Tel: 020 7935 6397 Fax: 020 7486 4578 — MB ChB Manch. 1981; BSc (Med. Sci.) St. And. 1978; FRCS Eng. 1988; FRCS (CTh) 1996. Cons. Cardiothoracic Surg. Barts & Lond. Chest Hosps. Specialty: Cardiothoracic Surg. Special Interest: Mitral Valve Repair; Surgery of the Aorta; Surgery of the Lung. Socs: BMA; Soc. Cardiothoracic Surgs. GB & Irel.

UPPAL, Sheila White City Health Centre, Australia Road, Shepherds Bush, London W12 7PH Tel: 020 8749 4145 — MB BS Lond. 1987; BSc (Hons.) Lond. 1984; Cert. Family Plann. JCC 1989; DRCOG 1989; MRCGP 1992. Specialty: Obst. & Gyn. Prev: SHO (Cas. & Orthop.) Poole Gen. Hosp.; SHO (O & G) Qu. Mary's Hosp. Lond.; SHO (Paediat.) Mater Childr. Hosp. Brisbane, Austral.

UPPALA, Raju Gudaru 37 Bron y Nant, Croesnewydd Road, Wrexham LL13 7TZ — MB BS Shivaji, India 1986.

UPPONI, Sara Suresh 128 Coventry Road, Nuneaton CV10 7AD — MB BS Lond. 1994.

UPPONI, Suresh Krishna 128 Coventry Road, Nuneaton CV10 7AD — MB BS Bombay 1956 (Grant Med. Coll. Bombay)

UPRICHARD, Andrew Charles Geoffrey 2 Park Street, Hillsborough BT26 6AL — MD Ed. 1988; MB ChB 1981; MRCP (UK) 1984. Research Fell. Dept. Therap. Belf. City Hosp.

UPRICHARD, William James Nicholas Flat 34, 99 Haverstock Hill, London NW3 4RR Email: jamesu@doctors.org.uk — MB BS Lond. 1996 (UCLMS) BSc 1993; MRCP (UK) 1999. Regist. (Haemat.) St Mary's Hosp. Lond. Specialty: Haematology. Prev: Research Fell. (Haemat.) Roy. Free Hosp. Lond.; SHO (Med.) Hammersmith Hosp. Lond.

UPRICHARD, William Owen Enderby Medical Centre, Shortridge Lane, Enderby, Leicester LE19 4LY Tel: 0116 286 6088 — MB BS Lond. 1968 (St. Geo.) MRCP (UK) 1973; DObst RCOG 1974; Dip. Pract. Dermat. Wales 1991; MRCGP 1992.

UPSDELL, Margaret Ann 85 Church Road, Woolton, Liverpool L25 6DB — MB ChB Liverp. 1965; Dip. Ven. Liverp. 1986.

UPSDELL, Mr Stephen Mark Noble's Hospital, Strang, Douglas IM4 4RJ Tel: 01624 650209 Fax: 01624 651231 Email: stephen.upsdell@nobles.chss.gov.im; Potter House Farm, Birdnest Lane, Cumberworth, Huddersfield HD8 8YF Tel: 01484 603187 — MD Lond. 1990 (Char. Cross) MB BS Lond. 1979; FRCS Eng. 1984; FRCS Ed. 1984; FEBU- Europe 1992. Cons. Urol. Noble's Hosp. Specialty: Urol. Socs: Fell. Europ. Bd. Urol. Prev: Sen. Regist. (Urol.) Manch.; Research Regist. (Nuclear Med. & Urol.) Manch. Roy. Infirm.; Cons. Urol. Huddersfield Roy. Infirm.

UPSHALL, Robert Thomas Percy Whinfield Surgery, Whinbush Way, Darlington DL1 3RT Tel: 01325 481321 Fax: 01325 380116 — MB BS Lond. 1976 (Univ. Coll. Hosp.) BSc (Hons.) Lond. 1973; MRCS Eng. LRCP Lond. 1976; DRCOG 1980. Clin. Asst. (Psychiat.) Durh. Priority Care NHS Trust; Med. Off. Hmyo Deerbolt, Barnard Castle; Forens. Med. Examr. Durh. Constab. Specialty: Occupat. Health. Socs: Brit. Soc. Med. & Dent. Hypn.; Soc. Occupat. Med. Prev: Trainee GP Redhill VTS; Ho. Phys. Basingstoke Dist. Hosp.; Ho. Surg. Qu. Alexandra Hosp. Portsmouth.

UPTHEGROVE, Rachel Anne 62 Coleshill Road, Curdworth, Sutton Coldfield B76 9HA — MB BS Lond. 1993.

UPTON, Alan Frazier (retired) 29 Barker Road, Sutton Coldfield B74 2NY Tel: 0121 354 1829 — MB ChB Birm. 1941; Cert. Av Med. MoD (Air) & Civil; Aviat. Auth. 1976. Prev: Ho. Surg. Birm. Matern. Hosp.

UPTON, Christopher Ernest 4/6 Longfleet Road, Poole BH15 2HX Tel: 01202 676111 — MB BS Lond. 1955 (King's Coll. Hosp.) DObst RCOG 1958; FRCGP 1982, M 1976. Jt. Course Organiser Dorset GP Train. Course. Prev: Med. Regist. Gen. Hosp. Poole; Obst.

Ho. Off. Camb. Matern. Hosp.; Ho. Phys. Diabetic Dept. & Ho.; Surg. Urol. & Orthop. Depts. King's Coll. Hosp.

UPTON, Christopher John Jenny Lind Children's Department, Norfolk and Norwich University Hospital, Colney Lane, Norwich NR4 7UY Tel: 01603 287544 Fax: 01603 287584 Email: chris.upton@nnuh.nhs.uk; Long Reach, 86 The St, Brundall, Norwich NR13 5LH Tel: 01603 717204 Email: chris.upton3@btopenworld.com — MB ChB (Hons.) Bristol 1981; DCH RCP Lond. 1984; MRCP (UK) 1984; DM Nottm. 1994; FRCP 1997; FRCPCH 1997. Cons. Paediat. Norf. & Norwich Hosps.; Hon. Sen. Lect. Univ. of E. Anglia. Specialty: Paediat.; Neonat.; Respirat. Med. Socs: Brit. Paediat. Respirat. Soc.; Brit. Assn of Perinatal Med.; Paediat. Research Soc. Prev: Sen. Regist. (Paediat.) Derby & Nottm.; Research Fell. Univ. Nottm.; Regist. Nottm. HA.

UPTON, Mr Julian John Mainwaring Somerset Nuffield Hospital, Staplegrove Elm, StapleGr., Taunton TA2 6AN Tel: 01823 286991 Fax: 01823 338951; Comeytrowe Lodge, Comeytrowe Lane, Taunton TA1 5JD Tel: 01823 283485 Fax: 01823 342168 — MB BChir Camb. 1962 (Guy's) MRCS Eng. LRCP Lond. 1962; MB Camb. 1963, BChir 1962; FRCS Eng. 1969; FRCS Ed. 1972. Cons. ENT Surg. Som. AHA. Specialty: Otorhinolaryngol. Socs: BMA; S. West. Laryngol. Assn.; (Ex-Pres.) W. Som. Med. Soc. Prev: Sen. Regist. (ENT) Yorks. RHA Train. Scheme; Regist. (ENT) Leeds Gen. Infirm.; Regist. (Gen. Surg.) Leeds Univ. Hosp.

UPTON, Karen Elizabeth 96 Grove Park, London SE5 8LE — MB BS Lond. 1982.

UPTON, Karina Mary The Amwell Practice, 4 Naoroji Street, London WC1X 0GB Tel: 020 7837 2020 — MB BS Lond. 1988; BSc (1st cl. Hons.) Lond. 1984; MRCP (UK) 1991; DCH RCP Lond. 1992; DRCOG 1993; MRCGP 1994. GP Lond. Prev: Trainee GP Lond.; SHO (Med.) Hammersmith & Roy. Free Hosps. Lond.; SHO (Paediat.) St. Mary's Hosp. Lond.

UPTON, Margaret Isabel (retired) 202 Attenborough Lane, Attenborough, Beeston, Nottingham NG9 6AL Tel: 0115 925 4305 — MB BS Lond. 1953 (King's Coll. Hosp.) MRCS Eng. LRCP Lond. 1952. Prev: Asst. Sec. S.E. Eng. BMA.

UPTON, Mark Neil Woodlands Family Medical Centre, 106 Yarm Lane, Stockton-on-Tees TS18 1YE — MB BS Lond. 1987; BSc Pharmacol. (1st cl. Hons.) Lond. 1982; MSc Epidemiol. Lond. 1995, MSc Human & Applied Physiol. 1985; DRCOG 1991; MRCGP 1993; DFFP 1996. GP, woodlands family Med. centre. Specialty: Gen. Pract.; Epidemiol. Prev: GP, Thornary & Barwick Med. Grp, Cleveland; Cons. Sen. Lect. in Clin. Epidemiol., univ. of Bris; GP/Regist. Northallerton.

UPTON, Mark William Martin — BM BCh 1985; DCH RCP Lond. 1987; MA Oxf. 1987; MRCGP 1990; MRCPsych 1994; ILTM 2002. Cons. (Pschiat. & Neuropsychiat.) Som. Partnership NHS Trust. Prev: SHO (Rotat.) Roy. Berks. Hosp. Reading.

UPTON, Neil The Gowerton Medical Centre, Mill Street, Gowerton, Swansea SA4 3ED Tel: 01792 872404 Fax: 01792 875170 — MB ChB Ed. 1969.

UPTON, Paul Martin The Old Vicarage, Church Road, Mabe, Penryn TR10 9JG — MB BS Lond. 1984; MRCP (UK) 1987; FRCA 1990. Cons. Anaesth. & ITU Roy. Cornw. Hosps. Trust Truro; Clin. Sub Dean for Roy. Cornw. Hosps., The Peninsula Med. Sch. Specialty: Anaesth. Socs: Assn. Anaesth.; SW Soc. Anaesth.; ASME. Prev: Sen. Regist. (Anaesth.) S. West. RHA.; Regist. (Anaesth.) Oxf. RHA.; SHO (Med.) S. West. RHA.

UPTON, Peter Gaunt 59 Kimbolton Road, Higham Ferrers, Wellingborough NN10 8DU — MB BS Lond. 1977; MA Camb. 1974, BA 1972.

UPTON, Susan Nancy Redlam Surgery, 62 Redlam, Blackburn BB2 1UW Tel: 01254 260051 Fax: 01254 691937; Bentham Road Health Centre, Mill Hill, Blackburn BB2 4PN — MB BS Newc. 1976; DCCH RCP Ed. 1986; MFFP 1997. Specialty: Gen. Pract. Prev: Clin. Med. Off. Burnley Health Dist.

UPTON, William Stuart Avenue Road Surgery, 3 Avenue Road, Dorridge, Solihull B93 8LH Tel: 01564 776262 Fax: 01564 779599; 5 Warren Drive, Dorridge, Solihull B93 8JY — MB ChB Birm. 1972; DObst RCOG 1974; MRCGP 1983.

UPWARD, James Walter 15 The Close, Royston SG8 7JT Tel: 01763 43327 — MB BS Lond. 1975; MRCS Eng. LRCP Lond. 1975; MRCP (UK) 1978.

UQLAT, Luay Nayel Eid c/o Student Cage, Level 6, Ninewells Hospital, Dundee DD1 9SY — MB ChB Dundee 1992.

URBANIAK, Professor Stanislaw Joseph 14 Earlspark Crescent, Bieldside, Aberdeen AB15 9AY — (Ed.) MB ChB Ed. 1970; MRCP (UK) 1972; BSc (Hons. Biochem.) Ed. 1967, PhD 1978; FRCP Ed. 1982; FRCPath 1994, M 1985; FRCP Lond. 1990. Prof. of Transfus. Med., Acad. Transfus. Med. Unit, Dept. Med. & Therap. Abdn. Univ. Med. Sch.; Hon. Cons. Grampian Univeristy Hosp. Trust, Abdn.; Nat. Advis. In ImmunohaemOtol., Scot. Nat. Blood Transfus. Serv., Edin. Specialty: Blood Transfus. Socs: Past Pres., Europ. Soc. Hemapheresis.; Brit. Soc. Haematol.; Brit. Blood Transfus. Soc. Prev: Dir. Aberd. & NE Scotl. Blood Transfus. Serv.; Sen. Regist. & Dep. Dir. Edin. & SE Scotl. Blood Transfus. Centre; MRC Jun. Research Fell. (Therap.) Roy. Infirm. Edin.

URCH, Catherine Elizabeth University College London, Department of Pharmacology, Gower Street, London WC1E 6BT Tel: 020 7679 3737 Email: c.urch@ucl.ac.uk — BM Soton. 1991; BSc (1st cl. Hons.) Soton. 1990; MRCP (UK) 1994; PhD (Pharmacol.) Lond. 2002. Cons. St Marys and Roy. Brompton Hosps., Lond. Specialty: Palliat. Med. Socs: Internat. Assn. Study of Pain. Prev: Hon. Sen. Lect. (Pharmacol.) Univ. Coll. Lond.; Sen. Regist. (Palliat. Med.) Trinity Hospice St. Thos. Hosp. Lond.

URE, David Stuart, MBE Department of Anaesthesia, Glasgow Royal Infirmary, Glasgow G4 0SF Tel: 0141 211 4621 Fax: 0141 211 4622; 244 Crow Road, Glasgow G11 7LA Tel: 0141 337 3274 — MB ChB Aberd. 1990 (Aberdeen) FRCA 1995. Specialist Regist. (Anaesth.) Glas. Roy. Infirm. Specialty: Anaesth. Socs: BMA; Assn. Anaesth. Prev: Career Regist. (Anaesth.) Glas. Roy. Infirm.

UREK, Fatma Hepgul 18 Oman Court, Oman Avenue, London NW2 6AY Tel: 020 8450 3552 — Tip Doktoru Istanbul 1968; MD Istanbul 1973; T(GP) 1991. Locum GP in N.-W. Lond. Specialty: Gen. Med. Socs: Med. Defence Union. Prev: GP Princip., Lond.; GP Lond.; Regist. (Haemat.) Southend Gen. Hosp.

UREN, Neal Gordon Royal Infirmary, Department of Cardiology, Little France Crescent, Edinburgh EH16 4SA Tel: 0131 242 1046 Fax: 0131 536 2021 — MB ChB Ed. 1984; BSc (Hons. Med. Sci.) Ed. 1981; MRCP UK 1987; MD (Hons.) Ed. 1994. Cons. Cardiol. Roy. Infirm. Edin.; Sen. Lect. (Cardiol.) Univ. Edin. Specialty: Cardiol. Special Interest: Interventional Cardiology. Socs: Fell. Europ. Soc. Cardiol.; Fell. Amer. Assn. Of Cardiol.; Fell. Amer. Coll.Cardiol. Prev: Sen. Regist. (Cardiol.) Glenfield Hosp. Leics.; Research Regist. & Regist. Hammersmith Hosp. Lond.; Sen. Interven. Fell. Stanford Univ. Hosp., Calif.

UREY, Michelle Roseanne Site 5 Royal Park Lane, Hillsborough BT26 6RG — MB BCh BAO Belf. 1993; DRCOG; MRCGP; DCH.

URICH, Henry 12 Moat Lodge, Harrow on the Hill, Harrow HA1 3LU Tel: 0208 422 6848 — MB ChB Polish Sch. Med. 1943 (Lwow & Polish Sch. Med. Ed.) MB ChB Polish Sch. of Med. 1943; FRCP Lond. 1973, M 1946; MRCS Eng. LRCP Lond. 1947; MD Bristol 1958; FRCPath 1972, M 1963. Prof. Emerit. Neuropath. Univ. Lond.; Cons. Neuropathol. Lond. Hosp. Specialty: Neuropath. Socs: Sen. Mem. Brit. Neuropath. Soc. & Assn. Brit. Neurols. Prev: Asst. Research Neuropathol. Frenchay Hosp. Bristol; Demonst. (Path.) Univ. Bristol; Resid. Path. Bristol Roy. Infirm.

URIDGE, Christopher Frank Ashlea, Cane Lane, Gr., Wantage OX12 0AA — MB BS Lond. 1983.

URMILA-RAO, Naraharisetty Grosvenor Medical Centre, 62 Grosvenor Street, Stalybridge SK15 1RZ Tel: 0161 303 7250 Fax: 0161 303 8377 — MB BS Osmania 1967; MB BS Osmania 1967.

URMSTON, John Hewlett Brabazon (retired) Ranchlands, Landford Wood, Landford, Salisbury SP5 2ES Tel: 01794 390354 — MRCS Eng. LRCP Lond. 1947 (Camb. & St. Thos.) Civil Aviat. Auth. Approved Examr. for Aircrew. Prev: Sen. Ho. Surg. St. Thos. Hosp.

URQUHART, Alexander (retired) Knapp Hill House, Bath Road, Wells BA5 3HT — MB ChB Glas. 1947; DPM Eng. 1965. Prev: Cons. Psychiat. Mendip Hosp. Wells, Som.

URQUHART, Alexander Scott Ridley Medical Group, Blyth Health Centre, Blyth NE24 1DX Tel: 01670 354417 — MB BS Durh. 1951; FRCGP 1977, M 1960.

URQUHART, Andrew Duncan 23 Notting Hill, Belfast BT9 5NS — BM BCh Oxf. 1992; MA Oxf. 1995, BA 1989; MRCP (UK) 1995. Hon. Clin. Lect. Qu. Univ. Belf.; Cons. Phys. Altnagelvin Area Hosp. Derry. Specialty: Gen. Med. Prev: Research Fell. (Geriat. Med.) Qu.

Univ. Belf.; Regist. (Gen. Med./Endocrinol.) Belf. City Hosp.; Regist. (Geriat. Med) Belf. City. Hosp.

URQUHART, Anne 2 Kinn Barns, New Hutton, Kendal LA8 0AZ Tel: 01539 720 357 — MB ChB Dundee 1976; DRCOG 1978; MRCGP 1981; DFFP 1998.

URQUHART, Calum Culloden Surgery, Keppoch Road, Culloden, Inverness IV2 7LL Tel: 01463 793400 Fax: 01463 793060 — MB ChB Ed. 1987; MRCGP 1993. GP Culloden, Inverness.

URQUHART, Craig Stirling 69 Shelley Drive, Bothwell, Glasgow G71 8TA — MB ChB Glas. 1998.

URQUHART, Daniel Rennie Forth Park Maternity Hospital, Kirkcaldy KY2 5RA; 19 Whytehouse Avenue, Kirkcaldy KY1 1UW Tel: 01592 263239 — MD Aberd. 1990; MB ChB 1981; MRCOG 1986. Cons. Forth Pk. Matern. Hosp. Kirkcaldy. Specialty: Obst. & Gyn.

URQUHART, George Edwin Duthie (retired) 26A Dundee Road, West Ferry, Dundee DD5 1LX — MB ChB Ed. 1960; FRCPath 1979, M 1967. Prev: Cons. Microbiol. (Virol.) Virus Unit Dept. Bact. Med. Sch. Ninewells Hosp. Dundee.

URQUHART, Graham Wylie Department of Clinical Radiology, Torbay Hospital, Lawes Bridge, Torquay TQ2 7AA Tel: 01803 614567; The Farm House, 4 Higher Alston Farm, Alston Lane, Churston Ferrers, Brixham TQ5 0HT Tel: 01803 842599 — MB BS Queensland 1973; DMRD Eng. 1981; FRCR 1990. Cons. Diag. Radiol. Torbay Hosp. Torquay. Specialty: Radiol. Prev: Clin. Asst. (Diag. Radiol.) Torbay Hosp. Torquay; Sen. Regist. St. Mary's Hosp. Lond.

URQUHART, Mr Hector Maconochie (retired) Killiganoon, 20 Culduthel Road, Inverness IV2 4AJ Tel: 01463 233142 — MB ChB Ed. 1940; FRCS Ed. 1947.

URQUHART, James Frederick 112 Brighton Road, South Croydon CR2 6AD — MB BS Lond. 1954.

URQUHART, James Macconnell (retired) 35 Albany Terrace, Dundee DD3 6HS Tel: 01382 322928 — (Glas.) MB ChB Glas. 1941; DPH Eng. 1950; FFPHM 1980, M 1972. Prev: Dist. Med. Off. Dundee Health Dist.

URQUHART, John Cameron, Maj. RAMC Retd. West Suffolk Hospital, Department of Anaesthetics, Bury St Edmunds IP33 2QZ Tel: 01284 713000 Fax: 01284 701993 Email: john.urquhart@wsh.nhs.uk — MB BS Lond. 1985 (St. Thos. Hosp. Lond.) DA (UK) 1989; Cert. Av. Med. 1990; FRCA 1993. Cons. Anaesth. W. Suff. Hosp. Bury St. Edmunds. Specialty: Anaesth. Prev: Sen. Regist. Rotat. (Anaesth.) E. Anglia; Hon. Regist. (Anaesth.) Qu. Charlottes & Chelsea Hosp. Lond.

URQUHART, Margaret McRobb (retired) 10 Atwater Court, Faversham Road, Lenham, Maidstone ME17 2PW — MB ChB Aberd. 1946. Prev: Sessional Clin. Med. Off. SE Thames HA.

URQUHART, Rachael 6 Swalcliffe Road, Tadmarton, Banbury OX15 5TE — MB ChB Liverp. 1991; DRCOG 1994; DFFP 1996; MRCGP 1996. GP (Locum); CMO in Family Plann. Specialty: Gen. Pract. Prev: GP Partner Walton Health Centre, Walton-on-Thames, Surrey.

URQUHART, Ronald Pirie Macdonald (retired) 12 Langbourne Avenue, London N6 6AL Tel: 020 8348 3693 — MB ChB Ed. 1952; DPM Eng. 1958; FRCPsych 1986, M 1971. Prev: Staff Mem. Brent Cons. Centre & Centre for Research into Adolesc Breakdown.

URRUTY, Jean-Pierre The White House, High St., Conisbourough, Doncaster DN6 9AF — MB ChB Leeds 1964.

URRY, Pauline Althea (retired) 67 Heathcroft, Hampstead Way, London NW11 7HL Tel: 020 8731 9145 — MB ChB Cape Town 1947 (UCT) Prev: Cons. Neuropath. Whittington Hosp. Lond., Roy. Free Hosp. Lond. & Camden & Islington AHA (T).

URSELL, Christine Emily Highfield Health, 31 University Road, Highfield, Southampton SO17 1BJ Tel: 023 8059 5545; Storn, Pinelands Road, Chilworth, Southampton SO16 7HH — MB BS Newc. 1974; DCH Eng. 1977; DRCOG 1978. Phys. Soton. Univ. Prev: Trainee GP Yeovil VTS; SHO (Med.) Coppetts Wood Hosp. Lond.; Ho. Phys. Roy. Vict. Infirm. Newc.

URSELL, Mrs Kathleen Mary (retired) 25 Southfield Approach, Charlton Kings, Cheltenham GL53 9LN Tel: 01242 526883 — MB ChB Birm. 1943; DCH Eng. 1948. Prev: Child Health Serv. Glos.

URSELL, Mr Paul Gerry Sutton Hospital, Roy Harfitt Eye Unit, Cotswold Road, Sutton SM2 5NF Tel: 01372 221452 Fax: 01372 221446 Email: paul@cataract-doctor.com — MB BS Lond. 1989 (St. Mary's) FRCOphth 1995; MD Lond 2000. Cons. Ophthal. Epsom & St Hellier NHS Trust. Specialty: Ophth. Special Interest: Cataract Surg.; Cataract Surg. Research; Refractive Surg. Socs: FRCOphth; MDU; ESCRS. Prev: IRIS Fund Research Fell. (Ophth.) St. Thos. Hosp. Lond.; Clin. Lect. Nuffield Dept. Ophth. Univ. Oxf.; Anterior segment Fell., Lions Eye Inst., Perth Austral.

URSELL, Mr William William Harvey Hospital, Kennington Road, Willesborough, Ashford TN24 0LZ — MB BS Lond. 1960 (St. Geo.) MRCS Eng. LRCP Lond. 1960; FRCS Eng. 1967; FRCOG 1982, M 1969. Cons. O & G William Harvey Hosp. Ashford, Roy. Vict. Hosp Folkestone, Buckland Hosp. Dover; Vict. Hosp. Deal & Kent & Canterbury Hosp.; Examr. Centr. Midw. Bd. Specialty: Obst. & Gyn. Socs: Fell. Roy. Soc. Med. Prev: Sen. Regist. (O & G) King's Coll. Hosp. Lond.; Resid. Med. Off. Qu. Charlotte's Matern. Hosp. Lond.; SHO Hosp. Sick Childr. Gt. Ormond St. Lond.

URWIN, Gillian Department of Microbiology, Colchester General Hospital, Colchester CO4 5JL; Churchgate House, Rectory Hill, East Bergholt, Colchester CO7 6TG — MB BS Lond. 1986 (St. Thos. Hosp. Med. Sch.) MSc Lond. 1991; MRCPath 1993. Cons. Microbiol. Essex Rivers Healthcare Trust Colchester. Specialty: Med. Microbiol. Prev: Sen. Regist. (Med. Microbiol.) SE Thames Region; Lect. (Med. Microbiol.) Lond. Hosp.

URWIN, Mr Graeme Henry York District Hospital, Department of Urology, Wigginton Road, York YO31 8HE Tel: 01904 725610 Fax: 01904 726886 Email: graeme.h.urwin@york.nhs.uk — MD Sheff. 1989 (St. Mary's) MRCS Eng. LRCP Lond. 1975; MB BS Lond. 1975; FRCS Eng. 1979; Dip HSM York 1992. Cons. Urol. York Dist. Hosp. Specialty: Urol. Prev: Sen. Regist. (Urol. Surg.) Roy. Hallamsh. Hosp. Sheff.; Wellcome Surgic. Research Fell. Univ. Sheff.; Regist. (Gen. & Urol Surg.) Roy. Hallamsh. Hosp. Sheff.

URWIN, Keith (retired) Westbrook, Maer Road, Exmouth EX8 2DB Tel: 01395 265618 Email: keithurwin@yahoo.com — MRCS Eng. LRCP Lond. 1960 (Birm.) Prev: GP Cwmbran Gwent.

URWIN, Olive Mary (retired) 2 Laxton Grove, Trentham, Stoke-on-Trent ST4 8LR Tel: 01782 641843 — MRCS Eng. LRCP Lond. 1962 (Manch.) DA Eng. 1965; DPM Eng. 1976; MRCPsych 1977. Prev: Cons. Child & Family Psychiat. N. Staffs. HA.

URWIN, Stephen Windhill Green Medical Centre, 2 Thackley Old Road, Shipley BD18 1QB Tel: 01274 584223 Fax: 01274 530182; Glenwood, Stubbings Road, Baildon, Shipley BD17 5DZ — MB ChB Leeds 1981; DRCOG 1984; MRCGP 1985. GP Shipley.

URWIN, Susan Christine Peterborough General Hospital, Peterborough; 18 Highland Avenue, Norwich NR2 3NP — MB BS Lond. 1990; BSc Basic Med. Scs. & Pharmacol. Lond. 1987; MRCP (UK) 1994; FRCA 1997. Specialist Regist. (Anaesth.) Norf. & PeterBoro. Hosp. Specialty: Anaesth. Prev: Specialist Regist. - Norf. & Norwich Hosp.; SHO (Anaesth.) Addenbrooke's Hosp. Camb. & Lister Hosp. Stevenage; Regist. (Gen. Med.) Princess Margt. Hosp. Swindon.

USBORNE, Caroline Margaret 54 Grange Cross Lane, Wirral CH48 8BQ Tel: 0151 625 5001 — MB ChB Liverp. 1993; BSc Liverp. 1988. SHO (Cardiol. & Med.) Wirral. Prev: SHO (Gen. Med.) Roy. Liverp. Hosp.; Ho. Off. Broadgreen Hosp.

USHA, Tindivandam Ramakrishnan 1 Clos Du Parcq, Richmond Road, St Helier, Jersey JE2 3GL — MB BS Madras 1974.

USHER, Alan Stanley Guy 14 Crabtree Drive, Norwood, Sheffield S5 7AZ — MB ChB Sheff. 1986.

USHER, James Richard Cumberland House, Jordangate, Macclesfield SK10 1EG Tel: 01625 428081 Fax: 01625 503128; Greenacres, 155 Langley Road, Langley, Macclesfield SK11 0DR Tel: 0126025 2038 — MB ChB Birm. 1981; DRCOG 1985; DCH RCP Lond. 1985; MRCGP 1986. Specialty: Gen. Pract.

USHER, John Leonard 58 Victoria Road, Crosby, Liverpool L23 7XZ — MB BS Lond. 1998.

USHER, Natasha Elizabeth Dunbeath Surgery, Achorn Road, Dunbeath KW6 6EZ Tel: 01593 731205 — MB ChB Glas. 1993. GP Princip. in Dunbeath. Specialty: Gen. Pract. Prev: GP Regist. Centr. Health Centre Cumbernauld; Trainee GP/SHO Monklands Hosp. Airdrie; Ho. Off. (Med.) Vict. Infirm. Glas.

USHER, Stephen Mark 31 Watson's Walk, St Albans AL1 1PO — MB BCh Wales 1995; FRCA 2002.

USHER-SOMERS, Nicholas Erdington Medical Centre, 103 Wood End Road, Erdington, Birmingham B24 8NT Tel: 0121 373 0085 Fax: 0121 386 1768 — MB ChB Birm. 1976; DRCOG 1982;

MRCGP 1985. Prev: SHO King Edwd. VII Hosp. Midhurst & Dudley Guest Hosp.; Ho. Surg. Gen. Hosp. Birm.

USHERWOOD, Martin McDougall Stoke Mandeville Hospital NHS Trust, Mandeville Road, Aylesbury HP21 8AL Tel: 01296 316550 Fax: 01296 316144; Hermit's Cottage, Dinton, Aylesbury HP17 8UP Tel: 01296 748129 Fax: 01296 747813 — (Lond. Hosp.) MB BS Lond. 1967; MRCS Eng. LRCP Lond. 1967; DObst RCOG 1969; FRCOG 1984, M 1972; MFFP 1993. Cons. O & G Stoke Mandeville Hosp. NHS Trust; Asst. Med. Dir. Aylesbury; Chairm. Thames Valley Cancer Network TSSG; Chairm. Four Counties Colposcopy Gp.; Regional Adviser for RCOG Oxf. Region. Specialty: Obst. & Gyn. Socs: Fell. Roy. Soc. Med.; Brit. Soc. Colpos. & Cerv. Path.; BMA. Prev: Teach. (Obst. & Gyn.) Lond. Univ.; Sen. Regist. (O & G Unit) Lond. Hosp.; Chairm. Oxf. Regional Gyn. Cancer Gp.

USISKIN, Sasha Isadora 17 Northmoor Road, Oxford OX2 6UW — MB BCh Wales 1997.

USMAN, Farina 101 Shakespeare Avenue, Bath BA2 4RQ — BM Soton. 1991.

USMAN, Mr Tamoor Princess Royal Hospital, Apley Castle, Telford TF1 6TF — MB ChB Manch. 1989 (St. And. & Manch.) BSc (Hons.) St. And. 1986; FRCS Ed. 1993; FRCS Ed (Gen. Surg.) 2000. Cons. Gen. & Breast Surg. Princess Roy. Hosp. Telford. Specialty: Gen. Surg. Socs: BMA; BASO; ASGBI. Prev: SPR (Gen. Surg.) City Hosp. Birm.; Specialist Regist. (Gen. Surg.) Heartlands Hosp. Birm.

USMANI, Imran 21 Rectory Park Road, Sheldon, Birmingham B26 3LJ — BM BS Nottm. 1996.

USMANI, Mr Islam Ahmed 29A Sweetcroft Lane, Hillingdon, Uxbridge UB10 9LE Tel: 01252 863291 Fax: 01252 863288 — MB BS Lucknow 1962 (K.G. Med. Coll. Lucknow) FRCS Ed. 1977. Sen. Med. Off. (Civil.) MoD S.E. Dist. Aldershot. Prev: Sen. Med. Off. (RAF); Surgic. Regist. Sefton Hosp. Liverp.; Surgic. Regist. Roy. Albert Edwd. Infirm.

USMANI, Mumtaz Parveen 29A Sweetcroft Lane, Hillingdon, Uxbridge UB10 9LE Tel: 020 7202 8304 Fax: 020 7202 8314 — MB BS Lucknow 1962 (King. Geo. Med. Coll. Lucknow) DObst RCOG 1974. Sen. Med. Off. (Civil.) Camb. Milit. Hosp. Aldershot. Prev: Sen. Med. Off. (RAF) M.O.D.; Regist. (O & G) Wigan.

USMANI, Omar Sharif — MB BS Lond. 1993 (King's Coll. Sch. Med. & Dent. Lond.) MRCP (UK) 1996; CCST 2003. Specialist Regist. (Thoracic Med.) Lond. Specialty: Respirat. Med.; Gen. Med. Prev: Clin. Research Fell. (Respirat. Med.) Nat. Heart and Lung Inst. Lond.

USSELMANN, Bernhard Michael Dept. of Gastroenterol., Warwick Hospital, Lakin Road, Warwick CV34 5BW Tel: 01926 495321 — MB BChir Camb. 1991 (Camb. Univ.) MRCP (UK) 1994; MD Warwick 2002. Cons. (Gastroenterol.) Warwick Hosp. Warwick. Specialty: Gastroenterol.; Gen. Med. Prev: SpR (Gastroenterol. & Gen. Med.) Selly Oak Hosp. Birm.; SpR (Hepat.) Qu. Eliz. Hosp. B'ham; Research Regist., Gastroenterol., Univ of Warwick, Coventry.

USSHER, Christopher William James, LVO (retired) Stonecroft, Myrtle Road, Crowborough TN6 1EY Tel: 018926 654628 — MRCS Eng. LRCP Lond. 1947 (St. Bart.) FRCP Ed. 1981, M 1965. Prev: Exec. Med. Adviser Private Pats. Plan Tunbridge Wells.

USSHER, Jonathan Howard Parade Surgery, The Parade, Liskeard PL14 6AF Tel: 01579 342667 Fax: 01579 340650; Polgray, Tregay Lane, Liskeard PL14 6RQ Tel: 01579 342960 — MB BS Lond. 1970 (St. Bart.) MRCS Eng. LRCP Lond. 1971; MRCGP 1975; DRCOG 1977. Specialty: Gen. Pract.

USTIANOWSKI, Andrew Peter Drusus de Sas — MB BS Lond. 1991; MRCP (UK) 1994; DTM & H RCP Lond. 1995; PhD (University of London) 2002; PCME (University of Brighton) 2003. SPR Medical Microbiology, Royal Free Hosp., London. Specialty: Infec. Dis.; Gen. Med.; Trop. Med. Prev: Regist. (Infec. Dis.) Harold Wood Hosp. Essex; Research Fell. & Hon. Lect. (Infec. Dis.s) Univ. Coll. Lond. Med. Sch.; Infec. Dis.s SpR, Univ. Coll. Lond.

USTIANOWSKI, Peter Andrew Swanfield Farm, Foots Lane, Burwash Weald, Etchingham TN19 7LE Tel: 01435 882797 Email: ustianowski_peter@hotmail.com — MB BS Lond. 1965 (Guy's) MRCS Eng. LRCP Lond. 1963; DObst RCOG 1965; Cert. Family Plann. JCC 1970; MFHom 1971; FFHom 2003. Cons. Phys. (Homeop. Med) Working from home & at Nelson's Clinic, Lond. Specialty: Homeop. Med. Socs: Assur. Med. Soc.; Brit. Soc. Med. & Dent. Hypn.; Fell.Roy.Soc.Med. Prev: Cons. Phys. (Homoeop. Med. & Hypnother.) Betteshanger, Near Deal, Kent; Resid. (O & G) Coventry Hosp. Gp.; Fell. & Clin. Asst. (Med. & Dermat.) Roy. Lond. Homoeop. Hosp.

USZYCKA, Barbara Stefania Aleksandra 15 The Greenway, Rayner's Lane, Pinner HA5 5DR — MB BS Lond. 1992.

UTHAYAKUMAR, Sundaralingam Department of Sexual Health and HIV, North Herts NHS Trust, Lister Hospital, Woodlands Clinic, Correys Mill Lane, Stevenage SG1 4AB Tel: 01438 314333 Ext: 4548 Fax: 01438 781545 Email: di.ithayakumai@nhs.net — MB BS Ceylon 1983; MRCS Eng. LRCP Lond. 1987; MRCOG 1993; MFFP 1994. Cons. Genito-Urin. Phys. Lister Hosp. Stevenage Herts. Specialty: Genitourinary Medicine. Special Interest: Bacterial Vaginosis; Vulval Dermatosis. Socs: BAASH.

UTIDJIAN, Haig Leon Dikran (retired) 3 The Spinney, Sudbury Hill Close, Wembley HA0 2QS Tel: 020 8904 3996 — MB BS Lond. 1954 (Univ. Coll. Hosp.) Prev: GP Wembley.

UTIDJIAN, Margaret Rosemary Anahid (retired) Maternity Unit, Harold Wood Hospital, Gubbins Lane, Romford RM3 0BE Tel: 01708 345533; 20 Harrow Drive, Hornchurch RM11 1NU Tel: 01708 470694 — MB BS Lond. 1960 (Univ. Coll. Hosp.) MRCS Eng. LRCP Lond. 1960; FRCOG 1979, M 1966, DObst 1964. Cons. O & G Havering Hosps. NHS Trust. Prev: Regist. (O & G) Hackney Hosp.

UTTING, Helen Jessica Wakelin Anaesthetic Department, Basildon Hospital, Basildon SS16 5NL Tel: 01268 593422 Fax: 01268 593948 — FRCA; MB BS Queensland 1964; FFA RCS Eng. 1969. Cons. Anaesth. Basildon & Thurrock Gen. Hosps. Trust. Specialty: Anaesth. Socs: Roy. Soc. Med.; BMA. Prev: Sen. Regist. Manch. Region & Roy. Lond. Hosp.

UTTING, John Arthur Broomfield Hospital, Chelmsford CM1 7ET Tel: 01245 440761 — MB BS Western Australia 1965 (W. Austral.) FRCP Lond. 1987, M 1969. Cons. Phys. Broomfield Hosp. Chelmsford. Specialty: Gen. Med. Socs: Fell. Roy. Soc. Med. Prev: Sen. Med. Regist. Baguley Hosp. Manch.

UTTING, Matthew Robert 84 Heyscroft Road, Manchester M20 4UZ — MB ChB Manch. 1997.

UTTING, Sarah Michele — MB ChB Birm. 1991; DRCOG 1994; MRCGP 1995. GP Princip., WaterLa. Surg., Brixton Water La., Lond. Specialty: Gen. Pract. Prev: VTA, St Geo.s Hosp. Med. Sch.; Trainee/Regist. G,P Morden Hall Med. Centre.; SHO (O & G & Paediat.) St. Geo. Hosp. Lond.

UTTLEY, Mr David (retired) Burrellhill, Skirwith, Penrith CA10 1RL Tel: 01768 88669 — MB ChB Leeds 1958; FRCS Ed. 1965; FRCS Glas. 1966. Prev: 1st Asst. Dept. Neurosurg. Nat. Hosp. Qu. Sq. Lond.

UTTLEY, Joanna Mary Clare 2 Clarendon Crescent, Edinburgh EH4 1PT Tel: 0131 332 6780 — MB ChB Glas. 1961; DObst RCOG 1963; Dip Occ Med 1995; Dip Occ Med London 1995. Specialty: Occupat. Health; Gen. Med. Prev: Lect. & Regist. (Path.) Univ. Edin.; Occupat. Phys. Roy. Infirm. Edin.

UTTLEY, William Richard Morningside Medical Practice, 2 Morningside Place, Edinburgh EH10 5ER Tel: 0131 332 6780 Email: billutt.comm.msn; Whakapapa Ski Field, Top of the Bruce, National Park North Island, New Zealand Tel: 00 64 07 892 3738 — MB ChB Ed. 1991; DRCOG 1994; MRCGP 1996. Whakapapa Ski Doctor New Zealand. Specialty: Sports Med. Prev: Whakapara Ski Doctor, NZ; GP Trainee Aberd.

UTTLEY, William Sutcliffe (retired) 2 Clarendon Crescent, Edinburgh EH4 Tel: 0131 332 6780 — MB ChB Ed. 1961; DObst RCOG 1963; DCH Eng. 1964; FRCP Ed. 1976, M 1965. Prev: Ho. Phys. & Ho. Surg. Edin. Roy. Infirm.

UWECHUE, Mr Joseph Lawrence Emeka — Lekarz Krakow 1972; Lekarz Krakow, Poland 1972; FRCS Ed. 1979; Dip Urol. . Lond. 1990. Cons. Surg. Milit. Hosp. Benin City, Nigeria. Specialty: Gen. Surg. Prev: Sen. Regist. (Surg.) Univ. Benin Teach. Hosp. Benin City, Nigeria.

UZOCHUKWU, Boniface Chidi 8 Holt Way, Leeds LS16 7QP — MB BS Ibadan 1977; MRCOG 1987. Regist. (O & G) Dewsbury Dist. Hosp. Specialty: Obst. & Gyn. Prev: Regist. (O & G) Forth Pk. Hosp. Kirkcaldy; Acting Regist. (O & G) Worcester Roy. Infirm.; SHO (O & G) New Cross Hosp. Wolverhampton.

UZOHO, Mr Rufus 10 Grove Place, Hartspring lane, Aldenham, Watford WD25 8AH Mob: 07958 973690 Fax: 020 8869 2864 Email: uzoho@hotmail.com — MB BS Nigeria 1976. Assoc.

Specialist (Obst. & Gyn.) Northwick Pk. Hosp. Harrow. Specialty: Obst. & Gyn. Special Interest: Urogynaecology.

UZOIGWE, Augustine Onuoha Department of Anaesthetics, Pontefract General Infirmary, Pontefract WF8 1PL Tel: 01977 792361 — MB BS Ibadan 1971; DA Eng. 1982.

UZOKA, Anthony Anene Eworitsemogha Grovemead Health Partnership, 67 Elliot Road, Hendon, London NW4 3EB Tel: 020 8203 4466 Fax: 020 8203 1682; No. 1 Jones Cottage, Barnet Road, Arkley, Barnet EN5 3LH Tel: 020 8441 8554 Fax: 020 8441 8554 — MB BCh BAO NUI 1992 (University College Dublin) DRCOG 1994; MRCGP 1997. GP Princip. Specialty: Paediat. Dent.

UZOKA, Kenneth Amechi Oritsetimeyin 30 Harcourt Road, London E15 3DU — MB BCh BAO NUI 1990.

UZOKWE, Christopher Osita King Fahad Hospital, PO Box 204, Al Baha, Saudi Arabia Tel: 00 966 7 7254000 — MB BS Lagos 1982; MRCP (UK) 1991. Cons. Emerg. Med. King Fahad Hosp. Al Baha, Saudi Arabia. Specialty: Accid. & Emerg. Prev: Regist. Trafford Gen. Hosp. Manch., Preston Roy. Infirm. & Manch. Roy. Infirm.

VAAL, Michiel Franciscus Rothwell & Desborough Health Care Group, 35 High St., Desborough, Kettering NN14 2NB — Artsexamen Rotterdam 1989.

VACHHANI, Maganlal Khimchand 103 Doris Road, Spark Hill, Birmingham B11 4ND — MB BS Gujarat 1969 (M.P. Shah Med. Coll. Jamnagar) SHO (Urol.) Vict. Hosp. Burnley.

VADEYAR, Hemant Jitendra North Manchester General Hospital, Delauneys Road, Crumpsall, Manchester M8 5RB Tel: 0161 720 2573 Fax: 0161 720 2228 Email: hemant.vadeyar@mail.nmanhe-tr.nwest.nhs.uk — MB BS Bombay 1988 (Univ. of Bombay) MS 1990; FRCS 1996; FRCS (Gen.) 2000. Cons. Hepato-Pancreato-Biliary Surg., N. Manch. Gen. Hosp. Specialty: Gen. Surg. Special Interest: Hepato-Pancreato-Biliary Surgery. Socs: ASGBI; AVGIS; IMPBA. Prev: Specialist Regist. Gen. Surg., Sherwood Forest Hosp.; Specialist Regist. Gen. Surg., UHB; Specialist Regist. Gen. Surg., Derby City Hosp.

VADGAMA, Bhumita Great Ormond Street Hospital for Sick Children, Department of Histopathology, Camella-Botnar Labratories, Great Ormond Street, London WC1N 3JH Tel: 020 7829 8663 Fax: 020 7829 7875 — MB ChB Leic. 1992; MRCPath 2002.

VADGAMA, Professor Pankaj Maganlal Interdisciplinary Research Centre (IRC) in Biomedical Materials, Queen Mary Unv. London, Mile End Road, London E1 4NS Tel: 020 7882 5151 Fax: 020 8983 1799 — MB BS Newc. 1971; Cphys FInstP; PhD Newc. 1984, BSc (1st cl. Hons.) Chem. 1976; FRCPath 1988, M 1977; CChem 1996; FRSC 1996. Prof. Clin. Biochem. & Hon. Cons. Chem. Path. Qu. Mary Univ. Lond. Barts & Roy. Lond. Specialty: Chem. Path. Socs: Assn. Clin. Biochem. Prev: Prof. Clin. Biochem. & Hon. Cons. Chem. Path. Univ. Manch.; Hon. Cons. Chem. Path. Roy. Vict. Infirm. Newc.; MRC Train. Fell.

VADGAMA, Sanjay 70 Brampton Road, London NW9 9DD; 9 Cranleigh Gardens, Harrow HA3 0UP — MB BS Lond. 1996.

VADHER, Sapna 5 Roydale Close, Loughborough LE11 5UW — MB ChB Sheff. 1998; MB ChB Sheff 1998.

VAFAIE, Kasra 27 Warneford Street, London E9 7NG — MB BS Lond. 1993.

VAFIDIS, Gillian Clare 23 Hurst Avenue, London N6 5TX — MB BS Lond. 1978 (Guy's) FRCS Eng. 1985; FCOphth 1989. Cons. Ophth. Edgware Gen. Hosp. Specialty: Ophth.

VAFIDIS, Mr Jonathan Anthony 8 Albert Crescent, Penarth CF64 Tel: 029 2070 3702 — MB Camb. 1977 (Guy's) MA Camb. 1976, MB 1977, BChir 1976; FRCS Eng. 1981. Cons. Neurosurg. Univ. Hosp. Wales. Specialty: Neurosurg. Socs: Soc. Brit. Neurol. Surg. Prev: Sen. Regist. & Regist. (Neurosurg.) Radcliffe Infirm. Oxf.

VAGGERS, Stewart David St George's Hospital, The Hatherton Centre, Corporation Street, Stafford ST16 3AG Tel: 01785 221342 Fax: 01785 221371 Email: dr.vaggers@ssh-tr.nhs.uk — MB ChB Leeds 1985; BSc (Psychol.) Leeds 1982; MRCPsych 1990; LLM (Legal Aspects of Med. Pract.) Cardiff 2001. Cons. Forens. Psychiat. S. Staffs. Healthcare NHS Trust. Specialty: Forens. Psychiat. Special Interest: Medicine & the Law. Prev: Regist. (Psychiat.) Glenside Hosp. Bristol.

VAGHADIA, Himat Department of Anaesthetics, Vancouver General Hospital, 855 West 12th Avenue, Vancouver BC V5Z 1M9, Canada Tel: 604 875 4575 Fax: 604 875 5209; 21 Crescent Drive S., Woodingdean, Brighton BN2 6RA Tel: 01273 306974 — MB BS Lond. 1979 (St. Bart.) BSc (Special) Lond. 1976, MB BS 1979; FFA RCS Eng. 1984; LMCC 1985; FRCPC 1986. Head Div. (Ambulatory Anaesth.) Vancouver Gen. Hosp. Surgic. Day Care Centre; Cons. Staff Anaesth. Vancouver Gen. Hosp. & Assoc. Anaesth. Servs.; Prof. Anaesth. Univ. Brit Columbia; Assoc. Staff (Anaesth.) P. Geo. Region Hosp., Richmond Gen. Hosp; Peace Arch Hosp., Mt. St. Josephs Hosp. & St. Vincent Hosp. Brit. Columbia. Specialty: Anaesth. Socs: Canad. Anaesth. Soc. & Brit. Columbia Asnaesth. Assn. Prev: Regist. (Anaesth.) Roy. Free, Middlx., Qu. Charlotte's, Soho & Eastman Dent. Hosps. Lond.; Clin. & Research Fell. (Anaesth.) Vancouver Gen. Hosp. & Univ. Brit. Columbia Canada; Resid. (Anaesth.) Vancouver Gen. Hosp., St. Paul's Hosp., Grace Matern. Hosp. & Brit. Columbia Childr. Hosp. Canada.

VAGHANI, Jethalal Tapubhai The Health Centre, High Street, Dodworth, Barnsley S75 3RF Tel: 01226 203881 — MB BS Saurasthra 1978. GP Barnsley, S. Yorks.

VAGHELA, Harkishan Kanji Malabar Road Medical Centre, 60 Malabar Road, Leicester LE1 2PD Tel: 0116 251 8047; 26 Mount Pleasant, Oadby, Leicester LE2 4UA Tel: 0116 271 8381 — MB ChB Leic. 1981; BSc (Hons.) Leic. 1979. Specialty: Gen. Pract.

VAGHELA, Hersad Mohan 51 Trowell Avenue, Nottingham NG8 2DW — MB BS Lond. 1997; BSc Lond. 1994; MRCSEd 2001; MRCS Eng. 2001; DLO R.C.S.Eng. 2002.

VAGHELA, Naresh Narshi Loughborough University Medical Centre, Loughborough University of Technology, Loughborough LE11 3TU Tel: 01509 222061 — MB ChB Leic. 1985 (Leicester) BSc Leic. 1983; DRCOG 1988. GP Princip. Med. Centre LoughBoro. Univ.; Hosp. Prat. Diabetes. Socs: BMA.

VAGHMARIA, Anil Birches Head Medical Centre, Diana Road, Birches Head, Stoke-on-Trent ST1 6RS Tel: 01782 286843 — MB ChB Birm. 1973 (Godfrey Huggins Med. Sch. Salisbury) DCH S. Afr. 1976; MSc (Primary Med. Care) Keele 1992. GP on flexible career scheme. Specialty: Rheumatol.; Educat. Prev: Regist. (Paediat.) N. Staffs. Matern. Hosp.; SHO (Paediat.) Birm. Childr. Hosp.; SHO (Paediat.) Hammersmith Hosp. Lond.

VAHDATI-BOLOURI, Mitra 13 Woodside Grove, Henbury, Bristol BS10 7RF Tel: 07876 744716 — MB BS Lond. 1996 (Charing Cross and Westminster) BSc Lond. 1995. Locum Medical Registrar. Specialty: Gen. Med. Prev: Ski Field Doctor, New Zealand; Medical Registrar, New Zealand; Clinical Fellow Acute Medicine, Bristol Royal Infirmary.

VAHID ASSR, Mohammad Djamel Site 56, Bradford Heights, Carrickfergus BT38 9EB Tel: 01960 360829; 25 Red Fort Drive, Bradford heights, Carrickfergus BT38 9EB Tel: 01960 360829 Email: djamelvahidassr@hotmail.com — MB BCh BAO Belf. 1991 (Queen's University Belfast) MRCP (UK) 1994; MD Belf. 1997. Specialist Regist. Specialty: Gen. Med.; Care of the Elderly. Socs: BGS.

VAID, Jaishi The Oaks, 5 Blakebrook, Kidderminster DY11 6AP Tel: 01562 755119 — MB BS Osmania 1971; MD (Paediat.) Osmania 1976; DCH RCPS Glas. 1977; Dip. Community Paediat. Warwick 1983; FRCPCH 1997. Cons., Community Paediat., Telford and Wrekin Primary Care Trust. Specialty: Paediat. Socs: Kidderminster Med. Soc.; Brit. Assn. of Community Child Health; Roy. Coll. of Paediat. and Child Health. Prev: SCMO (Child Health) Kidderminster Health Care NHS Trust & Kidderminster Gen. Hosp.; Regist. (Paediat.) Geo. Elliott Hosp. Nuneaton; Resid. Postgrad. Inst. Child Health Niloufer Hosp. Hyderabad.

VAID, Muhammad Ashraf Ebrahim 234 Arbroath Road, Dundee DD4 7SB — MB BS Karachi 1979; MRCP (UK) 1989.

VAID, Sudha Clare Street Surgery, 6 Clare Street, Riverside, Cardiff CF11 6BB Tel: 029 2066 4450 Fax: 029 2066 6466; 6 Clare Street, Riversdale, Cardiff CF11 6BB Tel: 029 2066 4450 — MB BS Punjab (India) 1961. Socs: Assoc. Mem. Fac. Hom. NHS Med. Pract.; Med. Protec. Soc.

VAID, Sundar Jaishi Alexander Road Surgery, 32 Alexander Road, Darlaston, Wednesbury WS10 9LJ Fax: 0121 526 2546; The Oaks, 5 Blakebrook, Kidderminster DY11 6AP — MB BS Madras 1976; BSc (Chem.) Madras 1970; DA (UK) 1980. Socs: Fac. Fam. Plann. & Reproduc. Health Care. Prev: Trainee GP Wolverhampton.

VAID, Vrunda 51 Kendal Drive, Gatley, Cheadle SK8 4QJ Tel: 0161 611 9023; The Oaks, 5 Blakebrook, Kidderminster DY11 6AP Tel: 01562 755119 — MB ChB Manch. 1998; DRCOG 2000; MRCGP 2002. HO, Med., Withington Hosp. Manch. Prev: HO, Surg. Roy. Oldham Hosp. Oldham.

VAIDYA, Abhay Chorley and South Ribble Hospital, Department of Anaesthetics, Preston Road, Chorley PR7 1PP Tel: 01257 245771 Fax: 01257 245776 — MB BS Bombay 1982; MD (Anaesth); FRCA. Cons. (Aneasth.) Chorley & S. Ribble Hosp. Specialty: Anaesth.

VAIDYA, Ashwinkumar Liladhar 128 Wigan Road, Ormskirk L39 2BA — MB BS Bombay 1980; FRCA 1993. Staff Grade (Anaesth.) Ormskirk Dist. & Gen. Hosp. Lancs. Specialty: Anaesth. Socs: BMA.

VAIDYA, Mr Dinesh Vithal Department of Urology, Treliske Hospital, Treliske, Truro TR1 3LJ — MB BS Bombay 1986; FRCS Ed. 1991.

VAIDYA, Gunvantrai Ambaram 140 Newdegate Road, Bedworth, Nuneaton CV12 8EP — MB BS Bombay 1947 (Grant Med. Coll.) Clin. Med. Off. Nuneaton (N. Warks.) Health Dist.

VAIDYA, Rajnikant Babubhai (retired) 18 Infield Park, Barrow-in-Furness LA13 9JL — MB BS Bombay 1954 (G.S. Med. Coll.) MRCOG 1967, DObst 1962. Prev: SHO (Gen. Surg.) Gen. Hosp. Burnley.

VAIDYA, Shashikant Mohanlal Faifield General Hospital, Roch House, Faifield General Hospital, Rochdale Old Road, Bury BL9 7TD Tel: 0161 778 3509 Email: drsmvaiaya@hotmail.com — MB BS Gujerat 1976; DGP Keele 1998; DPM Ireland 1998. Cons. Psychiat. Pennine Care NHS Trust, Bury. Specialty: Gen. Psychiat. Special Interest: Affective Disorders. Socs: Affective Disorders Gp.; Manch. Med. Soc. Prev: Povincial Psychiat. in Zimbabwe.

VAIDYANATHAN, Subramanian Regional Spinal Injuries Centre, District General Hospital, Town Lane, Kew, Southport PR8 6PN Tel: 01704 547471 — MB BS Madras 1970; MS Post. Inst. Med. Educ. & Res. Chandigash India 1974; MCh Post. Inst. Med. Educ. & Res., Chandigash India 1976; Dip Urol New Delhi India 1978; PhD Post. Inst. Med. Educ. & Res., Chandigash India 1984. Staff Grade Regional Spinal Injuries Centre Southport. Specialty: Orthop. Socs: BMA; Inter. Med. Soc. Paraplegia. Prev: Trust Doctor Regional Spinal Injuries Centre, Southport; Vis. Prof. to the Univ. of Mass., Worcester, MA, USA.

VAILE, Elizabeth City Medical Services Ltd., 17 St Helen's Place, London EC3A 6DE Tel: 020 7638 3001 — MB BS Lond. 1962 (King's Coll. Hosp.) MRCS Eng. LRCP Lond. 1962; DObst RCOG 1965; T(GP) 1991. Med. Off. City Med. Servs. Ltd. Specialty: Occupat. Health. Prev: Ho. Phys. King's Coll. Hosp. Lond.; Ho. Surg. S. Lond. Hosp. Wom.; Ho. Off. (Obst.) Roy. Vict. Hosp. Bournemouth.

VAILE, Howard Graham (retired) 27 Woodlands, Pickwick, Corsham SN13 0DA Tel: 01249 715035 Email: hgv@bigfoot.com — MB BS Lond. 1962 (King's Coll. Hosp.) MRCS Eng. LRCP Lond. 1962; DIH Soc. Apoth. Lond. 1969; FFOM RCP Lond. 1990, M 1978; T(OM) 1991; FRCP Lond. 1999. p/t Cons. Occupat. Med. Prev: Chief Med. Off. BBC Lond.

VAILE, Julian Charles 16 Sycamore Road, Bournville, Birmingham B30 2AD — MB ChB Birm. 1991; ChB Birm. 1991; MRCP (UK) 1994. Regist. (Cardiol.) Qu. Eliz. Hosp. Birm. Specialty: Cardiol.

VAILE, Michael Steel Berkeley 63 Joy Lane, Whitstable CT5 4DD Tel: 01227 272058 — MB BS Lond. 1962 (St Thos.) DA Eng. 1964; DObst RCOG 1965; MRCGP 1976; FFPHM RCP (UK) 1987; FRCP 1998. Specialty: Pub. Health Med. Socs: Fell. Roy. Soc. Med. Prev: Dir. (Pub. Health Med.) W. Kent HA.

VAILLANT, Charles Harry Cavendish Medical Centre, 214 Park Road North, Birkenhead CH41 8BU Tel: 0151 652 1955; 88 Shrewsbury Road, Birkenhead CH43 6TF — MB ChB Liverp. 1978; PhD Liverp. 1971, BSc (Hons.) 1968; MRCS Eng. LRCP Lond. 1978; DRCOG 1983. Specialty: Gen. Med.

VAIRAVAN, Mr Manickam Sandwell & West Birmingham Hospitals NHS Trust, Sandwell Hospital, West Bromwich B71 4HJ Tel: 0121 607 3219 Fax: 0121 607 7970; 2 Warren House Walk, The Avenue, Walmley, Sutton Coldfield B76 1TS — MB BS Madras 1984; FRCS Glas. 1990; FRCS Ed. 1990; FRCS (Ins. Collegiate) 2000; Specialist Register 2001. Cons. Surg. Sandwell & W. Birm. Hosps. NHS Trust. Specialty: Gen. Surg. Socs: FICS 1995; Assn. Surg.; BMA. Prev: Regist. (Surg.) Neath Gen. Hosp., Mt. Vernon Hosp. Middlx. & Nevill Hall Hosp. Abergavenny; Staff Surg. St Mary's Hosp. Newport, I. of Wight; Regist. Surg. Nevill Hall Hosp. Abergavenny.

VAIZEY, Ms Carolynne Jane St Mark's Hospital, Watford Road, Harrow HA1 3UJ Tel: 020 8235 4132 Fax: 020 8235 4277 Email: carolynne.vaizey@nwlh.nhs.uk — MB ChB Cape Town 1982; FCS South Africa; MD Lond.; FRCS (Gen.) 1994. Clin. Sen. Lect. & Hon. Cons. St Mark's Hosp. Harrow. Specialty: Gen. Surg. Special Interest: Anal problems; Colorectal cancer; Faecal incontinence. Socs: Assn. Colorectal Surg. Prev: Cons. Colorectal Surg., The Middlx. Hosp.; Hon. Sen. Lect., Univ. Coll. Lond.

VAIZEY, Mary Jane (retired) Drove House, Gipsey Bridge, Boston PE22 7DB Tel: 01205 280388 Fax: 01205 280388 Email: mjvaizey@doctors.org.uk — (Oxf.) BM BCh Oxf. 1965; MA Oxf. 1965; DCH Eng. 1968; MRCP (UK) 1970; FRCP Lond. 1989; FRCPCH 1997. Prev: Cons. Paediat. Pilgrim Hosp. Boston.

VAJA, Kanji Harji (retired) — MB BS Gujarat 1963 (B.J. Med. Coll. Ahmedabad) Prev: Salaried G.P (PMS Pilot) Heart of Birm., PCG.

VAJA, Rakesh 44 Cross Road, Croydon CR0 6TA — MB ChB Leeds 1994. SHO (Anaesth.) Mayday Univ. Hosp. Thornton Heath. Prev: SHO (A & E Med.) Colchester Gen. Hosp.; Ho. Off. (Surg.) Leicester Gen. Hosp.; Ho. Off. (Med.) Leeds Infirm.

VAKHARIA, Bipin Ramaniklat Galleries Health Centre, Washington Centre, Washington NE38 7NQ Tel: 0191 416 1841 — MB BS Gujarat 1972. GP Washington, Tyne & Wear.

VAKIL, Anita Sandhurst Group Practice, 72 Yorktown Road, Sandhurst GU47 9BT Tel: 01344 777015 Fax: 01344 777226 — MB BS Lond. 1991 (Charing Cross & Westminster) DCH RCP Lond. 1995; DRCOG 1995; MRCGP 1996; DFFP 1996. GP Princip.

VAKIL, Mary Alice Osborne (retired) 54 Bonser Road, Twickenham TW1 4RG Tel: 020 8892 8659 — MB BCh BAO Belf. 1949 (Queen's Univ.) Prev: SCMO (Child Health) Wandsworth Community Health.

VAKIL, Pervez Ardeshir Friars Walk, 29 Cedar Road, Farnborough GU14 7AU — MB BS Bombay 1957; DObst RCOG 1970.

VAKIL, Sarosh Dhunjishaw (cons. rooms), 11 Moor Park Avenue, Preston PR1 6AN; Fiddlers Green, Walker Lane, Fulwood, Preston PR2 7AP — MB BS Lond. 1959; FRCP Lond. 1979, M 1967; FRCP Ed. 1980.

VAKIS, Mr Stelios 117 More Close, St Pauls Court, London W14 9BW; 21 Hann Road, Rownhams, Southampton SO16 8LN — MB BS Lond. 1989; FRCS Ed. 1994.

VALABHJI, Prassankumar (retired) The Paddock, 124A Heol Isaf, Radyr, Cardiff CF15 8EA — MB BCh Wales 1960 (Cardiff) MRCP (U.K.) 1964; FRCP Lond. 1981. Cons. Phys. E. Glam. Gen. Hosp. Prev: Med. Regist. Miners Treatm. Centre Llandough Hosp.

VALDEZ, Frederick Neville 8 Hillside View, Denton, Manchester M34 7EZ Tel: 0161 320 5419 — M.B., Ch.B. Manch. 1945.

VALDIMARSSON, Professor Helgi Department Immunology, Landspitalinn, The National University Hospital, Reykjavik 101, Iceland Tel: 00 354 543 5800 Ext: 5814 Fax: 00 354 5434828 Email: helgiv@landspitali.is; [New Address]; Laekjaras 16, Reykjavik 101, Iceland Tel: 00 354 5 572381 — Cand Med et Chir Reykjavik 1964 (Univ. Iceland) FRCPath Lond. 1991, M 1986. Director & Prof. Immunol. Univ. Iceland; Vis. Prof. Immunol. St. Mary's Hosp. Med. Sch. Lond. Specialty: Immunol.; Allergy. Socs: FRCPath; Icelandic Med. Soc.; Icelandic Assn. Allergy & Clin. Immunol. Prev: Sen. Lect. & Hon. Cons. (Immunol.) St. Mary's Hosp. Med.; Hon. Lect & Regist. Roy. Postgrad. Med. Sch.

VALE, John Allister City Hospital NHS Trust, Birmingham B18 7QH Tel: 0121 507 4123 Fax: 0121 507 5580 — MB BS Lond. 1968 (Guy's) MRCS Eng. LRCP Lond. 1968; MRCP (UK) 1973; MD Lond. 1980; FRCP Lond. 1984; FFOM RCP Lond. 1992; FRCP Ed. 1994; FRCP Glas. 1997. Dir. Nat. Poisons Informat. Serv. & W. Midl. Poisons Unit & Cons. Clin. Pharmacol. City Hosp. NHS Trust; Examr. MRCP (UK) & AFOM; Chairm. MRCP (UK) Part 1 Exam. Bd. & Sec. MRCP (UK) Policy Comm.; Censor Roy. Coll. of Physicians of Lond. Specialty: Pharmacology; Gen. Med.; Occupat. Health. Socs: Brit. Pharm. Soc.; Fell. Amer. Acad. Clin. Toxicol. 1988; (President-elect) Brit. Toxicol. Soc. Prev: Co-Dir. Centre for Chem. Incidents Birm.; Trustee Amer. Acad. Clin. Toxicol.; Pres. Europ. Assn. Poisons Centres & Clin. Toxicol.

VALE, Mrs Joyce Cecile, MBE (retired) 7 Glebe Field, Georgeham, Braunton EX33 1QL — MB BS Lond. 1959. Cytologist Guy's Hosp. Lond.

VALE, Mr Justin Alastair Department of Urology, St. Mary's Hospital, Praed St., London W2 1NY; 76 The Avenue, London W13 8LB — MB BS Lond. 1984; FRCS Eng. 1988; BSc Lond. 1981,

MS 1992; FRCS (Urol.) 1993. Cons. Urol. Surg. St. Mary's Hosp. Lond. Specialty: Urol. Prev: Sen. Regist. (Urol.) St. Mary's Hosp. Lond.

VALE, Kathryn Elliott Old Orchard, Chapel Hill, Sedlescombe, Battle TN33 0QX — BM BCh Oxf. 1974; DRCOG 1977; MRCPsych 1979; MRCGP 1981.

VALE, Philip Temple The Beeeches, School Lane, Bronington, Whitchurch SY13 3HN — MB BS Durh. 1960; DIH Soc. Apoth. Lond. 1972; FFOM RCP Lond. 1990, MFOM 1978. Specialty: Occupat. Health. Prev: Sen. Employm. Med. Adviser EMAS.

VALE, Raymond John 7 Clebefield, Georgeham, Braunton EX33 1QL Tel: 01271 890684 Email: rayvale@aol.com — MB BS Lond. 1948 (Guy's) MRCS Eng. LRCP Lond. 1948; DA Eng. 1950; FFA RCS Eng. 1954; FRCP Ed. 1969, M 1954. Emerit. Cons. Anaesth. Guy's Hosp. & Chelsea Hosp. for Wom. Lond. Specialty: Anaesth. Socs: Assn. Anaesth.; Fell. Roy. Soc. Med. (Mem. Sect. Anaesth.). Prev: Res. Anaesth. Guy's Hosp. & Maxillo-Facial & Plastic Surg. Unit E.; Grinstead.

VALE, Simon Sebastian Harley House Surgery, 2 Irnham Road, Minehead TA24 5DL Tel: 01643 703441 Fax: 01643 704867 — MB BS Lond. 1988; BSc Lond. 1979; MRCGP 1992. GP Harley Ho. Surg. Minehead; Hosp. Practioner Accdent and Emergncy Minehead; Clin. Asst. Som. Drugs Serv. Taunton. Specialty: Gen. Pract. Socs: MRCGP.

VALEINIS, Mara 332 Oakwood Lane, Leeds LS8 3LF Tel: 0113 248 7407 — MRCS Eng. LRCP Lond. 1967.

VALENTE, Jane Elizabeth The Old Rectory, 1 Church St., Fen Ditton, Cambridge CB5 8SU Tel: 01223 292234 — MB BS Lond. 1987; MRCP (UK) 1993. Paediat. Cons. Hinchingbrooke Hosp. Huntingdon. Specialty: Paediat.; Respirat. Med. Prev: Sen. Regist. (Paediat.) Camb.

VALENTINE, Amor Adam (retired) 9 Towers Drive, Kirby Muxloe, Leicester LE9 2EW Tel: 0116 239 2234 — MB ChB St. And. 1940 (Dundee) DPM Lond. 1951; FRCPsych 1971. Prev: Med. Supt. & Cons. Psychiat. Glenfrith Hosp. Leic.

VALENTINE, Mr Brian Harvey (retired) The Paddock, 96 High St, Westham, Pevensey BN24 5LJ Tel: 01323 768070 — MB BS Lond. 1966 (Guy's) MRCS Eng. LRCP Lond. 1966; DObst 1973; FRCOG 1991, M 1975; FRCS Ed. 1975. Locum (Ret.). Prev: Cons. Adviser & Chairm. Asst. Conception Unit Esperance Private Hosp. Eastbourne.

VALENTINE, Christopher Brett Department of Genitdurinary Medicine, Ravenscraig Hospital, Inverkip Road, Greenock PA16 9HA Tel: 01475 656308 Email: chris.valentine@renver-pct.scot.nhs.uk — MB ChB Leeds 1986; BSc Leeds 1983; MRCP (UK) 1990; Dip. GU Med. Soc. Apoth. Lond. 1994; DFFP 1995; FRCP, (Lond) 2001. Cons.Genito. Urin. Med. renver Primary Care NHS Trust. Specialty: Genitourinary Medicine. Socs: Soc. Study VD; Internat. AIDS Soc.; Brit. Soc. Colposc. & Cervic. Pathol. Prev: Lect. (Genitourin. Med.) Univ. Liverp.; Research Fell. MRC HIV Clin. Trials Centre (Clin. Epidemiol.) Roy. Brompton & Nat. Heart & Lung Inst. Lond.; Research Fell. (Clin. Immunol.) St. Mary's Hosp Lond.

VALENTINE, David Angus (retired) Filey Surgery, Station Avenue, Filey YO14 9AE Tel: 01723 515881 Fax: 01723 515197; The Low Barn, Hunmanby, Filey YO14 0JY Tel: 01723 890308 Fax: 01723 891309 — MB ChB Leeds 1962; BSc (1st cl. Hons. Physiol.) Leeds 1962; MB ChB (Distinc.) Leeds 1964.

VALENTINE, David Edward West Harwood Crofts, West Calder EH55 8LF — MB BCh BAO NUI 1982.

VALENTINE, David Thomas Bryn Cross Surgery, 246 Wigan Road, Ashton-in-Makerfield, Wigan WN4 0AR Tel: 01942 727270 Fax: 01942 272197 — MB ChB Liverp. 1993. GP Principal.

VALENTINE, James Low Wood, Ben Rhydding, Ilkley LS29 8AZ Tel: 01943 609491 — MB ChB Glas. 1929; DPM Lond. 1933; FRCPsych 1971. Specialty: Gen. Psychiat. Socs: BMA. Prev: Hon. Cons. Psychiat. Scalebor Pk. Burley-in-Wharfedale & Leeds Gen.; Phys. Supt. & Cons. Psychiat. Scalebor Pk. Burley-in-Wharfedale; Cons. Psychiat. Leeds Univ. Dept. Stud. Health.

VALENTINE, Jane Louise Linden Medical Centre, 9A Linden Avenue, Maidenhead SL6 6HD Tel: 01628 20846 Fax: 01628 789318 — MB ChB Manch. 1985 (Manchester) DRCOG 1988. GP Maidenhead.

VALENTINE, John Carpenter Water Meadows, Harrold, Bedford MK43 7DE Tel: 01234 720383 Email: jackval@lineone.net — MB ChB (2nd cl. Hons.) Bristol 1941; FRCPath 1963. Prev: Cons. Morbid Anat. & Histopath. N. Beds. HA; Capt. IMS/IAMC; Lect. (Path.) Univ. Bristol.

VALENTINE, John Paul St Chads Surgery, Gullock Tyning, Midsomer Norton, Bath BA3 2UH Tel: 01761 413334 Fax: 01761 411176 — BM BCh Oxf. 1972; MA Oxf. 1972, BSc 1970, BM BCh 1972; DCH Eng. 1975; DRCOG 1977; MRCGP 1977. Course Organiser Bath & Swindon VTS. Prev: Trainee GP Swindon-Cirencester VTS; Ho. Surg. Roy. United Hosp. Bath; Ho. Phys. Radcliffe Infirm. Oxf.

VALENTINE, Jonathan Michael James Pain Management Centre, Bowthrope Road, Norwich NR2 3TU Tel: 01603 288453 Fax: 01603 288553 Email: john.valentine@nnuh.nhs.uk; 23 Dyers Yard, Norwich NR3 3QY Email: jmj.valentine@btopenworld.com — MB ChB Leeds 1986. Consultant in pain Management, Norfolk and Norfolk Hospital, Norwich; Cons., Pricilla Bacon Lodge Hospice, Norwich. Specialty: Anaesth. Special Interest: Palliat. Care. Socs: Chairm., Anglian Pain Soc.; Chairm. UK and Irel. Chapter of the Internat. Neuromodulation Soc. Prev: Sen. Regist. (Anaesth.) Yorks. Region; Sen. Regist. Melbourne, Austral.; Regist. (Anaesth.) St. Jas. Univ. Hosp. Leeds.

VALENTINE, Laurence 28 Emlyn Road, London W12 9TD Tel: 020 8743 5287 — MB BS Lond. 1954 (Univ. Coll. Hosp.)

VALENTINE, Linda Church Plain Surgery, Loddon, Norwich NR14 6EX Tel: 01508 520222 — MB ChB Leeds 1987; DRCOG 1991; DCH RCP Lond. 1991. GP Asst. Ch. Plain Surg. Loddon Norwich. Specialty: Gen. Med.; Family Plann. & Reproduc. Health; Paediat. Prev: GP Warrengate Surg. Wakefield; Trainee GP Wakefield VTS.

VALENTINE, Malcolm Jack Brimmond Medical Group, 106 Inverurie Road, Bucksburn, Aberdeen AB21 9AT Tel: 01224 713490 Fax: 01224 716317; 104 Desswood Place, Aberdeen AB15 4DQ — MB ChB Aberd. 1982; DRCOG 1985; MRCGP 1986; FRCGP 1997; MD 2001. Gen. Practitioner, Aberd.; Occupat. Phys. Schlumberger, Aberd.; Hon. Senior Lect. (Gen. Pract.) Univ. Aberd.; Asst. Director PostGrad. CP Educat. Specialty: Occupat. Health. Socs: National Association of Primary Care Education. Prev: Hon. Clinician Hyperbaric Unit Grampian HB; Trainee GP NE Scotl. VTS.

VALENTINE, Mary Josephine New Court Surgery, Borough Fields, Wootton Bassett, Swindon SN4 7AX Tel: 01793 852302 Fax: 01793 851119 — MB ChB Bristol 1980; MRCP (UK) 1984; DA (UK) 1986; MRCGP 1987. GP Wootton Bassett; Hosp. Pract. (Endocrinol. & Gen. Med.) Princess Margt. Hosp. Swindon. Specialty: Endocrinol.

VALENTINE, Mr Neil Wilson Stracathro Hospital, Brechin DD9 7QA Tel: 01356 647291 Fax: 01356 665101; 78 Lour Road, Forfar DD8 2AZ Tel: 01307 463427 Fax: 01307 467836 Email: nwvalentine@compuserve.com — MB ChB Glas. 1980; FRCS Glas. 1984. Cons. Orthop. Surg. Stracathro Hosp. Brechin; Hon. Sen. Lect. Univ. Dundee. Specialty: Orthop. Socs: Fell. Brit. Scoliosis Soc.; Fell. BOA; Fell. Europ. Spine Soc. Prev: Sen. Regist. (Orthop.) Oswestry & Stoke-on-Trent; Research Fell. (Spinal) Hartshill Orthop. Hosp. Stoke on Trent; Regist. (Orthop.) Vict. Infirm. & Glas. Roy. Infirm.

VALENTINE, Nicola Jane 121 Hale Drive, London NW7 3EJ — MB BS Lond. 1990; BSc Lond. 1987; DRCOG 1993; MRCGP 1994. Asst. GP Lond. Prev: Trainee GP Lond.

VALENTINE, Mr Peter William Martin The Guildford Nuffield Hospital, Stirling Road, Guildford GU2 7RF Tel: 01483 555946 MB BS Lond. 1990; FRCS Eng. 1995. Cons. ENT Surg.. The Roy. Surrey Co. Hosp. Guildford; Ashford & St. Peter's Hosps. Prev: Specialist ENT Regist., N. Thames Rotat.

VALENTINE, Prudence (retired) 11 Stancomb Avenue, Ramsgate CT11 0EX Tel: 01843 592039 — MB BS Lond. 1952; MRCS Eng. LRCP Lond. 1952; DObst RCOG 1955.

VALENTINE, Simon Hugh Charles — MB BS Lond. 1985; MRCGP 1989; Dip Sports Med Bath 2001. Specialty: Sports Med.

VALENTINI, Patrizia 80 Plumstead Common Road, London SE18 3RD — Laurea Milan 1995. Specialty: Cardiol.

VALERIO, Mr David Grantham & District NHS Trust, 101 Manthorpe Road, Grantham NG31 8DG Tel: 01476 565232 Fax: 01476 590441; 138 Manthorpe Road, Grantham NG31 8DL Tel: 01476 571611 — MB ChB Sheff. 1970; FRCS Eng. 1975; FRCS Ed. 1975; MS Sheff. 1982. Cons. Gen. Surg. Grantham & Kesteven Gen. Hosp. Specialty: Gen. Surg. Prev: Sen. Regist. (Gen. Surg.) Aberd. Roy. Infirm.

VALERIO, Dorando (retired) 97 Prince of Wales Road, Sheffield S2 1EZ Tel: 0114 397124 — LRCS Ed. 1939 (St. Mungo's Coll. Glas.) L.R.C.P., L.R.C.S. Ed., L.R.F.P.S. Glas. 1939. Prev: Clin. Asst. Out-pats. South. Gen. Hosp. Glas.

VALI, Ahmed Mohamed North Glamorgan NHS Trust, Prince Charles Hospital, Merthyr Tydfil CF49 9DT — MB BChir Camb. 1980; MA Camb. 1981; FRCR 1986. Cons. (Radiol.) P. Chas. Hosp. Specialty: Radiol. Prev: Sen. Regist. (Radiol.) NW Regional HA.

VALLANCE, Barry Daniel Hairmyres Hospital, Eaglesham Road, East Kilbride, Glasgow G75 8RG Tel: 01355 584476 Fax: 01355 584473 Email: barry.vallance@lanarkshire.scot.nhs.uk; Faraways, 5 Sandringham Avenue, Newton Mearns, Glasgow G77 5DU Tel: 0141 639 1962 Fax: 0141 639 6775 — MB ChB Glas. 1973 (Glasgow University) FRCP Edin.; FRCP Glas. 1987. Cons. Phys. & Cardiol. Hairmyres Hospital,. NHS Lanarksh.. Specialty: Cardiol. Special Interest: Interventional Cardiol. Socs: Brit. Cardiac Soc.; Scott. Cardiac Soc.; Brit. Cardaic Interven. Soc. Prev: Lect., Sen. Regist. & Regist. (Med. Cardiol.) Glas. Roy. Infirm.; Hon. Research Regist. (Med.) South. Gen. Hosp. Glas.

VALLANCE, Harry David Anaesthetic Department, North Manchester General Hospital, Delauneys Road, Crumpsall, Manchester M8 5RL Tel: 0161 795 4567 — MB ChB Leeds 1984; DA (UK) 1987; FRCA 1993. Cons. (Anaesth.) N. Manch. Gen. Hosp. Specialty: Anaesth. Socs: Assn. Anaesth.; Manch. Med. Soc.; Obst. Anaesth. Assn. Prev: Sen. Regist. (Anaesth.) Booth Hall Childr. Hosp. Manch.

VALLANCE, James Howard 12 Lumley Road, Durham DH1 5NP — MB ChB Ed. 1997.

VALLANCE, Kevin Andrew George Eliot Hospital NHS Trust, College Street, Nuneaton CV10 7DJ Tel: 024 7635 1351 — MB ChB Birm. 1980; FRCR 1986. Cons. Radiol. Geo. Eliot Hosp. NHS Trust Nuneaton. Specialty: Radiol. Prev: Sen. Regist. & Regist. (Radiol.) W. Midl. RHA; SHO (Cardiothoracic Surg.) Coventry HA.

VALLANCE, Norma Bryan 56 Russell Drive, Bearsden, Glasgow G61 3BB — MB ChB Glas. 1970.

VALLANCE, Patrick John Thompson 28 Bushnell Road, London SW17 8QP Tel: 020 8675 2267 — MB BS Lond. 1984; MRCP (UK) 1987; BSc Lond. 1981, MD 1990; FRCP 1995; FMedSci 1999. Prof. & Hon. Cons. Clin. Pharmacol. Univ. Coll. Hosp. Lond. Specialty: Pharmacology. Prev: Sen. Lect. & Hon. Cons. Clin. Pharmacol. St. Geo. Hosp. Med. Sch. Lond.; Lect. (Clin. Pharmacol.) & Hon. Regist. (Med.) St. Geo. Hosp. Med. Sch. Lond.; Wellcome Clin. Fell.

VALLANCE, Mr Ramsay 56 Russell Drive, Bearsden, Glasgow G61 3BB — MB ChB Glas. 1969; FRCS Glas. 1973; FRCR 1976; DMRD Eng. 1977. Cons. Radiol. Gartnavel Gen. Hosp. Glas.; Hon. Clin. Sen. Lect. (Radiol.), Univ. of Glas. Specialty: Radiol. Prev: Regist. (Diag. Radiol.) South. Gen. Hosp. Glas.; Sen. Regist. (Diag. Radiol.) & Jun. Ho. Phys. West. Infirm. Glas.

VALLANCE, Reuben Leon Brunswick Health Centre, Brunswick St., Hartfield Close, Chorlton on Medlock, Manchester M13 9YA Tel: 0161 273 4901; 4 Singleton Close, Salford M7 4NF — LRCP LRCS Ed. 1949 (Anderson Coll. Glas.) LRCP LRCS Ed. LRFPS Glas. 1949; MRCGP 1976. Prev: Capt. RAMC; Ho. Phys. & Ho. Obstetr. Crumpsall Hosp. Manch.

VALLANCE, Tony Roger Leicester General Hospital, Gwendolen Road, Leicester LE4 5PW Tel: 0116 249 0490; 20 Gloucester Crescent, Melton Mowbray LE13 0AQ Tel: 01664 64791 — MB BS Lond. 1972 (Westm.) MRCS Eng. LRCP Lond. 1972; MRCP (UK) 1977. Cons. Phys. in Geriat. Med. Leicester Gen. Hosp. Specialty: Care of the Elderly.

VALLANCE-OWEN, Mr Andrew John BUPA, BUPA House, 15-19 Bloomsbury Way, London WC1A 2BA Tel: 020 7656 2037 Fax: 020 7656 2708 Email: vallanca@bupa.com; 13 Lancaster Avenue, Hadley Wood, Barnet EN4 0EP Tel: 020 8440 9503 Fax: 020 8364 8770 — MB ChB Birm. 1976; FRCS Ed. 1982; MBA Open 1994. Gp. Med. Dir. BUPA Lond.; Non-executive director, Outcome Technologies. Specialty: Gen. Surg.; Medical management. Special Interest: Healthcare Strategy; Professionalism, Communication. Socs: Worshipful Soc. Apoth.; Roy. Soc. Med.; BMA. Prev: Med. Dir. BUPA Health Servs.; Under Sec. & Scott. Sec. BMA; Provin. Sec. N. of Eng. BMA.

VALLANCE-OWEN, John 10 Spinney Drive, Great Shelford, Cambridge CB2 5LY Tel: 01223 842767; 17 St. Matthews Lodge, Oakley Square, London NW1 1NB Tel: 020 7388 3644 — (Camb. & Lond. Hosp.) FRCP Lond. 1962, M 1946; MB BChir Camb. 1946; MA Camb. 1946, BA (Hons.) 1943, MD 1951; FRCPI (Hon.) 1970; FRCPath 1971. Vis. Prof. Imperial Coll. of Sc. Technol. & Med. Hammersmith Hosp. Lond. Specialty: Gen. Med.; Endocrinol. Socs: Assn. Phys.; Med. Res. Soc.; Roy. Soc. Med. Prev: Prof. Med. Qu.'s Univ. Belf. & Cons. Phys. Roy. Vict. Hosp. Belf.; Reader (Med.) Univ. Newc. & Cons. Phys. Roy. Vict. Hosp. Newc.; Foundat. Prof. & Chairm. Dept. Med., Chinese Univ. Hong Kong.

VALLE, Anne McKay (retired) 1/4 Greenhill Court, Edinburgh EH9 1BF Tel: 0131 447 4286 — (Univ. & St. Mungo's Coll. Glas.) LRCP LRCS Ed., LRFPS Glas. 1950; DObst RCOG 1955; FFCM 1984, M 1974. Prev: SCM. Hull HA.

VALLE, Juan William Department of Medical Oncology, Christie Hospital NHS Trust, Manchester M20 4BX Tel: 0161 446 8106 Fax: 0161 446 3299 Email: juan.valle@christie-tr.nwest.nhs.uk — MB ChB Sheff. 1989; MRCPI 1994; MSc (Oncology) Univ. of Manch. 2000. Sen. Lect./ Hon. Cons. (Med. Oncol.) Christie Hosp. NHS Trust; Hon. Cons. (Med. Oncol.) N. Manch. Gen. Hosp. NHS Trust. Specialty: Oncol. Socs: BMA; ASCO; UKCCR. Prev: Specialist Regist. (Med. Oncol.) Christie Hosp. NHS Trust Manch.; Research Regist. (Med. Oncol.) Christie Hosp. NHS Trust Manch.; SHO (Gen. Med.) Walsgrave Hosp. Coventry.

VALLELY, Andrew John Brian 29 Earl Road, Northfleet, Gravesend DA11 7AE — MB BS Lond. 1990 (Roy. Free Hosp. Sch. Med.) DTM & H RCP Lond. 1992; MRCP (UK) 1994. Dist. Med. Off. Rabaraba Dist. & Diocese of Dogura, Milne Bay Province, PNG.

VALLELY, Carolyn Teresa Joan Andress, Annaghmore, Portadown, Craigavon — LRCPI & LM, LRSCI & LM 1962; LRCPI & LM, LRCSI & LM 1962.

VALLELY, Stephen Ronald Department of Radiology, Belfast City Hospital, Lisburn Road, Belfast BT7 9AB Tel: 02890 263840 Fax: 02890 263790 Email: stephen.vallely@bch.n-i.nhs.uk — MB BCh BAO Belf. 1985 (Qu. Univ. Belf.) FRCR 1991; MD Belf. 1993; FFR RCSI 1996. Cons. Radiol. Belf. City Hosp. Specialty: Radiol.; Nuclear Med. Prev: Cons. Radiol. Ulster Hosp. Dundonald.

VALLET, Elspeth Anne Woodlands Surgery, 24 Woodlands, Meeting House Lane, Balsall Common, Coventry CV7 7FX Tel: 01676 532587 Fax: 01676 535154; 73 Old Station Road, Hampton in Arden, Solihull B92 0HA Tel: 01676 32213 — MB BS Lond. 1976 (Roy. Free) MRCS Eng. LRCP Lond. 1976; DRCOG 1981. GP Balsall Comon.

VALLI, Paola 31 Wises Lane, Sittingbourne ME10 1YN Email: PaolaValli@doctors.org.uk — State Exam Brescia 1992; MA (Palliat. Care) Italy 2001. GP Train. (Gen. Pract. O & G, Community Med.). Specialty: Gen. Pract.; Family Plann. & Reproduc. Health.

VALLIS, Christopher John Department of Paediatric Anaesthesia, Royal Victoria Infirmary, Newcastle upon Tyne NE1 4LP Tel: 0191 232 5131 Fax: 0191 282 5376 Email: c.j.vallis@ncl.ac.uk — MB BS Lond. 1975 (Univ. Coll. Hosp.) BSc Lond. 1972, MB BS 1975; FRCA 1980; DCH Eng. 1981; FRCPCH 1997. Cons. Paediat. Anaesth. Roy. Vict. Infirm. Newc. u. Tyne; Hon. Clin. Lect. Univ. Newc. Specialty: Anaesth. Socs: Assn. Paediat. Anaesth. Prev: Sen. Regist. (Anaesth.) St. Thos. Hosp. & Hosp. for Sick Childr. Lond.

VALLIS, Katherine Anne 37 Beech Croft Road, Oxford OX2 7AY — MB BS Lond. 1981 (St. Bart.) MRCP (UK) 1984; FRCR 1988. Prev: Clin. Research Fell. ICRF Molecular Pharmacol. Gp.; Sen. Regist. (Clin. Oncol.) Hammersmith Hosp. Lond.

VALLIS, Mr Martin Philip — MB BS Lond. 1979; FRCS Glas. 1985; DRCOG 1987; MRCGP 1988. GP LoW.oft.; Hosp. Practitioner (ENT) Jas. Paget Hosp. Gorleston Norf.

VALLON, Alan Geoffrey Crawley Hospital, West Green Drive, Crawley RH11 7DH Tel: 01293 527866 — MB ChB Manch. 1972; MRCP (UK) 1976; T(M) 1991; FRCP Lond. 1994. Cons. Phys. With Responsibil. c/o Elderly Crawley & Horsham Hosps.; Dir. Of Med. Educat., Surrey & Sussex healthcare NHS Trust. Specialty: Gen. Med.; Gastroenterol. Socs: Brit. Soc. Gastroenterol. & Brit. Geriat. Soc. Prev: Sen. Regist. (Med. & Geriat. Med.) Middlx. Hosp. Lond.; Regist. (Med. & Gastroenterol.) Middlx. Hosp. Lond.; SHO (Med. & Gastroenterol.) Manch. Roy. Infirm.

VALLOW, Peter Warneford (retired) 38 Ashbourne Avenue, Cleckheaton BD19 5JJ Tel: 01274 873585 — MB ChB Leeds 1951. Prev: GP Heckmondwike, W. Yorks.

VALLOW, Mrs Rachel Betty (retired) 38 Ashbourne Avenue, Cleckheaton BD19 5JJ — MB ChB Leeds 1950. Prev: Ho. Surg. (O & G) Leeds Gen. Infirm.

VALLS BALLESPI, Jordi 10 Harefield Close, Enfield EN2 8NQ — LMS Barcelona 1989. SHO (Med.) Southend Hosp. Specialty: Gen. Med. Socs: Assn. Study Obesity. Prev: SHO (Geriat.) Rochford Hosp. Southend Healthcare NHS Trust; Ho. Off. (Med.) Peterboro. Dist. Hosp.

VALLURI, Parthasarathy The Medical Centre, 32 High Street, Rishton, Blackburn BB1 4LA Tel: 01254 884226 Fax: 01254 726190 — MB BS Madras 1973; MB BS Madras 1973.

VALMAN, Hyman Bernard 105 Bridge Lane, London NW11 0EU Tel: 020 8458 1951 Fax: 020 8458 1951 — (Camb. & Westm.) MB BChir Camb. 1958; DCH Eng. 1963; DObst RCOG 1963; FRCP Lond. 1978, M 1967; MA Camb. 1958, MD 1974; FRCPCH 1996. Cons. Paediat. Northwick Pk. Hosp. Harrow; Archiv. Roy. Coll. of Paediat. and Child Health. Specialty: Paediat. Socs: Fell. Roy. Soc. Med. Prev: Sen. Regist. Hosp. Sick Childr. Gt. Ormond St. Lond.; Regist. (Paediat.) Qu. Eliz. Hosp. Childr. Hackney; Cas. Off. Westm. Hosp.

VALMIKI, Vidyasagar Halappa 2 Hall Drive, Oadby, Leicester LE2 4HE — MB BS Poona 1978; LRCP LRCS Ed. LRCPS Glas. 1983.

VALORI, Mr Alexander Maxim Harleston Doctors Surgery, Bullock Fair Close, Harleston IP20 9AT Tel: 01379 853217 Fax: 01379 854082; Kingsland Farm, Denton, Harleston IP20 0AH Tel: 01986 788767 Email: alex.valori@nhs.net — MB ChB Manch. 1975; BSc (Med. Sci.) St And. 1972; FRCS Ed. 1981. GP Harleston; Hosp. Pract. (Migraine Clinic) Norf. & Norwich Univ. Hosp. NHS Trust. Special Interest: Cervico-Trigeminal Pain Managem. Socs: Cervicogenic Headache Int. Study Gp.; Brit. Assn. Study of Headache. Prev: Regist. Orthop. Surg. St Geo. Hosp. Lond.; Regist. (Surg.) King Edwd. VII Hosp. Windsor; SHO (Surg.) Roy. Marsden Hosp. Lond.

VALORI, Roland Mark Glocestershire Royal Infirmary, Great Western Road, Gloucester GL1 3NN Tel: 0845 422 6620 Fax: 0845 422 6892 Email: roland.valori@btopenworld.com — MB BS 1976; MRCP (UK) 1978; MD Lond. 1984; T(M) 1989; MSc (Oxon.) 2000. Cons. Phys. & Gastroenterol. Glos. Roy. Hosp.; Nat. Clin. Lead, Endoscopy Servs. Specialty: Gastroenterol. Prev: Cons. Phys., Univ. Coll. and Middlx. Hosps. 1989-93.

VALSALAN, Umadevi The Surgery, 122 Sutton Road, Erdington, Birmingham B23 5TJ Tel: 0121 373 0056 Fax: 0121 382 3212; 22 Sir Alfreds Way, Sutton Coldfield B76 1ES Tel: 0121 329 3076 — MB BS Mysore 1966 (Kasturba Med. Coll. Mangalore) MRCOG 1974, DObst 1970. Prev: Regist. (Ment. Subnorm.) Chelmsley Hosp. Birm.; SHO (Gyn. & Obst.) Leicester Gen. Hosp.; Ho. Off. (Gen. Surg.) S. Middlx. Hosp. Isleworth.

VALSALAN, Velandy Coombil 22 Sir Alfreds Way, Sutton Coldfield B76 1ES Tel: 0121 329 3076 — MB BS Karnatak 1961 (Kasturba Med. Coll. Mangalore) BSc (Zool.) Madras 1955; DPM RCPSI 1972. Cons. Psychiat. (Ment. Subn.) Chelmsley Hosp. Birm. Specialty: Gen. Psychiat. Socs: Inst. Ment. Subn. Prev: Sen. Regist. Chelmsley Hosp. Birm.; Regist. Towers Hosp. Leicester & Cane Hill Hosp. Coulsdon.

VAMADEVA, Praba 1 Maes yr Ysgol, Peniel, Carmarthen SA32 7BT Tel: 01267 238615 — MB BS Peradeniya 1985; MRCP (UK) 1991.

VAN AMERONGEN, Andre Jacques, DFC (retired) Grafton House, Blisworth, Northampton NN7 3BN Tel: 01604 858208 — MB BCh Witwatersrand 1950; FRCOG 1966, M 1958. Prev: Sen. Cons. (O & G) Govt. Rhodesia & Nyasaland.

VAN ARENTHALS, Adriana Johanna Sandrina Kenwood, Main Road, Bosham, Chichester PO18 8PH Tel: 01243 572727 — Artsexamen Free U Amsterdam 1990; Artsexamen Free Univ Amsterdam 1990; DCH RCP Lond. 1993.

VAN ASCH, Patti Fishponds Health Centre, Beechwood Road, Fishponds, Bristol BS16 3TD; The Sign of the Dolphin, Westerleigh, Bristol BS37 8QQ Tel: 01454 312122 — MB BS Lond. 1964 (St. Mary's) MRCS Eng. LRCP Lond. 1964; DObst RCOG 1966. Prev: Ho. Surg. Addenbrooke's Hosp. Camb.; Regist. (Anaesth.) Southmead Hosp. Bristol.

VAN BEINUM, Michael Elias Child & Family Clinic, 194 Quarry Street, Hamilton Tel: 01698 426753 — MB ChB Ed. 1983 (Edinburgh) SAPP; BSc (Hons.) Sussex 1974; MRCPsych 1988; MPhil Ed. 1991; PhD Glas. 2003. Cons. Child & Adolesc. Psychiat., Hamilton, Larnarkshire; Hon. Sen. Lect. Univ. Glas.; Vis. Schol., MRC Social & Pub. Hlth Sci. Resrch Unit Univ. of Glas. Specialty: Child & Adolesc. Psychiat.; Psychother.; Gen. Psychiat. Socs: (Scott. Exec.) Roy. Coll. Psychiat. (Child & Adolesc. Sect.).; Clin. Tutor, Roy. Coll. of Psychiat.s. Prev: Cons. Adolesc. Psychiat. PossilPk. Health Centre Glas.

VAN BESOUW, Jean-Pierre William Gerard St. George's Hospital, Department of Anaesthesia, London SW17 0QT Tel: 020 8725 3317 Email: jean-pierre.vanbesouw@stgeorges.nhs.uk — MB BS Lond. 1981 (St. Barts.) BSc (Hons.) Lond. 1978, MB BS 1981; FRCA 1985. Cons. Anaesth. St. Geo. Hosp. Lond.; Examr. Roy. Coll. of Anaesth.; Regional Adviser Roy. Coll. Anaesth. Specialty: Anaesth. Socs: Assn. Cardiothoracic Anaesth.; Assn. Anaesth.; Europ. Assn. Cardiothoracic Anaesth. Prev: Sen. Regist. (Anaesth.) St. Bart., Hosp. for Sick Childr. & Whipps Cross Hosps. Lond.; Regist. (Anaesth.) St. Geo. Hosp. Lond.; SHO Rotat. (Med. Intens. Ther. Unit & Anaesth.) Whittington Hosp. Lond.

VAN BOXEL, Pieter Jacobus Willem Berkshire Healthcare NHS Trust, Wokingham Hosptial RG41 2RE — MB ChB Cape Town 1972; MRCPsych. 1977; FRCP (Psych) 1999. Cons. (Child & Adolesc. Psychiat.) Child & Adolesc. Ment. Helth Serv. Specialty: Child & Adolesc. Psychiat. Prev: Sen. Regist. (Child & Adolesc. Psychiat.) Guys Hosp. Lond.

VAN BUREN, Alison Elizabeth Town Gate Practice, Chepstow Community Hospital, Tempest Way, Chepstow NP16 5XP Tel: 01291 636444 Fax: 01291 636465; Sylvian Cottage, Glyn Road, Tintern Parva, Chepstow NP16 6TH Tel: 01291 689315 — MB ChB Bristol 1988; MRCP (UK) 1992; DFFP 1995. Specialty: Gen. Pract. Socs: BMA. Prev: Trainee GP Chepstow; SHO Rotat. (Gen. Med.) E. Birm. Hosp.; Family Pract. Residency Progr. Denver Colorado, USA.

VAN BUREN-SCHELE, Michael Northern Devon Healthcare, North Devon District Hospital, Raleigh Park, Barnstaple EX31 4JB Tel: 012713 22665 Fax: 012713 11523 — MB ChB Leic. 1982 (Leicester) MRCPsych. 1988. Cons. Psychiat. N. Devon Healthcare Barnstaple. Gen. Adult Psychiat. & Psychiat. of old age. Specialty: Gen. Psychiat.; Geriat. Psychiat. Prev: Sen. Regist. (Psychiat.) St. Bart. & Homerton Hosps. Lond.; Sen. Regist. (Psychiat.) Warley Hosp. Brentwood.

VAN BUUREN, Caspar Maurits Dieuwert The Close, Wingate TS28 5LS — Artsexamen Amsterdam 1986.

VAN COOTEN, Sarah Eileen Jenner Practice, 21 Stanstead Road, Forest Hill, London SE23 1HN — MB BS Lond. 1991 (Univ. Coll. Lond.) DRCOG 1994. Specialty: Gen. Pract. Socs: MRCGP.

VAN DE PETTE, John Edward William Royal South Hampshire Hospital, Romsey Road, Winchester SO22 5DG — MB BS Lond. 1977 (Guy's) BSc (Hons.) Lond. 1974; MRCS Eng. LRCP Lond. 1977; FRCP Lond. 1991; FRCPath 1994. Cons. Roy. S. Hants. Hosp. Winchester. Specialty: Haematology. Prev: Cons. Haemat. Frimley Pk. Hosp. & Farnham Hosp.; Hon. Cons., Roy. Surrey Co. Hosp.; Speciality Lead Haematologist, Partnership Path.

VAN DE VELDE, Robert Ijntze 2 Harthill Avenue, Gildersome, Morley, Leeds LS27 7EY — Artsexamen Amsterdam 1992.

VAN DEN BENT, Paul Jacques Gordon and Partners, 1 North Street, Peterborough PE1 2RA Tel: 01733 312731 Fax: 01733 311447 — Artsexamen Rotterdam 1986 (Erasmus Univ. Rotterdam) MRCGP 1990. Specialty: Gen. Pract.

VAN DEN BERGHE, Rosalind Cathryn 12 Woodland Close, Marlow SL7 3LE — BM BS Nottm. 1980; BMedSci 1978.

VAN DEN BERK, Joannes Catharine Leon Marie Grantham Health Centre, Beckett House, Grantham Road, London SW9 9DL — Artsexamen Nijmegen 1989. GP Princip. Specialty: Gen. Pract.

VAN DEN BOSCH, Cornelia Anne Department of Public Health, West Surrey Health Protection Unit, The Ridgeway, Old Bisley Road, Frimley, Camberley GU16 5QE Tel: 01276 605540 Fax: 01276 605402 — MB BS Lond. 1968 (St Mary's) MRCS Eng. LRCP Lond. 1968; DCH Eng. 1977; MRCP (UK) 1978; Cert JCC Lond. 1980; MSc Distinc. (Clin. Trop. Med.) Lond. 1984; MD Lond. 1994; FRCPCH 1994; MD Lond. 1994; FRCPCH 1994. Cons. Communicable Dis. Control, Surrey Health Protec. Unit; Hon. Sen. Lect. (Microbiol.) Roy. Lond. Med. Coll.; Hon. Lect. St. Bart. Med. Coll. Specialty: Infec. Dis. Socs: Fell. Roy. Soc. Trop. Med. & Hyg.; Brit. Paediat. Assn.; British Infection Society. Prev: Sen. Med. Off. DoH Lond.; Sen. Research Fell. (Virol.) Roy. Postgrad Med. Sch. &

Hon. Cons. Hammersmith Hosp. Lond.; Sen. Lect. & Hons. Cons. Paediat. Dept. Trop Paediat. Liverp. Sch. Trop. Med.

VAN DEN BROEK, Adrianus Johannes Cornelis Maria 2 The Green, Somerleyton, Lowestoft NR32 5PX Tel: 01502 730513 — Artsexamen Leiden 1993.

VAN DEN BROEK, Alyson ELizabeth Laburnum House, Hinders Lane, Gloucester GL19 3EZ Tel: 01452 830424 — BM BS Nottm. 1990; MRCGP. Specialty: Gen. Pract. Socs: Fac. Fam. Plann. & Reproduc. Health.

VAN DEN BRUL, Karen Ann Health Centre, Bishops Close, Spennymoor DL16 6ED Tel: 01388 811455 Fax: 01388 812034 — MB BS Newc. 1982; DRCOG 1985; MRCGP 1986. Gen. Practitioner, Spennymoor, C.Durh. Prev: Clin. Asst. (Diabetes) Bishop Auckland Gen. Hosp.

VAN DEN BRUL, Peter John (retired) Haverigg, The Park, Drinkstone, Bury St Edmunds IP30 9ST Tel: 01359 270384 — (St. Thos.) MB BS Lond. 1952; DA Eng. 1959; FFA RCS Eng. 1968. Prev: Cons. Anaesth. Bury St. Edmunds Health Dist.

VAN DEN DWEY, Katia Sandwell Heath Care NHS Trust, Hallam St., West Bromwich B71 4HJ — MD Ghent 1991.

VAN DEN HURK, Peter Johannes Department of Obstetrics & Gynaecology, 7th Floor, N. Wing, St Thomas' Hospital, Lambeth Palace Road, London SE1 7EH; 53 Celestial Gardens, Lewisham, London SE13 5RP Tel: 020 8297 9842 — Artsexamen Amsterdam 1992; DRCOG - RCOG 1995. Specialist Regist. (O & G), St. Thomas' Hosp., Lond., SE1. Specialty: Obst. & Gyn. Prev: Lewisham Hosp.; Stoke-on-Trent Hosp.

VAN DER HAUWAERT, Nicolas The Medical Specialist Group, PO Box 113, Alexandra House, St Martin's, Guernsey GY1 3EX — MD Louvain 1988.

VAN DER HEIJDEN, Ludovicus Petrus Johannes Heathcliffe, Main St., Palterton, Chesterfield S44 6UR — Artsexamen Nijmegen 1985.

VAN DER KNAAP, Jill (retired) 9 Elmwood Avenue, London N13 4HG — MB BS Lond. 1967 (Lond. Hosp.) DPM Eng. 1971; MRCPsych 1972. Prev: Clin. Asst. Eric Shepherd Unit Leavesden Hosp. Herts.

VAN DER LEE, Aileen Janet The Surgery, Station Road, Bridge of Weir PA11 3LH Tel: 01505 612555 Fax: 01505 615032 — MB ChB Ed. 1983.

VAN DER LINDEN, Harald Harry Emanuel M Trent Vale Medical Practice, 876 London Road, Trent Vale, Stoke-on-Trent ST4 5NX Tel: 01782 746898 — Artsexamen Nijmegen 1989; Artsexamen Nijmegen 1989.

VAN DER MEULEN, Jacobus Josephus Nicolaas Marie 14 Sunbury Road, Eton, Windsor SL4 6BA — Artsexamen Rotterdam 1995.

VAN DER MOST, Renee Nathalie Primavera, Wheatsheaf Enclosure, Liphook GU30 7EJ — MB BS Lond. 1998; BA (Hons) Camb 1989; PhD Cambridge 1993. Specialty: Gen. Surg.

VAN DER PLAS, Frank Peter Wish Valley Surgery, Talbot Road, Hawkhurst, Cranbrook TN18 4NB Tel: 01580 753211 Fax: 01580 754612 — Artsexamen Amsterdam 1990.

VAN DER PUTT, Rohan Patrick 24 Kenwood Gardens, Ilford IG2 6YQ — MB BS Lond. 1992.

VAN DER STAR, Richard John Department of Clinical Neurophysiology, Wessex Neurological Centre, Southampton General Hospital, Southampton SO16 6YD Tel: 023 8079 6786 Fax: 023 8079 8557; 27 Satchell Lane, Hamble, Southampton SO31 4HF — BM Soton. 1980; FRCP Lond. 2000. Cons. Clin. Neurophysiol. Wessex Neurol. Centre Soton. Gen. Hosp. Specialty: Clin. Neurophysiol. Prev: Sen. Regist. (Clin. Neurophysiol.) Wessex Neurol. Centre; Regist. (Med.) Soton. Gen. Hosp. & Qu. Alexandra Hosp. Portsmouth.

VAN DER VOET, Johannes Cornelis Maria The James Cook University Hospital, Marton Road, Middlesbrough TS4 3BW Tel: 01642 850850 Fax: 01642 854940 — Artsexamen Amsterdam 1989 (Univ. Amsterdam) Cons. Clin. Oncol. S. James Cook Univ. Hosp.. Middlesbrough; Specialist in Radiother. 1995. Specialty: Oncol.; Radiother. Prev: Sen. Regist. (Clin. Oncol.) Christie Hosp. Manch.

VAN DER VOORT, Judith Henriette 23 Pontcanna Street, Cardiff CF11 9HQ — Artsexamen Utrecht 1988; MRCP (UK) 1993.

VAN DER WALT, Lona Basement Flat 1, 72 Denbigh St., London SW1V 2EX — MB ChB Stellenbosch 1991.

VAN DER WEYDEN, Barendina Johanna (retired) The Hollies, 11 Albion Hill, Loughton IG10 4RA Tel: 020 8508 6540 Fax: 020 8508 6540 — MB BS Lond. 1963 (Lond. Hosp.) MRCS Eng. LRCP Lond. 1963; DObst RCOG 1966. Prev: Assoc. Specialist (Ultrasound & Echocardiogr.) & Hon. Clin. Asst. (Gen. Med.) Whipps Cross Hosp. Lond.

VAN DESSEL, Michael Gerard The Spinney Medical Centre, 23 Whittle Street, St Helens WA10 3EB Tel: 01744 758999 Fax: 01744 758322; Aisling, 16 Elm Grove, Eccleston Park, Prescot L34 2RX Tel: 0151 426 6501 — MB BCh BAO NUI 1982; BSc NUI 1984. Socs: Liverp. Med. Inst.; St. Helens Med. Soc.

VAN DIEPEN, Hendrikus Reinder 6 Butler Gardens, Market Harborough LE16 9LY — Artsexamen Groningen 1988.

VAN DOORN, Ms Catharina Adriana Maria Great Ormond Street Hospital for Children, Cardiac Wing, Great Ormond Street, London WC1N 3JH Tel: 020 7405 9200 Fax: 0113 392 8056 — Artsexamen Utrecht 1984 (State Univ. Utrecht, Netherlands) FRCS Ed. 1990; FRCS Eng. 1991; FRCS (CTh) 1997; MD Leeds 1998. Sen. Clin. Lect. in Cardiothoratic Surg. Specialty: Cardiothoracic Surg. Prev: Sen. Regist. (Paediat. Cardiothoracic Surg.) Birm. Childr.'s Hosp.; Sen. Regist. (Cardiothoracic. Surg.) Leeds Gen. Infirm.; Cons., (Adult & Paediat. Cardiothoracic Surg.), Leeds Gen Infirm.

VAN DORP, Francoise Anne Oaks Cottage, Enton, Godalming GU8 5AG — BM BCh Oxf. 1990.

VAN DORP, Maria Hester Oaks Cottage, Enton Green, Godalming GU8 5AG Tel: 01483 416605 — Artsexamen Leiden 1963. Assoc. Specialist (Geriat. Med.) NW Surrey HA.

VAN DUIJN, Niklaas (retired) The Grange Practice, Allerton Clinic, Bell Dean Road, Allerton, Bradford BD15 7NJ Tel: 01274 541696 — Artsexamen Groningen 1990. GP Bradford, W. Yorks.

VAN ESSEN, Janet Clark (retired) Laurel Bank Nursing and Residential Home, Westbourne Road, Lancaster LA1 5EF Tel: 01524 388980 — MB ChB Ed. 1941. Prev: Ho. Surg. (O & G) Roy. Infirm. & Simpson Matern. Hosp. Edin.

VAN EVERY, Thomas Hugo 28 Chantry View Road, Guildford GU1 3XS — MB ChB Birm. 1995; ChB Birm. 1995. SHO (O & G) Chelsea & Westminster Hosp. Specialty: Obst. & Gyn.

VAN GEENE, Mr Peter Academic Department of Obstetrics & Gynaecology, Northern Road Hospital, Herries Road, Sheffield S5 7AU — MB BS Lond. 1981 (Char. Cross) FRCS Ed. 1985; MRCOG 1991. Birthright Research Fell. (Gyn. Oncol.) Acad. Dept. O & G Dudley Rd. Hosp. Birm. Specialty: Obst. & Gyn. Prev: Regist. (O & G) Southmead Hosp. Bristol; Regist. (Surg.) King Edwd. VII Hosp. Windsor.

VAN GELDEREN-SWART, Adriana Geertje 23 Fulmar Drive, East Grinstead RH19 3XL — Artsexamen Amsterdam 1992.

VAN GRUTTEN, Mary (retired) 88 Gove Hill Road, Tunbridge Wells TN1 1ST — (Roy. Free) MB BS Lond. 1950; MRCS Eng. LRCP Lond. 1950. Prev: Cons. Dermat. Dartford & Gravesham, & Medway Health Dists.

VAN HAGEN, Thomas Christopher 319 Muswell Hill Broadway, London N10 1BY — MB BS Lond. 1995.

VAN HAMEL, Jennifer Clare Margaret The Great Western Hospital, Marlborough Road, Swindon SN9; The Old Rectory, 36 The Street, Hullavington, Chippenham SN14 6DU — MB BS Lond. 1987; FRCA 1992. Cons. Anaesth. Princess Margt. Hosp. Swindon. Specialty: Anaesth.

VAN HASSELT, Gillian Louise Mary 6 Dunkeld Road, Bournemouth BH3 7EN Tel: 01202 291666 Fax: 01202 292039 Email: gillvh@netcomuk.co.uk — MB BCh Witwatersrand 1976; FFA RCS Eng. 1982. Cons. Anaesth. Poole Gen. Hosp. Trust. Specialty: Anaesth.

VAN HEEL, David Alexander 149 Avondale Road, Shipley BD18 4QZ — BM BCh Oxf. 1993; MRCP (UK) 1993; MA Cantab. 1994. Specialty: Gastroenterol.

VAN HEYNINGEN, Charles Clinical Laboratories, University Hospital Aintree, Lower Lane, Liverpool L9 7AL Tel: 0151 529 3907 Fax: 0151 529 3310 Email: charles.vanheyningen@aht.nwest.nhs.uk; 3 Grosvenor Close, Southport PR8 2TJ — MB BS Lond. 1973 (St Bartholomew's Hosp. Lond.) BSc Biochem. Lond. 1970; ECFMG Lond. 1974; FRCPath 1996, M 1983. Cons. Chem. Path. Aintree Hosps. (NHS) Trust &

Southport & Ormskirk (NHS) Trust; Hon. Lect. (Clin. Chem.) Univ. Liverp. Specialty: Chem. Path. Socs: Assn. Clin. Biochem.; Roy. Coll. Pathol.; HEART UK. Prev: Sen. Regist. (Chem. Path.) Westm. Hosp. Lond. & Kingston Hosp. Surrey; Regist. (Chem. Path.) St. Geo. Hosp. Lond.

VAN HILLE, Mr Philip Thomas Department of Neurosurgery, General Infirmary at Leeds, Great George St., Leeds LS1 2EX Tel: 0113 392 6648 Fax: 0113 392 6315; Grange House, 203 Shay Lane, Walton, Wakefield WF2 6NW Tel: 01924 253686 — MB ChB Cape Town 1972; FRCS Eng. 1980. Cons. Neurosurg. Gen. Infirm. Leeds. Specialty: Neurosurg. Prev: Cons. Sen. Regist. (Neurosurg.) Leeds West. HA.

VAN HOOGSTRATEN, Johannes Wilhelmus Antonius Petrus Friarage Hospital, Northallerton DL6 1JG — Artsexamen Groningen 1989.

VAN IDDEKINGE, Basil Department of Obstetrics & Gynaecology, Hammersmith Hospital, Du Cane Road, London W12 0NN — MB BCh Witwatersrand 1966; FCOG S. Afr. 1972; MRCOG 1973. Sen. Lect. (O & G) Hammersmith Hosp. Lond. Prev: Cons. (O & G) Baragwanath Hosp. Johannesburg, S. Africa; Regist. (O & G) Hammersmith Hosp. Lond. & Johannesburg Gen.; Hosp., S. Africa.

VAN KAMPEN, Maria Northumbria Healthcare NHS Trust, Orthopaedics Department, North Tyneside General Hospital, Rake Lane, North Shields NE61 2DL — Artsexamen Nijmegen 1987. Cons. Orthop. Surg. Northumbria Healthcare NHS Trust. Specialty: Trauma & Orthop. Surg.

VAN KEMPEN, Christopher Edward Meddygfa Wdig, Main Street, Goodwick SA64 0BN Tel: 01348 872802 Fax: 01348 874717 Email: chris@goodwicksurgery.co.uk; 1 & 2 Rhoslannog Cottages, Mathry, Haverfordwest SA62 5HG Tel: 01348 872802 Fax: 01348 874717 Email: chris@goodwicksurgery.co.uk — BM Soton. 1983. Specialty: Acupunc.; Palliat. Med. Prev: SHO (A & E) Weymouth & Dist. Hosp.; SHO (Orthop.) Weymouth & Dist. Hosp.; Ho. Surg. Dorset Co. Hosp. Dorchester.

VAN LANY, Peggy 79 Barrowby Gate, Grantham NG31 8RA — MD Louvain 1996 (K.U. Leuven) SHO (O & G) P'boro. Dist. Hosp. Specialty: Obst. & Gyn.

VAN LIESHOUT, Theodorus Antonius 4/14A Turner Street, London E1 2AS — MB BS Queensland 1987.

VAN LOO, Greet North Tees General Hospital, Hardwick, Stockton-on-Tees TS19 8PE — MD Louvain 1992.

VAN LOO-PLOWMAN, Ingrid Helen Geraldine 139 Hemingford Road, Islington, London N1 1BZ Tel: 0207 607 5307 — Artsexamen Leiden 1992. Specialty: Occupat. Health.

VAN MAARSEVEEN, Petrus Leonardus Newland Health Centre, 187 Cottingham Road, Hull HU5 2EG Tel: 01482 492219 Fax: 01482 441418 — Artsexamen Nijmegen 1985 (Katholieke Univ. Nijmegen) DRCOG 1992. GP Hull.

VAN MARLE, William 18 St Mary's Road, Harborne, Birmingham B17 0HA — MB ChB Birm. 1978.

VAN MIERT, Matthew Marinus 18 Layfield Road, Brunton Park, Newcastle upon Tyne NE3 5AA; 9 Saxon Road, Hoylake, Wirral CH47 3AE — MB BS Lond. 1984 (St. George's London) MA Camb. 1985; FRCA 1990. Cons. Anesth. Wirral Trust. Specialty: Anaesth.

VAN MOURIK, Indra Darmini Maria Liver Unit, Birmingham Children's Hospital, Steelhouse Lane, Birmingham B4 6NH Tel: 0121 333 8255 Fax: 0121 333 8251 — Artsexamen Amsterdam 1988 (Univ. Amsterdam) MRCPI 1995. — Cons. (Paediatric Hepatologist) Liver Unit, Birm. Children's Hosp. NHS Trust. Specialty: Paediat. Socs: MRCPCH; KNMG (Dutch Royal College of Medicine); BSPGHAN (Brit. Soc. Paed. Gastr. Hepatol. & Nutrition). Prev: Specialist Regist. (Paediat.) City Hosp. NHS Trust, Birm.; Clin. Research Fell. & Hon. Regist. Liver Unit Birm. Childr. Hosp.

VAN NIMMEN, Bart Royal Devon & Exeter Hospital (Wonford), Barrack Road, Exeter EX2 5DW — MD Louvain 1992.

VAN OLDENBEEK, Carolus Johannes Jacobus Maria Trafford Healthcare NHS Trust, Moorside Road, Davyhulme M41 5SL Tel: 0161 746 2301 Fax: 0161 746 2287 Email: carl.vanoldenbeek@trafford.nhs.uk; 76 Claude Road, Manchester M21 8DF — Artsexamen Rotterdam 1988; CCST Anaesth. 1998. Cons. in Anaesth. & Critical Care, Trafford Healthcare NHS Trust, Manch. Specialty: Anaesth. Special Interest: Acute Pain; Critical Care; Total Intravenous Anaesth. Socs: Fell. of the Roy. Coll. of Anaesth.

VAN OLDENBORGH, Mr Hermanus Marius 12 Upper Wimpole Street, London W1G 6LW Tel: 020 7935 3289 — MB ChB Cape Town 1965; FRCS Ed. 1972; DO Eng. 1975; FRCSI 1977. Socs: Ophth. Soc. UK & Mem. Oxf. Ophth. Congr. Prev: Sen. Regist. Moorfields Eye Hosp. Lond.

VAN OSS, Helen Georgina Park Lane Surgery, Park Lane, Woodstock OX20 1UD Tel: 01993 811452 — MB BS Lond. 1978; MRCGP 1982; DRCOG 1982.

VAN PAESSCHEN, Wim Epilepsy Research Group, 33 Green Square, London WC1N 3BG — MD Antwerp 1984.

VAN PELT, Howard John Ferdinand London Road South Surgery, 366 London Road South, Lowestoft NR33 0BQ Tel: 01502 573333 Fax: 01502 581590; 53 Walmer Road, Lowestoft NR33 7LE Tel: 01502 568625 — MRCS Eng. LRCP Lond. 1968 (Leeds) DObst RCOG 1971.

VAN REENEN, Samantha 12 Rothesay Court, Harleyford Road, London SE11 5SU — MB BCh Witwatersrand 1997.

VAN RHIJN, Maarten Flat 3, Priscilla House, Sunbury Cross Centre, Sunbury-on-Thames TW16 7BG — Artsexamen Rotterdam 1986.

VAN ROOYEN, Elise 45 Kipling Road, Cheltenham GL51 7DG — MB ChB Pretoria 1980.

VAN ROSS, Ernest Rodney Edward Disablement Services Centre, Withington Hospital, Cavendish Road, Manchester M20 1LB Tel: 0161 611 3763 — MB BS Bangalore 1973 (St. Johns, Bangalore) FRCS Eng. 1979; MCh (Orth) Liverp. 1983; FRCP Lond 2000. Cons. Rehabil. Med. Withington Hosp. & Manch. Roy. Infirm.; Cons. in Rehabil. Med., Centr. Manch. Univ. Hosp. Trust; Cons. to Pace Rehabil., 36 Brook St., Cheadle, Chesh. Specialty: Rehabil. Med. Socs: Brit. Soc. Rehabil. Med. (Exec. Comm); International Society for Prosthetics and Orthoidis.

VAN ROSS, Rosemary Theresa Goretti Park Green House, Sunderland Street, Macclesfield SK11 6HW Tel: 01625 429555; 12 Butley Lane, Prestbury, Macclesfield SK10 4HU Tel: 01625 820956 — MB BCh Cork 1981; DCH; DRCOG; MRCGP. GP, Macclesfield.

VAN RYSSEN, John Stephen Michael William Peter The Seven Dials Medical Centre, 24 Montpelier Crescent, Brighton BN1 3JJ Tel: 01273 773089 Fax: 01273 207098 — MRCS Eng. LRCP Lond. 1969.

VAN RYSSEN, Maureen Ellen Philomena (retired) Dobbins, Castle Lane, Bramber, Steyning BN44 3FB Tel: 01903 879051 — MB BS Lond. 1965 (Roy. Free) MRCS Eng. LRCP Lond. 1964; FFA RCS Eng. 1972. Cons. Anaesth. Worthing & Southlands Hosp. Trust. Prev: Sen. Regist. Dept. Anaesth. Guy's Hosp. Lond.

VAN SAENE, Hendrik Karel Firminus Department of Medical Microbiology, University of Liverpool, PO Box 147, Liverpool L69 3GA Tel: 0151 706 4399 Fax: 0151 706 5805 Email: h.c.kelly@liv.ac.uk; 321 The Colonnades, Albert Dock Village, Liverpool L3 4AB — MD Louvain 1973; PhD Groningen 1982; FRCPath 1997, MRCPath 1987. Reader (Med. Microbiol.) Univ. Liverp.; Hon. Cons. Microbiol. Roy. Liverp. Childr. NHS Trust Alder Hey. Specialty: Med. Microbiol. Socs: Eur. Soc. Clin. Microbiol. & Infect. Dis.; Brit. Assn. Med. Microbiols.

VAN SCHAICK, Suzanna Hilary Bakersfield Medical Centre, 141 Oakdale Road, Nottingham NG3 7EJ Tel: 0115 940 1007; 131 Winchester Street, Nottingham NG5 4DR Tel: 0115 924 5101 — BM BCh Oxf. 1976; BA Oxf. 1972; MRCP (UK) 1978.

VAN SCHAYK, Marjolein Scapa Medical Group, Health Centre, New Scapa Road, Kirkwall KW15 1BQ Tel: 01856 885445 Fax: 01856 873556.

VAN SEENUS, Theodora Edith Community Child Health, Birling Ward, Preston Hall, Maidstone ME20 7NY — Artsexamen Leiden 1971 (Leiden, The Nethrlands) DCH RCP Lond. 1986. Clin. Med. Off. (Community Child Health) Maidstone. Specialty: Community Child Health.

VAN SOMEREN, Robert Niall Melville 13 The Close, London N14 6DP — MB ChB Ed. 1979; MRCP (UK) 1985; MD Ed. 1988. Cons. Phys. Chase Farm Hosp. Enfield. Specialty: Gastroenterol.

VAN SOMEREN, Vivienne Hazel Department of Child Health, Royal Free Hampstead NHS Trust, Pond St., London NW3 2QG Tel: 020 7794 0500 Ext: 3066 Fax: 020 7830 2210 Email: vivienne.vansomeren@royalfree.nhs.uk — MB ChB Ed. 1976; FRCPCH; MRCP (UK) 1979; MD Ed. 1985; FRCP Eng. 1985. Cons. Paediat. & Sen. Lect. (Child Health) Roy. Free Hosp. Lond. Specialty:

Paediat.; Neonat. Socs: Resusitation Counc.; Neonat. Soc. Prev: Lect. (Paediat.) UMDS Guy's & St. Thos. Hosps. Lond.

VAN SPELDE, Johannes Franciscus Petrus Standish Medical Practice, Rodenhurst, Church Street, Standish, Wigan WN6 0JP Tel: 01257 421909 Fax: 01257 424259 — Artsexamen Nijmegen 1988.

VAN STADEN, Gavin Nicholas 167 Hamlin Lane, Exeter EX1 2SQ — MB BCh Witwatersrand 1996.

VAN STEENIS, Dick (retired) — MB BS Adelaide 1959. Prev: Clin. Asst. (Oncol.) St. Richards Hosp. Chichester.

VAN STIGT, Elisabeth Saskia Langford Medical Practice, 9 Nightingale Place, Bicester OX26 6XX Tel: 01869 245665 — MB BS Lond. 1989; MRCGP 1994; DFFP 1994. GP Princip. Specialty: Gen. Pract.

VAN'T HOFF, Hugh Colin Betworthy Cottage, Trenley Road, Coaley, Dursley GL11 5AZ Tel: 01453 860006 Mob: 07753 727678 Email: clogs@doctors.org.uk — MB BS Lond. 1985 (Guys Medical School) BSc (Hons.) Lond. 1982, MB BS 1985; DTM & H Liverp. 1990; MRCGP 1993. Self Employed Gen. Practitioner (locum). Specialty: Gen. Pract. Prev: GP Partner, Malago Surg., Bedminster.

VAN'T HOFF, William Gordon Great Ormond Street Hospital, Great Ormond St., London WC1N 3JH Tel: 020 7405 9200 Fax: 020 7829 8841 — MB BS Lond. 1983 (Guy's) MRCP (UK) 1986; BSc (1st cl. Hons.) Lond. 1980, MD 1994; FRCPH 1999. Cons. Paediat. Nephrol. Gt. Ormond St. Hosp. for Childr. NHS Trust. Specialty: Paediat. Prev: Lect. (Paediat. Nephrol.) Inst. Child Health Lond.; Lect. (Paediat.) Guy's Hosp. Lond.; Regist. (Paediat.) John Radcliffe Hosp. Oxf.

VAN TERHEYDEN, Kenneth Malcolm René The Health Centre, Melbourn Street, Royston SG8 7BS Tel: 01763 242981 Fax: 01763 249197 — MB BS Lond. 1977 (Roy. Free) MRCS Eng. LRCP Lond. 1977.

VAN TERHEYDEN, Nicolas John Eskdale René 11 Oaklands, Westwood Drive, Ilkley LS29 9RE — MB BS Lond. 1986. Specialty: Paediat.

VAN TOOREN, Richard 25 Greville House, Kinnerton St., London SW1X 8EY — MB BS Lond. 1966; MRCS Eng. LRCP Lond. 1966.

VAN TWUYVER, Paulien 20 Elie Avenue, Barnhill, Dundee DD5 3SF — MB ChB Dundee 1986; FRCA 1992. Specialty: Anaesth. Prev: Sen. Regist. (Anaesth.).

VAN VELSEN, Cleo Lorely John Howard Centre, 2 Crozier Terrace, Hackney, London E9 6AT Tel: 020 8919 8562 Fax: 020 8919 8421 — MB BS Lond. 1984 (Kings Coll. Hosp. Lond.) MRCPsych 1989. Cons. Forens. Psychotherapist John Howard Centre Lond.; Hon. Cons. Psychotherapist Maudsley Hosp. Lond.; Hon. Cons. Psychotherapist Gt. Ormond St. Lond. Specialty: Psychother.; Medico Legal. Socs: Founder Mem. Internat. Assn. Forens. Psychother.; Assoc. Mem. Brit. Inst. Psychoanal. Prev: Cons. Psychother. Maudsley Hosp. Lond.; Sen. Regist. (Psychother.) Maudsley Hosp. Lond.; Exam. Doctor Med. Foundat. c/o Victims of Torture.

VAN VELZEN, Professor Dick Fetal & Infant Pathology, Department of Pathology, Royal Liverpool Children's Hospital Alder Hey, Eaton Road, Liverpool L12 2AP Tel: 0151 707 0414 — Artsexamen Free U Amsterdam 1979; Artsexamen Free Univ Amsterdam 1979. Prof. Fetal & Infant Path. Univ. Liverp.; Head Dept. Fetal & Infant Path. (Histopath.) Roy. Liverp. Childr. Hosp. Alder Hey; Research Cons. CIBA-GEIGY Pharmaceut. Horsham & CIBA-GEIGY Forschungs Inst. Basle. Switz. Specialty: Histopath. Socs: Soc. Paediat. Path. USA & Paediat. Path. Soc. Europe (Comm.). Prev: Head Electron Microscopy Dept. & Head Dept. Paediat. Path. SSDZ Delft,The Netherlands.

VAN WOERDEN, Hugo Cornelis Temple of Peace and health, Cathays Park, Cardiff CF10 3NW — MB ChB Aberd. 1987 (Aberdeen) MRCGP 1991; DGM RCP Lond. 1992; DRCOG 1993. Specialty: Gen. Pract.

VAN WOERKOM, Arthur Ernest 304 Pickhurst Lane, West Wickham BR4 0HT — BChir Camb. 1978.

VAN WYK, André Louis Royal Berkshire & Battle Hospital, Elderly Care Medicine Department, London Road, Reading RG1 5AN Tel: 0118 963 6290 Email: andre.vanwyk@rbbh-tr.nhs.uk — MB ChB Cape Town 1983. Cons. (Elderly Med.) Berksh. & Battle Hosp. Specialty: Gen. Med.; Care of the Elderly. Special Interest: Stroke Med. Socs: FRCP(UK).

VAN WYK, Gerrit Jacobus Anaestetics Deptartment, Maidstone Hospital, Hermitage Lane, Maidstone ME16 9NN Tel: 01622 29000; 20 Chapmill, St. Quentins Road, Capetown 8001, South Africa — MB ChB Stellenbosch 1979; BSc Stellenbosch 1974; DA (UK) 1990.

VAN ZINDEREN BAKKER, Rindert Dirk (retired) 70 Bradbourne Road, Sevenoaks TN13 3QA Tel: 01732 464772 Fax: 01732 464772; 70 Bradbourne Road, Sevenoaks TN13 3QA Tel: 01732 464772 Email: rbakker@aol.com — MB ChB Pretoria 1968 (Cape Town Pretoria)

VAN ZWANENBERG, Timothy David Adelaide Medical Centre, Adelaide Terrace, Newcastle upon Tyne NE4 8BE; 8 Queens Road, Jesmond, Newcastle upon Tyne NE2 2PP — MRCS Eng. LRCP Lond. 1971; MB Camb. 1972, BChir 1971; DRCOG 1973; MRCGP 1977. Sen. Lect. Dept. Family & Community Med. Univ. Newc. upon Tyne. Prev: Med. Supt. Nonga Base Hosp. Rabaul, Papua New Guinea; Provin. Health Off. E. New Brit. Papua New Guinea.

VAN ZYL, Jacobus Eduard The Head and Neck Unit, The Royal Marsden Hospital, Fulham, London SW3 6JJ — MB ChB Stellenbosch 1981.

VAN ZYL, Margaret Elizabeth Newlands, Cud Lane, Edge, Stroud GL6 6ND Tel: 01452 812773 — MB ChB Aberd. 1955; MA Aberd. 1949, MB ChB 1955.

VANAT, Tarala Mohamedhusein (retired) 68 Wyatts Drive, Thorpe Bay, Southend-on-Sea SS1 3DE Tel: 01702 585912 — MB BS Gujarat 1969 (M.P. Shah Med. Coll. Jamnagar)

VANCE, Gillian Helen Sarah Southampton General Hospital, Tremona Road, Southampton SO16 6YD Tel: 023 8077 7222; 12 Lansdowne Park, Lisburn BT27 5DJ Tel: 01846 601858 — MB BChir Camb. 1993; MRCP (UK) 1995. Clin. Research Fell. Soton. Gen. Hosp. Specialty: Paediat. Socs: BMA; MDU. Prev: SHO (Paediat. Cardiol.) Soton. Gen. Hosp.

VANCE, John Peden (retired) Traquair, Holmwood Avenue, Uddingston, Glasgow G71 7AJ Tel: 01698 813134 — MD Glas. 1975, MB ChB 1960; DObst RCOG 1962; FRCA 1965; FRCP Glas. 1987. Hon. Snr. Clin. Lect. (Anaesth.) Univ. Glas. Prev: Cons. Anaesth. Roy. Infirm. Glas.

VANDEBERG, Colette Rosine Elise Hanna Lodge, Hamm Court, Weybridge KT13 8YF — MD Liege 1985.

VANDENBERGHE, Elisabeth Anne Michelle Haematology Department Floor A, Royal Hallamshire Hospital, Glossop Road, Sheffield S10 2JA; The Barn, 23 Millhouses Lane, Sheffield S7 2HA — MB BCh BAO NUI 1983 (Univ. Coll. Dub.) MRCPI 1985; PhD Leuven 1992; MRCPath 1993. Cons. Haemat. Roy. Hallamsh. Hosp. & Sheff. Childr. Hosp.; Hon. Lect. Sheff. Univ. Specialty: Haematology. Socs: Brit. Soc. Haematol.; Eur. Haematol. Assn. (Mem. Eur. Bone Marrow Transpl. Gp.). Prev: Sen. Regist. Rotat. (Haemat.) Univ. Coll. Hosp. Middlx.; Research Fell. Haemat. Malig. Cytogenetics Catholic Univ. of Louvain, Belgium; Regist. (Haemat.) Mater Miser. Hosp. Dub.

VANDENBURG, Malcolm John Consultrum Psychiatric, Clinical Trials, Florence Nightingale Clinic Chelsea, 7 Radnor Walk, London SW3 4PB Tel: 020 7349 3917 Fax: 020 7351 7564; 26 Christchurch Hill, Hampstead, London NW3 1LG Tel: 020 7435 9386 Fax: 020 7435 2672 — MB BS Lond. 1973 (St. Bart.) BSc (Hons.) Lond. 1970; FFPM RCP (UK) 1994; FRCP Lond. 1996. Pharmaceut. Dir. & MD, Positive under Pressure; Clin. Advantage Phaemacutical Servs.; Dir. Positive Solutions. Help with Addic.. Specialty: Gen. Med.; Pharmaceutical Medicine; Psychother. Socs: Med. Res. Soc.; Fell. Amer. Coll. Clin. Pharmacol.; Amer. Acad. Pharmacat. Phys. Prev: Pres. & CEO IBRD-Rostrum Global Ltd. Romford; Dir. Clin. Research Merck Sharpe & Dohme UK; Lect. (Med.) & Hon. Sen. Regist. Lond. Hosp.

VANDENDRIESSCHE, Marianne Adrien Withelmina London Vein Institute, 4 Upper Wimpole Street, London W1G 6LF Tel: 020 7224 2830/020 7323 2830 Fax: 020 7224 2930 Email: mvandendriessche@hotmail.com — MD Ghent 1978 (Ghent University Medical School Belgium) FRCS (Belg.); Dip. Surg. Spec Belgium 1984. Cons. Vasc. Surg. Gen. Hosp. Jan Palfyn Ghent, Belgium; Cons. Vasc. Surg. Wellington Hospital London NW6; Private Pract. Lond.; Cons. Vasc. Surg. St Vincent's Hosp. Ghent, Belgium. Specialty: Gen. Surg.; Vasc. Med. Socs: Fell. Roy. Soc. Surg. Belgium; Fell. Roy. Belgium Soc. Vasc. Surg.; Benelux Soc. Phlebology. Prev: Cons. Vasc. Surg. Institut Moderne Ghent,

Belgium; Surg. Asst. Hopital Hotel Dieu, Rouen; Surg. Asst Hopital Notre Dame de Bon Secours, Paris.

VANDENWIJNGAERDEN, Stany 29 Banner Way, Stone Cross, Pevensey BN24 5FE — MD Louvain 1989.

VANDERPUIJE, John Abraham 6 Hedgerley Gardens, Greenford UB6 9NT — MB BS Lond. 1970; MRCS Eng. LRCP Lond. 1970.

VANDERPUMP, Mark Patrick John Royal Free Hospital, Department of Endocrinology, Pond Street, London NW2 2QG Tel: 0207 472 6280 Fax: 0207 472 6487 Email: mark.vanderpump@royalfree.nhs.uk — MB ChB Birm. 1987 (Birmingham) MRCP (UK) 1990; MD Birm. 1995. Cons. Phys. & Hon. Sen. Lect. Endocrinol. & Diabetes Roy. Free Hosp. Lond. Specialty: Endocrinol.; Diabetes. Socs: Soc. Endocrinol.; Brit. Thyroid Assn.; Brit. Diabetic Assn. Prev: Cons. Phys. (Endocrinol. & Diabetes) N. Middlx. Hosp. NHS Trust; Sen. Regist. (Endocrinol., Diabetes & Gen. Med.) N. Staffs. Roy. Infirm. Stoke-on-Trent; Regional Research Fell & Regist. Rotat. (Gen. Med., Diabetes & Endocrinol.) North. RHA.

VANDERVELDE, Elise Mimi 25 Sinclair Grove, London NW11 9JH Tel: 020 8455 9190 — MB BS Durh. 1961 (Newc.) Dip. Bact. Lond 1966. Prev: Sen. Microbiol. Pub. Health Laborat. Serv. Lond.

VANDYK, Edward (retired) PO Box 5569, Newbury RG20 8YY — MB BS Lond. 1970; MRCS Eng. LRCP Lond. 1970; MRCGP 1980.

VANEZIS, Professor Peter Department of Forensic Medicines & Science, University of Glasgow, Glasgow G12 8QQ Tel: 0141 330 4573 Fax: 0141 330 4602; 17 Thornly Park Avenue, Paisley PA2 7SD — MB ChB Bristol 1972 (Univ. Bristol) DMJ (Path.) Soc. Apoth. Lond. 1976; FRCPath 1990, M 1978; MD Bristol 1985; PhD Lond. 1990; FRCP (Glas) 1998, M 1996. Regius Prof. Forens. Med. & Sci. & Head Dept. Univ. Glas.; Hon. Cons. Forens. Med. to Army; Hon. Cons. Forens. Med. Gtr. Glas. HB, & Govt. RePub. Cyprus & Medico-Legal Inst Santiago, Chile. Specialty: Forens. Path. Socs: Fell. (Counc.) Brit. Assn. Forens. Med.; BMA; (Pres.) Brit. Acad. Forens. Scis. Prev: Reader & Head (Forens. Med. & Toxicol.) Char. Cross & Westm. Med. Sch. Lond.; Sen. Lect. (Forens. Med.) Lond. Hosp. Med. Coll.

VANGIKAR, Madhusoodan Baburao (retired) 12 Summerfield Drive, Tyldesley, Manchester M29 7PQ Tel: 01942 894046 — (Poona) MB BS Poona 1954.

VANGIKAR, Michael Milind 4 Wendover Close, Noctorum, Birkenhead CH43 9HU Tel: 0151 652 5974 — MB ChB Liverp. 1991; FRCA 1997. Specialist Regist. (Anaesth.) Mersey Deanery. Specialty: Anaesth.

VANHEGAN, Gillian Margaret 79 Harley Street, London W1G 8PZ Tel: 020 7486 1586 Fax: 020 7486 0397; Westbourne, 9 Alverstone Rd, London NW2 5JS Tel: 020 8459 2311 Fax: 020 7486 0397 Email: gillian.vanhegan@virgin.net — MB BS Lond. 1970 (St. Bartholomew's Hospital Medical School) MRCS Eng. LRCP Lond. 1970; DObst RCOG 1972; MFFP 1993. p/t Med. Dir. & Cons. In Med. Gyn. & Psychosexual Med., Lond. Brook Advisory Centres; Cons. Psycho-Sexual Med. BUPA Lond.; Cons. Psychosexual Med. Riverside H.A. Lond. Specialty: Family Plann. & Reproduc. Health; Genitourinary Medicine; Psychosexual Med. Special Interest: Contraceptive Implants; Persistent Candida; Erectile Dysfunction. Socs: Brit. Menopause Soc.; Lond. Soc. Family Plann. Doctors; Inst. Psychosexual Med. Prev: Sessional Med. Off. Camden & Islington AHA (T); SHO (Obst. Unit) Roy. Free Hosp. Lond.; Ho. Phys. St. Bart. Hosp. Lond.

VANHEGAN, Mr John Andrew David (retired) 79 Harley Street, London W1G 8PZ Tel: 020 7487 4278 Fax: 020 7486 0397 Email: john.vanhegan@virgin.net; 9 Alverstone Road, London NW2 5JS Tel: 020 8459 2311 — MB BS Lond. 1970 (St. Bart.) MRCS Eng. LRCP Lond. 1970; FRCS Eng. 1976; Cert. Higher Surgic. Train. RCS Eng. 1982. Cons. Orthop. Surg. Lond. Prev: Sen. Regist. (Orthop.) Hammersmith Hosp. Lond.

VANHEGAN, Robert Ian Swindon Private Histopathology, 83 London Street, Faringdon SN7 8AA Tel: 01367 242368 Fax: 01367 244037 Email: vanheganri@doctors.org.uk — BM BCh Oxf. 1970; DPhil Oxf. 1969, MA 1968; FRCPath 1991, M 1979. Specialty: Histopath.; Pathology, General; Medico Legal. Special Interest: Surgic. Path. & Morbid Anat. Socs: Expert Witness Inst.; Path. Soc; Assn of Clin. Pathol. Prev: Cons. Path. Princess Margt. Hosp. Swindon.; Clin. Tutor (Path.) Univ. Oxf.; Lect. (Physiol.) Lady Margt. Hall.

VANHOUSE, Sheila Hazel Meadowside Family Health Centre, 30 Winchcombe Road, Solihull B92 8PJ Tel: 0121 743 2560/742 5666 Fax: 0121 743 4216; 8 Burgess Croft, Hampton Coppice, Solihull B92 0QJ — BM BS Nottm. 1984; DRCOG 1988; MRCGP 1989. GP Solihull.

VANIA, Abdul-Kader Arrazi Medical Centre, 1 Evington Lane, Leicester LE5 5PQ Tel: 0116 249 0000 Fax: 0116 249 0088 Email: vandoc27@yahoo.co.uk — MB ChB Leic. 1987; MRCP (UK) 1990; DFFP 1995. Regist. (Thoracic Med. & Neurol.) Centr. Middlx. Hosp. Lond.; Clin. Asst. Dept. Endocrinol. LRI. Specialty: Gen. Pract.; Endocrinol.; Acupunc.; Medico Legal. Prev: SHO (Endocrinol., Neurol., Dermat. & Haemat.) Leic. Roy. Infirm.

VANIER, Therese Marie (retired) 12 Chestnut House, Barston Road, London SE27 9HD Tel: 020 8761 4670 — MB BChir Camb. 1953; FRCP Lond. 1978, M 1959. Prev: Cons. Phys. St. Christopher's Hospice Lond.

VANITA, Dr 29 West End, Sherborne St John, Basingstoke RG24 9LE — MB BS Panjab 1970.

VANN, Adrian Michael 14 Ecton Lane, Sywell, Northampton NN6 0BA — MB ChB Liverp. 1993.

VANN, James Anthony St Thomas Court Surgery, St. Thomas Court, Church Street, Axminster EX13 5AG Tel: 01297 32126 Fax: 01297 35759 — MB BS Lond. 1978; MA Oxf. 1972; DRCOG 1982.

VANNER, Anne Marie Narvik Ho., Princess Alexander Hosp., Addison House, Fourth Avenue, Harlow CM20 1DS; 21 Rowney Gardens, Sawbridgeworth CM21 0AT Tel: 01279 723431 Fax: 01279 724151 — MB BCh Wales 1967 (Cardiff) MRCGP 1981; AFOM RCP Lond. 1993. Occupational Health Phys.; Company Med. Off. Nortel Networks & Merck Sharpe & Dohme Harlow; Occupat. Health Phys. Princess Alexandra Hosp. NHS Trust Harlow; Sen. Occupat. Health Adviser to Harlow Occupat. Health Serv.; Health & Safety Apptd. Doctor for Lead Asbestos & Ionising Radiat.; Occupational Health Phys, to N.I.B.S.C.; Sen. Clin. Fell. in OCI Med. Addenbrookes Hosp., Camb. Specialty: Occupat. Health. Socs: BMA; Soc. Occupat. Med.; Assoc. Mem. Fac. Occupat. Med. Prev: Retd. G.P. Addison Ho. Harlow.

VANNER, Richard Guy Gloucestershire Royal NHS Trust, Great Western Road, Gloucester GL1 Tel: 01452 528555 — MB BS Lond. 1981; FRCA 1986. Cons. Anaesth. Glos. Roy. NHS Trust. Specialty: Anaesth.

VANNER, Tracey Frances Margaret Good Hope Hospital, Rectory Road, Sutton Coldfield B75 7RR — MB BCh Wales 1987; MRCOG 1993. Cons. Obst. & Gynaecologist, Good Hope Hosp. NHS Trust, Sutton, Coldfield. Specialty: Obst. & Gyn. Socs: Brit. Fetal Matern. Med. Soc.; Birm. & Midl.s Obst. & Gyn. Soc.

VANNIASEGARAM, Mr Iyngaran The Willows, St. George's Hospital, 117 Suttons Lane, Hornchurch RM12 6RS Tel: 01708 465462 Fax: 01708 465158 — MB BS Sri Lanka 1977; DLO RCS Eng. 1984; FRCS Ed. (Orl.) 1987; MSc (Med.) Lond. 1991. Cons. Audiological Med. Barking & Dagenham (BOD) PCT; Med. Director BO PCT. Specialty: Audiol. Med. Socs: BMA; Brit. Assn. Audiol. Phys.; Internat. Assn. Phys. in Audiol. Prev: Sen. Regist. (Audiological Med.) Nat. Hosp. Neurol. & Neurosurg., Roy. Nat. Throat, Nose & Ear Hosp. & Gt. Ormond St. Hosp.; +Lond.

VANSTRAELEN, Michel 55 Castleton Road, Ilford IG3 9QW — MD Louvain 1986.

VAQUAS, Shah Muhammad Louth County Hospital, High Holme Road, Louth LN11 06U Fax: 01507 602195 — MB BS Karachi 1982; MRCPI 1993. Specialty: Gen. Med.; Care of the Elderly. Special Interest: Falls Syncope.

VAQUAS, Shams 10 Canonsfield Road, Welwyn AL6 0QH — MB BS Karachi 1985; FRCS Ed. 1990.

VARA, Roshni 120 Central Road, Worcester Park KT4 8HT — MB BS Lond. 1998.

VARADA REDDY, Peta Srinivasulureddy Department of Radiology, Medway Hospital, Windmill Road, Gillingham ME7 5NY — MB BS Sri Venkateswara 1973 (Kurnool Med. Coll.) BSc Sri Venkateswara 1967, MB BS 1973; DMRD Madras 1976; DMRD Eng. 1979; FRCR 1982. Cons. Radiol. Medway Hosp. Specialty: Radiol. Prev: Cons. (Radiol.) St. John's Hosp. Livingston; Sen. Regist. Roy. Infirm. Edin.; Regist. (Radiol.) Roy. Infirm. Edin. & St. Peter's Hosp. Chertsey.

VARADARAJAN, Chathapurum Ramanathan 2 Daphene Gardens, Limavady Road, Waterside, Londonderry BT47 6LX Tel:

01504 44707 — MB BS Mysore 1969 (Kasthurba Med. Coll. Mangalore) BSc Kerala 1962; FFA RCSI 1974. Cons. Anaesth. Altnagelvin Hosp. Londonderry. Specialty: Anaesth. Socs: Intractable Pain Soc. Gt. Brit. & Irel. Prev: Tutor & Regist. Dept. Anaesth. S. Belf. Gp. Hosps.; Cons. i/c Pain Relief Clin. Altnagelvin Hosp. Lond.derry.

VARADARAJAN, Mr Raghu Tudor Cottage, 63 Borrowcop Lane, Lichfield WS14 9LS — MB BS Madras 1988; FRCS Ed. 1992. Regist. (HPB Surg.) St. Vincent's Hosp. Elm Pk. Dub. Specialty: Gen. Surg. Prev: Regist. (Vasc. Surg.) Galway; Regist. (Gen. Surg.) Princess Margt. Hosp. Swindon.

VARADHARAJAN, Subbaraman 14 New Heath Close, Wednesdfield, Wolverhampton WV11 1XX — MB BS Madras 1988.

VARAH, Sri Sleaford Road Surgery, 1 Sleaford Road, Heckington, Sleaford NG34 9QP — MB BS Sri Lanka 1978.

VARATHARAJ, Jayaratnam 22 Allens Road, Enfield EN3 4PN — MB BS Sri Lanka 1976; LRCP LRCS Ed. LRCPS Glas. 1985.

VARAWALLA, Nermeen Yunus 14 Ashworth Mansions, Elgin Avenue, London W9 1JL — MB BS Bombay 1985; MD Bombay 1988; DPhil Oxf. 1992; MRCOG 1993. Sen. Regist. Rotat. (O & G) W. Midl. Specialty: Obst. & Gyn. Prev: Regist. Rotat. Oxf.; Rhodes Research Fell. Univ. Oxf.; Lect. (O & G) Univ. Bombay.

VARCHEVKER, Jose Arturo 27 Dunstan Road, London NW11 8AG Tel: 020 8381 4555 Fax: 020 8381 4477 — Social Psych. Buenos Aires 1967; Medico Buenos Aires 1968. Assoc. Specialist (Psychiat.). Specialty: Gen. Psychiat.; Psychother. Socs: Brit. Psychoanal. Soc.; Brit. Inst. Psychoanal.; Fell. Lond. Centre of Psychotherap. Prev: Clin. Asst. MarlBoro. Family Serv.; Cons. N.W. Thames RHA; Regist. Cassel Hosp. Richmond & Henderson Hosp. Sutton.

VARDE, Kishor Department of Obstetrics & Gynaecology, East Glamorgan General Hospital, Church Village, Pontypridd CF38 1AB — MB BS Durham 1959.

VARDI, Glen Droitwich Knee Clinic, St Andrew's Road, Droitwich WR9 8YX Tel: 01905 794558 Fax: 01905 795916; 80A Southover, London N12 7HB — MB ChB Pretoria 1984.

VARDILL, David Melbury, Broad Oak, Sturminster Newton DT10 2HG — MB BCh Wales 1998.

VARDON, Valerie Mary Elderly Health Services, Queen Alexandra Hospital, Cosham, Portsmouth PO6 3LY Tel: 023 92 286 059; 12 Dornmere Lane, Waterlooville PO7 8QH Tel: 023 9226 3723 — MB BS Newc. 1972; MRCP (UK) 1977. Assoc. Specialist (Elderly Health Serv.) Qu. Alexandra Hosp. Portsmouth. Specialty: Palliat. Med. Prev: Sen. Community Med. Off. (c/o Elderly) Newc. HA; Sen. Regist. (Geriat.) Newc. Gen. Hosp.

VARDY, Dulcie Lucia Fieldway, West Strand, West Wittering, Chichester PO20 8AU — MB ChB Leeds 1956; DPH Lond. 1963.

VARDY, Emma Rachael Louise Cunningham Academic Unit Molecular Vascular Medicine, G. Floor, Martin Wing, Leeds General Infirmary, Leeds LS1 3EX — MB ChB Sheff. 1998; MB ChB Sheff 1998. Clin. Research Fellow/ Hon. Specialist Regist., Leeds Gen. Infirm. Specialty: Accid. & Emerg. Prev: HO, Rotat. Northern Gen. Hosp.; Sho, (A & E) Northern Gen. Hosp. Sheff..; SHO Rotat. in Medicine,St. James' Univ. Hosp., Leeds.

VARDY, Jennifer Margaret 1/L 5 Peel Street, Glasgow G11 5LL — MB ChB Glas. 1994.

VARDY, Peter Ivan War Pensions Agency, Norcross, Blackpool FY5 3TA Tel: 01253 333134 — (Westm.) AKC 1962; MB BS Lond. 1962; DObst RCOG 1964; MRCGP 1971. Med. Adviser War Pens. Agency Blackpool. Specialty: Civil Serv. Prev: GP Runcorn; Ho. Surg. & Ho. Phys. St. Stephen's Hosp. Chelsea; Ho. Surg. (O & G) & Ho. Phys. (Paediat.) Chester City Hosp.

VARDY, Sarah Brigitte c/o Mr R Vardy, 4 Bracken Lane, Retford DN22 7EU — MB BS Lond. 1992.

VARDY, Mr Stephen James, Wing Cdr. RAF Med. Br. Retd. Ophthalmic Department, Peterborough District General Hospital, Thorpe Road, Peterborough PE3 6DA Tel: 01733 875730 Fax: 01733 874939 — MB ChB 1982 (Birmingham) FRCS Ed. 1990; FRCOphth 1993. Cons. Ophth. PD Hosp.s Trust; Cons. Adviser (Ophth.) RAF; Cons. Ophth. MDHU P'boro. Specialty: Ophth. Socs: UK Soc. Cataract & Refractive Surg.; RCM; Brit. Oculoplastic Surg. Soc. Prev: Fell. Moorfields Eye Hosp. Lond.; Sen. Regist. The Eye Hosp. Soton.

VAREY, Nicolas Calvert (retired) Caduceus, Main St., Knedlington, Goole DN14 7EU Tel: 01430 430833 — (St. And.) MB ChB St. And. 1965; FFPM 1994, M 1990. Chairm. Tees E. & N. Yorks. NHS Ambul. Trust. Prev: Med. Dir. Reckitt & Colman Ltd. Hull.

VARGHESE, Chirakal Mathai 47 Winterfield Drive, Bolton BL3 4TE — MB BS Kerala 1972; DCH; MRCP 1 1985; DCCH Edin 1986; DTM & H Liverp. 1986; MSc Manchester, 1991. Cons., Community Pediatrician, in Audiol. Specialty: Audiol. Med.

VARGHESE, David 12 Abbey Drive, Church Lane, London SW17 9PN — MB ChB Liverp. 1995.

VARGHESE, Manalil Alexander High Street Medical Centre, 91/91A High St., Wrekenton, Gateshead NE9 7JR Tel: 0191 491 0666 — MB BS 1975 Kerala. GP Gateshead, Tyne & Wear.

VARGHESE, Mathew Moyle Hospital, Gloucester Avenue, Larne BT40 1RP Tel: 028 2827 5431; 69A Carrickfergus Road, Larne BT40 3JX Tel: 028 2827 0283 — MB BS Nagpur 1974 (Govt. Med. Coll. Nagpur) MRCP (UK) 1977; FRCP Lond. 1997. Cons. Phys. Moyle Hosp. Larne; Fell. Ulster Med. Soc. Specialty: Gen. Med.; Care of the Elderly; Diabetes. Socs: Brit. Geriat. Soc. Prev: Sen. Regist. (Geriat. Med.) Roy. Vict. Hosp. Belf.

VARGHESE, Mr Soonu West Cumberland Hospital, Hensingham, Whitehaven CA28 8JG Tel: 01946 693181; Willowdene, Little Broughton, Cockermouth CA13 0YG Tel: 01900 824914 — MB BS Mysore 1973; DO RCS Eng. 1978; FRCS Ed. 1983. Cons. Ophth. W. Cumbld. Hosp. Whitehaven. Specialty: Ophth. Special Interest: Diabetic Retinopathy. Socs: Eur. Soc. Cataract & Refractive Surg.; Roy. Coll. of Ophthalmologists; Amer. Acad. Prev: Cons. & Sen. Regist. Al-Qassimi Hosp. Sharjah UAE; Regist. South. Gen. Hsop. Glas.

VARIA, Haren Nitin 3 Calderburn Close, The Meadows, Horwich, Bolton BL6 6RL Tel: 07968 824549 Email: harenvaria@hotmail.com — MB ChB Leicester 1997; FRCR 2004. Specialist Regist., Diagnostic Radiol., N. Manch. Train. scheme. Specialty: Radiol.

VARIAN, John Anthony 7B Follet Road, Toposham, Exeter EX3 0JP — MB BCh BAO NUI 1979; MRCPsych 1985.

VARIEND, Sadick 94 Ashdell Road, Broomhill, Sheffield S10 3DB Tel: 0114 266 0404 — MD Cape Town 1979; MB ChB 1965; DCH Eng. 1971; MRCP (UK) 1972; FRCPath 1989, M 1977; FRCP Lond. 1990. Cons. Histopath. Sheff. Childr. Hosp.; Hon. Clin. Lect. (Path. & Paediat.) Univ. Sheff. Specialty: Histopath.

VARKER, Jonathon Andrew 376 St Helens Road, Bolton BL3 3RR Tel: 01204 62418; 11 Newstead Drive, Bolton BL3 3RE Tel: 01204 64123 — MB ChB Manch. 1989; MRCGP 1993.

VARKEY, Arun Thomas Roche House, 33 Eastfield Crescent, Laughton, Sheffield S25 1YT — MB BS Berhampur 1981.

VARKEY, Sujatha Roche House, 33 Eastfield Crescent, Laughton, Sheffield S25 1YT — MB BS India 1985; MRCP (UK) 1990.

VARKEY, Thoppil Antony Willenhall Medical Centre, Croft/Gomer Street, Willenhall WV13 2DR Tel: 01902 600833 Fax: 01902 609403; 76 Bilston Road, Willenhall WV13 2JL Tel: 01902 636840 — MB BS Mysore 1972 (Kasturba Med. Coll. Mangalore) GP Willenhall. Prev: Regist. (Psychiat.) Worcester Roy. Infirm. (Newton Br.) & Towers Hosp. Leics.; Regist. (Psychiat.) Stallington Hosp. Stoke-on-Trent.

VARLEY, Bruce Quinton 5 Albion Mews, Thornhill Road, London N1 1JX Tel: 020 7607 5723 Fax: 020 7607 5723 — MRCS Eng. LRCP Lond. 1976 (St. Bart.) BSc (Physiol.) Lond. 1970, MB BS 1976; FFA RCS Eng. 1980. Cons. Anaesth. St. Bart. Hosp. Lond.; Cons. Anaesth. King Edwd. VII Hosp. for Offs. Lond. Specialty: Anaesth. Socs: Fell. Roy. Soc. Med.; Assn. Anaesth. GB & Irel. & Harveian Soc. Lond. Prev: Cons. Anaesth. St. Marks Hosps. Lond.; Cons. Anaesth. & Hon. Lect. Groote Schuur Hosp. Univ. Cape Town.

VARLEY, Edith Mary (retired) 7 Melrose Crescent, Hale, Altrincham WA15 8NN Tel: 0161 980 6437 — BM BCh Oxf. 1957; DA Eng. 1961; FFA RCS Eng. 1965. Prev: Cons. Anaesth. Wythenshawe Hosp. Manch.

VARLEY, Gordon Jesse (retired) 9 Sycamore Crescent, Macclesfield SK11 8LL Tel: 01625 425741 — (Birm.) MB ChB Birm. 1955. Prev: Ho. Phys. & Ho. Surg. (Obst.) Solihull Hosp.

VARLEY, Gordon Ward 23 Old North Road, Wansford, Peterborough PE8 6LB — MB ChB Leeds 1983.

VARLEY, Ruth 41 Tower Street, Barnsley S70 1QS — MB ChB Leeds 1995.

VARLEY, Simon Charles 129 Regent Road, Lostock, Bolton BL6 4DX — MB BS Lond. 1988; FRCA 1993. Cons. (Anaesth.) Manch. Roy. Infirm. Specialty: Anaesth.

VARLEY, Yvonne Worth 261 New hey Road, Huddersfield HD3 4GH Tel: 01484 648967 — BM Soton. 1977; BSc Lond. 1966; DCH RCP Lond. 1984; DCCH RCP Ed. 1984; DOccMed 1998; DFFP 1998. Occupational ed. Private Provides. Specialty: Occupat. Health; Gen. Pract. Socs: Soc. Occupat. Med.; Hudds. Med. Soc. (Pres. 1999-2000). Prev: Occupational ed. Adviser Univ. Huddersfield HD1 3DH; Princip. GP The Univ. Huddersfield HD1 3DH.

VARMA, Aarti 42 Alwen Avenue, Huddersfield HD2 2SJ — MB ChB Leeds 1992. Specialty: Gen. Surg. Prev: SHO (Orthop.) Castle Hill Hosp. Cottingham; SHO (Gen. Surg.) Castle Hill Hosp.

VARMA, Alakh Niranjan (retired) Rauceby Hospital, Sleaford NG34 8PP Tel: 01529 416048 Fax: 01529 488239; 149 Grantham Road, Sleaford NG34 7NR Tel: 01529 303681 — MB BS Patna 1956 (Med. Coll. Patna) BSc Patna 1949; DPM Eng. 1971; DPM Ed. 1971; MRCPsych 1972. Cons. Child Psychiat. S. Lincs. Health Dist. Prev: Sen. Med. Off. Min. of Health, Ghana.

VARMA, Aloke 9 Stone Street, Southsea PO5 3BN — MB ChB Manch. 1996.

VARMA, Bhola Nath 32 Brookfield Drive, Boothstown, Worsley, Manchester M28 1JY — MB BS Patna 1954; TDD Wales 1958. Socs: BMA. Fell. Amer. Coll. Chest Phys. Prev: Regist. Chest Dis. E. Birm. Hosp. Birm. & Birm. Chest Clinic, Manch.; Chest Clinic & Monsall Hosp Manch.

VARMA, Chetan 95 Montbelle Road, London SE9 3NY — MB BS Lond. 1992; BSc Hons. Lond. 1989, MB BS 1992.

VARMA, Mr Jagmohan Singh Department of Surgery, The Medical School, The University, Newcastle upon Tyne NE2 4HH Tel: 0191 282 4384 Fax: 0191 282 0330 Email: j.s.varma@ncl.ac.uk; The West Wing, Netherton Hall, Nedderton Village, Bedlington NE22 6AS Tel: 01670 823185 Fax: 01670 821274 Email: j.s.varma@ncl.ac.uk — MB ChB Ed. 1977; BSc (Hons.) Ed. 1974; FRCS Ed. 1982; MD 1988; FRCP Ed. 2003. Sen. Lect. & Hon. Cons. Surg. Med. Sch. Newc. upon Tyne Hosps. NHS Trust; Vis. Lect. (Surg.) P. Wales Hosp, Chinese Univ. Hong Kong, 1988. Specialty: Gen. Surg. Special Interest: Laparoscopic Surg.; Anorectal Physiol.; Colorectal Cancer. Socs: Surgic. Research Soc. UK; Assn. Coloproctol.; Brit. Soc. Gastroenterol. Prev: Sen. Regist. (Gen. Surg.) Teachg. Hosp. Edin.; Wellcome Trust Surgic. Research Fell. Univ. Edin. Dept. Surg. & Urol. West. Gen. Hosp. Edin.; SHO (Path.) Edin.

VARMA, Kailash Behari Colinton Road Surgery, 163 Colinton Road, Edinburgh EH14 1BE — MB BS Patna 1962. GP Edin.

VARMA, Mahendra Pratap Singh Erne Hospital, Cornagrade Rd, Enniskillen BT7 6AY Tel: 02866 382431 Fax: 02866 382657; Sionghasan, Bellanleck, Enniskillen BT92 2BA Tel: 02866 348770 — LRCPI & LM, LRSCI & LM 1969 (RCSI) PhD 1975; MRCP (UK) 1977; FRCPI 1984; FCCP 1987; FRCP Glas. 1988; FESC 1989; FRCP Lond. 1996. Cons. Phys. & Cardiol. Erne Hosp. Enniskillen. Specialty: Cardiol.; Diabetes. Socs: Irish Cardiac Soc.; Fell. Roy. Acad. Med. Dub.; Fell. Amer. Coll. Chest Phys.

VARMA, Meena Colinton Road Surgery, 163 Colinton Road, Edinburgh EH14 1BE; (Surgery), 30 Chesser Crescent, Edinburgh EH14 1SB Tel: 0131 443 2456 — MB BS Ranchi 1966 (Rajendra Med. Coll.) DObst RCPI 1975.

VARMA, Munivenkatappa Ravindra 43 Fairholme Avenue, Eccleston Park, Prescot L34 2RN.

VARMA, Paula Nina Ty-Newydd Farmhouse, Sigingstone, Cowbridge CF71 7LP — MB BCh Wales 1994; BSc Ed. 1989. SHO (Med.) Pontypridd. Specialty: Gen. Med.

VARMA, Rajesh Dept. of Obs & Gyn, Queens Medical Centre, Nottingham NG7 2UH — MB ChB Aberd. 1995. Specialist Regist., Dept. of Obs. & Gyn. Qu.s Med. Centre, Notts. Specialty: Obst. & Gyn.

VARMA, Mr Rajesh Birmingham Women's Hospital, Academic Department of Obstetrics & Gynaecology, 2nd Floor, Edgbaston, Birmingham B15 2TG Tel: 0121 607 4751 Email: r.varma@bham.ac.uk — MB BS (Hons.) Lond. 1995 (Guy's & St Thos.) BA (Hons.) Camb. 1992; MA Camb. 1997; DFFP 1998; MRCOG 2000. Lect. in Obst. and Gyn.; MRC Clin. Fell. Academic Dept. Obst. & Gyn. Birm. Wom. Hosp. Specialty: Obst. & Gyn.; Research. Special Interest: Genetic and molecular pathogenesis of endometriosis; Ectopic Pregn.; Vaginal birth after caesarean Sect. Socs: Med. Protection Soc.; BMA; Brit. Adolesc. & Paediat. Gyn. Prev: Specialist Regist. (Obst. & Gyn.) Bedford Hosp. NHS Trust & Luton & Dunstable NHS Trust; Sen. SHO (Obst. & Gyn.) Qu. Med. Centre Nottm.; SHO (Obst. & Gyn.) Qu. Med. Centre Nottm., Derby City Hosp. & North. Gen. Hosp. Sheff.

VARMA, Rajiv Linden Lea, Hillwood Grove, Hutton Mount, Brentwood CM13 2PD — MB BS Delhi 1980; MRCOG 1987.

VARMA, Rashmi Bala 95 Montbelle Road, London SE9 3NY — MB BS Lond. 1993.

VARMA, Mr Ravi 8 Rosemary Drive, Redbridge, Ilford IG4 5JD Tel: 020 8550 5593 — MB BS Bihar 1963 (Darbhanga Med. Coll.) MS Bihar 1966. Clin. Asst. Minor Injuries Unit St. Leonards Hosp. Lond. Socs: BMA. Prev: Clin. Asst. (Orthop. & A & E) Whipps Cross Hosp. Lond.; Regist. (Orthop.) Whipps Cross Hosp. Lond.

VARMA, Sandeep Queen's Medical Centre, Department of Dermatology, B Floor South Block, Nottingham NG7 2UH Tel: 0115 924 9924 Ext: 42114 Fax: 0115 849 3299 Email: sandeep.varma@mail.qmcuh-tr.trent.nhs.uk — MB BCh Wales 1993; BMedSc (Hons.) Path. Sci. Wales 1991; MRCP (UK) 1996. Cons. Dermatol. Queens Med. Centre Nottm. Specialty: Dermat. Socs: BMA; Brit. Assn. of Dermat.; Brit. Soc. of Dermatologic Surg. Prev: Specialist Regist. (Dermat.) Univ. Hosp. Wales.

VARMA, Sanjay 163 Colinton Road, Edinburgh EH14 1BE — MB ChB Ed. 1991.

VARMA, Mr Sanjay Kumar Leicester Royal Infirmary, Infirmary Square, Leicester LE1 5WW Tel: 0116 254 1414 Fax: 0116 258 5852 Email: sanjay.varma@uhl-tr.nhs.uk — MB BS All India Inst. Med. Sciences 1977 (All India Inst. Med. Sci., New Delhi, India) MS 1979; FRCS Ed. 1981; FRCS (Plast) Ed. 1992. Cons. Plastic Surg. University Hospitals of Leicester NHS Trust, Leicester. Specialty: Plastic Surg. Socs: BAPS; BAAPS; Expert Witness Institute. Prev: Sen. Regist. (Plastic Surg.) Leeds & Bradford; Regist. (Plastic Surg.) Leicester.

VARMA, Mr Thelekat Raman Kerala The Walton Centre for Neurology and Neurosurgery, Fazakerley, Liverpool L9 7LJ — MB BS Bangalor 1972 (Bangalore Med. Coll.) MB BS Bangalore 1972; FRCS Ed. 1979. Cons. Neurosurg. The Walton Centre for Neurol. & Neurosurg. Liverp. Specialty: Neurosurg. Prev: Cons. Neurosurg. Dundee Roy. Infirm.; Sen. Regist. (Neurosurg.) Univ. Hosp. Wales Cardiff; Regist. (Neurosurg.) Hallamsh. Hosp. Sheff. & Walton Hosp. Liverp.

VARNAM, Michael Adrian Windmill Practice, Sneinton Health Centre, Beaumont Street, Nottingham NG2 4PJ Tel: 0115 950 5426; 73 Stanton Road, Ilkeston DE7 5FW Tel: 0115 932 2639 — (Lond. Hosp.) MB BS Lond. 1967; DObst RCOG 1969; FRCGP 1980, M 1972; DM Nottm. 1988; MFPHM 2000; FRIPHH 2001. Mem. City Counc. Area Comm.; Vice Chairm. PEC Nottm. PCT, Non Exec. Bd. Health Developm. Agency. Specialty: Alcohol & Substance Misuse. Prev: Assoc. Advisor Gp.; Chairm. RCGP Educat. Div.; Course Organiser VTS Nottm.

VARNAM, Robert Michael 73 Stanton Road, Ilkeston DE7 5FW — MB ChB Manch. 1995.

VARNAVA, Amanda Maria Deborah 53 Etchingham Park Road, London N3 2EB; 9 St Mark's Place, London W11 1NS — MB BS Lond. 1990 (Oxford and St Bartholomew's) BA Oxf. 1987; MRCP Lond. 1993. Research Regist. (Cardiol.) St Geo.'s Hosp. Lond. Specialty: Cardiol. Prev: Regist. (Cardiol.) Roy. Brompton & St Geo.'s Hosps. Lond.

VARNAVIDES, Christakis Kyriacos Dib Lane Practice, 112A Dib Lane, Leeds LS8 3AY Tel: 0113 295 4650 Fax: 0113 295 4663; 40 North Park Avenue, Leeds LS8 1EJ Tel: 0113 266 2132 Fax: 0113 266 2132 — (Leeds) BSc (Hons.) Leeds 1967; MB ChB Leeds 1970; DObst RCOG 1972; FRCGP 1987, M 1977; Cert. Family Plann. JCC 1979. Tutor (Gen. Pract.) Univ. Leeds; Examr. Roy. Coll. Gen. Pract.; Trainer (Gen. Pract.) Leeds AHA (T); Clin. Asst. (Dermat.) Leeds Gen. Infirm. Specialty: Dermat. Prev: Chairm. Yorks. Fac. RCGP; Regist. (Med. & Mineral Metab.) & Ho. Phys. Leeds Gen. Infirm.; SHO (Obst.) Leeds Matern. Hosp.

VARNEY, Angela Dawn The Thatched Cottage, Hill St., Calmore, Southampton SO40 2RX — MB ChB Liverp. 1985; DRCOG 1990. GP Soton.

VARNEY, Mrs Patricia Ann (retired) Riverthatch, The Abbotsbrook, Bourne End SL8 5QU Tel: 01628 521077 — MRCS Eng. LRCP Lond. 1974; Dip. GU Med. Soc. Apoth. Lond. 1992;

MFFP 1993. Prev: Clin. Asst. (Genitourin. Med.) Char. Cross Hosp. Lond. & Vict. Clinic for Sexual Health.

VARNEY, Paul Ronald Lilac Cottage, Buttons Lane, West Wellow, Romsey SO51 6BR — MB BCh Wales 1971; DObst RCOG 1974; MRCGP 1975. Prev: Hon. Clin. Tutor Univ. Soton. Med. Sch.

VARNEY, Veronica Ann St Helier NHS Trust, Wrythe Lane, Carshalton SM5 1AA; 59 Meadow Walk, Epsom KT19 0AX — MB BS Lond. 1983; MD; MRCP (UK) 1987; FRCP 2000. Regist. (Med., Clin. Allergy & Immunol.) Roy. Brompton Papworth Hosp.; Gen. med.; Resp. med.; Immunol. & allergy (CCST). Specialty: Respirat. Med. Prev: Regist. & Research Regist. Roy. Brompton Hosp. Lond.; Regist. (Chest Med. & Intens. Care Med.) Papworth Hosp. & AddenbrookesHosp. Camb.

VARSANI, Gattotkutch Bhimji 7 Compton House, 4 Carlisle Road, Shirley, Southampton SO16 4BS — BM Soton. 1998.

VARSHNEY, Giriraj Kishore Rhys House Family Health Care, Rhys House, James St, Ebbw Vale NP23 6JG Tel: 01495 307407; 4 Pant-y-Fforest, New Town, Ebbw Vale NP23 5FR Tel: 01495 308821 — MB BS Lucknow 1968 (K.G. Med. Coll. Lucknow) BSc Agra 1962; DTCD Wales 1995. Specialty: Psychother. Socs: Med. Protec.

VARSHNEY, Mahavir Prasad Riverbank Medical Centre, Walford Avenue, Worle, Weston Super Mare BS22 7YZ Tel: 01934 521133 Fax: 01934 522226 — LMSSA Lond. 1979 (J.N. Medical Coll., Aligarh, India) BSc Aligarh 1964, MB BS 1969; DTM & H Liverp. 1974; DCH Dub. 1977. Specialty: Paediat.; Dermat.

VARTAN, Charles Philip Westbourne Medical Centre, Milburn Road, Bournemouth BH4 9HJ Tel: 01202 752550 Fax: 01202 769700; 18 Fairview Park, Overbury Rd, Poole BH14 9JZ Tel: 01202 741517 — (St. Bart.) MB BS Lond. 1966; MRCS Eng. LRCP Lond. 1966; MRCP (UK) 1970; FRCP 1999. GP Bournemouth; Hosp. Pract. (Gastroenterol., Endoscopy. & Biliary Endoscopy) Bournemouth Gen. Hosp.

VARTIKOVSKI, Rolland Flat 40, 250 Camphill Avenue, Glasgow G41 3AS — Vrach Kishinev Medical Inst. USSR 1968.

VARTY, Christopher Paul The Orchard Surgery, Penstone Park, Lancing BN15 9AG Tel: 01903 843333 Fax: 01903 843332 — MB BS Lond. 1989 (St. Geo. Lond.) DCH RCP Lond. 1994. Specialty: Gen. Pract.

VARTY, Mr Kevin Department of Surgery, Addenbrookes NHS Trust, Box 201, Hills Road, Cambridge CB2 2QQ Tel: 01223 216992 Fax: 01223 216015 — BM BCh Oxf. 1985; BA (Hons.) Oxf. 1985, BM BCh Oxf. 1985; FRCS Eng. 1989; MD 1994; FRCS (Gen.) 1997. Cons. (Vasc. Surg.) Camb. Specialty: Gen. Surg. Special Interest: Deep Vein Thrombosis & Venous Insufficiency; Diabetic Foot; Limb Ischaemia & Bypass Surg. Socs: Vasc. Surg. Soc.; Assn. of Surgeons of Gt. Britain & Irel. (ASGBI); Europ. Vasc. Soc. Prev: SHO (Gen. Surg.) Wonford Hosp. Exeter.; Regist. Nottm. Derby; Sen. Regist. Leics.

VARUGHESE, Mohini Anna 38 West Way, Shirley, Croydon CR0 8RB — MB BS Lond. 1998.

VARUGHESE, Punnackattu Scaria 16 Methuen Road, Edgware HA8 6EX — MB BS Kerala 1972.

VARUGHESE, Reuben Thomas Jacob 116 Chesterfield Gardens, London N4 1LR — MB BS Lond. 1988.

VARVEL, David Adrian Brundall Medical Centre, The Dales, Brundall, Norwich NR13 5RP Tel: 01603 712255 Fax: 01603 712156; 3 Brandon Court, Brundall, Norwich NR13 5NW — MB BS Lond. 1967 (Univ. Coll. Hosp.) DObst RCOG 1971. Socs: BMA. Prev: SHO (O & G) W. Suff. Gen. Hosp. Bury St. Edmunds; Ho. Phys. (Gen. Med.) & Ho. Surg. (Gen. Surg.) Princess Margt. Hosp. Swindon.

VARVINSKY, Andrey Torbay Hospital, Department of Anaesthesia, Lawes Bridge, Torquay TQ2 7AA Tel: 01803 654310 Fax: 01803 654312 Email: andrey.varvinsk@nhs.net — Vrach Archangel Med. Inst. 1986; DA 1996; FRCA 1999. Cons. Anaesth. S. Devon Healthcare NHS Trust. Specialty: Anaesth. Special Interest: Difficult Airways; Ophth. Anaesth.; Regional Anaesth. Socs: Brit. Ophth. Anaesth. Soc.; Europ. Soc. Anaesth.; Assn. Anaesth. GB & Irel. Prev: SpR Univ. Hosp. Wales Cardiff; SpR Univ. Roy. Gwent Hosp. Newport.

VAS FALCAO, Custodio Mariano Gustavo Withybush General Hospital, Fishguard Road, Haverfordwest SA61 2PZ Tel: 01437 773189; Rushacre House, Redstone Road, Narberth SA67 7ES Tel: 01834 861322 — MB BS Bombay 1982; DCH RCP Lond. 1985; FRCPCH 1996. Cons. Paediat. Withybush Gen. Hosp. HaverfordW. Specialty: Paediat.

VASA, Mr Sanjiv Arunchandra 12 Dorset Road, Altrincham WA14 4QN — MB BS Gujarat 1973 (N.H.L. Municip. Med. Coll.) MB BS Gujarat. 1973; FRCS Ed. 1979; FRCS Glas. 1979. Cons. Plastic Surg. Ahmedabad, India. Specialty: Plastic Surg.

VASANTH, Esther Chandrika Bag Lane Surgery, 32 Bag Lane, Atherton, Manchester M46 0EE Tel: 01942 896489 Fax: 01942 888793 — MB BS Bangalore 1970; MB BS Bangalore 1970.

VASANTHAKUMARI, Somasundaramurthy c/o Dr Meena Choksi, 20 Penrhos, Radyr, Cardiff CF15 8RJ — MB BS Madras 1977; MRCOG 1988.

VASANTHI-SREENIVASAN, Pudiya 30 Green Pastures, Stockport SK4 3RA — MB BS Mysore 1974; DObst RCPI 1983.

VASEY, David Whitby Group Practice, Spring Vale Medical Centre, Whitby YO21 1SD Tel: 01947 820888 Fax: 01947 824100 — MB ChB Liverp. 1967 (Camb. & Liverp.) GPwSI Opthal.; MB BChir Camb 1967; MA Camb. 1968; DObst RCOG 1969. Clin. Asst. (Ophth.) Whitby Hosp. Prev: Squadron Ldr. RAF Med. Br., Specialist O & G; SHO W. Suff. Gen. Hosp. Bury St. Edmunds; Ho. Off. Southport Gen. Infirm.

VASEY, David Peregrine The Ipswich Hospital, Department of Obstetrics & Gynaecology, Heath Road, Ipswich IP4 5PD Tel: 01473 703011 Fax: 01473 703018 Email: david.vasey@ipswichhospital.nhs.uk — MB BCh Wales 1969 (Welsh Sch. of Med.) FRCOG 1988, M 1975; FRCS (C) 1981. Cons. Gyn. Oncologist. Specialty: Obst. & Gyn.; Oncol. Socs: Brit. Soc. for Colposcopy and Cervical Path.; Brit. Gyn. Cancer Soc. Prev: Specialist in O & G Univ. Alberta Hosp. Edmonton Alberta; Canada.

VASEY, Jean Margaret (retired) 104 Hayes Road, Bromley BR2 9AB Tel: 020 8460 5631 — MB BS Lond. 1963 (St. Thos.) DO Eng. 1966. Assoc. Specialist Moorfields Eye Hosp. Lond. & Bromley Hosp. Prev: Cons. (Ophth.) Cane Hill Hosp. Coulsdon.

VASEY, Joyce Lilly (retired) Frieldhurst Farm, Frieldhurst Road, Cornholme, Todmorden OL14 8JL Tel: 01706 814036 — MB BS Durh. 1950 (Newc.)

VASEY, Paul Austin Beatson Oncology Centre, Western Infirmary, Glasgow G11 6NT Tel: 0141 2112318 Fax: 0141 2111869 Email: pav1y@clinmed.gla.ac.uk — MB ChB Dundee 1988; MRCP (UK) 1991; MSc Glas. 1994; MD Dundee 1996. Sen. Lect. & Hon. Cons. (Med. Oncol.) Beatson Oncol. Centre, West. Infirm. Glas. Specialty: Oncol. Socs: (Comm.) Assn. Cancer Phys. Prev: Lect. & Hon. Sen. Regist. (Med. Oncol.) Beatson Oncol. Centre West. Infirm. Glas.; Research Fell. & Hon. Regist. (Med.) Beatson Oncol. Centre Glas.; SHO Rotat. (Gen. Med.) Stobhill Gen. Hosp. Glas.

VASEY, Ronald Owen Offerton Health Centre, 10 Offerton Lane, Offerton, Stockport SK2 5AR Tel: 0161 480 0324; 56 Higher Hill Gate, Stockport SK1 3PZ Tel: 0161 480 2352 Fax: 0161 480 3158 — LMSSA Lond. 1970; MRCS Eng. LRCP Lond. 1972.

VASEY, Sarah Elyse 8 Winchester Drive, Exmouth EX8 5QA — MB ChB Birm. 1996.

VASFALCAO, Isabel Ignatius Rushacre House, Redstone Road, Narberth SA67 7ES Tel: 01834 861322 — MB BS Bombay 1982. Assoc. Psychiat. Derwen NHS Trust Carmarthen. Specialty: Gen. Psychiat.

VASHISHT, Rajiv Cromwell Hospital, Cromwell Road, London SW5 0TH Tel: 020 7460 5661 Fax: 020 7460 5728 Email: r_vashisht19@hotmail.com — MB BS Poona 1981; FRCS Eng.; FRCS Glas.; FICS; MPhil Lond. Cons. Surg., W. Middlx. Univ. Hosp., Isleworth; Sen. Lect., Imperial Coll.; Cons. Surg., Cromwell Hosp. Lond.; Cons. Surg., Clementine Churchill Hosp., Harrow; Cons. Surg., Lister Hosp. Lond. Specialty: Gen. Surg. Special Interest: Breast, Laparoscopic and Venous Surg. Socs: ASGBI; BASO. Prev: Sen. Regist., Char. Cross Hosp.

VASHISHT, Sohan Lal Warrior Square Surgery, 61 Warrior Square, Southend-on-Sea SS1 2JJ Tel: 01702 618411 Fax: 01702 464163 — MB BS Gujarat 1971.

VASHISHT, Sudha Rani 6 Beaufort Gardens, Ilford IG1 3DB Tel: 020 8544 4636 — MB BCh Wales 1985; DRCOG 1989. SHO (Paediat.) Lond. Hosp. Specialty: Community Child Health; Family Plann. & Reproduc. Health; Homeop. Med. Prev: Trainee GP Chelmsford; SHO (O & G) Rush Green Hosp. Romford; SHO (Geriat.) Hillingdon Hosp. Uxbridge.

VASI, Surendrakumar Chhotubhai (retired) 51 Grassmoor Road, Birmingham B38 8BU — (Bombay) MB BS Bombay 1966. GP Birm.; Hosp. Pract. Selly Oak Hosp. (Varicose Veins Clinic) Birm. Prev: Ho. Surg. (Gen. Surg.) Manor Hosp. Walsall.

VASI, Varsha 26 Coventon Road, Aylesbury HP19 9JL — MB ChB Leeds 1998.

VASIDYA, Shridhar Vasudeo — MB BS Poona 1981. Staff Phys. (Integrated Med.) Grantham & Dist. Gen. Hosp. Specialty: Gen. Med. Special Interest: Acute Med.; Endoscopy (GI).

VASISHTA, Sanjeev — MB BS Delhi 1982 (Mavlana Azad Coll. Delhi) MRCP (UK) 1989. Specialist Regist. (Gen. & Geriat. Med.) Glan Hafren NHS Trust; Cons. Phys., Roy. Gwent & St. Woolos Hosp., Newport. Specialty: Gen. Med. Prev: Regist. (Gen. Med.) Herefordsh. HA.; SHO (Gen. Med.) Gravesend & N. Kent. Hosps.; SHO (Gen. & Geriat. Med.) Herts. & Essex Gen. Hosp.

VASKOVIC, Tania 61 Carlisle Place, London SW1P 1HZ — LRCP LRCS LRCPS Ed., Glas. 1998; LRCP Ed LRCS Ed LRCPS Glas 1998.

VASS, Alexander Dimitri 14 Holt Drive, Kirby Muxloe, Leicester LE9 2EX — MB BS Lond. 1994.

VASS, Neil Norroy The Surgery, 1 Binfield Road, London SW4 6TB Tel: 020 7622 1424 Fax: 020 7501 1891 — MB BS Lond. 1981 (St Thos. Hosp. Lond.) DRCOG 1985; DPD 1990; MSc Lond. 1994; MRCGP 1997; DFFP 1997; DipDrug Addiction 2002. Edit. Bd. Palliat. Care Today; Clin. Asst. Dermat. Sutton Hosp. Specialty: Gen. Pract. Prev: Gen. Practitioner, Battersea, 1985-98; Trainee GP St. Thos. Hosp. VTS, 82-85.

VASSALL-ADAMS, Nicola Irene High Hedges, Brookthorpe, Gloucester GL4 0US Tel: 01452 813656 — MB BS Lond. 1967 (Middlx.) Assoc. Specialist (Psychiat./Psychother.) Glos. HA. Prev: Ho. Surg. Tilbury Hosp.; Ho. Phys. St. And. Hosp. Billericay; SHO (Psychiat.) Middlx. Hosp. Lond.

VASSALLO, Alison Ann The Lennard Surgery, 1-3 Lewis Rd, Bedminster Down, Bristol BS13 75D Tel: 0117 964 2211 Fax: 0117 987 3227 — MB BS Lond. 1991 (St. Bart. Med. Coll.) DRCOG 1994; DFFP 1994; MRCGP 1995; DCH RCP Lond. 1996.

VASSALLO, Catherine Maria Littlemore Hospital, Sandford Road, Oxford OX4 4XN Tel: 01865 223036 — MB BS Lond. 1991; MA Oxon 1994; MSc. London 1997; MRCPsych 1997. Rot. Specialist Regist., Oxf. Specialty: Gen. Psychiat. Socs: MRCPsych. Prev: Regist. Rotat. (Psychiat.) Oxf.; SHO Rotat.(Psychiat.)UCL.

VASSALLO, Mr David John, Lt.-Col. RAMC Royal Hospital Haslar, Gosport PO12 2AA Tel: 02392 762118 Fax: 02392 762960 — MRCS Eng. LRCP Lond. 1981; FRCS Ed. 1985. Cons. Gen. Surg. Roy. Hosp. Haslar. Gosport; Hon. Sen. Lect., Leonard Chesh. Centre for Conflict Recovery, Univ. Coll., Lond. Specialty: Gen. Surg. Socs: Roy. Soc. of Med. Prev: Cons. Gen. Surg. Duke of Connaught Unit, Musgrave Pk. Hosp. Belf.; Cons. Gen. Surg. Camb. Milit. Hosp. Aldershot; Sen. Regist. (Gen. Surg.) Camb. Milit. Hosp. Aldershot, St. Bart. Hosp. Lond. & St. Peter's Hosp. Chertsey.

VASSALLO, Michael Royal Bournemouth Hospital, Castle Lane East, Bournemouth BH7 7DW Tel: 01202 704590 Fax: 01202 704542 Email: michael.vassallo@rbch-tr.swest.nhs.uk — MD Malta 1986; FRCP Lond.; DGM Lond.; PhD Soton.; MPhil Soton. Cons. Phys., Roy. Bournemouth Hosp. Specialty: Gen. Med. Socs: BMA; BGS; MPS.

VASSERMAN, David The Surgery, 66 Long Lane, London EC1A 9EJ Tel: 020 7600 9440 — MB ChB Manch. 1982; MRCPsych 1988; MRCGP 1990.

VASSILAS, Christopher Alexander Department of Old Age Psychiatry, West Suffolk Hospital, Hardwick Lane, Bury St Edmunds IP33 2QZ Tel: 01284 763131 — MD Bristol 1994; MB ChB Liverp. 1980; MPhil Ed. 1988. Specialty: Geriat. Psychiat. Socs: Roy. Coll. Psychiat. Prev: Lect. (Ment. Health) Univ. Bristol.

VASSILIADIS, Helena Sophie Nottingham Psychotherapy Unit, 114 Thorneywood Mount, Nottingham — BM BS Nottm. 1990; MRC Psych. Cons., Psychother. Specialty: Gen. Psychiat.; Psychother.

VASSILIADIS, Nikolaos Department of Forensic Medicine, Guy's Hospital, St Thomas St., London SE1 9RT — Ptychio Iatrikes Thessalonika 1974.

VASSILIOU, George Steliou Hammersmith Hospital, Du Cane Road, London W12 0HS; 10 Goodrich House, Sewardstone Road, London E2 9JN Email: georger@lineone.net — MB BS Lond. 1994; BSc (1st cl. Hons.) Pharmacol. Lond. 1991; MB BS (Distinc.) Lond. 1994; MRCP (UK) 1997. Specialist Regist. (Haemat.) N. Thames Deanery Centr. Middlx. Hosp., Hammersmith Hosp., Roy. Free Hosp., Gt. Ormond St. Hosp. for Sick Childr. Specialty: Haematology. Socs: Hellenic Med. Soc.; Regist. Train. RCPath.; Brit. Soc. Haematol. Prev: SHO (Haemat.) Addenbrooke's Hosp. Camb.

VASU, Makakkath (retired) — MB BS Mysore 1970.

VASU, Vimal Whitecroft, Glynogwr, Blackmill, Bridgend CF35 6EL — MB BS Lond. 1998.

VASUDAVEN, Bhargawa King's Drive Surgery, 2 King's Drive, Gravesend DA12 5BG Tel: 01474 560717; 359 Singlewell Road, Gravesend DA11 7RL — (Grant Medical College Bombay, India) MBBS Bombay 1976; FRCS Ed 1984. Sector GP in local PCG (responsible for 34 GPs in 10 different Pract.s); GP Chairm. Local Community Hosp. Project. Prev: Chm Jt. Commissioning Gp. Dartford Dist.

VASUDEV, Kadaba Srinath Department of Pathology, Victoria Hospital, Blackpool FY3 8NR Tel: 01253 300000 Fax: 01253 303675; 10 Silverdale Road, Lytham St Annes FY8 3RE Tel: 01253 720747 Fax: 01253 720747 Email: vasudev@globalnet.co.uk — (Bangalore Med. Coll.) MB BS Bangalore 1967; FRCPath 1976. Cons. Histopath. Vict. Hosp. Blackpool. Specialty: Histopath. Socs: BMA (Sec. Blackpool & Fylde Div.); Overseas Doctors Assn.; Assn. Clin. Path. & Internat. Acad. Path. Prev: Postgrad. & Undergrad. Tutor Univ. Manch.

VASUDEV, Naveen Srinath 10 Silverdale Road, Lytham St Annes FY8 3RE — MB ChB Dundee 1998; BMSc (Hons.) Dundee 1995. Specialty: Gen. Med.

VASUDEVA, Arvind Kumar Kingston Hospital NHS Trust, Galsworthy Road, Kingston-upon-Thames KT2 7QB Tel: 0208 5467 711 — BM BCh Oxf. 1987; MA Camb. 1988; DRCOG 1990; DCH RCP Lond. 1991; MRCGP 1991; MRCP (UK) 1992. Cons. Cardiol. Kingston & St George's Hosp. Specialty: Cardiol.; Gen. Med. Special Interest: Echocardiography. Socs: Brit. Cardiac Soc.; Europ. Cardiac Soc. Prev: Research Fell. (Cardiol.) St. Geo. Hosp. Med. Sch. Lond.

VASUDEVA KAMATH, Surathkal Scholes, Wigan WN1 3NH — MB BS Mysore 1974; MB BS Mysore 1974.

VASUDEVAN NAIR, Devakiamma Chandrasekharan Willenhall Health Centre, Field Street, Willenhall WV13 2NZ Fax: 01902 634448 — MB BS Kerala 1973.

VATER, Mairlys Derby City General Hospital, Anaesthetic Department, Southern Derbyshire Acute Hospitals NHS Trust, Derby DE22 3NE Tel: 01332 340131 Fax: 01332 290559 Email: mairvater@hotmail.com; The Grange, Packhorse Road, Melbourne, Derby DE73 1EG Tel: 01332 863653 — MB BCh Wales 1975; DA Eng. 1978; FFA RCS Eng. 1980. Cons. Anaesth. Southern Derbysh. Acute NHS Trust. Specialty: Anaesth.

VATERLAWS, Albert Lynwood — MB BCh Wales 1964; MRCP (U.K.) 1971; DCMT . Lond. 1972. Cons. Llandudno Gen. Hosp. Wales. Specialty: Rheumatol. Special Interest: Bone Disorders.

VATERLAWS, Albert Lynwood Llandudno General Hospital, Llandudno LL30 1LB Tel: 01492 862 343 Fax: 01492 877 818 Email: lyn.vaterlaws@nww-tr.wales.nhs.uk — MB BCh Wales 1964; MRCP Lond. 1971; DCMT 1972; FRCP 1988 (Welsh Nat. Sch. of Med.) Specialty: Gen. Med. Special Interest: Bone Diseases; Rheum. Socs: Welsh Soc. of Physicians; Brit. Soc. of Rheum.; Nat. Osteoporosis Soc. Prev: Lecturer/ Acting Assoicate Prof., Univ., Kuala Lumpar; Sen. Lect. in Med. Univ., New Guinea.

VATHENEN, Santi Cardiorespiratory Department, Alexandra Hospital, Woodrow Drive, Redditch B98 7UB Tel: 01527 503030 Fax: 01527 503881 — BM Soton. 1980 (Southampton) MRCP (UK) 1983; DM Soton. 1989; T(M) 1992; FRCP (Lond) 1998. Cons. Phys. Respirat. & Gen. Med. Alexandra Hosp. Redditch. Specialty: Respirat. Med.; Gen. Med. Special Interest: Asthma. Socs: Brit. Thorac. Soc. & Amer. Thorac. Soc. Prev: Sen. Regist. (Respirat. & Gen. Med.) Killingbeck Hosp. Leeds; Research Fell. (Respirat. Med.) City Hosp. Nottm.; Regist. (Gen. Med.) Glenfield Hosp. Leicester.

VATISH, Manu 94 Clough Road, Rotherham S61 1RF — BChir Camb. 1994; M.A. Oxon 1989; DPhil Oxon 1992; MBCamb. 1994. Specialist Regist., (O & G) Oxf. Rotat.; Clin. Lect. Warwick Univ. 1999. Specialty: Obst. & Gyn. Prev: SHO Qu. Charlotte's Hosp. O & H; SHO John Radcliffe Hosp. O&H.

VATISH, Ravi Kumar Kirpal Medical Practice, Soho Health Centre, Louise Road, Handsworth, Birmingham B21 0RY Tel: 0121 554 0033 — MB ChB Sheffield 1976; MB ChB Sheffield 1976.

VATSALA, Chandakacherla Narasimha c/o Drive B. Shah, 73 Lakeside Gardens, Merthyr Tydfil CF48 1EW — MB BS Sri Venkateswara 1985.

VAUDREY, Barbara Wood Hall, Stoke Ash, Eye IP23 7ES — MB BS Lond. 1953 (St. Bart.) LMSSA Lond. 1953.

VAUGHAN, Andrew Richard Sinclair Snaefell Surgery, Cushag Road, AnaghCoar, Douglas IM2 2SU Tel: 01624 676622 Fax: 01624 674515; 72 Ard Reayrt, Ramsey Road, Laxey IM4 7QU — MB ChB Dundee 1989; DFFP 1994; DRCOG 1994; (Hon. Fac. of Homeopothy) 1998. Socs: BMA.

VAUGHAN, Antony Rathbone Bron Derw Surgery, Bron Derw, Garth Road, Bangor LL57 2RS Tel: 01248 370900 Fax: 01248 370652; Perfeddgoed Bach, Caerhun, Bangor LL57 4DS Tel: 01248 370350 — MB BS Lond. 1972 (Lond. Hosp.) DObst RCOG 1974; MRCGP 1980. Med. Adviser N. Wales Health Auth. Prev: SHO Copthorne Hosp. Shrewsbury; Ho. Off. Neurosurg. Unit Lond. Hosp.; Resid. King Edwd. VII Memor. Hosp., Bermuda.

VAUGHAN, David Atkinson 29 Mile End Road, Norwich NR4 7QX Tel: 01603 443300 Fax: 01603 446012 — MB BS Lond. 1979; DCH RCP Lond. 1983; DRCOG 1983; MRCGP 1984.

VAUGHAN, David Hughes (retired) Mill Hill Cottage, 190 Woodford Road, Poynton, Stockport SK12 1EH — MB ChB Ed. 1950; DPH Manch. 1958; FFCM 1977, M 1974; FFPHM 1989. Prev: Cons. Pub. Health Med. N. West. RHA.

VAUGHAN, David John Adrian Northwick Park Hospital, Watford Road, Harrow HA1 3UJ Tel: 020 8869 3969 Fax: 020 8869 3975 — MB BS Lond. 1991 (St Marys) FRCA 1996. Cons. Anaesth., N. W. Lond. NHS Trust, Northwick Pk. Hosp., Harrow. Specialty: Anaesth. Socs: Anaesth. Res. Soc.; Obst. Anaesth. Assn.; Eur. Anaesthesiologists Assn. Prev: Regist. (Anaesth.) St. Mary's Hosp. Lond.; Lect. in Anaesth. and ITU, Imperial Coll., Lond.

VAUGHAN, Deborah Laura Jane Wentloog Road Health Centre, 98 Wentloog Road, Rumney, Cardiff CF3 3XE Tel: 029 2079 7746 Fax: 029 2079 0231 — MB BCh Wales 1988. Specialty: Obst. & Gyn.

VAUGHAN, Donna Athena Waverley Medical Centre, Dhrymple Street, Stranraer DG9 7DW — MB BCh BAO Belf. 1984; DMH Belf. 1992. Med. Off. Ekwendeni Hosp., Malawi.

VAUGHAN, Gerard Joseph Bewicke Health Centre, 51 Tynemouth Road, Wallsend NE28 0AD Tel: 0191 262 3036 Fax: 0191 295 1663 — MB BCh BAO NUI 1980. GP Wallsend, Tyne & Wear.

VAUGHAN, Jenny Rosemary 58 Shorrolds Road, Fulham, London SW6 7TP — BM BS Nottm. 1992; MRCP MRCP, PL.D.

VAUGHAN, John Anthony 9 The Lees, Malvern WR14 3HT — MB BCh Wales 1980; MRCPsych 1985. Cons. Psychiat. Worcester & DHA. Specialty: Gen. Psychiat. Prev: Cons. Psychiat. Leics. HA.

VAUGHAN, John Martin Measham Medical Unit, High Street, Measham, Swadlincote DE12 7HR Tel: 01530 270667 Fax: 01530 271433; 39 Burton Road, Ashby-de-la-Zouch LE65 2LF Tel: 01530 412220 — MB ChB Liverp. 1971; DObst RCOG 1973; DCH Eng. 1973; FRCGP 1987, M 1975.

VAUGHAN, Mr John Michael Martin Shell Centre, London SE1 7NA Tel: 0207 934 5864 Fax: 0207 934 7046 Email: michael.j.vaughan@shell.com; 28 Huntingdon Gardens, London W4 3HX Tel: 020 8742 3009 Fax: 020 8742 3009 — MB Camb. 1973 (Camb. & St. Mary's) BChir Camb. 1973; MA Camb. 1973; FRCS Eng. 1979; Cert. Av. Med. 1991; AFOM RCP Lond. 1996. Sen. Med. Adviser, Shell Internat. Health Services-Europe. Specialty: Gen. Surg.; Occupat. Health. Socs: Fell. Roy. Soc. Med.; Soc. Occupat. Med. Prev: Chief Med. Off. Shell Nigeria; Sen. Med. Adviser Shell UK; Surg. Shell Petroleum Developm. Company Lagos, Nigeria & Brunei.

VAUGHAN, Professor John Patrick Department of Public Health & Policy, London School of Hygiene & Tropical Medicine, Gower St., London WC1E 7HT Tel: 020 7636 8636 Fax: 020 7637 5391 — MB BS Lond. 1961 (Guy's) MRCS Eng. LRCP Lond. 1961; DObst RCOG 1963; DCMT . Lond. 1964; FRCP Ed. 1982, M 1965; DTPH Lond 1969; FFPHM RCP (UK) 1988, M 1974; MD Lond. 1978. Prof. Health Care Epidemiol. Lond. Sch. Hyg. & Trop. Med.; Hon. Cons. Pub. Health Med. N. Thames RHA. Specialty: Pub. Health Med. Socs: Fell. Roy. Soc. Trop. Med. & Hyg. Prev: Sen. Lect. (Trop. Epidemiol.) Lond. Sch. Hyg. & Trop. Med.; Sen. Lect. Community Health (Epidemiol.) Univ. Nottm.; Sen. Lect. (Community Med.) Univ. Dar es Salaam, Tanzania.

VAUGHAN, Joseph (retired) 5 Clumber Road, Sheffield S10 3LE Tel: 0114 230 1736 — MD Czechoslovakia 1942 (Prague & Cardiff) Prev: Ho. Surg. Lister Hosp. Hitchin.

VAUGHAN, Kevin Francis The Smethwick Medical Centre, Regent Street, Smethwick, Warley B66 3BQ Tel: 0121 558 0105 Fax: 0121 555 7206; 104 Wentworth Road, Harborne, Birmingham B17 9SY Tel: 0121 427 6420 — MB Camb. 1972; MB BChir Camb. 1972; MA Camb. 1972; DObst RCOG 1973; DA (UK) 1976; MRCGP 1988. Prev: Med. Supt. Kisiizi Hosp, Uganda.

VAUGHAN, Mark Owen Avenue Villa Surgery, Brynmor Road, Llanelli SA15 2TJ Tel: 01554 774401 Fax: 01554 775229 — MB BCh Wales 1979 (University of Wales College of Medicine) MRCGP (Distinc.) 1983; FRCGP 1997. Chair. Carmarthenshire Local Health Gp.; Chair Carmarthenshire health and social care partnership Bd. Prev: PostGrad. Organiser, P. Philip Hosp., Llanelli.

VAUGHAN, Matthew Mountfort 5 Manby Road, Malvern WR14 3BD Email: matthewmvaughan@yahoo.com — MB ChB Sheff. 1991; FRCR, 1997; MMedSc, Keele 1998. Attend. Radiologist, Virginia Mason Med. Centre, Seattle, Washington. Specialty: Radiol. Special Interest: MRI of the Abdomen and Pelvis. Prev: SR, Radiol., John Radcliffe Hosp. Oxf..; Fell. in Radiol., Carnell Univ. Med. Center, New York Presbyt. Hosp. Cornell.

VAUGHAN, Merrell Sandra Thame Health Centre, East Street, Thame OX9 3JZ Tel: 01844 261066 — MB BS Lond. 1991.

VAUGHAN, Michael Crofton Health Centre, Slack Lane, Crofton, Wakefield WF4 1HJ Tel: 01924 862612 — MB ChB Manch. 1970; BSc Manch. 1967, MB ChB 1970; MRCP (U.K.) 1973. Prev: SHO Med. Univ. Hosp. of S. Manch.

VAUGHAN, Mrs Naomi Victoria MASU St Marys Hospital, Norfolk Place, London W2 Tel: 020 7886 6666 Email: n.v.vaughan@ic.ac.uk; 28A Lime Grove, London W12 8EA Tel: 020 7749 9812 — MB BS Lond. 1991; FRCS Eng. 1997. Research Fell. (Gen. Surg.) Acad. Specialty: Gen. Surg.

VAUGHAN, Nicholas John Ashton Royal Sussex County Hospital, Eastern Road, Brighton BN2 5BE Tel: 01273 696955 Fax: 01273 676345 Email: nvaughan@mistral.co.uk; The Hundred, Brighton Road, Woodmancote, Henfield BN5 9RT — MB BChir Camb. 1975; MB BCh Camb. 1975; MA Camb. 1975; MRCP (UK) 1977; MD Camb. 1985; FRCP Lond. 1991. Cons. Phys. & Clin. Dir. (Med.) Roy. Sussex Co. Hosp. Brighton & Hove Gen. Hosp.; Hon. Sen. Lect. KCL. Specialty: Gen. Med.; Diabetes; Endocrinol. Socs: Brit. Diabetic Assn.; Eur. Assn. for Study Diabetes. Prev: Sen. Regist. (Med.) St. Geo. Hosp. Lond.; Regist. (Med.) Middlx. Hosp. Lond.; SHO Hammersmith Hosp. Lond.

VAUGHAN, Pamela Kathleen 1 Stormont Villas, Massey Avenue, Belfast BT4 2JT — MB BCh BAO Belf. 1975.

VAUGHAN, Paul Howard The Medical Centre, Station Road, Haydock, St Helens WA11 0JN Tel: 01744 734419 Fax: 01744 454875; 3 Pike House Road, Eccleston, St Helens WA10 5JZ Tel: 01744 755258 — MB ChB Liverp. 1971. GP Princip. Specialty: Gen. Pract.

VAUGHAN, Philip Joseph The Surgery, Bridge St., Polesworth, Tamworth B78 1DT Tel: 01827 330269; The Magnolias, Curlew Close, Warton, Tamworth B79 0HL Tel: 01827 892893 — MRCS Eng. LRCP Lond. 1964 (Leeds) Socs: BMA. Prev: Ho. Surg. & Ho. Phys. Clayton Hosp. Wakefield; SHO Obst. Doncaster Roy. Infirm.; RAF Med. Br.

VAUGHAN, Ralph Stephens 17 Ash Tree Close, Radyr, Cardiff CF15 8RX — MB BS Lond. 1966 (Middlx.) DA Eng. 1968; FFA RCS Eng. 1970. Cons. Anaesth. Univ. Hosp. Wales & Hon. Clin. Teach. Univ. Wales Coll; Med. Cardiff. Specialty: Anaesth. Socs: Assn. Anaesths. Prev: Ho. Phys. Middlx. Hosp. Lond.; Ho. Surg. St. And. Hosp. Billericay; Lect. Anaesth. Welsh Nat. Sch. Med. Cardiff.

VAUGHAN, Robert King Cross Surgery, 199 King Cross Road, Halifax HX1 3LW Tel: 01422 330612 Fax: 01422 323740 — MB ChB Leeds 1989.

VAUGHAN, Mr Roger Norfolk & Norwich Hospital, Brunswick Road, Norwich NR9 5BP Tel: 01603 286395 — MB ChB Leeds 1974; BSc (Hons.) Leeds 1971, MB ChB 1974; FRCS Eng. 1979. Cons. Cardiothoracic Surg. E. Anglia RHA. Specialty: Cardiothoracic Surg. Prev: Sen. Regist. (Cardiothoracic Surg.) S. Manch. Health

Dist.; SHO (A & E) Frenchay Hosp. Bristol; Demonst. Anat. Leeds Univ.

VAUGHAN, Roger John (retired) 43 Kings Road, Emsworth PO10 7HW Tel: 01243 375638 — MB BChir Camb. 1953 (Camb. & Middlx.) MA Camb. 1953; MRCGP 1973. GP Horndean. Prev: Ho. Phys. Lister Hosp. Hitchin.

VAUGHAN, Simon Timothy Andrew Blackpool Victoria Hospital, Whinney Heys Road, Blackpool FY3 8NR Tel: 01253 303499 Email: dr.vaughan@bfwhospitals.nhs.uk — MB ChB Manch. 1989; BSc (Hons.) Manch. 1986; MRCP Ed. 1993; FRCA 1997. Cons. in Anaesth. & Intens. Care Med. Specialty: Anaesth.; Intens. Care. Special Interest: Critical Care. Prev: Specialist Regist. (Anaesth.) N. W. (East) Deanery Rotat.; SHO (Gen. Med.) Blackburn Roy. Infirm. & Qu. Pk. Hosp. Blackburn; SHO (Anaesth. & A & E) Roy. Preston Hosp.

VAUGHAN, Susan Jacqueline Trinity Street Surgery, 1 Trinity Street, Norwich NR2 2BG Tel: 01603 624844 Fax: 01603 766829; Hatherley Farm House, Mill Road, Little Melton, Norwich NR9 3NZ Tel: 01603 810581 — MB Camb. 1971 (St. Mary's) BChir 1970; DObst RCOG 1972; DCH Eng. 1974; MRCP (UK) 1978.

VAUGHAN-DAVIES, Sophie Louise 3 Chestnut Drive, Egham Hill, Egham TW20 0BJ — MB BS Lond. 1998.

VAUGHAN HUDSON, Gillian Rose (retired) Owls Hatch Cottage, Seale, Farnham GU10 1JD Tel: 01252 782456 — (Middlx.) MB BS Lond. 1961; FRCP 1997. Trustee of Lymphoma Research Trust & Lymphoma Assn. Prev: Dir. of BNLI.

VAUGHAN-HUGHES, Richard Gareth (retired) 32 Heath Farm Road, Codsall, Wolverhampton WV8 1HT Tel: 01902 842818 — MB ChB Liverp. 1959. Prev: Regist. (Paediat.) St. Catherine's Hosp. Birkenhead.

VAUGHAN-JONES, Neal Dalton Square Surgery, 8 Dalton Square, Lancaster LA1 1PN Tel: 01524 842200 — MB ChB Birm. 1985; MRCP (UK) 1988; DRCOG 1990; MRCGP 1992; T(GP) 1992. Specialty: Gen. Pract. Prev: SHO Rotat. (Med.) Preston; Trainee GP Keighley & Addingham.

VAUGHAN-JONES, Mr Richard Henry Linden Suite, Worcester Royal Hospital, Worcester — MB BS Lond. 1983 (Charing Cross) BSc Biochem. Lond. 1980; FRCS Ed. 1987; FRCS Eng. 1989; FRCS (Orl.) 1995. Cons. Worcester Roy. Infirm., Worcester; Mid./Sth. Staffs. Deaf Childr.'s Soc. Pres. Specialty: Otolaryngol. Socs: Brit. Assn. Otol.; Scott. Otolaryngol. Soc. Prev: Sen. Regist. (ENT) N. Riding Infirm. Middlesbrough Cleveland; Sen. Regist. Ninewells Hosp. Med. Sch. Dundee; Cons. Stafford Dist. Gen. Hosp. & Cannock.

VAUGHAN JONES, Samantha Anne St Peter's Hospital, Ashford & St Peter's NHS Trust, Guildford Rd, Chertsey KT16 0PZ — MB BS Lond. 1988 (St. Thomas's) MRCP (UK) 1992; MD Lond. 1997; MD 1998. p/t Cons. (Dermat.) St. Peter's Hosp. Chertsey Surrey. Specialty: Dermat. Socs: Roy. Soc. Med. & BMA; Brit. Assn. Dermat. Prev: Specialist Regist. (Dermat.) St. John's Inst. Dermatol.; Regist. (Gastroenterol. & Cardiol.) St. Peters Hosp. Chertsey; SHO (Gen. Med.) Kingston Hosp.

VAUGHAN-LANE, Mr Timothy Hinchingbrooke Hospital, Hinchingbrooke Park, Huntingdon PE29 6NT Tel: 01480 416416; Elms Farm, 111 Great North Road, Eaton Socon, St Neots, Huntingdon PE19 8EL Tel: 01480 477475 — MB ChB Birm. 1971; FRCS Eng. 1977. Clin. Dir. Trauma & Orthopaedics Hinchingbrooke Hosp. Huntingdon. Specialty: Orthop.; Trauma & Orthop. Surg. Socs: Fell. BOA; Mem. BASK. Prev: Cons. Orthop. Surg. RAF; Sen. Regist. (Orthop.) Addenbrooke's Hosp. Camb.; Sen. Regist. (Orthop.) Newmarket Gen. Hosp.

VAUGHAN-SMITH, Stephen Uxbridge Health Centre, George St., Uxbridge UB8 1UB Tel: 01895 231925 Fax: 01895 813190; Brickfield Cottage, Knighton Way Lane, New Denham, Uxbridge UB9 4EQ Tel: 01895 273517 — MB BS Lond. 1983 (St. Marys London) BSc Nottm. 1967; PhD Birm. 1971, MSc 1968; DRCOG 1987. Clin. Asst. (A & E) Wexham Pk. Hosp. Slough.; Sect. 12 Approved Doctor, Ment. Health Act. Socs: Brit. Assn. Immed. Care Schemes.

VAUGHAN WILLIAMS, Catherine Ann (retired) Starting Haw, Low St, Austwick, Lancaster LA2 8BN Tel: 015242 51714 Fax: 015242 51714 Email: c.a.v-w@ntlworld.com — MB ChB Liverp. 1970 (Liverpool) FRCOG 1993, M 1976; MD Liverp. 1981. Prev: Cons. O & G Dumfries & Galloway HB.

VAUGHAN WILLIAMS, Professor Edward Miles 153 Woodstock Road, Oxford OX2 7NA Tel: 01865 515839 Fax: 01865 515839 Email: edward.vaughanwilliams@hertford.ox.ac.uk — (Oxf.) DSc Oxf. 1961, BSc 1946, DM 1953, BM BCh 1947; FRCP Lond. 1984, M 1979. Specialty: Pharmacology. Socs: Hon. Fell. Doctor Honoris Causa, Paris 1982 & Amer. Coll. Clin.; Emerit. Fell. Hertford Coll. Oxf.; Pharmacol., Physiol. & Cardiac Socs. Prev: Creasy Vis. Prof. Clin. Pharmacol. Chicago Med. Sch. 1990; Fell. Rockefeller Foundat. 1951.; Schorstein Research Fell. Univ. Oxf. 1950.

VAUGHTON, Mr Keith Chivers Morriston Hospital, Swansea SA6 6NL Tel: 01792 703591 Fax: 01792 796438 Email: keith.vaughton@swansea-tr.wales.nhs.uk — BM BCh Oxf. 1971 (Oxf. Univ.) MA Oxf. 1971; DObst RCOG 1973; FRCS Eng. 1976. Cons. Urol. Surg.Swansea NHS Trust; Regional speciality Adviser for Wales to the Roy. Coll. of Surg.s; Regional Adviser to Brit. Assn. of Urological Surg.s; Honarary Sen. Lect. to Univ. of Wales Coll. of Med. Specialty: Urol. Socs: Brit. Assn. Urol. Surg.; Welsh Urol. Soc.; Welsh Surgic. Soc.

VAUSE, Michael Harold 90 Bloom Street, Edgeley, Stockport SK3 9LH Tel: 0161 480 2726 — MB ChB Manch. 1956. Prev: Ho. Surg. Bolton Roy. Infirm.; Ho. Phys. Birch Hill Hosp. Rochdale; Asst. Res. Surg. Off. Stockport Infirm.

VAUSE, Sarah Helen St. Mary's Hospital, Hathersage Road, Manchester M13 0JH Tel: 0161 276 6426 — MB ChB Manch. 1987; MRCOG 1993; MD 1997. Cons. in Feto material Med., St. Mary's Hosp., Manch. Specialty: Obst. & Gyn.

VAUTREY, Richard Mark Meanwood Group Practice, 548 Meanwood Road, Leeds LS6 4JN Tel: 0113 295 1737 Fax: 0113 295 1736 — MB ChB Manch. 1988; DRCOG 1991; DCH RCP Lond. 1991; MRCGP 1994.

VAUX, Alison (retired) Silvretta, 23 Went Hill Close, Ackworth, Pontefract WF7 7LP Tel: 01977 704962 — MB BS Lond. 1962 (St. Bart.) MRCS Eng. LRCP Lond. 1962; DObst RCOG 1966. Prev: BMA.

VAUX, David John Talbutt Lincoln College, Oxford OX1 3DR — BM BCh Oxf. 1984; MA, DPhil. Oxf. 1982. Lect. (Experim. Path.) Univ. Oxf. Specialty: Pathology, General.

VAUX, Richard Hugh Cutcliffe The Surgery, Yeoman Lane, Bearsted, Maidstone ME14 4DS Tel: 01622 37326; Greenhill House, Otham, Maidstone ME15 8RR Tel: 01622 861245 — MB BChir Camb. 1960 (Guy's) MA Camb. 1961; DCH Eng. 1963; DObst RCOG 1964.

VAVASOUR, Simon Mark Andrew Paston Surgery, 9-11 Park Lane, North Walsham NR28 0BQ Tel: 01692 403015 Fax: 01692 500619 Email: simon.vavasour@nhs.net; 5 Mile End Road, Norwich NR4 7QY Tel: 01603 457961 Email: simon.vavasour@nhs.net — MB BS Lond. 1991 (Char. Cross & Westm.) MRCGP 1996. GP N. Walsham. Specialty: Gen. Pract.; Urol. Prev: PCG Bd. Mem., N. Norf.

VAVRECKA, Milan John Frank The Surgeries, Grafton Road, Canvey Island SS8 7BT Tel: 01268 682277; 16B Grafton Road, Canvey Island SS8 7BT Tel: 01268 692280 — MUDr Prague 1953; LMSSA Lond. 1975.

VAZ, Francis Guilherme South Warwickshire General Hospitals NHS Trust, Lakin Road, Warwick CV34 5BW — MB BS Bangalor (St John's Med. Coll.) FRCP Lond. 1996, M (UK) 1981; FRCP Edin 2000. Cons. Phys. (Med. & Care of Elderly) S. Warks. Gen. Hosps. NHS Trust. Specialty: Care of the Elderly. Special Interest: Orthogeriatric Rehabil.; Stroke. Socs: Brit. Geriat. Soc.

VAZ, Mr Francis Melvin 46 Norwood Park Road, London SE27 9UA — MB BS Lond. 1994; BSc (Hons.) Lond. 1991; FRCS 1998; FRCS (Oto) 1999. Specialty: Otorhinolaryngol.

VAZ, Olive Kathleen 11A Eton Place, Eton College Road, London NW3 2BT Tel: 020 7722 3242 — MB BS Calcutta 1956 (Nilratan Sarkar Med. Coll.) DCH Lond. 1964.

VAZ PATO, Maria Department of Clinical Neurophysiology, The National Hospital for Neurology & Neurosurgery, Queen Square, London WC1N 3BG — Lic Med Coimbra 1988.

VAZE, Bhaskar Chintaman Waterloo Road Surgery, 279 Waterloo Road, Cobridge, Stoke-on-Trent ST6 3HR Tel: 01782 279915 — MB BS Nagpur 1963.

VAZE, Nirmala Ramesh Weston super Mare General Hospital, Grange Road, Weston Super Mare BS23 4TQ — MB BS Ranchi 1971.

VAZIR, Muhummmad Hasan Althagelvin Hospital, Londonderry BT47 6SB Tel: 02871 345171 Ext: 4175 Fax: 02871 611259; 8 Clarenence Avenue, Londonderry BT48 7NH — MB BS Karachi 1979 (Dow Med. Coll. & Civil Hosp., Karachi) MRCPath 1991; T(Path) 1991; FRCP (Path) 2000. Cons. Histopath./Cytopath. Altivagelvin Hosp. Specialty: Histopath. Socs: BMA; ACP; Roy. Soc. Med. Prev: Cons. Path. Antrim Hosp.; Cons. Path. & Head Path. Shaukat Khanum Memor. Cancer Hosp., Lahore, Pakistan; Higher Specialist Trainer Progr. Univ. Coll. Hosp. Galway & St Vincents Hosp. Dub.

VAZIRI, Katherine 45 Milner Drive, Whitton, Twickenham TW2 7PH — MB ChB Manch. 1995.

VAZIRI, Mr Manoocher Accident & Emergency Department, Prince Philip Hospital, Bryngwyn Mawr, Dafen, Llanelli SA14 8QF; 16 King George Court, Derwen Fawr, Swansea SA2 8AR — MD Tehran 1962; LMSSA Lond. 1968; FRCS Ed. 1969. Cons. A & E P. Philip Hosp. Llanelli. Specialty: Accid. & Emerg. Socs: Brit. Assn. Accid. & Emerg. Med.; BMA. Prev: Cons. Surg. Nat. Iranian Oil Co. Hosp., Abadan; Regist. (Surg.) Mansfield Gp. Hosps.; SHO St. Helier Hosp. Carshalton.

VEAL, Christopher Trevor 3 Oak Vale, Bosillion Lane, Grampound, Truro TR2 4QY Tel: 01726 882220 — MB BS Newc. 1972; MRCGP 1976; MPH Leeds 1992; MFPHM UK 1993; FFPHM UK 2000; DFFP 2004. Med. Dir. & Cons. (Pub. Health Med.) Calderdale & Kirklees Health Auth.. Cons. in Pub. Health Med. Cornw. and the Isles of Scilly Health Auth.; GP & Director S. W. Breast Screening Quality Assur. Team. Specialty: Pub. Health Med.; Gen. Pract.

VEALE, David Mikael William de Coverly The Priory Hospital North London, The Bourne, Southgate, London N14 6RA Tel: 020 8882 8191 Fax: 020 8447 8138 — MB BS Lond. 1982 (Roy. Free) MRCPsych 1987; Dip.CACP 1990; MPhil Lond. 1989, BSc 1979, MD 1995; FRCPsych 2003. Cons. Psychiat., The Priory Hosp. N. Lond., Lond.; Hon. Sen. Lect. Univ. Dept. Psychiat. Roy. Free and Univ. Coll. Med. Sch. Specialty: Gen. Psychiat. Special Interest: Body Dysmorphic Disorder; Cognitive Behaviour Ther.; Obsessive Compulsive Disorder. Socs: (Ex Treas.) Brit. Assn. Behavioural & Congnitive Psychotherapies; Ex Chairm. OCD Action. Prev: Lect. (Behavioural Psychother.) Inst. Psychiat. Lond.; Sen. Regist. (Psychiat.) Maudsley Hosp. Lond.; Regist. (Psychiat.) Roy. Free Hosp. Lond.

VEALE, Michael Joseph Jessop Medical Practice, 24 Pennine Avenue, Riddings, Alfreton DE55 4AE Tel: 01773 602707 Fax: 01773 513502 — MB BCh Wales 1979.

VEALL, Guy Richard Quentin 34 Ranmoor Road, Ranmoor, Sheffield S10 3HG — MB BS Lond. 1986; FRCA. 1992.

VEALL, Roger Martin (retired) 1 Plant's Close, East Wellow, Romsey SO51 6AW Tel: 01794 22192 — MRCS Eng. LRCP Lond. 1965 (Univ. Coll. Hosp.) MPhil Lond. 1970, MB BS 1965; MRCP Lond. 1967; MRCPsych 1972. Prev: Cons. (Ment. Handicap) Tatchbury Mt. Hosp.Calmore.

VEASEY, Duncan Andrew Rectory Farm, East Chaldon Road, Winfrith Newburgh, Dorchester DT2 8DJ Tel: 01305 852457 — MB BS Lond. 1977 (St. Bart.) BSc (Biochem.) Lond. 1975; LMSSA Lond. 1977; DPM 1982; MRCPsych 1983. Private Pract. Medico-Legal Cons. Specialty: Gen. Psychiat. Socs: Liveryman Worshipful Soc. Apoth.; Founder Mem. Soc. Expert Witnesses; Foundat. Mem. Expert Witness Inst. Prev: Cons. Psychiat. Avalon NHS Trust Yeovil; Cons. (Psychiat.) W. Dorset Ment. Health NHS Trust; Med. Dir. Huntercombe Manor Maidenhead.

VEASEY, Keith Alan Rose Cottage, 14 Nichols St., Desborough, Kettering NN14 2QU Tel: 01536 710061 — MB ChB Leic. 1981; BA (Hons.) Stirling 1976.

VECHT, Mr Joshua Andrew — MB BS Lond. 1997 (Roy. Free Hosp.) MRCS Eng. 2001.

VECHT, Romeo Jacques The Wellington Hospital, Circus Road, London NW8 9JG Tel: 020 7328 4105 Fax: 020 7328 0463 Email: r.vecht@virgin.net; 118 Maida Vale, London W9 1PT Tel: 020 7328 4105 Fax: 020 7328 0463 — MB ChB Bristol 1962; MRCP (UK) 1973; FACC 1983; FRCP Lond. 1991; FESC 1994. Cons. Cardiol. Wellington Hosp. Lond.; Cons. Cardiol.Roy. Brompton Hosp., Lond. Specialty: Cardiol. Socs: Brit. Cardiac Soc.; FACC; Fell. Europ. Soc. Cardiol. Prev: Cons. Cardiol. Harley St. Clinic, Lond.; Cons. Cardiol. Heart Hosp., Lond.; Hon. Cons. Cardiol. Acad. Surg. & Cardiovasc. Units St. Mary's Hosp. Lond.

VEDI, Krishan Kumar 7 Pexwood, Chadderton, Oldham OL1 2TS Tel: 0161 624 3302 — MB ChB Sheff. 1966; MRCP (UK) 1971; FRCP Lond. 1988. Cons. Phys. (Gen. Med., Diabetes & Endocrinol.) Roy. Oldham Hosp. Specialty: Endocrinol. Prev: Regist. (Neurol.) Roy. Hosp. Sheff. (Fulwood Annexe); Sen. Regist. (Gen. Med., Neurol. & Nephrol.) Withington Hosp. Manch.; Sen. Regist. (Gen. Med., Diabetes & Endocrinol.) Manch. Roy. Infirm.

VEDI, Mr Vikas 5 Shelley Crescent, Hounslow TW5 9BQ Email: v.vedi@redinet.freeserve.co.uk — MB BS Lond. 1989 (Univ. Coll. and Middlx. Hosp. Med. Sch.) BSc (Hons.) Biochem. & Immunol. Lond. 1989; MB BS Lond. 1992; FRCS Eng 1997. Specialist Regist. (Orthop.) S. W. Thames Region. Specialty: Orthop. Socs: BOTA; BMA; Asso. Mem. Brit. Orthopaedic Assoc. Prev: Football Assn. Research Fell. (Orthop. & IMR) St. Mary's Hosp. Lond.; SHO Rotat. (Surg.) St. Peters NHS Trust Chertsey; SHO (Orthop.) Soton. Gen. Hosp.

VEDPATHAK, Vinit Sheshnath Department of Anaesthetics, Glan Clwyd Hospital, Rhyl LL18 5UJ — MB BS Bombay 1983.

VEEDER, Arthur Saul, OStJ 56 Montagu Avenue, Gosforth, Newcastle upon Tyne NE3 4JN Tel: 0191 285 8484 — (Manchester) MRCS Eng. LRCP Lond. 1941, DMJ; FRSA. Police Surg. Newc. Specialty: Forens. Psychiat. Socs: Brit. Acad. Forens. Sci.; BMA; (Counc.) Assn. Police Surgs. Prev: Ho. Surg. (Neurol.) Winwick E.M.S. Hosp. Warrington; Cas. Off. & Ho. Phys. Burton-on-Trent Gen. Infirm.; Capt. RAMC.

VEEN, Mr Harald Gilbert Baid Hospital, South Road, Lerwick ZE1 0TB Tel: 01595 743000 Fax: 01595 743097. Gen. Surg. Cons. Surg., G ilbert Bain Hosp.; Honorary Consultant Surgeon, Lerwick, Shetland. Specialty: Gen. Surg.

VEENHUIZEN, Paul Gerrit The Manor Clinic, 31 Manor Road, Folkestone CT20 2SE Tel: 01303 851146 Fax: 01303 220914 — Artsexamen Utrecht 1989. GP. Specialty: Gen. Surg.

VEENHUIZEN, Philippa Anne Manor Road Surgery, 31 Manor Road, Folkestone CT20 2SE Tel: 01303 851122 Fax: 01303 220914; 2 Cliff Road, Folkestone CT20 2JD — MB ChB Leeds 1982; DCH RCP Glas. 1990; MRCGP 1991; DRCOG 1991; DTM & H Liverp. 1993.

VEERABANGSA, Mohamed 124 Buckswood Drive, Gossops Green, Crawley RH11 8JG Tel: 01293 535615 & profess. 527866 — MB BS Ceylon 1968 (Peradeniya) DPM Eng. 1977; MRCPsych 1978. Cons. Psychiat. (Ment. Illness) with s/i in Psychogeriat. Crawley Hosp. & Horsham Hosp. Specialty: Geriat. Psychiat. Socs: BMA. Prev: Sen. Regist. (Adult Psychiat.) Acad. Dept. Univ. Leicester; (W.cotes Hosp.) & Leicester Roy. Infirm.; Sen. Regist. PsychoGeriat. Assessm. Unit Leicester Gen. Hosp.

VEERAMANI, Ramasamy Broadmoor Hospital, Crowthorne RG45 7EG Tel: 01344 773111; 74A New Wokingham Road, Crowthorne RG45 6JP — MB BS Madras 1970; DPM Univ Madras, 1977; B.Clin Psych. Lond 1992. Assoc. Specialist in Forens. Psychiat. Broadmoor Hosp. Crowthorpe Berks. Specialty: Gen. Psychiat.; Forens. Psychiat. Socs: Affil. The Roy. Coll. of Psychiat.s Lond.; BMA.

VEERAVAHU, Mylvaganam St Luke's Hospital, Genitourinary Medicine, Little Horton Lane, Bradford BD5 0NA Tel: 01274 365511 Email: mylvaganam.veeravahu@bradfordhospitals.nhs.uk — MB BS Ceylon 1969. Locum Cons. (Genitourin. Med.) St Luke's Hosp. Bradford. Specialty: Genitourinary Medicine. Special Interest: Chlamydia. Socs: BMA; Brit. Assn. for Sexual Health & HIV Med. Prev: Cons. (Genitourin. Med.) Halton Gen. Hosp. Runcorn.

VEERAVAHU, Ratneswary Mathura, 14 Barford Close, Westbrook, Warrington WA5 8TL — MB BS Ceylon 1969 (Univ. Ceylon, Colombo) Clin. Med. Off. St. Helens & Knowsley Community Health Trust; Clin. Med. Off. (Occupat. Health) St. Helen's & Knowsley Hosps. Trust. Specialty: Community Child Health. Prev: Clin. Med. Off. S. Birm. HA; Clin. Med. Off. W. Birm. Auth.

VEGA, Eileen Joyce (retired) 9 Auden Close, Lincoln LN2 4BS Tel: 01552 22126 — MB ChB Liverp. 1958; DLO Eng. 1967. GP Lincoln.

VEGA ESCAMILLA, Ignacio 66 Hazel Drive, Woodley, Reading RG5 3SA — LMS Oviedo 1991.

VEIDENHEIMER, Malcolm Charles Health Care International, Beardmore St., Clydebank G81 4HX Tel: 0141 951 5660 Fax: 0141

951 5744 — L Newfoundland Med. Bd. 1957; MD CM Qu. Univ. Canada 1954; FRCSC 1961. Vice-Chairm. Surg. & Chief Div. Gen. Surg. Health Care Internat. Scotl. Specialty: Gen. Surg. Prev: Ex-Chairm. Sect. Colon & Rectal Surg. Lahey Clinic Foundat. Burlington, Mass, USA; Lect. (Surg.) Harvard Med. Sch. Boston, Mass., USA.

VEIRAS, Maria Bernadette 121 All Souls Avenue, Willesden, London NW10 3AT — MB BS Lond. 1996.

VEITCH, Donald 19 Stokesley Road, Marton, Middlesbrough TS7 8DT — MB BS Durh. 1949; LM Dub. 1955.

VEITCH, Elizabeth Mary Helen Coldstream Health Centre, Kelso Road, Coldstream TD12 4LQ Tel: 01890 882711 Fax: 01890 883547; Monument Cottage, Coldstream TD12 4AT — MB BS Lond. 1979 (Roy. Free) MRCGP 1991. Specialty: Gen. Pract.

VEITCH, Graeme Reston (retired) May Trees, 12 Davenham Avenue, Northwood HA6 3HN Tel: 01923 822361 — (Glas.) MB ChB Glas. 1951; DObst RCOG 1956; DA Eng. 1963; FFA RCS Eng. 1970. Prev: Cons. Anaesth. Mt. Vernon Hosp. Northwood Middlx.

VEITCH, Ian Henry Mitford (retired) 200 Brooklands Road, Sale, Manchester M33 3PB — MB BChir Camb. 1954 (Camb. & Newc.) DObst RCOG 1960; FFCM 1977, M 1974. Prev: Area Med. Off. Salford AHA (T).

VEITCH, John William Beech House Group Practice, Beech House Medical Centre, St Bridgets Lane, Egremont CA22 2BD Tel: 01946 814488 Fax: 01946 820372; Beech House Medical Group, St. Bridgets Lane, Egremont CA22 2B Tel: 01946 820692 Fax: 01946 820372 — MB ChB Ed. 1965; FRCGP 1988, M 1975. Asst. Med. Off. BNFL Sellafield; Div. Police Surg. Whitehaven; Med. Off. Cumbria Rubgy Union. Specialty: Sports Med.; Cardiol.; Diabetes. Socs: (Ex-Sec.) W. Cumbld. Med. Soc.; Ex. Provost Cumbria Fac. of RCGP. Prev: Regist. (Anaesth.) W. Cumbld. Hosp. Hensingham; SHO (Anaesth.) East. Gen. Hosp. Edin. & Leith Hosp. Edin.

VEITCH, Tanya Muirhead Medical Centre, Muirhead, Dundee DD2 5NH Tel: 01382 580264 Fax: 01382 581199; 1 Norwood Crescent, Dundee DD2 1PD — MB ChB Dundee 1984; DRCOG 1987.

VEITCH, Yvonne Pinfold Medical Practice, The Health Centre, Pinfold Gate, Loughborough LE11 1DQ Tel: 01509 263753 Fax: 01509 264124 — MB BS Newc. 1972; BSc (Hons.) Physiol. Newc. 1969, MB BS 1972; MRCGP 1991; DFFP 1993. GP LoughBorough.; Hosp. Practitioner (Genito-urin. Med.) Leicester Roy. Infirmy.

VEKES, Katalin Cherry Lodge, 29 Byerley Way, Crabbet Park, Crawley RH10 7YU Tel: 01293 884733 — MRCS Eng. LRCP Lond. 1981; MD Semmelwis, Hungary 1965; DCH Lond. 1983. SCMO (Community Child Health) Wandsworth HA. Specialty: Community Child Health. Socs: BMA & Brit. Paediat. Assn.

VELAMAIL, Vetrivel Morthen Road Surgery, 2 Morthen Road, Wickersley, Rotherham S66 1EU Tel: 01709 549711; 3 First Lane, Wickersley, Rotherham S66 1DU — MB ChB Sheff. 1986.

VELAMATI, Mohan Das Medway Hospital, Gillingham ME7 5NY Tel: 01634 46111 — MB BS Osmania 1971 (Gandhi Med. Coll.) DMRD Eng. 1978; FFR RCSI 1979. Cons. Radiol. Medway Hosp. Gillingham. Specialty: Radiol. Prev: Sen. Regist. (Radiol.) Leeds AHA (T); Regist. (Radiol.) Aberd. Roy. Infirm.

VELANGI, Mark Rajan Haematology Department, Royal Victoria Infirmary, Newcastle upon Tyne Tel: 0191 232 5131 — MB ChB Edin. 1991; MRCP (UK) 1996; MRCPath 2003. Specialist Regist. (Haemat.) Newc. Specialty: Haematology. Prev: SHO (Med.) New Cross Hosp. Wolverhampton.

VELANGI, Shireen Sarita Department of Dermatology, Sunderland Royal Hospital, Kayll Road, Sunderland SR2 7TP Tel: 0191 569 9004 Fax: 0191 569 9201 — MB ChB Ed. 1991; MRCP (UK) 1995. Cons. Dermatol. N. Durh. NHS Trust. Specialty: Dermat. Socs: Roy. Coll. of Phys.s; Brit. Assn. of Dermatol.s; Internat. Soc. for the Study of Vulvo-Vaginal Dis.s.

VELASCO, Nestor Mayday University Hospital, London Road, Thornton Heath, Croydon CR7 7YE Tel: 020 8401 3572 Fax: 020 8401 3570 — Medico Cirujano U National de Colombia 1975. Cons. (Nephrol.) Mayday Univ. Hosp. Lond. Specialty: Nephrol. Special Interest: Dialysis; Hypertens.

VELAUDAPILLAI, Chitra Priyadharshini Brindhavan, Stow Road, Sturton by Stow, Lincoln LN1 2BZ — MB BS Sri Lanka 1977; LRCP LRCS Ed. LRCPS Glas. 1984; FRCS Ed. 1988; FRCOphth 1992. Regist. (Ophth.) Co. Hosp. Lincoln; Ophth. Med. Practitioner; Indep. and self employed. Specialty: Ophth.

VELAZQUEZ GUERRA, Maria Dolores 15 Lynton Mansions, McAuley Close, London SE1 7BW — LMS U Autonoma Madrid 1992.

VELDTMAN, Gruschen Rodney Department Paediatric Cardiology, Leeds General Infirmary, Great George St., Leeds LS1 3EX Tel: 0113 243 2799; 2 Crofthouse Grove, Morley, Leeds LS27 8PA Tel: 0113 253 3461 — MB ChB Cape Town 1991; Dip. Obst. 1992; MRCP(UK) 1995. Specialist Regist. (Paediat. Cardiol.) Leeds Gen. Infirm.; Fell. Adult Congen. Cardiol.; for 1999 & 2000, Toronto Canada. Specialty: Paediat. Cardiol. Socs: BPEG; BPCA. Prev: SHO (Gen. Paediat.) Roy. Hosp. for Sick Childr., Yorkill Glas.

VELDTMAN, Ursula Margarete 5C Orchard Court, The Royal National Orthopaedic Hospital, Brockley Hill, Stanmore HA7 4LP — State Exam Med Gottingen 1990.

VELINENI, Mr Venkat Eswarlu Alexandra Hospital, Woodrow Drive, Redditch B98 7UB Tel: 01527 503030 Fax: 01527 512002 — MB BS Banaras Hindu 1973 (Institute of Medical Sciences) FRCS Ed. 1983. Cons. Surg. - ColoProctol., Worcs. Acute Hosp.s NHS Trust. Specialty: Gen. Surg.

VELKES, Valerie Liebe 20 Wilton Row, London SW1X 7NS — MB ChB Cape Town 1959.

VELL, Tracey Jayne Surrey Lodge Group Practice, 11 Anson Road, Victoria Park, Leicester LE1 7RY Tel: 0161 224 2471 Fax: 0161 257 2264 — MB ChB Leic. 1991; DCH RCP Lond. 1993; MRCGP Lond. 1996. GP Princip. Specialty: Gen. Pract.

VELLA, Anton 7, Ellesboro Road, Harborne, Birmingham B17 8PU Tel: 0121 426 5365 Email: anton.vella@swbh.nhs.uk — MD Malta 1972 (Roy. Univ. of Malta) DA UK 1988. Cons. Anaesthestist, City Hosp., Birm. Specialty: Anaesth. Special Interest: Pain and Hypnosis.

VELLA, Ivan Flat 10, 21/22 Lilley Road, Liverpool L7 OLP — MRCS Eng. LRCP Lond. 1983.

VELLA, Mark Anthony William Harvey Hospital, Willsborough, Ashford TN24 0LZ Tel: 01233 616767 Fax: 01233 616049 Email: mark.vella@ekht.nhs.uk — MRCS Eng. LRCP Lond. 1979 (Guy's) MRCP (UK) 1982; MPhil Lond. 1985; FRCP (UK) 1998. Cons. Phys., Diabetes and Lipid Disorders; Sub Dean GKT Med. Sch. Specialty: Gen. Med.; Diabetes. Prev: Sen. Regist. Guy's Hosp. Lond.; Regist. (Med.) Whittington Hosp. Lond.; Regist. (Med.) Univ. Coll. Hosp. Lond.

VELLA, Ray The Surgery, 14 Manor Road, Beckenham BR3 5LE Tel: 020 8650 0957 Fax: 020 8663 6070; 21 Aldersmead Road, Beckenham BR3 1NA Tel: 020 8778 2859 — MRCS Eng. LRCP Lond. 1981 (Guy's) MRCGP 1986.

VELLA, Victoria Mary Patricia Simmonds Accident & Emergency Department, Worcester Royal Hospital, Worcester Tel: 01905 763333 — MB BCh Wales 1986; FRCS (A&E). Staff Grade (A&E), Worcester Roy. Hosp.; Sen. Trust Grade (A & E). Specialty: Accid. & Emerg. Prev: Clin. Asst. (A & E) Selly Oak Hosp. Birm.

VELLA BONELLO, Louise Martha 37 Flood Street, London SW3 5ST — MRCS Eng. LRCP Lond. 1978; FFA RCS Eng. 1982. Cons. Anaesth. Roy. Free Hosp. Lond. Specialty: Anaesth. Prev: Vis. Asst. Prof. Anaesth. & ITU John Hopkins Hosp. Baltimore; Lect. & Sen. Regist. St. Thos. Hosp.; Regist. Guy's Hosp. Lond.

VELLACOTT, Ian Diarmid The Croft, Middle St., Dunston, Lincoln LN4 2EW — MB BCh Wales 1977; FRCOG 1996, M 1983. Cons. O & G Lincoln Co. Hosp.; Clin. Teach., Univ. of Nottm. Specialty: Obst. & Gyn. Prev: Lect. & Sen. Regist. (O & G) Roy. Free Hosp. Lond.; Regist. (O & G) Middlx. Hosp. & Woms. Hosp. Soho Sq. Lond.; Research Regist. (O & G) St. Thos. Hosp. Lond.

VELLACOTT, Mr Keith David Royal Gwent Hospital, Cardiff Road, Newport NP20 2UB Tel: 01633 234112 Fax: 01633 234252; Glasllwch House, 4 Glasllwch Crescent, Newport NP20 3SE Tel: 01633 252303 Fax: 01633 223127 Email: k.d.vellacott@btinternet.com — MB BS Lond. 1972 (Lond. Hosp.) MRCS Eng. LRCP Lond. 1972; DCH Eng. 1975; FRCS Eng. 1977; DM Nottm. 1981. Cons. Surg. Roy. Gwent Hosp. Newport; Hon. Sen. Lect. Univ. Wales Coll Med. Specialty: Gen. Surg. Socs: Assn. Surg.; Assn. Coloproctol. Prev: Sen. Regist. (Surg.) Bristol & Weston HA; Wellcome Research Fell. Nottm. Univ. Regist. Cheltenham Gen. Hosp.; SHO United Bristol. Hosps.

VELLACOTT, Michael Nelson Plas y Bryn Surgery, Chapel Street, Wrexham LL13 7DD Tel: 01978 351308 Fax: 01978 312324;

Cottsmoor House, Ruthin Road, Wrexham LL11 3BP Tel: 01978 354260 — MB BS Lond. 1972; MRCS Eng. LRCP Lond. 1970; AFOM RCP Lond. 1988. Fact. Doctor Tetra Pak, Pouvair Ltd; Apptd. Doctor under Lonising Radiat. Regulator 1985, Pirelli Cables Ltd (Wrexham & Prescott), Rescam Image Products, Hoyalens Ltd. Specialty: Occupat. Health.

VELLACOTT, William Noel (retired) Long Cottage, Stonebarrow Lane, Charmouth, Bridport DT6 6RA Tel: 01297 560381 — MRCS Eng. LRCP Lond. 1950 (Guy's) LMSSA Lond. 1939; MA Camb. 1940; DA Eng. 1946; FFA RCS Eng. 1954; FRCA 1965. Prev: Cons. Anaesth. Worcester Roy. Infirm.

VELLANI, Zarina Iqbal Ramzan (retired) 138 Bawnmore Road, Rugby CV22 6JT Tel: 01788 813869 — MB BS Lond. 1959 (Roy. Free) MRCS Eng. LRCP Lond. 1959; DObst RCOG 1961; MFCM RCP (UK) 1985. Prev: Dir. Pub. Health Harrow HA.

VELLENOWETH, Sarah Margaret The Almshouse Surgery, Trinity Medical Centre, Thornhill Street, Wakefield WF1 1PG Tel: 01924 327150 Fax: 01924 327165; 16 Bottom Boat Road, Bottom Boat, Stanley, Wakefield WF3 4AY Tel: 01924 820486 Email: 113045.2124@compuserve.com — MB ChB Leeds 1989; DRCOG 1992; DFFP 1993; MRCGP 1995. Princip. GP. Prev: Trainee GP Wakefield VTS.

VELLODI, Ashok Metabolic Unit, Great Ormond St. Hospital for Children NHS Trust, Great Ormond St., London WC1N 3JH Tel: 020 7405 9200 Fax: 020 7813 8597; 55 Georges Wood Road, Brookmans Park, Hatfield AL9 7BX — MB BS Poona 1976; MD (Paediat.) All India Inst. Med. Scs. 1979; FRCP 1995, MRCP 1982; FRCPCH 1997. Cons. Paediat. & Hon. Sen. Lect. Metab. Unit Gt. Ormond St. Hosp. Childr. NHS Trust. Specialty: Paediat. Prev: Sen. Regist. (Paediat.) St. Thos. Hosp. Lond.; Lect. (Child Health) Westm. Childr. Hosp. Lond.; Regist. Alder Hey Childr. Hosp. Liverp.

VELLODI, Chandrika Barnet General Hospital, Wellhouse Lane, Barnet EN5 3DJ Tel: 020 8440 5111; 55 Georges Wood Road, Brookmans Park, Hatfield AL9 7BX — MB BS Lond. 1978 (St. Bart.) MRCP (UK) 1982. Cons. Phys. (Geriat. Med.) Barnet Gen. Hosp. Specialty: Care of the Elderly. Socs: Brit. Geriat. Soc. Prev: Sen. Regist. (Geriat. & Med.), Roy. Liverp. Hosp.; Regist. (Med.) Walton Hosp. Liverp.

VELUPILLAI, Suntheralingam 113 Balaam Street, London E13 8AF Tel: 020 8472 1238 Fax: 020 8470 1739; 39 Knighton Road, London E7 0EE — MB BS Ceylon 1962. Socs: BMA; Roy. Soc. Med. Prev: Regist. (Venereol.) St. Bart. Hosp. Lond. & Homerton Gr. Clinics E. Hosp. Lond.; SHO (Venereol.) St. Bart. Hosp. Lond. & P. of Wales Hosp. Lond.

VELUSAMI, Othimalaigounder Gaer Medical Centre, 71 Gaer Road, Newport NP20 3GX Tel: 01633 840827 — MB BS Madras 1974 (Madras University) BSc 1967; DA (UK) 1982. GP A & E Gen. Surg., Psychiat. Anaesth. & O & G; Police Surg.; Examg. Med. Practitioner EMP for DLA. Specialty: Gen. Pract. Socs: LMC.

VEMPALI, Venkata Madhava Rao The Princess Alexandra Hospital NHS Trust, Eye Unit, Hamstel Road, Harlow CM20 1QX Tel: 01279 827905 Fax: 01279 793719 — MB BS Andhra 1986; MD; FRCS Ed. 1993; FRCOphth 2003. Cons. Ophth. Surg.; Lead Doctor for Head and Neck Directorate. Specialty: Ophth. Special Interest: Cataract Surgery; Ocular Motility. Socs: BMA; Amer. Acad. Ophth.; Amer. Assn. Paediat. Ophth.

VENABLES, Andrew John The Elms Resource Centre, Odsal Clinic, Odsal Road, Bradford BD6 1PR — MB BS Newc. 1979; MRCGP 1985; MRCPsych 1988; M.Med. Sci. (Clin. Psych.) 1989.

VENABLES, Mr Christopher Wilfred 57 Hackwood Park, Hexham NE46 1AZ Tel: 01434 608277 Fax: 01434 608277 — (Westm.) MB BS Lond. 1958; MRCS Eng. LRCP Lond. 1958; FRCS Eng. 1961; MS Lond. 1970. Emerit. Cons. Surg. (Gastroenterol.) Freeman Hosp. Newc.; Locum Cons. (Endoscopy) Northumbria NHS Trust; Med. Advis. NHS Informat. Auth. Specialty: Gen. Surg.; Gastroenterol. Special Interest: Healthcare Computing. Socs: Fell. Roy. Soc. Med.; NE Surgic. Soc.; Brit. Soc. Gastroenterol. Prev: Hon. Lect. & Sen. Lect. (Surg.) Univ. Newc.; Research Fell. Mt. Sinai Hosp. New York, USA; Cons. in Surgic. Gastroenterol. Freeman Hosp.: Newc.

VENABLES, Elizabeth Mary Charing Cross Hospital, Earling, Hammersmith & Fulham Mental Health Trust, Fulham Place Road, London W6 8RF Tel: 020 8846 1509 Fax: 020 8846 1133; Flat 2, 131 Hammersmith Grove, London W6 0NJ Tel: 020 8563 7106 — MB BS Adelaide 1992; MRCPsych Dec. 1999. Specialist Regist., Pychogeriats. Specialty: Gen. Psychiat.

VENABLES, Graham Stuart Royal Hallamshire Hospital, Sheffield S10 2JF Tel: 0114 2712197 Fax: 0114 271 2441 Email: graham.venables@sth.nhs.uk — BM BCh Oxf. 1973 (Camb. & Oxf.) Dip. Phil & Health Care Swansea; BA (MA) Camb 1970; MRCP (UK) 1976; DM Oxf. 1984; FRCP Ed. 1989; FRCP Lond. 1991; FRCOPhth 1999. Cons. Neurol.Sheff. Teachg. hosp. NHS Trust; Clin. Director Neurosci.s, Sheff. Teachg. Hosp. Specialty: Neurol. Socs: Europ. Stroke Counc. Prev: Sen. Lect. (Med. Neurol.) Dept. Neurosci. Univ. Edin.; 1st Asst. (Neurol.) Univ. Newc.; Assoc. Post Dean Sheff. Med. Sch.

VENABLES, Katherine Margaret Department of Occupational & Environmental Medicine, Imperial College School of Medicine, National Heart & Lung Institute, Dovehouse St., London SW3 6LR Tel: 020 7351 8328 Fax: 020 7351 8336; 32 Franconia Road, Clapham, London SW4 9ND Tel: 020 7720 2481 — MB BS Lond. 1973 (St. Bart.) MRCP (UK) 1977; BSc Lond. 1970, MD 1987, MSc (Distinc.) Occupat. Med. 1980; MFOM RCP Lond. 1988, FFOM 1993; FRCP Lond. 1994; MSc 1995; MFPHM RCP (UK) 1996. Univ. Lect.Iniv.Oxf; Hon. Cons. Pub. Health Kensington, Chelsea & Westm. HA; Sen. Lect. Imperial Coll. Sch. Med. Nat. Heart & Lung Inst. Lond. & Hon. Cons. Phys. Brompton Hosp. Lond. Specialty: Occupat. Health; Epidemiol. Socs: Chairm. Sci. Comm. Epidemiol.; Internat.Commiss. Occupat.Health; Res. Comm. Brit. Thoracic Soc. Prev: Lect. Lond. Sch. Hyg. & Trop. Med.; Lect. Cardiothoracic Inst. Lond.; Regist. St. Geo. Hosp. & St. Thos. Hosp.Lond.

VENABLES, Malcolm Crown Street Surgery, 17 Crown Street, Swinton, Rotherham S64 8LY Tel: 01709 583862; Brookside, Manor Lane, Adwick-upon-Dearne, Mexborough S64 0NN Tel: 01709 583677 — MB ChB Sheff. 1982. Socs: MRCGP.

VENABLES, Martin Geoffrey Malcolm Hillside Farm, Ireton Wood, Idridgehay, Belper DE56 2SD Tel: 01335 370532 — BM BCh Oxf. 1948. Prev: Ho. Surg. ENT Dept. Roy. Hosp. Sheff.; Ho. Phys. Roy. Infirm. Sheff.

VENABLES, Michael Thomas CAMHS, Horsham Hospital, Hurst Road, Horsham RH12 2DR Tel: 01403 227014 — MRCS Eng. LRCP Lond. 1980 (Middlesex Hosp.) BA Oxf. 1973; MRCPsych 1984. Cons. Child & Adolesc. Psychiat. SurAd NHS Trust, Horsham Hosp. Specialty: Child & Adolesc. Psychiat. Socs: Assn. Child Psychol. & Psychiat.

VENABLES, Paul Andrew 11A Pheasant Walk, Littlemore, Oxford OX4 4XX — BM Soton. 1998.

VENABLES, Peter (retired) 29 The Avenue, Andover SP10 3EP — (Middlx.) MB BChir Camb. 1944; MRCS Eng. LRCP Lond. 1944; MRCP Lond. 1945. Prev: Cas. Med. Off. & Med. Regist. Middlx. Hosp.

VENABLES, Thomas Leopold Salterford House, Calverton, Nottingham NG14 6NZ Tel: 0115 965 5316 Fax: 0115 965 5627 — MB BChir Camb. 1965 (Camb. & Westm.) MB Camb. 1965, BChir 1964; MA CAmb. 1965; FRCGP 1980, M 1972; FRCP 1997. Specialty: Acupunc.; Medico Legal. Socs: (Pres.) Nottm. M-C Soc.; Osler Club Lond.; Nottm. Medico-Legal Soc. Prev: Upjohn Trav. Fell.; Med. Specialist RAF.; Lect. (Gen. Pract.) Nottm. Univ. Med. Sch.

VENESS, Alan Maurice (retired) Sandwell and West NHS Trust, Dudley Road, Birmingham B18 7QH Tel: 0121 554 3801; 43 Pilkington Avenue, Sutton Coldfield B72 1LA Email: alanv@care4free.net — (Birmingham) MB ChB Birm. 1964; FRCA Eng. 1970. Cons. Anaesth. Birmingham Hosp. NHS Trust Birm. Prev: Sen. Regist. (Anaesth.) St. Geo. Hosp. Lond. & Hosp. Sick Childr. Gt. Ormond St.

VENETO, Bruno The Thatches, Crossing Road, Palgrave, Diss IP22 1AW Tel: 01379 643314 — State DMS Padua 1989. Prev: SHO (Cas., Gen. Surg. & Orthop.) Hammersmith Hosp. Lond.; Demonst. (Anat.) St. Geo. Hosp. Med. Sch. Lond.; Cas. Off. St. Helier Hosp. Carshalton.

VENISON, Tania Dawn Station Rd Surgery, 74 Station Rd, West Wickham BR4 Tel: 020 8777 8245 — MB BS Lond. 1996 (Royal London Hospital Medical College) DRCOG. SHO (Gen. Med.). Specialty: Gen. Med. Prev: SHO (Oncol.); Ho. Off. (Gen. Surg.); Ho. Off. (Gen. Med.).

VENKAT, Kandasami Ramaswamy Eastgate, Gillott Road, Edgbaston, Birmingham B16 0EU Tel: 0121 454 1712; Srisai, 40 Selwyn Road, Edgbaston, Birmingham B16 0SN Tel: 0121 454 4721

— MB BS Madras 1964 (Madural Med. Coll.) MRCGP 1974; Diploma in Acupunc. UK 1996; Diabetes & ITS Managem. Warwick 2000. Socs: BMA; FRSM 1998. Prev: Regist. (A & E) Vict. Hosp. Blackpool; SHO (Cas. & Gen. Surg.) St. Jas. Hosp. Tredegar; Asst. Med. Off. (Surg.) South. Rly. HQ Hosp. Mysore.

VENKAT-RAMAN, Gopalakrishnan Queen Alexandra Hospital, Renal Unit, Sotuwick Hill Road, Portsmouth PO6 3LY Tel: 023 9228 6000 Fax: 023 9228 6461 Email: gvr@porthosp.nhs.uk — MB BS Poona 1974; MD Delhi 1978; MNAMS (India) 1979; MRCP (UK) 1980; FRCP Lond. 1992; Dip Med Educat Dundee 2002. Cons. Nephrol. Wessex Regional Renal & Transpl. Unit. Specialty: Nephrol.; Gen. Med.; Medical Education. Special Interest: Hypertens.; Transpl.

VENKAT RAMAN, Mr Narayanaswamy Department of Fetomaternal Medicine, Maternity Day Care Unit, St Mary's Hospital, Praed St., London W2 1NY Tel: 020 7886 6691 Fax: 020 7886 2169; House 5, Kershaw Close, Langton Gate, 118 North St, Hornchurch RM11 1SW Tel: 01708 459276 — MB BS Osmania 1980 (Osmania Med. Coll., Hyderabad, India) MD Osmania 1985; Dip Nat Bd Examin (NBE), New Delhi, 1986; MRCOG 1992; Cert. Adv Ultrasound RCOG/RCR Lond. 1997. Staff Grade Specialist Feto-Matern. Med. Dept. of Obst. St Mary's Hosp. Lond. Specialty: Obst. & Gyn. Socs: BMA; Fell. Roy. Soc. Med. Lond. Prev: Regist. O & G, The Jessop Hosp. Hosp. For Wom., Sheff.. UK; Regist. O & G, the Doncester Roy. Infirm. & Montagu Hosp. NHS Trust, Doncester, S.Yorks. UK.

VENKATA RAMA SASTRY, Kolluri c/o Professor A. D. Medelow, Department of Neurosurgery, Newcastle General Hospital, Westgate Road, Newcastle upon Tyne NE4 6BE — MB BS Sri Venkateswara 1969.

VENKATACHALAM, Dhanvanti Narayan Department of Anaesthetics, Medway Maritime Hospital, Windmill Road, Gillingham Kent Tel: 01634 833722 Fax: 01634 833856 Email: gasdoc@blueyonder.co.uk; Almond Lodge, 46 Almond Grove, Hempstead, Gillingham ME7 3SE Tel: 01634 234365 — MB BS Mysore 1981 (Kasturba Medicial Coll.) DA Eng. 1983; DObst RCPI 1987; FFARCSI Irel. 1988. Cons. Anaesth., Medway Maritime Hosp., Kent. Specialty: Anaesth.; Intens. Care. Special Interest: Head & Neck Surg.; Obst. Anaesth.; Regional Anaesth. Socs: Hosp. Consultants and Specialists Assn.; BMA; Roy. Coll. Of Anaesthetics. Prev: GP Princip. Sittingbourne Kent; Sen. Regist. in Anaesth., Kings Coll. Hosp.

VENKATARAMAN, Geetha Department of Obstetrics & Gynaecology, West Middlesex University Hospital, Twickenham Road, Isleworth TW7 6AF Tel: 020 8565 5435 Fax: 020 8565 5973; 53 The Beeches, 200 Lampton Road, Hounslow TW3 4DF Tel: 020 8577 9007 — MB BS Madras 1975; MD Madras 1985; MRCOG 1993. Clin. Asst. (O & G) W. Middlx. Univ. Hosp.

VENKATARAMAN, Marakatham c/o Mrs H. Faulkner, Personnel Department, Maternity Unit, Walsgrave Hospital NHS Trust, Clifford Bridge Road, Coventry CV2 2DX — MB BS Madras 1983; MRCP (UK) 1989.

VENKATARAMANAN, Mr Palgudi Ramaswamy Flat 710, Block 7 Friars Field, Royal Gwent Hospital, Newport NP20 4EZ; 3 Townsend Close, Woodloes Park, Warwick CV34 5TT Tel: 01926 497620 — MB BS Madurai 1978; FRCS Ed. 1987. Regist. (Orthop.) Roy. Gwent Hosp. Newport. Specialty: Transpl. Surg. Prev: Regist. (Orthop.) Furness Gen. Hosp. Barrow in Furness.

VENKATARATNAM BABU, Kari 95 Park Way, Crawley RH10 3BS — MB BS Sri Venateswara 1973.

VENKATESAN, Mr Dhamaraikulam 24 Landseer Close, Liberty Avenue, Hamilton Gardens, London SW20 2UT — MB BS Bangalor 1970 (Bangalore Med. Coll.) MB BS Bangalore 1970; FRCS Ed. 1976. Regist. (Gen. Surg.) Horton Gen. Hosp. Banbury. Specialty: Gen. Surg. Prev: SHO (Thoracic Surg.) St. Helier Hosp. Carshalton; Rotating SHO (Surg.) Taunton & Som. Hosp. (MusGr. Pk. Br.); SHO (Gen. Surg. & Cas.) Dreadnought Seamen's Hosp. Greenwich.

VENKATESAN, Pradhib Bimingham Heartlands Hospital, Birmingham B9 5SS Tel: 0121 766 6611; 11 Mossdale Road, Nottingham NG5 3GX — MB BChir Camb. 1984 (Univ. Camb.) MRCP (UK) 1986; DTM & H RCP Lond. 1994; PhD Nottm. 1996. Clin. Lect. (Infec.) Univ. Birm. Specialty: Infec. Dis. Prev: Wellcome Research Fell. (Microbial Dis.) Univ. Nottm.; Regist. (Med.) City Hosp. Nottm.; SHO (Cardiol.) Hammersmith Hosp. Lond.

VENKATESH, Maya Nayak 12 Shetland Drive, Glendale Estate, Nuneaton CV10 7LA — MB BS Mangalore 1988; FRCS Ed. 1993.

VENKATESH, Udupa Rajagopal St Lukes Hospital, Department of Paediatrics, Little Horton Lane, Bradford BD6 1RG — MB BS Madras 1983; MRCPI 1991.

VENKATESHAM, Guduguntla Chiswick Health Centre, Fishers Lane, London W4 1RX Tel: 020 8321 3551 Fax: 020 8321 3556 — MB BS Osmania 1974; MFFP 1993. CMO (Family Plann.) & Instruc. Dr. Specialty: Gen. Pract. Socs: Overseas Doctors Assn. (Ex-Treas. NW Thames Div.); Osmania Med. Grad. Assn. (Ex-Treas.); SHRI Venkateswere (Balaji) Temple of UK (Ex-Fund Raising Sec.).

VENKATESWARLU, Vasantham District General Hospital, Town Lane, Kew, Southport PR8 6NJ; 10 Wennington Road, Southport PR9 7EU — MB BS Sri Venkateswara 1971 (Kurnool Med. Coll.) DA Eng. 1976. Clin. Med. Off. (Anaesth.) Dist. Gen. Hosp. S.port. Prev: Regist. (Anaesth.) Gem. Hosp. Jersey.

VENKATRAMAN, Thondiculum Bhaskaran Bawtry Road Surgery, 171 Bawtry Road, Brinsworth, Rotherham S60 5ND Tel: 01709 828806 — MB BS Delhi 1975.

VENKITESWARAN, Nemmara Thiruvenkitanathan Parkgate Medical Centre, Netherfield Lane, Parkgate, Rotherham S62 6AW Tel: 01709 514500 Fax: 01709 514490 — MB BS Bangalore 1967.

VENKITESWARAN, Ramachandran (retired) 2A Bradpole Road, Strouden Park, Bournemouth BH8 9NX Tel: 01202 532253; 11 William Road, Queens Park, Bournemouth BH7 7BB Tel: 01202 246719 — MB BS Karnatak 1964; DCH RCP Lond. 1971; DRCOG 1974; MRCGP 1975.

VENN, Carl Stuart Abertillery Health Centre, Abertillery; 15 Alma Street, Brynmawr, Ebbw Vale NP23 4DZ — MB ChB Bristol 1983; BSc Bristol 1980, MB ChB 1983; DRCOG 1988; MRCGP 1990.

VENN, Mr Graham Erskine London Bridge Hospital, Suite 305, Emblem House, 27 Tooley Street, London SE1 2PR Tel: 020 7378 6566 Fax: 020 7378 8156 Email: graham@gvenn.demon.co.uk; Flat 106, The Listed Building, 350 Highway, London E1W 3HU Tel: 020 7790 2257 — MB BS Lond. 1977; FRCS Ed. 1981; FRCS Eng. 1982; FICS Chicago 1990; MS Lond. 1991; FETCS 1998. Cons. Cardiothoracic Surg. Guy's & St. Thos. Hosp.; Hon. Cons. Cardiac Surg. to Brit. Army; Hon. Sen. Lect. Univ. Lond. Specialty: Cardiothoracic Surg.; Cardiol.; Gen. Surg. Socs: Brit. Cardiac Soc.; Eur. Assn. Cardiothoracic Surg.; Roy. Soc. Med. (Past Pres. Cardiothoracic Sect.). Prev: Sen. Regist. (Cardiothoracic Surg.) Middlx., Hammersmith & Harefield Hosps. Lond.

VENN, Michael George Pierre, OBE, Air Commodore RAF Med. 51 Willoughby Drive, Empingham, Oakham LE15 8PY Tel: 01780 460602 Fax: 01780 460602 — MB BS Lond. 1955 (Middlx.) DAvMed Eng. 1968; MRAeS 1976; FFOM RCP Lond. 1994, MFOM 1980. Indep. Cons. Aviat. & Occupat. Med.; Aviat. Med. Gp. Roy. Aeronautical Soc. Specialty: Occupat. Health. Socs: Fell. Aerospace Med. Assn.; Soc. Occupat. Med. Prev: Dep. Head. Med. Servs. John Lewis Partnership plc Lond.; Commandant RAF Centr. Med. Estab. RAF Kelvin Hse. Lond.; Aerospace Med. Staff. Off. Brit. Defence Staff Washington, USA.

VENN, Paul Hex (retired) Milber Down, 7 Selwyn Road, Eastbourne BN21 2LD — MRCS Eng. LRCP Lond. 1948 (St. Bart.) DA Eng. 1953; FFA RCS Eng. 1954. Prev: Cons. Anaesth. Eastbourne Dist. Gen. Hosp.

VENN, Peter John Clare House, Lewes Road, East Grinstead RH19 3SY — MB BS Lond. 1979; FFA RCS Eng. 1984. Cons. Anaesth. Qu. Vict. Hosp. E. Grinstead; Examr. Roy. Coll. Anaesth. Specialty: Anaesth. Socs: Fell. Roy. Soc. Med.; Assn. Anaesth.; Plastic Surg. & Burns Anaesth. Assn. Prev: Sen. Regist. Nuffield Dept. Anaesth. Oxf. RHA; Lect. (Anaesth.) Nat. Hosp. Nerv. Dis. Qu. Sq. Lond.; Regist. (Anaesth.) Char. Cross Hosp. Lond.

VENN, Philippa Mary Cleveland Clinic, 12 Cleveland Road, St Helier, Jersey JE1 4HD Tel: 01534 722381/734121 — BM Soton. 1989; MRCP (UK) 1992; MRCGP 1994. GP Jersey Chanel. Prev: Trainee GP Chelmsford; SHO (O & G) St. Johns Hosp. Chelmsford; SHO (Gen. Med.) Qu. Eliz. Hosp. Birm.

VENN, Richard Mark 7 New Road, Forest Green, Dorking RH5 5SA — MB BS Lond. 1987. Specialty: Anaesth.

VENN, Mr Robin John (retired) 32 Whiting Street, Bury St Edmunds IP33 1NP Tel: 01284 755093 Email: robin.venn@virgin.net — (Middlx.) MB BS Lond. 1951; FRCOG 1973, M 1960; MMSA 1963. Prev: Cons. O & G Bury St. Edmunds.

VENN, Sarah Joanna The Bridge Centre, Foundry Bridge, Abertillery NP13 1BQ Tel: 01495 322682 Fax: 01495 322686; 15 Alma Street, Brynmawr, Ebbw Vale NP23 4DZ Tel: 01495 313541 — (Bristol) MB ChB Bristol 1983; DGM RCP Lond. 1986; MRCGP 1989; DCH RCP 1995. GP & Specialist Regist. (Pub.h Health) Gwent. Specialty: Pub. Health Med. Prev: Volunteer Action Health S. India; GP Princip.; Staff Grade (Community Paediat.).

VENN, Mrs Suzanne Nicola St Richard's Hospital, Chichester PO19 4SE — MB BS Lond. 1987; FRCS Eng. 1992; MS 1996; FRCS (Urol) 1999. Cons. Urological Surg., St Richard's Hosp., Chichester; Sen. Lect. Inst. of Urol., UCLH. Specialty: Urol.

VENN-TRELOAR, Josephine Mary Community Child Health Services, Memorial Hospital, Shooters Hill, Woolwich, London SE18 3RZ — MB BS Lond. 1984; AKC 1984; DRCOG 1987; MRCGP 1988. Clin. Med. Off. (Child Health) Greenwich Healthcare NHS Trust. Specialty: Community Child Health. Prev: GP Asst. Vanburgh Hill Health Centre; GP Assist. Ingleton Ave. Surg. Welling.

VENNAM, Mr Ramesh Babu 3 Maes Celyn, Wrexham LL13 7QG — MB BS Nagarjuna India 1979; FRCS Glas. 1989. Regist. (Gen. Surg.) Blackburn Roy. Infirm. Specialty: Gen. Surg.

VENNER, Elizabeth Anne Tredale Cottage, Tregunna, St Breock, Wadebridge PL27 7HX Tel: 01208 813114 — MB BS Lond. 1992; BSc (Hons.) Lond. 1989; MRCP (UK) 1995.

VENNER, Mr Robert Martin Whincorft, 288 Glasgow Road, Waterfoot, Eaglesham, Glasgow G76 0EW — MB ChB Birm. 1968; FRCS Ed. 1975.

VENNING, Geoffrey Richard 14 Lucas Road, High Wycombe HP13 6QG Tel: 01494 526543; Malastreges, Cuzance, par Martel Lot 46600, France Tel: 00 33 65 327536 — BM BCh Oxf. 1944; FRCP Lond. 1973, M 1949. Dir. Pharmaceut. Research Serv. Specialty: Pharmacology. Socs: Founder Fell. Fac. Pharmaceut. Med.; Fell. Roy. Soc. Med.; Airborne Med. Soc. Prev: Vice-Pres. Janssen Pharmaceutica N.V. Belgium, & Dir. of Research & Developm. UK; Sen. Med. Off. Med. Div. DHSS; Sen. Regist. (Med.) Univ. Dept. Med. Manch. Roy. Infirm. & Manch. RHB.

VENNING, Helen Elizabeth Paediatric Rheumatology Clinic, Department of Child Health, University Hospital, Nottingham NG7 2UH Tel: 0115 924 9924 Ext: 43442 Fax: 0115 849 3313 Email: helen.venning@qmcuh-tr.trent.nhs.uk — BM BS Nottm. 1977; BMedSci Nottm. 1975; MRCP (UK) 1981; FRCP Lond. 1994; FRCPCH 1997. Cons. Paediat. Rheum. Univ. Hosp. Nottm. Specialty: Paediat.; Rheumatol. Prev: Cons. Paediat. (Rheum. & Community) Nottm. Community Unit.

VENNING, Mary Ruth (retired) 14 Lucas Road, High Wycombe HP13 6QG Tel: 01494 526543 — BM BCh Oxf. 1944; CPH Wales 1951. Prev: SCMO Bucks. CC.

VENNING, Michael Charles Teaching Unit 6, University Hospital of South Manchester, Nell Lane, Didsbury, Manchester M20 2LR Tel: 0161 291 3667 Fax: 0161 291 3670 Email: mike.venning@smuht.nwest.nhs.uk; 12 Kingston Road, Didsbury, Manchester M20 2RZ Tel: 0161 445 7238 — BM BCh Oxf. 1979 (Oxford) PhD Cornell 1976; BA Oxf. 1969, BM BCh 1979; MRCP (UK) 1981; FRCP (UK) 1996. Cons. Renal & Gen. Phys. Univ. Hosp. S. Manch.; Hon. Lect. Univ. Manch. Med. Sch.; Roy. Coll. Tutor, Smith Manch. Univ. Hosp. Specialty: Nephrol.; Gen. Med.; Immunol. Socs: Renal Assn.; Internat. Soc. Nephrol.; Internat. Soc. Peritoneal Dialysis. Prev: Lect. (Med.) Univ. Newc.; Research Regist. Hammersmith Hosp. Lond.; Sen. Ho. Off. Brompton Hosp.

VENNING, Molly Anne (retired) 4 Buckstone Close, London SE23 3QT — MB BS Lond. 1974 (Middlx. Hosp.) MRCPsych 1985. Prev: Sen. Regist. (Psychother.) Bethlem Roy. & Maudsley Hosps.

VENNING, Stephanie Louise The Wheatcroft, Weasenham, King's Lynn PE32 2SW — MB BS Newc. 1998.

VENNING, Vanessa Ann Department of Dermatology, Churchill Hospital, Old Road, Headington, Oxford OX3 7LJ Tel: 01865 228274 Fax: 01865 228260 Email: vanessa.venning@orh.nhs.uk — BM BCh Oxf. 1978 (Oxford) MRCP (UK) 1980; BA Oxf. 1975, DM 1994; FRCP 1997. Cons. Dermat.Ch.ill Hosp. Oxf. Specialty: Dermat. Prev: Sen. Regist. (Dermat.) Slade Hosp. Oxf.; Cons. Dermat., N. Hants. Hosp.s.

VENTERS, Brian Parkgrove Terrace Surgery, 22B Parkgrove Terrace, Edinburgh EH4 7NX Tel: 0131 312 6600 Fax: 0131 312 7798; 4 East Barnton Gardens, Edinburgh EH4 6AR Tel: 0131 336 3553 — MB ChB Ed. 1975; BSc (Med. Sci.) Ed. 1972. Specialty: Hypnother.; Acupunc. Prev: Ho. Off. (Orthop. Surg.) Roy. Infirm. Edin.; Ho. Off. (Respirat. Unit) North. Gen. Hosp. Edin.; Clin. Asst. Beechmont Hosp. Edin.

VENTERS, Gregor Lachlan Pentland Medical Centre, 44 Pentland View, Currie EH14 5QB Tel: 0131 449 2142 Fax: 0131 451 5855 — MB ChB Ed. 1984.

VENTERS, Nicholas David 48 Brantwood Road, Bradford BD9 6QA — MB ChB Liverp. 1998.

VENTHAM, Peter Anthony Anaesthetics Department, Poole Hospital Trust, Longfleet Road, Poole BH15 2JB Tel: 01202 665511 Fax: 01202 442672; The Old Barn, Millhams St, Christchurch BH23 1DN Tel: 01202 484307 — BM Soton. 1976; BSc (Hons.) Biochem. Wales 1969; FFA RCS Eng. 1984. Cons. Anaesth. Dorset HA. Specialty: Anaesth. Socs: Assn. Anaesth. & Pain Soc. Prev: Sen. Regist. (Anaesth.) Roy. Free & Northwick Pk. Hosps.

VENTON, Tamsin Jayne Riverside Surgery, Albion St., Shaldon, Teignmouth TQ14 0DF Tel: 01626 873331 Fax: 01626 772107; Glendevon Medical Centre, 3 Carlton Place, Teignmouth TQ14 8AB Tel: 01626 770955 Fax: 01626 772107 — MB BS Lond. 1988; MRCGP 1993; DFFP 1994. Prev: Trainee GP Torbay HA VTS.

VENTRESCA, Giampietro 15 Steele Road, London W4 5AB Tel: 020 8987 8810 — State DMS Milan 1983; MD Milan 1988; MSc Aberd. 1991; MFPM RCP (UK) 1996. Specialty: Pharmaceutical Medicine. Socs: Scott. Soc. Experim. Med.; Brit. Pharm. Soc. (Clin. Sect.).

VENTRESS, Michael Andrew 76 Moorside Crescent, Fishburn, Stockton-on-Tees TS21 4DH — MB ChB Liverp. 1993.

VENUGOPAL, Janardanan Bransholme South Health Centre, Goodhart Road, Bransholme, Hull HU7 4DW Tel: 01482 831257; 61 The Dales, Cottingham HU16 5JS — MB BS Kerala 1968 (Trivandrum Med. Coll.) Prev: Regist. (Psychiat.) Walsgrave Hosp. Coventry; SHO (Geriat.) Alexandra Hosp. Barnstaple; SHO (Geriat.) De Lancey Hosp. Cheltenham.

VENUGOPAL, Ramaswamysetty Esk Road Medical Centre, 12 Esk Road, London E13 8LJ Tel: 020 7474 9002 Fax: 020 7473 1917.

VENUGOPAL, Sriramashetty, OBE (retired) Aston Health Centre, 175 Trinity Road, Aston, Birmingham B6 6JA Tel: 0121 328 3597 Fax: 0121 327 1674; 24 Melville Road, Edgbaston, Birmingham B16 9JT Tel: 0121 454 1725 — MB BS Osmania 1960 (Osmania Med. Coll. Hyderabad) DMRD Madras 1965; FRIPHH 1988; FRCGP 1997, M 1990; FRSH 1997; MFPHM (RCP) 1998. Mem. Local Med. Comm. & Dist. Med. Comm.; Nat. Pres. Brit. Minority Ethnic Health Professional Assn. (BMEHPA). Prev: Hosp. Pract. (Psychiat.) All St.s Hosp. Birm.

VENUS, Matthew Robert 43A Settles Street, London E1 1JN — MB BS Lond. 1997.

VERBER, Ian Graham North Tees General Hospital, Stockton-on-Tees TS19 8PE Tel: 01642 617617 Fax: 01642 624940; Old School House, Bentley Wynd, Yarm TS15 9BS Tel: 01642 788992 — MB BCh Wales 1974; DCH Eng. 1977; MRCP (UK) 1980; FRCP Lond. 1995; FRCPCH 1997. Cons. Paediat. N. Tees Health Trust; Clin. Lect. Univ. Newc. Specialty: Paediat.; Neonat. Socs: BMA; Brit. Assn. Perinatal Med.; N. Eng. Paediatric Soc. (Sec.). Prev: Lect. (Child Health) St. Geo. Hosp. Med. Sch. Lond.; Research Fell. Roy. Manch. Childr. Hosp.; Ho. Off. Hosp. Sick Childr. Lond.

VERBORG, Stefan Andreas Department of Postgraduate Medicine, Thornburrow Drive, Stoke-on-Trent ST4 7QB; 87 Aberporth Road, Llandaff, Cardiff CF14 2PQ — State Exam Med Dusseldorf 1986; FRCPS Glas. 1993.

VERBOV, Professor Julian Lionel 31 Rodney Street, Liverpool L1 9EH Tel: 0151 703 2900 Fax: 0151 703 2930 Email: verbov@blueyonder.co.uk; 38 Montclair Drive, Liverpool L18 0HB Tel: 0151 722 0074 — (Liverp.) MB ChB Liverp. 1959; MRCS Eng. LRCP Lond. 1959; FRCP Lond. 1978, M 1965; MD Liverp. 1971; FIBiol 1985, M 1979, C 1979; FRCPCH 1991; FLS 2001. p/t Hon. Prof. Dermat. Univ. Liverp.; JP; Cons. Paediat. (Dermat.) Roy. Liverp. Childr. Hosp. NHS Trust Alder Hey; Cons. Fingerprint Soc. Specialty: Dermat. Special Interest: Comparative Med.; Dermatoglyphics; Genodermatoses. Socs: Fell. Roy. Soc. Med.; Fell. Zoolog. Soc. Lond.; Past-Exec. Mem. Brit. Assn. Dermat. Prev: Edr. Brit. Jl. Dermat.; Cons. Dermat. I. of Man; Sen. Regist. (Dermat.) St. Bart. Hosp. Lond.

VERCOE, Michael George Skinner (retired) 20 Allington Mead, Exeter EX4 5AP Tel: 01392 256479 — MB BS Lond. 1950 (St. Bart.) MRCS Eng. LRCP Lond. 1950; DObst RCOG 1954.

VERCOE, Stephen Ide Lane Surgery, Ide Lane, Alphinton, Exeter EX2 8UP Tel: 01392 439868 Fax: 01392 493513; Hillpark, Christow, Exeter EX6 7NP — MB BS Lond. 1983 (Camb. & Univ. Coll. Hosp.) MA Camb. 1984; DRCOG 1986; Cert. Family Plann. JCC 1986; MRCGP 1987. Socs: BMA. Prev: Trainee GP Exeter VTS; Ho. Phys. Whittington Hosp. Lond.; Ho. Surg. Northampton Gen. Hosp.

VERCOE-ROGERS, John Patrick 9 Brookvale, Broughshane, Ballymena BT43 7JQ — MB BCh BAO NUI 1991.

VERDI, Kumud Gibson Lane Practice, Kippax, Leeds LS25 7JN — MB BS Newc. 1991; DCH RCP 1997; DRCOG 1998; MRCGP 1998. Specialty: Gen. Pract. Prev: GP Regist. Northumbria VTS; SHO (Med.) Sunderland HA.

VERDIN, Stuart Michael Edge Grove School, Aldenham, Radlett — MB BS Lond. 1991; DA (UK) 1995. Clin. Research Fell. Roy. Free Hosp. Specialty: Obst. & Gyn.

VERDON, Jonathon Hendley Cranleigh Health Centre, 18 High Street, Cranleigh GU6 8AE Tel: 01483 273951 Fax: 01483 275755 — MB BS Lond. 1974; MRCS Eng. LRCP Lond. 1974; DRCOG 1978. Prev: GP Trainee Brighton VTS; SHO (Anaesth.) Hammersmith Hosp.; Ho. Surg. Roy. Free Hosp. Lond.

VERE, Duncan Wright (retired) 14 Broadfield Way, Buckhurst Hill IG9 5AG — (Lond. Hosp.) MB BS (Hons.) Lond. 1952; FRCP Lond. 1968, M 1954; MD Lond. 1964; Hon FFPM RCP (UK) 1994. Prev: Emerit. Prof. of Therap. Lond. Univ.

VERE-HODGE, Mr Nicholas (retired) Watersmead, Donhead Saint Mary, Shaftesbury SP7 9DP Tel: 01747 728 — MB BChir Camb. 1938 (St. Geo. & Camb.) MRCS Eng. LRCP Lond. 1938; FRCS Eng. 1940. Prev: Hon. Cons. Orthop. Surg. E. Dorset Health Dist.

VEREL, Agnes Cobden Miller (retired) 7 Warren Rise, Coal Aston, Dronfield S18 2EB — MB ChB Aberd. 1947. Prev: Co. Med. Off. Union Carbide UK Ltd., Carbon Products Div. Sheff.

VEREL, David (retired) 1 Mussons Close, Corby Glen, Grantham NG33 4NY Tel: 01476 550083 — (Camb & Lond. Hosp.) MB BChir Camb. 1943; FRCP Lond. 1967, M 1945; MD Camb. 1948. Prev: Regional Cardiol. Trent.

VERGANI, Professor Diego Institute of Liver Studies, King's College Hospital, Denmark Hill, London SE5 9RS Tel: 020 7346 3303 Ext: 3695 Fax: 020 7346 3700 Email: diego.vergani@kcl.ac.uk; 14 Crab Hill, Beckenham BR3 5HE Tel: 020 8658 6003 Fax: 020 8658 6211 Email: diego@vergani.demon.co.uk — MD Milan 1971; FRCP Lond.; FRCPath Lond.; State Exam Milan 1972; Dip. Internal Med. Milan 1976; Dip. Clin. Immunol. Milan 1979; PhD Lond. 1990. Prof. of Liver Immunopathology, Guy's, Kings and St. Thomas Sch. of Med., Lond.; Hon. Cons. Physicians, Kings Coll. Hosp., Lond. Socs: Fell. Roy. Coll. Path.; Amer. Assn. for the study of liver diseases; Europ. Assn. for the study of the liver. Prev: Prof. & Hon. Cons. (Immunol.) King's Coll. Sch. Med. & Dent. Lond.; Cons. Immunol., Camberwell HA.

VERGANO, James Bruno (retired) 3 Beltane Drive, Wimbledon, London SW19 5JR Tel: 020 8946 3189 — MB BChir Camb. 1952 (Guy's & Camb.) BA (Nat. Sc. Trip.) Camb. 1948, MA 1951; LMSSA Lond. 1951; FRCGP 1979, M 1962. Prev: GP Kensington Lond.

VERGHESE, Anthony Richard Sundon Medical Centre, 142-144 Sundon Park Road, Sundon Park, Luton LU3 3AH Tel: 01582 571130 Fax: 01582 564452 — MB ChB Leeds 1978; DRCOG 1985; MRCGP 1987.

VERGHESE, Chandy Intensive Care Unit, Royal Berkshire Hospital, Reading RG1 5AN Tel: 01734 875111; 6 The Mount, Reading RG1 5HL Tel: 01734 310234 — MB BS Madras 1974; DA (UK) 1978; FFA RCS Eng. 1982. Cons. Anaesth. (Intens. Care) Roy. Berks. Hosp. & Battle Hosp. Reading. Specialty: Anaesth. Socs: Intens. Care Soc.; Assn. Anaesth.; Founder Mem. Soc. Airway Managem. Prev: Sen. Lect. & Hon. Cons. Lond. Hosp. Med. Coll. & Newham HA; Lect. & Hon. Sen. Regist. (Anaesth.) The Lond. Hosp. Whitechapel; Lect. & Hon. Sen. Regist. Whipps Cross Hosp. Lond.

VERGHESE, Gigi Sara Carnarvon Road Surgery, 7 Carnarvon Road, Southend-on-Sea SS2 6LR Tel: 01702 466340 Fax: 01702 603179 — MB BS Kerala 1977; MB BS Univ. Kerala 1977; MD Dermat. Calicut 1981; DTM & H 1986.

VERGHESE, Rachel 27 Mill Road, Cambridge CB1 2AB — MB BS Kerala 1981; MRCOU UK 1993. Specialty: Obst. & Gyn.

VERGNAUD, Stephanie 15 Buchanan Gardens, London NW10 5AD — MD Paris 1988; MRCPsych 1994.

VERHEUL, Meindert Roger Kings Family Practice, 30-34 Magpie Hall Road, Chatham ME4 5JY — MB BS Lond. 1984; DRCOG 1988; DCH RCP Lond. 1989. GP Chatham Kent.

VERIKIOU, Katherine 18 Canterbury House, Royal St., London SE1 7LN — Ptychio Iatrikes Athens 1988.

VERINDER, Mr David George Reginald West Cumberland Hospital, Hensingham, Whitehaven CA28 8JG Tel: 01946 693181 Fax: 01946 523532; Sanderson House, Summerhill, Sandwith, Whitehaven CA28 9UP Tel: 01946 690429 — (Sheff.) MRCS Eng. LRCP Lond. 1968; MB ChB Sheff. 1968; FRCS Eng. 1973. Cons. Orthop. Surg. W. Cumbria Health Care NHS Trust W. Cumbld. Hosp. Whitehaven. Specialty: Orthop. Prev: Cons. Orthop. Surg. Bassetlaw HA; Cons. Orthop. Surg. Worksop & Retford Health Dists.; Sen. Regist. Rotat. (Orthop.) Sheff. AHA (T).

VERITY, Christopher Michael The Child Development Centre, Addenbrooke's Hospital, Box 107, Hills Road, Cambridge CB2 2QQ Tel: 01223 216662 Fax: 01223 242171; The White Cottage, 67 High St, Grantchester, Cambridge CB3 9NF Tel: 01223 840227 — (St. Thos.) BM BCh Oxf. 1970; MA Oxf. 1972; MRCP (UK) 1974; DCH RCP Lond. 1978; FRCP Lond. 1990; FRCPCH 1997. Cons. Paediat. Neurol. Addenbrooke's Hosp. Camb.; Assoc. Lect. Med. Sch. Univ. Camb. Specialty: Paediat. Neurol. Socs: Brit. Paediat. Neurol. Assn.; Assn. Brit. Neurol.; Internat. League Against Epilepsy, Brit. Br. Prev: Lect. (Child Health) Bristol Roy. Hosp. Sick Childr.; Fell. (Paediat. Neurol.) Univ. Brit. Columbia, Vancouver Canada; Ho. Phys. Hosp. Sick Childr. Gt. Ormond St. Lond.

VERITY, David Harding Moorfields Eye Hosptial, London EC1V 2PD; 10 Sandhills, Walton St, Walton on the Hill, Tadworth KT20 7PJ — BM BCh Oxf. 1991; BA (Hons.) Physiol. Oxf. 1989; FRCOpth 1996; MA Oxf. 2000. Fell.(Ophth.) Moorfields Eye Hosp. Lond. Specialty: Ophth. Socs: Christ. Med. Fellowsh.; Soc. Apoth.; ARVO. Prev: SHO (Ophth.) St. John Ophth. Hosp. Jerusalem; SHO (Ophth.) Salisbury Dist. Hosp.; SHO (Neurosurg.) Soton.

VERITY, Donald Wrathall, TD (retired) Blea Busk, Nr. Askrigg, Leyburn DL8 3JD Tel: 01969 650742 — MRCS Eng. LRCP Lond. 1950 (Oxf. & St. Geo.)

VERITY, Henry John, TD Heathcote Medical Centre, Heathcote, Tadworth KT20 5TH Tel: 01737 360202 Fax: 01737 370119; 10 Duffield Road, Walton-on-The-Hill, Tadworth KT20 7UQ Tel: 01737 814242 Fax: 01737 279555 Email: hjverity@doctors.org.uk — (Trinity Coll. Camb. & St. Thos.) LMSSA Lond. 1964; MB BChir Camb. 1965. Prev: Surg. Lt. RN; Supt. St. Michaels Miss. Hosp. Kuruman, S. Afr.; Sen. Med. Off. Fogo Cott. Hosp. Newfld.

VERITY, Jennifer Catherine Terry The Castle Practice, Health Centre, Central Street, Ludgershall, Andover SP11 9RA Tel: 01264 790356 Fax: 01264 791256; Fleetwood, Cow Lane, Kimpton, Andover SP11 8NY — MB BS Lond. 1971 (St. Bart.) MRCS Eng. LRCP Lond. 1971; DObst RCOG 1974; Cert. FPA 1975; MFFP 1994. GP Ludgershall; Clin. Asst. i n Psychiat. at Andover CMHT. Prev: Ho. Off. (Obst.) St. Bart. Hosp. Lond.; Ho. Surg. N. Middlx. Hosp. Lond.; Ho. Phys. St. Leonard's Hosp. Lond.

VERITY, Lisa Jane 39 Midge Hall Drive, Rochdale OL11 4AX — MB ChB Leic. 1993.

VERITY, Richard Henry Edenfield Road Surgery, Cutgate Shopping Precinct, Edenfield Road, Rochdale OL11 5AQ Tel: 01706 344044 Fax: 01706 526882; 39 Midge Hall Drive, Bamford, Rochdale OL11 4AX Tel: 01706 31942 — MB BS Lond. 1969 (Roy. Free) DObst RCOG 1971.

VERITY, Robert Gavin 137 Sheffield Road, Woodhouse, Sheffield S13 7ER — MB ChB Sheff. 1998.

VERITY, Tara 33 Manor Road, Caddington, Luton LU1 4EE — MB BChir Camb. 1991; DCH RCP Lond. 1993; DRCOG 1994; MRCGP 1995. Specialty: Gen. Pract. Socs: BMA; Christ. Med. Fellowsh. Prev: Trainee GP/SHO Whittington Hosp. Lond. VTS.

VERJEE, Salim Abdulmahmed Kassam Suleman Coplow, Main Road, Fyfield, Abingdon OX13 5LN Tel: 01865 390716 — MB ChB East Africa 1969 (Makerere Univ. Coll.) MRCGP 1975. Staff Grade (Blood Trans.) NBS John Radcliffe Hosp. Oxf. Specialty: Blood Transfus. Prev: Clin. Asst. (Blood Trans.) John Radcliffe Hosp. Oxf.; SHO (Paediat.) Newc. Gen. Hosp.; SHO (Med.) Ashington Hosp.

VERMA, Ajit Kumar The Childrens Centre, Lowestoft Road, Gorleston, Great Yarmouth NR31 6SQ; 12 Wyngates, Blofield, Norwich NR13 4JG Tel: 01603 716509 — MB BS Patna 1974; DCH RCPS Glas. 1981; MRCPI 1983; FRCPCH (UK) 1997; FRCP (L) 1999. Cons. Paediat. (Community Paediat.) Childr. Centre Gt. Yarmouth. Specialty: Paediat. Socs: BMA; RCP; Brit. Assn. Comm. Child Health; Roy. Coll. of Paediat. & Child Health.

VERMA, Amar Nath The Surgery, 302 Vicarage Road, King's Heath, Birmingham B14 7NH Tel: 0121 444 5959 Fax: 0121 441 4050 — MB BS Bihar 1972 (DMC Darbhanga, Bihar, India)

VERMA, Amarjit Newhall Street Surgery, 14-16 Newhall Street, Cannock WS11 1AB Tel: 01543 506511 Fax: 01543 462356 — MB BS Punjabi 1972. Socs: Cannock Med. Soc.

VERMA, Arpana 100 Moorcroft Road, Moseley, Birmingham B13 8LU — MB ChB Manch. 1995.

VERMA, Dev Kumar 119 Old Park Ave, Enfield EN2 6PP — MB BS Lond. 1997.

VERMA, Hira Lal Verma, Meir Health Centre, Saracen's Way, Meir, Stoke-on-Trent ST3 7DS Tel: 01782 319321; 4 Pine Tree Drive, Stoke-on-Trent ST11 9HF Tel: 01782 397856 — MB BS Bihar 1966.

VERMA, Mahipal Singh Hartley Road Medical Centre, 91 Hartley Road, Radford, Nottingham NG7 3AQ Tel: 0115 942 2622 Fax: 0115 924 9150; 3 Dormy Close, Bramcote, Nottingham NG9 3DE Tel: 0115 925 7007 Fax: 0115 925 7007 — MB BS Lucknow 1967 (G.S.V.M. Med. Coll. Kanpur) Dip. Orthop. Lucknow 1968; MS (Orthop.) Kanpur 1970; DObst RCOG 1974. Clin. Asst. (Rheum.) Univ. Hosp. Nottm. Specialty: Rehabil. Med.; Rheumatol. Socs: Overseas Doctors Assn. Prev: Med. Off. Dept. of Sch. Health; Demonst. (Orthop.) Med. Coll. Meerut, India; Resid. SHO (Orthop. & Cas.) Qu. Eliz. Hosp. Gateshead.

VERMA, Narinder Kumar c/o Little Plumstead Hospital, Hospital Road, Little Plumstead, Norwich NR13 5EW; 6 Blofield Road, Brundall, Norwich NR13 5NN — MB BS Punjab 1974 (Govt. Med. Coll. Patiala) DPM Lond. 1979; MRCPsych 1982; T(Psych) 1991. Cons. Psychiat. Little Plumstead Hosp. Norwich. Specialty: Gen. Psychiat.

VERMA, Neelam The Crown Wood Medical Centre, 4A Crown Row, Bracknell RG12 0TH Tel: 01344 310310 Fax: 01344 310300; Poney's Close Surgery, Broad Lane, Bracknell RG12 9BY Tel: 01344 424070 — MB BS Jammu & Kashmir 1967 (Med. Coll. Srinagar) Socs: Windsor & Dist. Med. Soc.

VERMA, Raj Kumar Victoria Hospital, Whinney Heys Road, Blackpool FY3 8NR — MB BS Magdhu Univ. 1986; MRCP (UK); DCH; MRCPCH (UK); MD (Paediat.). Cons. Paediat. Specialty: Paediat. Special Interest: Neurodisability.

VERMA, Raman Kumar 4 Pinetree Drive, Blythe Bridge, Stoke-on-Trent ST11 9HF — MB BS Lond. 1993 (St. Geo. Hosp. Med. Sch.) SHO (Intens. Care) Addenbrooke's Hosp. Camb. Specialty: Anaesth. Socs: Train. Mem. Assn. Anaesth. Prev: SHO Rotat. (Anaesth.) Northwick Pk., St. Mark's Hosps. Middlx. & Mt. Vernon Hosp. N.wood, Middlx.; Ho. Off. (Surg.) Walsgrave NHS Trust; Ho. Off. (Med.) N. Staffs. NHS Trust.

VERMA, Ranjeet Gorleston Medical Centre, Stuart Close, Gorleston-on-Sea, Great Yarmouth NR31 7BU Tel: 01493 650490 — MB BS Patna 1979; MB BS Patna 1979.

VERMA, Ranjit Derby City General Hospital, Uttoxeter Road, Derby DE22 3NE Tel: 01332 625549 Fax: 01332 625583; Oak Lodge, 43 Farley Road, Derby DE23 6BW Tel: 01332 603585 Fax: 01332 295128 — MB ChB Manch. 1975; DA Eng. 1978; FRCA Eng. 1980. Cons. Anaesth. Southern Derbysh. Acute NHS Trust. Specialty: Anaesth. Socs: Derby Med. Soc.; Assn. Anaesth.; Obst. Anaesth. Assn. (ex. Comm. Mem. & Treas.). Prev: Sen. Regist. (Anaesth.) Nottm. HA; Regist. & SHO (Anaesth.) Liverp. HA.

VERMA, Ratan Kumar 4 Pine Tree Drive, Blythe Bridge, Stoke-on-Trent ST11 9HF — MB BS Lond. 1991; BSc (Hons.) Physiol. Lond. 1988; MRCP (UK) 1995. Regist. (Radiol.) Leicester Roy. Infirm. Specialty: Radiol. Prev: Regist. (Med.) Neath Gen. Hosp.; SHO (Med.) Univ. Hosp. Wales, Cardiff Roy. Infirm. & Llandough Hosps. Cardiff; Ho. Surg. Westm. Hosp.

VERMA, Rinku 6 Blofield Road, Brundall, Norwich NR13 5NN — MB BS Lond. 1998.

VERMA, Santosh Kumar The Surgery, 192 Charles Road, Small Heath, Birmingham B10 9AB Tel: 0121 772 0398 Fax: 0121 772 4268 — MB BS Ranchi 1973; MB BS Ranchi 1973.

VERMA, Mrs Savitri (retired) 7 Charlotte Grove, Beeston, Nottingham NG9 3HU — MB BS Punjab 1942 (Lady Hardinge Med. Coll. New Delhi)

VERMA, Sonia Sujata Samantha 18 Lyndhurst Court, Albert Rd, Stoneygate, Leicester — MB ChB Bristol 1997.

VERMA, Sonu Geetanjali 34 Green Street, Fallowfield, Manchester M14 6TJ — MB ChB Manch. 1996.

VERMA, Sudershan Kumar Cornerways Medical Centre, 27 Woolfall Heath Avenue, Huyton, Liverpool L36 3TH Tel: 0151 489 4444 Fax: 0151 489 0528 — MB BS Punjabi Univ. 1968.

VERMA, Sunil Regional Secure Unit, St. Bernards Hospital, Uxbridge Road, Southall UB1 3EU — MB BS Ranchi 1983; MRCPsych 1994.

VERMA, Upender Kumar High Road Surgery, 136 High Road, Leytonstone, London E15 1UA — MB BS Lond. 1985 (Guy's) MRCGP. GP. Prev: Trainee GP; SHO (Psychiat.) Claybury Hosp. Woodford Bridge; SHO (Acute Med. for Elderly & A & E) Whipps Cross Hosp. Lond.

VERMAAK, Zoe Alberta Gwent Community Health, Oakfield House, Llanfrechfa Grange, Cwmbran NP44 8YN Tel: 01633 623497 Fax: 01633 623508 — MB ChB Cape Town 1971; Dip. Child Health 1978; Dip. Trop Med. & Hyg 1979; Dip. Pub Health 1980; MSc Louisianna 1994. Cons. Paediat.Gwent Community Health Wales; Postgrad. Lect. (Community Health) Cardiff Univ. Specialty: Community Child Health. Socs: Fell. Roy. Soc. Trop. Med. & Hyg.; Fell. RCP & CH; Fell. Roy. Inst. Pub. Health. Prev: Dep. Dir. Pub. Health I. of Man; Sen. Med. Off. Cape Div. Counc.; Sen. Med. Off. CMR Infec. Dis. Hosp., Johannesburg.

VERMEULEN, Jan Willem Broadmoor Hospital, Crowthorne RG45 7EG Tel: 01344 773111 Fax: 01344 773327 — MB ChB Cape Town 1968; MRCPsych 1979; DPM Eng. 1979; BA (Hons.) Univ. S. Afr. 1976, BSc (Hons.) 1985. Cons. Forens. Psychiat. Broadmoor Hosp. Crowthorne. Specialty: Forens. Psychiat. Prev: Cons. Forens. Psychiat. HM Prison Norwich; Hon. Lect. (Forens. Psychiat.) Univ. Zimbabwe; Cons. Psychiat. (Forens. Psychiat.) Min. Health, Zimbabwe.

VERNE, Julia Elvira Caroline Wanda Government Office for the South West, 2 Rivergate, Temple Quay, Bristol BS1 6ED Tel: 0117 900 3539 Email: jverne.gosw@go-regions.gsi.gov.uk — MB BS Lond. 1986; FFPHM; MSc; PhD. Director S. W. Pub. Health Observatory.

VERNEY, Geoffrey Ivan 87 Barton Road, Cambridge CB3 9LL Tel: 01223 352526 — MB BChir Camb. 1952 (Camb. & St. Bart.) MA Camb. 1959, MB BChir 1952; DMRD Eng. 1959; FFR 1963; FRCR 1975. Cons. (Diag. Radiol.) Addenbrooke's Hosp. Camb. & Papworth Hosp. Socs: BMA & Roy. Soc. Med. Prev: Maj. RAMC (TAVR) Cons. Radiol.; Squadron Ldr. RAF Med. Br.; Sen. Regist. (Diag. Radiol.) Roy. Vict. Infirm. Newc. upon Tyne &.

VERNHAM, Guy Anthony Department of ENT, Victoria Infirmary, Langside, Glasgow G42 9TY Tel: 0141 649 4545; 33 Queensberry Avenue, Clarkston, Glasgow G76 7DU Tel: 0141 571 8827 — BM Soton. 1981; FRCS (Otol.) Ed. 1990; Cert. Specialist Train. (Otolaryngol) Europe 1994. Staff Grade (OtoLaryngol.) Vict. Infirm. Glas. Specialty: Otolaryngol.

VERNON, Anthony Richard Wallingford Medical Practice, Reading Road, Wallingford OX10 9DU Tel: 01491 835577 Fax: 01491 824034; Mill Lodge, Reading Road, Cholsey, Wallingford OX10 9HG Tel: 01491 651355 — MB BS Lond. 1978 (St. Mary's) DRCOG 1984; MRCGP 1989.

VERNON, Clare Christine Department of Clinical Oncology, Hammersmith Hospital, Du Cane Road, London W12 0NN Tel: 020 8383 3170 Fax: 020 8383 1789; 18 Brookfield Avenue, Ealing, London W5 1LA Tel: 020 8997 1786 — MB BChir Camb. 1977; MA Camb. 1977; FRCR 1983. Cons. Radiother. & Oncol. Hammersmith Hosp. Lond.; Vis. Prof. Radiat. & Oncol. Qu. Mary Hosp. Univ. Hong Kong; Sec. Radiother. Club. Specialty: Oncol.; Radiother. Socs: (Pres.) Europ. Soc. Hyperthermic Oncol.; (Counc.) Roy. Soc. Radiol. Prev: Sen. Lect. (Hyperthermia) MRC Hammersmith Hosp. Lond.; Sen. Regist. (Radiother.) Middlx. Hosp. Lond. & Mt. Vernon Hosp. Northwood; Regist. (Radiother.) Middlx. & Roy. Free Hosps. Lond.

VERNON, David Russell Henderson Medical Directorate, Victoria Infirmary, Langside, Glasgow G42 9TY Tel: 0141 201 6000 Fax: 0141 201 5206; 73 Woodside Drive, Waterfoot, Eaglesham, Glasgow G76 0HD — (Guy's) MB BS Lond. 1967; MRCS Eng. LRCP Lond. 1967; MRCP (UK) 1972; FRCP Glas. 1987; FRCP Lond. 1998. Cons. Phys. Vict. Infirm. Glas. Specialty: Respirat. Med. Socs: Brit. Soc. Allergy & Clin. Immunol.; Brit. & Scott. Thoracic Socs.; Eur. Respirat. Soc. Prev: Sen. Regist. (Respirat. & Gen. Med.) Gtr. Glas. HB; Regist. (Med.) Glas. Roy. Infirm. & Raigmore Hosp. Inverness.

VERNON, Fiona Hyslop Health Centre, Thornhill DG3 5AA Tel: 01848 330208 Fax: 01848 330223; Cairnview, Waulkmill Park, Carronbridge, Thornhill DG3 5BA — MB ChB Glas. 1982; DRCOG 1984. GP Thornhill Dumfriessh. Prev: GP Dumfries & Galloway VTS.; GP Cumnock.

VERNON, Gordon Richard Peter Aufrere 25 Lennox Gardens, Knightsbridge, London SW1X 0DE Tel: 020 7589 3103 — MRCS Eng. LRCP Lond. 1952 (St. Mary's) Surg. Lt. RNVR. Mem. BMA. Prev: Ho. Surg. Epsom Dist. Hosp.; Res. Med. Off. Stafford Gen. Infirm.

VERNON, Jane Evelyn The Old Court House Surgery, Throwley Way, Sutton SM1 4A Tel: 020 8643 8866 — MB BS Lond. 1979 (Univ. Coll. Hosp.) DRCOG 1981.

VERNON, Jane Melanie 24 Woodside Road, Downend, Bristol BS16 2SL Tel: 0117 956 5510 — BM Soton. 1985 (Southampton) DRCOG 1989; MRCGP 1990; FRCA 1995. Cons. Anaesth. Nottm. City Hosp. Specialty: Anaesth. Prev: Specialist Regist. (Anaesth.) Nottm.; Trainee GP Torbay Hosp. VTS; SHO (Anaesth.) Roy. Devon & Exeter Hosp.

VERNON, Jennifer Alexandra 5 Alfred Salter House, Longfield Estate, Fort Road, London SE1 5PS Tel: 020 7231 7801 — MB BChir Camb. 1978 (St. Geo.) MA, MB Camb. 1978, BChir 1977.

VERNON, John David Sidney (retired) Crugmawr Cottage, Pemparc, Cardigan SA43 1RE Tel: 01239 613649 — (St. Bart.) BA Camb. 1950; MB BChir Camb. 1954. Prev: Assoc. Specialist Spinal Unit Stoke Mandeville Hosp. Aylesbury.

VERNON, John Gervase John Tasker House Surgery, 56 New Street, Great Dunmow, Dunmow CM6 1BH Tel: 01371 872121 Fax: 01371 873793; Martingales, Causeway End Road, Felsted, Dunmow CM6 3LU Tel: 01371 820481 — MB BS Lond. 1977 (Univ. Coll. Hosp.) MA Camb. 1975; MB BS Lond. Lond. 1977; DRCOG 1979; DCH RCP Lond. 1979; MRCP (UK) (Paediat.) 1984; FRCGP 1995, M 1985; MSc (GP) 2001. Specialty: Gen. Pract. Prev: Clin. Asst. (Diabetes) Herts & Essex Hosp. Bishop's Stortford.

VERNON, John Parry Hawkhill Medical Centre, Hawkhill, Dundee DD1 5LA Tel: 01382 669589 Fax: 01382 645526; 31 The Logan, Liff, Dundee DD2 5PJ Tel: 01382 580176 — MB ChB Dundee 1977; MRCGP 1982.

VERNON, John Paxton (retired) Tinshill Lane Surgery, 8 Tinshill Lane, Leeds LS16 7AP Tel: 0113 267 3462 Fax: 0113 230 0402; 2 Adel park Court, Leeds LS16 8HS — MB ChB Leeds 1964.

VERNON, Kevin Grant Flat 3, 76 Castle Road, Southsea PO5 3AZ Tel: 023 9287 1812 — BM Soton. 1994. SHO (A & E) Poole Gen. Hosp. Prev: SHO (O & G) & Ho. Off. (Med.) St. Mary's Hosp. Portsmouth; Ho. Off. (Surg.) Qu. Alexandra's Hosp. Portsmouth.

VERNON, Margaret Mathews Hawkhill Medical Centre, Hawkhill, Dundee DD1 5LA Tel: 01382 669589 Fax: 01382 645526; 31 The Logan, Liff, Dundee DD2 5PJ Tel: 01382 580176 — MB ChB Dundee 1978.

VERNON, Michael Seymour (retired) Chasefield, Braiswick, Colchester CO4 5BQ Tel: 01206 853318 — (Guy's) MRCS Eng. LRCP Lond. 1965; MB BS Lond. 1966; FFA RCS Eng. 1970. Prev: Cons. Anaesth. Essex Rivers Healthcare Trust, Colchester.

VERNON, Peter Heygate (retired) 66 Collington Avenue, Bexhill-on-Sea TN39 3RA Tel: 01424 216112 — (St. Thomas' Hospital London) MRCS Eng. LRCP Lond. 1945; DPH Lond. 1950; MFOM RCP Lond. 1981. Prev: Sen. Med. Off. SE Region Brit. Gas Corp.

VERNON, Peter Leslie Humphrey (retired) 21 Moorfield, St. Stephens, Canterbury CT2 7AN Tel: 01227 450192 — (Guy's) MB BS Lond. 1960; MRCS Eng. LRCP Lond. 1960; DObst RCOG 1963. Med. Mem. Tribunal Serv. Prev: Obst. Ho. Surg. & Ho. Phys. Buckland Hosp. Dover.

VERNON, Phillip Raymund Acumedic, 101-105 Camden High Street, London NW1 7JN Tel: 020 7388 6704 Fax: 020 7387 8081 — MRCS Eng. LRCP Lond. 1977 (Sheff.) Cert Prescribed Equival Exp JCPTGP 1981; Dip. Med. Acupunc. 1998; DCM Beijing 1998. Specialist in Chinese Med. (Acupunc. and Chinese Herbal Med.) Lond.; Specialist in Chinese Med. Acumedic Foundat. Lond.; Asst. GP to Dr. Ko, Lond.; Specialist in Chinese Med., ChristCh. Hall Surg., Crough End, Lond. Socs: Brit. Med. Acupunct. Soc.; Chinese Med. Inst. and Register (Lond.). Prev: Indep. Acupunc. Liverp.; GP Gold Coast Queensland, Austral.; Specialist in Acupunc. Dept. Neurol. Walton Hosp. Liverp.

VERNON, Stephen Andrew University Hospital NHS Trust, University Hospital, Nottingham NG7 2UH Tel: 0115 924 9924 Ext: 44645 — MB ChB Bristol 1978; DO Eng. 1982; FRCS Eng. 1982; FRCOphth 1988; DM Nottm. 1994. Cons. Ophth. Univ. Hosp. Nottm.; Cons. Ophth., The Pk. Hosp., Sherwood Lodge Drive, Nottm. Specialty: Ophth. Socs: Eur. Glaucoma Soc.; Midl. Ophth. Soc. (Pres. 2000 -2001); UK & Eire Glaucoma Soc. (Counc. Mem.). Prev: Sen. Regist. Oxf. Eye Hosp.; Regist. Bristol Eye Hosp.; Ho. Phys. Profess. Med. Unit Bristol Roy. Infirm.

VERNON-PARRY, James, RD (retired) Breck House, Carlton Forest, Worksop S81 0TR Tel: 01909 730560 — MB ChB Manch. 1951; Cert Av Med MoD (Air) & CAA; D. Orth 1948; FRCOG 1974, M 1961, DObst 1957; MMSA Lond. 1962; Aviat Auth. 1974. Sen. Cons. O & G Bassetlaw DHA; Hon. Clin. Lect. (Obst. & Gyn.) Univ. Sheff.; Examr. RCOG & Univ. Sheff.; Authorised Med. Examr. Bd. of Trade & Civil Aviat. Auth. Prev: Sen. Regist. O & G S. Belf. Hosp. Gp. & Hon. Sen. Tutor (O & G) Qu.s's Univ. Belf.

VERNON-PARRY, Kathleen Claire (retired) Breck House, Carlton Forest, Worksop S81 0TR Tel: 01909 730560 — MB ChB Manch. 1953; DA Eng. 1957. Prev: Assoc. Specialist in Anaesth. Worksop & Retford Hosp. Gp.

VERNON-ROBERTS, Mark (retired) Widegate Cottage, Widegate, Swansea SA3 2AB Tel: 01792 232126 — MB BS Lond. 1968 (Char. Cross) DObst RCOG 1970.

VERNON-SMITH, Jillian Wendy Seven Posts Surgery, Prestbury Road, Prestbury, Cheltenham GL52 3DD Tel: 01242 244103 — MB BS Lond. 1990 (GUYS Hosp.) Specialty: Gen. Pract.

VEROW, Peter Graham Occupational Health Unit, 30 Hallam Close, Hallam St., West Bromwich B71 4HU Tel: 0121 607 3417 Fax: 0121 607 3420; 54 Sandhills Lane, Barnt Green, Birmingham B45 8NX Tel: 0121 445 1181 Email: petelsport@aol.co — MB BS Lond. 1977 (St. Mary's) MRCS Eng. LRCP Lond. 1976; DA Eng. 1980; Cert. Family Plann. JCC 1981; Dip. Sports Med. Lond 1983; MFOM RCP Lond. 1990, AFOM 1987; FFOM 1997. Cons. Occupat. Health Phys. Sandwell HA; Hon. Sen. Lect. Birm. Univ. Specialty: Occupat. Health. Socs: Soc. Occupat. Med.; (Chairm.) Assn. NHS Occupat. Phys. Prev: Occupat. Phys. Rover Gp. Ltd. Birm.

VEROW, Peter William (retired) The Old Rectory, Bugthorpe, York YO41 1QG Tel: 01759 368444 Email: peter_verow@hotmail.com — MB BCh Wales 1966 (Cardiff) DMRD Eng. 1971; Lic. Roy. Inst. Chem. 1971; FRCR 1974. Prev: Cons. Radiol. Dist. Gen. Hosp. York.

VERRICO, Joseph Anthony Alexander (retired) 26 Glenville Avenue, Giffnock, Glasgow G46 7AH — MB ChB Glas. 1944.

VERRIER JONES, Edward Roger (retired) Greenfields, Newport Road, St Mellons, Cardiff CF3 5TW Tel: 029 2036 1941 — MB Camb. 1962 (Camb. & Univ. Coll. Hosp.) MA Camb. 1967, BA 1958, MB 1962, BChir 1961; DCH Eng. 1965; FRCP Ed. 1978, M 1967; FRCP Lond. 1979, M 1968; Hon. FRCPCH 2001. Prev: Cons. Paediatr. Llandough Hosp. NHS Trust.

VERRIER JONES, Kate KRUF Children's Kidney Centre for Wales, University Hospital of Wales, Heath Park, Cardiff CF14 4XN Tel: 029 2074 4919 Fax: 029 2074 4822 Email: verrier-jones@cf.ac.uk — MB BCh Wales 1969 (Welsh National School Of Medicine) MRCP (UK) 1972; FRCP Lond. 1987; FRCPCH 1997. Laura Ashley Reader, Paediat. Nephrol. Dept. of Child Health Univ. of Wales Coll. of Med. Specialty: Paediat. Socs: Brit. Assn. Paediat. Nephrol. & Europ. Soc. Paediat.; Nephrol. Sec. Gen.; Internat. Paediatric Nephol. Assn., Ass. Sec. 1997-2000. Prev: Cons. Paediat. Nephrol. Cardiff Roy. Infirm; Sen. Regist. (Paediat. Nephrol.) Cardiff Roy. Infirm.; Regist. Hammersmith Hosp. Lond. & Soton. Gen. Hosp.

VERRILL, Peter John Alde Reach, Saxmundham Rd, Aldeburgh IP15 5PD Tel: 01728 454177 — MB BS Lond. 1953 (Univ. Coll. Hosp.) DA Eng. 1957; FFA RCS Eng. 1959. Emerit. Cons. UCL Hosps. Specialty: Anaesth. Socs: Fell. Univ. Coll. Lond. Prev: Cons. Anaesth. Univ. Coll. Hosp.; Fell. Anesthesiol. Mayo Clinic Rochester, USA; Dean Fac. Clin. Scis. Univ. Coll. Lond.

VERRILL, Richard Peter Framfield House Surgery, 42 St. Johns Street, Woodbridge IP12 1ED Tel: 01394 382157; Little Red House, Hasketon, Woodbridge IP13 6JA — MB BS Lond. 1981; DRCOG 1986; MRCGP 1986.

VERRINDER, Christian John Langworthy Kate's Cottage, 128 Botley Road, Chesham HP5 1XN — BM BS Nottm. 1996.

VERSO, Nancy Elizabeth 19 Brindley Quays, Braunston, Daventry NN11 7AN — MB ChB Liverp. 1998.

VERSTRATEN, Leendert Department of Orthopaedic Surgery, Mayday University Hospital, London Road, Croydon CR7 7YE Tel: 020 8684 6999 — Artsexamen Rotterdam 1988. SHO (Orthop.) Mayday Univ. Hosp. Thornton Heath. Specialty: Orthop. Prev: SHO (Gen. Surg.) Soton. Gen. Hosp.; SHO (Orthop. Surg.) Lord Mayor Treloar Hosp. Alton; SHO (A & E) Soton. Gen. Hosp.

VERSTREKEN, Patrick 15 Morcroft Road, Huyton, Liverpool L36 8BG — MD Ghent 1991.

VESELY, Mr Martin Jacob John 103 Lincoln Park, Amersham HP7 9HF — BM BCh Oxf. 1991; MA Camb. 1992; FRCS Eng. 1995. Specialty: Plastic Surg.

VESEY, Jennifer Springfield Surgery, Park Road, Bingley BD16 4LR Tel: 01274 567991 Fax: 01274 566865; 5 Pennygate, Spring Lane, Eldwick, Bingley BD16 3BN — MB ChB Birm. 1972; DObst RCOG 1974; MRCP (UK) 1975. GP Princip. Prev: Regist. (Paediat.) Auckland Hosp. Bd. N.Z.; SHO (Neonat. Paediat.) John Radcliffe Hosp. Oxf.

VESEY, Richard John Springfield Surgery, Park Road, Bingley BD16 4LR Tel: 01274 567991 Fax: 01274 566865 — MB ChB Birm. 1972; MRCGP 1979. G.P Princip.; Trainer Airedale Vocational Train. Scheme. Prev: Anaesth. Regist. Auckland Hosp. Bd. New Zealand; Res. Med. Off. Warwick Gen. Hosp.

VESEY, Mr Sean Gerard Tara Hall, 54 Westbourne Road, Birkdale, Southport PR8 2JB — MB BCh BAO NUI 1979; FRCSI 1983; FEBU 1992; FRCS (Eng.) 2001. Cons. Urol. Southport & Ormskirk Hosps. Specialty: Urol. Socs: Fell. Roy. Soc. Med.

VESSELINOVA-JENKINS, Chrisso Kolevo 118 Harley Street, London W1N 1AG Tel: 020 7935 5635 Fax: 020 7487 5595; 24 Albany Road, Blackwood NP12 1DZ Tel: 01495 224725 Fax: 01495 228330 — State Exam. Med. Pavlov Higher Inst. Med. Plovdiv 1956. Med. Dir. Nikolai Sleep Monitoring Clinic St Luke's Hosp. Lond. Specialty: Immunol. Socs: Fell. Roy. Soc. Med. Prev: Asst. Prof. Dept. Epidemiol. Med. Acad. Sofia, Bulgaria; Clin. Asst. P.H.L.S. Cardiff; Mem. Roy. Coll. Pediat. Child Health.

VESSEY, Professor Martin Paterson, CBE University of Oxford, Unit of Health Care Epidemiology, Old Road Campus, Headington, Oxford OX3 7LF Tel: 01865 227030 Fax: 01865 226993 Email: martin.vessey@dphpc.ox.ac.uk; Clifden Cottage, Burford Road, Fulbrook, Burford OX18 4BL Tel: 01993 824985 — MB BS Lond. 1959 (Univ. Coll. Hosp.) MB BS (Hons. Applied Pharmacol. & Therap.) Lond. 1959; MD Lond. 1971; FFPH 1974; MA Oxf. 1974; FRCP Ed. 1979, M 1978; FRCGP 1983; FRCP Lond. 1987; FRCOG 1989; FRS 1991; FFFP 1994. p/t Emerit. Prof. Pub. Health Univ. Oxf.; Fell. St. Cross Coll. Oxf. Specialty: Pub. Health Med.; Epidemiol.; Family Plann. & Reproduc. Health. Socs: BMA; British Breast Group; Soc. for Social Med. Prev: Lect. Dept. Regius Prof. Med. Radcliffe Infirm. Oxf.; Mem. Scientif. Staff, MRC Statistical Research Unit; Ho. Off. Barnet Gen. Hosp.

VESSEY, William Clifford Remillo, Orford Road, Binbrook, Market Rasen LN8 6DU — MB ChB Ed. 1998.

VESTEY, James Patrick Department of Dermatology, Raigmore Hospital, Perth Road, Inverness IV2 3UJ Tel: 01463 704000 — BM Soton. 1978; MRCP (UK) 1982; DM Soton. 1990; T(M) 1991; FRCP Ed. 1996. Cons. Dermat. Raigmore Hosp. Specialty: Dermat. Prev: Cons. Dermat. Roy. Hull Hosps.; Lect. (Dermat.) Roy. Infirm. Edin.

VESTEY, Miss Sarah Brunhilde Longcourt Cottage, Randwick, Stroud GL6 6HJ Tel: 01453 757770 — MB BS Lond. 1990 (UCL) FRCS. Breast ell. Regis. Chelterham Gen. Hosp. Specialty: Gen. Surg. Socs: FRCS.

VETHANAYAGAM, Seemampillai Gatwick Park Hospital, Povey Cross Road, Horley RH6 0BB — MB BS Ceylon 1971; FRCOG; MSOG (Sri Lanka); T(OG) 1994.

VETHANAYAGAM, Stephen Vetharatnam St Annes Centre, 729 The Ridge, St Leonards-on-Sea TN37 7PT Tel: 01424 754889 Fax: 01424 754130 — MB BS Colombo 1974. Assoc. Specialist (Psychogeriat.) E. Sussex County Healthcare NHS Trust. Specialty: Geriat. Psychiat.; Gen. Psychiat.; Care of the Elderly. Socs: Fell. RSM; Internat. PsychoGeriat. Assoc. Prev: Staff Grade Psychiat. (Psychogeriat.) Hastings & Rother NHS Trust.; Regist. (Forens. Psychiat.) Hellingly Hosp. Hailsham.

VETPILLAI, Mr Muruguppillai 52 North Way, London NW9 0RB — MB BS Ceylon 1970; FRCS Ed. 1978; FRCS Eng. 1980. Staff Grade Surg. (A & E) Watford Gen. Hosp. Specialty: Accid. & Emerg. Prev: Sen. Lect. (Surg.) Univ. Jaffna, Sri Lanka.

VETPILLAI, Soranambigai 52 North Way, London NW9 0RB — MB BS Ceylon 1970; DPath Eng. 1980. Staff Grade (Haemat.) N. Lond. Blood Transfus. Serv. Edgware. Specialty: Blood Transfus. Prev: Lect. (Microbiol.) Univ. Jaffna, Sri Lanka.

VETTER, Norman John Donan Dêg, 31 Heol Isaf, Radyr, Cardiff CF15 8AG — MB ChB Ed. 1967; Dip. Community. Med. Ed. 1975; MD Ed. 1976; MFCM 1977. Sen. Lect. (Pub. Health Med.) Dept. Epidemiol. & Community Med. Univ. Wales. Socs: Brit. Geriat. Soc. & Cardiff Med. Soc. Prev: Dir. Research Team for c/o Elderly Welsh Nat. Sch. Med. Cardiff; Fell. (Community Med.) Edin. Univ.; Research Fell. Lipids in Cardiol. & Mobile Intens. Care.

VETTIANKAL, Giby George 4 School Road, Newry BT34 5QA — MB BCh BAO Belf. 1994.

VETTRAINO, Mark Damian 51 Brendan Road, Nottingham NG8 1HX — MB ChB Ed. 1990.

VETTUKATTIL, Joseph John Southampton University Hospitals NHS Trust, Tremona Road, Southampton SO16 6YD Tel: 02380 796944 Email: joseph.vettukattil@suht.swest.nhs.uk; 3 Hookwater Road, Chandlers Ford, Eastleigh SO53 5PQ — DNB; MD; MRCPCH; CCST; MB BS Bangalore 1988. Specialty: Paediat.; Cardiol.

VEVERS, Geoffrey William Gwynne Thatcham Medical Practice, Bath Road, Thatcham RG18 3HD Tel: 01635 867171 Fax: 01635 876395 Email: geoffrey.vevers@gp-k81073.nhs.uk — MB BS Lond. 1977 (Guy's) MRCS Eng. LRCP Lond. 1976; DOCC MED 1999. Socs: Roy. Soc. of Med. Prev: SHO (Neurol. & Dermat.) Guy's Hosp. Lond.

VEVERS, Jeremy Jock Moatfield Surgery, St Michael's Road, East Grinstead RH19 3GW Tel: 01342 327555 Fax: 01342 316240; The Hollies, East Hill Lane, Copthorne, Crawley RH10 3JA Tel: 01342 716238 — MB BS Lond. 1974 (St. Bart.) DRCOG 1977; DCH Eng. 1978; DA Eng. 1979. Specialty: Psychother.

VEYS, Charles Arthur, OBE (retired) 11 Pearce's Orchard, Henley-on-Thames RG9 2LF Tel: 01491 579557 — (Liverp.) MFOH (Ret); MB ChB Liverp. 1956; DPH 1962; DIH Soc. Apoth. Lond. 1963; Cert. Occupat. Hyg. 1969; MD Liverp. 1973; FFOM RCP Lond. 1979. Prev: Hon Sen. Research Fell. Sch. Postgrad. Med. Univ. Keele, Staffs.

VEYS, Paul Anthony Great Ormond Street, Hospital for Children NHS Trust, London WC1N 3JH Tel: 020 7813 8335 Fax: 020 7829 8640; 13 Eyot Gardens, London W6 9TN Tel: 020 8748 6729 — MB BS Lond. 1983 (St. Barts. Hosp.) MRCP (UK) 1986; MRCPath 1991. Cons. Paediat. (Bone Marrow Transpl.) Gt. Ormond St. Hosp. for Childr. NHS Trust. Specialty: Paediat.; Haematology; Immunol.

VEYSEY, Sian Louise 1 Newland Street, Rugby CV22 7BJ Tel: 01788 536616 — MB BS Lond. 1993 (St. Geos. Hosp.) Specialty: Accid. & Emerg.

VEYSI, Veysi Tuna Department of Anatomy, University of Leeds, Leeds LS1; 113 Belmont Avenue, Cockfosters, Barnet EN4 9JS Tel: 020 8449 1493 — MB ChB Leeds 1993; BSc Leeds 1992, MB ChB 1993. Demonst. (Anat.) Univ. Leeds.

VHADRA, Elizabeth Mary Tall Pines, Haytor, Newton Abbot TQ13 9XY Tel: 01364 661274 — MB BS Lond. 1994 (St. Bart. Hosp. Med. Coll. Lond.) BSc (Hons.) Anthropol. Lond. 1991; DCH 1996; DRCOG 1997; MRCGP 1998; DFFP 1999. Locum. Specialty: Gen. Pract. Prev: GP Regist. Heavitree, H. C. Exeter; SHO (Psychiat.) Wonford Hse. Hosp. Exeter; SHO (O & G) Whittington Hosp. Lond.

VHADRA, Mr Ranjan Kumar Heyburn Farm, Glossop Road, Little Hayfield, High Peak SK22 2NR Tel: 01663 749477 — MB BS Lond. 1992 (St Bartholomews) FRCS Eng 1997. Specialist Regist. in Trauma Orthop., N. W. Rotat. Specialty: Orthop. Socs: FRCS - Roy. Coll. at Surg.s at Eng. (Fell.); BOA - Brit. Orthopaedic Assn. (Assoc. Mem.).

VIALE, Jean Paul Nuffield Department of Anaesthetics, University of Oxford, Radcliffe Infirmary, Oxford OX2 6HE — MD Lyons 1976.

VIALE, Nicholas John Norfolk Mental Health Care NHS Trust, Julian Hospital, Bowthorpe Rd, Norwich NR2 3TD Tel: 01603 421834 Fax: 01603 421831 — MB BS Lond. 1984 (Univ. of Lond.)

MRCPsych 1994. Cons. In Geriat. Psychiat. Specialty: Geriat. Psychiat. Prev: Trainee GP Twickenham Lond.; Sen. Regist. (Psychiat.) Roy. Free & Assoc. Hosps. Lond.

VIAN, Andrew Stanley The Sidings, Dicks La, Westhead, Ormskirk L40 6JA — MB BCh Wales 1997.

VIAPREE, Mr Roger Oliver 78 Ridgeview Road, London N20 0HL — MB ChB Glas. 1974; DLO RCS Eng. 1982; FRCS Ed. 1985. SHO (Plastic Surg.) Manor Hosp. Nuneaton. Prev: SHO (ENT) St. Margt. Hosp. Epping & Bedford Gen. Hosp.; SHO (ENT) & (Gen. Surg.) Luton & Dunstable Hosp. Luton.

VIBERTI, Professor Giancarlo Francesco Unit for Metabolic Medicine, 5th Floor Thomas Guy House, GKT School of Medicine, KCL Guy's Hospital, London SE1 9RT Tel: 020 7955 4826 Fax: 020 7955 2985 Email: giancarlo.viberti@kcl.ac.uk — (Univ. Milan & Turin) Dip. Endocrinol. Turin 1971; MD Milan 1969, State DMS 1975; MRCP (UK) 1985; FRCP Lond. 1990. Prof. Diabetes & Metab. Med., Head Unit Metab. Med. & Cons. Phys. GKT Sch. of Med. King's Coll. Lond. Specialty: Gen. Med. Special Interest: Diabetic Vasc. complications. Socs: Internat. Soc. Nephrol.; Eur. Assoc. Study Diabetes; Amer. Diabetes Assoc.

VIBHUTI, Ravi Churchill Clinic, 94 Churchill Avenue, Chatham ME5 0DL Tel: 01634 842397 — MB BS Karnatak 1974; T(GP) 1991. Vasectomy Surg. & Family Plann. Cons. Specialty: Gen. Pract.; Family Plann. & Reproduc. Health. Socs: Sec. BMA Dartford Gravesend & Medway Div.; Conserv. Med. Soc.

VICARAGE, Philip Harrison Wharfside Family Practice, Canal Road, Tavistock PL19 8AR Tel: 01822 616131 Fax: 01822 616404; The Tiles, Wrotham Road, Culverstone Meopham, Gravesend DA13 0RE Tel: 01732 822653 — MB ChB Manch. 1979; BSc St. And. 1976. Sen. Partner Gen. Pract., Tavistoke, Devon; Occupat. Phys. Socs: Fell. Roy. Soc. Med.; Kent Local Med. Comm. Prev: Sen. Partner Gen. Pract. Meopham, Kent; Clin. Asst. (Haemat.); Palliat. Care Phys.

VICARY, David John (retired) The Health Centre, Castleton Way, Eye IP23 7DD Tel: 01379 870689; Park Farm, Brome, Eye IP23 8AH Tel: 01379 870550 — MB BChir Camb. 1973 (Cambridge and Kings College Hospital London) DCH Eng. 1974; DObst RCOG 1974; MRCP (UK) 1975; FRCP 1997. Prev: Ho. Phys. Nottm. Gen. Hosp.

VICARY, Frederick Robin Highgate Hospital, 17 View Road, London N6 4DJ Tel: 020 8341 6989 Fax: 020 8348 7205 Email: vicaryassist@aol.com — MB BS Lond. 1969 (Westm.) MRCP (UK) 1971; FRCP Lond. 1984. Cons. Phys. (Gen. Med. & Gastroenterol.) Whittington Hosp. Lond. Specialty: Gen. Med.; Gastroenterol. Prev: Sen. Regist. Westm. Hosp. Lond.; Med. Off. Salvation Army Hosp. Chikankata, Zambia; Regist. (Med.) Univ. Coll. Hosp. Lond.

VICCA, Anthony Francis Microbiology Department, Diana Princess of Wales Hospital, Scartho Road, Grimsby DN33 2BA Tel: 01472 874111 — MB ChB Aberd. 1987; MRCPath 1996, D 1992. Const. Microbiol., Diana Princess of Wales Hosp. Grimsby. Specialty: Med. Microbiol. Prev: Sen. Regist. (Microbiol.) Leics. Path. Serv.; Reg. (Microbiol.) Centr. MicroBiol. Labs Edin.

VICE, Patricia Ann Royal Preston hospital, Sharoe Green Lane, Fulwood, Preston PR2 9HT Tel: 01772 710811 Fax: 01772 712944; 35 Dukes Meadow, Ingol, Preston PR2 7AS Tel: 01772 731931 Email: vicepa@websurf.co.uk — MB ChB Leeds 1969; BSc Leeds 1966; MRCP (UK) 1972; FCRP Lond. 1989. Cons. Phys. Roy. Preston Hosp. s/i Endocrinol. & Diabetes. Specialty: Endocrinol.

VICK, John Alexander Stewart (retired) The Pines, 7 Wymondley Close, Hitchin SG4 9PW Tel: 01462 432904 Fax: 01462 459591 Email: john.vick@btinternet.com — (Lond. Hosp.) MB BS Lond. 1960; MRCS Eng. LRCP Lond. 1960; DObst RCOG 1963; MRCGP 1971. Hon. Hosp. Pract. (Paediat.) Lister Hosp. Prev: GP Hitchin.

VICKERS, Alison Ruth Gill Street Health Centre, 11 Gill Street, London E14 8HQ Tel: 020 7515 2211 — MB BS Lond. 1990 (Charing Cross & Westminster) BSc Lond. 1987; DROG 1994; MRCGP 1995; Dip (Primary Care Therapeutics) 1997; MSc Public Health London School Hygiene and Tropical Medicine 1999. GP Princip. (3/4 Time).

VICKERS, Andrew Philip Humble Bee Nest, Littedale Road, Quernmore, Lancaster LA2 9EP — MB BS Lond. 1977 (St. Thomas') MRCS Eng. LRCP Lond. 1977; FFA RCS Eng. 1982. Cons. (Anaesth.) Morcambe Bay Acute Hosps. Trust. Specialty: Anaesth. Socs: Counc. Mem. The Pain Soc.

VICKERS, Anthony Adrian (retired) Highfield, Brook Bank, Broadwas-on-Teme, Worcester WR6 5NE Tel: 01886 821471 Email: avickers@onetel.net.uk — MB BS Lond. 1942 (St. Mary's) ADMR 1944; FFR 1950; FRCR 1975. Prev: Cons. Radiol. Worcester Roy. Infirm.

VICKERS, Beatrice Ann Josephine 32 Graceland Gardens, London SW16 2ST — MB BS Lond. 1991.

VICKERS, Professor Christopher Francis Howard Bronallt, Dyffryn Ardudwy LL44 2BE Tel: 01341 247784 — MB ChB Manch. 1950; FRCP Ed. 1970, M 1956; FRCP Lond. 1971, M 1958; MD Manch. 1960. Emerit. Cons. Dermat. Roy. Liverp. Hosp. Broadgreen Gen. Hosp. & Roy. Liverp Childr. Hosp. (Alder Hey); Emerit. Prof. (Dermat.) Univ. Liverp. Specialty: Dermat. Socs: (Ex-Pres.) N. Eng. Dermat. Soc.; Hon. Mem. Brit. Soc. Paediat. Dermat.; Hon. Mem. Amer. Soc. Dermat. Prev: Prof. Dermat. Univ. Liverp.; Cons. Dermat. Roy. Liverp., Newsham Gen. & Alder Hey Childr. Hosps. Liverp.; Assoc. Prof. West. Reserve Univ. Cleveland, USA.

VICKERS, David Michael Stockport NHS Trust, The Path Lab., Poplar Grove, Stockport SK2 7JE Tel: 0161 419 5607; Booth Farm Cottage, Kinder Road, Hayfield, High Peak SK22 2LJ Tel: 01663 746009 — MB ChB Liverp. 1967; FRCPath 1976. Cons. Histopath. Stepping Hill Hosp. Stockport. Specialty: Histopath. Prev: Sen. Regist. (Histopath.) N. West. RHA; Regist. (Path.) Whiston Hosp.; SHO (Path.) & Ho. Off. Broadgreen Hosp. Liverp.

VICKERS, David William Community Child Health, Ida Darwin, Fulbourn, Cambridge CB1 5EE Tel: 01223 884160 Fax: 01223 884161 Email: david.vickers@lifespan-tr.anglox.nhs.uk; The Mill, The Mill, Abington Pigotts, Royston SG8 0SA Tel: 01763 853424 Email: dwvickers@doctors.org.uk — BM BCh Oxf. 1982; MA Oxf. 1983; MRCP (UK) 1986; FRCPCH 1997. Cons. Community Paediat. S. Cambs.; Hon. Cons. Paediat. Addenbrooke's Hosp. NHS Trust; Assoc.s Univ. Lect., Univ. of Cambs. Specialty: Community Child Health.

VICKERS, Gareth Andrew 4 Kenilworth Close, Wistaston, Crewe CW2 6SN — MB ChB Manch. 1992.

VICKERS, James Roderick 38 Brook Street, Benson, Wallingford OX10 6LH Tel: 01491 833583; Neb Corner, Neb Lane, Oxted RH8 9JN Tel: 01883 713741 — MB BS Lond. 1988; MRCGP 1994; DRCOG 1994. Socs: Med. Protec. Soc.

VICKERS, Jean Elizabeth Wigan & Bolton Health Authority, Bryan House, 61 Standishgate, Wigan WN1 1AH Tel: 01942 772868; 46 Albert Road W., Bolton BL1 5HG Tel: 01204 840367 — MB BS Lond. 1972 (Univ. Coll. Hosp.) MRCGP 1984; MFPHM RCP (UK) 1992. Cons. Pub. Health Med. Wigan & Bolton HA. Specialty: Pub. Health Med. Prev: Med. Dir. Coll. Health Serv. Bloomsbury HA; Ho. Phys. & Ho. Surg. St. Chas. Hosp. Lond.

VICKERS, John Cedric Earnswood Medical Centre, 92 Victoria Street, Crewe CW1 2JR Tel: 01270 257255 Fax: 01270 501943 — MB ChB Liverp. 1972; DObst RCOG 1975; MRCGP 1977.

VICKERS, Mr Jonathan Hayward 70 Chesterfield Road, St Andrews, Bristol BS6 5DP Tel: 0117 924 3356 Email: atonks@bmj.com — MB ChB Bristol 1986; BSc (Hons.) Bristol 1983; FRCS Eng. 1991; FRCS Gen. Surg. 1998. Specialist Regist. (Surg.) Univ. Bristol. Specialty: Gen. Surg.

VICKERS, Julie Patricia Castleside Farm, Tattenhall Lane, Beeston, Tarporley CW6 9UA — MB ChB Dundee 1997.

VICKERS, Kenneth Whitley Road Medical Centre, 1 Whitley Road, Collyhurst, Manchester M40 7QH Tel: 0161 205 4407 Fax: 0161 203 5269 — MB ChB Manch. 1984; DRCOG 1987; DCH RCP Lond. 1987; MRCGP 1988. Med. Ref. for UK Sports Diving Med. Comm. Specialty: Gen. Pract.

VICKERS, Lewis Edward 8 Almond Drive, East Kilbride, Glasgow G74 2HX Tel: 0141 222898 Email: lewvickers@aol.com — MB ChB Glas. 1990; MRCP 1994. Specialist Regist. (Cardiol. & Gen. Med.) W. Scotl.. Specialty: Cardiol.; Gen. Med. Prev: research fell. (Cardiol.), Glas. Roy. Infirm.; SHO (Cardiol.) Glas. Roy. Infirm.; SHO (Gen. Med.) The Ayr Hosp.

VICKERS, Mark Adrian Rothley, 3 Gowanbrae Road, Bieldside, Aberdeen AB15 9AQ Email: m.a.vickers@abdn.ac.uk — BM BCh Oxf. 1983; BA Camb. 1980; MRCP (UK) 1986; DM Oxf. 1992; MRCPath 1995. Sen. Lect. (Haemat.) Aberd. Univ. Specialty: Haematology. Prev: Sen. Regist. (Haemat.) Roy. Berks. Hosp. Reading & John Radcliffe Hosp. Oxf.; Regist. (Haemat.)

Hammersmith Hosp. Lond.; MRC Train. Fell. John Radcliffe Hosp. Oxf.

VICKERS, Martin John Bridge Road Surgery, 66-88 Bridge Road, Litherland, Liverpool L21 6PH Tel: 0151 949 0249 Fax: 0151 928 2008 — BM BCh Oxf. 1985; MA Oxf. 1990, BA 1982; DGM RCP Lond. 1989. Mem. Sefton LMC. Prev: GP Auckland NZ; Trainee GP Cumbria.

VICKERS, Professor Michael Douglas Allen, OBE (retired) North Pines, 113 Cyncoed Road, Cardiff CF23 6AD Tel: 029 2075 3698 Email: mdvickers@doctors.org.uk/michael@mdvickers.plus.com — (Guy's) MB BS Lond. 1955; MRCS Eng. LRCP Lond. 1955; DA Eng. 1957; FFA RCS Eng. 1959; Hon. FFA RACS 1976. Emerit. Prof. Anaesth. Univ. of Wales Coll. Med. Cardiff. Prev: Pres. World Federat. of Anaesthesiologists.

VICKERS, Phillip James High Street Surgery, High Street, Pewsey SN9 5AQ Tel: 01672 563511 Fax: 01672 563004 Email: phillip.vickers@gp-j83017.nhs.uk; Mead House, Milton Lilbourne, Pewsey SN9 5LJ Tel: 01672 562358 Email: vickers48@btinternet.com — MB BS Lond. 1971 (Westm.) MRCS Eng. LRCP Lond. 1971; DObst RCOG 1976. PEC Mem., Kennet and N. Wilts PCT. Specialty: Gen. Pract. Prev: Regist. (Microbiol. & Immunol.) Westm. Hosp. Lond.; SHO (A & E) Qu. Mary's Hosp. Roehampton; Ho. Surg. Profess. Unit. Westm. Hosp. Lond.

VICKERS, Rachel Jane Anaesthetic Department, Queen's Hospital, Belvedere Road, Burton-on-Trent DE13 0RB — MB ChB Bristol 1987; FRCA 1993. Cons. Anaesth., Queen's Hosp., Burton-on-Trent. Specialty: Anaesth. Prev: Sen. Regist. (Anaesth.) Midls. RHA.; Regist. (Anaesth.) Leicester Roy. Infirm.

VICKERS, Mr Roger Henry 149 Harley Street, London W1G 6BN Tel: 020 7935 4444 Fax: 020 7935 5742; 11 Edenhurst Avenue, London SW6 3PD Tel: 020 7736 1065 — BM BCh Oxf. 1970 (St. Thos.) MA Oxf. 1970; FRCS Eng. 1975. Orthop. Surg. to HM The Qu.; Cons. Orthop. Surg. St. Geo. Hosp. & K. Edwd. VII Hosp. for Offs. Lond.; Civil. Cons. Orthop. Surg. to the Army. Specialty: Orthop. Socs: Apptd. Mem. Counc. Med. Defence Union; Mem. of Advis. Bd. Prev: Sen. Regist. (Orthop.) Char. Cross Hosp. Lond.; Regist. (Surg.) Watford Gen. Hosp.; SHO (Orthop.) Rowley Bristow Orthop. Hosp. Pyrford.

VICKERS, Miss Sarah Frances Sussex Eye Hospital, Eastern Road, Brighton BN2 5BF Tel: 01273 606126 Fax: 01273 69 36 74 — MB BS Lond. 1976 (St. Thos.) FRCOphth; FRCS Eng. 1983. Cons. Ophth. Sussex Eye Hosp. Brighton & Hurstwood Pk. Hosp. Haywards Heath. Specialty: Ophth. Socs: FEU. Roy. Con. Ophlnalmdogist; Fell., Roy. Coll. of Ophth.s; Amer. Acad. Ophth. Prev: Resid. Surg. Off. Moorfields Eye Hosp. Lond.; Strabismus Fell. Moorfield Eye Hosp.

VICKERS, William John, CMG (retired) 174 Ashby Road, Burton-on-Trent DE15 0LG — MRCS Eng. LRCP Lond. 1922; C St J; DPH Camb. 1924, DTM & H 1930; Barrister at Law Inner Temple 1938. Prev: DMS Singapore.

VICKERSTAFF, Helen Jane 5 Aldermoor Avenue, Storrington, Pulborough RH20 4PT Tel: 01903 743346; 5 Aldermoor Avenue, Storrington, Pulborough RH20 4PT Tel: 01903 743346 — MB BS Lond. 1998 (St Geo.) BSc Lond. 1995. A & E Roy. Perth Hosp. Western Australia. Specialty: Accid. & Emerg.

VICKERSTAFF, Kirsten Moraich 1 Ferrars Court, Huntingdon PE29 3BU — BA (Hons.) Camb. 1987, MB BChir 1991; DCH RCP Lond. 1993; DRCOG 1994.

VICKERY, Christopher James 31 Kings Avenue, Bishopston, Bristol BS7 8JL Tel: 0117 944 5870 — MB ChB Bristol 1988; BSc (Biol.) Lond. 1982; FRCS Eng. 1992. Rotat. Surg. Regist. SW Surg. Rotat. Specialty: Gen. Surg. Prev: Regist. (Surg.) Derriford Plymouth; Regist. (Surg.) Frenchay.

VICKERY, Mr Craig William 10 Linden House, Barkley's Hill, Stapleton, Bristol BS16 1FB Tel: 0117 965 3192 Email: craig.w.vickery@bristol.ac.uk — BM BCh Oxf. 1993; MA Cantab 1994; FRCS Eng. 1997. Clin. Research Fell. Bristol Roy. Infirm. Specialty: Gen. Surg. Socs: Surgs. in Train.; Eur. Org. Research & Treatm. of Cancer. Prev: SHO (Gen. Surg.) Frenchay Hosp. Bristol; SHO (Neurosurg.) Frenchay Hosp. Bristol; SHO (Orthop.) Frenchay Hosp. Bristol.

VICKERY, Heather Felicity Ann (retired) Glebe Cottage, Church Lane, Baylham, Ipswich IP6 8JS — MB BS Lond. 1953 (Roy. Free) MRCS Eng. LRCP Lond. 1954; DPM Eng. 1967. Prev: Med. Off. (Psychol. Med.) Middlx. Hosp. Lond.

VICKERY, Ian Malcolm Newman Oral Surgery Clinic, 35 Lower Redland Road, Redland, Bristol BS6 6TB Tel: 0117 946 6188 Fax: 0117 946 6177 Email: ivickery@aol.com — MRCS Eng. LRCP Lond. 1967 (Bristol) MB ChB Bristol 1967, BDS 1958; FDS RCS Eng. 1970, L 1958. Cons. Oral Surg. Newman Oral Surg. Clinic Bristol. Specialty: Oral & Maxillofacial Surg. Socs: Brit. Assn. Oral & Maxillo-Facial Surgs.; Brit. Assn. OGL & Maxillo. Surgs. Prev: Cons. Oral Surg. Southmead HA; Sen. Regist. United Bristol Hosps.; Specialist RAF Hosp. Changi, Singapore.

VICKERY, Kenneth, OStJ 18 Ravens Croft, Mount Road, Eastbourne BN20 7HX Tel: 01323 724315 — (St. Bart.) MRCS Eng. LRCP Lond. 1941; MB BS Lond. 1943; DPH Eng. 1947; MD Lond. 1947; FFPHM RCP (UK) 1975. Specialty: Pub. Health Med. Prev: Med. Ref. Eastbourne Crematorium; Hon. Cons. Pub. Health Eastbourne; MOH Co. Boro. Eastbourne.

VICKERY, Michael Hadden (retired) 5 Westgrove, Fordingbridge SP6 1LS Tel: 01425 652492 — MB BS Lond. 1950 (St. Thos.) MRCS Eng. LRCP Lond. 1950; DObst RCOG 1954.

VICKERY, Sheena Helen Elizabeth — MB BS Lond. 1982 (Guy's) DRCOG 1986. Prev: Princip. Gen. Pract., Banks Surg., 272 Wimborne Rd., Bournemouth, BH3 7AT; GP Trainee Ealing Hosp. VTS.

VICTOR-BEZA, Miriam GA Marine Gate, Marine Drive, Brighton BN2 5TN Tel: 01273 621655 — Medic Bucharest 1961; FRIPHH (London). Specialty: Gen. Pract.; Family Plann. & Reproduc. Health; Community Child Health. Socs: Mem. Fac. Child Health; Fell. Inst. Hyg. & Pub. Health. Prev: GP Principal; GP Locum; CMO Child Health.

VICTORATOS, George Department of Neurosurgery, Hope Hospital, Salford M6 8HD Tel: 0161 206 4340 Fax: 0161 795 9902 Email: gvictorato@aol.com — MD Athens 1965; FRCS 1973. Cons. Neurosurg., Hope Hosp. Salford; Cons. Neurosurg., Roy. Manch. Children's Hosp. Specialty: Neurosurg. Socs: Soc. of Brit. Neurol. Surgeons.

VICTORIA, Bernadette Anne Department of Anaesthetics, Lincoln County Hospital, Greetwell Road, Lincoln LN2 5QY Tel: 01522 573690 Email: anne.victoria@ulh.nhs.uk — MB BS Rajasthan 1982; FRCA 1994. Cons. Anaesth., Lincoln Co. Hosp. Specialty: Anaesth.

VIDGEON, Steven David 41 Great Thrift, Petts Wood, Orpington BR5 1NE — MB BS Lond. 1998.

VIDHANI, Kim Sleepy Hollow, Halloughton, Southwell NG25 0QP Tel: 01636 814147; 13 Arlington Drive, Mapperley Park, Nottingham NG3 5EN Tel: 0115 960 2091 — MB ChB Leeds 1990. Specialist Regist. (Anaesth.) Nottm. Specialty: Anaesth. Socs: Intens. Care Soc.; Assn. Anaesth. & BMA. Prev: SHO (Anaesth.) Nottm.; SHO (Cardiol.) Northern en. Hosp. Sheff.; SHO (Renal Med.) Northern Gen. Hosp. Sheff.

VIDHYADHARAN, Anitha 15 Bartle Avenue, London E6 3AJ — MB BS Lond. 1993.

VIDYASAGAR, Halevoor Nagabhushan St. Georges Hospital, Corporation St., Stafford ST16 3AG Tel: 01785 57888 — MB BS Bangalor 1979; MB BS Bangalore 1979; MRCPsych 1987. Cons. Psychiat. (special responsibil. Forens. Psychiat.) St. Geo. Hosp. Stafford. Specialty: Gen. Psychiat.

VIDYAVATHI, Manthravadi 5 Broadhalgh, Rochdale OL11 5LX — MB BS Andhra 1981; MRCP (UK) 1990.

VIEGAS, Marisa 36 Queen's Gate Place Mews, London SW7 5BQ Tel: 020 7589 6473 Fax: 020 7589 7176 — MB BS Lond. 1980; MRCP (UK) 1983.

VIEL, Maurizio 15 Harley Street, London W1N 1DA; Flat 2, 27 Hyde Park Gardens, London W2 2LZ — State DMS Milan 1984.

VIEL, Roberto 15 Harley Street, London W1G 9QQ Tel: 020 7636 4272 Fax: 020 7436 1677; Flat 10, 28 Hyde Park Gardens, London W2 2NB Tel: 020 7724 9269 — State Exam Milan 1984. Socs: Brit. Assn. Cosmetic Surg.; Amer. Acad. Cosmetic Surg.; Società Italiana Di Chirurgia Estetica.

VIETEN, Daniela Bristol Royal Hospital for Children, Paul O'Gorman Building, Upper Maudlin Street, Bristol BS2 8JE Email: danielav@doctors.org.uk; 38B Durdham Park, Bristol BS6 6XB — MB BCh Wales 1997 (Univ. of Wales Coll. of Med.) BSc (Basic Orthop. Sci.) Lond. 1996; MRCPCH 2000. Clin. Research Fell. Paediatric Surg., Bristol Roy. Hosp. for Childr., Bristol. Specialty: Paediat. Surg.; Research. Socs: Roy. Coll. of Paediat. and Child Health (Ordinary); Roy. Coll. of Surgeons of Eng. (Affiliate); Roy.

Coll. of Surgeons of Edin. Prev: Sen. Ho. Off. Plastic Surg., Frenchay Hosp., Bristol; Sen. Ho. Off. Orthopaedic Surg., Frenchay Hosp., Bristol; Sen. Ho. Off. Gen. Surg., Frenchay Hosp., Bristol.

VIEWEG, Reinout 181 Laburnum Grove, Portsmouth PO2 0HE — BM BS Nottm. 1988; DRCOG 1991.

VIG, Stella 84 Tewkesbury Street, Cardiff CF24 4QT — MB BCh Wales 1991; BSc (Hons.) Wales 1988; FRCS Ed. 1995; FRCS Eng. 1995. Calman Specialist Regist. Rotat. (Gen. Surg.) Llandough Hosp. Cardiff. Specialty: Gen. Surg.

VIGANO, Paola Clelia 12 Falkland Avenue, London N3 1QR — MB BS Lond. 1994.

VIGGERS, Jennifer Mary Royal Marsden Hospital, Fulham Road, London SW3 6JJ; 30 Smith Square, Westminster, London SW1P 3HF — MB BS Lond. 1967 (St Thos.) MRCS Eng. LRCP Lond. 1967; DA Eng. 1970. Clin. Asst. Early Diag. Unit Roy. Marsden Hosp. Lond. Specialty: Oncol. Prev: SHO (Anaesth.) & Ho. Phys. Kingston Hosp.; Ho. Surg. Qu. Alexandra Hosp. Portsmouth.

VIGUSHIN, David Michael Department of Cancer Medicine, 6th Floor MRC Cyclotron Building, Imperial College of Science, Technology & Medicine, Hammersmith Hospital Campus, Du Cane Road, London W12 0NN — MB BCh Witwatersrand 1986; MRCP Eng. 1990; PhD Lond. 1995. Sen. Lect. in Cancer Med., Imperial Coll. of Sci., Technol. & Med., Lond.; Hon. Cons. in Med. Oncol. Hammersmith Hosps. NHS Trust, Lond. Specialty: Oncol. Socs: Mem. of Brit. Med. Assn.; Mem. of Assn. of Cancer Phys.s; Active Mem. of Amer. Assn. for Cancer Research. Prev: Clin. Lect. (Hon. Sen. Regist.) Med. Oncol., Imperial Coll. of Sci., Technol. & Med., Hammersmith Hosps. NHS Trust Lond.; Research Fell. (Hon. Regist.) Immunol. Med., Roy. Postgrad. Med. Sch. & Hammersmith Hosp., Lond.; Sen. Ho. Off. in Gen. Med. Geo. Eliot Hosp. Nuneaton.

VIIRA, David John 59 Pangfield Park, Coventry CV5 9NN — MB BS Lond. 1993.

VIJAYA, Vipran 42 Shakespeare Crescent, London E12 6LN — MB ChB Liverp. 1994.

VIJAYA BHASKAR, Pothapragada 13 Bryn Rhedyn, Coed-Y-Cwm, Pontypridd CF37 3DP — MB BS Andhra 1974.

VIJAYA GANESH, Thulasiraman 4 Bonrek Close, Hainault, Ilford IG6 2QL — MB BS Madurai-Kamaraj, India 1988.

VIJAYA KUMAR, Marithammanahally Nanjundiah Ground Floor Flat, 69 Swanmore Road, Ryde PO33 2TG — MB BS Bangalor 1979; MB BS Bangalore 1979; MRCPI 1985.

VIJAYADURAI, Pavaladurai Department of Immunology, Lancashire Teaching Hospital, Sharoe Green Lane N,.Fulwood, Preston PR2 9HT Tel: 01772 522130 Fax: 01772 710021 — MB BS Colombo 1982; MRCP (UK) 1990; DRCPath 1993; MRCPath 1997. Cons. (Immunol.), Roy. Preston Hosp. Preston & Hope Hosp. Salford, Manch. Specialty: Immunol. Socs: Brit. Soc. Immunol.; BMA; MRCPath. Prev: Sen. Regist. (Immunol.) Roy. Liverp. Univ. Hosp.; Regist. & SHO (Immunol.) Qu. Med. Centre Nottm.; Regist. Stepping Hill Hosp. Manch. & Halifax Gen. Hosp.

VIJAYAKULASINGAM, Vijayaluxumidevi 36 Stanstead Manor, St James Road, Sutton SM1 2AZ — MB BS Colombo, Sri Lanka 1983; FRCA 1992.

VIJAYAKUMAR, Kodali 15 Speedwell Crescent, Scunthorpe DN15 8UP — MB BS Andhra 1973.

VIJAYAKUMAR, Marimuthu 4 Stonefield, Six Acres, London N4 3PG — LRCP LRCS Ed. LRCPS Glas. 1994.

VIJAYAKUMAR, Narayanaswami Leicester General Hospital NHS Trust, Gwendolen Road, Leicester LE5 4PW Tel: 0116 258 4052 Fax: 0116 258 4666 — MB BS Madras 1981; MRCP MRCPS 1992 Dublin. Assoc. Specialist (Integrated Med.) Leicester Gen. Hosp. Specialty: Gen. Med.; Care of the Elderly. Special Interest: Gastroenterol.

VIJAYAKUMAR, P Hirwaun Health Centre, Hirwaun, Aberdare CF44 9NS Tel: 01685 811999 Fax: 01685 814145.

VIJAYAN, Kesava Pillai Royal National Orthopaedic Hospital, Stanmore HA7 4LP Tel: 020 8954 2300 — MB BS Madurai Kamaraj 1983; MSc Orthop. Lond. 1989. Regist. (Orthop.) Roy. Nat. Orthop. Hosp. Stanmore.

VIJAYANATHAN, Sanjay 2 Irvine Avenue, Harrow HA3 8QE — MB BS Lond. 1991.

VIJAYARAGHAVAN, Shanti Newham General Hospital, Glen Road, Plaistow, London E13 8SL Tel: 020 7476 4000 Fax: 020 7368 8002; 202 East End Road, London N2 0PZ Tel: 020 8883 1214 — MB BS Bombay 1986 (Grant Med. Coll. Bombay) MD Bombay 1988; MRCP (UK) 1991; MPhil Lond. 1995. Cons. Phys. (Diabetes & Endocrinol.) Newham Gen. Hosp.; Hon. Sen. Lect. (Med.) Roy. Lond. & St. Bart. Sch. Med. & Dent. Lond. Specialty: Endocrinol. Prev: Lect. (Med.) Roy. Lond. & St. Bart. Sch. Med. & Dent. Lond.

VIJAYARAGHAVAN, Srinivasan 6 Clover Road, Etherley Dene, Bishop Auckland DL14 0TT — MB BS Madurai Kamaraj Univ. 1975; FRCA 1993.

VIJAYARATNAM, Deena Dayalan 147 Helmsley Road, Newcastle upon Tyne NE2 1RE — MB BS (Merit) Newc. 1998.

VIJAYASIMHULU, Gorjala Thirumala Lincoln County Hospital, Department of Radiology, Greetwell Road, Lincoln LN2 5QY Tel: 01522 512512 Email: g.vijay@ulh.nhs.uk; Sai Nivas, Grayingham Road, Kirton in Lindsey, Gainsborough DN21 4EL Tel: 01652 640158 — MB BS Sri Venkateswara 1971 (Kurnool Med. Coll.) DMRD Madras 1974; FRCR 1979; Dip HSM York 1995. Cons. Radiol. Lincoln Co. Hosp. Specialty: Radiol. Special Interest: Ultrasound & CT Imaging. Prev: Cons. Radiol. Scunthorpe & Goole Hosps.; Cons. Radiol. Shotley Bridge Gen. Hosp.; Sen. Regist. Newc. Teach. Gp. Hosps.

VIJAYKUMAR, Mr Annaswami Royal Infirmary, Bolton Road, Blackburn BB2 3LR Tel: 01254 294000 Fax: 01254 294050; Logan House, Main Road, Eastburn, Keighley BD20 7SJ Tel: 01535 633356 Fax: 01535 633356 — MB BS Madras 1972 (Madras Medical College) DO RCPSI 1976; FRCS Ed. 1989; FRCOphth 1990. Cons. Ophth. Blackburn, Hyndburn & Ribble Valley Healthcare NHS Trust & Burnley Health Care NHS Trust. Specialty: Ophth. Socs: N. Eng. Ophthalmol. Soc.; UK & Irel. Soc. Cataract & Reractive Surg.; Internat. Mem. Amer. Acad. Opth. Prev: Assoc. Specialist (Ophth.) Huddersfield NHS Trust; Regist. (Ophth.) Newc. Gen. Hosp., Hull Roy. Infirm. & Huddersfield Roy. Infirm.; SHO (Ophth.) Newc. Gen. Hosp.

VIJAYKUMAR, Usha Logan House, Main Road, Eastburn, Keighley BD20 7SJ — MB BS Madras 1973 (Madras Med. Coll.) Clin. Med. Off. (Child Health & Family Plann.) Bradford HA. Specialty: Community Child Health. Socs: Fac. Community Health; Soc. Pub. Health. Prev: SHO (Geriat. Med.) Castle Hill Hosp. Cottingham; SHO (Gen. Med.) Qu. Eliz. Hosp. Gateshead; Ho. Off. (Gen. Med.) Dunston Hill Hosp. Gateshead.

VIJEYASINGAM, Mr Rajasingham 58 Cholmley Gardens, Fortune Green Road, Hampstead, London NW6 1AJ — MB BS Lond. 1984; FRCS Ed. 1989; FRCS Eng. 1990. Specialty: Gen. Surg.

VIJH, Meena 188 Creynolds Lane, Solihull B90 4ES — MB BS Himachal Pradesh 1985; MRCP (UK) 1995.

VIJH, Mr Vikram 54 Paxford Road, Wembley HA0 3RQ — MB BS Lond. 1988; FRCS Eng. 1992; FRCS Ed. 1992; FRCS (Plast) 2002. Locum Cons. Chelsea & Westm. Hosp. Specialty: Plastic Surg. Socs: Fell. Roy. Soc. Med.; BMA. Prev: Regist. Plastic Surg. St Andrews, Billcieay; Research Regist. (Plastic Surg.) Mt. Vernon Hosp. Northwood; Regist. (Plastic Surg.) Pan Thames.

VILAPLANA CANNON, John Paul 30 Mossywood Place, Cumbernauld, Glasgow G68 9DS — LMS U Autonoma Barcelona 1991.

VILARINO-VARELA, Maria Jose 10B Antill Road, London E3 5BP — MB BS Lond. 1993.

VILCHES MORAGA, Arturo 38 Healdwood Drive, Burnley BB12 0EA — MB BS Madrid, Spain 1993; MRCP UK 1999; PGM Lond. 2000. Specialty: Care of the Elderly. Socs: BMA; MDU. Prev: SHO & Ho. Off. (Gen. Med.) Burnley Gen. Hosp.; SHO (Gen. Med.) Roy. Preston Hosp.; SHO (Gen. Med. & MFE) Roy. Preston.

VILE, Kathryn Sarah Marjorie Okethampton Medical Centre, East Street, Okehampton EX20 1AY Tel: 01837 52233; Middle Gooseford, Whiddon Down, Okehampton EX20 2QH Tel: 01647 231210 Fax: 01647 231210 — MB ChB Bristol 1985; MRCGP 1989; Cert. Family Plann. JCC 1989. Prev: Trainee GP Exeter HA VTS; Ho. Surg. Torbay Hosp. Torquay; Ho. Phys. Ham Green Hosp. S.mead.

VILLAGE, Anne Lesley 64 Hillside Road, Beeston, Nottingham NG9 3AY — MB ChB Sheff. 1976; MFFP 1993. Prev: Nottingham GP Retainer Scheme.

VILLAGRAN MORENO, Jose Maria 9 Dalegarth, Hurst Park Avenue, Cambridge CB4 2AG Tel: 01223 322745 — LMS Cadiz 1983.

VILLAQUIRAN URIBE, Jaime Alberto 40 Beaumont Terrace S., Gosforth, Newcastle upon Tyne NE3 1AS — Medico y Cirujano Univ. del Valle 1982; Medico y Cirujan Univ. del Valle 1982.

VILLAR, B Louise Bell The Vineyard, Windmill Hill, Saffron Walden CB10 1RR — MB ChB Aberd. 1974; DRCOG 1978; MRCP (UK) 1982; MRCGP 1984.

VILLAR, Monica Tracey Anne Poole Hospital NHS Trust, Longfleet Road, Poole BH15 2JB Tel: 01202 665511 Fax: 01202 442993 — MB BS Lond. 1983 (New Hall, Camb. Univ. & King's Coll. Hosp. Med. Sch.) MA Camb. 1984; MRCP (UK) 1986; DM Soton 1997; FRCP 1998. Cons. Phys. (Med. for Elderly) Poole Hosp. NHS Trust. Specialty: Care of the Elderly. Socs: Brit. Geriat. Soc. Prev: Sen. Regist. (Gen. Med. & Geriat.) Roy. Bournemouth Gen. Hosp. & S. Hants. Hosp. Soton.

VILLAR, Mr Richard Neville Cambridge Hip & Knee Unit, BUPA Cambridge Lea Hospital, 30 New Road, Impington, Cambridge CB4 9EL Tel: 01223 235888 Fax: 01223 235884 Email: rvillar@uk-consultants.co.uk — MB BS Lond. 1977 (St. Thos. Hosp.) BSc (Anat.) Lond. 1974; FRCS Eng. 1982; MS Soton. 1987; MA Camb. 1997. p/t Cons. Orthop. Addenbrooke's Hosp. Camb.; Assoc. Lect. Univ. Camb. Specialty: Orthop. Socs: Fell. BOA; Eur. Hip Soc.; Eur. Soc. Knee Surg. & Arthroscopy. Prev: Sen. Regist. (Orthop.) Addenbrooke's Hosp. Camb.; Regist. (Orthop.) Soton. Gen. Hosp.; Capt. RAMC.

VILLENEAU, Alexandre Georges (retired) Mutton's Farm, Ashington RH20 3AJ Tel: 01903 892640 — (St. Geo.) MB BS Lond. 1952. Prev: Ho. Phys. St. Geo. Hosp. Lond. & Atkinson Morley's Hosp. Lond.

VILLIERS, Christopher Tile House Surgery, 33 Shenfield Road, Brentwood CM15 8AQ Tel: 01277 227711 Fax: 01277 200649; 104 Chelmsford Road, Shenfield, Brentwood CM15 8RL Tel: 01277 227219 — MB BS Lond. 1988 (London) MA Oxf. 1989; DRCOG 1991; DGM RCP Lond. 1991; MRCGP 1993. GP Princip.; Bd. Mem. Brentwood PCG. Specialty: Gen. Pract. Socs: (Sec.) Brentwood Dist. Med. Soc. Prev: GP/Regist. Harold Hill, Romford; SHO (O & G, Med. & Rheum.) Harold Wood Hosp. Romford.

VILLIERS, Gertrude Isobel Lamb (retired) Bell Cottage, 29 Dean St., Brewood, Stafford ST19 9BU Tel: 01902 850905 — (Univ. Coll. Dub.) MB BCh BAO Dub. 1952; LLB Wolverhampton University 1980. SCMO Mid Staffs. HA. Prev: Anaesth. Wolverhampton AHA.

VIMALACHANDRAN, Chandrakumar Dale 306 Wood Lane, Heskin, Chorley PR7 5NT — MB ChB Liverp. 1997.

VINAYAGAMOORTHY, Chelliah 371 Watford Road, St Albans AL2 3DD — MB BS Ceylon 1966; MRCP (UK) 1975. Sen. Regist. (Haemat.) Qu. Eliz. Hosp. Birm. Specialty: Haematology.

VINAYAGAMOORTHY, Pushpam Medical Centre, 2 Birchwood Lane, South Normanton, Derby DE65 3D Tel: 01773 862907; Birindavanam, Leavale, Broadmeadows, South Normaton, Alfreton DE55 3NA Tel: 01773 863291 — LRCP LRCS Ed. 1978; LRCP LRCS Ed. LRCPS Glas. 1978.

VINAYAGUM, Sandra Rita 62 Hamilton Road, Golders Green, London NW11 9EJ — MB ChB Manch. 1985.

VINAYAK, Mr Bippon Chander 190 Goodman Park, Slough SL2 5NL — MB BS Lond. 1986; FRCS Ed. 1990; FRCS Eng. 1992. Clin. Lect. & Hon. Sen. Regist. (Otolaryngol.) Univ. Oxf. Specialty: Otorhinolaryngol. Prev: Regist. (ENT) Oxf.; Regist. & SHO (ENT) St. Mary's Hosp. Lond.

VINAYAK, Inder Paul Victoria Medical Centre, 12-28 Glen Street, Hebburn NE31 1NU Tel: 0191 483 2106 Fax: 0191 428 5270 — MB BS Panjab 1964. GP Hebburn, Tyne & Wear.

VINAYAK, Veena Victoria Medical Centre, 12-28 Glen Street, Hebburn NE31 1NU Tel: 0191 483 2106 Fax: 0191 428 5270 — MB BS Rajasthan 1974. GP Hebburn, Tyne & Wear.

VINCE, Mr Alastair Stuart Northampton General Hospital, Department of Orthopaedics, Cliftonville, Northampton NN1 5BD Tel: 01604 544467 — MB ChB Birm. 1986; FRCS Glas. 1992; FRCS (Orth) 1998. Cons. Trauma & Orthopaedic Surg. Northampton Gen. Hosp. Specialty: Trauma & Orthop. Surg. Special Interest: Hip & Knee Surg. Socs: RSM - Counc. Orthopaedic Sect.; Brit. Hip. Soc.

VINCE, Frank Peter — MB Camb. 1963 (Lond. Hosp.) BChir 1962; FRCP Lond. 1979, M 1966. Cons. Phys. Coventry Gp. Hosps.; Chief Med. Off. Axa Sun Life Insur. Co. Specialty: Endocrinol.; Gen. Med.; Diabetes. Socs: Fell. Roy. Soc. Med.; Fell. Assur. Med. Soc.; Soc. Endocrinol. Prev: Lect. (Endocrinol.) Lond. Hosp.; Regist. Addenbrooke's Hosp. Camb.; Ho. Off. Lond. Hosp.

VINCE, Jonathan Department of Forensic Psychiatry, Shaftesbury Clinic, Springfield Hospital, Glenburnie Road, London SW17 7DJ Tel: 020 8682 0033 Fax: 020 8682 3450 Email: jvince@swlstg-tr.nhs.uk — MB BS Lond. 1986 (Univ. Coll. Lond.) BSc (Hons.) Lond. 1983; MRCPsych 1991; Dip FMH 1997. Cons. Forens. Psychiat. & Hon. Sen. Lect., S. W. Lond. & St. Geo. NHS Trust. & St Geo.'s Hosp. Med. Sch. Specialty: Forens. Psychiat.

VINCENT, Andrew Patrick Les Saisons Surgery, 20 David Place, St Helier JE2 4TD Tel: 01534 720314 Fax: 01534 733205; La Meadowbank, Rue de la Vallee, St Mary, Jersey JE3 3DL Tel: 01534 484490 Email: andy@localdial.com — BM Soton. 1987; MRCGP 1992. Specialty: Gen. Pract.

VINCENT, Professor Angela Carmen Weatherall Institute of Molecular Medicine, John Radcliffe Hospital, Oxford OX3 9DU Tel: 01865 222321 Fax: 01865 222402 Email: angela.vincent@imm.ox.ac.uk; Taverners, Woodeaton, Oxford OX3 9TH Tel: 01865 559636 — MB BS Lond. 1966 (Westm.) MRCS Eng. LRCP Lond. 1966; MSc (Biochem.) Lond. 1969; MRCPath 1991; FRCPath 1997. Univ. Lect. (Clin. Neuroimmunol.) Univ. Oxf.; Hon. Cons. Immunol. John Radcliffe Hosp. Oxf.; Prof. Neuroimmunol. Univ. Oxf. Specialty: Immunol. Socs: Assn. Brit. Neurol.; Brit. Soc. Immunol.; Amer. Neurol. Assn. Prev: Reader (Neurol.) Molecular Med. John Radcliffe Hosp. Oxf.; Univ. Research Lect. Inst. Molecular Med. John Radcliffe Hosp. Oxf.; Research Assoc. Roy. Free Hosp. Lond.

VINCENT, Angus 24A Eslington Terrace, Newcastle upon Tyne NE2 4RL Tel: 0191 212 0621 Fax: 0191 212 0621 — MB ChB Glas. 1994. Specialist Regist. Rotat. (Anaesth.) N.en Region.; SHO Rotat. (Anaesth. & Gen. Med.) Wansbeck Hosp. Ashington & Freeman Hosps. Newc. Specialty: Anaesth. Socs: BMA; Intens. Care Soc.; Assn. of Anaesth. GB & Irel.

VINCENT, Christian Mervyn Abiodun 25 Wyatt Park Road, London SW2 3TN — MRCS Eng. LRCP Lond. 1969.

VINCENT, Doris Susan Downfield Medical Practice, 325 Strathmartine Road, Dundee DD3 8NE Tel: 01382 812111 Fax: 01382 858315; 1 Station Brae, Newport-on-Tay DD6 8DQ Tel: 01382 543156 — MB ChB St. And. 1968; MRCGP 1979; FRCGP 1998.

VINCENT, Elizabeth Clare The Doctors House, Victoria Road, Marlow SL7 1DN Tel: 01628 484666 Fax: 01628 891206; 9 Claremont Road, Marlow SL7 1BH — BM BS Nottm. 1980.

VINCENT, Emma Jane Barn Close Surgery, 38-40 High Street, Broadway WR12 7BT — MB ChB Birm. 1997; DCH; DFFP; MRCGP; DRCOG.

VINCENT, James Christian 11 Garden Lane, Southsea PO5 3DP — BM Soton. 1986; DA (UK) 1990; MRCP (UK) 1991; FRCA 1994. Cons. Anaesth. Portsmouth Hosp. NHS Trust. Specialty: Anaesth.

VINCENT, John Anthony West Timperley Medical Centre, 21 Dawson Road, Altrincham WA14 5PF Tel: 0161 929 1515 Fax: 0161 941 6500; 9 Charter Close, Sale M33 5YG Tel: 0161 969 6861 — MB ChB Leeds 1986; DRCOG 1992. Prev: Sen. Med. Off. RAF Newton; Trainee GP/SHO RAF (H) Wroughton VTS; Jun. Med. Off. RAF Lyneham.

VINCENT, Mark Aidan (retired) The Orchard, 6B High St, Henlow SG16 6BS Tel: 01462 814460 Fax: 01462 814460 — BM BCh Oxf. 1978; MA Oxf. 1980, BA (Hons.) 1975; BMM BCh Oxf. 1978; DRCOG 1980; FRCGP 1995, M 1983.

VINCENT, Michael Edwin 43 Tinsley Road, London E1 3DA — MB BS Lond. 1981; DGM RCP Lond. 1985; DCH RCP Lond. 1985; DRCOG 1986; MRCGP St. Bart 1987. Prev: GP Esher, Surrey.

VINCENT, Michael Leonard Briardene, Wylam Wood Road, Wylam NE41 8HX — MB ChB Manch. 1994.

VINCENT, Nicholas Robert John The Writtle Surgery, 16A Lordship Road, Writtle, Chelmsford CM1 3EH Tel: 01245 421205 Fax: 01245 422094; 18 Little Meadow, Writtle, Chelmsford CM1 3LG Tel: 01245 421523 — MB BS Lond. 1982; DRCOG 1986. Clin. Asst. (Colposcopy) St. Johns Hosp. Chelmsford. Socs: BMA; Christ. Med. Fellowsh. Prev: Trainee GP Eastbourne VTS; Ho. Phys. BromsGr. & Redditch Hosp.; Ho. Surg. Ipswich Hosp.

VINCENT, Paul William Birtley Medical Group Practice, Birtley Medical Group, Durham Road, Birtley, Chester-le-Street DH3 2QT Tel: 0191 410 3421 Fax: 0191 410 9672 — MB BS Lond. 1982

(King's College London) MRCGP 1986; DRCOG 1986; DCCH RCP Ed. 1987; DA (UK) 1989; D.Occ.Med. RCP Lond. 1995. Specialty: Gen. Pract.; Occupat. Health. Socs: Christian Med. Fellowsh.

VINCENT, Philippa Jane Stockbridge Surgery, New St., Stockbridge SO20 6HG; 78 Stockbridge Road, Winchester SO22 6RL — MB BS Lond. 1996 (Univ. Coll. Lond.) BSc Hons (Psychol.) 1993; DCH, RCP Lond. 1998; DROG, RCOG 1998; DFFP RCOG 1998. GP Regist., VTS Winchester. Specialty: Gen. Pract.

VINCENT, Professor Richard Royal Sussex County Hospital, Cardiac Department, Eastern Road, Brighton BN2 5BE Tel: 01273 696955 Fax: 01273 684554 Email: r.vincent@brighton.ac.uk; 53 Hill Drive, Hove BN3 6QL Tel: 01273 558714 Fax: 01273 298644 — MB BS Lond. 1970 (King's Coll. Hosp.) MRCS Eng. LRCP Lond. 1970; MRCP (UK) 1973; BSc (Pharmacol.) Lond. 1967, MD 1984; FRCP Lond. 1985. Cons. Cardiol. Roy. Sussex Co. Hosp. Brighton; Assoc. Dean, Brighton and Sussex Med. Sch.; Prof. Med. Sci. Sussex Univ.; Head Med. Univ. Brighton; prof. Med., Univ. Brighton; Hon. Cons. Cardiol. KCH Lond. Specialty: Cardiol. Socs: Brit. Cardiac Soc.; Roy. Soc. Med.; Exec. Mem., Resusc. Counc. (UK).

VINCENT, Stephen Hereward, Surg. Cdr. RN Retd. Hawthorns, East End, Lymington SO41 5SY Tel: 01590 626370 Fax: 01590 626491 Email: steve@hawthorns3.demon.co.uk — MB BS Lond. 1970 (St. Thos.) MA Camb. 1970; MRCS Eng. LRCP Lond. 1970; DCH Eng. 1978; MRCGP 1979; FRCGP 1997. Cons. Adviser in Gen. Pract. to Med. Director Gen. (Naval). Specialty: Gen. Pract. Socs: BMA; ASME; Roy. Naval Med. Club. Prev: Course Organiser Soton. Day Release Course; Assoc. Adviser (Gen. Pract.) Soton. & SW Hants. Health Dist.

VINCENT-BROWN, Amanda Meredith Barclay The Bridge Practice, The Health Centre, Stepgates, Chertsey KT16 8HZ; 2 Lady Place Barns, Church Hill, Pyrford, Woking GU22 8XJ — MRCS Eng. LRCP Lond. 1976; C.I.D.C. 2002. G.P. Princip. Chertsey.

VINCENT-KEMP, Ruth (retired) Dunwood Hall, Longsdon, Leek ST9 9AR Tel: 01538 385071 — MRCS Eng. LRCP Lond. 1947 (Roy. Colls. Ed.) DCH Eng. 1953. Prev: Clin. Asst. (Paediat.) N. Staffs. Gp. Hosps.

VINCENT-SMITH, Lisa Mayling 37 Roslea Drive, Dennistoun, Glasgow G31 2QR — MB ChB Glas. 1997.

VINCENTI, Gareth Edward Paul The Harrogate Clinic, 23 Ripon Road, Harrogate HG1 2JL Tel: 01609 778730 Fax: 01609 778730 — MB BS Newc. 1981; MRCPsych 1988; FRCPsych 2000. Cons. Psych. in Private Pract.; Force Psychiat., Gtr. Manch. Police; Medical Director Harrogate Clinic. Specialty: Gen. Psychiat. Socs: Marcé Soc.; Seasonal Affective Disorder Assn.; Roy. Soc. Med. Prev: Cons. Psychiat. Northallerton Health Serv. NHS Trust; Dir. Postgrad. Educat. Northallerton; Vis. Cons. Psychiat., Northallerton Remand Centre.

VINCHENZO, A Stanley Road Surgery, 204 Stanley Road, Bootle L20 3EW Tel: 0151 922 5719.

VINCINI, Cornelio 21 Bridge Street, Driffield YO25 6DB — MB BS Lond. 1980; MRCGP 1984; DRCOG 1984.

VINDEN, Sybil Rosemary (retired) Heathfield House, Cale Green, Stockport SK2 6RA; 53 Clothorn Road, Didsbury, Manchester M20 6BP — MB ChB Cape Town 1961. Clin. Asst. (Psychiat. & Rehabil.) Stockport. Prev: GPVTS.

VINDLA, Mona Sherrington Park Medical Practice, 402 Mansfield Rd, Sherwood, Nottingham NG5 2EJ — MB BS Lond. 1988; DRCOG 1991; MRCGP 1992; Docc Med 2001. GP Princip. Nottm.; Health Adviser for health at work, providing Ocupational health advice. Specialty: Gen. Pract.; Occupat. Health. Socs: Soc. of Occupat.al Med. Prev: Trainee GP Gt. Yarmouth & Waveney VTS; Ho. Phys. Orsett Hosp.; Ho. Surg. Whipps Cross Hosp. Lond.

VINDLA, Srinivas North Derbyshire Royal Hospital, Calon S44 5BL Tel: 01246 512707 — MB BS Lond. 1989; BSc (Hons.) Zool. Lond. 1986. Specialist Regist., Dept. of Obs.& Gyn. Qu.s Med. Centre, Notts. Specialty: Obst. & Gyn. Prev: SHO (O & G) Nottm.; SHO (O & G) Jas. Paget Hosp. Gt. Yarmouth.

VINDLACHERUVU, Madhavi Flat 15, Lyndhurst, London Road, Leicester LE2 2AP — BChir Camb. 1995. Ho. Off. (Gen. Surg.) Ipswich Hosp. Specialty: Gen. Surg. Prev: Ho. Off. (Gen. Med.) Qu. Eliz. Hosp. King's Lynn.

VINDLACHERUVU, Mr Raghu Ram 47 Grosvenor Avenue, Jesmond, Newcastle upon Tyne NE2 2NP Tel: 0191 281 7328 — MB BChir Camb. 1994; MA Camb. 1995; FRCS Lond. 1997. Specialist Regist. in Neurosurg., Newc. Gen. Hosp., Westgate Rd., Newc. Specialty: Neurosurg. Prev: Sen. Ho. Off. (Gen. Surg.) Chase Farm Hosp. Enfield Lond.; SHO (Gen. Surg.) Roy. Free Hosp. Lond.; Sen. Ho. Off. (Neurosurg.) Atkinson Morley's Hosp. Lond.

VINE, Alison Mary Immunology Department, ICSM St Mary's, Norfolk Place, London W2 1PG Tel: 020 7594 3731 Fax: 020 7402 0653 — MB BS Lond. 1990 (Char. Cross and Westm. Med. Sch.) DPhil Oxon. 1996. Wellcome Postdoctoral Fell.; Speciality: Immunogenetics of HTLV-I Infect.; Immunol. Dept. I.C.S.M. at St. Mary's Lond. Specialty: Immunol. Prev: Wellcome Clin. Train. Fell. Dep. Human Anat. Oxf.

VINE, David John West Wirral Group Practice, 33 Thingwall Road, Irby, Wirral CH61 3UE Tel: 0151 648 1846 Fax: 0151 648 0362 — MB ChB Liverp. 1974; DObst RCOG 1976; MRCGP 1978; DCH RCPS Glas. 1978. GP. Specialty: Gen. Pract. Socs: BMA; Christian Med. Fell.ship.

VINE, Pauline Rosemary Anaesthetic Department, Bromley Hospital, Cromwell Avenue, Bromley BR2 9AJ — MB BS Lond. 1977 (Univ. Coll. Hosp.) BSc (1st cl. Hons.) Lond. 1974, MB BS 1977; MRCP (UK) 1980; FFA RCS Eng. 1982. Cons. Anaesth. Bromley Hosps Trust. Specialty: Anaesth.

VINE, Richard John Assynt Medical Practice, The Health Centre, Lochinver, Lairg IV27 4JZ — MB BCh BAO Belf. 1977; DRCOG 1980.

VINE, Sydney Maudsley (retired) 2 Woolven Close, Parkstone, Poole BH14 0QT Tel: 01202 730330 — MB BChir Camb. 1947 (Camb. & Guy's) MRCS Eng. LRCP Lond. 1943; BA Camb. 1940, MA, MB BChir 1947; FRCP Lond. 1974, M 1952. Mem. Med. Counc. on Alcoholism. Prev: Phys. i/c Dept. Geriat. Med. Reading Area Hosps.

VINEN, Catherine Susanna Department of Renal Medicine, St. George's Hospital, Medical School, Cranmer Terrace, London SW17 — BChir Camb. 1990; MRCP 1994. Clin. Res. Fell. Dept. of Renal Med. St. Geo.'s Hosp. Med. Sch. Specialty: Rheumatol.

VINER, Anthony Sidney (retired) Castle Cottage, Creech Heathfield, Taunton TA3 5EH Tel: 01823 443905 — (St. Mary's) MRCS Eng. LRCP Lond. 1952. Prev: Med. Off. DHSS.

VINER, Clare Rachel 4 Florence Road, Southsea PO5 2NE — MB ChB Leeds 1997.

VINER, Michael Anthony The Oaklands Practice, Yateley Medical Centre, Oaklands, Yateley GU46 7LS Tel: 01252 872333 — MB BS Lond. 1975 (Camb. & St. Mary's) MRCS Eng. LRCP Lond. 1975; MA Camb. 1976; Cert JCC Lond. 1979; DRCOG 1979. Prev: SHO (O & G), (A & E) & (Paediat.) Berks. AHA.

VINES, Benjamin Homfray 17 Chivenor Grove, Kingston upon Thames KT2 5GE — BM Soton. 1998.

VINES, Jill Rachel Long Street Practice, 51 Long Street, Cerne Abbas, Dorchester DT2 7JG Tel: 01300 341666 Fax: 01300 341090; Frome Farrow, 7B Dorchester Road, Frampton, Dorchester DT2 9NB — MB BS Lond. 1975; MRCS Eng.; LRCP Lond. 1975; DRCOG 1977; MRCGP 1981; MFHom 1998. GP; Homeop. Clinic. Specialty: Homeop. Med.; Dermat.; Family Plann. & Reproduc. Health. Prev: GP Dorchester & Falmouth.

VINESTOCK, Morris David Section of Forensic Psychiatry, St. Georges Hospital Medical School, Jenner Wing, Cranmer Terrace, London SW17 0RE Tel: 020 8725 5567 Fax: 020 8725 2475 — MB ChB Ed. 1979; MRCPsych 1992. Lect. (Forens. Psychiat.) St. Geo. Hosp. Med. Sch. Univ. Lond.

VINEY, Deirdre Bradley Cote Cottage, Cote, Bampton, Oxford OX18 2EG — MB BCh BAO Dub. 1957 (T.C. Dub.) FRACS (Primary); BA Dub. 1955, MB BCh BAO 1957; DA Eng. 1961.

VINEY, Mark Trevor Balmoral Surgery, 1 Victoria Road, Deal CT14 7AU Tel: 01304 369880 — MB BS Lond. 1989; AKC Lond. 1989; Cert. Family Plann. JCC 1991; DRCOG 1992; Cert. Prescribed Equiv. Exp. JCPTGP 1993; MRCGP 1993; DFFP 1993. GP Trainer; Clin Assist. Vict. Hosp. Deal. Prev: Trainee GP Tunbridge Wells HA VTS.

VINEY, Michael James (retired) 59 Thorogate, Rawmarsh, Rotherham S62 7HN — MB ChB Manch. 1955. Prev: Ho. Surg. Crumpsall Hosp. Manch. & Burton-on-Trent Infirm.

VINEY, Paul Leonard 75 Wiltshire Road, Salisbury SP2 8HT — MB BS Lond. 1996.

VINEY, Rebecca Margaret Morris Globe Town Surgery, 82-86 Roman Road, London E2 0PG; 84 Cloudesley Road, London N1 0EB

— MB BS Lond. 1986 (St. Bart. Hosp.) Dip OCC MED 1997. GP Tutor & Course Organiser GP Non-Princip. & Asst. GP, Globe Town Surg. Socs: Soc. Occupat. Med.; BMA. Prev: Princip. GP Jubilee St. Pract. Lond.

VINEY, Richard Philip Charles 11 Don Close, Edgbaston, Birmingham B15 3PN — MB ChB Birm. 1995.

VINIKER, Mr David Alan Private Office, c/o Holly House Hospital, High Road, Buckhurst Hill IG9 5HX Tel: 020 8504 6886 Fax: 020 8504 6678 — MB BS Lond. 1971 (Univ. Coll. Hosp.) FRCOG 1995, M 1976; MD Lond. 1983. Cons. O & G Whipps Cross Hosp.; Hon. Sen. Lect. Univ of Lond. Specialty: Obst. & Gyn. Socs: Amer. Soc. Reproduc. Med.; Brit. Fertil. Soc.; Brit. Menopause Soc. Prev: Sen. Regist. (O & G) Leicester Roy. Infirm.; Research Sen. Regist. (O & G) Univ. Coll. Hosp. Lond.; Regist. (O & G) Lond. Hosp.

VINING, David (retired) 141 Wigton Lane, Alwoodley, Leeds LS17 8SH — MB ChB Leeds 1941. Prev: Police Surg.

VINING, Roy MacDona Herringfleet, Heath Road, St. Olaves, Great Yarmouth NR31 9HL Tel: 01493 488385 Fax: 01493 488385 — MB BS Lond. 1953 (St. Mary's) Specialty: Gen. Pract.

VINITHARATNE, Juwundara Kankanamalage Padmasiri Department of Anaesthetics, Aldermaston Road, Basingstoke RG24 9NA; 55 Linden Avenue, Old Basing, Basingstoke RG24 7HS Tel: 01256 473651 — MB BS Ceylon 1967. Staff Grade (Anaesth.) N. Hants. Hosp. Basingstoke. Specialty: Anaesth. Socs: BMA.

VINNICOMBE, Mr John Hindon House, Havant Road, Emsworth PO10 7JE Tel: 01243 372528 — MB BChir Camb. 1956 (St. Thos.) MChir Camb. 1966, MA 1956; FRCS Eng. 1958. Cons. Urol. Surg. Portsmouth Hosp. Gp.; Clin. Teach. Soton. Univ. Med. Sch.; Cons. Urol. Surg. King Edwd. VII Hosp. Midhurst. Specialty: Urol. Prev: Sen. Surg. Regist. & Sen. Cas. Off. St. Thos. Hosp. Lond.; Research Fell. Stanford Univ. Med. Center, Calif., USA; Hon. Sec. & Treas. Brit. Assn. Urol. Surgs.

VINNICOMBE, Sarah Jane Department of Radiology, St Bartholomew's Hospital, West Smithfield, London EC1A 7BE; Flat 2, 16 Lorn Road, Stockwell, London SW9 0AD — MB BS Lond. 1984 (St. Thos.) BSc (Hons.) Lond. 1981; MRCP (UK) 1987; FRCR 1993. Cons. Diagn. Radiol. St. Bart. Hosp. Lond. Specialty: Radiol. Prev: Sen. Regist. & Regist. (Diagn. Radiol.) St. Geo. Hosp. Lond.; Regist. (Med.) Univ. Coll. Hosp. Lond.

VINOD KUMAR, Indu 7 Crowden Walk, Pogmoor, Barnsley S75 2LU — MB BS Osmania 1978.

VINOD KUMAR, Mr Puzhankara Ambalavattah Whiston Hospital, Department of Plastic Surgery, Prescot L35 5DR Tel: 0151 430 1401 Fax: 0151 430 1855 — (Armed Forces Med. Coll.) MB BS Poona 1970; MS Chandigarh 1975, MCh 1979, MNAMS 1979; FRACS 1992. Cons. Plastic & Hand Surg. Whiston Hosp. Specialty: Plastic Surg. Socs: Plastic Surg. Soc. & Brit. Assn. Plastic Surgs.; Brit. Assn. Aesthetic Plastic Surgs.; Indian Assoc. of Ophthalmol. Prev: Cons. Plastic Surg. Pinderfields Gen. Hosp. Wakefield; Sen Research Fell. St. Vincents Hosp. Melbourne, Austral.; Assoc. Prof. Jipmer Pondicherry.

VINSON, Marianne Claire Argyll & Clyde Health Board, Ross House, Hawkhead Road, Paisley PA2 7BN Tel: 0141 842 7230 Email: marianne.vinson@achb.scot.nhs.uk; 9 Novar Drive, Glasgow G12 9PX Email: marianvin@aol.com — MB ChB Birm. 1987; MFPHM RCP (UK) 1995. p/t Cons. Pub. Health Med. Argyll & Clyde HB. Specialty: Pub. Health Med. Prev: Sen. Regist. (Pub. Health Med.) Oxf. RHA.

VINSON, Paul Selby The Surgery, 50 The Glade, Furnace Green, Crawley RH10 6JN Tel: 01293 612741; 5 River Mead, Crawley RH11 0NS — (Univ. Coll. Med. Sch.) MB BS Lond. 1991; MRCGP 1995; DRCOG 1995. GP Princip. Specialty: Gen. Pract. Prev: Trainee GP Crawley VTS; Ho. Off. (Surg.) Stoke-on-Trent; Ho. Off. (Med.) Warwick.

VINT, David Geoffrey Dyson (retired) Riverside Farm, Wooton Courtenay, Minehead TA24 8RE — MB BChir Camb. 1952 (Camb. & Lond. Hosp.) MA, MB BChir Camb. 1952. Prev: Surg. Lt. RNVR.

VIPOND, Amanda Jane 15 Queen's Down, Creech St Michael, Taunton TA3 5QY — BM Soton. 1990; MRCP (UK) 1995. SHO (Anaesth.) Exeter.

VIPOND, Mr Mark Neil Gloucestershire Royal Hospital, Gloucester GL1 3NN Tel: 01452 394675 Fax: 01452 394813 — MB BS Lond. 1983; FRCS Ed. 1987; FRCS Eng. 1987; MS Lond. 1991. Cons. Gen. Surg. Glos. Roy. Hosp. Specialty: Gen. Surg. Socs: Assn. Surg.; Surgic. Research Soc.; Brit. Soc. Gastroenterol. Prev: Sen. Regist. (Gen. Surg.) Bristol Roy. Infirm.; Lect. (Surg.) Univ. Bristol.

VIPULENDRAN, Velupillai Department of Child Health and Paediatrics, Withybush General Hospital, Fishguard Road, Haverfordwest SA62 2PZ Tel: 01437 773848 Fax: 01437 773848 Email: v.vipulendran@virgin.net; Redhill House, Camrose, Haverfordwest SA62 6HU Tel: 01437 764668 — MB BS Peredeniya 1974; FRCP (UK) & FRCPCH; Cert. Community Paediat. Warwick 1988; Dip. Community Paediat. Nottm. 1989. Cons. Community Paediat. Pembrokesh. NHS Trust. Specialty: Paediat. Prev: Regist. (Community Paediat.) Nottm. HA; Med. Off. (Clin.) Centr. Birm. HA; Regist. (Neonat. & Gen. Paediat.) Selly Oak Hosp. & Sorrento Matern. Hosp. Birm.

VIRAPEN, Matthew Peter The Country Medical Centre, 122 Ballinlea Road, Armoy, Ballymoney BT53 8TY Tel: 028 2075 1266 Fax: 028 2075 1122; 58 Boyland Road, Ballymoney BT53 8LJ — MRCS Eng. LRCP Lond. 1970.

VIRCHIS, Andres Eliseo Dept. of Haematology, Barnet Hospital, Wellhouse Lane, Barnet EN5 3DN Tel: 020 8216 4383 Fax: 020 8216 4837 Email: andres.virchis@barnet-chase-tr.nhs.uk — MB BS Lond. 1988 (Univ. Coll. Lond.) BSc Lond. 1985; MRCP (UK) 1991; DRCPath 1995; MRCPath 1999. Cons. Haemat. Barnet Hosp, Herts.; Hon. Cons. Haemat. Univ. Coll. Lond. Hosps. Lond. Specialty: Haematology. Socs: BMA; Brit. Soc. Haematol.; Amer. Soc. Haemat. Prev: Sen. Regist. (Haemat.) Roy. Free Hosp.; Sen. Regist. (Haemat.) Hillingdon Hosp.; Regist. (Haemat.) Hammersmith Hosp. & Northwick Pk. Hosp.

VIRDEE, Bhagwant Singh Kiran Virdee Medical Centre, Sultan Road, Lordswood, Chatham ME5 8TJ Tel: 01634 669221 Email: bhagwant.virdee@gp-g82664.nhs.uk — MB BS Bombay 1972 (Seth G S Med. Coll.) Gen. Practitioner, Chatham, kent. Specialty: Gen. Pract.

VIRDEE, Dara Singh Baxters Close Surgery, 2 Baxters Close, Beaumont Leys, Leicester LE4 0QR Tel: 0116 235 3579; 244 Astill Lodge Road, Leicester LE4 1EF Tel: 0116 236 6333 — BM BS Nottm. 1985 (Nottm. Univ.) DCH RCP Lond. 1988; DRCOG 1990; MRCGP 1990.

VIRDEE, Manjit Singh 39 Tenby Road, Moseley, Birmingham B13 9LX — MB ChB Leic. 1983.

VIRDEE, Munmohan Singh 529 Hurst Road, Bexley DA5 3JS — MB BS Lond. 1994 (UMDS of GUY's & St Thomas') BSc Hons. 1991; MRCP Uk 1997. BHF Jun. Research Fell., Dept. of Cardiol. St Geo.'s Hosp. Lond. Specialty: Cardiol.

VIRDEE, Tejinder Singh 128 Pinner Hill Road, Pinner HA5 3SH — MB ChB Manch. 1979. Clin. Med. Off. (Paediat. Home Care) St. Mary's Hosp. Lond. Prev: Regist. (Paediat.) Whipps Cross Hosp. Lond.; SHO (Cardiol.) Hosp. Sick Childr. Gt. Ormond St. Lond.

VIRDEN, Joy Collins Yalding Surgery, Burgess Bank, Benover Road, Yalding, Maidstone ME18 6ES Tel: 01622 814380 Fax: 01622 814549; The Court Lodge, Yalding, Maidstone ME18 6HX Tel: 01622 814509 Fax: 01622 814962 Email: joyvirden@aol.com — MB BChir Camb. 1971; MA Camb. 1972; DObst RCOG 1973. Specialty: Gen. Pract.

VIRDI, Deshminder Singh Central Hill Practice, 60 Central Hill, London SE19 1DT Email: g3vgh@clara.net — MB BS Lond. 1994 (St. Geos. Hosp. Med. Sch.) Specialty: Gen. Pract.

VIRDI, Mr Jaspal Singh Princess Alexandra Hospital, Hamstel Road, Harlow CM20 1QX Tel: 01279 827092 Fax: 01279 827093 — MB BS Kanpur 1970; FRCS (Urol.); FRCS Eng.; MS; FEBU (Fell. Europ. Bd. Urol.); MCh (Urol.). Cons. Urol. Surg. Specialty: Urol. Special Interest: Incontinence; Prostate Diseases (Cancer); Urin. Stones. Socs: Brit. Assn. Urol. Surg.; Europ. Assn. Urol.; Amer. Urol. Assn.

VIRDI, Rajiv Pritpal Singh Montague Health Centre, Oakenhurst Road, Blackburn BB2 1PP Tel: 01254 268416 Fax: 01254 268450; 2 Gib Lane, Livesey, Blackburn BB2 5BP Email: virdi@easynet.co.uk — MB BS Poona 1974. p/t Clin. Assit. (Endoscopy) Blackburn. Specialty: Gastroenterol. Socs: Fell. Roy. Soc. Med.

VIRGO, Fiona Emma Pettetts Farm House, East Green, Great Bradley, Newmarket CB8 9LU — MB BS Lond. 1997.

VIRGO, Morag Anne c/o D. Small, 26 Mansionhouse Road, Edinburgh EH9 2JD — MB ChB Glas. 1984; MRCGP 1988; T(G) 1991.

VIRJEE, James Pesi Directorate of Clinical Radiology, Bristol Royal Infirmary, Bristol BS2 8HW Tel: 0117 928 2729 — MB ChB Bristol 1970; FRCR 1976. Cons. Radiol. United Bristol Healthcare Trust. Specialty: Radiol.

VIRJEE, Shareen 157 Kyverdale Road, Stoke Newington, London N16 6PS Tel: 020 8806 3786 — MB ChB Ed. 1993 (Edinburgh) MRCP Ed. 1996. Specialist Regist. Rotat. (Diabetes & Endocrinol.) N. W. Thames; Specialist Regist. St Mary's Hosp. Specialty: Endocrinol.; Gen. Med. Socs: MRCP; Brit. Endocrine Societies; Diabetes UK. Prev: Specialist Regist. Rotat. Watford Gen. Hosp.; Specialist Regist. Rotat. Hemel Hempstead & Chelsea & Westminster Hosps.; Specialist Regist. Rotat. Chelsea & Westminster Hosps.

VIRJI, Abbas Abdulhussein Nasser St Giles Surgery, 40 St. Giles Road, London SE5 7RF Tel: 020 7252 5936; 40 Winterbrook Road, Herne Hill, London SE24 9JA Tel: 020 7737 3352 Fax: 020 7642 5946 — MB ChB Liverp. 1969; MRCGP 1974; MSc Lond. 1990. LMC. Specialty: Rehabil. Med.; Rheumatol. Prev: GP Tutor St. Thos. Dist.; Clin. Asst. (Rheum.) King's Healthcare.

VIRR, Mr Andrew Jonathan 10 Margaret Road, Headington, Oxford OX3 8NG Email: virr@btinternet.com — MBBchir, Camb 1995 (Univ. Camb. & Addenbrooke's Hosp.) BA (Hons.) Camb. 1993; MA Camb. 1997; MRCS 1999; MSC Birmingham 2000. SPR, (A&E) Oxf. Deanery. Specialty: Accid. & Emerg. Socs: BMA; FAEM; BAEM. Prev: SHO (Orthop.) Nuffield Orthop. Centre Oxf.; SHO (Urol.) Churchill Hosp. Oxf.; SHO (A & E) John Radcliffe Hosp. Oxf.

VIS-NATHAN, Sreeni Ravensworth Surgery, Horsley Hill Road, South Shields NE33 3ET Tel: 0191 428 0606 Fax: 0191 427 6159 — MB BS Kerala 1974.

VISAVADIA, Bhavin Gordhan 94 Marlborough Road, London N22 8NN — MB BS Lond. 1998.

VISHU (VISHWANATH), Mudigere Channaveerappa Western Isles Hospital, Stornoway, Isle of Lewis HS1 2AF Tel: 01851 704704 Fax: 01851 706240; 20 Braighe Road, Stornoway, Isle of Lewis Tel: 01851 702762 — MB BS Mysore 1974; MD; MRCP. Cons. Phys. (Cardiol.). Specialty: Gen. Med.; Neurol. Socs: Brit. Cardiac Soc.; BMA; Brit. Soc. Heart Failure.

VISHWABHAN, Mr Satya Prakash 103 Porlock Avenue, Weeping Cross, Stafford ST17 0HT — MB BS Lucknow 1969; FRCS Glas. 1987. Specialty: Orthop.

VISHWANATH, Luna Sharmila 22 Swallowdale, Wolverhampton WV6 8DT — MB BS Dacca 1983; FRCS Ed. 1991.

VISHWANATH, Mandagere Ramamurthy 10 Windermere Avenue, Eastern Green, Coventry CV5 7GP — MB BS Mysore 1987.

VISHWANATH, Mr Mayasandra Subramanyam 22 Swallowdale, Wolverhampton WV6 8DT — MB BS Bangalore 1979; FRCS Ed. 1987.

VISHWESHWAR RAO, Mr Vunnam Tyrone County Hospital, Omagh BT79 0AP Tel: 01662 45211 — MB BS Nagpur 1962; MS Andhra 1966; FRCS Glas. 1981; FRCS Ed. 1981. Assoc. Specialist Tyrone Co. Hosp. Omagh. Specialty: Urol. Socs: BMA.

VISICK, James Hedley (retired) Sherbrooke, Chandler Road, Stoke Holy Cross, Norwich NR14 8RQ Tel: 01508 494474 — (St. Bart.) MB BS Lond. 1961; DMRD Eng. 1967; FFR 1969; FRCR 1975. Prev: Cons. Radiol. Norf. & Norwich Hosp.

VISICK, Julia 134 Millstream Way, Leegomery, Telford TF1 6QT — MB ChB Birm. 1996.

VISICK, Robert Hedley (retired) 3 Lloyd Close, Heslington, York YO10 5EU Tel: 01904 411138 — MB BS Lond. 1957 (St. Bart.) DObst RCOG 1962; DCH Eng. 1964. Prev: SHO (Child Health) St. Bart. Hosp. Lond.

VISSER, Michael James Dixton Surgery, Dixton Road, Monmouth NP25 3PL Tel: 01600 712152 Fax: 01600 772634 — MB BS Lond. 1989; BSc Lond. 1986, MB BS 1989. GP Partnership, 3/4 Time. Prev: SHO (Anaesth.) Gloucester Roy. Hosp.

VISUVANATHAN, Shikandhini Princess Alexandra Hospital, Pathology Laboratory, Department of Microbiology, Hamstel Road, Harlow CM20 1QX Fax: 01279 416846 — MB BS Lond. 1983 (Middlx.) MSc Lond. 1991; MD Lond. 1992; MRCPath 1992; FRCP (Path) 2001. Cons. Microbiol. Princess Alexandra Hosp. Harlow. Specialty: Med. Microbiol. Socs: BMA; Hosp. Infec. Soc.; Assn. Med. Microbiologists. Prev: Sen. Regist. (Microbiol.) Univ. Coll. Hosp. Lond.

VISVA NATHAN, Sivapragasam Gosbury Hill Health Centre, Orchard Gardens, Chessington KT9 1AG Tel: 020 8397 2142 Fax: 020 8974 2717; Halton House, 22 Pelhams Walk, Esher KT10 8QD — MB ChB Glas. 1964; MRCP (UK) 1970; MRCGP 1980; FRCP Glas. 1989; FRCP Lond. 2002. Clin. Asst. (Thoracic & Gen. Med.) Kingston Hosp. Kingston u. Thames; Med. Off. Surbiton Gen. Hosp. Specialty: Cardiol.

VISVANATHAN, Shyamala Padmini — MRCS Eng. LRCP Lond. 1978; CCST; MRCPsych. Cons. (Psychiat.) Harperbury. Prev: SHO (Anaesth.) Wexham Pk. Hosp.; Ho. Off. (Med.) Law Hosp.; SHO (Anaesth.) Hull Roy. Infirm.

VISWALINGAM, Niramala Devi Moorfields Eye Hospital, City Road, London EC1V 2PD Tel: 020 8946 6407; 2 Peek Crescent, Wimbledon, London SW19 5ER — MB BS Madras 1967 (Christ. Med. Coll. Vellore) DO RCS Eng. 1970. Assoc. Specialist Moorfields Eye Hosp. Lond.; Clin. Research Assoc. Inst. Ophth. Socs: Fac. Ophth.; Fell. Roy. Soc. Med. Prev: Regist. & SHO Kings Coll. Hosp. Lond.

VISWAN, Anjiparampil Kumaran Warwick Hospital, Lakin Road, Warwick CV34 5BW Tel: 01926 495321 Fax: 01926 403715 Email: vis.viswan@swh.nhs.uk — MB BS Kerala 1965 (Trivandrum Med. Coll.) DCH RCPS Glas. 1970; MRCP (UK) 1975; FRCP Lond. 1988; FRCP Ed. 1992. Cons. Phys. S. Warks. Gen. Hosps. NHS Trust. Specialty: Gen. Med.; Care of the Elderly. Socs: BMA. Prev: Sen. Regist. (Geriat. Med.) E. Birm. Hosp.

VISWANATH, Immaneni King George Hospital, Goodmayes, Ilford IG3 8YB Tel: 020 8983 8000 — MB BS Banaras Hindu 1968; MD Banaras Hindu 1973; MRCP (UK) 1980. Cons. Phys. in Acute Med. King Geo. Hosp. Ilford. Specialty: Gastroenterol. Prev: Assoc. Specialist (Med. & Gastroenterol.) King Geo. Hosp. Ilford; Sen. Regist. (Med.) Armed Forces Hosp. Riyadh, Saudi Arabia; Regist. (Med. & Gastroenterol.) Dudley Hosp.

VISWANATHAN, Ananth Chitur Moorfields Eye Hospital, City Road, London EC1V 2PD Tel: 0207 5662625 Fax: 0207 5662972 — MB BS Lond. 1989; BSc (Hons.) Lond. 1986; FRCOphth 1994; MD London 2001. p/t Consultant Surgeon. Specialty: Ophth. Prev: SHO (Ophth.) St. Thos. Hosp. Lond.; Specialist Regist. Rotat. (Ophth.) N. Thames; Internat. Glaucoma Assn. Research Fell. Inst. Ophth. Lond.

VISWANATHAN, Manickam The Surgery, 20 Kendal Parade, Silver Street, Edmonton, London N18 1ND Tel: 020 8803 0020; 2 Crowland Gardens, Southgate, London N14 6AP — MB BS Ceylon 1968.

VISWANATHAN, Palamiswamy Urology Department, Pontefract General Infimary, Friarwood Lane, Pontefract WF8 1PL — MB BS Madras 1971.

VISWESVARAIAH, Manickam The Clinic, Barbers Avenue, Rawmarsh, Rotherham S62 6AD Tel: 01709 522831 — MB BS Madras 1974.

VITAL, Marcos Freddy Dean Cross Surgery, 21 Radford Park Road, Plymstock, Plymouth PL9 9DL Tel: 01752 404743 — MRCS Eng. LRCP Lond. 1971; DObst RCOG 1973. GP Princip. Plymouth (Senior Partner); Adjudicating Med. Practitioner BAMS; Occ. Health Physician Med. Adviser Tecalemit Plymouth, Gleason Work Ltd. Plymouth; Ldr. RAF St. Mawgan Cornw.; Med. Adviser Becton Dickinson Ltd. Plymouth; Med. Adviser Gleason Works Ltd.; Examr. Norwegian Med. Directorate. Socs: Pres. Plymouth Med. Soc. & Sec. Exchange with France. Prev: Civil. Med. Pract. & Sen. Med. Off. RAF Mt.batten Plymouth.; Sen. Med. Off. No. 3 MHU RAF St. Mawgan at Rank of Sqad.

VITES, Jillian 56 Belsize Road, London NW6 4TG Tel: 020 7372 6845 — MB ChB Manch. 1973; MRCPsych 1977. Clin. Asst., Adolesc. Dept. Tourstoch Clinic. Specialty: Gen. Surg.; Psychother. Socs: Assoc. Mem. Inst. Psychoanal., RCPsych.

VITES, Nicholas Paul Naylor Street Surgery, 4 Naylor Street, Manchester M40 7JH Tel: 0161 205 3177 Email: nick.vites@lineone.net — MB ChB Manch. 1978; MRCP (UK) Glas. 1982.

VITHANA, Tilaka Alderney Hospital, Poole BH12 4NB Tel: 01202 735537 Fax: 01202 730657; 63A Cynthia Road, Parkstone, Poole BH12 3JE Tel: 01202 380643 — MB BS Ceylon 1967 (Colombo) Assoc. Specialist (Ment. Illness) Alderney Hosp. Poole. Specialty: Geriat. Psychiat. Socs: Affil. Roy. Coll. Psychiat. Prev: Clin. Asst. (Psychogeriat.) Alderney Hosp. Poole; Regist. (Psychiat.) Herrison Hosp. Dorchester.

VITHAYATHIL, Kurian Joseph Genitourinary Clinic Leatherhead Hospital, Polar Road, Leatherhead KT22 8SD Tel: 01372 362845 Fax: 01372 378498 — MB BS Poona 1979; MRCP (UK) 1985. Cons. Phys. (Genitourin. Med.) Leatherhead Hosp. Specialty: Genitourinary Medicine; HIV Med. Socs: BMA; Med. Soc. Study VD. Prev: Sen. Regist. (Genitourin. Med.) Soton. Univ. NHS Trust; Regist. Genitourin. Med. Roy. Berks. Hosp. Reading.

VITTLE, June Emily (retired) Pwllderi, 13 Rock House Est., Letterston, Haverfordwest SA62 5SQ Tel: 01348 451 — MB BCh Wales 1957 (Cardiff) Prev: Med. Asst. (Geriat.) Withybush Gen. Hosp. HaverfordW.. Assoc. Mem.

VITTY, Frederick Peeter Meldrum, Vitty and Pfeiffer, 40-42 Kingsway, Waterloo, Liverpool L22 4RQ Tel: 0151 928 2415 Fax: 0151 928 3775; Oakley, 4 Abbotsford Road, Blundellsands, Liverpool L23 6UX — MB Camb. 1980 (Camb. & St. Geo.) BChir 1979. Prev: Ho. Off. (Surg.) Ashford Gen. Hosp. Middlx.; Ho. Off. (Med.) St.Geo. Hosp. Lond.; Trainee GP Chester VTS.

VIVA, Mr Charles Middlesbrough General Hospital, Ayresome Green Lane, Middlesbrough TS5 5AZ Tel: 01642 850850 Fax: 01642 854136 — MB BS Punjab 1961; FRCS Ed. 1968; FRCS Eng. 1969; T(S) 1991. Sen. Cons. Plastic, Aesthetic & Hand Surg. Middlesbrough Gen. Hosp.; DL. Specialty: Plastic Surg.

VIVE, Jeremy Utaman c/o X-Ray Department, Crawley Hospital, West Green Drive, Crawley RH11 7DH Tel: 01293 527866 — MB BS Lond. 1982 (St. Thos.) BSc (Hons.) Lond. 1979, MB BS 1982; FRCR 1990; T(R) (CR) 1991. Cons. Radiol. Mid Downs HA. Specialty: Radiol. Prev: Sen. Regist. Rotat. (Diag. Radiol.) Leicester Roy. Infirm.; Regist. Rotat. (Radiol.) Qu. Med. Centre Nottm.; SHO Rotat. (Gen. Med.) City Hosp. Nottm.

VIVEKANANDA, Chatchithanantham The Surgery, 42 Central Road, Morden SM4 5RT — MB BS Sri Lanka 1976; LRCP LRCS Ed. LRCPS Glas. 1985; DGM RCP Lond. 1985. Trainee GP Purley. Prev: SHO (Geriat. Med.) St. Helier Hosp. Carshalton & Sutton Hosp.; SHO (A & E) N. Middlx. Hosp. Lond.; SHO (Dermat.) Grimsby Dist. Gen. Hosp.

VIVEKANANDAMURTY, Kadiyala 36 Braithwaite Road, Lowton, Warrington WA3 2AY Tel: 01942 718221 — MB BS Andhra 1975.

VIVEKANANTHAN, Malarvizhi 188 Ashbourne Road, Mitcham CR4 2DQ — MB BS Lond. 1993.

VIVIAN, Charles Trevarthen Benedict, Squadron Ldr. RAF Med. Br. Retd. Adastral Health Ltd., 1 Woodside Business Park, Whitley Wood Lane, Reading RG2 8LW Email: charlievivian@adastral.co.uk — MB BS Lond. 1988 (St. Thos. Hosp. Lond.) MRCGP 1994; DFFP 1996; Dip CPC 1996; AFOM 2003. Occupat. Med. Socs: Christ. Med. Fellowsh.; Soc. Occup. Med. Prev: Princip. GP; GP RAF Mt. Pleasant, Falkland Is.s & RAF High Wycombe; Trainee GP RAF Gutersloh VTS.

VIVIAN, Patrick Cyril (retired) Pumney, Drayton Road, Sutton Courteney, Abingdon OX14 4AJ Tel: 01235 848205 — MB BChir Camb. 1953 (Westm.) MA Camb. 1958, MB BChir 1953; DObst RCOG 1958. Prev: GP Abingdon.

VIVIAN, Peter Graham (retired) 21 Southern Lane, Barton-on-Sea, New Milton BH25 7JA — MB ChB Liverp. 1952.

VIVIERS, Louis Flat 2, Clare Court, 54 Clarendon Road, London W11 2HJ Email: louistin@dircon.co.uk — MB ChB Stellenbosch 1988.

VIVORI, Elena (retired) 7 Dudlow Grange, Green Lane, Liverpool L18 2EP — MD Genoa 1958 (University of Genoa) LRCP LRCS Ed. LRCPS Glas. 1966; DA Eng. 1969; FFA RCS Eng. 1972. Prev: Cons. Paediat. Anaesth. Alder Hey Childr.'s Hosp., Liverp.

VIZE, Mr Charles Edward (retired) 1 Mornington Villas, Manningham, Bradford BD8 7HB Tel: 01274 546861 Fax: 01274 487705; Cotswold, 18 Southfield Road, Burley-in-Wharfedale, Ilkley LS29 7PA Tel: 01943 863198 — BSc (Hons.) NUI 1969, MB BCh BAO 1967; FRCS Ed. 1973. Prev: Lect. (Otorhinolaryng.) Univ. Liverp. & ENT Infirm. Liverp.

VIZE, Christine Mary Avon and Wiltshire Mental Health Partnership NHS Trust, Green Lane Hospital, Devizes SN10 5DS Tel: 01380 731200 Fax: 01380 731308 Email: christine.vize@awp.nhs.uk — MB BChir Camb. 1986; MA Camb. 1987; MRCPsych 1990. Cons. Gen. Adult Psychiat. & Dep. Med. Director, Avon & Wilts. Partnership. Specialty: Gen. Psychiat. Prev: Lect. & Hon. Sen. Regist. St. Mary's Hosp. Med. Sch. Lond.; Hon. Regist. (Psychiat.) Addenbrooke's Hosp Camb.; Regist. (Psychiat.) Fulbourn Hosp. Camb.

VIZE, Mr Colin John 3 St Chads Grove, Headingley, Leeds LS6 3PN — MB BS Newc. 1993 (Newc. Upon Tyne) FRCPath. Coll of Ophchalmology, 1998. Specialist Regist. (Ophth.), Yorks., Deanery. Specialty: Ophth. Prev: SHO (Ophth.) St James Univ. Hosp. Leeds; SHO (Ophth.) Sunderland Eye Infirm.; SHO (Neurosurg.) Regional Neurosci. Centre Newc. Gen. Hosp.

VIZZA, Enrico Royal Free Hospital, Department of Obstetrics & Gynaecology, Minimally Invasive Therapy Unit, Pond St., London NW3 2QG — State DMS Rome 1994.

VLACHOU, Paraskevi 35 Oliver Court, London Rd, Leicester LE2 2PQ — MB ChB Leic. 1997.

VLACHTSIS, Helen 22 Heycroft, Gibbet Hill, Coventry CV4 7HE Tel: 024 76 414463; Flat 1, 1 Gillbrook Road, Didsbury, Manchester M20 6WH Tel: 0161 448 7246 — MB ChB Manch. 1995; FRCA; BSc (Hons) Physiol. Manch. 1992. SHO (Anaesth.) Roy. Oldham Hosp.; Cons. Anaesth. & Intens. Care Wytheshawe Hosp. Specialty: Anaesth. Socs: Fell. Manch. Med. Soc.; MRCAnaesth.; BMA. Prev: SHO (Chest Med./Cardiol.) Wythenshawe Hosp.; Ho. Off. (Surg.) MRI; Ho. Off. (Med.) Hope Hosp. Salford.

VLASTO, Mr Philip (retired) Little Ham, The Common, Child Okeford, Blandford Forum DT11 8QY Tel: 01258 861359 — BM BCh Oxf. 1943 (Lond. Hosp.) FRCS Eng. 1979. Prev: Mem. Med. & Survival Comm. & Med. Ref. RNLI.

VLIES, Margaret Joan Hillcrest Medical Centre, Holt Road, Wrexham LL13 8RG; 3 Croeshowell Court, Croeshowell Hill, Rossett, Wrexham LL12 0AA Tel: 01244 571307 — (Guy's) MB BS Lond. 1975; MRCS Eng. LRCP Lond. 1975; DRCOG 1979; MRCGP 1981. Asst. GP Wrexham. Prev: Trainee GP Carshalton VTS.

VLIES, Mr Philip Robin 3 Croeshowell Court, Croeshowell Hill, Rossett, Wrexham LL12 0AA Tel: 01244 571307 — MB BChir Camb. 1971 (Camb. & St. Mary's) MA, MB Camb. BChir 1971; FRCOG 1989, M 1976; FRCS Ed. 1977. Cons. O & G Wrexham Maelor Hosp. NHS Trust. Specialty: Obst. & Gyn. Prev: Lect. & Sen. Regist. (O & G) Middlx. Hosp. Lond.; Sen. Regist. Nat. Wom.'s Hosp. Auckland, New Zealand; Resid. Med. Off. Qu. Charlotte's Hosp. Lond.

VLISSIDES, Dimitrios Nikolaos 239 School Road, Sheffield S10 1GN Tel: 0114 266 4110 — Ptychio Iatrikes Athens 1972 (Athens Med. Sch.) PhD Sheff. 1976. Lect. Dept. Psychiat. Univ. Sheff. & Roy. Hallamshire Hosp. Socs: Roy. Coll. Psychiat. (Mem. Collegiate Trainees' Comm. & Represen. Coll. Educat. Comm.). Prev: Sen. Regist. Fulbourn Hosp.; Clin. Research Asst. Univ. Sheff.

VODDEN, Ms Julie Jane — MB ChB Bristol 1986; DA (UK) 1988; DRCOG 1991; MRCGP 1992; (FRCS Ed.) 1999. Staff Grade (Ophth.) MusGr. Pk. Hosp. Taunton. Specialty: Ophth. Socs: Roy. Coll. Ophth.

VOETEN, F Danetre Medical Practice, The Health Centre, London Road, Daventry NN11 4EJ Tel: 01327 703333 Fax: 01327 311221 — Artsexamen Nijmegen 1991 (Univ. Katholieke Nijmegen) DRCOG 1995.

VOGEL, Louis (retired) 25 Sandringham House, Windsor Way, London W14 0UD Tel: 020 7603 5581 Email: louis.vogel@ntlworld.com — MB BS Lond. 1945 (St. Bart.) DCP Lond 1950; FRCPath 1976, M 1964. Prev: Cons. Path. Newham HA & Roy. Lond. Hosp.

VOGEL, Markus Werner Flat 1, 13 Essendine Road, London W9 2LT — State Exam Med Frankfurt 1993.

VOGEL, Mary Louise William Harvey Hospital, Kennington Road, Ashford TN24 0LZ — MB ChB Bristol 1981; MRCPsych 1986. Cons. Psychiat. E. Kent Partnership Trust. Specialty: Gen. Psychiat. Prev: Cons. Psychiat. S. Kent Community Healthcare Trust; Sen. Regist. E. Anglian RHA; Regist. & SHO Barrow Hosp. Bristol.

VOGEL, Melanie 286A The Broadway, London NW9 6AE — State Exam Med Berlin 1994.

VOGELZANG, Sophia Antonia Mitchell and Partners, New Chapel Surgery, High Street, Long Crendon, Aylesbury HP18 9AF Tel: 01844 208228 Fax: 01844 201906 — MB BChir Camb. 1992. Trainee GP/SHO Stoke Mandeville Hosp. Specialty: Ment. Health. Prev: Ho. Off. St. Thos. & Roy. Sussex Co. Hosps.; Ho. Off. (Oncol. & Radiother.) Northampton Gen. Hosp.

VOGLER, Eleanor Jillian Arnott (retired) — (Bristol) MB ChB Bristol 1961; DPM Eng. 1965; MRCPsych 1972; MA Peace Studies Bradford 1994. Prev: Cons. Psychiat. Rehabil. Lynfield Mt. Hosp.

VOGT, Julie 71 Rodenhurst Road, London SW4 8AF — MB BS Lond. 1991 (St. Thomas' Hospital London) Specialist Regist. (Paediat.) Barnet Gen. Hosp. Specialty: Paediat.

VOGT, Stephen 101 Manthorpe Road, Grantham NG31 8DG Tel: 01476 565 232 Fax: 01476 567 567 — MB BChir Camb. 1978 (St. Mary's) BChir 1977; MA Camb. 1978; MRCOG 1986; FRCOG 1998. Cons. O & G Grantham & Dist. Gen. Hosp. Lincs. Specialty: Obst. & Gyn. Special Interest: Infertil. Prev: Sen. Regist. Queens Mary's Hosp. Roehamton.

VOGT MANDUCA, Ursula Western Eye Hospital, Marylebone Road, London NW1 Tel: 020 7935 0886 Email: uvogt1@aol.com — State Exam Med Dusseldorf 1978 (Univ. Dusseldorf) MD Ophth. Dusseldorf 1980. Assoc. Specialist West. Eye Hosp. Lond.; Med. Ophth. & Contact Lens Pract. Harley St. Specialty: Ophth. Special Interest: Contact Lens Work; Diabetes; General Ophthalmology. Socs: Eur. Contact Lens Soc. Ophth.; Roy. Coll. Ophth.; Roy. Soc. of Med. Prev: Clin. Asst. West. Ophth. Hosp. Lond.; Clin. Asst. Moorfields Eye Hosp.; Resid. Asst. Univ. Clinic Dusseldorf, Germany.

VOGWELL, Paul Charles 37 Rosemount Close, Oxton, Birkenhead CH43 2LR — MB BS Lond. 1988; BSc Lond. 1985, MB BS 1988. Regtl. Med. Off. Roy. Army Med. Corps.

VOHRA, Akbar Department of Anaesthesia, Manchester Royal Infirmary, Oxford Road, Manchester M13 9WL Tel: 0161 276 4552 Fax: 0161 276 8027; Squirrels Chase, Lea Bank Close, Macclesfield SK11 8PU — MB ChB Manch. 1983 (Manchester) DA (UK) 1985; FCAnaesth 1989. Cons. Anaesth.(Cardiac Anaesth. and Intens. Care) Manch. Roy. Infirm. Specialty: Anaesth. Socs: Assn. Anaesth. Gt. Brit. & Irel. & Anaesth. Research Soc.; Assn. of Cardiothoracic Anaesth.s; Soc. of Critical Care Med. Prev: Sen. Regist. (Anaesth.) NW RHA; Regist. Rotat. (Anaesth.) Wigan Hosp. & Manch. Roy. Infirm.; SHO (Neonat. Med.) St. Mary's Hosp. Manch.

VOHRA, Ameet Oak Lodge, Lee Chapel Lane, Basildon SS16 5NX — MB BS Lond. 1993.

VOHRA, Anjna Devi c/o P. Vohra, 115 Arundel Drive, Harrow HA2 8PW Tel: 020 8864 1343 — MB BS Punjab 1943 (Lady Hardinge Med. Coll. New Delhi)

VOHRA, Jatinder Paul Singh 7 Edlington Drive, Nottingham NG8 2TD — MB ChB Sheff. 1993.

VOHRA, Shashi West Sussex Health & Social Care NHS Trust, Martyn Long Centre, 78 Crawley Road, Horsham RH12 4HN Tel: 01403 266966 Fax: 01403 272140; 2 Wells Close, Horsham RH12 1US Tel: 01403 265296 — MB BS Delhi 1965 (Lady Hardinge Med. Coll.) DGO Delhi 1968; DObst RCOG 1970; Cert. JCC Lond. 1977; DFFP 1993. Assoc. Specialist (Learning Disabil.) Martyn Long Centre Horsham. Specialty: Ment. Health; Family Plann. & Reproduc. Health. Prev: SHO (Obst.) Bushey Matern. Hosp. & City of Lond. Matern. Hosp.; Med. Off. Birm. Family Plann. Assn.

VOHRA, Shiv Lal PO Box 626, Horsham RH12 1YP; 2 Wells Close, Horsham RH12 1US Tel: 01403 265296 — MB BS Delhi 1964 (Maulana Azad Med. Coll.) DPM Eng. 1969. Cons. Psychiat. W. Sussex Health & Social Care NHS Trust. Specialty: Ment. Health. Prev: Sen. Regist. (Psychiat.) Chelmsley Hosp. Birm. & Child Guid. Centre Covenrty; Regist. (Psychiat.) Centr. Middlx. Hosp. Lond.; Med. Off. (Psychiat.) Maulana Azad Med. Coll. & Assoc. Hosps. New Delhi, India.

VOHRA, Suleman 5 Roundwood Avenue, Reedleu, Burnley BB10 2LH — MB BS Karachi 1962.

VOHRA, Sumeet Abbey Lane Surgery, 23 Abbey Lane, Sheffield S8 0BJ Tel: 0114 274 5360 Fax: 0114 274 9580 — MB BS Lond. 1990 (Charing Cross & Westminster) MBBS Lond. 1992; MRCGP 1992. GP Princip.; Dir. Sheff. GP Co-op. Specialty: Gen. Pract. Socs: Sheff. Medicolegal Soc.

VOHRAH, Anil Raj Walsgrove Hospital, Clifford Bridge Road, Coventry — MB BS Lond. 1986; MRCP (UK) 1989; FRCR 1994. Cons. Walsgrave Hosp. NHS Trust. Specialty: Radiol.

VOHRAH, Ram Chand The Surgeries, Lombard Street, Newark NG24 1XG Tel: 01636 702363 Fax: 01636 613037; 25 Greet Lily Mill, Station Road, Southwell NG25 0GL — MB BS Lond. 1986 (Westm.) MRCGP 1994. Specialty: Dermat.

VOICE, Allan Flaxmead House, Chesterfield Road, Tibshelf, Derby — MB BS Lond. 1974 (St. Mary's) MRCS Eng. LRCP Lond. 1974; FFA RCS Eng. 1981. Cons. Centr. Notts. HA. Specialty: Anaesth.

VOICE, Elizabeth Andrea St Michael's Hospital, C E D U, Trent Valley Road, Lichfield WS13 6EF — MB ChB Leeds 1988; MRCGP 1992; DCCH Warwick 1996. Staff Grade (Comm. Paediat.) SE Staffs. Specialty: Community Child Health. Prev: Locum GP Lichfield; SHO (Palliat. Med.) Derbysh. Roy. Infirm.; Trainee GP Westgate Pract. Lichfield.

VOICE, Sally-Anne Mathers Townhead Practice, Links Health Centre, Marine Avenue, Montrose DD10 8TR Tel: 01674 76161 Fax: 01674 673151 — MB ChB Dundee 1992; DRCOG 1995; DFFP 1995. Partner, Townhead Practice . Montrose. Socs: BMA; MDU.

VOIGHT, Mary (retired) 33 Mereheath Park, Knutsford WA16 6AS Tel: 01565 632846 — (Liverp.) MB ChB Liverp. 1962. Prev: Sen. Med. Off. DSS.

VOISEY, Miss Sarah Carolyn 16 Port Lane, Hursley, Winchester SO21 2JS Tel: 01962 775447 — BM Soton. 1993; FRCS 1998. SHO Anaesth. St Richards Hosp. Chichestr. Specialty: Intens. Care; Anaesth. Socs: BMA. Prev: Regist. Paediat. Surg., Soton., Gen. Hosp.; SHO Intens. Care, Qu. Alexandra Hosp. Portsmouth; SHO (Gen. Surg.) N. Hants. Hosp. Basingstoke, Poole Hosp, Dorset & Qu. Alexandra Hosp. Portsmouth.

VOKE, Jennifer Mary Haematology Department, Queen Elizabeth II Hospital, Welwyn Garden City AL7 4HQ Tel: 01707 365209; 16 Hollybushh Lane, Harpenden AL5 4AT Tel: 01582 460739 — (Univ. Coll. Hosp.) FRCPath; MRCS Eng. LRCP Lond. 1968; MB BS Lond. 1968; MRCPath 1975. Cons. Haemat. Luton & Dunstable Hosp. NHS Trust, Beds. Specialty: Haematology. Prev: Sen. Regist. (Haemat.) Roy. Free Hosp. Lond.; Regist. (Haemat.) Univ. Coll. Hosp. Lond.; Leukaemia Research Fell. Hosp. Sick Childr. Gt. Ormond St. Lond.

VOKINS, Amanda Jane Oakleigh House, Low Road, Strumpshaw, Norwich NR13 4HU Tel: 01603 715966 — MB BS Lond. 1989 (Middlx. Hosp.) DCH RCP Lond. 1991; DRCOG 1992; MRCGP 1995. GP on Retainer Scheme, Norwich. Prev: Salaried Gen. Practitioner Norwich.

VOKINS, Colin Guy The Surgery, 42 Upper Rock Gardens, Brighton BN2 1QF Tel: 01273 600103 Fax: 01273 620100 — (St. Thos.) MB BS Lond. 1966; DObst RCOG 1969.

VOLANS, Mr Andrew Philip Accident & Emergency Department, Scarborough Hospital, Woodlands Drive, Scarborough YO12 6QL Email: andrew.volans@acute.sney.nhs.uk; Chestnut Cottage, Bridge Close, Burniston, Scarborough YO13 0HS — MB ChB Leeds 1983; BSc (Hons.) Leeds 1978; DA (UK) 1986; FRCS Ed. 1988; FFAEM 1996. Cons. (A & E) ScarBoro. Hosp. Specialty: Accid. & Emerg. Socs: BMA & Fac. Accid. & Emerg. Med.; Roy. Coll. Surg. Edin. Prev: Sen. Regist. (A & E) Roy. Hallamsh. Hosp. Sheff.; Regist. (Neurosurg.) Maudsley Hosp. Lond.; Regist. (Orthop.) & SHO Rotat. Airedale HA.

VOLANS, Glyn Noel — BSc (Hons. Physiol.) Durham. 1965; MB BS Newc. 1968; MRCP (UK) 1972; MD Newc. 1975; FRCP Lond. 1984. Dir. Med. Toxicology Unit & Cons. Phys. Guy's & St. Thomas' Hosp. Trust; Hon. Sen. Lect. UMDS. Specialty: Gen. Med. Socs: Fell. Roy. Soc. Med.; Brit. Toxicol. Soc.; Brit. Pharmacol. Soc. Prev: SHO Artific. Kidney Unit & Gen. Med. Roy. Vict. Infirm. Newc.; Regist. (Gen. Med.) Newc. Gen. Hosp.; Research Fell. Clin. Pharmacol. & Migraine Clinic St. Bart. Hosp.

VOLGER, Annette Jacqueline 9 Woodthorpe Road, Putney, London SW15 6UQ — MB BS Lond. 1985; FRCA 1991. Sen. Regist. Rotat. (Anaesth.) Char. Cross Hosp. Lond. Specialty: Anaesth. Socs: BMA & Roy. Soc. Med.

VOLIKAS, Ingrid 44 Greenhill Gdns, Merrow Park, Guildford GU4 7HH — MB BS Lond. 1993.

VOLK, Heather Margaret Jean Jaguar Cars halewood, Halewood, Liverpool L24 Tel: 0151 443 4320; 46 Heyes Lane, Alderley Edge SK9 7JY Tel: 0151 485 6320 — MB BS Lond. 1976 (Guy's) MRCS Eng. LRCP Lond. 1976; MRCGP 1982; MFOM RCP Lond. 1994, AFOM 1987. Sen. Med. Off. Jaguar Cars Ltd.; Med. Adviser John Lewis Partnership. Specialty: Occupat. Health. Socs: Soc. Occupat. Med.

VOLKERS, Mr Robert Charles 29 Hans Place, London SW1X 0JY Tel: 020 7584 7435 Fax: 020 7225 2816; Penleigh Mill, Dilton Marsh, Westbury Tel: 01373 822142 — MB BS Lond. 1967 (St. Bart.) MRCS Eng. LRCP Lond. 1967; FRCS Eng. 1973. Prev: Regist. Plastic Surg. Frenchay Hosp. Bristol.

VOLLUM, Dorothy Isabella (retired) Flat 1, 15 St Germans Place, London SE3 0NN Tel: 020 8858 3741 — MB BS Lond. 1960 (St.

Bart.) DCH Eng. 1964; FRCP Lond. 1979, M 1965; AMQ 1966; UKCP 2000; MSc 2000. Prev: Cons. Dermat. Lewisham Hosp.

VOLPE, Nicola 50 Castle Road, Mount Sorrel, Loughborough LE12 7EU — State Exam Rome 1980.

VON ARX, Mr Derek Peter Maxillofacial Unit, Luton and Dunstable Hospital, Lewsey Road, Luton LU4 0DZ Tel: 01582 497333 Fax: 01582 718069 Email: derek.vonarx@nhs.net; Westwood House, 19 Highfields, Bedford MK45 5GN Tel: 01525 714039 Email: derekvonarx@66sisters.freeserve.co.uk — MB BS Lond. 1993 (Kings Coll. Lond.) BDS Lond. 1978; FDS RCS Ed. 1984; FRCS Ed. 1997; FRCS (OMFS) 2000. Cons. (Oral & Maxillofacial Surg.) Luton and Dunstable Hosp.; Cons. (Oral & Maxillofacial Surg.) The Lister Hosp., Stevenage. Specialty: Oral & Maxillofacial Surg. Socs: BMA; Fell. Brit. Assn. Oral & Maxillofacial Surg. Prev: Specialist Regist. (Oral & Maxillofacial Surg.) Kent and Canterbury Hosp., Guy's Hosp. Lond., St. Geo.s Hosp., Lond.

VON BACKSTROM, Andre George 20 Lackford Road, Coulsdon CR5 3TA Tel: 01737 552785 Fax: 01737 556945 Email: avonb@aol.com; 20 Lackford Road, Coulsdon CR5 3TA Tel: 01737 552785 Fax: 01737 556945 Email: avonb@aol.com — MB ChB Pretoria 1988 (University of Pretoria) Sedationist in NHS Dent. Pract.s. Specialty: Anaesth. Socs: Social Coordinator for S.O.C.S. (Soc. for Conscious Sedation); SAAD (Soc. for Advancem. of Anaesth. in Dent.); ADA (Assn. of Dent. Anaesthestists). Prev: Hon. Clin. Asst. Anaesthetic Dept. Roy. Berks. Hosp. Reading.

VON BERGEN, Julian Edward (retired) Hatch Green Lodge, Hatch Beauchamp, Taunton TA3 6TN Tel: 01823 480884 — BM BCh Oxf. 1949 (St. Bart.) BM BCh Oxon. 1949. Prev: Capt. RAMC.

VON BERGEN, Mrs Sheila (retired) Hatch Green Lodge, Hatch Beauchamp, Taunton TA3 6TN Tel: 01823 480884 — BM BCh Oxf. 1949 (St. Bart.) BM BCh Oxon. 1949.

VON BERTELE, Michael James, OBE(Mil), OBE, Brigadier Ministry of Defence, Defence Medical Services Department , Floor 7 Zone G, Main Building, Whitehall, London SW1A 2HB Tel: 0207 8070471 Fax: 0207 2181447 Email: mike.vonbertele344@mod.uk — MB BCh Wales 1979 (WNSM Cardiff) DAvMed FOM RCP Lond. 1986; DIH RCP Lond. 1989; MFOM RCP Lond. 1992. Cons. (Occupat. Med.) Army. Specialty: Occupat. Health. Socs: Soc. Occupat. Med.

VON BIEL, Thomas Arnim 11 Newling Way, High Salvington, Worthing BN13 3DG — MB ChB Otago 1986.

VON EICHSTORFF, Peter Daniel George Dr Robson and Partners, Manzil Way, Cowley Road, Oxford OX4 1XD Tel: 01865 242109; 60 Bagley Wood Road, Kennington, Oxford OX1 5LY — MB ChB Dundee 1988; MA (Hons.) Dundee 1982. Specialty: Gen. Pract. Socs: Roy. Coll. Gen. Pract.; BMA. Prev: Ships Med. Off. Actaeon Shipping.

VON FRAGSTEIN, Martin Franz Frederick Prestwood House Surgery, 74 Midway Road, Midway, Swadlincote DE11 7PG Tel: 01283 212375 Fax: 01283 551923 — BM BS Nottm. 1984; BMedSci Nottm. 1982; DGM RCP Lond. 1987; MRCGP 1988; T(GP) 1991; MMedSci Nottm. 1998. Lect. (Gen. Pract.) Univ. Nottm.; Hon. Sec. Nottm. Guild Catholic Doctors. Specialty: Palliat. Med.

VON FRAUNHOFER, Michael Anthony Heald Green Health Centre, Finney Lane, Heald Green, Stockport SK7 3JD Tel: 0161 436 8384 Fax: 0161 493 9268 — MB ChB Manch. 1990; MRCGP 1994; T(GP) 1994; D.Occ.Med. RCP Lond. 1996. Occupat. Health Phys. Tameside Gen. Hosp.; Med. Off. St Anne's Hospice; Med. Off. Francis Ho. Specialty: Gen. Pract.; Occupat. Health; Palliat. Med. Socs: Fac. Occupat. Med.

VON FRAUNHOFER, Nicola Anne Merton Child & Family Service, Cricket Green Polyclinic, Birches Close, Cricket Green, Mitcham CR4 4LQ Tel: 020 8770 8828 Fax: 020 8770 8848 — (Bristol) MB ChB Bristol 1988; MRCPsych 1993. Cons. (Child & Adolesc. Psychiat.) Merton Child Guid. Clinic. Specialty: Child & Adolesc. Psychiat. Prev: St. Geo. Hosp. Train. Schemes (Psychiat./Child & Adolesc. Psychiat.).

VON GOETZ, Therese Campbell Bolling Chesterhill, Newport-on-Tay DD6 8QY — MB ChB Dundee 1987; BA Oxf. 1984; FRCS Eng. 1993. Research S. Thames Deaner. Specialty: Neurosurg. Socs: BMA (Jun. Doctor Comm.); Med. Wom. Federat.; Guild Catholic Doctors. Prev: Regist. (Neurosurg.) Atkinson Morley's Hosp.; SHO (Gen. Surg.) Basingstoke Dist. Hosp.; SHO (Gen. Surg.) Roy. Berks. Hosp. Reading.

VON KAISENBERG, Constantin Sylvius Leopold Research Centre for Foetal Medicine, Kings College Hospital, Denmark Hill, London SE5 9RS — State Exam Med Heidelberg 1990.

VON OPPELL, Professor Ulrich Otto Cardiff & Vale NHS Trust, Department of Cardiothoracic Surgery, University Hospital of Wales, Heath Park, Cardiff CF14 4XW Tel: 029 2074 2944 Fax: 029 2074 5439 Email: uvonopp@cardiffandvale.wales.nhs.uk; 12 Ty Gwendoline, Sophia Mansions, Marconi Avenue, Penarth CF64 1SS — MB BCh S. Africa 1977 (Univ. of the Witwatersrand) FCS (Cardiothoracic Surg.) Coll. of Med., S. Africa 1986; PhD (Cardiothoracic Surg.) Univ. of Cape Town, S. Africa 1993; FETCS 2001. Cons. Cardiac Surg., Univ. Hosp., Wales, Cardiff; Prof. of Cardiuothoracic Surg., Univ. of Cardiff, Wales. Specialty: Cardiothoracic Surg. Special Interest: Mitral & tricuspid valve repair Surg., coronary artery bypass graft Surg., arrhythmia Surg., aortic Surg. Socs: Europ. Assoc. of Cardiothoracic Surg.; Soc. of Thoracic Surgeons (USA); Soc. of Heart Valve Dis. Prev: Prof. of Cardiothoracic Surg., Univ. of Cape Town, S. Africa.

VON SCHREIBER, Simon Krishna 42 Queen Victoria Road, Sheffield S17 4HT — MB BS Lond. 1992.

VON WIDEKIND, Mr Clemens Heinrich Erich Northampton General Hospital NHS Trust, Cliftonville, Northampton NN1 5BD Tel: 01604 544301 Fax: 01604 544497 — MPH 1988 (Freie) DM 1989; MRCOG 2002. Consultant Obstetrician Gynaecologist, Northampton General Hospital, Northampton. Specialty: Obst. & Gyn. Prev: Cons. Obst. & Gyn., Leverkusen, Germany; Specialist Obst. & Gyn., Berlin, Germany.

VONAU, Barbara Ursula — State Exam Med Erlangen 1991; MD Erlangen 1992; MRCOG 1997; Dip Genitourin Med. 1999. p/t Cons. Specialty: Genitourinary Medicine; HIV Med. Special Interest: Colposcopy & Genital Herpes. Socs: BMA; MSSVD. Prev: Specialist Registrar (Genitorurin. & HIV) Chelsea & Westm. Hosp. Lond.; Specialist Train. Regist. GUM/HIV Char. Cross & Chelsea & Westm. Hosp.; Research Regist. (Genitourin. Med.) Chelsea & Westm. Hosp. Lond.

VORA, Ajay Jaikishore Department of Paediatric Haematology, Sheffield Children's Hospital, Sheffield S10 2TH Tel: 0114 271 7358 Fax: 0114 276 2289 Email: a.j.vora@sheffield.ac.uk — MB BS Bombay 1985; MD Bombay 1986; MRCP (UK) 1989; MRCPath 1991. Cons. Paediat. Haemat. Sheff. Childr. Hosp.; Hon. Lect. Univ. Sheff. Specialty: Haematology; Paediat. Prev: Sen. Regist. Haemat. Sheff.; Regist. Haemat. Leicester.

VORA, Ajaykumar The Medical Centre, 34 Victoria Road, Barnetby DN38 6JR Tel: 01652 688203 Fax: 01652 680841 — MB ChB Manch. 1983; MRCGP 1987; DRCOG 1987. GP Barnetby. Prev: Trainee GP Bury VTS; Ho. Off. (Med.) Bury HA; Ho. Off. (Surg.) Oldham HA.

VORA, Ashok Kumar West Heath Surgery, 196 West Heath Road, Northfield, Birmingham B31 3HB Tel: 0121 476 1135 Fax: 0121 476 1138; 94 Rednal Road, Kings Norton, Birmingham B38 8DU Tel: 0121 459 2431 — MB BS Lond. 1977 (St. Mary's) DRCOG 1982. Specialty: Gen. Pract. Prev: Trainee GP Birm. VTS; SHO (A & E) Hillingdon Hosp. Uxbridge; SHO (Paediat., Geriat. & O & G) VTS Selly Oak Hosp. Birm.

VORA, Girish Jay Cottage, 79 Straight Road, Old Windsor SL4 2NW Tel: 01753 868 383 Fax: 01753 868 398 Email: girishvora@hotmail.com — MB BS Bombay 1976 (Topiwala Nat. Med. Coll.) Cons. Anaesth., & Intens. Care, Ashford & St Peters Hosp., NHS Trust, Ashford & Chertsey. Specialty: Anaesth. Special Interest: Intensive Care. Socs: Intens. Care Soc., UK; Europ. Soc. of Intens. Care & Emerg.; Assn. of Anaesth. of UK & Irel. Prev: Cons. Anaesth., Johannesburg Gen. Hosp., Johannesburg.

VORA, Jitendu Popatlal Dept. of Diabetes & Endocrinology, Royal Liverpool University Hospitals, Liverpool L7 8XP Tel: 0151 706 3470 Fax: 0151 706 5877 Email: jiten.vora@rlbuh-tr.nwest.nhs.uk — BChir Camb. 1978 (Univ of Cambridge) MB Camb. 1978; MD 1991; FRCP 1996. Cons. (Diabetes & Endocrinol.) Roy. Liverp. Univ. Hosp.; Hon. Sen. Lect. (Med.) Univ. Liverp. Specialty: Gen. Med. Socs: Fell., Roy. Coll. of Med.; Mem. Diabetes UK; Mem. Soc. of Endocrinol.

VORA, Mahendra Shamji 18 Elgin Avenue, Kenton, Harrow HA3 8QL Tel: 020 8909 2579 — MB BS Bombay 1970. Socs: Defence Union.

VORSTER, DeWet Stockstrom Santa Maria, Santa Maria, Wrangaton, South Brent TQ10 9HJ Tel: 01364 73286; Santa Maria,

Wrangaton, South Brent TQ10 9HJ Tel: 01364 3286 — MB ChB Cape Town 1953; DPM Eng. 1959; DPsych McGill 1959; FRCPsych 1968. Cons. Child & Adolesc. Psychiat. MT Gould Hosp. Plymouth CHRN (SW); Cons. Mt Stuart Hospital Torquay; Cons. Duchy Hospital, Truro; Health Centre, Hitchin; Committee Rethink, Southwest, Taunton. Specialty: Child & Adolesc. Psychiat. Socs: Assn. Child Psychol. & Psychiat. Chairm. SW Br. & Amer Psychiat Assn. Prev: Cons. Psychiat. Johannesburg Gen. Hosp., Tara Hosp. & Johannesburg; Child Guid. Clinic S. Afr.; Cons. Child & Adolesc. Psychiat. Staines & Godalming Child Guid.

VORSTER, Mr Mark Andrew Regal Chambers, Bancroft, Hitchin SG5 1LL Tel: 01438 812494 Fax: 01438 816497 — MB BS Lond. 1982 (Westminster) BSc Lond. 1979; DRCOG 1989; FRCS Eng. 1990; MRCGP 1993. GP; Clin. Asst. (Colonscopy) Lister Hosp. Stevenage. Prev: Trainee GP Ivybridge VTS; Regist. (Surg.) Groote Schuur Hosp. Cape Town, S. Afr.; SHO (O & G) Freedom Fields Hosp. Plymouth.

VORUGANTI, Usha Rani Upper Parliament Street Surgery, 334 Upper Parliament Street, Liverpool L8 3LD Tel: 0151 709 1263.

VOS, Adrian Lawrence 39 Hargrave Road, London N19 5SH — MB BS Lond. 1996.

VOS, Helen Patricia (retired) — MB BChir Camb. 1984 (Cambridge) MA Camb.; DCH RCP Lond. 1987; Cert. Family Plann. JCC 1987; DRCOG 1988; MRCGP 1988. Prev: Trainee GP Oxf.

VOSE, Helen Clare Bishop Auckland General Hospital, Cockton Hill Road, Bishop Auckland DL14 6AD — MB BS Newc. 1998.

VOSE, Mark Anthony Frome Medical Practice, Health Centre, Park Road, Frome BA11 1EZ Tel: 01373 301300 Fax: 01373 301313; Innox Hill Cottage, 35 Innox Hill, Frome BA11 2LN Tel: 01373 467993 — MB BS Lond. 1986; DRCOG 1989; MRCGP 1990.

VOSS, Harold James, ERD (retired) Walnut Cottage, 10 Corby Road, Cottingham, Market Harborough LE16 8XH Tel: 01536 771787 — MRCS Eng. LRCP Lond. 1939 (Guy's) FRCPath 1963; MPhil Leic. 1987, BA 1981. Cons. Path. Kettering & Dist. Hosp. Gp. Prev: Asst. Path. Withington Hosp. Manch.

VOSS, Susan Barbara c/o Dr B. D. Sharpe, Magill Department of Anaesthesia, Chelsea & Westminster Hospital, 369 Fulham Road, London SW10 9NH — MB BS Sydney 1986.

VOTRUBA, Marcela School of Optometry & Vision Sciences, Redwood Building, Cardiff University, Cardiff CF10 3M Tel: 02920 870 134 Email: votrubam@cf.ac.uk; 74 Trinity Road, Wimbledon, London SW19 8QZ Tel: 020 8542 0483 — BM BCh Oxf. 1987 (University of Oxford Medical School) BA Oxf. 1984; MA 1987; FRCOphth 1992; PhD 1999. MRC Clin. Scientist Hon. Cons. Sen. Lect. Specialty: Ophth. Socs: Fell. Roy. Soc. Med. Lond.; Assn. for Research in Vision & Ophth.; Brit. Soc. of Human Genetics. Prev: Cons. (Ophth.), Moorfields Eye Hosp., Lond.; Wellcome Research Fell. Inst. Opth.; Hon. Regist., Moorfields Eye Hosp.

VOUGAS, Vassilios Liver Transplant Surgery Department, Kings College Hospital, Denmark Hill, London SE5 9RS — Ptychio Iatrikes Athens 1982. Sen. Regist. (Liver Transpl. Surg.) King's Coll. Hosp. Lond.

VOUSDEN, James Ernest Health Centre, New Street, Beaumaris LL58 8EL Tel: 01248 810818 Fax: 01248 811589; Hafod Wen, Llanddona, Beaumaris LL58 8UU Tel: 01248 811566 — MB BCh Wales 1984 (Welsh Nat. Sch. Med.) Clin. Asst. (Oncol.) Llandudno Gen. Hosp. Gwynedd. Socs: Roy. Coll. Gen. Practs.

VOWDEN, Mr Peter Bradford NHS Hospital Trust, Bradford Royal Infirmary, Duckworth Lane, Bradford BD9 6RJ Tel: 01274 364466 Fax: 01274 364807 Email: peter.vowden@bradfordhospitals.nhs.uk; Broxholme, 13 Staveley Road, Nab Wood, Shipley BD18 4HD Tel: 01274 585043 Fax: 01274 825367 Email: peter.vowden@blueyonder.co.uk — MD Leeds 1984; MB ChB 1976; FRCS Eng. 1980. Cons. Surg. Vasc. & Gen. Surg. Bradford Roy. Infirm.; Head of Serv. Surg. Specialty: Gen. Surg. Special Interest: Wound care. Socs: Vasc. Soc. of GB and Irel.; Surg. Research Soc.; Eur. Vasc. Soc.

VOWLES, Hilary Anne John Denmark Unit, Prestwich Hospital, New Bury Road, Manchester M25 3BL Tel: 0161 772 3400 Fax: 0161 798 5853; 34 Egerton Street, Prestwich, Manchester M25 1FQ Tel: 0161 798 7180 — MB BS Lond. 1986. Staff Grade Psychiat. John Denmark Unit Prestwich Hosp. Manch. Specialty: Gen. Psychiat. Prev: Regist. (Psychiat.) Borders Health Auth.

VOWLES, Julie Elizabeth Flat 11, The Grange, 114 Avenue Road, Acton, London W3 8QL Tel: 020 8993 3702; 3 The Pastures, Llanyravon, Cwmbran NP44 8SR Tel: 01633 482765 — MB BS Lond. 1991; BSc (Hons.) Lond. 1988; MRCP (UK) 1994. Specialist Regist. (Geriat. & Gen. Med.) Univ. Coll. & St Pancras Hosp. Lond. Specialty: Care of the Elderly. Prev: Regist. (Geriat. & Gen. Med.) Northwick Pk. Hosp. Harrow; Regist. (Geriat. & Gen. Med.) Centr. Middlx. Hosp. NHS Trust.

VOWLES, Mr Keith Douglas John (retired) Bridge House, Dunsford, Exeter EX6 7DB Tel: 01647 252200 — (Bristol) MB ChB (Gold Medal) Bristol 1946; FRCS Eng. 1953. Prev: Cons. Surg. Roy. Devon & Exeter Hosp.

VOWLES, Rosalind Elizabeth 12 Englewood Road, London SW12 9NZ — MB ChB Birm. 1993; ChB Birm. 1993; FRCS Eng. 1997. Specialty: Gen. Surg.

VOWLES, Stuart Cooper Lemon Street Surgery, 18 Lemon Street, Truro TR1 2LZ Tel: 01872 273133 Fax: 01872 260900 — MB BCh Wales 1974; DCH Eng. 1979; FRCGP 1995, M 1981. Specialty: Gen. Pract. Socs: BMA. Prev: SHO (Psychiat.) St. Lawrence's Hosp. Bodmin; SHO (Paediat.) Roy. Cornw. Hosp. (City & Treliske) Truro.

VOYCE, Christine Eirwen (retired) The Health Centre, High St., Redbourn, St Albans AL3 7LZ; 47 The Ridgeway, Marshalswick, St Albans AL4 9NR Tel: 01727 835824 — MB BS Lond. 1986 (Westminster Medical School) DCH RCP Lond. 1988; MRCGP 1990; Dip. Family Plann. JCC 1990. Clin. Asst. (A & E) Luton & Dunstable Hosp. NHS Trust; Clin. Med. Off. (Family Plann. & Reproductive Health Care) S. Beds. Community Health Care Trust. Prev: GP Welwyn Garden City & Hatfield.

VOYCE, Margaret Elizabeth Brighton General Hospital, Elm Grove, Brighton BN2 3EW Tel: 01273 696955 — MB BS Lond. 1977 (King's Coll. Hosp.) DRCOG 1980; Dip. Scientif. Basis Dermat. (Merit) 1993. Assoc. Specialist (Dermat.) Brighton & Sussex Universities NHS Trust. Specialty: Dermat. Socs: Brit. Assn. Dermat. Prev: GP Haywards Heath.

VOYCE, Michael Albert (retired) Chyvogue Cottage, Perranwell Station, Truro TR3 7JX — MB ChB Bristol 1959; FRCP Ed.; DCH Eng. 1962; MD Bristol 1968; FRCP Lond. 1989; FRCPCH 1997. Cons. Paediat. & Med. Dir. Roy. Cornw. Hosp. Trust. Prev: Lect. (Child Health) Univ. Bristol.

VOYSEY, Joanna Rachel The Mortimer Medical Practice, Croase Orchard Surgery, Kingsland, Leominster HR6 9QL Tel: 01568 708214 — BM BS Nottm. 1986.

VOYSEY, Margaret Mary (retired) 9 Reading Street Road, St. Peters, Broadstairs CT10 3EA Tel: 01843 863019 — MB BS Lond. 1954 (St. Bart.) DA Eng. 1956; FFA RCS Eng. 1961. Prev: Unit Gen. Manager Canterbury & Thanet HA.

VRANAKIS, Konstantinos Flat 8, 17 Inverness Terrace, London W2 6JE — Ptychio Iatrikes Athens 1977.

VRANJKOVIC, Vera — MB BS Lond. 1996 (Univ. Coll. Lond.) GP Locum Edin. Specialty: Accid. & Emerg. Prev: Ho. Off. (Gen. Med.) Taunton-MusGr. Hosp.; Ho. Off. (Gen. Surg.) Cheltenham Gen. Hosp.; SHO (A & E) Vict. Hosp. Kirkcaldy.

VREEDE, Eric 61A Quinton Street, London SW18 3QR Tel: 07919 791669 Email: ericvreede@compuserve.com — Artsexamen Amsterdam 1983 (University of Amsterdam) FFA RCSI 1994. Specialty: Anaesth. Prev: Regist. Rotat. (Anaesth.) St. Geo. Hosp. Lond.; Sen. Regist. (Anaesth.) Roy. Brompton Hosp.; Sen. Regist. Rotat. (Anaesth.) Chelsea & Westminster Hosp.

VRIONIDES, Yianis 14 Ronneby Close, Oatlands Chase, Weybridge KT13 9SB Tel: 01932 248484 — Ptychio Iatrikes Athens 1968 (Univ. Athens) MRCP (UK) 1974. Cons. Phys. Hillingdon Hosp. Uxbridge. Specialty: Gen. Med.

VROEGOP, Paul Gilles 142 Wellesley Road, London W4 3AP — MB ChB Auckland 1995.

VU, Thai Quoc 50 Bankfield Avenue, Lonasight, Manchester M13 0ZP — MB BS Lond. 1998.

VUCEVIC, Michael Anaesthetics Department, D Floor, Jubilee Wing, Leeds General Infirmary, Leeds LS1 3EX — MB ChB Birm. 1980; FFA RCS Eng. 1987. Cons. Anaesthetics & Intens. Care, Leeds Gen. Infirm. Specialty: Anaesth. Prev: Hon. Cons. & Sen. Lect. (Anaesth.) Univ. Leeds.; Sen. Regist. Rotat. (Anaesth.) Leeds RHA; Regist. (Anaesth.) Centr. & N. Birm. HAs.

VUCEVIC, Ranko 9 St Mildreds Road, Chelmsford CM2 9PU — MB BS Lond. 1995.

VUJANIC, Gordan Department of Pathology, University of Wales College of Medicine, Heath Park, Cardiff CF14 4XN Tel: 029 2074 2706 Fax: 029 2074 4276 — PhD Belgrade, Yugoslavia 1989, DS (Path.) 1983, MD 1978. Specialty: Histopath.

VULLIAMY, Christopher Benjamin Brecon War Memorial Hospital, Brecon LD3 7NS Tel: 01874 622443 Fax: 01874 610233; Lower Gaer Farm House, Tretower, Crickhowell NP8 1SB Tel: 01874 730859 — MB BS Lond. 1972 (Guy's) MRCS Eng. LRCP Lond. 1970; DObst RCOG 1973; DA Eng. 1973; DCH Eng. 1974; MRCP (UK) 1977; T(M)(Paediat.) 1991; FRCPCH 1997, M 1996; FRCP Lond. 1996. Cons. Paediat. (Community) Powys Health Care NHS Trust; Cons. Paediat. Nevill Hall & Dist. Trust. Specialty: Community Child Health. Socs: Welsh Paediat. Soc.; Brit. Assn. Community Child Health. Prev: Sen. Regist. (Paediat.) Bristol Childr. Hosp. & Southmead Hosp.; Sen. Regist. (Paediat.) Exeter Hosp.; Regist. (Paediat.) Southmead Hosp. Bristol.

VULLIAMY, David Gibb (retired) The Old School House, Lower Bockhampton, Dorchester DT2 8PZ — MB BChir Camb. 1942 (Camb. & Guy's) MRCS Eng. LRCP Lond. 1941; DCH Eng. 1948; MD Camb. 1952; FRCP Lond., M 1949 1970; FRCPCH (Hon) 1997. Prev: Cons. Paediatr. W. Dorset Hosps.

VULPE, Anna-Maria 11 Birch House, Lingwood Close, Southampton SO16 7GH — BM Soton. 1983.

VUPPALAPATI, Mr Gunasekar — MB BS Gulbarga 1996. SHO (Plastic Surg.) Roy. Preston Hosp. Specialty: Plastic Surg.

VUYLSTEKE, Alain Papworth Hospital, Department of Anaesthesia , Cambridge CB3 8RE Tel: 01480 830541 Fax: 01480 364936 Email: alain.vuylsteke@papworth.nhs.uk — MD Louvain 1991. Cons. in Cardiovasc. Anaesth. and Intens. Care; Lead Clinician for Critical Care; Director of Anaesthetic Research Unit. Specialty: Anaesth.; Intens. Care. Socs: EACTA; ICS; BMA.

VUYYURU, Sivakumari Rao and Vuyyuru, Howard Medical Practice, Howard Street, Glossop SK13 7DE Tel: 01457 854321 — MB BS Andhra 1971; MB BS Andhra, India 1971.

VYAS, Aashish 63 Hatch Road, London SW16 4PW — MB ChB Manch. 1990.

VYAS, Bhupendra Shambhuprasad 15 Barclay Close, Hertford Heath, Hertford SG13 7RW — MB BS Poona 1967 (B.J. Med. Coll. Poona) DPM Eng. 1972.

VYAS, Deborah Ruth Shirley Health Centre, Grove Road, Shirley, Southampton SO15 3 Tel: 023 8078 3611 — BM Soton. 1986; DRCOG 1988; MRCGP 1993. Prev: SHO Soton. & SW Hants. HA VTS.

VYAS, Dharmendra Kantilal Ballards Lane Surgery, 209 Ballards Lane, London N3 1LY Tel: 020 8346 0726 — MB BS Saurashtra 1970; MB BS Saurashtra 1970.

VYAS, H D Melbourne Road Health Centre, 63 Melbourne Road, Leicester LE2 0GU Tel: 0116 254 5301 — MB BS Baroda 1964; MB BS Baroda 1964.

VYAS, Harish Gunvantrai University Hospital, Queens Medical Centre, Nottingham NG7 2UH Tel: 0115 924 9924 Email: harish.vyas@mail.gmcuh-tr.trent.nhs.uk — MB BS Lond. 1975 (Guy's) MRCP (UK) 1978; DM Nottm. 1986; FRCP Lond. 1996; FRCPCH 1997. Cons. Paediat. (Intens. Care & Respirat. Med.) Qu. Med. Centre Nottm. Specialty: Intens. Care. Socs: Amer. Thoracic Soc.; Paediat. Intens. Care Soc.; Soc. Critical Care Med. Prev: Research Fell. (Child Health) Univ. Nottm.

VYAS, Mr Janardan Kantilal Basildon Hospital, Basildon SS16 5NL Tel: 01268 533911; 165 Waldegrave, Kingswood, Basildon SS16 5EJ Tel: 01268 533763 — MB BS Saurashtra 1972 (Shri M.P. Shah Med. Coll. Jamnagar) FRCS Glas. 1983; MSc (Orthop.) Lond. 1985. Assoc. Orthop. Surg. Basildon Hosp.; Hon. Lect. Lond. Sch. Osteop. Specialty: Orthop. Socs: BMA; Overseas Doctors Assn.; Brit. Orthop. Assn. Prev: Regist. (Orthop.) Basildon Hosp., OldCh. Hosp. Romford & Qu. Eliz. II Hosp. Welwyn Gdn. City.

VYAS, Julian Ramesh Department of Child Health, University of Leicester, Leicester LE1 7RH; 28 Old Road, Walgrave, Northampton NN6 9QW Tel: 01604 781683 — MB BS Lond. 1988 (Guy's Hosp. Med. Sch. Univ. Lond.) MRCP (UK) 1993. Clin. Lect. & Hon. Regist. (Child Health) Univ. Leicester & Leicester Roy. Infirm. Specialty: Paediat. Socs: Roy. Coll. Paediat. & Child Health. Prev: Regist. Northampton Gen. Hosp.; SHO Rotat. (Paediat.) Birm. Childr. Hosp.; SHO (Med.) Jas. Paget Hosp. Gt. Yarmouth.

VYAS, Jyotsana Belmont Health Centre, 516 Kenton Lane, Kenton, Harrow HA3 7LT Tel: 0208 427 1213; 29 Broadhurst Avenue, Edgware HA8 8TP — BM Soton. 1979. GP - Harrow. Specialty: Obst. & Gyn.; Paediat.; Family Plann. & Reproduc. Health.

VYAS, Kshama Hemant Old Station Road Surgery, 157 Old Station Road, Hayes UB3 4NA Tel: 020 8573 2037 Fax: 020 8813 7552 — MB BS Delhi 1975 (New Delhi, India) DRCOG 1982. Socs: Med. Protec. Soc.

VYAS, Paresh Paresh Vyas, Institute of Molecular Medicine, John Radcliffe Hospital, Oxford OX3 9DU Tel: 01865 222309 Fax: 01865 222500 — BM BCh Oxf. 1986 (Oxford) MRCP (UK) 1989; MRCPath 1996; FRCPath 2002. Wellcome Trust Sen. Clin. Fell., John Radcliffe Hosp. Oxf. Specialty: Haematology. Prev: Wellcome Sen. Clin. Fell. Childrs. Hosp. Harvard Med. Sch. Boston, MA, USA; Sen. Regis. (Heanatology), Roy. Free. Hosp.; SHO (Gen. Med./Haemat.) Univ. Coll. Hosp.

VYAS, Rashmikant Bhogilal Gallowhill Surgery, 4-6 Gallowhill, Larkhall ML9 1EX Tel: 01698 884082 Fax: 01698 889211 — MB BS Calcutta 1972. Clin. Asst. (A & E) Lanarksh. Specialty: Accid. & Emerg. Socs: Med. Defence Union.

VYAS, Samir Kumar Salisbury District Hospital, Odstock Road, Salisbury SP2 8BJ Tel: 01722 336262 Fax: 01722 332606; Clearbury Lodge, Nunton Lane, Nunton, Salisbury SP5 4HZ — BM Soton. 1986; MRCP (UK) 1989; DM 1997. Cons. Phys. & Gastroenterol. Salisbury Dist. Hosp. Specialty: Gastroenterol. Socs: BMA; Brit. Assn. Studies Liver; Pancreatic Soc. Prev: Sen. Regist. (Gen. Med. & Gastroenterol.) Soton. Gen. Hosp.; Brit. Dig. Foundat. Research Train. Fell. & Hon. Regist. Soton. Gen. Hosp.; Regist. (Med.) Soton. Gen. Hosp.

VYAS, Mr Sanjay Kumar Southmead Hospital, Westbury-on-Trym, Bristol BS10 5NB Tel: 0117 959 5156 Fax: 0117 959 5158 — MB BS Lond. 1985; MRCOG 1991; MD Lond. 1992. Cons. O & G Southmead Hosp. Bristol. Specialty: Obst. & Gyn. Prev: Sen. Regist. (O & G) St. Michael's Hosp. Bristol; Research Fell. (O & G) King's Coll. Hosp. Lond.

VYAS, Sunil 60 Abbey Avenue, Wembley HA0 1LL — MB ChB Glas. 1992.

VYAS, Mr Vinod Chimanlal 37 Green Street, Forest Gate, London E7 8DA Tel: 020 8472 0170 — MB BS Bombay 1953 (Grant Med. Coll.) BSc (Hons.) Bombay 1946. p/t Indep. Privat. Practitioner in Orthop. Med. Specialty: Orthop. Socs: BMA; Fell. Roy. Soc. Med. Prev: Cons. Orthop. Surg. E. Ham Mem. Hosp. Lond.; Cons. Orthop. Surg. Qu. Mary's Hosp. Lond.; Cosn. Orthop. Surg. St And. Hosp. Lond.

VYRAMUTHU, Navaratnam 282 Cassiobury Drive, Watford WD17 3AP — MUDr Prague 1972; FFR RCPI 1986.

VYRNWY-JONES, Peter, Maj. RAMC 5 Stoke Farthing Courtyard, Broadchalke, Salisbury SP5 5ED — MSc Occupat. Med. Lond. 1983, BSc (Hons.) 1973, MB BS 1975; DAvMed RCP Lond. 1980; MFOM RCP Lond. 1985, AFOM 1981. Cons. in Aviat. Med. (Army) attached USAARL Alabama, USA. Specialty: Aviat. Med. Socs: Soc. Occupat. Med.; Roy. Aeronaut. Soc. Prev: Cons. Aviat. Med. (Army) RAF Inst. Aviat. Med.; Specialist Aviat. Med. (Army) BAOR.

VYSE, Timothy James Rheumatology Department, ICSM, Hammersmith Campus, London W12 0NN Tel: 020 8383 2339 Email: t.vyse@ic.ac.uk — MA Camb. 1982; MB BS Lond. 1985; MRCP (UK) 1989; PhD 1994. Wellcome Trust Sen. Fell. Imperial Coll., Lond. Specialty: Rheumatol. Prev: Fulbright research fell.; Nat. Jewish Center for Immunol., Denver, USA.

VYSE-PEACOCK, Alicca 232 Queens Promenade, Blackpool FY2 9HA — MB ChB Manch. 1991.

VYVYAN, Henry Arthur Luke Department of Anaesthetics, St George's Hospital, Blackshaw Road, London SW17 0QT Tel: 020 8672 1255 — MB BS Lond. 1985; FRCA 1990. Sen. Regist. (Anaesth.) St. Geo. Hosp. Lond. Specialty: Anaesth. Prev: Sen. Regist. (Anaesth.) Roy. P. Alfred Hosp. Sidney, Austral.

WAAS, Moderage Joseph Heron Bernard The Surgery, Sturton Road, North Leverton, Retford DN22 0AB Tel: 01427 880223 Fax: 01427 880927; Hillcrest, Gainsborough Road, Saundby, Retford DN22 0AB Tel: 01427 848816 — MB ChB Sheff. 1974; MRCOG 1982, DRCOG 1980; MFFP 1993; FRCOG 1998. Princip. GP N. Leverton Notts.

WACE, Jocelyn Richard Department of Anaesthetics, Queen Alexandra Hospital, Portsmouth PO6 3LY Tel: 023 92 286279 Fax:

023 92 286681 — BM BCh Oxf. 1986; MA Camb. 1986, BA 1983; FRCA 1992. Cons. (Anaesth.) Portsmouth. Specialty: Anaesth.

WACE, Malini Rookery Medical Centre, Rookery House, Newmarket CB8 8NW Tel: 01638 665711 Fax: 01638 561280; Boyarin Lodge, Bury Road, Newmarket CB8 7BT Tel: 01638 664848 — MB Camb. 1984; MA Camb. 1985, MB 1984, BChir 1983; DRCOG 1986; MRCGP 1988. Prev: GP Camb.

WACE, Rupert Orlando Orchard House Surgery, Fred Archer Way, Newmarket CB8 8NU Tel: 01638 663322 Fax: 01638 561921 — MA Camb. 1985, MB 1984, BChir 1983; DCH RCP Lond. 1987; DRCOG 1987; MRCGP 1988. Prev: Trainee GP Newmarket VTS; SHO (Paediat.) Heath Rd. Hosp. Ipswich.

WACHSMUTH, Rachel Caroline Dermatology Dept., Leeds General Infirmary, Leeds LS1 3EX — BChir Camb. 1992 (Univ. Camb. & Addenbrooke's) MRCP 1996. Specialist Regist. (Dermat.) St. James & Leeds Gen. Infirm. Specialty: Dermat. Prev: SHO (Gen. Med.) St. Jas. Univ. Hosp. Leeds.

WACHTEL, Sean Lawrence 42 Hullmead, Shamley Green, Guildford GU5 0UG — MB ChB (Hons) Leic. 1994; BSc (Hons.)Leic. 1991; MRCP (UK) Ed. 1997; DFFP 2001; DTM & H Liverpool 2001; MRCGP 2002. GP Princip. Specialty: Gen. Pract. Prev: GP Regist. Gillingham Dorset.

WACKS, Harvey 24 Danesway, Prestwich, Manchester M25 0FS — MB ChB Manch. 1959; BSc Manch. 1954, MB ChB 1959; FRCPath. 1982, M 1969. Cons. Pathol. Sunderland Hosp. Gp. Specialty: Pathology, General. Prev: Regist. Path. Withington Hosp. Manch. & Roy. Lancaster Infirm.; Regist. Surg. Vict. Hosp. Blackpool.

WACLAWSKI, Eugene Raphael Renfrewshire & Inverclyde Primary Care NHS Trust, Occupational Health Service, The Hollybush, Dykebar Hospital, Grahamston Road, Paisley PA3 7AD Tel: 0141 884 9080 Fax: 0141 884 9061; 1 Novar Drive, Hyndland, Glasgow G12 9PX Email: ewaclaws@ewem.net — MD Glas. 1990; MB ChB 1981; MRCP (UK) 1984; MFOM RCP Lond. 1990; FRCP Glas. 1994; FFOM 1995. Cons. Occupat. Phys. & Dir. Occupat. Health Renfrewsh. Healthcare NHS Trust; Hon. Clin. Sen. Lect. Univ. Glas. Specialty: Occupat. Health. Socs: Soc. Occupat. Med.; Brit. Occupat. Hyg. Soc. Prev: Cons. Occupat. Phys. Inst. Occupat. Med. Ltd. Edin.

WACOGNE, Ian David 30 Green Street, Milton Malsor, Northampton NN7 3AT — BM BCh Oxf. 1993; BA (Hons.) Oxf. 1990; MRCP (UK) 1996. SHO (Paediat.) Birm. Childr. Hosp. Specialty: Paediat. Prev: SHO (Paediat.) Northampton Gen. Hosp.; Ho. Off. (Gen. Med.) John Radcliffe Hosp. Oxf.; Ho. Off. (Gen. Surg.) Derriford Hosp. Plymouth.

WADAMS, Stephen John Frederick 68 Browning Avenue, Bournemouth BH5 1NW — MB BS Lond. 1996.

WADD, Nicholas James — MB BS Newc. 1990; FRCR; MRCP. Cons. Clin. Oncol. Jas. Cook Univ. Hosp. Middlesbrough.

WADDELL, Andrew Michael Park Surgery, 278 Stratford Road, Shirley, Solihull B90 3AF Tel: 0121 241 1700 Fax: 0121 241 1821; 35 Manor Road, Solihull B91 2BL — MB ChB Birm. 1984.

WADDELL, Mr Angus Neil 7 Longfield Road, Bishopston, Bristol BS7 9AG Email: anguswaddell@compuserve.com — MB BS Lond. 1990; FRCS Eng. 1994. Specialty: Otorhinolaryngol.

WADDELL, Christine Agnes Pathology Department, Birmingham Women's Hospital, Edgbaston, Birmingham B15 2TG Tel: 0121 627 2723 Fax: 0121 627 2624 Email: christine.waddell@bham-womens.thenhs.com; 29 Elmdon Road, Selly Park, Birmingham B29 7LF Tel: 0121 472 7668 — MB ChB Sheff. 1970; DObst RCOG 1972; MSc (Clin. Cytopath.) Lond. 1993. Assoc. Specialist (Cytopath.) Birm. Wom. Hosp. Specialty: Pathology, General. Socs: Internat. Acad. Cytol.; Internet. Acad; Assn. Clin. Path. Prev: Regist. (Path.) Sheff. AHA (T).

WADDELL, Fiona Margaret Corbridge House, Corbridge-on-Tyne, Corbridge NE45 5LE Tel: 01434 633012 — MB BS Durh. 1957 (Newc.) Clin. Asst. Orthop. Surg. Hexham Gen. Hosp.; Assoc. Specialist Blood Transfus. Centre Newc. Prev: Ho. Off. Roy. Vict. Infirm. Newc.; SHO & Ho. Off. Princess Mary Matern. Hosp. Newc.

WADDELL, Mr Gordon Alex Bryce The Glasgow Nuffield Hospital, Glasgow G12 0PJ — MB ChB Glas. 1967; DSc Glas. 1992, BSc (Hons.) Physiol. 1964; FRCS Ed. 1971; MD Glas. 1976; FRCS Glas. 1983. Cons. Surg. (Orthop.) Glas. Nuffield Hosp.; Hon. Prof. Rheum. Univ. Manch. 1996; Hon. Prof. Orthop. Univ. Glas. 1992. Specialty: Orthop.

WADDELL, James, OBE (retired) Glengarry, 2 Cottesmore Gardens, Hale Barns, Altrincham WA15 8TS Tel: 0161 904 9050 — LRCP LRCS Ed. 1945 (Anderson Coll. Glas.) LRCP LRCS Ed. LRFPS Glas. 1945; MRCGP 1957; MFOM RCP Lond. 1981. Prev: Cons. Med. Advis. to Kellogg Co. (GB) Ltd.

WADDELL, James Alexander Rooks Nest, Somerford Road, Cirencester GL7 1TX Tel: 01285 651079 — MB ChB Ed. 1956; FRCP Ed. 1970, M 1960; FRCP Lond. 1974, M 1963. Specialty: Gen. Med.; Respirat. Med. Prev: Cons. Phys. Princess Margt. Hosp. Swindon & Cirencester Hosp.; Sen. Regist. Med. Westm. Hosp. Gp.; Brit. Postgrad. Med. Federat. Trav. Fell.

WADDELL, James Lindsay (retired) 11 Station Avenue, Haddington EH41 4EG Tel: 01620 823322 — MB ChB Ed. 1960; DPM RCPS Glas. 1963; FRCP Ed. 1990, M 1967; MRCPsych 1971. Prev: Phys. Supt. Hermanflat Hosp. Haddington.

WADDELL, Joanne Elisabeth 35 Manor Road, Solihull B91 2BL — MB ChB Birm. 1985. Partner in General Practice.

WADDELL, John Michael Northumberland Community Health, The Health Centre, Civic Precinct, Forum Way, Cramlington NE23 6QN Tel: 01670 713021 Fax: 01670 735880 — MB ChB Birm. 1981 (Birmingham) BSc Birm. 1978; DRCOG 1984; DCH RCP Lond. 1987; MRCGP 1988. GP Cramlington, N.d.; Clin. Asst. (Urol.).

WADDELL, Michael Osborne, MC (retired) North Side, Wall, Hexham NE46 4DU Tel: 01434 681904 — MB BS Durh. 1952; MD Vermont 1967.

WADDELL, Myra McInnes Buckingham Terrace Medical Practice, 31 Buckingham Terrace, Glasgow G12 8ED Tel: 0141 221 6210 Fax: 0141 211 6232 — MB ChB Glas. 1975; DRCOG 1977; MRCP (UK) 1979; MRCGP 1983.

WADDELL, Nicholas John Hamilton 20 Alderbrook Road, Solihull B91 1NN — MB ChB Birm. 1983.

WADDELL, Nicola Margaret Russell The Palatine Centre, 63/65 Palatine Road, Manchester M20 3LJ Tel: 0161 434 3555; 38 Kings Road, Wilmslow SK9 5PZ — MB BS Lond. 1987; MA Oxf. 1984; DCH RCP Lond. 1990; DRCOG 1990. Clin. Med. Off. (Family Plann. & Reproduc. Health Care) Palatine Centre Manch. Specialty: Family Plann. & Reproduc. Health. Prev: Trainee GP N.ants.; SHO (Paediat.) Northampton Gen. Hosp.

WADDELL, Turner Raith (retired) Fairways, Andover Down, Andover SP11 6LJ — MRCS Eng. LRCP Lond. 1944 (St Bart.) Prev: Med. Off. Enham-Alamein Village Settlem.

WADDELOW, Mrs Janet (retired) 30 Fearnville Mount, Leeds LS8 3DL Tel: 0113 265 3909 — MB ChB Leeds 1951; FRCOG 1989, M 1961, DObst 1954. Prev: Clin. Asst. (O & G) St. Jas. Univ. Hosp. Leeds.

WADDINGHAM, Rosemary Tadley Medical Partnership, Holmwood Health Centre, Franklin Avenue, Tadley RG26 4ER Tel: 01189 816661 Fax: 01189 817533; Blandford Hithe, Brimpton, Reading RG7 4TD Tel: 0118 971 3332 Fax: 0118 971 3332 — MB ChB Leeds 1977; DRCOG 1981; Family Plann. JCC Cert. 1981; MRCGP 1994. GP Princip. Specialty: Gen. Pract.; Family Plann. & Reproduc. Health.

WADDINGTON, Christopher Ware Road Surgery, 59 Ware Road, Hoddesdon EN11 9AB Tel: 01992 463363 Fax: 01992 471108 — MB BS Lond. 1980; BA (Oxf.) 1977; DRCOG 1984.

WADDINGTON, Derek (retired) 53 Southway Lane, Plymouth PL6 7DL Tel: 01752 773926 — MB ChB Sheff. 1951.

WADDINGTON, Duncan Calderdale & Huddersfield, NHS Trust, St. Lukes Hospital, Blackmoorfoot Road, Crosland Moor, Huddersfield HD4 5RQ Tel: 01484 343588 — MB BS Newc. 1986; MMedSc (Leeds) 1994. Cons. (Psychiat.) Calderdale & Huddersfield NHS Trust,Huddersfield. Specialty: Gen. Psychiat. Socs: Roy. Coll. Psychiat. Prev: Sen. Regist. Manch. Train. Scheme (Psychiat.); Regist. W. Yorks. Train. Scheme (Pschiatry); Regist. Newc. Train. Scheme (Psychiat.).

WADDINGTON, Gerald Eugene Stoneham Lane Surgery, 6 Stoneham Lane, Swaythling, Southampton SO16 2AB Tel: 023 8055 5776 Fax: 023 8039 9723; GP Practice Address, 6 Stoneham Lane, Swaythling, Southampton SO16 2AB Tel: 02380 555776 Fax: 023 803 99723 — MB ChB Bristol 1972; MRCGP 1978; D OCC MED 1995; DFFP RLOG 1997. Fleet Med. Adviser Cunard Line Ltd. Soton. Specialty: Occupat. Health. Prev: Surg. Lt.-Cdr. RNR.

WADDINGTON, Michael Hugh Guy (retired) Stonecott, 18 Chappell Road, Hoylandswaine, Sheffield S36 7JD — MB ChB Leeds 1951.

WADDINGTON, Richard John 34A Government Row, Enfield EN3 6JN — MB BS Lond. 1994 (Univ. Coll. Lond. Med. Sch.) MA Oxf. 1991. SpR (Anaesth.) Barts & the Lond. Hosps. Specialty: Anaesth.

WADDINGTON, Mr Richard Turner Golden Cross, Cawthorne, Barnsley S75 4HR — MB ChB Sheff. 1963; FRCS Ed. 1969; FRCS Eng. 1970. Cons. Surg. (Gen. Surg.) Barnsley Dist. Gen. Hosp. Specialty: Gen. Surg. Socs: Sheff. Med. Soc. Prev: Flight Lt. RAF Med. Br., Med. Off. Princess Mary's RAF Hosp. Halton; Sen. Regist. (Gen. Surg.) Roy. Hosp. Sheff.

WADDINGTON, Sara Jane Dept. Of Clinical Oncology, Royal South Hants Hospital, Southampton; Oak Tree House, Wangfield Lane, Curdridge, Southampton SO32 2DA — MB BS Lond. 1980; BSc. (Hons.) Pharmacol. Lond. 1973; DRCOG 1982; MRCGP 1984.

WADDY, Elizabeth Mary Bridge Surgery, St Peters Street, Stapenhill, Burton-on-Trent DE15 9AW Tel: 01283 563451 Fax: 01283 500896; 45 Tower Road, Burton-on-Trent DE15 0NH Tel: 01283 547322 — BM BS Nottm. 1977; DCH RCP Lond. 1981; DRCOG 1981; MRCGP 1982. Prev: SHO Burton-on-Trent VTS; SHO (Rheum.) Middlx. Hosp.; Ho. Off. (Med.) Nottm. Gen. Hosp. & (Surg.) Hillingdon Hosp. Uxbridge.

WADDY, Ethel Hunter (retired) 2 Pine Court, Little Brington, Northampton NN7 4EZ Tel: 01604 770255 — MB ChB Sheff. 1930. Prev: Anaesth. Manfield Orthop. Hosp.

WADDY, George William (retired) The Old Hall, Pitsford Road, Moulton, Northampton NN3 7SS Tel: 01604 405757 — MB BS Lond. 1952 (St. Bart.) MRCS Eng. LRCP Lond. 1952. Prev: Mem. N.ants. Local Med. Servs. Comm. & BMA.

WADDY, Rosemary Stacy, OStJ AXA PPP Healthcare OHS, MIS House, 23 St Leonards Road, Eastbourne BN21 3PX Tel: 01323 724889 Fax: 01323 721161; 4 Evelyn Way, Stoke D'Abernon, Cobham KT11 2SJ Tel: 01932 864458 Fax: 01932 864458 — MB BS Newc. 1970 (Newc. u. Tyne) DObst RCOG 1973; DA Eng. 1973; MFOM RCP Lond. 1985, AFOM 1981; DIH Eng. 1981; Cert. Av. Med. 1989; DAvMed 1994. Cons. Ocupational Health, AXA PPP Healthcare OHS; Area Surg. St. John Ambul. Specialty: Occupat. Health. Socs: Soc. Occupat. Med. Prev: Sen. Med. Off. Brit. Airways; SMO John Lewis Partnership; Med. Off. Ascension Is.

WADE, Abdel Aziz Hussien Coventry & Warwickshire Hospital, Stoney Stanton Road, Coventry CV1 4FH Tel: 024 76 844163/4 Fax: 024 76 844168; 1 Tintagel Grove, Kenilworth CV8 2PG Tel: 01926 512862 — MB BCh Cairo 1965; MRCOG 1975. Cons. Genitourin. Med. Coventry & Warks. Hosp.; Hon. Sen. Lect. Birm. Med. Sch. Specialty: Genitourinary Medicine. Socs: (Pres.) Midl. Soc. Genitourin. Med. Prev: Sen. Regist. (Genitourin. Med.) Manch. Roy. Infirm.; Lect. (Gyn. & Obst.) Benghazi Univ., Libya; Regist. (O & G) Mid-Staffs. HA.

WADE, Alan Grierson Clydebank Health Centre, Kilbowie Road, Clydebank G81 2TQ Tel: 0141 531 6410 Fax: 0141 531 6413; Cintra, 15 Edgehill Road, Bearsden, Glasgow G61 3AB Tel: 0141 942 3589 Fax: 0141 951 1931 — MB ChB Glas. 1969; FRCA Eng. 1973. Dir. Community Pharmacol. Serv. Ltd. Glas.; Chairm. Gen. Pract. Research Clydebank. Specialty: Pharmaceutical Medicine.

WADE, Andrew 9 Royal Garth, Beverley HU17 8NL — MB ChB Leeds 1971; T(Psych) 1991.

WADE, Andrew Orlando — MB BS Lond. 1994 (Charing Cross & Westm.) BSc (Biochem.) Lond. 1991; MRCP 2000.

WADE, Catherine Bernadette Court Yard Surgery, John Evans House, 28 Court Yard, London SE9 5QA Tel: 020 8850 1300 Fax: 020 8294 2378; Reeves House, The Street, Horton Kirby, Dartford DA4 9BY Tel: 01322 860225 — MB BS Lond. 1980 (Guy's Hospital) DRCOG 1983.

WADE, Charlotte Gillian Bradburn Winglock House, 40 Seymour Road, Newton Abbot TQ12 2PU — MB BS Lond. 1998; MB BS Lond 1998.

WADE, Courtenay Chirgwin, TD (retired) c/o The Royal Bank of Scotland, 38 Park St., Croydon CR9 1YS — (St. And.) MB ChB St. And. 1956, DPH 1963. Hon. Cons. Phys. (Community Med.) Char. Cross Hosp. Lond. Prev: Dist. Community Phys. S. Hammersmith Health Dist. (T).

WADE, David Charles County Surgery, 202-204 Abington Avenue, Northampton NN1 4QA Tel: 01604 632918 Fax: 01604 601578 — MB ChB Leic. 1987 (Leicester) BSc (Hons) Med. Sci. Leic. 1984; DRCOG 1991. Clin. Asst. (Epilepsy) Northampton.

WADE, Professor Derick Treharne Oxford Centre for Enablement, Windmill Road, Oxford OX3 7LD Tel: 01865 737306 Fax: 01865 737309 Email: derick.wade@dial.pipex.com; 28 Polstead Road, Oxford OX2 6TN Tel: 01865 556031 Email: derick.wade@dial.pipex.com — MB BChir Camb. 1974 (St. Thos.) MRCP (UK) 1976; MA Camb. 1974, MD 1985; FRCP Lond. 1994. Cons. (Neurol.) Oxf. Centre for Enablement; Edr. Clin. Rehabil. Specialty: Neurol.; Disabil. Med.; Rehabil. Med. Socs: (Counc.) Soc. Research in Rehabil.; Brit. Assn. Neurol.; Brit. Soc. Rehabil. Med. Prev: Cons. Neurol. Rivermead Hosp. Oxf.; Regist. (Clin. Neurophysiol.) Nat. Hosp. Nerv. Dis. Lond.; Regist. (Neurol.) & SHO (Neurosurg.) Frenchay Hosp. Bristol.

WADE, Elizabeth Clare 55 Withdean Crescent, Brighton BN1 6WG — MB BS Lond. 1996 (St. Bart.) BA (Hons.) Brighton 1988. SHO (Psychiat.) Homerton Hosp. Lond.; Staff Grade A & E Roy. Lond. Hosp; SHO Paediat Roy. Alexandra. Hosp. Brighton; SHO A & E Rotat. Roy. Sussex Co. Hosp. Brighton. Specialty: Accid. & Emerg. Prev: SHO (A & E) Roy. Lond. Hosp.

WADE, Isobel Renwick 112 Leylands Lane, Heaton, Bradford BD9 5QU — (Glas.) MB ChB Glas. 1969; DA Eng. 1971; Dip. Palliat. Med. Wales 1993. Assoc. Specialist Palliat. Med. Manorlands Hospice. Oxenhope. W. Yorks. Specialty: Palliat. Med. Socs: Assoc. of Palliat. Med.; BMA. Prev: Clin. Asst. (Anaesth.) Bradford AHA; Regist. Soton. Univ. Hosps.; Regist. & SHO (Anaesth.) Portsmouth Gp. Hosps.

WADE, Jane Rosanne (retired) Port Reeve, East Street, Mayfield TN20 6TZ Tel: 01435 873535 — MB BChir Camb. 1962 (Camb. & St. Bart.) DPH Liverp. 1965. Prev: Cons. Community Paediat. S. Downs Health NHS Trust.

WADE, Jeremy James Dulwich Public Health Laboratory & Medical Microbiology, King's College School of Medicine & Dentistry, King's College Hospital, Denmark Hill, London SE5 9RS Tel: 020 7346 3033 Fax: 020 7346 3404 — MB BS Lond. 1983 (Univ. Lond.) MSc Lond. 1990; MRCPath 1993; MD Lond. 1997. Cons. & Hon. Sen. Lect. (Med. Microbiol.) Dulwich Pub. Health Laborat. & Med. Microbiol. King's Coll. Sch. Med. & Dent. Specialty: Med. Microbiol. Socs: Hosp. Infec. Soc.; Brit. Soc. Antimicrob. Chemother.; Path. Soc. Prev: Lect. & Hon. Sen. Regist. (Med. Microbiol.) King's Coll. Sch. Med. & Dent. Lond.

WADE, Mr John David Throckenholt, Cranes Lane, Kingston, Cambridge CB3 7NJ Tel: 01233 262275 — MB BChir Camb. 1939 (Camb. & Univ. Coll. Hosp.) MRCS Eng., LRCP Lond. 1938; MA, MB BChir Camb. 1939; FRCS Eng. 1941; FRCS Ed. 1959. Socs: Assn. Thoracic Surgs. Gt. Brit. & Assn. Surgs. Gt. Brit. Prev: Cons. Thoracic Surg. Roy. Infirm. Edin.; Dorothy Temple Cross Fell.; Clin. & Research Fell. Mass. Gen. Hosp.

WADE, John Kennington (retired) Manor Cottage, Potterhanworth, Lincoln LN4 2DN Tel: 01522 791288 — MB BS Lond. 1962 (King's Coll. Hosp.) MRCS Eng. LRCP Lond. 1962. Prev: Hosp. Pract. (ENT) Co. Hosp. Lincoln.

WADE, John Philip Huddart Hammersmith Hospitals Trust, Charing Cross Hospital, Fulham Palace Road, London W6 8RF Tel: 020 8846 1303 Fax: 020 8846 7487 Email: jwade@hhnt.org; 11 Gardnor Road, Hampstead, London NW3 1HA Tel: 020 7431 2900 — MD Camb. 1982; MB 1975, BChir 1974, BA 1971; MRCP (UK) 1976; FRCP Lond. 1991. Cons. Neurol. Char. Cross Hosp. Lond. & Wexham Pk. Hosp. Slough. Specialty: Neurol. Prev: Sen. Regist. (Neurol.) Nat. Hosps. Nerv. Dis. & St. Bart. Hosp. Lond.; Fellowship Ontario Heart & Stroke Foundat. Univ. Hosp. Lond. Ontario.

WADE, Kim 37 Station Road, Skelmanthorpe, Huddersfield HD8 9AU — BM BS Nottm. 1992.

WADE, Malcolm John Windy Ridge, 112 Leylands Road, Bradford BD9 5QU Tel: 01274 499703 — MB BS Lond. 1968 (Lond. Hosp.) MRCS Eng. LRCP Lond. 1968; DObst RCOG 1970; DA Eng. 1971; FFA RCS Eng. 1973. Cons. Anaesth. Bradford Roy. Infirm. Specialty: Anaesth. Socs: Fell. Roy. Soc. Med.; Assn. Anaesths. Prev: Sen. Regist. Rotat. Soton. & Westm. Hosps.; Regist. (Anaesth.) Portsmouth Hosp. Gp.; Obst. Off. St. Mary's Matern. Hosp. Portsmouth.

WADE, Mary Ward Pickering (retired) 22 Hill Top Avenue, Cheadle Hulme, Cheadle SK8 7HY Tel: 0161 485 2228 — MB ChB Manch. 1943; MRCS Eng. LRCP Lond. 1943.

WADE, Nigel Ross Jubilee Surgery, Barrys Meadow, High St Titchfield, Fareham PO14 4EH Tel: 01329 844220 Fax: 01329 841484 — MB ChB Birm. 1987; MRCGP 1991; DRCOG 1991.

WADE, Mr Peter John Fraser Oak House, Eastwood Business Village, Binley Business Park, Binley, Coventry CV3 2UB Tel: 024 7656 1900 Fax: 024 7656 1901; Sedgemere, Fernhill Lane, Fen End, Kenilworth CV8 1NU Tel: 01676 532114 Fax: 01676 535448 Email: peterwade@sedgemere.freeserve.co.uk — MB BS Lond. 1971 (St. Thos.) LMCC 1974; FRCS Eng. 1976. Cons. Orthop. & Hand Surg. Clinic. Dir. Trauma & Orthop. Coventry; Clin. Dir. Trauma Univ. Coventry & Warwicks. NHS Trust; Counc. Mem., Brit. Soc. of Surg. for the hand. Specialty: Orthop. Socs: Coun. Mem. Brit. Orthopaedic Assoc.; Coun. Mem. Brit. Soc. Surg. of Hand; Coun. Mem. BMA. Prev: Clin. Tutor Coventry & Warks. Hosp.; Sen. Regist. (Orthop. S. E. Thames Rha; Sen. Research Regist. (Orthop.) St. Thomas Hosp. Lond.

WADE, Richard Geoffrey Huddart Albany Surgery, Albany Street, Newton Abbot TQ12 2TX Tel: 01626 334411 Fax: 01626 335663; Wingelock House, 40 Seymour Road, Newton Abbot TQ12 2PU Tel: 01626 54459 — MB ChB Manch. 1971; DObst RCOG 1973; MRCGP 1979; FRCGP 1999. NHS Direct Advis. Prev: Sen. Ho. Phys. (Paediat.) Roy. Manch. Childr. Hosp.; Ho. Phys. & Ho. Surg. Manch. Roy. Infirm.

WADE, Robin Moorlands Surgery, 139 Willow Road, Darlington DL3 9JP Tel: 01325 469168; 26 Linden Avenue, Darlington DL3 8PP — MB ChB Sheff. 1976; DRCOG 1982.

WADE, Roger Hedley 350 Telegraph Road, Heswall, Wirral CH60 6RW — MB ChB Liverp. 1992; FRCS Ed. 1996. Specialist Regist. (Orthop.). Specialty: Orthop.

WADE, Rosemary Verity — MB BS Lond. 1985 (Middlx. Hosp.) MRCGP 1994. Locum Cons. Palliat. Med. Prev: Sp. Regist. (Palliat. Med.), St. Nicholas Hospice, Bury St. Edmunds.

WADE, Rowena Juliet Rowan House, Crooks Lane, Studley B80 7QX — MB BS Lond. 1996.

WADE, Sally Jane 26 Linden Avenue, Darlington DL3 8PP — MB BS Newc. 1980; MRCGP 1984.

WADE, Simon The Medical Centre, Forest Gate Road, Corby NN17 1TR Tel: 01536 202507 Fax: 01536 206099; 18 Brunswick Gardens, Corby NN18 9ER Tel: 01536 746067 — MB BS Lond. 1986 (Kings College School of Medicine and Dentistry) DCH RCP Lond. 1989; MRCGP 1990; DRCOG 1990. GP Princip. Socs: BMA; Med. Protec. Soc.

WADE, Thomas Henry Hanbury 54 Harley Street, London W1N 1AD Tel: 020 7580 7558 — MB BChir Camb. 1949 (Univ. Coll. Hosp.) MA MB BChir Camb. 1949. Med. Adviser To Embassy of RePub. of Congo; Med. Represen. in Lond. For Abu Dhabi. Socs: BMA. Prev: Surg. Regist. Qu. Mary's Hosp. Childr. Carshalton; Asst. Lect. Anat. Univ. Coll. Cardiff; Clin. Asst. St. John's Hosp. Dis. of Skin Lond.

WADE-EVANS, Elizabeth Marion (retired) Ebenezer House, Orcop, Hereford HR2 8SD — MB BS Lond. 1950 (Roy. Free)

WADE-EVANS, Tom (retired) Ebenezer House, Orcop, Hereford HR2 8SD — MRCS Eng. LRCP Lond. 1948 (Westm.) BSc Wales 1945; MD Lond. 1961, MB BS 1951; FRCPath 1977, M 1965. Cons. Pathol. Birm. Wom. Hosps.; Hon. Cons. Path. Centr. Birm. HA. Prev: Ho. Phys. & Ho. Surg. O & G Depts. Westm. Hosp.

WADE-EVANS, Victoria Jane Ebenezer House, Orcop, Hereford HR2 8SD — MB BS Lond. 1981.

WADE-WEST, Susan Charis Bishops Waltham Surgery, Lower Lane, Bishops Waltham, Southampton SO32 1GR Tel: 01489 892288 Fax: 01489 894402; The Surgery, Lower Lane, Bishops Waltham, Southampton SO32 1GR Tel: 01489 892288 Fax: 01489 894402 — MB BS (Hons.) Lond. 1977 (Roy. Free) DRCOG 1982; MRCP (UK) 1983. GP Bishops Waltham. Prev: Research Regist. (Paediat.) Soton. Gen. Hosp.; SHO (Med. & O & G) Soton. Gen. Hosp.

WADE WEST, Thomas (retired) Wayside, Kew Lane, Old Bursledon, Southampton SO31 8DG Tel: 023 8040 3136 Fax: 023 8040 3136 — (St. Thos.) MRCS Eng. LRCP Lond. 1949; MB BS Lond. 1953; DObst RCOG 1953. Prev: Ho. Phys. (Obst.) St. Thos. Hosp.

WADEHRA, Vineet Flat 1, 2 Marchmont Road, Edinburgh EH9 1HZ; 34 Hadrian Court, Darras Hall, Newcastle upon Tyne NE20 9JU — MB ChB Ed. 1998; BSc (Med. Sci.) Ed. 1995. Specialty: Gen. Med.

WADERA, Satish Prakash Wadera, 478 Landseer Road, Ipswich IP3 9LU Tel: 01473 274494 Fax: 01473 727742 Email: michele.abson@gp-d83614.nhs.uk — (Darbhanga Med. Coll., Darbhanga (Bihak), India) MB BS 1966; DA (Lond.) 1970. Gen. Med. Practitioner, Ipswich. Specialty: Anaesth.; Alcohol & Substance Misuse; Sports Med.

WADEY, Lee Paul 84 Park Lane, Wallington SM6 0TL — MB BS Lond. 1989; MRCPCH; MRCP. Cons. Paediat. Epsom Gen. Hosp. Dorking Rd. Epsom Surrey.

WADGAONKAR, Pushkar Surendra Flat 76, Grosvenor Towers, Broadway, Belfast BT12 6HG — MB BS Bombay 1989; MRCP (UK) 1995.

WADGE, Dennis Allen (retired) Wellspring Lodge, Wellspring Road, Southrepps, Norwich NR11 8XA Tel: 01263 833603 — MB BS Lond. 1955 (St. Bart.) Prev: Ho Surg. Redhill Co. Hosp.

WADGE, Ernest John, OStJ (retired) Rowanwood, Bell Lane, Lower Broadheath, Worcester WR2 6RR — MB ChB Birm. 1944. Prev: Ho. Surg. Gen. Hosp. Birm.

WADGE, Valerie Anne Jesmond Clinic, 48 Osborne Road, Jesmond, Newcastle upon Tyne NE2 2AL Tel: 0191 281 4060 Fax: 0191 281 0231; 80 Moor Road North, Gosforth, Newcastle upon Tyne NE3 1AB Tel: 0191 213 2362 — MB BS Newc. 1978 (Newcastle Upon Tyne) Cert. JCC Lond. 1980; MRCGP 1982; DFFP 1997. Tutor (Gen. Pract.) Newc. u. Tyne; Gen. Practitioner.

WADGE, Winifred Joan (retired) 28 Church Street, Great Missenden HP16 0AZ Tel: 01240 64943 — MB BS Lond. 1936 (Univ. Coll. Hosp.) MA Camb. 1930; MRCS Eng. LRCP Lond. 1934; FRCS Eng. 1939. Prev: Surg. ENT Dept. Univ. Coll. Hosp.

WADHWA, Harish Kumar The Surgery, 191 Barrows Lane, Yardley, Birmingham B26 1QS Tel: 0121 783 2719 — MB BS Delhi 1971.

WADHWA, Pradeep 5 St Michael's Road, London NW2 6XD — MB BS Lond. 1979; DRCOG 1982; DCH RCP Lond. 1982; MRCGP 1983.

WADHWA, Vivek Kumar 241 Ainsworth Road, Bury BL8 2SQ — MB ChB Manch. 1998.

WADHWANI, Gulab Harjasram 1C Western Road, Sutton SM1 2SX — MB BS Bombay 1965.

WADLEY, Mr John Patrick University Department Neurosurgery, Institute of Neurology, Queen Square, London WC1N 3BG Tel: 020 7837 3611; Flat 501, The Beaux Arts Building, Manor Gardens, London N7 6JX Tel: 020 7272 0621 — MB ChB Liverp. 1989; FRCS Ed. 1994. Clin. Lect./Research Fell. (Neurosurg.) Inst. Neurol. Lond. Specialty: Neurosurg. Socs: Assoc. Mem. Soc. Brit. Neurol. Surgs.; Fell. Roy. Soc. Med.; Brit. Stereotactic and Image Guided Neurosurg. Gp. Prev: Regist. (Neurosurg.) Char. Cross Hosp. Lond.; Regist. (Neurosurg.) Roy. Free Hosp. Lond.; Demonst. (Anat.) Univ. Liverp. Sch. of Med.

WADLEY, Martin Stuart c/o 2 Wimsland Court, Holcot, Northampton NN6 9SA — MB ChB Sheff. 1990.

WADMAN, Simon Mark The Surgery, High Street, Heathfield TN21 8JD Tel: 01435 864999/862192 Fax: 01435 867449; Albury Cottage, Hadlow Down, Uckfield TN22 4HS — MB BS Lond. 1982.

WADROP, Thomas Anthony Middle House, 2 Box Drive, Nunthorpe, Middlesbrough TS7 0RH Tel: 01642 324679 Fax: 01642 317339 — MB ChB Ed. 1967; MRCGP 1980; DMJ 1995. GP; Princip. Police Surg. Cleveland. Socs: Assn. Police Surg.; RSM. Prev: Gen. Pract. Coveby Newham, Cleveland.

WADSLEY, Jonathan Charles 15 Onley Street, Norwich NR2 2EA Tel: 01603 766522 — BChir Camb. 1995; MB BChir Camb. 1996; MA Camb. 1997. SHO (Renal Med.) Norf. & Norwich Hosp. Specialty: Gen. Med. Prev: Ho. Off. (Surg.) Milton Keynes Gen. Hosp.; Ho. Off. (Med.) Addenbrookes Camb.; SHO (Med.) Norf. & Norwich Hosp.

WADSWORTH, Arthur Mayow (retired) 35 Glyn Garth Court, Menai Bridge LL59 5PB Tel: 01248 715269 — MB ChB Birm. 1938; MRCS Eng. LRCP Lond. 1938. JP.

WADSWORTH, Bridget Ann Littlegates, Hinton St George TA17 8SN — MB BS Lond. 1977.

WADSWORTH, George Reginald (retired) Beech House, Barrule Park, Ramsey IM8 2BR Tel: 01624 815471 — MB ChB Liverp. 1940 (University of Liverpool) MD Liverp. 1952. Prev: Prof. Physiol. Univ. Singapore.

WADSWORTH, Julian Ashley 16-18 Foster Lane, Hebden Bridge HX7 8HF — MB ChB Leeds 1994.

WADSWORTH, Mark Ronald The Surgery, 28 Holes Lane, Woolston, Warrington WA1 4NE Tel: 01925 653218 Fax: 01925 244767 — MB ChB Manch. 1984; DCH RCP Lond. 1986; Cert. Family Plann. JCC 1987; DRCOG 1988. GP Warrington.

WADSWORTH, Mr Paul Vincent (retired) 61 Dyke Road Avenue, Hove BN3 6DA Tel: 01273 507074 — (Oxf.) MA Oxf. 1948, BM BCh 1944; DObst RCOG 1949; FRCS Eng. 1951. Prev: Cons. ENT Surg. Roy. Sussex Co., Sussex Throat & Ear, Roy. Alexandra Childr., Haywards Heath & Cuckfield Hosps. & Chailey Heritage.

WADSWORTH, Richard Department of Anaesthesia, Manchester Royal Infirmary, Oxford Road, Manchester M13 9WL Tel: 0161 276 4033 Fax: 0161 273 6211; Harley Bank South, Victoria Road, Todmorden OL14 5LD — MB BChir Camb. 1986 (Univ. Camb.) BSc St. And. 1983; FRCA 1992. Cons. Anaesth. Manch. Roy. Infirm. Specialty: Anaesth. Socs: Assn. Anaesth.; Manch. Med. Soc.; BMA. Prev: Sen. Regist.(Anaesth.), Regist. & SHO NW RHA.

WADSWORTH, Susan Margaret Lakeside Surgery, Cottingham Road, Corby NN17 2UR Tel: 01536 204154; Riverbanks, Caldecott, Market Harborough LE16 8RU — MA Oxf. 1986, BM BCh 1984; DRCOG 1987; MRCGP 1988; FRCGP 1999. Specialty: Obst. & Gyn.

WADSWORTH, Timothy Mayow The Church Street Practice, David Corbet House, 2 Callows Lane, Kidderminster DY10 2JG Tel: 01562 822051 Fax: 01562 827251; Comely Bank, Lowe Lane, Wolverley, Kidderminster DY11 5QP Tel: 01562 850210 — MB ChB Birm. 1970 (Birm) BSc Ed. 1964; MRCGP 1979. Clin. Asst. Kidderminster Hosp.

WADZISZ, Faustyna Jowita 10 Dorchester Court, Wray Common Road, Reigate RH2 0UD — MB BCh BAO NUI 1955; DPM Eng. 1963. Assoc. Specialist (Psychiat.) Epsom Dist. Hosp. Socs: BMA.

WAGG, Adrian Stuart Department of Geriatric Medicine, University College Hospital, 25 Grafton Way, London WC1E 6AU Tel: 020 7380 9910 Fax: 020 7380 9652 Email: a.wagg@ucl.ac.uk; 13 Selwyn Road, Bow, London E3 5EA Tel: 020 8981 7909 — (Lond. Hosp. Med. Coll.) MB BS Lond. 1988; MRCP (UK) 1991; FRCP 2001. Sen. Lect. (Med.) Univ. Coll. Lond.; Hon. Cons. Camden & Islington Community Health Serv. NHS Trust; Cons. Phys. & Geriatician Univ. Coll. Lond. Hosp.; Clin. Director, Med. and Emerg. Serv.s UCLH. Specialty: Care of the Elderly; Gen. Med. Socs: Brit. Geriat. Soc. & Amer. Geriat. Soc.; Internat. Continence Soc. Prev: Sen. Regist. Camden & Islington Health Serv. NHS Trust; Sen. Regist. Northwick Pk. Hosp.; Regist. (Med.) Roy. Lond. Hosp.

WAGG, Michael George (retired) Treeton House, Redesmouth Road, Bellingham, Hexham NE48 2EH Tel: 01434 220358 — MB ChB St. And. 1950; DA Eng. 1959; FFA RCS Eng. 1962. Prev: Cons. Anaesth. Sunderland Hosp. Gp.

WAGHORN, Alison Jane Royal Liverpool University Hospita, Prescot Street, Liverpool L7 8XP — MB ChB Birm. 1986; FRCS Ed. 1990; FRCS Eng. 1992; FRCS Gen Ssurg 1999; MD 1999. Cons. Endocrine & Breast. Surg. Roy. Liverp. Univ. Trust. Specialty: Gen. Surg. Prev: Anat. Demonstr. Univ. Coll. Lond.; SHO Rotat.Kent & Cantebury Hosp.; Regist. Rotat. NW Thames.

WAGHORN, David John Wycombe Hospital
, Department of Microbiology, Queen Alexandra Road, High Wycombe HP11 2TT Tel: 01494 425246 Fax: 01494 425090 Email: david.waghorn@sbucks.nhs.uk; 40 Kinghorn Park, Maidenhead SL6 7TX — MB BS Lond. 1980 (Char. Cross) DRCOG 1983; MSc Lond. 1988; FRCPath 1996, M 1989. Cons. Microbiol. Wycombe Gen. Hosp. High Wycombe. Specialty: Med. Microbiol. Socs: Assn. Med. Microbiol.; Hosp. Infec. Soc.; Roy. Soc. Med. Prev: Lect. & Hon. Sen. Regist. (Microbiol.) St. Thos. Hosp. Lond.

WAGHORN, Geoffrey Bernard Merryhill House, 73 High Street, Braunston, Daventry NN11 7HS Tel: 01788 890698 — MB BS Lond. 1974 (Char. Cross Hosp. Med. Sch.) MRCS Eng. LRCP Lond. 1974; MRCGP 1979.

WAGHORNE, Nigel Julian Prince Philip Hospital, Dafen, Llanelli SA14 8QF Tel: 01554 756567; Towy Cottage, Ferryside SA17 5ST — MB BCh Wales 1992. Staff Grade Doctor, A & E, P. Philip Hosp., LLa.lli. Carmasthenshire. Specialty: Accid. & Emerg.

WAGLE, Ashish Umakant Royal Glamorgan Hospital, Ynys Maerdy, Llantrisant CF72 8XR Tel: 01443 443600 Fax: 01443 443468 Email: awagle@pr-tr.wales.nhs.uk — MB BS Bombay 1986; DA India 1987; MD India 1989; FRCA 1997. Cons. Anaesth. Specialty: Anaesth. Special Interest: Pain Managem. Socs: Pain Soc.; BMA; Anaesth. in Managem. (AIM).

WAGLE, Sudhir Ghanashyam Maldon Road Surgery, 39 Maldon Road, Danbury, Chelmsford CM3 4QL Tel: 01245 225868 Fax: 01245 224253; 6 Mill Lane, Danbury, Chelmsford CM3 4LF — MB BS Bombay 1974. Specialty: Gen. Pract. Socs: BMA; MDU. Prev: SHO (Gen. Med. & Cardiol.) Rush Green Hosp. Romford.

WAGMAN, Lyndon Lane End Medical Group, 25 Edgwarebury lane, Edgware HA8 8LJ Tel: 020 8958 4233 Fax: 020 8905 4657 — MB BS Lond. 1989; BSc Lond. 1986; DRCOG 1992; MRCGP 1993. Mem. W. Barnet PCG; GP Regist. Trainer. Prev: Clin. Asst. (Oncol.) Roy. Free Hosp. Lond.; Trainee GP Edgware VTS.

WAGNER, Alan John Woodlands Medical Centre, Woodland Road, Didcot OX11 0BB Tel: 01235 511355 Fax: 01235 512808 — MB BS Lond. 1966 (Middlx.) DAvMed Eng. 1970. Specialty: Aviat. Med. Prev: Ho. Off. Middlx. Hosp. Lond.

WAGNER, Catharine Helen — MB ChB Liverp. 1974 (Liverpool) DRCOG 1976; MRCGP 1978. Specialty: Gen. Pract. Socs: Roy. Coll. Gen. Pract.

WAGNER, Helga Rising Brook Surgery, Merrey Road, Stafford ST17 9LY Tel: 01785 251134 Fax: 01785 222441 — MB ChB Cape Town 1985.

WAGNER, Margaret Marian Fennell (retired) Basement Flat, 10 Frederick Place, Weymouth DT4 8HQ — MB BS Lond. 1948 (Roy. Free) MRCS Eng. LRCP Lond. 1947; FRCPath 1975, M 1964. Prev: Scientist MRC Pneumoconiosis Unit.

WAGNER, Nicholas Alan Giles Department of Mental Health for Older People, Stonebow Unit, The County Hospital, Union Walk, Hereford HR1 2ER Tel: 01432 355444 — (St. Bart.) MRCS Eng. LRCP Lond. 1969; MB BS Lond. 1970; DPM Eng. 1974; MRCPsych 1975; FRCPsych 2000. Cons. Psychiat. Hereford; Second Opinion Apptd. Doctor Ment. Health Act Commiss.; Med. Mem. Ment. Health Review Tribunal. Prev: Cons. Psychiat. W. Middlx. Univ. Hosp.; Hon. Sen. Lect. (Psychiat.) Char. Cross & Westm. Med. Sch. Lond.; Cons. Ment. Health Older People Herefordsh. Primary Care NHS Trust.

WAGNER, Peter Robinson (retired) Spindrift, 39 Duport Bay, St Austell PL26 6AQ Tel: 01726 63167 — MB BS Lond. 1948 (Guy's) MRCS Eng. LRCP Lond. 1948; DObst RCOG 1966; MD Lond. 1967. Prev: Cons. Aviat. Med. ASP EC Systems Ltd. Yeovil.

WAGNER, Robert Michael Cheviot Way Health Centre, Cheviot Way, Bourtreehill South, Irvine KA11 1JU Tel: 01294 211993 Fax: 01294 218461; 78 Kilnford Drive, Dundonald, Kilmarnock KA2 9ET Tel: 01563 851126 — MB ChB Bristol 1970; DObst RCOG 1974. Prev: Med. Off. Grenfell Assn. Labrador & Newfld.; SHO (Anaesth.) Roy. Devon & Exeter Hosp.; Med. Off. Parbatti S. Himalayan Expedit.

WAGNER, Simon David 3 Elmfield Road, London N2 8EB — MB BS Lond. 1984.

WAGSTAFF, Alison 13 Cleveden Gardens, Kelvinside, Glasgow G12 0PU — BM BS Nottm. 1979; FFA RCS Eng. 1985. Cons. Inst. Neurol. Sc. Glas. Specialty: Anaesth. Prev: Sen. Regist. North. RHA.

WAGSTAFF, Anthony Edward 1 Rayleigh Close, Newton Road, Cambridge CB2 2AZ Tel: 01223 357175 — MB BChir Camb. 1952 (Westm.) MA, MB BChir Camb. 1952; DIH Soc. Apoth. Lond. 1964; DAvMed Eng. 1971; MFOM RCP Lond. 1978. Indep. Cons. Occupat. Health Phys. Camb. Specialty: Occupat. Health. Socs: Internat. Acad. Aviat. & Space Med.; Fell. Roy. Soc. Med.; Soc. Occupat. Med. Prev: Sen. Med. Off. Civil Aviat. Auth.; Squadron Ldr. RAF Med. Br.; Chief Med. Off. Gulf Air Bahrain.

WAGSTAFF, Dorothea Primrose (retired) 7 Saxon Place, Lower Buckland Road, Lymington SO41 9EZ Tel: 01590 671975 — (Camb. & Univ. Coll. Hosp.) BA Camb. 1946; MB BChir Camb. 1949; MA Camb. 1998. Prev: Jun. Hosp. Med. Off. N. Lond. Blood Transfus. Centre.

WAGSTAFF, Elizabeth (retired) Willowbank House, Wear View, Durham DH1 1LW Tel: 0191 386 9367 — (Durh.) MB BS Durh. 1943; MRCOG 1949. Prev: Sen. Regist. St. Mary's Hosps. Manch.

WAGSTAFF, Professor John South West Wales Cancer Institute, Singleton Hospital, Sketty, Swansea SA3 1NR Tel: 01792 285299

Fax: 01792 285201 Email: john.wagstaff@swan.ac.uk; Musketierslaan 7, Maastricht 6213 BR, Netherlands Tel: 00 31 43 326 3977 — MB ChB Manch. 1976 (Manchester) MRCP (UK) 1979; MD Manch. 1986; FRCP (Lond.) 1996. Prof. and Hon. Cons. in Med. Oncol., S. Wales Cancer Inst., Swansea; Growth and Developm., Univ. Maastrichot; Bd. Mem. Dutch Soc. of Med. Oncol.; Hon. Prof. at the Univ. of Maastricht, The Netherlands. Specialty: Oncol. Socs: Assn. Cancer Physicians, UK; Europ. Soc. Med. Oncol.; Amer. Assn. Cancer Research. Prev: Prof. (Med. Oncol.) Vrije Univ. Ziekenhuis Amsterdam, Netherlands; Sen. Lect. (Med. Oncol.) Vrije Univ., Amsterdam; Lect. & Hon. Sen. Regist. (Med. Oncol.) Univ. Manch. & Christie Hosp. Manch.

WAGSTAFF, John Kenneth (retired) Willowbank House, Wear View, Durham DH1 1LW Tel: 0191 386 9367 — (Lond. Hosp.) MD Camb. 1953, MB BChir 1942; MRCS Eng. LRCP Lond. 1942; FRCP Lond. 1970, M 1948. Prev: Clin. Tutor Sussex Postgrad. Med. Centre.

WAGSTAFF, Miles Harvey Gloucestershire Hospitals NHS Trust, Gloucestershire Royal Hospital Childrens Services, Great Western Road, Gloucester GL1 3NN Tel: 08454 225188 Fax: 08454 225540 — MB BChir Camb. 1992; MRCP (Paeds.) 1995. Cons. Paediat., Gloucestershire Hosps. NHS Trust. Specialty: Paediat.; Neonat. Socs: RCPCH; BAPM.

WAGSTAFF, Peter John Castlecroft Medical Practice, 104 Castlecroft Road, Castlecroft, Wolverhampton WV3 8LU; The Old Smithy, Ebstree Road, Seisdon, Wolverhampton WV5 7ES — MB ChB Birm. 1986; DCM 1989. Princip. Gen. Pract. Specialty: Gen. Pract. Prev: SHO (Paediat.) Worcester Roy. Infirm.; SHO Rotat. (Surg.) Worcester Roy. Infirm.; SHO (A & E) Wolverhampton Hosp.

WAGSTAFF, Rebecca Jane Croftlands, Castle Carrock, Brampton CA8 9LT Tel: 01228 70409 Email: rebecca.wagstaff@ncha.nhs.uk — MB ChB Liverp. 1985; MSc Newc. 1991; MFPHM 1992. Cons. in Pub. Health Med., Dept Pub. Health Med., N. Cumbria Health Auth., Carlisle, Cumbria. Specialty: Pub. Health Med. Prev: Sen.Regist. (Pub. Health Med.) North. RHA.

WAGSTAFF, Thomas Ian Newcastle upon Tyne Hospitals NHS Trust, Freeman Hospital, Queen Victoria Road, Newcastle upon Tyne NE1 4LP Tel: 0191 232 5131 Fax: 0191 227 5173; 9 King John's Court, Darras Hall, Ponteland, Newcastle upon Tyne NE20 9AR Tel: 01661 823329 — MB BS Lond. 1965 (Univ. Coll. Hosp.) MRCS Eng. LRCP Lond. 1965; FRCOG 1983, M 1970; BSc (Special. Anat.) Lond. 1962, MD 1979. p/t Cons. Emerit., Freeman Hosp., Newc. upon Tyne. Specialty: Obst. & Gyn. Socs: Scientif. Fell. Zool. Soc. Lond.; Blair Bell Res. Soc.; Liveryman Worshipful Soc. Apoth. Prev: Cons. O & G & Clin. Dir. Roy. Vict. Infirm. Newc. u. Tyne; Regist. (O & G) Luton & Dunstable Hosp.; Lect. & Sen. Regist. (Obst. Unit) & Ho. Surg. & Ho. Phys. Univ. Coll. Hosp. Lond.

WAGSTAFF, William (retired) 8 Longacre Road, Dronfield, Sheffield S18 1UQ — (Manch.) MB ChB Manch. 1957; DTM & H Eng. 1960; FRCPath 1980, M 1968; FRCP Ed. 1988; FRCP Lond. 1990. Prev: Dir. Regional Transfus. Centre Sheff.

WAGSTYL, Jan Wendel St James's Practice, 138 Croydon Road, Beckenham BR3 4DG Tel: 020 8650 0568 Fax: 020 8650 4172; 138 Croydon Road, Beckenham BR3 — MB ChB Birm. 1983; DRCOG 1986; DCH 1986; MRCGP 1987. Princip GP Birm.

WAGSTYL, Sabina 8 Vicarage Road, Harborne, Birmingham B17 0SP — MB BCh BAO NUI 1954 (Galway) Asst. MOH Pub. Health Dept. Birm. Prev: Ho. Phys. & Ho. Surg. Roy. Infirm. Huddersfield; Ho. Phys. Paediat. City Gen. Hosp. Stoke-on-Trent; SHO Cas. Selly Oak Hosp. Birm.

WAH, Tze Min 44 Sudbury Heights Avenue, Greenford UB6 0LX — MB ChB Leeds 1995.

WAHAB, Mr Mohammed Adel Parkwood Health Centre, Long Catlis Road, Parkwood, Gillingham ME8 9PR — MB BCh Alexandria 1971; FRCS Glas. 1979. Specialty: Gen. Surg.

WAHAB, Mumtaz Abdul Lister Hospital, Coreys Mill Lane, Stevenage SG1 4AB Tel: 01438 314333; 1 Bassetts Close, Farnborough, Orpington BR6 7AQ — MB BS Osmania 1981; MB BS Osmania Univ. India 1981; MRCS Eng. LRCP Lond. 1988; DRCOG 1993. Staff Grade Doctor (O & G) Lister Hosp. Stevenage.

WAHBA, Mr Hany Fahmy St Marks Medical Centre, 24 Wrottesley Road, Plumstead, London SE18 3EP Tel: 020 8854 6262 Fax: 020 8317 3098 — MB BCh Cairo 1978; MRCS Eng. LRCP Lond. 1979; FRCS Ed. 1985. Clin. Asst. (Gen. Surg.) Greenwich Health Care Trust. Specialty: Gen. Surg. Prev: SHO (Gen. Surg.) Roy. Liverp. Hosp.; SHO Rotat. (Surg.) Univ. Hosp. Wales & Cardiff Roy. Infirm.; SHO (Orthop. Surg.) P'boro. HA.

WAHBA, Nabil Youssef 16 Kings Avenue, Eastbourne BN21 2PF Tel: 01323 724062 — MB ChB Alexandria 1970; Dip Psychother BHR 1989; Dip Counsel CSCT 1998; MLCOM (Med. Osteo.) 2002. Psychotherapist, Counsellor, Osteopath, Pain Managem. Specialty: Psychother.; Anaesth. Socs: Accred. Mem. Med. & Den. Soc.Hypn.; Retd. Mem. Assn. Anaesth.; Brit. Med. Accup. Soc. Prev: Assoc. Specialist in Anaesth., Dist. Gen. Hosp., Eastbourne; Staff Grade in Pyschiatry, Ticehurst; Private Counsellor & Psychotherapist.

WAHBY, Cesar Cesai Tawfiq 16 Chervilles, Maidstone ME16 9JE — MB ChB Baghdad 1955; LMSSA Lond. 1961; DPM Eng. 1965. Med. Asst. Long Gr. Hosp. Epsom. Socs: Roy. Med.-Psych. Assn. Prev: Ho. Surg. Hammersmith Hosp. & Roy. Marsden Hosp. Chelsea; Cas. Off. W. Lond. Hosp.

WAHEDNA, Irfan Barnsley District General Hosptial, Gawber Road, Barnsley S75 2EP — MB BS Karachi 1983; MRCP (UK) 1988; FRCP 1999. Cons. Phys. Barnsley Dist. Gen. Hosp. Specialty: Respirat. Med. Prev: Sen. Regist. Univ. Coll. Hosp. Lond.; Research Fell. (Respirat.) City Hosp. Nottm.; Regist. (Respirat. Gen. Med.) Lodge Moor Hosp. Sheff.

WAHEED, Abdul Pontllanfraith Health Centre, Off Blackwood Road, Pontllanfraith, Blackwood NP12 2YU Tel: 01495 227131 Fax: 01495 220361 — MB BS Peshawar, Pakistan 1978; MRCS Eng. LRCP Lond. 1984.

WAHEED, Muhammad (retired) 30 Woodstock Close, Upton, Macclesfield SK10 3DZ — MB BS Punjab 1965.

WAHEED, Nosheen 30 Woodstock Close, Macclesfield SK10 3DZ — MB ChB Manch. 1992.

WAHEED, Mrs Waheeda Fields House, Fields Park Avenue, Newport NP18 2JS Tel: 01633 211703 — MB BS Punjab 1959 (King. Edwd. Med. Coll. Lahore) MB BS Punjab (Pakistan) 1959; DPM Eng. 1969; MRCPsych 1972. Cons. Psychiat. St. Cadoc's Hosp. Caerleon. Specialty: Gen. Psychiat. Prev: SHO (Cas.) St. Peter's Hosp. Chertsey & King's Lynn Gen. Hosp.; Res. Med. Off. Vict. Hosp. Woking.

WAI, Angela Sin-Yi 58 Bancroft Avenue, London N2 0AS — MB ChB Dundee 1982; DA Eng. 1985. Regist. (Anaesth.) Roy. Free Hosp. Lond. Specialty: Anaesth. Prev: Regist. (Anaesth.) Southend HA.

WAIGHT, Catherine Teresa Trinity Hospice, 30 Clapham Common, Northside, London SW4 0RN; 17 St Georges Court, Garden Row, London SE1 6HD — BM BS Nottm. 1987; MRCGP 1992. Specialty: Palliat. Med.

WAIN, Asghar Ali Downe Hospital, Pound Lane, Downpatrick BT30 6JA Tel: 028 4461 3311 Email: ali_wain@dltrust.n-i.nhs.uk — MB BS Punjab 1984; FRCS Eng., Glas., Ire. Locum Cons. (A & E Med) Downe Hosp. Downpatrick. Specialty: Accid. & Emerg.

WAIN, Eileen Anne (retired) Brander Lodge, Tripp Lane, Linton, Wetherby LS22 4HX Tel: 01937 581157 — MB ChB Glas. 1960; DObst RCOG 1963; DPH Leeds 1978; FFPHM RCP (UK) 1991. Prev: Dir. Pub. Health Leeds HA.

WAIN, Elizabeth Mary St Thomas' Hospital, St John's Institute of Dermatology, Lambeth Palace Road, London SE1 7EH Tel: 020 7928 9292 Fax: 020 7922 8138 — MB BS Lond. 1997. Research Fell. St Johns Inst. of Dermat. Lond.

WAIN, Emma Charlotte Elizabeth 19 Sandfield Road, Headington, Oxford OX3 7RN — MB BS Lond. 1996.

WAIN, Mark Owen The Surgery, Bull Yard, Simpson Street, Spilsby PE23 5LG Tel: 01790 752555 Fax: 01790 754457 — MB BS Lond. 1978; BSc Lond. 1975; BSc Lond. 1975; FRCS Ed. 1983; MRCGP 1987.

WAIN, Michael Louis Whitstable Health Centre, Harbour Street, Whitstable CT5 1BZ Tel: 01227 794555 Fax: 01227 794677; Little Hall Farm, Alcroft Grange, Tyler Hill, Canterbury CT2 9NN Tel: 01227 463824 — MB BChir Camb. 1973 (St. Mary's) MA Camb. 1974, BA (Hons.) 1969, MB BChir 1973; MRCP (UK) 1975.

WAIN, Sarah Helen 87 St Cyrus Road, Colchester CO4 4LR — MB ChB Birm. 1998.

WAIND, Catherine Mary (retired) 14 Woodland Road, Ulverston LA12 0DX Tel: 01229 583086 — MB ChB Leeds 1947. Prev: Sen. Med. Off. Family Plann. SW Cumbria.

WAINE, Colin, OBE Sunderland Health Authority, Durham Road, Sunderland SR3 4AF Tel: 0191 565 6256 Fax: 0191 528 3455; 42 Etherley Lane, Bishop Auckland DL14 7QZ Tel: 01388 604429 — MB BS Durh. 1959 (King's Coll. Univ. Durh.) MB BS (2nd cl. Hons.) Durh. 1959; FRCGP 1976, M (Distinc.) 1968; FRCPath 1992. Dir. Health Progr. & Primary Care Developm. Sunderland HA. Specialty: Cardiol. Socs: (Ex-Chairm.) Roy. Coll. Gen. Pract.; Assoc. Mem. BPA; N. Eng. Med. Soc. Prev: Hosp. Pract. (Paediat.) Bishop Auckland Gen. Hosp.; Chairm. Clin. & Research Div. RCGP; Cons. & Brit. Delegate to Europ. Health Comm. Primary Care & Preven. Gp.

WAINE, Julie Marie 3 Sycamore Cottages, Frimley Road, Camberley GU15 2RA — BM Soton. 1994.

WAINFORD, Claire Michele 18 The Gardens, London SE22 9QE — MB BS Lond. 1988; BSc Anat. Lond. 1985, MB BS 1988.

WAINHOUSE, Catherine Louise Flat 1, 41 Achillies Road, London NW6 1DZ — MB ChB Leic. 1991.

WAINSCOAT, James Stephen 14 Woodlands Close, Headington, Oxford OX3 7RY Tel: 01865 220330 Fax: 01865 221778 — MB ChB Liverp. 1972; MSc (Immunol.) Birm. 1975; MRCP (UK) 1976; FRCPath 1992, M 1980; FRCP Lond. 1991. Cons. Haemat. John Radcliffe Hosp. Oxf.; Hon Director CRF Molecular Haemat. Specialty: Haematology. Prev: MRC Clin. Sc. Nuffield Dept. Clin. Med. Oxf.; Sen. Regist. (Haemat.) John Radcliffe Hosp. Oxf.

WAINSCOTT, Gillian Rose Darville Queen Elizabeth Psychiatric Hospital, Vincent Drive, Edgbaston, Birmingham B15 2QZ Tel: 0121 678 2010 Fax: 0121 678 2208 Email: gillian.wainscott@bsmht.nhs.uk — MB ChB Bristol 1968; DCH RCP Lond. 1972; MRCPsych 1992. Cons. Psychiat., Perinatal Psychiat., Birm. & Solihull Ment. Health NHS Trust; Hon. Sen. Clin. Lect., Univ. for Birm. Specialty: Gen. Psychiat. Prev: SHO (Paediat.) Hammersmith Hosp. Lond.; SHO (Paediat.) Brompton Hosp. Lond.; SHO (Med.) Bristol Roy. Infirm.

WAINSTEAD, Harold (Surgery), 1 Highdown Avenue, Worthing BN13 1PU Tel: 01903 65656; 17 Romney Court, Winchelsea Gardens, Worthing BN11 5EU — MRCS Eng. LRCP Lond. Lond. 1946 (Camb. & St. Geo.) MRCS Eng. 1945 LRCP Lond. 1946; BA, MB BChir Camb. 1949. Prev: Res. Med. Off. Roy. Vict. Hosp. Folkestone; Ho. Surg. St. Geo. Hosp.; Squadron Ldr. RAF.

WAINWRIGHT, Alexandra Jeannette Rosalind Rothschild House Surgery, Chapel Street, Tring HP23 6PU Tel: 01442 822468 Fax: 01442 825889; 14 Hillside, Cheddington, Leighton Buzzard LU7 0SP — BM Soton. 1983; MRCGP 1987. GP Tring. Prev: Trainee GP Lincoln VTS.

WAINWRIGHT, Mr Andrew Morris Nuffield Orthopaedic Centre, Oxford OX3 9DU Tel: 01865 741155 — MB ChB Leic. 1990; BSc (Hons.) Leic. 1987; FRCS Eng. 1994; FRCS (Trauma & Orth.) 2000. Specialist Regist. (Trauma & Orthop.) Nuffield Orthop. Centre Oxf. Specialty: Orthop. Special Interest: Paediatric Orthop. Socs: Girdlestone Orthop. Soc.; Brit. Orthop. Trainees Assn.; Brit. Orthop. Assn. Prev: Clin. Fell. Hosp. Sick Childr. Toronto Canad.; SHO (Plastic Surg.) Exeter; SHO (Orthop. & Gen. Surg.) Bristol.

WAINWRIGHT, Andrew Tristan Staff and Partners, Queensway Medical Centre, Olympic Way, Wellingborough NN8 3EP Tel: 01933 678767 Fax: 01933 676657; 4 The Paddocks, Orlingbury, Kettering NN14 1JU — MB ChB Manch. 1983; DRCOG 1986.

WAINWRIGHT, Anthony Christopher Southampton General Hospital, Tremona Road, Southampton SO16 6YD Tel: 023 8079 6720 Fax: 023 8079 4348 — MB BS Lond. 1967 (St. Thos.) FRCA 1971. Cons. Anaesth. Soton. Univ. Hosps. NHS Trust. Specialty: Anaesth. Special Interest: Ophth. Anaesth. Socs: Assn. Anaesth.; BOAS. Prev: Lect. Univ. Bristol; Sen. Regist. Univ. Hosp. of Wales Cardiff.

WAINWRIGHT, Anthony John Neuadd Felin, Talgarth, Brecon LD3 — MB ChB Birm. 1953.

WAINWRIGHT, Christian Thomas New House, College Rd, Denstone, Uttoxeter ST14 5HR — MB ChB Leic. 1997.

WAINWRIGHT, Christopher John Mount Pleasant Farm, Chalvington, Hailsham BN27 3TB — MB ChB Sheff. 1987.

WAINWRIGHT, Christopher John-Paul 21 Ratcliffe Road, Haydon Bridge, Hexham NE47 6ER — BM BS Nottm. 1994; BMedSci (Hons.) Nottm. 1990. Research Fell.Qu. Eliz. Hosp. Specialty: Orthop. Prev: SHO (Orthop.) Tyneside; SHO (A&E) S. Tyneside; Ho. Off. (Med.) Freeman Hosp. Newc.

WAINWRIGHT, David Theodore Neaudd Felin, Talgarth, Brecon LD3 0BN — MB ChB Birm. 1984.

WAINWRIGHT, Mr Denys (retired) 101 Swains Lane, Highgate Village, London N6 6PJ Tel: 020 8340 2131 — MB ChB Liverp. 1932; MCh Orth. Liverp. 1934, MB ChB 1932; FRCS Ed. 1937; FRCS Eng. 1971; Hon. DSc Keele 1975. Cons. Orthop. Surg. Robt. Jones & Agnes Hunt Orthop. Hosp. Oswestry. Prev: Cons. Orthop. Surg. N. Staffs. Hosp. Centre.

WAINWRIGHT, Elizabeth Ann Carron Hill, 221 Wallasey Road, Wallasey CH44 2AD; 11 Gainsborough Road, Southport PR8 2EY Tel: 01704 565782 — MB ChB Liverp. 1985; DRCOG 1988; MRCGP 1989. GP S.port. Prev: Trainee GP/SHO Liverp. VTS.; Ho. Off. Roy. Liverp. Hosp.

WAINWRIGHT, Geoffrey Anson Oakengates Medical Practice, Limes Walk, Oakengates, Telford TF2 6JJ Tel: 01952 620077 Fax: 01952 620209 — MB BS Newc. 1968; DTM & H Liverp. 1972. Socs: BMA. Prev: Jun. Ho. Off. (Med.) Dryburn Hosp. Durh.; SHO (Paediat.) Bishop Auckland Gen. Hosp.; Med. Off. Brit. Solomon Is.s Protec.

WAINWRIGHT, James Russell Health Centre, Pen y Bont, The Roe, St Asaph LL17 0LU Tel: 01745 583208 Fax: 01745 583748 — MB ChB Liverp. 1990; BSc (Hons.) Med. Cell Biol. Liverp. 1987; MRCGP 1994. Specialty: Gen. Pract.

WAINWRIGHT, Jane Elizabeth Talwrn Farm, Talwrn Road, Rhostyllen, Wrexham LL14 4ER — MB ChB Ed. 1992; MRCP (UK) 1995; MD Ed. 1999. SpR (Neurol.) Hope Hosp. Salford. Specialty: Pharmacology. Prev: SpR (Neurol.) S. Thames Lond.; Clin. Research Fell./Hon. Regist. (Neurol.) King's Coll. Sch. of Med. & Dent. Lond.; Specialist Regist. (Clin. Pharmacol. & Therap.) Western Infirm. Glas.

WAINWRIGHT, Jennifer Rose 126 King George V Drive N., Heath, Cardiff CF14 4EL — MB ChB Sheff. 1990. Higher Professional Train. Fell. (Gen. Pract.) Univ. Glas. Specialty: Gen. Pract. Socs: RCGP; MDDUS.

WAINWRIGHT, John, OBE 8 Windsor Court, Warren Drive, Deganwy, Conwy LL31 9TN Tel: 01492 583259 — MB BS Lond. 1950 (St Bart.) MRCS Eng. LRCP Lond. 1950. Prev: Act. Squadron Ldr. RAF Med. Br.

WAINWRIGHT, Nicholas James Department of Dermatology, Monklands Hospital, Monkscourt Avenue, Airdrie ML6 0JS Tel: 01236 746162 Fax: 01236 746239 — MB BS Lond. 1986 (Univ. Coll. & Middlx. Hosp.) MA Oxon. 1977; MRCP (UK) 1990; FRCP (Edin) 2000. Cons. Dermat. Monklands & Belshill Hosps. Trust Airdrie; Hon. Clin. Sen. Lect. Univ. Glas. Specialty: Dermat. Socs: Brit. Assn. Dermat.; PhotoMed. Soc. Prev: Sen. Regist. (Dermat.) Ninewells Hosp. Dundee; Regist. (Dermat.) Ninewells Hosp. Dundee; Regist. (Gen. Med. & Endocrinol.) Leeds Gen. Infirm.

WAINWRIGHT, Raymond James Department of Cardiology, King's College Hospital, Denmark Hill, London SE5 9RS — (Guy's) MD Lond. 1982, MB BS 1971; MRCS Eng. LRCP Lond. 1971; MRCP (UK) 1973; FRCP Lond. 1993. Cons. Cardiol. King's Coll. Hosp. Lond. Specialty: Cardiol. Prev: Cons. Cardiol. Brook Gen. Hosp. Lond.; Sen. Regist. Dept. Cardiol. Guy's Hosp. Lond.

WAISE, Ahmed York Hospital, Wiggington Road, York YO31 8HE Tel: 01904 5855 Email: ahmed.waise@york.nhs.uk — MB ChB Baghdad 1973; MRCP (UK) 1982; LRCP LRCS Ed. LRCPS Glas. 1983; MRCPath 1989; FRCPath 1998; FRCP Lond. 1999. Chem. Path.York Hospital, York. Specialty: Chem. Path.; Endocrinol. Prev: Sen. Regist. & Regist. (Chem. Path.) N. West. RHA; SHO (Gen. Med.) Roy. Infirm. Blackburn; SHO (Gen. Med.) Yarmook Hosp., Baghdad.

WAIT, Christopher Martin Little Croft, Duns Tew, Bicester OX25 6JR — MB BCh Oxf. 1981; MA, MB BCh Oxf. 1981; FFA RCS Eng. 1986. Cons. Anaesth. Horton Hosp. Banbury Oxon. HA. Specialty: Anaesth. Prev: Research Regist. & Sen. Regist. (Anaesth.) Nuffield Hosp. Oxf.

WAIT, Hilary Jane 132 Grand Drive, London SW20 9EA; 22 Mossville Gardens, Morden SM4 4DG — MB BS Lond. 1983; DA (UK) 1986; DRCOG 1987; DCH RCP Lond. 1988. Prev: Trainee GP Lond.; SHO (Neonates) All St.s Hosp. Chatham; SHO (Paediat.) Maidstone Hosp.

WAITE, Alasdair 39 Nunholme Road, Dumfries DG1 1JW — MB ChB Aberd. 1994.

WAITE, Alison 45 Coach Road, Guiseley, Leeds LS20 8AY — MB ChB Manch. 1995.

WAITE, Anthony John 9 Kenwood Road, Shrewsbury SY3 8AH — LMSSA Lond. 1993.

WAITE, Christopher John 30 Bristol Avenue, Saltburn-by-the-Sea TS12 1BW — MB BCh Wales 1994.

WAITE, David William (retired) 63 Chazey Road, Caversham, Reading RG4 7DU Tel: 0118 947 5606 — MB ChB Manch. 1963; DObst RCOG 1965; DA Eng. 1967; DMRD Eng. 1971; FFR 1973; FRCR 1975.

WAITE, Frank Thomas John (retired) Waite, McFadden and Brown, 35 George Street, Dumfries DG1 1EA Tel: 01387 53724 Fax: 01387 259780; 39 Nunholm Road, Dumfries DG1 1JW Tel: 01387 255717 — (Edinburgh) MB ChB Ed. 1966; MRCP (UK) 1972; FRCP Ed 1999.

WAITE, Heather Claire Sunnybrook House, Llangoed, Beaumaris LL58 8NY — BM BS Nottm. 1995.

WAITE, Ian 12 Sedgefield Road, Radcliffe, Manchester M26 1YE; 31 Conningsby Close, Bromley Rise, Bromley Cross, Bolton BL7 9NY — MB ChB Manch. 1990; FRCA 1995. Cons. Anaesth. Pain Managem.Roy.Bolton.Hosp.Bolton. Specialty: Anaesth.

WAITE, Ian Joseph (retired) 35 Belmont Avenue, Baildon, Shipley BD17 5AJ Tel: 01274 586884 — (Sheff.) MB ChB Sheff. 1952; DObst RCOG 1953. Prev: Regist. Childr. Hosp. Bradford.

WAITE, Jonathan Queen's Medical Centre, The Courtyard, Nottingham NG7 2UH — MB ChB Ed. 1976; BSc (Hons. Pharmacol.) Ed. 1973; MRCPsych 1980; FRCPsych 1995; LIM (Mental Health Law) Northumbria 2001. Cons. Psychiat. Dept. Health c/o Elderly Qu. Med. Centre Nottm.; Lord Chancellor's Med. Visitor. Specialty: Gen. Psychiat.; Geriat. Psychiat. Socs: Fell. Roy. Med. Soc. Edin.; BNPA; BGS.

WAITE, Jonathan Chapman 152 Revelstoke Road, London SW18 5PA — MB BS Lond. 1994.

WAITE, Kathrin Elizabeth Airedale Hospital, Skipton Road, Steeton, Keighley BD20 6TD Tel: 01535 652511 — MB BChir Camb. 1981; MA Camb. 1981; FRCA 1989. Cons. Anaesth. Airedale Gen. Hosp. Keighley. Specialty: Anaesth. Special Interest: Obstetric Anaesth. Socs: Assn. Anaesth. Gt. Brit. & Irel.; Pain Soc. Prev: Cons. Anaesth. Ashford Hosp. Middlx.; Sen. Regist. (Anaesth.) Hammersmith Hosp. Lond.; Regist. (Anaesth.) St Peter's Hosp. Chertsey.

WAITE, Malcolm Austin (retired) 52 Woodbourne, Norfolk Road, Edgebaston, Birmingham B15 3PP Tel: 0121 454 4401 Mob: 07887 673974 Email: malcolm.waite@doctors.org.uk — MB ChB Leeds 1964; MRCP Lond. 1969; MD Leeds 1973; FRCP Lond. 1984. Prev: Cons. Phys. & Lect. (Med.) Qu. Eliz. Hosp. Birm.

WAITE, Norma Rosemary 22 Almatade Road, Bitterne, Southampton SO18 6AB Tel: 023 8032 7194 — BM Soton. 1983; DRCOG 1986.

WAITT, Dora Joy 15 Richmond Road, Thornton Heath, Croydon CR7 7QE — MB BS Lond. 1992.

WAITT, Roger Henry Francis Falstead House, The Street, HamSt., Ashford TN26 2HG Tel: 01233 732206 — MB BS Lond. 1963; LMSSA Lond. 1961; DObst RCOG 1963; DMRD Eng. 1968. Specialty: Radiol.

WAIWAIKU, Kokulo Nyanpee High Road Family Doctors, 119 High Road, Benfleet SS7 3LA Tel: 01268 753591 Fax: 01268 794585; 277 Hart Road, Thundersilly, Benfleet SS7 3UW Tel: 0116 875 5591 — MD Univ. Liberia 1980 (R M Doeliotti, Liberia) BSc Liberia 1973; DCCH Ed 1988; DTM & H Liverp 1989; MSc London 1990. GP Princip. Specialty: Gen. Pract.; Paediat. Socs: BMA.

WAJED, Mohammed Ali 220 Sandridge Road, St Albans AL1 4AL Tel: 01727 835505 Fax: 01727 835505 Email: mohammedwajed@hotmail.com — MB BS Dacca 1963 (Chittagong Med. Coll.) DPhysMed Eng. 1969; MRCP (UK) 1973; MRCS Eng. LRCP Lond. 1974; FRCP Lond. 1991. Cons. Rheum. & Rehabil. Hemel Hempstead Gen. Hosp., St. Albans City Hosp. & Garston Manor Med. Rehabil. Centre. Specialty: Rehabil. Med.; Rheumatol. Socs: Hosp. Cons. & Spec. Assn.; Brit. Soc. Rheum. & Mem. BMA. Prev: Sen. Regist. Norf. & Norwich Hosp.; Sen. Regist. (Rheum.) Lond. Hosp.; Regist. (Rheum.) King's Coll. Hosp. Lond.

WAJED, Mr Shahjehan Ali Dept. of Surgery, Royal Free Hospital, Pond Street, London NW3 2QG; 70 Blake Road, London N11 2AM Fax: 079 7071 8037 Email: swajed@hotmail.com — BM BCh Oxf. 1992; BA Camb. 1989, MA 1993; FRCS Eng. 1996. Specialist Regist. Rotat. (Gen. Surg.) N. Thames; Lect. in Surg., Roy. Free and VCL Med. Sch. Specialty: Gen. Surg. Prev: Research Fell. 1999-2000; Dept. of Surg., Univ. of South. Calif., Los Angeles, USA.

WAJID, Abdul 81 Havering Gardens, Chadwell Heath, Romford RM6 5BH Tel: 020 8590 4479 — MB BS Punjab 1962 (Nishtar Med. Coll. Multan) MB BS Punjab (Pakistan) 1962; DCH RCPS Glas. 1965. SCMO Redbridge HCT. Specialty: Community Child Health.

WAJID, Mohammad Abdul c/o 3 Woburn Grove, Hartlepool TS25 1HD — MB BS Punjab 1989.

WAKANKAR, Hemant Madhukar Department of Orthopaedics, Kent and Sussex Hospital, Mount Ephraim, Tunbridge Wells TN4 8AT Tel: 01892 526111; Flat 1, Derwent House, Barnet EN5 3HD Tel: 020 8440 3949 — MB BS Bombay 1988 (Bombay, India) MS (Orth) Bombay 1990; DNB (Orth) New Delhi 1991; FRCS Glas. 1995; MChOrth Liverp. 1996; FRCS (Orth) 1997. Jt. Revision Fell. (Orthop.) Kent & Sussex Hosp. Tunbridge Wells & Horder Centre for Arthritis CrowBoro. Specialty: Orthop.

WAKATSUKI, Mai Hylands, Harvest Hill, Bourne End SL8 5JJ Tel: 01628 525760 Email: m_wakatsuki@hotmail.com — BM BS Nottm. 1998; BMedSci 1996. SHO Oncological Mamatology Christie Hosp. Manch. Specialty: Gen. Med.

WAKE, Angela Margaret The Church Lane Practice, 2 Church Lane, Merton Park, London SW19 3NY Tel: 020 8542 1174 Fax: 020 8544 1583 — MB BS Lond. 1979 (Lond. Hosp.) BSc. (Biochem.) Lond. 1976.

WAKE, Anne Marian Royal Gwent Hospital, Cardiff Road, Newport NP20 2UB Tel: 01633 234321; 35 Bryn Glas, Thornhill, Cardiff CF14 9AA Tel: 01222 615322 — MB BCh Wales 1977; FRCR 1983. Cons. Radiol. Gwent NHS Healthcare Newport. Specialty: Radiol. Socs: Roy. Coll. Radiol. & Brit. Inst. Radiol.; BMA. Prev: Cons. Radiol. P. Chas. Hosp. Merthyr Tydfil; Sen. Regist. (Radiol.) Univ. Hosp. Wales Cardiff.

WAKE, Carie Ann — MB BS Lond. 1997; MRCP.

WAKE, Colin Reginald Manor House, Cross Lane, Holcombe, Bury CO8 5HR — MB ChB Manch. 1970; MRCOG 1977. Cons. (O & G) Fairfield Gen. Hosp. Bury. Specialty: Obst. & Gyn.

WAKE, Deborah Jane 4 Park Place, Lunanhead, Forfar DD8 3NA — MB ChB Ed. 1998.

WAKE, Mr Mark 1 Dartmouth Avenue, Pattingham, Wolverhampton WV6 7DP — MB ChB Birm. 1983; FRCS Ed. 1988; FRCS Eng. 1989.

WAKE, Martyn Charles The Surgery, 2 Church Lane, Merton Park, London SW19 3NY Tel: 020 8542 1174 Fax: 020 8544 1583 — MB BS Lond. 1979 (Guy's) BSc (Anat.) Lond. 1976, MB BS 1979; DRCOG 1982.

WAKE, Michael John Clayton Consulting Rooms, 38 Harborne Road, Edgbaston, Birmingham B15 3HE Tel: 0121 454 8899 Fax: 0121 454 1390 Email: mjcwake@compuserve.com; The Lodge, 30A Frederick Road, Edgbaston, Birmingham B15 1JN Tel: 0121 455 7654 Fax: 0121 455 8705 Email: mjcwake@compuserve.com — (Birmingham) BDS Birm. 1962; MB ChB Birm. 1969; FDS RCS Eng. 1972; FRCS(Edin) 2000. Private Surg. Pract. (Oral. & Maxil. Surg.) Edgbaston Birm.; Hon. Sen. Clin. Lect. Univ. Birm. Specialty: Oral & Maxillofacial Surg. Socs: Fell. Brit. Assn. Oral & Maxillofacial Surg. Pres. 1999; BMA. Prev: Hon. Edr. Brit. Jl. Oral & Maxillofacial Surg.; Cons. Craniofacial Surg. Birm. Childr. Hosp. NHS Trust; Cons. Oral & Maxillofacial Surg. Univ. Hosp. Birm. NHS Trust & Birm. Childr. Hosp. NHS Trust.

WAKE, Pamela Judith Knarsdale House, Roseworth Crescent, Newcastle upon Tyne NE3 1NR — BM BS Nottm. 1993.

WAKE, Mr Philip Nicholas 5 Ashbourne Avenue, Blundellsands, Liverpool L23 8TX — MB ChB Liverp. 1969; DCH Eng. 1973; FRCS Eng. 1974. Cons. (Vasc. & Gen. Surg.) Warrington Hosp. Specialty: Gen. Surg.; Surgery, Vascular.

WAKE, Suzanne Louise 43 Stamford Road, West Bridgford, Nottingham NG2 6GD Email: suzanne.wake@ntlworld.com — BM BS Nottm. 1994.

WAKEEL, Riadh Adil Petrous King George Hospital, Barley Lane, Goodmayes, Ilford IG3 8YB Tel: 020 8970 8064 Fax: 020 8970 8124; 17 Chigwell Park Drive, Chigwell IG7 5BD Tel: 020 8500 6424 Fax: 020 8281 9904 — (Baghdad University) MB ChB Baghdad 1969; Dip. Dermat. Lond. 1977; MRCPI 1985; MRCP (UK) 1985; FRCP Ed. 1997; FRCP Lond. 1998. Cons. Dermat. King Geo. Hosp. Ilford Essex. Specialty: Dermat. Socs: Brit. Assn. Dermat.; Fell. Roy. Soc. Med.; Amer. Acad. of Dermat. Prev: Sen. Regist. & Hon

Leecturer (Dermat.) Aberd. Roy. Infirm.; Regist. (Dermat.) Stobhill Gen. Hosp. Glas.; Regist. (Med.) Orpington Hosp.

WAKEFIELD, Catharine Jane Porchester Health Centre, Portchester, Fareham PO16 9TU — MB BS Lond. 1979; DRCOG 1982.

WAKEFIELD, Mr Christian Hamilton Royal Hampshire County Hospital, Romsey Road, Winchester SO22 5DG Tel: 01962 824830 Fax: 01962 824640 Email: christian.wakefield@weht.swest.nhs.uk — MD Lond. 1998; BSc Lond. 1988; MB BS Lond. 1989; FRCS Ed. 1996. Cons. (Surg.) Roy. Hants. Co. Hosp. Winchester. Specialty: Gen. Surg. Socs: AESGBI; EAES; SARS. Prev: Lect. (Surg.) Edin.; SHO (Surg.) Roy. Infirm. Edin.; Research Fell. (Surg.) Acad. Surg. Unit St. Mary's Hosp. Lond.

WAKEFIELD, Christopher John Wakefield and Partners, Lever Chambers Centre for Health, 1st Floor, Bolton BL1 1SQ Tel: 01204 360030/31 Fax: 01204 360033; The Lindens, 235 Greenmount Lane, Bolton BL1 5JB Tel: 01204 492957 — MB ChB Manch. 1971; DObst RCOG 1974.

WAKEFIELD, Deborah Ann The White Rose Surgery, Exchange Street, South Elmsall, Pontefract WF9 2RD Tel: 01977 642412 Fax: 01977 641290 — MB ChB Leeds 1986.

WAKEFIELD, Graham Stanley (retired) Dale Cottage, Charlcombe Lane, Bath BA1 8DR Tel: 01225 312248 Fax: 01225 312248 — MB BS Lond. 1953 (St. Mary's) FRCP Lond. 1971, M 1955. Prev: Cons. Neurol. Roy. United Hosp. Bath.

WAKEFIELD, Marion Ann Sue Nicholls centre, Manu House, Bierton Road, Aylesbury HP20 1EG Tel: 01296 489951 — MB BS Lond. 1969 (Lond. Hosp.) DCH Eng. 1972; MRCP (UK) 1975; FRCP Lond. 1994; FRCPCH 1997, M 1996. Cons. Paediat. Manor Ho. Hosp. Aylesbury. Specialty: Paediat. Socs: Fell. Roy. Soc. Med. Prev: Sen. Regist. (Paediat.) Aylesbury Health Dist. & Pk. Hosp. Childr. Oxf.; Regist. (Paediat.) Stoke Mandeville Hosp. Aylesbury; SHO (Paediat.) Aylesbury Health Dist.

WAKEFIELD, Mavis (retired) 5 The Grange, Chorleywood Close, Rickmansworth WD3 4EG — MB ChB Birm. 1951; MRCP Ed. 1955. Prev: SCMO (Community Health Servs.) Hillingdon HA.

WAKEFIELD, Peter Clive Whitehorse Vale Surgery, Whitehorse Vale, Barton Hills, Luton LU3 4AD Tel: 01582 490087 — MB BS Lond. 1967; MRCS Eng. LRCP Lond. 1967.

WAKEFIELD, Richard John 61 The Mount, Selby YO8 9BD — BM Soton. 1991 (Soton. Med. Sch.) Research Fell. in Rheumat. Leeds Gen. Infirm.

WAKEFIELD, Ruth Margaret Fairfield General Hospital, Rochdale Old Rd, Bury BL9 7TD — MB ChB Sheff. 1989 (Sheffield) MRCP (UK) 1994; MRCPCH 1997. Cons. (Paediat.) Fairfield Gen. Hosp. Lancs. Specialty: Paediat. Socs: Mem. of the Roy. Coll. of Paediat. And Child Health. Prev: Regist. Rotat. (Paediat.) St. Jas. Univ. Hosp. Leeds, Bradford Roy. Infirm. & St Luke's Bradford.; Specialist Regist. (Paediat.) St. Jas. Univ. Hosp., Leeds.

WAKEFIELD, Mr Simon Eyles James Cook University Hospital, Marton Road, Middlesbrough TS4 3BW — MB BS Lond. 1987; BSc (Hons.) Chem. Surrey 1982; FRCS Eng. 1991. Specialty: Gen. Surg. Prev: Lect. (Gen. Surg.) Trent RHA; Regist. (Gen. Surg.) Oxon. RHA.

WAKEFIELD, Susan Margaret Stockwell Lodge Medical Centre, Rosedale Way, Cheshunt, Waltham Cross EN7 6HL Tel: 01992 624408 Fax: 01992 626206; 61 Tolmers Road, Cuffley, Potters Bar EN6 4JG — MB BS Lond. 1976 (St. Thos.) BSc (Hons.) Lond. 1973; MRCP (UK) 1979. Prev: Regist. (Gen. Path.) & SHO (Gen. Med.) FarnBoro. Hosp., Kent.

WAKEFIELD, Valerie Ann Barnsley District General Hospital, Barnsley S75 2EP; Ringwood Cottage, Rails Road, Rivelin, Sheffield S6 6GF — MB ChB Sheff. 1977; MRCP (UK) 1982. Cons. Phys. i/c c/o Elderly. Specialty: Gen. Med.

WAKEFORD, Neil Anthony Andrew Neatenden Farm, New England Lane, Sedlescombe, Battle TN33 0RP — MB ChB Manch. 1992.

WAKEFORD, Timothy David Carpalla Villa, Carpalla, Foxhole, St Austell PL26 7TY — MB BS Lond. 1998.

WAKEHAM, Craig Timothy Long Street Practice, 51 Long Street, Cerne Abbas, Dorchester DT2 7JG Tel: 01300 341666 Fax: 01300 341090; Five Bells House, Piddletrenthide, Dorchester DT2 7QX Tel: 01300 348690 — BM BS Nottm. 1984; BMedSci. Nottm. 1982; DRCOG 1988; MRCGP 1989. Princip. GP Clin. Asst. (Diabetes) Dorchester.

WAKEHAM, Niklas Rufus 49 Chetwynd Road, London NW5 1BX — MB BS Lond. 1996.

WAKELEY, Mr Charles John Old Bittern Barn, West Harptree, Bristol BS40 6HQ — MB BS Lond. 1983; BSc Lond. 1980; FRCS Eng. 1987; FRCS Ed. 1987; FRCR 1991. Cons. Radiol. Bristol Roy. Infirm. Specialty: Radiol. Socs: BMA; RCR; BSSR. Prev: Sen. Regist. (Radiol.) Bristol Roy. Infirm.; SHO (Gen. Surg.) Mayday Hosp. Thornton Heath; SHO (A & E) Char. Cross Hosp. Lond.

WAKELEY, Sir John Cecil Nicholson, Bt, CStJ (retired) Mickle Lodge, Mickle, Trafford, Chester CH2 4EB Tel: 01244 300316 — MB BS Lond. 1950 (King's Coll. Hosp.) MRCS Eng. LRCP Lond. 1950; FRCS Eng. 1955; FACS 1973. Prev: Sen. Regist. (Surg.) King's Coll. Hosp. Lond. & Roy. Postgrad. Med. Sch. Hammersmith Hosp.

WAKELEY, Richard Michael (retired) Coves Cottage, High St, St Peters, Broadstairs CT10 2TH Tel: 01843 869478 — (Kings College Hospital) MB BS Lond. 1957.

WAKELIN, James Herbert Sydney (retired) Hollybanks, Old Peterston Road, Groes Faen, Pontyclun CF72 8NU Tel: 029 2089 1790 — MB BCh Wales 1948 (Cardiff) BSc Wales 1945, MB BCh 1948; DObst RCOG 1950; MRCGP 1989. Prev: Ho. Phys. & Ho. Surg. O & G E. Glam. Hosp. Pontypridd.

WAKELIN, Sarah Helen St Mary's Hospital, Department of Dermatology, Praed Street, London W2 1NY Tel: 020 7886 1083 Fax: 020 7886 1134 Email: sarah.wakelin@st-marys.nhs.uk — MB BS Lond. 1988 (King's Coll.) BSc (Hons.) Pharmacol. Lond. 1985; MRCP (UK) 1991; FRCP 2004. Cons. Derm. St Marys. Hosp; Hon. Sen. Lect. Imperial Coll. of Sci., Technol. and Med. Specialty: Dermat. Socs: Europ. Soc. of Contact Dermatitis; St John's Dermatological Soc. (Pres. 2004-05); Brit. Assn. Dermat. Prev: Sen. Regist. (Dermat.) St. John's Inst. St. Thos. Hosp. Lond.; Sen. Regist. (Dermat.) Amersham Hsop. Bucks.; Regist. (Dermat.) Roy. Berks. Hosp. Reading.

WAKELING, Anthony (retired) 59 Bishopsthorpe Road, London SE26 4PA Tel: 020 8778 6994 — MB ChB Birm. 1961; PhD Birm. 1966, BSc 1958, MB ChB 1961; DPM Lond. 1968; FRCPsych. 1979, M 1972. Emetitus Prof. Psychiat. Roy. Free Hosp. Sch. Med. Lond.; Hon. Cons. (Psychiat.) Roy. Free Hosp. & Friern Hosp. Lond. Prev: Sen. Lect. Psychiat. Roy. Free Hosp. Sch. Med. Lond.

WAKELING, Howard Grenville 15 Emmett Road, Rownhams, Southampton SO16 8JB — MB BS Lond. 1988 (Middlx. Hosp. Med. Sch. Lond.) BSc Lond. 1985, MB BS 1988; MRCP (UK) 1993; FRCA 1994. Specialist Regist. Wessex Rotat. Specialty: Anaesth. Prev: Rotat. Regist. Basingstoke & Soton.; Vis. Assoc. in Anaesth. Duke Univ. Med. Center N. Carolina; SHO (Anaesth.) Roy. United Hosp. Bath & Southmead Hosp. Bristol.

WAKELING, John Amaziah 70 Heol Isaf, Radyr, Cardiff CF15 8DZ — MB BCh Wales 1994.

WAKELING, Marilen (retired) 59 Bishopsthorpe Road, London SE26 4PA Tel: 020 8778 6994 — MB ChB Birm. 1961; DPM Eng. 1965. Community Med. Off. Lewisham & Guy's Health Dists.; Sen. Clin. Med. Off. (Family Plann.) Optimum Health Servs.; Family Plann. Instruct. Doctor. Prev: Regist. (Child Psychiat.) King's Coll. Hosp. Lond.

WAKELING, Zoe Claire 40 Dunholme Road, Newcastle upon Tyne NE4 6XE — MB BS Newc. 1998.

WAKELY, Catherine 15 Acacia Grove, London SE21 8ER — BM BS Nottm. 1994.

WAKELY, James Nicholas The Surgery, Chapel Lane, Plumstead Market, Colchester CO7 7AG — MRCS Eng. LRCP Lond. 1980; MA (Theol.) Camb. 1977, MB BChir 1983; DFFP 1993. GP Colechester; Dep. Police Surg. Chelmsford.; Clin. Asst. (Psychiat.) Clacton Hosp. Prev: SHO (O & G) Rush Green Hosp. Romford; SHO (Cas. & Orthop.) Herts & Essex Hosp. Bishops Stortford; SHO (Psychiat.) Princess Alexandra Hosp. Harlow.

WAKELY, John Henry (retired) Redcroft, Meols Drive, Hoylake, Wirral CH47 4AQ Tel: 0151 632 1777 — LRCP LRCS Ed. 1941 (Roy. Colls. Ed.) LRCP LRCS Ed. LRFPS Glas. 1941; DA Eng. 1948; FFA RCS Eng. 1954. Prev: Cons. Anaesth. Liverp. AHA (T) & St. Helens & Knowsley AHA.

WAKELY, Suzanne Louise — BM Soton. 1997; MRCP 2000. Specialty: Gen. Med.

WAKEMAN, Mr Robert Basildon Hospital, Nethermayne, Basildon SS16 5NL Tel: 01268 593742 — MB BS Lond. 1981; FRCS Eng. 1986; FCS(SA) Orth. 1992; T(S) 1994. Cons. Orthop. Basildon Hosp.

Specialty: Orthop. Prev: Regist. Rotat. (Orthop.) Roy. Free Hosp. Lond.

WAKERLEY, Mark Brice Flat 2, Penleys Court, Penleys Grove St., York YO31 7RW — MB BS Lond. 1992.

WAKERLEY, Rebecca Louise 6 Peacocks Close, Stokesley, Middlesbrough TS9 5QD Tel: 01642 713231 — MB BS Newc. 1996.

WAKES MILLER, Clive Hugh (retired) Moss Cottage, The Green, Thornham, Hunstanton PE36 6NIT Tel: 01485 512525 Email: wmclive@aol.com — MB BS Lond. 1962 (Guy's) MRCS Eng. LRCP Lond. 1962; MRCGP 1970; Cert. Av. Med. 1970; AFOM RCP Lond. 1982. Prev: Med. Examr. Benefits Norf.

WAKLEY, Gillian Margaret Kidsgrove Medical Centre, Mount Road, Kidsgrove, Stoke-on-Trent ST7 4AY Tel: 01782 784221 Fax: 01782 781703; 80 Sneyd Avenue, Newcastle ST5 2PY Tel: 01782 624447 Fax: 01782 624447 — MB ChB Bristol 1965; MFFP 1994. Sen. Clin. Lect. (Primary Care) Keele Univ. 1997. Socs: Inst. Psychosexual Med.

WAKTARE, Johan Esbjorn Patrik 103 Canbury Avenue, Kingston upon Thames KT2 6JR Tel: 020 8286 8021 — MB ChB Manch. 1989; MRCP 1993. Clin. Research Regist. (Cardiol. Scis.) St. Geos. Hosp. Med. Sch. Specialty: Cardiol.

WALAPU, Myanga Fumbanani Macdonald St Davids Hospital, Department of Public Health, PO Box 13, Carmarthen SA31 3YH Tel: 01267 234501 Fax: 01267 223337 — MB ChB Manch. 1978; DRCOG 1980; MSc Manch. 1985; MFCM RCP (UK) 1986. Cons. Pub. Health Med. Nat. Pub. Health Serv. for Wales. Specialty: Pub. Health Med.

WALAWENDER, Andrzej Josef c/o JAT, PO Box 367, Twickenham TW2 7TU Tel: 020 8898 7429 Fax: 020 8894 4335 Email: jatco@compuserve.com — MB BS Lond. 1985.

WALAYAT, Muhammed Department of Cardiology, Royal Hospital for Sick Children, Edinburgh EH9 1LF Tel: 0131 667 1991; 6/2 Dalrymple Crescent, Edinburgh EH9 2NU — MB BS Pakistan 1985; MRCP (UK) 1991.

WALBAUM, David William Flat 3/3, 1 Woodlands Drive, Glasgow G4 9EQ — MB ChB Glas. 1993; MRCP (UK) 1996. Specialty: Gen. Med.; Nephrol.

WALBAUM, Mr Philip Raby (retired) 10 Ravelston Heights, Ravelston House Park, Edinburgh EH4 3LX — MB ChB Ed. 1944 (Univ. Ed.) MB ChB (Hnrs.) Ed. 1944; FRCS Ed. 1948. Prev: Cons. Cardiothoracic Surg. Lothian HB.

WALBRIDGE, David Gerrard Department of Psychiatry, Royal South Hants Hospital, Graham Road, Southampton SO14 0YG Tel: 023 8063 4288 — MB ChB Bristol 1981; MRCPsych 1986; BSc Bristol 1978, MD 1993. Cons. Psychiat. Roy. S. Hants. Hosp. Soton.; Hon. Clin. Teach. Univ. Soton. Specialty: Gen. Psychiat. Prev: Sen. Regist. (Psychiat.) Warneford Hosp. Oxf.; Regist. & SHO (Psychiat.) Barrow Hosp. Bristol; SHO (Gen. Med.) Dist. Gen. Hosp. Gorleston.

WALBROOK, Emma Elizabeth 71 Earlswood Road, Redhill RH1 6HJ — MB BS Lond. 1997.

WALBY, Mr Anthony Peter 41 Derryvolgie Avenue, Belfast BT9 6FP — MB BCh BAO Belf. 1974; MB BCh Belf. 1974; FRCS Ed. 1979. Cons. Otorhinolaryng. Roy. Vict. Hosp., Roy. Belf. Hosp. for Sick Childr. & City Hosp. Belf. Specialty: Otorhinolaryngol.

WALBY, Ceri Woodlands Surgery, Woodlands Terrace, Caerau, Maesteg CF34 0SR Tel: 01656 734203; 7 Pen-y-Wain Road, Cardiff CF24 4GB — MB BCh Wales 1989 (Univ. Wales Coll. Med.) MRCP (UK) 1992; MRCGP 1996.

WALCZAK, Mr Jonathan Peter Beauchamp Princess Royal University Hospital, Farnborough BR6 8ND Tel: 01689 865702 Email: gluteusminimus@aol.com — MB BS Lond. 1987 (UMDS) BSc (Biochem.) Lond. 1984; FRCS Eng. 1992; FRCS (Orth.) 1998. Cons. Trauma. Orthop. Surg. Specialty: Orthop. Special Interest: Minimal Access Hip Replacement; sports injuries; Arthroscopic knee Surg. Socs: Mem. BOA. Prev: Treas. to S. E. Thames higher Train. Progr. in Orthopaedic Surg.

WALD, Professor Nicholas John Wolfson Institute of Preventive Medicine, Barts & The London, Queen Mary's School of Medicine & Dentistry, Charterhouse Square, London EC1M 6BQ Tel: 020 7882 6269 Fax: 020 7882 6270 Email: n.j.wald@qmul.ac.uk; 9 Park Crescent Mews East, London W1W 5AF Tel: 020 7636 2721 — (Univ. Coll. Hosp.) MB BS Lond. 1967; FPHM Lond. 1982; FRCP Lond. 1986; DSc (Med.) Lond. 1987; FRCOG 1992; F Med Sci 1998; Cbiol FiBiol 2000; FRS 2004. Prof. Environm. & Preven. Med. & Director of Wolfson Inst of Preven. Med.; Edr. Jl. Med. Screening; Hon Cons. Specialty: Pub. Health Med.; Epidemiol. Socs: Assn. Phys. Prev: Dep. Dir. ICRF Cancer Epidemiol. & Clin. Trials Unit Univ. Oxf.; Mem. Scientif. Staff Med. Research Counc. Northwick Pk. Hosp.; Regist. (Med.) Univ. Coll. Hosp. Lond.

WALDEK, Stephen Renal Unit, Hope Hospital, Salford M6 8HD Tel: 0161 789 7373 Fax: 0161 787 5775; 31 Harboro Road, Sale M33 5AN Tel: 0161 973 6275 Email: walkeks@compuserve.com — MB BCh Wales 1971; MRCP (UK) 1974; FRCP Lond. 1990. Cons. Nephrol. Salford, DHA; Med. Dir. Specialty: Nephrol. Prev: Sen. Regist. (Nephrol.) Sheff. AHA (T).

WALDEN, Amanda 1 Howe Close, Mudeford, Christchurch BH23 3JA — MB ChB Liverp. 1983; Cert. Family Plann. JCC 1986. Retainer Scheme in Gen. Pract. Bournemouth. Prev: SHO (O & G) Poole Gen. Hosp.; Community Med. Off. E. Dorset HA; Trainee GP Boscombe VTS.

WALDEN, Andrew Peter Flat B, 165 Battersea Rise, London SW11 1HP — MB BS Lond. 1994.

WALDEN, Anne Fiona Doreen 49 Barcombe Heights, Preston, Paignton TQ3 1PU — MB BS Lond. 1985; DRCOG 1989. Prev: Trainee GP CMH VTS.

WALDEN, Faye The Medical Centre, 143 Rookwood Avenue, Leeds LS9 0NL; 6 Wigton Grove, Leeds LS17 7DZ — (Leeds) MB ChB Leeds 1962.

WALDEN, Neil Patrick Michael Marazion Surgery, Gwallon Lane, Marazion TR17 0HW; Elm Cottage, Relubbus, Penzance TR20 9EP Tel: 01736 763417 — MB BS Lond. 1982.

WALDEN, Peter Alexander Mennie (cons. rooms), 15 Basil Mansions, Basil Street, London SW3 1QJ Tel: 020 7589 4781 Mob: 07860 170582 Fax: 020 7581 0244; 85 Rusthall Avenue, Chiswick, London W4 1BN Tel: 020 8994 4363 — MB BS Lond. 1964 (St. Geo.) MRCS Eng. LRCP Lond. 1963; DObst RCOG 1966; MRCP (UK) 1970; BAcC 1980. Specialty: Gen. Pract. Socs: Fell. Roy. Soc. Med.; BMA.

WALDEN, Richard John (retired) Bossall, 126 Bluehouse Lane, Limpsfield, Oxted RH8 0AR Tel: 01883 712952 Fax: 01883 712952 — MB BS Lond. 1963 (Guy's) MRCS Eng. LRCP Lond. 1963; Dip. Pharm. Med. RCP (UK) 1976; MD Lond. 1989. Prev: Sen. Res. Fell. Clin. Pharmacol. UCL.

WALDEN, Susan Jane, Maj. RAMC 85 Rusthall Avenue, London W4 1BN Tel: 020 8994 4363 — MB BS Lond. 1991 (King's Coll.) DRCOG 1995; DCCH 1995; MRCGP 1998.

WALDEN, Tracey Anne 8 Hartnell Court, Albert Road, Corfe Mullen, Wimborne BH21 3TY — MB BS Lond. 1992 (St. Bart.) Med. Off. Joseph Weld Hospice Dorchester (p/t). Specialty: Palliat. Med.; Gen. Pract. Prev: Princip. (Gen. Pract.) The Pk. Surg. Yeovil.

WALDENBERG-NAMROW, Caroline 39 Winding Way, Leeds LS17 7RG — MB ChB Manch. 1995; BA Hons. Oxf. 1993.

WALDER, Andrew David Anaesthetic Department, North Devon District Hospital, Raleigh Park, Barnstaple EX31 4JB — MB BS Lond. 1986; MRCP (UK) 1991; FRCA 1992. Clin. Dir. (Intens. Care) N. Devon Dist. Hosp. Specialty: Anaesth.

WALDER, Professor Dennis Neville (retired) 21 Osbaldeston Gardens, Gosforth, Newcastle upon Tyne NE3 4JE Tel: 0191 285 2327 — MB ChB Bristol 1940; FRCS Eng. 1954; FRCS Ed. 1954; MD Bristol 1947, ChM 1965; MFOM RCP Lond. 1980. Prev: Chairm. MRC Decompression Sickness Panel.

WALDER, Geoffrey Peter Lilliput Surgery, Elms Avenue, Lindisfarne, Poole BH14 8EE — MB BS (per GMC) Newcastle 1974. GP; Clin. Asst. in Opthalmology. Specialty: Ophth.; Diabetes.

WALDES, Mr Rodney Maxwell Greenford Avenue Medical Centre, 322 Greenford Avenue, London W7 3AH Tel: 020 8578 1880 Email: rodney.waldes@btinternet.com; 96 Church Road, Hanwell, London W7 3BE Tel: 020 8567 3665 Fax: 020 8567 3665 — MB ChB Manch. 1970; FRCS Eng. 1977. Prev: Regist. (Radiodiag.) Hammersmith Hosp. Lond.; Regist. (Surg.) Hammersmith Hosp. Lond.; Regist. (Surg.) King Edwd. Memor. Hosp. Ealing.

WALDIE, Mr Wilfrid (retired) Moorcroft, Old Whisky Road, Auchterhouse, Dundee DD3 0RD Tel: 01382 320232 — MB ChB Glas. 1947; FRCS Ed. 1960. Cons. Orthop. Surg. Dundee Roy. Infirm.; Hon. Sen. Lect. in Orthop. Surg. Univ. Dundee. Prev: Sen. Orthop. Regist. Bridge of Earn Hosp. Perth.

WALDIN, Ian Ernest Gwynne Gainford Surgery, Main Road, Gainford, Darlington DL2 3BE Tel: 01325 730204 — MB BS Lond. 1979 (St. Bart.) LMSSA Lond. 1977; DRCOG 1983; DCH RCP Lond. 1983; MRCGP 1985.

WALDMAN, Adam Daniel Bernard Department of Diagnostic Radiology, Middlesex Hospital, London W1N 8AA Tel: 020 7323 6772; 3 Davenant Road, London N19 3NW — MB BChir Camb. 1993; BSc (Hons.) Lancaster 1981; PhD Bristol 1985; MA Camb. 1994; MRCP (UK) 1995. Specialist Regist. (Diagnostic Radio.) UCL Hosps. Specialty: Radiol. Prev: SHO (Med.) Whittington & Hammersmith Hosps.; Ho. Off. (Surg.) W. Suff. Hosp.; Ho. Off. (Med.) Addenbrooke's Hosp. Camb.

WALDMAN, Brian Lewin (retired) Edgehill, Ogdens N., Fordingbridge SP6 2QD Tel: 01425 653660 — MB BS Lond. 1960 (St. Mary's) DObst RCOG 1964; FRCGP 1981, M 1973. Prev: Ho. Phys. & Ho. Surg. Roy. W. Sussex Hosp. Chichester.

WALDMAN, Ernest Isidor 16 Dorrington Road, Sale M33 5EB — MB ChB Liverp. 1951.

WALDMAN, Jack (retired) 62A Warren Drive, Wallasey CH45 0JT Tel: 0151 639 7091 — MRCS Eng. LRCP Lond. 1943 (Liverp.) MRCGP 1963.

WALDMAN, Louise Jane Stamford Hill Group Practice, 2 Egerton Road, Stamford Hill, London N16 6UA Tel: 020 8800 1000 Fax: 020 8880 2402 — MB ChB Bristol 1987; DGM RCP Lond. 1991; DFFP 1995; MRCGP 1999. GP Stamford Hill Lond. Specialty: Paediat. Prev: Staff Grade (Community Paediat.) City & E. Lond.; GP/Regist. Stamford Hill Gp. Pract. Lond.

WALDMAN, Nicola Sarah — MB BS Lond. 1990 (St. Mary's Hospital) DRCOG 1995; T(GP) 1996; MRCGP 1996; DFFP 1996. GP Princip. Merton Surg. Lond.

WALDMAN, Steven Joseph Ailsa Craig Medical Group, 270 Dickenson Road, Longsight, Manchester M13 0YL Tel: 0161 224 5555 Fax: 0161 248 9112; 61 Linksway, Gatley, Cheadle SK8 4LA Tel: 0161 491 2910 — MB ChB Liverp. 1972; DObst RCOG 1975; Cert FPA 1976; MRCGP 1976. GP Trainer. Prev: SHO (Paediat.) W. Middlx. Hosp. Isleworth; SHO (Med.) Hadassah Hosp. Jerusalem, Israel; SHO (O & G) St. Mary's Hosp. Lond.

WALDMANN, Carl Samuel, Squadron Ldr. RAF Med. Br. Retd. Intensive Care Unit, Royal Berkshire Hospital, Reading RG1 5AN Tel: 01189 877249 Fax: 01189 877250 Email: cswald@aol.com — MB BChir Camb. 1976 (Cambridge University and The London Hospital) MA, MB Camb. 1976, BChir 1975; DA Eng. 1978; FFA RCS Eng. 1980; Europ. Dip. Intens Care Med. 1993. Cons. Anaesth. & Dir. Intens. Care Units Roy. Berks. & Battle Hosps. Reading; Div. Director, Clin. Support Serv. at Royal Berks & Battle NHS Trust; Edr., JICS. Specialty: Anaesth.; Intens. Care. Socs: Assn. Anaesth.; Europ. Soc. of Intens. Care (Chairm. Sect. of Technol. Assessm.); Intens. Care Soc. (Counc. Mem.). Prev: Lect. Lond. Hosp. Med. Sch.; Sen. Regist. (Anaesth.) Gt. Ormond St. Hosp. Lond.; Sen. Regist. Lond. Hosp. Whitechapel.

WALDOCK, Mr Andrew Luton & Dunstable Hospital NHS Trust, Wewsey Road, Luton LU4 0DZ Tel: 01582 497174 Fax: 01582 497174 — BM BS Nottm. 1989; BMedSci Nottm. 1987; FRCOphth 1994; MD 1998. Cons. Ophth. Surg. Luton & Dunstable Hosp. Luton. Specialty: Ophth. Special Interest: Cornea & Extern. Eye Dis.; Glaucoma. Socs: Internat. Mem. of Amer. Acad. of Ophth.; Mem. of Europ. & UK Cataract & Refractive Societies. Prev: Specialist Regist. (Ophth.) Roy. Devon & Exeter Hosp.; Research Regist. (Ophth.) Bristol Eye Hosp.; Specialist Regist. Orpth. Torbay Hosp.

WALDON, Richard David Rowcroft Medical Centre, Rowcroft Retreat, Stroud GL5 3BE Tel: 01453 764471 Fax: 01453 755247; Woodlands, South Woodchester, Stroud GL5 5EQ Tel: 01453 872158 — MB BS Lond. 1986; BSc Lond. 1981; DCH RCP Lond. 1990. Prev: SHO & Clin. Med. Off. (Paediat.) Epsom Dist. Gen. Hosp. Surrey; SHO (A & E) St. Stephens Hosp. Lond.; SHO (Gen. Med.) Epsom Dist. Gen. Hosp. Surrey.

WALDRAM, Mr Michael Andrew Royal Orthopaedic Hospital NHS Trust, Woodlands, Northfield, Birmingham B31 2AP Tel: 0121 685 4223 Fax: 0121 685 4041 Email: michael.waldram@roh.nhs.uk — MB BS Lond. 1977 (Roy. Free) FRCS Ed. 1982; FRCS (Orth.) Ed. 1987. Cons. Orthop. & Hand Surg. Roy. Orthop. Hosp. Birm. & Selly Oak Hosp. Birm. Specialty: Orthop. Special Interest: Hand Surg. Socs: Brit. Orthop. Assn.; Brit. Soc. Surg. Hand; Christian Med. Fellowsh. Prev: Christine Kleinert Hand Fellowsh. Louisville, Kentucky; Sen. Regist. Roy. Orthop. Hosp. Birm.; Regist. (Surg.) Basingstoke Dist. Hosp.

WALDRON, Alexandra Catherine Houston 26 Graham Park Road, Gosforth, Newcastle upon Tyne NE3 4BH — MB ChB Sheff. 1995.

WALDRON, Brian Alan (retired) Long Acre Lodge, Flatts Lane, Calverton, Nottingham NG14 6JZ Tel: 0115 965 3283 — MB BS Lond. 1960 (St. Mary's) MRCS Eng. LRCP Lond. 1960; DObst RCOG 1963; DA Eng. 1964; MRCGP 1968; FFA RCS Eng. 1971. Prev: Cons. Anaesth. Nottm. City Hosp. & Univ. Hosp. Nottm.

WALDRON, Bryan Le Gros (retired) 51 Dunraven Drive, Derriford, Plymouth PL6 6AT Tel: 01752 792691 — MB BChir Camb. 1957 (St. Bart.) BA, MB Camb. 1958, BChir 1957; DA Eng. 1959; FFA RCS Eng. 1961. Cons. Anaesth. Plymouth Health Dist.

WALDRON, Felicity Mary The Surgery, Church Lane, Bishopthorpe, York YO60 6PS Tel: 01904 630918 — MB ChB Dundee 1976.

WALDRON, Gerard John Mark Northern Health & Social Services Board, County Hall, Galgorm Road, Ballymena BT42 1QB Tel: 028 2566 2207; 35 Sourhill, Ballymena BT42 2LG Tel: 028 2564 0606 Fax: 028 2564 8488 — MB BCh BAO NUI 1981 (Galway) MFPHM 1995. Cons. (Publ. Health Med.) N. Health & Socl Servs. Bd. Specialty: Pub. Health Med. Prev: Cons. Solihull HA; Sen. Regist. Dumfries & Galloway HB; Regist. & Sen. Regist. Croydon HA.

WALDRON, Gillian 31 Maidstone Road, Bounds Green, London N11 2TR Tel: 020 8888 4253 — MB ChB Birm. 1971; MRCPsych 1975; FRCPsych 2004. Cons. Psychiat. Grovelands Priory Hosp. Lond. Specialty: Gen. Psychiat. Prev: Cons. Psychiat. Tower Hamlets HA; Lect. (Psychiat.) Lond. Hosp.

WALDRON, Harry Arthur 31 Maidstone Road, London N11 2TR — MD Birm. 1977; PhD Birm. 1975, MD 1977, MB ChB 1971; DHMSA Lond. 1974; MRCP (UK) 1977; FFOM RCP Lond. 1980, M 1978; FRCP Lond. 1993. Cons. Phys. St. Mary's Hosp. Lond.; Research Fell. Inst. Archeology UCL; Edr. Brit. Jl. Indust. Med. Specialty: Gen. Med.; Occupat. Health. Socs: Soc. Occupat. Med.; Fell. Roy. Soc. Med. Prev: Sen. Lect. (Occupat. Med.) Lond.; Ho. Surg. & Ho. Phys. Gen. Hosp. Birm.

WALDRON, Jean Winifred (retired) 12 Park Road, Fowey PL23 1ED — MB ChB Leeds 1954; DCH Eng. 1963; MA 1996; M Th 1998.

WALDRON, Mr John ENT Department, Royal United Hospital, Bath BA1 3NG; 66 Murhill, Limpley Stoke, Bath BA2 7FQ — MB BS Lond. 1981; FRCS (Otol.) Eng. 1986. Cons. ENT Surg. Roy. United Hosp. Bath. Specialty: Otorhinolaryngol.

WALDRON, John Henry Mowbray House, Malpas Road, Northallerton DL7 8FW Tel: 01609 775281 Fax: 01609 778029 — MB BS Newc. 1982.

WALDRON, John Pius 19 Pembridge Crescent, London W11 3DX — MB BCh BAO NUI 1978; MRCPI 1980.

WALDRON, Martin Nigel Schering-Plough Ltd, Schering-Plough House, Shire Park, Welwyn Garden City AL7 1TW Tel: 01707 363780 Fax: 01707 363690; 24 Westlecote Gardens, Luton LU2 7DR — MB BS Lond. 1980. Med. Marketing Manager Schering-Plough Ltd. Specialty: Pharmaceutical Medicine. Prev: Sen. Med. Adviser Hoechst Roussel Ltd.; GP Luton; Ho. Surg. Roy. Free Hosp. Lond.

WALDRON, Mary Department of Child Health, Southampton General Hospital, Tremona Road, Southampton SO16 6YD Tel: 023 8079 8809 — MB BCh BAO NUI 1980 (Galway) MRCPI 1987. Cons. Paediat. Nephrol. Soton. Univ. Hosp. Specialty: Paediat.; Nephrol. Socs: Internat. Paediat. Nephrol. Assn.; Brit. Assn. Paediat. Nephrol.

WALDRON, Michael Jeremy Fowey River Practice, Rawlings Lane, Fowey PL23 1DT Tel: 01726 832451; Cedron House, 32 Tower Park, Fowey PL23 1JD Tel: 01726 833209 — BSc Wales 1978, MB BCh 1983; DCH RCP Lond. 1986; MRCGP 1988.

WALDRON, Michael John Caldbeck and Partners, Hurst Close, Gossops Green, Crawley RH11 8TY Tel: 01293 527138 Fax: 01293 522571 — MB BS Lond. 1987; DRCOG 1991. Prev: Trainee GP Eastbourne VTS; SHO (Gen. Med.) St. Marys Hosp. Eastbourne; Ho. Off. (Gen. Surg.) Eastbourne Dist. Gen. Hosp.

WALDRON, Murray Neil Houston 26 Graham Park Road, Gosforth, Newcastle upon Tyne NE3 4BH — BM BCh Oxf. 1992.

WALDRON, Richard William The Surgery, 102 Preston Road, Weymouth DT3 6BB Tel: 01305 832203; The Spinney, 97 Wyke Road, Weymouth DT4 9QS — MB BS Lond. 1980; DRCOG 1985; MBA Bournemouth 1999.

WALDRON, Susan May Graeme Medical Centre, 1 Western Avenue, Falkirk FK2 7HR Tel: 01324 624437 Fax: 01324 633737; 15 Panbrae, Boiness, Edinburgh EH51 0EJ Tel: 01506 824836 — MB ChB Manch. 1989; BSc (Med. Sci.) St. And. 1986; DRCOG 1992; MRCGP 1993; DCCH RCP Ed. 1994. GP. Specialty: Gen. Pract. Prev: Trainee (Community Paediat.) Sighthill Health Centre Edin.; Chief Med. Off. VRO Rajahmundry Andhra, Pradesh, India; SHO (A & E) Falkirk Roy. Infirm.

WALDRUM, Christopher Ian Greengate Medical Centre, 1 Greengate Lane, Birstall, Leicester LE4 3JF Tel: 0116 267 7901 — MB ChB Leic. 1989.

WALE, Jane Louise 33 Christchurch Lane, Lichfield WS13 8AY — MB ChB Birm. 1998; MRCP 2000. SHO (Anaesth.) Birm.

WALE, Laurence William 15 Pearman Street, London SE1 7RB — MB BS Lond. 1983.

WALE, Martin Charles Johnson CDSC (Trent), Public Health Laboratory, Queens Medical Centre, Nottingham NG7 2UH Tel: 0115 970 9048 Fax: 0115 970 9019 — BM BS Nottm. 1980; BMedSci (Hons.) Nottm. 1978; Dip. Bact. Manch. 1988; MRCPath 1990; FRCPath 1998. Cons. Regional Epidemiol. CDSC (Trent) Nottm.; Hon. Cons. Microbiol. PHLS Trent. Specialty: Epidemiol.; Med. Microbiol. Prev: Cons. Microbiol. & Communicable Dis. Control Soton.; Sen. Regist. Pub. Health Laborat. City Hosp. Nottm. & Hon. Regist. Pub. Health Laborat. Portsmouth; Med. Off. 40 Commando R.M.

WALE, Peter Frederick (retired) 202 Attenborough Lane, Beeston, Nottingham NG9 6AL Tel: 0115 9254 305 — MB BS Lond. 1955 (St. Geo.) MRCS Eng. LRCP Lond. 1955; DMRT Eng. 1960; FFR 1967. Cons. Radiother. Derbysh. Roy. Infirm. & Nottm. Gen. Hosp. Prev: Cons. Radiotherap. Romford Hosp. Gp.

WALES, Alan Christopher Bergamot House, 37 Long Meadows, Burley-in-Wharfedale, Ilkley LS29 7RY Tel: 01943 865139 — MB ChB Leeds 1965; DObst RCOG 1971; MRCGP 1980. Specialist (Disabil. Med.) W. Yorks. Specialty: Disabil. Med. Prev: Med. Adviser Teach.'s Pension Scheme; Med. Adviser Benefits Agency Med. Servs.; GP Penistone & Stannington Sheff.

WALES, Andrew Thomas Peggs La Cottage, Queniborough, Leicester LE7 3DF — MB BS Lond. 1998.

WALES, Deborah Anne Royal Lancaster Infirmary, Ashton Road, Lancaster LA1 4RP — MB ChB Leeds 1986; MRCP UK 1993; FRCA 1994. Cons. Respirat. Phys. Roy. Lancs. Infirm. Specialty: Respirat. Med. Special Interest: Non-invasive Ventilation. Socs: Brit. Thorac. Soc. Prev: Specialist Regist. (Respirat. Med.) Wythenshawe Hosp. Manch.; Regist. (Respirat. Med.) Roy. Lancs. Infirm.; Regist. (Respirat. Med.) Hope Hosp. Salford.

WALES, Elisabeth Lucy Hall Garth, Kingsley Road, Frodsham, Warrington WA6 6BB — MB ChB Bristol 1993.

WALES, Elizabeth 9 The Woodlands, Esher KT10 8DD — MB BS Durh. 1949; LMSSA Lond. 1947; DCH Eng. 1959; DPH Leeds 1961; DObst RCOG 1963; MFCM 1975. Prev: Sen. Med. Off. DHSS.

WALES, Emma Kathryn Hallgarth, Kingsley Road, Frodsham, Warrington WA6 6BB — MB BS Newc. 1994.

WALES, Ian Frederick Hall Lisburn Health Centre, Linenhall Street, Lisburn BT28 1LU; 33 Windsor Hill, Carnreagh, Hillsborough BT26 6RL Tel: 01846 683443 — MB BCh BAO Belf. 1982; DRCOG 1986; DCH Dub. 1986; MRCGP 1988. Specialty: Paediat.

WALES, Jeremy Kenneth Harvard c/o Academic Unitof Child Health, Sheffield Children's Hospital, Western Bank, Sheffield S10 2TH Tel: 0114 271 7508 Fax: 0114 275 5364 Email: j.k.wales@sheffield.ac.uk — BM BCh Oxf. 1979; MRCP; MA Oxf. 1980, DM 1990; FRCPCH 1997. Sen. Lect. (Paediat. Endocrinol.) & Hon. Cons. Paediat. Univ. Sheff. Specialty: Paediat. Socs: Eur. Soc. Paediat. Endocrinol.; Brit. Soc. Paediat. Endocrinol. Prev: Lect. (Paediat.) Sheff. Univ.; Regist. (Paediat.) Soton. & Basingstoke.

WALES, Joanne Elizabeth Jane Macclesfield District General Hospital, Victoria Road, Macclesfield SK10 3BL Tel: 01625 421000; 7 Moorlands Close, Tytherington, Macclesfield SK10 2TL Tel: 01625 428528 — MB ChB Liverp. 1986; DA (UK) 1989. Clin. Asst. (Anaesth.) Macclesfield Dist. Gen. Hosp. Specialty: Anaesth.

WALES, John Kenneth (retired) Academic Unit of Medicine, Martin Wing, The General Infirmary, Leeds LS1 3EX Tel: 0113 392 3470 Fax: 0113 242 3811; School House, Acaster-Selby, Appleton Roebuck, York YO23 7BP Tel: 01904 744220 — (Leeds) MB ChB Leeds 1960; MD Leeds 1965; M 1968; FRCP Lond. 1979. Sen. Lect. Univ. Leeds & Hon. Cons. Phys. Leeds Teach. Hosps. NHS Trust. Prev: Asst. Prof. Med. Geo. Washington Sch. Med. Washington, DC.

WALES, John Michael Glenfield General Hospital, Groby Road, Leicester LE3 9QP Tel: 0116 287 1471 Fax: 0116 255 6841; Peggs Lane Cottage, Pegg Lane, Queniborough, Leicester LE7 3DF Tel: 0116 260 5726 — MB BChir Camb. 1966 (St.Bart.) BChir 1965; MRCP (UK) 1970; FRCP Lond. 1981. Cons. Phys. (Gen. & Chest Med.) Glenfield Gen. Hosp. Leicester; Assoc. Med. Director, UHL Trust (Univ. Hosps. Leicester NHS Trust). Specialty: Gen. Med. Socs: BMA & Brit. Thoracic Soc. Prev: Sen. Regist. (Med.) Soton. Gp. Hosps.; SHO Warwick Hosp.

WALES, Nicholas Michael Chelsea and Westminster Hospital, 369 Fulham Road, London SW10 9NH Tel: 020 8746 8694 Email: nick.wales@chelwest.nhs.uk — MB BS Lond. 1991 (St Mary's Hosp. Paddington) BSc Lond. 1988; MRCOG 1997. Cons. Obst. and Gynaecologist, Chelsea and Westm. Hosp.; Cons. Obst. and Gynaecologist, Lister Hosp., Chelsea bridge, Lond.; Cons. Obst. and Gynaecologist, Princess Margt. Hosp., Windsor. Specialty: Obst. & Gyn. Special Interest: Cervical Sutures; Colposcopy; Reconstruction of the Cervix.

WALES, Raymond Mitchell Dumbarton Health Centre, Station Road, Dumbarton G82 1PW Tel: 01389 602655 Fax: 01389 602622 — MB ChB Glas. 1970.

WALES, Richard Michael Department of Psychiatry, St. Andrews Hospital, Yarmouth Road, Norwich NR7 0EW Tel: 01603 31122; 132 South Hill Road, Thorpe, Norwich NR7 0LR — MB ChB Aberd. 1982. SHO (Forens. Psychiat.) Norwich HA. Specialty: Forens. Psychiat. Prev: SHO (Radiother. & Oncol.) Norwich HA; Regist. (Chest, Gen. & Geriat. Med.) W. Essex HA.

WALESBY, Mr Robin Kingsley 88 Harley Street, London W1N 1AE Tel: 020 7486 4617; Fleur House, 7 The Drive, Coombe Hill, Kingston upon Thames KT2 7NY Tel: 020 8942 6368 Fax: 020 8949 6835 — MRCS Eng. LRCP Lond. 1970 (Roy. Free) MSc Lond. 1972, MB BS 1970; FRCS Eng. 1975. Sen. Lect. & Cons. Cardiothoracic Surg. Roy. Free & Univ. Colllege Hosp. Med. Sch. Specialty: Cardiothoracic Surg. Socs: Soc. Cardiothorac. Surg. GB & Irel.; Eur. Soc. Cardiothorac. Surg. Prev: Cons. Cardiothoracic Surg. Lond. Chest Hosp. Roy. Free Hosp. & Southend Health Auth.; Sen. Regist. (Cardiothoracex Surg.) Roy. Postgrad. Med. Sch. Lond. Hosp. Sick Childr. Lond. & Middlx. & Harefield Hosps. Lond.

WALEWSKA, Renata Janina Flat 35, Shore Court, Shore Lane, Sheffield S10 3BW — MB ChB Sheff. 1993.

WALFORD, Claire Susan Northwood Health Centre, Neal Close, Northwood HA6 1TQ Tel: 01923 820844; Heathbourne Lodge, Heathbourne Road, Bushey, Watford WD23 1PA Tel: 020 8950 0344 Fax: 020 8950 0344 — MB BS Lond. 1975 (Univ. Coll. Hosp.) DCH Eng. 1977; MRCGP 1987. Cons. Grade Specialist (Primary Care) A & E Dept. UCL Hosps Trust. Socs: BMA; Nat. Assn. Fundholding Pract. Prev: SHO (A & E) Univ. Coll. Hosp. Lond.; Trainee GP Harrow Weald Middlx.; Regist. (Paediat.) Northwick Pk. Hosp.

WALFORD, David Henry Howard 15 Shore Road, Little Bispham, Thornton-Cleveleys FY5 1PF — MB BChir Camb. 1948 (Camb. & St. Thos.) MA, MB BChir Camb. 1948. Prev: Ho. Phys. Grimsby & Dist. Hosp.

WALFORD, Diana Marion Public Health Laboratory Service, 61 Colindale Avenue, London NW9 5DF Tel: 020 8200 1295 Fax: 020 8358 3242 — MB ChB Liverp. 1968; MRCP (UK) 1972; FRCPath 1986, M 1974; BSc (1st cl. Hons) Liverp. 1965, MD 1976; MSc (Epidemiol.) Lond. 1987; FFPHM RCP (UK) 1995, M 1989; FRCP Lond. 1990. Dir. Pub. Health Laborat. Serv. Lond. Specialty: Pub. Health Med. Socs: Founder Mem. Brit. Blood Transfus. Soc.; Hon. Life Mem. Brit. Assn. Med. Managers. Prev: Dep. Chief Med. Off. DoH; Dir. NHS Managem. Exec.; Hon. Cons. (Haemat.) Centr. Middlx. Hosp.

WALFORD, Frank Roy (retired) 15 Grove Road, Chichester PO19 2AR Tel: 01243 533947 — (Birm.) MB ChB Birm. 1958; FRCPath 1980, M 1967. Prev: Cons. St. Wilfrids Hospice Chichester.

WALFORD, Geraldine Ann 65 Princetown Road, Bangor BT20 3TD — MB BS Lond. 1976.

WALFORD, Harriet Katherine — MB ChB Bristol 1986; MRCGP 1991; BA (Hons.) Brighton 1997. p/t GP Principal. Specialty: Gen. Pract. Prev: Locum GP & Asst. GP.

WALFORD, Linda Jane Leeds Psychotherapy Training Institute, 2A Weetwood Lane, Leeds LS16 5LS Tel: 0113 278 9953 — MB ChB Leeds 1980; MRCPsych 1985. Dir. (Clin. Train.) Leeds Psychother. Train. Inst. Specialty: Psychother.

WALFORD, Mrs Mary Elizabeth (retired) Sibford, Church Hill, Marnhull, Sturminster Newton DT10 1PU Tel: 01258 820201 — MB ChB St. And. 1948; FRCS Eng. 1956. Prev: Cons. Orthop. Surg. Portsmouth Gp. Hosps.

WALFORD, Norman Quentin 10 Queen Quay, Welshback, Bristol BS1 4SL — MB Camb. 1977; BChir 1976; MRCPath 1987. Sen. Lect. (Histopath.) Univ. Amsterdam. Prev: Lect. (Histopath.) Inst. Child Health; Regist. (Histopath.) Hammersmith Hosp.; Ho. Off. Liver Unit King's Coll. Hosp.

WALFORD, Rita (retired) Flat 42, The Four Tubs, Little Bushey Lane, Bushey Heath, Watford WD23 4SJ Tel: 020 8950 6950 — MB ChB Birm. 1938. Prev: RAF Med. Br. 1942-45.

WALFORD, Sally Anne 24 Victoria Place, Stirling FK8 2QT — MB ChB Sheff. 1985.

WALFORD, Simon Royal Wolverhampton Hospital NHS Trust, Clinical Sub-Dean, School of Medicine, University of Birmingham, Birmingham Tel: 01902 643007 Fax: 01902 643173 — MB BChir Camb. 1975; MA Camb. 1975; MRCP (UK) 1976; MD Camb. 1984; FRCP Lond. 1992. Cons. Phys. Roy. Wolverhampton Hosps. NHS Trust.; Clin. Sub-Dean, Univ. of Birm. Sch. of Med. Specialty: Gen. Med.; Diabetes; Endocrinol. Prev: Med. Director, Roy. Wolverhampton Hosps. NHS Trust; 1st Asst. (Med. Endocrinol.) Med. Sch. Univ. Newc.; Regist. & Novo Research Fell. (Med.) Univ. Hosp. Nottm.

WALGAMA, Suduweli Kondage Lettis 80 Countisbury Avenue, Bush Hill Park, Enfield EN1 2NN Tel: 020 8360 5179 — MB BS Ceylon 1968; MRCP (UK) 1978; DCH Eng. 1979; MRCS Eng. LRCP Lond. 1980. Clin. Med. Off. Enfield & Haringey AHA. Prev: SHO (Paediat., Gen. Med. & Geriat. Med.) St. Margt's Hosp. Epping.; SHO (Geriat. Med.) St. Geo. Hosp. HornCh..

WALI, Gitanath Druids Heath Surgery, 27 Pound Road, Druids Heath, Birmingham B14 5SB Tel: 0121 430 5461 — MB BS Mysore 1974; MB BS Mysore 1974.

WALI, Mr Jaweed General Surgery, Causeway Hospital, Coleraine BT52 1HS Tel: 028 7032 7032; 12 Castlewood Avenue, Coleraine BT52 1JR Tel: 028 7035 3746 — MB BS Karnatak 1977; FFAEM; FRCS Ed. 1985; FRCS Glas. 1985. Specialty: Accid. & Emerg.; Gen. Surg.

WALI, Jonathan David Higham Ferrers Surgery, 5 College Street, Higham Ferrers, Rushden NN10 8DX Tel: 01234 267652 — MB BS Lond. 1990. Prev: Trainee GP Bedford Gen. Hosp.

WALIA, Sandeep 774 Great West Road, Isleworth TW7 5NA — MB BS Lond. 1988.

WALIMBE, Sharadini Station Road Surgery, 269 Station Road, Sykehead, Shotts ML7 4AQ Tel: 01501 823490; 6 Camstradden Drive W., Bearsden, Glasgow G61 4AJ — MB BS Poona 1966; LRCP LRCS Ed. LRCPSI Glas. 1972; MRCOG 1972.

WALINCK, Jean Margaret (retired) The Latch, 9 Marine Parade, North Berwick EH39 4LD Tel: 01620 892760 — MB ChB Ed. 1954; DObst RCOG 1956; MRCGP 1965.

WALJI, Mohamed-Taki Ismail Walji, Balsall Heath Health Centre, 43 Edward Road, Birmingham B12 9LP Tel: 0121 446 2500 Fax: 0121 440 5861 — MB BS Lond. 1977; MRCS Eng. LRCP Lond. 1977; MRCGP Lond. 1982.

WALJI, Shahenaz Farouk Oakleigh, 24 Tring Avenue, Ealing Common, London W5 3QA — MB BS Lond. 1977 (Roy. Free) MRCP (UK) 1981. Specialty: Diabetes.

WALK, David Alexander (retired) 58 Foxley Lane, Purley CR8 3EE — (Roy. Free) MB BS Lond. 1957; MRCP Lond. 1961; DPM Eng. 1965; FRCPsych 1978, M 1971. Emerit. Hon. Cons. Child Psychiat. Pathfinder NHS Trust. Prev: Cons. Child Psychiat. St. Geo. Hosp. Lond.

WALKDEN, Diana Whitehouse Farm, Preston on the Hill, Warrington WA4 4LW Tel: 01928 714337 — MB ChB Liverp. 1960; MB ChB (Hnrs.) Liverp. 1960; MRCS Eng. LRCP Lond. 1960. Clin. Asst. Dept. A & E W. Chesh. Hosp. Specialty: Accid. & Emerg. Socs: Liverp. Med. Inst.; Chester & N. Wales Med. Soc. Prev: Hon. Phys. & Hon. Surg. Roy. Southern Hosp. Liverp.

WALKDEN, Mr John Alexander Denis Whitehouse Farm, Preston on the Hill, Warrington — MRCS Eng. LRCP Lond. 1957 (Liverp.) FRCS Eng. 1965; MB ChB Liverp. 1957, MChOrth 1967. Cons. Orthop. Surg. W. Chesh. & Centr. Wirral Hosps. Mem. Liverp.; Med. Inst. & Chester & N. Wales Med. Soc. Specialty: Orthop. Prev: Sen. Orthop. Regist. United Liverp. Hosps. & Liverp. RHB; Orthop. Regist. & Surg. Regist. Profess. Unit Broadgreen Hosp.; Liverp.

WALKDEN, Leon 1 Parkside, Hampton Hill, Hampton TW12 1NU Tel: 020 8943 3673 — MRCS Eng. LRCP Lond. 1946 (St. Geo.) FISM, 1991. Clin. Asst. W. Middlx. Univ. Hosp. & Hillingdon Hosp. Uxbridge. Socs: Sec. Brit. Assn. Traumatol. in Sport. Prev: Asst. Venereol. W. Middlx. Hosp. Isleworth, Hillingdon Hosp. & Centr.; Middlx. Hosp. Acton; Clin. Asst. Paediat. Dept. W. Middlx. Hosp.

WALKDEN, Susan Bridget X-Ray Department, Poole Hospital NHS Trust, Longfleet Road, Poole BH15 2JB Tel: 01202 665511; 39 Birchwood Road, Parkstone, Poole BH14 9NW Tel: 01202 747287 Email: sbwhnon.demon.co.uk — (Camb. & St. Thos.) MB BChir Camb. 1969; MA Camb. 1969; DMRD Eng. 1972; FFR 1974. Cons. Radiol. Wessex RHA. Specialty: Radiol. Socs: Fell. Roy. Soc. Med.; Fell. Roy. Soc. Radiol.; Brit. Inst. Radiol.

WALKDEN, Valerie Mary Department of Dermatology, Wexham Park Hospital, Slough SL2 4HL Tel: 01753 633108 Fax: 01753 633762; 2 Burlington Road, Burnham, Slough SL1 7BQ Email: valavwalkden.freeserve.co.uk — MB BS Lond. 1974 (Roy Free Lond.) BSc (Hons.) Lond. 1971; MRCS Eng. LRCP Lond. 1974; MRCP (UK) 1977; FRCP 1999. Cons. Demat. Wexham Pk. Hosp. Specialty: Dermat. Socs: Fell. Roy. Soc. Med.; Fell. St. John's Hosp. Dermat. Soc.; Brit. Assn. Dermat. Prev: Sen. Regist. (Dermat.) Amersham Gen. Hosp. Bucks.; Clin. Research Asst. Wycombe Gen. Hosp. High Wycombe; Regist. (Dermat.) Roy. Berks. Hosp. Reading.

WALKDEN, Walter James (retired) Arisaig, Water Lane, Eyam, Hope Valley S32 5RG — (Birm.) MB ChB Birm. 1944; FRCP Lond. 1973, M 1950. Prev: Cons. Phys. Sandwell HA.

WALKER, Abigail Helen Towerhurst, The Avenue, Collingham, Wetherby LS22 5BU — MB ChB Ed. 1997.

WALKER, Adrian Bernard Department of Endocrinology and Diabetes, Ward 60, Nines Block, City General Hospital, Stoke-on-Trent ST4 6QG — BM BCh Oxf. 1988 (Oxford) MA Oxf. 1989; DM Oxf. 2000; FRCP 2002. Cons. Phys. (Diabetes & Endocrinol.) N. Staffs. Hosp. Specialty: Gen. Med. Prev: Sen. Regist. (Gen. Med., Diabetes & Endocrinol.) Liverp.; Research Fell. (Diabetes) Univ. Liverp.; Regist. (Gen. Med., Diabetes & Endocrinol.) Roy. Liverp. Univ. Hosp.

WALKER, Adrian Kerr Yates Beaver's Lodge, Penpol, Devoran, Truro TR3 6NP Tel: 01872 864994 — (Guy's) MB BS Lond. 1968; MRCS Eng. LRCP Lond. 1968; DA Eng. 1970; DObst RCOG 1972; FFA RCS Eng. 1974. Cons. Anaesth. Roy. Cornw. Hosps. Trust. Specialty: Anaesth. Prev: Sen. Regist. Addenbrooke's Hosp. Camb.; Med. Off. Brit. Solomon Is.s; Med. Dir. Roy. Cornw.. Hosp. Trust.

WALKER, Adrian Mark NPHS Microbiology, YSBYTY Gwynedd, Bangor LL57 2PW Tel: 01248 384367 Fax: 01248 370163 Email: mark.walker@phls.wales.nhs.uk; Tyn Lon, Pentraeth LL75 8YH — MB Camb. 1974 (Middlx.) BChir Camb 1974; MA Camb. 1974; MRCPath 1982. Cons. Microbiol., Nat. Pub. Health Serv. for Wales, Bangor; Hon. Cons. Microbiol., N. W. Wales NHS Trust, Bangor. Specialty: Med. Microbiol. Socs: Brit. Med. Assn.; Assn. of Med. Microbiol. Prev: Cons. Communicable Dis. Control Gwynedd Health Auth.; Cons. Microbiol. Preston, Chorley & S. Ribble Health Dists.; Sen. Regist. (Microbiol.) Addenbrooke's Hosp. Camb.

WALKER, Aileen Elizabeth WS Atkins Healthcare, Clifton House, Clifton Place, Glasgow G3 7YY Tel: 0141 332 7030; 21 Blacklands Place, Lenzie, Kirkintilloch, Glasgow G66 5NJ Tel: 0141 776 0592 — MB ChB Glas. 1977; MPH Leeds 1984; MFPHM RCP (UK) 1988; MHSM 1990. Cons. Med. Planner WS Atkins Healthcare Glas. Specialty: Pub. Health Med. Prev: Cons. Pub. Health Med. Scott. CSA; Regist. (Psychiat.) N. Canterbury Hosp. Bd. ChristCh., NZ; Trav. Sec. Christian Med. Fellowship.

WALKER, Alan Kelvingrove Med. Centre, 28 Hands Rd., Heanor DE75 7HA Tel: 01773 713201; 28 Hands Road, Heanor DE75 7HA Tel: 01773 744067 — MB ChB Glas. 1978; MRCP (UK) 1982.

WALKER, Alan Eastfield Group Practice, 1 Eastway, Eastfield, Scarborough YO11 3LS Tel: 01723 582297 Fax: 01723 582528; May Dene, Beech Lane, West Ayton, Scarborough YO13 9JG Tel: 01723 862320 — MB ChB Leeds 1974; BSc (Hons.) (Anat.) Leeds 1971; DCH RCPS Glas. 1979; DRCOG Lond. 1981. Specialty: Anat. Prev: Lect. (Anat.) Univ. Leeds Med. Sch.

WALKER, Alan George (retired) 9 Croham Valley Road, South Croydon CR2 7JE — MB ChB Manch. 1945; BSc Manch. 1942, MB ChB 1945. Prev: GP S. Croydon, Chesh. & Manch.

WALKER, Mr Alasdair James, Surg. Capt. RN Department of Surgery, Derriford Hospital, Plymouth PL6 8DH Tel: 01752 763776 Fax: 01752 792537 Email: alasdair.walker@phnt.swest.nhs.uk — MB ChB Glas. 1979; FRCS Glas. 1985; T(S) 1991. Cons. Gen. & Vasc. Surg. & Div. Dir. Surg. Services Derriford Hosp. Plymouth & RN. Specialty: Gen. Surg. Socs: Fell. Roy. Soc. Med.; Vasc. Surg. Soc.; Brit. Assn. of Med. Managers. Prev: Hon. Sen. Regist. (Vasc. Surg.) Roy. Infirm. Edin.; Sen. Specialist (Surg.) RN Hosp. Plymouth & Haslar; Squad. Med. Off. HMS Plymouth.

WALKER, Alexander Gordon Rosedale Surgery, Ashburnham Way, Carlton, Lowestoft NR33 8LG Tel: 01502 505100; The Red House, North Cliff, Kessingland, Lowestoft NR33 7RA Tel: 01502 740397 — MB ChB Manch. 1978; DRCOG 1981; D.Occ Med. RCP Lond. 1995. Med. Adviser Birds Eye Walls Ltd.; G.P. Tutor, LoW.oft. Prev: Trainee GP Norwich VTS.

WALKER, Alexander Kirkland (retired) 15 West Mill Bank, Colinton, Edinburgh EH13 0QT — MB ChB Glas. 1955; DObst RCOG 1959; DIH Soc. Apoth. Lond. 1972; MRCGP 1975; AFOM 1981. Prev: Occupat. Health Phys. Co. Health Ltd. Tyne & Wear.

WALKER, Alexander Percy (retired) Bentfield, Maryborough Road, Prestwick KA9 1SW Tel: 01292 477876 Fax: 01292 678893 — (Univ. Glas.) MB ChB Glas. 1939; DObst RCOG 1947; MRCGP 1965. Dep. Lt. Ayr & Arran. Prev: Adj. Med. Off. DHSS.

WALKER, Alexander Peter (retired) 51 Netherblane, Blanefield, Nr. Glasgow, Glasgow G63 9JP — MB ChB Glas. 1952; DObst RCOG 1957; MRCGP 1968.

WALKER, Alison 138 Rosslyn Avenue, Rutherglen, Glasgow G73 3EX — MB ChB Dundee 1991; MRCP UK 1995; FRCA 2002.

WALKER, Alison C/o, A & E Department, Leeds General Infirmary, Gt. George St., Leeds LS1 3EX — BChir Camb. 1995 (Cambridge) BDS Ed. 1987; FDS RCS Eng. 1992; BA (Med. Sci.) Camb. 1992; MBBS Camb. 1995; FRCS Eng. 1998; Dip IMC RCS Edin. 1998. Specialty: Accid. & Emerg. Prev: Regist. (Oral & Maxillofacial Surg.) Pinderfields Hosp. Wakefield.

WALKER, Amanda Balmacaan Road Surgery, Balmacaan Road, Drumnadrochit, Inverness IV63 6UR Tel: 01456 450577 Fax: 01456 450799 — MB ChB Ed. 1986; DRCOG 1988; MRCGP 1991.

WALKER, Amy 28 Eastheath Avenue, Wokingham RG41 2PJ — MB ChB Leeds 1998.

WALKER, Andrew Allan (retired) Ladyacre Cottage, Old Park Lane, Farnham GU10 5AA — MB ChB Ed. 1956.

WALKER, Andrew Douglas William Schaw House, Stair, Mauchline KA5 5JA Tel: 01292 591213 — MB ChB Ed. 1978; MSc Ed. 1984, BSc 1975; MFCM 1989. Chief. Admin. Med. Off. & Dir. Health Plann. & Pub. Health Ayrsh. & Arran HB. Specialty: Pub. Health Med. Prev: Cons. Pub. Health Fife HB.

WALKER, Angela Hoyland Health Centre, 2 Duke St., Hoyland, Barnsley S74 9QS Tel: 01226 742915 Fax: 01226 745585; 6 Towngate, Thurlstone, Sheffield S36 9RH — MB ChB Leeds 1982.

WALKER, Angela 5 Osborne Road, Buckhurst Hill IG9 5RR — MB ChB Liverp. 1991.

WALKER, Angela Margaret 4 Copse View Cottages, Redenham, Andover SP11 9AT — MB BS Lond. 1970 (Guy's) MRCS Eng. LRCP Lond. 1970; DCH Eng. 1973; DObst RCOG 1973; MRCP (UK) 1976. Socs: BMA.

WALKER, Ann Elizabeth Norwood Road Surgery, 70 Norwood Road, Southall UB2 4EY Tel: 020 8574 4454 — MB ChB Bristol 1986 (Univ. Bristol) DCH RCP Lond. 1989; DRCOG 1991. GP S.all. Specialty: Gen. Pract. Prev: Clin. Asst. (Community Paediat.) W. Lond. Healthcare; Trainee GP Greenford Middlx.

WALKER, Ann Mary 12 Shire Oak Road, Leeds LS6 2DE — MB ChB Glas. 1973.

WALKER, Anna Krystyna Springfield House, Burnt House Lane, Preesall, Poulton-le-Fylde FY6 0PQ — MB ChB Glas. 1985; MRCGP 1989.

WALKER, Anne Catherine Pinhoe Surgery, Pinn Lane, Exeter EX1 3SY Tel: 01392 469666 Fax: 01392 464178; Egremont, Red Cross, Silverton, Exeter EX5 4DE Tel: 01392 860641 — MB ChB St. And. 1968. Prev: SHO (Anaesth.) United Birm. Hosps.; Ho. Off. King's Cross Hosp. Dundee; Ho. Surg. Selly Oak Hosp. Birm.

WALKER, Anne Elizabeth Stockett Lane Surgery, 3 Stockett Lane, Coxheath, Maidstone ME17 4PS Fax: 01622 741987 — MB BS Lond. 1980; DCH RCP Lond. 1983; Cert. Family Plann. JCC 1984; DRCOG 1984; MRCGP 1985. Gen. Pract.

WALKER, Anne Exley (retired) 39 Rectory Drive, Wingerworth, Chesterfield S42 6RU Tel: 01246 277021 — (Sheff.) MB ChB Sheff. 1958; MD Sheff. 1965; FRCP Ed. 1975, M 1966. Prev: Cons. Dermat. Roy. Hosp. Chesterfield & United Sheff. Hosps.

WALKER, Anne Muriel Zuill Sandyford Initiative, 6 Sandyford Place, Glasgow G3; 10 Royal Terrace, Glasgow G3 7NT — MB ChB Glas. 1963; DObst. RCOG 1965; Dip. Ven. Soc. Apoth. Lond. 1975. Clin. Asst. (Genitourin. Med.) Sandyford Initiative. Prev: Dir. Health Commiss. NSW Sexually Transm. Dis. Clinic Sydney, Austral.

WALKER, Annette 47 Harperley Gardens, Stanley DH9 8RZ; 24B Tasman Street, Nelson, New Zealand Tel: NZ (03)545 6167 Fax: NZ (03)545 9007 — MB ChB Leeds 1992. GP Locum. Specialty: Gen. Pract.

WALKER, Anthea Noel The Hollies, West Felton, Oswestry SY11 4JU — MB BS Lond. 1972; FRCS Eng. 1979.

WALKER, Mr Anthony Paul Laughton Hall, Laughton, Gainsborough DN21 3PP Tel: 01427 628688 — MB ChB Leeds 1973; FRCS Eng. 1978. Cons. Orthop. Surg. Scunthorpe Gen. Hosp. Specialty: Orthop. Socs: Fell. BOA. Prev: Sen. Regist. (Orthop.) Yorks. RHA.

WALKER, Antony Hayden 34 Newbould Lane, Sheffield S10 2PL — MB ChB Sheff. 1994.

WALKER, Archibald Brian Kilsyth Medical Partnership, Kilsyth Health Centre, Burngreen Park, Kilsyth, Glasgow G65 0HU Tel: 01236 822081 Fax: 01236 826231; Rosamar, Allanfauld Road, Kilsyth, Glasgow G65 9DE — MB ChB Glas. 1973; Dip. Sports Med. Scott. Roy. Med. Coll.; MD Glas. 1990. Hon. Sen. Lect. Glas. Univ. Specialty: Gen. Pract.; Sports Med. Socs: Brit. Assn. Sports Med.; Amer. Counc. Sports Med.

WALKER, Arthur Alexander (retired) Sarnia, Hernes Nest, Bewdley DY12 Tel: 01299 402363 — MB BS Durh. 1953.

WALKER, Audrey Mai 10 Oak Lane, Wilmslow SK9 6AA — MB ChB Sheff. 1956.

WALKER, Ava e80B Denton Road, London N8 9NT — MB BS Lond. 1979.

WALKER, Barrie Dr B Walker and Partners, Health Centre, Gosforth Road, Seascale CA20 1PN Tel: 01946 728101; Lyndale, Gosforth Road, Seascale CA20 1HA Tel: 0194 67 28551 — MB BChir Camb. 1972 (Middlx.) MA Camb. 1971; DObst RCOG 1974; FRCGP 1991, M 1978. Med. Off. DERAProof & Experim. Estab. Eskmeals; Chairm. Cumbria Primary Care Effectiveness Gp.; Mem. Northern & Yorks. Regional Cancer Working Gp.; Mem. & Clin. Governance Lead W. Cumbria PCG. Specialty: Gen. Pract. Prev: Trainee GP Guildford VTS; Ho. Surg. (Surg.) Middlx. Hosp. Lond.; Ho. Phys. Kettering Gen. Hosp.

WALKER, Barry Egerton St. James's University Hospital, Leeds LS9 7TF — MD Leeds 1971; MB ChB 1961; FRCP Lond. 1979, M 1966. Cons. Phys. & Lect. Med. St. Jas. Hosp. Leeds. Specialty: Gen. Med. Socs: BMA & Brit. Soc. Gastroenterol. Prev: SHO Chapel Allerton Hosp. Leeds; Ho. Off. (Gen. Surg.) Leeds Gen. Infirm.; Ho. Off. (Gen. Med.) Bradford Roy. Infirm.

WALKER, Bernard Hugh Bentham Medical Practice, Grasmere Drive, High Bentham, Lancaster LA2 7JP Tel: 01524 261202 Fax: 01524 262222905 — MB ChB Manch. 1968. Prev: Res. Clin. Pathol. Manch. Roy. Infirm. Ho. Surg. Ancoats Hosp. Manch.; Ho. Phys. Crumpsall Hosp. Manch.

WALKER, Beverley Jane Summerley House, Ellwood Road, Beaconsfield HP9 1EN Tel: 01494 670942 Fax: 01494 670698 — MB BS Lond. 1978 (King's Coll. Hosp.) AKC; MRCP (UK) 1981. Specialty: Diabetes. Socs: BDA. Prev: Lect. (Nephrol.) Inst. Urol.

WALKER, Professor Brian Robert University of Edinburgh, Endocrinology Unit, Medical Sciences Department, Western General Hospital, Edinburgh EH4 2XU Tel: 0131 537 1736 Fax: 0131 537 1012 Email: b.walker@ed.ac.uk — MB ChB Ed. 1986; MRCP (UK) 1989; BSc Ed. 1984, MD 1993; FRCP Ed. 1999. Prof. of Endocrinol.

Univ. Edin.; Hon. Cons. NHS Lothian Univ. Hosps. Div. Specialty: Endocrinol.; Diabetes. Socs: (Sec.) Caledonian Soc. Endocrinol. Prev: MRC Train. Fell. Univ. (Med.) West. Gen. Hosp. Edin.

WALKER, Brian William McWhirter (retired) 1 Wood Drive, St. Mellion, Saltash PL12 6UR — MB ChB Glas. 1960; DObst RCOG 1965.

WALKER, Bryan Alexander The Consultation Suite, Lourdes Hospital, Liverpool L18 1HQ Tel: 0151 733 7123 Fax: 0151 735 0446 — MD Liverp. 1969; MB ChB 1956; FRCP Lond. 1974, M 1965. Cons. Phys. Lourdes Hosp. Liverp.; Cons. Med. Off. Roy. Sun Alliance Ltd; Cons. Med. Off. Roy. Liver Assur. Specialty: Gen. Med. Socs: Assn. Phys.; Fell. Assur. Med. Soc.; Fell. Roy. Soc. Med. Prev: Cons. Phys. Roy. Liverp. Univ. Hosp. & Broadgreen Hosp.; Lect. Liverp. Univ.

WALKER, Carol Louise Market Street Health Group, 52 Market St., East Ham, London E6 2RA Tel: 020 8472 0202; 24 Lyal Road, Bow, London E3 5QG Tel: 020 8980 3836 — MB BS Lond. 1994; MA Camb. 1995; DRCOG 1996. GP Regist. Market St. Health Centre, E.ham Lond. Specialty: Gen. Pract. Prev: SHO (Psychiat.) E.ham Memor. Hosp.; SHO (Paediat.) Newham Gen. Hosp.; SHO (O & G) Newham Gen. Hosp.

WALKER, Carolyn Anne Peterlo Med. Centre, Middleton, Manchester; 1 Alkrington Green, Middleton, Manchester M24 1ED — MB ChB Leeds 1990 (Univ. Leeds) DCCH RCP Ed. 1993; MRCGP 1995.

WALKER, Charles Herbert (retired) Maple Down, 28 Blundellsands Road E., Blundellsands, Liverpool L23 8SQ — MD Aberd. 1958, MB ChB 1951. Prev: Ho. Off. Aberd. Roy. Infirm.

WALKER, Charles Victor Stuart Cavendish Medical Centre, 214 Park Road North, Birkenhead CH41 8BU Tel: 0151 652 1955 — MB ChB Liverp. 1982.

WALKER, Christine Ann — MB ChB Glas. 1994; DRCOG Lond. 1997; MRCGP Glasg. 2000. Specialty: Gen. Psychiat.

WALKER, Christine Anne Northampton General Hospital NHS Trust, Cliftonville, Northampton NN1 5BD Tel: 01604 544538 Fax: 01604 545988; The Walnuts, Church St, Blakesley, Towcester NN12 8RA Tel: 01327 860747 — BM BCh Oxf. 1983 (Oxford) BA (Hons. Physiol. Sci.) Oxf. 1980; DRCOG 1986; DCH RCP Lond. 1987; MRCP (UK) 1990. Cons. (Paediat.) Northampton Gen. Hosp. Specialty: Paediat. Socs: Fell. RCPCH. Prev: Sen. Regist. (Paediat.) Northampton Gen. Hosp.; Sen. Regist. (Paediat.) Roy. Hosp. Sick Childr. Edin.; Research Fell. (Child Life & Health) Univ. Edin.

WALKER, Christopher Prestwood Road West Surgery, 81 Prestwood Road West, Wednesfield, Wolverhampton WV11 1HT Tel: 01902 721021 Fax: 01902 306225; Chiviot House, 20 Stockwell Road, Tettenhall, Wolverhampton WV6 9PQ Tel: 01902 751197 — MB Camb. 1974 (St. Mary's) M 1973; BChir 1973; FRCGP 1994; MMed Sc 1999. Postgrad. Tutor S. Staffs Med. Centre.; Chairman Wolverhampton Local Medical Committee. Prev: SHO (Cas.) & Ho. Surg. St. Mary's (Harrow Rd. Br.) Hosp. Lond.; Ho. Phys. Qu. Eliz. II Hosp. Welwyn Gdn. City.

WALKER, Christopher Allan 8 Ratcliffe Drive, Huncote, Leicester LE9 3BA — MB ChB Manch. 1971; BSc (Hons. Physiol.) Manch. 1968, MB ChB 1971; MRCPsych 1975; DPM Eng. 1975. Cons. Psychiat. Towers Hosp. Leicester. Specialty: Gen. Psychiat. Prev: Lect. (Psychiat.) Univ. Leicester; Regist. & Sen. Regist. Univ. Hosp. S. Manch.

WALKER, Mr Christopher Charles 154 Hanging Hill Lane, Hutton, Brentwood CM13 2HG — MB BS Newc. 1968 (Newcastle Upon Tyne) FRCS Eng. 1974. Cons. Plastic Surg. St Andrews Centre for Plastic Surg. and Burns, Broomfield Hosp., Chelmsford; Cons. Plastic Surg. Whipps Cross Hosp. Lond.; Hon. Cons. Plastic Surg. Roy. Lond. Hosp.; Hon Sen. Lect. St Barts Med. Coll.; Med. Director, Mid Essex Hosps. Trust. Specialty: Plastic Surg. Socs: Fell. Roy. Soc. Med.; Brit. Ass. Plastic Surg. Hon Treas. & Coun. Mem.; Brit. burn ass Counc. Mem. Prev: Sen. Regist. (Plastic Surg.) Univ. Hosp. S. Manch., Christie Hosp. & Booth Hall Childr. Hosp. Manch.; Regist. (Plastic Surg.) Mt. Vernon Hosp. & Univ. Coll. Hosp. Lond.; Regist. MRC Burns Research.

WALKER, Christopher Darnton (retired) 9 Brit View Road, West Bay, Bridport DT6 4HY Tel: 01308 456267 Email: aunt94@dsl.pipex.com — (Camb. & St. Mary's) MRCS Eng. LRCP Lond. 1961; MB BChir Camb. 1962. Prev: Med. Ref. Eltham Crematorium.

WALKER, Christopher Francis Victoria Surgery, 5 Victoria Road, Holyhead LL65 1UD; Yeovil, The Mountain, Holyhead LL65 1YW Tel: 01407 764791 — MB ChB Birm. 1973; DRCOG 1979; MRCGP 1980; DA (UK) 1980.

WALKER, Christopher James Park Health Centre, 190 Duke Street, Sheffield S2 5QQ Tel: 0114 272 7768; 57 Meersbrook Road, Sheffield S8 9HU — MRCS Eng. LRCP Lond. 1979.

WALKER, Mr Christopher John Maidstone Hospital, Hermitage Lane, Barming, Maidstone ME16 9QQ Tel: 01622 729000 Ext: 4209; Chittenden House, Lovehurst Lane, Staplehurst, Tonbridge TN12 0EX Tel: 01580 891989 Fax: 01580 891989 — MB BS Lond. 1966 (St. Mary's) MRCS Eng. LRCP Lond. 1966; FRCS Eng. 1973. Cons. Orthop. Surg. The Maidstone Hosp. Specialty: Orthop. Socs: Brit. Orthopaedic foot Surg. Soc. Prev: Sen. Orthop. Regist. St. Mary's Hosp. Lond., Battle Hosp. Reading & Roy. Nat. Orthop. Hosp. Lond.; Surg. Regist. (Profess. Unit) St. Mary's Hosp. Lond.

WALKER, Christopher Peter Ravenscroft Department of Anaesthesia and Intensive Care, Royal Brompton and Harefield NHS Trust, Harefield, Uxbridge UB9 6JH — MB BS Lond. 1990 (University of London - Royal Free Hospital) FRCA 1996; CCST 1999. Cons. in Cardiothoriac Anaesth. and Intens. care, Harefield Hosp.; Roy. Coll. Anaesth. Tutor at Harefield Hosp.; Lead Cons. For acute pain and resesitation, at Harefield Hospital. Specialty: Anaesth. Socs: FRCAnaesth.; BMA; Assn. Anaesths. Prev: Spr Locum Cons., Roy. Brompton and Harefield Hosp.s; Vis. Sen. Regist., Univ. of Natal, Durban; Spr Hammersmith and Roy. Marsden Hosp.s.

WALKER, Mr Christopher Richard Department of Orthopaedic Surgery, Royal Liverpool University Hospital, Prescot St., Liverpool L7 8XP Tel: 0151 706 3440 Fax: 0151 706 2440 — MRCS Eng. LRCP Lond. 1981 (Liverpool) FRCS Ed 1986; FRCS Eng 1988; MCh (Orth.) Liverp. 1990; FRCS (Orth.) 1994. Cons. Trauma & Orthop. Surg. Roy. Liverp. Univ. Hosp. Specialty: Trauma & Orthop. Surg. Socs: Fell. BOA; Brit. Orthop. Foot Surg. Soc. Prev: Lect. (Orthop. & Accid. Surg.) Roy. Liverp. Univ. Hosp.; Regist. (Orthop.) Mersey RHA; Research Fell. Thackary Clin. Univ. Liverp.

WALKER, Clive Reece Weybridge Health Centre, 22 Church Street, Weybridge KT13 8DW Tel: 01932 853366 Fax: 01932 844902; 18 Mayfield Road, Weybridge KT13 8XD Tel: 01932 851100 — (St Georges Hosp Lond) MB BS Lond. 1968; MRCP (U.K.) 1972; FRCP 1998. GP & Hosp. Pract. Thoracic Med. Specialty: Respirat. Med. Prev: Regist. (Med.) & Resid. Med. Off. St. Geo. Hosp. Lond.; Clinician MRC Laborats., The Gambia.; Asst. Div. Med. Off. Weybridge.

WALKER, Mr Colin Burleigh Springbank House, School Lane, Boldre, Lymington SO41 5QE Tel: 01590 673718 — MB BChir Camb. 1949 (St. Thos.) MA Camb. 1958, MB BChir 1949; FRCS Eng. 1958. Socs: FCOphth. Prev: Emerit. Cons. Ophth. Surg. Soton. Univ. Hosp. Gp.; Sen. Regist. (Ophth.) St. Thos. Hosp. Lond.; Chief Clin. Asst. & Sen. Res. Off. Moorfields Eye Hosp. City Rd.

WALKER, Colin Cecil Russell (retired) Inglewood, Place Road, Melksham SN12 6JN Tel: 01225 707044 — MB ChB Ed. 1948. Prev: Ho. Phys. Edin. Roy. Infirm.

WALKER, Colin Dieppe (retired) Cranwill Dene, Cricket Hill Lane, Yateley GU46 6BQ Tel: 0125 870788 — MB BS Lond. 1959 (Westm.) Prev: Ho. Surg. & Res. Obst. Asst. Westm. Hosp. Lond.

WALKER, Colin Heriot MacDonald (retired) 61 Dalkeith Road, Dundee DD4 7JJ Tel: 01382 454323 Email: WalkerHeriot@aol.com — MB ChB Ed. 1946; FRCP Ed. 1963, M 1950; DCH Eng. 1951; MD Ed. 1952; FACC 1963; Hon. FRCPCH 1996. Hon. Reader (Child Health) Univ. Dundee. Prev: Cons. Paediat. Tayside HB.

WALKER, Colin Peter 41 The Delph, Lower Earley, Reading RG6 3AN — MB BS Lond. 1981; MRCP (UK) 1986. Regist. (Gen. Med.) Roy. Berks. Hosp. Reading. Specialty: Gen. Med. Prev: SHO (Gen. Med.) St. Helier Hosp. Carshalton; SHO (A & E) St. Bart. Hosp. Lond.

WALKER, Mr Colin Robert Connell Flat 4/3 Canada Court, 63 Miller St., Glasgow G1 1EB Tel: 0141 221 2554 — MB ChB Manch. 1987; FRCS Ed. 1992; FRCPS Glas. 1992. SHO (Orthop.) Vic. Infirm. Glas.

WALKER, David Airdrie Health Centre, Monkscourt Avenue, Airdrie ML6 0JU Tel: 01236 766446 Fax: 01236 766513; 18 Arthur Avenue, Airdrie ML6 9EZ Tel: 01236 762198 — MB ChB Glas. 1986; BSc Strathclyde 1981; DFM Glas. 1993. Dep. Police Surg. Specialty: Gen. Psychiat. Socs: Assn. Police Surg.; BMA.

WALKER, David Andrew 30 Victoria Springs, Holmfirth HD9 2 NB Tel: 01484 683196 Email: dawalker@doctors.org.uk — MD Liverp. 1979; MB ChB 1971; MRCP (U.K.) 1974; FRCP 1990. p/t Occupational Health Phys. Specialty: Gen. Med. Socs: BMA & SOM.

WALKER, David Austin Department of Child Health, University Hospital, Nottingham NG7 2UH Tel: 0115 924 9924 Fax: 0115 970 9382 Email: david.walker@nottingham.ac.uk; 92 Parkside, Wollaton, Nottingham NG8 2NN Tel: 0115 928 2635 — BM BS Nottm. 1977; Fell. Roy. Coll. Paediat. & Child Health; BMedSci Nottm. 1975; FRCP Lond. 1996. Sen. Lect. (Paediat. Oncol.) Univ. Hosp. Nottm.; Cons. Paediat. Oncol. Specialty: Paediat. Socs: UK Childh. Cancer Study Gp. (Chairm. Brain Tumour Comm.); FRCPCh.; Fell. RCP. Prev: Research Fell. Roy. Childr. Hosp. Melbourne, Austral.; Clin. Fell. Leukaemia Research Fund Hosp. for Sick Childr. Gt. Ormond St. Lond.

WALKER, David Douglas (retired) 12 Essex Brae, Edinburgh EH4 6LN — MB ChB Ed. 1959; DPH 1962; DIH Dund 1970; MFCM 1974; FFOM RCP Lond. 1994, M 1978. Cons. Ocxcupat. Health Phys. Edin. Prev: Med. Adviser Brit. Gas. (Scotl.).

WALKER, Mr David Ian (retired) Beechwood Consulting Rooms, The Highfield Hospital, Manchester Road, Rochdale LL11 4LZ Tel: 01706 766608 Fax: 01706 766602 — MB ChB Manch. 1965; FRCS Edin. 1971; F.Pod.A (Hon) 1994. private Orthopaedic Pract. and Medicolegal Reporting; Hon. Cons. Orthop. Surg. Penine Acute Hosps. NHS Trust. Prev: Cons. Orthopaedic Surg., Rochdale 1979-2002.

WALKER, David James The Halt, Myrtle Lane, Pen Y Maes, Holtwell, Chester CH8 7BT — MB ChB Manch. 1995. SHO (Orthop.) Surg. Chester Hosp.; Anat. Demonst. Univ. Liverp; Ho. Off. (Surg.) Hope Hosp. Manch.; Ho. Off. (Med.) Nobles Hosp. I. of Man. Specialty: Orthop.

WALKER, David John 36 Tapton Mount Close, Sheffield S10 5DJ — MB ChB Birm. 1994.

WALKER, David John 29 Bemersyde Drive, Jesmond, Newcastle upon Tyne NE2 2HL — MD Newc. 1986; MA Camb 1978, BA 1974; MB BS 1977; MRCP UK 1980; FRCP Uk 1993. Cons. Rheum. Newc. & Tyneside HA. Specialty: Rheumatol.

WALKER, David John Macclesfield District General Hospital, Victoria Road, Macclesfield SK10 3BL Tel: 01625 421000 — MB ChB Liverp. 1970; MRCP (UK) 1975; FRCP Lond. 1991. Cons. Phys. Macclesfield Dist. Gen. Hosp. Specialty: Care of the Elderly. Socs: Liverp. Med. Inst. & Brit. Geriat. Soc.; BMA. Prev: Sen. Regist. (Geriat.) Newsham Gen. Hosp. Liverp. & David Lewis North. Hosp. Liverp.; Regist. (Med.) Liverp. AHA (T).

WALKER, David John Royal United Hospital, Combe Park, Bath BA1 3NG Tel: 01225 824651 Email: walker@doctors.org.uk — MB ChB Birm. 1985; MRCOG 1990; MD Warwick 1994. Cons. O & G Roy. United Hosp. Bath. Specialty: Obst. & Gyn. Prev: Sen. Regist. Rotat. (O & G) W. Midl. RHA.; Research Regist. (O & G) Univ. Warwick; Regist. Rotat. (Obst.) W. Midl. RHA.

WALKER, David Martin — BM BS Nottm. 1975; DRCOG 1978; MRCGP 1980. Prev: Trainee GP/SHO Char. Cross Hosp. Lond. VTS; Asst. Lect. (Human Morphol.) Nottm. Univ. Med. Sch.; Cas. Off. Nottm. Gen. Hosp.

WALKER, David Michael Conquest Hospital, Department of Cardiology, The Ridge, St Leonards-on-Sea TN37 7RD Tel: 01424 755255 Ext: 6319 Fax: 01424 758132 — MB BChir Camb. 1985 (Camb. & St Thos.) BA (Hons.) Cantab. 1982; MA Camb. 1986; MRCP UK 1988; MD Camb. 1995; FRCP 2001. Cons. Cardiol. E. Sussex Hosps. NHS Trust; Cons. Cardiol. Roy. Sussex Co. Hosp. Brighton. Specialty: Cardiol.; Gen. Med. Special Interest: Heart Failure; Interventional Cardiol. Socs: Brit. Cardiac Soc.; Brit. Cardiac Intervention Soc.; Brit. Soc. Heart Failure. Prev: Hon. Cons. Cardiol. KCH Lond.; Sen. Regist. (Cardiol.) St. Mary's Hosp. & Hammersmith Hosp. Lond.

WALKER, David Ralph 13B St Thomas Street, Newcastle upon Tyne NE1 4LE Tel: 0191 261 5927 — MB BS Newc. 1987; MSc Newc. 1994, BMedSc 1986, MB BS 1987; MRCP (UK) 1991; MFPHM RCP (UK) 1994. Sen. Regist. (Pub. Health Med.) Centres for Dis. Control & Prevent. Atlanta, USA. Specialty: Pub. Health Med.

WALKER, Deborah Mary The Hawthorns, Burleigh Lane, Ascot SL5 8PF — MB BS Lond. 1978 (Roy. Free) MRCS Eng. LRCP Lond. 1978; DCH Eng. 1981; MRCGP 1982 DRCOG 1982. Non Princip., Gen. Pract., Ascot; Clin. Asst. Antenatal Clinic, King Edwd. VII Hosp., Windsor.

WALKER, Deirdre Susan 26 Grenville Drive, Cambuslang, Glasgow G72 8DS — MB ChB Ed. 1993.

WALKER, Dennis (retired) 27 Avenue Road, Doncaster DN2 4AE Tel: 01302 342181 — MB ChB Leeds 1951. Prev: Ho. Surg. (Orthop.) St. Jas. Hosp. Leeds.

WALKER, Derek Lindsay (retired) Ludloes, Gloucester Street, Painswick, Stroud GL6 6QR Tel: 01452 813253 — MRCS Eng. LRCP Lond. 1948 (King's Coll. Lond. & St Geo.) MD Lond. 1958, MB BS 1949; DPM Eng. 1954; FRCPsych 1971. Hon. Cons. Dept. Applied Neurophysiol. Gloucester Roy. Hosp. Prev: Cons. Psychiat. & Phys. Supt. Horton Rd. & Coney Hill Hosps.

WALKER, Desmond (retired) Wellfield House, Sunderland Bridge Vill., Croxdale, Durham DH6 5HB — MB BS Durh. 1952. Prev: G.P Durh. City.

WALKER, Dorothy Elizabeth Blackhall Medical Centre, 51 Hillhouse Road, Edinburgh EH4 3TH Tel: 0131 332 7696 Fax: 0131 315 2884; 110 Craigcrook Road, Edinburgh EH4 3PN — MB ChB Aberd. 1980; MRCGP 1984; DRCOG 1984; FRCGP 2002.

WALKER, Dorothy May 7 Hightown, Collieston, Ellon AB41 8RS — MB ChB Aberd. 1955. Prev: Sen. Med. Off. W. Suff. CC.

WALKER, Douglas Arthur Jack 65 Grove Road, Millhouses, Sheffield S7 2GY — BM BCh Oxf. 1980; DPhil Oxf. 1986, MA, BM BCh 1980; FFA RCS Eng. 1986. Sen. Regist. (Anaesth.) Roy. Hallamsh. & N. Gen. Hosps. Sheff. Specialty: Anaesth. Prev: Lect. Anaesth. Univ. Sheff.

WALKER, Douglas Ewen (retired) 51 Belgrave Road, Corstorphine, Edinburgh EH12 6NH Tel: 0131 334 4583 — MB ChB Aberd. 1943; DPH Aberd. 1948. Prev: Sen. Med. Off. Scott. Home & Health Dept.

WALKER, Douglas Robert Castlegait Surgery, Links Health Centre, Marine Avenue, Montrose DD10 8TR Tel: 01674 672554 Fax: 01674 675025; 10 Morven Avenue, Montrose DD10 9DL — MB ChB Dundee 1984. Specialty: Orthop.; Sports Med.

WALKER, Edward Corrie 4-6 Kirkgate, Hanging Heaton, Batley WF17 6DA — MB ChB Sheff. 1986; DA (UK) 1989; FRCA 1991. Staff Doctor (A & E) Dewsbury Health Care Trust. Specialty: Accid. & Emerg.

WALKER, Mr Edward Milnes Milton Keynes General NHS Trust, Saxon St., Eaglestone, Milton Keynes MK6 5LD Tel: 01908 243075 Fax: 01908 243075; Model Farm, 4 Brook End, North Crawley, Newport Pagnell MK16 9HH Tel: 01234 391781 — MB BS Lond. 1969 (Middlx.) MRCS Eng. LRCP Lond. 1969; FRCS Eng. 1974. Cons. Urol. Milton Keynes Hosp. Specialty: Urol. Socs: Assoc. Mem. BAUS. Prev: Sen. Regist. (Gen. Surg.) Nottm. Gen. Hosp.; Regist. (Surg.) Westm. Hosp. Lond. & Northampton Gen. Hosp.

WALKER, Elizabeth Harriet 11 Blackthorn Road, Kenilworth CV8 2DS; 11 Blackthorn Road, Kenilworth CV8 2DS — MB BS Lond. 1994 (KCSMD London) DCH 1998. GP Regist. Winchester.

WALKER, Elizabeth Helen 1 Hampton Mews, Stockport SK3 8SY Tel: 0161 487 3986 — MB BS Lond. 1996 (St. Georges Hospital Medical School) BSc Hons. St. George's Hosp Med. Sch. 1993. SHO Psychiat. Macclesfield Dist. Gen. Hosp. Specialty: Gen. Psychiat. Prev: SHO Psychiat. Stepping Hill hospital Stockport (p/t).

WALKER, Elizabeth Helen May 10 Curle Avenue, Lincoln LN2 4AN Tel: 01552 530777 — MB BChir Camb. 1953 (Univ. Coll. Hosp.) MA, MB BChir Camb. 1953; DCH Eng. 1955; FRCOG 1978, M 1965. Emerit. Cons. Lincoln Gp. Hosps. Specialty: Obst. & Gyn. Socs: N. Eng. Obst. & Gyn. Soc.; Wom. Gyn. Vis. Club. Prev: Lect. (O & G) Roy. Free Hosp. Lond.; Regist. (O & G) Newc. Gen. Hosp.; Med. Off. St. Luke's Hosp. Chabua, India.

WALKER, Elizabeth Jane 6 Bromyard Avenue, Sutton Coldfield B76 1RQ — MB ChB Birm. 1994; ChB Birm. 1994.

WALKER, Emma Jane (Surgery), 82 Little Road, London SW6 1TN; 21 Gastein Road, London W6 8LT — MB BS Lond. 1991; DRCOG 1995. Specialty: Gen. Pract.

WALKER, Emma Katherine Lucy BBC TV, White City, 201 Wood Lane, London W12 7TS Tel: 020 8752 6349 Email: emma.walker@bbc.co.uk — MB ChB Ed. 1987; BSc (Hons. Path.) Ed. 1985; BM ChB Ed. 1987. Producer BBC TV. Prev: Ho. Off. West. Gen. Hosp. Edin.

WALKER, Eric Department of Pathology, Crosshouse Hospital, Kilmarnock KA2 0BE Email: eric.walker@aaaht.scot.nhs.uk — MB

ChB Aberd. 1986; PhD Aberd. 1979, BSc (Hons.) 1975; MRCPath 1994. Cons. Path. CrossHo. Hosp. Kilmarnock. Specialty: Histopath. Prev: Sen. Regist., Regist. & SHO (Path.) Roy. Infirm. Glas.

WALKER, Evelyn Claire Eskbridge Medical Centre, 8A Bridge Street, Musselburgh EH21 6AG Tel: 0131 665 6821; 'Kirklands', Main St, Gullane EH31 2AL Tel: 01620 842879 Fax: 01620 842879 — MB ChB Ed. 1986 (Cambridge & Edinburgh) MA Cantab 1986; MA Cantab 1986; DRCOG 1988; DRCOG 1988; DRCOG 1988; MRCGP 2000. GP Retainer,; Represen. on Lotian Med. Comm. Specialty: Gen. Pract. Socs: MDDUS; BMA. Prev: Trainee GP at Eskbridge Med. Centre; SHO (Med. Paediat.) Roy. Hosp. Sick Childr. Edin.; SHO (O & G) Simpsons Mem. Matern. Hosp. Edin.

WALKER, Ewa Maria 17 Oakhill Avenue, London NW3 7RD Tel: 020 7431 3436 Fax: 020 7431 3436 — Lekarz Poland 1972. Indep. Psychother. Pract. Lond. Prev: SHO (Clin. Path. & Haemat.) St. Geo. Hosp. Lond.; Sen. Research Fell & Hon. Regist. BMT Unit Roy. Free Hosp. Lond.; Pharmaceut. Phys. Wellcome Foundat.

WALKER, Ewen Macaulay — MD Aberd. 1990; MB ChB (Commend.) 1977; MRCOG 1982; FRCOG 1997. Cons. Obst. and Gynaecologist, Crosshouse Hosp., Kilmarnock. Specialty: Obst. & Gyn. Socs: Brit. Gynaecol. Cancer Soc.; Brit. Soc. Colposcopy and Cervical Cytol. Prev: Regist. Edin. Roy. Infirm. & Simpson Memor. Matern. Hosp.; Lect. (O & G) Ninewells Hosp. Dundee.

WALKER, Fiona Amberley, Romsey Road, Cadnam, Southampton SO40 2NN — BM Soton. 1992.

WALKER, Fiona Christine 94 Roseburn Street, Netherlee, Edinburgh EH12 5PL — MB ChB Edin. 1989 (Univ. Ed.) MRCGP 1996. Staff Grade (Palliat. Med), Vict. Hospice, Kircaldy. Specialty: Palliat. Med. Prev: Clin. Asst. (Palliat. Med.) Cedar Hse., Kirkcaldy; GP Regist. Edin.

WALKER, Folliott Charles Edward Johnson and Partners, Langley House, 27 West Street, Chichester PO19 1RW Tel: 01243 782266/782955 Fax: 01243 779188 — MB BS Lond. 1982 (St. Thos.) BSc Hons. (Anat.) Lond. 1979; DRCOG 1985; MRCGP 1986. Prev: Trainee GP Basingstoke VTS; Ho Phys. Worthing Hosp. Lond.; Ho. Surg. St. Geo. Hosp. Lond.

WALKER, Professor Frederick Department of Pathology, University Medical Buildings, Foresterhill, Aberdeen AB25 2ZD Tel: 01224 681818 Fax: 01224 663002 — MB ChB Glas. 1958 (Univ. Glas.) MB ChB (Commend.) Glas. 1958; FRCPath 1978, M 1966; PhD Glas. 1966, MD (Hons. & Bellahouston Medal) 1971. Regius Prof. Path. Univ. Aberd.; Hon. Cons. Aberd. Roy. Hosps. NHS Trust. Specialty: Histopath. Socs: Chairm. & Gen. Sec. Path. Soc. GB & Irel.; Scott. Soc. Experim. Med. Prev: Foundat. Prof. Path. Univ. Leicester; Sen. Lect. (Path.) Univ. Aberd.; Lect. (Path.) Univ. Glas.

WALKER, Frederick Hughes (retired) Clifftops, 7 Sea Gate View, Sewerby, Bridlington YO15 1ET Tel: 01262 602223 — MB BS Lond. 1950 (Guy's) MRCS Eng. LRCP Lond. 1950.

WALKER, Gail Allison The Surgery, 62 Windsor Drive, Orpington BR6 6HD Tel: 01689 852204 Fax: 01689 857122; Treetops, 39 Oxenden Wood Road, Orpington BR6 6HP — MB BS Lond. 1979; MRCGP 1984.

WALKER, Geoffrey (retired) 27 Wollaton Hall Drive, Nottingham NG8 1AF Tel: 0115 916 0736 Email: walkerng81af@supanet.com — MB BS Lond. 1950 (Middlx.) MSc Lond. 1970, BSc 1947; FRCP Lond. 1983, M 1952; FRCPath 1977, M 1965; Hon. DSc CNAA 1991. Prev: Cons. Chem. Path. Univ. Hosp. Nottm.

WALKER, Mr Geoffrey Fleetwood (retired) 9D The Grove, Highgate Vill., London N6 6JU Tel: 020 8340 2313 Fax: 020 8340 2313 Email: geoffrey.walker@bigfoot.com — MB BS Lond. 1951 (Middlx.) FRCS Eng. 1958; FRCS Ed. 1958. Volun. Developing Country orthapaedic Teachg., Worl Orthapedic Concern (UK) in Africa and S.E. Asia. Prev: Prof. Univ. Addis Ababa.

WALKER, Geoffrey Robert Pease Way Medical Centre, 2 Pease Way, Newton Aycliffe DL5 5NH Tel: 01325 301888 — MB BS Lond. 1995 (Char. Cross & Westm.) BSc (Hons.) Westm. 1988. GP Partner Pease Way Med. Centre Newton Aycliffe Co. Durh. Specialty: Anaesth. Socs: Train. Mem. Assn. AnE.h. Prev: SHO (Anaesth.) St Peters Hosp. Chertsey; SHO (Anaesth.) Roy. Surrey, Hosp. Guilford; SHO (Acc. & Emerg.) Qu. Mary's Hosp. Koethampton.

WALKER, George Dymond WellCare Private General Practice, 8 Monmouth Place, Bath BA1 2AU Tel: 08700 105656 Fax: 01225 312040 — MB BChir Camb. 1960 (Lond. Hosp.) DObst RCOG 1962; Cert JCC Lond. 1976; MRCGP 1977. Socs: Soc. Occupat. Med.; Internat. Health Eval. Assn. Prev: GP Princip. Oldfield Surg. Bath.

WALKER, George Peter (retired) Kent House, 18 Redhills Road, Arnside, Carnforth LA5 0AU Tel: 01524 762156 Fax: 01524 762156 Email: peterwalker@doctors.org.uk — MB ChB Manch. 1954; FRCOG 1975, M 1961, DObst 1957. Prev: Cons. O & G Roy. Liverp. & Mill Rd. Matern. Hosp. Liverp.

WALKER, George Richard Leyburn Medical Practice, The Nurseries, Leyburn DL8 5AU Tel: 01969 622391 Fax: 01969 624446; Manor Barn, Harmby, Leyburn DL8 5PD — MB ChB Manch. 1969.

WALKER, Giles Austen 59 Clarendon Rise, London SE13 5EX — MB BS Lond. 1994.

WALKER, Gordon McPherson The Surgery, Station Road, Yarmouth PO41 0QP — MB ChB Sheff. 1984; DCH RCP Lond. 1987; MRCGP Lond. 1988. GP Yarmouth. Prev: GP Freshwater.

WALKER, Gordon Trevor 57 Newfield Lane, Dore, Sheffield S17 3DD; 98 Bents Road, Sheffield S11 9RL — MB ChB Sheff. 1965. SHO (Gen. Surg.) Derby City Hosp.; Company Med. Director. Socs: Counc. BMA. Prev: SHO (Orthop.) Roy. Infirm. Sheff.

WALKER, Graeme Alexander (3F1) 15 Livingstone Place, Marchmont, Edinburgh EH9 1PB — MB ChB Ed. 1996.

WALKER, Graham Duncan 3 West Hayes, Lymington SO41 3RL — MB BS Lond. 1982; MRCP (UK) 1985; FRCR 1991. Sen. Regist. (Diag. Radiol.) Wessex Train. Sch. Specialty: Radiol. Prev: Regist. (Gen. Med.) Guy's Hosp. Lond.; SHO (Rotat.) Gen. Med. E. Dorset HA.

WALKER, Graham John Northampton General Hospital NHS Trust, Cliftonville, Northampton NN1 5BD — MB ChB Dundee 1985; DA (UK) 1988; DRCOG 1989; FFA RCSI 1991; FCAnaesth 1991; MBA Heriat-Watt Univ. 1995. Cons. Anaesth. Northampton Gen. Hosp. Specialty: Anaesth. Prev: Sen. Regist. (Anaesth.) Roy. Infirm. Edin.; Regist. Rotat. (Anaesth.) Edin. Lothian HB; SHO (Anaesth. & O & G) Chester HA.

WALKER, Heather Ann Cameron c/o Anaesthetic Department, North Manchester General Hospital, Delaunays Road, Crumpsall, Manchester M8 5RB — MB ChB Ed. 1972; BSc (Med. Sci.) Ed. 1969, MB ChB 1972; DObst RCOG 1974; DA Eng. 1975; FFA RCS Eng. 1981; FFA RCSI 1981. Cons. (Anaesth.) N. Manch. Gen. Hosp. Specialty: Anaesth. Prev: Sen. Regist. (Anaesth.) Sheff. AHA; Regist. (Anaesth.) Derbysh. Roy. Infirm. Derby; Regist. (Anaesth.) Newc. AHA.

WALKER, Heather Jane 35 Addison Road, Hove BN3 1TQ — MB ChB Liverp. 1994.

***WALKER, Helen Joanne** Avon Croft, High Hawsker, Whitby YO22 4LH — MB ChB Liverp. 1998; MB ChB Liverp 1998. Pre Registration Howe Off. Whiston Hosp. Prescot.

WALKER, Herbert Alan Stephens (retired) Ferndale, 10 Newbridge Crescent, Wolverhampton WV6 0LN Tel: 01902 753316 — MB BS Durh. 1953. Prev: Asst. Resid. Med. Off. & Ho. Phys. (Childr.) Roy. Vict. Infirm. Newc.

WALKER, Iain William Caythorpe Surgery, 52-56 High Street, Caythorpe, Grantham NG32 3DN Tel: 01400 272215 Fax: 01400 273608; 9 Health Farm Close, Sudbrook, Grantham NG32 3SP Tel: 01400 230172 — BM BCh Oxf. 1989; MA Camb. 1990; DCH RCP Lond. 1991; Cert. Family Plann. JCC 1992; DRCOG 1993; MRCGP 1994. GP. Socs: Christ. Med. Fellowsh.; BMA. Prev: Trainee GP/SHO Nottm. VTS; Trainee GP/SHO Macclesfield Dist. Gen. Hosp. VTS; Ho. Off. (Surg.) Roy. United Hosp. Bath.

WALKER, Isabeau Alexandra Great Ormond Street Hospital, Great Ormond Street, London WC1 3JH — MB BChir Camb. 1984; FRCA 1990. Cons. Paediat. Anaesth. Gt. Ormond St. Hosp. NHS Trust Lond. Specialty: Anaesth.

WALKER, Isobel Deda Dept of Haematology, Glasgow Royal Infirmary, Glasgow G4 0SF Tel: 0141 552 5692 Fax: 0141 211 4919; 44 North Grange Road, Bearsden, Glasgow G61 3AF — (Glas.) MD Glas. 1983, MB ChB 1967; FRCPath 1984, M 1974; FRCP Ed. 1986. Cons. Haemat. Glas. Roy. Infirm. & Hon. Clin. Sen. Lect. Univ. Glas.; Chairm. Steering Comm. UK NEQAS Blood Coagulation. Specialty: Haematology. Socs: Brit. Soc. Haematol. (Ex-Pres.); Chairm. Brit. Comm. Standards in Haematol.; Internat. Soc. Thrombosis & Haemostasis. Prev: Sen. Regist., Regist. & SHO (Haemat.) Glas. Roy. Infirm.

WALKER, Jack (retired) Lincoln Road, Leasingham, Sleaford NG34 8JS Tel: 01529 302644 — MB ChB Birm. 1953; BSc (Hons.) Birm. 1950; DObst RCOG 1955; DA Eng. 1955; MRCGP 1973. Prev: Clin. Asst. (Anaesth.) Boston Hosp. Gp.

WALKER, Jacqueline 1 Witham Close, Chandler's Ford, Eastleigh SO53 4TJ — BM Soton. 1994. SHO (Gen. Med.) Yeovil Dist. Hosp. Specialty: Gen. Med. Prev: SHO (Gen. Med.) E. Surrey Hosp.; SHO (Gen. Med.) Salisbury Dist. Hosp.

WALKER, Jacqueline Rosemary Coldstone House, Shipton Road, Ascott-u-Wychwood, Chipping Norton OX7 6AG Tel: 01993 832708 Fax: 01993 832823; Coldstone House, Shipton Road, Ascott-u-Wychwood, Chipping Norton OX7 6AG Tel: 01993 832708 Fax: 01993 832823 — MRCS Eng. LRCP Lond. 1976 (Westm.) MSc Lond. 1981, MB BS 1976; FRCPath. 1982. Hon. Clin. Asst. Specialty: Pub. Health Med.; Virology. Prev: Cons. Communicable Dis. Control N.W. Surrey HA.; Cons. Virol. Pub. Health Laborat. Epsom; Asst. Microbiol. Pub. Health Laborat. New Addenbrookes Hosp. Camb.

WALKER, James 40 Sevenoaks Avenue, Heaton Moor, Stockport SK4 4AW Tel: 0161 432 7316 — MB ChB Aberd. 1938.

WALKER, James, DFC (retired) 23 Bellevale Avenue, Ayr KA7 2RP Tel: 01292 267184 — MB ChB St. And. 1951; FRCGP 1981, M 1971.

WALKER, James 23 St Johns Road, Ballygowan Road, Hillsborough BT26 6ED — MB BCh BAO Belf. 1977; DMRD RCP Lond. 1982; FRCR 1984. Cons. Radiol. Craigavon Area Hosp. Specialty: Radiol. Socs: Ulster Radiol. Soc. Prev: Sen. Regist. & Regist. (Radiol.) Belf. City Hosp. & Roy. Vict. Hosp.

WALKER, James Alexander Grasmere, Rowhorne Road, Nadderwater, Exeter EX4 2JE Tel: 01392 211895 — MB BS Lond. 1949 (Char. Cross) MRCGP 1963. Prev: Ho. Surg. Char. Cross Hosp.; Ho. Phys. Bridge of Earn Hosp.; Med. Off. RAF.

WALKER, James Campbell 10 Liberton Drive, Edinburgh EH16 6NN — MB ChB St. And. 1946; DPH 1963. Socs: BMA. Prev: Ho. Surg. Stracathro Hosp. Brechin; Asst. MOH Dundee Corp.; Dep. MOH & Dep. Princip. Sch. Med. Off. Co. Boro. Hartlepool.

WALKER, James David Medical Unit, ST Johns Hospital, Livingston EH54 6PP Tel: 0151 6419666 Fax: 0150 6417493 Email: james.walker@wlt.swt.nhs.uk; 109 Trinity Road, Edinburgh EH5 3JY Tel: 0131 551 1306 — MB BS Lond. 1982 (Middlx.) MRCP (UK) 1985; BSc (Hons.) Lond. 1979, MD 1994; FRCP Edin. 1999. Cons. Phys. St johns Hosp., Lond. Specialty: Gen. Med. Special Interest: Diabetes; Endocrinol. Socs: Brit. Diabetic Assn.; Amer. Diabetic Assn.; Eur. Assn. for Study Diabetes. Prev: Cons. Phys., Roy. Infirm. of Edin.; Sen. Regist., St. Bartholomews Hosp., Lond.

WALKER, Mr James Downie (retired) Lynton House, Parkside View, Leeds LS6 4NS Tel: 0113 278 7298 — MB ChB Leeds 1956; FRCS Ed. 1968. Prev: Commonw. Med. Off. Gympie Queensland Australia.

WALKER, Professor James Johnston St. James's University Hospital, Department of Obstetrics & Gynaecology, Beckett Street, Leeds LS9 7TF Tel: 0113 206 5872 Fax: 0113 234 3450 Email: j.j.walker@leeds.ac.uk; National Patient Safety Agency, 4-8 Maple Street, London W1T 5HD Tel: 020 7927 9352 Email: james.walker@npsa.nhs.uk; 12 Shire Oak Road, Headingley, Leeds LS6 2DE Tel: 0113 278 9599 Fax: 0113 234 3450 — MB ChB Glas. 1976; MRCP (UK) 1981; MRCOG Lond. 1981; FRCPS Glas. 1991; MD Glas. 1992; FRCOG 1994. Prof. O & G Univ. Leeds St. Jas. Univ. Hosp.; Clincal Specialty Adviser (Obstetrics) NPSA. Specialty: Obst. & Gyn. Special Interest: Computers in Med.; Pat. Safety; Risk Managem. Socs: Fell. Roy. Soc. Med.; Soc. of Matern. Fetal Med. (USA); Brit. Soc. of Matern. Fetal Med. Prev: Reader, Sen. Lect. & Lect. (O & G) Glas. Uiv.

WALKER, Mr James Montserrat (retired) 33 Chestnut Avenue, Southborough, Tunbridge Wells TN4 0BT Tel: 01892 535546 — (Belf.) MB BCh BAO Belf. 1957; FRCS Ed. 1964; FRCS Eng. 1964; DTM & H Liverp. 1967; FFAEM 1993. Prev: Cons. i/c Emerg. & Accid. Kent & Sussex Hosp. Tunbridge Wells.

WALKER, James Stewart (retired) Strathmore, 15 Dundas Crescent, Kirkwall KW15 1JQ — MB ChB St. And. 1962; DA Eng. 1967; DObst RCOG 1972.

WALKER, James William Berkshire Independent Hospital, Wensley Road, Coley Park, Reading RG1 6UZ Tel: 01189 560056; Kendrick House, 96 Kendrick Road, Reading RG1 5DW Tel: 01189 872191 Fax: 01189 756705 — (Char. Cross) MB BS Lond. 1958; DObst RCOG 1959; MRCGP 1967. Chief Med. Adviser South. Electric & Indep. Pract. Clin. Hypn. & Behaviour Ther.; Authorised Med. Examr. Civil Aviat. Auth.; Med. Adviser, John Lewis Ptnsp.Med. Adviser, hewlett Packard. Specialty: Occupat. Health; Psychother. Socs: Fell. Roy. Soc. Med.; Accred. Mem. Soc. Med. & Dent. Hypn.; Soc. Occupat. Med. Prev: Cons. Phys. (Occupat. Health) St. Mary's Hosp. Newport, I. of Wight; Med. Off. RAF.

WALKER, James William Simon Alison Lea Medical Centre, Calderwood, East Kilbride, Glasgow G74 3BE Tel: 01355 233653 Fax: 01355 261689; 69 East Kilbride Road, Busby, Glasgow G76 8HX Tel: 0141 644 5582 — (Glas.) MB ChB Glas. 1969; DObst RCOG 1971; FRCGP 1994, M 1976. Drs Walker, & Partners, Alison Lea Med. Centre, E. Kilbrike. Socs: (Ex-Pres.) E. Kilbride Med. Soc.; Glas. Midl. & West. Med. Assn. (Ex-Pres.). Prev: SHO (Med.) Stobhill Hosp. Glas.; Ho. Off. Glas. Roy. Matern. Hosp. & Roy. Hosp. Sick Childr. Glas.; Sen. Clin. Tutor, Dept. of Gen. Pract. Univ. Glasg.

WALKER, Jan Andrew Bernard Lumsden Wexham Park Hospital, Department of Clinical Biochemistry, Slough SL2 4HL Tel: 01753 633448 Fax: 01753 633448 Email: ian.walker@hwph-tr.nhs.uk — MB ChB Bristol 1987; MA Camb. 1985; MD Soton. 1997; MRCPath 1997. Cons. Chem. Path. Heatherwood & Wexham Pk. Hosps. Slough. Specialty: Biochem.; Endocrinol.; Diabetes. Socs: Assn. Clin. Biochem.; Brit. Hyperlip .Assn. Prev: Sen. Regist. (Biochem.ry) St. Mary's Hosp. Lond.; Reg. Biochemistry, Southampton Gen Hosp.; SHO (Gen. Med.) Roy. Gwent Hosp.

WALKER, Jane Royal Infirmary of Edinburgh, Simpson Centre for Reproductive Health , US Department, Little France, Edinburgh EH16 4SA Fax: 0131 242 2802 Email: jane.walker@luht.scot.nhs.uk — MB ChB Ed. 1986; BSc Ed. 1984; MRCP (UK) 1989; DMRD Ed. 1991; FRCR 1992. Cons. Radiol. Simpson Centre Reproductive Health Edin. Specialty: Radiol.

WALKER, Janet (retired) Ladyacre Cottage, Old Park Lane, Farnham GU10 5AA Tel: 01252 712107 — MB ChB Sheff. 1955.

WALKER, Janet Elizabeth Aldborough Forge, Boroughbridge, York YO51 9HG — MB BS Newc. 1994.

WALKER, Janet Margaret 10E Cross Lane, Lisburn BT28 2TH — MB BCh BAO Belf. 1986 (Qu. Univ. Belf.) MRCGP 1991; MFHom 1992; D.Occ.Med. RCP Lond. 1996. Specialty: Homeop. Med. Prev: GP Asst., Templemore Ave. HC Belf.; Trainee GP Newtownabbey; SHO (O & G) Mid-Ulster Hosp.

WALKER, Jason Michael 16 Crown Terrace, Dowanhill, Glasgow G12 9ES — MB ChB Glas. 1994.

WALKER, Jean Barbara 24 Sivermere Park, Shifnal TF11 9BN — MB ChB Leeds 1982.

WALKER, Jeanne Elizabeth (retired) 228 Upper Batley Low Lane, Batley WF17 0JF Tel: 01924 444365 — MB ChB Leeds 1948. Prev: Ho. Phys. & Asst. Cas. Off. Leeds Pub. Disp. & Hosp.

WALKER, Jeffery Miles (retired) Porchfield House, Mickleton, Chipping Campden GL55 6RZ Tel: 01386 438872 — (Birm.) MB ChB Birm. 1950; MRCS Eng. LRCP Lond. 1950; FRCP Ed. 1971, M 1957; FRCP Lond. 1975, M 1960. Prev: Cons. Phys. Salford HA.

WALKER, Jennifer Louise 50 Dorling Drive, Epsom KT17 3BH — BM BS Nottm. 1996.

WALKER, Jennifer Mary (retired) Rectory Farmhouse, Englishcombe, Bath BA2 9DU Tel: 01225 425073 Email: jennie@barnhire.com — (Lond. Hosp.) MB Camb. 1961, BChir 1960. Prev: Med. Adviser West. Nat. Adoption Soc. Bath.

WALKER, Jennifer Susan Department of Anaesthetics, L & IDGH, Glengallen Road, Oban PA34 4HH Tel: 01631 567500; Foothills, Ganavan, Oban PA34 5TU Tel: 01631 562827 Email: jennifer.walker2@virgin.net — MB ChB Ed. 1988; BSc (Hons.) St. And. 1985; DA (UK) 1991; FRCA 1994. Cons. Anaesth. Lorn & Is.s Dist. Gen. Hosp. Oban. Specialty: Anaesth. Socs: Pain Soc.; ESRA; Scott. Anaesth. Soc. Prev: Sen. Regist. (Anaesth.) Southern Gen. Hosp., Glas.; Career Regist. Rotat. (Anaesth.) West. Infirm. Glas.; SHO (Anaesth.) Law Hosp. Carluke & Glas. Roy. Infirm.

WALKER, Jenny Paediatric Surgical Unit, Sheffield Childrens Hospital, Western Bank, Sheffield S10 2TH Tel: 0114 271 7000 Fax: 0114 276 8419; Converted Garage, Carlton, Leyburn DL8 4AY Tel: 01969 640676 — MB ChB Leeds 1974; FRCS Ed. 1982; FRCS Eng. 1983; ChM Leeds 1986. Cons. Paediat. Surg. Sheff. Childr. Hosp. Sheff. Specialty: Paediat. Surg. Prev: Sen. Regist. (Paediat. Surg.)

Alder Hey Hosp. Liverp.; Research Regist. (Urol.) City Hosp. Nottm.; Gen. Med. Off. State Brunei.

WALKER, Jeremy David Saunders Church Street Medical Centre, 11B Church Street, Eastwood, Nottingham NG16 3BP Tel: 01773 712065 Fax: 01773 534295; 38 Central Avenue, Hucknall, Nottingham NG15 7JH Tel: 0115 955 0623 — BM BS Nottm. 1988 (Nottingham) BMedSci 1986; MRCGP 1993; T(GP) 1993. GP Princip. Prev: Trainee GP/SHO N. Notts. VTS; Ho. Off. (Surg.) Derbysh. Roy. Infirm.; Ho. Off. (Med.) City Hosp. Nottm.

WALKER, Joan Lyall (retired) 4 Moorway, Tranmere Park, Guiseley, Leeds LS20 8LB Tel: 01943 875324 — MB ChB Glas. 1948. Prev: Gen. Practitioner Bradford.

WALKER, Joanna Margaret Department of Paediatrics, St. Marys Hospital, Milton Road, Portsmouth PO3 6AD Tel: 023 92 866100 Fax: 023 92 866101 Email: joanna.walker@porthosp.nhs.uk — MB BS Lond. 1982 (Roy. Free) BA York 1977; MRCP (UK) 1985; FRCP 2003. Cons. Paediat. Portsmouth Hosps. NHS Trust. Specialty: Paediat. Socs: Diabetes UK; United Kingdom Childr.s Cancer Study Gp. (Assoc. Mem.); Brit. Soc. Paediatric Endocrinol. & Diabetes. Prev: Clin. Lect. (Paediat.) Camb. Univ.; Clin. Research Fell. Soton. Univ.; SHO Profess. Med. Unit Hosp. Sick Childr. Lond.

WALKER, Joanna Margaret 24 Kingsway, Scarborough YO12 6SG — MB ChB Ed. 1993; BSc (Hons.) Newc. 1988.

WALKER, Joanna Margaret 14 Hightree Drive, Henbury, Macclesfield SK11 9PD — MB ChB Dund. 1998.

WALKER, John Brian (retired) Quay House, Portscatho, Truro TR2 5HF Tel: 01872 580456; Thorne House, Silver Road, Burnham-on-Crouch CM0 8LA Tel: 01621 782545 — (Oxf. & Lond. Hosp.) BM BCh Oxf. 1947. Prev: Capt. RAMC, Jun. Ophth. Specialist.

WALKER, John Douglas c/o Mr J.P.D. Walker, 71 Granville St., Woodville, Swadlincote DE11 7JQ — MB BCh Witwatersrand 1956; FRCOG 1983, M 1964.

WALKER, John Edward Graham St Johns Hospital, Wood Street, Chelmsford CM2 9BG Fax: 01245 513695 Email: jegwalker@aol.com — MB BS 1972 (St Georges) BDS Manch. 1965; FDS Eng. 1974; MA Landegg 1998. Cons. Maxillo-Facial Surg., Middlx. Trust, Chelmsford; Hon. Cons. Maxillo-Facial Surg., Colchester. Specialty: Oral & Maxillofacial Surg. Special Interest: Oropharyngeal Oncology. Socs: BMA; BDA; BAHNO.

WALKER, John Edward Stuart Grebe House, 27 Westgate, Hornsea HU18 1BP Tel: 01964 533430 — MRCS Eng. LRCP Lond. 1963 (Leeds) DObst RCOG 1965. Socs: Brit. Assn. Sport & Med. Prev: SHO (Dermat.) Gen. Infirm. Leeds; Ho. Off. (Gen. Med. & Surg.) St. Jas. Hosp. Leeds; Ho. Off. St. Luke's Matern. Hosp. Bradford.

WALKER, John Geoffrey The Private Consulting Rooms, Lindo Wing, St Mary's Hospital, London W2 1NY; 42 Highgate High Street, London N6 5JG Tel: 020 8348 7955 — MD Lond. 1971 (Middlx.) MB BS (Hons.) 1958; FRCP Lond. 1974, M 1960. Hon. Cons. Phys. Gastroenterologist St. Mary's Hosp. Lond. Specialty: Gen. Med.; Gastroenterol. Socs: Assn. Phys. & Brit. Soc. Gastroenterol. Prev: Sen. Regist. Med. Gastroenterol. Unit Centr. Middlx. & Middlx. Hosps. Lond.; Lect. (Med.) Roy. Free Hosp. Lond.

WALKER, Professor John Hilton Low Luddick House, Woolsington, Newcastle upon Tyne NE13 8DE Tel: 0191 286 0551 — MD Durh. 1959. MB BS 1954; DPH Newc. 1964; FFCM 1976, M 1972; FRCGP 1977, M 1972; Hon. FRCPCH 1996. Emerit. Prof. Univ. Newc. Prev: Prof. & Head, Dept. Family & Community Med. Univ. Newc.; Chairm. Exam. Bd. Roy. Coll. Gen. Pract.; Mem. Soc. Social Med. & Brit. Paediat. Assn.

WALKER, John Malcolm University College Hospital, The Hatter Institute, Gower Street, London WC1E 6AU Tel: 020 7380 9756 Fax: 020 7388 5095 Email: malcolm.walker@uclh.org — MB ChB Birm. 1975; BSc (Hons. Anat.) Birm. 1972; MRCP UK 1978; MD Birm. 1984; FRCP 1991. Cons. Cardiol. Univ. Coll. Lond. Hosp. & The Heart Hosp. Lond.; Hon. Cons. Cardiol. St Luke's Hosp. for Clergy Lond.; Clin. Dir. Hatter Inst. Cardiol. Lond.; Hons. Cons. Cardiol. King Edw. VII Hosp. for Officers Lond. Specialty: Cardiol.; Gen. Med. Special Interest: Adult Cardiology & Intervention (PCI, Pacemakers); Cardiomyopathy of Haemaglobinopathies. Socs: Pres. Brit. Assn. Cardiovasc. Rehabil. (BACR); Brit. Cardiac Soc.; Fell. RSM. Prev: Clin. Lect. & Sen. Regist. (Cardiol.) John Radcliffe Hosp. Oxf.; Regist. (Cardiol.) St Thos. Hosp. Lond.

WALKER, John Yuill (retired) 47 Victoria Park Road, Exeter EX2 4NU Tel: 01392 496401 — MB ChB Ed. 1931. Prev: Ho. Phys. Edin. Roy. Infirm. & Leith Gen. Hosp.

WALKER, Jonathan 4 Chatsworth Close, Wistaston, Crewe CW2 6SW — MB ChB Liverp. 1993; BSc (Hons.) Physiol. Liverp. 1990; MRCP (UK) 1996; DTM & H Liverp. 1997. SHO Anaesth. Roy. Liverp. Univ. Hosp. Liverp. Specialty: Anaesth. Prev: SHO (Gen. Med.) Aintree Hosps. Liverp.

WALKER, Josephine Merrien Georgian House, 81 Carolgate, Retford DN22 6EH Tel: 01777 709543 Fax: 01777 709004; Welham Hall, Welham, Retford DN22 0SF Tel: 01777 701252 Fax: 01771 701252 — MB ChB Sheff. 1977. Indep. GP (Herbal Med., Acupunture, Complementary Therapies); Med. Adviser for EMP (UK) Ltd Aaron Assocs. Prev: Partner Drs Smith, Brown, Crooks & Walker Retford; Clin. Asst. GU Med. Dept. Bassetlaw Hosp.

WALKER, June Abercrombie 27 Finch Lane, Bushey, Watford WD23 3AJ — MRCS Eng. LRCP Lond. 1962 (Univ. Aberd. & Roy. Free) DA Eng. 1975; FFA RCS Eng. 1979. Specialty: Anaesth. Prev: Cons. Anaesth. Watford Gen. Hosp.; Sen. Regist. N. Middlx. & Roy. Free Hosps. Lond.

WALKER, Mrs June Margaret (retired) 20 Woolsington Park S., Newcastle upon Tyne NE13 8BJ — (Durh.) MB BS Durh. 1950. Clin. Med. Off. Newc. HA.

WALKER, Justin Robert Andrew 7 Sudbury Drive, Lostock, Bolton BL6 4PP — MB ChB Ed. 1993.

WALKER, Katherine Justice Ormiston East, Brittains La, Sevenoaks TN13 2NF — MB ChB Bristol 1997.

WALKER, Kathleen Rutledge Vinniehill, Gatehouse of Fleet, Castle Douglas DG7 2EQ — MB ChB Manch. 1949.

WALKER, Keith Sinclair 43 Station Road, Scalby, Scarborough YO13 0QA Email: keithwalker@tesco.net — MB ChB Glas. 1963; FRCGP 1985, M 1976. p/t Dep. Med. Ref., Woodlands Crematorium, Scarborough. Specialty: Gen. Pract. Prev: Regist. (Med.) Aberd. Gen. Hosp. Gp.; Asst. Resid. (Path.) Boston City Hosp., USA; Partner, Belgrave Surg., ScarBoro.

WALKER, Mr Kenneth Alexander Abbeylands, Abbots Drive, Virginia Water GU25 4SE Tel: 01344 843758 — MB BS Lond. 1960 (St. Bart.) MRCS Eng. LRCP Lond. 1960; FRCS Eng. 1972. Emerit. Cons. Surg. (Trauma & Orthop.) Ashford (Middlx.) Hosp.; Med. Cons. RAC Motor Sport Assoc. & RAC Med. Panel; Chairm.. Motor Sport assoc. Med. Panel. Specialty: Orthop. Special Interest: Medico-legal; Sports Injury; Trauma. Socs: Fell. BOA; Brit. Assn. Surg. Knee; Internat. Soc. Arthroscopy, Knee Surg. & Orthop. Sports Med. Prev: Chief Asst. (Orthop.) St. Thos. Hosp. Lond.; Asst. Prof. Orthop. Surg. Albert Einstein Med. Coll. New York; Regist. (Orthop.) Westm. Hosp. Lond.

WALKER, Kenneth Grant University Department of Surgery, Western Infirmary, Glasgow G11 6NT Tel: 0141 211 2163 Fax: 0141 334 1826; 108 Norse Road, Glasgow G14 9EQ — MB ChB Aberd. 1989. Clin. Research Fell. Univ. Glas. Specialty: Gen. Surg. Socs: Brit. Transpl. Soc. Prev: SHO (Paediat.) Roy. Hosp. Sick Childr. Glas.; SHO (A & E) West. Infirm. Glas.; SHO (Surg.) West. Infirm. Glas.

WALKER, Kenneth Peter, OBE, TD Executive Medical Centre, 24 Chatsworth Road, Croydon CR0 1HA Tel: 020 8688 3430 Fax: 020 8688 4150; Shalcombe Manor, Shalcombe, Yarmouth PO41 0UF Tel: 01983 531551 — (Guy's) LMSSA Lond. 1954; AFOM RCP Lond. 1978. Dir. Exec. Med. & Occupat. Health Centre Croydon; Med. Adviser to Schumberger, West. Geophyical, Halliburton, Brown & Roots, Kverner & Balfour Beatty Overseas, W.S. Atkins & RAC; Col. RAMC TA. Specialty: Occupat. Health. Socs: Soc. Occupat. Med.; Airbourne Med. Soc. Prev: Chief Med. Off. Nestles Gp.; Ho. Phys. & Ho. Surg. (Obst.) Redhill Co. Hosp.

WALKER, Kevin John Grianon, Dunbar Lane, Duffus, Elgin IV30 5QN — MB ChB Ed. 1998.

WALKER, Mr Lawrence Urology Department, Monklands District General Hospital, Monkscourt Avenue, Airdrie ML6 0JS Tel: 01236 712281; 14 Westbourne Crescent, Bearsden, Glasgow G61 4HD Tel: 0141 942 6462 Fax: 0141 942 2854 Email: lawriew87@hotmail.com — MB ChB Glas. 1997 (Glasgow) FRCS Glas. 1982; FRCS Eng. 1984; MD Glas. 1992; FRCS Glas. (Urol.) 1998. Cons. Urol. Monklands Hosp. Specialty: Urol. Prev: Sen. Regist. (Urol.) W. of Scotl. Rotat.

WALKER, Leighton James 23 Maybush Road, Wakefield WF1 5AZ — MB ChB Ed. 1996.

WALKER, Lewis Ardach Health Centre, Highfield Road, Buckie AB5 1JE Tel: 01542 831555 Fax: 01542 835799 — MB ChB Aberd. 1981; MRCP (UK) 1984; DRCOG 1988; FRCP Glasg. 1999. Specialty: Hypnother.

WALKER, Linda Jean Elizabeth Mid-Ulster Hospital, Magherafelt BT45 5EX — MD Belf. 1986; MB BCh BAO 1977; MRCP (UK) 1980. Cons. Phys. & Geriat. Mid-Ulster Hosp. Magherafelt. Specialty: Gen. Med.; Care of the Elderly.

WALKER, Linsey Anne — MB ChB Ed. 1998.

WALKER, Mair Bron Wylfa, Llangunnor Road, Carmarthen SA31 2PB Tel: 01267 236516 — MB BCh Wales 1959 (Cardiff) DCH Eng. 1972. Socs: Assoc. Mem. BPA; Fac. Comm. Health; FRCPCh. Prev: SCMO Carmarthen/Dinefwr Health Unit; Med. Off. Family Plann. Assn. Clinics; Asst. Med. Off. Pub. Health W. Glam. Div.

WALKER, Margaret (retired) 27 The Avenue Road, Doncaster DN2 4AE Tel: 01302 342181 — MB ChB Leeds 1951.

WALKER, Margaret Helen 36 Kilmardinny Gate, Bearsden, Glasgow G61 3ND — MB ChB Glas. 1951. Med. Bd. Pract. DSS. Prev: Med. Ho. Off. & Ho. Off. O & G Stobhill Hosp.

WALKER, Margaret Julia Bute Lodge, 182 Petersham Road, Richmond TW10 7AD — MB BS Lond. 1991.

WALKER, Margaret Mary 4 Chalfonts, York YO24 1EX — MB ChB Liverp. 1952.

WALKER, Margaret Mary (retired) 4 Glenpark Avenue, Giffnock, Glasgow G46 7JF Tel: 0141 638 3928 — MB ChB Glas. 1968 (Glasgow) DObst RCOG 1970; MRCPsych 1975. Prev: Sen. Regist. (Psychiat.) Gtr. Glas. HB.

WALKER, Marion Winifred 9 Swallow Craig, Dalgety Bay, Dunfermline KY11 9YR Tel: 01383 824278; Department of Radiology, Queen Margaret Hospital, Whitefield Road, Dunfermline KY12 Tel: 01383 623623 Fax: 01383 627072 — (RCSI) LRCPI & LM, LRCSI & LM 1969; DMRD Eng. 1976; FFR RCSI 1979. Cons. Radiol. Fife Acute Hosps. NHS Trust. Specialty: Radiol. Prev: Cons. Radiol. Hairmyres Hosp. E. Kilbride; Sen. Regist. & Regist. (Radiol.) Vict. Infirm. Glas.& Roy. Infirm. Glas.

WALKER, Marjorie Mary Department of Histopath., St Mary's Hospital, Praed St., London W2 1NY Email: mm.walker@ic.ac.uk — BM BS Nottm. 1976; MRCPath 1984; FRCPath 1996. Sen. Lect. & Hon. Cons. St. Mary's Hosp. Lond. Specialty: Histopath.

WALKER, Mark Department of Medicine, School of Clinical Medical Sciences, Floor 4, William Leech Building, Medical School, Framlington Place, Newcastle upon Tyne NE2 4HH Tel: 0191 222 7019 Email: mark.walker@ncl.ac.uk — MB BS Newc. 1983; MD Newc. 1992, BMedSci (1st cl. Hons.) 1980, MB BS 1983; FRCP 1997. Sen. Lect. & Hon. Cons. (Diabetes) Sch. Clin. Med. Scis. New. u. Tyne. Specialty: Gen. Med.; Endocrinol.; Diabetes. Prev: Regist. (Med.) Roy. Hallamsh. Hosp. Sheff.

WALKER, Mark Adam — MB ChB Ed. 1997. SHO Psychiat., Falkirk and Dist. Roy. Infirm., Forth Valley NHS Trust; PRHO Surg., Dumfries & Galloway Roy. Infirm. Prev: PRHO Med., Vict. Hosp., Kirkcaldy, Fife Acute NHS Trust.

WALKER, Mark Andrew (retired) Kilve Cottage, Maddocks Slade, Burnham-on-Sea TA8 2AN Tel: 01278 788209 — MB ChB Bristol 1966; DObst RCOG 1970; DA Eng. 1972; FFA RCS Eng. 1975.

WALKER, Mark Christopher Michael Lytham Road Surgery, 352 Lytham Road, Blackpool FY4 1DW Tel: 01253 402546 Fax: 01253 349637 — MB ChB Dundee 1986; MRCGP 1991. Specialty: Dermat.

WALKER, Marten James The Group Practice, Health Centre, Springfield Road, Stornoway HS1 2PS Tel: 01851 703145 Fax: 01851 706138; Ingleside, 75 Newvalley, Laxdale, Stornoway HS2 0DN — MB ChB Aberd. 1984; DCH RCP Lond. 1987; DRCOG 1988; Cert Family Plann. JCC 1989; MRCGP 1989. Specialty: Accid. & Emerg. Prev: Trainee GP Aboyne; SHO (O & G) Highland HB; SHO (Paediat.) Soton. & SW Hants. HA.

WALKER, Martin Bernard Derriford Hospital, Intensive Care Unit, Plymouth PL6 8DH Tel: 01752 792555 Fax: 01752 763287 Email: martin.walker@phnt.swest.nhs.uk; Didham Farm, Buckland Monachorum, Yelverton PL20 7NW Tel: 01822 854474 — MB BS Lond. 1984; FRCA 1989. Cons. Anaesth. Derriford Hosp. Plymouth. Specialty: Anaesth. Prev: Sen. Regist. (Anaesth.) Oxf. RHA; Regist. (Anaesth.) St. Bart. Hosp. Lond.; Asst. Prof. Univ. Texas.

WALKER, Martin Joseph Ryhope Health Centre, Black Road, Sunderland SR2 0RY Tel: 0191 521 0210 Fax: 0191 521 4235; 85 Ryhope Road, Sunderland SR2 7SZ — MB ChB Dundee 1978. Specialty: Gen. Pract.

WALKER, Martine Anne The Firs, Fulbourn Hospital, Cambridge CB1 5EF — MB BS Sydney 1987.

WALKER, Mary Alice 3 Baylie Street, Stourbridge DY8 1AZ Tel: 01384 379530 — MB BS Lond. 1974 (St. Mary's) MA Camb. 1973; DCH Eng. 1976.

WALKER, Mary Frances Laurel Bank Surgery, 216B Kirkstall Lane, Leeds LS6 3DS Tel: 0113 295 3900 Fax: 0113 295 3901; 6 Welburn Avenue, Leeds LS16 5HJ Tel: 0113 274 7661 — MB ChB Glas. 1968 (Glasgow) MFFPRHC; DCH 1972; MRCP (UK) 1972.

WALKER, Mary Patricia c/o The North Brink Practice, 7 North Brink, Wisbech PE13 1JR — MB BCh BAO NUI 1987; LRCPSI 1987.

WALKER, Matthew Charles 57 Loxley Road, London SW18 3LL — MB BChir Camb. 1990; BA Camb. 1986; MRCP (UK) 1992.

WALKER, Matthew Craig Middleton and Partners, Sele Gate Surgery, Hencotes, Hexham NE46 2EG Tel: 01434 602237 Fax: 01434 609496 — MB ChB Leeds 1989; DRCOG 1992; MRCGP 1993.

WALKER, Michael 24 Peterborough Close, Worcester WR5 1PW — MB ChB Birm. 1995; BSc (Hons.) Pharmacol. Birm. 1992. SHO (Gen. Surg.) Princess Roy. Hosp. Telford Shrops. Specialty: Gen. Surg. Prev: Ho. Off. (Surg.) Russells Hall Hosp. Dudley W. Midl.

WALKER, Mr Michael Alexander West Cumberland Hospital, Hensingham, Whitehaven CA28 8JG Tel: 01946 693181; How Garth, Pardshaw, Cockermouth CA13 0SP — MD Ed. 1989; MB ChB 1978; FRCS Ed. 1983. Cons. Gen. & Vasc. Surg W. Cumbld. Hosp. Whitehaven. Specialty: Gen. Surg.

WALKER, Michael Campbell The Surgery, 16 Windsor Road, Chobham, Woking GU24 8NA Tel: 01276 857117; Changan, Sendmarsh Road, Ripley, Woking GU23 6JN Tel: 01483 225987 — MB ChB Bristol 1990; MRCGP 1996. GP Partner Surrey. Socs: MDU. Prev: SHO (O & G) Frimley Pk. Hosp.; SHO (A & E) Frimley Pk. Hosp.

WALKER, Professor Michael Grant Department of Vascular Surgery, Manchester Royal Infirmary, Oxford Road, Manchester M13 9WL Tel: 0161 276 4525 Fax: 0161 276 8014 Email: mgwalker@fs3.scg.man.ac.uk; Manor Lodge, Mill Lane, Cheadle SK8 2NT Tel: 0161 428 0291 Fax: 0161 428 6202 — MB ChB Aberd. 1964; FRCS Ed. 1970; ChM Aberd. 1976. Prof. Vas. Surg. Manch. Roy. Infirm. Specialty: Vasc. Med. Prev: Cons. Vasc. Surg. Manch. Roy. Infirm.; Sen. Regist. (Surg.) Edin. Roy. Infirm.; Research Fell. (Vasc. Surg.), Ho. Surg. & Ho. Phys. Aberd. Roy. Infirm.

WALKER, Michael Peter (retired) Oak Tree House, 39 Oak Lodge Tye, White Hart Lane, Springfield, Chelmsford CM1 6GY Tel: 01245 466683 — MB ChB Bristol 1949. Prev: GP Chelmsford.

WALKER, Neal William Errigal Medical Centre, Old Dungannon Road, Ballygawley, Dungannon BT70 2EY Tel: 028 8556 8212 Email: nealww@doctors.org.uk — MB BCh BAO Belf. 1993; DGM RCPS Glas. 1995; DRCOG 1996; MRCGP 1997; DFFP 2003. p/t Salaried Gen. Practitioner. Specialty: Gen. Pract. Socs: Roy. Coll. of Gen. Practitioners.

WALKER, Neil Patrick John Department of Dermatology, Churchill Hospital, Headington, Oxford OX3 7LJ Tel: 01865 228237 Fax: 01865 228260; The Old Pottery, Coldstone House, Shipton Road, Ascott-u-Wychwood, Chipping Norton OX7 6AG Tel: 01993 832812 Fax: 01993 832832 — MB BS Lond. 1975 (Westm.) BSc Lond. 1972; MRCS Eng. LRCP Lond. 1975; MRCP (UK) 1978; FRCP Lond. 1993. Hon. Cons. Dermat. Churchill Hosp. Oxf. Specialty: Dermat. Socs: Brit. Assn. Dermat.; Brit. Soc. Dermat. Surg.; (Comm.) Eur. Soc. Micrographic Surg. Prev: Sen. Lect. St. John's Inst. Dermat. St. Thos. Hosp. Lond.; Sen. Regist. (Dermat.) Addenbrooke's Hosp. Camb.; Fell. Micrographic Surg. & Cutan. Oncol. Cleveland Clinic Ohio, USA.

WALKER, Nicholas Allen 11 Dochdwy Road, Llandough, Penarth CF64 2PB — MB BCh Wales 1970; MRCGP 1980. GP Cardiff.

WALKER, Nicholas David Fairfield Cottage, Macrae Road, Yateley GU46 6NQ — BM Soton. 1989; DRCOG 1992; DA (UK) 1993.

WALKER, Nicholas Lawrence 142 Main Street, Barton Under Needwood, Burton-on-Trent DE13 8AB — MB ChB Birm. 1981;

MRCP (UK) 1985. Med. Off. Occupat. Health Serv. Nottm. Specialty: Occupat. Health. Prev: Sen. Med. Off. GKN plc; Asst. Works Med. Off. Assoc. Octel Co. Ellesmere Port; SHO (Gen. Med.) Warneford Hosp. Leamington Spa.

WALKER, Nicholas Paul Ravenscraig Hospital, Inverkip Road, Greenock PA16 9HA Tel: 01475 502391/01475 633777 Ext: 62321 Email: nick.walker@nhs.net — MB ChB Auckland 1989 (Univ. Auckland, New Zealand) BHB Auckland 1986; MRCPsych 1995. Cons. (Gen. & Rehabil. Psychiat.) & Hon. Clin. Senical Sen. Lect. (Psychol. Med.) Revenscraig Hosp. & Univ. of Glas.; Coll. Tutor for Basic Psychiatric Train. Scheme in Inverclyde. Specialty: Gen. Psychiat. Socs: Roy. Coll. of Psychiat.s, Lond. Prev: Sen. Regist. & Clin. Regist., Roy. Cornhill Hosp. & Univ. of Aberd., Aberd. 1996-1999.

WALKER, Nigel George Grange Lea, 23 Hollingwood Lane, Bradford BD7 2RE Tel: 01274 571437 Fax: 01274 571437 — MB BS Lond 1978 (London) GP Bradford, W. Yorks.

WALKER, Norman Anthony (retired) 13 Brookside, Cambridge CB2 1JE Tel: 01223 351625 — MB BS Lond. 1947 (Lond. Hosp.) MRCS Eng. LRCP Lond. 1947. Prev: Ho. Phys. & Ho. Surg. Lond. Hosp.

WALKER, Norman Jan Piet, OBE Salisbury Medical Centre, 474 Antrim Road, Belfast BT15 5GF Tel: 028 9077 7905 — MB BCh BAO Belf. 1972 (Queen's University Belfast) MRCGP 1980. GP Trainer Belf.; JP. Socs: Fell. Ulster Med. Soc.; Irish Coll. of Gen. Pract.

WALKER, Patrick George 62 Wimpole Street, London W1G 8AJ Tel: 020 7224 3054 Fax: 020 7224 3086 Email: patrick.walker@royalfree.nhs.uk — MD Lond. 1984; MB BS 1973; FRCOG 1992, M 1980; T(OG) 1986. Cons. Gyn. Roy. Free Hosp. Lond.; Pres. of BSCCP 2003-2005; Mem. Exec. Bd. IFCPC 2003-2005; Chairm. Nat. Quality Assur. Gp. in Colposcopy 2002-2004. Specialty: Obst. & Gyn. Special Interest: Colposcolpy; Gyn. Cancer. Socs: Pres. Of Brit. Soc. Of Colposcopy & Cerv. Path.; BGCS. Prev: Florence & William Blair Bell Memor. Research Fell. RCOG.; Assistant Treasurer IFCPC 1999-2002; Vis. Gynaecologist HMP Holloway 1986-1991.

WALKER, Paul Crawford The Courtyard, Bronllys, Brecon LD3 0LU Tel: 01874 712726 Fax: 01874 712739 Email: paul.walker@nphs.wales.nhs.uk; 8 Church Avenue, Sneyd Park, Bristol BS9 1LD Tel: 0117 968 2205 Fax: 0117 968 2205 — MB BChir Camb. 1966 (Cambridge) Dip. Soc. Med. Ed. 1971; FFCM 1980; MA Camb. 1991. Director (Public Health) Powys Health Bd.; Vis. Fell. Univ. W. Eng. Specialty: Pub. Health Med.; Epidemiol.; Infec. Dis. Special Interest: Health Impact Assessm. Socs: Bristol M-C Soc.; BMA; Brit. Soc. Rehabil. Med. Prev: Sen. Lect. Univ. Wales Coll. Med. Cardiff; Dir. (Pub. Health) Norwich HA; Regional Med. Off. NE Thames RHA.

WALKER, Paul Phillip Department of Respiratory Medicine, University Hospital Aintree, Lower Lane, Liverpool L9 7AL; 38 Chandag Road, Keynsham, Bristol BS31 1NR — BM BS Nottm. 1992; BMedSci (Hons.) Nottm. 1990; MRCP (UK) 1995. Specialist Regist. (Respirat. Med.), Merseyside Region. Specialty: Respirat. Med.

WALKER, Peter Alan 99 Stamfordham Road, Fenham, Newcastle upon Tyne NE5 3JN — MB ChB Leeds 1983.

WALKER, Peter Irvine Tod 36 Kilmardinny Gate, Bearsden, Glasgow G61 3ND — MB ChB Glas. 1951. Med. Ref. Scott. Home & Health Dept. Prev: Regional Med. Off. Scott. Home & Health Dept.

WALKER, Peter James Willow Corner, Bendish, Hitchin SG4 8JH Tel: 01438 871350 — MB BS Lond. 1978 (Univ. Coll. Hosp.) PhD Lond. 1962; MA Camb. 1964; Cert. JCPTGP 1982. Princip. GP (Herts. & Beds.). Specialty: Gen. Pract. Socs: Fell. Roy. Soc. Trop. Med. & Hyg.

WALKER, Mr Philip Martin 22 Mossdale Avenue, Bolton BL1 5YA Tel: 01204 483122 Email: p.m.walker@btinternet.com — MB ChB Manch. 1992; FRCS Ed. 1997. Regist. (Gen. Surg.) Bury Gen. Hosp. Bury. Specialty: Gen. Surg. Socs: Manch. Med. Soc. Prev: SHO (Gen. Surg.) Birch Hill Hosp. Rochdale; SHO (Ear, Nose & Throat) Fairfield Hosp. Bury.

WALKER, Philippa Jane Ferndale, 10 Newbridge Crescent, Wolverhampton WV6 0LN — MB ChB Birm. 1993.

WALKER, Philippa May Riverside Medical Practice, Roushill, Shrewsbury SY1 1PQ Tel: 01743 352371 Fax: 01743 340269 — MB ChB Manch. 1980; DRCOG 1983; MRCGP 1987.

WALKER, Phillip Edward Court House, 42 Beaconsfield Road, Woolton, Liverpool L25 6EL — MB ChB Liverp. 1970.

WALKER, Phillip Roy (retired) Dunbelly Barn, Orlingbury Road, Isham, Kettering NN14 1HW Tel: 01536 726282 — BM BCh Oxf. 1951; MA Oxf. 1949.

WALKER, Phyllis Jane Learning Disabilities Service, Carseview Avenue, Medipark, Dundee DD2 1HN Tel: 01382 878711 — MB ChB Aberd. 1980 (Univ. Aberd.) DRCOG 1984; MRCPsych 1987. Cons. Psychiat. Roy. Dundee Liff Hosp. Specialty: Gen. Psychiat. Prev: Sen. Regist. (Psychiat.) Roy. Dundee Liff Hosp.

WALKER, Raymond Grant Drymen Road Surgery, 96 Drymen Road, Bearsden, Glasgow G61 2SY Tel: 0141 942 9494 Fax: 0141 931 5496 Email: ray.walker@gp40402.glasgow-hb.scot.nhs.uk; 52 North Grange Road, Bearsden, Glasgow G61 3AF — MB ChB Glas. 1979 (Glas. Univ.) Specialty: Gen. Pract.

WALKER, Richard Charles Michael Waterloo House Surgery, Waterloo House, 42-44 Wellington Street, Millom LA18 4DE Tel: 01229 772123 — MB ChB Birm. 1990; MRCGP 1993; DRCOG 1993.

WALKER, Richard Irving The Manor Street Surgery, Manor Street, Berkhamsted HP4 2DL Tel: 01442 875935; 72 Greenway, Berkhamsted HP4 3LF Tel: 01442 875614 — MB BS Lond. 1980; MRCGP 1986.

WALKER, Richard Mark Health Centre, Village Road, Llanfairfechan LL33 0NH Tel: 01248 680021 Fax: 01248 681711; Glanffrwd, Fernbrook Rd, Penmaenmawr LL34 6DE — MB ChB Manch. 1985; DRCOG 1988; MRCGP 1989.

WALKER, Richard Stephen Pain Clinic, Walsgrave hospital, UHCW NHS Trust, Coventry CV2 2DX Tel: 02476 538628 Fax: 02476 535218 Email: r.s.walker@virgin.net — MB BS Newc. 1982; FFA RCS Eng. 1988. Cons. in Anaesth.,Pain Managem. and Local Osteopath; Pain Managment Cons., Coventry Consg. Rooms. Specialty: Anaesth. Special Interest: Musculoskeletal Medicine; Osteopathy. Socs: Pain Soc. of Gt. Britain; Assn. of Anaesthetists; Assn. of Med. Osteopaths. Prev: Post Fellowship Regist. (Anaesth.) Coventry; Regist. (Anaesth.) Qu. Med. Centre Nottm.; SHO (Anaesth.) Roy. Vict. Infirm. Newc.

WALKER, Richard William Northumbria Healthcare NHS Trust, North Tyneside General Hospital, Rake Lane, North Shields NE29 8NH Tel: 0191 273 2709 Fax: 0191 293 2709 — MB BS Newc. 1982; MRCP (UK) 1985; DTM & H Liverp. 1989; FRACP 1991; FRCP 1999; FRCP Edin 2000; MD Newc. 2002. Cons. Phys. (Gen. Med. & Geriat.) N. Tyneside Gen. Hosp. Specialty: Gen. Med. Socs: Fell. Roy. Soc. Trop. Med. & Hyg.; Brit. Geriat. Soc.; African Gerontol. Soc. Prev: Research Assoc. Tanzanian Adult Morbidity & Mortality Project; Sen. Regist. Rotat. (Med. & Geriat.) North. Region; Sen. Regist. (Med.) Roy. Vict. Hosp. Banjul, The Gambia.

WALKER, Rita Cecily (retired) Foxgloves, 134 Eastmoor Park, Harpenden AL5 1BP — (St. Mary's) BSc Lond. 1954; MB BS Lond. 1958; MRCS Eng. LRCP Lond. 1958; DCH Eng. 1961; MRCP (UK) 1970; FRCP Lond. 1984. Prev: Cons. Geriat. Med. OldCh. Hosp. Romford & St. Geo. Hosp. HornCh..

WALKER, Robert Yew Tree Cottage Surgery, 15 Leyton Road, Harpenden AL5 2HX Tel: 01582 712126 Fax: 01582 462414; Pine Needles, 12 Roundwood Park, Harpenden AL5 3AB Tel: 01582 768720 — MB BCh Wales 1978; DRCOG 1983; MRCGP 1984. GP Trainer.

WALKER, Robert Alan 175 Lugtrout Lane, Solihull B91 2RU — MB ChB Birm. 1987.

WALKER, Robert Alistair 25 Slievenamaddy Avenue, Newcastle BT33 0DT — MB BCh BAO Belf. 1994.

WALKER, Robert Bernard William (retired) Blackford Grange, Flat 22, 39 Blackford Avenue, Edinburgh EH9 3HN Tel: 0131 667 0578 Email: rw@hebrides.u-net.com — MB ChB Ed. 1937. Prev: Med. Off. DGM Hosp. Livingstonia, Malawi.

WALKER, Robert Douglas Clifton House S., 8 Moor Road, Clifton, Workington CA14 1TS Tel: 01900 603762 — MB ChB Liverp. 1971; MRCS Eng. LRCP Lond. 1971; MRCP (UK) 1974; FRCGP 1992, M 1977; MICGP 1987; FRCP Ed. 1997. Dir. Primary Care N. Cumbria HA; Examr. Irish Coll. Gen. Pract. Prev: GP

Workington, Cumbria; Ho Off. Profess. Med. & Surg. Units & Regist. (Med.) Broadgreen Hosp. Liverp.

WALKER, Mr Robert Glyndwr 62 Kilburn Road, York YO10 4DE Tel: 01904 631468 — MB BS Lond. 1989 (Royal Free Hospital School of Medicine) MRCOG 1995. Specialist Regist. (O & G), Yorks. region; Locum Cons. (O & G), Friarage Hosp., Northallerton. Specialty: Obst. & Gyn. Prev: Regist. (O & G) Inverclyde Roy. Hosp. Greenock; SHO (O & G) Glas. Roy. Infirm. & Glas. Roy. Matern. Hosp.; SHO (O & G) Vict. Infirm. & Rutherglen Matern. Hosp.

WALKER, Robert James Cornerstone Surgery, 469 Chorley Old Road, Bolton BL1 6AH Tel: 01204 495426 Fax: 01204 497423; 22 Carlton Road, Bolton BL1 5HU Tel: 01204 491360 — MB ChB Manch. 1977; BSc (Med. Sci.) St. And. 1974.

WALKER, Robert Sibbald Rominar, Erskine Road, Whitecraigs, Glasgow G46 6TH Tel: 0141 639 4808 — MB BS Lond. 1945 (Anderson Coll. Glas.) LRCP LRCS Ed. LRFPS Glas. 1944; FRCP Ed. 1972, M 1949; MD Lond. 1949; FRCP Glas. 1967, M 1962. Cons. Phys. Glas. Specialty: Gen. Med. Socs: Scott. Soc. Phys.; Scott. Cardiac Soc. Prev: Cons. Phys. Law Hosp. Carluke; Capt. RAMC; Sen. Regist. (Med.) Roy. Infirm. Glas.

WALKER, Mr Robert Toby Peterborough District Hospital, Midland Road, Peterborough PE3 6DA Tel: 01733 874000; Holly House, High St, Morcott, Oakham LE15 9DN Tel: 01572 747429 — MB BS Lond. 1974 (St. Geo.) FRCS Eng. 1979; MS Lond. 1988. Cons. Gen. & Vasc. Surg., P'boro. Hosps. NHS Trust. Specialty: Gen. Surg. Prev: Sen. Regist. (Vasc. Surg.) Princess Alexandra Hosp. Queensland, Austral.; Sen. Regist., Gen. Surg., S.W. Thames.

WALKER, Robert William Mundell Royal Manchester Children's Hospital, Pendlebury, Manchester M27 4HA Tel: 0161 794 4696; 73 Church Road, Urmston, Manchester M41 9EJ — MB ChB Glas. 1984; DCH RCPS Glas. 1986; FRCA. 1989. Cons. Paediatric Anaesth., RMCH. Specialty: Anaesth. Socs: BMA; AAGBI; Assoc. of Paed. Anaesth.s. Prev: Regist. (Anaesth.) Trafford Gen. Hosp. & Hope Hosp. Salford; Regist. (Anaesth.) W.mead Hosp. Sydney, Austral.; Sen. Regist. (Anaesth.) N.W. RHA.

WALKER, Rodney William Hearn The Royal London Hospital, Whitechapel, London E1 1BB Tel: 020 7377 7359 — BM BCh Oxf. 1975; BA 1972,MA Camb. 1976; MRCP (UK) 1977; PhD Lond. 1986; FRCP Lond. 1993. Cons. Neurol. Barts and the Lond. NHS trust. Specialty: Neurol. Prev: Sen. Regist. (Neurol.) Nat. Hosp. for Nerv. Dis. & St. Bart. Hosp. Lond.; Regist. (Neurol.) Nat. Hosp. for Nerv. Dis. Lond.; Ho. Phys. Radcliffe Infirm. Oxf.

WALKER, Mr Roger Michael Haydn Department of Urology, Epsom & St Helier NHS Trust, Epsom Hospital, Dorking Road, Epsom KT18 7EG Tel: 01372 735106 Fax: 01372 735159 Email: rmhwalker@baus.org.uk; 52 Inglethorpe Street, Fulham, London SW6 6NT Tel: 0207 610 3354 Email: rmhwalker@baus.org.uk — MB BS Lond. 1989 (Charing Cross & Westminster Med School) FRCS Eng. 1993; FRCS FRCS (urol) 1999; FEBU 2001. Cons.Surg. (Urol.) Epsom & St Helier NHS Trust, Epsom & St Helier Hosp. Surrey. Specialty: Urol. Socs: Fell. Roy. Coll. Surgs.; Fell. Roy. Soc. Med.; Full Mem. BAUS. Prev: Regist. (Urol.) Char. Cross Hosp. Lond.; Regist. (Urol.) Hammersmith Hosp.; Regist (Urol.) N.wicck Pk. Hosp.

WALKER, Ronald James Friockheim Health Centre, Westgate, Friockheim, Arbroath DD11 4TX Tel: 01241 828444 Fax: 01241 828565; Three Trees, Redford, Carmyllie, Arbroath DD11 2RD Tel: 01241 860347 Fax: 01241 860347 — MB ChB Dundee 1977; MRCGP Ed. 1984. GP Friockheim Health Centre; Civil. Med. Off. Roy. Marines Condor.

WALKER, Rosalie Anne Betts Avenue Medical Centre, 2 Betts Avenue, Benwell, Newcastle upon Tyne NE15 6TD Tel: 0191 274 2767/2842 Fax: 0191 274 0244 — MB BS Lond. 1983; BSc Lond. 1980, MB BS 1983; MRCGP 1987; DRCOG 1987. Trainee GP Northumbria VTS; SHO (Dermat.) Roy. Vict. Infirm. Newc. Prev: SHO (Psychiat.) St. Geo. Hosp. Morpeth.; SHO (Cas.) Hexham Gen. Hosp.; SHO (O & G) S. Shields Gen. Hosp.

WALKER, Professor Rosemary Ann Dept. of Cancer Studies & Molecular Med., Robert Kilpatrick Clinical Sciences Building, Leicester Royal Infirmary, PO Box 65, Leicester LE3 9QP Tel: 0116 252 3224 Fax: 0116 252 3274 Email: raw14@ie.ac.uk — MB ChB Birm. 1971; FRCPath 1989, M 1977; MD Birm. 1980. Prof. of Path., Univ. of Leicester; Hon. Cons. Breast Histopath., Leicester. Specialty: Histopath. Special Interest: Breast. Socs: Brit. Assn. for Cancer Research; ACP; Path. Soc.

WALKER, Roy Oliver (retired) Dunkeld, 119 Worcester Lane, Pedmore, Stourbridge DY9 0SJ Tel: 01562 886542 — (Birm.) MB ChB Birm. 1956; DObst RCOG 1960. Prev: Chairm. Med. Bd.

WALKER, Mr Russell William Nevill Hall Hospital, Abergavenny NP7 7EG Tel: 01873 732732; Cwn Farm, Llangenny, Crickhowell NP8 1HD Tel: 01873 811230 — MB BS Lond. 1987 (St. George's Hospital Medical School) FRCS Eng. 1992; FRCS (Trauma & Orthop) 1999. Cons., Nevill Hill Hosp., Abergavenny. Specialty: Orthop. Socs: Brit. Trauma Soc.; BOA; BMA. Prev: Regist. (Orthop.) St. Geo. Hosp. Lond.; Ho. Phys. K. Edwd. VII Hosp. Midhurst; Ho. Surg. St. Geo.'s Hosp. Lond.

WALKER, Ruth Elizabeth White Lodge Medical Practice, 68 Silver Street, Enfield EN1 3EW Tel: 020 8363 4156 Fax: 020 8364 6295 — MB ChB St. And. 1966.

WALKER, Sally Elizabeth Dr. Rose and Partners, Spring Terrace Health Centre, Spring Terrace, North Shields NE29 0HQ Tel: 0191 296 1588 Fax: 0191 296 2901; 28 Beverley Terrace, North Shields NE30 4NU — MB BS Newc. 1991; MRCGP 1995. GP. Specialty: Gen. Pract.

WALKER, Samantha Anne 6 Bromyard Avenue, Sutton Coldfield B76 1RQ — MB ChB Birm. 1994; ChB Birm. 1994.

WALKER, Sara Child & Family Consultation Service, The Terraces, Mount Gould Hospital, Mount Gould Road, Plymouth PL4 7QD Tel: 01752 272325 Fax: 01752 272361 — MB BCh Wales 1976; MRCPsych 1992. Cons. Child & Adolesc. Psychiat. Plymouth NHS Hosps. Trust. Specialty: Child & Adolesc. Psychiat.

WALKER, Sarah Belle Chapel Cottage, Hamstead Marshall, Newbury RG20 0HP — MB ChB Aberd. 1991.

WALKER, Sarah Louise 177 Russell Road, Moseley, Birmingham B13 8RR — MB ChB Manch. 1979; FRCR 1985.

WALKER, Shona Ann Department old age Psychiatry, Clerkseat, Royal Cornhill Hospital, Aberdeen Tel: 01224 681818 Ext: 57285; 29 Osborne Place, Aberdeen AB25 2BX Tel: 01224 641582 — MB ChB Aberd. 1986; MRCGP 1990; MRCPsych 1992. Sen. Regist. (Psychiat.) Aberd. Specialty: Gen. Psychiat.; Geriat. Psychiat. Prev: Regist. & SHO (Psychiat.) Aberd.; Trainee GP Skene VTS.

WALKER, Sian Rebecca The Old Gaol, Temple St., Brill, Aylesbury HP18 9SX Tel: 01844 238762; Wyeth, Huntercombe Lane South, Taplow, Maidenhead SL6 0PM Tel: 01628 414976 Fax: 01628 414976 Email: walkers@wyeth.com — MB ChB Leeds 1984; Dip. Pharm. Med 1998 (RCP); Cert. Family Plann. JCC 1988; MRCGP 1988; DRCOG 1990; MFPM 2002. Head of Med. Affairs, Wyeth; Director of Immunol. and Transplantation. Specialty: Pharmaceutical Medicine.

WALKER, Mr Simon 3 Chedworth Drive, Old Hall Gardens, Baguley, Manchester M23 1LW Tel: 0161 945 8300 — MB ChB Sheff. 1993; FRCOphth 1998. Specialist Regist. Rotat. (Ophth.) Manch. Roy. Eye Hosp. Specialty: Ophth. Socs: Med. Protec. Soc. Prev: SHO Rotat. (Ophth.) W. Glas. Tennent Inst. Glas.; Hon. Off. Roy. Hallamsh. Hosp. Sheff.; Sen. Health Off. (A & E) Doncaster Roy. Infirm.

WALKER, Simon Charles 42 River Court, Upper Ground, London SE1 9PE — MB BS Lond. 1989.

WALKER, Simon Wyndham Department of Clinical Biochemistry, The Royal Infirmary, Edinburgh EH3 9YW Tel: 0131 536 2700 — MB BS Lond. 1977 (Middlx.) BA (1st cl. Hons.) Oxf. 1972, MA 1975, DM 1989. Sen. Lect. (Clin. Biochem.) Univ. Edin. & Hon. Cons. Lothian HB. Specialty: Chem. Path. Prev: Lect. (Clin. Chem.) Univ. Edin. & Hon. Sen. Regist. Lothian Health Bd.; Wellcome Research Fell. (Human Metab. & Clin. Biochem.) Univ. Sheff.; Lect. (Path.) Univ. Leicester.

WALKER, Stephanie 69 Sandown Road, Belfast BT5 6GU — MB ChB belf. 1998; MB ChB belf 1998.

WALKER, Stephen Eric Nene Valley Medical Centre, Clayton, Orton Goldhay, Peterborough PE2 5GP Tel: 01733 366600 Fax: 01733 370711 — MB BS Lond. 1986.

WALKER, Stephen Lloyd c/o 80 Parkside, Wollaton, Nottingham NG8 2NN — MB ChB Bristol 1991.

WALKER, Stuart Keith Flat 2, Cedar House, Elmbank, Barnet Road, Barnet EN5 3HD — MB BCh Wales 1990; MRCP (UK) 1993. Specialty: Gen. Med.; Cardiol.

WALKER, Mr Stuart Robert 8 Trefoil Close, Hamilton, Leicester LE5 1TF; 12 Lindisfarne Drive, Loughborough LE11 4FX Tel: 01509 844155 Email: stuart.walker@virgin.net — MB BS Lond. 1990; FRCS Eng. 1994. Regist. (Surg.) Leics. Specialty: Gen. Surg.

WALKER, Susan 112 West Street, Huddersfield HD3 3JX Fax: 01484 461113 Email: dr.suewalker@virgin.net — MB BS Newc. 1983 (Newcastle upon Tyne) DRCOG 1987; MRCGP 1988; DFFP 1994. Specialty: Trop. Med. Prev: Med. Off. St. Francis Hosp. Zambia, Afr.; GP Hartlepool; Med. Off. Raleigh Fitkin Memor. Hosp. Manzini Swaziland, (Afr.).

WALKER, Susan Hilda 76 Chadwick Street, Belfast BT9 7FD — MB BCh BAO Belf. 1990; DGM RCP Lond. 1992; DRCOG 1993; MRCGP 1994. Specialty: Gen. Pract.

WALKER, Susan Jane Box Surgery, London Road, Box, Corsham SN13 8NA Tel: 01225 742361 — MB BS Lond. 1979 (Char. Cross) DCH RCP Lond. 1983; MRCGP 1986; MFHom 1994. Socs: Inst. Psychosexual Med.

WALKER, Susan Mary 35 Daleside, Greetland, Halifax HX4 8QD — MB ChB Sheff. 1995.

WALKER, Suzanne Claire Worcester Royal Infirmary NHS Trust, Newtown Road, Worcester WR5 Tel: 01905 763333; 24 Peterborough Close, Worcester WR5 1PW Tel: 01905 767374 — MB ChB Birm. 1995; BSc (Hons.) Biochem. Birm. 1992. SHO (VTS) Wors. Roy. Infirm. Specialty: Pub. Health Med.; Paediat. Prev: SHO (Med.) Good Hope Hosp. NHS Trust Sutton Coldfield; Ho. Off. (Med.) Good Hope Hosp. NHS Trust Sutton Coldfield; Ho. Off. (Surg.) City Hosp. NHS Trust Birm.

WALKER, Tara 389 Upper Shoreham Road, Shoreham-by-Sea BN43 5NF; 271 Hadley Highstone, Hadley Green, Barnet EN5 4PU — MB BS Lond. 1993; MRCPath Lond. 2001. Locum Cons. Histopath., Qu. Alexander Hosp., Cosham, W. Sussex. Specialty: Histopath. Socs: RSM - Young Fell. Represen. within Path. Comm.; BMA. Prev: Specialist Regist. (Histopath.) Roy. Free Hosp. Hampstead.

WALKER, Thomas Hamilton (retired) 10 Golf Course Road, Knightsridge W., Livingston EH54 8QF Tel: 01506 38833 — LRCP LRCS Ed. 1949; LRCP LRCS Ed. LRFPS Glas. 1949. Prev: Ho. Surg. Bangour Gen. Hosp.

WALKER, Thomas Milnes 38 Redlands Road, Reading RG1 5HD — MB BS Lond. 1968 (Middlx.) DMRD Eng. 1975; FRCR 1976. Cons. Radiol. Roy. Berks. Hosp. Reading. Specialty: Radiol. Prev: Regist. (Radiol.) Bristol Roy. Infirm.; Lect. (Radiol.) Univ. W. Indies Kingston, Jamaica.

WALKER, Timothy Jonathan Dept. of Anaesthesia, Queen Elizabeth II Hospital, Howlands, Welwyn Garden City AL7 4HQ Tel: 01707 365445 Fax: 01707 365446 Email: tim.walker@qeii.enherts-tr.nhs.uk; 60 Uplands Road, Hornsey Vale, London N8 9NJ Fax: 020 8347 9574 — MB BS Lond. 1988 (Middlesex UCH) FRCA. Cons. Anaesth. Qu. Eliz. II Hosp. Welwyn Garden City herts. Specialty: Anaesth.

WALKER, Timothy Richard Wolfe The Park Medical Practice, Cannands Grave Road, Shepton Mallet BA4 5RT Tel: 01749 342350 Fax: 01749 346845 — MB ChB Dundee 1977. Hon. Med. Off. Rugby Football Union 1993 to present. Prev: Ho. Surg. Basingstoke Dist. Hosp.; Ho. Phys. Perth Roy. Infirm.; Med. Off. H.M. Prison Cornhill Shepton Mallet.

WALKER, Timothy Samuel John 179 Hillhall Road, Lisburn BT27 5JA — MB BCh BAO Belf. 1987.

WALKER, Valerie Chemical Pathology, Level D, South Block, Southampton General Hospital, Tremona Road, Southampton SO16 6YD Tel: 02380 796419 Fax: 02380 796 4339 Email: valerie.walker@suht.swest.nhs.uk — MB ChB Liverp. 1969; FRCPCH; BSc (Hons.) Liverp. 1966; MD 1976; FRCPath 1989, M 1977. Cons. Chem. Path. Soton. Gen. Hosp.; Hon. Clin. Sen. Lect. (Human Genetics) Fac. Med. Univ. Soton.; Head of Trace Element Unit, Soton.Gen.Hosp.; Cons. (Chem. Path.) BUPA Chalybeate Hosp., Soton. Specialty: Chem. Path. Socs: Soc. Study of inborn errors in Metab.; Mem. Brit. inherited Metab. Dis. Gp.; Mem. Assn. Clin. Biochem.s. Prev: Sen. Lect. (Clin. Biochem.) Fac. Med. Univ. Soton.; Hon. Cons. Chem. Path. Soton. Gen. Hosp.

WALKER, William Clark (retired) Saddlers Barn, 6 Chantry Court, Ripley, Harrogate HG3 3AD Tel: 01423 771026 — MB ChB Ed. 1950; FRCP Ed. 1971, M 1956; FRCP Lond. 1976, M 1963; MD Ed. 1966. Prev: Cons. Phys. Pinderfields Gen. Hosp. Wakefield.

WALKER, William Edward Broadmeadow Health Centre, Keynell Covert, Kings Norton, Birmingham B30 3QT Tel: 0121 458 1340 — MB BS Lond. 1981 (Char. Cross) Cert. Family Plann. JCC 1983; DRCOG 1983; DCH RCP Lond. 1984; MRCGP 1985. Prev: GP Hendon.

WALKER, Mr William Farquhar 438 Blackness Road, Dundee DD2 1TQ Tel: 01382 668179 — MB ChB St. And. 1948; MB ChB (Commend.) St. And. 1948; FRCS Ed. 1953; FRCS Eng. 1954; DSc St. And. 1975, ChM 1958; FRSE 1973; FIBiol. 1988. Emerit. Prof. Vasc. Surg. Univ. Dundee. Socs: (Ex-Pres.) Assn. Surgs.; (Ex-Pres.) Assn. Vasc. Surgs. GB & Irel. Prev: Cons. Surg. Ninewells Hosp. Dundee; Hon. Prof. Vasc. Surg. Univ. Dundee; Sen. Lect. (Surg.) Univ. St. And.

WALKER, William Henry Andrew Cherryvalley Health Centre, Kings Square, Belfast BT5 7AR — MB BCh BAO Belf. 1985; DRCOG 1988; MRCGP 1989; DCH Dub. 1989. Prev: SHO (Paediat., O & G & Med.) Ulster Hosp. Dundonald.

WALKER, William Izett (retired) 10 Ediscum Garth, Bishop Auckland DL14 6UH Tel: 01388 603143 — MD Glas. 1941 (Univ. Glas.) MB ChB 1930; MRad Liverp. 1948; DMRD Eng. 1948. Prev: Radiol. Gen. Hosp. Bishop Auckland & Memor. Hosp. Darlington.

WALKER, William Lumsden, SBStJ (retired) 6 Kellaway Crescent, Westbury-on-Trym, Bristol BS9 4TE Tel: 0117 942 4197 — (Aberd.) MB ChB Aberd. 1941; DPH 1947; DPM Roy. Med. Psych. Assn. 1953; MD Aberd. 1963; FRCPsych 1971. Prev: Cons. Child & Adolesc. Psychiat. Roy. Hosp. Sick Childr. Bristol, & Southmead Hosp.

WALKER, Mr William Martin (retired) Round Hill Lodge, Little Alne, Solihull B95 6HP Tel: 01564 793363 — MB ChB St. And. 1943 (Dundee) BSc St. And. 1943; DOMS Eng. 1947; FRCS Eng. 1950. Prev: Surg. Birm. & Midl. Eye Hosp.

WALKER, Mr William Stanley — MB BChir Camb. 1977; MA Camb. 1978; FRCS Ed. 1981; FRCS Eng. 1982; FETCS 2001. Cons. Cardiothoracic Surg. Lothian Health Bd. Edin. Specialty: Cardiothoracic Surg.

WALKER, Wilson David HM Prison, Southall St., Manchester M60 9AH Tel: 0161 834 8626 Fax: 0161 833 1864; 6 Goatscliffe Cottages, Main Road, Grindleford, Hope Valley S32 2HG Tel: 01433 631674 — MB ChB Birm. 1983; MRCPsych 1989; Dip. Addic. Behaviour Lond. 1992; Dip. Prison Med. (RCGP/RCP, London/RC Psych) Birm. 1998. Sen. Med. Off. Clin. Dir. HMP Manch. Specialty: Civil Serv. Prev: Med. Off. HM Y.O.I. Glen Parva Leic.; Regist. (Psychiat.) Co. Hosp. Lincoln; Regist. (Psychiat.) Nottm. Rotat. Train. Scheme.

WALKER, Woodruff John Royal Surrey County Hospital, Egerton Road, Guildford GU2 7XX Tel: 01483 464053 Fax: 01483 402712 — MB BS Lond. 1970; FRCR SA 1977; FRCR 1978. Cons. Radiol. Roy. Surrey Co. Hosp. Guildford.; Practitioner, Lond. Clinic, Guildford Nuffield, Mt. Alvernia, Ashtead Hosp. Specialty: Radiol. Special Interest: Fibroid Embolism. Socs: Roy. Soc. of Med.; Roy. Coll. of Radiologists; Soc. of Cardiovasc. Interventional Radiol. Prev: Regist. & Cons. Radiol. Groote-Schuur Hosp. Capte Town. S. Africa.

WALKER, Zoe Anne Manor Lodge, Middle St., Kilham, Driffield YO25 4RL — MB BS Newc. 1997.

WALKER, Zuzana Mental Health Unit, St Margaret's Hospital, The Plain, Epping CM16 6TN Tel: 01279 828793 Fax: 01992 571089 — MD Charles Univ. Prague 1983 (Charing Cross and Westminster) MRCS Eng. LRCP Lond. 1987; DGM RCP Lond. 1989; MRCPsych 1992; MD University of London 2002. Sen. Lect. (Old Age Psychiat.) Univ. Coll. Lond. Specialty: Geriat. Psychiat. Special Interest: Memory Clinic. Prev: Lect. (Old Age Psychiat.) Univ. Coll. Lond.; Research Fell. (Psychiat.) Univ. Coll. Lond.; Regist. Rotat. (Psychiat.) N. Lond. Train. Scheme.

WALKER-BAKER, Lee 139 Malefant Street, Cardiff CF24 4QF — MB BCh Wales 1995.

WALKER-BONE, Karen Elizabeth MRC Environmental Epidemiology Unit, Southern General Hospital, Tremona Road, Southampton SO16 6YD — BM 1991 (Soton.) MRCP 1995. Specialist Regist. Rheum; ARC Clin. Research. Fell. Specialty: Rheumatol. Socs: BMA; BSR.

WALKER-BRASH, Mr Robert Munro Thorburn (retired) Dene Cottage, 6 Ramley Road, Pennington, Lymington SO41 8GQ Tel: 01590 672215 — (St. Bart.) BM BCh Oxf. 1944; MA Oxf. 1945;

FRCS Eng. 1950. Surg. Orpington & Sevenoaks Hosps. Prev: Sen. Regist. & Ho. Surg. St. Bart. Hosp. Lond.

WALKER-DATE, Susan Elizabeth Adeline Road Surgery, 4 Adeline Road, Boscombe, Bournemouth BH5 1EF Tel: 01202 309421 Fax: 01202 304893 — MB BS Lond. 1989. Prev: Trainee GP Hatfield; SHO (O & G, Med. & Med. for Elderly) Qu. Eliz. II Hosp. Welwyn Gdn. City; Ho. Off. Frimley Pk. Hosp.

WALKER-KINNEAR, Malcolm Henry Royal Edinburgh Hospital, Morningside Park, Edinburgh EH10 5HF Tel: 0131 537 6000; 7 Lasswade Court, 32 School Green, Lasswade EH18 1NB — MB ChB Aberd. 1990; MRCPsych 1995. Specialist Regist. (Psychiat.) Lothian HB. Specialty: Gen. Psychiat. Socs: Roy. Coll. Psychiat.; Internat. Assn. Cognitive Psychother. Prev: Regist. (Psychiat.) Lothian HB; SHO (Psychiat.) Lothian & Grampian HBs.

WALKER-LOVE, May Pettigrew Leebank, 8 Garngaber Avenue, Lenzie, Glasgow G66 4LJ Tel: 0141 776 1623 — MB ChB Glas. 1975; DCH RCPS Glas. 1977; DRCOG 1977; MRCGP 1980; DA Eng. 1980. GP Lanarksh. Specialty: Gen. Pract. Socs: Lanarksh. LMC; BASICS; Brit. Menopause Soc. Prev: GP Kirkintilloch; Clin. Asst. (Geriat.) Stobhill Hosp. Glas.; Clin. Asst. (Anaesth.) Paisley.

WALKER-SMITH, Professor John Angus University Department Paediatric Gastroenterology, Royal Free Hospital, London NW3 2QG Tel: 020 7830 2779 Fax: 020 7830 2146; 16 Monkham's Drive, Woodford Green IG8 0LQ Tel: 020 8505 7756 Fax: 020 8505 7756 — MB BS Sydney 1960; FRCP Ed. 1978, M 1963; FRCP Lond. 1977, M 1964; FRACP 1972, M 1965; MD Sydney 1971; FRCPCH 1997. Emerit. Prof. Paediat. Gastroenterol Univ of Lond. Specialty: Gastroenterol. Socs: (Sec.) Europ. Soc. Pediat. Gastroenterol. (ESPGHAN); Brit. Soc. Gastroenterol.; Brit. Soc. Paediat. Gastroenterol. & Nutrit. Prev: Research Fell. Kinderklinik Zurich, Switz.; Staff Phys. (Gastroenterol.) Roy. Alexandra Hosp. Childr. Sydney, Austral.; Prof. Paediat. Gastroenterol. Med. Coll. St Bartholomew Hosp. Lond.

WALKINGTON, Robert Paul Emmanuel Northgate Medical Practice, 1 Northgate, Canterbury CT1 1WL Tel: 01227 463570 Fax: 01227 786147 — MB ChB Birm. 1990 (Birm) DRCOG 1993; MRCGP 1994. GP; Clin.Asst.GU.Med.

WALKINSHAW, Stephen Andrew Liverpool Womens Hospital, Crown St., Liverpool L8 7SS Tel: 0151 708 9988; 43 Menlove Avenue, Liverpool L18 2EH — MB ChB Glas. 1978; BSc (Hons. 1st Class, Genetics) Glas. 1975; MRCOG 1983; MD 1990; FRCOG 2003. Cons. Fetal Med. Liverp.; Hon. Lect. Univ. Liverp. Specialty: Obst. & Gyn. Prev: RCOG Train. Fell. (Fetal Med.) Newc.

WALKLEY, Jullien Hardie Caton Ladybarn Group Practice, 177 Mauldeth Road, Fallowfield, Manchester M14 6SG Tel: 0161 224 2873 Fax: 0161 225 3276; 34 Errwood Road, Manchester M19 2PH Tel: 0161 286 2574 — MB ChB Manch. 1984.

WALL, Anthony Robert James The Health Centre, Hermitage Road, St John's, Woking GU21 8TD Tel: 01483 723451 Fax: 01483 751879; Four Walls, Hook Hill Lane, Hook Heath, Woking GU22 0PT Tel: 01487 763150 Fax: 01483 724510 Email: afourwalls@aol.com — MB BS Lond. 1974 (St. Bart.) MRCS Eng. LRCP Lond. 1973; DCH Eng. 1977. GP; Team Med. Attendant Bisley Football Club & Woking Athletic Club; Dir. Clin. Trials Research Unit. Specialty: Gen. Pract.; Paediat. Socs: BSMA Guildford Med. Soc.; Brit. Assn. Sports Med. Prev: Regist. (Paediat.) North. Gen. Hosp. Sheff.; Regist. (Med. & Paediat.) Barnet Gen. Hosp.; SHO (Paediat.) Edgware Gen. Hosp. Lond.

WALL, Catherine Elizabeth York Road Group Practice, York Road, Ellesmere Port CH65 0DB — MB BS Lond. 1987; DRCOG 1991; DCH RCP Lond. 1992; MRCGP 1992; DA (UK) 1993. G.P. Princip.

WALL, Christina Mary Whitby Group Practice, 114 Chester Road, Whitby, Ellesmere Port CH65 6TG Tel: 0151 355 6151 Fax: 0151 355 6843; 9 Field Hey Lane, Willaston, Neston, South Wirral CH64 1TG Tel: 0151 327 4187 — MB BS Newc. 1981 (Newcastle upon Tyne) DRCOG 1983; DFFP 1998. Specialty: Gen. Pract.

WALL, David Anthony Rout and Partners, Kearsley Medical Centre, Jackson Street, Bolton BL4 8EP Tel: 01204 73164 — MB ChB Manch. 1981. Socs: Assoc. Mem. Roy. Coll. Gen. Pract.; Bolton & Dist. Med. Soc.

WALL, David William Ley Mill Surgery, 228 Lichfield Road, Sutton Coldfield B74 2UE Tel: 0121 308 0359 Fax: 0121 323 2682; 150 Lichfield Road, Four Oaks, Sutton Coldfield B74 2TF — MB ChB Birm. 1970; MRCP (U.K.) 1972; MRCGP 1976; FRCGP London 1986; FRCP London 1997; MMEd Dundee 1998. Dep. regional postGrad. dean (W.Midl.s Deanery) Birm. Prev: Regist. (Med.) Qu. Eliz. Hosp. Birm.; SHO (Med.) Univ. Rhodesia.

WALL, Ian Francis Gordon and Partners, The Redwell Medical Centre, 1 Turner Road, Wellingborough NN8 4UT Tel: 01933 400777 Fax: 01933 671959 Email: ian.wall@gp-k83011.nhs.uk — MB ChB Birm. 1977; MRCGP 1982; T(GP) 1991; D.Occ.Med. RCP Lond. 1994; DMJ(Clin) Soc. Apoth. Lond. 1994. Princip. Police Surg. N.ants. Police. Prev: Lect. (Anat.) Univ. Birm.; Ho. Phys. Selly Oak Hosp. Birm.; Ho. Surg. Gen. Hosp. Birm.

WALL, Ian John 39 Wilsden Way, Lyne Paddock, Kidlington OX5 1TN — MB BS Lond. 1985.

WALL, John Anthony (retired) 96 Merton Mansions, Bushey Road, London SW20 8DG Tel: 020 8540 9956 — MB BS Lond. 1959 (Guy's) MRCS Eng. LRCP Lond. 1959; DObst RCOG 1963. Prev: Chief Exec. Med. Defence Union.

WALL, Leslie Errol (retired) 23 Maida Avenue, London W2 1SR — MB ChB Birm. 1949; DObst RCOG 1962; MRCGP 1970. Prev: Outpat. Off. Roy. Throat, Nose & Ear Hosp.

WALL, Lucy Rosalind Western General Hospital, Edinburgh Cancer Centre, Crewe Road, Edinburgh EH4 2XU Tel: 0131 537 1029/0131 537 3916 — MB BS Lond. 1990; MRCP (UK) 1994; MSc Edinburgh 1998; MD London 2002. Cons. in Med. Oncol.; Cons. in Med. Oncol., Qu. Margt. Hosp., Dunfermline; Cons. in Med. Oncol., Borders Gen. Hosp., Melrose. Specialty: Oncol. Special Interest: Upper GI Cancers; Hepatobiliary Cancers; Neuroendocrine Tumours.

WALL, Lyndon Trevor Occupational Medical Consultancy, 52 Greenhill, Blackwell, Bromsgrove B60 1BL Tel: 0121 445 5251 Fax: 0121 445 6228 Email: lyndonpaula.omc@virgin.net — (Leeds) LMSSA Lond. 1969; DObst RCOG 1973; MRCGP 1975; MSc (Occupat. Med.) Lond. 1980; FFOM RCP Lond. 1994, MFOM 1987, AFOM 1981. Indep. Occupat. Phys. Specialty: Occupat. Health. Special Interest: Back Pain; Stress Managem. Socs: Soc. Occupat. Med.; British Institute of Musculoskeletal Medicine. Prev: Chief Med. Adviser Minerva Health Managem. Redditch; Sen. Med. Off. RAF Med. Br.; Sen. Employm. Med. Adviser.

WALL, Martyn Turner Caradoc Surgery, Station Approach, Frinton-on-Sea CO13 9JT Tel: 01255 850101 Fax: 01255 851004 — MB BS Lond. 1978.

WALL, Michael Keith South Staffordshire Strategic Health Authority, Mellor House, Corporation St., Stafford ST16 3SR Tel: 01785 252233 Fax: 01785 221131; The Beeches, 121 Walsall Road, Lichfield WS13 8AD Tel: 01543 258750 — MRCS Eng. LRCP Lond. 1975; MA Camb. 1974; MFCM 1986; FFPHM RCP (UK) 1996. Dir. Pub. Health & Strategy Policy S. Staffs. HA. Specialty: Pub. Health Med. Prev: Dir. Pub. Health & Plann. M. Staffs. HA; Cons. Pub. Health Med. SE Staffs. HA; Sen. Regist. (Community Med.) W. Midl. RHA.

WALL, Michele 11 Beaver Close, Lexden, Colchester CO3 9DZ — MB ChB Leic. 1993.

WALL, Owen Richard 32 Park Villa Court, Roundhay, Leeds LS8 1EB — MB ChB Leeds 1998.

WALL, Peter Robert The Nunhead Surgery, 58 Nunhead Grove, London SE15 3LY Tel: 020 7639 2715 Fax: 020 7635 6942 — MB ChB Otago 1981. GP Nunhead Surg. Lond.

WALL, Robert Anthony Sutton Community Mental Health Team, Patrick House, 5 Maney Corner, Birmingham Road, Birmingham B72 1QL Tel: 0121 685 6703 Email: wall.robert@bsmht.nhs.uk — MB ChB Birm. 1974 (Univ. of Birm.) MRCPsych 1979. Cons. Psychiat. Northern Birm. Ment. Health (NHS) Trust; Clin. Director, N. Locality, Birm. and Solihull Ment. health NHS Trust. Specialty: Gen. Psychiat. Prev: Chairm. Div. of Psychiat. N. Birm. HA; Chairm. Med. Advisery Comm. Northern Birm. Ment. Health Trust.

WALL, Tracey Jane Morriston Hospital, Morriston, Swansea SA6 6NL Tel: 01792 703280 — MB BCh Wales 1988 (University Hospital Wales) FRCA 1996. Cons. Anaesth. Moriston Hosp., Swansea. Specialty: Anaesth. Prev: Specialist Regist. (Anaesth.) Welsh Sch. of Anaesth.

WALL, William Henry Jeremy Radiology Department, Royal Lancaster Infirmary, Ashton Road, Lancaster LA1 4RP; 23a Lindeth Road, Silverdale, Carnforth LA5 0TT Tel: 01524 701083 — (Lond. Hosp.) MB BS Lond. 1965; DObst RCOG 1969; DMRD Eng. 1978;

FRCR 1980. Cons. Radiol. Roy. Lancaster & Westmorland Gen. Infirm. Hosp. Specialty: Radiol.

WALL, William Henry Jeremy Stoney End, 23A Lindeth Road, Silverdale, Carnforth LA5 0TT — MB BS Lond. 1965 (Lond. Hosp. Med. Coll.) DMRD 1978; FRCR 1980. Cons. Radiol., Roy. Lancaster Hosp.; Cons. Radiol., Westmorland Hosp., Kendal. Specialty: Radiol. Special Interest: Radionuclide Imaging. Socs: Roy. Coll. of Radiol.; Brit. Nuclear Med. Soc.

WALLACE, Alan Douglas Department of Radiology, Royal Alexandra Hospital NHS Trust, Corsebar Road, Paisley PA2 Tel: 0141 580 4335 — MB ChB Glas. 1987 (Univ. Glas.) MRCP (UK) 1991; FRCR 1996. Cons. (Radiol.) Roy. Alexandra Hosp. NHS Trust Paisley; Clin. Director, Diagnostics Directorate, RAH NHS Trust, Corsebar Rd, Paisley; Cons. Radiologist, Ross Hall Hosp., Crookston Rd, Glas. Specialty: Radiol. Socs: Roy. M-C Soc. Glas.; Scott. Radiol. Soc. Prev: Sen. Regist. (Diagnostic Radiol.) Glas. Roy. Infirm.; Regist. (Diagnostic Radiol.) Glas. Roy. Infirm.; Regist. (Med.) Univ. West. Infirm. Glas.

WALLACE, Alan Stewart (retired) Harmony House, 2 Harnham Road, Salisbury SP2 8JG Tel: 01722 334347 — MRCS Eng. LRCP Lond. 1944 (Univ. Coll. Hosp.) DObst RCOG 1948; DMJ (Clin.) Soc. Apoth. Lond. 1969. Prev: Div. Police Surg. Wilts Constab.

WALLACE, Alan Stewart Grangewood Surgery, Chester Road, Shiney Row, Houghton-le-Spring DH4 4RB Tel: 0191 385 2898; 31 Breamish Drive, Rickleton, Washington NE38 9HS Tel: 0191 415 3419 — MB ChB Manch. 1982 (Manchester) BSc (Med. Sci.) St. And. 1979; MB ChB (Hons.) Manch. 1982; MRCGP 1986. GP Princip. Specialty: Gen. Pract. Prev: Trainee GP Edin.; SHO (Paediat. & Med.) Roy. Albert Edwd. Infirm. Wigan; SHO (O & G) Billinge Hosp. Wigan.

WALLACE, Alison Rowena Builth & Llanwrtyd Wells Group Medical Practice, Glandwr Park, Builth Wells LD2 3DZ Tel: 01982 552207 Fax: 01982 553826; The Bage, Vowchurch, Hereford HR2 0RL Tel: 01981 550666 — MB BS Lond. 1987 (Univ. Coll. Lond./Middlx. Lond.) DRCOG 1991; MRCGP 1993.

WALLACE, Mr Andrew Lachlan St Mary's Hospital, Praed Street, London W2 1NY Tel: 020 7886 1627 Fax: 020 7886 1766; Hospital of St John & St Elizabeth, The Shoulder Unit, 60 Grove End Road, London NW8 9NH Tel: 020 7806 4044 Fax: 020 7289 4031 Email: shoulder.unit@hje.org.uk — MB BS (Hons.) New South Wales 1987; PhD Ed. 1992; FRACS (Orth.) 1997. Sen. Lect. & Hon. Cons. (Musculoskeletal Surg.) Imp. Coll. Lond. Specialty: Trauma & Orthop. Surg. Special Interest: Arthroscopic Surg.; Shoulder & Elbow Surg. Socs: Fell. Austral. Orthop. Assn.; Fell. Brit. Orthop. Assn.; Brit. Elbow & Shoulder Soc. Prev: Research Fell. McCaig Centre(Jt. Injury & Arthritis Research) Univ. Calgary Alberta, Canad.; Regist. Sydney Southside Orthop. Train. Scheme; Regist. Roy. Infirm. Edin.

WALLACE, Ann Christine Margaret 19 Moreton Road, Bosham, Chichester PO18 8LL — MB BS Lond. 1979; FRCPCH; BSc (Hons.) Lond. 1976, MSc (Distinc.) 1989, MB BS 1979; DCH RCP Lond. 1986. Cons. Paediat. Community Child Health Chichester. Specialty: Paediat.

WALLACE, Ann Kathleen Poole Farm, Poole Lane, Woolacombe EX34 7AP Tel: 01271 870817 — MB BS Lond. 1974 (Roy. Free) MRCS Eng. LRCP Lond. 1974; DCH Eng. 1976; DRCOG 1977. p/t Staff Grade Community Paediat., N. Devon Primary Care Trust. Specialty: Community Child Health. Prev: Community Med. Off. (Paediat.) N. Devon Healthcare Trust.

WALLACE, Anne Maree Lothian Health, 148 Pleasance, Edinburgh EH8 9RS Tel: 0131 536 9148 Fax: 0131 536 9164; 33 Malleny Millgate, Balerno, Edinburgh EH14 7AY — MB ChB Aberd. 1978; MSc Ed. 1983; MFCM 1985. Cons. (Pub. Health Med.) Lothian Health Bd. Specialty: Pub. Health Med. Socs: Fell. Fac. Pub. Health Med.

WALLACE, Mr Antony Francis, TD (retired) Mill Green Cottage, Mill Green, Ingatestone CM4 0HX Tel: 01277 353133 — (Univ. Coll. Hosp.) MB BS (Hons. Surg., Hyg. & Forens. Med.) Lond. 1950; FRCS Eng. 1955; DHMSA 1982. Hon. Cons. (Plastic Surg.) RAF; Emerit. Cons. (Plastic Surg.) to The Army & RN. Prev: Cons. Plastic Surg. St. Bart. Hosp. Lond., Regional Plastic Surg. Centre Billericay K. Edwd. VII Hosp. for Offs. Lond.

WALLACE, Archibald Duncan Lilybank House, Campbeltown PA28 Tel: 01586 52658 & profess. 52105 — MB ChB Glas. 1948. GP Campeltown. Prev: Unit Med. Off. Kintyre Unit Argyll & Clyde Health Bd.; Ho. Surg. & Asst. Cas. Surg. Glas. West. Infirm.

WALLACE, Betty Eileen (retired) Capons Farm, Cowfold, Horsham RH13 8DE Tel: 01403 864386 — MB BCh BAO Dub. 1952 (TC Dub.) MA, MD Dub. 1960; FRCPath 1969. Prev: Consult. (Microbiol.) Sussex Co. Hosp. Brighton.

WALLACE, Brian Anthony The Evelyn Hospital, Trumpington Road, Cambridge CB2 2AF Tel: 01223 303336 Fax: 01223 316068; Keffords, Barley, Royston SG8 8LB Tel: 01763 848287 — MB BS Lond. 1961 (Lond. Hosp.) MRCS Eng. LRCP Lond. 1960; DObst RCOG 1961. Aviat. Med. Examr. Civil Aviat. Auth. (UK) & Federat. Aviat. Auth. (USA). Specialty: Aviat. Med. Prev: Sen. Med. Off. Govt. Uganda; GP Royston, Herts.

WALLACE, Brian Bernard (retired) 12 Holly Grove, Lisvane, Cardiff CF14 0UJ Tel: 029 2075 3447 — MB BS Lond. 1961 (Middlx.) DObst RCOG 1963; FRCGP 1978, M 1969. Prev: Sen. Lect. (Gen. Pract.) Univ. Wales Coll. Med.

WALLACE, Catherine Jane 14 Mortonhall Park Loan, Edinburgh EH17 8SN — MB ChB Aberd. 1998.

WALLACE, Colin Andrew Fishponds Health Centre, Beechwood Road, Fishponds, Bristol BS16 3TD Tel: 0117 965 6281 — MB ChB Glas. 1975.

WALLACE, Mr Colin Ernest Cromwell Hospital, Cromwell Road, London SW5 0TU Tel: 020 7460 5700 Fax: 020 7460 5555 — MB BS Sydney 1963 (Sydney Australia) FRCS Ed. ENT 1970; T(S) 1991. Cons. ENT Surg. Cromwell Hosp. Lond. Specialty: Otorhinolaryngol. Socs: BMA; RSM; MDU.

WALLACE, Daphne Rowena Duckworth (retired) The Vicarage, Skipton Road, Earby, Barnoldswick BB18 6JL — MB ChB St. And. 1965; DPM Newc. 1972; FRCPsych 1994. M 1976; Dip. Psychother. Liverp. 1990. Prev: Cons. Psychiat. of Old Age Leeds Community & Ment. Health Trust.

WALLACE, Mr David Hamilton 35 Dunscore Brae, Hamilton ML3 9DH — MB ChB Ed. 1987; FRCS Glas. 1992. Specialty: Gen. Surg.

WALLACE, David Ian Ross St Brannocks Road Medical Centre, St. Brannocks Road, Ilfracombe EX34 8EG Tel: 01271 863840; Poole Farm, Poole Lane, Woolacombe EX34 7AP Tel: 01271 870817 — MB BS Lond. 1975 (Roy. Free) DRCOG 1979; MRCGP 1990.

WALLACE, David John Muirhead Medical Centre, Muirhead, Dundee DD2 5NH Tel: 01382 580264 Fax: 01382 581199; 34 Forest Park Place, Right Ground Floor Flat, Dundee DD1 5NT Tel: 01382 227687 — MB ChB Dundee 1976; DRCOG 1980; MRCGP 1982. Prison Med. Off.

WALLACE, Mr David Michael Alexander 7 Hermitage Road, Edgbaston, Birmingham B15 3UP — MB BS Lond. 1970; FRCS Eng. 1976. Cons. Urol. Qu. Eliz. Hosp. Birm. Specialty: Urol.

WALLACE, Donald (retired) The Surgery, 237 St Mary's Lane, Upminster RM14 3BX Tel: 01402 226626 — MB BS Lond. 1951 (Lond. Hosp.) MRCS Eng. LRCP Lond. 1951. Prev: GP Upminster.

WALLACE, Donald Angus 33 Burghley Street, Bourne PE10 9NS — BM BCh Oxf. 1986.

WALLACE, Donald Greer The Surgery, Erskine View, Old Kilpatrick, Glasgow G60 5JG Tel: 01389 874281 Fax: 01389 890919; 25 Morven Road, Gartconnell, Bearsden, Glasgow G61 3BY Tel: 0141 942 3546 — MB ChB Glas. 1971; DObst RCOG 1973; MRCGP 1976. Gen. Practitioner in Old Kilpatrick & Clydebank; Med. Off. c/o the Elderly Blawarthill Hosp. Glas. Prev: SHO (O & G) Vale of Leven Hosp. Alexandria; Ho. Off. (Gen. Surg. & Med.) Roy. Alexandra Infirm. Paisley.

WALLACE, Eda Jacqueline Queens House, Flat 2,7, Queens Hospital, Queens Road, Croydon CR9 2PQ — MB BS West Indies 1989.

WALLACE, Edwin Lindsay Markinch Medical Centre, 19 High Street, Markinch, Glenrothes KY7 6ER Tel: 01592 610640 Fax: 01592 612089 — MB ChB Aberd. 1978. GP Glenrothes, Fife.

WALLACE, Elisabeth Caroline Hall Farm, Coney Weston, Bury St Edmunds IP31 1HG — MB BS Lond. 1976 (St. Mary's) DRCOG 1978; DCH Eng. 1980.

WALLACE, Elizabeth Ann Hay Gowanpark, Sandyhill Road, Banff AB45 1BE Tel: 01261 22443 — MB ChB Aberd. 1965; DPH Glas. 1970; CIH Dund 1983. Socs: Soc. Occupat. Med.; BMA. Prev: Asst. Co. MOH Banffsh.; SHO (Geriat.) Ashludie Hosp. Dundee; Ho. Off. Craig Dunain Hosp. Inverness.

WALLACE, Elsie Lilian Mary 31 Grayscroft Road, London SW16 5UP Tel: 020 8764 2060 — LRCP Irel. 1954 (RCSI) LRCPI & LM, LRCSI & LM 1954; DPH Eng. 1967; MFCM 1972; MFOM RCP Lond. 1978; Specialist Accredit. (Occupat. Med.) RCP Lond. 1978; MFOM RCPI 1980; MFPHM 1989; F.FOM (RCPI) 1999. Specialty: Occupat. Health. Socs: Soc. Occupat. Med. Prev: Sen. Employm. Med. Adviser EMAS; PMO Lond. Boro. Ealing; Sen. Med. Off. & Med. Off. Lond. Boro. S.wark.;'Effects of n-Butyl Glycidyl Ether Exposure'.

WALLACE, Euan David Vine Cottage, East Harting, Petersfield GU31 5NQ Tel: 01730 825265 — MB Camb. 1965 (Camb. & St. Thos.) MA Camb. 1966, BChir 1964; MRCP U.K. 1969; DObst RCOG 1972. Assoc. Specialist, Macmillan Unit, King Edwd. VII Hosp. Maidhurst, W.Sussex GU29 OBL; Hosp. Pract., Med. Outpats., Petersfield Hosp. Petersfield, Hants.; Clin. Assist., Dermat., St. Mary's Hosp. Portsmouth. Specialty: Palliat. Med.; Gen. Med.; Dermat. Socs: Liveryman Worshipful Soc. Apoth. Lond.; BMA. Prev: GP Tutor & Regist. (Med.) Qu. Alexander Hosp. Cosham; Cas. Off. & Ho. Surg. Eye Dept. St. Thos. Hosp. Lond.

WALLACE, Ewan Donaldson Great Western Road Medical Group, 327 Great Western Road, Aberdeen AB10 6LT Tel: 01224 571318 Fax: 01224 573865; 14 Carnegie Crescent, Aberdeen AB15 4AE — MB ChB Aberd. 1983; DRCOG 1987; MRCGP 1987. GP Aberd.

WALLACE, Ewan Duncan 1A Aucharn, Sunnypark, Kinross KY13 8BX — MB ChB Glas. 1997.

WALLACE, Fiona 45 Stanley Street, Southsea PO5 2DS — MB BS Lond. 1992. Specialty: Accid. & Emerg.

WALLACE, Gillian Margaret Fleming 24 Corrennie Gardens, Edinburgh EH10 6DB — MB ChB Ed. 1993.

WALLACE, Hilda Rockcliffe (retired) East Leake Hall, East Leake, Loughborough LE12 6LQ — MB ChB Ed. 1922 (Univ. Ed.) Prev: Lect. in Health Educat. Leic.

WALLACE, Iain Wilson Greater Glasgow Primary Care Trust, Trust Headquarters, Gartnavel Royal Hospital, 1055 Great Western Road, Glasgow G12 0XH Tel: 0141 211 3658 Fax: 0141 211 3971 — MB ChB Glas. 1984; BSc (Hons.) Glas. 1981; DRCOG 1987; MBA 2001; FRCGP 2002. Med. Director Gtr. Glas. Primary Care Trust. Prev: Ho. Phys. & Ho. Surg. W. Infirm Glas.

WALLACE, Ian Muiredge Surgery, Buckhaven, Leven KY8 1HJ Tel: 01592 3299 — MB ChB St. And. 1959. Prev: Ho. Phys. & Sen. Ho. Off. Cas. Dept. Dundee Roy. Infirm.; Ho. Off. (O & G) Maryfield Hosp. Dundee.

WALLACE, Ian Robert (retired) 3 Saxon Close, Exning, Newmarket CB8 7NS Tel: 01638 577331 — MB BCh BAO Belf. 1954; DCH Eng. 1957; FRCGP 1986, M 1968.

WALLACE, Mr Ian William John, OStJ BUPA Murrayfield Hospital, Corstorphine Road, Edinburgh EH12 6UD Tel: 01506 419666 Fax: 01506 460386; Rivaldsgreen House, Friarsbrae, Linlithgow EH49 6BG Tel: 01506 845700 Fax: 01506 845100 — MB ChB Ed. 1964; BSc Ed. 1962; FRCS Ed. 1968. Cons. Surg. & Urol. St. John's Hosp. Howden; Dir. (Clin. Servs.) W. Lothian NHS Trust. Specialty: Urol. Socs: Assoc. Mem. BAUS. Prev: Cons. Surg. Bangour Gen. Hosp. Broxburn; Lect. (Clin. Surg.) Univ. Edin.; Regist. Rotat. (Surg.) Lothian HB.

WALLACE, Ingrid Maria Bassett Road Surgery, 29 Bassett Road, Leighton Buzzard LU7 1AR Tel: 01525 373111 Fax: 01525 853767; 4 Fortescue Drive, Shenley Church Road, Milton Keynes MK5 6BJ Tel: 01908 504339 Fax: 01908 504339 — MB BS Lond. 1989; DRCOG 1991; DCH RCP Lond. 1992; MRCGP 1993. Course Organiser, Aylesbury. Specialty: Gen. Pract.

WALLACE, James Gordon (retired) 2 Eastwood House, 2 Greetwell Road, Lincoln LN2 4AQ Tel: 01522 530654 — BM BCh Oxf. 1950 (Oxf. & St. Bart.) MA Oxf. 1950; DCP Lond 1956; Dip. Bact. Lond 1960; FRCPath 1977, M 1966. Prev: Cons. Bacteriol. & Dir. Pub. Health Laborat. Lincoln.

WALLACE, Mr James Randall (retired) Law Hospital NHS Trust, Carluke ML8 5ER Tel: 01698 361100; 5 Brierybank Avenue, Lanark ML11 9AN Tel: 01555 663490 — MB ChB Glas. 1966; FRCS Glas. 1970; FRCS Eng. 1971. Cons. Surg. Law Hosp. NHS Trust Carluke.; Locum Gen. Paediatric Surg.

WALLACE, James Richard Chapman (retired) Penwood, The Avenue, Ross-on-Wye HR9 5AW — LMSSA Lond. 1950 (St. Bart.)

WALLACE, James Thomas 40 Hadham Road, Bishop's Stortford CM23 2QT Tel: 01279 654053 — MB BS Lond. 1949 (Lond. Hosp.) MRCS Eng. LRCP Lond. 1949; Cert. Av Med. MoD (Air) & CAA 1973. Apptd. Examr. Min. of Civil Aviat. & Federal Aviat. Admin. USA. Specialty: Aviat. Med. Prev: Med. Off. Stansted Airport; Apptd. Med. Inspec. Commonw. Immigrants & Aliens; Ho. Surg. & Res. Anaesth. Roy. Berks. Hosp. Reading.

WALLACE, Jan Barbara Beatson Oncology Centre, Western Infirmary, Dumbarton Road, Glasgow Tel: 0141 211 2000; 90 Kessington Road, Bearsden, Glasgow G61 2QB Tel: 0141 563193 — MB ChB Leic. 1991 (Leicester) MRCP (UK) 1994; MSc (Oncol.) Glas. 1996; FRCR 1998. Specialist Regist. (Clin. Oncol.) BeatsonOncol.Centre Glas. Specialty: Oncol.

WALLACE, Jennifer Anne 8 Riverside, Craigends, Houston, Johnstone PA6 7DL — MB BS Lond. 1967; MRCS Eng. LRCP Lond. 1967; DA Eng. 1970; FFA RCS Eng. 1973. Specialty: Anaesth.

WALLACE, Mrs Jessie Stewart (retired) 94 Finnart Street, Greenock PA16 8HL Tel: 01475 803933 — MB ChB Glas. 1961. Clin. Med. Off. Gtr. Glas. HB. Prev: clin med off GGNB.

WALLACE, Mr John 209 Findhorn, Forres IV36 3YS — MB ChB Ed. 1963; FRCS Ed. 1970; FCOphth 1989. Hon. Sen. Lect. Univ. Aberd.; Cons. Ophth. Grampian Health Bd. Specialty: Ophth. Prev: Sen. Regist. Dept. Ophth. West. Infirm. Glas.; Research Fell. MRC Epidemiol. Research Unit Cardiff; Ho. Off. Metab. Unit West. Gen. Infirm. Edin.

WALLACE, John Alastair Kennedy 120 South Street, Armadale, Bathgate EH48 3JU — MB ChB Ed. 1942; DPH 1958; DIH Soc. Apoth. Lond. 1968. Prev: Maj. RAMC.

WALLACE, John Alexander Beech Lodge, 9 Enagh Road, Ballymoney BT53 7PN Tel: 012656 65591 — MB BCh BAO Belf. 1969; FRCOG 1988, M 1974. Cons. (O & G) Robinson Memor. & Route Hosps. Ballymoney & Coleraine Hosp. Specialty: Obst. & Gyn. Prev: Jun. Cons. (O & G) King Edwd. VIII Hosp. Durban, S. Africa.

WALLACE, Julia Dawn Woodside Medical Group A, 80 Western Road, Woodside, Aberdeen AB24 4SU Tel: 01224 492631 Fax: 01224 276173; 14 Carnegie Crescent, Aberdeen AB15 4AE Tel: 01224 324696 — MB ChB Aberd. 1983; DRCOG 1987; MRCGP 1988. Specialty: Accid. & Emerg. Prev: Regist. (A & E) Grampian HB.

WALLACE, Katherine Ann Gunn 8 Riverside, Houston, Johnstone PA6 7DL — MB ChB Ed. 1996.

WALLACE, Kenneth Robert 41 Church Pavement, Swine Gate, Grantham NG31 6RL Tel: 01476 560360 Email: kennethwallace@compuserve.com — (Camb. & Guy's) BA Camb. 1948; MB BChir Camb. 1948; Dip. Bact. Lond 1953; MFHom 1970. Prev: Ho. Surg. S. Hosp. Dartford; RAF Med. Br.; Sen. Bacteriol. Pub. Health Laborat. Serv.

WALLACE, Kim Deidre 6 Victoria Gardens, Marlow Road, High Wycombe HP11 1SY Tel: 01494 558022 Fax: 01494 511113 — MB BS Lond. 1983 (St Marys) DCH RCP Lond. 1985; DRCOG 1986; MRCGP 1987. Clin. Asst. Gen. Surg. Specialty: Gen. Surg. Prev: GP High Wycombe; Trainee GP Banbury VTS.

WALLACE, Margaret (retired) 9 Rochford Way, Bishopstone, Seaford BN25 2TA — MB ChB Glas. 1954; DCH RFPS Glas. 1958. Prev: Paediat. Regist. E. Riding Hosp. Gp. & Newc. Hosp. Gp.

WALLACE, Margaret Anne Florence (retired) 81 Sweep Road, Cookstown BT80 8JT — MB BCh BAO Belf. 1965.

WALLACE, Marina Helen Watford General Hospital, Vicarage Road, Watford WD1 8HB — MB BS Lond. 1990; FRCS Eng. 1994. Specialty: Gen. Surg.

WALLACE, Mark Jonathan Gosford Hill Medical Centre, 167 Oxford Road, Kidlington OX5 2NS Tel: 01865 374242 Fax: 01865 377826 — MB BS Lond. 1991; BSc (Hons.) Lond. 1988; DRCOG 1993; DCH RCP Lond. 1994; MRCGP 1995. GP Princip. Gosford Hill Med. Centre Oxf. Specialty: Gen. Pract. Prev: GP Regist. Lond. Acad. Trainee Scheme.

WALLACE, Mary Clark 18 The Walnuts, Branksome Road, Norwich NR4 6SR Tel: 01603 56005 — MB ChB Glas. 1947 (Univ. Glas.) Prev: Ho. Surg. Sorrento Matern. Hosp. Birm.; Ho. Phys. Alder Hey Childr. Hosp. Liverp. & Leicester Gen. Hosp.

WALLACE, Maureen Elizabeth Hamilton Willenhall Oak Medical Centre, 70 Remembrance Road, Coventry CV3 3DP Tel: 024 7663 9909 Fax: 024 7630 5312 — MB BCh BAO Belf. 1976; MRCGP 1980; ECFMG Cert. 1 9769.

WALLACE, Mr Murray Evelyn Queen's Hospital, Burton Hospital NHS Trust, Burton-on-Trent DE13 0RB Tel: 01283 566333 — MB

BCh Witwatersrand 1982; FCS(SA) Orth 1991; T(S) 1992. Cons. Orthop. Surg. Burton Hosp. NHS Trust; Hon. Clin. Sen. Lect. (Orthop.) Keele Univ. Stoke-on-Trent. Specialty: Orthop. Socs: Fell. BOA; BMA. Prev: Sen. Regist. Musgrave Pk. Hosp. Belf.

WALLACE, Nicola Suzanne 174 Bridge Street, Portadown, Craigavon BT63 5AS — MB BCh BAO Belf. 1994 (QUB) BSc 1992; FRCA 1999. Specialty: Anaesth.

WALLACE, Norman Walker Chinpark Medical Centre, 6 Saughton Road, Edinburgh EH11 3RA Tel: 0131 455 7999 Fax: 0131 455 8800 — MB ChB Ed. 1976; BSc (Med. Sci.) Ed. 1973; MRCGP 1981. Premises Adviser Lothian - Primar Care Unit. Specialty: Gen. Pract. Prev: Trainee (Paediat.) & SHO (Geriat.) Lothian HB; Obst. EMMS Hosp. Nazareth, Israel.

WALLACE, Olga Nanette Meadowbank, Warren Close, Payhembury, Honiton EX14 3NA — MB BS Lond. 1976; MRCS Eng. LRCP Lond. 1976. Specialty: Ophth.

WALLACE, Paul Anthony Castle Practice, 2 Hawthorne Road, Castle Bromwich, Birmingham B36 0HH Tel: 0121 747 2422 Fax: 0121 749 1196; 8 Wilkinson Croft, Birmingham B8 2RE — MB BCh BAO NUI 1984. Specialty: Obst. & Gyn.

WALLACE, Paul George 18 Dundonald Road, London NW10 3HR Tel: 020 8960 5278 — MB BS Lond. 1976; MSc Lond. 1985, BSc (Hons.) 1973, MB BS 1976; MRCGP 1982. Sen. Lect. Dept. Gen. Pract. St. Mary's Hosp. Med. Sch. Lond. W2. Prev: MRC Epidemiol. Train. Research Fell. Univ. Lond.; Sir Jules Thorn Fell. Gen. Pract.

WALLACE, Peter Gunn MacRae 8 Riverside, Craigends, Houston, Johnstone PA6 7DL — MB ChB Glas. 1968; DObst RCOG 1970; FFA RCS Eng. 1973. Cons. Anaesth. West. Infirm. Glas. Specialty: Anaesth.

WALLACE, Richard Barnes Towcester Medical Centre, Link Way, Towcester NN12 6HH Tel: 01327 359339 Fax: 01327 358944 — MB ChB Bristol 1972; MRCGP 1977.

WALLACE, Richard Brian — MB BCh BAO Dub. 1980 (Trinity Coll. Dub.) BA Dub. 1980; DRCOG 1983; MICGP 1987; MFOM RCPI 1997, LFOM 1995. Occupat. Health Phys. (Occupat. Health) N. Irel. Civil Serv. Belf.; Specialist Occupational Phys., BMI Health Servs. Specialty: Occupat. Health. Socs: Soc. Occupat. Med. Prev: GP BrookeBoro.; Univ. Phys. Univ. Ulster Coleraine; Indust. Med. Off. Harland & Wolff plc Belf.

WALLACE, Mr Richard Gilmore Hanna 8 My Ladys Mile, Holywood BT18 9EW Tel: 01232 425298 Fax: 01232 425298; 8 My Ladys Mile, Holywood BT18 9EW Tel: 01231 425298 Fax: 01231 425298 — MD Belf. 1987; MB BCh BAO 1975; FRCS Ed. 1982; MCh (Orth.) Liverp. 1984. Cons. Orthor. Surg. Musgrave Pk. Hosp. Belf. & Ulster Hosp. Dundonald. Specialty: Orthop. Prev: Sen. Regist. (Orthop. Surg.) Musgrave Pk. Belf.

WALLACE, Richard James Callon (retired) Rutherglen Health Centre, 130 Stonelaw Road, Rutherglen, Glasgow G73 2PQ Tel: 0141 531 6030 Fax: 0141 531 6031; 6 Central Avenue, Cambuslang, Glasgow G72 8AX Tel: 0141 641 4488 Email: rjcwallace@aol.com — MB ChB Ed. 1963; DObst RCOG 1965. Princip. GP Glas. Prev: Maj. RAMC.

WALLACE, Ronald Macdonald Oldmeldrum Medical Centre, The Meadows, Oldmeldrum, Inverurie AB51 0BF Tel: 01651 872239 Fax: 01651 872968 Email: ron.wallace@oldmeldrum.grampian.scot.nhs.uk; 27 Westbank Park, Oldmeldrum, Inverurie AB51 0DG Tel: 01651 872861 Email: ron@cofd.co.uk — MB ChB Aberd. 1978; FRCGP 1997, M 1982. Teach. Fell. (Gen. Pract.) Univ. Aberd.

WALLACE, Rosemary Margaret 39 Pemberley Avenue, Bedford MK40 2LE — MB ChB Glas. 1974; MRCOG 1980, DObst. 1976.

WALLACE, Sally Spencer Place Medical Practice, Chapeltown Health Centre, Chapeltown, Leeds LS7 4BB Tel: 0113 240 9090 — MB ChB Sheff. 1992; MRCGP 1996. p/t GP Retainer.

WALLACE, Simon Andrew 11 Golden Square, London W1F 9JB Tel: 020 766 6377 Fax: 020 7664 6372; 46 Eaton Place, Brighton BN2 1EG Tel: 01273 695671 — MB BS Lond. 1984 (Char. Cross Hosp.) DRCOG 1988; MFPHM RCP (UK) 1992. Med. Cons. World Care UK. Specialty: Pub. Health Med. Socs: BMA; Roy. Soc. Med. Prev: Locum Cons. (Pub. Health Med.) Fife HB; Trainee GP/SHO (Paediat., O & G, A & E & Orthop.) Brighton HA; Trainee Progr. (Pub. Health Med. S.Thames Region (E.).

WALLACE, Siobhan Lodge Health, 20 Lodge Manor, Coleraine BT52 1JX Tel: 028 7034 4494 Fax: 028 7032 1759; 86 Coolyvenny Road, Coleraine BT51 3SF — MB ChB Dundee 1992; DRCOG 1994; DFFP 1995; MRCGP 1996. GP. Specialty: Gen. Pract. Socs: (Comm.) North. Irel. Family Plann. Assn.; RCGP; NI Female GP Assn. Prev: GP/Regist. Coleraine.

WALLACE, Susan 32 Duchywood, Heights Lane, Bradford BD9 6DZ — MB ChB Ed. 1994.

***WALLACE, Suzanne Vera Frances** — BM BCh Oxf. 1997. PRHO (Gen. Med.) John Radcliffe Hosp. Oxf. Specialty: Obst. & Gyn. Prev: PRHO (Gen. Surg.) Roy. United Hosp. Bath; SHO Obys & Gyn Nottm. City Hosp.

WALLACE, Tara Mary Radcliffe Infirmary, Woodstock Road, Oxford OX2 6HE Tel: 01865 311188; 55 Islip Road, Oxford OX2 7SP — MB BS Lond. 1991 (Char. Cross & Westm.) MRCP (UK) 1995. Specialist Regist. (Diabetes & Endocrinol.) Radcliffe Infirm. Oxf. Specialty: Diabetes; Endocrinol.; Gen. Med. Socs: Brit. Diabetic Assn.; Brit. Endocrine Soc. Prev: Regist. (Diabetes, Endocrinol. & Med.) Roy. Berks. Hosp. Reading; SHO (Gen. Med.) Southmead Hosp. Bristol.

WALLACE, Victoria Ann 4 Bowes Lyon Place, Lytham St Annes FY8 3UE — MB BS Lond. 1997.

WALLACE, Wendy June Queenhill Medical Practice, 31 Queenhill Road, South Croydon CR2 8DU Tel: 020 8651 1141 Fax: 020 8651 5011; 15 Searchwood Road, Warlingham CR6 9BB Tel: 0188 362 5749 — MB BS Lond. 1973 (Roy. Free) MRCS Eng. LRCP Lond. 1973; DA S. Afr. 1976. Prev: Regist. (Anaesth.) Johannesburg Gen. Hosp. Univ. Witwatersrand.

WALLACE, William Andrew Hamilton Department of Pathology, Northern General Hospital, Herries Road, Sheffield S5 7AU — MB ChB (Hons.) Ed. 1986; BSc (Hons.) Ed. 1984; MRCP (UK) 1989; PhD Ed. 1995; MRCPath 1997, D 1996. Cons. (Histopath.) Northern Gen. Hosp. NHS Trust Sheff. Specialty: Histopath. Prev: Sen. Regist. (Path.) Roy. Infirm. Edin. NHS Trust; Postgrad. Research Fell. Edin. Univ. Fac. Med.; Regist. (Path.) Edin. Univ. Med. Sch.

WALLACE, Professor William Angus Division of Orthopaedic & Accident Surgery, University Hospital, Queens Medical Centre, Nottingham NG7 2UH Tel: 0115 970 9407 Fax: 0115 849 3282 Email: angus.wallace@nottingham.ac.uk; High Trees, Foxwood Lane, Woodborough, Nottingham NG14 6ED Tel: 0115 965 2372 Fax: 0115 965 4638 Email: angus.wallace@rcsed.ac.uk — MB ChB St. And. 1972 (St Andrews) FRCS Ed. 1977; FRCS (Orthop.) Ed. 1985; FRCS Eng. 1997. Prof. Orthop. & Accid. Surg. Univ. Nottm.; Hon. Cons. Orthop. Surg. Qu. Med. Centre; Nottm. & City Hosp. Nottm.; Hon. Cons. Surg. Portland Traing. Coll. Specialty: Trauma & Orthop. Surg.; Sports Med. Socs: Brit. Elbow & Sholder Soc. President (2001-3); Chairman Intercollegiate Speciality Board in Trauma & Orthopaedic Surgery (2002-5); Dean, Faculty of Medical Informatics RCS Ed (2000-3). Prev: Sen. Lect. (Orthop. Surg.) Univ. Manch. & Cons. Orthop. Surg. Hope; Hosp. Salford; Lect. (Orthop. Surg.) Univ. Nottm.; MRC Research Fell. (Orthop.).

WALLACE, William David 174 Bridge Street, Portadown, Craigavon BT63 5AS — MB BCh Belf. 1998.

WALLACE, William Forbes Pentland Medical Centre, 44 Pentland View, Currie EH14 5QB Tel: 0131 449 2142 Fax: 0131 451 5855; 11 Cherry Tree Park, Balerno EH14 5AQ Tel: 0131 449 2951 — MB ChB Glas. 1970 (Glasgow) DObst RCOG 1972; MRCGP 1974. GP Princip.; GP Trainer. Socs: Ed. Clin. Club; BMA; RCGP.

WALLACE, Professor William Frederick Matthew Dept of Physiology, Medical Biology Centre, 97 Lisburn Road, Belfast BT9 7BL Tel: 02890 335796 Fax: 02890 331838 Email: w.wallace@qub.ac.uk — MB BCh BAO Belf. 1961; FRCP Lond. 1981, M 1966; BSc (Physiol.) (1st cl. Hons.) Belf. 1958, MD 1966; FRCA 1991; FRCS (Ed) 2002; FCARCSI 2002. Prof. Emeritus Applied Physiol. Qu. Univ. Belf.; Examr., RCS Ed, CARCSI. Specialty: Clin. Physiol. Socs: Physiol. Soc. Prev: Regist. N. Irel. Hosps. Auth.; Vis. Prof. Physiol. Univ. Jos, Nigeria.; Cons. Physiol. Belf. City Hosp.

WALLACE, William Hamilton 4 Belmont Avenue, Uddingston, Glasgow G71 7AX Tel: 01698 2652 — MB ChB Ed. 1957. Prev: Orthop. Regist. Kilmarnock Infirm.; Med. Off. Ballochmyle Hosp. Mauchline; Surg. Ho. Off. Kilmarnock Infirm.

WALLACE, William Hamish Beith Royal Hospital for Sick Children, Sciennes Road, Edinburgh EH9 1LF Tel: 0131 536 0426 Fax: 0131 536 0430 Email: hamish.wallace@luht.scot.nhs.uk — MB BS Lond. 1980 (St Geo.) MRCP Uk 1985; MD Lond. 1992; FRCP Ed 1994; FRCS Ed. 2004. Cons. Paediat. Oncol. Roy. Hosp.

Sick Childr. Edin.; Sen. Lect. (Child Life & Health) Univ. Edin. Specialty: Paediat.; Oncol. Socs: Eur. Soc. Paediat. Endocrinol.; Soc. Internat. Oncol. Paediat. Prev: Sen. Regist. (Paediat.) Hosps. for Sick Childr. Gt. Ormond St. Lond.; Research Fell. (Paediat. Endocrinol.) Christie Hosp. & Radium Inst. Manch.; Regist. (Paediat.) Roy. Hosp. for Sick Childr. Edin.

WALLACE, William Morton Murray (retired) Rosalynn, Brodick KA27 8DP Tel: 01770 302306 — MB ChB Glas. 1951.

WALLACE, William Shaw (retired) Flat 2, Ascot House, Third Avenue, Hove BN3 2PD Tel: 01273 778 7114 — MB ChB Glas. 1942 (Univ. Glas.) MRCGP 1955. Prev: Ho. Phys. Glas. Roy. Infirm.

WALLACE, Wilson Macaulay, OStJ, Lt.-Col. RAMC Retd. 16 College Court, Royal Hospital, Chelsea, London SW3 4SR — MB BCh BAO Belf. 1964; FRCP Lond. 1998 M 1972. Ranald Martin Medal (Trop. Med.) & 2nd Montefiore Prize (Milit. Surg.) RAM Coll. Millbank; Cons. Phys. Roy. Hosp. Chelsea. Specialty: Care of the Elderly. Prev: Sen. Med. Off. RAF Innsworth; Cons. Phys. Brit. Milit. Hosp. Hong Kong; Cons. Phys. RAF Hosp. Wroughton & Qu. Eliz. Milit. Hosp. Woolwich.

WALLACE-JONES, Dudley Richard (retired) Little Garth, Wood Lane, Parkgate, Neston, South Wirral CH64 6QX Tel: 0151 336 4160 — (Univs. Camb. & Liverp.) MA Camb. 1948, BA 1944, MB BChir 1946; DMR Liverp. 1951; DMRD Lond. 1951; FRCR 1983. Prev: Cons. Radiol. Walton & Fazakerley Hosp. Liverp.

WALLAGE, Sarah Aberdeen Royal Infirmary, Foresterhill, Aberdeen AB25 2ZN — MB BS Lond. 1991; MRCOG 1997; MFFP 2003. Locum Cons. Gyn. Aberd. Roy. Infirm. Specialty: Obst. & Gyn. Prev: Clin. Research. Fell. Gyn. Dugald Baird Centre Aberd.; Specialist Regist. Rotat. W. Mids; Comm. Gyn. Trainee Aberd.

WALLAM, Timothy David Field House Surgery, Victoria Road, Bridlington YO15 2AT Tel: 01262 673362; The Forge, Middle St, Rudston, Driffield YO25 4UF Tel: 01262 420711 — BM BS Nottm. 1983; BMedSci (Hons.) Nottm. 1981, BM BS 1983; MRCGP 1987; DGM RCP Lond. 1986, DRCOG 1987. Prev: Ho. Off. (Med. & Surg.) Furness Gen. Hosp. Barrow-in-Furness; Trainee GP Notts. VTS.

WALLAT, Wolfgang Curran and Partners, Manor Health Centre, 86 Clapham Manor Street, London SW4 6EB Tel: 020 7411 6866 Fax: 020 7411 6857 Email: wolfgang.wallat@gp-g85708.nhs.uk; 211 Restons Crescent, Eltham, London SE9 2JZ — State Exam Med Hannover 1986; MD Hannover 1988; MRCGP 1995. GP Princip.; Formulary Comm. Mem., Guy's & St. Thomas' NHS Trust; Med.s Managem. Comm. Mem., N. Lamberth PCG.

WALLAT-VAGO, Susan Beatrice 40 Lake Road, London SW19 7EX — MB ChB Leic. 1985.

WALLBANK, Gail Rosemary Plas Newydd, Carno, Caersws SY17 5JR Tel: 01686 420212 — MB ChB Birm. 1971; DRCOG 1978. Specialty: Pub. Health Med. Prev: GP Newtown Pwys 2. GP Surgeries Newtown, Powys; Clin. Med. Off. (Community Health) Powys HA.; Med. Off. Family Plann. Clinics. Powys HA.

WALLBANK, Ian William 240 Minster Court, Liverpool L7 3QH — MB ChB Liverp. 1989.

WALLBANK, Nicola Jane 6 Walleys Drive, Newcastle ST5 0NG; The Tyles, 41 Montagu Road, Datchet, Slough SL3 9DT — MB BChir Camb. 1992 (Fitzwilliam Coll. Camb.) MA Camb. 1994; DCH RCP Lond. 1994; DRCOG 1995; DFFP 1997; MRCGP 1997; LoC C IUT 2000. GP. Specialty: Gen. Pract. Prev: GP Trainee Watford VTS.

WALLBANK, William Alistair Covenant House, Cider Mill Lane, Chipping Campden GL55 6HU — MB BS Lond. 1961 (Guy's) MRCS Eng. LRCP Lond. 1961; FFA RCS Eng. 1966. Cons. Anaesth. Univ. Hosp. of S. Manch. Specialty: Anaesth.

WALLBRIDGE, Christopher Martyn 304 Dobbin Hill, Sheffield S11 7JG — MB ChB Sheff. 1977; MRCPsych. 1982. Cons. Psychiat. Sheff. HA; Hon. Clin. Lect. Univ. Sheff. Specialty: Gen. Psychiat. Prev: Lect. Psychiat. Univ. Sheff.; Regist. (Psychiat.) Sheff. HA.

WALLBRIDGE, David Ross Royal Shrewsbury Hospital, Mytton Oak Road, Shrewsbury SY3 8DN Tel: 01743 261000 — MB ChB Birm. 1984; MRCP (UK) 1987; MD 1996. Cons. Phys. & Cardiol. Specialty: Cardiol.

WALLEN, Gerald Desmond Patrick (retired) Wonford House Hospital, Dryden Road, Exeter EX2 5AF Tel: 01392 403624 Fax: 01392 403477; Stavros, 18 Rydon Lane, Exeter EX2 7AW Tel: 01392 873138 — MB ChB Birm. 1957; MRCS Eng. LRCP Lond. 1957; DObst RCOG 1963; DPM Eng. 1966; FRCPsych 1984, M 1971. Cons. Psychiat. Exeter HA. Prev: Lect. (Psychiat.) Univ. Sheff.

WALLER, Christine Margaret 56 Percy Road, Ore, Hastings TN35 5AR — MB BS Melbourne 1985.

WALLER, Christopher John 90 Hazelhurst Road, Worsley, Manchester M28 2SP — MB ChB Bristol 1995.

WALLER, Deborah Jane Beaumont Street Surgery, 19 Beaumont Street, Oxford OX1 2NA Tel: 01865 240501 Fax: 01865 240503; Dean Court House, 89 Eynsham Road, Botley, Oxford OX2 9BY Tel: 01865 862017 — MB BChir Camb. 1985; DCH RCP Lond. 1987; MRCGP 1990. Socs: BMA. Prev: Clin. Lect. Wellcome Trust; Trainee GP Oxf. VTS.

WALLER, Deryk Pierre Edmund 3A Shrewsbury Road, Oxton, Wirral — MB ChB Sheff. 1989; MRCGP 1998.

WALLER, Dilys Claire Elizabeth The Surgery, Cockfield, Bishop Auckland DL13 5AF Tel: 01388 718202 Fax: 01388 710600; Burn Farm, Willington, Crook DL15 0HZ Tel: 01388 747484 — MB BS Newc. 1985; MRCP (UK) 1988; DCH RCP Lond. 1989; MRCGP 1990.

WALLER, James Otway DeWarrenne (retired) 3 Ironlatch Close, St Leonards-on-Sea TN38 9JQ Tel: 01424 429117 — MB BS Lond. 1963 (St.Bart.) MRCS Eng. LRCP Lond. 1963; MRCP Lond. 1965. Prev: Gen. Practitioner.

WALLER, Joanne Marie The Surgeries, Lombard St., Newark NG24 1XG Tel: 01636 702363 — MB ChB Leeds 1992; DRCOG 1996; MRCGP 1997; DCH 1997. GP. Specialty: Gen. Pract. Prev: GP Regist. Bridge St. Med. Pract. Otley; SHO (Paediat.) Airedale Gen. Hosp.; GP Regist. Grange Pk. Surg. Burley in Wharfdale.

WALLER, John Gamble, Col. late RAMC Retd. 20 Hartfield Road, Bexhill-on-Sea TN39 3EA Tel: 01424 843806 — MB ChB Ed. 1945 (Edin.) DTM & H RCP Lond. 1964; FRCGP 1980, M 1965; DCH RCP Lond. 1968; DObst RCOG 1971. Prev: Phys. Roy. Commiss. Jubail Project, Saudi Arabia; GP Oldham.

WALLER, Jonathan Francis 37 Church Hill, Epping CM16 4RA Tel: 01992 576649 — MB BS Lond. 1972; MRCP (UK) 1975; BSc (Anat., 1st cl. Hons.) Lond. 1969, MD 1982; FRCP Lond. 1992. Cons. Phys. Princess Alexandra Hosp. NHS Trust Harlow. Specialty: Gen. Med. Prev: Sen. Regist. (Gen. & Respirat. Med.) Roy. Free & Brompton Hosps.; Research Fell. Lung Func. Unit Brompton Hosps.; Regist. (Gen. Respirat. Med.) Lond. Hosp.

WALLER, Julian Ronald Lee — MB ChB Birm. 1998.

WALLER, Julie Alison 46 St Cadoc Road, Heath, Cardiff CF14 4NE — MB BCh Wales 1979; DRCOG 1982; MRCGP 1983; DCH RCP Lond. 1992. Specialty: Family Plann. & Reproduc. Health.

WALLER, Kathleen Grace Ealing Hospital, Uxbridge Road, Southall UB1 3HW Tel: 020 8574 2444; 34 Sunnyside Road, Ealing, London W5 5HU Tel: 020 8567 8195 — BM BCh Oxf. 1988; BA (2nd cl. Hons. Physiol.) Oxf. 1985; MRCOG 1993; DM 1997. Sen. Regist.Obyst.Gyn.Ealing Hosp. Specialty: Obst. & Gyn. Prev: Regist. (O & G) Watford Gen. Hosp. & Hammersmith Hosp.; Research Fell. (O & G) Univ. Wales Coll. Med. Cardiff; Sen. Regist. (O & G) Hammersmith Hosp.

WALLER, Patrick Charles 15 Tamella Road, Botley, Southampton SO30 2NY Tel: 01489 798107 Fax: 01489 690016 Email: patrick.waller@btinternet.com — MB ChB Sheff. 1980; MD Sheff. 1989, BMedSci. 1977; MRCP (UK) 1983; MPH Glas. 1988; FRCP Ed. 1993; FFPM RCP (UK) 1995. Cons. in Pharmacovigilance and Pharmacoepidemiology; Vis. Prof. (Pharmacological Scis.) Univ. of Newc.-upon-Tyne. Specialty: Pharmacology. Socs: Brit. Pharm. Soc.; Internat. Soc. Pharmacoepidemiol. Prev: Sen. Research Fell. Drug Safety Research Unit Soton.; Research Fell. Glas. Blood Pressure Clinic; Research Regist. (Cardiovasc. Dis.) Roy. Hallamsh. Hosp. Sheff.

WALLER, Robin Eric West child and fanily therapy team, Centenary house, 55 Albert Terrace Rd, Sheffield S6 3BR Tel: 0114 226 2034 — MB ChB Birm. 1972; MRCPsych 1984. Cons. Child & Adolesc. Psychiat. Sheff. HA. Specialty: Child & Adolesc. Psychiat. Prev: Sen. Regist. (Child & Adolesc. Psychiat.) Leics. HA.

WALLER, Rosalind Wye Surgery, 67 Oxenturn Road, Wye, Ashford TN25 5AY Tel: 01233 812414/812419 Fax: 01233 813236; Burnthouse Farm, Station Road, Chartham, Canterbury CT4 7HU — MB BS Lond. 1981 (Middlx.) BSc Bristol (Chem. Phys.) 1975; DCH RCP Lond. 1984. GP Ashford Kent. Specialty: Gen. Pract. Prev: SHO Qu. Eliz. Hosp. for Childr. Lond.; SHO (Neonat.) John Radcliffe Hosp. Oxf.; SHO (Paediat.) Northwick Pk. Hosp. Harrow.

WALLER, Sally Louise Nettleham Medical Practice, 14 Lodge Lane, Nettleham, Lincoln LN2 2RS Tel: 01522 751717 Fax: 01522 754474 — MB BS Newc. 1989; MRCGP 1994; DFFP 1994. Prev: Trainee GP Lincoln.

WALLER, Simon Charles 25 Thorncombe Road, London SE22 8PX — MB BS Lond. 1996. Socs: MRCPCH.

WALLER, Stella Mary Queen Elizabeth II Hospital, Essendon Ward, Howlands, Welwyn Garden City AL7 4HQ; 2 High Ash Road, Wheathampstead, St Albans AL4 8DY Tel: 01582 832465 Email: stella@aewaller.co.uk — MB BS Newc. 1978; DO Eng. 1982. Assoc. Specialist. Specialty: Ophth. Socs: MRCOphth. Prev: Regist. (Ophth.) Luton & Dunstable Hosp.

WALLERS, Kenneth John Department of Radiology, Monklands District General Hospital, Monkscourt Avenue, Airdrie ML6 0JS Tel: 01236 748748 Fax: 01236 746223 — MB ChB Dundee 1976; DMRD Eng. 1980; FRCR 1984. Cons. Radiol. Monklands Dist. Gen. Hosp. Airdrie. Specialty: Radiol.

WALLEY, Betty Margaret (retired) 49 Brean Down Avenue, Henleaze, Bristol BS0 4JE — MB BS Lond. 1948 (Univ. Coll. Hosp.) DPH Bristol 1963; DCH Eng. 1966. Prev: SCMO (Child Psychiat.) Avon AHA.

WALLEY, Denis Raymond Flat 3, 2 Selborne Road, Hove BN3 3AG — MB BCh BAO NUI 1987.

WALLEY, Kenneth (retired) 8 Valencia Road, Liverpool L15 8LL; 8 Valencia Road, Liverpool L15 8LL Tel: 0151 722 4778 — MB ChB Liverp. 1951; MFOM RCP Lond. 1978.

WALLEY, Margaret Ruth (retired) Dowles Croft, Greenacres Lane, Bewdley DY12 2RE Tel: 01299 400250 — MB ChB Manch. 1950; MB ChB Manch. 1950 DPM Durh. 1955; MRCPsych 1971. Prev: Cons. Psychiat. Durh. CC.

WALLEY, Professor Thomas Joseph Department Pharmacology & Therapeutics, University of Liverpool, PO Box 147, Liverpool L69 3BX — MD NUI 1990; MB BCh BAO 1980; FRCPI 1993, M 1982; MRCP (UK) 1984; FRCP (Lond.) 1995. Prof. Clin. Pharmacol. Univ. Liverp.; Hon. Cons. Phys. & Clin. Pharmacol. Roy. Liverp. Hosp.; Hon. Cons. Clin. Pharmacol. Mersey RHA. Specialty: Pharmacology. Socs: Assn. Phys. Prev: Sen. Lect. (Pharmacol. & Therap.) Univ. Liverp.; Lect. (Pharmacol. & Therap.) Univ. Liverp.

WALLICE, Malcolm Robert Bruce (retired) 20 Fforff-y-Dyffryn, Hermitage Park, Wrexham LL13 7GW Tel: 01978 313198; 20 Ffordd-y-Dyffryn, Hermitage Park, Wrexham LL13 7GW Tel: 01978 313198 — MB ChB Liverp. 1954; DObst RCOG 1956.

WALLICE, Patrick Donald Bruce (retired) 7 Willow Drive, Wrea Green, Preston PR4 2NT — MB ChB Liverp. 1955; DObst RCOG 1957; AFOM RCP Lond. 1982. Prev: SCMO (Occupat. Health) Preston DHA.

WALLING, Alice Elisabeth University of Durham, Student Health Centre, 42 Old Elvet, Durham DH1 3JF; 142 Gilesgate, Durham DH1 1QQ Tel: 0191 384 6076 — MB BS Newc. 1984; MRCGP 1988.

WALLING, Martyn Ronald Parkside Surgery, Tawney Street, Boston PE21 6PF Tel: 01205 365881 Fax: 01205 357583; Belmont, 23 Sibsey Road, Boston PE21 9QY — MB ChB Sheff. 1976; FRCGP 1994, M 1980; DRCOG 1980; MFFP 1994. Clin. Asst. (Obst. Ultrasound) Family Plann. Clinic Ment. Handicap Unit; Edit. Bd. Brit. Jl. Sexual Med. Specialty: Family Plann. & Reproduc. Health. Prev: Vis. Fell. Internat. Med. Mass. Gen. Hosp. Boston, USA; Trainee GP Boston, Lincs. VTS; Ho. Surg. Roy. Hosp. Sheff.

WALLINGTON, David Michael AON occupational health, 2 Circus Place, London EC2M 5RS Tel: 020 7628 0523 — MB BCh Wales 1976; DA Eng. 1981; DIH Lond. 1983; FFOM RCP Lond. 1995, MFOM 1987. Director Clin. Ocupational Med. AON Occupational Health. Specialty: Occupat. Health. Socs: Soc. Occupat. Med.; (Chairm.) Lond. GRP; Counc. SOM. Prev: Dir. of Occupat. Health Metropolitan Police Serv.; Chief Occupat. & Sen. Occupat. Health Phys. Wellcome Foundat. Ltd. Dartford Kent; Med. Off. & Sen. Med. Off. Rolls-Royce plc Derbysh.

WALLINGTON, Margaret 126 Chosen Way, Hucclecote, Gloucester GL3 3BZ — MB BCh Wales 1974; DObst. RCOG 1976; MRCOG 1979.

WALLINGTON, St Clair Hamilton Archer (retired) The Rectory, Langtree, Torrington Tel: 0180 55 273 — MB ChB Birm. 1927.

WALLINGTON, Timothy Baden Amesbury House, Gloucester Road, Almondsbury, Bristol BS32 4AA Tel: 01454 614192 Email: ac113@beeb.net — MB BChir Camb. 1970; BA (1st cl.) Camb. 1967; FRCP Lond. 1988; FRCPath 1995. Cons. Immunol. Nat. Blood Serv. Bristol & Southmead Hosp. Bristol. Specialty: Immunol. Prev: Sen. Regist. (Immunol.) Nottm. City Hosp.; Regist. (Med.) Southmead Hosp. Bristol; MRC Jun. Research Fell. Southmead Hosp. Bristol.

WALLIS, Andrew James Greenlanes, Ullenhall, Solihull B95 5NF — MB BS Lond. 1991.

WALLIS, Charles Burne Department of Anaesthetics, Western General Hospital, Edinburgh EH4 2XU Tel: 0131 537 1000 — MB ChB Ed. 1984; DRCOG 1986; FRCA. 1992. Cons. Anaesth. Specialty: Anaesth.; Intens. Care. Socs: Scott. Intens. Care Soc. & NE Scotl. Soc. Anaesth. Prev: Sen. Regist. Ninewells Hosp. Dundee; SHO (Anaesth.) West. Gen. Hosp. Edin.

WALLIS, Christopher Julian Andover Health Centre, Charlton Road, Andover SP10 3LD Tel: 01264 350270 Fax: 01264 336701 — MB ChB Bristol 1975; DRCOG 1980; DCH Eng. 1981; MRCGP 1982.

WALLIS, Clive Bernard Crown Street Surgery, 17 Crown Street, Swinton, Rotherham S64 8LY Tel: 01709 583862 — MB ChB Sheff. 1980. Prev: Trainee GP Burnley VTS.

WALLIS, Colin Erick Great Ormond Street Hospital, Great Ormond Street, London WC1N 3JH Tel: 020 7405 9200 — MB ChB Cape Town 1980; MD 1988; FCP SA 1990; FRCPCH 1996. Cons. Respirat. Paediat. Gt. Ormond St. Hosp. Lond. Specialty: Respirat. Med.

WALLIS, Daniel Nathan Accident & Emergency Department, St. Thomas' Hospital, Lambeth Palace Road, London SE1 7EH — MB BS Lond. 1981; DRCOG 1986; MRCP (UK) 1986; MRCGP 1988; DCH RCP Lond. 1989. cons. (A & E Med.) Guy's & St. Thomas' Hosp. Trust. Specialty: Accid. & Emerg.

WALLIS, Diane Elizabeth Park View Surgery, 24-28 Leicester Road, Loughborough LE11 2AG — MB ChB Dundee 1983; MRCGP 1988. Asst. GP. Specialty: Gen. Pract.

WALLIS, Elspeth Gordon The New Surgery, The Nap, Kings Langley WD4 8ET Tel: 01923 261035 Fax: 01923 269629 Email: epi.wallis@nhs.net — MB BS Lond. 1972 (Middlx.) DCH Eng. 1974; MRCP (UK) 1978. Prev: Regist. Radiother. Middlx. Hosp. Lond.; Regist. (Med. Oncol.) St. Bart. & Hackney Hosps.; Regist. (Med. & Paediat.) St. And. Hosp. Bow.

WALLIS, Erica Joy Room L100 Floor L, Ryal Hallamshire Hospital, Glossup Rd, Sheffield S10 2JF Email: e.j.wallis@sheffield.ac.uk — MB ChB Sheff. 1992 (Sheffield) Research Asst. (Clin. Pharmacol. & Ther.) Univ. Sheff. Specialty: Pharmacology.

WALLIS, Ethel Marjorie (retired) 38 Solent Way, Alverstoke, Gosport PO12 2NS — MB ChB Ed. 1948 (Univ. Ed.) DObst RCOG 1951; DPH Eng. 1957. Prev: SCMO (Child Health) Portsmouth & SE Hants. HA.

WALLIS, Geoffrey Garfit Casa Rohan, Longwood Hall, Bingley BD16 2RX Tel: 01274 568072 Fax: 01274 568072; Harrogate Clinic, 23 Ripon Road, Harrogate HG1 2JL Tel: 01423 500599 Fax: 01423 531074 — (Univ. Coll. Hosp.) MRCS Eng. LRCP Lond. 1941; MB BS Lond. 1942; DPM Eng. 1955; MD Lond. 1966; FRCPsych 1971; CCST 1996. Cons. Psychiat. Harrogate Clinic. Specialty: Gen. Psychiat. Socs: Fell. Roy. Soc. Med.; Leeds & W. Riding Medico-Legal Soc.; Soc. Clin. Psychiat. Prev: Cons. Psychiat. High Royds Hosp. Menston; Hon. Lect. Univ. Leeds; Adviser (Psychiat.) Med. Dir. Gen. (Naval).

WALLIS, Helen 27 Hampermill Lane, Oxhey, Watford WD19 4NS — MB ChB Leeds 1984.

WALLIS, Helen Louise 27 Sunny Bank Road, Liverpool L16 7PN — MB ChB (Hons.) Birm. 1992; MRCP (UK) 1995. Specialist Regist. Rotat. (Cardiol.) Wessex. Specialty: Cardiol.; Gen. Med.

WALLIS, James Fintan Edward Mary Aberdeen Royal Infirmary, Foresterhill, Aberdeen AB25 2ZN Tel: 01224 681818; The Lodge, Tornadee Hospital, Milltimber AB13 0HW Tel: 01224 869845 — MB BCh BAO NUI 1987 (Univ. Coll. Dub. Irel.) MRCPI 1990; FRCR 1994; FFR RCSI 1994. Sen. Lect. (MRI) Hon. Cons. Aberd. Roy. Infirm. Specialty: Radiol. Prev: Sen. Regist. (Diagnostic Imaging) Aberd. Roy. Infirm.; Regist. (Radiol.) St. Jas. Hosp. Dub.

WALLIS, Joanne — MB ChB Leic. 1985.

WALLIS, Mr John Department of Cardiothoracic Surgery, South Cleveland Hospital, Middlesbrough TS4 3BW Tel: 01642 850850; 64 Langbaugh Road, Hutton Rudby, Yarm TS15 0HL — BSc (1st cl.

Hons.) Lond. 1970; MRCS Eng. LRCP Lond. 1973; MB BS Lond. 1973; DA Eng. 1975; MRCP (UK) 1977; FRCS Eng. 1980; FRCP 2000. Cons. Cardiothoracic Surg. S. Cleveland Hosp. Middlesbrough. Specialty: Cardiothoracic Surg. Prev: Research Fell. (Cardiothoracic Surg.) Univ. Alabama, Birm., Alabama, USA.

WALLIS, John Harold Skirbeck House, 140 Spilsby Road, Boston PE21 9PE Tel: 01205 2320 — MB BS Lond. 1946 (Lond. Hosp.) Prev: Ho. Phys. & Ho. Surg. Lond. Hosp.

WALLIS, Jonathan Peter Department of Haematology, Freeman Hospital, Freeman Road, High Heaton, Newcastle upon Tyne NE7 7DN Tel: 0191 223 1285 Fax: 0191 223 1199 Email: jonathan.wallis@tfh.nuth.northy.nhs.uk — MB BS Lond. 1979; MRCP 1984; MRCPath 1989; FRCP 1998; FRCPath 1999. Cons. Haemat. Freeman Hosp. Newc. u. Tyne. Specialty: Haematology. Special Interest: Blood transfusion; Red Cell Disorders. Socs: BSH; BBTS; AABB.

WALLIS, Malcolm Montgomery (retired) 32 Strand Court, Topsham, Exeter EX3 0AZ — MB ChB Liverp. 1934. Prev: Ho. Phys. & Res. Anaesth. Roy. South. Hosp. Liverp.

WALLIS, Michael St Johns Street Surgery, 16 St. Johns Street, Kempston, Bedford MK42 8EP Tel: 01234 851323 Fax: 01234 843293 — MRCS Eng. LRCP Lond. 1972.

WALLIS, Michael Graham Staines Health Centre, Knowle Green, Staines TW18 1XD Tel: 01784 883620 Fax: 01784 441244; Walnut Tree House, 11 Lammas Close, Staines TW18 4XT — MRCS Eng. LRCP Lond. 1973 (St. Mary's) Socs: Brit. Med. Acupunc. Soc.

WALLIS, Michael Owen Wallis and Partners, The Health Centre, 5 Stanmore Road, Stevenage SG1 3QA Tel: 01438 313223 Fax: 01438 749734 — MB BS Lond. 1977; MRCS Eng. LRCP Lond. 1976.

WALLIS, Nicola Trudle Syngenta Central Toxicology Laboratory, Alderley Park, Macclesfield SK10 4TJ Tel: 01625 510927 Fax: 01625 517911 Email: nicola.wallis@syngenta.com — MB ChB Birm. 1987 (Birmingham) BSc ((Hons) Anat.) 1984; MRCPath 1987; Dip Pharm 2000; MFPP 2002. Head Endocrine & Reproductive Toxicology. Specialty: Histopath.; Pharmaceutical Medicine. Prev: Sen. Regist. (Histopath.) North. West. RHA.; Regist. (Histopath.) North. West. RHA; SHO (Path.) Centr. Birm. HA.

WALLIS, Patricia Gwendoline (retired) 44 Blackheath Park, London SE3 9SJ Tel: 020 8852 7110 Fax: 020 8852 7110 Email: pat-wallis@doctors.org.uk — MB BS Lond. 1953 (Char Cross) DCH Eng. 1955; DObst RCOG 1955; FRCP Lond. 1974, M 1958; FRCPCH 1997. Hon. Cons. Paediat. Lewisham Childr. Hosp. Prev: Cons. Paediat. Childr. Hosp. Sydenham & Lewisham Hosp.

WALLIS, Peter (retired) Abdy Cottage, The Green, Whiston, Rotherham S60 4JD — MRCS Eng. LRCP Lond. 1952.

WALLIS, Peter Barnham Medical Centre, 134 Barnham Road, Barnham, Bognor Regis PO22 0EH Tel: 01243 555829 Fax: 01243 554218 — MB BS Lond. 1965 (King's Coll. Hosp.) MRCS Eng. LRCP Lond. 1965. Socs: BMA. Prev: SHO (Path.) & Ho. Surg. (ENT Surg.) King's Coll. Hosp. Lond.; Ho. Phys. Dulwich Hosp.

WALLIS, Peter John Walker Department Geriatric Medicine, Boldesley Green East, Birmingham Heartlands Hospital, Yardley Green Road, Birmingham B9 5SS Tel: 0121 424 0769 Fax: 0121 753 0653; 38 Alderbrook Road, Solihull B91 1NN Tel: 0121 711 4078 Email: peterwallis@compuserve.com — MB BS Lond. 1977 (St. Mary's) BSc Lond. 1974; MB BS (Hons.) Lond. 1977; MRCP (UK) 1979; FRCP Lond. 1995. Cons. Phys. (Geriat. Med.) Birm. Heartlands Hosp.; Hon. Sen. Clin. Lect. Univ. Birm. Specialty: Care of the Elderly; Gen. Med. Prev: Sen. Regist. (Gen. & Geriat. Med.) W. Midl. Train. Scheme; Regist. (Med.) Westm. Hosp. Lond.; Research Fell. The Lond. Hosp. Whitechapel.

WALLIS, Ruth Mary 42 Stockwell Green, London SW9 9HX — BM Soton. 1980.

WALLIS, Sheila Mary Battle Hospital, Dingley Child Development Centre, Oxford Road, Reading RG30 1AG Tel: 0118 963 6213 Fax: 0118 963 6209 Email: sheila.wallis@rbbh-tr.nhs.uk — MB ChB Manch. 1969; DCH Eng. 1972; MRCP (UK) 1974; FRCP Lond. 1994; FRCPCH 1997. Cons. Paediat. (Neurodisability) Roy. Berks. & Battle Hosps. Reading. Specialty: Paediat. Socs: Neonat. Soc.; Brit. Paediat. Neurol. Assn.; Eur. Acad. Childh. Disabil. Prev: Sen. Regist. (Paediat.) Roy. Berks. Hosp. Reading & Wolfson Centre Inst. Child Health Lond.; Research Fell. (Paediat.) Qu. Charlotte's Hosp. Wom. Lond.

WALLIS, Simon Charles Chorley & South Ribble District General Hospital, Preston Road, Chorley; 33 Southport Road, Chorley PR7 1LF — MB BChir Camb. 1975 (Camb./Birm.) MRCP (UK) 1978; FRCP 1993. Cons. Phys. (Diabetes & Endocrinol.) Chorley & S. Ribble Dist. Gen. Hosp. Specialty: Endocrinol. Prev: Sen. Lect & Hon. Cons. Endocrinol. & Metab. Roy. Postgrad. Med. Sch. Hammersmith Hosp. Lond.; Clin. Sci. MRC Clin. Research Centre Harrow; MRC Research Fell. Recombinant DNA Technol. St. Marys & St. Bart. Lond.

WALLIS, Mr Simon William John H2 Ophthalmic Unit, Royal Bolton Hospital, Minerva Road, Farnworth, Bolton BL4 0JR Tel: 01204 390519 Fax: 01204 390554 — MB ChB Manch. 1980; DO RCS Eng. 1986; FRCS Ed. 1988; FCOphth. 1989. Cons. Ophth. Bolton Hosps. Specialty: Ophth. Prev: Sen. Regist. Manch. Roy. Eye Hosp.

WALLIS, Timothy David Nettleham Medical Practice, 14 Lodge Lane, Nettleham, Lincoln LN2 2RS Tel: 01522 751717; Kerio, 9 Chestnut Close, Sudbrooke, Lincoln LN2 2RD Tel: 01522 751211 — MB ChB Ed. 1965. p/t General Practice (Locum); HM Dep. Coroner Lincoln Dist.; Expert witness; Med. Practitioner Lincoln. Specialty: Gen. Pract. Prev: Clin. Asst. (Dermat.) Lincoln Co. Hosp.; Med. Off. Kapsowar Hosp. Kenya; Sen. Health Off. (Surg.) Mildmay Mission Hosp. Lond.

WALLIS, Toby David Fordingbridge Surgery, Bartons Road, Fordingbridge SP6 1RS Tel: 01425 653430 — MB BS Lond. 1997 (Char. Cross & Westm.) GP Princip. Hants. Specialty: Gen. Pract. Special Interest: Minor Surg. Socs: RCGP. Prev: Salaried GP Hadleigh Pract. Poole; SHO (Paediat., O & G, Accid. & Emerg. & Care of Elderly) Poole Hosp.; SHO (Orthop.) Frenchay Hosp. Bristol.

WALLIS, William Richard James 6A Mildford Place, London W1P 9HH — (St Thomas') MB Camb. 1987, BChir 1986; LMSSA Lond. 1986; MRCP Lond. 1990; PhD Lond. 1997. Regist. Cardiol. St. Barts. Specialty: Cardiol. Socs: Brit. Cardiac Soc.; Roy. Coll. Phys.; BCIS.

WALLOND, Julia Clare 4 Newcombe Street, Exeter EX1 2TG — MB ChB Bristol 1998.

WALLS, Mr Andrew David Finlay Uplands, 83 Edinburgh Road, Dumfries DG1 1JX Tel: 01387 252830 Fax: 01387 241741 — MB BS Lond. 1967 (St. Thos.) FRCS Eng. 1973; FRCS Ed. 1986. Cons. Surg. Dumfries & Galloway Acute & Matern. NHS Trust; Dir. Postgrad. Med. Educat. Dumfries & Galloway HB; Clin. Sen. Lect. Univ. Aberd.; Hon. Sen. Lect. Univ. Glas. Specialty: Gastroenterol. Socs: Brit. Soc. Gastroenterol.; BMA; Chairm. LREC. Prev: Sen. Regist. (Surg.) West. Gen. Hosp. Edin.; Ho. Surg. St. Thos. Hosp. Lond.; Lect. (Anat.) King's Coll. Lond.

WALLS, Anne Teresa Rose 37 Glenmaquill Road, Magherafelt BT45 5EW — MB BCh BAO NUI 1992.

WALLS, Dorothy Brown (retired) Hesslewood, The Orchard, Kitty Frisk House, Hexham NE46 1UN — MB BS Durh. 1949 (Kings College Newcastle Upon Tyne) Prev: Ho. Surg. & Ho. Phys. (Gyn. & Obst.) Roy. Vict. Infirm. Newc.

WALLS, Mr Eldred Wright 19 Dean Park Crescent, Edinburgh EH4 1PH Tel: 0131 332 7164 — MB ChB (Hons.) Glas. 1934; FRSE; BSc Glas. 1931, MD (Hons.) 1947; FRCS Eng. 1976; FRCS Ed. 1981. Emerit. Prof. Anat. Univ. Lond.; Hon. Cons. Anat. St Mark's Hosp. Lond.; Lect. (Anat.) Univ. Edin. (2003-). Specialty: Anat. Socs: (Ex-Pres.) Anat. Soc.; (Pres.) Assn. Blind Chartered Physiother. Prev: Dean Middlx. Hosp. Med. Sch.; Lect. (Anat.) Univ. Edin.; Sen. Lect. (Anat.) Univ. Wales.

WALLS, Elizabeth Cairns (retired) 40 Lake Avenue, Walsall WS5 3PA Tel: 01922 649749 — (Belf.) MB BCh BAO Belf. 1946.

WALLS, Fionnuala Bernadette 29 High Street, Draperstown, Magherafelt BT45 7AB Tel: 01648 28201 — MB BCh BAO NUI 1977; DRCOG 1981. GP Draperstown.

WALLS, Janet North Manchester General Hospital, Crumpsall, Manchester M8 6RL — MB ChB Liverp. 1986. Specialty: Gen. Surg.

WALLS, John Bradshaw 53 Church Road, Altofts, Wakefield WF3 4HR — MB ChB Leeds 1968; BSc (Anat.) Leeds 1965, MB ChB 1968; DMRD Eng. 1977. Cons. Radiol. Pinderfields Gen. Hosp. Wakefield. Specialty: Radiol.

WALLS, Marguerite Joan Church View House, Church Lane, Adel, Leeds LS16 8DG Tel: 0113 261 3882 — MB ChB Leeds 1947. Prev: Clin. Med. Off. Leeds E. & West. HA; Ho. Surg. (Obst.) St. Jas. Hosp. Leeds; Ho. Phys. Dewsbury Gen. Infirm.

WALLS, Maurice Youll 52 Woolsington Gardens, Woolsington, Newcastle upon Tyne NE13 8AR Tel: 0191 286 9999 — MB BS Durh. 1955; DPH Newc. 1966; MFCM 1974; MFPHM 1989. Assoc. Specialist Nat. Blood Transfus. Serv.; Mem. North. Regional Med. Comm.; Mem. North. Regional Manpower Comm. Socs: N.. Region Assoc. Specialist Gp. Prev: Sen. Med. Off. (Community Med.) Newc. AHA; GP Newbiggin-by-the-Sea; Ho. Off. Shotley Bridge Hosp.
WALLS, Ngaire Jean Chaldon Road Surgery, Chaldon Road, Caterham CR3 5PG Tel: 01883 345466 Fax: 01883 330942; Wood End, 80 Welcomes Road, Kenley CR8 5HE Tel: 020 8660 0770 — MB BS Lond. 1975 (St. Mary's) MRCS Eng. LRCP Lond. 1975; DRCOG 1977.
WALLS, Timothy John Newcastle General Hospital, Department of Neurology, Westgate Road, Newcastle upon Tyne NE4 6BE Tel: 0191 233 6161 Ext: 22460 Fax: 0191 272 4823 Email: t.j.walls@ncl.ac.uk; 18 Adeline Gardens, Gosforth, Newcastle upon Tyne NE3 4JQ Tel: 0191 285 8281 — MB BS (Hons) Newc. 1977; MD Newc. 1988, BMedSci (Hons.) 1974; MRCP (UK) 1979; FRCP Lond. 1994. Cons. Neurol. Newc. Gen. Hosp.; Hon. Clin. Sen. Lect. in Neurol. Univ. of Newc. Upon Tyne. Specialty: Neurol. Socs: Association of British Neurologists; Neuromuscular Disease. Prev: Cons. Neurologist Qu. Eliz. Hosp. Gateshead; Research Fell. & Fulbright Schol. Mayo Clinic Rochester, USA.
WALLS, William David Clayton Hospital, Northgate, Wakefield WF1 3JS Tel: 01924 214141; 98 Ouzlewell Green, Loft House, Wakefield WF3 3QW Tel: 0113 282 1376 — MB ChB Leeds 1960; FRCP Lond. 1979, M 1965; MD (Distinc.) Leeds 1969. Cons. Phys. Pinderfields & Clayton Hosps. Wakefield. Specialty: Gen. Med.; Gastroenterol. Socs: Brit. Soc. Gastroenterol.; Brit. Soc. Med. & Dent. Hypn. Prev: Sen. Regist. (Gen. Med.) Leeds RHB; Research Asst. (Med.) Univ. Leeds.
WALLS, William Kenneth Johnstone Church View House, Church View, Adel, Leeds LS16 8DG Tel: 0113 261 3882 — MB ChB Leeds 1940; MRCS Eng. LRCP Lond. 1941. Hon. Lect. (Anat.) & Life Fell. Univ. Leeds. Specialty: Anat. Socs: Anat. Soc.& BMA. Prev: Sen. Lect. (Anat.) Univ. Leeds; Instruc. Doctor (Family Plann.) Leeds AHA; Regist. (Surg. & Neurosurg.) Leeds Gen. Infirm.
WALLWORK, Professor John Department of Cardiothoracic Surgery, Papworth Hospital, Papworth Everard, Cambridge CB3 8RE Tel: 01480 364418 Fax: 01480 831281 Email: john.wallwork@papworth.nhs.uk; 3 Latham Road, Cambridge CB2 2EG Tel: 01223 352827 — MB ChB Edin. 1970 (Edinburgh) FMedSci; BSc (Hons.) Ed. 1967; FRCS Ed. 1974; FRCS (ad eund.) 1992; FRCP Edin 2000. Prof. Cardiothoracic Surg.; Dir. Transpl. Serv. Specialty: Cardiothoracic Surg.; Transpl. Surg. Special Interest: Cardiothoracic Surg. in the elderly; Research into xenotransplantation; Right heart failure and Eval. of left ventricular assist devices for long-term mobilisation and heart failure. Socs: Internat. Soc. Heart & Lung Transpl.; Internat. Transpl. Soc.; (Counc.) Europ. Soc. for Organ Transpl. Prev: Chief Resid. Cardiovasc. Surg. & Cardiac Transpl. Stanford Univ. Med. Sch., USA; Sen. Regist. (Cardiothoracic Surg.) St. Bart. Hosp. Lond.; Cons. Cardiothoracic Surg. Papworth Hosp. Camb.
WALLWORK, Lynne Louise 179 Forest Avenue, Aberdeen AB15 4UU — MB ChB Aberd. 1997 (Aberdeen) BSc Med. Sci 1995; MBchB 1997. GP Asst. Aberd. Specialty: Paediat. Dent. Prev: GP VTS SHO.
WALLWORK, Michael Anthony Health Services Centre, Shelley Lane, Kirkburton, Huddersfield HD8 0SJ Tel: 01484 602040 Fax: 01484 602012; Spinney Court, 3A Thorpe Lane, Almondbury, Huddersfield HD5 8TA Tel: 01484 304486 — MB ChB Leeds 1987; DRCOG 1991; MRCGP 1992. GP Huddersf. Specialty: Acupunc.; Paediat.; Gen. Pract. Socs: BMA; Brit. Med. Acupunct. Soc.
WALLWORTH, Roy Allen Peel House Medical Centre, Avenue Parade, Accrington BB5 6RD Tel: 01254 237231 Fax: 01254 389525; 58 Woodfield Avenue, Accrington BB5 2PJ — MB BS Lond. 1981; DRCOG 1985; MRCGP 1985.
WALMSLEY, Annabel Michaela 6 Windlesham Park, Woodlands Lane, Windlesham GU20 6AT — MB BS Lond. 1996.
WALMSLEY, Anona Elizabeth Lisburn Health Centre, Linenhall Street, Lisburn BT28 1LU Tel: 02892 603333 Fax: 02892 501503; Green Acres, 202 Belsize Road, Lisburn BT27 4DT Tel: 01846 670725 Fax: 01846 661119 — MB BCh BAO Belf. 1974 (Queens University Belfast) DRCOG 1976; MRCGP 1979.
WALMSLEY, Anthony John Department of Anaesthetics, Eastbourne DGH, Kings Drive, Eastbourne BN21 2NA Tel: 01323 417400; 3 Macmillian Drive, Eastbourne BN21 1SU Tel: 01323 643736 — MB BS Lond. 1978; FFA RCS Eng. 1982. Cons. Anaesth. Eastbourne DHA. Specialty: Anaesth.
WALMSLEY, Mr Byron Henry Baddeley House, Woodend, Wickham, Fareham PO17 6LB Tel: 01329 832811 — MB ChB Dundee 1974; BSc St. And. 1971; FRCS Eng. 1980. Cons. Urol. St. Mary's Hosp. Portsmouth. Specialty: Urol. Prev: Sen. Regist. (Urol.) St. Mary's Hosp. Portsmouth; Sen. Regist. Inst. Urol. Lond.
WALMSLEY, David Royal Lancaster Infirmary, Ashton Road, Lancaster LA1 4RP Tel: 01524 65944 Fax: 01524 846346 Email: david.walmsley@l.bay-tr.nwest.nhs.uk — MB ChB Birm. 1981 (Birmingham) BSc Birm. 1978; MRCP (UK) 1984; MD Birm. 1991; FRCP 1999. Cons. Phys. (Diabetes & Endocrinol.) Morecambe Bay Hosps. NHS Trust. Specialty: Endocrinol.; Diabetes; Gen. Med.
WALMSLEY, David Antony (retired) Willow House, School Lane, Great Leighs, Chelmsford CM3 1NL — (Lond. Hosp.) MB BS Lond. 1954; DA Eng. 1956; FFA RCS Eng. 1957. Prev: Cons. Anaesth. Mid Essex Hosps. Trust.
WALMSLEY, Felicity Jane 15 Riselaw Crescent, Edinburgh EH10 6HN — MB ChB Ed. 1974; MRCGP 1983.
WALMSLEY, Gerald Luke 22 Limehill Road, Tunbridge Wells TN1 1LL Tel: 01892 515344 — MB ChB Leeds 1973.
WALMSLEY, James Marcus Little Gables, Ewhurst Road, Cranleigh GU6 7AG Email: james.walmsley@pfizer.com — MB BS Newc. 1992; MFPM; MRCP UK 1997; Dip Pharm Med 2001. UK Med. Dir. Pfizer Consumer Healthcare.
WALMSLEY, Katharine Mary Department of Clinical Radiology, 2nd Floor Cecil Fleming House, UCLH NHS Trust, Grafton Way, London WC1E 6AU Tel: 020 7380 9648 Fax: 020 7388 2147 Email: kate.walmsley@uclh.org — MB ChB Bristol 1971; MB ChB (Hons.) Bristol 1971; DMRD Eng. 1976; FRCR 1977. Cons. Radiol. Univ. Coll. Lond. Hosps. & King Edwd. VII Hosp. for Offs. Lond. Specialty: Radiol. Prev: Sen. Regist. (Radiodiag.) Middlx. Hosp. Lond.
WALMSLEY, Paul Nigel Hudson 92 Kentmere Drive, Cherry Tree, Blackburn BB2 5HF — MB ChB Birm. 1980.
WALMSLEY, Phillip Jonathan 36 Lucerne Street, Sefton Park, Liverpool L17 8XT; Shireburn House, 236 Garstang Road, Fulwood, Preston PR2 9QB Tel: 01772 718785 — MB ChB Manch. 1995 (Univ. Manch.) Ho. Off. (Gen. Surg. & Orthop.) Hope Hosp. Salford. Specialty: Gen. Surg. Socs: BMA; MDU; Med. Sickness Soc.
WALMSLEY, Russell Stuart 28 Kidderminster Road, West Hagley, Stourbridge DY9 0QD — MB ChB Bristol 1986; MRCP (UK) 1991; MD Bristol 2000. Phys./Gastroenterologist; N. Shore Hosp., Auckland, New Zealand. Specialty: Gastroenterol.; Gen. Med. Socs: Brit. Soc. of Gastroenterol.; New Zealand Soc. of Gastroenterol.; Roy. Coll. of Phys. of Lond. Prev: Research Fell. (Gastroenterol.) Roy. Free Hosp. Med. Sch. Lond.; Regist. (Gastroenterol. & Gen. Med.) Gen. Hosp. & Qu. Eliz. Hosps. Birm.
WALMSLEY, Sarah Ruth 32 Edmund Road, Brandon IP27 0XA — MB ChB Ed. 1997.
WALMSLEY, Terry Ann Tonge Moor Health Centre, Thicketford Road, Bolton BL2 2LW Tel: 01204 365449 — MB ChB Manch. 1971; DObst RCOG 1973.
WALMSLEY, Thomas Osborn Clinic, Fareham PO16 7ES Tel: 01329 288331 Fax: 01329 825519 — MB ChB Dundee 1970; MRCPsych 1974; FRCPsych 1997. Cons. Psychiat. Portsmouth Healthcare NHS Trust; Clin. Teach. Soton. Univ. Specialty: Gen. Psychiat. Socs: Fell. Roy. Soc. of Med. Prev: Cons. Psychiat. Roy. Edin. Hosp.; Hon. Sen. Lect. (Psychiat.) Univ. Edin.
WALPOLE, Gerard Anthony Mary Operations Div., Maydown Works, PO Box 15, Londonderry BT47 1TU — MB BCh BAO NUI 1980; MRCGP 1984; DIH Lond. 1989; AFOM RCP Lond. 1989. Specialty: Occupat. Health.
WALPOLE, Rachel Helen Royal Gwent Hospital, Cardiff Road, Newport NP9 2UB — MB ChB Ed. 1991 (Edinburgh) FRCA Lond. 1996. Cons. Anaesth., Roy. Gwent Hosp., Newport. Specialty: Anaesth. Prev: SHO (Anaesth.) SE Scotl. Train. Scheme & Wansbeck Gen. Hosp. N.d.; Specialist Regist. (Anaesth.) SE Scotl. Sch. Anaesth.
WALPORT, Professor Mark Jeremy Division of Medicine, ICSM, Hammersmith Campus, Du Cane Road, London W12 0NN Tel: 020 8383 3299 Fax: 020 8383 2024 Email: m.walport@ic.ac.uk — MB

BChir Camb. 1977; PhD Camb. 1986, MA 1981; FRCP Lond. 1990; FRCPath 1997, M 1991; F Med Sci 1998. Prof.Imperial.Coll.Sch.Med./Chair.Div.Med;Hon.Cons.Hammersmith Hosp.; Regist. Acad. Med. Sci. Specialty: Rheumatol.; Immunol.; Gen. Med. Socs: (Counc.) Brit. Soc. Rheum. Prev: Prof. Med. Roy. Postgrad. Med. Sch. & Hon. Cons. Hammersmith Hosp. Lond.; MRC Train. Fell. MRC Mechanisms in Tumour Immunity Unit Camb.

WALPORT, Samuel (retired) 16 Grange Gardens, Pinner HA5 5QE Tel: 020 8868 3951 — (Anderson Coll. Glas.) LRCP LRCS Ed. LRFPS Glas. 1944. Prev: Capt. RAMC.

WALSH, Miss Aideen Kathleen Mary Room MO13, University Hospital of North Staffordshire - City General, Newcastle Road, Stoke-on-Trent ST4 6QG Tel: 01782 552176 — MB BCh BAO NUI 1984 (RCSI) LRCPI & LM, LRCSI & LM 1984; BSc NUI 1986; FRCS Ed. 1989; FRCS Eng. 1989; MD Leicester 1994. Cons. Gen. & Vasc. Surg. Univ. Hosp. N. Staffs.; Sen. Lect. (Med. Education) Keele Univ. Specialty: Gen. Surg.

WALSH, Alison Barbara 6 Partick Bridge Street, Glasgow G11 6PC — MB ChB Glas. 1998; DRCOG.

WALSH, Anthony Romney House Surgery, 39-41 Long Street, Tetbury GL8 8AA Tel: 01666 502303 Fax: 01666 504549 — MB ChB Manch. 1970; DObst RCOG 1972.

WALSH, Anthony Copleston 141A Harrowden Road, Bedford MK42 0RU Tel: 01234 262255 Fax: 01234 348885 Email: tony.walsh@shortstown.net — MB BS Lond. 1976; BA Oxf. 1970; DCH Eng. 1979; MRCGP 1981. GP Princip. Shortstown Health Centre. Specialty: Gen. Pract. Special Interest: Paediat. & Psychother. Socs: BMA; MDU. Prev: GP Princip. Kents Hill Surg. Milton Keynes; GP Princip. Walnut Tree Health Centre Milton Keynes.; GP Princip. Stirchley Health Centre Telford.

WALSH, Anthony Copleston 57 Frithwood Crescent, Kents Hill, Milton Keynes MK7 6HQ Tel: 01908 677451 — MB BS Lond. 1976; MRCGP.

WALSH, Mr Anthony Richard 44 Carpenter Road, Birmingham B15 2JJ — MB BChir Camb. 1977; FRCS Eng. 1981.

WALSH, Bartholomew 26 Grove Road, Barnes, London SW13 0HH Tel: 020 8876 6358 — MB BCh BAO NUI 1981; BA Lond. 1988; Dip. Clin. Microbiol. Lond 1989; MRCPath 1990; Dip. Hist. Med. Soc. Apoth. Lond. 1992; MSc Pub. Health Lond. 1995. Cons. Communicable Dis. Control Surrey. Specialty: Pub. Health Med. Prev: Sen. Regist. (Microbiol.) Wycombe Gen. Hosp. & John Radcliffe Hosp. Oxf.; Regist. N. Middlx. Hosp. Lond.; SHO St. Mary's Hosp. Lond.

WALSH, Catherine Mary S3, Box 175, Addenbrooke's Hospital, Hills Road, Cambridge CB2 2QQ — MB BCh BAO NUI 1984; MRCPsych. 1988. Cons. Psychiat. Addenbrooke's Hosp. Camb. Specialty: Gen. Psychiat.

WALSH, Christopher John Lytham The Health Centre, 80 Knaresborough Road, Harrogate HG2 7LU Tel: 01278 434293 Email: nick.airey@sompar.nhs.uk — MB ChB Leeds 1985; DRCOG 1988; MRCGP 1989.

WALSH, Mr Ciaran Joseph Wirral Hospital NHS Trust, Arrowe Park, Arrowe Park Road, Upton, Wirral CH49 5PE Tel: 0151 604 7052 Fax: 0151 604 1760 — MB BCh BAO NUI 1984; BSc Mch FRCSI (Gen); LRCPSI 1984. Cons. Colorectal & Gen. Surg. Specialty: Gen. Surg. Socs: BAPEN; Assn. of Colopractol, R.S.M..; (ASCRS - Pending).

WALSH, Colum 126 Edge Lane Drive, Liverpool L13 4AF — MB BS Newc. 1992.

WALSH, David Andrew Rheumatology Unit, City Hospital, Hucknall Road, Nottingham NG5 1PB Tel: 0115 969 1169 Ext: 46376 Email: david.walsh@nottingham.ac.uk; Department Rheumatolology, Kings Mill Centre, Mansfield Road, Sutton-in-Ashfield NG17 4JL Tel: 01623 22515 Ext: 3656 Fax: 01623 672348 — MB BS Lond. 1985; MA Camb. 1986; MRCP (UK) 1988; PhD Lond. 1994. Sen. Lect. & Hon. Cons. Nottm. Univ. Specialty: Rehabil. Med.; Rheumatol.

WALSH, David Anthony Priory Medical Group, Cornlands Road, Acomb, York YO24 3WX Tel: 01904 781423 Fax: 01904 784886 — MB BS Lond. 1971.

WALSH, David Brian (retired) Information Systems Department, Perth & Kinross Healthcare NHS Trust, Perth PH1 1NX Tel: 01738 623311 Fax: 01738 473244; The Whirlies, Kinnettles, Forfar DD8 1XF Tel: 01307 820367 — MB ChB Manch. 1965; MRCPath 1972. Project Doctor - IHIS Project. Prev: Cons. Dundee Teachg. Hosps. NHS Trust.

WALSH, David Ian Plantation House Medical Centre, 2-6 Austin Friars, London EC2N 2HE Tel: 020 7929 2733 Fax: 020 7628 6002 — MB BS Lond. 1985 (Roy. Free Hosp. Lond.) Indep. GP Lond. Specialty: Occupat. Health. Socs: Roy. Soc. Occupat. Md. Prev: SHO (Paediat.) Brook Gen. Hosp; SHO (Anaesth.) St. Mary's Hosp. Lond.; SHO (O & G) Fairfield Hosp. Sydney, Austral.

WALSH, David Michael 36A Methley Street, London SE11 4AJ — MB BS Lond. 1993.

WALSH, Deirdre Ann Department of Paediatrics, Causeway Hospital, 4 Newbridge Road, Coleraine BT52 1TP — MB BCh BAO NUI 1983.

WALSH, Dermot Simon Lawrence Hill Health Centre, Hassell Drive, Easton, Bristol BS2 0AN Tel: 0117 955 5241 Fax: 0117 941 1162; 42 Colthurst Drive, Hanham, Bristol BS15 3SG — MB BCh BAO NUI 1981 (Nat. Univ. of Irel.) DCH NUI 1983; DObst RCPI 1984; MRCGP 1986. Prev: SHO (Psychiat.) St. Vincent's Hosp. Dub.

WALSH, Eamonn John Mercheford House Surgery, Mercheford House, Elwyn Road, March PE15 9BT Tel: 01354 656841 Fax: 01354 660788 — MB BS Lond. 1980; MRCGP 1985; DRCOG 1985.

WALSH, Edward John (retired) Sandway, Thornton Gate, Thornton-Cleveleys FY5 1JN Tel: 01253 852704 — MRCS Eng. LRCP Lond. 1957 (Liverp.) DPH Liverp. 1963; MFCM 1974. Prev: Sen. Med. Off. DHSS.

WALSH, Edward Michael 7 Richmond PArk Road, Clifton, Bristol BS8 3AS — MB BS Lond. 1971 (St Bart.) BSc Lond. 1967; MRCS Eng. LRCP Lond. 1971; FFA RCS Eng. 1976. Cons. (Anaesth.) Southmead Hosp. Bristol. Specialty: Anaesth. Prev: Sen. Regist. (Anaesth.) Bristol Health Dist. (T); Cons. (Anaesth.) Oman Armed Forces; Lect. (Anaesth.) Lond. Hosp. Med. Coll.

WALSH, Eleanor Susan Torwold, 23 Ledcameroch Crescent, Bearsden, Glasgow G61 4AD — MB BCh BAO Dub. 1972; BA Dub. 1970; DA RCPSI 1974; FFA RCSI 1976. Cons. (Anaesth.) Stobhill Hosp., Glas. Specialty: Anaesth. Prev: Cons. (Anaesth.) Centr. Middx Hosp., Lond.; Sen. Regist. (Anaesth.) Hammersmith Hosp. Lond.

WALSH, Elizabeth Anna Maria 24 Warriner Gardens, London SW11 4EB — MB BCh BAO NUI 1991; DRCOG 1994; MRCGP 1995. Specialty: Gen. Pract.

WALSH, Elizabeth Maureen Fowberry House, The Green, Longframlington NE65 8AQ — MB BS Newc. 1975; DA Eng. 1980; MRCGP 1981.

WALSH, Geoffrey Parkin (retired) Winterton, Berrygate Lane, Sharow, Ripon HG4 5BJ Tel: 01765 605033 — MB ChB St. And. 1954; DObst RCOG 1955. Prev: Ho. Phys. Blackburn Roy. Infirm.

WALSH, Gillian Dianne Sutton Park Surgery, 34 Chester Road North, Sutton Coldfield B73 6SP Tel: 0121 353 2586 Fax: 0121 353 5289; 31 Marlpit Lane, Four Oaks, Sutton Coldfield B75 5PH — MB ChB Birm. 1984; BSc (Hons.) Birm. 1981; DRCOG 1988; MRCGP 1989. Prev: Trainee GP Sutton Coldfield VTS; SHO (O & G) Solihull Hosp.; SHO (Paediat.) Sandwell Dist. Gen. Hosp. Bromwich.

WALSH, Graham 3 Sunny Bank, Leeds LS8 4EB — MB BS Lond. 1998.

WALSH, Graham John Armada Surgery, 28 Oxford Place, Western Approach, Plymouth PL1 5AJ Tel: 01752 665805 Fax: 01752 220056 — MB ChB Bristol 1969; DFFP; D.Occ.Med.; DObst RCOG 1972. Gen. Practitioner - Plymouth; Occupational Health Pract. - Plymouth; Medico-Legal Reporting, Plymouth; Vasectomy Serv., Plymouth. Specialty: Family Plann. & Reproduc. Health; Occupat. Health. Socs: Plymouth Med. Soc.; Soc. Occupat. Med.; Plymouth Med. Centre Club. Prev: Accid. and Emerg. Dept., Plymouth; Family Plann. Clinic, Plymouth.

WALSH, Helen Margaret — MB ChB Sheff. 1988; DRCOG 1991; MRCGP 1993. GP Asst.

WALSH, Mr Henry Patrick John Lourde Hospital, Greenbank Road, Liverpool L18 1HQ — MB ChB Manch. 1978; FRCS Eng. 1982; MChOrth Liverp. 1985. Cons. Orthop. Surg. Alder Hey Childr. Hosp. & Fazakerley Hosp. Liverp. Specialty: Trauma & Orthop. Surg. Socs: Brit. Orthop. Assn; Foot & Ankle Soc.; Brit. Soc. Childr. Orthop. Surg. Prev: Sen. Lect. & Hon. Cons. (Orthop. & Accid. Surg.) Univ. Liverp.; Clin. Lect. & Hon. Sen. Regist. (Orthop. & Accid. Surg.) Univ. Liverp.; Regist. (Orthop.) Roy. Liverp. Hosp. & Alder Hey Childr. Hosp.

WALSH, Hilary Margaret The Doctors House, Victoria Road, Marlow SL7 1DN Tel: 01628 484666 Fax: 01628 891206; Jonquils, Frieth Road, Marlow SL7 2JQ Tel: 01628 486887 — MB ChB Liverp. 1971; DObst RCOG 1973.

WALSH, Ian 49 St Pauls Close, Farington Moss, Preston PR26 6RT — MB ChB Glas. 1998.

WALSH, Mr Ian Kinsella 3 Palace Gardens, Chichester Park, Belfast BT15 5DT — MB BCh BAO Belf. 1987 (Queens University of Belfast) FRCSI 1991; FRCPS Glas. 1991; MD Belf. 1998; FRCS (Urol) 1998. Cons. (Urol. & Neurol.) Belf. City Hosp. Specialty: Urol. Socs: Irish Radiat. Research Soc.; Assn. Surg. Train.; Brit. Assn. Urol. Surgs. Prev: Specialist Regist. (Urol.) Belf. City Hosp.; Vis. Asst. Prof. Dept. Urol. Univ. of Calif. Davis; Clin. Research Fell. & SHO (Urol.) Belf. City Hosp.

WALSH, Jacinta Marie 20 St Paul's Close, Adlington, Chorley PR6 9RS — MB BCh Wales 1993.

WALSH, James (retired) 53 Stockton Lane, York YO31 1BP Tel: 01904 424407 — (Cork) MB BCh BAO NUI 1943.

WALSH, James Bernard, OStJ 14 Ashley Park, Armagh BT60 1EU Tel: 028 3752 8332; 14 Ashley Park, Armagh BT60 1EU Tel: 028 3762 8332 — MB BCh BAO Belf. 1956; DPM RCPSI 1962; FRCPI 1986, M 1965; MRCPsych 1971. Private Pract. with some locum Appts. Specialty: Gen. Psychiat. Socs: BMA; R.Col. Psychiat.s. Prev: Cons. Psychiat. South. Health & Social Servs. Bd.; Cons. Psychiat. Tyrone & Fermanagh Hosp. Omagh; Sen. Regist. Purdysburn Hosp.

WALSH, James Michael Meade, RD, SBStJ Westcourt, 12 The Street, Rustington, Littlehampton BN16 3NX Tel: 01903 784311 Fax: 01903 850907; The Laurels, Ash Lane, Rustington, Littlehampton BN16 3BT Tel: 01903 773771 Fax: 01903 850907 — MB BS Lond. 1967 (Lond. Hosp.) MRCS Eng. LRCP Lond. 1967; DObst RCOG 1970. Med. Off. Littlehampton Hosp. & Zachary Merton Community Hosp. Rustington; Surg. Capt. RNR; Dep. Co. Surg. St. John Ambul. Brig. Sussex. Specialty: Gen. Pract. Socs: Fell. Roy. Soc. Med.; Assn. Police Surg.; BMA. Prev: Dir. Med. Reserves RNR; Regist. RN Matern. Unit Malta; Chairm. Social Servs. W. Sussex CC & Sussex Police Auth.

WALSH, James Sarto John 15 Broomyknowe, Edinburgh EH14 1JZ — LRCPI & LM, LRSCI & LM 1977; LRCPI & LM, LRCSI & LM 1977; FFR RCSI 1986; FRCR 1987.

WALSH, James Thomas 57 Station Road, Mickleover, Derby DE3 9GJ — MRCS Eng. LRCP Lond. 1969.

WALSH, Janet Elizabeth Richmond House, Grosvenor Road, Wrexham LL11 1BT Tel: 01978 350050 Fax: 01978 261243 — MB BS Lond. 1986; MRCPsych. Cons.. (Child & Adolesc. Psychiat.)Wrexham N.Wales. Specialty: Child & Adolesc. Psychiat.

WALSH, Jennifer Susan 39 Beauchief Rise, Sheffield S8 0EL — MB ChB Sheff. 1997. Clin. Res. Fel. Univ. Of Sheff.; Hon. SpR (Med.) North. Gen. Hosp. Sheff. Specialty: Gen. Med. Prev: SHO Med. Roy. Hallamshire Hosp. Sheff.

WALSH, Joanna Elizabeth Royal Alexandra Hospital, Corsebar Road, Paisley PA2 9PN Tel: 0141 314 6905 Email: jo.walsh@rah.scot.nhs.uk; Wellbank House, Campsie Glen, Glasgow G66 7AR — MB ChB Aberd. 1989; MRCP (UK) 1993. Cons. Paediat. + Paediat. Rheum. Roy. Alexandra Hosp. and Inverclyde Roy. Hosp.; Clin. Lect. Univ. of Glas. Specialty: Paediat. Socs: BMA; RCPCH; BSPAR. Prev: Specialist Regist. Paediat. (Rheum.) Gt. Ormond St. Hosp. Lond.; Specialist Regist. Paediat. (Rheum.) Birm. Childr.'s Hosp.; Regist. PICU Roy. Hosp. Sick Childr., Glas.

WALSH, Joanna Ismay 104 Howard Drive, Letchworth SG6 2DG — BM Soton. 1993; MRCP (paeds.) Lond. 1997; MRCGP UK 2000. GP Locum Bristol.

WALSH, Joanne The Health Centre, Back Hills, Botesdale, Diss IP22 4WG Tel: 01379 898295 — MB ChB Manch. 1992; DFFP; BSc St. And. 1989. Asst GP Botesdale Health Centre Botlesdale Diss (P/T). Specialty: Gen. Pract.

WALSH, John Christopher St. Stephen's Centre, 369 Fulham Road, London SW10 9TH Tel: 020 8746 8000 — MB BS Lond. 1989; MRCP (UK) 1994. Sen. Regist. (HIV & Genitourin. Med.) Chelsea & Westm. Hosp. Lond. Specialty: Genitourinary Medicine.

WALSH, Mr John Kingsley Princes Margaret Hospital, Osborne Road, Windsor SL4 3SJ Tel: 01753 841716 Fax: 01753 859407 Email: walsh@windsor91.fsnet.co.uk; 62 Kings Road, Windsor SL4 2AH Tel: 01753 840603 Email: walsh@windsor91.fsnet.co.uk — (University of Otago) MB ChB (Otago) 1962; FRCS (Ed) 1970; FRACS (Orth) 1971. Private Medico-Legal Cons., Princess Margt. Hosp., Windsor, SL4 3SJ; Medico-Legal Cons., 10 Harley St., Lond. W1G 3. Specialty: Orthop. Prev: Cons. Orhthopaedic Surg., Ashford Hosp. Middlx.

WALSH, John Paul Rosyth Surgery, 195 Queensferry Road, Rosyth, Dunfermline KY11 2LQ — MB BCh BAO Dub. 1990.

WALSH, John Terence — MB ChB Sheff. 1989; BMedSci. (Hons.) Sheff. 1988; MRCP (UK) 1992; FRCP 2003. Cons. Cardiol. Qu.s Med. Centre. Notts. Specialty: Cardiol. Socs: Brit. Cardiac Soc.; Brit. Soc. Heart Failure; Brit. Soc. Echocardiography. Prev: Research Fell. (Cardiol.) Qu. Med. Centre Nottm.; SHO (Gen. Med.) Roy. Hallamsh. Hosp. Sheff.; SHO (Gen. Med.) Qu. Med. Centre Nottm.

WALSH, Joseph Michael Greenfield House, 169 Kirk Road, Wishaw ML2 7BZ Tel: 01698 375544 Email: j.m.walsh@btinternet.com — MB ChB Glas. 1958. Prev: as below; Med. Mem. Indep. Tribunal Servs.; GP Princip. Health Centre Wishaw.

WALSH, Josephine Lynne Canute Surgery, 66A Portsmouth Road, Woolston, Southampton SO19 9AL Tel: 023 8043 6277 Fax: 023 8039 9751 — MB BCh Dublin 1974; MB BCh Dub. 1974. GP Soton.

WALSH, Joyce Bench Mark Barn, Elswick Lodge, Mellor, Blackburn BB2 7EX — MB ChB Ed. 1958.

WALSH, Kevin John Hinchingbrooke Hospital, Huntingdon PE29 6NT Tel: 01480 416416 Fax: 01480 416490; Orchard House, Bury Road, Ramsey, Huntingdon PE26 1NA Tel: 01487 815981 — BM BCh Oxf. 1979; MA Camb. 1980; DM Soton. 1992; FRCP Lond. 1998. Cons. Phys. Hinchingbrooke Healthcare NHS Trust Huntingdon. Specialty: Care of the Elderly. Socs: Brit. Geriat. Soc. Prev: Sen. Regist. (Geriat.) W. Midl. Regional Train. Scheme; Research Regist. MRC Soton.; Lect. (Rehabil.) Univ. of Soton.

WALSH, Lesley Jane 77 Wyatt Road, Sutton Coldfield B75 7NH Tel: 0121 378 4127 — MB ChB Bristol 1987; BA Open 1983; MRCP (UK) 1990. Regist. Rotat. (Gen. Med.) City Hosp. Nottm. Specialty: Gen. Med. Prev: SHO Rotat. (Gen. Med.) N. Birm. Gen. Hosp.; Ho. Off. (Geriat. Med.) Derbysh. Roy. Infirm.

WALSH, Mrs Margaret Litchfield Chingford Health Centre, 109 York Road, Chingford, London E4 8LF Tel: 020 8529 8655; 34 The Avenue, Loughton IG10 4PX Tel: 020 8508 6598 — MB ChB Sheff. 1965. SCMO Waltham Forest HA.

WALSH, Marie Therese Josephine 8 McLean Drive, Priorslee Grange, Priorslee, Telford TF2 9RT — MB BCh BAO NUI 1980; DCH RCPSI 1981; FRCR 1986. Cons. Radiol. Princess Roy. Hosp. Telford. Specialty: Radiol.

WALSH, Mark 121 Albert Drive, Sheerwater, Woking GU21 5QY — MB BS Lond. 1996.

WALSH, Martin Paul Seffield Occupational Health Service, Northern General Hospital, Herries Road, Sheffield S5 7AU Tel: 0114 271 4161 Fax: 0114 244 4470; 26 Stainmore Avenue, Sothall, Sheffield S20 2GN Tel: 0114 247 3845 — MRCS Eng. LRCP Lond. 1971; DObst RCOG 1974; MSc (Occupat. Med.) Lond. 1975; DIH Eng. 1976; DFFP 1996; DEBHC Oxf. 1998. Occupational hys., Sheff. Ocupational Health Serv., North. Gen. Hosp., Sheff.; Occupational hys., BMI Health Servs. Leeds. Specialty: Occupat. Health. Socs: Soc. of Occupat.al Med.; Assn. of NHS Occupat.al Health Phys.s. Prev: Trainee GP Neath VTS; Mem. Scientif. Staff MRC & DHSS Epidemiol. & Med. Care Unit Northwick Pk. Hosp. Harrow.; Gen. Practitioner, Birley Health Centre, Sheff. 1976-2000.

WALSH, Mary Clare Daintree Surgery, 98 Wentloog Road, Rumney, Cardiff CF3 8EU Tel: 029 2079 7746 Fax: 029 2079 0231 — MB BCh Wales 1985 (University of Wales College of Wales) DCH RCP Lond. 1988; DRCOG 1988. GP Princip.

WALSH, Mary Madeleine Theresa Women's Secure Services, Annesley House Hospital, Mansfield Rd, Annesley, Nottingham NG15 0AR Tel: 01623 727901 Fax: 01623 727927 — BM BS Nottm. 1978; MA Psychoanalytical Studies, Uni. Of E. London & Tavistock Clinic; BMedSci Nottm. 1976; MRCGP 1982; DCH RCP Lond. 1984; MRCPsych 1989. Cons. Forens. Psychiat. Wom.'s Secure Servs. Nottm. Specialty: Forens. Psychiat. Prev: Cons. Forens. Psychiat. Rampton Hosp. 1995-2001 Retford, Nottm.; Sen. Regist. Rotat. (Psychiat.) Nottm. Train. Scheme.

WALSH, Maureen Yvonne 30 Ravenhill Court, Belfast BT6 8FS — MB BCh BAO Belf. 1978.

WALSH, Melanie Frances Broadway Surgery, 2 Broadway, Fulwood, Preston PR2 9TH; 25 Bosburn Drive, Mellor Brook, Blackburn BB2 7PA — MB BCh BAO Belf. 1991; DRCOG 1993; MRCGP 1995.

WALSH, Mr Michael Edward Leeds Nuffield Hospital, 2 Leighton Street, Leeds LS1 3EB Tel: 0113 225 3823 Fax: 0113 225 3823 Email: mikewalsh@in2000.net; BUPA Hospital Leeds, Jackson Avenue, Leeds LS8 1NT Tel: 0113 269 3939; The Close, 7 Wetherby Road, Leeds LS8 2JU Tel: 0113 305 2459 — MB ChB Ed. 1978; FRCS Ed. 1984; MPhil Stathclyde 1989; FRCS (Orth.) Ed. 1992. Indep. Cons. Orthop. Surg. Specialty: Orthop. Special Interest: Rotator Cuff Tear; Shoulder Instability; Subacromial Impingment. Socs: Brit. Orthop. Assn. & Brit. Elbow & Shoulder Soc.; Brit. Soc. Surg. Hand. Prev: Cons. Orthopaedic & Upper Limb Surg., Gen. Infirm. at Leeds.

WALSH, Mr Michael Stephen Department of Surgery, The Royal London Hospital, London E1 1BB Tel: 020 7377 7723 Fax: 020 7377 7044; Fortune Cottage, Epping Green, Epping CM16 6QL Tel: 01992 577337 Fax: 01992 577337 — MB BS Lond. 1984 (St. Mary's) BSc Lond. 1981; FRCS Eng. 1988; MS Lond. 1996; FRCS 1997. Cons.Trauma Vasc. Surg. Roy. Lond. Hosp. Specialty: Gen. Surg. Socs: Vasc. Surg. Soc.; Assn. Surg.; Brit. Trauma Soc. Prev: Sen. Regist. (Vasc. Surg.) Univ. Coll. Hosp. Lond.; Sen. Regist. (Gen. Surg.) Southend Gen. Hosp.; Cons. (Gen. & Vasc. Surg.) Whipps Cross Hosp. Lond.

WALSH, Nigel Dennis 40A Apsley Road, Bristol BS8 2SS Tel: 01179 737450 — MRCS Eng. LRCP Lond. Lond. 1952 (St. Geo.) MRCGP 1970; FFM RCP UK 1989. Cons. pharmaceutical Phys.; The Med. expert partnership. Specialty: Pharmaceutical Medicine; Medico Legal. Socs: Fell. Roy. Soc. Med.; Brit. Assn. Pharmaceut. Phys. Prev: Med. Dir. Warner Lambert Internat.; Hon. Med. Off. Dorrigo Hosp., Austral.; Resid. Obst. Asst. St. Geo. Hosp. Lond.

WALSH, Patrick Francis 96 Brisbane Road, Largs KA30 8NN — MB ChB Glas. 1981; BSc Glas. (Immunol.) 1978, MB ChB 1981; FRCR 1987. Cons. Radiol. Inverclyde Roy. Hosp. Greenock. Specialty: Radiol. Prev: Regist/Sen. Regist. (Radiol.) Gtr. Glas. HB.; SHO (A & E/Orthop.) Hairmyres Hosp. E. Kilbride.

WALSH, Patrick Joseph Finton Millbrook, Little Malvern, Malvern WR14 4JP Tel: 01684 575554 — MB BS Lond. 1947 (Guy's) DPM Eng. 1955; DPM Eng. 1955; MRCPsych 1971; MRCPsych 1971. Specialty: Gen. Psychiat. Socs: Fell. Roy. Soc. Med.; BMA. Prev: Cons. Psychiat. S. Worcs. Hosp. Grp.; Asst. Psychiat. St. Bernard's Hosp. S.all; Sen. Regist. (Psychiat.) Warlingham Pk. Hosp.

WALSH, Patrick Martin (retired) 56 Main Street, Newcastle BT33 0AE Tel: 013967 23221; 3 The Fairways, Dundrum Road, Newcastle BT33 0RX Tel: 013967 24451 — MB BCh BAO Belf. 1953.

WALSH, Patrick Michael John 411 Allenby Road, Southall UB1 2HG — BM BCh Oxf. 1964; DPM Eng. 1967.

WALSH, Mr Patrick Vaughan Raigmore Hospital, Inverness IV2 3UJ Tel: 01463 704000 Fax: 01463 711322; Mid Feabuie, Culloden Moor, Inverness IV2 5EQ Tel: 01463 792534 — MB BS Lond. 1971 (Lond. Hosp.) FRCS Eng. 1977; MS Lond. 1983; FRCS Glas. 1993; FRCS Edin. 1999. Cons. Surg. Raigmore Hosp. Inverness. Specialty: Gen. Surg. Socs: Fell. Roy. Soc. Med.; BASO. Prev: Sen. Regist. (Surg.) Gtr. Glas. HB; Research Fell. (Surg.) Univ. Liverp.; Regist. (Surg.) Chester Roy. Infirm.

WALSH, Peter Alexander 12 Sykes Close, Greenfield, Oldham OL3 7PT — MB ChB Leeds 1991.

WALSH, Peter Roderick Steppes Mill House, Bodenham Moor, Hereford HR1 3HS — MRCS Eng. LRCP Lond. 1942 (Middlx.) MRCP Lond. 1952. Specialty: Cardiol.

WALSH, Raymond Staveleigh Medical Centre, King Street, Stalybridge SK15 2AE Tel: 0161 304 8009 Fax: 0161 303 7207; Fairhaven, 20 Werneth Road, Woodley, Stockport SK6 1HW — MB ChB Manch. 1972; DObst RCOG 1975.

WALSH, Redmond Clapham Family Practice, 51 Clapham High Street, London SW4 7TL Tel: 020 7622 4455 Fax: 020 7622 4466; 13 Brookwood Rise, Artane, Dublin 5, Republic of Ireland — MB BCh BAO NUI 1983; LRCPI & LM LRCSI & LM 1983.

WALSH, Richard Joseph 5 Kingsley Crescent, Long Eaton, Nottingham NG10 3DA Tel: 0160 76 62370 — MB BS Lond. 1973 (Guy's) MRCS Eng. LRCP Lond. 1973.

WALSH, Richard Nicholas 45 Dapdune Court, Woodbridge Road, Guildford GU1 4RU — MB ChB Birm. 1989.

WALSH, Mr Rory McConn Department Ear, Nose & Throat, Guy's Hospital, St Thomas St., London SE1 9RT; Flat 4, House 2, The Paragon, London SE3 0NX Tel: 020 8852 7505 — MB BCh BAO Dub. 1987; FRCS Eng. 1993. Regist. (ENT) Guy's & Lewisham Hosps. Lond. Specialty: Otolaryngol. Prev: SHO (ENT) Lewisham Hosp. Lond.; SHO (Gen. Surg.) Hammersmith Hosp. Lond.; Demonst. (Anat.) Trinity Coll. Dub.

WALSH, Ruth Clare Orchard House, 12A Station Road, Studley B80 7HS — MB BS Lond. 1998.

WALSH, Sarah Jane 13 York Street, Norwich NR2 2AN Tel: 01603 623461 — MB ChB Birm. 1992; FRCA 1998. Specialist Regist. Anglia Deanery. Specialty: Anaesth. Socs: Birm. Med. Res. Expeditionary Soc.; Intens. Care Soc. Prev: SHO (Anaesth.) Burton on Trent; SHO (ITU) Roy. Lond. Hosp.; SHO (Anaesth.) Birm. Heartlands Hosp.f.

WALSH, Simon James 1 Lagan Villas, Dromore BT25 1LN — MB BCh Belf. 1997.

WALSH, Simon James Meade The Laurels, 44 Ash Lane, Rustington, Littlehampton BN16 3BT — MB BS Lond. 1994 (Lond. Hosp.) MRCP(UK) 1999. Specialist Regist. (Accid. & Emerg. Med.) N. Thames E. Deanery. Specialty: Accid. & Emerg.; Gen. Med. Prev: SHO (Med.) Princess Alexandra Hosp. Harlow; SHO (Orthop.) Whipps Cross Hosp. Lond.; SHO (Elderly Med.) Whipps Cross Hosp. Lond.

WALSH, Simon Roy The Surgery, 2 Heathcote Street, Newcastle ST5 7EB Tel: 01782 561057 Fax: 01782 563907; Maple House, Church Road, Aston Juxta Mondrum, Nantwich CW5 6DR Tel: 01270 627868 — MB ChB Manch. 1979; Cert. FPA 1981.

WALSH, Stephanie 12 Church Lane, Nether Poppleton, York YO26 6LB — MB ChB Leeds 1985 (Univ. Leeds) MRCGP 1989. Clin. Asst. (Palliat. Med.) St. Leonards Hospice York. Specialty: Palliat. Med.

WALSH, Susan Jane Maple House, Church Road, Aston Juxta Mondrum, Nantwich CW5 6DR Tel: 01270 627868 — MB ChB Manch. 1981; DRCOG 1983; Cert. FPA 1985; MFFP 1994; Dip. Genito Urinary Med & Venerol 1999. SCMO (Family Plann.) Chesh. Community Healthcare Trust Nantwich; Clin.Asst.Genito-Urin. med.Roy.Liverp.Univ.Hosp. Specialty: Family Plann. & Reproduc. Health; Genitourinary Medicine.

WALSH, Terence John 19 Burrell Close, Prenton, Birkenhead CH42 8QE Tel: 0151 608 8353 — MRCS Eng. LRCP Lond. 1954.

WALSH, Mr Timothy Hays Roud Cottage, Roud, Ventnor PO38 3LH Tel: 01983 840675 — MB BS Lond. 1970 (Univ. Coll. Hosp.) BSc Physiol. 1966; FRCS Eng. 1975; MS Lond. 1984. Cons. Surg. St Mary's Hosp. Newport I. of Wight; Clin. Tutor I. of Wight; Mem. Ct. Examrs. RCS Eng. Specialty: Gen. Surg. Prev: Regist. (Surg.) Addenbrooke's Hosp. Camb.; Sen. Regist. (Surg.) Lond. Hosp.; Resid. Surg. Off. St. Mark's Hosp. Lond.

WALSH, Timothy Simon Lothian University NHS Trust/Lothian Health, New Edinburgh Royal Infirmary, Lauriston Place, Edinburgh EH3 9YW Tel: 0131 242 3136 Email: timothy.walsh@ed.ac.uk — MB ChB Ed. 1988 (Edin.) BSc (Hons.) Ed. 1986; MRCP (UK) 1991; FRCA 1994; MD (Edinburgh) 1999. Cons. Anaesth. IC RIE Edin; Hon. Sen. Lect. RIE. Specialty: Anaesth.; Intens. Care. Socs: Intens. Care Soc.; Scott. Intens. Care Soc.; BMA.

WALSH, William John St. Andrews at Harrow, Bowden House Clinic, London Road, Harrow-on-the-Hill, Harrow HA1 3JL Tel: 0208 966 7000 Fax: 0208 864 6092 — MB BS Queensland 1968 (University of Queensland, Australia) FRANZCP 1986; MRCPsych 1987. Cons. Psychiat., Bowden Ho. Clinic, Harrow on the Hill. Specialty: Gen. Psychiat. Special Interest: Adult Gen.; Forens. Socs: Australian and New Zealand College of Pychiatrists; Royal College of Psychiatry. Prev: Medical Director, P.I.C.U., Bowden House; Consultant Psychiatrist, West Herts NHS Trust; Consultant Psychiatrist, Ayesbury Vale NHS Tust.

WALSH, Mr William Kevin Plouer Hill House, Causey Hill, Hexham NE46 2DL — MB BS Newc. 1968; FRCS Eng. 1973. Orthop. Surg. Gen. Hosp. Hexham. Prev: Sen. Regist. Birm. Accid. Hosp.; Sen. Regist. (Orthop.) & Regist. (Orthop.) Robt. Jones & Agnes Hunt Hosp. OsW.ry.

WALSH, William Roger Lane End, Glen Auldyn, Lezayre, Ramsey IM7 2AD Tel: 01624 812213 — MB BChir Camb. 1948 (Guy's & Camb.) MA Camb. 1948.

WALSH-WARING, Mr Gerald Patrick (retired) Corace House, Broad St., East Isley, Newbury RG20 7LW — MB BS Lond. 1958 (St. Mary's) DLO Eng. 1962; FRCS Eng. 1964. Hon. Cons. ENT Surg. Hammersmith Hosp. Lond.; Cons. i/c Jt. St. Mary's & Hammersmith Hosps. Head & Neck Oncol. Serv.; Examr. for Fellowship Otolaryngol. RCS Eng. Prev: Sen. Regist. (ENT) St. Mary's Hosp. Lond.

WALSHAM, Anna Clare The Old Hall, 1 High St., Billingborough, Sleaford NG34 0QA — MB ChB Manch. 1997.

WALSHAW, Carol Anne Oakworth Health Centre, 3 Lidget Mill, Oakworth, Keighley BD22 7HN Tel: 01535 643306 Fax: 01535 645832 — MB ChB Liverp. 1974.

WALSHAW, Colin Francis Radiology Dept, Victoria Hospital, Blackpool FY3 8NR Tel: 01253 306912 Fax: 01253 306960 — MSc Manch. 1991, MB ChB 1984; MRCP (UK) 1987; FRCR 1994. Cons. Radiol. Vict. Hosp. Blackpool. Specialty: Radiol. Prev: Sen.Reg.Radiol.Univ.Hosp.Wales.Cardiff.

WALSHAW, Martin John 12 Moreton Road, Upton, Wirral CH49 6LL — MB ChB Liverp. 1978.

WALSHAW, Mr Nigel William David (retired) 10a Bosley Way, Christchurch BH23 2HF Tel: 01460 63359 — MRCS Eng. LRCP Lond. 1965 (Guy's) BChir 1965; LMSSA Lond. 1965; MA (Double 1st cl. Hons.) Camb. 1962, MB 1966; DO Eng. 1969; FRCS Eng. 1971. Prev: Cons. Ophth. Surg. Roy. Gwent Hosp. Newport.

WALSHAW, Russell John The Surgery, Manlake Avenue, Winterton, Scunthorpe DN15 9TA Tel: 01724 732202 Fax: 01724 734992 — MB ChB Sheff. 1966; MRCGP 1971. Med. Sec. N. Lincs. & E. Yorks. LMC; Mem. Gen. Med. Servs. Comm. Specialty: Gen. Pract. Socs: BMA. Prev: SHO (Obst.) Nether Edge Hosp. Sheff.; Ho. Surg. Sheff. Roy. Hosp.; Ho. Off. (Med.) Sheff. Roy. Infirm.

WALSHE, Adrian Dominic Flat 24, Elmwood Court, Pershore Road, Birmingham B5 7PD — MB BS Newc. 1985.

WALSHE, David Kevin 31 Cambridge Road, Linthorpe, Middlesbrough TS5 5NG Tel: 01642 88662 — MB BCh BAO Dub. 1943 (TC Dub.) BA, MB BCh BAO Dub. 1943. Police Surg. Co. Boro. Middlesbrough; Med. Off. Remand Home Middlesbrough. Socs: Assn. Med. Internat. de Notre Dame de Lourdes. Prev: Ho. Surg. Ho. Phys. & Res. Surg. Off. N. Ormesby Hosp. Middlesbrough.

WALSHE, Elaine Teresa 45 Ashwood Avenue, Bridge of Don, Aberdeen AB22 8XH — MB BCh BAO NUI 1985.

WALSHE, Ethna Ann (retired) Glencroft, 213 Wythenshawe Road, Manchester M23 9DB Tel: 0161 998 3511 — MB ChB Glas. 1952; DA Eng. 1956. Prev: Ho. Off. Redlands Hosp. Wom. Glas. & Stockton & Thornaby Hosp.

WALSHE, Geraldine Miriam (retired) 7 Minley Close, Cove, Farnborough GU14 9RT — MB BCh BAO NUI 1955.

WALSHE, John Michael Department Neurology, Middlesex Hospital, London W1N 8AA Tel: 020 7636 8333 Ext: 4873; Broom Lodge, 58 High Street, Hemingford Grey, Huntingdon PE28 9BN Tel: 01480 462487 — (Univ. Coll. Hosp.) MB BChir Camb. 1945; FRCP Lond. 1964, M 1949; MA Camb. 1945, ScD 1965; MD (hon. causa) Uppsala 1994. Hon. Sen. Lect. (Med.) UCL & (Neurol.) Middlx. Hosp. Lond. Socs: Assn. Phys. Prev: Bilton Pollard Trav. Fell. Boston City Hosp.; Reader (Metab. Dis.) Univ. Camb.; Hon. Cons. Phys. Addenbrooke's Hosp. Camb.

WALSHE, Kieran Gerard Dundrum Surgery, 14 Church View, Dundrum, Newcastle BT33 0NA Tel: 028 43751267 Email: dundrum@donardgroup.freeserve.co.uk — (Univ. Coll. Cork) MB BCh BAO Univ. Coll. Cork 1977; MD (NUI) 1985; MRCGP 1986; MICGP 1986. Eli Lilly Research Fell. (Metab. Unit) Roy. Vict. Hosp. Belf.; Specialist (Diabetes) Lagan Valley Hosp. Lisburn. Socs: Eur. Assn. Study Diabetes. Prev: Regist. (Med. & Endrocrinol.) Roy. Vict. Hosp. Belf.; Intern & SHO Limerick Regional Hosp.; Lilly Research Fell.

WALSHE, Margaret Mary (retired) 9 Church End., Haddenham, Aylesbury HP17 8AH Tel: 01844 291731 — MB BS Lond. 1956 (Roy. Free) MRCS Eng. LRCP Lond. 1956; DObst RCOG 1958; FRCP Lond. 1976, M 1962. Prev: Cons. Dermat. Aylesbury, Milton Keynes & Wycombe HAs.

WALSHE, Mary Bridget Anne 40 Spratt Hall Road, London E11 2RQ — MB BCh BAO Dub. 1978; MB BCh Dub. 1978.

WALSHE, Peadar Bernard Marybrook Medical Centre, Marybrook Street, Berkeley GL13 9BL Tel: 01453 810228 Fax: 01453 511778 — MB BCh BAO Dub. 1981. Socs: BMA (Counc. Mem. Glos. Br.).

WALSHE-BRENNAN, Kieran Stanislaus Apartment 9 Moygannon Court, Warrenpoint, Newry BT34 3JW Tel: 016937 52530; c/o Sir Patrick McKenna, 19 Barrule Park, Ramsey Tel: 01624 812071 — MSc Belf. 1949, MB BCh BAO 1957; DPH Belf. 1961; DPM Dub. 1965; MRCPsych 1971; MFCM 1974. Specialty: Gen. Psychiat.; Child & Adolesc. Psychiat.; Pub. Health Med. Socs: Fell. Roy. Soc. Health; Fell. Roy. Inst. Pub. Health & Hyg.; FRSS. Prev: Clin. Lect. Sheff. Univ. 1966-1971; Cons. Psychiat. Mersey RHA, Roy. Hallamsh. Hosp. Sheff. & Yorkton & Melville Hosps. Canada.; Lect. Keele Univ. 1975-1982 and Examr.

WALSMA, Pieter Whitefields Surgery, Hunsbury Hill Road, Camp Hill, Northampton NN4 9UW Tel: 01604 760171 Fax: 01604 708528 — Artsexamen Groningen 1976.

WALSTER, Verity Margaret Joanna Hedon Group Practice, Market Hill House, 4 Market Hill, Hull HU12 8JD — MB ChB Glas. 1991; DFFP 1994; MRCGP 1995. GP Princip. Hedon Gp. Pract., Hedon; Clin. Med. Off. (Reproductive & Sexual Health) E. Yorks. Community Healthcare Trust. Specialty: Family Plann. & Reproduc. Health; Diabetes. Prev: GP Asst. Old Fire Station Pract. Beverley.

WALSWORTH-BELL, Joanna Pierce South Staffordshire Health Authority, Mellor House, Corporation St., Stafford ST16 3SR Tel: 01785 52233; Junction House, Fradley Junction, Alrewas, Burton-on-Trent DE13 7DN Tel: 01283 791457 — MB BS Lond. 1971 (St. Bart.) MRCS Eng. LRCP Lond. 1971; DCH Eng. 1975; MSc (Social Med.) Lond. 1978; MFPHM Eng. 1981; MSSc Manchester 1992. Cons. Pub. Health Med. S. Staffs. HA. Specialty: Pub. Health Med. Socs: Fell. Fac. Pub. Health Med. Prev: Regional Specialist Pub. Health Med. NW RHA; Sen. Regist. (Community Med.) St. Thos. Hosp. Lond.; Regist. (Community Med.) Hants. AHA (T).

WALT, Helen J Yardley Green Medical Centre, 73 Yardley Green Road, Bordesley Green, Birmingham B9 5PU Tel: 0121 773 3838 Fax: 0121 506 2005; 48 Westfield Road, Edgbaston, Birmingham B15 3QG Tel: 0121 246 4649 Email: nikkiwalt@tiscali.co.uk — MB BS Lond. 1978 (Westm.)

WALT, Robert Peter Birmingham Heartlands Hospital, Bordesley Green E., Birmingham B9 5ST; 48 Westfield Road, Edgbaston, Birmingham B15 3QG — MB ChB Birm 1976; MRCP (UK) 1978; MD Birm. 1986; FRCP Lond. 1992. Cons. Phys. (Gastroenterol.) Birm. Heartlands Hosp. Specialty: Gastroenterol. Prev: Sen. Lect. & Hon. Cons. Dept. Med. Qu. Eliz. Hosp. Birm.; Lect. & Hon. Sen. Regist. (Therap.) Univ. Hosp. Nottm.; Regist. Acad. Dept. Med. Roy. Free Hosp. Lond.

WALTER, Christine Marian 1 Rye Gardens, Oakdale, Blackburn BB2 4HF — MB BS Lond. 1972; DObst. RCOG 1973; DCH RCP Lond. 1976. Prev: Clin. Med. Off. (Child Health.) Mid. Downs HA.

WALTER, Christopher John Stephen (retired) 326 Columbine Road, Ely CB6 3WR — MB BS Lond. 1960 (Lond Hosp.) DPM Eng. 1965; FRCPsych 1987, M 1971. Prev: Cons. Psychiat. Princess Alexandra Hosp. Harlow & Herts. & Essex Gen. Hosp. Bishop's Stortford.

WALTER, Mr Darren Paul South Manchester University Hospital, Southmoor Road, Manchester M23 9LT — MB ChB Manch. 1989; FRCS Ed. 1993; Dip. Immediate Med. Care RCS Ed. 1998; FFAEM 2000. Cons. (Emerg. Med.) S. Manch. Univ. Hosp. Specialty: Accid. & Emerg. Socs: Brit. Assn. Immed. Care Schemes. Prev: Specialist Regist. (Emerg. Med.) Yorks. Region; HEMS Regist. Roy. Lond. Hosp.

WALTER, Fiona Mary Mutlow Hall, Wendens Ambo, Saffron Walden CB11 4JL; Mutlow Hall, Wendens Ambo, Saffron Walden CB11 4JL Tel: 01799 540440 Email: fmw22@medschl.cam.ac.uk — MB BChir Camb. 1983 (St. Thos.) MA Camb. 1982; DCH RCP Lond. 1984; DRCOG 1985; FRCGP 1995, M 1987; MSC Lond. 2000. p/t Research Fell., GP & Primary Care Research Unit, Univ. of Camb.; GP. Asst.. Dr Stephens and Partners, Camb. Specialty: Gen. Pract.

WALTER, Hazel Pamela Steeple View, 3 Yarkhill Court Barns, Yarkhill, Hereford HR1 3TD Tel: 01432 890320 Fax: 01432 890360 Email: hazelwalter@compuserve.com — (Middlx.) MRCS Eng. LRCP Lond. 1968; MB BS Lond. 1968; DObst RCOG 1970; MRCGP 1980; DMJ(Clin) Soc. Apoth. Lond. 1994; DFFP 1994. p/t Forens. Phys. W. Mercia; Adviser in Clin. Forens. Med. to Gwent Constab. Specialty: Genitourinary Medicine; Family Plann. & Reproduc. Health; Alcohol

& Substance Misuse; Medico Legal. Special Interest: Clin. Forens. Med. aspects of sexual abuses assault. Socs: Roy. Soc. Med. (Counc. Clin. Forens. Med. Sect.); Assn. Police Surg.; Brit. Assn. Forens. Sci. Prev: Clin. Asst. (Genitourin. Med.) Ambrose King Centre, The Roy. Lond. Hosp.; Clin. Asst. Dermat. (Chace Wing) Enfield Dist. Hosp.; GP Trainer Palmers Green Lond.

WALTER, Ian McNeil 63 Thanet Road, Bexley DA5 1AP — MRCS Eng. LRCP Lond. 1947 (Lond. Hosp.)

WALTER, James Andrew Stokenview Medical Centre, Oxford Road, Stokenchurch, High Wycombe HP14 3SX Tel: 01494 483633 Fax: 01494 483690; Luke House, Water End, High Wycombe HP14 3XH — (St. Mary's) MRCS Eng. LRCP Lond. 1970; DCH Eng. 1973. Prev: Trainee Gen. Pract. Cirencester Vocational Train. Scheme; Med. Off. Tarawa, Kiribati.

WALTER, Joanna Clare 27 Vicarage Gardens, Scunthorpe DN15 7BA — MB BChir Camb. 1989.

WALTER, John Hugh The Cottage, 15 Blantyre Road, Swinton, Manchester M27 5ER — MB BS Lond. 1978 (St. Mary's) DCH RCP Lond. 1983; MRCP (UK) 1984; MSc Lond. 1987, MD 1990; FRCP Lond. 1996; FRCPCH Lond. 1997. Cons. Paediat. (Inherited Metab. Dis.) Roy. Manch. Childr. Hosp. Specialty: Paediat. Socs: Chair of Coun. of Soc. for the study of inborn errors of Metab.; Brit. inherited Metab. Dis. gp. Prev: Lect. (Child Health) Univ. Bristol; Clin. Research Fell. Inst. Child Health Lond.

WALTER, Lilian Starr (retired) 2 Searle Road, Farnham GU9 8LJ — MB BS Lond. 1950 (Roy. Free) DObst RCOG 1953.

WALTER, Margaret Valerie Church Farm House, Ripple, Deal CT14 8JL Tel: 01304 372113 — (Lond. Hosp.) MB BS Lond. 1958; MRCS Eng. LRCP Lond. 1959; DO Eng. 1966. Clin. Asst. (Ophth.) Kent & Canterbury Hosp. Specialty: Ophth. Prev: Clin. Asst. Ophth. Roy. Vict. Hosp. Folkestone & Vict. Hosp. Deal; Gyn. & Obst. Ho. Off. & Ho. Surg. Roy. Vict. Hosp. Folkestone.

WALTER, Michael The Surgery, 1 Arlington Road, Eastbourne BN21 1DH Tel: 01323 727531 Fax: 01323 417085; 16 Compton Drive, Eastbourne BN20 8BU — MB BS Lond. 1965 (Guy's) MRCS Eng. LRCP Lond. 1965; DObst RCOG 1968; FRCGP 1988, M 1975. Prev: SHO (Paediat.) St. Luke's Hosp. Guildford; Ho. Surg. & Ho. Phys. Roy. Surrey Co. Hosp.

WALTER, Nigel Richard The Surgery, 24 Albert Road, Bexhill-on-Sea TN40 1DG Tel: 01424 730456/734430 Fax: 01424 225615; 23 Little Twitten, Cooden, Bexhill-on-Sea TN39 4SS Tel: 01424 843394 — MB BS Lond. 1981; DRCOG 1986; MRCGP 1986.

WALTER, Norah (retired) 4 Sunbury Avenue, East Sheen, London SW14 8RA — MB BCh BAO Belf. 1943; DCH Eng. 1947; MFCM 1974. Prev: Princip. Med. Off. Richmond, Twickenham & Roehampton HA.

WALTER, Mr Pelham Howard Hurstwood Park Hospital, Haywards Heath RH16 7SJ Tel: 01444 441881 Fax: 01444 417995 — MB BS Lond. 1969 (Lond. Hosp.) BSc Lond. 1966, MB BS 1969; FRCS Eng. 1975. Cons. (Neurosurg.) Hurstwood Pk. Hosp., Haywards Heath. Specialty: Neurosurg. Socs: BMA. Prev: Sen. Regist. (Neurosurg.) Lond. Hosp. Whitechapel; Regist. (Neurosurg.) Brook Hosp. Lond.; Regist. (Neurosurg.).

WALTER, Rachel Mary 21 Weston Lea, West Horsley, Leatherhead KT24 6LG — MB ChB Sheff. 1989; DRCOG 1994; MRCGP 1994.

WALTER, Robert David Ellaslea, 29 Castle Douglas Road, Dumfries DG2 7PA — MB ChB Leic. 1994; MRCGP 1998. GP Reg Dunscore. Specialty: Gen. Pract.

WALTER, Timothy Neil The Falkland Surgery, Monks Lane, Newbury RG14 7DF Tel: 01635 40160 — MB BS Lond. 1985; MRCGP 1990. Specialty: Anaesth.

WALTERS, Alexander Demetrius West End Road Surgery, 62 West End Road, Bitterne, Southampton SO18 6TG Tel: 023 8044 9162 Fax: 023 8039 9742 — MB BS Lond. 1986. Specialty: Gen. Med.

WALTERS, Alun James (retired) Roseland, Poltimore, Exeter — MRCS Eng. LRCP Lond. 1949 (Guy's) LDS RCS Eng. 1942; BDS Lond. 1943. Prev: Dent. Surg. W. Eng. Sch. For Partially Sighted, Exeter.

WALTERS, Anita Sian Elm Lodge Surgery, 43 Gloucester Road North, Filton, Bristol BS7 0SN — MB ChB Bristol 1992; BSc Hons (Physiol.) Bristol 1988; MRCGP 1997.

WALTERS, Anna Ellen 24 Prenton Hall Road, Birkenhead CH43 0RA — BM BCh Oxf. 1990; BA (Hons.) Oxf. 1987; FRCS Ed. 1994. Specialist Regist. (Plastic Surg.)Norf. & Norwich Univ. Hosp. Specialty: Plastic Surg. Prev: SHO (Plastic) Qu. Mary's Univ. Hosp. Lond.; SHO (Gen. Surg. & A & E) Hammersmith Hosp. Lond.; SPR Plastics Addenbrookes.

WALTERS, Anne Marisia Wessex Renal Unit, Queen Alexandra Hospital, Cosham, Portsmouth PO6 3LY; 18 Park Crescent, Emsworth PO10 7NT — MB ChB Glas. 1982; FRCS Eng. 1986; FRCS Ed. 1986; FRCS Glas. 1986; MD Glas. 1994. Cons. (Gen. & Transpl. Surg.) Wessex Renal & Transpl. Unit Qu. Alexandra Hosp. Cosham Portsmouth. Specialty: Gen. Surg. Prev: Cons. Gen. & Transpl. Surg. Portsmouth Hosps. NHS Trust; Lect. (Surg.) Univ. Camb.; Career Regist. W. Yorks.

WALTERS, Antony Mayford House Surgery, Boroughbridge Road, Northallerton DL7 8AW Tel: 01609 772105 Fax: 01609 778553; 25 South Parade, Northallerton DL7 8SG Email: antony.walters@btinternet.com — MB ChB Liverp. 1983; Dip. Health Econ. Aberd 1990; Dip. In Travel Medicine Glasgow 1999. Princip. Gen. Pract., Northallerton, N. Yorks; Mem. N. Yorks. LMC. Special Interest: Med. in Motorsport; Travel Med. Socs: Internat. Soc. Travel Med. Prev: Team Doctor for Ford World Rally Team (2000); GP Ceduna, S. Australia (1988-1989); SHO (A & E) N. Manch. Gen. Hosp. (1984).

WALTERS, Audrey Marguerite Bedgrove Surgery, Brentwood Way, Aylesbury HP21 7TL Tel: 01296 330330 Fax: 01296 399179; Exwing Cottage, Meadway, Oving, Aylesbury HP22 4EX Tel: 01296 640867 — MB BS Lond. 1982 (St. Mary's) DRCOG 1985; MRCGP 1986.

WALTERS, Brian Tennant (retired) 43 Bennett Drive, Hove BN3 6US — LRCP LRCS Ed. LRFPS Glas. 1949 (Ed.) Prev: Resid. Med. Off. Profess. Orthop. Unit Roy. Infirm. Edin.

WALTERS, Carolyn Clare 15 Barnard Road, Leigh-on-Sea SS9 3PH — BM Soton. 1994 (Southampton) DRCOG 1998; DFFP 1998; MRCGP 2001. GP Rochford, Essex. Specialty: Gen. Pract.; Family Plann. & Reproduc. Health. Prev: Salaried Rotating Gen. Practitioner, C/o S. Essex Health Auth. Arcadia Ho., The Drive, Brentwood; GP Regist., N. St. Med. Care Rainsford; SHO (O & G) Southend Hosp.

WALTERS, Catherine Charlotte (retired) 4 Parsonage Close, Stratford-Sub-Castle, Salisbury SP1 3LP — MB ChB Bristol 1949.

WALTERS, Catrin Mallt Alder Hey Hospital, Community Paediatrics, Mulberry House, Eaton Road, Liverpool L12 2AP Tel: 0151 252 5252 Fax: 0151 252 5076 Email: mallt.walters@rlc.nhs.uk; 49 Menlove Avenue, Cauderstones, Liverpool L18 2EH — MB ChB Liverp. 1977; DRCOG 1979; DCH 1983; MRCP (UK) 1992. Cons. Community Paediat. Roy. Liverp. Childr. NHS Trust; Med. Off. (Paediat. A & E) Alderhey Hosp. Specialty: Paediat. Socs: MRCPCH. Prev: Cons. Community Paediat. W. Lancs. NHS Trust Ormskirk.

WALTERS, Constance (retired) 89 Regent Road, Leicester LE1 6YG Tel: 0116 256 4141 — MB BCh Wales 1924 (Cardiff) BSc Wales 1921, MB BCh 1924. Prev: Asst. Ophth. Leicester Roy. Infirm. & Sch. Clinics Leicester Co.

WALTERS, Professor Dafydd Vaughan Department of Child Health, St. George's Hospital Medical School, Cranmer Terrace, London SW17 0RE Tel: 020 8725 5973 Fax: 020 8725 2858 Email: dwalters@sghms.ac.uk — MB BS Lond. 1971 (Univ. Coll. Lond.) BSc (Physiol.) Lond. 1968; FRCP Lond. 1988, M 1974; FRCPCH 1997. Prof. Child Health St. Geo. Hosp. Med. Sch. Lond. Specialty: Paediat. Socs: Eur. Soc. Paed. Res.; Sec. Assoc. Clin. Profs. Paediat.; Dep. Chairm. of Exec. Comm.. Physiol. Soc. Prev: Reader & Hon. Cons. Paediat. Univ. Coll. Lond.; MRC Trav. Fell. CVRI Univ. Calif. Med. Centre San Francisco, USA.

WALTERS, Daniel Desmond Dept. of Paediatrics, Bronglais General Hospital, Aberystwyth SY23 1ER Tel: 019 7062 3131 Fax: 019 7063 — MB BCh Wales 1966; DCH Eng. 1969; MRCP (UK) 1973; MSc Lond. 1975; FRCP Lond. 1996; FRCPCH 1997. Cons. Paediat. Bronglais Gen. Hosp. Aberystwyth. Specialty: Paediat. Prev: Sen. Regist. (Paediat.) Oxf. RHA; Regist. Westm. Hosp. Lond.; Research Asst. Middlx. Hosp. Lond.

WALTERS, David Paul Salisbury District Hospital, Odstock Road, Salisbury SP2 8BJ; Flanders Field, Brook Street, Fovant, Salisbury SP3 5JB Tel: 01722 714896 Email: david.walters1@virgin.net —

LMSSA Lond. 1981 (Royal Free Hospital, London) MD Lond. 1992, MB BS 1982; MRCP (UK) 1986; FRCP 1997. Cons. Phys. Salisbury Dis. Hosp. Specialty: Rehabil. Med. Special Interest: Stroke Dis. Socs: Brit. Diabetic Assn. (Med. & Scientif. Sect.); Brit. Geriat. Soc. Prev: Sen. Regist. (Gen. & Geriat. Med.) Oxf.; BDA Research Fell. Poole Gen. Hosp.; Regist. Rotat. (Med.) Soton. & Salisbury.

WALTERS, Elizabeth Anne Child & Family Consultation Service, The Royal London Hospital, Whitechapel, London E1 1BB Tel: 020 7377 7390 Fax: 020 7247 3699 — MB ChB Glas. 1972; MRCPsych 1984. Cons. Child Psychiat.The Roy. Lond. Hosp. Whitechapel. Specialty: Child & Adolesc. Psychiat. Prev: Cons. Child Psychiat. Pk. Hosp. for Childr. Oxf.

WALTERS, Frances Judith Vale Pleasant, Silverdale, Newcastle ST5 6PS — MB BS London 1983; MB BS London 1983.

WALTERS, Mrs Frances Mary The Medical Centre, 377 Stamfordham Road, Westerhope, Newcastle upon Tyne NE5 2LH Tel: 0191 286 9178 Fax: 0191 271 1086; Lane End House, Main St, Corbridge NE45 5LE Tel: 0143 463 2281 — MB ChB Glas. 1965. Br. Med. Off. N.d. Red Cross; Chairm. New. LMC. Socs: BMA & Brit. Med. Pilots Assn. Prev: Regtl. Med. Off. 101 Fd. Regt. RA(V); Ho. Surg. Good Hope Hosp. Sutton Coldfield; Ho. Phys. Newc. Gen. Hosp.

WALTERS, Francis James MacDonald Frenchay Hospital, Anaesthetic Department, Bristol BS16 1LE Tel: 0117 970 2020 Fax: 0117 957 4414 Email: frank.walters@north-bristol.swest.nhs.uk; Parson's Well, Littleton-on-Severn, Bristol BS35 1NR Tel: 01454 412531 Fax: 0870 162 3992 Email: frank@drwalters.org.uk — (Univ. Coll. Hosp.) MB BChir Camb. 1970; MA Camb. 1971; FFA RCS Eng. 1974. Cons. Anaesth. Frenchay Hosp. Bristol. Specialty: Anaesth. Special Interest: Daycare Anaesth.; Neuroanaesthetics. Socs: (Past Pres.) Neuro Anaesth. Soc. Gt. Britain and Irel.; Assn. Anaesth.; (Past Pres.) Plastic Surg. & Burns Anaesth. Prev: Lect. (Anaesth.) Univ. Soton.; Clin. Fell. (Anaesth.) Hosp. Sick Childr. Toronto, Canada; Ho. Surg. Univ. Coll. Hosp. Lond.

WALTERS, Mr Gavin Harrogate District Foundation Trust, Lancaster Park Road, Harrogate HG2 7SX Tel: 01423 553580 — MB ChB Leeds 1990; MRCP (UK) 1993; FRCOphth 1996. Cons. Ophth. Surg., Harrogate/ York; Hon. Cons. Ophth., York. Specialty: Ophth. Special Interest: Age Related Mascular Degeneration; Small Incision Cataract Surg.; Diabetic Retinopathy.

WALTERS, Gerald Ernest (retired) Pine Trees, Forest Road, Grantown-on-Spey PH26 3JL — MB Calcutta 1949. Prev: Med. Off. Brit. Honduras.

WALTERS, Giles Desmond Department of Neptrology, Leicester General Hospital, Gwendolen Road, Leicester LE5 4PW Email: gilesw@doctors.net.uk — MB ChB Ed. 1990; BA Camb. 1987; MRCP (UK) 1993. Specialist Regist. (Renal Med.) Leic. Gen. Hosp. Specialty: Nephrol. Prev: Regist. Rotat. (Renal) Leicester Gen. Hosp.; SHO Rotat. (Gen. Med.) Lothian.; SHO (Gen. Med.) Falkirk & Dist. Roy. Infirm.

WALTERS, Glyn (retired) Rockhurst, Burwash, Etchingham TN19 7HW Tel: 01435 882525 — MB BS Lond. 1949 (Roy. Lond. Hosp.) MRCS Eng. LRCP Lond. 1949. Prev: Ho. Surg. Lond. Hosp.

WALTERS, Glyndwr (retired) 4 Parsonage Close, Stratford-Sub-Castle, Salisbury SP1 3LP — MD Bristol 1958, MB ChB 1949; FRCP Lond. 1971, M 1952; FRCPath 1970, M 1963. Prev: Cons. Chem. Pathol. Bristol Roy. Infirm.

WALTERS, Helen Mary Queenswood Surgery, 223 London Road, Waterlooville PO8 8DA Tel: 023 9226 3491; Rivendell, Hill House Hill, Liphook GU30 7PX Tel: 01428 751969 Email: charles.walters@which.net — MB ChB Leic. 1989 (Leicester University) DRCOG 1993; Dip Health Managem Keele 1996. GP Waterlooville; Primary Care Med. Adviser N. & Mid Hants HA; PCG Bd. Mem.

WALTERS, Huw Llewellyn 34 Alleyn Road, Dulwich, London SE21 8AL — MB BCh Wales 1966; DMRD Eng. 1975; FRCR 1978.

WALTERS, James Howard Parsons Well, The Village, Littleton-upon-Severn, Bristol BS35 1NR — MB BS Lond. 1998.

WALTERS, Joanne — MB ChB Sheff. 1988 (Sheffield) MRCP (UK) 1992; MRCGP 1995. Clin. Med. Off. (Family Plann.) E. Yorks. Specialty: Gen. Pract. Prev: Clin. Asst. Diabetes/Endocrinol.

WALTERS, John Christopher 4 The Old School, Whiteshill, Stroud GL6 6AB — MB ChB Ed. 1965; DO Eng. 1974. Specialty: Ophth.

WALTERS, John Duncan, OStJ, Surg. Capt. RN Retd. (retired) Two Ways, 30 St John's Road, Cosham, Portsmouth PO6 2DR Tel: 023 9237 6599 — MB BS Lond. 1951 (Univ. Coll. Hosp.) DIH Soc. Apoth. Lond. 1956; DPH 1959; MFCM 1974; MFOM RCP Lond. 1979. Prev: Cons. Pub. Health Med. St. Mary's Hosp. Portsmouth.

WALTERS, John Nicholas Whitfield, 26 Station Approach, Shepperton TW17 8AL Tel: 01932 231003 Email: nickwalters@medix-uk.com — MB BCh Wales 1978 (Welsh Nat. Sch. Med.) DA (UK) 1981; DRCOG 1983; MRCGP 1987; Dip Musculoskel Med. 1997; MLCOM 1997; MSc 1997. Civil. Med. Practitioner Defence Med. Servs. Train. Centre Aldershot; Private Pract. Osteop. & Orthop. Med. Specialty: Orthop. Socs: Fell. Roy. Soc. Med.; BMA. Prev: Squadron Ldr. RAF Med. Br.; Ships Surg. P & O Steam Navigation Co.; Surg. Lt. Cdr. RN.

WALTERS, Julian Roger Ford Imperial College London, Gastroenterology Section, Hammersmith Hospital, Du Cane Road, London W12 0NN Tel: 020 8383 2361 Fax: 020 8749 3436 Email: julian.walters@imperial.ac.uk — MB BChir Camb. 1975; MRCP 1977; FRCP 1993. Reader (Gastroenterol.) Imp. Coll. Lond.; Hon. Cons. Gastroenterol. Hammersmith Hosp. Lond. Specialty: Gastroenterol. Special Interest: Intestinal Diseases. Socs: Brit. Soc. Gastroenterol.; Amer. Gastroenterol. Assn.; Assn. Phys. Prev: Lect. (Gastroenterol.) Guy's Hosp. Lond.; Asst. Prof. State Univ. New York, Buffalo.

WALTERS, Katherine Rachel Dept of Primary Care Sciences, Royal Free & University College London Medical School, Archway Campus Holborn Union Building Highgate Hill, London N19 5NF Email: k.walters@ucl.ac.uk — BM BS Nottm. 1992; BMedSci (Hons.) Nottm. 1990; DCH RCP Lond. 1995; DFFP 1996; DRCOG 1996; MRCGP 1997. Clin. Lect. Primary Care UCL; GP Asst. Lond. Specialty: Gen. Pract. Socs: Mem. BMA; Fell.Roy.Soc.Med. Prev: Reg.Lond.Academ.Train.Scheme.

WALTERS, Mark Ian 24 Hayward Close, Walkington, Beverley HU17 8YB — MB ChB Sheff. 1988; MRCP (UK) 1992. Specialty: Gen. Med.

WALTERS, Martin David Stewart St. Mary's Hospital, South Wharf Road, London W2 1BL — MB BChir Camb. 1977; FRCP (UK) 1996. Sen. Lect.(Paedia Infec. Diseases) Imperial Coll. of Sci. & Med.; Hon. Cons. (Paedia.) St Marys Hosp. London. Specialty: Paediat.

WALTERS, Mary Elizabeth (retired) 2 Dollar Street, Cirencester GL7 2AJ Tel: 01285 2953 — MRCS Eng. LRCP Lond. 1948 (UCL and W. Lond.) BSc Lond. 1942; LLCO 1968. Prev: Clin. Asst. (Physical Med.) Princess Margt. Hosp. Swindon.

WALTERS, Matthew Robertson 98 Southbrae Drive, Glasgow G13 1TZ — MB ChB Glas. 1994.

WALTERS, Melvyn Terence Department of Rheumatology, Latilla Building, Royal Sussex County Hospital, Eastern Road, Brighton BN2 5BE Tel: 01273 696955 Ext: 4630 Fax: 01273 673466; Hundred Steddle Barn, Brighton Road, Woodmancote, Henfield BN5 9RT — MB ChB Manch. 1975 (Manchester) MRCP (UK) 1979; DCH RCP Lond. 1981; DM Soton. 1989; FRCP Lond. 1993. Cons. Rheum. Roy. Sussex Co. Hosp. Brighton. Specialty: Rheumatol.

WALTERS, Morgan De Parys Medical Centre, 23 De Parys Avenue, Bedford MK40 2TX Tel: 01234 350022 Fax: 01234 213402 — MB BCh Wales 1986.

WALTERS, Nigel Stewart Helmsley Medical Centre, Carlton Road, Helmsley, York YO62 5HD Tel: 01439 770288 Fax: 01439 771169 Email: nigel.walters@gp-b82068.nhs.uk; 4 Flatts Lane, Wombleton, York YO62 7RU Tel: 01751 431827 — MB BS Lond. 1971; BSc (Hons. Pharmacol.) Lond. 1968; DObst RCOG 1975.

WALTERS, Pamela Mary Bethel Villa, Llannon, Llanelli SA14 8JW — MB BCh Wales 1993.

WALTERS, Patricia Elizabeth Forge Road Surgery, Forge Road, Southsea, Wrexham LL11 5RR Tel: 01978 758311 Fax: 01978 752351 — MB ChB Manch. 1978. GP Wrexham.

WALTERS, Patricia Lynne Lane End House, Main St., Corbridge NE45 5LE — MB ChB Glas. 1995. Specialty: Gen. Pract.

WALTERS, Philip John Waterloo House Surgery, Waterloo House, 42-44 Wellington Street, Millom LA18 4DE Tel: 01229 772123; Wood House, The Hill, Millom LA18 5HG — MB ChB Liverp. 1983. Prev: SHO (Radiother. & Geriat.) Cumbld. Infirm. Carlisle.

WALTERS, Richard Bryn Builth Surgery, Glandwr Park, Builth Wells LD2 3TN Tel: 01246 568518 — MB BS Lond. 1992 (St. Geo.

Hosp. Med. Sch.) DRCOG 1994; Cert. Prescribed Equiv. Exp. JCPTGP 1996; DFFP 1996; MRCGP 1996. Specialty: Gen. Pract. Prev: Trainee GP N. Gwent VTS.

WALTERS, Richard Lewis Kettering General Hospital, Rothwell Road, Kettering NN16 8UZ Tel: 01536 492254; Cartref, Grafton Underwood, Kettering NN14 3AA — MB BS Lond. 1965 (St. Marys) FRCP Lond. 1971. Cons. Phys. (Geriat. & Gen. Med.) Kettering Health Dist. Specialty: Gen. Med.; Care of the Elderly. Socs: Roy. Coll. of Physicians; Brit. Geriat. Soc.

WALTERS, Mr Robert Frederick Cardiff Eye Unit, University Hospital of Wales, Cardiff CF14 4XW Tel: 029 2074 3862 — MB BS Lond. 1982 (Roy. Free Hosp. Sch. Med.) BSc (Hons.) Aberd. 1971; DO RCS Eng. 1986; FRCS Eng. 1986; FRCOphth 1988; FRCS Edin. 2003. Cons. Ophth. Univ. Hosp. Wales Cardiff. Specialty: Ophth. Socs: BMA; Roy. Soc. Med. Prev: Sen. Regist. (Ophth.) Soton & Portsmouth HAs; Sen. Regist. Moorfields Eye Hosp. Lond.

WALTERS, Roger Owen, Lt.-Col. RAMC Retd. Child Health, North Hampshire Hospital, Aldermaston Road, Basingstoke RG24 9NA Tel: 01256 314798 Fax: 01256 314796 Email: roger.walters@nhht.nhs.uk; 2 Vyne Meadow, Sherborne St. John, Basingstoke RG24 9PZ Tel: 01256 850457 — MB BS Lond. 1963 (St. Thos.) FRCPCH; DCH Eng. 1970; DTM & H Eng. 1971; MRCP (UK) 1975; FRCP Lond. 1987. Cons. Paediat.; Adoption Med. Adviser, Hants. CC. Specialty: Paediat. Socs: BMA. Prev: Cons. Paediat. Camb. Milit. Hosp. Aldershot; Cons. Paediat. Brit. Milt. Hosp., Hong Kong.; Med. Director, Loddon NHS Trust.

WALTERS, Sarah Department of Public Health & Epidemiology, Medical School, University of Birmingham, Birmingham B15 2TT Tel: 0121 414 6760 Fax: 0121 414 7788 Email: s.walters@bham.ac.uk — MB BS Lond. 1985 (St. George's Hosp. Med.Sch.) BSc (Hons.) Surrey 1980; MRCP (UK) 1988; MFPHM RCP (UK) 1992; FFPHM (UK) 1999; FRCP (UK) 1999. Sen. Lect. (Pub. Health & Epidemiol.) Univ. Birm. Med. Sch. Specialty: Pub. Health Med. Socs: Brit. Thorac. Soc. Prev: Lect. (Pub. Health Med.) Univ. Birm. Med. Sch.; Trainee (Pub. Health Med.) W. Midl. RHA; Regist. (Chest Med.) E. Birm. Hosp.

WALTERS, Sarah Elizabeth 14 Green Leys, St Ives, Huntingdon PE27 6SB — BChir Camb. 1996.

WALTERS, Susan Jayne 34 Alleyn Road, Dulwich, London SE21 8AL — MB BCh Wales 1966.

WALTERS, Miss Tena Kerry Kent House, Oast East, Court Lane, Hadlow, Tonbridge TN11 0PX — MB BS Lond. 1983 (St Bart.) FRCS Eng. 1987; MS Lond. 1994. Cons. (Gen. Surg./Breast) & Lead Clinician Qu. Mary's Sidcup. Specialty: Gen. Surg. Socs: RSM; Assn. Surg.; BASO. Prev: SHO Rotat. (Surg.) Kent & Canterbury Hosp; Sen. Regist. (Gen. Surg.) Welsh Train. Scheme; Lect. (Gen. Surg.) Profess. Unit Med. Coll. St Bart. Hosp. Lond.

WALTERS, Walter Duncan Alloa Health Centre, Marshill, Alloa FK10 1AB Tel: 01259 212088 Fax: 01259 724788; 18 Kellie Place, Alloa FK10 2DW Tel: 01259 215186 — MB ChB Glas. 1968. Socs: BMA. Prev: Ho. Off. (Surg.) Ballochmyle Hosp.; Ho. Off. (Med.) Roy. Alexandria Infirm.

WALTERSON, Laurence Imlach (retired) Craiglea, Biggar ML12 6RE Tel: 01899 221542 — MB ChB Aberd. 1957.

***WALTHER, Axel** Accident & Emergency Department, Addenbrooke's Hospital, Cambridge CB2 2QQ Tel: 01223 245151; Gluckstrasse 11, Hanau 63452, Germany — BM BCh Oxf. 1997 (Oxford) MA (Hons.) Camb. 1994. SHO (A & E) Addenbrooke's Hosp. Camb. Specialty: Accid. & Emerg.

WALTHEW, Richard Ian 13 Priory Road, Wilmslow SK9 5PS — MB BCh Wales 1992 (Univ. Wales Coll. Med. Cardiff) BSc (Hons) Wales 1989; MRCGP 1996.

WALTON, Alexander (retired) Stonegate Lodge, Love Lane, Spalding PE11 2PE Tel: 01775 724759 Fax: 01775 766168 — (Newc.) MB BS Durh. 1965; MRCGP 1975. Police Surg. Spalding; Med. Off. Johnson Hosp. Spalding; Clin. Asst. Welland Hosp. Spalding. Prev: SHO, Ho. Phys. & Ho. Surg., Newc. Gen. Hosp.

WALTON, Anna Marie 17 Rees Drive, Coventry CV3 6QF — BM Soton. 1995. SHO Rotat. (Gen. Med.) Princess Margt. Hosp. Swindon. Specialty: Gen. Med. Prev: RMO (Emerg. Med.) Fremantle Hosp., Australia.

WALTON, Anthony William James 18 Glebe Drive, Rayleigh SS6 9HJ — MB BCh Witwatersrand 1973; T(GP) 1991.

WALTON, Bryan 9 Loom Lane, Radlett WD7 8AA Tel: 0115 925 5542 Fax: 01923 853570; 9 Loom Lane, Radlett WD7 8AA Tel: 01923 853923 Fax: 01923 853570 — (Lond. Hosp.) MB BS Lond. 1966; FFA RCS Eng. 1970. Hon. Cons. Anaesth. & Intens. Care Roy. Lond. Hosp. Trust.; Adviser. Anaesth/Intens. care Princess Grace Hosp. Specialty: Anaesth.; Intens. Care. Prev: Cons. Anaesth. Roy. Lond. Hosp.

WALTON, Caroline Elizabeth Richmond Medical Centre, 462 Richmond Road, Sheffield S13 8NA Tel: 0114 239 9291 Fax: 0114 253 0737 — MB ChB Sheff. 1982; MRCGP 1986.

WALTON, Christopher 23 Ferriby High Road, North Ferriby HU14 3LD — MB BS Newc. 1974; MRCP (UK) 1977; FRCP Lond. 1993. Cons. Phys. (Gen. Med., Diabetes & Endocrinol.) Hull Roy. Infirm. Specialty: Endocrinol.; Diabetes; Gen. Med. Socs: Brit. Diabetic Assn. Prev: Sen. Regist. (Med.) Hull & Leeds Rotat. Hull Roy. Infirm. & Leeds Gen. Infirm.; Tutor (Med.) Manch. Roy. Infirm.; Regist. (Med. & Diabetes) St. Jas. Univ. Hosp. Leeds.

WALTON, Christopher James Fulwell Medical Centre, Ebdon Lane, off Dene Lane, Sunderland SR6 8DZ Tel: 0191 548 3635 — MB ChB Birm. 1980.

WALTON, David Alan Parkgate Health Centre, Park Place, Darlington DL1 5LW Tel: 01325 462396; 242 Carmel Road N., Darlington DL3 9TG — MB BS Durh. 1960. Socs: BMA. Prev: Squadron Ldr. RAF Med. Br.; SHO & Ho. Surg. (O & G) Newc. Gen. Hosp.

WALTON, David John O'Colmain and Partners, Fearnhead Cross Medical Centre, 25 Fearnhead Cross, Warrington WA2 0HD Tel: 01925 847000 Fax: 01925 818650; The Cottage, Bellhouse Lane, Grappenhall, Warrington WA4 2SG — BSc (Hons.) Manch. 1981, MB ChB 1984; DCH RCP Lond. 1986; DRCOG 1987; MRCGP 1989; Dip Occ Med 2000. Prev: Trainee GP; SHO (Cas.) Hope Hosp.; SHO (Psychiat.) Bridgewater Hosp.

WALTON, Dorothy Patricia Mayday Hospital, Thornton Heath, Croydon CR7 7YE Tel: 020 8401 3000; 3 Hoadly Road, Streatham, London SW16 1AE Tel: 020 8769 1791 — (Char. Cross) MB BS Lond. 1968; MRCS Eng. LRCP Lond. 1968; FFA RCS Eng. 1974. Cons. Anaesth. Mayday Hosp. Thornton Heath. Specialty: Anaesth. Prev: Regist. (Anaesth.) Westm. Hosp. Lond.; SHO (Anaesth.) St. Geo. Hosp. Lond. & St. Jas. Hosp. Lond.

WALTON, Douglas Ashley Hugh (retired) Sunnybank, Quarry Lane, Allithwaite, Grange-over-Sands LA11 7QJ Tel: 0153 95 32188 — MB Calcutta 1941; DMRD Eng. 1950. Prev: Cons. Radiol. Rochdale HA.

WALTON, Eileen Elizabeth Ty Mawr Gwyn, Flemingston, Barry CF62 4QJ Tel: 01446 750410 — MB BS Durh. 1957.

WALTON, Ernest Ward, TD (retired) 32 The Green, Norton, Stockton-on-Tees TS20 1DX Tel: 01642 554653 — MD Durh. 1957; MB BS 1949; FRCPath 1972, M 1963. JP. Prev: Chairm. Exec. Med. Dir., Cleveland Med. Laborat. Ltd.

WALTON, Gail Margaret Littlewick Medical Centre, 42 Nottingham Road, Ilkeston DE7 5PR Tel: 0115 932 5229 Fax: 0115 932 5413; 44 Church Lane, Cossall, Nottingham NG16 2RW — MB ChB Bristol 1983; DRCOG 1987; MRCGP 1988. Trainee GP Heanor VTS, Derbysh. Prev: SHO (Paediat. & O & G) S. Derbysh. HA.

WALTON, Gary Michael Appleby, 93 Knutsford Road, Row of Trees, Alderley Edge SK9 7SH — MB ChB Manch. 1995; BDS Manch. 1984; MDS Manch. 1989; FDS RCS Ed. 1989; MSc Manch. 1994; FRCS Eng. 1997; FRCS (OMFS) 2000. SpR Northwest Maxillofacial Surg. Rotat. Specialty: Oral & Maxillofacial Surg. Socs: BMA; Brit. Assn. Oral & Maxillofacial Surgs.; Brit. Assn. Head & Neck Oncologists. Prev: SHO (Gen. Surg.) Wythenshawe Hosp. Manch.; SHO Orthop. Wythenshawe Hosp. Manch.; Lect. & Hon. Regist. (Oral & Maxillofacial Surg.) Univ. Manch.

WALTON, Heather Ann Stewart The Allport Surgery, Treetops Primary Healthcare Centre, Bridle Road, Bromborough, Wirral CH62 6AR Tel: 0151 328 5630 — MB ChB Liverp. 1992; DRCOG 1996 Birm. GP; GP The Allport Surg., Treetops Primary Healthcare Centre, Bridle Rd., BromBoro., Wirral. Prev: SHO (Paediat.) Chester; GP/Regist. Neston; SHO (O & G) Wirral.

WALTON, Professor Henry John 38 Blacket Place, Edinburgh EH9 1RL Tel: 0131 667 7811 Fax: 0131 662 0337 — MB ChB Cape Town 1946; MD Cape Town 1954; DPM Lond. 1956; FRCP Ed. 1968, M 1966; PhD Ed. 1966; FRCPsych 1971; MD (Hons.)

Uppsala 1984; MD (Hons.) Lisbon 1990; MD (Hons.) Tucuman 1992. Prof. Emerit. Psychiat. & Internat. Med. Educat. Univ. Edin.; Edr. Med. Educat. Specialty: Gen. Psychiat. Socs: (Ex-Pres.) Assn. Med. Educat. Europe; (Ex-Pres.) World Federat. Med. Educat. Prev: Prof. Dept. Psychiat. Univ. Edin.; Sen. Regist. Maudsley Hosp. Lond.; Sen. Research Fell. (Psychiat.) Coll. Phys. & Surg. Columbia Univ. NY, USA.

WALTON, Ian James 14 Horseley Heath, Tipton DY4 7QU Tel: 0121 557 2027 Email: ianwalton@btinternet.com — MB BS Lond. 1980; MRCGP 1986. Hosp. Practitioner in Psychiat., Dudley Relief Cinic; Chair. Tipton Care Organisation PMS Project. Specialty: Gen. Pract.

WALTON, Ian Thomas Hallgarth Surgery, Cheapside, Shildon DL4 2HP Tel: 01388 772362 Fax: 01388 774150; The Beeches, West Layton, Richmond DL11 7PS Tel: 01325 718201 — MB ChB Dundee 1979.

WALTON, Ivan George Department of Medicine of Elderly, Charing Cross Hospital, Fulham Palace Road, London W6 8RF; 31 Grafton Square, London SW4 0DB — BM BCh Oxf. 1968; MA Oxf. 1968; MRCP (UK) 1974; MSc 1974; DObst RCOG 1976; FRCP Lond. 1990. Cons. Geriat. Char. Cross Hosp. Lond. Specialty: Care of the Elderly; Gen. Med. Special Interest: Dementia. Socs: Brit. Geriat. Soc.; Brit. Med. Assn. Prev: GP Teignmouth, Devon.

WALTON, James Hartley 20 Sinah Lane, Hayling Island PO11 0EY — MB BS Lond. 1968; MRCS Eng. LRCP Lond. 1967; DA Eng. 1979.

WALTON, Jane Catherine 10 Wolds Drive, Farnborough, Orpington BR6 8NS — MB BS Lond. 1992 (St. Mary's Hospital Paddington) BSc (Hons.) Lond. 1991. Specialist Regist. St. Geo.'s Rotat. Specialty: Anaesth.

WALTON, Jennifer Margaret 110 Monton Road, Eccles, Manchester M30 9HG — MB ChB Manch. 1979; DRCOG 1982.

WALTON, Jill Deirdre National Blood Service East Anglia Centre, Long Road, Cambridge CB2 2PT Tel: 01223 548000; Raggles, Noons Folly, Newmarket Road, Royston SG8 7NG Tel: 01763 244616 Email: jdh@raggles.fsnet.co.uk — MB BCh Witwatersrand 1965; FFA RCS Eng. 1971. Med. Off. Nat. Blood Trans. Serv. Specialty: Blood Transfus.

WALTON, John Alexander Walton and Partners, West Street Surgery, 12 West Street, Chipping Norton OX7 5AA Tel: 01608 642529 Fax: 01608 645066; New England, Hastings Hill, Churchill, Chipping Norton OX7 6NA Tel: 01608 658249 Email: jwalton@supanet.com — MB ChB Cape Town 1975; DRCOG 1981; MRCGP 1982; FRCGP 1999. GP Trainer Chipping Norton; PEC Chair, Cherwell Vale PCT. Specialty: Gen. Pract. Socs: BMA; RCGP. Prev: SHO (Paediat.) Red Cross Childr. Hosp. Cape Town; SHO (GP Linked) Horton Gen. Hosp. Banbury; Med. Supt. St. Matthews Gen. Hosp. Ciskei S. Afr.

WALTON, John Leaver Leicester Terrace Health Care Centre, 8 Leicester Terrace, Northampton NN2 6AL Tel: 01604 33682 Fax: 01604 233408 — BM BCh Oxf. 1972; MA, MSc; MRCGP 1977; FRCGP 1997. Prev: SHO Northampton Gen. Hosp.; Ho. Off. Radcliffe Infirm. Oxf.

WALTON OF DETCHANT, Right Honourable Lord John Nicholas, TD (retired) The Old Piggery, Detchant, Belford NE70 7PF Tel: 01668 213374 Fax: 01668 213012 Email: waldetch@aol.com — MB BS (1st cl. Hons.) Durh. 1945 (Newc.) Hon. FRCPC 1984; Hon. MD Sheff. 1987; Hon. DSc Hull 1988; Hon. DCL Newc. 1988; Laurea Hon. Causa Genea 1992; Hon. FRCPath 1993; Hon. FRCPsych 1993; Hon. DSc Oxf. Brookes 1994; FRCP Lond. 1963, M 1950; MD Durh. 1952; DSc Newc. 1972; Hon. Dr. de l'Univ. Aix-Marseille 1975; Hon. DSc Leeds 1979; Hon. DSc Leic. 1980; Hon. FACP 1980; Hon. FRCP Ed. 1981. Hon. Fell. (Ex-Warden) Green Coll. Oxf. Prev: Pres. Gen. Med. Counc. 1982-89.

WALTON, Jonathan James 34 Newbould Lane, Sheffield S10 2PL — MB ChB Sheff. 1994.

WALTON, Kenneth Robert 7 Leighton Avenue, Pinner HA5 3BW — MB BS Lond. 1976; MA Camb. 1973; MRCP (UK) 1979.

WALTON, Professor Kenneth Walter William Henry 7 Selly Close, Selly Park, Birmingham B29 7JG Tel: 0121 471 5223 Email: kwaltonb29@hotmail.com — MRCS Eng. LRCP Lond. 1942 (Univ. Coll. Hosp.) MD Lond. 1949, MB BS 1942; FRCPath 1965; PhD Birm. 1954, DSc 1976. Emerit. Prof. Birm. Univ.; Hon. Cons. Birm. AHA (T). Specialty: Pathology, General; Rheumatol.; Immunol. Socs: Fell. Roy. Soc. Med.; Path. Soc. Prev: Asst. Pathol. Dept. Morbid Anat. Univ. Coll. Hosp. Med. Sch.; Maj. RAMC, Specialist in Path. Army Path. Serv.

WALTON, Krystyna Floyd Unit for Neurological Rehabilitation, Birch Hill Hospital, Rochdale OL12 9QB Tel: 01706 754240 Fax: 01706 754241 Email: krystyna.walton@exchange.rhc-tr.nwest.nhs.uk — MB ChB Liverp. 1977; MRCP (UK) 1980; FRCP Lond. 1995; Europ. Dip. Phys. Med. & Rehab. 1995. Cons. Rehabil. Med. Rochdale healthcare NHS Trust; Cons. Rehabil. Med. Highbank Brain Injuiry Unit, Bury; hon cons in rehab, Salford Roy. Hosp.s NHS Trust. Specialty: Rehabil. Med. Prev: Sen. Regist. (Rheum. & Rehabil.) NW RHA; Regist. (Neurol.) N. Manch. Gen. Hosp.

WALTON, Linda Margaret 3 Beechwood Terrace, Newport-on-Tay DD6 8JG Tel: 01382 543194 — MB ChB Liverp. 1974; FFA RCS Eng. 1979. Assoc. Specialist (Anaesth.) Ninewells Hosp. Dundee. Specialty: Anaesth.

WALTON, Lynda Jane 32 Marton Drive, Wolviston Court, Billingham TS22 5BA Tel: 01642 553770 — BM BS Nottm. 1996; MRCPCH; BMedSci 1994. SpR Paediat. Nottm. Specialty: Paediat. Prev: Resid. Med. Off. Qu. Eliz. II Hosp. Brisbane Australia; SHO Paediat. Nottm.

WALTON, Margaret Jean 22 Chapel Street, Milborne St Andrew, Blandford Forum DT11 0JP — MRCS Eng. LRCP Lond. 1957; DCH Eng. 1964. Assoc. Specialist (Paediat.) Dorchester & W. Dorset Hosp. Gp. Prev: Res. Med. Off. Odstock Hosp. Salisbury; Paediat. Regist. Bournemouth & E. Dorset Hosp. Gp.

WALTON, Mark Ronald Yorkshire Street, 80 Yorkshire Street, Burnley BB11 3BT Tel: 01282 420141 Fax: 01282 832477 — MB ChB Leic. 1983.

WALTON, Melanie Jane 239 Hubert Road, Selly Oak, Birmingham B29 6ES — MB ChB Birm. 1995.

WALTON, Michael Robert High House, West Harsley, Northallerton DL6 2DR — MB BS Lond. 1969; FFA RCS Eng. 1975. Cons. Anaesth. Friarage Hosp. N.allerton. Specialty: Anaesth. Prev: Anaesth. Regist. Radcliffe Infirm. Oxf.; Sen. Regist. Addenbrooke's Hosp. Camb. & Norf. & Norwich Hosp.

WALTON, Neil Patrick 4 Tower Close, Horsham RH13 0AF — MB BS Lond. 1993.

WALTON, Nicolas 20 Bridgebank Road, Smithybridge, Littleborough OL15 8QU — MB ChB Leic. 1988.

WALTON, Nina Kylie Dorothy — MB ChB Leic. 1995. SPR Anaesth. Specialty: Anaesth.

WALTON, Paul Robert The Surgery, Cross Road, Sacriston, Durham DH7 6LJ Tel: 0191 371 0232; Ford House, Ford Road, Lanchester, Durham DH7 0SH Tel: 01207 521345 — MB ChB Manch. 1977; BSc St. And. 1974.

WALTON, Peter Kenneth Henry Playhatch Farmhouse, Foxhill Lane, Playhatch, Reading RG4 9QT — MB BChir Camb. 1982; MA Camb. 1985; MBA Lond. 1988. Managing Dir. Dendrite Clin. Systems Ltd. Lond. Prev: Sen. Managem. Cons. Internat. Hosps. Gp.; Resid. (O & G) Nat. Guard King Khalid Hosp. Jeddah.

WALTON, Rebecca Sarah High House Farm, West Harsley, Northallerton DL6 2DR — BM BS Nottm. 1994.

WALTON, Richard Stuart Castlecroft Medical Practice, 104 Castlecroft Road, Castlecroft, Wolverhampton WV3 8LU Tel: 01902 761629 Fax: 01902 765660 — MB ChB Birm. 1969.

WALTON, Robert Douglas 56 St Johns Crescent, Clowne, Chesterfield S43 4EB — MB ChB Manch. 1977.

WALTON, Robert John Grove Medical Practice, Shirley Health Centre, Grove Road, Shirley, Southampton SO15 3UA Tel: 023 8078 3611 Fax: 023 8078 3156; 21 Holly Hill, Southampton SO16 7ES Tel: 02380 769847 — MB BS Lond. 1968 (King's Coll. Hosp.) BSc (Physiol.) Lond. 1965; DPhil Oxf. 1979; MRCGP 1985; FRCP 2002. Prev: Lect. Univ. Soton.; Fell. Research Univ. Oxf.; Regist. (Med.) Radcliffe Infirm. Oxf.

WALTON, Robert Thompson Bury Knowle Health Centre, 207 London Road, Headington, Oxford OX3 9JA Tel: 01865 761651 Fax: 01865 768559; 24 Staunton Road, Headington, Oxford OX3 7TW — MB BS Lond. 1983 (St. Geo.) BSc Lond. 1980; MRCP (UK) 1986; DCH RCP Lond. 1986; MRCGP 1987; FRCGP 2000; FRCP 2001. Socs: Med. Protec. Soc. Prev: SHO (O & G) Ashford Hosp. Middlx.; SHO (Gen. Med.) St. Geo. Hosp. Lond.; Clin. Asst. (Gastroenterol.) Wycombe Gen. Hosp.

WALTON, Sharon Marie 166 Kirkham Road, Freckleton, Preston PR4 1HU — MB BS Newc. 1994; DFFP.

WALTON, Shernaz Department of Dermatology, The Princess Royal Hospital, Saltshouse Road, Hull HU8 9HE Tel: 01482 676794 Fax: 01482 676791 Email: shernaz.walton@hey.nhs.uk — MB BS Bombay 1973; DV & D Bombay 1974; MD Bombay 1976; MRCP UK 1980; FRCP Lond. 1999. Cons. Dermatol. Hul and E. Yorks. NHS Trust and York Med. Sch. Specialty: Dermat. Special Interest: Acne; Skin Cancers. Socs: Med. Protec. Soc.; N. of Eng. Dermatological Soc.; Brit. Assn. of Dermatologists. Prev: Cons. Dermatol. Scunthorpe; Locum Cons. Dermatol., Roy. Hull Hosps. NHS Trust; Sen. Regist., (Hull / Leeds).

WALTON, Simon Anthony 157 Chewton Street, New Eastwood, Nottingham NG16 3JR — MB BS Newc. 1992.

WALTON, Simon Murray Eastbourne District General Hospital, East Sussex Hospitals NHS Trust, Department of Anaesthesia, Kings Drive, Eastbourne BN21 2UD — MB BS Lond. 1994 (St Mary's Hosp. Med. Sch.) MA (Med. Ethics and Law) Keele 2004. Cons. in Anaesth. and Intens. Care. Specialty: Anaesth.; Intens. Care.

WALTON, Stephen 14 Whiteadder Way, Isle of Dogs, London E14 9UR — MD Manch. 1978; MB ChB 1973; MRCP (U.K.) 1976. Cons. Cardiol. Aberd. Roy. Infirm. Specialty: Cardiol.

WALTON, Stephen Frederick Stockwell Road Surgery, 21 Stockwell Road, Knaresborough HG5 0JY Tel: 01423 867433 Fax: 01423 869633 — BSc (Hons.) (Med. Biochem. Studies) Birm. 1976, MB ChB 1979; DRCOG 1982; DCH RCP Lond. 1982; MRCGP 1983. Prev: Trainee GP Harrogate; SHO Selly Oak Hosp. Birm.

WALTON, Stephen Robert Finlow Hill Cottage, Finlow Hill Lane, Over Alderley, Macclesfield SK10 4UG — MB ChB Sheff. 1995.

WALTON, Stuart Michael University Hospital of North Tees, Stockton-on-Tees TS19 8PE Tel: 01642 624218 Fax: 01642 624209 — MB BS Newc. 1968; FRCOG 1985, M 1973; MFFP 1993. Cons. O & G N. Stockton-on-Tees; Sen. Clin. Lect., Univ. of Newc. upon Tyne. Specialty: Obst. & Gyn. Special Interest: Hysteroscopic Surg.; Menstrual Disorders. Socs: Brit. Soc. of Gyn. Endoscopy. Prev: Regional Coll. Adviser; Lect. (O & G) Univ. Nairobi, Kenya.; Sen. Lect. (O & G) Wellington Clin. Sch. Med. Wellington, NZ.

WALTON, Susan Elizabeth The Surgery, Cross Road, Sacriston, Durham DH7 6LJ Tel: 0191 371 0232; Ford House, Ford Road, Lanchester, Durham DH7 0SH Tel: 0191 521345 — MB ChB Manch. 1979; BSc (Med. Sci.) St. And. 1976.

WALTON, Susan Elizabeth Community Health Office, Nuffield Health Centre, Welch Way, Witney OX28 6JQ Tel: 01993 776920; Minster Cottage, Church St, Charlbury, Oxford OX7 3PR Tel: 01608 811096 — MB ChB Bristol 1963; Dip. Community Paediat. Warwick 1983. Sen. Med. Off. (Child Health & Family Plann.) Oxf. Radcliffe Hosp. NHS Trust. Specialty: Family Plann. & Reproduc. Health. Socs: Brit. Paediat. Assn.; Foundat. Mem. Fac. Community Health; Fac. Family Plann. & Reproduc. Health Care. Prev: Hon. SHO (Paediat.) Radcliffe Infirm. Oxf.; Clin. Med. Off. Harrow Health Dist.; Asst. Sch. Med. Off. Salop CC.

WALTON, Suzanne Joy South Essex Health Authority, Arcadia House, The Drive, Warley, Brentwood CM13 3BE Email: suzanne.walton@sessex-ha.nthames.nhsuk — MB BS Lond. 1994 (UCMSM) BSc London 1991; MRCPH 1999; MSc London 2001. Specialty: Pub. Health Med.; Paediat. Prev: SpR Paediat. St John's Hosp. Chelmsford; SHO Gt. Ormond St. Hosp.; SHO (Paediat.) Princess Alexandra Hosp. Harlow Essex.

WALTON, Thomas James 5 Sandfield Close, Scunthorpe DN17 2XE Email: tjwalton@doctors.org.uk — BM BS Nottm. 1998.

WALTON, Wendy Jane Marden Medical Practice, 25 Sutton Road, Shrewsbury SY2 6DL Tel: 01743 241313; Holm House, Station Road, Pontesbury, Shrewsbury SY5 0QY Tel: 01743 792714 Email: wendy-jane@doctors.org.uk — MB BS Lond. 1982; DA Eng. 1984; DRCOG 1985; MRCGP 1987. GP.

WALTON-SMITH, Peter Russell (retired) 6 The Birches Close, North Baddesley, Southampton SO52 9HL Tel: 023 8073 3089 — (Camb. & St. Mary's) MB BChir Camb. 1958; MA Camb. 1958; DObst RCOG 1959. Prev: GP Soton.

WALUUBE, David Daniel Falijala William Harvey Hospital, East Kent Hospitals NHS Trust, Kennington Road, Ashford TN24 0LZ Tel: 01233 633331 Ext: 86041 Fax: 01233 616043; 6 Pennine Way, Downswood, Maidstone ME15 8YG — MB ChB Makerere 1970; DA UK 1985; MRCA 2002.

WALWYN, Jane Louise 51 Clovelly Avenue, Grainger Park, Newcastle upon Tyne NE4 8SE Tel: 0191 272 0889 — MB BS Newc. 1990; DRCOG 1993; MRCGP 1994. Trainee GP Northumbria VTS.

WALZMAN, Michael George Elliot Hospital NHS Trust, College St., Nuneaton CV10 7DJ — MB Dub. 1974 (Trinity College, Dublin) MB BCh BAO 1974; MRCOG 1979; MD Dub. 1985; FRCOG 1995. Clin. tutor Geo. Eliot Hosp Nuneaton. Specialty: Genitourinary Medicine.

WAMBEEK, Nicholas Dominic 24 Chestnut Road, Horley RH6 8PF Tel: 01293 786704 — MB BS West. Australia 1985.

WAMUO, Ihuoma Alozua — MB BS Ibadan 1988; MRCP (UK) 1994. Cons. in Rheum. and Gen. Med. Specialty: Rheumatol. Socs: RSM; BSR. Prev: Locum Cons., N. Middlx. Hosp.

WAN, Mr Andrew Chung Ting Flat 79, Consort Rise House, Buckingham Palace Road, London SW1W 9TB — MB BCh BAO NUI 1991; LRCP &S I 1991; FRCSI 1996. Specialist Regist. N.W. Thames; Research Fell. Specialty: Gen. Surg. Socs: Roy. Soc. of Med. - Fell.

WAN, Ka-Ming Bettina 13 Eleanor Close, Rotherhithe, London SE16 6PA Tel: 020 7237 2174 — MB BS Lond. 1996. Specialty: Gen. Med.

WAN, Sidney Kam Hung Ystrad Wrallt, Nantgaredig, Carmarthen SA32 7LG — MB BCh Wales 1979; MRCP (UK) 1982; FRCR 1989.

WAN FOOK CHEUNG, Wan Chung Hon A&E Department, Royal Surrey County Hospital, Egerton Road, Guildford GU2 7XX Tel: 01483 571122 Fax: 01483 406617 Email: alan.wan@royalsurrey.nhs.uk — MB ChB Leeds 1982 (leeds) FRCS 1986; DTM & H 1990; FFAEM 1994. Cons. in A&E Med., Roy. Surrey Co. Hosp., Guildford. Specialty: Accid. & Emerg. Socs: Britsh Assn. of Accid. and Emerg. Med.; Brit. Med. Assn.

WAN HO HEE, Horatio Tameside General Hospital, Ashton-under-Lyne OL6 9RW Tel: 0161 331 5151 Fax: 0161 331 5222; 2nd Floor, 16 Nicholas Street, Manchester M1 2TR Tel: 0161 228 2548 — (Hong Kong) MB BS Hong Kong 1969; MRCP (UK) 1975; MSc (Clin. Pharmacol.) Manch. 1977; FRCP Lond. 1992. Cons. Phys. Geriat. Med. Tameside Gen. Hosp. Ashton-under-Lyne. Specialty: Care of the Elderly. Socs: BMA. Prev: Lect. & Hon. Sen. Regist. (Geriat. Med.) Univ. Manch.; Med. Off. (Gen. Med.) Nethersole Hosp. Hong Kong; Regist. (Med.) S.E. Kent Health Dist.

WAN HUSSEIN, Husswan Yasmin 74 Humphrey Road, Manchester M16 9DF; 16 Monton Avenue, Eccles, Manchester M30 9HS — MB ChB Manch. 1997.

WANAS, Taha Mahmoud Department Genitourinary Medicine, New Cross Hospital, Wednesfield Road, Wolverhampton WV10 0QP Tel: 01902 644835 Fax: 01902 644830; 61 Sabrina Road, Wightwick, Wolverhampton WV6 8BP Tel: 01902 380424 Fax: 01902 762203 — (Univ. Cairo) MB BCh Cairo 1964; DS Cairo 1967; FRCOG 1991, M 1976; MFFP 1995. Cons. Phys. (Genitourin. Med.) Newcross Hosp. Wolverhampton & Hon. Sen. Clin. Lect. Univ. Birm. Med. Sch.; Cons. Phys. (Genitourin Med.) Sir Robt. Peel Tamworth Staffs. Specialty: Genitourinary Medicine; HIV Med.; Psychosexual Med. Socs: Med. Soc. Study VD; Counc. Brit. Erectile DysFunc. Soc.; Pres. Midl. Soc. Genitourin. Med. Prev: Sen. Regist. (Genitourin. Med.) North. RHA; Regist. (O & G) Bradford & Worthing HAs.

WAND, Mr Jonathan Sinclair Cheltenham General Hospital, College Road, Cheltenham GL53 7AN Tel: 01242 273245 — MB BS Lond. 1977 (St Bart.) BSc Lond. 1974; FRCS Eng. 1983. Cons. Orthop. Surg. Glos. Hosps. NHS Trust; Director J W Ortho Ltd Cheltenham & Lond. Specialty: Orthop. Special Interest: Upper Limb Surg. & Trauma. Socs: Fell. Brit. Orth. Assn. (BOA); Brit. Elbow & Shoulder Soc. Prev: Sen. Regist. (Orthop.) Westm. & Univ. Coll. Hosp. Lond.; MRC Train. Fell. (Bone Dis. Research Gp.) Northwick Pk. Hosp. Middlx.; Lect. (Anat.) St Bart. Med. Coll. Hosp. Lond.

WAND, Laurence Geoffrey Rowland, TD (retired) The Homestead, 19 Gidea Close, Gidea Park, Romford RM2 5NP Tel: 01708 745268 — (Camb. & St. Bart.) MRCS Eng. LRCP Lond. 1946; MB BChir Camb. 1947; MA Camb. 1947; FRCGP 1992, M 1967. Prev: Col. late RAMC (V).

WAND, Penelope Jane Marie Curie Centre, Caterham, Harestone Drive, Caterham CR3 6YQ Tel: 01883 832600 Fax: 01883 832633; Glebe House, Big Common Lane, Bletchingly, Redhill RH1 4QE Tel: 01883 744571 Fax: 01883 341992 — MB BS Lond. 1972; MRCP (UK) 1977; FRCR 1987; FRCP Lond. 1995. Cons. Palliat. Med. &

Med. Dir. Marie Curie Centre Caterham.; Hon. Cons. E. Surrey Healthcare Trust. Specialty: Palliat. Med. Prev: Sen. Regist. Roy. Marsden Hosp.; Regist. (Med.) St. Luke's Hosp. Guildford.

WANDER, Adam Paul Ampthill Square Medical Centre, 219 Eversholt St., London NW1 1DR Tel: 020 7387 0420 Fax: 020 7387 6161 Email: adam.wander@gp-f83006.nhs.uk — MB ChB Ed. 1992 (Edin) BSc 1990; DRCOG 1996; DFFP 1996; MRCGP 1997. GP; GP Tutor. Specialty: Gen. Pract. Socs: MPS.

WANDER, Mr Georges Charles Andrew — MB BChir Camb. 1979; FRCS Glas. 1985. Specialty: Gen. Surg. Prev: Regist. (Gen. Surg.) Torbay Hosp.; SHO (O & G) W. Suff. Hosp. Bury St. Edmunds.

WANDLESS, Gillian Mary Brookfield, Church Lane, East Norton, Leicester LE7 9XA Tel: 0116 259 8300 Email: gill.wandless@doctors.org.uk — MB BS Lond. 1967 (Roy. Free) MRCS Eng. LRCP Lond. 1967; DObst RCOG 1969; MFFP 1993. Cons. Family Plann. & Reproduc. Health Care, Univ. Hosps. Leicester NHS Trust. Specialty: Family Plann. & Reproduc. Health. Prev: SCMO Fosse Health NHS Trust Leics.; Clin. Asst. (Genitourin. Med.) Leicester Roy. Infirm. Trust; Sessional Med. Off. Univ. Leicester Stud. Health Serv.

WANDLESS, Irene (retired) — MD Newc. 1981; MB BS 1972; MRCP (U.K.) 1975.

WANDLESS, John Godfrey Brookfield, Church Lane, East Norton, Leicester LE7 9XA — (Roy. Free) BSc (Hons. Physiol.) Lond. 1965, MB BS 1968; MRCS Eng. LRCP Lond. 1968; FFA RCS Eng. 1973. Cons. Anaesth. Leicester Roy. Infirm. & Leicester Gen. Hosp. Specialty: Anaesth. Prev: Sen. Regist. (Anaesth.) Lond. Chest Hosp. & Middlx. Hosp. Lond.; Regist. (Anaesth.) Hosp. Sick Childr. Gt. Ormond St. Lond.

WANDLESS, Roger John c/o Mrs A. M. Wandless, 25 Parkside Avenue, Cockermouth CA13 0DR — MB ChB Birm. 1989; MRCP (UK) 1993.

WANDLESS, Stephen 5 Gosmore Road, Hitchin SG4 9AN — MB BS Lond. 1977 (The Lond. Hosp. Whitechapel) Specialty: Paediat.

WANG, Gordon Ka Pun Yateley Health Centre, Yateley GU46 7LS; 63 Willowmead Close, Woking GU21 3DN — MB BS Lond. 1988.

WANG, Mr Man Kin 25 Rothamstead Avenue, Harpenden AL5 2DN Tel: 01582 762233 — MB Camb. 1963 (Camb. & Univ. Coll. Hosp.) BChir 1962; DO Eng. 1967; FRCS Eng. 1969; FRCOphth 1994. Cons. Ophth. Luton & Dunstable Hosp. & Mid Herts Hosp. Gp. Specialty: Ophth. Socs: Assn. Eye Research & Oxf. Ophth. Congr. Prev: Sen. Regist. & Lect. Univ. Dept. Manch. Roy. Eye Hosp.; Research Asst. (Chem. Path.) Univ. Coll. Hosp. Med. Sch. Lond.; SHO Eye Dept. Univ. Coll. Hosp. Lond.

WANG, Mou Yee Ellen 1 Debden Close, Royal Park Gate, Kingston upon Thames KT2 5GD — MB BCh Wales 1986; FRCS (Ophth.) Ed. 1998. Specialty: Ophth.

WANG, Rong Zeng Chinese Medical Centre, 150 Station Road, Finchley Central, London N3 2SG Tel: 020 8343 4393 — MD Kweiyang, China 1950. Specialty: Urol. Socs: Chinese Med. Assn.; BMA. Prev: Dir. Surgic. Dept. Chui Yang Lin Hosp. Peking, China; Clin. Asst. (Urol.) Dept. Hammersmith Hosp. Lond.; Regist. Wessex Regional Transpl. Unit St. Mary's Hosp. Portsmouth.

WANG, Stephen Tao-Sing c/o Mr & Mrs M Wang, 5 Fairmead Walk, Waterlooville PO8 9AL — MB BS Lond. 1992.

WANG, Timothy Wai-Ming Frimley Park Hospital, Department of Clinical Biochemistry, Portsmouth Road, Frimley, Camberley GU16 7UJ Tel: 01276 604118 Fax: 01276 604924 Email: tim.wang@fph-tr.nhs.uk; Royal Surrey County Hospital, Egerton Road, Guildford GU2 7XX Tel: 01483 464121 Fax: 01483 464072 — MB ChB Sheff. 1983; PhD Open Univ. 1996; MRCPath 1998. Cons. Clin. Biochem. Frimley Pk. Hosp. Surrey & Roy. Surrey Co. Hosp.; Sen. Lect. Metab. Endocrine, Nutritional Med. Univ, Surrey. Specialty: Biochem. Special Interest: Lipidology; Metab. Med.; Renal Stones Dis.

WANGER, Karen Marie Health Care Centre, Penn Lane, Melbourne, Derby DE73 1EF — MB ChB Birm. 1992.

WANI, Mushtaq Ahmad Morriston Hospital NHS Trust, Morriston, Swansea SA6 6NL Tel: 01792 703246 — MB BS Jammu & Kashmir 1974 (Govt. Med. Coll. Srinagar Kashmir) MRCP (UK) 1986; MRCP(I) 1987. Cons. Phys. (Gen. & Geriat. Med.) Morriston Hosp. Swansea. Specialty: Care of the Elderly. Special Interest: Falls; Stroke; Syncope. Prev: Sen. Regist. Lister Hosp. Stevenage.

WANI, Mustaq Ahmad South Hornchurch Clinic, Southend Road, Rainham RM13 7XR Tel: 01708 557601 Fax: 01708 555945 — MB BS Jammu & Kashmir 1973; MB BS Jammu & Kashmir 1973.

WANIGARATNE, Dayananda Sirisena HM Prison Woodhill, Tattenhoe Street, Milton Keynes MK4 4DA — MB BS Ceylon 1969; Cert. Health Management Keele; DPM Eng. 1980. Sen. Med. Off. & Clin. Dir. HMP Woodhill. Specialty: Gen. Psychiat. Socs: Civil Serv. Med. Gp Comm. 1998/99. Prev: Sen. Med. Off. HMP Pentonville & Holloway; Med. Off. Durh. Prison; Regional Med. Off. (Malariol.) Matara, Sri Lanka.

WANKE, Miriam Eva Andrea 16 West Park Road, Smethwick, Smethwick B67 7JJ — State Exam Med Mainz 1990.

WANKLYN, Peter David Kimbolton 5 Prospect Place, Horsforth, Leeds LS18 4BW — MB ChB Birm. 1987; MB ChB (Hons.) Birm. 1987; MRCP (UK) 1990. Cons. Geriat. Leeds Gen. Infirm. Gt. Geo. St. Leeds. Specialty: Care of the Elderly. Socs: BMA & Brit. Geriat. Soc. Prev: SR Elderly Med. St. James Leeds; SR Med. St. James Leeds; SR Med. LGI, Leeds.

WANKOWSKA, Heather Claire Ipswich Hospital NHS Trust, Department of Sexual Health, Heath Road, Ipswich IP4 5PD Tel: 01473 703264 Fax: 01473 703121 Email: heather.wankowska@ipswichhospital.nhs.uk; Combs Hall, Combs, Stowmarket IP14 2EH Tel: 01449 676859 — MB BS Lond. 1974 (Univ. Coll. Hosp.) MRCGP 1978; Dip. Ven. Soc. Apoth. Lond. 1986; DFFP 1995. Cons. in Sexual Health. Specialty: Genitourinary Medicine; Family Plann. & Reproduc. Health; Psychosexual Med. Socs: BMA; BASHH; BHIVA. Prev: Hon. Cons. (Sexual Health) Ipswich Hosp.; Clin. Asst. (Genitourin. Med.) E. & W. Suff. AHA's; Trainee GP Ipswich VTS.

WANKOWSKI, Adam Franciszek Combs Ford Surgery, Combs Lane, Stowmarket IP14 2SY Tel: 01449 678333 Fax: 01449 614535; Combs Hall, Combs, Stowmarket IP14 2EH — MB BS Lond. 1974; MRCGP 1978.

WANNAN, Gary John Parkside Clinic, 63-65 Lancaster Road, London W11 1QG Tel: 020 8383 6126 Email: gary.wannan@nhs.net — MB ChB Ed. 1991; BSc (Med. Sci.) Ed. 1989; DCH Glas. 1994; MRCGP 1995; MRC Psych 1998; Dip FMS 2001; Dip Med Educat 2003. Cons. Child & Adolesc. Psychiat. Specialty: Child & Adolesc. Psychiat.; Gen. Pract.; Educat. Special Interest: Parental Ment. health; Ct. work; Family Ther.

WANSBROUGH-JONES, Mark Harding St. Georges Hospital Medical School, Cranmer Terrace, London SW17 0RE Tel: 020 8725 5828 Fax: 020 8725 3487 Email: wansbrou@sghms.ac.uk; 7 Highview Road, London SE19 3SS Tel: 020 8653 7968 — MB BS Lond. 1969 (St. Thos.) MSc (Immunol.) Lond. 1976, MB BS 1969; FRCP Lond. 1987, MRCP (UK) 1972. Cons. & Sen. Lect. (Infec. Dis.) St. Geo. Hosp. Lond. Specialty: Infec. Dis. Prev: Regist. (Med.) Hammersmith Hosp. Lond.; Lect. Liver Unit King's Coll. Hosp. Lond.

WANT, Ernest (retired) 1 The Pines, Cow Lane, Bramcote, Nottingham NG9 3BB — MB ChB Bristol 1936. Prev: Ho. Phys. Roy. Gwent Hosp. Newport.

WAPSHAW, Mr Henry (retired) 5 Whittingehame Drive, Glasgow G12 0XS Tel: 0141 339 7705 — MD Glas. 1947; ChM 1954, MB ChB 1933; FRCS Ed. 1940; FRCS Glas. 1962.

WAPSHAW, Jean Angus (retired) 5 Whittingehame Drive, Glasgow G12 0XS Tel: 0141 339 7705 — MB ChB Glas. 1942; MB ChB (Commend.) Glas. 1942. Prev: Assoc. Specialist Med. Computing, Glas. Blood Pressure Clinic.

WARAICH, Manprit Kaur 177 Southend Road, Stanford-le-Hope SS17 7AA — MB BS Lond. 1991; FRCA.

WARAICH, Mohammed Khalid — MB ChB Leic. 1998; MB ChB Leic 1998.

WARBEY, Victoria 26 Belsize Square, London NW3 4HU Tel: 020 7794 0194 — MB BS Lond. 1996 (Camb.) MA 1997. Med. SHO Rotat. at Hillingdon & Harefield Hosp.

WARBRICK-SMITH, David Warbrick-Smith and Partners, The Moat House Surgery, Beech Close, Warboys, Huntingdon PE28 2RQ Tel: 01487 822230 Fax: 01487 823721 Email: moat@wardoc.demon.co.uk; 4 Meadow Close, Hemingford Grey, Huntingdon PE28 9DN — MB BS Lond. 1972 (Middlx.) DObst RCOG 1976; DA Eng. 1978.

WARBURTON, Anne Louise Red Lion Surgery, 86 Hednesford Road, Cannock WS11 2LB Tel: 01543 502391; Cranmore, Longden Common Lane, Longden, Shrewsbury SY5 8AQ Tel: 01743 718513

— MB ChB Manch. 1985; BSc Manch. 1982; Cert. Family Plann. JCC 1989; MRCGP 1990; DRCOG 1990; DFFP 1995. Socs: St. Paul; BMA. Prev: Asst. GP Worthen, Shrops. & Long Stratton; GP Princip. Newport, Shrops.

WARBURTON, Carol Jill 2 Lavender Close, Rugby CV23 0XB — MB ChB Birm. 1993 (Univ. Birm.) MRCGP 1998. GP Princip. p/t, Rugby. Specialty: Gen. Pract.

WARBURTON, Christopher James Aintree Chest Centre, University Hospital Aintree, Lower Lane, Liverpool L9 7AL Tel: 0151 525 5980 Fax: 0151 529 2847; Wellfield House, 323 Mossy Lea Road, Wrightington, Wigan WN6 9SB Tel: 01257 422154 — MB ChB Manch. 1987; MRCP (UK) 1990; AFOM RCP Lond. 1993; MD Manch. 1996; FRCP (Lond.) 2001. Cons. Phys. (Respirat. & Gen. Med.) Univ. Hosp. Aintree Liverp.; Clin. Lect. Univ. Liverp.; Hon. Fell. Univ. Salford. Specialty: Respirat. Med. Socs: Brit. Thorac. Soc. Prev: Sen. Regist. (Thoracic Med.) Fazakerley Hosp. Liverp.; Sen. Regist. (Thoracic Med.) Freeman Hosp. Newc. u. Tyne.

WARBURTON, David John Robert Lutterworth Health Centre, Gilmorton Road, Lutterworth LE17 4EB Tel: 01455 553531; Wychwood, Dunton Lane, Ashby Parva, Lutterworth LE17 5HX Tel: 01455 209633 — MB ChB Manch. 1963; MRCS Eng. LRCP Lond. 1963; DObst RCOG 1965.

WARBURTON, Elizabeth Anne Addenbrokes Hospital, Box 83 Neuroscience, Cambridge CB2 2QQ Tel: 01223 217837 Email: eaw23@medschl.cam.ac.uk — MB BS Lond. 1987 (Oxford & Guys Hospital) BA Oxf. 1984; MA Oxf. 1986; MRCP (UK) 1990; DM Oxf. 1998. Cons. In Stroke Med. Addenbrookes Camb.; Camb. Nuffield Hosp. Socs: Brit. Assn. of Stroke Phys. (BASP); Association of British Neurologists (ABN); British Neuroscience Association (BNA). Prev: Regist. (Med.) Epsom & Char. Cross Hosp. Lond.; Research Regist. Char. Cross & Hammersmith Hosp. Lond.; MRC Train. Fell. RPMS Hammersmith Hosp. Lond.

WARBURTON, Ian Richard Ovoca, 460 Didsbury Road, Heaton Mersey, Stockport SK4 3BT Tel: 0161 432 2032 Fax: 0161 947 9689 — MB ChB Manch. 1979; MRCGP 1983.

WARBURTON, Michael Charles Health Centre, Windmill Avenue, Hassocks BN6 8LY — MB BS Lond. 1982; MBA 1999 Imperial College; DRCOG 1987; MRCGP 1990. Clin. Director, Modernisation Team, Brighton Healthcare; Dir. Mid Sussex Out of Hours CoOperat.; Med. Off. Brighton Rugby Club. Prev: Chairm. Mid Sussex PCG; Chairm. Prof. Exec. Mid Sussex PCT.

WARBURTON, Richard Croft Cottage, Hollins Lane, Forton, Preston PR3 0AB — MB BS Lond. 1964. Aviat. Med. Specialist Brit. Aerospace Warton. Specialty: Aviat. Med.

WARBURTON, Richard Alistair The Health Centre, Rydal Road, Ambleside LA22 9BP Tel: 015394 32693; Croft Cottage, Hollins Lane, Forton, Preston PR3 0AB — MB BS Newc. 1990. Specialty: Aviat. Med.

WARBURTON, Thomas Harold Martin (retired) 5 Bavant Road, Brighton BN1 6RD Tel: 01273 552294 Email: mrwarbur94@aol.com — (St. Bart.) MB BS (Hnrs.) Lond. 1953; MRCS Eng. LRCP Lond. 1953; DObst RCOG 1955. Prev: GP Peacehaven.

WARD, Adam Anthony Department of Musculosketal Medicine, Royal London Homoeopathic Hospital, University College London Hospitals Trust, Great Ormond Street, London WC1N 3HR Tel: 020 7837 8833 Fax: 020 7833 7229; 41 Frankfield Rise, Tunbridge Wells TN2 5LF Tel: 01892 525799 — MB BS Lond. 1972 (Westm.) Dip. Med. Ac.; MSc Lond. 1978; MRCGP 1982; Dip. Orth. Med. Paris 1983; MFHom 1984. Clin. director & Cons. Phys. Orthopaedic & Musculoskeletal Med.Roy. Lond. Homoeop. Hosp.; Examr. for Diploma in Musculoskeletal Med. Soc. of Apoth. of Lond. Specialty: Orthop.; Rheumatol.; Gen. Med. Socs: (Counc.) Brit. Inst. Musculoskeletal Med.; Brit. Med. Acupunct. Soc.; Fell. Fac. Homoeop. Lond. Prev: Phys. (Orthop. Med.) Hotel Dieu, Paris, France; Lect. & Hon. Sen. Regist. (Epidemiol.) Westm. Hosp. Med. Sch. Lond.; Edr. BRd.way.

WARD, Adrian Denis The Surgery, Lorne Street, Lochgilphead PA31 8LU Tel: 01546 602921 Fax: 01546 606735 — MB ChB Leeds 1984. GP Lochgilphead, Argyll. Prev: SHO (A & E) Huddersfield Roy. Infirm.; SHO (Chest Med.) Pontefract Gen. Hosp.; SHO (Anaesth.) Airedale Gen. Hosp. Keighley.

WARD, Adrian Lawrence Alloa Health Centre, Marshill, Alloa FK10 1AB Tel: 01259 212088 Fax: 01259 724788 — MB ChB Aberd. 1990; BMedBiol. (Hons.) Aberd. 1990; Cert. Family Plann. JCC 1992; DCH RCP Lond. 1993; DRCOG 1993; DFFP 1993; MRCGP 1994. GP Alloa; Med. Off. United Glass Alloa; Fact. Med. Off. Weir Pumps Alloa. Socs: Roy. Coll. Gen. Pract.; BMA.

WARD, Alan Blakey (retired) 21 Wadsworth Park, Branthwaite, Workington CA14 4SR — MB BS Durh. 1942 (Univ. Durh.) DA Eng. 1950; FFA RCS Eng. 1954. Prev: Cons. Anaesth. W. Cumbld. Gp. Hosps.

WARD, Alan Geoffrey 16 Pencepool Orchard, Plymtree, Cullompton EX15 2JG Tel: 01884 277582 — MB ChB Leic. 1981 (Leicester 1975-1981) Cert. Family Plann. JCC 1985; DRCOG 1985; DCH RCP Lond. 1985; MRCGP 1986. Research/Med. Journalism. Specialty: Community Child Health. Special Interest: Audit; Interagency working; Pat. centred care. Socs: Devon & Exeter Med. Soc. Prev: Trainee GP Plymouth VTS; GP Princip. (East Devon) 1986-2002.

WARD, Alan Robert Godfrey The Surgery, 16 Watford Road, Crick, Northampton NN6 7TT Tel: 01788 822203 Fax: 01788 824177 — MRCS Eng. LRCP Lond. 1970 (St. Mary's) Prev: Ho. Surg. Gulson Hosp. Coventry; Ho. Phys. & Regist. (Cas.) St. Cross Hosp. Rugby.

WARD, Alastair Hugh 2 Bindon Lane, Wool, Wareham BH20 6BN Tel: 01929 463597 — MB BS Lond. 1987 (Guy's Hosp. Med. Sch. Lond.) MRCP (UK) 1991; DRCOG 1994; DCH RCP Lond. 1994; MRCGP 1995; DTM & H 1998. Med. Co-Ordinator Farah, Afghanistan. Specialty: Gen. Pract. Prev: Med. Off. i/c Muthale Miss. Hosp., Kenya; Trainee GP Poole VTS; Regist. (Gen. & Renal Med.) Roy. Sussex Co. Hosp. Brighton.

WARD, Alexandra Monica Vivienne 7A Charmouth Grove, Poole BH14 0LP — MB BS Lond. 1992; MRCP (UK) 1995. Specialty: Diabetes.

WARD, Allan Edward Abbey Health Centre, East Abbey Street, Arbroath DD11 1EN Tel: 01241 872692; 15 Monkbarns Drive, Arbroath DD11 2DS — MB ChB Dundee 1980; MRCP (UK) 1983; DRCOG 1985; MRCGP 1986.

WARD, Andrea Susan Wadlerslade Surgery, Walderslade, 194 King Street, Barnsley S74 9LJ Tel: 01226 743221 Fax: 01226 741100 — MB ChB Sheff. 1989; DCH RCP Lond. 1991; MRCGP 1993. Specialty: Paediat. Socs: Christ. Med. Fellowsh.

WARD, Andrew South Wigston Health Centre, 80 Blaby Road, South Wigston, Leicester LE18 4SE Tel: 0116 210 0486 — MB ChB Leic. 1992 (Leicester) DRCOG. GP Princip. Specialty: Gen. Pract.

WARD, Andrew James Markham House, 140 Wyke Road, Weymouth DT4 9QR — MB BS Lond. 1998.

WARD, Ann Maureen (retired) Cherwell, Meadway, Berkhamsted HP4 2PN Tel: 01442 864968 — (Char. Cross) MB BS Lond. 1957; DObst RCOG 1958. Prev: Ho. Off. (Obst.) Kingsbury Matern. Hosp. Lond.

WARD, Anne Josephine Mary — MB BCh BAO Dub. 1986; MRCPI 1988; MRCPSYCH 1993; MD 1994. Cons. (Psychother.) Maudsley Hosp. Lond. Specialty: Gen. Psychiat.; Psychother.

WARD, Anthony Barrington, Maj. RAMC Retd. North Staffordshire Rehabilitation Centre, Haywood Hospital, High Lane, Stoke-on-Trent ST6 7AG Tel: 01782 556 226 Fax: 01782 556 165 Email: anthony.ward@uhns.nhs.uk; Bearstone Farm, Bearstone, Market Drayton TF9 4HG Tel: 01630 647135 Fax: 01630 647252 Email: anthony@bward2.freeserve.co.uk — MB ChB Dundee 1975; BSc St. And. 1972; MRCP (UK) 1981; FRCP Ed. 1992; FRCP Lond. 1994. Cons. & Sen. Lect. (Rehabil. Med.) Univ. Hosp. of N.Staffs Stoke-on-Trent; Sen. Lect. Postgrad. Med. Sch. Univ. Keele. Specialty: Rehabil. Med.; Rheumatol. Socs: (Pres.) Brit. Soc. Rehabil. Med; Brit. Soc. Rheum.; Roy. Coll. Phys. Edin. (Regional Advisor). Prev: Cons. Rheum. & Rehabil. Qu. Eliz. Milit. Hosp. Lond.; Sen. Regist. (Rheum.) St. Thos. Hosp. Lond.; Regtl. Med. Off. 50th Missile Regt. RA.

WARD, Mr Anthony Joseph Department of Orthopaedic Surgery, North Bristol NHS Trust, Frenchay Hospital, Bristol BS9 4BP Tel: 01179 701212 Ext: 6582 Fax: 01179 186641 — BM BS Nottm. 1981 (Nottm. Univ. Med. Sch.) BMedSci. (Hons.) Nottm. 1979; FRCS Eng. 1986. Cons. In Trauma & Orthop. Surg., N. Bristol NHS Trust, Bristol; Hon. Clincial Sen. Lect., Univ. of Bristol. Specialty: Trauma & Orthop. Surg. Special Interest: Arthritis Surgery; Knee Injuries; Multiple Trauma. Socs: Brit. Orthop. Assn.; Brit. Trauma Soc.; Brit. Hip Soc.

WARD, Anthony Milford Department of Immunology, PO Box 894, Sheffield S5 7YT Tel: 0114 271 5552 Fax: 0114 261 9893 Email: amw@immqas.org.uk; 19 Kerwin Drive, Dore, Sheffield S17 3DG Tel: 0114 236 6996 — (St. Bart.) MRCS Eng. LRCP Lond. 1963; MB BChir Camb. 1966; MA Camb. 1966; FRCPath 1982, M 1970. Hon. Cons. Clin. Immunol. Sheff. HA; Reader (Immunol.) Acad. Div. Med. Univ. Sheff.; Dir. Supraregional Specific Protein Ref. Unit.; Cons. Clin. Immunol. Rotherham DGH NHS Trust; Cons. Clin. Immunol. Doncaster & MexBoro. NHS Trust. Specialty: Immunol. Socs: Assn. Clin. Pathols. & Brit. Soc. Immunol.; Amer. Assoc. Clin. Chem. Prev: Lect. (Path.) Sheff. Univ.; Regist. (Clin. Path.) United Sheff. Hosps.; Resid. (Clin. Path.) St. Geo. Hosp. Lond.

WARD, Arthur John (retired) Hawthorne, Owler Park Road, Ilkley LS29 0BG — BSc (Hons. Physics) Durh. 1943; MB ChB Leeds 1952; DMRT Eng. 1955; FFR 1958. Sen. Clin. Lect. Univ. Leeds; Cons. Radiother, Leeds AHA (T). Prev: Regist. Radiother. Centre Leeds.

WARD, Barbara-Anne St Saviours Surgery, Merick Road, Malvern Link, Malvern WR14 1DD Tel: 01684 572323 Fax: 01684 891067 — MB BS Lond. 1981; DRCOG 1983.

WARD, Barnaby James Essex Lodge, 85 Chaveney Road, Quorn, Loughborough LE12 8AB — BChir Camb. 1995.

WARD, Brian Hermitage Green Lodge, Hermitage Green Lane, Winwick, Warrington WA2 8SJ Tel: 01925 26164 — MB ChB Manch. 1950; DPM Leeds 1958; FRCPsych 1972. Cons. Psychiat. Winwick Hosp. Warrington. Specialty: Gen. Psychiat. Socs: BMA. Prev: Med. Supt. Winwick Hosp.; Asst. Sen. Med. Off. Leeds RHB; Area Psychiat. RAMC.

WARD, Carol Patricia Royal South Hants Hospital, Brinton Terrace, off St Mary's Road, Southampton Tel: 023 8063 4288; 7 Dale Close, Littleton, Winchester SO22 6RA Tel: 01962 883185 — MB BS Lond. 1980 (Middlx.) MRCP (UK) 1983; DRCOG 1985; MRCGP 1986. Staff Grade Radiother. & Oncol. Roy. S. Hants. Hosp. Specialty: Oncol.; Radiother. Prev: GP Asst. Stockbridge; Trainee GP Lechlade; SHO (Gen. Med. & A & E) Princess Margt. Hosp. Swindon.

WARD, Caroline Sandra Nutt Radiology Department, Kingston Hospital NHS Department, Galsworthy Road, Kingston upon Thames KT2 7QB Tel: 020 8546 7711; 2 Coombe Rise, Kingston upon Thames KT2 7EX Tel: 020 8942 0222 — MB BCh BAO Dub. 1977 (Trinity Coll. Dub.) MRCPI 1980; DCH Univ. Coll. Dub. 1981; DMRD RCR 1984; FRCR 1985; FRCPI 1992. Cons. Radiol. Kingston Hosp. Kingston u. Thames. Specialty: Radiol. Socs: Roy. Coll. Radiol.; Brit. Inst. of Radiol.; Roy. Coll. Phys.s of Irel. Prev: Cons. Radiol. Ashford Hosp. Middlx.; Sen. Regist. (Radiol.) St. Geo. Hosp. Lond.

WARD, Catherine Joyce 61 Hallam Grange Road, Sheffield S10 4BL — MB ChB Sheff. 1980; DCH RCP Lond. 1987.

WARD, Catherine Sarah Flat 4, 13 Lavender Gardens, Battersea, London SW11 1DH Tel: 020 7350 2722 — MB BS Lond. 1994; BSc (Hons.) Lond. 1991; MRCP 1999; DRCOG 1999; MRCGP 2001. GP Assoc., SLOVTS, Lond. Specialty: Gen. Pract.

WARD, Catherine Theresa 80 Old Street, Hill Head, Fareham PO14 3HN — MB BS Lond. 1997.

WARD, Cecilia Caroline (retired) Grange Park, Moy, Dungannon BT71 7EQ Tel: 02887 784238 Fax: 01868 784238 — MB BCh BAO Belf. 1957; DCH RCP Lond. 1961; MFFP 1993. Prev: SHO Roy. Belf. Hosp. for Sick Childr. & Roy. Vict. Hosp. Belf.

WARD, Christine Joan Garden Flat, 33 Cathcart Road, London SW10 — MB BS Lond. 1982.

WARD, Christopher Albert The Clayton Medical Centre, Wellington Street, Clayton le Moors, Accrington BB5 5HU Tel: 01254 383131 Fax: 01254 392261 — MB ChB Dundee 1974; BSc St. And. 1971. Clin. Asst. (Cardio.) DHA Represent.

WARD, Christopher Charles Brockwell Medical Group, Brockwell Centre, Northumbrian Road, Cramlington NE23 1XZ Tel: 01670 392700 Fax: 01670 392701; 17 Yarmouth Drive, Westwood Grange, Cramlington NE23 1TL Tel: 01670 732211 — MB BS Newc. 1978.

WARD, Professor Christopher David University of Nottingham, Rehabilitation Research Unit, Derby City General Hospital, Uttoxeter Road, Derby DE22 3NE Tel: 01332 625680 Fax: 01332 625681 Email: c.d.ward@nottingham.ac.uk; 82 Edward Road, West Bridgford, Nottingham NG2 5GB Tel: 0115 981 2238 — MD Camb. 1983; FRCP (1992); MB BChir 1977. Head Div. of Rehabil. & Ageing Univ. of Nottm.; Hon. Cons. (Rehabil. Med. & Neurol.) S. Derbsh. Hosps. NHS Trust. Specialty: Neurol.; Rehabil. Med. Special Interest: Progressive Neurol. diseases. Socs: Brit. Soc. Rehab. Med.; Assn. Brit. Neurols.; Fell. Roy. Soc. Med. Prev: Sen. Lect. Univ. Dept. Rehabil. & Cons. Neurol. Soton Gen. Hosp.; Clin. Lect. Dept. Neurol. Oxf. Univ.

WARD, Christopher John The Surgery, 54 Thorne Road, Doncaster DN1 2JP Tel: 01302 361222 — MB ChB Leeds 1982.

WARD, Mr Christopher Margrave (retired) Knollbury, West End, Chadlington, Chipping Norton OX7 3NJ Tel: 01608 676265 — (Lond. Hosp.) MA Lond. 1992, BSc 1962; MRCS Eng. LRCP Lond. 1965; MB BS Lond. 1966; FRCS Eng. 1972. Prev: Hon. Cons. Plastic & Reconstruc. Surg. Char. Cross Hosp. & W. Middlx. Hosp.

WARD, Christopher Raymond 66 Woodlea, Middlesbrough TS8 0TX — BM BS Nottm. 1985.

WARD, Daniela Antonia 71 Dan-y-Bryn Avenue, Radyr, Cardiff CF15 8DQ — MB ChB Ed. 1990; MRCGP 1994. Clin. Asst. Addic. Unit WhitCh. Hosp. Cardiff. Specialty: Alcohol & Substance Misuse. Prev: SHO (A & E) Wrexham Maelor NHS Hosp.; SHO (Psychiat.) Roy. Cornhill Hosp. Aberd.; SHO (Med. & Paediat.) Ninewells Hosp. Dundee.

WARD, David Anthony 3 Greenfield Road, Newcastle upon Tyne NE3 5TN Tel: 0191 219 5023 Fax: 0191 219 5022 — MB ChB Sheff. 1987; MRCPsych 1995. Cons. Adolesc. Psychiat. Specialty: Child & Adolesc. Psychiat.

WARD, Mr David Anthony Department of Orthopaedics, Kingston Hospital, Galsworthy Road, Kingston upon Thames KT2 7QB Tel: 020 8546 7711 Fax: 020 8355 2982; Weylands, Pyrford Road, West Byfleet KT14 6QY Tel: 01932 348282 Fax: 01932 336676 — MB BS Lond. 1985; FRCS Ed. 1989; FRCS Eng. 1989; FRCS (Orth.) 1994. Cons. Orthop. & Trauma Kingston Hosp. Kingston-upon-Thames. Specialty: Orthop. Socs: Fell. BOA; Roy. Soc. Med.; Brit. Trauma Soc. Prev: Cons. Orthop. & Trauma Qu. Mary's Univ. Hosp. Lond.; Sen. Regist. (Orthop.) Char. Cross Hosp. Lond.; Regist. Rotat. (Orthop.) St. Geo. Hosp. Lond.

WARD, David Arthur 6 St Wilfrids Road, Bessacarr, Doncaster DN4 6AA — MB ChB Manch. 1978; MRCP Lond. 1980; FRCR 1985. Cons. Radiol. Doncaster Roy. Infirm. Specialty: Radiol. Prev: Regist. (Radiol.) Gen. Infirm. & St. Jas. Hosp. Leeds; Regist. (Gen. Med.) Doncaster Roy. Infirm.

WARD, Mr David Christopher The Friarage Hospital, Northallerton DL6 1JG — MB BS Bangalore 1973; FRCS Ed. 1977; LRCP LRCS Ed. LRCPS Glas. 1979; ChM Leeds 1989. Cons. Surg. Northallerton HA. Specialty: Gen. Surg. Socs: Assn. Surg.; Assn. Coloproctol.; Assn. Upper G.I. Surg. Prev: Lect. (Surg.) Univ. Leeds & Hon. Sen. Regist. Leeds West. HA.

WARD, David Ernest 84 Harley Street, London W1G 7HW Tel: 020 7079 4290 Fax: 020 7079 4294 Email: dr.davidward@btopenworld.com — MRCS Eng. LRCP Lond. 1971 (Guy's) MD Lond. 1981, BSc (Physiol.) 1968, MB BS 1971; MRCP (UK) 1973; FRCP Lond. 1989. Cons. Cardiol. St. Geo. Hosp. Lond. Specialty: Cardiol. Special Interest: Coronary Interven.; Radiofrequency/cryothermal ablation. Socs: Fell. Amer. Coll. Cardio.; Brit. Cardiac Soc. Prev: Sen. Regist. (Cardiol.) Brompton Hosp. Lond.; Regist. (Cardiol.) St. Bart. Hosp. Lond.; Regist. (Med.) Char. Cross Hosp. Lond.

WARD, David Gareth 30 Bennett Park, London SE3 9RB — MB ChB Liverp. 1998.

WARD, David George The Surgery, Marlpits Lane, Honiton EX14 2NY Tel: 01404 41141 Fax: 01404 46621 — MB BS Lond. 1983 (St. Geo.) BSc Lond. 1980; MRCGP 1987; DRCOG 1988. Prev: Trainee GP VTS Univ. Exeter; Ho. Off. (Med.) St. Geo. Hosp. Lond.; Ho. Off. (Surg.) Derriford Hosp. Plymouth.

WARD, David James — MB ChB Dundee 1979; BSc (Hons.) Dund 1974; MRCGP 1989. Prev: Surg. Cdr. Rn.

WARD, Mr David Joseph Leicester Royal Infirmary, Department of Plastic Surgery, Leicester LE1 5WW Tel: 0116 258 5286 Fax: 0116 258 6082 Email: julie.a.green@uhl-tr.nhs.uk; Sauvey Castle Farm, Withcote, Oakham LE15 8DT Tel: 01664 454870 Fax: 01664 454880 Email: plastic.surgeon@virgin.net — MB BS Lond. 1976 (King's Coll. Hosp.) FRCS Eng. 1980; T(S) 1991; FRCS Ed. 2004. Cons. (Plastic Surg.) Leicester Roy. Infirm.; Professional Conduct Comm., Gen. Med. Counc. (Apptd. Mem.); Clin. Teach. Univ. Leic. Sch. Med.; Examr. Intercollegiate Bd. Plastic Surg. Specialty: Plastic Surg. Socs: Brit. Assn. Aesthetic Plastic Surgs.; Brit. Burns Assn.;

Brit. Soc. Surgen Hand Assoc. Prev: Mem. Ct. Examrs. RCS Eng.; Sen. Regist. (Plastic Surg.) Qu. Vict. Hosp. E. Grinstead; Regist. (Plastic Surg.) St. Geo. & Qu. Mary's Hosps. Lond.

WARD, David Michael The Surgery, 29 Chesterfield Drive, Ipswich IP1 6DW Tel: 01473 741349 — MB ChB Bristol 1984; BA (Hons.) Oxf. 1981; MB ChB (Hons.) Bristol 1984; DCH RCP Lond. 1987; DRCOG Lond. 1988; MRCGP 1989; T(GP) 1991.

WARD, Mr David Michael, OBE, KStJ (retired) The Hermitage, Ringmore, Shaldon, Teignmouth TQ14 0ET Tel: 01626 873392 Email: sonmikward@btinternet.com — MB ChB Birm. 1955; DObst RCOG 1959; DO Eng. 1962; FRCS Eng. 1965; FCOphth 1989. Prev: Cons. Ophth. Torbay Hosp. Torquay.

WARD, David Ralph Compton Health Centre, Compton, Ashbourne DE6 1GN Tel: 01335 300588; Lower Brook Barn, Snelston, Ashbourne DE6 2GP — MB ChB Birm. 1987; DRCOG 1991; DFFP 1997. GP Princip. Derbysh. Specialty: Pub. Health Med.

WARD, Deborah Louise 53 Blackstock Road, Sheffield S14 1AB — MB ChB Leic. 1992.

WARD, Debra Levenshulme Health Centre, Dunstable Street, Levenshulme, Manchester M19 3BX Tel: 0161 225 4033 Fax: 0161 248 8020 — MB ChB Manch. 1985; MRCGP 1989; DRCOG 1989.

WARD, Dermot Joseph 4 Jubilee Terrace, Chichester PO19 1XL Tel: 01243 778716 — LRCPI & LM, LRCSI & LM 1961; FRCPI 1972, M 1965; DPM Eng. 1965; FRCPsych 1984, M 1971. Indep. Cons. Psychiat., Chichester; Med. Mem., Ment. health review tribunal, Surbiton, Surrey; Second opinion advisary Phys. Ment. health act commision, Nottm. Specialty: Gen. Psychiat.; Psychother.; Geriat. Psychiat. Socs: Fell. Roy. Soc. Med.; BMA; Exec. Mem.Soc. of Clin. Psychiat.s. Prev: Cons. Psychiat. St David's Hosp. Carmathern & Graylingwell Hosp. Chichester; Cons. Psychiat. & Clin. Dir. St. Loman's Hosp. Dub.; Sen. Regist. (Psychiat.) Roundway Hosp. Devizes.

WARD, Derrick Edward Whitchurch Road Medical Centre, 210-212 Whitchurch Road, Heath, Cardiff CF14 3NB Tel: 029 2062 1282 Fax: 029 2052 0210; 41 Caegwyn Road, Whitchurch, Cardiff CF14 1TB — MB BCh Wales 1973 (Cardiff) Cert JCC Lond. 1978; DRCOG 1978; MRCGP 1979. Clin. Asst. (Genitourin. Med.) Cardiff Roy. Infirm.; Clin. Tutor, Coll. Med., Univ. of Wales. Prev: Surg. Lt. RN; Ho. Surg. Accid. Unit Cardiff Roy. Infirm.; Ho. Phys. Llandough Hosp. Penarth.

WARD, Dorothy May Blair 6 Ballantrae, Stewartfield, East Kilbride, Glasgow G74 4TZ Tel: 0141 248881 Fax: 0141248886 — (Glas.) MB ChB Glas. 1950; FRCGP 1999. Med. Mem. Disabil. Appeals Tribunal W. of Scotl.; Med. Assessor Indep. Tribunal Serv. W. of Scotl. Specialty: Obst. & Gyn. Socs: Fell. BMA; Fell. Roy. Soc. Med.; Med. Wom. Internat. Assn. Prev: GP Glas.; Hosp. Pract. (Geriat.) Cowglen Hosp. Glas.; Ho. Off. (Med.) Thoracic Surg. Unit, Woodend Hosp. Aberd.

WARD, Duncan Brand Grosvenor House Surgery, Grosvenor House, Warwick Square, Carlisle CA1 1LB Tel: 01228 536561 Fax: 01228 515786 — MB ChB Manch. 1979; DRCOG 1983; MRCGP 1984. Prev: SHO (O & G) Univ. Hosp. S. Manch.; SHO (Paediat.) St. Mary's Hosp. Manch.; SHO (Paediat.) Roy. Hosp. Sick Childr. Glas.

WARD, Edward (retired) Badger's Earth, Little Missenden, Amersham HP7 0RD — MB BCh BAO Dub. 1951; DPH Liverp. 1964; FFCM 1983, M 1974. Prev: Dir. Pub. Health Wycombe HA.

WARD, Eileen Gillian Marloes, 23 Avenue Road, Dorridge, Solihull B93 8LD Tel: 01564 772032 — MB ChB Birm. 1964 (Lond.) DO Eng. 1980; MRCOphth 1989.

WARD, Eileen Mary Claire Shakoor, Ward, Seery and Ahmad, Gardenia Surgery, 2A Gardenia Avenue, Luton LU3 2NS Tel: 01582 572612 Fax: 01582 494553 — MB BCh BAO NUI 1976 (Univ. Coll. Galway, Eire) DCH Eng. 1979; DRCOG 1980; MRCGP 1980. Socs: BMA. Prev: Duty Dep. Police Surg. (S. Bed.).

WARD, Elizabeth Sheffield 4 Patten Road, London SW18 3RH Tel: 020 8874 4938 Fax: 020 8874 4938 — MB BS Lond. 1967 (Middlx.) MBAcA 1992; LicAc 1992; MBAcC 1995. Med. Off. Family Plann. Clinics Lond.; Clin. Asst. (Dermat.) Hillingdon & Hounslow AHA. Specialty: Dermat. Prev: SHO (Paediat.) Mayday Hosp. Croydon; Ho. Phys. N. Middlx. Hosp. Lond.; Ho. Surg. Harefield Hosp.

WARD, Eric Townhead Surgeries, Townhead, Settle BD24 9JA Tel: 01729 822611 Fax: 01729 892916; Warrendale House, 2 Townhead Avenue, Settle BD24 9RQ Tel: 01729 823341 — MB ChB Manch. 1970; DObst RCOG 1972; MRCGP 1976. Specialty: Ment. Health. Prev: Trainee GP Airedale VTS; SHO (O & G) Withington Hosp. Manch.; Ho. Surg. Manch. Roy. Infirm.

WARD, Francis Gosman (retired) 37 High Street, Datchet, Slough SL3 9EQ — MB ChB St. And. 1959; MFOM RCP Lond. 1981; FCCP (USA) 1989; T(OM) 1992. Prev: Sen. Med. Adviser Benefits Agency Med. Servs. DSS.

WARD, Gemma Clare Central Clinic, Childrens Centre, Durham Road, Sunderland; 5 Thornhill Terrace, Sunderland SR2 7JL — MB BS Newc. 1983; DCCH RCP Ed. 1987; MSc (Community Paediat.) 1990. Assoc. Specialist (Community Child Health) Childr.'s Centre Sunderland. Specialty: Community Child Health. Socs: Reg. Rep. BACDA; BACCH; RCPCH. Prev: SHO (Haemat.) Roy. Infirm. Sunderland.; SHO (Psychiat.) Cherry Knowle Hosp. Sunderland.

WARD, Geoffrey David (retired) — (Univ. Coll. Hosp.) MB BS Lond. 1964; MRCS Eng. LRCP Lond. 1964; FRCOG 1982, M 1969. Prev: Cons. O & G Walsall Hosps. NHS Trust.

WARD, George Priestley (retired) 15 Wenthill Close, Ackworth, Pontefract WF7 7LP Tel: 01977 600370 — MB ChB Leeds 1952; FRCGP 1981, M 1965; DA Eng. 1970. Prev: Hosp. Pract. (Anaesth.) Pontefract Gen. Infirm.

WARD, Graham Gordon (retired) Ernespie, Longdogs Lane, Ottery St Mary EX11 1HX Tel: 01404 812621 Fax: 01404 812621 Email: graham_ward@talk21.com — MB BS Lond. 1960 (Guy's) MRCS Eng. LRCP Lond. 1959; DObst RCOG 1961; MRCGP 1968. Chairm. Ottery St. Mary Hosp. League of Friends. Prev: Ho. Surg. (Orthop.) Guy's Hosp. Lond.

WARD, Graham Russell Kennedy Way Surgery, Kennedy Way, Yate, Bristol BS37 4AA Tel: 01454 313849 Fax: 01454 329039 — MB BCh Wales 1983. GP Yate. Prev: SHO (Rotat.) (Gen. Med.) Walsgrave Hosp. Coventry; Ho. Off. (Gen. Med.) Roy. Gwent Hosp. Newport; Ho. Off. (Surg.) Univ. Coll. Hosp. Cardiff.

WARD, Mr Gregory Mayday University Hospital, 530 London Road, Croydon CR7 7YE Tel: 020 8401 3157 Fax: 020 8401 3681 Email: gregory.ward@mayday.nhs.uk — MB BS Sydney 1973 (Sydney Univ.) FRANZCP; FRCOG. Cons. (Obst. & Gyn.) Mayday NHS Trust; Train. Progr. Director, SW Thame Deanery. Specialty: Obst. & Gyn. Special Interest: Gynaecological Endcrinology; Maternal Medicine. Socs: RSM; Brit. Feto-maternal Med. Soc.; Internat. Soc. of Obst. Med.

WARD, Mr Harry Charles — MB BS Lond. 1975; FRCS Eng. 1979; MS Lond. 1992. Cons. Paediat. Surg. Uni. Hosp. Lewisham & Guy's & St. Thos. NHS Trust. Specialty: Paediat. Surg. Prev: Sen. Regist. (Paediat. Surg.) Hosp. Sick Childr. Lond.; Regist. (Paediat. Surg.) Qu. Eliz. Hosp. Sick Childr. Lond.; Research Fell. Acad. (Surg.) St. Mary's Hosp. Lond.

WARD, Helen Department of Epidemiology & Public Health, Imperial College London, London W2 1PG Tel: 020 7594 3303 Fax: 020 7402 2150 Email: h.ward@imperial.ac.uk — MB ChB Sheff. 1981 (Sheffield) MSc (Epidemiol. Distinc.) Lond. 1993; MFPHM RCP (UK) 1993; FFPHM RCP (UK) 1999. Sen. Lect. (Pub. Health Med.) Imperial Coll. Lond.; Hon. Cons. in Genitourin. Med. Specialty: Pub. Health Med.; Genitourinary Medicine. Socs: Soc. Study VD. Prev: Sen. Regist. (Pub. Health Med.) NW Thames RHA; Research Fell. (Epidemiol.) & Research Regist. (Genitourin. Med.) St. Mary's Hosp. Med. Sch. Lond.; Hon. Cons. Pub. Health Med. N. Thames RHA.

WARD, Helen Emily Middleton Lodge Surgery, New Ollerton, Newark NG22 9SZ Tel: 01623 860668 Fax: 01623 836073 — BM BS Nottm. 1980; MRCGP 1985; DRCOG 1985.

WARD, Helen Louise 3 Steeple Court, Coventry Road, London E1 5QZ — MB BS Lond. 1992.

WARD, Helen Mary Walls General Practice, Walls General Practice, Walls, Shetland ZE2 9PF Tel: 01595 809352; Anderville, Walls, Shetland ZE2 9PF — MB ChB Sheff. 1986; BSc Zool. Sheff. 1979; BMedSci Sheff. 1985; MRCGP 1996.

WARD, Hester Janet Teresa Lothian Health Board, 148 Pleasance, Edinburgh EH8 9RS Tel: 0131 536 9000; 7 Wardie Crescent, Trinity, Edinburgh EH5 1AF Tel: 0131 552 0519 — MB BS Lond. 1987 (Char. Cross & Westm.) MSc (Pub. Health Med.) Lond. 1993, BSc (Hons.) Biochem. 1984; MRCP (UK) 1991; MFPHM RCP (UK) 1995. Cons. (Pub. Health Med.) Lothian HB - on secondment to the Nat. CJD Surveillance Unit, Edin. Specialty: Infec. Dis. Prev: Sen. Regist. (Pub. Health Med.) Lothian HB; Regist. (Pub.

Health Med.) SE HA & SE Thames RHA; SHO (Med.) Char. Cross Hosp. Lond.

WARD, Ian James Ezzat and Partners, Phoenix Family Care, 35 Park Road, Coventry CV1 2LE Tel: 024 7622 7234 Fax: 024 7663 4816; 29 Coopers Walk, Bubbenhall, Coventry CV8 3JB — MB ChB Leeds 1980; DRCOG 1984.

WARD, Ian Roger 196 Foundry Lane, Southampton SO15 3LE — BM Soton. 1995. Specialty: Gen. Pract.

WARD, Ida Joyce (retired) Kirkvale, Lea, Matlock DE4 5JP Tel: 01629 534604 — MB ChB Leeds 1949; Cert Family Plann. RCOG, RCGP & Family Plann; MRCS Eng. LRCP Lond. 1949; Assn. 1976. Prev: GP Crich, Dethick, Lea & Holloway.

WARD, Iris Violet Irene (retired) 19 Knowle Village, Budleigh Salterton EX9 6AL Tel: 01395 442404 — MB BS (Hons.) Lond. 1925 (Lond. Sch. Med. Wom.) MD Lond. 1930; DCH Eng. 1950. Prev: Asst. Paediat. Research Unit Exeter City Hosp.

WARD, Jacqueline Anne 29 Coopers Walk, Bubbenhall, Coventry CV8 3JB — MB ChB Leeds 1980; DRCOG 1983; MRCGP 1984; D.Occ.Med. RCP Lond. 1995; DFFP 1995.

WARD, James (retired) Eildon, Murrell Hill, Grange-over-Sands LA11 7HN Tel: 015395 34425 — MB ChB Liverp. 1945; DCP Lond 1952; DPath Eng. 1957; FRCPath 1975, M 1963. Prev: Cons. Clin. Pathol. Scott. Borders Hosp. Gp.

WARD, James Christopher Rodney Flat 5 Collingwood House, 10 Collingwood Ter, Newcastle upon Tyne NE2 2JP — MB BS Newc. 1997.

WARD, James Robin 1 Farnham Lane, Ferrensby, Knaresborough HG5 9JG — MB ChB Sheff. 1965; DObst RCOG 1967. Prev: GP Richmond; Clin. Asst. (O & G & Radiol.) Darlington Memor. Hosp.; Ho. Obst. Off., Ho. Phys. & Ho. Surg. Maelor Gen. Hosp. Wrexham.

WARD, Jane King's College London, Division of Physiology, Guy's Campus, Shepherd's House, London SE1 1UL Tel: 020 7848 6304; Glenside, 45 Madeira Park, Tunbridge Wells TN2 5SY Tel: 01892 529199 — MB ChB Manch. 1977; BSc Manch. 1974, MB ChB 1977; PhD Lond. 1988. Sen. Lect. (Physiol.) UMDS Guy's & St. Thos. Hosp. Lond. Specialty: Anat.; Respirat. Med.

WARD, Janet Amelia The Surgery, Marlpits Lane, Honiton EX14 2NY Tel: 01404 41141 Fax: 01404 46621 — MB BS Lond. 1981; MRCGP 1987; T(GP) 1991.

WARD, Jean Lomax (retired) 27 Elms Drive, Bare, Morecambe LA4 6DG Tel: 01524 410657 — MB ChB Leeds 1955; DObst RCOG 1957; MRCGP 1968. Prev: GP Morecambe Health Centre.

WARD, Jean Paula Rock Hall, Nidd, Harrogate HG3 3BB Tel: 01423 770077 — MB BS Lond. 1949 (Roy. Free) MRCS Eng. LRCP Lond. 1948; DObst RCOG 1950; DA Eng. 1954. Anaesth. Harrogate & Ripon Hosp. Gp. Socs: BMA & Yorks. Soc. Anaesths. Prev: Gyn. & Obst. Ho. Surg. Roy. Free Hosp.; O & G Regist. Padd. Hosp.; SHO (Anaesth.) Addenbrooke's Hosp. Camb.

WARD, Jenifer Ann (retired) The Coach House, 1A Meadows Close, Portishead, Bristol BS20 8BU — MB ChB Birm. 1968. Prev: Sen. Med. Off. DHSS.

WARD, Mr Jeremy Bruce Department of Surgery, Royal Liverpool University Hospital, University of Liverpool, Liverpool L69 3BX Tel: 0151 706 4170; 16 Addingham Road, Liverpool L18 2EW Tel: 0151 475 0846 — MB ChB Ed. 1989; FRCS Ed. 1993. Lect. Dept. Surg. Roy. Liverp. Univ. Hosp. Specialty: Gen. Surg. Socs: Pancreatic Soc. Prev: Specialist Regist. (Gen. Surg.) Warrington Hosp.; Research Fell. (Surg. & Physiol.) Univ. of Liverp.; SHO (Surg.) Warrington.

WARD, John Dale (retired) Royal Hallamshire Hospital, Glossop Road, Sheffield S10 2JF Tel: 0114 271 2938 Fax: 0114 271 3708; 68 Dore Road, Sheffield S17 3NE Tel: 0114 236 4698 — (Lond. Hosp.) MB BS Lond. 1961; FRCP Lond. 1976, M 1965; BSc Lond. 1958, MD 1971. Cons. Phys. Roy. Hallamsh. Hosp. Sheff.; Prof. Diabetic Med. Univ. Sheff. Prev: Sen. Regist. Lond. Hosp.

WARD, John Edward Hendon Anaesthetic Department, Queen Medical Centre, Nottingham NG7 2UH Tel: 0115 924 9924 — BM BS Nottm. 1986 (Nottingham) FRCA 1994; CCST 1998. Cons. (Anaesth.) Sheff. Specialty: Anaesth. Socs: Vasc. Anaesth. Soc.; Brit. Soc. of orthopaedic Anaesth.s (ord-Mem.); ass of Anaesth.s of GB & I (ord-Mem.). Prev: Research Regist. (Anaesth.) Nottm. & Derby; Regist. Rotat. (Anaesth.) Nottm. & Mansfield; Regist. (A & E) Cairns Queensland, Austral.

WARD, John Kingsley 2 Meadway, Westcliff on Sea SS0 8PJ Tel: 01702 710810 — MB BS Durh. 1960; FRCOG 1980, M 1967, DObst 1962. Specialty: Obst. & Gyn. Socs: BMA. Prev: Cons. O & G Southend-on-Sea Hosp. Gp.; Ho. Phys. (Med.) Roy. Vict. Infirm. Newc.; SHO (Surg.) & Regist. (O & G) Newc. Gen. Hosp.

WARD, John Luzzi Campbell (retired) 22B Duchy Road, Harrogate HG1 2ER Tel: 01423 560299 — (Leeds) M.B., Ch.B. Leeds 1941. Prev: Ho. Phys. Leeds Gen. Infirm.

WARD, Mr John Peter (retired) Clematis Cottages, Boreham Lane, Boreham St., Nr. Herstmonceux,, Hailsham BN27 4SL Tel: 01323 832186 — MB BS Lond. 1962 (St Mary's) MRCS Eng. LRCP Lond. 1962; FRCS Eng. 1967; MS Lond. 1974; Specialist Accredit. (Urol.) RCS Eng. 1974; T(S) 1991. Hon. Cons. Urol. Eastbourne NHS Trust; Hon. Sen. Clin. Lect. Inst. Urol. Univ. Coll. Univ. Lond.; Examr. MD. Univ. Mansoura, Egypt; Examr. Inst. Urol. Univ. Lond. Prev: Sen. Regist. (Urol.) St Bart. Hosp. Lond.

WARD, John Philip Quarrier Woodgate Valley Practice, 61 Stevens Avenue, Woodgate Valley, Birmingham B32 3SD Tel: 0121 427 6174 Fax: 0121 428 4146; 15 Park Hill Road, Harborne, Birmingham B17 9SJ Tel: 0121 427 3169 — MB ChB Birm. 1983. Clin. Asst. Roy. Orthop. Hosp. Birm. Specialty: Orthop. Socs: Birm. Med. Inst.

WARD, John William 8 Lanes Avenue, Northfleet, Gravesend DA11 7HR Tel: 01474 59633 — MB BS Lond. 1975; FRCR 1983.

WARD, John William 85 Chaveney Road, Quorndon, Loughborough LE12 8AB Tel: 01509 412862 — MB ChB Sheff. 1968; BPharm Nottm. 1961; MRCP (UK) 1972; FRCP Lond. 1988. Cons. Clin. Pharmacol. Glenfield Gen. Hosp. Leicester; Prof. Clin. Pharmacy Univ. Nottm. Specialty: Pharmacology. Socs: Brit. Pharm. Soc.; Brit. Thorac. Soc. Prev: Lect. (Pharmacol. & Therap.) Univ. Sheff.

WARD, John William Keith (retired) Winton, Thame Lane, Culham, Abingdon OX14 3DS Tel: 01235 525364 Fax: 01235 525364 — MB ChB St And. 1972 (St Andrews) FRCP Ed. 2004; DObst RCOG 1974; Cert. JCC Lond. 1976; FRCGP 1995, M 1976; DFFP 1993. Prev: GP Partner Malthouse Surg. Abingdon Oxon.

WARD, Karen Louise 12 Poplar Place, Gosforth, Newcastle upon Tyne NE3 1DR — MB BS Newc. 1990; DFFP 1994; MRCOG 1996. Specialty: Obst. & Gyn.

WARD, Katherine Nora Department of Virology, Royal Free & University College London Medical School, Windeyer Institute for Medical Sciences, 46 Cleveland Street, London W1T 4JF Tel: 020 7679 9134/9490 Fax: 020 7580 5896 Email: k.n.ward@ucl.ac.uk — MB BChir Camb. 1983; PhD Lond. 1973, BSc 1969; FRCPath 1998, MRCPath 1989; MA Camb. 1990. Cons. & Hon. Sen. Lect. Univ. Coll. Lond. Hosps. Trust & Royal Free & Univ. Coll. Lond. Med. Sch. Specialty: Virology. Socs: Soc. Gen. Microbiol.; Eur. Soc. Clin. Virol.; Internat. Soc. Antiviral Research. Prev: Sen. Lect. & Hon. Cons. Imperial Coll. Sch. of Med. & Hammersmith Hosp.; Clin. Lect. (Path.) Univ. Camb.; Hon. Sen. Regist. (Virol.) Addenbrooke's Hosp. Camb. & Hon. Asst. Med. Microbiol. Pub. Health Laborat. Camb.

WARD, Kathleen Anne — MB BCh BAO Belf. 1987 (Queens university of Belfast) MRCP (UK) 1990; MD 1993; FRCP 2002. Cons. Derm. Cannock Chase Hosp. Staffs. Specialty: Dermat. Special Interest: Skin Cancer; Vulval Condits. Socs: Brit. Ass of Dermatol.s; Roy. Coll. Phys.s; Roy. Soc. Med.

WARD, Kathryn Louise 13 Chatsworth Avenue, Southwell NG25 0AE — MB BS Lond. 1992.

WARD, Kathryn Patricia Airedale General Hospital, Skipton Road, Steeton, Keighley BD20 6TD Tel: 01535 292178 Fax: 01535 292224 Email: kate.ward@anhst.nhs.uk; Glenaire, Green Lane, Glusburn, Keighley BD20 8RU Tel: 01535 632146 — MB ChB Birm. 1975; DCH Eng. 1978; MRCP (UK) 1979; FRCP Lond. 1995; FRCPCH 1999. Cons. Paediat. Airedale Gen. Hosp.; Designated Doctor Child Protec. N. Yorks PCT; Designated Doctor, Child Protec., Bradford and Airedale. Specialty: Paediat. Special Interest: Allergy; Child Protection; Nutrition. Socs: Brit. Soc. Paediat. Gastroenterol.; Roy. Coll. of Paediat. and Child Health; Roy. Soc. of Med. Prev: Cons. Paediat. Airedale Gen. Hosp.; Sen. Regist. (Paediat.) Roy. Aberd. Childr. Hosp.; Research Regist. Grampian HB.

WARD, Kaye Churchgate Surgery, 119 Manchester Road, Denton, Manchester M34 3RA Tel: 0161 336 2114 Fax: 0161 320 7045 — MB ChB Manch. 1989; MRCGP 1993.

WARD, Kevin Jason 7 Grosvenor Park, York YO30 6BX — MB BS Lond. 1994; MRCGP 1997. Cons. (Palliat. Med.) Mid Yorks. NHS

Trust Pontefract. Specialty: Palliat. Med. Prev: Specialist Regist. Palliat. Med, Leeds.

WARD, Kevin John 5 Elmton Lane, Eythorne, Dover CT15 4AR — MB BS Lond. 1991 (Kings Coll.Sch.Med.Dentist.Lond) BSc Lond. 1988, MB BS 1991; MRCP 1994. Specialty: Cardiol.

WARD, Kirsty Louise 16 Brookhouse Avenue, Leicester LE2 0JE — MB ChB Leic. 1992.

WARD, Lesley Monica Moir Medical Centre, Regent St., Long Eaton, Nottingham NG10 1QQ Tel: 0115 973 5820 Fax: 0115 946 0197; 20 Bostocks Lane, Risley, Derby DE72 3SX Tel: 0115 917 9738 — MB ChB Sheff. 1979 (Sheffield)

WARD, Lindsay Stuart Stirchley Medical Practice, Stirchley Health Centre, Stirchley, Telford TF3 1FB Tel: 01952 660444 Fax: 01952 415139 — BM (Hons.) Soton. 1978.

WARD, Lisabeth Lee Taylor and Partners, Shirehampton Health Centre, Pembroke Road, Shirehampton, Bristol BS11 9SB Tel: 0117 916 2233 Fax: 0117 930 8246 — MB BS Lond. 1984; DCH RCP Lond. 1989.

WARD, Lucy 4 Patten Road, London SW18 3RH — MB BS Lond. 1996.

WARD, Lucy Elizabeth Community Team, 3rd Floor, Shieldfield Health Centre, 4 Clarence Walk, Newcastle upon Tyne NE2 1AL Tel: 0191 232 2766 — MB ChB Manch. 1983; MRCGP 1990. Staff Grade (Social Paediat.) Community Team, Newc. u. Tyne; Lect. Dept. Primary Health Care, Newc. Specialty: Child & Adolesc. Psychiat.

WARD, Malcolm Gordon Crich Medical Practice Bulling Lane, Bulling Lane, Crich, Matlock DE4 5DX Tel: 01773 852966 Fax: 01773 853919 — MB ChB Leeds 1977; MRCGP 1981. Chairm. Dispensing Doctors' Assn. Socs: Co-opted Mem. GPC Rural Pract. Subcommittee; Mem. RGCP Rural Gp.

WARD, Mark Alistair Auckland Medical Group, 54 Cockton Hill Road, Bishop Auckland DL14 6BB Tel: 01388 602728 — MB BS Lond. 1982.

WARD, Mark Robert (retired) Norvic Clinic, Thorpe, Norwich NR7 0SS — MB ChB Birm. 1984. Cons. Forens. Psychiat. Norwich.

WARD, Martyn Lester 24 St James Road, Wokingham RG40 4RT Tel: 01734 732955 — MB BS Lond. 1978; FCAnaesth. 1990. Head of Project Developm. Sandoz Pharmaceut. Frimley; Clin. Asst. (Anaesth.) Frimley Pk. Hosp. Surrey. Specialty: Pharmaceutical Medicine.

WARD, Mr Martyn Wootton, OBE, Group Capt. RAF Med. Br. Retd. (retired) — (St. Geo.) MB BS Lond. 1964; FRCS Ed. 1974. Prev: Cons. Adviser Orthop. Surg. RAF Med. Br.

WARD, Mary McLelland 3 Spire Heights, Gilstead Lane, Gilstead, Bingley BD16 3LN Tel: 01274 566066 — (Glas.) MB ChB Glas. 1951; DObst RCOG 1953; DPM Eng. 1970; FRCPsych 1993, M 1972; Dip. Psychother. Leeds 1976. Hon. Cons. Child Psychiat. Bradford HA. Specialty: Child & Adolesc. Psychiat. Socs: Assn. Family Ther.; Assn. Child Psychol. & Psychiat. Prev: Cons. Child Psychiat. Bradford HA; Cons. Psychiat. Stud. Health Univ. Bradford; Sen. Regist. (Child & Adolesc. Psychiat.) St. Jas. Hosp. Leeds.

WARD, Matthew Margrave 15 Cumberland Road, Richmond TW9 3HJ — MB ChB Bristol 1997.

WARD, Maurice Alfred George (retired) Kelvin, 8 Penenden Heath Road, Maidstone ME14 2DA Tel: 01622 752760 — (Birm.) MB ChB Birm. 1937; DPH Eng. 1941. Prev: Hyg. Specialist RAMC.

WARD, Michael (retired) 13 The Quarries, Swindon SN1 4EX Tel: 01793 536030 — MB BS Durh. 1958; FRCGP 1981, M 1974.

WARD, Michael 1 Knapp Rise, Haslingfield, Cambridge CB3 7LQ — MB BS Lond. 1994.

WARD, Michael Conor St Helier Hospital, Wrythe Lane, Carshalton SN5 1AA Tel: 020 8296 2689 — MB BCh BAO NUI 1979; MD NUI 1987; FRCP 1995. Cons. Phys. & Sen. Lect. Geriat. St. Helier Hosp. Carshalton & St. Geo. Hosp. Med. Sch. Lond. Specialty: Gen. Med. Prev: Sen. Regist. (Geriat. Med.) St. Geo. Hosp. Lond.

WARD, Michael Elliott Nuffield Department of Anaesthetics, Oxford Radcliffe NHS Trust, Oxford OX3 9DU Tel: 01865 221587 Fax: 01865 220027 Email: michael.ward@nda.ox.ac.uk — (King's Coll. Hosp.) MB BS Lond. 1969; MRCS Eng. LRCP Lond. 1969; FFA RCS Eng. 1973. Cons. Anaesth. Nuffield Dept. Anaesth. John Radcliffe Hosp. Oxf.; Med. Dir. Oxon. Ambul. Serv.; Mem. Jt.Roy. Coll. & Ambul. Liaison Comm. Specialty: Anaesth. Prev: Company Sec. Resus. Counc. Trading Co.; Sen. Regist. (Anaesth.) Qu. Vict. Hosp. E. Grinstead; Lect. (Anaesth.) King's Coll. Hosp. Lond.

WARD, Michael James 86 Glenshan Road, Londonderry BT47 3SF — MB BCh BAO Belf. 1994.

WARD, Michael Jonathan King's Mill Hospital, Mansfield Road, Sutton-in-Ashfield NG17 4JL Tel: 01623 22515 — MB ChB Dundee 1976; MB ChB (Hons.) Dundee 1976; MRCP (UK) 1978; DM Nottm. 1983; FRCP Lond. 1994. Cons. Phys. Mansfield.; Clin. Tutor Univ. Nottm. Specialty: Respirat. Med. Socs: Brit. Thorac. Soc.; Amer. Thoracic Soc.

WARD, Michael Joseph 361 Methilhaven Road, Methil, Leven KY8 3HR Tel: 01333 426913 Fax: 01333 422300 — MB ChB Ed. 1978 (Edin.) LMCC Vancouver 1981. GP Clin. Asst. (Geriat.) Randolph Wemyss Hosp. Buckhaven. Prev: GP Clin. Asst. (Anaesth.) Randolph Wemyss Hosp. Buckhaven; GP Clin. Asst. (Cas.) Vict. Hosp. Kirkcaldy.

WARD, Michael Kingsley 11 Wilson Gardens, Newcastle upon Tyne NE3 4JA — MB BS (2nd Cl. Hons.) Newc. 1969; MRCP (U.K.) 1972; FRCP Lond. 1984. Cons. Nephrol. Roy. Vict. Infirm. Newc. upon Tyne; Sen. Lect. Med. Univ. Newc. Specialty: Nephrol. Prev: Lect. in Med. Univ. Newc.; Hon. Sen. Regist. Dept. Med. Roy. Vict. Infirm. Newc. upon Tyne; Regist. Dept. Med. Hammersmith Hosp. Lond.

WARD, Mr Michael Phelps, CBE (retired) Pheasant Hill, Lurgashall, Petworth GU28 9EP — MB BChir Camb. 1949 (Camb. & Lond. Hosp.) MRCS Eng. LRCP Lond. 1949; FRCS Eng. 1955; MA Camb. 1962, BA 1946, MD 1968. Emerit. Cons. Surg. St. And. Hosp. Bow & Newham Dist. Gen. Hosp.; Hon. Lect. (Surg.) Lond. Hosp. Med. Coll. Prev: Asst. Resid. Roy. Vict. Hosp. Montreal, Canada.

WARD, Michael Thomas (retired) Great Crabthorn, 80 Old St, Hill Head, Fareham PO14 3HN Tel: 01329 662581 Fax: 01329 662581 — MB BS Lond. 1958 (St. Mary's) MRCS Eng. LRCP Lond. 1958; DObst RCOG 1960; MRCGP 1996. Prev: Assoc. Dir. Postgrad. Gen. Pract. Educat. Wessex.

WARD, Mr Michael William Noel Chase Farm Hospital, The Ridgeway, Enfield EN2 8JL Tel: 020 8366 6600; 51 Lanchester Road, Highgate, London N6 4SX — BM BCh Oxf. 1972 (Univ. Coll. Hosp.) MA Oxf. 1972, MCh 1985, BM BCh 1972; FRCS Eng. 1978. Cons. Surg. Chase Farm & Highlands Hosp. Enfield. Specialty: Gen. Surg.

WARD, Morag Christine Lochee Health Centre, 1 Marshall Street, Lochee, Dundee DD2 3BR Tel: 01382 611283 — MB ChB Dundee 1984. GP Dundee.

WARD, Nicholas Alexander Lawton Bampton Surgery, Landells, Bampton OX18 2LJ Tel: 01993 850257; 9 Bushey Row, Bampton OX18 2JX Tel: 01993 851226 — MB BChir Camb. 1989; MA Camb. 1989; DRCOG 1991; DCH RCP Lond. 1991; MRCGP 1992. Socs: BMA.

WARD, Nicholas Charles The Grange Medical Centre, West Cliff Road, Ramsgate CT11 9LJ Tel: 01843 595051 Fax: 01843 591999 — MB BS Lond. 1986; DRCOG 1989.

WARD, Nicholas John Towcester Medical Centre, Link Way, Towcester NN12 6HH Tel: 01327 359953 Fax: 01327 358929 — MB BS Lond. 1986; DRCOG 1989; MRCGP 1991. Specialty: Gen. Med. Prev: Trainee GP Northampton VTS.

WARD, Nicholas Mark Carnwarth Health Centre, 7 Biggar Road, Carnwath, Lanark ML11 8HJ Tel: 01555 840214 — MB ChB Ed. 1988. SHO (Cas.) Hull Roy. Infirm. Specialty: Gen. Pract. Prev: SHO (A & E) Perth Roy. Infirm.

WARD, Nicholas Steven Institute of Neurology & National Hospital for Neurology & Neurosurgery, London WC1N Email: n.ward@fil.ion.ucl.ac.uk — MB BS Lond. 1989; BSc Lond. 1986; MRCP (UK) 1994. Clin. Fell. in Stroke Med. Inst. of Neurol. & Nat. Hosp. Neurol. & Neurosurg., Lond. Specialty: Neurol. Prev: Specialist Regist. (Neurol.) Roy. Lond. Hosp.; SHO Nat. Hosp. Neurol. & Neurosurg. Lond.; Specialist Regist. (Neurol.) Nat. Hosp. Neurol. & Neurosurg.

WARD, Nicolas Wyndham University Hospital of Wales, Heath Park, Cardiff CF14 4WZ; 10 Groveland Road, Birchgrove, Cardiff CF14 4QX — MB ChB Birm. 1990; ChB Birm. 1990. Specialist Regist. (Histopath.) Univ. Hosp. Wales. Specialty: Histopath. Prev: Lect. (Anat.) Birm. Univ. Med. Sch.

WARD, Nicole Low Heulah Cottage, Dunsley, Whitby YO21 3TL — MB ChB Manch. 1997.

WARD, Professor Owen Conor Maurice Kennedy Research Centre for Emeritus Staff, University College, Dublin H, Republic of Ireland; 18 Thamespoint, Teddington TW11 9PP Tel: 020 8977 0153 Fax: 020 8977 0153 — MB BCh BAO NUI 1947; DCH RCPSI 1948; DCH NUI 1949; MD (Paediat.) NUI 1951; FRCPI 1959, M 1952; FRCP Glas. 1983; FRCP Lond. 1995; FRCPCH (Hon.) 1997. Emerit. Prof. Paediat. Univ. Coll. Dub.; Adviser Emerit. Down Syndrome Assn. of Irel; Hon. Cons. Paediat., Kingston Hosp. NHS Trust. Specialty: Paediat.; Paediat. Cardiol. Socs: Eur. Assn. Paediat. Cardiols.; Fell. Roy. Soc. Med.; Scientif. Counc. Europ. Down Syndrome Assn. (Brussels). Prev: Cons. Paediat. Our Lady's Hosp. Sick Childr. Crumlin; Sen. Regist. (Child Health) Univ. Liverp.; Ho. Phys. Mater Miser. Hosp. Dub.

WARD, Pamela Mary St Ronans Health Centre, Innerleithen EH44 6QE — MB ChB Ed. 1996; DRCOG 1999; MRCGP 2000; DFFP 2000. p/t GP St Ronans Health Centre Innerleithen; Clin. Asst. Drug & Alcohol Misuse Castle Craig Hosp.; Med. Off. RSC Glencourse Carn. Specialty: Gen. Pract. Socs: Mem. Roy. Coll. Gen. Practitioners.

WARD, Patricia Ann St Mary's Hospital, Praed Street, London NW2 1NY; 2 Angel Cottages, Milespit Hill, Mill Hill, London NW7 1RD — MB BS Lond. 1988 (Univ. coll. and Middlx. Sch. of Med.) MRCP (UK) 1991; FRCS Ed. 1993; FFAEM 1997. Cons. (A & E Med.) St. Mary's Hosp. Praed St. Lond. Specialty: Accid. & Emerg. Socs: Fell. Fac. A&E Med.; Brit. Assn. Accid. & Emerg. Med. Prev: Regist. (A & E) St. Mary's Hosp. Lond.; Regist. Helicopter Emerg. Med. Serv. Chems. Roy. Lond. Hosp. Lond.; Specialist Regist. A & E Whipps Cross Hosp. Lond.

WARD, Patrick Gerald (retired) Dunturk, Castlewellan BT31 9PF Tel: 028 437 78461 — MB BCh BAO Belf. 1961. Prev: Ho. Off. Roy. Vict. Hosp. Belf. & Musgrave Pk. Hosp. Belf.

WARD, Patrick Joshua, MBE (Surgery) Wakefield House, Bessbrook, Newry BT35 7DA Tel: 028 3083 0400; Broomhill, 16 Goragh Road, Newry BT35 6PZ Tel: 028 3026 3470 — LRCPI & LM, LRSCI & LM 1954 (Roy. Coll. Surgs. Dub. & Qu. Univ. Belf.) DPH Belf. 1956; MRCGP 1968; AFOM RCP Lond. 1983. Occupat. Health; Staff Med. Offcer Daisy Hill Hosp. Newry; JP; Dep. Lt. Co. Armagh; Med. Adviser Norbrook Laborat. Ltd Newry. Specialty: Occupat. Health; Gen. Med. Socs: Fell. BMA. Prev: Chairm. Local Med. Comm. (South. Area); Hon. Treas. GMSC (N. Irel.); Chairm. BMA (N. Irel.) South. Div.

WARD, Paul John Whitby Group Practice, Spring Vale Medical Centre, Whitby YO21 1SD Tel: 01947 820888; Brook Cottage, Raw, Whitby YO22 4PP — MB ChB Leeds 1971; DObst RCOG 1973. Prev: Ho. Off. Bradford Roy. Infirm.; SHO (Obst.) Profess. Unit. Leeds Matern. Hosp.; SHO (Paediat.) Alder Hey Hosp. Liverp.

WARD, Paul Stanley Derriford Hospital, Department of Child Health, Brest Road, Plymouth PL6 8DH Tel: 01752 763454 Fax: 01752 763467 Email: paul.ward@phnt.swest.nhs.uk; 5 Raynham Road, Stoke, Plymouth PL3 4EU Tel: 01752 561744 Email: psward@tiscali.co.uk/wardps@lineone.net — MB ChB Bristol 1977; BSc (Med. Microbiol.) Bristol 1974; DCH Eng. 1979; FRCP Lond. 1995; FRCPCH 1997, M 1996. Cons. Paediat. Derriford Hosp. Plymouth. Specialty: Paediat. Special Interest: Paediatric Endocrinol., paediatric Oncol. Socs: Brit. Soc. Paediat. Endocrinol. & Diabetes; Assoc. Mem. UK Childr. Cancer Study Gp. Prev: Sen. Regist. (Paediat.) Addenbrooke's Hosp. Camb.; Sen. Regist. (Paediat.) Norf. & Norwich Hosp.; Research Fell. & Regist. (Paediat.) Bristol Roy. Hosp. for Sick Childr.

WARD, Penelope 13 Damask Close, West End, Woking GU24 9PD — MB BS Lond. 1978; MRCOG 1987. Clin. Research Asst. St. Mary's Hosp. Med. Sch. Lond.

WARD, Peter (retired) — MB BS Lond. 1950 (Westm.) DMRD Eng. 1957; FFR 1960. Prev: Cons. Radiol. Sheff. AHA.

WARD, Peter James Macready (retired) The King's House, 29 Keppel St., Dunston, Gateshead NE11 9AR Tel: 0191 460 7404 — MB BChir Camb. 1966; MA Camb. 1968; DCH Eng. 1968. Prev: GP Birtley.

WARD, Peter John 5 Firwood Stables, Bolton BL2 3AQ — MB ChB Bristol 1989.

WARD, Peter John (retired) Red Cow Byre, Watling St., Kensworth, Dunstable LU6 3QT Tel: 01582 840527 — (Univ. Coll. Hosp.) MB BS Lond. 1960. Prev: GP St. Albans.

WARD, Mr Peter John Princess Royal Hospital, Hurstwood Park Neurological Centre, Lewes Road, Haywards Heath RH17 7SJ Tel: 01444 441881 Fax: 01444 417995 — (Middlx.) BSc Lond. 1968; MB BS Lond. 1971; FRCS Eng. 1977. Cons. Neurosurg. Hurstwood Pk. Neurol. Centre Princess Roy. Hosp.; Cons. Neurosurg. Roy. Sussex Co. Hosp. Brighton. Specialty: Neurosurg. Socs: Mem. Soc. Brit. Neurol. Surgs.; Brighton & Sussex Medico-Chirurgical. Prev: Sen. Regist. (Neurosurg.) St. Bart. Hosp. Lond.; Regist. Inst. Neurol. Sci. Glas. & Nat. Hosp. Qu. Sq. Lond.; Ho. Phys. & Ho. Surg. Middlx. Hosp. Lond.

WARD, Peter John (retired) Pinfold Surgery, Station Road, Owston Ferry, Doncaster DN9 1AW Tel: 01427 728443 Fax: 01427 728558; Step Aside, North St, Owston Ferry, Doncaster DN9 1RT Tel: 01427 728445 Fax: 01427 28445 — MB BS Lond. 1958 (Lond. Hosp.) Prev: Clin. Asst. (Psychiat.) Scunthorpe Gen. Hosp.

WARD, Peter Michael Charing Cross Hospital, Fulham Palace Road, London W6 8RF Tel: 020 8846 1234 — MB BS Lond. 1986; BSc (Physiol.) Lond. 1979; FRCA 1990. Cons. Anaesth. Char. Cross Hosp. Lond. Specialty: Anaesth.

WARD, Peter Roger (retired) 260 Broomhill Road, Aberdeen AB10 7LP Tel: 01224 313804 Email: peruward@aol.com — MB ChB Manch. 1951; DMRD Eng. 1957; FFR 1961; FRCR 1975. Prev: Cons. Radiol. Roy. Infirm. Aberd.

WARD, Rachel Ann The Health Centre, Worcester Street, Stourport-on-Severn DY13 8EH Tel: 01299 827141 Fax: 01299 879074; Eardiston View, Menith Wood, Worcester WR6 6UD — MB ChB Liverp. 1986 (Liverpool) BSc Pharmacol. Liverp. 1981. Prev: SHO (Paediat.) Good Hope Hosp. Sutton Coldfield.

WARD, Rachel Ann Moorlands Medical Centre, Dyson House, Regent St., Leek ST13 6LU Tel: 01538 399008; Lower Brook Barn, Virgins Alley Lane, Snelston, Derby DE6 2GP — MB ChB Birm. 1987. Prev: Community Paediat. N. Staffs. HA GPVTS.

WARD, Richard Humphry Thomas (retired) University College Hospital, 25 Grafton Way, London WC1E 6AU Tel: 020 7383 7916 Fax: 020 7380 9816; Eagle House, Sulgrave, Banbury OX17 2SQ Tel: 01295 760296 Fax: 01295 768832 — (St. Bart.) MRCS Eng. LRCP Lond. 1962; MB BChir Camb. 1963; MA Camb. 1964; DObst RCOG 1964; FRCOG 1981, M 1968. Cons. & Sen. Lect. (O & G) Univ. Coll. Hosp. Lond. Prev: Lect. Univ. Coll. Hosp. Med. Sch. Lond.

WARD, Richard Leonard (retired) Clouds Hill, Mellor, Blackburn BB2 7HA Tel: 0125 481 2404 — (St. Mary's) MRCS Eng. LRCP Lond. 1942; MD Lond. 1950, MB BS 1943; FRCP Lond. 1970, M 1948. Prev: Cons. Phys. Blackburn Health Dist.

WARD, Richard William George Lower Loady Farm, Highweek, Newton Abbot TQ12 1QE Tel: 01626 367714 — MB ChB Birm. 1975; FP Cert Birm. 1975.

WARD, Robert Derek Markham House, 140 Wyke Road, Wyke Regis, Weymouth DT4 9QR — MB BS Lond. 1971 (Guy's) MRCS Eng. LRCP Lond. 1971; DObst RCOG 1975. Prev: SHO (O & G) & SHO (Paediat.) Salisbury Gen. Hosp. (Odstock; Br.); SHO (A & E) Hillingdon Hosp. Uxbridge.

WARD, Mr Robert Douglas 5 West Road, Kingston upon Thames KT2 7HA Tel: 020 8942 8884 Email: drrobertward@hotmail.com — (St Georges Hosp) MB BS Lond. 1994; FRCS (Eng.) 1998. Ho. Off. (Gen. Surg.) Ashford Hosp. Middlx. Specialty: Gen. Surg. Prev: Ho. Off. (Gastroenterol. & Gen. Med.) St. Richards Hosp. Chichester.; Ho. Off. (Gen. Surg.) Ashford Hosp. Middlx.; SHO A & E Worthing Hosp. W. Sussex.

WARD, Robert John The Surgery, 50 The Glade, Furnace Green, Crawley RH10 6JN Tel: 01293 612741 — BM BS Nottm. 1986; BM BS Nottm. 1986.

WARD, Roger Sidney Worcestershire Royal Hospital, Radiology, Charles Hastings Way, Worcester WR5 1DD Tel: 01905 763333 — MB ChB Birm. 1965; DMRD Eng. 1969; FFR 1971. Cons. Radiol. & Nuclear Phys. Worcester Roy. Infirm. Specialty: Radiol. Prev: Sen. Regist. (Radiol.) United Birm. Hosps.

WARD, Ronald Wilfred The Surgery, Snainton, Scarborough YO13 9AP Tel: 01723 859302 — MB BS Lond. 1972 (St. Thos.) BSc (Hons.) (Biochem.) Lond. 1969, MB BS 1972; MRCGP 1978.

WARD, Rosalind Frances 5 Rivers Edge, Charlton Marshall, Blandford Forum DT11 9PJ — MB ChB Glas. 1997.

WARD, Roselle Paulette Stephanie 33 Killeaton Crescent, Derriaghy, Belfast BT17 9HB — MB BCh BAO Belf. 1993.

WARD, Rosemary Virginia Hurst (retired) 5 Rosemont Road, Richmond TW10 6QN — MB BS Lond. 1959 (Roy. Free) MRCS Eng. LRCP Lond. 1959. Prev: GP Richmond.

WARD, Ruth The Health Centre, 20 Duncan Street, Greenock PA15 4LY Tel: 01475 724477; 107 Finnart Street, Greenock PA16 8HN — MB ChB Glas. 1978; DRCOG 1980. GP Greenock Health Centre.; Clin. Asst. Palliat. Care Ardgowan Hospice, Greenock.

WARD, Sarah Louise 71 Chandos Ave, London N20 9EG — MB BS Lond. 1993.

WARD, Mr Sean Edward Charles Clifford Dental Hospital, Wellesley Road, Sheffield S10 2SZ Tel: 0114 271 7810 — MB ChB Liverp. 1982; BDS Liverp. 1972; FFD RCSI 1985; FRCS Ed. 1988. Cons. Oral & Maxillofacial Surg. Sheff. HA; Cons. Maxillofacial Surg. AMI Thornbury Hosp. & Claremont Hosp. Sheff. Specialty: Oral & Maxillofacial Surg. Socs: Fell. Brit. Assn. Oral & Maxillofacial Surg.; BMA; Brit. Assn. Head & Neck Oncol. Prev: Sen. Regist. (Oral & Maxillofacial Surg.) Trent RHA.

WARD, Sheelagh Margaret Area Community Child Health Department, Stirling Royal Infirmary, Stirling FK8 2AU Tel: 01786 434000; 7 Manse Crescent, Stirling FK7 9AJ Tel: 01786 464321 — (Glas.) MB ChB Glas. 1969. Staff Grade (Community Paediat.) Forth Valley Primary Care NHS Trust. Specialty: Community Child Health. Prev: Clin. Med. Off. Forth Valley HB; Ho. Off. (Med.) Falkirk & Dist. Roy. Infirm.; Ho. Off. (Surg.) Stirling Roy. Infirm.

WARD, Shelley Jane 2 Ringstead Way, Aylesbury HP21 7ND — BChir Camb. 1988.

WARD, Simon Charles Department of Radiology, St. Mary's Hospital, Milton Road, Portsmouth PO3 6AD Tel: 023 92 866173 — MB BS Lond. 1984; BSc (Hons.) Lond. 1981; MRCP (UK) 1987; FRCR 1991; T(R) (CR) 1992. Cons. (Radiol.) Portsmouth Hosps. NHS Trust. Specialty: Radiol.

WARD, Simon Jeremy Churchside Medical Practice, Wood Street, Mansfield NG18 1QB Tel: 01623 664877 Fax: 01623 664878 — MB ChB Birm. 1985; DRCOG 1989; DFFP 1993; MRCGP 2002. Clin. Tutor (Gen. Pract.) Nottm. Specialty: Gen. Med. Socs: BMA; Mansfield Med. Soc. Prev: SHO (Med.) Staffs. Gen. Infirm.; SHO (Paediat. & O & G) Stafford Dist. Gen. Hosp.

WARD, Simon Jonathan 6 Cambridge Close, Sale, Manchester M33 4JY — MB ChB Ed. 1989.

WARD, Simon Joseph 32 Dovercourt Road, London SE22 8ST — MB BS Lond. 1986 (King's College) MA Camb. (1983); MRCP (UK) 1991; FRCS Ed. 1994; MSc (Paediat.) Lond. 1996; MPhil Camb. 1997. Cons. Paediatric A + E, King Geo. Hosp. Ilford. Specialty: Paediat.; Accid. & Emerg.; Educat. Socs: Assoc. Study Med. Ed. Prev: Hon. Regist. (Paediat., A & E) Alder Hey Childr. Hosp. Liverp.; Hon. Regist. (Paediat., Intens. Care) Gt. Ormond St. Childr. Hosp.; Resp. Fell. Gt.Ormond St. Child. Hosp.

WARD, Stephanie Department of Child Health, Tickhill Road Hospital, Tickhill Road, Balby, Doncaster DN4 8QL Tel: 01302 796246 Fax: 01302 796377; 31 Scaftworth Close, Bessacarr, Doncaster DN4 7RH — MB ChB Sheff. 1974; MFFP; MRCPCH; MMSc Leeds Univ. 1997. Assoc. Specialist (Paediat.)/Community Child Health Doncaster & Basset Law Hosps NHS Trust. Specialty: Community Child Health.

WARD, Stephen 7 August House, 17 Palmeira Avenue, Westcliff on Sea SS0 7RP — MB ChB Manch. 1974; FFA RCS Eng 1979. Cons. Anaesth. N.E. Thames RHA. Specialty: Anaesth.

WARD, Stephen Exmouth Health Centre, Claremont Grove, Exmouth EX8 2JF Tel: 01395 273001 Fax: 01395 273771; Caledon, Westbourne Terrace, Budleigh Salterton EX9 Tel: 01395 446276 — MB ChB Liverp. 1980; MRCP (UK) 1983; MRCGP 1987; DRCOG 1987. Trainer GP Pract.

WARD, Stephen Christopher 45 Stretton Road, Great Glen, Leicester LE8 9GN — MB BS Lond. 1996.

WARD, Stephen Patrick 30 Whyke Road, Chichester PO19 7AW; Flat 8 Jenner House, Restell Close, London SE3 7UW — MB BS Lond. 1990.

WARD, Stephen Thomas Sandy Lane Surgery, Sandy Lane, Leyland, Preston PR25 2EB Tel: 01772 909915 Fax: 01772 909911 — MB ChB Liverp. 1978.

WARD, Stuart Andrew Porteous Fryern and Millers Dale Partnership, Fryern Surgery, Oakmount Road, Chandlers Ford, Eastleigh SO53 2LH Tel: 023 8027 3252/3458 Fax: 023 8027 3459 — BM Soton. 1986; DRCOG 1989. Specialty: Gen. Pract. Prev: Trainee GP Portsmouth VTS.

WARD, Susan Clare Southwold, Wilmslow Road, Woodford, Stockport SK7 1RH Tel: 0161 439 4001; AEA International, 38 Russell St, Causeway Bay, Hong Kong Tel: 00 852 2528 9900 Fax: 00 852 2528 9933 — MB BS Lond. 1991; DCH RCP Lond. 1993; MRCGP 1995; DRCOG 1995. GP; Hon. Lect. (Gen. Pract.). Socs: BMA & MPS. Prev: GP Discovery Bay Med. Centre, Hong Kong; Lect. Gen. Pract. Roy. Free Sch. of Med.

WARD, Miss Susan Jennie Kings Mill Hospital, Sutton-in-Ashfield NG17 4JT; High Barn, 160 Edwards Lane, Sherwood, Nottingham NG5 3HZ — BM BS Nottm. 1980; BMedSci Nottm. 1978; FRCS Ed. 1986; FRCOG 1989; DM 1995; DM Nottm. 1995. Cons. (O & G) Kings Mill Hosp.; Dist. Tutor (Obst. & Gyn.) Mansfield; Pres. Med. Woms. Federat. E. Midl.s. Specialty: Obst. & Gyn. Socs: Fell. Birm. Midl. Obst. & Gyn. Soc. Prev: Sen. Regist. Nottm. Hosps.; Regist. (O & G) Leicester Gen. Hosp.; Regist. (Urol.) & SHO (O & G) Univ. Hosp. Nottm.

WARD, Susan Margaret Queen Mary's Sidcup NHS Trust, Haematology Department, Frognal Avenue, Sidcup DA14 6LT Tel: 020 8308 3023 — MB BS Lond. 1977 (St. Mary's) BSc (Med. Sci.) Lond. 1974; MRCP (UK) 1981; MRCPath 1988; FRCPath 1997; FRCP 1999. Cons. Haematologist Qu. Mary's Sidcup NHS Trust. Specialty: Haematology.

WARD, Susan Mary Eborall and Partners, Fountain Medical Centre, Sherwood Avenue, Newark NG24 1QH Tel: 01636 704378/9 Fax: 01636 610875 — MB ChB Liverp. 1974; DRCOG 1976.

WARD, Thomas County Practice, Barking Road, Needham Market, Ipswich IP6 8EZ Tel: 01449 720666 Fax: 01449 720030 — MB ChB Glas. 1966; DCH RCPS Glas. 1969. Prev: Regist. (Gen. Med.) Dept. Mat. Med. Glas. Univ.; Ho. Off. (Paediat.) & Ho. Phys. Stobhill Gen. Hosp. Glas.

WARD, Thomas Arthur Brook Cottage, Raw, Robin Hoods Bay, Whitby YO22 4PP — MB BS Lond. 1996.

WARD, Thomas William 155 Newton Drive, Blackpool FY3 8LZ Tel: 01253 392814 Fax: 01253 300261; 111 Newton Drive, Blackpool FY3 8LZ Fax: 01253 300261 — MB ChB Sheff. 1977; DCH Eng. 1979; DRCOG 1981; FRCGP 1996, M 1982; DFFP 1996. Fell. Higher Profess. Train. N. W. (E.) Region; Hon. Sen. Lect. Lanc. Postgrad. Sch. Med. Health. Prev: Course Organiser (Gen. Pract.) Blackpool VTS.; Clin. Asst. (Dermat.) Vict. Hosp. Blackpool.

WARD, Timothy Staveleigh Medical Centre, King Street, Stalybridge SK15 2AE Tel: 0161 304 8009 Fax: 0161 303 7207; 314 Stockport Road, Marple, Stockport SK6 6ET — MB BS Newc. 1978; DRCOG 1980; MRCGP 1982.

WARD, Timothy Mark Gordon French Weir Health Centre, French Weir Avenue, Taunton TA1 1NW Tel: 01823 331381 Fax: 01823 323689 — MB BS Lond. 1990; BSc Lond. 1987; MRCGP 1995; DFFP 1995. Specialty: Gen. Pract.

WARD, Timothy Peter 80 Old Street, Fareham PO14 3HN — MB BS Lond. 1993; BSc (Psychol.) Lond. 1992; MRCP (UK) 1998.

WARD, Tracey Jane Conquest Hospital, The Ridge, St Leonards-on-Sea TN37 7RD Tel: 01424 755255 — MB BS (Hons.) Lond. 1984; DRCOG 1987; MRCGP (Distinction) 1988; DCH RCP Lond. 1990; MRCP (UK) 1992; FRCPCH 1997; MSc Community Paediatrics 1997. Cons. Community Paediat. Hastings & Rother NHS Trust. Specialty: Community Child Health. Prev: Sen. Regist. (Communtiy Paediat.) Optimum Health Care Lewisham & S.wark; Regist. (Community Paediat.) Guy's & Lewisham Hosps.; Trainee GP Ipswich VTS.

WARD, Miss Victoria Mary Margaretha 1 Hamilton House, 8 Victory Place, Quayside, London E14 8BQ Email: vmmw@aol.com — MB ChB Leic. 1993; FRCSI 1997; FRCS (Oto) 1998. Specialist Regist. in OtoLaryngol., Guy's & St Thomas Trust, Lond. Specialty: Otorhinolaryngol.

WARD, Wendy Ann (Surgery), 1 Kew Gdns. Road, Richmond TW9 3HN Tel: 020 8940 1048 Fax: 020 8332 7644; 15

Cumberland Road, Richmond TW9 3HJ Tel: 020 8940 4252 Fax: 020 8332 7770 — (Bristol University) MB ChB Bristol 1970; DCH Eng. 1973; DRCOG 1978; MRCGP 1980; MSc Lond. 1996.

WARD, William (retired) 47 Marlow Road, Gainsborough DN21 1YG Tel: 01427 613873 — MB BCh BAO NUI 1949 (Univ. Coll. Dub.) DPH (2nd Cl. Hons.) 1954. Prev: MoH GainsBoro. UD & RD & Isle of Axholme RD.

WARD, William Christopher (retired) 19 Harperley, Astley Village, Chorley PR7 1XB Tel: 01257 271808 — MB ChB Manch. 1980; BSc (Hons.) Manch. 1977, MB ChB 1980. Prev: SHO (Geriat.) Bolton Gen. Hosp.

WARD, William Daniel 52 Wimpole Road, Colchester CO1 2DL Tel: 01206 794794 Fax: 01206 790403; 113 Prettygate Road, Colchester CO3 4DZ Tel: 01206 572705 — MB ChB Glas. 1963. Ex-Chairm. Essex LMC. Socs: Chairm. NE Essex Doctors Emerg. Serv. (BASICS). Prev: Ho. Surg. & Ho. Phys. Glas. Roy. Infirm.; Ho. Surg. (Obst.) Bushey Matern. Hosp.

WARD, William Duncan 67 The Avenue, Richmond TW9 2AH — MB BS Lond. 1994.

WARD-BOOTH, Ronald Patrick Brook Hill Surgery, 30 Brook Hill, Little Waltham, Chelmsford CM3 3LL Tel: 01245 360253 Fax: 01245 361343; Markhams Cottage, Pleshey, Chelmsford CM3 1HY Tel: 973 37 298 — MB BS Lond. 1974; BDS Birm. 1967.

WARD-BOOTH, Stephen 5 Ouston Road, Knossington, Oakham LE15 8LX — MB ChB Leic. 1997.

WARD-CAMPBELL, Gordon James 12 Rosset Green Lane, Harrogate HG2 — BM BS Nottm. 1994.

WARD-MCQUAID, John Michael Cherry Garth, 16 Humberston Avenue, Humberston, Grimsby DN36 4SJ — LRCPI & LM, LRSCI & LM 1969; LRCPI & LM, LRCSI & LM 1969; FFA RCS Eng. 1978. Cons. Anaesth. Grimsby Dist. Gen. Hosp. Specialty: Anaesth.

WARD PLATT, Martin Peter Royal Victoria Infirmary, Ward 35, Queen Victoria Road, Newcastle upon Tyne NE1 4LP Tel: 0191 282 5197 Fax: 0191 282 5038 Email: m.p.ward-platt@ncl.ac.uk — MB ChB Bristol 1979; MRCP (UK) 1983; MD Bristol 1989; FRCP Lond. 1994; FRCPCH 1998; FRCP Edin 2000. Cons. Paediat. Sen. Lect. (Child Health) Roy. Vict. Infirm. Newc. u. Tyne; Hon. Cons. Paediat., Northumbria Healthcare NHS Trust; Clin. Director, Regional Matern. Surg. Office. Specialty: Paediat.; Neonat. Special Interest: Cot death. Socs: Brit. Assn. Perinatal Med.; Soc. Reproduc. & Infant Psychol.; Internat. Assn. Study of Pain. Prev: Cons. Paediat. Clin. Sub-Dir. for Neonat. Servs. Princess Mary Matern. Hosp. Newc.; Sen. Regist. (Neonat.) Newc. HA; Fell. (Neonat.) Monash Med. Centre, Melbourne.

WARD PLATT, Patricia (retired) Greengates Cottage, Astley Burf, Stourport-on-Severn DY13 0SD Tel: 01299 879638 Email: patwp@fish.co.uk — BM BCh Oxf. 1947; DCH Eng. 1949. Prev: Stud. Health Phys. (Stud. Health Serv.) Liverp. Univ.

WARDALE, Janette Gibb Fender Way Health Centre, Fender Way, Birkenhead CH43 9QS Tel: 0151 677 9103 Fax: 0151 604 0392; 7 Barker Road, Irby, Wirral CH61 3XH Tel: 0151 648 5325 — MB ChB Glas. 1970; Cert. Family Pract. JCC 1976. Prev: Regist. (Path.) United Liverp. Hosps.; Ho. Off. (Med.) South. Gen. Hosp. Glas.; Ho. Off. (Surg.) Vict. Infirm. Glas.

WARDALL, Gordon James 11 Beechwood, Linlithgow EH49 6SD — MB ChB Ed. 1984; FRCA 1989; T(Anaesth.) 1993. Cons. Anaesth. Falkirk & Dist. Roy. Infirm. Specialty: Anaesth. Prev: Sen. Regist. (Anaesth.) Roy. Infirm. Edin.

WARDELL, Anthony Michael John — MB BChir Camb. 1987; MA Camb. 1981; MRCPsych 1991. Cons. (Child & Adolesc. Psychiat.) Invicta Community NHS Trust. Specialty: Child & Adolesc. Psychiat. Prev: Sen.Regist. (Child & Adolesc. Psychiat.) St. Geo. Hosp. Lond.; Cons (C&A psychiat) Instit ch Trust.

WARDELL-YERBURGH, John Gerald Oswald (retired) 6 Old Northwick Lane, Worcester WR3 7LY Tel: 01905 452518 Email: northwick6@aol.com — MB BChir Camb. 1949 (Camb. & St. Bart.) MA, MB BChir Camb. 1949; DPM Eng. 1954; MRCPsych 1972. Prev: Cons. Psychiat. John Connolly Hosp. Rednal.

WARDELL-YERBURGH, Sheena Jane 1 The Park, Kingscote, Tetbury GL8 8XY — MB BCh Wales 1987. Prev: GP Nailsworth Retainer Scheme.

WARDELL-YERBURGH, Tom Charles May Lane Surgery, Dursley GL11 4JN Tel: 01453 540540 Fax: 01453 540570 — MB BCh Wales 1987. Prev: Trainee GP Cheltenham; SHO (A & E) Glos. Roy. Infirm.; SHO (Dermat.) Glos. Roy. Hosp.

WARDEN, David John Collington Surgery, 23 Terminus Road, Bexhill-on-Sea TN39 3LR Tel: 01424 217465/216675 Fax: 01424 216675; 8 Meads Road, Bexhill-on-Sea TN39 4SY — MB BS Lond. 1985 (Lond. Hosp.) MA Camb. 1989, BA 1982. Clin. Asst. (Rheumat.) Conquest Hosp. Hastings. Specialty: Gen. Med.

WARDEN, Matthew Giles Top Flat, 347A New King's Road, London SW6 4RJ Tel: 020 7731 3435 — MB BS Lond. 1995 (UMDS Guy's & St. Thos. Lond.) SHO (Psychiat.) St. Bart. Hosp. Lond. Specialty: Gen. Psychiat.

WARDHAUGH, Allan Doyle The Lodge, Talygarn, Pontyclun CF72 9JT — MB ChB Ed. 1989.

WARDILL, Lesley Forster 9 May Fields, Sindlesham, Wokingham RG41 5BY Tel: 0118 978 3495 Email: lesley.wardill@virgin.net — (Liverpool University) MB ChB Liverp. 1957; DCH Eng. 1960; DPM Eng. 1973; MRCPsych 1982. Indep. Pract. Wokingham. Specialty: Psychother. Socs: Roy. Coll. Psychiats. Prev: Assoc. Specialist (Psychiat.) Wokingham Ment. Health Servs. & Eldon Day Hosp. Reading; Clin. Asst. (Psychiat.) Warneford Hosp. Oxf.

WARDLAW, Joanna Marguerite Western General Hospital, Department of Clinical Neurosciences, Crewe Road, Edinburgh EH4 2XU — MB ChB Ed. 1982; BSc (Hons.) Physiol. Ed. 1979, MB ChB (Hons.) 1982; MRCP (UK) 1986; DMRD 1987; FRCR 1988; MD 1994; FRCP 1998. Prof. of Radiol. Univ. Edin.; Hon. Cons. Neuroradiol. West. Gen. Hosp. NHS Trust Edin. Specialty: Radiol. Special Interest: Stroke Imaging. Prev: Cons. Neuroradiol. South. Gen. Hosp. NHS Trust Glas.

WARDLE, Albert Dennis (retired) 165 Moor Green Lane, Moseley, Birmingham B13 8NT Tel: 0121 449 0700; 165 Moor Green Lane, Moseley, Birmingham B13 8NT Tel: 0121 449 0700 — MB ChB Birm. 1953. Prev: GP Birm.

WARDLE, John Kenneth Pathology Department, Noble's Isle of Man Hospital, Douglas IM1 4QA Tel: 01624 642350 Fax: 01624 642180 Email: wardle@mcb.net; Cooyrt Vane, Ballamodha, Ballasalla IM9 3AY Tel: 01624 824316 Fax: 01624 827068 — MB BS Lond. 1975; FRCPath 1994, M 1982. Cons. Path. Noble's IOM Hosp. Douglas; Dir. I. of Man Blood Transfus. Serv. Specialty: Pathology, General. Socs: Brit. Soc. Antimicrob. Chemother.; Assn. Clin. Path. Prev: Cons. Microbiol. Wolverhampton Pub. Health Laborat.; Asst. Lect. (Path.) St. Thos. Hosp. Med. Sch. Lond.; Sen. Regist. (Microbiol.) Newc. Gen. Hosp.

WARDLE, Judith Cecilia Rosanne (retired) Fourwinds, 49a Union St., Hamilton ML3 6NA Tel: 01698 424926 — MB BS Lond. 1956 (Lond. Hosp.) MRCS Eng. LRCP Lond. 1958; DObst RCOG 1958; MMedSci. (Nottm.) 1981; MFPHM 1989. Prev: Cons. Pub. Health Med. Lanarksh. HB.

WARDLE, Nicholas Stuart 7 Chester Gardens, Morden SM4 6QL Email: nic@nwardle.freeserve.co.uk — MB BS Lond. 1998 (St George's Hospital Medical School) MB BS Lond 1998. Specialty: Gen. Surg.

WARDLE, Mr Peter Gordon Women's Health Services, The Cotswold Centre, Southmead Hospital, Bristol BS10 5NB Tel: 0117 959 5171; Roseacre, 15 Clevedon Road, Flax Bourton, Bristol BS48 1NQ — (Bristol) MB ChB Bristol 1975; FRCS Eng. 1982; FRCOG 1996, M 1983; MD Bristol 1988. Cons. O & G Wom.'s Health Servs. Bristol. Specialty: Obst. & Gyn. Special Interest: Reproductive Med. & Surg.; Female Reproductive Endocrinol.; Male & Female Infertil. Socs: Brit. Fert. Soc. Prev: Cons. & Sen. Lect. O & G Univ. Bristol; Dep. Dir. Univ. Bristol Centre for Reproductive Med.; RCOG Fell. (Reproduc. Med.) Univ. Bristol.

WARDLE, Robert Stanley (retired) Highfield, 23 Knoll Park, St Clement, Truro TR1 1FF Tel: 01872 242560 — MB BChir Camb. 1954 (Camb. & St. Thos.) MA Camb. 1955, MB BChir 1954; DObst RCOG 1958. Prev: Gen. Pract., Chard, Som.

WARDLE, Rosalind Mary The Medical Centre, Dobles Lane, Holsworthy EX22 6GH Tel: 01409 253692 Fax: 01409 254184 — MB ChB Bristol 1985; DCH RCP Lond. 1988; MRCGP 1989; Cert. Family Plann. JCC 1989; Dip. Ther. 1997; DRCOG 2001. Gen. Practitioners Holsworthy. Specialty: Gen. Pract. Prev: Trainee GP Plymouth VTS; SHO (O & G) Solihull Hosp.; SHO (Dermat.) Plymouth.

WARDLE, Stephen Paul Queen's Medical Centre, Neonatal Unit, University Hospital, Nottingham NG7 2UH Tel: 0115 924 9924 Fax:

0115 970 9903 Email: steve.wardle@mail.qmcuh-tr.trent.nhs.uk — MB ChB Liverp. 1990 (Liverpool) MRCPCH; MRCP (UK) 1993; MD Liverpool, 1999. Cons. Neonatologist Queen's Med. Centre Univ. Hosp. Nottm. Specialty: Neonat. Prev: Lect. (Neonatal Med.) Univ. Liverp.; Research Regist. Liverp. Wom. Hosp.; Regist. Rotat. (Paediat.) NW Region.

WARDLE, Terence David Sunnycroft, Clayhanger Lane, Mere, Knutsford WA16 6QG — BM BS Nottm. 1984; DM Nottm. 1992, BMedSci (Hons.) 1982; BM BS (Hons.) Nottm. 1984; MRCP (UK) 1987. Lect. (Med.) Hope Hosp. Manch. Specialty: Gastroenterol. Prev: Research Fell. Univ. Dept. Med. Hope Hosp. Manch.; Regist. Rotat. (Med.) N. Staffs. Med. Centre Stoke-on-Trent; SHO Rotat. (Med.) N. Staffs. Med. Centre Stoke-on-Trent.

WARDLEY, Andrew Michael Department of Medical Oncology, Greenlea Oncology Unit, Huddersfield Royal Infirmary, Huddersfield HD3 3EA Tel: 01484 482150 Fax: 01484 482187; Ash Tree Cottage, 72 The Village, Thurstonland, Huddersfield HD4 6XX Tel: 01484 666171 — MB ChB Manch. 1989; MRCP (UK) 1993. Specialist Regist. Med. Oncol. Leeds Rotat. Specialty: Oncol. Socs: Roy. Coll. Phys.; Assn. Cancer Phys. Prev: Research Regist. (Med. Oncol.) Christie Hosp. Manch.; Clin. Lect. (Hon. Regist.) Manch. Univ. in Med. Oncol.

WARDLEY, James Raymond 21 Broomfield Drive, Alderholt, Fordingbridge SP6 3HY — (Manch.) MD Manch. 1942, MB ChB 1935; MRCS Eng. LRCP Lond. 1935. Socs: Fell. Manch. Med. Soc. Prev: Ho. Surg. Roy. Infirm. Manch.; Phys. Lake Hosp. Ashton-under-Lyne; Med. Specialist, Maj. R.A.M.C.

WARDMAN, Andrew George Leigh Infirmary, The Avenue, Leigh WN7 1HS Tel: 01942 672333; 54 Albert Road W., Heaton, Bolton BL1 5HG — MB ChB Ed. 1976; MRCP (UK) 1980; MD Ed. 1986; FRCP Lond. 1995. Cons. Phys. Wigan & Leigh Health Servs. Trust. Specialty: Gen. Med. Prev: Sen. Regist. (Med.) Leeds & Bradford.

WARDMAN, Derek Graham — MB ChB Leeds 1981; MPH Leeds 1986; MFCM 1988; FFPHM RCP (UK) 1995. Dir. Of Pub. Health, Calderdale & Kirklees H.A; 5 River Pk., Honley, Holmfirth HD9 6PS. Specialty: Pub. Health Med.

WARDMAN, Lyn Elizabeth Heaton Medical Centre, 2 Lucy St., Bolton BL1 5PU Tel: 01204 843677 Fax: 01204 495485 — MB ChB Leeds 1980; MRCGP 1985.

WARDROP, Alan George Monk Street Health Centre, 74 Monk Street, Aberdare CF44 7PA Tel: 01685 875906 Fax: 01685 875906 — MB BS Monash 1978.

WARDROP, Charles Alexander James Broomhill, 111 Viewlands Road W., Perth PH1 1EH Tel: 01738 638588 — MB ChB St. And. 1962; FRCP Ed. 1982, M 1968; FRCPath 1982, M 1970. Hon. Cons. Haematol. Specialty: Haematology. Socs: Eur. Soc. Paediat. Research; UK Neonat. Soc. Prev: Lect. (Haemat.) Univ. Glas.; Ho. Phys. Dundee Roy. Infirm.; Ho. Surg. Maryfield Hosp. Dundee.

WARDROP, Mr Peter John Charles Department of ENT, Crosshouse Hospital, Kilmarnock KA2 0BE Tel: 01563 577326 Fax: 01563 577974 — MB BCh Wales 1988; FRCS Eng. 1992; FRCS Ed. 1994; FRCS (Orl.) Ed. 1998. Cons. ENT Ayrsh. & Arran NHS Trust CrossHo. Hosp. Kilmarnock. Specialty: Otolaryngol. Socs: ORS; BAOHNS - Brit. Assn. Otolaryngologists - Head Neck Surg.s; BCIG - Brit. Cochlear Implant Gp. Prev: Regist. (ENT) City Hosp. Edin.; SHO (Surg.) Qu. Med. Centre Nottm.; SHO (Plastics) St. Luke's Bradford.

WARDROPE, Mr James Accident & Emergency Department, Northern General Hospital, Herries Road, Sheffield S5 7AU Tel: 0114 271 4972 Fax: 0114 261 1897 — MB ChB Ed. 1978; FRCS Ed. 1982; FRCS Eng. 1983; FRCS (A&E) Ed. 1986; FFAEM 1993. Cons. A & E Med. N. Gen. Hosp. Sheff. Specialty: Accid. & Emerg. Socs: Brit. Assn. Accid. & Emerg. Med.; Fell. Fac. A&E Med. (President Elect.). Prev: Sen. Regist. (A & E) Roy. Hallamsh. Hosp. Sheff.; Research Regist. Univ. Leeds; Regist. Rotat. (Surg.) Leeds Gen. Infirm.

WARDROPPER, Alison Grace University Hospital of North Durham, North Road, Durham DH1 5TW Fax: 0191 333 6901 — BM BS Nottm. 1986; MRCP (UK) 1989. Cons. in Genitourin. Med.,Dryburn and Bishop Auckland Hosp.; Honourary Cons. Phys., Newc. Gen. Hosp. Specialty: Genitourinary Medicine. Socs: AGUM; MSSVD; FRCP(Lond.).

WARE, Anthony Wicks (retired) 1 Westgarth Gardens, Bury St Edmunds IP33 3LB Tel: 01284 754253 — MRCS Eng. LRCP Lond. 1955.

WARE, Mr Charles Francis Wakefield (retired) Old Manse, 147 Ballynahinch Road, Hillsborough BT26 6BD — MB BCh BAO Belf. 1958; FRCS Ed. 1965; DO RCS Eng. 1966; FRCSI 1974; FRCOphth 1991. Assoc. Specialist EHSSB/SHSSB N. Irel. Prev: Sen. Regist. Eye & Ear Clinic Belf.

WARE, Christopher John Grattan (retired) 6 The Green, Cuddesdon, Oxford OX44 9JZ — MB BS Lond. 1978; MRCGP 1985; DRCOG 1985; MRCPsych 1989. Prev: Sen. Regist. (Psychiat.) Warneford Hosp. Oxf.

WARE, Claire-Louise 22 Gnoll Cr, Neath SA11 3TF — BM Soton. 1997.

WARE, Clive Charles Newark Road Surgery, 501 Newark Road, South Hykeham, Lincoln LN6 8RT Tel: 01522 537944 Fax: 01522 510932 — MB ChB Liverp. 1985; DCH RCP Lond. 1988; DGM RCP Lond. 1988; DRCOG 1989; FRCGP 1997, M 1989; T(GP) 1991; MBA Leeds 1994.

WARE, Mr Colin Clement Tree Tops, 247 Thorpe Hall Avenue, Thorpe Bay, Southend-on-Sea SS1 3SG Tel: 01702 86797 — MB BS Lond. 1962 (Westm.) BSc Lond. 1954, MB BS (Hons.) 1962; FRCS Eng. 1965. Cons. Surg. Southend-on-Sea Gp. Hosps. Socs: Fell. Roy. Soc. Med.; Fell. Assn. Surg. Prev: Sen. Surg. Regist. Westm. Hosp.; Lect. in Surg. St. Thos. Hosp. Lond. Ho. Surg. St. Jas. Hosp. Balham.

WARE, Delyth Ann Pencoed and Llanharan Medical Centres, Heol-yr-Onnen, Pencoed, Bridgend CF35 5PF Tel: 01656 860270 Fax: 01656 861228; 6 Parklands, Corntown, Bridgend CF35 5BE Tel: 01656 662948 — MB BS Lond. 1977 (Guy's) BSc (Biochem.) Lond. 1974; MRCS Eng. LRCP Lond. 1977; DCH Eng. 1979; MRCGP 1991.

WARE, Mrs Jean Marian (retired) 4 Bearcroft Gardens, Mickleton, Chipping Campden GL55 6TY Tel: 01368 438988 — MB BS Lond. 1957 (St. Bart.) Family Plann. Med. Off. & Sessional Sch. Med. Off. Southend Health Dist. Prev: Clin. Med. Off. Lond. Boro. Havering.

WARE, Mr John Walter (retired) 152 Harley Street, London W1N 1HH Tel: 020 7935 8868; Oak Ridge, 30 Christchurch Crescent, Radlett WD7 8AJ Tel: 01923 857551 — MB ChB Bristol 1953; FRCS Ed. 1970. Prev: Cons. Traum. & Orthop. Surg.

WARE, Lynda Maria Morland House Surgery, 2 London Road, Wheatley, Oxford OX33 1YJ Tel: 01865 872448 Fax: 01865 874158; 6 The Green, Cuddesdon, Oxford OX44 9JZ Email: lyndaware@aol.com — MB BChir Camb. 1978 (Westm.) MA Camb. 1978; DRCOG 1980; MRCGP 1983. GP Wheatley, Oxf.; Clin. Tutor (Gen. Pract.) Univ. Oxf. Socs: Brit. Menopause Soc.

WARE, Robert John 1B Reddons Road, Beckenham BR3 1LY — MB BS Lond. 1972 (King's Coll. Hosp.) FFA RCS Eng. 1976. SHO (Anaesth.) King's Coll. Hosp. Lond. Specialty: Anaesth.

WARE, Ronald William (retired) Flat 2, The Willows, 83 Vincent Square, London SW1P 2PF Tel: 020 7828 2686 — MRCS Eng. LRCP Lond. 1952 (Westm.) DLO Eng. 1956; DObst RCOG 1958; DIH Soc. Apoth. Lond. 1961; DA Eng. 1969. Prev: Med. Dir. Mobil Saudi Arabia Inc.

WARE, Stephen John 74 Norsey Road, Billericay CM11 1AT Tel: 01277 58659 — MB BS Lond. 1967 (St. Thos.) DCH Eng. 1969; MRCP (UK) 1970. Cons. Paediat. Basildon & Southend Health Dists. Specialty: Paediat.

WAREHAM, Conrad Arthur 6 Peterborough Drive, Sheffield S10 4JB — BM Soton. 1984.

WAREHAM, Karen Patricia 7 Kipling Close, Yateley GU46 6YA — MB ChB Bristol 1995; MRCP 1998. SHO. Med.derriford.Hosp. Plymouth. Specialty: Gen. Med.

WAREHAM, Nicholas John Strangeways Research Labs, Worts Causeway, Cambridge CB1 8RN Tel: 01223 330315 Fax: 01223 330316 Email: njw1004@medschl.cam.ac.uk; 4 Kingfisher Close, Bourn, Cambridge CB3 7TJ — MB BS Lond. 1986; MRCP (UK) 1990; MSc Pub. Health Med. Lond. 1991; MFPHM RCP (UK) 1992; PhD Camb. 1997; FFPHM 2003; FRCP 2003. Director, MRC Epidemiol. Unit; Hon. Cons. Pub. Health Med., Addenbooke's NHS Trust. Specialty: Epidemiol. Prev: Sen. Regist. (Epidemiol. & Pub. Health Med.) Inst. Pub. Health Camb.; Sen. Clin. Fell., Wellcome Trust, Univ. Camb.; MRC Clinician Scientist Fell., Univ. Camb.

WAREING, Mr Michael John 18 Upper Wimpole Street, London W1G 6LX Tel: 020 7935 1304 Fax: 020 7224 1645 Email: mjw@orl-hns.co.uk; St Bartholomew's Hospital, ENT Department, West Smithfield, London EC1A 7BE Tel: 020 7601 7173 Email:

michaelwareing@bartsandthelondon.nhs.uk — MB BS Lond. 1988 (St Bart.) BSc Lond. 1985; FRCS Eng. 1992; FRCS (Otol.) Eng. 1993; FRCS (ORL-HNS) 1998. Cons. Otolaryngol. St Bart's & Roy. Lond. Hosp.; Assoc. Clin. Director St Bart's & Roy. Lond. Hosp. Specialty: Otolaryngol. Special Interest: Otol.; Paediatric Otolaryngol.; Surgic. Neurotology. Socs: BMA; Brit. Assn. Otol. Head & Neck Surg.; Roy. Soc. Med. Prev: Specialist Regist. Rotat. (Otolaryngol. Head & Neck Surg.) S. Thames (E.); Neurotological Fell. Addenbrookes Hosp. Camb.; TWJ Fell. (Otol.) Univ. Calif. San Francisco.

WARENIUS, Professor Hilmar Meek University of Liverpool, Oncology Research Unit, Department of Medicine, The Duncan Building, Daulby St., Liverpool L69 3GA Tel: 0151 706 4532 Fax: 0151 706 5802 Email: warenius@liverpool.ac.uk; 14 Delavor Road, Heswall, Wirral CH60 4RN Tel: 0151 342 3034 — (Camb. & Middlx.) MRCS Eng. LRCP Lond. 1968; MB BChir Camb. 1969; PhD Camb. 1980, MA 1970; MRCP (UK) 1971; DMRT 1973; FRCR 1975; FRCP Lond. 1987. Prof. & Dir. Oncol. Research Univ. of Liverp.; Hon. Prof, Guangxi Med. Univ., China; Chief Med. Off. & Dir. of R&D TheRyte Ltd. The Duncan Building Liverp. Specialty: Oncol.; Radiother.; Medico Legal; Research. Special Interest: Molecular Cell Biol. of Cancer; Proteomic Theranostics. Socs: Brit. Assn. Cancer Research; Roy. Coll. of Physicians; Roy. Coll. of Radiologists. Prev: Vis. Prof. & Hon. Cons. Clin. Oncol. Hammersmith Hosp. Lond.; Hon. Coordinator MRC Fast Neutron Studies Clatterbridge Hosp. Merseyside; Cons. Radiotherap. & Oncol. Newc. Gen. Hosp.

WARES, Alastair Neil Pendyffryn Medical Group, Ffordd Pendyffryn, Prestatyn LL19 9DH Tel: 01745 886444 Fax: 01745 889831; 6 The Circle, Prestatyn LL19 9EU — MB ChB Liverp. 1979; MPhil (Med. Law) Glasgow 2001. Partner in Howes, Jessup, Wares, Scriven, Williams, Phillips, Campbell, Popat & Morrison. Socs: Fell. Internat. Med. Law & Ethics Soc.

WARFIELD, Adrian Thomas Department of Cellular Pathology (Histopathology), The Medical School, Vincent Drive, Birmingham B15 2TT Tel: 0121 414 4012/0121 414 4016 Fax: 0121 627 2101 — MB ChB Birm. 1986; MRCPath 1994; FCPath 2002. Cons. Histopath. Univ. Hosps. NHS Trust; Hon. Sen. Clin. Lect. (Path.) Univ. of Birm.; Cons. Histopath. Birm. Heartlands Hosptial. Specialty: Histopath. Socs: Brit. Soc. Clin. Cytopath.; Assn. Clin. Path.; Path. Soc. Prev: Sen. Regist. (Histopath.) N. Staffs. Hosp. Centre & Birm. Heartlands Hosp.

WARIN, Andrew Peter The Royal Devon & Exeter Hospital (Wonford), Barrack Road, Exeter EX2 5DW Tel: 01392 402250 Fax: 01392 402210; The Gables, Priory Close, East Budleigh, Budleigh Salterton EX9 7EZ — (Guy's) MB BS Lond. 1967; MRCS Eng. LRCP Lond. 1967; MRCP (UK) 1970; FRCP Lond. 1983. Cons. Dermat. Roy. Devon & Exeter Hosp. Exeter. Specialty: Dermat. Socs: Fell. Roy. Soc. Med. (Dermat. Sect.); Brit. Assn. Dermat.; Amer. Acad. of Dermat. Prev: Cons. Dermat. St. John's Hosp. Dis. Skin Lond.; Sen. Lect. Inst. Dermat. Lond.; Assoc. Prof. Dermat. Pahlavi Univ. Med. Sch., Iran.

WARIN, Judith Mary Psychotherapy Department, Wonford House Hospital, Dryden Road, Exeter EX2 5AF Tel: 01392 403446; Maranatha, Rewe, Exeter EX5 4EU — MB BS Lond. 1968 (Guy's) BSc (Biochem.) Lond. 1965. Clin. Asst. (Psychother.) Wonford Hse. Hosp. Exeter. Specialty: Psychother. Prev: Clin. Asst. (Psychother. & Radiother.) Wonford Hosp. Exeter; Clin. Asst. Renal Unit Roy. Devon & Exeter Hosp. (Wonford); SCMO Lewisham Health Dist.

WARIN, William Arthur Southmead Health Centre, Ullswater Road, Bristol BS10 6DF Tel: 0117 950 7150 Fax: 0117 959 1110; 3 Burlington Road, Bristol BS6 6TJ — MB ChB Birm. 1979; DRCOG 1984; MRCGP 1986. Prev: Trainee GP Southmead Bristol.

WARING, Eileen (retired) 25 The Glen, Worthing BN13 2AD Tel: 01903 691027 Email: E.Waring@tesco.net — MRCS Eng. LRCP Lond. 1956 (Manch.) Prev: SCMO Worthing.

WARING, Howard Linton Ingersley Unit, Macclesfield District Hospital, Macclesfield SK10 3BL Tel: 01625 663722 Fax: 01625 663107 — MB ChB Ed. 1973; MRCPsych. 1978; MD Lond. 1988; MD Aberd. 1988. Cons. Psychiat. E. Chesh. Trust Macclesfield. Specialty: Gen. Psychiat. Socs: Roy. Coll. Psychiat.

WARING, Ian Stuart Tudor Lodge Health Centre, 3 Nithsdale Road, Weston Super Mare BS23 4JP Tel: 01934 622665 Fax: 01934 644332 — MB ChB Bristol 1965.

WARING, James Rodney (retired) War Memorial Health Centre, Crickhowell NP8 1AG Tel: 01873 810255 Fax: 01873 811949; 7 Park Drive, Llangattock, Crickhowell NP8 1PP — MB BS Durh. 1959; DObst RCOG 1966. Prev: GP. War Memor. Health Centre, Crickhowell.

WARING, John Richard Northgate Surgery, Northgate, Pontefract WF8 1NG Tel: 01977 703635 Fax: 01977 702562; Arncliffe, 110 Carleton Road, Pontefract WF8 3NQ Tel: 01977 600941 — (Manch.) MRCS Eng. LRCP Lond. 1969. Chairm. Wakefield LMC.

WARING, Mr Michael Room 684D, Skipton House, 80 London Road, Elephant & Castle, London SE1 6LH Tel: 020 7972 5120 Fax: 020 7972 5156; Hawk House, Church Lane, E. Haddon, Northampton NN6 8DB Tel: 01604 770369 — MB BChir Camb. 1972; MRCS Eng. LRCP Lond. 1971; MA Camb. 1972; FRCS Eng. 1978; BA (Hons.) Open 1988. Sen. Med. Off. DoH Elephant & Castle. Specialty: Gen. Surg.

WARING, Nicholas Anthony (retired) 12 Les Rosiers Grove, Cashs Park, Wincanton BA9 9NT Tel: 01963 33358 — MRCS Eng. LRCP Lond. 1955 (Camb. & Lond. Hosp.) MA Camb. 1973. Prev: Regional Med. Off. DHSS.

WARING, Nicholas John Gillies and Overbridge Medical Partnership, Brighton Hill, Sullivan Road, Basingstoke RG22 4EH Tel: 01256 479747; Spinney Cottage, North Waltham Road, Oakley, Basingstoke RG23 7EA Tel: 01256 780397 Email: nick@spinneyco.freeserve.co.uk — MB BCh Wales 1971 (Welsh Nat. Sch. Med.) MRCS Eng. LRCP Lond. 1972; DObst RCOG 1973; FRCGP 1987, M 1975. Socs: Worshipful Soc. Apoth. Lond.; Wessex Res. Netw. Prev: SHO (Paediat.) & Ho. Surg. Univ. Hosp. of Wales Cardiff; Ho. Phys. Roy. S. Hants. Hosp. Soton.

WARING, William Brian (retired) Durnford Medical Centre, 113 Long St., Middleton, Manchester M24 6DL Tel: 0161 643 2011; 1A Hardfield Road, Alkrington, Middleton, Manchester M24 1PQ Tel: 0161 643 2822 — MB ChB Manch. 1956. Prev: Ho. Surg. Manch. Roy. Infirm.

WARINTON, Andrew David Rakaia Lodge, Saxon Street, Lower Langford, Bristol BS40 5BP — MB BChir Camb. 1988; DRCOG, MRCGP, Dip Occ. Med.

WARIYAR, Unnikrishna Kundukulangara Varriyam Royal Victoria Infirmary, Neonatal Services, Leazes Wing, Newcastle upon Tyne NE1 4LP Tel: 0191 282 5156 Fax: 0191 282 5038 Email: u.k.wariyar@ncl.ac.uk — MB BS Kerala 1973 (Univ. of Kerala) BSc Kerala 1966; DCH Calcutta 1975; DCCH Edin. 1984; MRCP UK 1984; FRCPCH 1992; FRCP 1992; MD Newc. 1992. Cons. Paediat. / Neonatologist, Newc. Upon Tyne; Vis. Neonatologist - Wansbeck Hosp., Ashington; Clin. Sen. Lect. (Child Health) Univ. of Newc. Upon Tyne. Specialty: Neonat. Special Interest: Long Term Outcome; neuro Development. Socs: Roy. Coll. of Paediat. and Child Health; Neonat. Soc.; Brit. Assn. of Perinatal Med. Prev: Cons. Paediat., N. Tyneside Hosp.

WARK, Kathryn Jessie London Chest Hospital, Royal Hospitals NHS Trust, Bonner Road, London E2 9JX Tel: 020 8980 4433 — MB BS Queensland 1973 (Univ. Queensland) FFA RCS Lond. 1980. Cons. Anaesth. (Cardiothoracic Anaesth.) Lond. Chest & St. Bart. Hosps. Roy. Hosps. NHS Trust. Specialty: Anaesth. Socs: Anaesth. Res. Soc.; Assn. Cardiothoracic Anaesth. Prev: Cons. Anaesth. Guy's Hosp. Lond.; Sen. Regist. Lond. Hosp.

WARLAND, Jane Christine Grey Walls, Smith Hill, Bishopsteignton, Teignmouth TQ14 9QT Tel: 01626 773565; Flat 10, The Courtenay, Courtenay place, Teignmouth TQ14 8AY Tel: 01626 778543 — MB ChB Leeds 1995; BSc Leeds 1992; MRCP (Paeds) Lond. 1999. SHOA & E)Roy.Shrewsbury Hosp. Specialty: Accid. & Emerg.; Paediat. Socs: BMA; MDU.

WARLEY, Anthony Robert Holmes Salisbury District Hospital, Salisbury SP2 8BJ Tel: 01722 336262 — MB BS Lond. 1978 (Westm.) MRCP (UK) 1981; MD Lond. 1988; FRCP 1998. Cons. Phys. Gen. & Respirat. Med. Salisbury Dist. Hosp. Specialty: Gen. Med. Prev: Sen. Regist. (Med.) Frenchay Hosp. & Bristol Roy. Infirm.; Research Fell. Churchill Hosp. Oxf.; SHO MusGr. Hosp. Taunton.

WARLOW, Allan Llewellyn (retired) 14 Ocean Drive, Port Soif, Vale, Guernsey GY6 8AG — MRCS Eng. LRCP Lond. 1947 (Char. Cross)

WARLOW, Andrea Linda 4 Hayston Avenue, Hakin, Milford Haven SA73 3EB — MB BCh Wales 1979; DCH RCP Lond. 1983.

WARLOW, Professor Charles Picton Western General Hospital, Department of Clinical Neurosciences, Crewe Road, Edinburgh EH4 2XU Tel: 0131 537 2082 Fax: 0131 332 5150 Email: charles.warlow@ed.ac.uk — MB BChir Camb. 1968; BA Camb. 1965; MRCP (UK) 1970; MD Camb. 1975; FRCP Lond. 1983; FRCP Ed. 1987; FRCP Glas. 1993; FMEDSci 1998. Prof. Med. Neurol. Univ. Edin.; Hon. Cons. Neurol. Specialty: Neurol. Special Interest: Stroke; functional problems, Epidemiol. Socs: Fell. Acad. Med. Sci. (1998); Assn. Brit. Neurol. (Pres. 2001-3) & Amer. Neurol. Assn.; Brit. Assn. Stroke Phys. Prev: Clin. Reader (Neurol.) Univ. Oxf.; Lect. (Med.) Aberd. Univ.; Regist. & Sen. Regist. (Neurol.) Nat. Hosps. Nerv. Dis. Lond.

WARLOW, Colin Norman, Surg. Cdr. RN Retd. 27 Bellair Road, Havant PO9 2RG Tel: 023 9247 5447 Fax: 023 9247 5447 Email: colin.warlow@btopenworld.com — (Univ. Coll. Dub.) MB BCh BAO NUI 1960; DTM & H Eng. 1967; MRCGP 1974; Dip. GU Med. Soc. Apoth Lond. 1989. Locum Hosp. Practitioner Dept GU Med. St Mary's Hosp. Newport. Specialty: Genitourinary Medicine. Socs: Soc. Study of Sexually Transm. Dis.s of Irel.; Brit. Assn. Sexual Health HIV. Prev: PMO HMS Sultan, Mercury & Fearless; Adviser (Genitourin. Med.) MDG(N); Med. Off. (Genitourin.) HMS Nelson Portsmouth.

WARLOW, Jennifer Jane University of Bradford Health Centre, Laneisteridge Lane, Bradford BD5 0NH Tel: 01274 234979 Fax: 01274 235940 — MB ChB Leeds 1985; DRCOG 1988; DCCH 1993.

WARLOW, Mr Peter Frederick Maurice 16 The Crescent, Brixton, Plymouth PL8 2AP Tel: 01752 880946 — MB BS Lond. 1950; FRCS Ed. 1961.

WARLOW, Steven Rosemary Medical Centre, 2 Rosemary Gardens, Parkstone, Poole BH12 3HF Tel: 01202 741300; 9 Overbury Road, Parkstone, Poole BH14 9JL Tel: 01202 743495 — MB BS Lond. 1979 (Westm.) MA Camb. 1979; MRCS Eng. LRCP Lond. 1979; DRCOG 1981; MRCGP 1983.

WARLTIER, Betty Rosemary (retired) 19 Woodhall Avenue, Pinner HA5 3DY Tel: 020 8866 3985 — MB BChir Camb. 1952 (Camb. & Middlx.) MA Camb. 1952; MRCS Eng. LRCP Lond. 1952; DA Eng. 1954; FFA RCS Eng. 1955; DObst RCOG 1957. Cons. Anaesth. Mt. Vernon Hosp. Northwood. Prev: Sen. Regist. (Anaesth.) Char. Cross Hosp.

WARMAN, Linda Helen 19 Park Drive, London NW11 7SN — MB ChB Manch. 1972; DObst RCOG 1975.

WARNE, Roger William Department Geriatric Medicine, Royal Perth Hospital, Wellington St., Perth 6000, Australia Tel: 00 619 2242099 Fax: 00 619 2243339; 35 Elm Tree Park, Yealmpton, Plymouth PL8 2ED Tel: 01752 880457 — MB BS Lond. 1971 (FRCP Lond 1997) MRCS Eng. LRCP Lond. 1971; MRCP (UK) 1975; FRACP 1979; MMed Melbourne 1984; FRCP Ed. 1994. Phys. Bentley Health Serv. Aged Care Servs. Perth, Austral.; Assoc. Prof. Sch. Pub. Health. Curtin Univ of Tech. Australia. Specialty: Care of the Elderly; Gen. Med.; Epidemiol. Socs: State Comm. Austral. Assn. Gerontol.; Aus. Soc. Geriat.. Med; Brit.Geriat.s Soc. Prev: Phys. (Geriat. Med.) Roy. Perth Hosp. W. Austral.; Convenor Teach. Geriat. Med. Gp. & Federal Represen. Teach. & Research Austral. Geriat. Soc. West. Austral. Div.; Sen. Specialist Phys. (Geriat. Med.) Heidelberg Repatriation Hosp.

WARNE, Stephanie Anastasia 5 Summerhill, Prehen Park, Londonderry BT47 2PL Tel: 01504 347902 — MB BCh Wales 1995 (Univ. Wales Coll. Med.) SHO (Gen. Surg.) E. Glam. Hosp.; SHO (Paediat. Surg.) Gt. Ormond St Childr. Hosp. Lond. Specialty: Paediat. Surg.; Gen. Surg. Socs: MDU; Wom. in Surg. Train. Prev: SHO (Cardiothoracic Surg.) Univ. Hosp. of Wales Cardiff; SHO (Orthop.) E. Glam. Hosp. Pontypridd; SHO (Gen. Surg.) Univ. Hosp. Wales Cardiff.

WARNELL, Ian Haydn Department of Anaesthesia, Newcastle General Hospital, Newcastle upon Tyne NE6 4BE Tel: 0191 273 8811 — MB BS Lond. 1977; MRCP (UK) 1981; FFA RCS Eng. 1983. Cons. Anaesth. Newc. Gen. Hosp. Specialty: Anaesth.

WARNER, Adrian Anthony Little Acre, Ufford Road, Bainton, Stamford PE9 3BB — MB Camb. 1967 (Middlx.) BChir 1966; DMRD Eng. 1972; FFR 1974; Cert Amer. Bd. Radiol. 1975. Cons. Radiol. Hinchingbrooke Hosp. Huntingdon. Specialty: Radiol. Prev: Sen. Cons. Radiol. Nat. Guard K. Khalid Hosp., Saudi Arabia; Teach. (Radiol.) Univ. Camb. & Univ. Leicester; Cons. Radiol. P'boro. Dist. Hosp.

WARNER, Andrew Philip 54 Lemon Street, Truro TR1 2PE; 16 Shepherds Hill, Southam, Leamington Spa CV47 1GD Tel: 01926 811023 — MB BS Lond. 1995 (St. Georges Hospital) GP Regist. Kineton Surg. Socs: GP VTS Warwick Hosp.

WARNER, Barry Graham 2 Liquorstane, Falkland, Cupar KY15 7DQ; 8 Silver meadows, barton, Richmond DL10 6SL — MB ChB Dundee 1997. SHO Surgic. Rotat. Darlington Memor. Hosp.

WARNER, Cedric Martin Woodlands Health Centre, Allington Road, Paddock Wood, Tonbridge TN12 6AR Tel: 01892 833331; Pimms Place, Peckham Bush, Tonbridge TN12 5LL Tel: 01622 871736 — MB ChB Birm. 1963; DObst RCOG 1966; MRCGP 1969. Med. Off. Child Welf. Clinic Kent CC; Trainer GP SE Thames RHA. Specialty: Gen. Pract. Socs: BMA. Prev: Mem. Dist. Managem. Team Tunbridge Wells DHA; Clin. Asst. (Rheum.) Homoeop. Hosp. Tunbridge Wells; SHO (Trauma) Kidderminster Gen. Hosp.

WARNER, Christopher Eric James Osmaston Road Medical Centre, 212 Osmaston Road, Derby DE23 8JX Tel: 01332 346433 Fax: 01332 345854 — BM BS Nottm. 1989; BMedSci Nottm. 1987; MRCGP 1993. Specialty: Gen. Pract.

WARNER, Diana Lewen The Surgery, 43 Nevil Road, Bishopston, Bristol BS7 9EG Tel: 0117 924 5630 Fax: 0117 924 5630 — MB BS Lond. 1982. Prev: Trainee GP E. Glam. Gen. Hosp. VTS.

WARNER, Edward Maurice (retired) 204 Hall Green Road, West Bromwich B71 2DX Tel: 0121 588 2456 — MB ChB Birm. 1948.

WARNER, Graham Terrance Anthony — MB BS Lond. 1988 (Middlx.) BSc (Hons.) Lond. 1985; MRCP (UK) 1992; MD (Lond.) 1997. Specialty: Neurol. Socs: BMA; MDU; Assoc. Brit. Neurols. Prev: Cons. Neurol. Southend Hosp.; Specialist Regist. (Neurol.) Wessex Neuro Centre Soton. Gen. Hosp.; Research Regist. (Neurol.) Roy. Lond. Hosp.

WARNER, Gregory Nightingale Surgery, Greatwell Drive, Cupernham Lane, Romsey SO51 7QN Tel: 01794 517878 Fax: 01794 514236; 27 Raglan Close, Chandlers Ford, Eastleigh SO53 4NH Tel: 01703 255551 — MB BS Lond. 1985 (King's Coll. Hosp.) MA Camb. 1986; DRCOG 1987; DCH RCP Lond. 1987; MRCGP 1989.

WARNER, Mr James Garth Royal Bolton Hospital, Minerva Road, Farnworth, Bolton BL4 0JR Tel: 01204 390374 Fax: 01204 390344 — MB ChB Manch. 1987 (St. And. & Manch.) FRCS (Tr & Orth.) 1997 Intercoll Spec Bd.; BSc St. And. 1984; FRCS Eng. 1991. Cons. Orthopaedic and Trauma Surg., Roy. Bolton Hosp. Specialty: Trauma & Orthop. Surg. Prev: Sen. Regist. (Orthop. Surg.) Hope Hosp. Salford; Sir Harry Platt Research Fell. (Orthop.) & Hon. Sen. Regist. (Orthop. Surg.) Univ. Manch.; Regist. (Orthop.) Stockport Infirm.

WARNER, James Robert The Surgery, Park Lane, Stubbington, Fareham PO14 2JP Tel: 01329 664231 Fax: 01329 664958 — MB ChB Manch. 1976; BSc (Med. Sci.) St. And. 1973; DRCOG 1984. Hosp. Pract. (Endoscopy) RH Haslar Gosport; Vice-Chairm. Portsmouth & SE Hants. LMC; Hon. Lect. Soton. Med. Sch. Specialty: Gastroenterol. Prev: Surg. Lt. Cdr. RN.

WARNER, Jennifer Anne Anaesthetic Department, City Hospital, Hucknall Road, Nottingham NG5 1PB Email: jennifer.warner@ntlworld.com — MB BS Lond. 1978 (St. Mary's) FFA RCS Eng. 1982. Cons. Anaesth. City Hosp. Nottm.

WARNER, Professor John Oliver Southampton General Hospital, Infection, Inflammation and Repair Division, Child Health, MP 803, Level F South Academic Block, Tremona Road, Southampton SO16 6YD Tel: 023 8079 6160 Fax: 023 8079 6378 Email: jow@soton.ac.uk — (Sheff.) MB ChB Sheff. 1968; DCH Eng. 1970; MRCP (UK) 1972; MD Sheff. 1979; FRCP Lond. 1986; FRCPCH 1997; F Med Sci 1999; FAAAAI 2001. Prof. Child Health Univ. Soton.; Edr.-in-Chief Paediat. Allergy & Immunol. Specialty: Paediat.; Respirat. Med. Socs: (Ex-Sec.) Brit. Soc. Allergy & Clin. Immunol.; Eur. Respirat. Soc. (Ex-Head Paediat. Assembly 1993-97).; Amer. Thoracic Soc. Prev: Reader (Paediat.) Nat. Heart & Lung Inst. Lond. Univ.; Hon. Cons. Paediat. Brompton Hosp. & St. Mary's Hosp. Lond.; Sen. Regist., Research Fell. & Hon. Sen. Regist. Hosp. for Sick Childr. Gt. Ormond. St. Lond.

WARNER, Justin Tobias 15 Mafeking Road, Penylan, Cardiff CF23 5DQ Tel: 029 2048 7047 — MB BCh Wales 1989; BSc (Biochem.) 1984; MRCP (UK) 1992. Regist. (Paediat.) Llandough NHS Trust Hosp. Cardiff. Specialty: Paediat.

WARNER, Karen Lesley Worden Medical Centre, West Paddock, Leyland, Preston PR5 1HW Tel: 01772 423555 Fax: 01772 623878 Email: kl.warner@btinternet.com — MB ChB Manch. 1987 (Manchester) MRCGP 1991; DRCOG 1992. Specialty: Family Plann. & Reproduc. Health. Prev: Trainee GP Preston VTS; SHO (Paediat. & Psychiat.) Roy. Preston Hosp. Lancs.

WARNER, Katharine Jane Nightingale Surgery, Greatwell Drive, Cupernham Lane, Romsey SO51 7QN Tel: 01794 517878 Fax: 01794 514236; 27 Raglan Close, Chandlers Ford, Eastleigh SO53 4NH Tel: 01703 255551 — MB BS Lond. 1983 (King's Coll. Hosp.) MA Camb. 1984; DRCOG 1986; MRCGP 1988. Hon. Clin. Tutor Soton. Univ. Prev: Clin. Med. Off. (Child Health) Soton.

WARNER, Malcolm David Faringdon Medical Centre, Volunteer Way, Faringdon SN7 7YU Tel: 01367 242388 Fax: 01367 243394; Astley House, Market Place, Faringdon SN7 7HU Tel: 01367 240049 Email: malcolmwarner@compuserve.com — MB BS Lond. 1973 (Lond. Hosp.) DCH Eng. 1976.

WARNER, Michael Weston The Cottage, Royston Road, Wendens Ambo, Saffron Walden CB11 4JX — MB ChB Manch. 1995.

WARNER, Nicholas James Magnolia House, Summerlands, Yeovil Email: nick.warner@gwent.wales.nhs.uk — MB ChB Birm. 1981; FRCPsych. Cons. Psychiat. Old Age Som. Partnership NHS Trust. Specialty: Geriat. Psychiat. Prev: Sen. Regist. (Psychiat.) Worcester Roy. Infirm.; Regist. (Psychiat.) WhitCh. Hosp. Cardiff; SHO/Regist. (Psychiat.) St. Crispin Hosp. N.ampton.

WARNER, Nicola Jane Department Clinical Oncology, Churchill Hospital, Old Road, Headington, Oxford OX25 4RT Tel: 01865 225262 Fax: 01865 225559; Orchard House, Orchard Lane, Uppes Heyfard, Oxford OX25 5LD — BM Soton. 1985; MRCP (UK) 1988; FRCR 1995. p/t Cons. Clin. Oncol. Churchill Hosp. Oxf. Specialty: Oncol. Prev: Regist. Fell. W.mead Hosp. Sydney, Australia; Regist. (Radiother. & Oncol.) Churchill Hosp. Oxf.

WARNER, Orlando Jonathan Nuffield Department of Anaesthetics, The John Radcliffe Hospital, Oxford OX3 9DU — MB BS Lond. 1988 (The Lond. Hosp. Med. Centre, Univ. of Lond.) FRCA Roy. Coll. Of Anaesthetics (Eng) 1993; FRCS Roy. Coll. Of Surg. Of Eng. 1995; EDICM Euro. Dip. Of Intensive Care Med. 1999. Cons. Anaesthetist. Socs: Anaesthetic Research Soc.; Euro. Soc. Of Intensive Care; Difficult Airway Soc.

WARNER, Rachel Wynne Community Health Sheffield NHS Trust, Argyll House, 9 Williamson Road, Sheffield S11 9AR Tel: 0114 271 8656 Fax: 0114 271 6643 — MB BS Lond. 1985; MA Oxf. 1986; MRCGP 1989; MRCPsych 1992; MSc (Psychiat.) Manch. 1994. Cons. Psychiat. Community Health Sheff. Specialty: Gen. Psychiat.

WARNER, Richard Graham The Surgery, Kingstone, Hereford HR2 9HN Tel: 01981 250215 Fax: 01981 251171 — BM BCh Oxf. 1985; MA Oxf. 1987; DCH RCP Lond. 1988; MRCGP 1995. Specialty: Gen. Pract.

WARNER, Rodney Harry Lewen Practice A, Hinckley Health Centre, 27 Hill Street, Hinckley LE10 1DS; The Courtyard, Higham Lane, Stoke Golding, Nuneaton CV13 6EX Tel: 07771 983249 — MB BS Lond. 1979 (Middlx.) BSc Lond. 1976; DRCOG 1983; MRCGP 1984. Clin. Asst. (Orthop.) Leicester. Specialty: Diabetes.

WARNER, Stephen Terence The Health Centre, Doctor Lane, Mirfield WF14 8DU Tel: 01924 495721 Fax: 01924 480605 — MB ChB Leeds 1978; LicAc. 1992. Indep. Acupunc. W. Yorks. Specialty: Gen. Med. Socs: Hudds. Med. Soc.

WARNER, Sven Nicholas Banks Health Centre, Newgate Street, Worksop S80 1HP Tel: 01909 500266 Fax: 01909 478014; Brook House, Netherthorpe, Worksop S80 3JG Tel: 01909 483066 — MB ChB Sheff. 1981; DRCOG 1984; MRCGP 1985. Med. Off. Welbeck Coll. Worksop; Mem. N. Notts. N.Notts LMC. Prev: Trainee GP Kiveton Pk. Health Centre Sheff.; SHO (Paediat. & O & G) Bassetlaw Dist. Hosp. Worksop; SHO (A & E) Roy. Hallamsh. Hosp. Sheff.

WARNER, Thomas Treharne Department Clinical Neurosciences, Royal Free Hospital School of Medicine, Rowland Hill St., London NW3 2PF Tel: 020 7794 0500 Fax: 020 7431 1577 — BM BCh Oxf. 1987; BA Oxon 1984; MRCP (UK) 1990; PhD Lond. 1997; FRCP 2002. Reader (Neurol.) Hon. Cons. Neurol. Roy. Free Hosp. Sch. of Med. Liste Hosp. Stevenage Nat. Hosp. for Neurol. & Neurosurg. Lond. Specialty: Neurol. Prev: Lect. (Neurogenetics) Inst. Neurol. Lond.

WARNER, Zyta Lidia (retired) — MB BCh BAO NUI 1956. Prev: GP Harrow.

WARNER-SMITH, John Duff Wallis and Partners, The Health Centre, 5 Stanmore Road, Stevenage SG1 3QA Tel: 01438 313223 Fax: 01438 749734 — BM BS Nottm. 1975.

WARNES, Gordon David Caskgate Street Surgery, 3 Caskgate Street, Gainsborough DN21 2DJ Tel: 01427 612501 Fax: 01427 615459 — MB ChB Leeds 1984; DCH RCP Lond. 1987; MRCGP 1988.

WARNES, Professor Thomas Walter University Department of Gastroenterology, Manchester Royal Infirmary, Manchester M13 9WL Tel: 0161 276 4316 Fax: 0161 276 8779; Cotswold, 66 Moss Road, Alderley Edge SK9 7JB Tel: 01625 584310 — (Manch.) MB ChB Manch. 1962; FRCP 1980, M 1967; MD Manch. 1975. Cons. Phys. (Gastroenterol.) Manch. Roy. Infirm.; Hon. Lect. (Med.) Manch. Univ.; Vis. Pofessor, Dept. Biomolecular Sci., Univ. Manch. Inst. Sci. & Technol., July 1999. Specialty: Gastroenterol. Socs: Brit. Soc. Gastroenterol.; Assn. Phys.; Internat. Assn. Study of Liver. Prev: Sen. Regist. & Regist. (Med.) Univ. Coll. Hosp. Lond.; Tutor (Med.) Univ. Manch.

WARNKE, Peter Department of Neuroscience, The University of Liverpool, Lower Lane, Liverpool L9 7LJ Tel: 0151 529 5949 Fax: 0151 529 5465 Email: p.c.warnke@liv.ac.uk; 14 The Evergreens, Formby, Liverpool L37 3RW Tel: 01704 831462 — State Exam Med Freiburg 1983; MD. Prof. of Neurosurg., Univ. of Liverp.; Hon. Cons., The Walton Centre for Neurol. & Neurosurg., & Clatterbridge Centre for Oncol. Specialty: Neurosurg. Special Interest: Brain Tumours; Epilepsy; Radiosurgery. Socs: Amer. Assn. Neurol Surg.; Soc. Brit. Nerol. Surg.; Europ. Soc. Stereotactic & Functional Neurosurg. Prev: Vice-Chairman, Dept. of Stereotatic Neurosurg., Univ. of Freiburg, Germany.

WARNOCK, Ann Margaret Mary Quayside Medical Practice, 82-84 Strand Road, Londonderry BT48 7NN Tel: 028 7126 2790 Fax: 028 7137 3729 — MB BCh BAO Belf. 1983.

WARNOCK, Mr David Samuel Musgrave Park Hospital, Stockman's Lane BT9 7JB; 19 Ballymagin Road, Magheralin, Craigavon BT67 0RU Tel: 028 9090 2129 — MB BCh BAO Belf. 1991; MB BCh Belf. 1991; FRCS Ed. 1995; FRCS (TR & ORTH) 2001. Cons. Musgrave Pk. Hosp. Belf. Specialty: Trauma & Orthop. Surg. Socs: Ulster Med. Soc.; BOA (British Orthopaedic Assocn).

WARNOCK, Jessie Helen (retired) Ardmore, 8 Regent Place, West Ferry, Dundee DD5 1AT Tel: 01382 730299 — MB BCh BAO Belf. 1945 (Qu. Univ. Belf.)

WARNOCK, John Mathers Turnbull (retired) Kishmul, Burnside Road, Fettercairn, Laurencekirk AB30 1XX Tel: 01561 340366 — MB ChB Glas. 1953. Prev: Ho. Off. (Surg & Med.) Hairmyres Hosp. E. Kilbride.

WARNOCK, Monica Mary Stoke Gifford Medical Centre, Ratcliffe Drive, Stoke Gifford, Bristol BS34 8UE Tel: 0117 979 9430 — MB BCh BAO Belf. 1989 (QUB) DGM 1991; DRCOG 1992; MRCGP 1993; DCH 1996. GP; Clin. Asst. Palliat. med. St Peters Hosp. Bristol. Specialty: Gen. Pract.

WARNOCK, Niall Geoffrey York Hospital, Wigginton Road, York YO31 8HE Tel: 01904 726675 Fax: 01904 726825 — MB ChB Leeds 1983; MRCP (UK) 1986; FRCR 1990; T(R) (CR) 1992. Cons. Radiol. York Dist. Hosp. Specialty: Radiol. Prev: Asst. Prof. (Radiol.) Univ. Iowa.

WARNOCK, Sheila Mary 14 Avon Grove, Edinburgh EH4 6RF — MB BCh BAO Belf. 1980.

WARNOCK, William Alexander 215 Spring Grove Road, Isleworth TW7 4AF Tel: 020 8560 7750 Fax: 020 8232 8927 — MB BCh BAO Belf. 1964 (Qu. Univ. Belf.)

WARR, Carolyn Anne 14 Church Lane, Cliftonwood, Bristol BS8 4TR Tel: 0117 921 3117 — MB ChB Bristol 1993; MRCP Lond. 1997. SHO (Anaesth.) Gloucester Roy. Hosp. Specialty: Anaesth. Prev: SHO Rotat. (Renal Med./ITU/Anaesth.); SHO (Endocrine, Gen. Med. Neurol.) Frenchay Hosp. Bristol.

WARR, Edward Ernest 24 Leoplod Road, Bristol BS6 — MB ChB Bristol 1963.

WARR, Oenone Carol Clanricarde Surgery, Clanricarde Road, Tunbridge Wells TN1 4PJ — MB BS Lond. 1980 (St. Thos.) MRCGP 1985; DRCOG 1985. GP Tunbridge Wells Retainer Scheme; Clin. Asst. (Rheum.) Kent & Sussex Hosp. Trust Tunbridge Wells. Specialty: Gen. Pract.; Rheumatol.; Neurol. Prev: GP Lond.; SHO (Med.) The Amer. Hosp. Paris; SHO (Med.) St. Peter's Hosp. Chertsey.

WARR, Mr Robert Philip 14 Church Lane, Clifton, Bristol BS8 4TR Tel: 0117 921 3117 — BM Soton. 1989; FRCS Eng. 1995. Research Regist. (Plastic Surg.) Frenchay Hosp. Bristol. Prev: SHO Rotat. (Surg.) Frenchay Hosp. Bristol.

WARRACK, John Hyslop (retired) 37 Arlington Road, Littleover, Derby DE23 6NZ — MB ChB Aberd. 1947.

WARRAN, Patricia Chanterlands Avenue Surgery, 149-153 Chanterlands Avenue, Hull HU5 3TJ Tel: 01482 343614; 101 Ferriby High Road, North Ferriby HU14 3LA — MB ChB Manch. 1974; FFA RCS Eng. 1979; MRCGP 1991.

WARRANDER, Anna (retired) 4 Clark Place, Belford NE70 7LT Tel: 01668 213224 — MB BS Lond. 1959 (St. Bart.) MRCS Eng. LRCP Lond. 1959. Prev: Clin. Med. Off. N.d. HA.

WARRE, John Henry Devonshire House Surgery, Essington, North Tawton, Okehampton EX20 2EX Tel: 01837 82204 Fax: 01837 82459 — MB ChB Birm. 1971; DObst RCOG 1974. Specialty: Accid. & Emerg. Socs: BMA; BASICS. Prev: GP Tomintoul.

WARRELL, Professor David Alan University of Oxford, Nuffield Department of Clinical Medicine, John Radcliffe Hospital, Headington, Oxford OX3 9DU Tel: 01865 221332 Fax: 01865 220984 Email: david.warrell@ndm.ox.ac.uk — BM BCh Oxf. 1964 (Oxf & St. Thos.) MRCS Eng. LRCP Lond. 1965; FRCP Lond. 1977, M 1966; MA Oxf 1964, DSc 1990, DM 1970; F Med Sci 1998; FRCP Ed 1998. Dep. Head, Nuffield Dept. of Clin. Med. and Prof. Trop. Med. and Infect. Dis., Univ. Oxf.; Hon. Cons. Malaria to the Army; Hon. Clin. Dir. Alistair Reid Venom Research Unit Liverp. Sch. Trop. Med.; Hon. Cons. Phys., Oxf. Radcliffe NHS Hosps. Trust. Specialty: Trop. Med.; Gen. Med.; Immunol. Special Interest: Malaria; Relapsing Fevers; Toxicology. Socs: Hon. Mem.Amer. Soc. of Trop. Med Hygience; Hon. Fellow Ceylon College of Physicians; Pres. Roy. Soc. Trop. Med. & Hyg. Prev: Head, Nuffield Dept. of Clin. Med. Univ. Oxf.; Cons. Malaria, Snake Bite & Rabies WHO; Pro Bono Med. Panel, Foreign & Commonw. Office.

WARRELL, David Watson (retired) Beudy Ychain, Llanfaglan, Caernarfon LL54 5RA Tel: 01286 672710 — MB ChB Sheff. 1953; MRCS Eng. LRCP Lond. 1953; MD Sheff. 1964; FRCOG 1970. Prev: Urol. Gyn. Centr. Manch. Hosps. Trust.

WARRELL, Mary Jean 4 Larkins Lane, Old Headington, Oxford OX3 9DW Tel: 01865 220968 Fax: 01865 760683 — MB BS Lond. 1971 (St. Mary's) MRCP (UK) 1974; FRCPath 1990, M 1978. Specialty: Virology. Prev: Wellcome Research Fell. Sir William Dunn Sch. Path. Oxf.; Cons. Fac. Trop. Med. Mahidol Univ. Bangkok, Thailand; Sen. Regist. (Clin. Virol.) Churchill Hosp. Oxf.

WARRELL, Richard John Department of Health Care of the Elderly, Derriford Hospital, Derriford Road, Plymouth PL6 8DH Tel: 01752 792891 Fax: 01752 792894 — MB ChB Liverp. 1975; MRCP (UK) 1979. Cons. in Health Care for the Elderly, Plymouth Primary Health Care Trust, Plymouth, Devon. Specialty: Care of the Elderly. Prev: Sen. Regist. (Geriat. Med.) Wessex RHA.

WARREN, A Peter Medical Services, Sutherland House, 29-37 Brighton Road, Sutton SM2 5AN Tel: 020 8652 6000 Fax: 020 8652 6160; 21 Glengall Road, London SE15 6NJ Tel: 020 7237 2180 Fax: 020 7237 2180 — MB ChB St. And. 1968; DDAM 2000 (Faculty of Occupational Medicine); MRCGP 1987. Med. Adviser Med. Servs. Lond.; Hon. Med. Adviser Roy. Philharmonic Orchestra. Specialty: Gen. Pract.; Disabil. Med. Socs: Assn. Med. Advisers to Brit. Orchestras; Brit. Assn. Performing Arts Med.; Assur. Med. Soc. Prev: Clin. Asst. (Dermat.) Kings Coll. Hosp. Lond.; Clin. Asst. (Radiotherap.) Norf. & Norwich Hosp.; GP Norwich & Lond.

WARREN, Professor Alan John University of Cambridge, MRC Laboratory of Molecular Biology, Hills Road, Cambridge CB2 2QH — MB ChB Glas. 1986; BSc Glas. 1983; MRCP (UK) 1989; PhD Camb. 1995; MRCPath 1997; FRCP (UK) 2002. Prof. Haemo. MRC Lab. Mol. Biol. Camb. Uni. Specialty: Haematology. Special Interest: Myelodysplasia; Leukaemia; Aplastic Anaemia. Socs: Brit. Soc. of Haemat.; Amer. Soc. of Haemat.; Med. and Dent. Defence Union of Scotl. Prev: MRC Sen. Clin. Fell.; MRC Clin. Scientist & Hon. Sen. Regist. Camb.; MRC Train. Fell. LMB Camb.

WARREN, Angela Elizabeth The Forest Group Practice, The Surgery, Bury Road, Brandon IP27 0BU Tel: 01842 813353 Fax: 01842 815221; Hartley Place, Nursery Lane, Hockwold, Thetford IP26 4ND Tel: 01842 828824 — MRCS Eng. LRCP Lond. 1975 (Guy's Hosp.) BSc (Hons.) (Pharm.) Lond. 1972, MB BS 1975; DRCOG 1977; Cert JCC Lond. 1977; DCH Eng. 1980.

WARREN, Anna Kristin 1A Witherington Road, London N5 1PN Tel: 020 7607 2524 — MB BS Lond. 1991; BSc (Hons.) Lond. 1988; MRCP (UK) 1994. Lect. & Hon. Sen. Regist. (c/o Elderly) Qu. Mary & Westfield Coll. & Roy. Lond. Hosps. Lond. Specialty: Care of the Elderly. Prev: Regist. (Gen. Med. & c/o Elderly) Bromley Hosp. Kent.

WARREN, Anne Yvonne Addenbrooke's Hospital, Department of Histopathology, Box 325, Hills Road, Cambridge CB2 2QQ Tel: 01223 217163 — MB BS Lond. 1987 (Univ. Coll.) MRCPath 1995; MSc (Clin. Cytopath.) Lond. 1996. Cons. Histo/Cytopathologist, Addenbrookes Hosp. Cambs. Specialty: Histopath. Special Interest: Gyn. & Urological Path. & Cytol. Prev: Cons. Histopath. P'boro. Dist. Hosp.; Sen. Regist. (Histopath.) P'boro. Dist. Hosp.; Ho. Off. (Surg.) Univ. Coll. & Middlx. Hosps. Lond.

WARREN, Anthony John Cygnet Hospital Ealing, 23 Lorfton Road, Ealing, London W5 2HT Tel: 0208 991 6699 Fax: 0208 991 0440 Email: cygnetdoc@aol.com — MB BS Lond. 1972 (Middlx.) BSc Lond. 1969; MRCPsych 1977; Tpsych 1993. Cons. Pyshchiatrist; Vis. Cons. Psychiat., Bowden Ho. Clinic, Harrow. Specialty: Gen. Psychiat. Socs: Mem. BMA; Fell. RSM; Mem. RCPsych. Prev: Regist. (Psychiat.) St. Geo. Hosp. Med. Sch. & Atkinson Morley's; Sen. Regist. (Psychiat.) St. Geo. Hosp. Med. Sch.; Cons. Psychiat., Hillingdon Hosp.

WARREN, Antony Richard Lensfield Medical Practice, 48 Lensfield Road, Cambridge CB2 1EH Tel: 01223 352779 Fax: 01223 566930 Email: antony.warren@nhs.net — BM BCh Oxf. 1978; MA Oxf. 1980, BA (Hons.) 1975; DRCOG 1980; MRCGP 1982. Specialty: Gen. Pract. Socs: BMA. Prev: Trainee GP Rookery Med. Centre Newmarket; SHO (Geriat.) Chesterton Hosp. Camb.; SHO (Obst.) John Radcliffe Hosp. Oxf.

WARREN, Bryan Frederick Department of Cellular Pathology, John Radcliffe Hospital, Headington, Oxford OX3 9DU Tel: 01865 220510 Fax: 01865 220574 — MB ChB Liverp. 1981. Cons. Path. John Radcliffe Hosp. Oxf. Specialty: Histopath. Socs: Assn. Coloproctol.; Ct. of Examrs Roy. Coll. Surg. Eng.; Assn. Clin. Path. (Council. Mem.). Prev: Lect. (Path.) Bristol Univ.

WARREN, Carol Ann Department of Genito Urinary Medicine, Nottingham City Hospital Trust, Hucknall Road, Nottingham NG5 1PB Tel: 01159 627965; 15 Bradshaw Drive, Holbrook, Belper DE56 0SZ — MB ChB Manch. 1967; DObst RCOG 1969; MRCOG 1980. Staff Phys. (Genitourin. Med.) Nottm. City Hosp. Specialty: Genitourinary Medicine. Socs: Med. Soc. Study VD; Soc. Colposcopy & Cervical Path. Prev: Sen. Regist. (Genitourin. Med.) Nottm. Gen. Hosp. & Leicester Roy. Infirm; Regist. (Genitourin. Med.) Nottm. Gen. Hosp.; Regist. (O & G) Newc. Gen. Hosp.

WARREN, Caroline Jane 35 Kingsway, London SW14 7HL — MB BS Lond. 1985; MRCGP 1995. Specialty: Gen. Pract.

WARREN, Christine Anne Penarth Health Centre, Stanwell Road, Penarth CF64 3XE Tel: 029 2070 0911; 6 Thorn Grove, Penarth CF64 5BZ — MB BCh Wales 1984 (Welsh National School of Medicine) DCH RCP Lond. 1988; MRCGP 1991; Dip. Therap. Wales 1995. Med. Adviser Bro Taf HA. Specialty: Gen. Med.

WARREN, Christopher William Royal Hallamshire Hospital, Department of Histopathology, Sheffield S10 2JF Tel: 0114 271 2811 Fax: 0114 271 2200 Email: chris.warren@sth.nhs.uk; 333 Crimicar Lane, Sheffield S10 4EN Tel: 0114 263 0994 Email: chriswarren@onetel.com — MB ChB (Hons.) Sheff. 1988; BMedSci (1st cl. Hons.) Sheff. 1983; PhD Sheff. 1987; MRCPath 1996. Cons. Histopath./Cytopathol. Sheff. Teachg. Hosps. NHS Trust . Hosp. NHS Trust. Specialty: Histopath. Special Interest: Gyn. Path. and dermatopathology; Gyn. Path. & Dermatopath. Prev: Sen. Regist. & Regist. Rotat. (Histopath.) Leeds (N.. & Yorks. RHA); SHO Rotat. (Histopath.) Sheff. HA; Ho. Off. North. Gen. & Roy. Hallamsh. Hosps. Sheff.

WARREN, Clive Edwin John Stuart House Surgery, 20 Main Ridge West, Boston PE21 6SS Tel: 01205 362173 Fax: 01205 365710 — MB BS Lond. 1980 (Westm.) MA (1st Cl.) (Camb.) 1981; DRCOG 1983; MRCGP (Distinc.) 1984. Specialty: Accid. & Emerg. Prev: Trainee GP Pilgrim Hosp. Boston VTS; Ho. Surg. W. Suff. Hosp. Bury St. Edmunds; Ho. Phys. Westm. Hosp.

WARREN, Edward St leger Jubilee Avenue Surgery, 24 Jubilee Avenue, Whitton, Twickenham TW2 6JB Tel: 020 8893 8464 Fax: 020 8893 3954 — MB ChB Witwatersrand 1974. Accredit. Trainer (Gen. Pract.) Twickenham.

WARREN, Elisa Renee 12 Skippon Terrace, Thorner, Leeds LS14 3HA Email: elisa.warren@virgin.net — MB ChB Leeds 1990; FRCA Lond. 1997. Cons. Anaesth., St. James Univ. Hosp., Leeds. Specialty: Anaesth. Socs: Roy. Coll. Anaesth.; BMA; Assn. Anaesth.

WARREN, Elisabeth Central Cheshire Primay Care Trust, Barony Headquarters, Nantwich CW5 5QU Tel: 01270 415387; 64 Mountway, Waverton, Chester CH3 7QF Tel: 01244 332091 — State Exam Med Cologne 1978; MD Cologne 1979; DCCH RCP Ed. 1991. Specialty: Paediat. Prev: Community Paediat. & SCMO Chesh. Community Health Care Trust Nantwich; Clin. Med. Off. Wirral HA; SHO (Paediat.) Stäedt Krankenhaus Leverkusen, W. Germany.

WARREN, Elizabeth Jane Callington Health Centre, Haye Road, Callington PL17; Prospect Farm, Latchley, Gunnislake PL18 9AX — MB ChB Birm. 1978. Prev: Regist. (Anaesth.) Plymouth Gen. Hosp.; SHO (Anaesth.) N. Staffs. Hosp. Centre Stoke-on-Trent.

WARREN, Fiona Margaret Whitby Group Practice Surgery, Chester Road, Whitby, Ellesmere Port CH65 6TG Tel: 0151 355 6153 Fax: 0151 355 6843 — MB ChB Liverp. 1984 (Liverpool) DRCOG 1988; MRCGP 1989. Prev: SHO (A & E) & Ho. Off. Walton Hosp. Liverp.; Trainee GP Chester VTS.

WARREN, George Albert Ramsden Keystone, 47 Firle Road, Eastbourne BN22 8EE Tel: 01323 29492 — LRCPI & LM, LRSCI & LM 1932.

WARREN, Grace Chandrani Mental Health Unit, Rotherham District General Hospital, Moorgate, Rotherham S60 2UD Tel: 01709 820000 — MB ChB Sheff. 1984; MRCPsych 1991. Cons. (en. Adult Psychiat.) Rotherham Priority Health NHS Trust; Hon. Clin. Lect., Univ. of Sheff. Specialty: Gen. Psychiat. Socs: Roy. Coll. Psychiat.; BMA. Prev: Lect. Univ. Dept. Psychiat. Sheff.; Research Regist. (Psychiat.) Univ. Sheff.; Regist. (Psychiat.) Sheff. HA.

WARREN, Mr Hugh Walter Queen Elizabeth Hospital, Gayton Road, King's Lynn PE30 4ET — MB BS Lond. 1985; FRCS Eng. 1989; MS 1996; FRCS (Gen.) 1997. Cons. Gen. Surg. Socs: AUGIS. Prev: Regist. Glas. Roy. Infirm.

WARREN, Jill St. Michaels Hospice, Hornbeam Park Avenue, Harrogate HG2 8QL — MB BS Newc. 1984; DGM RCP Lond. 1988; MRCGP 1988; Dip. Palliat. Med. Wales 1994. Med. Dir. St. Michaels Hospice Harrogate. Specialty: Palliat. Med. Prev: Med. Dir. St. And. Hospice Grimsby.

WARREN, Joan Elizabeth (retired) 69 Marlborough Road, Worthing BN12 4HD Tel: 01903 246342 — (St. And.) MB ChB MB ChB St. And. 1952; DPH Eng. 1970. Prev: SCMO W. Sussex AHA.

WARREN, John Bowen D41 Odhams Walk, London WC2H 9SB — MB BS Lond. 1977 (Guy's) MRCP (UK) 1979; MD Lond. 1983; FRCP Lond. 1994. Med. Cons. Med. Control. Agency Lond.; Hon. Sen. Lect. (Clin. Pharmacol.) St. Thos. Hosp. Lond. Specialty: Pharmacology; Cardiol.; Pharmacology. Socs: Brit. Pharmacol. Soc.; Amer. Heart Assn.; Brit. MicroCirc. Soc. Prev: Sen. Lect. & Hon. Cons. Nat. Heart & Lung Inst. Lond.; Sen. Regist. (Clin. Pharmacol.) Hammersmith Hosp. Lond.

WARREN, John Pelham Princess Alexandra Hospital, Hamstel Road, Harlow CM20 1QX Tel: 01279 444455 Fax: 01279 827172 Email: john.warren@pah.nhs.uk — MB BChir Camb. 1967; MB Camb. 1967, BChir 1966; DCH Eng. 1968; MRCP (UK) 1970; FRCP Lond. 1987. p/t Cons. Phys. Princess Alexandra Hosp. Harlow; Cons. Phys., Rivers Hosp., Sawbridgeworth. Specialty: Respirat. Med. Socs: Brit. Med. Assn.; Brit. Thoracic Soc. Prev: Sen. Regist. (Med.) King's Coll. Hosp. Lond.; Ho. Phys. Lond. Hosp.

WARREN, Jonathan Sidney Nightingale Road Surgery, 1-3 Nightingale Road, London N9 8AJ Tel: 020 8804 3333 Fax: 020 8805 7776; 122A Wood Street, Barnet EN5 4DA — MB BS Lond. 1974 (St. Geo.) BSc (Hons.) (Pharmacol.) Lond. 1971; MRCGP 1981; DFFP 1993. Sen. Partner GP Edmonton; Clin Asst. (Ment. Handicap) Chase Farm Hosp. Enfield. Socs: Brit. Soc. Med. & Dent. Hypn. Prev: Clin. Asst. (Paediat.) N. Middlx. Hosp. Lond.; Clin. Asst. (Obst.) Whittington Hosp. Lond.; Cas. Off. & Ho. Off. (Surg.) St. Geo. Hosp. Tooting.

WARREN, Joseph Brian Nursery House, Forest Road, Ascot SL5 8QU Tel: 01344 885300 — (St. Mary's) MRCS Eng. LRCP Lond. 1958; DObst RCOG 1961; MA Camb. 1958, MB 1964, BChir 1963; FFA RCS Eng. 1971. Private Anaesth. Pract. Specialty: Anaesth. Prev: Cons. Heatherwood-Waxham Pk. Hosps. Trust; Sen. Regist. Char. Cross Hosp. Gp.; Regist. Groote Schuur Hosp. Cape Town, S. Afr.

WARREN, Lynn Margaret 164 Hazelwood Lane, London N13 5HJ — MB BS Lond. 1996.

WARREN, Marion Marjorie — MB ChB Ed. 1998.

WARREN, Martin John X-Ray Department, Luton & Dunstable NHS Trust, Lewsey Road, Luton LU4 0DZ Tel: 01582 718082 — MB BS Lond. 1978 (St. Thos.) FRCP; BSc Lond. 1975; MRCP (UK) 1982; FRCR 1987. Cons. Radiol. Luton & Dunstable NHS Trust. Specialty: Radiol.

WARREN, Mary Ethel St Helier Hospital, Wrythe Lane, Carshalton SM5 1AA Tel: 020 8296 3032 Fax: 020 8296 3013; 29 Send Barns Lane, Send, Woking GU23 7BS — BM BCh Oxf. 1975 (Oxf. & St. Bart.) BA 1969; BMCH 1973; FRCR 1991; MSc Nuclear Med. Lond. 1995; Cert. Adv Study Health Managem 1999. Cons. Radiol. St. Helier Hosp. Carshalton. Specialty: Radiol. Socs: BMA; BNMS; Fell. Roy. Coll. Radiols. Prev: Sen. Regist. (Radiol.) St. Geo. Hosp. Lond.; Regist. (Radiol.) Frimley Pk. Hosp. & St. Geo. Hosp. Lond.

WARREN, Matthew David 14 Henley Road, Ipswich IP1 3SL — MB BS Newc. 1994.

WARREN, Michael Donald (retired) 2 Bridge Down, Bridge, Canterbury CT4 5AZ Tel: 01227 830233 — (Guy's) MB BS Lond. 1946; MD Lond. 1952; DIH Eng. 1952; DPH (Distinc.) Lond. 1952; FRCP Lond. 1975, M 1969; FFCM RCP (UK) 1972; FFPHM 2000. Prev: Prof. & Dir. Health Servs. Research Unit Univ. Kent.

WARREN, Michael Robert Stoneleigh Surgery, Police Square, Milnthorpe LA7 7PW Tel: 015395 63307; Cairnsmore, Dugg Hill, Heversham, Milnthorpe LA7 7EF Tel: 0153 95 63536 — MB ChB Leeds 1967; MB ChB (Hons.) Leeds 1967. Prev: Ho. Surg. Profess. Surgic. Unit & Cas. Off. Gen. Infirm. Leeds; Ho. Phys. Chapel Allerton Hosp. Leeds.

WARREN, Mr Nicholas Paul Accident & Emergency Department, Northwick Park Hospital, Watford Road, Harrow HA1 3UJ — MB BS Lond. 1976; MA Oxf. 1977; FRCS Ed. 1982; FRCS Eng. 1982. Asso. Specialist Accidents & Emerg. Dept. Prev: Career Regist. (Surg.) N.W. Thames RHA.; SHO (Accid. Dept.) Lond. Hosp.

WARREN, Nigel Raymond 29 Send Barns Lane, Send, Woking GU23 7BS — MRCS Eng. LRCP Lond. 1977 (St. Bart.) BA Oxf. 1959; Dip. Addic. Behaviour Lond. 1991. Hon. Cons. Forens. Psychiat. Specialty: Forens. Psychiat. Socs: BMA. Prev: Sen. Med. Off. HM YOI & Remand Centre Feltham Middlx.; Regist. (Forens. & Gen. Psychiat.) Brookwood Hosp. Knaphill; Regist. (Psychiat. inc. Ment. Health) Rubery Hill Hosp. S. Birm.

WARREN, Paul Anthony Surrey Hampshire Borders NHS Trust, Bridge Centre, Basingstoke RG21 7PJ Tel: 01256 316303 Fax: 01256 316356 — BM Soton. 1980; MRCPsych 1985. Surrey Hamshire Borders NHS Trust. Specialty: Gen. Psychiat. Prev: Sen. Regist. (Psychiat.) Basingstoke Dist. Hosp.; Sen. Regist (Psychiat.) Roy. S. Hants Hosp. Soton.; Sen. Regist (Psychiat.) Wessex Regional Secure Unit.

WARREN, Peter Michael Ty'r Dderwen, Cwrt Henri, Dryslwyn, Carmarthen SA32 8RX Tel: 01558 668039 — MB ChB St. And. 1972; MRCP (UK) 1976.

WARREN, Mr Richard Anthony 152 Harley Street, London W1G 7LH Tel: 020 7935 3834 Fax: 020 7224 2574 Email: doctor.warren@virgin.net — (Liverp.) MB ChB Liverp. 1976; FRCS Ed. 1981; MD Sheff. 1988; FICS 1989; FFAEM 1993. Cons. Surg. Indep. & Medico Legal Pract. Lond. Clinic. Specialty: Orthop.; Medico Legal. Socs: Medico-Legal Soc.; Brit. Soc. Trauma; Brit. Inst. Musculosketal Med. Prev: Clin. Tutor & Sen. Examr. (Surg.) Univ. Lond.; Cons. Surg. Westm. & St. Stephens Hosp. Lond.

WARREN, Richard Charles Norfolk and Norwich Hospital, Brunswick Road, Norwich Tel: 01603 286286 Fax: 01603 286781; 14 Christchurch Road, Norwich NR2 2AE Tel: 01603 454173 Fax: 01603 454173 — MB BS Lond. 1977 (King's Coll. Hosp.) DRCOG 1979; DCH RCP Lond. 1980; FRCOG 1996, M 1983. Cons. O & G Norf. & Norwich Hosp.; Counc. RCOG; Counc. RCOG Med. workforce Advisery Comm. Specialty: Obst. & Gyn. Socs: Past Chairm. RCOG Med. Workforce Advisory Comm.; Chairm. RCOG Servs. Comm. Prev: Regional Adviser (Obst. & Gyn.) E. Anglia; Research Fell. & Clin. Sen. Regist. King's Coll. Hosp. Lond.; regional Adviser (obs+Gyn) E. Anglia.

WARREN, Roderic Ellis Microbiology Laboratory, Royal Shrewsbury Hospital, Shrewsbury SY3 8XQ Tel: 01743 261163 — MB BChir Camb. 1971; MA Camb. 1971; FRCPath 1988, M 1977. Cons. (Microbiologist) Roy. Shrewsbury Hosp.; Hon. Sen. Lect. (Infec.

Dis.) Univ. Birm.; Clin. Director, Shrewsbury & Telford Hosp. NHS Trust. Specialty: Med. Microbiol. Socs: Brit. Soc. Antimicrob. Chemother. Counc.; Hosp. Infec. Soc. Prev: Gp. Dir. PHLS Midl.; Cons. Microbiol. Addenbrooke's Hosp. Camb.; Sen. Regist. Camb. Health Dist. (T).

WARREN, Roderick Edward 11 St Swithuns Ter, Lewes BN7 1UJ — MB ChB Ed. 1997.

WARREN, Rosemary Jane (retired) Sandways Cottage, Bourton, Gillingham SP8 5BQ — MB BS Lond. 1970 (Middlx.)

WARREN, Ruth Mary Leigh Addenbrooke's Hospital, Cambridge CB2 2QQ Tel: 01223 217627 Fax: 01223 217886 Email: rmlw2@cam.ac.uk; 3 Watlington Road, Old Harlow, Harlow CM17 0DX Tel: 01279 419704 Fax: 01279 429771 — MB BChir Camb. 1967 (Camb. & Lond. Hosp.) DCH Eng. 1969; MRCP (UK) 1971; FRCR 1976; FRCP Lond. 1991; MA Camb. 1967, MD 1995. Cons. Radiol. Addenbrooke's Hosp. Camb. Specialty: Radiol. Prev: Med. Dir. & Cons. Radiol. Princess Alexandra Hosp. NHS Trust; Sen. Regist. (Radiol.) King's Coll. Hosp. Lond.; Ho. Phys. & Ho. Surg. Lond. Hosp.

WARREN, Stella Avis Frida (retired) 16 Ashdown Road, Portishead, Bristol BS20 8DP Tel: 0117 984 9081 — MB ChB Bristol 1957.

WARREN, Mr Stephen John Chase Farm Hospital, The Ridgeway, Enfield EN2 8JL; Pavilion, Roundhurst, Haslemere GU27 3BN Tel: 020 8967 5981 Fax: 020 8370 9043 — MB BS Lond. 1986 (London Hospital Medical College) BSc Hons Lond. 1983; FRCS (Ed.) 1991; FRCS (Gen. Surg.) 1999; MS Lond. 2000. Cons. Gen. Surg. with an interest in Coloproctol. & Laparoscopic Surg. Specialty: Gen. Surg. Socs: Assn. of Coloproctol.; Assn. of Endoscopic Surg.s; Assn. of Surg.s of GB & Irel. Prev: Lect. (Surg.), Roy. Lond. Hosp.; Specialist Regist. Univ. Coll. Hosp. & Middlx. Hosp.; Specialist Regist. Colchester Gen. Hosp.

WARREN, Stephen John Hyde Park Surgery, 2 Hyde Park Road, Mutley, Plymouth PL3 4RJ Tel: 01752 224437 Fax: 01752 217029; 33 Widey Lane, Crownhill, Plymouth PL6 5JS Tel: 01752 771991 — MB ChB Manch. 1977; MRCGP 1981; DCH RCP Lond. 1987. Specialty: Care of the Elderly.

WARREN, Stephen John CAMHS, Lennard Lodge, 3 Lennard Road, Croydon CR0 2UL Tel: 020 8700 8800 Fax: 020 8700 8809 — MB BS Lond. 1985 (Guy's Hosp.) DCH RCP Lond. 1987; MRCPsych 1990. Cons. Child & Adolesc. Psychiat. Croydon CAMHS; Hon. Cons. Psychiat. Roy. Marsden Hosp. Lond. Specialty: Child & Adolesc. Psychiat. Socs: ACPP. Prev: Sen. Regist. (Child & Adolesc. Psychiat.) St. Geo. Hosp. Lond.; Regist. (Psychiat.) Leeds HA.

WARREN, Stephen Willis Old Station Surgery, 39 Brecon Road, Abergavenny NP7 5UH Tel: 01873 859000 Fax: 01873 850163 — MB BS Lond. 1978 (St. Mary's) Prev: Ho. Phys. King Edwd. VIII Hosp. Windsor; Ho. Surg. St. Mary's Hosp. Lond.

WARREN, Susan West Wales General Hospital, Glangwili, Carmarthen SA31 2AF Tel: 01267 235151; Ty'r Derwen, Cwrt Henri, Dryslwyn, Carmarthen SA32 8RX Tel: 01558 668039 — MB ChB Dundee 1972; DCH Eng. 1974; MRCGP 1979; FRCPCH 1997. Cons. Paediat. (Community Child Health) Carmarthen & Dist. NHS Trust. Specialty: Paediat.

WARREN, Vanessa Jean 79 Westbourne Road, West Kirby, Wirral CH48 4DH — MB ChB Liverp. 1992.

WARREN, Virginia Jane BUPA, BUPA House, 15 Bloomsbury Way, London WC1A 2BA Tel: 020 7656 2049 Fax: 020 7656 2708 Email: warrenv@bupa.com — MB BChir Camb. 1981; MA Oxf. 1985, BA (Hons.) 1978; DHMSA 1981; MD Camb. 1987; MFPHM RCP (UK) 1993; FFPHM RCP (UK) 2000. Cons. Pub. Health Med. BUPA. Specialty: Pub. Health Med. Socs: Camb. Med. Grads Club. Prev: Sen. Regist. (Pub. Health Med.) Fac. Pub. Health Med. & E. Anglia RHA; Research Fell. (Gastroenterol.) Addenbrooke's Hosp. Camb.

WARREN, William Edward Burncross Surgery, 1 Bevan Way, Chapeltown, Sheffield S35 1RN Tel: 0114 246 6052 Fax: 0114 245 0276 — MB ChB Sheff. 1977; DRCOG 1979; MRCGP 1981.

WARREN-BROWNE, Caroline Yelverton The Willow Surgery, Coronation Road, Downend, Bristol BS16 5DH Tel: 0117 970 9500 — MB ChB Bristol 1979; MRCGP 1984.

WARREN-BROWNE, Muriel G (retired) The School House, Elsted, Midhurst GU29 0JY Tel: 01730 825297 — (Univ. Ed.) MB ChB Ed. 1946. Prev: Clin. Asst. (Dermat. & Rheum.) St. Richard's Hosp. Chichester.

WARRENDER, Thomas Stuart Mercheford House Surgery, Mercheford House, Elwyn Road, March PE15 9BT Tel: 01354 656841 Fax: 01354 660788; 8 Regent Avenue, Manchester PE15 8LN Tel: 0161 54928 — MB ChB Ed. 1971; BSc (Med. Sci.) Ed. 1968, MB ChB 1971; DObst RCOG 1973. Prev: SHO (O & G) Simpson Memor. Matern. Pavil. Roy. Infirm. Edin.; Surg. Ho. Off. Roodlands Hosp. Haddington.

WARRENDER, Tracey 29 Overhill Gardens, Bridge of Don, Aberdeen AB22 8QR — MB ChB Aberd. 1998.

WARRENS, Anthony Nigel Hammersmith Hospital, Imperial College Faculty of Medicine, Renal Unit, Du Cane Road, London W12 0NN Tel: 020 8383 3152 Fax: 020 8383 2788 — BM BCh Oxf. 1984; BSc Glas. 1981; MRCP (UK) 1987; PhD Lond. 1996; FRCP 2000; DM Oxf. 2003. Sen. Lect. & Hon. Cons. Phys. Renal Unit & Dept. Immunol. Imperial Coll. Hammersmith Hosp. Lond. Specialty: Nephrol.; Immunol.; Gen. Med. Socs: Renal Assn.; Collegiate Mem. RCP Lond.; Brit. Transpl. Soc. Prev: MRC Clinician Scientist & Hon. Sen. Regist. Hammersmith Hosp. Lond.; Regist. (Med.) Hammersmith & Ashford Middlx. Hosp.; SHO (Med.) Hammersmith & Brompton Hosps. & Nat. Hosp. Nerv. Dis. Lond.

WARRICK, Mr Charles Kay, CBE (retired) 5 The Fellside, Kenton, Newcastle upon Tyne NE3 4LJ Tel: 0191 285 5328 — MB BS Lond. 1940 (St. Bart.) MRCS Eng. LRCP Lond. 1939; DMR Lond 1941; FRCS Ed. 1946; FFR 1953; FRCP Lond. 1973, M 1966; FRCR 1975. Prev: Radiol. i/c Roy. Vict. Infirm. & Clin. Lect. Radiol. & Lect. Radiol.

WARRICK, John Walmsley (retired) Old Stables, Osmington, Weymouth DT3 6ET Tel: 01305 832113 — MRCS Eng. LRCP Lond. 1938 (King's Coll. Hosp.) DA Eng. 1944; FFA RCS Eng. 1954. Prev: Cons. Anaesth. W. Dorset Gp. Hosps.

WARRICK, Michael John Sewell Spa Road Surgery, Spa Road East, Llandrindod Wells LD1 5ES Tel: 01597 824291 / 842292 Fax: 01597 824503 — MB ChB Birm. 1977; DRCOG 1980; MRCGP 1981.

WARRICK, Stephanie Margaret Spa Road Surgery, Spa Road East, Llandrindod Wells LD1 5ES Tel: 01597 824291 / 842292 Fax: 01597 824503 — BSc (Hons.) Birm. 1973, MB ChB 1977; DRCOG 1989; DCH RCP Lond. 1992; MRCGP 1993.

WARRINER, Richenda Miriam (retired) Scorton, Lime Tree Close, East Preston, Littlehampton BN16 1JA Tel: 01903 770707 — MB BS Lond. 1956 (Guy's) LMSSA Lond. 1956; DObst RCOG 1959. Prev: Obst. Ho. Surg. Hillingdon Hosp.

WARRINER, Sara Elizabeth Ashcroft Road Surgery, 26 Ashcroft Road, Stopsley Green, Luton LU2 9AU Tel: 01525 872266; 26 Ashcroft Road, Luton LU2 9AU Tel: 01582 722555 — MB BS Lond. 1980 (Roy. Free Hosp.) Specialty: Obst. & Gyn. Prev: SHO Roy. Nat. Throat, Nose & Ear Hosp.; Cas. Off. Lond. Hosp. Whitechapel; Ho. Off. Roy. Free Hosp. Lond.

WARRINGTON, Bernadette Mary Veronica Health Centre, Rodney Road, Walton-on-Thames KT12 3LB Tel: 01932 228999 Fax: 01932 225586; 3 Sidney Road, Walton-on-Thames KT12 2NB — MB BS Lond. 1961 (Middlx.)

WARRINGTON, Dorothy Ruth 93 Newgate Street, Morpeth NE61 1BZ — MB ChB Manch. 1984; DRCOG 1986; MRCGP 1988. GP Ashington N.umberland. Prev: GP Sunderland; Trainee GP Bolton VTS.

WARRINGTON, Mr George Surrey and Sussex NHS Trust, East Surrey Hospital, Canada Avenue, Redhill RH1 5RH Tel: 01737 768511 — MD Malta 1971; FRCS Eng. 1978. Cons. ENT Surg. Crawley & Horsham Hosps. & New E. Surrey, Caterham & Oxted Hosps. Specialty: Otorhinolaryngol. Socs: Brit. Assn. Otol. Head & Neck Surg. Prev: Sen. Regist. Roy. Nat. Throat, Nose & Ear Hosp. Lond.; Sen. Regist. (ENT) St. Geo. Hosp. Lond.; Demonst. (Anat.) Univ. Leeds.

WARRINGTON, Jane Susan St Helena Hospice, Barncroft Close, Eastwood Drive, Colchester CO4 4SF Tel: 01206 845566 Fax: 01206 842445 — MB ChB Birm. 1978; MRCPsych 1983. Cons. Psychiat. Leicester Gen. Hosp. Specialty: Gen. Psychiat. Prev: Lect. Psychiat. Ment. Subnorm. Univ. Leic.; Hon. Sen. Regist. Leic. HA.

WARRINGTON, Jill Royal Cornhill Hospital, Cornhill Road, Aberdeen AB25 2ZH Tel: 01224 663131 — MB ChB Aberd. 1987;

MRCPsych 1991. Cons. (Psychiat. of Old Age) Roy. Cornhill Hosp. Specialty: Geriat. Psychiat.

WARRINGTON, Nigel John Netherton Health Centre, Halesowen Road, Dudley DY2 9PU Tel: 01384 254935 Fax: 01384 242468 — MB ChB Birm. 1980 (Birmingham) MRCGP 1985.

WARRINGTON, Rachel 59 Pettingale Road, Croesyceiliog, Cwmbran NP44 2NZ — MB BS Lond. 1998.

WARRINGTON, Robert The Health Centre, Rodney Road, Walton-on-Thames KT12 3LB Tel: 01932 228999 — MB BChir Camb. 1960 (Middlx.) BA Camb. 1960; DObst RCOG 1963.

WARRINGTON, Shirley Royal Victoria Infirmary, Queen Victoria Road, Newcastle upon Tyne NE1 4LP Tel: 0191 232 5131; 2 Beechfield Road, Gosforth, Newcastle upon Tyne NE3 4DR Tel: 0191 285 6310 — MB BS Newc. 1986; DRCOG 1989; DCH RCP Lond. 1990; MRCGP 1991; MRCP Ed. 1993; MRCPCH 1997. Regist. (Paediat.) Newc. Specialty: Paediat. Socs: N. Eng. Paediatric Soc. Prev: Regist. (Paediat.)Sunderland; Regist. (Paediat.) N.umberland; Regist. (Peadiat.) Gateshead.

WARRINGTON, Stephen 196 Harbour Lane, Milnrow, Rochdale OL16 4EL — MB ChB Manch. 1989. SHO Rotat. (Psychiat.) Salford Ment. Health Servs. Prestwich Hosp. Train Scheme.

WARRINGTON, Steven John Hammersmith Medicines Research Ltd., Central Middlesex Hospital, Acton Lane, London NW10 7NS Tel: 020 8961 4130 Fax: 020 8961 8665 Email: swarrinton@hmrlondon.com — MB BChir Camb. 1972 (St. Bart.) MRCP (UK) 1974; MA Camb. 1972, MD 1984; FRCP Ed. 1990; FFPM RCP (UK) 1991; FRCP Lond. 1991. Med. Dir. Hammersmith Med. Research Ltd.; Hon. Lect. (Clin. Pharmacol.) St. Bart. Hosp. Lond. Specialty: Pharmacology. Socs: Brit. Pharm. Soc. Prev: Research Regist. (Cardiol. & Clin. Pharmacol.) St. Bart. Hosp. Lond.; Lect. (Clin. Pharmacol.) St. Bart. Hosp. Med. Coll. Lond.; Resid. Med. Off. Nat. Heart Hosp. Lond.

WARRIS, Kauser Jabeen New Road Clinic, 114 New Road, Chingford, London E4 9SY Tel: 020 8524 8124; 71 Empress Avenue, Woodford Green IG8 9DZ Tel: 020 8505 6392 — MB BS Punjab 1984; DRCOG 1997; MRCGP 1999. GP Redbridge and Waltham Forest HA. Specialty: Family Plann. & Reproduc. Health.

WARSAP, Alan John, QHP, OStJ, Brigadier late RAMC Retd. Llaneth House, St. Margarets, Vowchurch, Hereford HR2 0RF — BM BCh Oxf. 1965; MA Oxf. 1965; FRCGP 1982, M 1973. Med. Mem.The Appeals Serv.; Civil. Med. Pract. (Gen. Pract.) MoD. Specialty: Gen. Pract. Socs: Fell. Med. Soc. Lond.; BMA. Prev: Dir. Army Gen. Pract.; Sen. Lect. (Gen. Pract.) RAMC; SMO Roy. Milit. Acad. Sandhurst.

WARSHOW, Usama Majid Mbarak 33 Sturdee House, Shipton St., London E2 7SA — MB BS Lond. 1998.

WARSOP, Andrew David 16 High Meadow, Tollerton, Nottingham NG12 4DZ — MB ChB Manch. 1989.

WARTAN, Sonia Wahan Anaesthetic Department, Epsom & St Helier NHS Trust, St Helier Hospital, Wrythe Lane, Carshalton SM5 1AA Tel: 020 8296 2444 — MB ChB Baghdad 1981; MB ChB Baghdad Iraq 1981; FFA RCS Eng 1993. Cons. Anaesth. Pain. Managem. Epsom. St Helier. NHS Trust. Specialty: Anaesth. Socs: Internat. Assn. Study of Pain; Pain. Soc; Assn. Anaesth. Prev: Sen.Reg.anaesth.Guys Hosp.; Research.Fell.Chronic Pain.Managem.Guys.Hosp.

WARTNABY, Helen Tamarisk, 12 Kingsham Avenue, Chichester PO19 8AN — MB BS Lond. 1988; MRCGP 1994.

WARTNABY, Kathleen Mary (retired) 11 Greenhurst Lane, Hurst Green, Oxted RH8 0LD Tel: 01883 714461 — (Roy. Free) MD Lond. 1965, MB BS 1955; MRCP Lond. 1958; DPM Eng. 1966; MRCPsych 1972. Prev: Cons. Psychiat. Netherne Hosp. Coulsdon, Redhill Gen. Hosp. & Oxted Hosps.

WARWICK, Adrian Paul Wordsley Hospital, Department of Obstetrics & Gynaecology, Stream Road, Wordsley, Stourbridge DY8 5QX Tel: 01384 456111; The Leys, The Shortyard, Wolverley, Kidderminster DY11 5XF — MB ChB Liverp. 1984; MRCOG 1990. Cons. O & G Dudley Gp. Hosps. NHS Trust. Specialty: Obst. & Gyn. Socs: Brit. Soc. Colpos. & Cerv. Path.; Brit. Gyn. Cancer Soc. Prev: Sen. Regist. City Hosp. & Birm. & Midl. Hosp. Wom.; Research Fell. N. Staffs. Matern. Hosp; Regist. Rotat. (O & G) W. Midl., Stoke-on-Trent, Stafford & Shrewsbury.

WARWICK, Mr David John Southampton University Hospitals, Southampton SO16 6UY Tel: 023 8025 8422/07887 651451 Fax: 023 8025 8446; Wessex Nuffield Hospital, Chandlers Ford, Southampton SO53 2DW — BM Soton. 1986; Dip. IMC RCS Ed. 1989; FRCS Eng. 1990; MD Bristol 1995; FRCS (Orth.) 1996. p/t Cons. Hand Surg. Soton. Univ. Hosps. NHS Trust Soton. Specialty: Orthop. Socs: Fell. BOA; Brit. Soc. Surg. Hand. Prev: Fell. (Hand Surg.) Roy. N. Shore Hosp. Sydney Australia; Lect. (Orthop.) Univ. Bristol & Sen. Regist. S & W RHA; Career Regist. (Orthop.) S. West. RHA.

WARWICK, Frederick (retired) — MB BChir Camb. 1959 (Camb. & Guy's) DCH Eng. 1964, DMRD 1966; FFR 1970. Prev: Cons. Radiol. Manch. Roy. Infirm.

WARWICK, Graham Lawrie Department of Nephrology, Leicester General Hospital, Glendolen Road, Leicester LE2 2FL Tel: 0116 258 8038; Stoctone House, 19A Gaulby Lane, Stoughton, Leicester LE2 2FL Email: graham_warwick1@excite.co.uk — MB ChB Glas. 1981; MRCP (UK) 1984; MD Glas. 1991; FRCP Lond. 1997. Cons. Nephrol. Leicester Gen. Hosp. Specialty: Nephrol. Prev: Sen. Regist. (Nephrol. & Gen. Med.) Roy. Infirm. Glas.; Hon. Regist. & Lect. Renal Unit & Inst. Biochem. Roy. Infirm Glas.; Regist. (Gen. Med. & Nephrol.) Glas. Roy. Infirm.

WARWICK, Helen Marie Levitts Surgery, Levitts Road, Bugbrooke, Northampton NN7 3QN Tel: 01604 830348 Fax: 01604 832785; 42 Pound Lane, Bugbrooke, Northampton NN7 3RH — BM BS Nottm. 1989; BMedSci 1987 Nottm.; DRCOG 1991 Lond.; MRCGP 1994 Lond.; DCH 1992 Glas. GP Princip. Specialty: Obst. & Gyn. Socs: BMA; MDU. Prev: SHO (Cas.) Northampton Gen. Hosp.; SHO GP Trainee N.ants.; SHO Palliat. Med. Cynthia Spencer Hospice N.ants.

WARWICK, Hilary Margaret Clare Department of General Psychiatry, St. George's Hospital Medical School, Cranmer Terrace, London SW17 0RE Tel: 020 8725 5543 — MB ChB Leeds 1980; MMedSci (Clin. Psychiat.) Leeds 1985, MB ChB 1980; MRCPsych 1984. Sen. Lect. (Psychiat.) St. Geo.'s Hosp. Sch. Lond. Specialty: Gen. Psychiat. Prev: Sen. Regist. Maudsley Hosp. Lond.

WARWICK, Jeremy Swain Fell Cottage Surgery, 123 Kells Lane, Low Fell, Gateshead NE9 5XY Tel: 0191 487 2656 — MB BS Newc. 1988.

WARWICK, John Richard Queenswood Surgery, 223 London Road, Waterlooville PO8 8DA Tel: 023 9226 3491; The Studio, Roberts Close, Wickham PO17 5HH Tel: 01329 835298 Email: john@warwi.freeserve.co.uk — MB ChB Manch. 1985 (St And. & Manch.) BSc (Med. Sci.) St. And. 1982, BSc (Astron./Physics) 1979; MRCGP 1989; T(GP) 1991; FRCGP 1998. p/t GP Partner & Principle; GP Appraiser; NCAA Assessor; QPA Assessor. Special Interest: GP assessing; GP training/education; Subst. misuse. Prev: GP Partner & Princip. Broughton Ho. Surg. Batley W. Yorks.

WARWICK, Jonathan Paul Nuffield Department of Anesthetics, Radcliffe Infirmary, Woodstock Road, Oxford OX2 6HE Tel: 01865 224774; Tudor Cottage, 144 Woodstock Road, Yarnton OX5 1PW Tel: 01865 379357 — MB ChB Birm. 1987; DA (UK) 1990; FRCA 1993. Cons. (Anaesth.) Radcliffe Infirm. Oxf. Specialty: Anaesth. Socs: Hon. Sec. Assn Burn & Reconstruc. Anaesth. Prev: Sen. Regist. (Anaesth.) John Radcliffe Hosp. Oxf.; Sen. Regist. (Anaesth.) Milton Keynes Gen. Hosp. NHS Trust; Regist. (Anaesth.) Princess Mary Hosp. RAF Akrotiri.

WARWICK, Lily Anne (retired) Newbattle Group Practice, Mayfield, Dalkeith EH22 — MB ChB Ed. 1965.

WARWICK, Malcolm Stewart (retired) Heron's Lea, 10 Longland Lane, Georgeham, Braunton EX33 1JR — MB ChB Birm. 1955; MRCS Eng. LRCP Lond. 1955; DPH Ed. 1957; DObst RCOG 1960. Med. Staff Ilfracombe & Dist. Cott. Hosp.; Police Surg.; Local Treasury Med. Off. Prev: Ho. Phys. & Ho. Surg. Qu. Eliz. Hosp. Birm.

WARWICK, Nicholas Graham 23 High Tree Drive, Earley, Reading RG6 1EU — MB BS Lond. 1986 (CXHMS) Specialty: Pharmaceutical Medicine; Gen. Pract.

WARWICK, Ralph Roderick Gardner (home) Fala House, 55 Eskbank Road, Dalkeith EH22 3BU — MB ChB Ed. 1966; BSc (Hons. Bact.) Ed. 1964; MRCP (U.K.) 1970; MRCGP 1977.

WARWICK, Ruth Marilyn North London Blood Transfusion Centre, Colindale Avenue, Edgware, London NW9 5BG — MB ChB 1973 (Bristol) MRCP UK 1977; MRCPath 1980; FRCPath 1992; FRCP 1997. Lead Cons., Tissue Servs., Nat. Blood Servs., Lond. Med. Advisor Lond. Cord. Blood Bank. Specialty: Haematology. Prev: Lead Cons. Tissue Services, National Blood Services; Sen. Regist.

(Haemat.) Roy. Free Hosp. Lond.; Cons. Haemat. Qu. Charlottes Hosp. Wom. Lond., RPGMS.

WARWICK, Wilfred James Greer (retired) Plas Gwyn, 257 Penn Road, Wolverhampton WV4 5SF Tel: 01902 341361 — MB BCh BAO Dub. 1937.

WARWICK-BROWN, Janet Margaret Denmead Health Centre, Hambledon Road, Denmead, Waterlooville PO7 6NR Tel: 023 9225 7112 Fax: 023 9225 7113; 7 Brent Court, Emsworth PO10 7JA Tel: 01243 371502 — MB BS Lond. 1980 (St. Bart.) BSc (Hons.) Lond. 1977; DRCOG 1984; MRCOG 1988. Hosp. Pract. Dept. Obst. & Gyn. St. Mary's Hosp. Portsmouth. Prev: Regist. (O & G) St. Mary's Hosp. Portsmouth.

WARWICK-BROWN, Mr Nigel Peter Southend Hospital, ENT Department, Prittlewell Chase, Westcliff on Sea SS0 0RY Tel: 01702 435555 Fax: 01702 221300 — MB BS Lond. 1978 (Lond. Hosp.) FRCSI 1984; FRCS Eng. 1985. Cons. Surg. (ENT) Southend Hosp. Specialty: Otorhinolaryngol. Socs: Fell. Roy. Soc. Med. Prev: Sen. Regist. (ENT) Radcliffe Infirm. Oxf. & Roy. Berks. Hosp. Reading; Regist. (ENT) Char. Cross Hosp. Lond.; SHO (ENT) Roy. Nat. Throat, Nose & Ear Hosp. Lond.

WARWICK-BROWN, Robert (retired) 47 Colts Bay, Craigweil, Bognor Regis PO21 4EH Tel: 01243 262457 — (Camb. & St. Bart.) MB BChir Camb. 1948; MA Camb. 1948; AFOM RCP Lond. 1981. Prev: Ho. Surg. Thoracic Unit & Lect. (Anat.) St. Bart. Hosp.

WARWICKER, Peter Maciej The Grove Medical Centre, Church Road, Egham TW20 9QJ Tel: 01784 433159 Fax: 01784 477208; 50 Simons Walk, Finglefield Green, Egham TW20 9SQ Tel: 01784 430090 — MB BS Lond. 1987; MRCGP (Distinc.) 1991; DRCOG 1991.

WASAN, Balvinder Singh 28 Charlbert Court, Charlbert St., London NW8 7BX Tel: 020 7722 9865 — MB BS Lond. 1994; BSc Lond. 1991. SHO (Med.) Hammersmith Hosp. Lond. Specialty: Gen. Med. Prev: SHO (Med.) Hillingdon & Harefield Hosps. Middlx.

WASAN, Harpreet Singh 16 Chesterfield Road, Chiswick, London W4 3HG Tel: 020 8 987 8807 Fax: 020 8383 4758; 6/E Haven Court, 128 Leighton Road, Hong Kong Tel: 00 852 5771386 Fax: 00 852 5597550 — MB BS Lond. 1986; MB BS (Hons.) Lond. 1986; MRCP (UK) 1990. Med. Research Counc. Train. Fell. Imperial Cancer Research Fund Lond.; Hon. Sen. Regist. (Med. Oncol.) Hammersmith Hosp. Roy. Postgrad. Med. Sch. Specialty: Oncol. Prev: Regist. Rotat. (Gen. Med.) Univ. Coll. Hosp., Middlx., Whittington., Lond. Chest Hosps.; SHO Rotat. (Gen. Med.) St. Geo. Hosp. Lond.; SHO (Med.) St. Mary's Hosp. Lond.

WASAN, Prabhjote Kaur 16 Chesterfield Road, Chiswick, London W4 3HG Tel: 020 8987 8807 — MB BS Lond. 1991. Trainee GP/SHO Ealing Hosp. Lond VTS.

WASFI, Fawzi Mahmood 392 Fulham Palace Road, London SW6 6HU — MRCS Eng. LRCP Lond. 1979.

WASHBROOK, Reginald Alfred Hryhoruk, TD 219 Lichfield Road, Rushall, Walsall WS4 1EA Tel: 01922 640384 — MB ChB St. And. 1956; DPM Lond. 1960; DPM Eng. 1962; MSc McGill 1967; FRCPsych 1992, M 1971; BTh (Hons.) Oxen 1999. Maj. RAMC (V). Socs: Internat. Soc. Criminols. & Brit. Counc. Alcoholism. Prev: Research Fell. (Foren. Psychiat.) Univ. McGill, Canada; Ho. Surg. Derbysh. Childr. Hosp. Derby; Ho. Phys. Dundee Roy. Infirm.

WASHINGTON, Avril Joan Dept. Paediatrics & Child Health, Homerton University Hospital NHS Trust, Homerton Row, London E9 6SR Tel: 020 8510 7876 Fax: 020 8510 7171 Email: avril.washington@homerton.nhs.uk — MB BS Lond. 1984 (Kings College Hospital) MRCP (UK) 1990. p/t Consultant Paediat., Dept. Paediat. & Child health, Homerton University Hosp., Hackney, Lond. (6 sessions); Consultant Paediatrician (Child in Mind Project) at RCPCH (PIT) (Secondment, 5 sessions). Specialty: Paediat. Special Interest: Child Ment. Health. Socs: Roy. Coll. Paediat. & Child Health (Fellow) (FRCPCH); Dep. Convenor, Brit. Paediatric Psychiat. and Psychol. Gp.; Brit. Med. Assn. Prev: Sen. Regist. (Paediat.) Roy. Free Hosp. Lond.; Regist. (Paediat. A & E) Qu. Eliz. Hosp. Childr. Lond. (P/T); Regist. Rotat. (Paediat.) Roy. Lond. Hosp.

WASHINGTON, James Stephen (retired) 8 Elliott Avenue, Frenchay, Bristol BS16 1PB Tel: 0117 956 7846 — (Leeds) MB ChB Leeds 1948; DIH Eng. 1962. Prev: Med. Adviser Hepworth Minerals & Chems. Ltd.

WASHINGTON, Mark Ian Neston Surgery, Mellock Lane, Little Neston, South Wirral CH64 4BN Tel: 0151 336 3951 Fax: 0151 353 0173 — MB ChB Liverp. 1989; DCH RCP Lond. 1992; DRCOG 1994. GP, Neston Surg., Neston. Specialty: Gen. Pract.

WASHINGTON, Robert John Mackenzie Womack, Elbury Lane, Churston Ferrers, Brixham TQ5 Tel: 01803 842117 — (Birm.) MB ChB Birm. 1961; DObst RCOG 1963. Asst. Surg. (Orthop. & Trauma) Torbay Hosp. Torquay. Socs: BMA. Prev: Ho. Surg. & Ho. Phys. Gen. Hosp. Birm.; Obst. Ho. Off. Dudley Rd. Hosp. Birm.; Cas. Surg. Regist. Gen. Hosp. Birm.

WASHINGTON, Stephen James — MB ChB Birm. 1998.

WASHINGTON, Suzanne Elizabeth Jayne 33 Fulmer Road, Sheffield S11 8UF Tel: 0114 266 0442; 244 Shear Brow, Blackburn BB1 8DS Tel: 01254 698501 — MB ChB Sheff. 1994. SHO (A & E) Chesterfield & N. Derbys. Roy. Hosp. NHS Trust. Prev: Ho. Off. (Gen., Renal & Cardiothoracic Surg.) North. Gen. Hosp. Sheff.; Ho. Off. (Gen. Med. & Dermat.) Chesterfield Hosp. Derbysh.

WASIM, Mohammad Glyn Ebwy Surgery, James Street, Ebbw Vale NP23 6JG Tel: 01495 302716 Fax: 01495 305166 — MB BS Patna 1974; MB BS Patna 1974.

WASON, Anne-Marie Bradford Hospitals NHS Trust, X-ray Department, Duckworth Lane, Bradford BD9 6RJ Tel: 01274 364543 — BM BS Nottm. 1986; BMedSci Nottm. 1983; MRCP (UK) 1989; FRCR 1993. Cons. Radiol. Specialty: Radiol.

WASPE, Sharon Rose 29 Atherstone Close, Oadby, Leicester LE2 4SP Tel: 0116 2711 059 — MB ChB Leic. 1998 (Leicester) SHO Burns & Plastic Surgery, Leicester Royal Infirmary. Specialty: Gen. Med.

WASS, Mr Alastair Roland Accident & Emergency Department, Pinderfields General Hospital, Aberford Road, Wakefield WF1 4DG Tel: 01924 212419 Fax: 01924 214840; Barn Moor, 1 Hungate Close, Dame Lane, Saxton, Tadcaster LS24 9TP Tel: 01937 557151 — MB BS Lond. 1987; FRCS Eng. 1992; FFAEM 1997. Accid. and Emerg. Cons., Pinderfields Hosp. Specialty: Accid. & Emerg. Special Interest: Maj. Trauma; Minor Fractures; Soft Tissue Injury.

WASS, Professor John Andrew Hall Department of Endocrinology, Churchill Hospital, Oxford OX3 7LJ Tel: 01865 227621 Fax: 01865 227938 Email: john.wass@noc.anglox.nhs.uk; Holmby House, Sibford Ferris, Banbury OX15 5RG Tel: 01869 350375 — MB BS Lond. 1971 (Guy's) MRCS Eng. LRCP Lond. 1971; MRCP (UK) 1973; MD Lond. 1980; FRCP Lond. 1986; MA Oxford 1995. Cons. Phys. (Endocrinol. & Metab.) Radcliffe Infirm. & Nuffield Orthop. Centre Oxf.; Prof. Endocrinol. Univ. Oxf. Specialty: Endocrinol. Socs: Amer. Endocrinol. Soc.; Soc. Endocrinol.; Assoc. Phys. Prev: Prof. Clin. Endocrinol. St. Bart. Hosp. Med. Sch. Lond.; Regist. Guy's Hosp. Lond. & King's Coll. Hosp. Lond.

WASS, Valerie Jean Lambeth Walk Group Practice, 5 Lambeth Walk, London SE11 6SP Tel: 020 7735 4412 Fax: 020 7820 1888 — MB BS Lond. 1972 (Guy's) BSc Lond. 1969; MRCS Eng. LRCP Lond. 1972; DCH Eng. 1974; MRCP Lond. 1982; FRCGP 1995. Sen. Lect. (Primary Health Care Med. Educat.) UMDS Lond. Prev: Regist. (Med.) Guy's Hosp. Lond.

WASSEF, Mouneer Abd-Elshahid Treloar Haemophilia Centre, Holybourne, Alton GU34 4EN Tel: 01420 88415; 6 Marshal Close, The Butts, Alton GU34 1RA — MB BCh Ain Shams 1962 (Cairo) SCMO Treloar Haemophilia Centre Alton & Basingstoke Dist. Hosp. Prev: Regist. (Haemat.) St. Mary's Hosp. Lond.; Regist. (Haemat.) N. Middlx. Hosp. Lond.; Regist. (Haemat. & Histopath.) Birch Hill Hosp. Rochdale.

WASSERBERG, Mr Jonathan Department of Neurosurgery, Queen Elizabeth Hospital, Birmingham; 1 The Stables, Sel Wick Road, Selly Park, Birmingham B29 7JW Tel: 0121 472 0520 — (Camb.) BSc (Hons.) Leic. 1983; MB BChir Camb. 1985; FRCS Eng. 1990. Sen. Lect. & Hon. Cons. Neurosurg. Qu. Eliz. Hosp. Birm.; Cons. Neurosurg., Qu. Eliz. Hosp. B'ham. Specialty: Neurosurg. Socs: Full Mem. Soc. Brit. Neurol. Surgs. Prev: Regist. (Neurosurg.) South. Gen. Hosp. Glas. & Hull Roy. Infirm.; Sen. Regist. (Neurosurg.) South. Gen. Hosp. Glas.

WASSIF, Wassif Samuel 9 Giles House, 158/160 Westbourne Grove, London W11 2RJ Tel: 020 7727 7835 Fax: 020 7221 7824 — MB ChB Assiut 1980; MB ChB Assiut Egypt 1980; MSc Lond. 1993. Sen. Regist. (Clin. Biochem.) King's Coll. Hosp. Lond. Specialty: Chem. Path. Prev: Regist. King's Coll. Hosp. Lond.; SHO Leicester Roy. Infirm.

WASSMER, Evangeline Birmingham Children's Hospital Neurology Dept, Steelhouse Lane, Birmingham B4 6NH — Artsexamen

Amsterdam 1994; DCH 1996; MRCP 1996. Cons. Birm. Children's Hosp. Specialty: Paediat. Neurol.; Paediat.; Child & Adolesc. Psychiat. Socs: RCPaed. Prev: Specialist Regist. (Paediat. Neurol.).

WASSON, Ciaran Whiterock Health Clinic, 6 Whiterock Grove, Belfast BT12 7RQ Tel: 028 9032 3153 Fax: 028 9061 9431; 181 Upper Lisburn Road, Belfast BT10 0LJ Tel: 01232 619431 — MB BCh BAO Belf. 1981 (Qus. Belf.) DFFP 1993. Socs: Fell. Ulster Med. Soc.; Assoc. Mem. Irish Otolaryngol. Soc.

WASSON, Colin Michael Alexander 14 Styal Road, Wilmslow SK9 4AE Email: colin.wasson@virgin.net — MB ChB Manch. 1992. Specialist Regist. (Anaesth.). Specialty: Anaesth.

WASSON, Jane Fulton McIlwaine The Health Centre, 20 Cleveland Square, Middlesbrough TS1 2NX Tel: 01642 245069 Fax: 01642 230388; 8 Morton Carr Lane, Nunthorpe, Middlesbrough TS7 0JU Tel: 01642 316112 — MB ChB Bristol 1975; Cert. Family Plann. JCC 1979.

WASSON, Lorraine Frances 91 Linn Road, Larne BT40 2BA — MB BCh BAO Belf. 1993.

WASSON, Sharon Jane 14 Styal Road, Wilmslow SK9 4AE — MB ChB Manch. 1992.

WASTELL, Professor Christopher Chelsea Westminster Hospital, Surgical Unit, Fulham Road, London SW10 9NH Tel: 020 8746 8463 Fax: 020 8746 8282; 7 Manor Way, Beckenham BR3 3LH Tel: 020 8650 5882 Fax: 020 8650 5882 Email: cwastell@globalnet.co.uk — (Guy's) MB BS Lond. 1957; MRCS Eng. LRCP Lond. 1957; FRCS Eng. 1960; MS Lond. 1966. Emerit. Prof. & Hon. Cons. (Gen. & Gastroenterol. Surg.) Chelsea Westm. Hosp., Imperial Coll. of Med. Lond. Specialty: Gen. Surg. Socs: Hellenic Soc. Experim. Med.; Hunt. Soc. (Ex-Pres.); Roy. Soc. Med. Prev: Lect. (Surg.) Westm. Med. Sch. Lond.; Hon. Cons. Surg. Roy. Hosp. Chelsea & Roy. Brompton Hosp. Lond.; Regist. (Surg.) Westm. Hosp. Lond.

WASTELL, Hilary Janet Department of clinical biochemistry, Freeman Hospital, High Heaton, Newcastle upon Tyne NE7 7BN Tel: 0191 223 1094 Fax: 0191 223 1292 — MB BS Newc. 1981; BSc (Hons.) Leeds 1972; MSc Newc. 1977; MRCPath 1988. Cons. Chem. Path. Freeman Hosp., Newc. Upon Tyne. Specialty: Chem. Path. Socs: Assn. Clin. Biochem.; Ass. Clin. Path. Prev: Sen. Regist. (Chem. Path.) Newc. Gen. Hosp.; Ho. Phys. & Surg. Roy. Vict. Infirm. Newc.

WASTIE, Jonathan Charles St. Peter's Med. Centre, 30-36 Oxford St., Brighton BN1 4LA; 37B Preston Park Avenue, Brighton BN1 6HG — MB BS Lond. 1992 (Charing Cross/Westminster) BSc (Hons.) Lond. 1986, MB BS 1992; Dip GUM 1998; DFFP 2000. Hosp. Practitioner GUM/HIV Sussex Co. Hosp. Specialty: HIV Med.; Pub. Health Med.; Genitourinary Medicine. Socs: BHIVA; MSSVD.

WASTY, Mr Syed Wajahat Hussain 1 Foxhome Close, Willow Grove, Chislehurst BR7 5XT — MB BS Karachi 1981; FRCS Glas. 1986.

WASU, Paramjit Singh The Surgery, 275A Kings Road, South Harrow, Harrow HA2 9LG Tel: 020 8866 0920 Fax: 020 8426 1104 — MB BS Banaras Hindu 1974; MB BS Banaras Hindu 1974.

WAT, Cynthia Kam Yin Roche Pharmaceuticals, 40 Broadwater Road, Welwyn Garden City AL7 3AY; 54 Cumberland Terrace, London NW1 4HJ — MB BS Lond. 1992; MRCP (UK). Specialty: Pharmaceutical Medicine; Infec. Dis.; Med. Microbiol.

WAT, Dennis Shu-Chang 1st Floor Flat, 77 Cowbridge Road, Canton, Cardiff CF11 9AF — MB BCh Wales 1998.

WATERER, Suzanne Cathryn Brunton Place Surgery, 9 Brunton Place, Edinburgh EH7 5EG Tel: 0131 557 5545 — MB ChB Dundee 1982; MRCGP 1986; DRCOG 1986; DFFP 1994.

WATERFALL, Joan Margaret (retired) 15 Remus Gate, Brackley NN13 7HY Tel: 01280 702812 — (Manch.) MB ChB Manch. 1946; DA Eng. 1953. Cons. Anaesth. P. Chas. Hosp. Merthyr & Cynon Valley Gp. Prev: Staff Asst. (Anaesth.) Mayo Clinic, USA.

WATERFALL, Mr Nicholas Brian 97 Bromham Road, Bedford MK40 4BS — MB BS Lond. 1969 (St. Bart.) FRCS Eng. 1975. Cons. Surg. Bedford Gen. Hosp. Specialty: Urol. Socs: Fell. Roy. Soc. Med.; Brit. Assn. Urol. Surg. Prev: Sen. Regist. (Surg.) Char. Cross Hosp. Lond.; Regist. (Surg.) Bedford Gen. Hosp.; Ho. Off. St. Bart. Hosp. Lond.

WATERFIELD, Mr Andrew Hamilton Princes Wing, Queen Elizabeth II Hospital, Welwyn Garden City AL7 4HQ Tel: 01707 365265 Fax: 01707 365244; Dairy Cottage, Lamer Lane, Wheathampstead, St Albans AL4 8RG Tel: 01582 831261 Fax: 01582 831262 Email: andrewhwaterfield@btopenworld.com — (St. Mary's); MB BS Lond. 1978; FRCS Ed. 1983; FRCS Eng. 1984. Cons. Surg. Orthop. & Trauma Qu. Eliz. II Hosp. Welwyn Gdn. City. Specialty: Orthop. Socs: Fell. BOA; BMA. Prev: Sen. Regist. & Regist. (Orthop.) Lond. Hosp. Whitechapel; Sen. Regist. (Orthop.) Roy. Nat. Orthop. Hosp. Stanmore; Chief Resid. (Orthop.) Mass. Gen. Hosp. & Clin. Fell. Harvard Med. Sch. Boston, USA.

WATERFIELD, Peter Hepburn (retired) Tregarne House, Mawnan Smith, Falmouth TR11 5JP — MB BS Lond. 1960 (Roy. Free) MRCS Eng. LRCP Lond. 1958; DObst RCOG 1960. Prev: Ho. Phys. St. Helen's Hosp. Hastings.

WATERHOUSE, Clive Yare Valley Medical Practice, 202 Thorpe Road, Norwich NR1 1TJ Tel: 01603 437559 Fax: 01603 701773 — MB ChB Leeds 1983; MRCGP 1989.

WATERHOUSE, David Graham Cornishway Medical Centre, 37 Cornishway, Woodhouse Park, Manchester M22 0LY Tel: 0161 437 1467 Fax: 0161 493 9043; 9 Turnberry Drive, Wilmslow SK9 2QW — MB BChir Camb. 1979; MA, MB Camb. 1979, BChir 1978; DRCOG 1982.

WATERHOUSE, Elizabeth Aileen (retired) Clare Farm, Dullingham, Newmarket CB8 9UJ Tel: 01638 507267 Fax: 01638 507267 — MB BS Durh. 1952. Prev: Sessional Med. Off. Region. Blood Transfus. Serv. Camb.

WATERHOUSE, Esther Tremaine 54 Grand Avenue, London N10 3BP — BM BS Nottm. 1991. Sen. Regist., Palliat. Med., Leicester.

WATERHOUSE, John Crichton Royal Hospital, Dumfries DG1 4TG Tel: 01387 244000 Fax: 01387 257735 — MB ChB Dundee 1976; MRCPsych 1983; MMedSci Leeds 1983; MD Dundee 1986. Cons. Psychiat. Crichton Roy. Hosp. Dumfries. Specialty: Alcohol & Substance Misuse.

WATERHOUSE, Mr Norman 55 Harley Street, London W1N 1DD Tel: 0207 636 4073 Fax: 0207 636 6417 Email: wtrhouse@globalnet.co.uk — MB ChB Birm. 1978 (Birmingham) FRCS Ed. 1982; FRCS Eng. 1982; FRCS (Plast Surg.) 1987. Cons. Plastic & Reconstruc. Surg. Chelsea & Westminster Hosp.; Pres. Brit. Assn. of Aesthetic Plastic Surgeons; Director and Trustees Med. Charity Facing The World. Specialty: Plastic Surg. Socs: Internat. Soc. of Craniofacial Surg.; Internat. Soc. of Aesthetic Surg.; Brit. Assn. of Aesthetic Plastic Surgeons.

WATERHOUSE, Paul White's Farm, Sampford, Arundel, Wellington TA21 9QN — MB BS Lond. 1990.

WATERHOUSE, Thomas Dennis (retired) Whites Farm, Sampford Arundel, Wellington TA21 9QN Tel: 01823 672435 Fax: 01823 673142 — MB ChB Bristol 1961; DA Eng. 1967; DObst RCOG 1967; FFA RCS Eng. 1970. Cons. Anaesth. S. Som. Clin. Area. Prev: Lect. Nuffield Dept. Anaesth. Radcliffe Infirm. Oxf.

WATERLOW, Professor John Conrad, CMG (retired) 15 Hillgate Street, London W8 7SP Tel: 020 7727 7456; Parsonage House, Oare, Marlborough SN8 4JA Tel: 01672 563464 — MB BChir Camb. 1942; ScD Camb. 1966, MD 1948; FRCP Lond. 1969; Hon. DSc W. Indies 1978; FRS 1982; Hon. DSc Reading 1983. Prev: Dir. MRC Trop. Metab. Research Unit Univ. W. Indies.

WATERLOW, John Kenneth (retired) 1 Springfield Road, Hinckley LE10 1AN Tel: 01455 446483 — MB BS Lond. 1945 (St. Bart.) Prev: GP Hinckley.

WATERMAN, David 24 Cowdray Court, Kingston Park, Newcastle upon Tyne NE3 2UA — MB BS Newc. 1995.

WATERMAN, Mark Rupert 7 Sandown Park, Belfast BT5 6HD — MB BCh BAO Belf. 1980.

WATERS, Mr Alan Addenbrooke's Hospital, Hills Road, Cambridge CB2 2QQ Tel: 01223 216676; Minglepen, Mingle Lane, Great Shelford, Cambridge CB2 5BG Tel: 01223 844160 Fax: 012230 842241 — MB ChB Ed. 1971; BSc (Med. Sci. Biochem.) (Hons.) Ed. 1968; FRCS Ed. 1975; FRCS Eng. 1976; MChir Camb. 1985, MA 1983. Cons. Neurosurg. Addenbrooke's Hosp. Camb. Specialty: Neurosurg. Socs: Soc. Brit. Neurol. Surgs. Prev: Lect. (Neurosurg.) Univ. Camb.; Sen. Regist. (Neurosurg.) Addenbrooke's Hosp. Camb.; Regist. (Surg. & Neurosurg.) Edin. Roy. Infirm.

WATERS, Alice May 21 Ingham Drive, Coldean, Brighton BN1 9GL Tel: 01273 66893 — MB BS Madras 1939; DGO 1940; DObst RCOG 1948. Prev: Asst. Surg. Govt. Gen. Hosp. Madras;

Graded Surg. & Gyn. IAMC; Specialist Trainee O & G W. Middlx. Hosp. Isleworth.

WATERS, Andrew Derek The Health Centre, Gibson Lane, Kippax, Leeds LS25 7JN Tel: 0113 287 0870 Fax: 0113 232 0746 — BM BS Nottm. 1983.

WATERS, Anthony Kevin 10 Chapel Close, Helmsley, York YO62 5BE Tel: 01439 771474 Email: akwaters@btinternet.com — (Camb. & St. Mary's) MA, MB Camb. 1969, BChir 1968; FRCP Lond. 1986, M 1972. Cons. Phys. Wharfedale Gen. Hosp. Otley; Clin. Lect. Univ. Leeds. Specialty: Gen. Med.; Diabetes; Endocrinol. Prev: Sen. Regist. Leeds AHA; Governors' Research Fell. & Med. Regist. Char. Cross Hosp. Lond.

WATERS, Brian Westbrook, Castle St., Rhuddlan, Rhyl LL18 5AB — MB ChB Liverp. 1973; DObst RCOG 1975; MRCP (UK) 1978; DA Eng. 1982; FFA RCS Eng. 1984. Specialty: Anaesth.

WATERS, Colin George (retired) Spinneys, Saunton, Braunton EX33 1LG Tel: 01271 812032 — MB BChir Camb. 1957 (St. Geo.) BA (1st cl. Hons.) Camb. 1953; DObst RCOG 1958; DA Eng. 1959; MRCGP 1969. Prev: Gen. Practitioner, Caen Health Centre,Braunton, N Devon.

WATERS, Deborah Jane — (Char. Cross Hosp. Med. Sch.) BSc Lond. 1983; MB BS Lond. 1985; DCH RCP Lond. 1987; DRCOG 1989; Cert. Family Plann. JCC 1989; MRCGP 1990. Gen. Practitioner. Specialty: Community Child Health; Gen. Pract. Prev: GP Barry; Trainee GP Ealing Hosp. Southall VTS; Staff Grade (Community Paediat.) Glan Hafren NHS Trust.

WATERS, Mr Eric Albert Heath Cottage, Clarendon Road, Alderbury, Salisbury SP5 3AT Tel: 01722 710069 Email: ericaw@doctors.org.uk; Salisbury Health Care NHS Trust, Salisbury District Hospital, Salisbury SP2 8BJ Tel: 01722 336262 Fax: 01722 331529 — BSc Leeds 1965, MB ChB 1968; FRCS Eng. 1974; FRCS Ed. 1984; FFAEM 1996. Cons. in A & E Salisbury Dist. Hosp.; Med. Dir. Salisbury Health Care. Specialty: Accid. & Emerg.

WATERS, Fiona Helen Drings Close Surgery, 1 Drings Close, Over, Cambridge CB4 5NZ Tel: 01954 231550 Fax: 01954 231573; Minglepen, 20 Mingle Lane, Great Shelford, Cambridge CB2 5BG Tel: 01223 844160 — MB ChB Ed. 1974; DObst RCOG 1976. Prev: GP Swavesey.

WATERS, Fiona Mary 147 Ruxley Lane, Epsom KT19 9EX — MB ChB Manch. 1992.

WATERS, Fiona Sarah Highlands, Old Lane, Stanningfield, Bury St Edmunds IP29 4SA — MB BS Lond. 1997.

WATERS, Harry 28 Castlenau, London SW13 9RU Tel: 020 8748 5512 — MB BCh BAO Dub. 1925; BA; LM Rotunda 1925. Lect. & Examr. Brit. Red Cross Soc.; Examr. in 1st Aid ILEA; Hon. Med. Off. Amateur Boxing Assn. Eng. Socs: Hunt. Soc. & W. Lond. M-C Soc. Prev: Med. Off. i/c West. Hosp. Mobile Unit; Surg. Clin. Asst. W. Lond. Hosp. Hammersmith; Capt. RAMC.

WATERS, Harry Jason (retired) Asian Leadership InStreet, Phuket 8300, Thailand; 12 Convent Gardens, Findon, Worthing BN14 0RZ — MB BS Lond. 1995 (St. Mary's) BSc Lond. 1992. Prev: Med. Dir. Asian Ldr.ship Inst. Thailand.

WATERS, Harry Richard Carna, 12 Covent Gardens, Findon, Worthing BN14 0RZ — MB BS Lond. 1964 (St. Mary's) MRCS Eng. LRCP Lond. 1964; DA Eng. 1966; DObst RCOG 1967; FFA RCS Eng. 1968. Cons. Anaesth. Worthing, Southlands & Dist. Gp. Hosps. Specialty: Anaesth. Socs: Assn. Anaesths. Prev: Sen. Regist. St. Thos. Hosp. Lond.

WATERS, Henry John Village Medical Centre, 400-404 Linthorpe Road, Middlesbrough TS5 6HF Tel: 01642 851234 Fax: 01642 820821; 45 Byemoor Avenue, Great Ayton, Middlesbrough TS9 6JP Tel: 01642 724291 — MB BS Newc. 1973; DCH RCPS Glas. 1976; MRCGP 1977. Clin. Asst. (Rheum.) S. Cleveland Hosp. Middlesbrough & N.; Tees Gen. Hosp. Stockton-on-Tees. Specialty: Rehabil. Med.; Rheumatol.

WATERS, Hilary Mary Eastdene, The Folly, Ditcheat, Shepton Mallet BA4 6QS — MB BS Lond. 1978.

WATERS, Ieuan Rhys 9 Heol Yr Onnen, Pencoed, Bridgend CF35 5PF — MB ChB Leeds 1989.

WATERS, Ifan Richard (retired) 15 Abbey House, Cirencester GL7 2QU — MRCS Eng. LRCP Lond. 1943 (Guy's) Prev: SCMO Wilts. HA. RAF Med. Br.

WATERS, Jennifer Kate 39 Stow Road, Stow-cum-Quy, Cambridge CB5 9AD — MB BS Lond. 1998.

WATERS, John (retired) 18 Bryony Road, Weoley Hill, Birmingham B29 4BU — MB ChB Birm. 1954; MRCS Eng. LRCP Lond. 1954; DPH Eng. 1958; DObst RCOG 1962; MRCGP 1969. Prev: GP Birm.

WATERS, John Mortimer J M Waters and Partners, 21 Beaufort Road, Southbourne, Bournemouth BH6 5AJ Tel: 01202 433081 Fax: 01202 430527; 58 Sopers Lane, Christchurch BH23 1JF — MB BS Lond. 1976 (St. Geo.) MRCS Eng. LRCP Lond. 1976; MRCGP 1984. GP Princip.; Hosp. Pract. Cardiac Dept. Roy. Bournemouth Hosp. Prev: Trainee GP Bournemouth VTS; Ho. Surg. St. Geo. Hosp. Tooting; Ho. Phys. Mayday Hosp. Croydon.

WATERS, Mr John Stephen (retired) The Coach House, Ufford Place, Lower Ufford, Woodbridge IP13 6DP — (Char. Cross) MB BS Lond. 1957; FRCS Eng. 1962; MS Lond. 1972. Prev: Cons. Surg. Singleton & Morriston Hosps. Swansea.

WATERS, Mr Kenneth John 84 Harley Street, London W1G 2HW Tel: 020 7079 4214 Fax: 020 7079 4215 — MB BS Newc. 1969; DObst RCOG 1971; FRCS Eng. 1975. Indep. Cons. Gen. & Vasc. Surg. Lond. Specialty: Gen. Surg. Socs: Vasc. Surg. Soc.; Brit. Assn. Day Surg.

WATERS, Margaret Joan 4 Ferndown, Claremont Road, Surbiton KT6 4RY Tel: 020 8390 2310 — MB BS Lond. 1940; MRCS Eng. LRCP Lond. 1937; DPH Ed. 1940.

WATERS, Margaret Ronaldson (retired) c/o Royal Bank of Scotland, Piccadilly Branch, Haymarket, London SW1Y 4SE — MB ChB Ed. 1924; DMRE Camb. 1925. Prev: Radiol. Gen. Hosp. Stroud.

WATERS, Maria Bernadette 6 Crescent Drive, Petts Wood, Orpington BR5 1BD — MB BS Lond. 1993.

WATERS, Marion Rosemary A&E Department, Countess of Chester Hospital, Liverpool Road, Chester CH2 1UL — MB ChB Manch. 1975; FRCS Eng. 1980.

WATERS, Mark Richard Cantilupe Surgery, 49-51 St. Owen Street, Hereford HR1 2JB Tel: 01432 268031 Fax: 01432 352584; 9 Clive Street, Hereford HR1 2SB Tel: 01432 267116 — BM Soton. 1987 (Southampton) DRCOG 1990; MRCGP 1991. GP Tutor Herefordshire; GP Trainer. Prev: Trainee GP/SHO Hereford Co. Hosp. VTS; Ho. Phys. Addenbrookes Hosp. Camb.; Ho. Surg. United Norwich Hosp.

WATERS, Michael Alan Turton (retired) 6 Golding Avenue, Marlborough SN8 1TH — MB BS Lond. 1951 (Char. Cross) MRCS Eng. LRCP Lond. 1951; DPM Eng. 1954; FRCP Ed. 1971, M 1957; FRCPsych 1972, M 1971. Prev: Cons. Psychiat. Swindon Health Dist.

WATERS, Ruth Anne Plastic Surgery & Burns Unit, Sellyoak Hospital, Raddlebarn Road, Birmingham B29 6JD Tel: 0121 627 8905 Fax: 0121 627 8782; 3 Church View Farm, Osgathorpe, Loughborough LE12 9SY — BM Soton. 1983; FRCS Eng. 1988; FRCS (Plast) 1996. Cons. Plastic Surg. Univ. Hosp. NHS Trust Birm. Specialty: Plastic Surg. Socs: Brit. Microsurgic. Soc. Prev: Hand Surg. Fell. Pulvertaft Hand Centre Derbysh. Roy. Infirm.; Sen. Regist. (Plastic Surg.) W. Midl.; Regist. (Plastic Surg.) W. Norwich Hosp.

WATERS, Ryan John 3 Florence Road, Fleet GU52 6LF — MB BS Lond. 1998.

WATERS, Simon Howard Wellands House, Town Gate, Cleckheaton W Yorkshire Email: simonwaters@doctors.org.uk — BM Soton. 1998.

WATERS, Stephen David 42 Longfields, Ongar CM5 9BZ — MB BS Lond. 1992 (London Hospital Medical College) Bsc (hons) Sociology applied to medicine 1989; MRCP (UK) 1998. Specialist Regist. in Gen. (internal) Med. & Geriat.s, W. Midl.s Rotat. Specialty: Gen. Med.; Care of the Elderly. Socs: W Midl.s Inst. Ageing & Health; Brit. Geriat. Soc.; BMA. Prev: SHO (Med. Rotat.) Colchester Gen. Hosp.; SHO (A+E) Southend Hosp.; HO (Surg.) Roy. Lond. Hosp.

WATERS, Stephen James Medical and Industrial Services Ltd, 23 St Leonard's Road, Eastbourne BN21 3UT Tel: 01323 724889 Fax: 01323 721161; 29 Chichester Drive E., Saltdean, Brighton BN2 8LD Tel: 01273 883689 — MB ChB Liverp. 1982; DRCOG 1985; DCCH RCGP 1986; T(GP) 1991; Dip. Occ. Med. Roy. Coll. Phys. 1998. Occupat. Phys. MIS Ltd Eastbourne; Comp.Med.Advis. Specialty: Occupat. Health. Socs: Soc. Occupat. Med.; Christ. Med. Fellowsh.; Fell. Roy. Soc. Med. Prev: GP Peacehaven; SHO (Community Child Health) Edin.; SHO (O & G, Psychiat., A & E) Liverp.

WATERS, Stuart Scott St James Surgery, Harold Street, Dover CT16 1SF Tel: 01304 225559 Fax: 01304 213070 — MB ChB

Manch. 1977. Prev: SHO (Gen. Med.) Manch. Roy. Infirm.; SHO (Chest Med.) Blackpool Vict. Infirm.

WATERS, Thomas Cyril Swallowfield, Wheelers Lane, Linton, Maidstone ME17 4BN — MB ChB Bristol 1957; DPM Eng. 1963; MRCPsych 1971. Cons. Psychiat. Maidstone Child Guid. Serv., Maidstone Hosp. Socs: BMA. Prev: Sen. Regist. Child Psychiat. Bristol Childr. Hosp. & Child & Family; Guid. Serv. Bristol & Tutor in Ment. Health Univ. Bristol; Regist. (Psychiat.) Littlemore Hosp. Oxf. & St. Crispin Hosp. Duston.

WATERS, Professor William Estlin Orchards, Broxmore Park, Sherfield English, Romsey SO51 6FT Tel: 01794 884254 — (St. Bart.) MB BS Lond. 1958; DIH St. And. 1965; FFCM 1976, M 1974; FFPHM RCP (UK) 1989. Emerit. Prof. Community Med. Univ. Soton. Specialty: Pub. Health Med. Prev: Sen. Lect., Reader & Prof. (Clin. Epidemiol. & Community Med.) Soton. Univ.; on Staff MRC Epidemiol. Unit (S. Wales) Cardiff; Sec. Internat. Epidemiol. Assn.

WATERSON, Imogen Margaret West Norfolk P.C.T., St. James, Extons Road, King's Lynn PE30 5NU Tel: 01553 816368 Fax: 01553 761104 Email: imogen.waterson@westnorfolk.pct-nhs.uk; The Old Rectory, Saxthorpe, Norwich NR11 7BJ Tel: 01263 587610 — MB BChir Camb. 1973 (Cambridge and St. Bartholomew's Hospital) MA Camb. 1974; DObst RCOG 1976; MRCP (UK) 1978; T(M)(Paediat.) 1992; FRCPCH 1997; FRCP 1997. Cons. Comm. Paediat. W. Norf. PCT, Kings Lynn; Trainer Assn. for Research in Infant & Child Developm. Specialty: Community Child Health. Socs: Brit. Assn. of Community Child Health (BACCH). Prev: SCMO (Comm. Paediat.) Norwich HA; Regist. (Paediat. & Gen. Med.) Shrewsbury.

WATERSON, Peter Graham Springfield Medical Practice, 9 Springfield Road, Bishopbriggs, Glasgow G64 1PJ Tel: 0141 772 4744 Fax: 0141 772 3035; 67 Stirling Drive, Bishopbriggs, Glasgow G64 3PG Tel: 0141 772 4642 — BM BCh Oxf. 1962; DObst 1966.

WATERSTON, Anthony John Ross Community Paediatric Department, Newcastle General Hospital, Newcastle upon Tyne NE4 6BE Tel: 0191 273 8811 Ext: 23362 Fax: 0191 219 5072 Email: a.j.r.waterston@ncl.ac.uk; 20 Burdon Terrace, Jesmond, Newcastle upon Tyne NE2 3AE Tel: 0191 281 6752 Email: a.j.r.waterston@acl.ac.uk — (St. And. & Dundee) MB ChB St. And. 1968; DObst RCOG 1971; DCH RCP Lond. 1971; MRCP (UK) 1976; MD Dundee 1990; FRCP Lond. 1993; MRCPCH 1996; FRCPCH 1997. Cons. Community Paediat. Newc. Gen. Hosp.; Hon. Sen. Lect., Univ. of Newc. Specialty: Community Child Health. Socs: (Pres.) N. Eng. Paediat. Soc.; FRCPCh. Prev: Convenor Brit. Assn. Community Child Health; Clin. Research Fell. & Hon. Cons. Paediat. Univ. Dundee; Cons. & Lect. (Child Health) Univ. Zimbabwe, Harare.

WATERSTON, Elizabeth Cartington Terrace Medical Group, 1 Cartington Terrace, Heaton, Newcastle upon Tyne NE6 5RS Tel: 0191 265 5755 Fax: 0192 276 2921; 20 Burdon Terrace, Jesmond, Newcastle upon Tyne NE2 3AE Tel: 0191 281 6752 — MB ChB St. And. 1968; Dip FPA. 1971; MRCGP 1986. Socs: Med. Wom. Federat.; BMA. Prev: Trainee GP Dundee VTS; Med. Off. (Geriat.) Parirenyetwa Hosp. Harare Zimbabwe; Regist. (Geriat.) Roy. Vict. Hosp. Dundee.

WATERSTON, Paul Fyfe Lochwinnoch Surgery, 31 Main Street, Lochwinnoch PA12 4AH Tel: 01505 842200 Fax: 01505 843144; 31 Main Street, Lochwinnoch PA12 4AH Tel: 01505 842200 — MB ChB Glas. 1975. GP Lochwinnoch, Renfrewsh.

WATERSTONE, John Justin Department of Obstetrics & Gynaecology, Kings College Hospital, Denmark Hill, London SE5 8RX; 90 Highlands Heath, Portsmouth Road, Putney, London SW15 3TY Tel: 020 8785 7887 — MB BCh BAO Dub. 1982; BSc Dub. 1976; DCH RCPSI Dub. 1984; MRCOG 1988. Research Regist. (O & G) Kings Coll. Med. Sch., Kings Coll. Hosp. Lond. Specialty: Obst. & Gyn.

WATERSTONE, Mark Peter Malcolm Department of Public Health, UMDS, Capital House, 42 Linton St., London SE1 3QD Tel: 020 8299 3480; 79c Overhill Road, London SE1 3QD Tel: 020 7955 4945 — MB BS Lond. 1990; MRCOG 1996. Specialist Regist. S. E. Thames & Research Fell. UMDS Guy's & St Thomas Hosp. Lond. Specialty: Obst. & Gyn. Socs: Fell. RSM.

WATERWORTH, Alison Margaret The Grange Medical Centre, Dacre Banks, Harrogate HG3 4DX Tel: 01423 780436 Fax: 01423 781416 Email: alison.waterworth@gp-b82004.nhs.uk — MB BS Newc. 1973 (Newcastle) DObst RCOG 1976.

WATERWORTH, Alison Sarah St. James's Hospital, Leeds; 46 George Street, Saltaire, Shipley BD18 4PT — BM BCh Oxf. 1997; MA Oxf. 1999. Trainee (Gen. Surg.(. Specialty: Gen. Surg. Prev: Anat. Demonst., Leeds Univ.; SHO (A&E), Bradford Roy. Infirm.

WATERWORTH, Susan Mary 28 Stanhope Road, Darlington DL3 7SQ — MB BS Newc. 1973; MFFP; DMJ. GP Principle.

WATERWORTH, Mr Thomas Alan, OStJ, RD, QHS (retired) Polmayne, Rock Road, Rock, Wadebridge PL27 6NW Tel: 01208 863295 — MB BS Lond. 1965 (St. Geo.) MRCS Eng. LRCP Lond. 1965; FRCS Eng. 1970. Cons. Surg. Hosp. Walsgrave Hosp. Coventry. Prev: Sen. Regist. United Birm. Hosps.

WATFORD, Norman Charles Trevor (retired) Martlets, East Wittering, Chichester PO20 8DU Tel: 01243 670110 — (Guy's) MB BS Lond. 1945; MRCP Lond. 1950. Prev: Ho. Surg. & Ho. Phys. Pembury Hosp.

WATHEN, Christopher George Department of Medicine, Wycombe Hospital, High Wycombe HP11 2TT — MB ChB (Hons.) Ed. 1979; LM Dub. 1980; DRCOG 1981; MRCP (UK) 1982; BSc (1st cl. Hons.) Ed. 1976, MD 1988; FRCP Ed. 1995; FRCP Lond. 1996. Cons. Phys. With an interest in Thoracic Med., Bucks. Hosps. NHS Trust; Cons. Phys. Stoke Mandeville Bucks. Specialty: Gen. Med. Socs: Amer. Thoracic Soc.; Brit. Thoracic Soc.; Amer. Heart Assn. Prev: Sen. Regist. (Gen. Respirat. Med.) City Hosp., Roy. Infirm. Edin. & North. Gen. Hosp.; Lect. (Med.) Univ. Edin.

WATHEN, David John The Surgeries, Lombard Street, Newark NG24 1XG Tel: 01636 702363 Fax: 01636 613037; 4 Speight Close, Winthorpe, Newark NG24 2PF — MB ChB Birm. 1984; DRCOG 1988; MRCGP 1989; DCH RCP Lond. 1991. Socs: BMA.

WATHEN, Susan Jane Crossroads Surgery, Church Road, Milford, Godalming GU8 5JD — MB BS Lond. 1987; DRCOG 1991; MRCGP 1992. GP Retainer. Specialty: Gen. Pract. Socs: BMA. Prev: Asst. GP The Surg. Burlington La., Lond.

WATKEYS, Jane Elizabeth Mary Central Clinic, Orchard Street, Swansea SA1 5AT Tel: 01792 517950 Fax: 01792 517042 Email: jane.watkeys@swansea-tr.wales.nhs.uk; 48 Rhyd y Defaid Drive, Swansea SA2 8AL Tel: 01792 208203 Email: janewatkeys@swansea-tr.wales.nhs.uk — MB BCh Wales 1968; DCH RCP Lond. 1970; MSc Lond. (Community Med.) 1981; FFPHM RCP (UK) 1994; FRCPCH 1997. Cons. Paediat. Swansea NHS Trust; Hon. Cons. Camden Primary Care Trust Lond. Specialty: Paediat. Special Interest: Child Protec. Socs: Roy. Soc. of Med. Prev: Cons. Community Paediat. Camden & Islington NHS Trust.; Hon. Cons. Univ. Coll. Hosps. Lond.; SCM (Child Health) & Cons. Community Paediat. S.Glam. HA.

WATKIN, Andrew Ross Amman Valley Medical Practice, Meddyga'r Waun Surgery, Graig Road, Ammanford SA18 1EG Tel: 01269 822231 — MB ChB Birm. 1984.

WATKIN, Bernard Curtis 62 Wimpole Street, London W1M 7DE Tel: 020 7486 8684 Fax: 020 7935 8269 — MB BS Lond. 1962 (St. Bart.) DPhysMed Eng. 1966. Scientif. Adviser (Orthop.) ICI Ltd.; Cons. IMG (Internat. Managem. Gp.). Specialty: Orthop. Socs: Brit. Assn. Manip. Med. & Soc. Orthop. Med. Prev: Hon. Clin. Asst. (Rheum.) St. Stephen's Hosp. Lond.; Regist. Arthur Stanley Inst. Rheum. Middlx. Hosp. Lond.; Regist. (Physical Med.) St. Thos. Hosp. Lond.

WATKIN, Mr David Francis Lloyd (retired) The Gables, 8 Knighton Rise, Oadby, Leicester LE2 2RE Tel: 0116 270 5855 — (Camb. & Westm.) MB BChir Camb. 1959; FRCS Eng. 1962; MA Camb. 1960, MChir Camb. 1965. Prev: Clin. Sub-Dean Univ. Leicester Sch. Med. Past Pres. Assn. Surgeons GB & Ireland.

WATKIN, Elisabeth Marian Radiology Department, Leicester General Hospital, Gwendolen Road, Leicester LE5 4PW Tel: 0116 249 0490 Fax: 0116 258 4525; The Gables, 8 Knighton Rise, Oadby, Leicester LE2 2RE Tel: 0116 270 5855 — (Westm.) MB BS Lond. 1960; MRCS Eng. LRCP Lond. 1960; DMRD Eng. 1970; FFR 1973; FRCR 1975. Cons. Radiol. Leicester Gen. Hosp. Specialty: Radiol. Socs: Brit. Inst. Radiol.; Brit. Soc. Interven. Radiol.; Brit. Nuclear Med. Soc. Prev: Sen. Regist. (Diag. Radiol.) Leics. AHA (T); Regist. (Diag. Radiol.) North. Gen. Hosp. Sheff.; Ho. Phys. & Ho. Surg. St. Stephen's Hosp. Lond.

WATKIN, Elizabeth Jane 29 Thornbeck Avenue, Hightown, Liverpool L38 9EX — MB ChB Liverp. 1987.

WATKIN, Frances Marguerite 49 Stroma Road, Allerton, Liverpool L18 9SN — MB ChB Liverp. 1996.

WATKIN, Mr Gwyn Thomas Ysbyty Gwynedd, Bangor LL57 2PW Tel: 01248 352994; Pant y Ddolen, Halfway Bridge, Bangor LL57 4AD Tel: 01248 352994 — MB BS Lond. 1974 (Middlx.) MS Lond. 1987, MB BS 1974; FRCS Eng. 1978. Cons. Gen. & Vasc. Surg. Gwynedd HA. Specialty: Gen. Surg. Socs: Fell. Roy. Soc. Med.; Vasc. Surg. Soc. Prev: Sen. Regist. (Surg.) Bloomsbury Vasc. Unit Middlx. Hosp. Lond.

WATKIN, Hywel Beech House Surgery, Beech House, 69 Vale Street, Denbigh LL16 3AU Tel: 01745 812863 Fax: 01745 816574 — MB BS Lond. 1978 (Guy's) BSc (Hons.) Phys. Med. Lond. 1975, MB BS 1978; DRCOG 1980; DCH Eng. 1981; MRCGP 1982; MLCOM 1997; M.Sc. (Musculoskelet. & Osteop. Med.) Lond. 1997; Dip M-S Med. SA 1997. Socs: Accred. Mem. Brit. Med. Acupunc. Soc.; Brit. Inst. Musculoskel. Med.

WATKIN, Janet Byron House Surgery, 30 Byron Road, Gillingham ME7 5QH Tel: 01634 576347 Fax: 01634 570159 — MB ChB Sheff. 1980.

WATKIN, John Ernest 68 Harley Street, London W1N 1AE Tel: 020 7935 3980 Fax: 020 7636 6262; Great Yard, Whitedown, Wootton St. Lawrence, Basingstoke RG23 8PF Tel: 01256 850678 — (Cardiff) BSc, MB BCh Wales 1952. Prev: Phys. E. India Clinic Calcutta, India; Maj. RAMC RARO.

WATKIN, John Ivan The Surgery, Highfield Road, North Thoresby, Grimsby DN36 5RT Tel: 01472 840202; The Maltings, Station Road, North Thoresby, Grimsby DN36 5QS Tel: 01472 840202 — MB ChB Sheff. 1959. Prev: Clin. Asst. (Anaesth.) Grimsby Gp. Hosps.; Regist. Anaesth. United Sheff. Hosps.; Ho. Surg. Sheff. Roy. Infirm.

WATKIN, Lucy Ann Chase Farm Hospital, 127 The Ridgeway, Enfield EN2 8JL — MB BS Lond. 1998.

WATKIN, Nicholas Andrew 15 St Mary's Road, Oxford OX4 1PX — BM BCh Oxf. 1989.

WATKIN, Peter Morton Homestead Cottage, 1 Occupation Lane, Shooters Hill, London SE18 3JH — MB BS Lond. 1972; MRCS Eng. LRCP Lond. 1972; DCH Eng. 1977; MSc Manch. 1988. Sen. Med. Off. (Audiol.) Redbridge & Waltham Forest HA; Head of Audiol. Serv. Redbridge & Waltham Forest HA. Specialty: Audiol. Med. Socs: Fac. Comm. Health. Prev: Sen. Med. Off. (Clin.) Redbridge HA.

WATKIN, Richard — MB ChB Birm. 1998.

WATKIN, Ross Rickard (retired) Orchard Cottage, Rectory Road, Mugswell, Coulsdon CR5 3SY Tel: 01737 557564 Email: rosswatkin@yahoo.co.uk — (Guy's) MB BS Lond. 1957; MRCS Eng. LRCP Lond. 1957; DObst RCOG 1960; DA Eng. 1961; FFA RCS Eng. 1964. Emerit. Cons. Anaesth. Guy's Hosp. Lond. Prev: Chairm. SE Thames RHA Anaesth. Specialty Sub-Comm.

WATKIN, Sara Louise Nottingham City Hospital, Neonatal Intensive Care Unit, Hucknall Road, Nottingham NG5 1PB Tel: 0115 969 1169 Fax: 0115 962 7926 Email: swatkin@ncht.trent.nhs.uk; Hillside House, Church View, Osgathorpe, Longbrough LE12 9XE — MB ChB Manch. 1986; MRCP (UK) 1989; MD Keele 1996; FRCPCH UK 1997. Cons. Neonatologist Nottm. City Hosp. Specialty: Neonat. Socs: BMA; Brit. Assn. Perinatal Med.; FRCPCh. Prev: Lect. & Hon. Sen. Regist. (Child Health) Qu. Med. Centre Nottm.; Research Regist. (Paediat.) Acad. Dept. Paediat. Univ. Keele; Regist. (Paediat.) Nottm. City Hosp.

WATKIN, Simon Wilfred Department of Respiratory Medicine, Norfolk & Norwich Hospital, Norwich NR4 7UY Tel: 01603 289644 Fax: 01603 289640 Email: simon.watkin@nnuh.nhs.uk; 26 Badgers Brook Road, Drayton, Norwich NR8 6EY Tel: 01603 262047 — MB ChB Liverp. 1983; BSc (Hons.) (Physiol.) Liverp. 1980, MD 1994; FRCP 1999. Cons. Respirat., HIV & Gen. Med. Norf. & Norwich Hosp. Trust. Specialty: Respirat. Med.; HIV Med.; Gen. Med. Socs: Brit. Thorac. Soc.; Roy. Soc. Med. Prev: Sen. Regist. (Respirat. & Gen. Med.) Roy. Liverp. Univ. Hosp.; Regist. (Respirat. Med.) Glas. Roy. Infirm.; CRC Clin. Research Fell. (Radiati. Oncol.) Clatterbridge Hosp.

WATKIN JONES, Andrew St James's University Hospital, Leeds LS9 7TF Tel: 0113 243 3144; 9 Woodlea Court, Woodlea Village, Meanwood Park, Leeds LS6 4SL — MB ChB Leeds 1997. Basic Surgic. Train. Rotat., St Jas. Univ. Hosp. Specialty: Gen. Surg.

WATKINS, Alistair James Hadleigh House, 20 Kirkway, Broadstone BH18 8EE Tel: 01202 692268 Fax: 01202 658954 — MB BS Lond. 1989; MRCGP 1995.

WATKINS, Armond Vincent 37 Addison Road, London W14 — MB BS Lond. 1960.

WATKINS, Beverley Joy Whittington Road Surgery, 9 Whittington Road, Norton, Stourbridge DY8 3DB Tel: 01384 393120 Fax: 01384 353636 — MB ChB Birm. 1983; DRCOG 1986; DCH RCP Lond. 1986; MRCGP 1987. Prev: Trainee GP Dudley VTS.

WATKINS, Christopher John The Surgery, 15 West Town Road, Backwell, Bristol BS48 3HA Tel: 0117 462026 Fax: 0117 795609; 2 The Green, West Town, Backwell, Bristol BS48 3BG Tel: 01275 464239 — MRCS Eng. LRCP Lond. 1967 (St. Bart.) PhD Lond. 1980, MB BS 1967; DA Eng. 1969; DObst RCOG 1970; FRCGP 1983, M 1971. Cons. Sen. Lect. Gen. Pract. Bristol Univ. Socs: BMA; AUDGP; Bristol M-C Soc. Prev: Reader Gen. Pract. United Med. & Dent. Sch. Lond.

WATKINS, Daphne Louisa (retired) Ty Newydd, Velindre, Crymych SA41 3XF — MB Camb. 1967 (St. Thos.) MA Camb. 1976, MB 1967, BChir 1966.

WATKINS, David 100 Newmarket Road, Norwich NR2 2LB — MB BS Lond. 1952 (St. Bart.) MRCS Eng. LRCP Lond. 1952. Hosp. Pract. (Chest) Norwich Health Dist.; Clin. Asst. (Continuing Care) Priscila Bacon Lodge Norwich.

WATKINS, David Ainsley (retired) — MRCS Eng. LRCP Lond. 1945 (St. Mary's) Prev: Ho. Phys. Swansea & Morriston Hosps.

WATKINS, David Charles 32 Ormiston Crescent, Knock, Belfast BT4 3TQ; 10 Barkers Lane, Sale M33 6RG — MB ChB Ed. 1991; MRCPCH 1996; MRCP Ed. 1996; Dip SEM (GB &I) 2000. Specialist Regist. (Paed.) Booth Hall Childr.'s Hosp, Man. Specialty: Paediat.; Sports Med.

WATKINS, David John The Portland Practice, St Paul's Medical Centre, 121 Swindon Road, Cheltenham GL50 4DP Tel: 01242 707792; The Surgery, Glebe Farm Court Road, Hatherley, Cheltenham GL51 3EB Tel: 01242 863333 — MB Camb. 1969; BChir 1968; DObst RCOG 1973.

WATKINS, David William 76 Corporation Road, Newport NP19 0AX — MB BCh Wales 1954.

WATKINS, Dorothy Caroline (retired) 2 Ffordd Gwern, Cwrt y Brenin, St Fagans, Cardiff CF5 6PB Tel: 029 2089 1537 — (Roy. Free) MRCS Eng. LRCP Lond. 1961; MFFP 1993. Prev: SCMO Gwent HA.

WATKINS, Eileen Dorothy (retired) Glaslyn, Riverside, Tiddington Road, Stratford-upon-Avon CV37 7BD Tel: 01789 298085 Fax: 01789 298085 Email: revdocmw@waitrose.com — MB ChB Leeds 1959.

WATKINS, Eileen Gertrude (retired) Glyn Heulog, Usk NP15 1HY — MB BCh BAO NUI 1952; MFCM 1955; DPH (Hons.) NUI 1955. Med. Off. DSS. Prev: Dep. Med. Off. Health & Dep. Sch. Med. Off. Rhondda Glam.

WATKINS, Eric Paul Holmes Kent Elms Health Centre, Rayleigh Road, Leigh-on-Sea SS9 5UU; 24 Kings Road, Westcliff on Sea SS0 8LL — MB BS Lond. 1980; MRCS Eng. LRCP Lond. 1979.

WATKINS, Professor Eric Sidney Department of Neurosurgery, The Princes Grace Hospital, 42-52 Nottingham Place, London W1U 5NY Tel: 020 7486 1234 Fax: 020 7232 0525; Belmont House, Lennel Road, Coldstream TD12 4ET Tel: 01890 882411 Fax: 01890 882007 — (Liverp.) BSc (Hons. Physiol.) Liverp. 1949, MD 1956, MB ChB 1952; FRCS Ed. 1969. Prof. Emerit. Neurosurg. Lond. Hosp. Med. Coll. & Hon. Cons. Neurosurg. Lond. Indep. Hosp. Specialty: Neurosurg. Socs: Soc. Brit. Neurosurgs. & Amer. Acad. Neurosurgs. Prev: Prof. Neurosurg. State Univ. New York Syracuse, USA; Clin. Neurosurgic. Research Asst. Middlx. Hosp. Lond.

WATKINS, Gareth David Coquet Medical Group, Amble Health Centre, Percy Drive, Morpeth NE65 0HD Tel: 01665 710481 Fax: 01665 713031; 6 Lingfield Close, Warkworth, Morpeth NE65 0YN — MB BS Newc. 1985 (Newcastle) MRCGP 1989; DRCOG 1989.

WATKINS, Gina Olwen 2 Dollis Road, Finchley, London N3 1RG — MB BS Lond. 1987; BSc Lond. 1984, MB BS 1987. Trainee GP Broomfield Hosp. Chelmsford VTS. Prev: Ho. Phys. Chase Farm Hosp. Enfield; Ho. Surg. Univ. Coll. Hosp. Lond.

WATKINS, Guy David 42 High Street, Melbourn, Royston SG8 6DZ — MB BS Lond. 1987; MRCGP 1991. Specialty: Gen. Pract.

WATKINS, Professor Hugh Christian John Radcliffe Hospital, University of Oxford, Cardiovascular Medicine, Oxford OX3 9DU Tel: 01865 220257 Fax: 01865 768844 Email: hugh.watkins@cardiov.ox.ac.uk — MB BS Lond. 1984 (St. Bartholomew's) FRCP 1997, M 1987; PhD Lond. 1995, BSc 1981,

MD 1995. Field Marshal Alexander Prof. Cardiovasc. Med. Univ. Oxf.; Hon. Cons. Cardiol. & Med. John Radcliffe Hosp. Oxf.; Prof.ial Fell. Exeter Coll. Oxf. Specialty: Cardiol.; Gen. Med. Special Interest: Cardiomyopathy; Inherited Heart Diseases. Socs: Assn. Phys.; Fell. Acad. Med. Sciences. Prev: Asst. Prof. Med. Harvard Med. Sch. Boston & Assoc. Phys. Brigham & Wom. Hosp. Boston, USA.

WATKINS, Jean Margaret Winton Health Centre, 31 Alma Road, Winton, Bournemouth BH9 1BP Tel: 01202 519311; 25 Copse Road, Burley, Ringwood BH24 4EG Tel: 01425 403224 Fax: 01425 402088 Email: jeanwatkins@compuserve.com — MB BS Lond. 1955 (Roy. Free) MRCS Eng. LRCP Lond. 1955; DObst RCOG 1957; DCH Eng. 1958; MRCGP 1976. Community Med. Off. (Family Plann.) Dorset HA. Prev: GP The Alma Partnership, Bournemouth; GP Lakeside Health Centre Thamesmead; Sen. Lect. (Gen. Pract.) Guy's & St. Thos. United Med. & Dent. Sch. Lond.

WATKINS, Joanne Department of Psychiatry, Hellesdon Hospital, Drayton Road, Norwich NR6 5BE — MB ChB Leic. 1995. SHO Rotat. (Psychiat.) Norwich Ment. Health Trust. Specialty: Gen. Psychiat. Prev: SHO Rotat. (Med.) Leicester Hosps.; Ho. Surg. (Gen. Surg. & Gyn.) Leic. Gen. Hosp.; Ho. Phys. (Ge. Med./Rheum.) Leic. Roy. Infirm.

WATKINS, John Ceri-Nant, 3 Cefn Buchan Close, Llangwm, Usk NP15 1HW; 38 Cotswold Way, Newport NP19 9DL Tel: 01633 270934 — MB BCh Wales 1981; BSc Wales 1975, MB BCh 1981; MRCGP 1985. 2nd Prize Nat. Syntex Award 1985.

WATKINS, John Department of Cardiology, St. Mary's General Hospital, Milton Road, Portsmouth PO3 6AD Tel: 02392 866051 Fax: 02392 866046 Email: jwat18@aol.com; 18 Cousins Grove, Southsea PO4 9RP Tel: 02392 739151 Fax: 02392 739151 Email: jwat18@aol.com — MRCS Eng. LRCP Lond. 1973 (St. Bart.) MB BS Lond. 1973, BSc 1970; MRCP (UK) 1976; FRCP Lond. 1990. Cons. Cardiol. Portsmouth Acute NHS Trust; Clin. Dir. For Cardiol. Specialty: Cardiol. Special Interest: Cardiovascular Pharmacology; Pacing. Socs: Brit. Cardiac Soc.; Brit. Pacing & Electrophysiol. Gp. Prev: Sen. Regist. Cardiol. John Radcliffe Hosp. Oxf.; Harkness Fell. (Cardiovasc. Pharmacol.) Univ. Calif., San Diego.

WATKINS, John Benjamin (retired) 2 Ffordd Gwern, Cwrt y Brenin, St Fagans, Cardiff CF5 6PB Tel: 029 2089 1537 — MB BS Lond. 1961 (Char. Cross) MFOM RCP Lond. 1982. Prev: Sen. Med. Off. Brit. Steel Corp. Llanwern Gp. Newport.

WATKINS, John Stirling (retired) — (Newc.) MB BS Newc. 1966; MRCP (UK) 1970; FRCP Lond. 1985. Prev: SHO (Neurol.) Newc. Gen. Hosp.

WATKINS, Kevin Paul Wadebridge Health Centre, Wadebridge PL27 7BS Tel: 01208 2222 — MB BS Lond. 1981.

WATKINS, Mr Laurence Dale Institute of Neurology, Queen Square, London WC1N 3BG Tel: 020 7837 3611 Fax: 020 7837 2458; 13 Wigan Road, Westhead, Ormskirk L40 6HY — MB Camb. 1984; BChir 1983; MA Camb. 1984; FRCS Eng. 1989. Clin. Lect. (Neurol. Surg.) Inst. Neurol. Lond. Prev: Regist. (Surg. Neurol.) Nat. Hosp. for Neurol. & Neurosurg. Lond.; Regist. (Neurosurg.) Hosp. for Sick Childr. Gt. Ormond St. Lond.

WATKINS, Mr Mark John Guy The Royal Hospital, Haslar, Gosport PO12 2AA Tel: 023 9276 2118 Fax: 023 9276 2960; 59 Western Way, Gosport PO12 2NF — MB Camb. 1978; BChir 1977; FRCS Ed. 1983. Cons. Gen. Surg. Roy. Hosp. Haslar. Specialty: Gen. Surg.

WATKINS, Mary Elana Greyston House Surgery, 99 Station Road, Redhill RH1 1EB Tel: 01737 761201 Fax: 01737 780510; 15 The Fairways, Somerset Road, Redhill RH1 6LP Tel: 01737 243882 — MB BS Lond. 1970 (St. Mary's) MRCS Eng. LRCP Lond. 1970; DObst RCOG 1974.

WATKINS, Mary Elizabeth Community Health Office, Ambulance Head Quarters, Ascots Lane, Stanstead Road, Welwyn Garden City AL7 4HL Tel: 01707 365229 Fax: 01707 365329; 81 Valley Road, Welwyn Garden City AL8 7DR Tel: 01707 338159 — MB BS Lond. 1967 (St. Geo.) SCMO Welwyn Gdn. City. Specialty: Community Child Health. Socs: Assoc. Mem. Coll. Paediat. Prev: Med. Off. Mzuzu Health Centre, Malawi; Med. Off. Mbabane Govt. Hosp., Swaziland.

WATKINS, Meredith Wynne (retired) Hafodwenog, Wellfield Place, Glynneath, Neath SA11 5EP — MB ChB Ed. 1960; DObst RCOG 1962. Prev: Ho. Surg., Ho. Phys. & SHO (O & G) Caerphilly Dist. Miner's Hosp.

WATKINS, Merryl Dilys Ada Roundwood Surgery, Wood St., Mansfield NG18 1QQ — MB BS Lond. 1992; BSc 1989; DCh 1994; DRCOG 1995; MRCGP 1998. GP. Prev: Ho. Phys. Harold Wood Hosp. Essex; Ho. Surg. Princess Alexandra Hosp. Harlow.; Trainee GP Mansfield VTS.

WATKINS, Nicholas Andrew North Hey, Mill St., Chagford, Newton Abbot TQ13 8AW — MB BS Lond. 1991.

WATKINS, Nigel Ross c/o 14 Bristol Terrace, Bargoed CF81 8RF; 12 Maelog Close, Pontyclun CF72 9AF — MB BCh Wales 1984.

WATKINS, Olga 24 Tulipan Crescent, Callander FK17 8AR Tel: 01877 330587 — MB ChB Glas. 1976; DRCOG 1978; Dip. Pract. Dermat. Wales 1995. Salaried GP Pk. Avenue Med. Centre Stirling; Clin. Asst. (Dermat.) Stirling Roy. Infirm. Specialty: Dermat.

WATKINS, Oswald Heath, MC (retired) Tymperleys, Crossway Green, Chepstow NP16 5LX Tel: 01291 623181 — MB BChir Camb. 1952 (St. Thos.) MA Camb. 1952, MB BChir 1952; DObst RCOG 1956. Prev: Ho. Surg. St. Thos. Hosp. Lond. & Sorrento Matern. Hosp. Birm.

WATKINS, Peter John King's Diabetes Centre, King's College Hospital, Denmark Hill, London SE5 9RS Tel: 020 73461737 Email: peter.watkins1@virgin.net; 31 Lancaster Avenue, London SE27 9EL Tel: 020 8761 8086 Email: peter.watkins1@virgin.net — MB BChir Camb. 1961 (St. Bart.) MB Camb. 1962, BChir 1961; FRCP Lond. 1975, M 1965; MD Camb. 1968. Hon Cons. (Gen. Med. & Diabetes) King's Coll. Hosp. Lond.; Edr., Clin. Med. Jl., Roy. Coll. of Physicians. Specialty: Diabetes; Gen. Med. Socs: Ass of Phys.s of Gt. Britain & Irel. Prev: Sen. Regist. (Med.) Gen. Hosp. Birm.; Research Fell. United Birm. Hosps.; Chairm. Med. & Scientif. Sect. Brit. Diabetic Assn. & Hon. Treas, Assn. Phys. GB & Irel.

WATKINS, Rhona 9G Hughenden Gardens, Glasgow G12 9XW — MB ChB Glas. 1977; FRCPath 1996, M 1983; MD Glas. 1987; Dip. Forens. Med. Glas 1995. Cons. W. Scotl. Blood Transfus. Serv.; Hon. Clin. Sen. Lect. Glas. Specialty: Haematology.

WATKINS, Rhys Mervyn Heathville Road Surgery, 5 Heathville Road, Gloucester GL1 3DP Tel: 01452 528299 Fax: 01452 522959; Villa Vinaria, 95 London Road, Gloucester GL1 3HH — MB BS Lond. 1979; DRCOG 1983; MRCGP 1984. Clin. Asst. (ENT) Glos. Roy. Hosp.; Police Surg. Glos. Constab. Specialty: Gen. Pract.

WATKINS, Roger Dexter (retired) 3 Kathleen Park, Helensburgh G84 8TH — MB ChB Aberd. 1968; MRCGP 1977. Prev: Ho. Surg. (Orthop.), Ho. Off. (Paediat.) & Ho. Off. (O & G).

WATKINS, Mr Roger Malcolm Derriford Hospital, Derriford Road, Plymouth PL6 8DH Tel: 01752 792108 Fax: 01752 517562 Email: roger.watkins@phnt.swest.nhs.uk; Bay Tree House, The Crescent, Crapstone, Yelverton PL20 7PS Tel: 01822 852504 — MB BChir Camb. 1976 (Camb. & Westm.) MA Camb. 1977; FRCS Eng. 1980. Cons. Surg. Derriford Hosp. Plymouth. Specialty: Gen. Surg. Special Interest: Breast Surg. Socs: Brit. Assn. Surg. Oncol.; Assn. Surg.Gt. Brit. & N. Ire.; BMA. Prev: Sen. Regist. (Surg.) Roy. Marsden Hosp. & Westm. Hosp. Lond.; Clin. Lect. (Surg.) Nuffield Dept. of Surg. John Radcliffe Hosp. Oxf.; Demonst. (Anat.) Univ. Camb.

WATKINS, Ronald Peter Sycamore, 33A Aylesbury Road, Wing, Leighton Buzzard LU7 0PD Tel: 01296 682556 Fax: 01296 682556 — MB ChB Liverp. 1949; DObst RCOG 1969; Cert. JCC Lond. 1980. Specialty: Obst. & Gyn.

WATKINS, Rosemary Anne 264 Rotton Park Road, Edgbaston, Birmingham B16 0LU Tel: 0121 429 2683; 12 Jasmin Croft, Kings Heath, Birmingham B14 5AX — MB ChB Birm. 1972 (Birmingham) DObst RCOG 1974. Asst. GP. p/t, Dr IS Marok, Birm. Specialty: Gen. Pract.

WATKINS, Russell Julian Department of Ophthalmology, West Norwich Hospital, Bowthorpe Road, Norwich NR2 3TU Tel: 01603 286286 Fax: 01603 288261 — MB ChB Leic. 1997; BSc (Hons) Bradford. 1985; MCOptom 1986; PhD Brad. 1991. Clin. Asst. (Ophth.), W. Norwich Hosp. (PT); Sen. Lect. Anglia Polytechnic Univ. Specialty: Ophth. Prev: SHO (Ophth.) W. Norwich Hosp.; Ho. Off. (Med. & Surg.) Leic. Hosps.

WATKINS, Ruth Primrose Felicity ICSM St Mary's Department of Microbiology, Wright Fleming Institute, Norfolk Place, London W2 1PZ Tel: 020 7886 1557 Email: r.watkins@ic.ac.uk; 11 Elborough Street, Southfields, London SW18 5DP Tel: 020 8874 2297 — MB BS Lond. 1973 (St. Bart.) MSc Lond. 1984, BSc (Hons.) 1970, MB BS 1973; MRCP (UK) 1977; MRCPath 1986. Sen. Lect. & Hon. Cons. Virol. Imperial Coll. Sci. Technol. & Med. &

St.Mary's Hosp. Lond. Specialty: Virology. Prev: Cons. & Sen. Research Fell. (Virol.) Hammersmith Hosp. Lond.; Sen. Regist. (Virol.) St. Geo. Hosp. Lond.; Regist. Med. Microbiol. Lond. Hosp.

WATKINS, Ryan Charles Brighton and Sussex University Hospitals NHS Trust, Royal Sussex County Hospital, Eastern Road, Brighton BN2 5BE Tel: 01273 696955 Ext: 4195 Email: ryanw@doctors.org.uk — BM BS Nottm. 1992; BMedSc 1990; MRCP (UK) 1996; MRCPCH 1999. Cons. Neonatol. Specialty: Paediat.

WATKINS, Sally Louise 3 Rushall Close, Walsall WS4 2HQ Tel: 01922 620583 — MB ChB Birm. 1997. SHO (Paediat.) Wolverhampton. Specialty: Paediat.; Gen. Surg. Prev: HO. Off. (Surg.) Good Hope Hosp. Sutton Coldfield; Ho. Off. (Med.) Walsall Manor Hosp. Walsall.

WATKINS, Sarah Catherine 18 Cousins Grove, Southsea PO4 9RP — MB BS Lond. 1998.

WATKINS, Sarah Elizabeth 7A High St. Mews, Leighton Buzzard LU7 1EA Tel: 01525 379769 Fax: 01525 377298; 1 Copper Beech Way, Leighton Buzzard LU7 3BD Tel: 01525 372524 — MB BS Lond. 1969 (St. Mary's) DObst RCOG 1972; MRCGP 1983. Med. Acupunc.; Police Surg. Beds. Socs: AFME Lond.

WATKINS, Sidney Maurice Kynoch (retired) 8 Airlie Court, Gleneagles Village, Auchterarder PH3 1SA — (Aberd.) MB ChB 1937. Prev: Ho. Surg. Roy. Hosp. Chesterfield.

WATKINS, Simon David 26 Hillside Crescent, Harrow HA2 0QX — BM Soton. 1993.

WATKINS, Stanley Albert South Burden Farm, Broadbury, Okehampton EX20 4LF Tel: 01837 87316 — MB BS Lond. 1953 (Westm.) Prev: Regist. Colindale Hosp.; Sen. Ho. Off. Lond. Chest Hosp. (Country Br.) & W. Lond. Hosp.

WATKINS, Stephen James David Bartley Green Health Centre, Romsley Road, Bartley Green, Birmingham B32 3PR Tel: 0121 477 4300 — MB BS Lond. 1988.

WATKINS, Stephen John Stockport Primary Care Trust, 8th Floor, Regent House, Stockport SK4 1BS Tel: 0161 4265031 Fax: 0161 4778272 Email: stephen.watkins@stockport-pct.nhs.uk; 1 Parklands, Shaw, Oldham OL2 8LW Tel: 01706 846017 — MB ChB Manch. 1974; MSc (Community Med.) Manch. 1982, BSc (Hons.) (Pharmacol.) 1971; FFPHM RCP (UK) 1993, M 1984. Dir. Pub. Health Stockport Primary Care Trust; Chairm. Transport & Health Study Gp.; Hon. Lect. Univ. Manch. Specialty: Pub. Health Med. Socs: BMA (Past Chairm. Comm. Pub. Health Med. & Community Health); Manch. Med. Soc.; (Past Pres.) Med. Practs. Union. Prev: SCM Oldham HA; Regist. (Med.) W. Pk. Hosp. Macclesfield; SHO (Geriat.) Wythenshawe Hosp. Manch.

WATKINS, Stephen John Owen Carnewater Practice, Dennison Road, Bodmin PL31 2LB Tel: 01208 72321 Fax: 01208 78478 — (Middlx.) MB BS Lond. 1970; DObst RCOG 1972; DCH Eng. 1973; FRCGP 1993, M 1980; Dip. Ther. (Cardiff). VTS Course organiser Cornw. Specialty: Gen. Pract. Prev: Research Fell. (Primary Health Care & Gen. Pract.) Postgrad. Med. Sch. Univ. Plymouth; VTS Course organiser Cornw.; Univ. Clin. Tutor (Gen. Pract.) Cornw.

WATKINS, Stuart Craig 5 Ebberston Road E., Rhos-on-Sea, Colwyn Bay LL28 4DP Tel: 01492 547889 Fax: 01492 534834 Email: stuartwatkins@hotmail.com — MB ChB Birm. 1995; ChB Birm. 1995. Reg.Emerg. Med. Liverp.Hosp Sydney Au. Specialty: Accid. & Emerg. Prev: SHO A & E Qu.ns Med.Centre.Notts; Surg.Reg.Roy.P..Alfred.Hosp.Camperdown.Sydney.Au.

WATKINS, Susan Mary Marchfield House, Church Road, Marlow SL7 3RZ; 2 Clipper View, Edgbaston, Birmingham B16 9DJ Tel: 0121 455 7829 Fax: 0121 454 8627 — MB BS Lond. 1990 (Royal Free Hospital School of Medicine) Dip. Anaesth. Roy. Coll. Anaesth. 1994. Specialist Regist. (Anaesth.) Coventry Sch. of Anaesth. Specialty: Anaesth. Socs: Assn. Anaesth.; MRCAnaesth.

WATKINS, Susan Patricia (retired) 9 Manor Drive, Bathford, Bath BA1 7TY Tel: 01225 858726 — MB ChB Birm. 1959; DObst RCOG 1961. Prev: GP N.ants.

WATKINS, Sylvia Madeleine Stonelegh, 13 Priory Way, Hitchin SG4 9BJ Tel: 01462 451775 — BM BCh Oxf. 1961 (Oxf. & St. Bart.) MA Oxf. 1961, DM 1973, BM BCh 1961; FRCP Lond. 1980, M 1964. Hon. Cons. Phys. & Med. Oncol. Lister Hosp. Stevenage. Specialty: Oncol. Socs: BMA. Prev: Sen. Regist. (Med.) Roy. Free Hosp. Lond.; Regist. Univ. Nervenklinik, Heidelberg, Germany; Ho. Phys. St. Bart. Hosp. Lond.

WATKINS, Thomas Irvin (retired) 41 Springfield Road, Ulverston LA12 0EJ Tel: 01229 582913 — MB ChB Leeds 1938; MRCGP 1976.

WATKINS, Timothy The Old Vicarage, Spilsby Road, Horncastle LN9 6AL Tel: 01507 522477 Fax: 01507 522997; Langton Hill Farm, Langton Hill, Horncastle LN9 5JP — MB ChB Sheff. 1983; MRCGP 1987; Dip. IMC RCS Ed. 1991. Socs: Lincs. LMC; Brit. Assn. Immediate Care Nat. Educat. Comm.

WATKINS, Tudno Gareth Lewis e31 Cae Rex, Llanblethian, Cowbridge CF71 7JS — MB BCh Wales 1971; FFA RCS Eng. 1975. Specialty: Anaesth.

WATKINSON, Mr Anthony Francis Royal Devon and Exeter Hospital, Exeter EX1 2ED Mob: 07932 605466 Email: melosborne@compuserve.com; Thorverton House, Thorverton House, Silver Street, Thorverton, Exeter EX5 5LT Tel: 01392 861948 Email: melosborne@compuserve.com — MB BS Lond. 1984 (Roy. Free Hosp. Lond.) MSc Oxf. 1979; FRCS Eng. 1988; FRCR 1991. Cons. (Radiol.) Roy. Devon & Exeter Hosp. Exeter. Specialty: Radiol. Special Interest: Interventional Radiol. Socs: BMA; Brit. Soc. Interven. Radiol.; Soc. Cardiovasc. & Interven. Radiol. Prev: Cons. & Hon. Sen. Lect. (Radiol.) Roy. Free Hosp. Lond.; Lect. (Interven. Radiol.) UMDS Guy's Hosp. Lond.; Fell. (Interven. Radiol.) Vancouver Gen. Hosp., Canada.

WATKINSON, Deborah Susan 28 Kensington Avenue, Watford WD18 7RY — MB BS Lond. 1988 (Univ. Coll. Lond.) BSc Lond. 1985; DRCOG 1991; MRCGP 1992; DTM & H Liverp. 1993; Dip Palliat Med 1997. Assoc. Spec. Florence Nightingale Ho. Hospice Aylesbury. Specialty: Palliat. Med. Prev: Spec. Reg. Palliat. Med. N. Thames.

WATKINSON, Geoffrey (cons. rooms), Nuffield McAlpin Clinic, Beaconsfield Road, Glasgow G12 0PJ Tel: 0141 334 9441; Glasgow Nuffield Hospital, Beaconsfield Road, Glasgow G12 0PJ — MRCS Eng. LRCP Lond. 1943 (St. Bart.) MD Lond. 1945, MB BS 1943; FRCP Lond. 1962, M 1944; FRCP Glas. 1971, M 1969. Examr. RCPS Glas. Specialty: Gastroenterol. Socs: (Ex-Pres.) Brit. Soc. Gastroenterol.; (Ex-Pres. & Ex-Sec.Gen.) Organisat. Mondial de Gastroenterol. Prev: Hon. Lect. (Med.) & Internal Examr. Univ. Glas.; Cons. Phys. & Gastroenterol. West. Infirm., Gartnavel Gen. & South. Gen. Hosps. Glas.; Cons. Phys. York Hosp. Gp.

WATKINSON, Hilary Leith Bonnyrigg Health Centre, High Street, Bonnyrigg EH19 2DA Tel: 0131 663 7272; 54 Grange Loan, Edinburgh EH9 2EP Tel: 0131 667 6360 — MB ChB Ed. 1971; DObst RCOG 1973; DA Eng. 1976. Med. Asst. (Anaesth.) Lauriston Dent. Centre Edin.

WATKINSON, Mr John Carmel ENT Department, Queen Elizabeth Hospital, Vincent Drive, Edgbaston, Birmingham B15 2TH Tel: 0121 627 2295 Fax: 0121 627 2291; 34 Wellington Road, Edgbaston, Birmingham B15 2ES Tel: 0121 440 1981 Fax: 0121 440 1981 — MB BS Lond. 1979 (Roy. Free) FRCS Glas. 1984; FRCS Ed. 1984; DLO RCS Eng. 1986; FRCS (Orl.) Eng. 1986; MS Lond. 1990, MSc (Nuclear Med.) 1987; FICS 1991. Cons. Otolaryngol. Qu. Eliz. Hosp. Birm. Specialty: Otolaryngol. Socs: Fell. Roy. Soc. Med.; Brit. Nuclear Med. Soc.; BMA. Prev: Sen. Regist. (Otolaryngol.) Guy's Hosp. Lond.; Sen. Regist. (Head & Neck & Plastics) Roy. Marsden Hosp. Lond.; SHO (Otolaryngol.) Roy. Free Hosp. Lond.

WATKINSON, Michael Neonatal Unit, Birmingham Heartlands Hospital, Bordesley Green E., Birmingham B9 5ST Tel: 0121 424 2719 Fax: 0121 424 2718 — MB BChir Camb. 1973; MRCP (UK) 1975; FRCP Lond. 1992; FRCPCH 1997. Cons. Paediat. Birm. Heartlands Hosp. Specialty: Paediat.; Neonat. Prev: Sen. Regist. (Paediat) St. Geo. Hosp. Lond.; Research Paediat. MRC Dunn Nutrit. Unit Keneba, The Gambia; Regist (Paediat.) Roy. Vict. Infirm. Newc. u. Tyne.

WATKINSON, Peter James 17 Warwick Street, Crookes, Sheffield S10 1LX — MB ChB Sheff. 1993.

WATKINSON, Peter Martin New Court Surgery, 39 Boulevard, Weston Super Mare BS23 1PF Tel: 01934 624242 Fax: 01934 642608; The Beeches, 11 Woodland Road, Weston Super Mare BS23 4HF Tel: 01934 417734 — MB ChB Manch. 1971; DObst RCOG 1975. Prev: Clin. Asst. (ENT) Weston Gen. Hosp.; SHO (Obst.) Southmead Hosp. Bristol; SHO (Gyn.) Ham Green Hosp. Pill.

WATKINSON, Sally Ann Pheasey Woodland View Surgery, Woodland View, West Rainton, Houghton-le-Spring DH4 6RQ Tel: 0191 584 3809; 11 Rosemount, Plawsworth Road, Durham

DH1 5GA — MB BS Newc. 1987 (Newcastle-u-Tyne) MRCGP 1991. Part. Gen. Pract. W. Rainton, Durh. Prev: Trainee GP Newc. u Tyne.

WATKINSON, Sally Jane 30 Deerlands Road, Chesterfield S40 4DF — MB BS Lond. 1997; BSc 1994. Specialty: Obst. & Gyn.

WATKINSON, Susan Elizabeth 2 Torridon Close, Sinfin, Derby DE24 9LJ — MB ChB Leeds 1977; FFA RCSI 1984. Specialty: Anaesth.

WATKINSON, William Michael Forbes (retired) Pinehill Surgery, Pinehill Road, Bordon GU35 0BS Tel: 01420 472113 — MB BS Lond. 1973 (St Bartholomews) MRCS Eng. LRCP Lond. 1973. Prev: Sen. Med. Off., Bordon Garrison, Bordon, Hants.

WATKISS, Jonathan Bruce Flat 29, The Lab Building, 177 Rosebery Ave, London EC1R 4TN — MB BS Lond. 1989; DRCOG 1992; MRCGP 1993; T(G) 1993; FRCA 1998. Consultant Anaesthetist, Guys & St Thomas, London. Specialty: Anaesth. Prev: Specialist Regist. (Anaesth.) Centr. N. Lond. Rotat. UCH/Roy. Free; Repatriation Med. SHO Anaesth. Barts/Roy. Lond.; Psychiat. SHO St Chas. Hosp. Lond.

WATMOUGH, David Dept. of Gastroenterol., Queens Hospital, Belvedere Road, Burton-on-Trent DE13 0RB Tel: 01283 566333 — MB ChB Sheff. 1986 (Sheffield) BMedSci Sheff. 1986, MB ChB 1986; FRACP 1997. Cons.(Gen. Med. & Gastroenterol.) Qu.s Hosp. Burton upon Trent, Staffs. Specialty: Gastroenterol. Socs: Gastroenterolog. Soc. Australia & W.Midl.s Phys. Assoc. Prev: Advanced Trainee (Gastroenterol.) Sir Chas. Gardiner Hosp. Perth, Australia; Regist. (Gen. Med.) Roy. Perth Hosp., Australia; Regist. Univ. Dept. Med. Roy. Perth Hosp. West. Austral.

WATMOUGH, Gerald Ian Ullapool Medical Practice, The Health Centre, Market Street, Ullapool IV26 2XE Tel: 01854 612015/612595 Fax: 01854 613025; 47 Forest View Road, Loughton IG10 4DY — MRCS Eng. LRCP Lond. 1973 (St. Bart.) BSc Lond. 1969, MB BS 1972. Prev: Regist. (Paediat.) Raigmore Hosp. Inverness; Regist. (Paediat.) & Regist. (Anaesth.) Palmerston N. Hosp., N.Z.

WATMOUGH, Patrick John 18 Millfield Road, Chorley PR7 1RE — MB ChB Dundee 1996.

WATNEY, Patsy Jeanne Moncaster (retired) Waterton, The Wad, West Wittering, Chichester PO20 8AH Tel: 01243 513592 — MB BChir Camb. 1956 (St. Thos.) FRCOG 1979, M 1964; MA Camb. 1956, MD 1972. Prev: Cons. O & G Sandwell Dist. Gen. Hosp. W. Bromwich.

WATRAS, Gregory Jan Maharishi Ayur Ved Health Centre, 3 Rowan Road, Ashurst, Skelmersdale WN8 6UQ Tel: 01695 51008; Evergreens, Allendale Drive, St. Ishmaels, Haverfordwest SA62 3TP Tel: 01646 636330 — MB ChB Sheff. 1973. Med. Dir. Maharishi Ayur-Ved Health Centre Skelmersdale. Prev: GP Milford Haven.

WATRASIEWICZ, Krystyna Ewa 30 Drayton Hill, London W13 0JF — MRCS Eng. LRCP Lond. 1961.

WATRELOT, Antoine Medicare Français, 3 Harrington Gardens, London SW7 4JJ Tel: 020 7370 4999; Cres, Le Britannia, 20 Blvd E. Deruelle, Lyon 69003, France Tel: 00 33 437 48 90 90 Fax: 00 33 437 48 90 94 Email: watrelot@wanadoo.fr — MD Grenoble 1978; DGO Grenoble 1979. Cons. IVF Clinic, Lyon. Specialty: Obst. & Gyn. Socs: Amer. Assn. Gyn. Laparoscopists.; (Pres.) Infertil. Centre of Lyons, France; IVF French Soc. Prev: Regist. & Head of Clinic. Grenoble Hosp., France; Sen. Regist. Hosp. St. Joseph, Lyon, France.

WATSHAM, Christine Mary Priscilla (retired) 46 High Street, Little Shelford, Cambridge CB2 5ES — MB BS Lond. 1963 (Roy. Free) MRCS Eng. LRCP Lond. 1963; DA Eng. 1965; DObst RCOG 1965; FFA RCS Eng. 1968. Prev: Cons. Anaesth. Bourn Hall Clinic Camb.

WATSON, Agnes Teak The Old Barn, 4 King St., Bishop's Stortford CM23 2NB — MB ChB Leeds 1990; FRCA 1997. Cons., Anaesthetics, St. Andrews, Broomfield Hosp., Chelmsford. Specialty: Anaesth. Prev: Regist. (Anaesth.) The Roy. Hosp. Lond. Sch. of Anaesth.; Regist. (Anaesth.) Qu.'s Med. Centre Nottm.

WATSON, Alan 286 Cottingham Road, Hull HU6 8QA — MB BS Newc. 1979; MRCOG 1986. Assoc Spec Obst & Gyn Roy Hull Hosp. Specialty: Obst. & Gyn. Prev: Staff Grade Roy Hull Hosp.

WATSON, Alan Rees Children & Young People's Kidney Unit, City Hospital, Hucknall Road, Nottingham NG5 1PB Tel: 0115 962 7961 Fax: 0115 962 7759 Email: awatson@ncht.trent.nhs.uk; 78 Lambourne Drive, Wollaton, Nottingham NG8 1GR — MB ChB Ed. 1973 (Edinburgh) MRCP (UK) 1976; FRCP Ed. 1988; FRCPCH 1997. Cons. Paediat. Nephrol. City Hosp. Nottm.; Special Sen. Lect., Sch. of Human Developm., Univ. of Nottm. Specialty: Paediat.; Nephrol. Special Interest: Antenatal Urin. tract abnormality; Chronic renal failure; Healthcare ethics. Socs: Convenor Europ. Paediatric Pertoneal Working Gp.; Chairm., UK Clinical Ethics Network; Pres. Nottm. Med-Chi Soc. Prev: Staff Nephrol. Hosp. Sick Childr. Toronto, Canada; Lect. (Child Health) Univ. Manch.; Regist. Paediat. Durban, S. Africa.

WATSON, Alan Spence (retired) — MB ChB Ed. 1950; MRCGP 1968. Chairm. Panel on Ethics. Edin. Indep. Ethics Comm. for Med. Research, Elphinstone Research Centre, Tranent, Scotl. Prev: GP Musselburgh.

WATSON, Alastair John Mackenzie Department of Medicine, University of Liverpool, Daulby St., Liverpool L69 3GA Tel: 0151 706 4074 Fax: 0151 706 5802 Email: alastair.watson@liv.ac.uk; 7 Ridgebourne Close, Warrington WA5 9YB Tel: 01925 574207 — MB BS Lond. 1980 (St. Thomas' London) MRCP (UK) 1983; MD Camb. 1989; FRCP 1999. Prof. (Med.) Univ. Liverp.; Hon. Cons. Phys. Roy. Liverp. Univ. Specialty: Gen. Med.; Gastroenterol. Socs: Brit. Soc. Gastroenterol.; Amer. Gastroenterol. Assn. Prev: Sen. Lect. (Med.) Univ. Manch.; Research Fell. (Gastroenterol.) John Hopkins Hosp., Baltimore, USA; Research Regist. St. Bart. Hosp. Lond.

WATSON, Alexander Davidson West Gate Health Centre, Charleston Drive, Dundee DD2 4AD Tel: 01382 632771 Fax: 01382 633839 Email: awatson@westgate2.tayside.scot.nhs.uk; 5 West Park Gardens, Dundee DD2 1NY Tel: 01382 667321 — MB ChB Dundee 1973; DObst RCOG 1975; MRCGP 1977; FRCGP 1999. Princip. in Gen. Pract. Westgate Health Centre Chas.ton Dr., Dundee; Hon. Sen. Lect., Dept. Gen. Pract., Univ. Dundee; Clin. Asst. Cardiovasc. Risk Clinic, Ninewells Hosp., Dundee. Specialty: Gen. Pract. Socs: Brit. Hypertens. Soc.; Scott. Thoracic Soc. Prev: Clin. Asst. Chest Unit, Kings Cross Hosp., Dundee.

WATSON, Alexander Stewart 12 Abbey Park, Auchterarder PH3 1EN — MB ChB Glas. 1949.

WATSON, Alexander William — MB ChB Leeds 1998; BSc Lond. 1997.

WATSON, Alison Jane 3 Bowtrees, Ashbrooke Range, Sunderland SR2 7TL Tel: 0191 510 9395 — MB ChB Dundee 1979; MFPHM 1990; MBA Durh. 1995. Specialty: Pub. Health Med. Prev: Cons. Pub. Health Med. Sunderland HA.

WATSON, Alison Margaret Copperstones, Little Lane, Upper Bucklebury, Reading RG7 6QX Tel: 01635 871871 — (Westm.) MRCS Eng. LRCP Lond. 1969; MB BS Lond. 1969; DObst RCOG 1971; FRCGP 1996, M 1975. Course Organiser Reading VTS. Prev: GP Thatcham Health Centre Berks.& Parkside Family Pract. Reading.

WATSON, Alison Mary Thornley Street Surgery, 40 Thornley Street, Wolverhampton WV1 1JP Tel: 01902 688500 Fax: 01902 444074; 40 Thornley Street, Wolverhampton WV1 1JP — MB ChB Birm. 1982.

WATSON, Allan John Stewart Field House Surgery, Victoria Road, Bridlington YO15 2AT Tel: 01262 623362; Chantry Cottage, West St, Flamborough, Bridlington YO15 1PH Tel: 01262 850501 — MB ChB Ed. 1963; DObst RCOG 1966.

WATSON, Mr Allan Philip Southport General Infirmary, The Eye Unit, Scarisbrick New Road, Southport PR8 6PH Tel: 01704 703446 Fax: 01704 703492 — MB BCh BAO NUI 1980; DO RCS Eng. 1983; FRCS Ed. 1984; FRCOphth 1989. Cons. Ophth. Surg. Southport & Ormskirk NHS Trust. Specialty: Ophth. Socs: United Kingdom and Irel. Soc. of Cataract and Refractive Surg.s; Europ. Soc. of Cataract and Refractive Surg.s.

WATSON, Andrew Brailsford Arbury Road Surgery, 114 Arbury Road, Cambridge CB4 2JG Tel: 01223 364433 Fax: 01223 315728; 17 Nursery Walk, Cambridge CB4 3PR Tel: 01223 323269 — MB BS Lond. 1983; DGM RCP Lond. 1986; DRCOG 1987; MRCGP 1989. SHO (O & G) Newmarket Gen. Hosp. Socs: RCGP; Primary Care Theum. Soc. Prev: SHO (A & E) Hinchingbrooke Hosp. Huntingdon.; Ho. Phys. Hartlepool Gen. Hosp.; Ho. Surg. Roy. Free Hosp. Lond.

WATSON, Andrew Henry Paediatric Department, St. Mary's Hospital, Newport PO30 5TG Tel: 01983 534343 Fax: 01983 530215 — MB BS Lond. 1974 (St. Geo.) MRCS Eng. LRCP Lond. 1974; DCH Eng. 1976; MRCP (UK) 1977; FRCP Lond. 1992; FRCPCH 1997. Cons. Paediat. I. of Wight. Specialty: Paediat. Prev: Lect. & Hon. Sen. Regist. (Paediat.) St. Bart., Lond. Hosp. & Qu.

Eliz. Hosp. Lond.; Regist. (Paediat.) Qu. Charlotte's Matern. Hosp. Lond.

WATSON, Andrew John Sowerby Department of Obstetrics and Gynaecology, Tameside General Hospital, Fountain St., Ashton-under-Lyne OL6 9RW Tel: 0161 331 6158 Fax: 0161 331 6074 Email: andy.watson@tgh.nhs.uk — MB ChB Leeds 1986; MRCOG 1991. Cons. in O & G; Hon. Clin. Lect. Obst. & Gyn. Manch. Univ. Specialty: Obst. & Gyn. Special Interest: Pelvic pain. Socs: Brit. Soc. Colpos. & Cerv. Path.; Brit. Fertil. Soc.; RCOG.

WATSON, Angela Station Road Surgery, 2 Station Road, Prestwick KA9 1AQ Tel: 01292 671444 Fax: 01292 678023; 3 Southpark Avenue, Prestwick KA9 1PY Tel: 01292 474042 — MB ChB Glas. 1970; DObst RCOG 1972; MRCGP 1975. Clin. Asst. (Haemat.) Ayr Hosp. Prev: Trainee GP N. Ayrsh. VTS.

WATSON, Mr Angus James Mackintosh No. 10, Sillerton House, 16 Albyn Terrace, Aberdeen AB10 1YP Tel: 01224 644929 Email: a.j.watson@abdn.ac.uk; No. 10, Sillerton House, 16 Albyn Terrace, Aberdeen AB10 1YP Tel: 01224 644929 Email: anguswatson@compuserve.com — MB ChB Manch. 1991 (St. And. & Manch.) BSc (Med. Sci.) St. And. 1988; FRCS Ed. 1995. Regist. (Gen. Surg.) Higher Surgic. Train. Scheme Grampian Region; Research Fell. (Surg.) Aberd. Univ. Specialty: Gen. Surg. Prev: SHO Rotat. (Surg.) Hope Hosp. Salford; SHO (A & E) & Demonst. (Anat.) Roy. Hallamsh. Hosp. Sheff.

WATSON, Ann Department of Haematology, Stoke Mandeville Hospital, Aylesbury HP21 8AL Tel: 01296 84111 Email: ann.watson@smh.nhs.uk; Gorwell Cottage, Gorwell, Watlington OX49 5JB Tel: 01491 613840 — MB BS Lond. 1975; BSc (Physiol.) Lond. 1972; FRCP (UK) 1978; FRCPath 1985. Cons. Haemat. Stoke Mandeville Hosp. Aylesbury. Specialty: Haematology. Prev: Sen. Regist. (Haemat.) Roy. Berks. Hosp. Reading; Regist. (Haemat.) Glas. Roy. Infirm.

WATSON, Anna Catherine 24 Kent Gardens, Ealing, London W13 8BU Tel: 020 8998 3283 — MB ChB Bristol 1989; FRCA 1995. Regist. (Anaesth.) St. Mary's Hosp. Lond. Specialty: Anaesth. Prev: SHO (Anaesth.) St. Bart. Hosp. Lond.

WATSON, Anne (retired) 15 Hurst Rise Road, Cumnor Hill, Oxford OX2 9HE — MRCS Eng. LRCP Lond. 1964 (Oxf. & Univ. Coll. Hosp.) MA, BM BCh Oxf. 1964; DFFP 1993; LF Hom 2000. Prev: GP.

WATSON, Anne McIntyre Maryfield Medical Centre, 9 Morgan Street, Dundee DD4 6QE Tel: 01382 462292 Fax: 01382 461052; 320 Blackness Road, Dundee DD2 1SD Tel: 01382 566429 — MB ChB Dundee 1982; DRCOG 1984; MRCGP 1986. Clin. Asst. (Palliat. Med.) Roxburghe Hse. Dundee.

WATSON, Annette Barbara Joiner's Cottage, Linton-on-Ouse, York YO30 2AS — MB ChB Leeds 1986.

WATSON, Anthony Hilltops Medical Centre, Kensington Drive, Great Holm, Milton Keynes MK8 9HN Tel: 01296 4235 — MB BS Lond. 1979; DRCOG 1981; MRCGP 1983; FRCGP 2001.

WATSON, Anthony The Cobham Health Centre, 168 Portsmouth Road, Cobham KT11 1HT Tel: 01932 867231 Fax: 01932 866874; 1 Randolph Close, Stoke D'Abernon, Cobham KT11 2SW Tel: 01932 862966 — MB BS Lond. 1971; Dip. Pharm. Med. RCP 1981.

WATSON, Anthony James (retired) Magali, Hook Road, Ampfield, Romsey SO51 9DB — MB BS Durh. 1949 (Newc.) DCH Eng. 1951; DA Eng. 1971. Hosp. Pract. (Anaesth.) Roy. Co. Hosp. Winchester. Prev: Regist. (Med.) & Ho. Phys. Childr. Dept. & Cardiovasc. Dept. Gen. Hosp. Newc.

WATSON, Anthony John (retired) Bewley Cottage, Ismays Road, Ightham, Sevenoaks TN15 9BE Tel: 01732 885337 — (St. Thos.) MA, MB Camb. 1957, BChir 1956; DObst RCOG 1960. Prev: Hosp. Pract. (ENT) Weald Kent Trust.

WATSON, Anthony Thayne (retired) 6 Princess Royal Close, Lincoln LN2 5RX Tel: 01522 523007 — (Univ. Ed.) MB ChB Ed. 1948; DObst RCOG 1951; MRCGP 1965. Prev: Resid. Ho. Off. (Obst.) City Gen. Hosp. Sheff.

WATSON, Mr Antony Charles Harington (retired) St Helens, Waverley Road, Melrose TD6 9AA Tel: 01896 822082 Email: tony@watson-36.fsnet.co.uk — (Ed.) MB ChB Ed. 1960; FRCS Ed. 1964. Prev: Cons. Plastic Surg. Roy. Hosp. for Sick Childr. Edin., St John's Hosp. Livingston.

WATSON, Arthur Barrie (retired) 83 Buckingham Road, Shoreham-by-Sea BN43 5UD — MB BS Lond. 1954 (Univ. Coll. Hosp.) DObst RCOG 1960.

WATSON, Arthur Vincent Reid, MBE (retired) The Rowans, Craigour Road, Torphins, Banchory AB31 4HE Tel: 01339 882140 — MB ChB Aberd. 1958; DObst RCOG 1961; MRCGP 1971. Prev: Ho. Phys. Roy. Aberd. Hosp. Sick Childr.

WATSON, Barbara (retired) 8 Culver Road, Winchester SO23 9JF — MB ChB Ed. 1950. Prev: Clin. Asst. in Psychiat. at the Dept. of Pyschiatry. Roy. S. Hants Hosp. Southampton.

WATSON, Beverley Jill 16 Gains Lane, Great Gidding, Huntingdon PE28 5NL — MB BS Lond. 1986 (Univ. Coll. Lond.) FRCA 1993. Cons. Anaesth. Qu. Eliz. Hosp. Kings Lynn. Specialty: Anaesth.

WATSON, Brian (retired) Theold Hay Barn, 1 Lineage Court, Burford, Tenbury Wells WR15 8HD Tel: 01584 781667 — MB ChB Birm. 1953. Prev: GP Handsworth Birm.

WATSON, Brian Granville 12 Westfield Avenue, Gosforth, Newcastle upon Tyne NE3 4YH Tel: 0191 285553 — MB BS Durh. 1965; FFA RCS Eng. 1969. Cons. Anaesth. Regional Cardiothoracic Surg. Centre Freeman Hosp. Newc. Specialty: Anaesth. Socs: Hon. Sec. N. Eng. Soc. Anaesth. Prev: Sen. Regist. (Anaesth.) Newc.; Sen. Med. Off. (Anaesth.) Baragwanath Hosp. Johannesburg; Regist. (Anaesth.) Alder Hey Childr. Hosp. Liverp.

WATSON, Mr Carl Memorial Hospital, Darlington DL3 6HX; Ingle Nook, 46 Cleveland Avenue, Darlington DL3 7HG — MB ChB Leeds 1981; FRCS Ed. 1986. Cons. ENT Surg. Memor. Hosp. Darlington. Specialty: Otolaryngol. Prev: Sen. Regist. (Otolaryngol.) Gen. Infirm. Leeds.

WATSON, Carole Anne Grove House Practice, St Pauls Health Centre, High St, Runcorn WA7 1AB Tel: 01928 566561 Fax: 01928 590212; 23 Sylvan Close, Selsdon, South Croydon CR2 8DS — MB BS Lond. 1990; DCH RCP Lond. 1992; DRCOG 1993; MRCGP 1994; DFFP 1994.

WATSON, Caroline Iylah Jane 7 Hawthorne Road, Stapleford, Cambridge CB2 5DU — MB BChir Camb. 1994; MRCGP.

WATSON, Caroline Jane The Medical Centre, The Meadows, Old Meldrum, Inverurie AB51 0BF Tel: 01651 872239; St Peters Brae, Peterwell Road, Fyvie, Turriff AB53 8RF — MB ChB Aberd. 1986.

WATSON, Catherine Julie — MB ChB Bristol 1993.

WATSON, Ceri Susan 38 Newport View, Heading Ley, Leeds LS6 3BX — MB ChB Leeds 1994. Specialty: Care of the Elderly.

WATSON, Christine Mary (retired) 36 Alleyn Road, West Dulwich, London SE21 8AL Tel: 020 8670 0444 Fax: 020 8670 0562 Email: jimw@casab.demon.co.uk — (King's Coll. Hosp.) MB BS Lond. 1961; MRCS Eng. LRCP Lond. 1961; DCH Eng. 1963; DObst RCOG 1963; MD Lond. 1973; MFFP 1993. Prev: Cons. Family Plann. & Reproduc. Healthcare Optimum Health Servs. Lond.

WATSON, Christopher Anthony The Health Centre, University of Sussex, Falmer, Brighton BN1 9RW Tel: 01273 249049 Fax: 01273 249040; 36 Chichester Drive E., Saltdean, Brighton BN2 8LB Fax: 01273 297218 — MB BS Lond. 1981 (St. Mary's) DRCOG 1983. Prev: SHO (Orthop. & Trauma & O & G) Roy. Sussex Co. Hosp. Brighton; SHO (Paediat. Surg.) Roy. Alexandra Childr. Hosp. Brighton.

WATSON, Christopher Greenhowe (retired) Flat 2 Windsor Court, 7 Cavendish Avenue, Harrogate HG2 8HX — (Sheff.) MB ChB Sheff. 1955. Prev: SHO City Gen. Hosp. Sheff.

WATSON, Mr Christopher John Edward Addenbrooke's Hospital, Department of Surgery, Hills Road, Cambridge CB2 2QQ — MB BChir Camb. 1984; FRCS Eng. 1988; MA Camb. 1985, BA (Hons.) 1981, MD 1994; FRCS (Gen.) 1995. Cons. Surg. Addenbrooke's Hosp. Camb. Specialty: Transpl. Surg. Special Interest: Aortic Surg.; Carotid Artery Surg.; Peripheral Vasc. Dis. Prev: Cons. (Transpl. Surg.) Churchill Hosp. Oxf.; Sen. Regist. (Transpl.) Addenbrooke's Camb.; Sen. Regist. (Gen. & Vasc. Surg.) John Radcliffe Hosp. Oxf.

WATSON, Christopher Neville (retired) The Moat House, Moor Lane, Keswick, Leeds LS17 9ET Tel: 01937 573344 — BM BCh Oxf. 1950 (Oxf. & Guy's) MA, BM BCh Oxon. 1950. Prev: Ho. Surg. Thoracic Unit, Guy's Hosp.

WATSON, Claire Green Lane Hospital, Devizes SN10 5DS Tel: 01380 731200 Fax: 01380 731308; 4 Stapleford Close, Chippenham SN15 3FZ — MB ChB Manch. 1974; MRCPsych 1985.

Cons. Psychiat. of Old Age Green La. Hosp. Devizes. Specialty: Geriat. Psychiat. Prev: Cons. Psychiat. of Old Age Roundway Hosp. Devizes; Sen. Regist. (Psychiat. Old Age) St. Martin's Hosp. Bath & Torbay Hosp.; Regist. (Gen. Psychiat.) St. John's Hosp. Bucks.

WATSON, Colin (retired) 8 Church View, Narborough, Leicester LE19 2GY Tel: 0116 286 5916 — MB ChB Leeds 1954; DObst RCOG 1956; FRCGP 1972, M 1961. Prev: Hon. Lect. (Obst. in Gen. Pract.) Univ. Leeds.

WATSON, Craig Fyvie Health Centre, Health Centre, 27 Parnassus Gardens, Turriff AB53 8QD Tel: 01651 891205 Fax: 01651 891834; St Peters Brae, Peterwell Road, Fyvie, Turriff AB53 8RD Tel: 01651 891430 — MB ChB Ed. 1984; DRCOG 1988; MRCGP 1989.

WATSON, Cyril Colin East Crest, Red Lane, Colne BB8 7JR — MB BS Lond. 1965 (Roy. Free) MRCS Eng. LRCP Lond. 1965; MRCP Lond. 1968. Cons. Phys. Burnley Gp. Hosps. Specialty: Gen. Med. Prev: Sen. Med. Regist. Derby Roy. Infirm.; Med. Regist. Nottm. Gen. Hosp.; Regist. (Cardiol.) Groby Rd. Hosp. Leicester.

WATSON, Dale Gary Flat 3, 74 Northumberland Road, Manchester M16 9PP — MB ChB Liverp. 1996.

WATSON, Danie-Marie Kim 150 Ruskin Park House, Champion Hill, London SE5 8TL — MB BS Lond. 1994.

WATSON, Daphne Alice Sutton (retired) Wrightington Hospital, Hall Lane, Appley Bridge, Wigan WN6 9EP Tel: 01257 256244; Tarnside, 44 Ruff Lane, Ormskirk L39 4QZ Tel: 01695 572120 — MB BChir Camb. 1967 (Camb. & Guy's) BA Camb. 1963; FFA RCSI 1973. Cons. Anaesth. Wrightington Hosp. for Jt. Dis. Prev: Cons. Anaesth. W. Lancs. NHS Trust.

WATSON, David — MB ChB Ed. 1983 (Ed. Univ.) BSc (Med. Sci.) Ed. 1980; DA (UK) 1986; FFA RCS Eng. 1988. Cons. Anaeth. Roy. Infirm Edin. Specialty: Anaesth.; Intens. Care. Socs: Scott. Soc. Anaesth. & Edin. & E. Scotl. Soc. Anaesth.; Scott. Intens. Care Soc.

WATSON, David Adams Brae Terrace Surgery, Brae Terrace, Munlochy IV8 8NG Tel: 01463 811200 Fax: 01463 811383; Tulach Ard, Munlochy IV8 8ND Tel: 01463 811430 — MB ChB Aberd. 1971. Prev: GP Arrochar; GP Glenrothes; SHO (O & G) Raigmore Hosp. Inverness.

WATSON, Mr David Anthony (retired) Darbys House, High St., Chipping Campden GL55 6AL Tel: 01386 841164 — MB BS Lond. 1946 (St. Bart.) MRCS Eng. LRCP Lond. 1945; FRCS Eng. 1955. Hon. Cons. Adviser Nat. Heart Research Fund. Prev: Cons. Cardiothoracic Surg. Gen. Infirm. & Killingbeck Hosp. Leeds.

WATSON, David Bruce Friarwood Surgery, Carleton Glen, Pontefract WF8 1SU Tel: 01977 703235 Fax: 01977 600527 — MB ChB Leeds 1985. Prev: SHO (Gen. Med.) Pontefract Gen. Infirm.; Ho. Off. (Gen. Med.) Pontefract Gen. Infirm.; Ho. Off. (Gen. Surg.) Harrogate Dist. & Gen. Hosps.

WATSON, David George Agar 3 Loris Road, Hammersmith, London W6 7QA — MB BS Sydney 1967; MRCP (UK) 1970; DCH RCP Lond. 1971.

WATSON, David Graham Central Surgery, Sussex Road, Gorleston-on-Sea, Great Yarmouth NR31 6QB Tel: 01493 414141 Fax: 01493 656253; Central Surgery, Sussex Road, Gorleston, Great Yarmouth NR31 6QB Tel: 01493 414141 Fax: 01493 656253 Email: watson@omsimedical.demon.co.uk — MB BS Lond. 1971 (St. Thos.) DObst RCOG 1973; AFOM RCP Lond. 1981. Specialty: Occupat. Health.

WATSON, David Howard Victoria Surgery, Victoria Street, Bury St Edmunds IP33 3BD Tel: 01284 725550 Fax: 01284 725551 — MB BS Lond. 1966 (Char. Cross) MRCS Eng. LRCP Lond. 1965. Prev: Regist. (Med.) W. Herts. Hosp. Hemel Hempstead; SHO (Anaesth.) Lincoln Co. Hosp.; SHO (Obst.) Hull Matern. Hosp.

WATSON, David James 71 New Edinburgh Road, Uddingston, Glasgow G71 6AB — MB ChB Manch. 1991.

WATSON, David Kay 20 Chester Road, Wrexham LL11 2SA — MB BS Newc. 1972; MRCPath 1980. Cons. Haemat. Maelor Gen. Hosp. Wrexham. Specialty: Haematology. Prev: Sen. Regist. (Haemat.) Gen. Infirm. Leeds; Regist. (Path.) Huddersfield Roy. Infirm.; SHO (Path.) Soton. Gen. Hosp.

WATSON, David Lister (retired) St. Mildred's, North St., Milverton, Taunton TA4 1LG Tel: 01823 400447 — MB ChB Manch. 1948; FRCGP 1983, M 1975. Prev: Sen. Ho. Off. & Ho. Phys. Manch. Roy. Infirm.

WATSON, David Lyndon Hyde Park Surgery, 3 Woodsley Road, Leeds LS6 1SG Tel: 0113 295 1235 Fax: 0113 295 1220 — MB ChB Leeds 1987.

WATSON, Mr David Malcolm, TD 115A Harley Street, London W1G 6AR Tel: 020 7935 8922 Fax: 020 7486 0211; 11 Meadway Close, Hampstead Garden Suburb, London NW11 7BA Tel: 020 8455 2507 — MB BS Lond. 1957 (St. Thos.) FRCS Eng. 1963; FRCOphth 1989. Emerit. Cons. Guy's & St Thos. Hosp. Lond.; Ophth. Surg. King Edwd. VII Hosp. Lond.; Ophth. Surg. Hosp. St. John & Eliz. Lond. Specialty: Ophth. Socs: Fell. Roy. Soc. Med.; Fell. Ophth. Soc. UK. Prev: Cons. Ophth. Surg. Guy's Hosp. Lond.; Chief Clin. Asst. Detachm. Unit Moorfields Eye Hosp. (High Holborn) Lond.; Ho. Surg. & Chief Asst. Eye Dept. St. Thos. Hosp. Lond.

WATSON, David Michael 1 Dunelm Street, South Shields NE33 3JT — MB ChB Leeds 1986.

WATSON, David Norman Stechford Health Centre, 393 Station Road, Stechford, Birmingham B33 8PL Tel: 0121 783 2109/0121 783 2893 Fax: 0121 785 0619 Email: david.watson@easternbirminghampct.nhs.uk; Stechford Health Centre, 393 Station Road, Stechford, Birmingham B33 8PL Tel: 0121 783 2109 — MB ChB Ed. 1980; BSc (Med. Sci.) Ed. 1977. GP. Specialty: Gen. Pract. Prev: GP Warks.; Community Child Health Off. Warks.

WATSON, Mr David Patrick Hubert Emergency Department, Royal United Hospitals, Bath BA1 3NG Tel: 01225 824002 Fax: 01225 825636 Email: david.watson@ruh-bath.swest.nhs.uk — MB BCh BAO NUI 1982; FRCSI 1987; FFAEM 1994. Cons. A & E Bath Roy. United Hosps. Specialty: Accid. & Emerg. Prev: Cons. A & E Guy's Hosp. Lond.; Sen. Lect. (A & E) Guy's Hosp. & Lewisham Hosp.

WATSON, Mr David Selby 27 Sunbury Avenue, West Jesmond, Newcastle upon Tyne NE2 3HD — MB ChB Ed. 1991; FRCS Ed. 1996. SpR (Gen. Surg.) Newc. upon Tyne. Specialty: Gen. Surg. Prev: Research Fell. (Surg.) Univ. Newc. u. Tyne.

WATSON, Miss Deirdre Clare Torbitt Thoracic Surgical Unit, Norfolk & Norwich Hospital, Brunswick Road, Norwich NR1 3SR Tel: 01603 286395 Fax: 01603 287882 — MB BS Lond. 1971 (Guy's) MRCS Eng. LRCP Lond. 1971; FRCS Eng. 1975; FRCS Ed. 1975. Cons. Thoracic Surg. Norf. & Norwich Hosp. Specialty: Cardiothoracic Surg. Socs: Soc. Cardiothoracic Surgs. GB & Irel.; Coun. Mem. Europ. Assn. for Cardiothoracic Surg. Prev: Cons. Thoracic Surg. Birm. Heartlands & Childr. Hosps.

WATSON, Mr Desmond John North Riding Infirmary, Newport Rd, Middlesbrough TS1 5JE Tel: 01642 850850 Fax: 01642 854070; 6 Ferguson Way, Redmarshall, Stockton-on-Tees TS21 1FB Tel: 01742 631031 — BM BCh Oxf. 1980; FRCS (Otol.) Eng. 1986; MA Oxf. 1988. Cons. Otolaryngolist S. Tees Acute Hosp.s HNS Trust. Specialty: Otorhinolaryngol.; Medico Legal. Prev: Cons. Otolaryngol. W. Suff. HA.; Regist. Sen. Regist. (Otolaryng.) Bristol & Bath Hosps.; SHO (Otolarnyg.) Roy. Nat. Throat Nose & Ear Hosp. Lond.

WATSON, Diane The Portland Road Practice, 16 Portland Road, London W11 4LA Tel: 020 7727 7711 Fax: 020 7226 6755; 17 Bloemfontein Road, London W12 7BH Tel: 020 8740 0765 — MB BS Lond. 1983; BA Camb. 1980; DRCOG 1986; MRCGP 1996. Cement Tutor Imperial Coll. & GP Princip. Lond. Prev: Ho. Surg. Guy's Hosp. Lond.; Ho. Phys. Lewisham Hosp. Lond.

WATSON, Doreen 7 Four Acres Drive, Kilmaurs, Kilmarnock KA3 2ND — MB ChB Glas. 1991.

WATSON, Dorothy Betty Dougal Corsenside, Cooden Close, Bexhill-on-Sea TN39 4TQ Tel: 0142 433014 — MB BS Lond. 1948 (Roy. Free) MRCS Eng. LRCP Lond. 1942. Prev: Ho. Surg. Roy. Free Hosp. Lond.; Capt. RAMC.

WATSON, Duncan MacDonald West Cumberland Hospital, Whitehaven CA28 8JG; Weston Lodge, 2 Brigham Road, Cockermouth CA13 0AX — MB BS Newc. 1976; FFARCS 1982. Cons. (Anaesth.) W. Cumbld. Hosp. Whitehaven. Specialty: Anaesth.

WATSON, Duncan McKenzie Ivy House, High St, Walton, Lutterworth LE17 5RG — MB ChB Leic. 1981; FFA RCSI 1988. Cons. Anaesth. Intens. Care Walsgrave Hosp. Trust Coventry. Specialty: Anaesth. Prev: Sen. Regist. (Anaesth.) Sheff.

WATSON, Edward Norton (retired) 42 Chester Close South., Regent's Park, London NW1 4JG Tel: 020 7486 6965 Email: ewat42@supanet.com — (St. Thos.) MRCS Eng. LRCP Lond. 1944;

MFOM RCP Lond. 1979. Prev: Chief Med. Off. Gen. Counc. Brit. Shipping & Merchant Navy Estab.

WATSON, Elizabeth Anne Woosehill Surgery, Emmview Close, Woosehill, Wokingham RG41 3DA Tel: 01896 830203 Fax: 01896 831202; Rowanburn, 146 Galashiels Road, Stow, Galashiels TD1 2RA Tel: 01578 730269 — MB ChB Bristol 1985; DCH RCP Lond. 1987; MRCGP 1990; DRCOG 1990. Partner GP St Ronan's Health Centre Innerleithen; Clin. Asst. Dingleton Hosp., Melrose. Prev: Med. Off. St. And. Nursing Home Drygrange; Trainee GP Earlston; SHO (O & G) Roy. Infirm. Edin.

WATSON, Elizabeth Anne 286 Cottingham Road, Hull HU6 8QA — MB BS Newc. 1980. Asst. EM.

WATSON, Elizabeth Thompson 111 Needless Road, Perth PH2 0LB — MB ChB St. And. 1939.

WATSON, Emma Jane 13 Grasleigh Way, Allerton, Bradford BD15 9AN — MB ChB Ed. 1993.

WATSON, Mr Eric Alan John 166 Dawlish Road, Selly Oak, Birmingham B29 7AR Tel: 0121 471 3617 Email: eaj.watson@virgin.net — MB ChB Birm. 1991; MRCOG 1998. Cons. Obst. & Gynaecologist, Wordsley Hosp., Dudley Gp. of Hosps. HNS Trust. Specialty: Obst. & Gyn.

WATSON, Eric Reed (retired) 27 Kilnford Drive, Dundonald, Kilmarnock KA2 9EU Tel: 01563 851458 — (Leeds) BSc Leeds 1947; MB ChB Leeds 1950; DMRT Eng. 1957; FFR 1964. Prev: Cons. Radiotherap. West. Infirm. Glas.

WATSON, Fiona Elizabeth Community Drug Problem Service, 22-24 Spittal St., Edinburgh EH3 9DU Tel: 0131 537 8345 Fax: 0131 537 8350; 22 Baberton Mains Loan, Edinburgh EH14 3EP — MB ChB Dundee 1982; MRCGP 1987; MRCPsych 1989. Cons. Psychiat. Drug Dependency Lothian Primary Care Trust. Specialty: Alcohol & Substance Misuse.

WATSON, Fiona Jane 219 Bellenden Road, London SE15 4DG Tel: 020 7277 6389 — MB BS Newc. 1992; DFFP 1997. Specialty: Gen. Pract. Socs: BMA.

WATSON, Fiona Lorraine 5 Magheralave Park N., Lisburn BT28 3NL — MB BCh Belf. 1998.

WATSON, Forbes Gordon 17 Kirkintilloch Road, Kirkintilloch, Glasgow G66 4RN — MB ChB Glas. 1989.

WATSON, Frederick James The Wooden Bungalow Medical Practice, Victoria St., Wrappy, Market Rasen LN8 5PF Tel: 01673 858880; Hilltop, Hameringham, Horncastle LN9 6PG Tel: 0165 888245 — MB BCh BAO Belf. 1978.

WATSON, Garron Maxwell Holmedene, Armthorpe, Doncaster DN3 3AB Tel: 01302 831200 — MB ChB Manch. 1950. Prev: SHO (O & G) Whitehaven Gen. Hosp.; SHO Cas., Gen. & Orthop. Surg. Gen. Hosp. Middlesbrough.

WATSON, Gavin Moffat The Surgery, 15 King Street, Paisley PA1 2PR Tel: 0141 889 3144 Fax: 0141 889 7134 — MB ChB Glas. 1967; DObst RCOG 1969; MRCGP 1972. Prev: Trainee Gen. Pract. Glas. Vocational Train. Scheme.

WATSON, Geoffrey Wilfred 42 Huckley Way, Bradley Stoke, Bristol BS32 8AR Tel: 0117 969 2893 — MB BS Lond. 1989; DA (UK) 1992. SHO Rotat. (Gen. Med.) Frenchay Hosp. Bristol. Prev: SHO (Anaesth., Trauma & Orthop.) Princess Margt. Hosp. Swindon.

WATSON, George Craig Shepperton Health Centre, Shepperton Court Drive, Laleham Road, Shepperton TW17 8EJ Tel: 01932 245289 — MB BS Lond. 1952 (Lond. Hosp.) Prev: Ho. Surg. Poplar Hosp.; Res. Anaesth. Lond. Hosp.; Sen. Ho. Phys. Nottm. Childr. Hosp.

WATSON, George Dickson Department of Radiology, Ninewells Hospital, Dundee Tel: 01382 660111 — MB ChB Glas. 1973; DMRD Eng. 1978; FRCR 1981. Consultant Radiologist.

WATSON, Georgina Mary 18 Ravelston Dykes, Edinburgh EH4 3ED Tel: 0131 332 2798 — MB ChB Glas. 1975; Cert. Family Plann. JCC 1977; DRCOG 1977. Prev: GP Glas & Bristol.

WATSON, Gerald Howard Vincent Strabane Health Centre, Upper Main Street, Strabane BT82 8AS Tel: 028 7138 4118; 8 Coach Road, Baronscourt, Newtownstewart, Omagh BT78 4BF Tel: 016626 61980 — MB BCh BAO Dub. 1976 (T.C. Dub.) DRCOG 1978; MRCGP 1983. Socs: Assoc. Mem. BMA.

WATSON, Mr Gerald Stewart (retired) 8 Cunning Park Drive, Doonfoot, Ayr KA7 4DT Tel: 01292 441989 — MB ChB Ed. 1966; FRCS Ed. 1970. Cons. Urol. Ayr Hosp. Prev: Sen. Regist. (Urol.) Roy. Infirm. Edin.

WATSON, Gillian Carol 73 Morven Road, Bearsden, Glasgow G61 3BY Tel: 0141 942 6724 — MB ChB Glas. 1997 (Glasgow Univ.) SHO (A&E), Blackburn Roy. Infirm. Prev: SHO (Paediat.), CrossHo. Hosp.; Jun. Ho. Off. (Surg.), Hairmyre Hosp.; Jun. Ho. Off. (Med.), Ayr Hosp.

WATSON, Graham Charles Maryfield Medical Centre, 9 Morgan Street, Dundee DD4 6QE Tel: 01382 462292 Fax: 01382 461052; 320 Blackness Road, Dundee DD2 1SD — MB ChB Dundee 1981. Socs: Roy. Coll. Gen. Pract.

WATSON, Graham David Almsford House Surgery, 1 Almsford House, Beckfield Lane, Acomb, York YO26 5PA Tel: 01904 799000 Fax: 01904 789407 — MB ChB Leeds 1969; DObst RCOG 1971.

WATSON, Mr Graham Michael Eastbourne District General Hospital, King's Drive, Hill, Eastbourne BN21 2UD Tel: 01323 417400 Fax: 01323 414954; Wannock Place, Jevington Road, Wannock, Polegate BN26 5NT Tel: 01323 487786 — MB BChir Camb. 1976; FRCS Eng. 1979; FRCS (Urol.) 1988; MD Camb. 1989. Cons. (Urol.) Eastbourne Dist. Gen. Hosp. Specialty: Urol. Prev: Sen. Regist. St. Peter's Hosp. Lond.; Sen. Lect. St. Peter's Hosp. Lond.; Cons. (Urol.) Whittington Hosp. Lond.

WATSON, Harold Kirk (retired) 30 Queensberry House, Friars Lane, Richmond TW9 1NU Tel: 020 8948 1190 — MB ChB Sheff. 1948. Prev: Med. Dir. Dome/Hollister-Stier.

WATSON, Mr Harold Preston (retired) 3 High Orchard, St. Clement's Road, St Helier, Jersey JE2 4PH — MB ChB St. And. 1938; FRCS Ed. 1947. Prev: Surg. Colonial Hosp. Port of Spain Trinidad.

WATSON, Heather Kay — MB ChB Ed. 1998; MRCPCH 2002; DRCOG 2004. Specialty: Paediat.

WATSON, Helen Deborah 106 Colne Road, Earby, Colne BB18 6XS — MB ChB Leeds 1987.

WATSON, Helen Jennifer Lutterworth Road Medical Centre, 58 Lutterworth Road, Blaby, Leicester LE8 4DN Tel: 0116 247 7828 — MB ChB Leic. 1980 (Leicester) Prev: SHO (Obst.) Leeds Gen. Infirm.; SHO (Gen. Med./Chest Dis.) Groby Rd. Hosp. Leics.

WATSON, Helen Mairi Stewart Northumberland Health Authority, Morley Croft, Loansdean, Morpeth NE61 2DL Tel: 01670 394400 Fax: 01670 394501; 11 Park Drive, Deuchar Park, Morpeth NE61 2SY Tel: 01670 513583 — MB ChB Aberd. 1974; MSc Dub. 1981; FFPHM 1994. Cons., Pub. Health Med., N.d. HA. Specialty: Pub. Health Med.

WATSON, Helen Mary 11 Brookfield, Mawdesley, Ormskirk L40 2QJ — BM BCh Oxf. 1990; DCH RCP Lond. 1993; DRCOG 1994. Prev: Trainee GP Northumbria VTS; SHO (Gen. Med.) S. Cleveland Hosp. Middlesbrough; SHO (Paediat.) Roy. Vict. Infirm. Newc.

WATSON, Helen Rosemary Lower Farm, Mabberley, Pontesbury, Shrewsbury SY5 0TP — MB BChir Camb. 1982; BSc (Hons.) St. And. 1978; FRCR 1989. Cons. Diag. Radiol. Roy. Shrewsbury Hosp. Specialty: Radiol. Prev: Sen. Regist. (Diag. Radiol.) Nottm. HA.

WATSON, Helen Susan 233 Bellenden Road, London SE15 4DQ — MB BS Lond. 1990; MRCOG 1996. Specialist Regist. (O & G) Maidstone Hosp. Maidstone, Kent. Specialty: Obst. & Gyn. Prev: Specialist Regist. (O & G) St Thos. & Guys Hosps.; Specialist Regist. (O & G) Pembury Hosp., Kent.

WATSON, Henry George Department of Haematology, Aberdeen Royal Infirmary, Aberdeen AB25 2ZN Tel: 01224 681818 Fax: 01224 840714 Email: henry.watson@arh.grampian.scot.nhs.uk — MB ChB Aberd. 1983 (Univ. Aberd.) MRCP (UK) 1988; MRCPath 1994; FRCP Ed 1997; MD 1997. Cons. Haemat. Aberd. Roy. Infirm. Specialty: Haematology. Prev: Sen. Regist. (Haemat.) Roy. Infirm. Edin.; Lect. (Haemat.) Univ. Edin.; Regist. (Haemat.) W. Midl. HA.

WATSON, Howard (retired) 8 Woodthorpe Lane, Sandal, Wakefield WF2 6JH — MB ChB Leeds 1956; DObst RCOG 1958. Prev: Ho. Phys. (Obst.) & Ho. Surg. Halifax Gen. Hosp.

WATSON, Howard Peter National Britiania occupational division, Britannia house, Caerphilly CF83 3GG; Linden House, 4 Woodland Close, St. Arvans, Chepstow NP16 6EF — MB ChB Leeds 1980; MRCGP 1988; AFOM RCP Lond. 1993. Occupat. Phys. and Med. director, Nat. Britannia Occupat. Health Div. Specialty: Occupat. Health. Prev: Med. Off. Brit. Steel plc Llanwern Works; Med. Off. Brit. Rail; Occupational hys. BUPA Ocupational health.

WATSON, Hugh Philipson 2 Burghley Road, Wimbledon, London SW19 5BH Tel: 020 8946 1245 — MB BS Lond. 1953 (St. Mary's)

MRCS Eng. LRCP Lond. 1953; MRCGP 1961. Specialty: Occupat. Health. Socs: Fell. Roy. Soc. Med. Prev: Regional Med. Off. Ranks Hovis McDougall Ltd.; Clin. Asst. Wilson Hosp. Mitcham; Ho. Surg. (ENT) St. Mary's Hosp. Lond.

WATSON, Hugh Stewart Kelso (retired) 45 Grange Road, Cheddleton, Leek ST13 7NP Tel: 01538 360210 — MB ChB Ed. 1951. Prev: GP Leek.

WATSON, Ian Alastair Ross, Col. late RAMC Retd. (retired) 16 Mill Rise, Mill Lane, Bourton, Gillingham SP8 5DH Tel: 01747 841387 Email: alastair.watson@btinternet.com — MB BS Durh. 1952 (Newc.) DTM & H Eng. 1969; MRCGP 1976. Prev: Ho. Phys. (Orthop.) & Ho. Surg. (ENT) Roy. Vict. Infirm. Newc.

WATSON, Ian Douglas 63-83 Hylton Road, Sunderland SR4 7AF Tel: 0191 567 9179 Fax: 0191 514 7452 — MB ChB Dundee 1979; DRCOG 1981; MRCGP 1983. GP.

WATSON, Ian Norman O'Colmain and Partners, Fearnhead Cross Medical Centre, 25 Fearnhead Cross, Warrington WA2 0HD Tel: 01925 847000 Fax: 01925 818650; Longford Street Surgery, Longford St, Warrington WA2 7QZ — MB ChB Liverp. 1982.

WATSON, Ian Peter Michael Saddleworth Medical Practice, The Clinic, Smithy Lane, Oldham OL3 6AH Tel: 01457 872228 Fax: 01457 876520 — MB ChB Leic. 1992; MRCGP 1997.

WATSON, Isabel Frances Well Close Square Surgery, Well Close Square, Berwick-upon-Tweed TD15 1LL Tel: 01289 356920 Fax: 01289 356939 — MB BS Newc. 1976; MRCGP 1980. GP Berwick upon Tweed. Prev: GP Asst. Durh. Univ. Health Centre; Clin. Med. Off. Sch. Health Serv. Morpeth.

WATSON, Ivan Robert George 17 Edenvale Park, Omagh BT78 5EB — MB BCh BAO Belf. 1992.

WATSON, James Bernard 86 Wateringpool Lane, Lostock Hall, Preston PR5 5UA — MB BS Lond. 1993.

WATSON, James David Intensive Care Department, Homerton Hospital NHS Trust, Homerton Row, London E9 6SR Tel: 020 8510 7303 Fax: 020 8510 7668 Email: j.d.watson@qmul.ac.uk; 41 Kingshurst Road, London SE12 9LD — MB BS Lond. 1977 (St. Bart.) BSc Lond. 1974, MB BS 1977; FRCA 1982. Cons. & Sen. Lect. (Intens. Care Med.)Barts and The Lond. NHS Trust Lond. Specialty: Intens. Care. Prev: Sen. Regist. (Anaesth.) Soton. & Poole Gen. Hosps.; Research Regist. (Anaesth. & ITU) St. Bart. Hosp. Lond.; Regist. (Anaesth.) Nat. Heart Hosp.

WATSON, Mr James Davidson 18 Ravelston Dykes, Edinburgh EH4 3ED Tel: 0131 332 2798 — MB ChB Glas. 1975; MB ChB (Commend.) Glas. 1975; FRCS Glas. 1979; FRCS Glas. (Plast) 1987; FRCS Ed. 1990. Cons. Plastic Surg. St. John's Hosp. W. Lothian NHS Trust.; Hon. Cons. in Burns & Plastic Surg. Brit. Army; Hon. Sen. Lect. in Surg., The Univ. of Edin. Specialty: Plastic Surg. Prev: Sen. Regist. (Plastic Surg.) Frenchay Hosp. Bristol; Regist. (Plastic Surg.) Canniesburn Hosp. Glas.; Regist. (Surg.) W. Scotl. Surgic. Train. Scheme.

WATSON, James Ingram The Taymount Surgery, 1 Taymount Terrace, Perth PH1 1NU Tel: 01738 627117 Fax: 01738 444713; 4 Hatton Mews, Perth PH2 7DR Tel: 01738 625069 — MB ChB Glas. 1963 (Glas) DObst RCOG 1965. Med Adviser Highland distillers Perth. Specialty: Gen. Pract.

WATSON, Professor James Patrick (retired) — (King's Coll. Hosp.) MB BChir Camb. 1960; DCH Eng. 1963; FRCP Lond. 1978, M 1964; Acad. DPM Univ. Lond. 1967; FRCPsych 1977, M 1971; MD Camb. 1974. Emerit. Prof. of Psychiat. GKT, King's Coll. Lond. Prev: Sen. Lect. & Cons. Psychiat. St. Geo. Hosp. Med. Sch. Lond.

WATSON, James Victor Little Hilden, London Road, Tonbridge TN10 3DD — MB BS Lond. 1964; DMRT Eng. 1969.

WATSON, Jane Christine Dolphin House Surgery, 6-7 East Street, Ware SG12 9HJ Tel: 01920 468777 Fax: 01920 484892; 2 Musleigh Manor, Widbury Gardens, Ware SG12 7AT Tel: 01920 469637 — MB BS Lond. 1983; DRCOG 1987; Cert. Family Plann. JCC 1987. Prev: Trainee GP Luton & Dunstable VTS; Ho. Phys. Luton & Dunstable Hosp.; Ho. Surg. Roy. Free Hosp.

WATSON, Jennifer Margaret Beaumaris, Church Avenue, Cardross, Dumbarton G82 5NS Tel: 01389 841387 — MB BS Lond. 1971 (St. Mary's Hosp. Lond.) MFFP 1993. Clin. Asst. (Colposcopy) West. Infirm. Glas. & Vale of Leven Alexandria; Instruc. Doctor Glas. Family Plann. Assn. Prev: SHO (Obst. & Anaesth.) & Ho. Phys. St. Mary's Hosp. Lond.

WATSON, Jennifer May Lennox and Partners, 9 Alloway Place, Ayr KA7 2AA Tel: 01292 611835 Fax: 01292 284982; 8 Cunning Park Drive, Doonfoot, Ayr KA7 4DT Tel: 01292 441989 — (Ed.) MB ChB Ed. 1966; Cert. FPA 1971; Cert. Prescribed Equiv. Exp. JCPTGP 1981. Prev: Trainee GP Ayr VTS; Regist. SE Scotl. Blood Transfus. Serv.; Ho. Off. (O & G) West. Gen. Hosp. Edin.

WATSON, Jeremy Neil Bewley Cottage, Ismays Road, Ightham, Sevenoaks TN15 9BE — MB BS Lond. 1985; DRCOG 1990; MRCGP 1990.

WATSON, Joanna The Surgery, Mount Avenue, Shenfield, Brentwood CM13 2NL Tel: 01277 224612 Fax: 01277 201218; 14 Surman Crescent, Hutton, Brentwood CM13 2PP — MB BS Lond. 1981; DRCOG 1984. Specialty: Gen. Pract.

WATSON, Mr John (retired) Iddons, Henleys Down, Catsfield, Battle TN33 9BN Tel: 01424 830226 Email: john.watson@iddons.demon.co.uk — MB BChir Camb. 1939 (Camb. & Guy's) MRCS Eng. LRCP Lond. 1938; MA Camb. 1939; FRCS Ed. 1947; FRCS Eng. (ad eund.) 1963. Hon. Cons. Plastic Surg. Qu. Vict. Hosp. E. Grinstead. Prev: Cons. Plastic Surg. Roy. Lond. Hosp. & King Edwd. VII Hosp. for Offs.

WATSON, John Essex House, Station Road, Barnes, London SW13 0LW Tel: 020 8876 9882 Fax: 020 8876 1033 — MB BS Lond. 1966; FRACGP 1974; DRCOG 1977. Med. Contributor Telemed Surrey; Co. Doctor ICL Windsor. Socs: BMA; Assoc. Mem. Roy. Soc. Med. Prev: Clin. Asst. (Obst.) Kingston Hosp.; SHO (O & G) Enfield Hosp.; Ho. Surg. & Ho. Phys. Hillingdon Hosp.

WATSON, Mr John Arthur Standish Pilgrim Hospital, Sibsey Road, Boston PE21 9QS; Tytton Hall, Wyberton, Boston PE21 7HT Tel: 01205 310305 — MB BS Lond. 1980; FRCS Ed. 1986. Cons. Orthop. Surg. Pilgrim Hosp. Boston. Specialty: Orthop.

WATSON, Professor John David Northern Health & Social Services Board, County Hall, Galgorm Road, Ballymena BT42 1QB Tel: 028 2566 2208 — LM Rotunda 1972; BA Dub. 1969, MB BCh BAO 1971; DObst RCOG 1973; Dip. Soc Med. Ed. 1974; MFCM 1977; FFCM 1986; FFPHM 1990; FRCP 1999. Dir. of Pub. Health NHSSB Ballymena.; Vis. Prof.Pub.Health Univ.Ulster. Specialty: Pub. Health Med. Prev: Asst. Chief Admin. Med. Off. EHSSB Belf.; Clin. Clerk Rotunda Hosp. Dub.; Ho. Off. Roy. Matern. Hosp. Belf.

WATSON, John Ernest (retired) Keogh and Keenleside, Beech House Surgery, 1 Ash Tree Road, Knaresborough HG5 0UB Tel: 01423 542564 — MB BCh BAO Belf. 1945. Treasury Med. Off.

WATSON, John Martin HPA Communicable Disease Surveillance Centre, 61 Colindale Avenue, London NW9 5EQ Tel: 020 8200 6868 Fax: 020 8200 7868 Email: john.watson@hpa.org.uk — MB BS Lond. 1979 (Med. Coll. St. Bart. Hosp. Lond.) MRCP (UK) 1982; MSc Lond. 1984; MFPHM RCP (UK) 1989; FRCP Lond. 1995; FFPHM RCP (UK) 1995. Cons. Clin. Epidemiol. & Head Respiratory Diseases Dept., Health Prot. Agency, Communeable Disease Surveillance Centre, Lond.; Hon. Sen. Lect. (Infec. & Trop. Dis.) Lond. Sch. Hyg. & Trop. Med. Specialty: Epidemiol.; Respirat. Med.; Infec. Dis. Socs: Jt. Tuberc. Comm. Brit. Thoracic Soc.; Internat. Union Against Tuberc. & Lung Dis. Prev: Hon. Sen. Lect. Nat. Heart & Lung Inst. Roy. Brompton & Nat. Heart Hosp. Lond.

WATSON, John Maxwell Wellclose Square, Berwick-upon-Tweed TD15 1LL Tel: 01289 306634; Windyridge, Scremerston, Berwick-upon-Tweed TD15 2RJ Tel: 01289 305201 — MB ChB Aberd. 1977; MRCP Ed. 1984.

WATSON, John Paul Leeds General Infirmary, Great George St., Leeds LS1 3EX Tel: 0113 392 5296 Fax: 0113 392 6316 — MB Camb. 1984; BA Camb. 1981; BChir Camb. 1983; MRCP (UK) 1987; DTM & H RCP Lond. 1989; CCST 1998; FRCP Lond. 2002. Cons. Phys. (Respiratory Medicine) Leeds Gen. Infirm.; Hon. Sen. Lect. Univ. of Leeds. Specialty: Respirat. Med.; Gen. Med. Special Interest: Non Invasive Ventilation; Tuberculosis. Socs: Brit. Thorac. Soc.; Europ. Respirat. Soc. Prev: Sen. Regist. Leeds Gen. Infirm./Killingbeck Hosp.; Research Fell. Worcester Roy. Infirm.; Phys. Tansen Hosp. United Mission Nepal.

WATSON, John Smyly (retired) 1 Alfreton Close, Wimbledon, London SW19 5NS Tel: 020 8946 5276 — MRCS Eng. LRCP Lond. 1943 (St. Mary's) MD Lond. 1950, MB BS 1943; MRCP Lond. 1949. Prev: Cons. Phys. (Geriat.) St. Geo. & Bolingbroke Hosps. Lond.

WATSON, Mr John Trevor (retired) 60 The Paddock, Busby, Glasgow G76 8SL — (Glas.) MB ChB Glas. 1961; FRCS Ed. 1966.

Cons. Orthop. Surg. Hairmyres Hosp. E. Kilbride. Prev: Resid. in Path. Boston City Hosp., U.S.A.

WATSON, John Ulric The Surgery, Fairfield Medical Centre, Lower Road, Great Bookham, Leatherhead KT23 4DP Tel: 01372 452755; The Flint House, 36 Middle Farm Place, Effingham, Leatherhead KT24 5LA Tel: 01372 454787 — MB BS Lond. 1962 (St. Bart.) DObst RCOG 1964; DA Eng. 1966. Vice-Chairm. Surrey FHSA; Chairm. Surrey LMC. Socs: BMA; BMAS. Prev: SHO (O & G) Redhill Gen. Hosp.; Ho. Surg. & Ho. Phys. Whipps Cross Hosp.; Ho. Surg. (O & G) St. Bart. Hosp.

WATSON, Jonathan Mark Grosvenor Medical Centre, Grosvenor Street, Crewe CW1 3HB Tel: 01270 256348 Fax: 01270 250786; 118 Waterloo Road, Haslington, Crewe CW1 5TA Tel: 01270 581269 — MB ChB Ed. 1984; MRCGP 1989.

WATSON, Jonathan Michael Silverdale, Fieldhouse Lane, Hepscott, Morpeth NE61 6LT — MB BS Newc. 1992. Specialist Regist. Anaesth. Specialty: Anaesth.

WATSON, Jonathan Peter 4 Fairville Close, Cramlington NE23 3GJ — BM BCh Oxf. 1989; MA Camb. 1990, BA 1986; MRCP (UK) 1992. Regist. (Gastroenterol.) N. Shields. Specialty: Gastroenterol. Prev: Traine Fell. Med. Research Counc.

WATSON, Joyce Macdonald (retired) 16 Montague Street, Broughty Ferry, Dundee DD5 2RD — MB ChB St. And. 1960 (Dundee) DObst RCOG 1964; FRCP Ed. 1981, M 1966. Prev: Cons. Phys. in Med. for the Elderly, Dundee.

WATSON, Joyce Margaret — MB ChB Glas. 1986 (Glasgow) DRCOG 1992; T(GP) 1993; DFFP 1999. GP Non-Princip. Specialty: Family Planning; Sports Med.; Trop. Med.

WATSON, Karen Alicia Robin Hood Surgery, 1493 Stratford Rd, Hall Green, Birmingham B28 9HT — MB ChB Liverp. 1989; DA (UK) 1995; DFFP 1995. GP Birm. Specialty: Gen. Pract. Prev: GP/Regist. Chessington; SHO (O & G) Epsom Hosp. Surrey; SHO (Paediat. & Anaesth.) Kingston Hosp.

WATSON, Keith John K12 Medical Centre, HMS Nelson, Queen St., Portsmouth PO1 3HH — MB ChB Birm. 1982; BSc Birm. 1979, MB ChB 1982. Civil. Med. Pract. Med. Centre HMS Nelson Portsmouth.

WATSON, Kenneth Melvyn The Manor House, Twigworth, Gloucester GL2 9PW; (Surgery), 16 Cheltenham Road, Gloucester GL2 0LS Tel: 01452 35959 — MB BS Lond. 1966 (King's Coll. Hosp.) MRCS Eng. LRCP Lond. 1967; DObst RCOG 1968. Prev: SHO King's Coll. Hosp. Lond.; Med. Off. Nkana Hosp. Kitwe, Zambia; Med. Off. Aberd. Hosp. New Glas., Nova Scotia, Canada.

WATSON, Kevin John Cohen and Partners, West Lodge Surgery, New Street, Farsley, Pudsey LS28 5DL Tel: 0113 257 0295 Fax: 0113 236 2509; The Barn, Holt Lane, Adel, Leeds LS16 7NN Tel: 0113 267 5733 — MB ChB Leeds 1969; DObst RCOG 1973; DA Eng. 1974.

WATSON, Laura Jane Radiology Department, West Suffolk Hospital, Hardwick Lane, Bury St Edmunds IP33 2QZ Tel: 01284 713376 — BM BCh Oxf. 1981 (Oxford) MA Oxf. 1982; FRCR 1987. Cons. Radiol. W. Suff. Hosps. NHS Trust. Specialty: Radiol. Socs: Brit. Inst. Radiol.; Brit. Med. Ultrasound Soc. Prev: Sen. Regist. (Diag. Radiol.) & Frenchay Hosp. Bristol & John Radcliffe Hosp. Oxf.

WATSON, Lawrence Joseph Castlegate Surgery, 42 Castle Street, Hertford SG14 1HH Tel: 01992 589928; 6 Park Road, Hertford SG13 7LF — MB BS Lond. 1973; DObst RCOG 1976.

WATSON, Leila Margaret (retired) 2 House o' Hill Brae, Edinburgh EH4 5DQ Tel: 0131 336 3750 — (Ed.) MB ChB Ed. 1947; DPH Ed. 1957; MFCM 1972. Prev: Community Med. Specialist Health Educat. Div. Common Servs. Agency.

WATSON, Lesley Jean — MB ChB Leeds 1992; FRCS 1999. SpR A&E Manch. Rotat.

WATSON, Lilla (retired) 4 Edgerton Road, Leeds LS16 5JD — MB BS Durh. 1957. Ref. Regional Med. Serv. Prev: GP Leeds.

WATSON, Linda Ann 127 York Road, (Chadwick House), Hartlepool TS26 9ND Tel: 01429 234646; 5 The Green, Elwick Village, Hartlepool TS27 3ED — MB BS Lond. 1987. Specialty: Gen. Pract.

WATSON, Louise 43 Westlands Avenue, Slough SL1 6AH — MB BCh Wales 1991.

WATSON, Lyal Clifton Albert (retired) 18 Hadley Heights, Hadley Road, Barnet EN5 5QH Tel: 020 8447 1825 — (Sydney) MB BS Sydney 1950; FRACP 1965, M 1953; FRCP Lond. 1975, M 1969. Prev: Cons. & Hon. Cons. Phys. Univ. Coll. Hosp. Lond.

WATSON, Malcolm John Wester Ballochearn Farm, Balfron, Glasgow G63 0QE Tel: 0141 860357 — MB ChB Glas. 1995 (Glasgow) SHO A&E Roy.Alex.Hosp. Paisley. Specialty: Gen. Med. Socs: Full Mem. MRCP Glas. Coll. Prev: SHO (Med.) Southern Gen. Hosp. Glas.; SHO (A & E) Glas. Roy. Infirm. & Western Infirm. Glas.

WATSON, Mr Mark Alexander Norfolk and Norwich Health Care Trust, Brunswick Road, Norwich NR1 3SR; 13 Chapel Lane, Thorpe St. Andrew, Norwich NR7 0EX Tel: 01603 702452 — MB BS Lond. 1991 (St. Thomas's Hospital) BSc (Hons) Lond. 1988; FRCS Eng. 1995.

WATSON, Mark Benjamin St Thomas Health Centre, Cowick Street, St. Thomas, Exeter EX4 1HJ Tel: 01392 676677 Fax: 01392 676677 — MB ChB Bristol 1989; MRCGP 1994; DRCOG 1994. Prev: Trainee GP Exeter VTS.

WATSON, Mark Edward James Cassio Surgery, 62-68 Merton Road, Watford WD18 0WL Tel: 01923 226011 Fax: 01923 817342 — MB BS Lond. 1982 (Char. Cross) DRCOG 1985. Socs: Fell. Roy. Soc. Med.; W Herts. & Watford Med. Soc. Prev: SHO (O & G) Char. Cross & W. Lond. Hosp.; SHO (A & E & Orthop.) Watford Gen. Hosp.; Ho. Surg. Char. Cross Hosp. Lond.

WATSON, Mr Mark Gordon ENT Department, Donacaster Royal Infirmary, Armthorpe Road, Doncaster DN2 5LT Tel: 01302 553197 Fax: 01302 381323 Email: mark.watson@dbh.nhs.uk; South View, Dame Lane, Misson, Doncaster DN10 6EB Tel: 01302 719179 Email: mark.watson@which.net — MB ChB Birm. 1981; FRCS (Orl.) Eng. 1986; T(S) 1991. Cons. Otolaryngologist, Head and Neck Surg., Doncaster Roy. Infirm.; Cons. Otolaryngologist, Head and Neck Surg., Bassetlaw Dist. Gen. Hospital,. Worksop. Specialty: Otorhinolaryngol. Socs: Otolaryngol. Research Soc. & Brit. Voice Assn. Prev: Sen. Regist. (Otolaryngol.) Freeman Hosp. Newc. & Sunderland Gen. Hosp.; Regist. (Otolaryngol.) Birm. HAs; Cas. Off. & SHO (Otolaryngol.) Dudley Rd. Hosp. Birm.

WATSON, Mark Robert Llwynbedw Medical Centre, 82/86 Caerphilly Road, Birchgrove, Cardiff CF14 4AG Tel: 029 2052 1222 Fax: 029 2052 2873 — MB BCh Wales 1983.

WATSON, Martha Huie (retired) 24 Hills Road, Strathaven ML10 6LQ Tel: 01357 521054 — MB ChB Glas. 1944. Prev: Cons. Phys. (Geriat.) Lanarksh. HB.

WATSON, Mary (retired) 21 Tretawn Gardens, London NW7 4NP — MB ChB Ed. 1933 (Univ. Ed.) Prev: Princip. Med. Off. Lond. Boro. Barnet. Ho. Surg. Vict. Infirm. Glas.

WATSON, Mary, SJM (retired) 9 Penn Lea Road, Bath BA1 3RF Tel: 01225 421754 — MB ChB New Zealand 1935 (Otago) DA Eng. 1947; FFA RCS Eng. 1954. Prev: Cons. Anaesth. Roy. United & St. Martin's Hosps. Bath & Bath & Wessex Orthop Hosp.

WATSON, Mary Aitken 57 Gartmore Road, Paisley PA1 3NG Tel: 0141 889 5880 — MB ChB Glas. 1967; DObst RCOG 1969; MRCP (UK) 1971; FRCP Glas. 1988; MPhil (Law & Ethics in Med.) Univ. Glas. 1998. Assoc. Specialist Renal Unit West. Infirm. Glas.

WATSON, Mary Eileen Campbell Trumpington Street Medical Practice, 56 Trumpington Street, Cambridge CB2 1RG Tel: 01223 361611 Fax: 01223 356837; 40 Plumian Way, Balsham, Cambridge CB1 6EG Tel: 01223 290905 — MB BChir Camb. 1988; MA Camb. 1989, BA Med. Sci 1985; MB BChir Camb. 1989; DCH RCP Lond. 1991; DRCOG 1992; MRCGP 1995. Prev: GP Rawdon, Leeds.

WATSON, Maureen Rachel Homefirst Community Health & Social Services Trust, Holywell Hospital, 60 Steeple Road, Antrim BT41 2RJ Tel: 02894 413191 Fax: 02894 413190 — MB BCh BAO Belf. 1976; FRCPsych; MRCPsych 1981; MA Belf. 1997. Cons. Psychiat. Holywell Hosp. Antrim; Head of Ment. Health Serv.s. Specialty: Gen. Psychiat.

WATSON, Maxwell Sheldrake 79 Northland Village, Dungannon BT71 6JN Tel: 028 8775 2832 — MB ChB Ed. 1985; DCH RCSI 1988; DRCOG 1988; MRCGP 1989; DMH QUB 1994; Dip Palliat Med Wales 2000. SpR (Palliative Med.) N. Irel. Socs: RCGP; BMA; APM. Prev: GP Dungannon.

WATSON, Melville Stuart Queens Road Medical Group, 6 Queens Road, Aberdeen AB15 4NU Tel: 01224 641560 Fax: 01224 659629 Email: stuart.watson@qrmg.grampian.scot.nhs.uk — MB ChB Aberd. 1988; MRCGP 1992; T(GP) 1992; MSc Aberd. 1995. Gen. Practitioner; Chairm. Aberd. Inner City Healthcare Co-op. Specialty: Gen. Pract.

WATSON, Michael (retired) Cherry Orchard, 50 Buxton Road, Weymouth DT4 9PN Tel: 01305 773885 — (Univ. Coll. Hosp.) MB BS Lond. 1961; MRCS Eng. LRCP Lond. 1961; DObst RCOG 1963; MRCGP 1974.

WATSON, Michael County Practice, Barking Road, Needham Market, Ipswich IP6 8EZ Tel: 01449 720666 Fax: 01449 720030 — MB BS Newc. 1971; DObst RCOG 1973. Prev: SHO (Paediat.) Univ. Hosp. W. Indies, Jamaica; SHO (Obst.) St. Mary's Hosp. Kettering.

WATSON, Michael David (retired) Estoril, 9 The Old Bath Road, Sonning, Reading RG4 6SZ Tel: 01189 693764 — (Univ. Coll. Med. Sch. Lond.) MB BS Lond. 1962; DTM & H Liverp. 1997. GP Reading. Prev: Med. Off. Jamaica.

WATSON, Mr Michael Ellis Department of Urology, Royal Preston Hospital, Sharoe Green Lane, Fulwood, Preston PR2 9HT Tel: 01772 522483 Fax: 01772 522946 Email: mike.watson@lthtr.nhs.uk — MB ChB (Commendation) Glas. 1968 (Glasgow University) FRCS Glas. 1975; PhD Glas. 1975. Cons. (Urol.) Roy. Preston Hosp. Specialty: Urol. Special Interest: Endourology; Stone Surgery. Socs: Brit. Assn. Urologic. Surgs.; BMA; Preston Medico-Ethical Soc. Prev: Sen. Regist. (Urol.) Roy. Hallamshire Hosp. Sheff.; Regist. (Urol.) Roy. Infirm. Glas.; Regist. (Surg.) Roy. Infirm. Glas.

WATSON, Michael James (retired) 29 Tower Road South, Warmley, Bristol BS30 8BJ Tel: 0117 967 4128 — MB ChB Bristol 1956; MRCS Eng. LRCP Lond. 1956. Prev: SHO (Gen. Surg.) Frenchay Hosp. Bristol.

WATSON, Michael Leonard Royal Infirmary, Edinburgh EH16 4SA Email: mike.watson@luht.scot.nhs.uk — MBChB 1973 (Edinburgh) BSc (Hons) Ed. 1970; FRCP Ed. 1986; MD 1986. Cons. Phys. Roy. Infirm. Edin.; Chief Med. Off. Scott. Provident Insur. co.; Chief Med. Off. Northern lightHo. Bd. Specialty: Gen. Med. Special Interest: Hypertens.; Nephrol. Socs: Dean Roy. Coll. Phys. Edin.

WATSON, Mr Michael Selby Suite 306, Emblem House, London Bridge Hospital, Tooley St., London SE1 2PN Tel: 020 7403 5858 Fax: 020 7357 8192 — MB BChir Camb. 1967 (Westm.) MRCS Eng. LRCP Lond. 1966; MB BChir (Distinc.) Camb. 1967; MA Camb. 1967; MRCP (UK) 1970; FRCS Eng. 1971. Cons. Orthop. Surg. Guy's Hosp. Lond. Specialty: Orthop. Socs: Fell. BOA; (Ex-Pres.) Europ. Soc. Surg. of Shoulder & Elbow; Corresp. Mem. Amer. Soc. of Shoulder & Elbow Surg. Prev: Lect. Inst. Orthop. Lond.; Regist. Westm. Hosp. Lond.

WATSON, Michael William Pasteur Mérieux MSD Ltd., Mallards Reach, Bridge Avenue, Maidenhead SL6 1QP Tel: 01628 587632 Fax: 01628 671722; 123 Stormont Road, London SW11 5EJ Tel: 020 7223 5958 — MB ChB Birm. 1988; MRCP (UK) 1992; Dip. Pharm. Med. RCP (UK) 1995. Med. Dir. Pasteur Mérieux MSD Ltd. UK. Specialty: Pharmaceutical Medicine. Socs: Brit. Assn. Pharmaceut. Phys.; Roy. Soc. Med. Prev: Clin. Project Scientist Takeda Euro R & D Centre GmbH; Med. Adviser Bristol-Meyers Squibb Pharmaceut. Ltd.; Regist. Rotat. (Gastroenterol.) Barking Hosp.

WATSON, Michael William St Isan Road Surgery, 46 St. Isan Road, Heath, Cardiff CF14 4UR Tel: 029 2062 7518 Fax: 029 2052 2886; 12 Mill Close, Lisvane, Cardiff CF14 0XQ Tel: 029 2076 3354 Fax: 029 2076 4777 — MB ChB Bristol 1964; DMJ (Clin.) Soc. Apoth. Lond. 1971; DCCH RCP Ed. RCGP & FCM 1983. Socs: Cardiff Med. Soc. Prev: Clin. Asst. (Psychiat.) Bristol Roy. Infirm.; Ho. Surg. Bristol Roy. Infirm.; Ho. Phys. Bristol Roy. Hosp. Sick Childr.

WATSON, Neale Ramsay The Hillingdon Hospital, Pield Heath Road, Uxbridge UB8 3NN Tel: 01865 279445 Fax: 01865 279444 Email: nrwatson@denham.demon.co.uk; Antiquities, Village Road, Denham Village, Uxbridge UB9 5BE Tel: 01865 834635 — MB BS Lond. 1983 (Roy. Free Hosp.) MRCOG 1992. Cons. O & G Hillingdon Hosp. Uxbridge. Specialty: Obst. & Gyn. Socs: Fell. Roy. Soc. Med. (Obst. & Gyn. Sect.). Prev: Regist. (O & G) King's Coll. Hosp. Lond.; Lect. (O & G) John Radcliffe Hosp. Oxf.

WATSON, Nicholas Alan Eastbourne District General Hospital, Eastbourne BN21 2UD Tel: 01323 417400; 15 The Grove, Patton Ratton, Eastbourne BN20 9DA — MB BS Lond. 1984; FRCA Eng. 1988. Cons. Anaesth. Eastbourne Dist. Gen. Hosp. Specialty: Anaesth.; Intens. Care. Socs: Assn. Anaesth.; Europ. Intens. Care Soc. Prev: Sen. Regist. (Anaesth.) St. Mary's Hosp. Lond.; Regist. (Anaesth.) St. Mary's Hosp. Lond.; SHO (Anaesth.) Eastbourne Dist. Gen. Hosp.

WATSON, Nicholas Andrew 30A Wimpole St, London W1G 8YA Tel: 07000 781687; Melmore, 10 Golf Road, Stanton-on-the-Wolds, Keyworth, Nottingham NG12 5BH Tel: 0160 773603 — BM BS Nottm. 1975; DCH Eng. 1979; MRCGP 1979; Cert. JCC Lond. 1980. Pres. Soc. Orthop. Med. Specialty: Orthop. Socs: Fell. (Pres.) Soc. Orthop. Med.; Brit. Inst. Orthop. Med. & Roy. Soc. Med. Prev: Treas. Inst. Orthop. Med.; Chairm. Soc. Orthop. Med.

WATSON, Nicholas Timothy Bryce 8 Corberry Avenue, Dumfries DG2 7QQ Email: brycewatson@compuserve.com — MB ChB St. And. 1972; DObst RCOG 1974; FFA RCS Eng. 1977. Cons. Anaesth. Dumfries & Galloway Health Bd. Specialty: Anaesth.

WATSON, Mr Nicolas James James Paget Hospital, Lowestoft Road, Great Yarmouth NR31 6LA Tel: 01493 452452; Bracken Hill, Priory Road, St. Olaves, Great Yarmouth NR31 9HQ — BM Soton. 1984; FRCS Eng. 1988; FRCOphth 1988. Cons. Ophth. Jas. Paget Hosp. Gt. Yarmouth. Specialty: Ophth.

WATSON, Nigel Frank Arnewood Practice, Milton Medical Centre, Avenue Road, New Milton BH25 5JP Tel: 01425 620393 Fax: 01425 624219; 8 Albert Road, New Milton BH25 6SP Tel: 01425 621130 Fax: 01425 621130 Email: nfwat@aol.com — MB BS Lond. 1982 (Westm.) DCH RCP Lond. 1985; DRCOG 1986; Cert. Family Plann. JCC 1986; MRCGP 1987. GP Princip. New Milton; Chairm. LMC Soton. & SW Hants.; GPC Wessex Regional Represen.; Bd. Mem. PCG. Prev: Trainee GP Rugby VTS; SHO Roy. Nat. Orthop. Hosp. Lond.; SHO (A & E) Univ. Coll. Hosp. Lond.

WATSON, Norman Philip (retired) Sandford St Martin, Chipping Norton OX7 7AG — MB ChB Liverp. 1945. Prev: Regist. (Med.) Roy. Infirm. Liverp.

WATSON, Norval 628 Fulwood Road, Sheffield S10 3QJ Tel: 0114 230 5102 — (Glas.) MB ChB Glas. 1946; DPH Glas. 1953. Emerit. Cons. Spinal Injuries Unit Lodge Moor Hosp. Sheff. Specialty: Orthop. Socs: Internat. Soc. Paraplegia. Prev: Dep. Phys. Supt. Lodge Moor Hosp. Sheff.; Regist. (Infec. Dis.) Ruchill Hosp. Glas.; Surg. Lt. RN.

WATSON, Patricia Mary School Clinic, Morley St., Brighton BN2 2RA Tel: 01273 693600; 4 Court Ord Road, Rottingdean, Brighton BN2 7FD — MB BS Newc. 1973. Specialty: Community Child Health.

WATSON, Paul Anthony Windrush Health Centre, Welch Way, Witney OX28 6JS Tel: 01993 702911 Fax: 01993 700931 — BM BCh Oxf. 1983 (Oxford, Cambridge) MA Camb. 1984; DRCOG 1985; DCH RCP Lond. 1986; MRCGP 1987. GP Princip. Windrush Health Centre Witney. Prev: Trainee GP Windsor VTS.; Ho. Phys. Horton Gen. Hosp. Banbury; Ho. Surg. Profess. Unit John Radcliffe Hosp. Oxf.

WATSON, Paul Stephen Essex Strategic Health Authority, Collingwood Road, Witham CM8 2TT Tel: 01376 302253; 40 Plumian Way, Balsham, Cambridge CB1 6EG Tel: 01223 290905 — MB BChir Camb. 1988 (Univ. Camb. Clin. Sch.) MA Camb. 1989; DCH RCP Lond. 1990; MFPHM RCP (UK) 1992; MPH Leeds 1992. Med. Dir. Essex Strategic Health Auth. Specialty: Pub. Health Med. Prev: Dir. of Acute Servs. Camb. & Hunt. HA; Cons. Pub. Health Med. Wakefield HA.

WATSON, Penelope Ann Dr I H McKee and Partners, Wester Hailes Health Centre, 7 Murrayburn Gate, Edinburgh EH14 2SS Tel: 0131 537 7300 Fax: 0131 537 7337; 37 Fernielaw Avenue, Edinburgh EH13 0EF Tel: 0131 441 5827 Fax: 0131 441 6253 — MB ChB Ed. 1972; DObst RCOG 1974; MRCGP 1984; MFFP 1993; M.Sc (Public Helath), Edin., 1999. Community Med. Off. (Family Plann.) Lothian HB; GP Mem. of S.W. Edin., LHCC for Clinic Effectiveness. Specialty: Family Plann. & Reproduc. Health; Pub. Health Med. Socs: BMA; Scott. Family Plann. Med. Soc.; GP Writers Assn. Prev: SHO Simpson Memor. Matern. Pavil. Ed.; Ho. Off. Roy. Infirm. Ed.; GP Locality Coordinator S. W. Edin. at Lothian Health.

WATSON, Peter (retired) Apartment 16, Martello Place, Golf Road, Felixstowe IP11 7NB Tel: 01394 276919 — MB ChB Liverp. 1955. JP. Prev: Sen. Med. Off. DHSS Centr. Office Norcross, Blackpool.

WATSON, Peter Greystones, 2 Main St., Newtown Linford, Leicester LE6 0AD — MB ChB Manch. 1958; DObst RCOG 1961; MRCGP 1971. Prev: Ho. Surg. Profess. Unit Manch. Roy. Infirm.; Ho. Phys. & Sen. Ho. Off. (Paediat.) Pk. Hosp. Davyhulme.

WATSON, Peter George Newcastle General Hospital, Department of Genitourinary Medicine, Westgate Road, Newcastle upon Tyne NE4 6BE Tel: 0191 256 3257 Fax: 0191 256 3256 — MB ChB Ed. 1979 (Univ. Ed.) BSc (Med. Sci.) (Hons.) Ed. 1976; MRCP (UK) 1982; DMRD Ed. 1984. Cons. Genitourin. Med. Newc. City Health NHS Trust & Northumbria Health Care NHS Trust; Clin. Lect. Infec. Dis.s & Trop. Med. Univ. Newc. u. Tyne. Specialty: Genitourinary Medicine. Socs: (Sec.) Assn. Genitourin. Med.; Med. Soc. Study of VD; Soc. Study Sexually Transm. Dis. Irel. Prev: Sen. Regist. (Genitourin. Med.) Glas. Roy. Infirm.; Regist. (Radiol.) Roy. Infirm. Edin.

WATSON, Professor Peter Gordon 17 Adams Road, Cambridge CB3 9AD Tel: 01223 353789 Fax: 01223 460910 — MB BChir Camb. 1957 (Univ. Coll. Hosp.) MRCS Eng. LRCP Lond. 1956; MA Camb. 1957; DO Eng. 1960; FRCS Eng. 1963; FRCOphth 1988. Boerhaave Prof., Univ. of Leiden, Netherlands; Chairm. Educat. Internat. Counc. Ophth.; Hon. Cons. Addenbrooke's Hosp. Camb; Hon. Cons., Moorfields Eye Hosp., Lond. Specialty: Ophth. Socs: Academia Ophthalmologica Internationalis; FRCOpth. (Honoris Causi). Prev: Sen. Lect. Inst. Ophth. & Moorfields Eye Hosp.; Sen. Resid. Ophth. Moorfields Eye Hosp.; Ho. Surg. & Ho. Phys. Univ. Coll. Hosp. Lond.

WATSON, Peter James Tanfield View Surgery, Scott Street, Stanley DH9 8AD Tel: 01207 232384; The Cardinals, Queens Road, Blackhill, Consett DH8 0BL Tel: 01207 509428 — (Nottm.) BMedSci Nottm. 1976; BM BS Nottm. 1978; MRCGP 1984.

WATSON, Mr Peter Sherratt (retired) 8 Stratton Place, Shop Lane, Wells-next-the-Sea NR23 1JR — MB BS Lond. 1948 (St. Mary's) MRCS Eng. LRCP Lond. 1949; FRCOG 1968, M 1954; FRCS Eng. 1957. Prev: Cons. Obstetr. & Gynaecol. Qu. Eliz. II Hosp. Welwyn Gdn. City.

WATSON, Mr Philip Charles (retired) 2 Station New Road, Brundall, Norwich NR13 5PQ Tel: 01603 712137 — MB BS Lond. 1942 (St. Bart.) MRCS Eng. LRCP Lond. 1941; FRCS Eng. 1946. Cons. Surg. Pilgrim Hosp. Boston. Prev: Surg. Tutor & Chief Asst. St. Bart. Hosp.

WATSON, Philippa Jane Quartly Department of Anaesthetics, Wycombe General Hospital, High Wycombe HP11 2TT Tel: 01494 426523 Fax: 01494 426524; Forge House, Coleshill, Amersham HP7 0LR Tel: 01494726736 — MB ChB Dundee 1973; FFA RCS Eng. 1978. Cons. Anaesth. Wycombe Gen. Hosp. Specialty: Anaesth.

WATSON, Rachel 58 Barons Mead, Southampton SO16 9TD — BM Soton. 1993.

WATSON, Rachel Halliwell Surgery, Lindfield Drive, Bolton BL1 3RG Tel: 01204 23642; 23 Third Street, Bolton BL1 7NN — BM BS Nottm. 1988; DFFP 1994; MRCGP 1994.

WATSON, Reginald Hubert (retired) Glendyne, Haygrove Road, Bridgwater TA6 7HZ — MB BCh BAO NUI 1938; DPH Leeds 1942; MFCM 1947. Med. Off. Health Bridgwater.

WATSON, Richard James Craigallian Avenue Surgery, 11 Craigallian Avenue, Cambuslang, Glasgow G72 8RW Tel: 0141 641 3129 — MB ChB Glas. 1983; MRCGP 1989; DCH RCP Lond. 1989; DRCOG 1990. GP Cambuslang Glas. Prev: GP Belén Nicaragua.

WATSON, Richard Marshall Manor House Surgery, Providence Place, Bridlington YO15 2QW Tel: 01262 602661 Fax: 01262 400891; Tara, Great Edstone, York YO62 6PB Tel: 01751 432036 — MB BS Lond. 1975. Specialty: Ophth.

WATSON, Richard Scott Hawthorne Cottage, 56 Ridge St., Stourbridge DY8 4QF — MB BS Lond. 1983.

WATSON, Robert Alistair Mackay Dr A Wilson and Partners, Sighthill Health Centre, 380 Calder Road, Edinburgh EH11 4AU Tel: 0131 537 7060; 1 Loaning Crescent, Peebles EH45 9JR — MB ChB Ed. 1976 (Edinburgh) DTCH Liverp. 1982; MRCP (UK) 1984; MRCGP 1986. Specialty: Community Child Health.

WATSON, Robert Anthony 16 Coplow Avenue, Tean, Stoke-on-Trent ST10 4JQ — MB ChB Leeds 1993.

WATSON, Robert Daniel Steadman 4 Richmond Hill Gardens, Edgbaston, Birmingham B15 3RW — MD Birm. 1981; BSc Birm. 1970, MB ChB 1973; MRCP (UK) 1976; FRCP Lond. 1989. Cons. Cardiol. City Hosp. Dudley Rd. Birm.; Hon. Sen. Lect. Univ. Birm.; Clin. Sub-dean Univ. Birm. Specialty: Cardiol. Socs: Brit. Cardiac Soc.; Brit. Cardiovasc. Interven. Soc. Prev: Cons. Cardiol. Dudley Rd. Hosp. Birm.; Lect. Dept. Med. Univ. Birm.; SHO (Med.) Llandough Hosp. Penarth.

WATSON, Robert Doré St Marys Road Surgery, St. Marys Road, Newbury RG14 1EQ Tel: 01635 31444 Fax: 01635 551316 — MB BS Lond. 1973; MRCGP 1978.

WATSON, Robert George Peter Grandview, 21 Ballymenoch Road, Holywood BT18 0HH Tel: 01232 426486 — MB BCh BAO Belf. 1977; BSc (Hons.) Physiol. Belf. 1974, MD 1985, MB BCh BAO 1977; MRCP (UK) 1981. Sen. Lect. & Cons. Phys. Med. Qu. Univ. Belf. & Roy. Vict. Hosp. Belf. Specialty: Gastroenterol. Prev: Sen. Regist. (Internal Med.) EHSSB.

WATSON, Robert Graham Dunblane Medical Practice, Heatlh Centre, Well Place, Dunblane FK15 9BQ Tel: 01786 822595 Fax: 01786 825298 — MB ChB Ed. 1983; Cert. Family Plann. JCC 1985; DRCOG 1985.

WATSON, Mr Robert John Four Trees, 159 Ribchester Road, Clayton Le Dale, Blackburn BB1 9EE Tel: 01254 245879 — MB BS Newc. 1977; FRCS Eng. 1981; ChM Manch. 1987. Cons. Surg. Blackburn Roy. Infirm. Specialty: Gen. Surg.

WATSON, Robin Joseph Derby Road Practice, 52 Derby Road, Ipswich IP3 8DN Tel: 01473 728121 Fax: 01473 718810; Tarnside Road, Witnesham, Ipswich IP6 9EH — BSc (1st cl. Hons.) Belf. 1973, MB BCh 1976; DRCOG 1982; MRCGP 1982.

WATSON, Ronald Innes Courtyard Surgery, The Courtyard, London Road, Horsham RH12 1AT Tel: 01403 253100 Fax: 01403 267480 — MB BS Lond. 1975 (Middlx.) DRCOG 1978. Prev: Resid. Med. Off. St. Margt.'s Hosp. Wom. Sydney & Mater Miser.; Childr. Hosp. Brisbane Australia; Resid. (Med.) Toronto E. Gen. Hosp. Canada.

WATSON, Sally Jane Collfryn, Bethesda Bach, Caernarfon LL54 5SH — MB ChB Manch. 1997.

WATSON, Sandra Jane Surrey Hampshire Borders NHS Trust, Farnham Road Hospital, Farnham Road, Guildford GU2 7LX Tel: 01483 443535 — MB BS Lond. 1978; MRCS Eng. LRCP Lond. 1978; Cert. Family Plann. JCC 1980; MRCPsych 1986. Cons. Psychiat. Surrey Hants. Borders NHS Trust Guildford. Specialty: Gen. Psychiat.

WATSON, Sarah Anne Mangrove Hall Farm Cottage, Mangrove Green, Cockernhoe, Luton LU2 8QE — MB ChB Cape Town 1988.

WATSON, Simon Dominic John Flat 4, 19-21Parkfield Road, Bradford BD8 7AA — MB BS Newc. 1988.

WATSON, Simon James Montalto Medical Centre, 2 Dromore Rd, Ballynahinch BT24 8AH — MB ChB BAO Belf. 1988; DMH Belf. 1991; DRCOG 1992; MRCGP 1993; DCH RCPI 1994; DFFP Belfast 1995. Dep. Forens. Med. Off.. Belf.

WATSON, Simon James William Phagocyte Laboratory, MRC Centre for Inflammation Research, 1st Floor, Medical School, Teviot Place, Edinburgh EH8 9AG Email: simon.watson@ed.ac.uk — MB ChB Liverp. 1996; BClinSci. (1st cl. Hons.) Liverp. 1995; MB ChB (Commendation) Liverp. 1996; MRCP UK Feb 1999. Clin. Research Fell. MRC Centre for Inflammation Research; Specialist Regist. (Nephrol. & Gen. Med.) Roy. Infirm. Edin. Specialty: Gen. Med. Socs: UK Renal Association. Prev: SHO (Gen. Med.) Queen's Med. Centre Univ. Hosp. Nottm.; Ho. Phys. & Surg. Roy. Liverp. Hosp.

WATSON, Simon Paul 34 Millfield Gardens, Nether Poppleton, York YO26 6NZ — MB ChB Leeds 1989; DRCOG 1992; DCH RCP Lond. 1994.

WATSON, Simon Peter Atter The Surgery, Worcester Road, Great Witley, Worcester WR6 6HR Tel: 01299 896370 Fax: 01299 896873 — MB BS Nottm. 1982; DRCOG 1985; MRCGP 1987.

WATSON, Stanley Valentine John (retired) 4 Edgerton Road, Leeds LS16 5JD — MB BS Durh. 1954. Prev: Ref. Div. Med. Serv.

WATSON, Stephen David Royal Albert Edward Infirmary, Wigan Lane, Wigan WN1 2NN Tel: 01942 244000; 1 Amber Grove, Westhoughton, Bolton BL5 3LE Tel: 01942 811707 — MB ChB Manch. 1985; BSc Manch. 1982; MRCP (UK) 1990; FRCR 1996. Cons. Radiol. Wigan & Leigh NHS Trust. Specialty: Radiol.

WATSON, Stephen John Lincoln Road Practice, 63 Lincoln Road, Peterborough PE1 2SF Tel: 01733 565511 Fax: 01733 569230 — MB ChB Dundee 1982; BSc (Hons.) Dund 1978, MB ChB 1982; DRCOG 1984; MRCGP 1986. Socs: BMA. Prev: Trainee GP Angus VTS; Jun. Med. Ho. Off. King's Cross Hosp. Dundee; Jun. Surg. Ho. Off. Ninewells Hosp. Dundee.

WATSON, Mr Stewart Fernleigh Consulting Centre, 77 Alderley Road, Wilmslow SK9 1PA Tel: 01625 536488 Fax: 01625 548348 — (Univ. Coll. Hosp.) MB Camb. 1971, BChir 1970; MRCP (UK) 1972; FRCS Eng. 1974. Cons. Plastic & Hand Surg. Wythenshaw Hosp., Manch. &Pendelbury Childr. Hosp. & Hope Hosp. Specialty: Plastic Surg. Socs: BSSH; BAPS; BAAPS. Prev: Cons. Plastic Surg. St. Lawrence Hosp. Plastic & Reconstruc. Surg. Centre Chepstow; Sen. Regist. (Plastic Surg.) Withington Hosp. Manch.

WATSON, Stuart Department of Psychiatry, Leazes Wing, RUI, Newcastle upon Tyne Email: stuart.watson@ncl.ac.uk — MB BS Newc. 1992 (Nescastle) MRCPsych 1997. Regist. (Psychiat.) Northern Regional Rotat. Specialty: Gen. Psychiat. Prev: SHO Rotat. (Psychiat.) N.d.

WATSON, Stuart Brown — MB ChB Aberd. 1984. Specialty: Plastic Surg.

WATSON, Susan Clare Stockwell Lodge Medical Centre, Rosedale Way, Cheshunt, Waltham Cross EN7 6HL Tel: 01992 624408 Fax: 01992 626206 — MB BS Lond. 1978 (Roy. Free) DRCOG 1981.

WATSON, Susan Victoria Worth Hall Paddock, Turners Hill Road, Worth, Crawley RH10 4PE Tel: 01293 883962 — MB BS Lond. 1984; BSc (Intercalated) Lond. 1981; Cert. Family Plann. JCC 1988; DRCOG 1988.

WATSON, Tara Elizabeth 49 Wilton Crescent, Southampton SO15 2QG — BM Soton l984; DCH RCP Lond. 1987; MRCGP 1988. GP Soton Retainer Scheme. Socs: BMA. Prev: Trainee GP Hants.

WATSON, Terence Mark (retired) 8 North Road, Builth Wells LD2 3BU Tel: 01982 552337 — MB BS Lond. 1970; DObst RCOG 1975. Chairm. & Powys Commissioning Gp. Prev: Ho. Surg. & Ho. Phys. King's Lynn Dist. Hosp.

WATSON, Theresa Olivia Tara, Great Edstone, York YO62 6PB Tel: 017514 32036 — MB ChB Birm. 1960; BA 1998. Prev: Med. Off. WHO Smallpox Progr. Bangladesh.

WATSON, Timothy Mark Furze Cottage, Cheriton Bishop, Exeter EX6 6HF — BM BS Nottm. 1994.

WATSON, Timothy Peter Flat 1, 52 West End Lane, West Hampstead, London NW6 2NE — MB BS Lond. 1997.

WATSON, Timothy Richard The Surgery, Village Hall, Worthen, Shrewsbury SY5 9HT Tel: 01743 891401 Fax: 01743 891668; Plox Cottage, Brockton, Worthen, Shrewsbury SY5 9HU — MB ChB Liverp. 1967.

WATSON, Tracey Elizabeth 14 Park View Avenue, Burley Park, Leeds LS4 2LH — MB ChB Leeds 1992; MRCP Glasgow 1999. Specialty: Accid. & Emerg.

WATSON, Veronica Frances 27 Well Orchard, Bamberbridge, Preston PR5 8HJ — MB ChB Glas. 1989.

WATSON, Wendy Anne 14 Granville Place, Aberdeen AB10 6NZ — MB ChB Aberd. 1995.

WATSON, William Forbes Beech House Surgery, 1 Ash Tree Road, Knaresborough HG5 0UB Tel: 01423 542564 — MB BCh BAO Belf. 1975; DRCOG 1977.

WATSON, William Frederick (retired) The Rose Garden, Oldlands Hall, Herons Ghyll, Uckfield TN22 3DA Tel: 01825 712369 Fax: 01825 712224 — D(OBST)RCOG 1950; LRCP LRCS Ed. LRCPS Glas. 1948.

WATSON, William Howison Haematology Department, Monklands District General Hospital, Airdrie ML6 0JS Tel: 01236 712099/01236 748748 Fax: 01236 746129 Email: william.watson@laht.scot.nhs.uk; Hundalee, Larch Avenue, Lenzie, Glasgow G66 4HX Tel: 0141 777 6405 — (Glasgow) BSc (Hons. Physiol.) Glas. 1966; MB ChB (Commend.) Glas. 1968; MRCP (UK) 1975; FRCPath 1987, M 1975; FRCP Glas. 1987. Cons. Haemat. Monklands Gen. Hosp. Airdrie; Hon. Clin. Sen. Lect. Univ. Glas. Specialty: Haematology. Prev: Lect. (Haemat.) Univ. Dept. Haemat. Glas. West. Infirm.

WATSON, William Humphreys, MBE, MC (retired) 17 St John's Hill, Shrewsbury SY1 1JJ Tel: 01743 231387 — (Guy's) MB BS Lond. 1950; MRCS Eng. LRCP Lond. 1950; DObst RCOG 1952; MRCGP 1967. Prev: Res. Obstetr. . Guy's Hosp.

WATSON, William Rowell (retired) The Little Manor House, 9 Manor Close, Tunbridge Wells TN4 8YB Tel: 01892 528261 — MRCS Eng. LRCP Lond. 1941 (Guy's) DA Eng. 1944; FFA RCS Eng. 1954. Hon. Cons. Anaesth. Eastbourne Health Dists.

WATSON, Winifred (retired) Melrose, Stapleton, Presteigne LD8 2LR Tel: 01544 267330 Fax: 01544 267330 — MB ChB Leeds 1954.

WATSON, Winifred Mary Bertha (retired) 17 St John's Hill, Shrewsbury SY1 1JJ — MB ChB Aberd. 1947.

WATSON, Yolanda Maria Rita 5 West Park Gardens, Dundee DD2 1NY — MB ChB Ed. 1973; BSc (Med. Sci.) Ed. 1970, MB ChB 1973. Clin. Asst. Gen. Adult Psychiat. Allardy Centre Dundee. Specialty: Gen. Psychiat.

WATSON-HOPKINSON, William Ian (retired) 12 Highclere Drive, Camberley GU15 1JY Tel: 01276 502222 — MB BS Lond. 1958; BSc (Anat.) Lond. 1955, MB BS 1958; MFOM RCP Lond. 1982. Prev: Centre for Human Sci. Defence Research Agency FarnBoro. Hants.

WATSON-JONES, Alan (retired) Gardener's Cottage, Airds Bay, Taynuilt PA35 1JR Tel: 01866 822356 — MB ChB Birm. 1942. Prev: Ho. Phys. Qu. Eliz. Hosp. Birm.

WATSON-JONES, Deborah Lindsay 12 Walden Lodge Close, Devizes SN10 5BU — BM BCh Oxf. 1988; BA (Hons.) Zool. Oxf. 1982; MRCP (UK) 1992; MSc (Communicable Dis. Epidemiol.) Lond. 1995; PhD Univ. Of Lond. 2001. Clin. Lect. Lond. Sch. Hyg. & Trop. Med. Lond. Socs: BMA; Study Soc. VD; Roy. Soc. Trop. Med. & Hyg. Prev: Research Fell. Lond. Sch. Hyg. & Trop. Med. Lond.

WATSON-JONES, Esther Margaret Christine 2 The Steadings, Clifton, Morpeth NE61 6AH — MB ChB Cape Town 1968.

WATT, Alan 74 St David's Way, Watford Farm, Caerphilly CF83 1EZ — MB ChB Aberd. 1986. Regist. (Geriat. Med.) Llandough Hosp. Cardiff. Specialty: Gen. Med. Prev: Regist. (Geriat. Med.) Caerphilly Miners Dist. Hosp.; SHO (A & E) N. Tees Gen. Hosp. Stockton-on-Tees; Ho. Off. (Med.) New Cross Hosp. Wolverhampton.

WATT, Alan Douglas Waddesdon Surgery, Goss Avenue, Waddesdon, Aylesbury HP18 0LY Tel: 01296 658585 Fax: 01296 658467; 2 Manor Gardens, Main St, Grendon Underwood, Aylesbury HP18 0UT — MB BS Lond. 1980 (Charing Cross) DRCOG 1983; MRCGP 1985. Gen. Med. Practitioner, Aylesbury, Bucks.

WATT, Alastair James 32 Bradley Street, Wotton-under-Edge GL12 7AR — MB BS Lond. 1996.

WATT, Alastair James McCurrach Worcester Street Surgery, 24 Worcester Street, Stourbridge DY8 1AW Tel: 01384 371616; 24 Worcester Street, Stourbridge DY8 1AW Tel: 01384 371616 — MRCS Eng. LRCP Lond. 1971 (Roy. Free) BSc (Biochem.) Lond. 1968, MB BS 1971; DRCOG 1977; MRCGP 1979. Assoc. RCPath. Lond.; Mem. Primary Health Care, Specialist Gp. Brit. Computer Soc. Prev: SHO (Paediat.) Wordsley Hosp. nr Stourbridge; Regist. (Path.) Bristol Roy. Infirm.; SHO (Psychiat.) Burton Rd. Hosp. Dudley.

WATT, Alastair McEwan Waterside Medical Centre, Court Street, Leamington Spa CV31 2BB Tel: 01926 428321 Fax: 01926 458350 — BM BS Nottm. 1985; BMedSci 1983; DCH RCP Lond. 1987; DRCOG 1988; MRCGP 1989.

WATT, Alexander John (retired) 32 Spoutwells Drive, Scone, Perth PH2 6RR Tel: 01738 551548 — MB ChB Aberd. 1956. Prev: Authorised Med. Examr. Civil Aviat. Auth.

WATT, Alison Margaret (retired) Tarrywood, Whitchurch, Tavistock PL19 9LE Tel: 01822 612304 Fax: 01822 612304 — (Westm.) MB BS (Hons.) Lond. 1955; FRCOG 1989, M 1960, DObst 1957. Prev: Assoc. Specialist (Colposcopy) Derriford Hosp. Plymouth.

WATT, Andrew Graeme 11 Draffen Mont, Stewarton KA3 5LG Email: 100743.3514@compuserve.com — MB ChB Glas. 1983; BSc (Hons.) Glas. 1979; MRCP (UK) 1989; DTM & H Liverp. 1990. Cons. Phys. and Geritatrician, Biggart and Ayr Hosps., Ayrsh. Prev: Med. Off. Lady Willingdon Hosp. Manali, India; Specialist Regist. (Gen. & Geriat. Med.) Glas.

WATT, Andrew James Bruce Dept. Of Diagnostic Imaging & Clinical Physics, The Royal Hospital for Sick Children, Dalnair Street, Yorkhill, Glasgow G3 8SJ Tel: 0141 201 0100 Fax: 0141 201 0098 — MB ChB Glas. 1990; MRCP Glas. 1993; FRCR 1997. Cons. Paediatric Radiologist, Roy. Hosp. for Sick Childr., Glas. Specialty: Radiol. Socs: Roy. Coll. Phys. & Surgs. Glas.; Fell. Roy. Coll. Radiols.

WATT, Andrew Niall Finlayson Street Practice, 33 Finlayson Street, Fraserburgh AB43 9JW Tel: 01346 518088 Fax: 01346 510015 — MB ChB Aberd. 1986; MRCGP 1992.

WATT, Anne Mure Strathbogie Cottage, Cormistone, Biggar ML12 6NS Tel: 0189 93 236 — MB ChB Ed. 1939; Dip. Soc. Med. 1970.

WATT, Archibald David Glasgow Occupational Health, Glasgow Royal Infirmary, Wishart Street, Glasgow G31 3HT Tel: 0141 211 0427 Email: david.watt@northglasgow.scot.nhs.uk; 15 Newtyle Road, Paisley PA1 3JU Tel: 0141 882 1078 Fax: 0141 882 1078 Email: d.watt@watt90.freeserve.co.uk — MB ChB Dundee 1973; DCH RCPS Glas. 1976; DRCOG 1977; MRCGP 1979; FFOM RCP Lond. 1993, M 1984, A 1983; FRCP Glas 1999; FRCP, RCP (Glas) 1999. Cons. Occupat. Med. Gtr. Glas. HB.; Hon. Sen. Lect. (Pub. Health) Univ. Glas.; Chairm. Scot-Gp. Soc. Specialty: Occupat. Health. Socs: Epilespy Assn. Scotl. Prev: Med. Off. The Post Office Glas.; Employm. Med. Adviser HSE Glas.; Train. Progr. Dir. In Ocupational Med. W. of Scotl. PostGrad. Med Educ. Bd.

WATT, Barry Bydand Medical Group, Jubilee Hospital, Bleachfield Street, Huntly AB54 8EX Tel: 01466 792116 Fax: 01466 794699 — MB ChB Aberd. 1989; MRCGP 1993. GP. Specialty: Gen. Pract. Prev: SHO (Orthop. & Cas.) Borders Gen. Hosp. Melrose.; Trainee GP Peebles.

WATT, Brian (retired) Mycobacteria Laboratory, City Hospital, Edinburgh EH10 5SB Tel: 0131 536 6357 Fax: 0131 536 6152; Silverburn House, Penicuik EH26 9LF Tel: 01968 672085 — MB ChB Ed. 1965; MD Ed. 1972; FRCPath. 1984; FRCP Ed. 1993. Dir. Scott. Mycobact. Ref. Laborat.; Cons. Bacteriol. City Hosp. Edin.; Pat. Servs. Dir. Med. Microbiol. Servs. Lothain Univ. Hosp. NHS Trust; Hon. Sen. Lect. (Bact.) Univ. Edin. Prev: Cons. Microbiol. West. Gen. Hosp. Edin.

WATT, Carolyn Susan St John's Hospice, Slyne Road, Lancaster LA2 6ST Tel: 01524 382538 — MB ChB Glas. 1982; DRCOG 1984; MRCGP 1986; Dip. Palliat. Med. Wales 1997. Assoc. Specialist (Palliat. Care) St John's Hospice Lancaster. Specialty: Palliat. Med. Socs: Assn. Palliat. Med.; BMA; Palliat. Care Forum. Prev: Palliat. Care Phys. Butterwick Hospice, Stockton-upon-Tees; Clin. Asst. Palliat. Med. St John's Hospice Slyne Lancaster; GP Irvine.

WATT, Cynthia Mary 50 Stockport Road, Marple, Stockport SK6 6AB Tel: 0161 426 0299 Fax: 0161 427 8112; 34 Townscliffe Lane, Mellor, Stockport SK6 5AP — MB ChB Manch. 1979; DRCOG 1981.

WATT, David Campbell (retired) 75 Wykeham Way, Haddenham, Aylesbury HP17 8BU Tel: 01844 291966 — (Glas.) MB ChB Glas. 1943; DPM Eng. 1948; BSc Glas. 1940, MD 1951; FRCPsych 1972. Prev: Hon. Cons. Med. Genetics Churchill Hosp. Oxf.

WATT, David Erickson Tollgate Health Centre, 220 Tollgate Road, London E6 5JS Tel: 0207 445 7700 Fax: 0207 445 7715; 70 Cadogan Terrace, London E9 5HP Tel: 020 8986 3420 Fax: 020 8986 3420 — MB ChB Sheff. 1983; BMedSci Sheff. 1980. Socs: (Hon. Sec.) Balint Soc. Prev: Trainee GP Birm. & Lond. VTS.

WATT, David Sproul Langaller, Pilcorn St., Wedmore BS28 4AP — MB ChB Glas. 1944.

WATT, Douglas Arthur Lawrence (retired) Sruthan House, Lochaline, Morvern, Oban PA34 5XT Tel: 01967 421632 — MB ChB Glas. 1956; DObst RCOG 1958; FRFPS Glas. 1959; FRCP Lond. 1975, M 1961; FRCP Ed. 1974, M 1962; FRCP Glas. 1972. Prev: Cons. Phys. & Med. Dir. Chorley & S. Ribble NHS Trust.

WATT, Douglas Burns Stewart (retired) 53 Christian Fields, Norbury, London SW16 3JU Tel: 020 8764 8450 — LRCP LRCS Ed. 1949; LRCP LRCS Ed., LRFPS Glas. 1949.

WATT, Elizabeth — MB BCh BAO Belf. 1992; DCH RCPS Glas. 1998. Staff Grade Paediat.Ulster Hosp. Specialty: Paediat.

WATT, Elizabeth Margaret Department of Reproductive Medicine, St. Michaels Hospital, Southwell St., Bristol BS2 8EG Tel: 01179 285767 Fax: 01179 285792; Felwood House, Stanshalls Lane, Felton, Bristol BS40 9UQ Tel: 01275 472519 — (Roy. Free) MB BS Lond. 1966; DObst RCOG 1968; MFFP 1994. SCMO (Reproduc. Med.) United Bristol Healthcare Trust; Sen. Clin. Med. Off. N. Bristol NHS Trust & Taunton PCT; Research Assoc. UK Family Plann. Research Network Univ. Exeter; Assoc. Specialist, Brook Advis. Centre Bristol; Specialist Asst. Dept. Reproduct. Med. St. Michaels Hosp. Bristol. Specialty: Family Plann. & Reproduc. Health. Socs: Brit. Fertil. Soc.; Brit. Menopause Soc.; Brit. Soc. Paed. Adolesc. Gyn. Prev: Ho. Surg. (Obst.) Whittington Hosp.; Ho. Surg. Roy. Free Hosp.

WATT, Fiona Elizabeth 20 Morland Avenue, Leicester LE2 2PE — MB BS Newc. 1998.

WATT, Florence Anne Glenside Hospital, Blackberry Hill, Stapleton, Bristol BS16 1ED — MB ChB Ed. 1983; DRCOG 1985; MRCPsych 1990. Regist. (Psychiat.) Train Scheme Glenside Hosp. Bristol. Specialty: Forens. Psychiat. Prev: SHO (Psychiat.) Torbay Hosp. Train. Sch. Torquay; GP Plymouth; Trainee GP Dumfries & Galloway VTS.

WATT, Frances Joan — BM BCh Oxf. 1996 (Oxford) GP Locum Oxf. Specialty: Gen. Med. Prev: SHO Rotat. (Gen. Med.) Princess Margt. Hosp. Swindon.

WATT, Frances Katherine Fishponds Health Centre, Beechwood Road, Fishponds, Bristol BS16 3TD Tel: 0117 908 2365 Fax: 0117 908 2377; 17 Fordington Dairy, Athelstan Road, Dorchester DT1 1FD — MB BS Lond. 1989 (St Bart.'s) DRCOG; DFFP; MRCGP.

WATT, Gavin Michael Cluness Fadlydyke, Muad, Peterhead AB42 5RY — MB ChB Aberd. 1990.

WATT, Gordon Lorimer (retired) Rosebank, 30 Main St., Alford AB33 8PX Tel: 0197 55 62172 — MB ChB Aberd. 1949. Prev: GP Aberd.sh.

WATT, Professor Graham Charles Murray Department General Practice, University of Glasgow, 4 Lancaster Crescent, Glasgow G12 0RR Tel: 0141 211 1682 Fax: 0141 576 2010 Email: g.c.m.watt@clinmed.gla.ac.uk; 15 Banavie Road, Glasgow G11 5AW Tel: 0141 576 2010 — MD Aberd. 1990, BMedBiol (Path) 1973; MB ChB Aberd. 1976; MRCP (UK) 1979; MRCGP 1986; MFCM 1987; FRCP Glas. 1990; FFPHM RCP (UK) 1994; FRCGP 1999; F.Med.Sci 2000. Prof. Gen. Pract. & Head of Dept.; Attached Worker MRC Pub. Health & Social Serv.s Unit. Univ. Glas. Specialty: Gen. Pract.; Pub. Health Med. Prev: Sen. Lect. (Pub. Health) Univ. Glas.; Sen. Med. Off. Scott. Home & Health Dept. Edin.; Head Glas. Monica Project Centre.

WATT, Graham Cheyne (retired) 1A Old Priory Road, Easton-in-Gordano, Bristol BS20 0PB Tel: 01275 372214 — MB ChB Ed. 1937; DTM Liverp. 1938.

WATT, Graham John 6 Meadow Bank, Stockport SK4 2HL — MB ChB Manch. 1991.

WATT, Gregor 37 Kirkhill Road, Edinburgh EH16 5DE Tel: 0131 662 9912 — MB ChB Ed. 1992; BSc (Hons.) Med. Sci. Ed. 1991; DCCH RCP Ed. 1995; MRCGP 1997. Paediat. Regist. (Gen. Pract.). Specialty: Gen. Pract. Prev: Regist. (A & E) Melbourne, Austral.; SHO (O & G) Roy. Infirm. Edin.; SHO (Paediat.) Roy. Hosp. Sick Childr. Edin.

WATT, Helen Patricia (retired) 23 Suffolk Place, 1 Lime kiln Quay Road, Woodbridge IP12 1XB Tel: 01394 384078 — MB ChB St. And. 1952. Prev: Sen. Med. Off. (Ment. Health) Doncaster Co. Boro.

WATT, Iain (retired) 8 Parrys Grove, Stoke Bishop, Bristol BS9 1TT Tel: 0117 968 7101 Email: iain.watt@doctors.org.uk — (Lond. Hosp.) MB BS Lond. 1966; DObst RCOG 1968; MRCP (UK) 1970; DMRD Eng. 1972; FFR 1974; FRCR 1975; FRCP Lond. 1996. Cons. Radiol. United Bristol Healthcare NHS Trust. Prev: Sen. Regist. (Diag. Radiol.) Bristol Health Dist. (T).

WATT, Mr Iain Inverclyde Royal Hospital, Larkfield Road, Greenock PA16 0XN Tel: 01475 37103 — MB ChB 1976; FRCS Glas. 1982; MD Aberd. 1987. Cons. Gen. Surg. Inverclyde Roy. Hosp. Greenock. Specialty: Gen. Surg. Socs: Fell. Roy. Coll. Phys.s & Surveyor of Glas.; Assn. of Surg. Gt. Britain & Irel.

WATT, Ian Alexander Kennaway 3 Richmond Road, Heaton Mersey, Stockport SK4 3BZ.

WATT, Ian Douglas Watt and Partners, Wargrave House, 23 St. Owen Street, Hereford HR1 2JB Tel: 01432 272285 Fax: 01432 344059; The Pines, 52 Southbank Road, Hereford HR1 2TL Tel: 01432 272904 — MB BS Lond. 1972 (Lond. Hosp.) DObst RCOG 1975; DA Eng. 1977. GP Trainer Hereford VTS. Specialty: Gen. Pract.

WATT, Professor Ian Scot University of York, Department of Health Sciences, York YO10 5DD Tel: 01904 321341 Email: isw1@york.ac.uk; 50 Frenchgate, Richmond DL10 7AG Tel: 01748 850 913 — MB ChB Manch. 1981 (St Andrew's & Manchester Univ.) MPH Leeds 1991; MFPHM RCP, UK 1993; FFPHM RCP, UK 1999. Prof. (Primary & Community Care) Univ. of York; Hon. Cons. Pub. Health Med.; GP Princip. (Job Share). Specialty: Pub. Health Med.; Gen. Pract. Prev: Sen. Regist. (Pub. Health Med.) Yorks. RHA; GP Lancs.; Vis. Lect. (Pub. Health Med.) Univ. Leeds.

WATT, Sir James, KBE, Surg. Vice-Admiral (retired) 7 Cambisgate, Church Road, Wimbledon, London SW19 5AL Tel: 020 8947 0146 — (Durh.) MB BS Durh. 1938; MS Durh. 1949; FRCS Eng. 1955; FICS 1963; MD Newc. 1972; FRCP Lond. 1975; Hon. FRCS Ed. 1976; Hon. DCh Newc. 1978. Prev: Med. Dir.-Gen. Navy.

WATT, James Affleck Gilroy (retired) 3 Middleton Drive, Helensburgh G84 7BE — (Ed.) MB ChB Ed. 1958; FRCP Ed. 1977, M 1963; DPM Eng. 1966; MD Ed. 1970; FRCPsych 1985, M 1973. Prev: Cons. Psychiat. Gartnavel Roy. Hosp. Glas.

WATT, James Miller 36 Westfield Road, Edgbaston, Birmingham B15 3QG — MB ChB Birm. 1970; DObst RCOG 1972; DA Eng. 1973; FFA RCSI 1974. Cons. (Anaesth.) Centr. Birm. Health Dist. (T). Specialty: Anaesth.

WATT, Jean Barbara Meole Cottage, Mill Road, Meole Brace, Shrewsbury SY3 9JT — MB ChB Birm. 1972; MRCP (UK) 1975; FRCP Lond. 1994; FRCPCH 1997. Cons. Paediat. Cross Ho.s Shrewsbury & Roy. Shrewsbury Hosp. Specialty: Paediat. Socs: Brit. Paediat. Assn. Prev: Sen. Regist. St. Mary's Hosp. Lond.; Regist. (Paediat.) Hosp. Sick Childr. Gt. Ormond St.

WATT, John A (retired) Hillwood Cottage, Newbridge EH28 8LU — MB ChB Ed. 1941 (Oxf. & Ed.) BA Oxf. 1936; MLCOM 1989; MRO 1990. Prev: Lect. (Physiol.) Univ. Edin.

WATT, John Newton Queensway Medical Centre, Doctors Surgery, Queensway, Poulton-le-Fylde FY6 7ST Tel: 01253 890219 Fax: 01253 894222 — MB ChB Manch. 1985; DRCOG 1988; MRCGP 1989. Prev: Trainee GP Stockport Chesh. VTS.

WATT, John William Heddle Southport & Ormskirk Hospital Trust, Town Lane, Southport PR8 6PN Tel: 01704 547471 Fax: 01704 543156 Email: john.watt@southportandormskirk.nhs.uk; 26 Yew Tree Road, Ormskirk L39 1NU Tel: 01695 578843 Email: johnwhwatt@mauriceg.demon.co.uk — MB ChB Liverp. 1973 (MB ChB Liverpool 1973) FRCA Lond. 1977; MD Liverpool 1981. Cons. Anaesth. Southport & Ormskirk Acute Hosp. Trust. Specialty: Anaesth.

WATT, Jonathan William Glendinning Salford Royal Hospitals NHS Trust, Hope Hospital, Stott Lane, Salford M6 8HD Tel: 0161 789 7373; 5 Warwick Drive, Hale, Altrincham WA15 9EA Tel: 0161 928 6717 Email: jon@watt.u-net.com — MB BS Lond. 1985; FRCA. 1992. Cons. Pain Managem. & Anaesth., Salford Roy. Hosp. Specialty: Anaesth. Socs: Assn. Anaesth.

WATT, Joyce Mary (retired) 26 Guildford Drive, Chandlers Ford, Eastleigh SO53 3PT; 26 Guildford Drive, Chandlers Ford, Eastleigh SO53 3PT Tel: 023 80266 536 — (Char. Cross) MB BS Lond. 1957. Prev: SHO Chest Clinic Plaistow Hosp. Lond.

WATT, Karen Patricia 23 Forbes Road, Edinburgh EH10 4EG — MB ChB Ed. 1996. Specialty: Obst. & Gyn.

WATT, Linda Janet Leverndale Hospital, 510 Crookston Road, Glasgow G53 7TU — MB ChB Aberd. 1978; MRCPsych 1983; FRCPsych 1999. Med. Director & Cons. Psychiat. Glas. Specialty: Gen. Psychiat. Prev: Med. Servs. Manager & Cons. Psychiat. Glas.

WATT, Lisbeth Lynda 34 Craignish Avenue, Norbury, London SW16 4RN — MB ChB Bristol 1978; DO RCS Eng. 1982; FRCS Eng. 1985. Assoc. Specialist Ophth. Qu. Mary's Hosp. Sidcup.

WATT, Lucinda Mary Johnstone 8 Broomhill Court, Londonderry BT47 6WP — MB BCh BAO Belf. 1984; DCH Dub. 1988; DRCOG 1988; MRCGP 1989. Staff Grade c/o the Elderley Altnagelvin Area Hosp. Londonderry; Assoc. Specialist (Care of Elderly) Altnagelvin Hosps. Trust. Londonderry. Specialty: Care of the Elderly. Socs: MRCGP. Prev: GP Retainer Scheme, Crumlin Co. Antrim; SHO (Psychiat.) Holywell Hosp. Antrim; Trainee GP. Co. Antrim N. Irel. VTS.

WATT, Margaret Jean Terrago Lodge, 46 West St., Easton-on-the-Hill, Stamford PE9 3LS Tel: 01780 765562; Terrago Lodge, 46 West St., Easton-on-the-Hill, Stamford PE9 3LS — MB BS Lond. 1959 (Lond. Hosp.) DA Eng. 1961; DObst RCOG 1961; FFA RCS Eng. 1965. Hon. Cons. Anaesth. Southend-on-Sea Hosps. Specialty: Anaesth. Socs: Assn. Anaesths. Prev: Cons. Anaesth. Southend-on-Sea Hosp. Gp.; Sen. Regist. (Anaesth.) Lond. Hosp. & Gen. Hosp. Southend; Regist. (Anaesth.) Lond. Hosp. & Poplar Hosp.

WATT, Mark James 18 Great Western Place, Aberdeen AB10 6QL — MB ChB Aberd. 1998.

WATT, Martin Monklands Hospital, Monkscourt Avenue, Airdrie ML6 0JS Tel: 01236 712186 Fax: 01236 713138 Email: martin.watt@laht.scot.nhs.uk — MB ChB Glas. (Glasgow) FFAEM; FRCS; Dip FMS. Cons. in Accid. and Emerg. Med., Monklands Hosp., Airdrie; Hon. Clin. Teach., Glas. Univ.; Regional Research Adviser, Fac. of Accid. and Emerg. Med. Specialty: Accid. & Emerg.; Sports Med. Socs: Internat. Soc. for study of Mountain Med.; Soc. of Wilderness Med.

WATT, Michael Ward 21, Royal Victoria Hospital, Grosvenor Road, Belfast BT12 6BA Tel: 01232 894921 Fax: 01232 235258; 20 Ashvale Drive, Hillsborough BT26 6DN Tel: 01846 689552 — MB BCh BAO Belf. 1985; BSc (Hons.) Physiol. Belf. 1982; MRCP (UK) 1988. Cons. Neurol. Roy. Vict. Hosp. Belf. Specialty: Neurol. Prev: Sen. Regist. & Regist. (Neurol.) Roy. Vict. Hosp. Belf.

WATT, Monika Martha — MB ChB Leeds 1976; MSc Aberd. 1993; FFOM RCP Lond. 1996. Cons. Occupational Phys. / Force Med. Adviser Grampian Police. Specialty: Occupat. Health. Prev: Force med. Advis. Grampian Police.

WATT, Nicola 11 Kilmaurs Drive, Giffnock, Glasgow G46 6ET — MB ChB Glas. 1993.

WATT, Nicola Karen Bury Farm House, Church La, Broxbourne EN10 7QF — MB ChB Sheff. 1997.

WATT, Mr Nigel Alan Roderick Departmentof Orthopaedic Surgery, University South Carolina, Two Richland Medical Park Suite 404, Columbia SC 29203, USA Tel: 00 1 803 7656812; 128 Broadwater Street W., Worthing BN14 9DJ Tel: 01903 36888 — MB BChir Camb. 1978 (King's Coll. Hosp.) MA Camb. 1979, MB BChir 1978; FRCS Ed. 1984; FRCS Eng. 1984; FRCS Ed. (Orth.) 1989. Sen. Regist. (Orthop. Surg.) Guy's & St. Thomas Hosp. Higher Train. Rotat.. Specialty: Orthop. Prev: Regist. (Orthop. Surg.) Princess Margt. Rose Orthop. Hosp. Edin.; Surgic. Regist. Addenbrookes Hosp. Camb.; Cas. Off. ChristCh. Pub. Hosp. New Zealand.

WATT, Penelope Ann Four Winds, 10 Andover Road N., Winchester Tel: 01962 880050 — MB BS Lond. 1960; MRCS Eng. LRCP Lond. 1960.

WATT, Peter Arbuthnot (retired) Tarrywood, Whitchurch, Tavistock PL19 9LE — (Lond. Hosp.) MA, MB BChir Camb. 1952; MRCS Eng. LRCP Lond. 1952; DObst RCOG 1956; MRCP Lond. 1960; FRCGP 1991. Prev: Ho. Phys. Ho. Surg. & Resid. Accouch. Lond. Hosp.

WATT, Peter John Four Winds, 10 Andover Road N., Winchester Tel: 01962 880050 — MB BS Lond. 1960; MD Lond 1969, MB BS 1960; MRCS Eng. LRCP Lond. 1960; MRCP Lond. 1962. Prof. of Microbiol. Soton. Univ.; Cons. Microbiol. Wessex RHB. Specialty: Med. Microbiol. Socs: Roy. Soc. Med. & Soc. Gen. Microbiol. Prev: Sen. Regist. Bacteriol. Hammersmith Hosp. Lond.; Sen. Lect. Bacteriol. St. Mary's Hosp. Med. Sch. Lond.

WATT, Robert MacKay, OBE (retired) — (Ed.) PhD Ed. 1972; MB ChB Ed 1966; BSc Ed 1963; Dip. Community. Med. Ed. 1976. Prev: Home Off. Chief Insp. Animals (Scientif. Procedures) Act 1986.

WATT, Roger William Royal Bolton Hospital, Minerva Road, Farnworth, Bolton BL4 0JR Tel: 01204 390546 Fax: 01204 390657; The Squirrels, 105 The Hall Coppice, Egerton, Bolton BL7 9UF — (St. Bart.) MB BS Lond. 1968; DCH Eng. 1970; MRCP (UK) 1975; FRCP Lond. 1990; FRCPCH 1997. Cons. Paediat. Bolton Hosps. NHS Trust. Specialty: Paediat. Prev: Sen. Regist. (Paediat.) Wigan & Roy. Manch. Childr. Hosp.; Tutor (Paediat.) Univ. Manch.; Regist. (Paediat.) St. Geo. Hosp. Lond.

WATT, Ruby Margaret Julie Elmbank Group, Foresterhill Health Centre, Westburn Road, Aberdeen AB25 2AY Tel: 01224 696949 Fax: 01224 691650 Email: ruby.watt@elmbank.grampian.scot.nhs.uk — MB ChB Aberd. 1980; BMedBiol Aberd. 1978; FRCGP 1994, M 1987; DRCOG 1989; MFHom 2002.

WATT, Sheila Margaret Raigmore Hospital, Inverness IV2 3UJ — MB ChB Aberd. 1990; DCCH Edin 1996; JCPTGP 1996. Assoc. Spec. Community Paediat. Inverness. Specialty: Gen. Pract.; Community Child Health; Paediat. Socs: BMA; BACCH; DSMIG.

WATT, Simon Geoffrey 126 Deepdale Drive, Rainhill, Prescot L35 4QJ — MB ChB Liverp. 1998.

WATT, Sioban Elizabeth Harewood Medical Practice, Richmond Road, Catterick Garrison DL9 3JD Tel: 01748 850913 — MB ChB Manch. 1981; DRCOG 1984; DCP Sheff. 1992. Specialty: Gen. Pract. Prev: SCMO Hull HA.

WATT, Stephanie Jane Department Anaesthetics, Barnet General Hospital, Wellhouse Lane, Barnet EN5 3DJ; 60 Kenerne Drive,

Barnet EN5 2NN — MB BS Lond. 1985; FRCA 1996. Cons. Anaesth. Barnet Gen. Hosp. Specialty: Anaesth.

WATT, Stephen James Quartains, Drumoak, Banchory AB31 5EP Tel: 01330 811636 — MB BS Lond. 1973 (St. Bart.) MRCS Eng. LRCP Lond. 1973; MRCP (UK) 1977; AFOM RCP Lond. 1988; FRCP Ed. 1990. Sen. Lect. Dept. Environm. & Occupat. Med. Univ. Aberd. Specialty: Occupat. Health; Respirat. Med. Prev: Lect. (Med.) Univ. Aberd.; Res. Fell. (Cardiovasc. Studies & Med.) Gen. Infirm. Leeds; Ho. Off. (Orthop.) St. Bart. Hosp. Lond.

WATT, Thomas Arthur (retired) 3 Southern Avenue, Rutherglen, Glasgow G73 4JN Tel: 0141 634 8737 — MB ChB Glas. 1943 (Univ. Glas.) MRCGP 1956.

WATT, Tracey Craven dept. Of Anaesthetics, Royal Oldham Hospital, Oldham OL1 2JH — MB ChB Manch. 1983; FCAnaesth. 1990; FRCA 1990. Specialty: Anaesth.; Intens. Care.

WATT, Victoria Beatrice Olive House, Black Lane, Loxley, Sheffield S6 6SE Tel: 0114 234 3082 — MB ChB Sheff. 1998.

WATT, William Alexander (retired) Cheriths Brook, Charlton Drive, Charlton Kings, Cheltenham GL53 8ES Tel: 01242 515642 — MB ChB Aberd. 1946; MRCGP 1953. Prev: Ho. Surg. Beckenham Hosp. & Aberd. Matern. Hosp.

WATT, William Morison Grosvenor Road Surgery, 17 Grosvenor Road, Paignton TQ4 5AZ Tel: 01803 559308 Fax: 01803_ 526702; Bardwell, Hookhills Road, Paignton TQ4 7NH — MB BS Lond. 1972 (St. Mary's) MSc (Health Care) Exeter 1991; FRCGP 2002. Assoc. Dir. GP Postgrad. Educat.. S. West. Deanery. Socs: BMA. Prev: PGEA Coordinator S. West. RHA; Clin. Tutor (Gen. Pract.) S. West. RHA.; Lect. Univ. Exeter.

WATT-SMITH, Jane Ann Anaesthetic Department, Queen Alexandra Hospital, Cosham, Portsmouth PO6 3LY Tel: 023 92 379451; Rose Cottage, Prinsted Lane, Prinstead, Emsworth PO10 8HT — MB BS Lond. 1971; FFA RCS Eng. 1976. Cons. Anaesth. Qu. Alexandra Hosp. Portsmouth. Specialty: Anaesth.

WATT SMITH, Stephen Richard maxillofacial Unit, John Radcliffe Hospital, Oxford OX3 9DU Tel: 01865 221400 Fax: 01865 22043 Email: steve.watt-smith@clinical-medicine.ox.ac.uk — MB BS Lond. 1982 (UCL Lond) MD Lond 1994. Cons. Maxillofacial. Surg. John Radcliffe Hosp. Oxf; Hon. Clin. Sen. Lect. Nuffield. Dept. Surg. Univ. Oxf. Specialty: Oral & Maxillofacial Surg.

WATT-SMYRK, Charles William c/o 2 Keswick Close, Cringleford, Norwich NR4 6UW — MB BS Lond. 1976. GP Maidenhead.

WATTERS, Mr Anthony Thomas Bradford Teaching Hospital NHS Trust, Bradford Royal Infirmary, Duckworth Lane, Bradford BD9 6RJ Tel: 01274 364552 Email: anthony.watters@bradfordhospitals.nhs.uk — MB ChB Glas. 1977; FRCS Ed. 1984. p/t Cons. Orthop. Trauma Bradford Roy. Infirm. Specialty: Trauma & Orthop. Surg. Socs: Brit. Orthop. Assn.; Brit. Trauma Soc.

WATTERS, Barbara (retired) Langside, Bassenthwaite, Keswick CA12 4QH Tel: 01768 76471 — MB BS Lond. 1948 (Roy. Free) MRCS Eng. LRCP Lond. 1947; DCH Eng. 1957.

WATTERS, Bernard Vincent Benbree, 67 Carrive Road, Forkhill, Newry BT35 9TE — MB BCh BAO Belf. 1992.

WATTERS, Elizabeth Ann The Orchards, Toft Road, Knutsford WA16 9EB Tel: 01565 632104 — MRCS Eng. LRCP Lond. 1960.

WATTERS, Fionnuala Mary (retired) 41 Ashley Park, Newry Road, Armagh BT60 1EU Tel: 01861 523656 — LRCPI & LM, LRCSI & LM 1961; DPH Belf. 1970; FFCM 1984, M 1975. Examg. Med. Practitioner DHSS. Prev: Cons. in Pub. Health Med., SHSSB Armagh HQ.

WATTERS, Mr Gavin William Roger Southend Hospital, Prittlewell Chase, Westcliff on Sea SS0 0RY — BM BCh Oxf. 1987; FRCS Eng. 1991; FRCS (ORL) 1997. Cons ENT Surg. Southend Hosp.; Cons ENT Surg. BUPA Wellesley Hosp. Specialty: Otolaryngol. Special Interest: Head & Neck Oncol.; Thyroid Surg. Socs: Brit. Assn. Otorhinolaryngol.; Brit. Assn. Head & Neck Oncol.; RSM. Prev: Sen. Regist. (Otolaryngol.) St Marys & Roy. Marsden Hosps. Lond.; Sen. Regist. Qu. Alexandra Hosp. Portsmouth.

WATTERS, James 109 Hodges Street, Wigan WN6 7JE Tel: 01942 493676 — MB ChB Ed. 1976; DCH RCP Lond. 1981; MRCPsych 1985. Clin. Med. Off. (Community Paediat.) Wigan. Specialty: Community Child Health.

WATTERS, Janet Patricia Donegall Road Surgery, 293 Donegall Road, Belfast BT12 5NB Tel: 028 9032 3973; 21 Beechlands, Belfast BT9 5HU — MB BCh BAO Belf. 1983 (Queens University Belfast) DGM RCP Lond. 1986; DCH Dub. 1988; DRCOG 1988; MRCGP 1989. Prev: Trainee GP HillsBoro.; GP Princip.

WATTERS, Joan Katherine Bridge House, Main St., Weeton, Leeds LS17 0AY — MB ChB Sheff. 1965; DMRD Eng. 1970; FFR 1972; FRCR 1975. Cons. Radiol. Leeds Gen. Infirm. Specialty: Radiol. Prev: Ho. Phys. Roy. Hosp. Sheff.; Regist. (Radiol.) United Sheff. Hosps.; Sen. Regist. (Radiol.) Nottm. Univ. Gp. Hosps.

WATTERS, John Gerald Houghton Health Centre, Church Street, Houghton-le-Spring DH4 4DN Tel: 0191 584 2154 — MB BS Newc. 1975. GP Hebburn, Tyne & Wear.

WATTERS, Julie Stirling Trust Hospital, Stirling Tel: 01786 434000; 28 Hawthorn Road, Prestonpans EH32 9QF — MB ChB Ed. 1986; DA (UK) 1989. SHO (Anaesth.) Stirling Trust Hosp. Specialty: Anaesth. Prev: SHO (A & E) Roy. Edin. Infirm.; SHO (A & E) Roy. Hosp. Sick Childr. Glas.

WATTERS, Kenneth John 27 Cheyne Row, London SW3 5HW — MB BCh BAO Dub. 1974 (Dublin University) VP Clin. Research Europe Covance; Clin. Asst. (Diabetes) Ealing Hosp. Trust. Specialty: Pharmaceutical Medicine. Prev: Dir. Med. Safety & Regulatory Affairs SmithKline Beecham Consumer Healthcare.

WATTERS, Malcolm Peter Raitt Warenne House, Great Coxwell, Faringdon SN7 7NB — MB BChir Camb. 1989; MRCP (UK) 1992; FRCA 1995. Cons. Anaaesthesia/ITU, Princess Margt. Hosp., Swindon. Specialty: Anaesth. Prev: Regist. SW Region Anaesth. Train. Scheme.

WATTERS, Margaret Mary 19 Blanchland Drive, Sunderland SR5 1PT — LRCP LRCS Ed. 1941 (Anderson & St. Mungo's Colls. Glas.) LRCP LRCS Ed. LRFPS Glas. 1941.

WATTERS, Norah Patricia (retired) Caladh Ur, Braes, Ullapool IV26 2SZ Tel: 01854 612098 — MB ChB Aberd. 1951; DObst RCOG 1954; DA Eng. 1957.

WATTERS, Oonagh Frances 29 Robin Hood Lane, Kingston Vale, London SW15 3PU — MB ChB Dundee 1976.

WATTERS, Patrick Thomas 10 The Grove, Radlett WD7 7NF Tel: 01923 855434 & profess. 081 954 5641 — MB BCh BAO NUI 1954 (Univ. Coll. Dub.) DA Eng. 1956; FFA RCS Eng. 1971. Cons. Anaesth. Edgware Gen. Hosp. & Colindale Hosp.; Hon. Cons. Anaesth. Hosp. St Johns's & St Eliz. Lond. Specialty: Anaesth. Socs: Assn. Anaesths. Prev: Wing Cdr. RAF Med. Br. Cons. Anaesth.; Anaesth. Regist. Roy. Nat. Orthop. Hosp. Stanmore; Hon. Research Fell. Dept. Anaesths. RCS Lond.

WATTERS, Sean Robert Watercress Medical Group, Mansfield Park Surgery, Lymington Bottom Road, Medstead, Alton GU34 5EW Tel: 01420 562922 Fax: 01420 562923 — MB BS Lond. 1984 (St. Thos.) FFA RCS Eng. 1988; MRCGP 1990; DRCOG 1990. Specialty: Gen. Pract. Socs: BMA. Prev: Trainee GP Poole VTS; Regist. (Anaesth.) Char. Cross & Hillingdon Hosps.

WATTERSON, Brian Robert Saintfield Health Centre, Fairview, Saintfield, Ballynahinch BT24 7AD Tel: 028 9751 2239 Fax: 028 9751 9040; 11 Linden Close, Saintfield, Ballynahinch BT24 7BH Tel: 01238 519040 — MB BCh BAO Belf. 1968; DObst RCOG 1972; MRCGP 1973. Specialty: Gen. Med.; Genetics. Prev: Hosp. Pract. (Geriat.) Ards & Bangor Hosps.

WATTIE, Mr James Alistair (retired) Belmont, Botcheston Road, Newtown Unthank, Leicester LE9 9FB — MB ChB Aberd. 1960; FRCS Eng. 1967; DMRD Ed. 1969. Prev: Cons. Radiol. Leicester Hosps. Gp.

WATTIE, John Nicholson (retired) Spindles Ridge, Old Farm Copse, West Wellow, Romsey SO51 6RJ Tel: 01794 322534 Email: jwattie@onetel.net.uk — MB ChB Aberd. 1947; DCH Eng. 1952; DObst RCOG 1953; FRCP Ed. 1980, M 1958. Prev: GP Romsey.

WATTIE, Moira Louise 5E Burston Road, London SW15 6AR — MB BS Lond. 1993; DA (UK) 1995. N. W. Thames Deanery Curr.ly at Ealing Hosp. NHS Trust. Specialty: Anaesth. Prev: SHO (Anaesth.) Char. Cross Hosp. Lond.; SHO (Geriat.) Univ. Coll. Lond. Hosps.

WATTIS, Professor John Philip St. Luke's Hospital, Blackmoorfoot Road, Huddersfield HD4 5RQ Tel: 01484 343451 Email: john.wattis@cht.nhs.uk — MB ChB Liverp. 1972; FRCPsych 1991, M 1978; DPM Eng. 1978. Cons. Psychiat. South West Yorkshire NHS Trust; Vis. Prof. of Old Age Psychiat., Huddersfield Univ. Specialty: Geriat. Psychiat. Prev: Med. Director, Leeds Community & Ment. Health NHS Trust; Sen. Lect. (Psychiat.) Univ.

Leeds Sch. Clin. Med.; Sen. Lect. & Cons. Psychiat. of Old Age Newsam Centre Seacroft Hosp. Leeds.

WATTON, Desmond 303 Hagley Road, Pedmore, Stourbridge DY9 0RJ — MB ChB Birm. 1952.

WATTON, Eric The Surgery, 24 Broadwater Road, Worthing BN14 8AB Tel: 01903 231701; Pine Tree Cottage, 60 Poulters Lane, Worthing BN14 7TA — MB BS Lond. 1963 (King's Coll. Hosp.) MRCS Eng. LRCP Lond. 1963; DObst RCOG 1965. Prev: Ho. Phys. & Ho. Surg. Dulwich Hosp.; Ho. Off. (Paediat.) Bristol Roy. Hosp. Sick Childr.

WATTON, Mary Joyce (retired) Southwood, Church Road, Purley CR8 3QQ Tel: 020 8660 3235 — MB ChB Leeds 1951.

WATTON, Richard John Whitehouse Surgery, 189 Prince of Wales Road, Sheffield S2 1FA Tel: 0114 239 7229 Fax: 0114 253 1650 — MB ChB Sheff. 1981; DCH RCP Lond. 1984; DRCOG 1985; MRCGP 1985.

WATTON, Robert William (retired) Southwood, Church Road, Purley CR8 3QQ Tel: 020 8660 3235 — (Lond. Hosp.) MB BS Lond. 1954; DCH RCP Lond. 1958; DPH Eng. 1957, DIH 1963; FFCM 1983, M 1972; AFOM RCP Lond. 1982; FFPHM 1987. Prev: Sen. Med. Off. DHSS.

WATTS, Andrew Charles Sarum House Surgery, 3 St. Ethelbert Street, Hereford HR1 2NS Tel: 01432 265422 Fax: 01432 358440 — MB BS Lond. 1985.

WATTS, Andrew John 36 Banbury Road, Kidlington OX5 2BU Tel: 01865 372656; 27 Salisbury Road, Crookes, Sheffield S10 1WA Tel: 0114 266 0487 — MB ChB Sheff. 1994. GP Locum. Specialty: Gen. Pract. Prev: GP/Regist. Barnsley Dist. Gen. Hosp. VTS; SHO (Gen. Med.) Barnsley Dist. Gen.; SHO (O & G) Barnsley Dist. Gen.

WATTS, Andrew Mark Honor Oak Health Centre, 20-21 Turnham Road, London SE4 2HH Tel: 020 7639 9797; Seasons, 40 Madeira Avenue, Bromley BR1 4AY — MB BS Lond. 1989 (Roy. Free Hosp. Sch. Med.) BSc (Hons.) Nursing CNAA 1983; DCH RCP Lond. 1992; DFFP 1993; MRCGP 1993. GP S. Lond. Homeless Team; RCGP/RCN/DoH Educat. Fellowship (Jt. Research Post Promoting Interprofessional Train. Between GP Regist & Community Nurses); Health Quality Serv.-Surveyor (King's Fund). Socs: (Bd.) Interprofessional Educat.

WATTS, Andrew Rodney 15 Druid Woods, Avon Way, Bristol BS9 1SX — MB ChB Sheff. 1992.

WATTS, Anne Elizabeth Downshire Hospital, Ardglass Road, Downpatrick BT30 6RA Tel: 02844 613311 Fax: 02844 612444 — MD Belf. 1988, MB BCh BAO 1970; DCH RCPS Glas. 1972; MRCPsych 1987. p/t Cons. Psychiat., Downshire Hosp., Downpatrick. Specialty: Gen. Psychiat. Special Interest: Psychiatric Intens. care. Socs: Roy. Coll. of Psychiatrists. Prev: Director, Carlisle Ho. Addic. Unit, Presbyt. Ch., Belf.

WATTS, Anthony James Caythorpe Surgery, 52-56 High Street, Caythorpe, Grantham NG32 3DN Tel: 01400 272215 Fax: 01400 273608; Ivy House, Dycote Lane, Welbourn, Lincoln LN5 0NJ — MB ChB Leic. 1984; DRCOG 1987; MRCGP 1988.

WATTS, Arthur Stanley (retired) The Frith, Mortimer, Reading RG7 2JL Tel: 01734 332487 — (Westm.) BSc (Hons. Physiol.) Lond. 1937, MD 1947, MB BS; MRCS Eng. LRCP Lond. 1940; MRCP Lond. 1943. Prev: Med. Regist. Westm. Hosp.

WATTS, Beverley Louise 18 Litchford Road, Ashley, New Milton BH25 5BQ Tel: 01425 621375; 15 Alresford Road, Winchester SO23 0HG Tel: 01962 870875 — MB BS Lond. 1993 (UMDS (Guy's)) BSc (Hons.) Lond. 1990; MRCP (Lond.) 1995. Specialist Regist. (A & E Med.) Wessex Region. Specialty: Accid. & Emerg. Socs: Roy. Coll. Phys. (Lond.); Brit. Assn. Accid. & Emerg. Med.; Fac. for Accid. & Emerg.

WATTS, Christopher Waterloo Surgery, 617 Wakefield Road, Waterloo, Huddersfield HD5 9XP Tel: 01484 531461 — MB ChB Manch. 1978.

WATTS, Christopher Cameron William 71 Christchurch Road, London SW14 7AT — MB BS Lond. 1998.

WATTS, Christopher John Barking and Havering Health Authority, Directorate of Public Health, The Clockhouse East St., Barking IG11 8EY Tel: 020 8532 6362 Fax: 020 8532 6354; 15 Cromwell Avenue, Highgate, London N6 5HN Tel: 020 8245 4135 Fax: 020 8245 4135 — MB BS Sydney 1971; BSc (Med.) Sydney 1968; DTM & H Sydney 1978; MSc (Soc. Med.) Lond. 1980; MFCM 1981; FFPHM RCP (Austral.) 1991; FFPHM RCP (UK) 1993; FRCP (UK) 1998. Dir. Pub. Health Barking & Havering HA. Specialty: Pub. Health Med. Socs: Assn. Directors of Pub. Health. Prev: Dir. Med. Serv. (Austral.); Specialist (Community Med.) Barking Havering & Brentwood HA; Sen. Regist. (Community Med.) City & E. Lond. AHA.

WATTS, Colin 58 Chiltern Road, Sheffield S6 4QX — MB BS Newc. 1991.

WATTS, Darren Paul 17 Brockridge Lane, Frampton, Cotterell, Bristol BS36 2HU — MB BS Lond. 1993.

WATTS, Darryl Russell Blackberry Hill Hospital, Manor Road, Bristol BS16 2EW — MB ChB Bristol 1984; MSc Bristol 1992, MB ChB 1984; MRCPsych. 1989. Cons. Gen. Psychiat. Blackberry Hill Hosp. Bristol. Specialty: Gen. Psychiat.

WATTS, David Anthony 8 Annandale Street, Edinburgh EH7 4AN — MB ChB Ed. 1992; MRCP 1998. SHO (Gen. Med.) Stirling Roy. Infirm. Stirling. Specialty: Gen. Med.

WATTS, Derrett James North Staffordshire Combined Healthcare Trust, Clydesdale Centre, 167 Queens Road, Penkhill, Stoke-on-Trent ST4 7LF Tel: 01782 427650 — MB BCh Wales 1987 (University of Wales) DRCOG 1992; MRCPsych 1997. Specialist Regist. Rotat. (Psychiat.) W. Midl. Specialty: Gen. Psychiat. Socs: Christian Med. Fellowsh.; BMA. Prev: Regist. Rotat. (Psychiat.) N. Staffs. Combined Healthcare Stoke-on-Trent; GP Stoke-on-Trent; Trainee GP/SHO N. Staffs. HA VTS.

WATTS, Edward Thomas Spinney View, Tebworth Road, Wingfield, Leighton Buzzard LU7 9QH — MB ChB Birm. 1973.

WATTS, Eric James Department Haematology, Basildon Hospital, Basildon SS16 5NL; Cherry Cottage, 11 Parkway, Shenfield, Brentwood CM15 8LH — MB ChB Glas. 1971; MRCP (UK) 1978; FRCPath 1996, M 1984; DM Soton 1988; FRCP Glas. 1995. Cons. Haemat. Basildon & Thurrock HA. Specialty: Haematology. Prev: Sen. Regist. (Haemat.) Soton. Hosp. & Portsmouth Hosp.; Regist. (Haemat.) Hammersmith Hosp.

WATTS, Erica Caroline 104 Chatto Road, Torquay TQ1 4HY — BM Soton. 1982; DCH RCPS Glas. 1985. GPTorquay; CA Oncol.; BA Doctor. Prev: Trainee GP Dawlish VTS; SHO (O & G & Paediat.) Plymouth HA; SHO (Cas.) Torbay HA.

WATTS, Mr George Thomas 4 Amesbury Road, Moseley, Birmingham B13 8LD Tel: 0121 449 2242 — (Birm.) ChM Birm. 1959, MB ChB 1944; FRCS Eng. 1950. Cons. Surg. United Birm. Hosps. Socs: Assn. Surg. & Moynihan Chir. Club. Prev: Lect. in Surg. Univ. Birm.; Res. Surg. Off. Qu. Eliz. Hosp. Birm.; Research & Clin. Fell. (Surg.) Mass. Gen. Hosp. Boston.

WATTS, Gillian Moir Royal Bolton Hospital, Minerva Road, Farnworth, Bolton BL4 0JR — BM Soton. 1984; FRCS Ed. 1991. Assoc. Specialist, Roy. Bolton Hosp. Prev: Regist. (Ophth.) Manch. Roy. Eye Hosp.; SHO Wythenshawe Hosp. Manch. & N. Manch. Gen. Hosp.; Tutor (Anat.) & SHO (Ophth.) Manch. Eye Hosp.

WATTS, Graham Vincent The Witterings Health Centre, Cakeham Road, East Wittering, Chichester PO20 8BH Tel: 01243 673434 Fax: 01243 672563 — BM Soton. 1977.

WATTS, Helen Rose Schlumberger-Sema Medical Services, Govt Buildings, Flowers Hill, Bristol BS4 Tel: 0117 971 8311 — MB BS Sydney 1971; DDAM 2002. Med. Adviser Schlumberger-Sema Bristol. Specialty: Disabil. Med. Socs: Roy. Inst. Pub. Health. Prev: Med. Adviser BAMS, Bristol; Acting SCMO E. Wilts. Health Care.

WATTS, James Christopher Anaestetic Department, Burnley General Hospital, Casterton Avenue, Burnley BB10 2PQ Tel: 01282 425071 — MB ChB Manch. 1989 (St. And. & Manch.) BSc (Med. Sci.) St. And. 1986; FRCA 1995. Cons. Anaesth. Burnley Gen. Hosp. Specialty: Anaesth. Socs: Intens. Care Soc.; Assn. Anaesth.; Difficult Airway Soc. Prev: Sen. Regist. (Anaesth.) Princess Roy. Hosp. Telford; Sen. Regist. Roy. Shrewsbury Hosp.; Sen. Regist. (Anaesth.) Stoke on Trent.

WATTS, Mrs Jennifer Anne Royal Hampshire County Hospital, Romsey Road, Winchester SO22 5DG Tel: 01962 863535 Fax: 01962 824429; Hollybank cottage, Row Hill, Bramshaw, Lyndhurst SO43 7JE Tel: 02380 812432 Fax: 02380 811371 — MB Camb. 1972; BChir 1971; DO Eng. 1974; FRCS Eng. 1981; FRCOphth 1988. Cons. Ophth. Roy. Hants. Co. Hosp. Winchester. Specialty: Ophth. Prev: Sen. Regist. (Ophth.) Roy. Vict. Hosp. Bournemouth.

WATTS, Jillian Patricia Tottington Health Centre, 16 Market Street, Tottington, Bury BL8 4AD — MB ChB Liverp. 1987; DRCOG 1991; MRCGP 1993; DFFP 1996. GP Princip. Tottington Health

Centre Bury Lancs. Specialty: Gen. Pract. Socs: BMA. Prev: GP Bury Retainer Scheme; Asst. (Chest Med.) Bury Gen. Hosp.

WATTS, Joanna Prudence 7 Little St. Johns Street, Woodbridge, Ipswich IP12 1EE Tel: 01394 382046; 7 North Close, Ipswich IP4 2TL Tel: 01473 254080 — BM BCh Oxf. 1977; MA Camb. 1979, BA 1974; DRCOG 1979; MRCGP 1981. GP Partner Ipswich. Prev: SHO (Accid. Serv.) Radcliffe Infirm. Oxf.; SHO (Rheum.) Battle Hosp. Reading; SHO (Obst.) John Radcliffe Hosp. Oxf.

WATTS, Mr John Aubrey Ewart (retired) Four Winds, Dartford Road, Horton Kirby, Dartford DA4 9JE Tel: 01322 863256 — MB BS Lond. 1940 (Guy's) MRCS Eng. LRCP Lond. 1940; FRCS Ed. 1942. Prev: Cons. Surg. Dartford Dist. Hosp.

WATTS, Professor John Cadman, OBE, MC, Col. late RAMC (retired) Grove Court, 17 Beech Way, Woodbridge IP12 4BW Tel: 01394 382618 — MB BS Lond. 1938 (St Thos.) MRCS Eng. LRCP Lond. 1936; FRCS Eng. 1949. Prev: Cons. Orthop. Surg. Bedford Gen. Hosp.

WATTS, John David Dundonald Medical Practice, 9 Main Street, Dundonald, Kilmarnock KA2 9HF Tel: 01563 850496 Fax: 01563 850426; 24 Main Street, Dundonald, Kilmarnock KA2 9HE Tel: 01563 850496 Fax: 01563 851349 — MB ChB Glas. 1963; MRCGP 1996. Chief Exec. Ayrsh. Doctors on Call; Sec. Ayrsh. & Arran LMC. Socs: BMA. Prev: Capt. RAMC; Ho. Off. Aberystwyth Gen. Hosp.

WATTS, John Ffrancon Worcester Royal Hospital, Charles Hastings Way, Worcester WR5 1DD; Stonehall farmhouse, Stonebow Road, Drakes Broughton, Worcester WR10 2AT — MD Wales 1985 (Welsh Nat. Sch. Med.) MB BCh Wales 1975; FRCOG 1993, M 1981. Cons. O&G Worcester acute Hosp. NHS trust. Specialty: Obst. & Gyn. Prev: Cons. O & G City Hosp. NHS Trust Birm.

WATTS, Julie Denise Anaesthetic Department, Royal Free Hospital, Pond St., London NW3 2GQ; 89 Chetwynd Road, London NW5 1DA — MB BS Monash 1978; FRCA 1992. Cons. Anaesth. & Hon. Sen. Lect. Roy. Free Hosp. Specialty: Anaesth. Socs: Roy. Soc. Med.; MRCAnaesth.

WATTS, Kathleen Alison (retired) — MB BS Newc. 1976 (University of Newcastle-upon-Tyne) FRCS Ed. 1981; FFAEM 1993. Prev: Cons. A & E City Hosp. NHS Trust Birm.

WATTS, Kathryn Anne 2 Nottingham Street, Cardiff CF5 1JP — MB BCh Wales 1977.

WATTS, Malcolm Richard Fernside, 9 North Road, Ormesby St.Margaret, Great Yarmouth NR29 3SA Tel: 01493 730537 — MB ChB Bristol 1974; MRCGP 1979.

WATTS, Margaret Ishbel 39 Monument Road, Ayr KA7 2QS — MB BS Lond. 1979; MRCS Eng. LRCP Lond. 1979; MRCGP 1985.

WATTS, Marjorie Emily The Maze, Boars Head, Crowborough TN6 3HE Tel: 01892 652407 — MB BS Lond. 1953 (Char. Cross) DObst RCOG 1955; DPH Eng. 1959; MFCM 1972. Dist. Med. Off. Greenwich HA. Specialty: Pub. Health Med. Socs: BMA. Prev: Dep. MOH Lond. Boro. Greenwich; Dep. MOH Metrop. Boro. Camberwell, Med. Off. LCC; Ho. Surg. Char. Cross Hosp. Lond.

WATTS, Mr Mark Thomas Arrowe Park Hospital, Eye Department, Arrowe Park Road, Upton, Wirral Tel: 0151 604 7186 Fax: 0151 604 7152 Email: mckevitt.sharon@wht.nhs.uk — MB ChB Birm. 1981 (Birmingham) DO RCS Eng. 1986; FRCS Eng. 1986; FRCOphth. 1988. Cons. Ophth. Surg. Wirral Hosps. NHS Trust; Hon. Sen. Lect. Roy. Liverp. Univ. Hosp.; Hon. Assoc. Clin. Prof. Univ. of Ohio; hon ass clin prof Geo. washington Univ. Specialty: Ophth. Special Interest: Cataract Surg.; Oculoplastic Surg. Prev: Sen. Regist. Roy. Hallamsh. Hosp. Sheff.; Fell. Moorfields Eye Hosp. Lond.; Regist. Birm. & Midl. Eye Hosp.

WATTS, Martin 14 Trenchard Avenue, Stafford ST16 3QB — MB ChB Leeds 1988.

WATTS, Martin Alan Waterloo Surgery, 191 Devonport Road, Stoke, Plymouth PL1 5RN Tel: 01752 563147 Fax: 01752 563304; Glencoe, 1 Glencoe Villas, Clearbrook, Yelverton PL20 6JB Tel: 01822 852400 — MB BS Lond. 1979; DRCOG 1982.

WATTS, Michael Barrett The Datchet Medical Centre, 4 Green Lane, Datchet, Slough SL3 9EX Tel: 01753 541268 Fax: 01753 582324 — MB BS Lond. 1985; MRCGP 1989. Prev: Ho. Phys. Char. Cross Hosp. Lond.; Ho. Surg. W. Herts. Hosp.; Trainee GP Edware Gen. Hosp. VTS.

WATTS, Michael Robin (retired) The Surgery, St. Mary St., Thornbury, Bristol BS35 2AT Tel: 01454 413691; The Winnocks, Thornbury Road, Alveston, Bristol BS12 2LJ — MB ChB Bristol 1961; DObst RCOG 1963. Police Surg. Prev: SHO (Obst.), Ho. Surg. & Ho. Phys. Southmead Hosp. Bristol.

WATTS, Michelle Christina Sanna House, Low Road, Westmuir, Kirriemuir DD8 5LN — MB ChB Aberd. 1991.

WATTS, Neera Public Health Sevices, Le Bas Centre, St Saviours Road, St Helier, Jersey JE1 4HR Tel: 01534 89933 — MB BS Mysore 1979; MRCS Eng. LRCP Lond. 1981. Clin. Med.Off. Specialty: Pub. Health Med.; Community Child Health; Pub. Health Med.

WATTS, Nita 23 Woodfall Avenue, Barnet EN5 2EZ — MB BS Lond. 1976.

WATTS, Paul Michael 12A Flodden Road, London SE5 9LH — MB BS Lond. 1990; BSc (Hons.) Lond. 1987, MB BS 1990; MRCP Lond. 1993. Specialty: Neurol.

WATTS, Richard Arthur Bury Hill House, Woodbridge IP12 1JD Tel: 01394 382422 Email: richard.watts2@btinternet.com — BM BCh Oxf 1982 (Oxf.) MRCS Eng. LRCP Lond. 1981; BM BCh Oxf. 1982; MRCP (UK) 1985; MA Oxf. 1982, DM 1991; FRCP Lond. 1999. Cons. Rheum. Ipswich Hosp.; Edr. Rheum. Specialty: Rheumatol. Socs: Fell. Amer. Coll. Rheum.; Brit. Soc. Rheum.; Brit. Soc. Immunol. Prev: Hon. Sen. Lect. Sch. Health. Univ.E. Anglia; Sen. Regist. (Rheum.) Norf. & Norwich Hosp.; Sen. Regist. (Rheum.) Addenbrooke's Hosp. Camb.

WATTS, Richard William Ernest Consulting Rooms, 5th Floor, 86 Harley Street, London W1 Tel: 020 7586 5959 Ext: 2572 Fax: 020 7226588; 86 Harley Street, London W1; 14 Holly Lodge Gardens, Highgate, London N6 6AA Tel: 020 8340 7725 Fax: 0208 340 5767 — MB BS (Hons.) Lond. 1945 (St. Bart.) M 1949; PhD Lond. 1953; MD 1960; FRCP Lond. 1967; FRSC (C.Chem) 1971; DSc Lond. 1975. Cons. Phys. (Gen. Med., Endocrinol., Metab. Dis. & Renal Dis.); Vis. Prof. Div. Med. Imperial Coll. of Sci., Technol. & Med. Hammersmith Hosp. Specialty: Gen. Med.; Endocrinol.; Nephrol. Special Interest: Metab. Diseases. Socs: Emerit. Mem. Biochem. Soc.; MRCP, Counsellor R & P Lond.; Brit. Postgrad. Med. Federat., Univ. Lond. Prev: Hon. Cons. Phys. Hammersmith Hosp.; Head Div. Inherited Metab. Dis. Asst. Dir. (Clin.) & Cons. Phys. MRC Clin. Research Centre & Northwick Pk. Hosp. Harrow; Examr., Lond.

WATTS, Roger (retired) Wilmercroft, Wilmerhatch Lane, Epsom KT18 7EQ Tel: 0137 272 0835 — (Guy's) MB BS Lond. 1953. Prev: Ho. Surg. Guy's Hosp. Lond.

WATTS, Ronald Williams (retired) Moor Cottage, Advie, Grantown-on-Spey PH26 3LP Tel: 01807 510241 — MB BChir Lond. 1937 (Camb. & St. Thos.) MB BChir. Camb 1937; MRCS Eng. LRCP Lond. 1937. Prev: Ho. Phys. & Cas. Off. St. Thos. Hosp. Lond.

WATTS, Shelagh Rosemarie (retired) Anglers Reach, 42 Hampton Park Road, Hereford HR1 1TH Tel: 01432 266430 — MB BS Lond. 1953 (Roy. Free) MRCS Eng. LRCP Lond. 1953; DA Eng. 1955; FRCA Eng. 1958.

WATTS, Simon George Thomas Avenue Road Surgery, 3 Avenue Road, Dorridge, Solihull B93 8LH Tel: 01564 776262 Fax: 01564 779599; 374 Station Road, Dorridge, Solihull B93 8ES — MB ChB Birm. 1983.

WATTS, Simon James 5 Edwards Lane, Sherwood, Nottingham NG5 3AA — MB BCh Witwatersrand 1989.

WATTS, Stephen James George Clare Surgery, Swan Drive, New Road, Chatteris PE16 6EX Tel: 01354 695888 Fax: 01354 695415 — MB BS Lond. 1979 (St. Marys) Cert. Family Plann. JCC 1986; JCPTGP 1987; Dip FP RCOG 1993. Gen. Practitioner, Geo. Clare Surg., Chatterls; Police Surg., Centr. Div., Camks Constab.; Prison Med. Off. Specialty: Med. Microbiol. Socs: Mem. Roy. Soc. Med. Prev: SHO (Paediat. Surg.) Hosp. Sick Childr. Lond.; Ho. Phys. St. Mary's Hosp. Lond. W9.

WATTS, Stephen John The New Surgery, 8 Shenfield Road, Brentwood CM15 8AB Tel: 01277 218393 Fax: 01277 201017; 19 Middleton Road, Shenfield, Brentwood CM15 8DL — MB BS Lond. 1973 (St. Geo.) BSc Lond. 1970; MRCGP 1981. Specialty: Gen. Pract.

WATTS, Toni Ivy House, Dycote Lane, Welbourn, Lincoln LN5 0NJ — MB ChB Leic. 1984; DRCOG 1987; MRCGP 1988. GP Lincoln.

WATTS, Uma 95 Hartfield Avenue, Elstree, Borehamwood WD6 3JJ Tel: 0208 953 7337 — MB BS Agra 1955.

WATTS, Vikram Kumar Priory Hospital N. London, The Bourne, Southgate, London N14 6RA Tel: 020 8882 8191 Fax: 020 8447

8138 — MB BS Lond. 1981 (St. Mary's) BSc (Hons.) Lond. 1977; MRCPsych 1989. Staff Cons.; Hon. Sen. Lect. Roy. Free Hosp. Lond. Specialty: Gen. Psychiat. Socs: MRCPsych. Prev: Sen. Regist. (Psychiat.) Maudsley Hosp. Lond.; Regist. (Psychiat.) St. Geo. Hosp. Lond.

WATTS-RUSSELL, Julian Victor André Biggin Hall, Benefield, Peterborough PE8 5AB Tel: 01832 205350 Fax: 01832 205350 Email: j.watts.russell@farmline.com — MB ChB Birm. 1966; DA W. Indies 1968; MRCP (UK) 1970; FFA RCS Eng. 1972. Specialty: Anaesth. Socs: BMA. Prev: Regtl. Med. Off. Coldstream Guards; Anaesth. Specialist RAMC; Regist. (Med.) St. Mary's Hosp. Lond.

WATTS-TOBIN, Mary Elizabeth Ann Blake 68 Rydal Road, Lancaster LA1 3HA — (Univ. Coll. Hosp.) MRCS Eng. LRCP Lond. 1965; MA, MB Camb. 1966, BChir 1965; DPM Eng. 1976; MRCPsych 1977; FRCPsych 1997. Cons. Psychiat. Lancaster Moor Hosp. Specialty: Gen. Psychiat.

WATTSFORD, Richard Haddon (retired) 40 Eastern Way, Ponteland, Newcastle upon Tyne NE20 9PF Tel: 01661 871749 — (Durh.) MB BS Durh. 1951; MRCGP 1966. Prev: Ho. Phys. & Ho. Surg. Roy. Vict. Infirm. Newc.

WATURA, Roland Department of Radiology, University of Wales College of Medicine, Cardiff CF14 4XN Tel: 01656 655469; 13 Yr Efail, Treoes, Bridgend CF35 5EG Tel: 029 2074 3028 Fax: 01222 743029 — MB BCh Wales 1986; MRCP (UK) 1990; FRCR 1994. Specialty: Radiol. Prev: Sen. Regist. (Radiol.) & Lect. (Diagn. Radiol.) Univ. Hosp. Wales Cardiff.

WATWOOD, Kenneth Bethel, Wildwood Drive, Stafford ST17 4PY — MB ChB Birm. 1961; MRCS Eng. LRCP Lond. 1961. Socs: BMA. Prev: Sen. Ho. Surg. (Obst & Gyn.) Groundslow Hosp. Tittensor; Ho. Surg. & Ho. Phys. Staffs. Gen. Infirm.

WAUCHOB, David William (retired) 4 Highfields, Heswall, Wirral CH60 7TF Tel: 0151 342 6858 — MB BCh BAO Belf. 1941 (Qu. Univ. Belf.) DPH Belf. 1948; FFCM RCP (UK) 1979, M 1972. Prev: MOH & Princip. Sch. Med. Off. Blackpool Co. Boro.

WAUCHOB, Todd Duncan Liverpool Women's Hospital NHS Trust, Department Anaesthesia, Crown St., Liverpool L8 7SS Tel: 0151 708 9988 — MB ChB Leeds 1978; FFARCS Eng. 1983; DRCOG 1984. Cons. Anaesth. Liverp. HA. Specialty: Anaesth. Socs: Obst. Anaesth. Assn.; Assn. Anaesths.; BMA. Prev: Sen. Regist. (Anaesth.) Trent RHA; Regist. (Anaesth.) Sheff. HA Trent Region; SHO (Anaesth.) York Dist. Gen. Hosp.

WAUDBY, Hectorina 35 Grigor Drive, Inverness IV2 4LS — MB ChB Aberd. 1951. Prev: Med. Off. Overseas Staff Leprosy Mission; Relieving Doctor Hayling Chau Leprosarium, Hong Kong; Med. Off. Itu Leprosy Colony, Nigeria.

WAUGH, Janet Gordon Stewart (retired) 2 Mill Lane, Wadenhoe, Peterborough PE8 5XD — (King's Coll.) MB BS Lond. 1946; MRCS Eng. LRCP Lond. 1946; Cert JCC Lond. 1967.

WAUGH, Martin Fenham Hall Surgery, Fenham Hall Drive, Fenham, Newcastle upon Tyne NE4 9XD — MB BS Newcastle 1980; MB BS Newc. 1980. GP Newc.

WAUGH, Michael Anthony Wellfield House, 151 Roker Lane, Pudsey LS28 9ND Tel: 0113 256 5255; Nuffield Hospital Leeds, 2 Leighton Street, Leeds LS1 3EB Tel: 0113 388 2000 Ext: 3882126 — MB BS Lond. 1966 (Char. Cross) DHMSA Lond. 1970; Dip. Ven. Soc. Apoth. Lond. 1974; FRCPI 1994, M 1993; FRCP Lond. 1995; FAChSHP 1997. Cons. Phys. (Genitourin.) Nuffield Hosp. Leeds. Specialty: Genitourinary Medicine. Special Interest: Dermatovenereology in the developing World. Socs: Internat. Union against Sexually Transm. Infecs. (Past Pres.); Founding Mem. Europ. Acad. Dermat. Venerol.; Roy. Soc. of Med. Sub Dean North. and Yorks. Prev: Cons. Phys. (Genitourin.) Gen. Infirm. Leeds.

WAUGH, Norman Robert Department of Public Health, University of Aberdeen, Foresterhill, Aberdeen AB25 2ZD — MB ChB Ed. 1972; DA Eng. 1974; MRCP (UK) 1979; MPH Dundee 1986; MFCM 1986; FRCP Glas. 1992; FFPHM RCP (UK) 1994; FRCP Ed. 1995. Prof. of Pub. health, Univ. of Aberd. Specialty: Pub. Health Med.; Epidemiol. Prev: Regist. (Med.) Dumfries & Galloway Roy. Infirm.; SHO (Anaesth.) East. Gen. Hosp. Edin.; Ho. Phys. Chalmers Hosp. Edin.

WAUGH, Paula Karen 40 Glendale, Belfast BT10 0NX — MB BCh BAO Belf. 1997.

WAUGH, Peter John Coultershaw Farm House, Petworth GU28 0JE Email: znm33@dial.pipex.com — MB BCh BAO NUI 1978; LRCPI & LM, LRCSI & LM 1978; DAvMed RCP Lond. 1982; MA Dub. 1984; MFOM RCP Lond. 1994, AFOM 1985. Specialty: Aviat. Med.; Occupat. Health. Socs: BMA; MRAeS.

WAUGH, Robert Edward Michael Market Street Health Group, 52 Market Street, East Ham, London E6 2RA Tel: 020 8548 2200 Fax: 020 8548 2288 — BM Soton. 1978; MRCGP 1983.

WAUGH, Walter Norman (retired) 34 St Baldreds Road, North Berwick EH39 4PY Tel: 01620 892454 — MB ChB St. And. 1956; DObst RCOG 1961; MRCGP 1968.

WAWMAN, Ronald John (retired) Stable Cottage, Lewdown, Okehampton EX20 4DQ — (Sheff.) MB ChB Sheff. 1957; DPM Eng. 1962; FRCPsych 1980, M 1971. Prev: PMO DHSS.

WAXMAN, Professor Jonathan Hugh Hammersmith Hospital, Department of Oncology, Du Cane Road, London W12 0NN Tel: 020 8383 1080 — MD Lond. 1986; BSc (Hons.) Lond. 1972, MD 1986, MB BS 1975; MRCP (UK) 1978; FRCP Lond. 1990. Prof. & Hon. Cons. Imperial Col, Hammersmith Hosp. Campus; Chairm. of the Proslzlz cancer charity. Specialty: Oncol. Socs: Assn. Phys.; Amer. Soc. Clin. Oncol. Prev: Sen. Regist. (Oncol.) St. Bart. Hosp. Lond.; Regist. (Med.) St. Mary's Hosp. Lond.; SHO Lond. Chest Hosp.

WAY, Adam Christian 16 Kenmore Court, 26 Acol Road, London NW6 3AG — MB ChB Sheff. 1998 (Sheffield) SHO Gen. Surgic., Northwick Pk. & St. Marys Hosp., Watford Rd., Harrow. Prev: Orthop., Northwick Pk. Hosp., Harrow; A & E, Northwick Pk. Hosp., Harrow; Orthop., Roy. Nat. Orthopaedic Hosp. (RNOH).

WAY, Mr Bernard Gordon Barnsley D & H, Gawber Road, Barnsley S75 2; 1 The Paddock, Woolley, Wakefield WF4 2LZ Tel: 01226 384641 — (Middlx.) MB BS Lond. 1963; FRCS Ed. 1972. Cons. Urol. Surg. Barnsley HA. Specialty: Urol. Socs: Brit. Assn. Urol. Surgs. Prev: Regist. (Surg.) Roy. Hosp. Wolverhampton; Surg. Regist. Crewe Memor. Hosp.; Regist. (Urol. Surg.) Newc. Univ. Hosps.

WAY, Bernard Philip James The Surgery, School Hill House, 33 High Street, Lewes BN7 2LU — MB ChB Birm. 1974; MRCP (UK) 1978. Hosp. Practioner Cardiac Dept. Roy. Sussex Co. Hosp. Brighton. Specialty: Gen. Pract.; Cardiol. Prev: Regist. (Cardiol.) Guy's Hosp. Lond.; SHO (Cardiol.) Lond. Chest Hosp.; SHO (Med.) Qu. Alexandra Hosp. & Wessex Regional Renal Unit Portsmouth.

WAY, Beryl Joy Broughton House Surgery, Redenhall Road, Harleston IP20 9AY Tel: 01379 852213; Beech Tree Cottage, Walpole, Halesworth IP19 9AU — MRCS Eng. LRCP Lond. 1973 (Guy's) Prev: Regist. (Psychiat.) Maudsley Hosp. Lond.; SHO (Psychiat.) FarnBoro. Hosp. Kent; Ho. Surg. Guy's Hosp. Lond.

WAY, Carolyn Frances Broadway Green Farm, Petham, Canterbury CT4 5RX Tel: 01227 700283; Homestead, Blackhill Road, Wellow, Romsey SO51 6AQ Tel: 01794 322493 — MB BS Lond. 1993 (King's Coll. Lond.) BSc Lond. 1990. SHO (Anaesth.) Soton. Gen. Hosp. Specialty: Anaesth. Prev: SHO (c/o Elderly) Eastbourne; SHO (A & E) Brighton; Ho. Off. (Surg.) Lond.

WAY, Geoffrey Leslie, OStJ (retired) Court Cottage, Milford, Godalming GU8 5HJ Tel: 01483 424548 — MRCS Eng. LRCP Lond. 1938 (St. Bart.) DA Eng. 1946; FFA RCS Eng. 1953. Prev: Cons. Anaesth. Guildford & Godalming Gp. Hosps. & King Edwd. VII Hosp. Midhurst.

WAY, Hedwig Marianne Martha (retired) 64 Bushmead Court, Hancock Drive, Luton LU2 7GY Tel: 01582 728037 — LRCP LRCS Ed. 1952; LRFPS Glas. Prev: Asst. GP Luton.

WAY, Marion Crosbie (retired) 5 Foxes Row, Brancepeth, Durham DH7 8DH — BM BCh Oxf. 1946 (Univ. Coll. Hosp. & Oxf.) MA, BM BCh Oxf. 1946; DTM & H Liverp. 1949; DCH Eng. 1949; DPM Eng. 1970; FRCPsych. 1980, M 1973. Mem. Ment. Health Commiss. Prev: Cons. Psychiat. Earls Ho. Hosp. Durh.

WAY, Mark Gregory — MB ChB Leic. 1998. Specialty: Anaesth.

WAY, Melanie Bentley Village Surgery, Bentley, Farnham GU10 5LP Tel: 01420 22106; Stonecroft, 8 Pottery Lane, Wrecclesham, Farnham GU10 4QG Tel: 01252 716327 — MB BS Lond. 1986; MRCGP 1990. Socs: BMA. Prev: Retainer Farnham Health Centre; Trainee GP Medway VTS.

WAYDENFELD, Stefan William (retired) 1 Tenterden Close, London NW4 1TJ Tel: 020 8203 5254 — LRCPI & LM, LRSCI & LM 1953 (Royal College of Surgeons, School of Surgery, Dublin) LRCPI & LM, LRCSI & LM 1953; MRCGP 1963. Prev: GP Lond.

WAYGOOD, Alistair Roy 1 Grove Park Terrace, London W4 3QG — MRCS Eng. LRCP Lond. 1970; MB BS Lond. 1970.

WAYMAN, Mr John 7 Bernard Close, Rackheath, Norwich NR13 6QS — MB BS Newc. 1991; FRCS Eng. 1995.

WAYMAN, Matthew James Calver 15 Northcliffe Avenue, Nottingham NG3 6DA — MB ChB Leeds 1992.

WAYMONT, Mr Brian Department of Urology, New Cross Hospital, Wolverhampton WV10 0QP Tel: 01902 307999 Fax: 01902 642872 — (Birm.) MB ChB Birm. 1980; FRCS Ed. 1985; MD Birm 1993; FRCS (Urol.) 1995. Cons. Urol. New Cross Hosp. Wolverhampton NHS Trust. Specialty: Urol. Prev: Sen. Regist. (Urol.) Mersey RHA; Regist. (Urol.) Selly Oak Hosp. Birm.; Research Regist. (Urol.) Qu. Eliz. Hosp. Birm.

WAYNE, Adrian Nicholas Brondesbury Medical Centre, 279 Kilburn High Road, London NW6 7JQ Tel: 020 7624 9853 Fax: 020 7372 3660 — MB BS Lond. 1981 (Univ. Coll. Hosp.) BSc (Hons.) (Biochem.) Lond. 1978; DCH RCP Lond. 1984; MRCGP 1985; DRCOG 1985. Socs: BMA. Prev: Trainee GP St. Bart. Hosp. VTS; Ho. Surg. Univ. Coll. Hosp. Lond.; Ho. Phys. St. Bart. Hosp. Lond.

WAYNE, Christopher John Wycombe Hospital, Queen Alexandra Road, High Wycombe HP11 2TT Tel: 01494 526161 Ext: 2279 Email: drcjwayne@aol.com — MB ChB Birm. 1989; MRCOG Lond. 1997. Cons. in Obst. and Gyn., Wycombe Hosp.; Cons. in Obst. and Gyn., Chiltern Hosp., Gt. Missenden; Cons. in Obst. and Gyn., Shelborne Hosp., High Wycombe. Specialty: Obst. & Gyn. Socs: Roy. Coll. of Obst. and Gyn.; Brit. Med. Ultrasound Soc.; Brit. Matern. Fetal Med. Soc. Prev: Specialist Regist. in Obst. and Gyn., Surrey Co. Hosp., Guildford; Specialist Regist. in Obst. and Gyn., St Georges Hosp., Lond.; Specialist Regist. in Obst. and Gyn., Kingston Hosp., Kingston Upon Thames.

WAYNE, David Johnson (retired) 39 Warkworth Street, Cambridge CB1 1EG Tel: 01223 352505 Fax: 01223 462508 Email: davidwayne@beeb.net — (Oxf. & Univ. Coll. Hosp. Lond.) BM BCh Oxf. 1958; MA Oxf. 1958; FRCP Lond. 1979, M 1963; FRCP Ed. 1976, M 1963. Prev: Cons. Phys. (Gen. Med. & Geriat. & Diabetes & Endocrinol.) Jas. Paget, Healthcare, NHS Trust Gt. Yarmouth.

WAYNE, Harold Leslie 93 Copeland Drive, Parkstone, Poole BH14 8NP — MB ChB Manch. 1948.

WAYTE, Christopher No 18 Surgery, 18 Upper Oldfield Park, Bath BA2 3JZ Tel: 01225 427402 — MB ChB Bristol 1980; BSc (Biochem.) Bristol 1977; DRCOG 1985; MRCGP 1987. G.P. Princip.; Clin. Asst., Breast Unit, Roy. United Hosp., Bath.

WAYTE, Donald Malcolm, Lt.-Col. RAMC 40 Ffriddoedd Road, Bangor LL57 2TW Tel: 01248 362865 Email: d@wayte1745.freeseve.co.uk; 40 Ffriddoedd Road, Bangor LL57 2TW Tel: 01248 362865 — MB BS Birm. 1957; MB ChB Birm. 1957; MRCS Eng. LRCP Lond. 1957; DTM & H Eng. 1959, DPath 1964; MRCPath 1967; FRCPath 1979, M 1967; MD Birm. 1969. p/t Forens. Path. Dist. Gen. Hosp. Bangor; Locum Cons. Histopath. and Cytologist. Specialty: Histopath. Socs: BMA; BAFM; IAP. Prev: Cons. Histopath. And Cytopathologist, N. W. Wales Hosp. Trust, Gwynedd LL57 2PW; Home Office Pathologist, North Wales.

WAYTE, Jeffrey Alan 11 Mortens Wood, Amersham HP7 9EQ — MB BS Adelaide 1983.

WEADICK, Paul Richard Stanhope Surgery, Stanhope Road, Waltham Cross EN8 7DJ Tel: 01992 635300 Fax: 01992 624292 — MB ChB Liverp. 1983.

WEALE, Mr Adrian Elliott Bristol Royal Infirmary, Department of Orthopaedics, Marlborough Street, Bristol BS2 8HW Tel: 0117 928 4966 Fax: 0117 928 2659 Email: adrian.weale@ubht.swest.nhs.uk — MB BS Lond. 1986 (St Mary's) FRCS Eng. 1991; FRCS (Orth.) 1996; FRCS Ed. 2000; MS Lond. 2001. Cons. Orthop. Surg. United Bristol Healthcare NHS Trust; Hon. Cons. Orthop. Surg. Avon Orthop. Centre Bristol. Specialty: Orthop. Special Interest: Knee Surg. & Jt. Replacement. Socs: Brit. Orthop. Assn.; Girdlestone Soc.; Brit. Assn. Surg. of the Knee. Prev: Biomet Research Fell. Univ. of Oxf.; Sen. Regist. (Orthop. & Traum. Surg.) Bristol Roy. Infirm.; Regist. (Orthop. & Traum. Surg.) Bristol Roy. Infirm.

WEALE, Andrew Robert 560 Warwick Road, Solihull B91 1AD — BM BS Nottm. 1996.

WEAR, Alan Nicholas — MB BS Lond. 1980 (Roy. Free) BSc (Biomed. Sci.) Lond. 1977; DRCOG 1984; MRCGP 1985; MRCPsych 1989. Cons. Psychiat. Marchwood Priory Hosp.; Clin. Teach. Soton. Med. Sch. Specialty: Gen. Psychiat. Socs: Assoc. Mem. Gp. Analytic Soc. Prev: Cons. St. James Hosp. Portsmouth; Sen. Regist. Wessex Regional Rotat. Portsmouth; Squibb Research Fell. Oxf. Univ.

WEAR, Ian Joseph Duke Street Surgery, 4 Duke Street, Barrow-in-Furness LA14 1LF Tel: 01229 820068 Fax: 01229 813840; The White Rose, 13 Walnut Hill, Holebeck, Barrow-in-Furness LA13 0JX Tel: 01229 839174 Fax: 01229 839174 — MB BS Newc. 1989; DRCOG 1993.

WEARDEN, David John Northfield & Mastrick Medical Practice, Quarry Road, Aberdeen AB16 5UW; 23 Cromar Gardens, Kingswells, Aberdeen AB15 8TF — MB ChB Aberd. 1985.

WEARING, Elizabeth Ann 38 Dukes Wood, Crowthorne RG45 6NF Tel: 01344 775653 — MB BS Newc. 1970; HFFP RCOG; DA Eng. 1972. Lead Clinician Family Plann. Surrey/Hants. Borders Trust; Clin. Asst. (Anaesth. St.Peter's Hosp. Chertsey. Specialty: Family Plann. & Reproduc. Health; Anaesth. Prev: Regist. (Anaesth.) St. Peters Hosp. Chertsey; Hon. Surg. & Hon. Phys. Princess Alexandra Hosp. Harlow.

WEARMOUTH, Elizabeth Margaret Fristan Ward, Eastbourne District General Hospital, Kings Drive, Eastbourne BN21 2UD Tel: 01323 435836 Fax: 01323 413751 — MB ChB Leeds 1980 (Leeds Med. Sch.) DCH RCP Lond. 1983; MRCP (UK) 1985; Cert. Family Plann. JCC 1985; MRCGP 1985; FRCPCH 1997. Cons. Paediat. Specialty: Paediat. Special Interest: Adoption & fostering; Community Child Health. Socs: BMA; Sec. S. Thames Paediat. Soc.; RCPCH.

WEARN, Andrew Mark The Laurie Pike Health Centre, 95 Birchfield Road, Handsworth, Birmingham B19 1LH Tel: 0121 554 0621 Fax: 0121 554 6163; 922 Bristol Road, Sellyoak, Birmingham B29 6NB — MB ChB Birm. 1990; MRCGP 1995; DFFP 1995; M.Med.Sci. Birm. 1998. Lect. (Gen. Pract.) Birm. Specialty: Gen. Pract. Socs: BMA; AUDGP; CMF.

WEARNE, Mr Iain Michael James Dept. of Ophth., Eastbourne District Hospital, Kings Drive, Eastbourne BN21 2UD — MB ChB Birm. 1991; ChB Birm. 1991; FRCOphth 1995. Cons. Opthalmic & Oculoplastic Surg., E. Sussex NHS Trust; Coll. Tutor. Special Interest: Refractive Cataract Surg. Prev: Secailist Regist., Moorfields Eye Hosp., Lond.; Oculoplastics Fell., Moorfields Eye Hosp., Lond.

WEARNE, John Penrose Great Sutton Medical Centre, Old Chester Road, Great Sutton, Ellesmere Port CH66 3PB Tel: 0151 339 3126 Fax: 0151 339 9225; 6 Dibbins Green, Wirral CH63 0QF Tel: 0151 334 7640 Fax: 0151 343 0313 Email: jwearne@compuserve.com — MB ChB Liverp. 1982; DRCOG 1985; FRCGP 1996, M 1986. Clin. Asst. (Ophth.) Arrowe Pk. Hosp. Birkenhead. Specialty: Ophth.

WEARNE, Simon 41 Boscathnoe Way, Heamoor, Penzance TR18 3JS; 92 Powdermill Lane, Tunbridge Wells Tel: 01892 619586 — MB BS Lond. 1998 (St Georges) MA(Oxon.) 1992.

WEARNE, Susan Marion South Bank Medical Centre, 175 Bishopthorpe Road, York YO23 1PD; 3 Longwood Link, York YO30 4UG — (Southampton) BM Soton. 1987; DCH RCP Lond. 1990; MRCGP 1991; DRCOG 1992; DFFP 1994. Hon. Sen. Clin. Lect. Leeds Univ. Prev: Trainee GP Kettering Dist. Gen. Hosp.; Ho. Off. Roy. S. Hants. Hosp.

WEARS, Robert Solihull Hospital, Lode Lane, Solihull B91 2JL Tel: 0121 711 4455 Fax: 0121 711 5057; 55 Links Drive, Solihull B91 2DJ — MB ChB Manch. 1986; MRCP (UK) 1990; MSc Lond. 1994; FRCP Lond. 1998. Cons. Phys. Gen. Med. (interest c/o elderly) Solihull Hosp.; Hon. Sen. Clin. Lect. Specialty: Gen. Med. Socs: Brit. Geriat. Soc.; W Midl. Inst. of Ageing and Health; Midl. Gastroenterol. Soc. Prev: Sen. Regist. (Gen. & Geriat. Med.) W. Midl. Regional Train. Scheme; Regist. Rotat. (Gen. & Geriat. Med.) N. & E. Birm.

WEATHERALL, Sir David John (retired) Weatherall Inst. of Molecular Medicine, University of Oxford, John Radcliffe Hospital, Headington, Oxford OX3 9DS Tel: 01865 222360 Fax: 01865 222501 Email: liz.rose@imm.ox.ac.uk; 8 Cumnor Rise Road, Cumnor Hill, Oxford OX2 9HD — Hon. FRCPCH 1996; Dec. Of Humane Letters, Johns Hopkins Univ. 1998; MD Liverp. 1962 FRCP FRCP Ed.; Hon. MD Leeds 1988; Hon. MD Sheff. 1989; Hon. DSc Ed. 1989; Hon. Imperial Coll. 1990; Hon. FACP 1991; Hon. DSc Aberd. 1991; Hon. DSc Leic. 1991; Hon. MD Leeds 1988, Hon. LLD Bristol 1994, Liverp. 1991; Hon. DSc Keele 1993; Hon. MD Nottm. 1993; Hon. DSc McGill, 1999; MB ChB (Hons.) Liverp. 1956; Hon. DSc Lond. 1993, Oxf. Brookes Univ. 1995; Hon. DSc Manch 1988,

South Bank Univ. 1995; Hon. DSc Exeter, 1999; FRCP Lond. 1969, M 1958; FRCPath 1978, M 1969; Hon. DSc Mahidol, Uni. Thailand, 1999; MA Oxf. 1974; FRS 1977; FRCP Ed. 1983; Hon. FRACP 1986; Hon. FRCOG 1988. Emerit. Regius Prof. Med. Univ. Oxf. Prev: Hon. Cons. Phys. Oxon. HA.

WEATHERALL, Josephine Alice Coreen (retired) Willows, Charlbury, Oxford OX7 3PX Tel: 01608 810200 — (Univ. Ed.) BSc 1944, MB ChB Ed. 1945; FFCM 1980, M 1973. Prev: Cons. Epidemiol. to EEC Concerted Action - EUROCAT.

WEATHERALL, Miles (retired) Willows, Charlbury, Oxford OX7 3PX — (Oxf.) DSc Oxf. 1966, DM 1952, BM BCh 1943. Prev: Dir. (Estab.) Wellcome Research Laborats. Beckenham.

WEATHERBY, Emma Dale 186 Grove Lane, Cheadle Hulme, Cheadle SK8 7NH — MB ChB Bristol 1992.

WEATHERBY, Stuart John 4 The Avenue, Alsager, Stoke-on-Trent ST7 2AN — MB ChB Bristol 1993.

WEATHERHEAD, Anne Elizabeth (retired) Newton Park, 59 Brechin Road, Kirriemuir DD8 4DE — MB ChB Ed. 1960; MRCPsych 1983. Prev: Med. Off. Ment. Welf. Commiss. for Scotl.

WEATHERHEAD, Martin Paul Southwick Health Centre, The Green, Southwick, Sunderland SR5 2LT Tel: 0191 548 6550 Fax: 0191 548 0867 — MB BS Newc. 1988.

WEATHERHEAD, Susan Margaret Central Milton Keynes Medical, 1 North Sixth Street, Saxon Gate West, Milton Keynes MK9 2NR Tel: 01908 605775 Fax: 01908 676752; 1 Abraham Close, Willen Park, Milton Keynes MK15 9JA — MB BS Lond. 1982; BA Oxf. 1979; DRCOG 1984; MRCGP 1986; DCH RCP Lond. 1987. Specialty: Dermat.

WEATHERILL, Barbara Ann Fforestfach Medical Centre, 118 Ravenhill Road, Fforestfach, Swansea SA5 5AA Tel: 01792 581666 Fax: 01792 585332; Sheraton House, Gowerton Road, Three Crosses, Swansea SA4 3PX Tel: 01792 872001 Fax: 01792 872001 — BM Soton. 1978; DRCOG 1980; MRCP (UK) 1981; MRCGP 1987. GP Principal; GP Trainer & Swansea VTS Course Organiser.

WEATHERILL, David 17 Blaidwood Drive, Durham DH1 3TD — MB ChB Leeds 1973; PhD Leeds 1982, BSc (Hons.) 1970; FFA RCS Eng. 1977. Cons. Anaesth. Dryburn Hosp. Durh. Specialty: Anaesth.

WEATHERILL, Mr John Randolph Springbank House, Menston Old Lane, Menston, Ilkley LS29 7QQ — MB BS Lond. 1961; DO Eng. 1964; FRCS Eng. 1967. Cons. Ophth. Bradford Roy. Infirm.; Hon. Vis. Prof. Ophth. Sci. Bradford Univ. Specialty: Ophth. Socs: Ophth. Soc. UK. Prev: Sen. Regist. Bristol Eye Hosp.

WEATHERILL, Julia 20 Meadows Lane, Darton, Barnsley S75 5PF — MB ChB Ed. 1996.

WEATHERILL, Walter Frederick 12 St Martin's Court, Lairgate, Beverley HU17 8JB — MRCS Eng. LRCP Lond. 1948 (Leeds) MRCGP 1966.

WEATHERLEY, Anne Ash Surgery, Chilton Gardens, Ash, Canterbury CT3 2HA Tel: 01304 812227; Longbrook, Church Hill, Elmstone, Preston, Canterbury CT3 1HL — MB ChB Leeds 1979; DRCOG 1983; DCH RCP Lond. 1983; MRCGP 1984.

WEATHERLEY, Mr Christopher Roy 1 The Quadrant, Wonford Road, Exeter EX2 4LE Tel: 01392 272951 Fax: 01392 421662 — MD Liverp. 1980; MB ChB 1968; FRCS Ed. 1973; FRCS Eng. 1974; FRCS (Orthop.) Ed. 1984. Cons. Spinal Surg. Princess Eliz. Orthop. Centre & Roy. Devon & Exeter Hosp. (Wonford). Specialty: Orthop.

WEATHERLEY, Pauline Logan 54 Grasmere Road, Muswell Hill, London N10 2DJ — MB ChB Aberd. 1972; DO RCS Eng. 1990.

WEATHERLEY, Rachel Ellen 16 Moorhouse Cl, Chester CH2 2HU — MB ChB Leeds 1997.

WEATHERSTONE, Robert MacKenzie 23 Chigwell Rise, Chigwell IG7 6AQ Tel: 020 8500 3280; Havering Hospitals Trust, Oldchurch Hospital, Romford RM7 0BE Tel: 01708 746090 — MB BChir Camb. 1971; MA, MB Camb. 1971, BChir 1970; MRCP (UK) 1974; FRCP Lond. 1989. Cons. Phys. Havering Hosps. Trust. Specialty: Gen. Med.; Respirat. Med.

WEATHERUP, Alan Salisbury Road Surgery, 98 Salisbury Road, Barry CF62 6PU Tel: 01446 720049 Fax: 01446 733691; 52 Picton Road, Rhoose, Barry CF62 3HU — MB BCh Wales 1983; MRCGP 1988. CME Tutor Vale Glam. Socs: BMA; Barry Med. Soc.; Cardiff Med. Soc.

WEATHERUP, Claire Helen Pershore Health Centre, Priest Lane, Pershore WR10 1EB — MB ChB Birm. 1988 (Birmingham) MRCGP 1993.

WEATHERUP, James (retired) 38 Malone Hill Park, Malone Road, Belfast BT9 6RE — MB BCh BAO Belf. 1954; DObst RCOG 1956.

WEATHERUP, John 1 Hoadly Road, London SW16 1AE — MB BCh BAO Belf. 1947.

WEAVER, Andrew John Radcliffe NHS Trust, Hedley Way, Headington, Oxford OX3 7LJ Tel: 01865 225681 Fax: 01865 225660 Email: andrew.weaver@orh.nhs.uk — MB BS Lond. 1985 (Westm.) MRCP (UK) 1989; FRCR 1993; MD Univ. Lond. 1997. Cons. (Clin. Oncol.) Oxf. Specialty: Oncol. Special Interest: Colorectal, Endocrine and Urological Cancer. Socs: Radiother. Vis. Soc.

WEAVER, Andrew Bernard Child & Adolescent Mental Health Service, Macclesfield DGH, Victoria road, Macclesfield SK10 33L Tel: 01625 663772 — (Manchester) MB ChB Manch. 1984; MRCPsych 1988. Cons. Child & Adolesc. Psychiat. E. Chesh. NHS Trust Macclesfield; Clin. Lect. Univ. Liverp. Specialty: Child & Adolesc. Psychiat. Socs: ACPP. Prev: Sen. Regist. (Child & Adolesc. Psychiat.) Manch.; Regist. Rotat. (Psychiat.) N. Manch.

WEAVER, Andrew John Winch Lane Surgery, Winch Lane, Haverfordwest SA61 1RN Tel: 01437 762333 Fax: 01437 766912 — MB ChB Bristol 1972; DObst RCOG 1974; MRCGP 1978; Dip. Ther. Wales 1995. Prev: SHO (O & G & Paediat.) W. Wales Gen. Hosp. Carmarthen; Ho. Surg. St. Martin's Hosp. Bath.

WEAVER, Ann Lynette Bartlett Winch Lane Surgery, Winch Lane, Haverfordwest SA61 1RN Tel: 01437 762333 Fax: 01437 766912; Redlands, 10 Merlins Hill, Haverfordwest SA61 1PQ — MB ChB Bristol 1972; MRCGP 1978; Dip. Ther. Wales 1995. Prev: SHO (O & G) W. Wales Gen. Hosp. Carmarthen; Ho. Surg. MusGr. Pk. Hosp. Taunton; Ho. Phys. Roy. United Hosp. Bath.

WEAVER, Miss Anne Elizabeth 4 Hazell Park, Amersham HP7 9AB Tel: 01494 729470 Email: aeweaver@bigfoot.com — BM BS Nottm. 1995 (Nottingham) BMedSci Nottm. 1993; MRCS Eng. 1998; Dip IMC (RCS Ed.) 2000. Specialist Regist. (A&E Med.), Merseyside Rot. Specialty: Accid. & Emerg.

WEAVER, Anthony David Odiham Health Centre, Deer Park View, Odiham, Hook RG29 1JY; Butterwood, The St, North Warnborough, Hook RG29 1BG Tel: 01256 703132 Fax: 01256 703508 — BM BCh Oxf. 1974 (Univ. Coll. Hosp.) MA Oxf. 1975; DCH Eng. 1977. Specialty: Acupunc.; Homeop. Med.; Occupat. Health. Socs: Assoc. Mem. Brit. Med. Acupunc. Soc.; Soc. Occupat. Med.

WEAVER, Christine Beverley 4 Hazell Park, Amersham HP7 9AB — MB ChB Birm. 1998.

WEAVER, Corinna Mary (retired) 15 Queenwood, Cyncoed, Cardiff CF23 9LE — (Cardiff) MB BCh Wales 1959; DCH Eng. 1961; DObst RCOG 1962; FRCP Ed. 1981, M 1968; FRCPCH 1994. Prev: Cons. Paediat. Univ. Hosp. of Wales Cardiff.

WEAVER, Hamilton Melville (retired) Croftcroy, Manse Road, Killin FK21 8UY Tel: 01567 820567 — MB ChB Ed. 1940. Prev: GP P'boro.

WEAVER, Helen 41 Bolton Road E., Wirral CH62 4RU — MB ChB Dundee 1994; DRCOG 1996.

WEAVER, Helen Paula Bicester Health Centre, Bicester OX26 6AT; Rivendell, 4 Old London Rd, Milton Common, Thame OX9 2JR — MB ChB Bristol 1988; DA (UK) 1991; DRCOG 1993; MRCGP 1995. Asst. GP Oxon. Specialty: Gen. Pract. Prev: SHO (A & E) Stockport Infirm.; Trainee GP Burton Rd. Family Pract. Manch. & Bridge St. Surg. W. Yorks.

WEAVER, John Andrew 37 Adelaide Park, Belfast BT9 6FY Tel: 01232 668789 — MD Belf. 1954; MB BCh BAO 1950; FRCP Lond. 1970, M 1954. Cons. Phys. Roy. Vict. Hosp. Belf.; Capt. RAMC, TA, Med. Off. N. Irish Horse. Specialty: Gen. Med. Prev: Med. Research Counc. Trav. Fell. in Med. (Eli Lilly Fell.) Endocrine; Dept. Johns Hopkins Hosp. Baltimore; Med. Regist. Roy. Vict. Hosp. Belf.

WEAVER, Mr John Patrick Acton (retired) 229 Strathmartine Road, Dundee DD3 8QQ Tel: 01382 889383 Fax: 01382 889383 — (Oxf. & Guy's) MA Oxf. 1950; BA (1st cl. Hons. Animal Physiol.) 1950; BSc 1952; BM BCh Oxf. 1954; FRCS Ed. 1960; FRCS Eng. 1961; DM MCh 1968. Prev: Cons. Urol. Roy. Dundee Infirm. & Hon. Sen. Lect. (Surg.) Univ. Dundee.

WEAVER, Jolanta Urszula St Annes Cottage, Church Chare, Whickham, Newcastle upon Tyne NE16 4SH Tel: 0191 488 2745 Fax: 0191 491394 Email: wju.weaver@virgin.net — MRCS Eng. LRCP Lond. 1984 (Lond. Hosp. Coll.) MRCP (UK) 1987; PhD Lond. 1993. Sen. Regist. (Diabetes, Endocrinol. & Gen. Med.) Freeman

Hosp. Newc. u. Tyne; Sen. Lect. (Diabetes Med.) Qu. Eliz. Hosp.; Dept. of Med. Univ. of Newc. Specialty: Endocrinol. Socs: Med. Res. Soc.; Soc. Endocrinol.; Brit. Diabetic Assn. Prev: Sen. Regist. (Diabetes, Endocrinol. & Gen. Med.) Roy. Vict. Infirm. Newc. & Middlesbrough Gen. Hosp.; Lect. (Endocrinol.) Roy. Hosp. Lond.

WEAVER, Judith Barbara 75 Hamilton Avenue, Harbourne, Birmingham B17 8AS — MB BS Lond. 1966 (Univ. Coll. Hosp.) MD Lond 1978, MB BS 1966; MRCS Eng. LRCP Lond. 1966; FRCS Ed. 1973; FRCOG 1986, M 1973. Cons. Obst. Birm. Matern. Hosp. Specialty: Obst. & Gyn. Prev: Lect. Dept. O & G Welsh Nat. Sch. Med. Cardiff; Regist. (O & G) United Birm. Hosps.; SHO Gyn. Univ. Coll. Hosp. Lond.

WEAVER, Kevin Nicholas John Happy House Surgery, Durham Road, Sunderland SR3 4BY Tel: 0191 528 2222; 15 Roker Park Terrace, Sunderland SR6 9LY — MB ChB Manch. 1982.

WEAVER, Professor Lawrence Trevelyan Department of Child Health, Yorkhill Hospitals, Dalnair St., Glasgow G3 8SJ Tel: 0141 201 0236 Fax: 0141 201 0837 — MB BChir Camb. 1973 (St. Thos.) MA Camb. 1973, MD Camb. 1986, BA Camb. 1970; MRCS Eng. LRCP Lond. 1973; DRCOG 1977; MRCP (UK) 1979; DCH Eng. 1979; FRCP Lond. 1994; FRCP Glas. 1994; FRCPCH 1998. Prof. Child Health Univ. Glas.; Hon. Cons. Paediat. Yorkhill Hosps. Glas. Specialty: Paediat. Socs: Counc. Europ. Soc. Paediat. Gastroenterol. Nutrit.; Nutrit. Soc.; Brit. Soc. Gastroenterol. Prev: Mem. Scientif. Staff MRC Dunn Nutrit. Unit. Camb.; MRC Research Fell. Dunn Nutrit. Unit Camb.; Fulbright Travel Schol. Harvard Univ. Med. Sch.

WEAVER, Michael Kenneth 47 Elsdon Road, Gosforth, Newcastle upon Tyne NE3 1HY; 47 Elsdon Road, Gosforth, Newcastle upon Tyne NE3 1HY — MB BS Newc. 1983.

WEAVER, Nicola Frances Parkway Medical Centre, 2 Frenton Close, Chapel House Estate, Newcastle upon Tyne NE5 1EH Tel: 0191 267 1313 Fax: 0191 229 0630 — MB BS Lond. 1987; BA Camb. 1984; MRCP (UK) 1991.

WEAVER, Mr Paul Cassford Queen Alexandra Hospital, Cosham, Portsmouth PO6 3LY Tel: 023 92 379451 Fax: 023 92 214162; 9 Sarum Close, Sarum Road, Winchester SO22 5LY Tel: 01962 863081 Fax: 01962 863081 Email: paulweave01@hotmail.com — (St. Bart.) MB BS Lond. 1960; MRCS Eng. LRCP Lond. 1960; FRCS Eng. 1967; FRCS Ed. 1967; MD Lond. 1970. Cons. Surg., Oncol. & Upper Gastrointestinal Portsmouth Hosps. NHS Trust; Clin. Teach. & Examr. Surg. Wessex Med. Sch. Univ. Soton; Sen. Lect. Med. Educat. Specialty: Gen. Surg.; Paediat. Socs: Fell. Brit. Assn. Surg. Oncol.; Fell. Assoc. Surgs. GB & Irel.; (Past Pres.) Wessex Surgs. Prev: Sen. Regist. (Surg.) Westm. Hosp. Lond. & Clin. Asst. St. Marks Hosp.; Regist. (Surg.) St. Bart. Hosp. Lond.; Ho. Off. (Gen. Surg. & Orthop.) Unit St. Bart. Hosp. Lond.

WEAVER, Mr Ralph Michael Hexham General Hospital, Hexham NE46 1QJ — MB BS Lond. 1970; BSc (Anat.) Lond. 1967; FRCS Eng. 1976. Cons. Gen. Surg.; Med. Dir. Hexham Gen. Hosp. Specialty: Gen. Surg. Prev: Sen. Surg. Regist. W. Midl. Regional Train. Scheme; Ho. Phys. Univ. Coll. Hosp. Lond.

WEAVER, Richard David Talbot Medical Centre, 63 Kinson Road, Bournemouth BH10 4BX Tel: 01202 523059 Fax: 01202 533239 — MB BCh BAO Belf. 1978 (Qu. Univ. Belf.) DRCOG 1981; MRCGP 1986; FRCGP 2000. GP; Assoc. Dir. Postgrad. GP Educat. (Dorset). Prev: Course Organiser Dorset VTS; Chairm. E. Dorset Non-Fundholders Gp.; Tutor (Gen. Pract.) Bournemouth & ChristCh.

WEAVER, Sean Anthony 4 Burford Road, East Harnham, Salisbury SP2 8AN — BM BCh Oxf. 1993; MRCP 1996. Research Fell.(Gastroenterol. & Gen. Med.). Specialty: Gastroenterol.

WEAVER, Simon Richard 7 Westville Road, Cardiff CF23 5DE — MB BCh Wales 1997.

WEAVERS, Barbara Janet St Michaels Hospice, Bartestree, Hereford HR1 4HA Tel: 01432 851000; The Villa Farm, Pendock, Staunton, Gloucester GL19 3PG — MB BCh Wales 1977. Sen. Med. Off. St. Michaels Hospice Hereford. Specialty: Palliat. Med.

WEAVIND, Glenn Peter 16 Taw Drive, Chandlers Ford, Eastleigh SO53 4SL — BM Soton. 1980; MRCPath. 1989.

WEAVING, Hester Claudia (retired) Rose Cottage, Station Road, Armathwaite, Carlisle CA4 9PL — MB BCh BAO Belf. 1949; DPM RCPSI 1952; MRCPsych 1972. Psychiat. Eden Valley Hospice Carlisle. Prev: Cons. Psychiat. Durh. Health Dist. & Co. Hosp. Durh.

WEAVING, Jennifer Elizabeth — MB ChB Manch. 1982; BSc (Med. Sci.) St. And. 1979; DRCOG 1985. Regist. In O&G, Carlisle. Prev: Trainee GP E. Cumbria VTS; Ho. Off. (Med./Surg.) Rochdale HA.

WEAVING, Peter Geoffrey Brampton Medical Practice, 4 Market Place, Brampton CA8 1NL Tel: 016977 2551 Fax: 016977 41944; Castellane House, Great Corby, Carlisle CA4 8NQ Tel: 0169 772551 — BM BS Nottm. 1981; BMedSci. Nottm. 1979, BM BS 1981; DRCOG 1985; MRCGP 1986. Prev: Trainee GP/SHO Brampton Cumbria; SHO (Gen. & Geriat. Med.) Birch Hill Hosp. Rochdale; Ho. Off. (Gen. Med.) Bury Gen. Hosp.

WEBB, Adrian Leslie 400 Bald Hill Road, Warwick RI 02886, USA; 3 Midhurst Close, Chilwell, Nottingham NG9 5FQ — MB BS Lond. 1980; MRCPsych 1984. Staff Psychiat. Harvard Community Health Plan of New Eng. Warwick, R hode. Is., USA; Clin. Asst. Prof. Brown Univ. Providence Rhode Is. USA. Specialty: Gen. Psychiat. Socs: Amer. Psychiat. Assn.; Roy. Coll. Psychiat. Prev: Med. Director E. Bay Ment. Health Center Inc. Barrington Rhode Is., USA; Staff Psychiat., Psychiat. Specialists Inc. Pawtucket Rhode Is., USA.

WEBB, Alan Edward Royal Hospital for Sick Children, Yorkhill, Glasgow G3 8SJ Tel: 0141 201 0000 — MB ChB Ed. 1989; MRCP Ed. 1994; CCST (Paediat.) 2003. Locum Cons. Paediat. Specialty: Paediat.

WEBB, Alan Terence 7 Myrtle Way, Brough HU15 1SR Tel: 01482 675080 — MB BS Lond. 1986; MRCP (UK) 1990; MD Lond. 1995. Cons. (Nephrol. & Gen. Med.) Hull Roy. Infirm. Specialty: Nephrol. Socs: BMA; Renal Assn. Prev: Cons. (Nephrol. & Gen. Med.) St. Luke's Hosp. Bradford; SpR W. Midlands Train. Progr.; Regist. (Nephrol. & Gen. Med.) Univ. Hosp. S. Manch.

WEBB, Alexandra Joan St. Wilfrid's Hospice, Grosvenor Road, Chichester PO19 2FP Tel: 01243 775302 Fax: 01243 538171 — MB ChB Ed. 1979; FFA RCSI 1987. Cons. Palliat. Med. St Wilfrid's Hospice Chichester.; Hon. Cons.(Palliat. Med.) St. Richard's Hosp. & Sussex, Weald & Down NHS Trusts Chichester. Specialty: Palliat. Med. Prev: Sen. Regist. (Palliat. Med.) St. Columba's Hospice Edin.; Sen. Regist. McMillan Fell. Chronic Pain & Palliat. Med. Bradford & Leeds HAs.

WEBB, Alison Dora (retired) Fernleigh, 4 Church Park, Newton Ferrers, Plymouth PL8 1AJ Tel: 01752 873033 — (W. Lond.) MRCS Eng. LRCP Lond. 1948; BM BCh Oxf. 1949; DPM Eng. 1972. Prev: Sen. Regist. (Child Psychiat.) Nuffield Child Psychiat.

WEBB, Andrew Arthur Charlton 3 Gwynne Park Avenue, Woodford Green IG8 8AB — MB BS Lond. 1992.

WEBB, Andrew John Elderly Care Unit, Dorset County Hospital, Williams Avenue, Dorchester DT1 2JY Tel: 01305 251150 Fax: 01305 254155 — MB BS Newc. 1975; MRCP (UK) 1979. Cons. Phys. c/o Elderly W. Dorset HA. Specialty: Care of the Elderly. Socs: Brit. Geriat. Soc.

WEBB, Andrew Michael Department of Anaesthesia, Lincoln County Hospital, Greetwell Road, Lincoln LN2 5QY Tel: 01522 512512 — MB ChB Leic. 1986; FRCA 1995. Cons. Anaesth., Lincoln Co. Hosp. Specialty: Anaesth. Socs: Pain Soc.

WEBB, Andrew Roy University College London Hospitals NHS Trust, Foley Street, London W1W 6DN — MB BCh Wales 1981 (Univ. Wales) MRCP (UK) 1984; MD Wales 1993; FRCP Lond. 1997. Med. Director and Cons. in Intens. Care Med. Specialty: Intens. Care. Socs: Fell. Roy. Soc. Med.; Eur. Soc. Intens. Care Med.; Intens. Care Soc. Prev: Cons. Phys. (ITU) Bloomsbury & Islington HA; Clin. Research Fell. & Lect. (Med.) St. Geo. Hosp. Med. Sch.; Regist. (Med.) S & W Glam. HA.

WEBB, Andrew Russell 11 Gilders, Sawbridgeworth CM21 0EE — MB BS Lond. 1990; BSc Lond. 1986; MRCP (UK) 1994. Research Fell. & Hon. Regist. Roy. Marsden Hosp. Specialty: Oncol. Prev: SHO Rotat. (Med.) Chase Farm.

WEBB, Anne Margaret Caroline Central Abacus, 40/46 Dale Street, Liverpool L2 5SF Tel: 0151 284 2500 Fax: 0151293 2005 — MB ChB Sheff. 1981; DRCOG 1983; MRCGP 1985; MRCOG 1988; MFFP 1993. Cons. Family Plann & Reproduc. Health Care N. Mersey Community NHS Trust; Regional Adviser (Mersey) Fac. of Family Plann. & Reproductive Health Care RCOG. Specialty: Family Plann. & Reproduc. Health. Socs: Bd. Mem. Fac. Family Plann & Reproduc. Health Care RCOG; (Bd. Mem.) Europ. Soc. Contracep. Prev: SCMO (Family Plann.) Centr. Manch. & S. Manch.; WHO Research Fell. Manch. Univ.

WEBB, Mr Anthony John (retired) Grange Park House, 10 Grange Park, Westbury-on-Trym, Bristol BS9 4BP Tel: 01179 629320 — (Bristol) MB ChB Bristol 1953; FRCS Eng. 1959; ChM Bristol 1974. Sen. Research Fell. Univ. Bristol; Sen. Clin. Lect. (Surg.) Univ. Bristol 1990. Prev: Cons. Surg. Bristol Roy. Infirm.

WEBB, Professor Anthony Kevin 50 Swann Lane, Cheadle Hulme, Cheadle SK8 7HU — MB BS Lond. 1972; FRCP Lond. 1990. Prof. of Thoriac Med.. Wythenshawe Hosp. Specialty: Respirat. Med. Prev: Cons. Phys. N. Manch. Gen. Hosp. & Monsall Hosp.; Sen. Regist. (Chest Med.) Wythenshawe Hosp. Manch.; Regist. (Med.) Whipps Cross Hosp. & Lond. Hosp.

WEBB, Antony Roger The Surgery, High Street, Cheslyn Hay, Walsall WS6 7AB Tel: 01922 701280 — MRCS Eng. LRCP Lond. 1975.

WEBB, Brendan Joseph Ampleforth Abbey, York YO62 4EN Tel: 01439 766810 Fax: 01439 766724 — (Camb. & St. Bart.) MRCS Eng. LRCP Lond. 1943; MA Camb. 1945. Prev: Surg. Lt. RNVR; Ho. Surg. St. Bart. Hosp.

WEBB, Brian Wykeham (retired) Nigella, West Monkton, Taunton TA2 8QT Tel: 01823 412442 — (Middlx.) MRCS Eng. LRCP Lond. 1945; MB BS Lond. 1946; DCH Eng. 1951; MD Lond. 1952; FRCP Lond. 1970, M 1953; FRCPCH 1997. Cons. Paediat. W. Som. Health Dist. Prev: Vis. WHO Prof. Paediat. & Child Health Univ. Khartoum.

WEBB, Carol Louise Ilkeston Health Centre, South Street, Ilkeston DE7 5PZ Tel: 0115 932 2933 — BM BS Nottm. 1987; DRCOG 1991.

WEBB, Carole Ann Queens Hospital Burton, Belvedere Road, Burton-on-Trent DE13 0RB Tel: 01283 566333; The Ridgeway, 46A Main St, Repton, Derby DE65 6FB Tel: 01283 704873 — MB ChB Sheff. 1984; FRCA 1991. Cons. Anaesth. & Intens. Care Qu. Hosp. Burton-on-Trent. Specialty: Anaesth.; Intens. Care. Prev: Sen. Regist. (Anaesth.) Midl. Train. Scheme; Regist. Rotat. (Anaesth.) Stoke-on-Trent.

WEBB, Cecil Hugh The Royal Hospitals NHS Trust, Grosvenor Road, Belfast BT12 6BA Tel: 02890 240503 Fax: 02890 311416 — MB BCh BAO Belf. 1985; BDS Belf. 1971; FRCPath 1991, M 1979; FFPath RCPI 1990. Cons. Clin. Bact. Roy. Hosps. NHS Trust. Specialty: Med. Microbiol. Prev: Sen. Lect. & Cons. Oral Med. & Path. Sch. Dent. Sci. Univ. Dub.; Lect. (Microbiol. & Immunobiol.) Qu. Univ. Belf.

WEBB, Christopher David Prospect House, Harmby, Leyburn DL8 5PE Tel: 01969 623199 — MB ChB Leeds 1993; DRCOG 1996; MRCGP 1997; DFFP 1997. GP Princip. Catterick Village Health Centre. Specialty: Gen. Pract. Prev: Harrogate VTS.

WEBB, Christopher James 5 Lawson Close, Woolston, Warrington WA1 4EG — MB ChB Liverp. 1994. SHO (ENT) Arrowe Pk. Hosp. Wirral Merseyside. Specialty: Otorhinolaryngol. Prev: SHO (Orthop.) Bury & Fairfield Hosp.; SHO (Ear, Nose & Throat) Roy. Liverp. Hosp.; SHO (Ear, Nose & Throat) N. Manch. Gen. Hosp.

WEBB, Christopher Lewis Wakely (retired) Stable Cottage, Frogmore, Kingsbridge TQ7 2PE Tel: 01548 531600 — MB BS Lond. 1960 (Lond. Hosp.) MRCS Eng. LRCP Lond. 1960; DObst RCOG 1962; DA Eng. 1964. Prev: SCMO Port & Environm. Health Soton. & SW Hants. HA (T).

WEBB, Clyde Bernard Park Street Practice, Park Street, Ripon HG4 2BE Tel: 01765 692366 Fax: 01765 606440 — MB BS Lond. 1979 (Roy. Free Hosp. Sch. Med.) MRCGP 1983; DRCOG 1983; Dip. Occ. Med. 1995. Specialty: Occupat. Health. Socs: SOM.

WEBB, David Brynley Picton House, Llanblethian, Cowbridge CF71 7JF Tel: 01656 752752 — MB BChir Camb. 1973; MA Camb. 1972, MD 1986; FRCP 1996. Cons. Phys. (Gen. Med.) Princess of Wales Hosp. Bridgend. Specialty: Gen. Med.; Nephrol. Socs: Sec. Dist. Gen. Nephrologists Soc. Prev: Lect. (Renal Med.) Cardiff Roy. Infirm.

WEBB, Professor David John Clinical Pharmacology Unit & Research Centre, University Department of Medicine, Western General Hospital, Edinburgh EH4 2XU Tel: 0131 537 2003 Fax: 0131 537 2003 Email: d.j.webb@ed.ac.uk; 26 Inverleith Gardens, Edinburgh EH3 5PS Tel: 0131 552 4518 Fax: 0131 552 4518 — MB BS Lond. 1977 (Lond. Hosp.) MRCP (UK) 1980; MD Lond. 1990; FRCP Ed. 1992; FFPM RCP (UK) 1993; FRCP Lond. 1994; F Med. Sci. 1999. Christison Prof. Therap. & Clin. Pharmacol. Univ. Edin. & Hon. Cons. Phys. Western Gen. Hosp. Edin.; Chairm. Univ. Dept. Med. W. Gen. Hosp. Edin.; Ldr. Centre for Research in Cardiovasc. Biol.; Dir. Clin. Research Centre Western Gen. Hosp. Edin.; Chairm. Lothian Area Drug & Therap. Comm. Specialty: Pharmacology. Socs: Brit. Hypertens. Soc.; Internat. Soc. Hypertens.; Brit. Pharm. Soc. (Sec. Clin. Sect.). Prev: Sen. Lect. (Med.) Univ. Edin.; Lect. (Clin. Pharmacol.) & Hon. Sen. Regist. (Med.) St. Geo. Hosp. Lond.; Clin. Scientist MRC Blood Pressure Unit Western Infirm. Glas..

WEBB, David Kenneth Humphries Department of Haematology, Great Ormond St. Children's Hospital, Great Ormond St., London WC1N 3JH Tel: 020 7829 8831 Fax: 020 7813 8410; Hognore Farm, Pilgrims Way, Wrotham, Sevenoaks TN15 7NN — MB BS Lond. 1978 (Guy's Hospital London) MRCP (UK) 1981; MD Lond. 1990; MRCPath 1990; FRCP (UK) 1995; MRCPCH 1996. Cons. (Paediat. Haemat.). Specialty: Haematology.

WEBB, David Robert 41 Upland Road, Selly Park, Birmingham B29 7JS — MB ChB Aberd. 1997.

WEBB, Donald Albert (retired) 1 Waterdale Close, Westbury-on-Trym, Bristol BS9 4QN Tel: 0117 962 2061 — MB ChB Sheff. 1956. Prev: Assoc. Specialist (Blood Transfus.) Southmead Hosp. Bristol.

WEBB, Elizabeth Mary Grove House Surgery, 18 Wilton Road, Salisbury SP2 7EE; Island Cottage, West Harnham, Salisbury SP2 8EU Tel: 01722 334537 — MB BS Lond. 1966 (St. Bart.) MRCS Eng. LRCP Lond. 1966; DObst RCOG 1968; DCH Eng. 1971; MRCGP 1979.

WEBB, Elspeth Valmai Jocelyn Department Child Health, University of Wales College of Medicine, Cardiff CF14 4XN Tel: 029 2053 6795 Fax: 029 2074 3359 — MB BS Lond. 1978 (St Geos. Hosp. Lond.) DTM & H RCP Lond. 1980; DCH RCP Lond. 1981; MRCP (UK) 1983; FRCP 1996; FRCPCH 1997. Hon. Cons. Paediat. Community Child Health Cardiff Community Health Care Trust; Sen. Lect. Child Health Univ. of Wales Coll. Med. Specialty: Paediat. Socs: Brit. Assn. of Community Child Health; Welsh Paediat. Soc.; RCPCH Child Pub. Health Gp. Prev: Lect. (Community & Child Health) Qu. Med. Centre Nottm.; Regist. (Paediat.) St. David's & Llandough Hosps. Cardiff; GP Trainee Isle of Skye VTS.

WEBB, Emma Jane Students Health Service, 25 Belgrave Road, Clifton, Bristol BS8 2AA Tel: 0117 973 7716; 1 Broadleys Avenue, Henleaze, Bristol BS9 4LY Tel: 0117 962 4800 Email: ejwebb@doctors.org.uk — MB ChB Bristol 1994; DRCOG 1998; DFFP 1999. GP, Univ. of Bristol, Bristol. Specialty: Gen. Pract. Prev: GP Regist.; GP Locum, Bristol.

WEBB, Eric John 9 Overend Close, Bradwell, Milton Keynes MK13 9EJ Tel: 01908 311981 Email: drericwebb@clara.co.uk — MB BChir Camb. 1976 (Camb. & Char. Cross) MA Camb. 1976; DCH Eng. 1979. p/t Asst. G.P. Watling Vale Med. Centre, Milton Keynes; Clinical Assistant G.U. Medicine, Milton Keynes Hospital; Private G.P. and Occupational Health Practitioner. Specialty: Gen. Pract.; Occupat. Health; Genitourinary Medicine. Special Interest: Male Menopause; Men's Health; Sexual Dysfunction. Socs: Nat. Assn. Non Principals; Medico-Legal Soc.; RSM. Prev: Partner Centr. Milton Keynes Med. Gp.

WEBB, Frances Maxine Urmston Group Practice, 154 Church Road, Urmston, Manchester M41 9DL Tel: 0161 755 9870; 2A Broadoak Park Road, Monton, Eccles, Manchester M30 9LQ Tel: 0161 787 8235 — MB ChB Manch. 1983; DCH RCP Lond. 1985; MRCGP 1988. Prev: SHO (O & G) St. Mary's Hosp. Manch.; SHO (Paediat.) Booth Hall Childr. Hosp. Manch.; SHO (A & E) Hope Hosp. Salford.

WEBB, Francis William Stanley, RD (retired) Glebe House, Church Lane, Baylham, Ipswich IP6 8JS Tel: 01473 830337 Fax: 01473 832854 — MB Camb. 1961 (Lond. Hosp.) BChir 1960; DObst RCOG 1964; FRCP Lond. 1984, M 1966. Cons. Rheum. Ipswich Hosp. Prev: Regist. Rheum. Middlx. Hosp.

WEBB, Frank Ewart (retired) 29 Augustus Road, Edgbaston, Birmingham B15 3PQ Tel: 0121 455 9440 — MB ChB Birm. 1946; MRCS Eng. LRCP Lond. 1946. Prev: GP Birm.

WEBB, Professor Hubert Eustace (retired) 56 Fairacres, Roehampton Lane, London SW15 5LY Tel: 020 8487 8391 — MA Oxf. 1948, DM 1961, BM BCh 1951; FRCP Lond. 1969, M 1954; FRCPath 1988; DSc Med. Lond. 1990. Cons. Phys. Dept. Neurol. & Prof. Neurovirol. St. Thos. Hosp. Lond.; Dir. (Neurovirol.) Unit Rayne Inst. Prev: Temp. Staff Mem. Rockefeller Foundat.

WEBB, Hugh Basil Graham (retired) Mistlemead, North Tawton, Okehampton EX20 2HB Tel: 01837 82603 — MRCS Eng. LRCP Lond. 1950 (Middlx.) DObst RCOG 1953. Prev: Med. Off. North. Provinces, Nigeria.

WEBB, Janet Elizabeth — MB ChB Sheff. 1980; DRCOG 1992; DCCH 1993; MRCGP 1994.

WEBB, Janet Lois Cheltenham Road Surgery, 16 Cheltenham Road, Gloucester GL2 0LS Tel: 01452 522575 Fax: 01452 304321; Longford Lodge, 109 Tewkesbury Road, Longford, Gloucester GL2 9BN — BM Soton. 1980; MRCP (UK) 1984; MRCGP 1987.

WEBB, Mr Jason Crispin John 1 Broadleys Avenue, Henleaze, Bristol BS9 4LY Email: jcwebb@doctors.org.uk; Flat 4, All Saints Court, All Saints Road, Clifton, Bristol BS8 2JE — MB ChB Bristol 1994; FRCS Eng; BSc (Hons.) Cell & Molecular Path. Bristol 1991; MB ChB (Hons.) Bristol 1994. SpR S.W.Deanery Rotation. Specialty: Orthop. Prev: SHO Rotat. (Surg.) Roy. Surrey Co. Hosp.; SHO Roy. Nat. Orthepaedic Hosp., Stanmore, Middlx.; SHO (A&E Med.) Bristol Roy. Infirm.

WEBB, Jennifer Neale Rushall House, Rushall Lane, Lytchett Matravers, Poole BH16 6AJ — MB ChB Bristol 1982; DRCOG 1984; MRCGP 1986; DCCH RCP Lond. 1987. Family Plann. Poole. Prev: GP Retainer Scheme Nottm. & Edin.

WEBB, Jill Barbara 13 Mill Way, Rickmansworth WD3 8QR — MB BS Newc. 1990; FRCS Eng. 1995. SHO (Plastic Surg.) Mid. Essex. Specialty: Plastic Surg. Prev: SHO (Gen. Surg.) Hillingdon Gen. Hosp.; SHO (Gen. & Plastic Surg.) Mt. Vernon Hosp.

WEBB, Joan Dorothy (retired) Rose Gardens, 15 Eynsham Road, Oxford OX2 9BS Tel: 01865 863851 — MB BS Lond. 1946 (Roy. Free) MRCS Eng. LRCP Lond. 1945; MRCP Lond. 1947. Prev: Clin. Asst. (Path.) King's Mill Hosp. Sutton-in-Ashfield.

WEBB, Joanna Heathcote Medical Centre, Heathcote, Tadworth KT20 5TH Tel: 01737 360202 — (St. Thos.) MB BS Lond. 1968; MRCS Eng. LRCP Lond. 1968; MRCGP 1983. Prev: Ho. Surg. Sutton Gen. Hosp.; Ho. Phys. St. Thos. Hosp. Lond.

WEBB, Mr John Beverley 64 Norton Road, Letchworth SG6 1AE Tel: 01462 675628 — (St. Mary's) MRCS Eng. LRCP Lond. 1969; FRCS Eng. 1974; FRCOG 1993, M 1980. Cons. O & G Lister Hosp. Stevenage. Specialty: Obst. & Gyn. Prev: Sen. Regist. (O & G) Hammersmith Hosp. Lond. & Northwick Pk. Hosp. Middlx.; GP/Surg. Austral. Inland Med. Serv.; Regist. (O & G) Roy. Free Hosp. & City of Lond. Matern. Hosp.

WEBB, John Francis, MC, Col. late RAMC Retd. (retired) 38 Westover Road, Fleet GU51 3DB Tel: 01252 613080 — (Newc.) MB BS Durh. 1940; MD Durh. 1956; FRCP Ed. 1972, M 1966. Prev: Phys. i/c MoD Sprue Research Team Hong Kong.

WEBB, John Gilbert Health Centre, Pwllheli Road, Criccieth LL52 0RR Tel: 01766 523451 Fax: 01766 523453; Erw Las, Penaber, Criccieth LL52 0ES Tel: 01766 522715 — MB BCh Wales 1975.

WEBB, Mr John Kenneth Harold Spinal Unit, D Floor, West Block, Queens Medical Centre, Nottingham NG7 2UH Tel: 0115 970 9761 Fax: 0115 970 9991 Email: johnkwebb@compuserve.com — MB BS Lond. 1966 (The Lond. Hosp.) FRCS Eng. 1971; Cert. Higher Educat. 1977. Cons., Spinal Surg., Univ. Hosp., Nottm.; Cons. Adviser, Spinal Surg., Roy. Air Force; Phys., to The P. of Wales & household. Specialty: Orthop. Socs: The Europ. Spine Soc.; The Scoliosis Research Soc. Prev: Past Chairm. of the Internat. AO Spine Bd.

WEBB, Professor John Kingdon Guy, OBE Fernleigh, 4 Church Park, Newton Ferrers, Plymouth PL8 1AJ Tel: 01752 873033 — (Oxf.) BM BCh Oxf. 1942; MA Oxf. 1947; FRCP Lond. 1967, M 1950. Emerit. Prof. Child Health Univ. Newc.; Hon. Cons. Paediat. Roy. Vict. Infirm. Newc. Specialty: Paediat. Socs: FRCPCh; Hon. Fell. Indian Acad. Paediat. Prev: James Spence Prof. Child Health Univ. Newc.; Prof. of Paediat. & Dir. Christian Med. Coll. & Hosp. Vellore, India.

WEBB, John Neville (retired) 56 St Albans Road, Edinburgh EH9 2LX Tel: 0131 667 2637 — MB BChir Camb. 1960 (Camb. & St. Thos.) MD Camb. 1969, MA, MB 1960, BChir 1959; DObst RCOG 1961; FRCP Ed. 1974, M 1964.

WEBB, Jonathan Roy Queen Elizabeth Hospital, Stadium Road, Woolwich, London SE18 4QH Tel: 0208 836 4095 Fax: 0208 836 4094 Email: jonathan.webb@nhs.net — MB BS Lond. 1968 (Guy's) MRCP (U.K.) 1973; FRCP Lond. 1987. Cons. Phys. Woolwich, Lond. SE18 4QH. Specialty: Gen. Med.; Respirat. Med. Special Interest: Sleep. Socs: British Thoracic Society; British Sleep Society.

WEBB, Judith Ann Westwood The London Clinic, Diagnostic Radiology Department, London W1G.6BW Tel: 020 7935 4444; 3 Sellers Hall Close, Finchley, London N3 1JL Tel: 020 8346 2705 Email: jawwebb@btopenworld.com — MB BS Lond. 1967 (St. Bart.) MD Lond. 1983, BSc (1st cl. Hons.) Physiol.) 1964; MRCP (UK) 1971; DMRD Eng. 1973; FRCR 1976; FRCP Lond. 1991. Cons. Diagn. Radiol. St. Bart. Hosp. Lond. Specialty: Radiol. Special Interest: Urin. Tract & Gyn. Imaging; Ultrasonography; Contrast Media. Socs: FRSM; Soc. Uroradiol.; Euro. Soc. Urogenital Radiol. (Past Pres). Prev: Sen. Regist. (Diagn. Radiol.) & Jun. Regist. (Med.) St. Bart. Hosp. Lond.; Instruc. (Diagn. Radiol.) Univ. Cal. San. Diego, USA.

WEBB, Mr Julian Francis Waldron St. Thomas Hospital, Lambeth Palace Road, London SE1 7EH; 14 Chatterton Road, Highbury, London N4 2DZ — MB BS Lond. 1987; FRCS Ed. 1994.

WEBB, Kenneth Rhys Hughes and Partners, 15 Dereham Road, Mattishall, Dereham NR20 3QA Tel: 01362 850227 Fax: 01362 858466; Southfield House, Common Road, East Tuddenham, Dereham NR20 3NF Tel: 01362 880216 — MB BS Lond. 1975.

WEBB, Kevin Iain Flat G, Alexandra Court, 10A Alexandra Road, Weymouth DT4 7QH — MB ChB Cape Town 1995.

WEBB, Mr Lennox Andrew Burnside Cottage, Kirk Road, Houston, Johnstone PA6 7HN — MB ChB Dundee 1987; FRCOphth 1993, M 1990; FRCS Ed. 1992. Cons. Roy. Alexandra Hosp. Paisley Scotl.; Hon. Sen. Clin. Lect. Glas. Caledonian Univ. Glas. Specialty: Ophth. Socs: BMA. Prev: Orbit Oculoplastic & Anterior Segment Fell. Eye Care Centre Univ. Brit. Columbia, Canada; Sen. Regist. Tennent Inst. Ophth. Glas.

WEBB, Lesley Ann 26 Brisbane Grove, Hartburn, Stockton-on-Tees TS18 5BW — MB ChB Dundee 1978; MRCP (UK) 1985. Regist. (Radiol.) Roy. Vict. Infirm. Newc. upon Tyne. Specialty: Radiol. Prev: SHO (Dermat.) Carter Bequest Hosp. Middlesbrough; SHO (Chest Med.) Poole Hosp. Middlesbrough; SHO (Gen. Med.) Hartlepool Gen. Hosp.

WEBB, Lindsay Joy Adshall Road Medical Practice, 97 Adshall Road, (off Councillor Lane), Cheadle SK8 2JN; 50 Swann Lane, Cheadle Hulme, Cheadle SK8 7HU — MB BS Lond. 1972 (Middlx. Hosp.) MRCP (UK) 1974; MD Lond. 1981. Prev: CMO Centr. Manch.; MRC Research. Fell. Roy. Free Hosp. Lond.

WEBB, Lynda Jane 28A Ongar Road, Fulham, London SW6 1SJ — MB BS Lond. 1989.

WEBB, Mark Robert 43 Cutsdean Close, Bishops Cleeve, Cheltenham GL52 8UT — MB BCh Witwatersrand 1992.

WEBB, Michael Alfred Healey, KStJ, OBE 48 Offington Avenue, Worthing BN14 9PJ Tel: 01903 260095 Fax: 01903 690934 — (King's Coll. Hosp.) MRCS Eng. LRCP Lond. 1961; DIH Soc. Apoth. Lond. 1978; FFOM RCP Lond. 1996, M 1980. Cons. Occupat. Health W. Sussex. Specialty: Occupat. Health. Socs: Soc. Occupat. Med. & Mem. BMA. Prev: Sen. Med. Adviser SE Area Post Off.; Med. Adviser Commonw. Smelting Ltd Avonmouth; Employm. Med. Adviser EMAS.

WEBB, Michael Stephen Carroll Department of Paediatrics, Gloucestershire Royal Hospital, Great Western Road, Gloucester GL1 3NN Tel: 08454 228493 Fax: 08454 228145 Email: mike.webb@glos.nhs.uk; Longford Lodge, Tewkesbury Road, Longford, Gloucester GL2 9BN Tel: 01452 730450 — MB ChB Bristol 1976 (Bristol Univ.) FRCP Lond. 1995; FRCPCH 1998. Cons. Paediat. Glos. Roy. Hosp.; RCPCH Regional Adviser, S. W. Specialty: Paediat. Prev: Sen. Regist. (Paediat.) Soton. & Portsmouth HAs; Clin. Research Fell. Dept. Child Health Univ. Hosp. Nottm.; SHO (Paediat.) Roy. Hosp. Sick Childr. Gt. Ormond St. Lond.

WEBB, Michelle Claire The Renal Unit, Guy's & St Thomas' Hospital Trust, St Thomas St., London SE1 9RT — BChir Camb. 1988; MA Camb. 1989, BChir 1988; MRCP (UK) 1991; MD (Camb.) 1997. Sen. Regist. Renal Med. Specialty: Nephrol.

WEBB, Nicholas John Alexander Department pf Nephrology, Royal Manchester Children's Hospital, Pendlebury, Manchester M27 4HA Tel: 0161 727 2435 Fax: 0161 727 2630 — BM BS Nottm. 1986; BMedSci Nottm. 1984, BM BS 1986; FRCPCH 1997; DM Nottm. 1998; FRCP 1999. Cons. Paediat. Nephrol. Roy. Manch. Childr. Hosp. Manch. Specialty: Paediat. Socs: Brit. Assn. Paediat. Nephrol.; Internat. Paediat. Nephrol. Assn. Prev: Sen. Regist.

(Paediat. Nephrol.) Roy. Manch. Childr. Hosp.; Clin. Fell. (Paediat. Nephrol.) Hosp. for Sick Childr. Toronto; Regist. (Paediat.) Roy. Childr. Hosp. Melbourne.

WEBB, Peta Sedgley The Seaton and Colyton Medical Practice, Seaton Health Centre, 148 Harepath Road, Seaton EX12 2DU Tel: 01297 20877 Fax: 01297 23031; Broadstone Farm House, Walditch, Bridport DT6 4LQ Tel: 01308 425665 — MB ChB Leic. 1984 (Leicester) BSc (Hons.) Lond. 1979; DRCOG 1991.

WEBB, Peter The Health Centre, Station Road, Haydock, St Helens WA11 0JN Tel: 01744 34419 — MB ChB Liverp. 1967; DObst RCOG 1969. Clin. Asst. (Rheum.) Whiston Hosp. Prescot. Specialty: Rehabil. Med.; Rheumatol.

WEBB, Mr Peter John The Old Farm, Gully Lane, Luppitt, Honiton EX14 4RZ Tel: 01404 891701 — MB BS Lond. 1969 (Univ. Coll. Hosp.) BSc Lond. 1965; MRCS Eng. LRCP Lond. 1969; FRCS Eng. 1974. Cons. Spinal Surg. MusGr. Pk. Hosp. Taunton. Specialty: Orthop. Prev: Cons. Orthop. Surg. Roy. Nat. Orthop. Hosp. Stanmore; Hon. Cons. Orthop. Surg. Italian Hosp. Lond.; Cons. Orthop. Surg. Hosp. Sick Childr. Lond.

WEBB, Mr Peter John Woodcut House, 238 Maidstone Road, Chatham ME4 6JN Tel: 01634 844755 Fax: 01634 844755 — MB BS Lond. 1972; FRCS Eng. 1977; MS Lond. 1985. Cons. Surg. Medway NHS Trust. Specialty: Gen. Surg. Socs: BMA; Assn. Surg.; Assn. Coloproctol. Prev: Sen. Regist. (Surgic.) King's Coll. Hosp. Lond.; Research Fell. Thrombosis Unit King's Coll. Hosp. Lond.; Ho. Surg. Profess. Unit Middlx. Hosp. Lond.

WEBB, Philip Guy Skellern and Partners, Bridport Medical Centre, North Allington, Bridport DT6 5DU Tel: 01308 421109 Fax: 01308 420869; Broadstone Farm House, Walditch, Bridport DT6 4LQ Tel: 01308 425665 — MB ChB Birm. 1980; MRCP (UK) 1984.

WEBB, Rachel Delyth 25 Park Street, Denbigh LL16 3DE — MB ChB Liverp. 1992.

WEBB, Ralph James 27 Harford Drive, Watford WD17 3DQ — MB BS Lond. 1981.

WEBB, Ray Talbot, Wing Cdr. RAF Med. Br. Retd. Trinity Surgery, Norwich Road, Wisbech PE13 3UZ Tel: 01945 476999 Fax: 01945 476900 — BM Soton. 1978; MRCGP 1983; DRCOG 1983; DAvMed FOM RCP Lond. 1988. Prev: Adviser (Gen. Pract.) RAF.; Ho. Surg. & Ho. Phys. Weymouth & Dist. Hosp.

WEBB, Rosemarie Felicity The Surgery, High Street, Epworth, Doncaster DN9 1EP Tel: 01427 872232 Fax: 01427 874944; 1 Mill Lane, Westwoodside, Doncaster DN9 2AF Tel: 01427 752193 — (Edinburgh) MB ChB Ed. 1971; DObst RCOG 1974; FRCGP 1995, M 1975; MFFP 1994. GP Princip.; Trainer GP Doncaster VTS. Prev: Trainee GP Doncaster VTS; Ho. Phys. & Ho. Surg. Hull Roy. Infirm.

WEBB, Samuel Wilson 26 Deramore Park S., Malone Road, Belfast BT9 5JY Tel: 01232 666543 — MB BCh BAO Belf. 1966; BSc (Hons. Anat.) Belf. 1963, MB 1974, MB BCh BAO 1966; MRCP (UK) 1970; MD Belf. 1974. Cons. Cardiol. Roy. Vict. Hosp. Belf. Specialty: Cardiol.

WEBB, Sarah Elizabeth (retired) 3 Abbey Street, Bath BA1 1NN Tel: 01225 464738 — MB BS Lond. 1970; DObst RCOG 1973; DCH RCP Lond. 1974; MRCGP 1979.

WEBB, Sheila Joy Bradford HA, New Mill, Victoria Road, Saltaire, Shipley BD18 3LD Tel: 01274 366007; Trevethick, Cragg Drive, Ilkley LS29 8BE Tel: 01943 603227 — MB ChB Sheff. 1974; DRCOG 1977; MRCGP 1978; MPH Leeds 1988; MFPHM RCP (UK) 1991; FFPHM 1998; Dip Ther Newc. 2001. Cons. Pub. Health Med. Bradford HA. Specialty: Pub. Health Med. Prev: GP Bradford Univ. & Birkenhead; Sen. Regist. (Pub. Health Med.) Yorks RHA.

WEBB, Spencer Edwin 10 Upgrove Manor Way, Chessingham Gardens, London SW2 2QX — MB BS Lond. 1996.

WEBB, Steven Anthony Rochford Flat 9, Bishopsbourne, 134-136 Westbourne Terrace, London W2 6QB — MB BS Western Australia 1988; FRACP 1995. Research Fell. Molecular Infec. Dis. Unit Dept. Paediat. St. Mary's Hosp. Med. Sch. Lond. Specialty: Intens. Care.

WEBB, Stuart Charles St Charles Hospital, Exmoor St., London W10 6DZ Tel: 020 8962 4126 Fax: 020 8962 4131; 43 Granville Road, Barnet EN5 4DS — MB BS Lond. 1974 (Univ. Coll. Hosp.) BSc (Physiol.) Lond. 1971, MB BS 1974; MRCP (UK) 1978; MD Lond. 1985; FRCP (Eng.) 1992. Cons. Phys. St Mary's Hosp. Lond. Specialty: Care of the Elderly. Socs: Brit. Cardiac Soc.; Brit. Pacing & Electrophysiol. Gp. Prev: Sen. Regist. (c/o the Elderly) Hammersmith Hosp. Lond.; Regist. (Cardiol.) Nat. Heart Hosp. Lond.; Regist. (Med.) Roy. Free Hosp. Lond.

WEBB, Timothy Birkett Nonesuch, 25 Park St., Denbigh LL16 3DE Tel: 01745 583910; 25 Park Street, Denbigh LL16 3DE — MB BCh Wales 1967 (Cardiff) DA Eng. 1969; FFA RCS Eng. 1972. Cons. Anaesth. Glan Clwyd Hosp.Conway and Denbighsh. NHS Trust. Specialty: Anaesth. Socs: Assn. Dent. Anaesth.; Pain Soc.; Age Anaesth. Assn. Mem.ship sec & Treas. Prev: Sen. Regist. (Anaesth.) Singleton Hosp. Swansea & Univ. Hosp. Wales Cardiff; SHO (Orthop. & Trauma) Morriston Hosp. Swansea; SHO (O & G) Mt. Pleasant Hosp.

WEBB, Timothy Ewart Department of Psychiatry, West Suffolk Hospital, Hardwick Lane, Bury St Edmunds IP33 2QZ Tel: 01284 713590 Fax: 01284 713694 — MB ChB Birm. 1977; MRCPsych 1983; FRCPsych 2001. Cons. Adult Psychiat. Local Health Partnerships NHS Trust; Director of Clin. Strategy, Local Health Partnership NHS Trust. Specialty: Gen. Psychiat. Prev: Cons. Psychiat. Plymouth HA.

WEBB, Timothy Richard 7 Erasmus Way, Lichfield WS13 7AW — MB ChB Birm. 1997; MRCP 2002. SHO (Med.) Soton. Gen. Hosp. Specialty: Cardiol. Prev: SHO (Med.) Roy. Shrewsbury Hosp. Shrewsbury; SHO (A. & E.) Halifax Roy. Infirm.

WEBB, William Bert (retired) Underwood, Portskwitt, Newport NP26 5UL Tel: 01291 420267 — MB BChir Camb. 1947 (Camb. & Guy's) Med. Off. Chepstow & Dist. Hosp.; Police Surg. Prev: Res. Med. Off. Surbiton Gen. Hosp.

WEBB, William Murcott William Harvey Hospital, Willesborough, Ashford TN24 0LZ Tel: 01233 633331; Ashley House, Swan Lane, Sellindge, Ashford TN25 6EB — MB ChB Birm. 1975; BSc (Physiol.) Birm. 1972; DMRD Eng. 1984; FRCR 1985. Cons. Radiologist, E. Kent Hosps. NHS Trust. Specialty: Radiol. Prev: Sen. Regist. & Regist. (Radiol.) Hull Roy. Infirm.; SHO Rotat. (Gen. Surg. & Orthop.) Chelmsford.

WEBB-PEPLOE, Katharine Mary Royal Brompton Hospital, Sydney St., London SW3 6NP Tel: 020 7352 8121; 29 Fentiman Road, London SW8 1LD — MB BChir Camb. 1988; BA Camb. 1985; MRCP (UK) 1991. Specialty: Cardiol.; Gen. Med. Prev: Research Regist. (Cardiol.) Roy. Brompton Hosp. & Nat. Heart & Lung Inst. Lond.

WEBB-PEPLOE, Michael Murray, OBE The Consulting Rooms, York House, 199 Westminster Bridge Road, London SE1 7UT Fax: 020 7922 8301 Email: m.webb-peploe@doctors.org.uk; 27 Torrington Road, Claygate, Esher KT10 0SA Tel: 01372 464879 — MB Camb. 1961 (Camb. & St. Thos.) BChir 1960; FRCP Lond. 1976, M 1963. Emerit. Cons. Cardiol., Guys and St Thomas NHS Trust. Specialty: Cardiol. Socs: Brit. Cardiac Soc.; Ass of Phys.s of Gt. Britain & Irel. Prev: Cons. Phys. Dept. Cardiol. St. Thos. Hosp. Lond; Research Assoc. Mayo Clinic Rochester, Minn., USA; Hon civil Cons. Cardiol. to the Army.

WEBB-WILSON, Gavin John Rood Lane Medical Centre, 10 Rood Lane, London EC3M 8BN Tel: 020 7283 4027 Fax: 020 7626 2184; Ash Tree House, Horton Kirby, Dartford DA4 9BY Tel: 01322 863349 — (St. Thos.) MA, MB Camb. 1970, BChir 1969; MRCOG 1978. Examr. Various Shipping & Insur. Companies & Banks City of Lond. Specialty: Obst. & Gyn. Socs: Fell. Assur. Med. Soc.; Med. Soc. Lond. Prev: Sen. Regist. (O & G) Nat. Wom. Hosp. Auckland, NZ; Regist. (O & G) St. Thos. Hosp. Lond.; Sen. Research Resid. Dept. Infertil. McGill Univ. Montreal.

WEBBER, Andrew Mark The Misbourne Surgery, Church Lane, Chalfont St. Peter, Gerrards Cross SL9 9RR Tel: 01494 874006 Fax: 01494 875455; 27 Kings Road, Chalfont St Giles HP8 4HS Tel: 01494 873117 — MB BS Lond. 1983 (Middlx.) BSc Lond. 1980. Prev: Trainee GP High Wycombe VTS; Ho. Phys. Qu. Eliz. II Hosp. Welwyn Garden City; Ho. Surg. Wycombe Gen. Hosp. High Wycombe.

WEBBER, Ian Trevor Aufrichtig 79A Belsize Park Gardens, London NW3 4JP — MB ChB Cape Town 1978; MSc Epidemiol. Lond. 1983.

WEBBER, Jane Elizabeth Ipswich General Hospital, Heath Road, Ipswich; 46 Brampton Road, Cambridge CB1 3HL Email: janew66@hotmail.com — MB BS (Hons) Lond. 1992 (St. Geo. Hosp. Med. Sch. Lond.) FRCS 1999. SpR (Trauma & Orthop.) Ipswich Gen. Hosp. Prev: SpR (Trauma & Orthop.) Luton &

Dunstable Hosp. Luton; SHO (Cardiothoracic Surg.) St. Geo. Hosp. Lond.; Demonst. (Anat.) St. Geo. Hosp. Lond.

WEBBER, Jonathan Selly Oak Hospital, Diabetes Centre, Raddlebard Road, Selly Oak, Birmingham B29 6JD; 99 Park Hill Road, Harborne, Birmingham B17 9HH — BM BCh Oxf. 1987; BA (Hons.) 1984; MA Camb. 1988; MRCP (UK) 1990; DM Nottm. 1994. Cons. (Diabetology) Diabetes Centre Selly Oak Hosp. Birm. Specialty: Dietetics/Nutrit.; Diabetes. Socs: Nutrit. Soc.; Ass for the study of obesity; Diabetes UK. Prev: Sen. Lect. in Clin. Nutrit. and Metab., Uni of Nottm.; Hon Cons. universsity Hosp. Nottm.; Sen. Regist. (Diabetes & Gen. Med.) City Hosp. Birm.

WEBBER, Lawrence Martin 17 Burdett Avenue, West Wimbledon, London SW20 0ST Tel: 020 8946 3243 Fax: 020 8542 6969 — (Westm.) MRCS Eng. LRCP Lond. 1960; MB BS Lond. 1961; DObst RCOG 1962. GP. Prev: Clin. Asst. Chest Clinic Kingston Hosp.; Med. Off. Nchanga Copper Mines Chingola, Zambia; Regist. (Med.) Qu. Mary's Hosp. Stratford.

WEBBER, Lisa Jan Imperial College London, Institute of Reproductive & Developmental Biology, Hammersmith Hospital, Du Cane Road, London W12 0NN Tel: 020 7594 2100 Fax: 020 7594 2111 Email: l.webber@imperial.ac.uk — BM BCh Oxf. 1991; BA (Physiol. Sc.) Oxf. 1988; MRCOG 1996. Clin. Lect. (O & G) Imperial Coll. Lond. & St Mary's Hosp. NHS Trust. Specialty: Obst. & Gyn. Special Interest: Reproductive Endocrinol.

WEBBER, Mr Mark Clifford Benjamin Withington Hospital, Nell Lane, West Didsbury, Manchester M20 2LR; 14 Beccles Road, Brooklands, Sale M33 3RP — MB ChB Manch. 1988; BSc St. And. 1986; FRCS Ed. 1992. SHO (Gen. Surg.) Trafford Gen. Hosp. Prev: SHO (Orthop. & Gen. Breast Surg.) Withington Hosp. Manch.

WEBBER, Michael George (retired) 21 Thornhill Close, Old Amersham, Amersham HP7 0EW Tel: 01494 431071 — MB BS Lond. 1951 (Middlx.) MRCGP 1965. Prev: Ho. Surg. Mt. Vernon Hosp. Northwood & Wembley Hosp.

WEBBER, Mr Peter Adrian ENT Department, Queen Elizabeth Hospital, King's Lynn PE30 4ET Tel: 01553 613724 Fax: 01553 613700 — MB BS Lond. 1977; FRCS (Orl.) Ed. 1984; MAE 1997. Cons. ENT Surg. Qu. Eliz. Hosp., Kings Lynn; ENT Cons. Norf. and Norwich Univ. Hosp. NHS Trust. Specialty: Otorhinolaryngol.

WEBBER, Richard James, Surg. Lt. RN Hewitt Croft, Threshfield, Skipton BD23 5HB Tel: 01756 753473 — MB BS Lond. 1994. Med. Off. HMS Vigilant. Socs: BMA; MDU. Prev: Med. Off. HMS Vanguard, HMS Neptune & HMS Collingwood.

WEBBER, Roger Hugh London School of Hygiene & Tropical Medicine, Keppel St., London WC1E 7HT Tel: 020 7927 2438 Fax: 020 7580 9075; Kiln Cottage, 45 North Lane, Buriton, Petersfield GU31 5RS Tel: 01730 266564 — MB BS Lond. 1967 (Roy. Free) MRCS Eng. LRCP Lond. 1967; DTM & H Liverp. 1969; DObst RCOG 1969; DTPH Lond. 1973; MSc Lond. 1980, MD 1976. Sen. Lect. Lond. Sch. Hyg. & Trop. Med.; Cons. & Hon. Sen. Lect. (Trop. Med.) UCL Hosps. Specialty: Epidemiol. Socs: Fell. Roy. Soc. Trop. Med. & Hyg. Prev: Med. Co-ordinator & Community Health Specialist UK/Tanzania Health Project Mbeya Tanzania; Chief Med. Off. (Communicable Dis.) Solomon Is.

WEBBER, Mrs Sally Margaret Royal United Hospital, Bath BA1 3NG — MB BS Lond. 1983; MRCP (UK) 1987; FCOphth 1989; DO RCS Eng. 1989. Cons. Ophth., Roy. United Hosp. Bath. Specialty: Ophth. Prev: Regist. (Ophth.) Roy. Hosp. Reading; Regist. K. Edwd. VII Hosp. Windsor; SHO & Regist. Rotat. Oxf. Eye Hosp.

WEBBER, Stephen John 280 Crookesmoor Road, Sheffield S10 1BE — MB ChB Sheff. 1993.

WEBBER, Suzanne Kim Royal Gwent Hospital, Cardiff Road, Newport NP20 2UB Tel: 01633 238444 Fax: 01633 656294; 33 Jenkyns Close, Southampton SO30 2UP Tel: 01489 790822 — MB ChB Leic. 1987; BSc (Hons.) Leic. 1984, MB ChB 1987; FRCOphth 1992. Cons. Ophth. Specialty: Ophth. Prev: Fell. (Corneal & Refractive Surg.) Sydney Refractive Surg. Centre, Sydney; Regist. (Ophth.) Roy. Vict. Infirm., Newc.; SHO (Ophth.) Birm. & Midl. Eye Hosp.

WEBBERLEY, Michael John Worcester Royal Infirmary, Ronkswood Branch, Newtown Road, Worcester WR5 1HN Tel: 01905 703333; Fort Royal House, 37 Fort Royal Hill, Worcester WR5 1BT — MB ChB Dundee 1982; MRCP (UK) 1985; MD Dundee 1991; FRCP UK 2000. Cons. Phys. (Gastroenterol.) Worcester Roy. Infirm. NHS Trust. Specialty: Gastroenterol. Socs: BSG. Prev: Sen. Regist. (Med. & Gastroenterol.) Qu. Eliz. Hosp. Birm.

WEBBORN, Anthony David John Department of Sports Medicine, London Hospital Medical College, Royal London Hospital, Bancroft Road, London E1 4DG Tel: 020 7377 7839 Fax: 020 8983 6500; Esperance Private Hospital, Hartington Place, Eastbourne BN21 3BG Tel: 01323 410717 Fax: 01323 730313 — MB BS Lond. 1979; MRCGP 1985; Dip. Sports Med. (Distinc.) Lond. 1993; MSc (Sports Med.) Lond. 1996. Clin. Research Fell. (Sports Med.) Lond. Hosp. Med. Coll. Specialty: Sports Med. Socs: Amer. Coll. Sports Med.; E.bourne Med. Soc.; Brit. Assn. Sport & Med. Prev: Med. Off RAF; GP Polegate.

WEBBORN, David John Pendle View Surgery, Arthur Street, Brierfield, Nelson BB9 5RZ Tel: 01282 614599 — MB ChB Bristol 1982; MRCGP 1986; DRCOG 1986. Course Organiser Burnley & Blackburn. Socs: BMA.

WEBER, Andrzej Marek 89 Southfield Road, Chiswick, London W4 1BB Tel: 020 8994 3099 Fax: 020 8747 8968; 14 North Avenue, Ealing, London W13 8AP Tel: 020 8997 2650 Fax: 020 8981 8020 Email: webers@keystone.demon.co.uk — MB BS Lond. 1981 (Roy. Free) DRCOG 1984. Assoc. Specialist Ealing Hosp. Specialty: Gen. Pract. Prev: Clin. Asst. Ealing Hosp.

WEBER, Beatrix Elisabeth Ocean's End Annexe, Rose Hill, Marazion TR17 0HB — State Exam Med. Munich 1988.

WEBER, Joelle 33 Cranbourne Gardens, London NW11 0HS — MB BS Lond. 1997.

WEBER, John Christian Peter (retired) The Ridings, Woodfield Lane, Brookmans Park, Hatfield AL9 6JJ Tel: 01707 650859 — (Guy's) MD Lond. 1949, MB BS 1944. Med. Cons. Pharmaceut. Indust. Lond. Prev: Sen. Med. Off. DHSS (Meds. Div.) Lond.

WEBER, Professor Jonathan Norden Wright-Fleming Institute, Jefferiss Research Trust Laboratories, Imperial College London, St. Mary's Campus, Norfolk Place, London W2 1PG Tel: 020 7594 3901 Email: j.weber@imperial.ac.uk — MB BChir Camb. 1979 (Cambridge) MA Camb. 1979; FRCP 1993, M (UK) 1983; FRCPath 1997; FMedSci 1999; PhD Camb. (Virology) 2003. Prof. (Genitourin. Med.) & Communicable Dis. Imperial Coll. Lond., St. Mary's Campus.; Hon. Cons. (Phys.) St. Mary's Hosp.; Dean (St. Mary's Campus), Faculty of Med., Imperial Coll. Lond. Specialty: Genitourinary Medicine; Infec. Dis.; Virology. Socs: Brit. Infec. Soc.; MSSVD Counc.; BASHH 2003. Prev: Sen. Lect. & Hon. Cons. (Phys.) Infec. Dis. Unit Roy. Postgrad. Med. Sch. Hammersmith Hosp. Lond.; Lect. Div. Cell & Molecular Biol. Chester Beatty Laboratories Inst. Cancer Research Lond.; Wellcome Research Fell. St. Mary's Hosp. Med. Sch. Lond.

WEBER, Maurice Emile (retired) 310 Pickhurst Lane, West Wickham BR4 0HT Tel: 020 8460 0234 — (St. Bart.) MRCS Eng. LRCP Lond. 1942. Prev: Clin. Asst. Bromley Hosp.

WEBER, Stephan Flat 4, Greentrees, 6 Lansdowne, Worthing BN11 4NA — State Exam Med Berlin 1991.

WEBLEY, Michael The Limes, 10 Churchway, Haddenham, Aylesbury HP17 8AA Tel: 01844 291356 — MB BS Lond. 1967 (Westm.) MRCS Eng. LRCP Lond. 1967; MRCP (UK) 1970; FRCP Lond. 1986. Cons. Rheum. Oxf. Regional Rheum. Dis. Research Centre Stoke Mandeville Hosp. Aylesbury. Specialty: Rheumatol. Socs: FRSM; Brit. Soc. Rheum. Prev: Sen. Regist. Westm. Hosp. & St. Stephens Hosp. Lond.; Resid. Med. Off. Brompton Hosp. Lond.

WEBSTER, Alan Rimmington (retired) 28 Castlegate, Helmsley, York YO62 5AB — (Leeds) MB ChB Leeds 1948; DObst RCOG 1949. Prev: Ho. Phys. Roy. Infirm. Bradford.

WEBSTER, Alison Glaxo Wellcome Research & Development, Greenford Road, Greenford UB6 0HE — MB BS Lond. 1982; MRCPath 1989; BSc Lond. 1979, MD 1994. Specialty: Virology.

WEBSTER, Amanda Jennifer 12 Shepherds Way, West Lulworth, Wareham BH20 5SL — MB BS Lond. 1985; FRCA. 1991. Anaesth. E. Dorset HA. Specialty: Anaesth.

WEBSTER, Andrew c/o Sushee Webster, 28A Queen St., Stirling FK8 1HN — MB ChB Glas. 1997.

WEBSTER, Andrew Patrick Stone Home, Alton, Stoke-on-Trent ST10 4AG — MB ChB Liverp. 1998.

WEBSTER, Andrew Royston 406 Winchester Road, Southampton SO16 7DH — BM BCh Oxf. 1987; FCOphth. 1991.

WEBSTER, Ann Margaret 3 Laurel Bank, Hamilton ML3 8EP — MB ChB Manch. 1990.

WEBSTER, Anna Louise 24 Bucklow Gardens, Lymm WA13 9RQ — MB ChB Manch. 1998.

WEBSTER, Anthony David Bonython Royal Free Hospital School of Medicine, Department of Clinical Immunology, Rowland Hill Street, London NW3 2PF Tel: 020 7830 2141 Fax: 020 7830 2224 — MB BChir Camb. 1965 (St Mary's) BA Camb. 1961; MA Camb. 1968; FRCP Lond. 1981; MD Camb. 1993; FRCPath 1996. Con. Immunol. & Sen. Lect. Roy. Free Hosp. Med. Sch. Lond.; Hon. Cons. Clin. Immunol. Roy. Free Hosp. Med. Sch. Lond. Specialty: Immunol. Socs: Brit. Soc. Immunol. & Assn. Phys. Prev: Hon. Cons. Immunol. Clin. Research Centre Northwick Pk. Hosp. Harrow.

WEBSTER, Antony Peter 52 Highfield Road, Cheadle Hulme, Cheadle SK8 6EP — MB ChB Birm. 1992.

WEBSTER, Claire Diana St. Johns House Surgery, 28 Bromyard Road, Worcester WR2 5BU — MB ChB Manch. 1987.

WEBSTER, David Woolton House Medical Centre, 4b Woolton Street, Woolton, Liverpool LL5 5JA; Aisburth Hall Cottage, Grassendale, Liverpool L19 9EA — MB ChB Liverp. 1989; MRCP (UK) 1992; MRCGP 1995. Assoc. Phys. NW Primary Care Initiative / GP Princip.; Liverp. Univ. Med. Sch. Specialty: Pub. Health Med.; Paediat.; Rheumatol. Socs: Liverp. Med. Inst.; Christian Med. Fell.ship. Prev: SHO (O & G) Liverp. Wom. Hosp. Trust; Assoc. Phys. N W Primary Care Initiative.

WEBSTER, David Anthony The Surgery, School Lane, Upton-upon-Severn, Worcester WR8 0LF Tel: 01684 592696 Fax: 01684 593122; The Grange, Hill End, Upton-on-Severn, Worcester WR8 0RN Tel: 01684 833239 — MB BS Lond. 1964 (St. Thos.) DObst RCOG 1967; DTM & H Eng. 1971; MRCGP 1979. Specialty: Community Child Health. Socs: BMA. Prev: Med. Off. i/c Amudat Hosp., Uganda; MOH Marsabit Dist., Kenya.

WEBSTER, Mr David John Tatchell University of Wales, College of Medicine, Heath Park, Cardiff CF4 4XM Tel: 029 2074 2020 Fax: 029 2074 3199; Sunnycroft, 25 St. Edeyrns Road, Cyncoed, Cardiff CF23 6TB Tel: 029 2075 7117 — MD Bristol 1986, MB ChB 1967; FRCS Eng. 1972. Sen. Lect. (Surg.) Univ. Wales Coll. Med. Cardiff; Hon. Cons. Surg. S. Glam. HA. Prev: Regist. Rotat. (Surg.) Univ. Hosp. Wales Cardiff; Lect. (Surg.) Welsh Nat. Sch. Med. Cardiff; Research Fell. Ohio State Univ. Columbus, USA.

WEBSTER, Deborah Jane Vesper Hawk Farm, Smarden, Ashford TN27 8PU — MB ChB Birm. 1997.

WEBSTER, Diana 36 Craignabo Road, Peterhead AB42 2YE; 31 Fairview Parade, Aberdeen AB22 8ZX Tel: 01224 706592 — MB ChB Aberd. 1997 (Aberdeen) BSc Med Sci Aberd. 1995.

WEBSTER, Diana Christina Shirley — MB ChB Leeds 1977; DRCOG 1980; MRCGP 1981; MPH Leeds 1982; MFCM 1988. Specialty: Pub. Health Med.

WEBSTER, Donald Drummond 7 Croft Hills, Stokesley, Middlesbrough TS9 5NW Tel: 01642 710088 — (Newc.) MB BS Durh. 1945; DPM 1950; FRCPsych 1976, M 1971. Prev: Cons. Psychiat. S. Tees Health Auth.

WEBSTER, Elizabeth (retired) 7 Croft Hills, Stokesley, Middlesbrough TS9 5NW Tel: 01642 710088 — (Newc. upon Tyne) M.B., B.S. Durh. 1945. Prev: Med. Off. Cherry Knowle E.M.S. Hosp. Sunderland.

WEBSTER, Elizabeth Ann Webster and Hanna, Newbury Park Health Centre, 40 Perrymans Farm Road, Ilford IG2 7LE Tel: 020 8518 2414 Fax: 020 8518 3194 — MB ChB Aberd. 1970; MRCGP 1975.

WEBSTER, Eric Marshall The Health Centre, Osborn Road, Fareham PO16 7ER Tel: 01329 823456 Fax: 01329 285772; Bay Tree Cottage, 18 Church Road, Locks Heath, Southampton SO31 6LU — MB ChB Aberd. 1979; D. Clin. Hyp London 1998-; LF Hom (Med.); MB ChB Aberdeen 1979.

WEBSTER, Fiona Barbara — MB BS Lond. 1970; MRCS Eng. LRCP Lond. 1970.

WEBSTER, Frances 2 Glebelands Avenue, South Woodford, London E18 2AB Tel: 020 8989 6272; 46 Malmesbury Road, London E18 2NN — BM BS Nottm. 1985; MRCGP 1990. Trainee GP/SHO Chase Farm Hosp. Enfield. Prev: Ho. Off. (Med.) St. Geo. Hosp. Lincoln; Ho. Off. (Surg.) N. Middlx. Hosp. Lond.

WEBSTER, Frederick Lawrence (retired) 25 Hanbury Road, Clifton, Bristol BS8 2EP Tel: 0117 973 8041 — MB ChB Bristol 1959; DA Eng. 1962; DObst RCOG 1963.

WEBSTER, George John Mitchell 47 North Road, London N6 4BE — MB BS Lond. 1991; BSc (Hons.) Lond. 1988; MRCP Lond. 1994. Regist. (Gasteroenterol.) Whittington Hosp. Lond. Prev: SHO (Cardiol.) Roy. Brompton Nat. Heart & Lung Hosp. Lond.; SHO (Neurol.) Hammersmith Hosp. Lond.

WEBSTER, George Waddell (retired) 15 Northcliffe Gardens, Broadstairs CT10 3AL — MB ChB Aberd. 1953; MRCGP 1965.

WEBSTER, Gillian Kelso The Mission Practice, 208 Cambridge Heath Road, London E2 9LS Tel: 020 8983 7300 Fax: 020 8983 6800 — MB ChB Liverp. 1970; DObst. RCOG 1972; MRCP (UK) 1974; DTM & H Liverp. 1979; MRCGP 1983. Gen. Practitioner Mission Pract. Lond. Prev: Clin. Asst., Dermat. Dept. St Andrews Hosp., Bow, Lond.; Med. Off. Magila Hosp. Tanga Region, Tanzania, E. Afr.; Dep. Sen. Med. Off. Nixon Memor. Methodist Hosp. Segbwema, Sierra Leone, W. Afr.

WEBSTER, Grace Alexandra Mary (retired) 9 Cleveland Court, Kent Avenue, London W13 8BJ Tel: 020 8998 5112 — MB ChB Aberd. 1947; DObst RCOG 1951; DPH Lond. 1960; MFCM 1973. Prev: Specialist Community Med. Hounslow & Spelthorne DHA.

WEBSTER, Graham David Woodeside Health Centre, Barr Street, Glasgow G20 7LR Tel: 0141 531 9570 Fax: 0141 531 9572; 9 Kingsborough Gardens, Glasgow G12 9NH — MB ChB Aberd. 1978.

WEBSTER, Mr Guy Michael Dept. of Urology, Worcester Royal Infirmary, Newtown Rd, Worcester WR5 — MB ChB Birm. 1988; FRCS Ed. 1992; FRCS 1997. Cons. Urol. N. Worcs. Acute NHS Trust. Specialty: Urol. Socs: Brit. Assn. of Urological Surg.s.

WEBSTER, Helen Louise — MB ChB Dundee 1995. GP Retainee, Rotherham. Specialty: Gen. Pract. Prev: GP Retainee, Cambs.

WEBSTER, James 6 Newburgh Drive, Middleton Park, Bridge of Don, Aberdeen AB22 8SR — MB ChB Aberd. 1969.

WEBSTER, James Bruce Lindsay (retired) 17 The Gorseway, St. Georges Road, Hayling Island PO11 0DR Tel: 023 9246 4103 Fax: 01705 464103 Email: bruce@linweb.fsnet.co.uk — MB BChir Camb. 1964 (St. Thos.) Prev: GP Hayling Is.

WEBSTER, Janet Patricia 21 Lloyd Street, Mareeba QLD 4880, Australia Email: janetross@bigfoot.com — MB ChB Leeds 1988 (Leeds Univ. Med. Sch.) FACR RM 1999; FRACGP 1999; Grad. Dip. Of Rural Gen. Pract., Australia 2000. Sen. Med.Off. Mareeba Hosp. Specialty: Gen. Pract.; Anaesth. Socs: Mem. Of far N. Old Rural Div. Of GP. Prev: GP Regist. Rockhampton, Queensland, Australia; GP Regist. Airlie Beach Queensland, Australia.

WEBSTER, Jennifer Ann Ward 30, Stirling Royal Infirmary, Livilands Gate, Stirling FK8 2AU Tel: 01786 434000 — MB ChB Dundee 1977; MRCPsych 1983. Cons. Psychiat. Stirling Roy. Infirm. Specialty: Gen. Psychiat. Prev: Cons. Psychiat. Hartwood Hosp. Shotts & Hairmyres Hosp. E. Kilbride; Sen. Regist. (Psychother.) Roy. Edin. Hosp.

WEBSTER, Joanne 247 Newbold Road, Chesterfield S41 7AQ — MB BS Newc. 1998.

WEBSTER, John Aberdeen Royal Infirmary, Aberdeen AB25 2ZN Tel: 01224 553718 Fax: 01224 553081 Email: j.webster@arh.grampian.scot.nhs.uk; Arisaig, Old Skene Road, Kingswells, Aberdeen AB15 8TA Tel: 01224 743828 — MB ChB Aberd. 1973; MRCP (UK) 1975; MD Aberd. 1981; FRCP Ed. 1988. Grampian Univ. Hosp.s trust, Aberd. Specialty: Gen. Med. Socs: Brit. Hypertens. Soc. & Brit. Pharmacol. Soc. Prev: Sen. Lect. (Med. & Therap.) Univ. Aberd.; MRC Fell. Roy. Postgrad. Med. Sch. Lond.; Cons. Phys. Aberd. Roy Hosps. NHS Trust.

WEBSTER, John Webster and Twomey, Rainford Health Centre, Higher Lane, St Helens WA11 8AZ Tel: 01744 882855 Fax: 01744 886559 — MB ChB Liverp. 1974; DRCOG 1977.

WEBSTER, John Cedar Cottage, 6 Main Street, Calverton, Nottingham NG14 6FQ — MB ChB Liverp. 1960; FRCOG 1989, M 1978.

WEBSTER, John Charles Thompson Lynfield Mount Hospital, Heights Lane, Bradford BD9 6DP Tel: 01274 494194 — MB BChir Camb. 1975 (Camb. Univ.) MA, MB Camb. 1975, BChir 1974; MRCPsych 1983; MMedSci Leeds 1984. Cons. Psychiat. Lynfield Mt. Hosp. Bradford. Specialty: Gen. Psychiat. Prev: Tutor (Psychiat.) Univ. Leeds; Sen. Regist. (Psychiat.) St. Jas. Hosp. Leeds.

WEBSTER, John Louis (retired) 285 Beverley Road, Kirkella, Hull HU10 7AQ Tel: 01482 652692 — (Birmingham) MB ChB Birm.

1955; DObst RCOG 1960; FRCA 1963. Prev: Cons. (Anaesth.) Hull & E. Yorks. HA.

WEBSTER, Jonathan Department of Diabetes & Endocrinology, Northern General Hospital, Herries Road, Sheffield S5 7AU Tel: 0114 226 6926 Fax: 0114 226 6924; 21 Cortworth Road, Ecclesall, Sheffield S11 9LN Tel: 0114 235 1637 — MB BS Lond. 1983 (Westminster Medical School London, Clare College Cambridge) MRCP (UK) 1986; MA Camb. 1985, MD 1993; FRCP FRCP (London) 2000. Cons. Phys. & Endocrinol. N. Gen. & Roy. Hallamsh. Hosps. Sheff. Specialty: Endocrinol. Socs: Soc. Endocrinol.; Eur. Neuroendocrine Assn.; Endocrine Soc. (USA). Prev: Lect. (Med. & Endocrinol.) Univ. Wales Coll. Med. Cardiff; Research Fell (Med.) Cedars-Sinai Med. Center UCLA Sch. Med. Los Angeles Calif., USA; MRC Train. Fell. Neuroendocrine Sect. (Med.) Univ Wales Coll of Med. Cardiff.

WEBSTER, Julie Anne Sleaford Medical Group, Riverside Surgery, 47 Boston Road, Sleaford NG34 7HD Tel: 01529 303301 Fax: 01529 415401; Belvoir Lodge, 71 Woolsthorpe Road, Woolsthorpe-by-Colsterworth, Grantham NG33 5NT Tel: 01476 860875 — MB BS Lond. 1982 (Guys Hospital) Prev: Trainee GP Pilgrim Hosp. Boston VTS.

WEBSTER, Karen 4 Old Clare Road, Tandragee, Craigavon BT62 2EX — MB BCh BAO Belf. 1991.

WEBSTER, Mr Keith University Hospital Birmingham, Department of Maxillofacial Surgery, Edgbaston, Birmingham B15 2DT Tel: 0121 627 8536 Email: k.webster@bham.ac.uk — MB BS Lond. 1991 (Guy's) BDS Liverp. 1983; FDS RCS Eng. 1990; FRCS Eng. 1993; FRCS 1997; MMEDSCI Birm 1999. Cons. Maxillofacial Surg., Univ. Hosp. Birm. NHS Trust; Cons. Maxillofacial Surg. Heartland and Solihull NHS Trust; Hon Sen. Lect. Birm. Dent. Sch. Specialty: Oral & Maxillofacial Surg. Socs: BAOMS; BAHNO; EORTC. Prev: Sen. Regist. (Oral & Maxillofacial Surg.) Roy. Hosp. Wolverhampton; Regist. (Oral Surg.) N. Staffs. NHS Trust; SHO (Surg.) St. Helier NHS Trust.

WEBSTER, Laura Helen 16 Inchcape Road, Broughty Ferry, Dundee DD5 2LL — MB ChB Dundee 1998.

WEBSTER, Louise Katherine c/o J C Webster, The Dennen, 59 Wilden Road, Renhold, Bedford MK41 0LY; Adel Manor Cottage, off Long Causeway, Adel, Leeds LS16 8EX — MB ChB Leic. 1993; FRCA Lond. 2001. Specialist Regist. Anaesth. N/W Yorks. Specialty: Anaesth.

WEBSTER, Lynne Department of Psychiatry, Manchester Royal Infirmary, Oxford Road, Manchester M13 9WL Tel: 0161 276 5365 Fax: 0161 276 5444 — MB ChB Manch. 1977; FRCPsych 1996, M 1983; BSc (Psychol.) Manch. 1974, MSc 1984. Cons. Psychiat. i/c Psychosexual Med. Manch. Roy. Infirm.; Hon. Lect. (Psychiat. & Obst. & Gyn.) Univ. Manch. Specialty: Psychosexual Med. Socs: Manch. Medico-Legal Soc.; Gen. Mem. Brit. Assn. Sexual & Marital Ther.; Fell. Prev: Sen. Regist. (Psychiat.) Univ. Hosp. S. Manch.

WEBSTER, Malcolm Long Lane Medical Centre, Long Lane, Liverpool L9 6DQ Tel: 0151 530 1009 — MB ChB Liverp. 1960; DObst RCOG 1963.

WEBSTER, Mark Frenchwood Avenue Surgery, 49 Frenchwood Avenue, Preston PR1 4ND Tel: 01772 254173 — MRCS Eng. LRCP Lond. 1982 (Liverp.)

WEBSTER, Martin Howard Glenside Practice, Castle Bytham Surgery, 12b High Street, Grantham NG33 4RZ Tel: 01780 410205 Fax: 01780 410817 — MB ChB Dundee 1979; DA Eng. 1982; MRCGP 1987. Prev: Med. Off. RAF.

WEBSTER, Mr Martyn Hector Cochrane Regional Plastic and Reconstructive Surgery Unit, Canniesburn Hospital, Bearsden, Glasgow G61 1QL Email: martynw@globalnet.co.uk; Trinity Chambers, 18 Woodside Terrace, Glasgow G3 7XH Tel: 0141 332 0035 Fax: 0141 332 0037 Email: mw@martynwebster.com — (Glasgow) MB ChB Glas. 1963; FRCS RCPS Glas. 1972. Cons. Plastic Surg. Golden Jubilee Hosp. Clydebank Glas. Specialty: Plastic Surg. Special Interest: Reconstruc. Plastic Surg. & Burns in Africa (Ghana). Socs: Brit. Assn. of Plastic Surgeons; Brit. Assn. of Aesthetic Plastic Surgeons (Past President); Europ. Assn. of Plastic Surgeons (Past President).

WEBSTER, Mary Augusta 6 Forest Lawns, 124 Streetly Lane, Sutton Coldfield B74 4TD Tel: 0121 353 2654 Fax: 0121 353 2654 — (Birm.) MB ChB Birm. 1949; MRCS Eng. LRCP Lond. 1949; DObst RCOG 1950. Cytol. & Menopause Councellor W. Midl.; Med. Examr. DSS - NDA Med. Servs. Specialty: Obst. & Gyn. Socs: Brit. Cytol. Soc.; Brit. Menopause Soc. Prev: Clin. Asst. Burton-on-Trent Gen. Hosp.; SCMO SE Staffs. HA; Med. Off. Selfridge Ltd. Lond.

WEBSTER, Mary Rosamund Lendal House, 91 Marton Road, Bridlington YO16 7PX Tel: 01262 672907 — MB BS Lond. 1938 (Roy. Free Hosp. Lond.) MRCS Eng. LRCP Lond. 1935; DPH Leeds 1939; FRCOG 1974, M 1942. Socs: N. Eng. O & G Soc. & BMA. Prev: Res. Obst. Off. St. Mary's Hosp. Manch.

WEBSTER, Michael Harvey Taunton & Somerset Hospital, Musgrove Park, Taunton TA1 5DA Tel: 01823 333444 Fax: 01823 342635 — MB ChB Bristol 1972; DCH Eng. 1974; FRCP Lond. 1995; FRCPCH 1997. Cons. Paediat., Taunton and Som. Hosp.; Cons. Paediat. Metab. Med., N. Bristol NHS Trust. Specialty: Paediat. Prev: Sen. Regist. (Paediat.) Birm. HA (T).

WEBSTER, Nigel Charles Harding Newcroft Surgery, Mill Street, Rocester, Uttoxeter ST14 5JX Tel: 01889 590208 Fax: 01889 590196 — MB ChB St. And. 1969; DCH Eng. 1972.

WEBSTER, Professor Nigel Robert Wickerinn Farmhouse, Banchory AB31 5QX — MB ChB Leeds 1977; PhD Leeds 1985, BSc (Hons.) (Pharmacol.) 1974; FFA RCS Eng. 1981; FRCP Ed. 1996. Specialty: Intens. Care.

WEBSTER, Nola Jean White Lodge Practices, 21 Grosvenor Street, St Helier, Jersey JE1 4HA Tel: 01534 23892 Fax: 01534 601955; 6 Vic Q Farm Close, Grouville JE3 9FL — MB ChB Birm. 1965; BSc Birm. 1962. GP Jersey. Socs: BMA. Prev: GP Birm.; Research Fell. (Pharmacol.) Birm. Med. Sch.; Ho. Phys. & Ho. Surg. E. Birm. Hosp.

WEBSTER, Patricia Alice Charlotte (retired) 285 Beverley Road, Kirkella, Hull HU10 7AQ Tel: 01482 652692 — (Char. Cross) MB BS Lond. 1955; DObst RCOG 1958; FRCPCH 1997. Prev: Clin. Asst. (Paediat.) Hull HA.

WEBSTER, Patricia Anne The Surgery, Manlake Avenue, Winterton, Scunthorpe DN15 9TA Tel: 01724 732202 Fax: 01724 734992; 8 North Street, Roxby, Scunthorpe DN15 9QN Tel: 01724 732461 — MB ChB Sheff. 1982; DRCOG 1986; MRCGP 1987. Prev: Trainee GP Scunthorpe HA VTS.

WEBSTER, Peter Mark Maudsley Hospital, Eating Disorder Out-Patients, Denmark Hill, London SE5 8AZ Tel: 020 7919 3180 Fax: 020 7919 2358 — MB BChir Camb. 1993 (Camb. & Roy. Lond.) MA Camb. 1992. Cons. (Psychiat.) Maudsley Hosp. Lond. Specialty: Gen. Psychiat. Special Interest: Cognative Analytic Thearpy. Socs: Med. Defence Union. Prev: Specialist Regist., Maudsley; SHO (Psychiat.) Maudsley Hosp. Lond.; Specialist Regist. (Psychiat.) Maudsley Hosp. Lond.

WEBSTER, Philip Powell Manselton Surgery, Elgin Street, Manselton, Swansea SA5 8QE Tel: 01792 653643 / 642459 Fax: 01792 645257 — MB BS Lond. 1975 (St. Geo. Hosp. Med. Sch.) DRCOG 1977. Specialty: Family Plann. & Reproduc. Health. Socs: MDU; BMA.

WEBSTER, Premila Nalini Division Of Public Health, Institute of Health Science, University of Oxford, Old Road, Headington, Oxford OX3 7LF Tel: 01865 226735 Email: premila.webster@dphpc.ox.ac.uk — MB BS Madras 1978 (Christian Medical College) DA Madras 1982; DA 1987; MSc Lond. 1993; MFPHM 1998. Director of Educat. & Train. in Pub. Health/ Cons./ Hon. SNR, Lect., Inst. of H.Sci.s, Univ. Oxf. Specialty: Pub. Health Med. Socs: Counc. Mem. of the Sect. of Epidemiol. & Pub. Health, The Roy. Soc. of Med., UK. Prev: Cons. WHO Health Cities Project Europ. Office, Copenhagen.

WEBSTER, Priscilla Jacqueline Russell 7 Wood Lane, Iver SL0 0LQ — MRCS Eng. LRCP Lond. 1981 (St. Bart.) BSc Lond. 1978, MB BS 1981. Regist. (Path.) St. Bart. Hosp. Lond. Specialty: Pathology, General. Prev: SHO (Path.) St. Bart. Hosp. Lond.; Ho. Surg. St. Bart. Hosp. Lond.; Ho. Phys. Whipp's Cross Hosp. Lond.

WEBSTER, Rae Elizabeth Department of Anaesthetics, Northampton General Hospital NHS Trust, Cliftonville, Northampton NN1 5BD Tel: 01604 545671 Fax: 01604 545672 — MB ChB Aberd. 1979; FFA RCS Eng. 1985; MBA (Open) 1997. Cons. Anaesth. & Intens. Care Northampton Gen. Hosp. NHS Trust. Specialty: Anaesth.; Intens. Care. Prev: Cons. Anaesth. & Intens Care. Dundee Teachg. Hosps. Trust; Clin. Fell. (Critical Care) Toronto Hosp. (W.. Div.) Toronto, Ontario.

WEBSTER, Reginald Christopher, TD 24 Lynwood Court, Middleton Road, Manchester M8 4JX — MB BCh BAO (Hons.) NUI 1928 (Cork & Manch.) LM Coombe 1932; BSc NUI 1927, MD 1933; DPH Manch. 1938; DCH Eng. 1947. Med. Asst. Calderstones

Hosp. Whalley; Corps. Surg. St. John Ambul. Brig. Socs: FRSH. Prev: Div. MOH Lancs. CC & Co. Dist.; Col. late RAMC; Div. MOH & Sch. Med. Off. W. Riding CC.

WEBSTER, Richard Hugh Longlevens Surgery, 19b Church Road, Longlevens, Gloucester GL2 0AJ Tel: 01452 522695 Fax: 01452 525547; Longlevens Surgery, 19b Church Road, Longlevens, Gloucester GL2 0AJ Tel: 01452 522695 — MB BChir Camb. 1988 (Cambridge and King's College London) MA Camb. 1989; MRCGP 1993. Prev: Trainee GP Cheltenham & Gloucester VTS; SHO (Med.) Univ. Hosp. of Wales Cardiff.

WEBSTER, Richard William (Surgery), 4 Londesborough Road, Market Weighton, York YO43 3AY; Totterdownhill Farm, Nunburnholme, York YO42 1QA — MB BS Newc. 1973; MRCGP 1977.

WEBSTER, Robert Anthony 1 Christina Street, Harrogate HG1 2DF — MB ChB Leeds 1993. Specialty: Gen. Pract.

WEBSTER, Robert Edward, Squadron Ldr. RAF Med. Br. Retd. National Blood Service, Trent Centre, Longley Lane, Sheffield S5 7JN Tel: 0114 203 4813 Fax: 0114 203 4811 — MB BS Lond. 1982 (St. Geo. Hosp. Med. Sch.) MRCPath 1992. Cons. Haemat. Nat. Blood Serv. Sheff. Specialty: Haematology. Prev: Cons. Haemat. RAF Inst. Path. & Trop. Med. Aylesbury; SHO (Path.) Roy. Liverp. Hosp. Liverp.; Ho. Phys. (Gen. & Geriat. Med.) St. Jas. Hosp. Lond.

WEBSTER, Robert William Johan 150 Claremont, Alloa FK10 2EG Tel: 01259 212088 — MB ChB Ed. 1964; DRCOG 1971.

WEBSTER, Sally Elizabeth The Old Post Office, 5 Ouston Road, Knossington, Oakham LE15 8LX — MB ChB Leic. 1997.

WEBSTER, Sara Wallace Aigburth Hall Cottage, 1A Aigburth Hall Avenue, Liverpool L19 9EA — MB ChB Liverp. 1992. Specialty: Dermat. Prev: SHO (Dermat.) Roy. Liverp. Univ. Hosp.

WEBSTER, Sarah Carolyn — MB ChB Birm. 1998.

WEBSTER, Stephen George Philip Ferry Corner, Water St., Old Chesterton, Cambridge CB4 1NZ Tel: 01223 359037 — MRCS Eng. LRCP Lond. 1964 (Lond. Hosp.) MA Camb.; MD Lond. 1973, MB BS 1964; FRCP Lond. 1988. Private Med. Practitioner; Assoc. Lect. (Med.) Univ. Camb; The Appeals Serv., GMC. Specialty: Gen. Med.; Care of the Elderly. Socs: Brit. Geriat. Soc.; Brit. Soc. Res. on Ageing. Prev: Sen. Regist. (Gen. & Geriat. Med.) United Oxf. Hosps.; Research Regist. & Regist. (Med.) Univ. Hosp. S. Manch.

WEBSTER, Stephen James Crossley Practice, 16 Henley Road, Coventry CV2 1LP Tel: 024 7668 9435 Fax: 024 7666 7127 — MB BS Durh. 1967 (Newc.) MRCP (U.K.) 1972.

WEBSTER, Victoria Jayne 25 St Edeyrn's Road, Cardiff CF23 6TB Email: v.j.webster@sheffield.ac.uk — MB ChB Sheff. 1992 (Sheffield) FRCA 1997. Specialty: Anaesth.

WEBSTER, Victoria Louisa Dept. Anaesthesia, Queen's Medical Centre, University Hospital, Nottingham NG7 2UH — MB BS Lond. 1993 (King's Coll. Lond.) DA (UK) 1996; FRCA Lond. 1999. Specialist Regist. (Anaesth.) Qu. Med. Centre Nottm. Specialty: Anaesth. Prev: SHO (Anaesth.) Qu. Med. Centre Nottm.; SHO (Anaesth.) W. Dorset Gen. Hosp.; SHO (A & E) Weymouth Hosp. Dorset.

WEBSTER, Vincent George The Stone House, Alton, Stoke-on-Trent ST10 4AG Tel: 01538 702210 Fax: 01538 703500 — LRCPI & LM, LRSCI & LM 1971; LRCPI & LM, LRCSI & LM 1971.

WEBSTER-HARRISON, Philip John Jackson and Partners, Port View Surgery, Higher Port View, Saltash PL12 4BU Tel: 01752 847131 Fax: 01752 847124 — MB BS London 1984; MB BS London 1984.

WEBSTER-SMITH, Claudia Suzanne Brockham Court Farm, Brockham Green, Brockham, Betchworth RH3 7JS — MB ChB Manch. 1998; DCH 2002.

WEDDELL, Craig Robert Esso Petroleum UK Ltd., Occupational Health, Fawley Refinery, Southampton S045 1TX Tel: 023 8089 6190 Fax: 023 8089 6234 — MB BS Lond. 1991; DRCOG 1995; MRCGP 1996; AFOM 2000. Med. Off. (Occupat. Health Physician) Esso Petroleum UK Ltd. Specialty: Occupat. Health. Socs: Mem. Roy. Coll. of Gen. Practitioners; Mem. of the Soc. of Occupat.al Med.; Fellow Royal Soc. Of Med.

WEDDELL, David John The Surgery, 2048 Bristol Road, Rubery, Birmingham B45 9JL Tel: 0121 457 7966 — MB ChB Birm. 1976.

WEDDELL, Jean Mary (retired) 8 Denny Crescent, London SE11 4UY Tel: 020 7735 9303 — MD Lond. 1972 (St. Thos.) MB BS 1953; FFCM 1977, M 1972; FRCP Lond. 1999. Prev: Sen. Lect. Dept. Community Med. St. Thos. Hosp. Lond.

WEDDERBURN, Mr Andrew Weir 22 Church Street, Romsey SO51 8BU — MB BS Lond. 1990; FRCS Eng. 1994; FRCS Urol 2000. Cons. Urol. Roy. Bournemouth Hosp. Prev: SpR Wessex Rotation; SR Perth W Australia.

WEDDERBURN, Clare 22 Church Street, Romsey SO51 8BU Tel: 01794 512852 — MB BS Lond. 1993 (UMDS) DA (UK) 1995; DCH 1997; MRCGP 1998. GP Retainer Scheme. Specialty: Gen. Pract. Prev: GP Regist. Blackfield Health Centre Soton.; SHO (O & G) Roy. Hampsh. Co. Hosp. Winchester; SHO (Paediat.) St. Richard's Hosp. Chichester.

WEDDERBURN, John Pyle (retired) 11 Carlidnack Close, Mawnan Smith, Falmouth TR11 5HF Tel: 01326 250522 — MB BS Durh. 1944 (Newc.) Prev: GP Wolverhampton & Hypnother.

WEDDERBURN, Lucy Rachel Imperial Cancer Research Fund, Lincoln's Inn Fields, London WC2A 3PX; 83 Listria Park, London N16 5SP — MB BS Lond. 1986; BA (Hons.) Camb. 1982; MRCP (UK) 1989. Clin. Research Fell. Imperial Cancer Research Fund Lond. Socs: Brit. Soc. Immunol. & Brit. Soc. Rheum. Prev: Regist. (Med.) The Roy. Lond. Hosp.; SHO Roy. Marsden Hosp.; SHO The Lond. Chest Hosp.

WEDDERBURN, Stephen Rubislaw Place Medical Group, 7 Rubislaw Place, Aberdeen AB10 1QB Tel: 01224 641968 Fax: 01224 627159 — MB ChB Aberd. 1979 (Aberd. Univ.) Cert. Family Plann. JCC 1983; MRCGP 1983; DRCOG 1984. Primary Care Dermatol. Kincardine Community Hosp. Stonehaven; Hosp. Practitioner, Woolmanhill Hosp., Aberd. Infirm.; Asst. Club Doctor Aberd. Football Club. Specialty: Dermat. Socs: Med. Chai Soc.; Primary Care Dermatol. Soc.

WEDDERSPOON, Andrew David 4 Heathwood Walk, Bexley DA5 2BP — MB BS Lond. 1961 (Lond. Hosp.) MRCS Eng. LRCP Lond. 1961. Prev: Ho. Surg. Poplar Hosp.; Ho. Phys. St. And. Hosp. Bow.

WEDELES, Elinor Holmes 5 Sharples Hall Street, London NW1 8YL Tel: 020 7722 4450 — MRCS Eng. LRCP Lond. 1942 (W. Lond.) Indep. Pract. (Psychoanal.) Lond. Specialty: Psychother. Socs: Brit. Psychoanal. Soc.

WEDGBROW, Cheryl Stephanie 1 Western Drive, Hanslope, Milton Keynes MK19 7LA Tel: 01908 510230; 7 Croft Lane, Roade, Northampton NN7 2QZ — MB BS Lond. 1991; BSc (Hons.) Lond. 1988; DRCOG 1994; MRCGP 1995. Clin. Asst. Family Plann. Specialty: Family Plann. & Reproduc. Health. Prev: Trainee GP Northampton Gen. Hosp.; SHO (A & E) Horton Gen. Hosp. Banbury; Ho. Off. (Surg.) Qu. Mary's Univ. Hosp. Lond.

WEDGWOOD, Mr Dennis Leveson Royal Shrewsbury Hospital, Copthorne, Mytton Oak Road, Shrewsbury SY3 8BR Tel: 01743 261151 Fax: 01743 261366 — MB BS Lond. 1970 (Westminster) BDS Lond. 1960; FDS RCS Eng. 1966; FRCD (C) 1978; FRCS Ed. 1985. Cons. Oral & Maxillofacial Surg. Roy. Shrewsbury Hosp., Robt. Jones & Agnes Hunt Orthop. Hosp. Oswestry & Princess Roy. Hosp. Telford. Specialty: Oral & Maxillofacial Surg. Socs: Fell. Brit. Assn. Oral & Maxillofacial Surg.; BMA. Prev: Chief Dent. Serv. Health Sci. Centre Winnipeg Manitoba, Canada; Prof. & Chairm. Oral & Maxillofacial Surg. Univ. Manitoba; Cons. Oral & Maxillofacial Surg. St. Boniface Hosp. Winnipeg.

WEDGWOOD, Frances 14 Raeburn Street, London SW2 5QU — MB BS Lond. 1994; MA Hons. Camb. 1991. Specialty: Paediat.

WEDGWOOD, Ivan Marston (retired) Beechwood, 25 Main St., Copmanthorpe, York YO23 3ST Tel: 01904 707660 — (Leeds) MRCS Eng. LRCP Lond. 1949. Prev: Ho. Surg. & Sen. Res. Anaesth. Off. Gen. Infirm. Leeds.

WEDGWOOD, John, CBE 156 Ashley Gardens, Thirleby Road, London SW1P 1HW Tel: 020 7828 8319 — (Camb. & Guy's) MRCS Eng. LRCP Lond. 1943; MA Camb. 1948, MD 1954, MB BChir 1948; FRCP Lond. 1968, M 1949. Chairm. RSAS Age Care; Vice-Pres. Roy. Hosp. for Neurodisabil. Lond. Specialty: Gen. Med. Socs: FRSM; Liveryman Soc. Apoth.; BMA. Prev: Cons. Phys. Geriat. Middlx. Hosp. Lond.; Dir. Med. & Research Servs. Roy. Home & Hosp. Putney Lond.; Sen. Med. Regist. Cardiol. Dept. St. Bart. Hosp. Lond.

WEDGWOOD, John Philip Brailsford Medical Centre, The Green, Church Lane, Ashbourne DE6 3BX Tel: 01335 360328 Fax: 01335 361095; Nether Cropper Farm, Back Lane, Sutton on The Hill, Derby

DE6 5JL Tel: 0128 373 4631 — MB ChB Leeds 1983; DRCOG 1986; MRCGP 1987. Prev: Trainee GP Derby VTS; Ho. Phys. (Gen. Med.) Roy. Halifax Infirm.; Ho. Surg. (Orthop./Gen. Surg.) St. Jas. Univ. Hosp. Leeds.

WEDGWOOD, Jonathan James 25 Main Street, Copmanthorpe, York YO23 3ST — MB BCh BAO NUI 1988; LRCPSI 1988; DA (UK) 1992; FRCA 1994. Regist. (Anaesth.) Roy. Infirm. Edin.; Cons. (Anaesth.) West. Gen. Hosp. Edin. Specialty: Anaesth. Prev: SHO (Anaesth.) Roy. Infirm. Edin.

WEDGWOOD, Kevin Roy 302 Beverley Road, Anlaby, Hull HU10 7BG Email: Kevwed@aol.com — MB ChB Leeds 1978; BSc (Hons.) (Biochem.) Leeds 1975; FRCS RCS Eng. 1982; MD Leeds 1987. Cons. Surg. Castle Hill Hosp. Cottingham. Specialty: Gen. Surg. Prev: Sen. Regist. Yorks. Rotat.; Surgic. Regist. United Norwich Hosps.; Research Regist. Univ. Dept. Surg. Univ. Missouri Columbia USA.

WEDLEY, John Raymond Royal Lancaster Infirmary, Pain Management Service, Ashton Road, Lancaster LA1 4RP Tel: 01524 583528 Fax: 01524 583519; Long Yocking How, Eskdale Green, Holmrook CA19 1UA — MB ChB Liverp. 1968; DA Eng. 1971; FFA RCS Eng. 1974. Cons. in Pain Med. Morcambe Bay Hosps. NHS Trust. Specialty: Anaesth. Special Interest: Interven. Treatm. of Chronic Pain; Neuromodulation & Radio Frequency Lesioning. Socs: BMA; Assn. Anaesth.; Pain Soc. Prev: Cons. Anaesth. & Pain Managem. Guy's & St Thos. NHS Trust Lond.; Sen. Lect. (Anaesth.) Guy's Hosp. Lond.

WEDLOCK, Karen 61 Woodhead Green, Hamilton ML3 8TJ — MB ChB Glas. 1998.

WEDZICHA, Professor Jadwiga Anna Academic Unit of Respiratory Medicine, Dominion House, St Batholomew's Hospital, London EC1A 7BE Tel: 020 8983 2219 Fax: 020 7601 8616 Email: j.a.wedzicha@qmul.ac.uk — MB BS Lond. 1978 (St. Bart.) BA Oxf. 1975; MRCP (UK) 1980; MD Lond. 1985; FRCP Lond. 1994. Prof. (Respirat. Med.) St. Bart.'s & Roy. Lond. Sch. Med. Dent.; Hon.Con.Phys Bart and the Lond. Trust; Editor in Chief, Thorax. Specialty: Respirat. Med. Special Interest: COPD Exacerbations; Domiciliary Ventilology; Support and Oxygen Ther. for Respiratory Failiure. Socs: Eur. Respirat. Soc.; Amer. Thoracic Soc.; Membe of Counc., Brit. Thorac. Soc. Prev: Sen. Regist. (Thoracic Med.) Lond. Hosp.; Regist. Lond. Chest Hosp.; SHO Brompton Hosp. Lond.

WEE, Alexander Andre Boon Liang 9 Arlington, London N12 7JR — MB BS Lond. 1993.

WEE, Bee Leng Sir Michael Sobell House, Churchill Hospital, Headington, Oxford OX3 7LJ — MB BCh BAO Dub. 1988 (Trinity Coll. Dub.) DCH RCP Lond. 1990; DObst RCOG 1991; MICGP 1992; Dip. Palliat. Med. Wales 1994; MRCGP 2001; PhD Univ. of Soton 2003. Sen. Clin. Lect. In Palliative Med. Sir Michael Sobell House, Oxford; Assoc. Dir. Clin. Studies Oxf. Univ. Specialty: Palliat. Med. Socs: Roy. Coll. Gen. Pract.; Assn. Palliat. Med.

WEE, Christine Eng Lin 67 Elmcroft Crescent, North Harrow, Harrow HA2 6HL — MB BS Lond. 1996.

WEE, Michael Yoong Kan Poole Hospital NHS Trust, Longfleet Road, Poole BH15 2JB — MB ChB Dundee 1978 (University of Dundee) BSc (1st cl. Hons. Biochem.) Dund 1978; MB ChB Dundee 1982; FFA RCS Eng. 1986. Lead Cons. Anaesth. (Obst.) Poole Hosp. Specialty: Anaesth. Special Interest: Informat. for Patients; Obst.; Research & Audit. Socs: Obst. Anaesth. Assn.; Assn. Of Anaesthetists of GB & Irel.; Roy. Coll. of Anaesthetists. Prev: Sen. Regist. (Anaesth.) Brit. Roy. Infirm. & Roy. Cornw. Hosp. Truro; Sen. Regist. (Anaesth.) Gentofte Hosp. Copenhagen, Denmark; Hon. Sec., obstretics Anaesth.s ass.

WEE, Sian-Choong Bushmills Medical Centre, 6 Priestland Road, Bushmills BT57 8QP Tel: 028 2073 1233 Fax: 028 2073 2810; The Old Quarry, 35 Craigaboney Road, Bushmills BT57 8XD — MB BCh BAO Belf. 1975; MRCOG 1982, D 1978. Specialty: Obst. & Gyn.

WEEDEN, Amanda Claire 47 New Street, Chagford, Newton Abbot TQ13 8BB — MB ChB Birm. 1994; ChB Birm. 1994. SHO (Anaesth.) The Dudley Gp. of Hosps. NHS Trust Dudley W. Midl. Specialty: Anaesth. Socs: MRCAnaesth.; BMA. Prev: SHO (A & E) Birm. Heartlands Hosp.

WEEDEN, Mr David Francis Norman Southampton General Hospital, Tremona Road, Southampton SO16 6YD Tel: 023 8079 6239 Fax: 023 8079 6277; Field House, Greenfield Close, Hedge End, Southampton SO30 4DN Tel: 023 8040 4850 Fax: 023 8040 4850 — MB BS Lond. 1972 (Roy. Free) MRCS Eng. LRCP Lond. 1972; FRCS Eng. 1977; FRCS (Cardiothor.) Ed. 1985. Cons. Thoracic Surg. Wessex Cardiothoracic Centre Soton. Specialty: Cardiothoracic Surg. Special Interest: Oesophagal Cancer; pectus deformity. Socs: Fell. Soc. Thoracic & Cardiac Surgs. Prev: Sen. Regist. & Regist. (Cardiothoracic) North. Gen. Hosp. Sheff.; Resid. Surg. Off. Brompton Hosp. Lond.

WEEDER, Raymond George Greenbank House, 24 Greenbank Road, Tunstall, Stoke-on-Trent ST6 7EY Tel: 01782 814177 — MB ChB Ed. 1958 (Edin.) Specialty: Respirat. Med.; Rheumatol.; Anat. Prev: Sen. Med. Off. 224 Field Ambul. RAMC (V); Regist. (Med.) E. Cumbld. Hosp. Gp.; Regist. (Respirat. Dis.) Stoke-on-Trent Hosp. Gp.

WEEKES, Clare Alison Old Station Surgery, 39 Brecon Road, Abergavenny NP7 5UH Tel: 01873 859000 Fax: 01873 850163; 64 Chapel Road, Abergavenny NP7 7DS — MB BS Lond. 1983; DRCOG 1985; DCH RCP Lond. 1986; MRCGP 1987.

WEEKES, Richard Duncan McCallum Tait and Partners, 68 Pipeland Road, St Andrews KY16 8JZ Tel: 01334 476840 Fax: 01334 472295; Loaning Hill, Kilmany, Cupar KY15 4PT Tel: 01382 330696 — (Aberdeen) MB ChB Aberd. 1990; Dip IMC RCS Ed. 1996; MRCGP Roy. Coll. of GP's 1997; DFFP 1998. Partner in Gen. Pract.; Hon. Lect. at St. And. Univ. Specialty: Gen. Pract.; Family Plann. & Reproduc. Health. Socs: Roy. Coll. Gen. Pract.; BMA; Brit. Assn. of Immed. Care Schemes. Prev: Regtl. Med. Off. Roy. Green Jackets & Coldstream Guards.

WEEKS, Andrew David Scunthorpe General Hospital, Cliff Gardens, Scunthorpe DN15 7BH Tel: 01724 282282; 20 Norwood Avenue, Scunthorpe DN15 7AR Tel: 01724 870392 Email: aweeks@doctors.org.uk — MB ChB Sheff. 1989 (Sheffield Univ.) DCH RCP Lond. 1992; MRCOG Lond. 1996. Specialist Regist. (O & G),Jessop Hosp.Wom..Sheff. Specialty: Obst. & Gyn. Prev: Research Regist., St Jas. Hosp., Leeds; SHO (O & G) Jessop Hosp., Sheff.; SHO (O & G) North. Gen. Hosp. Sheff.

WEEKS, Ann Kathleen Ellesmere Medical Centre, Stockport Road, Cheadle Heath, Stockport SK3 0RQ Tel: 0161 428 6729 — MB ChB Liverp. 1990; DCH RCP Lond. 1992; DRCOG 1992; MRCGP 1994. GP Stockport Retainer Scheme. Specialty: Gen. Pract.

WEEKS, David Cecil, Brigadier late RAMC Retd. (retired) 4 Fircroft, Branksomewood Road, Fleet GU51 4JF Tel: 01252 687205 Fax: 01252 687205 Email: david.weeks@ntlworld.com — (Bristol) MB ChB Bristol. 1957; DTM & H Eng. 1967; FFPHM 1988, M 1973. Prev: Sec. Gen. Counc. & Regist. of Osteopaths.

WEEKS, Ian Robert Bradley Shaw Health Centre, Crookesbroom Lane, Hatfield, Doncaster DN7 6JN; The Hawthorns, Churchill Avenue, Hatfield, Doncaster DN7 6LU Tel: 01302 350264 — MB ChB Aberd. 1980; MRCGP 1984; DRCOG 1984.

WEEKS, Jennifer Hilary 82 St Margaret's Street, Rochester ME1 3BJ Tel: 01634 841072 — MB BS Lond. 1981 (Lond. Hosp.) Breast Clinician N. Kent Consortium; Breast Clinician Maidstone & Tunbridge Wells. Prev: SHO (O & G) The Lond. Hosp.; SHO (Gen. Med.) Centr. Middlx. Hosp. Lond. & Roy. Cornw. Hosp. Truro.

WEEKS, Kenneth Frederick (retired) 2 Buckland Heights, Buckland Road, Newton Abbot TQ12 4DF — MB BS Lond. 1948 (King's Coll. Hosp.) DPM Eng. 1952; FRCPsych 1974, M 1971. Prev: Cons. Psychiat. Plymouth Clin. Area.

WEEKS, Michael Charles (Surgery), 205 Shard End Crescent, Shard End, Birmingham B34 7RE Tel: 0121 747 8291 Fax: 0121 749 5497; 78 Elmdon Lane, Marston Green, Birmingham B37 7EG Tel: 0121 779 2778 — MB ChB Birm. 1961; DCH Eng. 1964. Specialty: Paediat. Prev: Ho. Phys. & Ho. Surg. Hallam Hosp. W. Bromwich; Ho. Phys. Birm. Childr. Hosp.

WEEKS, Nicola Jane 109 Barkham Ride, Finchampstead, Wokingham RG40 4EP — MB BCh Wales 1998.

WEEKS, Paul Anthony 10 Johnson Street, Lemington, Newcastle upon Tyne NE15 8DL — MB BS Newc. 1977.

WEEKS, Peter Julien Harrodale, Grainbeck Lane, Killinghall, Harrogate HG3 2AA — MB ChB Liverp. 1994.

WEEKS, Philippe Harold 9 Upper Brighton Road, Surbiton KT6 6LQ — MB BS Lond. 1993; MRCGP.

WEEKS, Rachel Mary Brookside Group Practice, Brookside Close, Gipsy Lane, Reading RG6 7HG — MB ChB Ed. 1983; DRCOG 1986; MRCGP 1987; DCCH RCGP & FCM 1988; T(GP) 1991.

WEEKS, Reginald Frank (retired) Istana, 8 Gospond Road, Barnham, Bognor Regis PO22 0EU Tel: 01243 552917 Fax: 01243

552917 Email: reg.weeks@btinternet.com — MB ChB Bristol 1958. Prev: Emerit. Cons. A & E St. Richards Hosp. Roy. W. Sussex Trust (RTO).

WEEKS, Robert Anthony 1 The Whitehouse, Mardy, Abergavenny NP7 6LB — MB BCh Wales 1989.

WEEKS, Robert Victor Mill Road Surgery, Mill Road, Market Rasen LN8 3BP Tel: 01673 843556 Fax: 01673 844388; Walnut Cottage, Church St, Middle Rasen, Market Rasen LN8 3TR Tel: 01673 842474 — MB BS Lond. 1986; MRCGP 1992; DRCOG 1993. Prev: Maj. RAMC.

WEEKS, Roger Lewis Weeks and Rana, 2 Deanhill Road, London SW14 7DF Tel: 020 8876 2424 Fax: 020 8876 3249; 9 Upper Brighton Road, Surbiton KT6 6LQ Tel: 020 8390 0910 Fax: 020 8390 9273 — MB BS Lond. 1969 (Char. Cross) MRCS Eng. LRCP Lond. 1964; DObst RCOG 1971. Chairm. Safescript Ltd. Specialty: Gen. Med. Prev: Med. Author Cons. to NHS Centre for Coding & cl.ification; Gen. Med. Off. (for Min. of Overseas Developm.) Thakhek, Laos; Lect. (Anat.) King's Coll. Lond.

WEEKS, Victoria Christina 86 Barn Hill, Wembley Park, Wembley HA9 9LQ — MB BS Lond. 1980; BSc. Lond. 1977.

WEEKS, William Thomas Shaftesbury Avenue, 119 Shaftesbury Avenue, Southend-on-Sea SS1 3AN Tel: 01702 582687 Fax: 01702 589143— MB BS Lond. 1976.

WEEPLE, Joan Anne East Wing, Esk Medical Centre, Ladywell Way, Musselburgh EH21 6AB Tel: 0131 665 2267 Fax: 0131 653 2348; 19 Lauder Road, Edinburgh EH9 2JG Tel: 0131 668 1150 — MB ChB Glas. 1970. Prev: GP Glas. & N.olt; Ho. Phys. & Ho. Surg. Northwick Pk. Hosp. Harrow.

WEERA, Chitra Ranjan Waranakula 7 Millwell Crescent, Chigwell IG7 5HX Tel: 020 8500 6235 — MRCS Eng. LRCP Lond. 1959 (Middlx.)

WEERACKODY, Roshan Priantha 10 Balmoral Avenue, Glenmavis, Airdrie ML6 0PY — MB ChB Aberd. 1998.

WEERAKKODY, Chitra Sarojini 46 Caerphilly Close, Rhiwderin, Newport NP10 8RF Tel: 01633 894312 — MB BS Sri Lanka 1974; DTCD Wales 1983; MRCS Eng. LRCP Lond. 1991; DGM RCP Lond. 1993.

WEERAKONE, Ratna Susantha 30 Cadshaw Close, Blackburn BB1 8RN Tel: 01254 65077 — MB BS Ceylon 1951; DPH Ed. 1965. Sen. Med. Off. (Adult Health & Social Servs.) Blackburn Health Dist. Prev: Med. Off. Antifilariasis Campaign, Ceylon; MOH Matara, Ceylon & Moratuwa, Ceylon.

WEERAKOON, Bernard Stanley, Capt. RAMC Scarisbrick Centre, Ormskirk District General Hospital, Ormskirk L39 2AZ Tel: 01695 577111; 1 Fulford Park House, Main St, Fulford, York YO10 4PQ — MB BS Ceylon 1959; DPM RCPSI 1982; MRCPsych 1983. Cons. Psychiat. Ormskirk Dist. Gen. Hosp. Specialty: Gen. Psychiat. Socs: Roy. Soc. Health; Ceylon Med. Assn.

WEERAMANTHRI, Sunil Piyaratne (retired) 20 The Willows, Glinton, Peterborough PE6 7NE Tel: 01733 253717 — (Moscow) MD Moscow Peoples Friendship Univ. 1966; LMSSA Lond. 1979; MACF DAC Sri Lanka 1984; PhD (Alternative Med.) Sri Lanka 1986. GP Princip. Orton Malborne. Prev: Regist. (O & G) Muhimtrili Hosp. Dar-es-Salaam, Tanzania.

WEERAMANTHRI, Tara Bernice Camberwell Child & Adolescent Service, Lister Health Centre, 25 Commercial Way, London SE15 6DP Tel: 020 7701 7371 Fax: 020 7701 8697— MB BS Lond. 1978; MRCPsych 1985. Cons. (Child. & Adolesc. Psychiat.) S. Lond. & Mandsley NHS Trust, Lond. Specialty: Child & Adolesc. Psychiat. Prev: Cons. (Child & Adolesc. Psychiat.) Newham HA Lond.

WEERASENA, Lathika Queen Elizabeth Psychiatric Hospital, Mindelsohn Way, off Vincent Drive, Edgebaston, Birmingham B15 2QZ — MB BS Colombo 1985. Staff Grade (Psychiat.) Qu. Eliz. Psychiatric Hosp. Birm. Specialty: Geriat. Psychiat.

WEERASENA, Mr Nihal Anurakumar — MB BS Rajasthan 1979 (Jaipur India) FRCS Ed. 1986; FRCS (Cth) 1995. Cons. (Cardiothoracic Surg.) Leeds Gen. Infirm.; Hon. Sen. Lect. Specialty: Cardiothoracic Surg. Special Interest: Paediatric Cardiac Surgery. Socs: Soc. Cardiothoracic Surg. GB & Irel.; Fell. Internat. Coll. Surg.; Europ. Soc. Cardiac Surg. Prev: Divisional Chief Cardiovasc. Surg.; Assoc. Prof. of Surg. Univ. Ottawa Canada; Cons. Cardiovasc. Surg. Child. Hosp. E.. Ontario Canada.

WEERASINGHE, Mr Bodipaksa Piyasiri 43 Torrington Drive, Harrow HA2 8ND — MB BS Ceylon 1968; DLO RCS Eng. 1980; FRCS Eng. 1983. Assoc. Specialist (ENT Surg.) Conquest Hosp. St. Leonards on Sea. Prev: Clin. Asst. Hastings Roy. E. Sussex Hosp.; Regist. (ENT) Eastbourne Gen. Hosp.; Cons. Anuradhapura Gen. Hosp.

WEERASINGHE, Mr Buddhadasa Dharmawansa 10 Watling Road, Bishop Auckland DL14 6RP Tel: 01388 604338 — MB BS Ceylon 1955 (Colombo Med. Sch.) FRCS Ed. 1963; FRCS Eng. 1964. Cons. Orthop. Surg. SW Durh. Health Dist.; Emerit. Cons. Orthop. Surg. SW Durh. Health Dist. Specialty: Orthop. Socs: Sen. Fell. BOA; BMA. Prev: Regist. (Surg.) Gen. Hosp. Colombo, Ceylon; Regist. (Orthop.) Harlow Wood Orthop. Hosp. Mansfield; Clin. Asst. (Orthop. & Limb Surg.) Roy. Vict. Infirm. Newc. u. Tyne.

WEERASINGHE, Padma Malini 2 Mulgrave Road, Harrow HA1 3UF Tel: 020 8864 4933 — MB BS Ceylon 1968; DA Eng. 1976; FFA RCS Eng. 1980; FFA RCSI 1980. Assoc. Specialist (Anaesth.) Ealing Hosp. S.all. Specialty: Anaesth. Socs: Assn. Anaesth. Prev: Regist. (Anaesth.) S. Lond. Hosp. Wom.; SHO (Anaesth.) St. Margt. Hosp. Epping & Lister Hosp. Stevenage.

WEERASINGHE, Somaratna (retired) 52A Middleton Lane, Middleton St George, Darlington DL2 1AL — MB BS Ceylon 1966; DPM Eng. 1974; FRCPsych 1992, M 1976. Prev: Cons. Psychiat. Darlington Memor. Hosp.

WEERASINGHE, Yamuna Ninethrie 289B Alexandra Avenue, Harrow HA2 9DX — (Univ. Soton.) BM Soton. 1993; MRCP UK 1998. Specialist Regist. (Paediat.), Lond. Specialty: Paediat. Socs: Med. Defence Union; BMA. Prev: SHO (Paediat.) Gt. Ormond St. Hosp. Lond.; SHO (Neonat.) Hammersmith Hosp. Lond.

WEETMAN, Professor Anthony Peter The Medical School, Beech Hill Road, Sheffield S10 2RX Tel: 0114 271 2570 Fax: 0114 271 3960 — MB BS Newc. 1977; MRCP (UK) 1979; DSc Newc. 1993, MD 1983; FRCP Lond. 1990; FRCP Ed. 2004. Dean The Sch. of Med. Univ. Sheff.; Sir Arthur Hall Prof. Med. Univ. Sheff.; Prof. Med. Univ. Sheff. & Hon. Cons. Phys. N. Gen. Hosp. Sheff. Specialty: Endocrinol. Socs: Assn. Phys. & Europ. Thyroid Assn.; Fell., Acad. of Med. Sci.s. Prev: Lect. Univ. Camb.; Wellcome Sen. Research Fell. (Clin. Sc.) Univ. Camb.; MRC Trav. Fell. NIH Washington DC, USA.

WEETMAN, Jacqueline Patricia 9 William Street, Manchester M20 6RQ — MB ChB Manch. 1990.

WEETMAN, Myrna Gray Central Avenue Health Centre, Central Avenue, Ardrossan KA22 7DX Tel: 01294 463838 Fax: 01294 462798; 27 Caldwell Road, West Kilbride KA23 9LF Tel: 01294 823871 — MB ChB Sheff. 1966. Socs: BMA.

WEGNER, Matthias-Peter Paediatric Department, Poole Hospital NHS Trust, Longfleet Road, Poole BH15 2JB — State Exam Med Hamburg 1991. SHO (Paediat.) Poole Hosp. NHS Trust. Specialty: Paediat. Prev: SHO (Paediat.) Glos. Roy. Hosp.

WEGSTAPEL, Mr Hendrik 10 Mayfield Road, Bromley BR1 2HD — Artsexamen Groningen 1984; FRCS Ed. 1990.

WEHNER, Helen Elizabeth Hillview Family Practice, Hareclive Road, Hartcliffe, Bristol BS13 0JP Tel: 0117 9645588/9647925 Fax: 0117 964 9055; 70 Church Road, Horfield, Bristol BS7 8SE Tel: 0117 942 0998 — MB BS Lond. 1983 (Roy. Free Hosp. Sch. Med.) DCH RCP Lond. 1987; MRCGP 1989; MPH Wales 1998. Lect. (Pub. Health Med.) Univ. Bristol; Hon. Specialist Regist. (Pub. Health Med.) Avon HA. Specialty: Pub. Health Med. Prev: Med. Off. St. Martin Hosp. Oshikuku, Namibia; GP Warminster.

WEHNER, Mary Elizabeth (retired) 7 Church Road, Thorpeness, Leiston IP16 4PJ Tel: 01728 453215 — MB BChir Camb. 1943 (Camb. & W. Lond.) MRCS Eng. LRCP Lond. 1941; DCH Eng. 1946. Prev: Clin. Med. Off. SW Herts. Health Dist.

WEI, Chun Wilson 173A Lanark Road, London W9 1NX — MB BCh BAO NUI 1979; LRCPI & LM, LRCSI & LM 1979; DCH Dub. 1982; FRCS 1987.

WEI, Terence Chiu Man University Department Clinical Neurology, Institute of Neurology, Queen Square, London WC1N 3BG; 52 Eton Hall, Eton College Road, London NW3 2DR — MB Camb. 1987; MA Camb. 1988, MB 1987, BChir 1986; MRCP (UK) 1990. Specialty: Neurol. Prev: Research Fell. Univ. Bristol & Inst. Neurol. Lond.; Regist. (Med.) Qu. Eliz. II Hosp. Welwyn Gdn. City; SHO (Neurosurg.) & Regist. (Neurol.) OldCh. Hosp. Romford.

WEICH, Scott Richard University Department of Psychiatry, Royal Free Hospital School of Medicine, Rowland Hill St., London NW3 2PF Tel: 020 7794 0500 Email: scott@rfhsm.ac.uk — MB BS

Lond. 1987; MA Camb. 1988; MRCPsych 1991; MSc Lond. 1995. Sen. Lect. (Psychiat.) Roy. Free Hosp. Sch. Med. Lond.; Hon. Cons. Psychiat. Roy. Free Hosp. MHS Trust Lond. Specialty: Gen. Psychiat. Prev: Clin. Research & Lect. Inst. of Psychiat. Lond.; Regist. Bethlem Roy. & Maudsley Hosp. Lond.

WEIDMANN, Peter John Crispin Southampton University Hospitals Trust, Shackleton Department of Anaesthetics, Tremona Road, Southampton SO16 6YD Tel: 023 8079 6720 Email: crispin.widmann@suht.swest.nhs.uk — MB ChB Leic. 1991 (Leicester) FRCA Lond. 1996; FANZCA Australia 2001. Cons. Anaesth. (Cardiac., Neuro, Neurointensive care) SUHT Soton. Socs: ACTA; RCA; AACBI.

WEIDMANN, Sarah Jane Coach House Surgery, 12 Park Avenue, Watford WD18 7LX Tel: 01923 223178 Fax: 01923 816464 — MB BS Lond. 1980; DRCOG 1983; MRCGP 1985. Course Organiser Watford VTS.

WEIGHILL, Mr Francis James (cons. rooms), 15 St John St., Manchester M3 4DG Tel: 0161 834 7373 Fax: 0161 834 9294; The Firs,, Norley Road, Kingsley, Warrington WA6 6LS Tel: 01928 788190 — MB ChB Liverp. 1964; FRCS Ed. 1969; FRCS Eng. 1970; MChOrth Liverp. 1971. Cons. Orthop. Surg. Withington Hosp. & Wythenshawe Hosp. Manch.; Vis. Surg. Duchess of York Hosp. Babies Manch. Specialty: Orthop. Socs: Fell. BOA; BMA. Prev: Sen. Regist. (Orthop.) Liverp. Roy. Infirm.; Regist. (Surg.) Leith Hosp. Edin.; Clin. Research Fell. Hosp. Sick Childr. Toronto, Canada.

WEIGHILL, Mr John Stephen Sussex Throat & Ear Department, Royal Sussex County Hospital, Eastern Road, Brighton BN2 5BE Tel: 01273 69955 Fax: 01273 602730; 67 Wayland Avenue, Brighton BN1 5JL Tel: 01273 882527 — MB BS Lond. 1977 (Westm.) FRCS (Orl.) Eng. 1982. Cons. ENT Surg. Brighton Health Care Roy. Sussex Co. Hosp., Roy. Alexandra Childr. Hosp. & Worthing HA. Specialty: Otolaryngol. Socs: Roy. Soc. Med. (Sects. Otol. & Laryngol.); Brit. Assn. Otol. Prev: Sen. Regist. Manch. Roy. Infirm.; Interne D'Etranger Gustave Roussy Hosp., Paris.

WEIGHILL, Patricia Ann 21 Burton Avenue, Timperley, Altrincham WA15 6AQ Tel: 0161 969 1764 — MB ChB Liverp. 1982. SHO (O & G) Whiston Hosp. Merseyside.

WEIGHMAN, Maurice Alun Timothy 26 Cyprus Avenue, St Annes-on-Sea, Lytham St Annes FY8 1DY Tel: 01253 731067 Fax: 01253 300261 — MB BS Lond. 1985; MRCGP 1989.

WEIGHTMAN, Nigel Challoner Microbiology Department, Friarage Hospital, Northallerton DL6 1JG — MB BS Lond. 1981; MRCPath 1988; FRCPath 1997. Cons. Microbiol. Friarage Hosp. Northallerton. Specialty: Med. Microbiol. Prev: Sen. Regist. (Microbiol.) Pub. Health Laborat. Preston & Manch.; Regist. (Microbiol.) Bristol Roy. Infirm.

WEIL, Dolores Maria The Surgery, Gaywood House, North St, Bedminster, Bristol BS3 3AZ Tel: 0117 966 1412 Fax: 0117 953 1250; 40 Caledonia Place, Bristol BS8 4DN Tel: 0117 973 5958 — BM BS Nottm. 1983; MRCGP 1989.

WEIL, Eva (retired) 23 The Vale, Chelsea, London SW3 6AG Tel: 020 7352 2948 — MB BCh BAO Dub. 1949 (T.C. Dub.) Prev: Ho. Phys. Burnley Gen. Hosp. & Hope Hosp. Salford.

WEILER-MITHOFF, Mrs Eva Maria Glasgow Royal Infirmary, Canniesburn Plastic Surgery Unit, Jubilee Building, 84 Castle Street, Glasgow G4 0SF Tel: 0141 811 5798 Fax: 0141 211 5652 — State Exam Med Marburg 1984 (Marburg/Germany) FRCS Ed. 1992; FRCS (Plast) 1996. Cons. (Plastic Surg.) Glas. Roy. Infirm. Specialty: Plastic Surg. Socs: BMA; BAPS. Prev: Cons. (Plastic Surg.) Canniesburn Hosp. Glas.; Sen. Regist. (Plastic Surg.) Canniesburn Hosp. Glas.; Regist. (Plastic Surg.) Frenchay Hosp. Bristol.

WEINBREN, Henrietta 36 Canonbury Square, Islington, London N1 2AN — MB BS Lond. 1986; DRCOG 1991; DCH RCP Lond. 1991; MRCGP 1998. GP Asst. Lond.

WEINBREN, Herschell Kenneth 1 Kithurst Close, East Preston, Littlehampton BN16 2TQ — MB BCh Witwatersrand 1946; BSc Witwatersrand 1942; MD 1957. Prof. Experim. Path. Roy. Postgrad. Med. Sch. Lond. Prev: Reader in Experim. Path. Lond. Hosp. Med. Coll.; Prof. Path. Univ. Nottm.; Prof. Histopath. Roy. Postgrad. Med. Sch. Lond.

WEINBREN, Ian (retired) 18 Balmoral Road, St Annes, Lytham St Annes FY8 1ER Tel: 01253 720597 — MB BChir Camb. 1952 (Lond. Hosp.) FRCP Lond. 1974, M 1959. Prev: Cons. Phys. Blackpool & Fylde Hosp. Gp.

WEINBREN, Jeremy Hillingdon Hospital, Pield Heath Road, Uxbridge UB8 3NN Email: jeremy@weinbren.globalnet.co.uk — MB BS Lond. 1984; DA (UK) 1989; FRCA 1994. Specialty: Anaesth.

WEINBRENN, Gerald Hyman Department Radiology, Edgware General Hospital, Edgware HA8 0AD Tel: 020 8732 6720; Beechwood, 26A Rosecroft Avenue, London NW3 7QB — MB BCh Witwatersrand 1957; DMRD 1961; MSc (Nuclear Med.) Lond. 1976. Cons. Radiol. Edgware Gen. Hosp. Specialty: Radiol. Prev: Sen. Regist. (Radiol.) Westm., Brompton & St. Stephens Hosps. Lond.

WEINDLING, Professor Alan Michael Neonatal Unit, Liverpool Women's Hospital, Crown Street, Liverpool L8 7SS Tel: 0151 702 4055 Fax: 0151 702 4313 Email: a.m.weindling@liv.ac.uk — MB BS Lond. 1974 (Guy's) BSc 1971; MD 1986; FRCP 1991; MA 1991; FRCPCH 1999. Prof. Of Perinatal Med., Uni. Of Liverp.; Counc. Mem. Brit. Assn. Perinatal Med. & Neonat. Soc.; Hon. Cons. Paediat. Roy. Liverp. Childr.'s Hosp. Specialty: Paediat. Socs: Neonat. Soc.; Europ. Soc. of Paediatric Research; Brit. Assn. of Perinatal Med. Prev: Sen. Regist. (Paediat.) St. Mary's Hosp. Manch.; Research Fell. Univ. Dept. Paediat. John Radcliffe Hosp. Oxf.; SHO Hosp. Sick Childr. Gt. Ormond St. Lond.

WEINER, Christopher Andrew 3 Lynton Park Road, Cheadle Hulme, Cheadle SK8 6JA — MB ChB Birm. 1993.

WEINER, 0 Michael Wilton Villa, 103/105 Ashton Road, Denton, Manchester M34 3LW — (Liverpool) MB ChB 1967. Medico-Legal Expert Witness; Fact. Doctor. Specialty: Medico Legal. Prev: GP.

WEINER, Nathan (retired) Idle House, Eaton, Retford DN22 0PS Tel: 01777 869993 — MB ChB Glas. 1947.

WEINHARDT, Anne Barbara Department of Medical Microbiology, Glasgow Royal Infirmary, Castle St., Glasgow G4 0SF — MB ChB Leic. 1985.

WEINKOVE, Cyril — MB ChB Cape Town 1963; FCP (SA); PhD Cape Town.

WEINREB, Irene Rachel Imperial College Health Centre, Southside, Watt's Way, London SW7 1LU Tel: 020 7584 6301 Fax: 020 7594 9390 — MB BS Lond. 1976 (Roy. Free) MRCS Eng. LRCP Lond. 1976; DRCOG 1979; MBA DIC (Imperial Coll.) 2000. GP Imperial Coll. Univ. Lond. Specialty: Gen. Pract.

WEINSTEIN, Andrew Felix Chase Farm Hospital, Enfield EN2 8JL Tel: 020 8366 6600 — MB BChir Camb. 1978; BA 1975; MA Camb. 1979; MRCP (UK) 1983; FRCP 1997. Cons. Phys. Geriat. Med. Chase Farm Hosp. Specialty: Care of the Elderly. Prev: Sen. Regist. (Geriat. Med.) Westm. & Char. Cross Hosps.

WEINSTEIN, Charles Battle Hospital, Oxford Road, Reading RG30 1AG — MB BChir Camb. 1980; MA Camb. 1981, BA 1978, MB BChir 1980; FRCP 1997, MRCP (UK) 1984; MSc (Computer Sc.) Birm. 1985.

WEINSTEIN, Vivian Felix 22 Northumberland Road, Leamington Spa CV32 6HA Tel: 01926 424062 Fax: 01926 889135 — MB BCh Witwatersrand 1953; FRCP Lond. 1977, M 1957. Specialty: Gen. Med. Prev: Cons. Phys. S. Warks. Health Dist.

WEINSTOCK, Harold Steven Whitley Road Medical Centre, 1 Whitley Road, Collyhurst, Manchester M40 7QH Tel: 0161 205 4407 Fax: 0161 203 5269; 4 Pinfold Lane, Whitefield, Manchester M45 7JS — MB ChB Manch. 1975. Clin. Asst. (Gastroenterol.) N. Manch. Gen. Hosp.; Tutor (Gen. Pract.) Univ. Manch.; Bd. Mem. S. Manch. PCG; Med. Dir. Out of Hours CoOperat.

WEINSTOCK, Norman Graham 20 Acris Street, London SW18 2QP Tel: 020 8874 9423 — MB BCh Wales 1967; MRCP (UK) 1972; DPM Eng. 1972; MFPHM 1989. Prev: Regist. (Cardiol.) Char. Cross Hosp. Lond.; Regist. (Psychiat.) Char. Cross Hosp. Lond.; SHO (Med.) St. Francis Hosp. Lond.

WEINSTOCK, Samuel The Health Centre, 1A Fountayne Road, London N16 7EA Tel: 020 8806 3311; 29 Nottingham Place, London W1U 5LW Tel: 020 7935 7674 — MRCS Eng. LRCP Lond. 1936 (Lond. Hosp.)

WEIR, Adam 50 Tavistock Drive, Mapperley Park, Nottingham NG3 5DW — MB BS Newc. 1998. SHO A&E Dryburn Hosp., Durh. Specialty: Accid. & Emerg.

WEIR, Alan Duncan Kirriemuir Health Centre, Tannage Brae, Kirriemuir DD8 4DL Tel: 01575 573333 Fax: 01575 574230; Appin, 51 Brechin Road, Kirriemuir DD8 4DE — MB ChB Dundee 1980.

WEIR, Mr Alastair McLean 22 Moriston Drive, Livingston EH54 9HT — MB ChB Ed. 1980; BSc (Hons.) Ed. 1977, MB ChB 1980; FRCS Ed. 1985; MRCGP 1991; DMedRehab RCP Lond. 1992.

Sen. Regist. (Rehabil. Med.) Astley Ainslie Hosp. Edin. Specialty: Rehabil. Med.; Rheumatol. Socs: Scott. Soc. Rehabil. (Comm. Mem.); Brit. Soc. Rehabil. Med.

WEIR, Alistair William Goold (retired) Rose Cottage, Kippen, Stirling FK8 3DT Tel: 01786 870493 — (Glas.) MB ChB Glas. 1950; FRCOG 1971, M 1958. Prev: Cons. O & G Stirling Roy. Infirm.

WEIR, Andrew Ian Southern General Hospital , Institute of Neurological Sciences, 1345 Govan Road, Glasgow G51 4TF Tel: 0141 201 2480 Fax: 0141 201 2519 Email: andrew@neurophysglas.org; The Glasgow Nuffield Hospital, Nuffield House, 1000 Great Western Road, Glasgow G12 0PJ; 16 The Oaks, Killearn, Glasgow G63 9SF — MB ChB Glas. 1975 (Glas. Univ.) MSc Glas. 1977, BSc (Hons.) 1971, MB ChB 1975; MRCP (UK) 1978; FRCP Glas. 1988. Cons. Clin. (Neurophysiol.) Inst. Neurol. Sc. South. Gen. Hosp. Glas.; Hon. Sen. Lect. (Neurol.) Univ. of Glas. Specialty: Clin. Neurophysiol. Special Interest: Motor Neurone Diseases; Nerve Trauma and Entrapment; Neuromuscular Dis. Socs: Amer. Assn. of Neuromuscular and Electrodiagnostic Medicine; Brit. Soc. for Clin. Neurophysiology; Physiological Society; Internat. Alliance of ALS/MND Associations; Assn. of Brit. Neurologists. Prev: Sen. Clin. Reasearch Fell. (Wellcome Trust) Inst. Neurol. Sc. S.

WEIR, Andrew Wickham The Shaftesbury Practice, Abbey View Medical Centre, Salisbury Road, Shaftesbury SP7 8DH Tel: 01747 856700 Fax: 01747 856701; Pensbury Close, Shaftesbury SP7 8QJ Tel: 01747 852437 — MB BS Lond. 1971 (St. Bart.) MRCS Eng. LRCP Lond. 1971; DObst RCOG 1973; DA Eng. 1975. Med. Off. Westm. Memor. Hosp. Shaftesbury. Socs: BMA. Prev: Med. Off. Guys Marsh Youth Custody Centre; Clin. Asst. (Anaesth.) Salisbury Gen. Hosp.; Ho. Surg. St. Bart. Hosp. Lond.

WEIR, Basil (retired) 64 Doddington Road, Swallowbeck, Lincoln LN6 7EU — MB ChB St. And. 1956. Prev: SHO (Paediat.) St. Geo. Hosp. Lincoln.

WEIR, Cameron John Ninewells Hospital & Medical School, University Department of Anaesthesia, Dundee DD1 9SY Tel: 01382 660111; 43 Bay Road, Wormit, Newport-on-Tay DD6 8LW — MB ChB Glas. 1993; BSc 1988; FRCA 1997. Research Fell./Specialist Regist. Specialty: Anaesth. Socs: Scott. Soc. Anaesth.; Anaesth. Res. Soc.; Assn. of Anaesth.

WEIR, Clifford Ronald Tennet Institute of Opthalmology, Gartnavel General Hospital, Glasgow — MB ChB Glas. 1992; BSc (Hons.) Glas. 1989; FRCOphth 1996; MD Glasgow 2001. Tennent Inst. of Ophth., Gartnavel Gen. Hosp. Glas. Specialty: Ophth. Prev: Specialist Regist. Glas.; SHO Ophth., Glas.

WEIR, Mr Colin Derek Craigavon area hospital, 68 Lurgan Road, Portadown, Craigavon BT67 0QP Email: cdweir@dial.pipex.com; 36 Langtry Lodge, Moira, Craigavon BT67 0GT Tel: 02892 619638 Email: cdweir@dial.pipex.com — MB BCh BAO Belf. 1984 (Queens university, Belfast) FRCS Ed. 1988. Cons. Gen. & Vasc. Surg. Craigavon Area Hosp. Portadown; Honourary Clin. Lect. in Surg., Qu.s Univ., Belf. Specialty: Gen. Surg.; Vasc. Med. Socs: Nutrit. Soc.; Vasc. Surg. Soc. GB & Irel.; Eur. Soc. Vasc. Surg. Prev: Sen. Regist. Vasc. Surgic. Units Roy. Vict. & Belf. City Hosp.

WEIR, David Cuthbertson Chest Unit, North Manchester General Hospital, Manchester M8 5RB Tel: 0161 720 2077 Fax: 0161 720 2048; 10 Holmefield, Sale M33 3AN — MB ChB Ed. 1981 (Edinburgh) BA Oxf. 1978; MRCP (UK) 1984; MD Edin. 1995; FRCP Lond 1996. Cons. Phys. in Gen. Med. with an interest in Respirat. Med., N. Manch. Gen. Hsopital, Manch.; Hon. Clin. Lect., Univ. of Manch. Med. Sch.; Clin. Dir. Chest Directorate; Chairm. Clin. Audit Commitee. Specialty: Gen. Med. Socs: Eur. Respirat. Soc.; Inst. Health Serv. Manch. Prev: Research Fell. E. Birm. Hosp. & Solihull Hosps.

WEIR, Mr David John Freeman Hospital, Freeman Road, Newcastle upon Tyne NE7 7DN Tel: 0191 284 3111 Fax: 0191 223 1238 — MB ChB Dundee 1985; FRCS Eng. 1990; FRCS (Orth.) 1995. Cons. Orthop. Surg. Freeman Hosp. Newc. u. Tyne. Specialty: Orthop. Socs: Fell. BOA. Prev: Sen. Regist. (Knee Fell.) Freeman Hosp. Newc.; Regist. Rotat. (Orthop.) North. RHA; Regist. Rotat. (Surg.) Newc. u. Tyne.

WEIR, Desmond Atholl Duncan (retired) Twillick, Boscastle PL35 0AB Tel: 01840 250504 — MB BS Lond. 1954 (St. Bart.) Prev: Med. Regist. Dorset Co. Hosp. Dorchester.

WEIR, Diarmid James Grant Sutherland House, 209 Mayburn Avenue, Loanhead EH20 9ER Tel: 0131 440 0149 — MB ChB Manch. 1986; BSc St. And. 1983; DCH RCP Lond. 1993; DFFP 1994. Specialty: Cardiol. Socs: BMA. Prev: SHO (A & E) Warrington Dist. Gen. Hosp.; SHO (Gen. Med.) Walton & Fazakerley Hosps. Liverp.; SHO (Cardiol.) Broadgreen Hosp. Liverp.

WEIR, Professor Donald Mackay 36 Drummond Place, Edinburgh EH3 6PW Tel: 0131 556 7646 — MB ChB Ed. 1955; MD (Hons.) Ed. 1962; FRCP Ed. 1981, M 1976. Specialty: Immunol. Socs: Brit. Soc. Immunol.; Eur. Inflammation Soc. Prev: Prof. Immunol. Dept. Med. Microbiol. Univ. Edin. Med. Sch.; Hon. Cons. Lothian HB; Hon. Fell. (Med. Microbiol.) Edin. Med. Sch.

WEIR, Fiona Jean Trevor Mann Baby Unit, Royal Sussex County Hospital, Eastern Road, Brighton BN2 5BE — MB BS Lond. 1982 (King's Coll. Hosp. Lond.) MRCP (UK) 1986. Cons. Neonat. Roy. Sussex Co. Hosp. Specialty: Neonat.

WEIR, Gordon Boundary House Surgery, Boundary House, Mount Lane, Bracknell RG12 9PG Tel: 01344 483900 Fax: 01344 862203 — MB ChB Glas. 1984 (University of Glasgow) DRCOG 1986; MRCGP 1988. Prev: SHO Ayrsh. & Arran HB VTS; HO. Off. (Med. & Surg.) CrossHo. Hosp. Kilmarnock.

WEIR, Graeme 60 Whitless Court, Ardrossan KA22 7PB — MB ChB Ed. 1998; MB ChB Ed 1998.

WEIR, Iain Kirkland Ivry House - Child, Adolescent & Family Consultation Service, 23 Henley Road, Ipswich IP1 3TF Tel: 01473 214811 Fax: 01473 280809; Bramblewood, Leeks Hill, Melton, Woodbridge IP12 1LW Tel: 01394 385909 Fax: 01394 382992 Email: weirwizard@aol.com — MB BS Lond. 1968 (Guy's) MRCS Eng. LRCP Lond. 1968; MRCPsych 1975. Cons. Psychiat., Priv. Prac.; Cons. Psychiat. Ivy Ho. Child, Adolesc. & Fam. Consult. Serv. Local Health Partn. NHS Trust, Ipswich. Specialty: Child & Adolesc. Psychiat. Prev: Med. Dir. E. Suff.. Local Health Serv. NHS Trust; Clin. Dir. Child & Family Psychiat. E. Suff. Local Health Servs. NHS Trust; Cons. Child Psychiat. Guy's Hosp. & Lewisham Child & Family Psychiat. Clinic.

WEIR, Mr Ian George Cameron The Old Manse, Station Road, Friockheim, Arbroath DD11 4SE — MB ChB Glas. 1979; FRCS Ed. 1986.

WEIR, Ivan Richard Joseph Park Avenue Medical Centre, 9 Park Avenue, Stirling FK8 2QR Tel: 01786 473529; 10 Batter Flatts Gardens, Stirling FK7 9JU Tel: 01786 465630 — MB BCh BAO Belf. 1983 (Qu. Univ. Belf.) BSc (Hons. Biochem.) Belf. 1981; DRCOG 1986; DCH RCPSI 1986; MRCGP 1987.

WEIR, Jack, MC (retired) Marchfield, Port Glasgow Road, Kilmacolm PA13 4SG — MB ChB Glas. 1939.

WEIR, James Barclay De Vere The Surgery, 3 Glasgow Road, Paisley PA1 3QS Tel: 0141 889 2604 Fax: 0141 887 9039 — MB ChB Glas. 1975; DRCOG 1977; DCH RCP Lond. 1978; MRCGP 1980. GP Paisley, Renfrewsh.

WEIR, James Simon Leslie 4 Toll Bar Corner, Longwick, Princes Risborough HP27 9BN — MB BS Lond. 1997; MRCGP; DRCOG; BSc; DCH.

WEIR, James Thomson (retired) Rhana, 13 Hunters Grove, Hunters Quay, Dunoon PA23 8LQ — LRCP LRCS Ed. 1944 (Anderson's & St. Mungo's Colls.) LRCP LRCS Ed. LRFPS Glas. 1944; DTM & H Liverp. 1959. Sen. Med. Off. (Occupat. Health) Surrey CC Kingston upon Thames. Prev: Chief Med. Off. Kuwait Oil Co. K.S.C Ahmadi, Kuwait.

WEIR, Professor Jamie Aberdeen Royal Infirmary, Radiology Department, Foresterhill, Aberdeen AB25 2ZN Tel: 01224 554519; September Cottage, Skene, Westhill AB32 6UX — MB BS Lond. 1968; MRCP (UK) 1972; DMRD Eng. 1973; FRCR 1975; FRCP Ed. 1985; FRANZCR 1998. Cons. Radiol. Grampian HB; Clin. Prof. Radiol. Univ. Aberd. Specialty: Radiol. Special Interest: Cardiothoracic Radiol.

WEIR, Jane Jackson The Old Rectory Surgery, 18 Castle Street, Saffron Walden CB10 1BP Tel: 01799 522327 Fax: 01799 525436; 30 Saxon Way, Saffron Walden CB11 4EG — MB BChir Camb. 1982; BSc St. And. 1979; DRCOG 1986; MRCGP 1986. Specialty: Dermat.

WEIR, Jennifer Mary 50 Killead Road, Aldergrove, Crumlin BT29 4EN — BM BCh Oxf. 1992.

WEIR, John Alexander Bonnybridge Health Centre, Larbert Road, Bonnybridge FK4 1ED Tel: 01324 812315 Fax: 01324 814696 — MB ChB Manch. 1977; BSc St. And. 1974; DO RCS Eng. 1984.

Specialty: Ophth. Prev: Regist. (Ophth.) Westm. Hosp. Lond.; SHO (Neurol.) Middlx. Hosp. Lond.; Ho. Off. Manch. Roy. Infirm.

WEIR, John Anthony David Marfleet Group Practice, 350 Preston Road, Hull HU9 5HH Tel: 01482 701834 — MB ChB Leeds 1985.

WEIR, John Gordon 34E The Limes, Linden Gardens, London W2 4ET Tel: 020 7727 1315 — (Aberd.) MB ChB Aberd. 1952; DPM Eng. 1960; MA Aberd. 1945, MD 1964; FRCPsych 1977, M 1971. Specialty: Gen. Psychiat. Prev: Cons. Psychiat. St. Mary's Hosp. Lond. & Mildmay Mission Hosp.; Cons. Psychotherapist St. Bernard's Hosp. S.all.

WEIR, John Philip Dumbarton Road Surgery, 1398 Dumbarton Road, Glasgow G14 9DS Tel: 0141 959 1520 Fax: 0141 959 8463 — MB ChB Glas. 1971; Dip Forens. Med. 1988.

WEIR, June Marie Prouteaux Cloverlea, 24 Clonevin Park, Lisburn BT28 3BL Tel: 01846 673531 — MB BCh BAO Belf. 1954. Assoc. Specialist (ENT) Roy. Vict. Hosp. Belf. Specialty: Otolaryngol. Prev: JHMO (ENT) Daisy Hill Hosp. Newry.

WEIR, Karla Amanda Jane Bracken Ridge, Heath Ride, Finchampstead, Wokingham RG40 3QN — MB ChB Glas. 1984; DCH RCPS Glas. 1987; MRCGP 1988. GP Finchampstead Berks. Prev: Clin. Med. Off. Soton. HA; Trainee GP Ayr.

WEIR, Karoline Mary Elmwood Medical Centre, 7 Burlington Road, Buxton SK17 9AY Tel: 01298 23019 — MB ChB Liverp. 1984; FRCGP 1996, MRCGP 1988. GP; Cas. Off. Prev: Trainee GP (O & G/Dermat./Ophth./ENT) Hinchinbrooke Hosp. Huntingdon VTS; RMO 1 Roy. Scots. Werl W. Germany; Trainee GP Celle Med. Centre, W. Germany VTS.

WEIR, Margaret Jean Castle of Fiddes, Stonehaven AB39 2XX Tel: 0156 94 213; 14 Cowley Street, London SW1P 3LZ Tel: 020 7799 3269 — MB BS Lond. 1969 (Middx) MRCP (UK) 1974; FRCP 1999. Cons. Genitourin. Med./HIV Barnet NHS Trust Roy. Free NHS Trust; Hon. Sen. Lect. Roy. Free Hosp. Sch. Med. Specialty: Genitourinary Medicine. Socs: Assn. Genitourin. Med.; Med. Soc. Study VD. Prev: Sen. Med. Off. DoH; Sen. Regist. (Genitourin. Med.) Gtr. Glas. HB; Regist. (Dermat.) King's Coll. Hosp. Lond.

WEIR, Mr Neil Francis (cons. rooms) 2 West Road, Guildford GU1 2AU Tel: 01483 569719 Fax: 01483 306380 Email: neilweir@btinternet.com — MB BS Lond. 1965 (Westm.) MRCS Eng. LRCP Lond. 1965; FRCS Eng. 1971. Hon. Cons. Surg. (ENT) Roy. Surrey Co. Hosp. Guildford. Specialty: Otolaryngol. Special Interest: Otol., voice. Socs: Edr. Jl. of Laryngol. and Otol.; Director of Britain-Nepal Otol. Serv. (BRINOS); RSM (Past Vice-Pres.). Prev: Hon. Cons. Otol. Atkinson Morley's Hosp. Lond.; Cons. Surg. (ENT) Roy. Surrey Co. Hosp. Guildford.

WEIR, Nicholas Ulrick 17 Quillings Way, Borrowash, Derby DE72 3YA — MB ChB Sheff. 1991; MRCP (UK) 1994. SHO (Neurol.) West. Gen. Hosp. Edin.

WEIR, Patricia Margaret Paediatric Intensive Care Unit, Bristol Royal Hospital for Children, Upper Maudlin Street, Bristol BS2 8BJ Tel: 0117 342 8843 — MB ChB Glas. 1980; FFA RCS Eng. 1987. Cons. In Paediatric Anaesth. and Intens. Care. Specialty: Anaesth.

WEIR, Paul Edens Mater Hospital Trust, Crumlin Road, Belfast BT14 6AB Tel: 02890 803 507 Email: paul.weir@mater.n-i.nhs.uk; 11 Demesne Grove, Holywood BT18 9NQ Tel: 02890 426 887 — MB BCh BAO Belf. 1971 (Queens university of Belfast) FRCOG 1990, M 1977, DObst 1973; MD Belf. 1978. Cons. O & G Mater Hosp. Trust; N.I Rep. Hosp. Recognition Comm. RCOG. Specialty: Obst. & Gyn. Special Interest: Colposcopy; Oncol.; Reproductive Med. Socs: Fell. RCOG. Prev: Post Grad. Tutor Matern. Hosp. Trust; Chair. Med. Staff Matern. Hosp. Trust; Train. Progr. Dir. (Obst. & Gyn.) Northern Irel.

WEIR, Paul Samuel 3 Dufferin Villas, Groomsport Road, Bangor BT20 5PH Tel: 01247 456651 — MB BCh BAO Belf. 1987 (QUB) FFAR csi 1995; M Phil 1999. cons.Anaesth.Belf. city Hosp. Specialty: Anaesth.

***WEIR, Philip Ashley** Seven Oaks Farm, Artabrackagh Road, Portadown, Craigavon BT62 4HB Tel: 02838 354 164 Email: philipaweir@hotmail.com — MB BCh BAO Belf. 1998 (Queen's University Belfast) Dip. Mental Health (with distinction) 2003. p/t Sen. Ho. Off. In Psychiat., Whitabbey, Holywell Hosps..; Political Advisor. Socs: Northern Ireland Medical Soc. Prev: Senior House Officer in Paediatrics (Antrim Area Hospital); Senior House Officer in General Medicine (Antrim Area Hospital); Junior House Officer (South Tyrone Hospital).

WEIR, Mr Robert Desmond Belgrave Medical Centre, 22 Asline Road, Sheffield S2 4UJ Tel: 0114 255 1184 — BM BS Nottm. 1977; FRCS Ed. 1983. Specialty: Gen. Pract.

WEIR, Robert Edward Peter 31 Lauderdale Drive, Petersham, Richmond TW10 7BS — MB BS Lond. 1996.

WEIR, Robert John Stuart (retired) Timbers, 248 London Road, Withdean, Brighton BN1 6YA Tel: 01273 552743; 31 Gainsborough House, 4/6 Eaton Gardens, Hove BN3 3UA Tel: 01273 749033 — (T.C. Dub.) MB BCh BAO Dub. 1946; BA Dub. 1946. Prev: Capt. RAMC.

WEIR, Ronald John Glasgow Nuffield Hospital, Beaconsfield Road, Glasgow G12 0PJ Tel: 0141 334 9441 Fax: 0141 339 1150 Email: ron@weir01.fsnet.co.uk; White Lodge, 21a Thorn Road, Bearsden, Glasgow G61 4BS Tel: 0141 943 1367 — MB ChB Glas. 1960; FRCP Glas. 1976, M 1965; MD Glas. 1973. p/t Cons. Phys. Glas. Nuffield Hosp. Glas.; Cons. Med. Off. Abbey Nat. Life Glas. Specialty: Gen. Med. Socs: Internat. Soc. Hypertens.; Assn. Phys. GB & Irel.; Diabetes UK. Prev: Cons. Phys., W. Glas. Hosp. Univ. NHS Trust.

WEIR, Rosemary Radiology Department, Hairmyres Hospital, East Kilbride, Glasgow G41 4NL Tel: 01355 585780; 27 Fotheringay Road, Pollokshields, Glasgow G41 4NL Tel: 0141 423 6370 — MB ChB Ed. 1969; BSc (Med. Sc.) 1966; DMRD Eng. 1974; FRCR 1976. Cons. Radiol. Hairmyres Hosp. E. Kilbride. Specialty: Radiol.

WEIR, Roy Deans, OBE (retired) Creagan Gorm, Inverneil, Lochgilphead PA30 8ES Tel: 01546 606368 — MB ChB Aberd. 1950; MD Aberd. 1962, DPH 1955; FRCP Ed. 1979, M 1970; FFCM 1972; FRCP Lond. 1989. Prev: Prof. of Social Med. Univ. Aberd.

WEIR, Susanne Marlow and Partners, The Surgery, Bell Lane, Stroud GL6 9JF Tel: 01453 883793 Fax: 01453 731670 — MB ChB Sheff. 1986.

WEIR, Mr William Ian The London Chest Hospital, Bonner Road, London E2 9JX — MB BChir Camb. 1975 (Camb. & Lond. Hosp.) MA Camb. 1975; FRCS Eng. 1982; FRCS Ed. (Cth.) 1987. Cons. Cardiothoracic Surg. Barts & The Lond. NHS Trust. Specialty: Cardiothoracic Surg. Socs: Liverp. Med. Inst.; Soc. Cardiothor. Surg. Gt. Brit. & Irel. Prev: Cons. Cardiothoracic Surg. Cardiothoracic Centre Liverp.; Sen. Regist. (Cardiothoracic Surg.) Lond. Hosp.; Fell. (Surg.) Westmead Hosp. Sydney, NSW.

WEIR, William Malcolm Windmill Cottage, Whipsnade, Dunstable LU6 2LL Tel: 01582 873425 Fax: 01582 873309 — MB BS Lond. 1956 (Middlx.) MRCS Eng. LRCP Lond. 1957; DObst RCOG 1962. HM Coroner for Essex. Prev: Ho. Surg. & Ho. Phys. (Paediat.) Middlx. Hosp.; GP Beds.

WEIR, Winifred Isabella The Surgery, 15 King Street, Paisley PA1 2PR Tel: 0141 889 3144 Fax: 0141 889 7134; Mogarth, 62 Amochrie Road, Paisley PA2 0AH — MB ChB Glas. 1981; DRCOG 1984; MRCGP 1985; DCH RCPS Glas. 1985.

WEISBLATT, Emma Jane Louise Developmental Psychiatry Section, University of Cambridge, Douglas House, 186 Trumpington Road, Cambridge CB2 2AH Tel: 01223 746001 Fax: 01223 746002 Email: ejw44@cus.cam.ac.uk — MB BChir Camb. 1989 (Cambridge and the London Hospital) MA Camb. 1993, BA 1986; MRCPsych 1997; PhD 2002. Clin. Lect. in Developm. Psychiat. & Honarary specialist Regist. in Child & Adolesc. Psychiat., Camb. Specialty: Child & Adolesc. Psychiat. Socs: Brit. Neuropsychiat. Assn.; Tuberous Sclerosis Assn.; Br. Secret. Assoc of child Psychiat.s and Psychologists. Prev: SHO (Pschiatry) Addenbrooke's Hosp., Camb.; Research Regist. (Psychiat.) Addenbrooke's Hosp. Camb.; Hon. Cons. (Developm. Psychiat.) Camb.

WEISER, Richard Morriston Hospital, Ysbyty Treforys, Morriston, Swansea SA6 6NL Tel: 01792 702125 Fax: 01792 703249 — MB BCh Wales 1964 (Welsh Coll. Med.) MRCP (UK) 1971; FRCP Eng. 1983. Cons. Neurol. Morriston Hosp. NHS Trust Swansea; Hon. Sen. Lect. Univ. Coll. Swansea. Specialty: Neurol.; Clin. Neurophysiol. Socs: Assn. Brit. Neurol.; Med. Res. Soc. Prev: Sen. Regist. (Clin. Neurol. & Neurophysiol.) Regional Neurol. Centre Newc.; Regist. (Gen. Med.) Soton Gen. Hosp.; Eaton Research Fell. (Renal Dis.) Cardiff Roy. Infirm.

WEISL, Mr Hanus (retired) Cardiff Consulting Rooms, 128 Newport Road, Cardiff CF24 1DH Tel: 029 2046 4499 Fax: 029 2047 0309 — MB ChB Manch. 1948; MD (Commend.) Manch. 1953; FRCS Eng. 1957; MChOrth Liverp. 1958. Prev: Cons. Orthop. & Trauma Surg. S. Glam. AHA.

WEISS, Paul David Mitcheldean Surgery, Brook Street, Mitcheldean GL17 0AU Tel: 01594 542270 Fax: 01594 544897 — MB ChB Leeds 1993; DFFP 1996; DCH 1997; MRCGP 1998; D Med 2002. GP; Clin. Asst. in Endoscopy and Flexible Sigmoidoscopy and Occupational Health.

WEISSBERG, Alison Petersfield Medical Practice, Dr Farrant & Partners, 25 Mill Road, Cambridge CB1 2AB Tel: 01223 350647 Fax: 01223 576096; 118 Shelford Road, Trumpington, Cambridge CB2 2NF — MB ChB Birm. 1976.

WEISSBERG, Professor Peter Leslie Addenbroooke's Hospital, Cambridge CB2 2QQ Tel: 01223 331504 Fax: 01223 331505 Email: sgd21@medschl.cam.ac.uk — MB ChB Birm. 1976; MRCP (UK) 1978; MD Birm. 1985; FRCP Lond. 1992; FRCP Ed 1996; F Med Sci 1999. Hon. Cons. Cardiol. Addenbrooke's Hosp. Cambs. & Papworth Hosp. Camb.; BHF Prof. (Cardiovasc. Med.) Univ. Camb. Addenbrooke's Hosp. Specialty: Cardiol. Socs: Assn. Phys.; Brit. Cardiac Soc.; Brit. Atherosclerosis Soc. Prev: Lect. (Cardiovasc. Med.) Univ. Birm.; MRC Research Fell. Baker Inst. Melbourne, Austral.

WEISSEN, Pamela Rose Kinorth Medical Centre, 26 Abbotswell Crescent, Aberdeen AB12 5JW Tel: 01224 876000 Fax: 01224 899182; 4 Braeside Terrace, Aberdeen AB15 7TT Tel: 01224 321924 — MB ChB Aberd. 1990; MRCGP 1994. Specialty: Psychother. Prev: Trainee GP/SHO (Psychiat.) Grampian HB VTS.

WEISZ, Gabriela Maria 25 Park Avenue, London NW2 5AN — State Exam Med. Dusseldorf 1985.

WEISZ, Michael Tibor 3 The Paddocks, Carlby, Stamford PE9 4NH — MB ChB Birm. 1983; FCAnaesth 1990. Cons. Anaesth. P'boro. NHS Trust. Specialty: Anaesth.

WEITHAUS, Norbert Freeman Hospital, High Heaton, Newcastle upon Tyne NE7 7DN — State Exam Med Erlangen 1992.

WEITHERS, Mr Edghar Christopher North Middlesex Hospital, Sterling Way, Edmonton, London N18 1QX Tel: 020 8887 2000; 30 Courtland Avenue, Norbury, London SW16 3BE Tel: 020 8764 3362 — MRCS Eng. LRCP Lond. 1981; State Exam. Med. Heidleberg 1972; FRCS Ed. 1979.

WELARE-SMITH, Jayne Michele Spring Terrace Health Centre, Spring Terrace, North Shields NE28 0HQ Tel: 0191 296 1588; 5 Seaburn Grove, Seaton Sluice, Whitley Bay NE26 4HG Tel: 0191 237 0402 — MB BS Newc. 1991; MRCGP 1996, DRCOG 1993. Princip. GP N. Shields.

WELBOURN, Mr Charles Richard Burkewood Musgrove Park Hospital, Taunton TA1 5DA; 94 Princess Victoria Street, Clifton, Bristol BS8 4DB — MB BS Lond. 1983 (University College London) FRCS Ed. & Glas. 1988; MD Lond. 1991; FRCS (Gen) Ed. 1995; FRCS 1997. Cons. Surg. MusGr. Pk. Hosp. Taunton. Specialty: Gen. Surg. Prev: Sen. Regist. S. W. Region; Sen. Regist. Bristol Roy. Infirm.; Research Fell. Harvard Med. Sch.

WELBOURN, Professor Richard Burkewood 2 The Beeches, Tilehurst, Reading RG31 6RQ Tel: 01189 429258 — (Camb. & Liverp.) MB BChir Camb. 1942; FRCS Eng. 1948; MA Camb., BA 1940, MD 1953; Hon. MD Karolinska 1974; Hon. DSc Belf. 1985. Emerit. Prof. Surg. Endocrinol. Univ. Lond. Specialty: Gen. Surg. Socs: Hon. Fell. Amer. Surg. Assn.; Fell. W. Afr. Coll. Surgs. 1974; Fell. Internat. Surg. Soc. (Prize & Medal 1995). Prev: Vis. Schol. Univ. Calif., Los Angeles; Prof. Surg. & Dir. Dept. Surg. Roy. Postgrad. Med. Sch. & Hammersmith Hosp. Lond.; Prof. Surgic. Sc. Qu. Univ. Belf.

WELBOURNE, Arthur Sydney (retired) The Limes, Great Massingham, King's Lynn PE32 2JQ Tel: 01485 520422 — BM BCh Oxf. 1949; BA, BM BCh Oxon. 1949. Prev: Ho. Phys. (Paediat.) Radcliffe Infirm. Oxf.

WELBOURNE, Jill (retired) Burnaby House, 14 Greenway Road, Redland, Bristol BS6 6SG Tel: 0117 973 0183 Fax: 0117 923 9527 Email: jill@welbournes.freeserve.co.uk — BM BCh Oxf. 1963 (St. Mary's) Prev: Clin. Asst. (Psychiat.) Profess. Unit Glenside Hosp. Bristol.

WELBURY, Janet Central Clinic, The Childrens Centre, Durham Road, Sunderland SR3 4AF Tel: 0191 565 6256 Ext: 45274 Fax: 0191 569 9938 Email: jan.welbury@chs.northy.nhs.uk — MB ChB Sheff. 1975; FRCPCH; DRCOG 1977; MRCP (UK) (Paediat.) 1983. Cons. Paediat. 1993-. Specialty: Paediat.

WELBURY, Robert Richard Dental Hospital, Richardson Road, Newcastle upon Tyne NE2 4AZ Tel: 0191 232 5131 Fax: 0191 222 6137; 27 Swarland Avenue, Benton, Newcastle upon Tyne NE7 7TE Tel: 0191 266 3572 — MB BS Newc. 1984 (Newcastle upon Tyne) BDS 1978; PhD Newc. 1989, MB BS 1984; FDS RCS Eng. 1986. Regional Cons. Paediat. Dent. Surg. Newc. u. Tyne; Hon. Sen. Lect. Newc. Univ. Specialty: Paediat. Dent.

WELBY, Sharon Bianca 1 Stone Cottage, Bell Vale Road, Gateacre, Liverpool L25 2QB Tel: 0151 428 9224 — BM BS Nottm. 1985; MRCP (UK) 1988. Regist. (Haemat.) Broadgreen Hosp. & Roy. Liverp. Hosp. Specialty: Haematology. Prev: SHO (Infect. Dis.) Fazakerley Hosp.; Regist. Rotat. (Med.) North. Gen. Hosp. Sheff.

WELCH, Mr Andrew Robert ENT Department, Freeman Hospital, High Heaton, Newcastle upon Tyne NE7 7DN Tel: 0191 284 3111 Fax: 0191 223 1246; 12 Wilson Gardens, Gosforth, Newcastle upon Tyne NE3 4JA Tel: 0191 285 6514 Fax: 0191 285 5271 — MB BS Newc. 1976 (Newcastle-upon-Tyne) FRCS Eng. 1981. Cons. Otolaryngol. Freeman Hosp. Newc u. Tyne; Hon. Clin. Lect. (Otolaryngol.) Univ. Newc. Specialty: Otolaryngol. Prev: Sen. Regist. Roy. Vict. Infirm. Newc.; Regist. Leicester Roy. Infirm.

WELCH, Caroline Beatrice 1 Hoggarth Close, Petersfield GU31 4YY — MB BS Lond. 1984.

WELCH, Catherine Jane Cherry Croft, Grange Park, Swanland, North Ferriby HU14 3NA — MB ChB Manch. 1998; MB ChB Manch 1998.

WELCH, Mr Christopher Charles — MB ChB Manch. 1973 (Manchester) DObst 1975; FRCOG 1991, M 1979; FRCS Ed. 1981. Cons. O & G Basildon & Thurrock HA.; Clin. Director Obst., Gyn. and Paediat., B&T NHS Trust; Assoc. Med. Director, B&T NHS Trust. Specialty: Obst. & Gyn. Socs: BSCCP; BSGE; RSM.

WELCH, Christopher Ross Arrowe Park Hospital, Duchess of Westminster Wing, Upton, Wirral CH49 5PE Tel: 0151 604 7158 Fax: 0151 604 1552 Email: ross.welch@whnt.nhs.uk — MB BS Lond. 1981 (King's College Hospital Medical School) DA (UK) 1985; MRCOG 1989; MD Lond. 1994; FRCOG 2001. Cons. O & G Arrowe Pk. Hosp. Wirral. Specialty: Obst. & Gyn. Socs: Internat. Fetal Med. & Surg. Soc.; Pres. Internat. Fetal Med. and Surg. Soc. (1998-99); Brit. Matern. Fetal Med. Soc. Prev: Lect. (Fetal Med.) Birm. Matern. Hosp.; Sen. Regist. (Fetal Med.) Liverp. Matern. Hosp.; Research Fell. (Fetal Med.) RPMS Inst. & O & G Qu. Charlotte's Hosp. Lond.

WELCH, Coral Irmgard (retired) 27 The Glebe, Sudbury CO10 9SN; 16 Creffield Road, Colchester CO3 3JA — MB BS (Hons.) Lond. 1951 (King's Coll. Hosp.) DCH Eng. 1956. Prev: GP Colchester.

WELCH, David Macpherson (retired) 16 Kedleston Drive, Cringleford, Norwich NR4 6XN Tel: 01603 454996 — MB BS Lond. 1962 (St. Bart.) MRCS Eng. LRCP Lond. 1961; DObst RCOG 1964. Chairm. Norf. & Norwich Benevolent Med. Soc.

WELCH, Dilys Mary (retired) The Rookery, Scotland Lane, Horforth, Leeds LS18 5HP Tel: 0113 22049 — MB ChB Sheff. 1955. Princip. Gen. Pract. Leeds. Prev: Med. Regist. Gen. Hosp. S. Shields.

WELCH, Emma Felicity Jane Spinaway, The Droveway, St Margaret's Bay, Dover CT15 6DE — MB ChB Bristol 1994.

WELCH, Flora Mary Barnard Castle Surgery, Victoria Road, Barnard Castle DL12 8HT Tel: 01833 690707 — MB ChB Aberd. 1981; DRCOG 1984; MRCGP 1985. Prev: Ho. Off. (Med.) Aberd. Roy. Infirm.; Ho. Off. (Surg.) Darlington Memor. Hosp.; Trainee GP Northallerton VTS.

WELCH, Geoffrey Philip Freshfield Surgery, 61 Gores Lane, Formby, Liverpool L37 3NU Tel: 01704 879430 Fax: 01704 833883; Amazonas, Sandy Lane, Hightown, Liverpool L38 3RP Tel: 0151 929 3216 — MB ChB Liverp. 1980 (Liverpool) DRCOG Lond. 1984; Cert. Family Plann. JCC 1984; DFFP (Rcog) 1998. Cons. in Primary Care Southport & Formby Community NHS Trust; Clin. Asst. (Orthop. Surg.) Southport & Formby Dist. Gen. Hosp.; Med. Off. St. Joseph's Childr. Hosp. Formby.; Med. Assessor Independant Tribunal Serv.; Clin. ass Cardiol. Southport DGH. Prev: Princip GP. Liverp.

WELCH, George Hunter Southern General Hospital, Department of Surgery, Govan Road, Glasgow G51 4TF Tel: 0141 201 2731; Castlehill, 202 Nithsdale Road, Pollokshields, Glasgow G41 5EU Tel: 0141 422 1505 — MB ChB Glas. 1977 (Unvi. Glas.) FRCS Glas. 1981; MD Glas. 1987. Cons. Surg. (Vasc. Surg.) S. Glas. Uni. Hosp. NHS Trust; Hon. Sen. Lect., Dept. of Surg. Uni. Of Glas.; Bd. of Examr.s, Roy. Coll. Of Phys. And Surg. Glas. Specialty: Gen. Surg. Socs: Vasc. Surgic. Soc. GB & Irel.; Assn. Surg. Of GB & Irel.; Amer.

Coll. Of Angiology. Prev: Cons. Surg. (Gen. & Vasc. Surg.) S. Ayrsh. Hosp. NHS Trust; Sen. Regist. (Gen. Surg.) Gtr. Glas. HB; Regist. (Peripheral Vasc. Surg.) Glas. Roy. Infirm.

WELCH, Mr George Somerville, OBE, TD (retired) 63 Culduthel Road, Inverness IV2 4HQ — MB BS Lond. 1959 (Lond. Hosp.) MRCS Eng. LRCP Lond. 1959; FRCS Eng. 1963; FRCS Ed. 1988. Prev: Cons. Orthop. Surg. Highland HB.

WELCH, Mr Ian McLay South Manchester University Hospital NHS Trust, Manchester M23 9LT Tel: 0161 998 7070 Fax: 0161 291 6658 — MB ChB (Hons.) Sheff. 1991; BSc Sheff. 1983; PhD Sheff 1988; FRCS Eng. 1995; FRCS Ed. 1995; FRCS (Gen. Surg./Upper GI) 2000. Cons. (Oesophago-gastric Surg.) S. Manch. Univ. and Christie Hosps. Specialty: Gen. Surg. Prev: Specialist Regist. (Surg.) N. Trent.

WELCH, Jan Mary Department of Sexual Health, King's College Hospital, Denmark Hill, London SE5 9RS Tel: 020 7346 3852 Fax: 020 7346 3486 — MB BS Lond. 1980 (St. Thos.) BSc Lond. 1977; FRCP Lond. 1995. Cons. Genitourin. Med. King's Coll. Hosp. Lond.; Dir. Postgrad. Med. Ed. Kings Coll. Hosp.; Clin. Director of the Haven (King's Sexual Assault Referral Centre); Postgrad. Dean GKT Sch. of Med., Denmark Hill Campus. Specialty: Genitourinary Medicine; HIV Med. Socs: Med. Soc. Study VD. Prev: Sen. Regist. (Genitourin. Med.) St. Thos. Hosp. Lond.; Sen. Regist. (Clin. Virol.) St. Thos. Hosp. Lond.; Regist. (Med. & Infec. Dis.) Hither Green Hosp. Lond.

WELCH, Jennifer Christine Dept. of Haematology, Sheffield Children's hospital, Western Bank, Sheffield S10 2TH Fax: 0114 271 7477 Email: jenny.welch@sch.nhs.uk — BM BS Nottm. 1987; BMedSci Nottm. 1985; MRCP (UK) 1991; Dip RCPath 1999; MRCPath 2001. Cons. Paediatric Haematologist, Sheff. Childr.'s Hosp. Specialty: Haematology; Paediat. Socs: Roy. Coll. of Paediat. & Child Health; Brit. Soc. Haematol.; UKCCSG. Prev: Regist. (Haemat.) N.Trent Train. Scheme; Leukaemia Research Fund Regist. (Paediat. Haemat. & Oncol.) Childr. Hosp. Sheff.; Regist. (Paediat.) Trent Regional Train. Scheme.

WELCH, John Philip Lane (retired) 10 Maison Dieu, Richmond DL10 7AU — MB ChB St. And. 1955. Prev: Ho. Phys. Harrogate & Dist. Gen. Hosp.

WELCH, Judith Anne 1 St Georges Road, Hightown, Liverpool L38 3RY — MB ChB Liverp. 1978; MRCP Ed. 1981; DRCOG 1985.

WELCH, Kate Antonia Commercial Road Surgery, 75 Commercial Road, Leeds LS5 3AT Tel: 0113 275 2780; 18 Stanhope Avenue, Horsforth, Leeds LS18 5AR — MB BS Lond. 1984; DRCOG 1988. Clin. Asst. (Dermat.) Leeds Gen. Infirm. Prev: SHO (Dermat.) York Dist. Hosp.

WELCH, Lesley Jayne Strensall Medical Centre, Southfields Road, Strensall, York YO32 5UA Tel: 01904 490532 — MB ChB Liverp. 1983; DRCOG 1987; Cert. Family Plann. JCC 1987; MRCGP 1991. Prev: Trainee GP Henleaze Bristol VTS; SHO (O & G & Psych.) Doncaster Roy. Infirm.; Cas. Off. Doncaster Roy. Infirm.

WELCH, Mark Wythenshawe Hospital, Southmoor Road, Wythenshawe, Manchester M23 9LT — MB ChB Leeds 1984. Specialty: Gen. Surg. Prev: SHO (Cardiothoracic Surg.) Killingbeck Hosp. Leeds; SHO (ENT Surg.) Seacroft Hosp. Leeds; SHO (A & E) Leeds Gen. Infirm.

WELCH, Michael Thomas Christopher The Health Centre, Commercial Road, Skelmanthorpe, Huddersfield HD8 9DA Tel: 01484 862239; Denby Dale Surgery, 313 Wakefield Road, Denby Dale, Huddersfield HD8 8RX Tel: 01484 862239 — BM Soton. 1982. Prev: Clin. Asst. (Anaesth.) Dewsbury Gen Hosp.; Trainee GP Failsworth VTS; SHO (Anaesth., O & G & A & E) Oldham HA.

WELCH, Mr Neil Thomas Nottingham City Hospital, Nottingham NG5 1PB Tel: 0115 9691169 — MB BS Lond. 1984 (Lond. Hosp. Med. Coll.) BSc Lond. 1981; FRCS Ed. 1988; MS Lond. 1995; FRCS (Gen.) 1997. Cons. (Gen. Surg.) Nottm.. City hosp. Specialty: Gen. Surg. Socs: BMA. Prev: Sen. Regist. (Gen. Surg.) Liverp. Hosp., NSW, Austral.; Sen. Regist. (Gen. Surg.) W. Midl. RHA; Research Fell. (Surg.) St. Joseph Hosp. Omaha, Nebraska, USA.

WELCH, Nigel Charles Cunningham — MB BCh Wales 1973 (Welsh Nat. Sch. Med.)

WELCH, Nina Mary Waterfield House Surgery, 186 Henwood Green Road, Pembury, Tunbridge Wells TN2 4LR Tel: 01892 825488; 7 Heskett Park, Pembury, Tunbridge Wells TN2 4JF — MB BS Lond. 1989 (St George's London) Prev: Trainee GP & Ho. Surg. Frimley Pk. Hosp.; Ho. Phys. St. Geo. Hosp. Lond.

WELCH, Richard Arthur, CStJ Concept 2000, 250 Farnborough Road, Farnborough GU14 7LU Tel: 01252 528324 Fax: 01252 528325 Email: richard.welch@postoffice.co.uk; Toscanna, Soldridge Road, Medstead, Alton GU34 5JF Tel: 01420562228 Fax: 01252 528325 — (Glas.) ECFMG Cert 1969; MB ChB Glas. 1969; DObst RCOG 1971; MRCGP 1980; DIH Lond. 1984; MSc (Occupat. Med.) Lond. 1985; FFOM RCP Lond. 1991, M 1985. Chief Med. Adviser Post Office. Specialty: Occupat. Health. Socs: FRSM (Pres. Occupat. Med. Sect.); Soc. Occupat. Med. (Ex. Comm. Mem.); BMA (Ex-Comm. Mem. Occupat. Health Sect.). Prev: Med. Off. Talbot Ltd. Linwood; GP The Health Centre, Linwood; Regist. (Psychiat.) Stobhill Hosp. Glas.

WELCH, Robert Brian Commercial Road Surgery, 75 Commercial Road, Leeds LS5 3AT Tel: 0113 275 2780 — MB BS Durh. 1953. Prev: Ho. Phys. & Ho. Surg. Roy. Vict. Infirm. Newc.; Ho. Off. Gyn. & Obst. Dept. Matern. Hosp. Sunderland; RAF.

WELCH, Robert Gordon (retired) Hartdale, Queensberry Avenue, Hartlepool TS26 9NW Tel: 01429 274397 — (St. Thos.) MD Lond. 1951, MB BS 1945; FRCP Lond. 1973, M 1950. Prev: Cons. Paediat. Hartlepool, N. & S. Tees Dist. HAs.

WELCH, Robert James Royal Shrewsbury Hospital, Mytton Oak Road, Shrewsbury SY3 8XQ Tel: 01743 261000 Fax: 01743 261444 Email: bob.welch@rsh.nhs.uk; Wychwood, Bicton Lane, Bicton, Shrewsbury SY3 8EU Tel: 01743 850081 Email: wychwood.bicton@lineone.net — BSc Hons. Manch. 1976; MB ChB Manch. 1978; MRCP (UK) 1982; FRCPCH 1996. Cons. Neonat. Roy. Shrewsbury Hosp. Specialty: Neonat. Prev: Sen. Regist. (Neonat. Paediat.) Princess Mary Matern. Hosp. Newc.; Fell. (Neonat.) Univ. Alberta Hosps., Canada.

WELCH, Ronald Frank (retired) 20 Langton Avenue, Whetstone, London N20 9DB — MRCS Eng. LRCP Lond. 1940 (Westm.) MD Lond. 1946, MB BS 1940; FRCPath 1963. Prev: Hon. Cons. Path. Barnet Gen. Hosp.

WELCH, Rosemary Ann Beighton Health Centre, Queens Road, Beighton, Sheffield S20 1BJ Tel: 0114 269 5061 — MB BS Lond. 1984; MRCGP 1989; DRCOG 1989; DCH RCP Lond. 1990. Prev: SHO (Community/ Gen. Paediat.) Sheff. HA; GP Trainee Eckington Derbysh.

WELCH, Sarah Louise Marina House, Addiction Resource Centre, 63-65 Denmark Hill, London SE5 Tel: 020 7703 6333 Fax: 020 7740 5730; Addiction Research Unit, 4 Windsor Walk, London SE5 8LF Tel: 020 7703 6333 Fax: 020 7701 8454 — BM BCh Oxf. 1988 (Cambridge & Oxford) MA (Camb.) 1988; DPhil Oxf. 1994; MRCPsych 1994. Cons. Psychiat. in the Addic.s; Hon. Sen. Lect. Inst. Psychiat.1998. Specialty: Alcohol & Substance Misuse. Prev: Clin. Lect. in the Addic.s, Addic. Research Unit, Inst. Psychiat. & Hon. Sen. Regist. Bethlem & Maudsley NHS Trust; Regist. & SHO (Psychiat.) Maudsley Hosp. Lond.; Research SHO (Psychiat.) Univ. Oxf.

WELCH, Steven Brian 4 Porchester House, Philpot St., London E1 2JF — MB BS Lond. 1993.

WELCH, Mr Theodore Phillips (retired) 56 School Lane, Toft, Cambridge CB3 7RE Tel: 01223 263371 Fax: 01223 263371 — MB BS Lond. 1958 (Univ. Coll. Hosp.) MRCS Eng. LRCP Lond. 1958; FRCS Eng. 1964. Prev: Cons. i/c A & E Dept. Northwick Pk. Hosp. Harrow.

WELCHER, Eileen Mary (retired) Middle Coombe Farm, Huish Champflower, Taunton TA4 2HG Tel: 01984 624683 Email: ewelcher@talk21.com — MB BS Lond. 1947 (Roy. Free) DA Eng. 1957; FFA RCS Eng. 1963. Prev: Cons. Anaesth. Torbay Hosp. Gp.

WELCHEW, Edward Amin 201 Tom Lane, Fulwood, Sheffield S10 3PH — MB ChB Bristol 1974; FFA RCS Eng. 1979. Cons. Anaesth. Sheff. HA; Hon. Clin. Lect. Univ. Sheff.; Vis. Lect. Sheff. Polytechnic. Specialty: Anaesth. Socs: Anaesth. Research Soc. Prev: Lect. (Anaesth.) Univ. Sheff.

WELCHEW, Kathleen Lois Wadlerslade Surgery, Walderslade, 194 King Street, Barnsley S74 9LJ — MB ChB Bristol 1974; DRCOG 1977; MRCGP 1978.

WELCHMAN, Charlotte Louise Sundial House, Altrincham Road, Styal, Wilmslow SK9 4JE — MB BS Newc. 1998; MB BS Newc 1998.

WELDING, Ian Joseph The Elms, Crank Road, Billinge, Wigan WN5 7EX — MB ChB Manch. 1987.

WELDING, Robert Nigel 11 Polstead Road, Oxford OX2 6TW — MB BS Lond. 1990.

WELDON, Brian Dominic 11 Drake Close, Aughton, Ormskirk L39 5QL — MB ChB Liverp. 1974.

WELDON, David Philip 26 Hill Crest Drive, Beverley HU17 7JL — MB BS Newc. 1997; MRCS Ed. 2002.

WELDON, Jennifer Ruth 17 Devonshire Place, Jesmond, Newcastle upon Tyne NE2 2NB — MB BS Newc. 1998; MB BS Newc 1998.

WELDON, Michael John Stoke Mandeville Hospital, Mandeville Road, Aylesbury HP21 8AL Tel: 01296 315000; 19 Dovecote, Haddenham, Aylesbury HP17 8BP Tel: 01844 299049 — MB ChB Leeds 1986; BSc (Hons.) Leeds 1983; MRCP (UK) 1989; MD 1997. Cons. Phys. & Gastroenterol. Stoke Mandeville Hosp. Bucks. Specialty: Gastroenterol.; Gen. Med. Socs: Brit. Inflammation Research Assn.; Brit. Soc. Gastroenterol. Prev: Sen. Regist. St. Geo. Hosp. Lond.; Research Regist. (Gastroenterol.) St. Geo. Hosp. Med. Sch. Lond.; Regist. (Med.) North. Gen. Hosp. Sheff.

WELDON, Oliver George William 4 The Cloisters, Newcastle upon Tyne NE7 7LS Tel: 0191 284 2057 — MB BS Lond. 1973 (St. Bart.) MRCS Eng. LRCP Lond. 1973; FRCA 1978. Cons. Anaesth. Freeman Hosp. Newc. Specialty: Anaesth. Socs: Assn. Anaesth.; BMA. Prev: Sen. Regist. (Anaesth.) SW RHA; SHO (Anaesth.) St. Bart. Hosp. Lond.; Ho. Phys. Roy. Sussex Co. Hosp. Brighton.

WELDON, Rachel Henriette Small Isles Medical Practice, Isle of Eigg PH42 4RL Tel: 01687 482427 Fax: 01687 482422 — Artsexamen Utrect 1987.

WELEMINSKY, Antonin (retired) 45 Evesham Road, Middleton, Manchester M24 1QL — MD Prague 1933. Prev: Asst. Chest Phys. Pontefract.

WELFORD, James Richard Francis Carlton Medical Practice, 252 Girlington Road, Bradford BD8 9PB Tel: 01274 491448/9 Fax: 01274 483362 — MB ChB Leeds 1989. GP Partner; Clin. Asst. (Gastroenterol.) W. Yorks. Specialty: Gen. Pract.

WELFORD, Roy Audus Glastonbury Health Centre, 1 Wells Road, Glastonbury BA6 9DD Tel: 01458 834100 Fax: 01458 834371 — BM Soton. 1978; DRCOG 1982; MFHom 1987.

WELHAM, Judith Renal unit, Wrexham Maelor Hospital, Croesnewydd Road, Wrexham LL13 7TD Tel: 01978 291100 — MB BCh Wales 1986; MRCP (UK) 1989. Assoc. Specialist (Renal/Diabetes) Wrexham Maelor Hosp. Specialty: Nephrol. Prev: Staff Grade Phys. (Renal Med.) Wrexham Maelor Hosp.; Regist. (Renal) Univ. Hosp. S. Manch.

WELHAM, Katie Louise — BChir Camb. 1996; MA MB; MRCP.

WELHAM, Mr Richard Alexander Norton, ED 72 Berkeley Avenue, Reading RG1 6HY Tel: 0118 955 3457 Fax: 0118 955 3478 — MB ChB Leeds 1959; DO Eng. 1965; FRCS Eng. 1967. Cons. Ophth. Surg. Roy. Berks. Hosp. Reading. Specialty: Ophth. Socs: Reading Path. Soc.; RSM; Soc. of Apothcaries of Lond. Prev: Cons. Ophth. Surg. Moorfields Eye Hosp. Lond.; Pres. Reading Path.Soc.; Treas. Europ. Soc. Opth. Plastic & Reconstruct. Surg.

WELI, Tajana Dilini Snowdrop Hill, Glosthorpe Manor, Ashwicken, King's Lynn PE32 1NB — MB ChB Manch. 1998.

WELLAND, Hilary Ann 23 The Paddocks, Hempstead, Gillingham ME7 3NG — MB BS Lond. 1994.

WELLBELOVE, Pamela Anne 2 Forester Road, Southgate, Crawley RH10 6EQ Tel: 01293 522231 — MB BS Lond. 1962 (Westm.) MRCS Eng. LRCP Lond. 1962; DObst RCOG 1964; DFFP 1993. Socs: BMA.

WELLDON, Estela Valentina 121 Harley Street, London W1N 1DH Tel: 020 7935 9076; Portman Clinic, 8 Fitzjohns Avenue, London NW3 5NA Fax: 020 7447 3748 — Medico Univ. Nacional de Cuyo 1962; FRCPsych 1987, M 1973; DSc (Hon) Oxf. Brookes 1997. Cons. Psychother. & Clin. Tutor Portman Clinic Lond.; Dir. 1st. Dip. Course & Hon. Sen. Lect. (Forens. Psychother.) UCL; Mem. Bd. Dirs. Internat. Assn. Gp. Psychother.; Hon. Sen. Lect. UCL 1995. Specialty: Psychother. Socs: Internat. Assn. Forens. Psychother. (Pres.); BMA; Med. Protec. Soc. Prev: Postgrad. Fell. Menninger Sch. Psychiat. Topeka, USA.

WELLEN, Tamsyn 40 Hilda Wharf, Aylesbury HP20 1RJ — MB BCh Witwatersrand 1997.

WELLER, Claire Susan 12 Ashtree Cl, Newcastle upon Tyne NE4 6ST — MB BS Newc. 1997.

WELLER, Evelyn Mary (retired) Homecroft Surgery, Voguebeloth, Illogan, Redruth TR16 4ET Fax: 01209 843707 — MB BS Lond. 1974.

WELLER, Gillian de Mowbray Leigh (retired) 7 Cousins Grove, Southsea PO4 9RP Tel: 023 9273 2958 — MB BS Lond. 1957 (St. Thos.) Prev: Hosp. Pract. (Geriat.) St. Mary's Hosp. Portsmouth.

WELLER, Ian Vincent Derrick 63 Grimsdyke Road, Pinner HA5 4PP — MB BS Lond. 1974 (St. Bart.) MRCP (UK) 1977; BSc (1st cl. Hons.) Physiol. Lond. 1971, MD 1983. Wellcome Trust Sen. Lect. Infec. Dis.; Hon. Cons. Acad. Dept. Genitourin. Med. Middlx. Hosp. Med. Sch. Lond. Specialty: Genitourinary Medicine. Socs: Med. Soc. Study of VD; Brit. Assn. Study of Liver. Prev: Regist. (Med.) St. Mary's Hosp. Paddington, Lond.; MRC Train. Fell. Roy. Free Hosp. Lond.; Lect. Acad. Dept. Genitourin. Med. Middlx. Hosp. Med. Sch. Lond.

WELLER, Jennifer Margaret (retired) Moorside, Charles Lane, Old Glossop, Glossop SK13 7SF — MB BChir Camb. 1963; DMRD Eng. 1967; FRCR 1971. Prev: Cons. Radiol. N.E. Manch. Gp. Hosps.

WELLER, Professor Malcolm Philip Isadore 30 Arkwright Road, London NW3 6BH Tel: 020 7794 5804 Fax: 020 7431 1589 Email: mweller@onetel.net.uk — MB BS Newc. 1972 (Newcastle upon Tyne) C.Pysch; FBPsS 1986, AF 1980, M 1956; MA (Experim. Psychol.) Camb. 1959; FRCPsych 1987, M 1975. Emerit. Cons. Psychiat., Barnet, Enfield & Haringey NHS Mutual Health Trust; Hon. Prof. Middlx. Univ.; Extern. Examr. Manch. & Singapore Univs.; Chairm. N. Thames Regional Psychiat. Comm.; Hon. Med. Adviser,; Edr-in-Chief, Bailliers Clin. Psychiat. Series (II) Vols. Specialty: Gen. Psychiat. Socs: FRCPsych. FCINP; Emerit. Mem. Sci.; Founder Mem. Brit. Assn. Psychopharmacol. Prev: Vis. Fell. Fitzwilliam Coll. Camb.; Extern. Examr. Manch. & Singapore Univs.; Vice-Chairm. NE Thames Regional Comm. Hosp. Med. Servs.

WELLER, Matthew David 170 Dawlish Road, Selly Oak, Birmingham B29 7AR Tel: 0121 689 5573 — MB ChB Birm. 1997. SHO Orthop. & Trauma Worcester Hosp. Specialty: Orthop.

WELLER, Michael Arthur, OBE, KStJ (retired) Aldboro' Lodge, Park St., Thaxted, Dunmow CM6 2ND Tel: 01371 830780 — (St. Bart.) MRCS Eng. LRCP Lond. 1948; MB BS Lond. 1949; FRCGP 1970. Prev: Hon. Nat. Chairm. (Support Gps.) Research into Ageing Lond.

WELLER, Peter Herbert Department of Paediatric Respiratory Medicine, Birmingham Children's Hospital, Steelhouse Lane, Birmingham B4 6NH Tel: 0121 333 8205 Fax: 0121 333 8201 Email: peter.weller@bch.nhs.uk — MB BChir Camb. 1969 (St John's Camb. & St. Thos.) MA Camb. 1970; MRCP (UK) 1973; FRCP Lond. 1986; FRPCH 1997. Cons. Paediat. Chest Phys. Birm. Childr.s Hosp.; Clin. Director, Bimingham Childrens Hosp., Birm. Specialty: Paediat. Special Interest: Asthma; Cysilc Fibrosis. Socs: BTS; ERS; RSM. Prev: Cons. Paediat. Chest Phys. Birm. City Hosp.; Research Fell. & Sen. Regist. Hosp. Sick Childr. Gt. Ormond St. Lond.

WELLER, Mr Peter Jeremy Oral Maxillofacial Surgery Department, Southend Hospital Trust, Prittlewell Chase, Westcliff on Sea SS0 0RY Tel: 01702 221014; Bay Lodge, 501 Victoria Avenue, Prittlewell, Southend-on-Sea SS2 6NL Tel: 01702 352442 Fax: 01702 352442 — MB BS Lond. 1983 (Char. Cross Hosp.) BDS 1973; FDS RCPS Glas. 1985; FRCS Ed. 1988. Cons. Oral Surg. Southend Hosp. Trust, Basildon & Thurrock Hosps. Trust. Specialty: Oral & Maxillofacial Surg. Socs: Fell. Brit. Assn. Oral & Maxillofacial Surg.; Hosp. Cons. & Spec. Assn.; BMA. Prev: Sen. Regist. (Oral. & Maxillofacial Surg.) Westm. Hosp. Lond.; Sen. Regist. (Oral Surg.) Guy's Hosp.; Regist. (Oral Surg.) St. Barts. Hosp.

WELLER, Richard John Greenhill Eastfield House Surgery, 6 St. Johns Road, Newbury RG14 7LW Tel: 01635 41495 Fax: 01635 522751; 8 Buckingham Road, Newbury RG14 6DJ Tel: 01635 40739 — MB ChB Leeds 1969; DObst RCOG 1971; DA Eng. 1973.

WELLER, Richard Paul John Beresford University of Edinburgh, University Department of Dermatology, Lauriston Building, Lauriston Place, Edinburgh EH3 9HA Email: r.weller@ed.ac.uk — MB BS Lond. 1987 (St. Thos. Hosp.) MRCP (UK) 1990; MD London 2000. Sen. Lect. (Dermat.) Univ. Edin. Specialty: Dermat. Socs: Brit. Assn. Dermatol.; Brit. Soc. Investig. Dermat.; Eur. Soc. Dermat. Rese. Prev: Vis. Research Fell. Dept. of Surg. Univ. of Pittsburgh USA; Research Fell., immunBiol. abteiling,Hainrich-Heine univ, Germany; Regist. (Dermat.) Aberd. Roy. Infirm.

WELLER, Robin Moray, TD 2 Miles Road, Clifton, Bristol BS8 2JN — MB BS Lond. 1966 (St. Bart.) MRCS Eng. LRCP Lond. 1965; DA Eng. 1968; FFA RCS Eng. 1970. Cons. Anaesth. Frenchay Hosp. Bristol. Specialty: Anaesth. Socs: Past Pres. Bristol Medico-Legal Soc.; Pres. Soc. of Anaesth.s of S. W. Region; Past Pres. Cossham Med. Soc. Prev: Sen. Regist. (Anaesth.) Frenchay Hosp. Bristol & United Bristol Hosps.; Vis. Asst. Prof. Dept. Anaesth. Univ. Virginia Med. Center.

WELLER, Professor Roy Oliver 22 Abbey Hill Road, Winchester SO23 7AT Tel: 01962 867465 Email: row@soton.ac.uk; Qazvin, 22 Abbey Hill Road, Winchester SO23 7AT Tel: 01962 867465 — (Guy's) MRCS Eng. LRCP Lond. 1961; MB BS Lond. 1962; FRCPath 1982, M 1970; PhD Lond. 1967, BSc (Anat. Hons.) 1959, MD 1971. Course Director Path., Wessex Courses, Soton. Specialty: Neuropath. Special Interest: Brain Tumours; Neuroimmunology; Neuroregenerative Diseases. Socs: Path. Soc.; Neuropath. Soc.; Assn. of Brit. Neurol.s. Prev: Prof. & Cons. Neuropath. Fac. of Med. Soton. Univ. & Soton. Univ. Hosps. NHS Trust; vice Pres. of the Internat. Soc. of Neuropath.; Regional Adviser in Path. (99-03) Pres. of the Brit. NeuroPath. Soc.(01-02).

WELLER, Stanley Douglas Victor (retired) 18 Gerrard Buildings, Pulteney Mews, Bath BA2 4DQ Tel: 01224 420020 — (Univ. Coll. Hosp.) MB BS Lond. 1941; MRCS Eng. LRCP Lond. 1941; FRCP Lond. 1969, M 1947; MD Lond. 1947; DCH Eng. 1948; FRCP & CH 1998. Prev: Prof. of Child Health Makerere Univ. Coll. Kampala, Uganda.

WELLER, Stephan The Petersgate Medical Centre, 99 Amersall Road, Scawthorpe, Doncaster DN5 9PQ Tel: 01302 390490 — State Exam Med Bonn 1988 (Bonn, Germany) Med. Doctorate Bonn 1990; MRCGP 1995; DFFP 1995. Specialty: Gen. Pract.

WELLER, Timothy Mark Atticus Department of Medical Microbiology, City Hospital NHS Trust, Dudley Road, Birmingham B18 7QH — MB ChB Birm. 1988; ChB Birm. 1988; MRCPath 1997; MD Uni. Birm. 1999. Cons. Microbiologist - City Hosp. Birm. Specialty: Med. Microbiol.

WELLESLEY, Amanda Jane 8 Michaels Close, London SE13 5BP — MB ChB Leeds 1985; FRCS Ed. 1991.

WELLESLEY, Diana Gay Wessex Clinical Genetics Service, Princess Anne Hospital, Southampton SO16 5YA Tel: 023 8022 1716 Fax: 023 8079 4346 Email: dgw@soton.ac.uk; Tangley House, Southdown Road, Shawford, Winchester SO21 2BY Tel: 01962 712409 Fax: 01962 712049 — BM Soton. 1977 (Southampton) Assoc. Specialist (Clin. Genetics) Princess Anne Hosp. Soton., Head of Prenatal Genetics, PAH, Soton. Specialty: Genetics. Socs: BMA; Brit.Soc. Human Genetics; BINOCAR. Prev: Asst. (Genetics) Princess Margt. Hosp. Perth, W. Austral.; Med. Off. Auth. for Intellectual Handicap, Perth, W. Austral.; Fell. Clin. Genetics Univ. South. Calif., USA.

WELLESLEY, Hugo Arthur Lawrence — MB ChB Bristol 1998.

WELLINGHAM, Charles Bernard Lattice Barn Surgery, 14 Woodbridge Road East, Ipswich IP4 5PA — MB BS Lond. 1976; DCH Eng. 1980; DRCOG 1981; MRCGP 1981.

WELLINGS, Deborah Julie — MB ChB Birm. 1985; DRCOG 1988; DCH RCP Lond. 1989; MRCGP 1990. GP Retainer Scheme. Specialty: Palliat. Med.; Rehabil. Med.; Educat. Prev: GP Droitwich; Cons. in Rehabil. Med., Birm. Specialist Community Turst.

WELLINGS, Michael John 300 Fencepiece Road, Ilford IG6 2TA Tel: 020 8500 0066 Fax: 020 8559 8670; 4 The Green, Woodford Green IG8 0NF Tel: 020 8504 0407 — MB BS Lond. 1968 (St. Mary's) DObst RCOG 1970; MRCGP 1979. Clin. Asst. Surg. Forest Hosp. Buckhurst Hill. Socs: Brit. Soc. Allergy & Clin. Immunol.

WELLINGS, Mr Richard Matthew Coventry & Warwickshire University Hospitals NHS Trust, Coventry — MB ChB Birm. 1982; FRCS Ed. 1986; FRCR 1990. Cons. Radiol. Covntry & Warks. Univ. Hosps.. NHS Trust Coventry. Specialty: Radiol. Prev: Sen. Regist. (Radiol.) W. Midl. RHA; Regist. (Radiol.) W. Midl. Region.

WELLINGTON, Catherine Mary Sheet Street Surgery, 21 Sheet Street, Windsor SL4 1BZ Tel: 01753 860334 Fax: 01753 833696 — MB BS Lond. 1992 (Middlesex Hospital University College London) DRCOG; BSc Lond. 1989; MRCGP 1 9986. GP.

WELLINGTON, Mr Peter Ernest St Mary's Hospital, Accident and Emergency Department, Newport PO30 5TG Tel: 01983 534660 Fax: 01983 534642 Email: peter.wellington@iow.nhs.uk — MB BCh BAO Dub. 1973 (TC Dub.) FRCSI 1979. Cons. A & E St. Mary's Hosp. Newport, I. of Wight. Specialty: Accid. & Emerg. Special Interest: Orthopaedic Trauma. Prev: Regist. (Orthop.) Glas. Roy. Infirm.; Sen. Regist. Accid. and Emerg., Glas. Roy. Infirm.

WELLS, Mr Alan David 42 Exeter Gardens, Stamford PE9 2RN — MB BS Lond. 1974; MS Lond. 1985, MB BS 1974; FRCS Eng. 1979. Cons. Gen. Surg. P'boro. Dist. Hosp. Specialty: Gen. Surg. Prev: Sen. Regist. St. Thos. Hosp. Lond.; Regist. (Surg.) King's Coll. Hosp. Lond.; Research Fell. State Univ. New York, Buffalo USA.

WELLS, Alastair James The Moat House Surgery, Worsted Green, Merstham, Redhill RH1 3PN Tel: 01737 642207 Fax: 01737 642209 — MB BS Lond. 1983 (Roy. Free) DRCOG 1985; MRCGP 1987. Socs: Assur. Med. Soc. Prev: SHO Croydon VTS; Ho. Surg. Roy. Free Hosp. Lond.; Ho. Phys. Barnet Gen. Hosp.

WELLS, Albert Logan (retired) 71 Pennard Road, Southgate, Swansea SA3 2AJ Tel: 01792 233315 — MB BCh BAO Belf. 1945 (Qu. Univ. Belf.) DCP Lond 1948; MD Belf. 1951; MRCPI 1952; FRCPath 1966, M 1964. Prev: Cons. Path. Llanelli Hosp. & Min. of Home Affairs N. Irel.

WELLS, Alec Anthony 101 Montpelier Road, Brighton BN1 2LQ Tel: 01273 777807 Fax: 01273 777807; Braefield House, Southwell NG25 0PX Tel: 01636 813491 — MB ChB Sheff. 1964. Private GP. Prev: Cas. Off. Roy. Hosp. Sheff.; Ho. Phys. Profess. Unit Childr. Hosp. Sheff.; SHO O & G Scarsdale Hosp. Chesterfield.

WELLS, Alison Elizabeth Burnt Oak, Heath Drive, Walton-on-the-Hill, Tadworth KT20 7QQ Tel: 01737 812788 — MB BS Lond. 1985; DRCOG 1989. Specialty: Obst. & Gyn.

WELLS, Andrew David Gair Cottage, Lochgair, Lochgilphead PA31 8SD — MB ChB Aberd. 1984.

WELLS, Angus William Flat 2, 1 Grosvenor Villas, Grosvenor Road, Newcastle upon Tyne NE2 2RU — MB ChB Ed. 1990.

WELLS, Anthony Lethbridge 5 London Road, Beccles NR34 9TZ Tel: 01502 712024 — MB BChir Camb. 1949 (St. Bart.) BA, MB BChir Camb. 1949; DLO Eng. 1951; DObst RCOG 1953. Prev: Ho. Phys. St. Bart. Hosp.; Ho. Surg. Obst. Dept. Radcliffe Infirm. Oxf.; Capt. RAMC.

WELLS, Brian John 47 Devonshire Street, London W1G 7AW Tel: 020 7631 0160 Mob: 07803 130629 — MB BChir Camb. 1974 (Camb. & Middlx. Hosp.) MA Camb. 1973, BA 1970; FRCPsych 1996, M 1984. Med. Director Riverside Ment. Health Trust. Specialty: Gen. Psychiat.; Medico Legal. Socs: BMA; Soc. Study of Addic. Prev: Sen. Regist. Bethlem Roy. & Maudsley Hosps.; Cons. Psychait. & Lead Clin. Subst. Misuse Serv. Riverside Ment. Health Trust.

WELLS, Catherine Anne — BM Soton. 1997.

WELLS, Christine Anne Corney Place Medical Group, The Health Centre, Bridge Lane, Penrith CA11 8HW Tel: 01768 245226 Fax: 01786 245229; 10 Vestaneum, Crosby-on-Eden, Carlisle CA6 4PN Tel: 01228 573180 Email: wellsmustc@aol.com — MB BS Lond. 1994 (St. Bart. Hosp. Lond.) Dip Family Plann 1998 FFPA; PhD (Arts) London 1984; MB BS London 1994; MRCGP Royal College GPs 1998. Clin. Med.off.Wellwoman, Family Plann & youth Serv.Dumfries & Galloway. Specialty: Gen. Pract. Socs: FRSM; RCGPs; BMA. Prev: GP.

WELLS, Christopher William 97 The Wills Building, Wills Oval, Newcastle upon Tyne NE7 7RG — MB BS Newc. 1997.

WELLS, Clive Alan Department of Histopathology, St. Bartholomews Hospital, London EC1A 7BE — MB Camb. 1978; BChir 1977; MRCPath 1986. Cons. Path. St. Bart. Hosp. Lond.; Regional Co-ordinator Breast Screening Path. N.E. Thames RHA Region. Specialty: Pathology, General. Socs: RCPath. Advis. Gp. on Breast Cancer Screening.

WELLS, David Poulett (retired) Waterton Barn Cottage, Ampney Crucis, Cirencester GL7 5RR Tel: 01285 657863 Email: d@davidwells.freeserve.co.uk — BM BCh Oxf. 1958; DObst RCOG 1961; FRCGP 1988, M 1973.

WELLS, David Thomas, OStJ BUPA OH, Room 23, Wyvern House, Railway Terrace, Derby DE1 2RY Tel: 01332 714000 Fax: 01332 714601 Email: welssda@bupa.com; 14 Spenbeck Drive, Allestree, Derby DE22 2UH — MRCS Eng. LRCP Lond. 1971 (Sheffield) DIH Eng. 1980; MFOM RCP Lond. 1983. Cons. Occupat. Phys. (BUPA OH) Derby. Specialty: Occupat. Health. Socs: Soc. Occupat. Med. Prev: Sen. Med. Off. Brit. Railways Bd. Derby; Regist. (A & E Med.) & SHO (Hand Surg.) Derbysh. Roy. Infirm.

WELLS, Derek Geoffrey (retired) Bron Teigl, Cwm Teigl, Llan Ffestiniog, Blaenau Ffestiniog LL41 4RF — MB BS Lond. 1947 (Westm.) Prev: Ho. Phys. & Res. Obst. Asst. Westm. Hosp.

WELLS, Derek Geoffrey Ty-Fry Cottage, Cliff Road, Hythe CT21 5XL Tel: 01303 266469 — (Roy. Free) MB BS Lond. 1961; Dip. Biochem. Chelsea Coll. Sci. & Technol. 1970; FRCPath 1984, M 1972. Cons. Haemat. E. Rent health trust. Specialty: Haematology. Prev: Sen. Regist. (Clin. Path.) Roy. Marsden Hosp. Lond.; Regist. (Chem. Path.) Westm. Hosp. Lond.; Res. Pathol. Nat. Hosp. Qu. Sq. Lond.

WELLS, Duncan Lewis 241 Tubbenden La S., Orpington BR6 7DW — MB BS Lond. 1997.

WELLS, Fanny (retired) Logan Cottage, 74 Gloucester Road, London SW7 4QW Tel: 020 7584 8281 — MD Bari 1935.

WELLS, Mr Francis Charles Papworth Hospital, Department of Cardiothoracic Surgery, Papworth Everard, Cambridge CB3 8RE Tel: 01480 364421 Email: francis.wells@papworth.nhs.uk — MB BS Lond. 1975 (Char. Cross) BSc (Hons.) Lond. 1972; MRCS Eng. LRCP Lond. 1975; FRCS Eng. 1981; MS Lond. 1986; MA Camb. 1991. Cons. Cardiothoracic Surg. Papworth Hosp. Camb.; Assoc. Lect. Univ. Camb; Hons. Cons. Gt. Ormond St. Hosp. Lond. Specialty: Cardiothoracic Surg.; Transpl. Surg. Special Interest: Complex Valve Reconstruction; Thoracic Oncol. Socs: Fell. Roy. Soc. Med.; Cardiac Soc.; Europ. Assn. of Thoracic Surg. Prev: Sen. Research Fell. (Cardiac Surg.) Univ. Alabama, USA; Sen. Regist. (Cardiothoracic Surg.) Brompton. Hosp. Lond.; Regist. (Surg.) Addenbrooke's Hosp. Camb.

WELLS, Francis Owen (retired) Marix Drug Development, Rhodfa Marics, Ynysmaerdy, Llantrisant CF72 8UX Tel: 01443 234400 Fax: 01443 234401 Email: frankwells @matrix.co.uk; Old Hadleigh, London Road, Capel St Mary, Ipswich IP9 2JJ Tel: 01473 730101 Fax: 01473 730102 Email: fow5851@aol.com — MB BS Lond. 1960 (Lond. Hosp.) FFPM (Distinc.) RCP (UK) 1995; FRCP Ed 1998; FRCP (London) 1999. Cons. Pharmaceut. Phys. Medico-Legal Investig.s, Non-Exec. Director. Prev: Dir. Div. Med. Sci. & Technol. Assn. Brit. Pharmaceut. Industry.

WELLS, Francis Raymund (retired) The Magnolia Star, 8 Ballard Close, Poole BH15 1UH Tel: 01202 687359 — BM BCh Oxf. 1951. Prev: Brain Bank Co-ordinator & Pk.inson's Dis. Soc. Research Fell. Inst. Neurol. Lond.

WELLS, Gareth Edward 59 Daniel Hill Street, Sheffield S6 3JH — MB ChB Sheff. 1998.

WELLS, Geoffrey George (retired) Norsewood, Broomheath, Woodbridge IP12 4DL Tel: 01394 386375 — MB ChB Ed. 1945 (Univ. Ed.) AFOM RCP Lond. 1980. Employm. Med. Adviser EMAS; Clin. Asst. (Orthop.) Ipswich Hosp. Prev: Ho. Surg. Wingfield Morris Orthop. Hosp.

WELLS, Gillian Ruth Humberstone Park Surgery, 190 Uppingham Road, Leicester LE5 0QG Tel: 0116 276 6605; 3 Snowden's End, Wigston, Leicester LE18 1LG — MB ChB Leic. 1987; DRCOG 1991; MRCGP 1992. Princip. GP Leic. Specialty: Gen. Pract. Prev: Trainee GP Leicester VTS.

WELLS, Grahame John The Harrow Health Care Centre, 84-88 Pinner Road, North Harrow, Harrow HA1 4HZ; 4 Upper Lattimore Road, St Albans AL1 3TU Tel: 01727 830330 — MB BS Lond. 1979.

WELLS, Irving Pascoe Eydon Lodge, Yelverton PL20 6AS — MB BS Lond. 1972; MRCS Eng. LRCP Lond. 1973; FRCR 1978; FRCP Lond. 1994. Cons. Radiol. Plymouth Gen. Hosp. Specialty: Radiol. Socs: Brit. Soc. Intervent. Radiol. (Mem. Counc.); Eur. Soc. Uroradiol. Prev: Sen. Regist. (Diag. Radiol.) King's Coll. Hosp. Lond.

WELLS, Janet, OStJ (retired) 14 Spenbeck Drive, Allestree, Derby DE22 2UH Tel: 01332 552403 — MB ChB Sheff. 1970. Prev: Phys. (Occupat. Health) Derbysh. CC.

WELLS, Jason Mark 18 Firtree Avenue, Countesthorpe, Leicester LE8 5TH — MB ChB Sheff. 1993.

WELLS, Jean Mary Staines Health Centre, Knowle Green, Staines TW18 1XD — MB ChB Leeds 1967.

WELLS, Jennifer Margaret, OBE, Brigadier Army Medical Directorate, Former Army Staff College, Slim Road, Camberley GU15 4NP Tel: 01276 412702 Fax: 01276 412737 — MB ChB Glas. 1976; DRCOG 1982; MSc (Gen. Pract.) Lond. 1995; FRCGP 2000. Dir. Army Med. Pract.; Course Organiser Defence Med. Servs. GP Educat. Specialty: Gen. Pract. Prev: Serv. Gen. Pract.

WELLS, Joan Catherine 173 Ashley Gardens, Emery Hill St., London SW1P 1PD Tel: 020 7828 0985 Fax: 020 7931 7635 — MB BS Lond. 1948 (Roy. Free) MRCS Eng. LRCP Lond. 1948; MD Lond. 1950; MRCP Lond. 1950; DCH Eng. 1955; DPM Eng. 1966; MRCPsych 1972. Specialty: Child & Adolesc. Psychiat. Socs: FRSM. Prev: Cons. Psychiat. Qu. Mary's Hosp. Childr. & Merton HA; Sen. Regist. Maudsley Hosp. Lond.

WELLS, John Christopher Durant 45A Rodney Street, Liverpool L1 9EW Tel: 0151 708 9344 Fax: 0151 707 0609; Apt 311, The Colonnades, Albert Dock, Liverpool L3 4AB Tel: 0151 709 8180 Fax: 0151 707 0609 Email: cxwells@aol.com — (Liverp.) MB ChB Liverp. 1970; MRCS Eng. LRCP Lond. 1970; LMCC 1974; FRCA Eng 1978; FFA RCS Eng. 1978. Specialist (relief of Chronic Pain) Liverp.; Dir. Pain Relief (Research) Foundat.; Hon. Cons. (Pain Relief) Liverp. Marie Curie Home; Hon. Cons. (Pain Relief) Clatterbridge Centre for Oncol. Specialty: Anaesth.; Palliat. Med.; Disabil. Med. Socs: Hon. Asst. Sec., Pain Soc. GB & Irel.; Chairm. Scient. Comm. Pain Soc. GB & Irel.; Hon. Sec. World Soc. Pain Clinicians. Prev: Dir. Centre for Pain Relief, Walton Hosp.; Hon. Sen. Lect. Univ. of Liverp.

WELLS, John Kirkwood Gillman Department of Anaesthetics, North Hampshire Hospital, Aldermaston Road, Basingstoke RG24 9NA — MB BS Lond. 1971 (Westm.) DA Eng. 1974; FFA RCS Eng. 1979. Cons. Anaesth. Basingstoke & N. Hants. HA. Specialty: Anaesth. Socs: Intens. Care Soc. Prev: Sen. Regist. Char. Cross Hosp. Med. Sch.; Regist. Brompton Hosp. Lond.

WELLS, John Michael Weston (retired) 7 Ringstead Road, Heacham, King's Lynn PE31 7JA Tel: 01485 70219 — MRCS Eng. LRCP Lond. 1940 (Guy's) DMRD Eng. 1947. Prev: Cons. Radiol. W. Norf. & King's Lynn Gen. Hosp.

WELLS, Jonathan Joseph Hillview Medical Centre, 60 Bromsgrove Road, Redditch B97 4RN Tel: 01527 66511 — MB BS Lond. 1987; MRCP (UK) 1990; DRCOG 1992; T(GP) 1993; MRCGP 1993. Specialty: Gen. Med. Prev: Trainee GP Measham Med. Unit; Regist. (Gen. Med.) Leicester Roy. Infirm.; SHO (O & G) Leicester Gen. Hosp.

WELLS, Julie Alison 70 Mount Road, Canterbury CT1 1YF — MB BS Lond. 1996.

WELLS, Keith Marple Cottage Surgery, 50 Church Street, Marple, Stockport SK6 6BW Tel: 0161 426 0011 Fax: 0161 427 8160; 29 Hollins Lane, Marple Bridge, Stockport SK6 5BD Tel: 0161 449 8326 — MB ChB Manch. 1971 (Manchester) DCH RCPS Glas. 1973; DObst RCOG 1974; MRCGP 1976. Prev: SHO (O & G) Withington Hosp.; SHO (Paediat.) & SHO (Med.) Stepping Hill Hosp. Stockport.

WELLS, Laurence Gregory Warwickshire Health Authority, Westgate House, Market St., Warwick CV34 4DE Tel: 01926 493491 Fax: 01926 495074 — MB ChB Cape Town 1971; FFPHM RCP (UK) 1995. Dir. Pub. Health Warks. HA. Specialty: Pub. Health Med. Prev: SCM S. Warks. HA; Med. Off. & Med. Sup. Chas. Johnson Memor. Hosp., Zululand; Med. Off. German Inst. Med. Mission Tuebingen, W. Germany.

WELLS, Louise Claire Minton Altwood Close, Maidenhead SL6 4PP — MB BS Lond. 1993.

WELLS, Mark Philip Paul Wrythe Green Surgery, Wrythe Lane, Carshalton SM5 2RE.

WELLS, Martin David Cliftonville Road Surgery, 61 Cliftonville Road, Belfast BT14 6JN Tel: 028 9074 7361 — (Qu. Univ. Belf.) MB BCh BAO Belf. 1985; DRCOG 1988; Cert. Family Plann. JCC 1988; DCH RCP Glas. 1989; DMH RCP Lond. 1989; MRCGP 1991.

WELLS, Mary Beverley The Surgery, 160 Streetly Road, Erdington, Birmingham B23 7BD Tel: 0121 350 2323 Fax: 0121 382 0169; Forge Farm House, Forge Lane, Footherley, Lichfield WS14 0HU — MB ChB Birm. 1971.

WELLS, Mrs Meher Derek (retired) Ty-Fry Cottage, Cliff Road, Hythe CT21 5XL Tel: 01303 266469 — MB BS Osmania 1960; FRCSI 1968; FRCS Eng. 1970; MD Univ. Lond. 1990. Prev: Sen. Regist. Univ. Coll. Hosp. Lond.

WELLS, Professor Michael Department of Pathology, University of Sheffield Medical School, Beech Hill Road, Sheffield S10 2RX Tel: 0114 271 2397 Fax: 0114 278 0059 Email: m.wells@sheffield.ac.uk; 57 Ranmoor Crescent, Sheffield S10 3GW Tel: 0114 230 8260 Email: mike@mikewell.demon.co.uk — MB ChB Manch. 1976; FRCPath 1995, M 1983; BSc (Hons.) Manch. 1974, MD 1986. Hon. Cons. Path. Univ. Hosps. Centr. Sheff.; Prof.

Gyn. Path. Univ. Sheff. Specialty: Histopath. Socs: Brit. Gyn. Cancer Soc.; (Meeting Sec.) Path Soc. GB & Irel.; Internat. Acad. Path. (Ex-Hon. Sec. Brit. Div.). Prev: Prof. Gyn. Path. Univ. Leeds; Sen. Lect. Univ. Leeds; Lect. (Path.) Univ. Bristol.

WELLS, Michelle Lesley Launceston Medical Centre, Landlake Road, Launceston PL15 9HH Tel: 01566 772131 Fax: 01566 772223 — BM BS Nottm. 1989; BMedSci (Hons.) Nottm. 1986. Specialty: Gen. Pract.

WELLS, Nigel John Nether Leazes, Beech Hill, Hexham NE46 3AG — MB ChB Dundee 1997.

WELLS, Paula Department of Radiotherapy & Oncology, St Bartholomews Hospital, West Smithfield, London EC1A 7BE Tel: 020 7601 8044 Fax: 020 7601 8364 Email: paula.wells@bartsandthelondon.nhs.uk — MB BS Lond. 1986 (St Bartholomews Hospital London) MRCP (UK) 1989; FRCR 1994; PhD 2001. Cons. Clin Oncologist St Bartholomews Hosp Lond.. Specialty: Oncol.; Radiother. Prev: Sen. Regis. Clin. Oncol. Roy. Marsden Hosp. Lond.; Hon. Sen. Regist. & Research Sen. Regist. MRC Cyclotron Unit Hammersmith.

WELLS, Peter George (retired) High Trees, Dark Lane, Henbury, Macclesfield SK11 9PE Tel: 01625 420872 — MB ChB Sheff. 1954 (Univ. Sheff.) DObst RCOG 1956; DCH Eng. 1956; DPM Eng. 1965; FRCPsych 1979, M 1971; FRANZCP 1983, M 1981; T(Psychiat.) 1991. Lect. Univ. Manch. & Univ. Liverp.; Adviser to Visyon. Prev: Cons. Psychiat. (Adolesc. Servs.) Mersey & N. W. RHAs.

WELLS, Philip Andrew Gordon Street Surgery, Ashton-under-Lyne OL6 6PR Tel: 0161 330 5104 — MB ChB Leeds 1983; DGM RCP Lond. 1989; MRCGP 1991.

WELLS, Richard David 39 Regent Street, West End, Stoke-on-Trent ST4 5HQ — MB ChB Dundee 1995.

WELLS, Richard Douglas William The Castle Practice, Health Centre, Central Street, Ludgershall, Andover SP11 9RA Tel: 01264 790356 Fax: 01264 791256; 28 St. James Street, Ludgershall, Andover SP11 9QF Tel: 01264 790398 — MB BS Lond. 1973 (St. Bart.) BSc Lond. 1970; DObst RCOG 1976. GP Represen. Wilts LMC. Socs: Salisbury Med. Soc. Prev: Trainee GP Exeter VTS; Sen. Resid. Med. Off. (Obst.) Health Commiss. NSW, Austral.; Ho. Phys. St. Bart. Hosp. Lond.

WELLS, Robert Arthur Company Health Ltd., 335 Red Bank Road, Bispham Village Chambers, Bispham Village, Blackpool FY2 0HJ Tel: 01253 590555 Fax: 01253 590555; 43 Everest Drive, Bispham, Blackpool FY2 9DH — MB ChB Manch. 1978; BSc. (Hons.) Manch. 1976; MRCGP 1982; D.Occ.Med. RCO Lond. 1995; MBA Ed. 1995. Managing Dir. Co. Health Ltd.; Occupat. Phys.; Apptd. Doctor (Health & Safety Exec.) for Lead, Asbestos, Compressed Air Surveillance & Ionising Radiat; Trainer (Gen. Pract.) Blackpool VTS; Med. Adviser P & O CMW Laboratories Kerry Foods. Specialty: Occupat. Health. Socs: Soc. Occupat. Med. Prev: Med. Advisor to Tower & Winter Gdns. Blackpool; Med. Off. RAMC GSM (N. Irel.).

WELLS, Roger Augustus Elm House Surgery, 29 Beckenham Road, Beckenham BR3 4PR Tel: 020 8650 0173 — MB BS Lond. 1978 (St. Mary's) BSc (Hons.) Lond. 1975; DRCOG 1983; MRCGP 1986. GP Princip. Specialty: Gen. Pract. Special Interest: Respirat. Med.; Sexual Health. Socs: Christian Med. Fellowsh. Prev: Trainee GP St Peters Hosp. Chertsey.

WELLS, Ruth Blackbrook Surgery, Lisieux Way, Taunton TA1 2LB Tel: 01823 259444 Fax: 01823 322715; The Cottage, Goosenford, Cheddon Fitzpaine, Taunton TA2 8LH — MB BS Lond. 1979; DRCOG 1981; DCH Eng. 1981; MRCGP 1983; MFFP 1992. SCMO (Family Plann.) Som. HA.

WELLS, Sarah Louise Armitage 58 Byron Street, Hale, Altrincham WA14 2EL; 35 Weldale Drive, Stoney Gate, Leicester LE2 2AR Tel: 0116 270 9862 — MB ChB Liverp. 1994; DFFP 1996; DRCOG 1996. SHO Palliat. Med.Nottm. City Hosp. Specialty: Palliat. Med. Prev: SHO (Paediat.) Arrowe Pk. Hosp. Wirral; GP Regist. Bunbury Med. Pract.; SHO Psych.Rugby Hosp.

WELLS, Simon Kingsley X-Ray Department, Musgrove Park Hospital, Taunton TA1 5DA — MB BS Lond. 1976 (Middlx.) BA Oxf. 1973; FRCR 1983. Cons. Radiol. Taunton & Som. Hosp. Taunton. Specialty: Radiol. Prev: Sen. Regist. (Radiol.) Soton. Gen. Hosp.; SHO (Med.) Nevill Hall Hosp. Abergavenny; SHO (Orthop.) Yeovil Dist. Hosp.

WELLS, Stephen Department of Histopathology, Royal Bolton Hospital, Minerva Road, Farnworth, Bolton BL4 0JR Tel: 01204 390534 Fax: 01204 390946; 6 Oaker Avenue, Didsbury, Manchester M20 2XH — MB ChB Manch. 1975 (Manchester) FRCPath. 1993, M 1981. Cons. Histopath. Roy. Bolton Hosp. Specialty: Histopath. Prev: Sen. Regist. (Histopath.) Hope Hosp., Salford, Wythenshawe Hosp. Manch. & Univ. Manch.

WELLS, Mr Stuart Charles Somerset Nuffield Hospital, Stapelgrove Elm, Taunton TA2 6AN Tel: 01823 286991 Fax: 01823 250610; The Old School House, Otterford, Chard TA20 3QX Tel: 01823 601339 — MB BS Lond. 1972; MRCS Eng. LRCP Lond. 1972; FRCS Eng. 1979. Cons. & ENT Surg. Taunton & Som. Hosps. (MusGr. Pk. Br.) Taunton. Specialty: Otolaryngol.

WELLS, Susan Margaret West Kirby Health Centre, The Concourse, Grange Road, Wirral CH48 4HZ Tel: 0151 625 9171 Fax: 0151 625 9499; 11 Bertram Drive, Meols, Wirral CH47 0LG Tel: 0151 632 0539 Fax: 0151 632 6424 — MB BChir Camb. 1983 (Cambridge) MA Oxf. 1989, BA 1980; DRCOG 1986; FRCGP 1993, M 1987. GP Princip.; Clin. Asst. (Diabetes). Prev: Trainee GP Rotat. Chester VTS; Ho. Surg. Addenbrooke's Hosp. Camb.; Ho. Phys. Arrowe Pk. Hosp. Wirral.

WELLS, Timothy Alastair 7 Barbrook Close, Tilehurst, Reading RG31 6RT — MB BS Lond. 1996.

WELLS, Wilfrid Denys Edward Forge Farm House, Forge Lane, Footherley, Lichfield WS14 0HU — MB ChB Birm. 1974; BSc (Hons.) Wales 1969. Hon. Sen. Lect. (Gen. Pract.) Univ. Birm. Socs: (Sec.) W. Midl. Assn. Fundholding Practs.; Drug Utilization Res. Gp. UK. Prev: Clin. Chair Medicines Managem. Collaborative; Postgrad. GP Tutor Walsall Manor Hosp.; Regist. (Med.) Dudley Rd. Hosp. Birm.

WELLSTEED, Anthony John (retired) 18 New Close Road, Shipley BD18 4AU Tel: 01274 587558 — MB BS Lond. 1958 (Univ. Coll. Hosp.) FRCP Lond. 1982, M 1965. Prev: Cons. Infec. Dis. Bradford Roy. Infirm.

WELLSTOOD-EASON, Malcolm John Howard Queens Hospital, Belvedere Road, Burton-on-Trent DE13 0RB Tel: 01283 566333; The Old Forge, 7 Main St, Ravenstone, Coalville LE67 2AS — MB ChB Liverp. 1968; MRCS Eng. LRCP Lond. 1969; FFA RCS Eng. 1977. Cons. Qus. Hosp. Burton on Trent. Specialty: Anaesth. Prev: Cons. Leics. AHA (T).

WELLSTOOD-EASON, Susan Penelope Brandon Mental Health Unit, Leicester LE5 4PW; 53 Stamford Road, Oakham LE15 6HZ — MRCS Eng. LRCP Lond. 1970; MRCPsych 1982. Cons. Psychiat. Leicester Ment. Health Serv. Specialty: Gen. Psychiat. Prev: Clin. Lect. (Psychiat.) Univ. Leic.; Regist. (Psychiat.) Leics. AHA (T); Med. Dir. Leicester Ment. Health Serv. NHS TrustMed. Dir. Leicester Ment. Health Serv. NHS Trust.

WELLWOOD, Mr James McKinney 50 Clifton Hill, St. Johns Wood, London NW8 0QG Tel: 020 7625 5697 Fax: 020 7372 3406 Email: j.wellwood@btinternet.com; 50 Clifton Hill, St. Johns Wood, London NW8 0QG Tel: 020 7625 5697 — (Camb. & St. Thos.) MB BChir Camb. 1966; MChir Camb. 1978, MA 1966; FRCS Eng. 1970. p/t Cons. Surg. Whipps Cross Hosp. Lond.; Hon. Sen. Lect. St. Bart. Hosp. Med. Sch. Lond. Specialty: Gen. Surg. Socs: FRSM; Brit. Soc. Gastroenterol.; Assn. Endoscopic Surgs. Prev: Clin. Dir. (Surg.) Forest Healthcare Trust; Chief Asst. St. Bart. Hosp. Lond.; Hon. Sen. Regist. (Research) & Regist. (Surg.) St. Thos. Hosp. Lond.

WELLWOOD, Marion Rachel Three New Horizons Court, Brentford TW8 9EP Tel: 020 8975 2094 Fax: 020 8975 2499 Email: marion.r.wellwood@sb.com; 5 Hazell Park, Amersham HP7 9AB — MB ChB Ed. 1978 (Edinburgh University Medical School) BSc Ed. 1975, MB ChB 1978; FRCP Toronto 1984; FRCPC 1984. Vice Pres. & Dir. Med. Communication SmithKline Beecham Pharmaceut. Specialty: Pharmaceutical Medicine.

WELPLY, Mr Gilman Adrian Chinnery 1 Harley Street, London W1G 9QD Tel: 020 8947 8852 Fax: 01446 760 730 Email: gwelphy@doctors.org.uk; White Gate Lodge, St. Nicholas, Cardiff CF5 6SJ Tel: 01446 760730 Fax: 01446 760730 Email: gwelply@doctors.org.uk — MB BS Lond. 1964 (St. Geo.) MRCS Eng. LRCP Lond. 1964; FRCS Eng. 1968; FRCOG 1987, M 1971; T(OG) 1991. Private Practioner. Specialty: Obst. & Gyn. Socs: Minimal Access Surg.; Menopause. Prev: Cons. O & G St. Helier Hosp. Carshalton; Sen. Regist. (O & G) St. Geo. Hosp. Lond. & Soton. Gen. Hosp.; Regist. (O & G) St. Geo. Hosp. Lond.

WELSBY, Ann (retired) Millgarth, Kirklinton, Carlisle CA6 6DW Tel: 01228 75684 — LRCPI & LM, LRSCI & LM 1972; DObst RCOG 1975. Prev: GP E. Cumbria FPC.

WELSBY, Philip Douglas Infectious Disease Unit, Western General Hospital, Edinburgh EH4 2XU Tel: 0131 537 1000 Email: p.welsby@ed.ac.uk — (Roy. Free) MB BS Lond. 1970; MRCS Eng. LRCP Lond. 1970; MRCP (U.K.) 1973; FRCP Ed. 1984. Cons. Phys. in Communicable Dis. City Hosp. Edin. Specialty: Gen. Med. Prev: Sen. Regist. (Infec. Dis.) Roy. Free Hosp. Lond.; Med. Regist. S. Grampian Health Dist.; Med. Regist. St. Peter's Hosp. Chertsey.

WELSBY, Susan Mary 1708 Lanier Place, Washington DC NW20009, USA; 296 Singlewell Road, Gravesend DA11 7RF Tel: 01474 534648 — MB ChB Manch. 1978; DTM & H Liverp. 1985; MPH USA 1992. Internat. Cons. Washington DC, USA. Prev: Med. Off. Health Governm. Barbados.

WELSH, Bernard Mark Ardach Health Centre, Buckie; 1 Seafield Street, Elgin IV30 1QZ — MB ChB Aberd. 1987; MA (Psychol.) St. And. 1982; DTM & H Liverp. 1992; MRCGP 1992; MSc (Pub. Health & Health Servs. Research) 2000. Gen. Practitioner Ardach Health Centre Buckie. Prev: Med. Off. Medecins Sans Frontieres 1994,1995.

WELSH, Professor Christopher Lawrence Medical School, Beach Hill Road, Sheffield S10 2RX Tel: 0114 271 2668 Fax: 0114 271 3959; 38 Clarendon Road, Sheffield S10 3TR Tel: 0114 230 5782 Fax: 0114 230 5782 — MB BChir Camb. 1973; FRCS Eng. 1977; MA Camb. 1973, MChir 1986. Postgrad. Med. Dean Univ. Sheff.; Regional Postgrad. Dean NHSE Trent. Specialty: Gen. Surg. Prev: Cons. Vasc. Surg. North. Gen. Hosp. Sheff.; Clin. Dean Univ. Sheff.; Lect. & Sen. Regist. Surg. Profess. Unit St. Bart. Hosp. Lond.

WELSH, Colin David Eaton Road Surgery, 276 Eaton Road, West Derby, Liverpool L12 2AW Tel: 0151 228 3768 Fax: 0151 — MB ChB Liverp. 1986; DRCOG 1992. Specialty: Gen. Pract.

WELSH, Colin John Percy Huddersfield Royal Infirmary, Acre St., Lindley, Huddersfield HD3 3EA — MB ChB Glas. 1987; BSc (Hons) Glas. 1985; MRCP (UK) 1990. Cons. Gen. Med. & Cardiol. Huddersfield Roy. Infirm. Specialty: Cardiol.; Gen. Med. Prev: Regist. (Cardiol.) Leeds Gen. Infirm.; SHO Rotat. (Med.) Newc. u. Tyne.

WELSH, Miss Fenella Kate Sally Beechwood House, Offham, Lewes BN7 3QQ — MB BChir Camb. 1993 (Camb. & St. Mary's Lond.) FRCS 1997. Specialty: Gen. Surg.

WELSH, Geoffrey Hugh Student Health Centre, 42 Old Elvet, Durham DH1 3JF Tel: 0191 386 5081; Viewlands, Percy Terrace, Nevilles Cross, Durham DH1 4DY Tel: 0191 384 9824 — MB BS Newc. 1987; MRCGP 1991. Prev: GP Coxhoe, Durh.

WELSH, Harry (retired) Drumhella, Mainsforth, Ferryhill DL17 9AA Tel: 01740 652159 — MB ChB Leeds 1956.

WELSH, Janet Leila Graingerville Family Planning Clinic, 4 Graingerville North, Westgate Road, Newcastle upon Tyne NE4 6UJ Tel: 0191 219 5239; 73 Dunsgreen, Ponteland, Newcastle upon Tyne NE20 9EJ Tel: 01661 820358 Fax: 01661 820358 — MB BS Newc. 1980; BA (Hons.) York 1974; DCH RCP Lond. 1983; DRCOG 1984; MRCGP 1985; MFFP 1994. Sen. Med. Off. Contracep. & Sexual Health Serv. Newc. City Health NHS Trust. Specialty: Family Plann. & Reproduc. Health. Socs: Assoc. Mem. Inst. Psychosexual Med; BMA; Brit. Menopause Soc. Prev: Head Clin. Serv. (Family Plann. & Well Wom.) Newc. City Health NHS Trust; Lead Clinician (Audit) North. Region & Heads Serv. Gp. (Community Family Plann.) Newc. u. Tyne; GP Wylam.

WELSH, Kennedy Robert 30 Princess Drive, Kirby Muxloe, Leicester LE9 2DJ — MB BS Lond. 1980.

WELSH, Lawrence 28 Handly Cross, Manor Woods, Medomsly, Consett DH8 6TZ — MB BS Lond. 1984; BSc (Immunol.) Lond. 1981, MB BS 1984.

WELSH, Liz (retired) 22 Four Acres Close, Nailsea BS48 4YF Tel: 01275 851309 — (St. Bart.) MB BS Lond. 1966; DObst RCOG 1968; FFA RCS Eng. 1972; MFHom RCP Lond. 1986; MSc Exeter 1990. Prev: Specialist Regist. Pub. Health.

WELSH, Mary Annette The Lennard Surgery, 1-3 Lewis Road, Bishopsworth, Bristol BS13 7JD Tel: 0117 964 0900 Fax: 0117 987 3227; 83 Sommerville Road, St. Andrews, Bristol BS7 9AE — MB ChB Bristol 1978; MRCGP 1983; MRCOG 1985. Hosp. Pract. (Obst.) Bristol Matern. Hosp. & (Gyn.) St. Michael's Hosp Bristol; Course Organiser for Bristol GP Vocational Train. Scheme (2 sessions/week). Specialty: Obst. & Gyn.

WELSH, Mary Catherine 54 Ridge End Villas, Headingley, Leeds LS6 2DA — MB ChB Leeds 1968; DPM Leeds 1972; Dip. Psychother. Leeds 1983. Clin. Asst. Child & Family Serv. Airedale NHS Trust. Specialty: Child & Adolesc. Psychiat. Prev: Regist. (Psychiat.) Profess. Dept. Psychiat. Leeds Gen. Infirm.; Regist. (Child & Adolesc. Psychiat.) Highlands Adolesc. Unit; Regist. (Adult Psychiat.) Scalebor Pk. Hosp. Burley-in-Wharfedale.

WELSH, Peter Bryan (retired) Carabey House, Newbury Road, Lambourn, Hungerford RG17 7LL Tel: 01488 71914 Email: welsh.carabey@pop3.hiway.co.uk — MB ChB Birm. 1967. Prev: GP Argyll.

WELSH, Peter John Bodmin Road Health Centre, Bodmin Road, Ashton on Mersey, Sale M33 5JH Tel: 0161 962 4625 Fax: 0161 905 3317; Fern Bank, 34 South Grove, Brooklands, Sale M33 3AU Tel: 0161 962 6925 — MB ChB Manch. 1972. Specialty: Gen. Pract.

WELSH, Roger Randal (retired) Montagu Lodge, Church Street, Winkfield, Windsor SL4 4SF Tel: 01344 882716 Email: randrwelsh@aol.com — MB BS Lond. 1956 (St. Geo.) Cert. Av. Med. 1978; MRACGP 1984. Prev: Med. Dir. HRH Princess Christian's Hosp. Windsor.

WELSH, Sheila Lennox NHS Argyll and Clyde, Argyll Unit, Ravenscraig Hospital, Inverkip Road, Greenock PA16 9HA Tel: 01475 502326 Email: sheila.welsh57@ntlworld.com — MB ChB Glas. 1968; DObst RCOG 1970; DA Eng. 1971; MFFP 1993. Sen. Med. Off. (Family Plann. & Reproductive Health) Renfrewsh. & Inverclyde Primary Care NHS Trust. Specialty: Family Plann. & Reproduc. Health. Socs: BMA; Brit. Menopause Soc.; Scott. Family Plann. Med. Soc. Prev: Regist. (Anaesth.) West. Infirm. Glas.; Ho. Off. (Obst.) Qu. Mother's Hosp. Glas.; SCMO Glas. Family Plann. Clinic.

WELSH, Susan Hope 72 Quarry Avenue, Bebington, Wirral CH63 3HF Tel: 0151 645 6227 — MB ChB Glas. 1976. Assoc. Specialist (Dermat.) Wirral Hosp. Trust. Specialty: Dermat. Prev: Staff Grade (Dermat.) Wirrall Hosp. Trust.; Clin. Asst. (Dermat.) Chester Roy. Infirm. Wirral Hosp. Trust; GP Bebington.

WELTON, Edward John (retired) Tre-Llydiart, Chirbury Road, Montgomery SY15 6QP Tel: 01686 668313 — MB ChB Liverp. 1963; DObst RCOG 1965. Prev: GP Montgomery.

WELTON, Elizabeth Ann Tre-Llydiart, Chirbury Road, Montgomery SY15 6QP Tel: 01686 668313 Email: welton@dial.pipex.com — MB ChB Liverp. 1964; DObst RCOG 1966. Locum Gen. Practitioner. Prev: Clin. Asst. (Paediat. Orthop.) Roy. Shrewsbury Hosps.; Ho. Phys. & Ho. Surg. Liverp. Roy. Infirm.; Ho. Off. Mill Rd. Matern. Hosp. Liverp.

WELTON, Mark David Michael Trent Vale Medical Practice, 876 London Road, Trent Vale, Stoke-on-Trent ST4 5NX Tel: 01782 746898; 11 Sheridan Way, Stone ST15 8XG — MB ChB Birm. 1990 (Birmingham) MRCGP 1995. Specialty: Gen. Pract. Socs: (Pres.) Stoke Young Princips. Gp. Prev: Trainee GP N. Staffs. VTS.

WELTON, Robert (retired) Egerton House, Lees Road, Mossley, Ashton-under-Lyne OL5 0PQ Tel: 0145 783 3606 — MB ChB Manch. 1952; FRCGP 1989, M 1976.

WELTON, Trudy The Red House, 26 Keswick Road, Cringleford, Norwich NR4 6UG — MB BS Lond. 1976; MA Oxf. 1977. Prev: Med. Advisor Norf. FHSA; GP Norwich; Ho. Surg. St. Bart. Hosp. Lond.

WEMBRIDGE, Kevin Richard 26 Dover Road, Hunter's Bar, Sheffield S11 8RH — MB ChB Sheff. 1993; FRCS Eng. 1999. SSHO (Orthop.) Barnsley Dist. Gen. Specialty: Orthop. Socs: MDU; MSS; BMA.

WEMYSS-HOLDEN, Mr Guy David Department of Urology, Blackburn Royal Infirmary, Blackburn BB2 3LR Tel: 01254 263555; Four Acres, Shire Lane, Hurst Green, Clitheroe BB7 9QR Tel: 01254 826744 — MB BS Nottm. 1982; FRCS Ed. 1987; MD Nottm. 1993; FRCS (Urol.) 1994. Cons. Urol. Blackburn Roy. Infirm. Specialty: Urol. Prev: Sen. Regist. (Urol.) NW Region Manch.

WEMYSS-HOLDEN, Simon Andrew Garden House, Back St., Ilmington, Shipston-on-Stour CV36 4LJ — BM BS Nottm. 1988.

WENDON, Julia Alexis Institute of Liver Studies, Kings College Hospital, Bessemer Road, London SE5 9PJ Tel: 020 7346 3252 Email: julia.wendon@kcl.ac.uk; 74 Talfourd Road, London SE15 5NZ — MB ChB Dundee 1982; FRCP Lond. 1996. Sen. Lect. Inst. Liver Studies Kings Coll. Hosp. Lond. Specialty: Intens. Care.

WENGER, Mr Reginald Julien James (retired) Essex Nuffield Hospital, Brentwood CM15 8EN Tel: 01277 365134 Fax: 01277 365134; Fir House, 45 Great Stony Park, Ongar CM5 0TH Tel: 01277 365134 Fax: 01277 365134 — MB BS Lond. 1968 (St. Bart.) MRCS Eng. LRCP Lond. 1968; DObst RCOG 1970; FRCS Eng. 1973. Cons. Orthop. Surg. Prev: Sen. Regist. (Orthop.) King's Coll. Hosp. Lond.

WENGRAF, Carol Lindsay 47 St John's Park, London SE3 7JW Tel: 020 8858 4598 — MB BS Lond. 1962 (Guy's) MRCS Eng. LRCP Lond. 1962; FRCS Eng. 1967. Cons. ENT Surg. Greenwich, Lewisham & Woolwich Hosp. Gps. Specialty: Otolaryngol. Prev: Sen. Regist. ENT Dept. Guy's Hosp. Lond.; SHO ENT Dept. Westm. Hosp.

WENGROWE, Nolan Elliot Golders Hill Health Centre, Hillside, 151 North End Road, London NW11 7HX Tel: 020 8455 6886 Fax: 020 8201 9225; 13 Grey Close, London NW11 6QG Tel: 020 8455 9290 — MB ChB Cape Town 1978; MRCGP 1984. Prev: SHO (Neonat.) Whittington Hosp. Lond.; SHO (Paediat.) Northwick Pk. Hosp. Harrow & Brompton Hosp. Lond.

WENHAM, Geoffrey Andrew Department of Anaesthetics, University Hospital of Wales, Heath Park, Cardiff CF14 4XW Tel: 029 2074 3255; 7 Melin Dwr, Draethen, Newport NP10 8GL — MB BCh Wales 1975 (Welsh Nat. Sch. Med.) FFA RCS Eng. 1979. Cons. Anaesth. Univ. Hosp. Wales. Specialty: Anaesth.

WENHAM, John Timothy — MB ChB Manch. 1998. SHO (O & G), Roy. Bolton Hosp. Specialty: Obst. & Gyn. Prev: Ho. Off. (Med.), Roy. Bolton; Ho. Off. (Surg.), Roy. Bolton.

WENHAM, Josephine Anne 6 Laburnum Mews, Stonehouse GL10 2PW — MB ChB Sheff. 1998; MB ChB Sheff 1998.

WENHAM, Mr Peter William 31 Sutton Passeys Crescent, Wollaton Park, Nottingham NG8 1BX Tel: 0115 970 2481 — MB BChir Camb. 1973 (St. Thos.) FRCS Eng. 1978; MD Camb. 1985. Cons. Gen. Vasc. Surg. Nottm. Univ. Hosp. & Nottm. City Hosp. Specialty: Gen. Surg. Socs: Vasc. Soc. GB & Irel. Prev: Sen. Lect. Nottm. Univ.; Sen. Regist. Nottm. HA.

WENHAM, Sarah Julia X Ray Department, Ysbyty Gwynedd, Penrhosgarnedd, Bangor LL57 2PW Tel: 01248 384690 — MB ChB Leic. 1990; BSc Leic. 1986; MRCP 1992; FRCR 1997. Cons. Radiologist. Specialty: Radiol. Special Interest: Cross Sectional and Oncological Imaging. Socs: BMA; RCR.

WENHAM, Timothy Nigel 8 Ramsey Road, Sheffield S10 1LR — MB ChB Sheff. 1998.

WENHAM, Vivienne Caroline 2 Fl 1 Leamington Place, Edinburgh EH10 4JR — MB ChB Ed. 1998; MB ChB Ed 1998.

WENLEY, Mary Ruth Amwell Street Surgery, 19 Amwell Street, Hoddesdon EN11 8TS Tel: 01992 464147 Fax: 01992 708698; 108 High Street, Roydon, Harlow CM19 5EE — MB BS Lond. 1983; MRCGP 1987; DCH RCP Lond. 1987. Prev: Trainee GP W. Essex VTS.

WENSLEY, Richard Thomas 15 Cherington Road, Cheadle SK8 1LN — MB ChB Liverp. 1963; FRCPath. 1982, M 1970; MRCP (U.K.) 1973. Cons. Haemat. Manch. Roy. Infirm. & Manch. Regional Blood Transfus. Centre. Specialty: Blood Transfus. Prev: Sen. Regist. (Haemat.) Bristol Roy. Infirm.

WENSLEY, Susan Katherine Bristol Royal Infirmary, Marlborough St., Bristol BS2 8HW; 1 Fernbank Road, Redland, Bristol BS6 6QA Tel: 0117 907 1948 — MB ChB Bristol 1988; MRCP (UK) 1992. Staff Grade (Geriat. Med.). Specialty: Care of the Elderly. Socs: Brit. Geriat. Soc.; Brit. Soc. of Gerontology. Prev: Regist. (Geriat. Med.) Brist. Roy. Infirm.; SHO Rotat. (Gen. Med.) Gloucester HA.

WENSTONE, Richard 12th Floor, Department of Anaesthesia & Intensive Care, Royal Liverpool University Hospital, Liverpool L7 8XP Tel: 0151 706 3191 Fax: 0151 706 5646 Email: wenstone@liverpool.ac.uk — MB ChB Manch. 1983; DA (UK) 1985; FFA RCS Eng. 1988. Cons. Anaesth. & IC Roy. Liverp. Univ. Hosp. & Clin. Dir. IC; Hon. Clin. Lect. Univ. Liverp. Specialty: Intens. Care. Socs: Soc. Critical Care Med. & Intens. Care Soc.; Eur. Soc. Intens. Care Med. Prev: Sen. Regist. (Anaesth.) Mersey RHA; Fell. Critical Care Univ. Toronto; Regist. (Anaesth.) Liverp., St. Helens & Knowsley HA.

WENT, Emma Louise 4 Crown Point Drive, Bixley, Norwich NR14 8RR — MB BS Lond. 1993.

WENT, Janice (retired) 106 Upland Drive, Derriford, Plymouth PL6 6BG Tel: 01752 779786 — MB BCh BAO Dub. 1963; MSc Birm. 1968; FRCPath 1984, M 1970; MCB 1971. Cons. Chem. Path. Dept. Clin. Chem. Derriford Hosp. Prev: Sen. Regist. Clin. Chem. Guy's Hosp. Lond.

WENTEL, James Douglas — BM BS Nottm. 1995. Specialty: Anaesth.; Paediat.

WENZERUL, Alison Mary The Alderney Community Hospital, Ringwood Road, Parkstowe, Poole BH23 7JN — MB ChB Leeds 1977; MRCPsych 1982; MRCPsych 1982. Cons. Gen. Adult Psychiat. The Alderney Community Hosp., Pk.stowe, Poole. Socs: Roy. Coll. of Psychiatrisits; BMA. Prev: SPR Perinatal Psychiat., Old Manor Hosp., Salisbury; SPR Gen. Adult Psychiat., DOP, Soton.; SpR Gen. Adult Psych, Poole.

WEPPNER, Gregory John The Dene, Gatehouse Lane, Goddards Green, Hassocks BN6 9LE — MB BS Queensland 1980; MRCPsych. 1986; MPhil Ed. 1992; LLM (Master of Laws Degree) Univ. of Wales, Coll. of Cardiff 1995; LLM Univ. Of Wales, Col., Cardiff 1995. Cons. Forens. Psychiat., The Dene, Goddards Green. Specialty: Forens. Psychiat. Prev: Sen. Regist. (Psychiat.) WhitCh. Hosp. Cardiff.

WERB, Mr Abraham (retired) 9 Oak Lodge Close, Dennis Lane, Stanmore HA7 4QB Tel: 020 8954 1588 — MB ChB Cape Town 1945; DOMS Dub. 1956; DO Eng. 1956; FRCS Eng. 1970; FRCOphth 1989. Prev: Corneoplastic Unit Qu. Vict. Hosp. E. Grinstead.

WERCHOLA, Larysa Oksana (Surgery), 205 Russell Drive, Wollaton, Nottingham NG8 2BD Tel: 0115 928 3201 Fax: 0115 985 4981; Health Centre, 97 Derby Road, Stapleford, Nottingham NG9 7AT Tel: 0115 939 6111 Fax: 0115 970 9241 — MB BS Nottm. 1982; DObst 1985; MRCGP 1986.

WERNER, David John Siegmar Fforestfach Medical Centre, 118 Ravenhill Road, Fforestfach, Swansea SA5 5AA Tel: 01792 581666 Fax: 01792 585332; 10 Rhyd y Defaid Drive, Sketty, Swansea SA2 8AH Tel: 01792 454404 Fax: 01792 585332 — MB BS Lond. 1986 (Univ. Coll. Lond.) BSc Lond. 1983, MB BS 1986; MRCGP 1990. GP Trainer Swansea Bay VTS.

WERNHAM, Catherine Mary Batheaston Medical Centre, Batheaston Medical Centre, Coalpit Road, Bath BA1 7NP Tel: 01225 858686 Fax: 01225 852521 — MB ChB Birm. 1993; MA Camb. 1993, BA 1989; DRCOG 1995; DFFP 1995; MRCGP 1997. GP Partner. Specialty: Gen. Pract.

WERNICK, Simon Paul Cosham Health Centre, Vectis Way, Portsmouth PO6 3AW Tel: 023 9238 1117 Fax: 0223 9221 4266; Knudge Cottage, Wickham Common, Wickham, Fareham PO17 6JQ Tel: 023 92 833373 — MB ChB Bristol 1976; MRCGP 1980; DA (UK) 1981. GP Tutor Portsmouth.

WERNO, Anja Maria 31 Eltisley Avenue, Newnham, Cambridge CB3 9JG — State Exam Med Saarland 1993.

WERRETT, Gavin Charles 36 Longmead, Merrow, Guildford GU1 2HW — MB ChB Bristol 1995; MRCP. SHO Anasesth. Exeter. Socs: MRCP. Prev: Frenchay, Bristol; Qu. Alexandra Portsmaouth, Brighton.

WERRING, David John National Hospital for Neurology & Neurosurgery, Institute of Neurology, Queen Square, London WC1N 3BG — MB BS Lond. 1992 (Guy's) BSc Lond. 1989; MRCP (UK) 1995; PhD Lond. 2000. Cons. Neurologist, Nat. Hosp. for Neurol. and Neurosurg. (UCLH NHS Trust) and Watford Gen. Hosp. Specialty: Neurol. Special Interest: Stroke, structural and functional magnetic resonance imaging. Socs: Roy. Coll. Phys. Lond.; BMA; Assn. Brit. Neurol. Prev: Specialist Regist. (Neurol.) & Stroke Clin. Train. Fell. Inst. Neurol. Lond.; Specialist Regist. (Neurol.) St Thos. Hosp. Lond.; Soecialist Regist. (Neurol.) King's Coll. Hosp. Lond.

WERRY, Carol Ann 26 Fleet Avenue, Upminster RM14 1PY — MB BS Lond. 1977 (St. Geo.) Specialty: Med. Microbiol.

WERRY, Diana Mary (retired) 7 Almond Close, Old Basing, Basingstoke RG24 7DW — MB BS Lond. 1962 (Westm.) MRCS Eng. LRCP Lond. 1962; DObst RCOG 1965; DMRD Eng. 1969. Prev: Cons. Radiol. N. Hants. Hosp. NHS Trust & Bronglais Hosp. Aberystwyth.

WERTH, Fiona 46 Queen's Avenue, Muswell Hill, London N10 3BJ Tel: 020 8883 1846 — MB BS Lond. 1986.

WESBY, Roger David St Bernard's Hospital, Uxbridge Road, Southall UB1 3HW — MB ChB Sheff. 1978; DCH RCP Lond. 1986; DRCOG 1988; MRCPsych. 1991. Specialty: Gen. Psychiat.

WESLEY, Helen Mary Mallott (retired) Oxleas, Oxleas NHS Trust, Pinewood Bexley Hospital, Old Bexley's Lane, Bexley DA5 2BF Tel:

01322 526282 Fax: 01322 556531; Spark Haw, Froghole, Crockham Hill, Edenbridge TN8 6TD Tel: 01732 866242 Fax: 01732 867707 — (Sheff.) MB ChB Sheff. 1969; DCH Eng. 1971; MRCP (UK) 1975. Prev: Cons. Community Paediat. Ravensbourne NHS Trust Bromley.

WESS, Jennifer Mary Leasowe House, Northwood, Ellesmere SY12 0LU — MB ChB Liverp. 1986; MRCGP 1992.

WESSELL, Helen Naomi 12 Linton Grove, Leeds LS17 8PS — MB BS Sydney 1978.

WESSELS, Helen Mary Annette Hewson 574 Daws Heath Road, Hadleigh, Benfleet SS7 2NL — MB BCh BAO NUI 1955.

WESSELY, Kathryn Louise — BM BCh Oxf. 1997; BSc (1st cl.) Ed. 1994; MRCP 1999. Pre-reg Ho. Off. Jobs Aug 97-Feb 98 Med. (NDM) John Radcliffe, Oxf. Prev: SHO (Cardiol.) Roy. Brompton Hosp. Lond.; SHO (A&E) St. Thomas's Hosp. Lond.; Surg. Derriford Hosp. Plymouth.

WESSELY, Simon Charles 103 Denmark Hill, Camberwell, London SE5 8AZ Tel: 020 7848 5130 Fax: 020 7848 5129 Email: s.wessely@iop.kcl.ac.uk — BM BCh Oxf. 1981; FMed Sa; FRCPsych; MA, BA, Oxf. 1981; MSc Oxf. 1989; MD Oxf. 1993; FRCP 1997. (Psychiat.) SKT Sch. of Med. & Inst. Psychiat.; Director, King's Centre Milit. Health Research; Hon. Cons. Adviser Brit. Army Med. Servs.; Prof. (Psychol. Med.) Guy's, King's & St Thos. Sch. of Med. & Inst. of Psychiat. Specialty: Gen. Psychiat.; Epidemiol. Socs: Fell. Acad. Med. Sci.s. Prev: Sen. Regist. Bethlem & Maudsley Hosps. Lond. & Nat. Hosp. Lond.; SHO (Med.) Freeman Hosp. Newc.

WESSELY, Tessa Louise Fyfield House, Fyfield, Andover SP11 8EP — MB BS Lond. 1984.

WESSON, Colin Martin (retired) Wellspring, Old Rydon Lane, Exeter EX2 7JZ Tel: 01392 873015 — MB BS Lond. 1964 (St. Mary's & Roy. Dent.) BDS (Hons.) 1958; LDS RCS 1958; MRCS Eng. LRCP Lond. 1964; FDS RCS Eng. 1968. Cons. Oral & Maxillofacial Surg. Qu. Eliz. II Hosp. Welwyn Garden City. Prev: Sen. Regist. (Dent.) King's Coll. Hosp. & Qu. Vict. Hosp. E. Grinstead.

WESSON, Ian Mcmillan 59 Addiscombe Road, Croydon CR0 6SD Tel: 020 8688 6290 Fax: 020 8686 5818; Haling Croft, 61 St. Augustine's Avenue, South Croydon CR2 6JQ Tel: 020 8407 0970 Email: macwesson@aol.com — MB BS Lond. 1962 (St. Geo.) AKC. Socs: Croydon Med. Soc. & BMA. Prev: Ho. Phys., Res. Obst. Asst. & Sen. Cas. Off. St. Geo. Hosp. Lond.

WESSON, Michael Lloyd Hesketh Centre, 51-55 Albert Road, Southport PR9 0LT Tel: 01704 530940 — MB ChB Liverp. 1987. Cons. Psychiat. Southport & Formby Community (NHS) Trust. Specialty: Gen. Psychiat.

WEST, Alexander Glynn Medway Maritime Hospital, Windmill Road, Gillingham ME7 5NY — MB BS Lond. 1994; MRCP Lond. 1997.

WEST, Mr Andrew 1 White Cottages, Easby, Middlesbrough TS9 6JG Tel: 01642 724232 — MB BS Lond. 1976 (Guy's) MRCS Eng. LRCP Lond. 1976; FRCS Eng. 1981; FFAEM 1993. Cons. A & E Med. Darlington Memor. Hosp. Specialty: Accid. & Emerg. Socs: Brit. Assn. Emerg. Med. & BMA.

WEST, Andrew John Stoneybridge Farm, Latcham, Wedmore BS28 4SB — MB BS Lond. 1970; MRCS Eng. LRCP Lond. 1970.

WEST, Anne Prior The Manse, Old Walls, Llanrhidin, Gower, Swansea SA3 1HB — BM Soton. 1983; MSc Lond. 1976, BSc 1975; DRCOG 1985; DCH RCP Lond. 1986; MRCGP 1987. Specialty: Genetics. Prev: Trainee GP Soton VTS.

WEST, Barbara Anne Kathleen Drumchapel Health Centre, 80-90 Kinfauns Drive, Glasgow G15 7TS Tel: 0141 211 6100 Fax: 0141 211 6104; 139 Canniesburn Road, Bearsden, Glasgow G61 1HB — MB ChB Ed. 1972; FRCS Ed. 1977; MRCGP 1986.

WEST, Betty (retired) The Sett, 50 Eastfield Crescent, Badger Hill, York YO10 5JB Tel: 01904 412015 — BSc (Physiol.) Lond. 1949; MB ChB Manch. 1954. Prev: GP Chilwell.

WEST, Charles Archibald Easthope Road Health Centre, Easthope Road, Church Stretton SY6 6BL Tel: 01694 722127 Fax: 01694 724604; Gorswen, Sandford Avenue, Church Stretton SY6 7AB Tel: 01694 722674 — MB ChB Birm. 1973. Prev: Unit Gen. Manager Shropsh. HA; Ho. Surg. Gen. Hosp. Birm.; Ho. Phys. Copthorne Hosp. Shrewsbury.

WEST, Mr Charles George Hook Woodstock, Junction Road, Deane, Bolton BL3 4NE — MB BChir Camb. 1970 (Univ. Camb. & Guy's Hosp. Lond.) MA Camb. 1970; FRCS Eng. 1974. Cons. Neurol. Surg. Hope Hosp. Salford & Roy. Manch. Childr. Hosp.; Hon. Lect. (Neurosurg.) Univ. Manch. Specialty: Neurosurg. Socs: Fell. Coll. Surg. Hong Kong. Prev: Vis. Prof. Neurosurg. Chinese Univ. Hong Kong; Sen. Regist. (Neurosurg.) Roy. Vict. Hosp. Belf.

WEST, Christian Alexande 58 Seven Star Road, Solihull B91 2BY — MB ChB Leeds 1998.

WEST, Christine Parry 29 Polton Road, Loanhead EH20 9BU — MD Ed. 1989; MB ChB 1973; DCH Eng. 1976; FRCOG 1993, M 1979. Cons. O & G Edin. Roy. Infirm. & Simpson Memor. Matern. Pavil. Edin.; Sen. Lect. Univ. Edin. Specialty: Obst. & Gyn. Prev: Sen. Regist. (O & G) Simpson Memor. Matern. Pavil. & Roy. Infirm. Edin.; SHO (Paediat. Surg.) Roy. Hosp. Sick Childr. Edin.

WEST, Clive Henry Dartford East Health Centre, Pilgrims Way, Dartford DA1 1QY Tel: 01322 274211 Fax: 01322 284329; Fiacre, Ash Road, Ash, Sevenoaks TN15 7HJ — MRCS Eng. LRCP Lond. 1967; MB BS Rangoon 1963; DObst RCOG 1969. Prev: Squadron Ldr. RAF Med. Br., Sen. Med. Off. Regional Med. Centre RAF; Halton & Med. Centre RAF Episkopi, Cyprus.

WEST, Colin Andrew Clifton Road Surgery, 95 Clifton Road, Rugby CV21 3QQ Tel: 01788 578800/568810 Fax: 01788 541063 — MB ChB Birm. 1977; MA Oxf. 1982, BA 1968; DRCOG 1981; MRCGP 1982. GP Princip.; Clin. Asst. Rehabil. Med. Roy. Leamingston Sps Rehabil. Hosp.; Police Surg., Warks. Police. Socs: Rugby & Dist. Med. Soc. Prev: SHO (Paediat. & Obst. & Gyn) Brit. Milit. Hosp. Rinteln, BFPO 29.

WEST, Colin John The Surgery, Woolton Hill, Newbury RG20 9UL Tel: 01635 253324 — MB BS Lond. 1978; DRCOG 1982; MRCGP 1984; DCH RCP Lond. 1984. Prev: Asst. Lect. Bland Sutton Inst. Middlx. Hosp. Lond.

WEST, David John Ashley Farmhouse, School Lane, Ashley, Market Drayton TF9 4LF Tel: 0163 087 2540 — MB ChB Leeds 1979; DMRD 1985; FRCR 1986. Cons. Radiol. City Gen. Hosp. & N. Staffs. Roy. Infirm. Stoke on Trent. Specialty: Radiol. Prev: Lect. (Radiol. Sci.) United Med. & Dent. Schs. Guy's & St. Thos. Hosps. Lond.; Sen. Regist. N. Staffs. Roy. Infirm. Stoke-on-Trent.

WEST, David Martin (retired) — MB ChB Liverp. 1975; FFA RCS Eng. 1979. Prev: Cons. Anaesth. & IC W. Lancs. DHA.

WEST, David Reuben White Rose Cottage, Swettenham, Congleton CW12 2LE — MB BS Lond. 1991.

WEST, Deborah Rosemary Sarah Gorswen, Sandford Avenue, Church Stretton SY6 7AB Tel: 01694 722674 — MB ChB Birm. 1973. GP Princip. Broseley Shrops. Prev: Ho. Surg. Qu. Eliz. Hosp. Birm.; Ho. Phys. City Gen. Hosp. Stoke-on-Trent; Trainee Gen. Pract. Shrewsbury Vocational Train. Scheme.

WEST, Donald James 32 Fen Road, Milton, Cambridge CB4 6AD Tel: 01223 860308 Email: fad72@dial.pipex.com — MB ChB Liverp. 1947; DPM Lond. 1952; MD Liverp. 1958; FRCPsych 1986, M 1971; PhD Camb. 1967, Litt D 1979. Emerit. Prof. Clin. Criminology Univ. Camb.; Emerit. Fell. Darwin Coll. Camb. Specialty: Forens. Psychiat. Socs: World Psychiat. Assn.; Brit. Soc. Criminol. Prev: Ment. Health Act Commiss.er; Hon. Cons. Camb. Psychiat. Serv.; Sen. Regist. Forens. Unit Maudsley Hosp. Lond.

WEST, Dorothy Rutt House, Ivybridge PL21 0DQ Tel: 01752 892792 — MRCS Eng. LRCP Lond. 1958 (Univ. Coll. Hosp.) MFHom 1979. Indep. Pract. (Homoeop. Med.) Devon. Specialty: Homeop. Med. Prev: Ho. Surg. N. Middlx. Hosp. Edmonton; Ho. Phys. Co. Hosp. Hereford.

WEST, Elizabeth Alexandra The Old Rectory, Church St., Barkston, Grantham NG32 2NB — MB ChB Liverp. 1998.

WEST, Elizabeth Anne Priory Clinic, 14-18 New Church Road, Hove BN3 4FH Tel: 01273 747464 Fax: 01273 727321; Redleaf, 22 Steep Lane, Findon, Worthing BN14 0UE Tel: 01903 874140 Fax: 01903 877585 — MB BS Lond. 1984. Assoc. Specialist (Psychiat.) Priory Clinic Hove. Specialty: Gen. Psychiat.; Psychosexual Med. Prev: Clin. Asst. (Psychiat.) Brighton HA.

WEST, George Philip (retired) Mentley, Clare Drive, Farnham Common, Slough SL2 3LL Tel: 01753 643810 — (St. Mary's) MRCS Eng. LRCP Lond. 1943; MB BS Lond. 1944. Prev: Cas. Phys. St. Mary's Hosp.

WEST, Gerard Patrick Woodside Health Centre, Barr Street, Glasgow G20 7LR Tel: 0141 531 9521 Fax: 0141 531 9545 — MB ChB Glas. 1981; DRCOG 1983; MRCGP 1988; Dip. Pract. Dermat. 1991.

WEST, Gladys Mary Lesley (retired) Whipley Manor, Guildford Road, Normandy, Guildford GU3 2BE Tel: 01483 235198 — MRCS Eng. LRCP Lond. 1955 (Leeds) Prev: Asst. Psychiat. Abraham Cowley Unit St. Peters Hosp. Chertsey.

WEST, Hilary Department of General Practice, 5 Lambeth Walk, London SE11 6SP — MB BS Lond. 1998.

WEST, Mr James Department of Ophthalmology, The Royal Hallamshire Hospital, Glossop Road, Sheffield S10 2JF — MB BChir Camb. 1985; MA 1987; DO Glas. 1988; FRCOphth 1989; FRCS Glas. 1989. Cons. Ophth. Roy. Hallamshire Hosp. Sheff. Specialty: Ophth.

WEST, Janet Rae The Surgery, Frambury Lane, Newport, Saffron Walden CB11 3PY Tel: 01799 540696 Email: jan.west@gp-f81034.nhs.uk; 181 Monks Walk, Buntingford SG9 9DU Tel: 01763 273460 Email: janet@west181.fsnet.co.uk — MB ChB Dundee 1982; BMSc 1979; Dip. IMC RCS Ed. 1995; DRCOG 1997; MRCGP 1999. GP Princip.; Macmillan GP Facilitator, Palliat. Care, Uttlesford PCT. Specialty: Gen. Pract. Socs: BMA; RCGP. Prev: GP Regist. Royston Herts.

WEST, Joe Queen's Medical Centre, Division of Epidemiology & Public Health, University of Nottingham Medical School, Nottingham NG7 2UH — BM BS Nottm. 1995; MSc; MRCP.

WEST, John Nicholas Wayne Q Floor, Royal Hallamshire Hospital, Glossop Road, Sheffield S10 2JF Tel: 0114 271 2935 — MB BS Lond. 1981 (St.Thos. Hosp. Lond.) MRCP (UK) 1984; MD Lond. 1992; FRCP 1999. Cons. Cardiol. & Phys. Centr. Sheff. Univ. Hosp. Trust. Specialty: Cardiol. Socs: Brit. Hypertens. Soc. & Brit. Cardiac Soc. Prev: Lect. (Cardiol.) Qu. Eliz. Hosp. Birm.; Regist. (Med.) Qu. Eliz. Hosp. Birm.; Ho. Phys. St. Thos. Hosp. Lond.

WEST, John Ronald Crook West, Gillies and Steeden, 7 Stanhope Mews West, London SW7 5RB Tel: 020 7835 0400 Fax: 020 7835 0979; 9 Ullswater Road, Barnes, London SW13 9PL Tel: 020 8748 1912 — MB BChir Camb. 1970 (Camb. & St. Bart.) MRCS Eng. LRCP Lond. 1969; MB Camb. 1970, BChir 1969; MA Camb. 1970; MRCGP 1974.

WEST, Jonathan Alan 100 Clapham Common Westside, London SW4 9AZ — MB BS Lond. 1993; MRC Psych Part 1 1998. SHO Psychiat. Haudsley Hosp. Specialty: Gen. Psychiat.; Forens. Psychiat.

WEST, Jonathan David Peter 40 Bath Road, Banbury OX16 0TP Tel: 01295 255895 — MB BS Lond. 1995 (Trinity Hall, Cambridge/ London Hospital Medical School) BA Camb 1992; MA Cambridge 1998. Banbury Gen. Pract., VTS. Specialty: Gen. Pract.

WEST, Mr Jonathan Haden Royal Devon & Exeter Hospital, Exeter EX1 2ED Tel: 01392 411611; Riverview, Trews Weir Reach, Exeter EX2 4EG — MB BS Lond. 1978; MA Camb. 1979; FRCS Eng. 1983; MRCOG 1985. Cons. Gyn. Roy. Devon & Exeter Hosp. Specialty: Obst. & Gyn. Prev: Sen. Regist. Oxf. RHA.

WEST, Jonathan Joly McLaren (retired) 41 Five Mile Drive, Oxford OX2 8HT — MB Camb. 1958 (Middlx.) BChir Camb. 1957; BA Camb. 1954, MA 1958; DObst RCOG 1959. Prev: GP, Thatcham HC. Berks.

WEST, Mrs Judith Ann Opthalmology Department, The Royal Hallamshire Hospital, Glossop Road, Sheffield S10 2JF — MB BChir Camb. 1989; MA Camb. 1990; FRCOphth 1994, M 1993.

WEST, Judith Vivienne — MB ChB Birm. 1983; MRCP (UK) 1987; MD 1997; MD 1997. Cons. Paediat. Leics. & Rutland Healthcare Trust. Specialty: Paediat. Prev: Lect. (Child Health) Univ. Leicester; Fell. (Paediat. Thoracic Med.) Roy. Childr. Hosp. Melbourne, Vict., Austral.; Clin. Research Fell. Inst. Child Health & Hon. Lect. Univ. Birm.

WEST, Kevin John The Corner, 1 Prestwold Lane, Hoton, Loughborough LE12 5SH — MB BS Lond. 1979; FFA RCS Eng. 1984. Specialty: Anaesth.

WEST, Kevin Paul Department of Histopathology, Leicester Royal Infirmary, Leicester LE1 5WW — MB ChB Leic. 1981; MRCPath 1987; FRCPath 1998. Cons. Histopath. Univ. Hosps. of Leicester NHS Trust. Specialty: Histopath. Prev: Sen. Lect. (Path.) Univ. Leicester & Hon. Cons. Histopath Leics. HA.

WEST, Letitia Rozanne (retired) Nethercourt Lodge, Nethercourt Hill, Ramsgate CT11 0RZ Tel: 01843 586704 — (St. And.) MB ChB St. And. 1957; DPM Eng. 1966; MRCPsych 1973. Prev: Cons. Psychiat. St. Augustine's Hosp. Chartham Down.

WEST, Lydia Beatrice — MB ChB Leeds 1976; DRCOG 1980; MRCGP 1981; DFFP 1994. Specialty: Family Plann. & Reproduc. Health.

WEST, Margaret (retired) Walnut Tree Farm House, Main Road, Ashbocking, Ipswich IP6 9JX Tel: 01473 890623 — (Manchester) MB ChB Manch. 1960; DCH Eng. 1964; DPH Manch. 1968.

WEST, Mary Frances (retired) Fir Tree Cottage, The Common, Chipperfield, Kings Langley WD4 9BU Tel: 01923 260688 — (Univ. Coll. Lond. & W. Lond.) MB BS Lond. 1950; DA Eng. 1956; FFA RCS Eng. 1960. Prev: Cons. Anaesth. Watford & Hemel Hempstead Gen. Hosps.

WEST, Nicholas Cowie 'Pasture Gate', Ennerdale Bridge, Cleator CA23 3AR — MB Camb. 1978; BChir 1977; MRCP (UK) 1980; MRCPath 1984. Cons. Haemat. W. Cumbld. Hosp. Whitehaven. Specialty: Haematology.

WEST, Nicholas Edward John 58 Kenwood Drive, Shrewsbury SY3 8SY — MB BChir Camb. 1993.

WEST, Noreen Stephanie 37 Beechwood Road, Kings Heath, Birmingham B14 4AB — MB ChB Birm. 1991. SHO (Psychiat.) All St.s Hosp. Birm. Prev: SHO (Paediat., Neonatol. & Psychiat.) New Cross Hosp. Wolverhampton; Ho. Off. (Neurol & Gen. Med.) Qu. Eliz. Hosp. Birm.

WEST, Pamela Gillian Riverview, 2 Trews Weir Reach, Exeter EX2 4EG Tel: 01392 79610 — MB BS Lond. 1976; MRCS Eng. LRCP Lond. 1976. Private Asst. Nuffield Hosp. Exeter. Prev: Trainee GP Lond. (St. Thos.) VTS; Ho. Surg. (ENT) St. Thos. Hosp. Lond.; Ho. Phys. Kingston Hosp.

WEST, Pamela Karen Anne Central Dales Practice, Hawes DL8 3DR Tel: 01969 667200 Fax: 01969 667149 — MB ChB Leeds 1983; MRCGP 1987; DRCOG 1987. GP Hawes N. Yorks. Specialty: Gen. Pract. Prev: GP Wyke, Bradford.; GP Byfield, Normants.

WEST, Penelope Susan 12 Vicarage Gardens, Netheravon, Salisbury SP4 9RW — MB BS Lond. 1986; BSc Lond. 1983, MB BS 1986; DA (UK) 1989. SHO (Spinal Injuries) Duke of Cornw. Spinal Treatm. Centre Odstock Hosp. Salisbury. Prev: SHO (Anaesth.) Princess Margt. Hosp. Swindon Wilts; SHO (Anaesth.) William Harvey Hosp. WillesBoro.; Ho. Phys. Char. Cross Hosp. Lond.

WEST, Peter (retired) 27 Tilehouse Road, Guildford GU4 8AP Tel: 01483 566026 — MB BS Lond. 1944 (Oxf.) BM BCh Oxf. 1944; DPH Eng. 1949; DCH RCP Lond. 1950. Prev: Ho. Surg. Radcliffe Infirm. Oxf. & Hosp. Sick Childr. Gt. Ormond St.

WEST, Mr Peter Duncan Buller Queen Alexandra Hospital, Cosham, Portsmouth PO6 3LY Tel: 023 92 379451; Two School Cottages, School Lane, Bosham, Chichester PO18 8NY Tel: 01243 574175 — BM BCh Oxf. 1979; MA Oxf. 1980; FRCS Eng. 1985; MSc Manch. 1990. Cons. Audiol. Med. Qu. Alexandra Hosp. Portsmouth & St. Richard's Hosp. Chichester. Specialty: Audiol. Med.

WEST, Peter Guy Fortescue (retired) — MB BChir Camb. 1965; DPM Eng. 1970; MRCPsych 1972. Prev: Cons. Psychiat. Old Age Scalebor Pk. Hosp. Burley-in-Wharfedale.

WEST, Philip Boundaries Surgery, 17 Winchester Rd, Four Marks, Alton GU34 5HG Tel: 01420 563152 Fax: 01420 564172 — MB BS Lond. 1995. GP Asst.

WEST, Rebecca — MB BS Lond. 1994 (Char. Cross and Westm. Med. Sch.) DFFP 1997; DRCOG Lond 1999. SHO (O & G) St. Richards Hosp. Chichester. Specialty: Obst. & Gyn.; Family Plann. & Reproduc. Health. Socs: MDU.

WEST, Richard Clive The Surgery, Harborough Road N., Northampton NN2 8LL Tel: 01604 845144 — MB ChB Ed. 1963.

WEST, Richard James Queen Elizabeth Hospital, Birmingham B15 7UZ Tel: 0121 972 1311; 23 Oxford Road, Birmingham B13 9EH Tel: 0121 449 6700 — MB ChB Ed. 1967; DMRD Eng. 1971; FFR 1973; FRCR 1977. Cons. Radiol. Qu. Eliz. Hosp. Birm.; Hon. Sen. Lect. Birm. Univ. Specialty: Radiol. Socs: Sec. Brit. Soc. Interven.al Radiol. Prev: Sen. Regist. Dudley Rd. Hosp. & United Birm. Hosps.; Regist. (Radiodiag.) United Birm. Hosps.

WEST, Professor Richard John (retired) 4 Old Vicarage Place, Apsley Road, Bristol BS8 2TD Tel: 0117 973 8311 — (Middlx.) MB BS Lond. 1962; DObst RCOG 1964; MRCP (UK) 1967; DCH RCP Lond. 1969; MD Lond. 1975; FRCP Lond. 1979; FRCPCH 1997. Med. Postgrad. Dean S. West. Region & Hon. Prof. Med. Postgrad. Studies Univ. Bristol; Hon. Cons. Frenchay Hosp. Bristol; Hon. Cons.

Paediat. United Bristol Healthcare Trust; Gen. Sec. Inst. Med. Ethics Lond. Prev: Dean, Sen. Lect. & Cons. Paediat. St. Geo. Hosp. & Med. Sch. Lond.

WEST, Richard John Woolpit Health Centre, Heath Road, Woolpit, Bury St Edmunds IP30 9QU Tel: 01359 240298 Fax: 01359 241975; Saffron House, Saffron House, Old Stowmarket Road, Woolpit, Bury St Edmunds IP30 9QS Email: richard.west25@btinternet.com — MB ChB Manch. 1993; DCH RCP Lond. 1995; DGM RCP Lond. 1996; MRCGP RCGP Lond. 1997. GP Princip.; GP Tutor West Suffolk; GP Trainer. Specialty: Gen. Pract. Prev: SHO (Geriat., O & G, Paediat. & A & E) W. Suff. Hosp.; GP Reg.

WEST, Roger John (retired) 12 Redwing Road, Kempshott, Basingstoke RG22 5UP Email: rogerwest@doctors.org.uk — MB BS Lond. 1965 (Lond. Hosp.) MSc Manch. 1974; MRCS Eng. LRCP Lond. 1965; DObst RCOG 1968; MRCGP 1972; FFCM 1980, M 1974. Prev: Director (Pub. Health) Suff. HA.

WEST, Ruth Margaret (retired) 32 Mercian Court, Park Place, Cheltenham GL50 2RA Tel: 01242 577182 — (Birm.) MB ChB Birm. 1940; DObst RCOG 1942; DPH Eng. 1948. Prev: Sen. Med. Off. Surrey AHA.

WEST, Sheila Leslie Department of Anaesthesia, Cheltenham General Hospital, Sandford Park Road, Cheltenham GL53 7AN Tel: 01242 222222 Fax: 01242 273405 Email: sheila.west@egnhst.org.uk — MB BS Lond. 1976 (Guy's Hospital Medical School) MRCS Eng. LRCP Lond. 1975; DRCOG 1979; FFA RCS Eng. 1981. Cons. Anaesth. E. Glos. NHS Trust. Specialty: Anaesth.

WEST, Shirley Anne 4 Dilwyn Gardens, Bridgend CF31 3NT Tel: 01656 63930 — MB ChB Manch. 1972. Clin. Asst. Princess of Wales Hosp. Bridgend. Socs: Assn. Anaesths. Prev: Regist. (Anaesth.) Univ. Hosp. Wales Cardiff.

WEST, Siaron Mair Ty Bryn Surgery, The Bryn, Trethomas, Caerphilly CF83 8GL Tel: 029 2086 8011 — MB BCh Wales 1994 (univ.Wales) DRCOG 1999; MRCGP 2001. GP Retainer Ty Bryn Surg. Trethomas Newport. Specialty: Gen. Pract. Socs: Christ. Med. Fellowsh. Prev: SHO Paediat E. Glam..NHS.Trust; SHO O & G.E. Glam.. NHS. Trust; GP. Regist.

WEST, Simon Christopher 30 Topaz Street, Cardiff CF24 1PH — MB BCh Wales 1991. SHO (Urol.) Cardiff Roy. Infirm.

WEST, Siobhan Louise 23 Avon Road, Hale, Altrincham WA15 0LB — MB ChB Bristol 1993. Specialist Regist. Paediat. N. W. Region Rotat. Specialty: Paediat.

WEST, Stephen Edmund Corinthian Surgery, St Paul's Medical Centre, 121 Swindon Road, Cheltenham GL50 4DP Tel: 01242 707777 Fax: 01242 707776; Painters Cottage, Elkstone, Cheltenham GL53 9PV — MB BS Lond. 1976 (Guys Hospital) MRCS Eng. LRCP Lond. 1976; MRCOG 1982; MRCGP 1983. Clin. Asst. (Colposcopy) Cheltenham.

WEST, Susan Elizabeth The Ridgeway Surgery, 1 Mount Echo Avenue, Chingford, London E4 7JX Tel: 020 8529 2233 Fax: 020 8529 4484; Tailours, High Road, Chigwell IG7 6DL Tel: 020 8500 0293 Fax: 020 8500 1696 — MB BS Lond. 1978 (Middlx.) BSc Lond. 1973; DRCOG 1980; DMJ (Clin.) Soc. Apoth. Lond. 1992.

WEST, Susan Helen Cossham Hospital, Lodge Road, Kingswood, Bristol BS15 1LF Tel: 0117 975 8054 Fax: 0117 975 8034 Email: sue.west@awp.nhs.uk; 66 Woodstock Road, Redland, Bristol BS6 7ER — MB BS Newc. 1979; MRCPsych 1988. Cons. Psychiat., Old Age, Cossham Hosp., Bristol. Specialty: Geriat. Psychiat. Special Interest: Deliberate Self-harm; ECT.

WEST, Suzanne Catheryn The Health Centre, Queensway, Billingham TS23 2LA Tel: 01642 552700/552151 Fax: 01642 532908 — MB ChB Leic. 1995.

WEST, Terence Edward Timothy 58 Kenwood Drive, Shrewsbury SY3 8SY Tel: 01743 233697 Fax: 01952 242218 — MB BChir Camb. 1964 (St. Mary's) MD Camb. 1976, MA 1964; FRCP Lond. 1981, M 1967. Cons. Phys. Princess Roy. Hosp. Telford & Roy. Shrewsbury Hosp. Specialty: Endocrinol. Socs: Brit. Typhoid Assoc. Prev: Lect. (Med.) St. Thos. Hosp. Med. Sch. Lond.; Regist. (Med.) Middlx. Hosp. Lond.; Ho. Phys. Med. Unit St. Mary's Hosp. Lond.

WEST, Thomas Stephens, OBE (retired) 30 Pineheath Road, High Kelling, Holt NR25 6QF — MB BS Lond. 1957.

WEST, Timothy Peter The Surgeries, Lombard Street, Newark NG24 1XG Tel: 01636 702363 Fax: 01636 613037; 61 Milner Street, Newark NG24 4AA Tel: 01636 679751 — MB ChB Liverp. 1969; DObst RCOG 1971; DPM Eng 1978. Prev: Regist. (Psychiat.) Roundway Hosp. Devizes; Ho. Phys. Broadgreen Hosp. Liverp.

WEST-JONES, Jennifer Susan — MB ChB Leic. 1998; BSc Brunel 1989; MRCS Ed. 2003.

WESTABY, Catherine Alexandra Marie 5 Lawn Crescent, Richmond TW9 3NR — MB BS Lond. 1978; BSc (Psychol.) Durh. 1973; MRCS Eng. LRCP Lond. 1978; DRCOG 1980. Specialty: Gen. Pract.

WESTABY, Mr Stephen — MB BS Lond. 1972; FETCS; MS; BSc; PhD; FESC; FRCS Eng. 1978. Sen. Cons. Cardiac Surg. John Radcliffe Hosp. Oxf. Specialty: Cardiothoracic Surg.

WESTALL, Glen Philip 144 Melbourne Grove, London SE22 8SA — MB BS Lond. 1993.

WESTALL, William Graham Crwys Road Surgery, 151 Crwys Road, Cathays, Cardiff CF24 4XT Tel: 029 2039 6987 Fax: 029 2064 0523 — MB ChB Bristol 1962; DObst RCOG 1965; DPH Bristol 1974. Prev: Employm. Med. Adviser EMAS; SHO (Med.) E. Glam. Hosp. Pontypridd.

WESTAWAY, Christine Elizabeth The John Kelso Practice, Ball Haye Road, Leek ST13 6 — MB ChB Leic. 1985.

WESTBROOK, Anthony Paul Derbyshire Royal Infiirmary, London Road, Derby — BM BS Nottm. 1994. SHO Orthop. DRI Derby. Specialty: Orthop.

WESTBROOK, Freddie Kingshill Farm, Wishaw ML2 9PJ — MB ChB Manch. 1978; BSc St. And. 1975; MRCGP 1982. Med. Quality Manager -sema Med. Servs. Specialty: Disabil. Med.

WESTBROOK, Mark Andrew The Shrubbery, 65A Perry Street, Northfleet, Gravesend DA11 8RD Tel: 01474 356661 Fax: 01474 534542 — MB BS Lond. 1990. Specialty: Gen. Pract.

WESTBROOK, Patricia (retired) 19 Titchfield Road, Troon KA10 6AN — MB ChB Glas. 1961 (Glas.) Indep. GP & Hypnother. Troon; Cons. Lifestyle, AMI Ross Hall Hosp. Glas. Prev: Sen. Med. Off. (Family Plann.) Glas.

WESTBURY, Charlotte Beth Chester Beatty Laboratory, Institute Of Cancer Research, Fulham Road, London SW3 6JB Email: charlotte.westbury@icr.ac.uk — MB ChB Ed. 1994 (Univ. Ed.) BSc (Hons) Med. Sci. Edin. 1991; MRCP 1997; FRCR 2002. Clin. Research Fell. (Clin. Oncol.) Inst. of Cancer Research, Lond. Specialty: Oncol. Socs: FRSM. Prev: Specialist Regist. (Clin. Oncol.), The Roy. Marsden NHS Trust, Lond.

WESTBURY, Professor Gerald, OBE Apartment 4, 7 Cambridge Gate, London NW1 4JX — (Westm.) MB BS (Hons.) Lond. 1949; FRCP Lond. 1976, M 1951; FRCS Eng. 1952; Hon. FRCS Ed. 1993. Emerit. Prof. Surg. Univ. Lond. & Inst. Cancer Research. Specialty: Gen. Surg. Socs: FRSM. Prev: Hon. Cons. Surg. Roy. Marsden Hosp.; Cons. Surg. Westm. Hosp. Lond.; Ho. Surg. & Sen. Regist. (Surg.) Westm. Hosp.

WESTBURY, Harry (retired) 2A Brickwall Lane, Ruislip HA4 8JX Tel: 01895 673137 — MB BS Lond. 1956 (Westm.) MRCS Eng. LRCP Lond. 1956; MRCP Lond. 1961; DMRD Eng. 1963; FFR 1967; FRCR 1975. Cons. Radiol. Harefield & Mt. Vernon Hosps. Prev: Sen. Regist. (X-Ray) Soton. Gen. Hosp. & St. Mary's Hosp. Lond.

WESTCAR, Paul David Chapel Row Surgery, The Avenue, Bucklebury, Reading RG7 6NS Tel: 01189 713252 Fax: 01189 714161; Hidden Cottage, Rotten Row, Tutts Clump, Bradfield, Reading RG7 6LQ — MB BChir Camb. 1984 (Cambridge & Westminster) MA Camb. 1985; DRCOG 1989; MRCGP 1989. Sch. Med. Adviser Bradfield Coll. Bradfield, Berks. Socs: (Ex-Sec.) Newbury Med. Soc. Prev: Trainee GP W. Suff. VTS.

WESTCOTT, Edward Daniel Anders 11 Roberts Lane, Chalfont St Peter, Gerrards Cross SL9 0QR — MB BS Lond. 1996.

WESTCOTT, Godfrey Francis BM Box 7894, London WC1N 3XX — MB BS Lond. 1952.

WESTCOTT, Mr Mark Christopher 22 Fabian Road, London SW6 7TZ Tel: 020 7386 7803 — MB BS Lond. 1989 (St. Thos. Hosp. Med. Sch.) FRCOphth 1993. Specialist Regist. N. Thames Rotat.; Research Fell. at The Inst. of Ophth. & Moorfields Eye Hosp. Specialty: Ophth. Prev: SHO West. Eye Hosp. Lond.

WESTCOTT, Richard Howson East Street Surgery, East Street, South Molton EX36 3BU Tel: 01769 573811; 4 Paradise Lawn, South Molton EX36 3DJ Tel: 01769 572225 — BM BCh Oxf. 1973; MA Oxf. 1973; DCH Eng. 1976; FRCGP 1994, M 1977; DRCOG 1977. Lect. 1997; Fell. Inst. Gen. Pract. Univ. Exeter; Assoc. Adviser

Univ. Bristol; GP Trainer Devon. Prev: Trainee GP Exeter VTS; Ho. Phys. Radcliffe Infirm. Oxf.; Ho. Surg. Roy. United Hosp. Bath.

WESTCOTT, Tessa (retired) Pendle, Ledborough Wood, Beaconsfield HP9 2DJ Tel: 01494 674796 — MB BS Lond. 1960 (Roy. Free) MRCS Eng. LRCP Lond. 1960. Prev: Assoc. Specialist (Gen. Med.) Wycombe Gen. Hosp. High Wycombe.

WESTENSEE, Wilma Alma Road Surgery, 68 Alma Road, Portswood, Southampton SO14 6UX Tel: 023 8067 2666 Fax: 023 8055 0972; Denny Cottage, Denny Lodge, Lyndhurst SO43 7FZ — MB ChB Stellenbosch 1979. Prev: Trainee GP Bournemouth VTS; SHO (O & G, Rheum. & Rehabil.) Soton. Gen. Hosp.

WESTERHOLM, Ronald 9 Northway Court, Bishopston, Swansea SA3 3JZ — MB BS Lond. 1965 (Univ. Coll. Hosp.) DObst RCOG 1967; DPM Eng. 1970; FRCPsych 1993. Cons. Psychiat. Cefn Coed Hosp. Swansea. Specialty: Gen. Psychiat.

WESTERMAN, Roger Millfield Surgery, Millfield Lane, Easingwold, York YO61 3JR Tel: 01347 821557 — MB BCh Wales 1977.

WESTERMANN, Willem Barend Pangbourne Medical Practice, The Boat House Surgery, Whitchurch Road, Pangbourne, Reading RG8 7DP Tel: 0118 984 2234 Fax: 0118 984 3022; Juniper House, Beckfords, Upper Basildon, Reading RG8 8PB Tel: 01491 671400 — MB BChir Camb. 1972; BA Camb. 1968, MA, MB 1972, BChir 1971.

WESTERN, Hannah Ruth 22B Templars Avenue, London NW11 0NY — MB BS Lond. 1996.

WESTERN, Jane Margaret Beck House, 3 West Parade Road, Scarborough YO12 5ED Tel: 01723 352522 — MB BS Lond. 1982; MRCGP 1986; DRCOG 1986; Postgraduate Diploma in Clinical Psychiatry Leeds 2000. Staff Grade Child and Adolesc. Pschiatry Dept., ScarBoro.

WESTERN, Nicholas Vernon Blair South Ham House, 96 Paddock Road, Basingstoke RG22 6RL Tel: 01992 624408 Fax: 01992 626206; 8 Little Brook Road, Roydon, Harlow CM19 5LR Tel: 01279 792896 — MB BS Lond. 1987; BA (Physiol. Sci.) Oxf. 1983. Specialty: Gen. Pract.

WESTGARTH, David Station Medical Group, Gatacre Street, Blyth NE24 1HD Tel: 01670 396540 Fax: 01670 396517; 20 Esher Gardens, Sandringham Park, Blyth NE24 3RR Tel: 01670 354642 — MB ChB Liverp. 1972; MRCP (U.K.) 1975; MRCGP 1978. GP Blyth. Prev: Med. Regist. David Lewis North. Hosp. Liverp.; SHO (Gen. Med.) Whiston Hosp.; Ho. Surg. & Ho. Phys. Broadgreen Hosp. Liverp.

WESTGARTH, Sarah Elizabeth 43 Hillsden Road, Beaumont Park, Whitley Bay NE25 9XF — MB ChB Sheff. 1998; MB ChB Sheff 1998.

WESTGARTH, Thomas John Nelson Health Centre, Cecil Street, North Shields NE29 0DZ Tel: 0191 257 1204/4001 Fax: 0191 258 7191 — MB BS Newcastle 1969; MB BS Newc. 1969. GP N. Shields Tyne & Wear.

WESTGARTH, Trevor (retired) Dingli, 5 Pinewood Close, Ashton Road, Lancaster LA2 0AD Tel: 01524 68338 — MB BS Durh. 1957 (Newc.) DCP Lond 1963. Prev: Regist. N. Lancs. & S. W.mld. Gp. Path. Dept. & Roy. Postgrad. Med.

WESTGATE, Robert 1 Brunswick Street, Carlisle CA1 1ED — MB BS Newc. 1993; DRCOG; MRCGP. Special Interest: Diabetes; Health Informatics.

WESTHEAD, John Neil Trinity House Surgery, 17 Irish Street, Whitehaven CA28 7BU Tel: 01946 693412 Fax: 01946 592046; 25 The Crofts, St Bees CA27 0BH Tel: 01946 822674 — MB ChB Ed. 1970; DPM Eng. 1974; MRCPsych 1975; MRCGP 1977; MD Ed. 1983.

WESTHEAD, Matthew James Knowle House Surgery, 4 Meavy Way, Crownhill, Plymouth PL5 3JB Tel: 01752 771895 — MB Camb. 1966 (Camb. & St. Thos.) BChir 1965; DObst RCOG 1967.

WESTIN, Mr Thomas Royal Hallamshire Hospital, Department of Otolaryngology, Glossop Road, Sheffield S10 2JF Tel: 0114 226 1189 Fax: 0114 271 1985 Email: thomas.westin@broadbanddoctor.com — Lakarexamen Gothenburg 1980. Cons. (Otolaryngol.); Hon. Sen. Clin. Lect. Univ. Sheff. Specialty: Otolaryngol. Special Interest: Head & Neck Surg.

WESTLAKE, Anthony Charles 15 Ascot Close, Eastbourne BN20 7HL Tel: 01323 644584 Fax: 01323 644584 — MB ChB Liverp. 1972; DA Eng. 1977; AFOM RCP Lond. 1982. Company Med. Adviser Med. & Indust. Servs. Ltd. Eastbourne. Specialty: Occupat. Health. Socs: Soc. Occupat Med.; BMA; Fellow Roy. Soc. Med. Prev: Regional Med. Off. Brit. Rlys. Bd. Euston; Regist. (Anaesth.) Plymouth Gen. Hosp.; SHO (Anaesth.) IC Derbysh. Roy. Infirm.

WESTLAKE, Athene Sally Anaesthetic Department, St George's Hospital, Tooting, London SW17 0QT Tel: 020 8672 1255; 46 Seymour Walk, London SW10 9NF Tel: 020 7352 6768 — MB ChB Bristol 1989 (Bristol Univ.) FRCA 1994. Specialist Regist. (Anaesth.) St Geos. Hosp. Socs: BMA & Assn. Anaesth. Prev: Specialist Regist. (Anaesth.) Qu. Mary's Univ. Hosp. Lond.; Specialist Regist. (Anaesth.) Roy. Brompton Hosp. Lond.; Regist. St Geo's Hosp. Lond.

WESTLAKE, Helen Elizabeth 49 Earls Court Road, Penylan, Cardiff CF23 9DE — MB BCh Wales 1991; BSc (Hons.) Biochem. Wales 1986. Trainee GP Cardiff VTS.

WESTLAKE, John David Penylan Road Surgery, 100 Penylan Road, Roath Park, Cardiff CF23 5RH Tel: 029 2046 1100 Fax: 029 2045 1623 — MB BCh Wales 1988; DCH RCP Lond. 1991; DRCOG 1991; T(GP) 1992; MRCGP 1993. Prev: Trainee GP/SHO (Paediat. & O & G) Nevill Hall Hosp. Abergavenny; Ho. Off. (Gen. Med., Thoracic Med. & Gen. Surg.) Llandough Hosp.

WESTLAKE-GUY, Carol Howat Moston Lodge Children's Centre, Countess of Chester Health Park, Chester CH2 1UL Tel: 01244 364802; 13 The Spinney, Gayton, Wirral CH60 3SU Tel: 0151 342 4540 — MRCS Eng. LRCP Lond. 1961. SCMO (Community Child Health) Chester. Specialty: Paediat.

WESTMAN, Alison Jane Three Bridges Regional Secure unit, Ealing, Hammersmith & Fulham NHS Trust, Uxbridge Road, Southall UB1 3EU Tel: 020 8354 8200 Fax: 020 8967 5477; 1 Appletree Grove, Cumberland Drive, Redbourn, St Albans AL3 7PG — MB ChB Manch. 1983; DRCOG 1986; MRCPsych 1991. Cons. Child Psychiat. Ealing Hammersmith & Fulham NHS Trust. Specialty: Child & Adolesc. Psychiat. Prev: Sen. Regist. (Child & Adolesc. Psychiat.) NW Lond. RHA.

WESTMERLAND, Simon Peter 2 Aston Gardens, Glossop SK13 8PJ — MB ChB Sheff. 1993.

WESTMORE, Mr Graham Anthony 40 Littlemoor Lane, Sibsey, Boston PE22 0TU Tel: 01205 750912 Fax: 01205 750912 — MB BS Lond. 1970 (Univ. Lond., St. Geo. Hosp. Lond.) FRCS Eng. 1976. Cons. ENT, Head & Neck Surg. (Private Practice). Specialty: Otorhinolaryngol. Socs: Fell. Roy. Soc. Med.; Brit. Skull Base Soc.; Eur. Skull Base Soc. Prev: Cons. ENT Surg. Milton Keynes Hosp.; Sen. Regist. (ENT) St. Geo. Hosp. Lond.; Cons. ENT & Head & Neck Surg. Pilgrim Hosp. Boston.

WESTMORELAND, Diana University Hospital of Wales, NPHS Microbiology, Heath Park, Cardiff CF4 4XW Tel: 029 2074 2178 Fax: 029 2074 2178 Email: diana.westmoreland@nphs.wales.nhs.uk — BM BCh Oxf. 1984; BA (Hons. Biochem.) Camb. 1971; MA Camb. 1971; MSc (Virol.) Birm. 1972; DPhil (Virol) Oxf. 1974; FRCPath (Virol.) 1987; MRCPath 1988. Cons. Virol. Pub. Health Laborat. Serv. Cardiff.; Dep. Laborat. Dir. NPHS Cardiff. Specialty: Med. Microbiol. Prev: Asst. Microbiol. Pub. Health Laborat. Serv. Bristol.

WESTON, Adrian Hugh Spencer Llanfyllin Medical Centre, High Street, Llanfyllin SY22 5DG Tel: 01691 648054 Fax: 01691 648165; Tyn Llan, Llanfechain SY22 6UJ — MB BS Lond. 1979; DRCOG 1985; MRCGP 1987.

WESTON, Alasdair Neil Rubislaw Terrace Surgery, 23 Rubislaw Terrace, Aberdeen AB10 1XE Tel: 01224 643665 Fax: 01224 625197 — MB ChB Aberd. 1975.

WESTON, Anne Louise Chapeloak Practice, 347 Oakwood Lane, Leeds LS8 3HA Tel: 0113 295 3750 Fax: 0113 295 3460; 48 North Park Avenue, Roundhay, Leeds LS8 1EY — MB ChB Bristol 1984; DRCOG 1987; DCH RCP Lond. 1988; MRCGP 1989. GP Leeds. Prev: Partner in Gen. Pract. Bristol; GP Bristol; Trainee GP Nailsea VTS.

WESTON, Charles Elborough Dorset County Hospital, Renal Unit, Williams Avenue, Dorchester DT1 2JY Tel: 01305 255269 Fax: 01305 254756 Email: charles.weston@wdgh.nhs.uk — MB BS Lond. 1988 (Roy. Free Hosp.) MRCP (UK) 1993; USMLE (I, II, III) 1996. Cons. Phys. & Nephrol. Specialty: Nephrol. Special Interest: Acute Renal Failure. Socs: Renal Assn.; Amer. Soc. Nephrol. Prev: Regist. (Renal) King's Coll. Hosp. Lond.; Specialist Regist. (Nephrol. & Gen. Med.) St Helier Hosp.Carlshalton, Surrey; Specialist Regist. (Nephrol.) St Geo. Hosp. Lond.

WESTON, Christopher Graham Solihull Hospital, Lode Lane, Solihull B91 2JL Tel: 0121 424 5330 — MB ChB Birm. 1976; FFA RCS Eng. 1981. Cons. (Anaesth.) Birm. Heartlands & Solihull Hosp. NHS Trust. Specialty: Anaesth. Prev: Sen. Regist. (Anaesth.) W. Midl. RHA; Regist. (Anaesth.) Coventry AHA.

WESTON, Clive Frank Mantell Department of Cardiology, Singleton Hospital, Sketty, Swansea SA2 8QA Tel: 01792 205666 Fax: 01792 285354 — MB BCh Wales 1981; MRCP (UK) 1984; FRCP 1999. Cons. Cardiol. Singleton Hosp. Swansea; Hon. Sen. Lect., Univ. Wales Coll. of Med.; Dep. Director Swansea Clin. Sch. Specialty: Cardiol.; Educat. Socs: Brit. Cardiac Soc.; Resusc. Counc. Prev: Sen. Lect. (Cardiol.) Univ. Leeds; Lect. (Cardiol. Epidemiol.) Univ. Wales Coll. Med.; Regist. (Cardiol.) Univ. Hosp. Wales.

WESTON, David Andrew The Atherstone Surgery, 1 Ratcliffe Road, Atherstone CV9 1EU Tel: 01827 713664 Fax: 01827 713666; Schoonder Cottage, 1 Church Lane, Ratcliffe Culey, Atherstone CV9 3PA — MB ChB Leic. 1982. Specialty: Acupunc.; Research. Socs: The Brit. Med. Acupunc. Soc.

WESTON, Mr David Manfred Loddon Vale Practice, Hurricane Way, Woodley, Reading RG5 4UX Tel: 0118 969 0160 Fax: 0118 969 9103; Barn House, Tanners Lane, Chalkhouse Green, Reading RG4 9AB Tel: 0118 972 1878 Fax: 0118 972 2685 — MB BS Lond. 1966 (Char. Cross) MRCS Eng. LRCP Lond. 1966; FRCS Eng. 1971. Hosp. Pract. (Surg.) Roy. Berks. Hosp. Reading; Surg. Marie Stopes Clinic. Specialty: Gen. Pract.; Gen. Surg.

WESTON, Diane Helen 14 Aldridge Court, Baldock SG7 5TA — MB BS Lond. 1963 (Roy. Free) MRCS Eng. LRCP Lond. 1963; DPM Eng. 1966; MRCPsych 1973. Cons. Child & Adolesc. Psychiat. Child & Family Guid. Clinic, Lister Hosp., Stevenage. Specialty: Child & Adolesc. Psychiat. Prev: Ho. Surg. & Paediat. Ho. Phys. St. Albans City Hosp.; Sen. Regist.; Dept. Childr. & Parents Tavistock Clinic Lond.

WESTON, Jane Crawley Hospital, West Green Drive, Crawley RH11 7DH Tel: 01293 600300 Fax: 01293 600404 Email: jane.weston@sash.nhs.uk — BM BCh Oxf. 1988; MA Oxf. 1986, DPhil 1986; MRCPath 1994; FRCPath 2003. p/t Cons. Histopath. & Cytopath. Surrey & Sussex Healthcare NHS Trust. Specialty: Histopath. Socs: BMA; Brit. Soc. Clin. Cytol.; Assn. of Clin. Pathologists. Prev: Sen. Regist. (Histopath.) Hammersmith Hosp. Lond.; Sen. Regist. & Regist. Northwick Pk. Hosp. Harrow.

WESTON, John Arthur Barton The Abbey Practice, The Family Health Centre, Stepgates, Chertsey KT16 8HZ Tel: 01932 565655 Fax: 01932 501842; Chestnuts, Blackdown Avenue, Woking GU22 8QG — MB Camb. 1962 (St. Thos.) BChir 1961; DObst RCOG 1965; DCH Eng. 1966; FRCGP 1979, M 1971. GP Princip.; GP Tutor St. Peter's Hosp. Chertsey. Socs: BMA. Prev: GP Trainee Course Organiser SW Thames RHA.

WESTON, Judith Clare 164A Bellingham Road, London SE6 1EJ — MB ChB Liverp. 1993.

WESTON, Mark Elson (retired) Victoria House, Bluntisham Road, Needingworth, St Ives PE27 4TA Tel: 01480 466793 Fax: 01480 466755 — MRCS Eng. LRCP Lond. 1962 (St. Mary's) BA Oxf. 1959; DObst RCOG 1964. Prev: Ho. Phys. (Paediat.) St. Mary's Hosp. Lond.

WESTON, Michael Dennis 24 Plytree, Thorpe Bay, Southend-on-Sea SS1 3RA — MB BS Lond. 1980; FCAnaesth 1990. Specialty: Anaesth.

WESTON, Michael John Ultrasound Department, St James's University Hospital, Beckett St., Leeds LS9 7TF Tel: 0113 206 4330 Fax: 0113 206 5466 Email: micheal.weston@leedsth.nhs.uk — MB ChB Bristol 1984; MRCP (UK) 1987; FRCR 1990; T(R) (CR) 1992. Cons. Radiol. St. Jas. Univ. Hosp. Leeds. Specialty: Radiol. Socs: Brit. Inst. Radiol.; Brit. Med. Ultrasound Soc.; Brit. Med. Assn. Prev: Sen. Regist. (Radiodiag.) S. West. RHA.; Regist. (Radiodiag.) Bristol Roy. Infirm.

WESTON, Michael John 148 Harley Street, London W1G 7LG Tel: 020 7487 5020 Fax: 020 7224 1528; Brambles, Elm Green Lane, Danbury, Chelmsford CM3 4DR Tel: 01245 226445 — (Camb. & St. Thos.) MA, MB Camb. 1970, MD 1978, BChir 1969; FRCP Lond. 1982, M 1971. Cons. Phys. Gen. Med. Broomfield Hosp. Chelmsford; Hon. Cons. Nephrol. KCH Lond. Specialty: Gen. Med.; Nephrol. Socs: Renal Assn.; Med. Res. Soc. Prev: Cons. Phys. Gen. & Renal Med. King's Coll. Hosp. Lond.; Lect. (Med.) & Hon. Sen. Regist. King's Coll. Hosp. Lond.; Regist. (Med.) Roy. Sussex Co. Hosp. Brighton.

WESTON, Mr Neil Craig 7 Long Meadow, Gayton, Wirral CH60 8QQ Tel: 0151 342 4590 — MB BChir Camb. 1983; BA (Phys. Sci.) Oxf. 1980; FRCS Eng. 1989. Regist. (Gen. Surg.) Whipps Cross Hosp. Lond. Specialty: Urol. Prev: SHO (Urol.) Addenbrookes Hosp. Camb.; SHO (Gen. Surg.) Hinchingbrooke Hosp. Huntingdon.

WESTON, Penelope Mary East Barnet Health Centre, 149 East Barnet Road, Barnet EN4 8QZ Tel: 020 8440 7417 Fax: 020 8447 0126 — (Guy's) BSc (Food & Managem. Sc.) Lond. 1976, MB BS 1982; DRCOG 1984; DCH RCP Lond. 1986; MRCGP 1986. GP Princip. E. Barnet Health Centre.

WESTON, Peter (retired) 17 Cissbury Road, Worthing BN14 9LD — MB BChir Camb. 1958 (Middlx.) MA, MB Camb. 1958, BChir 1957; DObst RCOG 1963. Prev: GP Worthing.

WESTON, Mr Peter Alexander Murray (retired) Old Rectory, Church Town, Sebergham, Carlisle CA5 7HS Tel: 01697 476263 — MB BS Lond. 1951 (St. Bart.) MRCS Eng. LRCP Lond. 1947; FRCS Eng. 1952; LMCC 1953. Prev: Cons. Surg. S. Regions Health Project, Mbeya, Tanzania.

WESTON, Peter Godfrey Woodhouse (retired) Wednesday Cottage, Main St., Buchlyvie, Stirling FK8 3LR Tel: 01360 850408 — MB ChB Ed. 1949. Cons. Hypnother. Edin. Prev: GP Edin.

WESTON, Philip John 68 Evington Drive, Leicester LE5 5PD — MB ChB Leic. 1987.

WESTON, Philip John High Pastures, 138 Liverpool Road North, Liverpool L31 2HW Tel: 0151 526 2161 Fax: 0151 527 2377 — MB ChB Liverp. 1989; DCH RCP Lond. 1995; DRCOG 1995. Specialty: Gen. Pract. Prev: Trainee GP Southport Dist. Gen. Hosp. VTS; SHO (Orthop.) Whiston Hosp.; SHO (Gen. Surg.) Southport Hosp.

WESTON, Mr Philip Mark Tempest Pinderfields Hospital, Aberford Road, Wakefield WF1 4DG Tel: 01924 201688 Fax: 01924 212921 — MB BCh Wales 1980 (Welsh National School of Medicine) FRCS Ed. 1984; MCh Wales 1989; FRCS (Urol.) 1991. Cons. Urol. Surg. Pinderfields Hosp.; Roy. Coll. of Surg.s Tutor, Area Coordinator, Wakefield Div., Yorks. Sch. of Surg.. Specialty: Urol. Socs: Med. Res. Soc.; EORTC GU Gp.; Brit. Assn. Urological Surg.s. Prev: Cons. Urol. Surg. Clayton Hosp. Wakefield; Sen. Regist. (Urol.) W. Midl. RHA; Regist. (Urol.) Cardiff Roy. Infirm. & Univ. Hosp. Wales.

WESTON, Sandra Jane 8 Clarence Street, Richmond TW9 2SA — MB BS Lond. 1989; BSc Lond. 1986, MB BS 1989; DFFP 1993.

WESTON, Sian Nerys c/o Cefn Coed Hospital, Heol Waunarlwydd, Cockett, Swansea SA2 0GH Tel: 01792 561155 — MB BCh Wales 1995 (Univ. Wales Coll. Med.) SHOold Age Psychiat. Cefn Coed Hosp. Swansea; SHO (Psychiat.) Cefn Coed Hosp. Swansea. Specialty: Gen. Psychiat. Socs: Inceptor Roy. Coll. Psychiat. Prev: SHO (Child Psychiat.) Trehafod Unit Cefn Coed Hosp. Swansea; SHO (Adult Psychiat.) Cefn Coed Hosp. Swansea; SHO (Psychiat.) St. Jas. Univ. Hosp. Leeds.

WESTON, Theodore Paul Birbeck Medical Group, Penrith Health Centre, Bridge Lane, Penrith CA11 8HW Tel: 01768 245200 Fax: 01768 245295; The College, Tirrill, Penrith CA10 2JE Tel: 01768 245389 — MB BS Lond. 1982 (Char. Cross) DRCOG 1986; MRCGP 1990. Prev: Trainee GP Northampton VTS; SHO (Dermat. & A & E) Northampton HA.

WESTON, Trevor Edmund Thomas Robert Street Surgery, 89D Robert Street, London NW1 3QT Tel: 020 7387 4576 — MD Lond. 1962 (St. Bart.) MB BS 1951; MRCGP 1958. Butterworth Gold Medal Coll. GP 1959; Cons. Venereol. Roy. Surrey Co. Hosp., Woking Vict. Hosp. & Frimley Pk. Hosp; Med. Off. Daily Telegraph Benev. Fund; Cons. Med. Edr. Family Doctor Pub.ats. Socs: BMA (Chairm. St. Pancras Div.); Airborne Med. Soc. Prev: Regist. Guy's Hosp. Lond.; Sen. Regist . St. Thos. Hosp.; Clin. Asst. St. Bart. Hosp. Lond.

WESTON, Vivienne Clare Department of Microbiology & PHL, University Hospital, Queens Medical Centre, Nottingham NG7 2UH — MB BS Lond. 1987 (Roy. Free) MRCP (UK) 1990; MSc (Clin. Microbiol.) Lond. 1995; MRCPath 1998. Cons. (Microbiol) Qu. Med. Centre Nottm. Specialty: Med. Microbiol. Socs: RCPath; HIS; AMM. Prev: Sen. Regist. (Microbiol.) Qu. Med. Centre Nottm.; Regist. (Microbiol.) Leicester Roy. Infirm.; SHO (Renal Med.) Dulwich Hosp. Lond.

WESTON-BAKER, Elizabeth Jane North Road West Medical Centre, 167 North Road West, Plymouth PL1 5BZ Tel: 01752 662780 Fax: 01752 254541; Pamflete House, Holbeton, Plymouth PL8 1JR — (Guy's) MB BS Lond. 1977; MRCS Eng. LRCP Lond. 1977; MRCP (UK) 1979; MRCGP 1983.

WESTON-BURT, Paul Michael Woodlands Surgery, Tilgate Way, Tilgate, Crawley RH10 5BS Tel: 01293 525204 Fax: 01293 514778 — MB BChir Camb. 1966 (St. Bart.) MA, MB Camb. 1966, BChir 1965; MRCS Eng. LRCP Lond. 1965; DA Eng. 1968; DObst RCOG 1968.

WESTON-DAVIES, Mr Wynne Hurst, TD Evolutec Ltd., The Magdalen Centre, Oxford Science Park, Oxford OX4 4GA Tel: 01865 784070 Fax: 01865 399991 Email: wwd@evolutec.co.uk — MB BS Lond. 1967 (St. Mary's) MRCS Eng. LRCP Lond. 1967; FRCS Eng. 1972. Med. & Developm. Director, Evolutec Ltd., Oxf. Specialty: Pharmaceutical Medicine; Gen. Surg. Socs: FRCM. Prev: Med. Dir. Cutis Clin. Research Ltd.; Europ. Med. Dir. Bristol Myers Squibb Convatec; Asst. Dir.y Clin. Research Squibb Europe.

WESTON SMITH, Paul Andrew Littlewick Medical Centre, 42 Nottingham Road, Ilkeston DE7 5PR Tel: 0115 932 5229 Fax: 0115 932 5413 — MB ChB Birm. 1973; DRCOG 1978. Univ. Tutor (Gen. Pract.) Nottm. Med. Sch.; Chairm. Ilkeston Hosp. Med. Comm.; Exec. Mem. Erework, PCT. Specialty: Gen. Pract. Socs: BMA; Derbysh. LMC. Prev: Trainee GP Cardiff (Welsh Nat. Sch. Med.) VTS.

WESTON UNDERWOOD, Mr John The Old Mill, Tregoose, Newquay TR8 4NE Email: jwu@millstreet.demon.co.uk — MB BS Lond. 1968 (St. Geo.) BSc Lond. 1965; MRCS Eng. LRCP Lond. 1968; FRCS Eng. 1974. Cons. Surg. Benenden Hosp. Cranbrook. Specialty: Gen. Surg. Prev: Surg. 1st Asst. St. Geo. Hosp. Lond.; Regist. (Surg.) St. Jas. Hosp. Lond.

WESTON UNDERWOOD, Rosemary Ann (retired) Hampton, Hawkhurst Road, Kenley CR8 5DL Tel: 020 8660 7706 — MB BS Lond. 1967 (St. Geo.) MRCS Eng. LRCP Lond. 1967; DObst RCOG 1969; DCH Eng. 1970.

WESTPHAL-BURDON, Silke Ursula Steadings Home Farm, Bridle path, Newcastle upon Tyne NE3 5EU — State Exam Med Berlin 1988 (Berlin, Germany) MD Berlin 1990; MRCGP 1996. GP. Prev: GP Partner, 1 Cartingon Tce Med. Gp., Heaton Newc. upon Tyne, NE6 5RS.

WESTROP, Richard John — MB ChB Dundee 1978. GP Hull. Specialty: Gen. Pract. Socs: Soc. Med. & Dent. Hypn.

WESTWATER, Jason John Flat 2/4 Parsonage Square, Collegelands, Glasgow G4 0TA — MB ChB Glas. 1995.

WESTWELL, Diana Frances Albert Road Medical Centre, 60 Albert Road, Shrewsbury SY1 4HY Tel: 01743 281950 Fax: 01743 233198 — MB ChB Glas. 1987; DRCOG 1990; Cert. Family Plann. JCC 1991; T(GP) 1991.

WESTWICK, Rachel Jane 20 Brookway, London SE3 9BJ — MB ChB Liverp. 1996.

WESTWOOD, Mr Christopher Anthony The Laurels, Church Lane, Fotherby, Louth LN11 0UH — MB ChB Bristol 1968; FRCS Eng. 1974. Cons. (Gen. Surg. & Urol.) Grimsby & Louth Health Dist. Specialty: Urol. Prev: Sen. Regist. Leics. HA (T) & St. Peters Hosp. Lond.; SHO (Gen. Surg.) Frenchay Hosp. Bristol.

WESTWOOD, Christopher Norman Ridgeway Practice, Plympton Health Centre, Mudgeway, Plymouth PL7 1AD Tel: 01752 346634; Old Treby Farm, Yealmpton, Plymouth PL8 2LJ Tel: 01752 880409 — MB BS Lond. 1970 (Char. Cross) MRCS Eng. LRCP Lond. 1970; DObst RCOG 1973. Prev: Ho. Phys. & Ho. Surg. Char. Cross Hosp.; SHO (Obst.) & Cas. Off. Plymouth Health Dist.

WESTWOOD, Colin Timperley Health Centre, 169 Grove Lane, Timperley, Altrincham WA15 6PH Tel: 0161 980 3751 Fax: 0161 904 9678 — MB ChB Manch. 1973; DCH Eng. 1976; DObst RCOG 1976; MRCGP 1981.

WESTWOOD, Dawn Lesley Dalkeith Medical Practice, 24 St Andrew Street, Dalkeith EH22 1AP Tel: 0131 665 2267; Eskwood, Lasswade EH18 1EJ — MB ChB Ed. 1989. Trainee GP Musselburgh.

WESTWOOD, Gavin Ralph Peel House Medical Centre, Avenue Parade, Accrington BB5 6RD Tel: 01254 237231 Fax: 01254 389525; Brooklands, 110 Hollins Lane, Accrington BB5 2JS — MB ChB Manch. 1985; MRCGP 1989. Specialty: Gen. Pract. Prev: Trainee GP Blackburn VTS.

WESTWOOD, Louisa Katherine Martagon, Rimes Close, Kingston Bagpuize, Abingdon OX13 5AL — BM BS Nottm. 1994.

WESTWOOD, Mark Anthony The Village Green Surgery, The Green, Wallsend NE28 6BB Tel: 0191 295 8500 Fax: 0191 295 8519 — MB ChB Leic. 1984. GP Wallsend, Tyne & Wear SHO (Med. Rotat.) Freeman Hosp. Newc. Prev: Ho. Off. (Med.& Surg.) Leicester Roy. Infirm.

WESTWOOD, Paul Arthur Newcombes Surgery, Newcombes, Crediton EX17 2AR Tel: 01363 772263 Fax: 01363 775906; Weirholme, Half Moon, Newton, St Cyres, Exeter EX5 5AB Tel: 01392 851414 Fax: 01392 851414 — (Liverp.) MB ChB Liverp. 1967; DPM Eng. 1971; MRCPsych 1976; MRCGP 1981. Prev: SHO W. Chesh. Psychiat. Hosp. Chester; Ho. Phys. Walton Hosp. Liverp.; Ho. Surg. Broadgreen Hosp. Liverp.

WESTWOOD, Paul Richard Bodfeddyg, 102 High St., Glynneath, Neath SA11 5AL Tel: 01639 720311 Fax: 01639 722579 Email: pw@valeofneathgps.co.uk; Pwll Dylluan, Penderyn, Aberdare CF44 9QA — MB BCh Wales 1982 (Welsh National School of Medicine) DRCOG 1987; MRCGP 1991; DFFP 1996. GP Princip. Specialty: Gen. Pract. Prev: RN Med. Off.

WESTWOOD, Suzanne Louise 6 Moorlands Park, Cuddington, Northwich CW8 2LY — BM BCh Oxf. 1998.

WESTWOOD, Tina Louise The Surgery, Wharf Road, Gnosall, Stafford ST20 0DB — MB ChB Dundee 1990. Specialty: Gen. Pract.

WESTWOOD, William John Abbott (retired) 4 Church Lane, Lyddington, Oakham LE15 9LN Tel: 01572 822299 — (Birm.) BSc (Hons.) Birm. 1959, MB ChB (Hons.) 1962; DObst RCOG 1968; Cert. Family Plann. JCC 1976. Indep. Non-Princip. GP. Prev: GP Princip. Corby.

WESTWORTH, Betty Patricia (retired) 24 Virginia Beeches, Callow Hill, Virginia Water GU25 4LT Tel: 01344 843953 — MB ChB St. And. 1956; DObst RCOG 1957; DPH Lond. 1967; FFCM 1987. Prev: Specialist in Community Med. (Social Servs./Child Health) S.W. Surrey HA.

WETHERALL, Mr Anthony Philip Kidderminster General Hospital, Bewdley Road, Kidderminster DY11 6RJ — MB ChB Manch. 1978; FRCS Ed. 1983; FRCS Eng. 1984. Cons. Gen. Surg. Kidderminster Gen. Hosp. Specialty: Gen. Surg. Socs: Assn. Coloproctol. Prev: Cons. Gen. Surg. Roy. Air Force Med. Br.

WETHERALL, Linda Michelle 5 Farnham Park, Bangor BT20 3SR — MB ChB Manch. 1998.

WETHERALL, Michael Richard Brydges Department of Histopathology, Sunderland Royal Hospital, Kayll Road, Sunderland SR4 7TP Tel: 0191 565 6256 Fax: 0191 569 9230; 32 Oaklands, Gosforth, Newcastle upon Tyne NE3 4YP Tel: 0191 284 5932 — MB BS Newc. 1979; MA Camb. 1975; MRCPath 1989. Cons. Histopath. Sunderland Roy. Hosp. Specialty: Histopath. Prev: Sen. Regist. (Histopath.) Roy. Vict. Infirm. Newc.; Demonst. (Path.) Roy. Vict. Infirm. Newc.

WETHERED, Oliver James Courtney Warley, Links Road, Winchester SO22 5HP Tel: 01962 852962 Fax: 01962 855410 Email: oliver@wethered.clara.net — (Char. Cross) MA Oxf. 1964; MB BS Lond. 1969; MRCP (U.K.) 1975; DMRD Eng. 1977; FRCR 1980; FRCR 1980; FRCP 1999. Cons. Diag. Radiol. Roy. Hants. Co. Hosp. Winchester. Specialty: Radiol. Prev: Sen. Regist. (Diag. Radiol.) St. Geo. Hosp. Lond.; Regist. (Radiol.) Guy's Hosp. Lond.; Regist (Med.) W. Middlx. Hosp. Lond.

WETHERELL, Mr Geoffrey Alfred (retired) Poole House, 10 Albert Drive, Neston CH64 6QH Tel: 0151 353 8673 — MB ChB Liverp. 1943; FRCS Eng. 1952; MChOrth 1953. Prev: Cons. Orthop. Surg. Clatterbridge Gen. Hosp.

WETHERELL, Heather Caroline The Health Centre, Viewley Centre, Hemlington, Middlesbrough TS8 9JQ Tel: 01642 590500 Fax: 01642 591721; Grangecroft, Kirkby Lane, Great Broughton, Middlesbrough TS9 7HG — BM BS Nottm. 1988; BMedSci Nottm. 1986; DRCOG 1992; MRCGP 1993. Clin. Asst. (Anaesth.) Friarage Hosp. Northallerton. Prev: Trainee GP Northallerton VTS; SHO (Anaesth.) Friarage Hosp. Northallerton.

WETHERELL, Owen Charles (retired) Eden House, Old Malton, Malton YO17 6RT Tel: 01653 693243 — (Camb. & St. Mary's) MRCS Eng. LRCP Lond. 1961; MB BChir Camb. 1962; MA Camb. 1962; DObst RCOG 1964. Prev: SHO (Paediat.) York Co. Hosp.

WETHERELL, Mr Roderick Grant Kent & Canterbury Hospital, Ethelbert Road, Canterbury CT1 3NG; Waylands, Town Hill, Bridge,

Canterbury CT4 5AH — MB ChB Birm. 1978; FRCS Ed. 1984; MD Birm. 1992. Cons. Orthop. Surg. Kent & Canterbury Hosp. Specialty: Orthop. Prev: Sen. Regist. (Orthop.) SE. Thames RHA; Research Fell. (Orthop.) Rayne Inst. St. Thos. Hosp. Lond.

WETHERELL, Simon Charles Queen Square Surgery, 2 Queen Square, Lancaster LA1 1RP Tel: 01524 843333 Fax: 01524 847550; Moorgate Barn, Littledale Road, Brookhouse, Lancaster LA2 9PH Tel: 01524 771363 — BM BCh Oxf. 1985; MRCGP 1989; DRCOG 1989; MA Lancs. Uni 2000.

WETHERILL, Diana Mary Lynwood, 16 Oxford Road, Dewsbury WF13 4JT Tel: 01924 465889 Fax: 01924 519434 — (Leeds) MB ChB Leeds 1965; MMedSc Leeds 1985; DMJ (Clin.) Soc. Apoth. Lond. 1991. Police Surg. W. Yorks. Specialty: Forens. Path. Socs: FRSM (Pres. Sect. Clin. Forens. And Legal Med.); BMA; Assn. Police Surg. Prev: GP, Cleckheaton, W. Yorks; Med. Off. Fox's Biscuits Batley; Ho. Off. St. Jas. Hosp. Leeds.

WETHERILL, John Homer (retired) Lynwood, 16 Oxford Road, Dewsbury WF13 4JT Tel: 01924 465889 Fax: 01924 519434 — (Leeds) MB ChB (Hons.) Leeds 1959; FRCP Lond. 1981, M 1965. Prev: Cons. Phys. Dewsbury Health Care NHS Trust.

WETHERILL, Mr Martin Harry Shalstone Hill Farm, Shalstone, Buckingham MK18 5NB — MB BS Lond. 1973; MRCS Eng. LRCP Lond. 1973; FRCS Ed. 1980. Cons. Orthop. Surg. Qu. Eliz. Milit. Hosp. Lond. Specialty: Orthop. Prev: Hon. Sen. Regist. Nuffield Orthop. Centre Oxf.; Hon. Sen. Regist. Orthop. Dept. Hosp. for Sick Childr. Gt. Ormond St.; Lond.

WETHERLY, James Marshall Rennie (retired) 41 Great Southern Road, Aberdeen AB11 7XY Tel: 01224 585141 — MB ChB Aberd. 1951.

WETSON, Ronald Ernest Steyning Health Centre, Tanyard Lane, Steyning BN44 3RJ Tel: 01903 843400 Fax: 01903 812981 — MB ChB Birm. 1974; BSc (Hons.) (Biol. Scs.) Birm. 1969; DRCOG 1976; DCH Eng. 1977; MRCGP 1978.

WETTON, Charles William Neve 3 Rosedew Road, Hammersmith, London W6 9ET Tel: 020 8748 2867 — MB BS Lond. 1987; MRCP (UK) 1990; FRCR 1994. Sen. Regist. St. Mary's Hosp. Lond. Specialty: Radiol. Prev: SHO Westm., St. Stephens, Roy. Marsden, Roy. Brompton & Nat. Heart Hosps.

WEXLER, Mr David Mark Northern Penobscot Orthopaedics, Millinocket, Maine, USA; 54 Kingsmere Park, London NW9 8PL Tel: 020 8205 3912 — MB BS Lond. 1989 (St. Bart. Univ. Lond.) FRCS Glas. 1994; FRCS Tr & Orth 1999. SpR Trauma & Orthop. Surg. 2001. Specialty: Virology. Prev: SHO (A & E) Southend Gen. Hosp.; Demonst. (Anat.) Roy. Free Hosp. Lond.; Specialist Regist. Rotat. (Orthop.) N. Thames (W.).

WEXLER, Sarah Anne Royal United Hospital , Haematology Department, Combe Park, Bath BA1 3NG Tel: 01225 428331 Email: sarah.wexler@ruh-bath.swest.nhs.uk — MB BS Lond. 1989 (St. Bartholomews Hospital Medical School) MRCP Lond. 1995; MRCPath. 1999. Consultant Haematologist, Royal United Hospital, Bath. Specialty: Haematology.

WEY, Emmanuel Quintela 19 Norton Road, Leyton, London E10 7LQ — MB BS Lond. 1998 (St Georges) Paediat.SHO FarnBoro. Hosp. Specialty: Neuropath. Prev: Ho. Off. Gen.med St Geo.s Hosp.Lond.

WEYELL, Richard Stanley Charles Hicks Centre, 75 Ermine Street, Huntingdon PE29 3EZ Tel: 01480 453038 Fax: 01480 434104 — MB BS Lond. 1985; DCH RCP Lond. 1990; MRCGP 1991. Specialty: Community Child Health.

WEYHAM, Christopher John 19 Arlington Court, Stourbridge DY8 1NN — MB ChB Dund. 1998.

WEYMAN, Christine 14 Windsor Road, Finchley, London N3 3SS Tel: 020 8 349 1096; 1624 NW 12th Street, Gainesville FL 32609, USA Tel: 904 374882 — MB BS Lond. 1982; BSc NSW 1973; PhD Lond. 1977. Fell. (Paediat. Haemat. & Oncol.) Univ. of Florida.

WEYMES, Cameron, TD (retired) Mill Cottage, Mill Hall, Eaglesham, Glasgow G76 0PD Tel: 0135 532506 — (Univ. Ed..) MD Ed. 1963, MB ChB 1947; DPH Glas. 1955; FRCP Glas. 1971, M 1967; MSc Strathclyde 1969; FFCM 1972. Prev: Hon. Surg. To H.M. the Qu..

WEYNDLING, Jadwiga Magdalena (retired) Eastleigh, Stoke St Michael, Bath BA3 5JT Tel: 01749 840859 — MB ChB Ed. 1953 (Edin.) Prev: Princip. GP Gorebridge Gp. Pract. Midlothian.

WHALE, Christopher Ian 9 Folder Lane, Sprotbrough, Doncaster DN5 7PD Tel: 01302 850107 Email: chriswhale@hotmail.com — MB ChB Liverp. 1996. Jun. Ho. Off. Mackay Base Hosp. Queensland, Australia. Prev: Ho. Off. Arrowe Pk. Hosp. Wirral.

WHALE, Kathleen (retired) 30 Burlington Road, Altrincham WA14 1HR — MB ChB Manch. 1955; Dip. Bact. Manch. 1975; FRCPath 1988, M 1977; BA (Hons.) Manch. 1995; B Phil Manch. 1998. Prev: Cons. Med. Microbiol. Manch. AHA (T) (N. Dist.).

WHALE, Rowland 98 Cambridge Road, Great Shelford, Cambridge CB2 5JS Tel: 01223 842845 — MB BS Lond. 1977; MSc (Gerontol.) Lond. 1990, MB BS 1977; MRCP (UK) 1980. Cons. Phys. Redbridge Heath Trust. Specialty: Gen. Med. Prev: Clin. Tutor Univ. Camb.

WHALE, Sally Ann Orchard Street Health Centre, Ipswich IP4 2PU Tel: 01473 213261 — MB ChB Birm. 1985; DRCOG 1988; MRCGP 1998. GP. Specialty: Gen. Pract. Prev: Black Country VTS Course Organiser; W'ton N.E. PCG Bd. Mem.; GP Partner Wolverhampton.

WHALE, William Richard South Downs NHS Trust, Brighton General Hospital, Brighton Tel: 01273 696011 Email: s.whale@bton.ac.uk; 14 Portland Mansions, 134-1336 Marine Parade, Brighton BN2 1DF — MB BS Lond. 1990 (St. Geo.) Cons. Psychiat., S. Downs NHS Trust, Brighton; Sen. Lect. Pyschiatry Univ. of Brighton, Brighton. Specialty: Gen. Psychiat. Socs: MRCPsych. Prev: Sen. Regist. (Psychiat.) Haleacre Unit. Amersham; Sen. Regist. & Regist. (Psychiat.) Warneford Hosp. Oxf.; Clin. Research Fell., Univ. of Oxf.

WHALEN, Steven Howard Wessex Road Surgery, Wessex Road, Parkstone, Poole BH14 8BQ Tel: 01202 734924 Fax: 01202 738957; 14 Wynford Road, Poole BH14 8PG Tel: 01202 740119 — MB ChB Bristol 1975; DA Eng. 1978. Specialty: Gen. Pract.

WHALEY, Anne Patricia sir Humphrey Davy Dept Anaesthesia, Bristol Royal Infirmary, Bristol BS2 8HW Tel: 01179 282163 — MB BS Lond. 1986; MA (Med. Sci.) Camb. 1986; FRCA (UK) 1994, MRCP 1989. Cons. Anaesth. IC Bristol roy. Infirm. Specialty: Anaesth.; Intens. Care. Socs: Train. Mem. Assn. Anaesth. Prev: Spr Anaesth. S. W. Rotat.; Cons. (ITU and Anaesth.) Bristol Roy. Infirm.; Sen. Regist. (ICU) Roy. Shove & Roy. Alexandra Child. Hosp. Sydney.

WHALEY, Katherine Elizabeth 52 Alma Road, Carshalton SM5 2PF — MB ChB Leic. 1995.

WHALLETT, Andrew John The Guest Hospital, Dudley Group of Hospitals, Tipton Rd, Dudley DY1 4SE — MB ChB Birm. 1991; BSc (Hons.) Birm. 1988; MB ChB (Hons.) Birm. 1991; MRCP (UK) 1995. Cons. Rheumatologist. Specialty: Rheumatol.; Educat. Socs: Brit. Soc. for Rheum.; UK Behcet's Forum. Prev: SpR, West Midlands, 1995-2000; SHO (Med.) City Hosp. Birm.; SHO (Med.) Kidderminster Gen. Hosp.

WHALLETT, Diana Joan Thornbury Health Centre, Eastland Road, Thornbury, Bristol BS35 1DP Tel: 01454 412599 Fax: 01454 41911; Fairfield House, 58 Castle St, Thornbury, Bristol BS35 1HG Tel: 01454 412346 — MB ChB Birm. 1963; DObst RCOG 1965; Cert. Family Plann. JCC 1966; Cert. Contracep. & Family Plann. RCOG & RCGP 1974; Instruc. Cert. 1976; MFFP 1993. GP; Sen. Clin. Med. Off. Family Plann. Clinic N. Bristol NHS Trust. Prev: Ho. Phys. Qu. Eliz. Hosp. Birm.; Ho. Surg. (Obst.) Hallam Hosp. W. Bromwich.

WHALLETT, Miss Elizabeth Jane 58 Castle Street, Thornbury, Bristol BS35 1HG — MB ChB Birm. 1991; FRCS Ed. 1997. SHO (Plastic Surg. & Burns.) Northern Gen. Hosp. Sheff. Specialty: Plastic Surg. Socs: Med. Protec. Soc.; Surgic. Soc. Prev: SHO (Plastic Surg.) N. Staffs. Hosp., SHO (Plastic Surg.) Morriston Hosp. Swansea; SHO (Plastic Surg.) Sandwell Healthcare NHS Trust; SHO (Thoracic Surg.) Birm. Heartlands Hosp.

WHALLETT, Michael John (retired) Fairfield House, 58 Castle St, Thornbury, Bristol BS35 1HG Tel: 01454 412346 — (Birm.) MB ChB Birm. 1962; DObst RCOG 1964. Prev: Med. Off. Thornbury Hosp.

WHALLEY, Francis Edward Rutherford House, Langley Park, Durham DH7 9XD Tel: 0191 373 1386 Fax: 0191 373 4288 — MB BS London 1976; MB BS Lond. 1976. GP Brandon, Co Durh.

WHALLEY, Frederick Lawrence (retired) Range House, Salterns Road, Lee-on-the-Solent PO13 9NL Email: whalleymins@doctors.org.uk — MB BChir Camb. 1952 (St. Thos.) MA Camb. 1952; MRCS Eng. LRCP Lond. 1953; DObst RCOG 1956; MRCGP 1965. Prev: Mem. Hants. LMC.

WHALLEY, James Thomas 3 Merton Place, Birkenhead CH43 4XD — MB ChB Dundee 1989.

WHALLEY, John 22 Meadowcroft, Church Park N., Euxton, Chorley PR7 6BU — MB ChB Leeds 1970.

WHALLEY, John Andrew 12 The Gables, Cottam, Preston PR4 0LG — MB ChB Manch. 1995; MRCP (UK) 1999; DMRD 2001.

WHALLEY, Professor Lawrence Jeffrey Department of Mental Health, University Medical Buildings, Foresterhill, Aberdeen AB25 2ZD Tel: 01224 681818 Fax: 01224 663145; 16 Albert Terrace, Edinburgh EH10 5EA — MB BS Newc. 1969; DPM Edin. 1973; FRCPsych 1990, M 1974; MD Newc. 1976. Prof. Ment. Health Univ. Aberd.; Hon. Cons. Psychiat. Grampian HB. Specialty: Gen. Psychiat.; Geriat. Psychiat. Socs: BMA; Soc. for Neurosci. Prev: Sen. Lect. (Psychiat.) Univ. Edin.; Sen. Clin. Sc. MRC Brain Metab. Unit Roy. Edin. Hosp.; Sen. Regist. (Psychiat.) Lothian HB.

WHALLEY, Mary Jane 85 Hamilton Road, Reading RG1 5RB — MB BS Lond. 1974; MRCPsych 1978; FRCPsych 2003. Cons. Psychiat. W. Norf. PCT. Specialty: Gen. Psychiat. Prev: Sen. Regist. (Psychiat.) Littlemore Hosp. Oxf.; Ho. Off. Addenbrookes Hosp. Camb.

WHALLEY, Simon Adam Greenend, Coach Road, Ashover, Chesterfield S45 0JN — BM BS Nottm. 1990; BMedSci Nottm. 1988; MRCP (UK) 1993. Specialty: Gastroenterol.

WHAMOND, William Nelson, DFC Bishop's Barn, Cross Roads, Keighley BD22 9AQ Tel: 01535 642297 — MRCS Eng. LRCP Lond. 1950 (Guy's)

WHARFE, Simon Michael Webster Chartham Surgery, Parish Road, Chartham, Canterbury CT4 7JU Tel: 01227 738224 Fax: 01227 732115 — MB BS Newc. 1974; DRCOG 1976; MRCGP 1978; MA Cantab. 1999. Assoc. Med. Director E. Kent Community Trust. Specialty: Gen. Pract. Prev: Clin. Research Phys. Pfizer Cent. Research; Local Med. Off Civil Serv. Dept. Med. Advisory Serv.; Trainee GP Newc. VTS.

WHARIN, Fiona Jane (retired) 60 Headlands, Kettering NN15 6DG — MB BS Lond. 1972; MRCS Eng.; MRCP (UK) 1996, L. 1972; DRCOG 1977; DCH RCP Lond. 1992; MRCPCH 1997. Prev: Staff Grade Pract. Community Paediat.

WHARIN, Paul Douglas 60 Headlands, Kettering NN15 6DG — MB BChir Camb. 1972; MA, MB Camb. 1972, BChir 1971; DObst RCOG 1975. Locum GP; Clin. Asst. (Palliat. Care) Cransley Hospital Kettering.

WHARRAM, Jonathan The Surgery, 14 Queenstown Road, Battersea, London SW8 3RX Tel: 020 7622 9295 Fax: 020 7498 5206 — MB BS Lond. 1981; DRCOG 1983; DCH RCP Lond. 1984; MRCGP 1985; Cert. Family Plann. JCC 1986. Prev: GP Surrey.

WHARTON, Amanda Jane Nuffield Road Medical Centre, Nuffield Road, Chesterton, Cambridge CB4 1GL Tel: 01223 423424 — MB BChir Camb. 1995; BSc Bristol 1975; PhD Lond. 1985. Gen. Practitioner, Camb.; Camb. United Football Club Doctor, Camb. Specialty: Rheumatol.; Sports Med.; Educat.

WHARTON, Professor Brian Arthur MRC Childhood Nutrition Research Centre, Institute of Child Health, Guilford Street, London WC1N 1EH Tel: 020 7905 2143 Fax: 020 7831 9903 Email: bwharton@ich.ucl.ac.uk; School House, Belbroughton, Stourbridge DY9 9TF Tel: 01562 730243 Fax: 01562 730243 Email: brianawharton@onetel.com — (Birm.) MB ChB (Distinc. Social Med., Paediat. & Child Health) Birm. 1960; DCH Eng. 1962; FRCP Lond. 1979, M 1965; FRCP Ed. 1974, M 1965; DSc Birm. 1994, MD (Hons.) 1968; MBA Warwick 1990; FRCP Glas. 1991; FRCPCH 1997. Hon. Prof. Univ. Coll. Lond. Inst. of Child Health Lond. Specialty: Paediat. Socs: Nutrit. Soc. (UK, USA); Soc. for Paediat. Research (Europe and USA); Worshipful Soc. Apoth. Prev: Dir. Gen. Brit. Nutrit. Foundat. Lond.; Prof. Human Nutrit. Univ. Glas.; Cons. Paediat. Sorrento Matern. & Selly Oak Hosps. Birm.

WHARTON, Brian Kenneth, Wing Cdr. (retired) — MRCS Eng. LRCP Lond. 1952 (Lond. Hosp.) DPM Eng. 1960; FRCPsych 1983, M 1971. Prev: Vis. Cons. Psychiat. St. And. Hosp.

WHARTON, Christopher Frederick Percy Princess Royal University Hospital, The Medical Unit, Farnborough Common, Orpington BR6 8ND; 24-26 High Street, Chipstead, Sevenoaks TN13 2RP Tel: 01732 452906 Fax: 01732 452906 — BM BCh Oxf. 1964 (Oxf. & Guy's Hosp. Lond.) MRCS Eng. LRCP Lond. 1963; DM Oxf. 1972, MA 1964; FRCP Lond. 1980, M 1969. p/t Cons. Phys. Princess Roy. Univ. Hosp. Specialty: Gen. Med. Special Interest: Dysrhythmias; Heart Failure; Hypertension. Socs: Brit. Cardiac Soc.; Europ. Cardiac. Soc. Prev: Sen. Regist., Regist. (Med. & Cardiol.), Ho. Surg. & Ho. Phys. Guy's Hosp. Lond.

WHARTON, Elen Oak Street Surgery, Oak Street, Cwmbran NP44 3LT Tel: 01633 866719 Fax: 01633 838208 — MB BCh Wales 1981; MRCGP (Distinc.) 1987.

WHARTON, Elizabeth Valerie 60A Main Street, Donaghcloney, Craigavon BT66 7LR Tel: 01762 881225; 24 Ballymacormick Road, Dromore BT25 1QR Tel: 01846 692030 — MB BCh BAO Belf. 1969.

WHARTON, Iain Philip 10 Old Village Road, Little Weighton, Cottingham HU20 3US — MB BS Newc. 1997.

WHARTON, John Graham Burntwood Health Centre, Hudson Drive, Burntwood, Walsall WS7 0EN Tel: 01543 670162; 22 Footherley Road, Shenstone, Lichfield WS14 0NJ Tel: 01543 480890 — MB ChB Liverp. 1977; BSc (1st cl. Hons.) Chem. Nottm. 1971; MRCP (UK) 1979; MRCGP 1985. Specialty: Gen. Pract. Prev: Research Stud. (Chem.) Univ. Camb; Regist. (Med.) John Radcliffe Hosp. Oxf.

WHARTON, Lucy Helen St Michael's Cottage, Black Bull Lane, Fulwood, Preston PR2 9YB; 25 Marlborough Road, London W4 4EU — MB BS Lond. 1993.

WHARTON, Mr Malcolm Robert 11 Moor Park Avenue, Preston PR1 6AS Tel: 01772 555640 Fax: 01772 555640; St Michaels Cottage, Black Bull Lane, Fulwood, Preston PR2 9YB Tel: 01772 719202 — (Manch.) MB ChB Manch. 1962; DObst RCOG 1964; FRCS Ed. 1969; MChOrth Liverp. 1972. Cons. Orthop. Surg. Preston Health Dist. Specialty: Orthop. Socs: Fell. Manch. Med. Soc. & Brit. Orthop. Assn. Prev: Sen. Regist. (Orthop.) Manch. RHB; Regist. (Orthop.) Roy. South. Hosp. Liverp.; SHO (Surg.) Manch. Roy. Infirm.

WHARTON, Paul John 3 Norbury Crescent, Littleover, Derby DE23 2QT — MB ChB Manch. 1995.

WHARTON, Richard Lloyd Newbridge Surgery, 129 Newbridge Hill, Bath BA1 3PT Tel: 01225 425807 Fax: 01225 447776; Hamswell Farm, Hamswell, Bath BA1 9DG Tel: 01225 891234 Fax: 01225 892334 Email: richard@hamswellfarm.fsnet.co.uk — MB ChB Bristol 1976; DRCOG 1978; MRCGP 1984. Lect. (Gen. Pract.) Sch. of Postgrad. Med.; Tutor (Gen. Pract.) Bath Univ. Prev: Assoc. Tutor (Gen. Pract.) Bath.

WHARTON, Mr Richard Quartermaine 3 Hall Close, Harpole, Northampton NN7 4DY — MB BS Lond. 1991 (United Med. & Dent. Schs.) FRCS Eng. 1996; MS 2002; FRCS (GEN) 2003. Specialist Regist., Chelsea & Westm. Rotat. Specialty: Gen. Surg. Socs: RSM; Assn. of Coloproctology of GB & Irel.; Assn. of Surgeons of GB & Irel. Prev: Research Fell. (Gen. Surg.) Chelsea & Westm. Gen. Hosp. Lond.; Resid. Surgic. Off. St Marks Hosp., Harrow.

WHARTON, Simon Peter 43 Milton Road, Sheffield S7 1HP — MB BS Lond. 1992.

WHARTON, Stephen Barrie Neuropathology Laboratory, University of Edinburgh, Western General Hospital, Crewe Road, Edinburgh EH4 2XU Tel: 0131 537 1975 — MB BS Lond. 1988 (Charing Cross and Westminster London) BSc (Hons.) Lond. 1985; MSc Camb. 1995; MRCPath 1997. Sen. Lect. & Hon. Cons. Neuropath. Western Gen. Hosp. Edin. Specialty: Neuropath. Socs: Brit. Neuropath. Soc. Prev: Sen. Regist. (Neuropath.) Addenbrooke's Hosp. Camb.; Hon. Regist. (Histopath.) Addenbrooke's Hosp. Camb.; SHO (Histopath.) Addenbrooke's Hosp. Camb.

WHATLEY, Gregory Charles Anselm Tameside General Hospital, Fountain Street, Ashton-under-Lyne OL6 9RW — MB BS Lond. 1987 (Char. Cross and Westm.) MSc Med. Parasitol Lond. 1989; DTM & H RCP Lond. 1989; MRCP (UK) 1992. Cons. Phys. and Gastroenterologist. Specialty: Gastroenterol. Socs: Brit. Soc. of Gastroenterol.; Midl. Gastroenterol. Soc.; Midl. Phys. Soc. Prev: SHO Rotat. Leicester Gp. Hosp.s; SHO (Accid. & Emerg.) Northampton Gen. Hosp.; Ho. Phys. & Ho. Surg. Char. Cross Hosp. Lond.

WHATLEY, Roger John (retired) 496A Semington Road, Melksham SN12 6DX Tel: 01225 702436 — MB ChB Bristol 1960; DObst RCOG 1962; DCH Eng. 1962; MRCGP 1968.

WHATLEY, Sheila Ann (retired) 496A Semington Road, Melksham SN12 6DX Tel: 01225 702436 — MB ChB Bristol 1960.

WHATLING, Paul James Faculty of Medical Informatics, Royal College of Surgeons of Edinburgh, Nicolson Street, Edinburgh EH8 9DW Tel: 0131 527 3412 Fax: 0131 527 1746 Email: paul.whatling@rcsed.ac.uk — MB BCh Wales 1990; FRCS Ed.

1995; MD Wales 2003. Dir. Fac. of Med. Informatics, Roy. Coll. of Surg.s of Edin.; Vis. Sen. Lect. Inst. of Health & Med. Univ. of Bath. Specialty: Educat. Socs: Brit. Med. Informatics Soc. Prev: Specialist Regist. (Gen. Surg.) Roy. Berks. Hosp. Reading; Regist. (Gen. Surg.) Wexham Pk. Hosp. Slough; Research Regist. (Vasc. Surg.) Univ. Hosp. Birm. & Univ. Birm.

WHATMORE, Katherine Sarah Howard Cwmbran Village Surgery, Victoria Street, Cwmbran NP44 3JS Tel: 01633 871177 Fax: 01633 860234 Email: kathy.smith@ukgateway.net — MB ChB Bristol 1981; Cert. Family Plann. JCC 1985; DRCOG 1985; MRCGP 1986. GP Appraiser, Dept. Gen. Pract., Univ. Wales Coll. Med.; GP Retainer, Dr. Rowland & Partners, Cwmbran. Socs: BMA. Prev: Partner, Brookside Gp. Pract., Reading; Clin. Asst. (Psychiat.) I. of Wight HA; Trainee GP/SHO I. of Wight VTS.

WHATMORE, Peter Banks (retired) 101 Fairfield Park, Ayr KA7 2AU Tel: 01292 269603 — MRCS Eng. LRCP Lond. 1957 (Guy's) MB BS Lond. 1957, LLB 1951, DPM 1961; FRCPsych 1979, M 1970. Cons. Psychiat. i/c Admin. Douglas Inch Centre Glas. & Scott Home & Health Dept. (Prisons Div.). Prev: Cons. Psychiat. Murray Roy. Hosp. Perth.

WHATMORE, Mr William John The Barn, Vicarage Road, Stoneleigh, Coventry CV8 3DH Tel: 024 76 41470 — MB ChB Ed. 1961; FRCS Ed. 1965. Cons. Neurosurg. Coventry AHA & S. Warks. Health Dist. Specialty: Neurosurg. Socs: Soc. Brit. Neurol. Surgs. Prev: Sen. Regist. (Neurosurg.) Edin. Roy. Infirm.

WHATMOUGH, Philip Michael Ash Vale Health Centre, Wharf Road, Ash Vale, Aldershot GU12 5BA Tel: 01252 317551; 136 Shawfield Road, Ash, Aldershot GU12 6SG — MB BS Lond. 1982 (King's Coll. Hosp.) BSc Lond. 1979; DRCOG 1992; MRCGP 1992. Prev: SHO (Neonat. Intens. Care & Paediat.) St. Mary's Hosp. I. of Wight; Trainee GP Niton Ventnor I. of Wight; SHO (Gen. Med.) St. Mary's Hosp. Newport I. of Wight.

WHEAL, John Derek Launceston Medical Centre, Landlake Road, Launceston PL15 9HH Tel: 01566 772131 Fax: 01566 772223; Sheers Barton, Lawhitton, Launceston PL15 9NJ — MB BChir Camb. 1971 (Guy's) MA Camb. 1972, MB BChir 1971; DObst RCOG 1974; DCH Eng. 1976.

WHEAR, Mr Nicholas Michael Royal Wolverhampton Hospitals NHS Trust, New Cross Hospital, Wednesbury, Wolverhampton Tel: 01902 695405 — MB BS Lond. 1986 (Charing Cross) LDS RCS 1979; BDS (Hons.) Lond. 1978, MB BS (Hons.) 1986; FRCS Ed. 1989; FDS RCS Eng. 1989. Cons. Maxillofacial Surg. Dudley & Wolverhampton NHS Trust; Cons. Maxillofacial, Head & Neck Surg., Dudley NHS Trust. Specialty: Oral & Maxillofacial Surg. Special Interest: Head & Neck Oncol., Microvascular Surg., Salivary gland Surg. Socs: Fell. Brit. Assn. Oral & Maxillofacial Surg.; Brit. Microsurgic. Soc. Prev: Sen. Ho. Off., Neurosurg., Atkinson Morley's Hosp., Feb. 1988 - Aug. 1988; Regist. Oral & Maxillofacial Surg., St. Georges Hospital/Kings Coll. Hosp., Lond., Sep. 1988-Nov. 1990; Senior Registrar, Oral & Maxillofacial Surgery, SW & SE Thames Regional Health Authorities rotaiton, St. Richard's Hospital/St. Thomas' Hospital, Nov. 1990-Apr. 1993.

WHEATCROFT, David John The Coach House, Mill Lane, Stotfold, Hitchin SG5 4NU — MB ChB St. And. 1970. Letchworth Hosp.; Police Surg. Stevenage Div.; Research Asst. UK Prospective Diabetes Study; Clin. Asst. Diabetic Clinic Lister Hosp. Stevenage. Specialty: Diabetes. Socs: BMA. Prev: SHO (Obst.) Barrnurs Home Northampton Gen. Hosp.; Ho. Phys. Gloucester Roy. Hosp.; Ho. Surg. Maryfield Hosp. Dundee.

WHEATCROFT, Mary Susan The Town House, 123-125 Green Lane, Derby DE1 1RZ — MB BChir Camb. 1985; BSc Soton 1980; BA Oxf. 1983; MRCPsych 1991. Cons. Child & Adolesc. Psychiat. S. Derbysh., Ment. Health Trust. Specialty: Child & Adolesc. Psychiat.

WHEATCROFT, Stephen Bentley Dept. Of Cardiology, Kings College Hospital, London SE5 — MB ChB Birm. 1994; BSc (Hons.) Birm. 1991; MRCP 1997.

WHEATER, Andrew William 15 Milner Avenue, Bury BL9 6NG Tel: 0161 705 2850 — MB BS Newc. 1981; BSc (Med. Sci.) St. And. 1978; MRCOG 1989; MSc (Comp Sci.) Manch. 1995. Cons. Gyn. Merseyside Clinic Liverp. Specialty: Obst. & Gyn.

WHEATER, Mary Queen Elizabeth Hospital, Gayton Road, King's Lynn PE30 4ET — MB BChir Camb. 1988 (Cambridge) PhD Camb. 1970; MRCP (UK) 1992; FRCPCH 1997. Cons. Paediat. Qu. Eliz. Hosp. King's Lynn. Specialty: Paediat. Socs: Brit. Paediat. Neurol. Assn.; Fell. Coll. Paediat. & Child Health; Brit. Assn. Perinatal Med. Prev: Sen. Regist. Rotat. Addenbrooke's Hosp. Camb. & Norf. & Norwich Hosp.

WHEATER, Matthew James Abbots Gate, Abbotsbrook, Bourne End SL8 5QS — BM Soton. 1998.

WHEATER, Rebecca Anne 19 Moness Crescent, Aberfeldy PH15 2DL — MB ChB Manch. 1992.

WHEATLEY, Alexander Hugh ENT Department, Great Western Road, Gloucester GL1 3NN — MB ChB Birm. 1991; ChB Birm. 1991; FRCS 1995; FRCS 1996. Cons. ENT/ Head And Neck Surg.

WHEATLEY, Anna Marie Kingswood Health Centre, Alma Road, Kingswood, Bristol BS15 4EJ Tel: 0117 961 1774 Fax: 0117 947 8969 — MB ChB Bristol 1984. Specialty: Gen. Pract. Prev: Trainee GP Brighton HA VTS.

WHEATLEY, Mr Brian Eastfield House, Bellerby, Leyburn DL8 5QP — MB BS Durh. 1962; FRCS Ed. 1967. Dir. Research & Developm. Environm. Contaminants Med. Serv. Br. Dept. Nat. Health & Welf. Ottawa, Canada. Socs: Internat. Leprosy Assn. & BMA. Prev: Asst. Dep. Minister Health Servs. Developm. Dept. Health & Human Resources Yukon Govt., Canada; Assoc. Dir. Gen. Operat. Med. Servs. Br. Dept. Nat. Health & Welf., Canada; Dir. Environm. Contaminants Program, Med. Servs. Br. Dept. Nat. Health & Welf. Canada.

WHEATLEY, Charles Henry 18 Cedar Heights, Petersham, Richmond TW10 7AE — MB ChB Ed. 1946.

WHEATLEY, Christopher John Leyburn Medical Practice, The Nurseries, Leyburn DL8 5AU Tel: 01969 622391 Fax: 01969 624446 — MB BS Durh. 1965; MRCOG 1970; MFFP 1994. Trainer (Gen. Pract.) Leyburn. Prev: GP (Surg. Obst.) Frobisher Bay Gen. Hosp. Baffin Is., Canada; Regist. Leeds Matern. Hosp.; SHO Jessop Hosp. Wom. Sheff.

WHEATLEY, Professor David John Department of Cardiac Surgery, Glasgow Royal Infirmary, 10 Alexandra Parade, Glasgow G31 2ER Tel: 0141 211 4730 Fax: 0141 552 0987 — MD Cape Town 1979; ChM 1976, MB ChB 1964; FRCS Ed. 1969; Dip. in Higher Surgical Training in Cardiothoracic Surgery 1975; FRCS Glas. 1980; FRCP Edin. 1995; FRCS Eng. 1998; FMedSci 1998; FECTS 2002. Prof. Cardiac Surg. Univ. Glas. Specialty: Cardiothoracic Surg. Special Interest: Coronary Surg.; Vasc. Heart Dis. Socs: Eur. Assn. Cardiothoracic Surg.; Soc. Cardiothoracic Surgs. GB & Irel.; Amer. Assn. of Thoracic Surgeons. Prev: Sen. Lect. & Hon. Cons. Cardiac Surg. Univ. Edin.

WHEATLEY, David Pearse Department of Psychological Medicine, Royal Masonic Hospital, Ravenscourt Park, London W6 0TN Tel: 020 8740 9000 Fax: 020 8741 8290; 69 Broughton Avenue, Richmond TW10 7UL Tel: 020 8948 3659 Fax: 020 8948 3659 — MB BChir Camb. 1945 (Camb. & Guy's) MRCS Eng. LRCP Lond. 1945; MA Camb. 1945, MD 1951; FRCPsych 1982, M 1976. Cons. Psychiat. Roy. Masonic Hosp. Lond.; Head GP Research Gp. & Psychopharmacol. Research Gp.; Vis. Sci. (Psychiat.) Univ. S. Florida Tampa, USA; Med. Cons. Feighurer Research Inst. San Diego & Lond. Specialty: Gen. Psychiat. Socs: Hon. Mem. Brit. Assn. Psychopharmacol.; (Ex-Pres.) Internat. Soc. Investig. Stress. Prev: Hon. Med. Assoc. Maudsley Hosp. Lond. i/c Stress Clinic; Edr. Stress Med.; Mem. New Clin. Drug Eval. Unit Nat. Inst. Ment. Health, USA.

WHEATLEY, Donald Stewart Prospect House Surgery, Prospect House, King Street, Carlisle CA7 3AH Tel: 016973 20224 Fax: 016973 23624 — MB BChir Camb. 1971. GP Carlisle.

WHEATLEY, Duncan Angus Royal Cornwall Hospital, Truro TR1 3JW; 19 Knoll Park, Truro TR1 1FF — MB BS Lond. 1992; FRCR 2000.

WHEATLEY, Elizabeth Ann Picu, King's College Hospital, Denmark Hill, London SE5 9LS; 24 Philbeach Gardens, Earls Court, London SW5 9DY — MB BS Lond. 1984 (St. Marys) DA (UK) 1990; FRCA 1993. Cons. Anaesth. and Intens. Care. Specialty: Anaesth.; Intens. Care. Prev: Sen. Regist. Gt. Ormond St. Lond.

WHEATLEY, Emma Catherine Royal Bolton Hospital, Minerva Road, Farnworth, Bolton BL4 0JR Tel: 01204 390762 Fax: 01204 390640 — MB ChB Leeds 1988; MB ChB (Hons.) Leeds 1988; DA (UK) 1991; FRCA 1994. Cons. (Anaesth. & IC) Bolton. Specialty: Anaesth.; Intens. Care. Socs: Med. Protec. Soc.; Intens. Care Soc.

WHEATLEY, Graham, Maj. RAMC Munro Medical Centre, West Elloe Avenue, Spalding PE11 2BY Tel: 01775 725530 Fax: 01775 766168 — BM BS Nottm. 1986; BMedSci Nottm. 1984.

WHEATLEY, Ian Michael Hereward Medical Centre, Exeter Street, Bourne PE10 9XR Tel: 01778 393399 — MB ChB Leic. 1990 (Univ. Leicester) MRCGP 1994; DCH RCP Lond. 1994; (Dip. Primary Care Rheumat.) Bath 2000. Specialty: Gen. Pract. Socs: Primary Care Rheum. Soc.; Brit. Med. Acupunture Soc.

WHEATLEY, Kathleen Anne Wheatley and Macdonald, 163 Birmingham Road, Allesley Village, Coventry CV5 9BD Tel: 024 7640 3250 Fax: 024 7640 5009 — MB ChB Birm. 1976; BSc (Hons.) (Anat.) Birm. 1973; MRCGP 1984; MRCGP 1984; FRCGP 2002.

WHEATLEY, Mr Kevin Edward Sandwell General Hospital, Lyndon, West Bromwich B71 4HJ Email: kevin@wheat.demon.co.uk — MB BS Newc. 1979; FRCS Ed. 1984; FRCS Eng. 1985; MD Newc. 1993; MA (Educat.) Open 2004. Cons. Surg. (Gen. Surg.) Sandwell Gen. Hosp.; Hon. Sen. Lect., Univ. of Birm. Specialty: Gen. Surg. Special Interest: Colorectal. Prev: Career Regist. W. Midl.

WHEATLEY, Margaret (retired) Valley View, Canada Lane, Caistor, Lincoln LN7 6RN — MB ChB Sheff. 1963. Clin. Med. Off. Scunthorpe HA.

WHEATLEY, Peter Kenneth (retired) Southwold, The Plains, Wetheral, Carlisle CA4 8LA Tel: 01228 560610 — MB BS Lond. 1953 (St. Thos.) Prev: Clin. Asst. Whitehaven Hosp.

WHEATLEY, Richard John Old Station Surgery, 39 Brecon Road, Abergavenny NP7 5UH Tel: 01873 859000 Fax: 01873 850163 — MB ChB Bristol 1984; DRCOG 1986; MRCGP 1988. GP Abergavenny. Prev: Trainee GP Avon VTS.

WHEATLEY, Robert Central School Clinic, 158 Whitegate Drive, Blackpool FY3 9HG — MB BS Newc. 1986; MRCP (UK) 1990; MRCPCH 1996. Cons. Community Paediat. Centr. Sch. Clinic Blackpool. Specialty: Community Child Health. Socs: Brit. Assn. Community Child Health. Prev: Sen. Regist. (Community Child Health) Trent RHA, Derby & Leicester; Regist. (Paediat.) Stoke-on-Trent.

WHEATLEY, Robin The Surgery, Front Street, Pelton, Chester-le-Street DH2 1DE Tel: 0191 382 6703 Fax: 0191 382 6715; 26 Harthope Close, Rickleton Village, Washington NE38 9DZ Tel: 0191 417 7503 — MB BS Newc. 1983 (Newc. u. Tyne) MRCGP 1987. Specialty: Gen. Pract.

WHEATLEY, Sally-Anne John Radcliffe Hospital, Nuffield Department of Anaesthetics, Headley Way, Headington, Oxford OX3 9DU Tel: 01865 221590 — MB ChB Ed. 1983; FFARCSI 1991. Cons. Anaesth.

WHEATLEY, Susan Ruth 16 Mayfair Gardens, Boston PE21 9NZ — MB ChB Ed. 1986 (Edinburgh) MRCGP 1991. Prev: GP Lincs.; SHO (ENT & Ophth.) Pilgrim Hosp. Boston; Trainee GP Boston.

WHEATLEY, Trevor Princess Royal Hospital, Lewes Road, Haywards Heath RH16 4EX Tel: 01444 441885 Email: trevor.wheatley@mid-sussex.sthames.nhs.uic — MB BChir Camb. 1974; MA Camb. 1974; MRCP (UK) 1976; MD Camb. 1988; FRCP Lond. 1994. Cons. Phys. Princess Roy. Hosp. W. Sussex; Vis. Lect. (Biochem.) Univ. Sussex. Specialty: Endocrinol. Socs: Amer. Endocrine Soc.; N. Amer. Menopause Soc.; Nat. Osteoperosis Soc. Prev: Clin. Lect. (Med.) Camb. Univ.; Hon. Sen. Regist. Addenbrooke's Hosp. Camb.; Regist. (Med.) Addenbrooke's Hosp. Camb.

WHEATLEY, Victoria Jane 25 Woodleigh Avenue, Birmingham B17 0NW — MB ChB Birm. 1997. Specialty: Gen. Med.

WHEATLEY PRICE, Michael (retired) Manor Lodge, Chew Magna, Bristol BS40 8QE Tel: 01275 332488 — BM BCh Oxf. 1958 (Oxf., Vienna & Westm.) MA Oxf. 1957, BM BCh 1958; Dip. Ven. Soc. Apoth. Lond. 1976. Prev: Cons. Genitourin. Med. Avon AHA (T).

WHEATLEY PRICE, Nicola The Hedges Medical Centre, Eyres Monsell, Pasley Road, Leicester LE2 9BU Tel: 0116 225 1277 Fax: 0116 225 1477 — MB ChB Leic. 1992; DRCOG 1995. GP Leic. Specialty: Gen. Pract.

WHEATLY, Rachel Sarah Wythenshawe Hospital, Manchester M23 9LT Tel: 0161 998 7070 — MB ChB Manch. 1982; DA (UK) 1986; FCAnaesth. 1990. Cons. Anaesth. S. Manch. Univ. Hosps. NHS Trust. Specialty: Anaesth. Prev: Sen. Regist. & Regist. (Anaesth.) NW RHA; SHO (Anaesth.) Chester HA.

WHEBLE, Andrew Marcus North Devon District Hospital, Raleigh Park, Barnstaple EX31 4JB Tel: 01271 322786; Halsinger Farm, Halsinger, Braunton EX33 2NL Tel: 01271 814504 Fax: 01271 816139 — MB BS Lond. 1972 (Kings Coll. Hosp. Med. Sch.) MRCOG 1982; FRCOG 1996. Cons. O & G N. Devon Dist. Hosp. Barnstaple. Specialty: Obst. & Gyn. Prev: Sen. Regist. (O & G) N. West. RHA; Lect. Qu. Charlotte's Hosp. & Chelsea Hosp. for Wom.; Research Regist. John Radcliffe Hosp. Oxf.

WHEBLE, Suzanne Margaret Avicenna, High Street, Hopton, Diss IP22 2QX Tel: 01953 681303 Fax: 01953 681305; Northern House, Fakenham Magna, Thetford IP24 2QX Tel: 01359 268398 — MB BS Lond. 1975 (King's Coll. Hosp.) Prev: GP Knutsford Chesh.; Trainee GP S. Manch. VTS; SHO (Chest & Gen. Med.) Barrowmore Hosp. Gt. Barrow.

WHEBLE, Mr Victor Henry, SBStJ (retired) Spindrift, 4 Higher Ham, Georgeham, Braunton EX33 1JN Tel: 01271 890826 Fax: 01271 891066 — BM BCh Oxf. 1944 (Oxf. & King's Coll. Hosp.) MA Oxf. 1945, BA 1941, BM BCh 1944; FRCS Ed. 1947; DTM & H Antwerp 1947. Prev: Vis. Research Fell. Univ. UMIST & Salford.

WHEELAN, Lorna (retired) 71 Cottenham Park Road, London SW20 0DR Tel: 020 8946 6663 — MD Aberd. 1954; MB ChB 1948; DPM Lond. 1953; FRCPsych 1973. Prev: Cons. King's Coll. Hosp.

WHEELANS, John Craig 11 Ladylands Terrace, Selkirk TD7 4BB — MB ChB Glas. 1998.

WHEELDIN, William Chorley Road Surgery, 65 Chorley Road, Swinton, Manchester M27 4AF Tel: 0161 794 6287 Fax: 0161 728 3415 — MB ChB Manch. 1989; MRCGP 1993.

WHEELDON, Katy 83 Marlborough Avenue, Broomhill, Glasgow G11 7BT — MB ChB Glas. 1998.

WHEELDON, Professor Nigel Mark South Yorkshire Cardiothoracic Unit, Northern General Hospital, Herries Road, Sheffield S5 7AU Tel: 0114 243 4343 Fax: 0114 261 0350 — MB ChB Manch. 1986; MRCP (UK) 1989; MD Manch. 1993; FESC 2000; FRCP 2000. Cons. (Cardiol.) S. Yorks. Cardiothoracic Unit Sheff.; Hon. Prof. Of Internat. Cardiol. Beijing Univ. Beijing PR China; Vis. Prof. Dalian Med. Univ. Dalian PR China. Specialty: Cardiol. Socs: Internat. Fell. of the Hong Kong Coll. of Cardiol.; Brit. Cardiovasc Interven. Soc.; Brit. Cardiac Soc. Prev: Sen. Regist. (Cardiol.) Cardiothoracic Unit North. Gen. Hosp. Sheff.; Sen. Regist. & Lect. (Cardiovasc. Med.) Ninewells Hosp. & Med. Sch. Dundee; Research Regist. (Cardiovasc. Med.) Ninewells Hosp. Dundee.

WHEELDON, Roger St Annes Group Practice, 161 Station Road, Herne Bay CT6 5NF Tel: 01227 742226 Fax: 01227 741439 — MB ChB Sheff. 1968; DCH Eng. 1970. GP Herne Bay. Prev: Regist. (Paediat.) Sheff. Childr. Hosp.

WHEELDON, Veronica Catherine 83 Marlborough Avenue, Broomhill, Glasgow G11 7BT Tel: 0141 339 7099 — MB ChB Glas. 1972. Clin. Med. Off. E. Dist. Gtr. Glas. HB.

WHEELER, Alison West View Surgery, 9 Park Rd, Keynsham, Bristol BS31 1BX Tel: 0117 986 3063 Fax: 0117 986 5061 — MB BS Newc. 1979; DRCOG 1982; MRCGP 1983. GP Princip.

WHEELER, Alyson Jane John Radcliffe Hospital, Headington, Oxford OX3 9DJ; 42 Churchward Close, Grove, Oxford — MB BCh Wales 1992.

WHEELER, Anne Karen The Surgery, Miller Way, Wainscott, Rochester ME2 4LP Tel: 01634 717450; 11 Margetts Place, Lower Upnor, Rochester ME2 4XF — BM BS Nottm. 1985; Cert. Prescribed Equiv. Exp. JCPTGP 1989; DRCOG 1989; MRCGP 1996; DFFP 1998. GP Princip. Specialty: Gen. Pract.

WHEELER, Anthony John — MB BS Lond. 1994 (UCL) BSc (Physiol.) Lond. 1979, MB BS 1994; MRCPCH 1997; MRCP UK 1997. SHO (Paediat.) Roy. Free Hosp. Lond.; Specialist Regist., Donald Winnicott Centre, Coate St., Lond. Specialty: Paediat.

WHEELER, Daniel Wren 130 Victor Road, Penge, London SE20 7JT — BM BCh Oxf. 1994; MA Oxf. 1991; MRCP (Lond.) 1997. SHO (Anaesth.) Greenwich Hosp. Lond. Specialty: Anaesth. Socs: MDU. Prev: SHO (Gen. Med.) Poole Hosp.; SHO (Elderly Care) Poole Hosp.; SHO (A & E) John Radcliffe Hosp. Oxf.

WHEELER, David Collins — MB ChB Birm. 1980 (Birm. Univ.) MRCP (UK) 1984; MD Birm. 1991; FRCP 1999. Sen. Lect. (Nephrol.) Roy. Free & Univ. Coll. Med. Sch. Lond.; Hon. Cons. (Nephrologist) Roy. Free, Hampstead, NHS Trust. Specialty: Nephrol. Special

Interest: Cariovascular compuations of chronic kidney Dis. Prev: Cons. Nephrologist, Univ. Hosp., Birm., NHS Trust.

WHEELER, David Michael Gallions Reach Health Centre, Thamesmead, London SE28 8BE Tel: 020 8333 5000; 3 Gregor Mews, Langton Way, London SE3 7JX — AKC; BSc Lond. 1974, MB BS 1979; DCH RCP Lond. 1981; MRCP (UK) 1983; MRCGP 1987. Course Organiser Greenwich VTS. Prev: Lect. (Gen. Pract.) UMDS Guy's & St. Thos. Hosps. Lond.

WHEELER, David Victor (retired) Highbridge House, High Bridge, Dalston, Carlisle CA5 7DR Tel: 016974 76086 Email: davidwheeler@doctors.net.uk — MB BS Lond. 1967 (Roy. Free) Prev: Princip. GP Dalston Carlisle.

WHEELER, Mr James Malcolm Donald Dept. Of Surgery, Northampton General Hospital, Northampton; 42 Churchward Close, Grove, Wantage OX12 0QZ — MB BCh Wales 1992 (Univ. Wales Coll. Med.) FRCS Eng. 1996; MD Wales 2000. Specialty: Gen. Surg.

WHEELER, Jeremy Stuart The Symons Medical Centre, 25 All Saints Avenue, Maidenhead SL6 6EL Tel: 01628 626131 Fax: 01628 410051; The Coppice, Green Lane, Littlewick Green, Maidenhead SL6 3RH — MB BS Lond. 1981 (Char. Cross) MRCS Eng. LRCP Lond. 1981; DRCOG 1984; MRCGP 1985; DCH RCP Lond. 1985. Clin. Asst. (Paediat.) St. Marks Hosp. Maidenhead; Clin. Med. Off. Bramerton Ment. Handicap Resid. Homes. Specialty: Gen. Med.; Paediat. Socs: Windsor Med. Soc. Prev: Trainee GP Richmond VTS; SHO (Paediat., O & G & Accid.) Centr. Middlx. Hosp. Lond.

WHEELER, Mr John Howard 8 Little Brownings, Sydenham Rise, London SE23 3XJ Tel: 020 8699 1802 — MB BS Lond. 1963 (Char. Cross) FRCS Ed. 1967; FRCS Eng. 1970; LMCC 1985. Cons. Gen. Surg. P.. Rupert. Reg. Hosp. B.C., Canada. Specialty: Gen. Surg. Socs: BMA. Prev: Cons. Gen. Surg. G.R. Baker Hosp. Quesnel B.C., Canada; Cons. Gen. Surg. St. Nicholas Hosp. Lond.; Regist. (Surg.) Gen. Hosp. Nottm. & Char. Cross Hosp. Lond.

WHEELER, Julian Guy Sarum House Surgery, 3 St. Ethelbert Street, Hereford HR1 2NS Tel: 01432 265422 Fax: 01432 358440; Walnut House, Priors Frome, Mordiford, Hereford HR1 4EH — MB BS Lond. 1968 (Guy's) MRCS Eng. LRCP Lond. 1968; DObst RCOG 1970.

WHEELER, Kate Anne Hero Department of Paediatrics, Oxford Radcliffe Hospital, Headley Way, Oxford OX3 9DU Tel: 01865 741166 Fax: 01865 221083 Email: kate.wheeler@paediatrics.oxford.ac.uk; 6 Donnington Square, Newbury RG14 1PJ Tel: 01635 38310 — MB BS Lond. 1976; DRCOG 1978; MRCP UK 1980; MRCGP 1987. Cons. Paediat. (Paediat. Oncol.) Oxf. Radcliffe Hosp. Specialty: Paediat. Socs: FRCPCH; SIOP; BMA. Prev: Sen. Regist. (Paediat.) John Radcliffe Hosp. Oxf.; Leukaemia Research Fell. & Hon. Sen. Regist. (Oncol. & Haemat.) Hosp. Sick Childr. Lond.

WHEELER, Kenneth Mons (retired) Fulford, Tredegar NP22 4LP Tel: 01495 722592 — (Cardiff) BSc Wales 1937, MB BCh (Distinc. Surg. & Pub; Health) 1940. Prev: Med. Off. i/c Geriat. & Isolat. Units Ashvale Hse. Tredegar.

WHEELER, Professor Malcolm Hubert (retired) Aldbourne House, Cottrell Drive, Bonvilston, Cardiff CF5 6TY Tel: 01446 781126 Fax: 01446 781127 Email: m.h.wheeler@btinternet.com — (Wales) MB BCh Wales 1965; FRCS Eng. 1970; MD Wales 1973. Prof. & Cons. Surg. Univ. Hosp. Wales & Roy. Infirm. Cardiff. Prev: Sen. Lect. & Cons. Surg. Welsh Nat. Sch. Med. & Llandough Hosp. Penarth.

WHEELER, Murray Stuart 9 Birfed Crescent, Leeds LS4 2QF — BM Soton. 1993; MRCP 1996. Specialist Regist., Paediatric Intens. Care, Birm. Childrens Hosp. Specialty: Paediat. Prev: Specialist. Reg. Paediat.Hull. Roy. Infirm.

WHEELER, Patrick Clive Gage c/o The William Harvey Hospital, Ashford TN24 0LZ — BM BCh Oxf. 1968 (St. Thos.) DM Oxf. 1977, MA, BM BCh 1968; MRCP (UK) 1971; FRCP Lond. 1987. Cons. Phys. & Gastroenterol. SE kent Health Dist. Specialty: Gastroenterol. Socs: Brit. Soc. Gastroenterol.; BMA. Prev: Cons. Phys. SE Kent Health Dist.; Regist. (Med.) St. Thos. Hosp. Lond.; Lect. & Sen. Regist. King's Coll. Hosp. Med. Sch.

WHEELER, Patrick Crane 286 Victoria Park Road, Leicester LE2 1XE Email: patrickwheeler@doctors.org.uk — MB ChB Leic. 1998; DRCOG 2000; DFFP 2000; MRCGP (Merit) 2003. GPSI (Sports & Musculoskeletal Med.). Specialty: Gen. Pract. Special Interest: Sports & Musculoskeletel Med. Socs: BMA; MDU.

WHEELER, Peter John 82 Sloane Street, London SW1X 9PA Tel: 020 7245 9333 Fax: 020 7245 9232; 4 Chester Row, London SW1 9JH Tel: 0207 730 4727 — MB BS Lond. 1975 (Guy's & King's Coll. Hosp.) BSc (1st cl. Hons. Neurobiol.) Lond. 1971; MRCS Eng. LRCP Lond. 1975; MRCP (UK) 1978; DRCOG 1980; MRCGP 1981. Apoth. to HRH The P. of Wales; Vis. Med. Off. King Edwd. VII Hosp. for Offs. Lond. Socs: Worshipful Soc. Apoth. Prev: Regist. (Med.) King's Coll. Hosp. Lond.

WHEELER, Richard Alexander Edward Aldbourne House, Cottrell Drive, Bonvilston, Cardiff CF5 6TY Tel: 01446 781126 — MB ChB Birm. 1997 (Birmingham) SHO (Gen. Med.), Sutton Coldfield. Specialty: Gen. Med. Socs: BMA; MDU. Prev: Ho. Off. (Renal Med.) Qu. Eliz. Hosp. Edgbaston Birm.

WHEELER, Richard Handley (retired) Kingsclere, 14 Beacon Road, Ditchling, Hassocks BN6 8UL Tel: 01273 843173 — MB BChir Camb. 1942 (Lond. Hosp.) FRCP Lond. 1972, M 1948; DPM Lond. 1950; FRCPsych 1972. Prev: Cons. Psychiat. St. Francis Hosp. Haywards Heath.

WHEELER, Mr Robert Alec Consultant Paediatric Surgeon, Southampton General Hospital, Tremona Road, Southampton SO16 6YD Tel: 02380 794144 Email: robert.wheele@suht.swest.nhs.uk; Haisborough House, Furzey Lane, Brockenhurst SO42 7WB Tel: 01590 612266 — MB BS Lond. 1982 (Char. Cross Hosp. Lond.) FRCS 1988; MS Soton. 1992; FRCPCH 2001; LLB 2003. Cons. Paediat. And Neonat. Surg.; Med. Lawyer, Soton. Univ. Hosp. Trust. Specialty: Paediat. Surg. Socs: Brit. Assn. Paediat. Surg.; SIOP; IPSO. Prev: Resid. Asst. Surg. & (Paediat. Surg.) Gt. Ormond St. Lond.

WHEELER, Roger John Martonside Medical Centre, 1a Martonside Way, Middlesbrough TS4 3BY Tel: 01642 812266 Fax: 01642 828722; 5 Muirfield, Nunthorpe, Middlesbrough TS7 0JN Tel: 01642 300546 — BM BS Nottm. 1981; BMedSci Nottm. 1979; MRCGP 1985; DRCOG 1985; Dip. Ther. Newc. 1995. Prev: GP Princip. N. Ormesby Middlesbrough; GP Trainee Bassetlaw VTS.

WHEELER, Terence Keith (retired) Church Farm., Great Eversden, Cambridge CB3 7HU Tel: 01223 264264 Fax: 01223 264264 — MB BS Lond. 1961 (King's Coll. Hosp.) MRCS Eng. LRCP Lond. 1961; DMRT Eng. 1968; FFR (Rohan Williams Medal) 1970; FRCR 1975. Cons. Clin. Oncol. Addenbrooke's (NHS) Trust Camb. Univ. Teachg. Hosps. Trust Oxf. Anglia RHA. Prev: Sen. Asst. Radiother. Univ. Camb.

WHEELER, Timothy 5 Park Lane, Twyford, Winchester SO21 1QT — BM BCh Oxf. 1968 (St. Bart.) MRCS Eng. LRCP Lond. 1967; MRCOG 1974; DM Oxf. 1979. Sen. Lect. Dept. Human ReProduc. Soton. Univ. Fell. Roy. Soc. Socs: Blair Bell Research Soc.

WHEELER, Valerie Ann Linton Health Centre, Coles Lane, Linton, Cambridge CB1 6JS Tel: 01223 891456 Fax: 01223 890033; 2 Martins Lane, Linton, Cambridge CB1 6NG Tel: 01223 891774 — MB ChB Dundee 1984; DRCOG 1987.

WHEELER, William Frederick (retired) Pond Cottage, Toogoolawah, Partridge Lane, Newdigate, Dorking RH5 5EB Tel: 01293 862468 Fax: 01293 862169 — (St. Thos.) MRCS Eng. LRCP Lond. 1949. Prev: Asst. Chest Phys. (Thoracic Med.) Lond. Chest Hosp.

WHEELEY, Martin St George 3M Health Care Ltd, Morley St., Loughborough LE11 1EP Tel: 01509 613367 Fax: 01509 613030; Farthings Barn, Doctors Lane, Breedon on the Hill, Derby DE73 8AQ — MB BChir Camb. 1973 (Camb. & Guy's) MRCS Eng. LRCP Lond. 1972; MA Camb. 1973; Dip. Pharm. Med. RCP (UK) 1980; FFPM RCP (UK) 1992. Dir. of Pharmacovigilance, Europe. Specialty: Pharmaceutical Medicine. Socs: BMA. Prev: Dir. of Europ. Pharmacovigil.c.a. Wyeth, UK; Dir. Investig.al Drug Safety Bristol-Myers Squibb Brussels, Belgium; GP P'boro.

WHEELWRIGHT, Mr Eugene Frederick 2 Camstradden Drive E., Bearsden, Glasgow G61 4AH Tel: 0141 943 1236 Fax: 0141 557 0468 — MB BS Lond. 1980 (King's Coll. Hosp.) BSc (Pathol.) Lond. 1977; FRCS Eng. 1984. Cons. Orthop. Surg. Glas. Roy. Infirm. & Stobhill Gen. Hosp. Glas. Specialty: Orthop. Prev: Sen. Regist. (Orthop.) Princess Margt. Rose Orthop. Hosp. & Roy. Infirm. Edin.; Regist. (Surg.) Roy. Hallamsh. Hosp. Sheff.; SHO (Orthop.) Roy. Nat. Orthop. Hosp. Stanmore.

WHEILDON, Margaret Hilda Epsom and St Helier NHS Trust, St Helier Hospital, Wrythe Lane, Carshalton SM5 1AA Tel: 020 8296 2000 Fax: 020 8296 2962 Email: mwheildon@sthelier.sghms.ac.uk; Bourton, Blundel Lane, Stoke D'Abernon, Cobham KT11 2SE Tel: 01932 868000 Email: mwheilden@aol.com — (King's Coll. Hosp.) MB BS Lond. 1966; MRCS Eng. LRCP Lond. 1966; DObst RCOG 1968; DA Eng. 1970; FRCA Eng. 1979. Macmillan Cons. Palliat. Med. Epsom & St. Helier NHS Trust. Specialty: Palliat. Med. Prev: Med. Dir. St. Raphael's Hospice Cheam; SHO (Anaesth.) & Ho. Surg. (A & E) King's Coll. Hosp.; Ho. Phys. (Paediat.) Belgrave Hosp. Childr.

WHELAN, Diana Elizabeth Oakbridge, Three Oaks, Hastings TN35 4NG Tel: 01424 752577 — MB BS Lond. 1939; MRCS Eng. LRCP Lond. 1939.

WHELAN, Edmund 5 Stoneycroft Close, Liverpool L13 0AT Tel: 0151 228 6558 — MB ChB Liverp. 1981; FFA RCS Eng. 1985; MA (Med. Ethics) Keele 1993. Cons. Anaesth. St. Helens & Knowsley HA. Specialty: Anaesth. Prev: Sen. Regist. (Anaesth.) Mersey RHA; Research Fell. (Anaesth.) Vanderbilt Univ. Nashville, USA.

WHELAN, Jeremy Simon Department of Medical Oncology, The Middlesex Hospital, Mortimer St., London W1T 3AA Email: j.whelan@ucl.ac.uk; 43 Hillfield Park, Muswell Hill, London N10 3QU — MB BS Lond. 1984; MRCP (UK) 1988; MD Lond. 1993. Cons. Med. Oncol. Middlx. Hosp. Lond. Specialty: Oncol.

WHELAN, Joan Allan (retired) 49 North Castle Street, St Andrews KY16 9BG Tel: 01334 477734 — MB ChB St. And. 1948; DObst RCOG 1950; DA Eng. 1955; FFA RCS Eng. 1974. Prev: Cons. Anaesth. Dr. Grays Hosp. Elgin.

WHELAN, Katherine Manor Farm House, East Carlton, Yeadon, Leeds LS19 7BG Tel: 0113 250 4987 — MB BS Lond. 1971 (Univ. Coll. Hosp.)

WHELAN, Laura Majella 11 Primate's Manor, Armagh BT60 2LP — MB BCh BAO NUI 1980.

WHELAN, Michael Joseph 116 St Micheal's Road, Crosby, Liverpool L23 7UW — MB BCh Wales 1992.

WHELAN, Niall (retired) Arrochar, Meadow Lane, North Cockerington, Louth LN11 7ER — MRCS Eng. LRCP Lond. 1951 (St. Bart.) Clin. Asst. Alfred Morris Head Injury Rehabil. Unit MusGr. Pk. Hosp. Taunton. Prev: Police Surg. Leics. Constab.

WHELAN, Nicholas Hugh Danes Dyke Surgery, 463A Scalby Road, Newby, Scarborough YO12 6UA Tel: 01723 375343 Fax: 01723 501582; Top House, Newlands Road, Cloughton, Scarborough YO13 0AR — MB ChB Sheff. 1984; DRCOG 1988; MRCGP (Distinc.) 1992; Dip. Ther. (Distinc.) Newc. 1996.

WHELAN, Mr Peter Manor Farm House, East Carlton, Yeadon, Leeds LS19 7BG — MB BS Lond. 1971; MS Lond. 1981, MB BS 1971; FRCS Eng. 1975. Cons. Urol. St. Jas. Univ. Hosp. Leeds. Specialty: Urol. Prev: Sen. Regist. (Urol.) Leeds & Bradford; Wellcome Surgic. Research Fell. Nuffield Dept. Surg. Oxf.; John Marshall Fell. in Surg. Path. Univ. Coll. Hosp. Med. Sch. Lond.

WHELAN, Rachel Mary 31 Beehive Hill, Birmingham Rd, Kenilworth CV8 1BY — MB ChB Bristol 1997.

WHELAN, Roxana Josephine Hamilton Derby Road Health Centre, 336 Derby Road, Lenton NG7 2DW Tel: 0115 978 8587 — BM BS Nottm. 1995; BMedSci Nottm. 1993; DCH 1999; DRCOG 2000; MRCGP 2000; DFFP 2001. p/t GP Princip. Nottm. Specialty: Gen. Pract. Special Interest: Family Plann.; Pregn. Crisis; Stud. Teachg. Socs: RCGP; FFPRHC. Prev: SHO (Integrated Med.) Lincoln; SHO (A & E) Doncaster; Ho. Off. (Med.) Lincoln & Ho. Off. (Surg.) Banbury.

WHELAN, Timothy Ranger, Maj. RAMC Retd. Pyle Street Health Centre, The Dower House, 27 Pyle Street, Newport PO30 1JW Tel: 01983 523525 — MB BChir Camb. 1981 (St. Thos.) MA Camb. 1982; DLO RCS Eng. 1990; DGM RCP Lond. 1992; MRCGP 1993; Cert. Family Plann. JCC 1993. GP Princip. Newport Isle of Wight. Specialty: Gen. Pract. Socs: Airborne Med. Soc. Prev: Trainee GP I. of Wight HA; Specialist (ENT Surg.) RAMC.

WHELDON, David Bryant 74 Kimbolton Road, Bedford MK40 2NZ — MB ChB Bristol 1973.

WHELDON, Geoffrey Robert Ridge Garth, Briggswath, Whitby YO21 1RT Tel: 01947 810045 — MB BS Durh. 1945 (Newc. upon Tyne) Prev: Hon. Phys. to H.M. the Qu.; PMO RN Sick Quarters HMS Nelson Portsmouth; Surg. Capt. RN.

WHELDON, Philippa Mary 70 Stanley Road, Cambridge CB5 8LB — MB BS Lond. 1983 (St. Thomas) BA Oxf. 1976; MSc Surrey 1977.

WHELEHAN, Irene Maria 105 Banner Cross Road, Sheffield S11 9HQ Tel: 0114 236 3537 — MB BS Lond. 1990; BSc Lond. 1987; FRCOphth 1994. Regist. (Ophth.) Roy. Hallamsh. Hosp. Sheff. Specialty: Ophth. Prev: SHO Moorfields Eye Hosp. Lond.

WHELEHAN, Joseph Mary (retired) Hillworth Lodge, Devizes SN10 5ET — LRCPI & LM, LRSCI & LM 1947 (RCSI) LRCPI & LM, LRCSI & LM 1947. Prev: Clin. Asst. Roundway Hosp. Devizes.

WHETHAM, Jennifer Margaret School House, Ashmore, Salisbury SP5 5AA — BM BS Nottm. 1997.

WHETSTONE, Sarah Church Street Partnership, 30A Church Street, Bishop's Stortford CM23 2LY Tel: 01279 657636 Fax: 01279 505464 — MB BS Lond. 1983.

WHEYWELL, Roger (retired) Owls Lodge, Forton, Andover SP11 6NU Email: rogerwheywell@hotmail.com — MB ChB Sheff. 1967; FFPM RCP (UK) 1995. Prev: Dir. of Research & Developm. Bayer plc, Pharmaceut. Div.

WHIBLEY, Hannah Kathrine The Cottage, Astley Burf, Stourport-on-Severn DY13 0RX Tel: 01299 826191 — MB BS Lond. 1987 (St Georges.Hosp.Lond) FRCA 1995. Cons. Anaesth. Specialty: Anaesth.

WHICHELLO, Karen Jane The Nook, Withyham Road, Groombridge, Tunbridge Wells TN3 9QP Tel: 01892 863326; Glenandred Lodge, Corseley Road, Groombridge, Tunbridge Wells TN3 9PN Tel: 01892 863699 — MB BS Lond. 1988 (UMDS Guy's) DRCOG 1991; MRCGP 1993. GP Asst. Groombridge, E Sussex. Specialty: Gen. Pract. Prev: Trainee GP Cuckfield VTS; SHO (ENT) Kent & Sussex Hosp. Tunbridge Wells; Ho. Phys. Guy's Hosp. Lond.

WHICHER, Professor John Templeman Rush House, Deighton, York YO19 6HQ Tel: 01904 728237 Fax: 01904 728522 Email: jwhicher@compuserve.com — MB BChir Camb. 1970 (Westm.) MA Camb. 1970; FRCPath 1990, M 1977; MSc Lond. 1977. Indep. Cons. Laborat. Med. Specialty: Chem. Path. Socs: Assn. Clin. Biochems. Prev: Prof. Molecular Path. Experim. Cancer Research Univ. Leeds; Prof. Chem. Path. Univ. Leeds Cons. Chem. Path. Gen. Infirm. Leeds; Cons. Chem. Path. St. Jas. Univ. Hosp. Leeds.

WHILE, Mr Adrian Christopher Anthony Adzor House, Wellington, Hereford HR4 8AP — MB Camb. 1975; BChir 1974; FRCS Ed. 1982; FRCOphth 1992. Cons. Surg. (Ophth.) Vict. Eye Hosp. Hereford. Specialty: Ophth. Prev: Fell. in Vitreoretinal Surg. & Oculoplastic Surg. Moorfields Eye Hosp.; Lond.; Resid. Surgic. Off. Moorfields Eye Hosp. Lond.

WHILE, Janet Anne Newtons Surgery, The Health Centre, Heath Road, Haywards Heath RH16 3BB Tel: 01444 412280 Fax: 01444 416943 — MB BCh Wales 1980 (Welsh Nat. Sch. Med.) DRCOG 1983; MRCGP 1992; MFFP 1995. Specialty: Obst. & Gyn.; Family Plann. & Reproduc. Health.

WHILE, Robin Symington Armstrong Jubilee Field Surgery, Yation Keynell, Chippenham SN14 7EJ Tel: 01249 782204 Fax: 01249 783110 Email: robin.while@gp-j83603.nhs.uk; The Old School, Burton, Chippenham SN14 7NZ Tel: 01249 782959 Fax: 01249 783110 Email: robin.while@gp-j83603.nhs.uk — MB BS Lond. 1972 (St. Bart.) MRCS Eng. LRCP Lond. 1972; Cert. Family Plann. JCC 1975; DObst RCOG 1975; LMCC 1977; FRCGP 2000. Occupat. Health AdviserWavin Bldg. Products; Sen. Lect. Dept. Gen. Pract. Postgrad. Sch. Med. Univ. Bath; Assoc. Adviser (Gen. Pract.) Bath & Swindon; Team Doctor, Bath Rugby PLC. Specialty: Occupat. Health; Sports Med. Socs: Disp. Doctors Assn.; Bath Clin. Soc. Prev: SHO (Obst.) Roy. Berks. Hosp. Reading; SHO (Psychiat.) St. Bart. Hosp. Psychiat. Unit Lond.; SHO (Paediat.) Hillingdon Hosp. Uxbridge.

WHILLIER, David Edward The Surgery, The Pond, East Peckam, Tonbridge TN12 8LP Tel: 01892 833331 Fax: 01892 838269 — MB BChir Camb. 1969 (Camb. & St. Thomas) MA Camb. 1967; DObst RCOG 1972; FRCGP 1993, M 1975; MSc Lond. 1988. GP Princip. Drs Warner, D. Whillier, Anderson, Cheales, Potterton & V. Whillier, Paddock Wood, Kent; Examr. RCGP.; Clin. Goverance Lead & Bd. Mem. Kent Weald PCG. Socs: Counc. Represen. SE Thames Fac. RCGP. Prev: Asst. Dean (CME) S. Thames (E.); Chairm. Twerps Locality Commissioning Gp.; Course Organiser Tunbridge Wells VTS.

WHILLIS, David Radiotherapy Department, Raigmore Hospital, Inverness IV2 3UJ — MB BS Lond. 1978; MRCP (UK) 1983; FRCR

1988. Cons. Radiother. & Oncol. Highland HB. Specialty: Oncol.; Radiother.

WHILLIS, Joanna Elisabeth Helens Lodge, Inshes, Inverness IV2 5BG — MB ChB Sheff. 1980; BMedSci Sheff. 1978, MB ChB 1980; DA Eng. 1984; DRCOG 1986.

WHIMSTER, Jean Helen 15 Johnsburn Haugh, Balerno, Edinburgh EH14 7ND — MB ChB Glas. 1969.

WHINCUP, Graham Hastings District General Hospital, Hastings Tel: 01424 755255; Homestall, The Street, Sedlescombe, Battle TN33 0QD Mob: 07778 266211 Fax: 01424 758068 — MB ChB Bristol 1975; FRCPCH; FRCP Lond. 1981; MD Sheff. 1987. Cons. Paediat. Hastings HA. Specialty: Paediat. Socs: (Pres.) BMA; Chair LNC. Prev: Sen. Regist. (Paediat.) St. Mary's Hosp. Lond. & Northwick Pk. Hosp. Harrow.

WHINCUP, Peter Hynes St. George's Hospital Medical School, Department of Community Health Sciences, London SW17 0RE Email: p.whincup@sghms.ac.uk — MB BChir Camb. 1981; MRCP (UK) 1983; PhD (Epidemiol.) Lond. 1991; MFPHM 1993; FFPHM 1997; FRCP 1997. Prof. St. Geo.'s Hosp. Med. Sch. Specialty: Epidemiol.; Cardiol.; Pub. Health Med. Socs: Brit. Cardiac Soc.; Brit. Hypertens. Soc. Prev: Reader (Epidemiol.) Roy. Free Hosp. Sch. Med. Lond.; Brit. Heart Foundat. Research Fell. Roy. Free Hosp. Sch. Med. Lond.; Regist. (Med.) Ipswich Hosps.

***WHINN, Olivia Hannah** — MB ChB Birm. 1998.

WHINNEY, Mr David John Dickens 14 Osier Crescent, Muswell Hill, London N10 1QU Tel: 020 8442 2549 — MB BS Lond. 1989; FRCS Eng. 1994. Specialty: Otolaryngol.

WHIPP, Elisabeth Clare 25A Alma Road, Bristol BS8 2BZ — BM BCh Oxf. 1972; FRCR 1978; MA Oxf. 1981. Cons. (Radiother. & Oncol.) Bristol Roy. Infirm. Specialty: Oncol.; Radiother. Prev: Sen. Regist. (Radiother. & Oncol.) Hammersmith Hosp. Lond.

WHIPP, Rev. Margaret Jane Westlands, 12 St Charles Road, Tudhoe Village, Spennymoor DL16 6JY Tel: 01388 811461 — MB ChB Sheff. 1979; BA Oxf. 1976; MRCP (UK) 1982; FRCR 1986; FRCP 1988. Cons. (Palliat. Med.) Hartlepool Dist. Hospice; Med. Dir. Sunderland St. Benedict's Hospice. Specialty: Palliat. Med.; Oncol.; Radiother. Prev: Med. Dir. Hartlepool & Dist. Hospice; Regist. (Med. Rotat.) Roy. Hallamshire Hosp. Sheff.; Cons. (Clin. Oncol.) Weston Pk. Hosp. Sheff.

WHIPPLE, Sarah Jane Bridget Grove Medical Centre, Wantage Tel: 01235 770079; 21 Hampden Road, Wantage OX12 7DP Tel: 01235 770079 — MRCS Eng. LRCP Lond. 1980; Dip Family Plann. 1984. p/t Ptnr Grove Med. Centre, Wantage, Oxon; Asst. at N. Bicester Surg. Specialty: Gen. Pract.; Audiol. Med. Socs: BMA. Prev: Clin. Med. Off. (Community Child Health) W. Berks. Health Serv.; Resid. MO Camden Dist. NSW, Austral.; Clin. Asst. Chorleywood Elm Pract. Herts.

WHIPPMAN, Sarah Caroline Ranworth Surgery, 103 Pier Avenue, Clacton-on-Sea CO15 1NJ — MB ChB Liverp. 1995; BClinSci Liverp. 1994; DRCOG 1997; DFFP 2000. Salaried GP Tendring PCT. Specialty: Gen. Pract.

***WHISHAW, Evelyn Mary Watson** Mead, Meadrow, Godalming GU7 3BZ Tel: 01483 415026 — LMSSA Lond. 1960.

WHISKER, Lisa Jane 20 Windmill Drive, Croxley Green, Rickmansworth WD3 3FD — MB ChB Birm. 1998.

WHISKER, Richard Barrington 42 Shepherds Croft, Portland DT5 1DJ; 42 Shepherds Croft, Portland DT5 1DJ — MB ChB Leeds 1980. Assoc. Specialist Anaesth., W. Dorset Hosps.

WHISKER, William Barrington Pennine Lodge, Old Lane, Sowerby Bridge HX6 4PA — MB ChB Bristol 1957; DPH 1962; MFCM 1972. Cons. Community Phys. Oldham AHA & Proper Off. Oldham Metrop. DC. Specialty: Gen. Med. Prev: MOH Dewsbury Co. Boro.

WHISTLER, David Mark The Mote Medical Practice, St Saviours Road, Maidstone ME15 9FL Tel: 01622 756888 Fax: 01622 672573; Home Ville, Mill Bank, Headlorn, Ashford TN27 9RD Tel: 01622 891592 — MB ChB Cape Town 1979 (UCT) MRCGP 1986.

WHISTON, Rhona Jayne Grosvenor Medical Centre, Grosvenor Street, Crewe CW1 3HB — MB ChB Liverp. 1993.

WHISTON, Mr Richard John University Hospital of Wales, Heath Park, Cardiff CF14 4WZ Tel: 029 2074 3576; 18 Heol-y-Felin, Rhiwbina, Cardiff CF14 6NB Tel: 029 2052 2991 — BM BS Nottm. 1986 (University of Nottingham) BMedSci Nottm. 1984; FRCS Eng. 1991; DM Nottm. 1995. Cons. Gen. & Vasc. Surg. Univ. Hosp. Wales Cardiff. Specialty: Gen. Surg.; Vasc. Med. Prev: Regist. (Gen. Surg.) Univ. Hosp. Wales Cardiff.; SHO (A & E) Derbysh. Roy. Infirm.; SHO (Gen. Surg.) Nottm.

WHITAKER, Andrew Spencer — MB ChB Manch. 1980; DRCOG 1983; MRCGP 1984. Prev: Trainee GP Cumbria VTS; Ho. Phys. & Ho. Surg. Roy. Lancaster Infirm.

WHITAKER, Anthony John 123 Skegby Lane, Mansfield NG19 6PF — MRCS Eng. LRCP Lond. 1973 (Leeds) FRCA 1978. Cons. Anaesth. i/c Intens. Care Kings Mill Hosp. Mansfield. Specialty: Anaesth. Socs: Assn. Anaesths. & BMA; Intens. Care Soc.

WHITAKER, Mr Bernard Langdon (retired) Urquhart House, 71 High St., Buntingford SG9 9AE Tel: 01763 271293 — MB BS Lond. 1949 (Guy's) MRCS Eng. LRCP Lond. 1949; FRCS Eng. 1957; MS Lond. 1971. Prev: Cons. Surg. Co. Hosp. Hertford & Qu. Eliz. II Hosp. Welwyn Gdn. City.

WHITAKER, Brian Carrstones, Halifax Road, Ripponden, Sowerby Bridge HX6 4AH Tel: 01422 822444 — MB ChB Leeds 1957; DObst RCOG 1965. Med. Off. Overgate Hospice Elland. Specialty: Palliat. Med. Socs: MRCGP; Fell. BMA. Prev: GP W. Yorks.; Ho. Surg. Leeds Gen. Infirm.; Ho. Phys. & Ho. Off. (Obst.) Halifax Gen. Hosp.

WHITAKER, David Kenneth 22 Pine Road, Manchester M20 6UZ Tel: 0161 445 8474 — BM BS Nottm. 1975; BMedSci (Hons.) Nottm. 1973, BM BS 1975; FFA RCS Eng. 1980. Cons. (Anaesth.) Manch. Roy. Infirm. Specialty: Anaesth. Socs: Manch. Med. Soc.; FRSM. Prev: Sen. Regist. (Anaesth.) Roy. Perth Hosp. West. Australia; Regist. (Anaesth.) Wythenshawe Hosp. Manch.; Ho. Phys. Univ. Dept. Therap.

WHITAKER, Donald Callum 65 Marlborough Park Avenue, Sidcup DA15 9DL Tel: 020 8300 4970 Email: donald@doctors.org.uk — MB ChB Ed. 1993 (Edinburgh) FRCS (Ed.) 1997. Specialist Regist. (Cardiothoracic) S. Thames Rotat. Specialty: Cardiothoracic Surg. Prev: Res. Fell. (Cardiothoracic Surg.) Middlx. Hosp. Lond.

WHITAKER, Geoffrey Brian (retired) 25 Exeforde Avenue, Ashford TW15 2EF Tel: 01784 254408 — (Westm.) MB BS Lond. 1949; DObst RCOG 1951. Prev: Obst. Ho. Surg. New End Hosp. Hampstead.

WHITAKER, George Robert Bruce (retired) White Edge, The Bent, Curbar, Calver, Sheffield S32 3YD — MB ChB Sheff. 1947.

WHITAKER, Graham 14 St Fagans Drive, St. Fagans, Cardiff CF5 6EF — MB BS Lond. 1992.

WHITAKER, Helen Jane Eccleston Health Centre, 20 Doctors Lane, Eccleston, Chorley PR7 5RA Tel: 01257 451221 Fax: 01257 450911 — MB ChB Leic. 1988.

WHITAKER, Ian Michael 25 Fossway, York YO31 8SF — MB ChB Aberd. 1972; BMedBiol 1969; MRCPsych 1977. Assoc. Fac. Homoeop.

WHITAKER, James Alexander John Milford Crossroads Surgery, Church Rd, Godalming GU8 5QR Tel: 01483 414461 Email: hamish.whitaker@gp-h81031.nhs.uk; East Overton, Brook, Godalming GU8 5UH — MB BS Lond. 1981 (Lond. Hosp.) MA Camb. 1981; MRCGP 1987. GP Milford.; GP Tutor Guildford. Prev: Trainee GP Epsom Dist. Hosp. VTS.

WHITAKER, Joan Winfield 35 Mayfair Gardens, Woodford Green IG8 9AB Tel: 020 8504 0819 — LRCP LRCS Ed. 1952; Asst. MOH Waltham Forest; LRCP LRCS Ed. LRFPS Glas. 1952; DObst RCOG 1957. Prev: O & G Regist. Coventry & Warw. Hosp.; Ho. Surg. Simpson Memor. Pavil. Roy. Infirm. Edin.

WHITAKER, John Joseph Harrogate District Hospital, Lancaster Park Road, Harrogate HG2 7SX Tel: 01423 885959 Fax: 01423 881139 — MB ChB Ed. 1979; MRCP (UK) 1982; FRCP London 1996. Cons. Geriat. Med. Harrogate Healthcare NHS Trust. Specialty: Care of the Elderly.

WHITAKER, Jonathan Faraday (retired) Home Farmhouse, Puttenham, Guildford GU3 1AR Tel: 01483 810632 — (Univ. Coll. Hosp.) MB BS Lond. 1957; DObst RCOG 1963. Prev: Ho. Surg. Roy. North. Hosp.

WHITAKER, Margaret Rosevear (retired) 21 Dene Park, Didsbury, Manchester M20 2GF — MB ChB Manch. 1949. Prev: Med. Off. Regional Blood Transfus. Serv. Manch.

WHITAKER, Mark John Didsbury Medical Centre, 645 Wilmslow Road, Didsbury, Manchester M20 6BA Tel: 0161 445 1957 Fax: 0161 434 9931; 13 Pine Road, Didsbury, Manchester M20 6UY —

MB ChB Manch. 1982; BSc (Hons.) Manch. 1976. Hosp. Practitioner, Gastroenterol.

WHITAKER, Nicola Tracey Hall Floor Flat, 28 West Park, Bristol BS8 2LT — MB ChB Bristol 1985.

WHITAKER, Philip John 27 Beaumont Street, Oxford OX1 2NR Tel: 01865 311500 Fax: 01865 311720 — BM BS Nottm. 1990; MRCGP 1995; DFFP 1995; MA Univ. E. Anglia 1996. GP Princip. Oxf.; Forens. Med. Examr., Thames Valley Police, Oxf. Specialty: Gen. Pract.

WHITAKER, Mr Robert Henry (retired) 10 Summerfield, Cambridge CB3 9HE Tel: 01223 719340 Fax: 01223 719523 — MB BChir Camb. 1964 (Univ. Coll. Hosp.) MA Camb. 1964, MD 1986, MChir 1967; FRCS Eng. 1967. Asst. Clin. Anatomist Univ. Camb. Prev: Sen. Lect. (Urol.) Lond. Hosp. Med. Coll.

WHITAKER, Roger X-Ray Department, Derbyshire Royal Infirmary, Derby — MB ChB Manch. 1952; Cons. Radiol Derby Hosp. Gp; DMRD Eng. 1959; FFR 1961.

WHITAKER, Sarah Patricia Haslemere Health Centre, Church Lane, Haslemere GU27 2BQ — MB BS Lond. 1980.

WHITAKER, Simon Charles Department of Radiology, University Hospital, Nottingham NG7 2UH Tel: 0115 924 9924; The Hazels, Pk Avenue, Plumtree Park, Nottingham NG12 5LU Tel: 0115 937 2775 — MB BChir Camb. 1983 (Camb. & Middlx.) MA, MB Camb. 1983, BChir 1982; MRCP (UK) 1985; FRCR 1989. Cons. Radiol. Univ. Hosp. Nottm. Specialty: Radiol. Prev: Sen. Regist. (Radiol.) Univ. Hosp. Nottm.; SHO (Neurol.) The Brook Hosp. Lond.; SHO (Med.) Roy. Sussex Co. Hosp. Brighton.

WHITAKER, Stephen Gerard Dr Whitaker & Partners, Locks Road Surgery, 51 Locks Road, Locks Heath, Southampton SO31 7ZL Tel: 01489 583777 Fax: 01489 571374 Email: stephen.whitaker@gp-J82023.nhs.uk; Dr Whitaker & Partners, Whiteley Surgery, Yew Tree Drive, Whiteley, Fareham PO15 7LB Tel: 01489 881982 Fax: 01489 881980; 83 Raley Road, Locks Heath, Southampton SO31 6PB Tel: 01489 601272 Fax: 01489 601744 Email: sgwhit@ntlworld.com — MB ChB Ed. 1975; BSc Edin. 1972. Specialty: Gen. Pract. Socs: BMA. Prev: Trainee GP Dudley & Stourbridge VTS; Ho. Off. (Gen. Med.) Bangour Gen. Hosp. Broxburn; Ho. Off. (Gen. Surg.) Greenock Roy. Infirm.

WHITAKER, Stephen John 24 The Crescent, Belmont, Sutton SM2 6BJ — BM Soton. 1981; MRCP (UK) 1985; FRCR 1989.

WHITAKER, Tom (retired) 21 Dene Park, Didsbury, Manchester M20 2GF Tel: 0161 445 2560 — (Manch.) MB ChB Manch. 1949; LLB Lond. 1965. Prev: GP Manch.

WHITAKER, Valerie Suzanne Whitaker and Partners, 53 Bridge Street, Brigg DN20 8NS Tel: 01652 657779 Fax: 01652 659440; Blueberry House, 1 Maltkiln Lane, Brigg DN20 0RC — MB ChB Manch. 1980; BSc St. And. 1977; DRCOG 1982; MRCGP 1984; Member Institute of Psychosexual Medecine 1991. Socs: Inst. Psychosexual Med. Prev: GP Kirton Lindsey; Trainee GP E. Cumbrian VTS; Ho. Surg. Salford Roy. Hosp.

WHITAKER, William Stoke House, Bar Lane, Wakefield WF1 4AD Tel: 01924 372374 — (Leeds) MB ChB (Hons.) Leeds 1943; BSc (Hons.) Leeds 1941, MD 1946; FRCP Lond. 1963, M 1948. Emerit. Cons. Phys. Leeds Gen. Infirm. Specialty: Gen. Med. Socs: Assn. Phys. & Irel. & Cardiac Soc. Prev: Sen. Clin. Lect. (Med.) Univ. Leeds; Cons. Cardiol. United Leeds Hosps.; Cons. Phys. Leeds RHB.

WHITBREAD, Rhoderick Peter Wragby Surgery, Old Grammar School Way, Wragby, Market Rasen LN8 5DA Tel: 01673 858206 Fax: 01673 857622; 13 Minster Road, Lincoln LN2 1PW — MB BS Lond. 1976 (King's College Hosp.) FRCGP 1994. Princip. in GP; Adviser in BP Lincs.

WHITBREAD, Mr Timothy, Wing Cdr. Department of Surgery, Royal hospital Haslar, Haslar Road, Gosport PO12 2AA Tel: 02392 584255 Fax: 02392 762960 — MB BS Lond. 1982 (Guys hospital) FRCS Eng. 1990; FRCS Gen 1998. Cons. In Gen. And Vasc. Surg., Roy. Hosp. Halsar, Gosport, Hants..; Cons. Vasc. Surg., Qu. Alexandrra Hosp.; Roy. Coll. Surgic. tutor. Specialty: Gen. Surg.

WHITBY, Mr David Jonathan Palstic Surgery Department, BUPA Hospital, Russell Road, Whalley Range, Manchester M16 8AJ Tel: 0161 226 0312 — MB BS Lond. 1979 (Char. Cross) MRCS Eng. LRCP Lond. 1979; FRCS Eng. 1983; T(S) 1992. Cons. Plastic Surg. BUPA Hosp. Manch. Specialty: Plastic Surg. Socs: Brit. Assn. of Plastic Surg.s (BAPS); Brit. Assn. of Aesthetic Plastic Surg.s (BAAPS); Craniofacial Soc. of Gt. Britain & Irel. (- Hon. Edit. Represen.). Prev: Cons. Plastic Surg. Univ. Hosp. S. Manch.; Sen. Regist. (Plastic Surg.) St. Jas. Univ. Hosp. Leeds; Regist. (Plastic Surg.) Univ. Hosp. S. Manch.

WHITBY, Elizabeth Barbara Scarborough Hospital, Scarborough YO12 6QL — MB BS Lond. 1975; FRCS Eng. 1982. Cons. ENT ScarBoro. Dist. Gen. Hosp. Specialty: Otolaryngol.

WHITBY, James Douglas (retired) 127 Warkton Lane, Barton Seagrave, Kettering NN15 5AP — MRCS Eng. LRCP Lond. 1943; MA Camb. 1950, MB BChir 1947; DA Eng. 1949; FFA RCS Eng. 1954. Prev: Anaesth. Gen. Hosp. Newc.

WHITBY, Margaret Evelyn The Red Practice, Waterside Health Centre, Beaulieu Road, Hythe SO45 5WX Tel: 023 8084 5955 Fax: 023 8020 1292; Homefield, Fritham, Lyndhurst SO43 7HL Tel: 02380 812132 — MB ChB Sheff. 1983; MRCGP 1989; D.Occ.Med. Lond. 1996.

WHITBY, Peter James 1 Becontree Road, Liverpool L12 2BD — MB ChB Sheff. 1997.

WHITBY, Rachel Margaret John Anthony Centre, Newtown Road, Ronkswood, Worcester WR5 1HN — MB ChB Birm. 1979.

WHITBY, Robin James 3 Broom Way, Kettering NN15 7RB Tel: 01536 522133 — MB BS Lond. 1975 (Roy. Lond. Hosp. Med. Coll.) DRCOG 1977. GP Kettering. Socs: Kettering & Dist. Ethical Comm. Prev: Trainee GP Hemel Hempstead; SHO Rotat. (Surg.) Norf. & Norwich Hosp.; SHO (A & E) Harold Wood Hosp.

WHITBY, Ruth 991 Finchley Road, London NW11 7HB Tel: 020 8455 6710 Email: ruth.whitby@chello.at — MB BS Lond. 1989 (King's Coll.) BSc (1st cl. Hons.) Lond. 1989; DRCOG 1993; Japanese Med. Licence 1994. Well Woman Clinic Hillside Med. Centre. Special Interest: Well Woman Med. Prev: GP St Geo. Med. Centre Lond. NW4; SHO (Paediat.) St Mary's Hosp. Lond.; GP Tokyo 1994-97.

WHITBY, Sydney 37 Ravenscourt, Thornton Hall, Glasgow G74 5AZ Tel: 0141 644 5800 — LRCP LRCS Ed. 1951 (Anderson Coll. Med., Glas.) LRCP LRCS Ed. LRFPS Glas. 1951. Socs: BMA. Prev: Ho. Surg. Roy. Sussex Co. Hosp.

WHITBY, Thomas Edgar (retired) Tyddyn-y-Traeth, Broad Beach Road, Rhosneigr LL64 Tel: 01407 810392 — MB ChB Liverp. 1936; MRCS Eng. LRCP Lond. 1938.

WHITBY-SMITH, Brett James Wharf Road, Ash Vale, Aldershot GU12 5BA Tel: 01252 317551 Fax: 01252 338194 Email: brett.whitby-smith@gp-h81013.nhs.uk; Copse End, Glaziers Lane, Normandy, Guildford GU3 2EB — MB BS Lond. 1978 (Roy. Free) MRCS Eng. LRCP Lond. 1978; DRCOG 1981; MRCGP 1983.

WHITCHER, David Martin The Tollerton Surgery, 5-7 Hambleton View, Tollerton, York YO61 1QW Tel: 01347 838231 Fax: 01347 838699 — MB ChB St. And. 1971. Prev: Regist. (Med.) York Dist. Hosp.; SHO (Med.) Soton. Univ. Hosps.

WHITCHER, Harold Wray, OBE, TD 5 Broadlands, Farnborough GU14 7ER; 5 Broadlands, Farnborough GU14 7ER — MB ChB Ed. 1939 (Univ. Ed.) MA Oxf. 1954. Socs: Fell. Roy. Soc. of Med.

WHITCOMBE, Elizabeth Marion 44 Regent's Park Road, London NW1 7SX Tel: 020 7586 2436 — MB ChB Otago 1981; MA New Zealand 1960; MA Oxf. 1962; PhD Lond. 1967.

WHITCROFT, Ian Andrew 38 Sheerwater Close, Padgate, Warrington WA1 3JE — MRCS Eng. LRCP Lond. 1979; MD Liverp. 1986, MB ChB 1979; MRCP (UK) 1982; MD Washington DC 1984; Cert. Family Plann. JCC 1986; T(M) 1995. Reader (Dermat.) Univ. Brit. Columbia, Canada. Prev: Att. Phys. (Internal Med.) Pierce Co. Health Dept. Tachma Wash. USA; Att. Phys. (Internal Med. & Emerg.) Wentworth Douglas Hosp. Dover NH, USA.

WHITCROFT, Sovra Isabella Jan Department of Obstetrics & Gynaecology, Royal Surrey County Hospital, Egerton Road, Guildford GU2 7XX Tel: 01483 571122 — MB ChB Liverp. 1981; MRCOG 1989. Cons. O & G Roy. Surrey Co. Hosp. Guildford. Specialty: Obst. & Gyn. Prev: Sen. Regist. (O & G) John Radcliffe Hosp. Oxf.; Regist. & SHO (O & G) Southmead Hosp. Bristol; SHO (O & G) Gen. & Matern. Hosps. Bristol.

WHITE, Adrian Roger Peninsula Medical School, Room N32, ITTC Building, Tamar Science Park, Derriford, Plymouth PL6 8BX Tel: 01752 764448 Fax: 01752 764234 Email: adrian.white@pms.ac.uk; Acupuncture Clinic, 13 Peverell Park Road, Peverell, Plymouth Tel: 01752 764448 Mob: 07790 710497 Email: whitear@doctors.org.uk; 11 Essa Road, Saltash PL12 4ED Tel: 01752 843462 — BM BCh Oxf. 1972 (Oxf. & Middlx.) MA Oxf.

1972; DObst RCOG 1975; MD (Med. Studies) Peninsula Med. Sch., Exeter and Plymouth Universities 2004. Clin. Research Fell., Gen. Pract. and Primary Care, Peninsula Med. Sch., Universities of Exeter and Plymouth; Edr. Acupunc. Med. Brit. Med. Acupunc. Soc. Lond. Specialty: Acupunc.; Research. Special Interest: Acupunc.; Clin. Research. Socs: Brit. Med. Acupunct. Soc. Prev: Sen. Lect. (Complementary Med) Peninsula Med. Sch. Univ. Exter & Plymouth; Editor-in-chief Complementary Therapies in Med; Research Fell. (Complementary Med.) Postgrad. Med. Sch. Univ. Exeter.

WHITE, Aideen St Claire 44 Westwood Road, Beverley HU17 8EJ — MB BCh BAO Dub. 1979.

WHITE, Aileen Royal Alexandra Hospital, Corsebar Road, Paisley PA2 9PN Tel: 0141 880 4417 — MB ChB Aberd. 1978; FRCS Glas. 1983; FRCS Ed. 1984. Cons. Otolaryngologist, Roy. Alexandra Hosp., Paisley; Hon. Sen. Clin. Lect., Glas. Univ. Specialty: Otolaryngol. Special Interest: Head and Neck Surgical Oncology; laryngology. Socs: BMA; BAOHNS.

WHITE, Alan Anthony James Fullarton Practice, 40 Dalblair Road, Ayr KA7 1UL Tel: 01292 264260 Fax: 01292 292160; 8 Pattle Place, Alloway, Ayr KA7 4PS Tel: 01292 441402 — MB ChB Glas. 1983; DObst 1985; MRCGP 1987. GP Ayr. Prev: SHO (Dermat.) Glas. Roy. Infirm.; Trainee GP/SHO Monklands Dist. Hosp. VTS; Ho. Off. Glas. Roy. Infirm.

WHITE, Mr Alan Edward Thomas Department of Orthopaedics, Southend General Hospital, Prittlewell Chase, Westcliff on Sea SS0 0RY Tel: 01702 221063 — MB BCh Wales 1987; FRCS Ed. 1992; FRCS Eng. 1992; FRCS (Orth.) 1997. Cons. Orthop. Surg. Southend Hosp. Specialty: Orthop. Special Interest: Lower Limb Jt. Replacement. Prev: Sen. Regist. (Orthop.) Roy. Nat. Orthop. Hosp. Stanmore; Clin. Lect. Univ. Coll. Lond.; Regist. (Orthop.) Roy. Nat. Orthop. Hosp. Stanmore.

WHITE, Albert Edward (retired) 69 Park Parade, Whitley Bay NE26 1DU Tel: 01632 252 3135 — MB BS Durh. 1945. Prev: Ho. Surg. G.B. Hunter Memor. Hosp. Wallsendon-Tyne & Profess. Surg. Unit, Roy. Vict. Infirm. Newc.

WHITE, Alexander 5 Balgair Road, Glasgow G63 0PP — LRCP LRCS Ed. 1950 (St. Mungo's Coll. & Univ. Glas.) LRCP LRCS Ed. LRFPS Glas. 1950. Regist. Roy. Vict. Disp. Edin. Socs: BMA. Prev: Res. Med. Off. Honey La. Hosp. Waltham Abbey; Ho. Surg. Roy. Infirm. Glas.; Res. Asst. Phys. Belvidere Infec. Dis. Hosp. Glas.

WHITE, Alfred Charles Queen Elizabeth Psychiatric Hospital, Edgbaston, Birmingham B15 2QZ Tel: 0121 678 2014 Fax: 0121 678 2208 Email: alfred.white@6smht.nhs.uk — MB BS Lond. 1970 (King's) MRCS Eng. LRCP Lond. 1970; DPM Eng. 1973; FRCPsych 1991, M 1974; MD Lond. 1981. Cons. Psychiat. (Liaison Psychiat.) Qu. Eliz. Psychiat. Hosp. Birm. Specialty: Gen. Psychiat. Special Interest: Civil Forens. Psychiat.; Head Injury. Socs: Medico legal Soc.; Birm. Med. Inst.

WHITE, Andrew James 41 Fairview Street, Cheltenham GL52 2JF — MB BS Lond. 1988; BSc (Hons.) Lond. 1985; DTM & H Lond. 1991; MRCP Lond. 1998. SpR (Resp. Med.) W. Midlands. Prev: SHO (Med.) Cheltenham Gen. Hosp.; Tuberc. Prog. Coordinator East. Nepal Britain-Nepal-Med. Trust; Ho. Surg. Gloucester Roy. Hosp.

WHITE, Andrew John Crofton Health Centre, Slack Lane, Crofton, Wakefield WF4 1HJ Tel: 01924 862612 Fax: 01924 865519 — MB ChB Dundee 1975. Prev: Trainee GP Salisbury VTS; SHO (Gen. Med. & Geriat.) N.gate Hosp. Gt. Yarmouth.

WHITE, Andrew John 51 Clogher Road, Lisburn BT27 5PQ — BChir Camb. 1995.

WHITE, Andrew Mark — MB BCh Wales 1984 (Cardiff) Med. Advis. Drivers Med. Gp. DVLA Swansea. Prev: Med. Advis. SEMA; GP Pencoed, Bridgend.

WHITE, Andrew Peter Anaesthetic Department, Milton Keynes Hospital, Eaglestone, Milton Keynes MK6 5LJ Tel: 01908 660033 Fax: 01908 660033 — MB BS Lond. 1980 (Charing Cross) FFA RCS Eng. 1987. Cons. Anaesth. Milton Keynes Hosp. Specialty: Anaesth. Prev: Sen. Regist. Rotat. (Anaesth.) Oxf.; Regist. (Anaesth.) St. Bart. Hosp. Lond.

WHITE, Andrew William Ware Road Surgery, 77 Ware Road, Hertford SG13 7EE Tel: 01992 414500; 120 London Road, Ware SG12 9LY — MB BS Lond. 1983; MRCGP 1988; DRCOG 1991.

WHITE, Angela The Cripps Health Centre, University Park, Nottingham NG7 2QW Tel: 0115 950 1654 Fax: 0115 948 0347; 35 Prestwood Drive, Aspley, Nottingham NG8 3LY — MB ChB Birm. 1969; BA (Hons.) Open 1992. Phys. Univ. Health Serv. Nottm.

WHITE, Angela 16 Milton Avenue, Bath BA2 4QZ — MB ChB Bristol 1995. Specialty: Orthop.

WHITE, Ann Bernadette Lakeside Medicial Centre, Erne Hospital, Cornagrade Road, Enniskillen BT74 6AY Tel: 028 6632 7192 Fax: 028 6632 8686 — MB BCh BAO NUI 1984.

WHITE, Ann Catherine 2 Glebe Street, St Clements, Oxford OX4 1DQ; Appartment 12A, 929 Massachusetts Avenue, Cambridge MA02139, USA — BM BCh Oxf. 1996. Residency (Program in Paediats.) Massachussetts Gen. Hosp. Boston, USA. Specialty: Paediat. Socs: Amer. Acad. Paediat. Prev: Hse Off. (Med.) John Radcliffe, Oxf.; Hse Off. (Surg.) Torbay Hosp. Torquay.

WHITE, Anne Jean The Surgery, 3 Heyward Road, Southsea PO4 0DY Tel: 023 9273 7373; 72 Parkstone Avenue, Southsea PO4 0QZ Tel: 01705 731122 — MB ChB Manch. 1972; DObst RCOG 1974; FRCGP 1997. GP Tutor. Prev: SHO (Paediat.) & SHO (O & G) St. Mary's Hosp. Portsmouth; SHO (Med.) Roy. Portsmouth Hosp.

WHITE, Anthony Buckingham Terrace Surgery, 31 Buckingham Terrace, Glasgow G12 8ED Tel: 0141 221 6210 Fax: 0141 211 6232; 5 Arnwood Drive, Glasgow G12 0XY Tel: 0141 357 1921 — MB ChB Aberd. 1966.

WHITE, Anthony David Department of Medicine for the Elderly, Wrexham Maelor Hospital, Croesnewydd Road, Wrexham LL13 7TD; Ty r Pinwydd, Wesley Road, Bwlchgwyn, Wrexham LL11 5UY — MD Camb. 1991; MB 1975, BChir 1974; MRCP (UK) 1985; FRCP (Ed.) 1995; FRCP (Lond.) 1996. Cons. Phys. Med. for Elderly Wrexham Maelor Hosp. Wrexham. Specialty: Care of the Elderly. Socs: Brit. Geriat. Soc. Prev: R.I.D.E. Research Fell. & Hon. Sen. Regist. (Geriat. Med.) Univ. Hosp. Wales Cardiff; Regist. (Gen. Med.) Lister Hosp. Stevenage; Regist. (Geriat. Med.) Qu. Hosp. Croydon.

WHITE, Anthony George 152 Harley Street, London W1G 7LH Tel: 020 7935 8868 Fax: 020 7224 2574 — MB ChB Bristol 1959; FRCP Lond. 1980, M 1966; DPhysMed Eng. 1971. Cons. Rheum. Roy. Free Hosp. & Whittington Hosp. Lond.; Hon. Med. Dir. N. Lond. Sch. Physiother. & Hon. Sen. Lect. (Clin. Med.) Clin. Sc. UCL. Specialty: Rehabil. Med.; Rheumatol. Socs: FRSM; Brit. Soc. Rheum. Prev: Sen. Regist. Roy. Free Hosp. Lond.

WHITE, Anthony John Simon Rookery Medical Centre, Rookery House, Newmarket CB8 8NW Tel: 01638 665711 Fax: 01638 561280; Wayside, Fordham Road, Newmarket CB8 7AQ — MB BChir Camb. 1972; MA Camb. 1972; DCH Eng. 1973; MRCP (UK) 1974; MRCGP (Distinc.) 1980; FRCGP 1987. Approved Clin. Teach. & Trainer Camb. Univ. Med. Sch; Asst. Dir. (Gen. Pract.) Univ. Camb. Clin. Med. Sch. Specialty: Gen. Pract. Prev: Clin. Asst. (Paediat.) Newmarket.

WHITE, Ashley Margaret Woodlands Surgery, 146 Halfway Street, Sidcup DA15 8DF Tel: 020 8300 1680 Fax: 020 8309 7020 — MB ChB Aberd. 1968; FRCS; DCH. GP.

WHITE, Mr Barrie David Department of Neurosurgery, University Hospital, Queen's Medical Centre, Nottingham NG7 2UH Tel: 0115 970 9925 Fax: 0115 970 9104 — MB BS Lond. 1982 (King's Coll.) BSc (Hons.) Pharmacol. CNAA 1977; MRCP (UK) 1986; FRCS Lond. 1987; FRCS (SN) 1994. Cons. Neurosurg. Univ. Hosp. Qu. Med. Centre Nottm. Specialty: Neurosurg. Prev: Sen. Regist. & Regist. (Neurosurg.) Univ. Hosp. Qu. Med. Centre Nottm.; Regist. (Neurosurg.) Nat. Hosp. Nerv. Dis. Lond.; SHO (Surg. & Med.) Roy. United Hosp. Bath.

WHITE, Bronwen Myfanwy Dykes Hall Medical Centre, 156 Dykes Hall Road, Sheffield S6 4GQ Tel: 0114 232 3236; 138 Brooklands Crescent, Sheffield S10 4GG — MB ChB Ed. 1973; DObst RCOG 1976; MRCGP 1977.

WHITE, Caroline Claire 46 The Avenue, Ingol, Preston PR2 7AY — BM BS Nottm. 1998.

WHITE, Catharine Peta Department of Child Health, Morriston Hospital, Swansea SA6 6NL Tel: 01792 285047 Fax: 01792 285244; 45 Eaton Crescent, Uplands, Swansea SA1 4QL — MB BS Lond. 1980 (Guy's Hosp. Lond.) MRCP (UK) 1984; FRCPCH 1997; FRCP 1999. Cons. Paediat. Neurol. Swansea NHS Trust; Hon. Lect. (Child Health) Univ. of Wales Coll. of Med. Specialty: Paediat. Neurol. Prev: Sen. Regist. (Paediat. Neurol.) Liverp. Childr. Hosp.

WHITE, Catherine Elizabeth Princess Road Surgery, 471-475 Princess Road, Withington, Manchester M20 1BH Tel: 0161 445 7805 Fax: 0161 448 2419 — MB ChB Manch. 1987.

WHITE, Catherine Mary (retired) — MB ChB Glas. 1951; FRCPCH; DCH Eng. 1958; MRCP Lond. 1966; DTM & H Liverp. 1988. Prev: Cons. Paediat., Stockport & Macclesfield Dist. Hosp.s.

WHITE, Catherine Sylvia Northenden Health Centre, 489 Palatine Road, Northenden, Manchester M22 4DH Tel: 0161 998 3206 Fax: 0161 945 9173; 24 Atwood Road, Didsbury, Manchester M20 6TD Email: cathswhite@hotmail.com — MB ChB Liverp. 1988; DRCOG; DCH RCP Lond. 1991; MRCGP 1994; DMJ 1998. Forens. Phys. Manch.

WHITE, Chester, MBE, TD Darwin College, Cambridge CB3 9EU Tel: 01223 335660 Fax: 01223 335667; Grafton House, 22 Grafton St, Cambridge CB1 1DS Tel: 01223 356174 Fax: 01223 368 624 — (Oxf. & St. Mary's) BA 1956, BSc, MA 1959, BM BCh Oxf. 1960; PhD 1974, MA Camb. 1969; MSc Oxf. 1982. Praelector & Emerit. FELL Darwin Coll. Camb.; Med. Off. TWI Ltd; Med. Off. Camb. ACF. Specialty: Blood Transfus.; Occupat. Health; Haematology. Socs: FRSM; Harveian Soc.; BMA. Prev: Sen. Regist. (Path.) P'boro. Hosp.; Head Dept. Clin. Research Huntingdon Research Centre; Sen. Asst. Research (Med.) Univ. Camb.

WHITE, Christine Rosemary c/o Department of Childs Health, Pendragon House, Treliske Hospital, Truro TR1 3XQ — BChir Camb. 1971; MA, MB.

WHITE, Christopher James 1, The Paddocks, Lodge Hill, Caerleon, Newport NP18 3BZ — MB BCh Wales 1976; DRCOG 1979; MRCGP 1980. Sen. partner GP Princip.

WHITE, Christopher Paul The Surgery, Sydenham House, Mill Court, Ashford TN24 8DN Tel: 01233 645851 Fax: 01233 638281; (Surgery), Sydenham House, Church Road, Ashford TN24 8DN — MB BS Lond. 1970.

WHITE, Claire 8 Coolshinney Park, Magherafelt BT45 5JG — MB BCh Belf. 1998.

WHITE, Clement John (retired) 9 Church Side, Farnsfield, Newark NG22 8ET Tel: 01623 883152 — MB BS Lond. 1953 (Lond. Hosp.) DA Eng. 1959; FFA RCS Eng. 1963. Prev: Cons. Anaesth. Mansfield & Dist. Gen. Hosp. Harlow Wood Orthop. Hosp. & King's Mill Hosp. Sutton-in-Ashfield.

WHITE, Mr Clive Meldon Little Studley, Parkland, Bramhope, Leeds LS16 9AJ — MB BS Lond. 1970; FRCS Eng. 1975; MS Lond. 1983. Cons. Gen. Surg. Dewsbury Dist. Hosp. Specialty: Gen. Surg.

WHITE, Colin 35 Newington Road, Middlesbrough TS4 3EF — MB BS Newc. 1992.

WHITE, Colin Pontefract General Infirmary, Pontefract WF8 1PL Tel: 01977 606250; 43 Newgate, Pontefract WF8 1NG Tel: 01977 795074 Email: whitedrc@aol.com — MB ChB St. And. 1969; BSc (Biochem. & Physiol.) (1st cl. Hons.) St. And. 1966; MRCP (UK) 1972; FRCP Glas. 1984; FRCP Lond. 1990. Gen. Med. Diabetes & Endocrinol. Specialty: Diabetes; Endocrinol.; Gen. Med. Socs: BMA; Brit. Diabetic Assn. (Med. & Scientif. Sect.). Prev: Sen. Regist. (Med.) Manch. Roy. Infirm.; Lect. (Metab. Med.) Manch. Roy. Infirm.; Regist. (Med.) Glas. Roy. Infirm.

WHITE, Conor Vincent Health Centre, Great James Street, Londonderry BT48 7DH Tel: 028 7137 8522 — MB BCh BAO Belf. 1980; DRCOG 1983.

WHITE, Conrad North Durham Health Care NHS Trust, Department GU Medicine, University Hospital of North Durham, Durham DH1 5TW Tel: 0191 333 2660 Fax: 0191 333 6901 — MB ChB Ed. 1980 (Edinburgh) MRCOG 1986; Dip. GUM Soc. Apoth. Lond. 1989. Cons. Genitourin. Med. Durh. & Bishop Auckland. Specialty: Genitourinary Medicine. Socs: MSSUD (Mem. of Counc. 99/02); AGUM Prev: Sen. Regist. (Genitourin. Med.) Cardiff; Regist. (O & G) Ninewells Hosp. Dundee & Bangour Gen. Hosp. Broxburn.

WHITE, Craig Alisdair Summerpole, Brilley, Whitney-on-Wye, Hereford HR3 6JH — MB BS Lond. 1998.

WHITE, Craig Steven (retired) Aston Clinton Surgery, 136 London Road, Aston Clinton, Aylesbury HP22 5LB Tel: 01296 630241 Fax: 01296 630033 — MB BS Lond. 1990; DRCOG 1994; MRCGP 1995.

WHITE, Daniel Paul Department of Psychological Medicine, St. Bartholomew's Hospital, London EC1A 7BE Tel: 020 8510 8606 Fax: 020 8510 8716 — MB BS Lond. 1984; DA (UK) 1989; MRCPsych 1993. Cons. (Emerg. & Adult Psychiat.) St. Bart. & Homerton Hosps. Lond.; Clin. Tutor St Bart. SHO Rotat. Psychiat. Specialty: Gen. Psychiat. Prev: Sen. Regist. Rotat. (Adult Psychiat) St. Bart. Hosp. Lond.

WHITE, Daphne Winifred 27 The Green, Dunmurry, Belfast BT17 0QA — MB BCh BAO Belf. 1970; MRCP (UK) 1974.

WHITE, David Anthony Mulberry House, Castleford, Normanton & District Hospital, Lumley Street, Hightown, Castleford WF10 5LT Tel: 01977 605526 Fax: 01977 605501 — MB ChB Liverp. 1992; BSc (Hons.) 1989; MRCPsych 1997; Post Grad. Dip. Cog.Ther. Durham 1999; M Med Sci 1999; CCST 2001. Specialist Regist. Child & Adolesc. Psychiat. Specialty: Child & Adolesc. Psychiat. Socs: Roy. Coll. Psychiats.; ACPP; BMA.

WHITE, David Anthony 19 Chestnut Grove, Harrogate HG1 4HS — MB ChB Leeds 1994.

WHITE, David George Newpark Surgery, Talbot Green, Pontyclun CF72 8AJ Tel: 01443 228922 Fax: 01443 228319 — MB BCh Wales 1980; DRCOG 1984; MRCGP 1985. GP Talbot Green.

WHITE, David Harper Norton Medical Centre, Billingham Road, Norton, Stockton-on-Tees TS20 2UZ Tel: 01642 360111 Fax: 01642 558672; The Grove, Coal Lane, Wolviston, Billingham TS22 5LW Tel: 01740 644764 — MB BS Lond. 1980 (St. Mary's) DRCOG 1983; MRCGP 1986.

WHITE, David John Rosehill Surgery, 189 Manchester Road, Burnley BB11 4HP Tel: 01282 428200 Fax: 01282 838492; Kiddrow Lane Health Centre, Kiddrow Lane, Burnley — MB ChB Manch. 1988 (Oxford & Manchester) MA Oxf. 1989; MRCGP 1992; MFFP 1995. Princip. Gen. Pract.; PCG Bd. Mem. & Clin. Governance Lead (Caldicott Guardian); Bd. Mem. Deputising Serv.; Mem. Instruc. Doctor GP Clin. Trial Panel Fac. of Family Plann.; Broadcasting Dr. BBC Radio Lancs. Socs: BRd.casting Doctors; BMA; Soc. Occupat. Med.

WHITE, David John, MBE (retired) Placketts, High St., Adderbury, Banbury OX17 3LS Tel: 01295 812679 — MB BS Lond. 1959 (Univ. Coll. Hosp.) DObst RCOG 1962.

WHITE, David John Hawthorn House, Birmingham Heartlands Hospital, Birmingham B9 5SS Tel: 0121 424 3365 — MB ChB Sheff. 1983; FRCP 1997. Cons. Genitourin. Med. Birm. Heartlands Hosp.; Hon. Sen. Clin. Lect. Univ. Birm. Specialty: Genitourinary Medicine. Socs: Med. Soc. Study VD; Brit. Soc. Study Vulval Dis.

WHITE, David John Kalson 412 Whirlowdale Road, Sheffield S11 9NL Tel: 0114 236 8466 — MB BS Newc. 1963; FFA RCSI 1968; FFA RCS Eng. 1969. Cons. Anaesth. N. Gen. Hosp. Sheff. Specialty: Anaesth.

WHITE, Mr David Robert Dryburn Hospital, North Road, Durham DH1 5TW — MB BS Lond. 1977 (St. Mary's) BA Camb. 1974; FRCS Ed. 1983; FRCOG 1984. Cons. O & G N. Durh. Acute Hosps. Specialty: Obst. & Gyn. Prev: Sen. Regist. (O & G) Mersey RHA; Regist. (O & G) Aberd. Matern. Hosp. & St. Davids Hosp. Bangor.

WHITE, Davinia Marion 57 Dartmouth Road, Willesden, London NW2 4EP — MB ChB Otago 1979; FRACP 1987.

WHITE, Dawn Helen Brookside Health Centre, Brookside Road, Freshwater PO40 9DT Tel: 01983 753433 Email: rsimcock@doctors.org.uk — MB BS Lond. 1987; DRCOG 1994. GP. Specialty: Gen. Pract. Socs: Diplomate RCOG. Prev: Trainee GP/SHO Harold Wood Hosp. Romford VTS; Ho. Off. (Gen. Med.) Char. Cross Hosp. Lond.; Ho. Off. (Gen. Surg.) Hemel Hempstead Hosp.

WHITE, Deborah St Pauls Surgery, Orams Mount, Winchester SO22 5DD Tel: 01962 853599 — MB BCh Wales 1993; MRCGP 2000. GP St Pauls Surg. Winchester. Specialty: Gen. Pract.

WHITE, Denis Michael Drummond (retired) Dolbeau, 1 Wall Park Road, Brixham TQ5 9UE — MD Bristol 1970; MB ChB 1960; DPM Eng. 1963; FRCPsych 1984, M 1971. Prev: Cons. Psychiat. Dept. Ment. Health of Elderly Hereford HA.

WHITE, Denis Simpson, OBE Hill Medical Group, The Hill, 192 Kingsway, Belfast BT17 9AL Tel: 028 9061 8211 Fax: 028 9060 3911; Cosy Lodge, 23 Church Avenue, Dunmurry, Belfast BT17 9RS Tel: 01232 610540 — MB BCh BAO Belf. 1968; MICGP; DObst RCOG 1970; DCH RCPSI 1970; FRCGP 1986, M 1972. Socs: Ulster. Med. Soc; Provost NI Fac.RCGP; Lagan Valley GP Assn. (Ex-Chairm.). Prev: Ho. Off. Roy. Vict. Hosp. Belf. Roy. Matern. Hosp. Belf. & Roy. Belf.; Hosp. Sick Childr.

WHITE, Denise Mary Milton Keynes General Hospital, Standing Way, Eaglestone, Milton Keynes MK6 5LD Tel: 01908 243430; 11 Westbroke Gardens, Romsey SO51 7RQ Tel: 01794 523822 — BM

Soton. 1982; MRCP (UK) 1985; MRCPath 1992; DM Soton. 1995. Cons. Haematologist; Clin. Director Path. Specialty: Haematology. Special Interest: Thrombophilia. Socs: Brit. Soc. Haematol.; Roy. Coll. of Pathologists. Prev: Hon. Regist. Leukaemia Research Fund Clin. Train. Fellowship; Sen. Regist. (Haemat.) Bath HA.

WHITE, Derek Alexander British Telecommunications plc, BT Centre (pp A167), 81 Newgate St., London EC1A 7AJ Tel: 020 7356 4816 Fax: 020 7356 6047 — MB ChB Ed. 1966; BSc (Hons.) (Pharmacol.) Ed 1964; MRCGP 1972; DIH Soc. Apoth. Lond. 1977; FFOM RCP Lond. 1992, MFOM 1982, AFOM 1980. Chief Med. Off. BT plc. Specialty: Occupat. Health. Socs: FRSM; Soc. Occupat. Med. Prev: Med. Off. E. Scotl. Occupat. Health Serv.; Med. Off. Cape Industries Ltd.; GP Stirling.

WHITE, Diana Elizabeth Medical Centre, Cambridge Avenue, Bottesford, Scunthorpe DN16 3LG Tel: 01724 842415 Fax: 01724 271437; 70 West Common Gardens, Old Brumby, Scunthorpe DN17 1EH Tel: 01724 863481 — MB BS Newc. 1975; DRCOG 1980.

WHITE, Diana Gillian Department of Pathology, East Glamorgan NHS Trust, Pontypridd CF38 1AB Tel: 01443 218218 Fax: 01443 216040; Court Lea, Camerton Hill, Camerton, Bath BA2 0PS Tel: 01761 470782 — (Birmingham) MB ChB Birm. 1967; MSc (Med. Microbiol.) Lond. 1976; FRCPath 1989, M 1977. Cons. Microbiologist E. Glam. Gen. Hosp. Mid Glam. Specialty: Med. Microbiol. Socs: Assn. Clin. Path. & Brit. Soc. Antimicrobiol. Chemother.; Assn. Med. Microbiologists. Prev: Cons. Microbiol. & Dir. Pub. Health Laborat. Roy. United Hosp. Bath; Squadron Ldr. RAF Med. Br. Med. Off. (Path.) RAF Hosp. Cosford.

WHITE, Donna Ann 33 St Patrick's Way, Wigan WN1 3EJ — MB ChB Manch. 1993.

WHITE, Dorothy Gertrude 3 Fairholme Gardens, York Road, Farnham GU9 8JB Tel: 01252 737904 — MB BCh BAO Belf. 1968 (Qu. Univ. Belf.) FFA RCSI 1973. Cons. (Anaesth.) Frimley Pk. Hosp. Specialty: Anaesth. Prev: Sen. Regist. (Anaesth.) Roy. Vict. Hosp. Belf. & Craigavon Area Hosp.

WHITE, Dragana (retired) Watergore, 142 Busbridge Lane, Godalming GU7 1QJ Tel: 01483 421012 — MD Belgrade 1953; LRCP LRCS Ed. LRFPS Glas. 1959. Prev: Assoc. Specialist Milford Hosp. Godalming.

WHITE, Eileen (retired) Shere, 66 Parklands Road, Chichester PO19 3DU Tel: 01243 782055 — MB BCh BAO NUI 1961. Prev: Assoc. Specialist (Anaesth.) Roy. W. Sussex Hosp.

WHITE, Elizabeth Antonia Crouch Oak Family Practice, 45 Station Road, Addlestone, Weybridge Tel: 01932 840123; Stonehill Lodge, Stonehill Road, Ottershaw, Chertsey KT16 0EW Tel: 01932 875155 Fax: 01932 875303 — MB ChB Manch. 1972 (Manchester) MRCP (U.K.) 1974; DObst RCOG 1975; MRCGP 1986. Prev: Ho. Surg. & Ho. Phys. Withington Hosp. Manch.

WHITE, Elizabeth McCallum 4 Tremough Barton Cottages, Mabe, Penryn TR10 9EZ Email: drlizwhite@btopenworld.com; 4 Tremough Barton Cottages, Mabe, Penryn TR10 9EZ Email: drlizwhite@btopenworld.com — MB ChB Ed. 1962; DPH Lond. 1964; DCH Eng. 1967; MD Ed. 1973; FFPHM RCP (UK) 1989, M 1974. Indep. Cons.; Cons. Communiable DisCl. Control, Cornw. & Ios HA. Specialty: Pub. Health Med. Socs: FRSM. Prev: Cons. AIDS Task Force Europ. Community with Jamaican Nat. AIDS Control Progr.; Sen. Clin. Lect. (Internat. Community Health) Liverp. Sch. Trop. Med.

WHITE, Eric George — MB BS Newc. 1976; MRCP (UK) 1980.

WHITE, Fionuala Ann High Street Medical Group Practice, 29 High Street, Draperstown, Magherafelt BT45 7AB Tel: 028 7962 8201 Fax: 028 7962 7523 — MB BCh BAO NUI 1982.

WHITE, Frances Elizabeth Dept Radiology, Royal Liverpool Hospital, Prescot St., Liverpool L7 8XP Tel: 0151 706 2000; Pine Ridge, Dawstone Road, Heswall, Wirral CH60 0BT — MB BS Lond. 1972 (St. Bart) DMRD Eng. 1978; FRCR 1979; FRCP (U.K.) 1996. Med. Director Royal. L'pool. Univ. Hosp. Trust; Quality Assur. Radiologist NHSBSP NW. Region. Specialty: Radiol. Prev: Cons. Radiol. Freeman Rd. & Newc. Gen. Hosps.; Cons. Radiol. St. Bart. Hosp. Lond.

WHITE, Frances Mary 7 Marlborough Avenue, Bromsgrove B60 2PG Tel: 01527 72975 — MB ChB Leeds 1949; DObst RCOG 1951. JP; Med. Off. Dept. Surg. BromsGr. Gen. Hosp. Socs: Counc. BMA (Centr. Comm. Hosp. Med. Servs.).

WHITE, Gary John 19 Burgh Road, Prestwick KA9 1QU — MB ChB Glas. 1986.

WHITE, Gavin James 30 Southcroft Road, London SW17 9TR Tel: 020 8353 12893417 — MB BCh BAO Dub. 1992. SHO (Surg.) St. Geo. Hosp. Lond. Prev: Cas. Off. Lagan Valley Hosp. Lisburn; Anat. Demonst. Trinity Coll. Dub.; Ho. Off. (Surg.) Meath Hosp. Dub.

WHITE, Genie Yasmin The Surgery, Parkwood Drive, Warners End, Hemel Hempstead HP1 2LD Tel: 01442 250117 Fax: 01442 256185; Mentmore Views, Buckland Village, Aylesbury HP1 2LD — MB BS Lond. 1992; DRCOG 1995; MRCGP 1996. GP Princip. Specialty: Gen. Pract.

WHITE, George Baird 1 Sandleigh, Hoole, Chester CH2 3QN — MB ChB Aberd. 1968.

WHITE, George Malcolm James (retired) South Ryehill, Nunthorpe Village, Middlesbrough TS7 0NR Tel: 01642 316040 — MB ChB St. And. 1952; FFA RCS Eng. 1959. Indep. Cons. Anaesth. Cleveland. Prev: Anaesth. Specialist RAF Hosp. Halton.

WHITE, Gillian Mary 13 Princes Road, London SW19 8RQ — MB BS Lond. 1990.

WHITE, Gillian Patricia Windermere Health Centre, Goodley Dale, Windermere LA23 2EG Tel: 015394 42496; Lowthwaite Farm House, St. Johns in the Vale, Keswick CA12 4TS — MB BS Newc. 1985; DRCOG 1987; MRCGP 1989. Prev: Trainee GP Carlisle VTS.

WHITE, Gordon Bentley Bruce (retired) 5 Meadway, Upton, Wirral CH49 6JG Tel: 0151 677 4573 — MRCS Eng. LRCP Lond. 1946 (Univ. Coll. Hosp.) FRCPath; Dip. Bact. Lond 1950. Prev: Cons. Microbiol. PHLS Liverp.

WHITE, Graham Lingholme Health Centre, Atherton St., St Helens WA10 2HT Tel: 01744 22612 Fax: 01744 454493; Dial House, Higher Lane, Rainford, St Helens Tel: 01744 882734 — MB ChB Manch. 1959; DObst. RCOG 1962. Hosp. Pract. Rainhill Hosp. Socs: BMA & Vasectomy Advancem. Soc. Gt. Brit.

WHITE, H. John (retired) Himley Cottage, School Road, Himley, Dudley DY3 4LG Tel: 01902 893082 — MB ChB Birm. 1950; DObst. RCOG 1954. JP. Prev: Chairm. Dudley Family Pract. Comm. 1973-87.

WHITE, Harry Vere (retired) 14 Millfield Gardens, Hexham NE46 3EG — LMSSA Lond. 1949 (Camb. & Manch.) BA Camb. 1942; DPM Eng. 1966; MRCPsych 1972. Prev: Sen. Med. Off. HM Prison Maidstone.

WHITE, Mr Harvey 149 Harley Street, London W1G 6DE Tel: 020 7935 4444 Fax: 020 7616 7633; 7 Arlington Square, Islington, London N1 7DS Tel: 020 7226 4628 — BM BCh Oxf. 1961 (St. Bart.) MCh Oxf. 1970, DM 1967, MA 1961; MRCS Eng. LRCP Lond. 1962; FRCS Eng. 1970. Cons. Surg. Roy. Marsden Hosp. Lond. & King Edwd. VII Hosp. Offs. Lond. Specialty: Gen. Surg. Socs: Med. Soc. Lond. (Pres.); Hon. Mem. Edr. Roy. Soc. Med. 1990.; Chairm. Roy. Soc. Of Med. Press. Prev: SHO Hosp. Sick Childr. Gt. Ormond St. Lond.; Ho. Surg. Surgic. Unit & Sen. Regist. (Surg.) St. Bart. Hosp. Lond.

WHITE, Hazel Lorraine 58 Grimshaw Lane, Bollington, Macclesfield SK10 5LY — MB BChir Camb. 1993.

WHITE, Helen Dorothy 32 New La, Penwortham, Preston PR1 9JJ — MB ChB Liverp. 1997.

WHITE, Henry Gordon Budbrooke Medical Centre, Slade Hill, Hampton Magna, Warwick CV35 8SA Tel: 01926 403800 Fax: 01926 403855 — MB BS Lond. 1982 (St. Mary's Hosp.) BA Camb. 1979; DCH Lond. 1984; DRCOG Lond. 1986; MRCGP 1987. GP. Specialty: Gen. Pract.

WHITE, Henry Maxwell (retired) 7 Marlborough Avenue, Bromsgrove B60 2PG Tel: 01527 872975; 7 Marlborough Avenue, Bromsgrove B60 2PG Tel: 01527 872975 — (Leeds) MB ChB Leeds 1947; MRCS Eng. LRCP Lond. 1947; DObst RCOG 1951; MRCGP 1964. Prev: Mem. Bd. Sc. & Educat. (BMA). 1976-1988.

WHITE, Hugh Southmead Hospital, Southmead Road, Westbury-on-Trym, Bristol BS10 5NB Tel: 0117 959 5623; Old Garden House, Honey Hall Lane, Congresbury, Bristol BS49 5JX Tel: 01934 852230 — MB ChB Ed. 1975; BSc (Physiol.) Ed. 1972; FRCPath 1983; DMJ Path) Soc. Apoth. Lond. 1993. Cons. Histopath. Southmead Hosp. Bristol; Home Office Path. Avon & Som. Hants, Wilts. Specialty: Forens. Path. Socs: Brit. Assn. Forens. Med. Prev: Sen. Regist. (Path.) Edin. Univ.

WHITE, Iain Harvey Laich Medical Practice, Clifton Road, Lossiemouth IV31 6DJ Tel: 01343 812277 Fax: 01343 812396;

Traighean, Station Court, Burghead, Elgin IV30 — BSc (Med. Sci.) Ed. 1972, MB ChB 1975; DRCOG 1978; MRCGP 1980; DCH RCP Lond. 1985.

WHITE, Ian Leslie 23 Cross Lane, Frimley Green, Camberley GU16 6LP — MB BS Lond. 1991 (King's Coll. Sch. Med. & Dent. Lond.) Regist. Rotat. (Anaesth.) Hammersmith Hosp. Lond. Specialty: Anaesth. Socs: BMA; Assn. Anaesth.

WHITE, Ian Richard 152 Harley Street, London W1G 7LH Tel: 020 7935 3834 Fax: 020 7620 0890 — MRCS Eng. LRCP Lond. 1976 (Guy's) BSc Lond. 1973; MB BS Lond. 1976; MRCP (UK) 1978; DIH Lond. 1983; FRCP Lond. 1993; FFOM 2000; CChem. FRCS 2001; Cchem.FRCS 2001. Cons. Dermat. St. John's Inst. Dermat. St. Thos. Hosp. Lond.; Chairm. Scientif. Comm. for Cosmetic & Non- Food Prodicts. DG Sanco Europ. Commiss.; Mem. Scientif. Steering Comm. Europ. Commiss.; Advis. Comm. Borderline Substs Dept. of Health. (Chairm.). Specialty: Dermat. Socs: Europ. Soc. Contact Dermat.; Europ. Environm. & Contact Dermatitis research Gp.. Prev: Cons. & Sen. Regist. (Dermat.) St. John's Hosp. Dis. Skin Lond.; Regist. (Dermat.) Guy's Hosp. Lond.

WHITE, Ian Russell 9 Blinkbonny Avenue, Edinburgh EH4 3HT — MB ChB Aberd. 1994.

WHITE, Jacqueline Rosemary Phillips (retired) 55 Cumberland Street, Woodbridge IP12 4AQ — (Oxf.) BM BCh Oxf. 1959; MA Oxf. 1959. Prev: SCMO Dorset HA.

WHITE, Mr James Robertson Angus (retired) Trevear, The Saltings, Lelant, St Ives TR26 3DL — MB ChB St And. 1936; FRCS Ed. 1939. Prev: Cons. Surg. W. Cornw. Hosp. Penzance & St. Michael's Hosp. Hayle.

WHITE, Jane Caroline Gilbert Road Medical Group, 39 Gilbert Road, Bucksburn, Aberdeen AB21 9AN Tel: 01224 712138 Fax: 01224 712239 — MB ChB Aberd. 1988 (Univ. Aberd.) MRCGP 1992; DCCH RCP Ed. 1993; DFFP 1994; DRCOG 1994. Specialty: Gen. Pract. Prev: SHO (A & E) Stirling Roy. Infirm. & Raigmore Hosp. Inverness; SHO (Community Psychiat.) Dingleton Hosp. Melrose.

WHITE, Jane Crossman (retired) Bartestree House, Bartestree, Hereford HR1 4DT — MB ChB Birm. 1952; DObst RCOG 1954. Prev: Sen. Community Med. Off. (Family Plann.) HFDS Community Health NHS Trust.

WHITE, Janet Beryl Deliverance Church Medical Services, PO Box 1544, Mbale, Uganda; c/o Mr & Mrs V. Coles, 205 Farmers Close, Witney OX28 1NS Tel: 01993 772469 Fax: 01993 776073 Email: vernon.coles@btinternet.com — MB BS Lond. 1975 (St Mary's London) BSc (Hons.) (Psychol.) Lond. 1972; DA Eng. 1978; DRCOG 1979; MRCGP 1980. Dep. Director Med. Serv. Deliverance Ch. Uganda. Specialty: Gen. Pract. Prev: Doctor i/c King's Med. Centre, Nakuru, Kenya; GP Witney.

WHITE, Janet Fiona Church House, Condover, Shrewsbury SY5 7AA — BM Soton. 1987; MRCPsych 1993.

WHITE, Janet Mary (retired) 39 Sunnyfield, Mill Hill, London NW7 4RD Tel: 020 8959 6348 — MB BS Lond. 1952 (St. Mary's) DCH Eng. 1955.

WHITE, Janine Patricia Tyle House, Llanmaes, Llantwit Major CF61 2XZ — MB BCh Wales 1974; MRCP (UK) 1977; MD Wales 1988; FRCP Lond. 1994. Cons. Phys. Roy. Glamorgan Hosp. Specialty: Respirat. Med. Prev: Hon. Sen. Regist. (Med.) Llandough & Sully Hosps.; Research Fell. (Thoracic Med.) Guy's Hosp. Lond.; Lect. (Tuberc. & Chest Dis.) Wales.

WHITE, Jason Noble — MB ChB Glas. 1994; MRCGP.

WHITE, Jean Alexandra Finaghy Health Centre, 13-25 Finaghy Road South, Belfast BT10 0BX Tel: 028 9020 4444 — MB BCh BAO Belf. 1970; MRCGP 1985. Socs: RCGP; Ulster Med. Soc. Prev: Ho. Off. Roy. Vict. Hosp. Belf.; SHO Roy. Matern. Hosp. Belf.

WHITE, Jean Haddow (retired) 107 Marine Avenue, Whitley Bay NE26 3LW Tel: 0191 253 4710 — MB BS Durh. 1945 (Newc.) Prev: GP Whitley Bay.

WHITE, Jennifer Margaret Roxburgh House, Locharbriggs, Dumfries DG1 1RY — MB ChB Glas. 1991; MRCPsych 1999.

WHITE, Jessica Frances 23 Agate Road, London W6 0AJ — MB BChir Camb. 1994.

WHITE, Jill Barbara Department of Anaesthesia and Critical Care, Northampton General Hospital NHS Trust, Cliftonville, Northampton NN1 5BD Tel: 01604 545671 Fax: 01604 545670 Email: jill.white@ngh.nhs.uk; Beechwood, 1 Abington Park Crescent, Northampton NN3 3AD Tel: 01604 39253 — MB BS Lond. 1974 (St. Mary's) FFA RCS Eng. 1982. Cons. Anaesth. Northampton Dist. HA. Specialty: Anaesth.

WHITE, Jill Christine (retired) Applegarth, Legg Lane, Wimborne BH21 1LQ Tel: 01202 883933 — MB BS Lond. 1948; MRCS Eng. LRCP Lond. 1947; DCH Eng. 1950; DPH Leeds 1959. Prev: SCMO Dorset HA.

WHITE, Joanne Sally Orchard Surgery, Christchurch Medical Centre, Purewell Cross Road, Christchurch BH23 5ET Tel: 01202 481902 Fax: 01202 486887 — MB BS Lond. 1986; MRCGP 1993.

WHITE, Mr John — MB ChB Glas. 1946 (Univ. Glas.) FRCS Ed. 1952; FRCS Glas. 1970. Cons. Emerit. Roy. Infirm. Glas. Specialty: Orthop.

WHITE, John Bell Hill Medical Group, The Hill, 192 Kingsway, Belfast BT17 9AL — MB BCh BAO Belf. 1970; DCH RCPSI 1972; DObst RCOG 1972; FRCGP 1989, M 1974. Prev: Ho. Off. Roy. Vict. Hosp. Belf.; Ho. Off. Roy. Belf. Hosp. Sick Childr.; Ho. Off. Roy. Matern. Hosp. Belf.

WHITE, John Charles 6 Devonshire Road, Sheffield S17 3NT Tel: 0114 236 2542 — MB ChB (Hons.) Sheff. 1990; Dip. Legal Pract.; Post Grad. Dip. Law Nottm. Law Sch.; MRCP (UK) Ed. 1994; MRCGP 1995. Trainee Solicitor. Socs: Law Soc. Clin. Reg. Panel; S. Yorks. Medico-legal; Roy. Coll. Phys. Ed.

WHITE, John Christopher (retired) Health Centre, Ponteland, Newcastle upon Tyne NE16 4PD; Glenbriar, Grange Road, Stamfordham, Newcastle upon Tyne NE18 0PF — MB BS Durh. 1955 (Newc.) Prev: Ho. Phys. & Ho. Surg. Bishop Auckland Gen. Hosp.

WHITE, John Ernest Stephen Respiratory Medicine, York District Hospital, Wigginton Road, York YO31 8HE Tel: 01904 453481 Fax: 01904 454747 — BM BS Nottm. 1985; BMedSci Nottm. 1983, BM BS 1985; MRCP (UK) 1988. Cons. Phys. Specialty: Respirat. Med. Prev: Sen. Regist. (Respirat. Med.) Freeman Hosp. Newc.; Regist. (Chest. Med.) Freeman Hosp. Newc.; Regist. (Med.) Hexham Gen. Hosp.

WHITE, John Horder, Wing Cdr. RAF Med. Br. 6 Falkirk Road, Wroughton, Swindon SN4 9DU Tel: 01793 812821 — MB BS Lond. 1952 (St. Mary's) MRCS Eng. LRCP Lond. 1952. Prev: Gp. Capt. RAF.

WHITE, John Howard (retired) 27 Southill Road, Poole BH12 3AW — MB ChB Leeds 1957.

WHITE, John Jackson Barnard Castle Surgery, Victoria Road, Barnard Castle DL12 8HT Tel: 01833 690707 — MB BS Newc. 1975; DRCOG 1978; MRCGP 1979.

WHITE, Jonathan Atherley 44 Napier Street, Burton-on-Trent DE14 3LN Tel: 07751 190230; Sandon, Heath Road, Bradfield, Manningtree CO11 2HX — BM BS Nottm. 1982. Specialty: Care of the Elderly. Prev: SHO (Psychiat.) Walsgrave Hosp. Coventry; SHO (Geriat.) Northampton Gen. Hosp.; SHO (Gen. Orthop./A & E) Burton Dist. Hosp.

WHITE, Jonathan Celt Barton Health Centre, Short Lane, Barton-under-Needwood, Burton-on-Trent DE13 8LB Tel: 01283 712207 Fax: 01283 712116 — MB BS Lond. 1987; DRCOG 1991; MRCGP 1992.

WHITE, Jonathan Charles North Devon District Hospital, Barnstaple EX31 4JB Tel: 01271 22577; Tremethick, Trevance, Wadebridge PL27 7QF — MB ChB Bristol 1991; BSc (Hons.) Lond. 1982; MRCGP 1995.

WHITE, Mr Jonathan David Flat 4, Edward Court, Birmingham Road, Walsall WS1 2RF Tel: 01922 29959 — MB ChB Birm. 1990; ChB Birm. 1990; FRCS Ed. 1996.

WHITE, Jonathan Francis Middleton Penn Manor Medical Centre, Manor Road, Penn, Wolverhampton WV4 5PY Tel: 01902 331166 Fax: 01902 575078; 39 St. Philip's Avenue, Penn, Wolverhampton WV3 7DU — MB ChB Birm. 1978.

WHITE, Mr Jonathan Samuel 3 Rhanbuoy Close, Carrickfergus BT38 8FF — MB BCh BAO Belf. 1993; BMedSci (Hons) 1991; FRCSI 1997. Specialty: Gen. Surg.

WHITE, Julian Peter 186 Crofton Road, Orpington BR6 8JG; 186 Crofton Road, Orpington BR6 8JG Tel: 01689 54617 — MB BS Newc. 1981; MRCPsych 1986. Clin. Asst. (Psychogeriat.) Qu. Mary's Hosp. Sidcup. Prev: Med. Off. HM Youth Custody Centre Rochester; Regist. & SHO (Psychiat.) Maidstone HA.

***WHITE, Julie Anne** 5 Downside, Gosport PO13 0JS Tel: 01329 513519 — MB ChB Leic. 1998; MB ChB Leic 1998. Ho. Off. (Gen. Surg.) Geo. Eliot Hosp. Specialty: Gen. Surg. Socs: Med. Protec. Soc. Prev: Ho. Off. Gen. Med., Walsgrave Hosp.

WHITE, Julie Susan 19 Stockdale Avenue, Redcar TS10 5EF — MB BS Newc. 1992.

WHITE, Kalasyam Kochayyappan The Surgery, Low Moor Road, Kirkby-in-Ashfield, Nottingham NG17 7BG Tel: 01623 759447; La Vista, Coxmoor Road, Sutton-in-Ashfield NG17 5LF Tel: 01623 552612 — MB BS Karnatak 1964.

WHITE, Karen Jane Folkestone Community Mental Health Centre, 2-4 Radnor Park Avenue, Folkestone CT19 5BW Tel: 01303 222424 Fax: 01303 222444 — MB ChB Leeds 1982; MRCPsych 1987. Cons. Community Psychiat. E. Kent Community Trust. Specialty: Gen. Psychiat. Prev: Med. Dir. S. Kent Community Trust; Cons. & Sen. Lect. Community Psychiat. W. Lambeth Community Care Trust UMDS Lond.; Lect. (Community Psychiat.) UMDS Guys & St. Thomas Hosp. Lond.

WHITE, Kathleen Denise Department of neurology, Ninewells Hospital, Dundee DD1 9SY Tel: 01382 425720 Fax: 01382 425739 Email: kathleen.white@tuht.scot.nhs.uk — MB ChB Dundee 1987; BMSc (Hons) Path. Sci's. (Human Genetics) 1984; MRCP (UK) 1991; FRCP 2003. Cons. Neurol. Ninewells Hosp.s Dundee. Specialty: Neurol. Prev: part time Sen. Regist. (neurol) Manch. Roy. Infirm.; seb Regist. (neuro) Vict. Infirm., Newc. Upon Tyne; Regissst (neura) Notrh RHA.

WHITE, Lesley Jane 3 Ravelston Park, Edinburgh EH4 3DX — MB ChB Aberd. 1995.

WHITE, Lilian Freda 18 Beach Road, Tynemouth, North Shields NE30 2NS Tel: 0191 258 7505 — MB BS Durh. 1954 (Newc.) DPH Newc. 1968. Clin. Asst. Ashington Hosp.; Asst. Med. Off. Wallsend Municip. Boro. Prev: Ho. Phys. & Ho. Surg. Roy. Vict. Infirm. Newc.

WHITE, Lisa Antonia Marion 14 Leathwaite Road, London SW11 1XQ — BM BS Nottm. 1993.

WHITE, Liza Rebecca 41 Jenny Burton Way, Hucknall, Nottingham NG15 7QS — MB ChB Manch. 1995; BSc Open 1995. SHO (Gen. Med.) Nottm. City Hosp.

WHITE, Lorraine Andrea 21 Badger Wood Walk, Badger Hill, York YO10 5HN — MB BS Newc. 1993.

WHITE, Lucy Anne Whiteleaf, Crawley, Winchester SO21 2QD — MB BCh Oxf. 1988; MA Camb. 1985; MRCP (UK) 1992; FRCA 1995. Cons. (Anaesthetics) Soton. Gen. Hosp. Specialty: Anaesth. Prev: Regist. (Anaesth.) Portsmouth Hosps. Trust; SHO (Anaesth.) Soton. Gen. Hosp.; SHO (Gen. Med.) Basingstoke Dist. Hosp. & Soton. Gen. Hosp.

WHITE, Madeline Patricia Royal Hospital for Sick Children, Yorkhill NHS Trust, Glasgow G15 6PX — MB ChB Dundee 1973; MRCP (UK) 1980; FRCP Glas. 1994; FRCPCH 1998; FRCPCL 1998. Cons. Paediat. Gtr. Glas. HB. Specialty: Paediat.

WHITE, Mr Malcolm Edward Eales (retired) 1 Manor Farmhouse, Vicarage Road, Stoneleigh, Coventry CV8 3DH Tel: 024 7641 0014 — MB BChir Camb. 1947 (Camb. & Westm.) FRCS Eng. 1953. Prev: Cons. Surg. Walsgrave Hosp. Coventry.

WHITE, Malcolm Terence The Surgery, 18 Fouracre Road, Bristol BS16 6PG Tel: 0117 970 2033; 47 Church Road, Yate, Bristol BS37 5BH Tel: 01454 312155 — MB ChB Bristol 1956; DObst RCOG 1958.

WHITE, Margaret Mary Susan Brookfield Surgery, Whitbarrow Road, Lymm WA13 9DB Tel: 01925 756969 Fax: 01925 756173 — MB ChB Manch. 1979.

WHITE, Margaret Rose Mary (retired) Avondale, Pencader SA39 9AS — MB BCh Wales 1957 (Cardiff) BSc, MB BCh Wales 1957; DPM Eng. 1976. Prev: SCMO Gwent AHA.

WHITE, Margaret Stather 22 Upfield, Croydon CR0 5DQ Tel: 020 8654 1411 — MB ChB Sheff. 1943; DObst RCOG 1948. Prev: Asst. MOH Boro. Croydon; Ho. Surg. Infirm. Sheff.; Obst. Med. Off. St. Jas. Hosp. Balham.

WHITE, Marion Isobel Aberdeen Royal Infirmary, Foresterhill, Ward 29, Aberdeen AB25 9ZN — MB ChB Aberd. 1972 (Univ. of Aberd.) MRCP (UK) 1974; FRCP Glas. 1986; BA Open 1988. Cons. Dermat, Aberd. Roy. Infirm.; Hon. Sen. Lect., Aberd. Univ. Specialty: Dermat.

WHITE, Mark Andrew 16 Glenside Drive, Wilmslow SK9 1EH — MB ChB Manch. 1990; MRCP (UK) 1994; DA (UK) 1995; FRCA 1996; AFPM 1998. Pharmaceut. Phys. Chesh. Specialty: Pharmaceutical Medicine.

WHITE, Mark Thomas — MB ChB Manch. 1994.

WHITE, Martin Newlands, 122 Derwen Fawr Road, Derwen Fawr, Swansea SA2 8DP Tel: 01792 203248; St. David's House, 1 Uplands Terrace, Uplands, Swansea SA2 0GU Tel: 01792 472922 — MB BCh Wales 1975 (Cardiff) FRCR 1982. Cons. Radiol. Swansea NHS Trust Singleton Hosp. Specialty: Radiol. Prev: Sen. Regist. (Radiol.) Univ. Hosp. Wales Cardiff.

WHITE, Martin James Reeve University of Newcastle upon Tyne, School of Population and Health Sciences, The Medical School, Newcastle upon Tyne NE2 4HH Tel: 0191 222 6275 Fax: 0191 222 6461 Email: martin.white@newcastle.ac.uk — MB ChB Birm. 1983; MSc Newc 1989; MFPHM RCP, UK 1991; FFPHM RCP, UK 1997. Sen. Lect. & Cons. Pub. Health Med. Univ. Newc. u Tyne. Specialty: Pub. Health Med. Special Interest: Pub. Health Interven. Eval.; Social & Behavioural Epidemiol. Socs: Soc. Social Med.; BMA; Internat. Union Health Promotion & Educat. Prev: Lect. (Pub. Health Med.) & Hon. Sen. Regist. North. RHA.

WHITE, Martin John 160 Greenacres, Wetheral, Carlisle CA4 8LU Tel: 01228 561397; 160 Greenacres, Wetheral, Carlisle CA4 8LU Tel: 01228 561397 — MB BS Newc. 1983; FRCA 1989. Cons. Anaesth. Carlisle Hosps.; Lead clinician Intens. care unit, Cumbld. Infirm., Carlisle; Clin. Director- Anaesthetics, theatres and Intens. care, Cumbld. Infirm., Carlisle. Specialty: Anaesth.; Intens. Care. Prev: Sen. Regist. (Anaesth.) North. RHA.; Regist. S. Glam. HA.

WHITE, Mary Radiology Dept, Kingston University Hospital, Galsworthy Rd, Kingston upon Thames KT2 7QB Tel: 020 8546 7711; 19 Hollytree Close, London SW19 6EA Tel: 020 8789 4264 — MB BCh BAO NUI 1976; DCH 1978; MRCPI 1979; FRCR 1983. Cons. (Radiol.) Kingston Univ. Hosp. NHS Trust Kingston on Thames. Specialty: Radiol.

WHITE, Mary-Ellen The Ridings, Southlands Hospital, Shoreham-by-Sea Tel: 01273 455622 — MB BS Lond. 1991; MRCPsych 1995. Specialty: Gen. Psychiat.

WHITE, Matthew 8E Hayton Road, Aberdeen AB24 2QR — MB ChB Aberd. 1993.

WHITE, Maurice 17 Jeffreys Street, London NW1 9PS Tel: 020 7267 1444 — (T.C. Dub.) BA, MB BCh BAO Dub. 1956, DPM 1960. Specialty: Psychother. Socs: Brit. Psychoanal. Soc.

WHITE, Michael Joseph Stakes Lodge Surgery, 3A Lavender Road, Waterlooville PO7 8NS Tel: 023 9225 4581 Fax: 023 9235 8867 — MB BS Lond. 1981 (Lond. Hosp.) DCH RCP Lond. 1984; DRCOG 1985; MRCGP 1985. GP Princip. Drs. Boyle White Bateman King Burton. Prev: Trainee GP S. Gwent VTS.

WHITE, Michelle Claire — MB ChB Bristol 1994 (Univ. Bristol) DCH RCP Lond. 1996; FRCA Bristol 2002. SpR (Anaesth.) Bristol Sch. Specialty: Anaesth. Socs: Assn. Anaesth.; World Federat. of Anaesthetists; Internat. Soc. of Mountain Med. Prev: SHO (Paediat. & Neonat. Med.) Taunton & Som. Hosp.; SHO (A & E Med.) Frenchay Hosp. Bristol.

WHITE, Neil Morgan Lloyd The Mumbles Medical Practice, 10 West Cross Avenue, Norton, Swansea SA3 5UA Tel: 01792 403010 Fax: 01792 401934 — MB BCh Wales 1984; RCGP; MRCGP 1990.

WHITE, Nicholas The Chase, Glebe Lane, Burnham Overy Staithe, King's Lynn PE31 8JQ — MB ChB Manch. 1998.

WHITE, Nicholas Charles 74 Grange Road, Dudley DY1 2AW — MB ChB Birm. 1982.

WHITE, Professor Nicholas John, OBE Faculty of Tropical Medicine, Mahidol University, 420/6 Rajvithi Road, Bangkok 10400, Thailand Tel: 0066 2 460832 Fax: 0066 246 7795; Nuffield Department of Clinical Medicine, John Radcliffe Hospital, Headington, Oxford OX3 9DU Tel: 01865 220970 Fax: 01865 220984 — MRCS Eng. LRCP Lond. 1974; MD Lond. 1984, MB BS 1974; MRCP (UK) 1976; MA Oxf. 1986; FRCP 1989; DSc (Med.) Lond. 1995. Director Wellcome Trust Mahidol Univ. Oxf. Trop. Med. Research Prog.

WHITE, Nicholas Peter 12 Brackenway, Formby, Liverpool L37 7HG — MB BS Newc. 1993.

WHITE, Nicola Janine Alton Health Centre, Anstey Road, Alton GU34 2QX; Goldings, Worldham Hill, East Worldham, Alton GU34 3AT — MB BS Lond. 1981; MRCGP 1985; MRCGP 1985; DRCOG 1985; DRCOG 1985.

WHITE, Mrs Pamela (retired) 13 Barntongate Avenue, Edinburgh EH4 8BQ Tel: 0131 339 7530 — MB ChB Ed. 1950.

WHITE, Pamela Jean (retired) 4 Rectory Close, Lower Heswall, Wirral CH60 4TB — MRCS Eng. LRCP Lond. 1960. Prev: SCMO Liverp. HA.

WHITE, Pamela Olive (retired) 12 Hill Lane, Hartley, Plymouth PL3 5QX — (Roy. Free) MB BS Lond. 1964; DA Eng. 1967; FFA RCS Eng. 1970; BA Open 1987. Prev: Sen. Regist. (Anaesth.) Birm. Hosps.

WHITE, Patricia Clare West Kirby Health Centre, Grange Road, Wirral CH48 4HZ Tel: 0151 625 9171 Fax: 0151 625 9171 — MB ChB Liverp. 1988.

WHITE, Patricia Mary Bury Knowle Health Centre, London Road, Headington, Oxford OX3 9JA Tel: 01865 761651 Email: pat.white@gp-k84009.nhs.uk; Little Cranford, Moulsford, Wallingford OX10 9HU — MB BS Lond. 1976; MRCS Eng. LRCP Lond. 1976; DRCOG 1979; MRCGP 1982. Socs: Reading Path. Soc.

WHITE, Patrick Thomas Crown Dale Medical Centre, 61 Crown Dale, London SE19 3NY Tel: 020 8670 2414 Fax: 020 8670 0277 — MB BCh BAO NUI 1976 (Univ. Coll. Dub.) MRCP (UK) 1979; FRCGP 1995, M 1980. Sen. Lect. (Gen. Pract.) Guy's King's Sch. Med. Socs: BMA. Prev: Lect. (Gen. Pract.) King's Coll. Sch. Med. & Dent. Lond.; Research Fell. (Gen. Pract.) St. Geo. Hosp. Med. Sch. Lond.; Trainee GP Bangour VTS.

WHITE, Mr Paul Stephen Department of Otolaryngology, Ninewells Medical School, University of Dundee, Dundee DD1 9SY Tel: 01382 660111 Fax: 01382 632816 Email: paulw@doctors.org.uk; Brackenbrae, Emma Terrace, Blairgowrie PH10 6JA — MB ChB Otago 1982; FRACS 1990; T(S) 1991; FRCS Ed. 1995. Cons. Otolaryngolgist & Rhinologist, Tayside Univ. Hosps. NHS Trust; MATTUS Tutor (Otolaryngol.); Hon. Sen. Lect. Univ. Dundee; Cliincal Ldr. for ENT Serv.s,Tayside Univ. Hosp. NHS Trust; Hon. Sen. Lect. in Rhinology, Univ. of Dundee. Specialty: Otorhinolaryngol.; Gen. Surg. Socs: Brit. Assn. Otol.; Scott. Otolaryngol. Soc. (Counc. Mem.); Roy. Soc. Med. Prev: Cons. Otolaryngol. Lanarksh. HB; Sen. Regist. Glas. Roy. Infirm. & ChristCh. Hosp., NZ; Cons. Otolaryngol. Ninewells Hosp. Dundee & Perth Roy. Infirm.

WHITE, Peter Denton, OBE St. Bartholomew's Hospital , Department of Psychological Medicine, London EC1A 7BE Tel: 020 7601 8108 Fax: 020 7601 7969 Email: p.d.white@qmul.ac.uk — MB BS Lond. 1977 (St. Bart.) BSc (Psychol.) Lond. 1974; FRCPsych 1995, M 1983; MD Lond. 1993; FRCPsych 1995. Prof. of Psychol. Med., Bart's and the Lond., Qu. Mary's Sch. of Med. and Dent. Specialty: Gen. Psychiat. Special Interest: Chronic Fatigue & Pain; Mind Body Med. Socs: Internat. Coll. Psychosomatic Med.; Amer. Psychosomatic Assn. Prev: Lect. (Psychol. Med.) St. Bart. Hosp. Lond.; Ment. Health Foundat. Fell. St. Bart. Hosp. Lond.; Regist. Maudsley & Bethlem Roy. Hosp.

WHITE, Peter Gardner West End Medical Practice, 21 Chester Street, Edinburgh EH3 7RF Tel: 0131 225 5220 Fax: 0131 226 1910; 84 Craigcrook Road, Edinburgh EH4 3PN Tel: 0131 336 5505 — MB ChB Ed. 1970; BSc (Hons.) Ed. 1967; MRCP (UK) 1974. Prev: Regist. Roy. Infirm. Edin.; SHO West. Gen. Hosp. Edin.

WHITE, Peter James Nightingale Surgery, Greatwell Drive, Cupernham Lane, Romsey SO51 7QN Tel: 01794 517878 Fax: 01794 514236 Email: peterwhite@nightingalesurgery.com; Wealden, Chapel Lane, Timsbury, Romsey SO51 0NW Tel: 01794 367742 Email: peterwhite3@virgin.net — MB ChB Dundee 1974; BSc (Med. Sci.) St. And. 1971; MRCGP 1979; FRCGP 1998. GP Tutor Soton.; Chairm. Steering Gp. Wessex Research Network. Specialty: Gen. Pract. Socs: Nat. Assn. GP Tutors; RCGP; ILT.

WHITE, Peter Malcolm Castlehead Medical Centre, Ambleside Road, Keswick CA12 4DB Tel: 01768 772025 Fax: 01768 773862 — MB BS Lond. 1984; BSc (Hons.) Lond. 1981; DRCOG 1987; MRCGP 1988.

WHITE, Peter Noel Graham Sleaford Medical Group, Riverside Surgery, 47 Boston Road, Sleaford NG34 7HD Tel: 01529 303301 Fax: 01529 415401; Spring House, Leasingham, Sleaford NG34 — MB BS Lond. 1965 (Univ. Coll. Hosp.) MRCS Eng. LRCP Lond. 1965; DObst RCOG 1967. Clin. Asst. Clin. Immunol. Allergy Clinic Lincoln. Prev: Ho. Surg. Westm. Childr. Hosp.; Ho. Phys. Qu. Mary's Hosp. Roehampton; SHO Obst. Unit City Hosp. Nottm.

WHITE, Philip Graham Torbay Hospital, X-Ray Department, Torbay, Torquay TQ2 7AA Tel: 01803 655632 Email: philip.white3@nhs.net — MB BS Lond. 1984; BSc Lond. 1981; MRCP (UK) 1987; FRCR 1991; T(R) (CR) 1993. Specialty: Radiol. Prev: Cons. (Radiol.) Morriston Hosp. Swansea; Cons. (Radiol.) Neath Gen. Hosp.; Sen. Regist. (Radiol.) S. Glam. Health Auth.

WHITE, Philip Michael 41 Harker Park, Carlisle CA6 4HS — MB ChB Liverp. 1990; BSc (1st cl. Hons.) Liverp. 1988, MB ChB 1990. SHO (Med.) Roy. Liverp. Univ. Hosp.

WHITE, Philip Thomas 29 Blyth Hill Lane, London SE6 4UN — MB BCh Wales 1987.

WHITE, Philip Wayman Felinheli Surgery, 1 Felinheli Terrace, Y Felinheli LL56 4JF Tel: 01248 670423 Fax: 01248 670966; (Surgery), Coronation Road, Menai Bridge LL59 5BD Tel: 01248 712210 Fax: 01248 715829 — MB ChB Manch. 1976. Clin. Asst. (ENT) N. W. Wales Trust. Specialty: Otorhinolaryngol. Socs: BMA (Sec. N. W. Wales Div.).

WHITE, Philippa Jane Princess Anne Hospital, Coxford Road, Southampton SO16 5YA Tel: 023 8079 6041 — MB BS Lond. 1975; MRCOG 1980, D 1978; FRCOG 1995. Cons. Obst. Princess Anne Hosp. Soton. Specialty: Obst. & Gyn.

WHITE, Philippa Mary Bruce PHLS East, Directorate Office, Institute of Food Research, Norwich Research Park, Colney Lane, Norwich NR4 7UA Tel: 01603 506900 Fax: 01603 501188; 1 Carnation Cottage, 103 Dereham Road, Mattishall, Dereham NR20 3NU Tel: 01362 858494 — MB BS Lond. 1977 (Univ. Coll. Hosp.) MSc Lond. 1982, BSc (Hons.) 1974; MRCPath 1984; FRCPath 1995; MBA 1999. Gp. Dir. PHLS E.; Cons. Microbiol. (Virol.) Pub. Health Laborat. Norwich; Hon. Lect. Univ. E. Anglia. Specialty: Med. Microbiol. Prev: Dir. Pub. Health Laborat. Norwich; Assoc. Specialist Virus Refer. Laborat. Lond.; Sen. Regist. Pub. Health Laborat. Coventry.

WHITE, Phoebe Margaret (retired) 15a South Street, Totnes TQ9 5DZ Tel: 01803 864007 — MB ChB Ed. 1949; DCH Eng. 1953. Prev: SCMO Torbay.

WHITE, Priscilla Mary (retired) Hillside, Guineaford, Marwood, Barnstaple EX31 4EA Tel: 01271 371603 — MB Camb. 1965 (St. Thos.) BChir 1964; DCH Eng. 1967; DPM Eng. 1975; MRCPsych 1976. Prev: Cons. (Child Psychiat.) N. Devon Family Consultancy.

WHITE, Rachel Jane Crofton Surgery, 109A Crofton Road, Orpington BR6 8HU Tel: 01689 822266 Fax: 01689 891790; 74 Towncourt Crescent, Lee, Pettswood, Orpington BR5 1PJ — MB BS Lond. 1988. Specialty: Gen. Pract.

WHITE, Ralph William 18 Loxley View Road, Sheffield S10 1QZ — MB ChB Sheff. 1992.

WHITE, Randolph Wilbur (retired) — MD Toronto 1943 (Middlx. & Toronto) MCPS Alta 1946; FRCPath 1973, M 1964. Prev: Path. Reg. Q. Charlottes Hosp.

WHITE, Raymond George The Mater Hospital Trust, Crumlin Road, Belfast BT14 6AB, Ireland Tel: 02890 803505 Fax: 02890 802555 Email: rgwhite@mater.n-i.nhs.uk — MB BCh BAO Belf. 1976; MFFP; MRCOG 1981, D 1978; FRCOG 1986. Cons. Obst. and Gynaecologist The Mater Hosp. Trust, Belf.; Hon. Clin. Lect., Queens Univ., Belf. Specialty: Obst. & Gyn. Special Interest: Reproductive Endocrinol. Socs: Brit. Menopause Soc.; Ulster Obstetric and Gyn. Soc. Prev: Sen. Regist. (O & G) Centr. Hosp. Harare Zimbabwe; Regist. (O & G) Altnagelvin Hosp. Londonderry; Research Fell. Roy. Vict. Hosp. Belf.

WHITE, Raymund John Auchinairn Road Surgery, 127/129 Auchinairn Road, Bishopbriggs, Glasgow G64 1NF Tel: 0141 772 1808 Fax: 0141 762 1274 — MB ChB Glas. 1984. GP Glas. Prev: SHO (Dermat.) Stobhill Hosp. Glas.; SHO (Otolaryngol.) Stobhill Hosp. Glas.; SHO (Gen. Surg.) Monklands Dist. Gen. Hosp. Airdrie.

WHITE, Professor Richard Henry Reeve (retired) The Rye, 12 Cherry Hill Road, Barnt Green, Birmingham B45 8LJ Tel: 0121 445 4886 — (Guy's) MA Camb. 1951; MB BChir Camb. 1950; MRCS Eng. LRCP Lond. 1950; DCH Eng. 1952; FRCP Lond. 1972, M 1954; MD Birm. 1969; FRCPCH (Hon.) 1997. Prev: Emerit. Prof. Paediat. Nephrol. Univ. Birm.

WHITE, Richard Ian 23 St Johns Mansions, Clapton Square, London E5 8HT — MB BS Lond. 1978; MRCPsych 1985.

WHITE, Richard Patrick Walton Centre for Neurology & Neurosurgery, Lower Lane, Fazakerley, Liverpool L9 7LJ Tel: 0151 529 6260 Fax: 0151 529 5513 — MB ChB Leeds 1992; BSc

(Hons.) Leeds 1989; MRCP UK 1995; MD Lond. 1999. Cons. (Neurol.) Walton Centre Neurol. & Neurosurg. Liverp.; Cons. (Neurol.) Glan Clwyd Hosp. Denbighsh. Specialty: Neurol. Special Interest: Stroke. Socs: Assn. Brit. Neurol.; Brit. Assn. Stroke Phys. Prev: Specialist Regist. (Nerol.) NW. Lond. Neurosci. Rotat.

WHITE, Robert John 30 Kingsdown Road, Northfield, Birmingham B31 1AH — MB ChB Birm. 1978; MRCGP 1985. Trainee GP W. Cumbld. Hosp. Whitehaven VTS. Prev: Med. Regist. (Chest Dis.) Jersey Gen. Hosp.; SHO (Med.) Treliske Hosp. Truro; SHO (Med.) Tehidy Hosp. Camborne.

WHITE, Roderick John Stranraer Health Centre, Edinburgh Road, Stranraer DG9 7HG Tel: 01776 706566; Egmont, Larg Road, Stranraer DG9 — MB ChB Glas. 1976; DRCOG 1980; MRCGP 1981. Specialty: Gen. Pract.

WHITE, Roger George (retired) 101 Longdown Lane S., Epsom KT17 4JJ Tel: 01372 721001 — MB BS Lond. 1958 (St. Bart.) DObst RCOG 1961. Ex Med. Off. Epsom Coll.; Sen. Med. Off. to United Racecourses Ltd. Prev: Ho. Phys., Research Asst. & GP Clin. Asst. St. Bart. Hosp. Lond.

WHITE, Roger James Crosshouse Hospital, Kilmarnock KA2 0BE Tel: 01563 521133; 4 Macrae Drive, Prestwick KA9 1NY Tel: 01292 479752 Email: roger1402@aol.com — MB ChB Dundee 1975; FRCA 1980. Cons. Anaesth. CrossHo. Hosp. Kilmarnock. Specialty: Anaesth.

WHITE, Roger James (cons. rooms), Litfield House, Clifton, Bristol BS8 3LS Tel: 0117 973 1323 Fax: 0117 973 3303; 4 Church Avenue, Stoke Bishop, Bristol BS9 1LD Tel: 0117 968 4207 Email: roger.white4@virgin.net — (Camb. & St. Bart.) MA Camb. 1964, MD 1971, MB 1964, BChir 1963; FRCP Lond. 1980, M 1967. Sen. Lect. Med. Bristol Univ.; Cons. Phys. Frenchay Hosp. Bristol. Specialty: Gen. Med.; Respirat. Med. Prev: Research Asst. Cardiac Dept. St. Bart. Hosp.; Jun. Med. Regist. St. Bart. Hosp.; Sen. Med. Regist. St. Bart. Hosp. Lond.

WHITE, Roger William Barker (retired) 227 Park Road, Hartlepool TS26 9NG Tel: 01429 269395 — (Middlx.) MA, MB Camb. 1961, BChir 1960; FRCP Lond. 1979, M 1965. Prev: Cons. Gen. Phys. Cardiol. Hartlepool Gen. Hosp.

WHITE, Roma Shareen (retired) 4 Frances Street, Chesham HP5 3EQ Tel: 01494 784568 — MB BS Lond. 1961 (Roy. Free Hosp. Lond.) MRCS Eng. LRCP Lond. 1961; DObst RCOG 1963. Prev: SCMO Camden & Islington Community Trust.

WHITE, Ronald Bertie William (retired) Beech Hill, Flore, Northampton NN7 4LL Tel: 01327 340377 — MB ChB Sheff. 1959 (Sheffield) BA Open 1990. Prev: GP Flore, Northampton.

WHITE, Ronald James 19 Tyler Road, Limavady BT49 0DP — MB BCh BAO Belf. 1986.

WHITE, Ruth Elizabeth Bevis 51 Britannia Square, Worcester WR1 3HP — BM BCh Oxf. 1983; MA Camb. 1983; MRCPsych 1988; MPhil Lond. 1990. Cons. Psychiat. Worcester Roy. Infirm. NHS Trust. Specialty: Gen. Psychiat. Prev: Lect. (Psychiat.) St. Geo. Hosp. Lond.

WHITE, Ruth Robina Manor Farm House, 96 High St., Yelvertoft, Northampton NN6 6LQ — MB ChB Aberd. 1983.

WHITE, Sandra Katherine 4 High Ash Road, Wheathampstead, St Albans AL4 8DY Email: sandrawhite@doctors.org.uk — MB BS Lond. 1996 (St. Georges University of London) BSc Lond. 1995.

WHITE, Sarah Ann Bents Green Surgery, 98 Bents Road, Sheffield S11 9RL Tel: 0114 236 0641 Fax: 0114 262 1069; Bents Green Surgery, 98 Bents Road, Sheffield S11 9RL Tel: 0114 236 0641 — MB ChB Sheff. 1989 (Sheffield) DRCOG 1992; MRCGP Ed. 1994; DFFP 1996. GP; Family Plann. Doctor. Specialty: Gen. Pract.; Family Plann. & Reproduc. Health. Prev: Mem. BMA; Mem. RCGP; Mem. MPS.

WHITE, Sean Anthony 119 Harley Street, London W1G 6AN Email: seaniewhite@yahoo.co.uk — MB BS Lond. 1988 (The London Hospital Medical College) FRCA 1994. Cons. St Bart. Hosp. Lond. Specialty: Anaesth. Socs: Assn. Anaesth.; Pain. Soc; IASP. Prev: Regist. (Anaesth.) Roy. Lond. Hosp. Trust.

WHITE, Sheelagh Mary (retired) 1 Cathedral Square, Fortrose IV10 8TB — MB ChB Ed. 1964; DObst RCOG 1966; FFA RCS Eng. 1970. Prev: anaesthetics Cons., Inverness.

WHITE, Sheelagh McKie 7 Miller Street, Hamilton ML3 7EW — MB ChB Glas. 1977.

WHITE, Mr Stephen Howard Robert Jones & Agnes Hunt Orthop. & District Hospital NHS Trust, Oswestry SY10 7AG Tel: 01691 404093 Fax: 01691 404052 Email: george.pugh@rjah.nhs.uk — BM BS Nottm. 1980; BMedSci 1978; FRCS Eng. 1984; DM Nottm. 1993. Cons. Orthop. Surg. Robt. Jones & Agnes Hunt Orthop. & Dist. Hosp. Oswestry & Roy. Shrewsbury Hosp. NHS Trust; Cons. in Trauma and Orthopaedic Surg., Roy. Shrewsbury Hosp. NHS Trust; Cons. in Trauma and Orthopaedic Surg., Shrops. Nuffield Hosp. Specialty: Trauma & Orthop. Surg. Special Interest: Knee. Socs: Brit. Assn. Surg. Knee; Brit. Orthopaedic Assn.; Brit. Orthopaedic Research Soc. Prev: Sen. Regist. (Traum. & Orthop. Surg.) Oxf.

WHITE, Stephen Innes Department of Dermatology, Clatterbridge Hospital, Bebington, Wirral CH63 4JY Tel: 0151 482 7782 Fax: 0151 482 7785 Email: stephen.white@whnt.nhs.uk — MB ChB Manch. 1977; DRCOG 1979; MRCP (UK) 1981; MD Manch. 1990; FRCP Lond. 1996; FRCP Edin. 1996. Cons. Dermat. Wirral Hosp. Specialty: Dermat. Special Interest: Skin Cancer. Socs: Brit. Assn. of Dermatologists; Brit. Soc. of Dermatological Surg.; Birkenhead Med. Soc. Prev: Clin. Lect. (Dermat.) Univ. Glas. & Hon. Sen. Regist. West. Infirm. Glas.; Regist. (Dermat.) Roy. Vict. Infirm. Newc.; Ho. Phys. N. Manch. Gen. Hosp.

WHITE, Stephen Robert Broadway Surgery, 2 Broadway, Fulwood, Preston PR2 9TH Tel: 01772 717261 Fax: 01772 787652 — MB ChB Manch. 1986.

WHITE, Stephen Thomas Royal Victoria Hospital, Grosvenor Road, Belfast BT12 6BA — MB ChB Liverp. 1983; MB ChB (Hons.) Liverp. 1983; FRCOphth 1994.

WHITE, Mr Steven Alan St James University Hospital, Department of Hepatobiliary and Transplant Surgery, Beckett Street, Leeds LS9 7TF Tel: 0113 206 4890 Fax: 0113 243 3144 Email: steve_islets@hotmail.com — MB ChB Leic. 1992 (Leics) FRCS 1998; MD 1998. Lect.Surg. Univ. Leics; Moynihan Travel Fell.; Clin. Fell. HPB/transplant St James Leeds. Specialty: Transpl. Surg. Socs: Brit. Transpl..Soc; Pancreatic. Soc; Assoc.Surg. Prev: Hon. SHO (Surg.) Leicester Roy. Infirm.; Hon. Specialist Regist. S. Trent. Train. Scheme Gen. Surg; Clin. Research Fell. (Surg.) Univ. Leics.

WHITE, Steven Robert Department of Clinical Neurophysiology, Great Ormond Street Hospital for Children, London WC1N 3JH Tel: 020 7405 9200 — MB BChir Camb. 1978; BA (Psychol. & Phil.) Oxf. 1969, MA 1973, DPhil 1976; BA Camb. 1976; MRCPsych 1983; FRCP 2000. Cons. Neurophysiol. Gt. Ormond St. Hosp. For Childr. & St Mary's Hosp. Lond. Specialty: Clin. Neurophysiol. Socs: Fell. Roy. Soc. Trop. Med. & Hyg.; Brit. Psychol. Soc.; Ass of Brit. neUrol.s. Prev: Cons. Neurophysiol., Barts & The Lond. Hosp.; Cons. Neurophysiol. Middlx. Hosp. & Whittington Hosp. Lond.; Sen. Regist. (Clin. Neurophysiol.) Gen. Infirm. & St. Jas. Univ. Hosp. Leeds.

WHITE, Stuart Malcolm 63 Wilmington Way, Brighton BN1 8JG — MB BS Lond. 1994.

WHITE, Susan 141 Brigstock Road, Thornton Heath, Croydon CR7 7JN Tel: 020 8684 1128; 94 Pollards Hill N., Norbury, London SW16 4NZ Tel: 020 8679 8267 — (Newcastle) MB BS Newc. 1977; DRCOG 1981; MRCGP 1982; DCH RCP Lond. 1982. GP Princip.; Clin. Asst. Cardiol. Mayday Hosp. Thornton Health; GP Tutor Kings Coll. Med. Sch. Specialty: Cardiol.

WHITE, Susan Veronica c/o Dept. of Geriatric Medicine, University Hospital, Wales, Cardiff CF4 4XW Tel: 029 2074 3142 — MB BCh BAO NUI 1989; MRCPI 1992; DTM & H Liverp. 1995. SpR Geriat., Roy. Gwent Hosp., Newport. Specialty: Gen. Med.; Care of the Elderly. Socs: Brit. Geriat. Soc.

WHITE, Thomas State Hospital, Carstairs Junction, Lanark ML11 8RP Tel: 01555 840293 Fax: 01555 840112 Email: tomw@tsh.scot.nhs.uk; 33 Main St, Symington, Biggar ML12 6XP/ 01899 308235 — MB ChB Ed. 1983 (Edinburgh) BSc (Hons.) Ed. 1980; MRCPsych 1988; Dip. Forens. Med. Glas 1995. Cons. Forens. Psychiat. State Hosp. Specialty: Gen. Psychiat.; Forens. Psychiat. Prev: Cons. Psychiat. Forth Valley HB; Sen. Regist. (Gen. Adult Psychiat.) Gtr. Glas. HB.

WHITE, Thomas George Edward 22 Upfield, Croydon CR0 5DQ Tel: 020 8654 1411 — MD Belf. 1953 (Qu. Univ. Belf.) MB BCh BAO 1941; MRCOG 1947; MRCGP 1958. Socs: BMA; FRSM. Prev: Sen. Regist. Mayday Hosp. Croydon; Ho. Surg. Jessop Hosp. Wom. Sheff.; Maj. RAMC.

WHITE, Thomas John Clarence Avenue Surgery, 14 Clarence Avenue, Northampton NN2 6NZ Tel: 01604 718464 Fax: 01604 721589; 15 Park Avenue S., Northampton NN3 3AA Tel: 01604 633898 — MB BChir Camb. 1977 (Queens' Coll. Camb. & St. Bart. Lond.) MA, MB Camb. 1977, BChir 1976; DRCOG 1979; DCH Eng. 1980; MRCGP 1981. Specialty: Ment. Health. Socs: BMA; N.ampton Med. Assn. Prev: Ho. Off. (Surg. & Med.) & SHO (Paediat. & O & G) Northampton; Gen. Hosp.

WHITE, Thomas Milnes Fisher Medical Centre, Millfields, Coach Street, Skipton BD23 1EU; Westville, 17 West Bank Road, Skipton BD23 1QT Tel: 01756 700887 — MB BS Lond. 1983; MA Oxf. 1980; DRCOG 1986; DCH RCP Lond. 1986; MRCGP 1987. Prev: Trainee GP Reading VTS; Med. Off. Matlala Hosp. Lebowa, S. Afr.

WHITE, Timothy Clarke Fairfield Surgery, Station Road, Flookburgh, Grange-over-Sands LA11 7JY Tel: 015395 58307 Fax: 015395 58442; Pendlehurst, Ulverston LA12 7HD — MB BChir Camb. 1976; MA Camb. 1972; DRCOG 1978; MRCP (UK) 1982; MRCGP 1983; DTM & H RCP Lond. 1984; MPH Leeds 1992. Prev: Dir. Health Servs. Guadalcanal Province Sololom Is., Pacific Ocean.

WHITE, Timothy Joseph The Old Rectory, Macosquin, Coleraine BT51 4PN Tel: 01265 52640 — MB ChB Sheff. 1997; MRCS Part 1. SHO (Gen. Surg.), Hull Roy. Infirm. Specialty: Gen. Surg.

WHITE, Timothy Oliver 264 School Road, Crookes, Sheffield S10 1GP — MB ChB Sheff. 1995.

WHITE, Valerie Leonora (retired) Beech Hill, Flore, Northampton NN7 4LL Tel: 01327 340377 — MB ChB Sheff. 1956. Prev: GP Flore, Northampton.

WHITE, Veronica Lilian Coral — MB BS Lond. 1991; BSc (Pharmacol. & Basic Med. Sci.) Lond. 1988; MRCP (UK) 1995. p/t CCST General Internal & Respiratory Medicine; SPR North Thames (East). Specialty: Respirat. Med.; Gen. Med. Socs: Brit. Thorac. Soc.; FRSM; BMA. Prev: SHO Rotat. (Med.) Roy. Lond. Hosp.; Ho. Phys. OldCh. Hosp. Romford; Ho. Surg. Broomfield Hosp. Chelmsford.

WHITE, Wallace (retired) The Hill House, Holt Road, Letheringsett, Holt NR25 7YB Tel: 01263 713300 — MB BS Lond. 1954 (Lond. Hosp.) DObst RCOG 1961. Prev: Regist. & Ho. Off. (Dermat.) Lond. Hosp.

WHITE, William David Little Snakemoor, Sleepers Hill, Winchester SO22 4NA Tel: 01962 855888 — MB BS Lond. 1972 (St. Geo.) FRCA (Eng.) 1977. Cons. Anaesth. Roy. Hants. Co. Hosp. Winchester. Specialty: Anaesth. Socs: BMA; CCSC; Assn Anaesth. Prev: Sen. Regist. (Anaesth.) Westm. Hosp. & Soton. Gen. Hosp.; Regist. (Anaesth.) Bristol Roy. Infirm.; Ho. Surg. & Ho. Phys. Torbay Hosp.

WHITE, William Francis (retired) 4 Rectory Close, Lower Heswall, Wirral CH60 4TB Tel: 0151 342 8102 Fax: 0151 384 4398 — MB ChB Manch. 1956; FRCA Eng. 1965.

WHITE, William Frederick Department of Clinical Oncology, St Luke's Cancer Centre, Royal Surrey County Hospital, Guildford GU2 7XX Tel: 01483 406767 Fax: 01483 406827; The Shieling, Upper Guildown Road, Guildford GU2 4EZ Tel: 01483 39924 Fax: 01483 34191 — MB BS Lond. 1960 (Westm.) MRCS Eng. LRCP Lond. 1960; DMRT Eng. 1963; FFR 1965; FRCR 1975. Cons. Radiother. &Oncol.St. Luke's Hosp.Guildford; Hon. Cons. Roy. King Edwd. VII Hosp. Midhurst; Cons. St.Pete's Hosp. Specialty: Oncol.; Radiother.; Nuclear Med. Socs: Brit. Inst. Radiol.; Brit. Nuclear Med. Soc. Prev: Cons. Westminster Hosp. Lond.; Sen. Regist. Westminster Hosp.

WHITE, William Graham Meadowbank Health Centre, 3 Salmon Inn Road, Polmont, Falkirk FK2 0XF Tel: 01324 715540 Fax: 01324 716723; 1 Alexandra Park, Lenzie, Glasgow G66 5BH — MB ChB Glas. 1985; MRCGP 1990.

WHITE, William Joseph (retired) Sherwin House, Hillfarrance, Taunton TA4 1AP Tel: 01823 461306 — MB BS Lond. 1951 (Lond. Hosp.) MRCS Eng. LRCP Lond. 1951. Prev: Med. Off. Roy. Ordnance Explosives Div. Bridgwater.

WHITE, Mr William Leslie Rous Surgery, Rous Road, Newmarket CB8 8DH Tel: 01638 662018; Blantyre, 11 Rous Road, Newmarket CB8 8DH Tel: 01638 662033 — MB ChB Ed. 1959; FDS RCS Eng. 1954; FRCS Ed. 1968. Prev: Ho. Surg. Roy. Hosp. Sick Childr. Edin.; Regist. Gen. Surg. Newc. Gen. Hosp.

WHITE, Winston Timothy, OBE (retired) Wassledine, 4 Campton Road, Gravenhurst, Bedford MK45 4JB — (St. Bart.) MB BS Lond. 1951. Chairm. Luton & S. Beds. Hospice. Prev: Res. Ho. Off. Childr. Annexe & Res. Cas. Off. Luton & Dunstable Hosp.

WHITE-JONES, Robert Howel (retired) 38 Central Avenue, Eccleston Park, Prescot L34 2QP Tel: 0151 426 6885 — (Liverp.) MB ChB Liverp. 1938; DObst. RCOG 1940; DCH Eng. 1947; FRCP Lond. 1972, M 1948; MD Liverp. 1948. Prev: Cons. Paediat. St. Helens & Whiston Hosps.

WHITEAR, John Robert 13 Holland Dwellings, Newton St., London WC2B 5ES — MB BS Lond. 1992.

WHITEAR, Shah-naz 13 Holland Dwellings, Newton St., London WC2B 5ES — MB BS Lond. 1992.

WHITEAR, Mr William Patrick Department of Diagnostic Imaging, Ipswich Hospital, Heath Road, Ipswich IP4 5PD Tel: 01473 703364 Fax: 01473 270655 Email: patrick.whitear@ipswichhospital.nhs.uk; 37 Tuddenham Road, Ipswich IP4 2SN Tel: 01473 213362 — MB BS Lond. 1975 (St. Mary's) FRCS Eng. 1980; FRCR 1986. Cons. Radiol. Ipswich Hosp. Suff. Specialty: Radiol. Special Interest: Interventional Radiol.; Breast Imaging. Socs: BMA; Ipswich & Dist. Clin. Soc.; Brit. Inst. Radiol. Prev: Sen. Regist. (Radiol.) Univ. Coll. Hosp. Lond.; Regist. (Radiol.) St. Mary's Hosp. Lond.; Regist. Rotat. (Surg.) Manch. Roy. Infirm.

WHITECROSS, Susan Elizabeth Shiona Bradford Royal Infirmary, Radiology Department, Duckworth Lane, Bradford BD9 6RJ Tel: 01274 364123 Fax: 01274 364661 Email: shiona.whitecross@btopenworld.com — MB ChB Glas. 1978 (Glasgow) DRCOG 1980; FRCR 1985. Cons. Radiologist Bradford Teachg. Hosps. NHS & Pennine NHS Breast Screening Unit; Cons. Radiologist The Yorks. Clinic Bungley W Yorks; Cons. Radiologist The Highfield Hosp. Rochdale Lancs.; Hon. Lect. Health Care Studies Univ. of Bradford. Specialty: Radiol. Special Interest: Breast Radiol.; Musculoskeletal Radiol. Socs: Royal College of Radiologists; British Institute of Radiologists. Prev: Clin. Dir. (Radiol.) Oldham NHS Trust; Cons. Radiol. Airedale NHS Trust; Cons. Radiol. Oldham NHS Trust Oldham Lancs.

WHITEFIELD, Mr George Aaron 9A Belleisle Avenue, Uddington, Glasgow G71 7AP — LRCP LRCS Ed. 1948; LRCP LRCS Ed. LRFPS Glas. 1948; FRCS Ed. 1958.

WHITEFIELD, Mr Laurence Abraham Queen Mary's NHS Trust Sidcup, Frognal Avenue, Sidcup DA14 6LT Tel: 020 8302 2678 Fax: 020 8308 3089 Email: laurence.whitefield@qms.nhs.uk — MB BS Lond. 1989 (Char. Cross & Westm.) FRCOphth 1993. Cons. Ophth., Qu. Mary's Hos. Sidcup. Specialty: Ophth. Prev: Se. Regist., Moorfields Eye Hosp.

WHITEFIELD, Timothy David (retired) 8 Cock Pit Close, North Stainley, Ripon HG4 3HT Tel: 01765 635442 — MB BCh Wales 1969 (Cardiff) MRCGP 1977; AFOM RCP Lond. 1980. Medico-Legal Cons. & Publisher. Prev: GP Leeds.

WHITEFORD, David Mitchell — (Cambridge & St George's Hosp. London) MB BChir 1958; DObst RCOG 1960; DCH 1961; MA Camb. 1977. Princip. in Gen. Pract., Walthamstow, Lond., E17. Specialty: Gen. Pract. Socs: Walthamstow Med. Soc. (Pres.) '98-'99; Ex-Sec. Walthamstow Med. Soc.

WHITEFORD, Linda June 46 Elm Grove, Norton, Bromsgrove B61 0EJ Tel: 01527 875841 — (Oxford) BA Oxf. 1991; BM BCh Oxf. 1994; DCH (RCP) 1997. GP Regist. Nottm. Specialty: Gen. Pract.

WHITEFORD, Margo Lorraine Duncan Guthrie Institute of Medical Genetics, Yorkhill NHS Trust, Glasgow G3 8SJ Tel: 0141 201 0365 Fax: 0141 357 4277 Email: margo.whiteford@yorkhill.scot.nhs.uk; 27 Turnhill Avenue, Erskine PA8 7DL — MB ChB Dundee 1985; BSc (Pharmacol.) Dund 1980, MB ChB 1985; MRCP (UK) 1990. Cons. Clin. Geneticist. Specialty: Genetics. Prev: Sen. Regist. (Med. Genetics) Roy. Hosp. for Sick Childr. Glas.

WHITEHALL, Adrian Leslie Village Surgery, 233 Village Street, Derby DE23 8DD Tel: 01332 766762 Fax: 01332 272084 — MB ChB Leeds 1976; DRCOG 1978; MRCGP 1980; M.Med.Sci. Sheff. 1992. Prev: Trainee Gen. Pract. Derby Vocational Train. Scheme; Ho. Surg. & Ho. Phys. York Dist. Hosp.; SHO (O & G) Fulford Matern. Hosp. York.

WHITEHEAD, Anita Lilian Histopathology Department Box 235, Addenbrooke's Hospital, Hills rd, Cambridge CB2 2QQ Tel: 01223 217163 Fax: 01223 216980 Email: alw37@cam.ac.uk — MB BS Lond. 1978; BSc Bristol 1972; MRCPath 1987; FRCPath 1997.

Cons. In Paediat + Perinatal Path., Addenbrookes Hosp. Camb. Specialty: Histopath. Prev: Cons. Histopath. Hinchingbrooke Hosp. Huntingdon.

WHITEHEAD, Ann Penelope 19 Tring Avenue, Ealing, London W5 3QA Tel: 020 8992 1940 Fax: 020 8896 2922 — MB BS Lond. 1959 (Guy's) MRCS Eng. LRCP Lond. 1959; MFFP 1993. Specialty: Family Plann. & Reproduc. Health. Prev: SHO (Surg.) Dorking Gen. Hosp.; Asst. Hon. Surg. Cas. Off. & Hon. Phys. (Childr.s) Guy's Hosp. Lond.

WHITEHEAD, Anthony Martin Sanofi-Synthelabo, Guildford GU1 4YS Tel: 01483 554139 Fax: 01483 554829 Email: tony.whitehead@sanofi-synthelabo.com — MB ChB Liverp. 1979; DRCOG 1983; Dip. Pharm. Med. RCP (UK) 1986; MFPM RCP (UK) 1991; FFPM RCP UK 1999. Specialty: Pharmaceutical Medicine. Prev: Dir. (Clin. Dent.) Antisoma; Med. Dir. Pfizer Ltd. Kent; Med. Dir. Duphar Laborat. Ltd. Soton.

WHITEHEAD, Bruce Foster Cardiothoracic Unit, Great Ormond Street Hospital, for Children NHS Trust, London WC1N 3JH Tel: 020 7405 9200 Fax: 020 7813 8440; 27 Windsor Road, Wanstead, London E11 3QU — MB BS New South Wales 1979 (NSW,Aust.) MRCP (UK) 1986; FRCP Lond. 1996; FRCP 1996; FRCPCH 1997. Cons. Transpl. Phys. (Paediat. Cardiothoracic Transpl.) Gt. Ormond St. Hosp. Childr. Lond. Specialty: Paediat. Socs: Int. Soc. Heart & Lung Transpl..; ERS; Transpl. Soc. Prev: Clin. Research Fell. Stanford Univ. Med. Centre Stanford, Calif., USA.

WHITEHEAD, Claire Loraine 7 Rogers Ruff, Northwood HA6 2FD — MB ChB Sheff. 1993; BMedSci Sheff. 1992; MRCP (UK) 1997. Specialty: Care of the Elderly.

WHITEHEAD, Clare Elizabeth (retired) Dormans, Abbey Park, Burghfield Common, Reading RG7 3HQ — MB BChir Camb. 1959 (Camb. & Univ. Coll. Hosp.) MA Camb. 1960; MRCP (UK) 1974. Prev: Cons. Phys. Rehabil. Battle Hosp. Reading.

WHITEHEAD, David Mark The Glebe Surgery, Monastery Lane, Storrington, Pulborough RH20 4LR Tel: 01903 742942 Fax: 01903 740700; Hartswood House, Water Lane, Storrington, Pulborough RH20 3LY — MB BS Lond. 1980; DRCOG 1983; MRCGP 1985.

WHITEHEAD, Diane Yvonne Assumpta (retired) Wolsey Lodge, 1 St Mary's Road, Long Ditton, Surbiton KT6 5EU Tel: 020 8398 6286 — MB BS Lond. 1962 (Westm.) MRCS Eng. LRCP Lond. 1962; DObst RCOG 1964.

WHITEHEAD, Edna Marion (retired) Department Paediatrics & Child & Adolescent Psychiatry, Chaucer Unit, Northwick Park Hospital, Watford Road, Harrow HA1 3UJ Tel: 020 8869 2640; 34 Elstree Road, Bushey Heath, Watford WD23 4GL Tel: 020 8950 9262 — MB BCh Wales 1959; DObst RCOG 1961; Dip. FPA. 1964; DCH Eng. 1965; DA Eng. 1966; MRCPCH 1996. Assoc. Specialist (Community Paediat.) Northwick Pk. Hosp. Harrow. Prev: Med. Off. Lond. Boro. Islington.

WHITEHEAD, Mr Edward BUPA Hospital, Hull HU10 7AZ — MB ChB Ed. 1961; FRCS Ed. 1967; FRCS (C) 1969. Surg. (ENT) Hull Roy. Infirm. Prev: Active Staff Wellesley Hosp. Toronto, Canada; Asst. Prof. Univ. Toronto; Cons. ENT Surg. Doncaster Roy. Infirm.

WHITEHEAD, Elizabeth Monica Ealing Hospital NHS Trust, Uxbridge Road, Southall UB1 3HW Tel: 020 8574 2444 Fax: 020 8967 5630; Orford House, Chiswick Mall, Chiswick, London W4 2PS Tel: 020 8994 0671 — MB BS Lond. 1983 (King's Coll. Hosp.) BSc Lond. 1980; FRCA 1987. Cons. Anaesth. Ealing Hosp. Lond. Specialty: Anaesth. Socs: Roy. Soc. Med.; Assn. Anaesth.; Fell. Roy. Coll. Anaesth.s. Prev: Sen. Regist. (Anaesth.) Middlx. Hosp. Lond.

WHITEHEAD, Esme Mary 2 Printshop Road, Lylehill, Templepatrick, Ballyclare BT39 0HZ Tel: 028 9443 3351 — MB ChB (Hons) Manch. 1976; MRCP (UK) 1978; DCH RCPS Glas. 1983; BSc Hons. (Med. Biochem.) Manch. 1973, MD 1986; FRCP (Lond) 1997. Cons. Rheum. N. Bd. N. Irel. Specialty: Rheumatol. Prev: Sen. Regist. (Rheum.) Roy. Vict. Hosp. Belf.; Sen. Regist. (Pharmacol.) Belf. City Hosp.; Research Regist. (Endocrinol.) Christie Hosp. Manch.

WHITEHEAD, Evelyn Julie Hale Place, 29 Hale St., East Peckham, Tonbridge TN12 5HL Tel: 01622 871816 — MB ChB Manch. 1979; DRCOG 1982; DCH RCP Lond. 1983; DFFP 1996; RHC 1996. Specialty: Gen. Pract.

WHITEHEAD, Gail Ann 67 Appledore Avenue, Bexleyheath DA7 6QJ — MB BCh Wales 1994 (Univ. of Wales Coll. of Med.) MRCPCH (SPR Paed.) John Rodcliffe Hosp. Sen. SHO (Paediatr.) Blackpool Vict. Hosp. Specialty: Paediat. Prev: SHO (Paediatr.) Booth Hall Childr. Hosp. Manch.; SHO (Community Paediat.) N. Durh. NHS Trust; SHO (Neonat. Med.) St. Mary's Hosp. for Wom. & Childr. Manch.

WHITEHEAD, Helen Marie 2 Laurel Heights, Downpatrick BT30 6LH — MD Belf. 1990 (Queen's University Belfast) MB BCh BAO 1982; MRCP (UK) 1985; FRCP (Ed.) 1996; FRCP (Lond.) 1998. Cons. Phys. Internal Med. & Diabetes Down & Lisburn Community Trust. Specialty: Gen. Med.; Diabetes; Endocrinol. Socs: Diabetes UK; Irish Endocrine Soc.; BMA.

WHITEHEAD, John Ernest Michael (retired) Ashleigh Cottage, The St, Frampton on Severn, Gloucester GL2 7ED — MB BChir Camb. 1945 (Camb. & St. Thos.) MRCS Eng. LRCP Lond. 1944; MA Camb. 1946; Dip. Bact. Lond 1953; FRCPath 1970. Prev: Dir. Pub. Health Laborat. Serv. & Cons. Adviser (Microbiol.) DHSS.

WHITEHEAD, John Peter (retired) Yarde House, Combe Florey, Taunton TA4 3JB — MRCS Eng. LRCP Lond. 1943 (Lond. Hosp.) FRCPath. 1967, M 1964. Prev: Cons. Histopath. Basilden/Thurrock Dist.

WHITEHEAD, John Richard Edmund Barton Surgery, Barton Terrace, Dawlish EX7 9QH Tel: 01626 888877 Fax: 01626 888360 — (Bristol) BSc (1st cl. Hons. Psychol.) Bristol 1971; MB ChB 1977; MRCGP 1984. Hosp. Pract. (A & E) Roy. Devon & Exeter Hosp.; Force Med. Off. Devon & Cornw. Constab.; Hon. Research Fell. Dept. Police Studies Univ. Exeter. Specialty: Accid. & Emerg.; Occupat. Health. Socs: Soc. Occupat. Med. Prev: Trainee GP Univ. Exeter Postgrad. Med. Sch.; SHO (Anaesth.) Roy. Devon & Exeter Hosp. & Ho. Surg. Frenchay Hosp. Bristol; Ho. Phys. Roy. Devon & Exeter Hosp.

WHITEHEAD, Mr John Stanley Weston (retired) Ridgeway, Vicarage Lane, Burton-in-Kendal, Carnforth LA6 1NW — MB BChir Camb. 1947 (Camb. & Middlx.) MA, MChir Camb. 1954; FRCS Eng. 1951. Cons. Surg. Roy. Lanc. Infirm. Prev: Sen. Regist. (Surg.) Dudley Rd. Hosp. Birm.

WHITEHEAD, Judith Patricia Basildon Hospital, Basildon SS16 5NL Tel: 01268 533911 Fax: 01268 593948 — MB ChB Manch. 1981; FFA RCS Eng. 1986. Cons. Anaesth. Basildon Hosp. Specialty: Anaesth. Prev: Sen. Regist. Roy. Lond. Hosp.

WHITEHEAD, Malcolm Ian Department of Obst. & Gyn., King's College Hospital, Denmark Hill, London SE5 8RX Tel: 020 7387 8251 Fax: 020 7387 8252; 28 Parthenia Road, Fulham, London SW6 4BE Tel: Ex. Dir. — MB BS Lond. 1970 (Roy. Free) MRCS Eng. LRCP Lond. 1970; FRCOG 1989, M 1977, DObst 1973. Cons. O & G Kings Coll. Hosp. Lond. Specialty: Obst. & Gyn. Special Interest: Gynae-Endocrinology; Premature Menopause. Socs: Brit. Menopause Soc. (Ex-Chairm.). Prev: Lect. (O & G) Kings Coll. Hosp. Lond.; Regist. Inst. O & G Qu. Charlotte's Hosp. & Chelsea Hosp. Wom.

WHITEHEAD, Mary Anne Brigstock Medical Centre, 141 Brigstock Road, Thornton Heath CR7 7JN Tel: 020 8684 1128 Fax: 020 8689 3647 — MB BS Lond. 1973; BSc (Hons.) (Physiol.) Lond. 1970; DRCOG 1976; MRCGP 1977. Clin. Asst. Diabetic Dept. St. Geo. Hosp. Tooting. Specialty: Dermat.

WHITEHEAD, Mary Barbara (retired) 7 Rogers Ruff, Northwood HA6 2FD Tel: 01923 829314 — MB ChB Liverp. 1961; BSc (Hons. Physiol.) Liverp. 1956; DObst RCOG 1963. Prev: Lect. (Path.) Univ. Liverp.

WHITEHEAD, Michael James Department of Anaesthesia, Swansea NHS Trust, Singleton Hospital, Swansea SA2 8QA Tel: 01792 285427 Fax: 01792 208647; 19 Dysgwylfa, Sketty, Swansea SA2 9BG — MB ChB Bristol 1972; FFA RCS Eng. 1976. Cons. Anaesth. Swansea NHS Trust; Clin. Dir. Theatre Servs. Swansea NHS Trust. Specialty: Anaesth.

WHITEHEAD, Miranda Nialla New Forest District Council, Appletree Court, Lyndhurst SO43 7PA Email: miranda.whitehead@ntdc.gov.uk; Cleeves, Godshill Wood, Fordingbridge SP6 2LR Tel: 01425 652188 Email: miranda@bentinck2.freeserve.co.uk — MB BS Lond. 1973 (St. Bart.) MRCS Eng. LRCP Lond. 1973. Disabil. Employm. Cons., Disabil. Matters Ltd, Stockbridge. Special Interest: Disabil. and Employm.; Local Govt.; Pub. Health. Prev: GP Salisbury.; Med. Adviser to SOTS Progr. Portsmouth Primary Care Trust.

WHITEHEAD, Nicholas Francis Frome Medical Practice, Health Centre, Park Road, Frome BA11 1EZ Tel: 01373 301300 Fax:

01373 301313; 2 Raby Place, Bathwick Hill, Bath BA2 4EH — MB BS Lond. 1974 (Roy. Free) MRCS Eng. LRCP Lond. 1974; MRCGP 1978. Bd. Mem. Mendip PCG & Lead Clin. Governance. Specialty: Gen. Pract.

WHITEHEAD, Peter 190 King Street, Cottingham HU16 5QJ Tel: 01482 847250 — MB ChB Leeds 1964. Prev: Dir. Hull Emerg. Call Serv.; Jun. Receiv. Room Off. Leeds Gen. Infirm.; Ho. Surg. Hull Roy. Infirm.

WHITEHEAD, Peter Norman Dr M E Rouse and Partners, 24 St John's Avenue, Churchdown, Gloucester GL3 2DB Tel: 01452 713036 Fax: 01452 714726; Pegmore, Church Lane, Priors Norton, Gloucester GL2 9LS Tel: 01452 730352 — MB BS Lond. 1977 (Guy's) MRCS Eng. LRCP Lond. 1977; DRCOG 1980; DA Eng. 1982; MSc (Sports Med.) Nottm. 1995. Director of Sports Sci. & Med. for Brit. Equestrian Federat.; Chief Med. Off. Brit. Eventing. Specialty: Gen. Pract.; Sports Med. Socs: Med. Equestrian Assn. (Chairm.); FRSM. (Counc. Mem. Sect. Sports Med.).

WHITEHEAD, Peter Sinclair Fisher Medical Centre, Millfields, Skipton BD23 1EU Tel: 01756 799622 Fax: 01756 796194 — MB ChB Ed. 1981; MA Camb. 1974; DRCOG 1984; MRCGP 1985.

WHITEHEAD, Peter Thomas 19 Tring Avenue, Ealing, London W5 3QA Tel: 020 8992 1940 Fax: 020 8896 2922 — MB BS Lond. 1959 (Guy's) AFOM; MRCS Eng. LRCP Lond. 1959. Specialty: Occupat. Health. Prev: Ho. Surg. Cas. Off. & Ho. Phys. Guy's Hosp.

WHITEHEAD, Philip Jennings Church Road Surgery, 1 Church Road, Mitcham CR4 3YU Tel: 020 8648 2579 Fax: 020 8640 4013 — MB BS Lond. 1970 (St. Geo.) DObst RCOG 1972; DCH Eng. 1973. Tutor Div. Gen. Pract. St. Geo. Hosp. Med. Sch.; Apptd. Doctor EMAS Lead; Mem. Merton, Sutton & Wandsworth LMC. Prev: SHO (Obst.) St. Geo. Hosp. Lond.; SHO (Paediat.) Sydenham Childr. Hosp.

WHITEHEAD, Philip John (retired) Department of Pathology, Frenchay Hospital, Bristol BS16 1LE Tel: 0117 970 1212 Fax: 0117 957 1866; 10 Old Anst Road, Almondsbury, Bristol BS32 4HJ — MB ChB Bristol 1963; FRCPath 1982, M 1970. Cons. Haemat. N. Bristol NHS Trust. Prev: Cons. Path. W. Cumbld. Hosp. Gp.

WHITEHEAD, Robert Henry Brandwood Sean Yew Tree Cottage, 4 Butts Ash, Fawley Road, Hythe, Southampton SO4 — BM Soton. 1980. SHO (Anaesth.) W. Dorset Weymouth HA. Socs: Nat. Inst. Med. Herbalist.

WHITEHEAD, Stephanie Ann 28 The Crossways, Otley LS21 2AR Tel: 01943 466517 — BSc (Hons.) 1983; PhD. Microbiology 1988; MB ChB Leeds 1996. GP Regist.; SHO Paediat. Airedale W. Yorks. Specialty: Gen. Pract.

WHITEHEAD, Stephen Mark 39 Sunny Hill, Milford, Derby DE56 0QR — MB ChB Leeds 1975; DRCOG 1977; DTM & H Liverp. 1982; MFPHM 1988. Cons. Pub. Health Med. South. Derbysh. HA. Specialty: Pub. Health Med. Prev: Med. Off. Maua Methodist Hosp. Kenya.

WHITEHEAD, Mr Stephen Michael 34 Tower Road W., St Leonards-on-Sea TN38 0RG Tel: 01424 718059 — MB BChir Camb. 1973; MA Camb. 1973; FRCS Eng. 1977; MChir 1986. Cons. Surg., Conquest Hosp. Hastings & Rother NHS Trust. Specialty: Gen. Surg. Socs: Fell.of Assoc. of Surg. Of G.B. & Irel.; Vasc. Surg. Soc. GB & Irel.; Europ. Soc. Of Vasc. Surg. Prev: Sen. Regist. (Surg.) St. Thos. Hosp. Lond.; Regist. (Surg.) Kent & Canterbury Hosp.; Ho. Surg. St. Thos. Hosp. Lond.

WHITEHEAD, Susan Carol Elborough Street Surgery, 81-83 Elborough Street, Southfields, London SW18 5DS Tel: 020 8874 7113 Fax: 020 8874 3682 — MB BS Lond. 1971; DObst RCOG 1974; MRCGP 1976.

WHITEHEAD, Thomas Crosby The Close, Farnborough, Banbury OX17 1DZ — MB BS Lond. 1990.

WHITEHEAD, Timothy Robin Stuart Waterman 19 The Waterside, Hellesdon, Norwich NR6 5QN Tel: 01603 417099; The Health Centre, Adelaide St, Norwich NR6 4JL Tel: 01603 625015 Fax: 01603 766820 — MRCS Eng. LRCP Lond. 1974 (Westm.) Specialty: Gen. Pract.

WHITEHEAD, Vjera Brangjolica (retired) 18 Vineyard Road, London SW19 7JH — LAH Dub. 1965.

WHITEHEAD, William Harold Minfor Surgery, Park Road, Barmouth LL42 1PL Tel: 01341 280521 Fax: 01341 280912 — BM BCh Oxf. 1980; MA, BM BCh Oxf. 1980; MRCGP 1986. Course Organiser Gwynedd VTS.

WHITEHORN, Melanie White House Surgery, Weston Lane, Weston, Southampton SO19 9HJ Tel: 023 8044 9913 — BM Soton. 1981; DRCOG 1983; DCH RCP Lond. 1985; MRCGP 1985. GP. Special Interest: Geriat. Psychiat.

WHITEHOUSE, Alison Jayne 24 Chesford Crescent, Warwick CV34 5PR — MB ChB Leeds 1995.

WHITEHOUSE, Andrew Beckwith George Eliot Hospital, College Street, Nuneaton CV9 1BW Tel: 02476 865255 Email: andrews.whitehouse@geh.nhs.uk; 16 Coleshill Road, Atherstone CV9 1BW Tel: 01827 717755 Email: a.b.whitehouse@bham.ac.uk — MB BChir Camb. 1974 (Cambridge) MRCP (UK) 1976; MA Camb. 1990; FRCP Lond. 1993. Cons. Phys. Geo. Eliot Hosp. Nuneaton; Teach. Clin. Med. Leicester Univ. Med. Sch.; Director of Hosp. and Specialist Educat. at W. Midlands Postgrad. Deanery. Specialty: Gen. Med. Socs: Nat. Assn. Clin. Tutors (Counc.); Brit. Geriat. Soc.; ASME. Prev: Sen. Regist. Roy. Devon & Exeter Hosp.; Med. Off. Chas. Johnson Mem. Hosp. Nqutu, Kwazulu; SHO (Gen. Med.) Hillingdon Hosp. Uxbridge.

WHITEHOUSE, Andrew Michael Psychiatric Out Patients Department, B Floor, South Block, Queens Medical Centre, Nottingham NG7 2UH Tel: 0115 924 9924 — BM Soton. 1981; MPhil Ed. 1985; MRCPsych 1985; MA Camb. 1989. Cons. Psychiat. Qu.s Med. centre Nottm. Specialty: Gen. Psychiat. Socs: Brit. Med. Ass; Nottm.shire Medico-legal Soc. Prev: Clin. Lect. (Psychiat.) Addenbrookes Hosp. Camb.; Regist. (Psychiat.) Roy. Edin. Hosp.; Cons.(psychiat) bradgate Ment. health unit,Leics.

WHITEHOUSE, Anthony Richard Polkyth Surgery, 14 Carlyon Road, St Austell PL25 4EG Tel: 01726 75555; 4 Crinnis Wood Avenue, Carlyon Bay, St Austell PL25 3QD Tel: 01726 814415 — MB BS Lond. 1975 (St. Bart.) MRCS Eng. LRCP Lond. 1975. GP Princip.; Local Med. Off. for Civil Serv.; Dist. Med. Off. Brit. Red Cross; Med. Adviser St. Austell Brewery; Med. Off. Roach Foods Ltd.; Examr. Med. Pract. DSS. Specialty: Gen. Pract.

WHITEHOUSE, Professor Carl Raymond (retired) — MB BChir Camb. 1963 (Camb. & St Geo.) MA Camb. 1964; DObst RCOG 1965; FRCGP 1987, M 1969; DCH Eng. 1969. Prev: Prof. Teach. Med. in Community Univ. Manch.

WHITEHOUSE, Caroline Cheviot Road Surgery, 1 Cheviot Road, Millbrook, Southampton SO16 4AH Tel: 023 8077 3174 Fax: 023 8070 2748 — MB ChB Bristol 1987. Specialty: Gen. Pract.

WHITEHOUSE, David Haigh Health Centre, Redcar TS10 1SR Tel: 01642 475157; The Old Vicarage, Kirkleatham Village, Redcar TS10 5NN Tel: 01642 503250 — MB ChB Leeds 1954. Prev: Cas. Off. Bradford Roy. Infirm.; Ho. Phys. St. Luke's Hosp. Bradford; Med. Off. RAMC (Nat. Serv.).

WHITEHOUSE, David Roger 4 Lakeside, Little Aston Hall, Sutton Coldfield B74 3BJ — MB ChB Birm. 1954; MRCS Eng. LRCP Lond. 1954; DObst RCOG 1959.

WHITEHOUSE, Professor Graham Hugh 9 Belmont Road, West Kirby, Wirral CH48 5EY — MB BS (Hons.) Lond. 1965 (Westm.) MRCS Eng. LRCP Lond. 1965; FRCP Lond. 1983, M 1967; DMRD Eng. 1969; FFR 1971; FRCR 1975; DSc Lond. 2001. Emerit. Prof. Diagn. Radiol. Univ. Liverp. Specialty: Radiol. Special Interest: Breast Imaging; Diagnostic Radiol.; Magnetic Resanance Imaging. Socs: Roy. Soc. Med.; Brit. Med. Assn.; Brit. Inst. Of Radiol. Prev: Prof. pf Diagnostic Radiol., Univ. of Liverp.; Sen. Lect., Univ. of Liverp.; Asst. Prof., Univeristy of Rochester, New York, USA.

WHITEHOUSE, Joanna Louise — MB ChB Birm. 1992; MRCP (UK) 1995. Regist. (Respirat. Med.) St. Thos. Hosp. Lond. Specialty: Respirat. Med.; Gen. Med.

WHITEHOUSE, Pauline Amanda 27 The Foxgloves, Tanhouse Lane, Hedge End, Southampton SO30 0NG — MB BS Lond. 1996; MRCS Lond. 1999. Specialty: Gen. Surg.

WHITEHOUSE, Richard John 20 Brandy Hole Lane, Chichester PO19 5RY — MB BS Lond. 1992.

WHITEHOUSE, Richard William Manchester Royal Infirmary, Department of Clinical Radiology, Oxford Road, Manchester M13 9WL Tel: 0161 276 8590 Fax: 0161 276 4141 Email: richard.whitehouse@cmmc.nhs.uk — MB ChB Manch. 1981; BSc (Hons.) Manch. 1978; FRCR 1986; MD Manch. 1993. Cons. Musculoskeletal Radiologist NHS Manch.; Hon. Clin. Lect. (Diag. Radiol.) Univ. Manch. Specialty: Radiol. Special Interest: Musculoskeletal. Socs: Internat. Skeletal Soc.; Brit. Soc. of Skeletal Radiologists; Roy. Soc. of Med.

WHITEHOUSE, Susan Janina Main house, Hollymoorway, Northfield, Birmingham B31 5HE Tel: 0121 678 3630 — MB ChB Birm. 1986; MRCPsych 1992; MmedSci 1998. Locum Cons. Psychotherapist Main Ho. Therapeutic Community. Specialty: Psychother. Prev: Regist. Rotat. (Psychiat.) Birm.; Sen. Regist. Rotat. W. Mid. (Psychother.).

WHITEHOUSE, Tony — MB BS Lond. 1992; BSc Lond. 1989. Specialist Regist. (Anaesth.) N. Thames (Centr.) Sch. of Anaesth. Specialty: Anaesth.; Intens. Care.

WHITEHOUSE, William Patrick Audiffred Academic Child Health, E Floor / East Block, Queen's Medical Centre, Nottingham NG7 2UH Tel: 0115 924 9924 Fax: 0115 970 9382 — MB BS Lond. 1981 (Lond. Hosp.) BSc Lond. 1978; DCH Lond. 1983; FRCP 1997, MRCP (UK) 1986; FRCPCH 1997. Sen. Lect. In Paediat. Neurol., Univ. of Nottm.; Hon. Cons. Paediat. Neurol. Qu.'s Med. Centre, Nottm. Specialty: Paediat. Neurol.; Research. Socs: Brit. Paediat. Neurol. Assn. Counc. Mem.; Internat. League Against Epilepsy; Internat. Headache Soc. Prev: Cons. Paediat. Neurol. Childr. Hosp. Birm.; Sen. Regist. (Paediat. Neurol.) Childr. Hosp. Birm.; Research Fell. & Hon. Sen. Regist. (Paediat. Neurol.) Univ. Lond.

WHITEHURST, Antje Maria Florence Road Surgery, 26 Florence Road, Ealing, London W5 3TX — MB BS Lond. 1991 (St Mary's Hosp. Med. Sch. Lond.) MRCGP 1996. Princip. in Gen. Pract. Socs: Roy. Coll. of Gen. Practitioners.

WHITEHURST, Louise Mary Belgrave Medical Centre, 22 Asline Road, Sheffield S2 4UJ Tel: 0114 255 1184 — MB ChB Sheff. 1986 (Sheffield University) MRCGP 1990. GP. Prev: Trainee GP Oxf. VTS.

WHITEHURST, Philip Anaesthetics Department, Russells Hall Hospital, Dudley DY1 2HQ — MB ChB Aberd. 1976; FFA RCS Eng. 1980. Cons. Anaesth. Dudley Gp. Hosps. Trust. Specialty: Anaesth. Prev: Sen. Regist. (Anaesth.) Yorks. RHA; Regist. (Anaesth.) Univ. Coll. Hosp. Lond.

WHITELAW, Alan Stewart 9 Ambleside, East Kilbride, Glasgow G75 8TX — MB ChB Glas. 1998.

WHITELAW, Professor Andrew George Lindsay Neonatal Intensive Care Unit, Southmead Hospital, Southmead Road, Westbury-on-Trym, Bristol BS10 5NB Tel: 0117 959 5325 Fax: 0117 959 5324 Email: andrew.whitelaw@bristol.ac.uk — MB BChir 1971 (Cambridge & St. Marys) MRCP (UK) 1973; MD Camb. 1978; FRCP Lond. 1988; FRCPCH 1997. Prof. of Neonat. Med., Univ. of Bristol; Cons. neonatologist, N. Bristol and United Bristol NHS Trusts. Specialty: Paediat. Socs: Neonat. Soc.; Roy. Coll. Paediat. and child health; Europ. Soc. for paediatric research. Prev: Cons. Neonatol. Hammersmith Hosp. Lond.; Neonat. Fell. Hosp. Sick Childr. Toronto, Canada; Ho. Phys. Hosp. Sick Childr. Gt. Ormond St. Lond.

WHITELAW, Catherine Anne Meadowbank Health Centre, 3 Salmon Inn Road, Falkirk FK2 0XF Tel: 01324 715446 Fax: 01324 717986 — MB ChB Glas. 1977.

WHITELAW, Donald Crawford Bradford Hospital NHS Trust, Bradford Royal Infirmary, Duckworth Lane, Bradford BD9 6RS Tel: 01274 542200 — MB ChB Ed. 1985 (Edin.) MRCP (UK) 1989; MD Edin. 1998. Cons. Physician in Diabetes & Endocrinology, Bradford Hosp.s NHS Trust. Specialty: Diabetes; Endocrinol. Socs: Diabetes UK; Euro. Assoc. Study of Diabetes (EASD); Soc. For Endocrinology. Prev: Ho. Phys. Derriford Hosp. Plymouth; Ho. Off. Dept. Surgic. Neurol. West. Gen. Hosp. Edin.; SHO (A & E) Taunton & Som. Hosp. Taunton.

WHITELAW, Eileen Mary (retired) Laverock, 87 The Fairway, Aldwick Bay, Bognor Regis PO21 4EX — (Roy. Free) MB BS Lond. 1950.

WHITELAW, Elizabeth Anne Woodbridge Hill Surgery, 1 Deerbarn Road, Guildford GU2 8YB Tel: 01483 562230 Fax: 01483 452442 — BM Soton. 1992; MRCGP 1996. Specialty: Gen. Pract. Prev: Trainee GP Reading VTS.

WHITELAW, Fiona Margaret Elderslie House, Strathaven ML10 6PA — MB ChB Bristol 1990; DTM & H RCP Lond. 1993. SHO (Paediat.) Barnsley Dist. Gen. Hosp. Prev: SHO (Infec. Dis. & Trop. Med.) Coppetts Wood Hosp. Lond.

WHITELAW, Joan Meadowside, Brooke, Oakham LE15 8DE — (St. Thos.) MRCS Eng. LRCP Lond. 1963; MB BS Lond. 1964; DA Eng. 1972; DObst RCOG 1974; DCH RCPSI 1980. Clin. Asst. (Anaesth.) Leicester Gen. Hosp. Prev: SHO (Paediat.) & Ho. Off. (O & G) St. Luke's Hosp. Bradford; SHO (Anaesth.) York 'A' Gp. Hosps.

WHITELAW, John Deryk Atkinson (retired) Laverock, 87 The Fairway, Aldwick Bay, Bognor Regis PO21 4EX — (Univ. Coll. Hosp.) MB BS Lond. 1944; MRCS Eng. LRCP Lond. 1944. Prev: Sen. Med. Off. Home Office.

WHITELAW, Robert (retired) 36 Holmhead, Kilbirnie KA25 6BS Tel: 01505 683264 — MB ChB Glas. 1944; DPH (Commend.) St. And. 1948; DIH Eng. 1953; DIH Soc. Apoth. Lond. 1953; MFOM RCP Lond. 1978; Specialist Accredit. (Occupat. Med.) 1978. Prev: HM Med. Insp. Facts.

WHITELAW, Mr Stuart Charles 75 Hillfoot Drive, Bearsden, Glasgow G61 3QG — MB ChB Glas. 1981; FRCS Ed. 1987; FRCS Glas. 1988.

WHITELEY, Alan Mark 20 Sefton Drive, Mapperly Park, Nottingham NG3 5ER Tel: 0115 960 6514 Fax: 0115 960 6514 — MB BChir Camb. 1972 (Camb. & St. Bart.) MA, MB Camb. 1972, BChir 1971; FRCP 1988. Cons. Neurol. Nottm. & Mansfield Hosps. Specialty: Neurol. Prev: Sen. Regist. (Neurol.) St. Bart. Hosp. & Nat. Hosp. Qu. Sq. Lond.; Regist. Lond. Hosp.; SHO Centr. Middlx. Hosp. Lond.

WHITELEY, Andrew Michael The Medical Centre, Badgers Crescent, Shipston-on-Stour CV36 4BQ Tel: 01608 661845 Fax: 08700 553555 Email: andrew.whiteley@tmcc4.warwick-ha.wmids.nhs.uk — MB BS Lond. 1993 (St. Bart. Hosp. Lond.) Specialty: Gen. Pract.

WHITELEY, Elizabeth Anne (retired) Heatherdale, 6 Harrowby Lane, Grantham NG31 9HX Tel: 01476 564379 — MB ChB Sheff. 1954; MFCM 1972. Specialist Community Med. Community Servs. & Local Auth. Liaison S. Lincs. HA. Prev: Dep. Co. MOH & Dep. Princip. Sch. Med. Off. Parts of Kesteven, Lincs.

WHITELEY, Gillian Louise 57 Garstang Road W., Poulton-le-Fylde FY6 8AA — MB ChB Leeds 1984.

WHITELEY, Mr Graham Stuart Wynward Ysbyty Gwynedd, Penrhosgarnedd, Bangor LL57 2PW Tel: 01248 384777 Fax: 01248 384777 — MB BS Lond. 1980 (Royal Free Hospital School of Medicine) MS Lond. 1990, MB BS 1980; FRCS Eng. 1985. Cons. Surg. Gastroenterol. & Laparoscopic Surg. Ysbyty Gwynedd & Llandudno Gen. Hosp. Specialty: Gen. Surg. Socs: Assn. Surg.; Brit. Soc. Gastroenterol.; Assn. Coloproctol. Prev: Lect. (Surg.) Centr. Manch. Hosps.; Lect. (Surg.) Univ. Hosp. S. Manch. & Christie Hosp.; Lect. (Surg.) Hope Hosp. Salford.

WHITELEY, Jane Holly House, Sunderland, Cockermouth CA13 9SS — MB BS Lond. 1957 (Roy. Free)

WHITELEY, Joan E. (retired) 43 Cunliffe Close, Banbury Road, Oxford OX2 7BJ Tel: 01865 553240 — MB BChir Camb. 1945; PhD Camb. 1950. Prev: Asst. Dir. Research (Veterin. Clin. Med.) Sch. of Veterin. Med. Univ. Camb.

WHITELEY, Joanne Tracey Lordswood House, 54 Lordswood Road, Harborne, Birmingham B17 9DB Tel: 0121 426 2030 Fax: 0121 428 2658 — MB BS Lond. 1990.

WHITELEY, John David 44 Armstrong Road, Egham TW20 0RW — MB BS Lond. 1989.

WHITELEY, John Maxwell Flat 5, Summerfield Court, Edge Lane, Chorlton-Cum-Hardy, Manchester M21 9JN — MB ChB Manch. 1965.

WHITELEY, John Stuart The Wheelwrights Cottage, Wheelers Lane, Brockham, Betchworth RH3 7LA Tel: 0173 784 3446 Fax: 0173 784 3634 Email: stuart.whiteley@virgin.net — (Leeds) MB ChB Leeds 1950; DPM Eng. 1954; FRCP Ed. 1970, M 1961; FRCPsych 1982, M 1972; M. Inst GA (Hon.) 1993. p/t Indep. Cons. Psychother. Surrey. Specialty: Psychother. Socs: FRSM; Gp. Analyt. Soc.; Assoc. of Theraputic Communities. Prev: Cons. Psychiat. & Med. Dir. Henderson Hosp. Sutton; Cons. Psychiat. Warlingham Pk. Hosp.; Chief Asst. (Psychol. Med.) Westm. Hosp. Lond.

WHITELEY, Judith Chaelan, Irthington, Carlisle CA6 4NJ — MB ChB Dundee 1997.

WHITELEY, Mr Mark Steven Department of Vascular Surgery, Royal Surrey County Hospital, Egerton Road, Guildford GU2 7XX Tel: 01483 571122 — MB BS Lond. 1986 (St. Bart.) FRCS Eng. 1991; FRCS Ed. 1991; FRCS (Gen.) 1996; MS Bath 1998. Cons. Vasc. Surg. Roy. Surrey Co. Hosp.; Vis. Sen. Fell. Vasc. Surg. Univ. of Surrey. Specialty: Gen. Surg. Socs: Vasc. Surgic. Soc.; Assn. Surg.; Eur. Soc. Vasc. Surg. Prev: Clin. Lect. (Surg.) & Hon. Sen. Regist.

Univ. Oxf. Nuffield Dept. Surg. John Radcliffe Hosp. Oxf; Mem. Rouleaux Club (Vasc. Surgic. Trainee) Sec. 1994-1997; Lect. (Surg.) Univ. Bath & Roy. United Hosp. Bath.

WHITELEY, Michael Charles William Viewfield Medical Centre, 3 Viewfield Place, Stirling FK8 1NJ Tel: 01786 472028 Fax: 01786 463388 — MB BCh BAO Belf. 1983; DRCOG 1985; MRCGP 1987.

WHITELEY, Patricia Gideon Medical Centre, 10 Chapel Lane, Arnold, Nottingham NG5 7DR Tel: 0115 920 7988; Varenna, 70 Nottingham Road, Lowdham, Nottingham NG14 7AP — MB ChB Leeds 1970. Socs: Assoc. Mem. RCGP.

WHITELEY, Richard (retired) Austin and Partners, 4 Market Place, Billesdon, Leicester LE7 9AJ Tel: 0116 259 6206 Fax: 0116 259 6388 — MB ChB Manch. 1965.

WHITELEY, Simon Marcus Paediatric intensive care unit, St James University Hospital, Beckett Street, Leeds LS9 7TF Tel: 0113 243 3144 Fax: 0113 392 2645 Email: simon.whiteley@leedsth.nhs.uk — MB BS Lond. 1986 (The Middlx. Hosp. Med. Sch., Univ. of Lond.) FRCA 1992. Cons. (Paediat. Anaesth. & Paediat. IC) St James' Univ. Hosp. Leeds. Specialty: Anaesth.; Intens. Care.

WHITELEY, William Nichol Midway, Chapel Hill, Truro TR1 3BP — BM BCh Oxf. 1997.

WHITELOCK, David Ernest 52 High Street, Yelling, Huntingdon PE19 6SD — MB BS Lond. 1996.

WHITELOCKE, Mr Rodger Alexander Frederick 152 Harley Street, London W1G 7LH Tel: 020 7935 3834 Fax: 020 7224 2574; 19 Elvaston Place, London SW7 5QF Tel: 020 7584 9871 — MB BS Lond. 1968 (St. Bart.) MRCS Eng. LRCP Lond. 1968; PhD Lond. 1975; FRCS Eng. 1976; FRCOphth 1989. Cons. Ophth. Surg. St. Bart. Hosp. & Roy. Marsden Hosp. Lond.; Lead Clin. (Ophth) Bart's & The Lond. NHS Trust; Teach. (Ophth.) Univ. Lond. Specialty: Ophth. Socs: Fell. Roy. Soc. Med.; Assn. Eye Research; Brit. Microcirculat. Soc. Prev: Hon. Vis. Prof. Visual Sci. City Univ. Lond.; Sen. Regist. & Sen. Resid. Surg. Off. Moorfields Eye Hosp. (City Rd. Br.) Lond.; Research Asst. Inst. Ophth. Univ. Lond.

WHITEMAN, Helen Ruth Adelaide Medical Centre, Adelaide Terrace, Benwell, Newcastle upon Tyne NE4 8BE Tel: 0191 219 5599 Fax: 0191 219 5596 — MB BS Newc. 1990. GP Newc.

WHITEMAN, Ingrid Ann 31 Meadow Drive, Prestbury, Macclesfield SK10 4EY — MB ChB Manch. 1986; MRCGP 1990; T(GP) 1991.

WHITEMAN, Julia Ruth London Deanery, 20 Guilford Street, London WC1N 1DZ Tel: 020 7692 3166 Email: jwhiteman@londondeanery.ac.uk; 37 Fairfax Road, Teddington TW11 9DA — MB BS Lond. 1981 (Char. Cross Hosp.) MRCGP 1985; DRCOG 1985; MA Univ. Westminster 1998. Dep. GP Director Lond. Deanery. Prev: GP Sen. Partner Twickenham; GP Tutor W. Middlx. Hosp. & Hammersmith Hosp.; Assoc. Dean Postgrad. Gen. Pract.

WHITEMAN, Paul Donald Whiteladies, Cross Lane, Brancaster, King's Lynn PE31 8AE — MB BS Lond. 1967 (Westm.) MRCS Eng. LRCP Lond. 1967; MSc Lond. 1971, MD 1976. Specialty: Pharmaceutical Medicine. Prev: Dept. Head (Bioanalyt. Sci.s) Wellcome Foundat. Beckenham; Sen. Med. Off. (Nutrit.) DoH Lond.; Lect. (Paediat. Chem. Path.) Hosp. Sick Childr. Lond.

WHITEMAN, Sarah Jane Postgraduate Medical & Dental Education, 4th Floor Gateway House, Piccadilly South, Manchester M60 7LP Tel: 0161 237 2189 Fax: 0161 237 2108; General Medical Council, Barnett House, 53 Fountain Street, Manchester M2 2AN Tel: 07850 222 284 Email: sarah.whiteman@btinternet.com — MB BS Lond. 1986 (Roy. Free) MRCGP 1990; DRCOG 1992; DCH RCP Lond. 1993; Dip. IMC RCS Ed. 1994; FRCGP 1998; DMJ (Clin) 2001; DipMedEd 2003. p/t Assoc. Dean PGMD Noalwest Deanery Manc.; Case Examr. GMC Manc. Specialty: Educat.; Gen. Pract. Socs: Assn. Forens. Physicians; Roy. Coll. of Gen. Practitioners; Instituite Learning & Teachg. Prev: Assoc. Director GP Educat. Oxf.; Forens. Med. Examr. Beds, Northants, Thames Valley; GP Milton Keynes.

WHITEMAN, Sheila Mary (retired) Holyhead Surgery, 1 Chester St., Coundon, Coventry CV1 4DH — MB ChB Sheff. 1956.

WHITEN, Christopher John 45 Ernest Gardens, London W4 3QU — MB BS Lond. 1996.

WHITENBURGH, Martin John 38 Sandfield Road, Liverpool L25 3PE — MB ChB Liverp. 1991.

WHITEOAK, Karen Lynne Wallace Tattenhall Medical Practice, High St., Tattenhall, Chester CH3 9PX; Huntington Hall, Aldford Road, Chester CH3 6EA — MB ChB Manch. 1983; BSc (Med. Sci.) St. And. 1980. Specialty: Psychosexual Med.

WHITEOAK, Richard, Col. late RAMC The Royal Hospital, Haslar, Gosport PO12 2AA Tel: 02392 584255 Fax: 02392 762150 — MB BChir Camb. 1977 (St. Thos.) MB Camb. 1978, BChir 1977; MA Camb. 1978; MRCP (UK) 1981; FRCP Lond. 1995. Cons. Phys. Princess Mary's Hosp. RAF Akrotiri BFPO 57. Specialty: Gen. Med. Socs: Brit. Soc. Gastroenterol.; BMA. Prev: Sen. Specialist (Med.) Qu. Eliz. Milt. Hosp. Woolwich; Cons. Phys TMPH AKROTRI BFP057; Cons. Phys. BMH Rinteln BFPO 29.

WHITER, Alexandra Jane 10 Grange Avenue, London N20 8AD — BM BCh Oxf. 1996.

WHITER, Gaynor Lesley 10 Grange Avenue, Totteridge Village, London N20 8AD — MB BChir Camb. 1990; DRCOG 1991. SHO (Anaesth.) MusGr. Pk. Hosp. Taunton. Specialty: Anaesth. Prev: SHO (SCBU) Brighton; SHO (O & G) Brighton.

WHITESIDE, Anthony Health Centre, London St., Fleetwood FY7 6HD Tel: 01253 874486 & 0253 873312 — MB ChB Liverp. 1966; MRCS Eng. LRCP Lond. 1966; DObst RCOG 1970. Prev: SHO Med. Vict. Hosp. Blackpool; Cas. Off. Whiston Hosp. Prescot; Ho. Surg. David Lewis North. Hosp. Liverp.

WHITESIDE, Bernard Godfrey Hanham Surgery, 33 Whittucks Road, Hanham, Bristol BS15 3HY Tel: 0117 967 5201 Fax: 0117 947 7749; 46 Barry Road, Oldland Common, Bristol BS30 6QY Tel: 0117 932 8831 — MB BS Lond. 1975 (Guy's) MRCS Eng. LRCP Lond. 1974; DRCOG 1978; MRCGP 1979. Chairm. Assn. Fundholders Gp.; Mem. Avon LMC. Prev: Trainee GP Lond. (Brook Gen. Hosp.) VTS; Ho. Off. Orpington Hosp.

WHITESIDE, Catherine Elaine 6 Lawside Terrace, Dundee DD3 6EA — MB ChB Dund. 1998.

WHITESIDE, Christine Lesley 23 Alexandra Drive, Liverpool L17 8TB — MB ChB Liverp. 1982.

WHITESIDE, Mary Lorraine Whiteabbey Health Centre, 95 Doagh Road, Newtownabbey BT37 9QN Tel: 028 9086 4341 Fax: 028 9086 0443 — MB BCh BAO Belf. 1979.

WHITESIDE, Mr Michael Charles Richmond Antrim Area Hospital, 45 Bush Road, Antrim BT41 2RL; 1 The Orcuard, Circular Road, Belfast — MB BCh BAO Belf. 1986; FRCSI 1990; MD Belf. 1997. Cons. Surg. Specialty: Gen. Surg.

WHITESIDE, Michael William 7 Meadway, Bromborough, Wirral — MB BS Lond. 1970; MRCS Eng. LRCP Lond. 1970; DCH RCPS Glas. 1974.

WHITESIDE, Olivia Bedford House, 82 Cornwall Road, Harrogate HG1 2NE — MB BS Lond. 1998; MRCS (Eng).

WHITESIDE, Ralph Stephen 165 Cundy Street, Walkley, Sheffield S6 2WP — MB ChB Sheff. 1989.

WHITESIDE, Richard John 3 The Grange, Cairnburn Road, Belfast BT4 2PH — MB BCh BAO Belf. 1989.

WHITESIDE, Professor Thomas Charles Douay, MBE, Group Capt. RAF Med. Br. Retd. High Bank, Tighnabruaich PA21 2EB Tel: 01700 811600 — MB BCh Glas 1945; Psychologist; PhD (Hawthorne Prize) Glas. 1955; MRCP Lond. 1971; FRAeS 1971. Indep. Cons. Environm. Relations. Specialty: Aviat. Med. Socs: Brit. Psychol. Soc.; Internat. Acad. Aviat. Med.; Soc. Experim. Psychol. Prev: Hon. Lect. (Aviat. Med.) Univ. Glas.; Whittingham Prof. Aviat. Med.; OC RAF Aviat. Med. Train. Centre N. Luffenham.

WHITESIDE, William Noel, CStJ (Surgery) 10 Blyth Road, Bromley BR1 3RH Tel: 020 8460 7182; The House-on-the-Wall, Watts Lane, Chislehurst BR7 5PJ Tel: 020 8467 0958 — MB BCh BAO Dub. 1934; BA Dub. Dist. Surg. St. John Ambul. Brig. (Reserve); Hon. Vice-Pres. S.E. Sect. Lond. Br. Brit. Red Cross Soc. Socs: BMA & Harv. Soc. Prev: Wing Cdr. RAF Med. Br.

WHITESON, Adrian Leon, OBE 58A Wimpole Street, London W1M 7DE Tel: 020 7935 3351 Fax: 020 7487 2504; Pender Lodge, 6 Oakleigh Park N., London N20 9AR Tel: 020 8445 9365 — MB BS Lond. 1959 (St. Geo.) MB BS (Hons. Therap. & Pharm.) Lond. 1959; MRCS Eng. LRCP Lond. 1959. Indep. GP Lond. & Chief Med. Off. Brit. Boxing Bd. Control; Chief Med. Off. Providence Capitol & Liberty Life Assur. Companies; Sen. Med. Examr. Scott. Widows, Abbey Life & Other Insur. Companies; Chief Med. Adviser Trafalgar Hse. Gp.; Chairm. Med. Commiss. World Boxing Counc. Prev: Clin.

Asst. Diabetic Clinic St. Bart. Hosp. Lond.; Ho. Off. (Med.) & Cas. Off. St. Geo. Hosp. Lond.

WHITESON, Stephen Daniel 166 Kingsway, Gatley, Cheadle SK8 4NT — BM BS Nottm. 1986.

WHITEWAY, Miss Janet Elizabeth Department of Urology, South Cleveland Hospital, Middlesbrough TS4 3BW Fax: 01642 854708; 10 Cornfield Road, Middlesbrough TS5 5QL — BM BCh Oxf. 1974 (Oxf. & St. Thos.) MCh Oxf. 1985, BM BCh 1974; FRCS Eng. 1979. Cons. Urol. S. Cleveland Hosp. Middlesbrough; Adviser in Urol., Chief Med. Off./N.C.E.P.O.D. Specialty: Urol. Socs: Roy. Soc. Med. (Mem. Counc. Sect. Urol.) Brit. Assn. Urol. Surgs.; Epicurist N. Eng. Surg. Soc. Amer. Urol. Assoc. Prev: Sen. Regist. Freeman Hosp. Newc.; Regist. St Peter's Hosp. Lond.; Research Fell. St. Mark's Hosp. Lond.

WHITEWOOD, Colin Noel 18 Remburn Gardens, Lakin Road, Warwick CV34 5BW — MB BS Western Australia 1991.

WHITEWOOD, Felicity Jane 18 Remburn Gardens, Lakin Road, Warwick CV34 5BW — MB BS Western Australia 1991.

WHITFIELD, Andrea Marie 4 The Steeple, Caldy, Wirral CH48 1QE — MB ChB Bristol 1987.

WHITFIELD, Andrew John Lightwater Surgery, All Saints House, 39 All Saints Road, Lightwater GU18 5SQ Tel: 01276 472248 Fax: 01276 473873; 18 Walkers Ridge, Camberley GU15 2DF — MB ChB Sheff. 1985. Med. Adviser BOC Gp. Surrey. Specialty: Gen. Pract.

WHITFIELD, Ann (retired) 3 West Castle Road, Edinburgh EH10 5AT — MB BS Lond. 1959 (King's Coll. Hosp.) MRCS Eng. LRCP Lond. 1959; DA Eng. 1961; FFA RCS Eng. 1965. Prev: Cons. Anaesth. Edin. Roy. Infirm.

WHITFIELD, Mr Bernard Charles Stuart 7 Woodland Road, Kilner Park, Ulverston LA12 0DX Tel: 01229 582333 Fax: 01229 580934 — MB ChB Leeds 1979; BSc (Hons.) (Med. Microbiol.) Leeds 1976; FRCS (Gen. Surg.) Ed. 1983; FCS Otol. S Afr 1987; FRCS (Otol.) Ed. 1990. Cons. Otorhinolaryng. Morecambe Bay Hosp. Trust. Specialty: Otolaryngol. Socs: Brit. Assn. Otol.; N. Eng. ENT Soc.; Roy. Soc. Med. Prev: Clin. Lect. (Otolaryngol.) & Sen. Regist. Radcliffe Infirm. Oxf.; Clin. Lect. (Otolaryngol.) & Cons. Univ. Cape Town, SA.

WHITFIELD, Betty Elaine The Copse, Bannerdown Road, Baheaston, Bath BA1 7PL Tel: 01225 858855 — (Liverp.) MB ChB Liverp. 1950; DObst RCOG 1951.

WHITFIELD, Catherine Tracy Presteigne Medical Centre, Lugg View, Presteigne LD8 2RJ Tel: 01544 267985 Fax: 01544 267682; The Old Post Office, Byton, Presteigne LD8 2HS — MB BS Lond. 1980.

WHITFIELD, Professor Charles Richard (retired) 7 Grange Road, Bearsden, Glasgow G61 3PL Tel: 0141 942 5585 — MB BCh BAO Belf. 1950; FRCOG 1969, M 1959; MD Belf. 1965; FRCP Glas. 1981, M 1978. Prev: Regius Prof. Midw. Univ. Glas.

WHITFIELD, Christopher Digby (retired) 35 High View Road, London E18 2HL Tel: 020 8989 3816 — MB BCh BAO Dub. 1955.

WHITFIELD, Elizabeth Mary Derwent Clinic, Shotley Bridge General Hospital, Consett DH8 0NB — MB ChB Glas. 1985; MRCPsych 1990. Cons. Psychiat. of Old Age Shotley Bridge Hosp. Co. Durh. Specialty: Geriat. Psychiat.

WHITFIELD, Estelle — MB ChB Leeds 1998.

WHITFIELD, Frances Paston Surgery, 9-11 Park Lane, North Walsham NR28 0BQ Tel: 01692 403015 Fax: 01692 500619; Bradmoor Farm, North Walsham NR28 6BX — MB ChB Sheff. 1973 (Sheffield) FRCA Eng. 1978. GP North Walsham. Specialty: Gen. Pract. Prev: GP Tutor; Regist. (Anaesth.) Sheff. AHA (T).

WHITFIELD, George Thompson (retired) Cawood Croft, 471 Scalby Road, Newby, Scarborough YO12 6UA Tel: 01723 364847 — (Birm.) MB ChB Birm. 1957; MRCS Eng. LRCP Lond. 1957; DA Eng. 1962; FFA RCS Eng. 1969. Prev: Cons. Anaesth. ScarBoro. E. Yorks. Health Dists.

WHITFIELD, Gillian Anne Flat 3, 18 Smoke Lane, Reigate RH2 7HJ — MB BS Lond. 1998; MA CANTAB 1992; MB BS Lond 1998.

WHITFIELD, Grace Patricia The Surgery, 11-13 Charlton Road, Blackheath, London SE3 7HB Tel: 020 8858 2632 Fax: 020 8293 9286; 7 Woolacombe Road, London SE3 8QJ Tel: 020 8856 3677 — MB ChB Sheff. 1967. Socs: BMA.

WHITFIELD, Mr Hugh Newbold 43 Wimpole Street, London W1G 8AE Tel: 020 7935 3095 Fax: 020 7935 3147 Email: hughwhitfield@urologylondon.fsnet.co.uk — MB BChir Camb. 1969 (Camb. & St Bart.) MRCS Eng. LRCP Lond. 1968; MA Camb. 1969; FRCS Eng. 1973; MChir Camb. 1978. Cons. Urol. Roy. Berks. & Battle Hosps. NHS Trust; Hon. Cons. Urol. Northwick Pk. Hosp.; Hon. Cons. Urol. Gt. Ormond St. Hosp.; Hon. Cons. to the Army. Specialty: Urol. Special Interest: Endourology; Minimally Invasive Managem. of Benign Prostates; Upper Urin. Tract Obstruc. Socs: Brit. Assn. Urol. Surgs.; BMA; Roy. Soc. Med. Prev: Cons. Urol. St Bart. & Homerton Hosps. Lond.; Hunt. Prof. RCS Eng.; Chief Asst. (Urol.) St Bart. Hosp. Lond.

WHITFIELD, Juliette Jane The Burwell Surgery, Newmarket Road, Burwell, Cambridge CB5 0AE Tel: 01638 741234 Fax: 01638 743948; Lowfields, Lower End, Swaffham Prior, Cambridge CB5 0HT — BM Soton. 1987; DRCOG 1990; MRCGP 1992.

WHITFIELD, Kathleen Mary (retired) 35 High View Road, South Woodford, London E18 2HL — MB BCh BAO Dub. 1955; DA Eng. 1958.

WHITFIELD, Kevin John 16 Northumberland Gardens, Newcastle upon Tyne NE5 1PT Tel: 0191 267 4763 — MB BS Newc. 1994; BMedSc Newc. 1993. Specialty: Gen. Med.

WHITFIELD, Michael John (retired) 24 Hanbury Road, Bristol BS8 2EP Tel: 0117 973 8518 Email: m.whitfield@bris.ac.uk; Whiteladies Health Centre, Whatley Road, Clifton, Bristol BS8 2PU Tel: 0117 973 1201 Fax: 0117 946 7031 — MB BChir Camb. 1963 (Camb. & St. Thos.) MA, MB Camb. 1963, BChir 1962; MRCS Eng. LRCP Lond. 1962; DObst RCOG 1964; DCH Eng. 1965; FRCGP 1980, M 1969; DPH Bristol 1969. Prev: Sen.Lect.Univ.Bristol.

WHITFIELD, Mr Patrick John 17 Harley Street, London W1N 1DA Tel: 020 7580 6283; 3 Coombe Neville, Warren Road, Kingston upon Thames KT2 7HW Tel: 020 8949 4344 — (St. Geo.) MB BS Lond. 1958; MRCS Eng. LRCP Lond. 1958; FRCS Eng. 1963. Cons. Plastic Surg. Westm. Hosp. Lond., Qu. Mary's Hosp. Rosehampton &SW Thames RHA; Cons. Plastic Surg. Roy. Lond. Hosp. Trust, Lond. E1. Specialty: Plastic Surg. Socs: Fell. Roy. Soc. Med. (Pres. Plastic Surg. Sect.); Brit. Assn. Plastic Surg.; (Ex-Hon. Sec.) Brit. Assn. Aesthetic Plastic Surgs. Prev: Cons. Plastic Surg. Westm. Hosp. Lond., Qu. Mary's Hosp. Roehampton & SW Thames RHA; Resid. Asst. (Obst.) & Ho. Surg. (Gyn.) St. Geo. Hosp. Lond.; Sen. Regist. (Plastic Surg.) Burns & Oral Surg. Centre Qu. Mary's Hosp. Roehampton.

WHITFIELD, Paul Hudson York Hospital, Wiggington Road, York YO31 8HE Tel: 01904 726568 Fax: 01903 726346 Email: paul.whitfield@york.nhs.uk — MB BS Newc. 1991; FRCS; FDS Edin.; BDS Dundee 1983. Cons. Maxillofacial Surg., York NHS Trust, York; Cons. Maxillofacial Surg., Harrogate Dist. Hosp., Harrogate. Specialty: Oral & Maxillofacial Surg. Socs: BAOMS; BMA; BAHNO.

WHITFIELD, Paul Nicholas Kings Corner Surgery, Kings Road, Ascot SL5 0AE Tel: 01344 623181 Fax: 01344 875129 — MB BS Lond. 1981; BSc (Hons.) Physiol. Lond. 1978, MB BS 1981; DRCOG 1984; MRCGP 1986.

WHITFIELD, Mr Peter Cyril — BM (Distinc.) Soton. 1999; FRCS Eng. 1992; PhD Soton. 1998. Cons., Clin. Sen. Lect. Neurol. Surg. Grampain Univ. Hosps. Trust, Aberd. Specialty: Neurosurg. Socs: Soc. Brit. Neurosurg. Surg.; Fell. Roy. Coll. Surg.s (Eng.). Prev: Specialist Regist. (Neurol. Surg.) Addenbrooke's Hosp. Camb.; Med. Research Counc. Clin. Train. Fell. & Hon. Sen. Regist. (Neurosurg.) Addenbrooke's Hosp. Camb.; Regist. (Neurosurg.) Addenbrooke's Hosp. Camb.

WHITFIELD, Roseanne Louise 3 Coombe Neville, Warren Road, Kingston upon Thames KT2 7HW Tel: 020 8949 4344 — MB BS Lond. 1993; MFHom 1996; DRCOG 1997; MRCGP 1998. GP Non-Princip.; Homeop. Phys. Specialty: Gen. Pract.; Homeop. Med.

WHITFIELD, Ruth Jeanne Chest Clinic, Mayday University Hospital, London Road, Croydon CR7 7YE Tel: 020 8401 3138 Fax: 020 8401 3460 Email: ruth.whitfield@mayday.nhs.uk — MB BChir (Distinc. in Path.) Camb. 1970 (Westm.) MA Camb. 1970; MRCP (UK) 1973; FRCP 1998. Assoc. Specialist (Respiratory Med.), Croydon Chest Clinic Mayday Hosp. Specialty: Respirat. Med.; Diabetes. Special Interest: Tuberc. Prev: Med. Adviser Indep. Adopt. Serv. Lond.; Assoc. Specialist (Diabetes) KCH Lond.; Regist. (Diabetes) Kings Coll. Hosp. Lond.

WHITFIELD, Sarah Lucy — MB ChB Leeds 1997.

WHITFIELD, Stephen James Claypath Medical Practice, 26 Gilesgate, Durham DH1 1QW Tel: 0191 333 2830 Fax: 0191 333 2836 — MB ChB Aberd. 1987.

WHITFORD, David Leonard West Farm Avenue Surgery, 381 West Farm Avenue, Longbenton, Newcastle upon Tyne NE12 8UT Tel: 0191 266 1728 Fax: 0191 270 1488; 79 Jesmond Park W., Newcastle upon Tyne NE7 7BY Tel: 0191 281 1127 — MB BS Newc. 1982; MA Camb. 1983; DRCOG 1985; MRCGP 1986. GP Newc. upon Tyne. Prev: Trainee GP Northumbria VTS.

WHITFORD, John Herbert William (retired) The Anchorage, 43 Meols Drive, Hoylake, Wirral CH47 4AF Tel: 0151 632 3608 — MB ChB Liverp. 1962; DObst RCOG 1965; FFA RCS Eng. 1969. Prev: Cons. Anaesth. Wirral Hosp. Trust.

WHITFORD, Mrs Philippa Crosshouse Hospital, Level 4 West, Kilmarnock KA10 7AN Tel: 01563 577870 — MB ChB Glas. 1982; FRCS Glas. 1986; MD Glas. 1991. p/t Cons. Surg. (Breast Surg.) CrossHo. Hosp. Kilmarnock. Specialty: Gen. Surg. Special Interest: Breast Surg. Socs: Brit. Soc. Of Surg. Oncol.; Europ. Soc. Of Mastology. Prev: Sen. Regist. (Gen. Surg.) Aberd. Roy. Infirm.; Cons. Gen. Surg. Ahli Arab Hosp., Gaza Strip; Regist. (Gen. Surg.) Inverclyde Roy. Hosp.

WHITHAM, Graham Tweedie Braidcraft Medical Centre, 200 Braidcraft Road, Glasgow G53 5QD Tel: 0141 882 3396 Fax: 0141 883 3224; 4 Braehead Glebe, Stewarton, Kilmarnock KA3 5HG — MB ChB Dundee 1979; MRCGP 1986.

WHITING, Professor Brian Faculty of Medicine, University of Glasgow, Glasgow G12 8QQ Tel: 0141 330 4249 Fax: 0141 330 5440; 2 Milner Road, Jordanhill, Glasgow G13 1QL Tel: 0141 959 2324 Fax: 0141 959 2324 — MB ChB Glas. 1964; MRCP (UK) 1970; MD Glas. 1976; FRCP Glas 1979; FFPM (Distinc.) RCP UK 1989; FRCP Ed. 1996. Dean (Fac. Med.) Univ. Glas.; Titular Prof. Clin. Pharmacol. Med. & Therap. & Dean (Fac. Med.) Univ. Glas.; Cons. Phys. Med. & Therap. West. Infirm. Specialty: Pharmacology. Socs: Assn. Phys.; Brit. Pharm. Soc.; Found. Fell. Acad. Med. Sci. Prev: Reader & Sen. Lect. (Mat. Med.) Univ. Glas.; Cons. Phys. Univ. Med. Unit Stobhill Hosp. Glas.; Sen. Regist. (Med. & Clin. Pharmacol.) Univ. Med. Unit Stohill Hosp. Glas.

WHITING, Brian Hall Health Care Centre, HM Prison Elmley, Eastchurch, Sheppey, Sheerness ME12 4AY Tel: 01795 882143 Fax: 01795 882268 — MB ChB Glas. 1970; DObst RCOG 1972; MRCGP 1976; Cert JCC Lond. 1978. Specialty: Gen. Pract. Prev: SHO (Obst.) Falkirk Roy. Infirm.; esid. (Med.) & Resid. (Surg.) Stirling Roy. Infirm.; Squadron Ldr. RAF Med. Br. & Lt. Col. RAMC.

WHITING, Frances Elizabeth (retired) Swan Acre, All Saints Lane, Sutton Courtenay, Abingdon OX14 4AG Tel: 01235 848701 — MB BS Lond. 1970 (Roy. Free) MRCS Eng. LRCP Lond. 1970; DObst RCOG 1972. Clin. Med. Off. Oxf. HA. Prev: Ho. Phys. Luton & Dunstable Hosp.

WHITING, John Michael Sturge (retired) 27 Spindlewood, Elloughton, Brough HU15 1LL Tel: 01482 669486 — MB BS Lond. 1941 (Leeds) DA Eng. 1958; FRCGP 1980. Prev: Sen. Hosp. Med. Off. (Anaesth.) Beverley Dist. Hosps.

WHITING, Karen Alice Sunderland Royal Hospital, Kayll Road, Sunderland SR4 7TP Tel: 0191 565 6256; 1A Hillcrest, Durham DH1 1RB — MB ChB Manch. 1984 (Manchester) MB ChB (Hons.) Manch. 1984; MRCP (UK) 1990; FRCPCH 1997; MSc Warwick 1998. Cons. Paediat. (Neurodisabil.) Sunderland Roy. Hosp. Sunderland; Hon. Lect. Child Health Univ. of Newc. Specialty: Paediat. Socs: Brit. Paediat. Neurol. Assn. - Neurodisabil., Rep. on Exec. Counc.; Brit. Assn. Community Child Health - Neurodisabil. Rep. on CSAC; Child Developm. & Disabil. Gp. Roy. Coll. Paediat. & Child Health. Prev: Cons. Paediat. specialising in NeuroDisabil. E. Berks. Community NHS Trust & Coventry Healthcare NHS Trust; Cons. Paediat. specialising in Neurodisabil. N. Tees Gen. Hosp. Stockton-on-Tees.

WHITING, Martin Ross Collegiate Medical Centre, Brideoak St., Manchester M8 0AT Tel: 0161 205 4364 — MB ChB Manch. 1983; MRCGP 1987.

WHITING, Norman Richard (retired) 28 Henderson Close, Lichfield WS14 9YN — MRCS Eng. LRCP Lond. 1960 (Birm.) BSc (Hons. Physiol.) Birm. 1957, MB ChB 1960; DObst RCOG 1963. Prev: Ho. Phys. & Ho. Surg. N. Ormesby Hosp. Middlesbrough.

WHITING, Paul Charles 223 Walkley Road, Walkley, Sheffield S6 2XN — MB ChB Sheff. 1997.

WHITING, Simon Langton Trevithick Surgery, Basset Road, Camborne TR14 8TT Tel: 01209 716721 Fax: 01209 612488; 21 Trelawney Road, Falmouth TR11 3LT Tel: 01326 317817 Email: simonwhiting@dial.pipex.com — MB BChir Camb. 1978 (Camb. & Westm.) MA, MB Camb. 1979, BChir 1978; DRCOG 1982; MRCGP 1983; BA (OU) 1995. Clin. Asst. (A & E) Treliske Hosp. Truro. Prev: GP Burton-on-Trent; Trainee GP Derby VTS.

WHITING, Stephen William Shifnal Medical Practice, Shrewsbury Road, Shifnal TF11 8AJ Tel: 01952 460414 Fax: 01952 463192; Fernleigh, 25 Victoria Road, Shifnal TF11 8AE Tel: 01952 461640 — MB BS Lond. 1973; MRCS Eng. LRCP Lond. 1972; DObst RCOG 1975; MRCGP 1980. Prev: Ho. Surg. Redhill Gen. Hosp.; Ho. Phys. Metrop. Hosp. Lond.

WHITLEY, Alan John (retired) 74 The Balk, Walton, Wakefield WF2 6JX Tel: 01924 251467 Email: ajwhitley@doctors.org.uk MRCS Eng. LRCP Lond. 1958 (Leeds) DTM & H Liverp. 1960. Hosp. Pract. Seacroft Hosp. Leeds.

WHITLEY, Ian 21 Beechdale, Thwaite St., Cottingham, Hull — MB ChB Leeds 1983.

WHITLEY, Ian Graeme Leesbrook Surgery, Mellor Street, Lees, Oldham OL4 3DG Tel: 0161 621 4800 Fax: 0161 628 6717; 10 Treetops Close, Dobcross, Oldham OL3 5AS Tel: 01457 872522 — MB ChB Manch. 1988; MRCGP 1992.

WHITLEY, John Manners The Old Stables, Rowden Abbey Farm, Bromyard HR7 4LS Tel: 01885 483066 Fax: 01885 483066 — MB BS Lond. 1967; MRCS Eng. LRCP Lond. 1967. Lucum Cons. Anaesth. Worcester. Specialty: Anaesth.

WHITLEY, Linsey Louise Fairways, 8 Morlais, Conwy Marina, Conwy LL32 8GJ — MB BS Lond. 1998.

WHITLEY, Michael William St Triduanas Medical Practice, 54 Moira Park, Edinburgh EH7 6RU Tel: 0131 657 3341 Fax: 0131 669 6055; 4 CrookstonCt., Crookston Road, Inveresk, Musselburgh EH21 7TR — MB ChB Aberd. 1970; DObst RCOG 1972; MRCGP 1977.

WHITLEY, Simon Peter 11 Newlands Road, Newcastle upon Tyne NE2 3NT — MB BS Newc. 1997; BOS Newc. 1990; FOS RCPS Glas. 1994. Basic Surgic. Trainee, Northern region.

WHITLEY, Siobhan St Pauls Vicarage, Watling Avenue, Liverpool L21 9NU — MB BS Lond. 1998.

WHITLEY, Teresa Bridget Heath 300A Burdett Road, London E14 7DQ; Apartment 23, 5559 Hobart St, Pittsburgh PA 15217, USA — MB BChir Camb. 1989; MRCP (UK) 1993. Specialty: Gen. Med.

WHITLINGUM, Gabriel Lawrence 4 Seelig Avenue, London NW9 7BB — MB BS Lond. 1996.

WHITLOCK, Jennifer Anne 70 Cudham Lane N., Cudham, Sevenoaks TN14 7RA — MRCS Eng. LRCP Lond. 1959.

WHITLOCK, Mr Michael Roy 51 Ickenham Road, Ruislip HA4 7BZ Tel: 01895 674888 Email: whitlock@emergencies.fsnet.co.uk — MB BCh BAO Dub. 1975 (Dublin University) BA Dub. 1975; FRCSI 1981; FFAEM 1995; MD Birmingham 2000. Cons. A & E Barnet Hosp.; Clin. Dir. (A & E) WellHo. Trust Barnet, Edgware Hosps. Specialty: Accid. & Emerg. Socs: FRSM; BMA. Prev: Sen. Regist. (A & E) E. Birm. Hosp.; Regist. (A & E) Wexham Pk. Hosp. Slough.

WHITLOCK, Nicholas James Flat 4, 1 Surbiton Hill Park, Surbiton KT5 8EF Tel: 020 8339 9013 Mob: 07763 901333 — MB BS Lond. 1994 (Univ. Coll. & Middlx. Sch. Med.)

WHITLOCK, Paul Richard 42 Lucerne Road, Highbury, London N5 1TZ — MB BS Lond. 1994 (Univ. Coll. Lond. Med. Sch.) BSc (Hons.) Biochem. Liverp. 1989; FRCSI 1999. Research Fell. Cornell Univ. Med. Sch. New York. Prev: SHO (A & E) Univ. Coll. Hosp. Lond.; SHO (Cardiothoracic Surg.) Roy. Brompton Hosp. Lond.; SHO (Orthop. Surg.) Addenbrooke's Hosp. Camb.

WHITLOW, Barry John St Helier Hospital, Carshalton SM5 1AA — MB BS Lond. 1992; MRCOG 1999; MD Lond. 2000.

WHITLOW, Christine Michele Robin Hood Surgery, Robin Hood Lane, Sutton SM1 2RJ — MB BS Lond. 1992; MRCGP 1996.

WHITLOW, William Michael Boultham Park Medical Practice, Boultham Park Road, Lincoln LN6 7SS Tel: 01522 874444 Fax: 01522 874466 — MB BS Lond. 1981 (St. George Hospital Medical School) DRCOG 1984; MRCGP 1985; DA (UK) 1987.

WHITMARSH, Karen Ann Room 007, Doctors Residence, Cookridge Hospital, Cookridge, Leeds LS16 6QB — MB BS Lond. 1993. SHO (Oncol.and Radiother.) Cookridge Hosp. Specialty: Gen.

Med.; Oncol.; Radiother. Prev: SHO Rotat. (Med.) Roy. Berks. & Battle Hosps.; SHO (Gen. Surg.) Wycombe Gen. Hosp.

WHITMARSH, Simon Patrick Flat 2, 55 Woodlands Road, Isleworth TW7 6JT — MB ChB Manch. 1987; DRCOG 1992; T(GP) 1993; DFFP 1993; MRCP (UK) 1996. SHO (Paediat.) Kingston Hosp. Specialty: Paediat. Prev: SHO (Paediat.) St. Jas. Hosp. Leeds.; SHO (Neonatol.) Leeds Gen. Infirm.

WHITMARSH, Thomas Edward Glasgow Homoeopathic Hospital, 1053 Great Western Road, Glasgow G12 0XP Tel: 0141 211 1600 Fax: 0141 211 1631 — MB BS Lond. 1984; BA Camb. 1981; FFHom 1999; FRCP London 2001. Cons. Phys. (Homoeop.) Glas. Homoeop. Hosp. Specialty: Gen. Med.; Homeop. Med. Prev: Research Fell. (Neurosci.) Char. Cross & Westm. Med. Sch. Lond.; Sen. Regist. (Med. & Homoeop.) West. Infirm. Glas.; Regist. (Gen. Med.) West. Gen. Hosp. Edin.

WHITMARSH, Vincent Barrie (retired) The Vin Yard, Turners Hill Road, East Grinstead RH19 9LA Tel: 01342 328448 Fax: 01342 328448 — (King's Coll. Hosp.) MB BS Lond. 1966; MRCS Eng. LRCP Lond. 1966; FFPM RCP (UK) 1990. Cons. Pharmaceut. Phys. Sussex. Prev: Dir. & Vice-Pres. Clin. Safety & Pharmacoeconomics SmithKlein Beecham.

WHITMORE, Alan Victor Divisions of Pathology and Cell Biology, Institute of Opthalmology, 11-43 Bath Street, London EC1V 9EL Tel: 020 7608 6883 Fax: 020 7608 6862 Email: a.whitmore@ucl.ac.uk — BM BCh Oxf. 1996 (Univ. Oxford Clin. Med. & St. Johns Coll.) BSc Hons. Biol. Sci. with Computing Univ. Lond. Westfield Coll. 1984; PhD Visual Neurosci. Univ. Lond. Queen Mary Coll. 1987; BM BCh Clin. Med. Oxf. 1996. Clinical Lecturer in Ocular Pathology; Hon. Clin. Lect. and Histopath. Fell., Moorfields Hosp. NHS Trust; Vis. Investigator, The Jackson Laborat., 600 Main St., Bar Harbor, ME 04609-1500, USA. Specialty: Ophth.; Research. Special Interest: Ophth. neurodegeneration. Socs: Association for Research in Vision and Opthalmology (ARVO) - full member; Society for Neuroscience - foreign member. Prev: SHO Dept. of Ophthmalogy St. Thomas' Hosp. Lond.; SHO Dept. of Ophthmalogy W. Suff. Hosp. Bury St. Edmunds; MRC Clin. Research Fell. MRC Laborat. for Molecular Cell Biol. Univ. Coll. Lond.

WHITMORE, Alec Charles (retired) 29 Davies Avenue, Leeds LS8 1JZ Tel: 0113 266 3158/01972 500251 — MB BS Lond. 1956 (King's Coll. Hosp.) MRCS Eng. LRCP Lond. 1956. Indep. GP Leeds.

WHITMORE, Bethany Lucille Accident and Emergency Dept, St Thomas's Hospital, Lambeth Palace Road, London SE1 7EH Tel: 020 7928 9292; 33 Stangate, Royal St, London SE1 7EQ — MB BS Lond. 1994 (Univ. Coll. & Middlx. Hosp. Sch. Med. Lond.) BSc (Hons.) Med. Chem. Lond. 1989; AFRCS ED (A&E) 1998. Registr. (A&E). Specialty: Accid. & Emerg. Prev: SHO (Neurosurg.) Radcliffe Infirm. Oxf.; SHO (Gen. Med. & Haematol), W. Suff. Hosp.; SHO (A&E), John Radcliffe Hosp.

WHITMORE, David Noel 36 Parkhurst Road, Bexley DA5 1AR Tel: 01322 527471 — MB BChir Lond. 1955 (Camb. & Guy's) MRCS Eng. LRCP Lond. 1954; MB BChir Camb. 1955; MA Camb. 1955; FRCP Lond. 1979, M 1958; FRCPath 1976, M 1964. Specialty: Haematology. Prev: Clin. Asst. (Haemat.) Qu. Mary's Hosp. Trust Sidcup; Cons. Path. Lewisham Hosp. Lond.

WHITMORE, Ian Richard Spring Gardens Health Centre, Providence Street, Worcester WR1 2BS Tel: 01905 681781 Fax: 01905 681766; 1 The Orchards, Hatfield Lane, Hatfield, Worcester WR5 2PY Tel: 01905 820872 — BM BCh Oxf. 1974.

WHITMORE, Doctor/Professor Ian Vincent Laundry Cottage, Laundry Lane, Nazeing, Waltham Abbey EN9 2DY Tel: 01992 899206 Fax: 01992 899207 Email: iwhitmore@argonet.co.uk — MB BS Lond. 1968 (Guy's Hosp.) MRCS Eng. LRCP Lond. 1968; MD Lond. 1980. Prof. (Anat.) Stanford Univ. Med. Sch. Calif. USA (Sept-Mar each year). Specialty: Anat. Socs: FRSM; Fell. Brit. Assoc. Clin. Anat.; Anat. Soc. Prev: Lect. (Anat.) Manch. Univ.; Sen. Lect. (Topograph. Anat.) Qu. Mary & Westfield Coll.

WHITMORE, Jane Margaret St. Helens PCT, Cowley Hill Lane, St Helens WA10 2AP Tel: 01744 457271 — MB BS Lond. 1981; Mem. Inst. Of Psychosexual Med. 1993; MFFP 1993; DipVen (Liverpool) 1996. Cons. in family Plann. & reproductive health, St Helens PCT. Specialty: Family Plann. & Reproduc. Health; Genitourinary Medicine; Psychosexual Med.

WHITMORE, Thomas Kingsley (retired) 2 Reddings, Welwyn Garden City AL8 7LA Tel: 01707 325995 — (St. Bart.) MRCS Eng. LRCP Lond. 1944; DCH Eng. 1946. Prev: Research Paediat. (Community Paediat. Research) Westm. Childr. Hosp. Lond.

WHITNALL, Mr Mark — MB ChB Bristol 1994; BDS (Hons.) Cardiff 1987; FDS RCS Eng. 1992; FRCS Eng. 1998. Assoc. Specialist, OMFS, Bedford. Specialty: Oral & Maxillofacial Surg. Socs: Brit. Assn. Oral & Maxillofacial Surgs.

WHITNEY, John Deryck Wallace (retired) 11 Wellfield Road, Alrewas, Burton-on-Trent DE13 7HB Tel: 01283 792303 — MB BS Lond. 1954 (Lond. Hosp.) MRCS Eng. LRCP Lond. 1955; FRCGP 1978, M 1961; MFOM RCP Lond. 1983, AFOM 1980; DIH Eng. 1982; Accredit. Occupat. Med. RCP Lond. 1983. Prev: Occupat. Phys. Birm. City Counc.

WHITNEY, Peter George 79 Hunters Road, Spital Tongues, Newcastle upon Tyne NE2 4ND — MB BS Newc. 1998.

WHITNEY, Roger William X-Ray Department, Broomfield Hospital, Court Road, Broomfield, Chelmsford CM1 7ET Tel: 01245 514527 Fax: 01245 514979; Appletree Cottage, Hartford End, Chelmsford CM3 1LE — MB BCh BAO Dub. 1980. Cons. Radiol. Broomfield Hosp. Chelmsford. Specialty: Radiol. Prev: Sen. Regist. (Radiol.) N. Staffs. Roy. Infirm. Stoke-on-Trent.

WHITROW, William (retired) 6 Sorley Close, Marlborough SN8 1UH Tel: 01672 515448 — MB BS Lond. 1957 (Guy's) MRCS Eng. LRCP Lond. 1957; DCP Lond 1966; FRCPath 1982, M 1970. Prev: Med. Dir. N. Scotl. Blood Transfus. Serv.

WHITSON, Ann 26 Norfolk Road, Lytham, Lytham St Annes FY8 4JG — MB ChB Manch. 1977. Specialty: Haematology.

WHITTAKER, Alison Jean Chest Clinic, St Woolos Hospital, 131 Stow Hill, Newport NP20 4SZ Tel: 01633 234234 Ext: 6355 — BChir Camb. 1990; MB BChir Camb. 1990; MRCP UK 1993. Specialist Regist. (Respirat. Med.) N. E. Thames. Specialty: Gen. Med.; Respirat. Med. Socs: Brit. Thorac. Soc.; Europ. Thoracic Soc.

WHITTAKER, Andrew Rainbow Medical Centre, 333 Robins Lane, St Helens WA9 3PN Tel: 01744 811211; 41 Forest Grove, Eccleston Park, Prescot L34 2RY — MB ChB Liverp. 1977; DRCOG 1979.

WHITTAKER, Anne Margaret The Surgery, Denmark Street, Darlington DL3 0PD Tel: 01325 460731 Fax: 01325 362183; 3 Ashcroft Road, Darlington DL3 8PD Tel: 01325 468988 — MB BS Newc. 1974; DRCOG 1978; MRCGP 1978. GP Darlington. Prev: Clin. Asst. (Gen. Surg.) Friarage Hosp. Northallerton; GP Yarm; Trainee GP E. Cumbria VTS.

WHITTAKER, Bryony Eleanor 8 Lavant Road, Chichester PO19 5RH Tel: 01243 527264 Fax: 01243 530607; 7 Oldwick Meadows, Lavant, Chichester PO18 0BE — MB BS Lond. 1975 (Westm.) MRCS Eng. LRCP Lond. 1975; DRCOG 1977. Principle Gen. Pract. Chichester. Prev: SHO (Paediat.) & SHO (O & G) Roy. W. Sussex Hosp. St. Richard's Br.) Chichester; Ho. Surg. Westm. Hosp. Lond.

WHITTAKER, Caroline Anne Department of Dermatology, Amersham Hospital, Whielden St., Amersham HP7 0JD Tel: 01494 734600 Fax: 01494 734620; Roughacre, Chalfont Lane, Chorleywood, Rickmansworth WD3 5PP — MB BS Newc. 1984; MRCGP 1988; DRCOG 1989; Cert. Family Plann. JCC 1989; Dip. Pract. Dermat. Wales 1996. Clin. Asst. (Dermat.) Amersham Hosp. Specialty: Dermat. Prev: Regist. (Dermat.) Aberd. Roy. Infirm.; Clin. Lect. Aberd.; GP Retainer Elms Surg. Chorleywood.

WHITTAKER, Christine Margaret Hollyoaks Medical Centre, 229 Station Road, Wythall, Birmingham B47 6ET Tel: 01564 823182 Fax: 01564 824127; Chapel Green Farm, Chapel Lane, Wythall, Birmingham B47 6JX — MB ChB Birm. 1971. Clin. Asst. Oncol. Solihull Hosp.

WHITTAKER, David John Dormans Cross E., Hollow Lane, Dormansland, Lingfield RH7 6NU Tel: 01342 833449 Fax: 01342 836649 — MB BCh Wales 1983; DA (UK) 1986; Dip. Sports Med. Lond 1991. Specialist Anaesth. (Dent.) Poggo Anaesth. Gp. Prev: Chief Resid. King Edwd. VII Memor. Hosp. Bermuda; Dir. Diving Med. Serv. Cor-Brit. Diving Internat. Corfu.

WHITTAKER, Ian David Station Road Surgery, 74 Station Road, West Wickham BR4 0PU Tel: 020 8777 8245; 45 Steeple Heights, Biggin Hill, Westerham TN16 3UN — MB BS Lond. 1983. Prev: SHO (Paediat. & O & G) Shrodells Hosp. Watford; Ho. Phys. & Ho. Surg. Hartlepool Gen. Hosp.

WHITTAKER, James Anthony Cornerways, Woolfall Health Avenue, Huyton, Liverpool L36 3TH Tel: 0151 489 4444 — MB ChB Liverp. 1960.

WHITTAKER, Jane 44 Churchwood Road, Manchester M20 6TY — MB ChB Manch. 1990.

WHITTAKER, John Stuart (retired) 147 Grove Lane, Cheadle Hulme, Cheadle SK8 7NG Tel: 0161 440 0168 — MB ChB Manch. 1957; BSc (Hons. Anat.) Manch. 1954; FRCPath 1978, M 1965. Prev: Cons. Histopath. Wythenshawe Hosp. Manch.

WHITTAKER, Mr Jonathan David Accident and Emergency Department, Royal Preston Hospital, Sharoe Green Lane N., Fulwood, Preston PR2 9HT Tel: 01772 710303 Fax: 01772 716955; 11 Barnstaple Way, Cottam, Preston PR4 0LY Tel: 01772 732139 — MB ChB Manch. 1987; FRCS Ed. 1993; FFAEM 1998. Cons. (A & E Med.) Roy. Preston Hosp. Specialty: Accid. & Emerg. Socs: Brit. Assn. Accid. & Emerg. Med.; Fell. Fac. Accid. & Emerg. Med. Prev: Sen. Regist. (A & E Med.) Roy. Preston Hosp.

WHITTAKER, Julie Anne Teresa Patterdale Lodge Medical Centre, Legh Street, Newton-le-Willows WA12 9NA Tel: 01925 227111 Fax: 01925 290605 — MB ChB Manch. 1981.

WHITTAKER, Karen Burnley Wood Medical Centre, 50 Parliament St., Burnley BB11 3JX Tel: 01282 425521 Fax: 01282 832556; 8 Queens Road, Burnley BB10 1XX Tel: 01282 428391 — MB ChB Manch. 1988. Princip. in Gen. Pract. Specialty: Gen. Pract. Prev: Trainee GP/SHO Burnley Gen. Hosp.

WHITTAKER, Leslie Robert, OBE (retired) 56 Bollo Road, Chiswick, London W4 5LT Tel: 0208 995 5552 — MRCS Eng. LRCP Lond. 1945 (Char. Cross) DCH RCP Lond. 1949; DMRD 1955; FRCR 1964. Prev: Prof. Radiol. Fac. Med. Addis Ababa Univ.

WHITTAKER, Margaret Wardrop (retired) The Old Barn, Matthew Lane, Bradley, Keighley BD20 9DF Tel: 01535 633494 — MRCS Eng. LRCP Lond. 1945. Prev: Ho. Surg. & Ho. Phys. Wigan Infirm.

WHITTAKER, Mr Mark (retired) Hawthorn House, Ladderbanks Lane, Baildon, Shipley BD17 6RX Tel: 01274 583033 — MB BS Lond. 1965 (St. Bart.) MRCS Eng. LRCP Lond. 1965; FRCS Eng. 1971. Cons. Surg. Bradford AHA.; Clin. Tutor (Bradford) Univ. Leeds; Hon. Lect. Surg. Univ. Leeds. Prev: Ho. Surg. St. Bart. Hosp.

WHITTAKER, Mark Adrian, Surg. Cdr. RN Department of Pathology, The Royal Hospital, Haslar, Gosport PO12 2AA Tel: 023 9258 4255 Ext: 2816 Fax: 023 9276 2549; 15 Mansvid Avenue, East Cosham, Portsmouth PO6 2LX Tel: 023 9278 6703 Email: mark@whitbags.com — BM Soton. 1991 (Soton. Univ. Hosps. Med. Sch.) MRCPath 2001. Cons., Histopath., Roy. Hosp. Haslar, Gosport, Hants.; Hon. Cons., Histopath., Qu. Alexandra Hosp., Cosham, Portsmouth, PO6 3LX. Specialty: Histopath. Socs: Train. Mem. Assn. Clin. Path.; Brit. Div. Internat. Acad. of Path. Prev: SpR (Histopath), Soton. Gen. Hosp., Soton.; SHO (Histopath.) RN Hosp. Haslar Gosport; Med. Off. HMS Liverp. BFPO 327, HMS Dolphin Gosport & Inst. Naval Med. (Diving Med.) Gosport.

WHITTAKER, Mark David Gloucestershire Royal Hospital, Great Westem Road, Gloucester GL1 3NN Tel: 08454 222222 Ext: 5593 Email: Mark.Whittaker@glos.nhs.uk — BM BS Nottm. 1987; MRCOG. Cons. O & G. Specialty: Obst. & Gyn. Special Interest: Minimal Acess Surg.; Endometrial Ablation; Endometriosis Surg. Socs: British Society Gynaeclogical Endoscopy.

WHITTAKER, Nuala Ann 26 Crossland Road, Chorlton, Manchester M21 9DG — MB ChB Birm. 1995; DRGOG. GP Trainee. Specialty: Paediat. Dent.

WHITTAKER, Peter John Donald 8 Lavant Road, Chichester PO19 5RH Tel: 01243 527264 Fax: 01243 530607; 7 Oldwick Meadows, Lavant, Chichester PO18 0BE — MB BChir Camb. 1976 (Camb. & Westm.) MA Camb. 1982, BA 1972, MB 1976, BChir 1975; DCH Eng. 1977 DRCOG 1978; MRCGP 1980. GP Chichester. Specialty: Gen. Pract. Socs: BMA. Prev: SHO (Paediat.) & SHO (Med.) Roy. W. Sussex Hosp. (St. Richard's Br.) Chichester; Ho. Phys. Westm. Hosp. Lond.

WHITTAKER, Roger Graham 33 Hest Bank Lane, Hest Bank, Lancaster LA2 6DB — BChir Camb. 1994.

WHITTAKER, Russell Neil Lakeside Surgery, Cottingham Road, Corby NN17 2UR — MB BS Lond. 1981; MRCS Eng. LRCP Lond. 1981; DRCOG 1984; MRCGP 1985; FRCEP 1999.

WHITTAKER, Sean Jowett Royal Free Hospital, Pond St., London NW3 2QG Tel: 020 7830 2376 Fax: 020 7830 2247 — MB ChB Manch. 1981 (Manchester) MRCP (UK) 1984; MD Manch. 1994; FRCP (Lond.) 1998. Cons. Dermat. & Hon. Sen. Lect. Roy. Free Hosp. Lond.; Cons.Dermat and Sen. Lect. St. Johns Inst. of Dermat. St Thos. Hosp. Specialty: Dermat. Socs: Europ. org for research and Treatm. of cancer; Roy.Soc.Med; Brit.Soc.Dermat. Prev: Sen. Regist. St. John's Dermat. Centre St. Thos. Hosp. Lond.; Research Fell. (Molecular Genetics) RPMS Hammersmith Hosp. Lond.

WHITTAKER, Simon Mark 1 Maes Cadwgan, Creigiau, Cardiff CF15 9TQ — MB BCh Wales 1997.

WHITTAKER, Stanley James 4 Leyfield Road, Sheffield S17 3EE — MB ChB Manch. 1984; MRCGP 1988; DRCOG 1990; MRCOG 1995. Specialist Regist. (O & G) Sheff. Specialty: Obst. & Gyn. Prev: Regist. (O & G) Jessop Hosp. Wom. Sheff.

WHITTAKER, Wendy Elizabeth Abernethy House, 70 Silver Street, Enfield EN1 3EP Tel: 020 8366 1314 Fax: 020 8364 4176 — MB BS Lond. 1977; MRCS Eng. LRCP Lond. 1977.

WHITTAKER, William Ainsworth Highlands, Hadrian Way, Sandiway, Northwich CW8 2JR Tel: 01606 883396 — MB ChB Manch. 1951.

WHITTAKER, William McClure (retired) The Old Barn, Matthew Lane, Bradley, Keighley BD20 9DF Tel: 01535 633494 — MB ChB Manch. 1945. Prev: Ho. Phys., Ho. Surg. & Obst. Off. Withington Hosp. W. Didsbury.

WHITTAM, Mr David Elliott 37 Queens Road, Kingston upon Thames KT2 7SL Tel: 020 8549 4209 Fax: 020 8944 8059 — MB BS Lond. 1964 (St. Geo.) MRCS Eng. LRCP Lond. 1964; FRCS Eng. 1968. Cons. ENT Surg. St. Geo. Hosp. Lond. & Atkinson Morley's Hosp. Wimbledon; Hon. Cons. ENT Surg. Roy. Marsden Hosp. Sutton. Specialty: Otolaryngol. Socs: Brit. Assn. Otol.; Assn. Head & Neck Oncol. Prev: Sen. Regist. (ENT) St. Geo. Hosp. Lond.; Lect. (Anat. Med.) Sch. King's Coll. Univ. Lond.; Regist. (Neurosurg.) Atkinson Morley's Hosp. Lond.

WHITTAM, Lindsay Rosanne Kings College Hospital, Denmark Hill, London SE5; First Floor Flat, 70 Comeragh Road, London W14 9HR — MB BS Lond. 1990; MRCP (UK) 1992. Specialist Regist. (Dermat.) Kings Coll. Hosp. Specialty: Dermat.

WHITTARD, Brian Ralph (retired) 5 Woodleigh Park, Shaldon, Teignmouth TQ14 0BE Tel: 01626 873304 — (St. Bart.) MRCS Eng. LRCP Lond. 1951; MB BS Lond. 1953; FFA RCS Eng. 1960. Prev: Cons. Anaesth. Torbay Hosp.

WHITTARD, Shirley Frances (retired) 5 Woodleigh Park, Shaldon, Teignmouth TQ14 0BE Tel: 01626 873304 — MB BS Lond. 1953; MRCS Eng. LRCP Lond. 1953; FFA RCS Eng. 1957. Prev: Assoc. Specialist (Anaesth.) Torbay Health Dist.

WHITTEN, Lewis (retired) 11 Sandwick Court, Cyncoed Road, Cardiff CF23 6SS Tel: 029 2076 2572 — MB ChB Ed. 1927. Hon. Surg. St. John Ambul. Assn. Prev: Ho. Surg. & Ho. Phys. Vict. Hosp. Blackpool.

WHITTEN, Mark Peter 86 Cyncoed Road, Cyncoed, Cardiff CF23 5SH — MB BCh Wales 1966; FFA RCS Eng. 1970. Cons. Anaesth. Univ. Hosp. Wales Cardiff. Specialty: Anaesth.

WHITTEN, Sara Melissa 13 Linden Avenue, Ruislip HA4 8TW — MB BS Lond. 1993; MRCOG 1999.

WHITTER, Agnes Elizabeth (retired) 199 Queen's Road, Aberdeen AB15 8DB Tel: 01224 318627 — MB ChB Aberd. 1951; DObst RCOG 1957; DPH Ed. 1959. Prev: Assoc. Specialist Dept. Clin. Oncol. Grampian Health Bd.

WHITTET, Mr Heikki Bruce ENT Department, Singleton Hospital, Sketty Lane, Swansea SA2 8QA Tel: 01792 205666 Fax: 01792 208647 — MB BS Lond. 1980 (King's Coll. Hosp.) FRCS 1986. Cons. ENT Singleton Hosp. Swansea. Specialty: Otorhinolaryngol. Socs: Fell. Roy. Soc. Med.; Assoc. Mem. Brit. Assn. Otolaryngol. Prev: Sen. Regist. (ENT) Radcliffe Infirm. Oxf.; Regist. (ENT) Roy. Nat. Throat Nose & Ear Hosp. Lond.; SHO (ENT) Hosp. Sick Childr. Gt. Ormond St.

WHITTET, Martin Matthew, OBE (retired) — (Univ. Glas.) MB ChB Glas. 1942; DPM Lond. 1944; FRFPS Glas. 1945; FRCP Ed. 1960, M 1946; FRCP Glas. 1964, M 1962; FRCPsych 1971. JP. Inverness. Prev: Phys. Supt. Craig Dunain Hosp. & Cons. Psychiat. Highland HB & Hon. Sen. Clin. Lect. (Ment. Health) Univ. Aberd.

WHITTET, Sally Elizabeth The Surgery, 1 Binfield Road, London SW4 6TB Tel: 020 7622 1424 Fax: 020 7978 1436; 76 Whateley Road, London SE22 9DD Tel: 020 693 6482 — MB BS Lond. 1976; MRCGP 1982.

WHITTICASE, James Edward 52 Bennett Road, Sutton Coldfield B74 4TH — MB BS Lond. 1997.

WHITTINGHAM, Christopher George Nattrass 20 Hampton Road, Twickenham TW2 5QB Tel: 020 8898 3245 — MB BS Lond. 1974 (Lond. Hosp.)

WHITTINGHAM, David Beck (retired) Antron Lodge, Sithney, Helston TR13 0RJ Tel: 01326 573375 — MB BS Lond. 1963; MRCS Eng. LRCP Lond. 1963; FFA RCS Eng. 1967. Cons. Anaesth. St Michael's Hosp. Hayle Cornw. Prev: Cons. Anaesth. Cornw. & Isle of Scilly Hosp. Trust.

WHITTINGHAM, David Ivor (retired) Cotmandene, 41 Port Hill Road, Shrewsbury SY3 8RN Tel: 01743 235708 Email: david.whittingham@tesco.net — MB ChB Ed. 1962; DObst RCOG 1965. Med. Mem. Disabil. Appeals Tribunal. Prev: Gen. Practitioner Shrewsbury (Retd.).

WHITTINGHAM, Edward Beck (retired) Runkerry, Foxfields, West Chiltington, Pulborough RH20 2JQ — (Liverp.) M.B., Ch.B. Liverp. 1929; D.P.H. Liverp. 1931; F.R.C.S. Eng. 1934. Prev: Surg. Consult. OldCh. Hosp. Romford.

WHITTINGHAM, Fiona Gayle High House, Sandford, West Felton, Oswestry SY11 4EX Tel: 01691 610433 Fax: 01691 610433 — MB BCh Wales 1988; BSc Wales 1985; DCH RCP Lond. 1991; DRCOG 1992; MRCGP 1993. GP Shrops. Retainer Scheme; Clin. Asst. in Dermat., Wrexham Maelor Hosp.; Clin. Doctor, Sexual Health Servs., Shrops. Community & Ment. Health Trust, Cross Ho.s, Shrewsbury. Specialty: Dermat.; Family Plann. & Reproduc. Health. Prev: Trainee GP Shrewsbury; SHO (Accid & Emerg., O & G, Paediat. & Psychiat.) Roy. Shrewsbury Hosp.

WHITTINGHAM, George Edward (retired) Boundary Cottage, Dalbeattie DG5 4QS — MB BS Durh. 1960; MRCP Ed. 1966; FRCP Ed. 1985. Prev: Cons. (Geriat. Med.) Salford DHA (T).

WHITTINGHAM, Harold Warrender, OStJ, Group Capt. RAF Med. Br. Retd. 6 Oak Ash Green, Wilton, Salisbury SP2 0RR Tel: 01722 744539 — MB BChir Camb. 1939 (Camb. & Middlx.) MRCS Eng. LRCP Lond. 1939; MA Camb. 1940; DTM & H Eng. 1959. Prev: PMO Brit. Forces Gulf; Command Med. Specialist Middle E. Air Force; Ho. Phys. Middlx. Hosp.

WHITTINGHAM, Margaret Anne (retired) Beech Cottage, 20 Abbot's Ride, Farnham GU9 8HY — MB BS Durh. 1947 (King's College, University of Durham) MRCGP 1968. Prev: Ho. Phys. Newc. Gen. Hosp.

WHITTINGHAM, Vincent Mark — MB ChB Liverp. 1984; MRCPsych 1990. Cons(Psychiat. of Old Age) N. Derbysh. Specialty: Geriat. Psychiat.

WHITTINGHAM, Winifred Prudence Cotmandene, 41 Port Hill Road, Shrewsbury SY3 8RN Tel: 01743 235708 — MB ChB Ed. 1962.

WHITTINGTON, David Antony The Mission Practice, 208 Cambridge Heath Road, London E2 9LS Tel: 020 8983 7300 Fax: 020 8983 6800; 12 St. Johns Church Road, Hackney, London E9 6EJ Tel: 020 8986 9453 — MB ChB Birm. 1983; DCH RCP Lond. 1985; DRCOG 1986; MRCGP 1988. Prev: SHO (A & E) Roy. Free Hosp. Lond.; SHO (O & G) Solihull Hosp.; SHO (Paediat.) Sandwell Dist. Gen. Hosp. W. Bromwich.

WHITTINGTON, John MacRae Mitchell and Partners, New Chapel Surgery, High Street, Aylesbury HP18 9AF Tel: 01844 208228 Fax: 01844 201906; Manor Farm, Wotton Underwood, Aylesbury HP18 0SB Tel: 01844 237551 — MB BS Lond. 1976; MRCGP 1981; DRCOG 1981.

WHITTINGTON, John Richard Twyford Manor, Twyford, Buckingham MK18 4EL Tel: 01296 730225 Fax: 01296 738893 Email: john@mediscience.co.uk — MB BS Lond. 1973 (Westm.) BSc (Physiol.) Lond. 1970; MRCS Eng. LRCP Lond. 1973; MRCP (UK) 1978; MFPM RCP (UK) 1989; MSc (Applied Statistics) Sheff. 1994. Med. Dir. MediSci. Servs. Buckingham. Specialty: Pharmaceutical Medicine. Socs: Grad. Statistician Roy. Statistical Soc.; Brit. Assn. Pharmaceut. Phys. Prev: Hon. Sen. Research Assoc. (Cardiol.) Northwick Pk. Hosp.; Dir. Clin. Pharmacol. Advisory Servs. (Clin. & Gen.) Lond.

WHITTINGTON, Marc James 3 Langholme Close, Winstanley, Wigan WN3 6TT — MB ChB Manch. 1991.

WHITTINGTON, Richard Michael Coroner's Court, Newton St., Birmingham B4 6NE Tel: 0121 303 3228 Fax: 0121 233 4841; 3 Moreton Road, Oxford OX2 7AX Tel: 01865 556869 — (Oxf. & King's Coll. Hosp.) MA Oxf. 1957, BM BCh Oxf. 1955; DObst RCOG 1957; DCH Eng. 1958; DMJ(Clin) Soc. Apoth. Lond. 1972; MRCGP 1975; DSc (Hon.) Aston 1991; LLD (Hon.) B'Ham 1997. HM Coroner Birm. & Solihull; Hon. Teachg. Fell. Birm. Univ. Med. Sch. Socs: FRSM; Coroners Soc. Eng. & Wales. Prev: Pres. Coroners Soc. Eng. & Wales.; Pres. Birm. Med. Legal Soc.; Pres. Midl. Med. Soc.

WHITTINGTON, Timothy John 34 Knuston Spinney, Irchester, Wellingborough NN29 7ES — MB ChB Liverp. 1990.

WHITTLE, Andrew David Kelso Avenue Health Centre, Kelso Avenue, Thornton-Cleveleys FY5 3LF Tel: 01253 853992 Fax: 01253 822649 — MB ChB Liverp. 1982; DCH RCP Lond. 1985; DRCOG 1986; MRCGP 1988. GP Blackpool. Prev: Trainee GP Grimsby Dist. Gen. Hosp. VTS.

WHITTLE, Eileen Brookfields Health Centre, Seymour Street, Cambridge CB1 3DQ Tel: 01223 723160 Fax: 01223 723089; 10 Downham's Lane, Milton Road, Cambridge CB4 1XT — MB BS Lond. 1971 (Char. Cross) MRCS Eng. LRCP Lond. 1971; DObst RCOG 1974. Clin. Asst. (Geriat.) Brookfields Hosp. Camb. Prev: SHO (Dermat.) Nottm. Gen. Hosp.; SHO (Paediat.) Addenbrooke's Hosp. Camb.; Ho. Surg. (Obst.) St. Bart. Hosp. Lond.

WHITTLE, Elizabeth Jane Upper Aultvaich, Beauly IV4 7AN — MB ChB Manch. 1977; DRCOG 1979; MRCGP 1981.

WHITTLE, Elizabeth Ruth Anaesthetic Office, North Devon District Hospital, Raleigh Park, Barnstaple EX31 4JB Tel: 01271 22577; Southlands, Park Lane, Barnstaple EX32 9AL — MB ChB Bristol 1979; DRCOG 1981; FFA RCS Eng. 1984. Devon Dist. Hosp. Barnstaple. Specialty: Anaesth.

WHITTLE, Francis David (retired) Deanscourt, St Andrews KY16 9QT — MB BS Lond. 1956 (Middlx.) MA St. Andrew 2000.

WHITTLE, Professor Ian Roger, Maj. RAMC Retd. Department of Clinical Neurosciences, Western General Hospital, Crewe Road, Edinburgh EH4 2XU Tel: 0131 537 2103 Fax: 0131 537 2561 — MB BS Adelaide 1978; FRCS (Surg. Neurol.) Ed. 1985; FRACS 1985; MD Adelaide 1987; PhD Ed. 1990; FRCPE 1999. Cons. Neurosurg. West. Gen. Hosp. Edin. & Roy. Infirm. Edin.; Forbes Prof. Surgic. Neurol. Univ. Ed. Specialty: Neurosurg. Socs: Soc. Brit. Neurol. Surgs.; Eur. Soc. Sterotactic & Func.al Neurosurg. Prev: Regist. (Neurosurg.) Roy. P. Alfred & Roy. Alexander Hosp. for Childr. Sydney, Austral.; SHO (Surg.) Roy. Adelaide Hosp., Austral.

WHITTLE, Jocelyn Kay 1 Bessybrook Close, Lostock, Bolton BL6 4EA Tel: 01204 846796 — MB ChB Manch. 1997; BSc St. And. 1994. SHO O & G Billinge Hosp. Wigan. Specialty: Obst. & Gyn. Prev: SHO A & E Roy.Albert.Inf.Wigan; Ho. Off. (Gen. Med.) Roy. Albert Edwd. Infirm. Wigan; Ho. Off. Gen Surg. Lancaster.

WHITTLE, Jonathan Roydon Spencer Princess Alexandra Eye Pavilion, Chalmers St., Edinburgh EH3 9 Tel: 0131 536 1000; 40A Buckingham Terrace, Edinburgh EH4 3AP Tel: 0131 315 4756 Fax: 0131 315 4756 — MB ChB Ed. 1985 (Edin.) BSc (Hons.) Physiol. 1983; DORCS Eng. 1990; FRCS Ed. 1991; FRCOphth 1991. Head Acc. & Emerg. & Primary Care; Head of Serv., Electrodiagnostic Clinic Process Alexandra Eye Pavilion, Edin. Specialty: Ophth. Socs: Med. Protec. Soc. & Internat. Soc. Clin. Electrophysiol. of Vision. Prev: Regist. (Ophth) Princess Alexandra Eye Pavilion Edin.; Regist. (Ophth) Vict. Hosp. Kirkaldy; SHO (Ophth) Sussex Eye Hosp. Brighton.

WHITTLE, Kenneth George Phoenix Surgery, Rectory Road, Camborne TR14 7LA Tel: 01209 714876 Fax: 01209 612234 — MB BCh Wales 1967; DObst RCOG 1971. GP Cornw. Socs: BMA; W Penwith Med. Soc. Prev: SHO (Cardiothoracic Surg.) Sully Hosp.; SHO (Paediat.) United Cardiff Hosps.; SHO (Obst.) Yeovil Gen. Hosp.

WHITTLE, Professor Martin John Department of Fetal Medicine, Birmingham Womens Hospital, Birmingham B15 2TT Tel: 0121 627 2775 Fax: 0121 415 4837 Email: m.j.whittle@bham.ac.uk; Flat 28, 42 George Street, Birmingham B3 1QA Tel: 0121 684 3988 Fax: 0121 684 3988 — MB ChB Manch. 1972; MD Manch. 1980; FRCP Glas. 1988; FRCOG 1988; T(OG) 1991. Prof. Fetal Med. Univ. Birm.; Head Acad. Dept. of Obst. & Gyn. Specialty: Obst. & Gyn. Prev: Cons. O & G Gt. Glas. HB; SHO (O & G) St. Mary's Hosp. Manch.; Ho. Phys. & Ho. Surg. Manch. Roy. Infirm.

WHITTLE, Professor Michael William (retired) c/o Cob Cottage, Old Bosham, Chichester PO18 8HZ Email: Mike@crowaptok.com — MB BS (Hons.) Lond. 1965 (St Geo.) BSc (Hons.) Lond. 1962; PhD Surrey 1978, MSc (Distinc.) 1970. Prev: Prof. Rehabil. Technol. Univ. Tennessee, Chattanooga.

WHITTLE, Mr Richard John Miller (retired) 26 Howards Thicket, Gerrards Cross SL9 7NX — MB BS Lond. 1947 (St Bart.) MRCS

Eng. LRCP Lond. 1951; FRCS Eng. 1953; DMRT Eng. 1955; FFR 1960. Prev: Dir. Radiother. Dept. St. Bart. Hosp. Lond.

WHITTLE, Roger Anthony Sean Staunton & Corse Surgery, Corse, Staunton, Gloucester GL19 3RB Tel: 01452 840228 Fax: 01452 840072 — MB BS Lond. 1993 (Kings Coll. Lond.) DCH RCP 1995; DGM RCP 1996; DRCOG 1997; DFFP 1997; MRCGP 1998. Specialty: Gen. Pract. Prev: GP Regist. Cheltenham; SHO Rotat. Gloucs VTS.

WHITTLES, Susan Eleanor Rendcomb Surgery, Rendcomb, Cirencester GL7 7EY Tel: 01285 831257 — BM Soton. 1982; DCH RCP Lond. 1985; MRCGP 1986. Prev: Trainee GP Cirencester VTS.

WHITTLESTONE, Mr Timothy Harry Department of Urology, Bristol Royal Infirmary, Bristol B52 8HW — BM BCh Oxf. 1992; MA Camb. 1993; FRCS Eng. 1996; MD (Bristol) 2001. Consultant Urologist, Bristol Royal Infirmary; Hunt. Prof.ship RCS Eng. Specialty: Urol. Prev: Specialist Regist. Urol. Bristol Roy. Infirm.

WHITTON, Andrew Dean Charles Mechie and Partners, 67 Owen Road, Lancaster LA1 2LG Tel: 01524 846999 Fax: 01524 845174 — MB ChB Dundee 1981; DRCOG 1984; MRCGP 1986.

WHITTON, Ingrid Hall — MB ChB Glas. 1985 (Glasgow) MRCPsych 1990. Cons. Psychiat. St. Jas. Univ. Hosp. Leeds. Specialty: Gen. Psychiat.

WHITTON, Michael William Charles Hicks Centre, 75 Ermine Street, Huntingdon PE29 3EZ Tel: 01480 453038 Fax: 01480 434104 — MB ChB Leeds 1976; DRCOG 1982; Dip. Occ. Med. 1997; AFOM 1998. Occupational Health Phys. Socs: Soc. Occupat. Med.

WHITTON, Tessa Louise 12 The Maltings, Fairlawn Road, Bristol BS6 5BB — BM Soton. 1989; DA (UK) 1992; DTM & H Liverp. 1993. SHO (Paediat.) Roy. United Hosp. Trust Bath.

WHITTON, Theresa Jayne 156 Old Montague Street, London E1 5NA — MB BS Lond. 1997.

WHITTON, Tinku 18 Renters Avenue, London NW4 3RB Tel: 020 8202 9963 Fax: 020 8202 9963 — MB BS Lond. 1991; MRCP 1997. Specialty: Dermat.

WHITTY, Bryan Lawrence Broomhill Practice, 41 Broomhill Drive, Glasgow G11 7AD Tel: 0141 339 3626 Fax: 0141 334 2399; 126 Cleveden Road, Glasgow G12 0JT Tel: 0141 334 9857 — MB ChB Glas. 1964; DObst RCOG 1967; DA Eng. 1968. Apptd. Doctor (Lead Regulats.). Specialty: Occupat. Health. Prev: Med. Off. Nazareth Hosp., Israel; SHO (Anaesth.) West. Infirm. Glas.; Med. Off. Christian Hosp. Chandraghona, Bangladesh.

WHITTY, Christopher John MacRae — BM BCh Oxf. 1991; MA Oxf. 1991; MRCP (UK) 1995; MSc Lond. 1996; DTM & H RCP Lond. 1996; FRCP 2004. Sen. Lect. Lond. Sch. Hyg. & Trop. Med.; Hon. Cons. Phys. Hosp. Trop. Dis Lond. & UCLH; Hon. Cons., Hosp. Trop. Dis. Lond. & UCLH. Specialty: Trop. Med.; Epidemiol.; Infec. Dis. Prev: Sen. Regist., Guy's & St. Thomas's Hosp.s, Lond.; Sen. Regist. St. Geo.'s Hosp. Lond.; Clin. Lect. & Med. Spec. Coll. of Med.,Malawi Africa.

WHITTY, Margaret Mary (retired) 3 Cavendish Court, Hobson Road, Oxford OX2 7JU Tel: 01865 557916 — MB BS Lond. 1939 (Lond. Sch. Med. Wom.) MRCS Eng. LRCP Lond. 1939. Med. Off. Oxf. FPA. Prev: Asst. Med. Off. Chest Clinic, United Oxf. Hosps.

WHITTY, Paula Michelle Newcastle, North Tyneside & Northumberland Mental Health NHS Trust, 1st Floor, Milvain Building, Westgate Road, Newcastle upon Tyne NE61 2NU Tel: 0191 256 3881 Fax: 0191 273 2340 — MB ChB Leeds 1985 (University of Leeds) DA (UK) 1988; MSc (Distinc.) Lond. 1990; MFPHM RCP (UK) 1992; MD (Leeds) 2000. Specialty: Pub. Health Med.

WHITTY, Richard Terence 84 Davenport Avenue, Hessle HU13 0RW — BM BCh Oxf. 1968 (Lond. Hosp. & Oxf.) DA Eng. 1971; FFA RCS Eng. 1972. Cons. Anaesth. Hull Roy. Infirm. Specialty: Anaesth. Prev: Sen. Regist. Dept. Anaesth. Lond. Hosp.; Regist. Anaesth. Nat. Heart Hosp. Lond.; SHO Dept. Anaesth. St. Mary's Hosp. Lond.

WHITWELL, Duncan John 105 Western Avenue, Woodley, Reading RG5 3BL — BM BS Nottm. 1993.

WHITWELL, Elizabeth Anne (retired) 152 Bath Road, Banbury OX16 0TT Tel: 01295 266243 — (Roy. Free) MB BS Lond. 1962; MRCS Eng. LRCP Lond. 1962; DObst RCOG 1965; MFCH 1989. Prev: Staff grade Med. Off. community health.

WHITWELL, Francis David Southmead Hospital, Bristol BS10 5NB Tel: 0117 959 5898; 2 Goldney Avenue, Clifton, Bristol BS8 4RA Tel: 0117 974 1438 Email: davidwhitwell@btopenworld.com — MB BS Lond. 1968 (St. Thos.) BA Oxf. 1970; MRCPsych 1975; FRC Psych. 1995. Cons Psychiat. Southmead Hosps. Bristol; Hon. Sen. Clin. Lect. (Pyschiatry), Univ. Bristol. Specialty: Gen. Psychiat. Prev: Lect. (Ment. Health) Univ. Bristol; Regist. (Psychiat.) Warneford Hosp. Oxf.; SHO (Neurol. & Rheum.) Lambeth Hosp. Lond.

WHITWELL, George Steven Little Cherith, Manor La, Gerrards Cross SL9 7NJ Tel: 01753 884394 — MB ChB Leic. 1997. SHO (A&E) Leicester Roy. Infirm. Specialty: Accid. & Emerg. Socs: BMA; MPS. Prev: PRHO Gen. Med. Leic. Gen. Hosp.; PRHO Gen. Surg.Colology LR1.

WHITWELL, Joan Rosemary Liberton Hospital, Lasswade Road, Edinburgh EH16 6UB Tel: 0131 536 7828 Fax: 0131 536 7896; 5 Royal Circus, Edinburgh EH3 6TL Tel: 0131 225 1574 — MB ChB Ed. 1978; BSc (Mathematical Physics) Sussex 1968; PhD (Med. Physics) Leeds 1973; MRCP (UK) 1983. Cons. Geriat. Med. Liberton Hosp. Edin. Specialty: Care of the Elderly. Socs: Brit. Geriat. Soc. Prev: Sen. Regist. (Geriat. Med.) Roy. Vict. Hosp. Edin.; Research Regist. (Clin. Pharmacol.) Roy. Infirm. Edin.; Med. Physicist Leeds Gen. Infirm.

WHITWELL, Mr John Bagatelle, Burton Road, Branskome Park, Bournemouth BH1 6DU Tel: 01202 765678 — MB BS Lond. 1946 (Char. Cross) MS Lond. 1959, MB BS 1946; DO Eng. 1951; FRCS Eng. 1954; FCOphth 1988. Socs: FRSM; Ophth. Soc. Prev: Cons. Ophth. Surg. E. Dorset Health Dist.; Sen. Regist. Lond. Hosp. & Moorfields Eye Hosp.; Master Oxf. Ophth. Congr..

WHITWELL, Kerrie Ann — MB ChB Dundee 1992; FFAEM; FRCS Ed. Cons. (Emerg. Med.) Roy. Free Hosp. Lond. Specialty: Accid. & Emerg.

WHITWHAM, Marian (retired) Beckstones, Askham, Penrith CA10 2PG Tel: 01931 712499; Queen Street, Portsmouth — MB ChB Manch. 1960. Prev: Ho. Surg. & Ho. Phys. Roy. S. Hants. Hosp. Soton.

WHITWORTH, Alan (retired) Westbrae, 89 West St, Reigate RH2 9DA Tel: 01737 249888 — (St. Bart.) MB BChir Camb. 1959; DObst RCOG 1961; MA Camb. 1965. Prev: Princip. GP Reigate.

WHITWORTH, Alan Graham North Swindon Practice, Home Ground Surgery, Thames Avenue, Haydon Wick, Swindon SN25 1QQ Tel: 01793 705777 — MB BS Lond. 1985 (St. Mary's Lond.) PhD Manch. 1984; Dip Occ Med Birmingham 1988; LF Hom Faculty of Homeopathy 2001. GP Princip., Swindon; Clin. Asst. Dermat. P.s Margt. Hosp. Swindon. Specialty: Dermat.; Occupat. Health; Homeop. Med. Prev: GP Princip. S.sea Hants; Clin. Pharmacol. Hoechst UK Ltd.

WHITWORTH, Caroline Elizabeth Department of Renal Medicine, Royal Infirmary of Edinburgh, Little France, Edinburgh EH16 4SA Tel: 0131 242 1238 Fax: 0131 242 1233 — MB ChB Ed. 1988; MRCP (UK) 1991; BSc (Hons.) Pharmacol. Ed. 1985, MD 1995; FRCP (Edin) 2000. Cons. (Renal Med.); Hon. Clin. Sen. Lect. Dept. of Clin. & Surgic. Scis. Fac. of Med. Univ. of Edin. Specialty: Nephrol.; Gen. Med. Socs: Renal Assn.; Brit. Transpl. Soc. Prev: Lect. & Hon. Sen. Regist. (Nephrol. & Hypertens.) Univ. Leicester; Lect. & Hon. Regist. (Renal Med.) Edin. Roy. Infirm.; Research Fell. Centre for Genome Research Ed.

WHITWORTH, Christopher Martin Pengarth Road Surgery, Pengarth Road, St Agnes TR5 0TN Tel: 01872 553881 Fax: 01872 553885; 34 Vicarage Road, St Agnes TR5 0TF Tel: 01872 553130 — MB BS Lond. 1988 (St. Mary's) BSc Lond. 1985, MB BS 1988; MRCGP 1992. GP St. Agnes.

WHITWORTH, Diana Mary Dr A Wilson and Partners, Sighthill Health Centre, 380 Calder Road, Edinburgh EH11 4AU Tel: 0131 537 7060 Fax: 0131 537 7005 — MB ChB Ed. 1987; MA Oxf. 1989; DRCOG 1990; MRCGP 1991.

WHITWORTH, Mr George Robert Sydenham Green Health Centre, 26 Holmshaw Close, London SE26 4TH Tel: 020 8778 3358; 26 Perry Rise, Forest Hill, London SE23 2QL Tel: 020 8291 3416 — MB ChB Alexandria 1972; MRCS Eng. LRCP Lond. 1979; FRCS Eng. 1982. Prev: Regist. (Orthop. Surg.) Lewisham Hosp.; SHO (Gen. Surg.) Ipswich Gen. Hosp.; SHO (Orthop. Surg.) Crawley Gen. Hosp.

WHITWORTH, Helen Elizabeth Edenfield RSU, Prestwich Hospital, Bury New Road, Manchester M25 3BL; c/o 49 Overton Lane,

Hammerwich, Walsall WS7 0LQ — MB ChB Liverp. 1990; MRCPsych 1995. Specialist Regist. (Psychiat.) Manch. Specialty: Forens. Psychiat.

WHITWORTH, Henry, MBE (retired) 34 Vicarage Road, St Agnes TR5 0TF Tel: 01872 552239 — MB BS Lond. 1943 (Guy's) Prev: Sen. Res. Med. Off. Duchess of York Hosp. Babies Manch.

WHITWORTH, Mr Ian Howard Department of Plastic Surgery, Salisbury District Hospital, Salisbury SP2 8BJ Tel: 01722 336262 Email: ian.whitworth@salisbury.nhs.uk — MB BS Lond. 1988 (St. Bartholomews Hospital) BSc (Hons.) Pharmacol. Lond. 1985, MB BS 1988; FRCS Lond. 1992; MS (Lond) 1995; FRCS 1998. Cons. Plastic Surg.; Clin. Director Nat. Breast Implant Registry (UK). Specialty: Plastic Surg. Special Interest: Breast Surgery. Socs: Brit. Assn. of Aesthetic Plastic Surg.; Brit. Assn. Plastic Surg.

WHITWORTH, James Alexander Grover 23 Ingham Road, London NW6 1DG — MB ChB Liverp. 1979; MD Liverp. 1993; FRCP (UK) 1996; MFPHM (UK) 1999. Prof. (International Pub. Health). Prev: MRC Director Uganda.

WHITWORTH, Julia Caroline Helmford House Surgery, 283 High Street, London Colney, St Albans AL2 1EL Tel: 01727 823245; 23 Juniper Gardens, Shenley, Radlett WD7 9LA — MB BS Lond. 1981 (Roy. Free) MRCGP 1986. Prev: GP Lochmaddy, I. of N. Uist; SHO (Paediat. & Gen. Med.) Maidstone Gen. Hosp.; Ho. Off. (Gen. Surg. & Orthop.) Qu. Eliz. Hosp. & King's Lynn Hosp.

WHITWORTH, Magda Whitworth, 234 Baring Road, London SE12 0UL Tel: 020 8851 5212; 26 Perry Rise, Forest Hill, London SE23 2QL Tel: 020 8291 3416 — MB ChB Alexandria 1972; LMSSA Lond. 1978. Princip. Gen. Pract. Specialty: Gen. Pract. Socs: BMA.

WHITWORTH, Nina Helen Mount Pleasant Medical Centre, Ditherington Road, Shrewsbury SY1 4DQ Tel: 01743 235111 — MB BS Lond. 1991.

WHOLEY, Vivienne Gay Dept. of GU Medicine, Solway Suite, Cumberland Infirmary, Carlisle CA2 7HY Tel: 01228 814814 — MB BS Newc. 1991 (Newcastle Upon Tyne) Dip. GU Med. Soc. Apoth. Lond. 1995. Staff Grade (Genitourin. Med.). Specialty: Genitourinary Medicine; HIV Med.; Family Plann. & Reproduc. Health. Socs: Soc. Study VD; Assoc. GU Med. Prev: Regist. (Genitourin. Med.) Newc. & Sunderland Gen. Hosps.; SHO (Genitourin. Med.) King's Coll. Hosp. Lond. & Newc. & Sunderland Gen. Hosps.; SHO Rotat. (Med.) Tyneside Dist. Hosp. S. Shields.

WHONE, Alan Lane 31 Mangotsfield Road, Mangotsfield, Bristol BS16 9JJ — MB ChB Birm. 1994 (Birmingham University Hospital) ChB Birm. 1994; MRCP Lond. 1998. Research Fell.(Neurol.) Hammersmith Hosp., Lond. Specialty: Neurol. Socs: BMA. Prev: SHO (Neurol.) Kings Coll. Hosp. Lond.; SHO (Psychiat.) Maudsley Hosp. Lond.; SHO Rotat. (Gen. Med.) The Roy. Shrewsbury Hosp.

WHOOLEY, David John 82 College Road, London SE21 7LY — MB BCh BAO NUI 1990.

WHORWELL, Peter James Wythenshawe Hospital, Manchester M23 9LT Tel: 0161 291 5813 Fax: 0161 434 5194 — (Guy's) BSc (Hons.) Lond. 1970, MD 1979, MB BS 1969; MRCS Eng. LRCP Lond. 1969; MRCP (UK) 1972; FRCP Lond. 1988. Cons. Phys. & Sen. Lect. (Med.) Univ. Hosp. S. Manch. Specialty: Gastroenterol.

WHY, Howard John Francis Queen's Hospital Burton, Belevedere Road, Burton-on-Trent DE13 0RB Tel: 01283 566 333 Ext: 5541 Fax: 01283 593 027 — MB ChB Leeds 1983 (Leeds Univ.) MRCP (UK) 1988; FRCP 2000. Cons. Cardiol. Qu. Hosp. Burton-on-Trent; Hon. Cons. Cardiol. Glenfield Hosp. Leicester. Specialty: Cardiol. Special Interest: Cardiac Interven.; Cardiomyopathies. Socs: Brit. Soc. Echocardiogr.; Brit. Cardiac Soc. Prev: Research Fell. & Hon. Regist. (Cardiol.) King's Coll. Hosp. Lond.; Regist. (Med.) Basildon & Orsett Hosp. Grays.

WHYATT, Nicholas David (retired) Rose Cottage, Bowden Hill, Lacock, Chippenham SN15 2PW Tel: 01249 730516 — MB BS Lond. 1963 (St. Bart.) MRCS Eng. LRCP Lond. 1963; DObst RCOG 1965. Prev: Med. Off. St. And. Hosp. Chippenham.

WHYBREW, Katherine Joanna 19 Beaumont Street Surgery, Oxford SE11 5TN — BChir Camb. 1996. Specialty: Gen. Pract.

WHYBROW, Tracey Rebecca 23 Hobleythick Lane, Westcliff on Sea SS0 0RP — MB BS Lond. 1997 (St Barts Lond) BSc Lond. 1994; MRCP UK 2001. SHO Anaesthetics, Roy. Hants. Co. Hosp. Winchester. Specialty: Gen. Med. Prev: SHO Med. Soton. Gen Hosp. Soton.

WHYLER, David Keith Kinmel Bay Medical Centre, The Square, Kinmel Bay, Rhyl LL18 5AU Tel: 01745 353965 Fax: 01745 356407 — MB ChB Ed. 1984 (Edinburgh) Cert. Family Plann. JCC 1989; DFFP 1993. GP Rhyl; Clin. Med. Off. in Family Plann., Conwy and Denbighsh. Trust. Specialty: Community Child Health; Family Plann. & Reproduc. Health; Cardiol. Socs: Fell. (Ex-Pres.) Roy. Med. Soc. Edin. Prev: Trainee GP Clwyd FPC; Regist. Glan Clwyd Hosp. Bodelwyddan; Ho. Phys. & Ho. Surg. Roy. Infirm. Edin.

WHYMAN, Mr Mark Roy Cheltenham General Hospital, Department of Surgery, Sandford Road, Cheltenham GL53 7AN — MB BS Lond. 1984; FRCS Eng. 1988; MS Lond. 1992. Cons. Gen. & Vasc. Surg. Cheltenham Gen. Hosp. Specialty: Gen. Surg. Socs: Assn. Surg.; Vasc. Surg. Soc.; Eur. Soc. Vasc. Surg. Prev: Sen. Regist. S. W. Region; Regist. & Research Fell. Edin. Roy. Infirm.

WHYMARK, Andrew David 8 Cottesmore Drive, Loughborough LE11 2RL — MB ChB Sheff. 1995.

WHYMARK, Caroline Helen Ayr Hospital, Anaesthetics Department, Dalmellington Road, Ayr KA6 6DX — MB ChB Glas. 1995; FRCA. Cons. (Anaesth.) NHS Ayrsh. & Arran. Specialty: Anaesth. Prev: SHO (Anaesth.) Norf. & Norwich Hosp.

WHYTE, Augustine Patrick 21 Fitzwalter Road, Colchester CO3 3SY — MB BCh BAO Dub. 1943; DPM Eng. 1972; MRCPsych 1974. Cons. Psychiat. Severalls Hosp. Colchester. Specialty: Gen. Psychiat.

WHYTE, Barrie Glenlivet Community Surgery, Drumin, Glenlivet, Ballindalloch AB37 9AN Tel: 01807 590273 Fax: 01807 590411 — MB ChB Bristol 1968; DObst RCOG 1971; MRCGP 1976. Prev: Ho. Surg. (Obst.) Southmead Hosp. Bristol; Ho. Phys. Ham Geeen Hosp. Pill; Ho. Surg. Frenchay Hosp. Bristol.

WHYTE, Mr David Kirk 84 Balnakyle Road, Lochardil, Inverness IV2 4DJ Email: dkwhyte@aol.com — MD Dundee 1971 (St. And.) MB ChB St. And. 1963; DO Eng. 1965; FRCS Ed. 1968; FCOphth 1989. Cons. Ophth. Surg. Highland HB; Hon. Sen. Lect. (Ophth.) Univ. Aberd. Specialty: Ophth. Socs: Highland Med. Soc.; Scot. Ophth. Club. Prev: Anat. Demonst. Qu.'s Coll. Univ. St. And.; Regist. Ophth. & Sen. Regist. Ophth. Dundee Roy. Infirm.

WHYTE, George Cordner (retired) 10 The Boarlands, Port Eynon, Eynon, Swansea SA3 1NX Tel: 01792 391252 — (RCSI) LRCPI & LM, LRCSI & LM 1941. Prev: Med. Off. Pneumoconiosis Med. Panels DHSS.

WHYTE, Hugh Account Director Health, Hedra plc, 1 St. Colme Street, Edinburgh EH3 6AA Tel: 0131 220 8424 Fax: 0131 220 8201 Email: hugh.whyte@hedra.com; 24 Garvock Hill, Dunfermline KY12 7UU Tel: 01383 732235 — MB ChB Ed. 1979 (Edinburgh) DRCOG 1981; MRCGP 1983; FRCGP 1998. Sen. Med. Off. Scottish Executive Health Dept.; Hon. Lect. Univ. Dundee. Specialty: Pharmacology. Prev: Sen. Med. Off. Managem. Exec. Scott. Office Health Dept.; Med. Adviser (Primary Care) Tayside Health Bd.; Gen. Med. Practitioner.

WHYTE, Ian David King Street Surgery, King Street, Whalley, Blackburn BB7 9SL Tel: 01254 823273 Fax: 01254 824891; Longsight House, Longsight Road, Langho, Blackburn BB6 8AD Tel: 01254 245261 — MB ChB Liverp. 1979; DRCOG 1982; MRCGP 1989.

WHYTE, Mr Ian Ferguson 32 Crown Drive, Inverness IV2 3QG — MB ChB Dundee 1981; BMSc Dund 1978; DRCOG 1985; MRCGP 1986; DO RCS Dub. 1988; FRCS Ed. 1990; FRCOphth 1990. Ons. Ophth. Raigmore NHS Trust Inverness; Hon. Sen. Lect. Univ. Aberd. Specialty: Ophth. Socs: Brit. & Irish Assn. of Vitreoretinal Surgs. Prev: Sen. Regist. (Ophth.) Ninewells Teachg. Hosp. & Med. Sch. Univ. Dundee; Specialist Sen. Regist. (Vitreoretinal Surg.) Moorfields Eye Hosp. Lond.

WHYTE, Jennifer Anne 41 Gordon Road, Harborne, Birmingham B17 9HA — MB BCh BAO NUI 1988.

WHYTE, Judith Carol (retired) Humberstone Manor, 608 Gipsy Lane, Leicester LE5 0TB — MB ChB Leeds 1968; DPM Leeds 1973; MRCPsych 1977. Prev: Cons. Child Psychiat. S. Derbysh. HA.

WHYTE, Louis 325 Eaglesham Road, East Kilbride, Glasgow G75 8RW — (Univ. Glas.) M.B., Ch.B. Glas. 1946.

WHYTE, Professor Moira Katherine Brigid Academic Unit of Respiratory Medicine, M Floor, Royal Hallamshire Hospital, Sheffield S10 2JF Tel: 0114 271 2196 Fax: 0114 272 1104 Email: m.k.whyte@sheffield.ac.uk — MB BS Lond. 1984 (St. Bartholomew's Hospital Medical College) BSc (1st cl. Hons.) Lond.

1981; MRCP (UK) 1987; PhD Lond. 1994; FRCP 1998. Prof. Respirat. Med. & Hon. Cons. Phys. Univ. Sheff. & Roy. Hallamsh. Hosp. Sheff.; Hon. Cons. Physicians in Respiratory & Gen. Med, Sheffield Teaching Hosp.s NHS Trust. Specialty: Respirat. Med.; Gen. Med. Prev: Wellcome Advanced Fell. & Hon. Cons. Gen. & Respirat. Med. Univ. Hosp. Nottm.; Sen. Regist. (Respirat. & Gen. Med.) Hammersmith Hosp. Lond.; MRC Train. Fell. (Cell Biol.) Roy. Postgrad. Med. Sch. Lond.

WHYTE, Morag Duncan Ritchie 2 Barony Court, Ardrossan KA22 8DZ — MB ChB Ed. 1991.

WHYTE, Nicholas John Dixon 40 Wabingham Road, London E5 8NF — (St. Bart.) MA, MB Camb. 1972, BChir 1971. Prev: Ho. Phys. & SHO Qu. Eliz. Hosp. Childr. Lond.; Med. Regist. N. Middlx. Hosp. Lond.

WHYTE, Robert (retired) 3 Fitzroy Place, Glasgow G3 7RH Tel: 0141 248 5451 Fax: 0141 248 5451; Waverley, 70 East Kilbride Road, Busby, Glasgow G76 8HU Tel: 0141 644 1659 — MB ChB St. And. 1966; DPM Ed. & Glas. 1970; FRCPsych 1985, M 1972. Cons. Psychother. Parkhead Hosp. Glas.; Hon. Clin. Sen. Lect. in (Psychol. Med.) Univ. Glas. 1991-. Prev: Sen. Regist. Roy. Dundee Liff Hosp.

WHYTE, Ross Boyd 10 Calder Avenue, Troon KA10 7JT — MB ChB Glas. 1998.

WHYTE, Sean Paul 26 Ashdown Road, Chandlers Ford, Eastleigh SO53 5QW — BM BCh Oxf. 1996 (Oxford) MA Cantab) 1993. SHO (Psychiat.) Oxf.shire Ment. Healthcare NHS Trust Oxf. Specialty: Gen. Psychiat.

WHYTE, Simon David 110 Priors Grange, High Pittington, Durham DH6 1DB — MB BS Newc. 1994. Clin. Research Fell. (Neonat. IC) S. Cleveland Hosp. Middlesbrough. Specialty: Anaesth. Prev: SHO (Anaesth.) S. Cleveland Hosp. Middlesbrough; SHO (Anaesth.) Dryburn Hosp. Co. Durh.; SHO (Paediat. & Neonat.) Sunderland Dist. Gen. Hosp.

WHYTE, Stewart James Woodeside Health Centre, Barr Street, Glasgow G20 7LR Tel: 0141 531 9570 Fax: 0141 531 9572 — MB ChB Glas. 1980 (Glasgow) DRCOG 1981. Specialty: Gen. Pract.

WHYTE, Susan Frances Waverley, 70 East Kilbride Road, Busby, Glasgow G76 8HU — MB ChB St. And. 1969; DPM Ed. & Glas. 1972; MRCPsych 1973; FRCPsych 1988; FRCP Ed 1998. Cons. Psychiat. Leverndale Hosp.; Educational Co-ordinator Greater Glas. Comm. NHS Trust. Specialty: Gen. Psychiat. Prev: Regist. Roy. Dundee Liff Hosp.; Lect. in Psychiat. Univ. Dundee.

WHYTE, Ursula Mary (retired) 10 The Boarlands, Port Eynon, Swansea SA3 1NX Tel: 01792 391252 — (Roy. Free) MB BS Lond. 1949; MRCS Eng. LRCP Lond. 1949. Prev: Ho. Surg. Roy. Free Hosp. Lond.

WHYTE, William Giffen Rigislea, Neilston, Glasgow G78 3NY — MB ChB Glas. 1945 (Univ. Glas.) FRFPS Glas. 1950; FRCP Glas. 1967. Sen. Regist. (Med.) Roy. Infirm. Glas. Prev: Capt. RAMC; Ho. Phys. Glas. Roy. Infirm.

WHYTE-VENABLES, David Henry Tangley Medical Centre, 10 Tangley Park Road, Hampton TW12 3YH Tel: 020 8979 5056; Lansdowne, Priory Road, Hampton TW12 2PB Tel: 020 8979 5150 — MB Camb. 1959 (St. Geo.) BChir 1958. Prev: Ho. Surg. Gyn. Dept. & Res. Obst. Asst. Kersley Hosp. Coventry; Ho. Phys. & Ho. Surg. Epsom Dist. Hosp.

WHYTE-VENABLES, Michaela Brixton Hill Group Practice, 22 Raleigh Gardens, London SW2 1AE Tel: 020 8674 6376 Fax: 020 8671 0283 — MB BS Lond. 1991 (Roy. Free Med. Sch. Lond.) DRCOG 1995; DFFP 1995; MRCGP 1996. Hon. Research Fell. at Kings Coll. Hosp. Sch. of Med. & Dent. Specialty: Gen. Pract. Prev: Trainee GP/SHO St. Thos. Hosp. Lond. VTS.

WICKENDEN, David Hubert Hattersley Group Practice, Hattersley Road East, Hyde SK14 3EH Tel: 0161 368 4161 Fax: 0161 351 1989; 59 Dale Road, Marple, Stockport SK6 6NF Tel: 0161 427 2298 — MB BS Lond. 1961 (Lond. Hosp.) MRCS Eng. LRCP Lond. 1961; DObst RCOG 1964; DA Eng. 1967.

WICKENDEN, Gillian Hope Pringle Head, Pringle Bank, Warton, Carnforth LA5 9PW — MB ChB Manch. 1991; BA (Hons.) Manch. 1984. SHO (O & G). Specialty: Obst. & Gyn. Prev: SHO (Anaesth.) Roy. Lancaster Infirm.; SHO (Paediat.) Roy. Lancaster Infirm.

WICKENDEN, Peter Douglas, Brigadier late RAMC Retd. (retired) Whitehill Lodge, Portsmouth Road, Ripley, Woking GU23 6EW Tel: 01483 225282 — MB Camb. 1954 (Camb. & Univ. Coll. Hosp.) BChir 1953; DObst RCOG 1959; DPM Eng. 1966; FRCPsych. 1981, M 1971. Prev: Dir. Labwick Psychol. Assessm. Ltd.

WICKENS, Claire Louise 50 Gloucester Road, Dartford DA1 3DJ — MB ChB Dundee 1997.

WICKENS, Lissa Catharine 79 High Street, Orwell, Royston SG8 5QN — MB BS Lond. 1997.

WICKERT, Alison Jean St George Health Centre, Bellevue Road, St. George, Bristol BS5 7PH Tel: 0117 961 2161 Fax: 0117 961 8761; 91 Kennington Avenue, Bishopston, Bristol BS7 9EX — MB ChB Bristol 1980; BSc Bristol 1972; DRCOG 1983; MRCGP 1984.

WICKES, Alan Douglas Ashmore, 3 Miller St., Hamilton ML3 7EW Tel: 01698 425087 — MB ChB Glas. 1969; FFA RCSI 1977. Chief of Anaesth. & Dir. (Intens. Care) King Faisal Milit. Hosp.; Khamis Mushyat, Saudi Arabia. Specialty: Anaesth.

WICKHAM, Elizabeth Anne Medical Input, PO Box 246, Canterbury CT4 5YY Tel: 01227 700697 Fax: 01227 700697; Earley House, Petham, Canterbury CT4 5RY Tel: 01227 700434 — MB BS Lond. 1965 (Roy. Free) MRCS Eng. LRCP Lond. 1965. Indep. Pharm. Phys. Med. Input Canterbury. Specialty: Pharmaceutical Medicine. Socs: Fell. Fac. Pharmaceut. Phys.; FRSM. Prev: Sen. Med. Adviser Pfizer Ltd. Sandwich.

WICKHAM, Harvey Eugene Henry De La Vega 3A Hatherley Lane, Cheltenham GL51 6PN — MB BS Lond. 1994.

WICKHAM, Mr Henry (retired) The Oaks, 70 Victoria Road, Fulwood, Preston PR2 8NJ Tel: 01772 718197 — MB ChB Liverp. 1945; FRCS Eng. 1961. Prev: Cons. ENT Surg. Roy. Preston Hosp. & Chorley & Dist. Hosp.

WICKHAM, John Ewart Alfred — MB BS Lond. 1955.

WICKHAM, Louisa Jane — MB BS Lond. 1996; MRCOphth 2000.

WICKHAM, Mr Martin Henry Department Otolaryngology, Barnsley District General Hospital NHS Trust, Gawber Road, Barnsley S75 2EP Tel: 01226 777756 Fax: 01226 202859; 8 The Croft, West Bretton, Wakefield WF4 4LH — MB ChB Manch. 1977; FRCS Ed.DRL 1985. Cons. Otorhinolaryngol., Barnsley Gen. Hosp. NHS trust. Specialty: Otolaryngol.

WICKHAM, Michael, CStJ (retired) Hirsel Cottage, Town Yetholm, Kelso TD5 8RG Tel: 01573 420355 — MB ChB Birm. 1941. Prev: Co. Surg. St. John Ambul. Worcs. & Hereford.

WICKHAM, Timothy Andrew 34 Winifred Lane, Aughton, Ormskirk L39 5DJ — MB BS Lond. 1993.

WICKINS, Michael Charles Townsend House, 49 Harepath Road, Seaton EX12 2RY Tel: 01297 20616 Fax: 01297 20810; Kimaric, Elm Farm Lane, Colyford, Colyton EX24 6QS — MB BS Lond. 1973 (Univ. Coll. Hosp.) BSc (Hons.) (Physiol.) Lond. 1969; MRCGP 1979. Specialty: Gen. Pract.

WICKRAMASEKERA, Mr Dhammika c/o Mr. S. J. Onions, No. 93 Llandaff Drive, Prestatyn LL19 8TU Tel: 01745 854894; No 9/1 Rajagiriya Road, Rajagiriya, Kotte, Sri Lanka — MB BS Colombo 1984; FRCS Ed. 1992; LRCPS 1994; LMSSA Lond. 1994; LRCP 1994. Regist. (Surg.) Huddersfield Roy. Infirm. Specialty: Gen. Surg. Prev: Regist. (Surg.) Ysbyty Gwynedd Hosp. Bangor.

WICKRAMASINGHE, Kalutara Muhandiramge Susil Sumathi 14 Meadow Close, London Colney, St Albans AL2 1RQ — MB BS Ceylon 1958.

WICKRAMASINGHE, Lathika Skin Department, Oldchurch Hospital, Waterloo Road, Romford RM7 0BE Tel: 01708 756090 Ext: 3473; Serendip, 20 Newlands Close, Hutton, Brentwood CM13 2SD Tel: 01277 200371 Fax: 01277 202414 — MB BS Sri Lanka 1977. Staff Dermat. Old Ch. Hosp. Romford & Harold Wood Hosp. Essex. Specialty: Dermat. Prev: Regist. (Dermat.) Roy. Lond. & Whipps Cross Hosps. Lond.; Clin. Asst. (Gen. Med.) Barking Hosp. Essex; Regist. (Dermat.) Sunderland Roy. Infirm.

WICKRAMASINGHE, Liyanagae Sarath Piyatissa Harold Wood Hospital, Gubbins Lane, Harold Wood, Romford RM3 0BE Tel: 01708 708257 Fax: 01708 708283; Serendip, 20 Newlands Close, Hutton, Brentwood CM13 2SD Tel: 01277 200371 — MB BS Ceylon 1971; MRCP (UK) 1980; DGM RCP Lond. 1985; FRCP Lond. 1991. Cons. Phys. (Med. for Elderly) Harold Wood Hosp. Romford & High Wood Hosp. Brentwood. Specialty: Gen. Med. Prev: Sen. Regist. (Geriat. & Gen. Med.) Sunderland Hosp.; Regist. (Gen. Med.) Burnley Gen. Hosp.

WICKRAMASINGHE, Sudatta Gunamangala Maithri 130A Wood Street, Chelmsford CM2 8BL — MB ChB Aberd. 1996.

WICKRAMASINGHE, Sunitha Nimal 32 Braywick Road, Maidenhead SL6 1DA Tel: 01628 21665 — MB BS Ceylon 1964; ScD Camb. 1985, PhD 1968; FRCPath 1986, M 1975; MRCP (UK) 1987; FRCP Lond. 1991. Emerit. Prof. Haemat. St. Mary's Hosp. Med. Sch. Lond.; Hon. Cons. Haemat. St. Mary's Hosp. Lond. Specialty: Haematology. Prev: Lect., Sen. Lect. & Reader (Haemat.) St. Mary's Hosp. Med. Sch. Lond.

WICKRAMASURIYA, Boosabaduge Pujitha Nalin 16 Blackfen Road, Sidcup DA15 8SN — MB BS Lond. 1994.

WICKREMA, Felix Rajah De Silva 10 Moorlea Avenue, Dringhouses, York YO24 2PA Tel: 01904 702145 — MB BS Ceylon 1965; DRCOG 1981. Assoc. Specialist York Dist. Hosp.

WICKREMARATCHI, Mirdhu Mirmalani 34 Abbots Way, Bristol BS9 4SW — MB BCh Wales 1997.

WICKREMASINGHE, Amal Sarah Leeds General Infirmary, Great George St., Leeds LS1 3EX Tel: 0113 243 2799 — MB ChB Leeds 1998. SHO (O & G), Leeds Gen. Infirm., Leeds. Specialty: Obst. & Gyn.

WICKREMASINGHE, Sanjeewa Sudarshan Flat 21, Highgate Heights, 77 Shepherds Hill, London N6 5RF — MB BS Lond. 1996.

WICKREMASINGHE, Sarathchandra Piyasiri Newbury Group Practice, Newbury Park Health Centre, 40 Perrymans Farm Road, Barkingside, Ilford IG2 7LE Tel: 020 8554 3944 Fax: 020 8518 5911; 20 Greenleafe Drive, Barkingside, Ilford IG6 1LL Tel: 020 8550 3598 — MRCS Eng. LRCP Lond. 1959 (Univ. Coll. Lond. & W. Lond.) MRCP Lond. 1967. Rudolph Kohnstamm Prize (Med.) W. Lond. Hosp. Med. Sch. 1959. Prev: Ho. Phys. Ashford Hosp., Middlx.; SHO (Path.) Paddington Gen. Hosp.; Med. Regist. Wanstead Hosp.

WICKREMASINGHE, Sushila Malkanthi Newbury Group Practice, Newbury Park Health Centre, 40 Perrymans Farm Road, Barkingside, Ilford IG2 7LE Tel: 020 8554 3944 Fax: 020 8518 5911 — MB BS Ceylon 1958; MRCP Lond. 1964. Prev: Ho. Phys. Ashford Hosp., Middlx.; Med. Regist. Wanstead Hosp. Lond. & Connaught Hosp. Lond.

WICKREMESINGHE, Mr Sunanda Srilal 148 Burbage Road, Dulwich Village, London SE21 7AG — MB BS Ceylon 1967; FRCS Eng. 1972. Cons. (Surg. & Endoscopy) Mayday Univ. Hosp. Croydon. Prev: SHO (Surg.) St. Jas. Hosp. Balham; SHO (Orthop.) Rowley Bristow Orthop. Hosp. Pyrford & St. Peter's Hosp. Chertsey; SHO (Surg.) Hammersmith Hosp.

WICKS, Anthony Christopher Bateman 26 High Street, Kibworth Beauchamp, Leicester LE8 0HQ Tel: 0116 279 3562 — MB BCh BAO Dub. 1964 (TC Dub.) FRCP Lond 1982, M 1969; MD Birm. 1973. Cons. Phys. Gastroenterol. Leicester Gen. Hosp. Specialty: Gastroenterol. Socs: BMA & Brit. Soc. Gastroenterol. Prev: Regional Coll. Adviser, Roy. Coll. of Phys.s, S. Trent; Sen. Lect. (Med.) Univ. Rhodesia, Salisbury.

WICKS, Malcolm MacKenzie (retired) Yew Tree Cottage, Boreham Street, Hailsham BN27 4SF Tel: 01323 833910 — MB BS Lond. 1960 (Westm.) MRCS Eng. LRCP Lond. 1960; DObst RCOG 1963; MRCGP 1977. Prev: SHO (O & G) Dorking Gen. Hosp.

WICKS, Margaret Helen Lister House Surgery, Lister House, 53 Harrington Street, Pear Tree, Derby DE23 8PF Tel: 01332 271212 Fax: 01332 271939 — BM BS Nottm. 1983; MRCGP 1987. Prev: Trainee GP Derby VTS.

WICKS, Rachel Caldew House Cottage, Dalston, Carlisle CA5 7LL — MB ChB Birm. 1992.

WICKS, Robert MacKenzie Flat 2, 1 Handforth Road, London SW9 0LS — MB BS Lond. 1984.

WICKSTEAD, David Harold Corner Surgery, 99 Coldharbour Lane, London SE5 9NS Tel: 020 7274 4507 Fax: 020 7733 6545 — MB ChB Liverp. 1988 (Liverpool) T(GP) 1992; MSc (Health Care Ethics) 1992; DTM & H 1993; DFFP 1996. GP Princip. Lond. Prev: Trainee GP Whiston & St. Helens VTS.

WICKSTEAD, Mr Michael Ear, Nose and Throat Department, Norfolk and Norwich University Hospital, Colney Lane, Norwich NR4 7UY Tel: 01603 289718 Fax: 01603 287288 — MRCS Eng. LRCP Lond. 1978 (Camb. & St. Thos.) MA Camb. 1978, MB BChir 1979; FRCS (Orl.) Eng. 1983. Cons. ENT Surg. Norf. & Norwich Univ. Hosp. Specialty: Otolaryngol. Special Interest: otology; Paediatric ENT Surgery. Socs: Brit. Assn. of ENT and head and Neck Surgeons; Roy. Soc. of Med. Prev: Sen. Regist. (ENT Surg.) St. Thos. Hosp. Lond. & Hosp. for Sick Childr. Lond.

WICTOME, Jeffrey Southlea Surgery, 276 Lower Farnham, Aldershot GU11 3RB Tel: 01252 344868 Fax: 01252 342596; Brook House, Holbrook Close, Weybourne, Farnham GU9 9HS — MB ChB Liverp. 1971; MRCGP 1976; DRCOG 1977.

WIDAA, Abdel Rahman Bolton General Hospital, Minerva Road, Farnworth, Bolton BL4 0JR Tel: 01204 22444; Bolton General Hospital, Minerva Road, Farnworth, Bolton BL4 0JR — MB BCh Ain Shams 1970; DLO Eng. 1979. Clin. Asst. (ENT Surg. & Anaesth.) Bolton HA. Specialty: Anaesth. Prev: Regist. (ENT Surg. & Anaesth.) Bolton HA.

WIDD, Sarah Elizabeth Kent paediatric audiology service, Cobtree and Prestonhall Hospital, Maidstone; 5 The Gube, Egerton, Ashford TN27 9DH Tel: 01233 756460 — MB BS Lond. 1972 (Kings college hospital) MSO 2000. Clin. ass pred Audiol.; adjudicating Med off for benefits agency. Specialty: Community Child Health; Audiol. Med.; Disabil. Med. Prev: Sen. Clin. Med. Off. (Child Health Community) SE Kent HA.

WIDDERS, Jane Ashby Turn Primary Care Centre, The Link, Scunthorpe DN16 2UT Tel: 01724 842051 Fax: 01724 280346 — BM BS Nottm. 1988; MRCGP 1995. GP Ashby Turn Surg. N. Lincs.

WIDDICOMBE, Professor John Guy Sherrington School of Physiology, United Medical Dental School, St Thomas' Hospital, Lambeth Palace Road, London SE1 7EH Tel: 020 7928 9292 Fax: 020 7028 0729 — BM BCh Oxf. 1949 (Oxf. & St. Bart.) DPhil Oxf. 1953, MA 1950, BA 1946, DM 1967; FRCP Lond. 1977, M 1974. Emerit. Prof. Physiol. UMDS St. Thos. Hosp. Lond. Socs: Physiol. Soc.; Pharmacol. Soc. Prev: Emerit. Prof. Physiol. St. Geo. Hosp. Med. Sch. Tooting; Fell. Qu. Coll. Oxf., Nuffield Inst. Med. Research Oxf.; Sen. Lect. (Physiol.) St. Bart. Hosp. Lond.

WIDDICOMBE, Neil James 89 King Richard Drive, Bearswood, Bournemouth BH11 9UE — MB BS Lond. 1988.

WIDDISON, Mr Adam Lewis Department of Surgery, Royal Cornwall Hospital, Treliske, Truro TR1 3ST Tel: 01872 74242 — MB BCh Oxf. 1984 (Oxford Univ.) FRCS Eng. 1988; MA Oxf. 1985, DM 1991; PGCE 2002. Cons. Surg. Roy. Cornw. Hosp.; Hunt. Prof. 1995; Educational Supervision. Specialty: Gen. Surg. Socs: BMA; HCSA; RCS. Prev: Demonst. (Anat.) & Prospector Univ. Camb.

WIDDOWSON, David Jeremy 2 Bryn Avenue, Old Colwyn, Colwyn Bay LL29 8AL — MB BS Lond. 1980; MA (Cambs.) 1977; DMRD Liverp. 1984; FRCR Lond. 1986. Cons. Radiol. Glan Clwyd Hosp. Bodelwyddan. Specialty: Radiol.

WIDDOWSON, Eric Julian St Chads Surgery, Gullock Tyning, Midsomer Norton, Bath BA3 2UH Tel: 01761 413334 Fax: 01761 411176; Manor Farm House, The Green, Farmborough, Bath BA2 0BA — MB BS Lond. 1986 (Univ. Coll. Hosp.) BSc (Hons.) Manch. 1980; LMSSA Lond. 1985; DCH RCP Lond. 1989; DRCOG 1990; MRCGP 1990. Specialty: Sports Med. Socs: Brit. Assn. Sport & Med. Prev: Trainee GP/SHO (Paediat. & O & G) Roy. United Hosp. Bath VTS; Trainee GP/SHO (Gen. Med. & Geriat.) Jersey Gen. Hosp. VTS.

WIDDOWSON, Fiona Jean Myra Hoppersford Farm, Pimlico, Brackley NN13 5TN — MB ChB Bristol 1995; BSc Brighton 1989. SHO (A & E) Bedford Hosp. Prev: Ho. Off. (Surg.) MusGr. Pk. Hosp. Taunton; Ho. Off. (Med.) Roy. Cornw. Hosp. Treliske.

WIDDOWSON, Judith 1F1 5 Spittal Street, Edinburgh EH3 9DY — MB ChB Ed. 1998.

WIDDOWSON, Sally Melinda Sumner Health Centre, 35 Nayland Street, Christchurch 8008, New Zealand Tel: 00 64 3 326 6288 Fax: 00 64 3 326 5748; c/o Brow Head, Under Loughrigg, Ambleside LA22 9SB — MB ChB Sheff. 1986; DRCOG 1993; MRCGP 1995. Specialty: Gen. Pract.

WIDDRINGTON, Ian Harry South Hylton Surgery, 3-5 Cambria Street, South Hylton, Sunderland SR4 0LT Tel: 0191 534 7386 — MB ChB Leeds 1977; DRCOG 1982; MRCGP 1983.

WIDE, Jonathan Martin Dept. of Radiology, Whiston Hospital, Prescot; 8 Whitbarrow Road, Lymm WA13 9AE — MB BChir Camb. 1989; MA Camb. 1990, BA 1986; MRCP (UK) 1992; DMRD Liverp. 1995; FRCR 1996. Cons. (Radiol.) Whiston Hosp. Merseyside. Specialty: Radiol. Prev: Regist. (Radiodiagn.) Arrowe Pk. Hosp. Wirral; Regist. Roy. Liverp. Univ. Hosp.; SHO (Phys. & Renal Med.) Roy. Free Hosp. Lond.

WIDGINGTON, Nicola Jane The Simpson Health Centre, 70 Gregories Road, Beaconsfield HP9 1PS Tel: 01494 671571 Fax: 01494 680219; 21 Burkes Road, Beaconsfield HP9 1PB Tel: 01494

681235 — MB BS Lond. 1984; MRCGP 1988; DRCOG 1988; DCH RCP Lond. 1988.

WIECEK, Maryan Ryszard McNulty and Partners, Torkard Hill Medical Centre, Farleys Lane, Nottingham NG15 6DY Tel: 0115 963 3676 Fax: 0115 968 1957; 188 Papplewick Lane, Hucknall, Nottingham NG15 8EH — BM BS Nottm. 1977; MRCP (UK) 1981. Clin. Asst. (Dermat.) Kings Mill Hosp. Mansfield.

WIEJAK, Antoni Peter Atkinson Health Centre, Market Street, Barrow-in-Furness LA14 2LR Tel: 01229 822205 Fax: 01229 832938; Rampside Hall, Rampside, Barrow-in-Furness LA13 0PX — MB ChB Manch. 1979; DRCOG 1982; MRCGP 1983. Dir. Furness Emerg. Doctor Servs.; Med. Off. Barrow Lifeboat.

WIELAND, Satu Sinikka Lillian 33 Hichisson Road, London SE15 3AN — State Exam Med. Hamburg 1988. Specialty: Gen. Med.

WIELD, Cathryn Emily 432 Winchester Road, Southampton SO16 7DH — MB BS Lond. 1983; BSc (Hons.) Lond. 1980. Specialty: Accid. & Emerg.

WIELD, Thelma Dorothy (retired) 9 LangtonsCt., Alresford SO24 9UE Tel: 01962 732696 — (Roy. Colls. Ed.) LRCP LRCS Ed. LRFPS Glas. 1952; FFCM 1987, MFCM 1982. Prev: Cons. Pub. Health Med. Croyon DHA.

WIELEZYNSKI, Maurycy (retired) 7 Bryn Meadows, Newtown SY16 2DS — LMS Madrid 1960; LAH Dub. 1965; DObst RCOG 1966.

WIELINK, Roelien Cornelia Aliet Diana Chulmleigh Health Centre, Three Crossways, Chulmleigh EX18 7AA Tel: 01769 580269 Fax: 01769 581131 — Artsexamen Utrecht 1988.

WIELOGÓRSKI, Andrzej Krzysztof 5 Park Drive, London W3 8ND — MB BS Lond. 1974; FFA RCS Eng. 1980. Cons. Cardiothoracic Anaesth. St. Thos. Hosp. Lond. Guy's & St. Thos. Hosp. Trust. Specialty: Anaesth. Prev: Cons. Cardiothoracic Anaesth. Cardiothoracic Unit Brook Gen. Hosp. Lond.

WIENER, Andrew Julian Child & Adolescent Mental Health Service, Marlowes Health Centre, The Marlowes, Hemel Hempstead HP1 1HE Tel: 01442 251132 Fax: 01442 218310 Email: andrew.wiener@hpt.nhs.uk — MB ChB Ed. 1983; MA RCA 1986; MRCPsych 1993; MPhil 1996. Cons. (Child & Adolesc. Psychiat.) Child & Family Clinic Hemel Hempstead. Specialty: Child & Adolesc. Psychiat. Prev: Sen. Regist. (Child & Adolesc. Psychiat.) Tavistock Clinic. Lond.; Regist. & SHO Maudsley Hosp. Lond.

WIENER, Jarmila Josefa Department of Obstetrics & Gynaecology, Royal Gwent Hospital, Newport NP20 2UB Tel: 01633 234234 Fax: 01633 656111 Email: jo.weiner@gwent.wales.nhs.uk; 9 Cwrt Cefn, Lisvane, Cardiff CF14 0US Tel: 02920 759076 — MB BCh Wales 1971; Dobst RCOG 1973; MRCOG 1976; FRCOG 1995. Cons. O & G Roy. Gwent Hosp. Newport. Specialty: Obst. & Gyn. Socs: (Treas.) Treas. Welsh Obst. & Gyn. Soc.; Internat. Soc. Ultrasound in Obst. & Gyn.; Brit. Med ultrasound Soc. Prev: Sen. Regist. (O & G) Univ. Hosp. Wales Cardiff & W. Glam. HA; Assoc. Specialist (O & G) Roy. Gwent Hosp. Newport.

WIER, John 83 Nelson Road, Rayleigh SS6 8HQ — BM Soton. 1983.

WIERSEMA, Ubbo Frank 100G Richmond Hill, Richmond TW10 6RJ — MB BS Newc. 1991.

WIERZBICKI, Anthony Stanislaw St Thomas Hospital, Lambeth Palace Road, London SE1 7EH Tel: 020 7928 9292 Fax: 020 7928 4226; 6E Bedford Towers, Cavendish Place, Brighton BN1 2JG Tel: 01273 724378 — BM BCh Oxf. 1986; MA Camb. 1987, BA 1983; DPhil Oxf. 1993. Sen. Lect. & Hon. Cons. of Guy's & St Thos. Hosp. Lond. Specialty: Chem. Path. Socs: Amer. Soc. Human Genetics; Internat. Atherosclerosis Soc.; Brit. Hyperlipidaemia ass. Prev: Lect. & Hon. Sen. Regist. (Chem. Path.) Char. Cross & Westm. Med. Sch.; Regist. (Med. Biochem.) Univ. Hosp. Cardiff; MRC Research Fell. (Neurosci.s) Inst. Molecular Med. Oxf.

WIERZBICKI, Wladyslaw (retired) 7 Circle Court, Harrowdene Road, Wembley HA0 2JP Tel: 020 8902 0689 — MD Bologna 1947. Prev: Dent. Off. 11th Gen. Hosp. PRC LLa.rch Panna Camp nr. Wrexham.

WIESELBERG, H. Michael Paediatric Unit, Royal National Orthopaedic Hospital, Brockley Hill, Stanmore HA7 4LP Tel: 020 8954 2300 Fax: 020 8420 4566; 8 Broughton Avenue, London N3 3ER Tel: 01923 249244 — MB BChir Camb. 1970 (Camb. & St. Geo.) MA Camb. 1975, BA 1966; MRCS Eng. LRCP Lond. 1969; DCH Eng. 1973; MRCP (UK) 1975; MRCPsych 1976. p/t Cons. Child & Adolesc. Psychiat. Roy. Nat. Orthop. Hosp. Stanmore; Hon. Sen. Clin. Lect. Univ. Coll. & Middlsex Sch. Med. Lond. Specialty: Child & Adolesc. Psychiat. Prev: Regist. Bethlem Roy. & Maudsley Hosp. Lond.; Lect. Child Psychiat. Inst. Psychiat. Lond.; Cons. Middlx. & Univ. Coll. Hosps. Lond.

WIESEMANN, Peter 23 Blackstock Close, Headington, Oxford OX3 7JR Tel: 01865 771686 — State Exam Med Munich 1993 (University of Munich) DCH Lond. 1997.

WIESENDANGER, Peter Hans (retired) Tanner Brow, Bethesda Street, Upper Basildon, Reading RG8 8NU Tel: 01734 302513 — MRCS Eng. LRCP Lond. 1953 (King's Coll. Hosp.) MA Oxf. 1954, BM BCh 1953; DObst RCOG 1956.

WIESHMAN, Udo Carl Walton Centre for Neurology & Neurosurgery, Lower Lane, Fazakerley, Liverpool L9 7LJ Tel: 0151 529 5687 Email: udo.wieshmann@thewaltoncentre.nhs.uk — State Exam Med Berlin 1991. Cons. Neurologist, WCNN, Liverpool; Renacres Wall Hosp. Specialty: Neurol. Socs: ABN; RCP (afiliate mem.). Prev: WCNN.

WIESSLER, Regine Erika Holmwood Corner Surgery, 134 Malden Road, New Malden KT3 6DR Tel: 020 8942 0066 — MB ChB Cape Town 1990; BSc (Br. Col.) 1984; LMCC 1994; MSc Lond. 1995; DTM & H Lond. 1995; DRCOG 1998; MRCGP 1999. GP. Socs: BMA.

WIGDAHL, James Douglas (retired) High Orchard, Chequers Lane, North Runcton, King's Lynn PE33 0QN Tel: 01553 840352 — BM BCh Oxf. 1953 (Middlx.) MA 1953; DObst RCOG 1957; MRCGP 1966.

WIGFIELD, Arthur Salmon (retired) 35 Sandford Road, Mapperley, Nottingham NG3 6AL — MB BChir Camb. 1946 (Univ. Coll. Hosp.) MRCS Eng. LRCP Lond. 1936; MA, MD Camb. 1950, MB BChir 1946. Hon. Cons. Venereol. Newc HA (T). Prev: Cons. Venereol. Newc. Gen. Hosp.

WIGFIELD, Crispin Campbell 20 Montrose Avenue, Redland, Bristol BS6 6EQ — MB ChB Birm. 1993; BSc 1990; FRCS Eng. 1997. Specialist Regist. (Neuroserg.) S. W. Rotat. Frenchay Hosp. Bristol.

WIGFIELD, Mary (retired) 22 Tamarack Close, Eastbourne BN22 0TR Tel: 01323 506075 — MB BS Lond. 1953 (Roy. Free) MRCS Eng. LRCP Lond. 1953; DObst RCOG 1955; MFFP 1993. Sessional SCMO (Family Plann. & Psychosexual Med.) Eastbourne & Co. Healthcare NHS Trust. Prev: Sen. Clin. Off. (Family Plann.) Eastbourne Health Dist.

WIGFIELD, Miles Fraser Windrush Cottage, Itlay, Daglingworth, Cirencester GL7 7HZ — MB BS Lond. 1973; DCH Eng. 1976; DRCOG 1982.

WIGFIELD, Ruth Elizabeth Department of Child Health, North Hampshire Hospital, Aldermaston Road, Basingstoke RG24 9NA Tel: 01256 313688 Fax: 01256 314796 Email: ruth.wigfield@nhht.nhs.uk; The Hornbeams, Dever Close, Micheldever, Winchester SO21 3SR Tel: 01962 774817 Fax: 01962 774817 Email: ruthwigfield@doctors.org.uk — BM Soton. 1982; MRCPCH; MRCP (UK) 1987. p/t Cons. (Paediatr.), N. Hants. Hosp., Basingstoke. Specialty: Paediat.; Neonat. Socs: BAPM. Prev: Sen. Regist. (Paediat.) Soton. Univ. Hosps.; Research Fell. Inst. Child Health Bristol Univ.; Lect. & Hon. Regist. (Child Health & Neonat.) Bristol Univ.

WIGGAM, Malcolm Ivan Department of Health for the elderly, Royal Victoria Hospital, Grosvenor Road, Belfast BT12 6BA Tel: 028 9024 0503 — MB BCh BAO Belf. 1990 (Belfast) MRCP (UK) 1993; MB BCh BAO (Hons.) Belf. 1990, MD 1997. Cons. Phys., Med. for the elderly, Roy. Vict. Hosp Belf. Specialty: Care of the Elderly. Socs: Brit. Diabetes Assn.; Irish Endocrine Soc.; Brit. Geriat. Soc. Prev: Clin.Train. Fell. Stroke Med. Western Gen. Hosp. Edinb.; Research Fell. Metab. Unit Roy. Vict. Hosp. Belf.; Sen. Regist. (Geriat/Gen. (Internal) Med. N.Irel.

WIGGANS, Stephen Mark 17 Kirkstone Avenue, Cherry Tree, Blackburn BB2 5HJ — MB ChB Birm. 1996; FRCA.

WIGGINS, Betsy Linda 11 St Martins, Castle Bytham, Grantham NG33 4RH Tel: 01780 410433 — BM BCh Oxf. 1974; MRCPCH; MRCP (UK) 1977; DCH Eng. 1978; MRCGP 1981. Assoc. Specialist (Community Paediat.) United Lincs. Hosps. Specialty: Community Child Health. Prev: Clin. Med. Off. S. Lincs.

WIGGINS, Mr Brian Christopher (retired) Rookery Medical Centre, Rookery House, Newmarket CB8 8NW Tel: 01638 665711 Fax: 01638 561280; Drove End, Milburn Drove, Moulton, Newmarket CB8 8QW — BM BCh Oxf. 1967; FRCS Ed. 1972.

WIGGINS, Clive Andrew Thomas St. Johns Medical Centre, 287A Lewisham Way, London SE4 1XF Tel: 020 8692 2048 Ext: 1354 — MB BS Lond. 1989 (Licensed Associate Faculty Homeopathy) MRCGP 1996; DFFP 1997. Specialty: Gen. Pract. Socs: Assoc. Fac. Homeopathy; Brit. Acupunc. Soc. Prev: SHO (Med. Rheum.) Stoke Mandeville Hosp. Aylesbury; SHO (Med.) St. Thos. Hosp. Lond.; Ho. Phys. St. Peter's Hosp. Chertsey.

WIGGINS, Gillian Holt (retired) Keren, Kiln Lane, Winkfield, Windsor SL4 2DU Tel: 01344 884008 — MB ChB Birm. 1956. Prev: Assoc. Specialist Hillingdon Hosp. Uxbridge.

WIGGINS, John Wexham Park Hospital, Wexham, Slough SL2 4HL Tel: 01753 634464 Fax: 01753 634464; Standen, Longbottom Lane, Seer Green, Beaconsfield HP9 2UL Tel: 01494 676571 — MD Birm. 1985; MB ChB Birm. 1976; MRCP (UK) 1979; FRCP 1997. Cons. Phys. Wexham Pk. Hosp. Slough. Specialty: Gen. Med.; Respirat. Med. Socs: Brit. Thorac. Soc.; Amer. Thoracic Soc.; Eur. Respirat. Soc. Prev: Sen. Regist. (Gen. & Thoracic Med.) Brompton & Westm. Hosps. Lond.; Regist. (Gen. & Thoracic Med.) E. Birm. Hosp.; Sheldon Research Fell. W. Midl. RHA.

WIGGINS, Lisa Joyce 24 Woodland Way, London N21 3QA — MB ChB Liverp. 1994.

WIGGINS, Miriam Rose Birmingham Childrens Hospital, Ladywood, Birmingham B4 6; 24 Alexander Close, Bognor Regis PO21 4PL — MB ChB Birm. 1993. SHO (Paediat.) Birm. Childr. Hosp.

WIGGINS, Peter Sidney Castlemilk Health Centre, 71 Dougrie Drive, Glasgow G45 9AW Tel: 0141 531 8585 Fax: 0141 531 8596; 26 Braidpark Drive, Giffnock, Glasgow G46 6NB Tel: 0141 637 8281 — MB ChB Glas. 1979; DRCOG 1981; MRCGP 1983; MFHom RCP Lond. 1993. Specialty: Gen. Pract. Prev: Trainee GP Glas. VTS.

WIGGINS, Robert James Pathology Department, Hemel Hempstead General Hospital, Hillfield Road, Hemel Hempstead HP2 4AD Tel: 01442 213141 Fax: 01442 60253 — MB ChB Dundee 1981; BMSc (Hons.) Dund 1978; MSc Lond. 1988; MRCPath 1990; FRCPath 1998. Cons. MicroBiol. St Albans & Hemel Hempstead NHS Trust. Specialty: Med. Microbiol. Socs: FRSM; Assn. Clin. Paths.; Hosp. Infec. Soc. Prev: Sen. Regist. Whipps Cross Hosp. & St. Bart. Hosp. Lond.; Clin. Research Asst. St. Bart. Hosp. Med. Coll. Lond.; Regist. & SHO St. Bart. Hosp. Lond.

WIGGINS, William John Lutterworth Health Centre, Gilmorton Road, Lutterworth LE17 4EB Tel: 01455 553531; Swinford House, Swinford, Lutterworth LE17 6BJ Tel: 01788 860607 — (Guy's) MRCS Eng. LRCP Lond. 1968; MB BS Lond. 1968; DObst RCOG 1970; DCH Eng. 1971. Med. Adviser, Merck UK.; Med. Adviser, Blaby Dist. Counc.. Specialty: Gen. Pract.; Occupat. Health. Prev: Paediat. Canad. Forces Europe, Lahr, W. Germany.

WIGGLESWORTH, David Fearnley Bridge Street Practice, 21 Bridge Street, Driffield YO25 6DB Tel: 01377 253441 — MB ChB Leeds 1967. Chairm.PEC Yorks. Wolds & Coast, Primary Care Trust. Socs: BMA (Ex-Pres.) E. Yorks. Div. Prev: Ho. Phys. & Ho. Surg. Chapel Allerton Hosp. Leeds; SHO Hull Roy. Infirm.

WIGGLESWORTH, Professor Jonathan Semple (retired) Phelps House, Upper High St, Castle Cary BA7 7AT Tel: 01963 350360 Fax: 01963 359001 — (Univ. Coll. Hosp.) MB BChir Camb. 1960; MD Camb. 1964; FRCPath 1977, M 1965; FRCPCH 1997. Prev: Beit Memor. Fell. Graham Research Dept. & Graham Schol. in Path., Graham Research Dept. Univ. Coll. Hosp. Med. Sch.

WIGGLESWORTH, Mark David Flat 3, 29 Grosenvor Place, Jesmond, Newcastle upon Tyne NE2 2RD — MB BS Newc. 1993; Dip. IMC RCS Ed. 1996; DRCOG 1997; MRCGP 1998. SHO A&E Sunderland. Roy. Infirm. Specialty: Accid. & Emerg. Prev: GP/Regist. & SHO (O & G) Carlisle.

WIGHT, Ailsa Lockerbie Department of Health, Skipton House, 80 London Road, London SE1 6LH; 88 Shakespeare Road, London W3 6SN — MB BS Lond. 1981 (Middlx.) MSc Lond. 1987, MB BS 1981; FRCPath 1997. Sen. Med. Off. DoH Lond. Specialty: Med. Microbiol. Prev: Sen. Regist. (Med. Microbiol.) St. Mary's Hosp. Paddington Lond.; Asst. Lect. (Path.) Middlx. Hosp. Sch. Path. Univ. Lond.; Cas. Off. Univ. Coll. Hosp.

WIGHT, Alexander Muirhead 16-17 South Crescent, Ardrossan KA22 8EB Tel: 01294 463011 Fax: 01294 462790; Tamdhu, 11 Law Brae, West Kilbride KA23 9DD — MB ChB Glas. 1965.

WIGHT, Catherine Odessa 85 Washingborough Road, Heighington, Lincoln LN4 1QP — MB ChB Aberd. 1993.

WIGHT, David John 48 Greenhill Road, Alveston, Bristol BS35 3NA — MB ChB Manch. 1990.

WIGHT, Derek George Douglas Department of Histopathology, Addenbrooke's Hospital, Cambridge CB2 2QQ Tel: 01223 217168 Fax: 01223 216980; Rustat House, 32 Rustat Road, Cambridge CB1 3QT Tel: 01223 248087 Fax: 01223 248087 — MB BChir Camb. 1963 (Camb. & St. Thos.) MA Camb. 1970, BA 1960, MB BChir 1963; FRCPath 1982, M 1970. Cons. Pathol. Addenbrookes Hosp. Camb.; Assoc. Lect. (Path.) Univ. Camb; Fell. & Dir. of Studies in Path. & Clin. Med. St. John's Coll. Camb. Specialty: Histopath. Socs: Path. Soc.; Brit. Soc. Gastroenterol. Prev: Cas. Off. St. Thos. Hosp. Lond.; Lect. (Path.) St. Thos. Hosp. Med. Sch. & St. Geo. Hosp. Med. Sch. Lond.

WIGHT, Gillian Ruth Roulston Cottage, Sutton-under-Whitestone-Cliffe, Thirsk YO7 2PS Tel: 01845 597329 — MB BChir Camb. 1972 (Univ. Camb. & Middlx. Hosp. Med. Sch.) MA Camb. 1972; DCH Eng. 1973; DObst RCOG 1973; Cert. Family Plann. JCC 1974. SCMO (Family Plann. & Sexual Health) York & Northallerton HAs. Specialty: Family Plann. & Reproduc. Health. Socs: MFFP; York Med. Soc.; Assoc. Inst. Psychosexual Med. Prev: SHO (Paediat. & Anaesth.) & Ho. Off. (O & G) Hillingdon Hosp. Uxbridge.

WIGHT, Henry Stephen Christian (retired) 2 St Roman's Avenue, Duffield, Derby DE6 4HG — MRCS Eng. LRCP Lond. 1943 (St. Thos.)

WIGHT, Jane Alison Hoylake & Meols Medical Centre, 53 Birkenhead Road, Meols, Wirral CH47 5AF Tel: 0151 632 6660 Fax: 0151 632 5073 — MB BS Lond. 1987; MRCGP 1991; DRCOG 1991; T(GP) 1992; DFFP 1993. GP. Specialty: Gen. Pract. Prev: Trainee GP/SHO (O & G) Glos. Roy. Hosp. Gloucester & Cheltenham VTS; SHO (A & E) Cheltenham Gen. Hosp.; SHO (ENT) Roy. United Hosp. Bath.

WIGHT, Jeremy Peter North Sheffield PCT, Firth Park Clinic, Firth Park, Sheffield S5 6NU Tel: 0114 271 6330 Email: jeremy.wight@sheffieldn-pct.nhs.uk — MB BChir Camb. 1982; MB Bchir Camb 1982; MD Sheff. 1992; FFPHM 2001; FRCP 2002. Director of Pub. Health; Hon Sen. Lect., SCHARR, Sheff. Uni. Sheff. Specialty: Pub. Health Med. Prev: Sen. Regist. (Pub. Health Med.) Trent RHA; Regist. (Renal Unit) North. Gen. Hosp. Sheff.; Cons. & Dep. DPH Wakefield HA.

WIGHT, Katharine Clare Glenfield, Woodfarm Road, Malvern Wells, Malvern WR14 4PN — MB BCh Wales 1995.

WIGHT, Nicholas James Derek 32 Rustat Road, Cambridge CB1 3QT Tel: 01223 248087 — MB Camb. 1991; BChir 1990. Ho. Phys. Addenbrooke's Hosp. Cambs.

WIGHT, Mr Richard Graham North Riding Infirmary, Newport Road, Middlesbrough TS1 5JE Tel: 01642 854023 Fax: 01642 854064 — MB BS Newc. 1980; FRCS (Otol.) Ed. 1985; FRCS (Otol.) Eng. 1987. Cons. ENT Surg. N. Riding Infirm. Middlesbrough. Specialty: Otorhinolaryngol. Socs: Ord. Mem. Sect. of Larryngol. Roy. Soc. Med. Prev: Sen. Regist. (ENT) St. Mary's Hosp. Lond. & Roy. Marsden Hosp.

WIGHT, Rosalind Marie 25 Durham Road, Edinburgh EH13 0LD Tel: 0131 669 3633 — MB ChB Dundee 1988; T(GP) 1992. GP Princip. (at Durh. Rd. Med. Gp.). Prev: GP Cons. Edin. Homeless Pract.; Princip. Med. Off., MANGUZ1, S. Africa.

WIGHT, Vivien Laing Trevaylor Road Health Centre, Trevaylor Road, Falmouth TR11 2LH Tel: 01326 317317; Lamorna, Golladowr, Penhallow, Truro TR4 9LY Tel: 01872 573365 — MB ChB Dundee 1975. Gen. Practitioner; Doctor for Cornw. Brook; Community Hosp. Doctor, Falmouth Hosp., Falmouth.

WIGHT, William John Rustat House, 32 Rustat Road, Cambridge CB1 3QT — MB BS Newc. 1993.

WIGHTMAN, Archibald Ewart (retired) Cockburn House, 48 William St., Helensburgh G84 8XX — MB ChB Ed. 1958.

WIGHTMAN, Arthur James Alexander Royal Infirmary of Edinburgh, Little France, 51 Little France Crescent, Edinburgh EH16 9SH Tel: 0131 242 3765/3775 Fax: 0131 242 3776 — MB BS Lond. 1967 (St. Mary's) DMRD Eng. 1972; FFR 1974; FRCR 1975; FRCP Edin. 2002. Cons. Radiol. Roy. Infirm. Of Edin. Edin.;

Cons. Radiol. Min. of Defence; Cons. Radiologist, BUPA Murrayfield Hosp., Edin. Specialty: Radiol. Special Interest: Chest and ENT Radiol. Socs: Soc. Apoth.; Scott. Radiol Soc. Prev: Sen. Regist. (Radiodiagn.) Roy. Infirm. Edin.; Regist. (Diagn. Radiol.) King's Coll. Hosp. Lond.; Regist. (Diagn. Radiol.) Hammersmith Hosp. Lond.

WIGHTMAN, Douglas Howe of Fife Medical Practice, 27 Commercial Road, Ladybank, Cupar KY15 7JS Tel: 01337 830765 Fax: 01337 831658 — MB ChB Ed. 1971.

WIGHTMAN, Sheila (retired) 16 Brandy Hole Lane, Chichester PO19 4RY Tel: 01243 527125 — MB ChB Manch. 1953; DObst RCOG 1955. Prev: Assoc. Specialist (Psychogeriat.) Grayling Well Hosp. Chichester.

WIGHTMAN, Susan Jane Sharda, New Park Road, Cranleigh GU6 7HL — MB ChB Liverp. 1986; MRCGP 1990.

WIGHTON, Christopher James 444 West Wycombe Road, High Wycombe HP12 4AH — MB ChB Leic. 1998.

WIGLEY, Anne (retired) 90 Macklin Street, Derby DE1 1JX Tel: 01332 340381; 23 Ladycroft Paddock, Allestree, Derby DE22 2GA — MB BS Lond. 1957 (King's Coll. Hosp.) MRCS Eng. LRCP Lond. 1957; DObst RCOG 1960; FRCGP 1992. Prev: Ho. Surg. (Gyn.) & Ho. Phys. (Diabetic) King's Coll. Hosp. Lond.

WIGLEY, Antonia Mary 132 Pencisely Road, Cardiff CF5 1DR Tel: 029 2056 4469 — MB BCh Wales 1969.

WIGLEY, Elizabeth Janet Millennium Medical Centre, 121 Weoley Castle Road, Weoley Castle, Birmingham B29 5QD Tel: 0121 427 5201 Fax: 0121 427 5052; 36 Gleneagles Drive, Blackwell, Bromsgrove B60 1BD — MB ChB Birm. 1986. Prev: Trainee GP N.field Birm. VTS.

WIGMORE, John Sydenham (retired) 6 Laurel Drive, Burntwood, Walsall WS7 9BL Tel: 01543 682288 — MB ChB Birm. 1944. Prev: Ho. Surg. (Gyn. & Obst.) Roy. Berks. Hosp. Reading.

WIGMORE, Nicholas Paul Grosvenor House Surgery, Warwick Square, Carlisle CA1 1LB Tel: 01228 536561 — MB ChB Liverp. 1984. Specialty: Gen. Pract.

WIGMORE, Mr Stephen John University Department of Surgery, Royal Infirmary of Edinburgh, 1 Lauriston Place, Edinburgh EH3 9YW Tel: 0131 536 3830 Fax: 0131 228 2661 Email: s.wigmore@ed.ac.uk — MB BS Lond. 1989 (Univ. Lond.) BSc (1st. cl. Hons.) Lond. 1986; FRCS Ed. 1993; FRCS (Gen. Surg.) 2001. Sen. Lect., Wellcome Fell. & Hon. Cons. Surg. (Transplantation & HPB Surg.) Roy. Infirm. Edin. Specialty: Transpl. Surg.; Gen. Surg. Special Interest: HPB Surg.; Laborat. Research programmes into stress proteins and pre-conditioning; Transplantation. Socs: Brit. Med. Assn.; Brit. Transplantation Soc.; Soc. of Acad. Research Surg. (Council). Prev: Smith & Nephew Research Fell. (Surg.) Roy. Infirm. Edin.; Wilkis Scholar Univ. Edin.; Lect. (Surg.) Roy. Infirm. Edin.

WIGMORE, Timothy James 16 Tyndale Court, Wesferry Road, Isle of Dogs, London E14 3TQ; 84 Westville Road, Shepherds Bush, London W12 9BD Tel: 020 8740 8146 — BM BCh Oxf. 1994; BA Camb. 1991; FRCA 1999. Specialist Regist. (Anaesth.) Imperial Sch. of Anaesth. Specialty: Anaesth.

WIGNAKUMAR, Mr Velupillai 56 Twyford Road, West Harrow, Harrow HA2 0SL — MRCS Eng. LRCP Lond. 1988; LRCP LRCS Ed. LRCPS Glas. 1986; FRCS Eng. 1991; FRCS Ed. 1991.

WIGNALL, Brian Kay 126 Harley Street, London W1G 7JS — MB ChB Manch. 1958; DIH Eng. 1963; MRCP (UK) 1970; DMRD Eng. 1971; FFR 1973; FRCR 1975. Cons. Radiol. Char. Cross. Hosp. Lond. Specialty: Radiol. Socs: Roy. Soc. Med.; Med. Soc. Lond. Prev: Cons. Radiol. St. Geo. Hosp. Lond.

WIGNALL, Deborah Christine Southern Group Practice, Castletown Road, Port Erin IM9 6BD Tel: 01624 832226 — MB ChB Sheff. 1986; MRCGP 1991. GP South. Gp. Pract. Port Erin. Prev: GP Princip. Lowther Med. Centre Cumbria; Trainee GP W. Cumbria Scheme; Ho. Surg. & Ho. Phys. Nobles Hosp. Isle of Man.

WIGNALL, John Byron William Lytham Road Surgery, 2 Lytham Road, Fulwood, Preston PR2 8JB Tel: 01772 716033 Fax: 01772 715445 — MB ChB Manch. 1976; BSc St. And. 1973.

WIGNALL, John Rossall Nicholas Beechcroft, 2 Lynwith Court, Carlton, Goole DN14 9SB — MB ChB Leeds 1973.

WIGNALL, Oliver James West Suffolk Hospital, Hardwick Lane, Bury St Edmunds IP33 2QZ — MB BS Lond. 1998.

WIGNALL, Trudy Anne 5 Didsbury Park, Didsbury, Manchester M20 5LH Tel: 0161 445 6771 Fax: 0161 448 9085 Email: tpp@mcmail.com — MB ChB Liverp. 1984; FRCS Ed. 1988; FRCR 1994. Cons. Radiol., Warrington Hosp. NHS Trust (PT). Specialty: Radiol. Prev: Sen. Regist. (Radiol.) NW RHA; Regist. (Radiol.) NW RHA; Regist. (Gen. Surg.) Trafford Gen. Hosp.

WIGNARAJAH, Nandani Department of Anaesthetics, North Tees General Hospital, Hardwick, Stockton-on-Tees TS19 8PE Tel: 01642 617617; 33 Crooks Barn Lane, Norton, Stockton-on-Tees TS20 1LR Tel: 01642 554512 — MB BS Ceylon 1970 (Peradeniya) DA Eng. 1978; FFA RCS Eng. 1980. Cons. Anaesth. (long term locum) N. Tees Gen. Hosp. Specialty: Anaesth. Socs: Obst. Anaesth. Assn. Prev: Clin. Asst. (Anaesth.) N. Tees Gen. Hosp.; Regist. (Anaesth.) N. Tees Gen. Hosp., Yeovil Dist. Hosp. & Dryburn Hosp. Durh.; SHO (Anaesth.) Shotley Bridge Gen. Hosp. Consett.

WIGNELL, Debra Joan Windrush Surgery, 21 West Bar Street, Banbury OX16 9SA Tel: 01295 251491 — MB ChB Liverp. 1986; DRCOG 1989; MRCGP 1990; DCH RCP Lond. 1992. Sen. Partner Windrush Surg.; Community Med. Off. (Child Health) Stratford-upon-Avon. Specialty: Community Child Health. Prev: Trainee GP Blackpool VTS.

WIJAYAKOON, Amitha Punchikumari 51 Goodmayes Avenue, Goodmayes, Ilford IG3 8TN Tel: 020 8597 3740 — MB BS Ceylon 1967; DO RCS Eng. 1977. Clin. Asst. (Ophth.) Lond. Hosp. Whitechapel & Moorfields Eye Hosp. Lond. Socs: Coll. Ophth. Prev: SHO (Ophth.) Edgware Gen. Hosp.

WIJAYARATNA, Lilamani Olivia 4 South Gardens, Wembley HA9 9PG — MB BS Sri Lanka 1975; LMSSA Lond. 1992.

WIJAYARATNE, Wijayaratne Mudiyanselage TQP 14 Savannah Close, Kempston, Bedford MK42 8SH — MB BS Sri Lanka 1975; MRCS Eng. LRCP Lond. 1987.

WIJAYASINGHE, Mr Garumuni Emerson De Silva 9 Coombe Lane W., Kingston upon Thames KT2 7EW — MB BS Ceylon 1957; DO Eng. 1963; FRCS Eng. 1979; Dip. Amer. Bd. Ophth. 1980. Assoc. Specialist Moorfields Eye Hosp. Lond. Prev: Eye Surg. Govt. Gen. Hosps. Badulla, Anuradhapura & Ratnapura, Sri Lanka.

WIJAYATILAKE, Dhuleep Sanjay — MB BS Lond. 1996 (Charing Cross & Westminster Hospital) BSc (Neurosci.) 1995. Specialist Registrar (Anaesth. ICU). Specialty: Anaesth. Special Interest: Neuroanaesthetics. Prev: SHO (Anaesth.) Middlx. Hosp.; SHO (Neurosurg., Neuro-IC & A & E).

WIJAYATILAKE, Narada The Surgery, 2 Falconwood Parade, The Green, Welling DA16 2PL Tel: 020 7385 5728; 6 Mount Drive, Wembley HA9 9ED Tel: 020 8930 2323 — (Colombo) MB BS Ceylon 1966. Med. Off. Benefit Agency.

WIJAYAWARDENA, M A S S Halse Road Health Centre, Halse Road, Brackley NN13 6EJ Tel: 01280 703460 Fax: 01280 703460; Werney Lodge, 57A Manor Road, Brackley NN13 6ED Tel: 01280 700467 — MB BS Ceylon 1967 (Univ. Ceylon) DObst RCOG 1975; MRCOG 1981.

WIJAYAWARDHANA, Primrose Orpington Hospital, Orpington BR6 9JU Tel: 01689 27050; 18 Goddington Chase, Orpington BR6 9EA — MB BS Ceylon 1967; DCH RCP Lond. 1972; MRCP (UK) 1973; DGM RCP Lond. 1990. Research Regist. Orpington Hosp. Kent. Prev: Regist. St. Thos. Hosp. Lond.

WIJAYAWARDHANA, Upulranjan Dewamitta Grantham & District Hospital, Manthorpe Road, Grantham NG31 8DG Tel: 01476 565232 Fax: 01476 593512 Email: upul.wijayardhana@ulh.nhs.uk — MB BS Ceylon 1964; MD Ceylon 1967; FRCP Lond. 1984, M 1968; FACC 1985. Cons. Cardiol. Grantham & Dist. Hosp. Specialty: Cardiol. Special Interest: Heart Failure. Socs: (Vice-Pres.) Asian Pacific Soc. Cardiol.; Brit. Cardiac Soc. Prev: Sen. Cardiol. Gen. Hosp. Colombo, Sri Lanka.; Clin. Dir. Integrated Med.

WIJAYAWICKRAMA, Asoka 3 Libbards Gate, Solihull B91 3XQ — MB BS Lond. 1998.

WIJAYSINGHE, Druseela The Surgery, 96 Sirdar Road, London W11 4EG Tel: 020 7727 9238 Fax: 020 7460 7305 — MB BS Bombay 1971; MB BS Bombay 1971.

WIJEKOON, Janananda Banda The Surgery, 872 Green Lane, Dagenham RM8 1BX Tel: 020 8599 7151 Fax: 020 8983 8784 — MB BS Ceylon 1968.

WIJENDRA, Mr Somil Devendra Wijeratne and Partners, Belmont Health Centre, 516 Kenton Lane, Harrow HA3 7LT Tel: 020 8863 6863 Fax: 020 8863 9815; 56 Vernon Drive, Stanmore HA7 2BT Tel: 020 8427 1664 — MB BS Sri Lanka 1974 (Fac. Med. Univ. Ceylon Peradeniya, Sri Lanka) MRCS Eng. LRCP Lond. 1986; FRCS Ed. 1987; FRCS Eng. 1987. Forens. Med. Examr. Middlx. Specialty:

Plastic Surg.; Orthop. Prev: Regist. (Orthop.) Memor. Hosp. Darlington.

WIJERATNE, Jayantha Jayasiri Wijeratne and Partners, Belmont Health Centre, 516 Kenton Lane, Harrow HA3 7LT Tel: 020 8863 6863 Fax: 020 8424 0542 — MB BS Univ. Of Sri Lanka 1974; RCP & RCS London; LRCP, MRCS 1982; MRCP (UK) 1982; MD (Univ. Of Sri Lanka) 1983. Gen. Practitioner - Sen. Partner in Gp. Pract., Harrow Middx.; Police Surg. (Forens. Med. Examr.) Metrop. Police. Specialty: Gen. Med.; Gen. Pract. Socs: Roy. Coll. of Phys.s, Lond.; Roy. Coll. of Surg.s, Lond.; BMA.

WIJERATNE, Wijith Kumara 28 Blockley Road, Wembley HA0 3LR — BM Soton. 1995; MRCP (UK) 2001.

WIJESINGHE, Mr Lasantha Dinesh — MB BChir Camb. 1990; MA; MD; FRCS. Cons. Vasc. Surg. Roy. Bournemouth Hosp.; Vis. Research Fell. Bournemouth Univ. Specialty: Surgery, Vascular. Special Interest: Carotid Endarterectomy; Femorodistal Bypass; Hyperhidrosis. Prev: SpR Leeds Gen. Infirm.; SpR Hull Roy. Infirm.; SpR St James' Hosp. Leeds.

WIJESURENDRA, Chula Shrilal Stour Clinic, Kent & Canterbury Hospitals NHS Trust, Ethelbert Road, Canterbury CT1 3NG Tel: 01227 783120 Fax: 01227 783074; 43 Ethelbert Road, Canterbury CT1 3NF Tel: 01227 783120 Fax: 01227 783074 Email: 100775.3422@compuserve.com — MB BS Sri Lanka 1976; MRCP (UK) 1982; FRCP 1998. Cons. Genitourin. Med. Stour Clinic Kent & Canterbury NHS Trust & Qu. Eliz. The Qu. Mother Hosp.; Cons. Genitourin. Med. Sittingbourne Memor. Hosp. Specialty: Genitourinary Medicine. Socs: BMA; MSSVD; AGUM. Prev: Sen. Regist. (Genitourin. Med.) Cardiff Roy. Infirm.

WIJESURENDRA, Indrani Tilaka Department of Anaesthetics, Kent & Canterbury Hospital, Canterbury CT1 3NF Tel: 01227 766877; 43 Ethelbert Road, Canterbury CT1 3NF Tel: 01227 462287 — MB BS Ceylon 1971; FFA RCS Eng. 1980. Specialty: Anaesth. Prev: Regist. (Anaesth.) Rushgreen Hosp. Romford; Regist. Moorfields Eye Hosp., Roy. Nat. Orthop. Hosp., Roy. Nat. ENT Hosp. & Whittington Hosp. Lond.

WIJETHILLEKE, Mr Gigurawa Gamage Khemananda Medicare Unit, 1 Croston Road, Lostock Hall, Preston PR5 5RS Tel: 01772 620160 — MB BS Ceylon 1970; FRCS Eng. 1980. Princip. Gen. Pract., Medicare Unit, Lostock Hall, Preston; Clin. Assit. Haemat. Roy. Preston Hosp. Specialty: Medico Legal.

WIJETILLEKA, Ahangama Baduge Sunil Ananda Central Middlesex Hospital, Action Lane, Park Royal, London NW7 0NS; 332 Malden Road, New Malden KT3 6AU Tel: 020 8965 5733 — MB BS Sri Lanka 1975; FFA RCSI 1984. Cons. Anaesth. Centr. Middlx. Hosp. Lond. Specialty: Anaesth.

WIJETUNGE, Anil 13 Prout Grove, London NW10 1PU — MB BS Lond. 1988.

WIJETUNGE, Mr Don Bandula 51 New Caledonian Wharf, 6 Odessa St., London SE16 7TN Tel: 020 7394 9499 — MB BS Ceylon 1967; FRCS Ed. 1976. Cons. Surg. (A & E) St. Geo. Hosp. & Med. Sch. Lond. Specialty: Accid. & Emerg. Prev: Regist. Profess. Surgic. Unit Univ. Camb.; 1st Asst. Dept. Surg. St. Geo. Hosp. Lond.

WIJEWARDENA, Hattotuwa Chandrapala — MB BS Ceylon 1970 (Peradeniya Med. Sch. Ceylon) DPM Eng. 1980; MRCPsych 1981. Cons. Psychiat. Manor Hosp. Epsom. Specialty: Ment. Health. Prev: Sen. Regist. Cell Barnes Hosp. St. Albans; Regist. (Psychiat.) Walsgrave Hosp. Coventry; Regist. (Psychiat.) Dist. Hosp. Basingstoke.

WIJEWARDENE, Mr Primus Anura Sandwell General Hospital, West Bromwich B71 4HJ — MB BS Peradeniya 1980; FRCS Glas. 1988; Dip. Urol. Lond 1991. Regist. (Surg. & Urol.) Bangor Dist. Gen. Hosp. Prev: Regist. (Surg.) Llandudno Gen. Hosp.

WIJEYEKOON, Sanjaya Prabhath 12 The Herons, New Wanstead, London E11 2SD — MB BS Lond. 1996; MA Camb. 1997; MRCS Eng. 1999; MSc Lond. 2002. SHO Surg. Rotat. Whipps Crom Hosp. Lond.; Regist., Inst. of Liver Studies, Kings Coll. Hosp., Lond.

WIJEYESEKERA, Kamani Geshan Canterbury Road Surgery, 186 Canterbury Road, Davyhulril, Manchester — MB BCh Wales 1989 (Univ. Wales Coll. Med.) MRCP (UK) 1994; MRCGP 1999. Specialty: Gen. Pract.; Paediat.; Homeop. Med.

WIJNBERG, Andrew William Alberic The Surgery, 65 New Road, Rubery, Birmingham B45 9JT Tel: 0121 453 3591 Fax: 0121 457 7217 — MB ChB Cape Town 1981; MB ChB Cape Town 1981.

WIJNBERG, John Paul 65 Albany Road, Walton-on-Thames KT12 5QG — MB ChB Pretoria 1988.

WIKNER, Gavin Walford (retired) Linfords, Staithe Road, Repps with Bastwick, Great Yarmouth NR29 5JU Tel: 01692 670444 — MB BS Durh. 1943. Prev: Ho. Surg. Roy. Vict. Infirm. Newc.

WIKNER, Robert Anthony Potterells Medical Centre, Station Road, North Mymms, Hatfield AL9 7SN Tel: 01707 273338 Fax: 01707 263564; Agape, 11 Morven Close, Potters Bar EN6 5HE Tel: 01707 657767 — MRCS Eng. LRCP Lond. 1975 (Royal Free Hospital) BSc (Physiol.) Lond. 1970; MB BS Lond. 1975; DRCOG 1978; MRCGP 1979. Specialty: Gen. Pract.

WILBERFORCE, Barbara Doreen (retired) 11 Hawkins Close, Perry, Huntingdon PE28 0DQ Tel: 01480 811112 — MB ChB Birm. 1943; MRCS Eng. LRCP Lond. 1943. Prev: Wing Cdr. RAF Med. Br.

WILBOURN, Gary 6 Cobnar Drive, Dunston Estate, Newbold, Chesterfield S41 8DD — BM Soton. 1995.

WILBRAHAM, Darren George 215B Tooting High Street, London SW17 0SZ — MB BS Lond. 1996.

WILBRAHAM, Kim 190 Maldon Road, Colchester CO3 3AZ — MB ChB Liverp. 1989.

WILBUSH, Joel c/o Barclays Bank, 207-215 Glossop Road, Sheffield S10 2GX — MB ChB Sheff. 1943; FRCOG 1984, M 1950; Dip. Ethnol. Oxf. 1972; DPhil Oxf. 1980. Adjunct Prof. Univ. Alberta, Edmonton AB, Canada. Socs: Fell. Roy. Soc. Med.; Founder Mem. Internat. Menopause Soc. Prev: Regist. (O & G) N. Middlx. Hosp.; Regist. (Gyn.) Co. Hosp. Lincoln; Capt. RAMC.

WILCOCK, Andrew Hayward House, Nottingham City Hospital, Hucknall Road, Nottingham NG5 1PB — MB ChB Birm. 1987; MRCP (UK) 1991; DM Nottm. 1998; FRCP London 2000. Reader (Oncol. & Palliat. Med.) Nottm. City Hosp. Specialty: Palliat. Med. Prev: Sen. Regist. (Palliat. Med.) Oxf. Radcliffe NHS Trust; Research Fell. (Respirat. & Palliat. Med.) Nottm. City Hosp.; Sen. Lect. (Oncol. & Palliat. Med.) Nottm. City Hosp.

WILCOCK, Anthony Charles, Wing Cdr. RAF Med. Br. Gp Capt., Deputy Director Health Services, HQ PTC, RAF Innswotrh, Gloucester GL3 1EZ Tel: 01452 712612 Ext: 5820 — MB ChB Bristol 1983; MSc 1997 Aberdeen; MRCGP 1988; DRCOG 1989; DAvMed FOM RCP Lond. 1991; DFFP 1993; AFOM RCP Lond. 1994; MFOM 1998; FFOM 2003. Gp Capt, Dep. Med. Director Health Servs., RAF Innsworth, Glos. Specialty: Occupat. Health. Socs: Soc. Occupat. Med.

WILCOCK, Christian Jeremy Friends Road Medical Practice, 49 Friends Road, Croydon CR0 1ED Tel: 020 8688 0532 Fax: 020 8688 2165 — MB BS Lond. 1983; BSc Lond. 1980. GP Croydon.

WILCOCK, David John X-Ray Department, Royal Infirmary, University Hospital of North Staffordshire, Princes Road, Hartshill, Stoke-on-Trent ST4 7LN Tel: 01782 555246 Fax: 01782 747552 Email: david.wilcock@uhns.nhs.uk; University Department of Radiology, Leicester Royal Infirmary, Leicester LE1 5WW Tel: 0116 258 6719 — MB BChir Camb. 1984; MA (Hons.) Camb. 1981; MRCP (UK) 1988; FRCR 1992. Cons. Neuroradiologist, Univ. Hosp. of N. Staffs. Specialty: Radiol. Prev: Lect. Univ. Nottm.

WILCOCK, David John Pendlebury Health Centre, The Lowry Medical Centre, 659 Bolton Road, Manchester M27 8HP Tel: 0161 793 8686 Fax: 0161 727 8011; Didsbury House, 13 Ellesmere Road, Ellesmere Park, Eccles, Manchester M30 9JY — MB ChB Dundee 1980; MRCGP 1987.

WILCOCK, Florence Mary 6 Southfields Road, London SW18 1QN — BM BCh Oxf. 1993; BA (Hons.) Physiol. Sci. Oxf. 1990; DFFP 1996; MRCOG 2000. Specialist Regist. Flexible Trainee SPR since 1997(O & G) KSS Region currently Kingston Hospital, previously SPR Royal Free Hospital, Newham, Basildon. Specialty: Obst. & Gyn. Prev: SHO (Obst.) Whittington Hosp. Lond.; SHO (Paediat. Surg.) Gt. Ormond St. Hosp. Lond.; SHO (Gyn. & Neonat.) St. Mary's Hosp. NHS Trust.

WILCOCK, Gordon Keith Department of Care of the Elderly, University of Bristol, Frenchay Hospital, Bristol BS16 1LE Tel: 0117 975 3948 Fax: 0117 957 3955 Email: gordon.wilcock@bris.ac.uk — BM BCh Oxf. 1970; MRCP Lond. 1973; DM Oxf. 1977; FRCP 1984. Prof. in Care of the Elderly, Univ. of Bristol; Hon. Cons. Phys. in Care of the Elderly and Gen. Internal Med., Frenchay Hosp., Bristol. Specialty: Care of the Elderly. Special Interest: Alzheimers Disease and related disorders. Prev: Cons. Phys. to Dept. of Geriat. and Gen. Med., Oxon. Area Health Auth. 1976-1984; Clin. Lect. in

Geriat. and Gen. Med., Univ. of Oxf. 1978-1984; Sen. Regist. in Gen. Med. Camb. 1976.

WILCOCK, Jane Pendlebury Health Centre, The Lowry Medical Centre, 659 Bolton Road, Manchester M27 8HP Tel: 0161 793 8686 Fax: 0161 727 8011; Didsbury House, 13 Ellesmere Road, Ellesmere Park, Eccles, Manchester M30 9JY — MB ChB Manch. 1983 (Manchester) BSc (Hons.) 1980; MRCGP 1987; DRCOG 1988; DFFP 1997. GP & GP Trainer.

WILCOCK, Jonathan Michael Warbrick-Smith and Partners, The Moat House Surgery, Beech Close, Warboys, Huntingdon PE28 2RQ Tel: 01487 822230 Fax: 01487 823721 — MB ChB Leic. 1992; MRCGP 1996. GP Princip.

WILCOCK, Michael Alan Threshold Day Hospital, 4 Dudhope Terrace, Dundee DD3 6HG Tel: 01382 322026 — MB ChB Dundee 1978. Staff (Psychiat.) Tayside Primary Healthcare NHS Trust Dundee. Specialty: Gen. Psychiat. Prev: Regist. (Psychiat.) Ravenscraig Hosp. Greenock.

WILCOCKSON, Alastair Quentin Medical Centre, Whale Island, Portsmouth PO2 8ER Tel: 023 9254 7137 Fax: 023 9254 7138 — MB ChB Sheff. 1986; Dip. Sports Med. Lond. 1996. GP Med. Centre Whale Is. Portsmouth. Specialty: Sports Med. Prev: SMO HQ Garrison, Brunei; Regtl. MO 1 A & SH; SHO BMH Rinteln.

WILCOX, Adrian Hervey St Hellier Hospital, Department of Chemical Pathology, Carshalton SM5 1AA Tel: 020 8296 2661 Fax: 020 8641 2633 — MB BChir Camb. 1973; MA Camb. 1978; MRCP(I) 1982; MSc Lond. 1985; MRCPath 1986; FRCPath 1996; LLM Wales 2004. Cons. Chem. Path. St. Helier Hosp. Carshalton; Hon. Sen. Lect. St. Geo. Hosp. Med. Sch. Lond. Specialty: Chem. Path. Special Interest: Lipidology; Inborn errors of Metab. Socs: Assoc of Clin. Biochem.ry; Soc. For Study of Inborn Error of Metab.; Diabetes UK. Prev: Sen. Regist. (Chem. Path.) St. Geo. Hosp. Lond.

WILCOX, Alison Department of Pathology, Royal Infirmary, 84 Castle St., Glasgow G4; 1 Colonsay Drive, Newton Mearns, Glasgow G77 6TY — MB ChB Glas. 1977. Clin. Asst. (Cytol.) Roy. Infirm. Glas.; Med. Off. W. Scotl. Blood Transfus. Serv. Specialty: Blood Transfus.

WILCOX, Anne-Marie Carmel 105 First Avenue, Gillingham ME7 2LF — MB ChB Leic. 1998.

WILCOX, Bryan (retired) Pine End, Upper Cwmbran Road, Cwmbran NP44 5SN Tel: 01633 483606 — MB BCh Wales 1956 (Cardiff) Prev: GP Cwmbran.

WILCOX, Christine 11 Northfield Road, Kings Norton, Birmingham B30 1JD Tel: 0121 458 1597 — MB ChB Birm. 1974; Dip. Community Paediat. Warwick 1987. Clin. Med. Off. (Community Health Servs.) Birm. S. Health Dist.

WILCOX, Douglas Ewing Duncan Guthrie Institute of Medical Genetics, Royal Hospital for Sick Children, Yorkhill, Glasgow G3 8SJ Tel: 0141 201 0365 Fax: 0141 357 4277 Email: d.e.wilcox@clinmed.gla.ac.uk; 1 Colonsay Drive, Newton Mearns, Glasgow G77 6TY — MB ChB Glas. 1979 (Univ. Glas.) BSc (Hons.) Glas. 1976; MRCP (UK) 1982; FRCP Glas. 1996. Sen. Lect. & Hon. Cons. Roy. Hosp. Sick Childr. Glas. Specialty: Genetics. Prev: Lect. (Med. Genetics) & Clin. Research Asst. Duncan Guthrie Inst. Med. Genetics Univ. Glas.; SHO (Med.) West. Infirm. Glas.

WILCOX, Duncan Thomas Flat 21, Defoe House, Barbican, London EC2Y 8DN — MB BS Lond. 1987.

WILCOX, Fiona Jane Globetown Surgery, 82-86 Roman Road, London E2 0PG Tel: 020 8980 3023 Fax: 020 8983 4627; 80 Bonner Road, Bethanl Green, London E2 9JU Tel: 020 8981 6074 — MB BS Lond. 1986 (St. Barths. Hosp. Med. Sch.) BSc Lond. 1983, MB BS 1986; DCH RCP Lond. 1989; DRCOG 1990; MRCGP 1990.

WILCOX, Frank Leonard Blackpool Victoria Hospital NHS Trust, Whinney Heys Road, Blackpool FY3 8NR Tel: 01253 300000 Fax: 01253 303651 — (Manch. & St. And.) BSc St. And. 1974; MB ChB Manch. 1977; DRCOG 1979; FRCOG 1995, M 1982; MD Manch. 1983. Cons. O & G Blackpool Vict. NHS Trust. Specialty: Obst. & Gyn. Prev: Lect. St. Mary's Hosp. Manch.

WILCOX, Gregory Eugene Harold Road Surgery, 164 Harold Road, Hastings TN35 5NH Tel: 01424 720878/437962 Fax: 01424 719525; 24 Branksome Road, St Leonards-on-Sea TN38 0UA — MB BS Lond. 1981; DRCOG 1985; MRCGP 1986. Exec. Chairm., Hastings And St Leonards PCT Hastings.

WILCOX, Kay Elizabeth The Medical Centre, 32 London Road, Sittingbourne ME10 1ND Tel: 01795 472109/472100 — MB BS Lond. 1984; MRCGP 1992. Specialty: Gen. Med. Prev: SHO (O & G) All St.s Hosp. Chatham; SHO (Geriat. Med.) Kent & Canterbury Hosp.; SHO (Surg.) Qu. Eliz. Milit. Hosp. Lond.

WILCOX, Mark Anthony Pembury Hospital, Pembury, Tunbridge Wells TN2 4QS Tel: 01892 823535 Ext: 3181; Comptons, Down Lane, Frant, Tunbridge Wells TN3 9HP — MB ChB Bristol 1983; MRCOG 1989; DM Nottm. 1993; FRCOG 2002. Cons. O & G Pembury Hosp. Tunbridge Wells. Specialty: Obst. & Gyn. Socs: Hong Kong Coll. Obst. & Gyn. Prev: Sen. Regist. (O & G) Qu. Med. Centre Nottm.; Vis. Lect. Chinese Univ., Hong Kong; Research Fell. (O & G) City Hosp. Nottm.

WILCOX, Mark Harvey Department of Microbiology, University of Leeds & Leeds General Infirmary, Leeds LS2 9JT Tel: 0113 233 5595 Fax: 0113 233 5649 Email: markwi@pathology.leeds.ac.uk — BM BS Nottm. 1986; DM Nottm. 1990, BMedSci (Hons.) 1984; BM BS (Hons.) Nottm. 1986; MRCPath (Microbiol.) 1992. Sen. Lect. (Med. Microbiol.) Univ. Leeds & Hon. Cons. Leeds Gen. Infirm. Specialty: Med. Microbiol. Socs: Brit. Soc. Antimicrob. Chemother.; Sec. Hosp. Infec. Soc. Prev: Cons. Microbiol. Addenbrooke's Hosp. Camb. (PHLS); Clin. Lect. (Med. Microbiol.) Univ. Sheff. Med. Sch.; Clin. Research Fell. (Microbiol.) Univ. & City Hosps. Nottm.

WILCOX, Richard Gordon 89 Reservoir Road, Selly Oak, Birmingham B29 6SU — MB ChB Birm. 1997.

WILCOX, Richard Merlyn Laurence Wychall Lane Surgery, 11 Wychall Lane, Kings Norton, Birmingham B38 8TE Tel: 0121 628 2345 Fax: 0121 628 8282; 11 Northfield Road, Kings Norton, Birmingham B30 1JD Tel: 0121 458 1597 — MB ChB Birm. 1973; MRCGP 1985.

WILCOX, Professor Robert George Department of Cardiovascular Medicine, University Hospital, Nottingham NG7 2UH Tel: 0115 970 9343 Fax: 0115 970 9384; 33 Trent View Gardens, Radcliffe on Trent, Nottingham NG12 1AY Tel: 0115 933 3165 — (London Hospital Medical College) BSc (Hons.) Lond. 1967; MB BS Lond. 1970; MRCP (UK) 1973; DM Nottm. 1985; FRCP Lond. 1987. Prof. Cardiovasc. Med. & Hon. Cons. (Med.) Dept. Med. Univ. Hosp. Nottm. Specialty: Cardiol.; Gen. Med. Socs: Brit. Cardiac Soc.; Brit. Hypertens. Soc.; Assn. Phys. Prev: Reader & Sen. Lect. (Med.) Univ. Hosp. Nottm.; Lect. (Med.) Univ. Hosp. Nottm.; SHO (Med.) & Ho. Phys. & Ho. Surg. Lond. Hosp.

WILCOX, Tumini 162A High Road, London N2 9AS — LRCPI & LM, LRSCI & LM 1964; LRCPI & LM, LRCSI & LM 1964.

WILCZYNSKI, Peter Joseph George Lakeside Surgery, Cottingham Road, Corby NN17 2UR Tel: 01536 204154 Fax: 01536 748286; Wisteria Cottage, 36 High St, Stanion, Kettering NN14 1DF Tel: 01536 204004 Fax: 01536 204004 — MB BS Lond. 1980 (St. Bart.) MRCS Eng. LRCP Lond. 1980; DRCOG 1982. Chairm. CoOperat.; Police Surg. Northampton Police.

WILD, Adrian Graham Three Villages Medical Practice, Audnam Lodge, Wordsley, Stourbridge DY8 4AL Tel: 01384 395054 Fax: 01384 390969; 80 Bridgnorth Road, Wollaston, Stourbridge DY8 3PA Tel: 01384 395352 — BM Soton. 1982.

WILD, Alan Frederick Houldsworth Medical Centre, 1 Rowsley Grove, Stockport SK5 7AY Tel: 0161 442 3322 Fax: 0161 442 2594; 23 Douglas Road, Hazel Grove, Stockport SK7 4JG Tel: 0161 456 9080 — MB ChB Manch. 1974; DRCOG 1978. Socs: Assoc. Mem. Manch. Med. Soc. Prev: SHO (Med.) Bury Gen. Hosp; SHO (O & G) Oldham Gen. Hosp.; SHO (Anaesth.) Vict. Hosp. Blackpool.

WILD, Alfred Augustine — Cert Av Med MoD (Air) & CAA; MB ChB Ed. 1948; DMRD Ed. 1954; FFR 1961; FRCR 1975; Aviat. Auth. 1979. Specialty: Radiol. Socs: Brit. Inst. Radiol.; Roy. Coll. Radiol. Prev: Cons. Radiol. ScarBoro. Health Dist.; Sen. Regist. Edin. North. Hosps. Gp.; Capt. RAMC.

WILD, Anne-Marie Castlefields Health Centre, Chester Close, Castlefields, Runcorn WA7 2HY Tel: 01928 566671 Fax: 01928 581631; 20 Hilltop Road, Stockton Heath, Warrington WA4 2ED Tel: 01925 267500 — MB BCh Wales 1977; MRCGP 1987; DRCOG 1990. Specialty: Pharmacology.

WILD, David (retired) 16 Brandy Hole Lane, Chichester PO19 4RY Tel: 01243 527125 Email: david.wild2@btinternet.com — MB ChB Manch. 1953; DObst RCOG 1957; DPH Liverp. 1958; FFCM 1977, M 1974. Prev: Dir. Pub. Health Med. SW Thames RHA.

WILD, David Andrew Hebden Bridge Health Centre, Hangingroyd Lane, Hebden Bridge HX7 6AG Tel: 01422 842333 Fax: 01422 842404; Chapel House Farm, Grey Stone Lane, Todmorden OL14 8RN — MB ChB Leeds 1977; DRCOG 1979; MRCGP Lond. 1981.

WILD, Kathryn Airlie Dr Forbes and Partners, East Calder Medical Practice, 147 Main Street, Livingston EH53 0EW Tel: 01506 882882 Fax: 01506 883630; 14 Craigmount Terrace, Corstorphine, Edinburgh EH12 8BW Tel: 0131 339 2517 Email: wild7cc@aol.com — MB ChB Dundee 1987; MRCGP 1993; DCCH RCP Ed. 1993. GP. Specialty: Gen. Pract.

WILD, Nicholas James 179 Warton Terrace, Newcastle upon Tyne NE6 5DX — MB BS Newc. 1992.

WILD, Nicholas John Rolyan House, 20 Hill Top Road, Stockton Heath, Warrington WA4 2ED — MB BCh Wales 1977; DCH Eng. 1978; MRCP (UK) 1982. Cons. Paediat. Warrington Dist. Gen. Hosp.; Clin. Tutor Univ. Liverp. Specialty: Paediat.

WILD, Nicola Jane 45 Hartledon Road, Birmingham B17 0AA — MB ChB Birm. 1997.

WILD, Richard Norman Chiltern International Ltd, 171 Bath Road, Slough SL1 4AA Tel: 01753 216617 Fax: 01753 511116 Email: richard.wild@chiltern.com; 58 Bath Road, Chiswick, London W4 1LH — MB ChB Leeds 1969; DCH Eng. 1972; MRCP UK 1973; Dip Pharm Med Lond., Ed. & Glas. 1979; FFPM 1992, M 1989; FRCP Ed. 1995; FRCP Lond. 2004. Med. Director, Chiltern Internat., Slough. Specialty: Pharmaceutical Medicine. Socs: Fell. Roy. Soc. Med.; BrAPP; BMA. Prev: Med. Dir. Pharmacia Ltd.; Lect. (Child Health) Univ. of Soton.; Regist. (Paediat.) Roy. Liverp. Childr. Hosp.

WILD, Roger Essery (retired) The Lodge, 16 Gwydrin Road, Calderstones, Liverpool L18 3HA Tel: 0151 722 9264 — MB ChB Liverp. 1955; DObst RCOG 1960; DCH Eng. 1960; DMRD 1966; FFR 1970. Cons. Radiol. Warrington & Winwick NHS Trust.

WILD, Sarah Helen Health Care Research Unit, Leve B, South Academic Block, Southampton General Hospital, Southampton SO16 67D Tel: 02380 794774 — MB BChir Camb. 1987; MSc Lond. 1995, BSc 1984; MRCP (UK) 1989; DRCOG 1991; MRCGP 1992; MFPHM 2000; PLD 2000. Specialist Regist. (Pub. Health Med.) Univ. Of Southampton. Specialty: Pub. Health Med.; Epidemiol. Prev: Wellcome Clin. Research Fell. Lond. Sch. Hyg. & Trop. Med.; Posdoctoral Fell. Stanford Univ., Calif.; Trainee GP Camb.

WILD, Simon Mark 8 Percheron Way, Droitwich WR9 7RF — MB BCh Wales 1998.

WILD, Stephen Mark 28 Leadhall Lane, Harrogate HG2 9NE — MB ChB Leeds 1997; MSc Liverp. 1984, BSc (Hons.) 1992.

WILD, Stephen Roger 32 Alnwickhill Road, Liberton, Edinburgh EH16 6LN — MB ChB Ed. 1967; FRCR 1975; FRCP Ed. 1988.

WILD, Steven Peter Lower Gornal Health Centre, Bull Street, Gornal Wood, Dudley DY3 2NQ Tel: 01384 459621 Fax: 01384 359495 — MB ChB Manch. 1986; DCH RCP Lond. 1991. Specialty: Community Child Health. Socs: Assn. Res. Infant & Child Developm. Prev: Regist. (Paediat.) Alexandra Hosp. Redditch; SHO (O & G) Birm. Woms. Hosp.; SHO (Paediat.) Birm. Childr. Hosp.

WILDBORE, Patricia Moira Hazelwood Group Practice, 27 Parkfield Road, Coleshill, Birmingham B46 3LD Tel: 01675 463165 Fax: 01675 466253 — MB ChB Birm. 1988; DCH RCP Lond. 1992. GP. Specialty: Gen. Pract.

WILDBORE, Roger David Burnham Medical Centre, Love Lane, Burnham-on-Sea TA8 1EU Tel: 01278 795445 Fax: 01278 793024; 2 Brightstowe Road, Burnham-on-Sea TA8 2HW Tel: 01278 792110 — MB BChir Camb. 1963 (Camb. & Birm.) MA, MB Camb. 1963, BChir 1962; DObst RCOG 1964; DA Eng. 1965.

WILDE, Mr Adam David Royal Cornwall Hospital, Truro TR1 3JW Tel: 020 8225 0000; Mount Rose, Wheal Anna, Goonhavern, Truro TR4 9NW Tel: 01872 540567 — MB ChB Leeds 1987; FRCS (Eng) 1992; FRCS (Orl) 1997. Cons. ENT Surg. Specialty: Otorhinolaryngol.

WILDE, Arthur Harold (retired) 24 Woodside Drive, Shrewsbury SY3 9BW — MB ChB Liverp. 1952; DPH 1955; FFCM RCP (UK) 1984, MFCM 1972. Prev: Specialist Community Med. (Environm. Health) Shrops. HA.

WILDE, Mr Godfrey Philip John Radcliffe Hospital, Headington, Oxford OX3 9DU Tel: 01865 221177 Fax: 01865 221231 Email: phil.wilde@orh.nhs.uk — MB ChB Leeds 1980; FRCS Eng. 1985. Cons. Trauma & Orthop. Surg. John Radcliffe Hosp. Oxf.. Specialty: Trauma & Orthop. Surg. Socs: Fell. Roy. Soc. Med. & BOA; Brit. Trauma Soc. Prev: Cons. Orthop. Surg. Lister Hosp. Stevenage; Fell. (Arthroscopic Surg.) Toronto, Canada; Sen. Regist. (Orthop.) Nottm. Hosps.

WILDE, James Maxwell 4 Pierrepont Place, Bath BA1 1JX — MB BS Lond. 1993.

WILDE, Jane Crooks 53 Ballycoan Road, Purdysburn, Belfast BT8 8LL — MB BCh BAO Belf. 1973; MSc (Soc. Med.) Lond. 1977; MFCM 1980.

WILDE, Mr Jeremy Andrew 11 Glenmore Road, Salisbury SP1 3HF Tel: 01722 333191 — MB BChir Camb. 1974; MA, MB BChir Camb. 1974; FRCS Eng. 1978; MRCOG 1983; FRCOG 1996. Cons. (O & G) Salisbury Dist. Hosp. Specialty: Obst. & Gyn. Prev: Sen. Regist. Rotat. (O & G) Qu. Charlotte's Hosp. Lond.; Rotat. Regist. (O & G) St. Thos. Hosp. Lond. & Pembury Hosp.; Resid. Surgic. Off. (Gyn.) Chelsea Hosp. for Wom. Lond.

WILDE, Jonathan Thornton Department of Haematology, Queen Elizabeth Hospital, Queen Elizabeth Medical Centre, Edgbaston, Birmingham B15 2TH Tel: 0121 472 1311 — MB BChir Camb. 1980 (Guy's) MA, MB Camb. 1980, BChir 1979; MRCP (UK) 1984; MD Camb. 1989; MRCPath 1991; FRCP 1997; FRCPath 1999. Cons. Haemat. Qu. Eliz. Hosp. Birm. Specialty: Haematology.

WILDE, Julia Margaret (retired) Homewood, 1 Barlow Fold Road, Romiley, Stockport SK6 4LH — DCCH; MB ChB Manch. 1969. Prev: SCMO Community Child Health.

WILDE, Margaret Helen (retired) 13 Wyndham Crescent, Bridgend CF31 3DW Tel: 01656 653292 — MB ChB Aberd. 1948. Prev: Ho. Surg. (Gyn.) Aberd. Roy. Infirm.

WILDE, Neil Theodore 31 Grange Road, Bramhall, Stockport SK7 3BD — MB ChB Manch. 1995; BSc Lond. 1992.

WILDE, Robert Peter Havelock Department of Clinical Radiology, Bristol Royal Infirmary, Marlborough St., Bristol BS2 8HW Tel: 0117 928 2672 Fax: 0117 928 3267 — BM BCh Oxf. 1974; BSc (1st cl. Hons. Anat.) Liverp. 1970; MRCP (UK) 1977; FRCR 1980. Cons. Radiol. United Bristol Healthcare Trust. Specialty: Radiol. Socs: Brit. Cardiac Soc.; Brit. Soc. Echocardiogr.; Brit. Cardiovasc. Interven. Soc. Prev: Clin. Dir. Cardiac Servs. United Bristol Healthcare Trust; Fell. (Cardiovasc. Radiol.) Green La. Hosp., Auckland, NZ; Sen. Regist. (Radiol.) Bristol Roy. Infirm.

WILDE, Simon Marcus 2A Storer Road, Loughborough LE11 5EQ — BM BS Nottm. 1988; BMedSci Nottm. 1986; DCH RCP Lond. 1991; DRCOG 1992; MRCGP 1993. Prev: Clin. Asst. (Oncol.) Leics.; Trainee GP Lancaster VTS.

WILDE, Stephen Marek Julius Jozefowicz Marsh, Kennedy, Chapman, Wilde and Pathy, Netherfield Medical Practice, 2A Forester Street, Nottingham NG4 2NJ Tel: 0115 940 3775 Fax: 0115 961 4069 — MB BS Newc. 1985; MRCGP 1989.

WILDE, Susan 65 Rossall Grange Lane, Fleetwood FY7 8AA Email: wilde_sue@hotmail.com — MB ChB Manch. 1998.

WILDEN, Julie 47 Glenavon Road, Ipswich IP4 5QD — BM BS Nottm. 1995.

WILDEN, Simon Derek Taylor and Partners, The Surgery, Hexton Road, Barton-le-Clay, Bedford MK45 4TA Tel: 01582 528701 Fax: 01582 528714 — MB BS Lond. 1990 (Pembroke College Oxford and St Mary's Hospital London) MA Oxon. 1991; DRCOG 1992; Cert. Family Plann. JCC 1992; MRCGP 1994. Specialty: Gen. Pract. Socs: BMA; MRCGP. Prev: Trainee GP Bedford VTS.

WILDER-SMITH, Oliver Hamilton Gottwaldt 6C Sunnyside, Liverpool L8 3JD — MB ChB Liverp. 1980.

WILDERSPIN, Michael Piers Medical Department, Firth Rixson Forgings Ltd., Dale Road North, Darley Dale, Matlock DE4 2JB Tel: 01629 733621 Fax: 01629 734273; The Dell, 23 Clifton Road, Matlock Bath, Matlock DE4 3PW Tel: 01629 583190 Fax: 01629 583190 — MB BS Lond. 1959 (Guy's) MRCS Eng. LRCP Lond. 1958; FRCGP 1981, M 1968; Cert Family Plann 1976; AFOM RCP Lond. 1983; DFFP 1994. Company Med. Adviser Firth Rixson plc & P.P. Payne Ltd. Socs: Soc. Occupat. Med.; BMA; FRSM. Prev: Employ. Med. Advis. EMAS; Ho. Surg. (Orthop.) Guy's & New Cross Hosps.; Ho. Phys. (Experim. Med.) & Resid. Clin. Path. Guy's Hosp.

WILDGOOSE, Alastair David Dryland Surgery, 1 Field Street, Kettering NN16 8JZ Tel: 01536 518951 Fax: 01536 486200 — MB BS Newc. 1974; MRCGP 1978; AFOM RCP Lond. 1993. Specialty: Gen. Pract.

WILDGOOSE, Charlotte Dorothy Sighthill Health Centre, 380 Calder Road, Edinburgh EH11 4AU Tel: 0131 453 5335 — MB ChB Glas. 1977; DRCOG 1979.

WILDGOOSE, Nicholas William Endsleigh House, Clampitt Road, Ippleden, Newton Abbot TQ12 5RJ — MB ChB Sheff. 1980; MRCP (UK) 1984.

WILDIG, Catherine Elisabeth Child Development Centre, St Luke's Hospital, Little Horton Lane, Bradford BD5 0NA Fax: 01274 365010 Email: catherine.wildig@bradfordhospitals.nhs.uk — MB ChB Birm. 1989; Mmedsc 1999 Leeds; MRCP (UK) 1992; MRCPCH 1996; FRCPCH 2001. p/t Cons. Paediat. (NeuroDisabil.) Child Developm. Centre, St. Luke's Hosp. Bradford. Specialty: Community Child Health. Prev: Sen. Regist. Community Paediat. St. James' Univ. Hosp. Leeds; Sen. Regist. (Community Paediat.) Pinderfields Hosp. Wakefield; Regist. (Paediat. Vict. Hosp. Blackpool & Roy. Manch. Childr.'s Hosp.

WILDIN, Miss Clare Joanne 2 Cedar Cottages, Rolleston Road, Skeffington, Leicester LE7 9YD Tel: 0116 259 6430 — MB ChB Leic. 1991; FRCS Ed. 1995. Specialist Regist. (Orthop. Surg.) Leicester. Specialty: Orthop. Prev: SHO Rotat. (Surg.) Leicester; Demonst. (Anat.) Univ. Birm.

WILDIN, Helen Marie Runwell Hospital, The Chase, Wickford SS11 7QE — MB ChB Sheff. 1989. SHO (Psychiat.) Southend Community Care Trust. Specialty: Geriat. Psychiat.

WILDING, Alison Mary Clydebank Health Centre, Kilbowie Road, Clydebank G81 2TQ Tel: 0141 531 6475 Fax: 0141 531 6478 — MB ChB Glas. 1987; MRCGP 1991. Prev: Trainee GP Glas. VTS.

WILDING, Graeme 5 Gordon Rd, Surbiton KT5 9AR — MB BS Lond. 1997; MRCS.

WILDING, Huw Ioan Coach and Horses Surgery, The Car Park, St. Clears, Carmarthen SA33 4AA Tel: 01994 230379 Fax: 01994 231449; Green Acres, Laugharne, Carmarthen SA33 4QU Tel: 01994 427520 — MB BS Lond. 1974 (Westm.) MRCS Eng. LRCP Lond. 1974. Prev: Ho. Phys. Qu. Mary's Hosp. Roehampton; Ho. Surg. Westm. Hosp. Lond.

WILDING, John Paul Howard Clinical Sciences Centre, University Hospital Aintree, Longmoor Lane, Liverpool L9 7AL Tel: 0151 529 5885 Fax: 0151 529 5888 Email: j.p.h.wilding@liv.ac.uk — BM Soton. 1985; MRCP (UK) 1988; DM Soton. 1994. Reader (Diabetes, Endocrinol. & Gen. Med.) & Hon. Cons. Phys. Univ. Hosp. Aintree. Liverp. Specialty: Diabetes; Endocrinol. Socs: Brit. Diabetic Assn.; Assn. for Study Obesity; Eur. Assn. Study Diabetes. Prev: Sen. Regist. & MRC Train. Fell. (Med.) Hammersmith Hosp. Lond.; Regist. (Med.) Ealing & Hammersmith Hosp. Lond.

WILDING, Lucinda Jane 49 Woodlands Road, Surbiton KT6 6PR — MB BS Lond. 1996.

WILDING, Mr Robert Peter (retired) Maple Tree House, 68A Sedbergh Road, Kendal LA9 6BE — MB BChir Camb. 1959 (Lond. Hosp.) MA Camb. 1959; FRCS Eng. 1967. Prev: Cons. Gen. Surg. Orpington Hosp.

WILDMAN, Gillian Mary Florey Unit, Royal Berks Hospital, London Road, Reading RG1 5AN Tel: 0118 987 7213; 2 Bluecoat Walk, Harmans Water, Bracknell RG12 9NP — MB BCh Wales 1979. Staff Grade Genito Urin. Med. Roy. Berks. Hosp. Reading. Specialty: Genitourinary Medicine.

WILDMAN, Martin James 20 Watermill Close, Selly Oak, Birmingham B29 6TS — MB ChB Birm. 1989; BSc (Hons.) Physiol. Birm. 1986, MB ChB 1989; MRCP (UK) 1993; DTM & H Liverp. 1993; Dip. Evidence Based Medicare, Oxf. 2000; MPH Univ. Of Lond. 2001. Specialty: Respirat. Med.

WILDMAN, Martyn Andrew 10 New Road, Shenley, Radlett WD7 9EA — MB BS Lond. 1997 (UCL) BSc Pharm 1994; Dip IMC RCS Ed. 1999; FRCA (Primary) 2002. SpR (Anaesth. / Intens. Care) N. Thames Centr. Rotat. Specialty: Accid. & Emerg. Socs: BASICS. Prev: A & E SHO Barnet Gen. Hosp.

WILDMAN, Simone Marianne Chantel BUPA Wellness, 2-6 Austin Friars, London EC2N 2HD Tel: 020 7628 4001 — MB BS Queensland 1991. Lead Phys.

WILDMORE, Joan Christine High Stonecroft House, Newbrough, Hexham NE47 5AY — MB BS Newc. 1972. Clin. Med. Off. N.d. AHA.

WILDSMITH, Professor John Anthony Winston University Department of Anaesthesia, Ninewells Hospital & Medical School, Dundee DD1 9SY Tel: 01382 632427 Fax: 01382 644914 Email: j.a.w.wildsmith@dundee.ac.uk — (Ed.) FRCP Ed. 1996 (by election); MB ChB Ed. 1969; FFA RCS Eng. 1973; MD Ed. 1982. Prof. Anaesth. Univ. Dundee; Hon. Cons. Anaesth.Tayside univ hosp NHS trust. Dundee. Specialty: Anaesth. Special Interest: Allergy to anaesthetic/analgesic drugs; Dent. Anaesth. and sedation; Regional anaesthetic techniques. Socs: Edit. Bd. Brit. Jl. Anaesth.; Elec. Mem. Counc. Roy. Coll. Anaesths.; Chairm. Assn. of Professors of Anaesth. Prev: Vis. Lect. Brigham & Wom. Hosp. Harvard Med. Sch. Boston, USA; Lect. (Dent. Anaesth.) Univ. Edin.; Cons. Anaesth. & Clin. Dir. Roy. Infirm. Edin.

WILDSMITH, Patricia Helen Mather Avenue Practice, 584 Mather Avenue, Liverpool L19 4UG Tel: 0151 427 6239 Fax: 0151 427 8876 — MB ChB Liverp. 1990.

WILDY, Guy Stephen Ivy House Surgery, 27 The Parade, St Helier, Jersey JE2 3QQ Tel: 01534 728777 Fax: 01534 728977 — MB ChB Bristol 1979; MRCP (UK) 1983; DRCOG 1984; MRCGP 1985.

WILE, David Bowyer 97 Burtons Road, Hampton Hill, Hampton TW12 1DL — MB BCh Wales 1978; MSc Clin. Biochem. Lond. 1993. Staff Grade Chem. Path. Aintree Hosps. NHS Trust. Specialty: Chem. Path.; Diabetes. Socs: Brit. Soc. Human Genetics; Heart UK; Assn. Clin. Biochem. Prev: Regist. (Chem. Path.) Roy. Postgrad. Med. Sch. Lond.; Clin. Research Fell. Roy. Postgrad. Med. Sch. Hammersmith Hosp. Lond.

WILES, Benjamin George Robert Bridlington and District Hospital, Bridlington YO16 4BP — MB ChB Sheff. 2001. Sen. Ho. Off. Bridlington & Dist. Hosp.

WILES, Professor Charles Mark Department of Medicine (Neurol.), University of Wales Coll. of Med., Heath Park, Cardiff CF14 4XN Tel: 029 2074 3798 Fax: 029 2074 4091 — MB BS Lond. 1972 (St. Thos.) BSc Lond. 1969, PhD 1980, MB BS 1972; MRCP (UK) 1975; FRCP Lond. 1987. Prof. Neurol.& Head of Dept., Hon. Cons. Univ. Wales Coll. Med. Cardiff. Specialty: Neurol. Prev: Cons. Phys. Neurol. Nat. Hosp. For Nerv. Dis. Lond., Maida Vale & St. Thos. Hosps. Lond.; Sen. Regist. (Neurol.) Nat. Hosp. for Nerv. Dis. Qu. Sq. Lond. & St. Mary's Hosp. Lond.; Regist. (Neurol.) Nat. Hosp. Nerv. Dis. Qu. Sq. Lond.

WILES, Ian Derek Pulteney Practice, 35 Great Pulteney Street, Bath BA2 4BY Tel: 01225 464187 Fax: 01225 485305 — BM BCh Oxf. 1984; MA Camb. 1985 BM BCh 1984; DRCOG 1986; DCH RCP Lond. 1987; MRCP (UK) 1987; MRCGP 1988.

WILES, John Bromley Hospitals NHS Trust, Princess Royal University Hospital, Farnborough Common, Orpington BR6 8ND Tel: 01689 865667 Fax: 01689 864070; [New Address]; Harris HospisCare, Caritas House, Tregony Road, Orpington BR6 9XA/ 01689 825755/01689 892999; 418 Footscray Road, New Eltham, London SE9 3TU Tel: 0208 859 6512 — MB ChB Leeds 1972; DObst RCOG 1974; MRCP 2000. Cons. Palliat. Med. Bromley Hosp. NHS Trust; Med. Director, Harris HospisCare, Orpington; Hon Cons Palliat. Med., St Christophers Hospice, Lond. Specialty: Palliat. Med. Socs: BMA; Fell. Roy. Soc. Med.; Assn. Palliat. Med. Prev: Hon. Cons. Palliat. Med. King's Healthcare NHS Trust Lond.; Med. Direct. St. Catherine's Hospice, Crawley; Med. Direct. St. Joseph's Hospice Lond.

WILES, John Richard — MB BS Lond. 1978 (St. Geo.) FRCA 1984. Cons. Walton Centre for Neurol. & Neurosurg. NHS Trust Liverp. Specialty: Anaesth. Prev: Cons. Anaesth. & Pain Relief Walton Hosp. Liverp.

WILES, Philip Graham North Manchester General Hospital, Crumpsall, Manchester M8 5RB Tel: 0161 795 4567 Fax: 0161 720 2029; Elm Bank, Garth Road, Marple, Stockport SK6 6PB — MD Manch. 1985; BSc (Hons.) St. And. 1973; MB ChB 1976; MRCP (UK) 1980; FRCP 1996. Cons. Phys. N. Manch. Gen. Hosp.; Vis. Prof., Univ. of Salford, Sch. of Health Care Professionals. Specialty: Endocrinol. Socs: Brit. Diabetic Assn. (Mem. Med. & Scientif. Sect.); Med. Research Soc. Prev: Lect. & Hon. Sen. Regist. (Med.) Gen. Infirm. Leeds; Research Fell. (Diabetes) King's Coll. Hosp. Lond.; SHO (Med.) Manch. Roy. Infirm., N. Manch. Gen. & Altrincham Gen. Hosps.

WILEY, Charlotte Ann The Beeches, Bargate Street, Brewood, Stafford ST19 9BB — MB BS Lond. 1982 (St. Marys) BSc (Hons.) Lond. 1979, MB BS 1982; Cert. Family Plann. JCC 1984. GP Wolverhampton. Prev: SHO (Psychiat., O & G & Dermat.) Wolverhampton HA.

WILEY, David James (retired) 74 Pembroke Road, Clifton, Bristol BS8 3EG Tel: 0117 973 7962; 1 Brecon Close, Henleaze, Bristol BS9 4DG Tel: 0117 9625 004 — MB BCh BAO Belf. 1959; LAH Dub. 1959. Prev: Ho. Phys. & Ho. Surg. Belf. City Hosp.

WILEY, Paul Francis Wiley, Sinclair and Kettell, The Surgery, Pound Piece, Maiden Newton, Dorchester DT2 0DB Tel: 01300 320206 Fax: 01300 320399 — MB BS Newc. 1974; MRCP (UK) 1977; MRCGP 1980. Prev: Regist. (Paediat.) Roy. United Hosp. Bath; SHO (Paediat.) Newc. Gen. Hosp.; Ho. Surg. (Profess. Surg. Unit) Roy. Vict. Infirm. Newc.

WILFIN, Andrew Henry 10 Whirlowdale Cl, Sheffield S11 9NQ; 154 Beaufort Park, Beaufort Drive, London NW11 6DA Tel: 020 8905 5658 Email: andrew@wilfin.free-online.co.uk — MB ChB Manch. 1997. Psych. SHO St mary's Rotat. Ealing Hosp. Specialty: Accid. & Emerg.

WILFORD, Jane Mary 241 Wilton Street, Glasgow G20 6DE Tel: 0141 946 4332 Fax: 0141 3305018 Email: jw49a@clinmed.gla.ac.uk — MRCS Eng. LRCP Lond. 1991 (University College, Middlesex School of Medicine, London University) DTM & H RCP Lond. 1993; MRCGP 1996; AFOM 1998. Specialist. Occupat. Med. Salus; Lect. Occupat. Health Dept. Pub. Health Univ. Glas. Specialty: Occupat. Health. Socs: Soc. Occupat. Med.

WILFORD, Nicholas John 46 Brancepeth View, Brandon, Durham DH7 8TT Tel: 0191 378 4152 — MB BS Newc. 1993 (Newcastle upon Tyne) BMedSc (Hons.) Newc. 1990; DGM 1996; MRCGP 1997. GP. Specialty: Gen. Pract.; Sports Med. Socs: Brit. Assn. Sport & Med.

WILFORD, Peter John The Mote Medical Practice, St Saviours Road, Maidstone ME15 9FL Tel: 01622 756888 Fax: 01622 672573 — MB BS Lond. 1981; DCH RCP Lond. 1983; DRCOG 1985; MRCGP 1986.

WILKEN, Mr Bertie James, MBE Fockerby Hall, Garthorpe, Scunthorpe DN17 4SA Tel: 01724 798323 — MD Ed. 1967; MB ChB 1958; FRCS Ed. 1961; FRCS Eng. 1962; FRCP Ed. 1974, M 1963. Hon. Cons. Surg., Acad. Surgic. Unit, Uni. Of Hull. Specialty: Gen. Surg.; Gastroenterol. Socs: Brit. Soc. Gastroenterol.; Assn. Coloproctol. Prev: Surg. Specialist Centr. Hosp. Honiara, Solomen Is.; Cons. & Sen. Lect. (Surg.) Wessex RHA; Ho. Surg., Ho. Phys. & Cas. Off. Roy. Infirm. Edin.

WILKEN, Eric Howard (retired) 21 Leadhall Road, Harrogate HG2 9PE Tel: 01423 871329 — MB BS Durh. 1945 (King's Coll. Newc.) Prev: Ho. Phys. Gen. Hosp. Newc.

WILKERSON, John Noel Victoria Medical Centre, 7 Victoria Crescent West, Barnsley S75 2AE Tel: 01226 282758 Fax: 01226 729800; 1 Whinmoor Drive, Silkstone, Barnsley S75 4NR Tel: 01226 791164 — MB Camb. 1974; BA Camb. 1970, MB 1974, BChir 1973; DObst. RCOG 1975; FFA RCS 1980; Brit. Med. Acupuncture Soc. Dip. 1998. GP Princip.; Clin. Asst. (Palliat. Care) St Peter's Hospice Barnsley. Specialty: Gen. Pract.; Palliat. Med. Socs: Accred. Mem. BMAS.

WILKES, Anna 7 Ashley Close, Hendon, London NW4 1PH — MB BS Durh. 1947 (Newc.-On-Tyne) DPH 1954. Clin. Med. Off. Brent HA. Prev: Asst. Co. Med. Off. Herts. CC; Asst. Med. Off. Middlx. CC, E. Ham, Durh. Co.

WILKES, Deborah Ann — MB ChB Leic. 1986; MRCGP 1991; DRCOG 1991.

WILKES, Dennis 93 Witherford Croft, Solihull B91 1UA — MB ChB Liverp. 1978; MRCGP 1983.

WILKES, Professor Eric, MBE, OBE (retired) Curbar View Farm, Calver, Hope Valley S32 3XR Tel: 01433 631291 — MB BChir Camb. 1952 (St. Thos.) MA Camb. 1952; FRCP Lond. 1974, M 1954; DObst RCOG 1955; FRCGP 1973; FRCPsych 1980, M 1975; Hon. MD Sheff. 1986. Prev: Cons. Emerit. Trent Region Palliat. & Continuing Care Centre.

WILKES, Graeme Prospect House Medical Group, Prospect House, Prospect Place, Newcastle upon Tyne NE4 6QD Tel: 0191 273 4201 Fax: 0191 273 0129 — MB BS Newc. 1984; MRCP (UK) 1990; MRCGP 1993. Regist. (Cardiol.) GreenLa. Hosp. Auckland, NZ. Specialty: Cardiol. Prev: Regist. (Med.) Auckland Hosp. NZ.

WILKES, Heather Frances Briton Ferry Health Centre, Hunter Street, Briton Ferry, Neath SA11 5SF Tel: 01639 812270 Fax: 01639 813019 — MB ChB Bristol 1989; MRCGP 1993. Specialty: Gen. Pract.

WILKES, Jeannette Marie Delamere Practice, 257 Dialstone Lane, Great Moor, Stockport SK2 7NA Tel: 0161 445 5907 Fax: 0161 448 0466 — MB ChB Manch. 1985; DCH RCPS Glas. 1987; DRCOG 1988; MRCGP 1989.

WILKES, Judith Alison The Stanegate, Great Whittington, Newcastle upon Tyne NE19 2HA — MB BS Newc. 1981; FFA RCS 1988. Cons. Anaesth. Newc. Gen. Hosp. Specialty: Anaesth.

WILKES, Mark Peter Department of Anaesthesia and Intensive Care, Queen Elizabeth Hospital, Edgbaston, Birmingham Tel: 0121 472 1311; 91 Greenfield Road, Harborne, Birmingham B17 0EH Tel: 0121 426 2386 Fax: 0121 605 2009 Email: mark.wilkes@btinternet.com — MB ChB Birm. 1984 (Birmingham) FRCA 1991. Cons. Anaesth. Qu. Eliz. Hosp. Birm. Specialty: Anaesth.

WILKES, Michael Charles Thomas Worcestershire HA, Isaac Maddox House, Shrub Hill Road, Worcester WR4 9RW Tel: 01905 760019 Fax: 01905 28672 — MB BS Lond. 1959 (Univ. Coll. Hosp.) MRCS Eng. LRCP Lond. 1958; DObst RCOG 1960; DPH Lond. 1967; FFCM 1986, M 1973. Cons. Pub. Health Med. Worcs. HA. Specialty: Pub. Health Med. Prev: DPH Kidderminster HA; Dep. MOH Bath Co. Boro.; Surg. Lt. RN.

WILKES, Muriel Mary (retired) 21 College Hill, Sutton Coldfield B73 6HA Tel: 0121 355 2191 — MB BS Lond. 1944 (Lond. Sch. Med. Wom.) MRCS Eng. LRCP Lond. 1944; DA Eng. 1947. Prev: Resid. Anaesth. Birm. United Hosps. & Roy. W. Sussex Hosp. Chichester.

WILKES, Nicholas c/o Doctors Residence, Royal National Orthopaedic Hospital, Brockley Hill, Stanmore HA7 4LP — State Exam Med Hamburg 1986.

WILKES, Nicholas Andrew John (retired) The Stanegate, Great Whittington, Newcastle upon Tyne NE19 2HA — MB BS Lond. 1983 (Univ. Coll. Hosp.) MRCOG 1989; MFFP 1993; MA (Legal Studies) Newc. 1995. Solicitor Newc. u. Tyne. Prev: Regist. (O & G) Princess Mary Matern. Hosp. & Roy. Vict. Infirm. Newc.

WILKES, Nicholas Paul Fisher 14 Stack House, West Hill, Oxted RH8 9JA — MB BS Lond. 1979. Specialty: Cardiol.

WILKES, Peter Richard Balmacaan Road Surgery, Balmacaan Road, Drumnadrochit, Inverness IV63 6UR Tel: 01456 450577 Fax: 01456 450799; Balnacraig, Drumnadrochit, Inverness IV63 6UX — MB ChB Glas. 1983; BSc AKC Lond. 1973; MPhil Reading 1976; PhD Glas. 1980; DRCOG 1985; DCH RCPS Glas. 1986; MRCGP 1987. GP Culloden, Inverness.

WILKES, Robert Geoffrey 27B Warren Drive, Wallasey CH45 0JW Tel: 0151 639 6559 Fax: 0151 702 4006 — MB ChB Birm. 1966; FFA RCS Eng. 1972. Clin. Dir. (Intens. Care) Roy. Liverp. Univ. Trust Hosp. Specialty: Anaesth.

WILKES, Scott Coquet Medical Group, Amble Health Centre, Percy Drive, Morpeth NE65 0HD Tel: 01665 710481 Fax: 01665 713031 — MB ChB Leeds 1990; DFFP 1993; DRCOG 1993; MRCGP 1994. Specialty: Gen. Med. Prev: Trainee GP Morpeth & Durh.; SHO (Psychiat.) Sunderland.

WILKEY, Anthony Donald 63 Stonerwood Avenue, Hall Green, Birmingham B28 0AX — MB ChB Birm. 1980; FFA RCS Eng. 1985. Cons. Anaesth. Birm. Matern. & Qu. Eliz. Hosps. Birm. Specialty: Anaesth. Prev: Sen. Regist. (Anaesth.) Midl. Anaesth. Train. Sch.; Vis. Asst. Prof. Univ. Texas Med. Br. Galveston.

WILKEY, Brian Reginald (retired) 42 Tunwells Lane, Great Shelford, Cambridge CB2 5LJ Tel: 01223 843061 — BM BCh Oxf. 1958 (Univ. Coll. Hosp.) DA Eng. 1962; FFA RCS Eng. 1964. Cons. Anaesth. Addenbrooke's Hosp. Camb.; Assoc. Lect. Univ. Camb. Prev: Sen. Regist. (Anaesth.) Univ. Coll. Hosp. Lond.

WILKIE, Alexandra Wightman Quartercormick, Downpatrick BT30 — MB BCh BAO Belf. 1955; MFCM 1977.

WILKIE, Professor Andrew Oliver Mungo Weatherall Institute of Molecular Medicine, The John Radcliffe, Oxford OX3 9DS Tel: 01865 222619 Fax: 01865 222500 — BM BCh Oxf. 1983; MA Camb. 1984, BA 1980; MRCP (UK) 1986; DCH RCP Lond. 1987; MA Oxf. 1992, DM 1992; FRCP Lond. 1998; F Med Sci 2002. Nuffield Prof. of Path., Univ. of Oxf.; Hon. Cons. Clin. Genetics. Churchill Hosp. Oxf. & Oxf. Craniofacial Unit Radcliffe Infirm. Specialty: Genetics. Special Interest: Genetics of skull & limb malformation; Mutations in sperm. Socs: Ordinary Member Association of Physicians. Prev: Wellcome Sen. Research Fell. (Clin. Sci.) Weatherall Inst. Molecular Med. Oxf; Sen. Regist. (Clin.

Genetics) Univ. Hosp. Wales; Dysmorphol. Fell. (Paediat. Genetics) Inst. Child Health Lond.

WILKIE, Clare Elizabeth Brixton Hill Group Practice, 22 Raleigh Gardens, London SW2 1AE Tel: 020 8674 6376 Fax: 020 8671 0283 — MB BS Lond. 1984; BA Camb. 1976; DRCOG 1987; MRCGP 1989. Prev: Trainee GP St. Thos. Lond. VTS.

WILKIE, David John Port Glasgow Health Centre, 2 Bay Street, Port Glasgow PA14 5ED Tel: 01475 745321 — MB ChB Glas. 1980; DRCOG 1983; MRCGP 1984.

WILKIE, Douglas John Kenneth Rose Cottage, Lower Sandy Down Lane, Boldre, Lymington SO41 8PP — MRCS Eng. LRCP Lond. 1945; DOMS Eng. 1950.

WILKIE, Gail 16 Gartcows Road, Falkirk FK1 5QT — MB ChB Glas. 1994.

WILKIE, Irene Abercromby (retired) — MB ChB Aberd. 1959. Prev: Med. Off. Bd. of World Mission Ch. of Scotl. Edin.

WILKIE, Jill Nicola 116 Bellingdon Road, Chesham HP5 2HF Tel: 01494 792962 Email: jillwilkie@hotmail.com — MB BS Lond. 1991; BSc (1st. cl. Hons.) Pharm. 1988; MRCP (UK) 1994; FRCR 2000. Regist. (Radiol.) Roy. Lond. Trust. Specialty: Radiol. Socs: BMA; Roy. Coll. Phys.; Roy. Coll. Radiol. Prev: SHO Rotat. (Med.) Roy. Lond. Trust.; Ho. Off. (Gen. Med.) Chase Farm Hosp.; Ho. Off. (Gen. Surg. & Urol.) Edgware Gen. Hosp.

WILKIE, John Richard Fowey House, 108 Berrybrook Meadow, Exminster, Exeter EX6 8UA — MB BS Lond. 1966 (Lond. Hosp.) DMRT Eng. 1971; MSc (Social Med.) Lond. 1973. Staff Psychiat. Regional Secure Unit Langdon Hosp. Dawlish. Specialty: Gen. Psychiat. Socs: BMA; Affil. Roy. Coll. Psychiat.; Worshipful Soc. Apoth. Prev: Staff Psychiat. Cornw. & I. of Scilly HA; Regist. (Psychiat.) Exeter HA; Community Phys. Som. & Waltham Forest HAs.

WILKIE, Lesley McIntosh Ross House, Hawkhead Road, Paisley PA2 7BN Tel: 0141 842 7213 Fax: 0141 848 0165 — MB ChB Glas. 1975; MSc Community Med. Manch. 1988; MFCM 1989; FFPHM RCP (UK) 1996, M 1989; FRCP Glas. 2002. Dir. Pub. Health Argyll & Clyde HB. Specialty: Pub. Health Med. Prev: Cons. Pub. Health Med. Argyll & Clyde HB; Sen. Regist. (Community Med.) NW RHA.

WILKIE, Martin Erskine The Sheffield Kidney Institute, Northern General Hospital NHS Trust, Herries Road, Sheffield S5 7AU Tel: 0114 243 4343 Fax: 0114 256 2514 Email: martin.wilkie@sth.nhs.uk — MB ChB Manch. 1984 (St. And. & Manch.) BSc St. And. 1981; MRCP (UK) 1987; MD Manch. 1994; FRCP(Lond) 1999. Cons. Renal Phys. Sheff. Kidney Inst. Specialty: Nephrol. Socs: Brit. Transpl. Soc.; Renal Assn.; Eur. Dialysis & Transpl.Assn. Prev: Sen. Regist. (Nephrol.) Sheff. Kidney Inst; Research Fell. (Nephrol.) Lond. Hosp.; Regist. (Nephrol.) Univ. Hosp. S. Manch.

WILKIE, Mary (retired) 2 Northgate, Lincoln LN2 1QS Tel: 01522 523231 — MB ChB Sheff. 1956; DCH Eng. 1958. Prev: Ho. Phys. Roy. Hosp. Sheff. & Sheff. Childr. Hosp.

WILKIE, Michael John Broombank, Farr, Inverness IV2 6XJ Tel: 01808 521274 — MB ChB Aberd. 1995. Specialty: Anaesth.

WILKIE, Stewart Christopher 1/76 Kennishead Avenue, Thornliebank, Glasgow G46 8RT — MB ChB Glas. 1995.

WILKIE, Stuart The Surgery, Hemming Way, Chaddesley Corbett, Kidderminster DY10 4SF Tel: 01562 777239 Fax: 01562 777196; Ashcroft, Quarry Bank, Hartlebury, Kidderminster DY11 7TE — MB ChB Birm. 1987; ChB Birm. 1987; DCH RCP Lond. 1990; DRCOG 1991; DGM RCP Lond. 1992.

WILKIE, Veronica Mary Corbett Medical Practice, 36 Corbett Avenue, Droitwich WR9 7BE — MB ChB Birm. 1987; DPD Cardiff; Cert. EPCH, Oxford; DGM RCP Lond. 1989; DCH 1990; DRCOG 1991; MRCGP 1992; Dip. Occ. Med. 1996. Socs: Droitwich Med. Soc.

WILKIE, William Joseph Strone Place Surgery, Strone Place, Strone, Dunoon PA23 8RR Tel: 01369 840279 Fax: 01369 840664; Tandiwe, Shore Road, Strone, Dunoon PA23 8TB Tel: 01369 840556 — MB ChB Glas. 1968. GP & Clin. Asst. Geriat. Unit & Day Hosp. Dunoon & Dist. Gen. Hosp. Argyll. Specialty: Care of the Elderly. Socs: Founder Mem. Cowal Med. Soc.

WILKIESON, Carol Anne — MB ChB Glas. 1983 (Univ. of Glas.) MRCP (UK) 1986; FRCP Glas. 1997. Cons. Phys. Med for Elderly Roy. Alexandra Hosp. Paisley. Specialty: Care of the Elderly. Special Interest: geriatric - Orthopaedic Liason; Osteoparosis. Socs: Brit. Geriat. Soc.; Roy. Coll. of Physicians and Surgeons, Glas.; Scott. Soc. of Physicians. Prev: Sen. Regist. (Geriat. Med.) Vict. Geriat. Univ. Glas.; Sen. Regist. (Med.) Gartnavel Gen. Hosp. Glas. & Stobhill Hosp.

WILKIN, David John Whiteley 55 St Stephens Road, Ealing, London W13 8JA — MB BS Lond. 1970; MRCOG 1976.

WILKIN, Lucy Margaret (retired) 2 The Mews, Newton Park, Newton Solney, Burton-on-Trent DE15 0SU Tel: 01283 702168 — (Belf.) MB BCh BAO Belf. 1945. Community Med. Off. S.E. Staffs. HA.

WILKIN, Peter Michael Rowan 43 Charnmouth Court, St Albans AL1 4SJ — MB ChB Aberd. 1976; DRCOG 1980.

WILKIN, Professor Terence James University of Plymouth, Department Medicine, Buckland House, Drake Circus, Plymouth PL4 8AA Tel: 01752 232925 Fax: 01752 232925 — MD Dundee 1978; MB ChB St. And. 1969; MRCP (UK) 1972; MD (Commend.) Dundee 1978; FRCP Lond. 1988; FRCP (Ed) 1999. Prof. Med. Univ. Plymouth; Hon. Cons. Phys. SW Region. Specialty: Endocrinol. Socs: Assn. Phys. & Roy. Soc. Med.; Diabetes UK; Amer. Diabetes Ass. Prev: Reader (Med. Endocrinol.) Univ. Soton.; Wellcome Sen. Lect. (Endocrinol.) Univ. Soton.; Lect. (Therap.) Univ. Dundee.

WILKIN, William Mitchel (retired) 2 The Mews, Newton Park, Newton Solney, Burton-on-Trent DE15 0SU Tel: 01283 702168 — MB BCh BAO Belf. 1945. Prev: Ho. Surg. Belf. City Hosp. & Jubilee Matern. Hosp. Belf.

WILKINS, Alastair National Hospital for Neurology and Neurosurgery, Queen Square, London WC1N 3BG Tel: 0207 3873611 Email: aw255@cam.ac.uk — MB BChir Camb. 1994; MA (Hons.) Camb. 1995; MRCP (UK) 1996; PhD Camb. 2003. Specialist Regist. Nat. Hosp. Neurol. Specialty: Neurol. Socs: Assn. Brit. Neurol. Prev: Specialist Regist. Addenbrookes Hosp.Camb.; Specialist Regist. (Neurol.) Norf. & Norwich Hosp.; SHO Nat. Hosp. Neurol.

WILKINS, Alexandre 14 Kinnaird Av, Bromley BR1 4HG — MB ChB Birm. 1997. PRHO (Gen. Med.) Alexandra Hosp. Redditch.

WILKINS, Andrew Norman John 7 Abbey Meadow, Lelant, St Ives TR26 3LL; 9 Holmesland lane, Botley, Southampton SO32 1BY Tel: 01489 787901 Email: awilkins@clara.co.uk — MB ChB Manch. 1986 (Manchester) DA 1989; FRCA 1994. Cons. Anaesth., Southampton Gen. Hosp. Specialty: Anaesth.

WILKINS, Angela Cameron Anaesthetic Department, Queen Alexandra Hospital, Cosham, Portsmouth Tel: 02392 286279 Fax: 02392 286681; 9 Holmesland Lane, Botley, Southampton SO30 2EH Tel: 01489 787901 Email: awilkins@clara.co.uk — MB BS Adelaide 1987; FRCA 1995. Specialty: Anaesth.

WILKINS, Mrs Anne Hazel 1 Bearcroft Avenue, Worcester WR4 0DR Tel: 01905 754602 — MB ChB Ed. 1998. SHO (Med.) Worcester Roy. Infirm. Worcester GP VTS. Specialty: Infec. Dis.; Trop. Med. Prev: PRHO Gen surg Borders Gen Hosp.Melrose; PRHO Resp med.Roy.Infir.Edin; SHO (A. & E.) Kidderminster.

WILKINS, Anthony John The Cardinal Clinic, Oakley Green Road, Windsor SL4 5UL Tel: 01753 869755 Fax: 01753 842852; 14 Devonshire Place, London W1N 1PB Tel: 020 7935 0640 Fax: 020 7224 6256 — (Roy. Free) BSc Lond. 1975; MRCPsych 1983. Cons. Psychiat.heatherwood Hosp. Lond Rd, Ascot, Berks. SL5 8AA; Lect. (Forens. Psychiat.) Univ. Lond. Specialty: Gen. Psychiat.; Forens. Psychiat.

WILKINS, Bernard (retired) 52 Devonshire Court, New Hall Road, Salford M7 4JT — (Manch.) M.B., Ch.B. Manch. 1944.

WILKINS, Bridget Sally Pathology Department, Level E South Block, Southampton General Hospital, Tremona Road, Southampton SO16 6YD Tel: 023 8079 4946 Fax: 023 8079 6603 — (London and Cambridge) MB BChir Camb. 1983; MRCPath 1990; DM Soton. 1992; PhD Soton. 1996; FRCPath 1999. Sen. Lect. (Path.) Soton. Univ.; Honourary Cons. Histopath., Southampton Univ. Specialty: Histopath. Socs: Europ. Ass for haematoPath.; Brit. lymphoma pathologists gp.; Path. Soc. Prev: Clin. Research Fell. (Path.) Soton. Univ.; Lect. (Path.) Soton. Univ.; Regist. (Path.) Leeds Gen. Infirm.

WILKINS, Carolyn Anne 22 Devonshire Place, London W1 Tel: 020 7935 9366; The Coach House, 71 West Drive, Harrow HA3 6TX Tel: 020 8954 5175 — MB ChB Birm. 1968; DObst RCOG 1970. Specialist (Psychosexual Med.) Lond. Socs: Inst. Psychosexual Med. Prev: Research Fell. (Epidemiol.) Yale Univ., USA; Resid. (O & G) Univ. Miami, USA.

WILKINS, Christopher Jason 127 New Street, Andover SP10 1DR — BM BCh Oxf. 1992.

WILKINS, Christopher John The Oaks, 15 Barlaston Old Road, Trentham, Stoke-on-Trent ST4 8HD Email: cwilkins4@compuserve.com — MB ChB Bristol 1981; FFA RCS Eng. 1987. Cons. Anaesth. N. Staffs. HA.; RCA Coll. Tutor. Specialty: Anaesth. Prev: Sen. Regist. (Anaesth.) Yorks. RHA; Lect. (Anaesth.) Univ. Leic.

WILKINS, Daniel Christian 14 Belcombe Place, Bradford-on-Avon BA15 1NA — MB ChB Bristol 1995.

WILKINS, David Gordon (retired) Central Farm, Littleton On Severn, Bristol BS35 1NR Tel: 01454 412233 Fax: 01454 281529 Email: dgwilkins@compuserve.com — (Middlx.) MA, MB Camb. 1962, BChir 1961; DObst RCOG 1963; DA Eng. 1964; FFA RCS Eng. 1969. Prev: Cons. Anaesth. United Bristol Healthcare Trust.

WILKINS, Mr Denis Charles Nuffield Hospital, Plymouth PL6 8BG — MB ChB Liverp. 1966; FRCS Eng. 1973; MD Liverp. 1974. Cons. Gen., Vasc. & Endocrin. Surg. Derriford Hosp. Plymouth; Hon. Clin. Research Fell. Peninsular Med. Sch.; Examr. Intercollegiate Bd. of Surg. UK & Irel.; Chairm. Ct. of Examr. Roy. Coll. of Surg. Eng.; Non Exec. Dir. Brit. Antarctic Survey Med. Unit; Chair. SAC in Gen. Surg. GB & Irel. Specialty: Gen. Surg.; Transpl. Surg. Socs: Brit. Soc. Endocrine Surgs.; Mem. Vasc. Surg. Soc. GB & Irel.; Mem. Brit. Transpl. Soc. Prev: Chairm. Med. Staff Comm. Derriford Hosp. Plymouth; Chairm. Regional Train. Comm. in Gen. Surg., SW Region; Sen. Regist. (Surg.) Addenbrooke's Hosp. Camb.

WILKINS, Denise Elizabeth Maria Proctor and Partners, Doctors Surgery, 42 Heaton Road, Newcastle upon Tyne NE6 1SE Tel: 0191 265 5911 Fax: 0191 265 6974; 14 Elmfield Road, Gosforth, Newcastle upon Tyne NE3 4AY Tel: 0191 285 6228 — MB ChB Dundee 1977; DRCOG 1979; Cert. JCC Lond. 1979; MRCGP 1981.

WILKINS, Derek Charles, CBE Yew Tree Cottage, Webbs Green, Soberton, Southampton SO32 3PY Tel: 01489 877715; Yew Tree Cottage, Webbs Green, Soberton, Southampton SO32 2PY Tel: 01489 877715 — MB BS Lond. 1952 (Guy's) MRCS Eng. LRCP Lond. 1952; DObst RCOG 1955. Civil. Med. Pract. MoD (Army). Specialty: Gen. Pract. Prev: Brig. late RAMC (V); Ho. Phys., Asst. Ho. Surg. & Resid. (Obst.) Guy's Hosp.

WILKINS, Derrin Felicity 4 Sunnyside Cottages, Aldermaston Road, Basingstoke RG24 9LA — MB BS Lond. 1989.

WILKINS, Edmund Lygon North Manchester General Hospital, Delaunay's Road, Crumpsall, Manchester M8 6RL Tel: 0161 720 2733 Fax: 0161 720 2139 — MB BS Lond. 1977 (Middlx.) DTM & H Liverp. 1978; MRCP (UK) 1980; Dip. Bact. Manch. 1985; MRCPath 1987; FRCP Lond. 1996; FRCPath 1997. Cons. Phys. Infec. Dis. N. Manch. Gen. Hosp. Specialty: Infec. Dis. Prev: Sen. Regist. (Infec. Dis.) Northwick Pk. Hosp. Middlx.; Sen. Regist. (Med. Microbiol.) Pub. Health Laborat. Portsmouth; Regist. (Med. Microbiol.) Pub. Health Laborat. Liverp.

WILKINS, Elizabeth Ann Llwyn Brwydrau Surgery, 3 Frederick Place, Llansamlet, Swansea SA7 9RY Tel: 01792 771465 — MB BS Lond. 1983; MRCGP 1988.

WILKINS, Evelyn Margaret (retired) 78 Armorial Road, Styvechale, Coventry CV3 6GJ Tel: 024 76 414675 — MB ChB Birm. 1941; MB ChB (Hons.) Birm. 1941. Prev: Sen. Med. Off. Coventry AHA (Child Health).

WILKINS, Geoffrey Selwyn Flat 1, Merlewood, 17 Langham Road, Bowdon, Altrincham WA14 2HT — MB ChB Manch. 1963; DObst RCOG 1965. Locum GP Salford & Traford Suppl. List 2003-. Prev: NHS GP Salford from 1996.

WILKINS, Helen Margaret Ovoca, 460 Didsbury Road, Heaton Mersey, Stockport SK4 3BT — BM Soton. 1979; DRCOG 1982; MRCGP 1983. Gen. Practitioner.

WILKINS, Helen Mary Redwynde, 4 North Close, Bromborough, Wirral CH62 2BU Tel: 0151 334 5206 — MB ChB Liverp. 1982. SCMO Wom. Serv. Wirral Community Healthcare NHS Trust. Specialty: Family Plann. & Reproduc. Health. Socs: Accred. Mem. Brit. Assn. Sexual & Marital Ther. Prev: Trainee GP Ellesmere Port; SHO Arrowe Pk. Hosp. Upton; Ho. Off. Clatterbridge Hosp. Bebington.

WILKINS, Hubert Andrew (retired) 32 Overstrand Mansions, Prince of Wales Drive, Battersea Park, London SW11 4EZ — MB BChir Camb. 1964; MA, MB BChir Camb. 1964; DObst 1967; DTM & H Eng. 1968.

WILKINS, Ingrid Anne 103 Bromham Road, Bedford MK40 4BS; 253 Queen Edith's Way, Cambridge CB1 8NJ — MB BS Lond. 1994 (St. Bart. Hosp. Med. Sch.) BSc Lond. 1993; Dip. ATLS RCS Eng. 1995; ALS 1996; PALS 1997. SHO (Anaesth.) Camb. Specialty: Anaesth. Prev: SHO (Neonates.) Homerton Lond.; SHO Rotat. (Anaesth.) Nottm.; SHO (A & E) North. Gen. Hosp. Sheff.

WILKINS, Joanne Pembroke Road Surgery, 111 Pembroke Road, Clifton, Bristol BS8 3EU — BM BCh Oxf. 1985; MA; DRCOG 1987; MRCGP 1989. GP Retainee. Prev: Princip. in Gen. Pract., WhiteHo. Surg., Chipping Norton, Oxon.

WILKINS, Lisa Katherine Coldharbour, Sand Down Lane, Newton St Cyres, Exeter EX5 5DF — BM Soton. 1992; MRCP. Staff Grade Palliat. Med. St Annes Hosp Salford. Specialty: Palliat. Med. Prev: SHO (Haemat.) Univ. Hosp. Wales Cardiff; SHO (Med.) Roy. Devon & Exeter Hosp.; S. SHO (Med.) Roy. Gwent Hosp. Newport.

WILKINS, Margaret Caroline Village Surgery, Gillett Road, Poole BH12 5BF Tel: 01202 525252 Fax: 01202 533956 — MB ChB Bristol 1967; DObst RCOG 1969. Princip. In Gen. Pract. Village Surg. Poole; Clin. Asst. Breast Clinic Roy. Bournemouth Hosp. Specialty: Gen. Pract. Prev: Med. Off. Family Plann. Clinic Potters Bar; SHO (Obst.) City Matern. Hosp. Carlisle; Med. Off. Maseno Hosp., Kenya.

WILKINS, Margaret Freda West Wales General Hospital, Carmarthen SA31 2AF Tel: 01267 227616; 39 Llythrid Avenue, Uplands, Swansea SA2 0JJ Tel: 01792 297544 — MB ChB Bristol 1974; BSc Bristol 1971; FRCR 1984. Cons. Clin. Oncol. West. Wales Gen. Hosp. Carmarthen. Specialty: Oncol. Prev: Staff Grade (Radiother.) Singleton Hosp. Swansea; Sen. Regist. (Radiother.) Velindre Hosp. Cardiff.

WILKINS, Margaret Janet Elizabeth Department of Pathology, Bedford Hospital NHS Trust, Kempston Road, Bedford MK42 9DJ Tel: 01234 792094 Fax: 01234 795886 Email: margaret.wilkins@bedhos.anglox.nhs.uk; Yew Trees, Windmill Hill, Hitchin SG4 9RT Tel: 01462 432457 — MB BS Lond. 1984 (Roy. Free) MSc Lond. 1986; MRCPath 1992; FRCPath 2000. Cons. Histopath. & Cytopath., Bedford Hosp. Bedford. Specialty: Histopath. Prev: Sen. Regist. (Histopath.) St. Mary's Hosp. Lond.; Regist. (Histopath.) Hammersmith Hosp. Lond.; SHO/Regist. (Histopath.) Roy. Free Hosp. Lond.

WILKINS, Mark Richard Institute of Ophthalmology, Bath St., London EC1V 9EL Tel: 020 7608 6942 Fax: 020 7608 6887; Flat 2, 98 Greencroft Gardens, London NW6 3PH Email: mwilkins@easynet.co.uk — MB BS Lond. 1990; BA (Physiol. Sci.) Oxf. 1987; FRCOphth 1994. Research Fell. Inst. Ophth. Lond.; Research Regist. Moorfields Eye Hosp. Lond. Specialty: Ophth. Prev: SHO (Ophth.) King's Coll. Hosp., St. Geo. Hosp. & Frimley Pk. Hosp. Lond.

WILKINS, Martin Russell — MB ChB Birm. 1979.

WILKINS, Philip 78A New Dover Road, Canterbury CT1 3EQ — BChir Camb. 1990.

WILKINS, Philip Samuel Weston (retired) April Cottage, Prinsted Lane, Prinsted, Emsworth PO10 8HR Tel: 01243 377074 — MB ChB Birm. 1949; DCH Eng. 1954; FRCP Lond. 1974, M 1960. Prev: Cons. Phys. (Geriat.) Portsmouth & SE Hants. Health Dist.

WILKINS, Richard Anthony Cleveland House, 16 Spital Terrace, Gainsborough DN21 2HE Tel: 01427 613158 Fax: 01427 616644; 66 Willingham Road, Knaith Park, Gainsborough DN21 5ET Tel: 01427 810293 — MB ChB Dundee 1987; MRCGP Ed. 1993.

WILKINS, Robert Anthony Wellington Hospital, Wellington Place, London NW8 9LE Tel: 020 7483 5078 Email: xrawilkins@doctors.org.uk; The Coach House, 71 West Drive, Harrow HA3 6TX Tel: 020 8954 5175 — MB ChB Birm. 1964; BSc Birm. 1961; DMRD Eng. 1967; FFR 1969. Director of Radiol., Wellington Hosp. Specialty: Radiol. Prev: Cons. Radiol. Northwick Pk. Hosp. Harrow.

WILKINS, Sidney William (retired) Annedd Wen, Ruthin Road, Denbigh LL16 4RA Tel: 01745 812420 — MB ChB Birm. 1950; MRCS Eng. LRCP Lond. 1949. Prev: Clin. Asst. (Psychiat.) N. Wales Hosp. Denbigh.

WILKINS, William Edward The Elms, Pen-y-Fai, Bridgend CF31 4LS — MB BCh Wales 1972; MRCP (U.K.) 1976.

WILKINSON, Agnes Hallimond 54 Stokes Court, Diploma Avenue, East Finchley, London N2 8NX Tel: 020 8883 3680 — (Birm.) MB ChB Birm. 1939; MRCP Lond. 1942; FRCPsych 1985, M

1971. Profess. Mem. Soc. Analyt. Psychol. Socs: Gp. Analyt. Soc. Prev: Chairm. Med. Sect. Brit. Psychol. Soc.; Psychiat. Adviser Lond. Sch. of Economics; Phys. i/c Studs. Health Serv. Univ. Bristol.

WILKINSON, Alan Edward (retired) 22 Kingsend, Ruislip HA4 7DA Tel: 01895 635829 — (St. Mary's) MRCS Eng. LRCP Lond. 1939; MB BS Lond. 1951; FRCPath 1968. Prev: Director VD Refer. Laborat., The Lond. Hosp.

WILKINSON, Mr Alan James Belfast City Hospital, Lisburn Road, Belfast BT9 7AB Tel: 01232 263792; 16 Malone View Road, Belfast BT9 5PH Tel: 01232 616115 — MB BCh BAO Belf. 1973; FRCS Ed. 1978; MD Belf. 1984. Cons. Surg. Belf. City Hosp. Specialty: Gen. Surg. Prev: Cons. Surg. Roy. Vict. Hosp. Belf.; Sen. Surg. Tutor & Sen. Regist. Dept. Surg. Roy. Vict. Hosp. Belf.; Sen. Regist. Roy. Vict. Hosp. Belf.

WILKINSON, Mr Alan Royce (retired) Hull Royal Infirmary, Hull HU10 7TL Tel: 01482 653289; Springfield House, Rise Road, Skirlaugh, Hull HU11 5BH — MB ChB Sheff. 1967; FRCS Eng. 1973; FRCS Eng. 1973. Cons. Surg. Hull Roy. Infirm.; Clin. Dir. Critical Care. Prev: Lect. (Surg.) Qu. Eliz. Hosp. Birm.

WILKINSON, Alison Joan P.C.E.A. Chogoria Hospital, PO Box 35, Chogoria, Kenya; 70 Craigleith Hill Gardens, Edinburgh EH4 2JH — MB ChB Ed. 1976; DRCOG 1979; MRCOG 1991. Specialist Obst. & Gyn. Pcea Chogoria Hosp. Kenya. Specialty: Obst. & Gyn. Prev: Regist. (Obst. & Gyn.) Stirling Roy. Infirm.; SHO (Obst. & Gyn.) Furness Gen. Hosp. Barrow-in-Furness; SHO Regist. (Obst.) Nazareth Hosp. Israel.

WILKINSON, Alistair Thomas Great Western Road Medical Group, 327 Great Western Road, Aberdeen AB10 6LT Tel: 01224 571318 Fax: 01224 573865; 58 Cairnlee Avenue E., Cults, Aberdeen AB15 9NH — MB ChB Aberd. 1975; FRCGP; MRCGP 1979.

WILKINSON, Mr Alwyn (retired) 26 Selkirk Avenue, Oldham OL8 4DQ Tel: 0161 624 9029 — MB ChB Manch. 1949; FRCS Eng. 1961. Prev: Cons. Orthop. & Traum. Surg. Oldham Hosp.

WILKINSON, Andrea Janet Orchards Medical Centre, 10 Leigh Road, Boothstown, Worsley, Manchester M28 1CX; 65 Border Brook Lane, Worsley, Manchester M28 1XJ — MB ChB Manch. 1990 (Manchester) BSc (Hons.) Manch. 1987; MRCOG 1995; MRCOG 1997. GP Princip. Specialty: Gen. Pract.; Obst. & Gyn. Prev: Regist. NW Region; Clin. Research Fell.

WILKINSON, Andrew Cameron Howitt c/o Dr Martin Prior, 3 Rooke Way, London SE10 0JB — MB ChB New Zealand 1947; FRACP 1973, M 1956.

WILKINSON, Andrew John 93 Christchurch Street, Ipswich IP4 2DD Tel: 01473 212842 — MB BS Lond. 1966 (Lond. Hosp.) MRCGP 1978. Prev: SHO (Med.) Ipswich & E. Suff. Hosp.; SHO (Clin. Pathol.) Lond. Hosp.; Phys. Whipps Cross Hosp.

WILKINSON, Andrew Mark Charles Andrews Clinic, West End, Redruth TR15 2SF Tel: 01209 881810 Fax: 01209 881816 — MB BS Newc. 1984; MRCPsych 1988. Cons. Psychiat. of Old Age Cornw. Healthcare Trust. Specialty: Geriat. Psychiat. Prev: Cons. Psychiat. of Age Wirral Hosp. Trust; Sen. Regist. (Psychiat.) Mersey RHA; Regist. (Psychiat.) N. Yorks. GP VTS.

WILKINSON, Andrew Peter Descarrieres Castle Douglas Medical Group, Castle Douglas Health Centre, Academy Street, Castle Douglas DG7 1EE; Lochbank, Castle Douglas DG7 1TH Tel: 01556 503413 — (Edinbrugh) BSc (Med. Sci.) Ed. 1966; MB ChB Ed. 1969; DObst RCOG 1972. Brit. Med. Off. Brit. Red Cross Soc. Socs: BMA. Prev: Mem. & Vice-Chaim. Dumfries & Galloway HB; Mem. & Chairm. Dumfries & Galloway L.C.; Mem. SGMSC.

WILKINSON, Andrew Richard PO Box 31, Lechlade, Gloucester GL7 3YQ Mob: 07776 187502 Email: andrewwilkinson@oxfordmedicolegal.com — MB BS Lond. 1974 (Lond. Hosp.) BSc Lond. 1970; MRCS Eng. LRCP Lond. 1974; MRCGP 1978; DRCOG 1979; DFFP 1996; DMJ (Clin.) 1997; LLM 2002. Specialist Clin. Forens. & Legal Med. & Sen. Forens. Med. Examr., Oxon., Wilts. & Metrop. Police; Lect. Forens. Med., Univ. Coll. Dub.; Tutor Legal Med., Dept. Primary Health Care, Univ. Oxf. Specialty: Gen. Pract. Special Interest: Clin. Forens. & Legal Med.; Med. Educat. Socs: Oxf. Medico legal Soc. Prev: SHO (Med.) Warwick Hosp.; Sen. Partner, Dr Wilkinson & Partners, Broadshires Health Centre.

WILKINSON, Professor Andrew Robert University of Oxford, Neonatal Unit, Department of Paediatrics, John Radcliffe Hospital, Oxford OX3 9DU Tel: 01865 221355 Fax: 01865 221366 Email: andrew.wilkinson@paediatrics.ox.ac.uk — MB ChB Birm. 1968 (Birmingham) MRCP (UK) 1972; DCH Eng. 1972; FRCP Lond. 1986; MA Oxf. 1992; FRCPCH 1997. Prof. of Paediat. Univ. Oxf. John Radcliffe Hosp.; Hon. Cons. Paediat. Oxf. Radcliffe NHS Trust; Fell. All Souls Coll. Oxf. Specialty: Paediat.; Neonat. Socs: Pres. Neonatal Soc.; Past Pres. Brit. Assn. Perinatal Med.

WILKINSON, Anita Margaret Southgate Surgery, 2 Forester Road, Southgate, Crawley RH10 6EQ Tel: 01293 522231 Fax: 01293 515655 — MB ChB Manch. 1988; DCH RCP Lond. 1993; MRCP (UK) 1997. GP Crawley. Prev: Trainee GP/SHO (Geriat.) Crawley.

WILKINSON, Ann Fiona Rosemary 17 Austins Close, Market Harborough LE16 9BJ Tel: 01858 461910 — MB BS Lond. 1980; DRCOG 1983. Prev: GP Birm.

WILKINSON, Anna Louise Poverest Medical Centre, 42 Poverest Road, St Mary Cray, Orpington BR5 2DQ Tel: 01689 833643 Fax: 01689 891976 — BM BS Nottm. 1979; MRCGP 1983; Dip. Ther. Wales 1996.

WILKINSON, Anne Barbara Wonersh Surgery, The Sheilings, Wonersh, Guildford GU5 0PE Tel: 01483 898123 Fax: 01483 893104 — MB BS Lond. 1983; DCH Lond. 1988; DRCOG 1988; MRCGP 1993. GP Prinicipal. Socs: MDU. Prev: GP Princip. Pk.wood Drive Surg., Hemel Hempstead.

WILKINSON, Anne Marie 27 Waringfield Crescent, Moira, Craigavon BT67 0FG — MB BCh BAO Belf. 1994 (Queens - Belfast) DROG - 1996; MRCGP - 1998.

WILKINSON, Antony Edward Reid Hunter Health Centre, Andrew Street, East Kilbride, Glasgow G74 1AD Tel: 01355 906676 Fax: 01355 906676 — MB ChB Glas. 1987; DRCOG 1989; MRCGP 1991. Prev: Trainee GP Skelmorlie.

WILKINSON, Audrey 438 Blackmoorfoot Road, Crosland Moor, Huddersfield HD4 5NS Tel: 01484 653520 — (R.C.S.I.) LRCPI & LM, LRCSI & LM 1952; DPH Newc. 1966; MFCM 1972; MFCMI 1977. Specialty: Pub. Health Med.

WILKINSON, Beatrice Jean Hadrian Clinic, Newcastle General Hospital, Westgate Road, Newcastle upon Tyne NE4 6BE — MB BS Newc. 1980 (Univ. Newc. u. Tyne) DRCOG 1983; MRCPsych 1988. Cons. Psychiat. Hadrian Clinic Newc. Gen. Hosp. Specialty: Gen. Psychiat. Prev: Sen. Regist. (Psychiat.) Newc.; Trainee GP Newc. VTS.

WILKINSON, Beverley Anne 20 St Mary's Road, Worsley, Manchester M28 3RF — MB ChB Sheff. 1994.

WILKINSON, Brian Richard (retired) 22 Marlborough Road, Castle Bromwich, Birmingham B36 0EH Tel: 0121 747 8810 — (St. Bart.) MB BS Lond. 1951; MRCS Eng. LRCP Lond. 1951; DObst RCOG 1958; FRCGP 1986, M 1965. Prev: GP Shard End Birm.

WILKINSON, Bridget Ann 4 Londesborough Road, Market Weighton, York YO43 3AY Tel: 01430 873433 Fax: 01430 871466 — MB ChB Manch. 1988; BSc (Med. Sci.) St. And. 1985; DRCOG 1991; MRCGP 1992. Half time job-share Gen. Practitioner in Market Weighton. Specialty: Gen. Pract. Prev: Health Developm. Off. Nainital, India.

WILKINSON, Carole Dawn Old Hall Grounds Health Centre, Old Hall Grounds, Cowbridge CF71 7AH — MB BCh Wales 1990; DRCOG 1993; MRCGP 1994; DCH RCP Lond. 1995. Specialty: Gen. Pract.

WILKINSON, Charles Edward The Surgery, Chestnut Road, Sutton Benger, Chippenham SN15 4RP Tel: 01249 720244 Fax: 01249 721165 — MRCS Eng. LRCP Lond. 1975 (Middx Hosp. Med. Sch.) Cert. Family Plann. JCC 1978. Gen. Practitioner, Single Handed dispensing, Wilts. Health Auth.; Instruc. (Advanced Life Support in Obst.). Socs: Roy. Soc. Med.; CMAC Comm.; BMA. Prev: Police Surg. Chippenham Area; Clin. Asst. (PsychoGeriat.) Southmead Hosp.; Clin. Teach. Univ. Bristol.

WILKINSON, Charles Peter 19 Garland Road, Poole BH15 2LA — MB ChB Leic. 1997.

WILKINSON, Christopher David 135 Hubert Road, Selly Oak, Birmingham B29 6ET Tel: 0121 471 4645 — MB ChB Birm. 1988.

WILKINSON, Christopher Lindow Margaret Pyke Centre, 73 Charlotte Street, London W1T 4PL Tel: 020 7530 3620 — MB BS Lond. 1985; MFFP 1993. Cons. (Sexual & Reproduc. Health). Specialty: Womens Health.

WILKINSON, Clare Elizabeth 10 Mostyn Avenue, West Kirby, Wirral CH48 3HW — MB BCh Wales 1980; DRCOG 1984; MRCGP 1985. Prof. of Gen. Pract., 1998.

WILKINSON, Clare Elizabeth 30 Eborall Close, Warwick CV34 5QA — MB ChB Liverp. 1992 (Liverpool) BSc Liverp. 1989, MB ChB 1992; DRCOG 1995; MRCP 1997; DM 2003. Specialist Regist. Rheum. & Gen. Med. Specialty: Rheumatol.; Gen. Med.

WILKINSON, Darrell Sheldon (retired) Whitecroft, Hervines Road, Amersham HP6 5HT Tel: 01494 433940 — (St. Thos.) MRCS Eng. LRCP Lond. 1942; MB BS Lond. 1946; MD Lond. 1947; FRCP Lond. 1964, M. 1947. Prev: Cons. Dermat. Aylesbury & High Wycombe Health Dists.

WILKINSON, David (retired) Jelemy Tump, Ninevah Lane, Badsworth, Pontefract WF9 1AP Tel: 01977 643813 — MB ChB Aberd. 1956.

WILKINSON, Mr David 35 Moseley Wood Lane, Leeds LS16 7ER — MB ChB Leeds 1984; FRCS Eng. 1990; MD Leeds 1993. Cons. Gen. & Vasc. Surg. Bradford Hosps. NHS Trust. Specialty: Gen. Surg. Prev: Sen. Regist. North. & Yorks. RHA.

WILKINSON, David Andrew Charles 17 Stoke Paddock Road, Bristol BS9 2DJ — MB ChB Birm. 1993.

WILKINSON, David Colin Cae'r Berllan, Llangristiolus, Bodorgan LL62 5PS Tel: 01248 750524 — BM BCh Oxf. 1972; MA; DPM Lond. 1976; MRCPsych 1978. Cons. (Child & Adolesc. Psychiat.) Gwynedd AHA. Specialty: Child & Adolesc. Psychiat. Prev: Sen. Regist. (Child & Adolesc. Psychiat.) Roy. Manch. Childr. Hosp.

WILKINSON, David George Western Community Hospital, Walnut Grove, Millbrook, Southampton SO16 4XE Tel: 023 8047 5446 Email: dwilk2000@aol.com; 18 Cobbett Road, Southampton SO18 1HH — MB ChB Birm. 1975; MRCGP 1979; FRCPsych. 1994, M 1981. Cons. Old Age Psychiat. West. Community Hosp. Soton.; Hon. Sen. Lect. Univ. of Soton.; Director Memory Assessm. and Research Centre www.marc.soton.ac.uk. Specialty: Geriat. Psychiat.

WILKINSON, David Gregor Academic Department of Psychiatry, The London Hospital Medical College, Turner St., London E1 2AD Tel: 020 7377 7344 — MB ChB Ed. 1975; BSc Ed. 1973, MB ChB 1975; MRCP (UK) 1977; FRCPsych 1991, M 1980; MPhil (Psychiat.) Lond. 1981; FRCP Ed. 1989. Specialty: Gen. Psychiat. Prev: Dir. Acad. Sub-Dept. Psychol. Med. N. Wales Univ. Coll. of Med.; Hon. Cons. Psychiat. Clwyd HA; Resid. Psychiat. Med. Res. Counc. Unit Epidemiol. Studies Psychiat. Ed.

WILKINSON, David John Department of Anaesthesia, St. Bartholomew's Hospital, London EC1A 7BE Tel: 020 7601 7518 Fax: 020 7601 7520; High Willow, 49 Spring Grove, Loughton IG10 4QD Fax: 020 8502 3887 Email: davidwilkinson1@compuserve.com — MB BS Lond. 1972 (St. Bart.) MRCS Eng. LRCP Lond. 1971; DObst RCOG 1973; FRCA Eng. 1976; Hon. FCARCSI 2002. Cons. Anaesth. Barts and the Lond. NHS Trust & Homerton Univ. Hosp. Trust. Lond. Specialty: Anaesth. Socs: Dep. Sec. WFSA; Past Pres. CENSA; Vice Pres. Assn. Anaes. GB & Ire. Prev: Chairm. Dept of Anaesth. St. Bart. Hosp.; Med. Dir. Day Surg. Centre St. Bart. Hosp.

WILKINSON, David John Sheffield Teaching Hospitals NHS Trust, Herries Road, Sheffield S5 7AU Email: d.wilkinson@doctors.org.uk — MB ChB Sheff. 2003; BMedSci (Hons.) Sheff. 2000. Sheff. Basic Surgic. Train. Rotat. Specialty: Accid. & Emerg.

WILKINSON, Dawn Marsha St Mary's Hospital, Praed Street, London W2 1NY — MB BS Lond. 1993 (St Geo. Hosp.) MRCP Lond. 1996; Dip GU Med 2000; DFFP 2000. Cons. St Mary's Hosp. Lond. Specialty: Genitourinary Medicine. Prev: Specialist Regist. (GUM) Chelsea & Westm. Hosp. Lond.; Regist. (Genitourin. Med.) Chelsea & Westm. Hosp. Lond.; SHO (GUM), Chelsea & Westm. Hosp. Lond.

WILKINSON, Debra Blythe 4A The High Street, Great Ayton, Middlesbrough TS9 6NJ — MB BS Newc. 1993.

WILKINSON, Douglas Allan Outeniqua House, 313 Woodstock Road, Oxford OX2 7NY — MB ChB Cape Town 1985; BSc Cape Town 1980; DA (UK) 1988; MRCGP 1990; T(GP) 1991; FRCA 1993. Cons. Anaesth. Intens. Care Oxf. Specialty: Anaesth. Prev: Sen. Regist. Oxf.; Regist. Rotat. (Anaesth.) Bristol; GP Vocational Train. Scheme Taunton, Som.

WILKINSON, Edith Mary (retired) 5 Badcall, Scourie, Lairg IV27 4TH Tel: 01971 502206 — (Durham) MB BS Durh. 1942; DA Eng. 1951; FFA RCS Eng. 1954. Prev: Cons. Anaesth. Liverp. RHB.

WILKINSON, Elizabeth Jane The Health Centre, Midland St., Long Eaton, Nottingham NG10 1NY Tel: 0115 973 2370 Fax: 0115 946 3894; Grove House, 53 Grove Avenue, Chilwell, Nottingham NG9 4DZ Tel: 0115 925 5141 Fax: 0115 925 5141 — MB ChB Sheff. 1973; MRCGP 1977. Screening Phys. B.U.P.A. Socs: Nottm. M-C Soc. Prev: Trainee GP Doncaster VTS; Ho. Surg. Lincoln Co. Hosp.; Ho. Phys. Profess. Unit Sheff. Childrs. Hosp.

WILKINSON, Elizabeth Jane 3 Vale Court, Cowbridge CF71 7ES — MB BS Lond. 1985 (St. Mary's Hosp.) BSc Lond. 1982; DRCOG 1989; MRCGP 1990; MFPHM RCP (UK) 1994. Cons. in Pub. Health Nat. Pub. Health Serv. Socs: BMA. Prev: Sen. Regist. (Pub. Health Med.) Mid Glam. HA; Trainee GP Bridgend VTS; Sen. Med. Off. (Primary Healthcare Developm.) Welsh Off.

WILKINSON, Elizabeth Sarah PO Box 365, Harmondsworth, West Drayton UB7 0GB Tel: 020 8738 7745 Fax: 020 8738 7745 Email: elizabeth.s.wilkinson@britishairways.com; 3 Milton Road, Hampton TW12 2LL — MB ChB Manch. 1990 (St And. & Manch.) MRCGP 1995; AFOM 2000; MFOM 2003. Occupat. Phys. Brit. Airways Heathrow. Specialty: Occupat. Health.

WILKINSON, Ellen Jane Fromeside Clinic, Blackberry Hill Hospital, Stapleton, Bristol BS16 2ED Tel: 0117 958 3678 — BM Soton. 1987; MRCPsych 1993. Sen. Regist. (Psychiat.) Blackberry Hill Hosp. Bristol. Specialty: Gen. Psychiat.

WILKINSON, Elspeth Catto (retired) — MB BS Durh. 1943 (Newc.) MB BS (Hons.) Durh. 1943; DPM Lond. 1966. Prev: Cons. Child Psychiat. Qu. Eliz. Hosp. Gateshead.

WILKINSON, Emily Kate 8 Ember Lane, Esher KT10 8ER — MB BS Lond. 1998.

WILKINSON, Ewan Alastair John Central Liverpool PCT, 22 Pall Mall, Liverpool L3 6AL — MB ChB Ed. 1980; DRCOG 1983; DTM & H Liverp. 1984; MFPHM 1996. Cons. (Pub. Health Med.)Central Liverpool PCT. Specialty: Pub. Health Med. Prev: Dist. Health Off., Malawi.

WILKINSON, Frederick James (retired) The Stone Cottage, Gas House Lane, Morpeth NE61 1SR — MB BS Durh. 1950; FRCGP 1976, M 1969. Prev: GP N.d.

WILKINSON, Gemma 257 Hinton Way, Great Shelford, Cambridge CB2 5AN — BM BS Nottm. 1997.

WILKINSON, Mr Glen Alexander Low Department of Cardiothoracic Surgery, Northern General Hospital NHS Trust, Herries Road, Sheffield S5 7AU Tel: 0114 271 4951; 21 Mayfield Heights, Off Brook House Hill, Sheffield S10 3TT Tel: 01142 229 5202 — MB ChB Birm. 1973; FRCS Eng. 1978. Cons. Cardiothoracic Surg. N. Gen. Hosp. Sheff.; Hon Sen. Lect. Univ. of Sheff. Specialty: Cardiothoracic Surg. Socs: Soc. Cardiothor. Surg. GB & Irel. Prev: Sen. Regist. (Cardiothoracic Surg.) W. Midl. RHA; Sen. Fell. Acting Instruc. (Cardiothoracic Surg.) Univ. Washington Hosp. Seattle USA; Lect. (Cardiothoracic Surg.) Lond. Hosp. Whitechapel.

WILKINSON, Guy Matthew 13 Long Acre, Cuddington, Northwich CW8 2XP — MB ChB Liverp. 1992.

WILKINSON, Heather Louise 69 Lingmore Rise, Kendal LA9 7NR Tel: 01539 724767 — MB ChB Sheff. 1995 (Sheffield) Ho. Off. (Gen. Med.) Westmorland Gen. Hosp. Kendal Cumbria; GP Regist. Lancaster VTS. Specialty: Gen. Pract. Prev: SHO (Psychiat.) Ridge Lea Hosp. Lancaster; SHO (Paediat.) Roy. Lancaster Infirm.; GP Trainee Station Ho. Surg. Kendal.

WILKINSON, Helen Catrin 12 Woodkind Hey, Spital, Wirral CH63 9JZ — MB ChB Manch. 1991; DRCOG 1994. Trainee GP Wirral. Specialty: Gen. Pract.

WILKINSON, Helen Sarah Fisher Medical Centre, Millfields, Coach Street, Skipton BD23 1EU; 49 Otley Street, Skipton BD23 1ET Tel: 01756 69622 — MB BS Lond. 1984; DRCOG 1989; MRCGP 1989. Prev: Trainee GP Airedale VTS.

WILKINSON, Henry Charles 20 Gainsborough Drive, Lawford Dale, Manningtree CO11 2JU Tel: 01206 391877 — MB BS Lond. 1990 (Char., Cross & Westm. Med. Sch.) BSc (Marine Biol. & Zool.) Cardiff 1985; DCH RCP Lond. 1994. Specialty: Gen. Pract.

WILKINSON, Iain Michael Stewart (retired) 6 High Green, Great Shelford, Cambridge CB2 5EG Tel: 01223 843856 — MD Manch. 1970; BSc (Anat.) Manch. 1960, MD 1970, MB ChB 1963; FRCP Lond. 1981, M 1965; MA Camb. 1977. Prev: Univ. Lect. (Neurol.) & Hon. Cons. (Neurol.) Manch. Roy. Infirm.

WILKINSON, Ian Chadderton (Town) Health Centre, Middleton Road, Chadderton, Oldham OL9 0LH Tel: 0161 628 4543 Fax: 0161 284 1658 — MB ChB Bristol 1977. Clin. Asst. (A & E) Roy. Oldham Hosp.

WILKINSON, Ian Boden Department of Clinical Pharmacology, University of Cambridge, Addenbrookes Hospital, Cambridge CB22 QP Tel: 01222 336806 Fax: 0870 1269863; The Old School house, West Wickham, Cambridge CB1 6RY — BM BCh Oxf. 1993; MA Oxf. 1994, BA 1990; MRCP (UK) 1996; DM Oxf. 2004. Lect. clin, Pharm, Camb. unvi.; Hon. Cons. Phys., Addenbrookes Hosp. Cambr. Specialty: Gen. Med.; Pharmacology. Socs: Med. Res. Soc.; Brit. Pharmacological Soc.; Brit. Hypertens. Soc. Prev: Clin. Lecturesh. Med. Univ. Edin. West. Gen. Hosp. Edin.; Clin. Lect. John Radcliffe Hosp. Oxf.; SHO (Med.) Qu. Med. Centre Nottm.

WILKINSON, Ian Louttit (retired) 18 Woodfield, Nash Lane, Belbroughton, Stourbridge DY9 9SW — MB ChB Birm. 1948; MRCS Eng. LRCP Lond. 1948. Prev: Med. Off. Mary Stevens Matern. Home Stourbridge.

WILKINSON, James Robert Wyndham Eastbourne District General Hospital, Department of Respiratory Medicine, Kings Drive, Eastbourne BN21 2UD — MB BS Lond. 1983; MA Camb. 1983; MRCP (UK) 1986; MD Lond. 1993; FRCP Lond. 2000. Cons. (Respirat. & Gen. Med.) E. Sussex Hosps. NHS Trust. Specialty: Respirat. Med. Socs: Brit. Thorac. Soc. Prev: Research Regist. Guy's Hosp. Lond.; Sen. Regist. Sir Chas. Gairdner Hosp. Perth, West. Austral.; Sen. Regist. Soton. Gen. Hosp.

WILKINSON, Jane Dever Department of Child Health, Royal Hospital for Sick Children, Dalhair St, Yorkhill, Glasgow G3 8SJ Tel: 0141 201 0000 Fax: 0141 201 0837 Email: gcl159@clinmed.gla.ac.uk — MB ChB Aberd. 1985 (Aberdeen) MRCP (Ireland). Assoc. Specialist (Cystic Fibrosis); Hon. Clin. Lect., Dept of Child Health, Glas. Univ. Specialty: Paediat. Socs: BMA; MRCPCH; MRCP (Irel.).

WILKINSON, Jane Elizabeth Margery Valentine Cottage, Banbury St., Kineton, Warwick CV35 0JU — BM Soton. 1989.

WILKINSON, Jane Frances York Road Group Practice, York Rd, Ellesmere Port CH65 0DB — MB ChB Liverp. 1994; DCH RCP Lond. 1996; DRCOG Lond. 1998; DFFP Lond. 1998. Gen. Practitioner (Princip.), York Rd Gp. Pract., Ellesmere Port. Specialty: Gen. Pract. Prev: GP Regist. Wirral VTS.

WILKINSON, Jane Louise — MB ChB Manch. 1983. Cons. Child & Adolesc. Psychiat. Chesterfield and N. Derbysh. Roy. Hosp. NHS Trust. Specialty: Child & Adolesc. Psychiat. Prev: Sen. Regist. (Child & Adolesc. Psychiat.) Sheff.

WILKINSON, Jane Mary 14 Leswin Road, London N16 7NL — MB BChir Camb. 1993.

WILKINSON, Jane Sally Rosegarth House, Clifton Road, Tettenhall, Wolverhampton WV6 9AP Tel: 01902 759377 — MB ChB Manch. 1974 (St. And. & Manch.) BSc St. And. 1971; DObst RCOG 1976; DCH Glas. 1977; MRNZCGP 1978.

WILKINSON, Mr Jeremy Mark 9 Chorley Rd, Sheffield S10 3RJ — MB ChB Sheff. 1991; FRCS Eng. 1996; PhD Sheff. 2002. Specialist Regist. Orthop. Surg. N. Gen. Hosp. Sheff.

WILKINSON, Joan Oldham Family Health Services Authority, Lindley House, 1 John St., Oldham OL8 1DF Tel: 0161 626 4615 Fax: 0161 652 0182 — MB ChB Manch. 1957. Prev: Ho. Off. Oldham & Dist. Gen. Hosp. & Manch. Roy. Infirm.

WILKINSON, Joanna Ruth Rastrick Health Centre, Chapel Croft, Rastick, Brighouse HD6 3NA Tel: 01484 710853; 16 The Fairway, Fixby, Huddersfield HD2 2HU Tel: 01484 534763 — BM BS Nottm. 1981 (Nottingham) MRCGP 1986.

WILKINSON, Joanne Sarah 1 Sunscales Av, Cockermouth CA13 9DY — MB ChB Manch. 1997.

WILKINSON, John (retired) 70 Craigleith Hill Gardens, Edinburgh EH4 2JH Tel: 0131 332 2994 Email: jjwilkinson@doctors.org.uk — MB ChB Ed. 1941; MD Ed. 1956; DTM & H Ed. (Greig Medal) 1956; FRCP Ed. 1972, M 1957; MFCM 1979. Prev: SCM Lothian HB.

WILKINSON, John Darrell Department of Dermatology, Amersham General Hospital, Amersham HP7 0JD Tel: 01494 734600 Fax: 01494 734620; The Chiltern Hospital, London Road, Great Missenden HP16 0DG Tel: 01494 890890 Fax: 01494 890858 — MB BS Lond. 1972 (St. Thos.) MRCS Eng. LRCP Lond. 1972; FRCP UK 1988, M 1975. Cons. Dermat. & Assoc. Clin. Dir. S. Bucks. NHS Trust; Hon. Lect. Univ. Lond.; Chair. Euro. Environmental Contact Dermatitus Research Group; Cons. Dermatologist at the Chiltern Hosp., Great Nissendon, Bucks. Specialty: Dermat. Socs: Eur. Environm. Contact Dermat. Research Gp.; Eur. Soc. Contact Dermat.; Mem. Brit Assn. Dermatol. Prev: Sen. Regist. (Dermat.) St. Thos. Hosp. Lond.

WILKINSON, Mr John Leonard, OBE (retired) Quince Cottage, Llysworney, Cowbridge CF71 7NQ — MB ChB Manch. 1948; MRCS Eng. LRCP Lond. 1948; MD Manch. 1952; FRCS Eng. 1956; DTM & H Liverp. 1961. Prev: Sen. Lect. (Anat.) Univ. Coll. Cardiff.

WILKINSON, John Lindow (retired) Netherwood Cottage, Brookledge Lane, Adlington, Macclesfield SK10 4JU — MB ChB Leeds 1955. Prev: SHO (Paediat.) & Obst. Ho. Off. W. Pk. Hosp. Macclesfield.

WILKINSON, John Patrick Dinsmore Meadowside Family Health Centre, 30 Winchcombe Road, Solihull B92 8PJ Tel: 0121 743 2560/742 5666 Fax: 0121 743 4216 — MB ChB Birm. 1988; DGM RCP Lond. 1991; DRCOG 1992; MRCGP 1995. Prev: GP/SHO Ho. Med. Alexandra Hosp. Redditch; GP/SHO Bromsgrove & Redditch VTS Ho. Surg. Qu. Eliz. Hosp. Birm.; Trainee GP/SHO (Geriat.) Alexandra Hosp. Redditch VTS.

WILKINSON, Professor John Robert North East Public Health Observatory, Wolfson Research Institute, University of Durham Queen's campus, Stockton-on-Tees TS17 6BH Tel: 0191 334 0400 Fax: 0191 334 0392 Email: john.wilkinson@nepho.org.uk; Topside House, Marrick, Richmond DL11 7LQ Tel: 01748 884740 Fax: 01748 884975 Email: john.wilkinson@nepho.org.uk — MB ChB Ed. 1977 (Edinburgh) DRCOG 1980; MRCGP 1982; MFCM 1987; FFPHM 1994; MD Edin 2001. Director North East Pub. health observatory; Vis. Prof. of Pub. Health, Univ. of Teesside; Prof., Univ. of Durh.; Vis.. Sen. Lect. Nuffield Inst. Univ. Leeds 1994.; Visiting Fellow, University of York. Specialty: Pub. Health Med. Socs: BMA; Soc. for Social Med.; Fac. of Pub. health Med. Prev: Cons. Pub. Health S. Cumbria HA; Dir. Pub. Health Northallerton HA; Dep. Director of Pub. Health N. Yorks. Health Authority.

WILKINSON, Jonathan James Arthur Harbury Surgery, Mill Street, Harbury, Leamington Spa CV33 9HR Tel: 01926 612232 Fax: 01926 612991 — MB ChB Birm. 1988; MRCGP 1994. Specialty: Gen. Pract.

WILKINSON, Mr Jonathan Mark Orthopaedic Directorate, Lincoln Hospitals NHS Trust, County Hospital, Greetwell Road, Lincoln LN2 5QY Tel: 01522 573217 Fax: 01522 573080; The Hall, Norton Disney, Lincoln LN6 9JP Tel: 01636 892011 — MB BS Lond. 1965 (St. Bart.) MRCS Eng. LRCP Lond. 1965; FRCS Eng. 1972. Cons. Orthop. Surg. Lincoln Hosps. Specialty: Orthop. Prev: Sen. Regist. Rotat. (Orthop.) St. Bart. Hosp. Lond.; Regist. (Surg.) Ipswich Hosp.; Ho. Surg. St. Bart. Hosp. Lond.

WILKINSON, Julia Charlotte Fairfield, Bepton, Midhurst GU29 0NA — MB BCh BAO Dub. 1967; DPM Eng. 1972; MRCPsych 1973. Cons. Adult Ment. Illness Graylingwell Hosp. Chichester. Specialty: Gen. Psychiat. Prev: Sen. Psychiat. Regist. Roy. Edin. Hosp.; Sen. Psychiat. Regist. & Regist. (Psychiat.) Fulbourn Hosp. Camb.

WILKINSON, Kathleen Ann Norfolk & Norwich University Hospital NHS Trust, Colney Lane, Norwich NR4 Tel: 01603 287086 Fax: 01603 287886 Email: kathy.wilkinson@nnuh.nhs.uk; Manor Moorings, 10 Yarmouth Road, Thorpe St Andrew, Norwich NR7 0EF Tel: 01603 434116 — MB BS Lond. 1981 (Guys) DCH RCP Lond. 1983; FFA RCS Eng 1986; MRCP (UK) 1989; FRCPCH 1999. Cons. Paediat. Anaesth. Norf. & Norwich Health Care Trust. Specialty: Anaesth. Socs: Assoc. of Paediat. Anaesth. Prev: Cons. Paediat. Intens. Care Unit & Paediat. Anaesth. Hosp. Sick Childr. Gt. Ormond St. Lond.

WILKINSON, Keith Noble's Hospital, Douglas IM4 4EA — MB ChB Liverp. 1982; MRCP London 1986; FRCA London 1987. Cons. Anaesth., Braddan, Isle of Man. Specialty: Anaesth.

WILKINSON, Kenneth Norman 37 Aire Valley Drive, Bradley, Keighley BD20 9HY — MB ChB Leeds 1971; BSc Leeds 1968, MB ChB 1971; DCH Eng. 1974; MRCP (UK) 1975. Cons. Paediat. Airedale Gen. Hosp. Steeton. Specialty: Paediat.

WILKINSON, Laura Margaret West of Scotland Breast Screening Centre, Stock Exchange Court, Nelson Mandela Place, Glasgow G2 1QT Tel: 0141 572 5833 Fax: 0141 572 5801; Laigh Monkcastle, Dalry Road, Kilwinning KA13 6PN — MB ChB Glas.

1984; FRCR 1992. Cons. Radiol. West. Infirm. Glas. & Breast Screening Centre Glas.; Hon. Sen. Lect. Univ. Glas. Specialty: Radiol. Socs: Roy. Coll. Radiol. Prev: Sen. Regist. (Diag. Radiol.) West. Infirm. Glas.

WILKINSON, Louise Sarah Radiology Dept, St Georges Hospital, Blackshaw Road, London SW17 0QT Tel: 020 8672 1255 — BM BCh Oxf. 1987; BA Oxf. 1984; FRCR 1993. Cons. (diagnostic Radiol.) St Geo.s Hosp. Specialty: Radiol. Prev: Sen. Regist. (Diagn. Radiol.) Roy. Marsden Hosp.

WILKINSON, Lucille Marie 39 Christchurch Road, Norwich NR2 2BX — MB ChB Otago 1990.

WILKINSON, Marcia Isobel Pamela Gangies Farm, Gangies Hill, High Wych, Sawbridgeworth CM21 0LD Tel: 01279 721178 Fax: 01279 725724; Gangies Farm, Gangies Hill, High Wych, Sawbridgeworth CM21 0LD Tel: 01279 721178 — BM BCh Oxf. 1943; FRCP Lond. 1963, M 1946; MA Oxf. 1945, DM 1959. Specialty: Neurol.; Rehabil. Med. Socs: Fell. Roy. Soc. Med.; Assn. Brit. Neurols.; (Ex-Pres.) Internat. Headache Soc. Prev: Cons. Neurol. Eliz. G. Anderson Hosp. Lond. & Hackney Hosp.; Dir. Regional Neurol. Unit East. Hosp. Lond.; Sen. Regist. (Neurol.) Lond. Hosp.

WILKINSON, Margaret Anne (retired) 33 Summerhouse Avenue, Hounslow TW5 9DJ Tel: 0208 570 2831 — (Roy. Free) Acad. Dip. Gen. Biochem. Univ. Lond. 1966; MB BS Lond. 1970; DPM Eng. 1973; MSc (Neurochem.) Lond. 1974; MRCPsych 1977. Prev: Cons. Child & Adolesc. Psychiat. E. Berks. NHS Community Health Trust.

WILKINSON, Margaret Elizabeth The Coach House, Bolam, Morpeth NE61 3UA — MB ChB Ed. 1990; MRCP (UK) 1993.

WILKINSON, Mark 24 Grasmere Drive, Liverpool L21 5JJ — MB ChB Liverp. 1993.

WILKINSON, Mark Jonathan Department of Histopathology, Norfolk &Norwich University Hospital, Corley Lane, Norwich — MB ChB Birm. 1982; MRCPath 1990. Cons. Histopath Norf. & Norwich Univ. Hosp.. Specialty: Histopath. Prev: Lect. (Path.) Univ. Nottm.

WILKINSON, Mark Lawrence Guy's & St Thomas Hospital Trust, 1st Floor, College House, St Thomas' Hospital, London SE1 7EH Tel: 020 7188 2498 Fax: 020 7188 2484 Email: mark.wilkinson@gstt.nhs.uk — MB BS Lond. 1974 (Middlx. Hosp.) MRCP (UK) 1977; BSc Lond. 1971, MD 1985; FRCP Lond. 1992. Sen. Lect. & Cons. Gastroenterol. GKT Sch. Of Med. KCL. Guy's & St. Thos. Hosps. Lond. Specialty: Gastroenterol. Special Interest: ERCP. Socs: Brit. Soc. Gastroenterol. (Endoscopy Comm. Train. Off.); Internat. Assn. Study Liver; US. Soc.Gastrointestinal Endoscopy. Prev: Lect. Liver Unit King's Coll. Sch. Med. & Dent. Lond.; Regist. (Gastroenterol.) Middlx. Hosp. Lond.

WILKINSON, Martin John Brian The Harlequin Surgery, 160 Shard End Crescent, Shard End, Birmingham B34 7BP Tel: 0121 747 8291 Fax: 0121 749 5497; 249 Boldmere Road, Sutton Coldfield B73 5LL Tel: 0121 354 9973 — MB ChB Birm. 1982; DRCOG 1984; DCH RCP Lond. 1985; FRCGP 1993, M 1986; MMedSc Birm. 1994. Course Organiser E. Birm. VTS; Dep. Area Director Birm. Black Coventry & Solihull. Socs: Vice Chairm. Mid. Fac. Roy. Coll. GPs. Prev: Clin. Asst. (Paediat. Nephrol.) E. Birm. Hosp.; Trainee GP/SHO Centr. Birm. HA VTS; Trainee GP Sutton Coldfield & BromsGr..

WILKINSON, Mrs Mary Julia (retired) Rivermead House, Charmouth, Bridport DT6 6RR Tel: 01297 560683 — MB BS Lond. 1959 (Middlx.) DCH Eng. 1963; DObst RCOG 1964; MRCP (UK) 1977. Prev: Cons. Community Paediat. Thorpe Coombe Hosp. Lond.

WILKINSON, Matthew Blackbird Leys Health Centre, 63 Blackbird Leys Road, Oxford OX4 6HL Tel: 01865 778244; 93 Church Road, Sandford-on-Thames, Oxford OX4 4YA Tel: 01865 774178 — MB ChB Manch. 1976. Prev: Med. Off. Save the Childr. Fund Nepal.

WILKINSON, Matthew (retired) 3 Arnhall Gardens, Dundee DD2 1PH Tel: 01382 669320 — MB BChir Camb. 1949; FRCP Lond. 1972, M 1951; MD Camb. 1956; FRCP Ed. 1974, M 1969. Phys. Ninewells Hosp. Dundee; Lect. (Clin. Med.) Univ. Dundee. Prev: Phys. Ninewells Hosp. Dundee.

WILKINSON, Michael Boyd Department of Anaesthetics, Northampton General Hospital, Cliftonville, Northampton NN1 5BD Tel: 01604 545671 Fax: 01604 545672; Cherry Tree Cottage, 84 Billing Road, Brafield on The Green, Northampton NN7 1BL Tel: 01604 891509 — MB BS Lond. 1985 (St. Thos. Hosp. Lond.) LMSSA Lond. 1984; FCAnaesth 1990. Cons. Northampton Gen. Hosp. Trust. Specialty: Anaesth. Prev: Sen. Regist. Rotat. (Anaesth.) Newc.; Assoc. Prof. Duke Univ. Med. Center, USA.

WILKINSON, Mr Michael Charles Paul Department of Orthopaedic Surgery, King's College Hospital, Denmark Hill, London SE5 9RS Tel: 020 7346 3649 — MB BS Lond. 1982 (Westminster London) BSc (Hons.) Lond. 1979; FRCS Eng. 1986; FRCS (Orth.) 1994. Cons. Orthop. Surg. King's Coll. Hosp. Lond. Specialty: Trauma & Orthop. Surg. Socs: Fell. BOA; BASK. Prev: Sen. Regist. (Orthop.) Roy. N. Shore Hosp. Sydney NSW, Austral.; Sen. Regist. Rotat. (Orthop. Surg.) Char. Cross Hosp. Lond. & Regist. Rotat. (Orthop. Surg.) St Mary's Hosp. Lond.; SHO (Plastic Surg.) Qu. Mary's Hosp. Lond.

WILKINSON, Mr Michael James Swiers Royal Bolton Hospital, Minerva Road, Farnworth, Bolton BL4 0JR Tel: 01204 390538 Fax: 01204 390544; 8 Chelwood Mews, Chorley New Road, Lostock, Bolton BL6 4BF Email: mcquilk@doctors.org.uk — MS Lond. 1986 (Univ. Coll. Hosp.) BSc (Hons.) Lond. 1972, MS 1986, MB BS 1976; FRCS Eng. 1980. Cons. Surg. Roy. Bolton Hosp. Specialty: Gen. Surg. Socs: Fell. Assn. Surgs.; Fell. Assn. Upper G.I. Surg.; Fell. Roy. Soc. Med. Prev: Sen. Regist. (Surg.) NW Train. Scheme Salford HA; Research Fell. Christie Hosp. Manch.; Regist. Roy. Marsden Childrens Hosp.

WILKINSON, Nafisa Department of Histopathology, St. James's Hospital, Leeds LS9 7TF Tel: 0113 206 4196 Fax: 0113 206 5943 — MB BChir Camb. 1984; BA Camb. 1982; MRCPath 1993. Cons. in Gyn. Path. Specialty: Histopath. Prev: Lect. & Sen. Regist. (Histopath.) Univ. Leeds; Lect. & Sen. Regist. (Histopath.) Univ. Manch.; Regist. (Histopath.) NW RHA.

WILKINSON, Nicholas Mark Coleford Health Centre, Railway Drive, Coleford GL16 8RH Tel: 01594 598068; Millover, Main Road, Mile End, Coleford GL16 7BY Tel: 01594 810262 Email: nick@coleford.demon.co.uk — MB BS Lond. 1980 (Guy's) MRCGP 1984; DRCOG 1985; MSC Ther. Wales 2002. Princip. in Gen. Pract., Drs. Wilkinson, Longley, Cummins and Adams, Coleford Health Centre, Coleford, Gloucestershire; Clin. Asst. Endoscopy, Dilme Hosp., Cinderford, Gloucestershire. Specialty: Gen. Pract.

WILKINSON, Nicholas Michael Reginald 4 The Knoll, Billericay CM12 0NT — MB ChB Ed. 1990.

WILKINSON, Patricia Ann Stacksteads Surgery, 20 Farholme Lane, Stacksteads, Bacup OL13 0EX Tel: 01706 873122 Fax: 01706 874152 — MB ChB Manch. 1989. GP Princip. Specialty: Gen. Pract. Prev: GP Locum; GP Trainee, Burnley.

WILKINSON, Patricia Anne (retired) 45 Carsick Hill Crescent, Sheffield S10 3LS Tel: 0114 230 8612 — MB ChB Leeds 1972; FRCA 1976. Prev: Cons. Anaesth. Roy. Hallamsh. Hosp. Sheff.

WILKINSON, Paul Daryll Environmental Epidemiology Unit, London School of Hygiene and Tropical Medicine, Keppel St., London WC1E 7HT Tel: 020 7927 2444 Fax: 020 7580 4524; 31B Adolphus Road, Finsbury Park, London N4 2AT Tel: 020 8809 4309 — BM BCh Oxf. 1985; MRCP (UK) 1989; MSc Lond. 1991. Sen. Lect. (Environm. Epidemiol.) Lond. Sch. Hyg. & Trop. Med. Specialty: Epidemiol.

WILKINSON, Paul Oliver Douglas House, 146 Trumpington Road, Cambridge CB2 2AH — MA MB Bchir Camb. Camb. 1996; DCH; MRCPsych.

WILKINSON, Paul Robert — MB BS Newc. 1988; CCST (Anaesth.); T(GP); BMedSc Newc. 1987; MRCGP 1993; FRCA 1997. Cons. (Pain. Managem.) Roy. Vict. Infirm.; Hon. Sen. Lect. Univ. of Newc. Upon Tyne. Specialty: Anaesth. Prev: Specialist Regist. (Anaesth.) Roy. Vict. Infirm.; Pain Managem. Unit. Roy. Vict. Infirm; Trainee GP N.d. VTS.

WILKINSON, Pauline Belfast City Hospital, Lisburn Road, Belfast BT9 6NF Tel: 02890 882000 — MB BCh BAO Belf. 1987; MRCP (UK) 1991; MD Belf. 1995. Cons. Belfast City Hosp./ Marie Claire Centre. Specialty: Palliat. Med. Prev: Cons. Northern Irel. Hospice Belf.

WILKINSON, Professor Peter Charles 26 Randolph Road, Glasgow G11 7LG — (Lond. Hosp.) FRSE; MB BS Lond. 1956; MD Lond. 1967. Emerit. Prof. Cellular Immunol. Univ. Glas. Specialty: Immunol. Socs: Brit. Soc. Immunol. Prev: Vis. Prof. Rockerfeller Univ. New York; Lect. (Bact.) Lond. Hosp. Med. Coll.

WILKINSON, Peter John Health Protection Agency, HPA Corporate Affairs, 61 Colindale Avenue, London NW9 5DF Tel: 020 83276636 Email: peter.wilkinson@hpa.org.uk; Hambledon House,

Lodgefield Lane, Hoveringham, Nottingham NG14 7JQ Tel: 0115 966 4411 — MB BChir Camb. 1971 (Camb. & King's Coll. Hosp.) MA Camb. 1969; FRCPath 1988, M 1976. Head of Clin. Governance. Specialty: Med. Microbiol. Socs: Assn. Med. Microbiol.; Hosp. Infec. Soc.; Path. Soc. Prev: Regional Microbiol. E. Midlands; Cons. (Microbiol.) & Dir., Pub. Health Laborat. Nottm.; Cons. (Microbiol.) & Dir. Pub. Health Laborat. Plymouth.

WILKINSON, Peter Maurice 12 Ramsdale Road, Bramhall, Stockport SK7 2PZ — MRCS Eng. LRCP Lond. 1964 (Manch.) MSc (Clin. Pharmacol.) Manch. 1973, MB ChB 1964; MRCP (UK) 1974; FRCP Lond. 1985; FRCR (Hon.) 1993. Cons. Clin. Pharmacol. Christie Hosp. & Holt Radium Inst. Manch.; Lect. (Clin. Pharmacol.) Manch. Univ. Specialty: Pharmacology. Prev: Vis. Prof. (Med. Oncol.) Sidney Farber Cancer Inst. Boston, USA; Lect. (Med.) Harvard Med. Sch.

WILKINSON, Peter Raymond 90 Graham Avenue, Patcham, Brighton BN1 8HD — MB BS Lond. 1982 (Westm.) BSc (Hons.) Lond. 1979; MRCP (UK) 1987; MFPHM RCP (UK) 1996; Dipo.Tropical Med. And Hygiene Royal College of Physicians 1997. Cons. in Pub. Health Med., Brighton & Hove City PCT.

WILKINSON, Peter Roger Ashford Hospital, London Road, Ashford TW15 3AA Tel: 01784 884279 Fax: 01784 884612 Email: peterwilkinson@doctors.org.uk; St Peter's Hospital, Chertsey KT16 0PZ Tel: 01932 872000 Ext: 3988 — (Lond. Hosp.) MRCS Eng. LRCP Lond. 1969; MB BS Lond. 1969; DObst RCOG 1971; FRCP Lond. 1988, M 1973; MD Lond. 1985. Cons. Cardiol. Ashford & St Peter Hosps. NHS Trust; Dir. Clin. Studies Imperial Coll. Sch. Med. Specialty: Cardiol.; Gen. Med. Socs: Cardiac Soc. Prev: Sen. Regist. (Med.) Bristol Roy. Infirm.; Vis. Lect. Univ. Calif., San Francisco; Regist. (Med.) Northwick Pk. Hosp.

WILKINSON, Peter Stephen Bedford Road Surgery, 273 Bedford Road, Kempston, Bedford MK42 8QD Tel: 01234 852222 Fax: 01234 843558; 13 Cranfield Road, Wootton, Bedford MK43 9EB Tel: 01234 768434 — MB ChB Leic. 1981; DRCOG 1984; DCH RCP Lond. 1985; MRCGP 1985.

WILKINSON, Peter Winston (retired) Culross, 15 kingsway, Gayton, Wirral CH60 3SN Tel: 0151 342 6864 — MD Leeds 1977; MB ChB 1966; DCH Eng. 1968; FRCP Lond. 1988; FRCPCH 1997. Prev: Cons. Paediat. Arrowe Pk. Hosp. Wirral.

WILKINSON, Philip Ann 38 Oakwood Road, Sturry, Canterbury CT2 0LX — MB BS Lond. 1996.

WILKINSON, Philip Barr Oxfordshire Mental Healthcare NHS Trust, The Fulbrook Centre, Churchill Hospital, Old Road, Headington, Oxford OX3 7JU — BM BS Nottm. 1986.

WILKINSON, Raymond Walker (retired) 9 Granary Wharf, 57 Commercial Road, Weymouth DT4 8AL Tel: 01305 778967 Mob: 0779 509 4079 Email: ss9@btinternet.com — MB ChB Leeds 1945; DCH Eng. 1948; DMRD Eng. 1952; FFR 1956; FRCR 1975. Prev: Cons. Radiol. Reading Gp. Hosps.

WILKINSON, Richard David Churchfields Surgery, Recreation Road, Bromsgrove B61 8DT Tel: 01527 872163; Robins Meadow, 43 Hanbury Road, Stoke Prior, Bromsgrove B60 4DW — MB ChB Birm. 1965; MRCS Eng. LRCP Lond. 1965; DObst RCOG 1967. Hon. Phys. BromsGr. Cott. Hosp. Prev: Ho. Surg. & Ho. Phys. Qu. Eliz. Hosp. Birm.; Ho. Surg. Gen. Hosp. Birm.

WILKINSON, Richard Hanwell (retired) 26 Emden House, Barton Lane, Headington, Oxford OX3 9JU Tel: 01865 762973 — MB BChir Camb. 1946 (Lond. Hosp.) MRCS Eng. LRCP Lond. 1946; MA, MD Camb. 1952; FRCPath 1969, M 1964. Hon. Cons. Path. Oxf. HA. Prev: Cons. Chem. Path. Oxon. AHA (T).

WILKINSON, Robert Royal Infirmary, Blackburn BB2 3LR Tel: 01254 263555; (cons. rooms), Beardwood Hospital, Preston New Road, Blackburn BB2 7BG Tel: 01254 507607 — MB ChB (Hons) Leeds 1975; BSc (Pharm.) (Hons.) Leeds 1965; PhD Leeds 1972, BSc (Pharmacol.) (Hons.) 1966; MRCP (UK) 1978; FRCP Lond. 1992. Cons. Phys. (Gen. Med.) (s/i Endocrinol. & Diabetes) East Lancashire Hospitals Trust. Specialty: Endocrinol.; Diabetes; Gen. Med. Prev: Lect. (Clin. Med.) Univ. Birm. & Qu. Eliz. Hosp. Birm.; Regist. (Gen. Med.) Newc. AHA (T); Scientif. Staff MRC Mineral Metab. Unit Gen. Infirm. Leeds.

WILKINSON, Professor Robert Sunderland Royal Hospital, Renal Unit, Kayll Road, Sunderland SR4 7TP — MB BS (Hons.) Durh. 1963 (Newc.) BSc (Hons.) Durh. 1960; MRCP Lond. 1967; MD (Commend.) Newc. 1979; FRCP Lond. 1979. Locum Cons. Nephrol. Sunderland Roy. Hosps.; Prof. Emerit. Univ. Newc. Specialty: Nephrol. Special Interest: Hypertension. Socs: Nat. Assn. Phys. UK & Irel.; Renal Assn.; Brit. Hypertens. Soc. Prev: Prof. (Nephrol.) Univ. Newc.; Cons. Nephrol. Newc. Hosps. NHS Trust; Reader (Med.) Newc. Univ. Hosp.

WILKINSON, Sally Ann Southmead Hospital, Westbury-on-Trym, Bristol BS10 5NB Tel: 0117 950 5050 — MB ChB Bristol 1976; BSc (Hons.) Bristol 1973; MRCPsych 1983. Staff Grade (Psychiat.) Southmead Hosp. Bristol. Specialty: Gen. Psychiat. Prev: Clin. Asst. (Psychiat.) Southmead Hosp. Bristol.; Ho. Off. Southmead Hosp. Westbury-on-Trym & Ham Green Hosp. Bristol.

WILKINSON, Sarah Anne 8 Avondale Road, Ponteland, Newcastle upon Tyne NE20 9NA — BM BS Nottm. 1994.

WILKINSON, Sarah Louise 9 Gainsborough Road, Ipswich IP4 2UR — MB ChB Sheff. 1993.

WILKINSON, Sarah Louise 38 College Road, Upholland, Skelmersdale WN8 0PY — MB BS Lond. 1998.

WILKINSON, Simon David Midfield House, 75 Kidderminster Road, Hagley, Stourbridge DY9 0QN; 27 Hall Meadow, Hagley, Stourbridge DY9 9LE — MB ChB Birm. 1972. Socs: BMA. Prev: Trainee Gen. Pract. Abergavenny Vocational Train. Scheme; Ho. Phys. Worcester Roy. Infirm.; Ho. Surg. Gen. Hosp. Birm.

WILKINSON, Simon Malcolm 4 Londesborough Road, Market Weighton, York YO43 3AY Tel: 01430 873433 Fax: 01430 871466 — MB ChB Manch. 1988 (Manchester) DRCOG 1991; MRCGP 1992. Gen. Practioner, Marketweighton; PCT & Area Prescribing Comm. Specialty: Gen. Pract. Prev: Health Developm. Off. Nainital, India.

WILKINSON, Stephen Edward 18A North End, Durham DH1 4NJ — MB BS Newc. 1991; MRCPsych 1998.

WILKINSON, Stephen Mark Department of Dermatology, The General Infirmary, Leeds LS1 3EX — MB BChir Camb. 1984; MD Camb. 1995, BA 1982, MB BChir 1984; DRCOG 1987; MRCP (UK) 1989. Cons. Dermat. Leeds Gen. Infirm. Specialty: Dermat. Prev: Sen. Regist. (Dermat.) Skin Hosp. Manch.

WILKINSON, Stephen Paul Woodend Hospital, Aberdeen AB15 6XS Tel: 01224 556513 Fax: 01224 404019; 36 Brighton Place, Aberdeen AB10 6RS — MB BS Newc. 1979; MRCP (UK) 1982; FRCP Ed. 1999. Cons. Geriat. Med. Grampian HB; Hon. Clin. Sen. Lect. Univ. Aberd. Specialty: Care of the Elderly. Socs: Brit. Geriat. Soc.; Aberd. M-C Soc. Prev: Sen. Regist. (Geriat.) Grampian HB; Regist. (Geriat.) Tayside HB; Research Fell. Dept. Med. Ninewells Hosp. Dundee.

WILKINSON, Stephen Percy Derriford Hospital, Plymouth PL6 8DH Tel: 01752 792686; RidgeCt., Court Road, Newton Ferrers, Plymouth PL8 1DD Tel: 01752 873190 — (King's Coll. Hosp.) BSc (1st cl. Hons.) Lond. 1966, MD 1978, MB BS 1969; FRCP Lond. 1985. Cons. Phys. Derriford Hosp. Plymouth. Specialty: Gastroenterol. Socs: Brit. Soc. Gastroenterol. & Med. Res. Soc.; Assn. Phys. Prev: Cons. Phys. Glos. Roy. Hosp. Gloucester; Sen. Regist. Liver Unit King's Coll. Hosp. Lond.; SHO Radcliffe Infirm. Oxf.

WILKINSON, Tanya Sarah 27 Mucklestone Wood Lane, Loggerheads, Market Drayton TF9 4ED — MB ChB Manch. 1993.

WILKINSON, Theresa Dennis (retired) 128 Shepherds Bush Centre, London W12 8QX Tel: 020 8749 1882 — MB BS Lond. 1967 (Guy's) MRCS Eng. LRCP Lond. 1966.

WILKINSON, Timothy John McLaughlin and Partners, 27-29 Derby Road, North End, Portsmouth PO2 8HP Tel: 023 9266 3024 Fax: 023 9265 4991 — MB BS Lond. 1980.

WILKINSON, William Hardman (retired) Baringo, The Keep Gardens, Dartmouth TQ6 9JA — MRCS Eng. LRCP Lond. 1951 (St. Bart.) Prev: Wing Cdr. RAF Med. Br., Surg. Specialist RAF Hosp. Ely.

WILKS, David Michael Worsley 806 Duncan House, Dolphin Square, London SW1V 3PP Tel: 0207 798 5524 Email: michael@mwilks.demon.co.uk — MB BS Lond. 1972 (St. Mary's) DObst RCOG 1974. Princip. FME Metrop. Police. Socs: Assn. Police Surg. (Chairm. Metrop. & City Gp.); Chairm. Med. Ethics Comm. BMA; Dep. Chairm. Representative Body, BMA. Prev: GP Lond. & Richmond Surrey; Ho. Phys. & Ho. Off. (O & G) St. Mary's Hosp. Lond.; Ho. Surg. Wembley Hosp.

WILKS, David Peter Regional Infectious Diseases Unit, Western General Hospital, Crewe Road, Edinburgh EH4 2XU — MB BChir Camb. 1983; MRCP (UK) 1986; DTM & H RCP Lond. 1987; MA,

MD Camb. 1991; FRCP Edin. 2003. Cons. Phys. (Infec. Dis.) Western Gen. Hosp. Edin. Specialty: Infec. Dis. Socs: Fell. Roy. Soc. Trop. Med. & Hyg. Prev: Sen. Regist. (Infec. Dis. & Gen. Med.) Addenbrooke's Hosp. Camb.; Research Regist. (Immunol.) Clin. Research Centre Harrow; Regist. (Med.) Univ. Coll. Hosp. Lond.

WILKS, Diana Bramhall Health Centre, 66 Bramhall Lane South, Bramhall, Stockport SK7 2DY Tel: 0161 439 8213 Fax: 0161 439 6398; 9 Davenport Park Road, Davenport Road, Stockport SK7 6JU — MB ChB Manch. 1973.

WILKS, Mr John (retired) 15 Lostock Junction Lane, Bolton BL6 4JR — MB BS Lond. 1942 (Guy's) MRCS Eng. LRCP Lond. 1942; FRCS Eng. 1949. Cons. Surg. Bolton Hosp. Gp. Prev: Sen. Regist. Hosp. For Sick Childr. Gt. Ormond St.

WILKS, John Maurice (retired) The Spinney, Moult Hill, Salcombe TQ8 8LG Tel: 01548 842860 — MB BS Lond. 1946 (Guy's) MRCGP 1966.

WILKS, Mark Monkspath, Limerstone, Newport PO30 4AA Tel: 01983 740887 — MRCS Eng. LRCP Lond. 1942 (Guy's)

WILKS, Martin ZENECA Agrochemicals, Fernhurst, Haslemere GU27 3JE Tel: 01428 655041 Fax: 01428 657130 — State Exam Med Hanover 1983; MD Hanover 1986; PhD Surrey 1990. Med. Adviser, Zeneca AgroChem.s Fernhurst; Hon. Cons. Med. Toxicol. Guy's Hosp. Lond. Specialty: Occupat. Health. Prev: Clin. Toxicol. ICI Centr. Toxicol. Lab. Macclesfield.; Asst. (Intern. Med.) Med. Sch., Hannover.

WILKS, Peter Robert Witley Surgery, Wheeler Lane, Witley, Godalming GU8 5QR Tel: 01428 682218 Fax: 01428 682218; Sandhills Corner, Wormley, Godalming GU8 5UF Tel: 01428 683918 — MB Camb. 1978; MA Camb. 1980, MB 1978, BChir 1977; DRCOG 1981; MRCGP 1982. Specialty: Dermat. Prev: Trainee GP Norf. & Norwich Hosp. VTS; SHO (Path.) Char. Cross Hosp. Lond.; Ho. Surg. & Ho. Phys. Char. Cross Hosp. Lond.

WILL, Andrew Marshall Royal Manchester Childrens Hospital, Hospital Road, Pendlebury, Manchester M27 4HA Tel: 0161 727 2245 Fax: 0161 727 2545 Email: andrew.will@cmmc.nhs.uk — MD Manch. 1992; MB ChB 1978; MRCP (UK) 1983; MRCPath 1992. Cons. Paediat. Haemat. Roy. Manch. Childr. Hosp. Specialty: Haematology. Socs: N. W. Paediatric Assn.; N. W. Haemat. Assn.; BMA Paediatric CCSC.

WILL, David John The Young People's Unit, Royal Edinburgh Hospital, Tipperlinn Road, Edinburgh EH10 5HF Tel: 0131 447 2011; 5 Warrender Park Terrace, Edinburgh EH9 1JA — MB ChB Ed. 1972; MRCPsych 1977; FRCPsych 1995. Cons. Adolesc. Psychiat. Roy. Edin. Hosp. Specialty: Child & Adolesc. Psychiat. Socs: SAAP. Prev: Cons. (Child & Adolesc. Psychiat.) Roy. Infirm. Dundee; Asst. Prof. Dept. Psychiat. McMaster Univ. Canada; Sen. Regist. (Child & Adolesc. Psychiat.) Lothian Health Bd.

WILL, Eric John St James's University Hospital, Beckett Street, Leeds LS9 7TF Tel: 0113 206 4354 Fax: 0113 206 6216 — BM BCh Oxf. 1969 (Guy's) MA Oxf. 1972; FRCP Lond. 1989. Cons. Renal Med. St. Jas. Univ. Hosp. Leeds. Specialty: Nephrol. Socs: Roy. Soc. Med.; Eur. Renal Assn. Prev: Lect. (Med.) Nottm. Gen. Hosp.; Sen. Regist. (Med.) Nottm. City Hosp.; FUNGO Research Fell. Univ. Hosp. Leiden.

WILL, Malcolm Brodie 8 Alder Drive, Burghmuir, Perth PH1 1ER — MB ChB Glas. 1998.

WILL, Margaret 21 Berryhill Drive, Griffnock, Glasgow G46 7AS — MB ChB Glas. 1943 (Univ. Glas.) BSc Glas. 1940, MB ChB 1943. Med. Asst. Cytol. Roy. Samarit. Hosp. Glas. Prev: Ho. Surg. Glas. Roy. Infirm. & Roy. Matern. Hosp. Glas.

WILL, Richard Trenton, Ford Road, Lanchester, Durham DH7 0SN — MB BS Lond. 1972 (St. Geo.) FFA RCS Eng. 1977. Cons. (Anaesth.) Dryburn Hosp. Durh. Specialty: Anaesth.

WILL, Professor Robert George Department of Clinical Neurosciences, Western General Hospital, Edinburgh EH4 2XU; 4 St Catherine's Place, Edinburgh EH4 2XU Tel: 0131 667 3667 — MD Camb. 1985 (Lond. Hosp.) MA Camb. 1985, BA 1971, MB BChir 1974; MRCP (UK) 1978; FRCP(E) 1991; FRCP 1994. Prof. Cons. Neurol. West. Gen. Hosp. Edin. Specialty: Neurol. Special Interest: Jakob Disease. Socs: Scot. Soc. Phys.; Assn. Brit. Neurols. Prev: Sen. Regist. Guy's & Maida Vale Hosps. Lond.; Regist. (Neurol.) Nat. Hosp. Nerv. Dis. Lond.; Hon. Regist. (Neurol.) Dept. Clin. Neurol. Univ. Oxf.

WILL, Sheila Carol Catherine 1 Vale Road, Bowdon, Altrincham WA14 3JA — MB ChB Manch. 1978; BSc St. And. 1975; MFPHM 1992.

WILLAMUNE, Navaratne Bandara Northgate Hospital, Victoria Block, Great Yarmouth NR30 1BU Tel: 01493 337643 — MB BS Sri Lanka 1973 (Univ. of Ceylon) MRCPsych 1983. Cons., Locum Long Term; Psychiat., Old Age. Specialty: Gen. Psychiat. Socs: Brit. Med. Assn. Prev: Assoc. Specailist, Northgate Hosp.; Locum Cons., Northgate Hosp.; Regist., Brookwood Hosp., Woking Surrey.

WILLAN, Alison Louise York Road Group Practice, York Road, Ellesmere Port, South Wirral CH65 0DB Tel: 0151 355 2112 Fax: 0151 356 5512; 37 Heath Drive, Upton, Wirral CH49 6LE — MB ChB Manch. 1991 (Manch) MRCGP 1995.

WILLAN, John Curwen (retired) Health Centre, Carfax St., Swindon SN4 9LW Tel: 01793 692880 — MB BChir Camb. 1954 (St. Thos.) BA, MB BChir Camb. 1954; DObst RCOG 1955; MRCP Lond. 1957. Prev: Asst. Lect. Path. St. Thos. Hosp.

WILLAN, Professor Peter Leslie Terence 30 Coniston Road, Gatley, Cheadle SK8 4AP Email: pwillan@talk21.com — MB ChB Birm. 1970; FRCS Glas. 1976. Freelance Anat. Specialty: Anat.; Educat. Socs: Fell. Brit. Assn. Clin. Anat.; Anat. Soc. Prev: Prof. Anat. Univ. United Arab Emirates, Al-Ain; Sen. Lect. (Anat.) Univ. Manch.

WILLAN, William Kenneth (retired) 24 Longfield Road, Shaw, Oldham OL2 7HD — MB ChB Manch. 1953. Prev: Ho. Phys. Boundary Pk. Gen. Hosp. Oldham.

WILLARD, Christopher John Colston Arnewood Practice, Milton Medical Centre, Avenue Road, New Milton BH25 5JP Tel: 01425 620393 Fax: 01425 624219; Aubrey House, Keyhaven, Lymington SO41 0TL Tel: 01590 643219 — MB BS Lond. 1968 (Guy's) MRCS Eng. LRCP Lond. 1968; DObst RCOG 1971; DCH Eng. 1971. Trainer (Gen. Pract.) & Regist. Course Organiser Soton.; Med. Off. New Forest Marathon. Prev: SHO (Obst.) FarnBoro. Hosp. Kent; SHO (Paediat.) St. Albans City Hosp.

WILLARD, Hilary Louise 65 Forest Road, Worthing BN14 9LR — MB BS Lond. 1993.

WILLARS, Christopher Mark 39 Hantone Hill, Bathampton, Bath BA2 6XD; Flat 5, Towerfields, Westerham Road, Keston BR2 6HF — MB BS Lond. 1998.

WILLATT, Mr David Jonathan ENT Dept, Hope Hospital, Eccles Old Road, Salford M6 8HD Tel: 0161 787 4758 Fax: 0161 787 4723 — MB Camb. 1980; BChir 1979; FRCS Lond. 1985; MD Liverp. 1995. Cons. ENT Surg. Salford Roy. Hosps. NHS Trust & Centr. Manch. & Manch. Children's Hosps.; Hon. Clin. Lect. Univ. Sch. Med. Manch. Specialty: Otorhinolaryngol. Prev: Cons. ENT Surg. Hope & Roy. Manch. Childr. Hosps. Salford HA; Sen. Regist. (Otorhinolaryngol. Univ. Liverp.

WILLATT, Ian Duncan (retired) Crouch Readon, Rake Road, Liss GU33 7HE Tel: 01730 893316 — MD Ed. 1946; MB ChB 1939; FRCGP 1973, M 1960. Prev: Regist. (Med.) Roy. Infirm. Chester.

WILLATT, Jonathon Myles 13 Heyford Road, Steeple Aston, Oxford OX6 3SY — MB ChB Manch. 1997.

WILLATT, Richard Norman The Surgery, Southview Lodge, South View, Bromley BR1 3DR Tel: 020 8460 1945 Fax: 020 8323 1423; 9 Beadon Road, Bromley BR2 9AS — MB ChB Ed. 1973.

WILLATT, Ruth Annette Janie (retired) Crouch Readon, Rake Road, Liss GU33 7HE Tel: 01730 893316 — MB ChB Ed. 1939; BA (Hons.) Open 1977, BA 1974. Prev: Ho. Phys. E. Gen. Hosp. Leith.

WILLATTS, David George Six Bells Cottage, Upper Brailes, Banbury OX15 5AZ Tel: 01608 685363 — MB BS Lond. 1975; MA Camb.; MRCS Eng. LRCP Lond. 1975; FFA RCS Eng. 1980. Cons. Anaesth. Horton Hosp. Banbury. Specialty: Anaesth. Prev: Sen. Regist. (Anaesth.) St. Thos. Hosp. Lond.

WILLATTS, Sheila Margaret 6 Westbury Park, Durdham Down, Bristol BS6 7JB Tel: 0117 974 3447 Fax: 0117 946 6429 Email: swillatts@compuserve.com — (Univ. Coll. Hosp.) MRCS Eng. LRCP Lond. 1967; MB BS Lond. 1967; DA Eng. 1969; DObst RCOG 1969; FRCA Eng. 1973; MRCP (UK) 1974; FRCP Lond. 1988; MD Lond. 1994. GMC Assoc., Med. Vice Chair, S. and W. Regional Awards Comm. Specialty: Anaesth.; Intens. Care. Socs: Assn. Anaesth.; Anaesth. Sect. RSM; Anaesth. Res. Soc. Prev: Cons. Anaesth. Bristol Roy. Infirm.; Sen. Regist. (Anaesth.) King's Coll. & Brook Gen. Hosps. Lond.; SHO (Anaesth.) St. Helier Hosp. Carshalton.

WILLBY, Lesley Ann The Surgery, 59 Sheep St., Burford OX18 4LS — MB BS Lond. 1982 (St. Geo. Hosp. Med. Sch. Lond.) DRCOG 1986. p/t GP Partner Burford Surg. Oxf. Specialty: Paediat. Prev: GP Perth, Austral.

WILLCOCKS, Julian Anthony James 85A The Street, Basingstoke RG24 7BY — MB BS Lond. 1992.

WILLCOCKS, Lisa Claire 76 Bournemouth Road, Poole BH14 0EY — BM BCh Oxf. 1998.

WILLCOX, Christine Heather (retired) The Red House, Lower Flat, 32 Daglands Road, Fowey PL23 1JN — (Roy. Free) MB BS Lond. 1964; MRCS Eng. LRCP Lond. 1964. Occupat. Phys. Cornw. Healthcare Trust & Cornw. Co. Counc. Prev: Dist. Occupat. Health Phys. NW Herts. HA.

WILLCOX, Christopher Philip William (retired) Shaftgate, Paddock Lane, Selsey, Chichester PO20 9AZ — (Camb. & St. Mary's) MB BChir Camb. 1966; MA Camb. 1966; DObst RCOG 1967. Prev: Ho. Surg. St. Mary's Hosp.

WILLCOX, Denys Roy Calder (retired) 8 Lady JaneCt., Cavendish Avenue, Cambridge CB1 7UW — MB BS Lond. 1949 (Guy's Hosp.) MRCS Eng. LRCP Lond. 1939; FRCPath 1969. Prev: Cons. Chem. Path. Harlow Dist. Hosps.

WILLCOX, Professor Hugh Nicholas Anson Neurosciences, Weatherall Institute for Molecular Medicine, John Radcliffe Hospital, Oxford OX3 9DS Tel: 01865 222325 Fax: 01865 222402 Email: nick.willcox@imm.ox.ac.uk; 74 Crescent Road, Temple Cowley, Oxford OX4 2PD Tel: 01865 779123 — MB BChir Camb. 1968 (Middlx.) BA Camb. 1965, MA 1969; PhD CNAA 1975. Sen. Research Fell. (Neurosci.) Weatherall Inst. Molecular Med. John Radcliffe Hosp. Oxf.; Research Lect. (Neurosci.) Univ. Oxf. Specialty: Immunol. Special Interest: Protein evolution. Socs: Brit. Soc. Immunol. Prev: Lect. (Anat.) Newc.; Ho. Phys. Middlx. Hosp. Lond.

WILLCOX, Jeremy Robert Lower Newlands, Godwell Lane, Ivybridge PL21 0LE Tel: 01752 892600 — MB BS Lond. 1970 (St. Mary's) MRCS Eng. LRCP Lond. 1972; DCH Eng. 1973. Cons. Genitourin. Med. Plymouth Torquay Hosps. Specialty: Genitourinary Medicine. Socs: Med. Soc. Study VD; Assn. Genitourin. Med. Prev: Lect. (Genitourin. Med.) Acad. Unit Middlx. Hosp.; Sen. Regist. (Genitourin. Med.) St. Thos. Hosp.; Surg. to P & O SN Company.

WILLCOX, Merlin Luke 36 Hare Close, Buckingham MK18 7EW — BM BCh Oxf. 1998; BA 1995; DCH Lond. 1999; DGM 2000; DFFP 2000; DRCOG 2000; MRCGP 2003; LoC IUT 2003; DTM & H 2004. Locum GP; Clin. Researcher Antenna Technolgies Switz.; Sec. Research Initiative on Traditional Antimalarial Methods. Specialty: Gen. Pract. Prev: GP Regist. E. Oxf. Health Centre Oxf.; GP Regist. Masonic Ho. Surg. Buckingham; SHO (A & E) John Radcliffe Hosp. Oxf.

WILLCOX, Richard Neston Surgery, Mellock Lane, Little Neston, South Wirral CH64 4BN Tel: 0151 336 3951 Fax: 0151 353 0173; 26 Earle Drive, Parkgate, South Wirral CH64 6RZ Tel: 0151 336 6700 — MB ChB Liverp. 1970; DObst RCOG 1972; MRCGP 1977. Prev: Regist. (Med.) Walton Hosp. Liverp.; SHO (Obst.) Liverp. Matern. Hosp.; Ho. Off. Broadgreen Hosp. Liverp.

WILLCOX, Robert One Click Health, 59 Holmdene Avenue, London SE24 9LD Tel: 08707 606680 Email: info@oneclickhealth.co.uk; 39 Charlbury Road, Oxford OX2 6UX Tel: 01865 512660 — MB BS Lond. 1972 (Middlx.) DTM & H Liverp. 1980; FOM RCP Lond. 1999, AFOM 1983. Managing Dir. Specialty: Occupat. Health. Socs: Fell. Roy. Soc. Med.; Soc. Occupat. Med. Prev: Gp. Med. Off. Cable & Wireless; Med. Off. Brit. Petroleum; Med. Off. Brit. Airways Med. Serv.

WILLCOX-JONES, Colin 3 Old Rectory Ground, Church Road, Offham, West Malling ME19 5NY Tel: 01732 842665 — MB ChB Ed. 1968; DObst RCOG 1971; DCH Eng. 1972. Specialty: Gen. Pract. Prev: Ho. Off. Roy. Infirm. Edin.

WILLDIG, Kathryn Mary Holmes Chapel Health Centre, London Road, Holmes Chapel, Crewe CW4 7BB; Woodheath Cottage, Whitecroft Heath Road, Lower Withington, Macclesfield SK11 9DF — MB ChB Manch. 1977; BSc (Morbid Anat. Hons.) Manch. 1975; DRCOG 1980; DCH RCP Lond. 1981; MRCGP 1982.

WILLDIG, Paul John Chance, Congleton Lane, Siddington, Macclesfield SK11 9LE — MB ChB Manch. 1976; BSc (Physiol., Hons.) Manch. 1973, MB ChB 1976; MFOM RCP Lond. 1986, AFOM 1981; DIH Eng. 1981. Med. Off. West. Area NCB; Hon. Clin. Asst. Shelton Chest Clin. Stoke-on-Trent. Socs: Soc. Occupat. Med. Prev: Ho. Off. (Neurosurg.) & Ho. Phys. (Haemat.) Manch. Roy. Infirm.

WILLE, Richard William (retired) Sarum House, 3 St Ethelbert St., Hereford HR1 2NS Tel: 01432 267242; 25 Broomy Hill, Hereford HR4 0LJ Tel: 01432 267242 — MRCS Eng. LRCP Lond. 1960 (Guy's) DObst RCOG 1962. Prev: GP.

WILLEMS, Pierre Jacques Anthony St Marys House, Broad St., Wrington, Bristol BS40 5LA — LMSSA Lond. 1959 (Guy's) DPM Eng. 1966. Sen. Regist. (Psychiat.) Oxf. RHB; Med. Adviser Oxf & Dist. Counc. on Alcoholism. Specialty: Gen. Psychiat. Prev: Research Regist. (Alcoholism) Oxf. RHB.

WILLEMSE, Pierre Jules Andre Rotherham District General Hospital, Moorgate Road, Rotherham S60 2UD Tel: 01709 304270 Fax: 01709 304220 — DRS Groningen. Cons. Gastroenterologist. Specialty: Gastroenterol. Special Interest: Hepabiliarity; IBD. Socs: BSG; AGA; MDU.

WILLENBROCK, Philip Charles 13 Woodland Way, Wivenhoe, Colchester CO7 9AP Tel: 01206 823812 — BM BCh Oxf. 1968 (Lond. Hosp.) MA Oxf. 1968. Prev: GP Camborne; SHO (Neurol.) Churchill Hosp. Oxf.; Ho. Off. Lond. Hosp.

WILLENS, Marni Northcote Surgery, 2 Victoria Circus, Glasgow G12 9LD Tel: 0141 339 3211 Fax: 014 357 4480 — MB ChB Glas. 1990 (Glasgow) DRCOG 1993; MRCGP 1995. Partner N.cote Surg. Socs: Glas. LMC.

WILLERT, Emma Jane 17 Toucan Way, Basildon SS16 5ER — MB ChB Manch. 1997.

WILLETT, Christina Hill (retired) 75 Morven Road, Bearsden, Glasgow G61 3BY; 6 Yewtree Gardens, Forwich, Canterbury CT2 0DQ Tel: 01227 711695 — MB ChB Glas. 1959.

WILLETT, Claire Jeanette 28 Monro Drive, Guildford GU2 9PS — MB BCh Wales 1990; DCH RCP Lond. 1992; DRCOG 1993; MRCGP 1994. Specialty: Gen. Pract. Prev: Trainee GP Hinchingbrooke Hosp. Huntingdon.

WILLETT, Mr Keith Malcolm John Radcliffe Hospital, Headington, Oxford OX3 9DU Tel: 01865 220241 Fax: 01865 221231 — MB BS Lond. 1981 (Charing Cross) MRCS Eng. LRCP Lond. 1981; FRCS Eng. 1985. Prof. of Orthopaedic Trauma Surg.; Hon. Cons. Orthop. Trauma Surg. John Radcliffe Hosp. Oxf. Specialty: Trauma & Orthop. Surg. Socs: BOA; Brit. Trauma Soc.; OTA. Prev: Trauma Fell. Sunnybrook Health Sci. Centre Toronto, Canada; Sen. Regist. (Orthop.) Char. Cross Hosp. Lond.; SHO Rotat. St. Bart. Hosp. Lond.

WILLETT, Mark Old Mill Surgery, Marlborough Road, Nuneaton CV11 5PQ Tel: 024 7638 2554 Fax: 024 7635 0047 — MB ChB Birm. 1984.

WILLETTS, Geoffrey Thomas Shipley, TD (retired) Hanway, 22 Clarry Drive, Sutton Coldfield B74 2QT — MB ChB Birm. 1948. Prev: Ho. Phys. & Ho. Surg. Gen. Hosp. Birm.

WILLETTS, Mr Ian Edward 338 Halesowen Road, Cradley Heath, Warley B64 7JT — MB ChB Manch. 1988 (Manchester) BSc (Hons.) Anat. Manch. 1985; MB ChB (Hons.) Manch. 1988; FRCS Ed. 1993; FRCS Eng. 1993; DM Manchester 2000; FRCS (Paed. Surg.) 2003. Cons. Paediatric Surg. Bristol Roy. Hosp. Childr.; Hunt. Prof. RCS Eng. Specialty: Paediat. Surg. Special Interest: Paediatric Transplantation; Paediatric Urol.; Med. Educat. Socs: Assoc. Mem. Brit. Assn. Paediat. Surgs.; Fell. Roy. Soc. Med.; Internat. Paediatiec Transplantaion Assn. Prev: Specialist Regist. (Paediat. Surg.) Sheffield Childrens Hospital, Sheffield; Research Fell. (Paediat. Surg.) Nuffield Dept. Surg. Univ. Oxf.; Temp. Lect. (Anat.) Univ. Manch.

WILLETTS, Janet Margaret Shanklin Medical Centre, 1 Carter Road, Shanklin PO37 7HR Tel: 01983 862245 Fax: 01983 862310; Bagend, Slay Lane, Whitwell, Ventnor PO38 2QF Tel: 01983 730727 — MB BS Lond. 1979 (Guy's) BSc (Hons.) Lond. 1976; MRCS Eng. LRCP Lond. 1979. Prev: GP Newport, I. of Wight.

WILLETTS, Simon James Castlehill Health Centre, Castlehill, Forres IV36 1QF Tel: 01309 672233 — MB ChB Aberd. 1987 (Univ. Aberd.) MRCP (UK) 1993; MRCGP 1995. Unrestricted Princip. - Grampian H.B. Socs: BMA.

WILLEY, Mrs Muriel Gladys (retired) Heron Garth, Bleach Green, Egremont CA22 2NL Tel: 01946 820282 — MB BS Lond. 1945 (Roy. Free) DObst RCOG 1948. Prev: Med. Off. W. Cumbld. Family Plann. Clinics.

WILLEY, Richard Flynn Royal Lancaster Infirmary, Ashton Road, Lancaster LA1 4RP; Woodfield House, Moorside Road, Brookhouse, Lancaster LA2 9PN — MB ChB Ed. 1972; MRCP (UK) 1974; FRCP

Ed. 1988; FRCP 1991. Cons. Phys. Roy. Lancs. Infirm. & Westmorland Gen. Hosp. Kendal. Specialty: Gen. Med. Prev: Sen. Regist. (Gen. Med.) Roy. Infirm. Edin.

WILLIAMS, Adela Mary 41 Winchendon Road, Fulham, London SW6 5DH Tel: 020 7736 6234 — MB ChB Bristol 1984; DRCOG 1986. Prev: Trainee GP/SHO St. Albans VTS.

WILLIAMS, Professor Adrian Charles 53 Weoley Hill, Selly Oak, Birmingham B29 4AB Tel: 0121 472 0218 — MD Birm. 1978; MB ChB 1972; MRCP (UK) 1974; FRCP Lond. 1986. Bloomer Prof. Clin. Neurol. Univ. Birm. Prev: Cons. Neurol. Qu. Eliz. & Selly Oak Gen. Hosps. Birm. & Manor Hosp. Walsall; Regist. & Sen. Regist. Nat. Hosp. Nerv. Dis. Lond.; Vis. Fell. Nat. Insts. Health Bethesda, USA.

WILLIAMS, Adrian John Elgar House Surgery, Church Road, Redditch B97 4AB Tel: 01527 69261 Fax: 01527 596856; Rivendell, 58 Wellington Road, Bromsgrove B60 2AX Tel: 01527 79741 — MB ChB Bristol 1980; BSc (Hons. Pharmacol.) Bristol 1977, MB ChB 1980; MRCP (UK) 1984; Cert Family Plann. JCC 1984; DRCOG 1985. Socs: BMA & RCP. Prev: Trainee GP Worcester VTS; Ho. Phys. Profess. Med. Unit Bristol Roy. Infirm.

WILLIAMS, Adrian John Lane-Fox Respiratory Unit, St Thomas' Hospital, London SE1 7EH Tel: 020 7188 7188 Fax: 020 7922 8281 Email: asta@talk21.com; 8 Nightingale Square, London SW12 8QN Tel: 020 8673 4385 — (University College Hospital, London) MB BS Lond. 1969; MRCP (UK) 1971; FRCP Lond. 1989. Cons. Phys. & Clin. Dir. La.-Fox Respirat. Unit St. Thos. Respirat. & Sleep Med.; Hon. Sen. Lect. UMDS; Vis. Prof. UCLA. Specialty: Respirat. Med.; Intens. Care. Prev: Prof. Clin. Med. & Dir. Pulm. & Critical Care W. L.A. VA Med Center & UCLA Med. Center, Los Angeles, USA.

WILLIAMS, Adrian Tudor Annette Fox Haematology Unit, Bradford Royal infirmary, Duckworth Lane, Bradford BD9 6RJ Tel: 01274 364686 Fax: 01274 366925 Email: adrian.williams@bradfordhospitals.nhs.uk — MB BChir Camb. 1977 (St. Thos.) MA Camb. 1978; MRCP (UK) 1980; MRCPath 1986; FRCPath 1996; FRCP 1998. Cons. Haemat. Bradford Hosps. NHS Trust. Specialty: Haematology. Socs: BMA. Prev: Sen. Regist. (Haemat.) Guy's Hosp. Lond.; Regist. (Haemat.) King's Coll. Hosp. Lond.

WILLIAMS, Alan Clive Church View Surgery, Broadway Road, Broadway TA19 9RX Tel: 01460 55300 Fax: 01460 53999; Axhill House, Windmill Hill Lane, Ashill, Ilminster TA19 9NB Tel: 01823 480262 — MB BCh Wales 1960 (Welsh Nat. Sch. Med.) DObst RCOG 1963; MRCGP 1968. Specialty: Gen. Pract. Socs: BMA Chairm. Som. Div.; W Som. Med. Soc. Prev: Ho. Surg. (Urol.) United Cardiff Hosps.; Ho. Phys. E. Glam. Hosp.; Ho. Surg. (Obst.) Profess. Unit United Cardiff Hosps.

WILLIAMS, Alan Hugh Ferniehill Road Surgery, 8 Ferniehill Road, Edinburgh EH17 7AD Tel: 0131 664 2166 Fax: 0131 666 1075; 10 East Camus Road, Edinburgh EH10 6RE Tel: 0131 445 1223 — MB ChB Aberd. 1985; DCCH RCP Ed. 1990; Dip Occ Med 1996. Phys. (Occupat. Health) S. E. Scotl. Blood Trans. Serv. & Protein Fractionation Centre, Edin. Specialty: Paediat.

WILLIAMS, Alan John Ty-Elli Group Practice, Ty Elli, Llanelli SA15 3BD Tel: 01554 772678 / 773747 Fax: 01554 774476; Grey Gables, Heol Ddv, Llanelli SA15 4RN — MB BS Lond. 1982; MRCGP 1986.

WILLIAMS, Alan John Royal Bournemouth Hospital, Castle Lane E., Bournemouth BH7 7DW Tel: 01202 303626; Belle Heather, 166 Burley Road, Bransgore, Christchurch BH23 8DE — MB ChB Birm. 1975; MRCP (UK) 1978; MD Birm. 1987; FRCP Ed. 1994; FRCP Lond. 1995. Cons. Phys. Roy. Bournemouth Hosp.; Hon. Lect. UCL. Specialty: Gen. Med.; Respirat. Med. Socs: Brit. Thorac. Soc.& BMA. Prev: Sen. Regist. (Gen. Thoracic Med.) Mersey RHA; Sheldon Research Fell. E. Birm. Hosp.; Med. Regist. (Thoracic Med.) E. Birm. Hosp.

WILLIAMS, Alan Roy Macclesfield District General Hospital, Victoria Road, Macclesfield SK10 3BL Tel: 01625 421000/661820 Fax: 01625 661804 — MB ChB Liverp. 1975; MRCPath 1982; FRCPath 1992. Cons. Histopath. Macclesfield Dist. Gen. Hosp. & Home Office (Path.). Specialty: Histopath.; Forens. Path. Prev: Lect. (Path.) Univ. Liverp.; Regist. United Liverp. Hosps.

WILLIAMS, Mr Albert Frederick (retired) Pwll Crwn, Lon Yr Eglwys, Morfa Nefyn, Pwllheli LL53 6AR Tel: 01758 720285 — (Manch.) BSc Manch. 1936; MB ChB (2nd cl. Hons.) Manch. 1939; MRCS Eng. LRCP Lond. 1939; FRCS Eng. 1940. Prev: 1st Asst. Profess. Surgic. Unit, Manch. Roy. Infirm.

WILLIAMS, Aled (retired) Seawinds, 114 Ffordd Naddyn, Glan Conwy, Colwyn Bay LL28 5BJ — MB ChB Liverp. 1957; DObst RCOG 1960; FRCOG 1980, M 1967. Prev: Cons. O & G Maelor Gen. Hosp. Wrexham.

WILLIAMS, Alexander St Thomas Health Centre, Cowick Street, St. Thomas, Exeter EX4 1HJ Tel: 01392 676677 Fax: 01392 676677 — MB BS Lond. 1982; MRCP (UK) 1985; DRCOG 1989; MRCGP 1990. Clin. Asst. (Respirat. Med.) Winford Hosp. Specialty: Respirat. Med. Prev: Trainee GP Paignton; Regist. (Med.) Torbay Hosp.; SHO (O & G & ENT) Torbay Hosp.

WILLIAMS, Alexander Thomas Dunford 98 Harley Street, London W1G 7HZ Tel: 020 7629 8340; Ridge House, Ballantyne Drive, Kingswood, Tadworth KT20 6EA Tel: 01737 353995 — MB BS Lond. 1968 (Univ. Coll. Hosp.) MRCS Eng. LRCP Lond. 1965; DObst RCOG 1975; DIH Eng. 1976; MSc (Distinc.) Lond. 1976; MFOM RCP Lond. 1979. Med. Adviser Govt. Canada, Lond.; Med. Dir. Lond. Diagn. Centre; Assoc. Prof. Med. Univ. Nova Scotia. Specialty: Occupat. Health. Socs: Fell. Roy. Soc. Med.; Soc. Occupat. Med. Prev: Med. Dir., Arctic Health Serv. Canada; Dir. Occupat. Health, Nova Scotia, Canada; Lect. Lond. Sch. Hyg. & Trop. Med.

WILLIAMS, Alison Claire Claremont Surgery, 56-60 Castle Road, Scarborough YO11 1XE Tel: 01723 375050 — MB ChB Birm. 1988 (Birmingham) DRCOG 1991; MRCGP 1993. p/t GP, Scarborough.

WILLIAMS, Alison Jane — MB ChB Sheff. 1989; DRCOG 1992; MRCGP 1994.

WILLIAMS, Alistair Robert William Royal Infirmary of Edinburgh, Department of Pathology, 51 Little France Crescent, Edinburgh EH12 4SA Tel: 0131 242 7120 Fax: 0131 242 7169 Email: alistair.r.w.williams@ed.ac.uk; 11 Corremic Drive, Edinburgh EH10 6EQ Tel: 0131 447 1481 Fax: 0131 447 2500 — MD Ed. 1988; MB ChB Ed. 1979; MB CHB Ed 1979; MRCPath 1986; FRCPath 1997. Sen. Lect. (Path.) Univ. Edin. Specialty: Histopath. Socs: Path. Soc.; Brit. Gyn. Cancer Soc.; Internat. Soc. Gyn. Path.

WILLIAMS, Alun James The Practice Of Health, 31 Barry Road, Barry CF63 1BA Tel: 01446 700350 Fax: 01446 420795; Morfa, 12 Romilly Avenue, Barry CF62 6RB — MB BCh Wales 1979; DRCOG 1982; MRCGP 1987.

WILLIAMS, Alun Rhys Tan-Y-Bryn, Heol-Y-Bryn, Rhigos, Aberdare CF44 9DJ — BM BCh Oxf. 1994.

WILLIAMS, Mr Alun Tudno Old Royal Infirmary of Edinburgh, Lauriston Building, Lauriston Place, Edinburgh EH3 9HA Tel: 0131 536 3740 Fax: 0131 536 1001 — MB BS Lond. 1989 (St. Thos. Hosp. Lond.) BSc Lond. 1988; FRCS (Otol.) 1996; FRCS Eng. 1996; FRCS (ORL-HNS) 2001. Cons. (Ear Nose & Throat) Lothian Univ. Hosps. NHS Trust. Specialty: Otorhinolaryngol.

WILLIAMS, Alyn Christopher Prior Chapel Street Surgery, 93 Chapel Street, Billericay CM12 9LR Tel: 01277 622940/655134 Fax: 01277 631893; 8 The Knoll, Billericay CM12 0NT Tel: 01277 652841 — MB BS Lond. 1981; BSc (Physiol.) Lond. 1978. Clin. Asst. (Rheum.) Southend Hosp. Trust. Specialty: Gen. Pract.

WILLIAMS, Amanda Jane Melrose, Llwyncelyn Terrace, Nelson, Treharris CF46 6HF — MB BS Lond. 1989.

WILLIAMS, Andrew 39 Highfield Avenue, Appleton, Warrington WA4 5DX — MB ChB Birm. 1981; MRCGP 1987.

WILLIAMS, Andrew Anthony 29 Lambardes, New Ash Green, Longfield DA3 8HX — BM Soton. 1992; MRCP (UK) 1996. Regist. (Elderly & Gen. Med.) Dorset Co. Hosp. Dorchester. Specialty: Care of the Elderly; Gen. Med.

WILLIAMS, Andrew Brian 70C Old Dover Road, London SE3 8SY — MB BS Lond. 1991.

WILLIAMS, Andrew David 25 Westaway Drive, Hakin, Milford Haven SA73 3EQ — MB ChB Birm. 1993.

WILLIAMS, Andrew George Woodbury, Bromley Lane, Chislehurst BR7 6LE — MB BS Lond. 1985; MRCGP 1995. Clin. Commiss. Dir. Bromley Health. Specialty: Neurol. Socs: BMA & Christian Med. Fellowsh. Prev: SHO (Neurol.) Brook Gen. Hosp. Lond.; SHO (Gen. Med.) Orpington Hosp.

WILLIAMS, Andrew Ivor Lake Road Health Centre, Nutfield Place, Portsmouth PO1 4JT Tel: 023 9282 1201 Fax: 023 9287 5658 — MB BS Lond. 1987; DRCOG 1989; DGM RCP Lond. 1990; DCH RCP Lond. 1990; MRCGP 1991.

WILLIAMS, Andrew James Medical Research Department, Zeneca Pharmaceuticals, Alderley Park, Macclesfield SK10 4TG Tel: 01625 514348; 48 Legh Road, Prestbury, Macclesfield SK10 4HX — MB ChB Liverp. 1980; BSc (Hons.) Lond. 1971; PhD CNAA 1975. Chief Clin. Pharmacol. Zeneca Pharmaceut. Chesh.; Hon. Lect. (Med.) Manch. Univ. Med. Sch. Socs: Fell. Roy. Soc. Med.; Amer. Thoracic Soc.; (Meetings Sec.) Soc. Pharmaceut. Med. Prev: Sen. Clin. Pharmacol. Beecham Pharmaceut. Epsom; Lect. (Clin. Pharmacol.) St. Geo. Hosp. Med. Sch. Univ. Lond.

WILLIAMS, Andrew James Kevin Wester Marchbank, Mansfield Road, Balerno EH14 7JT — MB ChB Bristol 1980; MD Bristol 1988, BSc (Hons.) 1977; MRCP (UK) 1983; FRCP Ed. 1995. Cons. Phys. (Gastroenterol.) St. John's Hosp. Livingston. Specialty: Gastroenterol.

WILLIAMS, Andrew John Morriston Hospital, Heol Maes Eglwys, Cwmrhydyceirw, Swansea SA6 6NL Tel: 01792 703399 Fax: 01792 703716; Grove Cottage, Reynoldston, Gower, Swansea SA3 1AA Tel: 01792 390182 Email: ajwil52@lineone.net — (Lond. Hosp.) MB BS (Hons.) Lond. 1975; MRCP (UK) 1977; MD Lond. 1981; FRCP Lond. 1993. Cons. Phys. (Renal Med.) Morriston Hosp. Swansea. Specialty: Nephrol. Socs: Eur. Dialysis & Transpl. Assn.; Internat. Soc. Nephrol.; Renal ass. Prev: Sen. Regist. (Nephrol.) Lond. Hosp.; Lect. Cardiothoracic Inst. Lond.; Regist. (Med.) Qu. Mary's Hosp. Roehampton.

WILLIAMS, Mr Andrew Michael Royal National Orthopaedic Hospital, Brockley Hill, Stanmore HA7 4LP — MB BS Lond. 1987; FRCS Eng. 1991; FRCS (Orth.) 1995. SenLect/Hon cons. Roy.Nat.Ortop.Hosps. Tanmore. Specialty: Orthop. Socs: Fell. Roy. Soc. Med.; Brit. Orthop. Sports Trauma Assn.; Assoc. Brit. Orthop. Assn. Prev: Sen. Regist. Roy. Nat. Orthop. Hosp. Stanmore; Clin. Lect. Roy. Nat. Orthop. Hosp. Stanmore.

WILLIAMS, Andrew Nason Northampton General Hospital, Child Development Centre, Cliftonville, Northampton NN1 5BD Tel: 01604 544188 Fax: 01604 545988 Email: andrewnason.williams@ngh.nhs.uk — BM BCh Oxf. 1990; BA (Hons.) Oxf. 1987; MRCP UK 1994; MRCP 1997; MSc (Community Child Health) Warwick 1999. Cons. Community Paediat. Northants. Gen. Hosp.; Hon. Vis. Sen. Clin. Lect. Univ. Warwick; Hon. Research Fell. Centre for Historical Studies, Univ. Birm. Specialty: Paediat. Socs: Pres. 2005-07 Brit. Soc. for the Hist. of Paediat. & Child Health. Prev: Hon. Sen. Clin. Fell. Birm. Childr. Hosp.; Cons. Paediat. (Community Child Health) N. Warks. NHS Trust; Sen. Regist. Birm. Childr. Hosp.

WILLIAMS, Andrew Rhys Department of Anaesthetics, St George's Hospital, Blackshaw Road, Tooting, London SW17 0QT Tel: 020 8672 1255; 34 Beaufordt Avenue, Langland, Swansea SA3 4PB — MB BCh Wales 1981; DA (UK) 1985; FFA RCSI 1989. Sen. Regist. (Anaesth.) St. Geo., Atkinson Morley & Gt. Ormond St. Hosps. Specialty: Anaesth. Socs: Assn. Anaesth. Gt. Brit. & N. Irel. & Anaesth. Research Soc. Prev: Regist. (Anaesth.) Poole & Bournemouth Hosps.

WILLIAMS, Aneurin Gwyn Llanberis Surgery, High Street, Llanberis, Caernarfon LL55 4SU Tel: 01286 870634 Fax: 01286 871722; 3 Preswylfa, Llanberis, Caernarfon LL55 4LF Tel: 01286 870101 — MB BS Lond. 1983 (The London Hospital Medical College) Specialty: Gen. Pract. Prev: GP Canning Town Lond.; SHO (ENT & Paediat.) St. John's Hosp. Chelmsford; SHO (A & E) Broomfield Hosp. Chelmsford.

WILLIAMS, Angharad Wyn Parc Glas Surgery, Bodorgan LL62 5NL Tel: 01407 840294 — MB BCh Wales 1996 (Univ. Wales Coll. Med.) DFFP; DRCOG. GP, Anglesey. Specialty: Gen. Pract. Socs: BMA. Prev: Ho. Off. (Surg.); Ho. Off. (Med.); SHO (A & E).

WILLIAMS, Ann Athel The Medical Centre, Kingston Avenue, East Horsley, Leatherhead KT24 6QT Tel: 0148 654151; (resid.), Dytchley's, The St, West Horsley, Leatherhead KT24 6HS Tel: 0148 652487 — MB BS Lond. 1960 (Lond. Hosp.) MRCS Eng. LRCP Lond. 1960. Socs: BMA. Prev: Ho. Surg. & Ho. Phys. St. Luke's Hosp. Guildford.

WILLIAMS, Ann Elisabeth Wellers Cottage, Marringdean Road, Billingshurst RH14 9EJ — MB BS Lond. 1980.

WILLIAMS, Anne 33 Coalway Road, Penn, Wolverhampton WV3 7LU — MB BCh Wales 1965.

WILLIAMS, Anne Elizabeth Warstones Health Centre, Pinfold Grove, Penn, Wolverhampton WV4 4PS Tel: 01902 575012 — MB ChB Birm. 1983; MRCGP 1990. Specialty: Ophth.

WILLIAMS, Anne Marie Helene Thurston Road Surgery, 140 Thurston Road, Glasgow G52 2AZ Tel: 0141 883 8838 Fax: 0141 810 1511 Email: annemhwilliams@yahoo.co.uk; 5 Kirklee Gardens, Glasgow G12 0SG Tel: 0141 339 3234 Fax: 0141 586 7986 — MB BS Lond. 1981 (Guy's, London) DRCOG 1985; DCH RCP Lond. 1989; MRCGP 1990. GP Princip.; GP Clin. Undergrad. Tutor. Socs: World Federat. Doctors; Scott. Counc. on Human Bioethics. Prev: Trainee GP Kilburn Lond. VTS; Mother & Child Health (Pacarán) Canete Valley, Peru.

WILLIAMS, Anthony Longford Street Surgery, Longford Street, Heywood OL10 4NH Tel: 01706 621417 Fax: 01706 622915; Edgecroft, Manchester Road, Heywood OL10 2NL — MB BCh Wales 1974.

WILLIAMS, Anthony Brendon Flat 2, 13 Frederick Place, Bristol BS8 1AS — MB ChB Otago 1986.

WILLIAMS, Anthony Charles Côte De Neige, 19 Hillside Avenue, Worthing BN14 9QR — MB BS Lond. 1974; MRCS Eng. LRCP Lond. 1974; FFA RCS Eng. 1979. Cons. Anaesth. Worthing & Southlands Hosp. Specialty: Anaesth.

WILLIAMS, Rev. Anthony David Social Security Department, PO Box 55, St Helier, Jersey JE4 8PE Tel: 01534 280000; Spindrift, Lasrande Route de la Cote, La Mare, St Clement, Jersey JE2 6FS Tel: 01534 729540 Fax: 01534 863729 — MRCS Eng. LRCP Lond. 1963 (St. Mary's) DObst RCOG 1965; MRCGP 1968. Med. Off. Social Security Dept. St. Helier; Hon. Curate St. Helier Parish Ch. Socs: Jersey Med. Soc. Prev: GP Jersey; Obst. Jersey Matern. Hosp.

WILLIAMS, Anthony Ffoulkes Department of Child Health, St. George's Hospital Medical School, Cranmer Terrace, Tooting, London SW17 0RE Tel: 020 8725 2986 Fax: 020 8725 2858 — MB BS Lond. 1975 (Westm.) BSc Lond. 1972; MRCS Eng. LRCP Lond. 1975; MRCP (UK) 1978; DPhil Oxf. 1987; FRCP Lond. 1993; FRCPCH 1997. Cons. Neonat. Paediat. & Sen. Lect. St. Geo. Hosp. Med. Sch. Lond. Specialty: Neonat. Prev: Lect. (Child Health) Univ. Bristol; Research Fell. (Paediat.) Univ. Oxf.

WILLIAMS, Anthony Harold Elvin (retired) Cranesbie, 6 Dore Road, Dore, Sheffield S17 3NB — MB ChB Bristol 1956; FRCGP 1985, M 1962; MEd Warwick 1984. Hon. Lect. (Gen. Pract.) Univ. Sheff. Prev: Sen. Lect. (Postgrad. Med.) Univ. Warwick & Assoc. Adviser (Gen. Pract.) W. Midlands Regional Health Auth.

WILLIAMS, Anthony James Mounts Medical Centre, Campbell Street, Northampton NN1 3DS Tel: 01604 631952 Fax: 01604 634139; 17 Wymersley Close, Great Houghton, Northampton NN4 7PT — MB BS Lond. 1984.

WILLIAMS, Anthony John Barry Hospital, Colcot Road, Barry CF62 8YH Tel: 01446 704110 Email: anthony.williams.barry@cardiffandvale.wales.nhs.uk — (Lond. Hosp.) MB BS Lond. 1970; FRCPsych 1995, M 1975; LLM Wales 2001. Cons. Psychiat. Cardiff and Vale NHS Trust; Clin. Teach., Dept. of Psychol. Med., Univ. of Wales; Ment. Health Act Commr. Specialty: Geriat. Psychiat. Prev: Cons. Psychiat. St. Tydfils Hosp. Merthyr Tydfil & Towers Hosp. Leicester; Lect. (Psychiat.) Univ. Leicester.

WILLIAMS, Anthony John (retired) 68 Hest Bank Lane, Hest Bank, Lancaster LA2 6BS Tel: 01524 822200 — MB ChB Liverp. 1956. Prev: Partner, 2 Queen Sq. Lancaster.

WILLIAMS, Anthony Paul 6 Walnut Close, Miskin, Pontyclun CF72 8RZ Tel: 01443 230171 Fax: 01443 230172 — BSc Wales 1968; MB BCh Wales 1973; Cert. Family Plann. JCC 1976; MFCM 1989. Specialty: Community Child Health.

WILLIAMS, Anthony Peter — MB BS Lond. 1992 (Univ. Coll. Lond. & Middlx. Med. Sch.) BSc (Pharmacol.) Lond. 1989; MRCP (UK) 1995; MSc (Immunol.) Lond. 1998; MRCPath 2003. Wellcome Clinician Scientist Research Fell. Soton. Gen. Hosp. Specialty: Immunol.

WILLIAMS, Antony John City Surgery, 187 City Road, Roath, Cardiff CF24 3WD Tel: 029 2049 4250 Fax: 029 2049 1968 — MB BCh Wales 1957 (Cardiff)

WILLIAMS, Arfon Isfryn Surgery, Isfryn, Ffordd Dewi Sant, Nefyn, Pwllheli LL53 6EA Tel: 01758 720202 Fax: 01758 720083 — MB BCh Wales 1991; MRCGP 1995. Socs: BMA. Prev: Trainee GP Pwllheli; SHO (O & G & Paediat.) Ysbyty Gwynedd Bangor.

WILLIAMS, Arthur Alun (retired) 3 Sovereign Close, Kingsend, Ruislip HA4 7EF Tel: 01895 677570 — (Cardiff) MRCS Eng. LRCP Lond. 1938; MD Lond. 1948, MB BS 1946; FRCP Ed. 1962, M

1947. Hon. Cons. Phys. S. Tees Hosps. Prev: Cons. Phys. S. Teeside Hosps.

WILLIAMS, Arthur Hyatt, Maj. RAMC Retd. (retired) 29 St Johns Road, London NW11 0PE Tel: 020 8455 5682 Fax: 020 8458 2377; Jacob's Cottage, Jacob's Yard, Middle Barton, Oxford Tel: 01869 347387 — MD Liverp. 1949; MB ChB Liverp. 1938; DPM Eng. 1947; FRCPsych 1971. Prev: Hon. Dir. The Lond. Clinic of Psycho-Anal.

WILLIAMS, Arthur Jeffrey Department of Paediatrics, Glan Clwyd Dist. Hospital, Bodelwyddan, Rhyl Tel: 01745 583910 — MB ChB Birm. 1966; DCH Eng. 1971; MRCP (UK) 1974; FRCP Lond. 1989. Cons. (Paediat.) Glan Clwyd Dist. Hosp. Bodelwyddan. Specialty: Paediat. Prev: Maj. RAMC; Paediat. Regist. Burnley Gen. Hosp.; Lect. in Child Health Alder Hey Childr. Hosp. Liverp.

WILLIAMS, Arthur Llewelyn John (retired) 5 Minera Road, Ffirth, Wrexham LL11 5LR Tel: 01978 756614 — MB BS Lond. 1959 (King's Coll. Lond. & Westm.) AKC; FRIPHH; DObst RCOG 1962; DPH Wales 1966; FFPHM 1986. JP 1981-. Prev: Dir. Pub. Health Med. & Chief Admin. Med. Off. Clwyd HA.

WILLIAMS, Arthur Warriner, CBE (retired) Low Hollins, Cockermouth CA13 9UX Tel: 01900 85251 — MRCS Eng. LRCP Lond. 1929 (Camb. & Westm.) DTM & H 1931; MA Camb. 1934, BA 1926, MD 1938; FRCP Lond. 1955, M 1946. Prev: Prof. of Med. Makerere Coll. Univ. E. Africa.

WILLIAMS, Babatunde Olabode 1 Fox Gardens, Lymm WA13 9EY — MB BS Ibadan 1991.

WILLIAMS, Barbara Alice Reynolds (retired) 20 South Rise, Llanishen, Cardiff CF14 0RH — MB BCh Wales 1962; DObst RCOG 1967; DMRD Eng. 1975; FRCR 1978.

WILLIAMS, Barbara Anne Pavilion Family Doctors, 153A Stroud Road, Gloucester GL1 5JJ Tel: 01452 385555 Fax: 01452 531555 — MB BS Lond. 1986; DCH RCP Lond. 1989.

WILLIAMS, Barbara Anne Hill Brow, Main St., Tilton-on-the-Hill, Leicester LE7 9LF — MB ChB Dundee 1976; MRCGP 1981.

WILLIAMS, Barbara Mary (retired) Bicknor House, High St., Stevenage SG1 3BG Tel: 01438 729122 — MB ChB Birm. 1946. Prev: Anaesth., Lister Hosp., Stevenage.

WILLIAMS, Barbara Mary (retired) Little Debden, Petham, Canterbury CT4 5NN Tel: 01227 700154 — (St. Thos.) MB BS Lond. 1954; MRCS Eng. LRCP Lond. 1954; DObst RCOG 1956; DA Eng. 1957. Clin. Asst. Anaesth. Canterbury Hosp. Gp. Prev: Ho. Phys. Med. Unit, St. Thos. Hosp. Lond.

WILLIAMS, Benjamin James 50 Lady Edith's Avenue, Scarborough YO12 5RB; 212 Asmore Road, Queens Park, London W9 3DD Tel: 020 8969 1217 — MB BS Lond. 1993 (St Marys hosp) Specialist Regist. Anaesth. NW. Thames. Specialty: Anaesth. Socs: Assn. Anaesth.

WILLIAMS, Benjamin James Flat 18, Rochdale House, 19 Slate Wharf, Manchester M15 4SX — MB ChB Birm. 1995; ChB Birm. 1995.

WILLIAMS, Bernard Lincoln (retired) Brookfield, 23 Eyebrook Road, Bowdon, Altrincham WA14 3LH Tel: 0161 928 6016 — MB ChB Manch. 1948; MB ChB (Hnrs.) Manch. 1948; DPath Eng. 1957; FRCPath 1971, M 1963. Hon. Cons. Path. Pk. Hosp. Davyhulme. Prev: Lect. (Path.) Univ. Manch.

WILLIAMS, Beryl Wyn Brecon Medical Group Practice, Ty Henry Vaughan, Bridge Street, Brecon LD3 8AH Tel: 01874 622121 Fax: 01874 623742; 3 Buckingham Place, Glamorgan St, Brecon LD3 7DL — MB BCh Wales 1985; MRCGP 1989; DCH RCP Lond. 1989; DGM RCP Lond. 1991; DRCOG 1995. Specialty: Accid. & Emerg.

WILLIAMS, Bethan Sketty Surgery, De la Beche Road, Sketty, Swansea SA2 9EA Tel: 01792 206862; 10 Brynderi Close, Penllergaer, Swansea SA4 1AG — MB BCh Wales 1980 (Welsh Nat. Sch. of Med.) DRCOG 1982; MRCGP 1984.

WILLIAMS, Bethan Wyn 16 Belsize Road, Worthing BN11 4RH — MB BS Lond. 1987.

WILLIAMS, Bill Thomas Jordan 11 Northern Grove, West Didsbury, Manchester M20 8NL — MB ChB Manch. 1985. Regist. (Psychiat.) S. Manch. Univ. Dept., S. Manch. AHA. Specialty: Gen. Psychiat.

WILLIAMS, Billie Innes (retired) Court Yard House, Church End, Bletchington, Kidlington OX5 3DL Tel: 01869 350171 Fax: 01869 350789 — MB BChir Camb. 1949 (Roy. Free & Camb.) MA Camb. 1949; DO Eng. 1953; PhD Lond. 1975, MSc (Distinc.) 1967. Prev: Hon. Lect. in Ophth. (Leverhulme Fell.) St. Mary's Hosp. Lond.

WILLIAMS, Brian David Morgan (retired) White Lea, Beech Close, Stratford-upon-Avon CV37 7EB Tel: 01789 296555 — BM BCh Oxf. 1952 (Oxf. & Univ. Coll. Hosp.) MRCGP 1964. Prev: Resid. Med. Off. St. Pancras Br. Univ. Coll. Hosp.

WILLIAMS, Brian Emlyn Burney Hatfield Road Surgery, 70 Hatfield Road, Ipswich IP3 9AF Tel: 01473 723373; 52 Anglesea Road, Ipswich IP1 3PW Tel: 01473 216257 — (Middlx.) MRCS Eng. LRCP Lond. 1967; DO Eng. 1974; MRCOphth 1989. Attend. Ophth. Optimex Laser Eye Centre Lond.; Hosp. Pract. (Ophth.) Ipswich Dist. Gen. Hosp. Specialty: Ophth. Prev: Med. Off. Louise Margt. Matern. Hosp. Aldershot; Med. Off. Camb. Milit. Hosp. Aldershot.

WILLIAMS, Brian Melville Avon Partnership, Occupational Health Service, Southmead Hospital, Westbury on Trym, Bristol BS5 7BD Tel: 0117 959 5499 Email: brian.williams@north-bristol.swest.nhs.uk — MB ChB Liverp. 1982; AFOM RCP Lond. 1992; MFOM 1998. Cons. Ocupational Phys., Avon Partnership Occupational Health Serv., Bristol. Specialty: Occupat. Health. Prev: Med. Off. (Respirat. Dis.) Med. Bd.ing Centre Glas.

WILLIAMS, Brian Owen 15 Thorn Drive, High Burnside, Rutherglen, Glasgow G73 4RH Tel: 0141 634 4480 Fax: 0141 211 3465 — MB ChB Glas. 1970; MB ChB (Commend.) Glas. 1970; MRCP (UK) 1973; FRCP Glas. 1983; MD Glas. 1984; FRCP Lond. 1989; FRCP Ed. 1991. Clin. Dir. & Cons. Geriat. Gartnavel Gen. Hosp. Glas. Specialty: Care of the Elderly. Socs: FCPS (Pak) 1996; FRC SLT (Hon.) 1996; Sen. Mem. Scott. Soc. Phys. Prev: Sen. Regist. (Geriat. Med.) Vict. Infirm. Glas.; Sen. Regist. (Geriat. Med.) Stobhill Hosp. Glas.; Regist. (Med.) Vict. Infirm. Glas.

WILLIAMS, Brian Rees The Stewart Medical Centre, 15 Hartington Road, Buxton SK17 6JP Tel: 01298 22338 Fax: 01298 72678; Green Farm, King Sterndale, Buxton SK17 9SF Tel: 01298 70141 — BM BS Nottm. 1976; DRCOG 1980; DA Eng. 1981.

WILLIAMS, Brian Richard 2 Park Road N., Middlesbrough TS1 3LF Tel: 01642 247008 Fax: 01642 245748; Briary Cottage, 7 Maltby Road, Thornton, Middlesbrough TS8 9BU Tel: 01642 592693 — MB ChB Ed. 1971. Socs: BMA.

WILLIAMS, Brian Thomas (retired) Westover, Sheffield Road, Hathersage, Hope Valley S32 1DA — (Westm.) DPH Lond. 1964; DPM Eng. 1965; MD Sheff. 1973; FFPM RCP (UK) 1978, M 1974; FRCP Lond. 1990. Prev: Prof. Pub. Health Med. Univ. Nottm.

WILLIAMS, Professor Bryan Department of Medicine, Clinical Sciences Building, Leicester Royal Infirmary, PO Box 65, Leicester LE2 7LX Tel: 0116 252 3183 Fax: 0116 252 3273 Email: bw17@le.ac.uk — MB BS Lond. 1983 (St. Mary's Hosp. Med. Sch.) BSc (1st cl. Hons.) Lond. 1980; MRCP (UK) 1986; FRCP Lond. 1995; MD (Distinc.) Leicester 1996. Dir. Cardiovasc. Research Inst. Univ. Leicester. Specialty: Gen. Med.; Vasc. Med.; Nephrol. Special Interest: Hypertens. Socs: Fell. Amer. Counc. for High Blood Pressure Res.; Assn. Phys.; Internat. Soc. Hypertens. Prev: Sen. Lect. (Med.) Univ. Leicester; Lect. (Med.) & Hon. Sen. Regist. (Nephrol.) Leicester; Instruc. Med. Univ. of Colorado, Denver, USA.

WILLIAMS, Professor Bryan Davies Department of Rheumatology, University Hospital of Wales, Cardiff CF4 4XW Tel: 029 2074 3184 Fax: 029 2074 4388; Briar Bank, 18 Station Road, Dinas Powys CF64 4DF — MB BCh Wales 1966; MSc Birm. 1969; FRCP Lond. 1986, M 1969; FRCPath 1993, M 1992. Prof. & Cons. Rheum. Univ. Wales Coll. Med. Cardiff. Specialty: Rheumatol. Socs: Amer. Coll. Rheum.; Brit. Soc. Rheum.; Brit. Soc. Immunol.

WILLIAMS, Mr Bryn Terence Suite 204, Emblem House, London Bridge Hospital, 27 Tooley St., London SE1 2PR Tel: 020 7403 2150 Fax: 020 7403 4329; Kimberton, Warreners Lane, St. George's Hill, Weybridge KT13 0LH — MB ChB Birm. 1962; MRCS Eng. LRCP Lond. 1962; FRCS Eng. 1967. Specialty: Cardiothoracic Surg. Socs: Brit. Cardiac Soc.; Soc. Thoracic & Cardiovasc. Surgs.; Fell. Europ. Soc. Cardiol. Prev: Hon. Cons. Cardiothoracic Surg. to the Army; Cons. Cardiothoracic Surg. St. Thos. Hosp. Lond.; Sen. Regist. Nat. Heart & Chest Gp. Hosps. Lond.

WILLIAMS, Bryony Pauline Whitby Group Practice, Spring Vale Medical Centre, Whitby YO21 1SD Tel: 01947 820888 Fax: 01947 824100; Burnvale, Teapot Hill, Sandsend, Whitby YO21 3TF Tel: 01947 893004 — MB ChB Ed. 1983; MRCGP 1988; DRCOG 1989; Dip. IMC RCS Ed. 1992.

WILLIAMS, Mr Carl John (retired) Hope Hospital, Stott Lane, Salford M6 8HD Tel: 0161 789 7373; 69 Wardle Road, Sale M33 3DJ Tel: 0161 976 2660 — MB BS Lond. 1992 (UCL) BSc (Hons.) Med. Microbiol. Lond. 1989; FRCS 1997; FRCS 1998. Clin. Lect/Hon. Specialist Regist. Orthop. Surg. Prev: SHO (Gen. Surg.) Blackpool Vict. Hosp.

WILLIAMS, Carol Margaret Elizabeth (retired) Lime Tree Cottage, 19 Main St., Queniborough, Leicester LE7 8DB Tel: 0116 260 6228 — MB BS Lond. 1967 (Guy's) MRCS Eng. LRCP Lond. 1965; DObst RCOG 1969.

WILLIAMS, Caroline Emma Burway House, 61 High St., Kintbury, Hungerford RG17 9TL Tel: 01488 657730; 19 Laitwood Road, Balham, London SW12 9QN Tel: 020 8488 3381 — MB BS Lond. 1996 (Charring Cross & Westminster Medical School) SHO Med. St Geo.'s Hosp. Tooting Lond. Prev: SHO (A & E) W. Middlx. Univ. Hosp.

WILLIAMS, Caroline Jane 1 The Rowans, Aughton, Ormskirk L39 6TD — BM Soton. 1994 (Univ. Soton.) MRCP (UK) 1999.

WILLIAMS, Caroline Joy 1 Russell Close, Winford, Bristol BS40 8EF Tel: 01404 42080 — MB BS Lond. 1988; BSc (Nutrit.) Lond. 1985; DRCOG 1992. Trainee GP Harptree Pract. Bristol.

WILLIAMS, Catherine — MB BS Newc. 1988; MRCGP 1993; DCH RCP Lond. 1993.

WILLIAMS, Catherine Dilys 14 Kersley Road, London N16 0NP — MB BS Lond. 1987.

WILLIAMS, Catherine Elizabeth Mary c/o Bristol Eye Hospital, Lower Maudlin St., Bristol BS1 2LX Tel: 0117 923 0060 Fax: 0117 925 1421; 35 Haverstock Road, Knowle, Bristol BS4 2DA Tel: 0117 971666 — MB BS Lond. 1986; MPS; BMA; BSc Lond. 1983, MB BS 1986; FCOphth 1991; PhD 1998. Cons.; Sen. Ophth., ALSPAC study, Inst. of Child health,Univ. of Bristol. Specialty: Ophth. Prev: Sen. Regist. (Ophth.), S. W.; MRC Research Fell. Bristol Eye Hosp.; Regist. (Ophth.) Bristol Eye Hosp.

WILLIAMS, Catherine Shan Avonmead, Southmead Hospital, Westbury-on-Trym, Bristol BS10 5NB — MB BS Lond. 1985; BSc (Hons.) Lond. 1980; MRCPsych 2001.

WILLIAMS, Cecil William Llewelyn (retired) Lanreath, The Wigdale, Hawarden, Deeside CH5 3LL Tel: 01244 532557 — MB ChB Liverp. 1955; DObst RCOG 1958; MRCGP 1968. Hosp. Pract. (Psychiat.) Maelor Gen. Hosp. Wrexham. Prev: Ho. Surg. & Ho. Phys. David Lewis North. Hosp. Liverp.

WILLIAMS, Charles David The William Harvey Hospital, Ashford TN24 0LZ Tel: 01233 833331 Fax: 01233 616049; Stowting Court Stables, Stowting, Ashford TN25 6BA Tel: 01303 863344 — MB BChir Camb. 1978; MA Camb. 1979; FRCP (UK) 1997; MD(Camb.) 1999. Cons. Phys. Diabetes & Endocrinol. William Harvey Hosp. Ashford; Hon. Sen. Lect. (Med.) GKT St. Thos. Hosp. Lond. Specialty: Gen. Med. Prev: Lect. & Sen. Regist. UMDS St. Thos. Hosp. Lond.

WILLIAMS, Charles Edward University Department of Radiodiagnosis, Royal Liverpool Hospital, Liverpool L69 3BX Tel: 0151 709 0141 — MB BCh BAO Dub. 1978; FFR RCSI 1985; FRCR 1985. Sen. Clin. Lect./Hon. Cons. Radiol. Univ. Liverp. & Roy. Liverp. Hosp. Specialty: Radiol. Prev: Sen. Regist. (Diag. Radiol.) Leeds Gen. Infirm. & St. Jas. Hosp. Leeds.

WILLIAMS, Christina Janet Seymour 11 Frognal Way, London NW3 6XE Tel: 020 7435 4030 Fax: 020 7435 5636 Email: christopherwilliams@compuserve.com — (Guy's) MB BS Lond. 1965; MRCS Eng. LRCP Lond. 1965; MRCP (UK) 1970; FRCP Lond. 1992. p/t Cons. Adult Disabil. Med.; Med. Adviser SCOPE; Mem. Med. Appeal Tribunal Serv. Specialty: Disabil. Med.; Rehabil. Med. Special Interest: Profound brain damage, Congen. or acquired. Socs: BMA; Brit. Soc. Rehabil. Med.; Liveryman Worshipful Soc. Apoth. Lond. Prev: Cons. Rehabil. & Disabil. Med.; Cons. Rheum. & Rehabil. Nat. Hosp. Nerv. Dis. Lond. & Bloomsbury & Islington HA & Roy. Hosp. for Neurodisabil. Putney; Sen. Regist. (Rheum.) Middlx. Hosp. Lond.

WILLIAMS, Christine Maria Moorefields Eye Hospital, City Road, London EC1V 2PD Tel: 0207 566 2387 Fax: 0207 566 2435 Email: christina.moore@moorfields.nhs.uk; 5 Rodney Gardens, Pinner HA5 2RS — MB ChB Dundee 1978; FRCA 1990. Ophthalmic Anaesth. Moorfields Eye Hosp. Lond.; Cons. Anaesth. Specialty: Anaesth. Socs: Roy. Soc. of Med.; Brit. Ophthamic Anaesth. Soc.; Difficult Airway Soc. Prev: Sen. Regist. & Regist. (Anaesth.) Hammersmith Hosp. Lond.; SHO (Anaesth.) Northwick Pk. Hosp. Lond.

WILLIAMS, Mr Christopher Barrie The Park Hospital, Sherwood Lodge Drive, Arnold, Nottingham NG8 8RX Tel: 0115 978 7325; 25 Oundle Drive, Wollaton Park, Nottingham NG8 1BN Tel: 0115 978 7325 Fax: 0115 978 7325 — MB ChB Bristol 1962; FRCS Eng. 1966; MD Bristol 1968. Cons. Gen. Surg. Nottm. City Hosp.; Clin. Teach. Univ. Nottm. Med. Sch. Specialty: Gen. Surg. Socs: BMA. Prev: Sen. Regist. (Gen. Surg.) United Bristol Hosps.; Regist. (Surg.) Cardiff Roy. Infirm.; Ho. Surg. & Ho. Phys. Bristol Roy. Infirm.

WILLIAMS, Christopher Beverley 11 Frognal Way, Hampstead, London NW3 6XE Tel: 020 7435 4030 Fax: 020 7435 5636 Email: christopherwilliams@compuserve.com — BM BCh Oxf. 1964 (Univ. Coll. Hosp.) MA Oxf. 1964; MRCS Eng. LRCP Lond. 1965; FRCP Lond. 1979, M 1968; FRCS 1999. Specialty: Gastroenterol. Socs: Fell. Roy. Soc. Med.; Brit. Soc. Gastroenterol.; Liveryman Soc. Apoth. Prev: Cons. Phys. St. Mark's Hosp. for Intestinal & Colorectal Disorders Lond.

WILLIAMS, Christopher David Flat 2, 6 Jesmond Gardens, Jesmond, Newcastle upon Tyne NE2 2JN Tel: 0191 281 6721 — MB BS Newc. 1998; MRCP Edinburgh 2001. Specialty: Gen. Med.

WILLIAMS, Christopher John Psychological Medicine, Administration Building, Gartnaval Royal Hospital, 1055 Great Western Road, Glasgow G12 0XH Tel: 0141 211 3912 Email: chris.williams@clinmed.gla.ac.uk — MB ChB Leeds 1988 (Univ. of Leeds) BSc Leeds 1985, MMedSci (Clin. Psychiat.) 1994; MD Leeds 2001. Sen. Lect., Univ. Glasgow - Hon. Cons. Psychiat., Glas. - Director of Glas. Institute for Psychosocial Interven.s (GIPSI) Glas.; Hon. Cons. Psychiat. Specialty: Gen. Psychiat. Special Interest: Self-help stepped care models. Socs: Roy. Coll. Psychiat.; Brit. Psychol. Soc.; Brit. Assn. Behavioural & Cognitive Psychother. & UK Counc. Psychother. Prev: Lect. & Hon. Sen. Regist. (Psychiat.) Leeds Univ.; Regist. Rotat. (Psychiat.) Leeds HA.

WILLIAMS, Christopher John Royal United Hospital, Bath NHS Trust, Combe Park, Bath BA1 3NG Tel: 01179 685725 Fax: 01179 685725; Coombe Dene, 49 Coombe Lane, Stoke Bishop, Bristol BS9 2BL Tel: 01179 685725 Fax: 01179 685725 — MB BS Lond. 1996 (Kings College London) BSc Lond. 1993. SHO (Med.) Roy. United Hosp. Bath; Assoc. Coll. Tutor. Specialty: Gen. Med.

WILLIAMS, Christopher John Cole Leeds General Infirmary, Great George Street, Leeds — MB BS Lond. 1985; BSc Lond. 1982; MRCP (UK) 1990; DTM & H 1992. Cons. Paediatric Intensivist. Specialty: Paediat.; Intens. Care.

WILLIAMS, Christopher John Hacon Bristol Oncology Centre, Horfield Road, Bristol BS2 8ED Tel: 0117 928 3177 Email: christopher.williams@nbht.swest.nhs.uk; The Triangle, Sibford Road, Hook Norton, Banbury OX15 5JU Tel: 01608 737765 — MB BS Lond. 1971 (St. Mary's) MRCS Eng. LRCP Lond. 1971; MRCP (UK) 1974; DM Soton 1980; FRCP Lond. 1986. Cons. Med. Oncologist & Clin. Director, Bristol Haemat. & Oncol. Centre, Bristol. Socs: Amer. Soc. Clin. Oncol.; Assn. Cancer Phys.s; Eur. Soc. Med. Oncol. Prev: Sen. Lect. & Hon. Cons. Phys. CRC Med. Oncol. Unit Soton. Gen. Hosp.; Postdoctoral Fell. Div. Oncol. Stanford Univ. Med. Centre, USA; Vis. Cons. Med. Oncol. Gen. Hosp. St Helier Jersey.

WILLIAMS, Christopher John Harold Dr J M Beck and Partners, 21 Beaufort Road, Southbourne, Bournemouth BH6 5AJ Tel: 01202 433081 Fax: 01202 430527; Surf Sounds, 11 Percy Road, Bournemouth BH5 1JF Tel: 01202 398014 — MB ChB Birm. 1964; MRCS Eng. LRCP Lond. 1964; DPM Eng. 1968; MFCM 1974. Hosp. Pract. (Psychiat.) King's Pk. Community Hosp. Bournemouth. Prev: SCM (Social Servs.) Dorset AHA; Regist. (Psychiat.) St. Ann's Hosp. Poole.; SHO (O & G) Co. Hosp. Hereford.

WILLIAMS, Christopher Philip Richard 7 Pavan Gardens, Ensbury Park, Bournemouth BH10 5JH — MB BCh Wales 1995; MB BCh (Hons.) Wales 1995; MRCP (Lond.), 1998; MRCOphth 2000. SpR (Opth.) Wessex Rotat. Specialty: Ophth. Prev: SHO (Gen. Med.), E. Glam. Gen. Hosp.; SHO (Ophth.), Soton. Gen. Hosp.

WILLIAMS, Christopher Richard 35 Bryony Road, Birmingham B29 4BY — MB BCh Wales 1998.

WILLIAMS, Mr Christopher Richard Philip Orthopaedic Department, Royal Sussex County Hospital, Eastern Road, Brighton BN2 5BE Tel: 01273 696955 Fax: 01273 624297 — MB BS Lond. 1985 (St Georges Hosp. Lond.) FRCS Eng. 1989. Cons. Orthop.

Surg., Brighton. Specialty: Orthop. Special Interest: Hand Surgery. Socs: BSSH.

WILLIAMS, Christopher Robert Ashfield Surgery, Merthyr Mawr Road, Bridgend CF31 3NW Tel: 01656 652774 Fax: 01656 661187; Goodways, 78 Merthyr Mawr Road, Bridgend CF31 3NR Tel: 01656 653309 — MB Camb. 1977 (St. Mary's) MA Camb. 1977, BChir 1977; DRCOG 1982. GP Bridgend. Prev: Trainee GP Bridgend VTS; Ho. Phys. Harold Wood Hosp.; Ho. Surg. Northwick Pk. Hosp. Harrow.

WILLIAMS, Christopher Vawer Somers Town Health Centre, Blackfriars Close, Southsea PO5 4NJ Tel: 023 9285 1202 Fax: 023 9229 6380 — MB BS Lond. 1977 (Middlesex Hospital) Specialty: Gen. Pract.

WILLIAMS, Claire Ann 123 Southfield Road, Oxford OX4 1NY — MB BCh Wales 1997.

WILLIAMS, Clare Rosemary Anaesthetics Department, St Helier Hospital, Carshalton Tel: 020 8644 4343; 16 Mansel Road, Wimbledon, London SW19 4AA — BM BCh Oxf. 1971; BA, BM BCh Oxf. 1971; DObst RCOG 1973; FFA RCS Eng. 1977. Cons. Anaesth. St Helier Hosp. Carshalton. Specialty: Anaesth.

WILLIAMS, Mr Claude Arthur Kingsley 64 Langstone Close, Babbacombe, Torquay TQ1 3TY — MB ChB Birm. 1962; MRCS Eng. LRCP Lond. 1962; FRCS Ed. 1965.

WILLIAMS, Clive St Johns Lane Health Centre, St. Johns Lane, Bristol BS3 5AS Tel: 0117 966 7681 Fax: 0117 977 9676 — MB ChB Sheff. 1972.

WILLIAMS, Clive Propert The Grange, Vicarage Hill, Minera, Wrexham LL11 3YN — MD Liverp. 1978; MB ChB 1969; MRCPath 1980. Cons. (Chem. Path.) Maelor Gen. Hosp. Wrexham. Specialty: Chem. Path.

WILLIAMS, Colin 36 Albert Edward Road, Liverpool L7 8RZ — MB ChB Liverp. 1991.

WILLIAMS, Colin Anthony Portway Surgery, 1 The Portway, Porthcawl CF36 3XB Tel: 01656 304204 Fax: 01656 772605; 29 Danygraig Avenue, Porthcawl CF36 5AA Tel: 01656 784311 Fax: 01656 772605 — MB BCh Wales 1968 (Cardiff) DPD 1990. Prev: SHO (Med.) Nevill Hall Hosp. Abergavenny; Ho. Surg. & Ho. Phys. (Paediat.) United Cardiff Hosps.

WILLIAMS, Mr Colin Roger (retired) Nuffield Hospital, Wood Road, Tettenhall, Wolverhampton WV6 8LE Tel: 01902 741526/ 01902 754177 — MB BS Lond. 1963 (St. Bart.) FRCS Eng. 1967. Prev: Research Fell. (Dept. Path.) Univ. Birm.

WILLIAMS, Craig Lester Cranage Department of Microbiology, Royal Alexandra Hospital, Corsebar Road, Paisley PA2 9PN Tel: 0141 580 4453 Fax: 0141 580 4242 — MB ChB Liverp. 1982; MRCP (UK) 1986; MRCPath 1991; FRCP Ed. 1998; MD (Liverpool) 1999; FRCPath 2000. Cons. Microbiologist Roy. Alexandra Hosp. Paisley; Hon. Research Fell. Univ. Glas. Specialty: Med. Microbiol.

WILLIAMS, Dafydd Fon 30 Harthill Avenue, Leconfield, Beverley HU17 7LN — MB BS Nottm. 1982; BMedSci 1980.

WILLIAMS, Damian Carson Kings Norton Surgery, 6 Redditch Road, Kings Norton, Birmingham B38 8QS Tel: 0121 458 2550 Fax: 0121 459 2770 — MB ChB Birm. 1998; MRCGP 2004. GP Birm.

WILLIAMS, Dan Shannon Stamford Hill Group Practice, 2 Egerton Road, Stamford Hill, London N16 6UA Tel: 020 8800 1000 Fax: 020 8880 2402 Email: dan.williams@gp-f84013.nhs.uk — MB BCh Witwatersrand 1979. Princip., Gen. Pract.; Hosp. Practitioner Clin. Oncol., Chase Farm Hosp., Enfield, Middlx. Socs: Brit. Med.Assn. Prev: Lect. Gen. Med. Univ. Coll. Hosp. Lond.

WILLIAMS, Daniel Glyn Westcourt, 12 The Street, Rustington, Littlehampton BN16 3NX Tel: 01903 784311 Fax: 01903 850907 — MB BS Lond. 1990 (St Bartholomews) DRCOG 1993; MRCGP 1994. Specialty: Gen. Pract.

WILLIAMS, Professor Daniel Gwyn Department of Renal Medicine, Guy's Hospital, St Thomas St., London SE1 9RT — MD Wales 1974 (Cardiff) MB BCh 1963; FRCP Lond. 1978, M 1966. Prof. Med. UMDS Guy's & St. Thos. Hosp. Lond.; Cons. Phys. Renal Dis. Guy's Hosp. Lond. Specialty: Nephrol. Prev: SHO Med. Unit Cardiff Roy. Infirm.; Sen. Regist. Dept. Med. Radcliffe Infirm. Oxf.; Asst. Lect. (Med.) Roy. Postgrad. Med. Sch. Univ. Lond.

WILLIAMS, Daniel Harvey Redbrook, Llandevaud, Newport NP18 2AF — MB BCh Wales 1998.

WILLIAMS, David Catterick Garrison Family Practice, Catterick Garrison DL9 3JF Tel: 01748 833904; Strangford House, 11 The Village Farm, Middleton Tyas, Richmond DL10 6SQ — MB ChB Birm. 1986.

WILLIAMS, David (retired) The Old Orchard, Saintbury, Broadway WR12 7PX Tel: 01386 852318 — MB BCh BAO NUI 1951 (Cork) DA Eng. 1958. Prev: Assoc. Specialist (Anaesth.) Kidderminster Gen. Redditch Hosps.

WILLIAMS, David 45 James Street, Lossiemouth IV31 6BZ — MB ChB Dundee 1983; BMSc (Path.) Dund 1980; MRCP (UK) 1985; MD Ed. 1993; FRCP Ed. 1995. Cons. Med. & Gastroenterol. Doctor Gray's Hosp. Elgin. Specialty: Gen. Med.; Gastroenterol. Socs: Brit. Soc. Gastroenterol. Prev: Clin. Tutor Hope Hosp. Salford.; Lect. (Med.) Univ. Sheff.

WILLIAMS, David Alastair Wyndham Southover, Bronshill Road, Torquay TQ1 3HD Tel: 01803 327100 — MB BCh BAO Dub. 1958; MA. Prev: Regist. (Anaesth.) Torbay Hosp. Torquay; SHO (Anaesth.) Bristol United Hosps.; Surg. P. & O. Orient Lines.

WILLIAMS, David Anthony Blandford House Surgery, 7 London Road, Braintree CM7 2LD Tel: 01376 347100 Fax: 01376 349934; Boleyns, Church Lane, Bocking, Braintree CM7 5SE — MB BS Lond. 1978; DRCOG 1981.

WILLIAMS, David Anthony North Nottinghamshire Health, Ransom Hall, Southwell Road W., Rainworth, Mansfield NG21 0ER Tel: 01623 676026 Fax: 01623 414117; 18 Private Road, Sherwood, Nottingham NG5 4DB — MB ChB Sheff. 1980; MFPHM RCP (UK) 1995. CCDC. Specialty: Pub. Health Med. Prev: Train. Progr. Dir., Pub. Health. Med.

WILLIAMS, David Conon Compass House Centres, Brixham TQ5 9TF — MB ChB Birmingham 1971. Hosp. Practitioner in Endoscopy. Torbay Hosp. Prev: Med. Regist. Worcester Roy. Infirm.; Ho. Off. (O & G) Ronkswood Hosp. Worcester.

WILLIAMS, David Daniel Wyn Ingledene, Llandilo Road, Cross Hands, Llanelli SA14 6RR — MB BS Lond. 1962 (Lond. Hosp.) MRCS Eng. LRCP Lond. 1962. Prev: Gp. Orthop. Regist. Brentwood Hosps. Gp.; Ho. Off. (Midw. & Gyn.) St. And. Hosp. Lond.; Ho. Surg. & Cas. Off. Poplar Hosp. Lond.

WILLIAMS, David Donald Rhys Cefn Coed Hospital, Swansea SA2 0GH Tel: 01792 561155 Fax: 01792 516478 — (Lond. Hosp.) MRCS Eng. LRCP Lond. 1964; MD Lond. 1977, MB BS 1964; DPM Eng. 1968; MRCPsych 1972. Cons. Psychiat. W. Glam. HA. Specialty: Geriat. Psychiat. Socs: BMA; Welsh Med. Soc. (Y Gymdeithas Feddygol); IPA. Prev: Sen. Regist. WhitCh. Hosp. Cardiff & Morgannwg Hosp. Bridgend.

WILLIAMS, David Edward Sett Valley Medical Centre, Hyde Bank Road, New Mills, High Peak SK22 4BP Tel: 01663 743483; Dewsnaps, Chinley, High Peak SK23 6AW Tel: 01663 751175 — MB ChB Manch. 1973; DObst RCOG 1975.

WILLIAMS, David Edward 43 Marine Drive, Barry CF62 6QP Tel: 01831 527949 — MB BS Lond. 1985; BSc (Hons.) Biochem. Wales 1979. Med. Off. Subaru, Nissan & BMW Motor Racing Teams.

WILLIAMS, Mr David Gareth Holts Health Centre, Watery Lane, Newent GL18 1BA Tel: 01531 820689; Lower Farm House, Clifford's Mesne, Newent GL18 1JT Tel: 01531 821654 — MB BChir Camb. 1971 (Guy's) MA, MB BChir Camb. 1971; FRCS Eng. 1977. Family Plann. Surg. Glos. HA. Specialty: Gastroenterol.; Family Plann. & Reproduc. Health. Prev: Surg. Regist. Acad. Dept. Surg. Roy. Free Hosp. Lond.; SHO (Surg.) Roy. Cornw. Hosp. (City & Treliske) Truro; Surg. Regist. St. Helier Hosp. Carshalton.

WILLIAMS, David George 356 Crookesmoor Road, Crookes, Sheffield S10 1BH — MB ChB Sheff. 1995.

WILLIAMS, David Glyn 12 Green Park, Erodig, Wrexham LL13 7YE — MB BS Lond. 1990.

WILLIAMS, David Glyn Rushden Medical Practice, Adnitt Road, Rushden NN10 9TU Tel: 01933 412666 Fax: 01933 317666 — MB BS Lond. 1984.

WILLIAMS, David Hugh Eglwysbach Surgery, Berw Road, Pontypridd CF37 2AA Tel: 01443 406811 Fax: 01443 405457; 1 Tir-y-Coed, Parc Nant Celyn, Efail Isaf, Pontypridd CF38 1AJ — MB BCh Wales 1974; DRCOG 1976; DCH Eng. 1977; FRCGP 1994, M 1978. GP; Course Organiser; GP VTS.

WILLIAMS, Mr David Hugh Department of Orthopaedics, Hereford Hospitals NHS Trust, Stonebow Road, Hereford HR1 2ER Tel: 01432 355444 Ext: 5315 Fax: 01432 364425 Email: david.williams@hhtr.nhs.uk — MB BS Lond. 1974 (Univ. Coll. Hosp.) BSc (Hons.) Lond. 1971; FRCS Eng. 1979; MChOrth Liverp.

1986. Cons. Orthop. Surg. Hereford Hosps. & Robt. Jones & Agnes Hunt Orthop. Hosp. OsW.ry. Specialty: Orthop. Special Interest: Hip and Knee Arthroplasty; Orthopaedic Oncology. Socs: Brit. Orthopaedic Assn. Prev: Sen. Regist. Middlx. Hosp. & Roy. Nat. Orthop. Hosp. Lond.; Sen. Res. Harvard Combined Orthop. Train. Progr. Boston, U.S.A.

WILLIAMS, David Ian St Cadocs Hospital, Ty Bryn Adolescent Unit, Caerleon, Newport NP18 3XQ Tel: 01633 436944 Fax: 01633 436834 — BM Soton. 1988; MRCPsych 1994; MSc Wales 1995. Clin. Dir. Gwent Child Psychiat. Serv. Gwent Healthcare NHS Trust; Progr. Director - S. Wales Child Psychiat. Higher Train. Scheme. Specialty: Child & Adolesc. Psychiat. Socs: BMA; RSM; ACPP.

WILLIAMS, Sir David Innes (retired) 66 Murray Road, Wimbledon Common, London SW19 4PE Tel: 020 8879 1042 — MB BChir Camb. 1942 (Camb. & Univ. Coll. Hosp.) MRCS Eng. LRCP Lond. 1942; FRCS Eng. 1944; MA Camb. 1944, MD 1951, MChir 1945; Hon. FACS 1983; Hon. FRCSI 1984; Hon. FDS RCS Eng. 1986; Hon FRCPCH 1997. Prev: Cons. urological Surg., The Hosp. for sick Childr. Gt Ormond St.

WILLIAMS, Mr David James Old Canal Cottage, Dunkerton, Bath BA2 8BS — MB BS Lond. 1991 (The London Hospital Medical College) FRCS Eng. 1995; FRCS 2002. Spec. Regist. Rot. (Gen. Surg.) S. West. Specialty: Gen. Surg. Socs: Roy. Soc, Med.; Assn. Surg. Train.; Rouleaux Club. Prev: Research Fell. (Vasc. Surg.) Bath; SHO (Orthop. & Surg.) Swindon; SHO (Neurosurg. & A & E) Sheff.

WILLIAMS, Mr David John The White Cottage, 15 High Road, Essendon, Hatfield AL9 6HT — MB BS Lond. 1965 (St. Geo.) FRCS Eng. 1974. Cons. (Orthop. Surg.) BUPA Hosp. Harpenden. Specialty: Trauma & Orthop. Surg. Socs: Fell. Brit. Orthop. Assn.; Assoc. Fell. Brit. Soc. for Surg. of Hand; Fell. Roy. Soc. Med. Prev: Cons. Orthop. Surg. Qu. Eliz. II Hosp. Welwyn Gdn. City & Hertford; Cons. Orthop. Surg. N.W. Thames RHA; Sen. Regist. Rotat. (Orthop.) Char. Cross & St. Mary's Hosps. W2.

WILLIAMS, David John Longfleet House Surgery, 56 Longfleet Road, Poole BH15 2JD Tel: 01202 666677 Fax: 01202 660319 — BM Soton. 1979; DA Eng. 1981. Specialty: Gen. Pract.

WILLIAMS, David John 13 Spencer Hill, Wimbledon, London SW19 4PA Tel: 020 8946 3785 — MB BChir Camb. 1964 (St. Thos.) MA Camb. 1965; MRCP (UK) 1970; MRCGP 1972; FRCP Lond. 1982; FFAEM 1993; FRCS 1997; FRCP ED 1998; FRCS ED 1999; FRCA 2000. Clin. Adviser t the Health Serv. Commr. (Ombudsman); Mem. Of Criminal Injuries Compensation Appeals Panel. Specialty: Accid. & Emerg. Socs: Past Pres. Intercollegiate Fac. A & E Med.; (Ex-Pres.) Brit. Assn. for Accid. & Emerg. Med.; Vice-Pres. Europ. Soc. Emerg. Med. Prev: Cons. i/c A & E Middlx. Hosp. Lond.; Resid. Med. Off. Middlx. Hosp. Lond. & Nat. Heart Hosp. Lond.; Clin. Dir. A & E Guy's & St. Thos. Hosp. Lond.

WILLIAMS, David John Department of Obstretics and Gynaecology, Imperial College of Science, Technology and Medicine, Chelsea and Academic Westminster hospital, 369 Fulham Road, London SW10 9NH Tel: 020 8237 5175 Fax: 020 8237 5089 Email: david.williams@ic.ac.uk; 1 Hearne Road, London W4 3NJ — MB BS Lond. 1984 (The Royal London Hospital Medical College) MRCP (UK) 1987; PhD 2003. Sen. Lect./Honourary Cons., Matern. Med., Imperial Coll., Lond. Specialty: Obst. & Gyn.; Nephrol. Special Interest: Renal Dis. in Pregn.; Path. and Management of Pre-Eclampsia. Socs: Brit. Matern. and Fetal Med. Soc.; Sec. Macdonald Club Obst. Med. Gp.; Sec. Internat. Soc.Obstetric Med. Prev: Lect. & Hon. Sen. Regist. (Nephrol.) Univ. Coll. Lond. Med. Sch.; Research Fell. (Anat. & Developm. Biol.) Brit. Heart Foundat. Univ. Coll. Lond.; Regist. (Nephrol.) St. Peter's Hosp. Lond.

WILLIAMS, David John Morriston Hospital, Morriston, Swansea SA6 6NL — MB ChB Birm. 1990; DA (UK) 1996; FRCA (UK) 1997; DipDHM 2001; CCST 2002. Cons. Cardiothoracic Anaesth. Morriston Hosp. Swansea. Specialty: Anaesth. Prev: Clin. Fell. (Cardiac Anaesth.) Roy. Brompton Hosp. Lond.; Diving & Hyperbaric Med. Roy. Adelaide Hosp. Austral.

WILLIAMS, David John Michael Chalice Cottage, 90 The Street, Little Waltham, Chelmsford CM3 3NT Tel: 01245 360065 — MB BS Lond. 1976; FFA RCSI 1981; FFA RCS Eng. 1982; MBA Open Univ. 1995. Cons. Anaesth. Mid Essex Hosp. Chelmsford. Specialty: Anaesth. Prev: Cons. Anaesth. Broomfield Hosp. Chelmsford.; Sen. Regist. (Anaesth.) Lond. Hosp. Whitechapel; Sen. Regist. (Anaesth.) Hosp. for Sick Childr. Gt. Ormond St. Lond.

WILLIAMS, David Laurence Cherrybrook Medical Centre, Paignton TQ4 7SH Tel: 01803 844566 Fax: 01803 845244; 17 Oyster Bend, Paignton TQ4 6NL Tel: 01803 669183 — MB ChB Dundee 1978; DRCOG 1981; DA Eng. 1982. Socs: Torbay Med. Soc. Prev: Trainee GP Exeter VTS; SHO (O & G) W. Suff. Hosp. Bury St. Edmunds; SHO (Anaesth.) Torbay Hosp.

WILLIAMS, David Llewelyn Department of Clinical Biochemistry, Royal Berkshire Hospital, Reading RG1 5AN Tel: 0118 987 7709 Fax: 0118 987 7755 Email: sasdwill@cix.compulink.co.uk — MB Camb. 1972 (Camb. & Oxf.) MA Camb. 1987, BA 1961; PhD Reading 1966; MB BChir Camb. 1972; FRSC 1982; CChem 1982; FRCPath 1991. Dir. Path. & Cons. Chem. Pathol. Roy. Berks. & Battle Hosps. NHS Trust Reading; Vis. Prof. Univ. Reading. Specialty: Chem. Path. Socs: Assn. Clin. Biochems.; Assn. Clin. Paths. Prev: Cons. Chem. Pathol. St. Peter's Hosp. Chertsey & Ashford Hosp. Middlx.; Sen. Lect. (Clin. Biochem.) Univ. Surrey; Edr. Annals. Clin. Biochem.

WILLIAMS, David Lloyd The Surgery, 59 Sevenoaks Road, Orpington BR6 9JN Tel: 01689 820159 — MB BS Lond. 1978. Princip. Gen. Pract. Orpington. Prev: Ho. Surg. & Paediat. SHO Pembury Hosp.; Trainee Gen. Pract. Portsmouth Vocational Train. Scheme.

WILLIAMS, Mr David Lloyd Trelew, 73 Longogarth, Fferham, Benllech, Tyn-y-Gongl LL74 8TA Tel: 0124 88 52208 — MB BCh Wales 1965; FRCS Ed. 1975. Staff Grade (Orthop.) Glan Clwyd Hosp. St. Asaph. Specialty: Trauma & Orthop. Surg. Prev: Regist. (Orthop.) Withington Hosp. Manch.

WILLIAMS, David Mansell The Health Centre, Stanwell Road, Penarth CF64; 18 Victoria Square, Penarth CF64 Tel: 01222 702301 — MB BCh Wales 1965 (Cardiff) Prev: Sen. Ho. Phys. Profess. Med. Unit Cardiff Roy. Infirm.; Sen. Ho. Phys. Cardiothoracic Centre, Sully.

WILLIAMS, David Meredith (retired) Wycombe, Vaynor Road, Cefn Coed, Merthyr Tydfil CF48 2HE — MD Wales 1961 (Cardiff) BSc Wales 1942, MD 1961, MB BCh 1945; FRCP Lond. 1974, M 1952. Prev: Cons. Phys. Merthyr & Aberdare Hosps.

WILLIAMS, David Michael Jeremy, OStJ (retired) 6 Park Road, Barry CF62 6NU Tel: 01446 734925 Fax: 01446 734925 — MB BCh Wales 1960 (Cardiff) MD Wales 1978; FFOM 1992, MFOM 1981. Prev: Sen. Med. Off. B.P. Chem.s Ltd. Lond.

WILLIAMS, David Owen The Medical Centre, Kingston Avenue, E. Horsley, Leatherhead KT24 6QT Tel: 01483 284151 Fax: 01483 285814; Dytchleys, The St, West Horsley, Leatherhead KT24 6HS Tel: 0148 652487 — MB BS Lond. 1956 (Lond. Hosp.) MRCS Eng. LRCP Lond. 1956; DObst RCOG 1959. Socs: BMA (Ex-Chairm. Guildford Div.). Prev: Hosp. Pract. Accid. Centre Roy. Surrey Co. Hosp. Guildford; Receiv. Room Off., Ho. Surg. & Res. Accouch. Lond. Hosp.

WILLIAMS, David Owen 16 Mitchell Avenue, Jesmond, Newcastle upon Tyne NE2 3LA Tel: 0191 811410 — MB ChB Birm. 1964; MRCS Eng. LRCP Lond. 1964; FRCP Ed. 1983, M 1968; FRCP Lond. 1981, M 1968. Cons. Cardiol. Newc. HA. Specialty: Cardiol. Prev: Brit. Amer. Research Fell. Miami USA; Hon. Sen. Regist. Cardiol. Qu. Eliz. Hosp. Birm.; Regist. in Cardiol. Sully Hosp.

WILLIAMS, David Paul The Surgery, Marshall House, Bancroft Court, Hitchin SG5 1LH Tel: 01462 420740 — MB ChB Liverp. 1984. SHO (O & G) N.d. HA. Prev: Trainee GP N.d. VTS.

WILLIAMS, Professor David Robert Rhys Nuffield Institute for Health, 71-75 Clarendon Road, Leeds LS2 9PL Tel: 0113 233 3453 Fax: 0113 233 3952; 12 Ellis House, Ellis Court, Harrogate HG1 2SH Fax: 01423 875606 — MB BS Lond. 1972; MRCS Eng. LRCP Lond. 1972; PhD Durh. 1978; FFPHM RCP (UK) 1988, M 1982; MA Camb. 1988; FRCP Lond. 1993. Prof. Epidemiol. & Pub. Health Uni.Leeds. Specialty: Pub. Health Med. Socs: Mem. Bd. of Trustees, Diabetes UK; Vice-Pres. Int'l Diabetes Fed. Prev: Univ. Lect. Camb. Univ.; Addison Wheeler Research Fell. Univ. Durh.; MRC Train. Fell. Epidemiol. Dunn Clin. Nutrit. Centre Camb.

WILLIAMS, David Thomas Cascade Cottage, Pengam Road, Penpedairheol, Hengoed CF82 8BX — MB BCh Wales 1990.

WILLIAMS, David Thomas Victoria Surgery, 5 Victoria Road, Holyhead LL65 1UD; Bryn Teg, Gorad Road, Valley, Holyhead LL65 3BT Tel: 01407 742488 — MB BS Lond. 1982; DRCOG 1985; MRCGP 1987. GP Holyhead.

WILLIAMS, David Thomas Arthur, OStJ (retired) Nythfa, 11 Bishop's Grove, Sketty, Swansea SA2 8BE Tel: 01792 204321 — (Roy. Lond. Hosp.) MB BS Lond. 1956; DObst RCOG 1958.

WILLIAMS, David Tobias (retired) Tor-Na-Coille, 5 Walnut Grove, Kinfauns, Perth PH2 7UJ Tel: 01738 624629 — (St. And.) MB ChB St. And. 1961.

WILLIAMS, David Trevor Huxley Biffins, Lane End, Hambledon, Godalming GU8 4HD — MB BS Lond. 1970 (St Bart.) BDS Lond. 1966; MRCS Eng. LRCP Lond. 1970; DObst RCOG 1973; FFHom 1997. Specialty: Homeop. Med.; Acupunc.; Hypnother. Socs: Brit. Soc. Med. Dent. Hypn; Fell. Fac. Homeop.; Accred. Mem. Brit. Med. Acupunc.

WILLIAMS, David Vaughan South Forest Centre, 21 Thorne Close, Leytonstone, London E11 4HU Tel: 020 8535 6480 Fax: 020 8535 6481 Email: Vaughan.Williams@nelmht.nhs.uk — MB BCh Wales 1985 (University of Wales College of Medicine) MRCPsych 1990. Cons. Gen. Adult Psychi. NE Lon Ment. Health NHS Trust. Specialty: Gen. Psychiat. Prev: Regist. (Psychiat. & Ment. Handicap) Mid. Glam. HA; Clin. Asst. (Psychiat.) Claybury Hosp. NE Thames RHA; Ho. Off. (Gen. Med.) Clwyd HA.

WILLIAMS, Dean Thomas 37 Heath Park Avenue, Cardiff CF14 3RF — MB BS Lond. 1990.

WILLIAMS, Deborah (retired) Lonkeda, Pen-y-Walln, Pentyrch, Cardiff CF15 9SJ Tel: 029 2089 2398 — MB BS Newc. 1981. Retainer GP WhitCh. Cardiff. Prev: Trainee GP Ystrad Myroch.

WILLIAMS, Deborah Elizabeth Marine Surgery, 29 Belle Vue Road, Southbourne, Bournemouth BH6 3DB Tel: 01202 423377 Fax: 01202 424277 — MB BS Lond. 1974; DRCOG 1977; MRCGP 1978. GP Bournemouth. Prev: Trainee GP Bath VTS; Ho. Phys. Univ. Coll. Hosp. Lond.

WILLIAMS, Deborah Innes The Lawson Unit, The Royal Sussex County Hospital, Eastern Road, Brighton BN2 5BE; 60 Osmond Road, Hove BN3 1TF — MB ChB Sheff. 1984; MRCP (UK) 1987; DTM & H Lond. 1992. Cons. (GUM & HIV) The Roy. Sussex Co. Hosp. Brighton. Specialty: Genitourinary Medicine; HIV Med.

WILLIAMS, Deborah Lynne 8 Harold Hicks Place, Percy St., Oxford OX4 3OS — MB BCh Wales 1987; MRCPsych 1992.

WILLIAMS, Denise Karen Birmingham Women's Hospital, Department of Clinical Genetics, Edgbaston, Birmingham B15 2TG Tel: 0121 627 2630 Fax: 0121 627 2618 Email: denise.williams@bwhct.nhs.uk; 18 Dark Lane, Stoke Heath, Bromsgrove B60 3BH Tel: 01527 872293 Email: moloneydenise@hotmail.com — MB BCh Wales 1987 (University of Wales, College of Medicine) MRCP (UK) 1990; Dip. Human & Clin. Genetic Lond. 1992. Cons. Clin. geneticist, Birm. Specialty: Genetics. Prev: Sen. Regist. Rotat. Trent Clin. Genetics Leicester Roy. Infirm. & City Hosp. Nottm.; Regist. Clin. Genetics Birm. Matern. Hosp.; Regist. (Paediat.) Leic. Roy. Infirm.

WILLIAMS, Denise Mary Box 181, Addenbrooke's Hospital, Hill Road, Cambridge CB2 2QQ Tel: 01223 245151 Fax: 01223 216966 Email: denise.williams@addenbrookes.nhs.uk — MB BCh Wales 1980; MRCPCH; FRCP Lond, 1997,MRCP (UK) 1983. p/t Cons. Paediat. (Oncol.) Addenbrooke's Hosp. Camb. Specialty: Paediat.

WILLIAMS, Dennis Kenneth Treflan Surgery, Treflan, Lower Cardiff Road, Pwllheli LL53 5NF Tel: 01758 701457 Fax: 01758 701209 — MB ChB Liverp. 1975; DRCOG 1979; DCH RCP Lond. 1982; MRCGP 1983. Gen. Practitioner; Clin. Director; Project Director N. Wales Telemed. Project. Prev: Assoc. Post Grad. Organiser.

WILLIAMS, Denys Ian (retired) The Wheelhouse, 4 Kilburn Court, Kilburn, York YO61 4AW Tel: 01347 868696 Fax: 01347 868037 Email: doctorianwilliams@btinternet.com — (Ed.) MB ChB Ed. 1956.

WILLIAMS, Derek Owen Chest Clinic, Ealing Hospital, Uxbridge Road, Southall UB1 3HW Tel: 020 8967 5381 Fax: 020 8967 5660; 31 Pinn Way, Ruislip HA4 7QG — MB BS Lond. 1972 (Middlx.) MRCP (UK) 1977. Assoc. Specialist (Respirat. Med.) Chest Clinic Ealing Hosp. Southall & Chest & Allergy Clinic St. Mary's Hosp. Lond. Specialty: Respirat. Med. Socs: Brit. Thorac. Soc.; Amer. Thoracic Soc.; Eur. Respirat. Soc. Prev: Research Fell. & Hon. Sen. Regist. (Respirat. Med.) Hammersmith Hosp. Lond.; Instruc. (Med.) N. West. Memor. Hosp. Chicago, USA; Pulm. Fell. NW Univ. Chicago, USA.

WILLIAMS, Derfel Health Centre, Pen y Bont, The Roe, St Asaph LL17 0LU Tel: 01745 583208 Fax: 01745 583748; Bryn Arlais, Ffordd-Y-Bryn, Llanelwy, St Asaph LL17 0DD — BM Soton. 1986 (Southampton) PhD Liverp. 1979, BSc (Hons.) 1974; Dip. Palliat. Med. Wales 1993; MRCGP 1994. Prev: SHO (Paediat.) Ysbyty Glan Clwyd; Clin. Med. Off. (Community Paediat.) Clwyd N. HA; Trainee GP Clwyd N. VTS.

WILLIAMS, Deric Haydn The Health Centre, Fender Way, Noctorum, Birkenhead CH43 9QS Tel: 0151 677 1034 Fax: 0151 604 0392; Crud y Mynydd, 4 Glas Goed, Cilcain, Mold CH7 5PP Tel: 01352 741765 — MB BS Lond. 1954 (Guy's) MRCS Eng. LRCP Lond. 1954; DObst RCOG 1958; DPH Liverp. 1965; MRCGP 1980. Socs: Wirral Local Med. Comm. & Birkenhead Med. Soc. Prev: Sen. Asst. Div. Med. Off. Lancs. CC & Dep. MOH Kirkby UD; JHMO (Psychiat.) N. Wales Hosp. Denbigh; Ho. Surg. (O & G) Chester City Hosp.

WILLIAMS, Deryk John 8 The Knoll, Beckenham BR3 5JW — MB BS Lond. 1985; BSc (Hons.) Lond. 1982, MB BS 1985.

WILLIAMS, Mr Desmond Patrick Commins 25 Antringham Gardens, Westfield Road, Edgbaston, Birmingham B15 3QL Tel: 0121 455 0025 — MB ChB Liverp. 1947; DLO Eng. 1954; FRCS Ed. 1960. Cons. ENT Surg. Birm. & Midl. ENT Hosp.; Sen. Sen. Clin. Lect. Birm. Univ.; Adviser Otolaryng. & Assessor RCS Eng. Socs: Fell. Roy. Soc. Med.; Counc. Brit. Assn. Otolaryng. Prev: Demonst. Physiol. Liverp. Univ. & Hon. Demonst. (Anat.) Camb. Univ.; Sen. Regist. United Bristol Hosps.; Cons. ENT Surg. Maidstone & Medway Hosps.

WILLIAMS, Dewi Rheinallt Cons. Anaesthetist, Dumfries & Galloway Royal Infirmary, Dumfries DG1 4UP Tel: 01387 246246; Little Garth, 8 Castle Douglas Road, Dumfries DG2 7NX — (Ed.) MB ChB Ed. 1987; FRCA 1993. Cons. Anaesth. Dumfries & Galloway Roy. Infirm. Dumfries. Specialty: Anaesth.; Intens. Care. Socs: Intens. Care Soc.; Assn. Anaesth.; ESICM. Prev: SHO (Anaesth.) Ninewells Hosp. Dundee; Sen. Regist. (Anaesth.) Ninewells Hosp. Dundee.

WILLIAMS, Dominica Gale Old Road Surgery, Old Road, Abersychan, Pontypool NP4 7BH Tel: 01495 772239 Fax: 01495 773786; 7 Lime Trees Avenue, Llangattock, Crickhowell NP8 1LB Tel: 01873 810110 Fax: 01873 811606 — MB ChB Bristol 1965; DObst RCOG 1967. GP Princip.; Clin. Asst. Co. Hosp. Pontypool. Socs: Fac. Fam. Plann. & Reproduc. Health Care; Fac. Fam. Plann. & Reproduc. Health Care. Prev: GP Kingston & Richmond FPC; Clin. Med. Off. Gwent AHA.

WILLIAMS, Doris (retired) 7 Pencoed Avenue, Pontypridd CF37 4AN — MB BS Lond. 1926 (Cardiff & Westm.) MRCS Eng., LRCP Lond. 1923; DPH Wales 1926. Prev: Asst. Co. Sch. Med. Off. Glam. CC.

WILLIAMS, Dorothea Mary Oxford Street Surgery, Oxford Street, Aberaeron SA46 0JB Tel: 01545 570273 Fax: 01545 571625; Drefnewydd Farm, Aberaeron SA46 0JR Tel: 01545 570024 — MB ChB Birm. 1965.

WILLIAMS, Duncan Andrew Hannage Brook Medical Centre, Hannage Way, Wirksworth, Derby DE4 4JG — MB ChB Birm. 1992.

WILLIAMS, Duncan Howard Department of Anaesthetics, Christchurch Hospital, Private BAG 4710, Christchurch, New Zealand; Quarry Dene, 36 Church Lane, Bardsey, Leeds LS17 9DP Tel: 01937 572153 — MB ChB Sheff. 1983; FANZCA; DRCOG 1986. Cons. (Anaesth.) ChristCh. Hosp. Specialty: Anaesth. Socs: Fell. Australia & New Zealand Coll. Of Anaesth. Prev: Regist. (Anaesth.) Waikato Hosp. Hamilton, NZ.

WILLIAMS, Duncan Meredydd Amman Valley Medical Practice, Graig Road Surgery, Gwann-Cae-Gurwen, Ammanford SA18 Tel: 01269 822231; Oaklands, Derwydd Road, Derwydd, Ammanford SA18 2TT Tel: 01296 850785 — MB BCh Wales 1984; DRCOG 1987; MRCGP 1988. Specialty: Forens. Path.

WILLIAMS, Dylan Williams, O'Connor and Morgan, New Quay Surgery, Church Road, New Quay SA45 9PB Tel: 01545 560203 Fax: 01545 560916; Lake View, Oakford, Llanarth SA47 0RW Tel: 01545 580042 — MB BS Lond. 1978; BSc Lond. 1975; DA (UK) 1984.

WILLIAMS, Dylan Wyn 36 Holland Street, Ebbw Vale NP23 6HZ — MB BCh Wales 1990.

WILLIAMS, Dylan Wynne Department of Histopathology, Swansea NHS Trust, Singleton Hospital, Swansea SA2 8QA — MB BS Lond.

1983; BSc (Hons.) Lond. 1980, MB BS 1983; PhD Wales 1988; FRCPath 1999; MBA 2002. Cons. Histopath. Specialty: Histopath.
WILLIAMS, Earl Jon 20 Kingsley Avenue, Cannock WS12 4EA — MB ChB Leic. 1994.
WILLIAMS, Edna May Community & Mental Health Trust, St. Mary's Hospital, Greenhill Road, Armley, Leeds LS12 3QE Tel: 0113 279 0121; 8 St. Winfreds Road, Harrogate HG2 8LN Tel: 01423 883404 — MB ChB Aberd. 1976. Assoc. Specialist Community & Ment. Health Trust Leeds. Specialty: Community Child Health. Prev: SCMO Clwyd DHA.
WILLIAMS, Professor Sir Edward Dillwyn Thyroid Carcinogenesis Research Group, Strangeways Research Laboratories, Wort's Causeway, Cambridge CB1 8RN Tel: 01223 740180 Fax: 01223 411609 Email: dillwyn@srl.cam.ac.uk; Burford House, Hildersham, Cambridge CB1 6BU Tel: 01223 893316 — (Lond. Hosp.) MD Camb. 1983, MB BChir 1953; FRCPath. 1977, M 1965; FRCP Lond. 1977, M 1973. Emerit. Prof. Histopath. Univ. Camb; Director, Thyroid Carcinogenesis Research Gp., Strangeways Laborat., Camb. Specialty: Histopath. Special Interest: Carcinogenesis, especially thyroid & radiat.; Consequences of the Chernobyl Accid. Socs: Europ. Thyroid Assn. (Past Pres.); Roy. Coll. Path. (Past Pres.); BMA (Past Pres.). Prev: Prof. Path. Univ. Wales Coll. Med.; Reader (Morbid Anat.) Roy. Postgrad. Med. Sch. Lond.
WILLIAMS, Professor Edward Idris, OBE (retired) Morecambe Bay Hospitals NHS Trust, Trust HQ, Westmorland General Hospital, Burton Road, Kendal LA9 7RG Tel: 01539 795366 Fax: 01539 795313 Email: idris.williams@k.bay-tr.nwest.nhs.uk — MB ChB Manch. 1954; DObst RCOG 1961; FRCGP 1976, M 1965; MD Manch. 1973. Emerit. Prof. Gen. Pract. Univ. Nottm.; Chairm. Morecambe Bay Hosp.s NHS Trust. Prev: Sen. Lect. (Gen. Pract.) Univ. Manch.
WILLIAMS, Edward James (retired) 24 Birkett Drive, Ulverston LA12 9LS Tel: 01229 583746 — MB ChB Leeds 1960; DPM Leeds 1971; MRCPsych 1973. Prev: Hon. Cons. Psychiat. St. Luke's Hosp. for Clergy Lond.
WILLIAMS, Mr Edward John, RD Upper Meadow, Hedgerley Lane, Gerrards Cross SL9 7NP Tel: 01753 882651 — MB BS Lond. 1950 (Lond. Hosp.) MS Lond. 1965, MB BS 1950; FRCS Eng. 1958. Cons. Surg. St. Mary's Hosp. Lond. & Wexham Pk. Hosp. Slough. Socs: Pres. Vasc. Surg. Soc. Gt. Brit. & Irel.; Europ. Soc. Vasc. Surg.; Assn. Surgs. Gt. Brit. & Irel. Prev: Asst. Dir., Surg. Unit St. Mary's Hosp. Lond.; Sen. Regist. (Surg.) Lond. Hosp.; Surg. Fell. Presbyt. St. Luke's Hosp. Chicago, USA.
WILLIAMS, Edward Robert (retired) Croft Cottage, West End, Bitteswell, Lutterworth LE17 4UX Tel: 01455 557020 — MB BChir Camb. 1961 (Westm.) FRCP Lond. 1980, M 1963; MA, MD Camb. 1971. Prev: Sen. Regist. (Med.) Bristol Roy. Infirm.
WILLIAMS, Professor Edward Sydney (retired) Little Hollies, The Close, Wonersh, Guildford GU5 0PA Tel: 01483 892591 — MB BS Lond. 1957 (Middlx.) FRCP Lond. 1979, M 1970; PhD Lond. 1963, BSc 1950, MD 1971; FRCR 1983. Prev: Prof. Nuclear Med. Univ. Lond.
WILLIAMS, Edwin Market Street Surgery, 3-5 Market Street, Caernarfon LL55 1RT Tel: 01286 673224 Fax: 01286 676405 — MB BS Lond. 1988 (Guy's) Socs: Cymdeithas Feddygol. Prev: Trainee GP Awdurdod Iechyd Gwynedd VTS.
WILLIAMS, Edwina Rachel Louise Department of Liaison Psychiatry & ICRF Psychosocial Ongology, 3rd Floor, Riddell House, St Thomas's Hospital, Lambeth Palace Rd, London SE1 7EH Email: edwina.williams@kcl.ac.uk; 266 Camberwell New Road, London SE5 0RP Email: erlw@lineone.net — MB BCh Wales 1988; Msc (Manch). Specialty: Gen. Psychiat. Socs: MRCPsych.
WILLIAMS, Mr Eifion Vaughan 25 Heol-y-Coed, Rhiwbina, Cardiff CF14 6HQ — MB BCh Wales 1988; FRCS Glas. 1994. SHO E. Glam Ch. Village. Specialty: Gen. Surg. Prev: SHO (Gen. Surg.) Roy. Gwent Hosp.
WILLIAMS, Eileen Gibson Neish Glan Clywd Hospital, Conwy and Denbighshire NHS Trust, Rhyl LL18 5UJ Tel: 01745 534969 — MB ChB Glas. 1977; FFA RCS Eng. 1982. Cons. Anaesth. Glan Clwyd Hosp. Rhyl. Specialty: Anaesth. Prev: Sen. Regist. (Anaesth.) Mersey RHA; Sen. Regist. (Anaesth.) Ysbyty Glan Clwyd Hosp. Rhyl.; Sen. Regist. (Anaesth.) Countess of Chester Hosp.
WILLIAMS, Eirlys Jean (retired) Broadway, 43 Southgate Road, Southgate, Swansea SA3 2DA Tel: 01505 2207 — LRCP LRCS Ed. 1951; LRCP LRCS Ed. LRFPS Glas. 1951. Prev: Govt. Med. Off. Paediat. Unit Colon. War Memor. Hosp. Suva, Fiji.
WILLIAMS, Eleanor Mair Tabernacle Street Surgery, 4 Tabernacle Street, Skewen, Neath SA10 6UF Tel: 01792 817009 / 817573 Fax: 01792 321029; Ty-Gwyn, 33A Penywern Road, Neath SA10 7AW — MD Wales 1981; BSc (Hons.) (Genetics) Wales 1971, MB BCh 1976; MRCGP 1991. Hon. Lect. (Med. Genetics) Welsh Nat. Sch. Med.; Hosp. Pract. (Med. Genetics) Welsh Nat. Sch. Med. Cardiff & Singleton Hosp. Swansea.; Med. FHSA. Specialty: Genetics. Prev: Ho. Off. Dept. Med. Llandough Hosp. Cardiff & Dept. Surg. Univ. Hosp. Wales Cardiff.
WILLIAMS, Eleri Catherine 30 Esher Avenue, Walton-on-Thames KT12 2TA — MB BS Lond. 1991.
WILLIAMS, Elisabeth Dorothy The Coach House, 31A Park Hill, Moseley, Birmingham B13 8DR Tel: 0121 449 0123 — MB ChB Birm. 1960.
WILLIAMS, Elisabeth Ruth 19 Allt-Yr-Yn Close, Newport NP20 5ED — BM Soton. 1995. SHO (Paediat.) Roy. Gwent Hosp. Newport. Specialty: Paediat.
WILLIAMS, Elizabeth Ann — BChir Camb. 1986; MB 1987; MChir 1997; FC (Cardio) SA 2000.
WILLIAMS, Elizabeth Ann The Gillies Health Centre, Sullivan Rd, Brighton Hill, Basingstoke RG22 4EH Tel: 01256 479747 Fax: 01256 320627; Sherfield End, Reading Rd, Sherfield on Loddon, Hook RG27 0JG — BM BCh Oxf. 1978; MA Camb. 1978; DRCOG 1981; MRCGP 1982; MRCP (UK) 1982. Gen. Practitioner The Gillies & Overbridge Med. Partnership Basingstoke. Specialty: Gen. Pract. Prev: Clin. Asst. (Oncol.) Basingstoke Dist. Hosp.; Non-Princip. GP Basingstoke.
WILLIAMS, Elizabeth Anne Intake Farm, Chevin End Road, Menston, Ilkley LS29 6BP — MB ChB Leeds 1975. Assoc. Specialist Yorks. Regional Blood Transfus. Serv.
WILLIAMS, Elizabeth Anne Trinity Street Surgery, 20 Trinity Street, Dorchester DT1 1TU Tel: 01304 251545; West Knighton House, West Knighton, Dorchester DT2 8PF — MB BS Lond. 1978 (Middlx.) MRCP (UK) 1981; MRCP (UK) 1981; DCH RCP Lond. 1984; DCH RCP London 1984. Princip. in Gen. Pract.
WILLIAMS, Elizabeth Carol The Surgery, Captain French Lane, Kendal LA9 4HR Tel: 015394 42496 Fax: 015394 48329; Old Heathwaite, Pk Road, Windermere LA23 2DH Tel: 015394 44740 — MB BS Newc. 1975; DRCOG 1978; MRCGP 1979; MFFP 1993. GP Tutor Kendal. Specialty: Pub. Health Med. Socs: Brit. Med. Soc.; (Comm. Mem.) NW Soc. Sexual Med. & Family Plann. Prev: GP Sale; GP Trainee Newc. VTS; Clin. Med. Off. (Train., Family Plann. & Well Wom. Servs.) Manch.
WILLIAMS, Elizabeth Jane The Clapham Park Surgery, 72 Clarence Avenue, London SW4 8JP Tel: 020 8674 0101 Fax: 020 8674 2941 — MB BS Lond. 1982; DTM & H RCP Lond. 1989; DRCOG 1993.
WILLIAMS, Elizabeth Jane Geufron, Llangollen LL20 8DY — MB ChB Birm. 1969; DMRT Eng. 1972. SCMO (Radiother.) N. Staffs. Infirm. Prev: Sen. Regist. (Radiother.) N. Staffs.Infirm.; Clin. Asst. (Radiother.) N. Staffs. Infirm.; Regist. & Research Regist. Cookridge Hosp. Leeds.
WILLIAMS, Elizabeth Jean 8 Catalina Drive, Poole BH15 1UZ — BM Soton. 1990; BSc Psychol. (1st. cl. Hons.) 1989; MRCP (UK) 1993; PhD Soton. 2001. SpR Gastroenterol. & Gen. Med. Wessex. Specialty: Gastroenterol. Prev: MRC Clin. Research Fell. Dept. Med. Univ. Soton.; Regist. Rotat. (Gastroenterol. & Gen. Med.) Soton.; SHO Rotat. (Med.) Bournemouth & Poole.
WILLIAMS, Elizabeth Joan Department of Chemical Pathology, Princess of Wales Hospital, Coity Road, Bridgend CF31 1RQ Tel: 01656 752337 — MB BCh Wales 1981 (Welsh National School Medicine) PhD (Med. Biochem.) Wales 1975, BSc (Hons.) Biochem. 1971; MRCPath 1986; LLM 1993. Cons. Chem. Path. Princess of Wales Hosp. Bridgend.; Clin. Dir. (Pathol.) 1995-; PostGrad. Organiser/Clin. Tutor 1994-. Specialty: Chem. Path. Prev: Sen. Regist. (Med. Biochem.) Univ. Hosp. Wales. Cardiff.
WILLIAMS, Elizabeth Mary (retired) Land Farm, Blackshaw Head, Hebden Bridge HX7 7PJ Tel: 01422 842240 Fax: 01422 842260 — (Newc.) MB BS Durh. 1963; DCH Eng. 1965.
WILLIAMS, Elizabeth Mary White Posts, Charlton All Saints, Salisbury SP5 4HQ — MB ChB Bristol 1970; DObst RCOG 1972; DCH Eng. 1973. Specialty: Community Child Health.

WILLIAMS, Elwyn Brinley (retired) 4 Birch Tree Lane, Goostrey, Crewe CW4 8NS — MB BCh Wales 1968; Cardiff); MFPM RCP (UK) 1991. Prev: Clin. Asst. (Diabetes) Manch. Roy. Infirm.

WILLIAMS, Emily Margaret Nuffield Department Anaesthetics, John Radcliffe Hospital, Headley Way, Oxford OX3 9DU — BM Soton. 1982; DCH RCP Lond. 1987; FCAnaesth 1989. Cons. Anaesth. John Radcliffe Hosp. Oxf. Specialty: Anaesth. Prev: Sen. Regist. (Anaesth.) Roy. Free Hosp. Lond.

WILLIAMS, Emlyn 71 Rodney Street, Liverpool L1 9EX Tel: 0151 708 8300 Fax: 0151 707 2047 — (Char. Cross) MB BS Lond. 1967; FRCP Lond. 1989, M 1971. Cons. Phys. (Rheum. & Rehabil.) Roy. Liverp. Univ. Hosp. & The Univ. Hosp. at Aintree; Cons. in Rehabil. Med. Roy. Preston Hosp., Preston. Specialty: Rheumatol.; Rehabil. Med. Socs: Brit. Soc. Rheum.; Brit. Soc. Rehabil. Med.

WILLIAMS, Emma Elizabeth Ellen — MB BS Lond. 1992 (Univ. Coll. & Middlx. Hosp. Med. Sch.) BSc (Physiol.) Lond. 1989; DCH RCP Lond. 1995; MRCGP London 1999; DFFP 2000. Gen. Practitioner Retainer Scheme, Wickham Gp. Surg., Hants. Specialty: Gen. Pract.; Family Plann. & Reproduc. Health.

WILLIAMS, Erbin Hughes Llanishen Court Surgery, Llanishen Court, Llanishen, Cardiff CF14 5YU Tel: 029 2075 7025 Fax: 029 2074 7931; Llanishen Court Surgery, Llanishen, Cardiff CF14 5YU Tel: 01222 757025 — MB BCh Wales 1973; Cert Contracep. & Family Plann. RCOG, RCGP &; DObst RCOG 1975; Cert FPA 1976; MRCGP 1977. Princip. in Gen. Pract.

WILLIAMS, Evan (retired) Cartref, Tudweiliog, Pwllheli LL53 8NA Tel: 01758 770329 — (Guy's) MRCS Eng. LRCP Lond. 1942; DPH Birm. 1947; MFCM 1974.

WILLIAMS, Evan David Glyndwr 10 Hillside Park, Bargoed CF81 8NL Tel: 01443 831009 — MRCS Eng. LRCP Lond. 1961 (King's Coll. Hosp.) MB Camb. 1961, BChir 1960.

WILLIAMS, Evelyn May Isobel Department of Public Health, Quadrangle, University of Liverpool, Liverpool L69 3GB Tel: 0151 794 5690 Fax: 0151 794 5700 Email: emiw@liv.ac.uk; 6 Chestnut Avenue, Crosby, Liverpool L23 2SZ — MD Lond. 1989; MB BS 1978; MA Camb. 1979; MFCM 1989; FFPHM 1996. Sen. Lect. (Pub. Health) Univ. Liverp. Specialty: Pub. Health Med. Prev: Cons. Pub. Health Med. Oxf. RHA.

WILLIAMS, (Evelyn) Moira (retired) 7 Bennetts Copse, Chislehurst BR7 5SG Tel: 020 8467 9809 — MB BCh Wales 1962; MRCPath 1974. Prev: Cons. Haemat. S. Lond. Blood Transfus. Serv.

WILLIAMS, F Gail Welsh Blood Service, Ely Valley Road, Talbot Green, Pontyclun CF72 9WB Tel: 01443 622016 Fax: 01443 622028 Email: gail.williams@wbs.wales.nhs.uk; The Hollies, 52 Kelston Road, Whitchurch, Cardiff CF14 2AH Tel: 02920 610158 — MB BS Lond. 1972; MRCS Eng. LRCP Lond. 1972; Cert. Family Plann. JCC 1976; FRCPath 1991, M 1979; LLM 1994. Dir. Welsh Blood Serv. Specialty: Blood Transfus. Socs: Fell. Roy. Soc. Med.; Hon. Sec. Brit. Blood Transfus. Soc. Prev: Cons. Blood Transfus. Welsh Regional Transfus. Centre Cardiff; Cons. Haemat. P. Chas. Hosp. Merthyr Tydfil; Lect. (Haemat.) St. Mary's Hosp. Lond.

WILLIAMS, Ffion Eleri 19 Parc Gwelfor, Dyserth, Rhyl LL18 6LN — MB ChB Liverp. 1998; MB ChB Liverp 1998.

WILLIAMS, Fiona Clare Stoke Mandeville Hospital, Chest Department, Aylesbury HP21 8AL — MB ChB Aberd. 1989; MRCP (UK) 1994; MFPM 2000. Chest Specialist Staff Grade Stoke Mandeville Hosp. Specialty: Pharmaceutical Medicine; Gen. Med. Socs: Brit. Thorac. Soc. Prev: Med. Adviser Pharmaceut. Div. Bayer plc Newbury.; Clin. Asst. Stoke Mandeville Hosp.; Regist. & SHO (Med.) Stoke Mandeville Hosp. Aylesbury.

WILLIAMS, Frances 9 Pearson Road, Cleethorpes DN35 0DR — MB ChB Manch. 1988; FRCA 1994. Assoc. Specialist (Anaesth.) Jas. Paget Hosp. Specialty: Anaesth. Prev: Regist. (Anaesth.) Aberd. Roy. Infirm.; SHO (Anaesth.) Bradford Roy. Infirm.; SHO (Paediat.) Leeds Gen. Infirm.

WILLIAMS, Frances Mary Kingsley 75 Bennerley Road, London SW11 6DR Fax: 020 7223 8364; Research Haematology, 4th Floor North Wing, St. Thomas' Hospital, Lambeth Palace Road, London SE1 7EH Tel: 020 7928 9292 1439 Fax: 020 7928 5698 — MB BS Lond. 1992 (St. Mary's Hosp. Med. Sch.) BSc Lond. 1991; MRCP (UK) 1995. ARC Clin. Fell. Lupus Research Unit Rayne Inst. St. Thomas' Hosp. Lond. Specialty: Rheumatol.

WILLIAMS, Frances Watcyn Hillside, Friog, Fairbourne LL38 2NX — MB BChir Camb. 1982; MA Camb. 1982, MB BChir 1982; MRCP (UK) 1986; DTM & H Lond. 1991; MRCPCH 1997.

WILLIAMS, Frank Brynawel, LLangattock, Crickhowell NP8 1PY — MB BCh Wales 1973 (Cardiff) FRCR 1979; MA Wales 1994. Cons. Radiol. Nevill Hall Hosp. Abergavenny. Specialty: Radiol.

WILLIAMS, Frank Aldwyn Benedict Melrose Surgery, 73 London Road, Reading RG1 5BS Tel: 0118 950 7950 Fax: 0118 959 4044 — MRCS Eng. LRCP Lond. 1968.

WILLIAMS, Frank Middleton Warner (retired) 3 Tudor Gardens, London W3 0DT Tel: 020 8993 2034 — MB BS Lond. 1949 (Lond. Hosp. Med. Coll.) MRCP Ed. 1954; FRCP Ed. 1982. Prev: Cons. Phys. & Paediat. Med. Arts Centre, Geo.town, Guyana.

WILLIAMS, Frank Richard Seafield of Raigmore, Inverness IV2 7PA Tel: 01463 711205 Fax: 01463 711205 — (Ed.) AKC; BA Lond. 1962; BSc Ed. 1966; MB ChB Ed. 1969; DMRD 1973; FRCR 1976. Cons. Radiol. Highland HB. Specialty: Radiol. Socs: Highland Med. Soc., Scott. Radiol. Soc. & BMA.

WILLIAMS, Gabrielle Joan Village Surgery, Station Road, Southwater, Horsham RH13 9HQ Tel: 01403 730016 Fax: 01403 730660; 5 Kingsfold Close, Billingshurst RH14 9HG Tel: 01403 784401 — MB ChB Leeds 1970; DObst. RCOG 1972.

WILLIAMS, Gareth Heol Fach Surgery, Heol Fach, North Cornelly, Bridgend CF33 4LD Tel: 01656 740345 Fax: 01656 740872; Stormybrook Surgery, Waunbant Road, Kenfig Hill, Bridgend CF33 6DE Tel: 01656 746611 — MB BCh Wales 1977; MRCGP 1981.

WILLIAMS, Professor Gareth University of Bristol, Senate House, Tyndall Avenue, Bristol BS8 1TH Tel: 0117 928 8834 Fax: 0117 934 9854; Vellows, Rockhampton, Berkeley GL13 9DY Tel: 01454 260940 Email: gareth.williams@bristol.ac.uk — MB BChir Camb. 1977; FRCP Lond. 1991 (resigned 1998); MRCP (UK) 1979; MD Camb. 1986; FRCP Edin. 1999; ScD 2003. Dean Fac. Med. & Dent. Univ. Bristol & Hon. Cons. Phys. (Med.) United Bristol Healthcare Trust. Specialty: Diabetes. Socs: Amer. Diabetes Assn.; Anglo-French Med. Soc.(Past-Pres.). Prev: Prof. Med. Univ. Liverp. & Hon. Cons. Phys. (Med.) Aintree Hosps. Liverp.; R.D. Lawrence Research Fell. Roy. Postgrad. Med. Sch. Lond.

WILLIAMS, Gareth David 95 Regent Road, Leicester LE1 7AX — MB BS Lond. 1992 (St. Thos. Hosp. Med. Sch.) Specialist Regist. Anaesth. Leicester Teachg. Hosps. Specialty: Anaesth.

WILLIAMS, Gareth David Vaughan Old Fire Station, Albert Terrace, Beverley HU17 8JW Tel: 01482 862236 Fax: 01482 861863 — MB ChB Leeds 1985; DRCOG 1987; DCH Glas. 1988; BSc Leeds 1988; MRCGP 1989; FRCGP 1998.

WILLIAMS, Gareth Vaughan Darlington Memorial Hospital, Hollyhurst Road, Darlington DL3 6HX — MB BS Lond. 1973; MRCP (UK) 1975; FRCP Lond. 1991. Cons. Phys. Darlington Memor. Hosp. Specialty: Gen. Med. Prev: Cons. Phys. Qu. Eliz. Hosp. Gateshead.

WILLIAMS, Gaynor Caroline Holycroft Surgery, The Health Centre, Oakworth Road, Keighley BD21 1SA Tel: 01535 602010 Fax: 01535 691313; Holycroft Surgery, Oakworth Road, Keighley BD21 1SA — MB ChB Leeds 1982; BSc (Hons.) Leeds 1979, MB ChB 1982. Partner Gen. Pract.

WILLIAMS, Geoffrey Wynne Western Elms Surgery, 317 Oxford Road, Reading RG30 1AT Tel: 0118 959 0257 Fax: 0118 959 7950 — MB BCh Wales 1977; DRCOG 1980; MRCGP 1981.

WILLIAMS, George (retired) 14 Tiverton Drive, Sale M33 4RJ — MB ChB St. And. 1949; MD St. And. 1957; FRCPath 1973, M 1964; PhD Manch. 1965. Prev: Reader (Path.) Univ. Manch. & Hon. Cons. Path. Manch. Roy. Infirm.

WILLIAMS, Georgina Mary Court Road Surgery, Court Road, Malvern WR14 3BL Tel: 01684 573161; Hazeldene, 29 Richmond Road, Malvern WR14 1NE Tel: 01684 568297 — MB ChB Birm. 1991; ChB Birm. 1991; DRCOG 1994; MRCGP 1996. GP Princip.; Sch. Med. Off. Malvern Girls Coll.; Clin. Asst. Gyn. Specialty: Gen. Pract.; Obst. & Gyn. Prev: SHO (O & G) Worcester HA; SHO (Paediat.) Sandwell HA; SHO & Ho. Off. (Med.) E. Birm. Hosp.

WILLIAMS, Geraint Llwyd, TD 20 South Rise, Llanishen, Cardiff CF14 0RH — MD Wales 1970; MB BCh 1956; FRCOG 1977, M 1964.

WILLIAMS, Geraint Trefor 11 Cyncoed Crescent, Cyncoed, Cardiff CF23 6SW — MB BCh Wales 1973; BSc (Hons.) Wales 1970, MD 1981, MB BCh (Hons.) 1973; MRCP (UK) 1975; FRCPath

1991, M 1979; FRCP Lond. 1991; F Med Sci 2002. Prof. Path. Univ. Wales Coll. Med. Cardiff; Hon. Cons. Path. Univ. Hosp. Wales Cardiff. Specialty: Histopath. Socs: Path. Soc. Gt. Brit. & Irel.; Brit. Soc. Gastroenterol. Prev: Lect. (Path.) St. Bart. Hosp. & St. Mark's Hosp. Lond.

WILLIAMS, Mr Gerard Trevor N. Manch. Gen. Hosp., Pelaways Road M8 5RB Tel: 0161 720 2253 — MB ChB Bristol 1979; FRCS Eng. 1983; ChM Manchester 1990. Cons. Vasc. & Gen. Surg., N. Manch. Gen. Hosp. Specialty: Gen. Surg. Special Interest: Laparoscopic Hernia Repair. Socs: Vasc. Surgic. Soc.

WILLIAMS, Gethin Llewelyn Glan Aber, Llanrhaeadr, Denbigh LL16 4LN — MB BCh Wales 1994.

WILLIAMS, Gillian The Beeches, 67 Lower Olland Street, Bungay NR35 1BZ Tel: 01986 892055 Fax: 01986 895519; The Buck, Low Road, Earsham, Bungay NR35 2AG Tel: 01986 788470 — MB ChB Manch. 1971. Specialty: Palliat. Med.

WILLIAMS, Gillian Ann The Surgery, Bramblys, Basingstoke RG24 8ND Tel: 01256 467778; The Surgery, Bramblys Grange, Basingstoke RG21 8UW Tel: 01256 467778 Fax: 01256 842131 — MB BS Lond. 1962 (Westm.) MRCS Eng. LRCP Lond. 1962. Prev: SHO (O & G), & Cas. & Admissions Off. Roy. W. Sussex Hosp. Chichester; Ho. Phys. Rush Green Hosp. Romford.

WILLIAMS, Gillian Barbara Glyn The Surgery, Rockliffe Court, Hurworth Place, Darlington DL2 2DS Tel: 01325 720605 — MB ChB Liverp. 1980; DRCOG 1983; MRCGP 1984; DCH RCS Lond. 1984. GP Darlington.

WILLIAMS, Gillian Rhiannon North West London Hospitals Trusts, Department of Cellular Pathology, Watford Road, Harrow HA1 3UJ; 17 Dalmeny Road, London N7 0HG — MB BS Lond. 1987; MRCPath 1996, D 1992; MD 1998. Cons. Histopath. ICRF Lond. Specialty: Histopath. Socs: Path. Soc. Internat. Assn. Path. Prev: Lect. (Histopath.) UMDS Lond.; ICRF Research Fell. Colorectal Unit St. Marks Hosp. Lond.; Regist. (Histopath.) Soton. Gen. Hosp.

WILLIAMS, Glennis Monisola Cecilia — MB BS Newc. 1986; MRCP (UK) 1992; MRCGP 1993; JCPT 1993; DFFP 1993; (Diabetes) GPWSI 2004. Advanced Ldr. Warwick Univ. (Distance Delivery Course in Diabetes); Accredit. Trainer Insulin Ther. in Type 2 Diabetes. Specialty: Gen. Pract. Socs: Med. Protec. Soc. & BMA. Prev: Clin. Asst. (Diabetes) W. Middlx. Univ. Hosp.; Trainee GP Lond.; SHO (Obst. & Gyn., Paediat. & Geriat. Med.) W. Middlx. Univ. Hosp.

WILLIAMS, Glenwynne (retired) 6 Houndean Rise, Lewes BN7 1EG Tel: 01273 475952 — (St. Mary's) MB BS Lond. 1958; MRCS Eng. LRCP Lond. 1958; DObst RCOG 1961; DPH Sydney 1963; MPH Calif. 1968; FFCM 1981, M 1976. Ref. Crematorium. Prev: Dep. Dir. Pub. Health E. Sussex HA.

WILLIAMS, Glyn Roger The Knowe, Templehill, Troon KA10 6BH — MB BS Lond. 1971; DTM & H Eng. 1973; MRCP (UK) 1976. Cons. Phys. (Infec. Dis.) CrossHo. Hosp. Kilmarnock. Specialty: Infec. Dis. Prev: Lect. (Infec. Dis.) Univ. Glas.; Regist. (Microbiol.) Hammersmith Hosp. Lond.; Regist. (Infec. Dis.) Coppetts Wood Hosp. Lond.

WILLIAMS, Mr Gordon 12 Derwent Road, Twickenham TW2 7HQ Email: gwilliams@hhnt.org — MB BS Lond. 1968 (Univ. Coll. Hosp.) FRCS Eng. 1973; MS Lond. 1987; FRCS Ed. 2000; FRCSP Glas. 2005. Cons. Surg. Urol. & Transpl. Unit Hammersmith Hosp.; Hon Sen. Lect. Inst. of Urol., Middlx. Hosp. Specialty: Urol. Socs: SAC Urol. (Ex-Chairm.); RSM (Ex-Pres. Urol. Sect.); Chairm. Jt. Comm. for Higher Surgic. Train. Prev: Sen. Regist. (Urol. & Transpl.) Hammersmith Hosp. Lond.

WILLIAMS, Gordon Henry Gortnacally, Florence Court, Enniskillen BT92 1DB — MB ChB Liverp. 1975; DCH Eng. 1978; DRCOG 1981.

WILLIAMS, Gordon John Yorkshire Heart Centre, Leeds General Infirmary, Great George St., Leeds LS1 3EX Tel: 0113 392 5794 Fax: 0113 392 5265; Kinvara, 8 Thorp Arch Park, Thorp Arch, Wetherby LS23 7AN Tel: 01937 844516 Fax: 01937 541137 — MB BCh Wales 1967 (Cardiff) FRCP Lond. 1988; FACC 1988. Cons. Cardiol. Regional Cardiothoracic Centre Killingbeck Hosp. & Seacroft Hosp. Leeds; Hon. Sen. Lect. Med. Univ. Leeds. Specialty: Cardiol. Socs: Med. Research Soc. & Mem. Brit. Cardiac Soc. Prev: Ho. Phys. Med. Unit Cardiff Roy. Infirm.; Lect. (Cardiol.) Univ. Hosp. Wales Cardiff; Fell. (Paediat. Cardiol.) Hosp. Sick Childr. Toronto, Canada.

WILLIAMS, Graham Percival The Medical Centre, Badgers Crescent, Shipston-on-Stour CV36 4BQ Tel: 01608 661845; Home Farm, Cherington, Shipston-on-Stour CV36 5HS Tel: 01608 686414 — MB BS Lond. 1961 (Guy's) MB BS (Hons. Distinc. Surg.) Lond. 1961; MRCS Eng. LRCP Lond. 1961; DObst RCOG 1963; MRCGP 1972. Clin. Asst. Ellen Badger Hosp. Shipston-on-Stour; Med. Off. Brit. Schs. Exploring Soc. Expedition. Socs: BMA. Prev: Ho. Off. (O & G) Lambeth Hosp.; Ho. Phys. Orpington Hosp.; Ho. Surg. Guy's Hosp.

WILLIAMS, Graham Richard Molecular Endocrinology Group, Imperial College School Science, Hammersmith Hospital, Du Cane Road, London W12 0NN Tel: 020 8383 3014 Fax: 020 8383 8306 Email: graham.williams@ic.ac.uk — MB BS Lond. 1984 (St. Thos.) BSc Lond. 1981; MRCP (UK) 1987; PhD Birm. 1993; FRCP 1999. Reader in Trdociology, Imperial Coll. Humesintl Hosp.; Cons. Phys. Hammersmith Hosp. Lond. Specialty: Endocrinol. Prev: Lect. & Regist. (Med.) Qu. Eliz. Hosp. Birm.; Fell. Endocrinol. Harvard Univ. USA.

WILLIAMS, Mr Grant Burkhill — (Lond. Hosp.) MRCS Eng. LRCP Lond. 1956; MB BS Lond. 1957; FRCS Eng. 1961; MSc Lond. 1965, MS 1969. Cons. (Urol.) Char. Cross & Roy. Marsden Hosps. Lond.; Cons. Urological Surg. Lond. & Huntingdon. Specialty: Urol. Socs: Soc. of Apoth.; Expert Witness Inst.; Brit. Prostate Gp. Prev: Cons. Urol. Char. Cross Hosp. & Roy. Marsden Hosp. Lond.; Sen. Regist. Lond. Hosp. & Inst. Urol. Lond.; Med. Cons. HM Inspretorate of Prisons.

WILLIAMS, Gregory 27 Blacon Point Road, Chester CH1 5LD — MB ChB Leic. 1989.

WILLIAMS, Mr Gregory Joel Peter 210 Castellain Mansions, Castellian Road, London W9 1HD — MB BS W. Indies 1990; FRCS Eng. 1995.

WILLIAMS, Gwenlais Mary 14 Forest Close, Wendover, Aylesbury HP22 6BT — MB BS Lond. 1980; MRCP (UK) 1984; MRCGP 1990; DRCOG 1990; Cert. Family Plann. JCC 1991. GP Principle, Aston Clinton Surg., Aston Clinton, HP22 5LB. Prev: SHO (Neonat.) Oxf.; Regist. Rotat. (Paediat.) Bristol; SHO (O & G) Bath.

WILLIAMS, Gwilym Rees (retired) Hedgerows, 20 Bramley Close, Ledbury HR8 2XP Tel: 01531 2990 — MB BCh Wales 1943.

WILLIAMS, Harry 62 Old Edinburgh Road, Inverness IV2 3PG Tel: 01463 33536 — MB ChB St. And. 1945; MD St. And. 1956, MB ChB 1945. Cons. Bacteriol. N. RHB (Scotl.). Specialty: Med. Microbiol. Socs: Soc. Gen. Microbiol.; Path. Soc. Gt. Brit. Prev: Asst. Lect. Univ. St. And.; Lect. Univ. Durban.

WILLIAMS, Mr Harry William George, OBE (retired) School Cottage, Gattonside, Melrose TD6 9NB Tel: 01896 823263 — MRCS Eng. LRCP Lond. 1939 (Lond. Hosp.) FRCS Ed. 1947. Prev: Med. Adviser to Salvation Army.

WILLIAMS, Haydn John Sundon Medical Centre, 141/144 Sundon Park Rd, Luton LU3 3AH — MB BS Lond. 1993 (St. Mary's) BSc Lond. 1990; DGM RCP Lond. 1995; DRCOG 1996; MRCGP 1997. Gen. Practitioner. Specialty: Gen. Pract. Prev: SHP Palliat. Med., Isabel Hospice Welwyn Garden City; Trainee GP/SHO Lister Hosp. Stevenage VTS; Ho. Off. (Med., Surg. & Orthop.) Heatherwood & Wrexham Pk. Hosp.

WILLIAMS, Helen Catherine 180 Whitchurch Road, Tavistock PL19 9DF — MB BS Lond. 1993 (Charing Cross and Westminster) MRPharmS 1988; DRCOG 1991; MRCGP 1992. Specialty: Gen. Pract.

WILLIAMS, Helen Diane The Manor House, Clifton-on-Teme, Worcester WR6 6EN — BSc (Hons.) Lond. 1977; MB BS Lond. 1981; FFA RCS Eng. 1988. Cons. Anaesth. Worcester Roy. Infirm. Specialty: Anaesth. Prev: Cons. Anaeth. Hereford; Sen. Regist. (Anaesth.) Qu. Eliz. Hosp. Birm.; Sen. Regist. Brighton HA.

WILLIAMS, Helen Elizabeth 106 Heol Isaf, Radyr, Cardiff CF15 8EA — MB BS Lond. 1992.

WILLIAMS, Helen June 69 Clarence Road, Harborne, Birmingham B17 9JY — MB ChB Birm. 1995; MB ChB (Hons.) Birm. 1995. SHO (Paediat.) Birm. Childr. Hosp. Specialty: Paediat.

WILLIAMS, Helen Mary Sefton Dept. Of Microbiology, Norfolk & Norwich NHS Trust, Bowthorpe Road, Norwich NR2 3TX Tel: 01603 611816 Fax: 01603 620190 Email: hwilliams@nhs.phls.uk; Bramley, Chapel Street, Barford, Norwich NR9 4AB — MB BCh Wales 1979; MRCPath 1987; FRCPath 1997. Cons. Microbiologist PHLS Norwich.

Specialty: Med. Microbiol. Socs: Regist. RCPath; Dir. Clin. Audit & Effectiveness RCPath (95-99).

WILLIAMS, Henrietta Megan c/o 41 Chandos Avenue, Ealing, London W5 4EP — MB BS Lond. 1985; DRCOG 1988; DCH RCP Lond. 1990; MRCGP 1990; MFFP 1995; Dip GU Med. 1997. Specialty: Gen. Pract.; Genitourinary Medicine; HIV Med. Prev: Regist. Genito Urin. Med. Radcliffe Infirm. Oxf.; GP Middlx. Lond.; GP Fell. HIV Barnet Frisa Lond.

WILLIAMS, Hilary Frances 23 Castle Hill Avenue, Berkhamsted HP4 1HJ Tel: 01442 865291 — (Middlx.) MB BS Lond. 1954; DObst RCOG 1956.

WILLIAMS, Hilary Jane Ground Floor Flat, 1 Learmonth Gardens, Edinburgh EH4 1HD Tel: 0131 315 4173 — MB ChB Sheff. 1994. Specialist Regist. Infec. Dis. Specialty: Infec. Dis.; Gen. Med. Socs: MRCP (Ed.).

WILLIAMS, Mrs Honour Cynthia Imogen (retired) St Mary's, High Street, Bures CO8 5HZ Tel: 01787 227449 — MB ChB Birm. 1947; MRCS Eng. LRCP Lond. 1948. Assoc. Specialist (Haemat.) Broomfield Hosp. Chelmsford. Prev: Ho. Phys. Mile End Hosp. Lond.

WILLIAMS, Howard Owen (retired) Roundwood, 3 Ashlyns Road, Frinton-on-Sea CO13 9ET Tel: 01255 672917 — (Cardiff) BSc (Anat. & Physiol.) Wales 1941, MB BCh 1944. Prev: Cons. Phys. Whittington Hosp. Lond.

WILLIAMS, Hugh Iestyn Department of Clinical Pathology, General Hospital, Middlesbrough TS1 5JE — MB BChir Camb. 1948; DCP Lond 1958; FRCPath 1977, M 1965. Cons. Path. S. Tees Health Dist. Specialty: Pathology, General. Socs: Path. Soc. Gt. Brit.; Fell. Roy. Soc. Med. Prev: Sen. Pathol. Inst. Med. Research, Kuala Lumpur, Malaya.

WILLIAMS, Hugh Jeremy Hyatt Grove Court, Upstreet, Canterbury CT3 4DD — MB BS Lond. 1970 (Guy's) MB BS (Hons.) Lond. 1970; MRCP (U.K.) 1973; MRCPath 1977. Cons. (Haemat.) Maidstone Health Dist. Specialty: Haematology. Prev: Sen. Regist. (Haemat.) & Med. Regist. Guy's Hosp. Lond.; Asst. Lect. Dept. Pathol. Middlx. Hosp.

WILLIAMS, Mr Hugh Marshall Wayside, Worcester Road, Salford, Chipping Norton OX7 5YJ Email: hmw@fish.co.uk — MB BS Lond. 1962 (Char. Cross) MRCS Eng. LRCP Lond. 1962; FRCS Ed. 1969; FRCS Eng. 1970; MChOrth Liverp. 1971. Cons. Orthop. Surg. BUPA Hosp. Elland. Specialty: Orthop. Prev: Cons. Orthop. Surg. Huddersfield Roy. Infirm.

WILLIAMS, Mr Hugh Patrick 5 Harmont House, 20 Harley Street, London W1G 9PH Tel: 020 7636 4406 Fax: 020 7636 5150 — MB ChB NZ 1961; DO RCS Eng. 1967; FRCS Eng. 1970; FCOphth Eng. 1990; FRCOphth 1990. Cons. Ophth. Surg. Moorfields Eye Hosp. Lond.; Cons. Ophth. St. John & St. Eliz. Hosp. Lond.; Hon. Cons. Ophth. Surg. Moorfields Eye Hosp. Lond. Specialty: Ophth. Socs: Fell. Roy. Soc. Med.; Amer. Soc. Cataract & Refractive Surg.; UK & Irel. Soc. Cataract & Refractive Surg. Prev: Cons. Ophth. Surg. N. Middlx. Hosp. Lond.; Sen. Regist. Moorfields Eye Hosp. Lond.; Sen. Regist. Roy. Lond. Hosp.

WILLIAMS, Mr Huw Owain Llewellyn Royal Glamorgan Hospital, Llantrisant, Pontyclun CF72 8XR — MB BCh Wales 1982; FRCS Ed. (Orl.) 1988; FRCS Eng. (Orl.) 1989. Cons. ENT Roy. Glam. Hosp. M. Glam. Specialty: Otolaryngol. Prev: Sen. Regist. (ENT) St. Bart. Hosp. Lond.; Regist. (ENT) Roy. Nat. Throat Nose & Ear Hosp. Lond.

WILLIAMS, Huw Powell Mistletoe Cottage, 24 High Street, Steeple Ashton, Trowbridge BA14 6EL Tel: 01225 354604 Fax: 01225 775445 — MB BS Lond. 1976 (St. Mary's) BSc Lond. 1973; MRCP (UK) 1980; DRCOG 1981; MRCGP 1982. Partner at Adcroft Surgery, Trowbridge, Wiltshire; Clin. Asst. (Cardiol.) Roy. United Hosp. Bath. Specialty: Gen. Pract.; Cardiol. Special Interest: Echocardiography. Socs: Spencer Wells Soc. Prev: Vice Chairm. Wilts. Health Auth.; SHO (Med.) Hammersmith Hosp. Lond.; Vis. Assoc. Prof. Dept. Family Med. Ohio State Univ. Coll. Med. Columbus, USA.

WILLIAMS, Hywel Glan Nant, 70 Cemetery Road, Porth CF39 0BL — MB BS Lond. 1972; BSc Lond. 1969, MB BS 1972; DObst RCOG 1974; DCH Eng. 1975; MRCP (UK) 1978.

WILLIAMS, Professor Hywel Charles Centre of Evidence-Based Dermatology, Queen's Medical Centre, Nottingham NG7 2UH Tel: 0115 924 9924 Ext: 43000 Fax: 0115 970 9003 Email: hywel.williams@nottingham.ac.uk — MB BS Lond. 1982 (Charing Cross Hospital Medical School) BSc Lond. 1979; MSc Lond. 1991; PhD Lond. 1995; FRCP 1997. Prof. (Dermat.-Epidemiol.) Nottm.; Hon. Clin. Dermat. Cons. at Queens Med. Centre. Specialty: Dermat. Special Interest: Atopic eczema. Socs: Brit. Assn. Dermat.; Chairm. Brit. Epidermo-Epidemiol. soc.; Assn. of Physicians. Prev: Sen. Lect. (Dermat.) Nottm.; Wellcome Research Fell. (Dermato-Epidemiol.) St John's Dermat. Centre; Director of Trent Institute for Health Services Research.

WILLIAMS, Hywel Gareth Morris (retired) Craig Yr Wylan, Llanaber, Barmouth LL42 1AJ Tel: 01341 280226 — MB ChB Liverp. 1961; DObst RCOG 1969. Sessional Med. Off. Roy. Aero Estab. Llanbedr. Prev: Ho. Phys. & Ho. Surg. Liverp. Roy. Infirm.

WILLIAMS, Hywel Nicholas (retired) Bettws, Parrog, Newport SA42 0RX Tel: 01239 820559 Fax: 01239 820000 — MB BCh Wales 1961 (Cardiff) DObst RCOG 1963; FRCGP 1983, M 1975. Prev: Sen. Med. Off. Health Profess. Gp. Welsh Off. Cardiff.

WILLIAMS, Mr Hywel Rhys Dept. of Orthopaedics, York District Hospital, Wiggenton Road, York YO31 8HE — MB BCh Wales 1987 (Univ. Wales Coll. Med.) BSc (Hons.) Wales 1984; FRCS Eng. 1992; FRCS 1997; FRCS ORTH 1997. Cons. Dept. Orthop., York Dist. Hosp., York. Specialty: Orthop.; Trauma & Orthop. Surg. Socs: Elbow & Shoulder Soc.; Brit. Orthop. Assn. Prev: Sen. Regist. St. James Univ. Hosp. Leeds & Leeds Gen. Infirm.; Fell. (Shoulder Surg.) Roy. Berks. Hosp. Reading; Sen. Regist. (Orthop.) St. Jas. Univ. Hosp. Leeds & Leeds Gen. Infirm.

WILLIAMS, Mr Hywel Thomas Whitbourne, 226 Malvern Road, St John's, Worcester WR2 4PA — MB BChir Camb. 1962 (Westm.) MChir Camb. 1976, MA, MB 1962, BChir 1961; FRCS Eng. 1967. Cons. Urol. Worcester Roy. Infirm. Specialty: Urol.

WILLIAMS, Ian Medical Centre, 12A Greggs Wood Road, Tunbridge Wells TN2 3JL Tel: 01892 541444 Fax: 01892 511157; 33 Dornden Drive, Langton Green, Tunbridge Wells TN3 0AE Tel: 01892 863040 — BM BCh Wales 1982; MRCGP 1986; DRCOG 1986.

WILLIAMS, Ian Colin Martin The Health Centre, Green Lane, Corwen LL21 0AR Tel: 01490 412362 Email: ian.williams1@virgin.net — MB BCh Wales 1989 (University of Wales Coll. of Med.) DA; MRCGP, 1984. GP Princip.; Clin. Asst. (Anaesth.). Specialty: Gen. Pract.; Anaesth.

WILLIAMS, Ian Geoffrey Centre for Sexual Health & HIV Research, Royal Freeand University College Medical School, Mortimer Market Centre, Mortimer Market, London WC1E 6AU Tel: 020 7380 9893 Fax: 020 7380 9669 — MB ChB Manch. 1980; BSc (Hons.) (Physiol.) Manch. 1977; MRCP (UK) 1984; FRCP 1998. Sen. Lect. (Genitourin. Med.) Roy. Free & Univ. Coll. Med. Sch. Camden PCT & Univ. Coll. Lond. Hosps. Specialty: HIV Med.; Genitourinary Medicine. Socs: (Exec. Comm.) BHIVA; BASHH. Prev: Lect. (Genitourin. Med.) Univ. Coll. & Middlx. Hosp. Med. Sch. Lond.; Regist. (Med.) Qu. Alexandra & St Mary's Hosps. Portsmouth; SHO (Med.) Univ. Hosp. S. Manch.

WILLIAMS, Ian Grindon Wellside Surgery, 45 High Street, Sawtry, Huntingdon PE28 5SU Tel: 01487 830340 Fax: 01487 832753; 22 Highfield Avenue, Alconbury Weston, Huntingdon PE28 4JS Tel: 01480 890002 — MB BChir Camb. 1980; MA Camb. 1982; DRCOG 1984; MRCGP 1985; AFOM RCP Lond. 1992. Div. Surg. St. Johns Ambul.; (Occupat. Health Phys.) Hinchingbrooke Healthcare NHS Trust. Specialty: Gen. Pract. Socs: BMA; Soc. Occupat. Med.; Soc. Internet. in Med. Prev: Trainee GP P'boro. VTS; SHO (A & E) P'boro. Dist. Hosp.; Ho. Off. Addenbrooke's Hosp. Camb. & Huntingdon Co. Hosp.

WILLIAMS, Ian Lear Department of Cardiology, King's College Hospital, Denmark Hill, London SE5 9RS; 55 Nightingale Road, Farncombe, Godalming GU7 2HU Tel: 01483 420568 Fax: 01483 420568 Email: ilw1167@aol.com — MB BChir Camb. 1993 (Camb. & St. Geo.) MRCP (UK) 1995. Specialist Regist. Rotat. (Cardiol.) Roy. Sussex Co. Hosp. Brighton. Specialty: Cardiol. Prev: research fell. (Cardiol.) King's Coll. Hosp. Lond.; SHO (Cardiol.) Soton. Gen. Hosp.; SHO Rotat. (Gen. Med.) St. Richard's Hosp. Chichester.

WILLIAMS, Ian Michael 15 Spowart Avenue, Llanelli SA15 3HY — MB BCh Wales 1986.

WILLIAMS, Ian Peter Argraig, Ael Y Garth, Caernarfon LL55 1HA — MB BCh Wales 1991.

WILLIAMS, Ian Richard c/o Crofton Cottage, Broad St., Cuckfield, Haywards Heath RH17 5DX — MB ChB Bristol 1988.

WILLIAMS, Ian Richard 10 Chepstow Close, Chippenham SN14 0XP — MB ChB Leic. 1993.

WILLIAMS, Ian Roger 18 Montagu Road, Formby, Liverpool L37 1LA — MB ChB Ed. 1966; FRCP Lond. 1983, M 1969.

WILLIAMS, Ian Thomas Lloyd's Bank Ltd., 25 Camberwell Green, London SE5 7AB — MB BS Lond. 1966 (King's Coll. Hosp.) MRCS Eng. LRCP Lond. 1966.

WILLIAMS, Ifor Pennant (retired) Primrose Cottage, Walberswick, Southwold IP18 6UP — MB BCh Camb. 1945 (Westm.) MRCP Lond. 1947; DMRD Eng. 1952.

WILLIAMS, Ingeborg Eveline Ilse (retired) 6 Southcliff, Cliff Road, Falmouth TR11 4LY Tel: 01326 314676 — MD Hamburg 1945; MRCS Eng. LRCP Lond. 1957; DPM Eng. 1964; MRCPsych 1973. Prev: Cons. Psychiat. (Psychogeriat. Med.) Barncoose Hosp. Redruth & St. Lawrence's Hosp. Bodmin.

WILLIAMS, Iola Ann Arrowe Park Hospital, Arrowe Park Road, Upton, Wirral CH49 5PE Tel: 0151 678 5111 — MB BCh Wales 1978; MRCOG 1984; FRCOG 1997. Cons. O & G Arrowe Pk. Hosp. Merseyside. Specialty: Obst. & Gyn. Prev: Sen. Regist. (O & G) Roy. United Hosp. Bath & Bristol Matern. Hosp.; Research Regist. (Reproduc. Endocrinol.) Roy. Free Hosp. Lond.; Regist. (O & G) Princess Anne Hosp. Soton.

WILLIAMS, Isobel Petrie (retired) — (St. Geo.) MD Lond. 1983, MB BS 1965; DCH Eng. 1968; MRCP (UK) 1971; FRCP 1987. Private Work at BUPA Harpenden Herts. Prev: Cons. Phys. St. Albans & Hemel Hempstead NHS Trust.

WILLIAMS, Ivan Arthur (retired) Bucklands, Buckland-tout-Saints, Kingsbridge TQ7 2DS Tel: 01548 853141 — (Middlx.) MB BS Lond. 1956; FRCP Lond. 1975, M 1959; DPhysMed. Eng. 1959. Prev: Cons. Rheum. & Rehabil. Tunbridge Wells HA.

WILLIAMS, Ivon The Hermitage, 32-34 Preston St., Shrewsbury SY2 5NY — MB BS Lond. 1962 (St. Mary's) DA Eng. 1965; FFA RCS Eng. 1971. Cons. (Anaesth.) Roy. Shrewsbury Hosp. Specialty: Anaesth. Prev: Regist. (Anaesth.) Char. Cross Hosp. Lond.; Sen. Regist. (Anaesth.) Char. Cross Hosp. Lond.; Specialist Anaesth. Groote Schuur Hosp. Cape Town.

WILLIAMS, Jacqueline Sheila Corner Cottage, Stretton on Fosse, Moreton-in-Marsh GL56 9SD Tel: 01608 664205 — MB ChB Birm. 1989; DRCOG 1991; MRCGP 1993. GP Partner Chipping Camden. Specialty: Gen. Pract. Socs: BMA. Prev: GP Retainer; Trainee GP Harrogate; SHO (Gen. Med., Paediat., O & G & Psychiat.) Dumfries & Galloway Roy. Infirm.

WILLIAMS, Mr James Leigh Department of Ortho, Northern General Hospital, Herries Road, Sheffield S5 7AV; 40 Winchester Road, Sheffield S10 4EE Tel: 01142 302120 Fax: 01142 302120 — MB ChB Sheff. 1992; BMedSci 1991; FRCS 1997; FRCS (Ed.) 1997. Specialist Regist. Orthop. Surg. Northern Gen. Hosps. hef. Specialty: Orthop.; Trauma & Orthop. Surg. Socs: BOA.

WILLIAMS, Jane Mary 184 Norton Leys, Hillside, Rugby CV22 5RY — MB ChB Manch. 1979; BSc St. And. 1976; MBA (Pub. Sector Managem.) Aston 1994.

WILLIAMS, Jane Stanley (retired) 2 Mallard Way, Rest Bay, Porthcawl CF36 3TS Tel: 0165 671 4031 — MB BCh Wales 1951 (Cardiff) BSc. MB BCh Wales 1951; DA Eng. 1954. Prev: Sessional Clin. Med. Off. Mid Glam. Health Auth.

WILLIAMS, Janet Chelsfield Surgery, 62 Windsor Drive, Chelsfield, Orpington BR6 6HD — MB BS Lond. 1979. GP Orpington. Prev: Trainee GP Portsmouth VTS; Ho. Phys. Pembury Hosp.; Ho. Surg. Orpington Hosp.

WILLIAMS, Janet Barton House Health Centre, 233 Albion Road, London N16 9JT Tel: 020 7249 5511 Fax: 020 7254 8985 — MB ChB Manch. 1985; MRCPsych 1991; MRCGP 1993.

WILLIAMS, Jason David Louis Dermatology Registrar, hope Hospital, Salford M6 8HD — MB ChB Manch. 1997; BSc (Hons) Manch. 1994; MRCP 2000.

WILLIAMS, Jean Olwen (retired) — MB Camb. 1966 (St. Thos.) BChir 1965; MRCP Lond. 1968; MSc (Nuclear Med.) Lond. 1972. Prev: Cons. Clin. Audit E. Anglia Region.

WILLIAMS, Jeffrey Collwyn Richmond Clinic, 172 Caerleon Road, Newport NP19 7FY — MB BCh Wales 1991; MRCGP 1995; DRCOG 1995. Specialty: Gen. Pract.

WILLIAMS, Mr Jeremy Howard Accident and Emergency Department, West Wales General Hospital, Docgwili Road, Carmarthen SA31 2AF Tel: 01267 227007 Fax: 01267 227307 Email: jeremy.williams@carmarthen.wales.nhs.uk — MB BS Lond. 1986 (St Bart.) MA Oxf. 1983; FRCS 1992; FFAEM 1997; Dip Sports Med 2003. Cons. (A & E) W. Wales Gen. Hosp.; Honourary Sen. Lect., Swansea Unviversity. Specialty: Accid. & Emerg. Socs: Brit. Assn. Accid. & Emerg. Med.; BMA. Prev: Sen. Regist. (A & E) Morriston Hosp. Swansea; Regist. (A & E) Russells Hall Hosp.; Regist. (A & E) Hosp. Birm.

WILLIAMS, Joanne Marie Clarendon House, Clarendon St., Hyde SK14 2AQ — MB ChB Manch. 1987.

WILLIAMS, John (retired) Holeyn Hall, Wylam NE41 8BQ Tel: 01661 853673 — MD Newc. 1964; MB BS Durh. 1955; FRCGP 1980, M 1973. Prev: Hosp. Pract. Newc. Gen. Hosp.

WILLIAMS, John Arfon The Newlands, Penglais Road, Aberystwyth SY23 2EU — MB BS Lond. 1941 (Guy's) MRCS Eng. LRCP Lond. 1941; MRCOG 1952, DObst 1948. Prev: Ho. Surg. Preston Hall Hosp. Maidstone; Ho. Phys. Joyce Green Hosp. Dartford; Squadron Ldr. RAFVR.

WILLIAMS, John Arthur 22 Severn Street, Welshpool SY21 7AD Tel: 01938 552222 — MB BS Lond. 1977 (St. Bart.) MRCS Eng. LRCP Lond. 1977; LDS RCS Eng. 1980; FDS RCPS Glas. 1980; BDS 1980.

WILLIAMS, John Benedict 22 Bright Trees Road, Geddington, Kettering NN14 1BS — MB ChB Ed. 1996.

WILLIAMS, Professor John David Institute of Nephrology, University of Wales College of Medicine, Heath Park, Cardiff CF14 4XN Tel: 02920 748432 Fax: 02920 748470 Email: williamsjd4@cf.ac.uk — MB BCh Wales 1973; MRCP (UK) 1977; MD Wales 1985; FRCP Lond. 1988. Prof. Nephrol. & Hon. Dir. Inst. Nephrol. Univ. Wales Coll. Med. Specialty: Nephrol. Prev: Postdoctural Research Fell. Harvard Med. Sch. Boston, USA.

WILLIAMS, John David Queen Elizabeth Hospital, Gayton Road, King's Lynn PE30 4ET Tel: 01553 613726; The Pightle, Leziate Drove, Ashwicken, King's Lynn PE32 1LT — MB BChir Camb. 1977 (Camb. & St. Bart.) MB BChir Camb. 1976; MA Camb. 1977; FRCP 1997, MRCP 1980. Cons. Rheum. Qu. Eliz. Hosp. King's Lynn. Specialty: Rehabil. Med.; Rheumatol. Socs: Brit. Soc. Rheum. Prev: Sen. Regist. (Rheum.) Roy. Free & N. Middlx. Hosps. Lond.; Wellcome Research Fell. St. Bart. Hosp. Lond.; SHO Roy. Postgrad. Med. Sch. Lond.

WILLIAMS, John David 69 Victoria Park Road, London E9 7NA Tel: 020 8986 7046 — MD Liverp. 1964; BSc Lond. 1951; MB ChB 1956; DCP Lond 1961; FRCPath 1981, M 1965; MRCP (UK) 1986. Emerit. Prof. (Med. Microbiol.) The Univ. Lond.; Edr. Antibiotics Chemother. & Internat. Jl. Antimicrobial Agents. Specialty: Med. Microbiol. Socs: Past Pres. Internat. Soc. Chemother.; Past Pres. Federat. Europ. Soc. Chemother. & Infect.; Past Pres. Brit. Soc. Chemother. Prev: Prof. (Med. Microbiol.) Lond. Hosp. Med. Coll.

WILLIAMS, John David Gwynne (retired) 9 Castle Street, Ruthin LL15 1DP Tel: 01824 703242 Email: johndgwilliams@hotmail.com — MB ChB Manch. 1958; DObst RCOG 1962. p/t Examg. Med. Practitioners, Disbility Med., Benefit Agency, N. Wales.

WILLIAMS, John Desmond Stablehouse, Wilderness Road, Chislehurst BR7 5EY Tel: 020 8467 3896 — MB BS Lond. 1949 (Guy's) MRCS Eng. LRCP Lond. 1949; FRCP Lond. 1973, M 1954. Cons. Phys. Qu. Mary's Hosp. Sidcup & Orpington Hosp. Specialty: Gen. Med. Prev: Sen. Med. Regist., & Ho. Phys. & Asst. Ho. Surg. Guy's Hosp.; Research Assoc. in Med. Univ. Illinois Chicago U.S.A.

WILLIAMS, John Ellis 15 Edward Nicholl Court, Waterloo Road, Cardiff CF23 9BW Tel: 029 2049 3715 — MB BS Lond. 1985; FRCA 1991. Cons. Anaesth. & Pain Managem. Roy. Marsden Hosp. Lond. Specialty: Anaesth. Prev: Sen. Regist. (Anaesth.) Oxf. RHA; Vis. Asst. Prof. Dept. Anaesth. Univ. Maryland Hosp. Baltimore, Maryland, USA; Regist. (Anaesth.) St. Thos. Hosp. Lond.

WILLIAMS, John Frederick 62 West Stockwell Street, Colchester CO1 1HE Tel: 01206 369249 Fax: 01206 710661 — MB BS Lond. 1951 (Westm.) MRCS Eng. LRCP Lond. 1951; BA Open 1991.

WILLIAMS, John Gareth Tan Yr Onnen, Lon Graig, Llanfairpwllgwyngyll LL61 5AX Tel: 01248 714831 — MB ChB Liverp. 1966; MRCS Eng. LRCP Lond. 1966; DMRD Liverp. 1970; FFR 1972. Cons. Radiol. Ysbyty Gwynedd, Bangor. Specialty: Radiol. Prev: Sen. Regist. (Radiol.) Univ. Hosp. of Wales Cardiff; Sen. Regist. Radiol. Alder Hey Childrs. Hosp. Liverp.

WILLIAMS, John Gareth The Grange Medical Centre, 39 Leicester Road, Nuneaton CV11 6AB Tel: 024 7632 2810 Fax: 024 7632

2820 — MB ChB Leic. 1986; DCH RCP Lond. 1991. Specialty: Paediat.

WILLIAMS, John Gordon Halton General Hospital (NHS Trust), Runcorn WA7 2DA Tel: 01928 714567 Fax: 01928 753119 — MB ChB Liverp. 1975; MRCP (UK) 1978; MD Liverp. 1982; FRCP Lond. 1993. Cons. Phys. Halton Hosp. Runcorn. Specialty: Respirat. Med.; Gen. Med. Socs: Y Gymdeithas Feddygol & Brit. Thoracic Soc. Prev: Sen. Regist. Broadgreen Hosp. Liverp.; Univ. Research Regist. Liverp. Univ.

WILLIAMS, Professor John Gordon School of Postgrad. Studies in Med. & Health Care, Maes-y-Gwernen Hall, Morriston Hospital, Swansea SA6 6NL Tel: 01792 703531 Fax: 01792 797310; Harford House, 3 Richmond Villas, Ffynone, Swansea SA1 6DQ Tel: 01792 462424 — MB BChir Camb. 1971 (St. Thos.) MA Camb. 1971; MRCP (UK) 1972; MSc Lond. 1978; FRCP Lond. 1984. Prof. & Dir. Sch. of Postgrad. Studies Med. & Health Carelechyd Mogannwg Heath Auth., Univ. Wales Swans.; Cons. Gastroenterol. Neath Gen. Hosp.; Hon. Assoc. (Postgrad. Studies) Univ. Wales Coll. of Med. Specialty: Gastroenterol. Socs: Brit. Soc. Gastroenterol.; Amer. Gastroenterol. Assn. Prev: Prof. of Naval Med. & Cons. Phys. RN Hosp. Haslar Gosport; Cons. Phys. RN Hosp. Plymouth; Hon. Sen. Regist. St. Thos. Hosp. Lond.

WILLIAMS, John Gordon St Lukes Surgery, Warren Road, Guildford GU1 3JH Tel: 0870 4173979 Fax: 0870 4173978; 148 London Road, Guildford GU1 1UF Fax: 0870 0514626 Email: j.g.williams@surrey.ac.uk — MB BChir Camb. 1972 (Guys/Camb.) MRCP (UK) 1974; FRACP 1978; MRCGP 1990; FRCGP 2001. Specialty: Gen. Pract.; Health Informatics. Prev: Regist. (Med.) Roy. Brisbane Hosp. Queensland, Austral.; Ho. Off. (Med.) Hillingdon Hosp. Middlx.; Ho. Surg. Guy's Hosp. Lond.

WILLIAMS, Mr John Graham New Cross Hospital, Wolverhampton WV10 0QP Tel: 01902 643131 Fax: 01902 642971 — MB BCh Wales 1981; BSc (Human Anat.) Wales 1978; FRCS Eng. 1985; MCh Wales 1989. Cons. Surg. Roy. Wolverhampton Hosps. NHS Trust. Specialty: Gen. Surg. Special Interest: Anal Sepsis; Functional Bowel Disorders; Inflammatory Bowel Disease. Socs: Assn. Coloproct. GB & Irel.; Assn. of Surg. BrSoc GI. Prev: Lect. (Surg.) Univ. Birm. Qu. Eliz. Hosp.; Research Fell. Div. Colon & Rectal Surg. Univ. Minnesota, USA; Regist. (Surg.) Univ. Hosp. Wales Cardiff.

WILLIAMS, John Griffith Uplands Surgery, 48 Sketty Road, Uplands, Swansea SA2 0LJ Tel: 01792 298554 / 298555 Fax: 01792 280416; 145 Derwen Fawr Road, Swansea SA2 8ED — MB BCh Wales 1961; DObst RCOG 1966.

WILLIAMS, John Haydn (retired) Y Bwthyn, Warwick Road, Leek Wootton, Warwick CV35 7QR Tel: 01926 853071 — (St. Thos.) MB BS Lond. 1952; DIH Soc. Apoth. Lond. 1959; MFOM RCP Lond. 1979. Prev: Regional Med. Off. Lond. Midl. Region BR.

WILLIAMS, John Henry Marlborough Medical Practice, The Surgery, George Lane, Marlborough SN8 4BY Tel: 01672 512187 Fax: 01672 516809 — MB BS Lond. 1991 (St. George's) DRCOG 1994; DFFP 1994; MRCGP 1995. Specialty: Gen. Pract. Prev: GP/Regist. Market HarBoro.; SHO (Paediat. & Med.) Leicester Roy. Infirm.; SHO (Rheum.) Leicester Gen. Hosp.

WILLIAMS, John Holman Bentley (retired) Eastbourne House, 118 Eastbourne Road, St Austell PL25 4SS Tel: 01726 65094 — (Oxf.) MA BM BCh Oxf. 1957; DObst RCOG 1959; FRCGP 1982, M 1965. Prev: Med. Dir. Mt. Edgcumbe Hospice St. Austell.

WILLIAMS, John Humphrey Countess of Chester NHS Trust, Liverpool Road, Chester CH1 2BQ; The Spinney, Dicksons Drive, Newton, Chester CH2 2BR Tel: 01244 365000 — MB ChB Liverp. 1968; FRCOG 1988, M 1975. Cons. (O & G) Chester HA. Specialty: Obst. & Gyn.

WILLIAMS, John Justin Caedre House, 38 Park St., Bridgend CF31 4AX Tel: 01656 2721 — MB BS Lond. 1953 (St. Geo.) Prev: Ho. Surg. Chase Farm Hosp. Enfield; Res. Obst. Off. & Ho. Phys. Neath Gen. Hosp.

WILLIAMS, Mr John Leighton (retired) White Croft, 170 Watt Lane, Sheffield S10 5QW Tel: 0114 230 4568 Email: johnleig@waitrose.com — MB BS Lond. 1949 (Guy's) FRCS Eng. 1954. Prev: Cons. Urol. Surg. Roy. Hallamsh. Hosp. Sheff.

WILLIAMS, John Llewellyn Bronglais General Hospital, Aberystwyth, Aberystwyth Tel: 01970 672 3131 — MB BChir Camb. 1990; MRCP (UK) 1992. Cons. Paediat. Specialty: Paediat.

WILLIAMS, Mr John Llewellyn, CBE Nuffield Hospital, Broyle Road, Chichester PO19 4BE Tel: 01243 775952 Fax: 01243 831531 Email: williams.cookscroft@virgin.net — (Guy's) FDS RCS Eng. 1966, LDS 1961; BDS Lond. 1961; MB BS Lond. 1967; MRCS Eng. LRCP Lond. 1967; FRCS Ed. 1991; FRCS 1997; FRCA 1999. Hon. Cons. Maxillofacial Surg. Emerit.; Hon. Cons. Oral & Maxillofacial Surg. Qu. Mary's Hosp. Roehampton; Hon. Cons. Maxillofacial Surg. King Edwd. VII Hosp. Midhurst; Cons. Oral & Maxillofacial Surg Roy.W. sussex NHS Trust, Worthing & Southlands NHS Trusr; Chairm. Commitee Safety of Devices (NHRA). Specialty: Oral & Maxillofacial Surg. Socs: Pres Europ. Assn. Cranio-Maxillofacial Surg.; Pres. Brit. Assn. Oral.& Maxillofacial Surg.; Sec. Lister.Club. Prev: Vice-Pres. RCS Eng.; Dean Fac. Dent. Surg. RCS Eng.; Edr. Brit. Jl. Oral & Maxillofacial Surg.

WILLIAMS, John Parry 33 Durley Dean Road, Selly Oak, Birmingham B29 6SA — MB ChB Birm. 1995.

WILLIAMS, John Penfold Sheepmarket Surgery, Ryhall Road, Stamford PE9 1YA Tel: 01780 753151; Glebe Cottage, 45 West Street, Easton on The Hill, Stamford PE9 3LS Tel: 01780 481175 — MB BChir Camb. 1981 (Camb. & St. Barts.) MA Camb. 1982, BA 1978; DCH RCP Lond. 1984; DRCOG 1985; MRCGP 1986. GP Stamford. Specialty: Gen. Pract. Prev: Chief Medic Raleigh Expedition Patagonia; Trainee GP Overton, Hants.

WILLIAMS, Mr John Peter Rhys, MBE Princess of Wales Hospital, Bridgend CF31 1RQ; Llansannor Lodge, Llansannor, Cowbridge CF71 7RX Tel: 01446 772590 — MB BS Lond. 1973 (St. Mary's) MRCS Eng. LRCP Lond. 1973; FRCS Ed. 1980. Cons. Trauma & Orthop. Princess of Wales Hosp. Bridgend. Specialty: Orthop. Socs: Brit. Orthop. Assn.; BASK; BOSTA. Prev: Sen. Regist. (Orthop.) St. Mary's Hosp. Lond.; Regist. (Orthop.) & Regist. (Gen. Surg.) Univ. Hosp. Wales Cardiff.

WILLIAMS, Mr John Pritchard, RD (retired) 1 Woodfold, Fernhurst GU27 3ET Tel: 01428 654916 — MB BChir Camb. 1950 (St. Mary's) MChir Camb. 1959, MB BChir 1950; FRCS Eng. 1956. Hon. Cons. Urol. the Army. Prev: Cons. Urol. St. Peter's Hosps. & Greenwich Dist. Hosp. Lond. & King Edwd. VII Hosp. Off. Lond.

WILLIAMS, John Pritchard Gwernhefin, Glanhwfa Road, Llangefni LL77 7FA Tel: 01248 723260 — MB BCh Wales 1962 (Cardiff) MRCOG 1969, DObst 1964; FRCOG 1982. Cons. O & G St. David's Hosp. Bangor. Specialty: Obst. & Gyn. Socs: Welsh Obst. & Gyn. Soc. Prev: Regist. HM Stanley Hosp. St. Asaph & South. Gen Hosp. Glas.; Sen. Regist. St. David's Hosp. Bangor.

WILLIAMS, John Rainsbury Erne Hospital, Enniskillen BT74 6AY Tel: 028 6632 4711 Fax: 028 6638 2657; Rossfad House, Ballinamallard, Enniskillen BT94 2LS Tel: 02866 388505 — MB BCh BAO Dub. 1966; MRCP (UK) 1971; FRCP Lond., FRCP Ed. 1988. Cons. Phys. Erne Hosp. Enniskillen. Specialty: Gen. Med. Prev: Med. Specialist Kilimanjaro Christian Med. Centre Moshi, Tanzania.

WILLIAMS, Mr John Richard Department of Trauma and Orthopaedics/Surgery, The Medical School, Newcastle upon Tyne NE2 4HH Tel: 0191 222 5659 Fax: 0191 222 5659 Email: j.r.williams@ncl.ac.uk; 5 The Orchard, Coylam, Wylam NE41 8BS Tel: 01661 853649 Email: williams_john@msn.com — BM BCh Oxf. 1986 (Oxford) FRCS Eng. 1990; FRCS (Orth.) Eng. 1997; MA Oxf. 1983, BM BCh 1986, DM 1997. Sen.Lect.Trauma.Orthop.Surg.; Hon. Cons. Orthop. Surg. Newc. upon Tyne Hosp. NHS Trust. Specialty: Trauma & Orthop. Surg. Socs: Brit. Orthop. Assn.; Brit. Orthop. Research Soc.; Brit. Soc. Surg. Hand. Prev: Fell. Wrightington Hosp.; Regist. Nuffield Orthop. Centre NHS Trust Oxf.; Regist. (Orthop.) Stoke Mandeville Hosp. Aylesbury.

WILLIAMS, John Richard The Surgery, The Street, Holbrook, Ipswich IP9 2QS Tel: 01473 328263 Fax: 01473 327185; Broadacres, Shotley Road, Chelmondiston, Ipswich IP9 1EE — MB BS Lond. 1975 (Char. Cross) MRCS Eng. LRCP Lond. 1975.

WILLIAMS, John Richard Burton (retired) The Old Bell House, London Road, St Ippolyts, Hitchin SG4 7NE Tel: 01462 454198 — MB BS Lond. 1946 (St. Bart.) MRCS Eng. LRCP Lond. 1946; MD (Path.) Lond. 1952; FRCPath 1969, M 1964. Hon. Cons. Haemat. Lister Hosp. Stevenage. Prev: Cons. Haemat. Lister Hosp. Stevenage & Luton & Dunstable Hosp.

WILLIAMS, Mr John Sheldon The Health Centre, 10 Gresham Road, Oxted RH8 0BQ Tel: 01883 714361 Fax: 01883 722679 — MB BS Lond. 1979 (Kings Coll. Lond.) FRCS Eng. 1984; DRCOG

1985; DMJ (Clin.) 1996. Prev: Surg. Regist. W. Middlx. Univ. Hosp. Hounslow.; SHO (Med.) S. Middlx. Hosp.

WILLIAMS, Mr John Tanat 33 Coalway Road, Penn, Wolverhampton WV3 7LU Tel: 01902 341187 — MB BCh Wales 1966; FRCS Ed. 1972. Cons. Surg. Russells Hall Hosp. Dudley. Specialty: Gen. Surg. Socs: Fell. Assn. Surgs. Gt. Brit. & Irel.; Brit. Soc. Gastroenterol. Prev: Resid. Surgic Off. St. Marks Hosp. Lond.; Sen. Regist. Middlx. Hosp. Lond.; Post Grad. Fell. Univ. Calif. San Francisco.

WILLIAMS, John Tudor Borth Surgery, High Street, Borth SY24 5JE Tel: 01970 871475 Fax: 01970 871881 — MB BS Lond. 1962. Specialty: Gastroenterol.

WILLIAMS, John Walter Trades Lane Health Centre, Causewayend, Coupar Angus, Blairgowrie PH13 9DP Tel: 01828 627312 Fax: 01828 628253 — MB ChB St. And. 1968; DObst RCOG 1969; DCH RCPS Glas. 1971; MRCGP 1975.

WILLIAMS, Mr John Wyn 104 Ffordd Naddyn, Glan Conwy, Colwyn Bay LL28 5BJ — MB BChir Camb. 1982; MA Camb. 1984, MB BChir 1982; FRCS Lond. 1986; FRCR 1990.

WILLIAMS, Jonathan Adam Galloway Horse Fair Surgery, 12 Horse Fair, Banbury OX16 0AJ Tel: 01295 259484 Fax: 01295 279293; Holly Tree Farm House, Horley, Banbury OX15 6BJ — MB BS Lond. 1981; Dip Occ Med; DCH RCP Lond. 1985; DRCOG 1987.

WILLIAMS, Jonathan Craig 4 Bryn Celyn, Pontardawe, Swansea SA8 4LG — MB BCh Wales 1993.

WILLIAMS, Jonathan David Portishead Health Centre, Victoria Square, Portishead, Bristol BS20 6AQ Tel: 01275 847474 — MB ChB Bristol 1985; DCH RCP Lond. 1987; DRCOG 1988; MRCGP 1989; LF Hom (Med) 2001.

WILLIAMS, Jonathan Graham 8 Mellor Court, NHS Trust, Longridge, Preston PR3 3SD Tel: 01772 782360 — MB BChir Camb. 1974 (Kings Coll. Hosp.) MRCS Eng. LRCP Lond. 1973; MA Camb. 1974; FFA RCS Eng. 1979. Cons. Anaesth. Lancashire Teaching Hospitals, NHS Trust. Specialty: Anaesth. Prev: Sen. Regist. (Anaesth.) NW RHA; Lect. (Anaesth.) Univ. Calgary, Canada.

WILLIAMS, Jonathan Hyatt 43 Dyke Road Avenue, Hove BN3 6QA Tel: 01273 555284 Fax: 01273 563155 — MB BS Lond. 1967 (Guy's) MRCS Eng. LRCP Lond. 1967; DA Eng. 1969; FFA RCS Eng. 1971. Cons. Anaesth. Brighton Health Dist. Specialty: Anaesth. Socs: Assn. Anaesths.; BMA; Brit. Soc. Study Addic. Prev: Asst. Prof. Anaesth. Pk.land Hosp. Dallas, USA; Sen. Regist. King's Coll. Hosp. Lond.

WILLIAMS, Jonathan Owen Heaton 20 Wharton Street, London WC1X 9PT — MB BS Lond. 1992 (St Barts Lond) BSc 1980; MSC 1982; MRCGP 1996. Hon Research Fell. UCL. Specialty: Gen. Psychiat.

WILLIAMS, Jonathan Paul 24 Railway Drive, Sturminster Marshall, Wimborne BH21 4DQ — BM Soton. 1986. SHO (Paediat.) Poole Gen. Hosp.

WILLIAMS, Jonathan Wyn Meddygfa'r Llan, Church Surgery, Portland Street, Aberystwyth SY23 2DX Tel: 01970 624855 Fax: 01970 624855 — MB BS Lond. 1980; DCH RCP Lond. 1983; DRCOG 1984; MRCGP 1991.

WILLIAMS, Joseph Brian (retired) 3 Maeshendre, Waunfawr, Aberystwyth SY23 3PR Tel: 01970 612210 — MB BCh Wales 1957 (Cardiff) DObst RCOG 1961. Prev: Ho. Surg. & Ho. Phys. Caerphilly & Dist. Hosp.

WILLIAMS, Joyce Kathleen Kingsfield Medical Centre, 146 Alcester Road South, Kings Heath, Birmingham B14 6AA Tel: 0121 444 2054 Fax: 0121 443 5856 — MB ChB Birm. 1985; DRCOG 1989; DCH RCP Lond. 1990.

WILLIAMS, Judith Department of Paediatrics, Birmingham Heartlands Hospital Trust, Bordesley Green E., Birmingham B9 5SS Tel: 0121 766 6611 Fax: 0121 773 6458; The Dog House, 101 Old Station Road, Solihull B92 0HE Tel: 01675 443704 — MB ChB Liverp. 1977 (Liverpool) DRCOG 1979; MRCP (UK) 1981; MD Liverp. 1993. Cons. Paediat. Birm. Heartlands Hosp. Trust. Specialty: Paediat. Socs: BTS; BMA; RCPH. Prev: Sen. Regist. (Paediat.) W. Midl. RHA; Hon. Research Fell. Roy. Childr. Hosp. Melbourne, Austral.

WILLIAMS, Mr Julian Peter 15 Clifton Street, Alderley Edge SK9 7NW — MB ChB Manch. 1989; FRCS Ed. 1993. Specialist Regist. (Gen. Surg.) S. Manch. NW Region. Specialty: Gen. Surg.

WILLIAMS, June Elizabeth Alice Earnswood Medical Centre, 92 Victoria Street, Crewe CW1 2JR Tel: 01270 257255 Fax: 01270 501943 — MB BS Lond. 1987; DRCOG 1991. Specialty: Gen. Pract.

WILLIAMS, Justin Marc 22 Park Terrace, Burry Port SA16 0BW — MB ChB Leic. 1994.

WILLIAMS, Karen Jayne Addiction Treatment Unit, 44 London Road, Gloucester GL1 3NZ Tel: 01452 891260 Fax: 01452 891261 — MB ChB Dundee 1986 (Univ. Dundee) MRCPsych 1990. Cons. Psychiat. (Subst. Misuse) Addic. Treatm. Unit Glos. Specialty: Gen. Psychiat. Prev: Sen. Regist. Rotat. (Psychiat.) W. Midl.; Regist. Rotat. All Birm. Psychiat. Scheme; SHO Rotat. Gloucester Psychiat. Scheme Coney Hill Hosp. Glos.

WILLIAMS, Katharine Nola (retired) Y Bryn, Beaumaris LL58 8EE Tel: 01248 810257 — MB ChB Birm. 1944. Prev: Assoc. Specialist (Geriat.) Gwynedd AHA.

WILLIAMS, Katherine Lorraine Remote Health, Alice Springs NT 0870, Australia — MB ChB Leic. 1995. Dist. Med. Off. (Remote Health) Alice Springs NT 0870 Australia. Prev: Princip. Ho. Off. IC Unit Mt. Isa Base Hosp. Queensland, Australia.

WILLIAMS, Kathryn Esther Washington House Surgery, 77 Halse Road, Brackley NN13 6EQ Tel: 01280 702436; Hill House, Wrightons Hill, Helmdon, Brackley NN13 5UF — MB BS Lond. 1980; DA Eng. 1983; MFFP 1993. SCMO (Family Plann.) Oxf. Community NHS Trust.

WILLIAMS, Kathryn Mary 104 Cemetery Road, Porth CF39 0BH Tel: 01443 683501 — MB BCh Wales 1987.

WILLIAMS, Kathryn Vivienne 29 Hazel Grove, Bacup OL13 9XT Tel: 01706 873212 — MB ChB Bristol 1977; DA Eng. 1979.

WILLIAMS, Kaye Llewellyn 92 Victoria Road, Warminster BA12 8HG Tel: 01985 212672 — MRCS Eng. LRCP Lond. 1959 (W. Lond.) DObst RCOG 1970. Hon. Clin. Teach. (Primary Med. Care) Med. Sch. Univ. Soton. Socs: Salisbury Med. Soc. Prev: Lt.-Col. RAMC.

WILLIAMS, Keith 7 Harbourside, Tewkesbury GL20 5DT — BM BS Nottm. 1979; BMedSci (Hons.) 1977; MFCM 1984; FFPHM 1991, M 1989; FRCP Nottm. 1998.

WILLIAMS, Keith Nigel Anaesthetic Department, St. Thomas' Hospital, Lambeth Palace Road, London SE1 7EH Tel: 020 7928 9292 Fax: 020 7922 8079; 16 Mansel Road, Wimbledon, London SW19 4AA — MB BS Lond. 1980 (St. Thos.) MA Camb. 1979; MRCS Eng. LRCP Lond. 1979; FFA RCS Eng. 1985. Cons. Anaesth. St. Thos. Hosp. Lond. Specialty: Anaesth. Socs: Brit. Computer Soc. Prev: Sen. Regist. Brompton Hosp.; Sen. Regist. Northwick Pk. Hosp.

WILLIAMS, Kelvyn Parry (retired) Wenallt, Capel Dewi Road, Llangynnwr, Carmarthen SA32 8AA — MB BCh Wales 1947; MRCS Eng. LRCP Lond. 1947; DA Eng. 1956.

WILLIAMS, Kelwyn Daniel Norquay 18 Denmark Road, Gloucester GL1 3HZ Tel: 01452 891220 Fax: 01452 891333 Email: kelwyn.williams@glospart.nhs.uk — MB BS Lond. 1987; BSc Lond. 1984; MRCGP 1992; DCH 1992; MrCPsych. 1997. Cons. Psychi. Glouc. Specialty: Gen. Psychiat. Socs: BMA; MPS. Prev: Specialist Regist. (Psych.) Wotton Lawn Hosp. Gloucester; Specialist Regist. Adult Psychiat. Barrow Hosp. Bristol.

WILLIAMS, Kenneth Gabriel 7 Crofton Court, Wellington Road, Bournemouth BH8 8JH — MRCS Eng. LRCP Lond. 1950.

WILLIAMS, Mr Kenneth Gwylym David 72 Wickham Way, Park Langley, Beckenham BR3 3AF — MB BS Lond. 1961 (Char. Cross) MRCS Eng. LRCP Lond. 1961; FRCS Eng. 1970.

WILLIAMS, Kevin Rhydderch Willowbrook Health Centre, Cottingham Road, Corby NN17 2UR Tel: 01536 260747 Fax: 01536 402153; 7 Larkwood Close, Kettering NN16 9NQ Tel: 01536 511156 Fax: 01536 525684 Email: doctorw@aol.com — MB BS Lond. 1981 (St. George's) GP; Forens. Med. Examr. N.ants Police. Prev: Trainee GP Kettering VTS; Regist. (Med.) St. Albans City Hosp.

***WILLIAMS, Kimberley Jane** 106 Penland Road, Haywards Heath RH16 1PH — MB BS Lond. 1998 (St Barts) BSc; MB BS Lond 1998. Respirat. Med Ho. Off. Whitechapel. Specialty: Respirat. Med. Prev: Orthop. Ho. Off. Basildon; Gen. Surg. Ho. Off. Basildon; A & E SHO Whittington Hosp. Lond.

WILLIAMS, Kyra Ann 33 Chiswick Quay, Hartington Road, Chiswick, London W4 3UR — MB BS Lond. 1960 (Char. Cross) MRCP (UK) 1980. Cons. Rehabil. Parkside Health Trust & Cons. Younger Disabled Unit Willesden Hosp.; Assoc. Specialist Rheum. &

Rehabil. Northwick Pk. Hosp. Specialty: Rehabil. Med.; Rheumatol. Prev: Clin. Asst. (Rheumat.) Char. Cross Hosp., Ealing Hosp., St. Peter's Hosp. Chertsey & Vict. Hosp. Woking.

WILLIAMS, Lars 13 Kierhill Road, Cumbernauld, Glasgow G68 9BH — MB ChB Aberd. 1991.

WILLIAMS, Laurence Glyn St Thomas Surgery, Rifleman Lane, St. Thomas Green, Haverfordwest SA61 1QX Tel: 01437 762162 Fax: 01437 776811 — MB BS Lond. 1990; BSc (Hons.) 1978; PhD Lond. 1981; DRCOG 1993; DFFP 1993; MRCGP 1994; DCH RCP Lond. 1995. Specialty: Gen. Pract. Prev: Trainee GP W. Wales; Research Fell. (Med.) Profess. Unit. St. Barts. Hosp. Lond.; Ho. Off. (Med.) Wexham Pk. Hosp. Slough.

WILLIAMS, Layton Roy The Surgery, 560 Stratford Road, Sparkhill, Birmingham B11 4AN Tel: 0121 772 0284 — MB BCh Wales 1962 (Cardiff.)

WILLIAMS, Leanne Marie 26 High Street, Abercarn, Newport NP11 5GQ — MB BCh Wales 1995.

WILLIAMS, Leith Department of Surgery, St Helens & Knowsley NHS Trust, Warrington Road, Prescot L35 5DR Tel: 0151 426 1600; 45 Stonebridge House, Cobourg Street, Manchester M1 3GB Tel: 0161 236 0852 Email: leith.a@virgin.net — MB ChB Liverp. 1994; BClinSci (Hons.) Liverp. 1993; FRCS 1999; FRCS (Ed) 1999. Specialist Regist. (Gen. Surg.) Whiston Hosp. Specialty: Gen. Surg. Prev: Specialist Regist. (Gen. Surg.) Macclesfield DGH; Clin. Research Fell., (Gen. Surg.), Leeds Gen. Infirm.; SHO Rotat. (A & E) Whiston Hosp.

WILLIAMS, Leonard (retired) 11 Stanhope Road, Croydon CR0 5NS Tel: 020 8688 5957 — (St. Thos.) MB BS Lond. 1952; MRCGP 1976. Prev: Ho. Phys. Mayday Hosp. Croydon.

WILLIAMS, Leonard Hugh Paul 4 Highland Grove, Worksop S81 0JN Tel: 01909 484742 — BChir Camb. 1970; MB 1971; MRCP (UK) 1972. Cons. Paediat. Worksop Hosp. Specialty: Paediat.

WILLIAMS, Lesley The Mote, Moat Lane, Taynton, Gloucester GL19 3AW — MB ChB Leic. 1985; BA (Biol. Chem.) Essex 1975. SHO (O & G) Sheff. HA. Prev: Ho. Surg. & Ho. Phys. Kettering Gen. Hosp.

WILLIAMS, Lesley Seonaid Wellway Medical Group, Wellway, Morpeth NE61 1BY — MB ChB Aberd. 1993; DRCOG 1999; MRCGP 2000. Specialty: Gen. Pract. Prev: GP Regist., Northumbria VTS, Newc., 1997-99; SHO Paediat., N. Tyneside Hosp., Newc.; SHO Paediat., Newc. Gen. Hosp., Newc.

WILLIAMS, Mr Leslie Arnold (retired) 1 High Street, Solva, Haverfordwest SA62 6TF Tel: 0115 960888/01437 720169 — MB BCh Wales 1964; FRCS Ed. 1969; DMRD Eng. 1970; FFR 1972. Prev: Cons. Radiol. Dept. Radiodiag, Univ. Hosp. of Wales Cardiff & Cardiff Roy. Infirm.

WILLIAMS, Leslie Brian Department Radiology, Velindre Hospital, Whitchurch, Cardiff CF14 2TL; 13 Park Fields, Penyfai, Bridgend CF31 4NQ — MB BCh Wales 1977; MA Camb. 1981; MRCP (UK) 1981; FRCR 1985. Cons. Radiol. Velindre Hosp. Cardiff. Specialty: Radiol.

WILLIAMS, Lewis John Furness General Hospital, Dalton Lane, Barrow-in-Furness LA14 4LF Tel: 01229 870870; Stank Villa, Stank, Barrow-in-Furness LA13 0LR Tel: 01229 831791 Email: docsw@globalnet.co.uk — (Univ. Dundee) MB ChB Dundee 1970; FFA RCS Eng. 1975. Cons. Anaesth. Furness Gen. Hosp.; Lead Clinician Furness Gen. Hosp.; Med. Advis. Furness Mt.ain Rescue Team. Specialty: Anaesth. Socs: Fell.of the Roy. Coll. of Anaesth.s; Assn. Day Surg.

WILLIAMS, Mr Lewis Percival c/o Dr G Rebello, 9 Blackford Hill View, Edinburgh EH9 3HD — MB BS Madras 1963 (Stanley Med. Coll.) Dip. Orthop. Madras 1969; FRCS Ed. 1977. Regist. (Orthop. Surg.) Fife Health Bd. Specialty: Orthop.

WILLIAMS, Linda Kennedy The Surgery, 8 Lavant Road, Chichester PO19 5RH Tel: 01243 527264 Fax: 01243 530607 — MB BS Lond. 1990 (St Bartholomews Hospital Medical College) PhD Lond. 1985, BSc 1978; MRCP (UK) 1994; DA (UK) 1995; MRCGP 1996. Princip. GP; Clin. Asst. (Cardiol.) St Richards Hosp. Cichester. Specialty: Gen. Pract. Socs: BMA; RCEP; RCP. Prev: GP/Regist. Chichester; SHO (Anaesth. & Med.) St. Richards Hosp. Chichester.

WILLIAMS, Lisa The Turret Medical Centre, Catherine Street, Kirkintilloch, Glasgow G66 1JB Tel: 0141 211 8260 Fax: 0141 211 8264 — MB ChB Manch. 1990.

WILLIAMS, Lisa Amri — MB BCh Wales 1993.

WILLIAMS, Lisa Gwenan 15B Glenrafon Street, Bethesda, Bangor LL57 3AL — MB ChB Liverp. 1993.

WILLIAMS, Lisa Jane — MB ChB Leic. 1994; MRCPsych; MSc Liverp. 2002. SpR Psychiat. - Merseyside Train. Scheme. Prev: SHO (Psychiat.) Fazakerley Hosp. Liverp.; SHO (A & E) Southport Dist. Gen. Hosp.; Ho. Off. (Surg.) Geo. Eliot Hosp. Nuneaton.

WILLIAMS, Lora Young (retired) Quarry Dene, 36 Church Lane, Bardsey, Leeds LS17 9DP Tel: 01937 572153 — MB ChB Aberd. 1954; MA Aberd. 1949, MB ChB 1954; DA Eng. 1958. Prev: Med. Off. Cancer Families Studies Epidemiol. Dept. Leeds Univ.

WILLIAMS, Louise Patricia 38 Salisbury Crescent, Oxford OX2 7TL — MB BS Melbourne 1987.

WILLIAMS, Luke Robert 18 Rowan Lane, Skelmersdale WN8 6UL — MB ChB Manch. 1998.

WILLIAMS, Lynn Accident & Emergency Department, Queens Medical Centre, Nottingham NG7 2UH Tel: 0115 970 9153 — MB BCh Wales 1980; BA Wales 1974, MB BCh 1980; FRCS Ed. 1987; FFAEM 1993. Cons. A & E Qu.s Med. centre. Specialty: Accid. & Emerg.

WILLIAMS, Mani Prabha HMP Bristol Prison, Cambridge Road, Bristol BS7 8PS Tel: 0117 942 6661 — MB BS Kakatiya, India 1978; MB BS Kakatiya India 1978; LRCP LRCS Ed. LRCPS Glas. 1984; FRCS Ed. 1985.

WILLIAMS, Margaret Ashfield, Merthyrmawr Road, Bridgend CF31 3NW — MB ChB Manch. 1945. Socs: Coll. GP. Prev: Asst. Res. Med. Off. Crumpsall Hosp. Manch.; Asst. Res. Med. Off. Midw. & Gynaecol. Dept. Withington Hosp. Manch.

WILLIAMS, Margaret Eleanor 9 Llwyndern Drive, West Cross, Swansea SA3 5AP — MB BCh Wales 1993; BSc Physiol. (1st cl. Hons.) Wales 1990. SHO (Cas.) Morriston Hosp. Swansea. Specialty: Accid. & Emerg. Prev: SHO (Intens. Care) Univ. Hosp. Wales; SHO (Paediat.) Cardiff Roy. Infirm.; Ho. Off. (Neurol.) Univ. Hosp. Wales.

WILLIAMS, Margaret Elizabeth Marion Maple house, East Surrey Hospital, Canada Avenue, Redhill RH1 5RH — MB BS Lond. 1969 (King's Coll. Hosp.) MRCS Eng. LRCP Lond. 1969; DObst RCOG 1971; MRCP (U.K.) 1973. Cons. community Paediat., Surrey and Sussex healthcare trust. Specialty: Paediat. Prev: SCMO (Community Child Health) Merton & Sutton HA.

WILLIAMS, Margaret Frances (retired) 4 Carlton Bank, Harpenden AL5 4SU Tel: 01582 763383 — MB BS Lond. 1963 (Univ. Coll. Hosp.) MB BS (Distinc. Surg., Obst. & Gyn.) Lond. 1963; MRCS Eng. LRCP Lond. 1963; DObst RCOG 1965. Prev: Ho. Surg. Univ. Coll. Hosp.

WILLIAMS, Margaret Louise Princess Road Surgery, 471-475 Princess Road, Withington, Manchester M20 1BH Tel: 0161 445 7805 Fax: 0161 448 2419; 15 The Lawns, Belgrave Road, Bowdon, Manchester WA14 2YA Tel: 0161 929 8388 — MB ChB Manch. 1986. Prev: Trainee GP Wythenshawe VTS; SHO (Paediat.) Stockport.

WILLIAMS, Margaret Novello 52 Merthyr Mawr Road, Bridgend CF31 3NR — MB BCh Wales 1954.

WILLIAMS, Margaret Selina Isabel (retired) Birch Cottage, Torrington Close, Claygate, Esher KT10 0SB — (Roy. Free) MB BS Lond. 1953; MRCS Eng. LRCP Lond. 1953; DCH Eng. 1955. Prev: Med. Off. Europ. & Asian Hosp. Kampala, Uganda.

WILLIAMS, Margaret Valerie (retired) 6 Park Road, Barry CF62 6NU Tel: 01446 734925 — MB BCh Wales 1960 (Cardiff) Prev: GP Barry.

WILLIAMS, Marian 66 Mill Hill, Waringstown, Craigavon BT66 7QP — MB BCh Belf. 1997; MRCPCH.

WILLIAMS, Marie Elena South King Street Medical Centre, 25 South King Street, Blackpool FY1 4NF Tel: 01253 26637 — MB ChB Manch. 1987 (Univ. Manch.) MRCGP 1991. GP. Specialty: Gen. Pract.

WILLIAMS, Marion Sheila 15 High Street, Yarm TS15 9BH — MB ChB Dundee 1995; BMSc Dund 1992.

WILLIAMS, Marion Siobhan Mengage Street Surgery, 100 Mengage Street, Helston TR13 8RF — MB ChB Bristol 1978; MRCGP 1984. Prev: SHO (Psychiat., Cas. & ENT) Roy. Cornw. Hosp. Treliske.

WILLIAMS, Marjorie Martin (retired) 1 Witham House, St. George's Avenue, Northampton NN2 6SF Tel: 01604 715364 — MB ChB Birm. 1927. Prev: Sen. Asst. MOH Northampton.

WILLIAMS, Mark Aveley Medical Centre, 22 High Street, Aveley, South Ockendon RM15 4AD Tel: 01708 865640 Fax: 01708 891658; 18 St George Avenue, Grays RM17 5XB Tel: 01375 407493 Fax: 01708 891658 — BM Soton. 1983. GP S. Ockendon. Specialty: Otorhinolaryngol.; Forens. Psychiat. Prev: Trainee GP Ryde VTS; SHO (ENT) Luton Gen. Hosp.; SHO (Psych.) Worcester Newton Hosp.

WILLIAMS, Mark Andrew 23 Southcliffe Road, Christchurch BH23 4EN — MB BChir Camb. 1990; MA Camb. 1991; MRCP (UK) 1993; FRCA 1997. Specialist Regist. Dept. Anaes. Soton. Specialty: Intens. Care. Prev: SHO Nuffield Dept. Anaesth. Oxf.; SHO (Intens. Care) Middlx. & Univ. Coll. Hosp. Lond.

WILLIAMS, Mark David Ardroy, 49 Summerhill, Kingswinford DY6 9JG — BM BS Nottm. 1994.

WILLIAMS, Mark Edward Beech Tree Surgery, 68 Doncaster Road, Selby YO8 9AJ — MB ChB Liverp. 1983; DRCOG 1985; DCH RCP Lond. 1987; MRCGP 1990; MSc 2000.

WILLIAMS, Mark Gill Wareham Surgery, Streche Road, Wareham BH20 4PG Tel: 01929 553444; 1 Woodlake Cottage, Bloxworth, Wareham BH20 7ET — MB BS Lond. 1989 (St. George's Hospital, London) DFFP 1993; DRCOG 1994; MRCGP 1994. GP Wareham Surg., Dorset; Clin. Asst., Accid. & Emerg., Poole Hosp. NHS Trust, Poole.

WILLIAMS, Mark Howard 3 Saffron Close, Taunton TA1 3XW Tel: 01823 327863 Fax: 01823 327863 — MB BChir Camb. 1981 (Camb. & St. Mary's) MB BChir Camb. 1980; BA (Hons.) Camb. 1977, MA 1981; DCH RCPS Glas. 1984; DRCOG 1985; MRCGP 1988; DGM RCP Lond. 1988; MFPHM RCP (UK) 1993. Cons. & Sen. Lect. (Epidemiol. & Pub. Health Med.) Univ. Bristol; Hon. Cons. (Pub. Health Med.) SW RHA. Specialty: Pub. Health Med. Socs: BMA; Fell. Roy. Soc. Med. Prev: Lect. (Epidemiol. & Pub. Health Med.) Univ. Bristol; Ho. Surg. Profess. Surg. Unit & Cardiovasc. Unit St. Mary's Hosp. Lond.

WILLIAMS, Mark Rees 1 Cheshire Close, Madeley, Telford TF7 5SP — MB BS Lond. 1997.

WILLIAMS, Martin 56 Northern Road, Cosham, Portsmouth PO6 3DP Tel: 023 92 373321 — MB BCh BAO Dub. 1963 (Trinity Coll. Dub.) DObst RCOG 1966. Specialty: Gen. Pract.

WILLIAMS, Martin Bodreinallt Surgery, Bodreinallt, Conwy LL32 8AT Tel: 01492 593385 Fax: 01492 573715 — MB ChB Bristol 1974; DRCOG 1978; DA Eng. 1978.

WILLIAMS, Martin James (retired) The Cumbrian Clinic, West Cumberland Hospital, Whitehaven CA28 8JG Tel: 01946 523380; Low Hollins, Cockermouth CA13 9UX Tel: 01900 85251 — MB BChir Camb. 1965 (St. Thos.) FRCP Lond. 1980, M 1968. Cons. Phys. The Cumbrian Clinic W. Cumbld. Hosp. Whitehaven. Prev: Cons. Phys. W. Cumbld. Hosp.

WILLIAMS, Martin James Ladywell Medical Centre, West Wing, Edinburgh EH12 7TB Tel: 0131 334 3602; 63 Park Grove, Edinburgh EH4 7QF Tel: 0131 558 9190 — MB ChB Ed. 1991; BSc Ed. 1989; FRCS (A&E) Ed. 1997; MRCGP 1999; DCH (RCP) 2000. Gen. Practitioner Ladywell Med. Centre W. Edin. Specialty: Gen. Med. Prev: SHO (Intens. Care) Qu. Margt. Hosp. Dunferline; SHO (A & E) Qu. Margt. Hosp. Dunfermline; Regist. (A & E) Roy. Infirm. of Edin.

WILLIAMS, Martin Kenneth 30 Brill Close, Maidenhead SL6 3EJ — MB BS Lond. 1994.

WILLIAMS, Mr Martyn Peter Lees Addenbrooke's Hospital, Box 43, Hills Road, Cambridge CB2 2DD — MB BS Lond. 1979; FRCS Ed. 1984; FRCS (Paediat.) 1994. Cons. Paediat. Surg. & Paediat. Urol. Addenbrooke's Hosp. Camb. Specialty: Paediat. Surg. Socs: Brit. Assn. Paediat. Surg.; Brit. Assn. Paediat. Urol.; Eur. Soc. Paediat. Urol. Prev: Sen. Regist. (Paediat. Surg.) Roy. Vict. Infirm. Newc.; Regist. (Paediat. Surg.) Roy. Liverp. Childr. Hosp.; Research Fell. Smith & Nephew Research Roy. Childr. Hosp. Melbourne, Austral.

WILLIAMS, Mary Angela Theresa ICRF, Ashley Wing, St James Univesity Hospital, Beckett St., Leeds LS9 7TF Tel: 0113 283 7089 — MB ChB Cape Town 1970.

WILLIAMS, Mary-Claire 17 Bradfield Avenue, Bridgend CF31 4HL — MB BCh Wales 1998.

WILLIAMS, Mary Llywela Oakley House, Maesycwmmer, Hengoed CF8 — MB BCh Wales 1944 (Cardiff) DObst RCOG 1947. Asst. Med. Off. Mon. CC. Prev: Obst. Regist. St. Davids Hosp. Cardiff; Res. Med. Off. Derby City Hosp.; Ho. Surg. Warneford Gen. Hosp. Leamington Spa.

WILLIAMS, Matthew 106 Bowes Hill, Rowlands Castle PO9 6BS Tel: 023 9241 2565; 18 Barham Road, Petersfield GU32 3EX Tel: 01730 231610 — MB ChB Bristol 1993; DCH RCP Lond. 1995; DA (UK) 1996. Specialist Regist. anaesth. Q A Hosp. Portsmouth. Specialty: Anaesth. Socs: BMA; Train. Mem. Assn. AnE.h. Prev: SHO (Anaesth.) Roy. Devon & Exeter Hosp.; SHO (Paediat.) Taunton & Som.; Ho. Phys. Taunton.

WILLIAMS, Matthew Luke Llewelyn 41 Christchurch Road, Reading RG2 7AP — BChir Camb. 1996.

WILLIAMS, Medwyn Parc Glas, Bodorgan LL62 — MB ChB Liverp. 1981; DCH RCP Lond. 1984; DRCOG 1984; MRCGP 1985. Prev: Trainee GP Gwynedd HA.

WILLIAMS, Melanie Microbiology Department, Frimley Park Hospital, Portsmouth Road, Frimley, Camberley GU16 7UJ Tel: 01276 604604 Fax: 01276 21547 — MB BS Lond. 1967 (Char. Cross) MRCS Eng. LRCP Lond. 1967; MRCS Eng. LRCP Lond. 1967; M 1980; FRCPath 1992, M 1980; MD Lond. 1982; MD Lond. 1982; FRCPath 1992. Cons. Med. Microbiol. Frimley Pk. Hosp. Specialty: Med. Microbiol. Prev: Cons. Med. Microbiol. St. Jas. Hosp. Lond.; Sen. Lect. (Med. Microbiol.) St. Geo. Med. Sch. Lond.; Sen. Regist. (Bacteriol.) Glas. Roy. Infirm.

WILLIAMS, Merion Gwynne 45 Nursery Gardens, Staines TW18 1EJ — MB BS Lond. 1986.

WILLIAMS, Mr Michael Andrew Mayday University Hospital, Mayday Road, Croydon CR7 7YE Tel: 020 8401 3000; Wood End, 80 Welcomes Road, Kenley CR8 5HE Tel: 020 8660 0770 — MB BS Lond. 1975 (St. Mary's) MRCS Eng. LRCP Lond. 1975; FRCS Eng. 1979. Cons. Gen. & Vasc. Surg. Mayday Univ. Hosp. Croydon. Specialty: Gen. Surg. Prev: Research Regist. (Vasc. Surg.) St. Mary's Hosp. Med. Sch.; Sen. Regist. (Vasc. Surg.) St. Mary's Hosp. Harvard Schol.sh. Mass. Gen. Hosp., Boston.

WILLIAMS, Michael Andrew 22 Glencraig Park, Holywood BT18 0BZ — MB BCh Belf. 1998.

WILLIAMS, Michael Anthony Ashfield Surgery, Merthyr Mawr Road, Bridgend CF31 3NW Tel: 01656 652774 Fax: 01656 661187; Sudeley, Glanogwr Road, Bridgend CF31 3PF Tel: 01656 646861 — MB BS Lond. 1979 (St. Mary's Hospital London) DRCOG 1982; Dip. Med. Acupunc. BMAS 1998; Dip Sports Med Bath 1999. Specialty: Sports Med.; Acupunc. Socs: Brit. Med. Acupunct. Soc.; BMA; Brit. Assn Of Sports and Exercise Med.

WILLIAMS, Michael David Department of Haematology, Birmingham Children's Hospital, Steelhouse Lane, Birmingham B4 6NH Tel: 0121 333 9999 Fax: 0121 333 9841 — MD Liverp. 1987; MB ChB 1977; FRCP 1997; FRCPath 1997. Cons. Haemat. Childr. Hosp. Birm. Specialty: Haematology.

WILLIAMS, Michael David Royal Hospital Haslar, Haslar Rd, Gosport PO12 2AA — MB ChB Sheff. 1997.

WILLIAMS, Michael Gill, Surg. Capt. RN 6 Queen Anne's Drive, Bedhampton, Havant PO9 3PG Tel: 023 9248 2647 — MB BChir Camb. 1957 (St. Mary's) MA, MB Camb. 1957, BChir 1956; MRCS Eng. LRCP Lond. 1956; DObst RCOG 1958; DO Eng. 1962.

WILLIAMS, Michael James (retired) 48 Oakhill Road, Aberdeen AB15 5ES Tel: 01224 208046 — MB ChB Aberd. 1954; FRCP Lond. 1976, M 1959; MD Aberd. 1965; FRCP Ed. 1993. Prev: Cons. Phys. Aberd. Gen. Hosps.

WILLIAMS, Michael James Howard Watford General Hospital, Vicarage Road, Watford WD18 0HB Tel: 01923 217391 Fax: 01923 217279 Email: 101462.1205@compuserve.com — MB BS Lond. 1970 (St. Bart.) MRCS Eng. LRCP Lond. 1970; DCH Eng. 1973; MRCP (UK) 1973; FRCP Lond. 1990. Cons. Paediat. (s/i Newborn) Matern. Wing Watford Gen. Hosp.; Clin. Dir. (Family Servs.) Mt. Vernon & Watford Hosps. NHS Trust; Dir. (Childr. Servs.) W. Herts.; Chairm. Exam. Bd. Dip. in Child Health RCP Lond. Specialty: Paediat. Socs: Roy. Coll. Paediat. & Child Health. Prev: Sen. Regist. (Paediat.) St. Mary's Hosp. Lond.; Chief Resid. (Paediat.) Childr. Hosp. Med. Centre, Boston, USA; Instruc. (Paediat.) Harvard Med. Sch. Boston, USA.

WILLIAMS, Michael John (retired) Stretton House, Church Oakley, Basingstoke RG23 7LJ Tel: 01256 780635 — MB BS Lond. 1957 (Guy's) MRCS Eng. LRCP Lond. 1956; DObst RCOG 1958. Dep. Med. Ref. Basingstoke Crem. Prev: GP Basingstoke.

WILLIAMS, Michael Kingsley (Surgery), Gilbert House, 39 Woodfield Lane, Ashtead KT21 2BT Tel: 01372 276385; Sharston Lodge, Fortyfoot Road, Leatherhead KT22 8RN Tel: 01372 373315 — BM BCh Oxf. 1958 (St. Mary's) DObst RCOG 1959; DIH Soc. Apoth. Lond. 1962; MA (Engin. Sci.) Oxf. 1956, DM 1968; MRCGP 1980. Med. Off. Exide Batteries Ltd. Dagenham Dock. Specialty: Occupat. Health. Prev: Sen. Lect. (Occupat. Health) Lond. Sch. Hyg. & Trop. Med.; Indust. Med. Off. Electric Power Storage Co. Swinton; Ho. Phys. (Med.) St. Mary's Hosp.

WILLIAMS, Michael Philip Department of Radiology, Derriford Hospital, Plymouth; Yeoland Down, Golf Links Road, Yelverton PL20 6BN — BM BCh Oxf. 1979; MA Oxf. 1981; FRCR 1984; MBA (Health Exec.) Keele 1996. Cons. Radiol. Plymouth Hosps. NHS Trust. Specialty: Radiol. Prev: Clin. Tutor Univ. Bristol; Sen. Lect. (Radiol.) Roy. Marsden Hosp. Lond.; Sen. Regist. Addenbrooke's Hosp. Camb.

WILLIAMS, Mr Michael Richard Cumberland Infirmary, Carlisle CA2 7HY Tel: 01228 23444; The Old Vicarage, Rosley, Wigton CA7 8AU Tel: 016973 44255 — MB BS Lond. 1977 (The London Hospital Whitechapel) FRCS Eng. 1982; FRCS Ed. 1982; DM Nottm. 1988. Cons. Surg. Cumbld. Infirm. Carlisle. Specialty: Gen. Surg. Socs: Surg. Research Soc.; Brit. Assn. Endocrin. Surgs.; Assn. Breast Surgs. Prev: Sen. Regist. (Surg.) W. Midl. RHA; Regist. (Surg.) Nottm. & Dudley Rd. Hosp. Birm.; Tenovus Research Fell. City Hosp. Nottm. Breast Unit.

WILLIAMS, Michael Thomas Sweet Briars, East Dean Road, Lockrley, Romsey SO51 0JQ — MB BS Lond. 1991 (St. Geo.) MRCP (UK) 1994. Specialty: Anaesth.

WILLIAMS, Michael Vaughan Addenbrooke's Hospital, Oncology Centre, Box 193, Hills Road, Cambridge CB2 2QQ Tel: 01223 217020 Fax: 01223 217094 Email: michael.williams@addenbrookes.nhs.uk — MB BChir Camb. 1974 (Lond. Hosp.) MD Camb. 1984, MA 1974; MRCP (UK) 1975; FRCR 1982; FRCP 1997. Cons. Clin. Oncol. Addenbrooke's Hosp. Camb.; Regist., Fac.Oncology, Roy. Coll Radiologists. Specialty: Oncol. Prev: Med.Director, W.Anglia Cancer Network; Clin. Director, Oncol. Centre, Addenbrooke's; Sen. Regist. (Radiother.) Velindre Hosp. WhitCh. Cardiff.

WILLIAMS, Michael Wyn 9 East Avenue, Porthmadog LL49 9EN — MB BCh Wales 1982.

WILLIAMS, Michelle Lola 68 Rugby Avenue, Greenford UB6 0EZ — MB BS Lond. 1993.

WILLIAMS, Miriam Ann Smeeton Road Health Centre, Smeeton Road, Kibworth, Leicester LE8 0LG Tel: 0116 279 3308 Fax: 0116 279 3320; 87 Weir Road, Kibworth, Leicester LE8 0LQ Tel: 0153753 3864 — MB BCh BAO NUI 1971; MRCGP 1975; DCH RCPSI 1975.

WILLIAMS, Moira Anne Commins 3 Bryn-y-Coed, Hwfa Road, Bangor LL57 2BN Tel: 01248 361345; 25 Antringham Gardens, Edgbaston, Birmingham B15 3QL — MB ChB Birm. 1986. Community Child Health Med. Off. (Paediat.) Gwynedd Community Child Health Trust Caernarfon; Clin. Asst. (Haemat.) Ysbyty Gwynedd. Specialty: Community Child Health. Prev: Cas. Off. Ysbyty Gwynedd; SHO (Neurosurg.) Midl. Centre for Neurosurg. & Neurol. Smethwick; SHO (Otorhinolaryng.) Selly Oak Hosp. Birm.

WILLIAMS, Molly Therese (retired) 25A Chase Green Avenue, Enfield EN2 8EA — (Univ. Coll. Hosp.) MB BS Lond. 1949; DObst RCOG 1951. Prev: Hon. Med. Off. GP Unit St. Michael's Hosp. Enfield.

WILLIAMS, Namor Wyn Department of Pathology, Singleton Hospital, Sketty, Swansea SA2 8QA Tel: 01792 205666; 24 Alexandra Road, Canton, Cardiff CF5 1NS — MB BS Lond. 1983 (St. Bart.) BSc (Hons.) Lond. 1980; MRCPath 1992. Cons. Histopath. Swansea NHS Trust. Specialty: Histopath. Prev: Sen. Regist. (Histopath.) S. Glam. HA; Ho. Off. (Gen. Surg.) Crawley Hosp.; Ho. Off. (Gen. Med.) Whipps Cross Hosp. Lond.

WILLIAMS, Nefyn Howard Health Centre, Village Road, Llanfairfechan LL33 0NH Tel: 01248 680021 Fax: 01248 681711; Northcote, Pk Road, Llanfairfechan LL33 0AE — BM BCh Oxf. 1985; MA Oxf. 1982; DRCOG 1987; DCH RCP Lond. 1988; MRCGP 1991.

WILLIAMS, Neil Ashley 9 Bittell Road, Barnt Green, Birmingham B45 8LP — MB ChB Birm. 1989.

WILLIAMS, Neill Roger Dr N R Williams and Partners, Egginton Road, Etwall, Derby DE65 6NB Tel: 01283 732406 Fax: 01283 731200; 19 Willington Road, Etwall, Derby DE65 6JG Tel: 01283 732213 — MB BS Lond. 1971 (Univ. Coll. Hosp.) DObst RCOG 1973; DFFP 1999. Socs: Derby Med. Soc. Prev: Ho. Surg. Univ. Coll. Hosp. Lond.; SHO (O & G) Burton-on-Trent Gen. Hosp.

WILLIAMS, Nerys Rhiannon — MB ChB Manch. 1984; DCH RCP Lond. 1986; DRCOG (Silver Medal) 1987; DGM RCP Lond. 1987; MRCGP 1988; FFOM RCP Lond. 1995, MFOM, 1993, AFOM 1990; FRCP Lond. 1999. Sen. Med. Insp. & Head of EMAS; Mem. Edit. Panel Jl. Soc. Occupat. Med.; AFOM Examr. RCP Lond; Dep. Chief Examr. Fom RCP Lond.; Consg Occupat. Toxicol.. Dudley Rd. Hosp. Specialty: Occupat. Health. Socs: Soc. Occupat. Med. Prev: Sen. Employm. Med. Advisor Health & Safety Exec.; Employm. Med. Advisor Health & Safety Exec.; Occupat. Phys. Wellcome Foundat. Ltd. Beckenham.

WILLIAMS, Mr Nicholas Department Plastic Surgery, Royal Victoria Infirmary, Queen Victoria Road, Newcastle upon Tyne NE1 4LP — MB ChB Leeds 1988; BSc (Hons.) Leeds 1985; FRCS Eng. 1993; PHD 1999; FRCS 1999. Cons. Plastic, Recontructive and Hand Surg., Roy. Vict. Infirm., Newc. upon Tyne. Specialty: Plastic Surg. Socs: Full Mem. Brit. Soc. Surg. Hand; Full Mem. Brit. Soc. Aesthetic Plastic Surg.s; Full Mem. Brit. Assn. of Plastic Surgeons. Prev: Specialist Regist. Plastic Surg. North. Gen. Hosp. Sheff.; Specialist Regist. Plastic Surg.Roy.Vict..Infirm.Newc.; Hand Fell., St.Jas. Uni. Hosp, Leeds.

WILLIAMS, Nicholas James April Cottage, South Lane, Sutton Valence, Maidstone ME17 3AZ — MB BS Lond. 1994; FRCS Eng. 1999.

WILLIAMS, Nicola Moor Park Surgery, 49 Garstang Rd, Preston PR1 1LB Tel: 01772 252077 — MB ChB Dundee 1994; DFFP 1999; MRCGP 2001. GP Princip. Moor Pk. Surg. Preston; GP Assoc. at Lostock Hall Med. Centre, Leyland Rd, Lostock Hall, Preston. Specialty: Gen. Pract.

WILLIAMS, Nicola Jane 21 Heol Aradur, Llandaff, Cardiff CF5 2RE; Ty Cornel, 21 Hedl Aradur, Llandaff, Cardiff CF5 2RE Tel: 01222 552249 Fax: 01222 308195 — MB BCh Wales 1977 (welsh nat.Sch.med) DRCOG 1979. Specialty: Gen. Psychiat.; Palliat. Med.

WILLIAMS, Nicola Jane Anaesthetic Department, Gloucestershire Royal Hospital, Great Western Road, Gloucester GL1 3NN — MB BS Lond. 1983 (Roy. Free Hosp. Sch. of Med.) BSc Lond. 1980; FRCA 1991. Cons. (Anaesth.) Gloucester Healthcare Trust. Specialty: Anaesth.

WILLIAMS, Nicola Mary Flat 1, 163 New Kings Road, London SW6 4SN — MB BS Lond. 1994.

WILLIAMS, Nicolette 48 Ludlow Avenue, Luton LU1 3RW — MB BS Lond. 1991.

WILLIAMS, Mr Nigel University Hospitals Coventry & Warwickshire, Clifford Bridge Road, Walsgrave, Coventry LE2 4TG Tel: 024 76 602020 — BM BS Nottm. 1986 (Nottingham) BMedSci Nottm. 1984; FRCS 1991; ChM Manch. 1994; FRCS (Gen.) 1997. Cons.Surg.; Sen. Lect., Univ. of Warwick. Specialty: Gen. Surg. Socs: Assn. Surg.; Assn. Coloproctol. Prev: Tutor (Surg.) Univ. Manch.; Regist. Rotat. (Surg.) Leics.; SHO Rotat. (Surg.) Nottm.

WILLIAMS, Nigel Christopher Clarkson Surgery, De-Havilland Road, Wisbech PE13 3AN Tel: 01945 583133 Fax: 01945 464465; Dunnerdale House, 92 Church Road, Emneth, Wisbech PE14 8AF Tel: 01945 463446 — MB ChB Liverp. 1975; DCH Eng. 1979; MRCGP 1982. Socs: BMA. Prev: Trainee GP King's Lynn VTS; SHO (Med.) & Ho. Off. Walton Hosp. Liverp.

WILLIAMS, Nigel Dill 23 High Street, Wolstanton, Newcastle ST5 0EU — MB BCh BAO Belf. 1972. Cons. Microbiol. N. Staffs HA. Specialty: Med. Microbiol. Prev: Sen. Regist. (Med. Microbiol.) North. Gen. Hosp. Sheff.; Regist. (Med. Microbiol.) & SHO (Path.) Roy. Vict. Hosp. Belf.; Ho. Off. Belf. City Hosp.

WILLIAMS, Nina Sunthankar CPHM NPHS, 36 Orchard street, Swansea SA1 5AQ Tel: 01792 607 367 Fax: 01792 607 533 Email: nina.williams@nphs.wales.nhs.uk — MB BCh Wales 1983 (Univ. Wales Cardiff) DCH RCP Lond. 1988; DRCOG 1990; MFCH 1996; MSc (Community Child Health) Warwick 1996; MFPH (Lond.) 2002. Specialist Regist. (Pub. Health). Specialty: Pub. Health Med. Socs: Fac. Community Health; Soc. Pub. Health; BAACH. Prev: Acting SCMO (Child Health) DHSS I. of Man; Trainee GP Hants.

WILLIAMS, Noël (retired) — MB BCh BAO NUI 1947 (N.U.I Coric Ireland) Prev: SCMO N. Yorks. AHA.

WILLIAMS, Noreen Helen Walkley House Medical Centre, 23 Greenhow St., Walkley, Sheffield S6 3TN; 6 Hoober Road, Eccleshall, Sheffield S11 9SF — MB ChB Sheff. 1979. Prev: GP Trainee Sheff. VTS.

WILLIAMS, Norman Brian Department of Anaesthetics, Bristol Royal Infirmary, Marlborough St., Bristol BS2 8HW Tel: 0117 928 2163; 32 Old Sneed Park, Bristol BS9 1RF — MB BCh Wales 1961; DObst RCOG 1963; FFA RCS Eng. 1969. Cons. Anaesth. Bristol Health Dist. (T). Specialty: Anaesth. Socs: Fell. Roy. Soc. Med.; Assn. Anaesths. Prev: Sen. Regist. (Anaesth.) Bristol Health Dist. (T); Cons. Anaesth. Nchanga Consolidated Copper Mines Ltd. Kitwe, Zambia.

WILLIAMS, Norman Eric The Limes, Main St., Tinwell, Stamford PE9 3UD Tel: 01780 757273 Fax: 01780 757370 — (St. Thos.) MB (Distinc.) Camb. 1968, BChir 1967; MA Camb. 1968; MRCP (UK) 1971; FRCP Lond. 1995. Cons. Rheum. & Rehabil. P'boro. Hosp. & Addenbrooke's Hosp. Camb. Specialty: Rheumatol. Socs: BMA (Camb. Br.); BSR; NOS. Prev: Regist. (Rheum.) St. Thos. Hosp. Lond.; Regist. (Neurol.) & Ho. Phys. St. Thos. Hosp. Lond.

WILLIAMS, Professor Norman Stanley Centre for Academic Surgery, Institute of Cell and Molecular Science, Barts & The London Queen Mary's School of Medicine & Dentistry, The Royal London Hospital, Whitechapel, London E1 1BB Tel: 020 7377 7079 Fax: 020 7377 7283 Email: n.s.williams@qmul.ac.uk — MB BS Lond. 1970 (Lond. Hosp.) MRCS Eng. LRCP Lond. 1970; FRCS Eng. 1975; MS Lond. 1982. Prof. Surg. St Bart. & The Roy. Lond. Sch. of Med. & Dent.; Hon Cons. Surg. Barts & Lond. NHS Trust. Specialty: Gen. Surg. Socs: (Pres.) Ileostomy Assn. GB & Irel.; Chairman, QUASAR Steering Committee. Prev: Research Fell. Univ. Calif., Los Angeles, USA; Sen. Lect Univ. Leeds.

WILLIAMS, Norton Elwy (retired) 80 Whitefield Road, Walton, Warrington WA4 6NB Tel: 01925 265889 — MB ChB Liverp. 1956; FFA RCS Eng. 1963. Prev: Sen. Regist. (Anaesth.) United Sheff. Hosps.

WILLIAMS, Olivia Anna 12A Southway, Lewes BN7 1LU — BM Soton. 1983.

WILLIAMS, Olivia Eugenie Flat 2, 22 Upper Tichbourne St., Leicester LE2 1GJ — MB ChB Leic. 1995.

WILLIAMS, Olwen (retired) 36 Millfields, Pentlepoir, Kilgetty SA68 0SA — MB BCh Wales 1940 (Cardiff) Deptm. Med. Off. Glam. CC. Prev: Ho. Phys. Med. Unit, & Ho. Surg. Gyn. & Obst. Unit. Roy. Infirm.

WILLIAMS, Olwen Elizabeth Department of Genitourinary Medicine, Wrexham Maelor Hospital, Croesnewydd Road, Wrexham LL13 7TD Tel: 01745 582314 Fax: 01745 582314 — MB ChB Liverp. 1983; MRCP (UK) 1988; Dip. Ven. Liverp. 1989. Cons. Genitourin. Med. Wrexham Maelor & Glan Clwyd, Rhyl; Hon. Lect. Univ. Hosp. Of Wales; Hon. Lect. Liverp. Univ. Specialty: Genitourinary Medicine; HIV Med. Socs: Hon. Asst. Sec. - Med. Soc. for the Study of Venereal Dis.s (MSSVD). Prev: Sen. Regist. & Regist. (Genitourin. Med.) Roy. Liverp. Hosp.; Lect. (Genitourin. Med.) Univ. Liverp.

WILLIAMS, Owain Aled Drury Cottage, Bilden End, Chrishall, Royston SG8 8RE — BChir Camb. 1994.

WILLIAMS, Owen Glynn (retired) Limeslade House, Limeslade Bay, Mumbles, Swansea SA3 4JE Tel: 01792 366652 — MB BS Lond. 1945 (Cardiff) BSc Wales 1942; FRCP Lond. 1975, M 1948; MD Lond. 1951; FCPath 1965. Home Off. Path. S. Wales & Mon.; Cons. Path. & Dir. of Laborat. Swansea Gen. & Singleton Hosps. Prev: Demonst. (Path. & Bact.) Welsh Nat. Sch. Med. Cardiff.

WILLIAMS, Owen Martin Chingola, Tycroes LL63 5SW — MB BCh Wales 1994.

WILLIAMS, Patricia, MBE Riverside Medical Practice, Ballifeary Lane, Inverness IV3 5PW; Seafield of Raigmore, Inverness IV2 7PA Tel: 01463 711205 — MB ChB Ed. 1968; MFFP 1993. Prev: SCMO (Family Plann.) Highland HB.

WILLIAMS, Patricia Grace Shiellow Grag, Sheillow Wood, Belford NE70 7PH — MB BS Newc. 1975.

WILLIAMS, Patricia Jill HMP Lewes, Brighton Road, Lewes BN7 1EA Tel: 01273 477331 — MB BS Lond. 1976 (Roy. Free) MRCS Eng. LRCP Lond. 1976; MRCPsych. 1981. Vis. Psychiat. HM Prison Lewes. Specialty: Gen. Psychiat. Prev: GP Fordingbridge; Trainee GP Hants., FPC; Regist. (Psychiat.) Roy. Free Hosp. Lond.

WILLIAMS, Patrick Gilbert Noel Godolphin, Surg. Lt.-Cdr. RN Retd. Monteagle Surgery, Tesimond Drive, Monteagle Park, Yateley GU46 6FE Tel: 01252 878992 Fax: 01252 860677; 7 Knowles Avenue, Crowthorne RG45 6DU Tel: 01344 751290 Email: patwilliams77@hotmail.com — MB ChB Leeds 1975; BSc (Hons.) (Physiol.) Leeds 1972; MRCGP 1984. Med. Director, Blackwater Valley Doctors Co-op.; Med. Director, Blackwater Valley Co-op.; Now former Hon. Tutor (Gen. Pract.) St. Geo. Hosp. Lond. Prev: Specialist in Med. RN.

WILLIAMS, Paul Anthony Debyshire Constabullary, Butterly Hall, Ripley DE5 3RS Email: williamspaul@doctors.org.uk — MB ChB Leeds 1987; DRCOG 1991; MRCGP 1992; DMJ 2000; LF Hons. (Med.) 2001. Occupational Health Physcian; Homoeopathy. Specialty: Occupat. Health; Medico Legal; Homeop. Med. Socs: Police Surgs. Assn.; BMA; Fac. Med. Accupuncture Soc.

WILLIAMS, Paul Daniel — MB BS Newc. 1996; MRCGP 2000; DCH 2000; DFFP 2001; DTM & H Liverpool 2001. Locum Gen. Practitioner, Alma St. Med. Centre, Stockon-on-Teel. Specialty: Gen. Pract.

WILLIAMS, Paul Eirian University Hospital of Wales, Medical Biochemistry & Immunology, Cardiff CF14 4XN Tel: 029 2074 8358 Fax: 029 2074 8331 — BM BCh Oxf. 1979; MRCP (UK) 1983; MA Oxf. 1979, BA 1976, DM 1989; MRCPath 1993; FRCP 1998; FRCPath 2002. Cons. Clin. Immunol. Univ. Hosp. Wales. Specialty: Immunol.; Allergy. Socs: Brit. Soc. Immunol.; Internat. Soc. Analyt. Cytol.; Brit. ass for allergy and Clin. Immunol. Prev: Sen. Regist. (Immunol.) W. Midl. HA; Research Regist. Blood Transfus. Centre Roy. Infirm. Edin.; Regist. (Thoracic Med.) Llandough Hosp. Penarth.

WILLIAMS, Paul Ford Dialysis Unit, Ipswich NHS Hospital Trust, Heath Road, Ipswich IP4 5PO Tel: 01473 704117 Fax: 01473 704117; 15 Broughton Road, Ipswich IP1 3QR Email: pwilliams@anglianet.co.uk — BM BCh Oxf. 1976 (Oxford) FRCP Lond.; MA Oxf. 1977, BM BCh 1976; MRCP (UK) 1978; FRCP Ed. 1991. Cons. Gen. Med. (Nephrol.) Ipswich NHS Hosp. Trust Ipswich & Addenbrooke's Hosp. Camb. Specialty: Gen. Med.; Nephrol.

WILLIAMS, Paul Graham St Sampson's Medical Centre, Grandes Maisons Road, St. Sampson, Guernsey GY2 4JS Tel: 01481 245915 Fax: 01481 243179; Tyndale House, Les Vardes, St Peter Port, Guernsey GY1 1BH — MB ChB Leic. 1983; BSc Leic. 1981; DRCOG 1987; DCH RCP Lond. 1988; MRCGP 1989. GP Guernsey. Specialty: Rheumatol.; Sports Med. Socs: Brit. Inst. Musculoskel. Med. Prev: SHO (Rheum.) Rotherham HA.

WILLIAMS, Paul Howard Pendyffryn Medical Group, Ffordd Pendyffryn, Prestatyn LL19 9DH Tel: 0174 56 86444 — MB ChB Liverp. 1981; DCH RCP Lond. 1985. GP Prestatyn. Prev: Trainee GP Clwyd N. VTS; SHO (Gen. Med.) Whiston & St. Helens Hosps.; Ho. Off. (Gen. Med., Geriat., Gen. Surg. & Orthop.) Roy. Liverp. Hosp.

WILLIAMS, Paul Howard 11 High Street, Barford, Warwick CV35 8BU — BM BCh Oxf. 1984; MA Camb. 1985. Specialty: Radiol.

WILLIAMS, Paul Martyn Medway Maritime Hospital, Windmill Road, Gillingham ME7 5NY Tel: 01634 830000; Keites Styles, Munns Lane, Hartlip, Sittingbourne ME9 7SY — BM BCh Oxf. 1984; MA Camb. 1985; MRCP (UK) 1988. Cons. (Paediat.) Medway NHS Trust. Specialty: Paediat. Prev: Sen. Regist. (Paediat.) Mersey RHA.; Regist. (Paediat.) Adelaide Childr. Hosp. Adelaide, S. Austral.; Regist. (Paediat.) St. Jas. Univ. Hosp. Leeds.

WILLIAMS, Paul Raymond Upwell Health Centre, Townley Close, Upwell, Wisbech PE14 9BT Tel: 01945 773671 Fax: 01945 773152; Cartref, Town St., Upwell, Wisbech PE14 9AD Tel: 01945 772946 — MB BS Lond. 1982 (St. Geo.) BSc (Hons.) Lond. 1979, MB BS (Distinc.) 1982; DGM RCP Lond. 1986; MRCGP 1989. GP Wisbech.; Prescribing Lead Fenland PCG; GP Endoscopist Wisbech. Prev: Regist. (Gen. Surg.) Soton. Gen. Hosp.; SHO (Cardiothoracic Surg.) Brompton Hosp. Lond.; Anat. Prosector St. Thomas Hosp. Med. Sch.

WILLIAMS, Mr Paul Roger 94 Dogfield Street, Cardiff CF24 4QZ — MB BCh Wales 1990; BSc (Physiol) UCC 1987; FRCS Eng. 1995. Specialty: Orthop.

WILLIAMS, Paul Simon Camlet Lodge RSU, Chase Farm Hospital, The Ridgeway, Enfield EN2 8JL — MB BS Lond. 1996; MRCPsych 2000. SpR (Forensic Psychiat.) Chase Farm Hosp. Enfield.

WILLIAMS, Paul William The Church Street Practice, David Corbet House, 2 Callows Lane, Kidderminster DY10 2JG Tel: 01562 822051 Fax: 01562 827251 — MB ChB Birm. 1992.

WILLIAMS, Pauline Margaret Clinical Pharmacology Department, Greenford Road, Glaxo Wellcome plc, Greenford UB6 0HE Tel: 020 8966 3331 Fax: 020 8426 9383; Willow Barn, Elms Court, Little Wymondley, Hitchin SG4 7HP Tel: 01438 750340 — MB BCh Wales 1990; Dip. Pharm. Med. RCP (UK) 1995. Sen. Research Phys. (CNS, Clin. Pharmacol.) Glaxo Wellcome plc Greenford. Specialty: Pharmaceutical Medicine.

WILLIAMS, Penelope Susan Bridgegate Medical Centre, Winchester Street, Barrow-in-Furness LA13 9SH Tel: 01229 820304 Fax: 01229 836984 — MB ChB Dundee 1970; DObst RCOG 1972.

WILLIAMS, Peter Peverell Park Surgery, 162 Outlands Road, Peverell, Plymouth PL2 3PR Tel: 01752 791438 Fax: 01752 783623; Home Park House, Landrake, Saltash PL12 5EN — MB BS Lond. 1980; MRCP (UK) 1985.

WILLIAMS, Peter Bacup Health Centre, Bacup OL13 9AL Tel: 01706 876644 — MB ChB Bristol 1977; DRCOG 1982. Prev: Chairm. Rossendale PCG.

WILLIAMS, Peter Alexander Meredith 73 Mumbles Road, West Cross, Swansea SA3 5AA — MB BCh Wales 1991.

WILLIAMS, Peter Ashley — MB BCh Wales 1978; MRCPsych 1982; MRCP (UK) 1982. Cons. Psychiatrist; Cons. Gen. Psychiat. & Community Psychiat. WhitCh. Hosp. Cardiff. Specialty: Gen. Psychiat. Prev: Lect. Univ. Wales Coll. Med.; Wellcome Research Fell. & Hon. Sen. Regist. Univ. Hosp. Wales Cardiff; Regist. (Psychiat.) WhitCh. Hosp. Cardiff.

WILLIAMS, Peter David The Surgery, Butts Road, Bakewell DE45 1ED Tel: 01629 812871 Fax: 01629 814958 — MB BS Lond. 1997; DFFP Cert CLAM; MRCGP Lond. 1997. GP Partner. Specialty: Gen. Pract.

WILLIAMS, Peter George The Surgery, 1 Arlington Road, Eastbourne BN21 1DH Tel: 01323 727531 Fax: 01323 417085 Email: peter.williams@gp-G81050.nhs.uk/ peter.williams12@virgin.net; The Holt, 1 Ashburnham Road, Eastbourne BN21 2HU Tel: 01323 728317 — MB BCh Wales 1972 (Welsh Nat. Sch. Med. Cardiff) DObst RCOG 1976; MRCGP 1977; DFFP 1994; FRCGP 1999. GP; Tutor & Trainer (Gen. Pract.) Eastbourne; RCGP Coll. Represen.; LMC Chairm. Specialty: Gen. Pract. Socs: Assn. BRd.casting Doctors. Prev: Med. Off. RAF; SHO (Cas. & Accid. Surg.) Cardiff Roy. Infirm.; SHO (O & G) Univ. Hosp. of Wales Cardiff.

WILLIAMS, Peter Graham Castle Street Surgery, 39 Castle Street, Luton LU1 3AG Tel: 01582 729242 Fax: 01582 725192 — MB BS Lond. 1974 (Char. Cross) PhD Lond. 1972, BSc (Physiol.) (1st cl. Hons.) 1969; MRCS Eng. LRCP Lond. 1974. Stud. Health Phys. Univ. Luton. Specialty: Gastroenterol. Prev: Resid. Med. Off. Lond. Clinic; SHO (Med.) Hammersmith Hosp.; SHO (Obst. & Med.) Brighton Health Dist.

WILLIAMS, Peter Howard Eaton Socon Health Centre, 274 North Road, Eaton Socon, Huntingdon PE19 8BB Tel: 01480 477111 Fax: 01480 403524; 54 High Street, Yelling, Huntingdon PE19 6SD — MB Camb. 1975; MA Camb. 1975, MB 1975, BChir 1974; MRCGP 1986. Socs: MRCGP. Prev: GP Trainer Eaton Socon.

WILLIAMS, Peter Hugh Northenden Health Centre, 489 Palatine Road, Northenden, Manchester M22 4DH Tel: 0161 998 3206 Fax: 0161 945 9173; 28 Beech Avenue, Gatley, Cheadle SK8 4LS Tel: 0161 428 4464 — MB ChB Manch. 1967.

WILLIAMS, Peter Ian — MB ChB Liverp. 1986; FRCA 1993; MSc 2001. Specialty: Anaesth.

WILLIAMS, Peter Iorwerth 19 Bassaleg Road, Newport NP20 3EB Tel: 01633 267856 — MB BCh Wales 1965 (Cardiff) MRCS Eng. LRCP Lond. 1965; MRCP (UK) 1971; MD Wales 1981; FRCP Lond. 1993. Cons. Phys. Roy. Gwent Hosp. Newport; Private Pract. Newport; Expert Witness (Rheum.) Orthop. Med. Specialty: Rehabil. Med.; Rheumatol. Socs: Inst. Expert Witnesses.

WILLIAMS, Peter John Auchinlea House, Auchinlea Road, Easterhouse, Glasgow G34 9PA Tel: 0141 232 7200 — MB BChir Camb. 1969; MA Camb. 1970; MRCP (U.K.) 1975; MRCPsych 1980; FRCP Ed. 1999. Cons. Psychiat., Parkhead Hosp. Glas. Specialty: Gen. Psychiat. Prev: Staff Psychiat., Alberta Hosp., Edmonton, Canada; Cons. Psychiat. Dingleton Hosp. Melrose.

WILLIAMS, Peter Leslie Medway Hospital, Windmill Road, Gillingham ME7 5NY Tel: 01634 833904 Fax: 01634 833904; 11 Officers Terrace, Historic Dockyard, Chatham ME4 4LJ — MB BChir Camb. 1974 (St Thomas') BA Camb. 1970; MRCP (UK) 1977; FRCP Lond. 1994. Cons. Rheum. Medway Maritime Hosp., Gillingham. Specialty: Rheumatol. Prev: Sen. Regist. (Rheum.) Middlx., Northwick Pk. Harrow & Roy. Nat. Orthop. Hosps. Lond.

WILLIAMS, Peter Michael Gwynne Tinkers Lane Surgery, High Street, Wootton Bassett, Swindon SN4 7AT; The Shieling, Stoneover Lane, Wootton Bassett, Swindon SN4 8QX Tel: 01793 850157 Fax: 01793 848891 — MB ChB Liverp. 1974; DRCOG 1978; Cert. JCC Lond. 1979; MRCGP 1980. Trainer (Gen. Pract.) Wootton Bassett. Socs: MRCGP. Prev: Med. Off. Maj. RAMC; Med. Off. (Family Plann.) Wilts. AHA; Ho. Phys. & Ho. Surg. Whiston Hosp.

WILLIAMS, Peter Orchard, CBE (retired) Courtyard House, Bletchingdon, Kidlington OX5 3DL Tel: 01869 350171 — (St. Mary's & Camb.) MB BChir Camb. 1950; MA Camb. 1950; MRCS Eng. LRCP Lond. 1950; FRCP Lond. 1970, M 1952; Hon. DSc Birm. 1989; Hon. DM Nottm. 1990; Hon. DSc Univ. W. Indies 1991; Hon. DSc Glas. 1992; Hon. DM Oxf. 1992. Prev: Dir. The Wellcome Trust.

WILLIAMS, Peter Randall North Oxford Medical Centre, 96 Woodstock Road, Oxford OX2 7NE Tel: 01865 311005 Fax: 01865 311257; Alan Court, 13 Mill Lane, Old Marston, Oxford OX3 0PY — MB BChir Camb. 1971 (Univ. Coll. Hosp.) MA (Zool.) Nat. Sc. Trip.; MRCGP 1975. Bd. of Dirs. Med. Defence Union. Prev: Partner Kentish Town Health Centre; Hon. Sen. Lect. (Gen. Pract.) Univ. Coll. Hosp. Lond.; Course Organiser Oxf. VTS.

WILLIAMS, Peter Richard 29 Huntley Crescent, Winlaton, Blaydon-on-Tyne NE21 6EU — MB ChB Liverp. 1998.

WILLIAMS, Philip David Rhodes Ashfield Surgery, Merthyr Mawr Road, Bridgend CF31 3NW Tel: 01656 652774 Fax: 01656 661187 — MB BS Lond. 1975 (St. Mary's) MA Camb. 1975; MRCS Eng. LRCP Lond. 1975; MRCGP 1980. GP Mid. Glam. FPC; Mem. M. Glam. LMC. Prev: Cas. Off. & Ho. Phys. St. Mary's Hosp. Harrow Rd.; SHO (Gastroenterol.) Centr. Middlx. Hosp. Lond.

WILLIAMS, Mr Philip Mark Chesterfield Royal Hospital, Calow, Chesterfield S44 5BL Tel: 01246 513117 Fax: 01246 512660 Email: philip.williams@chesterfieldroyal.nhs.uk — MB BS Lond. 1986 (St Geo.) FRCS Eng. 1990; FRCS (Orth.) 1996. Cons. Orthopaedic Surg., Chesterfield and N. Derbysh. Roy. Hosp. Specialty: Orthop. Prev: Cons. (Orthop.) Law Hosp. NHS Trust; Sen. Regist. Dundee Teachg. Hosps.; Clin. Fell. (Paediat. Orthop. & Trauma) Birm. Childr. Hosp. & Roy. Orthop. Hosp. Birm.

WILLIAMS, Portia Louise 42 Seagrove Road, Portsmouth PO2 8AZ — MB BS Lond. 1998.

WILLIAMS, Priscilla Ashfield Surgery, Merthyr Mawr Road, Bridgend CF31 3NW; Llansannor Lodge, LLansannor, Cowbridge CF71 7RX Tel: 01446 772590 — MB BS Lond. 1973 (St. Mary's) DFFP; MRCS Eng. LRCP Lond. 1973; DObst RCOG 1976; DA Eng. 1977. GP Bridgend. Specialty: Gen. Pract.; Family Plann. & Reproduc. Health. Socs: St Mary's Cambrian Soc. Prev: Research Asst. Orthop. Dept. Welsh Nat. Sch. Med. Cardiff.

WILLIAMS, Rachel Angharad 43 Hempstead Lane, Potten End, Berkhamsted HP4 2RZ — MB ChB Manch. 1997; DRCOG 2001; MRCGP 2002.

WILLIAMS, Rachel Margaret Ysbyty Gwynedd, District General Hospital, Bangor LL57 2PW Tel: 01248 384431; Bryn Goleu, Penmaen Park, Llanfairfechan LL33 0RL Tel: 01248 681742 Email: bryn@goleu.u-net.com — MB BS Lond. 1981 (Guy's) MRCP (UK) 1985. Assoc. Specialist Ysbyty Gwynedd Dist. Gen. Hosp. Specialty: Haematology.

WILLIAMS, Raymond Iver John 26 Broomfield Road, Bexleyheath DA6 7PA Tel: 01322 21385 — MRCS Eng. LRCP Lond. 1950.

WILLIAMS, Raymond Stainton Tros y Gors, Waenfawr, Caernarfon LL55 4SD Tel: 01286 650317 Fax: 01286 650714; Liverpool House, Waenfawr, Caernarfon LL55 4YY Tel: 01286 650223 Fax: 01286 650714 — MB ChB Liverp. 1968; MRCGP 1971. Socs: BMA.

WILLIAMS, Rebecca Elizabeth Morlais The Spence Practice, Westcliff House, 48-50 Logan Rd, Bristol BS7 8DR — BA Cantab. 1991 (Cambridge '88-'91, Oxford '91-'94) MRCGP; BM BCh Oxf. 1994. GP Locum, Scott. Borders. Specialty: Gen. Pract. Socs: MRCGP.

WILLIAMS, Rex Darcy Alston 2 Penpoll Road, London E8 1EX — MB BS West Indies 1983.

WILLIAMS, Rhiannon Eluned Wyn Llwyn Onn, Llangollen Road, Trevor, Llangollen LL20 7TF — MB ChB Liverp. 1989; AFOM; DDAM.

WILLIAMS, Rhoda 31 East Street, Tewkesbury GL20 5NR; 62 High Street, Weston, Bath BA1 4DB — BM (Hons.) Soton. 1994; DCH RCP Lond. 1998; DRCOG 1999. Specialty: Gen. Pract.

WILLIAMS, Mr Rhodri John Llewellyn Royal Glamorgan Hospital, Llantrisant, Pontypridd CF72 8XR Tel: 01443 443539; Hafod-Y-Fro, Sigingstone, Cowbridge CF71 7LP Tel: 01446 775326 — MB BCh Wales 1978; FRCS Eng. 1982; MCh Wales 1988. Cons. Gen. Surg. Roy. Glam. Hosp. & Breast Test Wales. Specialty: Gen. Surg. Prev: Sen. Regist. (Gen. Surg.) Middlx. Hosp. Lond.; Lect. (Gen. Surg.) St. Mary's Hosp. Lond.; Clin. Research Fell. The Inst. Cancer Research.

WILLIAMS, Rhodri Wyn 50 Reedley Road, Bristol BS9 3SU — MB ChB Bristol 1997; BDS Birm. 1990; FDS RCS Ed. 1994. SHO(ENT) Southmead Hosp. Specialty: Oral & Maxillofacial Surg.; Gen. Surg.; Orthop. Prev: SHO (Gen. Surg.) Weston Gen. Hsopital, Weston Super Mare; SHO (Orthop.) Weston Gen. Hosp. Weston Super Mare; Ho. Off. (Med.) Weston Gen. Hosp.

WILLIAMS, Mr Rhys Llewellyn Cardiff and Vale NHS Trust, University Hospital Of Wales, Cardiff CF14 4XW Tel: 02920 745049 — MB BS Lond. 1988; FRCS Ed. 1992; FRCS (Orth) Edin. 1996. Cons. Orthpaedic Surg.; Hon. Clin. Tutor, UWCM. Specialty: Trauma & Orthop. Surg. Prev: Ho. Off. (Surg./Orthop.) Luckfield Hosp. Haywards Heath; Ho. Off. (Med.) St. Helens Hosp. Hastings.; SHO (A & E/Orthop.) Brighton HA.

WILLIAMS, Rhys Meyrick (retired) Nethertor, 15 West Cliff, Southgate, Swansea SA3 2AN Tel: 01441 283423 — MB BS Lond. 1939 (King's Coll. Hosp.) MRCS Eng. LRCP Lond. 1937; FRCOG 1965, M 1948. Prev: Cons. O & G Singleton, Mt. Pleasant & Gorseinon Hosps.

WILLIAMS, Rhys Tudor (retired) (cons. rooms), 23 Anson Road, Manchester M14 5BZ Tel: 0161 224 2000; 39 Pine Road, Manchester M20 6UZ Tel: 0161 445 5985 — MB BChir Camb. 1951 (Univ. Coll. Hosp.) FRCP Lond. 1972, M 1957. Prev: Med. Dir. Chesh. Community Healthcare Trust.

WILLIAMS, Richard Aelwyn Department of Rheumatology, Derbyshire Royal Infirmary, London Road, Derby DE1 2QY Tel: 01332 347171 Fax: 01332 254989; 31 Penny Long Lane, Derby DE22 1AX — BSc (Hons.) Lond. 1969, MB BS 1972; MRCP (UK) 1976; FRCP Ed. 1989. Cons. Rheumat. & Rehabil. Derby. Specialty: Rheumatol. Prev: Sen. Regist. (Rheum.) Middlx. Hosp. Lond.; Regist. (Med.) Univ. Hosp. Wales Cardiff; SHO (Paediat.) Cheltenham Gen. Hosp.

WILLIAMS, Richard Bartholomew Department of Rheumatology, Hereford County Hospital, Hereford HR1 2ER Tel: 01432 355444 Fax: 01432 364020; Stoke View, Shucknall Hill, Hereford HR1 3SL Tel: 01432 851438 — MB BS Lond. 1980; DRCOG 1985; MRCGP 1985; FRCP 1997. Cons. Rheum. & Phys. Hereford Hosps. NHS Trust. Specialty: Rheumatol.; Gen. Med. Socs: Brit. Soc. Rheum. Prev: Sen. Regist. (Rheum.) Roy. Lond. Hosp.

WILLIAMS, Richard Charles Melville Street Surgery, 17 Melville Street, Ryde PO33 2AF Tel: 01983 811431 Fax: 01983 817215; Millbank Cottage, Horringford, Newport PO30 3AP Tel: 01983 865130 — MB ChB Liverp. 1974; MRCGP 1980; DRCOG 1980; DAvMed. FOM RCP Lond. 1983. GP Princip.; Trainer (Gen. Pract.) Ryde I. of Wight. Specialty: Gen. Pract. Prev: Sen. Med. Off. RAF.

WILLIAMS, Richard Edward Alban Plas Afon, Glan-yr-Afon, Holywell CH8 9BQ — BM BS Nottm. 1982; BMedSci (Hons.) Nottm. 1980; FRCP Lond. 1997. Cons. Dermat. Glan Clwyd Dist. Gen. Hosp. Bodelwyddan. Specialty: Dermat. Prev: Clin. Lect. (Dermat.) Univ. Glas.; Regist. (Dermat.) West. Infirm. Glas.; Regist. (Gen. Med.) Clwyd N. HA.

WILLIAMS, Mr Richard Gareth University Hospital of Wales, Heath Park, Cardiff CF14 4XW Tel: 029 2074 2583; 16 Health Park Avenue, Cardiff Tel: 01752 769557/02920 751718 — MB BCh Wales 1983; FRCS Ed. 1988; MPhil Wales 1990; FRCS Eng. 1990. Cons. Otolaryngol. Univ. Hosp. Wales Cardiff. Specialty: Otolaryngol. Prev: Cons. Groote Schuur Hosp. Cape Town; Sen. Regist. (ENT) Univ. Hosp. Wales; Regist. Roy. Gwent Hosp. Newport.

WILLIAMS, Richard Glyn 10 Priory Gardens, Bridgend CF31 3LB — MB BCh Wales 1991.

WILLIAMS, Mr Richard Guilfoyle, TD (retired) 49 Manor Court Road, Hanwell, London W7 3EJ — MB BS Lond. 1949 (St. Mary's) DLO Eng. 1954; FRCS Eng. 1955. Hon. Cons. ENT Surg. Hull Roy. Infirm.; Hon. Cons. (Oto-Rhino-Laryng.) Duchess Kent's Milit. Hosp. Catterick. Prev: Regist. Roy. Nat. Throat, Nose & Ear Hosp.

WILLIAMS, Richard James Willson 17 Westover Road, Westbury-on-Trym, Bristol BS9 3LY — MB ChB Birm. 1972; MRCPsych 1976; DPM Eng. 1976. Cons. Child. & Adolsc. Psychiat. Roy. Hosp. Sick Childr. Bristol. Specialty: Child & Adolesc. Psychiat. Prev: Sen. Regist. Child & Adolsc. Psychiat. S. Glam. AHA.

WILLIAMS, Richard John Restalrig Park Medical Centre, 40 Alemoor Crescent, Edinburgh EH7 6UJ Tel: 0131 554 2141 Fax: 0131 554 5363; 3 Durham Road, Edinburgh EH15 1NU — MB ChB Ed. 1983; MRCGP 1987.

WILLIAMS, Mr Richard John Niall Norwich — MB BS Lond. 1990; FRCS Lond. 1994. Specialty: Cardiothoracic Surg.

WILLIAMS, Richard Michael Riverside Surgery, 525 New Chester Road, Rockferry, Birkenhead CH42 2AG Tel: 0151 645 3464 Fax: 0151 643 1676; Wilmar Lodge, Gayton Lane, Gayton, Wirral CH60 3SH — MB ChB Liverp. 1982; DRCOG 1984; DCH RCP Glas. 1986; MRCGP 1987. GP Wirral, Merseyside. Prev: SHO (Geriat. & Paediat.) Arrowe Pk. Hosp. Wirral.; SHO (O & G) Fazakerley Hosp.

WILLIAMS, Richard Michael Joseph Brookway, Sandylane, Oxted RH8 9LU Tel: 01883 712417 — BM BCh Oxf. 1987; BA Oxf. 1984, BM BCh 1987; MRCP (UK) 1993.

WILLIAMS, Mr Richard Shôn The Old Boathouse, Faenol Park, Bangor LL57 4BP Email: shon.williams@breathe.com; 12 Ffordd Gwyndy, Penrhos, Bangor LL57 2EX Tel: 01248 355381 Fax: 01248 355381 Email: gwilli1056@aol.com — MB BS Lond. 1989 (UCMHMS) FRCS FRCS. Specialty: Otolaryngol. Prev: Special Regist. Mersey Deanery.

WILLIAMS, Richard William St Annes Road East, 24 St. Annes Road East, Lytham St Annes FY8 1UR Tel: 01253 722121 Fax: 01253 781121; 3 Shalbourn Road, St Annes-on-Sea, Lytham St Annes FY8 1DN — MB ChB Manch. 1983; MRCGP 1988. Clin. Asst. (Ophth.) Vict. Hosp. Blackpool.

WILLIAMS, Richard Wyn Llidiart Gwyn, Bontnewydd, Caernarfon LL54 5TY — MB ChB Liverp. 1972.

WILLIAMS, Robat Ap-Iestyn Watkin, TD HM Prison Durham, Old Elvet, Durham DH1 3HU Tel: 0191 386 2621 ext 2339; 2 Pierremont Drive, Darlington DL3 9LZ Tel: 01325 252584 Email: dr.robat@dial.pipex.com — MB BS Lond. 1970 (Lond. Hosp.) LMSSA Lond 1970. Med. Off. HM Prison Durh. Socs: Brit. Soc. Med. & Dent. Hypn. & Int. Soc. Hypn. Prev: Dir. Healthcare Purchasing S. Durh. HA; Unit Gen. Manager Community Unit Darlington HA.; Maj. RAMC (TA).

WILLIAMS, Mr Robert (retired) Southdowns House, 48 West Street, Storrington, Pulborough RH20 4EE Tel: 01903 742266 Fax: 01903 746395 — MB BS Lond. 1977 (St. Bart.) MRCP (UK) 1980; DO RCS 1981; FRCS Eng. 1982; DPMSA 1982; FCOphth 1989. Cons. Ophth. S.downs Med. Gp. Storrington, W. Sussex. Prev: Cons. Ophth. W. Sussex Eye Unit Worthing Hosp.

WILLIAMS, Robert Allen Mile Oak Clinic, Chalky Road, Portslade, Brighton BN41 2WF Tel: 01273 417390/419365 Fax: 01273 889192 Email: robert.williams@nhs.net; Barrow Hill Farm, Barrow Hill, Henfield BN5 9DN Tel: 01273 491081 — MRCS Eng. LRCP Lond. 1975 (St. Bart.) DA Eng. 1981. Specialty: Gen. Pract. Prev: Regist. (Anaesth.) Roy. Sussex Co. Hosp. Brighton.

WILLIAMS, Robert Alun Menai Buckhurst Copse, Maiden Erlegh Drive, Reading RG6 7HP Tel: 0118 966 4959 — BM BCh Oxf. 1972; BSc (Hons.) Wales 1966; PhD Lond. 1970; MRCP (UK) 1975; MRCPath 1979; FRCPath 1991. Cons. (Histopath.) Roy. Berks. Hosp. Reading. Specialty: Histopath. Prev: SHO (Gen. Med.) Northwick Pk. Hosp. Harrow; Lect. (Clin. Path.) Univ. Oxf. Med. Sch.

WILLIAMS, Robert Clive 47 Anstruther Road, Edgbaston, Birmingham B15 3NW — MB ChB Bristol 1958; MRCS Eng. LRCP Lond. 1957; DAvMed Eng. 1969; DIH Eng. 1974; MSc Lond. 1974; FFOM RCP Lond. 1997, M 1981. Specialty: Occupat. Health. Socs: Soc. Occupat. Med. Prev: Chief Med. Off. GKN plc; Wing Cdr. RAF.

WILLIAMS, Robert Clive Anaesthetic Dept, Hermitage Lane, Maidstone ME16 9QQ Tel: 01622 729000 — MB BS Lond. 1989; FRCA 1996. Anaesth. Specialty: Anaesth.

WILLIAMS, Robert Delwyn, Capt. West Wirral Group Practice, 530 Pensby Road, Thingwall, Wirral CH61 7UE Tel: 0151 648 1174 Fax: 0151 648 0644; Heath Moor, 15 Beacon Lane, Heswall, Wirral CH60 0DG Tel: 0151 342 3276 — MB ChB Liverp. 1956 (Liverpool) DObst RCOG 1962. Socs: BMA. Prev: SHO (O & G)

Sharoe Green Hosp. Preston; Capt. RAMC; Ho. Surg. & Ho. Phys. Clatterbridge Gen. Hosp.

WILLIAMS, Robert Desmond (retired) Bicknor House, High St., Stevenage SG1 3BG — MB BChir Camb. 1948 (St. Bart.) MRCS Eng. LRCP Lond. 1946. Prev: Ho. Phys. Mansfield & Dist. Gen. Hosp.

WILLIAMS, Robert Fraser (retired) 95 Moss Lane, Sale M33 5BS Tel: 0161 973 6046 — MB ChB Ed. 1955; FRCPath 1975, M 1964. Prev: Cons. Microbiol. Monsall Hosp. Manch., Booth Hall Childr. Hosp. Manch. & Roy. Manch. Childr. Hosp. Pendlebury.

WILLIAMS, Robert Henry Morrah The Health Centre, Elm Grove, Mengham, Hayling Island PO11 9AP Tel: 023 9246 8413 Fax: 02392 637013 — MRCS Eng. LRCP Lond. 1974 (Guy's) BSc (Physiol.) Lond. 1971, MB BS 1974. Prev: Ho. Surg. Greenwich Dist. Hosp.; Ho. Phys. Poole Gen. Hosp.; Trainee Gen. Pract. Portsmouth Vocational Train. Scheme.

WILLIAMS, Robert Ian Treflan Surgery, Treflan, Lower Cardiff Road, Pwllheli LL53 5NF Tel: 01758 701457 Fax: 01758 701209; Bryn Eithin, Caernarfon Road, Pwllheli LL53 5YB Tel: 01758 701561 — MB BCh Wales 1982; MA Camb. 1981; Cert. Family Plann. JCC 1984.

WILLIAMS, Robert Ian 21 Coryton Rise, Whitchurch, Cardiff CF14 7EJ Tel: 029 2069 2919 Fax: 029 2069 2919 Email: frondeg1@aol.com; University Hospital of Wales, Cardiff CF14 4WZ Tel: 029 2074 7747 — MB BCh Wales 1991 (Univ of Wales Coll.Med) MRCP (UK) 1995. Specialist Regist. (Cardiol.) Univ. Wales Coll. Med. Cardiff. Specialty: Cardiol.; Gen. Med. Prev: Regist. (Cardiol.) Roy. Gwent Hosp. Newport; SHO (Gen. Med.) Morriston Hosp. Swansea.

WILLIAMS, Robert John Grove Surgery, Grove Lane, Thetford IP24 2HY Tel: 01842 752285 Fax: 01842 751316 — LMSSA Lond. 1971 (Leeds) DObst RCOG 1973. Prev: Regist. (O & G) Basildon Hosp.

WILLIAMS, Robert Kenneth Talbot Elderly Care Unit, Dorset County Hospital, Williams Avenue, Dorchester DT1 2JY Tel: 01305 263123; West Knighton House, West Knighton, Dorchester DT2 8PF Tel: 01305 852466 — MB BS Lond. 1976 (Middlx.) MRCP (UK) 1980. Cons. Phys. (Geriat. Med.) Dorset Co. Hosp. Dorchester. Specialty: Gen. Med. Prev: Sen. Regist. Northwick Pk. & Middlx. Hosp. Lond.; Regist. Selly Oak Hosp. Birm.

WILLIAMS, Mr Robert Lloyd 30 Devonshire Street, London W1G 6PU Tel: 020 7908 2300 Fax: 020 7908 2400 — MB BS Lond. 1986 (St. Bart.) FRCS Eng. 1990; FRCS (Orth.) 1996. p/t Cons. Orthop. Surg. Univ. Coll. Lond. NHS Trust; Cons. Orthopaedic Surg., Roy. Ballet Company, Lond. Specialty: Orthop.; Trauma & Orthop. Surg. Socs: Fell. Roy. Soc. Med.; Fell. BOA; BOFSS. Prev: Sen. Regist. (Orthop.) Middlx. Hosp. Lond.; Regist. (Orthop.) Roy. Nat. Orthop. Hosp. Stanmore & Chase Farm Hosp.; Ho. Surg. St. Bart. Hosp. Lond.

WILLIAMS, Robert Meirion LLwyn-Y-Fedw, Tyla, Govilon, Abergavenny NP7 9RU Tel: 01873 831824 — MB BCh Wales 1957 (Cardiff) DPH 1962; MFCM 1972. Cons. Pub. Health Med. M. Glam. HA. Specialty: Pub. Health Med. Prev: Med. Off. Health Merthyr Tydfil CBC.

WILLIAMS, Robert Pryce (retired) 273 Dobcroft Road, Sheffield S11 9LG Tel: 0114 236 2103 — MB BS Lond. 1958 (St. Mary's) MRCS Eng. LRCP Lond. 1957; FRCP (UK) 1982, M 1970. Cons. Phys. (Geriat. Med.) N. Gen. Hosp. Sheff.; Hon. Lect. Dept. Med. Sheff. Univ. Prev: Med. Asst. (Geriat.) & Regist. (Path. & Med.) North. Gen. Hosp.

WILLIAMS, Robert Stephen 106 Heol Isaf, Radyr, Cardiff CF15 8EA — MB BS Lond. 1992 (UCMSM) MRCP (UK) 1996. Specialist Regist. (Paediat.) S. W. Region. Specialty: Paediat.

WILLIAMS, Robin Edward Thomas Sidelands, Little Olantigh Rd, Wye, Ashford TN25 5DQ — BM BS Nottm. 1997.

WILLIAMS, Roger 64 Park Road., Hampton Hill, Hampton TW12 1HP — MB BS Lond. 1955 (St. Geo.) Capt. RAMC, RARO. Prev: Asst. Med. Off. Area 10 Middlx.; Ho. Surg. & Ho. Phys. Whipps Cross Hosp. Lond.; Capt. RAMC.

WILLIAMS, Professor Roger, CBE Institute of Hepatology, University College London, 69-75 Chenies Mews, London WC1E 6HX Tel: 020 7679 6510 Fax: 020 7380 0405 Email: roger.williams@ucl.ac.uk; 8 Eldon Road, Kensington, London W8 5PU Tel: 020 7937 5301 — MB BS Lond. 1953; MRCS Eng. LRCP Lond. 1953; MB BS (Hons. Distinc. in Med.) 1953; FRCP Lond. 1969, M 1957; MD Lond. 1960; FRCS Eng. 1988; FRCP Ed. 1990; FRACP 1991; Hon. FACP 1992; Ac Med Sci 2000; Hon. FRCPI 2001. Dir. Inst. Hepatol. Univ. Coll. Lond.; Hon. Cons. Med. UCH.; Cons.Foundat. for Liver Research; Dir. Liver Unit Cromwell Hosp. Lond. Specialty: Gastroenterol. Socs: Assn. Phys.; (Ex-Pres.) Brit. Soc. Gastroenterol.; (Ex-Pres.) Brit. Assn. Study of Liver. Prev: Cons. Phys. King's Coll. Hosp. & Dir. Inst. Liver Studies King's Coll. Hosp. Med. Sch.; Prof. Hepatol. King's Coll. Sch. Med. & Dent. Lond.; Lect. (Med.) Roy. Free Hosp. Lond.

WILLIAMS, Roger Breeze Geufron Hall, Llangollen LL20 8DY Tel: 01978 860676 — MB ChB Birm. 1969; BSc (Hons.) Sheff. 1964; MRCPath 1982. Cons. Histopath. Maelor Gen. Hosp. Wrexham Clwyd. Specialty: Histopath. Prev: Sen. Regist. (Histopath.) W. Midl. RHA.; Sen. Regist. (Chem. Path. & Histopath.) Leeds AHA (T); Sen. Regist. (Paediat. Path.) Sheff. AHA (T).

WILLIAMS, Roger Glyn (retired) Perivale, Higher Metherell, Callington PL17 8DD Tel: 01579 350737 Email: o+g@ukgateway.net — MB BS Lond. 1947 (Manch.) Prev: GP Bolton.

WILLIAMS, Mr Roger James Acresfield, Beechfield Road, Alderley Edge SK9 7AU Tel: 01625 582325 — MD Manch. 1976; MB ChB 1967; FRCS Ed. 1973; FRCS Eng. 1974. Cons. Surg. N. Manch. Gen. Hosp.; RCS Eng. Tutor. Specialty: Gen. Surg. Prev: Sen. Surg. Regist. & Tutor in Clin. Surg. Manch. Roy. Infirm.; Surg. Regist. Stepping Hill Hosp. Stockport.

WILLIAMS, Roger John The Chapel House, Mill Lane, Cloughton, Scarborough YO13 0AB — MB Camb. 1976; BChir 1975; MRCP (UK) 1980; MRCPsych 1985. Cons. Child & Adolesc. Psychiat. Beck Ho. ScarBoro.. Specialty: Child & Adolesc. Psychiat. Prev: Sen. Regist. (Child & Adolesc.) Psychiat. Oxf. Regional Train. Scheme; Regist. Paediat. John Radcliffe Hosp. Oxf.

WILLIAMS, Mr Roger Meyrick Horseleas, Bradfield, Reading RG7 6JA — BM BCh Oxf. 1971; FRCS Ed. 1976; FRCS Eng. 1977; FRCOG 1991, M 1978. Cons. O & G Roy. Berks. Hosp. Reading. Specialty: Obst. & Gyn. Prev: Sen. Regist. (O & G) John Radcliffe Matern. Hosp. Oxf.; Resid. Med. Off. Qu. Charlottes Matern. Hosp. Lond.; Regist. (O & G) King's Coll. Hosp. Lond.

WILLIAMS, Ronald Dennis Holton Road Medical Centre, 232 Holton Road, Barry CF63 4HS Tel: 01446 420222 Fax: 01446 749003 — MB BCh Wales 1974; BSc Wales 1971, MB BCh 1974; DRCOG 1976; MRCGP 1980.

WILLIAMS, Ronald Edward (retired) 8 Heidegger Crescent, London SW13 8HA Tel: 020 8748 8137 — MA, MB Camb. 1954, BChir 1953 (St. Mary's) MRCP Lond. 1957. Sen. Med. Adviser, Min. Div., Ch. Eng. Lond.; Regional Med. Admissions Off.; Emergency Bed Service. Prev: G.P Lond.

WILLIAMS, Rosemary Gwendoline Orchard Cottage, Fownhope, Hereford HR1 4PJ — MB ChB Birm. 1975; DRCOG 1978. Prev: Sen. Regist. (Community Med.) Paddington & N. Kensington Health Dist.

WILLIAMS, Rosemary Sian Risca Surgery, St. Mary Street, Risca, Newport NP11 6YS Tel: 01633 612666 — MB BCh Wales 1990; MRCGP 1996.

WILLIAMS, Mr Rowland James, OBE (retired) Llysfaen, Cardiff Road, Creigiau, Cardiff CF15 9NL Tel: 029 2089 0469 — MB BChir Camb. 1946 (Camb. & Univ. Coll. Hosp.) MRCS Eng. LRCP Lond. 1944; BA Camb. 1941, MA, MB BChir 1946; FRCS Eng. 1948. Prev: Hon. Cons. Surg. E. Glam. Gen. Hosp.

WILLIAMS, Roy Stephen 2 Cefn Cantref, Brecon LD3 8LT — MB BCh Wales 1995.

WILLIAMS, Royston Frank Woodview Medical Centre, 26 Holmecross Road, Thorplands, Northampton NN3 8AW Tel: 01604 670780 Fax: 01604 646208 — MB BS Lond. 1979; MRCGP 1983.

WILLIAMS, Ruth Wells Park Practice, 1 Wells Park Road, London SE26 6JD Tel: 020 8699 2840 Fax: 020 8699 2552; 147 St. Leonards Road, Clarendon Park, Leicester LE2 3BZ — MB ChB Leic. 1989; DRCOG 1993; MRCGP 1995.

WILLIAMS, Ruth Elizabeth Guy's Hospital, Department of Paediatric Neurology, 11th Floor, Guy's Tower, St Thomas Street, London SE1 9RT Tel: 020 71884004 Fax: 020 71880851 Email: ruth.williams@gstt.nhs.uk; 137 Wembley Hill Road, Wembley HA9 8DT Tel: 020 8902 5245 Email: ruth.williams@doctors.org.uk — BM BS Nottm. 1985; DCH RCP Lond. 1989; MRCP (UK) 1990; DM Nottm. 1995; FRCPCH 2004. p/t Cons. Paediat. Neurol.

Specialty: Paediat. Prev: Sen. Regist. (Paediat. Neurol.) Gt. Ormond St. Hosp. Childr. Lond.; Clin. Lect. (Paediat.) Univ. Coll. Lond. Med. Sch.; Wellcome Med. Grad. Research Train. Fell. Univ. Coll. Lond. Med. Sch.

WILLIAMS, Ruth Glyn Furnace House Surgery, St Andrews Road, Carmarthen SA31 1EX Tel: 01267 236616 Fax: 01267 222673 — MB BCh Wales 1982; DRCOG 1985; MRCGP 1986.

WILLIAMS, Ruth Laura Lodge Surgery, Normandy Road, St Albans AL3 5NP Tel: 01727 853107 Fax: 01727 862657 — MB BS Lond. 1993 (St. Mary's) BSc Lond. 1990; DGM RCP Lond. 1995; DRCOG 1996; MRCGP 1997. GP Partner The Lodge Surg. St. Albans. Specialty: Gen. Pract. Prev: GP Regist. Portmill Surg. Hitchin; SHO Lister Stevenge VTS; Ho. Off. (Surg. & Orthop.) Wexham Pk. & Heatherwood Hosp.

WILLIAMS, Sally Anne Orchard Medical Practice, Orchard Street, Ipswich IP4 2PU Tel: 01473 213261 — MB BS Lond. 1975 (Char. Cross) MRCS Eng. LRCP Lond. 1975; MRCGP 2003; Postgrad. Cert. of Med. Educat. Camb. 2004. GP Tutor Univ. of E. Anglia Med. Sch. Specialty: Gen. Pract.

WILLIAMS, Sally Wynne — MB BCh Wales 1988 (Wales College of Medicine) MRCPsych 1994. Specialty: Geriat. Psychiat. Prev: N. Birm. Ment. Health Trust.

WILLIAMS, Samuel Jonathan Selly Oak Hospital, Raddlebarn Road, Selly Oak, Birmingham B29 6JD Tel: 0121 627 1627 — Vrach Inst. of Paediat., Leningrad 1973; Vrach Leningrad Inst. of Paediatrics USSR 1973; DTM & H Liverp. 1974; DPH Lond. 1978; MMedSci (Surg. & Trauma) Birm. 1996. A&E Practitioner,Medicine/Care Univ. Hosp. NHS Trust (Selly Oak Birm.); Hon. Fell. Inst. Accid. Surg. Birm.; Forens. Med. Examr., (Clinical) police Surg., Health call Forens. Med. Servs., Coventry Midlands. Specialty: Accid. & Emerg. Socs: Fell. Roy. Inst. Pub. Health & Hyg.; Fell. Roy. Soc. Med. Prev: Lect. Teach. Hosp. Coll. Health Sc. Univ. Sokoto, Nigeria; Clin. Asst. (Orthop. Surg. & Traumatol.) S. Birm. HA; Lect. (Med. Sc.) Univ. Jos., Nigeria.

WILLIAMS, Sandra Jane Kingswood Surgery, Kingswood Road, Tunbridge Wells TN2 4UH Tel: 018920 511833; 85 Longmeads, Langton Green, Tunbridge Wells TN3 0AU Tel: 01892 863361 — MB BS Lond. 1986 (Char. Cross) DRCOG 1988; Cert. Family Plann. JCC 1988; MRCGP 1991.

WILLIAMS, Sara Catrin Rhydyfirian, Rhydyfelin, Aberystwyth SY23 4LU — BChir Camb. 1992.

WILLIAMS, Sarah 13 Aylestone Drive, Hereford HR1 1HT — BM BS Nottm. 1992.

WILLIAMS, Sarah Elin Wingfield, Penny Long Lane, Derby DE22 1AX — MB BCh Wales 1998.

WILLIAMS, Sarah Elizabeth c/o 20 Swisspine Gardens, St Helens WA9 5UE — MB BS Lond. 1998.

WILLIAMS, Sarah Jane Riverside Surgery, 48 Worthing Road, Horsham RH12 1UD Tel: 01403 264848 — MB BS Lond. 1989 (Charring Cross & Westminster) DRCOG 1993.

WILLIAMS, Sarah Jane 7 Kynnersley Lane, Leighton, Shrewsbury SY5 6RS — MB ChB Birm. 1998.

WILLIAMS, Sarah Sian Occupational Health and Safety Unit, Royal Free Hospital, London NW3 2QG Tel: 020 7830 2509 Fax: 020 7830 2512 Email: sian.williams@royalfree.nhs.uk — MB BS Lond. 1984 (Univ. Coll. Hosp.) MRCP (UK) 1987; MFOM RCP Lond. 1995; MD 1997. Cons. Occupat. Med. Roy. Free Hosp. Lond. Specialty: Occupat. Health.

WILLIAMS, Sean Roderick Rhys 32 Ealing Park Gardens, Ealing, London W5 4EU — MB ChB Leic. 1994; BSc Leic. 1992; FRCS 1999.

WILLIAMS, Sharmistha Karina c/o Mrs. K. De Silva, 11 Caroline Close, Croydon CR0 5JU — MB BS Lond. 1988.

WILLIAMS, Sharon Louise 5 Altwood Bailey, Maidenhead SL6 4PQ — MB BS Lond. 1989.

WILLIAMS, Sian The Knowe, 43 Queen St., Perth PH2 0EJ — MB BCh BAO Belf. 1978; DRCOG 1982. Staff Grade (Haemat.) Perth Roy. Infirm. Specialty: Care of the Elderly. Prev: Clin. Asst. (Geriat. Med.) Perth Roy. Infirm.

WILLIAMS, Sian Emma 11 Percy Road, Boscombe, Bournemouth BH5 1JF Tel: 01202 398014; 27 Lander Close, Baiter Park, Poole BH15 1UL Tel: 01202 469446 — MB BS Lond. 1997 (St Mary's Hospital) BSc 1996. SHO (Paediat.). Specialty: Paediat. Prev: SHO (ENT), Poole; PRHO (Med.), Winchester; PRHO (Surg.), Chichester.

WILLIAMS, Sian Lloyd 9 Holroyd Road, Putney, London SW15 6LN — MB BS Lond. 1978 (St. Bart.) DRCOG 1982; MRCGP 1982; DCH RCP Lond. 1983; DFFP 1995. GP Lond. Prev: Redhill GP VTS; Clin. Med. Off. (Child Health) Camberwell HA; Clin. Med. Off. (Family Plann.) Norwich.

WILLIAMS, Sian Mia 6 Honeys Green Lane, Liverpool L12 9EW — MB BCh Wales 1998.

WILLIAMS, Simon David St. Stephens House, 102 Woodfield Lane, Ashtead KT21 2DP Tel: 01372 272069 Fax: 01372 279123; 11 Homelands, Leatherhead KT22 8SU — MB BS Lond. 1983 (St. Bart. Hosp.) MRCGP 1989; DRCOG 1989.

WILLIAMS, Simon Edward Beechlawn, 35 Woodthorpe Lane, Sandal, Wakefield WF2 6JG Tel: 01924 253685 — MD Lond. 1980 (King's Coll. Hosp.) MB BS 1970; MRCP (UK) 1975; FRCP 1992. Cons. Phys. Med. & Respirat. Dis. Pinderfields Hosps. NHS Trust Wakefield. Specialty: Respirat. Med. Socs: Brit. Thorac. Soc. Prev: Sen. Regist. Rotat. (Med. & Respirat. Dis.) Leeds & Bradford; Tutor (Med.) Hope Hosp. & Manch Univ.

WILLIAMS, Simon Graham John Ipswich Hospital NHS Trust, Deptartment of Medicine, Heath Road, Ipswich IP4 5PD Email: simon.williams@ipswichhospital.nhs.uk — MB BS Lond. 1986; MA Cantab 1987; MD Lond. 1995; FRCP 2000. Cons. Ipswich Hosp. NHS Trust. Specialty: Gastroenterol. Prev: Sen. Regist. W. Middlx., Chelsea & Westm. Hosps.

WILLIAMS, Simon Haydn 137 New Hey Road, Wirral CH49 7NE — MB ChB Sheff. 1994.

WILLIAMS, Simon Timothy 4 Heron Close, Great Glen, Leicester LE8 9DZ — BM BS Nottm. 1991.

WILLIAMS, Simon Timothy Bowen 25 Loop Road, Beachley, Chepstow NP16 7HE — MB BCh Wales 1997.

WILLIAMS, Sindy The Moorings, Peak Lane, East Preston, Littlehampton BN16 1RN — MB BS Lond. 1990; MRCGP 1994.

WILLIAMS, Siôn Austin Gwynfa, Groesfawr, Llandyrnog, Denbigh LL16 4NB — MB BCh Wales 1986; MRCGP 1993.

WILLIAMS, Sioned 65 Glan-y-Mor Road, Llandudno LL30 3PF — MB BCh Wales 1994.

WILLIAMS, Stanley Robert (retired) 32 Hill Drive, Hove BN3 6QL — (Guy's) MB BS Lond. 1957; MRCS Eng. LRCP Lond. 1957; FFA RCS Eng. 1964.

WILLIAMS, Stephanie Jane Morecambe Health Centre, Hanover Street, Morecambe LA4 Tel: 01524 405765 — MB ChB Ed. 1992 (Edinburgh) GP Princip., Morecambe Health Centre. Specialty: Gen. Pract. Prev: GP Regist. Roy. Lancaster Infirm.

WILLIAMS, Stephen The Larches, Wetherby Road, Bardsey, Leeds LS17 9BB — MB ChB Bristol 1979; FFA RCS Eng. 1986.

WILLIAMS, Stephen Aled Runnymede Medical Practice, Newton Court Medical Centre, Burfield Road, Old Windsor, Windsor SL4 2QF Tel: 01753 863642 Fax: 01753 832180 — MB BCh Wales 1980; DCH RCP Lond. 1983; DRCOG 1985; MRCGP 1990.

WILLIAMS, Stephen Gareth 2 Elm Cottages, Burleigh Lane, South Huish, Kingsbridge TQ7 3EF — MB BS Lond. 1985; DCH RCP Lond. 1988; DRCOG 1990; MRCGP 1994. Prev: Ho. Phys. Qu. Eliz. II Hosp. Welwyn Garden City; Ho. Surg. Gloucester Roy. Hosp.

WILLIAMS, Stephen John Stoke Mandeville Hospital, Aylesbury HP21 8AL — MB BCh Wales 1969; MRCP (U.K.) 1974. Specialty: Respirat. Med. Prev: Sen. Regist. (Thoracic Med.) Brompton Hosp. Lond.; Regist. (Thoracic Med.) Brompton Hosp. Lond.; Regist. (Med. & Thoracic) S. Glam. AHA (T).

WILLIAMS, Stephen John Thompson Topsham Drive, Hill Road, Kilgetty SA68 — MB BS Lond. 1980.

WILLIAMS, Stephen Mark 63 Minny Street, Cathays, Cardiff CF24 4ET — MB BCh Wales 1998.

WILLIAMS, Stephen Morriss The Garth Surgery, Rectory Lane, Guisborough TS14 7DJ Tel: 01287 632206 Fax: 01287 635112; The Spinney, Hutton Village, Guisborough TS14 8ER Tel: 01287 637416 — MB BS Newc. 1972; MRCGP 1977; MRCP (UK) 1978. Princip. (Gen. Pract.) GuisBoro.; Cognitive Therapist The Whitecliffe Centre, E. Cleveland Hosp. Prev: Trainee Gen. Pract. Cleveland Vocational Train. Scheme; Ho. Phys. Cumbld. Infirm. Carlisle; Regist. (Med.) Palmerston N. Pub. Hosp., N.Z.

WILLIAMS, Stephen Padgett 179 Hubert Road, Selly Oak, Birmingham B29 6ET — MB ChB Birm. 1986.

WILLIAMS, Stephen Richard Station Road Surgery, 15-16 Station Road, Penarth CF64 3EP — MB BCh Wales 1985; BSc Wales 1980, MB BCh 1985. Trainee GP Newport Gwent. Prev: SHO (Cas.) Cardiff Roy. Infirm.

WILLIAMS, Stephen Richard The Health Centre, Lawson Street, Stockton-on-Tees TS18 1HX Tel: 01642 672351 Fax: 01642 618112 — MB ChB Leeds 1982; DRCOG 1984; DCH RCP Lond. 1986; MRCGP 1986.

WILLIAMS, Stuart Andrew Somerden Green, Chiddingstone, Edenbridge TN8 7AL Tel: 01892 870381 — BM Soton. 1989. SHO (A & E) W. Cornw. Hosp. Socs: BMA.

WILLIAMS, Stuart Michael 29 Purcell Road, Marston, Oxford OX3 0HB — BM BCh Oxf. 1992 (Univ. Oxf.) MRCP (UK) 1995. Regist. (Radiol.) John Radcliffe Hosp. Oxf. Specialty: Radiol.

WILLIAMS, Mr Stuart Rhys ENT Department, Poole Hospital NHS Trust, Longfleet Road, Poole BH15 2JB Tel: 01202 665511 — MB BS Lond. 1976; MRCS Eng. LRCP Lond. 1976; FFA RCS Eng. 1980; FRCS Ed. 1984; FRCS Eng. 1988. Specialty: Otorhinolaryngol.

WILLIAMS, Susan Department of Histopathology, Singleton Hospital, Sketty, Swansea SA2 8QA; 13 Parkfields, Peny Fai, Bridgend CF31 4NQ — MB BCh Wales 1977; MRCPath 1985. Cons. Histopath. Singleton Hosp. Swansea NHS Trust. Specialty: Histopath.

WILLIAMS, Susan Anne Roathwell Surgery, 116 Newport Road, Roath, Cardiff CF24 1YT Tel: 029 2049 4537 Fax: 029 2049 8086 — BM Soton. 1989; DRCOG 1991; MRCGP 1994. GP Roath Cardiff; GP Trainer; Clin. Asst. (A & E) Cardiff Roy. Infirm. Prev: Asst. GP Penylan, Cardiff.

WILLIAMS, Susan Beris 35/7 Wood Lane, Beverley HU17 8BS — MB BS Lond. 1994 (Cambridge and London) MA Camb. 1993. Research Fell. (Paediat. Surg.) Inst. of Child Health Lond. Specialty: Paediat. Surg. Prev: SHO (Cariothoracic Surg.) Roy. Brompton Hosp. Lond.

WILLIAMS, Susan Ebsworth High Street Surgery, 87 High Street, Abbots Langley WD5 0AJ Tel: 01923 262363 Fax: 01923 267374; Ashcroft, 186 Abbots Road, Abbots Langley WD5 0BL Tel: 01923 267840 — MB BS Lond. 1983; DCH RCP Lond. 1985; DRCOG 1985; MRCGP 1988. Prev: Trainee GP Watford VTS.

WILLIAMS, Susan Elizabeth Leasowes, Clun, Craven Arms SY7 8QA — MB ChB Dundee 1997. SHO A & E. Princess Roy. Hosp., Telford, Shrops. Specialty: Accid. & Emerg. Socs: Med. Defence Union. Prev: SHO Psychiat. Abeyshwym; SHO Med. Telford; SHO Surg. Telford.

WILLIAMS, Susan Elizabeth Long Barn Lane Surgery, 22 Long Barn Lane, Reading RG2 7SZ Tel: 0118 987 1377 Fax: 0118 978 0378 — MB ChB Sheffield 1968.

WILLIAMS, Susan Gladys Kippax Hall Surgery, 54 High Street, Kippax, Leeds LS25 7AB Tel: 0113 286 2044 Fax: 0113 287 3970 — MB ChB Ed. 1989 (Edinburgh)

WILLIAMS, Susan Jane Armstrong and Partners, Morrab Surgery, 2 Morrab Road, Penzance TR18 4EL Tel: 01736 363866 Fax: 01736 367809; St Michaels, Trenow, Long Rock, Penzance TR20 8YQ Tel: 01736 710184 — MB BS Lond. 1985; DRCOG 1989.

WILLIAMS, Susanne Maria (retired) Briar House, Weston Road, Bath BA1 2XT Tel: 01225 421509 — MB BS Lond. 1950 (Roy. Free) MRCS Eng. LRCP Lond. 1950; DObst RCOG 1954. Prev: Clin. Med. Off. Child Health Bristol.

WILLIAMS, Tania Montgomery House Surgery, Piggy Lane, Bicester OX26 6HT Tel: 01869 249222 — MB ChB Liverp. 1979; MSc Oxf. 1973; Cert. Prescribed Equiv. Exp. JCPTGP 1983.

WILLIAMS, Tegwyn Mel Caswell Clinic, Glanrhyd Hospital, Bridgend CF31 4LN Tel: 01656 662179 — MB BS Lond. 1983; MRCPsych 1987. Cons. Forens. Psychiat. Bridgend & Dist. NHS Trust. Specialty: Forens. Psychiat. Socs: Sec. Internat. Assn. Forens. Psychother. Prev: Sen. Regist. (Forens. Psychiat.) Wessex RHA.

WILLIAMS, Mrs Thelma (retired) Silverbrook, 50 Rhiwbina Hill, Rhiwbina, Cardiff CF14 6UQ Tel: 029 2062 6935 — MB BCh Wales 1957.

WILLIAMS, Thomas Darlington Dewdown, Nempnett Thrubwell, Chew Stoke, Bristol BS40 8YF — MD Liverp. 1954; BSc (Hnrs.) 1948, MB ChB 1951. Sen. Lect. Physiol. Univ. Bristol; Cons. (Med. Sc.) Bristol Health Dist. (T). Specialty: Clin. Physiol. Socs: Physiol. Soc. Prev: Holt Fell. 1951; Med. Research Counc. Stud. 1951-3; Specialist Physiol. RAMC, At Army Operat.al Research Gp.

WILLIAMS, Thomas Dewi Meurig Prince Philip Hospital, Bryngwynmawr, Dafen, Llanelli SA14 8QF Tel: 01554 756567 Fax: 01554 749410; Llandeilo yr Ynys, Nantgaredig, Carmarthen SA32 7LQ Tel: 01267 290151 Fax: 01267 290102 Email: meurigwill@aol.com — MB BCh Wales 1977; MA Oxf. 1976; MRCP (UK) 1980; MD Wales 1987; FRCP Lond. 1996. Cons. Phys. & Endocrinol. Carmarthenshire NHS Trust. Specialty: Gen. Med.; Diabetes; Endocrinol. Socs: Soc. Endocrinol. Prev: Lect. (Med.) Char. Cross & Westm. Med. Sch. Lond.; Research Fell. (Neuroendocrinol.) St. Mary's Hosp. Med. Sch. Lond.; SHO Roy. Postgrad. Med. Sch. Lond.

WILLIAMS, Thomas Henry Currer Nevill Hall Hospital, Abergavenny NP7 7EG Tel: 01873 732 482 — MB BS Lond. 1972; BSc (Hons.) Lond. 1969; MRCP (UK) 1976; FRCP Lond. 1995; FRCPCH 1997. Cons. Paediat. Nevill Hall Hosp. Abergavenny. Specialty: Paediat. Prev: Sen. Regist. (Paediat.) Leic. Roy. Infirm.

WILLIAMS, Thomas Ian Robertson Tregarthens, Little Weighton Road, Walkington, Beverley HU17 8TA — MB ChB St. And. 1970; FFA RCS Eng. 1974. Cons. Anaesth. Hull & Beverley Health Dists. Specialty: Anaesth. Prev: Anaesth. Sen. Regist. West. Infirm. Glas.

WILLIAMS, Thomas Neil 67 King George V Drive W., Cardiff CF14 4EF — MB BS Lond. 1985; DCH RCP Lond. 1988; DTM & H Lond. 1988; MRCP (UK) 1990; PhD 1999. Research.Fell.Wellcome Trust.Nuffield.Dept.Med.Oxf/Rearch. Unit.Kenya; Lect. Paediat. Infect. Dis. St Marys. Hosp. Lond. Specialty: Paediat. Prev: Malaria Research North. Dist. Hosp. Vanuatu, SW Pacific; Regist. (Paediat.) Whittington Hosp. Lond.

WILLIAMS, Mr Timothy Gabe The BUPA Hospital, Fordcombe Road, Fordcombe, Tunbridge Wells TN3 0RD Tel: 01892 740040; Burnt Oak, Back Lane, Waldron, Heathfield TN21 0NN Tel: 014 353 2273 — MB BChir Camb. 1970; MA, MChir Camb. 1983, MB 1970, BChir 1969; FRCS Eng. 1974. Cons. Surg. Kent. & Sussex Hosp. Tunbridge Wells. Specialty: Gen. Surg. Prev: Sen. Surg. Regist. St. Thos. Hosp. Lond.; Ho. Surg. Surgic. Unit St. Thos. Hosp. Lond.; Surg. Regist. Ipswich Gp. Hosps.

WILLIAMS, Timothy John Department of Respiratory Medicine, Kettering General Hospital, Rothwell Road, Kettering NN16 8UZ; Willow House, 27A Warkton Lane, Kettering NN15 5AB — MB ChB Cambridge 1969; MB ChB Cambridge 1969. Specialty: Respirat. Med.

WILLIAMS, Timothy Laurence 20 Clayworth Road, Newcastle upon Tyne NE3 5AB — MB BS Newc. 1990; MB BS (Hons.) Newc. 1990, BMedSc (Hons.) 1987; MRCP (UK) 1993; PhD Newc. 2000. Hon. Research Regist. (Neurosci.s) Univ. Newc. u. Tyne.; Consultant Neurologist, Royal Victoria Infirmary, Newcastle. Specialty: Neurol. Prev: SHO Rotat. (Med.) Newc.; Ho. Phys. Newc. Gen. Hosp.; Ho. Surg. Roy. Vict. Infirm. Newc. u. Tyne.

WILLIAMS, Tracey Elizabeth Jane Doctors Surgery, 40 St. Georges Crescent, Wrexham LL13 8DB Tel: 01978 290708 — MB ChB Manch. 1986 (Manch) DRCOG 1990. Specialty: Gen. Pract.

WILLIAMS, Trevor Dawson Oakengates Medical Practice, Limes Walk, Oakengates, Telford TF2 6JJ Tel: 01952 620077 Fax: 01952 620209 — MB BCh BAO Dub. 1982; DCH Dub. 1985; MRCGP 1988.

WILLIAMS, Valerie 8 Ashdale Close, Alsager, Stoke-on-Trent ST7 2EN — MB ChB Manch. 1979; FFA RCS Eng. 1983. Cons. Anaesth. Univ. Hosp. N. Staffs. Stoke-on-Trent; Sen. Lect. (Med. Educat.) Keele Univ. Specialty: Anaesth.; Intens. Care.

WILLIAMS, Valerie Susan 19 The Demesne, North Seaton, Ashington NE63 9TW — MB BS Lond. 1965 (Roy. Free) MRCS Eng. LRCP Lond. 1965; DCH Eng 1968; DObst RCOG 1968; MRCGP 1973.

WILLIAMS, Vicki Erica Ilse of Egg — MB ChB Manch. 1991. Specialty: Gen. Pract.

WILLIAMS, Mrs Victoria Louise The Park Medical Group, Fawdon Park Road, Newcastle upon Tyne NE3 2PE Tel: 0191 285 1763 Fax: 0191 284 2374 — MB BS Newc. 1989.

WILLIAMS, Vivien Nicola Thatcham Medical Practice, Bath Road, Thatcham RG18 3HD Tel: 01635 867171 Fax: 01635 876395 — MB BS Lond. 1979 (St. Thos.) DCH RCP Lond. 1983; DRCOG 1983; MRCGP 1984. Special Interest: Train. Socs: BMA; RCGP.

WILLIAMS, Wadad Tebeldy, 2 Cae Mawr, Penrhyncoch, Aberystwyth SY23 3EJ Tel: 01970 820060 — MRCS Eng. LRCP

Lond. 1957. Specialty: Gen. Med. Prev: Dir. Khartoum Clinic & Harper Nursing Home Khartoum; Med. Off. Civil Hosp. Khartoum.

WILLIAMS, Walter (retired) Ty-Draw House, Blaencwm, Treherbert, Treorchy, Cardiff CF42 5DP Tel: 01443 771238 — MB BCh Wales 1951 (Cardiff) Prev: Gen. Practitioner.

WILLIAMS, William 35 Abbey Gardens, London W6 8QR — MB BS Lond. 1993.

WILLIAMS, William David Cyril Dunns Lane Cottage, Evenjobb, Presteigne LD8 2SG — MB BS Lond. 1968; FFA RCS Eng. 1974. Specialty: Anaesth.

WILLIAMS, William Hugh (retired) Eelburn House, Westerdunes Park, Abbotsford Road, North Berwick EH39 5HJ Tel: 01620 892035 Fax: 01620 892035 — MB ChB Ed. 1960; LRCP LRCS Ed. LRFPS Glas. 1960; DObst RCOG 1963. Prev: Med. Off. Fairmile Marie Curie Centre.

WILLIAMS, Mr William Wood Broomfield Hospital, Court Road, Chelmsford CM1 7ET Tel: 01245 514824 Email: william.williams@meht.nhs.uk; 132 Broomfield Road, Chelmsford CM1 1RN — MB BS Lond. 1982 (St Marys Lond.) BSc Lond. 1979; FRCS Eng. 1986; FRCS ((Orth.)) 1993. Cons. Orthop. Surg. Broomfield Hosp. Chelmsford. Specialty: Trauma & Orthop. Surg. Socs: BMA; RSM; BOA.

WILLIAMS, Wyn Rowland Highways, Cayley Promenade, Rhos on Sea, Colwyn Bay LL28 4DU Tel: 01492 548268 Fax: 01745 534693 Email: wyn_r_williams@lineone.net — (Middlx.) MB BS Lond. 1967; MRCS Eng. LRCP Lond. 1967; MRCP (UK) 1972; FRCP Lond. 1990. Cons. Rheum. Glan Clwyd Hosp. NHS Trust. Specialty: Rheumatol. Socs: Brit. Soc. Rheum.& BMA. Prev: SHO, Regist. & Sen. Regist. Rheum. Dept. Middlx. Hosp. Lond.

WILLIAMS, Yvonne Failsworth Health Centre, Ashton Road W., Failsworth, Manchester M35 0HN Tel: 0161 682 6297 Fax: 0161 683 5861; 61 Redfearn Wood, Rochdale OL12 7GA — MB BCh Wales 1987 (Univ. Wales Coll. Med.) DRCOG 1990; MRCGP 1991; Cert. Prescribed Equiv. Exp. JCPTGP 1991; Cert. Family Plann. JCC 1991. Clin. Asst. (Gen. Med.) Bury Gen. Hosp. Prev: Trainee GP Wrexham VTS; Resid. Med. Off. (Cas.) Katoomba NSW, Austral.; SHO (Cas.) Bury Gen. Hosp.

WILLIAMS, Yvonne Frances Saunders Grove Court, Upstreet, Canterbury CT3 4DD — MB BS Lond. 1970 (Guy's) MB BS (Hons.) Lond. 1970; MRCS Eng. LRCP Lond. 1970; MRCP (UK) 1973; FRCPath 1989, M 1977; FRCP Lond. 1992. Cons. Haemat. Canterbury & Thanet Health Dist. Specialty: Haematology.

WILLIAMSON, Alastair David Bamford Dept of Anaesthesia, Good Hope Hospital NHS Trust, Rectory Rd, Sutton B75 7RR Tel: 0121 378 2211 Email: alastair.williamson@goodhope.nhs.uk — MB ChB Birm. 1990; MA Camb. 1990, BA (Hons.) 1987; DA (UK) 1993; FRCA 1996. Cons. Anaesth., Good Hope Hosp. NHS Trust; Nat. Clin. Anaesthetic Lead to Theatre and pre-Operative Assessm. Project of NHS modernisation Agency. Specialty: Anaesth.

WILLIAMSON, Andrea Elizabeth 23 Lochgreen Place, Kilmarnock KA1 4UY — MB ChB Glas. 1995.

WILLIAMSON, Andrew David 38 Crewe Road, Alsager, Stoke-on-Trent ST7 2ET Tel: 01270 882004 — MB ChB Manch. 1988; BSc (Experim. Immunol. & Oncol.) Manch. 1985; DRCOG 1991; MRCGP 1992. Prev: Trainee GP Stockport; SHO Stepping Hill Hosp. Stockport.

WILLIAMSON, Andrew Rowan (retired) 8 Sutton Road, Howden, Goole DN14 7DJ Tel: 01430 430834 — MB ChB Ed. 1951; DObst RCOG 1955; DCH Eng. 1957. Prev: Clin. Asst. (Psychogeriat.) Goole & Dist. Hosp.

WILLIAMSON, Ann Helena Mary Pennine Medical Centre, 193 Manchester Road, Mossley, Ashton-under-Lyne OL5 9AJ Tel: 01457 832590 Fax: 01457 836083 Email: ann@annwilliamson.co.uk; Hollybank House, Lees Road, Mossley, Ashton-under-Lyne OL5 0PL Tel: 0145 783 2604 Fax: 0145 783 9363 Email: ann.williamson@zen.co.uk — MB ChB Bristol 1972. GP Partner. Specialty: Gen. Pract. Socs: Chair of Accred. Mem. Brit. Soc. of Med. & Dent. Hypn.; Mem. Brit. Soc. Of Experim. & Clin. Hypn. Prev: Ho. Off. (Surg. & Med.) Oldham Roy. Infirm.; Ho. Off. (O & G) Oldham & Dist. Gen. Hosp.

WILLIAMSON, Mr Arthur William Rowe (retired) Cobden, Clarence Road, Tunbridge Wells TN1 1HE Tel: 01892 530509 — MB BS Lond. 1948 (Guy's) MB BS (Hnrs.) Lond. 1948; FRCS Eng. 1953. Hon. Surg. Tunbridge Wells Health Dist. Prev: Sen. Regist. Gen. Surg. & Urol. Guy's Hosp. Lond.

WILLIAMSON, Barbara Helen The Old Manor Barn, 2 Leatherbarrows Lane, Maghull, Liverpool L31 1AD — MB ChB Liverp. 1971. Staff Grace Doctor (Community Child Health) Roy. Liverp. Childr. Hosp.& Community Trust. Specialty: Community Child Health. Prev: Clin. Med. Off. S. Sefton HA.

WILLIAMSON, Mr Barry William Alexander Royal Alexandra Hospital, Department of General Surgery, Corsebar Road, Paisley PA2 9PN Tel: 0141 887 9111 — MB ChB Ed. 1972; BSc (Hons.) Ed. 1970; FRCS Ed. 1978; MD Ed. 1980. Cons. Surg. Roy. Alexandra Hosp. Paisley. Specialty: Gen. Surg.

WILLIAMSON, Mr Bruce Christopher MacGregor (retired) Penarth, Nottingham Road, Melton Mowbray LE13 0NT Tel: 01664 565127 Email: bcmcgw@eurobell.co.uk — (Middlx.) MB BS Lond. 1959; FRCS Eng. 1965. Prev: Surg. Asst. Melton & Dist. Memor. Hosp.

WILLIAMSON, Catherine Hammersmith Hospital, Institute of Reproductive & Developmental Biology, Imperial College London, Du Cane Road, London W12 0NN — MB ChB Manch. 1990; MRCP (UK) 1993; MD (Manch.) 2005. Sen. Lect. (Obstetric Medicine) Hammersmith Hosp. Lond.; Wellcome Advanced Clinic Fell. (Ostetric Med./Endocrinol.) Hammersmith Hosp., Lond. Specialty: Endocrinol.; Obst. & Gyn. Prev: Specialist Regist. (Endocrinol./Diabetes) Centr. Middlx. Hosp., Lond.; Lect. Endocrinol., St. Mary's Hosp., Lond.

WILLIAMSON, Catherine 12 Cranberry Rise, Loveclough, Rossendale BB4 8FB Tel: 01706 231677 — MB ChB Liverp. 1989. Staff Grade Phys. (Adult Med.) Roy. Oldham Hosp. Specialty: Gen. Med. Prev: Regist. (Elderly Care) Burnley Gen. Hosp. & Hope Hosp. Salford; SHO (Med. & Elderly Care) Tameside Hosp.

WILLIAMSON, Charles James Francis Lloyd (retired) The Moorings, 14 Russells Crescent, Horley RH6 7DN Tel: 01293 785371 Fax: 01293 785371 — MB BChir Camb. 1960 (Camb. & St. Bart.) MA Camb. 1960; MRCS Eng. LRCP Lond. 1961; DObst RCOG 1961; DA Eng. 1961. GP Adviser Surrey Oaklands NHS Trust. Prev: SHO (Anaesth.) Roy. Sussex Co. Hosp. Brighton.

WILLIAMSON, Colin MacGregor Felpham and Middleton Health Centre, 109 Flansham Park, Felpham, Bognor Regis PO22 6DH Tel: 01243 582384 Fax: 01243 584933 — MB BChir Camb. 1963 (Westm.) BA, MB Camb. 1963, BChir 1962. Prev: Ho. Phys. (Med. & Paediat.) & Jun. Cas. Off. Westm. Hosp.

WILLIAMSON, David Alexander James (retired) Rose Cottage, Woodside Lane, Lymington SO41 8FL Tel: 0159 673937 Email: davidwilliamson@onetel.net.uk — MD L Lond. 1946 (St. Barts.) MD Lond. 1946, MB BS 1940; DCH Eng. 1947; FRCP Lond. 1968; FRCPCH (Hon.) 1997. Prev: Chief Asst. Med. Unit St. Bart. Hosp.

WILLIAMSON, David James The Surgery, 1 Crawley Lane, Pound Hill, Crawley RH10 7DX Tel: 01293 549916 Fax: 01293 615382; 11 Selbourne Close, Pound Hill, Crawley RH10 3SA — MB ChB Bristol 1982; MRCGP 1986; DRCOG 1986. GP Crawley; Clin. Asst. (Diabetes) Brighton HA. Prev: SHO Som. VTS; SHO (Accid & Emerg.) Southmead HA; Ho. Phys. Southmead HA.

WILLIAMSON, Mr David Martin Department of Orthopaedics, Great Western Hospital, Marlborough Road, Swindon SN3 6BB Tel: 01793 604890; 17 Coxwell Road, Faringdon SN7 7EB Tel: 01367 240033 — BM BCh Oxf. 1980; MA Oxf. 1981; FRCS Eng. 1984. Cons. Orthop. Gt. West. Hosp. Swindon. Specialty: Orthop. Prev: Sen. Regist, (Orthop.) Nuffield Orthop. Centre & John Radcliffe Hosp. Oxf.; Regist. (Orthop.) Nuffield Orthop. Centre Oxf.; SHO (Surg.) Roy. United Hosp. Bath.

WILLIAMSON, David Philip Harvey Grosvenor Medical Centre, Grosvenor Street, Crewe CW1 3HB Tel: 01270 256348 Fax: 01270 250786; 496 Crewe Road, Wistaston, Crewe CW2 6PZ — MB ChB Manch. 1976.

WILLIAMSON, David Watson Clifton Surgery, 151 Newport Road, Cardiff CF24 1AG Tel: 029 2049 4539 — MB ChB Ed. 1954; DObst RCOG 1956; FRCGP 1981. Prev: Resid. Obst. Off. Cheltenham Matern. Hosp.; Ho. Phys. Chalmers Hosp. Edin.; Ho. Surg. Cheltenham Gen., Eye & Childr. Hosp.

WILLIAMSON, Deborah Kristine Thornborough House, South Kilvington, Thirsk YO7 2NP — MB ChB Manch. 1998.

WILLIAMSON, Diane Jane — MB ChB Ed. 1990; MRCP (UK) 1994. Clin. Fell. in Dermat., Sunnybrook and Wom.s Coll. health Sci., Toronto, Ontario, Canada. Specialty: Dermat. Prev: Regist.

(Dermat.) Univ. Hosp. Wales, Cardiff; SHO (Med.) Countess of Chester Hosp.; Sen. Regist. (Dermat.) Univ. Hosp. Wales, Cardiff.

WILLIAMSON, Dominic Brown House, Station Road, Eynsham, Oxford OX8 1HX — BM Soton. 1990; MRCP 1993; DA 1994; FFAEM 2001. Specialty: Accid. & Emerg.

WILLIAMSON, Dorothy Eliza (retired) 67 Fenwick Road, Giffnock, Glasgow G46 6AX Tel: 0141 569 5017 — MB ChB Glas. 1952.

WILLIAMSON, Douglas John Eli Lilly and Co Ltd., Dextra Court, Chapel Hill, Basingstoke RG21 5SY Tel: 01256 315999 Email: d.williamson@lilly.com — MB ChB Ed. 1986; MRCPsych. 1990. Assoc. Med. Dir. Eli Lilly & Co Ltd. Specialty: Pharmaceutical Medicine. Prev: Clin Research Phys. Lilly Industries Ltd.; Research Psychiat. MRC & Hon. Sen. Regist. Oxf. RHA; Research Regist. Crichton Roy. Hosp.

WILLIAMSON, Douglas MacGregor (retired) 46 BornCt., New St., Ledbury HR8 2DX Tel: 01531 635445 — MB ChB Aberd. 1941.

WILLIAMSON, Elizabeth J South Queensferry Medical Practice, 41 The Loan, South Queensferry EH30 9HA Tel: 0131 331 1396 — MB ChB Ed. 1977; BSc Ed. 1974; DRCOG 1979; MRCGP 1981. GP Princip.

WILLIAMSON, Mrs Elspeth Mary (retired) Rose Cottage, Woodside Lane, Lymington SO41 8FL Tel: 01590 673937 — MB BS Lond. 1946 (King's Coll. Hosp.) DCH Eng. 1949. Prev: SCMO (Med. Genetics) Soton. Gen. Hosp.

WILLIAMSON, Ernest Robert Desmond (retired) 10/1 St Margaret's Place, Thirlstane Road, Edinburgh EH9 1AY Tel: 0131 446 9125 — MB BCh BAO Dub. 1949 (TC Dub.) BA Dub. 1947. Prev: Partner in GP in Braintree, Essex.

WILLIAMSON, Esther Jennifer Elizabeth 68 Westfield Road, Edgbaston, Birmingham B15 3QQ — MB BCh BAO Belf. 1975; DRCOG 1977; DCH RCP Lond. 1981.

WILLIAMSON, George Henry (retired) 28A Moorend Park Road, Cheltenham GL53 0JY Tel: 01242 255388 — (Belf.) MB BCh BAO Belf. 1947; DPH Belf. 1967. Prev: Med. Off. DHSS.

WILLIAMSON, Gillian Florence Royal Marternity Hospital, Grosvenor Road, Belfast BT12 6BB — MB BCh BAO Belf. 1982; MRCOG 1987. Assoc. Specialist Roy. Matern. Hosp. Belf. Specialty: Obst. & Gyn. Prev: Regist. Craigavon Area Hosp. & Lagan Valley Hosp.

WILLIAMSON, Grace 25 Ballygomartin Road, Belfast BT13 3LA Tel: 01232 718841 — MB BCh BAO Belf. 1994. Specialty: Gen. Med.

WILLIAMSON, Mr Ian George Aldermoor Health Centre, Aldermoor Close, Southampton SO16 5ST Tel: 023 8079 7700 Fax: 023 8079 7767 — MD Ed. 1992; MB ChB 1975; FRCS Ed. 1979; MRCGP 1986. Sen. Lect. (Primary Care) Univ. Soton.

WILLIAMSON, Ian James Royal Gwent Hospital, Gwent Healthcare NHS Trust, Newport NP20 2UB; 26 The Shires, Marshfield, Cardiff CF3 2AX — MB ChB Ed. 1986; BSc (Hons.) Ed. 1984; MRCP (UK) 1989; MD Ed. 1999; FRCP Ed. 1999; FRCP Lond. 2000. Cons. Gen. Med. (Respirat. Med.) Roy. Gwent Hosp. Newport. Specialty: Respirat. Med. Prev: Sen. Regist. (Respirat. Med.) S. Glam.; Career Regist. (Respirat. Med.) Gtr. Glas. HB; Regist. (Respirat. Med.) North. Gen. Hosp. Edin.

WILLIAMSON, Professor James, CBE 8 Chester Street, Edinburgh EH3 7RA — MB ChB Glas. 1943; FRCP Ed. 1959, M 1949; DSc (Hons.) Rochester NY, USA 1989. Emerit. Prof. Geriat. Med. Univ. Edin. Specialty: Care of the Elderly.

WILLIAMSON, James Frith The Brownhill Surgery, 2 Brownhill Road, Chandlers Ford, Eastleigh SO53 2ZB Tel: 023 8025 2414 Fax: 023 8036 6604; 3 Hawkers Paddock, Knapp Lane, Ampfield, Romsey SO51 9BT Tel: 01794 368084 — MB ChB Bristol 1975; FFA RCS Eng. 1982. GP Chandlers Ford; Hosp. Practitioner, Dept. Anaesth., Southampton Univ. Hosp. Trust. Specialty: Anaesth. Prev: Trainee GP Soton.; Regist. (Anaesth.) Guy's Hosp. & Lewisham Hosp. Lond.; SHO (Anaesth.) Poole Gen. Hosp. Dorset.

WILLIAMSON, James McIntyre (retired) 4 Castleton Crescent, Newton Mearns, Glasgow G77 5JX Tel: 0141 616 0204 — MB ChB Glas. 1953; FRFPS Glas. 1958; FRCP Ed. 1975, M 1962; FRCP Glas. 1971, M 1962.

WILLIAMSON, James Sinclair (retired) Linden Lea, Middle Road, Lytchett Matravers, Poole BH16 6HJ Tel: 01202 625278 — (Glas.) MB ChB Glas. 1964. Prev: Regist. (Clin. Med.) Stobhill Gen. Hosp. Glas.

WILLIAMSON, Jean 18 Grange Street, York YO10 4BH — MB BCh BAO Dub. 1955 (T.C. Dub.)

WILLIAMSON, Mr John Ross Hall Hospital, 221 Crookston Road, Glasgow G52 3NQ; Highfield, 4 Balfleurs St., Milngavie, Glasgow G62 8HW Tel: 0141 955 0321 — MB ChB 1959 (Edin.) DO Eng. 1961; FRCS Glas. 1965; MD Ed. 1970; FCOphth. 1989. Cons. Opth- Ross Hall Hosp.; Examr. Ophth. Fell. Glas. Specialty: Ophth. Socs: BMA; Scott. Optical Club. Prev: Ho. Off. Stirling Roy. Infirm.; SHO & Regist. Glas. Eye Infirm. Glas.; Cons. Ophth. Vict. & South. Gen. Hosps. Glas.

WILLIAMSON, John 90 Lane Crescent, Drongan, Ayr KA6 7AH — MB ChB Glas. 1984.

WILLIAMSON, John Bernard The MDU, 230 Blackfriars Road, London SE1 8PJ Tel: 020 7202 1500 Fax: 020 7902 5920 Email: williamsonj@the-mdu.com; 51 Astonville Street, Southfields, London SW18 5AW — MB BS Lond. 1975 (Guy's) MRCS Eng. LRCP Lond. 1975; MRCGP 1980; Dip Community Emerg. Med. Auckland 1998; MA (Med. Ethics & Law) Lond. 2003. Sen. Med. Caims Hndler & Medico-legal Adviser. Socs: Medico-Legal Soc. Prev: GP Auckland; GP Bury St. Edmunds; Clin. Asst. (Geriat.) W. Suff. Hosp.

WILLIAMSON, John Boyd, DSC Mainbrace, Druidstone Road, St Mellons, Cardiff CF3 6XD Tel: 029 207 7563 — MB ChB Ed. 1952; Apptd. Fact. Doctor; Med. Off. Min. of Labour Rehabil. & Resettlem; Unit, Cardiff.

WILLIAMSON, John Bradley Royal Manchester Children's Hospital,, Pendlesbury, Manchester M27 8HA Tel: 0161 727 2170 — MB ChB Manch. 1980; FRCS Eng. 1984. Cons. In Spinal Surgery RMCH & Hope Hosp. Salford; Sen. Lect., Paediatric Neurology, Leeds General Infirmary. Socs: Fell. Scoliosis Research Soc.(Sec. & Treasurer); Brit. Assoc. of Spinal Surgery. Prev: Sen. Lect. (Orthop. Surg.) Manch. Univ.; Fell. (Spinal Surg.) Univ. of Hong Kong.

WILLIAMSON, John Charles Murdishaw Health Centre, Gorsewood Road, Murdishaw, Runcorn WA7 6ES Tel: 01928 712061 Fax: 01928 791988 — MB ChB Leeds 1974.

WILLIAMSON, John David (retired) 9 Pembroke Crescent, Hove BN3 5DH Tel: 01273 776491 Fax: 01273207235 Email: jdw@pavilion.co.uk — (Sheff.) MB ChB Sheff. 1968; DObst RCOG 1970; MRCGP 1975; MFCM 1980; DSc Sheff. 1988; FFPHM RCP (UK) 1993. Hon. Fell. Univ. Brighton; Trustee Standing Conf. on Pub. Health. Prev: Princip. Research Fell. (Pub. Health & Epidemiol.) Univ. Brighton.

WILLIAMSON, John Michael Steele Department of Pathology, The Hillingdon Hospital, Uxbridge UB8 3NN Tel: 01895 279562 — MB ChB Bristol 1980; MRCPath 1986. Histopath. Hillingdon Hosp. NHS Trust. Specialty: Histopath. Prev: Sen. Regist. (Histopath.) Yorks. RHA; Lect. (Histopath.) Leeds Univ.

WILLIAMSON, John Richard Healdswood Surgery, Mansfield Road, Skegby, Sutton-in-Ashfield NG17 3EE Tel: 01623 513553 — MB ChB Sheff. 1986 (Sheffield) Cert. Family Plann. JCC 1989. GP. Specialty: Gen. Pract. Prev: GP Princip. Retford Notts; GP Trainee Alford Lincs.; SHO (Geriat.) St. Geo. Hosp. Lincoln.

WILLIAMSON, Mr John Robert William Glover Department of Obstetrics & Gynaecology, Rosie Unit, Addenbrooke's Hospital, Hills Road, Cambridge CB2 2QQ Tel: 01223 216221 Fax: 01223 586591 Email: john.will@ntlworld.com; 8 Chaucer Road, Cambridge CB2 2EB Tel: 01223 360380 Fax: 01223 510021 — MB BCh BAO Dub. 1963 (T.C. Dub.) MA Dub. 1967, BA 1963; FRCSI 1967; FRCOG 1983, M 1970; MAO Dub. 1971. Cons. Addenbrookes Hosp. Camb.; Assoc. Lect. Camb. Univ. Specialty: Obst. & Gyn. Special Interest: Urogynaecology. Socs: Brit. Fertil. Soc.; Internat. Continence Soc. Prev: Sen. Regist. John Radcliffe Hosp. Oxf.; Regist. Rotunda Hosp. Dub.; Ho. Off. Roy. City of Dub. Hosp.

WILLIAMSON, Julia Mary 84 Steepside, Radbrook Grove, Shrewsbury SY3 6DR — MB ChB Sheff. 1985.

WILLIAMSON, Julie Catherine 249 Hale Road, Hale, Altrincham WA15 8RE — MB ChB Glas. 1990.

WILLIAMSON, Karen Marie Department of Obstetrics & Gynaecology, Nottingham City Hospital, Hucknall Road, Nottingham NG5 1PB Tel: 0115 969 1169 Fax: 0115 962 7920 Email: kwillia2@ncht.org.uk — MB ChB Dundee 1983 (Dundee Univ.) FRCS Ed. 1988; MRCOG 1989; FRCOG 2002. Cons. Gynecological Oncdogist Nottm. City Hosp. Specialty: Gynaecology. Socs: Brit. Gyn. Cancer Soc.; Int. Gyn. Cancer Soc. Prev: Sub-Specialty Trainee (Gyn. Oncol.) Leicester Roy. Infirm.

WILLIAMSON, Katharine Frances 66 Cranmore Road, Chislehurst BR7 6ET — MB BCh Wales 1973; DO Eng. 1978. Assoc. Specialist (Ophth.) Moorfields Eye Hosp. Lond.; Clin. Asst. (Diabetic Ophth.) FarnBoro. Hosp. Specialty: Ophth. Socs: MRCOphth.; Coll. Ophth. 1989. Prev: Clin. Asst. (Ophth.) Bromley Hosp.; SHO (Ophth.) Eye, Ear & Throat Hosp. Shrewsbury & St. Woolos Hosp. Newport.

WILLIAMSON, Katherine Mary Queen Alexandra hospital, Southwick Hill Road, Cosham, Portsmouth PO6 3LY Tel: 02392 286279; Holmsleigh, 4 Leith Road, Havant PO9 2ET Tel: 02392 477212 Fax: 02392 475974 — MB BS Lond. 1987; DA (UK) 1990; FFA RCSI 1992. Cons. Anaesth., Portsmouth Hosp. NHS Trust. Specialty: Anaesth. Prev: Specialist Regist. (Anaesth.) Univ. Hosp. Wales. Cardiff; Asst Prof. Anaesth. Indiana Univ. Div. of Pediatric Anesthesia & Critical Care Indianapolis, USA; Fell. (Paediat. Anaesth.) Childr. Nat. Med. Center Washington DC, USA.

WILLIAMSON, Kathryn Department of Elderly Psychiatry, Risca Health Centre, Risca, Newport NP11 6YF Tel: 01633 618060 — MB BS Lond. 1984 (St Mary's Hospital Medical School London) DRCOG 1987; MRCPsych 1991. Cons. Psychiat. St. Cadoc's Hosp. Caerleon Newport. Specialty: Geriat. Psychiat. Prev: Sen. Regist. Rotat. (Psychiattry) S. Wales; Regist. Rotat. (Psychiat.) Bridgend; Trainee GP Bridgend VTS.

WILLIAMSON, Kelly Michelle 14 Blackthorn Crescent, Aberdeen AB16 5LU — MB ChB Aberd. 1993.

WILLIAMSON, Kenneth Noel Bamford Williamson and Partners, Jericho Health Centre, Walton Street, Oxford OX2 6NW Tel: 01865 429993 Fax: 01865 458410; 56 Parktown, Oxford OX2 6SJ Tel: 01865 310624 — BM BCh Oxf. 1969. Tutor Univ Oxf. Dept of Primary Care. Prev: SHO (Accid. Serv.) Radcliffe Infirm. Oxf.; Gen. Med. Off. Govt. Seychelles; SHO (Obst.) John Radcliffe Hosp. Oxf.

WILLIAMSON, Kenneth Samuel Little Friars, Morning Thorpe, Long Stratton, Norwich NR15 2QL Tel: 01508 530373 — MB ChB Manch. 1957; MSc Manch. 1960, MD 1970; FFOM RCP Lond. 1979. Specialty: Occupat. Health. Socs: Fell. Roy. Soc. Med.; Soc. Occupat. Med. Prev: Dir. Occupat. Health & Hyg. Servs. Ltd.; Dir. Med. Servs. ICI plc.

WILLIAMSON, Lorna McLeod 157 High Street, Harston, Cambridge CB2 5QD — MB ChB Ed. 1987; MRCP (UK) 1980.

WILLIAMSON, Lyn 17 Coxwell Road, Faringdon SN7 7EB Tel: 01367 240033 — BM BCh Oxf. 1980; MA Oxf. 1981; DRCOG 1982; DCH RCP Lond. 1983; MRCP (UK) 1983; MRCGP 1987. Cons. Rheum., The Gt. West. Hosp. Swindon. Specialty: Rheumatol. Prev: GP Eynsham Oxf.; Regist. (Med.) Roy. United Hosp. Bath; Sen. Register in Rheum., Nuffield Orthop. Centre Oxf.

WILLIAMSON, Mark Roy The Medical Centre, Hall Close, Marske-by-the-Sea, Redcar TS11 6BW Tel: 01642 482725; Beechwood, Victoria Terrace, Saltburn-by-the-Sea TS12 1HN Tel: 01287 622822 Fax: 01287 483334 — MB BS Lond. 1983; MRCGP 1989.

WILLIAMSON, Mhari Bell The Health Centre, Charles Street, Langholm DG13 0JY Tel: 01387 380355 Fax: 01387 381211; 19 Whitaside, Langholm DG13 0JS — MB ChB Ed. 1978; DRCOG 1991; MRCGP 1994. GP Princip.; Train. E. Cumbria VTS.

WILLIAMSON, Mr Michael Edward Ross Royal United Hospital Bath NHS Trust, Combe Park, Bath BA1 3NG — MB BCh Wales 1987; BSc (Hons.) Wales 1984; FRCS Eng. 1991; FRCS 1997; MD 2000. Consultant Colorectal Surgeon. Specialty: Gen. Surg. Prev: Hon. Regist. & Research Fell. Univ. Leeds.

WILLIAMSON, Norman (retired) 1 Queen Square, Lancaster LA1 1RP; 6 Church Court, Bolton-le-Sands, Carnforth LA5 8EB — MB BS Lond. 1960 (St Geo.) MRCS Eng. LRCP Lond. 1960; DObst RCOG 1962. Prev: Cons. Immunol. Lancs. Immunol. Serv. Preston.

WILLIAMSON, Mr Peter Anthony St. George Hospital, Blackshaw Road, London SW17 0QT Tel: 020 87252052 Fax: 020 87253306 Email: peterawilliamson@yahoo.com — MB BS Lond. 1988 (Middlesex Hospital) FRCS Ed. 1994; FRCS ORL - NHS 1998. Cons. Surg., OtoLaryngol., St Geo.s Hosp. Lond.; Cons. Surg. OtoLaryngol., ST Helier Hosp., Carshalton, St Anthonys Hosp., Cheam, Parkside Hosp. Wimbledon, Ashtead Hosp. Ashtead; Hon. Cons. Surgeon, Head and Neck Surg., Roy. Marsden Hosp. Specialty: Otorhinolaryngol. Socs: Brit. Assn. Of Otorhinolaryngology - Head & Neck Surg.; Brit. Assn. Of Head and Neck Oncologists. Prev: Specialist Regist. (ENT) S. and W. of Eng.; Fell. Head and Neck Surg., Roy. Marsdon Hosp. Lond.

WILLIAMSON, Peter David The Randolph Surgery, 235A Elgin Avenue, London W9 1NH Tel: 020 7286 6880 Fax: 020 7286 9787; 26 Kelly Street, Kentish Town, London NW1 8PH Tel: 020 7267 3135 — MB BS Lond. 1980; MRCGP 1987.

WILLIAMSON, Richard Douglas Charles Wayside Surgery, 12 Russells Crescent, Horley RH6 7DN Tel: 01293 782057 Fax: 01293 821809 — MB ChB Leic. 1992. Specialty: Gen. Pract.

WILLIAMSON, Professor Robin Charles Noel Department of Surgery, Imperial College School of Medicine, Hammersmith Hospital, London W12 0NN Tel: 020 8383 3941 Email: r.williamson@ic.ac.uk/robin.williamson@rsm.ac.uk; The Barn, 88 Lower Road, Gerrards Cross SL9 8LB Tel: 01753 889816 — MB BChir Camb. 1968 (Camb. & St. Bart.) FRCS Eng. 1972; MA Camb. 1968, BA (1st cl. Hons.) 1964, MD 1983, MChir 1978; Hon. FRCS Thailand 1992; Hon. PhD Mahidol Univ. 1994. Cons. Surg. Hammersmith Hosp. Lond.; Assoc. Dean Roy. Soc. of Med.; Prof. Surg. Imp. Coll. Sch. Med; Examr. in Primary FRCS Exam 1981-1988 & Intercollegiate FRCS Exam 1994-; Mem. Advisery Comm. Mason Med. Research Foundat. 1999; Mem. Intercollegiate Bd. in Gen. Surg. 1998. Specialty: Gen. Surg. Socs: (Ex-Pres.) Pancreatic Soc.; (Ex-Pres.) Assn. Surgs. GB & Irel. (Chairm. Scientif. Comm.); (Pres) Europ. Soc. Surgs. Prev: Prof. Surg. Univ. Bristol & Hon. Cons. Surg. Avon HA & SW RHA; Sen. Regist. (Surg.) United Bristol Hosps. & SW RHB; Clin. & Research Fell. (Surg.) Mass. Gen. Hosp. & Harvard Med . Sch. Boston, USA.

WILLIAMSON, Rodney Medlock Vale Medical Practice, 58 Ashton Road, Droylsden, Manchester M43 7BW Tel: 0161 370 1610 Fax: 0161 301 4182 — MB ChB Manch. 1971. GP Manch.

WILLIAMSON, Roland Hugh Bamford, Lt.-Col. Job Hole, Kirbymoorside, York YO62 6AZ Tel: 01751 431520 Email: hugh.williamson@dsl.pipex.com — (Univ. Ed.) MRCGP 1990; MSc (Occupat. Health) Aberd. 1994; MFOM 1998. Occupat. Med. (Army). Specialty: Occupat. Health. Socs: Soc. of Occup. Med.; Roy. Soc. Med. Prev: RMO 1QO HLDRS./2SG; Ho. Off. (Gen. Med., Gen. Surg. & Orthop.) Bangour Gen. Hosp. W. Lothian; Occ Med Trainee (army).

WILLIAMSON, Ruth Hammersmith Hospital Imaging Department, Du Cane Road, London W12 0NN Tel: 020 8383 3389; 14 Brisbane Avenue, Wimbledon, London SW19 3AG Tel: 020 8540 3079 Email: ruth@williamson.demon.co.uk — MB BS Lond. 1989; BSc Lond. 1986, MB BS 1989; MRCP (UK) 1992; FRCR 1997. Specialty: Radiol.

WILLIAMSON, Sally Suzanne Hardwicke House Surgery, Hardwicke House, Stour Street, Sudbury CO10 2AY Tel: 01787 370011 Fax: 01787 376521; Churchside Cottage, Little Waldingfield, Sudbury CO10 0SW Tel: 01787 247934 — MB BS Lond. 1981 (St. Thos.) DRCOG 1984. Clin. Med. Off. Mid. Anglia Community Trust. Prev: SHO (O & G) St. Thos. Hosp. Lond.; Cas. Off. St. Peter's Hosp. Chertsey; Ho. Surg. St. Thos. Hosp. Lond.

WILLIAMSON, Sean Francis 9 Cringle Moor Chase, Great Broughton, Middlesbrough TS9 7HS — MB ChB Ed. 1988; DA (UK) 1990; FRCA 1994. Cons. NeuroAnaesth. S. Cleveland Hosp. Middlesbrough. Specialty: Anaesth.

WILLIAMSON, Sheila Anne Higgen (retired) 4 Castleton Crescent, Newton Mearns, Glasgow G77 5JX Tel: 0141 616 0204 — MB ChB Glas. 1956. Prev: Assoc. Specialist Ultrasonics Paisley Matern. Hosp.

WILLIAMSON, Shona Margaret Health Clinic, Mid Street, Bathgate EH48 1PT Tel: 01506 655155; 11 Riselaw Road, Edinburgh EH10 6HR Tel: 0131 447 5854 — MB ChB Ed. 1986; DRCOG 1989; MRCGP 1991.

WILLIAMSON, Sigrun Karin Albertville Surgery, 16 McCandless Street, Crumlin Road, Belfast BT13 1RU Tel: 028 9074 6308 Fax: 028 9074 9847; 13 Strathyre Park, Belfast BT10 0AZ Tel: 01232 601730 — MB BCh BAO Belf. 1973 (QUB)

WILLIAMSON, Sophia Louisa Harriet Queen Elizabeth Hospital, Gateshead NE9 6SX — BM Soton. 1989; MRCPath 1998. Cons. Histopath., Qu. Eliz. Hopital, Gateshead. Specialty: Histopath.

WILLIAMSON, Stuart William Harvey Hospital, Ashford TN24 0LZ Tel: 01233 633331 — MB ChB Sheff. 1967; DCH Eng. 1969; MRCP (UK) 1972; FRCP Lond. 1996; FRCPCH 1997. Cons. Paediat. E. Kent Hosp.NHS Trust. Specialty: Paediat. Prev: Sen. Regist. King's Coll. Hosp. Lond.; Jun. Regist. (Paediat.) St. Thos. Hosp. Lond.

WILLIAMSON, Thomas Arthur (retired) 44 Erridge Road, London SW19 3JB Tel: 020 8540 7935 — MB BS Lond. 1947 (Lond. Hosp.) MRCS Eng. LRCP Lond. 1947; MRCGP 1973. Prev: Div. Surg. St. John's Ambul. Assn.

WILLIAMSON, Mr Thomas Hardie Ophthalmology, St Thomas' Hospital, Lambeth Palace Road, London SE1 7EH Tel: 020 7928 9292 Fax: 020 7922 8157 — MB ChB Glas. 1984 (Univ. Glas.) FRCS Glas. 1988; FRCOphth 1988; MD Glas. 1995. Cons. (Ophth.) St Thomas Hosp. Lond.; Hon. Sen. Lect. KCL. Specialty: Ophth. Prev: SHO (Ophth.) Aberd. Roy. Infirm.; SHO (Ophth.) Addenbrooke's Hosp. Camb.; Sen. Regist. Tennent Inst. Glas.

WILLIAMSON, Timothy James 9 Calton Road, Bath BA2 4PP Tel: 01225 420905 — MB Camb. 1969 (St. Thos.) BChir 1968; DObst RCOG 1971; MSc (Audiological Med.) 1995. Cons. Community Paediat. (Audiology). Specialty: Community Child Health. Socs: Brit. Assn. Community Child Health; Brit. Assn. Community Drs in Audiol. Prev: SCMO Bath & W. Community NHS Trust; SHO (Geriat.) St. Martin's Hosp. Bath; GP Bath.

WILLIAMSON, Vincent Charles Department of Radiology, Arrowe Park Hospital, Upton, Wirral CH49 5PE Tel: 0151 678 5111 — MB ChB Wales 1983 (Cardiff) DMRD Aberd. 1987; FRCR 1989; BSc (HonsOpen) 2000. Cons. Diagn. Radiol. Wirral Hosps. Merseyside. Specialty: Radiol. Socs: Assn. Chest Radiol.; Brit. Med. Assn.; Roy. Coll. of Radiologists. Prev: Sen. Regist. (Diagn. Radiol.) Liverp.; Regist. (Diagn. Radiol.) Aberd. Roy. Infirm.; SHO (Gen. Med.) Bishop Auckland Gen. Hosp.

WILLIAMSON, Walter (retired) Castle Hill House, Middleham, Leyburn DL8 4QW Tel: 01969 623302 — MRCS Eng. LRCP Lond. 1959 (Trinity College Dublin) DObst RCOG 1963.

WILLIAMSON DUFFY, Lorraine Murray Flat 1/Left, 353 West Princes St., Woodlands, Glasgow G4 9EZ — MB ChB Glas. 1998.

WILLICOMBE, Peter Richard Havant Health Centre, Civic Centre Road, Havant PO9 2AQ Tel: 023 9248 2124 Fax: 023 9247 5515 — MB BChir Camb. 1974 (Camb. & Guy's) MA Camb. 1975; MRCP (UK) 1977; DRCOG 1982. Hosp. Pract. (Med.) St. Mary's Hosp. Portsmouth. Specialty: Respirat. Med. Prev: Regist. (Med.) St. Thos. Hosp. Lond.; SHO (Thoracic Med.) Brompton Hosp. Lond.; Ho. Off. (Med.) Guy's Hosp. Lond.

WILLIETS, Trevor Herbert (retired) 87 Kirklake Road, Formby L37 2DA — MB ChB Birm. 1958; MRCPath 1969. Prev: Regist. (Path.) Birm. Childr. Hosp. & Worcester Roy. Infirm.

WILLIMOTT, Edith Jane Young Peoples Department, Newberry Centre, West Lane Hospital, Middlesbrough TS5 4EE Tel: 01642 352113 — MB ChB Aberd. 1981; MRCPsych 1985. Cons. (Adolesc. Psychiat.) Newbury Centre, W. Lane Hosp., M'Boro. Specialty: Child & Adolesc. Psychiat. Prev: Regist. (Child & Adolesc. Psychiat.) Crichton Roy. Hosp. Dumfries.; Sen. Regist. (Child & Family Psychiat.) Fleming Nuffield Unit Newc.

WILLINGTON, Frederick Lane (retired) Innisfree, 40 Plymouth Road, Buckfastleigh TQ11 0DG Tel: 01364 642802 — (T.C. Dub.) MB BCh BAO (Hons.) Dub. 1939; MD Dub. 1960. Vis. Prof. (Geriat. Med.) Univ. West. Ontario, Canada; Recognised Clin. Teach. (Geriat. Med.) Welsh Nat. Sch. Med. Cardiff. Prev: Cons. Phys. (Geriat. Med.) Univ. Hosp. Wales, Cardiff & St. David's Hosp. Cardiff.

WILLIS, Allan Trevor (retired) 16 Biddenham Turn, Biddenham, Bedford MK40 4AT — MD Melbourne 1962; MB BS 1952; PhD Leeds 1956; FRCPath 1976, M 1963; MCPA 1963; FRACP 1974, M 1966; DSc 1971; FRCPA 1972. Prev: Dir. Pub. Health Laborat. Luton.

WILLIS, Andrew Charles The Diabetes Centre, Queen's Hospital, Belvedere Road, Burton-on-Trent DE13 0RB Tel: 01283 566333 Fax: 01283 593056 — MB BS Lond. 1987 (St. Thomas' Hospital Me. School) MRCP (UK) 1991; FRCP Lond. 2003. Cons. Phys. in Gen. Med., Diabetes & Endocrinol., Burton Hosps. NHS Trust. Specialty: Endocrinol.; Gen. Med.; Diabetes. Prev: Specialist Regist. (Diabetes & Endocrinol.) Walsgrave Hosp. Coventry; Specialist Regist. (Diabetes & Endocrinol.) Univ. Hosp., Birm.; Research Fell. (Diabetic Med.) Generla Hosp., Birm.

WILLIS, Andrew Peter David 8 Coombe Park, Sutton Coldfield B74 2QB — MB BS Lond. 1997.

WILLIS, Andrew William Dr A Willis and Partners, King Edward Road Surgery, Christchurch Medical Centre, Northampton NN1 5LY Tel: 01604 633466 Fax: 01604 603227; 19 Thorburn Road, Northampton NN3 3DA Tel: 01604 513187 Fax: 01604 513189 — MB BS Lond. 1970 (Middlx.) DObst RCOG 1972; DCH Eng. 1973; FRCGP 1995, M 1975; MSocSc (Health Serv. Managem.) Birm. 1991. Prev: Liaison GP N.ants. HA; GP Computer Facilitator N.ants. FHSA; Chairm. Nat. Assn. Commiss. GPs.

WILLIS, Anthony John Percival (retired) 49 Crowstone Road, Westcliff on Sea SS0 8BG Tel: 01702 45974 — MB BS Lond. 1954 (Lond. Hosp.) MRCP Lond. 1959. Prev: Cons. Phys. Southend Hosp. Gp.

WILLIS, Audrey Spencer (retired) 2 Grovelands, Lower Bourne, Farnham GU10 3RQ — (Univ. Coll. Hosp.) MRCS LRCP 1943; MB BChir Camb. 1945; FRCP Lond. 1980, M 1954; DCH Eng. 1962. Prev: Emerit. Cons. Phys. (Geriat. Med.) W. Surrey & NE Hants. HA.

WILLIS, Brian Alexander Anaesthetic Department, University Hospital of Wales, Heath Park, Cardiff CF14 4WZ Tel: 029 2074 3255; 14 Heol Isaf, Radyr, Cardiff CF15 8AL — MB BCh Wales 1981; PhD Wales 1968, BSc 1965, MB BCh 1981; FFA RCS Eng. 1985. Cons. Anaesth. Cardiff & Vale Trust; Clin. Dir. For Anaesth. Cardiff & Vale Trust, Cardiff. Specialty: Anaesth. Prev: Sen. Regist. (Anaesth.) Univ. Hosp. Wales Cardiff.

WILLIS, Bryony Margaret Royal Berkshire Hospital, London Road, Reading RG1 5AN; Heather House, 21 Wantage Road, Wallingford OX10 0LR — MB BS Newc. 1975; DRCOG 1978. p/t Assoc. Specialist (Fertil.) Roy. Berks NHS Trust; Clin. Asst. (Fertil.) Oxf. Radcliffe Hosps. NHS Trust. Specialty: Obst. & Gyn. Socs: British Fertility Society.

WILLIS, Charlotte Helen 1 Stafford Road, Brighton BN1 5PE — MB BS Lond. 1992.

WILLIS, Claire Elizabeth 9 St Ellens, Edenderry, Belfast BT8 8JN — MB BCh BAO Belf. 1991.

WILLIS, Claire Joanne 28 Wenden Road, Newbury RG14 7AE — MB BS Lond. 1996.

WILLIS, David Andrew Ware Road Surgery, 59 Ware Road, Hoddesdon EN11 9AB Tel: 01992 463363 Fax: 01992 471108 — MB BS Lond. 1979 (Char. Cross) BSc (Hons.) Lond. 1970, MB BS 1979; DRCOG 1982. Prev: Trainee GP Welwyn Garden City VTS; Ho. Phys. St. Albans City Hosp; Ho. Surg. Wembley Hosp.

WILLIS, David Michael Ferryhill Medical Practice, Durham Road, Ferryhill DL17 8JJ Tel: 01740 651238 Fax: 01740 656291 — MB BS Newc. 1987; DRCOG 1990; MRCGP 1991; DCH RCP Lond. 1991. Socs: BMA. Prev: Trainee GP Ulverston, Cumbria FPC.

WILLIS, Derek 41 Stutton Road, Tadcaster LS24 9HE — MB ChB Birm. 1993 (Birmingham) MB ChB (Hons.) Birm. 1993. Specialty: Palliat. Med.; Gen. Med. Socs: Roy. Coll. Phys. (Edin.).

WILLIS, Eunice Mary Weston Favell Health Centre, Weston Favell Centre, Northampton NN3 8DW Tel: 01604 409002 Fax: 01604 407034; 19 Thorburn Road, Weston Favell, Northampton NN3 3DA — MB BS Lond. 1970 (Middlx.) MB BS (Hons.) Lond. 1970. Clin. Asst. (Infertil.) N.ants. Gen. Hosp. Prev: SHO (Paediat.) Northampton Gen. Hosp.; Ho. Phys. (Gen. Med.) Salisbury Gen. Hosp.

WILLIS, Fenella Mai St George's Hospital, Blackshaw Rd, London SW17 0QT; 29 Alverstone Avenue, Wimbledon Park, London SW19 8BD — MB BS Lond. 1993 (Roy. Free Hosp.) BSc 1990; MRCP 1996; DipPCPath 2000. Specialist Regist. (Haemat.) St. Geo.'s Hosp., Tooting. Specialty: Haematology. Socs: Roy. Coll. Phys.; BMA; Brit. Soc. Haematol. Prev: Specialist Regist. (Haematol.) Mayday Hosp.; Specialist Regist. (Haematol.) St Helier's Hosp..; Specialist Regist. (Haemat.) Marsden Hosp.

WILLIS, Francis Peter (retired) Westow Lodge, Westow, York YO60 7LQ Tel: 01653 618204 Fax: 01653 618204 — (St. Mary's) MB BS Lond. 1950. Prev: Ho. Off. St. Mary's Hosp. & Roy. North. Hosp. Lond.

WILLIS, Francis Robert Renal Unit, Royal Hospital for Sick Children, Yorkhill, Glasgow G3 8SJ Tel: 0141 201 0000 Fax: 0141 201 0859 — MB BS West. Austral. 1987; DCCH RCP Ed. 1990; DCH RCP Glas. 1990; FRACP 1994. Sen. Regist. (Paediat. Nephrol.) Roy. Hosp. Sick Childr. Glas. Specialty: Paediat. Prev: Chief Regist. Princess Margt. Hosp. Childr. Perth, West. Austral.

WILLIS, Geoffrey Mark 12 Myrdle Court, Myrdle St., London E1 1HP — MB BS Lond. 1982.

WILLIS, Jacob (retired) The Studio, 46 Myrtlefield Park, Belfast BT9 6NF Tel: 028 667221 — MD Belf. 1960; MB BCh BAO 1956; FRCPath 1978, M 1966. Prev: Cons. Path. E. Health & Social Servs. Bd.

WILLIS, James Alexander Ratcliffe Alton Health Centre, Anstey Road, Alton GU34 2QX Tel: 01420 84676 Fax: 01420 542975; Greenacre, 28 Borovere Lane, Alton GU34 1PB Tel: 01420 83416 Fax: 01420 83416 Email: jarwillis@compuserve.com — MB BS Lond. 1967 (Middlx.) DObst RCOG 1969; DCH Eng. 1970; FRCGP 1996, M 1973. Specialty: Gen. Med. Prev: Ho. Phys. Middlx. Hosp.; Ho. Surg. Mt. Vernon Hosp. Northwood; Ho. Phys. (Paediat.) Whittington Hosp. Lond.

WILLIS, James Herbert Patrick c/o Lionel J. Lewis & Company, 117 Burnt Ash Road, London SE12 8RA — MB BS Lond. 1954; MRCS Eng. LRCP Lond. 1954; FRCP Ed. 1972, M 1960; FRCPsych 1975.

WILLIS, Janet 1 Dunluce Avenue, Belfast BT9 7HR — MB BCh BAO Belf. 1978; DCH Dub. 1984; MRCGP 1984.

WILLIS, Jennifer Mary Rae (retired) 5 Fenwick Close, Jesmond, Newcastle upon Tyne NE2 2LE — (Ed.) MB ChB Ed. 1957; DObst RCOG 1960; Cert FPA 1975. Prev: Clin. Med. Off. (Family Plann.) N. Tyneside AHA.

WILLIS, John Hodgson (retired) Wressle House, Brigg DN20 0BU — MB BS Lond. 1952 (St. Mary's) Prev: GP Brigg.

WILLIS, Kathryn Ann Marine Surgery, 29 Belle Vue Road, Southbourne, Bournemouth BH6 3DB Tel: 01202 486456 — BM Soton. 1985. Prev: Trainee GP Bournemouth; SHO (Paediat.) Soton HA; SHO (Psychiat.) Salisbury HA.

WILLIS, Keith James 16 Southsea Avenue, Goring-bySea, Worthing BN12 4BN — MB ChB Birm. 1968; MRCP (UK) 1972.

WILLIS, Kenneth Maddern 42 Great Bushey Drive, London N20 8QL Tel: 020 8445 2263 — MB ChB Liverp. 1939. Prev: Med. Off. Roy. Infirm. Liverp. & Clatterbridge EMS Hosp.; RAFVR.

WILLIS, Laura Kathryn 27 Crawford Gardens, Horsham RH13 5AZ — MB BS Lond. 1998.

WILLIS, Linda Gertrude Francis Eglwysbach Surgery, Berw Road, Pontypridd CF37 2AA Tel: 01443 406811 Fax: 01443 405457; 14 Heol Isaf, Radyr, Cardiff CF15 8AL Tel: 01222 844459 Fax: 01222 844459 — MB BCh Wales 1968 (Cardiff) Dip. Palliat. Med. Wales 1991. Hosp. Pract. (Anaesth.) E. Glam. Hosp. Pontypridd; Hosp. Pract. (Palliat. Med.) Y. Bwthyn Continuing Care Unit Pontypridd. Specialty: Anaesth.

WILLIS, Malcolm David Fergus, Maj. RAMC Retd. Long Stratton Health Centre, Flowerpot Lane, Long Stratton, Norwich NR15 2TS Tel: 01508 530781 Fax: 01508 533030; Tawny Lodge, The Green, Wacton, Norwich NR15 2UN Tel: 01508 532358 Fax: 01508 530848 Email: malcwillis@hotmail.com — MB BS Lond. 1979 (St. Mary's) MRCGP 1984. Specialty: Gen. Pract. Prev: SHO (ENT, Dermat., Ophth., Accid & Emerg. & O & G) Camb. Milit. Hosp.

WILLIS, Marcia Pearl Louise 27 Winterbourne Road, Thornton Heath, Croydon CR7 7QX — MB BS Lond. 1996 (Royal Free Hospital London) BSc Hons. (Neurosci.) 1993. Specialty: Gen. Psychiat. Prev: SHO (A & E Med.) Chase Farm Hosp. Enfield; Ho. Off. (Orthop. & Gen. Surg.) Roy. Free Hosp.; Ho. Off. (Gen. Med. & c/o the Elderly) QE II Hosp. Kings Lynn Norf.

WILLIS, Mark Howard George Child and Family Clinic, St Peters House, Bricket Road, St Albans AL1 3JW — MB BS Lond. 1993; BSc Lond. 1990, MB BS 1993.

WILLIS, Michael John 85 Castlecroft Road, Finchfield, Wolverhampton WV3 8BY — MB ChB Birm. 1985; ChB Birm. 1985.

WILLIS, Peter Sunnybank, Stourbridge Road, Penn, Wolverhampton WV4 5NF — MB ChB Birm. 1978; BSc (Hons.) Birm. 1973, MB ChB 1978.

WILLIS, Peter (retired) Burn Brae Surgery, Hencotes, Hexham NE46 2ED Tel: 01434 603627 Fax: 01434 606373; Wall Station, Wall, Hexham NE46 Tel: 01434 681045 — MB BS Newc. 1967; DObst RCOG 1969; DCH Eng. 1970.

WILLIS, Peter Frederick (retired) 9 Westleigh Road, Barton Seagrave, Kettering NN15 5AJ Tel: 01536 514 615 — MRCS Eng. LRCP Lond. 1950 (St. Bart.) DA Eng. 1957; FFA RCS Eng. 1963. Cons. Anaesth. Kettering & Northampton Area Dept. Prev: Anaesth. Regist. Roy. Nat. Throat, Nose & Ear Hosp. & Whittington.

WILLIS, Peter John Valiant (retired) 44 Hemingford Road, London N1 1DB Tel: 020 7609 2479 — MB BS Lond. 1967 (Middlx.) MRCS Eng. LRCP Lond. 1966; DObst RCOG 1969. Prev: GP Lond.

WILLIS, Mr Ralph Glen Woodfield, Whitchurch Road, Chester CH3 6AE Tel: 01244 335756 — MB ChB Leeds 1983 (Univ. Leeds) FRCS Ed. 1991; DA (UK) 1994; DRCOG 1995.

WILLIS, Richard John Salisbury Independent Medical Practice, 5 Wyndham Road, Salisbury SP1 3AA Tel: 01722 415444 Fax: 01722 415454; Felthams, Coombe Bissett, Salisbury SP5 4LE Tel: 01722 718512 — BM BCh Oxf. 1972 (Oxf. & St. Bart.) BA (Hons. Sch. Natural Sc.) 1969; MA Oxf. 1972. InDepend. Gen. Practitioner. Prev: Regist. (Med.) Prof. Unit St. Barts. Hosp. Lond.; GP Tutor Salisbury HA; Mem. Wessex RHA Med. Advisery Comm.

WILLIS, Mr Robert Geoffrey Department of Urology, Royal Cornwall Hospital, Treliske, Truro TR1 3LJ Tel: 01872 252719 Email: robert.willis@rcht.swest.nhs.uk — MB ChB Bristol 1975; FRCS Eng. 1980; MD Bristol 1989. Cons. Urol. Roy. Cornw. Hosp. Truro. Specialty: Urol. Socs: Full Mem. Assn. Urological Surg.s; Mem. Brit. Med. Assn. Prev: Cons. Urol. Cumbld. Infirm. Carlisle.; Sen. Regist. (Urol.) Yorks. RHA.; Regist. (Urol.) Freeman Hosp. Newc. upon Tyne.

WILLIS, Robert Geoffrey Bainbridge (retired) 57 Green Lane, Buxton SK17 9DL Tel: 01298 24133 — MB ChB Liverp. 1951; MRCS Eng. LRCP Lond. 1951; DObst RCOG 1956; DCH Eng. 1957; MRCGP 1971. Prev: SHO (Paediat.) Duchess of York Hosp. Babies Manch.

WILLIS, Stephen Arthur 25 Myers Road, Hillmorton, Rugby CV21 4BY — MB BChir Camb. 1993; MA Camb. 1993; DRCOG 1998.

WILLIS, Thomas James (retired) Mellingey, Constantine, Falmouth TR11 5QH — (Lond. Hosp.) MB BChir Camb. 1960; DA Eng. 1965; DObst RCOG 1965. Prev: Ho. Phys. & Ho. Surg. Lond. Hosp.

WILLIS, Tracey Anne Neurology Department, Birmingham Children's Hospital, Steel House Lane, Birmingham B4 6NH; 180 Hole Lane, Northfield, Birmingham B31 2DB — MB ChB Birm. 1994; ChB Birm. 1994; MRCPI 1998. Specialty: Paediat.

WILLIS-OWEN, Julia 8 Kashmir Close, New Haw, Addlestone KT15 3JD — MB BS Lond. 1993; DFFP 98; MRCGP 98; DRCOG 97. Locum GP Surrey.

WILLISON, Professor Hugh John Neurology Block, Ground Floor, University of Glasgow, Department of Neurology, Southern General Hospital, Glasgow G51 4TF Tel: 0141 201 1100 Fax: 0141 201 2993 Email: h.j.willison@clinmed.gla.ac.uk — MB BS Lond. 1980 (Middlesex Hosp.) MRCP (UK) 1983; PhD Lond. 1987; FRCP (UK) 1998; FRCP (Glas.) 1999. Prof. (Neurology) Univ. Glas. & South. Gen. Hosp. Glas. Specialty: Neurol. Special Interest: Peripheral Nerve Disorders. Prev: Wellcome Sen. Research Fell. (Clin. Sci.) Southern Gen. Hosp. Glas.; Fogarty Fell. Nat. Inst. of Health, USA; Clin. Lect. (Neurol.) Southern Gen. Hosp. Glas.

WILLISON, Jean Campbell (retired) 1/1 Fettes Rise, East Fettes Avenue, Edinburgh EH4 1QH — MB ChB Ed. 1941; DPH Glas. 1947; DCH Eng. 1948; MFCM 1972. Prev: Community Med. Specialist Lothian Health Bd.

WILLISON, Katherine Anna 23 The Rotyngs, Rottingdean, Brighton BN2 7DX — MB BS Lond. 1998.

WILLISON, Robert Gow (retired) 4 Nourse Close, Woodeaton, Oxford OX3 9TJ Tel: 01865 559109 Fax: 01865 559109 — BM BCh Oxf. 1951 (Oxford & Middlesex) FRCP Ed. 1971, M 1954; MA Oxf. 1951, DM 1968; MRCP Lond. 1978. Prev: Cons. Clin. Neurophysiol. Nat. Hosp. Nerv. Dis. Qu. Sq. Lond.

WILLITS, David Glen Staithe Surgery, Lower Staithe Road, Stalham, Norwich NR12 9BU Tel: 01692 582000 Fax: 01692 580428; Pond Farm, Staithe Road, Sutton, Norwich NR12 9QU Tel: 01692 580616 — MB BS Lond. 1960 (Lond. Hosp.) FRCGP 1990, M 1981.

WILLMAN, Alan (retired) Middle Filham, Ivybridge PL21 0LR Tel: 01752 690011 — MB BS Durh. 1956; DObst RCOG 1962. Prev: GP Ivybridge.

WILLMAN, Antony Sean, Maj. RAMC Garrison Medical Centre, Salamanca Barracks BFPO 53 Tel: 00 357 263255 — MB BS Lond. 1990. GP Regist. BFPO 53. Specialty: Accid. & Emerg.

WILLMER, Barbara Jane (retired) 60 Pine Avenue, West Wickham BR4 0LW Tel: 020 8777 3544 — (St. Mary's) MRCS Eng. LRCP Lond. 1958; MB BS Lond. 1959; DObst RCOG 1960. Prev: GP Croydon.

WILLMER, Jennifer Mary Barton Surgery, Lymington House, Barton Hill Way, Torquay TQ2 8JG Tel: 01803 323761 Fax: 01803

316920 — BM BCh Oxf. 1984 (Oxford University Medical School) DCH RCP Lond. 1986; DRCOG 1986; MRCGP 1988.

WILLMER, Katherine Anne West Cumberland Hospital, Whitehaven CA28 8TG Tel: 01946 523016 Fax: 01946 523 504 Email: kate.willimer@ncumbria_acute.nhs.uk — MB BS Lond. 1990 (St Mary's Hosp. Med. Sch.) MRCP (UK) 1993; CCST (Cardiology & General (Internal) Medicine) 2000. Cons. Cardiol. & Gen. Phys. N. Cumbria Acute Hosps. NHS Trust Whitehaven; Hon. Cons. Cardiol. James Cook Univ. Hosps. Middlesbrough. Specialty: Cardiol.; Gen. Med. Special Interest: Cardiac Rehabil. Socs: Brit.Soc.Echocardio.; Brit. Assn. Cardiac Rehabil. Prev: Cardiol. Regist. Dudley Gp. of Hosps. 1999 - 2000; Cardiol. Regist. City Gen. Hosp. Stoke on Trent 1996 - 1999.

WILLMOT, Mark Robert 69 Victoria Road, Harborne, Birmingham B17 0AQ — MB ChB Birm. 1996.

WILLMOTT, Anne Margaret 86 Lorne Road, Leicester LE2 1YG Tel: 0116 270 0983 — MB ChB Leic. 1991; MRCP (UK) 1995. Regist. (Paediat.) P'boro. Dist. Hosp.

WILLMOTT, Frederick Edwin Department of Genitourinary Medicine, Royal South Hants Hospital, Southampton SO14 0YG Tel: 023 8082 5438 — MB BS Lond. 1964 (Guy's) MCRS Eng. LRCP Lond. 1964; Dip Ven Liverp. 1970; MRCP (Hon.) 2000. Cons. Genitourin. Med. Roy. S. Hants. Hosp. Soton. Specialty: Genitourinary Medicine. Prev: Cons. Venereol. Leicester Roy. Infirm.; Cons. Venereol. Auckland Hosp. New Zealand.

WILLMOTT, Nicholas John Castle Mead Medical Centre, Hill Street, Hinckley LE10 1DS Tel: 01455 637659 Fax: 01455 238754 — BM BS Nottm. 1975; BMedSci (Hons.) Nottm. 1974, BM BS 1975; DRCOG 1978; MRCGP 1981. Prev: Trainee Gen. Pract. Nottm. Vocational Train. Scheme; Brit. Red Cross Thailand 1979/1980.

WILLMOTT, Philip Andrew Penton House, Queen Anne St., Shelton, Stoke-on-Trent ST4 2EQ Tel: 01782 848642 Fax: 01782 747617; 10 Sutherland Drive, Newcastle ST5 3NB Tel: 01782 614879 — MB BS Lond. 1963 (King's Coll. Hosp.) MRCS Eng. LRCP Lond. 1963; DObst RCOG 1965. Prev: Ho. Phys. King's Coll. Hosp.; Ho. Surg. Crewe & Dist. Memor. Hosp; Rural Leprosy Control Off. Princess Zenebe Work Hosp., Addis Ababa.

WILLMOTT, Sara Louise Lawrence Hill Health Centre, Hassell Drive, Bristol BS2 0AN Tel: 0117 955 5241 Fax: 0117 941 1162 — MB BCh BAO Dub. 1966; DA (UK) 1969.

WILLOCKS, Clare Margaret Glasgow Royal Maternity Hospital, 146-163 Rottenrow, Glasgow G4 0NA Tel: 0141 211 5400 Fax: 0141 211 5399 — MB ChB Glas. 1992; BSc (Hons.) Glas. 1989. Specialist Regist. (O & G) W. of Scotl. Train. Scheme. Specialty: Obst. & Gyn. Prev: SHO Glas. Roy. Infirm.

WILLOCKS, Lorna Jane CDSC (Eastern), Institute of Public Health, University Forvie Site, Robinson Way, Cambridge CB2 2SR Tel: 01223 762037 Fax: 01223 331865 — MB ChB Glas. 1983; MRCP (UK) 1986; MFPHM RCP (UK) 1995; MD Glas. 1995; FRCP 1998. Cons. Epidemiolog. (Communicable Dis.) CDSC (E.ern) Camb. Specialty: Infec. Dis.; Epidemiol. Socs: Brit. Infec. Soc.; Pub. Health Med. Environm. Gp.; Assn. Pub. Health. Prev: Sen. Regist. (Communicable Dis. & Epidemiol.) Oxf.; Research Regist. Med. Research Counc. City Hosp. Edin.; Regist. (Infect. Dis.) City Hosp. Edin. & Ruchill Hosp. Glas.

WILLOCKS, Timothy — MB BS Lond. 1984.

WILLOTT, Joanna Clare 32 Homefield Road, Exeter EX1 2QU — MB ChB Bristol 1998.

WILLOUGHBY, Bruce Jamieson Biermont, Bingley Road, Menston, Ilkley LS29 6BD — MB BS Newc. 1993.

WILLOUGHBY, Cathryn Maria Northumberland Child Health Centre, John Street, Ashington NE63 0JE Tel: 01670 395706 — MB BCh Wales 1993.

WILLOUGHBY, Charles Peter 42 West Park Crescent, Billericay CM12 9EG Tel: 01277 656302 — BM BCh Oxf. 1972; BA (Physiol.) (1st cl. Hons.) 1969; MA 1972; MRCP (UK) 1975; DM Oxf. 1980; FRCP Lond. 1992. Cons. Phys. & Gastroenterol. Basildon & Thurrock Gen. Hosps. Trust. Specialty: Gastroenterol. Socs: Brit. Soc. Gastroenterol. Prev: Hon. Sen. Regist. (Gastroenterol.) Nuffield Dept. Clin. Med. John Radcliffe Hosp. Oxf.; Jun. Research Fell. Linacre Coll. Oxf.

WILLOUGHBY, Colin Eric 19 Shona Green, Ballymena BT42 4AT — MB ChB Liverp. 1991 (Liverpool) BSc (1st cl. Hons. Anat.) Liverp. 1988; MB ChB (Hons.) Liverp. 1991; FRCOphth 1996. Specialist Regist. (Ophth.) Mersey Region. Specialty: Ophth.

WILLOUGHBY, John Michael Tait, RD (retired) — (St. Thos.) DM Oxf. 1974, MA, BM BCh 1962; MRCS Eng. LRCP Lond. 1962; FRCP Lond. 1979, M 1966. Prev: Chief Med. Off. Nat. Mutual Life Assur. Soc.

WILLOUGHBY, Roger Alastair Guy d'Eresby The Surgery, Mortimer, Reading RG7 3SQ Tel: 01734 332436 — MB BS Lond. 1960 (St. Bart.) DA Eng. 1963. Prev: SHO (Anaesth.) Bromley Hosp.; Ships Surg. P & O Orient Line. & Union Castle SS Co.

WILLOUGHBY, Sara Jane Bandele Haematology Dept, Hereford County Hospital, Union walk, Hereford HR1 2ER Tel: 01432 355444 Ext: 4435 — MB BS Lond. 1988 (Roy. Free Hosp. Sch. of Med.) MRCP 1992; MRCPath 1997. Specialty: Haematology.

WILLOUGHBY, Sarah Jane 7 Haughton Road, Woodseats, Sheffield S8 8QH — BM BCh Oxf. 1994 (OXF.) MA Oxf. 1996, BA 1991. GP Regist. Sheff. VTS. Specialty: Obst. & Gyn. Prev: SHO (O & G) Jessop Hosp. Sheff.; Ho. Off. (Med.) City Gen. Hosp. Stoke-on-Trent; Ho. Off. (Surg.) John Radcliffe Hosp. Oxf.

WILLOWS, Helen Plas Ffynnon Medical Centre, Middleton Road, Oswestry SY11 2RB Tel: 0151 526 1121 Fax: 0151 527 2631; 16 Hallmoor Close, Aughton, Ormskirk L39 4UQ Tel: 01695 571617 — BM Soton. 1987; BSc (Biochem.) Hull 1979; DRCOG 1990; Cert. Family Plann. JCC 1990; MRCGP (Distinc) 1992. Prev: Trainee GP Havant Health Centre.

WILLOWS, Mary Anona 17 Lower Road, Milton Malsor, Northampton NN7 3AW — MB BS Lond. 1974. Staff Phys. (Palliat. Med.) Northampton. Specialty: Palliat. Med.

WILLOWS, Richard Ian Reid Delapre Medical Centre, Gloucester Avenue, Northampton NN4 8QF Tel: 01604 761713 Fax: 01604 708589; 17 Lower Road, Milton Malsor, Northampton NN7 3AW Tel: 01604 858653 Email: rickwill@nccnet.co.uk — MB Camb. 1975; BChir 1974; DRCOG 1978; MRCGP 1978; FRCGP 1998. Course Organiser Northampton VTS.

WILLOX, David George Addison Croftfoot Road Surgery, 44 Croftfoot Road, Glasgow G44 5JT Tel: 0141 634 6333; 14 Bradda Avenue, Burnside, Glasgow G73 5DE Tel: 0141 634 4566 — MB ChB Glas. 1981; DRCOG 1984; MRCGP 1985. Exam. Phys. BUPA Med. Centre Glas. Socs: S.. Med. Soc. Glas.

WILLOX, Joanne Christine 74 Weymouth Drive, Glasgow G12 0LY — MD Glas. 1984; MB ChB 1978. Prev: Clin. Asst. Cytopath., Vale of Leven Hosp., Alexandria.

WILLOX, Margaret Fairlie Carraig House, Snape, Bedale DL8 2TF — MB ChB Glas. 1982; DCH RCP Lond. 1986; DRCOG 1986; MRCGP 1987.

WILLS, Adrian Jonathan 13A Kingsdown Road, Upper Holloway, London N19 4LT — MB BS Lond. 1986; MRCP (UK) 1990; MD Lond. 1995. Specialty: Neurol.

WILLS, Alan Robert — BM BCh Oxf. 1973; BA Oxf. 1970, BM BCh 1973; MRCPath. 1980. Cons. Microbiol. Macclesfield Dist. Gen. Hosp. Specialty: Med. Microbiol.

WILLS, Andrew Donald 24 Hazel Street, Leicester LE2 7JN — MB ChB Leic. 1998; MB ChB Leic 1998.

WILLS, Bridget Ann The Copse, 22 Welcomes Road, Kenley CR8 5HD — BM BS Nottm. 1982; MRCP (UK) 1985. Regist. (Med.) St. Geo. Hosp. Lond.

WILLS, Carole Irene The Surgery, 1 Uxendon Crescent, Wembley HA9 9TW Tel: 020 8904 3883 Fax: 020 8904 3899 — MB ChB Manch. 1969; BSc Manch. 1966, MB ChB 1969.

WILLS, Catherine Jane Queens Medical Centre, Nottingham NG7 2UH Tel: 0115 924 9924; 37 Moore Road, Mapperley, Nottingham NG3 6EF Tel: 0115 969 1176 — MB BS Lond. 1991 (Char. Cross Hosp. & West. Med. Sch.) BA Oxf. 1988; MRCP (UK) 1994. Specialty: Diabetes.

WILLS, Desiree Pamela (retired) 33 Comely Bank, Edinburgh EH4 1AJ Tel: 0131 343 2533 — MB ChB Glas. 1964 (Univ. Glas.) DPM Eng. 1972; MRCPsych 1973. Nat. Mem. Criminal Injuries Compensation Appeal Panel. Prev: Cons. Child & Adolesc. Psychiat. W. Lothian Health Dist. & Roy. Hosp. Sick Childr. Edin.

WILLS, Diana Rosemary Child & Family Guidance Centre, Tanner St., Winchester SO23 8AD — MB ChB Liverp. 1979; DCH RCP Lond. 1982.

WILLS, Dilys (retired) 131 Carisbrooke Way, Cyncoed, Cardiff CF23 9HU — (Cardiff) MB BCh Wales 1954; DCH Eng. 1962,

DMRD 1968; FRCR 1970; FFR RCSI 1971. Prev: Cons. Radiol. Bridgend Gen. Hosp.

WILLS, Emily The Surgery, 42 The Street, Uley, Dursley GL11 5SY Tel: 01453 860459; 18 High Furlong, Cam, Dursley GL11 5UZ Tel: 01453 544171 — MB ChB Bristol 1982; DCH RCP Lond. 1985; MRCGP 1986. Asst. (Gen. Pract.). Socs: BMA. Prev: Trainee GP N. Devon VTS; Dist. Health Off. Rumphi, Malawi.

WILLS, Frances Anne Connaught House, Winchester & Eastleigh Healthcare NHS Trust, Ronsell Road, Winchester SO22 5DE Tel: 01962 824262 — MB BS Lond. 1981; MRCPsych 1989. Cons. Psych. Winchester & E.leigh NHS Trust. Specialty: Gen. Psychiat.

WILLS, George Thomas The Old Court House, 4 Throwley Way, Sutton SM1 4AF Tel: 020 8643 8866; 36 The Avenue, Tadworth KT20 5AT Tel: 01737 3321 — MB BS Lond. 1959 (St. Bart.) DObst RCOG 1961.

WILLS, Hugh Graham 85 Wigton Road, Carlisle CA2 7EP — MB BS Newc. 1967. Prev: Ho. Phys. Vict. Hosp. Blackpool; Ho. Surg. Roy. S. Hants. Hosp. Soton.

WILLS, Janet Frances 9 Leman Drive, Houston, Johnstone PA6 7LN — MB ChB Glas. 1979; MRCGP 1983.

WILLS, John (retired) 50 Green Street, Hazlemere, High Wycombe HP15 7RA Tel: 01494 524181 — (Guy's) MB BS Lond. 1940; MRCS Eng. LRCP Lond. 1940; DObst RCOG 1946. JP. Prev: GP High Wycombe.

WILLS, Jonathan Stewart 37 Moore Road, Mapperley, Nottingham NG3 6EF Email: jswills@lineone.net — BM BCh Oxf. 1991 (Oxford) BA (Hons.) Oxf. 1988; FRCA 1997. Regist. (Anaesth.) Qu. Med. Centre Nottm. Specialty: Anaesth. Socs: Assn. Anaesth. Prev: Regist. (Anaesth.) Exeter; SHO (Anaesth.) Bristol; ITU SHO Nottm.

WILLS, Judith Claire 1 Hartley Avenue, Whitley Bay NE26 3 NS; 37 Keyes Gardens, Jesmond, Newcastle upon Tyne NE2 3RA — MB ChB Leeds 1993; DRCOG 1996; MRCGP 1997.

WILLS, Mr Leslie Charles (retired) Compton Randle, Compton Dundon, Somerton TA11 6PR Tel: 01458 445927 — MB ChB Aberd. 1966; FRCS Ed. 1972. Cons. ENT Surg. Aberd. Roy. Infirm.; Sen. Lect. ENT Aberd. Univ. Prev: Sen. Regist. ENT Dept. Aberd. Roy. Infirm.

WILLS, Mr Michael Ian University Hospitals Coventry & Warwickshire NHS Trust, Walsgrave Hospital, Clifford Brinde Road, Coventry CV2 2DX Tel: 024 7653 8946; Darracott, School Street, Churchover, Rugby CV23 0EG — MB ChB Bristol 1977; FRCS Eng. 1982. Cons. Urol. Walsgrave Hosp. Coventry. Specialty: Urol. Socs: Brit. Assn. Urol.; Bristol. Urol. Inst.

WILLS, Patricia Mary Bellbrooke Surgery, 395 Harehills Lane, Leeds LS9 6AP Tel: 0113 249 4848; 14 Ivy Lane, Boston Spa, Wetherby LS23 6PD Tel: 01937 844 3118 — MB ChB Ed. 1975; BSc (Med. Sci.) Ed. 1972; DA Eng. 1978; Cert. Family Plann. 1979. Asst. GP, Bellbrooke Surg., 395 Harehills La., Leeds; Locum Clin. Med. Off., Family Plann., York Health Trust. Specialty: Gen. Pract.; Family Plann. & Reproduc. Health.

WILLS, Patrick Charles Carisbrooke Health Centre, 22 Carisbrooke High Street, Newport PO30 1NR Tel: 01983 522150; 115 Durham Road, Bromley BR2 0SP — MB BS Lond. 1989 (King's Coll. Lond.) DGM RCP Lond. 1991; MSc Lond. 1993; MRCP (UK) 1995; DFFP 1996; MRCGP 1997. GP Princip.; Clin. Asst. (GU Med.) St. Mary's Hosp. Newport IoW. Specialty: Gen. Pract. Socs: BMA. Prev: Clin. Asst. (Genitourin. Med.) Beckenham Hosp.; GP/Regist. Bromley VTS; SHO (Med.) Bromley Hosp.

WILLS, Peter John Hillingdon Hospital, Pield Heath Road, Uxbridge UB8 3NN Tel: 01895 279266 Fax: 01895 279890 Email: peter.wills@thh.nhs.uk — MB ChB Birm. 1987; PhD; MRCPath 1984; MA Oxf. 1988; MRCP (UK) 1990. Cons. Phys., Respirat. and Gen. Med. Specialty: Respirat. Med. Prev: Regist. (Med.) Bournmouth Gen. & Westm. Hosps.; SHO (Infec. Dis.) St. Ann's Hosp. Tottenham; SHO (Gen. Med.) Russells Hall Hosp. Dudley.

WILLS, Rachel Emma Hawthorn Cottage, Bovey Tracey, Newton Abbot TQ13 9PT — MB ChB Birm. 1994.

WILLS, Simon John 18 Tanfield Road, Newcastle upon Tyne NE15 7DT — MB ChB Dundee 1993. Specialty: Gen. Pract.

WILLSDON, Helen Francis The Doctors House, Victoria Road, Marlow SL7 1DN Tel: 01628 484666 Fax: 01628 891206; Kings Dial Cottage, Medmenham, Marlow SL7 2EU — MB ChB Leeds 1975; MRCOG 1982; MRCGP 1986.

WILLSHAW, Mr Harry Edward BUPA Parkway Hospital, Damson Parkway, Solihull B91 2PP Tel: 0121 704 1451; Burtons Farm Cottage, Malthouse Lane, Earlswood, Solihull B94 5DU Tel: 01564 702438 Fax: 01564 702438 — MB ChB Leeds 1971; BSc Leeds 1967; FRCS Ed. 1977; FCOphth 1990. Cons. Ophth. Childr. Hosp. & Birm. & Midl. Eye Hosp.; Hon. Lect. Univ. Birm. Med. Sch. Specialty: Ophth.

WILLSHER, Thomas 99 Hopton Road, London SW16 2EL — MB BS Lond. 1996.

WILLSON, Garth 101 Christchurch Place, Peterlee SR8 2NS — MRCS Eng. LRCP Lond. 1978; MA Cantab.

WILLSON, Gordon Frederick (retired) 7 Horncastle Road, Louth LN11 9LB Tel: 01507 609144 — MB BS Lond. 1943 (Lond. Hosp.) MRCS Eng. LRCP Lond. 1942; MD Lond. 1948; DPH Lond. 1953; FFCM 1977, M 1974. Prev: Area Med. Off. Dorset AHA.

WILLSON, Heather Jane Shepherd Spring Medical Centre, Cricketers Way, Andover SP10 5DE Tel: 01264 361126 Fax: 01264 350138; 10 Kingsmead, Anna Valley, Andover SP11 7PN — MB ChB Sheff. 1982; DCH RCP Lond. 1986. Prev: SHO (Paediat.) Epsom Dist. Hosp.; SHO (Geriat.) Newmarket Gen. Hosp.; SHO (O & G) Addenbrooke's Hosp. Camb.

WILLSON, Jeremy David — MB ChB Birm. 1998.

WILLSON, John Christopher Cottingham Medical Centre, 17-19 South Street, Cottingham HU16 4AJ Tel: 01482 845078 Fax: 01482 845078; 25 St Barnabas Drive, Swanland, North Ferriby HU14 3RL — MB ChB Liverp. 1981.

WILLSON, Lionel Arthur Herbert 23 The Avenue, Wanstead, London E11 2EE Tel: 020 8989 1245 — MRCS Eng. LRCP Lond. 1942 (Lond. Hosp.) Socs: BMA. Prev: Ho. Phys., &c. Roy. Sussex Co. Hosp. Brighton; Ho. Surg. Mile End Hosp.

WILLSON, Mr Peter David Department of Surgery, Kingston Hospital, Galsworthy Road, Kingston upon Thames KT2 7QV Tel: 020 8934 2734 Fax: 020 8934 3268 Email: peter.wilson@kingstonhospital.nhs.uk — MB BS Lond. 1985 (Char. Cross & Westm.) BSc Lond. 1982; FRCS Eng. 1989; FRCS (Gen.) 1997. Cons. (Surg.) Kingston Hosp. Qu. Mary's Hosp.; Hon. Lect. (Anat.) Imperial Coll. Lond.; Lead Clinician in General Surgery; Lead Clinician in Upper GI Cancer. Specialty: Gen. Surg. Socs: Fell. Roy. Soc. Med.; Assn. Endoscopic Surgs.; Assn. Surg.

WILLSON, Sarah Ann Culm Davy House, Henyock, Cullompton EX15 3UT — MB BS Lond. 1977 (St. Bart.) MRCP (UK) 1979; FRCR 1983. Cons. Radiol. MusGr. Pk. Hosp. Taunton. Specialty: Radiol. Prev: Sen. Regist. (Radiol.) Middlx. Hosp. Lond.; Fell. Univ. Hosp. UCSD Med. Centre, San Diego, Calif., USA.

WILLSON, Thomas Hugh Burvill House Surgery, 52 Dellfield Road, Hatfield AL10 8HP Tel: 01707 269091 — MB BS Lond. 1984 (Roy. Free) MA Oxf. 1983, BA 1979; DRCOG 1988. Prev: SHO St. Albans GP VTS.

WILLSON, William Wynne (retired) Hurst, Green Lane, Henley-on-Thames RG9 1LS Tel: 01491 573024 — BM BCh Oxf. 1937 (Oxf. & St Mary's) BA Oxf. 1937; LMSSA Lond. 1937; DObst RCOG 1946; MRCGP 1959. Prev: Ho. Phys., Ho. Surg. & 3rd Asst. (Path.) St. Mary's Hosp. Lond.

WILLSON-LLOYD, Joanne Mary 170 Dawlish Road, Birmingham B29 7AR Tel: 0121 689 5573 — MB ChB Birm. 1997. GP VTS Redditch. Specialty: Paediat.

WILLY, Diana Margaret Mitchell Manor Farm Medical Centre, Mangate Street, Swaffham PE37 7QN Tel: 01760 721700 Fax: 01760 723703; Hill House, North Pickenham, Swaffham PE37 8JZ Tel: 01760 440679 — MB BS Lond. 1970 (Roy. Free) MRCS Eng. LRCP Lond. 1970; DObst RCOG 1973.

WILM, Ann Ranghild Hawthorn Bank, 27 Glasgow Road, Denny FK6 5DW — MB ChB Glas. 1990.

WILMALASUNDERA, Neil Flat 17, Falconet Court, Wapping High St., London E1W 3NX — MB BS Lond. 1996.

WILMINGTON, Andrew Macgregor Church Road Surgery, 261 Church Road, Stannes on Sea, Lytham St Annes FY8 3NP Tel: 01253 728911 Fax: 01253 732114; 14 Arundel Road, Ansdell, Lytham St Annes FY8 1AF Tel: 01253 730301 — MB ChB Aberd. 1984; DRCOG 1987; MRCGP 1988. Prev: Trainee GP Inverclyde Dist. Argyll & Clyde HB; Ho. Off. Co. Hosp. Oban.; Ho. Off. Woodend Hosp. Aberd.

WILMINGTON, Sheila MacIntosh 532 Paisley Road W., Glasgow G51 1RN; 16 Avondale Drive, Paisley PA1 3TN — MB ChB Glas. 1960; DObst RCOG 1962.

WILMOT, Elizabeth Frances St. Michael's Hospital, St. Michaels Road, Warwick CV34 5QW Tel: 01926 406733 Fax: 01926 406702 — MB ChB Birm. 1973; DObst RCOG 1975; MRCPsych 1984. Cons. Psychiat. St. Michaels Hosp. Specialty: Gen. Psychiat. Prev: Sen. Regist. Midl. Nerve Hosp. Birm.; Sen. Regist. Centr. Hosp. Warwick; Sen. Regist. Uffculme Clinic Birm.

WILMOT, John David Charles Beechwood Surgery, 57 John Street, Workington CA14 3BT Tel: 01900 64866 Fax: 01900 871561; 2 Greenside Cottages, Tallentire, Cockermouth CA13 0PR Tel: 01900 824774 — MB BS Newc. 1976; DCH RCPS Glas. 1979; FRCGP 1993, M 1980; DRCOG 1980. Provost, Cumbria Fac. RCGP; Clin. Asst., Drugs and Alcohol, N. Cumbria Addictive Behaviour NHS Trust. Specialty: Gen. Pract.

WILMOT, John Fabian Clarendon Lodge Medical Practice, 16 Clarendon Street, Leamington Spa CV32 5SS Tel: 01926 422094 Fax: 01926 331400 — MB ChB Birm. 1971; MB ChB (Distinc. Psychiat.) Birm. 1971; DObst RCOG 1973; DCH Eng. 1974; FRCGP 1988, M 1975. Sen. Lect. (Primary Care) Sch. Postgrad. Med. Educat. Univ. Warwick Coventry; Vice-Chairm. Warks. MAAG Edit. Bd. Brit. Jl. of Gen. Pract. Specialty: Gen. Pract. Socs: BMA; AUDGP; EGPRW. Prev: Sec. Gen. Pract. Research Club; Vis. Asst. Prof. Family Med. Univ. West. Ontario, Canada; Course Organiser Coventry & Warks. VTS.

WILMOT, Rosalind Anne Oundle Surgery, Glapthorne Road, Oundle, Peterborough PE8 4JA Tel: 01832 273408; Town Farm House, Old Weston, Huntingdon PE28 5LL — MB ChB Liverp. 1975 (Liverpool) DRCOG 1978. Socs: BMS. Prev: GP Cambs. & Soton.; Trainee GP Liverp. VTS.

WILMOT, Mr Thomas James (retired) Rathmore, 1A Knocksilla Park, Omagh BT79 0AR Tel: 01662 242244 — MB BS Lond. 1944 (Middlx.) DLO Eng. 1948; FRCS Eng. 1950; MS Lond. 1950; FRCSI 1980. Cons. ENT Surg. Omagh Co. Tyrone & Co. Fermanagh; Cons. Neuro-otol. Claremont St. Hosp. Belf. & Altnagelvin Hosp. Londonderry.

WILMSHURST, Mr Andrew David Department of Plastic Surgery, Ninewells Hospital, Dundee DD1 9SY; 19 Hallowhill, St Andrews KY16 8SF — MB BS Lond. 1974 (Univ. Coll. Hosp.) FRCS Eng. 1980. Cons. Plastic Surg. Ninewells Hosp. Dundee; Hon. Sen. Lect. Dundee Med. Sch. Specialty: Plastic Surg. Prev: Sen. Regist. (Plastic Surg.) Salisbury Dist. Hosp.

WILMSHURST, Andrew Peter Kirriemuir Health Centre, Tannage Brae, Kirriemuir DD8 4ES Tel: 01575 753333 Fax: 01575 574230 — MB BChir Camb. 1989 (Cambridge University) MRCP (UK) 1993; DRCOG 1997; MRCGP 1999. Specialty: Gen. Pract.

WILMSHURST, Joanne Madeleine 133A Greenwich High Road, Greenwich, London SE10 8JA Tel: 020 8305 1694; Carters Cottage, Hangersley, Ringwood BH24 3JN Tel: 01425 473586 — MB BS Lond. 1989; MRCP (UK) 1994. Specialist Regist. (Paediat. Neurol.) Guys Hosp. Specialty: Paediat. Neurol. Prev: Lect. (Paediat.) Guys Hosp. Lond.; Regist. (Paediat.) Lewisham; Regist. (Paediat.) Canterbury.

WILMSHURST, Mark John The Priory Surgery, 326 Wells Road, Bristol BS4 2QJ Tel: 0117 949 3988 Fax: 0117 778250 — MB ChB Sheff. 1989; MRCGP 1993; DRCOG 1993. Trainee GP Lincoln VTS.

WILMSHURST, Peter Thomas Royal Shrewsbury Hospital NHS Trust, Shrewsbury SY3 8XQ Tel: 01743 261108 Fax: 01743 261374 — MB ChB Manch. 1974; BSc (Hons.) Manch. 1971; MRCP (UK) 1976. Cons., Cardiol. Specialty: Cardiol.

WILMSHURST, Sally Louise 115 Stallards Close, Old Road, Bromyard HR7 4AX — MB ChB Manch. 1995.

WILNE, Brian David Harbury Surgery, Mill St., Harbury, Leamington Spa CV33 9HR Tel: 01926 612232 Fax: 01926 612991; Temple Cottage, Temple End, Harbury, Leamington Spa CV33 9NE — MB ChB Birm. 1962; DObst RCOG 1965. Specialty: Gen. Med. Socs: BMA. Prev: SHO St. Geo. Hosp. Lincoln; Ho. Surg. Ipswich & E. Suff. Hosp. & Hull Matern. Hosp.

WILNER, John Marston The Church Street Practice, David Corbet House, 2 Callows Lane, Kidderminster DY10 2JG Tel: 01562 822051 Fax: 01562 827251; The Limes, Long Bank, Bewdley DY12 2QS Tel: 01299 405375 — MB ChB Birm. 1962; MRCP (UK) 1967; FRCP Ed. 1994. Prev: Regist. (Med.) N. Staffs. Roy. Infirm. Stoke-on-Trent; Ho. Phys. & Regist. (Med.) Gen. Hosp. Birm.

WILSDON, Ralph Bernard Nevil (retired) Easby House, Easby, Great Ayton, Middlesbrough TS9 6JQ Tel: 01642 722473 — MRCS Eng. LRCP Lond. 1940 (Univ. Coll. Hosp.) MD Lond. 1950, MB BS 1941; FRCP Lond. 1971, M 1948. Prev: Cons. Phys. Middlesbrough Area (Newc. RHB).

WILSHAW, Mrs Hilary Anna Elmes Prospect House, 48 South St., Manningtree CO11 1BG — MB Camb. 1963, BChir 1962.

WILSKI-JALOSZYNSKI, Andrew Pembury Hospital, Tunbridge Wells TN2 4QJ; 4 Berkeley Road, Mount Sion, Tunbridge Wells TN1 1YR — Lekarz Warsaw 1971; DPM Lond. 1975; MRCPsych 1977. Med. Dir. Invicta NHS Trust. Specialty: Gen. Psychiat. Prev: Cons. (Psychiat.) Invicta NHS Trust; Lect. (Psychother.) Herts. Coll. Art; Sen. Regist. (Psychiat.), Westm. Hosp., Lond.

WILSON, Mr Adrian James Park View Cottage, Wash Hill, Wooburn Town, High Wycombe HP10 0JA — MB BS Lond. 1994 (St. Bart.) BSc (Biochem.) Manch. 1989; FRCS Pt. I Eng. 1996; FRCS Pt 2 1998. SHO (Surg.) Wycombe Gen. Hosp. Bucks.; Specialist Regist. Orth. Northwick Pk. Prev: SHO (Orthop.) Roy. Berks.; SHO (Orthop.) Roy. Nat. Orthop. Hosp.; Demonst. (Anat.) Univ. Camb.

WILSON, Aileen Johnston (retired) 23 Beechlands Avenue, Glasgow G44 3YT — MB ChB Glas. 1964; DObst RCOG 1966; DPH Glas. 1967; MRCGP 1975. Prev: GP Glas.

WILSON, Alan (retired) 260 Brooklands Road, Manchester M23 9HD Tel: 0161 962 2124 — MB ChB Manch. 1952. Sch. Med. Off. William Hulmes Grammar Sch. Manch. Prev: SHO (Med.) Wythenshawe Hosp. Manch.

WILSON, Alan George (retired) The Old Mill, Mill Lane, Adderbury, Banbury OX17 3LW Tel: 01295 810340 — (St. Geo.) BSc (Special Physiol.) Lond. 1958, MB BS 1961; MRCS Eng. LRCP Lond. 1961; FRCP Lond. 1985, M 1964; DMRD Eng. 1970; FFR 1972; FRCR 1975. Prof. (Diagnostic Radio.) Univ. Lond. Prev: Prof. (Diagnostic Radio.) St Geo.'s Hosp. Lond.

WILSON, Alan Graham McTurk Summervale Medical Centre, Wharf Lane, Ilminster TA19 0DT Tel: 01460 52354 Fax: 01460 52652 — MB BS Lond. 1981 (Royal Free Hospital School Medicine) MB BS London 1981; MA Cambridge 1982; MRCP (UK) 1985. Specialty: Gen. Pract.

WILSON, Alan Hamilton 89 Bawtry Road, Bessacarr, Doncaster DN4 7AG — MB BS Lond. 1954; DPM Eng. 1964; FRCPsych 1990, M 1972. Cons. Psychiat. Doncaster Roy. Infirm. & Loversall Hosp. Doncaster. Specialty: Gen. Psychiat. Prev: Sen. Regist. Leeds Gen. Infirm. & St. Jas. Hosp. Leeds.

WILSON, Mr Alan James St. Mary's Wing, Whittington Hospital, Highgate Hill, London N19 5NF — MB ChB Birm. 1971; FRCS Glas. 1976; MSc Glas. 1977; MD Birm. 1983. Cons. Surg. Whittington Hosp. Lond. Specialty: Gen. Surg. Socs: Surg. Research Soc. Prev: Lect. Surg. King's Coll. Hosp. Lond.; CRC Research Fell. King's Coll. Hosp. Med. Sch. Lond.

WILSON, Alan Oliver Arneil (retired) 14 Cammo Hill, Barnton, Edinburgh EH4 8EY Tel: 0131 339 2244 Fax: 0131 339 2244 Email: o.wilson@virgin.net — (Ed.) MB ChB Ed. 1952; DPM Eng. 1960; FRCPsych 1976, M 1971. Cons. (Scotl.) Ex-Servs. Ment. Welf. Soc. Prev: Cons. Psychiat. Murrayfield BUPA Hosp. Edin.

WILSON, Alan Robin Muir Nottingham Breast Institute, City Hospital, Hucknall Road, Nottingham NG5 1PB Tel: 0115 969 1689 Fax: 0115 962 7707 Email: rwilson@ncht.trent.nhs.uk — MB ChB Dundee 1979; MRCP (UK) 1982; FRCR 1987; FRCP Ed. 1993. Cons. Radiol. City Hosp. Nottm.; Clin. Director, Breast Directorate, City Hosp., Nottm. Specialty: Radiol. Socs: Roy. Coll. Radiol. (Sec. Breast Gp.); (Past Sec.) Europ. Gp. for Breast Cancer Screening.; Brit. Breast Gp. Prev: Cons. Radiol. Univ. Hosp. Nottm.; Lect. (Radiol.) Univ. Hosp. Nottm.

WILSON, Mr Alan William 79 Tremona Road, Southampton SO16 6HS — BM Soton. 1993; BDS Ed. 1985; FDS Ed. 1987; FRCS Lond. 1997. Specialist Regist. (Maxillofacial) QA Portsmouth. Specialty: Oral & Maxillofacial Surg.

WILSON, Mr Alastair 4 Halland Close, Crawley RH10 1SD — MB ChB Ed. 1976; FRCS Ed. 1983; FRCS Eng. 1983. Regist. (Surg.) Roy. E. Sussex Hosp. Hastings. Socs: Fell. Roy. Soc. Med. Lond.; Fell. Roy. Med. Soc. Edin. Prev: SHO Emerg. & Accid. Dept. Lond. Hosp. Whitechapel; SHO (Gen. Surg.) United Norwich Hosps.

WILSON, Mr Alastair Osborne (retired) 211 Henley Road, Ipswich IP1 6RL — MB ChB Ed. 1947 (Univ. Ed.) BSc Ed. 1946; FRCS Ed. 1953; FRCS Eng. 1961. Cons. Surg. Dudley Rd. Hosp. Birm. Prev: Sen. Regist. (Surg.) United Birm. Hosps.

WILSON, Mr Alastair Walter Rutique, Nethergate St., Harpley, King's Lynn PE31 6TW Tel: 01485 520914 Fax: 01485 520885 Email: alastair.wilson@btinternet.com — MB ChB Aberd. 1973; FRCS Eng. 1980; FFAEM 1994. Clin. Dir. (A & E & Helicopter Emerg. Med. Serv.) Barts & the Lond. Specialty: Accid. & Emerg. Socs: Brit. Trauma Soc. - Ex Pres.; Europ. Assoc. for Trauma and Emerg. Surg. - Vice Pres.(EATES). Prev: Sen. Regist. (Gen. Surg.) Lond. Hosp. Whitechapel & Old Ch. Hosp. Romford; Regist. (Gen. Surg.) Univ. Coll. & Brompton Hosps. Lond.

WILSON, Alexander John — MB ChB Zimbabwe 1985; BSc Natal 1980; LRCP LRCS Ed. LRCPS Glas. 1987; FFA RCSI 1992. Cons. Anaesth. W. Dorset Hosp. NHS Trust Dorchester. Specialty: Anaesth. Prev: Sen. Regist. (Anaesth.) W. Midl.

WILSON, Alexander Murray (retired) 87 Stumperlowe Hall Road, Sheffield S10 3QS Tel: 0114 230 1220 Email: a.m.wilson@sheffield.ac.uk — (Brist.) MB ChB Bristol 1959; DRCOG 1961; FFA RCS Eng. 1966; Cert. Av Med. 1983. Emerit. Hon. Sen. Clin. Lect., Univ. of Sheff.; Mem. Air Transport Users Co. C.A.A.; Hon. Clin. Lect. Univ. Sheff.; Assoc., Gen. Med. Counc. Prev: Cons. Anaesth. Sheff. Plastic Surg. Unit N. Gen. Hosp.

WILSON, Mrs Alison Margaret — MB BChir Camb. 1990; BA (Hons.) Camb. 1988; MRCOG 1996. Flexible Trainee Specialist Regist. (O & G) Rosie Matern. Hosp., Camb., W. Suff. Hosp., Bury St Edmunds. Specialty: Obst. & Gyn. Prev: Specialist Regist. (O & G), W. Suff. Hosp.; Regist. (O & G) Rosie Matern. Hosp. Camb.; SHO (Surg.) Chesterfield & N. Derbysh. Roy. Hosp.

WILSON, Alister Bryan Gartnavel Royal Hospital, Great Western Road, Glasgow G12 0XH — MB BCh BAO Belf. 1982; MB BCh Belf. 1982.

WILSON, Amanda Jane The Health Centre, Canterbury Way, Stevenage SG1 1QH Tel: 01438 357411 Fax: 01438 720523 — MB BS Lond. 1984. Prev: Trainee GP N. Middlx. Hosp. VTS; Ho. Phys. Edgware Gen. Hosp.; Ho. Surg. Chase Farm Hosp. Enfield.

WILSON, Amanda Margaret Kilbowie Road, Clydebank G81 2TQ; 42 Upper Glenburn Rd, Glasgow G61 4BN Tel: 0141 942 5043 — MB ChB Glas. 1991. SHO (Cas.) Leeds Gen. Hosp. Prev: Ho. Off. (Surg.) Vict. Infirm. Glas.; Ho. Off. (Med.) Roy. Infirm. Glas.

WILSON, Andrew Alexander (retired) 45 Bothwell Road, Hamilton ML3 0BB Tel: 01698 281866 — MB ChB Glas. 1947 (Univ. Glas.)

WILSON, Andrew Carl Edenfield Centre, Prestwich Hospital, Bury New Rd, Prestwich, Manchester M25 3BL Tel: 0161 772 3684 Fax: 0161 772 3446 — MB ChB Leeds 1985; MRCPsych 1989. Cons. Forens. Psychiat. N. Western Regional Forens. Serv.; Cons. Forens. Psychiat. Edenfield Centre,Bolton,Salford & Trafford Ment. health Partnership. Specialty: Forens. Psychiat. Prev: Sen. Regist. (Forens. Psychiat.) Reaside Clinic Birm.; Regist. Rotat. (Psychiat.) Merseyside RHA.

WILSON, Andrew Douglas Saffron Group Practice, 509 Saffron Lane, Leicester LE2 6UL Tel: 0116 244 0888 Fax: 01162 831405 — MB BS Newc. 1977; DRCOG 1979; MD Newc. 1991; FRCGP 1999. Reader Dept. Gen. Pract. & Primary Health Care Univ. of Leicester. Prev: Lect. (Gen. Pract.) Univ. Nottm.; GP North. Med. Unit Univ. Manitoba.

WILSON, Mr Andrew Douglas Harold Blond McIndoe, Royal Free Hospital, Hampstead, London NW3 2QG Tel: 020 7794 0500; 19 Drumgoose Road, Portadown, Craigavon BT62 1PH Tel: 0141 337 2064 — MB ChB Glas. 1997 (Glasgow) MRCS Glasgow 2000. Plastic Surg. Research Fell., Blond McIndoe, Roy. Free Hoepital. Specialty: Plastic Surg.

WILSON, Andrew Edgar James North Queen Street Surgery, 257 North Queen Street, Belfast BT15 1HS Tel: 028 9074 8317 Fax: 028 9075 4438; 3 Cricklewood Park, Belfast BT9 5GU Tel: 01232 663504 — MB BCh BAO Belf. 1989 (Queen's University Belfast) DCH RCP Lond. 1993; DRCOG 1994; DFFP 1995; MRCGP 1995.

WILSON, Andrew Gilmour Clark 147 Cregagh Road, Belfast BT6 0LB Tel: 028 457947 — MB BCh BAO Belf. 1952. Prev: Ho. Surg. & Ho. Phys. Belf. City Hosp.; Res. Med. Off. Roy. Lond. Homoeop. Hosp.

WILSON, Andrew Gordon, Capt. RAMC Murrayfield Medical Centre, 35 Sangton Crescent, Edinburgh EH12 5SS — MB ChB Ed. 1992. Specialty: Gen. Pract.

WILSON, Andrew Kevin 34 School Lane, Brereton, Sandbach CW11 1RN — MB ChB Birm. 1996.

WILSON, Andrew Malcolm University of East Anglia, Population Health Group, Faculty of Medicine, Health Policy & Practice, Norwich NR4 7TJ Email: a.m.wilson@uea.ac.uk — MB ChB Ed. 1992; MRCP (UK) 1996. Clin. Sen. Lect. Specialty: Respirat. Med. Socs: BMA; STS; MDU. Prev: Clin. Lect. Univ. of Dundee; Research Fell. Univ. Dundee; SHO (Med.) Hope Hosp. Manch. & Halifax Gen. Hosp.

WILSON, Andrew Peter Richard Department of Clinical Microbiology, University College Hospital, Grafton Way, London WC1E 6DB Tel: 020 7380 9516 Fax: 020 7388 8514 Email: peter.wilson@uclh.org — MB BS Lond. 1981 (Univ. Coll. Hosp.) MA Camb. 1981; MRCP (UK) 1984; MD Lond. 1987; MRCPath 1989; FRCPath 1997; FRCP (UK) 2000; FRCP FRCP (uk) 2000. Cons. & Hon. Sen. Lect. (Microbiol.) Univ. Coll. Lond. Hosps.; Hon. Sen. Lect. Lond. Sch. Hyg. & Trop. Med.; Hon. Cons. Whittington Hosp. Specialty: Med. Microbiol. Socs: Fell. Roy. Soc. Med.; Brit. Soc. Antimicrob. Chemother.; Hosp. Infec. Soc. Prev: Lect. & Hon. Sen. Regist. (Microbiol.) Univ. Coll. & Middlx. Hosps. Lond.; Research Regist. (Microbiol.) Univ. Coll. Hosp. Lond.; SHO (Med.) Northwick Pk. Hosp. Lond.

WILSON, Andrew Richard The Wilsden Medical Practice, 2 Lingbob Court, Wilsden, Bradford BD15 0NG Tel: 01535 273227 Fax: 01535 274860 — MB ChB Leeds 1985; DRCOG 1988; MRCGP 1991. GP Bradford, W. Yorks. Prev: Trainee GP Bradford HA VTS.

WILSON, Andrew Stuart Parker Temple Cowley Health Centre, Templar House, Temple Road, Oxford OX4 2HL Tel: 01865 777024 Fax: 01865 777548 — BM Soton. 1989; DFFP 1993; DRCOG 1993; MRCGP 1994. Specialty: Gen. Pract. Prev: Trainee GP/SHO Soton. VTS.

WILSON, Andrew Thomas Schopwick Surgery, Everett Court, Romeland, Borehamwood WD6 3BJ Tel: 020 8953 1008 Fax: 020 8905 2196; Donard, Letchmore Heath, Watford WD2 8EW Tel: 01923 854611 Fax: 01923 854611 — MRCS Eng. LRCP Lond. 1978 (Westminster) DFFP; LRCP; BSc, MB BS Lond. 1978; DRCOG 1981; FRCGP 1994. GP; Examr. Roy. Coll. Gen. Pract.; Assoc. Dean (Postgrad. Gen. Pract.) N. Thames (W.); Mem. Edit. Bd. Ed. Postgrads. GP. Specialty: Educat.; Gen. Pract. Special Interest: Med. Educat. Prev: GP Course Organiser Northwick Pk. Hosp. Harrow.

WILSON, Andrew Timothy Anaesthetic Department, Leeds Gen. Inf., Leeds LS1 3EX — MB ChB Leeds 1985; FRCA 1991. Cons. Anaesth. & Intensivist, Leeds Gen. Inf. Specialty: Anaesth. Socs: FRCA. Prev: Regist. Rotat. (Anaesth.) Sheff.

WILSON, Angela 42 South Avenue, Buxton SK17 6NQ — MB ChB Dundee 1988.

WILSON, Angela Dorothy The Writtle Surgery, 16A Lordship Road, Writtle, Chelmsford CM1 3EH — BM BS Nottm. 1997 (Nottingham) BMedSci Nottm. 1995.

WILSON, Angela Ruth 20 Lidgett Park Road, Leeds LS8 1JN — MB BS Lond. 1975; DRCOG 1977; MRCPsych 1983.

WILSON, Ann (retired) Health Centre, Academy St., Castle Douglas DG7 1EE Tel: 01556 2067; Lochaber, 65 Academy St., Castle Douglas DG7 1EE Tel: 01556 2656 — LRCPI & LM, LRSCI & LM 1965 (RCSI) LRCPI & LM, LRCSI & LM 1965; FRCOG 1989, M 1970, DObst 1967.

WILSON, Ann Ray Tamara (retired) 11 Larkswood Rise, Pinner HA5 2HH — MB BS Lond. 1961 (Univ. Coll. Hosp.) DPH 1964.

WILSON, Anna Stephenie The Gratton Surgery, Sutton Scotney, Winchester SO21 3LE Tel: 01962 760267 Fax: 01962 761138; Tioman, Stratton Road, St. Giles Hill, Winchester SO23 0JQ Tel: 01962 864102 Fax: 01962 877260 Email: dwilson155@aol.com — BM BCh Oxf. 1971 (St. Mary's and Oxf.) BSc (1st cl. Hons.) Lond. 1968; DObst RCOG 1973; DCH RCP Lond. 1974; MRCGP 1978; DTM & H RCP Lond. 1979; DFFP 1995; FRCGP 1998. GP Trainer; Med. Stud. Teach. Soton. Univ.; Dep. Police Surg.; GP SHO VTS Progr. Organiser and Wessex VTS; Sexual Heath and Child Protec. Local and Hants PCT; GP Mem. Hants. ACPC. Special Interest: Womens Health,Medical Educat. Socs: Assoc. Mem. Inst. Psychosexual Med.; Fac. Community Health. Prev: Clin. Med. Off.

(Community Health Serv.) Winchester HA & Wolverhampton HA; Chairm. Wessex Fac. Roy. Coll. GPs; Diplomat Bd. of Mem. Fac. of Family Plann. and Reproductive Health Counc.

WILSON, Anne Merrall (retired) Kinnaird, London Road, Poulton, Cirencester GL7 5JQ — (St. Mary's) MB BS Lond. 1957; MRCS Eng. LRCP Lond. 1957; DPM Eng. 1970; FRCPsych 1986, M 1972. Second Opinion Apptd. Dr Ment. Health Act Commiss.; Ment. Health Act Commision. Prev: Cons. Psychiat. E. Glos. NHS Trust.

WILSON, Anne Moya Yatton Family Practice, 155 Mendip Road, Yatton, Bristol BS49 4ER Tel: 01934 832277 Fax: 01934 876085 — MB ChB Glas. 1973; DRCOG 1976; MRCGP 1977; DCH RCPS Glas. 1977. Specialty: Gen. Pract. Socs: Roy. Coll. Gen. Pract.

WILSON, Anthony Ernest 8 The Paddock, Appleton Wiske, Northallerton DL6 2BE — MB BS Durh. 1965; AFOM RCP Lond. 1984. Sen.Med. Off. CORUSCRI Teeside. Specialty: Occupat. Health. Socs: BMA; BASICS; Soc. Occupat. Med. Prev: Regist. (A & E) Dundee Roy. Infirm.; Demonst. (Anat.) Dundee Univ.; Regist. (Cas. & Orthop.) Durh. Co. Hosp.

WILSON, Anthony Gerard Division of Genomic Medicine, University of Sheffield, Sheffield S10 2JF Email: a.g.wilson@shef.ac.uk; 1 Gladstone Mews, Ranmoor, Sheffield S10 3HS Tel: 01142 731402 Fax: 01142 712882 Email: a.g.wilson@sheffield.ac.uk — MB BCh BAO Belf. 1983; MRCP (UK) 1986; DCH RCPSI 1988; PhD Sheff. 1995; FRCP 2002. Sen. Lect. in Molecular Med/Rheum.; Reader in Molecular Med. / Rheum. 2002. Specialty: Gen. Med.; Rheumatol. Socs: Roy. Coll. Phys. Lond. & Brit. Soc. Rheum. Prev: ARC Research Fell. (Med. Fac.) Univ. Sheff.; Regist. & Lect. (Rheum.) North. Gen. Hosp. Edin.; SHO (Cardiol., Neurol. & Rheum.) Roy. Vict. Hosp. Belf.

WILSON, Anthony James Thomas Drayton Medical Practices, The Health Centre, Cheshire Street, Market Drayton TF9 3BS Tel: 01630 652158; 60 Main Road, Norton-in-Hales, Market Drayton TF9 4AT Tel: 01630 653426 — MB BS Lond. 1973 (Char. Cross) Prev: Trainee Gen. Pract. PeterBoro. Vocational Train. Scheme; Ho. Off. (Surg.) Profess. Unit Surg. & Ho. Off. (Med.) Char. Cross; Hosp. Lond.

WILSON, Anthony Robert (retired) Cedar House, Behoes Lane, Woodcote, Reading RG8 0PP Email: a.r.wilson@amserve.net — MB ChB Ed. 1956; DAvMed Eng. 1969; MFCM 1974; MRCGP 1975. Prev: GP Woodcote Reading.

WILSON, Arthur Claude (retired) Wateredge, Crosthwaite, Kendal LA8 8HX — MB ChB Glas. 1952; FRCOG 1974, M 1959. Prev: Cons. O & G North. Sefton Health Dist. (S.port).

WILSON, Barbara Elizabeth Chapel Cottage, Chieveley, Newbury RG16 8XG — MB ChB Leeds 1944.

WILSON, Bernard Gerard 15 Windsor Park, Belfast BT9 6FQ — MB BCh BAO Belf. 1979.

WILSON, Betty Nicol Child Development Centre, Bridgeton Health Centre, Abercromby St., Glasgow; 10 Ellergreen Road, Beardsen, Glasgow G61 2RJ — MB ChB Ed. 1979; BSc (Med. Sci.) Ed. 1976, MB ChB 1979; DRCOG 1982; MRCGP 1983; LF (Hom.) Glas. 1995. Cons. (Com. Paed.) Yorkhill NHS Trust. Specialty: Community Child Health. Socs: Chairperson BAAF (Scottish) Med. Advisers Gp. Prev: SCMO (Child Health) Gtr. Glas. Health Bd.; Clin. Med. Off. Forth Valley HB; Trainee GP S. Lothian VTS.

WILSON, Brian Andrew Langham Place Surgery, 11 Langham Place, Northampton NN2 6AA Tel: 01604 38162 Fax: 01604 602457 — MB BS Lond. 1985; DRCOG 1987 GUYS. Specialty: Gen. Pract.

WILSON, Bridget Elizabeth Birmingham Childrens' Hopsital, Steelhouse Lane, Birmingham B4 6NH — MB ChB Sheff. 1987 (Sheffield) MRCP (UK) 1992. Cons. In Paediatric Accid. & Emerg. Med. Birm. Childr.s' Hosp. Birm. Specialty: Paediat.; Accid. & Emerg. Socs: Roy. Coll. Of Paediat. & Child Health. Prev: SHO Rotat. (Paediat.) Qu. Med. Centre Nottm. & Derby Childr. Hosps.; SHO Rotat. (Paediat.) Leicester; Trainee GP Redditch VTS.

WILSON, Callum Stephen Greenpark Healthcare Trust, Musgrave Park Hospital, Stockman's Lane, Belfast BT9 7JB Tel: 02890 902000 Fax: 02890 902222 Email: callum.wilson@greenpark.n-i.nhs.uk — MB ChB Dundee 1990 (Univ. of Dundee) FRCA 1995. Cons. Anaesth. Specialty: Anaesth.

WILSON, Cameron MacKinnon Deepdale Road Healthcare Centre, Deepdale Road, Preston PR1 5AF Tel: 01772 655533 Fax: 01772 653414; 40 Preston Road, Grimsargh, Preston PR2 5SD Tel: 01772 651243 — MB ChB Glas. 1982; DCH RCP Lond. 1988. Prev: Med. Off. RN.

WILSON, Carol Mildred 16 Cleaver Park, Belfast BT9 5HX — MB BCh BAO Belf. 1979; MRCP (UK) 1983; MD Belf. 1986; FRCP Ed. 1995. Cons. Cardiol. Roy. Vict. Hosp. Belf. Specialty: Cardiol. Socs: Brit. Cardiac Soc.; (Treas.) Irish Cardiac Soc.; (Hon. Sec.) Ulster Med. Soc.

WILSON, Caroline Jane c/o Gransha Hospital, Clooney Road, Londonderry BT47 6TF Tel: 01504 860261; Northfield House, Gransha Hospital, Clooney Road, Londonderry BT47 6TF Tel: 01504 860261 — MB ChB Stellenbosch 1996 (University of Stellenbosch) SHO (Psychiat.) Gransha Hosp. Londonderry. Specialty: Gen. Psychiat. Prev: Jun. Ho. Off. Tygerberg Hosp. Western Cape, S. Africa.

WILSON, Caroline Lesley Department of Dermatology, St. James's University Hospital, Leeds LS9 7TF Tel: 0113 206 4900 Fax: 0113 206 4805 Email: caroline.wilson@leedsth.nhs.uk — MB BS Lond. 1982 (Westm.) MRCP (UK) 1986; BSc (1st cl. Hons.) Lond. 1979, MD 1995; FRCP (UK) 1999. Cons. Dermat. St. Jas. & Seacroft Univ. Hosp. NHS Trust Leeds. Specialty: Dermat. Prev: Sen. Regist. (Dermat.) Oxf. RHA & Hon. Regist. (Dermat.) Slade Hosp. Oxf.; Regist. (Med. & Dermat.) Stoke Mandeville Hosp.; SHO (Oncol.) Roy. Marsden Hosp.

WILSON, Mrs Caroline Samantha Grovehurst, Middle Lane, Denbigh LL16 3UW — MB ChB Birm. 1989; MRCGP 1995. Asst. in Gen. Pract.

WILSON, Catherine Mary 33 Tweskard Park, Belfast BT4 2JZ — MD Belf. 1987; MB BCh BAO 1976; FFA RCSI 1980. Cons. (Anaesth.) Ulster Hosp. Dundonald. Specialty: Anaesth.

WILSON, Catherine Mary Pathhead Medical Practice, 210 Main Street, Pathhead EH37 5PP Tel: 01875 320 302 Fax: 01875 320494; 8 Fala, Blackshiels, Pathhead EH37 5SY Tel: 01875 833296 — MB ChB Ed. 1977; BScMedSc 1974; BSc Ed. 1974; Dip. Occ. Med. RCP Lond. 1997; PG Dip Palliat. Care Glas. 2002; Cert. Diabetes Care, Warwick 2003. GP Partner Pathmead Med. Pract. Pathmead, Midlothian; Occupat. Health Phys. Lothian NHS Occupat. Health Serv. Morelands, Astley-Ainslie Hosp. Edin. Specialty: Gen. Pract.; Occupat. Health. Prev: Trainee GP Edin. VTS; Regist. (Psychiat.) Roy. Edin. Hosp.; SHO (Psychiat.) Roy. Edin. Hosp.

WILSON, Catherine Sara Plot 7, Summerfield, Wattisfield Road, Walsham-Le-Willows, Bury St Edmunds IP31 3BD — MB BS Lond. 1982.

WILSON, Catherine Stewart Abington, 37 Ayr Road, Prestwick KA9 1SY — MB ChB Glas. 1977; FFA RCSI 1981. Assoc. Specialist (Anaesth.) Ayrsh. & Arran Trust. Specialty: Anaesth.

WILSON, Catriona Edith Armadale Group Practice, 18 North Street, Armadale, Bathgate EH48 3QB Tel: 01501 730432 — MB ChB Glas. 1987. Specialty: Gen. Pract.

WILSON, Cedric James (retired) Thirty One, Beacon Road, Walsall WS5 3LF — MB BChir Camb. 1946 (Camb. & Birm.) MRCS Eng. LRCP Lond. 1946. Prev: Res. Surg. Off., Ho. Surg. & Anaesth. W. Bromwich & Dist. Gen. Hosp.

WILSON, Charles (retired) 25 Bog Road, Ballymena BT42 4HH Tel: 02825 649260 — MB BCh BAO Belf. 1965 (Qu. Univ. Belf.) MRCP (UK) 1970; FACC 1992; FRCP Lond. 1994. Prev: Cons. Cardiol. Antrim Hosp.

WILSON, Charles Alexander PO Box 164, Manchester M28 2XE Tel: 0161 7935006 — MB ChB Sheff. 1991 (Sheffield) MRCPath 1997; DRCPath (Forensic) 1998. Home Office Pathologist, Manch. Specialty: Forens. Path. Socs: Assn. Clin. Path; Brit. Assn. Forens. Med. Prev: Regist Rotat. (Histopath.) North. RHA; Lect. (Forens. Path.) Univ. Liverp.; Hon. Sen. Regist. (Histopath.) Roy. Liverp. Univ. Hosp.

WILSON, Charles Bernard Joseph Howitt Dept. of Oncol., Addenbrooke's NHS Trust, Hills Road, Cambridge CB2 2QQ Tel: 01223 217110 Fax: 01223 274409 — MRCS Eng. LRCP Lond. 1980 (Westm.) MD Lond. 1994, MB BS 1981; MRCP (UK) 1984; FRCR 1990; T(R) (CO) 1991. Cons. Clin. Oncol. Addenbrooke's Hosp. Camb.; Clin. Director Dept. of Oncol. Specialty: Oncol. Special Interest: Breast; Maligancies.

WILSON, Charles Frederick (Surgery), 178 Roe Lane, Southport PR9 7PN Tel: 01704 28439; 50 Ryder Crescent, Hillside, Southport PR8 3AF Tel: 01704 78304 — MB ChB Liverp. 1962. Socs: BMA &

S.port Med. Soc. Prev: SHO Clatterbridge Hosp. Bebington; Regist. Cas. Roy. Liverp. Childr. Hosp.

WILSON, Charles Nicholas Farnham Medical Centre, 435 Stanhope Road, South Shields NE33 4JE Tel: 0191 455 4748 Fax: 0191 455 8573 — MB ChB Dundee 1971; DObst RCOG 1974.

WILSON, Christina Isabella (retired) 75 Stewarton Drive, Cumbuslang, Glasgow G72 8DQ Tel: 0141 641 2195 — MB ChB Glas. 1948. Prev: SCMO Gtr. Glas. Health Bd.

WILSON, Christine Elizabeth Schopwick Surgery, Everett Court, Romeland, Borehamwood WD6 3BJ Tel: 020 8953 1008 Fax: 020 8905 2196; Donard, Alderham Road, Letchmore Health, Watford WD25 8EW — BM Soton. 1976 (Southampton) DRCOG 1979; MRCGP 1982. Specialty: Gen. Pract.

WILSON, Christine Hilary Castledawson Surgery, Station Road, Castledawson, Magherafelt BT45 8AZ Tel: 028 7938 6237 Fax: 028 7946 9613 — MB BCh BAO Belf. 1973; DRCOG 1977.

WILSON, Christine Shearer Auchinairn Road Surgery, 127/129 Auchinairn Road, Bishopbriggs, Glasgow G64 1NF Tel: 0141 772 1808 Fax: 0141 762 1274; 13 Ledcameroch Crescent, Bearsden, Glasgow G61 4AD — MB ChB Glas. 1983 (Glasgow) MRCGP 1987; DRCOG 1988; DCCH RCP Ed. 1988. Specialty: Gen. Pract. Prev: Trainee GP Livingston VTS; SHO (O & G) Stirling Roy. Infirm.; SHO (Infec. Dis.) Ruchill Hosp. Glas.

WILSON, Christopher Orthopaedic Department, BUPA Hospital, Cardiff CF23 8XL Tel: 029 2054 2655; 7 Palace Road, Cardiff CF5 2AF Tel: 029 2057 7117 Fax: 01222 577844 Email: chriswilson@cwilson.net — MB BS Lond. 1984 (Univ. Coll. Lond.) BSc (Hons.) Lond. 1981, MB BS 1984; FRCS Ed. 1989; FRCS Orth. 1996. Cons. Trauma & Orthop. Surg. Specialty: Orthop.

WILSON, Christopher Claud Stevenson Cedarhill, Auchencloch, Banknock, Bonnybridge FK4 1UA Tel: 01324 840227 — MB ChB Aberd. 1991; LR Hom Faculty homocop, June 1999. SHO Rotat. (Med.) Roy. United Hosp. & Roy. Nat. Hosp. Rheum. Dis. Bath. Specialty: Gen. Med.; Homeop. Med. Prev: SHO Rotat. (Med.) Worcester Roy. Infirm.; SHO (Neurosurg.) Radcliffe Infirm. Oxf.

WILSON, Christopher Edward Plympton Health Centre, Plympton, Plymouth PL7 2PS Tel: 01752 341474; Mansion 5, Mounthaven Village, Bitta Ford, Plymouth PC21 0XF Tel: 01752 345040 — MB BS Nottm. 1982; BMedSci Nottm. 1980, MB BS 1982; MRCGP 1986.

WILSON, Christopher John Thurlow, 9 Finchdean Road, Rowlands Castle PO9 6DA Tel: 023 9241 2350; Thurlow, 9 Finchdean Road, Rowlands Castle PO9 6DA Tel: 023 9241 2350 Email: wilson@thurlow.vispa.com — MB BS Lond. 1975 (Lond. Hosp.) DRCOG 1977. Prev: Regist. (Paediat.) St. Mary's Hosp. Lond.; SHO Qu. Eliz. Hosp. Childr. Lond.; SHO (O & G) Lond. Hosp.

WILSON, Christopher John Francis Broomlands Brae, Stirches Road, Hawick TD9 7HF — MB ChB Sheff. 1995.

WILSON, Mr Christopher Reid 8A Ailsa Drive, Glasgow G42 9UL — MB ChB Glas. 1990; FRCS Glas. 1994.

WILSON, Christopher Sean Church Walk Surgery, 28 Church Walk, Lurgan, Craigavon BT67 9AA Tel: 028 3832 7834 Fax: 028 3834 9331; 43 Kilmore Road, Lurgan, Craigavon BT67 9HT Tel: 02838 324789 Email: kilmorerd@supanet.com — MB BCh BAO Belf. 1979; DRCOG 1982; DCH RCPS Glas. 1982. Gen. Pract. Princip.; Jt. Med. Dir. Craigavon & Banbridge Community Trust.

WILSON, Christopher William Homecroft Surgery, Voguebeloth, Illogan, Redruth TR16 4ET Fax: 01209 843707; Chy Bean, Harris Mill, Illogan, Redruth TR16 4JE Tel: 01209 213207 Fax: 01209 213207 — MB BS Lond. 1974 (Westm.) MRCS Eng. LRCP Lond. 1973; DObst RCOG 1975; DA Eng. 1977. Prev: SHO (Cas. & Anaesth.) Roy. Cornw. Hosp. (Treliske) Truro; SHO (Gyn.) Camborne-Redruth Hosp.

WILSON, Claire Louise The Surgery, 66 Crown Road, Twickenham TW1 3ER Tel: 020 8546 1407 Fax: 020 8547 0075; 12 Norman Avenue, St. Margaret's, Twickenham TW1 2LY Tel: 020 8892 3072 — MB ChB Bristol 1985; DRCOG 1988; MRCGP 1989; DCH RCP Lond. 1989. Socs: BMA.

WILSON, Colin The Corners, 11 West End, Guisborough TS14 6NN — MB BCh BAO Belf. 1985 (Qu. Belf.) DRCOG 1988; DCH Dub. 1988; MRCGP 1989; MPH Leeds 1994. Med. Dir. Langbough PCG. Socs: Local Med. Comm.

WILSON, Mr Colin The Ayr Hospital, Dalmellington Road, Ayr KA6 6DX Tel: 01292 610555 Fax: 01292 288952; 8 Southpark Road, Ayr KA7 2TL Tel: 01292 260772 — MB ChB Glas. 1979; FRCS Glas. 1983; MD Glas. 1989; T(S) 1995. Cons. Surg. Ayr Hosp. Specialty: Gen. Surg. Socs: Assn. & Surgs. GB & Irel.; Brit. Soc. Gastroenterol. Prev: Sen. Regist. (Gen. Surg.) Roy. Infirm. Glas.; Jun. Cons. Surgic. Gastroenterol. Groote Schuur Hosp., Cape Town, S. Afr.

WILSON, Colin Alexander Hunter Health Centre, Andrew Street, East Kilbride, Glasgow G74 1AD Tel: 01355 906622 Fax: 01355 906629 — MB ChB Glas. 1983; Cert. Family Plann. JCC 1986; DRCOG 1986; MRCGP 1987.

WILSON, Colin Bryce Hollands and Partners, Bridport Medical Centre, North Allington, Bridport DT6 5DU Tel: 01308 421896 Fax: 01308 421109 — MB BS Lond. 1979 (Westm.) MRCGP; DO RCS Eng. 1984; DRCOG 1985. Trainee GP Mullion VTS. Prev: SHO/Regist. Oxf. Eye Hosp.; SHO (Obst.) John Radcliffe Hosp. Oxf.; Ophth. Roy. Commonw. Soc. Blind, Grenada.

WILSON, Colin Moffat Lorn Medical Centre, Soroba Road, Oban PA34 4HE Tel: 01631 563175 Fax: 01631 562708; Clachbheo, Glenmore Road, Oban PA34 4NB Tel: 01631 562418 — MB ChB Glas. 1978; FFA RCS Eng. 1982. Ltd. Specialist (Anaesth.) Lorn & Is.s Dist. Gen. Hosp. Specialty: Anaesth.; Sports Med. Prev: Regist. (Anaesth.) Vict. Infirm. Glas.

WILSON, Colin Rhodri Mactaggart, TD The Gateway, 4 Raynsford Road, Dallington, Northampton NN5 7HP — MB BS Lond. 1963 (St. Thos.) DPM Eng. 1968; MRCPsych 1972. Cons. Psychiat. St. And. Hosp. Northampton; Lt-Col. RAMC TA. Specialty: Gen. Psychiat. Socs: Med. Soc. Lond.; (Pres.) N.ampton Med. Soc.; Yeoman Soc. of Apoth. Prev: Sen. Regist. (Psychiat.) Univ. Coll. Hosp. & Maudsley Hosp. Lond.; Research Sen. Regist. Univ. Coll. Hosp. & Hosp. Trop. Dis. Lond.; Regist. (Psychiat.) Univ. Coll. Hosp. Lond.

WILSON, Daniel Timothy Richardson Mill Stream Surgery, Mill Stream, Benson, Wallingford OX10 6RL Tel: 01491 838286; 2 Eyres Close, Ewelme, Wallingford OX10 6LA Tel: 01491 833556 — BM BS Nottm. 1986; MPhil Nottm. 1985, BMedSci 1984; DRCOG 1989; FRCGP 1995, M 1990; DCH RCP Lond. 1990. Prev: Trainee GP N. Lincs. HA VTS.

WILSON, David Blackthorn Surgery, 73 Station Road, Netley Abbey, Southampton SO31 5AE Tel: 023 8045 3110 Fax: 023 8045 2747 — MB ChB Bristol 1968; DObst RCOG 1970.

WILSON, David Bennett 30 Deramore Park S., Malone Road, Belfast BT9 5JY — MB BCh BAO Belf. 1971; DObst RCOG 1973; FFA RCSI 1977. Specialty: Anaesth.

WILSON, David Charles Department of Child Life and Health, University of Edinburgh, 20 Sylvan Place, Edinburgh EH9 1UW — MB BCh Belf. 1984; MB BCh (Hons.) Belf. 1984; DCH RCP Lond. 1986; MRCP (UK) 1987.

WILSON, David Colin 164 Peel Brow, Ramsbottom, Bury BL0 0AX — MB ChB Ed. 1994.

WILSON, David Harold Grove House Practice, St Pauls Health Centre, High St, Runcorn WA7 1AB Tel: 01928 566561 Fax: 01928 590212 — MRCS Eng. LRCP Lond. 1982. Specialty: Dermat. Prev: Trainee GP Halewood; SHO (A & E) Broadgreen Hosp.; Ho. Off. St. Helen's Hosp.

WILSON, Mr David Hedley (retired) Lower Ackhill, Presteigne LD8 2ED Tel: 01544 267456 Email: d.h.wilson@btinternet.com — (Leeds) MB ChB Leeds 1951; DTM Antwerp 1954; FRCS Ed. 1964; FRCS Eng. 1988; FFAEM 1993. Prev: Dean Postgrad. Med. Educat. Univ. Leeds & Hon. Cons. Surg. A & E Leeds Gen. Infirm.

WILSON, Professor David Ian — MB BS Newc. 1984; BA Oxf. 1981; MRCP (UK) 1987; PhD Newc. 1996. Prof. of Human Developm. Genetics, Soton. Univ., Soton.; Hon. Cons. in Clin. Genetics, Soton. Univ. Hosp. Trust. Specialty: Genetics. Socs: Brit. Soc. Human Genetics. Prev: MRC Clin. Scientist; Univ. of Newc.; Sen. Lect. (Med. Genetics) Dept. Human Genetics & Med. Univ. of Newc.

WILSON, Mr David Ian Burns Unit, City Hospital, Hucknall Road, Nottingham NG5 1PB Tel: 0115 969 1169 Fax: 0115 840 2601 Email: dwilson@ncht.trent.nhs.uk — MB BS Lond. 1985 (St. George's Hospital Medical School) FRCS Eng. 1990; FRCS (Plast.) 1998. Cons. Burns & plastic Surg. City Hosp. Notts. Specialty: Plastic Surg. Socs: Brit. Burn Assoc. & Europ. Burn Assoc.; Amer. Burn Assoc.; Brit. Assoc. of Plastic Surg.s. Prev: Regist. (Burns & Plastic Surg.) City Hosp. Nottm.; Regist. (Plastic Surg.) Leicester Roy.

Infirm.; SHO (Plastic Surg.) Sub-Regional Burns & Plastic Surg. Unit Plymouth.

WILSON, David Ian Talbot, MBE (retired) Quackers, Duck St., Child Okeford, Blandford Forum DT11 8ET Tel: 01258 861338 — MB ChB Ed. 1949; FRCGP 1980, M 1965. Med. Adviser Hall & WoodLa. Ltd. Prev: Chairm. Assn. GP Community Hosp. (Eng. & Wales).

WILSON, David John Nuffield Orthopaedic Centre, Windmill Road, Headington, Oxford OX3 7LD Fax: 01865 227347 Email: david.wilson@noc.anglox.nhs.uk — MB BS Lond. 1976 (King's Coll. Hosp.) BSc. (Human Physiol.) Lond. 1973; MRCP (UK) 1980; FRCR 1983; Hon. MA Oxf. 1985. Cons. Radiol. Nuffield Orthop. Centre & John Radcliffe Hosp. Oxf.; Sen. Clin. Lect. Univ. Oxf.; Deputy Edr. Clinical Radiol. Specialty: Radiol. Special Interest: Vertebroplasty, MSK ultrasound. Socs: Internat. Skeletal Soc.; British Medical Ultrasound Society; British Institute of Radiology. Prev: Regist. & Sen. Regist. (Diag. Radiol.) John Radcliffe Hosp. Oxf.; SHO (Gen. Med.) Good Hope Hosp. Sutton Coldfield & MusGr. Pk. Hosp. Taunton.

WILSON, David Livingstone (retired) Cornerstone, 11 St Micheal Drive, Helensburgh, Glasgow G84 7SF Tel: 01436 677933 — MB ChB Glas. 1948 (Univ. Glas.) DTM & H Liverp. 1951; DPH Durh. 1962; FFPHM RCP (UK) 1981, M 1974. Prev: Dist. Med. Off. Newc. HA.

WILSON, David Neill Rampton Hospital, Retford, Nottingham DN22 0PD Tel: 01777 247703 Fax: 01777 247737 Email: david.wilson2@nottshc.nhs.uk; Halam House, Halam, Newark, Nottingham NG22 8AG Tel: 01636 812177 Fax: 01636 812177 — MB BS Lond. 1970; LMSSA Lond. 1970; DPM Eng. 1978; FRCPsych 1993, M 1979. Cons. Psychiat. Specialty: Ment. Health. Prev: Sen. Lect. & Hon. Cons. Psychiat. Nottm. Univ.; Cons. Psychiat. (Ment. Handicap) Gloucester HA; Sen. Regist. Lea Hosp. BromsGr. & Lea Castle Hosp. Kidderminster.

WILSON, David Roy (retired) 75 Middlecave Road, Malton YO17 7NQ Tel: 01653 692207 — MB BS Lond. 1964 (Guy's) MRCS Eng. LRCP Lond. 1963; DObst RCOG 1965. Prev: Regist. (Neurol.) Pinderfields Gen. Hosp. Wakefield.

WILSON, David Tinsley (retired) 15 Meadow Grove, Crawfordsburn, Bangor BT19 1JL — LRCP LRCS Ed. 1946 (Qu. Univ. Belf.) LRCP LRCS Ed. LRFPS Glas. 1946.

WILSON, Deborah County Durham Health Authority, Appleton House, Lanchester Road, Durham DH1 5XZ — MB BS Newc. 1990; MSc (Pub. Health) Newc. 1995; MFPHM 1997. Cons.Pub.healthMed.Communical Dis.Centro 1 Co. Durh. health Auth. Specialty: Pub. Health Med.

WILSON, Deborah Margaret 24 St Clair Tarrace, Edinburgh EH10 5NW — MB ChB Ed. 1992.

WILSON, Derek (retired) Môr Isaf, Hardwicke, Hay-on-Wye, Hereford HR3 5HA Tel: 01497 831253 Fax: 01497 831599 — (Guy's) MB BS Lond. 1956; MRCS Eng. LRCP Lond. 1956; DObst RCOG 1960; FRCGP 1977, M 1968. Prev: GP Hay-on-Wye.

WILSON, Diana Frances St. Columba's Hospice, 15 Boswall Road, Edinburgh EH5 3RW Tel: 0131 551 1381 Fax: 0131 552 3955 — MB BS Lond. 1977 (St. Bart.) MRCS Eng LRCP Lond. 1977; MRCP (UK) 1981; FRCR 1985. Cons. Palliat. Med. St. Columba's Hospice Edin. Specialty: Palliat. Med. Prev: Cons. Palliat. Med. Winchester HA; Sen. Regist. St. Columba's Hospice Edin.

WILSON, Diane Margaret — MB BCh Belf. 1998. Specialty: Gen. Med.

WILSON, Dirk Guy — MB BCh Wales 1989. Cons. Paed.Cardiolog. Uni. Hosp. Wales, Cardiff. Specialty: Paediat.; Cardiol.

WILSON, Doreen Mary (retired) Clunch Cottage, Lodge Road, Feltwell, Thetford IP26 4DL — MB BS Lond. 1954 (St. Bart.) Prev: Ho. Surg., Ho. Phys. & Cas. Off. Norf. & Norwich Hosp.

WILSON, Douglas George 11 Garden Street, Padiham, Burnley BB12 8NP — MB ChB Manch. 1985.

WILSON, Douglas Scott MacGregor c/o The Practice Manager, The Queens Road Medical Practice, The Queens Road, St Peter Port, Guernsey GY1 1RH; Grange End Medical Practice, St. Peter Port, Guernsey — MB ChB Aberd. 1979; MRCGP 1984.

WILSON, Duncan Henry The Village Surgery, 24-28 Laughton Road, Thurcroft, Rotherham S66 9LP Tel: 01709 542216 Fax: 01709 702356 — MB ChB Manch. 1984; BSc (Med. Sci.) St. And. 1981. Prev: Trainee GP Preston Lancs.

WILSON, Duncan Robertson, Maj. RAMC Royal Brompton Hospital, Sydney St., London SW3 6NP; 11 Coldstream Gardens, Putney, London SW18 1LJ Tel: 020 8877 9553 — MB ChB Dundee 1989; MRCP (UK) 1994. Specialist Regist. Roy. Brompton Hosp. Lond. Specialty: Respirat. Med.; Gen. Med. Socs: Brit. Thorac. Soc. Prev: Specialist Regist. Frimley Pk. Hosp. Surrey; Specialist (Gen. Med.) Camb. Milt. Hosp. Aldershot; SHO (ICU) Roy. Brompton Hosp.

WILSON, Edward 29 Kirk Road, Newport-on-Tay DD6 8JD — MB ChB Glas. 1981; FFA RCSI 1987. Cons. Anaesth. Ninewells Hosp. Dundee. Specialty: Anaesth.

WILSON, Edward Adrian 23 Plymouth Road, Penarth CF64 3DA — MB ChB Manch. 1994.

WILSON, Edward Harold (retired) 67 Cwtr Sant Tudno, Llandudno LL30 1BZ Tel: 01492 874060 — MB ChB Liverp. 1946; MD Liverp. 1954. Prev: Cons. Phys. (Geriat) Lancaster & E. Cumbria Health Dists.

WILSON, Eileen Cuthbertson 8 Barnford Crescent, Alloway, Ayr KA7 4UP — MB ChB Glas. 1978.

WILSON, Eileen Margaret (retired) 2 Earlspark Drive, Bieldiside, Aberdeen AB15 9AH Tel: 01224 869279 — MB ChB Aberd. 1958; DA Eng. 1961. Prev: SCMO Tayside HB.

WILSON, Elaine Health Centre, Wardles Lane, Great Wyrley, Walsall WS6 6EW Tel: 01922 415515 — MB BS Lond. 1981; DRCOG 1985; MSc Community Paediat. Warwick 1992; DFFP 1993. Prev: SCMO M. Staffs. HA.

WILSON, Elaine Anne Epilepsy Research Unit, Western Infirmary, Glasgow G11 6NT Tel: 0141 211 1925 Fax: 0141 211 1925; 4 Fife Crescent, Bothwell, Glasgow G71 8DG — MB ChB Glas. 1988; MRCGP 1994. Assoc. Specialist, Epilepsy Research Unit (Med.) W.. Infirm. Glas.

WILSON, Eleanor Mary Clachbeo, Glenmore Road, Oban PA34 4NB — MB ChB Glas. 1976. Clin. Med. Off. Family Plann. Clinic, W. Highland Hosp. Oban. Prev: Regist. (O & G) Rutherglen Matern. Hosp. Glas.; SHO (Anaesth.) Stobhill Hosp. Glas.

WILSON, Elena Macnaught Groves Orchard, The Common, Chipperfield, Kings Langley WD4 9BY — MB BS Lond. 1990 (University College and The Middlesex London) BSc (Pharmacol.) Lond. 1987; MRCP (UK) 1993; FRCR 1998. Regist. (Clin. Oncol.) Mt. Vernon Hosp. Northwood Middlx. Specialty: Oncol. Prev: Regist. (Clin. Oncol.) Char. Cross Hosp. Lond.; SHO (Med.) The Whittington Hosp. Lond.

WILSON, Elizabeth Anne 46 Bryansglen Park, Bangor BT20 3RS — MB BCh BAO Belf. 1983.

WILSON, Elizabeth Anne Ringwood Health Centre, The Close, Ringwood BH24 1JY Tel: 01425 478901; 17 Shelley Close, Ashley Heath, Ringwood BH24 2JA — BM Soton. 1983; DRCOG 1993. Clin. Med. Off. (Family Plann.) Hants. Prev: Trainee GP Ringwood Health Centre; SHO (O & G), Princess Anne Hosp., Soton; SHO (A & E) & (Radiother. & Oncol.) Poole Hosp.

WILSON, Elizabeth Booth Galpins Road Surgery, 6 Galpins Road, Thornton Heath CR7 6EA Tel: 020 8684 3450 Fax: 202 8683 0439 — MB BChir Camb. 1962 (St. Geo.) MA, MB Camb. 1962, BChir 1961; DObst RCOG 1963. Socs: BMA. Prev: Ho. Phys. Croydon Gen. Hosp.; Ho. Surg. Vict. Hosp. Childr. Lond. & Mayday Hosp. Croydon.

WILSON, Elizabeth Jean University Hospital Lewisham, Department of Histopathology, Lewisham High Street, London SE13 6LH Tel: 020 8333 3000; 21 Parkside, Vanbrugh Fields, London SE3 7QQ — MB BS Lond. 1976 (Lond. Hosp.) BSc Lond. 1973; MRCP UK 1979; FRCR 1983. Specialist Regist. (Histopath.). Specialty: Histopath. Prev: Sen. Med. Off. DoH; Sen. Regist. (Radiother. & Oncol.) Lond. Hosp.; Regist. (Radiother. & Oncol.) Lond. Hosp.

WILSON, Elizabeth Margaret 12 Charter Approach, Warwick CV34 6AE — BM BS Nottm. 1996. SHO Med. Warwick Hosp. Specialty: Gen. Med.

WILSON, Elizabeth Marion 3 Little Heath Close, Audlem, Crewe CW3 0HX — MB ChB Manch. 1976; BSc St. And. 1973.

WILSON, Elizabeth Mora Joan 9 Lindisfarne Road, Jesmond, Newcastle upon Tyne NE2 2HE Tel: 0191 281 0398 — MB ChB Aberd. 1968; DObst RCOG 1970; Cert. Family Plann. JCC 1977; MFFP 1993. SCMO (Contracep. & Sexual Health), Gateshead

Primary Care Trust; Clin. Asst. (Colposcopy) Newc. u. Tyne & Gateshead HAs. Specialty: Pub. Health Med. Prev: GP Woking & Newc.; SHO (Gyn.) Roy. North. Hosp. Lond.; SHO (Obst.) City of Lond. Matern. Hosp.

WILSON, Mrs Elizabeth Stanfield Bell (retired) 11 Westbourne Gardens, Glasgow G12 9XD Tel: 0141 334 3287 Email: libby@ewilson.fsnet.co.uk — (King's Coll. Hosp.) MB BS Lond. 1949; MRCS Eng., LRCP Lond. 1949; FFFP 1993. Prev: Area Co-Ordinator Family Plann. Servs. (Incl. Domiciliary) Gtr. Glas. HB:.

WILSON, Elizabeth Sylvia 83 Carnbee Avenue, Liberton, Edinburgh EH16 6GA Email: libbyirishrover@hotmail.com — MB ChB Glas. 1988 (St And. & Glas.) BSc (Hons.) St. And. 1984; FRCS Glas 1992; FRCA Lond 1999. Cons., Roy. Infirm., Edin. Specialty: Anaesth. Prev: Specialist Regist. Western Infirm. Glas.; SHO III (Gen. Surg.) West. Infirm. Glas.; SHO Surg. Specialties Rotat. West. Infirm. Glas.

WILSON, Emma Georgina 66 Polwarth Ter, Edinburgh EH11 1NJ — MB ChB Birm. 1997.

***WILSON, Emma Jane** 10 Nea Road, Highcliffe, Christchurch BH23 4NA — MB ChB Manch. 1997; BSc St. And. 1994. Ho. Off. (Med.) N. Manch. Gen. Hosp. Prev: Ho. Off. (Surg.) Roy. Preston Hosp.

WILSON, Ena (retired) Holywood Road Surgery, 54 Holywood Road, Belfast BT4 1NT Tel: 028 9065 4668; The Shieling, 6 Old Dundonald Road, Belfast BT16 2EG — MB BCh BAO Belf. 1960. Hosp. Pract. (ENT) Ulster Hosp. Dundonald.

WILSON, Eoin David Shiplett Court Farm, Shiplate Road, Bleadon, Weston Super Mare BS24 0NY; Shiplett Court Farm, Shiplate Road, Bleadon, Weston Super Mare BS24 0NY — MB BS Lond. 1998 (University College and Meddlesex School fo Medicine) BSc Human Biol & Basic Med Scis, Lond, 1995. RMO1 A&E(ITU)Gen. Med., Hornsby, Ku-Ring-Gai Hosp., Sydney, NSW, Australia. Specialty: Accid. & Emerg.; Intens. Care; Gen. Med. Socs: MPS and BMA; BMA.

WILSON, Esther Kencia, Cocklebury Road, Chippenham SN15 3NS — MB ChB Liverp. 1996.

WILSON, Esther Teresa — MB ChB Aberd. 1983. Clin. Med. Off. (Family Plann.) Dundee. Specialty: Gen. Pract. Prev: GP Fraserburgh; Trainee GP Forresterhill & Peterhead; Clin. Asst. (Ment. Handicap) Ladysbridge Hosp. Banff.

WILSON, Ewen Hugh Charles 1/L, 52 White Street, Glasgow G11 5EA — MB ChB Glas. 1994.

WILSON, Fay Wand Medical Centre, 279 Gooch Street, Highgate, Birmingham B5 7JE Tel: 0121 440 1561 Fax: 0121 440 0060; 179 St. Andrews Road, Birmingham B9 4NB — MB ChB Birm. 1980 (Birmingham) DRCOG 1984; DCH RCP Lond. 1985; MRCGP 1986. Med. Dir. Badger GP Out of Hours Co-op. Specialty: Gen. Pract.

WILSON, Fiona Ann TIL, 19 Roxborough St., Glasgow G12 9AP — MB ChB Glas. 1998. PRHO Surg., Stobhill Trust, Glas. Prev: PRHO Med., Stirling Roy. Infirm.

WILSON, Fiona Margaret (retired) 14 Cammo Hill, Edinburgh EH4 8EY Tel: 0131 339 2244 — MB ChB Glas. 1955. Prev: Sen. Med. Off. (Community Ment. Health) Lothian HB.

WILSON, Fiona Munro Chertsey Lane Surgery, 5 Chertsey Lane, Staines TW18 3JH Tel: 01784 454164 Fax: 01784 440522 — MB ChB Birm. 1990.

WILSON, Frances Olwen (retired) Beulah, 7 Herevale Grange, Ellenbrook, Worsley, Manchester M28 1ZA Tel: 0161 799 3640 — MB ChB Birm. 1954. Prev: GP Manch.

WILSON, Francis William Govanhill Health Centre, 233 Calder Street, Glasgow G42 7DR Tel: 0141 531 8370 Fax: 0141 531 4431; 26 King's Park Avenue, Glasgow G44 4UP Tel: 0141 636 6836 — MB ChB Glas. 1962; DObst RCOG 1964; FRCGP 1985, M 1976. Socs: S.. Med. Soc. & Roy. M-C Soc. Glas. Prev: Assoc. Adviser Univ. Glas.; Hosp. Pract. Cowglen Hosp. Glas.; Ho. Phys. Glas. Roy. Infirm.

WILSON, Mr Frank Dudley Group of Hospitals NHS Trust, Russells Hall Hospital, Dudley DY1 2HU Tel: 01384 244168 Fax: 01384 244169 Email: mr.wilson@dgoh-tr.nhs.uk — MB BS Newc. 1971 (Newcastle) FRCS Edin. 1975; FRCS Lond. 1976. Cons. Otolaryngol. Dudley NHS Hosps. Trust & Roy. Wolverhampton Hosps. Trust; Regional Speciality Adviser in Otolaryngol. to W. Midlands. Specialty: Otolaryngol. Socs: Roy. Soc. Med.; Brit. Assoc. of Otolaryngol. & Head/Neck Surg. Prev: Sen. Regist. (Otolaryngol.) Univ. Hosp. Wales Cardiff; TWJ Clin. & Research Fell. Univ. Calif. San Francisco, USA.

WILSON, Frank David (retired) The Old Chapel, Kingsdon, Somerton TA11 7LN — (St. Thos.) MB BS Lond. 1956; MRCS Eng. LRCP Lond. 1956.

WILSON, Geoffrey David St Dunstan's Park Health Centre -, St Dunstan's Park, Melrose TD6 9RX Tel: 01896 822161 Fax: 01896 823151; Bridlewood, Fishers Lane, Darnick, Melrose TD6 9AS Tel: 0189682 3143 — MB ChB Ed. 1983; DRCOG 1987; MRCGP 1988. Prev: Trainee GP Northumbria VTS.

WILSON, Geoffrey Donald — (Oxf. & St. Thos.) MA Oxf. 1954, BM BCh 1952. Socs: BMA (late Chairm.); (late Pres.) E.bourne Med. Soc.; Fell. Roy. Soc. Med. Prev: Ho. Surg. & Ho. Phys. St. Mary's Hosp. E.bourne.

WILSON, Geoffrey Keith Greenshadows, Hancocks Mount, Ascot SL5 9PQ — MB ChB Birm. 1975.

WILSON, Mr Geoffrey Ross — MB BChir Camb. 1976 (St. Geos. Hosp.) BA Camb. 1973; MA Camb. 1977; FRCS Eng. 1981; FRCS (Plast) 1991. Cons. Plastic Surg., Reconstruc. & Hand Surg., Chelsea & Westm. Hosp., Lond.; Hon. Cons., Plastic Surg., St Georges Hosp., Lond.; Hon. Cons., Plastic Surg., Epsom Gen. Hosp., Epsom. Specialty: Plastic Surg. Special Interest: Hand Surg. Socs: Brit. Assn. of Plastic Surg.; Brit. Assn. of Aesthetic Plastic Surg.

WILSON, George (retired) 50 Rowallan Drive, Kilmarnock KA3 1TU Tel: 01563 24892 — MB ChB Glas. 1950; DA Eng. 1957. Prev: Cons. (Anaesth.) Ayrsh. & Arran Health Bd.

WILSON, George Martin 39 Carnreagh, Hillsborough BT26 6LJ — MB BCh BAO Belf. 1976; DRCOG 1978; MRCGP 1981.

WILSON, George Morrison The Surgery, School Lane, Upton-upon-Severn, Worcester WR8 0LF Tel: 01684 592696 Fax: 01684 593122; Buryfield, School Lane, Upton on Severn, Worcester WR8 0LD Tel: 01684 592390 — (St. And.) MB ChB St. And. 1964. Specialty: Accid. & Emerg. Prev: SHO Radcliffe Infirm. & Nuffield Orthop. Centre Oxf.; Demonst. (Anat.) Univ. St. And.; Ho. Surg. & Ho. Phys. Dundee Roy. Infirm.

WILSON, George Stephen (retired) 1 Gorse Road, Blackburn BB2 6LY Tel: 01254 56664 — MB ChB Liverp. 1955. Prev: Assoc. Specialist (Genitourin. Med.) Bolton & Wigan AHAs.

WILSON, Georgina Harriette Mary 199 Victoria Rise, London SW4 0PF — MB BS Lond. 1995.

WILSON, Gerald Anthony 58 Priory Park, Belfast BT10 0AE Tel: 01232 627478 — MB BCh BAO Belf. 1992; DGM RCPS Glas. 1994; DRCOG 1995; MRCGP 1996. Specialty: Gen. Pract. Socs: BMA.

WILSON, Gerald Kingsley (retired) 32 St David's Road, Otley LS21 2AW Tel: 01943 464988 — MB BS Durh. 1957; MB BS Durh., 1957; DPhysMed Eng. 1972. GP S. Shields. Prev: Med. Regist. Bradford Gp. Hosps.

WILSON, Gillian Elizabeth Royal Cornhill Hospital, Young People's Department, Garden Villa, Aberdeen AB25 2ZH Tel: 01224 557268 — MB ChB Glas. 1974; MRCPsych 1978; Dip. Psychother. Aberd. 1981. Cons. Adolesc. Psychiat. NHS Grampian. Specialty: Child & Adolesc. Psychiat.

WILSON, Gillian Mary (retired) Dewsbury District Hospital, Healds Road, Dewsbury WF13 4HS Tel: 01924 512000 Fax: 01924 512025; 77 High St, Thornhill Edge, Dewsbury WF12 0PS Tel: 01603 250662/01924 455082 Fax: 01603 250662 Email: alaeddinhatoum@hotmail.com — (St. Mary's) MRCS Eng. LRCP Lond. 1965; FRCPCH 1997; MRCP (UK) 1972; FRCP 1988. Cons. (Paediat.) Dewsbury Health Dist., Dewsbury. Prev: Sen. Regist. (Paediat. & Developm. Med.) Northampton Health Dist.

WILSON, Gillian Sara The Scancentre, 277 Dunhill Road, Coleraine BT51 3QT Tel: 028 70321234 — MB ChB Sheff. 1989; MRCGP 1994. Clin. Director The Scan Centre, Coleraine. Specialty: Gen. Pract. Prev: GP Retainer in Med. Centre in Portrush.

WILSON, Gillian Susan Lizbeth Northgate Surgery, Northgate, Pontefract WF8 1NG Tel: 01977 703635 Fax: 01977 702562; 3 The Coppice, Sherburn-in-Elmet, Leeds LS25 6LU Tel: 01977 685412 Fax: 01977 684804 Email: atulpatel@supanet.com — MB ChB Bristol 1983; BSc Bristol 1980; DA (UK) 1985; Cert. Family Plann. JCC 1988; DRCOG 1988. Princip. GP. Dr. J.R.Waring & Partners, Pontefract. Specialty: Gen. Pract.; Genitourinary Medicine. Socs: Local Med. Comm. -Nominee on.; Area Child Protec. Comm. Prev: GP Princip., Allerton Bywater, Castleford, Yorks; Retainer GP,

N.gate Surg., Pontefract; Trainee GP Rawtenstall Health Centre Rossendale.

WILSON, Glenys Ruth Worcester Street Surgery, 24 Worcester Street, Stourbridge DY8 1AW Tel: 01384 371616; Rokeby, 62 Worcester Road, Hagley, Stourbridge DY9 0LD — MB BS Lond. 1987. Specialty: Family Plann. & Reproduc. Health.

WILSON, Godfrey Everett Department of Histopathology/Cytopathology, 1st Floor, Clinical Sciences Building, Manchester Royal Infirmary, Manchester M13 9WL Tel: 0161 276 8812 Email: godfrey.wilson@cmmc.nhs.uk — MB BCh BAO Dub. 1982 (TC Dub.) MRCPath 1992. Cons. Histopath. Centr. Manch. Healthcare Trust. Specialty: Histopath.

WILSON, Graeme Bond Flat 1, 1 Highbury Road, Manchester M16 8PT — MB ChB Leeds 1994.

WILSON, Graeme Eric Newham General Hospital, Plaistow, London E13 8SL — MB BCh Wales 1988 (UWCM) MRCP (UK) 1992. Cons., Newham Healthcare Trust, Lond. Specialty: Respirat. Med. Socs: Brit. Thoracic Soc. Prev: Regist. (Respirat.) Cardiothoracic Centre Liverp.; Sen. Regist. (Respirat.) Guy's & St. Thos. Hosp. Lond.; Hon. S.R., Roy. Brompton.

WILSON, Graham Allan Maclean 4 St Martins Avenue, Otley LS21 2AN — MB ChB Ed. 1991; FRCA 1996. Specialty: Anaesth.

WILSON, Graham Black Caldicot Medical Group, Gray Hill Surgery, Woodstock Way, Caldicot, Newport NP26 4DB Tel: 01291 420282 Fax: 01291 425853; 6 Queens Gardens, Magor, Newport — MB BCh Wales 1979; MRCGP 1983.

WILSON, Graham Martin Ramsey Group Practice Centre, Grove Mount South, Ramsey IM8 3EY Tel: 01624 813881 Fax: 01624 811921; Ben Gairn, Lheaney Road, Ramsey IM8 2JF — MRCS Eng. LRCP Lond. 1977 (St. Mary's) BSc (Hons.) Lond. 1974, MB BS 1977; DRCOG Lond. 1980; MRCGP 1981.

WILSON, Graham Miller St Catherine's Surgery, St Pauls Medical Centre, 121 Swindon Road, Cheltenham GL50 4DP Tel: 01242 580668 Fax: 01242 707699 — MB ChB Birm. 1984; MRCP (UK) 1987; MRCGP 1990.

WILSON, Guy (retired) Woodlands, 15 Pear Tree Lane, Maidstone ME15 9QY Tel: 01622 744660 — (Guy's) LMSSA Lond. 1934.

WILSON, Harold (retired) 1 ErringtonCt., Alma Road, Aigburth, Liverpool L17 6DP Tel: 0151 427 0275 — (Liverp.) MB ChB Liverp. 1950; PhD Liverp. 1955, MD 1959. Prev: Sen. Lect. (Pharmacol.) Univ. Liverp.

WILSON, Harry (retired) Ling House, 130 Skipton Road, Keighley BD21 3AN Tel: 01535 605747; Morningside, St. Mary's Road, Riddlesden, Keighley BD20 5PA — MB ChB Sheff. 1959. Prev: Ho. Surg. O & G Vict. & St. John's Hosps. Keighley.

WILSON, Hayley Jo Anne 244 Goodyersend Lane, Bedworth, Nuneaton CV12 0HM — MB ChB Bristol 1992.

WILSON, Hazel Mary 18 Eastern Way, Elmswell, Bury St Edmunds IP30 9DP — MRCS Eng. LRCP Lond. 1954; DCH Eng. 1959; DTM & H Liverp. 1961.

WILSON, Heather Norah University Health Service, University of Southampton, Building 48, Southampton SO17 1BJ Tel: 023 8055 7531 Fax: 023 8059 3259; Oakdene, 16 Brookvale Road, Highfield, Southampton SO17 1QP Tel: 02380 584681 — MB BS Lond. 1979 (Char. Cross) DRCOG 1983; FRCA Eng. 1984; MRCGP 1988. Specialty: Gen. Pract. Socs: BMA. Prev: Trainee GP Soton.; Regist. (Anaesth.) Bristol HA.

WILSON, Herbert Martin The Byre, Stonehouse Farm, Main St., Carlton, Nuneaton CV13 0AG — MB ChB Leic. 1980; BSc (Hons.) Manch. 1974.

WILSON, Herbert William (retired) 43 Bamford Way, Bamford, Rochdale OL11 5NB Tel: 01706 640991 — MB ChB Manch. 1947; FRCOG 1968, M 1954, DObst 1951. Prev: Cons. O & G Bury Dist. HA.

WILSON, Hilary (retired) 1 Golf Links Crescent, Newcastle BT33 0BE Tel: 01396 724029 — MB BCh BAO Belf. 1940; MB BCh BAO (Hnrs.) Belf. 1940. Prev: Med. Asst. West. Special Care Serv. Londonderry.

WILSON, Hilary Elaine Centre for Rheumatic Diseases, Royal Infirmary, Glasgow G4 0SF; 11 Falkland Street, 1/L, Hyndland, Glasgow G12 9PY Tel: 0141 339 3396 Email: hilary@jings.com — MB ChB Glas. 1991. Clin. Research Fell. Specialty: Rheumatol. Socs: Brit. Med. Acupunc. Soc.; Roy. Coll. of Phys.s, Glas.; Brit. Soc. Rheum.

WILSON, Hilda Mary (retired) 56 Castle Grove Avenue, Leeds LS6 4BS Tel: 0113 275 2494 — MB ChB Leeds 1952. Prev: Sen. Med. Off. (Child Health) Leeds E. HA.

WILSON, Hugo Oliver 25 Harwood Close, Tewin, Welwyn AL6 0LF — MB BS Lond. 1997.

WILSON, Iain Henry Royal Devon and Exeter Hospital, Exeter EX2 5DW — MB ChB Glas. 1978; FFA RCS Eng. 1983. Cons. Anaesth. Roy. Devon & Exeter Hosp. Specialty: Anaesth. Prev: Lect. (Anaesth.) Lusaka, Zambia.

WILSON, Ian Wolverhampton Road Surgery, 13 Wolverhampton Road, Stafford ST17 4BP Tel: 01785 258161 Fax: 01785 224140 — MB ChB Birm. 1973. Med. Pract. (Gastroenterol. Endoscopy) Mid Staffs. HA. Specialty: Gastroenterol. Socs: Midl. Gastroenterol. Soc.; Primary Care Soc. Gastroenterol.

WILSON, Mr Ian Clark Queen Elizabeth Hospital, Edgbaston, Birmingham B15 2TH Tel: 0121 697 8309 Fax: 0121 697 8329 Email: ian.c.wilson@uhb.nhs.uk; University Hospital Birmingham NHS Trust, Queen Elizabeth Hospital, Edgbaston, Birmingham B15 2TH Tel: 0121 697 8309 — MB ChB Birm. 1982; FRCS Lond. 1987; FRCS Ed. 1987; FRCS (CTh) 1994; MD Birm. 1995. Cons. Cardiothoracic Surg. Qu. Eliz. Hosp. Birm.; Cons. Cardiothoracic Surg., Priory Hosp., Edgbaston, Birm. Specialty: Cardiothoracic Surg. Special Interest: Coronary Artery Revascularisation; Valve Repair. Socs: Soc. Cardiothoracic Surg. of GB & Irel.; Internat. Soc. Heart & Lung Transpl. Prev: Research Fell. Johns Hopkins Hosp. Baltimore, USA; Transpl. Fell. (Cardiothoracic Surg.) Freeman Hosp. Newc.; Sen. Regist. (Cardiothoracic Surg.) W. Midl.

WILSON, Ian David 16 Corrie Court, Hamilton ML3 9XE — MB ChB Glas. 1991; FRCS 1997. Specialty: Urol.

WILSON, Ian David 9 Maxwell Road, London SW6 2HT — MB ChB Cape Town 1985.

WILSON, Ian Donald Cwrt-y-Cadno, Plwmp, Llandysul SA44 6HL — MB BS Lond. 1972; MRCS Eng. LRCP Lond. 1972; MRCPsych 1977.

WILSON, Ian Douglas (retired) Clova, 2 Lynwood Drive, Stalmine, Poulton-le-Fylde FY6 0PZ Tel: 01253 701282 — MB ChB St. And. 1955. Prev: Med. Off. DSS Blackpool.

WILSON, Ian George Department of Anaesthesia, St. James University Hospital, Leeds LS9 7TF Tel: 0113 243 3144 — MB ChB Dundee 1979; DRCOG 1982; DA (UK) 1984; FFARCS Eng. 1988. Cons. Paediat. Anaesth. St. Jas. Univ. Hosp. Leeds.; Lead Clinician Anaesth. Specialty: Anaesth. Prev: Lect. & Sen. Regist. (Anaesth.) Leicester; Trainee GP Airdrie VTS & Hawick VTS; SHO & Regist. (Anaesth.) Derbysh. Hosps.

WILSON, Ian John Pawaroo and Partners, The Old Forge Surgery, Pallion Pk, Sunderland SR4 6QE Tel: 0191 510 9393 Fax: 0191 510 9595 — MB ChB Leeds 1984.

WILSON, Ian Martin Shotfield Health Centre, Shotfield, Wallington SM6 0HY Tel: 020 8647 0031; 2A Court Hill, Chipstead, Croydon CR5 3NQ — MB BS Lond. 1980.

WILSON, Ian Robert Pain Management Service, Dewsbury & District Hospital, Halifax Rd, Dewsbury WF13 4HS Tel: 01924 512 058 — MB BS Newc. 1991; FRCA 1998; PG Dip 2001. Cons. in Pain Managem. & Anaesth.; Assn. Anaesth. GB & Irel. Specialty: Anaesth. Socs: BMA (Counc. Mem. & Pain Soc.); CCSC Member Chair Organisation Committee. Prev: SHO (Anaesth.) Hope Hosp. & N. Manch. Gen. Hosp.; SHO (Anaesth.) Roy. Oldham NHS Trust; SpR (Anaesth.) Yorks. Deanery.

WILSON, Ian Stuart Guardian Street Medical Centre, Guardian Street, Warrington WA5 1UD Tel: 01925 650226 Fax: 01925 240633; 15 Francis Road, Stockton Heath, Warrington WA4 6EB — MB ChB Manch. 1981; DRCOG 1984.

WILSON, Isabel Claire Welsh hearing Institute, Heath Hospital, Cardiff Tel: 029 2074 3471 — MB BCh Wales 1991; FRCS (Orl.) Eng. 1996; MSc (Audiological Med.) UCL 1999. Specialist Regist. (Audiol. & Med.) Univ. Hosp. Wales. Specialty: Audiol. Med. Socs: BMA. Prev: SHO (ENT) Roy. Gwent Hosp.; SHO ENT St Michaels Hosp. Bristol.

WILSON, Isabel Lilias (retired) 7 Ben Nevis Place, Kirkcaldy KY2 5RQ — MB ChB St. And. 1957; MRC Schol. 1958-59; MB ChB (Commend.) St. And. 1957, DPH 1960. Prev: SCMO Fife Health Bd.

WILSON, Isobel Margaret Morningside Medical Practice, 2 Morningside Place, Edinburgh EH10 5ER Tel: 0131 452 8406 Fax: 0131 447 3020; 100 Morningside Drive, Edinburgh EH10 5NT Tel:

0131 447 1653 — MB ChB Ed. 1976; BSc (Med. Sci.) Ed. 1973. GP; Med. Off. Geo. Watson's Coll. Edin. Specialty: Paediat.; Obst. & Gyn.; Diabetes. Socs: BMA. Prev: SHO (Paediat.) Roy. Hosp. Sick Childr. Edin.; SHO (Obst.) Elsie Inglis Matern. Hosp. Edin.; SHO (Cas.) Roy. Infirm. Edin.

WILSON, Ivor Vivian (retired) Anglers Lodge, Cliff Road, Hythe CT21 5XH Tel: 01303 268360 — (Newc.) MB BS Durh. 1951; FRCP Lond. 1974, M 1958. Prev: Cons. Phys. & Clin. Tutor SE Kent HA.

WILSON, Ivy Josephine Ama — BM BS Nottm. 1998.

WILSON, James (retired) 15 Campbell Road, Edinburgh EH12 6DT Tel: 0131 337 6763 — MB ChB Ed. 1952; DObst RCOG 1956; BChir FFA RCS Eng. 1967. Cons. Anaesth. Roy. Infirm. Edin. Prev: Cons. Anaesth. Leeds Matern. Hosp. & United Leeds Hosps.

WILSON, James Campbell (retired) 10 Widewell Road, Roborough, Plymouth PL6 7DN Tel: 01752 787299 Fax: 01752 787299 — MB BCh BAO NUI 1952; DTM & H Eng. 1967; DCH Eng. 1968; MRCP (UK) 1970; FRCP Lond. 1983.

WILSON, James Harold Epsom General Hospital, Dorking Road, Epsom KT18 7EG Tel: 01372 204195 Fax: 01372 204199 — MB ChB Bristol 1972; MRCPsych 1980. Cons. Psychother. Surrey Oaklands NHS Trust. Specialty: Psychother. Socs: Assoc. Mem. Lond. Centre for Psychother.; Inst. Gp. Anal. Prev: Cons. Psychother. Henderson Hosp. & Sutton Hosp.; Sen. Regist. (Psychother.) Henderson Hosp. & St. Geo. Hosp. Lond.; Regist. & Sen. Regist. (Psychiat.) Bethlem & Maudsley Hosp. Lond.

WILSON, Mr James Hubbard 101 Woodsford Square, London W14 8DT — MB BS Lond. 1985; FRCS Eng. 1991. Specialty: Orthop.

WILSON, James Maxwell Glover (retired) Millhill House, 77 Millhill, Musselburgh EH21 7RP Tel: 0131 665 5829 — MB BChir Camb. 1938 (Camb. & Univ. Coll. Hosp.) MRCS Eng. LRCP Lond. 1937; FRCP Lond. 1966, M. 1947; FFPHM 1972; FRCP Ed. 1981. Prev: Sen. PMO DHSS.

WILSON, James Moffett Templemore Avenue Health Centre, 98A Templemore Avenue, Belfast BT5 4GR Tel: 028 9020 4151; 18 Hampton Park, Belfast BT7 3JL — MB BCh BAO Belf. 1980; DRCOG 1983; MRCGP 1985.

WILSON, Mr James Noel, OBE (retired) The Chequers, Waterdale, Watford WD25 0GP Tel: 01923 672364 — (Birm.) MB ChB (Hons.) Birm. 1943; MRCS Eng. LRCP Lond. 1943; FRCS Eng. 1948; ChM Birm. 1949. Hon. Cons. Orthop. Surg. Roy. Nat. Orthop. Hosp. Lond. & Nat. Hosps. Nerv. Dis. Qu. Sq. & Maida Vale; Vice-Chairm. IMPACT (UK). Prev: Prof. Orthop. Addis Ababa Univ. 1989.

WILSON, James Richard Maughan Red House, Rectory La, Hethel, Norwich NR14 8HD — MB ChB Bristol 1997.

WILSON, Mr James Russell Department of Urology, York District Hospital, Wigginton Road, York YO31 Tel: 01904 631313 — MB ChB Sheff. 1992 (Sheffield) FRCS Glas. 1997; MD Sheffield 2000. Specialist Regist. (Urol.) York Dist. Hosp. York. Specialty: Urol. Prev: Specialist Regist. (Urol.) Bradford Roy. Infirm., Bradford.

WILSON, Jane Gillian (retired) 2 Brettenham Crescent, Ipswich IP4 2UB — (Roy. Free) MB BS Lond. 1956; MRCS Eng. LRCP Lond. 1956; DCH Eng. 1959; BA Hons. Open Univ. 1990.

WILSON, Jane Karen 250 Sandycombe Road, Kew, Richmond TW9 3NP — MB BS Lond. 1982 (St. Thos. Univ. Lond.) FRCOG 1988; MD Lond. 1992. Cons. O & G Kingston Hosp. NHS Trust. Specialty: Obst. & Gyn. Prev: Sen. Regist. (O & G) Qu. Charlotte's & Chelsea Hosp. Lond.; Regist. (O & G) Guys Hosp. Lond. & Roy. Co. Hosp. Brighton.

WILSON, Jane Margaret 33 Hartington Grove, Cambridge CB1 7UA Tel: 01223 241587 Email: wilson.howarth@virgin.net — BM Soton. 1985; BSc Plymouth 1975; MSc Oxf. 1979; DCH RCP Lond. 1992; DCCH RCP Ed. 1992; DFFP 2001. GP Non-Princip.; Clinical Medical Officer Family Planning; Trainer Register of Engineers for Disaster Relief. Specialty: Trop. Med.; Gen. Pract. Socs: Fell. Roy. Soc. Trop. Med. & Hyg.; Brit. Travel Health Assn. Member; International Society of Travel Medicine. Prev: Med. Assoc. AVSC Internat., Nepal; Health Adviser Water Aids, ASIA; Trainee GP Camb.

WILSON, Professor Janet Ann Department of Otolaryngology Head & Neck Surgery, Freeman Hospital, Newcastle upon Tyne NE7 7DN Tel: 0191 284 3111 Fax: 0191 223 1246 Email: janet.wilson@nuth.northy.nhs.uk; Oak House, 1 Jesmond Dene Road, Newcastle upon Tyne NE2 3QJ — MB ChB Ed. 1979; FRCS Ed. 1983; FRCS Eng. 1984; BSc Ed. 1976, MD 1989; T(S) 1991. Prof. Otolaryngol. Head & Neck Surg. Univ. Newc. u. Tyne; Hon. Cons. Otolaryngol. Freeman Hosp. Newc. Specialty: Otorhinolaryngol.; Otolaryngol. Socs: Roy. Soc. Med.; Brit. Assn. Otol.; Head and Neck Surgs. Prev: Cons. Otorhinolaryng. Roy. Infirm. Glas.; Lect. (Otolaryngol.) Roy. Infirm. Edin.

WILSON, Janet Diane Leeds General Infirmary, Department of Genitourinary Medicine, Great George Street, Leeds LS1 3EX; 66 Main Street, Thorner, Leeds LS14 3BU — MB ChB Bristol 1980; MRCP (UK) 1983; FRCP Lond. 1994. Cons. Genitourin. Med. Gen. Infirm. Leeds. Specialty: Genitourinary Medicine.

WILSON, Janet Elizabeth 4 Grand Prix Grove, Dundonald, Belfast BT16 2BD — MB ChB Ed. 1991.

WILSON, Janet Margaret Tamnaharrie, 41 Ballyhanwood Road, Dundonald, Belfast BT5 7SN — MB BCh BAO Belf. 1979; DRCOG 1981; MRCOG 1984; MFFP 1993. Clin. Med. Off. E. Health & Social Servs. Bd.; Sen. Clin. Med. Off. Colposcopy Clinic Roy. Vict. Hosp. Belf.; Clin. Asst. (Genitourin. Med.) Roy. Vict. Hosp. Belf. Specialty: Obst. & Gyn.

WILSON, Janie Margaret Cantilupe Surgery, 51 St Owen St., Hereford HR1 2JB — MB ChB Birm. 1979; DRCOG 1983; MRCGP 1985; DFFP 1997.

WILSON, Jaqueline Ann St Johns Medical Centre, 62 London Rd, Grantham NG31 6HR Tel: 01476 590055; Chestnut House, 4 Manor Drive, Long Bennington, Newark NG23 5GZ Tel: 01400 282335 Fax: 01400 282335 — BM BS Nottingham 1988; DRCOG 1991. GP.

WILSON, Jason Alexander Dept of Anaesthetics, Charing Cross Hospital, Fulham palace Road, London W6 8RF Tel: 020 8846 7017 — MB BS (Hons. I) Sydney 1986; FRCA 1994. Cons. Anaesth. Char. Cross Hosp. Lond; Hon. Sen. Lect., Imperial Coll. Med. Sch. Lond. Specialty: Anaesth.

WILSON, Jean Freda 27 Marton Road, Bridlington YO16 7AQ Tel: 01262 73578 — MRCS Eng. LRCP Lond. 1939; BA Camb. 1936, MB BChir 1940; DObst RCOG 1941; DPH Leeds 1942.

WILSON, Jean Margaret (retired) Pond Cottage, Hoxne, Eye IP21 4LZ — MRCS Eng. LRCP Lond. 1945; MB BS Lond. 1946.

WILSON, Jean Sandra Nicol Street Surgery, 48 Nicol Street, Kirkcaldy KY1 1PH Tel: 01592 642969 Fax: 01592 643526 — MB ChB Ed. 1985; DRCOG 1987; MRCGP 1990.

WILSON, Jeanie Livingston Darling (retired) 27 Gogo Street, Largs KA30 8BU Tel: 01475 672238 — MB ChB Glas. 1921. Prev: Ho. Surg. W. Norf. Hosp. King's Lynn & Roy. Infirm. Glas.

WILSON, Jennifer Jane Morris and Partners, 93 Queens Drive, Bedford MK41 9JE Tel: 01234 360482 Fax: 01234 219361; 2 Cornwall Road, Bedford MK40 3DH Tel: 01234 356644 Email: andy.jenny@tesco.net — MB ChB Leeds 1986; DRCOG 1989; DTM & H Liverp. 1990; MRCGP 1990. Prev: Miss. with Baptist Miss. Soc.; Trainee GP Bradford VTS.

WILSON, Jeremy Ian 144 Howard Road, Leicester LE2 1XJ Tel: 0116 270 0825 — MB ChB Leic. 1998. Specialty: Diabetes. Prev: PRMO Surg. Walscrane NHS Trust Aug 98 - Feb99; PRMO Med. Leisester Gen. Hos. Feb99-Aug99.

WILSON, Mr Jeremy Paul 2, West Hill Lane, Budleigh Salterton EX9 6AA Tel: 01395 443302 Email: hipjpw@aol.com — (Middlx.) MB Camb. 1958, BChir 1957; MA Camb. 1958; FRCS Eng. 1963; BA (Hons) York. 1996; MA Soton 1997. Socs: Fell. Roy. Soc. Med. (Ex-Mem. Counc. Sect. Coloproctol.)

WILSON, Jillian Elizabeth Summervale Medical Centre, Wharf Lane, Ilminster TA19 0DT Tel: 01460 52354 Fax: 01460 52652; Ilford Bridges Farm, Stoklinch, Ilminster TA19 9HZ Tel: 01460 259266 — MB Camb. 1985 (Cambridge and St Thomas' London) BChir Camb. 1984; DRCOG 1987; MRCGP 1988. GP Princip.

WILSON, Joan 7 Cumnor Rise Road, Cumnor Hill, Oxford OX2 9HD Tel: 01865 862521; 2 Warblers Close, Constantia, Cape Town 7806, South Africa Tel: 0027 21 794 7984 Fax: 0027 21 794 3331 — MB BS Lond. 1969 (University of London) Paediat. Pract., Cape Town, S. Africa. Specialty: Paediat. Prev: Cons. Paediat., J.G. Stiijdon Hosp., Johannesburg; Regist. Paediat., J.G. Stiijdon Hosp., Johannesburg; Regist. Paediat., Red Cross Childr.'s Hosp. Cape Town.

WILSON, Joan Mowbray (retired) 16 Larchfield, Colquhoun Street, Helensburgh G84 9JG Tel: 01436 676393 — MB ChB Ed.

1949 (Edinburgh) MRCGP 1969. Prev: Assoc. Specialist (Genitourin. Med.) Roy. Infirm. Glas.

WILSON, Joanne Clare Culduthel Road Health Centre, Ardlarich, 15 Culduthel Road, Inverness IV2 4AG Tel: 01463 712233 Fax: 01463 715479; Tanela More, 45 Henrietta St, Avoch IV9 8QT Tel: 01381 620279 — MB ChB Liverp. 1991 (Liverpool) DRCOG; MRCGP. GP Job Sharing Princip. Specialty: Gen. Pract. Socs: BMA.

WILSON, Jocelyn Ann The Hildenborough Medical Group, Westwood, Tonbridge Road, Hildenborough, Tonbridge TN11 9HL — MB BS Lond. 1983 (Univ. Coll. Hosp.) BSc Lond. 1980, MB BS 1983; DRCOG 1986; MRCGP 1987. GP Dartford. Prev: Trainee GP Qu. Marys Hosp. Sidcup.

WILSON, John (retired) Belair, 2 Cable Road, Whitehead, Carrickfergus BT38 9PX Tel: 01960 373458 — MB BCh BAO Belf. 1956; FRCGP 1982, M 1968. Prev: GP Carrickfergus.

WILSON, John (retired) 8 Hunter Road, London SW20 8NZ Tel: 020 8946 8103 — MB BS Durh. 1956; BSc (Hons.) Durham. 1953; MB BS (Hons.) 1956; FRCP Lond. 1972, M 1958; PhD Lond. 1965; FRCPCH 1997. Prev: Hon. Cons.Paediat. Neurol. Gt. Ormond St. Childr. Hosp. NHS Trust Lond.

WILSON, John Alasdair Victoria Hospital, Hayfield Road, Kirkcaldy KY2 5AH Tel: 01592 643355 Fax: 01592 648049 Email: ja.wilson@faht.scot.nhs.uk; Capelrig, Station Road, Kingskettle, Cupar KY15 7PX Tel: 01337 831262 Fax: 01592 648049 Email: wilson.capelrig@virgin.net — MB ChB Ed. 1974; MRCP (UK) 1979; MD Ed. 1988; FRCP Ed. 1990. Cons. Phys. (Gen. Med. & Gastroenterol.) Vict. Hosp. Kirkcaldy; Hon. Sen. Lect. (Biol. & Preclin Med.) Univ. St. And.; Univ. Clin. Teach. (Med.) Univ. Manch.; Mem. Clin. Teach. Staff (Fac. Med. Univ. Edin.). Specialty: Gastroenterol. Socs: Brit. Soc. Gastroenterol.; Scott. Soc. Phys.; Scottish Soc. Gastroenterol. Prev: Sen. Regist. (Gen. Med.) Ninewells Hosp. Dundee; Clin. Research Fell. McMaster Univ. Canada; Lect. (Clin. Pharmacol.) Univ. Dundee.

WILSON, John Allan 1 Forbes Road, Edinburgh EH10 4EF Tel: 0131 229 3786 — MB ChB Dundee 1980; DRCOG 1982; MRCP UK 1985; FRCP Ed. 1995. Cons. Phys. Gen. & Geriat. Med. St. John's Hosp. Livingston.; Cons. Phys. Gen. Med. BUPA Murrayfield Hosp. Edin. Specialty: Gen. Med. Socs: Mem. Intercollegiate Acad. Bd. of Sports and Exercise Med..; Locality co-ordinator diploma exam in sports and exercise Med..; Fell. and Examr. Roy. Coll. of Phys.s of Edin.. Prev: Cons. Phys. Gen. & Geriat. Med. Bangour Gen. Hosp. Broxburn; Sen. Regist. (Geriat. & Gen. Med.) City Hosp. Edin.; Regist. (Geriat. Med.) City Hosp. Edin.

WILSON, John Andrew 34 West Mill Rise, Walkington, Beverley HU17 8TP — MB ChB Leeds 1979; BSc (Hons.) (Anat.) Leeds 1976; Dip. Bact. Manch. 1984; MRCPath 1986. Cons. Med. Microbiol. Pub. Health Laborat. Hull Roy. Infirm. Specialty: Med. Microbiol. Prev: Sen. Regist. Stoke Pub. Health Laborat.; Regist. Newc. Pub. Health Laborat.

WILSON, John Anthony Clark (retired) 7 Herevale Grange, Ellenbrook, Worsley, Manchester M28 1ZA Tel: 0161 799 3640 — MB ChB Ed. 1941; FRCP Ed. 1971, M 1950; FRCP Lond. 1973, M 1952. Prev: Hon. Cons. Phys. Hope Hosp. Salford & Salford Roy. Hosp.

WILSON, John Atkinson (retired) 42 Childwall Park Avenue, Liverpool L16 0JQ Tel: 0151 722 2952 — MD Liverp. 1967; MB ChB 1958; FRCP Lond. 1974, M 1962. Prev: Cons. Phys. Roy. Liverp. Hosp.

WILSON, John Beattie (retired) The Whins, Kinnel Banks, Lochmaben, Lockerbie DG11 1TD Tel: 01387 810679 — MB ChB Ed. 1943; BSc (Hons. Path.) Ed. 1948, MD 1949; FRCP Ed. 1971, M 1949. Prev: Mem. Dumfries & Galloway HB 1976-1987.

WILSON, John Briddon (retired) Lovaine, Vendace Drive, Lochmaben, Lockerbie DG11 1QN Tel: 01387 810598 Email: j7aw@easicom.com — (Ed.) MB ChB Ed. 1964; MRCP (U.K.) 1971; FRCP Ed. 1982. Locum. Prev: Cons. Geriat. Dumfries & Galloway Roy. Infirm.

WILSON, John Campbell Grove Farm, 173 Dromore Road, Hillsborough BT26 6JA — MB BS Lond. 1996.

WILSON, John David (retired) 52 Jensen Road, Bracebridge Heath, Lincoln LN4 2QU Tel: 01522 524944 — MB ChB Manch. 1958; DPM Eng. 1963; MRCPsych 1984. Prev: Cons. Psychiat. Cheadle Roy. Hosp.

WILSON, John Fairlie Selkirk Health Centre, Viewfield Lane, Selkirk TD7 4LJ Tel: 01750 21674 Fax: 01750 23176 — MB ChB Birm. 1972; MRCP (UK) 1976; MRCGP 1980.

WILSON, John Frederick Millbarn Medical Centre, 34 London End, Beaconsfield HP9 2JH Tel: 01494 675303 Fax: 01494 680214 — MB ChB Bristol 1976; MRCGP 1983. Clin. Asst. (Rheum.) Wycombe Gen. Hosp.

WILSON, John Gordon Gilbert Road Medical Group, 39 Gilbert Road, Bucksburn, Aberdeen AB21 9AN Tel: 01224 712138 Fax: 01224 712239; 9 Glen Road, Dyce, Aberdeen AB21 7FB — MB ChB Aberd. 1979; MRCGP 1983.

WILSON, John Greer McTurk The Wooda Surgery, Clarence Wharf, Barnstaple Street, Bideford EX39 4AU Tel: 01237 471071 Fax: 01237 471059; Cross Fell, Raleigh Hill, Bideford EX39 3NX Tel: 01237 247 0082 Email: jgmwilson@cix.co.uk — MB BS Lond. 1976; MRCGP 1981; FRCGP 1999. GP Tutor N. Devon. Prev: Ho. Surg. Roy. Free Hosp. Lond.

WILSON, John Ian Pinderfields Hospital NHS Trust, Wakefield WF1 4DG Tel: 01924 201688; 21 Fieldhead Paddock, Boston Spa, Wetherby LS23 6SA Tel: 01937 845778 — MB BS Lond. 1979 (Guy's) MRCP (UK) 1983; BSc (Hons.) Lond. 1976, MD 1990; FRCP Lond. 1995. Cons. Cardiol. Pinderfields Hosp. Wakefield; Hon. Cons. Cardiol.Yorks. Heart Centre, Leeds; Hon. Sen. Lect. (Univ. of Leeds). Specialty: Cardiol. Socs: Brit. Cardiac Soc. & Brit. Pacing & Electrophys. Gp.; Brit. Cardiovasc. Interven. Soc. Prev: Sen. Regist. (Cardiol.) Leeds Gen. Infirm.; Research Fell. Univ. Leeds; Regist. (Med.) Centr. Middlx. Hosp. Lond.

WILSON, John Kenneth 27 Cambridge Road, Middlesbrough TS5 5NG Tel: 01642 88102 — LMSSA Lond. 1943 (Univ. Coll. Lond.) Prev: Ho. Phys., Res. Anaesth. & Cas. Off. Stockton & Thornaby Hosp.; Sen. Ho. Surg. Gen. Hosp. Middlesbrough.

WILSON, John Lindsay 101 Woodsford Square, London W14 8DT Tel: 020 7603 6118; 101 Woodsford Square, London W14 8DT Tel: 020 7603 6118 — MB BS Lond. 1953 (Lond. Hosp.) DPM Eng. 1956; FRCPsych 1974. Cons. Psychiat. Tavistock Clinic & Inst. Human Relats. Lond.; Sen. Tutor Inst. Psychiat. (Univ. Lond.); Hon. Cons. Maudsley Hosp. Lond. Specialty: Gen. Psychiat. Prev: Clin. Fell. & Sen. Regist. Tavistock Clinic Lond.; Research Asst. Med. Research Counc.; Regist. Maudsley Hosp.

WILSON, John Malcolm Apartment 7, Great Bowden Hall, Leicester Lane, Market Harborough LE16 7HP — MB BChir Camb. 1977; MA, MB Camb. 1977, BChir 1976; MRCP Ed. 1980.

WILSON, John Marshall (retired) The Health Centre, Priest Lane, Pershore WR10 1DR Tel: 01386 554567 — (Oxf. & St. Thos.) BM BCh Oxf. 1957; MA Oxf. 1957; DObst RCOG 1960; MRCGP 1969. Prev: Ho. Surg. Wom. Hosp. Wolverhampton.

WILSON, John Patrick 25 Brooklands Gardens, Whitehead, Carrickfergus BT38 9RS — MB BCh BAO Belf. 1996.

WILSON, John Robert Willoughby Larne Health Centre, Gloucester Avenue, Larne BT40 1PB Tel: 028 2826 1922 Fax: 028 2827 9560; 41 Wheatfield Heights, Ballygally, Larne BT40 2RT — MB BCh BAO Belf. 1984; DCH RCPI 1986; DRCOG 1987; MRCGP 1988. Prev: Trainee GP Belf.; SHO (Gen. Med. & O & G) Craigavon Area Hosp.; SHO (Gen. Surg. & Paediat.) Craigavon Area Hosp.

WILSON, John Robertson Avon Medical Centre, Academy Street, Larkhall ML9 2BJ Tel: 01698 882547 Fax: 01698 888138; 7 Karadale Gardens, Larkhall ML9 1BE Tel: 01698 884873 — MB ChB Aberd. 1977; MRCGP 1981.

WILSON, John Roslyn Muir (retired) Glenshee Cottage, Boquhan, Balfron, Glasgow G63 0RW — MB ChB Glas. 1949; DMRD Liverp. 1963; DMRD Eng. 1963; FFR 1971. Prev: Cons. Radiol. Stobhill Gen. Hosp. Glas.

WILSON, John Russell Greyston House Surgery, 99 Station Road, Redhill RH1 1EB Tel: 01737 761201 Fax: 01737 780510 — MB BS Lond. 1974 (St.Mary's Lond.) MRCGP 1981. Princip. GP. Prev: Trainee GP Brook Gen. Hosp. Woolwich VTS.

WILSON, Mr John Samuel Pattison (cons. rooms) Cromwell Hospital, Cromwell Road, London SW5 Tel: 020 7370 4233; 16 Smith Street, Chelsea, London SW3 4EE Tel: 020 7636 5186 — LRCP LRCS Ed. 1946; LRCP LRCS Ed. LRFPS Glas. 1946; FRCS Ed. 1959; FRCS Eng. 1973. Socs: Brit. Assn. Aesthetic Plastic Surgs. & Brit. Assn. Plastic; Fell. Roy. Coll. Med. Prev: Cons. Plastic. Surg. St. Geo., Westm., Roy. Marsden & Qu. Mary's Hosps. Lond.

WILSON, John Stanley (retired) Blairgarry, Callander FK17 8HP Tel: 01877 330121 — MB ChB Ed. 1944.

WILSON, John Trevor Elgin Medical Centre, 10 Victoria Crescent, Elgin IV30 1RQ Tel: 01343 547512 Fax: 01343 546781 — MB ChB Aberd. 1976; DRCOG 1980; MRCGP 1981.

WILSON, John Wardlaw 12 Glenorchil Place, Auchterarder PH3 1LR — MB ChB Glas. 1968; DObst RCOG 1970; Cert. Family Plann. JCC 1982. Area Med. Adviser Benefits Agency. Edin. Specialty: Disabil. Med. Prev: Med. Off. DHSS Lancs.; Gen. Pract. Auckland, New Zealand.

WILSON, John William 18 Carcluie Cresent, Ayr KA7 4SS — MB ChB Aberd. 1982; MRCGP 1987; DRCOG 1987. Prev: SHO (O & G) HM Stanley Hosp. Clwyd; Trainee GP E. Cumbria HA.

WILSON, Jonathan Mark 3 Windsor Road, Blackpool FY3 7SQ — MB ChB Manch. 1990; BSc St And. 1987.

WILSON, Jonathan Nicholas 8 Hunter Road, London SW20 8NZ — MB BS Newc. 1994; BMedSci (1st cl. Hons.) 1993; MRCP 1997. Specialist Registr. (Paediat.), John Radcliffe Hosp., Oxf. Specialty: Paediat.

WILSON, Jonathan Urquhart Department of Anaesthetics, Bedford Hospital, Kempston Road, Bedford MK42 9DJ Tel: 01234 355122; 26 Franklyn Gardens, Biddenham, Bedford MK40 4QE Tel: 01234 262966 Email: juw@doctors.org.uk — MB BS Lond. 1980 (St. Mary's) FFA RCS Eng. 1987. Cons. Anaesth. Bedford Hosp. NHS Trust. Specialty: Anaesth. Prev: Cons. Anaesth. Princess Mary's RAF Hosp. Halton; Squadron Ldr. RAF Med. Br.

WILSON, Joseph Rockfield Medical Centre, Doury Road, Ballymena BT43 6JD Tel: 028 25 638800 Fax: 028 25 633633 Email: dm.hopkins@p309.gp.n-i.nhs.uk — MB BCh BAO Belf. 1974.

WILSON, Joyce Isobel (retired) — MB ChB Bristol 1979; MSc Palliative Med. (Wales) 2002; BSc (Hons.) Exeter 1965; DRCOG 1982; MRCGP 1983. Prev: Princip. GP Welwyn Garden City.

WILSON, Joyce Whitelaw Barrhead Health Centre, Barrhead, Glasgow; 30 Glenfield Avenue, Paisley PA2 8JH Tel: 0141 884 8245 — MB ChB Glas. 1983.

WILSON, Judith Ann Paediatric Unit, Northwick Park Hospital, Watford Road, Harrow HA1 3UJ Tel: 020 8869 2640 — MB BS Lond. 1965 (St. Mary's) MRCS Eng. LRCP Lond. 1965; DCH Eng. 1967; FRCP Lond. 1987, M 1969. Cons. Paediat. Northwick Pk. Hosp.; Hon. Clin. Sen. Lect. ICMS. Specialty: Paediat. Prev: Sen. Regist. (Paediat.) & Regist. (Paediat.) St. Mary's Hosp. Lond.; Sen. Resid. Childr. Hosp. Med. Center Boston & Teach. Fell. Harvard; Med. Sch., U.S.A.

WILSON, Judith Frances (retired) Wyken, 173 Lache Lane, Chester CH4 7LU — MB ChB Birm. 1974. Prev: Lect. W. Chester Coll.

WILSON, Judy Ann (retired) Martins, School Lane, North Mundham, Chichester PO20 6LA Tel: 01243 785698 — MB BS Lond. 1957 (St. Bart.) DA Eng. 1959. Med. Asst. (Anaesth.) St. Richards Hosp. Chichester. Prev: Ho. Phys. & Ho. Surg. Southlands Hosp. Shoreham-by-Sea.

WILSON, Julian Michael Overton Park Surgery, Overton Park Road, Cheltenham GL50 3BP Tel: 01242 580511; 64 Andover Road, Cheltenham GL50 2TN — MB BS Lond. 1987; DRCOG 1991; MRCGP 1992; Dip. Palliat. Med. Wales 1994. Clin. Asst. in Palliat. Med. Prev: Cons. Palliat. Med. St. Davids Foundat. Newport, Gwent; Regist. (Palliat. Med.) Holme Tower Marie Curie Centre, Penarth; SHO (Palliat. Med.) St. Peter's Hospice Bristol.

WILSON, Julie Diane 3 Stockdam Glen, Lisburn BT28 3YS Tel: 02892 672848 — MB ChB Bristol 1990; DRCOG 1994; DCH RCPSI 1995; DMH Belf. 1995; DFFP 1996; MRCGP 1996. GP Lisburn. Specialty: Gen. Pract. Socs: BMA. Prev: Forens. Med. Off. Belf.

WILSON, Justin Edward Howitt 6 Doone Close, Teddington TW11 9AG — MB BS Lond. 1996.

WILSON, Karen Ann Clach na Croise, Sollas, Lochmaddy HS6 5BU — MB ChB Aberd. 1994; DRCOG 1997; MRCGP 1998. GP Retainee. Socs: RCGP. Prev: GP Locum; GP Regist. Inverness; SHO (Psychiat.) Craig Dunvain Hosp. Inverness.

WILSON, Karen Geraldine Alma Cottage, Baldhoon Road, Laxey IM4 7NE — MB ChB Manch. 1991; BSc (Hons.) Manch. 1988; DRCOG 1994; MRCGP 1995.

WILSON, Katharine Louise Springfield House, Bridge St., New Mills, High Peak SK22 4DN — MB ChB Leeds 1991.

WILSON, Katherine Ruth Henley (retired) 93 Stone Meadow, Oxford OX2 6TD Tel: 01865 510262 — MB BS Lond. 1967 (Roy. Free) MRCS Eng. LRCP Lond. 1967; DA Eng. 1970. Med. Off. (Disabil. Med.) Mary MarlBoro. Centre Oxf. Prev: Ho. Surg. Roy. Free Hosp. Lond.

WILSON, Kathleen Elizabeth Monklands District General Hospital, Pathology Department, Airdrie ML6 0JS Tel: 01236 748748 Fax: 01236 770117; The Gables, Stonebyres, Kirkfieldbank, Lanark ML11 9UW — MB ChB Aberd. 1977. Assoc. Specialist Histopath. Monklands Hosp. Aidrie. Specialty: Histopath.

WILSON, Kathryn Jane DME Box 135, Addenbrookes Hospital, Hills Road, Cambridge CB2 2QQ Tel: 01223 217785 Fax: 01223 217782 Email: jane.wilson@addenbrookes.anglox.nhs.uk — MB BS Lond. 1990 (Roy. Free Hosp.) MRCP Lond. 1994. Cons. Phys. Dept of Med. for the elderly. Specialty: Care of the Elderly; Gen. Med. Prev: Locum Cons. DME Addenbrookes Hosp.

WILSON, Keith McIver O'Neil Department of Haematology, University of Wales College of Medicine, Heath Park, Cardiff CF14 4XN Tel: 029 2074 4327 Fax: 029 2074 5442 Email: keith.wilson@wbs.wales.nhs.uk — MB BS West Indies 1985 (Univ. West Indies) MRCP (UK) 1993; DRCPath 1996; MRCPath 1997; FRCPath Lond. 2004. Clin. Sen. Lect. (Haemat.) Director (Blood & Marrow Transpl. Unit) Univ. of Wales Coll. of Med.; Hon. Cons. Haematologist, Univ. Hosp. of Wales & Welsh Blood Serv.; Cons. Haematologist; Lead Clinician (Apheresis); Med. Director Welsh Bone Marrow Donor Registry. Specialty: Haematology; Gen. Med. Special Interest: Transplantation & Transfus. Med. Socs: Brit. Soc. Haematol.; Brit. Blood Transfus. Soc.; Brit. Soc. for Blood & Marrow Transplantation. Prev: Sen. Regist. (Haemat.) The Roy. Marsden Hosp. NHS Trust Surrey; Sen. Regist. (Haemat.) St. Geo.'s Hosp. & Med. Sch. Lond.; Sen. Regist. (Haemat.) St.Helier NHS Trust.

WILSON, Kenneth Charles Malcolm, Capt. RAMC Royal Liverpool Hospital, Prescot St., Liverpool L7 — MB ChB Liverp. 1978; MRCPsych 1985; MPhil Lond. 1987. Cons. (Psychiat. of Old Age) Roy. Liverp. Hosp. Specialty: Geriat. Psychiat.

WILSON, Mr Kenneth William (retired) — MB ChB St. And. 1955; FRCS Eng. 1962. Prev: Cons. Surg. Roy. Halifax Infirm. & Halifax Gen. Hosp.

WILSON, Kirsty Madeleine 20 Alder Avenue, Fenham, Newcastle upon Tyne NE4 9TB — MB BS Newc. 1996.

WILSON, Laurence Anthony Department of Neurology, Royal Free Hospital, Pond St., London NW3 2QG Tel: 020 7794 0500 — MB ChB Otago 1967; FRACP 1978; FRCP Lond. 1989. Cons. Neurol. Roy. Free Hosp. & Barnet Gen. Hosp. Lond. Specialty: Neurol. Prev: Cons. Neurol. Centr. Middlx. Hosp. Lond.; Sen. Regist. (Neurol.) Guy's Hosp. & Nat. Hosps. Nerv. Dis. Lond.; Regist. (Neurol.) Middlx. Hosp.

WILSON, Lawrence Joseph 1 Manor Av, Penwortham, Preston, Preston PR1 0XE — MB ChB Manch. 1997.

WILSON, Lesley The Poplaces, Westmount, St. Helier, Jersey JE2 3LP Tel: 01534 624832 Fax: 01534 624860 — MB BS Lond. 1976; MRCPsych Lond. 1984. Cons. Old Age Psychiat. St. Helier, Jersey. Specialty: Geriat. Psychiat. Prev: Cons. Old Age Psychiat. Colindale & Napsbury Hosps.

WILSON, Mr Lester Francis Flat 5, 14 Dawson Place, London W2 4TJ — MB BS Lond. 1982; BSc Lond. (Hist. Med.) 1979; FRCS Eng. 1987; FRCS (Orth.) 1994. Cons. Orthop. & Spinal Surg. Whittington Hosp. Lond. Specialty: Orthop. Prev: Sen. Regist. Roy. Nat. Orthop. Hosp. Stanmore; Regist. Univ. Hosp. Nottm.; Spinal Research Fell. Univ. Hosp. & Harlow Wood Orthop. Hosps. Nottm.

WILSON, Lewis Andrew The Health Centre, Victoria Road, Ulverston LA12 0EW Tel: 01229 582223; Schiehallion, 22 Fell View, Swarthmoor, Ulverston LA12 0XF Tel: 01229 584208 — MB BS Lond. 1980 (Univ. Camb. Lond. Hosp. Med. Coll.) BA Lond. 1977; DRCOG 1982; Cert. Family Plann. JCC 1982; MRCGP 1984; DPM Wales 2001; Dip Palliat Med University of Wales 2001; CMDM 2002.

WILSON, Lockhart Lindsay 10 Highfield Road, Magherafelt BT45 5JD — MB BCh BAO Belf. 1986.

WILSON, Louisa Emma 29 Castle View Road, Canvey Island SS8 9FD — MB BS Lond. 1993 (St Mary's London) BSc Lond. 1992, MB BS 1993; MRCP(Paed) 1996. Sydney Childr.'s Hosp., High St, Randwick, Sydney, NSW, Australia 2031(Paediat. Regist.). Specialty: Paediat.

WILSON, Louise The Surgery, Recreation Drive, Billinge, Wigan WN5 7LZ Tel: 01744 892205; 58A Wigan Road, Standish, Wigan WN6 0BA Tel: 01942 425618 — MB ChB Liverp. 1979; DRCOG 1981.

WILSON, Louise 56 Melbourne Street, Leicester LE2 0AS — MB ChB Leic. 1993.

WILSON, Louise Caroline Unit for Clinical Genetics, Institute of Child Health, 30 Guilford St., London WC1N 1EH Tel: 020 7905 2607 Fax: 020 7813 8141 Email: l.wilson@ich.ucl.ac.uk — MB ChB Manch. 1987; BSc Biochemistry Manch. 1984; MRCP (UK) 1991; Dip. Clin. Genetics Lond. 1992. Cons. (Clin. Genetics) Gt. Ormond St. Hosp., Lond. Specialty: Genetics.

WILSON, Louise Elizabeth 6 Carolsteen Avenue, Helens Bay, Bangor BT19 1LJ — MB ChB Ed. 1986. Paediat. Intensivist Roy. Hosp. Sick Childr. Edin.; Sen. Lect. Fac. Med. Univ. Edin. Specialty: Paediat.

WILSON, Lucy Lillian 9 Laggan Road, Newton Mearns, Glasgow G77 6LP Email: luce3@hotmail.com — MB ChB Manch. 1998; BSc (Hons) Met. Biol St And 1995.

WILSON, Lynda Mary Norwood Medical Centre, 360 Herries Road, Sheffield S5 7HD Tel: 0114 242 6208 Fax: 0114 261 9243; 27 Carsick View Road, Sheffield S10 3LZ — MB ChB Dundee 1978; DRCOG 1981.

WILSON, Lynn 40 Sandhill Parade, Belfast BT5 6FH — MB BCh Belf. 1997.

WILSON, Lynn Margaret McIntosh, Gourlay and Partners, Stockbridge Health Centre, 1 India Place, Edinburgh EH3 6EH Tel: 0131 225 9191 Fax: 0131 226 6549; 95 Ravelston Dykes, Edinburgh EH12 6EY — MB ChB Ed. 1977; BSc Ed. 1974, MB ChB 1977.

WILSON, Madeleine Ann Ambrose Avenue Surgery, 76 Ambrose Avenue, Colchester CO3 4LN Tel: 01206 549444 Fax: 01206 369910; 7 Richardson Walk, Colchester CO3 4AJ Tel: 01206 765510 — MB ChB Bristol 1983; MB ChB Brist. 1983; DCH RCP Lond. 1986; MRCGP 1987. Prev: GP Manch.; Trainee GP Kenilworth; SHO (A & E & Geriat.) Dudley Rd. Hosp. Birm.

WILSON, Mairi Elizabeth Scott Burlington Road Surgery, 12/14 Burlington Road, Ipswich IP1 2EU; 48 Prittlewell Close, Ipswich IP2 9SP — MB ChB Aberd. 1980.

WILSON, Malachy Gerard Lister House Surgery, 35 The Parade, St Helier JE2 3QQ Tel: 01534 36336 Fax: 01534 35304 — MB BCh BAO Dub. 1980.

WILSON, Mr Malcolm Sapte — MB BS Lond. 1986 (Lond. Hosp.) FRCS Eng. 1990; MD Lond. 1994. Cons. Colorectal Surg. Christie Hosp. & S. Manch. Univ. Hosp. Wythenshawe. Specialty: Gen. Surg. Special Interest: Colorectal Cancer; Pelvic Surg.; Pseudomyxoma Peritoneii. Socs: Brit. Assn. Surg. Oncol.; Assn. Surg.; Assn. Coloproctol. Prev: Cons. (Gen. Surg.) Macclesfield Dist. Gen. Hosp. & Stepping Hill Stockport; Sen. Regist. (Gen. Surg.) NW RHA.

WILSON, Margaret (retired) 11 Bellevue Road, Kirkintilloch, Glasgow G66 1AL Tel: 0141 776 4229 — MB BS Lond. 1960 (Roy. Free) MSc (Physiol.) Lond. 1958; DCH Eng. 1963; MRCP (UK) 1970. Prev: Gen. Practitioner Glas. G64 2AA.

WILSON, Margaret Cunningham Gibb Charlotte Street Surgery, 1 Charlotte Street, Dumfries DG1 2AQ Tel: 01387 267626 Fax: 01387 266824; Riverside Cottage, Kelton, Dumfries DG1 4UA — MB ChB Aberd. 1971; DObst RCOG 1974; MRCGP 1986. Med. Off. Occupat. Health Dept. Crighton Roy. Hosp. Dumfries.

WILSON, Margaret Lynne Brendon Hills Surgery, Torre, Washford, Watchet TA23 0LA Tel: 01984 640454 Fax: 01984 641164 — BM Soton. 1984; MRCGP 1990.

WILSON, Marie Benedicta St David's Clinic, 2 Bramley Road, Ealing, London W5 4SS Tel: 020 8579 0165 Fax: 020 8579 0424; St. David's, 2 Bramley Road, London W5 4SS Tel: 020 8579 0165 — MB BS Madras 1956; DCH Eng. 1960; DObst RCOG 1961; MRCP Lond. 1965. Specialty: Cardiol.; Diabetes; Respirat. Med. Socs: Assoc. Mem. BMA; Med. Soc. Lond.; Hunt. Soc. Prev: SHO Glan Ely Hosp. Cardiff; SHO Acton Hosp. Lond.; Regist. Centr. Middlx. Hosp. Lond.

WILSON, Marie Elizabeth Easterhouse Health Centre, 9 Auchinlea Road, Glasgow G34 9HQ Tel: 0141 531 8150 Fax: 0141 531 8110; 2 Oban Drive, Glasgow G20 6AF — MB ChB Glas. 1981 (Glasgow) MRCOG 1986; MRCGP 1991. GP Partner; Vocat. Studies Glas. Univ. Specialty: Obst. & Gyn. Socs: Med. Wom. Federat. Prev: Trainee GP Kirkintilloch VTS; Regist. (O & G) W. Scotl.

WILSON, Mark Lower Street Health Centre, Lower Street, Tettenhall, Wolverhampton WV6 9LL Tel: 01902 444550/1 — MB BChir Camb. 1975 (Char. Cross) MB Camb. 1975, BChir 1974; MA Camb. 1975; DRCOG 1978. Socs: BMA; Wolverhampton Med. Inst. Prev: SHO (Geriat. Med., O & G & A & E) Plymouth Gen. Hosp. (Freedom Fields Br.).

WILSON, Martin 312 Alcester Road S., Birmingham B14 6EN — BM BS Nottm. 1994.

WILSON, Mr Martin Cooper Homewood, 1 Barlow Fold Road, Romiley, Stockport SK6 4LH Tel: 0161 494 8634 — MB ChB Manch. 1969; FRCS Eng. 1973; MD Manch. 1976. Cons. Gen. Surg. Tameside Gen. Hosp. Lancs. Specialty: Gen. Surg. Prev: Lect. in Clin. Surg. Univ. Edin.

WILSON, Martin Geoffrey Cleveland The Surgery, Station Road, Great Massingham, King's Lynn PE32 2JQ Tel: 01485 520521 Fax: 01485 520072; Red House Farm, Little Massingham, King's Lynn PE32 2JU Tel: 01485 520572 — MB BS Lond. 1974. Prev: Trainee GP/SHO King's Lynn Gen. Hosp. VTS; Ho. Phys. Whittington Hosp. Lond.; Ho. Surg. Dreadnought Seamans Hosp. Lond.

WILSON, Martin Thomson Vennel Street Health Centre, 50 Vennel Street, Dalry KA24 4AG — MB ChB Dundee 1978; DRCOG 1982.

WILSON, Mary 23 Brackley Road, Monton, Eccles, Manchester M30 9LG Tel: 0161 281 2262; Department of Radiology, Withington Hospital, Nell Lane, Manchester M20 2LR Tel: 0161 291 4079 — MB BS Lond. 1978 (St. Bart.) MRCS Eng. LRCP Lond. 1978; FRCR 1985. Cons. Radiol. S. Manch. Univ. Hosp. Trust. Specialty: Radiol. Prev: Sen. Regist. (Radiol.) N.W. RHA; Sen. Regist. (Radiol.) Nottm. HA.; Regist. (Radiol.) Nottm. HA.

WILSON, Mrs Mary Alexandra Marshall Chandos. 12 Parkside Mews, Hurst Road, Horsham RH12 2SA Tel: 01403 248747 — MB BS Lond. 1953 (Char. Cross) MRCS Eng. LRCP Lond. 1953; DObst RCOG 1954. Specialty: Gen. Pract. Prev: Ho. Surg. Harrow Hosp.; Resid. Obst. Off. Char. Cross Hosp. Lond.

WILSON, Mary Shelagh The Health House, 1 Wootton Street, Cosham, Portsmouth PO6 3AP Fax: 023 9232 6379; Brooklyn Cottage, Commonside, Westbourne, Emsworth PO10 8TD Tel: 01243 375633 — BM Soton. 1982.

WILSON, MattJames 52 Abbotswood Road, London SW16 1AW Tel: 020 8769 4020 — MB BS Lond. 1997 (St Bartholomews Hospital) SHO Rotat. (Surgic.) Roy. Berks. Hosp. Lond. Rd. Berks. Specialty: Gen. Surg. Prev: Ho. Off. (Med.) Colchester; Ho. Off. (Surgic.) Roy. Berks.

WILSON, Mrs Maureen Elizabeth (retired) Leewood, Leewood Road, Dunblane FK15 0DR Tel: 01786 822161 — MB ChB Glas. 1965.

WILSON, Melanie Patricia Bristol PHL, Department of Microbiology, Bristol Royal Infirmary, Bristol BS2 8HW Tel: 0117 928 2514; Hall Floor Flat, 32 Royal York Crescent, Bristol BS8 4JU — MB BS Lond. 1991 (St. Geo. Hosp. Med. Sch.) DRCPath 1998. Regist. (Microbiol.) Bristol Pub. Health Laborat. Specialty: Med. Microbiol. Socs: Hosp. Infec. Soc.; Brit. Soc. Antimicrob. Chemother. Prev: SHO (Med. Microbiol.) Bristol Roy. Infirm. & Good Hope Hosp. NHS Trust Sutton Coldfield; SHO (Biochem.) Good Hope Hosp. NHS Trust Sutton Coldfield; Ho. Off. (Gen. Med.) Qu. Alexandra's Hosp. Cosham.

WILSON, Michael Anthony Longueville, Mill Hill, Huntington, York YO32 9PY Tel: 01904 768861 Fax: 01904 762012 Email: postmaster@michaelwilson.plus.com — MB ChB Leeds 1958; DObst RCOG 1961; FRCGP 1979, M 1966. GP; Mem. A.B.P.I. Code of Pract. Appeal Bd. Socs: York Med. Soc.; Vice Pres. BMA. Prev: Chairm. Gen. Med. Servs. Comm.; Dep. Chairm. Standing Med. Advis. Comm.; Mem. Gen. Med. Council.

WILSON, Michael Anthony 11 The Comyns, Bushey Heath, Watford WD23 1HN Tel: 020 8950 3677 — MB BS Lond. 1950 (Middlx.) Med. Off. Bushey & Dist. Hosp.; Hosp. Pract. (Orthop.) Watford Gen. Hosp. & W. Herts. Hosp. Hemel; Med. Off. St. Margt.'s Sch. Bushey. Prev: GP Watford; SHO (Orthop.) Roy. Vict. Hosp. Bournemouth; Flight Lt. RAF.

WILSON, Michael David 25 Birch Polygon, Manchester M14 5HX — MB BS New South Wales 1990.

WILSON, Mr Michael George (retired) Litfield House, Litfield, Clifton, Bristol BS8 3LS Tel: 0117 973 1323; The Red House, 40 Coombe Lane, Westbury-on-Tym, Bristol BS9 2BJ Tel: 0117 968 2320 — (Leeds) MB ChB Leeds 1940; MRCS Eng. LRCP Lond. 1942; FRCS Eng. 1949; ChM Leeds 1957. Hon. Cons. Surg. Southmead Hosp. Bristol, Wells & Dist. Hosp. & Clevedon Cott Hosp. Prev: Lect. (Clin. Surg.) Univ. Bristol.

WILSON, Michael John 37 The Ridgeway, Fleetwood FY7 8AH — MB ChB Manch. 1973.

WILSON, Michael Raymond 51 Carlton House, Western Parade, Southsea PO5 3ED Tel: 023 9286 3222 — BM Soton. 1981.

WILSON, Michael St George 9A Wilbraham Place, London SW1X 9AE Tel: 020 7730 5119; 2 Stanford Road, London W8 5QJ Tel: 020 7937 6973 — MB BChir Camb. 1959 (Westm.) MRCS Eng. LRCP Lond. 1959; DObst RCOG 1963. Clin. Asst. (Dermat.) St. Mary's Hosp. Lond. Prev: Clin. Asst. Rheum Dept. Westm. Hosp. Lond.; Med. Off. Anaesth. Dept. Qu. Mary's Hosp. Hong Kong; Clin. Asst. ENT Dept. Westm. Hosp. Lond.

WILSON, Michael St George Kershaw Newtown Surgery, Park Street, Newtown SY16 1EF Tel: 01686 626221/626224 Fax: 01686 622610; 8 Meadow Lane, Newtown SY16 2DU Tel: 01686 628786 — MB Camb. 1973 (St. Thos.) BA Camb. 1969, MB 1973, BChir 1972; DCH Eng. 1974; DRCOG 1977. Prev: Ho. Surg. St. Thos. Hosp. Lond.; Ho. Off. (Paediat.) Essex Co. Hosp. Colchester; Ho. Surg. (Obst.) Roy. United Hosp. Bath.

WILSON, Michael Stanley (retired) Wycherts, West Hagbourne, Didcot OX11 0ND — MB BS Lond. 1953 (St. Bart.) LMSSA Lond. 1952; DO Eng. 1958. Prev: Dir. Contact Lens Servs. & Assoc. Specialist Ophth. West. Ophth. Hosp. Lond.

WILSON, Michael Stewart Dalkeith Medical Practice, 24 St Andrew Street, Dalkeith EH22 1AP Tel: 0131 561 5500 Fax: 0131 561 5555; 17 Lasswade Road, Eskbank, Dalkeith EH22 3EE Tel: 0131 663 8845 — MB ChB Ed. 1973; DCH RCPS Glas. 1975; DRCOG 1977; LMCC 1979; MRCGP 1981. GP Trainer (Paediat.) Sch. Community Paediat. Edin. Socs: Brit. Soc. Study of Infec.; Assoc. Mem. Fac. Homoeop.; Assn. Mem. Roy. Coll. Paediat. & Child Health. Prev: Regist. (Paediat.) Kingston Gen. Hosp. Kingston Ont. Canada; SHO (Med.) Roy. Hosp. Sick Childr. Edin.; Ho. Off. (Med.) West. Gen. Hosp. Edin.

WILSON, Morven Patricia Flat 0/2, 4 Vinicombe St., Glasgow G12 8BG — MB ChB Glas. 1997.

WILSON, Neil Department of Cardiology, Royal Hospital for Sick Children, Yorkhill, Glasgow G3 8SJ Tel: 0141 201 0246 Fax: 0141 201 0853 Email: wilsonneil@aol.com; Beechwood, Bridge of Weir Road, Kilmacolm PA13 4NN Tel: 01505 874324 Fax: 01505 874324 Email: 100441.2742@compuserve.com — MB BS Lond. 1978 (St. Thomas') DCH Glas. 1981; MRCP (UK) 1982; FRCP Ed. 1995; FRCP Ed. 1996. Cons. (Cardiol.) Roy. Hosp. For Sick Childr. Glas. Specialty: Cardiol.; Paediat. Cardiol. Prev: Cons. (Paediat. Cardiol.) King Faisal Specialist Hosp. Riyadh, Saudi Arabia; Cons. (Paediat. Cardiol.) Killingbeck Hosp. Leeds; Sen. Regist. (Paediat. Cardiol.) Killingbeck Hosp. Leeds.

WILSON, Neil David Holycroft Surgery, The Health Centre, Oakworth Road, Keighley BD21 1SA; The Old Vicarage, Lothersdale, Keighley BD20 8EQ Tel: 01535 634952 — MB ChB Birm. 1975. GP Keighley.

WILSON, Mr Neil Imray Livingstone 92 Inveroran Drive, Bearsden, Glasgow G61 2AT — MB ChB Glas. 1977; BSc Glas. 1975, MB ChB 1977; FRCS Glas. 1981; Dip Biomech (strath) 1987. Cons. and orthopaedic Surg.,Roy. Hosp. for sick Childr. and Western Infirm., Glas. Specialty: Orthop.; Trauma & Orthop. Surg. Socs: BMA; Assoc. Mem. Brit. Orthop. Assn.; Mem. Brit. Scoliosiss Soc. Prev: Sen. Regist. (Orthop. Surg.) Vict. Infirm. Glas.; Regist. (Orthop. Surg.) Univ. Dept. West. Infirm. Glas.; Jun. Ho. Off. (Med.) Profess. Unit. Stobhill Hosp. Glas.

WILSON, Niall Joseph Elliott Royal Liverpool & Broadgreen University Hospitals, Thomas Drive, Liverpool L14 3LB Tel: 0151 282 6856 Fax: 0151 282 6899 — MB ChB Liverp. 1991; BSc (Hons.) Liverp. 1988; FRCP 2004. Cons. Dermat. Roy. Liverp. Univ. Hosp.; Hon. Clin. Lect. (Med.) Univ. Liverp. Specialty: Dermat. Socs: Brit. Assn. Dermat.; Liverp. Med. Inst.; Dowling Club. Prev: SHO (Histopath. & Med.) Roy. Liverp. Univ. Hosp.; Ho. Off. Roy. Liverp. Hosp.; Regist. (Dermat.) Roy. Liverp. Univ. Hosp.

WILSON, Nicholas Hedley Helios Medical Centre, 17 Stoke Hill, Stoke Bishop, Bristol BS9 1JN Tel: 0117 982 6060 Email: nicholas.wilson@gp-l81622.nhs.uk; 15 Normanton Road, Clifton, Bristol BS8 2TY — MB BS Lond. 1985 (Westm.) BSc Lond. 1982; DA (UK) 1989; DCH RCP Lond. 1990; MRCGP 1993. Asst. GP; Sch. Doctor. Specialty: Gen. Pract. Prev: Trainee GP Bristol.; Research Fell. Univ. Westminster Lond.

WILSON, Nicholas James Helmsley Medical Centre, Carlton Road, Helmsley, York YO62 5HD Tel: 01424 219323 — MB BS Lond. 1988; DRCOG 1992.

WILSON, Mr Nicholas Muir Royal Hampshire County Hospital, Romsey Road, Winchester SO22 5DG Tel: 01962 825055 Fax: 01962 824640 — MB BS Lond. 1981 (St. Thos.) FRCS Eng. 1985; FRCS (Gen. Surg.) 1993; BSc (Hons.) Lond. 1978, MS 1994. Cons. Gen. Surg. Roy. Hants. Co. Hosp. Winchester; Arris & Gale Lect. RCS Eng; Edr. Thrombosis, Gen. Surg. & Curr. Med. Literature. Specialty: Gen. Surg.; Vasc. Med. Socs: Fell. Roy. Soc. Med.; Fell. Assn. Surgs.; Fell. Vasc. Surgic. Soc. Prev: Sen. Regist. St. Thomas's Hosp. Lond.; Lect. St. Thos. Hosp. Lond.; Regist. Lond. Chest Hosp. & Westm. Hosp. Lond.

WILSON, Nicholas Stephen Market Deeping Health Centre, Godsey Lane, Market Deeping, Peterborough PE6 8DD — MB ChB Leic. 1986; DTM & H Liverp. 1988. Socs: Fell. Roy. Soc. Trop. Med.

WILSON, Nicola Jane 12 Rectory Road, Gosforth, Newcastle upon Tyne NE3 1XR — MB BS Lond. 1996.

WILSON, Nicola Margaret Royal Brompton Hospital, Paediatrics Department, Sydney St., London SW3 6NP Tel: 020 7351 8232 Fax: 020 7351 8763 Email: n.wilson@rbh.nthames.nhs.uk; The Old Mill, Mill Lane, Adderbury, Banbury OX17 3LW Tel: 01295 810340 — MRCS Eng. LRCP Lond. 1964 (St. Geo.) MB BS 1964; DCH Eng. 1967; MD Eng. 1987; FRCPCH 1997. p/t Hon. Cons. Paediat. Specialty: Paediat.

WILSON, Nigel Leith Stoneycroft Medical Centre, Stoneville Road, Liverpool L13 6QD Tel: 0151 228 1138 Fax: 0151 228 1653; 68 Winifred Lane, Aughton, Ormskirk L39 5DL Tel: 01695 423497 — MB BChir Camb. 1982; MB BChir Camb. 1981; MA Camb. 1982; DRCOG 1985; Cert. Family Plann. JCC 1985; MRCGP (Distinc.) 1987; AFOM RCP UK 1994. Occupat. Phys. Liverp. Univ. Specialty: Occupat. Health. Prev: GP Bishop Auckland.

WILSON, Nigel Walton (retired) 14 Treadgold Street, London W11 4BP; 17 Pallinghurst Road, Parktown, Johannesburg 2193, South Africa — MB BS Lond. 1980; MA 1976.

WILSON, Mr Noel Vivian Department of Surgery, Kent & Canterbury Hospital, Ethelbert Road, Canterbury CT1 3NG Tel: 01227 766877; Horsehead Farm, Green Hills, Barham, Canterbury CT4 6JY — MB BS Lond. 1981 (St. Thos.) MB BS Lond. 19; FRCS Eng. 1986; MS Lond. 1992. Cons. Gen. & Vasc. Surg. Kent & Canterbury Hosp. Specialty: Gen. Surg. Socs: Vasc. Surg. Soc. GB & Irel.; Assn. Surg. Prev: Sen. Regist. & Regist. (Gen. Surg.) King's Coll. Hosp. Lond.; Sen. Fell. (Vasc.) St. Mary's Hosp. Lond.

WILSON, Norman Graham Michael Hungerford Medical Centre, School Crescent, Crewe CW1 5HA Tel: 01270 582589 Fax: 01270 216330; The Warren, Berkeley Crescent, Wistaston, Crewe CW2 6QA Tel: 01270 568735 — MRCS Eng. LRCP Lond. 1966 (Liverp.) DA (UK) 1969; DRCOG 1970. GP. Specialty: Gen. Pract. Socs: BMA (Pres Crewe Div.); Assoc. RCGP. Prev: Scheme Organiser S. Chesh. VTS; Hon. Clin. Tutor (Primary Care) Univ. of Liverp.; Mem. GPs in Asthma Gp.

WILSON, Mrs Olive Eversfield, Rockcliffe, Dalbeattie DG5 4QF Tel: 0155 663334 — (Univ. Ed.) M.B., Ch.B. Ed. 1943. Socs: BMA.

WILSON, Pamela Edith The Health Centre, Station Road, Haydock, St Helens WA11 0JN Tel: 01744 734419 Fax: 01744 454875 — MB ChB Manch. 1974 (Manchester) DObst RCOG 1976; Cert. Family Plann. JCC 1983. Prev: SHO (Paediat.) & SHO (O & G) Wigan AHA.

WILSON, Mrs Patricia Caroline Gladwyns House, Sheering Road, Hatfield Heath, Bishop's Stortford CM22 7LL Tel: 01279 730184 Fax: 01279 739053; Gladwyns House, Sheering Road, Hatfield Heath, Bishop's Stortford CM22 7LL Tel: 01279 730256 Fax: 01279 739053 — MB ChB Birm. 1970; MB ChB (Hons.) Birm. 1970; FRCOG 1990, M 1978. Consg. Gyn., Private Pract. At The Rivers Hosp., Herts. & St. John & St. Eliz., Lond. Specialty: Obst. & Gyn. Socs: Counc. Mem. Of Indep.Doctors Forum; Brit. Soc. Colpos. & Cerv. Path.; Brit. Soc. Gyn. Endoscopy. Prev: Sen. Regist.

Addenbrooke's Hosp. Camb.; Clin. Lect. (O & G) Clin. Sch. Camb.; Cons. O & G Essex & Herts. Health Servs.

WILSON, Patrick Antony Joseph 3 Mill Hill Road, Norwich NR2 3DP — MB BS Lond. 1984; MRCP (UK) 1987; FRCR 1991.

WILSON, Patrick John Kevin 59 Myrtlefield Park, Malone Road, Belfast BT9 6NG Tel: 01232 660083; 19 Winston Drive, Portstewart BT55 7NW Tel: 0126583 3022 — MB BCh BAO Belf. 1945 (Qu. Univ. Belf.) FRCGP 1980, M 1953; Assoc. Fac. Occupat. Med. RCP Lond. 1979; Lic. Fac. Occupat. Med. RCPI 1979. Hosp. Pract. Purdysburn Hosp. Belf. Med. Off. Bass Brewing Ltd.; Med. Off. DHSS Fell. Ulster Med. Soc. Socs: Soc. Occupat. Med. Prev: Clin. Asst. Med. Mater Infirm. Hosp. Belf.

WILSON, Patrick Pownall Bonnar and Partners, Sunnyside Surgery, Hawkins Road, Penzance TR18 2PJ Tel: 01736 63340 Fax: 01736 332116; 3 St Michael's Terrace, Penzance TR18 2JP Tel: 01736 366234 — MB BS Lond. 1979 (St. Thos.) DA Eng. 1982; DRCOG 1985; MRCGP 1986. Prev: Trainee GP Truro; SHO (Anaesth. & O & G) Treliske Hosp. Truro; SHO. (Cas.) Leicester Roy. Infirm.

WILSON, Paul Marybrook Medical Centre, Marybrook Street, Berkeley GL13 9BL Tel: 01453 810228 Fax: 01453 511778; The Bungalow, Canonbury Hill, Berkeley GL13 9BE Tel: 01452 810678 Email: paul.wilsondr@btinternet.com — MB ChB Bristol 1972; MRCGP 1976; DObst RCOG 1976; Diploma in Prision Medicine 2001. Med. Off. HM Prisons Leyhill & E.wood Pk.; Hon. Treas. Jenner Trust.; Apptd. Doctor to Health & Safety Exec. Ionising Radiat.s & Asbestosis. Socs: Roy. Soc. of Med. Prev: Trainee GP Teesside VTS; Ho. Surg. Bristol Roy. Infirm.; Ho. Phys. Cheltenham Gen. Hosp.

WILSON, Mr Paul Department of General Surgery, Royal Lancaster Infirmary, Lancaster LA1 4RP; Wood House, Wennington Road, Wray, Lancaster LA2 8QQ — MB ChB Birm. 1986; MB ChB (Hons.) Birm. 1986; FRCS Ed. 1990; FRCS (Gen.) 1996. Roy. Lancaster Infirm. Specialty: Gen. Surg. Prev: Cons. (Vasc. & Gen. Surg.) N. Manch. Gen. Hosp.; Sen. Regist. (Gen. Surg.) Roy. Oldham Hosp.; Sen. Regist. (Vasc. Surg.) Withington Hosp. Manch.

WILSON, Paul Anthony Department of Anaesthesia, Crosshouse Hospital, Kilmarnock KA2 0BE Tel: 01563 577172 Fax: 01563 577171 Email: paul.wilson@aaaht.scot.nhs.uk — MB ChB Glas. 1976 (University of Glasgow) FRCA 1982. Cons. Anaesth. N. Ayrsh. & Arran Trust. Specialty: Anaesth.; Intens. Care. Socs: Assn. Anaesth.; Scott. Soc. Anaesth.; Intens. Care Soc.

WILSON, Paul Bryan The Surgery, 232-234 Milton Road, Weston Super Mare BS22 8AG Tel: 01934 625022 Fax: 01934 612470; Shiplett Court Farm, Shiplate Road, Bleadon, Weston Super Mare BS22 0NY Tel: 01934 813412 — MB BS Lond. 1972 (Univ. Coll. Hosp.) DObst RCOG 1974. Prev: Trainee GP Univ. Coll. Hosp. Lond. VTS.

WILSON, Paul Douglas The Surgery, Field Road, Stainforth, Doncaster DN7 5AF Tel: 01302 841202; The Lodge, St. Bartholomews Rise, Cantley Lane, Doncaster DN4 6LS Tel: 01302 533318 — MB ChB Ed. 1979; BSc (Hons.) Ed. 1976; DRCOG 1984; MRCGP 1984. Lect. (Gen. Pract.) Sheff. Univ.

WILSON, Paul Frederick Dodington Surgery, 29 Dodington, Whitchurch SY13 1EL Tel: 01948 662033 Fax: 01948 663428; Alport House, Alport Road, Whitchurch SY13 1NR Tel: 01948 662676 — MB BS Lond. 1971. Socs: BMA. Prev: SHO (O & G, Paediat. & Psychiat.) N. Middlx. Hosp. Lond.

WILSON, Paul Gerard City Hospital NHS Trust, Dudley Road, Birmingham B18 7QH Tel: 0121 507 4952 Email: wilsonpg@globalnet.co.uk — MB ChB Birm. 1988 (Birmingham) MRCP (UK) 1992. Cons. Phys. and Gastroenterologist. Specialty: Gastroenterol. Special Interest: ERCP/Paucreatic Dis. Socs: Brit. Soc. of Gastroenterol. Prev: Regist. Rotat. (Gen. Med. & Gastroenterol.) Worcester Roy. Infirm. Selly Oak Hosp. Birm. & Qu. Eliz. Hosp. Birm.; SHO Rotat. (Med.) Chesterfield Roy. Hosp.; Research Fell., Univ. of Birm.

WILSON, Mr Paul Stephen (retired) ENT Department, North Staffordshire Hospitals NHS Trust, Newcastle Road, Stoke-on-Trent ST4 6QG Tel: 01782 552077 Fax: 01782 552895 — FRCS Eng. 1989; MB ChB Birm. 1983; FRCS (Orl.) Eng. 1993. Cons. (ENT Surg.) N. Staffs. Hosp. Trust.

WILSON, Paula Caroline 15 Quadrant Road, Glasgow G43 2QP — MB ChB Manch. 1993; FRCR; MRCP; BSc. Cons. Clin. Oncologist, Bristol Haemat. and Oncol. Centre. Specialty: Oncol. Prev: Specialist Regist. Clin. Oncol. The Roy. Marsden Hosp Lond.

WILSON, Pauline — MB ChB Aberd. 1998.

WILSON, Mr Peter Kinnesswood, Withybush Road, Haverfordwest SA62 4BN — MB ChB Ed. 1956; FRCS Ed. 1963; FRCS Eng. 1979. Cons. Withybush Gen. Hosp. HaverfordW.. Prev: Sen. Regist. in Gen. Surg. United Cardiff Hosps.

WILSON, Peter St Bartholomew's Hospital, 2nd Floor Pathology Block, West Smithfield, London EC1A 7BE Tel: 0207 601 8417 Fax: 0207 601 8409 Email: peter.wilson@bartsandthelondon.nhs.uk; 23 The Warren Drive, Wanstead, London E11 2LR — MB BChir Camb. 1975; MRCPath 1981. Cons. Med. MicroBiologist, St. Batholomews Hosp. & Newham; Sen. Lect. & Hon. Cons. Lond. Hosp. Med. Coll. & Newham Healthcare NHS Trust. Specialty: Med. Microbiol. Socs: (Exec. Counc. & Mem. Sec.) Assn. Clin. Path. Prev: Clin. Dir. Newham Healthcare; Gen. Manager (Acute Unit) Newham HA.

WILSON, Peter Charles 25 Bog Road, Ballymena BT42 4HH; 30 Linney Road, Bramhall, Stockport SK7 3JW Tel: 0161 439 7799 — MB ChB Manch. 1991. Specialist Regist. (O & G) N. W. Region. Specialty: Obst. & Gyn.

WILSON, Peter David 27 Marton Road, Bridlington YO16 7AQ — MB ChB Leeds 1972; BSc (Hons.) Leeds 1969, MB ChB 1972; MRCP (UK) 1976. Sen. Regist. (Dermat.) West. Infirm. & Stobhill Hosp. Glas. Specialty: Dermat. Prev: Ho. Off. Profess. Med. Unit. St. Jas. Hosp. Leeds; Regist. (Dermat.) Roy. Vict. Infirm. Newc.; Research Fell. Dermat. Univ. Pennsylvania, PA, USA.

WILSON, Peter Edward Albion Road Surgery, 30 Albion Road, St Peter's, Broadstairs CT10 2UP Tel: 0870 890 2477 Fax: 0870 890 2478 Email: peter@albionroadsurgery.com — MB BS Lond. 1979; DRCOG 1982. GP; Med. Director of StourCare Ltd. Specialty: Gen. Pract.

WILSON, Mr Peter Ernest Heaton (retired) 5 Davenport Road, Coventry CV5 6QA Tel: 024 7667 7838 Fax: 024 7671 3822; Millside, Little Shrewley, Hatton, Warwick CV35 7HN Tel: 01926 484400 Fax: 01926 484399 — MB BS Lond. 1956 (St. Thos.) FRCS Eng. 1966. Prev: Cons. Orthop. & Trauma Walsgrave Hosps NHS Trust.

WILSON, Peter Graham Torbay Hospital, Department Child Health, Vowden Hall, Lawes Bridge, Torquay TQ2 7AA Tel: 01803 655824 Fax: 01803 617174; Millcroft, Aish, Stoke Gabriel, Totnes TQ9 6PS Tel: 01803 782450 — MB ChB Birm. 1975; BSc Oxf. 1970; MRCGP 1979; MFPHM 1997. Community Paediat. & Child Health, Torbay Hosp., Torquay. Specialty: Community Child Health. Socs: Brit. Assn. Community Drs in Audiol. Prev: SCMO (Child Health) S. Devon Healthcare NHS Trust Torbay; Sen. Regist. (Pub. Health) Bristol & Weston HA.

WILSON, Peter James Ligoniel Health Centre, 74A Ligoniel Road, Belfast BT14 8BY Tel: 028 9039 1690; 25 Broomhill Park, Belfast BT9 5JB Tel: 01232 660841 — MB BCh BAO Belf. 1978; DRCOG 1983; MRCGP 1983.

WILSON, Mr Peter John Edgar Malyan (retired) Swallowshaw, The Street, Walberton, Arundel BN18 0PQ Tel: 01243 551316 — MB BS Lond. 1956 (Guy's) MRCS Eng. LRCP Lond. 1956; FRCS Ed. 1962; FRCS Eng. 1962. Prev: Cons. Neurosurg. Morriston Hosp. Swansea.

WILSON, Peter Nicholas North End Medical Centre, 211 North End Road, West Kensington, London W14 9NP Tel: 020 7385 7777 Fax: 020 7386 9612 — MB BChir Camb. 1982; MA, BChir Camb. 1981, MB 1982; MRCGP 1987.

WILSON, Peter Robert County Hospital, Hereford HR1 2ER; Stoneleigh, Bodenham, Hereford HR1 3HS — MB BS Lond. 1982; MRCP (UK) 1985; FRCR 1989. Cons. Radiol. Co. Gen. Hosp. Hereford; Clin. Director for Radiology. Specialty: Radiol. Prev: Regist. Lond. Hosp. Whitechapel; SHO (Med.) OldCh. Hosp. Romford; SHO (Med.) Qu. Mary's Hosp. Sidcup.

WILSON, Philip Osmund Gill Cellular Pathology, St. George's Hospital, London SW17 0QT Tel: 020 8725 2663 Fax: 020 8767 Ext: 7984 Email: p.wilson@sghms.ac.uk — BM Southampton 1981; MRCPath 1989; FRCPath 1995. Cons. Cellular Pathologist, St. George's Hosp., Lond. Specialty: Pathology, General. Socs: BSCC.

WILSON, Philip Andrew Brendon Hills Surgery, Torre, Washford, Watchet TA23 0LA Tel: 01984 640454 Fax: 01984 641164 — BM Soton. 1984; DRCOG 1988; MRCGP 1989.

WILSON, Philip Melvin Dunellan, Station Road, St Cyrus, Montrose DD10 0BQ — MB ChB Aberd. 1969.

WILSON, Philip Michael John Battlefield Road Surgery, 148 Battlefield Road, Glasgow G42 9JT Tel: 0141 632 6310 Fax: 0141 636 1180 — MB BChir Camb. 1984; MB Camb. 1984, BChir 1983; DPhil Oxf. 1984, MA 1984; MRCGP 1987; DCH RCP Lond. 1988; MRCP (UK) 1988; FRCGP 1997. Research Fell. (Gen. Pract.) Glas. Univ.

WILSON, Piers Timothy John Anaesthetic Department, North Hampshire Hospital, Basingstoke RG24 9NA; Crocus Cottage, 10 Basingstoke Road, Ramsdell, Tadley RG26 5RB — MB BS Newc. 1983; FFA RCS Eng. 1988. Cons. Anaesth. N. Hants. Hosp. Basingstoke. Specialty: Anaesth. Prev: Sen. Regist. Rotat. (Anaesth.) Soton. & Basingstoke; Regist. (Anaesth.) Gt. Ormond St. Hosp. Lond. & Soton. Gen. Hosp.; SHO (Neonat. Med.) Princess Anne Hosp. Soton.

WILSON, Ralph Noble, SBStJ (retired) Duffield House, Blind Lane, Breaston, Derby DE72 3BS Tel: 01332 875790 — (Durh.) MB BS Durh. 1943; DPH Lond. 1949; DIH Soc. Apoth. Lond. 1961. Prev: Med. Off. Stanton & Staveley Ltd.

WILSON, Raymond Gerrard 111 Moss Lane, Sale M33 5BU — MB BCh BAO NUI 1979; MRCGP 1984; DCH RCP Lond. 1984.

WILSON, Reginald John Lyons (retired) Ballyward, Castlewellan BT31 9PS Tel: 01820 650203 — (Belf.) MD Belf. 1946, MB BCh BAO 1940 Belf.

WILSON, Mr Richard Henry 9 Cranmore Gardens, Belfast BT9 6JL — MB BCh Belf. 1984; MBC BCh BAO (Hons.) Belf. 1984; DRCOG 1987; FRCSI 1988.

WILSON, Richard Jeremy Malcolm Clydebank Health Centre, Kilbowie Road, Clydebank G81 2TQ Tel: 0141 531 6400 Fax: 0141 531 6336; 11A Westbourne Gardens, Glasgow G12 9XD Tel: 0141 357 0827 — MB ChB Dundee 1982.

WILSON, Richard John Health Clinic, 407 Main Road, Dovercourt, Harwich CO12 4ET Tel: 01255 201299 Fax: 01255 201270 — MB ChB Glas. 1985.

WILSON, Richard John Wellspring Surgery, St. Anns Health Centre, St. Anns, Well Road, Nottingham NG3 3PX Tel: 0115 9505907/8 Fax: 0115 988 1582.

WILSON, Richard Jonathan Terry 7 New Walk Terrace, York YO10 4BG — MB ChB Manch. 1984 (Manch. & St. And.) BSc St. And. 1981; DA (UK) 1989; FRCA 1992. Cons. Anaesth. & Intens. Care York Dist. Hosp. Specialty: Anaesth.; Intens. Care. Socs: Assn. Anaesth.; Intens. Care Soc.; BMA. Prev: Sen. Regist. (Anaesth.) York, Hull & Leeds; Regist. (Anaesth.) Leeds Gen. Infirm. & York Dist. Hosp.; SHO (Anaesth.) Camb. Milit. Hosp. Aldershot.

WILSON, Richard Raymond, VRD (retired) 5 Marks Mews, Castle Lane, Warwick CV34 4BQ Tel: 01926 493375 — (St. Thos.) MRCS Eng. LRCP Lond. 1942.

WILSON, Mr Richard Yelverton Department of Surgery, Furness General Hospital, Dalton Lane, Barrow-in-Furness LA14 4LF Tel: 01229 870870 Email: richard.y.wilson@fgh.mbht.nhs.uk; Ashlands, Church Walk, Ulverston LA12 7EW Tel: 01229 586704 — (West. Austral.) MB BS Western Australia 1967; FRCS Eng. 1972. Cons. Urol. Furness Gen. Hosp. Cumbria, Westmorland Gen. Hosp. Kendal Cumbria and Roy. Lancaster Infirm., Lancaster. Specialty: Urol. Socs: Brit. Assn. Surgic. Oncol. (Full Mem.); Brit. Assn. Urol. Surg.; Brit Assoc. Urol.Surg. (Sect. of Oncol.). Prev: Lect. & Resid. Asst. (Surg.) Univ. Coll. Hosp. Lond.; SHO Univ. Hosp. S. Manch.; Ho. Phys. & Ho. Surg. Roy. Perth. Hosp., Austral.

WILSON, Robert (retired) 14 Forsyth Street, Greenock PA16 8DT Tel: 01475 27547 — MB ChB Glas. 1957. Prev: Cons. Clin. Biochem. Renfrewsh. Laborat. Serv.

WILSON, Robert Royal Brompton Hospital, Sidney Street, London SW3 6NP Tel: 020 7351 8338 Fax: 020 7351 8331 — MRCS Eng. LRCP Lond. 1979; MA Camb. 1980, MD 1987, MB 1979, BChir 1980; MRCP (UK) 1983; FRCP Lond. 1995. Reader & Cons. Phys. Nat. Heart & Lung Inst. & Roy. Brompton Hosp. Lond. Specialty: Respirat. Med. Socs: Mem. of Brit. Thoracic Soc.; Mem. of Europ. Respirat. Soc.; Mem. of Amer. Thoracic Soc.

WILSON, Robert Alistair 10 Lisnagarvey Drive, Lisburn BT28 3DW — MB BCh BAO Belf. 1990; MB BCh Belf. 1990.

WILSON, Robert Blue (retired) 15 Daleview Avenue, Glasgow G12 0HE Tel: 0141 576 1666 — MB ChB Glas. 1949.

WILSON, Robert Charles Duncan (retired) Old Dairy Cottage, Nutbourne Village, Pulborough RH20 2HE Tel: 01798 815294 Fax: 01798 815294 — MB ChB Aberd. 1956 (Univ. Aberd.) MD Canada 1960; LMCC Canada 1960; CCFP Canada 1972. Prev: Cons. Menopause & PMS Clinic Portland Hosp. Lond.

WILSON, Mr Robert George 7 Daltry Close, Yarm TS15 9XQ Tel: 01642 854841 — MB BS Newc. 1979; FRCS Eng. 1984; FRCS Ed. 1984; MD Newc. 1987. Cons. Surg. S. Cleveland Hosp. Middlesbrough. Specialty: Gen. Surg. Socs: Assn. Coloproctol.; Surgic. Research Soc.; BSG. Prev: Sen. Regist. North. RHA; Sen. Research Assoc. & Demonst. (Anat.) Univ. Newc.; SHO (Gen. Surg.) Roy. Vict. Infirm. Newc.

WILSON, Mr Robert Graeme 25 Swanston Terrace, Edinburgh EH10 7DN — MB ChB Aberd. 1980; FRCS Ed. 1984; ChM Aberd. 1991; FRCS (Gen.) 1995. Cons. Surg. West. Gen. Hosp. Edin. Specialty: Gen. Surg. Prev: Sen. Regist. (Gen. Surg.) Lothian HB.

WILSON, Mr Robert Irvine, MBE (retired) Spinney Cottage, 184 Finaghy Road Sth., Belfast BT10 0DH — MB BCh BAO Belf. 1938; MB BCh BAO. Belf. 1938; FRCS Ed. 1947; FRCSI (ad eund.) 1974. Prev: Emerit. Prof. Qu. Univ. Belf.

WILSON, Robert James, Surg. Lt.-Cdr. RN Retd. 2 Old School Close, Birdham, Chichester PO20 7ER Tel: 01243 513859 — MB BS Lond. 1973 (Guy's) MRCS Eng. LRCP Lond. 1973; MRCGP 1979.

WILSON, Robert James (retired) 1371 Warwick Road, Knowle, Solihull B93 9LW Tel: 01564 774412 — MB ChB Ed. 1957; MD Ed. 1973, BSc (Hons. Physiol.) 1954; MB ChB (Hons.) Ed. 1957; FRCP Ed. 1974, M 1962; FRCP Lond. 1982, M 1965. Prev: Cons. Phys. Solihull Hosp.

WILSON, Robert John Director of Public Health, West Lincolnshire Primary Care Trust, Cross O'Cliffe, Bracebridge Heath, Lincoln LN4 2HN Tel: 01522 515376 Fax: 01522 515364 — MB ChB Glas. 1986 (Glasgow) MRCGP 1990; MFPHM 1997. Cons. (Pub. Health Med.) Lincs. HA. Specialty: Pub. Health Med. Prev: Regist. (Pub. Health Med.) Leics. HA.

WILSON, Robert Richard 27 Iniscarn Park, Lisburn BT28 2BL — MB BCh BAO Belf. 1995.

WILSON, Robert Stanley Edward Lower Wood House, Lower Common, Longden, Shrewsbury SY5 8HB Tel: 0174 373657 — MB ChB Bristol 1968; BSc (Hons.) Bristol 1965, MB ChB (Hons.) 1968; MRCP (UK) 1972; FRCP Lond. 1985; MA Wales 1990. Gen. Phys. Roy. Shrewsbury Hosp.; Unit. Med. Advis. W. Unit. Shrops.; Chairm. Dist. Audit Comm. Shrops. HA. Prev: Sen. Med. Regist., SHO (Med.) & Ho. Phys. & Ho. Surg. United Bristol; Hosps.

WILSON, Robin Butler The Health Centre, Banks Road, Haddenham, Aylesbury HP17 8EE Tel: 01844 291874 Fax: 01844 292344 — Lekarz Lodz 1976; Lekarz Lodz 1976; MRCS Eng. LRCP Lond. London 1980.

WILSON, Robin John Abbey Surgery, 28 Plymouth Road, Tavistock PL19 8BU Tel: 01822 612247 Fax: 01822 618771 — MB BChir Camb. 1970 (St. Thos.) MB BChir Camb. 1969; MA Camb. 1969; MRCP (UK) 1972; DCH Eng. 1973; DObst RCOG 1974; MRCGP 1982. Prev: Regist. (Paediat.) Plymouth Gen. Hosp.; Resid. Med. Off. Westm. Childr. Hosp. Lond.

WILSON, Rodney Pearson North Lane, Navenby, Lincoln LN5 0EH Tel: 01522 810221 — MB BS Lond. 1964 (Lond. Hosp.) DObst RCOG 1966. Prev: Ho. Off. (Gen. Med. Surg. & O & G) Qu. Eliz. II Hosp. Welwyn Gdn. City; Ho. Off. (Gen. Surg.) Lond. Hosp.

WILSON, Roger Kyle 43 Surrey Street, Belfast BT9 7FR — MB BCh Belf. 1997.

WILSON, Mr Roger Stafford East Surrey Hospital, Canada Avenue, Redhill RH1 5RH Tel: 01737 768511; Ridge Green Farm, Kings Cross Lane, South Nutfield, Redhill RH1 5RL Tel: 01737 823200 Fax: 01737 823200 — MB ChB Birm. 1978; FRCS Eng. 1983; FRCOphth 1989. Cons. Ophth. E. Surrey HA; Cons. Adviser Ophth. Civil Aviat. Auth. Specialty: Ophth. Socs: Fell. Roy. Soc. Med.; UK Intraocular Implant Soc. Prev: Sen. Regist. (Ophth.) West. Ophth. Hosp. & Moorfields Eye Hosp. Lond.; SHO (Ophth.) Birm. & Midl. Eye Hosp.; Ho. Phys. Good Hope Gen. Hosp. Sutton Coldfield.

WILSON, Mr Ronald George (retired) Quality Assurance Reference Centre for Screening, General Hospital, West Gate Road, Newcastle upon Tyne NE4 6BE Tel: 0191 273 8811; 14 Hudshaw Gardens, Hexham NE46 1HY Tel: 01434 606180 Fax: 01434 606180 — MB ChB Aberd. 1961; FRCS Ed. 1970; MD Aberd.

1977. Prev: Cons. Surg. & Surg. Oncol. Gen. Hosp. Newc. & Newc. Breast Screen. Unit.

WILSON, Rosalind Mary (retired) Culm Park, Old Willand, Cullompton EX15 2RD Tel: 01884 33344 — MB BS Lond. 1951.

WILSON, Rowan Clare Department of Anaesthesia, St. James University Hospital, Beckett St., Leeds LS9 7 Tel: 0113 243 3144 Email: rwilson@epicure.u-net.com; Eltofts House, Carr Lane, Thorner, Leeds LS14 3HF Tel: 0113 289 3107 Fax: 0113 289 3800 — MB BS Lond. 1980 (Univ. Coll. Hosp.) MRCP (UK) 1984; FRCA 1989. Cons. Anaesth. St. James Univ. Hosp. Leeds.; Hon. Sen. Lect. Univ. Leeds. Specialty: Anaesth. Prev: Sen. Med. Off. Med. Educat., Train. & Staffing Div. Healthcare Directorate NHS Exec; Sen. Regist. Rotat. (Anaesth.) Yorks.

WILSON, Rowan Nicholas 12 St James Road, Prescot L35 0PF — MB BCh Wales 1991.

WILSON, Ruth Epsom District Hospital, Dorking Road, Epsom KT18 7EG; 91 College Road, Epsom KT17 4HH — MB ChB (Hons.) Leeds 1973; BSc (Anat.) Leeds 1970; DObst RCOG 1975; MRCGP 1977. Staff Grade (Neurol.) Epsom Dist. Hosp. Epsom.

WILSON, Mrs Ruth Audrey (retired) Charnock Green, Wigan Lane, Heath Charnock, Chorley PR7 4DD Tel: 012572 63250 — MB ChB Manch. 1946; MRCS Eng. LRCP Lond. 1946. Prev: Clin. Asst. Paediat. Roy. Albert Edwd. Infirm. Wigan.

WILSON, Ruth Edna Mary William Street Surgery, 67 William ST., Herne Bay CT6 5NR Tel: 01227 740000 Fax: 01227 742729; 33 Canterbury Road, Herne Bay CT6 5DQ Tel: 01227 368013 — MB ChB Glas. 1972; DObst RCOG 1975; DCH RCPS Glas. 1976. Breast linician Nat. Breast Screening Progr. Kent & Canterbury Hosp.; Clin. Asst. (Oncol.) Kent & Canterbury Hosp.

WILSON, Ruth Pauline Elspeth Temple Cowley Health Centre, Templar House, Temple Road, Oxford OX4 2HL Tel: 01865 777024 Fax: 01865 777548 — MB ChB Leeds 1985.

WILSON, Sally Ann 48 St Nicholas Drive, Shepperton TW17 9LD — MB ChB Bristol 1996.

WILSON, Sally-Anne 12 Limetrees Gardens, Gateshead NE9 5BE — MB BS Newc. 1994. SHO (A & E) Western Bay Tauranga NZ. Specialty: Accid. & Emerg. Socs: BMA; WIST. Prev: SHO (Med.) S. Tyneside Gen. Hosp.; SHO (A & E) N. Tyneside Gen. Hosp.; SHO (Urol. & Orthop.) Sunderland Dist. Gen. Hosp.

WILSON, Sally Ruth National Hospital for Neurology and Neurosurgery, Queen Square, London WC1N 3BG; 20 Oakington Road, London W9 2DH — MB BS Lond. 1983; BSc (Hons.) Lond. 1980, MB BS 1983; FRCA 1988. Specialty: Anaesth.

WILSON, Sam CNR Main & Centre STS, PO BOX 158, Pahiatua, New Zealand Tel: 00646 376 6466 Fax: 00646 376 6429; 110 Earlswood Road, Dorridge, Solihull B93 8RW — MB ChB Leeds 1976; FRNZCGP; (Otago) Dip. GP 2000. GP Pahiatua, Woodville & Eketakune, NZ. Prev: Med. Off. Suri Seri Begawan Hosp. Kuala Belait, Brunei; GP Coventry.

WILSON, Samuel John Simpson Lorna Doone, Praa Sands, Penzance TR20 9TQ — MB BS Lond. 1998.

WILSON, Sarah Stoneleigh, Bodenham, Hereford HR1 3HS — MB BS Lond. 1983; MSc. Community Med. Off. Hereford Community Trust. Specialty: Community Child Health.

WILSON, Sarah Harriet 8 Meadow Way, Kinoulton, Nottingham NG12 3RE — MB ChB Dundee 1979; BSc (Hons.) Dund 1974, MMSc 1976; MFCM 1989; MFFP 1993; FFPHM 1998. Dir. Pub. Health Nottm. HA. Specialty: Pub. Health Med. Prev: Sen. Lect. (Pub. Health Med.) Univ. Nottm. Med. Sch.; Regist. (Community Med.) Trent RHA.

WILSON, Sarah Juliet Royal Victoria Hospital, Grosvenor Road, Belfast BT12 6BA Tel: 01232 240503; Thornhill Gardens, 111 Marlborough Park South, Belfast BT9 6HW — MB BCh BAO Belf. 1994; MRCOphth 1998. SHO Ophth. Roy. Vict. Hosp. Belf. Specialty: Ophth.

WILSON, Sheena McRae 11 Inver Terrace, Muirhead, Dundee DD2 5LS Tel: 01382 580479 — MB ChB Dundee 1978. Staff Grade O & G Ninewells Hosp. Dundee.

WILSON, Simon James Percy The Surgery, 1-3 Chequers Drive, Prestwood, Great Missenden HP16 9DU Tel: 01494 862858; Roseberry, Broombarn Lane, Great Missenden HP16 9JD Tel: 01494 864737 — MB BS Lond. 1991 (Charing Cross & Westminster) DRCOG 1996; MRCGP 1998.

WILSON, Simon Paul Forensic Outreach Service, Clinical Treatment Centre, Maudsley Hospital, Denmark Hill, London SE5 8AZ Email: dr_simon_wilson@yahoo.co.uk — MB ChB Leeds 1995; MA (Phil.) Leeds 1993, BSc (Chem Path.) 1991; MRCPsych 1999. Cons. Forens. Psychiat., Maudsley Hosp. Specialty: Forens. Psychiat. Prev: Cons. Forens. Psychiat. HMP Brixton; Regist. (Psychiat.) Bethlem & Maudsley Hosps. Lond.

WILSON, Simon Russell "Fellside", Hale, Milnthorpe LA7 7BL Tel: 015395 63327 Fax: 015395 64059; Fellside, Hale, Milnthorpe LA7 7BL — MB ChB Manch. 1981. Prev: SHO Westmorland Co. Hosp. Kendal & Lancaster Infirm.; Ho. Off. Vict. Hosp. Blackpool; GP Princip., Milnthorpe, Cumbria.

WILSON, Stanley Darrin 132 Upper Newtownards Road, Belfast BT4 3EQ — MB BCh BAO Belf. 1989.

WILSON, Stephanie Margaret (retired) 14 St Thomas Gardens, London NW5 4EX — MD Dub. 1964 (T.C. Dub.) MB BCh BAO 1954; FRCPath 1976, M 1964. Prev: Cons. Histopath. St. Mary's Hosp. Lond.

WILSON, Stephen Geoffrey 91 College Road, Epsom KT17 4HH Tel: 01372 721062 Email: stephen.wilson@doctors.org.uk; 91 College Road, Epsom KT17 4HH Tel: 01372 721062 Fax: 01372 721062 Email: s.wilson@doctors.org.uk — MB ChB (Hons.) Leeds 1973; BSc (1st cl. Hons.) Physiol. Leeds 1970; MRCP (UK) 1975; Dip Immunol Chelsea 1977; MD 1981; FRCP Lond. 1990. p/t Cons. Neurol. St George's Hosp.Lond.; Cons. & Hon. Sen. Lect. St. Geo. Hosp. Lond. Specialty: Neurol. Special Interest: Parkinsons Dis.; Stroke. Prev: Cons. Neurol. Atkinson Morley's & Epsom Dist. Gen. Hosps.

WILSON, Stephen Jack — MB ChB Birm. 1995; MRCP Lond. 2002.

WILSON, Stephen John Rosemount Medical Practice, 1 View Terrace, Aberdeen AB25 2RS Tel: 01224 638050 Fax: 01224 627308 — MB ChB Aberd. 1979; MRCGP 1983. Specialty: Gen. Pract. Prev: Offshore Doctor OMS Aberd.

WILSON, Stephen John Nuffield Dept. Of Anaesthetics, Oxford, John Radcliff Hospital, Headington, Oxford OX3 9DU Tel: 01865 741166 — MB ChB Bristol 1990; FRCA 1999. Specialist Regist. (Anaesth.) Oxf. Specialty: Anaesth.; Intens. Care. Socs: BMA; Assn. Of Anaesth. G. Brit.; Fell. Of Roy. Coll. Of Anaesth. Prev: Regist. (Anaesth.) Northampton Gen. Hosp.

WILSON, Stephen Michael 6 Beaufort Grove, Morecambe LA4 6UF — MB ChB Ed. 1998.

WILSON, Stephen Robert C/o ISIS Centre, Little Clarendon St., Oxford OX1 2HS Tel: 01865 310744 Fax: 01865 310744 — MRCS Eng. LRCP Lond. 1968 (Roy. Free) DPM Eng. 1972; FRCPsych 1985, M 1974; MSc (Economics) Lond. 1974; MSc (Clin. Med.) Oxf. 1978. Hon. Cons. Psychother. Ment. Healthcare Trust; Hon. Research Fell. Centre for Psychonalytic Studies Univ. Kent; Cons. Psychotherapist, Dept. Psychother. Northamptonshire. Specialty: Psychother. Prev: Cons. Psychotherapist Warneford Hosp. Oxf.; Cons. Psychiat. (Psychother.) Littlemore Hosp. Oxf.; Hon. Sen. Clin. Lect. (Psychiat.) Univ. Oxf.

WILSON, Stuart Jonathan 8 Selm Park, Livingston EH54 5NU — MB ChB Aberd. 1993 (Aberdeen) Specialty: Gen. Med.

WILSON, Mr Stuart William Wythenshawe Hospital, Department of Plastic Surgery, Southmoor Road, Wythenshawe, Manchester M23 9LT — MB ChB Sheff. 1986; FRCS Glas. 1990; FRCS Eng. 1990; FRCS (Plast) 1997. Cons. Plastic Surg., Withington Hosp. Specialty: Plastic Surg. Prev: Sen. Regist. (Plastic Surg.) Pinderfield Hosp. Wakefield; Ho. Off. (Surg.) Roy. Hallamsh. Hosp. Sheff.; Ho. Phys. Lodge Moor Hosp. Sheff.

WILSON, Miss Susan Elaine 45A Samos Road, Anerley, London SE20 7TX Tel: 020 8325 3092; Department of Vascular Surgery, Leeds General Infirmary, Leeds LS1 — MB BS Lond. 1991 (Royal Free Hospital) BSc Lond. 1988; FRCS Eng. 1995. Research Regist. (Vasc. Surg.) Leeds Gen. Infirm. Specialty: Gen. Surg. Prev: Regist. (Gen. Surg.) Guy's Hosp. Lond.

WILSON, Susan Jane Vonda Queens Road Medical Practice, The Grange, St. Peter Port, Guernsey GY1 1RH Tel: 01481 724184 Fax: 01481 716431; Les Ruettes Farm, Les Ruettes, St. Andrews, Guernsey GY6 8UQ Tel: 01481 37142 — MB ChB Aberd. 1979; MRCGP Ed. 1983.

WILSON, Susannah Louise 40 Ashford Drive, Ravenshead, Nottingham NG15 9DE Tel: 01623 794341 — BM BS Nottm.

1995. SHO (Gen. Med.) Nottm. City Hosp. VTS; SHO (Obst. & Gyn.) Grantham & Dist. Hosp.; SHO (Paediat.) Qu. Med. Centre Nottm.. Specialty: Paediat. Prev: Ho. Off. (Gen. Surg. & Urol.) Nottm. City Hosp.; Ho. Off. (Gen. Med.) King's Mill Hosp. Mansfield.

WILSON, Suzannah Yvonne 25 Lime Close, Harrow HA3 7JG — MB BS West Indies 1993. SHO (Gen. Med.) Watford Gen. Hosp. Specialty: Cardiol.

WILSON, Suzanne Denise 2 Hockley Cottages, The Heath, Hatfield Heath, Bishop's Stortford CM22 7EA — MB ChB Sheff. 1991.

WILSON, Tamsin Margaret Newbiggin Hall Farmhouse, Hexham NE46 1TA — MB BS Newc. 1984. Clin. Asst. (Anaesth.) Hexham Gen. Hosp.

WILSON, Teresa Anne Howitt Meadowbank, 12 Woodland Way, Weybridge KT13 9SW — MB BCh Wales 1998.

WILSON, Thomas Daniel Partington 60 Binswood Avenue, Leamington Spa CV32 5RX — BChir Camb. 1995.

WILSON, Thomas Kyle Dr Clark's Practice, Kenilworth Avenue, Wishaw ML2 7BQ Tel: 01698 372201 Fax: 01698 371051; 22 Brownhill View, Newmains, Wishaw ML2 9QJ — MB ChB Glas. 1979; MRCGP 1984.

WILSON, Thomas MacSkimming (retired) Benvenuti, 4 King Street, Oldmeldrum, Inverurie AB51 0EQ Tel: 01651 873091 — MB ChB Aberd. 1944. Prev: Principle in Gen. Pract., Bucksburn Aberd. 68/88.

WILSON, Thomas Scott (retired) 75 Stewarton Drive, Cambuslang, Glasgow G72 8DQ Tel: 0141 641 2195 — (Univ. Glas.) MD Glas. 1951, MB ChB 1944; DPH Glas. 1949; DIH RFPS Glas. 1949; DPA Glas. 1959; FFCM 1974; FRCP Glas. 1979, M 1976. Prev: SCM Greater Glas. Health Bd.

WILSON, Thomas Scott (retired) Tanglewood, St. Clements Hill, Truro TR1 1NU Tel: 01872 73719 — MD Belf. 1947; MB BCh BAO 1940. Prev: Cons. Geriat. Phys. Cornw.

WILSON, Thomas Stephen (retired) 34 Malone Heights, Belfast BT9 5PG Tel: 02890 610042 — MB BCh BAO Belf. 1955; FRCPI 1987, M 1963; FRCPath 1977, M 1965. Prev: Cons. Bacteriol. Laborat. Belf. City Hosp.

WILSON, Timothy James Medway NHS Trust, Windmill Road, Gillingham ME7 5NY — MB BS Lond. 1973; MRCS Eng. LRCP Lond. 1971; FFA RCS Eng. 1978. Cons. Anaesth. Medway Health Dist. Specialty: Anaesth.

WILSON, Valerie Elizabeth Kensington Street Health Centre, Whitefield Place, Girlington, Bradford BD8 9LB Tel: 01274 499209; 26 Carrbottom Road, Greengates, Bradford BD10 0BB Tel: 01274 619184 Email: neasha@globalnet.co.uk — MB ChB Aberd. 1977. Clin. Asst. (Anaesth.) Leeds Gen. Infirm.

WILSON, Victor 1 James Close, Woodlands, Golders Green, London NW11 9QX Tel: 020 8458 6730 — MB BS Lond. 1952 (Char. Cross) Locum GP. Special Interest: Dermat. Socs: Ins. Med. Soc. Prev: Hosp. Pract. Dept. Dermat. Mt. Vernon Hosp. Northwood; Regist. & Ho. Phys. Dept. Dermat. Guy's Hosp. Lond.; Med. Off. Dept. Dermat. Hosp. Sick Childr. Gt. Ormond St.

WILSON, Virginia Sonia 49 Ovington Street, London SW3 2JA — MB BS Lond. 1980; DCH RCP Lond. 1983.

WILSON, Mr William (retired) 34 Calderwood Road, Glasgow G43 2RU Tel: 0141 637 4898 — MB ChB Glas. 1952; FRCS Ed. 1958; DO Eng. 1958; FRCOphth. 1990. Ophth. Surg. Glas. Roy. Infirm. & Canniesburn Hosp. Glas. Prev: Ophth. Surg. Vict. Infirm. Glas. Ophth. Inst. & South. Gen. Hosp. Glas.

WILSON, William Adamson Melvin Charlotte Street Surgery, 1 Charlotte Street, Dumfries DG1 2AQ Tel: 01387 267626 Fax: 01387 266824; Riverside, Kelton, Dumfries DG1 4UA — MB ChB Aberd. 1972; MRCGP 1977; Dip. Forens. Med. Glas 1991. Specialty: Gen. Pract.

WILSON, William Alan (retired) Rubislaw Place Medical Group, 7 Rubislaw Place, Aberdeen AB10 1QB Tel: 01224 641968 Fax: 01224 645738 — MB ChB Aberd. 1968; MRCGP 1974.

WILSON, William George The Retreat, Stourton Candle, Sturminster Newton DT10 2JN — MB BS Lond. 1990; DCH; MRCGP. Princip. Gen. Pract. Essex Ho. Med. Centre Chard Somerst.

WILSON, William John Chesney Portglenone Health Centre, 17 Townhill Road, Portglenone, Ballymena BT44 8AD Tel: 028 2582 1551 Fax: 028 2582 2539 — MB BCh BAO Belf. 1977 (Queens Univ. Belfast) DRCOG 1980; MRCGP 1981. Specialty: Gen. Pract.

WILSON, William Neil Willowfield Surgery, 50 Castlereagh Road, Belfast BT5 5FP Tel: 028 9045 7862 Fax: 028 9045 9785 — MB BCh BAO Belf. 1979; MRCGP 1989.

WILSON, William Richard — MB BCh Belf. 1998; BSC (Hons) Belf 1996; MB BCh Belf 1998. Anaesth. SHO., Altnagelvin Area Hsopital. Specialty: Anaesth. Prev: Jun. Ho. Off., Belf. City Hosp.

WILSON, William Scott (retired) 20 Dingley Road, Edgerton, Huddersfield HD3 3AY — MB ChB Glas. 1942; DPH 1947; MRCGP 1953. Prev: Res. Med. Off. Isolat. Hosp. & Sanat. Brighton & Roy. Infirm.

WILSON, Mr William Weatherston Charnock Green, Wigan Lane, Heath Charnock, Chorley PR7 4DD Tel: 012572 63250 — MRCS Eng. LRCP Lond. 1938 (Manch.) ChM Manch. 1959, MB ChB 1938; FRCS Eng. 1947. Surg. Emerit. Roy. Albert Edwd. Infirm. Wigan. Socs: Fell. Assn. Surgs. Gt. Brit. & Irel. & Manch. Med. Soc. Prev: Surgic. Chief Asst. Christie Hosp. & Manch. Roy. Infirm.; Mem. Ct. Examrs. RCS Eng.; Capt. RAMC.

WILSON, Yvonne Teresa 34 Malone Heights, Belfast BT9 5PG — MB ChB Dundee 1984; FRCS Glas. 1988; FRCS (Plast.) 1996. Cons. Plastic Surg. Birm. Childr.'s Hosp. B'ham. Specialty: Plastic Surg. Prev: Cons. (Plastic Surg.) St. Johns Hosp. Livingston & Roy. Hosp. for Sick Childr. Edin.; Sen. Regist. (Plastic Surg.) St. Johns Hosp. Livingston.; Regist. (Plastic Surg.) North. Gen. Hosp. Sheff.

WILSON-CROOME, Jonathan Iona, Smugglers Lane, Furzehill, Wimborne BH21 4HB — MB BS Lond. 1975 (Char. Cross) DRCOG 1981; MRCGP 1982. Non-Principal GP. Socs: Roy. Coll. Gen. Pract. & BMA. Prev: Med. Off. RAF.; CMO, Prime Med., Bournemouth.

WILSON-DAVIS, Margaret Lilian 14 Ballygallum Road, Downpatrick BT30 7DA Tel: 01396 615168 — MB BS Newc. 1965; FFA RCSI 1969; FFA RCS Eng. 1969. Specialty: Anaesth. Prev: Cons. (Anaesth.) Whiteabbey Hosp.; Sen. Regist. (Anaesth.) Roy. Vict. Hosp. Belf.; Sen. Regist. (Anaesth.) Sheff. HA.

WILSON-HAFFENDEN, Carolyn Fay Cambridgeshire and Peterborough Public Health Network, West Anglia Cancer Network, Kingfisher House, Hinchingbrooke Business Park, Huntingdon PE29 398500 Tel: 01480 398500 — MB ChB Ed. 1976. Cons. Pub. Health Med. NW Anglia Health Auth. Specialty: Pub. Health Med. Socs: Fac. Pub. Health Med. Prev: Sen. Regist. (Pub. Health Med.) Beds.

WILSON-HOLT, Mr Nicholas John Royal Cornwall Hospital, Treliske, Truro TR1 3JW Tel: 01872 253903; Duchy Hospital, Penventinnie Lane, Pen, Truro TR1 3UP Tel: 01872 226100 — MB BS Lond. 1982; BSc (Hons.) Lond. 1979; FRCS (Ophth.) Glas. 1986; FRCOphth 1989. Cons. Ophth. Surg. Roy. Cornw. Hosp. Trust.; Freeman Scholsh. Middlx. Hosp. Med. Sch. Specialty: Ophth. Prev: Sen. Regist. & Vitroretinal Fell Moorfields Eye Hosp. Lond.; Resid. Surgic. Off. Moorfields Eye Hosp.

WILSON JONES, Alexander Catherine Rose Longfield, Fairfield Lane, West End, Woking GU24 9QX — MB ChB Bristol 1995. Prev: Ho. Off. (Med.) Treliske Hosp. Cornw.; Ho. Off. (Surg.) Southmead Hosp. Bristol.

WILSON JONES, Charlotte Frances The Maudsley Hospital, Denmark Hill, London SE5 8AZ — MB BCh Wales 1991 (Univ. Wales Coll. Med.) MRCPsych 1996. Specialist Regist. Comm. Psychiat. The Maudsley Hosp Lond.; Hon. SOR liaison Psychiat. to St. Christophers Hospice, Sydenham, Lond. Specialty: Gen. Psychiat. Socs: BMA; Roy. Coll. Psychiat. Prev: Sen. Regist. Bethlem & Maudsley Adult Psychiat. NHS Trust, Lond.; Clin. Research Fell.Psychiat. Kings Coll. Lond. & Inst. of Psychiat.; Regist. (Psychiat.) Bethlem & Maudsley NHS Trust.

WILSON JONES, Nicholas Anthony Hugh Joseph Longfield, Fairfield Lane, Woking GU24 9QX — MB BCh Wales 1996.

WILSON-MACDONALD, Mr James St. Luke's Hospital, Latimer Road, Headington, Oxford OX3 7PF Tel: 01865 288866 Fax: 01865 744520 Email: jwmac@onetel.net.uk — MB ChB Bristol 1978; FRCS Eng. 1982; MCh 1990. p/t Cons. Orthopaedic Surg., Nuffield Orthopaedic Centre, Oxf. OX3 7LD. Specialty: Orthop. Socs: Brit. Scolosis Soc.-Exec.; Brit. Cervical Spine Soc.; Brit. Orthopaedic Assn. Prev: Cons. Orthop. Surg. Norf. & Norwich Hosp.

WILSON-NUNN, David Laurence Norfolk & Norwich University Hospital NHS Trust, Department of Anaesthesia, Norwich NR4 7UY Tel: 01603 287086 Fax: 01603 287886 Email: david.wilson-nunn@nnuh.nhs.uk — MB BChir Camb. 1992; BA Oxf. 1987; PhD

Camb. 1990; FRCA 1997. Cons. Specialty: Anaesth. Special Interest: Vasc. Anaesth.

WILSON-SHARP, Cecil Derek (retired) St. Peter's Croft, 4 Charles Moor, Stockton Lane, York YO31 1BE Tel: 01904 33890 — MB BS Lond. 1945 (Univ. Coll. Lond. & St. Bart.) DMRD 1950. Prev: Cons. Radiol. in Admi/c Essex Co. Hosp. & Others.

WILSON-SHARP, Rosalind Claire Pinderfields General Hospital, Aberford Road, Wakefield WF1 4DG Tel: 01924 201688 — MB BS Lond. 1975; MRCP (UK) 1979; FRCR 1983. Cons. Radiol. Pinderfields Gen. Hosp. Wakefield. Specialty: Radiol.

WILSON-STOREY, Mr Derrick Royal Hospital for Sick Children, Sciennes Road, Edinburgh EH9 1LF Tel: 0131 536 0000 Fax: 0131 536 0665 Email: derrickwilson-storey@luht.scot.nhs.uk — MD Sheff. 1988 (Sheffield) MB ChB Sheff. 1978; FRCS Ed. 1983. Cons. Paediat. Surg. Roy. Hosp. Sick Childr. Edin.; Clin. Sub Dean (Paedistrics), Univ. of Edin. Specialty: Paediat. Surg. Socs: Brit. Assn. Paediat. Surg.; Scott. Soc. Paediat. Surg.; Brit. Med. Assn. Prev: Sen. Regist. & Clin. Tutor (Paediat. Surg.) Childr. Hosp. Sheff.; Regist. (Paediat. Surg.) Edin.; Regist. (Gen. Surg.) Barnsley HA.

WILTER, Pierre Hendrik Willow Court, Marsham Lane, Gerrards Cross SL9 8HD Tel: 01753 899096 Fax: 01753 899095 Email: pierre@wa-global.com — MB ChB Cape Town 1980; BSc (Med.) Cape Town 1975; MBA Open 1991. Cons. Health Care Managem. PriceWaterHo.Coopers Lond. Prev: Med. Dir. HM YO1 & RC Feltham Middlx.; Clin. Asst. (Forens. Psychiat.) Regional Secure Unit St. Bernards Hosp. Lond.; Regist. (Psychiat.) Middlx. Hosp. & St. Bernards Hosp. Lond.

WILTON, Alison Yvonne Department of Community Paediatrics, 3/5 Craven Road, Reading RG1 5LF Tel: 01734 862277 Fax: 01734 750297; 7 St. Johns Road, Mortimer, Reading RG7 3TR Tel: 01734 331201 — MB ChB Birm. 1982; MRCP (UK) 1987. Cons. Paediat. (Community Child Health) Reading. Specialty: Pub. Health Med. Prev: Sen. Regist. (Community Paediat.) E. Anglia RHA; Clin. Research Regist. Univ. Birm.; Hon. Regist. (Paediat.) Dudley Rd. Hosp. Birm.

WILTON, Anthony 47 Caemawr Gardens, Porth CF39 9DB — MB BCh Wales 1982.

WILTON, Howard John West View House, 26 Callis Court Road, Broadstairs CT10 3AF Tel: 01843 862624 — MB BS Lond. 1971 (King's Coll. Hosp.) FFA RCS Eng. 1977. Cons. Anaesth. Canterbury & Thanet DHA. Specialty: Anaesth. Socs: Obst. Anaesth. Assn.; BMA (Hon. Sec. E. Kent Div.). Prev: Anaesth. Sen. Regist. Portsmouth & Soton. Health Dist.

WILTON, Joseph Frederick Lisson Grove Health Centre, Gateforth St, London NW8 8EG Tel: 020 7262 1366 Fax: 020 7258 1943; 28 Winscombe Street, London N19 5DG — MB BS Lond. 1977 (St. Bart.) BSc (Microbiol.) Reading 1969; MRCS Eng. LRCP Lond. 1977; DCH Eng. 1979; DRCOG 1980; MRCGP 1982. GP Princip. Lisson Gr. Health Centre Lond.; Course Organiser GP Ho. Off. in Gen. Pract.; Coordinator Further Educat. & Support for Non-Princip. KCW Health Auth. Prev: Trainee GP Kentish Town Health Centre.

WILTON, Mr Timothy James 81 Friargate, Derby DE1 1FL; Hillcrest, 22 Castle Hill, Duffield, Belper DE56 4EA — MB BS Lond. 1978 (University College Hospital) BA (Hons.) Oxf. 1975; FRCS Eng. 1983; MA Oxf. 1995. Cons. Orthop. Surg. Derbysh. Roy. Infirm.; Clin. Teach. Nottm. Uni. Med. Sch. Specialty: Trauma & Orthop. Surg. Socs: Fell. Orthop. Assn.; Treas. Brit. Assn. Surg. Knee. Prev: Sen. Regist. (Orthop.) Derbysh. Roy. Infirm. & Harlow Wood Orthop. Hosp.; Regist. (Orthop.) Univ. Hosp. & Harlow Wood Orthop. Hosp. Nottm.; Regist. Surg. Train. Scheme Welsh Nat. Sch. Med. Cardiff.

WILTSHAW, Eve, OBE (retired) The Cottage, Overnoons, Bexley Hill, Petworth GU28 9DZ — MB BCh Wales 1951 (Cardiff) MD Wales 1969; FRCP Lond. 1981, M 1971; FRCOG 1990. Prev: Cons. Phys. Roy. Marsden Hosp. Lond.

WILTSHIRE, Christopher Robert (retired) Dairy Farmhouse, Somersham Road, Bramford, Ipswich IP8 4NN Tel: 01473 832559 Fax: 01473 832559 — MB BS Lond. 1970 (Roy. Free) MRCP (UK) 1973; FRCR 1976; FRCP Lond. 1993. Prev: Regist. (Radiother.) Middlx. Hosp. Lond.

WILTSHIRE, Edwin Julian Mark Whitchurch Road Medical Centre, 210-212 Whitchurch Road, Heath, Cardiff CF14 3NB Tel: 029 2062 1282 Fax: 029 2052 0210 — MB BCh Wales 1984; DRCOG 1987; MRCGP 1988; Docc Med 1998.

WILTSHIRE, Robin James Abbott Laboratories, Abbott House, Norden Road, Maidenhead SL6 4XE Tel: 01628 644322 Fax: 01628 644185; 1 Hayward Place, Hedsor rd, Bourne End SL8 5EP Tel: 01628 526074 — MB ChB Birm. 1992 (Birmingham) BSc (Pharm.) Birm. 1989; Msc Aberdeen 1999. Med. Advisor Abbot Laboratories Maidenhead. Specialty: Pharmaceutical Medicine. Socs: BRAPP. Prev: Med. Off. Brit. Antarctic Survey.

WILTSHIRE, Susan Jane Department of Anaesthesia, The Ipswich Hospital NHS Trust, Heath Road, Ipswich IP4 5PD Tel: 01473 712233; Dairy Farm House, Somersham Road, Bramford, Ipswich IP8 4NN Tel: 01473 832559 — (Roy. Free) MB BS Lond. 1970; FFA RCS Eng. 1975. Cons. Anaesth. Ipswich Hosp. Specialty: Anaesth. Prev: Sen. Regist. (Anaesth.) Ipswich Hosp. & Addenbrooke's Hosp. Camb.; Regist. (Anaesth.) Lond. Hosp.

WIMALARATNE, Bala Manage Daya Sisil — MB BS Sri Lanka 1977; DA Eng. 1980; FFA RCS Eng. 1986. Specialty: Anaesth.

WIMALASIRI, Robert Wijepala 5 Grove Lane, Kingston upon Thames KT1 2SU — MB BS Ceylon 1962; MRCP (UK) 1987.

WIMALASUNDERA, Herbert Harischandra Gordon House Surgery, 78 Mattock Lane, Ealing, London W13 9NZ Tel: 020 8567 0631 — MB BS Ceylon 1961. Specialty: Care of the Elderly; Gen. Med.

WIMALASUNDERA, Ruwan Chinthaka 43 Tudor Drive, Kingston upon Thames KT2 5NW — (King's College Hospital) BSc Lond. 1988; MB BS Lond. 1991; MRCOG Lond. 1996. Clin. Research Fell. Imperial Coll. Med. Sch. Nat. Heart & Lung Inst.; Dept. Clin. Pharmacol. St Mary's Hosp. Lond. Specialty: Obst. & Gyn.

WIMALASURIA, Sarath Bandula 2 Firsby Avenue, Croydon CR0 8TL Tel: 020 8654 5003 — MBBS Celon; DTM & H Liverp.

WIMBLETON, Penelope Ann 14 Stanley Road, Bournemouth BH1 4SB — MB ChB Manch. 1989.

WIMBORNE, Jonathan Mark York Bridge Surgery, 5 James Street, Morecambe LA4 5TE — MB ChB Manch. 1988; MRCGP 1993.

WIMHURST, Mr James Anthony Department of Orthopaedics, Level 4, Bice Building, Royal Adelaide Hospital, Adelaide 5000, Adelaide CB5 8DW, Australia Email: woodwim@hotmail.com — MB BChir Camb. 1992 (Cambridge) MA Camb. 1992; FRCS (Eng.) 1996; MChir 2000; FRCS (Tr. & Orth.) 2001. Lect. in Orthop., Roy. Adelaide Hosp.; Jt. Replacement Fell., Dept. of Orthop., Roy. Adelaide Hosp. Specialty: Orthop. Special Interest: Hip and knee replacement Surg. Socs: Assoc. Mem. BOA; Brit. Orthop. Train. Assn. Prev: Specialist Regist. (Trauma & Orthop.) Addenbrooke's; Specialist Regist. (Trauma & Orthop.) Ipswich; Specialist Regist. (Trauma & Orthop.) Addenbrooke's.

WIMHURST, John Alan (retired) The Warren, Elmcroft Lane, Felixstowe IP11 9LX — (Lond. Hosp.) MB BS Lond. 1962; DObst RCOG 1964. Clin. Asst. Bartlet Hosp. Felixstowe. Prev: Clin. Asst. (A & E) Ipswich Hosp.

***WIMPENNY, Joanne Louise** 27 Aston Hill Drive, Aston-on-Trent, Derby DE72 2DD — MB ChB Birm. 1998.

WIMPERIS, Jennifer Zeala Norfolk & Norwich Hospital, Colney Lane, Norwich NR4 7UY Tel: 01603 289979 Fax: 01603 286918 Email: jennie.wimperis@nnuh.nhs.uk; 420 Unthank Road, Norwich NR4 7QH — MB BS Lond. 1979 (Oxf. & Middlx.) FRCP; FRCPath; BA Oxf. 1976; DM Oxf. 1987. p/t Cons. Haemat. Norf. & Norwich Hosp. (9 sessions). Specialty: Haematology.

WIN, Aung Zaw Hull Royal Infirmary, Anlaby Road, Hull HU3 2JZ Email: aungzawwin@aol.com. SHO (Med. Rotat.) Hull Roy. Infirm.

MYA THAN WIN, June Coggeshall Road Surgery, 9 Coggeshall Road, Braintree CM7 9DD Tel: 01376 552508 Fax: 01376 552690 — MB BS Med Inst (I) Rangoon 1975.

WIN, Maung Tun c/o Lloyds Bank, 6 Pall Mall, London SW1Y 5NG — MB BS Rangoon 1949.

WIN, Swe Swe Family Health Care Centre, 1 East Anglian Way, Gorleston-on-Sea, Great Yarmouth NR31 6TY Tel: 01493 662130 — MB BS Med Inst (I) Rangoon 1972; MB BS Med Inst (I) Rangoon 1972.

WIN HLAING, Dr Burma Hills Surgery, Ashridge Road, Wokingham RG40 1PH Tel: 01189 785854 Fax: 01189 893902 — MB BS Med. Inst. (I) Rangoon 1975.

WIN KO, Dr 38 Woolaston Avenue, Cardiff CF23 6HA — MB BS Med. Inst. Rangoon 1973.

WIN MAUNG, Dr HMP Whitmoor, March Tel: 01354 660653 — MB BS Med. Inst. (III) Mandalay 1967; MRCP (UK) 1973; FRCP Ed. 1987. Sen. Med. Off. HMP Whitmoor, March. Prev: Sen. Med. Off. HMP Full Sutton York.; Med. Off. HM Prison Serv. Hull; Cons. Phys. & Med. Supt. Toungoo, Burma.

WINARSO, Paulus 15 Lowerfold Way, Rochdale OL12 7HX — MB ChB Birm. 1976; DMRD 1981; FRCR 1983.

WINAYAK, Kamal 92 Heston Road, Heston, Hounslow TW5 0QP — MB BS Lond. 1987.

WINAYAK, Varendar Kumar The Medical Centre, 192 Twickenham Road, Hanworth, Feltham TW13 6HD Tel: 020 8979 3058 — MB BS Lond. 1978 (Univ. Coll. May. Med. Sch. Lond.) DRCOG 1982; MFFP 1982. GP Lond. Specialty: Family Plann. & Reproduc. Health. Prev: SCMO Margt. Pyke Centre Lond.; Med. Off. Marie Stopes Hse. Lond.; Cons. Phys. BUPA Med. Centre Lond.

WINBOW, Adrian John Godden Green Clinic, Godden Green, Sevenoaks TN15 0JR Tel: 01732 763491 Fax: 01732 763160 — MB BS Newc. 1969; DPM Eng. 1975; MRCPsych 1976; T(Psych) 1991; FRCPsych 1998. Cons. Psychiat, Godden Green Clinic; Cons. Psychiat. Hartswood Hosp. Brentwood; Cons. Psychiat. Shirley Oaks Hosp., Croydon; Cons. Psychiat. Nuffield Hosp., Tunbridge Wells. Specialty: Gen. Psychiat.; Psychother.; Hypnother. Socs: BMA & Brit. Soc. Med. & Dent. Hypn. Prev: Sen. Regist. (Psychiat.) Leics. DHA (T); Regist. (Psychiat.) St. Nicholas' Hosp. Newc.; Ho. Surg. & Ho. Phys. Roy. Vict. Infirm. Newc.

WINBURN, Philip E I 26 Oakhurst Drive, Newcastle upon Tyne NE3 4JS — MB BS Durh. 1947 (Newc.) Prev: Hosp. Pract. (Orthop.) Ashington Hosp.; Asst. Lect. (Anat.) Roy. Free Hosp. Med. Sch. Lond.; Ho. Surg. Roy. Vict. Infirm. Newc.

WINCESLAUS, Soosaipillai Joseph Kent & Sussex Hospital, Mount Ephraim, Tunbridge Wells TN4 8AT Tel: 01892 26111; 31 Byng Road, Tunbridge Wells TN4 8EG — MB BS Ceylon 1969; FRCOG 1993, M 1978. Cons. Genitourin. Med. Kent & Sussex Hosp. Tunbridge Wells; HIV Phys., Kent & Sussex Hosp. Tunbridge Wells. Specialty: Genitourinary Medicine; HIV Med. Prev: Sen. Regist. (Genitourin. Med.) Lond. Hosp.

WINCEWICZ, Andrzej Marian 92 Harley Street, London W1G 7HU; 119 Hatherley Court, Hatherley Grove, London W2 5RG Tel: 020 7229 5691 — MB BS Med. 1967; MB BS Med. Acad. Bialystok 1967; LMSSA Lond. 1977; DRCOG 1983. Specialty: Obst. & Gyn. Prev: Regist. (O & G) Newham Matern. Hosp. Lond. & St. Mary's Hosp. Wom. Lond.; Regist. (O & G) Qu. Mary's Hosp. Sidcup.; Asst. (O & G) City Hosp. Torun, Poland.

WINCH, Timothy Miller's Cottage, Ratham Lane, West Ashling, Chichester PO18 8DL — MB ChB Aberd. 1987.

WINCHESTER, Elizabeth Natalie Marten (retired) 4 Brook Manor, Turners Hill Road, East Grinstead RH19 4 LX — MB ChB Sheff. 1962 (Sheffield) MRCPsych. 1982. Prev: Ass. Specialist Child Psychiat., Coventry, Rugby, Nuneaton.

WINCHESTER, John Paul Theale Medical Centre, Englefield Road, Theale, Reading RG7 5AS Tel: 0118 930 2513 Fax: 0118 930 4419; 64 Horseshoe Road, Pangbourne, Reading RG8 7JL Tel: 01734 984 2583 — MB BS Lond. 1986 (University College London) DCH RCP Lond. 1989; MRCGP 1991. Clin. Asst. (Rheum.) Battle Hosp. Reading. Prev: Trainee GP Hay-on-Wye & Talgarth; SHO (O & G) Hillingdon Hosp.; SHO (A & E) Whittingdon Hosp. Lond.

WINCHESTER, John Sefton (retired) 4 Brook Manor, Turners Hill Road, East Grinstead RH19 4LX Tel: 01342 301645 — MB ChB Sheff. 1962; MRCPath 1982. Prev: GP, Covent.

WINCHESTER, Sandra Lesley (retired) 31 Montclair Drive, Liverpool L18 0HD Tel: 0151 722 6395 — (Liverp.) MB ChB Liverp. 1967; DObst RCOG 1969. Prev: SCMO (Community Child Health - Special Needs) Roy. Liverp. Childr. NHS Trust.

WINCHURCH, Stuart Ronald Carlton Street Surgery, Carlton Street, Horninglow, Burton-on-Trent DE13 0TE Tel: 01283 511387 Fax: 01283 517174; The Barn, Sutton on the Hill, Ashbourne DE6 53A Tel: 01283 733283 — MB ChB Liverp. 1979 (Liverpool) MB ChB (Hons.) Liverp. 1979; DRCOG 1981; DA (UK) 1986. GP; Hypnother. Counselling. Specialty: Gen. Pract.; Psychother. Prev: Anaesth./ITU Gen. Med.

WINDALL, Karen Margaret Tyn PwllBank, Bodedern, Holyhead LL65 3PB — MB ChB Leeds 1981; DA (UK) 1985. GP David Lewis Centre for Epilepsy Chesh.

WINDEBANK, Kevin Patrick Department of Child Health, Sir James Spence Institute, The Royal Victoria Infirmary, Newcastle upon Tyne NE1 4LP Tel: 0191 202 3026 Fax: 0191 202 3060 Email: k.p.windebank@ncl.ac.uk — BM BCh Oxf. 1977; MRCP (UK) 1983; MA Oxf. 1987; DM Oxf. 1999. Sen. Lect. in Child Health Univ. of Newc. upon Tyne; Hon. Cons. Paediat. Oncol. Roy. Vict. Infirm. Newc. Upon Tyne. Specialty: Paediat. Socs: Fell. RCP; Fell.RCPCH; Histocytosis Assn. Prev: Lect. (Paediat. Oncol.) Dept. Child Health Med. Sch. Newc.; Fell. (Paediat. Haemat. Oncol.) Mayo Clinic Rochester Minnesota, USA.

WINDEBANK, William John, SBStJ Derbyshire Royal Infirmary, London Road, Derby DE1 2QY Tel: 01332 347141 — MB ChB Glas. 1966; BSc (Hons. Physiol.) Glas. 1963; MRCP (UK) 1970; FRCP Glas. 1980; FRCP Lond. 1994. Cons. Phys. (Thoracic Med.) Derbysh. Roy. Infirm. Derby. Specialty: Gen. Med. Socs: Europ. Resusc. Counc.; Scott. Thoracic Soc.; Brit. Thorac. Soc. Prev: Regist. (Med.) Med. Centre Respirat. Investig. Roy. Infirm. Glas.; Ho. Phys & Ho. Surg. Glas. Roy. Infirm.

WINDER, Professor Anthony Frederick Department of Molecular Pathology and Clinical Biochemistry, Royal Free & University College Medical School, UCL, Pond St., London NW3 2QG Tel: 020 7830 2258 Fax: 020 7830 2235 Email: tony_w@rfhsm.ac.uk; Burtons Wood, Burtons Lane, Chalfont St Giles HP8 4BA Tel: 01494 763522 — BM BCh Oxf. 1963 (Oxf. & St. Mary's) PhD Lond. 1971; BA (Hons.) Oxf. 1959, MSc 1962, MA 1963, DM 1982; FRCPath 1985; FRCP 1997, M 1988. Prof. Chem. Path. & Human Metab. Univ. Lond.; Hon. Cons. Roy. Free Hampstead NHS; Hon. Chairm. Family Heart Assn. Specialty: Chem. Path. Socs: (Ex-Pres.) Assn. Clin. Path.; Assn. Clin. Biochem.; Brit. Hyperlipid. Assn. Prev: Chairm. RSM Forum on Lipids in Clin. Med.; Sen. Lect. (Chem. Path.) Inst. Ophth. Univ. Lond.; Hon. Reader (Path. & Med.) Univ. Leics.

WINDER, John Hugh (retired) 13 Westbourne Crescent, Highfield, Southampton SO17 1EA Tel: 023 8055 6514 — MB ChB Leeds 1956; DObst RCOG 1958; DA Eng. 1962; FFA RCS Eng. 1965. Prev: Cons. Anaesth. Soton Univ. Gp. Hosps.

WINDER, Stephen Royal Hallamshire Hospital, Eye Department A Floor, Glossop Road, Sheffield S10 2JF Tel: 0114 271 3381 Email: stephen.winder@sth.nhs.uk; 12 Petworth Drive, Sheffield S11 9QU Tel: 0114 235 6601 — MB BS Lond. 1987 (St Thos.) FRCOphth 1992. Cons. (Ophth) Roy. Hallmamsh. Hosp. Specialty: Ophth. Special Interest: Vitreoretinal Surg. Prev: Vitreoretinal Fell. Moorfields Lond.; Regist. (Ophth.) Aberd. Roy. Infirm.; SHO (Ophth.) Univ. Hosp. Nottm.

WINDHABER, Robin Alan James 37 Allensbank Road, Heath, Cardiff CF14 3PN — MB BCh Wales 1998.

WINDLE, Mary Frances Staunton Group Practice, 3-5 Bounds Green Road, Wood Green, London N22 8HE Tel: 020 8889 4311 Fax: 020 8826 9100 — MB BS Lond. 1976; BSc Lond. 1973; DRCOG 1982; MRCGP 1983.

WINDLE, Mr Richard Department of Surgery, Glenfield General Hospital, Groby Road, Leicester LE3 9 — MD Bristol 1979; MB ChB 1969; FRCS Eng. 1974. Cons. Surg. Leics. HA. Specialty: Gen. Surg.

WINDLE-TAYLOR, Mr Paul Carey Nuffield Hospital, Plymouth PL6 8BG Tel: 01752 775861 Fax: 01752 768969 — MB BChir Camb. 1972 (St. Thos.) MRCS Eng. LRCP Lond. 1972; MA Camb. 1972; FRCS Eng. 1976; MBA Plymouth 1994. Cons. Otolaryngol.Derriford Hosp., Plymouth. Specialty: Otolaryngol.; Medico Legal. Socs: Corr. Mem. Amer. Acad. Otolaryngol. Head & Neck Surg. Prev: Sen. Regist. Roy. Lond. Hosp. Whitechapel; Sen. Regist. Roy. Nat. Throat, Nose & Ear Hosp. Lond.; Regist. Gough Cooper Dept. Neurol. Surg., Nat. Hosp. Nerv. Dis.

WINDMILL, Maria Elaine 97 Princes Avenue, Walderslade, Chatham ME5 8AY — MB ChB Dundee 1995.

WINDRAM, Jonathan David 7 The Oval, Hartlepool TS26 9QH — MB ChB Glas. 1998.

WINDROSS, Peter Michael Chelsea and Westminster Hospital, 369 Fulham Road, London SW10 9NH Tel: 020 8746 8000; Flat 12, 697 Garratt Lane, London SW17 0PD Tel: 020 8947 6856 — MB BS Lond. 1996 (Charing Cross & Westminster Med. Sch.) SHO (Trauma & Orthop.) Chelsea & Westminster Hosp. Lond. Specialty: Trauma & Orthop. Surg.; Paediat. Prev: SHO (A & E) Char. Cross & Hammersmith Hosps. Lond.

WINDRUM, Philip 47 Vara Drive, Belfast BT13 3BY — MB BCh BAO Belf. 1994.

WINDSOR, Mr Alastair Colin James St Mark's Hospital, Watford Road, Harrow HA1 3UJ Tel: 020 8235 4020 Fax: 020 8235 4001 Email: alwindsor@aol.com — MB BS Lond. 1986 (St. Marys Hospital London) FRCS Ed. 1990; FRCS Eng. 1991; MD Lond. 1995. Cons. Surg., St Mark's Hosp.; Chairman, Dept. of Surgery, St. Mark's. Specialty: Gen. Surg. Socs: AAS; Nutrician Soc.; EACP. Prev: Sen. Lect. & Hon. Surg. St. James Hosp. Leeds.

WINDSOR, Alastair Macdonald 13 Cherry Street, Stratton Audley, Bicester OX27 9AA — MB BCh Wales 1985; MRCP (UK) 1989; FRCA 1993.

WINDSOR, Angus Cameron MacDonald Roseville, Fresh Water East Road, Lamphey, Pembroke SA71 5JX — MB BCh Wales 1961 (Cardiff) FRCP Glas. 1981, M 1966; MRCP Lond. 1967; FRCP Lond. 1994. Cons. Phys. Bristol Roy. Infirm. Specialty: Gen. Med.; Care of the Elderly. Socs: Brit. Soc. Research on Ageing; Brit. Geriat. Soc. Prev: Hon. Sen. Lect. Med. Brist. Roy. Infirm.

WINDSOR, Barry Patrick George (retired) 25 Keith Road, Bournemouth BH3 7DS Tel: 01202 527102 — MB BS Lond. 1960 (Middlx.) DObst RCOG 1962. Prev: Ho. Surg. Middlx. Hosp. Lond.

WINDSOR, Mr Colin William Ombler (retired) Willow House, The Common, Lower Broadheath, Worcester WR2 6RH — MB ChB Birm. 1956; MRCS Eng. LRCP Lond. 1956; FRCS Eng. 1962; ChM Birm. 1968. Cons. Surg. Worcester Roy. Infirm. Prev: Surg. Lt. RN.

WINDSOR, Hugh (retired) 57 Main Street, Hanworth, Feltham TW13 6SZ Tel: 020 8893 8151 — MB BS Lond. 1970; LRCPI & LM, LRCSI & LM 1970; DCH RCPSI 1972. Prev: Chief Med. Off. Salvation Army Chikankata Hosp. Mazabuka, Zambia.

WINDSOR, Jeremy Flat 2, St James' School, Georges Road, London N7 8HD — MB ChB DCH, Sheff. 1998.

WINDSOR, John Peter Walter 38 St Philip's Road, London E8 3BP — MB BS Lond. 1975; FFA RCS Eng. 1981. Cons. Anaesth. Whipps Cross Hosp. Lond. Specialty: Anaesth. Prev: Sen. Regist. Lond. Hosp.

WINDSOR, Katherine Twyn Simon Farm, Argoed, Blackwood NP12 0JA — MB BCh Wales 1989.

WINDSOR, Margaret Joan (retired) Willow House, The Common, Lower Broadheath, Worcester WR2 6RH Tel: 01905 333651 Fax: 01905 333382 — MB ChB Birm. 1956; MRCS Eng. LRCP Lond. 1956; MFFP 1993. Prev: Clin. Dir. (Family Plann.) Worcester & Dist. HA.

WINDSOR, Patricia Ann Roseville, Fresh Water East Road, Pembroke SA71 5JX — (Cardiff) MB BCh Wales 1963.

WINDSOR, Phyllis Margaret — (St. Mary's Hospital Medical School, London) MB BS Lond. 1977; MB BS Lond. 1977; FRCR 1984; BSc (Hons.) Lond. 1974, MD 1986; MSc ((Sports Medicine)) Glasgow 2002. Cons. & Hon. Sen. Lect. Dept. Radiother. & Oncol. Ninewells Hosp. Dundee; Club doctor Dundee Football club, Dundee. Specialty: Oncol.; Radiother.; Sports Med. Socs: Fell. of Roy. Coll. of Radiol.; Scott. Radiological Soc.; Europ. Soc. for Therapeutic Radiol. and Oncol. Prev: Lect. (Clin. Oncol.) Univ. Edin.

WINDSOR, Rachael Elizabeth 86 Westcombe Hill, Blackheath, London SE3 7DT — MB BS Lond. 1994 (St Georges Hospital) BSc Hons 1991; MRCP 1997. Specialist Regist. (Paediat.). Specialty: Paediat.

WINEARLS, Christopher Good Oxford Kidney Unit, The Churchill, Oxford Radcliffe Hospital Trust, Oxford OX3 7LJ Tel: 01865 225804 Fax: 01865 225773 — MB ChB Cape Town 1973 (Univ. Cape Town) DPhil Oxf. 1979; FRCP Lond. 1992. Cons. Nephrol. Churchill Hosp. Oxf. & Clin. Dir. of Oxf. Renal Unit; Hon. Sen. Clin. Lect. Univ. of Oxf. Specialty: Nephrol. Special Interest: Myeloma kidney; Adult Polycystic Kidney Dis. Socs: Renal Assn.; Assn. Phys.; Internat. Soc. Nephrol. Prev: Sen. Lect. (Med.) Roy. Postgrad. Med. Sch. Lond.; Sen. Regist. (Renal Med.) Hammersmith Hosp. Lond.; Regist. (Renal Unit) Churchill Hosp. Oxf.

WINER, John Boyle Department of Neurology, Queen Elizabeth Hospital, Edgbaston, Birmingham B15 2TH Tel: 0121 472 1311 — MB BS Lond. 1978 (Middlx.) MRCP (UK) 1980; MD Lond. 1986, MSc (Immunol.) 1985; FRCP Lond. 1995. Cons. Neurol. Univ. Hosp. NHS Trust Birm.; Sen. Lect. Univ. Birm. Specialty: Neurol. Socs: Fell. Roy. Soc. Med.; Brit. Soc. Immunol.; Assn. Brit. Neurol. Prev: Sen. Regist. Nat. Hosp. Nerv. Dis. & St. Mary's Hosp. Lond.; Regist. (Neurol.) Guy's Hosp. Lond.

WINFIELD, Christopher Raymond, Col. late RAMC 41 Wilhelm Raabe Strasse, Bielefeld 33604, Germany — BM BCh Oxf. 1969; MA Oxf. 1966, BM BCh 1969; FRCP Lond. 1988, M (UK) 1975; DCH Eng. 1977. Cons. Phys. Brit. Forces Germany; Command. Off. BMH Rinteln. Specialty: Gen. Med.

WINFIELD, David 2 Becketts Stables, Shrivenham, Swindon SN6 8EY — BM BS Nottm. 1996 (Nottingham) BMedSci Nottm. 1994.

WINFIELD, David Alfred 1 Chorley Drive, Sheffield S10 3RQ — MB ChB Sheff. 1967; FRCPath 1986, M 1973; MRCP (UK) 1974; FRCP Ed. 1985; FRCP Lond. 1986. Cons. Haemat. Sheff. Health Auth. (T). Specialty: Haematology. Socs: Brit. Soc. Haematol. & Assn. Clin. Path. Prev: Cons. Haemat. Derbysh. AHA; Sen. Regist. (Haemat.) United Sheff. Hosps.

WINFIELD, David Anthony, Wing Cdr. — MB ChB Bristol 1987; MSc Lond. 1973, BSc (Hons.) 1972; DPhil Oxf. 1977; DRCOG 1992; DCH RCP Lond. 1993; MRCGP 1993; Dip. Occ. Med. RCP Lond. 1995; DAvMed. RCP Lond. 1998. Specialty: Aviat. Med.

WINFIELD, Frances Isabel Buchanan (retired) 20 Foxgrove Avenue, Beckenham BR3 5BA — (Ed.) MB ChB Ed. 1936. Prev: Med. Off. Lond. Boro. Greenwich & Inner Lond. Educat. Auth.

WINFIELD, Jane The Surgery, 3 Heyward Road, Southsea PO4 0DY Tel: 023 9273 7373; 13 Selsey Avenue, Southsea PO4 9QL Tel: 01705 755812 — BM Soton. 1976; DRCOG 1978; DCH Eng. 1979; MRCGP 1983; MFHom Lond. 1992.

WINFIELD, John Little Gatehouse, Gatehouse Lane, Hathersage, Sheffield S32 1BQ — FREP; MB ChB Leeds 1972; MRCP (U.K.) 1975. Cons. Rheum., Roy. Hallamshire Hosp., Sheff.; Lect. in Rheumatolgy, Univ. of Sheff. Specialty: Rheumatol.; Rehabil. Med. Socs: BMA; Brit. Soc.Rheumatol.; Midl. Rhuematol. Soc.

WINFIELD, Philip John Wright Westgate Medical Practice, Braddon Close, Morecambe LA4 4UZ Tel: 01524 832888 Fax: 01524 832722 — MB ChB Manch. 1981 (Manchester)

WINFREY, Peter Marsden 5 Manor Farm Lane, Castos, Peterborough PE5 7BW Tel: 01733 380 481 — MB BS Lond. 1985 (St Mary's, London) MRCGP 1989; DObst Otago 1990; DTM & H Lond. 1992. Specialty: Gen. Pract.; Trop. Med. Socs: BMA; RCGP. Prev: SHO (Anaesth.), Peterboro., UK; Med. Sup. Kisiizi Hosp. Uganda; GP Train. Peterboro. UK.

WING, Antony John (retired) 16 Fairacres, Roehampton Lane, London SW15 5LX Tel: 020 8878 8824 Fax: 020 8878 6332 — BM BCh Oxf. 1958 (St. Thos.) FRCP Lond. 1976, M 1965; MA Oxf. 1958, DM 1969. Prev: Cons. Renal Phys. St. Geo.'s Hosp. Lond.

WING, Professor John Kenneth, CBE (retired) — (Univ. Coll. Hosp.) MB BS Lond. 1952; DPM 1956; PhD Lond. 1959, MD 1960; FRCPsych 1972. Emerit. Prof. Social Psychiat. Univ. Lond. Prev: Cons. Research Unit Roy. Coll. Psychiat.

WING, Lorna Gladys National Autistic Society, SCD Centre, Elliot House, 113 Masons Hill, Bromley BR2 9HT Tel: 020 8466 0098 Fax: 020 8466 0118 — MB BS Lond. 1952 (Univ. Coll. Hosp.) MRCS Eng. LRCP Lond. 1952; DPM Eng. 1956; MD Lond. 1965; FRCPsych 1980, M 1972. Cons. Nat. Autistic Soc. Lond. Specialty: Ment. Health. Prev: Hon. Cons. Maudsley Hosp. Lond.; Mem. Scientif. Staff Med. Research Counc.

WINGATE, Professor David Lionel G1 Science Research Unit, 26 Ashfield St., London E1 2AJ Tel: 020 7377 0977 Fax: 020 7375 2103 Email: d.l.wingate@mds.qmw.ac.uk; Sydney House, 7 Pilgrims Lane, London NW3 1SJ Tel: 020 7435 6101 Fax: 020 7419 7066 — BM BCh Oxf. 1960 (Oxf. & Middlx.) MSc Oxf. 1959, DM 1979, MA 1960; FRCP Lond. 1979, M 1967. Prof. Gastrointestinal Sci. Univ. Lond.; Dir. Gastrointestinal Sci. Research Unit St. Bart. & Roy. Lond. Hosps. Sch. Of Med. Specialty: Gastroenterol. Socs: Brit. Soc. Gastroenterol. & Amer. Gastroenterol. Assn.; Fell. Roy. Soc. of Arts. Prev: Sen. Lect. (Physiol.) Lond. Hosp. Med. Coll.; Reader (Gastroenterol.) Univ. Lond.; Research Asst. Gastroenterol. Unit Mayo Clinic Rochester, USA.

WINGATE, John Peter City Hospital, Dudley Road, Birmingham B18 7QH Tel: 0121 554 3801 — MB BS Newc. 1973; FRCR 1982. Cons. Radiol. City Hosp. Birm.; Hon. Sen. Clin. Lect. Univ. Birm. Specialty: Radiol. Prev: Sen. Regist. (Radiol.) Birm. Hosps.; SHO (Med.) Hull Gp. Hosps.; Ho. Off. Newc. Gen. Hosp.

WINGATE, Verity Anne (Surgery), 21 Woodthorpe Road, Kings Heath, Birmingham B14 6EF Tel: 0121 444 2054 Fax: 0121 443

5856; 35 Selly Wick Road, Selly Park, Birmingham B29 7JJ Tel: 0121 471 4896 — MB ChB Birm. 1979.

WINGATE-GRAY, Elisabeth 1 South Side, Shadforth, Durham DH6 1LL — MB BS Newc. 1968.

WINGFIELD, Caroline Ann The Avenue Surgery Partnership, 14 The Avenue, Warminster BA12 9AA — BM BCh Oxf. 1988; MA Oxf. 1988; DRCOG 1991; Cert. Family Plann. JCC 1991; MRCGP 1992; DFFP 1993.

WINGFIELD, David John Charles The Brook Green Medical Centre, Bute Gardens, London W6 7EG Tel: 020 7471 3333 Fax: 020 7471 3311; 5 Poplar Grove, London W6 7RF Tel: 020 7603 4200 — MB BS Lond. 1985 (St. Mary's Lond. & St. Peter's Coll. Oxf.) MA Oxf. 1987; DRCOG 1988; MRCGP 1989; DCH RCP Lond. 1989. GP Princip. Specialty: Gen. Pract. Socs: BMA; Brit. Hypertens. Soc. Prev: Trainee GP St. Stephen's & Westm. Hosps. Lond. VTS; Research Ldr. for W. Lond. Research Network; Research Fell. (Gen. Pract.) Char. Cross & Westm. Med. Sch.

WINGFIELD, John George (retired) Glandur, 15 Upper Hale Road, Farnham GU9 0NN — (Cardiff) MB BCh Wales 1959; MRCS Eng. LRCP Lond. 1960; FRCOG 1981, M 1967; MRCOG 1967. Prev: Sen. Regist. W. Middlx. Hosp. & Char. Cross Hosp. Gp.

WINGFIELD, Susan Nicola Adnitt Road, Rushden NN10 9TR Tel: 01933 460807 — MB ChB Sheff. 1985; MRCGP 1989; DRCOG 1989. GP Principle. Socs: BMA. Prev: SHO (O&G) Northampton; SHO (Radiother.) Leics. HA; SHO (Med.) Sheff. HA.

WINKLER, John Lewis 4 Kensington Mansions, Trebovir Road, London SW5 9TF Tel: 020 7373 2029 — MB BS Lond. 1944 (Lond. Hosp.) MRCS Eng. LRCP Lond. 1944. Clin. Asst. (Psychiat) St Mary Abbot's Hosps. Lond. Specialty: Gen. Med. Socs: W Lond. M-C Soc. Prev: Clin. Asst. (Med. & Surg.) Westm. Childr. Hosp.

WINKLEY, Linda Mary Oaklands Centre, Child & Adolescent Department, Selly Oak, Birmingham B29 6JD Tel: 0121 627 8321 Fax: 0121 627 8684 — MB ChB Birm. 1965 (Birm.) MRCS Eng. LRCP Lond. 1965; DObst RCOG 1967; DCH Eng. 1967; DPM Eng. 1972; FRCPsych 1989, M 1973. Cons. Psychiat. Birm. Childr. Hosps.; Hon. Sen. Clin. Lect. Univ. Birm. Specialty: Child & Adolesc. Psychiat.

WINN, Caroline Rachel York House, Romsey Road, Awbridge, Romsey SO51 0HG Tel: 01794 340139; York House, Romsey Road, Awbridge, Romsey SO51 0HG Tel: 01794 340139 — MB BCh Wales 1998. SHO (Med.) Princess of Wales Hosp., Bridgend, Cardiff. Specialty: Otorhinolaryngol. Prev: Ho. Off. Med. (Llandough, Cardiff); Ho. Off. Surg. (Morriston, Swansea).

WINN, John Henry Royal Victoria Hospital, Belfast BT12 6BA — MB BCh BAO Belf. 1988 (Qu. Univ. Belf.) MB BCh Belf. 1988; FFA RCSI 1996. Cons. (Anaesth.) in Trauma. Roy. Vict. Hosp. Belf. Specialty: Anaesth. Socs: BMA; Assn. Anaesth. Prev: Locum Cons. Card. Anaesth. St. Geo. Hosp. Lond.; Clin. Fell. Cardiac Anaesth. Harefield Hosp. Middlx.

WINN, Neil Barrie 111 Albion Road, Idle, Bradford BD10 9QL Tel: 01274 620375 — MB ChB Sheff. 1975; DRCOG 1977; MRCGP 1979.

WINN, Pauline Imogen Margaret (retired) 32 Nero Court, Justin Close, Brentford TW8 8QA — MB ChB Ed. 1950; DPM Eng. 1960; MRCPsych 1973. Prev: Assoc. Specialist St. Bernard's Hosp. S.all.

WINNARD, James Alan 21 Station Road, Eston, Middlesbrough TS6 9EW Tel: 01642 467093 — MB ChB Manch. 1995 (Univ. Manch.) Specialty: Accid. & Emerg.

WINNER, Simon Jeremy Department of Clinical Geratology, The Radcliffe Infirmary, Oxford OX2 6HE Tel: 01865 311188 Fax: 01865 224815 Email: simon.winner@geratol.ox.ac.uk — MB BChir Camb. 1975 (Univ. Coll. Hosp.) MB BChir Camb. 1974; MA Camb. 1975; MRCP (UK) 1977; FRCP Lond. 1997. Cons. Phys. (Gen. Med. & Clin. Geratol.) Radcliffe Infirm. & John Radcliffe Hosps. Oxf.; Hon. Sen. Clin. Lect. Univ. Oxf. Med. Sch. Specialty: Care of the Elderly. Prev: Clin. Lect. (Geriat. Med.) Nuffield Dept. Clin. Med. Univ. Oxf.; Specialist Phys. Papua New Guinea; Regist. (Med.) Univ. Coll. Hosp. Lond. & Whittington Hosp. Lond.

WINNETT, Andrew Robert Douglas 5/3 Arlington Road, Mornington Crescent, London NW1 7ER — MB BS Queensland 1990.

WINNEY, Robin John Department of Renal Medicine, Edinburgh Royal Infirmary, 51 Little France Crescent, Edinburgh EH3 9YW Tel: 0131 242 1246 Fax: 0131 242 1233 Email: robin.winney@fuht.scot.nhs.uk; 74 Lanark Road W., Currie EH14 5JZ Tel: 0131 449 2382 — MB ChB Ed. 1968 (Edin. Univ.) MRCP (UK) 1971; FRCP Ed. 1980. Cons. (Renal Phys.) Edin. Roy. Infirm. Specialty: Gen. Med. Special Interest: Managem. of Chronic Renal Failiure Including Renal Replacement. Socs: Brit. Renal Assn.; Europ. Renal Assn.; Brit. Transpl. Soc. Prev: Lead Renal Serv.s Edin. Roy. Infirm.

WINNICOTT, Harry David (retired) 1 Mallender Drive, Knowle, Solihull B93 9BX Tel: 01564 774265 — (St. Geo.) MB BS Lond. 1958. Prev: GP Birm.

WINNIFRITH, Tabitha Jessie Ann 10 Stockmore Street, Oxford OX4 1JT — MB BS Camb. 1993 (Roy. Lond. Hosp.) MA Camb. 1994, BA (Hons.) 1990; MRCP (UK) 1996; MRCGP (UK) 1999. GP Retainer in Oxf. Specialty: Gen. Pract. Prev: SHO (Old Age Psychiat.) Fulbrook Centre Oxf.; Med. SHO Leics.

WINNING, Andrew James West Middlesex University Hospital, Twickenham Road, Isleworth TW7 6AF Tel: 020 8565 5337/8 — BM BCh Oxf. 1977 (Oxf. & Lond.) DPhil Oxf. 1974, BA 1970, MA, BM BCh 1977; MRCP (UK) 1979; FRCP Lond. 1993. Cons. Phys. W. Middlx. Univ. Hosp. Isleworth & Ashford Hosp. Middlx. Specialty: Gen. Med. Socs: Med. Res. Soc. & Brit. Thoracic Soc. Prev: Lect. & Hon. Sen. Regist. Char. Cross & Westm. Med. Sch. Lond.; Regist. St. Thos. Hosp. Lond.; Med. Research Counc. Schol. Univ. Laborat. of Physiol. Oxf. & Inst. Physiol. Milan, Italy.

WINNING, Timothy John Berato, Barrs Brae, Kilmacolm PA13 4DE Tel: 01505 874473 — MB ChB Aberd. 1970; FFARCS Eng. 1975. Cons. Anaesth. Inverclyde Roy. Hosp. Greenock. Specialty: Anaesth. Socs: Assn. Anaesth. Gt. Brit. & Irel. Prev: Cons. Anaesth. E. Gen. Hosp. Edin.; Hon. Lect. Univ. Zimbabwe.

WINOCOUR, Bertram (retired) Flat 6, The Hollows, Ayr Road, Giffnock, Glasgow G46 7JB — LRCP LRCS Ed. 1948; LRCP LRCS Ed. LRFPS Glas. 1948.

WINOCOUR, Peter Howard Department of Medicine, Queen Elizabeth II Hospital, Welwyn Garden City Tel: 01707 328111 Fax: 01707 365306 — MB ChB Glas. 1979; MRCP (UK) 1982; MD Glas. 1989; FRCP Lond. 1998. Cons. Phys. N. Herts NHS Trust; Hon. Sen. Lect. Roy. Free Hosp. Sch. Med. Specialty: Endocrinol. Socs: Brit. Diabetic Assn.; Comm. Mem. Brit. Hyperlipidaemia Assn. (Ex-Off.); Hon. Secretary. Assn. Brit. Clin. Diabetesl. Prev: Lect. Univ. Newc.; Tutor (Med.) Hope Hosp. Manch.; Research Fell. Univ. Manch.

WINOKUR, Benjamin (retired) 8 Highwood Avenue, Leeds LS17 6ES Tel: 0113 268 8536 — MB BCh Witwatersrand 1949; DPM Eng. 1968. Prev: Cons. Psychiat. (Ment. Handicap) Meanwood Pk. Hosp. & Fieldhead Hosp.

WINPENNY, Helen Claire 143A Kingston Road, London SW19 1LJ — MB BS Lond. 1993; BSc Lond. 1990, MB BS (Distinc. Med.) 1993.

WINROW, Adrian Mark Fieldhead Hospital, Ouchthorpe Lane, Wakefield WF1 3SP Tel: 01924 327000 — MB ChB Leeds 1993; MRCPSych. Specialist Regist. (Psychiat. Geriat.) Fieldham Hosp. Wakefield. Specialty: Geriat. Psychiat. Prev: Trainee Psychiat. Leeds.

WINROW, Andrew Philip Department of Paediatrics, Kingston Hospital, Galsworthy Road, Kingston upon Thames KT2 7QB Tel: 020 8546 7711 Fax: 020 8934 3249 Email: andrew.winrow@kingstonhospital.nhs.uk — MB BS Lond. 1986 (Char. Cross & Westm.) FRCPCH; BSc (Hons.) Lond. 1983; MRCP (UK) 1990. Cons. Paediat. Kingston Hosp. Kingston upon Thames. Specialty: Paediat. Prev: Sen. Regist. (Paediat.) St. Mary's Hosp. Lond.; Med. Dir. Kingston Hosp. NHS Trust.

WINSEY, Audrey Mackay (retired) 4 Cambridge Road, Langland, Swansea SA3 4PE — MB ChB Aberd. 1959; DA Eng. 1963. Prev: Anaesth. Regist. King Geo. Hosp. Ilford.

WINSHIP, Anna Zuleika 1 Dudley Road, London N3 2QR — BM BS Nottm. 1992.

WINSHIP, Kulsum Abdulla (retired) 1 Dudley Road, Finchley, London N3 2QR Tel: 020 8346 3829 Fax: 020 8346 3829 — LRCPI & LM, LRSCI & LM 1956; LRCPI & LM, LRCSI & LM 1956; DCH Eng. 1958; MRCP Ed. 1965; FFPHM RCP (UK) 1988, M 1972; FRCP Ed. 1988; FFPM 1989. Prev: Sen. Med. Off. Med. Control Agency DoH.

WINSHIP, Shelagh Mary c/o Department of Anaesthesia, Perth Royal Infirmary, Perth PH1 1NX; 23 Muirton Bank, Perth PH1 5DW — MB ChB Sheff. 1985; FFA RCSI 1991; FRCA. 1992; FANZCA

1996. Cons., Perth Roy. Infirm. Specialty: Anaesth. Socs: Anaesthetic Research Soc.; Intens. Care Soc. Prev: Specialist Regist. (Anaesth.) Merseyside; Ltd. Specialist Belford Hosp. Fort William.

***WINSLADE, Claire Georgina** Scania, Links Road, Lowestoft NR32 4PQ — MB ChB Manch. 1998 (St Andrews/manchester) BSc 1995; MB ChB Manch 1998; MRCPCH 2001. SHO (Pub. Health) Felixstowe, Suff. Specialty: Gen. Surg. Prev: PRHO paediat.burnley; PRHO med.Burnley; SHO (Paediat.) Ashford Kent.

WINSLET, Professor Mark Christopher University Dept Surgery, Royal Free Hospital, Pond Street, London NW3 2QG — MB BS Lond. 1981 (Roy. Free Hosp. Sch. Med.) FRCS Eng. 1985; FRCS Ed. 1985; MS Lond. 1988. Prof. Surg. & Hon. Cons. Surg. Roy. Free Hosp. Sch. Med. Lond. Specialty: Gastroenterol.; Gen. Surg. Socs: Fell. Roy. Soc. Med.; BMA; Counc. Mem. Assn. Coloprotol. GB & Irel. Prev: Sen. Lect. & Hon. Cons. Surg. Roy. Free Hosp. Sch. Med. Lond.; Lect. & Sen. Regist. (Surg.) Univ. Birm. & United Birm. Hosps.; Regist. (Surg.) Leics. Hosps.

WINSLOW, George Stewart Stratheden Hospital, Cupar KY15 5RR — MB ChB Glas. 1971; MRCPsych 1981. Cons. Fife Psychiat. Serv. Specialty: Gen. Psychiat. Prev: Cons. Psychiat. Stratheden Hosp. Cupar.

WINSLOW, Lee Manchester Royal Infirmary, Oxford Road, Manchester M13 9WL Tel: 0161 276 1234 — MB ChB Leeds 1988; FRCA 1993. Cons. cardiothoraic Anaesth., Manch. Roy. Infirm. Specialty: Cardiol.; Anaesth.

WINSLOW, Nicholas Robert Scots Gap Surgery, Scots Gap, Morpeth NE61 4EG Tel: 01670 74216 Fax: 01670 774388 — MB BS Newc. 1982; BMedSc Newc. 1979, MB BS 1982; MRCP (UK) 1985; DGM RCP Lond. 1986; MRCGP 1987; DRCOG 1988. Socs: Brit. Geriat. Soc. Prev: Trainee GP Coldstream; Research Fell. Univ. Newc. upon Tyne.

WINSNES, Paul Frederick Rose Cottage, Chapel Lane, Rolleston-on-Dove, Burton-on-Trent DE13 9AG Tel: 01283 812686 — MB Camb. 1973 (St. Thos.) BA Camb. 1969, MB 1973, BChir 1972; DRCOG 1978. Prev: Ho. Off. (O & G), Ho. Off. (Paediat.) & SHO (Psychiat.) St.; Thos. Hosp. Lond.

WINSON, Mr Ian Geoffrey South Mead Hospital, Westbury-on-Trym, Bristol BS10 5NB Tel: 0117 9595197 Fax: 0117 9595924 Email: ian.winson@north-bristol.swest.nhs.uk — MB ChB Sheff. 1978; FRCS Ed. 1983. Cons. Orthop. & Trauma Surg. Southmead Hosp. Bristol. Specialty: Orthop. Special Interest: Foot & Ankle. Socs: Fell. BOA. Prev: Lect. & Sen. Regist. (Orthop.) Sheff.; Regist. (Orthop.) Brist. Roy. Infirm.; Regist. (Gen. Surg. & Orthop.) Cardiff.

WINSON, Maxwell David Woodside Cottage, Marsh Lane, Acton, Nantwich CW5 8PH Tel: 01270 628915 — MB ChB Liverp. 1967; BSc (1st cl. Hons.) Liverp. 1967; MB ChB (Hons.) Liverp. 1970; MRCP (UK) 1974; FRCP Lond. 1990. Cons. Phys. Leighton Hosp. Crewe. Specialty: Gen. Med. Socs: Brit. Thoracic Soc. Prev: Sen. Regist. (Gen. & Thoracic Med.) Llandough Hosp. Cardiff; Regist. (Gen. Med.) Nottm. City Hosp.; Lect. (Path.) Univ. Liverp.

WINSPEAR, Michael The Laurels Medical Practice, 28 Clarendon Road, St Helier, Jersey JE2 3YS Tel: 01534 733866 Fax: 01534 769597 — MB ChB Ed. 1988; BSc (Hons.) Salford 1982; MSc Newc. 1983; DRCOG 1991; MRCGP 1992.

WINSPUR, Mr Ian Hand Clinic, 29-31 Devonshire St., London W1N 1RF Tel: 020 7486 7131 Fax: 020 7486 0090; 8 Tennyson Court, 12 Dorset Square, London NW1 6QB Tel: 020 7402 6308 Fax: 020 7402 6308 — MB ChB Ed. 1969; FRCS Ed. 1974; FACS 1981; LLM 2000. Cons. Hand. Surg. King Edwd. VII Hosp. Midhurst & Devonshire Hosp. Lond. Specialty: Plastic Surg. Socs: Brit. Hand Soc.; Amer. Soc. Surg. Hand. Prev: Asst. Clin. Prof. Plastic Surg. Univ. Colorado; Cons. Hand Surg. Cottage Hosp. Santa Barabara, Calif., USA.

WINSTANLEY, Alison Michelle 6 New Street, Tiddington, Stratford-upon-Avon CV37 7DA — MB BS Lond. 1998.

WINSTANLEY, Claire Sophia Timbers, Warwick Road, Stratford-upon-Avon CV37 0NR — MB BS Newc. 1993.

WINSTANLEY, David Pierre (retired) 63 Weald Road, Brentwood CM14 4TN Tel: 01277 226809 Email: translations@davidwinstanley.plus.com — (Oxf. & Guy's) BM BCh Oxf. 1948; MRCP Lond. 1953; MRCPath 1963.

WINSTANLEY, Mr John, MC, TD (retired) The Old Post Office, 1 The Square, Brill, Aylesbury HP18 9RP Tel: 01844 238226 — MB BS Lond. 1951 (St. Thos.) FRCS Eng. 1957; FRCOphth 1988. Hon. Cons. Ophth. Surg. St. Thos. Hosp. Lond. Prev: Hon. Cons. Ophth. MoD (Army).

WINSTANLEY, Mr John Henry Robert Royal Bolton Hospital, Farnworth, Bolton BL4 0JR; 50 Crossfield Drive, Manchester M28 2QQ Tel: 0161 790 2070 — MB ChB (Hons.) Liverp. 1981; BDS Liverp. 1974; FDS RCPS Glas. 1978; FRCS Glas. 1985; FRCS Eng. 1987; MD Liverp. 1992. Specialty: Gen. Surg. Socs: Surgic. Research Soc. & Brit. Assn. for Cancer Research. Prev: Cons. Surg. Roy. Liverp. Univ. Hosp. & Broadgreen Hosp. Liverp.; Sen. Regist. (Gen. Surg.) Mersey Region.

WINSTANLEY, Maria Therese — MB ChB Liverp. 1979; MRCP (UK) 1982; DTM & H Liverp. 1989.

WINSTANLEY, Peter Andrew Department of Pharmacology and Therapeutics, University of Liverpool, Liverpool L69 3GE Tel: 0151 794 5544 Fax: 0151 794 5540 Email: peterwin@liv.ac.uk; 105 Druids Cross Road, Liverpool L18 3HN Tel: 0151 722 2710 — MB ChB Liverp. 1979 (Liverpool) MB ChB (Hons.) Liverp. 1979; MRCP (UK) 1982; DTM & H Liverp. 1988; MD Liverp. 1989; FRCP (UK) 1997. Reader Clin. Pharmacol. Univ. of Liverp. Specialty: Gen. Med. Socs: Fell. Roy. Soc. Trop. Med.; Brit. Pharm. Soc. Prev: Sen. Lect. (Clin. Pharmacol.) Univ. Liverp.; Clin. Lect. Nuffield Dept. Med. Oxf.

***WINSTANLEY, Ronald Peter** 1 Pine Road, Manchester M20 6UY Tel: 0161 445 6480 — (Roy. Free) LDS Manch. 1951; FDS RCS Eng. 1955; MRCS Eng. LRCP Lond. 1959. Specialty: Oral & Maxillofacial Surg. Prev: Cons. Hope Hosp. Salford; Sen. Regist. & Chief Asst. Maxillofacial Unit Withington Hosp. Manch.

WINSTOCK, Adam Rohan National Addiction Centre, Institute of Psychiatry, Addiction Science Building, 4 Windsor Walk, London SE5 Tel: 020 7703 6333 Fax: 020 7703 6333 — MB BS Lond. 1991; BSc Lond. 1988; MRCP (UK) 1994; MRCPsych 1997; MS Lond. 1999. SpR S. Lond. & Maudsley; Clin. Lect. NAC, IOP, KCL; SpR in Med. Educat. GK Med. Sch. 99/2000. Specialty: Alcohol & Substance Misuse; Gen. Psychiat. Socs: Roy. Soc. Study of Addic. & Alcohol; Lond. Toxicology Gp.; Int. Harm Reduction Alliance. Prev: Regist. (Pscyhiatry) Maudsley Hosp. Lond.; Regist. Nat. Alcohol Unit Bethlem Roy. Hosp.; SHO (Med.) Hammersmith.

WINSTOCK, Mr Donald (retired) 33 West Heath Avenue, London NW11 7QJ Tel: 020 8455 0619 — (St. Bart.) BDS (Hons.) Lond. 1948; MB BS Lond. 1956; MRCS Eng. LRCP Lond. 1956; FDS RCS Eng. 1959; FRCS Ed. 1985. Hon. Cons. Oral Surg. St. Bart. Hosp., Middlx. Hosp. & Edgware Gen. Hosp Lond; Sen. Lect. & Hon. Cons. Oral Surg. UMDS Guy's & St. Thos. Hosps. Lond. Prev: Sen. Regist. (Oral Surg.) St. Thos. Hosp. Lond.

WINSTOCK, Grant Bruce Milo 249 Garratt Lane#, London SW18 4UE Tel: 020 8870 1341/020 8870 8907 — MB BS Lond. 1982 (London) DMJ; MRCGP. Forens. Med. Examr. Specialty: Gen. Pract.

WINSTON, Alan 11 Fruin Avenue, Newton Mearns, Glasgow G77 6HA — MB ChB Glas. 1994.

WINSTON, Christopher Mark — MB BS Lond. 1980 (Char. Cross Hosp.) BSc Lond. 1977; MRCPsych 1987; T(Psych) 1992. Cons. Psychiat. St. Tydfil's Hosp. Merthyr Tydfil. Specialty: Gen. Psychiat. Prev: Lect. (Psychiat.) Med. Sch. Harare, Zimbabwe; Sen. Regist. (Psychiat.) WhitCh. Hosp. Cardiff & E. Glam. Hosp. M. Glam.

WINSTON, Ian 137 Camberwell New Road, London SE5 0SU — MB BS Lond. 1998.

WINSTON, Mr Maurice Elyis (retired) 16 St John Street, Manchester M3 4EA Tel: 0161 834 4282 Fax: 0161 835 1465; 2 Thorngrove Hill, Wilmslow SK9 1DF Tel: 01625 528882 — MB ChB Ed. 1938 (Univ. Ed.) FRCS Ed. 1945. Cons. Orthop. Surg. Manch. Prev: Cons. Orthop. Surg. Bolton Gp. Hosps.

WINSTON, Michael Patrick 43 Hilbre Road, Wirral CH48 3HB — MB BChir Camb. 1994.

WINSTON, Raymond (retired) 211 Battersea Bridge Road, London SW11 3AP Tel: 020 7223 5579 — MRCS Eng. LRCP Lond. 1942; FRCGP 1985. Prev: Capt. RAMC.

WINSTON, Professor Robert Maurice Lipson Hammersmith Hospital, Du Cane Road, London W12 0HS Tel: 020 8383 4152 Fax: 020 8749 6973 — MB BS Lond. 1964; MRCS Eng. 1964 LRCP Lond. 1964; FRCOG 1983, M 1971. Prof. Fertil. Studies Roy. Postgrad. Med. Sch. Lond.; Cons. Gyn. & Obst. Hammersmith Hosp. Lond. Specialty: Obst. & Gyn. Socs: Fell. Roy. Soc. Med.; Comm. Mem. Brit. Fertil. Soc.; Fell. Acad. Med. Prev: Reader (Fertil. Studies) Inst. O & G 1981-86; Prof. (Gyn.) Univ. Texas, USA.

WINSTON, Sarah Rosemary 43 Hilbre Road, Wirral CH48 3HB — MB BChir Camb. 1993.

WINTER, Adrienne Elisabeth (retired) Mickledore, 25 The Whiteway, Cirencester GL7 2ER Tel: 01285 655929 Fax: 01285 655929 Email: awinter@mickledore.com — MB BChir Camb. 1964 (Camb. & St. Thos.) MA Camb. 1964; DObst RCOG 1966. Prev: Cas. Off. St. Thos. Hosp. Lond.

WINTER, Miss Alison — MB ChB Glas. 1993; FRCS Ed 1998. Specialist Registr Gen. Surg., W. of Scotl. Specialty: Gen. Surg. Socs: Med. & Dent. Defence Union Scotl.; BMA; Assn. Surg.s in Train. Prev: SHO (Surg.) W. Glas. Hosp. Univ. NHS Trust; Sen. Health Off. (Accid. & Orthop. Surg.) Glas. Roy. Infirm.; Sen. Health Off. (Surg.) Hairmyres Hosp. Co. Kilbride.

WINTER, Andrew John Department GU Medicine, Sandyford Iniative, 6 Sandyford Place, Glasgow G3 7NB Tel: 0141 211 8608 Fax: 0141 211 8609 Email: andy.winter@glacomen.scot.nhs.uk — BM BCh Oxf. 1989; MRCP (UK) 1992; PhD (Birm.) 1997. Cons. In Genito-Urin. Med. and HIV, Glas. Specialty: Genitourinary Medicine; HIV Med. Prev: Clin. Research Fell. (Infec.) Univ. Birm.; Specialist Regist. (Med.) W. Midl.

WINTER, Angela The Cambridge Medical Group, 10A Cambridge Road, Linthorpe, Middlesbrough TS5 5NN Tel: 01642 851177 Fax: 01642 851176; 12 Rosemoor Close, Marton-in-Cleveland, Middlesbrough TS7 8LQ — MB BS Newc. 1987; MA (Med. Sci.) Camb. 1988; DRCOG 1991; MRCGP 1991. Specialty: Obst. & Gyn. Prev: Trainee GP Cleveland VTS.

WINTER, Christina Wei Mei Global Clinical Safety & Pharmacovigilance, Glaxo Wellcome Research & Development, Greenford Road, Greenford UB6 0HE Tel: 020 8966 3240 Fax: 020 8423 2097; 15 Woodbank Avenue, Gerrards Cross SL9 7PY Tel: 01753 888118 — MB BCh BAO Dub. 1975 (TC Dub.) MD Dub. 1984; Dip Pharm Med Facult Pharm Med London 1996; MFPM Lond. 2003. Med. Director, Med. Review Gp., Global Clin. Safety and Pharmacovigilance, GSK. Specialty: Pharmaceutical Medicine. Socs: Brit. Assn. Pharmaceut. Phys.; Med. Res. Soc. Prev: Lect. (Cardiovasc. Studies) Univ. Leeds; Safety Coordinator Aire Study (Clin. Trial); Demonst. (Physiol.) TC Dub.

WINTER, Craig David 87 Mayflower Way, Ongar CM5 9BB — MB BChir Camb. 1992; BSc Lond. 1989; FRCS (Eng.) 1996; FRCS (SN) 2002.

WINTER, David Paul (retired) Little Lea, Turners Hill Road, East Grinstead RH19 4LX Tel: 01342 325374; 9 Bodged Lane, Melcombe Bingham, Dorchester DT2 7UJ Tel: 01258 881645 — MB BS Lond. 1960 (King's Coll. Hosp.) MSc Lond. (Occupat. Med.) 1982, MB BS 1960; DObst RCOG 1962; DIH Eng. 1981; MFOM RCP Lond. 1985, A 1981; Specialist Accredit. Occupat. Med. JCHMT 1986. Prev: Med. Adviser Rentokil Gp. plc E. Grinstead.

WINTER, Emma 4 The Open, Leazes Square, Newcastle upon Tyne NE1 4DB — MB BS Newc. 1996.

WINTER, Gordon Robert (retired) Pennyroyal, 11 Pipers Close, Cobham KT11 3AU Tel: 01932 864622 — (St. Mary's) MRCS Eng. LRCP Lond. 1962; LMSSA Lond. 1962; DObst RCOG 1964. Prev: Ho. Surg. O & G Epsom Dist. Hosp.

WINTER, Heather Rosemary Department of Public Health & Epidemiology, The Medical School, University of Birmingham, Edgbaston, Birmingham B15 2TT Tel: 0121 414 6761 — MB BCh BAO Belf. 1982; MRCOG 1987; MD Belf. 1995. Sen. Clin. Lect. (Pub. Health & Epidenuol.) Univ. Birm. Specialty: Pub. Health Med. Prev: Sen. Regist. W. Midl. RHA.

WINTER, Helen Livingstone 10 Hillneuk Avenue, Bearsden, Glasgow G61 3PZ — MB ChB Glas. 1970. Clin. Med. Off. (Community Child Health) Yorkhill Trust. Specialty: Community Child Health.

WINTER, Henry Allan Graham (retired) Pilmer House, London Road, Crowborough TN6 2HZ Tel: 01892 662573 — MRCS Eng LRCP Lond. 1943.

WINTER, Jack Westwood 10 Hillneuk Avenue, Bearsden, Glasgow G61 3PZ — MB ChB Glas. 1997.

WINTER, John (retired) 39 The Downs, Blundellsands, Liverpool L23 6XS — MD Liverp. 1956; MB ChB 1941, MRad 1948; DMRD Eng. 1948. Prev: Cons. Radiol. Mersey RHA.

WINTER, John Anthony Cooper Wingate Medical Centre, 79 Bigdale Drive, Northwood, Liverpool L33 6YJ Tel: 0151 546 2958 Fax: 0151 546 2914 — MB ChB Liverp. 1969; MRCGP 1980; DIH Soc. Apoth. Lond. 1981; AFOM RCP Lond. 1982. Med. Adviser Brooke Bond Foods Manch.; Med. Adviser Samuel Banner & Co. Ltd., Balfour Beatty Ltd., BASF Liverp., Rathbone PLC. Socs: Soc. Occupat. Med. Prev: Med. Adviser Birds Eye Walls Ltd. Liverp.

WINTER, John Barry Mark Kent & Canterbury Hospital, Haemophilia Centre, Ethelbert Road, Canterbury CT1 3NG Tel: 01227 766877 Fax: 01277 783167 Email: mark.winter@ekht.nhs.uk — MB BS Lond. 1973 (Guy's) MRCS Eng. LRCP Lond. 1973; MRCP (UK) 1976; FRCPath 1992, M 1980; FRCP Eng. 1991. Cons. Haemat. & Dir. Haemophilia Centre Canterbury & Thanet HA; Hon. Sen. Lect. Univ. Kent. Specialty: Haematology. Socs: Brit. Soc. Haematol.; World Federat. Haemophilia; Brit. Soc. Haemostasis & Thrombosis. Prev: Lect. (Haemat.) Middlx. Hosp. Med. Sch. & Hon. Sen. Regist. Middlx. Hosp. Lond .; Lect. (Haemat.) Guy's Med. Sch. & Hon. Sen. Regist. Guy's Hosp. Lond.

WINTER, John Hirst Ninewells Hospital, Dundee DD1 9SY Tel: 01382 496457 Fax: 01382 496548 Email: john.h.winter@tuht.scot.nhs.uk — MB ChB Birm. 1974; MRCP (UK) 1978; BSc Birm. 1971, MD 1983; FRCP Glas. 1995; FRCP Ed. 1996. Cons. Phys. Dundee Teachg. Hosps. NHS Trust. Specialty: Respirat. Med.

WINTER, John Keith Joshua 26 Orchard Lane, Newtownards BT23 7PQ Tel: 01247 822427 — MB BCh BAO Belf. 1978 (Queens Univesity Belfast) DGM RCPS Glas. 1998.

WINTER, John Malcolm Salters Meadow Centre, Rugely Road, Chase Terrace, Burntwood W57 8AQ Tel: 01543 682611 Fax: 01543 675391 — MB ChB Manch. 1971. GP; Bd Mem. Lichfield & Burntwood PCG. Socs: Lichfield.Med.Soc.

WINTER, John Michael Cirencester Hospital, The Querns, Tetbury Road, Cirencester GL7 1UY Tel: 01285 655711 Fax: 01285 884623; Mickledore, 25 The Whiteway, Cirencester GL7 2ER Tel: 01285 655929 Fax: 01285 655929 — MB BS Lond. 1962 (St Bart.) MRCS Eng. LRCP Lond. 1962; DObst RCOG 1964; DCH Eng. 1966; MRCP (UK) 1973; FRCP 2003. p/t Trust Doctor (Med.) Cirencester Hosp. Specialty: Gen. Med. Socs: Christian Med. Fellowsh.; Roy. Soc. Med.; Brit. Med. Assoc. Prev: GP (Princip. & Trainer) St Peter's Rd. Surg. Cirencester, 1974-2000; Regist. (Med.) Hull Hosp. 1972-1974; Med. Off. Ngora (Ch. of Uganda) Hosp. 1966-1968.

WINTER, Julian Peter — MB ChB Leeds 1995 (Leeds Univ.) MRCP (UK), 1999. SpR Cardiol. (Yorkshire). Specialty: Gen. Med. Prev: SHO (A & E) Leeds Gen. Infirm.; SHO (Med. for Elderly) St. Jas. Univ. Hosp. Leeds; SHO (Gen. Med.) Leeds Gen. Infirm.

WINTER, Lee Nigel Palace Road Surgery, 3 Palace Road, London SW2 3DY Tel: 020 8674 2083 Fax: 020 8674 6040 Email: lee.winter@gp-g85041.nhs.uk; 3 Palace Road, Streatham Hill, London SW2 3DY — MB BS Lond. 1990 (St. Geo.) Specialty: Gen. Pract. Prev: Trainee GP Mayday Hosp. Croydon VTS.

WINTER, Lesley Joy Abigail — MB ChB Leeds 1995; DFFP 2000; DRCOG 2000; MRCGP 2001. p/t GP Princip. Windhill Green Med. Centre Shipley; Family Plann. Off. Bradford Community Ct. Specialty: Gen. Pract. Prev: GP Asst., Bradford - Family Plann. Off., Densbury.

WINTER, Margaret Elizabeth 146 East Street, Olney MK46 4BT — MB BS Lond. 1996.

WINTER, Michael David Whitburn Health Centre, 1 Weavers Lane, Whitburn, Bathgate EH47 0SD Tel: 01501 740297 Fax: 01501 744302; 2 Craigmount Court, Edinburgh EH4 8HL — MB ChB Ed. 1980; DRCOG 1982; MRCGP 1984; MRCPsych 1986. Socs: Chairm. Lothian LMC. Prev: Regist. (Psychiat.) Bangour Village Hosp. Broxburn.

WINTER, Peter John (retired) Angel Farm, Newland St., Coleford GL16 8NA Tel: 01594 837036; Angel Farm, Newland St, Coleford GL16 8NA — MB BS Lond. 1961 (Guy's) MA Camb. 1961; FRCP Lond. 1981, M 1968; DMRT Eng. 1970; FFR 1972; FRCR 1975; T(R) (CO) 1991. Prev: Cas. Off. & Ho. Phys. Guy's Hosp.

WINTER, Philippa Rachel Xanthe Shrewsbury Road Surgery, 20 Shrewsbury Road, Craven Arms SY7 9PY Tel: 01588 672309 Fax: 01588 673943 — MRCS Eng. LRCP Lond. 1976; DFFP 1997.

WINTER, Richard Keith Department of Radiology, Royal Glamorgan Hospital, Ynysmaerdy, Llantrisant, Pontyclun CF72 8XR Tel: 01443 443371 Fax: 01443 443367; 12 Cae Garw, Thornhill, Cardiff CF14 9DX Tel: 02920 522924 Email:

rkwinter@doctors.org.uk — MB BCh Wales 1977; FRCS Eng. 1982; FRCR 1986. Cons. Radiol. Roy. Glam. Hosp. RCT. Specialty: Radiol.

WINTER, Robert James University Hospital, Queen's Medical Centre, Nottingham NG7 2UH Tel: 0115 924 9924 Fax: 0115 970 9910 Email: bob.winter@nottingham.ac.uk; The Old Byre, Farmer Street, Nottingham NG11 6PE Tel: 0115 984 8023 — BM BS Nottm. 1982; DM Nottm. 1995, BMedSci (Hons.) 1980; MRCP (UK) 1986; FFA RCS Eng. 1987. Cons. Intens. Care Med. Univ. Hosp. Nottm. Specialty: Intens. Care. Prev: Sen. Regist. (Anaesth.) Trent RHA; Research Fell. Bristol Roy. Infirm.

WINTER, Robert James David Respiratory Medicine Unit, Box 40, Addenbrooke's Hospital, Cambridge CB2 2QQ Tel: 01223 217079 Fax: 01223 216 953 — MB BS Lond. 1977; MRCP (UK) 1979; BSc (Hons.) Lond. 1974, MD 1987; FRCP Lond. 1995. Cons. Phys. Addenbrooke's Hosp., Camb. Specialty: Respirat. Med. Prev: Cons. Phys. Barnet & Edgware Gen. Hosp.; Sen. Regist. (Respirat. Div.) Hammersmith Hosp. Lond.; MRC Train. Fell. Lond. Chest Hosp. & St. Mary's Hosp. Lond.

WINTER, Roger Andrew The Avenue Surgery, 1 The Avenue, South Moulsecoomb, Brighton BN2 4GF Tel: 01273 604220/606214 Fax: 01273 685507; 10 Deans Close, Woodingdean, Brighton BN2 6RN — MB ChB Birm. 1986 (Birmingham) DCH RCP Lond. 1989; DRCOG 1990; Cert. Family Plann. JCC 1990. Specialty: Gen. Pract. Prev: Trainee GP Kidderminster VTS; SHO (Paediat., O & G, A & E) Birm.

WINTER, Steven Michael Jarvis and Partners, Westbrook Medical Centre, 301-302 Westbrook Centre, Warrington WA5 8UF Tel: 01925 654152 Fax: 01925 632612 — MB ChB Sheff. 1983; DRCOG 1987; MRCGP 1988; DTM & H (Univ Liverpool) 2000. Prev: Trainee GP Wirral VTS; Ho. Off. (Surg. & Med.) Chesterfield & N. Derbysh. Roy. Hosp.

WINTER, Stuart Charles Alec 6 Ashbury Cl, Henley-in-Arden, Solihull — MB ChB Bristol 1997.

WINTER-BARKER, John Paul St Mary's Surgery, Applethwaite, Windermere LA23 1BA — MB ChB Glas. 1985.

WINTERBORN, Claire Justine — MB BS Lond. 1998.

WINTERBORN, Rebecca Jane 29 Monk Road, Bishopston, Bristol BS7 8LE Tel: 0117 924 8678 — MB ChB Bristol 1998.

WINTERBOTTOM, Keith Frederick (retired) Doctor's Corner, 205 Russell Drive, Wollaton, Nottingham NG8 2BD Tel: 0115 928 3201 — MB BChir Camb. 1968 (Univ. Coll. Hosp.) MA Camb. 1968.

WINTERBOTTOM, Paul Michael Heathfield, 30 Denmark Road, Gloucester GL1 3HZ Tel: 01452 891350 Fax: 01452 891341 — MB ChB Leeds 1985; MRCPsych 1992. Med. Dir. Gloucestershire Partnership NHS Trust; Cons Psychiat. in the Psychiat. of Learning Disabil. W. Gloucestershire; Cons Psychiat. to Relate Gloucestershire. Specialty: Ment. Health. Prev: Sen Reg S W. RHA; Regist. (Gen. Psychiat.) Yorks. RHA.; Clin. Dir Severn NHS Trust Learning Disabil. Directorate.

WINTERBOTTOM, Peter Mark 65 Oxford Street, Woodstock OX20 1TJ Tel: 01993 811291 Fax: 01993 811291 Email: fatboyblim@hotmail.com — MB BS Newc. 1996 (newcastleupon tyne) SHO A&E W.Cumbld..Hosp.Whitehaven.

WINTERBURN, Ruth Bewley Drive Surgery, 79 Bewley Drive, Liverpool L32 9PD Tel: 0151 546 2480 Fax: 0151 548 3474 — MB ChB Liverp. 1975; DCH Eng 1978; MRCGP 1982.

WINTERINGHAM, Tresca 6 Knoll Court, Knoll Hill, Bristol BS9 1QX — BM BCh Oxf. 1961.

WINTERS, Miss Zoe Ellen Bristol Royal Infirmary, Division of Surgery, Marlborough Street, Bristol BS2 8HW — MB BCh Witwatersrand 1983; FRCS Ed.; DPhil Oxon.; FRS SA. Specialty: Gen. Surg. Special Interest: Breast Surg.

WINTERSGILL, Eleanor Mary (retired) Severn NHS Trust, Rikenel, Montpellier, Gloucester GL1 1LY Tel: 01452 891023 Fax: 01452 891020; 10 The Cherry Orchard, Staverton, Cheltenham GL51 0TR — MB BS Lond. 1967 (St. Bart.) MB BS (Hons.) Lond. 1967; MRCS Eng. LRCP Lond. 1967; DCH RCP Lond. 1985; DCCH RCP Ed. 1985. Prev: Cons. Paediat. (Community Child Health) Severn NHS Trust Glos.

WINTERSGILL, Peter (retired) 28 Westfield Avenue, Oakes, Huddersfield HD3 4FN — MRCS Eng. LRCP Lond. 1951 (Camb. & Middlx.) Prev: Sen. Med. Off. Huddersfield HA.

WINTERTON, Anthony John (retired) Greystones, Greenway Park, Chippenham SN15 1QG Tel: 01249 443144 — MB BS Lond. 1954 (St. Mary's) MRCS Eng. LRCP Lond. 1954; DObst RCOG 1955; DCH Eng. 1956; MRCGP 1965. Locum GP. Prev: GP Chippenham.

WINTERTON, Elizabeth Anne Tretherres, St. Allen, Truro TR4 9QX — MB BS Lond. 1974 (King's Coll. Hosp.) Assoc. Specialist in Rehabillitation Med. St. Michael's Hosp. Hayle. Prev: Clin. Med. Off. Cornw. & Isles of Scilly HA.; Ho. Phys. Plymouth Gen. Hosp. (Greenbank Sect.); Ho. Surg. Roy. Cornw. Hosp. (Treliske) Truro.

WINTERTON, Helen Muriel 21 Westbrook Road, Milton, Weston Super Mare BS22 8JX Email: helen@mwinterton. fsnet. co.uk. — MB BS Lond. 1996 (Lond. Hosp. Med. Coll.) BSc (Hon.) King's College, London 1993; MRCP Lond. 2001; DRCOG 2003. GP Trainee. Specialty: Gen. Med. Socs: CMF.

WINTERTON, Ian Stewart Gosforth Memorial Medical Centre, Church Road, Gosforth, Newcastle upon Tyne NE3 1TX Tel: 0191 285 1119 — MB BS Newc. 1971; DObst RCOG 1973; MRCGP 1975; FRCGP 1999. Prev: Trainee GP Newc. VTS; Ho. Surg. Newc. Gen. Hosp.; Ho. Phys. Roy. Vict. Infirm. Newc.

WINTERTON, Michael Charles Tretherres, St. Allen, Truro TR4 9QX Tel: 01872 540354 — MB BS Lond. 1959 (King's Coll. Hosp.) MRCS Eng. LRCP Lond. 1959; FRCP Lond. 1979, M 1966. Cons. Phys. Roy. Cornw. Hosp. Treliske Truro. Specialty: Gen. Med.

WINTERTON, Sandra Gosforth Memorial Medical Centre, Church Road, Gosforth, Newcastle upon Tyne NE3 1TX Tel: 0191 285 1119 — MB BS Newc. 1971. Prev: Ho. Phys., Ho. Surg. & SHO (O & G) Hexham Gen. Hosp.

WINTERTON, Simon John Dorset County Hospital, Williams Avenue, Dorchester DT1 2JY Tel: 01305 255114 Fax: 01305 254778; Elwell Lea, 710 Dorchester Road, Upwey DT3 5LA Tel: 01305 813000 Fax: 01305 816100 Email: simon.winterton@talk21.com — MB BS Lond. 1982 (St. Mary's) BA Oxf. 1979; MRCP (UK) 1986; FRCP 1998. Cons. Cardiol. Dorset Co. Hosp. Dorchester. Specialty: Cardiol. Socs: Brit. Cardiac Soc. & Brit. Cardiovasc. Interven. Soc.; Brit. Pacing & Electrophysiol. Gp. Prev: Regist. (Cardiol.) Lond. Chest Hosp.; Research Fell. & Hon. Regist. (Cardiac) St. Mary's Hosp. Lond.; Regist. (Gen. Med.) Hillingdon Hosp.

WINTLE, Christopher James The Rogerstone Practice, Chapel Wood, Western Valley Road, Rogerstone, Newport NP10 9DU Tel: 01633 893272 Fax: 01633 895079; The Limes, Fields Pk Road, Newport NP20 5BH — MB BCh Wales 1968 (Cardiff) Prev: GP Trainee GP Unit Welsh Nat. Sch. Med. Cardiff; SHO (Gen. Med.) St. David's Hosp. Cardiff; Ho. Surg. Dept. Urol. & Ho. Phys. Cardiff Roy. Infirm.

WINTLE, Fiona Caroline 2 Aspland Road, Hyde SK14 5LS — MB ChB Manch. 1998.

WINTLE, Jennifer Margaret The Limes, Fields Park Road, Newport NP1 5BH — MB BCh Wales 1970; DObst RCOG 1972. Prev: SHO (O & G) & Ho. Phys. Roy. Gwent Hosp. Newport; Ho. Surg. & Ho. Phys. St. Woolos Hosp. Newport.

WINTLE, Matthew Edward 17 Picton Street, Kenfig Hill, Bridgend CF33 6EF — MB BCh Wales 1997.

WINTON, Donald Bain The Love Street Medical Centre, 40 Love Street, Paisley PA3 2DY Tel: 0141 889 3355 Fax: 0141 889 4785; 8 Hawick Avenue, Paisley PA2 9LD Tel: 0141 884 4999 — MB ChB St. And. 1961. Sen. Partner. Specialty: Gen. Pract.

WINTON, Elizabeth The Sheiling, 6 Bryntirion Hill, Bridgend CF31 4DA Tel: 01656 653818 — MB BCh BAO Belf. 1944; MB BCh BAO (Hnrs.) Belf. 1944. Prev: Sen. Extern Surg. & Ho. Surg. Roy. Vict. Hosp. Belf.

WINTON, Francis Edgar Phoenix Day Hospital, Hospital Rd, Bury St Edmunds IP33 3NR Tel: 01284 725333 x 2385 — MB BS Lond. 1980; BSc. Lond. 1977; FRCPsych FRCPsych, 1980; MRCPsych 1984. Cons. Rehabil. & Gen. Psychiat. W. Suff. Hosp. Specialty: Gen. Psychiat. Socs: Hon. Sec. of Rehabil. and social phychiatry Sect. of Roy. Coll. of Psychiat.s. Prev: Cons. Lincoln. Co. Hosp.; Sen. Regist. Maudsley Hosp. Lond.; Hon. Sen. Regist. Inst. Psychiat. Maudsley Hosp. Lond.

WINTON, Margaret (retired) Green Lane House, 1 Green Lane, Davenham, Northwich CW9 8HT — MB ChB Leeds 1949. Prev: SCMO Crewe Health Dist.

WINTON, Pamela Elizabeth 6 Sycamore Way, Moulsham Lodge, Chelmsford CM2 9LZ Tel: 01245 281403 — MB ChB Aberd. 1997; BSc Med Sci, 1995.

WINTOUR, David Ian Denburn Health Centre, Rosemount Viaduct, Aberdeen AB25 1QB — MB ChB Aberd. 1974.

WINWARD, John McGregor The Atherstone Surgery, 1 Ratcliffe Road, Atherstone CV9 1EU Tel: 01827 713664 Fax: 01827 713666 — MB BS Lond. 1982; DRCOG 1986; Cert. Family Plann JCC 1986.

WINWOOD, Paul John Royal Bournemouth Hospital, Castle Lane E., Bournemouth BH7 Tel: 01202 303626 Fax: 01202 704909 Email: paul.winwood@rbch-tr.swest.nhs.uk — MB BS Lond. 1985 (London Hospital Medical College) BSc (Hons.) Lond. 1984; MRCP (UK) 1988; DM Soton. 1994; FRCP Edin 2000; FRCP 2000. Cons. Phys. & Gastroenterol. Roy. Bournemouth Hosp.; Hon. Sen. Lect. Univ. Soton.; Clinical Tutor, Royal Bournemouth Hospital. Specialty: Gastroenterol. Socs: Brit. Soc. Gastroenterol.; Brit. Assn. for Study Liver; BMA. Prev: Lect. & Hon. Sen. Regist. (Med. & Gastroenterol.) Soton. Gen. Hosp.; MRC Trav. Fell. Liver Center Laborat. Univ. Calif. San Franciso, USA; Regist. Rotat. (Gen. Med. & Gastroenterol.) Soton. & Bournemouth Gen. Hosps.

WINWOOD, Robert Sidney (retired) Mellstock, 18 Dale Gardens, Woodford Green IG8 0PB — MB BS Lond. 1957 (Lond. Hosp.) FRCP Lond. 1978, M 1964. Prev: Cons. Phys. Whipps Cross Hosp. Lond. & Hon. Vis. Cardiol. St. Bart. Hosp. Lond.

WINYARD, Graham Peter Arthur NHS Management Executive, Quarry House, Quarry Hill, Leeds LS2 7PD; 15 Clifton Road, Winchester SO22 5BP — BM BCh Oxf. 1971; MRCP (UK) 1975; FFPHM 1987, M 1981; FRCP Lond. 1989. Med. Dir. NHS Managem. Exec. Leeds. Prev: Regional Med. Dir. & Dir. Pub. Health Wessex RHA.

WINYARD, Paul Julian Douglas Nephro-Urology Unit, ICH/605, 30 Guilford Street, London WC1N 1EH Tel: 020 7905 2116 Fax: 020 7905 2133 — BM BCh Oxf. 1986; MA Camb. 1987, BA (Med. Sci.) 1983; MRCP (UK) 1990. Sen. Lect. Inst. Child Health Lond.; Hon. Sen. Regist. (Nephrol.) Hosp. Childr. Gt. Ormond St. Lond. Specialty: Paediat. Prev: Regist. Qu. Eliz. Hosp. Childr. Hackney; Regist. (Paediat. Haemat & Oncol.) Hosp. Sick Childr. Gt. Ormond St. Lond.; Exchange Regist. Childr. Hosp. Philadelphia, USA.

WIRTH, Maria Alexandra Dumbarton Road Surgery, 1215 Dumbarton Road, Glasgow G14 9UT Tel: 0141 211 9045 Fax: 0141 211 9047 — MB ChB Glas. 1982; MRCOG 1983.

WISBY, Lee Robert 3 Cherry Cottages, School Road, Hastings TN35 5BQ — BM Soton. 1995.

WISCOMBE, Kieron Aubrey Raymond Munro Medical Centre, West Elloe Avenue, Spalding PE11 2BY Tel: 01775 725530 Fax: 01775 766168 — MB BS Lond. 1985 (St. Mary's Hosp. Lond.) DCH RCP Lond. 1987; DRCOG 1988; MRCGP 1989; Dip. IMC RCS Ed. 1989; FImcRCSEd 2000. GP Princip. Lincs Clin. Asst. (Acc. & Emerg.); PCG Exec. Bd. Mem. Socs: BASICS. Prev: Trainee GP Windsor VTS.

WISDOM, Anthony Rodwell Genitourinary Medicine, Newham Hospital, London E13 8SL Tel: 020 7363 8146; 24 St. Albans Road, London NW5 1RD Tel: 020 7482 2442 — (Lond. Hosp.) MB BS Lond. 1954. Cons. Genitourin Med. Newham Hosp. Lond. Specialty: Genitourinary Medicine. Socs: Fell. Hunt. Soc.; Med. Soc. Study VD. Prev: Cons. Genitourin Med. Barking, Havering & Brentwood HAs; Sen. Regist. (VD) St. Mary's Hosp. Lond.; Surg. Lt. RNVR.

WISDOM, Rosemary Jean (retired) Wykeham House, 11 Mill Hill, Alresford SO24 9DD Tel: 01962 732237 — MB BS Lond. 1953 (Univ. Coll. Hosp.)

WISDOM, Stephen John Dumfries and Galloway Royal Infirmary, Bankend Road, Dumfries DG1 4AP Tel: 01387 246246 — MB ChB Ed. 1982; BSc (Med. Sci.) Ed. 1980; MRCOG 1989; FRCOG 2001. Cons. (O & G) Dumfries & Galloway Roy. Infirm. & Cresswell Matern. Hosp. Specialty: Obst. & Gyn. Socs: Brit. Med. Ultrasound Soc.; Brit. Matern. and Foetal Med. Soc. Prev: Regist. (O & G) Glas. Roy. Matern. Hosp. & Glas. Roy. Infirm.

WISE, Arlene 146 Archerhill Road, Knightswood, Glasgow G13 3JH — MB ChB Glas. 1998.

WISE, Christopher Foston Longrigg Medical Centre, Leam Lane Estate, Gateshead NE10 8PH Tel: 0191 469 2173 Fax: 0191 495 0893; 16 Moor Place, Gosforth, Newcastle upon Tyne NE3 4AL — MB BS Newc. 1984; Cert. Family Plann. JCC 1987; MRCGP 1988; DRCOG 1988.

WISE, David (retired) 10 Gretaside, Keswick CA12 5LG; 7 Six Bells Lane, Sevenoaks TN13 1JE Tel: 01732 458032 — MB BChir Camb. 1952 (Camb. & St. Thos.) FRCP Lond. 1980, M 1954; MD Camb. 1960. Prev: Cons. Phys. W. Hill Hosp. Dartford.

WISE, David 75 Arlington Avenue, London N1 7BA — MB ChB Manch. 1991; BSc (Psychol.) 1st cl. Hons. CNAA Lond. 1985. SHO (Surg.) W. Cornw. Hosp. Penzance. Specialty: Accid. & Emerg. Prev: SHO (Med.) W. Cornw. Hosp. Penzance; SHO (A & E, Trauma & Orthop.) Treliske Hosp. Truro & Leighton Hosp. Chesh.; Lect. (Anat.) Manch. Univ. Med. Sch.

WISE, David Graham Denham Grove Medical Centre, 3 Vale Avenue, Grove, Wantage OX12 7LU Tel: 01235 770140 Fax: 01235 760027; 14 Truelocks Way, Charlton Heights, Wantage OX12 7EG Tel: 01235 768606 — MB ChB Bristol 1977; MB ChB (Hons.) Bristol 1977; DObst. RCOG 1980; DCH Eng. 1981; MRCGP 1981.

WISE, Mr David Ian (retired) Orchard Cottage, St Mary's Road, Dinton, Salisbury SP3 5HH Tel: 01722 716600 — MB BS Lond. 1966 (Lond. Hosp.) MRCS Eng. LRCP Lond. 1966; FRCS Eng. 1972. Prev: GP Worthing.

WISE, Mr David Ian Huddersfield Royal Infirmary, Acre Street, Lindley, Huddersfield HD3 3EA Tel: 01484 342214; The Old Inn, Flush House Lane, Holmbridge, Holmfirth, Huddersfield HD9 2QY Tel: 01484 682713 — MB ChB Leic. 1982; FRCS Glas. 1987; FRCS Eng. 1988; FRCS (Orth.) 1993. Cons. Orthop. Surg. Huddersfield Roy. Infirm. Specialty: Orthop.

WISE, Helen Jayne 13 Market St, Poole BH15 1NA — BM Soton. 1994. Specialist Regist. (Anaesth.). Specialty: Anaesth.; Intens. Care. Socs: Assn. of Anaesth.s; Intens. Care Soc. Prev: SHO (Anaesth.).

WISE, Mr Kenneth Stanley Hadyn The Chiltern Hospital & The Shelburne Hospital, Great Missenden HP16 0EN Tel: 01494 890890 Email: k.wise@dial.pipex.com — (St. Bart.) MB BS Lond. 1963; FRCS Eng. 1970. Specialty: Orthop. Socs: Fell. BOA & Brit. Soc. Surg. Hand.; World Orthopaedic Concern. Prev: Sen. Cons. (Orthop.) S. Bucks Trust; Sen. Regist. (Orthop.) Wessex Orthop. Train. Scheme; Asst. Lect. St. Bart. Hosp. Med. Coll.

WISE, Lindsay Karen 8 Cottesmore Gardens, Leigh-on-Sea SS9 2TG — MB BCh Wales 1993.

WISE, Mr Martin Portsmouth Hospitals NHS Trust, Queen Alexandra Hospital, Cosham, Portsmouth PO3 6QS Tel: 023 92 286000; Chellow Bank, 4 Ranvilles Lane, Catisfield, Fareham PO14 3DS Tel: 01329 842768 — MB ChB Bristol 1973; FRCS Eng. 1977; MD Bristol 1986. Cons. Surg. Specialty: Gen. Surg. Socs: Assn. Surg.; Brit. Assn. Surg. Oncol.; Brit. Transpl. Soc.

WISE, Matthew Peter 17 Hobart Close, High Wycombe HP13 6UF — MB BChir Camb. 1990; MA Camb. 1991, MB BChir 1990; MRCP (UK) 1993; DPhil Oxon. 1998. Specialty: Gen. Med.; Intens. Care.

WISE, Michael Erwin Jan Pitt House, North End Avenue, London NW3 7HP Email: j@wisepsych.freeserce.co.uk — MB BS Lond. 1992 (UMDS) MRCPysch 1997; MSc 1998. Specialist Regist. Hammersmith Hosp. Specialty: Gen. Psychiat. Socs: BMA; Jun. Doctors Negotiating Comm.; Comm. on Community Care. Prev: Research Fell. Lewisham & Guy's MHT; Regist. (Psychiat.) Guys & Lewisham MHT; SpR BKC&W MHT.

WISE, Raymond Percy (retired) Holmfield House, Farnham, Blandford Forum DT11 8DE Tel: 01725 516436 — MB BS Lond. 1952 (Westm.) MRCS Eng. LRCP Lond. 1952; DA Eng. 1954; FFA RCS Eng. 1956. Cons. Anaesth. St. Thos. Hosp. Lond. Prev: Sen. Regist. (Anaesth.) St. Thos. Hosp. Lond.

WISE, Professor Richard Health Protection Agency, c/o University of Birmingham, Edgbaston, Birmingham B15 2TT Tel: 01432 342767 — MB ChB Manch. 1966; FRCPath 1986, M 1974; MD Manch. 1981; FRCP (Hon) 1998; FMedSci 2003. Non Exe. Director Health Protec. Agency; Chair Specialist Adv. Comm. Antimicrobial Resistance; Civil. Cons. Army; Hon. Prof. Clin. Microbiol. Univ. Birm. Specialty: Med. Microbiol. Prev: Non Exec. Director, Centre for Applied Micro. Research; Cons. Med. Microbiol. City Hosp. Trust Birm.; Research Fell. (Microbiol.) Univ. Brit. Columbia.

WISE, Valerie Anne Helvellyn, Clovelly Road, Beacon Hill, Hindhead GU26 6RW — MB ChB Manch. 1982. Specialty: Blood Transfus.

WISELKA, Martin Joseph Department of Infection and Tropical Medicine, Leicester Royal Infirmary, Leicester LE1 5WW — BM BCh Oxf. 1982 (Oxford) MRCP (UK) 1985; MA Camb. 1983, MD 1992; PhD 1995; FRCP (uk) 1999. Cons. Infec. Dis. Leicester Roy. Infirm.; Sen. Lect. Dept. of Microbiol. and Immunol. Uiversity of Leicester.

Specialty: Infec. Dis.; Gen. Med.; Trop. Med. Socs: Brit. Infec. Soc.; Brit. HIV Assn.; Soc. for Gen. MicroBiol. Prev: Wellcome Trust Clin. Research Fell. & Sen. Regist. (Infec. Dis.) Univ.Leics.; SHO (Med.) Qu. Med. Centre Nottm.

WISELY, Catherine Macdonald (retired) 5 Hillway, Westcliff on Sea SS0 8QA Tel: 01702 76505 — MB ChB Ed. 1956; DA Eng. 1960; FFA RCS Eng. 1966. Prev: Cons. Anaesth. S. Essex Hosp. Gp.

WISELY, Mr Edward Hugh (retired) 5 Hillway, Westcliff on Sea SS0 8QA Tel: 01702 476505 — (Lond. Hosp.) FDS RCS Eng. 1960, LDS 1946; LRCP Lond. MRCS Eng. 1957. Prev: Cons. Oral Surg. Southend-on-Sea Hosp.

WISELY, Ivan Charles Fraser Brimmond Medical Group, 106 Inverurie Road, Bucksburn, Aberdeen AB21 9AT Tel: 01224 713869 Fax: 01224 716317; 1 Rubislaw Den N., Aberdeen AB15 4AL Tel: 01224 317750 Fax: 01224 322004 — MB ChB Aberd. 1967; DA Eng. 1970.

WISELY, Joanna 5 Hillway, Westcliff on Sea SS0 8QA Tel: 01702 76505; 3f2 80 Montrose Park, Edinburgh EH10 4NG Tel: 0131 228 6588 — MB ChB Ed. 1994 (Edin) DRCOG 1998. GP Reg. Specialty: Gen. Pract.

WISELY, Nicholas Alexander Wythenshawe Hospital , Department of Anaesthesia, Southmoor Road, Wythenshawe, Manchester M23 9LT Tel: 0161 291 5710 Email: nickwisely@yahoo.co.uk — MB ChB Ed. 1992 (Univ. Ed.) FRCA 1998. Consult. Anaes. S. Manch. Uni. Hosps. Specialty: Anaesth. Socs: Fell. Roy. Med. Soc.; Scott. Soc. Anaesth.; Fellow Royal Col. Anaesth. Prev: SHO Rotat. (Anaesth.) SE Scotl. Sch. Anaesth.; Specialist Regist. Train. Rotat. N. W. Region; Reg. Christchurch Hosp. NZ (Anaeasth).

WISEMAN, Alfred Malcolm (retired) 10 Shilton Garth Close, Old Earswick, York YO32 9SQ — MB BS Lond. 1970.

WISEMAN, Ann Juliet 3 Holmdene Avenue, Mill Hill, London NW7 2LY — MRCS Eng. LRCP Lond. 1961 (Guy's) DPH Eng. 1965; MFCM 1974; AFOM RCP Lond. 1978. Sessional Occupational Health Med. Off. Socs: Hunt. Soc. Prev: Sen. Med. Off. Barnet AHA; Deptm. Med. Off. Lond. Boro. Enfield; Med. Off. Blood Transfus. Serv.

WISEMAN, Aviva Woodrow Farm Cottages, Woodrow, Amersham HP7 0QH Tel: 01494 724734 Email: avivawiseman@compuserve.com — (King's Coll. Hosp.) MRCS Eng. LRCP Lond. 1945.

WISEMAN, Claire Elizabeth Worthing & Southlamds Hospitals NHS Trust, Worthing BN16 2JH — MB ChB Sheff. 1985; DFFP 1996. Staff Grade Family Planning & Reprod. Healthcare; Worthing Priority Care NHS Trust Worthing W. Sussex. Specialty: Family Plann. & Reproduc. Health. Prev: Clin. Med. Off. Contracep. & Sexual Health Dept.

WISEMAN, Denis Buchanan (retired) 32 Freemans Close, Stoke Poges, Slough SL2 4ER Tel: 01753 663543 — MB ChB Ed. 1941 (Univ. Ed.) Prev: Resid. Phys. Roy. Infirm. Edin.

WISEMAN, Elizabeth Claire 10 Priory Close, Ruskington, Sleaford NG34 9ED; 142 Howard Road, Leicester LE2 1XJ — MB ChB Leic. 1997. Specialty: Accid. & Emerg.

WISEMAN, Elizabeth Sarah 78 Poole Crescent, Birmingham B17 0PB — MB ChB Birm. 1995; ChB Birm. 1995.

WISEMAN, Hazel Gwendoline (retired) Chenoweth, Love Lane, Bodmin PL31 2BJ Tel: 01208 76049 — MB ChB Glas. 1949; DObst RCOG 1954; DCH Eng. 1966; DIH Eng. 1982; MFOM RCP Lond. 1984. Prev: Dist. Occupat. Health Phys. City & Hackney HA.

WISEMAN, Janet The Hollies, Griffiths Green, Claverley, Wolverhampton WV5 7BG — MB ChB Birm. 1977.

WISEMAN, Jennifer Ruth 15 Back Lane, Haslingfield, Cambridge CB3 7JN Tel: 01223 871635; 29 St Chad's Rise, Headingley, Leeds LS6 3QE Tel: 0113 278 0418 — MB BS Newc. 1988; MRCGP 1994; Dip. Palliat. Med. Wales 1997. Locum Cons. (Palliat. Med.) Dewsbury NHS Trust. Specialty: Palliat. Med. Prev: Specialist Regist. Rotat. (Palliat. Med.) Yorks.

WISEMAN, Louise Catherine 24 College Road, Ardingly, Haywards Heath RH17 6TY — MB BS Lond. 1997 (St marys hosp.Imperial.Coll) BSc 1994. GP Registrar, Haywards Heath. Specialty: Anaesth.

WISEMAN, Malcolm Raymond Lewisham Park Child and Family Therapy Centre, 78 Lewisham Park, London SE13 6QJ — MB Camb. 1977; BA 1973; MA Camb. 1976; MRCPsych 1982. Cons. Child & Adolesc. Psychiat., S. Lond. and Maudsley NHS Trust. Specialty: Child & Adolesc. Psychiat.

WISEMAN, Martin Fitzalan Medical Centre, Fitzalan Road, Littlehampton BN17 5JR Tel: 01903 733277 Fax: 01903 733773 — MB BS Lond. 1984.

WISEMAN, Oliver 166 Maygrove Road, London NW6 2EP — MB BChir Camb. 1995 (Addenbrooke's Hosp. Camb.) MA Camb. 1996; FRCS (Eng.) 1999. SpR (Urol.) Harold Wood Hosp. Romford Essex. Specialty: Anat. Prev: SpR & Research Fell. (Uro-Neurology) The Nat. Hosp. Qu. Sq. Lond.; SHO (Surg.) Norf. & Norwich Hosp.; SHO (A & E) Watford Gen. Hosp.

WISEMAN, Paul Jeremy Talbot Hampstead Group Practice, 75 Fleet Road, London NW3 2QU Tel: 020 7435 4000 Fax: 020 7435 9000; The Cromwell Hospital, Cromwell Road, London SW5 0TU Tel: 020 7370 4233 — MB BS Lond. 1982; Cert. Family Plann. JCC 1985; MRCGP 1987.

WISEMAN, Penelope Anne Barnet & Chase Farm NHS Trust, Barnet General Hospital, Wellhouse Lane, Barnet EN5 3DJ Tel: 020 8732 6718 — MB BS Lond. 1981 (Oxford) FRCP; MA Oxf. 1978; MRCP (UK) 1984; FRCP 1998. Cons. in Med. for the Elderly, Barnet Hosp., Barnet. Specialty: Care of the Elderly.

WISEMAN, Raymond (retired) 2 St Baldred's Crescent, North Berwick EH39 4PZ Tel: 01620 892775 — MB ChB Aberd. 1964; FRCPath 1982, M 1970; Dip. Bact. Lond 1970. Cons. Bact. St. John's Hosp. Livingston; Hon. Sen. Lect. (Bact.) Edin. Univ. Prev: Cons. Bact. Bangour Gen. Hosp. Broxburn.

WISEMAN, Richard Ansel Slough Place, Cuckfield, Haywards Heath RH17 5JD Tel: 01444 454312 Fax: 01444 416609 — MRCS Eng. LRCP Lond. 1960; DObst RCOG 1961; DTM & H Eng. 1964; PhD Lond. 1969; FFPM RCP (UK) 1991. Managing Dir. HOGENS Ltd. W. Sussex; Hon. Sen. Lect. Dept. of Epidemiol. & Populat. Health; Lond. Sch. Hyg. & Trop. Med. Lond. Specialty: Pharmaceutical Medicine; Epidemiol. Socs: Fell. Roy. Soc. Med. Prev: Managing & Med. Dir. Schering Chems. Ltd. W. Sussex; Lect. Lond. Sch. Hyg. & Trop. Med; Research Fell. Med. Unit Hosp. Trop. Dis. Lond.

WISEMAN, Simon Martin St. Paul's Road Medical Centre, 248-250 St Paul's Road, Canonbury, London N1 2LJ Tel: 020 7226 6333 — MB BS Lond. 1972 (Univ. Coll. Hosp.) MRCGP 1991. Gen. Practitioner St. Pauls Rd. med. Centre Lond. N1 2LJ; GP Tutor Whittington Hosp. Lond.; Hon. Clin. Lect. Dept. Primary Care & Populat. Sci. Roy. Free & Univ. Coll. Med. Sch. Lond. Specialty: Gen. Pract. Prev: Hosp. Pract. Regional Alcoholism & Drug Dependence Unit St. Bernards Wing Ealing Hosp. Lond.; SHO Shenley Hosp.; Ho. Surg. King Geo. Hosp. Ilford.

WISHART, Eva Hanna 99 Oakfield Road, Birmingham B29 7HW Tel: 0121 472 1768 — MB BS Lond. 1957 (Univ. Coll. Hosp.) MRCS Eng. LRCP Lond. 1957; DObst RCOG 1960; MFFP 1993. SCMO S. Birm. HA; Clin. Asst. (Ultrasound) Sandwell Hosp. Socs: BMA. Prev: Research Fell. (Med.) Qu. Eliz. Hosp. Birm.; Regist. (Microbiol.) Hosp. Sick Childr. Gt. Ormond St. Lond.

WISHART, Mr Gordon Cranston Cambridge Breast Unit, Box 97, Addenbrooke's Hospital, Hills Road, Cambridge CB2 2QQ Tel: 01223 216315 Fax: 01223 586932 Email: gordon.wishart@addenbrookes.nhs.uk — MB ChB Ed. 1983; FRCS Glas. 1987; MD Ed. 1992; FRCS (Gen.) 1995; FRCS Eng. 2001. Cons. Breast and Endocrine Surg., Addenbrook's Hosp., Camb. Specialty: Gen. Surg. Socs: Assn. Surg.; Brit. Assn. Surg. Oncol. (BASO); BASO Breast Gp. Prev: Cons. Gen. Surg. Princess Roy. Hosp. Haywards Heath; Sen. Regist. (Gen. Surg.) W. Scotl. Higher Surgic. Train. Scheme; Sen. Regist. (Surg.) West. Infirm. Glas.

WISHART, Ian Herbert The Health Centre, Crieff PH7 3SA Tel: 01764 2283; Woodhaven, East Craigmuir, Madderty, Crieff PH7 3NZ Tel: 01764 683396 — MB ChB St. And. 1959; DObst RCOG 1971; MRCGP 1974. Hon. Med. Off. Crieff & Dist. Hosp. & Glenalmond. Coll. Prev: SHO (Gen. Med.) Murray Roy. Hosp. Perth; Ho. Phys & Ho. Surg. Perth Roy. Infirm.; Ho. Surg. Forth Pk. Matern. Hosp. Kirkcaldy.

WISHART, Katharine Cecilia Hainton House, 66 West St., Kings Cliffe, Peterborough PE8 6XA — MB BS Lond. 1985. Socs: RCGP.

WISHART, Mrs Manijeh Seradji Warrington District General Hospital, Lovely Lane, Warrington WA5 1QG Tel: 01925 35911; North Cheshire Hospital, Stretton, Warrington WA4 4LU Tel: 01925 265000 — MD Teheran 1973; FRCS Eng. 1983; FCOphth 1988.

Cons. Ophth. Surg. Warrington Dist. Gen. Hosp. Specialty: Ophth. Socs: Oxf. Ophth. Soc. & Overseas Doctors Assn. Prev: Clin. Research Asst. Inst. Ophth. Moorfields Eye Hosp. Lond.; Regist. (Ophth.) OldCh. Hosp. Romford; SHO (Ophth.) Manch. Roy. Eye Hosp.

WISHART, Maria Olivia 3 Victoria Road, Cambridge CB4 3BW Email: maria.o.wishart@gsk.com — BChir Camb. 1992.

WISHART, Marion Gardiner (retired) Flat 6 Arbrook Hall, Church Road, Claygate, Esher KT10 0AR Tel: 01372 462406 — (Univ. Ed.) MB ChB Ed. 1947; DA Eng. 1950; FFA RCS Eng. 1954. Prev: Assoc. Specialist (Anaesth.) Poole Gen. Hosp.

WISHART, Mary (retired) Lower Sent, Oakwood Hill, Dorking RH5 5NB — MB ChB Glas. 1954; BSc Glas. 1950, MB ChB 1954. Prev: Asst. Lect. Physiol. Univ. Glas.

WISHART, Mr Peter Knight St. Pauls Eye Unit, Royal Liverpool Hospital, Prescot St., Liverpool L7 8XP Tel: 0151 706 3968 Fax: 0151 706 5861; Lourdes Hospital, 57 Greenbank Road, Liverpool L18 1HQ Tel: 0151 733 7123 Fax: 0151 735 0446 — MB ChB Aberd. 1976; DO Eng. 1980; FRCS Glas. 1982; FCOphth 1988. Cons. Ophth. Surg. St. Paul's Eye Unit Roy. Liverp. Univ. Hosp. Trust. Specialty: Ophth. Socs: N. Eng. Ophth. Soc. Prev: Resid. Surgic. Off. Moorfields Eye Hosp. Lond.; Sen. Regist. King's Coll. Hosp. Lond.

WISLEY, Alexander Barclay Finlayson Street Practice, 33 Finlayson Street, Fraserburgh AB43 9JW Tel: 01346 518088 Fax: 01346 510015; Craigielea, Commerce Lane, Fraserburgh AB43 9LF Tel: 01346 516738 Fax: 01346 510015 — MB ChB Aberd. 1975 (Aberdeen University) Phys. Fraserburgh Hosp. Specialty: Accid. & Emerg.; Alcohol & Substance Misuse; Gen. Psychiat.

WISMAYER, Emma Cecile Datchet, St. Georges Lane, Sandwich CT13 9JS — MB BCh Wales 1990.

WISSA, Atef Halim 10 Creek Road, South Woodham Ferrars, Chelmsford CM3 5GU — MB BCh Ain Shams 1975; LRCP LRCS Ed. LRCPS Glas. 1983.

WISTOW, Trevor Edwin William Flat A, 39 Mount Adon Park, Dulwich, London SE22 0DS Tel: 020 8693 9567; 44 Mile End Road, Godmanchester, Norwich NR4 7QX Tel: 01480 219743 Fax: 01603 504627 — MB BS Lond. 1986 (The Royal Free Hospital) BSc Lond. 1983, MB BS 1986; MRCP (UK) 1989. Cons. Cardiol. Norf. & Norwich Hosp., Norwich. Specialty: Cardiol. Prev: Sen. Regist. (Med.) Toowoomba, Queensland, Austral.

WISZNIEWSKA, Ruth Heather 42 Arnall Drive, Henbury, Bristol BS10 7AP — MB ChB Bristol 1994; DRCOG 1996. Specialty: Gen. Pract. Prev: SHO (Psychiat.) Weston Gen. Hosp. Weston Super Mare; SHO (ENT & O & G) St. Michaels Hosp. Bristol; SHO (Ophth.) Bristol Eye Hosp.

WITANA, Jaika Sali Department Audiological Medicine, Royal Hallamshire Hospital, Glossop Road, Sheffield S10 2JF Tel: 0114 271 1853 Fax: 0114 271 1855 — MB BS Sri Lanka 1979 (University of Sri Lanka, Colombo) FRCSI 1990; MS Sri Lanka 1991. Cons. Audiological Phys. Roy. Hallamshire Hosp. Sheffield. Specialty: Audiol. Med.; Otorhinolaryngol. Socs: Brit. Assn. Audiol. Phys. (Full); Brit. Soc. Audiol.; MPS. Prev: Specialist Regist. (Audiological Med.).

WITCHALLS, James Raymond Department of Health Screening, The London Clinic, 149 Harley Street, London W1N 2DE Tel: 020 7616 7746 Fax: 020 7381 9636; Maddox Farm, Little Bookham St, Little Bookham, Leatherhead KT23 3BU Tel: 01372 454197 — MB BS Lond. 1967 (St. Bart.) MRCS Eng. LRCP Lond. 1968; DObst RCOG 1972. Gen. Phys. Health Screening Dept. The Lond. Clinic 149 Harley St Lond.; Chairm. Pioneer Health Centre Ltd.; Governor Albert Schweitzer Hosp. Lambarene Gabon; Con. Health Servs. Dept. Shell Internat. PLC. Specialty: Gen. Med. Socs: Pres. Internat. Assn. Friends Albert Schweitzer; Roy. Soc. Med. Prev: Sen. Phys i/c BUPA Health Screening Centre Lond.; Med. Off. Albert Schweitzer Hosp. & Leprosarium Lambarene Gabon; Med. Cons. to the Juno Mission.

WITCHER, John William National Blood Service, Southmead Road, Bristol BS10 5ND Tel: 0117 950 7777; 4 Anchor Way, Pill, Bristol BS20 0JY — MB ChB Bristol 1969; DA Eng. 1973. Specialty: Blood Transfus. Socs: Fac. Anaesth. Prev: GP Bristol; Clin. Asst. (Anaesth.) Bristol.

WITCOMB, Alexandra Helen 50 Falmouth Road, Evington, Leicester LE5 4WH — MB BS Lond. 1989. SHO (Paediat.) Centr. Middlx. Hosp. Lond.

WITCOMBE, John Brian Bradstone House, Amberley, Stroud GL5 5AQ Tel: 01453 872220 — MB BS Lond. 1966 (St Thos.) MRCS Eng. LRCP Lond. 1966; DCH Eng. 1969; DMRD Eng. 1973; FRCR 1975. Cons. Radiol. Glos. Roy. Hosp. Specialty: Radiol. Prev: Sen. Regist. (Radiol.) Radcliffe Infirm. Oxf.; Vis. Asst. Prof. Radiol. Univ. Colorado Med. Center, Denver, USA; Sen. Lect. (Paediat. Radiol.) Univ. Manch.

WITCOMBE, Shirin (retired) 7 Longdown Lane N., Ewell, Epsom KT17 3HY Tel: 01372 815297 — MRCS Eng. LRCP Lond. 1949.

WITHAM, Elizabeth Alice (retired) 31 Egerton Road, Lymm WA13 0PA Tel: 01925 754707 — MB ChB Liverp. 1955. Prev: SHO (Med.) War Memor. Hosp. Scunthorpe.

WITHAM, Fiona Mary Queen Alexandra Hospital, Cosham, Portsmouth PO6 3LY Tel: 023 92 286030 Fax: 023 92 286895 Email: fiona.witham@porthosp.nhs.uk; 63 Lower Mead, Petersfield GU31 4NR — MB BS Lond. 1988; BSc Lond. 1985; MRCP (UK) 1991; FRCR 1994. Cons. Radiol. Qu. Alexandra Hosp. Portsmouth. Specialty: Radiol. Socs: BMA; BSSR; ESSR. Prev: Sen. Regist. (Radiol.) Soton. Univ. Hosp.; Regist. (Radiol.) Kings Coll. Hosp. Lond.; SHO (Diabetes, Endocrinol., Metab. Med. & Chest Med.) St. Thos. Hosp. Lond.

WITHANA, Kithsiri Amarananda Chase Farm Hospital NHS Trust, The Ridgeway, Enfield EN2 8JL Tel: 020 8967 5903; 27 Westpole Avenue, Cockfosters, Barnet EN4 0AX Tel: 020 8292 6873 — MB BS Ceylon 1962; DCH RCP Lond. 1971; MRCP (UK) 1973; DTCH Liverp. 1980; FRCP (L) 1996; FRCPCH 1997. Cons. Paediat. Chase Farm Hosps. Specialty: Paediat.

WITHECOMB, Julie Louise 25 Southdown Road, Brighton BN1 6FH — MB BS Lond. 1986.

WITHERINGTON, Elizabeth Mary Angela 190 Melton Road, Nottingham NG2 6FJ Tel: 01329 847015 — MB BChir Camb. 1986; MA Camb. 1986; DRCOG 1989; DGM RCP Lond. 1989; MRCGP 1990. Specialty: Care of the Elderly. Prev: GP Jubilee Surg. Titchfield Hants; Clin. Asst. (Geriat.) Qu. Alexandra Hosp. Portsmouth; Trainee GP Portsmouth VTS.

WITHEROW, Helen 98B Richmond Hill, Richmond TW10 6RJ — MB ChB Bristol 1993; BDS Birm. 1984.

WITHEROW, Mr Peter James (retired) Litfield House, 1 Litfield Place, Clifton, Bristol BS8 3LS Tel: 0117 973 1323 Fax: 0117 973 3303; 9 Cook's Folly Road, Sneyd Park, Bristol BS9 1PL Tel: 0117 968 2542 — MB ChB Birm. 1958; FRCS Eng. 1966. Prev: Cons. Orthop. Surg. Bristol Roy. Childr. Hosp., Southmead Hosp.

WITHEROW, Mr Ross O'Neill 16 Harmont House, 20 Harley St., London W1G 9PJ Tel: 020 7255 1623 Fax: 020 7323 3418 — MB BS Lond. 1968 (Univ. Coll. Hosp.) FRCS Eng. 1973; MS Lond. 1981; FEBU 1992. Cons. Urol. St. Mary's Hosp. Lond.; Sen. Clin. Lect. St. Mary's Hosp. Univ. Lond. Specialty: Urol. Socs: Fell. Roy. Soc. Med.; BAUS. Prev: Lect. & Hon. Sen. Regist. (Urol.) Lond. Hosp.; Resid. Surg. Off. St. Peters Hosps.; Postgrad. Research Fell. (Urol.) Univ. Calif. San Francisco, USA.

WITHERS, Andrew Walter James Grange Practice, Allerton Health Centre, Bell Dew Road, Bradford BD15 7NJ Tel: 01274 541696; 3 Kendal Avenue, Moorhead, Shipley BD18 4DU Email: andy-withers@compuserve.com — MB ChB Leeds 1982; DRCOG 1985; MRCGP 1986. Prev: Trainee GP Bradford VTS; Ho. Surg. Pinderfields Gen. Hosp. Wakefield; Ho. Phys. Bradford Roy. Infirm.

WITHERS, Anthony Francis Dennis Royal Crescent Surgery, 11 Royal Crescent, Cheltenham GL50 3DA Tel: 01242 580248 Fax: 01242 253618 — MB BChir Camb. 1965 (Camb. & Lond. Hosp.) MA Camb. 1968, MB BChir 1965.

WITHERS, Mr David Geoffrey (retired) The Sign of the Dolphin, Westerleigh, Bristol BS37 8QQ Tel: 01454 312122; (Surgery), Witney Mead, Frampton Cotterell, Bristol — MB ChB Bristol 1964; FRCS Ed. 1969; DObst RCOG 1970.

WITHERS, David James Warren Lodge, The Roundway, Rustington, Littlehampton BN16 2BW — MB BChir Camb. 1982.

WITHERS, Digby Paul The Health Centre, White Hart Close, Buntingford SG9 9DQ Tel: 01763 271362 Fax: 01763 272878; Woodstock, Hare St, Buntingford SG9 0EQ — MB BS Newc. 1972; BSc Newc. 1968; DTM Antwerp 1981; DRCOG 1985. Specialty: Gen. Pract. Socs: Fell. Roy. Soc. Med. Prev: SHO (Obst. & Paediat.) Leicester Gen. Hosp.; Med. Off. Hôpital de la CBFZ, Pimu, Zaïre; Ho. Phys. & Ho. Surg. Roy. Vict. Infirm. Newc.

WITHERS, Dominic John 15 Kersley Road, London N16 0NP — MB BS Lond. 1987.
WITHERS, Eleanor Jane Arbury Road Surgery, 114 Arbury Road, Cambridge CB4 2JG Tel: 01223 364433 Fax: 01223 315728 — MB BCh Wales 1985; DCH RCP Lond. 1989; MRCGP 1989; DRCOG 1991.
WITHERS, Keri Jane — MB BS Lond. 1987 (Roy. Free Hosp. Sch. Med.) DCH RCP Lond. 1990; MRCPsych 1994; DFFP 1997; DRCOG 1997; MRCGP 1998. GP Princip. Specialty: Gen. Pract. Prev: Sen. Regist. (Child & Adolesc. Psychiat.) Tavistock Clinic Hampstead; Regist. (Psychiat.) P. Henry Hosp. Sydney, Austral.; SHO (Paediat.) Chase Farm Hosp. Enfield.
WITHERS, Mark Richard 323 Brincliffe Edge Road, Sheffield S11 9DE — MB ChB Leic. 1988.
WITHERS, Michelle 42 Frensham Road, Crowthorne RG45 6QH — MB BS Lond. 1998.
WITHERS, Nicholas John Department of Respiratory Medicine, Royal Devon And Exeter Hospital, Barrack Rd, Exeter Ex2 5DW Tel: 01392 402827 Fax: 01392 402828 — MB BS Lond. 1988; MRCP (UK) 1991; DM Soton. 1998. Cons. Phys. with an interest in Respirat. Med., Roy. Devon And Exeter Hosp., Exeter. Specialty: Gen. Med. Prev: Sen. Registra, Respirat./Gen. Med., Bristol Hosp.
WITHERS, Peter Anthony 54 Churston Close, Westbury Park, Newcastle ST5 4LP — BM Soton. 1987; T(GP) 1993.
WITHERS, Richard Alan Yaxley Group Practice, Yaxley Health Centre, Landsdowne Road, Peterborough PE7 3JL Tel: 01733 240478 Fax: 01733 244645; Field Farm House, Bullock Road, Washingley, Peterborough PE7 3SJ Tel: 01733 244780 — MB BS Lond. 1983 (Univ. Coll. Hosp.) BSc Lond. 1978; DCH RCP Lond. 1986; DRCOG 1986; MRCGP 1988; AFOM RCP Lond. 1995. Force Med. Adviser Cambs. Constab. Specialty: Occupat. Health. Prev: Trainee GP P'boro. VTS; Ho. Surg. Northampton Gen. Hosp.; Ho. Phys. Whittingdon Hosp. Lond.
WITHERS, Ronald John Adams and Partners, The Health Centre, Tavanagh Avenue, Portadown, Craigavon BT62 3BU Tel: 028 3835 1393 — MB BCh BAO Belf. 1978; MRCGP 1982.
WITHERSPOON, Edward William (retired) 25 Potwell Gardens, The Hooks, Henfield BN5 9UY Tel: 01273 494979 Email: willeww00@aol.com — MB ChB Birm. 1949; FRSH 1970; DTM & H RCPS 1969; FFPM RCP (UK) 1990. Prev: Med. Dir. Warner Lambert/Pk.e Davis UK, Europe, Afr.
WITHERSPOON, Paul Flat 6 Kensington Court, 20 Kensington Road, Hyndland, Glasgow G12 9NP — MB ChB Glas. 1997.
WITHEY, John Sandford (retired) Lane End Farm, Hightown, Ringwood BH24 3DY Tel: 01425 472036 — MB BS Lond. 1955 (Char. Cross) DObst RCOG 1959.
WITHEY, Josephine Mary Heavitree Health Centre, South Lawn Terrace, Exeter EX1 2RX Tel: 01392 281100 Fax: 01392 281150 — MB BS Lond. 1977 (St Marys Hospital Medical School) DA 1980. Princip. Gen. Pract.,.
WITHINGTON, Brian Richard Hebburn Health Centre, Campbell Park Road, Hebburn NE31 2SP Tel: 0191 483 5533 Fax: 0191 428 1826 — MB BS Newcastle 1977; MB BS Newc. 1977. GP Hebburn, Tyne & Wear.
WITHINGTON, Brian Stephen Hull Royal Infirmary, Anlaby Road, Hull HU3 2JZ — MB BCh BAO Belf. 1989; FRCA. Cons. (Anaesth.) Hull Roy. Infirm. Anlaby Rd. Hull N. Humberside. Prev: SHO (Anaesth.) Princess Mary's RAF Hosp. Halton.
WITHINGTON, Peter Stuart Department of Anaesthetic and Intensive Care, The Royal London Hospital, Whitechapel, London E1 1BB Tel: 020 7377 7725 Fax: 020 7377 7126 Email: p.s.withington@qmul.ac.uk; 29 Meynell Road, Hackney, London E9 7AP Tel: 020 8533 4051 Fax: 020 8533 4051 Email: psw@hackney.u.net.com — MB BS Lond. 1979 (The London Hospital Medical College) FFA RCS Eng. 1983; FRCA Lond. 1984. Director of Intens. Care, The Roy. Lond. Hosp., Whitechapel, Lond.; Med. lead, N. E. Lond. Critical Care Network. Specialty: Anaesth. Special Interest: Critical Care. Socs: Assn. Anaesth.; Intens. Care Soc.
WITHNALL, David Mersea Road Surgery, 272a Mersea Road, Colchester CO2 8QY Tel: 01206 517 100 Fax: 01206 765667 — MB BS Lond. 1974 (St. Bart.) FRCGP 1997, M 1979. Prev: Trainee GP Colchester VTS; Ho. Phys. Connaught Hosp. Lond.; Hosp. Practitioner (Endoscopy) Colchester Gen. Hosp.
WITHNELL, Allan (retired) Compton Court, Compton Green, Redmarley, Gloucester GL19 3JB Tel: 01531 822330 — (Manch. & Leeds) MB ChB Manch. 1951. Prev: Area Med. Off. Glos. AHA.
WITHRINGTON, Robin Henry 45 The Street, Ash, Canterbury CT3 2EN Tel: 01304 812080 — MB BCh BAO Dub. 1973; BA Dub. 1971; MRCP (UK) 1978. Cons. (Rheum.) Canterbury & Thanet DHA. Specialty: Rheumatol. Prev: Sen. Regist. St. Marys Hosp. Lond. & Roy. Nat. Orthop. Hosp. Lond.
WITKIEWICZ, Tadeusz Stefan Department of Anaesthesia, Hairmyres & Stonehouse Hospitals NHS Trust, East Kilbride, Glasgow G75 8RG Tel: 0141 220292; 21 George Allan Place, Strathaven ML10 6EH Tel: 01357 521145 — Lekarz Warsaw 1978. Staff Grade Anaesth. Hairmyres & StoneHo. Hosps. NHS Trust E. Kilbride; Specialist Anaesth. (Poland) 1985. Specialty: Anaesth. Socs: Dip. Europ. Acad. Anaesthesiol. Prev: Staff Grade Anaesth. Law Hosp. Carluke.
WITNALL, Albert Peter (retired) Ysgubor Wen, Machynlleth SY20 8JA Tel: 01654 702228 — MB ChB Birm. 1961.
WITNEY, Raymond Lamprey (retired) 59 Northwood Road, Whitstable CT5 2HA Tel: 01227 272094 — MRCS Eng. LRCP Lond. 1938 (Camb. & St. Thos.) BA Camb. Prev: Temp. Capt. RAMC.
WITT, Jacqueline Middleton Blackthorn Medical Centre, St Andrews Road, Barming, Maidstone ME16 9AN Tel: 01622 726277 Fax: 01622 725774; Yard Cottage, Fant Farm, Maidstone ME16 8DE Tel: 01622 728008 — MB ChB Sheff. 1982; DRCOG 1986; MRCGP 1987. Prev: SHO (O & G) North. Gen. Hosp. Sheff.; SHO (Gen. Med.) Southport Gen. Infirm.
WITT, Mr Johan Delf The Middlesex Hospital, Department of Orthopaedics, Mortimer Street, London W1N 8AA Tel: 020 7380 9293 Email: johan.witt@uclh.org; 110 Sutherland Avenue, Maida Vale, London W9 2QP — MB BS Lond. 1983; FRCS Eng. 1987; FRCS (Orth.) 1992. Cons. Orthop. Surg. Univ. Coll. Lond. Hosps.; Clin. Director, Dept. of Orthop., Univ. Coll. Lond. Hosps. Specialty: Orthop. Socs: Fell. BOA; Brit. Hip Soc.; Brit. Orthopaedic Oncol. Soc. Prev: Sen. Regist. (Orthop. Surg.) King's Coll. Hosp. Lond.; Sen. Resid. Mass. Gen. Hosp., USA; Clin. Fell. Harvard Med. Sch., USA.
WITT, Judith Karen — MB ChB Liverp. 1998.
WITT, Margaret June 116 Harley Street, London W1G 7JL Tel: 020 7935 0588 Fax: 020 8505 2868; 21 The Albany, Sunset Avenue, Woodford Green IG8 0TJ Tel: 020 8505 8253 Fax: 020 8505 2868 — (St. Bart.) BSc (Physiol.) Lond. 1952; MB BS 1955; FRCS Eng. 1961; FRCOG 1979, M 1966. Cons. Obst. & Gyn. N. Middlx. Hosp. Lond.; Hon. Cons. Gyn. Endocrinol. St. Bart. Hosp. Lond.; Hon. Cons. St. Luke's Nursing Home for Clergy Lond.; Hon. Sen. Lect. St. Bart. Hosp. & Roy. Free Hosp.; Hon. Lect. City Univ. Specialty: Obst. & Gyn. Socs: Harv. Soc.; Med. Soc. Lond. Prev: Res. Surg. Off. Qu. Charlotte's Hosp. Lond. & Hosp. Wom. Soho Sq.; Regist. (Surg.) Peace Memor. Hosp. Watford; Sen. Regist. (Obst. & Gyn.) St. Bart. Hosp. Lond.
WITTE, Klaus Karl August 129 Port Road E., Barry CF63 9PX — MB BS Lond. 1994 (King's Coll.) MRCP (UK) 1997. Specialist Regist. (Cardiol.) Roy. Gwent Hosp. Newport. Specialty: Cardiol. Prev: SHO (Cardiol.) UHW NHS Trust Cardiff; SHO (Chest Med.) Llandough Hosp.
WITTEK, Mrs Irena Hanna 21 Streatham Close, Leigham Court Road, London SW16 2NQ — MB ChB Poland 1948; MB ChB Polish Sch. of Med. 1948; DCH Eng. 1953.
WITTELS, Peter Louis 6 Whitwick Moor, Thringstone, Coalville LE67 8NS — (Lond. Hosp.) MB BS Lond. 1970; MRCS Eng. LRCP Lond. 1970; MRCGP 1975. Non-Princip. Locum in GP & Med. Examr. in the Benefits Agency. Prev: SHO A & E Unit St. Leonard's Hosp. Lond.; Trainee GP Boston Lincs. VTS.
WITTMANN, Frederick William (retired) Burley, 22 The Chase, Reigate RH2 7DH Tel: 01737 762141 — MB ChB Glas. 1959; DA Eng. 1962; FFA RCS Eng. 1964. Cons. (Anaesth.) New E. Surrey Hosp. Prev: Regist. (Anaesth.) Redhill Gen. Hosp. & United Birm. Hosps.
WITTRAM, Conrad Magnolia, Old Shaw Lane, Shaw, Swindon SN5 5PH Tel: 01793 772751 Email: cwittram@partners.org — MB ChB Liverp. 1986; DMRD Liverp. 1991; FRCR 1993; FRANZCR 1998; American Board Radiol 1998; USMLE Step 1 & Step 2 1999; USMLE Step 3 2000. Asst. Prof. Thoracic Radiol. Mass. Gen. Hosp. / Harvard Med. Sch. Specialty: Radiol. Prev: Fell. (Thoracic

Radiolology) Univ. Toronto, Canda; Fell. (Clin. Radiol.) Univ. Alberta Hosp., Canada; Lect. (RadioDiag.) Univ. Liverp.

WITTS, Emma Jane 15 Beech Av, Chichester PO19 3DR — MB ChB Manch. 1997.

WITTS, Helena Maria The Three Swans Surgery, Rollestone Street, Salisbury SP1 1DX Tel: 01722 333548 Fax: 01722 503626 — MB BS Lond. 1991 (Char. Cross & Westm.) MRCGP 1996 (Distinc.); DRCOG 1993. Partner, GP Salisbury. Specialty: Gen. Pract. Socs: Wessex Fac. of Coll. of GPs Salisbury Med. Soc.; Salisbury LMC Represent. Wiltsh. LMC. Prev: SHO (Psychiat.) Old Manor Hosp. Salisbury; SHO (Paediat.) St. Mary's Hosp. Portsmouth; SHO (O & G) Princess Anne Hosp. Soton.

WITTS, Simon James Grovehurst Surgery, Grovehurst Road, Kemsley, Sittingbourne ME10 2ST Tel: 01795 430444 Fax: 01795 410539 — MB BS Lond. 1989; DTM & H Liverp. 1991; MRCGP 1995. Specialty: Trop. Med. Prev: Trainee GP Maidstone Hosp.; Resid. Med. Off. Hauyra Khassa Hosp. Cochabamba, Bolivia.

WLODARCZYK, Krzysztof Kazimierz King Street Surgery, King Street, Whalley, Blackburn BB7 9SL Tel: 01254 823273 Fax: 01254 824891; 34 Straits Lane, Read, Burnley BB12 7PQ Tel: 01282 770052 — MB ChB Manch. 1986 (Manchester) Cert. Family Plann. JCC 1988; DCH RCP Lond. 1988; MRCGP 1990; DRCOG 1990.

WOBER, Hilali Antony 18 Boathouse Reach, Henley-on-Thames RG9 1TJ Tel: 01491 578117 Fax: 01491 636271 Email: wm@doctors.org.uk — MB BS Lond. 1965 (St. Mary's) DRCOG 1969; DAvMed FOM RCP Lond. 1972; MFOM RCP Lond. 1981. Cons. Occupat. Phys.Univ Coll Lond. Chasefarm Hosp Enfield, CMO QBE Health; Dir. of WM Health Internat. Ltd. Specialty: Occupat. Health. Socs: Roy. Aeronaut Soc.; Aerospace Med. Assn. Prev: Med. Off. Roy. Air Force Med. Br.

WOBI, Bukar Diana, Princess of Wales Hospital, Grimsby DN33 2BA Tel: 01472 874111/01472 875595 Fax: 01472 875382 Email: bukar.wobi@nlg.nhs.uk; 2 Larchwood, Heatherwood, London Road, Ascot SL5 8AA Tel: 01334 27874 — MB BS Nigeria 1979 (Abu Zaria, Nigeria) MRCPCH; DTCH Liverp. 1985; MRCP (UK) 1991. Paediatric Cons., Diana, Princess of Wales Hosp., Grimsby. Specialty: Paediat. Special Interest: Infec. Diseases; Neprhology; Trop. Med. Socs: Roy. Coll. of Physicians of Eng. Prev: Regist. Heatherwood & Wexham Pk.; SHO (Paediat.) Chesterfield & N. Derbysh. Roy. Hosps.; SHO (Paediat.) Macclesfield.

WOFFENDEN, Laura Rachel Dodbrook House, Millbrook, Torpoint PL10 1AN — MB ChB Leeds 1998.

WOFFINDIN, Joyce Lowther Medical Centre, 1 Castle Meadows, Whitehaven CA28 7RG — MB ChB Dundee 1985; MRCGP 1990; Dip. Sports Med. Lond. 1990.

WOGU, Godwin Udo Ezechuku 41 Lynne Way, Northolt UB5 5UP — MB BCh BAO Dub. 1972.

WOHL, Miriam Ann 132 Victoria Park Road, Leicester LE2 1XD Tel: 0116 240 4243 Email: miriamwohl@hotmail.com; Reservoir View, Saddington, Leicester LE8 0QH Tel: 0116 240 4243 — MB ChB Glas. 1972 (Glas. Univ.) MSTAT; Cert. Family Plann. JCC 1981. Med. Off. BAMS Midl.; Medico-legal Expert; Mem. Disabil. Living Alswana Advis. Bd. Specialty: Rehabil. Med.; Rheumatol.; Alexander Technique. Socs: Soc. Of Teach. Of Alexander Technique. Prev: Med. Off. Brit. Red Cross Soc.; Med. Off. Pregn. & Gyn. Advis. Serv. Lond.; Med. Off. Pregn. Advis. Serv. Lond.

WOHL, Myer (retired) 86 Alexandra Park Road, London N10 2AD Tel: 020 8883 4800 — MRCS Eng. LRCP Lond. 1942 (St. Bart.)

WOJCIUK, Jerzy 35 Breck Road, Blackpool FY3 9DL — LRCP LRCS Ed. LRCPS Glas. 1997.

WOJNAROWSKA, Fenella Theta Department of Dermatology, Churchill Hospital, Old Road, Headington, Oxford OX3 7LJ — BM BCh Oxf. 1973 (St. Mary's) MA Oxf. 1972, MSc 1971, BM BCh 1973; FRCP Lond. 1993; DM Oxf. 1995. Prof. Of Dermat. & Cons. Dermatol. Oxf. Radcliffe Hosp. Oxf.; Cons. Dermatologist, Oxford Radcliffe Hosp.s, NHS Trust. Specialty: Dermat. Socs: Royal Soc. Med.; Royal Coll. Physicians; Brit. Assoc. Dermatology. Prev: Reader Dermat. Univ. Oxf.; Regist. (Dermat.) St. Mary's Hosp. Lond.; Sen. Clin. Lect. (Dermat.) Univ. Oxf.

WOJTULEWSKI, Jan Andrzej 16 Cranborne Avenue, Eastbourne BN20 7TS — MB BS Lond. 1963 (Westm.) MRCS Eng. LRCP Lond. 1963; MRCP (U.K.) 1971; FRCP Lond. 1987. Cons. Rheum. Eastbourne Health Dist. Specialty: Rheumatol. Prev: Sen. Regist. Westm. Hosp. Lond.; Med. Regist. Roy. Masonic Hosp. Lond.; Res. Med. Off. Amer. Hosp. Paris.

WOKO, Ellis Chinatu 77 Burnley Road, London NW10 1EE — MB BS Lond. 1996.

WOKO, Mr Samuel Chinatu The Surgery, 77 Burnley Road, London NW10 1EE Tel: 020 8452 7689 — MB BCh BAO Dub. 1960; FRCS Ed. 1969.

WOLANCZYK, Witold Jozef (retired) Eldene Health Centre, Eldene, Swindon SN3 3RZ — MB BCh BAO NUI 1955. Prev: Ho. Off. Roy. Matern. Hosp. Belf. & Roy. Belf. Hosp. Sick Childr.

WOLDMAN, Simon Jack 23 Poplar Avenue, Glasgow G77 5QZ; 53 Grampian Gardens, Dyce, Aberdeen AB21 7LF — MB ChB Glas. 1989; MRCP 1993. Specialist Regist. Cardiol. West. Scot. Rotat.

WOLF, Professor Andrew Robert West Hay Cottage, West Hay Road, Wrington, Bristol BS40 5NR Tel: 0117 928 2163 Email: andrew.r.wolf@bris.ac.uk — MB BChir Camb. 1980; FFA RCS Eng. 1985. Prof. of Anaesth. & Critical Care; Cons. (Paediat. Cardiac Anaesth. & Paediat. Intens. Care). Specialty: Anaesth. Special Interest: Paediatric Cardiac Anaesth.; Paediatric Intens. Care.

WOLF, Anton Lilac Cottage, 147 Waddicar Lane, Melling, Liverpool L31 1DS Tel: 0151 546 3377 — LRCP LRCS Ed. 1955; LRCP LRCS Ed. LRFPS Glas. 1955. Prev: Ho. Phys. Mill La. Hosp. Wallasey & Vict. Centr. Hosp. Wallasey; Sen. Ho. Off. O & G Gen. Hosp. Ashton-under-Lyne.

WOLF, Mr Bernhard Raigmore Hospital, Old Perth Road, Inverness IV2 3yw Tel: 01463 706127 Fax: 01463 704544 Email: bwolf@doctors.org.uk — State Exam Med Erlangen 1990 (Erlangen, Germany) FRCS Ed. 1995; Intercollegiate Exam 2001. Cons. Surg. (Gen. & Vasc. Surg.). Specialty: Gen. Surg. Special Interest: Vasc. Surg. Socs: Vasc. Surgic. Soc. of GB & Irel.; Europ. Soc. for Vasc. Surg.; BMA.

WOLF, Paulus A 10 Hayden Walk, Oadby, Leicester LE2 4TL — Artsexamen Maasricht 1988; Artsexamen Maastricht 1988.

WOLF, Rebecca Cassandra — MB ChB Sheff. 1997.

WOLFE, Carey Spencer Vine Surgery, Hindhayes Lane, Street BA16 0ET Tel: 01458 841122 Fax: 01458 840044; Welham Rise, Charlton Mackrell, Somerton TA11 7AJ — MB BChir Camb. 1981 (St. Thos.) MRCP (UK) 1984; DRCOG 1989. GP Practitioner Princip.; GP Orthopaedic Specialist Meridip PCT. Specialty: Gen. Pract.; Orthop. Socs: Brit. Soc. Rheum.; Roy. Coll. Phys.; Brit. Assn. for Sport in Med. Prev: Regist. (Med.) Soton. HA; Regist. (Rheum.) St. Thos. Hosp. Lond.

WOLFE, Charles David Alexander Division of Public Health Sciences, GRT School of Medicine Guy's Campus, London SE1 3QD Tel: 020 7955 5000 Fax: 020 7403 4602 Email: charles.wolfe@kcl.ac.uk; 48 West Square, London SE11 4SP — MB BS Lond. 1978 (Roy. Free Medical and Dental School London) MRCS Eng. LRCP Lond. 1978; FRCOG 1988; MD Lond. 1990; FFPHM RCP (UK) 1996. Reader (Pub. Health Med.) Guy's, King's & St Thomas' Sch. of Med. Lond.; Dir. Of Research and Developm., Guy's & St Thomas Hosp. Specialty: Pub. Health Med.

WOLFE, Ingrid Johanna Flat 7, 19 Frognal, London NW3 6AR — MB BS Lond. 1997.

WOLFE, James Godiva Cottage, Evesham Road, Salford Priors, Evesham WR11 8UU — MB ChB Liverp. 1996.

WOLFE, Jason — MB BS Lond. 1993; MRCS Roy. Coll. of Surgeons of Eng. (London) 1999. Sen. Ship's Phys., Carnival Cruise Lines; SHO (Intens. Care) Lewisham Hosp.; SHO (Anaesthetics) Southend Hosp. Specialty: Gen. Surg.; Trauma & Orthop. Surg.; Plastic Surg.; Accid. & Emerg. Socs: BAEM. Prev: LAS Accid. & Emerg. Med., Soton. Hosp.; SHO (Plastic Surg.) St Andrew Unit Chelmsford; SHO Rotat. (Surg.) Hammersmith Hosp. Lond.

WOLFE, Mr John Henry Nicholas 66 Harley Street, London W1G 7HD Tel: 020 7580 5030 Fax: 020 7631 5341 Email: jwolfe@uk-consultants.co.uk — MB BS Lond. 1971 (St. Thos.) FRCS Eng. 1975; MS Lond. 1981. Cons. Surg. St. Mary's Hosp. Lond.; Hon. Sen. Lect. Roy. Postgrad. Med. Sch. Hammersmith; Hon. Cons. (Surg.) Roy. Brompton Hosp.; Cons. Surg. Edwd. VII Hosp. for Off. Lond.; Mem. Edit. Bd. Europ. Jl. Vasc. Surg.; Vice Pres. Vase Div. UEMS. Socs: (Counc.) Vasc. Soc. GB & Irel. (Chairm. Vasc. Advis. Comm.); (Counc.) Assoc. Surg. GB & Irel.; Hon. Corr. Mem. Soc. Vascula Surg. USA. Prev: Sen. Regist. (Surg.) St. Thos. Hosp. Lond.; Research Fell. Harvard Med. Sch. Boston, USA; SHO St. Jas. Hosp. Balham.

WOLFE, Rev. Kenneth Wesley (retired) 40 Greenfield Avenue, Spinney Hill, Northampton NN3 2AF Tel: 01604 406369 — MB BCh BAO Belf. 1942. Prev: Cas. Off. Radcliffe Infirm. Oxf.

WOLFE, Martin James The Medical Specialist Group, PO Box 113, Alexandra House, Les Frieteaux, St Martin's, Guernsey GY1 3EX — MB BS Lond. 1973 (Middlx.) FFA RCS Eng. 1978. Specialty: Anaesth. Prev: Cons. Anaesth. N. Derbysh. HA & Rampton Hosp. Notts.; Cons. Anaesth. Bassetlaw HA.

WOLFE, Ronald Rutland Place Surgery, 21 Rutland Place, Glasgow G51 1TA Tel: 0141 427 3121 Fax: 0141 427 7600 — MB ChB Ed. 1977.

WOLFE, Samantha Sarah Braeside, Main St., Thornton le Moor, Northallerton DL7 9EA — MB ChB Leic. 1997.

WOLFENDALE, Katherine Dilys 115 Station Road, Marple, Stockport SK6 6PA — BM BS Nottm. 1997.

WOLFENDALE, Margaret Rose 19 Lower Way, Great Brickhill, Milton Keynes MK17 9AG Tel: 01525 261647 — MB BS Lond. 1956 (Roy. Free) MRCS Eng. LRCP Lond. 1955; MD Lond. 1980. Prev: Cons. Cytopath. Stoke Mandeville Hosp. Aylesbury.

WOLFENDALE, Richard Ellis (retired) 42 Grafton Street, Cambridge CB1 1DS Tel: 01223 464287 — MB BChir Camb. 1952; MRCS Eng. LRCP Lond. 1952. Prev: Ho. Surg. Manch. Roy. Infirm.

WOLFENDEN, Brian Anthony (retired) Field End, 2 Manor Farm Cottages, Marsworth, Tring HP23 4LN Tel: 01296 661698 — MB ChB Manch. 1949; MRCGP.

WOLFF, Anna Layla — MB ChB Manch. 1987 (Manchester) Specialty: Gen. Pract.

WOLFF, Anthony Herbert 26 Quernmore Road, London N4 4QX Tel: 020 8340 9510 — MB BS Lond. 1980 (Univ. Coll. Hosp.) BSc Lond. 1977, MB BS 1980; MRCP (UK) 1985; FCAnaesth. 1989. Sen. Regist. (Anaesth.) Roy. Free Hosp. Lond. Prev: SHO (Gen. Med.) Lond. Hosp.; Lect. (Physiol.) Lond. Hosp. Med. Coll.; Regist. (Gen. Med.) Lond. Hosp.

WOLFF, Antonia The Children's Centre, City Hospital Campus, Hucknall Road, Nottingham NG5 1PB Tel: 0115 962 7658 — BSc Lond. 1978, MB BS 1981; DCH RCP Lond. 1983; MRCP (UK) 1987. Cons. Community Paediat. Child & Family Centre Birm. Specialty: Paediat.

WOLFF, Christopher Bancroft 52 Victoria Park, Cambridge CB4 3EL Fax: 01462 742893 — MB ChB Sheff. 1962 (Univ. Sheff.) MRCP Lond. 1969; PhD Lond. 1975; FRCP 1998. Hon. Cons. Clin. Physiol. Guy's Hosp. Lond./Cons. St. Thomas's Hosp, Sherrington Sch.; Hon. Clin. Research Fell. Clin. Phys. Balts & the Lond. Specialty: Respirat. Med.; Intens. Care; Cardiol. Socs: Physiol. Soc.; Med. Res. Soc.; Int. Soc. For Oxygen transport to tissues. Prev: Clin. Research Fell. Kings Coll. Hosp. Lond.

WOLFF, Elizabeth Patricia Fay Bridge Lane Health Centre, 20 Bridge Lane, Battersea, London SW11 3AD Tel: 020 7585 1499 Fax: 020 7978 4707 — MB ChB Sheff. 1993; DRCOG 1995; MRCGP 1998. GP Battersea Lond.; Clin. Asst. Genito-Urin. Med. Specialty: Gen. Pract.

WOLFF, Geoffrey Simon MRC Social, Genetic & Develop. Psychiatry Research Centre, Institute of Psychiatry (Social Psychiatry Section), De Crespegny Park, London SE5 8AF — MB ChB Manch. 1985; BSc (Hons) (Anat.) Manch. 1982; MRCPsych 1990; MD Manch. 1995; DCBT 1997. Sen. Regist. Gen. Adult Psychiat. (Eating Disorders Unit) Bethlem & Maudsley (NHS) Trust Lond.; Attached worker, MRC Social, Genetic & Developm. Psychiat. Research Centre (Social Psychiat. Sect.), Inst. of Psychiat. Lond. Specialty: Gen. Psychiat. Socs: MRCPsych. Prev: Clin. Scientist, MRC Social, Genetic & Developm. Psychiat. Research Centre; +Inst. Psychiat. Lond.; Hon. Sen. Regist. Maudsley & Bethlem (NHS) Trust Lond.

WOLFF, Isidor (retired) Flat 7, The Apartments, Milverton Road, Whitecraigs, Glasgow G46 7JT Tel: 0141 6381512 — LRCP LRCS Ed. LRFPS Glas. 1942 (Anderson & St. Mungo's Colls. Glas.)

WOLFF, Linda Elisabet Bonnybridge Hospital, Falkirk Road, Bonnybridge FK4 1BD Tel: 01324 814685 Fax: 01324 815652; 19 Castle Road, Dollar FK14 7BE — MB ChB Ed. 1982; DRCOG 1985; MRCPsych 1987. Cons. Psychiat. (Old Age Psychiat.).

WOLFF, Professor Otto Herbert, CBE (retired) 53 Danbury Street, London N1 8LE Tel: 020 7226 0748 — MB BChir Camb. 1943 (Univ. Coll. Hosp.) MRCS Eng. LRCP Lond. 1943; FRCP Lond. 1962, M 1948; DCH Eng. 1949; MD Camb. 1954; BM BS FRCPCH (Honorary) 1996. Emerit. Prof. Child Health & Dean Inst. Child Health Lond. Prev: Cons. Phys. Hosp. Sick Childr. Gt. Ormond St. Lond.

WOLFF, Sulammith (retired) 38 Blacket Place, Edinburgh EH9 1RL Tel: 0131 667 7811 Fax: 0131 662 0337 Email: h.walton@ed.ac.uk — (Oxf.) BM BCh Oxf. 1947; DCH Eng. 1949; MA Oxf. 1950; FRCP Lond. 1972, M 1951; DPM Lond. 1958; FRCPsych 1972. Prev: Cons. Child. Psychiat. Roy. Hosp. Sick Childr. Edin.

WOLFF-MACDONALD, Elisabeth Marie 3 Dawson Place, London W2 4TD — MD Amiens 1983.

WOLFLE, Andrew Donald The Nook Surgery, Withyham Road, Groombridge, Tunbridge Wells TN3 9QP Tel: 01892 863326 Fax: 01892 863985 — MB BS Lond. 1988; MRCGP 1993; DRCOG 1993. Partnership - Wolfle & Barnaby, Br. Surg., Hartfield. Prev: Trainee GP Roy. Tunbridge Wells VTS; Ho. Phys. Guys Hosp.; Ho. Surg. Greenwich Dist. Hosp.

WOLFMAN, Leonard Charles Underlea Stables, North Sudley Road, Mossley Hill, Liverpool L17 6BT — MB ChB Liverp. 1947. Hon. Capt. RAMC; Hosp. Pract. Psychiat. Liverp. Drug Dependency Clinic. Socs: Liverp. Med. Inst.

WOLFMAN, Michael John Longrove Surgery, 70 Union Street, Barnet EN5 4HT Tel: 020 8441 9440/9563 Fax: 020 8441 4037; 9 Park Road, New Barnet, Barnet EN4 9QA — MB ChB Liverp. 1982; Cert. Family Plann. JCC 1988; DRCOG 1988. Clin. Asst. (A & E) Barnet Gen. Hosp.; Clin. Asst. Lond. Hospice; Club Doctor Barnet FC; Vice-Chairm. Williams Foundat.; Mem. Idiopathic Infantile Hypercalcaemia Foundat. (Mem. Med. Comm.). Specialty: Gen. Psychiat.

WOLFMAN, Stuart Samuel Underlea Stables, North Sudley Road, Mossley Hill, Liverpool L17 6BT — MB ChB Liverp. 1978; MRCP (UK) 1981.

WOLFSON, Martin Stephen Claremont Medical Centre, 2A Glenbuck Road, Surbiton KT6 6BS Tel: 020 8399 2280 Fax: 020 8390 0371; 11 St Leonards Road, Surbiton KT6 4DE Tel: 020 8399 7484 — MB BS Lond. 1974 (Westm.) BSc Lond. 1971, MB BS 1974; MRCP (UK) 1977; DRCOG 1981; MRCGP 1982. Occupat. Health Cons. St. Anthonys Hosp. Prev: Regist. (Med.) Guy's Hosp. Lond.; SHO (O & G) Dulwich Hosp. Lond.; SHO (Med.) St. Thomas Hosp. Lond.

WOLFSON, Richard, KStJ, Capt. RAMC Retd. (retired) 7 Eglinton Drive, Giffnock, Glasgow G46 7NQ Tel: 0141 638 4220 Fax: 0141 638 4222 Email: dick@jenniwolfson.fsnet.co.uk — LRCP LRCS Ed. LRFPS Glas. 1947 (Glasgow) BCH Ed. 1960; DA Eng. 1963. Anaesth. StoneHo. Hosp. Prev: Clin. Asst. (Anaesth.) Edin. Roy. Infirm.

WOLINSKI, Alexander Peter X-Ray Department, Russells Hall Hospital, Dudley Tel: 01384 456111; Gorse Green Cottage, Gorse Green Lane, Belbroughton, Stourbridge DY9 9UH Tel: 01562 730939 — MB ChB Birm. 1978; FRCR 1984. Cons. Radiol. Dudley Hosps. Specialty: Radiol. Socs: Brit. Inst. Radiol.; Brit. Soc. Interven.al Radiol. Prev: Sen. Regist. (Radiol.) Plymouth Gen. Hosp. & Bristol Roy. Infirm.; Regist. (Radiol.) Bristol Roy. Infirm.

WOLKIND, Stephen Nathaniel Flat 2, Helmsley, 7 Cleveland Road, London E18 2AY — MB BS Lond. 1962 (Middx.) DPM Eng. 1966; MD Lond. 1972; FRCPsych 1979, M 1973. Specialty: Child & Adolesc. Psychiat. Prev: Sen. Lect. (Clin. Psychiat.) Lond. Hosp. Med. Coll.; Sen. Regist. (Psychiat.) Lond. Hosp.; Regist. (Psychiat.) United Camb. Hosps.

WOLL, Professor Penella Jane Weston Park Hospital, Cancer Research Centre, Whitham Road, Sheffield S10 2SJ Tel: 0114 226 5235 Fax: 0114 226 5678 — MB BS Newc. 1980; BMedSci (Hons.) Newc. 1977; PhD Lond. 1990; FRCP 1998. Prof. (Med. Oncol.) Univ. Sheff. & Cons. Med. Oncol. Sheff. Teachng. Hosps. Specialty: Oncol. Socs: Assn. Cancer Phys. (Sec.). Prev: Reader (Clin. Oncol.) Univ. Nottm. & Hon. Cons. (Med. Oncol.) City Hosp. Nottm.; Lect. (Med. Oncol.) Univ. Manch. & Christie Hosp.; Clin. Research Fell. Imperial Cancer Research Fund & Guys Hosp. Lond.

WOLLASTON, John Francis The Tower, Elsdon, Newcastle upon Tyne NE19 1AA Tel: 01830 520179 Fax: 01830 520904 — MB BS Newc. 1969 (Newcastle Upon Tyne) DIH Soc. Apoth. Lond. 1978; MFOM RCP Lond. 1997, A 1980. Cons. Occupat. Phys. Indust. & Organisational Health. Specialty: Occupat. Health. Socs: Soc. of Occup. Med.; Roy. Soc. Of Med. Prev: Managing Dir. & Princip. Med. Advisor AMARC Occupat. Health & Safety Serv.; Chief Med.

Off. & Dir. Occupat. Health & Safety Servs. Brit. Ship Builders; Med. Off. RN.

WOLLASTON, Oenone Hilda (retired) The Staithe, 38 Cross Lane, Mossley, Congleton CW12 3JX Tel: 01260 271318 Email: oenonew@tinyworld.co.uk — MB BS Lond. 1958 (Lond. Hosp.) Cert. Family Plann. JCC 1960; MRCGP 1975. GP Amea Health Auth.; GP Stoke-on-Trent; Family Plann. Prev: Child Med. Off. AHA.

WOLLASTON, Sarah Chagford Health Centre, Chagford, Newton Abbot TQ13 8BW Tel: 01647 433320 Fax: 01647 432452 — MB BS Lond. 1986 (UMDS (Guys)) BSc (Path.) Lond. 1983; DRCOG 1991; MRCGP 1992. p/t Princip. in Gen. Pract.; GP Trainer. Prev: Trainee GP Bristol.

WOLLASTON, Sophie Leonora River Place Group Practice, River Place, Essex Road, London N1 2DE Tel: 020 7530 2100 Fax: 020 7530 2102 — MB BS Lond. 1988; BSc Lond. 1985; DCH 1991; DRCOG 1992; MRCGP 1994. Specialty: Gen. Pract.

WOLLNER, Leo (retired) 16 Blenheim Drive, Oxford OX2 8DG Tel: 01865 557109 — MB BS Lond. 1951 (Guy's) MRCS Eng. LRCP Lond. 1951; FRCP Lond. 1974, M 1957. Hon. Cons. Phys. Oxf. HA (T). Prev: Cons. Phys. (Gen. & Geriat. Med.) John Radcliffe Hosp. & Radcliffe Infirm. Oxf.

WOLLNER, Sylvia Helen (retired) 16 Blenheim Drive, Oxford OX2 8DG Tel: 01865 557109 — MB BS Lond. 1952 (Roy. Free) Prev: Assoc. Specialist (Geriat. Med.) Radcliffe Infirm. Oxf.

WOLMAN, Basil (retired) 29 Ashfield Lodge, Palatine Road, Didsbury, Manchester M20 2UD Tel: 0161 445 3500 — (Manch.) MB ChB Manch. 1941; MRCS Eng. LRCP Lond. 1942; FRCP Lond. 1972, M 1944; DCH Eng. 1947; MD Manch. 1951; FRCPCH 1997. Prev: Sub Dean Postgrad. (Med. Educat.) Univ. Manch.

WOLMAN, David (retired) 48 Hall Road E., Liverpool L23 8TU — MB ChB Manch. 1950; MRCGP 1965. Prev: SHO (Phys.) Roy. Albert Edwd. Infirm. Wigan.

WOLMAN, Richard Ian 1/3 Wilton Cresent, London SW1X 8RN Tel: 020 7235 1711 Fax: 020 7235 1681 — MB ChB Cape Town 1981 (Cape Town and St. Georges Tooting) Inceptor Roy. coll. Psychiat.; DPM (S. Afr.) Cape Town 1981. Private Cons. Med. Psychotherapist. Specialty: Gen. Psychiat.; Psychother.; Gen. Med. Socs: BMA.

WOLMAN, Roger Louis Royal National Orthopaedic Hospital, Brockley Hill, Stanmore HA7 4LP Tel: 020 8954 2300 — MB ChB Manch. 1981; MRCP (UK) 1984; MD Manch. 1990; FRCP (UK) 1998. Cons. Sports Med. & Rheum. Roy. Nat. Orthop. Hosp. Lond.; Cons. Brit. Olympic Med. Centre. Specialty: Rheumatol.; Sports Med. Socs: BSR; BIMM; BASEM. Prev: Sen. Regist. (Rheum. & Rehabil.) Roy. Nat. Orthop. Hosp. Lond.; Regist. Brit. Olympic Med. Centre Northwick Pk. Hosp. Middlx.; Regist. (Gen. Med. & Rheum.) Middlx. Hosp. Lond.

WOLPE, Alexander Paul Gudgeheath Lane Surgery, 187 Gudgeheath Lane, Fareham PO15 6QA Tel: 01329 280887 Fax: 01329 231321 — MB ChB Birm. 1982; DRCOG 1985; MRCGP 1987.

WOLSEY, Lotte Andrea Frolund 5 Coventry Road, Newton Hall, Durham DH1 5XD Tel: 0191 386 1610 — MB ChB Sheff. 1995 (Sheffield) DCH 1998; DRCOG 1998; DFFP 1999; MRCGP (Distinc.) 1999. Specialty: Gen. Pract. Socs: Med. Defence Union; BMA. Prev: SHO (Obstretics & Gyn.) Centr. Middlx. Hosp.

WOLSLEY, Karen 8 Belmont Park, Belfast BT4 3DU — MB BCh BAO Belf. 1992.

WOLSTENCROFT, Philip John, Surg. Lt. RN 36 Smithy Croft, Houghton, Carlisle CA3 0NS Tel: 01228 28098 — MB ChB Birm. 1989. Squadron Med. Off. RN. Prev: Ho. Phys. RNH Haslar; Ho. Surg. Birm. Accid. Hosp.

WOLSTENCROFT, Rachel Frances Cober View, Old Hill, Helston TR13 8HT Tel: 01326 565766 — MB ChB Manch. 1997. Specialty: Gen. Med.

WOLSTENHOLME, Allan Grant (retired) Airlie Cottage, Mayfield TN20 Tel: 01435 3169 — LMSSA Lond. 1944 (Guy's) Prev: Med. Regist. Hellingly Hosp. Hailsham.

WOLSTENHOLME, James Henry 18 Scammerton, Wilnecote, Tamworth B77 4LA — MB ChB Birm. 1996.

WOLSTENHOLME, Roger James Royal Albert Edward Infirmary, Wigan WN1 2NN Tel: 01942 822979/01942 822980 — MB BS Lond. 1974 (Westm.) BSc (Hons.) (Pharmacol.) Lond. 1971; MRCS Eng. LRCP Lond. 1974; MRCP (UK) 1978; DTM & H Eng. 1979; FRCP Ed. 1985; Dip. Sports Med. Scotl. 1993; FRCP Lond. 1994. Cons. Phys. Roy. Albert Edwd. Infirm. Wigan. Specialty: Gen. Med.; Respirat. Med. Special Interest: Respiritory. Socs: Brit. Thorac. Soc.; Brit. Soc. Clin. Allergy & Immunol.; Brit. Assn. Sport & Med. Prev: Assoc. Prof. Aga Khan Univ. Hosp. Karachi, Pakistan; Lect. (Respirat. Dis.) Univ. Edin.; Med. Off. (Min. Overseas Developm.) Maldive Is.s.

WOLSTENHOLME, Virginia 45 St Lukes Avenue, London SW4 7LG — BM Soton. 1993.

WOLTON, Ann Dorothy Maple Cottage, Water Lane, Somerton TA11 6RG — MB ChB Sheff. 1986.

WOLVERSON, Keith 33 Hobby Close, East Hunsby, Northampton NN4 0RN — MB BS Lond. 1996.

WOLVERSON, Mr Richard Lane City Hospital, Birmingham B18 7QH Tel: 0121 554 3801 Ext: 4749 Email: richard.wolverson@swbh.nhs.uk — MB BS Lond. 1974; MS Lond. 1986, MB BS 1974, BDS 1970; FRCS Eng. 1978. Cons. Gen. Surg. City Hosp. Birm.; Clin. Sen. Lect. Univ. Birm. Med. Sch.; Surg. Examr. Roy. Coll. of Surgeons of Eng. Specialty: Gastroenterol.; Paediat. Surg. Special Interest: Gen. & colo- rectal Surg. Socs: Fell. Assn. Surgs. Prev: Arris & Gale Lect. RCS Eng; Cons. Gen. Surg. Dudley Rd. Hosp. Birm.; Sheldon Clin. Research Fell. Dudley Rd. Hosp. Birm.

WOMACK, Christopher Department of Pathology, Peterborough District Hospital, Thorpe Road, Peterborough PE3 6DA Tel: 01733 874648 Fax: 01733 874791 Email: chris.womack@pbh-tr.nhs.uk — MB BS Lond. 1978; FRCPath 1996, M 1984; T(Path) 1991. Cons. Path. P'boro. Dist. Hosp. Specialty: Histopath.; Pathology, General. Socs: Assn. Clin. Paths.; Brit. Soc. Clin. Cytol.; Internat. Acad. Path. Prev: Sen. Regist. (Histopath.) Univ. & City Hosp. Nottm.; Regist. (Histopath.) St. Mary's Hosp. Manch.; SHO (Path.) Manch. Roy. Infirm.

WOMACK, Mr Nigel Richard Pinderfields Hospital, Aberford Road, Wakefield WF1 4DG; Kingswood House, 3 The Drive, Adel, Leeds LS16 6BG Tel: 0113 261 3198 — MB BS Lond. 1978 (Guy's) BSc (Hons.) Lond. 1975; MRCS Eng. LRCP Lond. 1978; FRCS Eng. 1981; MS Lond. 1988. Cons. Gen. Surg. Pinderfields Hosp. Wakefield. Specialty: Gen. Surg. Prev: Sen. Regist. (Surg.) Leeds; Lect. (Surg.) Lond. Hosp.; MRC Research Fell. Leeds Gen. Infirm.

WOMERSLEY, Adrienne Margaret Elizabeth (retired) Barns Close House, Amberley, Stroud GL5 5AG Tel: 01453 874100 Fax: 01453 874104 — MB BCh BAO Belf. 1979 (Queen's Belfast)

WOMERSLEY, Barbara Jean 37 Shakespeare Road, Acton, London W3 6SF — MB BS Lond. 1956 (St. Bart.) BSc (Physiol.) Lond. 1953, MB BS 1956.

WOMERSLEY, Deborah Susan 8 School Road, Himley, Dudley DY3 4LG — BM BS Nottm. 1988.

WOMERSLEY, Hester Clare Kohinur, Old Mill Road, Chelston, Torquay TQ2 6HW Tel: 01803 605508 — MB ChB Manch. 1991; BSc (Med. Sci.) 1st cl. Hons. Physiol. St. And. Univ. 1988; MRCPsych, June 1998. Specialist Regist. in Old Age Psychiat. Shelton Hosp. Specialty: Gen. Psychiat.; Geriat. Psychiat. Prev: Regist. (Gen. Psychiat.) WhitCh. Hosp. Cardiff; SHO (Old Age Psychiat.) Chorley Dist. Gen. Hosp.; SHO (Gen. Psychiat.) Roy. Oldham Hosp.

WOMERSLEY, John Greater Glasgow Health Board, 350 St Vincent St., Glasgow G3 8YU Tel: 0141 201 4815 Fax: 0141 201 4733; 22 Lochend Road, Bearsden, Glasgow G61 1DX Tel: 0141 942 7149 Email: john@womet.freeserve.co.uk — MB ChB Glas. 1966; PhD Glas. 1974, BSc 1963; DPH Glas. 1976; FFCM 1985, M 1977; FRCPS Glas. 1991. Cons. Pub. Health Med. Gtr. Glas. HB; Hon. Clin. Lect. Pub. Health Glas. Univ. Specialty: Pub. Health Med. Socs: BMA. Prev: SCM Gtr. Glas. HB & Lanarksh. HB; Lect. (Physiol.) Univ. Glas.

WOMERSLEY, John Samuel Bassett St Brannocks Road Medical Centre, St. Brannocks Road, Ilfracombe EX34 8EG Tel: 01271 863840 — MB BCh BAO Belf. 1981; MRCGP 1986.

WONG, Alexander Kai Ming 5 Bournbrook Road, Selly Oak, Birmingham B29 7BL — MB ChB Birm. 1994.

WONG, Alice Khin Mar Win 70 Norwood Road, Southall UB2 4EY; 162 Shakespear Avenue, Hayes UB4 0BP — MB BS Rangoon 1970; MB BS Rangoon, Burma 1970; DRCOG 1979.

WONG, Alison Po Ling Falmouth Road Surgery, 78 Falmouth Road, London SE1 4JW Tel: 020 7407 4101/0945 Fax: 020 7357 6170 — MB BS Lond. 1990; DRCOG 1993; MRCGP 1994.

WONG, Andrew No. 9, Andrew St., Liverpool L4 4DS Tel: 01510284 7850 — MB BS Singapore 1987 (Nat. Univ. Singapore) M Med (Anaesth.) 1996; FRCA 1997. Specialist Regist. (Anaesth.).

WONG, Aric Shiu-Quan Castle House, Castle Road, Horsell, Woking GU21 4ET — MB BS Lond. 1984; MRCGP 1989. Trainee GP Horsley VTS.

WONG, Cheong Yee The Surgery, 105 Carslake Road, London SW15 3DD Tel: 020 8785 6440 Fax: 020 8788 2063 — (Univ. Coll. Hosp.) MB BS Lond. 1969; DCH Eng. 1971; DObst RCOG 1972. Prev: SHO (Paediat.) N. Middlx. Hosp. Edmonton; SHO (O & G) Princess Alexandra Hosp. Harlow; SHO (Anaesth.) King Edwd. Memor. Hosp. Ealing.

WONG, Chi Chown 16 Russell Court, Cambridge CB2 1HW — BChir Camb. 1996.

WONG, Mr Chi Ho Department of Cardiothoracic Surgery, University Hospital Birmingham, Queen Elizabeth Medical Centre, Edgbaston, Birmingham B15 2TH Tel: 07050 609664 Fax: 0121 627 2542 Email: c.h.wong@bham.ac.uk; 116 Preston Road, Standish, Wigan WN6 0HY Tel: 01257 400919 Fax: 0121 627 2542 — MB BChir Camb. 1992 (Univ. Camb.) MA Camb. 1992, BA 1989; FRCS Ed. 1996; FRCS Eng. 1996. Regist., Dept. of Cardiothoracic, Univ. Hosp., Birm.; RCS Eng. Research Fellowship; Fell. MRC Cyclotron Unit, Hammersmith Hosp. Lond. Specialty: Cardiothoracic Surg. Socs: Fell. Roy. Soc. Med. Mem. Heart Surg. Forum; Fell. Soc. Cardiothoracic Surgs. GB & Irel.; Heart Surg. Forum. Prev: SHO Regional Spinal Unit, Roy. Orthop. Hosp.; Research Fell. (Surg.) Dept. of Cardiothoracic Surg. Univ. Birm.; SHO Rotat. (Surg.) Univ. Birm. Hosp. Trust.

WONG, Chi-Hung 28 Ferndale View, Doncaster DN5 8HG — MB ChB Sheff. 1990.

WONG, Chi Kuen Oxford Road Medical Centre, 25 Oxford Road, Burnley BB11 3BB Tel: 01282 423603 Fax: 01282 832827; 78 Lindsay Park, Worsthorne, Burnley BB10 3SQ — MB ChB Manch. 1979.

WONG, Chieh Lee 72 Beckhill Walk, Leeds LS7 2RW — MB ChB Leeds 1997.

WONG, Chin Yuan 9 Gateside Close, Cardiff CF23 8PB — MB BCh Wales 1990; MRCOG 1996.

WONG, Chiu Ming The Surgery, 105 Bellenden Road, London SE15 4QY Tel: 020 7639 9622 Fax: 020 7732 0870 — MB BS Lond. 1988.

WONG, Chiung Ing 72 Beckhill Walk, Meanwood, Leeds LS7 2RW — MB ChB Manch. 1998.

WONG, Chong Peng 14 St Kildas Road, Harrow HA1 1QA — MB BS Lond. 1967 (Roy. Free) DObst RCOG 1972. Prev: Ho. Off. (O & G) Lewisham Hosp.; Ho. Phys. (Paediat.) Roy. Free Hosp.; Obst. Ho. Surg. Roy. Free Hosp. Lond. (Liverp. Rd. Br.).

WONG, Mr Christopher Kwan Ming c/o C P Armstrongs Secretary, Frenchay Hospital, Frenchay Park, Bristol; 29 Cefn Onn Meadows, Lisvane, Cardiff CF14 0FL Tel: 01222 689674 — MB BCh Wales 1992; FRCS (Eng.) 1996. Specialist Regist. Rotat. SW Region. Specialty: Gen. Surg. Socs: BMA; Fell. RCS; ASIT. Prev: Specialist Regist. (Gen. & Vasc. Surg.) Treliske Hosp. Truro; SHO (Gen. Surg.) Univ. Hosp. Wales Cardiff; SHO (Trauma & Orthop. & A & E) Cardiff Roy. Infirm.

WONG, David Chuen Ho 11 Wolfe Crescent, London SE16 6SF — MB BS Lond. 1992.

WONG, David Jungmain Flat 11, 6 Riverview Place, Glasgow G5 8EB — MB ChB Glas. 1992.

WONG, Ee-Min — MB BS Lond. 1988 (London Hospital Medical College) FRCA 1993. Cons. Anaesth. Specialty: Anaesth. Prev: Sen. Registr., St Bart's; Regist. (Anaesth.) St Bart. Hosp. Lond.; SHO (Anaesth.) Whipps Cross Hosp. & Roy. Lond. Hosp.

WONG, Elizabeth Mandarin, Pewley Point, Pewley Hill, Guildford GU1 3SP; Dermatology Department, Royal Surrey County Hospital, Guildford GU2 7XX — MD Lond. 1987 (Univ. Coll. Hosp.) MB BS 1976; MRCP (UK) 1979; Specialist Accredit. Dermat. JCHMT 1984; FRCP 1997. Cons. Dermat. Roy. Surrey Co. Hosp. & Haslemere Hosps. Specialty: Dermat. Socs: Fell. Roy. Soc. Med.; Brit. Assn. Dermat.; BMA. Prev: Sen. Regist. & Lect. St. John's Hosp. Dis. Skin & Inst. Dermat. Lond.; Regist. (Med. & Dermat.) FarnBoro. Hosp.; Regist. (Dermat.) Guy's Hosp. & St. John's Hosp. Lond.

WONG, Felicia Cox Lane Surgery, Cox Lane, West Ewell, Epsom KT19 9PS — MB BS UMDS 1992 (St. Thos. Hosp. Lond.) DRCOG 1995; MRCGP 1996. Research Fell. The Toronto Hosp./P.ss Margt. Hosp./Ontario Cancer Inst., Toronto, Canada. Specialty: Gen. Pract. Socs: RCGP. Prev: GP/Regist. King's Coll. Hosp. VTS.

WONG, Folk-Man Apt. 3, 110 Palace Garden Terrace, London W8 4RT Tel: 020 7221 9337 Email: fmwong_md@yahoo.com — MB BS Lond. 1996; BSc 1992; MPH 2001.

WONG, Gavin Anthony Ernest Kai-Cheung Flat 2 Albert Court, 7 Elm Grove, Didsbury, Manchester M20 6PQ — MB ChB Dundee 1993; MRCP (UK) 1996. Specialty: Dermat.

WONG, Gen Tat 4 Cotlands Green, Dunmurry, Belfast BT17 0BF Tel: 01232 626279 Fax: 01232 626279 — MB BCh BAO Belf. 1992.

WONG, Geoffrey Richard Chee Keong — MB BS Lond. 1993 (UMDS) MA Camb. 1990; MRCGP 1999. GP Principal; Clin. Lect., Roy. Free & Univ. Coll. Med. Sch., UCL. Specialty: Gen. Pract. Prev: GP Asst.; Research Fell. Roy. Free & Univ. Coll. Med. Sch. UCL.

WONG, Grace Elaine Royal Surrey County Hospital, Egerton Road, Guildford GU2 7XX — MB BS Lond. 1993; MRCP. Specialty: Neurol.; Gen. Pract.

WONG, Grace Josephine Wing San 10 Aylmer Road, London N2 0BX — MB BS Lond. 1990.

WONG, Hoi Shing 15 Morningside, Washington NE38 9JH — MB ChB Manch. 1993.

WONG, Hok John Department of Clinical Biochemistry and Immunology, Kingston Hospital, Galsworthy Road, Kingston upon Thames KT2 7QB Tel: 020 8934 3292 Email: john.wong@kingstonhospital.nhs.uk — MB BCh BAO Dub. 1976 (Trinity College, Dublin University) MA Dub. 1980, MB BCh 1976; MSc Surrey 1980; MRCPath. 1984; FRC Path 1996. Cons. Chem. Path. Kingston Hosp. Specialty: Chem. Path. Prev: Sen. Regist. (Chem. Path.) Char. Cross Hosp.

WONG, Ismail Kien Chiong 73 Denison Road, London SW19 2DJ — MB BS Lond. 1998.

WONG, Mr Jackson Yan Wing Department of Paediatrics, Leicester Royal Infirmary, Leicester LE1 5WW Tel: 0116 541414; 11 Devonia Road, Oadby, Leicester LE2 4UJ Tel: 0116 271 2808 Fax: 0116 271 2808 — (St. Mary's Hosp. Med. Sch. Univ. Lond.) MB BS Lond. 1987; MB BS Lond. 1987; DCH RCP Lond. 1993; DCH RCP Lond. 1993; MRCP (UK) 1993; MRCP (UK) 1993; MRCPCH 1995; FHKAM (Paediat.) 1998; MHKCPaediat. 1998. Specialist Regist. (Paediat.) Leicester Roy. Infirm. Specialty: Paediat. Socs: BMA; Brit. Respirat. Soc.; Fell. Hong Kong Acad. Med. (Paediat.). Prev: Clin. Research Fell. (Paediat. Respirat. Med.) Dept. Child Health Univ. Leicester & Hon. Sen. Regist. Leicester Roy. Infirm.; Regist. (Paediat.) Hammersmith Hosp. & Qu. Charlotte & Chelsea Hosp. Lond.; Regist. (Paediat.) Lewisham Hosp. Lond.

WONG, Jacqueline Michelle Flat 5, 2 Lancaster Grove, London NW3 4NX — MB BChir Camb. 1990; MB Bchir (Cantab) 1990; MA (Cantab) 1991.

WONG, Jason Kar Wai 6 St. Paul's Walk, Cambridge CB1 2EX — MB BChir Camb. 1998; PhD Camb. 1998.

WONG, Jason Kin Fai 178 Whitehouse Road, Barnton, Edinburgh EH4 6DB — MB ChB Aberd. 1998.

WONG, John Soo Kiam Ashlea Medical Practice, 30 Upper Fairfield Road, Leatherhead KT22 7HH; 6 Grantham Avenue, Hartlepool TS26 9QT — MB ChB Aberd. 1983; MRCP (UK) 1988. Prev: Regist. (Gen. Med.) CrossHo. Hosp. Kilmarnock & Aberd. Roy. Infirm.; SHO (Med.) St. Luke's Hosp. Huddersfield.

WONG, Kayan Catherine Fazakerley Hospital, Longmoor Lane, Liverpool L9 7AL Tel: 0151 525 5980; 2A The Fairway, Alsager, Stoke-on-Trent ST7 2AZ Tel: 01270 872544 — MB ChB Liverp. 1991; BSc (Hons.) Liverp. 1986. SHO (Med. & Rheum.) Fazakerley Hosp. Liverp. Specialty: Gen. Med. Prev: Ho. Off. (Med., Surg., Geriat. & Urol.) Fazakerley Hosp. Liverp.

WONG, Kenneth Kak Yuen 37 Mount Pleasant Road, London NW10 3EG — MB ChB Ed. 1992. SHO (Urol.) Freeman Hosp. Newc. u. Tyne. Specialty: Urol.

WONG, Kirstin Elizabeth Brown Rigg, Halton Hall Gardens, Halton, Lancaster LA2 6LP — MB BS Lond. 1992 (Imperial College

London) DCH 1995; DRCOG 1996; MRCGP 1997; DFFP 1997. Specialty: Gen. Pract.

WONG, Lai Hong 4 The Leazes, Sunderland SR1 3SW — MB ChB Sheff. 1997; MRCS Ed. 2001.

WONG, Lin Hieng Walsgrave Hospital, Clifford Bridge Road, Coventry CV2 2DX — MB BCh Wales 1993; MRCP 1997; CCST (Gen. (Internal) Med. & Gastroenterol.) 2004. Cons. Walsgrave Hosp. Specialty: Gastroenterol.; Gen. Med. Prev: Specialist Regist. Gastroenterol. W. Midl. Traing. Scheme.

WONG, Mr Ling Sen 21 Furrows Close, Littlethorpe, Leicester LE9 5JR Tel: 0116 275 2228 Fax: 0121 627 2449 Email: lswong@hotmail.com; 14 Barclay Square, Renfrew PA4 8DY Tel: 0141 886 5381 — MB ChB Glas. 1989 (Glasgow) FRCS Ed. 1993; MD 1998. Specialist Regist. Qu. Eliz. Hosp. Birm.; Specialist Regist. Selly Oak Hosp. Birm. Specialty: Gen. Surg. Socs: Brit. Assn. Sugic. Oncol.; Assn. Surg. Train.; Assn. Coloproctol. Prev: Specialist Regist. (Gen. Surg.) Walsgrave Hosp. NHS Trust; Specialist Regist. Geo. Eliot Hosp. Nuneaton; Research Regist. (Gen. Surg.) Walsgrave Hosp. Coventry.

WONG, Locke Tse 30D South Hill Park, London NW3 2SB — MB BS Lond. 1996.

WONG, Man Kit Faith House Surgery, 723 Beverley Road, Hull HU6 7ER Tel: 01482 853296 Fax: 01482 855235; Shalom, 40 Badgers Wood, Cottingham HU16 5ST Tel: 01482 843293 — MB ChB Glas. 1987.

WONG, Margaret Mary Eye Unit, The Ayr Hospital, Dalmellington Road, Ayr KA6 6DX Tel: 01292 442384; 1 Knowle Road, Maidstone ME14 2BA — MB BS Med. Inst. (I) Rangoon 1985; FRCS Ed. 1995; FRCOphth 1995. Staff Ophth. Ayr Hosp. Specialty: Ophth. Prev: SHO Kent & Sussex Hosp., Kent Co. Ophth. Hosp. Maidstone & Roy. Eye Infirm. Plymouth.

WONG, Maria Ka Yee Flat 9 Albert Court, 20 Stoneygate Road, Leicester LE2 2AD — MB ChB Leic. 1993.

WONG, Mary Fiona Ming Chi Latham House, Sage Cross Street, Melton Mowbray LE13 1NX Tel: 01664 854949 Fax: 01664 501825 — MB BChir Camb. 1994 (Univ. Camb.) DGM; MA; MRCGP; DCH RCP Lond. 1996. GP Princ.; SHO (Rheum.) Leicester Gen. Hosp. Specialty: Rehabil. Med.; Rheumatol.; Gen. Pract. Prev: GP Regist.; SHO (Gen. Med.) Glenfield Gen. Hosp.; SHO (Paediat.) Northampton Gen. Hosp.

WONG, Matthew Chi-Chung 21 Weald Lane, Harrow HA3 5EU — MB BS Lond. 1998.

WONG, Michael — MB ChB Manch. 1991; DFFP 1994; DRCOG 1994; MRCGP 1995. Specialty: Gen. Pract. Prev: GP Ripley; Trainee GP Oldham; SHO (O & G) Bolton HA.

WONG, Michael Kwai Yew Brownrigg, Halton Hall Gardens, halton, Lancaster LA2 6LP Tel: 01524 811358 Fax: 01524 811358 — MB BS Lond. 1992 (Imperial College) DRCOG 1996; DCH 1996; MRCGP 1997; DFFP 1997. GP Assoc. Specialty: Gen. Pract.

WONG, Nelson Chi-Kit 11 Greemwood Close, Ashwellthorpe, Norwich NR16 1HB — MRCS Eng. LRCP Lond. 1978; MB BS Lond. 1978; MRCP (UK) 1981.

WONG, Newton Alexander Chiang Shuek Department of Pathology, University of Edinburgh Medical School, Teviot Place, Edinburgh EH8 9AG Tel: 0131 650 3001 — MB ChB Bristol 1993; MRCP 1996. Specialty: Histopath.

WONG, Nga Chung 4 The Leazes, Sunderland SR1 3SW Email: wongnc@netvigator.com — MB BS Newc. 1993. GP & Res. Med. Off. Union Hosp., Hong Kong. Socs: BMA.

WONG, Nyet Song Theresa 32 Barshaw Gardens, Appleton, Warrington WA4 5FA Tel: 01925 604035 Fax: 01925 604035 — MB BCh Wales 1994 (Univ.Wales.Coll.Med) AFRCS. SHO Gen. Surg. Countess of Chester. Hosp. Specialty: Gen. Surg. Prev: SHO (Gen. Surg.) Warrington. Gen. Hosp.; SHO (Plastics) Whiton Hosp.; SHO (Orthop.) Roy. Liverp. Univ. Hosp.

WONG, Oi Yee 16 The Beeches, Off Woodhead Drive, Cambridge CB4 1FY — MB BChir Camb. 1994. SHO Rotat. (Paediat.) Addenbrooke's Hosp. Camb. Specialty: Paediat.

WONG, Patricia Agnes Crabbs Cross Surgery, 38 Kenilworth Close, Crabbs Cross, Redditch B97 5JX Tel: 01527 544610 Fax: 01527 540286 — MB BS Lond. 1982. Specialty: Obst. & Gyn. Prev: Trainee GP Redditch; SHO (Gen. Psychiat.) Barnsley Hall Hosp. BromsGr.; SHO (Geriat. & A & E) Dudley Rd. Hosp. Birm.

WONG, Patricia Che 4 Hayfield Gardens, Birmingham B13 9LE — MB ChB Birm. 1995; ChB Birm. 1995.

WONG, Patrick Department of Anaesthetics, Queen Victoria Hospital, Holtye Road, East Grinstead RH19 3DZ — MB BS Lond. 1993. Specialty: Anaesth.

WONG, Paul Tong Yin Victoria Health Centre, 5 Suffrage Street, Smethwick, Warley B66 3PZ Tel: 0121 429 1373 & 021 420 2727 Fax: 0121 434 4549; 14 Greening Drive, Edgbaston, Birmingham B15 2XA — MB ChB Birm. 1978; MRCS Eng. LRCP Lond. 1978.

WONG, Quintin Kwing Kee North Brink Practice, 7 North Brink, Wisbech PE13 1JR Tel: 01945 585121 Fax: 01945 476423; The Old Vicarage, Barton Road, Wisbech PE13 4RP Tel: 01945 585121 Fax: 01945 476423 — MB BS Lond. 1985 (Royal Free Hospital School of Medicine, London) DRCOG 1989; MRCGP 1990. Princip. Gen. Pract. Prev: Trainee GP. Qu. Eliz. Hosp. King's Lynn Norf.

WONG, Richard Chiang Wen Flat 2, 8 Rooney Mansions, Clifton, Bristol BS8 4HY — MB ChB Bristol 1989; MB ChB (Hons.) Bristol 1989.

WONG, Richard Keng Mun — MB BChir Camb. 1995; MA 1996; MRCP (UK) 1998. Specialist Registar (Med.) Leicester Roy. Infirm. Specialty: Gen. Med.; Care of the Elderly. Prev: SHO (Derm) Leicester Roy. Infirm.; SHO (Endocrine) Leicester Roy. Infirm.; SHO (Neurol.) Leicester Roy. Infirm.

WONG, Roger Anthony Counselling & Support Team, Brownlee Centre, 1053 Great Western Road, Glasgow G12 0YN Tel: 0141 211 1085 Fax: 0141 211 1097; 6 Ellon Way, Paisley PA3 4BW Tel: 0141 887 9997 — MB ChB Glas. 1983; MRCPsych 1988. Clin. Coordinator, HIV Counselling & Support Team Glas. Specialty: Gen. Psychiat. Prev: Clin. Med. Off. HIV Counselling Clinic Edin.; Regist. (Psychiat.) Gartloch Hosp. Glas.

WONG, Mr Sai Hung David BUPA Murrayfields Wirral Hospital, Wirral CH61 1AU Tel: 0151 648 7000 — MB ChB Liverp. 1978; MRCS Eng. LRCP Lond. 1978; MRCP Lond. 1981; FRCS Eng. 1983; FRCOphth. 1989; FRCP 2000. Cons. Ophth. St. Paul's Eye Hosp. Liverp.; Hon. Clin. Lect. (Ophth.) Univ. Liverp. Specialty: Ophth. Prev: Sen. Regist. & Regist. Moorfields Eye Hosp. & St. Thos. Hosp. Lond.; Regist. & SHO St. Pauls Eye Hosp. Liverp.; Ho. Off. Roy. Liverp. Hosp.

WONG, Sarah Jane 11 Cullera Close, Northwood HA6 3SE — MB BS Lond. 1998.

***WONG, Selena** 47 Hough Road, Kings Heath, Birmingham B14 6HL — MB BS Lond. 1998; MB BS Lond 1998. Specialty: Gen. Med.

WONG, Simon Chi On Flat 2/L, 25 Queensborough Gardens, Hyndland, Glasgow G12 9QP — MB ChB Glas. 1995.

WONG, Siu Ling 3 Harvesters Way, Weavering, Maidstone ME14 5SH — MB BS Lond. 1986 (Lond. Hosp. Med. Coll.) DCH RCP Lond. 1988; DRCOG 1989; MRCGP 1990.

WONG, Smeeta Lirn Liih — MB ChB Sheff. 2003; BMedSci. PRHO (Gen. Surg.) Roy. Hallamsh. Hosp. & PRHO (Cardiol.) North. Gen. Hosp. Sheff.

WONG, Soo Kim 95-97 Crawford Street, London W1H 2HJ — MB BS Lond. 1985; DRCOG 1988; MRCGP 1989. Socs: BMA; Roy. Coll. of Gen. Practitioners. Prev: Trainee GP Edgware Gen. Hosp. VTS.

WONG, Stephen Phooi Yew 5 Chancellor's Walk, Cambridge CB4 3JG — BM BS Nottm. 1994.

WONG, Suzanne Yuk Siu 37 Whiteacre Close, Thornhill, Cardiff CF14 9DG — MB BS Lond. 1997.

WONG, Sze Chai Peter Department of Cardiology, University Hospital Aintree, Lower Lane, Liverpool L9 7AL Tel: 0151 529 2383 Fax: 0151 529 2724 Email: peter.wong@aht.nwest.nhs.uk — MB BS Lond. 1989 (The London Hospital Medical College) BSc Lond. 1986; MRCP UK 1993; MD London 2000. Cons. Cardiol. & Phys. in Gen. Med. Specialty: Cardiol.; Gen. Med. Socs: Med. Defence Union; Brit. Cardiovasc. Interven. Soc.; Brit. Soc. Of Echocardiography. Prev: SpR Train. -W. Midl.s; SHO Rotat. (Med. & Dermat.) Hull HA.; Ho. Off. (Surg.) Broomfield Hosp. Chelmsford Hosp.

WONG, Terence Hor Ga Institute of Liver Studies, King's College Hospital, Bessemer Road, London SE5 9PJ — MB BChir Camb. 1991; MA Camb. 1991. MB BChir 1991; MRCP (UK) 1993. Specialist Regist. Inst. Liver Studies King's Coll. Hosp. Lond. Specialty: Gastroenterol.; Gen. Med. Prev: Specialist Regist. Guildford Roy. Surrey Co. Hosp. Guildford; Clin. Research Fell. Inst.

Liver Studies King's Coll. Hosp.; SHO (Med.) St. Bartholomews Hosp. Lond.

WONG, Timothy Hong Tak Flat 9, Blair Court, Boundary Road, London NW8 6NT Tel: 020 7586 4827 — BChir Camb. 1986; MB 1987.

WONG, Tui Iar 14 Strutt Road, Sheffield S3 9AG — MB ChB Sheff. 1986. Regist. Rotat. (Psychiat.) Sheff. HA Train. Scheme; Regist. (Acute Adult Psychiat.) Middewood Hosp. Sheff. Specialty: Gen. Psychiat.

WONG, Tung-Shing 13 Parkside, Finchley, London N3 2PJ — MB BS Hong Kong 1976; DPM Eng. 1982. Staff Grade Psychiat. S. Lond. & Maudsley NHS Trust. Specialty: Gen. Psychiat. Socs: Affil. Roy. Coll. Psychiats. Prev: Staff Grade Psychiat. Lambeth Healthcare NHS Trust.

WONG, Voi Shim Department of Gastroentrology, Whittington Hospital, Highgate Hill, London Tel: 020 7288 5569 Email: voishim.wong@whittington.nhs.uk; Wollaston House, 25 Southwood Lane, Highgate, London N6 5ED Tel: 020 8348 6990 Email: info@woolastonhouse.com — MB ChB Manch. 1987; BSc St. And. 1984; MRCP (UK) 1991; MD 1998; FRCP 2004. Cons. Phys. / Gastroenterologist, Whittington Hosp., Lond. Specialty: Gastroenterol.; Gen. Med. Socs: Brit. Soc. of Gastroenterol.

WONG, Way Main Southend Hospital, Prittlewell Chase, Westcliff on Sea SS0 0RY Fax: 01702 221049 — MB BChir Camb. 1984; BA (Hon.) Camb. 1981; MRCP (UK) 1987. Cons. Rheumatologist. Specialty: Rheumatol. Socs: Brit. Soc. for Rheum.

WONG, Wilson Guy's Hospital, Department of Nephrology & Transplantation, 5th Floor, St Thomas Street, London SE1 9RT Tel: 020 7855 5000 — MB BS Lond. 1988; BSc (1st cl. Hons.) Lond. 1985; MRCP (UK) 1991; DPhil 1997. Sen.Lect.Hon.Cons.Nephrol.

WONG, Mr Wing Zou York District Hospital, Wigginton Road, York YO31 8HE — MB ChB Glas. 1988; FRCS Ed. 1992. Specialty: Gen. Surg. Prev: Regist. (Surg.) Higher Surgic. Trainee, Qu. Eliz. Hosp.; Regist. (Surg.) Higher Surgic. Trainee Dudley.

WONG, Yat Wing Room 64, Musgrave & Clark House, Royal Victoria Hospital, Grosvenor Road, Belfast BT12 6BA; 23 Upper Malone Park, Belfast BT9 6PP — MB BCh BAO Belf. 1995.

WONG, Mr Yin Lun Allen 2 High Street, Baldock SG7 6AR — MB ChB Glas. 1985; FRCS Ed. 1990; FRCS Glas. 1990.

WONG, Yuen Fong Solomon 14 Wigton Green, Leeds LS17 8QR — MB ChB Dundee 1988.

WONG, Yuk Ki 8 Deanfield Close, Hamble, Southampton SO31 4JJ — MB ChB Manch. 1990; BSc (Hons.) Manch. 1987, MB ChB 1990; MRCP (UK) 1993. Specialist Regist. (Cardiol.) Soton Gen. Hosp. Specialty: Cardiol. Prev: Regist. (Cardiol. & Med.) St. Mary's Hosp. Portsmouth; SHO (Med.) Birch Hill Hosp. Rochdale.

WONG CHING HWAI, Shim Yan Walton Hospital, Rice Lane, Liverpool L9 1AE — MB ChB Manch. 1984; MRCP (UK) 1988.

WONG CHUNG, Mr Kiang Kong Jean Marie (John) Department of Orthopaedic Surgery, Altnagelvin Hospital, Londonerry BT47 2AG Tel: 028 7134 5171; 5 The Haven, Texas Lane, Malahide, Dublin, Republic of Ireland — MB BCh BAO NUI 1978; LRCPI & LM, LRCSI & LM 1978; MCh NUI 1991, MB BCh BAO 1978; FRCSI 1982. Cons., Trauma & Orthopaedic Surg., Altnagelvin Hosp., Londonerry. Specialty: Trauma & Orthop. Surg. Special Interest: Foot & Ankle Soc. Socs: Brit. Orthopaedic Assn.

WONG HONG CHAI, Mr Flat 4, 26 Elsham Road, London W14 8HB — MB Camb. 1977; BChir 1976; MRCP (UK) 1980; FRCS Ed. 1982. Francis & Renee Hock Fell. Retinal Dis. Moorfields Eye Hosp. Lond. Prev: Resid. Surgic. Off. Moorfields Eye Hosp. Lond.

WONG KAM-KEE, Simon 10 Aylmer Road, Hampstead Garden Suburb, London N2 0BX Tel: 020 8340 9371 — MB BS Hong Kong 1960; DCH RCPS Glas. 1964; MRCP Ed. 1965.

WONG LAI CHENG, Dr 13 Hitherwood Drive, College Road, London SE19 1XA — MB BS Lond. 1979.

WONG LUN SANG, Angela San-Youn 143 Balls Pond Road, London N1 4BG — MB BS Lond. 1994.

WONG-LUN-SANG, Stella 53 Atkins Road, London SW12 0AH — MB BS Lond. 1998; MB BS Lond 1998.

WONGTSCHOWSKI, Karl Georg Julius 20 Tarranbrae, Willesden Lane, London NW6 7PL Tel: 020 8459 3649 — MD Berlin 1924.

WONKE, Beatrix Department of Haematology, Whittington Hospital, Highgate Hill, London N19 5NF — MD Zurich 1964; LMSSA Lond. 1970; FRCPath 1988, M 1976; FRCP FRCP 1999. Cons. Del The Whitlingttonn Hosp. NHS Trust; Clin. tutor UCLH. Specialty: Haematology. Socs: Roy. Coll. Pathol.; Roy. Coll. Phys.s. Prev: Hon. Cons. Roy. Free Hosp. Lond.

WONTUMI, Joseph Asiedu c/o Miss Parbury, T.A.T.D., British Council, 65 davies St., London W1Y 2AA — MB BS Lond. 1966.

WOO, Dominique Grace Department of Cardiology, Glenfield Hospital, Groby Road, Leicester LE3 9QP Tel: 0116 287 1471 — BM BS Nottm. 1990; BMedSci (Hons.) Nottm. 1988. Clin. Asst. (Cardiol.) Glenfield Hosp. Specialty: Palliat. Med. Prev: SHO Retainer Scheme (Cardiol.) Glenfield Hosp.; Staff Grade Phys. (Palliat. Med.) Sue Ryder Palliat. Care Home Staunton Harold; Clin. Asst. Palliat. Med. Marie Curie Centre Caterham.

WOO, Ka Chung Dawson 3 Belgrave Square, London SW1X 8PH — MB BS Lond. 1988.

WOO, Martin Payen Red Lion House Surgery, 86 Hednesford Road, Heath Hayes, Cannock WS12 5EA Tel: 01543 502391 Fax: 01543 573424; The Grange, Cannock Wood Street, Rawnsley, Hednesford, Cannock WS12 5PW Tel: 01543 685573 — MB ChB Birm. 1978; DRCOG 1982.

WOO, Michael Ting Chung Red Roofs, 31 Coton Road, Nuneaton CV11 5TW Tel: 024 7635 7100 Fax: 024 7664 2036 — MB BChir Camb. 1975; BA, MB BChir Camb. 1975; MRCP (UK) 1978; MRCGP 1980.

WOO, Professor Patricia Mang Ming, CBE Windeyer Institute of Medical Sciences, UCL, 46 Cleveland St., London W1T 4JF Tel: 020 7679 9148 Fax: 020 7679 9255 Email: patricia.woo@ucl.ac.uk; 319 Lonsdale Road, Barnes, London SW13 9PY — MB BS Lond. 1972 (Char. Cross) BSc Lond. 1969; MRCP (UK) 1975; PhD Camb. 1979; FRCP Lond. 1991; FRCPCH 1997; FMedSci 2001. Prof. Paediat. Rheum. Univ. Coll. Lond.; Hon. Cons. Phys. Hosp. for Sick Childr. & Univ. Coll. Hosp. Lond.; Vis. Prof. to ARC Epidemiol. Unit, Univ. of Manch. Specialty: Paediat. Socs: Pres. Paediat. Rheum. Europ. Soc.; Fell. RSM; Acad. Med. Sci. Prev: Head Molecular Rheum. MRC Clin. Research Centre Lond.; Research Fell. Div. Cell. Biol. Childr. Hosp. Med. Centre Boston, USA; Sen. Regist. (Med. & Rheum.) Guy's Hosp. Lond.

WOO, Yook Mun Renal Unit, Western Infirmary, Dunbarton Road, Glasgow G11 6NT; T/L Flat, 21 Queensborough Gardens, Glasgow G12 9PP — MB BS Sydney 1992; MRCP (UK) 1996. Regist. (Nephrol.) West. Infirm. Glas. Specialty: Nephrol. Socs: Scott. Renal Assn.; Renal Assn.

WOOD, Adrian Robert (retired) 5 Cross Road, Birchington CT7 9HN Tel: 01843 841661 — (St. Thos.) MB BS Lond. 1938; MRCS Eng. LRCP Lond. 1938.

WOOD, Agnes Pool Penicuik Health Centre, 37 Imrie Place, Penicuik EH26 8LF Tel: 01968 672612 Fax: 01968 671543; Martyrs Cross, Penicuik EH26 0NJ Tel: 01968 73799 — MB ChB Ed. 1976; DRCOG 1979; MRCGP 1980. Socs: Mem. of the Soc. of orthopaedic Med.

WOOD, Alan Edward (retired) 31 St Margaret's Street, Rochester ME1 1TU Tel: 01634 400358 Email: aewood1@tinyworld.co.uk — MB BS Lond. 1953 (Lond. Hosp.) FRCGP 1973, M 1960. Prev: Sen. Med. Off. DHSS.

WOOD, Mr Alan Jeffrey The Royal Hospitals Trust, St. Bartholomew's Hospital, West Smithfield, London EC1A 7BE Tel: 020 7601 7119 Fax: 020 7601 7117; 34 Circus Road, St Johns Wood, London NW8 9SG — MB BS Lond. 1975 (St. Bart.) MRCS Eng. LRCP Lond. 1975; FRCS Eng. 1980. Cons. Cardiothoracic Surg. St. Bart. Hosp. Lond.; Cons. Cardiothoracic Surg. Lond. Chest Hosp. & Roy. Lond. Hosp. Specialty: Cardiothoracic Surg.

WOOD, Alasdair Guy Park Lane Surgery, 8 Park Lane, Broxbourne EN10 7NQ Tel: 01992 465555; 1 Long Grove Close, Broxbourne EN10 7NP Tel: 01992 441649 — MB ChB Leic. 1989; DFFP 1995. Gen. Pract. Princip., Pk. La. Surg., Broxbourne. Specialty: Gen. Pract. Prev: Clin. Asst., Psychiat.

WOOD, Alison Jane Department of Child & Adsolescent Psychiatry, Duchess of York Childrens Hospital, Nell Lane, West Didsbury, Manchester M20 Tel: 0161 447 3131; 26 Moorfield Road, West Didsbury, Manchester M20 2UY Tel: 0161 434 5155 — MB ChB Leeds 1984; MRCPsych 1988; DRCOG 1990; DCH RCP Lond. 1990; MSc Psychiat. Manch. 1992; (Dip HSM) Open Univ. 1995; MD Manchester 1999. Cons. & Hon. Clin. Lect. (Child & Adsolesc. Psychiat.) S. Manch. Univ. Hosps. NHS Trust. Specialty: Child & Adolesc. Psychiat. Socs: Roy. Coll. Psychiat. Prev: Tutor &

Hon. Sen. Regist. (Child & Adolesc. Psychiat.) Roy. Manch. Childr. Hosp.; Sen. Regist. (Child & Adolesc. Psychiat.) NW RHA Train. Scheme; Trainee GP Macclesfield Dist. Gen. Hosp.

WOOD, Alison Janet Strathpeffer Medical Practice, The Medical Centre, Strathpeffer IV14 9AG Tel: 01997 421455 Fax: 01997 421172 — MB ChB Aberd. 1983; DRCOG 1984; MRCGP 1986.

WOOD, Alison Karen — MB ChB Manch. 1995; (Physics BSC I) London 1985. Sen. Ho. Officier, CHS, Sheff. Specialty: Gen. Psychiat. Socs: MDU.

WOOD, Amanda Catherine 23 Beaumont Road, St. Judes, Plymouth PL4 9BL; 20 Torr Crescent, Hartley, Plymouth PL3 5TW — MB ChB Manch. 1984.

WOOD, Andrea Amersham Health Centre, Chiltern Avenue, Amersham HP6 5AY Tel: 01494 434344 — MB ChB Leic. 1985.

WOOD, Andrew Mayne University Hospital of Wales, Department of Radiology, Heath Park, Cardiff CF14 4XW Tel: 029 2074 3955 Fax: 029 2074 3029; Fernbank, The Common, Dinas Powys CF64 4DL — MB BS Lond. 1983; BSc Lond. 1980; MRCP UK 1987; FRCR 1990. Cons. Radiol. Specialty: Radiol. Special Interest: Cardiac, Vasc. & Interventional Radiol. Socs: BMA; BSIR; CIRSE.

WOOD, Andrew Michael The Health Centre, Bunny Lane, Keyworth, Nottingham NG12 5JU Tel: 0115 937 3527 Fax: 0115 937 6781; 35 Selby Lane, Keyworth, Nottingham NG12 5AQ Tel: 0115 937 2406 — MB ChB Glas. 1979; BSc Glas. 1976; MRCGP 1983.

WOOD, Angela Clare Haematology Department, James Cook University Hospital, Marton Road, Middlesbrough T34 3BW — MB BS Newc. 1987; MRCP 1991; MRCPath 1998; MD Newcastle 1999. Cons. Haemat. James Cook Univ. Hosp., MiddlesBoro. Specialty: Haematology. Socs: Med. Soc. Haematol.

WOOD, Angus Donald Graham Poole Hospital NHS Trust, Longfleet Road, Poole BH15 2JB Tel: 0116 274 5003 Email: angns.wood@poole.nhs.uk; 36 Seafield Road, Friars Cliff, Christchurch BH23 4ET — MB BS Lond. 1985 (Westm. Med. Sch.) MRCP (UK) 1988; FRCR 1993. Cons. Radiol. Poole Hosp. Specialty: Radiol. Prev: Lect. (Magnetic Resonance Imaging) Lond. Hosp. Med. Coll.; Sen. Regist. (Radiol.) Soton. Gen. Hosp.

WOOD, Ann Mabel North Ridge Medical Practice, North Ridge, Rye Road, Hawkhurst, Cranbrook TN18 4EX Tel: 01580 753935 Fax: 01580 754452 — MB ChB Glas. 1981; MRCPsych 1986. Gen. Practitioner; Sch. Med. Off.

WOOD, Anna Francesca 41 Eaton Road, Alsager, Stoke-on-Trent ST7 2BQ — BM BS Nottm. 1994.

WOOD, Annette Lynne Heart of Birmingham Tpct, 142 Hagley Road, Birmingham B16 9PA Tel: 0121 695 2350 — MB BCh Wales 1986; MRCGP 1990; DRCOG 1990; MFPHM RCP (UK) 1995; FFPHM 2002. Cons. Pub. Health Med. Heart of Birm. Tpct. Specialty: Pub. Health Med. Prev: Sen. Regist. (Pub. Health Med.) W. Midl. RHA.

WOOD, Anthony Millard (retired) Spindrift, 101 Orchary Avenue, Parkstone, Poole BH14 8AN Tel: 01202 740695 — (Middlx.) MB BS Lond. 1955. Prev: GP Colchester.

WOOD, Antony John (retired) 26 Bentley Way, Stanmore HA7 3RP — MB BS Lond. 1956 (Westm.) DPH Bristol 1965; MFCM 1973. Prev: PMO (Health Educat.) Brent & Harrow AHA.

WOOD, Armorel Wendy Tulscroft, Poplar Lane, Bransgore, Christchurch BH23 8JE Tel: 01425 674415 — MB BS Lond. 1986; MA Oxf. 1983; Cert. Family Plann. JCC 1989. Clin. Asst. (Rheum. & Rehabil.) Roy. Bournemouth Hosp. Specialty: Rehabil. Med.; Rheumatol. Prev: SHO (Psychiat.) City Hosp. Truro; SHO (Med. for Elderly) York Dist. Hosp.; SHO (Cas.) Winchester.

WOOD, Arthur Brian (retired) 31 Heights Drive, Linthwaite, Huddersfield HD7 5SU — MRCS Eng. LRCP Lond. 1944 (St. Bart.) MRCGP 1959.

WOOD, Barbara Louise Psychotherapy Department, Maudsley Hospital, Denmark Hill, London SE5 8AZ Tel: 020 7919 2384/5 — MB BS Lond. 1987; MRCP (UK) 1991; MRCPsych 1994. Cons. Psychiatrist, Psychotherapy, Maudsley Hosp., Lond. Specialty: Psychother. Prev: Sen. Regist. (Psychother.) Maudsley Hosp. Lond.

WOOD, Beatrice Gillian Starcross, Great Austins, Farnham GU9 8JG Tel: 01252 715272 — MB ChB Aberd. 1962. Health Screening Phys. Parkside Suite Frimley Pk. Hos. NHS Trust. Prev: Occupat. Health Phys. Frimley Pk. Hosp. NHS Trust; Sen. Clin. Med. Off. Well Wom. & Family Plann. Clinics N.; Downs Community Health Unit.

WOOD, Benjamin Stuart Blachford (retired) 3 Kingsfield, Lymington SO41 3QY Tel: 01590 672967 — BM BCh Oxf. 1941 (Oxf. & St. Thos.) DM Oxf. 1951, BA, BM BCh 1941; FRCP Lond. 1966, M 1948; DCH Eng. 1948. Prev: Cons. Paediat. Birm. Centr. Health Dist. (T).

WOOD, Brian Robert Craigmillar Medical Group, 106 Niddrie Mains Road, Edinburgh EH16 4DT Tel: 0131 536 9500 Fax: 0131 536 9545 — MB ChB Ed. 1975.

WOOD, Bridget Caroline Oakhaven Hospice, Lower Pennington Lane, Lymington SO41 8ZZ Tel: 020 7249 8336 Email: beckywilliams@breathemail.net; 36 Seafield Road, Friars Cliff, Christchurch BH23 4ET — MB BS Lond. 1984; BA Camb. 1981; DRCOG 1986; MRCGP 1988; FRCR 1993. Cons. Palliat. Med. & Med. Dir. Oakhaven Hospice Lymington. Specialty: Palliat. Med. Prev: Sen. Regist. (Palliat. Med.) Wessex Region; Regist. (Radiother. Oncol.) Roy. S. Hants. Hosp.; Regist. (Palliat. Care) St. Christophers Hospice Lond.

WOOD, Bridget Mary (retired) Dormington House, Dormington, Hereford HR1 4ES Tel: 01432 850543 Fax: 01432 850543 — MB BS Lond. 1960 (Roy. Free) MB BS Lond. 1960; MRCS Eng. LRCP Lond. 1960; DA Eng. 1964; FFA RCS Eng. 1977. Prev: Clin. Dir. (Critical Care) & Cons. Anaesth. Sandwell Dist. Gen. Hosp.

WOOD, Carine Henriette Guy's Hospital, Department of Anaesthetics, St Thomas Street, London SE1 9RT Fax: 020 7955 8844 Email: carine.wood@gstt.sthames.nhs.uk; 36 Earl's Court Square, London SW5 9DQ Tel: 020 7370 6939 Fax: 020 7835 2081 Email: carine.wood@doctors.org.uk — MD Paris 1980; FFA RCSI Dub. 1985; FRCA 1987. Cons. Paediatric Anaesth. Guy's & St. Thos. NHS Trust Lond. Specialty: Anaesth. Socs: Fell. Roy. Soc. Med.; Soc. Clin. Française.; Fell. Roy. Coll. Anaesth. Prev: Sen. Regist. Char. Cross & Westm. Hosps.; Regist. Hammersmith & Edgware Hosps.; Regist. Northwick Pk. Hosp.

WOOD, Charles Geoffrey Millard The Surgery, Roman Way, Billingshurst RH14 9QZ Tel: 01403 782931 Fax: 01403 785505; Beke Glade, Marringdean Road, Billingshurst RH14 9HF Tel: 01403 782440 Fax: 01403 786691 — MB BS Lond. 1978 (St. Mary's Hosp.) Clin. Asst. (Dermat.) Worthing Hosp.

WOOD, Charles Roger (retired) Ethnam Cottage, Ethnam Lane, Sandhurst, Cranbrook TN18 5PS Tel: 0158 085 850 360 — (Lond. Hosp.) MRCS Eng. LRCP Lond. 1942. Prev: O & G Ho. Surg. King Edwd. VII Hosp. Windsor.

WOOD, Charlotte Elizabeth Brooklea Health Centre, Wick Road, Brislington, Bristol BS4 4HU Tel: 0117 971 1211; 4 Napier Road, Bristol BS6 6RT Tel: 0117 973 3572 — MB BS Lond. 1981; BA Oxf. 1978; DRCOG 1985; MRCGP 1986; DFFP 1996. Prev: GP Bedminster; Trainee GP Avon VTS.

WOOD, Christina Clare 3 Bassingham Road, London SW18 3AF — MB ChB Leic. 1991.

WOOD, Christine Bernadette Ashville Medical Centre, 430 Doncaster Road, Barnsley S70 3RJ Tel: 01226 216000; 96 Bluebell Ave, Penistone, Sheffield S36 6LQ Tel: 01226 765644 Email: barry@knee.demon.co.uk. — MB ChB Sheff. 1976.

WOOD, Christine Dorothy Salisbury Palliative Care Services, Salisbury District Hospital, Salisbury SP2 8BJ Tel: 01722 336262 Fax: 01722 338015 — MB BCh Wales 1978; FRCP (UK) 1981. Cons. Palliat. Med. Salisbury Dist. Hosp. Specialty: Palliat. Med. Prev: Med. Dir. Salisbury Macmillan Unit; Research Fell. Med. Coll. & Sen. Regist. (Med. Oncol.) St. Bart Hosp. Lond.; Hosp. Rotat. (Med.) Lond. Hosp.

WOOD, Mr Christopher Barry Department of Surgery, Wexham Park Hospital, Slough SL2 4HL Tel: 01753 633000 Fax: 01753 691343 — MD Wales 1984; MB BCh 1970; FRCS Ed. 1974. Hon. Cons. Surg. Wexham Pk. Hosp. Slough. Specialty: Gen. Surg. Prev: Sen. Lect. (Surg.) Roy. Postgrad. Med. Sch. Lond.; Lect. (Surg.) Roy. Infirm. Glas.; Research SHO (Surg.) Univ. Hosp. Wales Cardiff.

WOOD, Christopher Bryan Somerset 38 Church Crescent, Whetstone, London N20 0JP Tel: 020 8368 6951 Fax: 020 8368 6951 Email: christopher@christaret.demon.co.uk — MB BChir Camb. 1958 (Camb. & St Bart.) DCH Eng. 1959; FRCP Lond. 1973, M 1963; FRCPCH 1997. Emerit. Prof. Child Health Barts and The Lond. Qu. Mary's Sch. of Med. and Dent.; Hon. Cons. Paediat. Homerton Univ. Hosp. NHS Foundat. Trust. Specialty: Paediat. Socs:

Fell. Roy. Soc. Med.; BMA; Brit. Thorac. Soc. Prev: Lect. & Sen. Lect. (Child Health) Univ. Bristol; Research Fell. Paediat. Research Unit Guy's Hosp. Lond.; Regist. Evelina Childr. Hosp. (Guy's Hosp.) Lond.

WOOD, Christopher Holman (retired) Small Acres, Poplar Lane, Bransgore, Christchurch BH23 8JE Tel: 01425 672747 Fax: 01425 674941 — MB ChB Bristol 1956. Prev: Ho. Surg. & Ho. Phys. Bristol Roy. Infirm.

WOOD, Christopher John Michael St John's Surgery, Main Road, Terrington St. John, Wisbech PE14 7RR Tel: 01945 880471 Fax: 01945 880677 — MB BS Lond. 1972 (St. Bart.) MRCS Eng. LRCP Lond. 1972; DPM Eng. 1976; MRCPsych 1977.

WOOD, Christopher Mark Clarendon Wing, Belmont Grove, Leeds LS2 9 Tel: 0113 243 2799; 7 Laurel Hill Grove, Colton, Leeds LS15 9EL Tel: 0113 260 3874 — MB BS Lond. 1986; BA Camb. 1983; MRCP (UK) 1990. Lect. & Hon. Sen. Regist. (Paediat.) Leeds Gen. Infirm. Specialty: Paediat. Socs: Paediat. Research Soc. Prev: SHO (Paediat. Cas.) St Thos. Hosp. Lond.; SHO (Paediat.) St. Jas. Univ. Hosp. Leeds.

WOOD, Mr Christopher Patrick Langton Wrenwood, Park Avenue, Hartlepool TS26 0DZ — MB BS Lond. 1969 (St. Bart.) FRCS Eng. 1976. Specialty: Gen. Surg.

WOOD, Christopher Robert 442 Blackness Road, Dundee DD2 1TQ Tel: 01382 667547 — BM BS Nottm. 1995. SHO Surgic. Rot., Dorset Co. Hosp. Prev: Emerg. Med. Re. (Newc.); SHO (A&E) Leeds Gen. Infirm.; SHO (A&E) W. Cumbld. Hosp.

WOOD, Clare Mairi Park Avenue Medical Centre, Park Avenue, Dundee DD4 6PP Tel: 01382 462222 Fax: 01382 452866 — MB ChB Dundee 1992.

WOOD, Colin Samuel (retired) Crumlin medical centre, Crown st, Crumlin NP11 4PQ Tel: 01495 244633 Fax: 01495 249118; North Downs Hospital, 46 Tupwood Lane, Caterham CR3 6DP Tel: 01883 348981 — MB BCh Wales 1974 (Welsh National School of Medicine Cardiff) MSc Surrey 1981. Staff Phys. N. Downs Hosp. Caterham. Prev: Specialist (Disabil. Med.) Benefits Agency Med. Serv. DSS Sutton.

WOOD, Damian Mark St mary's Hospital, Hathforsage Road, Manchester M13 0JH — MB ChB Manch. 1995; DCH 1998. Clin. Fell. Paediat. St Mary's Hosp. Manch. Specialty: Paediat.

WOOD, Mr Daniel Nigel 32 Westcliff Drive, Leigh-on-Sea SS9 2LB Tel: 01702 715022 — MB BS Lond. 1994 (St. Bart.) FRCS Eng. 1998. Research Fell.Instit.Oncol. Lond. Specialty: Urol. Prev: SHO (Gen. Surg.) Southend Gen. Hosp.; SHO (Intens. Care) Qu. Alexandras Hosp. Portsmouth; SHO (A & E) Roy. Surrey Co. Hosp. Guildford.

WOOD, Professor David Allan Imperial College of Science, Technology and Medicine, National Heart & Lung Institute, Charing Cross Hospital, Fulham Palace Road, London W6 8RF Tel: 020 8846 7157 Fax: 020 8383 5513 — MB ChB Dundee 1974; MRCP (UK) 1979; MSc (Epidemiol.) Lond. 1981; FRCP Lond 1991; FRCP Ed. 1991. Prof. Clin. Epidemiol. Nat. Heart & Lung Inst. Univ. Lond.; Hon. Cons. Cardiol. Roy. Brompton & Bromley Hosps. Specialty: Cardiol. Prev: Sen. Lect. (Med.) Univ. Soton.; Wellcome Research Fell. (Clin. Epidemiol.) Cardovasc. Research Unit Univ. Edin.

WOOD, David Cecil The Surgery, Station Road, Knebworth SG3 6AP Tel: 01438 812494 Fax: 01438 816497; 29 Heath Lane, Codicote, Hitchin SG4 8YE Tel: 01438 820824 — MB ChB Aberd. 1972.

WOOD, David George Edwin The Cottage, Eglwysbach, Colwyn Bay LL28 5UD — MB ChB Bristol 1970; MRCS Eng. LRCP Lond. 1969; MRCGP 1977.

WOOD, David James Doncaster Royal Infirmary, Armthorpe Road, Doncaster DN2 5LT — MB BS Lond. 1988. Specialty: Anaesth.

WOOD, David Michael Department of Pharmacology, Jenner Wing, St George's Hospital Medical School, London SW17 0RE — MB ChB Bristol 1997 (Univ. of Bristol) MB ChB (Hons.) Bristol 1997; MRCP (UK) 2000. Clin. Pharmacol. and Therapeutics/Gim SpR St George's Hosp. Lond. Specialty: Gen. Med. Prev: Med. SHO Rotat. St George's Hosp. Lond.; John Racliffe Med. SHO Rotat. Oxf.; Ho. Phys. Bristol Roy. Infirm. Bristol.

WOOD, David Nugent 17 New Road, Brixham TQ5 8BL Tel: 01803 2731 — MB BS Lond. 1958 (St. Geo.) MRCS Eng. LRCP Lond. 1958; MRCGP 1970; AKC 1988. Prev: Ho. Phys. Stoke Mandeville Hosp. Aylesbury; Ho. Surg. St. Geo. Hosp. Lond.; Med. Off. Mildmay Miss. Hosp. Lond.

WOOD, David Richard Ellern Mede Centre for Eating Disorders, 31 Totteridge Common, London N20 8LR Tel: 020 8959 7774 Fax: 020 8959 6311 Email: david.wood@ellernmede.org — MB BS Lond. 1975 (Char. Cross) DRCOG 1978; MRCPsych 1984. Cons. Child & Adolesc. Psychiat. & Psychotherap. Specialty: Child & Adolesc. Psychiat. Socs: Inst. Gp. Anal.; Family Systems Div. Tavistock Soc. Psychother.; Assn. Child Psychol. & Psychiat. Prev: Cons. Child Psychiat. Hemel Hempstead; Sen. Regist. Tavistock Clinic Lond.; Regist. (Psychiat.) The Lond. Hosp. Whitechapel.

WOOD, David Robin Priory Hospital, Hayes Grove, Prestons Road, Hayes BR2 7AS Tel: 020 8462 7722 Fax: 020 8462 5028 — (Ed.) MB ChB Ed. 1962; MRCP Ed. 1967; MRCP Lond. 1969; MRCPsych 1972; DPM Eng. 1972; FRCP Ed 1996; FRCPsych. 1997. Cons. Psychiat. & Asst. Med. Dir. Priory Hosp. Bromley, Kent. Specialty: Gen. Psychiat. Socs: Fell. Roy. Soc. Med. Prev: Cons. Psychiat. & Med. Dir. Ravensbourne NHS Trust; Sen. Regist. Maudsley Hosp. Lond.; Regist. (Neurol.) North. Gen. Hosp. Edin.

WOOD, David Stanley, MBE (retired) 36 Highfields, Llandaff, Cardiff CF5 2QB Tel: 029 2056 6248 — (Cardiff) BSc Wales 1947; MB BCh Wales 1951. Prev: Ho. Phys., Cas. Off. (Surg.) & Ho. Surg. (O & G) Cardiff Roy. Infirm.

WOOD, David Wildman (retired) The Health Centre, High Street, Bedworth, Nuneaton CV12 8NQ — MRCS Eng. LRCP Lond. 1953 (Sheff.)

WOOD, David William 12 Cedar Drive, Durham DH1 3TF — MB ChB St. And. 1971; FRCA 1975. Cons. Anaesth. Durh. HA. Specialty: Anaesth. Prev: Sen. Regist. (Anaesth.) North. RHA; Regist. (Anaesth.) Cardiff.

WOOD, Dawn Agnes Avonmead Ward, Southmead Hospital, Westbury on Trym, Bristol BS10 5NB — MB BCh Wales 1989; T(GP) 1993. Staff Grade Psychiat. (Psychiat. of Old Age) Southmead Hosp. Bristol. Specialty: Geriat. Psychiat. Prev: Trainee GP W. Glam. VTS.

WOOD, Diana Frances University of Cambridge, School of Clinical Medicine, Addenbrooke's Hospital, Box 111, Cambridge CB2 2SP — MB ChB Birm. 1980; MRCP (UK) 1983; MD Birm. 1992; FRCP 1996; ADHES Lond. 1998. Director of Med. Educat. / Clin. Dean, Clin. Med., Univ. of Camb.; Hon. Cons. Phys., Addenbrooke's Hosp. Camb. Specialty: Endocrinol.; Gen. Med. Special Interest: Med. Educat. Prev: Dep. Dean for Educat., Reader in Med. Studies & Hon. Cons. Physcian Barts & The Lond. NHS Trust; Sen. Lect. Med., Barts & The Lond. NHS Trust; Lect. in Endocrinol. & Gen. Med., St Marys Hosp., Lond.

WOOD, Diana Frances Warden Lodge Surgery, 63 Albury Ride, Cheshunt, Waltham Cross EN8 8XE Tel: 01992 441649; 1 Long Grove Close, Broxbourne EN10 7NP — MB BS Lond. 1989; DFFP 1994. Gen. Practitioner.

WOOD, Dorothy Anne School Lane Surgery, School Lane, Washingborough, Lincoln LN4 1BN Tel: 01522 792360 Fax: 01522 794144; The Old Barn, Manor Road, Washingborough, Lincoln LN4 1BQ Tel: 01522 792360 — MB ChB Ed. 1978; DRCOG 1981; DCH Eng. 1982; MRCGP 1982.

WOOD, Mr Edward Hamilton (retired) 7 Maes Rhosyn, Rhuddlan, Rhyl LL18 2YW — MB ChB Birm. 1961; DObst RCOG 1963; FRCS Ed. 1968. Cons. Surg. Clwyd N. Health Dist.

WOOD, Edward Vaughan 101 Lightwater Meadow, Lightwater GU18 5XJ — MB ChB Liverp. 1996.

WOOD, Edwin Charles The Writtle Surgery, 16A Lordship Road, Writtle, Chelmsford CM1 3EH Tel: 01245 421205 Fax: 01245 422094 — MB BS Lond. 1985; DRCOG 1989; MRCGP 1990.

WOOD, Elizabeth Moody 95 Dulwich Village, London SE21 7BJ Tel: 020 8693 3836 — MB BS Lond. 1968 (Middlx.) MRCS Eng. LRCP Lond. 1968; DCH Eng. 1972; DTM & H Liverp. 1976; MRCP (UK) 1979; FRCP 2003; FRCPCH 2005. Staff Grade Paediat. Qu. Mary's Hosp. Sidcup. Prev: SHO (Paediat.) & Regist. (Paediat.) St. Mary's Hosp. Portsmouth.

WOOD, Emma Frances 105a Kilburn Park Road, London NW6 5LB — MB BS Lond. 1997.

WOOD, Emma Jane (nee Davis) 10 Cornwall Road, Cheam, Sutton SM2 6DR — MB BS Lond. 1997.

WOOD, Eric (retired) 286 Frederick Street, Oldham OL8 4HG Tel: 0161 624 6179 — MB ChB Manch. 1945.

WOOD, Eric Robert Miller 3 Lovers Walk, Dumfries DG1 1LR — MB BS Newc. 1975.

WOOD, Fiona Jane — MB ChB Liverp. 1986. Staff Grade (Community Paediat.). Specialty: Community Child Health.

WOOD, Frances Ann The Surgery, Gaywood House, North St, Bedminster, Bristol BS3 3AZ Tel: 0117 966 1412 Fax: 0117 953 1250; 17 Cricklade Road, Bishopston, Bristol BS7 9EW — MB ChB Bristol 1976; DRCOG 1980.

WOOD, Fraser Thomas 3 Kingswood Grove, Kingswells, Aberdeen AB15 8AH — MB ChB Glas. 1993.

WOOD, Frederick Brian Gaylor (retired) Jacaranda, Chapel Lane, Bransgore, Christchurch BH23 8BN — MB ChB Sheff. 1955 (Leeds) DPH Leeds 1967. Prev: Cons. Communicable Dis. Control Kent.

WOOD, Geoffrey Campbell Dale View Health Centre, Dale View, Caistor, Market Rasen LN7 6NX Tel: 01472 851203 Fax: 01472 852495 — MB BS Lond. 1981 (St Georges) Prev: Trainee GP Carshalton VTS; Med. Off. & Dist. Med. Off. St. Francis Hosp. Katete, Zambia.

WOOD, Geoffrey Holman (retired) Polmener, Mullion, Helston TR12 7DH Tel: 01326 240308 — MB ChB Bristol 1952. Prev: Hon. Med. Adviser (Lizard-Cadgwith Lifeboat) RNLI.

WOOD, Geoffrey Michael 341 Marine Road, Morecambe LA4 5AB — MB ChB Manch. 1957.

WOOD, Gillian Elizabeth Woodhouse Medical Centre, 7 Skelton Lane, Woodhouse, Sheffield S13 7LY Tel: 0114 269 0025 — MB ChB Sheff. 1988; MRCGP 1992.

WOOD, Gordon McKenzie George Eliot Hospital, Nuneaton CV10 7DJ — (Leeds) MB ChB Leeds 1977; MRCP (UK) 1980; BSc Leeds. 1974, MD 1989; FRCP Lond. 1995. Cons. Phys. Geo. Eliot Hosp. Nuneaton. Specialty: Gen. Med. Prev: Sen. Regist. (Gen. & Geriat. Med.) Dudley Rd. Hosp. Birm.; Regist. Profess. Med. Unit St. Jas. Univ. Hosp. Leeds.

WOOD, Graham Colin Avondale Unit, Royal Preston Hospital, Sharoe Green Lane, Preston PR2 9HT Tel: 01772 716565 — MB ChB Ed. 1979; BSc (Hons.) Ed. 1976; MRCGP 1983; MRCPsych 1989; MPsychMed Liverp. 1992. Cons. Psychiat. Lancashire Care NHS Trust. Prev: GP Newton-le-Willows Merseyside.

WOOD, Graham John (retired) 4 Cobden Crescent, Southampton SO18 4EW — MB BS Lond. 1973; FFA RCS Eng. 1978; T(Anaes.) 1991. Prev: Cons. Anaesth. King Faisal Specialist Hosp. Riyadh, Saudi Arabia.

WOOD, Greg 49 Chandos Road, East Finchley, London N2 9AR — MB BS Lond. 1988. Princip. Med. Off., HMS Neptune. Specialty: Gen. Psychiat. Prev: Princip. Med. Off., HMS Fearless; Princip. Med. Off. HMS Osprey Portland.

WOOD, Harry Joseph (retired) Holly Court, Kenyon Close, Stratford St Mary, Colchester CO7 6LJ Tel: 01206 322574 — MB BChir Camb. 1954 (Camb. & Lond. Hosp.) MRCS Eng. LRCP Lond. 1954; DObst RCOG 1956.

WOOD, Hazel Anne Queen Elizabeth II Hospital, Howlands, Welwyn Garden City AL7 4HQ Tel: 01707 328111 — MB ChB Leeds 1979; MRCPsych 1984. Cons. Psychiat. Old Age Qu. Eliz. II Hosp. Welwyn Garden City. Specialty: Geriat. Psychiat. Prev: Sen. Regist. (Psychiat.) Parkside HA.; Sen. Regist. (Psychiat.) Yorks. RHA.; Regist. (Psychiat.) Leeds Rotat. Train. Scheme.

WOOD, Helen Mary Borras Park Surgery, Borras Park Road, Wrexham LL12 7TH Tel: 01978 352341 Fax: 01978 310294 — MB BCh Wales 1983.

WOOD, Helen Mary Plas Goulbourne Farmhouse, Holt Road, Llan-Y-Pwll, Wrexham LL13 9SA — MB BCh Wales 1983; DRCOG 1985.

WOOD, Ian Hendrie Young Townhead Surgery, 6-8 High St., Irvine KA12 0AY Tel: 01294 73131; Kincraig, Kilwinning Road, Irvine KA12 8SU — MB ChB Glas. 1959; DObst RCOG 1961.

WOOD, Ian Robertson St Andrews Hospital, Billing Road, Northampton NN1 5DG Tel: 01604 629696 — BM BCh Oxf. 1975; BS Yale 1968; MA Oxf. 1970; MRCP (UK) 1976; MRCPsych 1980. cons. Psychiat. (Adult Ment. Health) St And. Hosp. Northampton. Specialty: Gen. Psychiat. Prev: Cons. Psychiat. Aylesbury Vale.

WOOD, James Graham Top Flat, 10 North Road, West Kirby, Wirral CH48 4DF — MB ChB Ed. 1994. Ho. Off. (Gen. Med.) Roy. Infirm. Edin. Prev: Ho. Off. (Paediat. Surg.) Roy. Hosp. Sick Childr. Edin.

WOOD, Mr James Jeremy The North London Nuffield Hospital, Cavell Drive, Uplands Park Road, Enfield EN2 7PR Tel: 020 8366 2122; 35 Muswell Road, Muswell Hill, London N10 2BS Tel: 020 8442 0472 — BM BCh Oxf. 1974; FRCS Eng. 1980; MA Oxf. 1974, DM 1988. Cons. Enfield & Haringay Breast Screening Progr. Specialty: Gen. Surg. Socs: Brit. Assn. Surg. Oncol. Prev: Sen. Regist. (Gen. Surg.) St. Bart. Hosp. Lond.; Regist. (Gen. Surg.) Whipps Cross Hosp. Lond; Research Fellowship Harvard Med. Sch. Boston, USA 1983-5.

WOOD, Jane Diana Dudley (retired) Vrogain, Park St., Denbigh LL16 3DE — MB BS Lond. 1961; FRCP Glas. 1985, M 1965; FRCP Lond. 1994. Prev: Cons. Phys. c/o Elderly Glan Clwyd Dist. Gen. Hosp. Trust.

WOOD, Jason Mortimer 6 Whiteway Drive, Heavitree, Exeter EX1 3AN — MB BS Lond. 1993 (Roy. Lond. Hosp.) BSc (Hons.) Lond. 1990; DCH Lond. 2001.

WOOD, Jennifer Mary (retired) 6 Keelam Lane, Keighley BD20 6DE — MB ChB Liverp. 1963; DTM & H Liverp. 1964.

WOOD, Jeremy Paul Royal Bolton Hospital, Minerva Road, Farnworth, Bolton BL4 0JR; 12 Churchwood Road, Didsbury, Manchester M20 6TY Email: jezden@hotmail.com — MB ChB Manch. 1992 (Manchaster) FRCA, 1998. Cons. Anaesth. with an interest in Intens. Care Roy. Bolton Hosp. Specialty: Anaesth. Socs: Intens. Care Soc. Mem. Assn. of Anaesth.s Mem. Prev: N.est Regional Specialist Regist.

WOOD, Joanne 541 Acklam Road, Acklam, Middlesbrough TS5 7HH — MB ChB Ed. 1996.

WOOD, Joanne Morag 48 Roman Way, Dunblane FK15 9DJ — MB ChB Glas. 1980; DA (UK) 1985. Staff Grade (Anaesth.) Falkirk & Dist. Roy. Infirm. Specialty: Anaesth.

WOOD, Johanna Mary 10 The Woodlands, Chelsfield Park, Orpington BR6 6HL Tel: 01689 851054 — MB ChB Manch. 1979. GP Retainer, Chelsfield, Kent; Health Correspondent Woman Alive; Health/Media Speaker Premier Radio. Specialty: Gen. Pract.; Med. Publishing. Socs: GPWA.

WOOD, John (retired) 16 Park Road, Deeping St James, Peterborough PE6 8ND — MB ChB Ed. 1954. Prev: Dir. Med. Dept. Brit. Counc.

WOOD, John Albert St Elizabeth's Medical Centre, Netherhall Road, netherhall, Leicester LE5 1DR Tel: 0116 241 6392 — MB BS Lond. 1966; MRCS Eng. LRCP Lond. 1966; DObst RCOG 1969; FRCGP 2002. Br. Med. Off. Leics. Br. Brit. Red Cross. Specialty: Gen. Pract. Prev: Asst. Br. Med. Off. Leics. Br. Brit. Red Cross Soc.; SHO (Paediat.) Leicester Roy. Infirm.; SHO (O & G) Good Hope Hosp. Sutton Coldfield.

WOOD, John Battersby (retired) Dormington House, Dormington, Hereford HR1 4ES Tel: 01432 850543 Fax: 01432 850543 Email: john.b.wood@lineone.net — (Oxf. & St. Mary's) BM BCh Oxf. 1960; FRCP Lond. 1979, M 1966. Prev: Cons. Phys. Hereford Co. Hosp.

WOOD, Mr John Bernard Flat 22, 1 Stewart St., London E14 3EX Tel: 020 7538 4951 — MB BS Lond. 1991; BSc (Hons.) Basic Med. Sci. & Anat. Lond. 1987; FRCS Ed. 1995. Career Regist. Rotat. (Orthop. Surg.) Guy's Hosp. Lond. Specialty: Orthop. Socs: Brit. Assn. Sport & Med.; Brit. Assn. Immed. Care Schemes; Brit. Orthop. Train. Assn. Prev: SHO (Gen. Surg.) Joyce Green Hosp. Kent; SHO (Cardiothoracic Surg.) Roy. Brompton Nat. Heart & Lung Hosp. Lond.; SHO (Plastic Surg.) St. Thos. Hosp. Lond.

WOOD, John Gervase (retired) Pinkneys Farm House, Fressingfield, Eye IP21 5SA Tel: 01379 586504 — BM BCh Oxf. 1958; MA Oxf. 1958. Prev: Princip. GP Oxf.

WOOD, John Hay (retired) 24 The Villas, London Road, Stoke-on-Trent ST4 5AQ Tel: 01782 411700/44237 — MB ChB Aberd. 1942; DPH 1947.

WOOD, John Kevin Yardley Wood Health Centre, 401 Highfield Road, Yardley Wood, Birmingham B14 4DU Tel: 0121 474 5186 Fax: 0121 436 7648; 83 St. Bernards Road, Solihull B92 7DF — MB ChB Birm. 1973.

WOOD, John Ramsay The Hollies, Auchenblae, Laurencekirk AB30 1XR Tel: 0156 12 220 — MB ChB Aberd. 1953; Dip. Soc. Med. Ed. 1968; FRSE 1980. Prev: Wing Cdr. RAF Med. Br.

WOOD, John Reginald Pinecones, Salisbury Road, St Margaret's Bay, Dover CT15 6DP Tel: 01304 853386 Fax: 01304 853686 Email: pinecones@compuserve.com/jrwpinecones@cs.com — MB BChir Camb. 1954 (Guy's) MRCS Eng LRCP Lond. 1953; DObst RCOG 1955; MRCGP 1963; DIH Soc. Apoth. Lond. 1971; MFOM RCP Lond. 1980; BA Camb. 1950, MA 1980. Med. Off. (Occupat. Health) Medway Hosp. Specialty: Occupat. Health; Gen. Pract. Socs:

Soc. Occupat. Med.; W Kent M-C Soc.; Roy. Soc. Med. Prev: Course Organiser Lond. (Brook Hosp.) VTS; Med. Off. Woolwich Bldg. Soc.; Apptd. Fact. Doctor Greenwich Dist.

WOOD, John Richard 63 Hemingford Gardens, Leven Park, Yarm TS15 9ST Tel: 01642 786895 — MB ChB Dundee 1980; DRCOG 1983; MRCGP 1984; Dip Occ Med 1997.

WOOD, John Roland Gastrointestinal & Metabolic diseases, Glaxowellcome R & D, Stockley Park W., Uxbridge Tel: 020 8990 8201 Fax: 020 8990 8150; Linden House, 4 Fulmer Drive, Gerrards Cross SL9 7HJ — MRCS Eng. LRCP Lond. 1978 (King's Coll. Hosp.) FFPM RCP; PhD Lond. 1988, BSc (Hons.) 1973, MB BS 1978. Dir Therapeutic Develop & product Strategy; Hon. Sen. Lect. Roy. Free Hosp. Sch. Med. Lond. Specialty: Pharmaceutical Medicine. Socs: Brit. Soc. Gastroenterol. & Physiol. Soc. Prev: Regist. Liver Unit King's Coll. Hosp. Lond.; SHO Brompton Hosp. Lond.; SHO Nat. Hosp. for Nerv. Dis. Lond.

WOOD, John Vaughan 101 Lightwater Meadow, Lightwater GU18 5XJ — MB ChB Manch. 1998.

WOOD, Jonathan Altham Brooklea Health Centre, Wick Road, Brislington, Bristol BS4 4HU Tel: 0117 711211 — BChir Camb. 1981; DCH RCP Lond. 1985; DRCOG 1985; Dip in Med Sci (Gen Practt) Birm. 1999. Specialty: Community Child Health; Gen. Pract.; Alcohol & Substance Misuse.

WOOD, Jonathan Mark David 16A Harriotts Lane, Ashtead KT21 2QH — MB ChB Manch. 1998.

WOOD, Jonathan Stuart Square Surgery, 66 The Square, Hartland, Bideford EX39 6BL Tel: 01237 441200; Burley House, 10 Tudor Close, Northam, Bideford EX39 3QD Tel: 01237 421138 — MB ChB Sheff. 1987; MRCGP 1992; DRCOG 1994. GP Hartland. Prev: SHO Barnsley Dist. Gen. Hosp. VTS; Ho. Off. (Gen. Med. & Surg.) Barnsley Dist. Gen. Hosp.

WOOD, Joseph Keith Department of Haematology, BUPA Hospital, Gartree Road, Leicester LE2 2FF Tel: 0116 265 3663 Fax: 0116 265 3673; Porters, Bowden Road, Thorpe Langton, Market Harborough LE16 7TP Tel: 01858 540225 Email: jkwood@home.gb.com — MB ChB Manch. 1962; FRCP Ed. 1978, M 1969; FRCPath 1982, M 1970; MRCP (UK) 1971; FRCP Lond. 1985. Cons. Haemat.Bupa and Nuffield Hosp.s Leicester; Hon. Sen. Lect.Path.. Univ. of Leicester. Specialty: Haematology. Socs: Mem.(Chairm. & Past Pres.) Leicester Med. Soc.; Brit. Soc. Haematol. Prev: Lect. (Haemat.) Univ. Edin.; Regist. (Haemat.) Univ. W. Indies; Regist. (Clin. Haemat.), Ho. Phys. & Ho. Surg. Roy. Infirm. Manch.

WOOD, Joyce Dorothy (retired) Garth Soar, Talsarnau LL47 6UW Tel: 01766 770227 — MB BS Lond. 1952 (Guy's) MRCS Eng. LRCP Lond. 1952; DCH Eng. 1956; DObst RCOG 1956; DPH Lond. 1960; MFCM 1974.

WOOD, Julie Anne 8 Friars Close, Colchester CO4 0SA — MB BS Lond. 1994.

WOOD, Katie Anne 45A Uplands Road, London N8 9NN — MB BS Lond. 1996.

WOOD, Katrina Mackay 4 Borras Park Road, Wrexham LL12 7TG — BM BCh Oxf. 1989.

WOOD, Kenneth Albert Carrick CMHT, 57 Pydar Street, Truro TR1 2SS Tel: 01872 356000 — MB ChB Bristol 1983; MRCPsych 1987; MSc Keele 1992; FRCPsych 2002. Cons. Psychiat. Cornw. Healthcare NHS Trust. Specialty: Gen. Psychiat. Socs: Brit. NeuroPsychiat. Assn. Bioethics. Prev: Cons. Psychiat. Highland HB; Lect. (Psychogeriat.) Univ. Newc.; Cons. Psychiat. Grampian Primary Care Trust.

WOOD, Kenneth Duncan (retired) Bridge House, Snape, Bedale DL8 2SZ Tel: 01677 470529 — MB ChB Leeds 1939. Prev: GP Spennymoor.

WOOD, Mr Kenneth Fowler (retired) 26 Southernhay Road, Leicester LE2 3TJ Tel: 0116 270 3081 — (Leeds & Washington Univ. St. Louis) MB ChB (Hons.) Leeds 1946; MD Washington Univ. St. Louis 1947; FRCS Eng. 1952; ChM Leeds 1961; DSc Leic 1980. Edr. of Bull. of the Med. Sch. Univ. of Leicester. Prev: Emerit. Cons. Surg. Roy. Infirm. Leicester & Leicester Gen. Hosp.

WOOD, Mr Laurence Edward Peter Walsgrave Hospital, Coventry; 6 Dalton Road, Earlsdon, Coventry CV5 6PB Tel: 0121 777 8550 — MB ChB Liverp. 1976; FRCS Eng. 1981; DTM & H Liverp. 1982; MRCOG 1990. Cons. (O & G) Univ. Hosp.s of coventry & Warks.; Hon. Sen. Lect., Univ. of Warwick; O & G Train. Progr. Director Univ. Hosp. of Coventry & Warks.; Assoc. Postgrad. Dean for Med. Educat. W. Midl.s Region. Specialty: Obst. & Gyn. Prev: Director of Educat. Nat. Counc. Governance Support Team.

WOOD, Margaret Columbia University, College of Physicians & Surgeons, 630 West 168th Street, P & S Box 46, New York 10032, USA Tel: 00 1 212 3053117 Fax: 00 1 212 3053296; 77 Strathern Road, Broughty Ferry, Dundee DD5 1PG — MB ChB St. And. 1970; FFARCS Eng. 1974; Dip. Amer. Bd Anaesth. 1996. Prof. & Chairm. Dept. Anesthesiol. Columbia Univ. Coll. Phys. & Surgs. NY, USA. Specialty: Anaesth. Socs: Pres. Assn. Univ. Anaesth. 1996-1998; Anaesth. Res. Soc. & Amer. Soc. Anaesth. Prev: Prof. Anesthesiol. Vanderbilt Univ., Nashville, TN, USA.

WOOD, Margaret Ann Wilverley, 22 High St, Castor, Peterborough PE5 7BB — BM BS Nottm. 1987; BMedSci Nottm. 1985. Clin. Asst. (Rheum.) P'boro. Specialty: Rehabil. Med.; Rheumatol. Prev: Trainee GP P'boro. VTS; Ho. Off. (Med. & Surg.) Roy. Vict. Hosp. Bournemouth.

WOOD, Margaret Caie (retired) 7 Pinefield, Inchmarlo, Banchory AB31 4AF Tel: 01330 825952; 21 Whinnyfold Village, Peterhead AB42 0QH Tel: 01779 812330 — MB ChB Aberd. 1947; DObst RCOG 1952; MFCM RCP (UK) 1973. Prev: Community Phys. (Child Health) Wirral HA.

WOOD, Margaret Elizabeth Ramblin, Yearngill, Aspatria, Carlisle CA7 3JX Tel: 0169 73 21161 — MB BS Lond. 1975 (Univ. Coll. Hosp.) MRCS Eng. LRCP Lond. 1975; DRCOG 1978.

WOOD, Margaret Laura Rotherham District General Hospital, Moorgate Road, Oakwood, Rotherham S60 2UD Tel: 01709 304160 Fax: 01709 304481 — MB ChB (Hons.) Sheff. 1977; MRCP 1980; FRCP Lond. 1995. Cons. Dermat. Rotherham Dist. Gen. Hosp. Specialty: Dermat.

WOOD, Marion Elizabeth Department of Haematology, Colchester General Hospital, Turner Road, Colchester CO4 5JL — MB BS Lond. 1980; FRCP 1998; FRCPath 2000. Cons. Haemat. Colchester Gen. Hosp. Specialty: Haematology. Prev: Sen. Regist. (Haemat.) Roy. Free Hosp. Lond.

WOOD, Mark Bailey 118 Ringwood Road, Christchurch BH23 5RF — MB BChir Camb. 1990; MA Camb. 1989, MB BChir 1990.

WOOD, Mark Edward Newcastle General Hospital, Westgate Road, Newcastle upon Tyne NE4 6BE — MB BChir Camb. 1996 (Cambridge) MRCPCH 2000. Specialist Regist. Newc. Specialty: Paediat. Prev: SHO (Paediat.) Newc.

WOOD, Martin James 118 Craigmount Avenue N., Edinburgh EH4 8HJ — MB ChB Aberd. 1997.

WOOD, Mr Martin Keith West Suffolk Hospital, Hardwick Lane, Bury St Edmunds IP33 2QZ Tel: 01284 713000 — MB BS Lond. 1987; BA (Oxf.) 1984; FRCS Eng. 1992; FRCS 1998. Cons. Orthopaedic Surg., W. Suff. Hosp., Bury St Edmunds. Specialty: Orthop. Prev: SHO (Plastic Surg.) Char. Cross Hosp. Lond.; Ho. Off. (Surg.) St. Mary's Hosp. Lond.; SHO (Orthop.) Northwick Pk. Hosp. Harrow.

WOOD, Mary Polmener, Mullion, Helston TR12 7DH — MB ChB Bristol 1952. Prev: Cas. Off. Southmead Hosp. Bristol; Res. Med. Off. Bruce Melville Wills Memor. Hosp. Bristol; Civil Med. Pract. Depot. King's Afr. Rifles Nakuru, Kenya.

WOOD, Mary Elspeth (retired) Eastlea, Harlow Road, Roydon, Harlow CM19 5HE — (King's Coll. Hosp.) MSc (Physiol.) Lond. 1950, MB BS 1955; MRCS Eng. LRCP Lond. 1955; DCH Eng. 1959. Prev: Regist. (Paediat.) Southend Gen. Hosp.

WOOD, Mary Margaret (retired) 38 Church Crescent, Whetstone, London N20 0JP Tel: 020 8368 6951 Fax: 020 8368 6951 Email: margaret@christaret.demon.co.uk — BM BCh Oxf. 1957 (Oxf. & St. Bart. Hosp.) Prev: Assoc. Specialist (Microbiol.) Watford Gen. Hosp.

WOOD, (Mary) Philippa Woodview Medical Centre, 26 Holmecross Road, Thorplands, Northampton NN3 8AW Tel: 01604 670780 Fax: 01604 646208 — MB BS Newc. 1977; DA Eng. 1980; MRCGP 1984. Specialty: Gen. Pract. Prev: Clin. Med. Off. (Child Health) Newc.; Regist. (Geriat. & Gen. Med.) Dryburn Hosp. Durh.; Regist. (Anaesth.) Dryburn Hosp. Durh.

WOOD, Matthew John Andrew Universtiy of Oxford, Department of Human Anatomy, South Parks Road, Oxford OX1 3QX — MB ChB Cape Town 1987.

WOOD, Matthew Laurence Berry Anaesthetic Department, Queen Alexandra Hospital, Cosham, Portsmouth PO6 3LY — MB ChB Manch. 1984; MRCP (UK) 1988; FRCA 1988. Cons. Anaesth.

Qu. Alexandra Hosp. Portsmouth. Specialty: Anaesth.; Paediat.; Vasc. Med. Socs: Assn. Anaesth. & Obst. Anaesth. Soc.; Assn Dent. Anaesth. Prev: Sen. Regist. (Anaesth.) St. Geo. Hosp. Lond.; Regist. (Anaesth.) Char. Cross Hosp. Lond.

WOOD, Melanie 118 Acre Lane, Brixton, London SW2 5RA; 75b Nightingale Lane, London SW12 8LY — MB BS Lond. 1996 (Charing Cross & Westminster) MRCP 1999. Specialty: Gen. Med.

WOOD, Michael Charles Ridgeways, The Stream, Catsfield, Battle TN33 9BD — MD Dub. 1941 (T.C. Dub.) MA Dub. 1947, BA 1936, MB BCh BAO 1937; DMR Lond 1947. Emerit. Cons. Croydon AHA. Prev: Cons. Radiol. Lewisham Hosp. Gp.; Dep. Dir. X-Ray Dept. Roy. Marsden Hosp. Lond.; Surg. Lt.-Cdr. RNVR.

WOOD, Michael Johnson Dundonald Medical Practice, 9 Main Street, Dundonald, Kilmarnock KA2 9HF Tel: 01563 850496 Fax: 01563 850426; 15 Kilnford Crescent, Dundonald, Kilmarnock KA2 9DW — MB ChB Glas. 1985; MRCGP 1989.

WOOD, Michael Keith 11 Fortinbras Way, Chelmsford CM2 9JA — MB BS Lond. 1992; BSc (Hons) 1989; MRCP 1996. Specialist Regist. (Thoracic Med.) N. E. Thames Region. Specialty: Respirat. Med.; Gen. Med. Prev: SHO (A & E) Mayday Univ. Hosp. Thornton Heath.

WOOD, Michael Richard Duncan Spennymoor Health Centre, Bishops Close, Spennymoor DL16 6ED Tel: 01388 811455 Fax: 01388 812034 — MB BS Newc. 1974; MRCGP 1978; MA Durham 1999. GP Sen. Partner; Company Med. Off. Weardale Railway Company Ltd. Co. Durh. Socs: BMA; Roy. Coll. Gen. Pract. Prev: Company Med. Off. Black & Decker Ltd. Co. Durh.

WOOD, Michael William Wellesley (retired) Wickham Orchard, Overdale Road, Willaston, Neston, South Wirral CH64 1SZ Tel: 0151 327 4779 Fax: 0151 327 4779 — MB BChir Camb. 1940 (St. Mary's) MRCS Eng. LRCP Lond. 1940; FRCP Lond. 1970, M 1947; MD Camb. 1949. Cons. Phys. Clatterbridge Hosp. Bebington; Vis. Cons. Phys. Hoylake Cottage Hosp. Prev: Chief Asst. (Med.) W. Middlx. Hosp.

WOOD, Miriam Anne Mount Street Surgery, 69 Mount Street, Coventry CV5 8DE Tel: 024 7667 2277 Fax: 024 7671 7352 Email: miriam.wood@nhs.net; 6 Dalton Road, Earlsdon, Coventry CV5 6PB Tel: 024 76 673841 — MB ChB Liverp. 1977; DTM & H Liverp. 1982. GP Coventry.

WOOD, Monica Jane School Lane Surgery, School Lane, Washingborough, Lincoln LN4 1BN Tel: 01522 792360 Fax: 01522 794144; Woodlands, Barff Road, Potterhanworth, Lincoln LN4 2DU Tel: 01522 791726 — MB BS Lond. 1980. Prev: Trainee GP Lincoln VTS.

WOOD, Nicholas James 19 Ivygreen Road, Manchester M21 9FF — MB BS Lond. 1994.

WOOD, Nicholas John — MB ChB Manch. 1991; MRCGP 2001. GP Locum; Clin. Asst. (Psychiat.) Westmorland Gen. Hosp. Kendal; Med. Mem. Appeals Tribunal. Specialty: Gen. Pract.

WOOD, Nicholas Simon 55 Brighton Terrace Road, Crookes, Sheffield S10 1NT Tel: 0114 266 3479 — MB ChB Sheff. 1991; MRCP (UK) 1997. Clin. Research Fell. - Neonatology Univ. Nottm. Dept. Child Health City Hosp. Nottm. Specialty: Neonat.

WOOD, Professor Nicholas William National Hospital for Neurology & Neurosurgery, Queen Square, London WC1N 3BG Tel: 020 7837 3611 Fax: 020 7278 5616 Email: n.wood@ion.ucl.ac.uk — MB ChB Birm. 1986; MRCP (UK) 1989; PhD Camb. 1995; FRCP 2000. Prof. & Hon. Cons. Neurol. Nat. Hosp. Neur. Hosp. Lond. Specialty: Neurol. Socs: Assn. Brit. Neurols.; Edit. Bd. Mem. Movement Disorder Soc.; Amer. Soc. Human Genetics. Prev: Sen. Lect. & Hon. Cons. Neurol. Nat. Hosp. Neurol. & Neurosurg. Lond.; Regist. (Neurol.) Nat. Hosp. Neurol. & Neurosurg. Lond. & Addenbrooke's Hosp. Camb.; Lect. (Neurol.) Inst. Neurol. Nat. Hosp. Neurol. & Neurosurg. Lond.

WOOD, Nicola Rachel Watermeadow Surgery, 31A Red Lion Street, Chesham HP5 1ET — MB ChB Bristol 1998. GP Chesham. Specialty: Gen. Pract. Socs: Exec. Comm. BMA Bucks.Div. Prev: PRHO High Wycombe Stoke Mandeville Hosp.

WOOD, Mr Nigel The Great Sutton Medical Centre, Old Chester Road, Great Sutton, South Wirral CH66 3PB Tel: 0151 339 2424; Jalna, Upper Raby Road, Neston, South Wirral CH64 7TZ — MB ChB Liverp. 1979; BSc (Hons.) Anat. Liverp. 1975, MB ChB 1979; FRCS Ed. 1984; DRCOG 1989; Cert. Family Plann. JCC 1989; MRCGP 1990.

WOOD, Nigel Charles Arden Medical Centre, Albany Road, Stratford-upon-Avon CV37 6PG Tel: 01789 414942 Fax: 01789 296427; Park House, Clopton House Gardens, Stratford-upon-Avon CV37 0QR Tel: 01789 296993 — MB BS Lond. 1978 (St. Thos.) MRCP (UK) 1981; DRCOG 1985. Prev: Regist. (Med.) Leeds Infirm.; SHO (Med.) Kidderminster & Dist. HA.

WOOD, Nigel Ewart (retired) Timbers, Sandy Bank, Riding Mill NE44 6HU Tel: 01434 682457 — MB BS Durh. 1944; DObst RCOG 1949; MRCGP 1953. Prev: Orthop. Ho. Surg. & Ho. Phys. Hexham Gen. Hosp.

WOOD, Nigel Ian Jaunty Springs Health Centre, 53 Jaunty Way, Sheffield S12 3DZ Tel: 0114 239 9453; 100 Howard Road, Sheffield S6 3RW Tel: 0114 234 4142 — MB ChB Sheff. 1977; DRCOG 1980.

WOOD, Nigel Robert The Wood Medical Practice, Strathbrock Partnership Centre, 189a West Main Street, Broxburn EH52 5LH Tel: 01506 771800 Fax: 01506 771920; Millburn Cottage, Burnbridge, Linlithgow EH49 6JF — MB ChB Ed. 1976; BSc (Med. Sci.) Ed. 1973, MB ChB 1976; DRCOG 1978; MRCGP 1980. Specialty: Gen. Pract.; Occupat. Health.

WOOD, Patrick Arthur Terence (retired) Coopers, 9 St Edmunds Place, Ipswich IP1 3RA Tel: 01473 230262 — MD Lond. 1961 (St. Bart.) MB BS 1944; DObst RCOG 1951. Prev: Nuffield Trav. Fell. For Gen. Practs. 1961-62.

WOOD, Paul Albert Avery Hodson and Partners, Park Farm Medical Centre, Allestree, Derby DE22 2QN Tel: 01332 559402 Fax: 01332 541001 — BM BS Nottm. 1988; BMedSci (Hons.) 1986; DRCOG 1991.

WOOD, Paul Louis Edward Rockingham Wing, Kettering General Hospital, Rothwell Road, Kettering NN16 8UZ Tel: 01536 492900 Fax: 01536 492871; The Old Vicarage, Dingley Road, Great Bowden, Market Harborough LE16 7ET Tel: 01858 432069 Fax: 01858 431746 Email: plwoldvic@compuserve.com — MB ChB Liverp. 1980; Dip Ven Liverp. 1983; MRCOG 1985; MD Leic. 1990; FRCOG 1998. Cons. O & G Kettering & Dist. Gen. Hosp.; Hon. Sen. Lect. Leicester/Warwick Med. Sch. Specialty: Obst. & Gyn. Special Interest: Minimal Access Surg.; Paediatric & Adolesc. Gyn.; Prenatal Screening. Socs: Expert Witness Inst. Prev: Lect. & Hon. Sen. Regist. (O & G) Univ. Leic.

WOOD, Paul Raymond Major Injuries Unit, Birmingham General Hospital, Steelhouse Lane, Birmingham B4 6NH — MB BCh Wales 1980; FFA RCS Eng. 1986. Specialty: Anaesth.

WOOD, Pauline Elizabeth Ann (retired) Heather Lodge, 87 Gartree Road, Oadby, Leicester LE2 2FE Tel: 0116 270 7888 — MB BS Lond. 1963 (Roy. Free) DA Eng. 1967. Assoc. Specialist (Anaesth.) Leicester Roy. Infirm. Prev: Clin. Asst. Leics. Hospice.

WOOD, Penelope Clare 8 Balmoral Terrace, Heaton, Newcastle upon Tyne NE6 5YA — MB BS Newc. 1996.

WOOD, Peter 4 Orchard Court, Longniddry EH32 0PE — MB ChB Ed. 1970; BDS 1964; FDS RCS Ed. 1973. Lect. Oral Med. & Oral Path. Univ. Sch. Dent. Edin. Socs: BMA; Roy. Odonto-Chir. Soc. Scotl. Prev: Lect. (Oral Med.) Univ. Edin.; Ho. Off. Roy. Infirm. Edin.; Regist. Edin. Dent. Hosp.

WOOD, Peter John Caldwell 8 Ravensbourne Drive, Chelmsford CM1 2SJ; Beauchamp House Surgery, 37 Baddow Road, Chelmsford CM2 0DB Tel: 01245 262255 Fax: 01245 262256 — MB BS Lond. 1983 (Middlx.) DRCOG 1987; DTM & H Liverp. 1988. GP Principal since 1997. Prev: Med. Dir. Kisiizi Hosp. Kabale, Uganda; SHO (Med. for Elderly) Airedale Gen. Hosp. Steeton.

WOOD, Peter John Watson The Grange Consulting Rooms, 92 Whitcliffe Road, Cleckheaton BD19 3DR Tel: 01274 878600 Fax: 01274 869898 Email: drwood@the-grange.org.uk — MB BS Lond. 1971 (St. Bart.) MRCS Eng. LRCP Lond. 1971; MRCPsych 1978; DPM Eng. 1978; FRCP FRCPsych 2000. Indep. Cons. Forens. Psychiat. Bradford. Specialty: Forens. Psychiat.

WOOD, Mr Peter Laurence Rolls Wrightington Hospital, Wigan WN6 9EP Tel: 0125725 6232 Fax: 0125725 6292 Email: peter.wood@wwi.nhs.uk; Orchard Cottage, 25 Canal Bank, Lymm WA13 9NR Email: plrwood@yahoo.com — MB BS Lond. 1971 (Char. Cross) MRCS Eng. LRCP Lond. 1971; FRCS Eng. 1976. Cons. Orthop. Surg. Wrightington Hosp. Wigan. Specialty: Orthop. Special Interest: Surg. for Arthritis of the Foot & Ankle; Total Ankle Replacement; Total Knee Replacement. Socs: Fell. BOA; BMA;

BOFSS. Prev: Fell. Orthop. Surg. St. Luke's Episcopal Hosp. Houston, Texas; Sen. Regist. (Orthop.) NW RHA.

WOOD, Peter Trevor, MBE, Maj. RAMC Retd. Chagford Health Centre, Chagford, Newton Abbot TQ13 8BW Tel: 01647 433320 Fax: 01647 432452 — MB ChB Bristol 1983; DA (UK) 1987; MRCGP 1988; DRCOG 1989; DCCH RCP Ed. 1993; DFFP 1994; Dip. Pract. Dermat. Wales 1994; Dip. IMC RCS Ed. 1994. Prev: Sen. Med. Off. SHAPE BFPO 26 & Family Med. Centre BFPO 23; SHO (O & G) Roy. Shrewsbury Hosp.; Trainee GP/SHO (Anaesth., Paediat. & Geriat.) Roy. Devon & Exeter Hosp.

WOOD, Philip Frank Brambles, 15A Townside, Haddenham, Aylesbury HP17 8BQ Tel: 01844 290878 — MB BCh Wales 1966; DCH Eng. 1968; DObst RCOG 1969; MRCGP 1970; Dip. Pharm. Med. RCP (UK) 1980; FFPM RCP (UK) 1992. Med. Dir. Teva Pharmaceut. Ltd. Specialty: Pharmaceutical Medicine. Prev: Med. Dir. Wellcome UK & Bristol-Myers Squibb Pharmaceut.; Med. Dir. Anthra Pharmaceut. Europe.

WOOD, Philip Fraser Anderson Union Brae Surgery, Union Brae, Tweedmouth, Berwick-upon-Tweed TD15 2HB Tel: 01289 330333 Fax: 01289 331075 — MB ChB Dundee 1982; MRCGP 1987; LFHom RCP Lond. 1996. Socs: Brit. Med. Acupunct. Soc.

WOOD, Philip Henry Nicholls Bephillick, Duloe, Liskeard PL14 4QA Tel: 01503 264635 — (St. Bart.) MB BS Lond. 1955; FRCP Lond. 1978, M 1971; FFCM 1972; FFPHM 1989. Emerit. Dir. Arthritis & Rheum. Counc. Epidemiol. Research Unit Univ Manch. Prev: Hon. Prof. Community Med. Univ. Manch.; Asst. Research Prof. Med. State Univ. N.Y. Buffalo, USA; Ho. Phys. Brompton Hosp. Lond.

WOOD, Philip Meldrum Laurel House Surgery, 12 Albert Road, Tamworth B79 7JN Tel: 01827 69283 Fax: 01827 318029 — MB BS Lond. 1967; MRCS Eng. LRCP Lond. 1967; MRCP (UK) 1972.

WOOD, Philip Michael Dawson Department of Clinical Chemistry and Immunology, Leeds General Infirmary, Great George Street, Leeds LS1 3EX Tel: 0113 392 2340 — MB BS Newc. 1991; BMedSc (Hons.) Newc. 1988; MRCP (UK) 1994; DPhil Oxon. 1997; MRCPath 2001. Specialist Regist. (Clin. Immunol.) Birm. Heartlands Hosp. Birm.; Cons. Immunol., Leeds Teachg. Hosp. Specialty: Immunol. Prev: Research Fell. Molecular Immunol. Gp. Nuffield Dept. Med. Oxf.; SHO (Med.) Newc. Hosps.; Clin. Lect. in Immunol., Birm. Univ.

WOOD, Philip Milton Wood, The Surgery, Chapel Road, Norwich NR11 7NN Tel: 01263 768602 Fax: 01263 761340; Smithy Cottage, The Loke, Bessingham, Norwich NR11 7JR — MB BChir Camb. 1984; MA Camb. 1985, BA 1981. Prev: SHO Gt. Yarmouth & Waveney, Norwich & P'boro. HAs.

WOOD, Philippa Jane University Hospital of North Durham, North Road, Durham DH1 5TW Tel: 0191 333 2333 Email: philippa.j.wood@lineone.net; 3 Rose Acre, Shincliffe, Durham DH1 2NT Tel: 0191 383 2410 — MB BS Lond. 1985 (Char. Cross & Westm.) DA (UK) 1987; FRCA 1990. Cons. Anaesth. Univ. Hosp. of N. Durh. Specialty: Anaesth. Socs: Mem. of Obstetric Assn. of Anaesth.s. Prev: Sen. Regist. (Anaesth.) Middlx. Hosp. Lond.

WOOD, Rachel Mary Flat 10, Arundel House, 21 Lawn Road, Portswood, Southampton SO17 2ER; 1 Hunters Mead, Hawkesbury Upton, Badminton GL9 1BL — BM Soton. 1998. PRHO Gen.Med.Roy.Bournemouth.Hosp. Prev: PRHO Gen.Surg.Poole.Gen.Hosp.

WOOD, Rachel Sarah 15 Wasley Close, Fearnhead, Warrington WA2 0DH — MB BS Newc. 1998.

WOOD, Raymond Anthony Berry Wraysdale House Surgery, Wraysdale House, Coniston LA21 8ES Tel: 015394 41205 — LRCPI & LM, LRSCI & LM 1971 (RCSI) DObst RCOG 1974. GP Coniston. Socs: Irish Coll. Gen. Pract.; BMA; Assoc. Mem. RCGP. Prev: Princip. GP Merseyside; Ho. Off. (Med. & Surg.) & SHO (O & G) Birch Hill Hosp. Rochdale; GP & GP Tutor King Fahd Milit. Hosp. Jeddah, Saudi Arabia.

WOOD, Rebecca Jane 103 Hunter House Road, Sheffield S11 8TX Tel: 0114 268 2159 — MB ChB Sheff. 1991; DRCOG 1996. Specialty: Gen. Pract.

WOOD, Rhian Copper Beeches, Theescombe Lane, Amberley, Stroud GL5 5AZ Tel: 01453 872671 — MB BS Lond. 1976; MRCS Eng. LRCP Lond. 1976.

WOOD, Richard Hamilton (retired) The Surgery, Moor View, Hinderwell, Saltburn-by-the-Sea TS13 5HH — MB BS Lond. 1971 (St. Mary's) Prev: GP Saltburn-by-the-Sea.

WOOD, Richard Holman (retired) Morva, Gillan, Manaccan, Helston TR12 6HG Tel: 01326 231560 — MB ChB Bristol 1948. Prev: Clin. Asst. Chelmsford & Essex Hosp.

WOOD, Richard John Rhinns Medical Centre, Port Charlotte, Isle of Islay PA48 7UD Tel: 01496 850210 Fax: 01496 850511; Coultorsay House, Isle of Islay PA49 7UN Tel: 01496 850298 — (Lond. Hosp.) MB BS Lond, 1966; MRCS Eng. LRCP Lond. 1966; DObst RCOG 1968. GP Princip. Prev: SHO (Obst.) St. John's Hosp Chelmsford; Ho. Phys. & Ho. Surg. Roy. Cornw. Hosp. Treliske.

WOOD, Mr Richard Mountford Thellusson 1 Plough Court, Roskrow, Penryn TR10 9AP Tel: 01326 378298 Fax: 01326 375622 Email: rmtwood@aol.com — (St. Bartholomews Hospital) MB BS Lond. 1966; FRCS Ed. 1973. Specialty: Gen. Pract.; Psychother. Prev: GP Hong Kong.

WOOD, Richard Neil Ashley Gateacre Brow Surgery, 1 Gateacre Brow, Liverpool L25 3PA Tel: 0151 428 1851 — MB ChB Bristol 1983; DA (UK) 1986; DRCOG 1991; MRCGP 1992. Prev: Trainee GP Blackpool VTS; S.C.C. Roy. Navy.

WOOD, Robert Allen Heady Hill Surgery, Heys Lane, Heywood OL10 3RB Tel: 0161 761 1775; 10 Mount Pleasant, Nangreaves, Bury BL9 6SP — MB ChB Manch. 1988; MRCGP 1993; DFFP 1993.

WOOD, Professor Robert Anderson (retired) Ballomill House, Abernethy, Perth PH2 9LD; Ballomill House, Abernethy, Perth PH2 9LD Tel: 01738 850201 — MB ChB Ed. 1963; BSc (Hons.) Ed. 1961; FRCP Ed. 1976, M 1966; FRCS Ed. 1994; FRCP Glas. 1997; FRCPsych 1999. Treas. RCP Edin.; Head of Counc. & Managem. Comm. MODUS; Mem. Criminal Injuries Compensation Appeal Panel. Prev: Cons. Phys. Perth & Kinross Health Dist.

WOOD, Mr Robert Anthony Bowness Ward 10, Ninewells Hospital and Medical School, Dundee DD1 9SY Tel: 01382 660111 Fax: 01382 633994; Lubnaig, 442 Blackness Road, Dundee DD2 1TQ Tel: 01382 667547 — MB ChB Leeds 1965; MRCP (London) 1969; FRCS Eng. 1971; FRCS Ed. 1981. Cons. Surg. Dundee Teachg. Hosp. Trust; Hon. Sen. Lect. (Surg.) Ninewells Hosp. Dundee. Specialty: Gen. Surg. Socs: Surgic. Research Soc.; Brit. Soc. Gastroenterol. Prev: Lect. (Surg.) Univ. Hosp. of Wales Cardiff; Regist. (Surg.) Norf. & Norwich Hosp.; SHO (Med.) York City Hosp.

WOOD, Mr Robert Anthony Bowness Ward 10, NineWells Hospital DD1 9SY Tel: 01382 660 111 Fax: 01382 633 994 — MRCP Lond. 1969; MB ChB Leeds 1965; FRCS Eng. 1970; FRCSE Edin. 1981. Gen. Surg.. Ninewells Hosp., Dundee; Clin. Ldr., Gen. Surg. UK; Intercollieciate Examr., Gen. Surg.. UK. Specialty: Gen. Surg. Special Interest: Breast; Colon. Socs: Severe Acute Respirat. Syndrome; Brit. Soc. of Gastroenterol.; Assn. of Surg., Gt. Britian & Irel.

WOOD, Robin UKAEA, Harwell, Didcot OX11 0RA Tel: 01235 435296 Fax: 01235 435018; 6A Gravel Lane, Drayton, Abingdon OX14 4HY — MB ChB Sheff. 1971; DIH Eng. 1980; MFOM Eng. 1982. Chief Med. Adviser Ukaea. Specialty: Occupat. Health. Socs: Soc. Occupat. Med.

WOOD, Robin Gaythorn Bramma Drayton Medical Practices, The Health Centre, Cheshire Street, Market Drayton TF9 3BS Tel: 01630 652158 — MB ChB Manch. 1971; DObst RCOG 1973.

WOOD, Rosemary Ann (retired) 1 Blenkarne Road, London SW11 6HZ Tel: 020 7228 9071 — MB ChB Bristol 1962.

WOOD, Sally Margaret Westway Surgery, 1 Wilson Road, Ely, Cardiff CF5 4LJ Tel: 029 2059 2351 Fax: 029 2059 9956 — MB BS Lond. 1982; MRCGP 1986. Forens. Med. Examr. Socs: Assn. Forens. Physicians; Wales Medico-Legal Soc.; Cardiff Med. Soc.

WOOD, Sarah Augusta Claremont Clinic, 459-463 Romford Road, Forest Gate, London E7 8AB Tel: 020 8522 0222 Fax: 020 8522 0444 Email: gussett74@yahoo.co.uk — MB BS Lond. 1980 (London) BSc Lond. 1977, MB BS 1980.

WOOD, Sarah Elizabeth 'Woodbank', Slades Road, Golcar, Huddersfield HD7 4NE Tel: 01484 652659 Fax: 01484 845080 — MB ChB Leeds 1996. SHO/GP Registr. (O & G), HGH. Prev: SHO (A&E), Ryde Hosp.; SHO (Paediatr.), Huddersfield.

WOOD, Miss Sarah Jane Yaveside, Herring Lane, Coston, Norwich NR9 4DT Email: woodwin@hotmail.com — MB BChir Camb. 1992 (Cambridge) MA Camb. 1992; FRCS (Eng.) 1996;

MChir 2000. Specialist Regist. (Urol.) Inst. Urol. & Nephrol. Lond. Specialty: Urol. Socs: BAUS; RCS (Eng.). Prev: SHO (Gen. Surg. & Urol.) Hinchingbrooke Hosp. Huntingdon.

WOOD, Sarah Morwenna — MB BS Lond. 1991; BA Oxf. 1983; MRCP (UK) 1994. Cons. & Hon. Sen. Lect. Specialty: Nephrol.; Gen. Med. Prev: Clin. Lect./Hon SpR Univ. of Edin. S. E. Scotl. Postgrad. Med. Educat. Bd. Roy. Infirm. of Edin.

WOOD, Sheila Alice (retired) 10 Grange Road, Bushey WD23 2LE — MB BS Lond. 1954 (Roy. Free) MRCS Eng. LRCP Lond. 1954; DObst RCOG 1956. Prev: Late GP Hemel Hempstead.

WOOD, Sheila Margaret Ballomill, Abernethy, Perth PH2 9LS Tel: 0173 885201 — MB ChB St. And. 1965. Regist. (Med.) Perth & Kinross Health Dist. Prev: Ho. Phys. St. Chas. Hosp. Lond.; Ho. Surg. Vict. Centr. Hosp. Wallasey; Asst. Lect. in Path. Univ. Dundee.

WOOD, Mr Simon Harold Charing Cross Hospital, Fulham Palace Road, London W6 8RF Tel: 020 8846 1720 — MB BS Lond. 1986; FRCS ed. 1990; FRCS ((Plast.)) 1997. Cons. Plastic Surg., Char. Cross Hosp., Lond.; Cons. Plast. Surg., St Mary's Hosp., Paddington, Lond. Specialty: Plastic Surg.; Paediat. Socs: Brit Assn. Of Plastic Surg.; Brit. Assn. Of Head & Neck Oncologists. Prev: Sen Regist. (Plastic Surg.) Addenbrookes. Camb.

WOOD, Simon Jon 18 Mardley Hill, Welwyn AL6 0TN; 17 Sandfield Road, Gateacre, Liverpool L25 3PE Tel: 0151 421 1245 — MB ChB Liverp. 1990 (Liverpool) MRCOG 1995. Research Fell. Reproductive Med. Unit Liverp. Wom.s Hosp. Specialty: Obst. & Gyn.

WOOD, Simon Marshall (retired) 3 St Leonards Road, Exeter EX2 4LA Tel: 01392 437435 — MB BChir Camb. 1964 (Camb. & Guy's) MRCS Eng. LRCP Lond. 1963; FRCOG 1981, M 1968, DObst 1966; MD Birm. 1974. Prev: Cons. O & G Roy. Devon & Exeter Hosp.

WOOD, Simon Morley 3 Barmby Avenue, York YO10 4HX — MB ChB Leeds 1980; MRCPsych 1984; MMedSc Leeds 1985.

WOOD, Simon Murray 9 Heathfield Road, Chelmsford CM1 7BZ — MB BS Lond. 1993; BSc (Hons. Human Genetics) Lond. 1992. SHO (Med. for Elderly People) Whipps Cross Hosp. Lond. Prev: SHO (A & E) Basildon Hosp. Essex; SHO (Psychiat.) E. Ham Memor. Hosp.; Ho. Off. (Surg.) Homerton Hsop. Lond.

WOOD, Stephanie Joan Northfield Health Centre, Northfield Road, Narberth SA67 7AA Tel: 01834 860316 Fax: 01834 861394; 4 Minwear Wood, Martletwy, Narberth SA67 8AA Tel: 01437 541305 — MB ChB Bristol 1983. GP Narberth. Prev: Trainee GP Withybush Hosp. HaverfordW..

WOOD, Stephen 4 Jubilee Cottages, Throwley Forstal, Faversham ME13 0PJ; 4 Jubliee Cottages, Throwley Forstal, Faversham ME13 0PJ Tel: 01795 890485 — MB BS Lond. 1979 (Guy's) BSc Lond. 1976, MB BS 1979; MRCPsych 1983. Sen. Lect. (Psychiat.) UMDS Guy's Hosp. Lond. & Acad. Psychiat. Unit Canterbury; Med. Dir. Canterbury & Thanet Community Healthcare NHS Trust; Cons. Psychiat. St Martin's Hosp. Canterbury. Specialty: Gen. Psychiat. Prev: Cons. Psychiat. Ment. Health Advice Centre Lewisham.

WOOD, Stephen Donnington Health Centre, 1 Henley Avenue, Oxford OX4 4DH Tel: 01865 771313; 12 Old High Street, Headington, Oxford OX3 9HN Tel: 01865 741211 — BM BCh Oxf. 1971 (St. Thos.) Tutor (Gen. Pract.) Oxf. Univ. Prev: SHO Cheltenham Gen. Hosp. & Churchill Hosp. Oxf.; Ho. Surg. St. Thos. Hosp. Lond.

WOOD, Stephen Jarvis Tyndale Oak Lodge, Lower Shockerwick, Bath BA1 7LW Tel: 01225 742376 — MB ChB Birm. 1977. Cons. Med. Advisor to Brit. Inst. for Brain Injured Childr. Bridgewater Som. Specialty: Occupat. Health. Prev: GP Wells Som.; Occupat. Health Phys. Herrison Hosp. Dorchester; Occupational Health Phys., Brit. Aerospace, Bridgewater, Som.

WOOD, Mr Stephen John ENT Department, Wrexham Park Hospital, Slough SL2 4HL; 9 Park Lane, Beaconsfield HP9 2HR — MB ChB Bristol 1987; FRCS Ed. 1992; FRCS Eng. 1992; FRCS Eng. 1994; FRCS (ORL) 1998. Specialist Regist. Rotat. (Otolaryngol.) SW Region/ Cons. Sen. Lect. & Hon. Cons. Otolaryngol., Head & Neck Surg.; Fell. in Head & Neck Surg., Toronto Gen. Hosp.; Cons. Otolaryngologist, Head and Neck Surgeon. Specialty: Otorhinolaryngol. Prev: Clin. research fell., Bristol Roy. Infirm.; SHO Rotat. (Surg.) Bristol Roy. Infirm.; Demonst. (Anat.) Bristol Univ.

WOOD, Mr Stephen Keith (retired) 4 Hook Water Close, Chandlers Ford, Eastleigh SO53 5PS Email: skwchf@compuserve.com — MB ChB Manch. 1958; FRCS Glas. 1965; FRCS Ed. 1968. Prev: Hon. Cons. Soton. Univ. Hosp. Trust.

WOOD, Stuart Fotheringham Dumbarton Road Surgery, 1264 Dumbarton Road, Glasgow G14 9PS Tel: 0141 959 6311 Fax: 0141 954 9759 — MD Glas. 1985; MB ChB 1973; FRCGP 1986, M 1978. Sen. Lect. Gen. Pract. Univ. Glas.; GP Glas. Prev: SHO (Med.) Stobhill Gen. Hosp. Glas.; Ho. Surg. Glas. Roy. Infirm.; Ho. Phys. Stobhill Gen. Hosp. Glas.

WOOD, Suzanne 62 Priory Road, Linlithgow EH49 6BS — MB ChB Glas. 1997; DFFP 2000; DRCOG 2000; MRCGP 2002. GP Slamannan Surgery. Specialty: Paediat. Socs: BMA. Prev: PRHO (Med./Surg.) St Johns Hosp. Livingston; SHO (A+E) St Johns Hosp. Livingston; SHO (Paediat.) St Johns Hosp. Livingston.

WOOD, Suzanne Anne c/o Doctors Mess, Chesterfield and North Derbyshire Royal Hospital, Calow, Chesterfield S44 5BL — MB ChB Sheff. 1997.

WOOD, Sylvia Allena (retired) Chimes Cottage, Sandside, Kirkby-in-Furness LA17 7UA Tel: 01229 889133 — MB ChB Manch. 1959. Prev: Regist. (O & G) Mpilo Hosp. Bulawayo, Rhodesia.

WOOD, Terence Alwyn The Health Centre, Testwood Lane, Totton, Southampton SO40 3ZN Tel: 023 8086 5051 Fax: 023 8086 5050; Rackenford, Pikes Hill Avenue, Lyndhurst SO43 7AX — MB ChB Bristol 1966; MRCGP 1976. Prev: Ho. Phys. & SHO Dept. Path. Southmead Hosp. Bristol; Ho. Surg. Roy. Infirm. Bristol.

WOOD, Thomas Alan 11 Reece Mews, London SW7 3HE Tel: 020 7584 0650 — MB Camb. 1967 (Camb. & St. Bart.) BChir 1966; FRCPath 1987, M 1974. Med. Dir. Selfusion Autologous Blood Serv. Prev: Dep. Dir. S. Lond. Blood Transfus. Centre; Hon. Cons. (Blood Transfus.) St. Geo. Hosp. Lond.; Lect. (Haemat.) St. Geo. Hosp. Med. Sch. Lond.

WOOD, Timothy Charles Anthony The Barn Surgery, Newbury, Gillingham SP8 4XS Tel: 01747 824201 Fax: 01747 825098 — BM Soton. 1986; MRCGP 1992; DRCOG 1992.

WOOD, Vernon (retired) Oratava, Castle Douglas DG7 1PE Tel: 01556 600221 Email: dr.wood@tesco.net — MB ChB St. And. 1966 (St Andrews) Private Involvem. in sports Med. Prev: GP Clifton Nottm. & Mansfield Notts.

WOOD, Wendy Elizabeth Ann The Garden Flat, 1 Talbot Place, Blackheath, London SE3 0TZ — MB BS Lond. 1968; MRCPath 1982; FRCPath 1994. Assoc. Specialist in Chem. Path. Greenwich Dist. Hosp. Specialty: Chem. Path.

WOOD, William Matthew 5 Cavensish Street, Chorley PR6 0RU — MB ChB Ed. 1968.

WOOD-ALLUM, Clare Alison 29 Matchless Close, Northampton NN5 6YE — BM BCh Oxf. 1997.

WOODALL, Nicholas Alexander 94 Kestrel View, Weymouth DT3 5QZ Tel: 01305 814352 Fax: 01305 814352 — MB BS Lond. 1995 (St George's Hosp. Med. Sch., Lond.) Locum GP. Specialty: Gen. Pract.

WOODALL, Nicholas Mark 9C Upton Close, Norwich NR4 7PD — MB ChB Liverp. 1980; FFA RCS Eng. 1985. Cons. Anaesth. Norf. & Norwich Hosp. Specialty: Anaesth. Prev: Sen. Regist. (Anaesth.) Middlx. Hosp. Lond.; Clin. Instruc. Univ. Calif., USA.

WOODALL, Peter Lyndon South Liverpool Child & Family Consultation Team, T Ward, Alder Hey Children's Hospital, Eaton Road, Liverpool Tel: 0151 228 4811 — MB ChB Manch. 1985; Dip. Psychother. Liverp. 1991; MRCPsych 1991. Cons. Child & Adolesc. Psychiat. Roy. Liverp. Childr. NHS Trust. Specialty: Child & Adolesc. Psychiat.

WOODBRIDGE, Kenneth (Surgery), 6 Townsend Road, Southall UB1 1EX Tel: 020 8574 2794 Fax: 020 8893 5463; 13 Lodge Close, Englefield Green, Egham TW20 0JF Tel: 01784 435232 Fax: 01784 893 5463 — (Cardiff) MB BCh Wales 1960. Med. Off. Ultra Electronics. Greenford (Communicats.) & Ultra (Loudwater). Specialty: Gen. Med. Socs: Assoc. Mem. RCGP; Assoc. Mem. Soc. Occupat. Med.

WOODBRIDGE, Kevin Francis Linklet House, North Ronaldsay, Orkney KW17 2BE Tel: 01857 633226 Fax: 01857 633207 — MB ChB Manch. 1972. Prev: SHO (Med.) Withington Hosp. Manch.

WOODBRIDGE, Sylvia (Surgery), 2 Baxters Close, Leicester LE4 0QR Tel: 0116 235 3579; 302 Leicester Road, Cropston, Leicester LE7 7GT Tel: 0116 235 6574 — MB BS Lond. 1951 (Roy. Free) MRCS Eng. LRCP Lond. 1951; CPH 1953.

WOODBURN, Alastair George Medical Centre, 12 East King Street, Helensburgh G84 7QL Tel: 01436 673366 Fax: 01436 679715; 55 John Street, Helensburgh G84 9LZ Tel: 01436 3366 — MB ChB Glas. 1971; BSc Glas. 1967, MB ChB 1971; DObst RCOG 1973; MRCGP 1975.

WOODBURN, Caroline Boreland Farm, Hollybush, Ayr KA6 7ED — MB ChB Glas. 1998.

WOODBURN, Elizabeth Mary Alice Ballyalbana, Ballyclare BT39 — LRCP LRCS Ed. 1962; LRCP LRCS Ed. LRFPS Glas. 1962.

WOODBURN, Kirstie Jane Roayl Victoria Hospital, Craigleith Road, Edinburgh EH4 2DN Tel: 0131 537 5000 — BM BCh Oxf. 1988; MA Oxf. 1985; MRCPsych 1993; MD Ed. 1997. Cons. in Old Age Psychiat. Edin. Specialty: Geriat. Psychiat. Prev: Wellcome Clin. Research Train. Fell. (Psychiat.) Univ. Edin.

WOODBURY-SMITH, Marc Ronald c/o Medical Personnel Department, Tatchbury Mount, Calmore, Totton, Southampton SO40 2RZ — MB ChB Dundee 1993.

WOODCOCK, Arthur Sutton (retired) Dale Garth, 12 Queens Drive, Heswall, Wirral CH60 6SH Tel: 0151 342 4378 — MB ChB Leeds 1944; MD (Distinc.) Leeds 1955; FRCPath 1970, M 1964; FRCOG (ad eundem) 1984.

WOODCOCK, Professor Ashley Arthur North West Lung Centre, Wythenshawe Hospital, Manchester M23 9LT Tel: 0161 291 2398 Fax: 0161 291 5020 — MB ChB Manch. 1975; MRCP (UK) 1977; BSc (1st cl. Hons. Physiol.) Manch. 1972, MD 1982; FRCP Lond. 1992. Cons. Phys. Wythenshawe Hosp. Manch./Prof. Resp. Med. Uni. Manch.; Dir. Regional Dept. of Respirat. Physiol. & Sleep Laborat. Specialty: Respirat. Med. Socs: Eur. Respirat. Soc.; Chairm. Clin. Assembly. Prev: Cons. Phys. Manch. Roy. Infirm.; Sen. Regist. Brompton Hosp. Lond.; Specialist Phys. Gen. Hosp. Bandar Seri Begawan, Brunei.

WOODCOCK, Barrie Ewart University Hospital Aintree, Longmoor Lane, Liverpool L9 7AL; 12 Hartley Road, Birkdale, Southport PR8 4SA — MB ChB Birm. 1977; MA (Physiol. Scs.) Oxf.; MRCP (UK) 1980; FRCPath 1996, M 1984; FRCP Lond. 1995. Cons. haematologist, Aintree Hosps. NHS Trust; Hon. Lect. Univ. Liverp. Specialty: Haematology. Prev: Cons. Haemat. Southport & Ormskirk NHS Trust; Sen. Regist. Rotat. (Haemat.) Sheff. HA; Regist. (Haemat.) Roy. Hallamsh. Hosp. Sheff.

WOODCOCK, Barrington Morton The Oaklands, Liverpool Road, Fiveways, Neston, Wirral CH62 6EL — MB ChB Bristol 1968; DCH Eng. 1973.

WOODCOCK, Clive John Longfield Road Surgery, 1 Longfield Road, Hartshill, Stoke-on-Trent ST4 6QN Tel: 01782 616587 Fax: 01782 719108; 54 The Avenue, Hartshill, Stoke-on-Trent ST4 6DA Tel: 01782 614272 — MB BS Lond. 1978 (St. Bart.) BSc Lond. 1975; DRCOG 1981; FRCGP 1995, M 1984; Dip. Sports Med. Glas. 1992. Specialty: Sports Med.

WOODCOCK, David Roy Peel House Medical Centre, Avenue Parade, Accrington BB5 6RD Tel: 01254 237231 Fax: 01254 389525; 61 Tarn Avenue, Lynwood Park, Clayton-le-Moors, Accrington BB5 5XT Tel: 01254 386064 — MB ChB Manch. 1984; BSc (Med. Sci.) St. And. 1981; DRCOG 1986; Cert. Family Plann. JCC 1987.

WOODCOCK, Justine Frances Namwen, Hoyle Hill, Beare Green, Dorking RH5 4PS — MB BS Lond. 1992. GP Princip., Steying Health Centre, W. Sussex, BN44 3SB. Specialty: Gen. Pract.

WOODCOCK, Kevin Rowland Royal Hampshire County Hospital, Winchester SO22 5DG Tel: 01962 824608 Fax: 01962 825308 Email: kevin.woodcock@weht.swest.nhs.uk — MB BS Lond. 1965 (St Mary's) MSc (Social Med.) Lond. 1973; MFPHM RCP (UK) 1974; MFPM RCP (UK) 1989; FRCP 2002. Cons. Genitourin. Med. Roy. Hants. Co. Hosp. Winchester. Specialty: Genitourinary Medicine; Pub. Health Med.; Pharmaceutical Medicine. Socs: Fell. Roy. Soc. Med.; Brit. Soc. of Sexual Health & HIV; Brit. Soc. of Antimicrobial Chemother. Prev: Pharmaceut. & Medico-Legal Cons. Serenissima Medica Winchester; Cons. & Sen. Lect. (Venereol.) Soton. Univ. Hosps.; Community Med. Specialist (Informat. & Plann.) Kensington, Chelsea & Westm. HAs.

WOODCOCK, Malcolm Gareth Lewin, Flight Lt. RAF Med. Br. MDHU Peterborough Eye Department, Peterborough District Hospital, Peterborough Tel: 01733 874000; 42 Empingham Road, Stamford PE9 2RH Tel: 01780 482268 — BM Soton. 1995 (University of Southampton) BSc (Hons.) Soton 1994. SHO (Opthalmology) PeterBoro. Dist. Hopsital. Specialty: Ophth. Prev: Jun. Med. Off. RAF Laarbruch, Germany.

WOODCOCK, Nicholas Paul 37 Leadley Croft, Copmanthorpe, York YO23 3YX — MB ChB Leeds 1994.

WOODCOCK, Patrick Willis 66 Tachbrook Street, London SW1V 2NA Tel: 020 7834 0654 — MB ChB Birm. 1943; MRCS Eng. LRCP Lond. 1944.

WOODCOCK, Peter James Ribblesdale House Medical Centre, Market Street, Bury BL9 0BU Tel: 0161 764 7241 Fax: 0161 763 3557 — MB ChB Manch. 1973. GP Bury.

WOODCOCK, Peter John 14 Laverdene Drive, Sheffield S17 4HH — MB ChB Sheff. 1989.

WOODCOCK, Thomas Edward Critical Care Directorate, Southampton General Hospital, Tremona Road, Southampton SO16 6YD — MB BS Lond. 1978 (Char. Cross Hosp.) FFA RCS 1982; Mphil Glas. 2002. Cons., Critical Care, Soton. Univ. Hosps. NHS Trust. Specialty: Anaesth. Special Interest: Intens. Care Med. Socs: Assn. of Anaesth.; Europ. Soc. of Intens. care Med.; Soc. of Critical Care Med.

WOODCOCK, Vanessa Emma — MB ChB Liverp. 1997.

WOODD-WALKER, Robert Basil (retired) 35 Lexden Road, Colchester CO3 3PX Tel: 01206 571896 — (St. Mary's) MB BChir Camb. 1959; MRCS Eng. LRCP Lond. 1960; DCH Eng. 1964; FRCP Lond. 1982, M 1966; FRCPCH 1997. Prev: Cons. Paediat. Gen. Hosp. Colchester.

WOODER, Margaret Louise (retired) The Limpet, 6 Overcliff, Port Isaac PL29 3RZ — BM Soton. 1976; MRCOG 1982. Resid. Med. Off. Duchy Hosp. Truro Cornw. Prev: Resid. Med. Off. Portland Hosp. Wom. & Childr. Lond.

WOODFIELD, Martyn Stillmoor House Surgery, Dennison Road, Bodmin PL31 2JJ; Stillmoor House, Bodmin PL31 2QP Tel: 01208 79059 — MB BCh Wales 1984; BSc Wales 1979, MB BCh 1984; MRCGP 1989.

WOODFORD, Ann Riverside, Nesfield Road, Ilkley LS29 0BE Tel: 01943 608193 Fax: 01943 608193 — MB ChB Manch. 1962. Clin. Asst. (Anaesth.) Airedale Gen. Hosp. Specialty: Anaesth. Socs: BMA. Prev: Ho. Surg. & Ho. Phys. Kingston Hosp.

WOODFORD, Charles Philip 2 Deepfields, Radbrook, Shrewsbury SY3 6DP — MB BS Lond. 1974 (Lond. Hosp.) DRCOG 1980; DCH RCP Lond. 1983.

WOODFORD, Derek The Surgery, Church Lane, Elvington, York YO41 5AD; The Old Rectory, Elvington, York YO4 5AD Fax: 01904 608710 — MB BS Lond. 1965 (King's Coll. Hosp.) MRCS Eng. LRCP Lond. 1965; DObst RCOG 1968.

WOODFORD, Henry John 41 Coniston Avenue, West Jesmond, Newcastle upon Tyne NE2 3EY Email: hw002b4614@blueyonder.co.uk — MB BS Lond. 1996; BSc; MRCP.

WOODFORD, Sarah Louise — BChir Camb. 1996; MB 1997.

WOODFORDE, Alec Robert (retired) Knowlewood, 4 Warren Close, Ringwood BH24 2AJ — MRCS Eng. LRCP Lond. 1933 (St. Bart.)

WOODFORDE, Christopher Simon John Peelhouse Medical Plaze, Peelhouse Lane, Widnes WA8 6TN Tel: 0151 424 6221 Fax: 0151 420 5436 Email: csjwoodforde@doctors.org.uk — MB ChB Liverp. 1991; BSc (Hons.) Liverp. 1986. Gen. Pract. Widnes; G.P. Fell. In Resp. Health for Halton P.C.T., Chesh..; Director of R.E.A.C.H. Progr. (Resp. Excellence Across Clin. Care in Halton). Socs: Med. Protec. Soc.; BMA; BASICS.

WOODGATE, Donald John Cardiac Department, Basildon Hospital, Basildon SS16 5NL Tel: 01268 533911 Fax: 01268 520392 — MB BS Lond. 1958 (Lond. Hosp.) DA Eng. 1961; FRCP Lond. 1979, M 1964. Cons. Phys. & Cardiol. & Clin. Dir. Cardiol. & Pharmaceut. Servs. Basildon & Thurrock HA. Specialty: Cardiol. Socs: Brit. Cardiac Soc. Prev: Sen. Regist. (Med.) Roy. Free Hosp. Lond.; Sen. Regist. (Cardiol. & Thoracic Med.) Roy. Free Hosp. Lond.; Ho. Surg. Lond. Hosp.

WOODGATE, Jane Elizabeth Woodgate and Packham, Fairfield Surgery, High Street, Etchingham TN19 7EU Tel: 01435 882306 Fax: 01435 882064; Cople Cottage, Burwash Weald, Etchingham TN19 7LA — MB BS Lond. 1981. Prev: Trainee GP Tunbridge Wells VTS.

WOODGATE, Mark 25B Brighton Road, Stoke Newington, London N16 8EQ — MB BS Lond. 1992. Regist. (Psychiat.) Roy. Lond.

Hosp. Lond. Specialty: Gen. Psychiat. Socs: Inceptor Roy. Coll. Psychiat.

WOODGATE, Mrs Moira Margaret (retired) 12 School Street, Hillmorton, Rugby CV21 4BW Tel: 01788 579170 — (Trinity Coll. Dub. Univ.) MB BCh BAO Dub. 1940. Prev: GP, Surbiton, Surrey.

WOODGER, Bruce Arthur 53 Dowanside Road, Glasgow G12 9DW Tel: 0141 339 1092 — MB ChB Glas. 1946; DPath Eng. 1954; FRCPath 1968; FRIC 1972. Cons. Path. Monklands Dist. Gen. Hosp. Coatbridge. Specialty: Pathology, General. Socs: Assn. Clin. Pathols. & Assn. Clin Biochems. Prev: Capt. RAMC; Cons. Path. Hairmyres Hosp. E. Kilbride; Sen. Lect. Path. Univ. Nairobi, Kenya.

WOODHALL, Andrew John Vernon House, Vernon Road, Heckmondwike WF16 9LU Tel: 01924 402091 — MB BS Lond. 1976 (Roy. Free) BSc Bristol 1967; MSc Lond. 1970, MB BS 1976; DRCOG 1979.

WOODHALL, Cynthia Ruth Whiston Hospital, Warrington Road, Prescot L35 5DR Tel: 0151 430 1452 Fax: 0151 430 1902 — MB ChB Manch. 1971; DRCOG 1977; MRCP (UK) 1979; MRCPCH 1979; FRCP Lond. 1995. Cons. Paediat. Whiston & St. Helens Hosps. Merseyside. Specialty: Paediat. Socs: Liverp. Paed. Soc.; Manch. Med. Soc. Prev: Sen. Regist. (Paediat.) NW RHA; Fell. (Neonat. Paediat.) Dalhowsie Univ. Halifax, Canada; Tutor (Child Health) Manch. Univ.

WOODHAM, Michael John 16 Tyrone Road, Southend-on-Sea SS1 3HF — MB BS Newc. 1980; FFA RCS Lond. 1986. Cons. Anaesth. Southend Hosp. Southend-on-Sea. Specialty: Anaesth. Prev: Sen. Regist. (Anaesth.) St. Geo. Hosp. Lond.

WOODHAM, Sarah Ellen The Hillingdon Hospital, Pield Heath Road, Uxbridge UB8 3NN Tel: 01895 279682 Email: sarah.woodham@thh.nhs.uk — MB BS West Indies 1992; MRCP; MSc 2003. Cons. Rheumat. Specialty: Rheumatol. Socs: RSM; BSR; Brit. Soc. Paediat. & Adolesc. Rheum. (BSPAR).

WOODHAMS, Anna Mary 50 Beverley Terrace, Cullercoats, North Shields NE30 4NU — MB BS Newc. 1996.

WOODHAMS, Lara Jessica The Brambles, 6 Carline Court, Northampton NN3 3RJ — MB BS Lond. 1998.

WOODHAMS, Simon David Worthing Hospital, Lyndhurst Road, Worthing BN11 2DH Tel: 01903 205111 — MB BS Lond. 1990 (St Thomas' Hosp. Lond.) FRCS; FRCS (Urol); MSc. Cons. Urological Surg. and Urological Oncologist. Specialty: Urol.

WOODHEAD, Anne Elizabeth 25 Drakes Way, Portishead, Bristol BS20 6LD Tel: 01272 844594 — MB ChB St. And. 1972; DObst RCOG 1974.

WOODHEAD, Christopher James Department of ENT, Leeds General Infirmary, Great George Street, Leeds LS1 3EX Tel: 0113 392 8034 Fax: 0113 392165 — MB ChB Birm. 1982; FRCS (ENT) Lond. 1988. Cons. in Otolaryngol., Head and neck Surg., Leeds Gen. Infirm.; Cons. in Otolarygology, BUPA Hosp. Leeds. Specialty: Otolaryngol. Special Interest: Otology; Thyroid Disorders.

WOODHEAD, David Magnus John Meopham Medical Centre, Wrotham Road, Meopham, Gravesend DA13 0AH Tel: 01474 814811/814068 Fax: 01474 814699 — MB ChB Manch. 1990.

WOODHEAD, Jill Louise 28 Hungerford Road, Bournemouth BH8 0EH — MB ChB Sheff. 1997.

WOODHEAD, Jonathan Wickham (retired) Upper Magdalen, Allington Park, Bridport DT6 5DD Tel: 01308 423365 — (Lond. Hosp.) MRCS Eng. LRCP Lond. 1951. Prev: SHO (Obst.) Newmarket Hosp.

WOODHEAD, Mark Andrew Manchester Royal Infirmary, Oxford Road, Manchester M13 9WL Tel: 0161 276 4381 Fax: 0161 276 4989 — MB BS Lond. 1979 (King's Coll. Hosp.) BSc (1st cl. Hons.) Lond. 1976; MRCP (UK) 1982; DM Nottm. 1988; FRCP Lond. 1996. Cons. Phys. (Respirat. & Gen. Med.) Manch. Roy. Infirm.; Hon. Lect. Univ. of Manch. Specialty: Respirat. Med. Special Interest: Pneumonia; Respirat. Infec. Socs: Brit. Thorac. Soc. (Sec. Research Comm. 1993-1996); Eur. Respirat. Soc. (Head Respirat. Infec. Sect. 1997-2001). Prev: Sen. Regist. (Respirat. & Gen. Med.) St. Geo. & Brompton Hosps. Lond.; Research Regist. Notts. HA; Ho. Phys. King's Coll. Hosp. Lond.

WOODHEAD, Nicholas Jesse Uplands Medical Practice, Bury New Road, Whitefield, Manchester M45 8GH Tel: 0161 766 8221 Fax: 0171 796 2417 — MB ChB Manch. 1969.

WOODHEAD, Nicola Jane Valkyrie, Whitepost Lane, Meopham, Gravesend DA13 0TH — MB ChB Manch. 1990. SHO (Psychiat.) Maidstone Priority Care Trust. Specialty: Geriat. Psychiat. Prev: SHO (O & G) St. Mary's Hosp. Manch.

WOODHEAD, Patricia Jane Weston General Hospital, Uphill, Weston Super Mare BS23 4TQ — BM Soton. 1979; MRCP (UK) 1982; FRCR 1986; MBA University of Bath 2000. Cons. (Radiol.) Weston Gen. Hosp. Weston Super Mare; Exec. Med. Director, Weston Health Trust. Specialty: Radiol. Prev: Regist. & Sen. Regist. (Radiol.) Univ. Coll Hosp. Lond.; Vis. Lect. Univ. Michigan, USA.

WOODHEAD, Peter Michael Hainslack Farm, Skipton Old Road, Colne BB8 7ER — MB BS Lond. 1983. Regist. Dept. Radiol. Leicester Roy. Infirm. Specialty: Radiol.

WOODHEAD, Richard Leslie (retired) 6 Bankfield Drive, Nab Wood, Shipley BD18 4AD — BM BCh Oxf. 1966 (Univ. Coll. Hosp.) MA Oxf. 1966; FRCP Lond. 1984, M 1969. Prev: Cons. Phys. Roy. Infirm. & St. Luke's Hosp. Bradford.

WOODHEAD, Robert Barry Croft House Surgery, 5 Croft House, 114 Manchester Road, Huddersfield HD7 5JY Tel: 01484 842652 Fax: 01484 348223 — MB ChB Manch. 1975; DRCOG 1978; MRCGP 1987.

WOODHEAD, Roderick John Group Surgery, Normans Place, Off Regent Road, Altrincham WA14 2AB Tel: 0161 928 2424; 9 Thorley Lane, Timperley, Altrincham WA15 7BJ Tel: 0161 980 5011 — MB ChB Manch. 1963.

WOODHEAD, Roxie 15 Moorfield Gardens, Chapeltown, Pudsey LS28 8BW Tel: 0113 256 5477 — MB ChB Leeds 1948. Socs: Bradford M-C Soc. Prev: Med. Off. Community Health Serv. Bradford HA; Ho. Phys. & Ho. Phys. Med. Profess. Unit, St. Jas. Hosp. Leeds; Ho. Phys. Paediat. Dept. Leeds Gen. Infirm.

WOODHEAD, Zoe Mary Surgery, Normans Place, Off Regent St., Altrincham WA14 2AB Tel: 0161 928 2424; 9 Thorley Lane, Timperley, Altrincham WA15 7BJ Tel: 0161 980 5011 — MB ChB Manch. 1963.

WOODHOUSE, Bruce Andrew Dyneley House Surgery, Newmarket Street, Skipton BD23 2HZ Tel: 01756 799311 Fax: 01756 707203; Newton Head, Bank Newton, Gargrave, Skipton BD23 3NT Tel: 01756 749421 Email: bwoodhouse@totalise.co.uk — BMedSci Nottm. 1987; BM BS Nottm. 1989; MRCGP (Distinc.) 1993. GP Skipton. Specialty: Gen. Pract. Prev: Trainee GP Airedale VTS; SHO (Orthop.) Airedale Gen. Hosp.; Ho. Off. (Med.) Nottm. Univ. Hosp.

WOODHOUSE, Carolyn Mary 22 Dennyview Road, Abbots Leigh, Bristol BS8 3RB Tel: 01275 373726 — MB ChB Bristol 1971; MRCGP 1977; D.Occ.Med. RCP Lond. 1996; DDAM 2001. Med. Team Ldr. Med. Serv. Schlumberger SEMA Grp. Specialty: Disabil. Med.; Occupat. Health.

WOODHOUSE, Christopher John Hulme Medical Centre, 175 Royce Road, Hulme, Manchester M15 5TJ Tel: 0161 226 0606 Fax: 0161 226 5644; 44 Kingston Road, Didsbury, Manchester M20 2SB — MB BCh BAO Belf. 1982; DCH RCP Lond. 1987; DRCOG 1987; MRCGP 1991.

WOODHOUSE, Mr Christopher Richard James (Lord Terrington) The Institute of Urology, 48 Riding House Street, London W1W 7EY Tel: 020 7679 9541 Fax: 020 7679 9542 Email: bjui@ucl.ac.uk — MB BS Lond. 1970 (Guy's) MRCS Eng. LRCP Lond. 1970; FRCS Eng. 1975; FEBU 1993. Reader in Adolesc. Urol. & Hon. Cons. Urol. Inst. Urol. Middlx. Hosp. Lond.; Cons. Urol. Roy. Marsden Hosp. Lond.; Hon. Cons. Urol. Hosp. for Childr. Gt. Ormond St.; Hon. Cons. Urol. UCL Hosp. Specialty: Urol. Socs: Fell. Roy. Soc. Med.; Brit. Assn. Urol. Surg.; Soc. Pelvic Surg. Prev: Cons. Urol. St. Geo. Hosp. Lond.; Sen. Regist. (Urol.) St. Peter's Hosps. (Inst. Urol.) Lond.; Regist. (Surg.) Lond. Hosp.

WOODHOUSE, John Government Office for the North East, Citygate House, Gallowgate, Newcastle upon Tyne NE1 4WH; 2 Highbury, West Jesmond, Newcastle upon Tyne NE2 3BX — MB BS Newc. 1984; MA Oxf. 1980; DRCOG 1987; MRCGP 1988; MSc (Pub. Health) Newc. 1991; MFPHM RCP (UK) 1992. Dep. RDPH for N. E., Govt. Office for the N. E., Newc. Specialty: Pub. Health Med. Prev: Cons. Pub. Health Phys. North. & Yorks. RHA; Sen. Regist. (Pub. Health Med.) North. RHA.

WOODHOUSE, Josephine Cecilia 3 Grimston Park Mansion, Grimston Park, Tadcaster LS24 9DB Tel: 01937 835360 — MB ChB Leeds 1975.

WOODHOUSE, Julian Isidoro Jose Antonio — MB BS Lond. 1992 (Roy. Free Hosp. Med. Sch.) MRCGP Lond. 1992; DFFP Roy

Free Hosp. Sch. Med. 1998. RMO 2nd BN The Roy. Gurkha Rifles. Specialty: Gen. Pract. Prev: Resid. Med. Off. & Dep. Post Master; S. Georgia (Brit. Antarctic Territory); Regtl. Med. Off. The Roy. Dragoon Guards.

WOODHOUSE, Kenneth Walter University Department of Geriatric Medicine, Llandough Hospital, Cardiff Tel: 029 2071 6985 Fax: 029 2071 1267 Email: woodhousekw@cardiff.ac.uk — MD Newc. 1985; BM (Hons.) Soton 1977; MRCP (UK) 1979; FRCP Lond. 1990; T(M) 1991. Prof. Geriat. Med. & Vice Dean Med. Univ. Wales Coll. Med. Cardiff. Specialty: Care of the Elderly. Socs: Brit. Pharm. Soc. & Brit. Geriat. Soc. Prev: Cons. Phys. & Sen. Lect. in Med. (Geriat.) & Clin. Pharmacol. Roy. Vict. Infirm. & Univ. Newc.; MRC Trav. Fell. Dept. Clin. Pharmacol. Karolinska Inst. Stockholm; MRC Train. Fell. Depts. Med. & Clin. Pharmacol. Univ. Newc.

WOODHOUSE, Mark Noel 86 Crosby Street, Cale Green, Stockport SK2 6SP — MB ChB Manch. 1988.

WOODHOUSE, Mervyn Ashley (retired) Well Cottage, 43 Dorchester Road, Frampton, Dorchester DT2 9NF; 13 Farfrae Cres, Dorchester DT1 2SR — (Birm.) MB ChB Birm. 1955; FRCPath 1977, M 1965. Prev: Cons. Pathologist, W. Dorset Gen. Hosp.s NHS TRUS.

WOODHOUSE, Monica Mary (retired) Well Cottage, 43 Dorchester Road, Frampton, Dorchester DT2 9NF; 13 Farfrae Cresc, Dorchester DT1 2SR — (Guy's) MRCS Eng. LRCP Lond. 1956; MB BS Lond. 1957. Prev: Clin. Asst. in Psycho-Geriat. W. Dorset HA.

WOODHOUSE, Paul Anthony Old Barn, Pond Farm, East Peckham, Tonbridge TN12 5NA — MB ChB Ed. 1986; BA Oxf. 1983.

WOODHOUSE, Peter Robert Norfolk and Norwich University Hospital, Colney Lane, Norwich NR4 7UY Tel: 01603 288002 Fax: 01603 288571 Email: peter.woodhouse@nnuh.nhs.uk — BM Soton. 1983; MRCP (UK) 1989; DM Soton. 1995; FRCP Lond. 1999. Cons. Geriat. Med. Norf. & Norwich Healthcare Trust; Hon. Sen. Lect. Univ. of E. Anglia. Specialty: Care of the Elderly. Socs: Brit. Geriat. Soc. Prev: Sen. Regist. (Gen. & Geriat. Med.) & Research Fell. (Clin. Gerontol.) Addenbrooke's Hosp. Camb.; Lect. (Physiol.) Lond. Hosp. Med. Coll.

WOODHOUSE, Phillip 22 Grinton Road, Stockton-on-Tees TS18 5HE — MB ChB Leic. 1998.

WOODHOUSE, Wendy Jane Child & Adolescent Psychiatry Department, Princess Margaret Hospital, Okus Road, Swindon SN1 4JU Tel: 01793 536231 — MB BS Lond. 1986; MRCP (UK) 1990; MRCPsych 1992. Cons. Child & Adolesc. Psychiat. Princess Margt. Hosp. Swindon. Specialty: Child & Adolesc. Psychiat. Prev: Sen. Regist. (Child Psychiat.) Maudsley Hosp. Lond.

WOODIER, Neville Christopher (retired) Pencefn, Llanddona, Beaumaris LL58 8UB Tel: 01248 811282 — (Liverp.) MB ChB (2nd Cl. Hnrs.) Liverp. 1954. Prev: Ho. Surg. & Ho. Phys. Liverp. Roy. Infirm.

WOODING, Clifford Desmond The Caludon Centre, Clifford Bridge Road, Walsgrave, Coventry CV2 2TE Tel: 024 7660 2020 — MB BS Lond. 1956 (Guys) MRCS, LRCP 1956; Dobst RCOG Lond. 1958; MPH (Columbia Univ.) New York 1967; MRCPsych Coventry 1985. p/t Locum Consultant/Adult Psychiat., The Caludon Centre, Clifford Bridge Rd., Coventry. Prev: Locum Cons., Old Age Psychiat., Caludon Centre, Nuneaton; Regist. & HO Old Age Psychiat., Walsgrave Hosp. & St. Mathew's Hosp., Burntwood.

WOODING, Daniel Francis Peter (retired) Mansion House Surgery, Abbey St., Stone ST15 8YE Tel: 01785 815555; Stoneygate House, Eccleshall Road, Walton, Stone ST15 0HN Tel: 01785 815533 — (St. Bart.) MB BS Lond. 1954; DObst RCOG 1957.

WOODING, Nicholas James 8 Barkers Lane, Wythall, Birmingham B47 6BU Tel: 01564 823539 — BM BCh Oxf. 1990; BA Oxf. 1987; DRCOG 1993; BA Open 1996; MRCGP 1996; DTM & H Liverpool 1996; MA Oxford 1997. Specialty: Gen. Med.; Community Child Health; Palliat. Med. Socs: Christian Med. Fellowsh. Prev: GP Trainee, Sydenlam Green Health Centre; GP VTS, Lewisham Hosps.

WOODING, Regan Mary Susan Well Close Square Surgery, Well Close Square, Berwick-upon-Tweed TD15 1LL Tel: 01289 356920 Fax: 01289 356939 — MB BS Lond. 1981; DRCOG 1983. GP Berwick upon Tweed.

WOODING, Simon Charles Long Clawson Medical Practice, The Surgery, The Sands, Melton Mowbray LE14 4PA Tel: 01664 822214/5 — BM BS Nottm. 1987; MRCGP 1992; DCH 1993. GP Melton Mowbray.

WOODING, Stephen James 14 Eccleshall Road, Walton, Stone ST15 0HN — MB BS Lond. 1983; BSc (Pharmacol.) Lond. 1980.

WOODINGS, David Francis Medicines Control Agency, Market Towers, 1 Nine Elms Lane, London SW8 5NQ Tel: 020 7273 0148 Fax: 020 7273 0190; Eastweald, 59 Valley Road, Ipswich IP1 4EG Tel: 01473 254220 — MB BChir Camb. 1969 (Camb. & Middlx.) MA, MB Camb. 1969, BChir 1968; MRCP (UK) 1971; FRCPath 1986, M 1974; FFPM 1989; FRCPS Glas. 1991; FRCP Lond. 1997. Sen. Med. Off. Med. Control Agency Lond. Specialty: Haematology. Socs: Fell. Roy. Soc. Med.; Brit. Soc. Haematol. Prev: Med. Dir. Schwarz Pharmaceut. Ltd. Chesham; Sen. Research Phys. Glaxo Gp. Research Ltd. Ware; Lect. (Haemat.) St. Geo. Hosp. & Med. Sch. Lond.

WOODINGS, John Trevor (retired) London Road Medical Centre, 2 London Road, Uppingham, Oakham LE15 9TJ Tel: 01572 823531; 56 Leicester Road, Uppingham, Oakham LE15 9SD Tel: 01572 822556 — MB ChB Ed. 1965; DA Eng. 1967.

WOODLAND, John Rheumatology Department, Standish Hospital, Stonehouse GL10 3DB; The Stocks., 5 Cleeve Road, Gotherington, Cheltenham GL52 9EW — MB BS Lond. 1969 (Guy's) MRCS Eng. LRCP Lond. 1969; MRCP (UK) 1972; FRCP Lond. 1989; T(M) 1991. Cons. Rheum. Glos. HA. Specialty: Rheumatol. Socs: Brit. Soc. Rheum. Prev: Sen. Regist. (Rheum.) Lond. Hosp.

WOODLAND, John Michael 18 Common Road, Wincanton BA9 9HU — MB ChB Birm. 1995.

WOODLEY, Alan George Grove Health Centre, 129 Dundee Road, Broughty Ferry, Dundee DD5 1DU Tel: 01382 778881 Fax: 01382 731884; 67 Marlee Road, Broughty Ferry, Dundee DD5 3EU Tel: 01382 739820 — MB ChB Dundee 1976; MRCP (UK) 1982; DCH RCP Lond. 1982. Hon. Med. Adviser, Dundee Br. RNLI. Specialty: Paediat.

WOODLEY, Helen Elizabeth Leeds General Infirmary, Great George St., Leeds LS1 3EX; The Cottage, Mill Lane, Pool-in-Wharfedale, Otley LS21 1LR Tel: 0113 284 3401 — MB BChir Camb. 1991; BA (Hons.) Camb. 1987, MA, MB 1991, BChir 1990. SHO Rotat. (Gen. Med., Radiother. & Oncol.) Cookridge Hosp.

WOODLEY, Joan Margaret 2 Manor Road, Ipswich IP4 2UX Tel: 01473 251210 — MB BS Lond. 1954; MRCS Eng. LRCP Lond. 1954.

WOODLIFF, Hugh Jackson Markholme, Keswick CA12 5PW — MB ChB Ed. 1950; MRCP (UK) 1954; FRCPath 1974, M 1963; FRCP Ed. 1971.

WOODMAN, Alastair Michael 19 Quarry Road, Belfast BT4 2JD — MB BCh Belf. 1998.

WOODMAN, Professor Ciaran Bernard John Centre for Cancer Epidemiology, Kinnaird Road, Manchester M20 — MB BCh BAO NUI 1977; MRCOG 1986; MFPHM 1988; MD 1990. Prof. Cancer Epidemiol. Univ. Manch. Specialty: Pub. Health Med. Prev: Sen. Lect. (Cancer Epidemiol.) Univ. Birm.; Lect. ((Social Med.) Univ. Birm.

WOODMAN, Geoffrey Francis Gordon (retired) Farrowsheals, 16 Linden Acres, Longhorsley, Morpeth NE65 8XQ Tel: 01670 788229 Email: gfwoodman77@hotmail.com — MB BS Durh. 1952; MRCGP 1970. Prev: Hosp. Pract. (Geriat.) Morpeth Cottage Hosp.

WOODMAN, Graham John Bronllys Hospital, Bronllys, Brecon L03 0LU Tel: 01874 711255; Vale Barn, Lower Chapel, Brecon LD3 9RE — MB ChB Birm. 1980; BSc Bristol 1970; DRCOG 1982; MRCGP 1984. Specialty: Care of the Elderly; Palliat. Med.; Rehabil. Med. Prev: DRS Ksiff, Woodman & Cross; Wylcwh St Surg.; Powys LD7 1AD.

WOODMAN, Jacqueline Rachel 22 Eden Drive, Oxford OX3 0AB — MB ChB Stellenbosch 1991.

WOODMAN, Michael John The Health Station Ltd, 21 Standhill Road, Hitchin SG5 1JE Tel: 01462 459595 Fax: 01462 435373 Email: mike.woodman@tesco.net — MB BS Lond. 1970 (St. Mary's) DRCOG 1972; DFFP 1994. Director The Health Station Ltd. Special Interest: Med. Examinations. Socs: Assur. Med. Soc.; Nat. Assn. Family Plann. Doctors; Brit. Travel Health Assn.

WOODMAN, Miriam Manchester Health Authority, Gateway House, Piccadilly S., Manchester M60 7LP Tel: 0161 237 2812 Fax: 0161 237 2813 — MB BCh BAO NUI 1978; MFPHM RCP (UK) 1987. Cons. Pub. Health Manch. Health Auth.; Hon. Clin. Lect. Univ. Manch. Specialty: Pub. Health Med. Prev: Cons. Pub. Health

Kidderminster Health Auth.; Sen. Regist. (Community Med.) Centr. Birm. Health Auth..

WOODMAN, Timothy John The Health Centre, Holding Street, Rainham, Gillingham ME8 7JP Tel: 01634 262333 — MB BS Lond. 1981; DRCOG 1984. SHO (Paediat.) S. W. Surrey HA. Prev: Trainee GP Witley; SHO (O & G) Medway HA; SHO (A & E) Cuckfield Hosp.

WOODMANSEY, Annica Louise 23 Weeping Cross, Stafford ST17 0DG Email: pacdwoodm@aol.com — MB ChB Sheff. 1986; DCH RCPS Glas. 1989. Specialty: Paediat. Prev: Staff Grade Paediat. (A & E) Sheff. Childr. Hosp. NHS Trust.; Staff Grade, Community Paediat., S. Staffs. Healthcare NHS Trust, Stafford Centr. Clinic.

WOODMANSEY, Paul Arnold Staffordshire General Hospital, Weston Road, Stafford ST16 3SA Tel: 01785 230677 Fax: 01785 230677 — MB ChB Sheff. 1986; MD Sheff. 1995, BMed Sci. (Hons.) 1983; MRCP (UK) 1989; FRCP Lond 2000. Cons. Cardiol. M. Staffs. NHS Trust; Hon. Cons. Cardiol. N. Staffs. NHS Trust. Specialty: Cardiol.; Gen. Med. Socs: Brit. Cardiac Soc.; Brit. Soc. of Echocardiography; Brit. Pacing & Electrophysiol. Gp. Prev: Regist. (Cardiol.) Leeds Gen. Infirm.; Research Regist. (Cardiol.) Roy. Hallamsh. Hosp. Sheff.

WOODNUTT, Mr David John 8 Talygarn Street, Heath, Cardiff CF14 3PT Tel: 029 2038 7092 Fax: 029 2038 7092 — MB BS Lond. 1990; BSc (Hons.) Bristol 1982; MPhil Open 1993; FRCS Eng. 1994. Regist. (Orthop.) Cardiff Roy. Infirm. Specialty: Orthop. Prev: SHO (A & E) Derbysh. Roy. Infirm.; Ho. Off. Char. Cross Hosp. Lond. & Barnstaple & N. Devon Dist. Hosps.

WOODROFFE, David (retired) 57 Wensleydale Road, Hampton TW12 2LP — (St. Geo.) MB BS Lond. 1954. Prev: GP Middlx.

WOODROFFE, Frederick James (retired) Swanton Lodge, Swanton St, Bredgar, Sittingbourne ME9 8AS Tel: 01622 884434 Email: f.woodroffe@btclick.com — (King's Coll. Hosp.) MSc (Gen. Biochem.) Lond. 1975, MB BS (Hons.); MRCS Eng. LRCP Lond. 1961; FRCP Lond. 1978, M 1966. Prev: Phys. Chase Farm Hosp. Trust.

WOODROFFE, Guy Campbell Ravenswood Surgery, New Road, Forfar DD8 2AE Tel: 01307 463558 Fax: 01307 468900 Email: drwoodroffe@ravenswood.finix.org.uk; Rockcliffe, 2 Bankhead Road, Forfar DD8 3JP Tel: 01307 467596 Email: guycw@supanet.com — MB ChB Ed. 1985; MRCGP 1989; DObst RCPI 1990; DFFP 1996. Princip. GP. Socs: Life Mem. Roy. Med. Soc. Prev: SHO (Paediat.) Burnley Gen. Hosp.; Trainee GP Hawick VTS; SHO (Med.) Edenhall Hosp. Musselburgh.

WOODROFFE, Janet Betty Seamura, Smallwood Hey Road, Pilling, Preston PR3 6HJ Tel: 01253 790109 — MB ChB Liverp. 1943; DA Eng. 1954. Socs: Fell. Manch. Med. Soc.; Liverp. Med. Inst. Prev: Cons. Anaesth. Preston HA; Regist. (Anaesth.) Chester Hosp. Gp.; Res. Anaesth. Preston Roy. Infirm.

WOODROFFE, Robert William North End Surgery, High Street, Buckingham MK18 1NU Tel: 01280 818600 Fax: 01280 818618; Hanover Barn, Hanover Farm, Addington, Buckingham MK18 2JW Tel: 01296 715607 Fax: 01296 711075 Email: roffe@globalnet.co.uk — MB BS Lond. 1971 (St. Thos.) BSc (Hons.) Lond. 1968, MB BS 1971; MA Keele Univ. 1993; LLM Cardiff 2002. Med. Off. Buckingham Hosp.; Deputy Coroner (Milton Keynes); Asst. Deputy Coroner (Bedford). Special Interest: Medico Legal. Socs: BMA. Prev: SHO (Med. & Oncol. & O & G) I. of Thanet HA; SHO (Cas.) St. Thos. Hosp. Lond.

WOODROFFE, Susan Aileen Rockcliffe, 2 Bankhead Road, Forfar DD8 3JP Tel: 01307 467596 Email: guycw@supanet.com — MB ChB Ed. 1985; DRCOG 1988; MRCGP 1989. GP Retainer, Ravenswood Surg., Forfar, Scot. Socs: Life Mem. Roy. Med. Soc. Prev: Trainee GP Edin.; SHO (Med.) Edenhall Hosp. Musselburgh; SHO (Cas., O & G, Paediat. & Psychiat.) West. Gen. Hosp. Edin.

WOODROOF, Gerard Martin Fenwick Chipton Barton, Dittisham, Dartmouth TQ6 0HW Email: gerard.woodroof@sdevonhc-tr.swest.nhs.uk — MB BS Lond. 1979 (Guy's) MSc Lond. 1984, BSc (Hons.) 1976; MRCS Eng. LRCP Lond. 1979; FFOM RCP Lond. 1995, MFOM 1987, AFOM 1985. Cons. Occupat. Phys. Torbay Hosp. Torquay & Derriford Hosp. Plymouth. Specialty: Occupat. Health.

WOODROW, Charles Jonathan 94 Milton Park, London N6 5PZ Tel: 020 8341 9780; Division of Infectious Diseases, St. George's Hospital Medical School, London SW17 0RE Tel: 020 8725 5834 Fax: 020 8725 3487 — MB BS Lond. 1993; BA (Hons.) Camb. 1990; MRCP Lond. 1996. Clin. Research Fell. St Geo.'s Hosp. Med. Sch. Lond. Specialty: Infec. Dis. Socs: BMA. Prev: SHO (Renal) St. Mary's Hosp. Lond.; SHO (Respirat. Med.) The Lond. Chest Hosp.; SHO (Rheumat. & Neurol.) Hammersmith Hosp. Lond.

WOODROW, David Frederick (retired) 47 Shooters Hill, Pangbourne, Reading RG8 7EA — MB BS Lond. 1969; MRCS Eng. LRCP Lond. 1969; FRCPath 1994. Prev: Sen. Lect. (Histopath.) Char. Cross & Westm. Med. Sch. Lond.

WOODROW, Elizabeth Ann 21Cyprus Avenue, Belfast BT5 5NT — MB BCh BAO Belf. 1988 (Queen's University Belfast) DRCOG 1992; MRCGP Belf. 1993; DCCH 1995; DFFP 1998. Clin. Med. Off. (Community Paediat.) Glengormley. Specialty: Community Child Health; Family Plann. & Reproduc. Health. Socs: BMA; Fac. Fam. Plann. & Reprod. Health Care. Prev: Asst. GP Whiteabbey Health Centre.

WOODROW, Graham Renal Unit, Leeds General Infirmary, Great George St., Leeds LS1 3EX Tel: 0113 392 2375 Fax: 0113 392 6560 — MB ChB Leeds 1986; MRCP (UK) 1989; MD Leeds 1997; FRCP 2001. Cons. (Renal Med.) Leeds Gen. Infirm.; Hon. Sen. Clin. Lect. Univ. of Leeds. Specialty: Nephrol. Socs: Brit. Renal Assn.; Eur. Dialysis & Transpl. Assn.; International Society of Peritoneal Dialysis. Prev: Sen. Regist. (Renal & Gen. Med.) Withington Hosp. Manch.; Research Regist. & Regist. (Med.) Leeds Gen. Infirm.; Regist. (Renal) Nottm. City Hosp.

WOODROW, Janice Marian Health Centre, Lake Lock Road, Stanley, Wakefield WF3 4HS Tel: 01924 822328 Fax: 01924 870052; The Poplars, Aberford Road, Stanley, Wakefield WF3 4AG — BM BS Nottm. 1980; BMedSci. Nottm. 1978, BM BS 1980; MRCGP 1984.

WOODROW, Joseph Charles Woak Hill, St. Davids Lane, Noctorum, Birkenhead CH43 9UD Tel: 0151 652 4989 — (Leeds) MB ChB Leeds 1948; FRCP Lond. 1971, M 1953; MD Leeds 1961. Emerit. Prof. Dept. Med. Univ. Liverp. Specialty: Rheumatol. Socs: Assn. Phys. & Brit. Soc. Rheum.; Liverp. Med. Inst. Prev: Hon. Cons. Phys. Roy. Liverp. Hosp. & Broadgreen Hosp. Liverp.; Prof. Rheum. Univ. Liverp.

WOODROW, Sarah Louise 41 Orchard Street, Cambridge CB1 1JS — MB BS Lond. 1991 (Char. Cross & Westm. Hosp. Lond.) BSc (1st cl. Hons.) Lond. 1988; MRCP (UK) 1993. Regist. (Dermat.) Addenbrooke's Hosp. NHS Trust Camb. Specialty: Dermat. Socs: BMA; Train. Mem. Brit. Assn. Dermat. Prev: SHO (Dermat.) Ealing Hosp.; SHO (Endocrinol. & Geriat.) Roy. Free NHS Trust.

WOODROW, Susan Patricia 5 Westfield Lane, Wigginton, York YO32 2FZ — MB ChB Leeds 1977. SCMO (Occupat. Health) York Dist. Hosp. Specialty: Occupat. Health. Prev: Princip. GP Easingwold Health Centre.

WOODRUFF, Mr Geoffrey Harold Addison Department of Ophthalmology, Leicester Royal Infirmary, Leicester LE1 5WW — MB BS Lond. 1976; BSc (Hons.) Lond. 1973; FRCS Ed. 1983; FRCOphth 1988. Cons. Ophth. Univ. Hosps. Leicester; Hon. Sen. Lect. Univ. Leicester. Specialty: Ophth. Socs: Fell. Roy. Coll. Ophth.; Roy. Soc. Med. Prev: Sen. Regist. (Ophth.) Tennent Inst. Glas.; Fell. (Paediat. Ophth.) Hosp. for Sick Childr. Toronto, Canada.

WOODRUFF, Michael James Flat 8, Kennedy Court, Tapton Crescent Road, Sheffield S10 5DA — MB ChB Sheff. 1994.

WOODRUFF, Professor Peter Waller Rolph University of Sheffield, Academic Clinical Psychiatry, The Longley Centre, Norwood Grange Drive, Sheffield S5 7JT — MB BS Newc. 1981; MRCP (UK) 1985; MRCPsych 1991; PhD (Lond) 1998. Prof. (Gen. Adult Psychiat.) Univ. of Sheff.; Hon. Cons. (Psychiat.) Sheff. Healthcare Trust. Specialty: Gen. Psychiat. Socs: Liveryman Worshipful Soc. Apoth.; Fell. Med. Soc. Lond. Prev: Asst. Prof. Univ. Maryland USA; Lect. King's Coll. Hosp. Med. Sch. Lond.; Regist. Maudsley Hosp. Lond.

WOODRUFF, Simon Addison 7 Hazlitt Road, London W14 0JY — MB BS Lond. 1991.

WOODS, Alexander Jamison 8 Meadow Park, Crawfordsburn, Helens Bay, Bangor BT19 1JN Tel: 0289 185 3376 — MB BCh BAO Belf. 1952; LM Coombe 1953; DA Eng. 1961. Mem. Fac. Anaesth. RCS Eng. Prev: Ho. Off. Moyle Hosp. Larne & Belf. City Hosp.; Sen. Ho. Off. Whiteabbey Chest Hosp.

WOODS, Alison Hellier 35 Highfield Road, Dunkirk, Nottingham NG7 2JE — BM BS Nottm. 1996.

WOODS, Amanda Jane Silverton Surgery, Silverton, Exeter EX5 4HX Tel: 01392 860176; Bridel Cottage, Shobrooke, Crediton EX17 1AZ — MB ChB Dundee 1979; BSc St. And. 1974.

WOODS, Amanda Louise 5 Melville Avenue, Wimbledon, London SW20 0NS Tel: 020 8946 9870 — MB BS Lond. 1986; MRCP (UK) 1989.

WOODS, Andrew Duncan 81 Shakespeare Way, Taverham, Norwich NR8 6SL — MB BS Lond. 1992. Ho. Phys. Heatherwood Hosp. Ascot.

WOODS, Brian Terence Annandale Surgery, 239 Mutton Lane, Potters Bar EN6 2AS Tel: 01707 644451; 69 Calder Avenue, Brookmans Park, Hatfield AL9 7AJ Tel: 01707 664822 — (Lond. Hosp.) MB BS Lond. 1966; MRCGP 1975. Potters Bar Hosp. Specialty: Orthop. Prev: Hosp. Pract. (Orthop.) Barnet Gen. Hosp.; Regist. (Accid. & Orthop.) Barnet Gen. Hosp.; Ho. Surg. (Gyn.) Chase Farm Hosp. Enfield.

WOODS, Caroline Mary The Surgery, High Street, Heathfield TN21 8JD Tel: 014246 3559; 96-98 High Street, Heathfield TN21 8JD Tel: 014352 4999 — BM Soton. 1979; DRCOG 1983. Prev: Trainee GP Hastings HA VTS.

WOODS, Christopher James Locking Hill Surgery, Locking Hill, Stroud GL5 1UY Tel: 01453 764222 Fax: 01453 756278; 22 Paul's Rise, North Woodchester, Stroud GL5 5PN — MRCS Eng. LRCP Lond. 1978; BSc (Pharm.) Lond. 1975, MB BS 1978; DA (UK) 1981; DRCOG 1985.

WOODS, Christopher John The Halliwell Surgery, Lindfield Drive, Bolton BL1 3RG Tel: 01204 523642 Fax: 01204 384204; 103 Holcombe Old Road, Holcombe, Bury BL8 4NF — MB ChB Manch. 1976; MRCGP 1984. Specialty: Gen. Pract.

WOODS, Claire Lisa — MB ChB Ed. 1993; FRCA 2000. SpR (Anaesth) Northern School of Anaesthesia. Specialty: Anaesth. Prev: SHO (Anaesth.) Sunderland Roy. Hosp. Sunderland; SHO (Med.) Wansbeck Gen. Hosp. N.umberland; SHO (Anaesth.) Wansbeck Gen. Hosp. N.umberland.

WOODS, Colin Gerard (retired) 22 Kirk Close, Oxford OX2 8JN Tel: 01865 554516 — MB ChB Leeds 1951; BSc (Hons.) Leeds 1948; FRCPath 1975, M 1964. Prev: Cons. Path. Nuffield Orthop. Centre Oxf.

WOODS, Colin John (retired) 19 Sandringham Road, Lytham St Annes FY8 1EZ Tel: 01253 725545 — MB ChB Liverp. 1962; FRCP Lond. 1981, M 1968. Prev: Cons. Paediat. Vict. Hosp. Blackpool.

WOODS, Mr David Anthony Great Western Hospital, Department of Orthopaedics, Marlborough Road, Swindon SN3 6BB Tel: 01793 604906 Email: david.a.woods@lineone.net/ davidwoods@smnhst.swest.nhs.uk; Tanyard House, Chilton Foliat, Hungerford RG17 0TG Tel: 01488 683830 Email: david.awoods@lineone.net — MB ChB Sheff. 1986; BMedSci Sheff. 1985; FRCS Eng. 1991; FRCS Glas. (Orth.) 1996. Cons. Orthop. Surg. Great Western Hosp. Swindon. Specialty: Trauma & Orthop. Surg. Special Interest: Shoulder Surg. Socs: Girdlestone Orthop. Soc.; BOA.

WOODS, David Granville St Marys Surgery, 37 St. Mary's Street, Ely CB7 4HF; 25 Fieldside, Ely CB6 3AT Tel: 01353 663554 — MB BS Lond. 1973 (Westm.) MRCS Eng. LRCP Lond. 1973; MRCGP 1978; DRCOG 1978. Prev: Sen. Med. Off. RAF Binbrook; SHO (O & G) RAF Hosp. Wegberg; Unit Med. Off. RAF Wildenrath.

WOODS, David Mack Forest Road Health Centre, 8 Forest Road, Hugglescote, Coalville LE67 3SH Tel: 01530 832109 — MB BS Lond. 1977 (Guys Hospital Medical School) MRCS Eng. LRCP Lond. 1976.

WOODS, David Richard 207 Cardigan Lane, Leeds LS6 1DX Tel: 0113 278 4685 — MB ChB Leeds 1990. Prev: Ho. Off. (Surg.) Camb. Milit. Hosp.; Ho. Off. (Med.) St. Jas. Hosp. Leeds.

WOODS, Declan John bVine Cottage, 3 Hallaton Road, Medbourne, Market Harborough LE16 8DR Tel: 0185 883776 — MB ChB Leeds 1975; FRCR 1983. Cons. Radiol. Kettering Gen. Hosp. Specialty: Radiol. Prev: Sen. Regist. (Radiol.) W. Midl. RHA.

WOODS, Donald Pierpoint (retired) Sweet Briar, Ovington, Alresford SO24 0RE Tel: 01962 732729 — BM BCh Oxf. 1954 (Oxf. & Lond. Hosp.) MA Oxf. 1954; DObst RCOG 1956; FRCGP 1981, M 1963; Cert. Av. Med. 1987. Prev: Ho. Phys., Ho. Surg. & Res. Accouch. Lond. Hosp.

WOODS, Elizabeth Anne — MB ChB Leeds 1981; DCH RCP Lond. 1985; DRCOG 1987; MRCGP 1990; Cert. Community Paediat. Sheff. 1990. Specialty: Community Child Health. Socs: BMA; RCGP; Soc. Orthop. Med. Prev: SHO (O & G) Luton & Dunstable Hosp.; SHO & CMO (Paediat.) Community Child Health Sheff. HA; SHO (Geriat. Med.) Univ. Manch.

WOODS, Hubert Frank, CBE Division of Clinical Sciences South, School of Medicine & Biomedical Sciences, Sheffield S10 2RX Tel: 0114 271 2475 Fax: 0114 271 1711; Aston Lane, Hope, Hope Valley S33 6RA Tel: 01433 623337 — BM BCh Oxf. 1965; BSc Leeds 1962; MRCP (UK) 1968; DPhil Oxf. 1971; FRCP Lond. 1978 FFPM RCP UK 1989; FRCP Ed. 1991. Prof. Clin. Pharmacol. & Therap. Univ. Sheff.; Sir Geo. Franklin Prof. Med.; Cons. Phys. Sheff. Teachg. Hosp. NHS Trust. Specialty: Pharmacology. Prev: Hon. Cons. Phys.

WOODS, Ian Yungarra, Ferryman's Walk, Nether Poppleton, York YO26 6HZ — MB ChB Manch. 1979; FFA RCS Eng. 1983. Cons. Anaesth. York HA. Specialty: Intens. Care. Socs: Brit. Assn. Anaesth.; Intens. Care Soc. Prev: Sen. Regist. (Anaesth.) N. West. RHA; Regist. (Anaesth.) Roy. Cornw. Hosp. Truro; SHO (Anaesth.) Withington Hosp. Manch.

WOODS, Ian Malcolm McClure Long Lane Medical Centre, Long Lane, Liverpool L9 6DQ Tel: 0151 530 1009 — MB ChB Dundee 1976. Hon. Med. Adviser Liverp. City Mission.

WOODS, Jacqueline Lee Penelope Isogroup International, 33 rue Arsène Houssaye, Paris 75008, France Tel: 00 33 1 53 53 53 00 Fax: 00 33 1 42 89 64 70; Pooh Corner, Loudwater Lane, Loudwater, Rickmansworth WD3 4HX Tel: 01923 896717 Fax: 01923 896818 — MB BS Lond. 1987; MA Camb. 1988; MBA Insead 1992.

WOODS, James Crerar Dr Moss and Partners, 28-38 Kings Road, Harrogate HG1 5JP Tel: 01423 560261 Fax: 01423 501099 — MB ChB Dundee 1982; MRCGP 1988.

WOODS, James Patrick 35 Ailesbury Crescent, Belfast BT7 3EZ — MB BCh BAO Belf. 1984; BSc (Hons.) Belf. 1981; MRCGP 1990; DRCOG 1990. Med. Off. DHSS Belf. Specialty: Civil Serv.

WOODS, Jennifer Mary Department Anaesthetics, Level 04, Derriford Hospital, Derriford Road, Plymouth PL6 8DH Tel: 01752 792691 Fax: 01752 763287 — MB BS Lond. 1973 (Roy. Free) Cert. Family Plann. JCC 1976; DObst RCOG 1976; DA Eng. 1977; FFA RCS Eng. 1981. Cons. Anaesth. SW RHA. Specialty: Anaesth. Socs: Assn. Anaesth. Gt. Brit. & Irel. & Soc. Anaesth. SW Region. Prev: Sen. Regist. (Anaesth.) Bristol & Weston HA.

WOODS, Jill Kathryn High Street Surgery, 60 High Street, Lurgan, Craigavon BT66 8BA Tel: 028 3832 4591 — MB BCh BAO Belf. 1992.

WOODS, John Declan 18 Harberton Park, Belfast BT9 6TS — MB BCh BAO Dub. 1986; BA Dub. 1986, MB BCh BAO 1986; MRCP (UK) 1990.

WOODS, John Joseph (retired) Ridge Farm, Brinscombe Lane, Membury, Axminster EX13 7JP Tel: 01297 33046 — MB BCh BAO NUI 1941 (Cork) Prev: Cons. Anaesth. Airedale Gen. Hosp.

WOODS, John Oliver (retired) The Mall, Armagh BT61 9AU Tel: 01861 523165; 11 Beresford Row, The Mall, Armagh BT61 9AU — (Qu. Univ. Belf.) MD Belf. 1967, MB BCh BAO 1959; DObst RCOG 1961; DCH RCPS Glas. 1966; FRCGP 1979, M 1968. Prev: Provost NI Fac. RCGP.

WOODS, Jonathan Philip — MB ChB Manch. 1981; BSc (Med. Sci.) St. And. 1978; DRCOG 1984; MRCGP 1986; MRCPsych 1988. Specialty: Geriat. Psychiat.

WOODS, Katherine Mary Department of Anaesthetics, University Hospital of Wales, Heath Park, Cardiff CF14 4XW Tel: 029 2074 7747; 4 Cyncoed Crescent, Cyncoed, Cardiff CF2 5SW Tel: 029 2075 7357 — MB BChir Camb. 1988; MA Camb. 1988, MB BChir Camb. 1988; FRCA 1992. Sen. Regist. (Anaesth.) Univ. Hosp. Wales Cardiff. Specialty: Anaesth. Prev: Regist. Rotat. (Anaesth.) Bloomsbury HA.

WOODS, Kathryn Anne 19 Hill Top Road, Oxford OX4 1PB — MB BS Lond. 1988 (St. Bart.) MB BS Lond. (Hons.) 1988; MRCP (UK) 1991. Lect. (Paediat. Endocrinol.) & Hon. Sen. Regist. Oxf. Univ. & John Radcliffe Hosp. Specialty: Paediat. Prev: Research Fell. (Paediat. Endocrinol.) St. Bart. Hosp. Lond.; Regist. (Paediat.) Qu. Eliz. & Gt. Ormond St. Hosps. for Sick Childr. Lond.

WOODS, Professor Kent Linton Medicines & Healthcare Products Regulatory Agency, Market Towers, 1 Nine Elms Lane, London SW8 5NQ Tel: 020 7084 2100 Fax: 020 7084 2548 Email:

kent.woods@mhra.gsi.gov.uk; Department of Cardiovascular Sciences, Clinical Sciences Building, Leister Royal Infirmary, Leicester LE2 7LX Tel: 0116 252 3126 Fax: 0116 252 3108 Email: klw@le.ac.uk — MB BChir Camb. 1972 (Camb. & Birm.) MRCP (UK) 1974; MA Camb 1973, MD 1980; MS Harvard 1983; FRCP Lond. 1988. Chief Exec. Medicines & Healthcare Products Regulatory Agency; Cons. Phys. Leics. Roy. Infirm.; Prof. Therap. Univ. Leicester. Specialty: Gen. Med. Socs: Assn. Phys.; Brit. Cardiac Soc.; Brit. Pharm. Soc. Prev: Dir. NHS Heath Techn. Asses. Prog; Lect. (Therap. & Clin. Pharmacol.) Univ. Birm.; MRC/Lilly Internat. Trav. Fell. (Epidemiol.) Harvard Univ.

WOODS, Lesley Anne Department of Anaesthetics, City Hospital Trust, Hucknall Road, Nottingham — MB ChB Manch. 1984; FCAnaesth 1990. Cons. Anaesth. City Hosp. Trust Nottm. Specialty: Anaesth. Socs: Assn. Anaesth.; Obst. Anaesth. Assn. Prev: Sen. Regist. (Anaesth.) Roy. Hallamsh. Hosp. Sheff.; Fell. (Intens. Care) Academisch Ziekenhuis Groningen, Netherlands; Regist. (Anaesth.) Roy. Hallamsh. Hosp. Sheff.

WOODS, Lynne Church Close Surgery, 3 Church Close, Boston PE21 6NB Tel: 01205 311133 Fax: 01205 358986 — MB ChB Sheff. 1977.

WOODS, Mary Rosaleen Cheadle Hospital, Royal Walk, Cheadle ST10 1NS Tel: 01538 487546 Fax: 01538 487530 — MB ChB Ed. 1980; BSc Ed. 1977; DRCOG 1983; MRCGP 1984; MRCPsych 1987. Specialty: Geriat. Psychiat. Prev: Sen. Regist. (Psychiat.) N. Staffs.; Regist. (Psychiat.) Roy. Edin. Hosp.

WOODS, Michael John West Bridgford Health Centre, 97 Musters Road, West Bridgford, Nottingham NG2 9PX Tel: 0115 9811858/5666 Fax: 0115 982 6448; The Willows, 43 Jessops Lane, Gedling, Nottingham NG4 4BQ Tel: 0115 952 5114 — BM BS Nottm. 1979; MRCGP 1984. Hon. Lect. Dept. of Gen. Pract.

WOODS, Paul Julian Church Close Surgery, 3 Church Close, Boston PE21 6NB Tel: 01205 311133 Fax: 01205 358986 — MB ChB Sheff. 1977; MRCGP 1981.

WOODS, Paul Michael Holbrook Surgery, Bartholomew Way, Horsham RH12 5JL Tel: 01403 755900 Fax: 01403 755909 — MB BS Lond. 1991 (Roy. Lond. Hosp. Med. Coll.) DFFP 1995; MRCGP 1995. Specialty: Gen. Pract. Socs: Med. Defence Union; BMA. Prev: Trainee GP Horsham.

WOODS, Peter Michael 52 Wimpole Road, Colchester CO1 2DL; Yew Tree House, Higham Road, Stratford St. Mary, Colchester CO7 6JU — MRCS Eng. LRCP Lond. 1976 (Westm.) BSc (Hons. Biochem. & Physiol.) Lond. 1972, MB BS 1976.

WOODS, Mr Robert Rex Church View Surgery, 30 Holland Road, Plymstock, Plymouth PL9 9BW Tel: 01752 403206; Barn Farm House, Barn Wood, Plymstock, Plymouth PL9 9NH — MB BS Lond. 1978 (St. Bart.) MA Oxf. 1973; FRCS Ed. 1982. GP; Hosp. Practitioner (Endoscopy), Derriford Hosp., Plymouth.

WOODS, Rosemary Coxhoe Medical Practice, 1 Lansdowne Road, Cornforth Lane, Coxhoe, Durham DH6 4DH Tel: 0191 377 0340 Fax: 0191 377 0604 — MB BS Newc. 1978; DRCOG 1981; MRCGP 1982. GP Coxhoe Co. Durh.

WOODS, Sheelagh Catherine Patricia Deeny Anaesthetics Department, University College Hospital, Gower St., London WC1E 6AU Tel: 020 7387 9300 Fax: 020 7380 9816; 16 Sudeley Street, London N1 8HP Tel: 020 7837 3981 — MB BCh BAO NUI 1966; FFA RCS Eng. 1973; FFA RCSI 1973. Cons. Anaesth. Univ. Coll. Hosp. Lond. Specialty: Anaesth. Socs: Obst. Anaesth. Assn. & Europ. Soc. Regional Anaesth. Prev: Sen. Regist. (Anaesth.) Univ. Coll. Hosp. & Hosp. Sick Childr. Gt. Ormond St.; Regist. (Anaesth.) St. Mary's Hosp. Lond. & Univ. Coll. Hosp. Lond.

WOODS, Sheelagh Kathleen Mary (retired) Armagh Health Centre, Dobbin Lane, Armagh BT61 1ER Tel: 01861 522663; 23 Newry Road, Armagh BT60 1ER Tel: 01861 522663 — MB BCh BAO Belf. 1930.

WOODS, Sheila Mary 3 Gainsborough Court, Skipton BD23 1QG — MB ChB Manch. 1982; BSc St. And. 1979; MB ChB (Hons.) Manch. 1982; MRCP (UK) 1985; DRCOG 1990; MRCGP 1991. GP Skipton. Prev: Med. Off. St. Paul's Hosp. Kashikishi, Zambia.

WOODS, Susan Elizabeth 4 Frenchs Road, Cambridge CB4 3LA — MB BChir Camb. 1993.

WOODS, Susan Elizabeth Hartington Surgery, Dig Street, Hartington, Buxton SK17 0AQ Tel: 01298 84315 Fax: 01298 84899; 2 Goldhill Cottages, Goldhill, Tansley, Matlock DE4 5FG Tel: 01629 56378 Fax: 01629 56378 Email: barmosley@aol.com — MB ChB Liverp. 1978; DRCOG 1983.

WOODS, Tracey Oriole Child & Family Services, (North West Team) Seymour House, 41-43 Seymour Terrace, Seymour St., Liverpool L3 5TE Tel: 0151 707 0101 Fax: 0151 708 9200 — MB ChB Liverp. 1985; MRCPsych 1990; MSc. Manch. 1995. Cons. Child & Family Psychiat. Alder Hey Roy. Liverp. Childr. NHS Trust. Specialty: Child & Adolesc. Psychiat. Prev: Sen. Regist. (Child & Adolesc. Psychiat.) Manch.; Research Regist. (Child & Adolesc. Psychiat.) Univ. Manch.; Regist. Rotat. (Psychiat.) Manch.

WOODS, William Graham Kilkeel Health Centre, Knockchree Avenue, Kilkeel, Newry BT34 4BS Tel: 028 4176 2601 Fax: 028 4176 3308 — MB BCh BAO Belf. 1973.

WOODS, Mr William Gustave Arnold Worthing Hospital, Lyndhurst Road, Worthing BN11 2DH — BM BCh Oxf. 1974; MA Oxf.; FRCS Eng. 1978; DM Oxf. 1987. Specialty: Gen. Surg.

WOODSFORD, Paul Vincent Ty-Cerdd, 29 Cae Rex, Llanblethian, Cowbridge CF71 7JS Tel: 0144 63 773305 & profess 0443 218218 — MB BS Lond. 1973 (St. Mary's) FFA RCS Eng. 1979. Dir. Intens. Care Unit & Cons. Anaesth. Roy. Glam. Hosp. Specialty: Anaesth. Socs: Fell. Fac. Anaesth. RCS Eng.; Assn. Anaesth. & Welsh Intens. Care Soc. Prev: Sen. Regist. (Anaesth.) Nottm. HA (T); Sen. Specialist (Anaesth.) Princess Alexandra Hosp. RAF Wroughton.

WOODSIDE, Robert, RD (retired) Flat 10 Wallace Court, 39 Wallace Road, Broadstone BH18 8NF Tel: 01202 691132 — MB BS Lond. 1951 (Lond. Hosp.) MRCS Eng. LRCP Lond. 1951. Prev: Sen. Med. & Health Off. Hong Kong Govt.

WOODSIDE, Robert Monckton (retired) Healdswood House, Skegby, Sutton-in-Ashfield NG17 3FR — MRCS Eng. LRCP Lond. 1943 (Guy's) Prev: Med. Off. Leicester & Nottm. Racecourses.

WOODWARD, Mr Alan Royal Glamorgan Hospital, Ynysmaerdy, Llantrisant CF72 8XR Tel: 01443 443541 Fax: 01443 223434 Email: alanwoodward@uk-herniasurgeon.co.uk — MB BCh Wales 1983; FRCS Ed. 1987; MCh Thesis 1993. Cons. Gen. Surg.,Royal Glam. Hosp., Llantrisant; Cons. Gen. Surg., BUPA Hosp. Cardiff; Cons. Gen. Surg., Llwynypia Hosp., Rhondda. Specialty: Gen. Surg. Special Interest: Hernia Surgery; laparoscopic Surgery; Surgical Gastroenterology. Socs: Assn. Surgeons GB and NI; Assn. Coloproctologists GB & NI; Bariatric Obesity Surg. Soc. Prev: Sen. Regist., Gen. Surg., Singleton Hosp., Swansea; Regist. Gen. Surg., Llandough Hosp., Cardiff; Regist. Gen. Surg., Nevill Hall Hosp., Abergavenny.

WOODWARD, Albert Kenneth (retired) Fleetwith, 29 Suckling Green Lane, Codsall, Wolverhampton WV8 2BP Tel: 01902 843747 Email: kandjwoodward@waitrose.com — (Birm.) MB ChB Birm. 1957; DObst RCOG 1959.

WOODWARD, Alison Jane Rothschild House Surgery, Chapel Street, Tring HP23 6PU Tel: 01442 822468; The Old House, 38 Station Road, Ivinghoe, Leighton Buzzard LU7 9EB Tel: 01296 668444 — MB BS Lond. 1976 (Middlesex) Princip., Gen. Pract. Rothscild Ho. Surg., Tring Herts. Prev: SO Empangeni Provin. Hosp. Empangeni Natal SA; Phys. & Surg. Chas. Johnson Memor. Hosp. Nqutu, Kwazulu, S. Afr.; SHO (ENT) Cheltenham Gen. Hosp. / A+E Cheltenham Roy. Hosp.

WOODWARD, Mrs Audrey Mary (retired) Woodlands, Swainsea Lane, Pickering YO18 8NF — MB ChB Leeds 1951; DCH Eng. 1954; MRCP Ed. 1956. SCMO ScarBoro. HA. Prev: Asst. Res. Med. Off. Birm. Childr. Hosp.

WOODWARD, Catherine Mary Department of Public Health Medicine, Avon Health Authority, King Square House, King Square, Bristol BS2 5EE — BSc (Biochem.) Leeds 1982, MB ChB 1985; DCH RCP Lond. 1987; MFPHM RCP (UK) 1994. Cons. in Pub. Health Med., Avon Health Auth.; Lect. (Pub. Health Med.) Univ. Cape Town. Specialty: Pub. Health Med. Socs: BMA & Soc. Social Med. Prev: Wessex Region Train. Scheme in Pub. Health Med.; Winchester DHA VTS.

WOODWARD, Cathryn Louise Queen Elizabeth Hospital, Edgbaston, Birmingham B15 2T Tel: 0121 472 1311 — MB ChB Birm. 1992; MRCP (UK) 1995; FRCR (UK) 2001. Regist. (Clin. Oncol.) Qu. Eliz. Hosp. Birm. Specialty: Oncol.; Radiother. Prev: SHO (Gen. Med.) Sandwell Hosp. Birm.; SHO (Oncol. & Radiother.) Cookridge Hosp. Leeds; SHO (A & E) City Hosp. Birm.

WOODWARD, David Keith Department of Anaesthetics, Northern General Hospital, Herries Road, Sheffield S5 7AU Tel: 0114 243

4343 — MB ChB Leeds 1986 (Univ. Leeds) MRCP (UK) 1989; FRCA 1994. Cons. Anaesth.,N.. Gen. Hosp. Sheff. Specialty: Anaesth. Prev: Sen.Reg. (Anaesth) The Alfred Hosp.Melbourne; Lect.,P. of Wales Hosp. Shatin,Hong Kong.

WOODWARD, Elisabeth Anne The Surgery, 20 Westdale Lane, Gedling, Nottingham NG4 3JA; 10 Retford Road, Sherwood, Nottingham NG5 1FZ Tel: 0115 960 5743 — BM BS Nottm. 1988; BMedSci Nottm. 1986; MRCGP 1992.

WOODWARD, Jeremy Mark 'Appletrees', Padlock Road, Westwratting, Cambridge CB1 5LS — MB BChir Camb. 1990; MA Camb. 1990; MRCP PL 2000. Cons. Gastroenterol. & Gen. Med. Addenbrookes Hosp. Camb. Prev: Ho. Phys. St. Thos. Hosp.; SHO (Cardiol.) Hammersmith Hosp. Lond.

WOODWARD, John 57 Greenville Drive, Maghull, Liverpool L31 7DF — MB ChB Liverp. 1978.

WOODWARD, John Wakerley Sidcup Health Centre, 43 Granville Road, Sidcup DA14 4TA Tel: 020 8302 7721 Fax: 020 8309 6579; 33 Rectory Lane, Sidcup DA14 4QN Tel: 020 8302 9970 Fax: 020 8302 2224 — MB BS Lond. 1962 (St. Thos.) DObst RCOG 1964; DCH Eng. 1965; FRCGP 1985, M 1974. Specialty: Gen. Med. Socs: BMA. Prev: Ho. Surg. Roy. Waterloo Hosp.; Ho. Phys. W. Kent Hosp. Maidstone; Ho. Off. (Obst.) Brit. Hosp. Mothers & Babies Woolwich.

WOODWARD, Mr Mark Nicholas Long Acre, Alveston, Stratford-upon-Avon CV37 7QN Tel: 01789 293780 — BM (Hons.) Soton. 1992; FRCS Eng. 1996. Specialty: Paediat. Surg.

WOODWARD, Nicholas Arthur (retired) Long Acre, Alveston Leys Park, Alveston, Stratford-upon-Avon CV37 7QN Tel: 01789 293780 — MB ChB Birm. 1962; MRCS Eng. LRCP Lond. 1962; DObst RCOG 1964; DA Eng. 1965; FFA RCS Eng. 1968. Prev: GP Bridge Ho. Med. Centre Stratford-upon-Avon.

WOODWARD, Philippa Jane 12 Mayfield Close, Walton-on-Thames KT12 5PR — BChir Camb. 1991.

WOODWARD, Rosalind Mary 8 Brookfield Gardens, Sarisbury Green, Southampton SO31 7DT — MB BS Lond. 1967.

WOODWARD, Roy Bennett Spread Initiative Department, Liverpool Health Authority, Hamilton House, 24 Pall Mall, Liverpool L3 6AL Tel: 0151 236 4620 Fax: 0151 258 1264 Email: spreadini@yahoo.com; 4 Butterfield Gardens, Aughton, Ormskirk L39 4XN Tel: 01695 576965 Email: roy@butterfield4.demon.co.uk — (Liverp.) MB ChB Liverp. 1969; FRCGP 1995, M 1978. Princip. Maghull Merseyside; Spread Initiative Co-ord. NW Region. Prev: Med. Adviser Sefton HA.

WOODWARD, Siân Glasfryn, Pentre Cilcain, Mold CH7 5PE — MB BCh Wales 1981. GP Trainee Clwyd HA.

WOODWARD, William Marshall Royal Cornwall Hospitals Trust, Treliske Hospital, Department of Anaesthesia, Treliske, Truro TR1 3LJ Tel: 01872 253134 Fax: 01872 252480 Email: william.woodward@rcht.swest.nhs.uk; Primrose Cottage, Greenwith Road, Perranwell Station, Truro TR3 7LU Tel: 01872 864104 — MB ChB Sheff. 1985 (Sheffield) DA (UK) 1988; FRCA 1992. Cons. (Anaesth./IC) Roy. Cornw. Hosp. Truro, Cornw. Specialty: Intens. Care. Prev: Sen. Regist. Rotat. (Anaesth.) Bristol; Lect. (Anaesth.) Univ. Sheff.; Regist. Rotat. (Anaesth.) Sheff.

WOODWARD-COURT, Rodney Ian The Phoenix Surgery, 64 Sea Lane, Goring-by-Sea, Worthing BN12 4PY Tel: 01903 240568 Fax: 01903 247099; 33 Lansdowne Road, Worthing BN11 4NF Tel: 01903 502135 — MB BS Lond. 1972 (Char. Cross) GP Goring-by-Sea. Prev: Med. Off. Ngora (Ch. of Uganda) Hosp.; SHO (Geriat.) Char. Cross Hosp. Lond.; Ho. Surg. W. Lond. Hosp.

WOODWARDS, Mr Robert Timothy Michael Maxillofacial Unit, North Manchester NHS Trust, Central Drive, Manchester M8 5RB Tel: 0161 720 2143 Fax: 0161 720 2284; 210 The Grand, 1 Aytoun St, Manchester M1 3DA Tel: 0161 236 7090 Fax: 0161 236 7090 — MB BCh Wales 1987 (Univ. Wales) FRCS Eng.; MD Manch.; BDS Birm. 1978; FDS RCS Eng. 1983; FRCS Ed. 1990. Cons. Oral & Maxillofacial Surg. Manch. NHS Trust & Rochdale NHS Trust. Specialty: Oral & Maxillofacial Surg. Socs: Liveryman Worshipful Soc. Apoth. City of Lond.; BMA; Brit. Assn. Oral & Maxillofacial Surg. Prev: Sen. Regist. (Oral & Maxillofacial Surg.) Qu. Mary's Univ. Hosp. Lond.

WOODWARK, Catherine 24 Cunningham Hill Road, St Albans AL1 5BY — MB ChB Bristol 1981.

WOODWORTH, Andrea Elizabeth 83 Griffiths Close, Swindon SN3 4NP — MB BCh Wales 1985; MRCGP 1990. Trainee GP Nevill Hall Hosp. Abergavenny. Prev: SHO (c/o Elderly) Nevill Hall Hosp. Abergavenny.

WOODYARD, Mr John Edward (retired) 32 Knowle Road, Stafford ST17 0DP Tel: 01785 665941 — (Westm.) MB Camb. 1956, BChir 1955; DObst RCOG 1957; FRCS Ed. 1961; FRCS Eng. 1961. Prev: Cons. Orthop. Surg. Dist. Gen. Hosp. Stafford.

WOODYATT, Christopher Prust 53 Church Street, South Cave, Brough HU15 2EP Tel: 01430 423173 — MB ChB Leeds 1969; BSc (Hons.) Leeds 1966; MB ChB (Hons.) Leeds 1969; DCH Eng. 1971; DObst RCOG 1972; FRCGP 1993, M 1974. Prev: Ho. Phys. Profess. Unit Birm. Childr. Hosp.; Concise Organiser Hull GP VTS Scheme.

WOODYER, Mr Anthony Bartlam Windy Harbour Cottage, Woodhead Road, Glossop SK13 7QE Tel: 01457 855239 Fax: 01457 855239 — MB ChB Ed. 1972; FRCS Ed. 1977; FRCS Eng. 1978; ChM Ed. 1985. Cons. Surg. Tameside Gen. Hosp. Ashton-under-Lyne. Specialty: Gen. Surg. Special Interest: Vasc.

WOOF, Alison Mary Haresfield House Surgery, 6-10 Bath Road, Worcester WR5 3EJ Tel: 01905 763161 Fax: 01905 67016; 3 Gargen Cottages, Marlbrook Lane, Sale Green, Droitwich WR9 7LW — MB ChB Birm. 1984; DCH RCP Lond. 1987; DRCOG 1988; MRCGP 1988; M.Med. Sci. Birm. 1998.

WOOF, William Richard Corbett Medical Practice, 36 Corbett Avenue, Droitwich WR9 7BE Tel: 01905 795566 Fax: 01905 796984; 7 Richmond Hill, Worcester WR5 1DP — MB BS Lond. 1986; MRCGP 1991; M Med.Sci. Birm. 1998. Clin. Lect, (Gen. Pract.) Univ. Brimingham; Clin. Asst. St. Richards Hospice Worcester. Specialty: Gen. Pract.; Palliat. Med. Prev: Clin. Research Fell. (Gen. Pract.) Univ. Birm.; Trainee GP Harefield Ho. Surg. Worcester; SHO (O & G) Worcester Roy. Infirm. VTS.

WOOFF, Derek James Stranraer Health Centre, Edinburgh Road, Stranraer DG9 7HG Tel: 01776 706566; Lochwood, 36 Larg Road, Stranraer DG9 0JE Tel: 01776 705778 — MB ChB Glas. 1980 (Glasgow) MRCGP 1984; DCH RCP Lond. 1984; DRCOG 1987. Specialty: Gen. Pract.

WOOKEY, Brian (retired) Pontcae Surgery, Dynevor Street, Georgetown, Merthyr Tydfil CF48 1YE Tel: 01685 723931 Fax: 01685 377048 — MB BCh Wales 1961; MRCGP 1980.

WOOKEY, Brian Eric Penny Liquorpond Street Surgery, 10 Liquorpond Street, Boston PE21 8UE Tel: 01205 362763 Fax: 01205 358918 — MB BS Lond. 1961 (Middlx.) DObst RCOG 1963; FRCGP 1980, M 1969. Chairm. Trent Regional Med. & Dent. Comm. Socs: BMA; Counc. Nat. Assn. of HAs.

WOOKEY, Sarah Lucy Mary West Bar Surgery, 1 West Bar Street, Banbury OX16 9SF Tel: 01295 256261 Fax: 01295 756848; Waggonners Cottage, Sandford Common Farm, Sandford St. Martin, Chipping Norton OX7 7AE Tel: 0160 863673 Fax: 0160 863417 Email: sarahw@andromedalight.co.uk — MB BCh BAO Belf. 1983; DRCOG 1985; DCH RCP Lond. 1985; MRCGP 1988; MRCP (UK) 1990; DFFP 1997. GP Banbury. Specialty: Gen. Pract.

WOOL, Rosemary Jane, CB Wicken House, 105 Weston Road, Aston Clinton, Aylesbury HP22 5EP Tel: 01296 630448 Fax: 01296 632448 — (Char. Cross) MB BS Lond. 1960; DObst RCOG 1965; DPM Eng. 1973; FRCPsych 1987, M 1974. Hon. Sec. Gen. Internat. Counc. Prison Med. Servs.; Med. Adv. To Dept. Leg. Affairs, Counc. Of Europe. Specialty: Gen. Psychiat.; Forens. Psychiat. Socs: Roy. Soc. Med., Internat. Counc. Prison Med. Servs.; BMA. Prev: Head of Educ. & Train. Dept of Addict. Behaviour, St. Geo.s's Hosp. Med. Sch.; Dir. of Health Care Prison Serv.

WOOLARD, Fiona Elizabeth Kennoway Medical Group, Jordan Lane, Kennoway, Leven KY8 5JZ Tel: 01333 350241 Fax: 01333 352884 — MB ChB Manch. 1987; BSc (Med. Sci.) St. And. 1984.

WOOLAS, Mr Robert Philip Gayfield, Portsdown Hill Road, Cosham, Portsmouth PO6 1BE Tel: 023 92 375178 — MB BS Lond. 1982; FRCS Glas. 1987; FRCS Ed. 1987; MRCOG 1990; MRACOG 1991; MD Lond. 1995. Cons. Gyn. Oncol. St. Mary's Hosp. Portsmouth. Specialty: Obst. & Gyn. Socs: Fell. Roy. Soc. Med.; Coun. Mem. Brit. Gyn. Cancer Soc.; Internat. Gyn. Cancer Soc. Prev: Fell. Roy. Marsden Hosp.; Regist. Roy. Lond. Hosp.; Resid. Med. Off. Qu. Charlottes Hosp.

WOOLCOCK, Jacqueline Anne New Pond Row Surgery, 35 South St., Lancing BN15 8AN Tel: 01903 752265; 6 Beach Road, Shoreham-by-Sea BN43 5LJ Tel: 01273 453540 — MB BChir

Camb. 1963 (New Hall Cambridge, Westminster Hospital) MRCS Eng. LRCP Lond. 1963; MRCP (UK) 1965; T(GP) 1993. GP Partner; Family Plann. Doctor Worthing Priority Care NHS Trust. Specialty: Gen. Pract.; Family Plann. & Reproduc. Health. Prev: SHO (Med.) Manch. Roy. Infirm.; Med. Off. Dohnavur Fellowship Hosp. Dohnavur Tirunelveli Dist. Tamil Nadu, India.

WOOLDER, Sara Louise The Coatham Surgery, 18 Coatham Road, Redcar TS10 1RJ Tel: 01642 483495; 'Edinbane', 11 Cringle Moor Chase, Great Broughton, Middlesbrough TS9 7HS Tel: 01642 710684 — BM BS Nottm. 1988 (Nottingham) BMedSci 1986; MRCGP 1992; DRCOG 1992.

WOOLDRIDGE, Wilfred John 3 Lyndhurst Drive, Hale, Altrincham WA15 8EA — MB ChB Manch. 1984; DA (UK) 1989; FRCA 1992. Cons. Cardiothoracic Anaesth. Wythenshawe Hosp. Manch. Specialty: Anaesth. Socs: BMA. Prev: Sen. Regist. (Anaesth.) NW Region.

WOOLER, Mr Geoffrey Hubert, TD, Lt.-Col. RAMC (retired) Shaw Grange, 19 Shaw Lane, Headingley, Leeds LS6 4DH Tel: 0113 275 9356 — (Camb. & Lond. Hosp.) MRCS Eng. LRCP Lond. 1937; MD Camb. 1947, MA, MB BChir 1938; FRCS Eng. 1941; Hon. MD Szeged Univ. Hungary 1983. Hon. Thoracic Surg. Leeds Gen. Infirm. Prev: Thoracic Surg. United Leeds Hosps.

WOOLF, Adrian Spencer Developmental Biology Unit, Institute of Child Health, 30 Guildford St., London WC1N 1EH; 15A Hanley Road, London N4 3DU — MB BS Lond. 1981; MB BS (Hons. Med.) Lond. 1981; MA Camb. 1982; MRCP (UK) 1984; MD Lond. 1989. Cons. & Sen. Lect. Inst. Child Health Lond. Specialty: Nephrol. Socs: Internat. Soc. Nephrol.; Amer. Soc. Nephrol. Prev: Research Fell. Div. Nephrol. UCLA Sch. Med. Los Angeles, USA; Regist. (Med.) Middlx. Hosp. Lond.

WOOLF, Alison Mary North Cardiff Medical Centre, Excalibur Drive, Thornhill, Cardiff CF14 9BB Tel: 029 2075 0322 Fax: 029 2075 7705; 3 Clun Terrace, Cathays, Cardiff CF24 4RB Tel: 029 2038 2614 — MB BCh Wales 1988; MRCP (UK) 1991; MRCGP Lond. 1996. GP N. Cardiff Med. Centre Cardiff. Specialty: Gen. Pract. Socs: BMA; MDU. Prev: GP Regist. Cardiff; Regist. (Haemat.) W. Midl.; SHO (Med.) W. Glam. HA.

WOOLF, Professor Anthony Derek Duke of Cornwall Rheumatology Department, Royal Cornwall Hospital, Truro TR1 3LJ Tel: 01872 253792 Fax: 01872 222857 Email: Anthony.woolf@btopenworld.com; Rope House, Point, Devoran, Truro TR3 6NS Tel: 01872 864442 Fax: 01872 870099 — MB BS Lond. 1975 (Lond. Hosp.) BSc Lond. 1972; MRCP (UK) 1979; FRCP Lond. 1994. Cons. Rheum. Cornw. & I. of Scilly HA; Hon. Prof. Peninsula Med. Sch., Univ. of Exeter & Plymouth. Specialty: Rheumatol. Socs: Brit. Soc. Rheum.; Eur. League Against Rheumatism (Mem. Exec. Comm.); Bone & Jt. decade int. Steering Comm. & Tresur. Prev: Sen. Regist. (Rheum.) Roy. Nat. Hosp. Rheum. Dis. Bath & Bristol Roy. Infirm.; Regist. (Gen. Med. & Rheum.) Guy's Hosp. Lond.; Hon. Prof. Postgrad. Med. Sch. Univ. of Plymouth.

WOOLF, Mr Anthony John (retired) 51 Maresfield Gardens, Hampstead, London NW3 5TE Tel: 020 7794 6365 Fax: 020 7431 9286 — MB BS Lond. 1956 (St. Mary's) MRCS Eng. LRCP Lond. 1948; FRCOG 1969, M 1956, DObst 1949; FRCS Eng. 1959. Hon. Lect. (Obst. & Gyn.) St. Bart. Hosp. Med. Coll. Lond.; Examr. RCOG; Examr. & Lect. Centr. Midw. Bd.; Examr. Obst. & Gyn. Conj. Bd. & Univ. Lond. Prev: Hon. Cons. Gyn. Homerton Hosp.

WOOLF, David Andrew Peterborough District Hospital, Thorpe Road, Peterborough PE3 6DA Tel: 01733 874246 Fax: 01733 874326 — MB BS Lond. 1983 (St. Thos.) BSc (1st cl. Hons. Physiol.) Lond. 1980; MRCP (UK) 1986; FRCPCH 1997. Cons. Paediat. P'boro. Dist. Hosp.; Honourary Cons. paeditrician Respirat. Med., Gt Ormond St Hosp. Specialty: Paediat.; Neonat. Socs: FRCPCh. Prev: Sen. Regist. (Paediat.) Hosp. Sick Childr. Gt. Ormond St. Lond.; Lect. (Child Health) & Hon. Sen. Regist. Inst. Child Health & Hosp. Sick Childr. Gt. Ormond St. Lond.; Regist. Rotat. (Paediat.) Lond. Hosp. & Newham Gen. Hosp.

WOOLF, Jesmond Clive (retired) 21 Cremorne Road, Chelsea, London SW10 0NB Tel: 020 7352 6505 — (St. Bart.) MB BS Lond. 1950. Prev: RAF Med. Br., Ho. Surg. St. Mary Abbots Hosp. Kensington.

WOOLF, Josephine Kay Scratchwood House, Barnet Lane, Elstree, Borehamwood WD6 3QU Tel: 020 8953 0900 — BM BCh Oxf. 1975 (Univ. Coll. Hosp.) MA Oxf. 1975; DRCOG 1978; MRCGP 1979. Specialist (Psychosexual Med.) Roy. Free Hosp. & Caryl Thos. Clinic. Harrow Wealdstone; Clin. Asst. Roy. Free Hosp. Sexual Problems Clin. Socs: Inst. Psychosexual Med. Prev: Trainee GP Lond. VTS; GP Twickenham; Med. Edr. Matern. & Child Health.

WOOLF, Margery Philippa Sidney (retired) Doctor's House, Leighland, Roadwater, Watchet TA23 0RP — (Oxf.) BM BCh Oxf. 1950; MA Oxf. 1955. Indep. Pract. Psychiat. Som. Prev: Cons. Psychiat. (long term locum) Yeovil Dist. Hosp.

WOOLF, Professor Neville (retired) 53 Dunstan Road, London NW11 8AE — MB ChB Cape Town 1952; FRCS Eng. 2001; M Med (Path) 1957; PhD Univ. Lond. 1961; FRCPath 1976, M 1964. Prev: Vice-Dean Fac. Clin. Sci. Univ. Coll. Lond.

WOOLF, Patricia Mollie (retired) 122 Elmer Road, Bognor Regis PO22 6LJ Tel: 01243 586870 — (Trinity Coll.) MB BCh BAO Dub. 1951; DCH Eng. 1954. Prev: Regist. Qu. Eliz. Hosp. Childr. Lond.

WOOLF, Peter Grahame 2A Vanbrugh Hill, London SE3 7UF Tel: 020 8858 5798 Fax: 020 8293 9998 — MRCS Eng. LRCP Lond. 1952 (Middlx.) DPM Eng. 1955; FRCPsych 1979, M 1971. Edr. Brit. Jl. Soc. & Clin. Psychiat. & www.scpnet.com. Specialty: Forens. Psychiat. Socs: Soc. of Clin. & Social Psychiat. Prev: Cons. Psychiat. Darenth Pk. Hosp. Dartford; Med. Mem. Ment. Health Rev. Tribunal.; Vis. Psychother. HM Youth Custody Centre Rochester & HM Prison Cookham Wood.

WOOLF, Rex Lee 48 Broxash Road, London SW11 6AB; Pegtyles, 14 Penington Road, Beaconsfield HP9 1ET Tel: 01494 670490 — MB BS Lond. 1988; FRCA 1993; CCST 1997. Cons. Anaesth. Wrexham Pk. hosp. Bucks; Hon. Cons. UCLH. Specialty: Anaesth.; Intens. Care. Socs: BMA; ICS; ACTA.

WOOLF, Simon Mitchley Avenue, 116 Mitchley Avenue, Sanderstead, South Croydon CR2 9HH Tel: 020 8657 6565 — BM Soton. 1979; MRCGP 1985. GP Croydon.

WOOLF, Mr Victor John North Middlesex University Hospital, Sterling Way, London N18 1QX Tel: 020 8887 2000 Email: victorwoolf@aol.com; 94 Bickenhall Mansions, Baker Street, London W1U 6BS Tel: 020 7935 9086 Fax: 020 7935 9086 — MB BS Lond. 1981 (Univ. Coll. Hosp.) FRCS Eng. 1988; FRCS Ed. 1988; FRCS Orth 1997. Cons. (Orthop. Surg.) N. Middlx. Hosp.; Mem. Panel of Examiners, Intercollegiate Speciality Bd. in Trauma & Orthopaedic Surg.; Mem. Ct. of Examiners Roy. Colleges of Surgeons of Edin. & Eng. Specialty: Orthop.; Trauma & Orthop. Surg. Special Interest: Extern. Fixation Techniques. Socs: Fell. Roy. Soc. Med.; Fell. BOA. Prev: Sen. Regist. Rotat. (Orthop.) Middlx., Stanmore & Gt. Ormond St. Hosps.; Regist. Rotat. (Orthop.) Roy. Free Hosp. Lond.

WOOLFALL, Philip 18 Marlbourough Ave, Newcastle upon Tyne NE3 2HT; 18 Marlbourough Ave, Newcastle upon Tyne NE3 2HT — MB ChB Leeds 1992; MRCP(UK) London 1996. Specialist Regist. Diagnostic Radiol., Freeman Hosp., Newc. Specialty: Radiol.

WOOLFENDEN, Emma Catherine O'Connell Street Medical Practice, O'Connell Street, Hawick — MB ChB Sheff. 1991; DCH; DTM & H; MRCGP.

WOOLFENDEN, Mr Kenneth Alan 48 Rodney Street, Liverpool L1 9AA Tel: 0151 709 2079; Riverside, Manorial Road, Parkgate, South Wirral CH64 6QW Tel: 0151 336 7229 — MB ChB Liverp. 1973; FRCS Eng. 1978; FEBU 1992. Cons. Urol. Roy. Liverp. Hosp. Specialty: Urol. Socs: Assoc. Mem. Liverp. Med. Inst.; Birkenhead Med. Soc. Prev: Ho. Phys. & Ho. Surg. Sefton Gen. Hosp. Liverp.; Sen. Demonst. (Anat.) Univ. Liverp.; Regist. (Urol.) Roy. Liverp. Hosp.

WOOLFENDEN, Margaret (retired) 795 Liverpool Road, Ainsdale, Southport PR8 3NU Tel: 01704 578383 Email: m.parker@merseymail.com — MB ChB Liverp. 1942. Prev: Resid. Med. Off. Southport E.M.S. Hosp.

WOOLFORD, David John 23 Burley Road, Oakham LE15 7BZ Tel: 01572 2449 — BM BCh Oxf. 1949 (Lond. Hosp.) MA, BM BCh Oxon. 1949; DObst RCOG 1950. Med. Off. Rutland Memor. Hosp. Oakham; Local Treasury Med. Off.; Anaesth. Off. Rutland Memor. Hosp. Oakham. Prev: Capt. RAMC; Clin. Obst. Off., Ho. Phys. & Ho. Surg. Lond. Hosp.

WOOLFORD, Marcus Christian David Park Drive Health Centre, 2A Park Drive, Leicester Forest East, Leicester LE3 3FN Tel: 0116 289 8111; 18 Faire Road, Glenfield, Leicester LE3 8EA Tel: 0116 231 1899 — MB ChB Leic. 1985; DRCOG 1988; MRCGP 1989.

Prev: Trainee GP Syston; SHO (A & E) Leic. Roy. Infirm.; SHO (O & G) Leic. Gen. Hosp.

WOOLFSON, Gerald 97 Harley Street, London W1N 1DF Tel: 020 7935 3400 Fax: 020 7487 3834; 16 Church Row, London NW3 6UP Tel: 020 7794 1974 — (Cape Town) MB ChB Cape Town 1954; DPM Eng. 1958; FRCP Glas. 1980, M 1963; FRCPsych 1979, M 1971. Cons. Psychiatr. St. Chas. Hosps. Lond.; Cons. Psychotherap. HM Prison Holloway; Hon. Cons. Psychiat. & Sen. Lect. Hammersmith Hosp. & Roy. Postgrad. Med. Sch. Lond. Specialty: Gen. Psychiat. Socs: Fell.Roy. Soc. Med.; Fell. Roy. Soc. Med. Prev: Cons. Psychiat. W. Pk. Hosp. Epsom; 1st Asst. Dept. Psychiat. St. Geo. Hosp. Lond.; Regist. Depts. Surg. & Neuropsychiat. Groote Schuur Hosp. Cape Town.

WOOLFSON, Harold (retired) 19 Chessington Lodge, Regents Park Road, London N3 3AA Tel: 020 8343 0551 Email: sashaharold@btinternet.com — LRCP LRCS Ed. LRFPS Glas. 1950; DCH RCPS Glas. 1964; MRCP (Glas.) 1967; FRCP Glas. 1979; FRCP Ed. 1980; FRCP Lond. 1989. Prev: Hon. Cons. Dermat. Brook Gen. Hosp. Lond.

WOOLFSON, Julian Department of Obstetrics & Gynaecology, Queen Mary's Hospital, Sidcup — MB ChB Birm. 1971; LLM; MRCOG 1978; FRCOG 1991. Cons. (O & G) Qu. Mary's Hosp. Sidcup. Specialty: Obst. & Gyn. Prev: Sen. Regist. Oxf. RHA; Regist. Matern. Dept. Roy. Berks. Hosp. Reading.

WOOLFSON, Peter Ivor Trafford General Hospital, Moorside Road, Davyhulme M41 5SL Tel: 0161 746 2206 Email: peter.woolfson.trafford.nhs.uk; 4 Barbondale Close, Whittle Hall, Warrington WA5 3HU — MB ChB Manch. 1989; BSc 1986; MRCP 1992; MD 1999. Cons. Cardiologist/ Phys., Trafford Gen. Hosp., Manch. Specialty: Cardiol.; Gen. Med. Socs: Brit. Soc. Echocardiogr.; Med. Research Soc.; Brit. Cardiac Soc. Prev: SpR Cardiol., Rochdale Infirm., Rochdale; SpR Cardiol., Manch. Roy. Infirmmary, Manch.; SpR Cardiol., Roy. Bolton Hosp., Bolton.

WOOLFSON, Robin Gideon — (Cambridge University, St. Thomas' Hospital Medical School) MB BChir Camb. 1984; MRCP (UK) 1987; MD Camb. 1991; FRCP Lond. 1999. Cons. Nephrologist, UCLH; Cons. Nephrologist Whittington Hosp. Trust. Specialty: Nephrol.; Gen. Med.

WOOLFSON, Stephen Benjamin 11Midhurst Avenue, London N10 3EP — MB BS Lond. 1988.

WOOLGAR, Justin David 96 Lyes Green, Corsley, Warminster BA12 7PA — MB ChB Leeds 1990.

WOOLGAR, Melanie Joy 16 Great Bounds Drive, Southborough, Tunbridge Wells TN4 0TP — MB ChB Bristol 1983.

WOOLGROVE, Cyril George Tresco, 4 Priorfields, Ashby-de-la-Zouch LE65 1EA Tel: 01530 412320 — MB ChB Birm. 1939; DPH Manch. 1946; FFCM RCP (UK) 1974, M 1964. MOH SE Derbysh. RDC & Long Eaton UDC; Sch. Health Serv. & Environm. Refer. to Handicaps, Housing & Family Health. Specialty: Pub. Health Med.; Occupat. Health. Socs: Fell. Soc. MOH & Manch. Med. Soc. Prev: Med. Off. Birm. RHB; Sen. Asst. MOH & Sen. Sch. Med. Off. Coventry; Dep. MOH & Dep. Sch. Med. Off. Co. Boro. Reading.

WOOLHOUSE, Ian Stewart 2 Mill Rise, South Gosforth, Newcastle upon Tyne NE3 1QY — MB BS Newc. 1993.

WOOLICH, John Gevenson The Surgery, 26A Park Road, Harlesden, London NW10 8TA Tel: 020 8965 5255 Fax: 020 8965 9080; 24 Sidmouth Road, London NW2 5JX Tel: 020 8459 4661 — MB BS Lond. 1959 (Westm.) MRCS Eng. LRCP Lond. 1960; DObst RCOG 1962; MRCGP 1975. Socs: BMA. Prev: Resid. Med. Off. Watford Matern. Hosp.; Ho. Phys. & Ho. Surg. St. Albans City Hosp.

WOOLLACOTT, Morvarid The Surgery, 57 Dowsett Road, Tottenham, London N17 9DL — MRCS Eng. LRCP Lond. London 1967.

WOOLLACOTT, Susan 89 Highgate West Hill, London N6 Tel: 020 8340 8228 — MB ChB Leeds 1965; DPM Eng. 1970; MRCPsych 1972.

WOOLLAM, Christopher Henry Morgan Department of Anaesthetics, Norfolk & Norwich University Hospitals HCT, Colney Lane, Norwich NR4 7UY — MB BS Lond. 1968 (St. Thos.) FFA RCS Eng. 1973. Cons. Anaesth. Norf. & Norwich Hosp. Specialty: Anaesth. Socs: Hosp. Cons. & Specialists Assn. & Assn. Anaesth. GB & Irel; RSM; AAGBI. Prev: Sen. Regist. Berks. AHA; Sen. Regist. & Regist. Nuffield Dept. Anaesth. Radcliffe Infirm. Oxf.

WOOLLAM, Victoria Anne Morgan Downing Street Surgery, 4 Downing Street, Farnham GU9 7NX Tel: 01252 716226 Fax: 01252 322338; Sandhills Corner, Wormley, Godalming GU8 5UF Tel: 01428 683 3618 — MB BS Lond. 1979 (Char. Cross) Clin. Asst. (Dermat.) Farnham Hosp. Specialty: Dermat.

WOOLLANDS, Ian Gordon Scunthorpe General Hospital, Cliff Gardens, Scunthorpe DN15 1BP Tel: 01724 290420 Email: iangwoollands @doctors.net.uk — MB ChB Leic. 1983; BSc Sheff. 1977; MRCGP 1987; AFOM RCP Lond. 1989. Dir. Kaizen Med. Serv. Ltd. Specialty: Occupat. Health; Gen. Pract. Socs: Soc. Occupat. Med.; Brit. Register of Complementary Practitioners - Chinese Med.; ISSSEEM. Prev: Chief Medical Officer, Corus plc.

WOOLLARD, Adrian John 9 Oaklands Drive, Penwortham, Preston PR1 0XY — MB ChB Manch. 1998.

WOOLLARD, Ann Elizabeth Merton Lodge Surgery, West Street, Alford LN13 9HT Tel: 01507 463262 Fax: 01507 466447; Claythorpe Manor, Claythorpe, Alford LN13 0DU Tel: 01507 450042 — MB BS Lond. 1981 (Royal Free Hospital) MRCGP 1985. Clin. Asst. (Dermat.) Louth Co. Hosp. Lincs. Specialty: Dermat. Prev: Trainee GP Pilgrim Hosp. Boston VTS; Ho. Surg. MusGr. Pk. Hosp. Taunton; Ho. Phys. Treliske Hosp. Truro.

WOOLLARD, Bruce Pargeter Pennys Lane Surgery, Pennys Lane, Cranborne, Wimborne BH21 5QE Tel: 01725 517272 Fax: 01725 517746; Lower Meadow Cottage, Tarrant Launceston, Blandford Forum DT11 8BY Tel: 01258 830511 Fax: 01258 830511 Email: brucewoollard@compuserve.com — MB BS Lond. 1988 (St. Mary's Hospital Paddington) DFFP 1994; DRCOG 1994. Clin. Asst. (Obst. & Gyn.) Blandford Hosp. Specialty: Gen. Pract. Prev: SHO (O & G) W. Dorset Hosp.; Trainee GP Wimborne Dorset; Clin. Asst. (Dermat.) Poole Gen. Hosp.

WOOLLARD, Christopher Mark 9 Oaklands Drive, Penwortham, Preston PR1 0XY — MB ChB Liverp. 1995.

WOOLLARD, Susan Jane Community Child Health, Mulberry House, Alder Hey Childrens Hospital, Eaton Road, Liverpool L12 2AP Tel: 0151 228 4811 — MB ChB Manch. 1978; FRCPCH; DCH Eng. 1981. Cons. Community Paedaiat. Roy. Liverp. Childr. Hosp. Specialty: Community Child Health. Socs: Fac. Comm. Health. Prev: SCMO (Child Health) Liverp.; Clin. Med. Off. (Child Health) Salford.

WOOLLASTON, Kevin Alan Harold Yardley Green Medical Centre, 75 Yardley Green Road, Bordesley Green, Birmingham B9 5PU Tel: 0121 773 3737; 16 Arnold Grove, Shirley, Solihull B90 3JR — MB ChB Manch. 1984.

WOOLLASTON, Marion Ethel Frances Four Vine Place, Brighton BN1 3HE Tel: 01273 737578 — MRCS Eng. LRCP Lond. 1942 (King's Coll. Hosp.) BSc Lond. (Physiol.) 1938; DPM Eng. 1952; FRCPsych. 1981, M 1972. Hon. Cons. Psychiat. Char. Cross Hosp. Lond. Specialty: Gen. Psychiat. Socs: Fell. Roy. Soc. Med. Prev: Cons. Psychiat. Char. Cross. Hosp. Lond.; Regist. (Psychiat.) St. Ebba's Hosp. Epsom & Banstead Hosp. Sutton.

WOOLLER, David Michael Whalebridge Practice, Health Centre, Carfax Street, Swindon SN1 1ED Tel: 01793 692933; 10 Callas Rise, Wanborough, Swindon SN4 0AQ Tel: 01793 790528 — MB ChB Sheff. 1966. Clin. Asst. (A & E) Princess Margt. Hosp. Swindon; Med. Off. Pinewood Sch. Bourton. Prev: Doctor to Brit. Men's Alpine Ski Team; Ho. Phys. & Cas. Off. & SHO (Orthop.) Roy. Hosp. Sheff.; SHO (Orthop.) King Edwd. VII Orthop. Hosp. Sheff.

WOOLLER, Dennis John Alfred The Whittington Hospital, Highgate Hill, London N19 5NF Tel: 020 7288 5464 Fax: 020 7288 5417 Email: dennis.wooler@whittington.thenhs.com; 65 Dresden Road, London N19 3BG Tel: 020 7272 2413 Fax: 020 7686 0967 Email: djawooller@aol.com — MB BS Queensland 1981; DA (UK) 1986; FANZCA 1992; FFARACS 1992. Cons. Anaesth. & Dir. (Day Surg.) Whittington Hosp. Lond. Specialty: Anaesth. Socs: Austral. Soc. Anaesth.; Assn. Anaesth.; BMA. Prev: Cons. Anaesth. Gold Coast Hosp. Southport, Austral.

WOOLLETT, Richard John Manor Brook Medical Centre, 117 Brook Lane, London SE3 0EN Tel: 020 8856 5678 Fax: 020 8856 8632 — MB BS Lond. 1984.

WOOLLEY, Andrew Charles Springfield, Street Road, Glastonbury BA6 9EG — BM BCh Oxf. 1996; MA Camb. 1997; MRCP 1999. SpR (Gen. Med. & Resp. Med.) Salisbury Dist. Hosp. Specialty: Gen. Med. Prev: SHO (Med.) Soton. Gen. Hosp.

WOOLLEY, Birgit Victoria Road Surgery, 50 Victoria Road, Worthing BN11 1XB Tel: 01903 230656 Fax: 01903 520094; 30 Nutbourne Road, Worthing BN14 7HS Tel: 01903 204710 Email: birgit@birgit.freeserve.co.uk — State Exam Med Heidelberg 1992; Dip. Psychol. Heidelberg 1977; DRCOG 1996; MRCGP 1997. GP Princip. Specialty: Paediat. Dent. Socs: Med. Protec. Soc.; BMA; RCGP. Prev: GP Regist. Sompting; SHO (Gen. Med.) Worthing Hosp. VTS.

WOOLLEY, Christopher Michael 24 Newfoundland Road, Gabalfa, Cardiff CF14 3LA Tel: 029 2052 2796 — MB BCh Wales 1994. Prev: Ho. Off. (Surg.) Neville Hall Hosp.; Ho. Off. (Med.) E. Glam. Hosp.

WOOLLEY, Jacqueline Louise 21 Lon Y Bryn, Eitminog, Bangor LL57 2LD — MB BCh Wales 1996. Med. SHO Rotat. Cardiff & E. Glam. Hosp. Specialty: Gen. Med. Socs: Med. Protec. Soc. Prev: Med. Ho. Off. E. Glam. Hosp.; Surg. Ho. Off. P. Chas. Hosp.

WOOLLEY, James Barry Senior House Officer, The Maudsley Hospital, Denmark Hill, London SE5 8AZ — MB BS Lond. 1996 (St. Mary's Hosp. Med. Sch.) BSc (Hons.) Lond. 1995. SHO (Psychiat.), The Maudsley Hosp., Lond. Specialty: Gen. Psychiat. Prev: SHO (Med.) Roy. Free Hosp. Lond.; Ho Surg. Northwick Pk. & St. Mark's Hosp., Harrow, Middlx.; Ho. Off. Med. Ealing Hosp. Middlx.

WOOLLEY, Michael James The Medical Centre, 37A Heaton Road, Heaton, Newcastle upon Tyne NE6 1TH Tel: 0191 265 8121 Fax: 0191 276 6085; 8 Bath Terrace, Tynemouth, North Shields NE30 4BL — MB ChB Liverp. 1982. Specialty: Gen. Pract.

WOOLLEY, Paul David Rosebank, Temple St, Padfield, Glossop SK13 1EL — MB ChB Sheff. 1981; DRCOG 1984; MRCP (UK) 1985; DFFP 1996; FRCP Lond. 1996. Cons. Genitourin Med. Withington Hosp. Manch. Specialty: Genitourinary Medicine. Prev: Sen. Regist. & Research Regist. (Genitourin. Med.) Roy. Hallamsh. Hosp. Sheff.

WOOLLEY, Sarah Louise Birmingham Childrens Hospital, Edgbaston, Birmingham B4 6; 11 Lapwing Drive, Hampton-in-Arden, Solihull B92 0BF Tel: 01675 443385 — MB ChB Birm. 1990; MRCP (UK) 1995; MRCPCH 1996. SHO (Paediat.) Birm. Childr. Hosp. Specialty: Paediat. Socs: Brit. Diabetic Assn. Prev: SHO (Paediat. & Neonat.) Addenbrooke's Hosp. Camb.; SHO (Paediat. & Neonat.) New Cross Hosp. Wolverhampton; Regist. (Diabetes & Endocrinol.) Singleton Hosp. Swansea.

WOOLLEY, Steven Michael 46 Riley Road, Yard Wood, Birmingham B14 4JH Tel: 0121 474413 — MB ChB Birm. 1997. SHO Gen. Surg., Birm. Heartlands Hosps. Specialty: Gen. Surg.; Cardiothoracic Surg.; Accid. & Emerg. Prev: SHO (A & E) Birm. Heartlands Hosp.; Ho. Off. (Surg.) Birm. Heartlands Hosp.; Ho. Off. (Med.) Alexandra Hosp. Redditch.

WOOLLEY, Vivian Lloyd (retired) Y Ddol, 21 Lon-y-Bryn, Eithinog, Bangor LL57 2LD Tel: 01248 352158 — MB BCh Wales 1964 (Cardiff) DCH Eng. 1969; MRCP (UK) 1970; FRCP Lond. 1990; FRCPCH 1997. Cons. Paediat. Gwynedd Hosp. Prev: Sen. Regist. (Paediat.) United Cardiff Hosps.

WOOLLEY, Wendy (retired) 45 Stanneylands Drive, Wilmslow SK9 4EU Tel: 01625 523553 — (Roy. Free) MB BS Lond. 1947. Prev: Clin. Asst. Dept. Rheum. Withington Hosp. Manch.

WOOLLONS, Andrew David The Surgery, 75 Longridge Avenue, Saltdean, Brighton BN2 8LA Tel: 01273 305723 Fax: 01273 300962 — MB ChB Bristol 1987; DCH RCP Lond. 1990; DRCOG 1991; MRCGP 1993. Specialty: Gen. Pract.

WOOLLONS, Arjida Department of Dermatology, Worthing and Southlands NHS Trust, Lyndhurst Road, Worthing BN11 2DH Tel: 01903 205111 Fax: 01903 823721 — MB BS Lond. 1987 (Guy's, London) MRCP (UK) 1993; MD 2001. Cons. Dermatol., Worthing & Southlands NHS Trust. Specialty: Dermat. Socs: BAD; BSID; BSPD. Prev: Specialist Regist. (Dermat.) Brighton Health Care NHS Trust & St. John's Inst. Dermat. Lond.; Regist. (Neurol.) Hurstwood Pk. Neurol. Centre; SHO Rotat. (Gen. Med.) Kent & Canterbury Hosp.

WOOLLONS, Martin John Pensby Road Surgery, 349 Pensby Road, Pensby, Wirral CH61 9NL Tel: 0151 648 1193 Fax: 0151 648 2934 — MB BS Lond. 1992.

WOOLMORE, Michael John Frank (retired) 457 Wellingborough Road, Northampton NN3 3HW Tel: 01604 713908 Email: michael@woolymed.demon.co.uk — (St. Bart.) MB BS Lond. 1959; MRCS Eng. LRCP Lond. 1959; DObst RCOG 1964; MRCGP 1975. Prev: GP Northampton.

WOOLNER, Catherine Anne University Health Service, University of Southampton, Building 48, Highfield, Southampton SO17 1BJ Tel: 023 8055 7531 Fax: 023 8059 3259 — MB ChB Birm. 1987.

WOOLNER, Harold William (retired) 4/1 Craufurdland, Braepark Rd, Edinburgh EH4 6DL Tel: 0131 317 7596 — LRCP LRCS Ed. 1944; LRCP LRCS Ed. LRFPS Glas. 1944; DPH Ed. 1952. Med. Off. Scott. Home & Health Dept. seconded to Ment. Welf. Commiss. Scotl. Prev: Sen. Health Off. West. Region Nigeria.

WOOLNOUGH, Melanie Jane Heatherlea, 5 Lucas Road, High Wycombe HP13 6QE — MB ChB Sheff. 1998.

WOOLRICH, Louise Helen 21 Haddon Crescent, Beeston, Nottingham NG9 5JU — MB ChB Bristol 1992.

WOOLRYCH, Jonathan Michael 20 Nightingale Road, Godalming GU7 3AG — MB BChir Camb. 1990.

WOOLRYCH, Michael Ernfrid (retired) 20 Nightingale Road, Godalming GU7 3AG — BM BCh Oxf. 1958 (Oxf. & St. Bart.) Prev: Ho. Off. (Paediat.) Radcliffe Infirm. Oxf.

WOOLRYCH, Rachel Susan Breaconside Farm, Moniaive, Thornhill DG3 4DZ — BChir Camb. 1994; BA Camb. 1992.

WOOLSEY, Siobhan Marie 12 McGreavy Drive, Lurgan, Craigavon BT66 6LS Tel: 01762 342030 — MB BCh BAO Belf. 1995; MB BCh Belf. 1995. Specialty: Gen. Surg.

WOOLTERTON, Mark Clive Avenue Road Surgery, 2 Avenue Road, Warley, Brentwood CM14 5EL Tel: 01277 212820 Fax: 01277 234169; 114 Woodman Road, Brentwood CM14 5AL — MB BChir Camb. 1989; MA Camb. 1990; MRCP (UK) 1992; MRCGP 1994.

WOOLTORTON, Mr Stephen John St Thomas Road Health Centre, St. Thomas Road, Newquay TR7 1RU Tel: 01637 878599; Tregosse, Wheal Friendly, St Agnes TR5 0SR Tel: 01872 552601 — MB BS Lond. 1974 (Westm.) BSc (Physiol.) Lond. 1970; MRCS Eng. LRCP Lond. 1974; DRCOG 1976; FRCS Eng. 1979. Specialty: Gen. Pract. Prev: GP. I. of Scilly; Med. Off. & Sen. Med. Off. St. Helena.

WOOLVEN, David William Brading (retired) The Glebe House, Clothall, Baldock SG7 6RE Tel: 01462 790335 — (Liverp.) MB ChB (1st Cl. Hons.) Liverp. 1952; DObst RCOG 1954.

WOON, Mr Wai Hong — MB BChir Camb. 1982; MRCP (UK) 1984; FRCS Ed. 1988; FRCOphth 1990. Cons. Ophth. Leeds Gen. Infirm. Specialty: Ophth. Special Interest: Vitreo-retinal Surgery.

WOOSNAM, Larissa Diana, Princess of Wales Hospital, Scartho Road, Grimsby DN33 2BA Tel: 01472 874111 Ext: 7103 Fax: 01472 875418 Email: larissa.woosnam@nlg.nhs.uk — Vrach 1974 (Kalinin State Med. Inst.) MRCP UK 1996. Cons. Phys. with a special interest in care of the elderly and osteoporosis, N.E. Lincs. NHS Trust, Grimsby. Specialty: Care of the Elderly. Socs: BGS; NOS; RCP.

WOOSTER, Edgar Gerald 28 Holly Grove, London SE15 5DF Fax: 020 7635 0448/020 7732 8517 — MB BChir Camb. 1957 (St. Bart.) MRCP Lond. 1960; DPM Lond. 1963; FRCPsych 1981, M 1971. Specialty: Psychother. Socs: Assoc. Mem. Brit. Psychoanalyt. Soc.; Mem. Gp. Analytic Soc. (Lond.). Prev: Cons. Psychiat. Lond. Univ. Centr. Inst. Stud. Health Serv.; Cons. Psychotherapist St. Geo. Hosp. Lond.; Sen. Regist. (Psychother.) Maudsley Hosp. Lond.

WOOSTER, Sarah Louise 28 Hawthorn Road, Hale, Altrincham WA15 9RG — MB ChB Sheff. 1988. Regist. Rotat. (Med. Microbiol.) NW RHA. Specialty: Med. Microbiol.

WOOTHIPOOM, Wit 28 Princes Gate, London SW7 — MB BS Lond. 1973; MRCP (UK) 1977.

WOOTLIFF, Alan Brian 10 St Regis Heights, Firecrest, West Heath Road, London NW3 7NE — (Manch.) MB ChB Manch. 1956. Prev: Clin. Asst. Dept. Rheum. E. Lond. Gp. Hosps.; Ho. Phys. Memor. Hosp. Darlington; Ho. Surg. St. Mary Abbot's Hosp. Lond.

WOOTTON, Alan (retired) Redwood House, Fiery Lane, Uley, Dursley GL11 5DA — MB ChB Birm. 1956; DObst RCOG 1963. Prev: GP Dursley.

WOOTTON, Alison Catherine The Surgery, Station Road, Langbank, Port Glasgow PA14 6YA; Newton Farm, Kilmacolm PA13 4TE — MB BS Newc. 1973. Prev: SHO (Obst.) Forth Pk. Matern. Hosp. Kirkcaldy; Regist. (Geriat.) Bridge of Weir Hosp.; Ho. Surg. Gt. Yarmouth & Gorleston Gen. Hosp.

WOOTTON, Ian David Phimester (retired) Cariad Cottage, Cleeve Road, Goring, Reading RG8 9DB Tel: 01491 873050 — MB BChir Camb. 1945 (St. Mary's) MA Camb. 1945; PhD Lond. 1950; FRSC

1956; FRCPath 1972, M 1963; FRCP Lond. 1974, M 1969. Prev: Univ. Lond. Prof. Chem. Path. Roy. Postgrad. Med. Sch. Lond.

WOOTTON, Mr James Robert Maelor General Hospital, Croesnewydd Road, Wrexham LL13 7TD — MB BS Lond. 1981 (St. Bart.) BSc (Hons. Pharmacol.) Lond. 1979, MB BS 1981; FRCS Eng. 1985. Regist. (Orthop. Train. Scheme) Robt. Jones & Agnes Hunt Orthop.; Hosp. OsW.ry. Specialty: Orthop. Prev: Regist. (Orthop.) Gwynedd Hosp. Bangor.

WOOTTON, Julia Clare St. Nicholas Hospice, Macmillan Way, Hardwick Lane, Bury St Edmunds IP33 2QY Tel: 01284 766133 Fax: 01284 752709 — BM Soton. 1985 (Southampton) BEd Lancaster 1972; Dip. Palliat. Med. Cardiff 1996. Med. Dir. St. Nicholas Hospice; Cons. Palliat. Med. W. Suff. Hosp., Hardwick La., Bury St. Edmunds, IP33 2QY. Specialty: Palliat. Med. Socs: Assn. for Palliat. Med.; Fell. Roy. Soc. of Med.; Brit. Med. Assn. Prev: Assoc. Specialist St. Lukes Hospice Basildon Essex.; G.P. Princip., Bournemouth, Dorset.

WOOTTON, Leslie William 15 Mamignot Close, Bearstead, Maidstone ME14 4PT Tel: 01622 735939 — MRCS Eng. LRCP Lond. 1967 (Sheff.) DObst RCOG 1969; DO Maidstone 1994. Lect. NESCOT. Specialty: Gen. Pract.; Osteop. Socs: Fell. Roy. Soc. Med. Prev: Ho. Surg. Wharncliffe Hosp. Sheff.; Ho. Phys. (Neurol.) Fulwood Annexe Roy. Hosp. Sheff.; Ho. Off. (Obst.) Jessop. Hosp. Sheff.

WOOTTON, Mary (retired) Redwood House, Fiery Lane, Uley, Dursley GL11 5DA Tel: 01453 860371 — (Birm.) MB ChB Birm. 1956. Prev: GP Dursley & Cas. Off. Stroud Gen Hosp.

WOOTTON, Matthew Alan Dept. Of Anaesthetics, Yeovil District General Hospiatal, Higher Kingston, Yeovil BA21 4AT Tel: 01935 384246 — MB BS Lond. 1990; BSc (Hons. Physiol.) Newc. 1984; FRCA 1996. Cons. Anaesth. Yeovil Dist. Gen. Hosp. Som. Specialty: Anaesth.

WOOTTON, Oonagh Rosemary The Doctors Centre, 41 Broomwood Road, Orpington BR5 2JP Tel: 01689 832454 Fax: 01689 826165; 20 Hamilton Road, Sidcup DA15 7HB Tel: 020 8302 5942 — MB ChB Sheff. 1965. Clin. Asst. (Haemat.) Qu. Mary's Hosp. Sidcup. Prev: Asst. MOH & Sch. Med. Off. Sheff.; Cas. Off. Roy. Hosp. Sheff.; Ho. Phys. (Dermat.) Sheff. Roy. Infirm.

WOOTTON, Romola Isabel (retired) Harvington, 10 Bell Road, Walsall WS5 3JW Tel: 0121 357 2067 — MB ChB Birm. 1959. Prev: Cons. Pub. Health Med. Walsall HA.

WOOTTON, Russell Philip New Surgery, Bridge of Weir Road, Kilmacolm PA13 4AP Tel: 01505 872844 Fax: 01505 872299; Newton Farm, Kilmacolm PA13 4TE — MB BS Newc. 1972. Med. Off. Epileptic Centre Quarriers Homes Bridge of Weir. Specialty: Gen. Pract. Prev: Cas. Off. Vict. Hosp. Kirkcaldy; Ho. Off. Sunderland Gen. Hosp.

WORAH, Rekha Church Lane Medical Centre, Orchid Rise, Off Church Lane, Scunthorpe DN15 7AN Tel: 01724 864341 Fax: 01724 876441 — MB BS Patna 1977. Trainee GP Hull.

WORBY, Malcolm Eric (retired) New Road Surgery, New Road, Brighstone, Newport PO30 4BB Tel: 01983 740219 Fax: 01983 741399; Rainsgrove, Chilton Lane, Brighstone, Newport PO30 4DS — MB BS Lond. 1970 (Guy's) MRCS Eng. LRCP Lond. 1970. Prev: Sen. Med. Off. UK Atomic Energy Auth.

WORDEN, Richard John Wayfarers, Pilgrims Way, Broad St., Hollingbourne, Maidstone ME17 1RB — MB BS Lond. 1961 (Guy's) MRCS Eng. LRCP Lond. 1961; DObst RCOG 1963. Med. Adviser Appeals Serv., tribunel appeals for Disabil. awareness. Specialty: Disabil. Med. Prev: GP Chatham; Ho. Off. (Obst.) Mile End Hosp.; Ho. Surg. & Ho. Phys. St. Olave's Hosp. Lond.

WORDEN, Timothy William John The Docs, 55-59 Bloom Street, Manchester M1 3LY Tel: 0161 237 9490 Fax: 0161 228 3164 — BM BS Nottm. 1979 (Nottingham) Specialty: Gen. Pract.

WORDLEY, Anthony Richard Ivy Grove Surgery, 1 Ivy Grove, Ripley DE5 3HN Tel: 01773 742286 Fax: 01773 749812; The Kennels, Alderwasley, Belper DE56 2RB Tel: 01629 822315 — MB BS Lond. 1979 (St. Thos.) Cert Family Plann. JCC 1984. Socs: Derby Med. Soc.

WORDSWORTH, Andrew Damian Trinty Surgery, Norwich Road, Wisbech PE13 3UZ Tel: 01945 436999 — BM BS Nottm. 1988; DGM; BMedSci, Nottm, 1986. GP Princip. Cambs Fens; Med. Examr; Police Surg. Cambridgeshire Constab.

WORDSWORTH, Professor Bryan Paul Seddon Ward, Nuffield Orthopaedic Centre, Oxford OX3 7LD Tel: 01865 741155 Fax: 01865 227 876 Email: paul.wordsworth@noc.anglox.nhs.uk; Tollgate Cottage, Lower Heyford, Bicester OX25 5PE Tel: 01869 340794 — MB BS Lond. 1975 (Westm. Med. Sch. Lond. Univ.) MRCP (UK) 1978; FRCP Lond. 1996. Clin. Reader (Rheum.) Nuffield Dept. Clin. Med. Univ. Oxf. & Hon. Cons. Rheum.; Prof. (Rheumatol.) Univ. Oxf. Specialty: Rheumatol. Socs: Brit. Soc. Rheum.; UK Skeletal Dysplasia Gp.; Med. Genetic Counc. Roy. Soc. Med. Prev: Sen. Regist. (Rheum. & Rehabil.) Nuffield Orthop. Centre Oxf.; Regist. (Rheum.) Middlx. Hosp. Lond.; Regist. (Med.) Mayday Hosp.

WORDSWORTH, Jennifer Mary — MB ChB Sheff. 1965; MFFP 1993. Cons. Family Plann. & Reproduc. Health Care. Specialty: Family Plann. & Reproduc. Health. Socs: Brit. Menopause Soc. (Counc. Mem.). Prev: GP Tideswell Derbysh.; Dir. Sexual & Reproduc. Health Sheff. NHS Trust.

WORDSWORTH, Matthew Thomas 50 Cork Lane, Glen Parva, Leicester LE2 9JS — MB ChB Birm. 1991; ChB Birm. 1991.

WORDSWORTH, Ruth Frances (retired) St. Marys Convent, Wantage OX12 9DJ Tel: 01235 771053 — MRCS Eng. LRCP Lond. 1937; DTM Calcutta 1939. Prev: Med. Miss. USPG Diocese, Poona.

WORDSWORTH, Victor Pargiter (retired) 11 Fiddicroft Avenue, Banstead SM7 3AD Tel: 01737 211762 — MRCS Eng. LRCP Lond. 1948 (St. Mary's) DA Eng. 1953; FFA RCS Eng. 1954. Prev: Cons. Anaesth. Croydon Gp. Hosps.

WORGAN, Mr Douglas Heath House, Minstead, Lyndhurst SO43 7GP Tel: 023 8081 2311 — MRCS Eng. LRCP Lond. 1960; MB BCh Wales 1960; FRCS Ed. 1966; FRCS Eng. 1969. Cons. ENT Surg. Soton. Univ. Gp. Hosps. Specialty: Otolaryngol. Socs: (Counc.) Roy. Soc. Med.; Brit. Assn. Otol. Prev: Sen. Regist. (ENT) Char. Cross Hosp. Gp.; Ho. Surg. St. Jas. Hosp. Balham & Birm. Accid. Hosp.

WORKMAN, Alan Robert Heol Fach Surgery, Heol Fach, North Cornelly, Bridgend CF33 4LD Tel: 01656 740345 Fax: 01656 740872; Montrose, Heol-Yr-Orsaf, Kenfig Hill, Bridgend CF33 6EQ Tel: 01656 746135 — MB BCh Wales 1984; DRCOG 1987.

WORKMAN, Alexander James Gordon Health Centre, 14 Market Place, Carluke ML8 4BP Tel: 01555 771012; Wintons, 33 West Avenue, Carluke ML8 5AE Tel: 01555 771877 — MB ChB Ed. 1972 (Edinburgh) Prev: SHO (Cas.) Derbysh. Roy. Infirm. Derby; Ho. Off. (O & G) East. Gen. Hosp. Edin.; Ho. Off. (Med. Paediat.) Leith Hosp. Edin.

WORKMAN, Clare Louise Nether Shannochill, Aberfoyle, Stirling FK8 3UZ Tel: 01877 382924 — MB ChB Leeds 1979 (Leeds Univ.) BSc (Hons.) Leeds 1976; D.Occ.Med. RCP Lond. 1995. Occupat. Health Phys., Lothian Primary Healthcare NHS Trust; Occupat. Health Phys. (PT), Company Health Ltd., Blackpool. Specialty: Occupat. Health. Socs: Soc. Occupat. Med.; BMA. Prev: Occupat. Health Phys., Salus, Lanarksh.; Occupat. Health Phys. Preston NHS Trust; Med. Off. DSS Leeds.

WORKMAN, Irvin Clarence Eugene Department Child & Family Psychiatry, London Road, Canterbury CT1 8LZ — MB BS Bangalor 1977; MB BS Bangalore 1977; MRCPsych 1985. Cons. Child & Adolesc. Psychiat. Canterbury Kent. Specialty: Child & Adolesc. Psychiat.

WORLEY, George Anthony 51 Ravenscroft Street, London E2 7QG — MB BS Lond. 1990.

WORLOCK, Frederick Cecil (retired) Brooklands, Fladbury, Pershore WR10 2QP — MB BChir Camb. 1958 (St. Thos.) MRCS Eng. LRCP Lond. 1957; MA Camb. 1958.

WORLOCK, Michael Stanley Gould (retired) Watersmeet, Cackle St., Nutley, Uckfield TN22 3DU Tel: 0182 571 2740 — MRCS Eng. LRCP Lond. 1949 (Camb. & St. Thos.)

WORLOCK, Mr Peter Harrison Trauma Service, John Radcliffe Hospital, Headington, Oxford OX3 9DU Tel: 01865 221177 Fax: 01865 221231 — MB BS Newc. 1976 (Univ. Newc. u. Tyne) FRCS Eng. 1981; FRCS Ed. 1981; DM Nottm. 1987. Cons. Trauma Surg. John Radcliffe Hosp. Oxf.; Civil Cons. Orthop. Trauma RAF. Specialty: Trauma & Orthop. Surg.; Medico Legal. Socs: Fell. BOA; Brit. Orthop. Research Soc. (Mem.); Brit. Trama Soc. (Mem.). Prev: Cons. Orthop. Surg. Sunderland Dist. Gen. Hosp.; Lect. (Orthop. & Accid. Surg.) Univ. Nottm. & Hon. Sen. Regist. Univ. Hosp. Nottm. & Harlow Wood Orthop. Hosp. Mansfield; Clin. Fell. (Orthop. &

Trauma Surg.) Sunnybrook Med. Centre & Regional Trauma Unit Univ. Toronto, Ontario, Canada.

WORMALD, John Leathard (retired) 95A Coniscliffe Road, Darlington DL3 7ES Tel: 01325 464378 — MB BS Durh. 1940 (Newc.) Prev: Orthop. Ho. Surg. Roy. Vict. Infirm. Newc.

WORMALD, Peter John (retired) Kasauli Pines, Highwood, Ringwood BH24 3LZ — MRCS Eng. LRCP Lond. 1938 (Middlx.) MA Camb. 1947, MD 1954, MB BChir 1938; FRCPath 1969. Prev: Dir. Pub. Health Laborat. Odstock Hosp. Salisbury.

WORMALD, Philip Nigel 37 Elm Grove Road, Exeter EX3 0EJ — MB ChB Birm. 1953; BSc (Hons.) Birm. 1950, MB ChB 1953; DObst RCOG 1958. Prev: SHO Med. Profess. Unit & Ho. Phys. & Ho. Surg. Qu. Eliz. Hosp. Birm.; SHO City Birm. Fev. Hosp.

WORMALD, Mr Richard Piers Leslie Department of Ophthalmic Epidemiology, Moorfields Eye Hospital, 162 City Road, London EC1V 2PD Tel: 020 7566 2818 Fax: 020 7608 6925; 35 Ellington Road, London N10 3DD — MB BChir Camb. 1977; BA Camb. 1974, MB 1978 BChir 1977; FRCS Glas. (Ophth.) 1985; MSc (Epidemiol.) Lond. 1989. Hon. Cons. & Sen. Lect. Moorfields Eye Hosp. Lond. Specialty: Epidemiol. Prev: Sen. Lect. & Hon. Cons. West. Ophth. Hosp. & St. Mary's Med. Sch. Lond.; Sen. Regist. & Regist. Moorfields Eye Hosp. Lond.; Lect. (Preven. Ophth.) Inst. Ophth. Lond.

WORMAN, Audrey June (retired) 3 Wilmot Cottages, Park Road, Banstead SM7 3DH — MB BS Lond. 1947 (Lond. Sch. Med. Wom.) MRCS Eng. LRCP Lond. 1946; DCH Eng. 1951.

WORMINGTON, Elsie Marjorie (retired) Westgrove, Banbury Lane, Culworth, Banbury OX17 2AX — MB ChB Birm. 1949.

WORMLEY, Robert Lee Derby Medical Centre, 8 Derby Square, Epsom KT19 8AG Tel: 01372 726361 — MB BS Lond. 1989.

WORMSLEY, Kenneth Geoffrey (retired) 12 Cherry Tree Close, High Salvington, Worthing BN13 3QJ Tel: 01903 693031 Fax: 01903 261789 — MB BS Lond. 1961 (Guy's) DSc Lond. 1974, BSc (Hons.) 1947, MD 1961, MB BS 1951; FRCP Lond. 1973, M 1956. Prev: Cons. Phys. Dundee Teach. Hosps.

WOROPAY, Sarah Jane Cannonhill Lane Medical Practice, 153 Cannon Hill Lane, Raynes Park, London SW20 9DA Tel: 020 8542 5201 Fax: 020 8540 9049 — MB BS Lond. 1982 (St. Geo. Hosp. Med. Sch.) DRCOG 1985; MRCGP 1986.

WORRALL, Anne-Marie — MB BS Lond. 1974 (St. Mary's) MRCS Eng. LRCP Lond. 1974; DRCOG 1978; Dip. Med. Educat. Dund 1991; MMedSci Nottm. 1993; MPH Nottm. 1995; Dip. Health Mgt. Keele 1996; DFPHM 1999. Specialty: Pub. Health Med.

WORRALL, Anthony (retired) Hillcrest, 83 Town End, Cheadle ST10 1PG Tel: 01538 756731 Email: antworrall@supanet.com — MB ChB Birm. 1960. Prev: Police Surg. Cheale.

WORRALL, Ernest Paterson 11 Upper Bourtree Drive, Burnside, Rutherglen, Glasgow G73 4EJ — MB ChB Glas. 1966; DPM Ed. & Glas. 1971; FRCPsych 1988, M 1973. Cons. Psychiat. In Indep. Pract. Specialty: Gen. Psychiat. Prev: Med. Dir. The Priory Hosp. Glas.; Cons. Psychiat., Southern Gen. Hosp., Glas.; Lect. (Psychiat.) Univ. Dundee.

WORRALL, Jennifer Garner Rheumatology Department, Whittington Hospital NHS Trust, Highgate Hill, London N19 5NF Tel: 020 7288 5740 Fax: 020 7288 5550; 10 Carysfort Road, London N8 8RB Tel: 020 7348 9454 — MB BS Lond. 1979; BSc (Econ) Lond. 1972; MD 1993; FRCP (UK) 2000. Cons. Whittington Hosp. Lond. Specialty: Rheumatol.; Gen. Med. Prev: Sen. Regist. Northwick Pk. Hosp.; Wellcome Clin. Research Fell. Middlx. Hosp. Lond.; Sen. Regist. Middlx. Hosp. Lond.

WORRALL, Margaret Ann Cunningham Oldham and Partners, Manor House Surgery, Manor Street, Glossop SK13 8PS Tel: 01457 860860 Fax: 01457 860017; 3 Blackshaw Road, Old Glossop, Glossop SK13 7SL — MB ChB Glas. 1965.

WORRALL-DAVIES, Anne Elizabeth Academic Unit of Child & Adolescent Mental Health, 12A Clarendon Road, Leeds LS2 9NN Tel: 0113 295 1760 Fax: 0113 295 1761 — MB ChB Leeds 1985; MRCPsych 1989; MD Leeds 1996, MMedSci 1990. Sen. Lect. (Child & Adolesc. Psychiat.) Leeds; Hon. Cons. Child Psychiat. Leeds. Specialty: Child & Adolesc. Psychiat. Prev: Sen. Regist. (Child & Adolesc. Psychiat.) Yorks. RHA; Tutor (Psychiat.) Univ. Leeds; Regist.& SHO Rotat. (Psychiat.) St. Jas. Univ. Hosp. Leeds.

WORRALL-KENT, Lindsey Sian University of Cambridge, Cambridge CB2 2AH — MB ChB Aberd. 1989; MRCPsych 1995; Phd Birm. 1998. Univ. Lect. Specialty: Child & Adolesc. Psychiat. Prev: Research Fell. Univ. Birm.

WORSDALL, Andrea Kate 49 Chaldon Road, London SW6 7NH — MB ChB Bristol 1989.

WORSDALL, Guy Mark Westfield Surgery, Waterford Park, Radstock, Bath BA3 3UJ Tel: 01761 436333; 36 Furlong Close, Midsomer Norton, Bath BA3 2PR — MB ChB Bristol 1982; DA (UK) 1985; DRCOG 1988.

WORSELL, Karen Elizabeth Castleton Health Centre, 2 Elizabeth Street, Castleton, Rochdale OL11 3HY Tel: 01706 658905 Fax: 01706 343990; 22 Wheelwright Drive, Smallbridge, Rochdale OL16 2QQ — MB ChB Birm. 1980 (Birmingham) MRCGP 1984. GP Rochdale.

WORSEY, Catherine Juliet 6 Exton Road, Nottingham NG5 1HB Tel: 0115 960 6851 — MB ChB Liverp. 1992. SHO (Cas.) Kings Mill Hosp. Mansfield, Notts. Specialty: Accid. & Emerg. Prev: SHO (Health c/o Elderly) Nottm. City Hosp.; SHO (Psychiat.) Mapperly Hosp. Nottm.; Ho. Off. (Med. & Surg.) Arrowe Pk. Hosp. Merseyside.

WORSFOLD, Belinda Jane — MB ChB Bristol 1995; MA Oxf. 1986; DRCOG 1997. Specialty: Gen. Pract.

WORSLEY, Adrian Paul Kings Mill Centre for Health Care Services NHS Trust, Sutton-in-Ashfield NG17 4JL Tel: 01623 25515 — BSc (Hons.) Lond. 1977; MB BS Lond. 1980; DCH RCP Lond. 1982; MRCP (UK) 1984. Specialty: Paediat. Prev: Sen. Regist. (Paediat.) Roy. Alexandra Hosp. Sick Childr. Brighton; Lect. (Neonat.) Bristol Matern. Hosp.; Sen. Regist. (Paediat.) King's Coll. Hosp. Lond.

WORSLEY, Alison Margaret 4 Seacombe Road, Sandbanks, Poole BH13 7RJ — MB BS Lond. 1975 (Middlx.) BSc Lond 1972; MRCP (UK) 1978; MRCPath 1984. Cons. Haemat. Poole Gen. Hosp. Specialty: Haematology. Prev: Sen. Regist. (Haemat.) Hammersmith Hosp. Lond.; Leukaemia Research Fund Clin. Train. Fell. MRC Leukaemia Unit; Hammersmith Hosp. Lond., Fell. (Haemat.) Mt. Sinai Hosp. NY.

WORSLEY, Andrew Peter Lewisham Hospital, Diabetic Department, Lewisham High Street, London SE13 6LH Tel: 020 8333 3000; Beechwood Lodge, Shire Lane, Orpington BR6 7EU — MB BS Lond. 1979; MRCP (UK) 1984; MD Lond. 1993. Cons. Phys. Lewisham Hosp. Lond.; Hon. Sen. Lect. Guy's & St Thos. Lond. Specialty: Gen. Med.; Diabetes. Prev: Sen. Regist. (Gen. Metab. & Molec. Med.) Clin. Research Centre Northwick Pk. Hosp. Harrow; Sen. Clin. Research Fellowsh. (Diabetes) Middlx. Hosp. Lond.

WORSLEY, David Eric, Brigadier late RAMC Retd. (retired) 10 Old College Close, Beccles NR34 9LY Tel: 01502 718151 — MB ChB Bristol 1952; FFCM 1979, M 1975; FFOM 1982, M 1981. Prev: Col. Commandant RAMC.

WORSLEY, Gillian Elizabeth Whitchurch Health Centre, Armada Road, Bristol BS14 0SU Tel: 01275 832285 Fax: 01275 540035 — MB ChB Bristol 1981; DRCOG 1983; MRCGP 1985.

WORSLEY, Mark Henry 6 Melville Terrace, Stirling FK8 2ND — MB ChB Glas. 1982; FFA RCS Eng. 1986. Cons. Anaesth. Stirling Roy. Infirm. Specialty: Anaesth.; Intens. Care. Prev: Sen. Regist. (Anaesth.) Roy. Infirm. Edin.

WORSLEY, Richard (retired) 12 King Edward Avenue, Lytham St Annes FY8 1DP Tel: 01253 725050 — LMSSA Lond. 1947 (Leeds) MRCGP Leeds 1961. Prev: Ho. Surg. St. Jas. Hosp. Leeds.

WORSLEY, Simon David — MB ChB Bristol 1976; BSc (Hons.) (Cell. Path.) Bristol 1976; DRCOG 1985. Prev: GP. HM Forces VTS.; Sen. Med. Off., HQ Hereford Garrison.

WORSLEY-WINTERINGHAM, Rosemary Jeannette (retired) Glannant, Gwernogle, Carmarthen SA32 7RZ Tel: 01267 202390 — MB BS Lond. 1967 (St Georges Hosp. Univ of Lond.) Drug & Alcohol Abuse Counsellor Washoe Med. Centre Reno, USA.

WORSSAM, Anthony Ralph Holtby (retired) Yearnor Mill, Worthycombe, Porlock, Minehead TA24 8JL — MB BChir Camb. 1948 (Guy's) FRCP Lond. 1977, M 1953; FRCPath 1970, M 1963. Prev: Sen. Regist. Path. St. Bart. Hosp.

WORSTMANN, Therese Queen's Hospital, Belvedere Road, Burton-on-Trent DE13 0RB Tel: 01283 566333 Fax: 01283 593014 — MB BS Lond. 1977 (St. Bart.) MRCS Eng. LRCP Lond. 1977; DO RCS Eng. 1982; FRCS Ed. (Ophth.) 1983; FRCOphth 1989. Cons. Ophth. Burton Hosps. Trust. Specialty: Ophth. Prev: Sen. Regist. (Ophth.) E. Anglian RHA; Regist. (Ophth.) Roy. Hallamsh. Hosp. Sheff.

WORSWICK, John Cowgill 108 St Mark's Road, Bush Hill Park, Enfield EN1 1BB — MRCS Eng. LRCP Lond. 1953; MA Camb. 1948.

WORT, Ian (retired) Wystra Del, Coverack, Helston TR12 6TH Tel: 01326 280501 — MB ChB Liverp. 1954; DObst RCOG 1956. Prev: Research Regist. (Dermat.) Truro, Penzance, Redruth & Helston Gp. Hosps.

WORT, Margaret Elizabeth (retired) 9 Leonard Court, Edwardes Square, London W8 6NL Tel: 020 7603 9636 — MB BS Lond. 1949 (Roy. Free) DObst RCOG 1953. Prev: Ho. Surg. Roy. Free Hosp. Lond.

WORT, Michael John — BM BS Nottm. 1977; BMedSci Nottm. 1975; FFA RCS Eng. 1983. Cons. Anaesth. & Pain Relief Withybush Gen. Hosp. HaverfordW.. Specialty: Anaesth. Prev: Cons. (Anaesth.) RAF Hosp. Halton; Cons. (Anaesth.) RAF Hosp. Wegberg; Hon. Sen. Regist. & Hon. Regist. (Anaesth.) Frenchay Hosp. Bristol.

WORT, Rosalyn Louise Occupational Health Department, Withybush General Hospital, Fishguard Road, Haverfordwest Tel: 01437 773217 Email: rosalyn.wort@pdt-tr.wales.nhs.uk — BM BS Nottm. 1977 (Nottingham university medical school) BMedSci Nottm. 1975; DRCOG 1982; MRCGP 1983; AFOM RCP Lond. 1995; MFOM RCP Lond. 1998. Cons.Occup.Phys. Withybush Gen. Hosp. HaverfordW. Pembrokesh. Specialty: Occupat. Health. Socs: Chairman to Welsh Groups of ANHOPS; Assn. Local Auth. Med. Advis.; Soc. Occupat. Med.

WORT, Stephen John 107 King's Road, Higher Bedington, Wirral CH63 8LX — MB BS Lond. 1993.

WORTERS, Alastair Robin (retired) Linthill Farmhouse, Eyemouth TD14 5TG Tel: 01890 752045 — MB BS Lond. 1952 (St. Thos.) MRCS Eng. LRCP Lond. 1952; DPM Eng. 1958; FRCPsych. 1981, M 1971. Prev: Cons. Psychiat. Manor Hosp. Epsom; Regist. Dept. Applied.

WORTERS, Jonathan Robin 69 Pickering Road, West Ayton, Scarborough YO13 9JE — MB BS Lond. 1978 (Middlx.) MRCP (UK) 1980; DRCOG 1987; MRCGP 1989.

WORTH, Austen Jonathan Jacob 2 Orchard Close, Oxton, Southwell NG25 0SR — BM BCh Oxf. 1997 (Oxford) BA Oxf. Spr (Paediat.) Crawley Hospital. Specialty: Paediat.; Neonat. Prev: Ho. Off. (Surg.) Cumbld. Infirm. Carlisle; Ho. Off. (Med.) John Radcliffe Hosp. Oxf.; SHO (Neonatocogy) St Geo.'s Lond.

WORTH, Christopher Thomas Janssen-Cilag Ltd, PO Box 79, Saunderton, High Wycombe HP14 4HJ Tel: 014894 567000 — BM BS Nottm. 1983; BMedSci Nottm. 1981; MRCGP 1987; MFPHM RCP (UK) 1991; T(GP) 1991; T(PHM) 1992; FFPHM RCP (UK) 1997; MFPM (Pharmaceutical Med.) Lond. 2004. Head (Med. Affairs) Janssen-Cilag Ltd. Specialty: Pub. Health Med.; Pharmaceutical Medicine. Prev: Dir. Pub. Health Calderdale & Kirklees HA; Dir. (Pub. Health) W. Yorks. HA; Lect. (Pub. Health Med.) Univ. Nottm.

WORTH, David Philip York District Hospital, Wigginton Road, York YO31 8HE; York Email: david.p.worth@excha.yhs-tr.northy.nhs.uk — MD Sheff. 1987; MB ChB Sheff. 1975; DCH Eng. 1977; MRCP (UK) 1978; FRCP Lond. 1994. Cons. Phys. York Dist. Hosp. Specialty: Gen. Med.; Nephrol. Prev: Sen. Regist. (Med.) Yorks. RHA.

WORTH, Jean Margaret Moston Lodge Childrens Centre, Countess of Chester Hospital, Liverpool Road, Chester CH2 1UL Tel: 01244 364801 — MB ChB Sheff. 1972; MSc (Com. Child Health) Warwick 2001. Assoc. Specialist (Community Paediat.) Countess of Chester Hosp. Specialty: Community Child Health. Socs: Assoc. Mem. Coll. Paediat. & Child Health. Prev: Trainee GP Hull VTS; Ho. Phys. North. Gen. Hosp. Sheff.; Ho. Surg. Hull Roy. Infirm.

WORTH, Karen Vivien St Luke's Surgery, Radford Health Centre, 1 Ilkeston Road, Radford, Nottingham NG7 3GW; 54 Watcombe Circus, Sherwood, Nottingham NG5 2DT Tel: 0115 969 1830 Email: shalom@zetnet.co.uk — BM BS Nottm. 1988; BMedSci Nottm. 1986; MRCGP 1993. Lect. Divison GP Nottm. Med. Sch. Specialty: Gen. Pract. Special Interest: Drug Misuse; Homeopathy.

WORTH, Penelope Jane Thornfield House, Hodgson Lane, Upper Poppleton, York YO26 6DY — MB ChB Leeds 1979.

WORTH, Mr Peter Herman Louis (retired) Broad Eaves, Mill Lane, Broxbourne EN10 7AZ Tel: 01992 309414/462827 Fax: 01992 309414 — MB Camb. 1961 (Middlx.) BChir 1960; FRCS Eng. 1967. Cons. Urol. Surg. Univ. Coll. Lond. Hosp. Trust & King Edwd. VII Hosp.; Hon. Sen. Lect. Inst. Urol. Lond. Prev: Sen. Regist. St. Paul's Hosp. Lond.

WORTH, Richard Christopher Countess of Chester Hospital, Liverpool Road, Chester CH2 1UL Tel: 01244 366441 Fax: 01244 366455 — MB ChB Sheff. 1971; DObst RCOG 1973; MRCP (UK) 1974; MD Sheff. 1983; FRCP Lond. 1989. Cons. Phys. Countess of Chester Hosp. NHS Trust. Specialty: Gen. Med.; Diabetes; Endocrinol. Socs: Fell. Roy. Soc. Med.; Brit. Diabetic Assn.; Soc. Endocrinol. Prev: Sen. Regist. (Med.) Sheff. HA; Research Fell. Roy. Vict. Infirm. Newc.; Regist. (Med.) Newc. HA.

WORTH, Mr Richard William 1A Gwendolen Avenue, Putney, London SW15 6EU — BM BCh Oxf. 1975; MA. DPhil Oxf. 1973, BM BCh 1975; FRCS Eng. 1979; MRCOG 1981. Cons. (O & G) Epsom Dist. Gen. Hosp. Specialty: Obst. & Gyn. Prev: Sen. Lect. (O & G) Char. Cross & Westm. Med. Sch. Lond.; Cons. (O & G) Qu. Mary's Univ. Hosp. Lond.; Sen. Regist. (O & G) Chelsea Hosp. Wom. & Qu. Charlotte's Hosp. Wom. Lond.

WORTHINGTON, Andrew Ralph (retired) Abbotswood, Sandy Lane, West Runton, Cromer NR27 9NB Tel: 01263 837545 — MB ChB Leeds 1952; DTM & H Eng. Lond. 1963; MFCM RCP (UK) 1972. Prev: Brigadier late RAMC Retd.

WORTHINGTON, Professor Brian Stewart (retired) c/o Academic Radiology, University Hospital, Queens Medical Centre, Clifton Boulevard, Nottingham NG7 2UH; Cliff Cottage, Belper Road, Shirland, Alfreton DE55 6AG Tel: 01773 834096 — (Guy's) FRS (1998); BSc (Hons. Physiol.) Lond. 1960; MB BS Lond. 1963; MRCS Eng. LRCP Lond. 1963; DMRD Eng. 1967; FFR (Rohan Williams Medal) 1969; F.Med Sci 1998. Emerit. Prof. Diagn. Radiol. Univ. Nottm.; Examr. Roy. Coll. Radiol. & DMRD Univ. Liverp.; Hon. Cons. Neuroradiol. Univ. Hosp. NHS Trust. Prev: Sen. Regist. (Diag. Radiol.) Lond. Hosp.

WORTHINGTON, Cathryn Anne Avondale Surgery, 3-5 Avondale Road, Chesterfield S40 4TF Tel: 01246 232946 Fax: 01246 279803; 14 Southfield Avenue, Chesterfield S41 0LX — MB ChB Liverp. 1990.

WORTHINGTON, Edmund Guy Barker (retired) Langley House, Hutton Buscel, Scarborough YO13 9LN Tel: 01723 864512 — MRCS Eng. LRCP Lond. 1952 (Camb. & Lond. Hosp.) DObst RCOG 1954; MRCGP 1960. Prev: Cas. Off. Leeds Pub. Disp. & Hosp.

WORTHINGTON, Jonathan Mark 15 Greenland Crescent, Larne BT40 1HE — MB BCh BAO Belf. 1995.

WORTHINGTON, Joy 34C Albyn Court, Tradespark, Nairn IV12 5PY — MB ChB Glas. 1995.

WORTHINGTON, Karen Anne The Rowans Surgery, 1 Windermere Road, Streatham, London SW16 5HF Tel: 020 8764 0407 Fax: 020 8679 4149 — MB BS Lond. 1986.

WORTHINGTON, Ross Charles Stourview Medical Centre, Crown Passage, High Street, Haverhill CB9 8BB Tel: 01784 437671; Surridges Farm, Hanchett End, Haverhill CB9 7RP — BM BCh Oxf. 1979; MA Oxf. 1983.

WORTHINGTON, Sidney Wonersh Surgery, The Sheilings, Wonersh, Guildford GU5 0PE Tel: 01483 898123 Fax: 01483 893104; Mulberry Cottage, Wonersh, Guildford GU5 0PB Tel: 01483 892676 — MB BChir Camb. 1967 (Guy's) MA Camb, 1967; DObst RCOG 1969; DCH Eng. 1971. Prev: Ho. Phys. (Gen. Med. & Infec. Dis.) Hither Green Hosp.; Ho. Surg. (Gen. Surg.) Kent & Sussex Hosp. Tunbridge Wells; Ho. Surg. (O & G) N. Middlx. Hosp.

WORTHINGTON, Mr Tim Rees 2 Rectory Close, Church Lane, Farndon, Chester CH3 6PS — MB ChB Birm. 1993; FRCS 1997. SpR S. Thames NHS Trust. Specialty: Gen. Surg. Prev: Simpson Research Fell. Roy. Coll. of Surgs. Hammersmith Hosp.

WORTHLEY, Paul Burrswood, Groombridge, Tunbridge Wells TN3 9PY Tel: 01892 863637 — MB BS Lond. 1976; DCH RCP Lond. 1989; Dip. Palliat. Med. Wales 1996. Resid. Phys. Burrswood Christian Hosp. & Pl. of Healing. Prev: Regist. (Paediat.) Adelaide Childr. Hosp.

WORTHY, Eric (retired) 28 Burnt Stones Drive, Sheffield S10 5TT — MB BChir Camb. 1963; BMedSci Sheff. 1968; FRCPath 1987, M 1969. Prev: Cons. Chem. Path. Sheff. Childr. Hosp.

WORTHY, Sylvia Anne Radiology Dept, Royal Victoria Infirmary, Queen Victoria Road, Newcastle upon Tyne NE1 4LP Tel: 0191 232 5131 — MB BS Newc. 1986; MRCP (UK) 1989; DMRD Liverp. 1991; FRCR 1992. Cons.Radiol.Roy.Vict.,InfirmNewc. Specialty: Radiol. Socs: RCR. Prev: Regist. (Radiol.) Merseyside & W. Midl.

RHAs; SHO Rotat. (Gen. Med.) Durh.; Sen. Regist. Rotat. (Radiol.) North. RHA.

WORTHY, Thomas Stanley 3 Little Dene, Lodore Road, Newcastle upon Tyne NE2 3NZ Tel: 0191 284 9122 — MB BChir Camb. 1957 (Camb. & Middlx) PhD Camb. 1957; DMRT Eng. 1960; FFR 1962. Specialty: Oncol.

WORTLEY, Pamela Mary Church View Medical Centre, Silksworth Terrace, Silksworth, Sunderland SR3 2AW Tel: 0191 521 1753 Fax: 0191 521 3884; 9 Thornhill Terrace, Sunderland SR2 7JL Tel: 0191 510 2456 — MB BS Newc. 1970; MRCGP (Distinc.) 1989; MFFP 1991. Trainer (Gen. Pract.) Sunderland; Mem. Sunderland LMC. Prev: Non Exec. Dir. Sunderland HA & Health Commiss.; SCMO Sunderland HA; Chairm. Sunderland LMC.

WORWOOD, Graham 17 Celyn Gr, Cardiff CF23 6SH — MB BCh Wales 1997.

WOSORNU ABBAN, Dzifa The Alexandra Hospital, Woodrow Drive, Redditch B98 7UB Tel: 01527 503030 Fax: 01527 512000 — MB ChB Glas. 1984; MRCP (UK) 1987; MD Glas. 1995; FRCP (Glas) 2000; FRCP (Lon) 2000. Cons. Gen. Med. & Cardiol. Alexandra Hosp. Redditch. Specialty: Cardiol. Socs: Collegiate Fell.. RCPS Glas.; BMA; Brit. Cardiac Soc. Prev: Sen. Regist. Vict. Infirm. Glas.; Clin. Research Fell. Univ. Birm.; Career Regist. (Cardiol.) Selly Oak Hosp.

WOSTENHOLM, David Kenneth The Annunciation Vicarage, 89 Washington St., Brighton BN2 2SR Tel: 01273 681341 Email: hanover@mistral.co.uk — MB ChB Ed. 1980; BTh (Hons.) Soton. 1988. Parish Priest Ch. of the Annunciation Brighton. Prev: Curate St. Margts. Ch. Leytonstone, Lond.

WOTHERSPOON, Andrew Charles Department of Histopathology, Royal Marsden NHS Trust, Fulham Road, London SW3 6JJ Tel: 020 7352 7348 Fax: 020 7352 7348 — MB BCh Wales 1984. Cons. Histopath. Roy. Marsden NHS Trust Lond. Specialty: Histopath. Prev: Sen. Lect. (Histopath.) Roy. Postgrad. Med. Sch. Lond.; Lect. (Histopath.) Univ. Coll. Lond. Med. Sch.; Sir Jules Thorn Fell. (Histopath.) Univ. Coll. & Middlx. Sch. Med.

WOTHERSPOON, Fiona 37 Cumberland Court, Festing Road, Southsea, Portsmouth PO4 0NH — BM Soton. 1994 (Southampton University) MRCP (UK) 1997. Specialist Regist. & Research Fell. (Diabetes & Endrocrinol.) QA Hosp., Portsmouth. Specialty: Diabetes; Endocrinol.; Gen. Med. Prev: Specialist Regist. (Diabetes & Endocrinol.) Treuske Hosp Truro Cornw.

WOTHERSPOON, John Phoenix Medical Centre, 28 Duke Street, St Helens WA10 2JP — MB ChB Liverp. 1986.

WOTHERSPOON, Mark Gavin Kingsclere Health Centre, Kingsclere, Newbury RG20 5UX Tel: 01635 296000 Fax: 01635 299282; Berthas Cottage, Hannington, Basingstoke RG26 5UA Tel: 01635 297867 — MB BS Lond. 1985; Dip. Sports Med. Lond 1992. Specialty: Sports Med.

WOTHERSPOON, Matthew 2 Longrigg, Wardley, Felling, Gateshead NE10 8QJ — LRCP LRCS Ed. 1949; LRCP LRCS Ed., LRFPS Glas. 1949.

WOTHERSPOON, William Campbell Northumbria Healthcare NHS Trust, Wansbeck General Hospital, Ashington NE63 9JJ Tel: 01670 521212 — MB ChB Aberd. 1974; DMRD Aberd. 1978; FRCR 1981. Cons. (Radiol.) Wansbeck Gen. Hosp. Specialty: Radiol. Socs: Fell. Roy. Coll. Radiols.; Brit. Med. Ultrasound Soc. Prev: Sen. Regist. (Diag. Radiol.) Newc. AHA; Trainee Regist. (Diag. Radiol.) Aberd..

WOTTON, Linde Diana Goddards Green, Angley Road, Cranbrook TN17 3LR Tel: 01580 715507 — MB BChir Camb. 1979; MRCPsych 1982.

WOTTON-MCTURK, Peter Howard 26 Raven Court, Hatfield AL10 8QN — MB ChB Ed. 1964; DPM Eng. 1970. Cons. Child Psychiat. Warwick Health Dist. Specialty: Child & Adolesc. Psychiat.

WOULDS, Merla 9 St Faiths Ct, West Pde, Lincoln LN1 1QZ — MB ChB Sheff. 1997.

WOWKONOWICZ, Krystyna (retired) 79b Englewood Road, London SW12 9PB Tel: 020 8673 4674 — Med. Dipl. Warsaw 1945; DMRD Eng. 1949. Prev: Cons. Radiol. Qu. Mary's Hosp. Sidcup.

WOYKA, Winifred Jane Graham Harrow Health Care Centre, 84-88 Pinner Road, Harrow HA1 4HZ Tel: 020 8861 1221 Fax: 020 8427 4915; 52 Pebworth Road, Harrow HA1 3UD — MB BChir Camb. 1979 (Cambridge) MA Camb. 1980; MRCGP 1983. Assoc.Specialist Menopause, Northwick Park Hosp. Specialty: Gen. Med. Socs: BMA. Prev: Trainee GP Roy. Free Hosp. Lond. VTS; Ho. Phys. Addenbrooke's Hosp. Camb.; Ho. Surg. P'boro. Dist. Hosp.

WOZENCROFT, David Wilfred Edward Jenner Unit, Peterborough District Hospital, Thorpe Road, Peterborough PE3 6DA Tel: 01733 874696 Fax: 01733 875802 — (Westm.) MRCS Eng. LRCP Lond. 1971; MB BS Lond. 1971; DA Eng. 1975; MRCPsych 1978. Cons. Child & Adolesc. Psychiat. P'boro. Dist. Hosp. Specialty: Child & Adolesc. Psychiat.

WOZENCROFT, Enid Myra (retired) Croftwold, 42b West Common, Harpenden AL5 2JW Tel: 01580 4330; Burvill House, Dellafield Road, Hatfield — MB BS Lond. 1954 (Roy. Free.) MRCS Eng. LRCP Lond. 1954; DObst RCOG 1955. Prev: Med. Off. Harpenden Family Plann. Clinic.

WOZNIAK, Mr Andrew Peter 40 Braeside, Beckenham BR3 1SU — MB BS Lond. 1976 (Guy's) MRCS Eng. LRCP Lond. 1975; FRCS Ed. 1984.

WOZNIAK, Edward Richard St Mary's Hospital, Milton Road, Portsmouth PO3 6AD Tel: 023 92 286000 Fax: 023 92 866101 — MB BS Lond. 1974 (Lond. Hosp.) BSc Lond. 1971; MRCP (UK) 1978; DCH Eng. 1979; FRCP Lond. 1993; FRCPCH 1997. Cons. Paediat. St. Mary's Hosp. Portsmouth. Specialty: Paediat. Socs: Regional Adviser Roy. Coll. Paediat. and Child Health; Examr. Councillor, former. Prev: Research Fell. (Child Health) Inst. Child Health; Hon. Sen. Regist. Hosp. Sick Childr. Gt. Ormond St. Lond.; Sen. Regist. (Child Health) Soton. Gen. Hosp.

WOZNIAK, Irena Anna 31 Elizabeth Road, Moseley, Birmingham B13 8QH — MB ChB Birm. 1978.

WOZNIAK, Janusz Tadeusz Kingsfield Medical Centre, 146 Alcester Road South, Kings Heath, Birmingham B14 6AA Tel: 0121 444 2054 Fax: 0121 443 5856; 7 Carpenter Road, Edgbaston, Birmingham B15 2JT — MB ChB Birm. 1971; MRCP (U.K.) 1974.

WOZNIAK, Sarah Woodgate Valley Practice, 61 Stevens Avenue, Woodgate Valley, Birmingham B32 3SD Tel: 0121 427 6174 Fax: 0121 428 4146; 7 Carpenter Road, Edgbaston, Birmingham B15 2JT — MB ChB Birm. 1974; DObst RCOG 1976.

WOZNIAK, Teresa Crown St Surgery, 1-23 Crown St, Alton W3 8SA Tel: 020 8992 1963 — MB BChir Camb. 1982; MA Camb. 1982; DRCOG 1985; MRCGP 1989. GP.

WRAGG, Andrew 61 The Chine, London N21 2EE Tel: 020 8360 6629 — MB BS Lond. 1994; BSc (1st cl. Hons.) Pharmacol. Lond. 1991. Ho. Off. St. Bart. & Homerton Hosps. Lond. Prev: Ho. Off. Bath.

WRAGG, Christopher Michael 5 Dunstan Hill, Kirton in Lindsey, Gainsborough DN21 4DU — MB ChB Liverp. 1976; DRCOG 1979; DCH Eng. 1980; DTM & H 1980.

WRAGG, Mr Peter George Doctors Surgery, Forge Close, Hayes, Bromley BR2 7LL Tel: 020 8462 1601 Fax: 020 8462 7410; 91 Hayes Road, Bromley BR2 9AE Tel: 020 8460 2933 — MRCP Eng. LRCP Lond. 1968; BSc (Anat.) Lond. 1964, MB BS 1968; FRCS Eng. 1975. Socs: BMA; Roy. Coll. of Surg.s; Med. Defense Union. Prev: Surg. Hôpital Protestant Dabou, Ivory Coast; Sen. Regist. (A & E) Portsmouth HA.; Princip. GP, Burford, Oxf.shire.

WRAIGE, Elizabeth Anne 62 St James's Avenue, Beckenham BR3 4HG — MB BS Lond. 1990.

WRAIGHT, Edwin Philip (retired) 51 Glisson Road, Cambridge CB1 2HG Tel: 01223 52610 — (Middlx.) PhD Camb. 1970, MA 1965; MB BChir Camb. 1966; DMRT Eng. 1971; FRCR 1990. Prev: Cons. Nuclear Med. Addenbrooke's Hosp. Camb.

WRAIGHT, Sara Katherine Firs House Surgery, Station Road, Impington, Cambridge CB4 9NP Tel: 01223 234286 Fax: 01223 235931; 51 Glisson Road, Cambridge CB1 2HG Tel: 01223 526210 — MB BChir Camb. 1983; MA Camb. 1969; DRCOG 1985; MRCGP 1987.

WRAIGHT, William John Stable House, Winkfield Road, Brookside, Ascot SL5 7LT Tel: 01344 882082 — MB BS Lond. 1973; MRCS Eng. LRCP Lond. 1973; DObst RCOG 1975; FFA RCS Eng. 1978. Cons. Anaesth. E. Berks. Health Dist. Specialty: Anaesth. Prev: Sen. Regist. (Anaesth.) Roy. Free Hosp. Lond.; Regist. (Anesth.) Birm. Health Dist. (T); Regist. (Anaesth.) Plymouth Gen. Hosp.

WRAITH, James Edmond Royal Manchester Children's Hospital, Willink Biochemical Genetics Unit, Manchester M27 4HA Tel: 0161 922 2137 Fax: 0161 922 2303 Email: ed.wraith@cmmc.nhs.uk;

Westfield, 257 Worsley Road, Swinton, Manchester M27 0YE Tel: 0161 281 2206 Email: ed.wraith@ntlworld.com — MB ChB Sheff. 1977; MRCP (UK) 1980; FRCPCH 1998. Cons. Paediat. Roy. Manch. Childr. Hosp. Specialty: Paediat. Prev: Clin. Fell. Murdoch Inst. Roy. Childr. Hosp. Melbourne, Austral.; Dir. Willink Biochem. Genetics Unit Roy. Manch. Childr. Hosp.

WRATHALL, Gareth James Frenchay Hospital, Frenchay Pk Road, Bristol BS16 1LE Email: gareth.wrathall@north-bristol.swest.nhs.uk — MB BS Lond. 1988; FRCA 1994. Cons. (Anaesth. & IC Med.) Frenchay Hosp. Hosp. Specialty: Anaesth.; Intens. Care. Socs: BMA & Assn. Anaesth.; Intens. Care Soc. Prev: Sen. Regist. (Anaesth. & Intens. Care Med.) S. & W. RHA; Regist. & SHO (Anaesth.) S. Birm. HA; SHO (Med.) Swindon HA.

WRATTEN, Juliette Claire Little Pixhall, Hawkhurst, Cranbrook TN18 4XT — MB ChB Ed. 1998.

WRAY, Mr Arnold Richard 13 Dunnwood Park, Prehen, Londonderry BT47 2NN — MB BCh BAO Belf. 1973; FRCS Ed. 1977; FRCS Eng. 1978; FRCS Ed. (Orth.) 1982. Cons. (Orthop. Surg.) Altnagelvin Hosp. Lond.derry. Specialty: Orthop.

WRAY, Mr Christopher Charles Airedale General Hospital, Steeton, Keighley BD20 6TD Tel: 01535 651308; Westfield House, Marton Road, Gargrave, Skipton BD23 3NL Tel: 01756 749303 — MB ChB Leeds 1976; FRCS Ed. 1981. Cons. Orthop. Surg. Airedale Gen. Hosp. Specialty: Orthop.; Trauma & Orthop. Surg. Socs: BOA; Brit. Soc. Surg. Hand. Prev: Sen. Regist. (Orthop.) Leicester Roy. Infirm.

WRAY, Professor David MacFarlane Glasgow Dental Hospital & School, 378 Sauchiehall St., Glasgow G2 3JZ Tel: 0141 2119700 Fax: 0141 211 9834 Email: d.wray@dental.gla.ac.uk; 2 Queensgate, 125 Dowanhill street, Glasgow G12 9DN Tel: 0141 334 0021 — MB ChB Glas. 1976; FDS RCPS Glas. 1979, BDS 1972; MD Glas. 1982; FDS RCS Ed. 1987; F. Med Sci 1998. Prof. Oral Med. & Dean of Dent. Sch. Univ. Glas.; Hon. Cons. Gtr. Glas. HB. Prev: Sen. Lect. (Oral Med. & Oral Path.) Univ. Edin.

WRAY, Mr Denis Gage (retired) 11 Clifford Road, Poynton, Stockport SK12 1HY Tel: 01625 872537 Fax: 01625 872537 — MB ChB Ed. 1950; FRCS Ed. 1960; MCh Orth. Liverp. 1961. Prev: Cons. Orthop. & Traum. Surg. Stockport AHA.

WRAY, Donald George Salisbury House Surgery, Lake St., Leighton Buzzard LU7 1RS Tel: 01525 373139 Fax: 01525 853006; The Craddocks, Heath Road, Leighton Buzzard LU7 3BW Tel: 01525 377153 — (Ed.) MB ChB Ed. 1959; DObst RCOG 1961. Socs: BMA. Prev: SHO (Paediat.) Shrodells Hosp. Watford.; Ho. Phys. East. Gen. Hosp. Edin.; Resid. Med. Off. Watford Matern. Hosp.

WRAY, Gillian Mary Helen 35 Merrivale, London N14 4TE — MB BS Lond. 1988.

WRAY, Gordon 10 Penleonard Close, Exeter EX2 4NY Tel: 01392 59506 — MB ChB St. And. 1958; MB ChB (Commend.) St. And. 1958; FFA RCS Eng. 1965. Cons. Anaesth. Roy. Devon & Exeter Hosp. Specialty: Anaesth.

WRAY, Heather Ann 78 Westfield Drive, Loughborough LE11 3QL Tel: 01509 550133 — MB ChB Manch. 1974; DObst RCOG 1976.

WRAY, John Robert Edward 12 Hillside Road, Southport PR8 4QB — MB ChB Liverp. 1985; Dip. IMC RCS Ed. 1989; Cert. Av. Med. 1989; DRCOG 1990.

WRAY, Kenneth Alexander Armitage (retired) 1 Southern Dene Close, Tilehurst, Reading RG31 6ND Tel: 0118 425748 — MB BChir Camb. 1945 (Lond. Hosp.) MRCS Eng. LRCP Lond. 1945; MRCP Lond. 1946. Indep. Lect. Health & Retirement. Prev: Ho. Phys. & Path. Asst. Lond. Hosp.

WRAY, Pamela Mary (retired) 30 Constable Road, Ipswich IP4 2UW Tel: 01473 258071 — MB ChB Sheff. 1946; MRCS Eng. LRCP Lond. 1946; FRCOG 1982, M 1954, DObst 1948; MD Sheff. 1959. Prev: Venereol. Ipswich & E. Suff. Hosp.

WRAY, Richard 8 The Dene, Chowns Hill, Hastings TN35 4PD Tel: 01424 752021; Conquest Hospital, The Ridge, St Leonards-on-Sea TN37 7RD Tel: 01424 755255 — MB ChB Leeds 1967; MRCP (UK) 1970; FRCP Lond. 1988. Cons. Cardiol., E. Sussex Hosps. NHS Trust; Hon. Cons. Cardiol., Kings Coll. Hosp. Lond. Specialty: Cardiol. Socs: Brit. Cardiac. Soc.; Brit. Assn. Med. Managers. Prev: Sen. Regist. (Cardiol.) Leeds Gen. Infirm.; MRC Jun. Research Fell. & Hon. Regist. & Ho. Phys. Hammersmith Hosp.

WRAY, Robert Harold Mount Baker, Moneymore, Magherafelt BT45 7TX — MB BCh BAO Belf. 1981; DRCOG 1984; DObst RCPI 1985; MRCGP 1985; MICGP 1985. GP Cookstown.

WRAY, Ruth Mary 25 Lyme Regis Road, Banstead SM7 2EY Tel: 01737 356814 — MB ChB Liverp. 1956; MRCPath 1976. Med. Off. Banstead FPA Clinic Surrey. Prev: Assoc. Specialist (Haemat.) St. Helier Hosp. NHS Trust Carshalton; Regist. (Path.) St. Helens & Croydon Hosp. Gps; SHO (Surg. & Orthop.) Mossley Hill Hosp. Liverp.

WRAY, Sarah Lesley 142 Russell Ct., Woburn Place, London WC1H 0LP — MB BS Lond. 1998; MB BS Lond 1998. PRHO.Gen.Surg.Mt. Vernon.Watford.Hosps. Prev: PRHO.Gen.med.Chase.Farm.Hosp.Enfield.

WRAY, Stephen Queens Road Medical Practice, St Peter Port, Guernsey GY1 1RH; Vieux Port, Le Rocher Road, St. Martins, Guernsey GY4 6EL — MB ChB Leic. 1984; DCH RCP Lond. 1988; MRCGP 1989. Prev: Med. Off. Popondetta, Papua New Guinea; Trainee GP Aberystwyth VTS.

WREDE, Mr Casper David Hamlett Taunton and Somerset NHS Trust, Taunton and Somerset Hospital, Musgrove Park, Taunton TA1 5DA Tel: 01823 333444 Email: david.wrede@tst.nhs.uk — MB BChir Camb. 1984 (Camb. & St. Thos.) BA Camb. 1980; MA Camb. 1984; FRCS (Eng.) 1990; MRCOG 1995. Cons. in Obst. and Gyn., Taunton, Som. Specialty: Obst. & Gyn. Special Interest: Colposcopy; Gynaecological Oncology; Minimal Access Surgery. Socs: Fell. Roy. Soc. Med.; Brit. Gyn. Cancer Soc.; Brit. Soc. for Colposcopy and Cervical Path. Prev: Cons. in Obst. and Gyn., Forth Pk. Hosp., Kirkcaldy, Fife 2000-2004; Sen. Regist. in Obst. and Gyn., W. Midlands Rotat. 1995-1999.

WREFORD, Jonathan Moore Health Centre, Moore Road, Bourton on the Water, Cheltenham GL54 2AZ Tel: 01451 820 242 Fax: 01451 820532 — MB BS Lond. 1987 (St. Bart.) DRCOG 1992. Specialty: Gen. Pract.

WREGLESWORTH, Janet Kay Grove House, St. Paul's Health Centre, High St., Runcorn WA7 1AB Tel: 01928 566561; 2 Hunts Lane, Grappenhall, Warrington WA4 2DT Tel: 01925 266094 — MB ChB Liverp. 1988; T(GP) 1993; Cert. Family Plann. JCC 1994. Prev: Ho. Off. (Gen. Med. & Gen. Surg.) Clatterbridge Hosp. Merseyside.

WREN, Alison Margaret 73 Heaton Street, Prestwich, Manchester M25 1HH — MB BS Newc. 1993.

WREN, Christopher Department of Paediatric Cardiology, Freeman Hospital, Newcastle upon Tyne NE7 7DN Tel: 0191 223 1082 Fax: 0191 213 2167 Email: christopher.wren@tfh.nuth.northy.nhs.uk — MB ChB Birm. 1975; MRCP (UK) 1978. Cons. Paediat. Cardiol., Freeman Hosp & GOSH. Specialty: Paediat. Cardiol.

WREN, Damian Richard Atkinson Morleys Hospital, Copse Hill, Wimbledon, London SW20 0NE Tel: 020 8946 7711; Vynes Cottage, The Green, Pirbright, Woking GU24 0JE — BM BCh Oxf. 1979; BA Oxf. 1976, DM 1988, BM BCh 1979; MRCP 1982; FRCP 1999. Cons. Neurol. Atkinson Morleys Hosp. & Frimley Pk. Hosp. Specialty: Neurol. Prev: Sen. Regist. Nat. Hosp. Neurol. & Neurosurg. Qu. Sq. & Kings Coll. Hosp. Lond.

WREN, Esmé Maria 21 Amber Court, Holland Road, Hove BN3 1LU Tel: 01273 771133 — (Liverp.) MB ChB Liverp. 1945; DObst RCOG 1947; FRCP Lond. 1972, M 1949; MD Liverp. 1953. Mem. Brighton & Hove Med. Clinic. Socs: BMA. Prev: Cons. Phys. Hove Gen. Hosp., Brighton Gen. Hosp., Bevendean Hosp. Brighton & Lady Chichester Hosp. Hove; Regist. (Med.) Liverp. United Hosps. & Nat. Heart Hosp. Lond.; Research Fell. Med. Liverp. Univ.

WREN, Marie Elizabeth Lister Fertility Unit, Lister Hospital, Chelsea Bridge Road, London SW1W 8RH — MB BS Lond. 1980; MRCOG 1985. Fertil. Specialist Lister Fertil. Unit Lister Hosp. Lond.

WREN, Mary Catherine Gleadless Medical Centre, 636 Gleadless Road, Sheffield S14 1PQ — MB ChB Sheff. 1987. Specialty: Dermat. Prev: Trainee GP Sheff. VTS.

WREN, Maurice William Godfrey, RD (retired) 43 Links Lane, Rowlands Castle PO9 6AE — MRCS Eng. LRCP Lond. 1960; MB ChB Liverp. 1960, DMRD 1964; FFR 1967; FRCR 1975. Cons. Radiol. Portsmouth & S.E. Hants. Health Dist.

WREN, Peter John James, VRD, OBE, KStJ 8 Wardle Court, Whittle Hall Farm, Whittle-le-Woods, Chorley PR6 7DQ — MD Liverp. 1967; FRCGP 1971. DL; JP.; Med. Off. Eaves La. Geriatr. Hosp. Chorley; Responsible Med. Off. Lisieux Hall Ment. Nurs.

Home; Co. Commr. Duke of Lancaster Dist. St. John Ambul. Brig. Socs: MIBiol; Genetical Soc.; C.Biol. Prev: Surg. Lt.-Cdr. RNR; Ho. Phys. Sefton Gen. Hosp. Liverp.; Nuffield Research Asst. Univ. Liverp. Med. Sch.

WREN, Siobhan Mairead Elizabeth Alencon, 43 Links Lane, Rowlands Castle PO9 6AE — MB BS Lond. 1996.

WRENCH, Ian James Royal Hallamshire Hospital, Sheffield S10 Tel: 0114 2711 900 — MB ChB Sheff. 1987; BMedSci Sheff. 1983; PhD Sheff. 1987; FRCA 1994. Cons. Roy. Hallamsh. Hosp. Sheff. Specialty: Anaesth. Socs: BMA & Med. Defence Union; FRCA Anaesth. Prev: Sen. Regist. Sheff.; Regist. (Anaesth.) Nottm.; SHO (Med.) York Dist. Hosp.

WRENCH, James Ross Edwin Hay-on-Wye Surgery, Forest Road, Hay-on-Wye, Hereford HR3 5DS Tel: 01497 822100 — MB BS Lond. 1991; MRCGP U.K 1999 (Univ. Lond. & Char. Cross & Westm. Hosp.) BSc (Immunol.) Lond. 1988; MRCP (UK) 1996; Dip Child Care Roy Coll. Child Health + Paed 1999. GP Princip. Hay on Wye & Talgorth. Specialty: Cardiol.; Gen. Pract.; Immunol. Socs: Scott. Heart and Arterial Dis. Risk Protec. Prev: Resid. Regist. (Med. & ITU) Som. Hosp. Greenpoint, Cape Town, S. Afr.; Cardiac Fell. Papworth Hosp. Camb.; SHO (Med.) Addenbrooke's Hosp. Camb.

WRENCH, John Gibson NHS Highland, Assynt House, Beechwood Park, Inverness IV2 3HG; 17 Bonaly Terrace, Edinburgh EH1 3C — MB ChB Ed. 1970 (Edinburgh) MSc (Community Med.) Ed. 1985, BSc (Med. Sci.) 1967; MRCP (UK) 1973; DObst RCOG 1975; MRCGP 1976; FFPHM RCP (UK) 1996, M 1988; FRCP (Ed) 1997; FRCP (Glas) 2001. Director of Pub. Health & Health Policy, NHS Highland, Inverness; Hon. Sen. Lect. (Pub. Health Med.) Univ. Edin.; Hon. Sen. Lect. (Pub. Health) Univ. of Aberd. Specialty: Pub. Health Med. Socs: Convenor Scott. Affairs Comm.; Fac. Pub. Health Med. Prev: Cons. Pub. Health Med. Forth Valley HB; Hon. Clin. Tutor (Med.) Univ. Edin.; GP Livingston.

WRENCH, Rosanne — MB BChir Camb. 1981; PhD Aston Univ. 1973, BSc 1970.

WRENN, Paul Anthony Michael The Ashes, Tamworth Road, Over Whitacre, Coleshill, Birmingham B46 2PG — MB ChB Birm. 1978.

WRESSELL, Susan Elizabeth Newcastle, North Tyneside & Northumberland Mental Health Trust, Fleming Nuffield Unit, Burdon Terrace, Newcastle upon Tyne NE2 3AE Tel: 0191 219 6429; 44 St. Georges Terrace, Jesmond, Newcastle upon Tyne NE2 2SY — MB BS Newc. 1983; MRCPsych 1987. Cons. Child & Adolesc. Psychiat. Fleming Nuffield Unit Newc. u. Tyne; Hon. Lect. (Child Health) Newc. Specialty: Child & Adolesc. Psychiat.

WRIDE, Jonathan Peter Home Farm, Oxton, Kenton, Exeter EX6 8EX — MB BCh Wales 1987; BSc (Hons) Wales 1982; MRCGP 1992. SCMO Addic.s Serv. Community Trust Exter. Specialty: Alcohol & Substance Misuse. Prev: Trainee GP Torbay VTS; Clin. Med. Off. Community Ment. Health Team Paignton.

WRIGGLESWORTH, Peter Bennet (retired) 186 Warbeck Hill Road, Blackpool Tel: 01253 51611 — MB ChB Manch. 1958; DCH Eng. 1963; DObst RCOG 1964. Prev: Capt. RAMC (Nat. Serv.) Hong Kong.

WRIGHT, Alan Charlton (retired) — MB ChB Ed. 1950; DIH Soc. Apoth. Lond. 1964. Prev: GP Worksop.

WRIGHT, Alan Duncan George Anaesthetic Department, Law Hospital, Carluke ML8 5ER Tel: 01698 361100; 466 Lanark Road W., Balerno, Edinburgh EH14 5AE Tel: 0131 449 4500 — MB ChB Ed. 1973 (Edinburgh) FFA RCS Eng. 1979. Cons. Anaesth. Law Hosp. Carluke. Specialty: Anaesth.

WRIGHT, Alan Finlay 5 Lynedoch Place, Edinburgh EH3 7PX — MB ChB St. And. 1971; MRCPsych 1980.

WRIGHT, Alan John Hudshaw House, Hexham NE46 1HZ — MB BS Lond. 1975; MRCS Eng. LRCP Lond. 1975; MRCP (UK) 1979. Cons. Phys. Gen. Hosp. Hexham. Specialty: Gen. Med. Socs: Assn. Phys. (N.. Br.) & Brit. Geriat. Soc. Prev: Sen. Regist. (Gen. & Geriat. Med.) Newc. HA.

WRIGHT, Alan John Benefits Agency, Arden House, Gosforth, Newcastle upon Tyne NE3 3BP Tel: 0191 223 3064; 88 Stoneybeck, Bishop Middleham, Ferryhill DL17 9BN Tel: 01740 651319 — MB BS Newc. 1976; MRCGP 1980. Med. Adviser NE Benefits Agency. Specialty: Civil Serv. Prev: Med. Servs. Manager NE Benefits Agency; Med. Off. Benefits Agency DSS Newc. u. Tyne; GP Ferry Hill Chilton.

WRIGHT, Alasdair Ross Greasby Health Centre, Greasby Road, Greasby, Wirral CH49 3AT Tel: 0151 678 3000 Fax: 0151 604 1813 — MB ChB Manch. 1994; BSc (Hons.) Phys. & Sports Sci. Glas. 1989; Dip. Sports Med. RCS Ed. 1997; DFFP 1998; DCH RCP Lond. 1998; DRCOG 1998; MRCGP 1999. G.P Pricipal, Greasby Health Centre, Greasby Rd, Greasby, Wirral. Specialty: Sports Med.; Paediat. Socs: BMA. Prev: GP/Regist. Guildford; G.P Princip., Linden Hall Surg., Newport, Shrops.

WRIGHT, Alexander David Manor Hospital, Moat Road, Walsall WS2 9PS; 72 Fitzroy Avenue, Harborne, Birmingham B17 8RQ Tel: 0121 427 7406 — MB BChir Camb. 1962; MRCS Eng. LRCP Lond. 1961. Hon. Cons. (Phys.) Univ. Hosp. Birm. Specialty: Diabetes. Prev: Sen. Lect. (Med.) Univ. Birm.; Cons. Phys. Walsall Hosp. Trust.

WRIGHT, Alexander Justin 210 Welford Road, Leicester LE2 6BD — MB ChB Leic. 1995.

WRIGHT, Alison Lesley Flat C, 232 Otley Road, Leeds LS16 5AB — MB ChB Leeds 1990.

WRIGHT, Alison Margaret Department of Genitourinary Medicine, Royal Hallamshire Hospital, Glossop Road, Sheffield S10 2JF Tel: 0114 271 3528 Email: alison.wright@sth.nhs.uk — MB BS Western Australia 1980; DRCOG 1989; MRCOG 1994; MFFP 1996; Dip GU Med 1998. Consultant in Genitourinary Medicine. Socs: BASHH; BHIVA.

WRIGHT, Alistair Kenneth John Roxburgh Street Surgery, 10 Roxburgh Street, Galashiels TD1 1PF Tel: 01896 752557 Fax: 01896 755374 — MB ChB Ed. 1981.

WRIGHT, Alwyn Peter (retired) 7 Grey Towers Drive, Nunthorpe, Middlesbrough TS7 0LS — MB BS Lond. 1952 (Univ. Coll. Hosp.) DObst RCOG 1954; DIH Soc. Apoth. Lond. 1959; FFOM RCP Lond. 1983, M 1979. Prev: Cons. Occupat. Phys.

WRIGHT, Mr Andrew Accident & Emergency Department, Doncaster Royal Infirmary, Doncaster DN2 5LT Tel: 01302 366666; 17 Poppyfields Way, Branton, Doncaster DN3 3UA — MB ChB Baghdad 1974; FRCS Ed. 1986; LMSSA Lond. 1986. Cons. A & E Med. Doncaster Roy. Infirm. Specialty: Accid. & Emerg. Socs: Brit. Assn. Accid. & Emerg. Med.; BMA; Med. Protec. Soc.

WRIGHT, Andrew David Priory Fields Surgery, Nursery Road, Huntingdon PE29 3RL Tel: 01480 52361 Fax: 01480 434640 — MB BS Lond. 1993 (University College and Middlesex School of Medicine) MA Cantab. 1994; DGM 1996; DCH 1997; DFFP 1997; MRCGP 1998; DRCOG 1998. Specialty: Gen. Pract.

WRIGHT, Andrew Hugh Ravenswood Doctors Surgery, Thomson Avenue, Johnstone PA5 8SU Tel: 01505 331979 Fax: 01505 323444 — MB ChB Glas. 1984; DRCOG 1987; MRCGP 1988. Prev: Trainee GP Paisley VTS; Ho. Surg. Hairmyres Hosp. E. Kilbride Glas.; Ho. Phys. Roy. Alexandra Infirm. Paisley.

WRIGHT, Andrew John Ladybridge Surgery, 10 Broadgate, Ladybridge, Bolton BL3 4PZ Tel: 01204 653267 Fax: 01204 665350; 1 The Hoskers, West Houghton, Bolton BL5 2DW — MB ChB Sheff. 1983; DRCOG 1986; MRCGP 1989; DCH RCP Lond. 1990.

WRIGHT, Andrew John Hampton Hill Medical Centre, 23 Wellington Road, Hampton TW12 1JP Tel: 020 8977 0043 Fax: 020 8977 8691 — MB ChB Bristol 1976; DCH Eng. 1980; MRCGP 1981. Socs: Med. Ass. Soc. Prev: IT Dir. Kingston & Richmond Multifund; Cons. NHS Centre for Clin. Coding Middlx.; Tainee GP Kettering VTS.

WRIGHT, Andrew Leslie Yeadon Health Centre, 17 South View Road, Yeadon, Leeds LS19 7PS Tel: 0113 295 4040 Fax: 0113 295 4044 — MB ChB Leeds 1981; BSc (Hons.) Physiol. Leeds 1978; DRCOG 1987. GP Leeds.

WRIGHT, Andrew Leslie St. Lukes Hospital, Little Horton Lane, Bradford BD5 0NA Tel: 01274 365547 Fax: 01274 365529 — MB ChB Sheff. 1981; BMedSci (Hons.) Sheff. 1979; MRCS Eng. LRCP Lond. 1981; MRCP (UK) 1984; FRCP Lond. 1995. Cons. Dermat. Bradford Roy. Infirm. & Airedale Hosp. Steeton. Specialty: Dermat. Prev: Sen. Regist. (Dermat.) Rupert Hallam Dept. Dermat. Sheff. HA; Hon. Clin. Tutor Univ. Sheff.; Regist. (Dermat.) Edin. Roy. Infirm.

WRIGHT, Andrew Martin The Surgery, 34 Teme Street, Tenbury Wells WR15 8AA Tel: 01584 810343 Fax: 01584 819734 — MB Camb. 1973; BChir 1972; MRCP (UK) 1977; DRCOG 1978.

WRIGHT, Andrew Ronald Department of Radiology, St Mary's Hospital, Praed St., London W2 1NY Tel: 020 7886 6363 Fax: 020 7886 6363 — MB BS Lond. 1981 (University College Hospital

London) MA Oxf. 1976; MRCP (UK) 1985; FRCR 1989; T(R) (CR) 1991. Specialty: Radiol. Prev: Cons. Radiol./Sen. Lect. Western Gen. Hosp. Edin.

WRIGHT, Andrew Timothy Wright and Partners, Heald Green Medical Centre, Finney Lane, Heald Green, Cheadle SK8 3JD Tel: 0161 436 8384 Fax: 0161 493 9268 — MB ChB Manch. 1985; BSc (Med. Sci.) St. And. 1982; MRCGP 1990; AFOM 1997. Specialty: Palliat. Med.; Occupat. Health. Socs: Brit. Med. Acupunct. Soc.; Soc. Occupat. Med. Prev: Princip. GP; Trainee GP Stockport VTS; SHO (O & G) Tameside Gen. Hosp.

WRIGHT, Ann Compton Crosburn House, Main Road, Long Bennington, Newark NG23 5DJ — MB BS Lond. 1962 (Roy. Free) MRCS Eng. LRCP Lond. 1962; DObst RCOG 1964.

WRIGHT, Ann Margaret 8 Croft Gardens, Holywood BT18 0PD — MB BS Lond. 1986.

WRIGHT, Ann Penelope (retired) The Moor, Westfield, Hastings TN35 4QR Tel: 01424 754913 — MB BS Lond. 1956 (Middlx.) Prev: Childr. Ho. Off. Radcliffe Infirm. Oxf.

WRIGHT, Anna Jane Highfield Health Centre, 2 Proctor Street, off Tong Street, Bradford BD4 9QA Tel: 01274 227700 Fax: 01274 227900 — MB ChB Leeds 1980; BSc (Hons.) Leeds 1977; DRCOG 1982; DCH RCP Lond. 1984; MRCGP 1984.

WRIGHT, Anthony Quarry Ground Surgery, Broadway, Edington, Bridgwater TA7 9JB Tel: 01278 722077 Fax: 01278 722352 — BM Soton. 1978; MRCP (UK) 1982; DRCOG 1985; MRCGP 1986; FRCGP 1998.

WRIGHT, Anthony (retired) Health & Safety Executive, Kiln House, Pottergate, Norwich NR2 1DA Tel: 01603 615711 Fax: 01603 761436; Cantley House, Cantley Lane, Cringleford, Norwich NR4 6TF Tel: 01603 452041 — MB BChir Camb. 1964 (Camb. & St. Bart.) MA, MB Camb. 1964, BChir 1963; DObst RCOG 1966; DIH 1981; MFOM RCP Lond. 1989; FFOM 1999. Prev: Sen. Med. Insp. Health & Safety Exec. Norwich.

WRIGHT, Professor Anthony Institute of Laryngology & Otology, 330 Grays Inn Road, London WC1X 8EE Tel: 020 7915 1308 Fax: 020 7837 9279 Email: anthony.wright@ucl.ac.uk; 150 Harley Street, London W1G 7LQ Tel: 020 7935 4579 Fax: 020 7935 3635; 4 Grange Road, Highgate, London N6 4AP Tel: 020 8340 5593 — MRCS Eng. LRCP Lond. 1974; DM Oxf. 1986, BM BCh 1974; FRCS Ed. 1979; LLM Wales 1995; FRCS Eng. 1995. Prof. Otorhinolaryng. & Dir. Inst. Laryngol. & Otol. Univ. Coll. Lond.; Hon. Cons. Otol. Roy. Nat. Throat, Nose & Ear Hosp. Lond. Specialty: Otolaryngol. Prev: Cons. Otol. Roy. Free Hosp. Lond.

WRIGHT, Anthony Thomas Stanley Hathaway Surgery, 32 New Road, Chippenham SN15 1HR Tel: 01249 447766 Fax: 01249 443948; The Stable House, Rowden Lane, Chippenham SN15 2NN Tel: 01249 447994 Email: tony.wright@nhs.net — MB ChB Sheff. 1979; DRCOG 1982; DCH RCP Eng. 1982; DA Eng. 1983; MRCGP 1987. Clin. Med. Off. Chippenham Community Hosp. Specialty: Paediat.

WRIGHT, Antony Marcus Bourne Galletly Practice Team, 40 North Road, Bourne PE10 9BT Tel: 01778 562200 Fax: 01778 562207; 34 Grampian Way, Grantham NG31 8FY Tel: 01476 564255 — MB BS Newc. 1992; BMedSc. Newc.; DFFP 1997; MRCGP 1997.

WRIGHT, Arthur Edwin, TD (retired) The Old Smithy, Westboat, Warden, Hexham NE46 3SB Tel: 01434 605847 — MB BS Durh. 1948 (Newc.) DPH Durh. 1954; MD Durh. 1957; Dip. Bact. Lond 1958; FRCPath 1973, M 1964. Hon. Cons. Newc. HA (T); Hon. Lect. (Microbiol.) Univ. Newc. Prev: Dir. Pub. Health Laborat. Newc.

WRIGHT, Barbara Yvonne The Beeches, 6 Westbury Gardens, Higher Odcombe, Yeovil BA22 8UR — MB BS Lond. 1971; MRCS Eng. LRCP Lond. 1971; DObst RCOG 1974; DA Eng. 1978.

WRIGHT, Barrie James Pettigrew (retired) 31 High Street, Dorchester-on-Thames, Wallingford OX10 7HN Tel: 01865 340029 — MRCS Eng. LRCP Lond. 1958 (St. Mary's) LMSSA Lond. 1956. Prev: Cas. Off. & Ho. Phys. & Ho. Surg. Harold Wood Hosp.

WRIGHT, Benjamin Accident & Emergency Department, Westminster Hospital, Dean Ryle St., London SW1P 2AP — MB BS Lond. 1991.

WRIGHT, Brian Eric Morden (retired) The Hermitage, Metheringham, Lincoln LN4 3HA Tel: 01526 320 569 — MRCS Eng. LRCP Lond. 1957 (St. Thos.) GP Principle. Prev: Ho. Surg. Vict. Hosp. Swindon.

WRIGHT, Brian John (retired) 13A Ashburton Road, Gosport PO12 2LH Tel: 023 9258 0106 — (King's Coll. & St. Geo.) MB BS Lond. 1951; DObst RCOG 1958; FRCGP 1983, M 1968. Prev: Ho. Phys. (Gen. Med. & Neurol.) & Ho. Surg. St. Geo. Hosp.

WRIGHT, Bryan Keith 17 Stanley Grove, Ruabon, Wrexham LL14 6AH — MB ChB Birm. 1991; ChB Birm. 1991.

WRIGHT, Camilla Jane Evelyn 26 Everington Street, London W6 8DU — MB ChB Leeds 1994.

WRIGHT, Carl Houghton Department of Diagnotic Imaging, Glan Clwyd Hospital, Bodelwyddan, Clwyd KK18 5UJ Tel: 01745 534512 Fax: 01745 534512 — MB ChB Liverp. 1970; DMRD Liverp. 1973; FRCR 1976. Cons. Radiol. Glan Clwyd Hosp. Bodelwyddan. Specialty: Radiol. Socs: BMA; Brit. Inst. Radiol.; BMUS. Prev: Sen. Research Fell. X-Ray Dept. St. Thos. Hosp. Lond.; Sen. Fell. (Diag. Radiol.) Univ. Kansas Med. Centre.

WRIGHT, Carol Jane 143 Portland Road, Bournemouth BH9 1NG — MB BS Lond. 1988; MRCP (UK) 1993.

WRIGHT, Caroline Isobel (retired) Flat 3, 9 Pembroke Avenue, Hove BN3 5DA — MD Lond. 1927 (Char. Cross) MB BS 1923; MRCS Eng. LRCP Lond. 1922, DPH 1924. Prev: Med. Insp. Childr. Dept. Home Office.

WRIGHT, Caroline Jane 55 Church Road, Wickham Bishop's, Witham CM8 3JZ — MB BChir Camb. 1993; MA.

WRIGHT, Catherine Jane Norwich Primary Care Trust, Little Plumstead Hospital, Norwich NR13 5EW Tel: 01603 711227 Fax: 01603 711202 Email: catherine.wright@norwich-pct.nhs.uk — BM Soton. 1987; MRCPsych 1992; Cert. MHS 1999. Cons. (Psychiat.) Learning Disabilities. Specialty: Ment. Health. Special Interest: Autistic Spectrum Disorders.

WRIGHT, Charles Edward Doctors Surgery, Pembroke Road, Framlingham, Woodbridge IP13 9HA Email: charles.wright2@virgin.net — MB BS Lond. 1992 (London Hosp) BSc Lond. 1989, MB BS 1992; MRCGP 1998. Specialty: Gen. Pract. Socs: BMA & MDU; RCGP.

WRIGHT, Charles Mark Vernon Portslade Health Centre, Church Road, Portslade, Brighton BN41 1LX Tel: 01273 422525/418445 Fax: 01273 413510 — MB BS London 1974; MRCS Eng LRCP Lond 1974. GP Brighton.

WRIGHT, Charles Richard Longshaw House, Billinge, Wigan WN5 7JA Tel: 01744 892417 — MB ChB Liverp. 1933; MRCS Eng. LRCP Lond. 1933. Prev: Ho. Surg. Stanley Hosp. Liverp.; Res. Med. Off. Mill Rd. Infirm. Liverp.; Maj. RAMC.

WRIGHT, Charles Stewart Weatherley 37 Corfton Road, Ealing, London W5 2HR Tel: 020 7935 2477 — MB BChir Camb. 1969 (Camb. & St. Mary's) MA, MB Camb. 1969, BChir 1968; MRCS Eng. LRCP Lond. 1968; FRCOG 1987, M 1973. Cons. (O & G) Hillingdon Hosp. Uxbridge; Hon. Sec. Spencer Wells Soc. Specialty: Obst. & Gyn. Socs: Fell. Roy. Soc. Med. (Hon. Sec. Sect. Obst. & Gyn.). Prev: Sen. Regist. St. Mary's Hosp. Lond.; Res. Surg. Off. Hosp. Wom. Soho Sq. Lond.; Res. Med. Off. Qu. Charlottes Matern. Hosp. Lond.

WRIGHT, Charles William The Medical Centre, 2 Frances Street, Doncaster DN1 1JS Tel: 01302 349431 Fax: 01302 364558; Estate Cottage, 6 Mosham Road, Blaxton, Doncaster DN9 3AZ Tel: 01302 770345 — MB BS Lond. 1974 (St. Bart.) MRCS Eng. LRCP Lond. 1974; BSc (Hons.) Lond. 1977; FRCS Eng. 1981; MRCGP 1988. Specialty: Disabil. Med.

WRIGHT, Charlotte Margaret Yorkhill Hospital, Peach Unit, QMH Tower, Glasgow G3 8SJ Tel: 0141 201 6927 Fax: 0141 201 6943 Email: charlotte.wright@clinmed.gla.ac.uk; 1 Moray Place, Strathbungo, Glasgow G41 2AQ — BM BCh Oxf. 1982; BMedSc Newc. 1979; MRCP (UK) 1987; MSc Lond. 1992; MD Newc. 1996. Sen. Lect. (Community Child Health) Glas. Univ.; Hon. Cons. (Community Child Health) Yorkhill Child Health Care Trust. Specialty: Community Child Health; Epidemiol.; Research. Socs: Fell. Roy. Coll. Paediat. & Child Health; Paediat. Research Soc.; Soc. for Social Med. Prev: 1st Asst. / Sen. Regist. Newc. Univ.; Sen. Lect. / Cons. Newc. Univ.; Wellcome Train. Fell. (Child Health) Newc.

WRIGHT, Christine Janet City Hospital, Haematology Department, Dudley Road, Birmingham B18 7QH Tel: 0121 507 6042 — MB ChB Bristol 1986; MRCP (UK) 1991; Dip RCPatch 1998; MRCPath 1999. Cons. Haemat. City Hosp. Birm. Specialty: Haematology. Prev: Regist. (Haemat.) Birm. Hosp.; Sen. Regist. (Haemat.) Uni. Hosp. Birm.

WRIGHT, Christopher Dept. of Pathology, Royal Victoria Infirmary, Newcastle upon Tyne NE1 4LP Tel: 0191 282 4362 — MB BS Newc. 1983; PhD Newc. 1994, MB BS 1983, BMedSci 1980; MRCPath 1990. Cons. Perinatal Pathologist. Specialty: Histopath.

WRIGHT, Christopher James (retired) 2 Old Hall Croft, Gargrave, Skipton BD23 3PQ Tel: 01756 749699 Email: cjwright@doctors.org.uk — MB ChB Leeds 1965; DA Eng. 1967; FFA RCS Eng. 1969. Prev: Sen. Regist. (Anaesth.) Leeds RHB.

WRIGHT, Christopher John George Deerbrook Surgery, 114-116 Norwood Road, London SE24 9BB Tel: 020 8674 4623 Fax: 020 8678 6236; 56 Amberley Gardens, Stoneleigh, Epsom KT19 0NG — MB ChB Ed. 1985 (Edinburgh) BSc Ed. 1984.

WRIGHT, Christopher Mark 5 Gorsewood Drive, Hakin, Milford Haven SA73 3EP — MB BS Lond. 1994; FRCA 2001.

WRIGHT, Colin Ernest (retired) 55 South Road, South Ockendon RM15 6NX — MB BS Lond. 1953.

WRIGHT, David, MC (retired) 28 Manor Road, Hemingford Grey, Huntingdon PE28 9BX — (Glas.) MB ChB Glas. 1941.

WRIGHT, David Department of Haematology, Pontefract General Infirmary, Pontefract WF8 1PL — MB BCh Wales 1983; BSc Wales 1980; MRCP (UK) 1987; MRCPath 1994; MD 1998. Cons. Haemat. Pontefract Gen. Hosp. Specialty: Haematology. Prev: Sen. Regist. (Haemat.) Roy. Liverp. Univ. Hosp.; Research Regist. UK REF Laborat. Withington Hosp. Manch.

WRIGHT, David Arthur (retired) Flat 4 Penthouse, 3 Bryanston Place, London W1H 2DE — MB BS Lond. 1952 (Univ. Coll. Hosp.) MRCS Eng. LRCP Lond. 1952. Med. Off. Foster Wheeler Ltd. Prev: Clin. Asst. ENT St. Mary's Hosp. & Paddington Green Childr. Hosp.

WRIGHT, Mr David Arthur (retired) Mount Alvernia Hospital, Harvey Road, Guildford GU1 3LX Tel: 01483 561315 Fax: 01483 538230 Email: davidwright400@aol.com; Eastbury Farm House, Compton, Guildford GU3 1EE Tel: 01483 810343 Fax: 01483 538230 Email: davidwright400@aol.com — MB BChir Camb. 1960 (Camb. & Guy's) MRCS Eng. LRCP Lond. 1959; MA Camb. 1960; FRCS Eng. 1966. ENT Surg. Mt. Alverna Hosp. Guildford.; Cons. ENT Surg. King Edwd. VII Hosp. Midhurst; Civil. Cons. ENT. Advis. to the Army. Prev: Pres.Brit.Assn.Otol, Head & Neck Surg.

WRIGHT, David Graham (retired) 29 Bloomfield Avenue, Bath BA2 3AB Tel: 01225 427920 — MB BS Lond. 1963 (Westm.) MRCS Eng. LRCP Lond. 1963; FRCP Lond. 1981, M 1967. Prev: Cons. Geriat. St. Martins Hosp. Bath.

WRIGHT, David Harold, CBE East Backstonegill Farm, Dent, Sedbergh LA10 5TE Tel: 01539 625073 — (St. Thos.) MSc Lond. 1989, MB BS 1970; MFOM RCP Lond. 1993, A 1989; FFOM RCP Lond 1999. Cons. Ocupational Phys. Post Office Employee Health Servs.; Mem. Ct. of Governers Lond. Sch. of Hyg. & Trop. Med. Specialty: Occupat. Health. Socs: Fell. Roy. Soc. Med.; Soc. Occupat. Med.- Hon Sec. Prev: Regtl. Med. Off. Roy. Scots Dragoon Guards; Chief Med. Off. UN Protec. Force, Yugoslavia.

WRIGHT, David James Thomas Gillies and Overbridge Medical Partnership, Brighton Hill, Sullivan Road, Basingstoke RG22 4EH Tel: 01256 479747; Yew Tree House, Long Parish, Andover SP11 6PT Tel: 01264 720598 — MB BS Lond. 1978 (Guys) MRCS Eng. LRCP Lond. 1977; DRCOG 1982; DCH Lond. 1982; MRCGP 1985. Prev: Trainee GP Brighton VTS.

WRIGHT, David John Donnington Medical Practice, Wrekin Drive, Donnington, Telford TF2 8EA Tel: 01952 605252 Fax: 01952 677010 — MB ChB Manch. 1989; BSc (1st cl. Hons.) Med. Biochem. Manch. 1986; DRCOG 1991; DCH RCP Lond. 1992; MRCGP 1993.

WRIGHT, David John Anaesthetic Department, Western General Hospital, Edinburgh EH4 2XU Tel: 0131 537 1661 Fax: 0131 537 1021; 20 Lennox Row, Edinburgh EH5 3JW Tel: 0131 552 3439 — MB BS Lond. 1968 (St. Bart.) MRCS Eng. LRCP Lond. 1968; DA Eng. 1971; FFA RCS Eng. 1974. Cons. Anaesth. West. Gen. Hosp. Edin. Specialty: Anaesth.

WRIGHT, David John 10 Rollesbrook Gardens, Southampton SO15 5WA — MB BS Lond. 1992 (UMDS (Guy's & St. Thomas))

WRIGHT, David Julian Maurice (retired) — MB BS Lond. 1961 (Middlx.) MD Lond. 1973; FRCPath 1991, M 1982. Prev: Cons. Microbiologist Char. Cross Hosp. Lond.

WRIGHT, David Justin Cardiothoracic Centre, Thomas Drive, Liverpool L14 3PE Email: david.wright@ctc.nhs.uk — MB ChB Leeds 1990; MRCP (UK) 1994. Cons. (Cardiol.). Specialty: Cardiol. Prev: Research Fell. (Cardiol.) Killingbeck Hosp. Leeds.

WRIGHT, Mr David Malcolm Southern General Hospital, Govan Road, Glasgow G51 4RF — MB ChB Glas. 1989; BSc (Hons.) Glas. 1986; FRCS Ed. 1993. Specialty: Gen. Surg. Prev: Specialist Regist. (Gen. Surg.) W. of Scotl. Higher Surgic. Train. Scheme; SHO West. Infirm. Glas.

WRIGHT, David Poulter (retired) The Butts, High Bank, Porlock, Minehead TA24 8NS Tel: 01643 862975 — MB ChB Leeds 1948; MRCGP 1964. Prev: Princip. GP Nailsea.

WRIGHT, David Robert 8 Maris Green, Great Shelford, Cambridge CB2 5EE — BM Soton. 1990.

WRIGHT, David Sheldon The Surgery, April Cottage, High Street, Uckfield TN22 4LA Tel: 01825 732333 Fax: 01825 732072 — MB BS Lond. 1987; BSc (Biochem.) Lond. 1984; DGM RCP Lond. 1989; MRCGP 1991. Prev: Trainee GP Whipps Cross Hosp. Lond. VTS.

WRIGHT, David Smethurst Inzievar Surgery, 2 Kenmore Street, Aberfeldy PH15 2BL Tel: 01887 820366 Fax: 01887 829566 Email: dr.dwright@inzievar.finix.org.uk; Tigh N'Acheonan, Dull, Aberfeldy PH15 2JQ Tel: 01887 820465 Email: drdwright@hotmail.com — MB ChB Dundee 1973; MRCP Edinburgh, UK 1976. GP Aberfeldy, Perthsh.; Sessional paynet for 'c/o the elderly' Aberfeldy Community Hosp.

WRIGHT, David Stephen, OBE, OStJ, Surg. Capt. RN Retd. (retired) 9 Ashburton Road, Alverstoke, Gosport PO12 2LH Tel: 023 9258 2459 Email: dswright@talk21.com — MB BS Lond. 1959 (St. Bart.) DPH Lond. 1967; DIH Soc. Apoth. Lond. 1968; MSc Salford 1973; MFCM RCP (UK) 1974; FFOM RCP Lond. 1983, M 1978; FRCP Lond. 1989. Prev: Cons. Occupat. Phys. Hants.

WRIGHT, David Wood Whitefriar's Surgery, Whitefriar's Street, Perth PH1 1PP Tel: 01738 627912 Fax: 01738 643969; 8 Strathearn Terrace, Perth PH2 0LS — MB ChB Dundee 1973; BSc Ed. 1968; DRCOG 1976; MRCGP 1978. Prev: SHO (Anaesth.) Ninewells Hosp. Dundee.

WRIGHT, Deirdre Jane 6 Manland Avenue, Harpenden AL5 4RF — MB BS Lond. 1981; BSc Lond. 1978, MB BS 1981; MRCP (UK) 1986; FRCR 1988. Cons. Radiol. Luton & Dunstable Hosp. Specialty: Radiol. Prev: Sen. Regist. (Radiol.) Guy's Hosp. Lond.

WRIGHT, Professor Dennis Howard (retired) Brae House, 31 Chilbolton Avenue, Winchester SO22 5HE Tel: 01962 863778 Fax: 01962 869530 Email: denniswright@totalise.co.uk — MB ChB Bristol 1956; BSc (Physiol. Hons.) Bristol 1953, MD 1964; FRCPath 1977, M 1965. Emerit. Prof. (Path.) Univ. Soton.; Hon. Cons.(Haematopath.) Roy. Bournemouth & ChristCh. Hosps. NHS Trust. Prev: Reader (Path.) Univ. Birm. & Makerere Univ. Coll., Uganda.

WRIGHT, Derek Geoffrey Green Lane Surgery, 2 Green Lane, Belper DE56 1BZ Tel: 01773 823521 Fax: 01773 821954 Email: dgw1962@aol.com — MB ChB Leeds 1985; DA (UK) 1987; DCH RCP Lond. 1989; DRCOG 1990; MRCGP 1991. Hosp. Practitioner; Babington Hosp., Belper, Derbysh. Socs: Derby Med. Soc. Prev: GP Wirksworth Health Centre Derbysh.; Trainee GP Colchester Gen. Hosp. VTS; Ho. Off. Rotat. (Anaesth.) St. Jas. Univ. Teach. Hosp. & York Dist. Hosp.

WRIGHT, Derek Halton Highfield, 14 Queen's Park Road, Burnley BB10 3LB Tel: 01282 424736 — (Manch.) MB ChB Manch. 1947. Prev: Ho. Surg. Gen. Surgic. Unit & Radium Inst. Burnley Vict. Hosp.; Med. Off. Prestwich Hosp.

WRIGHT, Donald Geoffrey 33 Mount Pleasant Road, Newtownabbey BT37 0NQ — MB BCh BAO Belf. 1986.

WRIGHT, Donald Robert (retired) 5 Meadow Lane, Milton Keynes Village, Milton Keynes MK10 9AZ Tel: 01908 661960 — BM BCh Oxf. 1954 (Oxf. & Univ. Coll. Hosp.) MA, BM BCh Oxf. 1954; MRCGP 1967. GP Cons. Med. Defence Union. Prev: Resid. Med. Off. St. Pancras Hosp. & Univ. Coll. Hosp. Lond.

WRIGHT, Dorothy Elizabeth 3 Kingswood Avenue, London NW6 6LA — MB BS Lond. 1952 (Roy. Free) MRCS Eng. LRCP Lond. 1951. Prev: Ho. Off. Univ. Coll. Hosp. W. Indies, Jamaica; Ho. Surg. Roy. Free Hosp. Lond.

WRIGHT, Douglas 7 Wake Green Road, Moseley, Birmingham B13 9HD Tel: 0121 449 0300; 3 St. Agnes Road, Moseley, Birmingham B13 9PH Tel: 0121 449 4870 — MB ChB Birm. 1956; MRCS Eng. LRCP Lond. 1956; DObst RCOG 1957; DMJ Soc. Apoth. Lond. 1969.

WRIGHT, Douglas David Wye Valley Surgery, 2 Desborough Avenue, High Wycombe HP11 2BN Tel: 01494 521044; 16 Abbots Way, High Wycombe HP12 4NR Email: dougw@vossnet.co.uk — BM Soton. 1988; DCH RCP Lond. 1993; MRCGP 1994.

WRIGHT, Douglas Milne Kirkham Health Centre, Moor Street, Kirkham, Preston PR4 2DL Tel: 01772 683420 — MB ChB Dundee 1978; MRCGP 1983.

WRIGHT, Edwina Caroline 119A Cumnor Hill, Oxford OX2 9JA — MB BS Lond. 1998.

WRIGHT, Elaine Catherine 15 Woodcote Park Avenue, Purley CR8 3ND Tel: 020 8660 4220 — MRCS Eng. LRCP Lond. 1955; MD Lond. 1980, MB BS 1955; DPM Eng. 1961; FRCPsych 1984, M 1971. Cons. Psychiat. St. Lawrence's Hosp. Caterham. Specialty: Gen. Psychiat. Prev: Cons. Psychiat. Fountain & Carshalton Hosp. Gp.

WRIGHT, Elizabeth 5 Lynedoch Place, Edinburgh EH3 7PX — MB ChB Dundee 1973; DCH RCPS Glas. 1975.

WRIGHT, Elizabeth Ann Department of Radiology, Countess of Chester Hospital, Liverpool Road, Chester CH2 1UL Tel: 01244 365285; Sakura, 2 Demage Lane S., Upton-by-Chester, Chester CH2 1EQ Tel: 01244 380711 — MB BCh BAO Belf. 1976; DMRD Liverp. 1987; FRCR 1990. Cons. Radiol. Chester Hosp. Specialty: Radiol. Prev: Sen. Regist. (Radiol.) Mersey Region; Regist. (Radiol.) Roy. Liverp. Hosp.

WRIGHT, Elizabeth Dorothy Department Microbiology, West Suffolk Hospital, Department of Microbiology, Hardwick Lane, Bury St Edmunds IP33 2QZ Tel: 01284 713000 Email: liz.wright@wsh.nhs.uk — MB BS Lond. 1981 (Roy. Free) MSc Lond. 1986, BSc 1971; PhD Glas. 1975; MRCPath 1986; FRCP FRCPath 1997. Cons. MicroBiol. W. Suff. Hosp. Bury, St Edmunds. Specialty: Med. Microbiol. Prev: Sen. Regist. (MicroBiol.) Qu. Mary's Hosp. & St. Geo.'s Hosp. Lond.; Cons. Microbiologist Worthing Hosp. Worthing.

WRIGHT, Elizabeth Julie Department of Anaesthesia, University Hospital Aintree, Longmoor Lane, Liverpool L9 7AL Tel: 0151 525 5153 — MB BS Newc. 1980 (Newcastle Upon Tyne) DA (UK) 1982; FFA RCS Eng. 1985. Cons. Anaesth. Aintree Hosp. Liverp. And Walton Centre for Neurol. and Neurosurg. Specialty: Anaesth.

WRIGHT, Ellen Sylvia Vandrugh Hill Health Centre, Vandrugh Hill, Greenwich, London SE10 9HA Tel: 0208 312 6095 Email: eswright@doctors.org.uk — (Barts Lond.) MA Oxf. 1980; MB BS Lond. 1985; FRCA 1990; MRCGP 2002. GP Partner. Vandrugh Hill Health Centre, Vandrugh Hill, Greenwich SE10; Hon. Cons.(Pain Phys.) Qu. Eliz. Hosp. Woolwich. Specialty: Anaesth.; Gen. Pract. Special Interest: Pain Managem. Socs: FRCA; BSMDH; BMAS. Prev: Cons. (Pain Managem.) Qu. Eliz. Hosp.; SR (Pain Managem.) St Thomas' Hosp.

WRIGHT, Eluned Marion Department of Anaesthetics, Llandough Hospital, Penlan Road, Penarth CF64 2XX Tel: 029 2071 1711 — BM BCh Oxf. 1983; BA Oxf. 1980; FRCA 1988. Cons. Anaesth. Llandough Hosp. Cardiff. Specialty: Anaesth. Prev: Sen. Regist. (Anaesth.) Univ. Hosp. Wales Cardiff.

WRIGHT, Eric Arthur (retired) 5 Sion Hill, Bath BA1 2UF Tel: 01225 420851 — MB BS Lond. 1944 (Guy's) LMSSA Lond. 1944; FRCP Lond. 1974, M 1949; DSc Lond. 1976, MD 1952; FRCPath 1966, M 1954. Emerit. Prof. Univ. of Lond. Prev: Prof. Morbid Anat. King's Coll. Hosp. Med. Sch. & Cons. Path. Kings Coll. Hosp.

WRIGHT, Eric Paul Department of Microbiology, Conquest Hospital, The Ridge, St Leonards-on-Sea TN37 7RD Tel: 01424 755255 Fax: 01424 758022 Email: paul.wright@esht.nhs.uk — MB ChB Liverp. 1975; Dip. Bact. (Distinct.) . Manch. 1980; FRCPath 1993, M 1982. Cons. Microbiol. Conquest Hosp. St. Leonards-on-Sea. Specialty: Med. Microbiol. Socs: BMA; Assn. Med. Microbiol.; Hosp. Infect. Soc. Prev: Asst. Med. Microbiol. Luton Pub. Health Laborat.; Trainee Med. Microbiol. Liverp. Pub. Health Laborat.; Ho. Off. (Med. Surg.) Fazakerley Hosp. Liverp.

WRIGHT, Eric Walter (retired) 3 Queen's Avenue, Woodford Green IG8 0JE Tel: 020 8504 2016 — (Univ. Ed.) MB ChB Ed. 1947; DPH Ed. 1952; FFCM 1979, M 1972; FFPHM 1989. Prev: Area Med. Off. Redbridge & Waltham Forest HA.

WRIGHT, Ernestine Abioseh 3 Penroy Avenue, Manchester M20 2ZH — MB ChB Manch. 1990. SHO (Gen. Med.) Wythenshawe Hosp. Manch. Specialty: Gen. Med. Socs: BMA.

WRIGHT, Ethel May 7 Church Farm Garth, Leeds LS17 8HD Tel: 0113 273 7472 — MB ChB Leeds 1951; DCH Eng. 1957.

WRIGHT, Fiona 36 Burnside Court, Bearsden, Glasgow G61 4QD — MB ChB Glas. 1994.

WRIGHT, Fiona Alison 102A Osbaldeston Road, London N16 6NL Tel: 020 8806 8574 — MB ChB Bristol 1987. Sen. Regist. (Pub. Health Med.) N. Thames Region. Specialty: Pub. Health Med. Socs: BMA. Prev: Research Asst. (Social Policy) Univ. Bristol; SHO (A & E) Cardiff Roy. Infirm.; Ho. Phys. Southmead Hosp. Bristol.

WRIGHT, Fiona Alison 3 St Margaret's Road, Swindon SN3 1RU — BM Soton. 1998.

WRIGHT, Fiona Judith 30 Kingsway, Waterloo, Liverpool L22 4RQ — MB ChB Aberd. 1991; MRCGP.

WRIGHT, Francine Joy Lodge Medical Centre, 1A Grange Park Avenue, Leeds LS8 3BA Tel: 0113 265 6454 Fax: 0113 295 3710 — MB ChB Leeds 1986; DRCOG 1990. Prev: Trainee GP Bradford VTS.

WRIGHT, Francis George de Longsden Norfolk Clinical Research, Staithe House, East Harbour Way, Burnham Overy Staithe, King's Lynn PE31 8JE Tel: 01328 730064 Fax: 01328 730064; Staithe House, Burnham Overy Staithe, King's Lynn PE31 8JE Tel: 01328 738236 — (St. Mary's) LMSSA Lond. 1958; MB BChir Camb. 1959. Socs: BMA. Prev: Med. Off. Uganda Med. Serv.

WRIGHT, Frank William, MBE Norfolk Park Health Centre, Tower Drive, Sheffield S2 3RE Tel: 0114 276 9661 Fax: 0114 276 9471; 72 Grove Road, Sheffield S7 2GZ Tel: 01442 362569 Fax: 01442 362569 Email: drfwright@blueyonder.co.uk — (Univ. Sheff.) MB ChB Sheff. 1960. Trainer (Gen. Pract.) Sheff.; Clin. Asst. Dermat. Roy. Hallamsh. Hosp. Sheff. Socs: Sheff. M-C Soc. (Pres. Elect). Prev: Clin. Asst. Renal Unit Lodgemoor Hosp. Sheff.; Regist. Birm. Accid. Hosp.; SHO (Gen. Surg.) N. Gen. Hosp. Sheff.

WRIGHT, Fraser George Dunblane Medical Practice, Heatlh Centre, Well Place, Dunblane FK15 9BQ Tel: 01786 822595 Fax: 01786 825298 — MB ChB Aberd. 1987; BSc Hons. Aberd. 1982. SHO (A & E) Stirling Roy. Infirm. Prev: Ho. Off. (Surg.) Stirling Roy. Infirm.; Ho. Off. (Med.) Raigmore Hosp. Inverness & Belford Hosp. Fort William.

WRIGHT, Frederick Keith (retired) Bron y Garth, 31 Ffforddlas, Prestatyn LL19 9SG Tel: 01745 854358 Email: fkwright@doctors.org.uk — (Birm.) MB ChB (Hons.) Birm. 1959; FRCP Lond. 1979, M 1965. Appeals Serv. (p/t). Prev: cons phys Glan Clywd Hosp. NHS Trust.

WRIGHT, Frederick Richard (retired) Pasir Pandang, 20A Grey Point, Helen's Bay, Bangor BT19 1LE Tel: 02891 853727 Fax: 02891 853727 Email: fredrwright@utvinternet.com — MB BCh BAO Belf. 1953 (Queens Belfast) DMRD Eng. 1960; FFR 1966; FRCR 1975; FFR RCSI 1981. Hon. Cons. Ulster Hosp. Dundonald. Prev: Cons. Radiol. Ulster, N. Down & Ards Hosps. Unit.

WRIGHT, Frederick Wynn (retired) Charfield, Cassington Road, Eynsham, Oxford OX29 4LH Tel: 01865 881496 — BM BCh Oxf. 1954; MRCP Lond. 1958; DMRD Eng. 1958; FFR 1961; DM Oxf. 1974; FRCR 1975; FRCP Lond. 1996. Prev: Consg. Rediologist, Oxf. Redcliffe Hosps. Trust.

WRIGHT, Gary David Department of Rheumatology, Royal Victoria Hospital, Belfast Tel: 02890 240503 — MB BCh BAO Belf. 1987; BSc (Hons.) 1985; MRCP 1990; MD 1992; FRCP 2002; FRCPI 2002. Cons. Rheumatologist. Specialty: Rheumatol. Socs: FRCP; BSR; ISR.

WRIGHT, Gavin Anthony Keaton 19 Caversham Avenue, London N13 4LL — MB BS Lond. 1996.

WRIGHT, Geoffrey David Stamp East Dean Cottage, East Dean, Salisbury SP5 1HH — MB ChB Birm. 1973; BSc Birm. 1970, MB ChB 1973; MRCP (UK) 1978; DM Soton. 1986; FRCP 1999. assoc. med. Dir. Glaxo Wellcome UK; Hon. Cons. Neurol. Raddclife Infirm.Oxf. Specialty: Neurol. Socs: BMA, N. Eng. Neurol. Assn. & S. Eng. Neurol. Assn. Prev: Sen. Regist. (Neurol.) Radcliffe Infirm. Oxf.; Regist. (Neurol.) Radcliffe Infirm. Oxf.; Research Regist. Wessex Neurol. Centre Soton. Gen. Hosp.

WRIGHT, Geraldine Margaret Queen Mary's University Hospital, Roehampton Lane, Roehampton, London SW15 5PN; 21 Devonhurst Place, Heathfield Terrace, London W4 4JB — MB BS Lond. 1978 (Roy. Free) BSc Lond. 1975; MRCP (UK) 1983; FRCP (UK) 1997. Sen. Lect. Char. Cross & Westm. Med. Sch. Lond. Specialty: Care of the Elderly.

WRIGHT, Gillian Ruth (retired) Glen Alainn, Treaslane, Portree IV51 9NX Tel: 01470 532392 — (Roy. Free) MB BS Lond. 1957; DObst RCOG 1959.

WRIGHT, Gladys Frances Ballymena Health Centre, Cushendall Road, Ballymena BT43 6HQ Tel: 028 2564 2181 Fax: 028 2565 8919; 57 Tullygarley Road, Ballymena BT42 2JA — MB BCh BAO Belf. 1983; DCH Dub. 1990; DRCOG 1990; MRCGP 1992. Prev: GP Smithfield Med Centre, Ballymena.

WRIGHT, Gordon Herbert (retired) 68 de Freville Avenue, Cambridge CB4 1HU — MRCS Eng. LRCP Lond. 1942 (Camb. & Lond. Hosp.) MB BChir Camb. 1951; MB BChir Camb. 1951; MB BChir Camb. 1951; MD Camb. 1954. Fell. Clare Coll. Prev: Lect. (Anat.) Univ. Camb.

WRIGHT, Grace Elliot (retired) 7 Rothley Close, Ponteland, Newcastle upon Tyne NE20 9TD Tel: 01661 22118 — MB BS Durh. 1926 (Newc.) Prev: Med. Off. Wom. Welf. Clinic (Family Plann. Assn.) Newc. &.

WRIGHT, Graham 17 Greenwood, 31 Princes Way, Wimbledon, London SW19 6QH — MB BS Lond. 1977; BSc Lond. 1974, MB BS 1977. SHO (Ophth.) Mayday Hosp. Thornton Heath. Prev: Ho. Surg. Frimley Pk. Hosp.; Ho. Phys. Roy. Hants. Co. Hosp. Winchester.

WRIGHT, Graham Alexander Craignean Surgery, Dunkeld PH8 0AD Tel: 01350 727269 Fax: 01350 728555; Mansewood, Oak Road, Birnam, Dunkeld PH8 0BL Tel: 01350 727135 — MB ChB Ed. 1982; MRCGP 1986. Clin. Asst. (Gastroenterol.) Perth Roy. Infirm. Prev: GP Fife; SHO (Paediat. Med.) Law Hosp. Carluke Lanarksh.; Cas. Off. (SHO) Vict. Hosp. Kirkcaldy.

WRIGHT, Mr Graham Charles Stairhill Farm, Moorlake, Crediton EX17 5EL — MB BS Lond. 1980; FRCS (Ophth.) Ed. 1990; FCOphth 1991. Specialty: Ophth.

WRIGHT, Graham Robert Riverton Medical Centre, 145 Palmerston St., Riverton, Southland 9654, New Zealand Tel: 0064 3 2348990 Fax: 0064 3 2348990; 17 Lime Grove, Royston SG8 7DJ Tel: 01763 246800 Email: graham.wright@dial.pipex.com — BM BS Nottm. 1989; MRCGP 1995; T(GP) 1995. GP Princip. Riverton Med. Centre. Prev: Partner Donneybrook Med. Centre.

WRIGHT, Hayley Suzanne The Surgery, East Lea, Humshaugh; Honeysuckle House, Oakwood, Hexham NE46 4LE — MB ChB Leic. 1987 (GP Retainer) MRCGP 1991; DRCOG 1991. GP Principal. Specialty: Obst. & Gyn. Prev: Trainee GP Northumbria VTS; GP Retainer.

WRIGHT, Helen 18 Grosvenor Terrace, Bootham, York YO30 7AG Tel: 01904 621679 — MB BS Lond. 1973 (Guy's)

WRIGHT, Helen Gail 5 Chandos Terrace, Avington, Winchester SO21 1DD Email: helenwright@chandosterrace.freeserve.co.uk — MB ChB Manch. 1993; BSc (Med. Sci.) St. And. 1990; MRCGP 1999. GP Locum. Specialty: Gen. Pract. Socs: (Treas.) Basingstroke Sessional GPs Gp.

WRIGHT, Helen Mary Inzievar Surgery, 2 Kenmore Street, Aberfeldy PH15 2BL Tel: 01887 820366 Fax: 01887 829566 — MB ChB Aberd. 1976; DRCOG 1979.

WRIGHT, Helen Mary Bridgemill Farmhouse, Beal, Berwick-upon-Tweed TD15 2RN Tel: 01289 381300; P.O. Box 2887, Pertu, Western Australia WA 6001, Australia — MB ChB Glas. 1995; DCH Glas. 1996; MRCP Glas. 1998. Paediat. Regist. Princess Margt. Hosp. Childr. Perth. W. Australia. Specialty: Paediat. Prev: SHO (Paediat.) CrossHo. Hosp. Kilmarnock; Ho. Off. (Gen. Med.) Ayr Hosp.; SHO Roy. Hosp. For Sick Childr. Yorkhill, Glas.

WRIGHT, Helen Patricia Roborough Surgery, 1 Eastcote Close, Southway, Plymouth PL6 6PH Tel: 01752 776930 — BM Soton. 1989; DRCOG 1993; MRCGP 1994. Specialty: Gen. Pract.

WRIGHT, Helena Margaret Elizabeth 6 Starborough Cottages, Station Road, Dormansland, Lingfield RH7 6NL — MB ChB Leic. 1989.

WRIGHT, Mr Henry Beric (retired) Brudenell House, Quainton, Aylesbury HP22 4AW Tel: 01296 655250 Fax: 01296 655250 — MB BS Lond. 1942 (Univ. Coll. Hosp.) MRCS Eng. LRCP Lond. 1942; FRCS Eng. 1955; MFOM RCP Lond. 1978. Lect. Retirem. & Ageing Problems. Prev: Chairm. BUPA Med. Centre & Governor BUPA.

WRIGHT, Henry John (retired) Kekewich House, 1 View Road, London N6 4DL — MB BCh BAO NUI 1939 (Univ. Coll. Dub.) MRCGP. Prev: Gen. Practitioner Nuneaton Warks.

WRIGHT, Henry William Newton Port Surgery, Newton Port, Haddington EH41 3NF Tel: 01620 825051 Fax: 01620 824622 — MB ChB Ed. 1983 (Edinburgh) Dip. Obst Otago 1986; MRCGP 1988. Specialty: Gen. Pract.

WRIGHT, Hugh Edward Maida Vale Medical Centre, 40 Biddulph Mansions, Elgin Avenue, London W9 1HT Tel: 020 7286 6464 Fax: 020 7266 1017; 112 Hamilton Terrace, St John's Wood, London NW8 9UP Tel: 020 7289 6413 — MB BS Lond. 1984 (St Mary's London) CDAF Eng. 1997; MRCGP 1998; DGM RCP Lond. 1999; DRCOG 1999. GP Princip. Maida Vale Med. Centre Lond.; Clin. Med. Off. Parkside Health. Specialty: Gen. Pract.; Ment. Health; Otorhinolaryngol. Socs: Fell.Roy. Soc. of Med. Prev: Private GP Wright Private Med. Pract. Lond.; SHO O & G Crawley Hosp. Sussex; SHO OtoLaryngol. Centr. Middlx. Hosp. Lond.

WRIGHT, Ian Alec 34 Beacon Square, Emsworth PO10 7HU — MB BS Lond. 1976; DRCOG 1979; MRCGP 1980.

WRIGHT, Ian Conrad Kings House, 14 New Road, Romsey SO51 7LN Fax: 01794 517875 — MB ChB Bristol 1992. Specialty: Anaesth.

WRIGHT, Ian Cosmo Institute of Psychiatry, De Crespigny Park, Denmark Hill, London SE5 8AF Tel: 020 7919 3535 — MB BChir Camb. 1990; MA Camb. 1991, MB BChir 1990; MRCP (UK) 1992; MRCPsych 1995; MSc Lond. 1995. Wellcome Clin. Train. Fell. Inst. of Psychiat.; Hon. Sen. Regist. Maudsley Hosp. Specialty: Gen. Psychiat. Prev: Lect. Inst. of Psychiat.; Regist. (Psychiat.) Maudsley Hosp.; SHO (Neurol.) Radcliffe Infirm. Oxf.

WRIGHT, Ian Gavin Department of Anaesthetics, Harefield Hospital, Harefield, Uxbridge UB9 6JH Tel: 0189 582 3737 — MB ChB Rhodesia 1977; LRCP LRCS Ed. LRCPS Glas. 1977; FFA SA 1983. Cons. (Anaesth.) Harefield Hosp. Specialty: Anaesth. Prev: Cons. (Anaesth.) Groote Schuur Hosp. & Red Cross Childr. Hosp. Cape Town.

WRIGHT, Mr Ian Peter 2 painters Place, Shrewsbury SY3 5PT Email: ipwright@globalnet.co.uk — MB ChB Manch. 1994; BSc (Immunol. & Oncol.) Manch. 1991; FRCS Eng. 1998. Specialist Regist. Trauma Orthop. Oswestry Rotat. Specialty: Trauma & Orthop. Surg. Socs: BOA. Prev: SHO (Surg.) Whiston Hosp. Merseyside; Ho. Off. Wythenshawe Hospial Manch.; SHO Orthop.Alder Hey Childr.s Hosp.

WRIGHT, Jacqueline Fiona Triscombe, Roslyn Road, Wellington TF1 3AX — MB ChB Manch. 1989; DCH RCP Lond. 1992; MRCGP 1993; DRCOG 1993; DFFP 2002. GP Lawley Medical Centre, Telford. Specialty: Gen. Pract.; Rheumatol. Prev: Clin. Asst. (Rheum.) P.s Roy. Hosp.; Retainee in Gen. Pract., Sutton Hill Surg.

WRIGHT, James Alexander Morrison (retired) Haslemere House, Golf Links Road, Yelverton PL20 6BN Tel: 01822 852323 — MB BCh BAO NUI 1957; FRCP Lond. 1982, M 1969.

WRIGHT, James Courtney (retired) 22 Briercliffe Road, Stoke Bishop, Bristol BS9 2DB Tel: 0117 968 6142 — LRCP LRCS Ed. 1949 (Glas.) LRCP LRCS Ed. LRFPS Glas. 1949.

WRIGHT, James Duncan (retired) c/o St Anne's Surgery, 161 Station Road, Herne Bay CT6 5NF Tel: 01227 361114; 5 Dence Park, Herne Bay CT6 6BG Tel: 01227 372529 — MB ChB Liverp. 1952; MRCS Eng. LRCP Lond. 1952.

WRIGHT, James Michael 246 Springfield Road, Chelmsford CM2 6BS — MB BS Lond. 1998.

WRIGHT, Jane Catherine 114 Wickham Avenue, Cheam, Sutton SM3 8EA — MB ChB Bristol 1988. SHO (Radiother. & Oncol.) Roy. Hosp. Wolverhampton. Specialty: Palliat. Med.

WRIGHT, Jane Elizabeth Mary Moreton Health Clinic, 8-10 Chadwick Street, Wirral CH46 7XA Tel: 0151 677 1207 Fax: 0151 604 0372 — MB ChB Liverp. 1983; DRCOG 1987.

WRIGHT, Janet Barbara Bradford Royal Infirmary, Maternity Unit, Duckworth Lane, Bradford BD9 6RJ Tel: 01274 542200 — MB BS Lond. 1991 (St Geo.) BSc Lond. 1988; MRCOG 1997. Cons. (O & G) Bradford Roy. Infirm. Specialty: Obst. & Gyn.

WRIGHT, Janet Ruth Fernville Surgery, Midland Road, Hemel Hempstead HP2 5BL Tel: 01442 213919 — MB BS Lond. 1980 (King's Coll. Hosp.) MRCGP 1984; DRCOG 1985. GP Hemel Hempstead. Specialty: Gen. Pract. Prev: GP Cirencester; Volunteer Community Health Project South. India; Regist. (Terminal Care) St. Joseph's Hospice Lond.

WRIGHT, Janine Louisa Basement Flat, 79 Barnsbury Street, Islington, London N1 1EJ Email: janine.wright@virgin.net — MB BS

Lond. 1990; MRCP (UK) 1995. Regist. (Med. & Gastroenterol.) Middlx. Hosp. Specialty: Gastroenterol.; Gen. Med. Socs: BMA. Prev: SpR Med. & Gastroenterol., King Geo. Hosp.; Spr Med. & Gastroenterol., Middlx. Hosp.

WRIGHT, Jayne Margaret 45 Donaghaguy Road, Warrenpoint, Newry BT34 3PR — MB BCh BAO Belf. 1981; FFA RCSI 1985. Cons. Anaesth. Daisy Hill Hosp. Newry. Specialty: Anaesth.

WRIGHT, Jean Margaret (retired) 11 Elms Avenue, Lytham St Annes FY8 5PW Tel: 01253 735673 — MB ChB Liverp. 1956; DObst RCOG 1960. Prev: SCMO Blackpool Child Developm. Centre.

WRIGHT, Jeremy Torquil St. Peter's Hospital, Guildford Road, Chertsey KT16 0PZ Tel: 01932 872000 Fax: 01483 875462; SIGIRI, College Lane, Woking GU22 0EW Tel: 01483 715699 Fax: 01483 724833 Email: jwrighta@cix.compulink.co.uk — MB BS Lond. 1971 (Univ. Coll. Hosp.) MRCS Eng. LRCP Lond. 1971; FRCOG 1991, M 1977; MBA 1996. Cons. O & G St. Peter's Hosp. Chertsey; Comm. Mem. BSGE. Specialty: Obst. & Gyn. Prev: Sen. Regist. (O & G) W. Middlx. Univ. Hosp. & Char. Cross Hosp. Lond.; Regist. (O & G) Whipps Cross Hosp. Lond.; Resid. Med. Off. Qu. Charlotte's Matern. Hosp. Lond.

WRIGHT, Joan Mary Birmingham University Medical Practice, Elms Road, Edgbaston, Birmingham B15 2SE Tel: 0121 414 5111; Cowsden Croft, Upton Snodsbury, Worcester WR7 4NX Tel: 01905 60515 — MRCS Eng. LRCP Lond. 1955 (Birm.) GP Birm. Univ. Health Centre; Med. Off. Family Plann. Assn. Clinics. Prev: Ho. Phys. & Ho. Surg. Little Bromwich Hosp.; Med. Off. Blood Transfus. Serv. Birm.

WRIGHT, Joan Patricia (retired) The Castle, Castle Edge, New Mills, High Peak SK22 4QF Tel: 01663 742364 — MB ChB Manch. 1952; DCH Eng. 1954; FRCP Ed. 1985, M 1962. Prev: Cons. Paediat. Cardiol. Manch. Roy. Infirm. & St. Mary's Hosp. Manch.

WRIGHT, Joanna Mary St Matthews Medical Centre, Prince Phillip House, Malabar Road, Leicester LE1 2NZ Tel: 0116 295 4700 — MB ChB Leic. 1991; MRCGP; DFFP 1997. GP Locum Non-Princip. Specialty: Gen. Pract.

WRIGHT, John (retired) The Garth, 10 Tynedale Terrace, Benton, Newcastle upon Tyne NE12 8AY — MB BS Durh. 1955. Prev: GP Walker Medical Group, Newcastle-Upon-Tyne.

WRIGHT, John Alan West Wirral Group Practice, Winterdyne, Rocky Lane, Heswall, Wirral CH60 0BY Tel: 0151 342 2557 Fax: 0151 342 9384 — (Liverp.) MB ChB Liverp. 1965; DTM & H Liverp. 1966; DObst RCOG 1967. Prev: Ho. Surg. (O & G) Chester City Hosp.; Ho. Phys. (Trop. Dis.), Ho. Phys. & Ho. Surg. Sefton Gen. Hosp.

WRIGHT, John Barry Debenham Limetrees Child & Family Unit, 31 Shipton Road, York YO30 6RF Tel: 01904 652908 Fax: 01904 632893 — MB BS Lond. 1985 (St. Bartholomew's Hospital) DCH RCP Lond. 1989; MRCGP 1989; MRCPsych 1991; MMedSc Leeds 1994; MD Lond. 2000. Cons. Child & Family Psychiat. York. Specialty: Child & Adolesc. Psychiat. Socs: York Med. Soc. Prev: Sen. Regist. Rotat. (Child Psychiat.) Leeds.

WRIGHT, John Brennan 202 Camberwell Grove, London SE5 8RJ Tel: 020 7733 0104 Fax: 020 7733 0104; 202 Camberwell Grove, London SE5 8RJ Tel: 020 7733 0104 Fax: 020 7733 0104 — LAH Dub. 1959.

WRIGHT, John Brian (retired) 8 Windsor Road, Chorley PR7 1LN Tel: 01257 265419 Email: jondoc.wright@vlrgin.net — MB ChB Manch. 1963. Prev: Ho. Off. Manch. Roy. Infirm., Leigh Infirm. & Bishop Auckland Gen. Hosp.

WRIGHT, John David (retired) 26 Highgate Avenue, Fulwood, Preston PR2 8LL — MB ChB Manch. 1963; FRCOG 1981, M 1968, DObst. 1965; MSc Manch. 1972. Prev: Clin. Tutor (Obst.) Univ. Manch.

WRIGHT, John Denham, MBE (retired) 21 Waterdale, Compton, Wolverhampton WV3 9DY Tel: 01902 422564 Fax: 01902 422564 — MB BS Lond. 1962; DCH Eng. 1964; DPH Lond. 1966; FFPHM RCP (UK) 1983, M 1972. Prev: Cons. Pub. Health Med. Wolverhampton HA.

WRIGHT, Mr John Edward 44 Wimpole Street, London W1 7DG Tel: 020 7580 1251 — MD Liverp. 1962; MB ChB 1956; DO Eng. 1965; FRCS Eng. 1967. Cons. Ophth. Surg. Moorfields Eye Hosp. City Rd. Lond.; Cons. Ophth. Surg. Roy. Nat. Throat Nose & Ear Hosp. Lond. Specialty: Ophth. Socs: Fell. Roy. Soc. Med.; Amer. Acad. Ophth. Prev: Cons. Ophth. Surg. St. Mary's Hosp. Lond.; Res. Surg. Off. Moorfields Eye Hosp. City Rd. Br. Lond.; Capt. RAMC.

WRIGHT, John Francis The Health Centre, Melbourn Street, Royston SG8 7BS Tel: 01763 242981 Fax: 01763 249197 — MB BS Lond. 1984 (Churchill Camb. & St.Thos.) MA Camb. 1985, BA 1981; MRCGP 1991; Dip. Occupat. Med. 1997; DFFP 1998.

WRIGHT, John Geoffrey Charles Heart Unit, Birmingham Children's Hospital, Steelhouse Lane, Birmingham B4 6NH Tel: 0121 333 9443 Fax: 0121 333 9441 — MB BChir Camb. 1975; MA Camb. 1972; MRCP (UK) 1977; FRCP Lond. 1994; FRCPCH 1996. Cons. Paediat. Cardiol. Childr. Hosp. Birm.; Hon. Sen. Lect. Univ. Birm.; Cons. Cardiol. (Fetal Med.) Univ. Birm. Specialty: Cardiol. Prev: Sen. Regist. (Paediat. Cardiol.) Roy. Liverp. Childr. Hosp.; Resid. Med. Off. Nat. Heart Hosp. Lond.

WRIGHT, John Henry (retired) 5 Haywards Close, The Heath, Glossop SK13 7AZ — MB ChB Liverp. 1957; FFA RCS Eng. 1963. Cons. Anaesth. Withington & The Christie Hosp.

WRIGHT, Mr John James 55 Robyns Way, Sevenoaks TN13 3ED — MB BS Lond. 1966; FRCS Eng. 1975. Prev: Regist. (Neurosurg.) Roy. P. Alfred Hosp., Sydney; SHO (Gen. Surg.) Redhill Gen. Hosp.; Ho. Phys. Norwich Hosp.

WRIGHT, Mr John Lawson William, RD 152 Harley Street, London W1G 7LH Tel: 020 7935 0444 Fax: 020 7224 2574; Winsland Mews House, Branstone Rd, Richmond TW9 3LB Tel: 020 8948 3968 Fax: 020 8940 0708 — MB ChB Bristol 1964; DObst RCOG 1966; FRCS Ed. 1968; FRCS Eng. (Orl.) 1971; MBA Open 1992. Hon. Cons. Surg. Otolaryngol. St. Mary's Hosp. Lond.; Civil. Cons. Otolaryngol. RN; Cons. Otolaryngol. to Gibraltar Govt. Specialty: Otolaryngol. Prev: 1st Asst. (Otolaryngol.) Radcliffe Infirm. Oxf.; Clin. & Research Fell. Harvard Med. Sch.

WRIGHT, John Patrick — (Nat. Univ. Irel. RCSI) MB BCh BAO NUI 1986; LRCPSI 1986; MRCPsych 1993; MD NUI 1995. Head Clin. Neurosci.,Eli Lilly Ltd. Europe; Sen. Lect. City & Hackney Community Serv. NHS Trust (Oct. 1997 to date); Sen. Lect. Inst. Psychiat. Univ. Lond. (April 1997 to 2000). Specialty: Gen. Psychiat.; Pharmaceutical Medicine; Genetics. Socs: Fell. Roy. Soc. Med.; Brit. Assn. Psychopharmacol.; World Psychiat. Assoc. Immunol. in Psychiat. (Comm. Founder).

WRIGHT, John Paul 38 Streatham Common N., London SW16 3HR — MB ChB Leeds 1993.

WRIGHT, John Paul Bradford Royal Infirmary, Duckworth Lane, Bradford BD9 6RJ; 6 Esholt Avenue, Guiseley, Leeds LS20 8AX — MB ChB Leeds 1987; BSc (Hons.) Leeds 1987; MRCP (UK) 1990; MPH Leeds 1994; MFPHM RCP (UK) 1996. Cons. Clin. Epidemiol. Bradford Roy. Infirm.; Edr. Brit. Jl. of Clin. Governance. Specialty: Pub. Health Med. Prev: Sen. Regist. (Pub. Health Med.) York; Med. Off. Good Shepherd Hosp., Swaziland.

WRIGHT, John Rodney 59 Deighton Lane, Batley WF17 7EU — MB ChB Leeds 1965.

WRIGHT, John Stephen (retired) 11 Elms Avenue, Lytham St Annes FY8 5PW — MD Liverp. 1972; MB ChB 1958; DObst RCOG 1963; FRCP Lond. 1979, M 1966. Prev: Cons. Cardiol. Vict. Hosp. Blackpool.

WRIGHT, John Steven Eastville Health Centre, East Park, Bristol BS5 6YA Tel: 0117 951 1261 Fax: 0117 935 5056 — MB ChB Bristol 1987; BSc Sheff. 1971; MB ChB (Hons.) Bristol 1987; DRCOG 1991. Specialty: Gen. Med.

WRIGHT, John Trevillian (retired) Silverthorn, Blocks Corner, Hatfield Heath, Bishop's Stortford CM22 7AX Tel: 01279 730366 — BM BCh Oxf. 1945 (Oxf. & Lond. Hosp.) FRCP Lond. 1964, M 1947; DM Oxf. 1953. Prev: Cons. Phys. (Gen. Med. & Gastroenterol.) Lond. Hosp.

WRIGHT, John Watson Cowdenbeath Medical Practice, 173 Stenhouse Street, Cowdenbeath KY4 9DH Tel: 01383 518500 Fax: 01383 518509 — MB ChB St Andrews 1970; MB ChB St And. 1970. GP Cowdenbeath, Fife.

WRIGHT, John William Royal Surrey County Hospital, Guildford GU2 7XX Email: john.wright@surrey.ac.uk; 8 Critchmere Vale, Haslemere GU27 1PS Tel: 01428 642142 — MB BS Lond. 1967 (Guy's) FRCP; MRCS Eng. LRCP Lond. 1967; MRCP (U.K.) 1971; MSc (Clin. Biochem.) Surrey 1974; MRCPath 1976. Cons. (Clin. Biochem.) Roy. Surrey Co. Hosp., Guildford; Reader in Metab. Med., Univ. of Surrey, Guildford GU2 7XH. Specialty: Biochem.; Diabetes; Endocrinol. Socs: Assn. of Clin. Biochem.s; Diabetes UK; Brit.

Hyperlipidaemia Assn. (Hon. Treas.). Prev: Regist. (Med.) St. Luke's Hosp. Guildford; Resid. (Med.) Penna. Hosp. Philadelphia, U.S.A.; Ho. Surg. Guy's Hosp. Lond.

WRIGHT, Jonathan Graham 17 Battersby Close, Yarm TS15 9RX — MB BS Newc. 1983; DRCOG 1986.

WRIGHT, Jonathan Mark — MB ChB Birm. 1982; DCH RCP Lond. 1987; DRCOG 1988; MRCGP 1988; MPhil 2000. Gen. Practitioner. Specialty: Gen. Pract.

WRIGHT, Judith Ann Reading Room Cottage, Shilton, Oxford — BM BCh Oxf. 1972.

WRIGHT, Judith Anne Cropredy Surgery, Claydon Road, Cropredy, Banbury OX17 1FB Tel: 01295 758372 Fax: 01295 750435; Magpies, Lower Farm Lane, Mollington, Banbury OX17 1BJ Tel: 01295 750724 — MB ChB Leic. 1982; DRCOG 1987.

WRIGHT, Judith Anne Gillian 30 Smith Street, London SW3 4EP Tel: 020 7352 6860 — MB BS Lond. 1958 (Guy's) MRCS Eng. LRCP Lond. 1958. Clin. Med. Off. Parkside. Specialty: Community Child Health. Socs: BMA. Prev: Clin. Med. Off. Kensington, Chelsea & Westm. AHA; Ho. Phys. Sheff. Roy. Infirm.; Ho. Surg. Wharnecliffe Hosp. Sheff.

WRIGHT, Judith Clare 35 Moor Road, Prudhoe NE42 5LL — MB ChB Leic. 1993; FRCA Lond. 1997. Specialist Regist. (Anaesth.) Glas. Roy. Infirm. Specialty: Anaesth.

WRIGHT, Judith Margaret Saddleworth Medical Practice, The Clinic, Smithy Lane, Oldham OL3 6AH Tel: 01457 872228 Fax: 01457 876520 — MB ChB Manch. 1975; MRCGP 1987. GP Uppermill.

WRIGHT, Julia Vanessa Cross Plain Surgery, 84 Bulford Road, Durrington, Salisbury SP4 8DH — BM Soton. 1991; MRCGP 1996; DFFP 1996. Partner in Gen. Pratice. Specialty: Gen. Pract.

WRIGHT, Julian Francis Hawthorn Medical Centre, May Close, Swindon SN2 1UU; Beechcroft, Common Platt, Lydiard Millicent, Swindon SN5 5LB — MB ChB Manch. 1972; DObst RCOG 1974; LF Hom 1997; MRCGP 2003. Specialty: Gen. Pract. Prev: SHO Cheltenham Childr. Hosp.; Ho. Phys. Univ. Hosp. S. Manch.; Ho. Surg. Manch. Roy. Infirm.

WRIGHT, Julian Robert 148 Weaste Lane, Salford M5 2JJ — MB BS Lond. 1994; BSc (Hons.) Lond. 1991; MRCP 1998. Locum. Reg. Nephrol. Gen. Med.Hope Hosp. Salford. Specialty: Nephrol.; Gen. Med. Socs: MDU & BMA; RCP. Prev: Ho. Off. (Renal & Gen. Med.) Withington Hosp. Manch.; Ho. Off. (Surg.) Barnet Gen. Hosp. Lond.; SHO Rotat. (Gen. Med.) N. Staffs. Hosps. Trust Stoke-on-Trent.

WRIGHT, Juliet Elizabeth — MB BS Lond. 1994 (UMDS Guy's & St. Thos. Hosp.) Specialty: Gen. Med.

WRIGHT, Justine Anne Mona Cottage, Hughes Lane, Harvington, Evesham WR11 5NH Tel: 01386 870324 — MB ChB Leic. 1993. Regist. (Anaesth.) Waikato Hosp. Hamilton NZ. Specialty: Anaesth. Prev: SHO (Anaesth.) Harrogate Dist. Hosp.; SHO (Anaesth.) Waikato Hosp. Hamilton, NZ.

WRIGHT, Kavin John Cricketfield Surgery, Cricketfield Road, Newton Abbot TQ12 2AS Tel: 01626 208020 Fax: 01626 333356 — MB BS Lond. 1970 (St. Geo.) DRCOG 1977; DCH Eng. 1977; MRCGP 1978.

WRIGHT, Kelso Cooper NHS Argyle & Hospital, 29B Esplanade, Greenock PA16 7RU Tel: 01475 725112 — LRCP LRCS Ed. LRFPS Glas. 1960. Prev: Princip. GP Port Glas. 1965-1997; NHS Argyll & Clyde Hosp. Board Supplementary Med. List from May 2003.

WRIGHT, Kelvin Donald A&E Dept, Wexham park Hospital, Wexham St., Slough SL2 4HL Tel: 01753 634022; Wycombe General Hospital, Queen Alexandra Road, High Wycombe HP11 2TT Tel: 01494 526161 — MB BS Lond. 1992 (King's Coll. Lond.) FRCS Eng. 1997; Dip. IMC RCS Ed. 1998. Specialist Regist. (A & E) Wexham Pk. Hosps.lough; St. John Ambul. Brig. Divisional Surg. St. Pancras Div.; Trauma Instruc. Two Shires Ambul. NHS Trust; Immediate Care Doctor-Berks. Ambul. Specialty: Accid. & Emerg. Socs: Brit. Assn. Immed. Care Schemes. Prev: SHO (Intens. Therap.) Char. Cross Hosp. Lond.; SHO (Surg.) Roy. Lond. Hosp.; SHO (Orthop.) Homerton Hosp. Lond.

WRIGHT, Kenneth James Thomas 6 Queen Street, Hadleigh, Ipswich IP7 5DZ Tel: 01473 828976 Fax: 01473 829059 Email: kenwright@doctors.org.uk — BM BCh Oxf. 1961 (Oxf. & Middlx.) BA (Animal Physiol., 1st cl. Hons.) Oxf. 1959; MPhil (Psychiat.) Lond. 1969; MRCPsych 1973. Specialty: Psychother.; Gen. Psychiat. Socs: Assoc. Mem. Brit. Psychoanalyt. Soc. Prev: Cons. Psychiat. Severalls Hosp. Colchester; Sen. Lect. & Hon. Cons. Psychother. Acad. Dept. Psychiat. Middlx. Hosp. Lond.; Sen. Regist. (Adult Psychiat.) Tavistock Clin. Lond.

WRIGHT, Mr Kenneth Urquhart University Hospital of North Durham, North Road, Durham DH1 5TW Tel: 0191 333 2333; 3 Park View, Oakenshaw, Crook DL15 0ST — MB ChB Manch. 1984 (Univ. Manch.) BSc St. And. 1981; FRCS Ed. 1990; FRCS (Orth.) 1996. Cons. Orthop. Surg. Dryburn Hosp. Durh. Specialty: Orthop. Prev: Sen. Regist. & Regist. (Orthop.) North. Region; PeriFellowsh. Regist. Wolverhampton.

WRIGHT, Lesley Anne Somerville Medical Practice, 4 Somerville, Poulton Road, Wallasey CH44 9ED Tel: 0151 638 9333 Fax: 0151 637 0291 — MB ChB Manch. 1979.

WRIGHT, Linda Toryglen Medical Centre, 20 GlenmoreAvenue, Toryglen, Glasgow G42 0EH — MB ChB Glas. 1992. GP Toryglen. Specialty: Gen. Pract.

WRIGHT, Linda The Consulting Rooms, 21 Neilston Road, Paisley PA2 6LW; Strathmore, 24 Donaldfield Road, Bridge of Weir PA11 3JG — MB ChB Glas. 1984 (Glasgow) DCH RCPS Glas. 1987; DRCOG 1987; MRCGP 1988. Prev: GP Glas. N. VTS; Ho. Phys. Hairmyres Hosp. E. Kilbride; Ho. Surg. Stobhill Gen. Hosp. Glas.

WRIGHT, Lionel Percy John (retired) Drumkeeran, 333 Ewell Road, Surbiton KT6 7BX Tel: 020 8399 1192 — (Guy's) MRCS Eng. LRCP Lond. 1942; MB BS Lond. 1948; Foundat. MRCGP 1953. Prev: SHO (Surg.) St. John's Hosp. Lewisham.

WRIGHT, Lucille Patricia BP PLC, Breakspear Park, Breakspear Way, Hemel Hempstead HP2 4UL Tel: 01442 225097 Fax: 01442 223878 Email: wrightlp@bp.com — BM BS Nottm. 1984 (Nottingham) BMedSci Nottm. 1982; MFOM RCP Lond. 1994, AFOM 1992. Regional Med. Director, BP plc. Specialty: Occupat. Health. Prev: Sen. Employm. Med. Adviser Health & Safety Exec. Luton.; Employm. Med. Adviser Health & Safety Exec. Luton.

WRIGHT, Lynn Mary 6 Dunning Drive, Westwood, Cumbernauld, Glasgow G68 0FN Tel: 01236 728649 — MB ChB Manch. 1996. Specialty: Obst. & Gyn.

WRIGHT, Lynne Marie Pencester Surgery, 10/12 Pencester Road, Dover CT16 1BW Tel: 01304 240553; Cherry Tree Cottage, West Hougham, Dover CT15 7AT — MB ChB Liverp. 1986; BSc Liverp. 1981, MB ChB 1986; DRCOG 1990.

WRIGHT, Malcolm (retired) 87 Belfield Road, Epsom KT19 9TF Tel: 020 8394 2728 — MB ChB Leeds 1951; MRCS Eng. LRCP Lond. 1951; DPM Eng. 1961; FRCPsych 1987, M 1971. Prev: Cons. Psychiat. Long Gr. Hosp. Epsom & Roy. Hosp. Richmond.

WRIGHT, Malcolm Harold George Cedar House Surgery, 14 Huntingdon Street, St. Neots, Huntingdon PE19 1BQ Tel: 01480 406677 Fax: 01480 475167; Tudor House, Eynesbury, St. Neots, Huntingdon PE19 2TA — MB ChB Liverp. 1969; MRCGP 1975. GP Cedar Ho. Surg.; Course Organiser VTS Hinchin Brooke Hosp. Socs: Brit. Med. & Dent. Hypn. Soc. Prev: Ho. Phys. & Ho. Surg. Roy. South. Hosp. Liverp.; SHO (O & G) & SHO Renal Unit Sefton Gen. Hosp. Liverp.

WRIGHT, Mr Malcolm Oliver (retired) 72 Cammo Grove, Barnton, Edinburgh EH4 8HA Tel: 0131 339 7005 — MB ChB Manch. 1966; FRCS Ed. 1987; FDS RCS Ed. 1993. Prev: Ho. Phys. & Ho. Surg. Manch. Roy. Infirm.

WRIGHT, Maree 11 Durham Close, Paignton TQ3 2QN Tel: 01803 663156 — BM BS Nottm. 1989; FRCA 1996. Specialty: Anaesth.

WRIGHT, Margaret Elizabeth Abermed Industrial Doctors Ltd, 56 Carden Place, Aberdeen AB10 1UP Tel: 01224 624314 Fax: 01224 626095 Email: dr.wright@industrialdoctors.co.uk — MB ChB Glas. 1980 (Univ. Glas.) MFOM RCP Lond. 1996, AFOM 1993; AFOM 1993; MSc Aberd. 1994; MSc Aberd. 1994; MFOM 1996; FFOM RCP Lond. 2002. Sen. Cons. Occupatonal Phys. Abermed Indust. Doctors Ltd. Aberd.; Clin. Lect. (Environm. & Occupat. Med.) Univ. Aberd.; hon Cons. in Ocupational Med. Grampian Univ., Aberd. Specialty: Occupat. Health. Socs: Soc. Occupat. Med.; Inst. Occupat. Safety & Health. Prev: Occupat. Phys. Grampian Healthcare NHS Trust.

WRIGHT, Margaret Mary James Paget Hospital, Gorleston, Great Yarmouth NR31 6LA Tel: 01493 600611 Fax: 01493 452753 Email: maggie.wright@jpaget.nhs.uk; 127 Corton Road, Lowestoft NR32 4PR Tel: 01502 561834 Fax: 01493 432753 Email: maggie.wright@jpaget.nhs.uk — MB ChB Dundee 1978; BSc

(Hons.) Dund 1973, MB ChB 1978; FFA RCS Eng. 1982. Cons. Anaesth. Gt. Yarmouth & Waveney HA. Specialty: Anaesth.; Intens. Care. Prev: Hon. Cons. (Anaesth.) Jas. Paget Hosp. Gorleston Gt. Yarmouth; Sen. Regist. (Anaesth.) Hammersmith Hosp. Lond.; Regist. (Anaesth.) Ninewells Hosp. Dundee.

WRIGHT, Marie Helen Isobel (retired) 10 Rutland Terrace, Stamford PE9 2QD Tel: 01780 755718 — MB ChB Glas. 1942 (Univ. Glas.) Prev: Clin. Asst. PeterBoro. Dist. Hosp.

WRIGHT, Marjorie Frances Lind (retired) The Firs, Reynoldston, Swansea SA3 1BR Tel: 01792 390188 — MB ChB St. And. 1962; DObst RCOG 1964; DA Eng. 1965. Prev: Med. Advis. Dept. Transport.

WRIGHT, Mark 44 Sleigh Road, Sturry, Canterbury CT2 0HT; Flat 1, 15 Milton Avenue, Highgate, London N6 5QF Tel: 020 8348 6786 Email: mwright433@aol.com — MB BS Lond. 1994 (St Bart.) BSc 1991; MRCP 1997. Specialist Regist. (Gastroenterol.). Specialty: Gastroenterol.

WRIGHT, Mark John 22 Brentford Road, Birmingham B14 4DQ — MB ChB Sheff. 1991; MRCP (UK) 1995. Regist. (Renal Med.) Leeds Gen. Infirm. Specialty: Nephrol. Prev: Regist. (Renal Med.) Hull Roy. Infirm.

WRIGHT, Mr Mark Philip James Department of Urology, Bristol Royal Infirmary, Bristol BS2 8HU Tel: 0117 928 4225 Fax: 0117 928 4225 Email: mpjwright@bristolurology.com — MB BS Lond. 1990 (St. Thos. Hosp. Lond.) FRCS Eng. 1994; MD Bristol 2001; FRCS 2001. Cons. Urological Surg. Specialty: Urol. Special Interest: Laparoscopic Urooncology. Socs: Sen. Urol. Regist. Gp.; Assoc. Mem. BAUS; Assn. Surg. Train.

WRIGHT, Mr Mark Renouf Princess Alexandra Eye Pactice, Chalmers Street, Edinburgh EH3 Fax: 0131 536 1674; 15 John Street, Edinburgh EH15 2EB Tel: 0131 669 1760/01865 557693 — MB ChB Aberd. 1985; FRCS Ed. 1993. Cons. Ophth. PAEP & St John's Hosp., Livingston. Specialty: Ophth.

WRIGHT, Martin Portugal Place Health Centre, Portugal Place, Wallsend NE28 6RZ Tel: 0191 262 5252 Fax: 0191 262 5252 — BM BS Nottm. 1986; BMedSci 1983; MRCGP 1991. GP Wallsend Tyne & Wear Trainee GP N.d. VTS.

WRIGHT, Martin Wilden (retired) Downsview, 59 High St., Chipstead, Sevenoaks TN13 2RW — MB ChB Manch. 1963; DObst RCOG 1965; DPH Eng. 1966. Prev: Sen. Med. Off.and SCMO and Sen. Med. Off. (Occupat. Health) E. Surrey HAFPC Oxted Health Centre Surrey.

WRIGHT, Mary Elizabeth Clark (retired) Burcot House, Blunsdon St Andrew, Swindon SN25 2DY Tel: 01793 721487 — MB ChB St. And. 1953.

WRIGHT, Mary Frances (retired) Flat 58 Watersedge Court, 1 Wharfside Close, Erith DA8 1QW — M.B., B.S. Lond. 1943.

WRIGHT, Maureen Edith St Johns Lane Health Centre, St. Johns Lane, Bristol BS3 5AS Tel: 0117 966 7681 Fax: 0117 977 9676; 40 Somerset Road, Knowle, Bristol BS4 2HU Tel: 0117 971 6940 — BM BCh Oxf. 1974; Cert. Family Plann. JCC 1976. Prev: Community Med. Off. (Family Plann.) Southmead HA.; Clin. Asst. (Genitourin. Med.) Bristol Roy. Infirm.; Princip. GP Lambeth, Southwark & Lewisham FPC.

WRIGHT, Mea Wallace (retired) The Butts, High Bank, Porlock, Minehead TA24 8NS Tel: 01643 862975 — MB BCh BAO Belf. 1950; DObst RCOG 1953. Prev: GP Nailsea.

WRIGHT, Michael George 10 Harley Street, London W1G 9PF Tel: 020 7467 8345 Fax: 020 7467 8312; 12 Den Close, Beckenham BR3 6RP Tel: 020 8658 3201 Fax: 020 8658 3201 — (Lond. Hosp.) MB BS Lond. 1963; MRCS Eng. LRCP Lond. 1963; MRCP (UK) 1973; FRCP Lond. 1994. Cons. Rheum. & Rehabil. Newham Health Dist. & Roy. Lond. Hosp.; Cons. Rheum. & Rehabil. Nat. Dock Labour Bd. Specialty: Rehabil. Med.; Rheumatol. Socs: Brit. Assn. Rheum. & Rehabil.; BMA; BIMM. Prev: Sen. Regist. King's Coll. Hosp. Lond.; Resid. Med. Off. Westm. Hosp. Lond.; Ho. Surg. Lond. Hosp.

WRIGHT, Michael James Institute of Human Genetics, International Centre for Life, Central Parkway, Newcastle upon Tyne NE1 3BZ — MB ChB Ed. 1987; MRCP (UK) 1990; MSc Univ. Newc. 1994. Cons. in Clin. Genetics Newc. upon Tyne NHS Trust. Specialty: Genetics. Prev: Clin. Fell. Centre for Med. Genetics Johns Hopkins Hosp. Baltimore, USA; Research Regist. (Human Genetics) Newc.

WRIGHT, Michael John Countesthorpe Health Centre, Central Street, Countesthorpe, Leicester LE8 5QJ Tel: 0116 277 6336; 15 Cosby Road, Countesthorpe, Leicester LE8 5PD — MB BS Lond. 1969 (Char. Cross) MRCS Eng. LRCP Lond. 1969; DObst RCOG 1971; DA Eng. 1974.

WRIGHT, Michael John Croft House Surgery, Croft House, 1145 Manchester Road, Slaithwaite, Huddersfield HD7 5JY Tel: 01484 842652 Fax: 01484 348223; Stoneycroft, 21 Rumbold Road, Edgerton, Huddersfield HD3 3DB Tel: 01484 532168 — MB BChir Camb. 1973 (Camb. & Middlx. Hosp.) MA Camb. 1973; DObst RCOG 1974. GP. Specialty: Gen. Pract. Socs: Hudds. Med. Soc.; BMA (Treas. Huddersfield Div.). Prev: Clin. Asst. (Dermat.) Huddersfield Roy. Infirm.; Trainee GP Huddersfield VTS; Ho. Phys. & Ho. Surg. Bedford Gen. Hosp.

WRIGHT, Michael Joseph (retired) 22 Doves Yard, London N1 0HQ — MB BCh BAO Belf. 1955 (Queens Univ. Belfast) DObst RCOG 1959; DA Eng. 1960; MRCGP 1971. Prev: Locum GP.

WRIGHT, Michelle 1 Barns Road, Budleigh Salterton EX9 6HJ — MB BS Lond. 1989; DA (UK) 1992.

WRIGHT, Nathanael Marcus James University of Leeds, Centre for Research in Primary Care, Clarendon Way, Leeds LS2 9NL — MB ChB Leeds 1989.

WRIGHT, Nathaniel James Selborne Flat 25, Ravenswood, 1 Spath Road, Manchester M20 2GA — MB ChB Manch. 1995.

WRIGHT, Neil John Mayfield Surgery, 54 Trentham Road, Longton, Stoke-on-Trent ST3 4DW Tel: 01782 599147 — MB ChB Bristol 1984; Cert. Family Plann. JCC 1987; DRCOG 1987. Specialty: Gen. Pract. Prev: Trainee GP Stockport; SHO (Elderly Med.) Bolton Gen. Hosp.; SHO (O & G & A & E) Wythenshawe Hosp. Manch.

WRIGHT, Neil Peter — MB BChir Camb. 1989; MRCP (UK) 1992. Cons. Paediat. Endocmology and Diabetes Sheff. Childrens Hosp. Specialty: Paediat.

WRIGHT, Neil Richard 53 Dudsbury Road, West Parley, Wimborne — MB ChB Leic. 1987; BSc Leic. 1984, MB ChB 1987.

WRIGHT, Neville Bryce X-Ray Department, Royal Liverpool Children's NHS Trust, Alder Hey, Eaton Rd, Liverpool Ll2 2AP — MB ChB Liverp. 1986; DMRD Liverp. 1991; FRCR 1992. Cons. Paediat. Radiol. Liverp. Childr. Hosp. Specialty: Radiol. Socs: Fell. Roy. Coll. Radiol.; BMA; Brit. Soc. of Paediatric Radiol. Prev: Sen. Regist. (Radiol.) North. Region; Research Fell. (Paediat. Radiol.) Univ. Liverp.; Regist. (Radiol.) Mersey Region.

WRIGHT, Nicholas 9 Burnett Close, Winchester SO22 5JQ Tel: 01962 866626 Fax: 01962 866626 — (St. Thos.) MB BChir Camb. 1957; DPM Eng. 1959; FRCP Lond. 1987, M 1961; FRCPsych 1983, M 1971. Cons. Forens. Psychiat. Private Pract., Winchester. Specialty: Forens. Psychiat. Prev: Cons. Psychiat. Marchwood, Priory Southampton; Cons. Psychiat. Wessex RHA; Sen. Regist. (Psychol. Med.) & Regist. (Neurol. & Psychol. Med.) St. Thos. Hosp. Lond.

WRIGHT, Nicola Jane Friarsgate Practice, Friarsgate Medical Centre, Friarsgate, Winchester SO23 8EF Tel: 01962 853599 Fax: 01962 849982 — BM Soton. 1987; DRCOG 1990. GP. Socs: MRCGP. Prev: SHO (A & E) Salisbury Gen. Infirm.; SHO (O & G, Paediat.) Roy. Hants. Co. Hosp.; Ho. Off. (Med.) Roy. Hants. Hosp.

WRIGHT, Noel Diamond, OBE (retired) 1 Upper Croft Road, Holywood BT18 0HJ Tel: 02890 422308 — (Belf.) MB BCh BAO Belf. 1945; FRCGP 1967. Prev: Mem. Gen. Med. Counc.

WRIGHT, Mr Norman Lesley The Dove House, Old Pembroke Farm, High St., Burwell, Cambridge CB5 0HB — MB BCh BAO Belf. 1953; Dobest RCOG 1955; MD Belf 1957; MRCP Lond 1959; FRCS Edin 1961. Specialty: Cardiothoracic Surg.

WRIGHT, Olwen Louise 14 Ardmore Heights, Holywood BT18 0PY — MB ChB Ed. 1994.

WRIGHT, Pamela Louise East Hill Surgery, 78 East Hill, Colchester CO1 2RW; Beech House, Church Road, Layer De La Haye, Colchester CO2 0EN Tel: 01206 734074 — MB BS Lond. 1982 (St Mary's Lond.) DRCOG 1986; MSc 2002. Specialty: Gen. Pract. Socs: Colchester Med. Soc. Prev: Trainee GP Colchester VTS; Hon. Off. Edgware Gen. Hosp. & Wexham Pk. Hosp.

WRIGHT, Patricia Augusta Pathology Department, University of Wales College of Medicine, Heath Park, Cardiff CF14 4XN Tel: 029 2074 7747; 26 Windsor Avenue, Radyr, Cardiff CF15 8BY Tel: 029 2084 3720 — MB BS Lond. 1987; BSc (1st cl. Hons.) Lond. 1984, MB BS 1987. Lect. (Path.) Univ. Wales Coll. Med. Cardiff. Specialty: Histopath. Socs: Path. Soc.; Amer. Assn. Advancem. Sci.

WRIGHT, Patrick James The Medical Health Centre, Gray Avenue, Sherburn, Durham DH6 1JE — MB ChB Dundee 1981; DRCOG 1983; DCCH Ed. 1984. Trainee GP Cleveland VTS. Socs: Assoc. Mem. RCGP.

WRIGHT, Paul Barnaby Plas Gwyn, Gannock Park, Deganwy, Conwy LL31 9PZ — MB ChB Bristol 1998.

WRIGHT, Paul Francis Cornwall Road Surgery, 15 Cornwall Road, Dorchester DT1 1RU Tel: 01305 251808 — MB BS Lond. 1973 (The London Hospital) BDS 1968; DRCOG 1977. Assoc. Dir. For GP Postgrad. Educat. Wessex; Course Organiser & Trainer GP Dorset VTS. Socs: Fell. Roy. Soc. Med.; Exec. Mem. Nat. Assn. Course Organisers. Prev: Lect. (Dent. Anat.) 1967; Lect. (Oral Path.) 1968; Sen. Lect. (Primary Care).

WRIGHT, Paul Hastings Holts Health Centre, Watery Lane, Newent GL18 1BA Tel: 01531 820689 — MB ChB Liverp. 1968; DObst RCOG 1971. Prev: Ho. Surg. & Ho. Phys. Leicester Roy. Infirm.; SHO O & G MusGr. Pk. Hosp. Taunton.

WRIGHT, Paul Kingsley 41 Well Lane, Heswall, Wirral CH60 8NQ — MB ChB Aberd. 1998.

WRIGHT, Paul Richard 22 Brentford Road, Birmingham B14 4DQ — MB ChB Leic. 1994.

WRIGHT, Pauline Montgomery 24 Ayr Road, Giffnock, Glasgow G46 6RY — MB ChB Glas. 1991.

WRIGHT, Penelope Jane Wapping Health Centre, 22 Wapping Lane, London E1W 2RL Tel: 020 7481 9376 — MB BS Lond. 1985; MA Camb. 1986; DRCOG 1987; MRCGP 1991.

WRIGHT, Peter Andrew Public Health Laboratory, Royal Preston Hospital, Preston PR2 9HG Tel: 01772 710113 Fax: 01772 710166 — MB ChB Manch. 1968; FRCPath 1988, M 1976. Cons. Microbiol. Pub. Health Laborat. Serv. Specialty: Med. Microbiol. Socs: Assn. Clin. Path.; Assn. Med. Microbiol. Prev: Cons. Microbiol. Blackburn; Cons. Bact. Glas. Roy. Infirm.; Hon. Clin. Lect. Univ. Glas.

WRIGHT, Mr Peter Dennis (retired) 30 Elmfield Road, Gosforth, Newcastle upon Tyne NE3 4BA — MD Newc. 1974; MB BS 1967; FRCS Eng. 1971. Prev: Cons. Surg. & Sen. Lect. Dept. Surg. Univ. Newc. Freeman Hosp.

WRIGHT, Peter George Yardley Hackwood Partnership, Essex House, Worting Road, Basingstoke RG21 8SU Tel: 01256 470464 Fax: 01256 357289; Fenimore, 61 Northfield Road, Sherfield-on-Loddon, Hook RG27 0DS — MB BS Lond. 1981 (Univ. Coll. Hosp. Med. Sch.) BSc Lond. 1978; MRCGP 1985; DRCOG 1985.

WRIGHT, Peter Henry Room 632, The Adelphi, 1-11 John Adam Street, London WC2N 6HT Email: peter.wright4@virgin.net; 23 Gordon Mansions, Torrington Place, London WC1E 7HF — MB BS Lond. 1968 (Univ. Coll. Hosp.) MRCS Eng. LRCP Lond. 1968; MRCP (UK) 1971; MSc (Occupat. Med.) 1982; MFOM RCP Lond. 1988, AFOM 1986. Med. Policy Adviser, Dept. for Work and Pens; Cons. Occupat. Specialty: Gen. Med.; Respirat. Med.; Occupat. Health. Prev: Sen. Lect. in Occupational Med., Lond. Sch. of Hyg. and Trop. Med.; Hon. Cons. Occupational Phys., Bloomsbury Health Auth.; Cons. Phys. & Chest Phys. Sandwell DHA.

WRIGHT, Peter James Department of Anaesthetics, Daisy Hill Hospital, Hospital Road, Newry BT35 8DR Tel: 028 3083 5000 — MB ChB Sheff. 1976; FFA RCS Eng. 1980; MSc Cardiff 2000. Cons. (Anaesth.) Daisy Hill Hosp. Newry. Specialty: Anaesth.; Acupunc. Socs: Pain Soc.; Brit. Med. Acupunct. Soc. Prev: Cons. & Regist. (Anaesth.) Roy. Hallamsh. Hosp. Sheff.; Sen. Regist. (Anaesth.) Roy. Vict. Hosp. Belf.; Research Fell. Montreal Neurol. Hosp. Canada.

WRIGHT, Peter John The Surgery, Greenwich Avenue, Hull HU9 4UX Tel: 01482 374415 Fax: 01482 786462; 20 Spencer Close, Hedon, Hull HU12 8HE — MB ChB Leeds 1983; DRCOG 1986.

WRIGHT, Peter Louis 11 Albion Hill, Loughton IG10 4RA Tel: 020 8508 6540 Email: drplwright@doctors.org.uk — MB BChir Camb. 1960 (Lond. Hosp.) FRCP Lond. 1978, M 1963; MA Camb. 1964. Hon. Cons. Phys. Whipps Cross Hosp., Leytonstone. Specialty: Gen. Med.; Gastroenterol. Socs: BMA. Prev: Lect. Med. Unit Lond. Hosp.; Cons. Phys. Whipps Cross Hosp., Leytonstone.

WRIGHT, Peter Norman Gladwick Medical Practice, Barley Clough Medical Centre, Hugget Street, Oldham OL4 1BN Tel: 0161 909 8370 Fax: 0161 909 8414; 18 Lincoln Close, Ashton-under-Lyne OL6 8BS Tel: 0161 339 2885 — MB ChB Manch. 1978; DRCOG 1982. Specialty: Gen. Pract.

WRIGHT, Mr Peter Randell (retired) 20 Streatley Lodge, Whitehouse Road, Oxford OX1 4QF Tel: 01865 726630 — (Oxf.) BM BCh Oxf. 1942; MA Oxf. 1942; FRCS Eng. 1948. Prev: Cons. Orthop. Surg. Canterbury & Thanet & SE Kent Health Dist.

WRIGHT, Richard Edward Caterham Valley Medical Practice, Eothen House, Eothen Close, Caterham CR3 6JU Tel: 01883 347811 Fax: 01883 342929; 12 Manor Avenue, Caterham CR3 6AN Tel: 01883 345182 — MB BS Lond. 1990 (St. Thomas's Hospital Medical School) DRCOG 1994; MRCGP 1996. Specialty: Gen. Pract. Prev: Trainee GP/SHO E. Surrey Hosp. Redhill VTS; SHO (Med.) & Ho. Phys. Battle Hosp. Reading; Ho. Surg. Basingstoke Dist. Hosp.

WRIGHT, Richard Geoffrey Department of Occupational Health, Carmarthen & District NHS Trust, West Wales General Hospital, Carmarthen SA31 2AF Tel: 01267 235151 Fax: 01267 227427; Berwyn, 71 Saron Road, Saron, Ammanford SA18 3LH Tel: 01269 595478 — MRCS Eng. LRCP Lond. 1970 (Guy's) FRCS Ed. 1977; AFOM RCP Lond. 1981; FRSH 1982; FRIPHH 1982. Sen. Occupat. Phys. & Dir. Occupat. Health Serv. Carmarthen & Dist. NHS Trust; Occupat. Health Co-ordinator Welsh Water Auth.; Med. Adviser Fire Brig., Co. Counc. & W. Wales Ambul. Trust. Specialty: Occupat. Health. Socs: Fell. Roy. Soc. Med. (Sect. Occupat. Med.); Fell. Roy. Soc. Health; Soc. Occupat. Med. Prev: Sen. Med. Off. Gp. Occupat. Health Centre, BP Research Centre Sunbury; Sen. Med. Off. BP Petroleum Developm. (UK) Ltd. Aberd.; Regist. (Surg.) Bradford Roy. Infirm.

WRIGHT, Richard Michael 52 Avondale Road, Gorleston, Great Yarmouth NR31 6DN — MB ChB Leic. 1991.

WRIGHT, Richard William Maylin 18 Grosvenor Terrace, York YO30 7AG — MRCS Eng. LRCP Lond. 1972 (Guy's) MRCP (UK) 1978. Med. Off. Bootham Sch. York.; Clin. Asst. (Haemat.) York Dist. Hosp. Socs: Brit. Soc. of Med. and Dent. Hypn. Prev: Med. Off. Coll. Ripon & York St. John.

WRIGHT, Robert (retired) 6 Ashlong Grove, Halstead CO9 2QH Tel: 01787 472468 — MB BChir Camb. 1940 (Camb. & Manch.) BA Camb. 1936. Prev: Ho. Phys. Manch. Roy. Infirm. & Crumpsall Hosp. Manch.

WRIGHT, Robert Anthony Dept. Of Cardiology, South Cleveland Hospital, Marton Road, Middlesbrough TS4 3BW Tel: 01642 282491 — MB ChB Ed. 1985 (Univ. Ed.) MRCP (UK) 1988; MD Ed. 1996; FRCP Lond. 2003; FRCP Edin. 2003. Conds. Cardiol. S. Cleveland Hosp. Specialty: Cardiol. Socs: Bris. Cardiac Soc.; Brit. Cardiovasc. Interven. Soc. Prev: Cons.Phys.The Ayr Hosp.; Sen. Regist. (Cardiol. & Gen. Med.) Roy. Infirm. Edin. & West. Gen. Edin.; Lect. (Cardiol.) Univ. Edin. & Roy. Infirm. Edin.

WRIGHT, Robert Edward Richard The Ulster Community Hospitals Trust, Belfast BT16 1RH Tel: 02890 484511; 171 Ballylesson Road, Belfast BT8 8JU Tel: 02890 826905 — MB BCh BAO Belf. 1985 (Queen's Univ. Belfast) FFR RCSI 1991; FRCR 1992. Cons. Radiol. Clin. Director, Clin. Diagnostics Directorate. Specialty: Radiol.; Paediat. Socs: Ulster Radiological Soc.; Ulster Med. Soc.; Europ. Assoc. of Radiol. Prev: Sen. Roy. Vict. Hosp. Belf.

WRIGHT, Robert William Ormskirk Street Surgery, 51A Ormskirk Stret, St Helens WA10 2TB Tel: 01744 29209 — MB ChB Liverp. 1988; DRCOG 1992.

WRIGHT, Ruth The Maternity Unit, Ipswich Hospital, Heath Road, Ipswich IP4 5PD Tel: 01473 703016/7; Bryher, St. Mary's Park, Bucklesham, Ipswich IP10 0DY Tel: 01473 659434 — MB BS Lond. 1953 (Roy. Free) SCMO Ipswich Hosp. Family Plann. Serv.; Dep. Police Surg. E. Suff.; Instruc. Doctor Nat. Assn. Family Plann. Doctors. Specialty: Obst. & Gyn.; Paediat. Prev: Clin. Asst. Ipswich Hosp. Family Plann. Serv.; Dept. Med. Off. Suff. AHA.

WRIGHT, Simon Andrew Hodge Road Surgery, 2 Hodge Road, Worsley, Manchester M28 3AT Tel: 0161 790 3615 Fax: 0161 703 7638 — MB BS Lond. 1987; MA Camb. 1988; MRCP (UK) 1990.

WRIGHT, Simon Ralph Rotherham General Hospital, Moorgate Road, Rotherham S60 2UD — MB ChB Sheff. 1983; MRCPsych 1988. Cons. Psychiat. (Older People) Rotherham Gen. Hosp. Prev: Clin. Lect. (Psychiat.) Univ. Sheff.

WRIGHT, Simon Ronald Aspley Medical Centre, 511 Aspley Lane, Aspley, Nottingham NG8 5RW Tel: 0115 929 2700 Fax: 0115 929 8276 — MB ChB Dundee 1980; DRCOG 1983; DCH RCP Lond. 1984; MRCGP 1984.

WRIGHT, Stanley Charles Falkirk & District Royal Infirmary, Major's Loan, Falkirk FK1 5QE Tel: 01324 624000 Fax: 01324 616020 Email: stan.wright@fvah.scot.nhs.uk; 4 Coxburn Brae, Bridge of Allan, Stirling FK9 4PS Tel: 01324 624000 — MB BCh BAO Belf. 1977; MRCP (UK) 1982; DRCOG 1983; MD Belf. 1988; FRCP Ed. 1999. Cons. (Gen. (Int.) Med. & Resp. Med.) Falkirk Roy. & Dist. Roy. Infirm.; Hon. Sen. Lect. Univ. Edin. Specialty: Respirat. Med. Socs: Brit. Thorac. Soc.; Scott. Thoracic Soc.

WRIGHT, Stephen Alexander 3 Culcavey Bridge, Hillsborough BT26 6RY — MB BCh (Hons) Belf. 1998; MRCP 2001.

WRIGHT, Stephen David 7 Byron Road, London W5 3LL — MB ChB Dundee 1985; MSc (Haemat.) Lond. 1991. Specialty: Biochem. Socs: Assoc. Mem. Clin. Path.

WRIGHT, Stephen Edward 26 Pinegarth, Ponteland, Newcastle upon Tyne NE20 9LF — MB ChB Sheff. 1997; MRCP 2001. Europ. SHO exchange scheme (Gen. Med.), St. Bartholomews Hosp., Lond. & L'Hopital Cantonale de Geneve, Geneva. Prev: SHO Rotat. (Gen. Med.) Roy. Vict. Infirm. Newc.

WRIGHT, Stephen Geoffrey Hospital for Tropical Diseases, Mortimer Market, off Capper St., Tottenham Court Road, London WC1E 6AU Tel: 020 7387 9300 Ext: 5968 Fax: 020 7380 9761 Email: stephen.wright@ishtm.ac.uk — MB BS Lond. 1968; MRCS Eng. LRCP Lond. 1968; DCMT . Lond. 1971; MRCP (UK) 1973; FRCP Lond. 1991. Cons. Phys. Hosp. Trop. Dis.; Phys. King Edwd. VII's Hosp.; Hon. Sen. Lect. (Infectious & Trop. Diseases) Lond. Sch. Hyg. & Trop. Med. Specialty: Trop. Med. Prev: Sen. Regist. Hosp. Trop. Dis. Lond.; SHO Northwick Pk. Hosp. Harrow; Ho. Off. (Neurosurg. Studies) Nat. Hosp. Nerv. Dis. Lond.

WRIGHT, Prof Stephen Geoffrey Faculty of Health, St Martin's College, Lancaster LA1 3JD — MB ChB Liverp. 1985.

WRIGHT, Stephen John Seacroft Road Surgery, Seacroft Road, Mablethorpe LN12 2DT Tel: 01507 473483 Fax: 01507 478865 — MB ChB Leic. 1986; MRCGP 1990.

WRIGHT, Stewart John Willow Green Surgery, Station Road, East Preston, Littlehampton BN16 3AH Tel: 01903 785152 Fax: 01903 859986 — MB BS Lond. 1983 (St Mary's) DRCOG 1986; DCH RCP Lond. 1987. GP Princip. Specialty: Gen. Pract. Special Interest: Audit; Prescribing. Prev: Trainee GP Thanet VTS.; SHO (A & E) Roy. Berks. Hosp. Reading; Ho. Surg. Hillingdon Hosp. Uxbridge.

WRIGHT, Stuart Lloyd 184 Park Road, Bearwood, Smethwick B67 5HU — MB ChB Birm. 1989. Med. Off. (Cas.) Geo. Town Hosp., Cayman Is.s.

WRIGHT, Susan Frances Jane — MB BChir Camb. 1989; DRCOG 1992; MRCGP 1994. GP Princip. Alresford. Specialty: Gen. Pract. Prev: Trainee GP Winchester VTS.

WRIGHT, Suzanne Gaenor 17 Battersby Close, Yarm TS15 9RX — MB BS Newc. 1984; DRCOG 1986. Trainee GP Cleveland VTS. Socs: BMA & Med. Defence Union. Prev: SHO (A & E) Qu. Eliz. Hosp. Gateshead; SHO (O & G) N. Tees Gen. Hosp. Stockton-on-Tees; SHO (Psychiat.) St. Lukes Hosp. Middlesbrough.

WRIGHT, Tanya Ruth 115 Coleraine Road, Portstewart BT55 7HR; 116 High Street, Uttoxeter ST14 7JH — MB ChB Dundee 1996.

WRIGHT, Thomas John Wyatt Alexander 35 Highgrove Drive, Ballyclare BT39 9XH Tel: 0196 03 42011 — MB BCh BAO Belf. 1981 (Belfast) DCH Dub. 1985; MRCGP 1986.

WRIGHT, Thomas Paul Markethill Health Centre, Newry Street, Markethill, Armagh BT60 1TA Tel: 028 3755 1306 Fax: 028 3755 2148; 62 Ballyloughan Road, Ahorey, Portadown, Craigavon BT62 3TA — MB BCh BAO Belf. 1985; DCH Dub. 1988; DRCOG 1989; MRCGP 1990.

WRIGHT, Timothy Freeman Scapa Medical Group, Health Centre, New Scapa Road, Kirkwall KW15 1BQ Tel: 01856 885445 Fax: 01856 873556; Westbank, St. Ola, Kirkwall KW15 1TR Tel: 01856 872606 — MB BS Lond. 1971 (Roy. Free) DObst RCOG 1976. Clin. Asst. (Obst.) Balfour Hosp. Kirkwall; Obst. Ultrasound Balfour Hosp. Kirkwall; Mem. Scott. Auth. Airmed. Examrs. Socs: Brit. Med. Ultrasound Soc. Prev: SHO (Obst.) Vale of Leven Hosp. Alexandria.

WRIGHT, Timothy Grant Sigiri, College Lane, Woking GU22 0EW — MB BS Lond. 1972; MCRS Eng. LRCP Lond. 1972; MRCP 1977.

WRIGHT, Timothy Samuel 22 Telegraph Lane, Claygate, Esher KT10 0DU — MB BS Lond. 1998.

WRIGHT, Trevor (retired) Fields Farm, Ashford Road, Bakewell DE45 1GL Tel: 01629 813966 — MD Belf. 1946, MB BCh BAO 1940; DCH Univ. Lond. 1947. Prev: Cons. Phys. (Handicap. Childr.) Childr. Hosp. Sheff.

WRIGHT, Vanessa Mary Barts & The London NHS Trust, Royal London Hospital, Whitechapel Road, London E1 1BB Tel: 020 7377 7000 Ext: 7799 Fax: 020 7377 7710; 28 Empire Wharf, 235 Old Ford Road, London E3 5NQ Tel: 020 8981 5844 — MB BS Lond. 1966; FRCS Eng. 1972; FRACS (Paed. Surg.) 1976. Cons. Paediat. Surg. Barts & The Lond. Hosp.; Cons. Paediat. Surg. UCL Hosp. Specialty: Paediat. Surg. Prev: Sen. Regist. Roy. Childr. Hosp. Melbourne, Austral.; Regist. Qu. Mary's Hosp. for Childr. Carshalton & Univ. Coll. Hosp. Lond.

WRIGHT, William Millfield Medical Centre, 63-83 Hylton Road, Sunderland SR4 7AF Tel: 0191 567 9179 Fax: 0191 514 7452; 7 McLaren Way, West Herrington, Houghton-le-Spring DH4 4NP Tel: 0191 584 0717 — MB BS Newc. 1977; DRCOG 1980; MRCGP 1981. GP Sunderland FPC. Socs: BMA.

WRIGHT, William Bryce (retired) Mill End Cottage, Northleach, Cheltenham GL54 3HJ Tel: 01451 860681 — MB ChB Glas. 1950; FRCP Ed. 1971, M 1955; FRCP Lond. 1979, M 1966. Prev: Cons. Geriat. S. West. RHA.

WRIGHT, William Michael Antony (retired) The Moor, Westfield, Hastings TN35 4QR Tel: 01424 754913 — MB BChir Camb. 1956 (Middlx.) MA, MB Camb. 1957, BChir 1956. Prev: Obst. Ho. Surg. St. Paul's Hosp. Hemel Hempstead.

WRIGHTON, Mr John Derek (retired) Cleaves Cliff, 39 Bowleaze Coveway, Preston, Weymouth DT3 6PL Tel: 01305 832418 Fax: 01305 832418 — MB BS Lond. 1956 (Char. Cross) DObst RCOG 1958; FRCS Eng. 1967. Hon. Cons. Orthop. W. Dorset Gp. Hosps. & Weymouth & Dist. Hosp. Prev: Sen. Regist. (Orthop.) Princess Eliz. Orthop. Hosp. Exeter & City.

WRIGHTON, Ronald John (retired) Stream House, Cootham, Storrington, Pulborough RH20 4JT Tel: 01903 742909 — MB BS Lond. 1959 (St. Thos.) MRCP Lond. 1963; FFPHM 1983. Prev: Dir. Pub. Health Mid Downs HA.

WRIGHTSON, Fiona Michelle 48 Cumberland Avenue, Goring-by-Sea, Worthing BN12 6JX — MB ChB Leic. 1998.

WRIGHTSON, Lynne Bartholomew Medical Group, The Health Centre, Bartholomew Avenue, Goole DN14 6AW Tel: 01405 767711 Fax: 01405 768212 — MB ChB Aberd. 1983; DRCOG 1986; MRCGP 1989.

WRIGLEY, David George — MB ChB Sheff. 1997 (Sheffield) MRCGP 2001. Princip. Specialty: Gen. Pract. Special Interest: Med. Politics. Prev: Non-Princip. GP, Carnforth, Lancs.; Non-Princip. GP, Morecambe Bay.; Ho. Off. (Surg.), Chesterfield.

WRIGLEY, Edward Thornton Freshfields, Keepers Lane, Codsall, Wolverhampton WV8 — MB BS Lond. 1971; DObst RCOG 1974.

WRIGLEY, Edwin John (retired) White Walls, Golf Links Lane, Selsey, Chichester PO20 9DP Tel: 01243 602426 — MB BS Lond. 1954 (St. Thos.) Prev: Dist. Med. Off. N. Nigeria.

WRIGLEY, Emma Caroline Farndon, 15 Riddings Road, Hale, Altrincham WA15 9DS — MB ChB Manch. 1986; MRCOG 1991; MFFP 1995. Cons. (O & G) Wythenshawe Hosp. Specialty: Obst. & Gyn. Prev: Specialist Regist. (O & G) Roy. Surrey Co. Hosp.; Research Fell. (Gyn. Oncol.) Christie Hosp. Manch.; Regist. (O & G) Mersey RHA.

WRIGLEY, Fenella Kate — MB BS Lond. 1996 (St. Geo. Hosp. Med Sch.) BSc (Hons.) Clin. Sci. Lond. 1995; MRCPCH 2000. SHO Paediat. Specialty: Paediat.; Accid. & Emerg.

WRIGLEY, Mr James Hall (retired) Walnut Tree Cottage, Church Hill, Marnhull, Sturminster Newton DT10 1PU Tel: 01258 820265 — (Ed.) MB ChB Ed. 1944; FRCS Ed. 1948. Prev: Cons. Surg. Bishop Auckland Gen. Hosp.

WRIGLEY, Katrin University Health Service, University of Southampton, Building 48, Highfield, Southampton SO17 1BJ Tel: 023 8055 7531 Fax: 023 8059 3259; 35 Hursley Road, Chandlers Ford, Eastleigh SO53 2FS — MB ChB Bristol 1972. GP Univ. Soton. Health Serv. Specialty: Gen. Med. Prev: GP Portswood Soton.; Trainee GP Bristol VTS; SHO (Psychiat.) Glenside Hosp. Bristol.

WRIGLEY, Mark William c/o Department of Anaesthesia, The Central Middlesex Hospital, Abbey Road, Park Royal, London NW10; 18 May Road, Twickenham TW2 6QP Tel: 020 8894 3432 — MB BS Lond. 1982; FFA RCS Eng. 1987. Cons. Anaesth. Centr. Middlx. NHS Trust. Specialty: Anaesth. Socs: Assn. Anaesth. Prev: Sen.

Regist. Middlx. Hosp. Lond.; Regist. (Anaesth.) Qu. Charlottes Matern. & Middlx. Hosps. Lond.

WRIGLEY, Peter Francis Martyn (retired) Old College House, All Saints Court, Church Lane, Pannal, Harrogate HG3 1NH Tel: 01423 879442 Fax: 01423 879442 Email: peter@wrigley.net — BM BCh Oxf. 1964 (Univ. Coll. Lond. & Magdalen Oxf.) PhD Lond. 1970, BSc 1961; FRCP Lond. 1979, M 1967. Prev: Cons. Phys. (Med. Oncol.) St. Bart. Hosp. Lond.

WRIGLEY, Richard Alan Waterloo Health Centre, 5 Lower Marsh, London SE1 7RJ Tel: 020 7928 4049 Fax: 020 7928 2644 — MB BS Lond. 1986.

WRIGLEY, Sophia Ruth Derriford Hospital, Derriford Road, Plymouth PL6 8DH Tel: 01752 777111 — MB ChB Bristol 1983; DRCOG 1985; DCH RCP Lond. 1986. Cons. Anesthetist Derriford Hosp., Plymouth. Specialty: Anaesth. Socs: Anaesth. Res. Soc.& Assn. Anaesth.; Assn. Paediat. Anaesth. Prev: Cons. Anaesth. Roy. Lond. Hosp.; Sen. Regist. Rotat. (Anaesth.) Univ. Coll. Hosp. Lond.

WRIGLEY, Susan Margaret 187 Moorgate Road, Rotherham S60 3AX Tel: 01709 382852 — MB ChB Birm. 1974; BSc (Med. Biochem.) Birm. 1971; MRCGP 1979. Specialty: Family Plann. & Reproduc. Health. Socs: BMA. Prev: Trainee GP Rotherham VTS; SHO (Med.) Qu. Alexandra Hosp. Cosham; Ho. Off. (Surg.) Halifax Gen. Hosp.

WRITER, Martin Darrell Levett Park Practice, 12 Brodrick Close, Hampden Park, Eastbourne BN22 9NQ — MB BS Lond. 1991 (St. Bart.) DCH RCPS Glas. 1994; DRCOG 1995; DFFP 1996. Socs: Roy. Coll.

WROBLEWSKA, Maria Helena Bennett Street Suregery, Stretford, Manchester M32 8SG — MB BS UC Lond. 1996; DFFP Lond. (Univ. Coll. Lond.) BSc (Hons. Psychol.) UC Lond. 1990. GP Regist. Edgeware Lond; GP Princip., Manch. Specialty: Gen. Pract. Prev: SHO, Palliat. Care, N. Lond. Hospice; SHO, Obst. & Gyn., Barnet Gen. Hosp.; SHO, Paediat., Barnet Gen. Hosp.

WROBLEWSKI, Professor Boguslaw Michael Centre for Hip Surgery, Wrightington Hospital, Wigan WN6 9EP Tel: 01257 256286 Fax: 01257 256291; The Coach House, Tan House Close, Parbold, Wigan WN8 7HH — MB ChB Leeds 1960; FRCS Ed. 1966. Cons. Orthop. Surg. Centre for Hip Surg. Wrightington Hosp. Wigan; Prof. Orthop. BioMech. Univ. Leeds 1992. Specialty: Orthop. Special Interest: Primary & Revision Hips. Socs: Fell. BOA; Internat. Hip Soc.; (Pres.) Brit. Hip Soc. Prev: Regist. (Surg.) Leeds Gen. Infirm.; Regist. Robt. Jones & Agnes Hunt Orthop. Hosp. OsW.ry. Sen. Orthop.; Regist. Birm. Roy. Orthop. Hosp.

WROE, Anna Caroline The Freeman Hospital, High Heaton, Newcastle — MB ChB Birm. 1997. Specialist Regist. Renal Med. Specialty: Endocrinol. Prev: Med. HO. Off.

WROE, Stephen John New Southgate Surgery, Buxton Place, off Leeds Road, Wakefield WF1 3JQ Tel: 01924 334400 Fax: 01924 334439; Midsett Cottage, Brockswood Court, Walton, Wakefield WF2 6RD — BM BCh Oxf. 1985; MA Oxf. 1988; DRCOG 1988.

WROE, Stephen Joseph National Hospital for Neurology & Neurosurgery, Department of Neurology, Box 98, Queen Square, London WC1N 3BG Tel: 0207 405 2882 Mob: 07850 226 473 Fax: 0207 061 9899 Email: sjwroe@ntlworld.com; 31 Graham Road, Ipswich IP1 3QE Tel: 01473 413451 — MB ChB Liverp. 1979; MRCP (UK) 1983; MD Liverp. 1993; FRCP Lond. 1996. Cons. Neurologist, Nat. Hosp. for Neurol. and Neurosurg., Qu. Sq., Lond. Specialty: Neurol. Special Interest: Neurodegenerative Disorders (Prion diseases), Epilepsy, Head injury, Trauma, Multiple Sclerosis, Medico-Legal Pract. Socs: Roy. Soc. of Med.; Assn. of Brit. Neurologists; Amer. Acad. of Neurol. Prev: Cons. Neurol., Ipswich; Cons. in Neurophysiology, Ipswich; Sen. Regist. in Neurol., Nat. Hosp., Queens Sq., Lond.

WRONG, Professor Oliver Murray Flat 8, 96-100 New Cavendish St., London W1W 6XN Tel: 020 7637 4740 — (Oxf.) BM BCh Oxf. 1947; FRCP Lond. 1967, M 1951; DM Oxf. 1964; FRCP Ed. 1970. Emerit. Prof. Med. Univ. Coll. Lond.; Vis. Prof. Med. Univs. Harvard & Sherbrooke 1974, Toronto & McGill 1976. Specialty: Gen. Med.; Nephrol. Socs: (Ex-Sec.) Renal Assn. Prev: Prof. Med. Univ. Dundee; Sen. Lect. (Med.) Roy. Postgrad. Med. Sch. Lond.; Chairm. Nat. Kidney Research Fund.

WROTH, Richard Peter Chesterfield Royal Hospital, Chesterfield S44 5BL Tel: 01246 552284 — BM Soton. 1987; FRCA 1994. Cons.(Anaesth.), Chesterfield Rjoyal Hosp. Specialty: Anaesth.; Intens. Care. Prev: Sen. Regist. (Anaesth.) N. Trent Region; Research Regist. (Anaesth.) Roy. Hallamsh. Hosp. Sheff.

WROUGHTON, Marjorie Anne (retired) 30 Royal Standard House, Standard Hill, Nottingham NG1 6FX Tel: 0115 941 7771 Fax: 0115 941 7771 Email: wroughton@standardhill.com — MB ChB Sheff. 1955. Prev: Assoc. Specialist (Dermat.) Univ. Hosp. Nottm.

WROUT, John Dawson Taunton Road Medical Centre, 12-16 Taunton Road, Bridgwater TA6 3LS Tel: 01278 720 000 Fax: 01278 423691; Willow House, Ham, Creech St Michael, Taunton TA3 5NZ Tel: 01823 443055 Email: jdwroot@cix.co.uk — BM BCh Oxf. 1971 (Guy's) MA Oxf. 1971; DObst RCOG 1973; FRCGP 1997, MRCGP 1976; MICGP 1988; DFFP 1993; FRCGP 2002. Princip. GP; Examr. MRCGP; Extern. Examr Cert. Fam.pract.Kuwait; Internat. Developm. Adviser RCGP Kuwait. Specialty: Rehabil. Med.; Rheumatol. Socs: W Som. Med. Club. Prev: Course Organiser Som. VTS; Examr. DRCOG & MICGP; RCGP Coll. Tutor Som.

WU, Alexandra 1 Meadow Bank, Primrose Hill, London NW3 3AY — MB BS Lond. 1983.

WU, Felix Siu-Man 6B Peak Hill Gardens, London SE26 4LE — MB ChB Sheff. 1992.

WU, Frederick Chung-Wei Manchester Royal Infirmary, Department of Endocrinology, Manchester M13 9WL Tel: 0161 276 8750 Fax: 0161 276 8019 Email: frederick.wu@man.ac.uk — MB ChB Ed. 1972; MRCP (UK) 1974; BSc (Hons.) Ed. 1970, MD 1983; FRCP Ed. 1989; FRCP Lond. 1995. Sen. Lect. (Endocrinol.) Univ. & Roy. Infirm. Manch.; Hon. Cons. Phys. Manch. Roy. Inifrm. & St. Mary's Hosp. Manch. Specialty: Endocrinol. Prev: MRC Clin. Sci. MRC Reproduc. Biol. Univ. Edin.; Sen. Regist. (Endocrinol. & Diabetes) Roy. Infirm. Edin.; Hon. Sen. Regist. (Endocrinol.) & MRC Clin. Research Fell. (O & G) Univ. Edin.

WU, Gladys (retired) 9 Craven Lodge, 15-17 Craven Hill, London W2 3EN — Medico Cirujano Peru 1970.

WU, Kenneth Hoong Jee 37 Ashburton Road, Birkenhead CH43 8TN — MB ChB Liverp. 1997.

WU, Kin-Chung 155 Trehafod Road, Pontypridd CF37 2LL — MB BCh Wales 1997.

WU, Wing Cheng Kenneth 71 New Edinburgh Road, Uddingston, Glasgow G71 6AB — MB ChB Manch. 1991.

WUBETU, Tebabu 37 Merley Gate, Morpeth NE61 2EP — MB BCh BAO Belf. 1984; MRCOG 1989. SHO Belf. City Hosp. Socs: BMA.

WOJCLK, Mr Andrzej Hinchingbrooke Hospital, Hinchingbrooke Park, Huntingdon PE18 8NT Tel: 01480 416471 Fax: 01480 416561 Email: andrew.wojclk@hinchingbrooke.nhs.uk — DM 1974 (Warsaw) FRCS 1991. Cons. Orthopaedic Surgeon/Spinal Surg., Hinchingbrooke Hosp.; Hon. Cons. Spinal Surg., Addenbrookes Hosp., Camb. Specialty: Orthop. Socs: BSS; BAO. Prev: Hon. Cons. Spinal Surg., Addenbrookes Hosp., Camb.

WULFF, Christian Hertel Department of Clinical Neurophysiology, Poole Hospital, Longfleet Road, Poole BH15 2JB Tel: 01202 442965 Fax: 01202 442762 Email: christian.wulff@poole.nhs.uk; 39 Dunkeld Road, Talbot Woods, Bournemouth BH3 7EW Tel: 01202 763293 — MD Copenhagen 1971. Cons. Clin. Neurophysiol. Poole Hosp. Dorset. Specialty: Clin. Neurophysiol.; Neurol.

WULFF, Douglas Edward 12 Hollyfield Road, Sutton Coldfield B75 7SG — MB BCh Witwatersrand 1975.

WUNNA, R The Surgery, 148 Castleford Road, Normanton WF6 2EP Tel: 01924 223636 Fax: 01924 220252 — MB BS Rangoon 1973; MB BS Med Inst (I) Rangoon 1973. GP Normanton, W. Yorks.

WUNSCH, Claire Margaret Abbotswood Medical Centre, Defford Road, Pershore WR10 1HZ Tel: 01386 552424; 27 Head Street, Pershore WR10 1DA — MB ChB Manch. 1983; MRCP (UK) 1987; DRCOG 1991; MRCGP 1992. Prev: Trainee GP Pershore; Regist. (Paediat.) E. Glam. Hosp. Pontypridd & Wellington Hosp., NZ; SHO (O & G) Worcs. Roy. Hosp.

WURM, Reinhard Engelbert 5 All Saints Road, Sutton SM1 3DA — MD Essen 1990; State Exam Med. 1984.

WURR, Catherine Jane West Leeds Child & Adolescent Mental Health Team, Cringlebar House, 415 Bradford Road, Leeds LS28 7HQ Tel: 0113 295 4111 — MB ChB Leeds 1987; MMedSci. Leeds 1992; MRCPsych. 1992; MD 2001. Cons. Child Adolesc. Psychiat. Child & Adolesc. Ment. Health Serv.s, Leeds; Sen. Clin. Lect. Univ. Leeds. Specialty: Child & Adolesc. Psychiat. Socs: East

Leeds Primary Care Trust. Prev: Sen. Regist. (Child Adolesc. Psychiat.) Yorks. RHA; Trainee Gen. Psych. Bootham Pk. Hosp. York VTS; Ho. Phys. Leeds Gen. Hosp.

WURR, Elizabeth Mary (retired) 70 Melrose Road, Norwich NR4 7PW — (Birm.) MB ChB Birm. 1966; BA (Hons.) Open 1989, BA 1984.

WUSU, Oladipo Olusegun Hunponu 76 Dobbies Road, Bonnyrigg EH19 2AZ — MB ChB Glas. 1962; MD Glas. 1970, MB ChB 1962; DPH Glas. 1967; MFCM RCP (UK) 1974; FRCP Glas. 1979, M 1977.

WYATT, Ann (retired) 9 Vancouver House, 44 Barrack Road, Christchurch BH23 1PF — (King's Coll. Hosp.) MRCS Eng. LRCP Lond. 1946; MB BS Lond. 1947; FRCGP 1983, M 1953. Prev: GP Princip. 1955-85.

WYATT, Mr Arthur Powell (retired) The Cottage, 72 Camden Pk Road, Chislehurst BR7 5HF Tel: 020 8467 9477 — MB BS Lond. 1955 (St. Bart.) FRCS Eng. 1960. Prev: Cons. Surgic. Greenwich healthcare Trust.

WYATT, Ben Timothy Brig Royd Surgery, Brig Royd, Ripponden, Sowerby Bridge HX6 4AN Tel: 01422 822209 — MB BS Lond. 1985; BSc Lond. 1982; DCH RCP Lond. 1989; DRCOG 1990; MRCGP 1992. Hosp. Pract. (Clin. Haemat.) Halifax.

WYATT, Caroline Marie 2 Garden Close, Givens Grove, Leatherhead KT22 8LU — BM BCh Oxf. 1998.

WYATT, Edward Henry (retired) 16 St James Road, Melton, North Ferriby HU14 3HZ Tel: 01482 633606 — (Lond. Hosp.) MB BS Lond. 1951; MRCS Eng. LRCP Lond. 1951; DObst RCOG 1953; DTM Antwerp 1954; FRCP Ed. 1977, M 1967; FRCP Lond. 1991. Prev: Cons. Dermat. Roy. Hull Hosps. Trust.

WYATT, Elma Priscilla (retired) 16 Casterbridge Road, Dorchester DT1 2AQ — MB BChir Camb. 1957 (St Mary's) MRCS Eng. LRCP Lond. 1957; DObst RCOG 1964. GP Dorchester Dorset.

WYATT, Geoffrey Paul Meadowville, 13 Guisborough Road, Great Ayton, Middlesbrough TS9 6AA Tel: 01642 722379 — MB ChB Liverp. 1973; DCH Eng. 1976; MRCP (UK) 1978. Cons. Paediat. Middlesbrough Gen. Hosp. Specialty: Paediat. Prev: Sen. Regist. (Paediat.) Soton. & Portsmouth Hosps.; Clin. Tutor (Child Health) Univ. Manch.; SHO (Paediat.) Coronation; Hosp. Univ. Witwatersrand, Johannesburg, S. Africa.

WYATT, George Bernard (retired) 9 Adelaide Terrace, Liverpool L22 8QD Tel: 0151 474 5661 Email: wyatt9@blueyonder.co.uk — MB BS Lond. 1957 (Univ. Coll. Hosp.) MRCS Eng. LRCP Lond. 1957; FFPH 1989; DCH Eng. 1959; FRCP Lond. 1977, M 1961; DTM & H Liverp. 1964; FFCM 1980, M 1974. Prev: Sen. Lect. (Trop. Med.) Liverp. Sch. Trop. Med.

WYATT, Hilary Anne Dept of Child Health, Kings College Hospital, Denmark Hill, London SE5 9RS Email: hilary.wyatt@kcl.ac.uk — MB BS Lond. 1984 (Westm.) MRCPCH; DCH RCP Lond. 1988; MRCP (UK) 1988. Cons. (Cystic Fibrosis) Kings Coll. Hosp. Lond. Specialty: Paediat. Prev: Clin. & Research Fell. (Cystic Fibrosis) King's Coll. Hosp. Lond.; Regist. (Child Health) All St.s Hosp. Chatham & King's Coll. Hosp. Lond.; Assoc. Specialist (Cystic Fibrosis) Dept. Child Health King's Coll. Hosp. Lond.

WYATT, James Andrew (retired) 24 Sheendale Road, Richmond TW9 2JJ — MB BCh Wales 1958; DCH Eng. 1963.

WYATT, Jean Louise (retired) 9 Adelaide Terrace, Waterloo, Liverpool L22 8QD Tel: 0151 474 5661 — (Bristol) MB ChB (Hons.) Bristol 1960; DTM & H Liverp. 1964; DCH Eng. 1978; MRCGP 1983. Occasional Locums. Prev: GP Princip.

WYATT, Jeremy Crispin School of Public Policy, University College London, 29 Tavistock Square, London WC1H 9EZ Tel: 020 7504 4986 Fax: 020 7504 4998 Email: jeremy.wyatt@ucl.ac.uk; 12 Greville Park Road, Ashtead KT21 2QT Tel: 01372 273634 — MB BS Lond. 1980 (Oxf. & Westm.) MRCP (UK) 1983; BA Oxf. 1977, DM 1991; FRCP 1999. Sen. Fell. Health Policy; Dir. Knowledge Managem. Centre; Sen. Research Fell. Centre for Statistics in Med. Univ. Oxf. Specialty: Epidemiol. Socs: (Pres.) Europ. Soc. Artific. Intelligence Med.; (Vice Chairm.) Brit. Med. Informatics Soc.; Fell. Amer. Coll. Med. Informatics. Prev: Med. Informatics Cons. ICRF, 1992-97; MRC Train. Fell. Stanford Univ. 1991-92; Lect. (Med. Informatics) Nat. Heart & Lung Inst. Lond.

WYATT, John Douglas (retired) 4 Cringleford Chase, Cringleford, Norwich NR4 7RS Tel: 01603 501939 — MRCS Eng. LRCP Lond. 1958 (Camb. & Westm.) MA Camb. 1961, MB 1958, BChir 1957; DObst RCOG 1960; LMCC 1975; Cert. Av. Med. 1975; Cert. Family Plann. JCC 1977. GP Locum. Prev: Sen. Med. Off. H.M. Prison Norwich.

WYATT, Professor John Stephen Department of Paediatrics, University College London Medical School, Rayne Institute, 5 University St., London WC1E 6JJ Tel: 020 7209 6113 Fax: 020 7209 6103 Email: j.wyatt@ucl.ac.uk; 84 Queens Drive, Finsbury Park, London N4 2HW — MB BS Lond. 1978 (St. Thos. Hosp., Univ. Lond.) BSc Lond. 1975; MRCS Eng. LRCP Lond. 1978; MRCP (UK) 1981; DCH RCP Lond. 1984; FRCP Lond. 1993; FRCPCH 1997. Hon. Cons. & Prof. Neonat. Paediat. Univ. Coll. Lond. Specialty: Neonat. Prev: Sen. Lect. & Lect. (Paediat.) Univ. Coll. Lond.

WYATT, Mr Jonathan Paul Forensic Medicine Unit, Medical School, Teviot Place, Edinburgh EH8 9AG Tel: 0131 650 3288 Fax: 0131 650 6529 — MB ChB Sheff.; BMedSci (Clin. Physiol.) Sheff. 1984; MB ChB Sheff. 1986; FRCS Ed. 1992. Research Fell. (Forens. Med.) Univ. Edin.; Mem. Fac. A & E Med. (Mem. Represen. Bd.). Specialty: Accid. & Emerg. Socs: Brit. Accid. & Emerg. Trainees Assn. (Scott. Represen.). Prev: Sen. Regist. (A & E) Roy. Infirm. Edin.; Regist. (A & E) West. Infirm. Glas.; Regist. (Surg.) Edin. Roy. Infirm. Assoc. Hosps.

WYATT, Judith Irene Pathology Department, St. James's University Hospital, Beckett St., Leeds LS9 7TF Tel: 0113 206 4571 Fax: 0113 206 5429 Email: judy.wyatt@leedsth.nhs.uk — MB ChB Bristol 1979; MRCPath 1986. Cons. Histopath. St. Jas. Hosp. Leeds. Specialty: Histopath.

WYATT, Martin Thomas Tree Lodge, 40 Brean Down Avenue, Weston Super Mare BS23 4JQ — MB ChB Bristol 1974.

WYATT, Megan Glen Bridgegate Medical Centre, Winchester St, Barrow-in-Furness LA13 9SH — MB BCh Witwatersrand 1989.

WYATT, Mr Michael Graham Freeman Hospital, High Heaton, Newcastle upon Tyne NE7 7DN Tel: 0191 284 3111 Fax: 0191 213 1968; 22 Adeline Gardens, Gosforth, Newcastle upon Tyne NE3 4JQ Tel: 0191 285 6858 Email: mikewyatt@lineone.net — MB BS Lond. 1982 (Newcastle 77/82) MSc (Med. Sci.) Glas. 1985; FRCS Eng. 1987; MD Newc. 1993; T(S) 1994. Cons. Gen. & Vasc. Surg. Freeman Hosp. Newc. u. Tyne. Specialty: Gen. Surg. Socs: Vasc. Surg. Soc.; Eur. Soc. Vasc. Surg.; Assn. Surg. Prev: Sen. Regist. (Gen. Surg.) SW HA; Research Fell. Bristol Roy. Infirm.; Regist. Frenchay Hosp. Bristol & Derriford Hosp. Plymouth.

WYATT, Miss Michelle Elizabeth 44 Broomwood Road, London SW11 6HT — MB BChir Camb. 1993 (Camb. Univ.) MA Camb. 1993; FRCS Eng. 1996; FRCS (Oto.) Eng. 1997. Specialist Regist. N. Thames Region. Specialty: Otorhinolaryngol.

WYATT, Miriam Louise The Abbey Practice, The Family Health Centre, Stepgates, Chertsey KT16 8HZ Tel: 01932 561199 Fax: 01932 571842 — BM BS Nottm. 1990; DGM RCP Lond. 1991; DRCOG 1994; MRCGP 1995.

WYATT, Nell Victoria Station Approach Health Centre, Station Approach, Bradford-on-Avon BA15 1DQ Tel: 01225 866611; Brew Cottage, Green Lane, Turleigh, Bradford-on-Avon BA15 2HH — MB BS Lond. 1992 (Univ. Coll. & Middlx. Sch. Med. Lond) MRCGP 1995; DCH RCP Lond. 1995; DRCOG 1996. GP Princip. Bradford-on-Avon.

WYATT, Paul Henry Glenside, Allendale Road, Hexham NE46 2NB — MB ChB Sheff. 1994; MRCPsych 2000.

WYATT, Richard, RD Glenfield Hospital, Groby Road, Leicester LE3 9QP Tel: 0116 287 1471; 40 Fairfield Crescent, Glenfield, Leicester LE3 8EH Tel: 0016 287 0170 Fax: 0116 287 0170 — MB BS Lond. 1966 (St. Mary's) MRCS Eng. LRCP Lond. 1966; DA Eng. 1969; FFA RCS Eng. 1973. Cons. Anaesth. Glenfield Trust Hosp. Leicester. Specialty: Anaesth. Socs: Vice-Pres. BAODA; Assn. Anaesths.; Pain Soc. Prev: Sen. Regist. (Anaesth.) Sheff. AHA (T); Ho. Off. St. Mary's Hosp. Lond.; Surg. Lt. RN (Anaesth. Specialist).

WYATT, Richard Damon 3 Orchard Close, March PE15 9DF — MB BS Lond. 1998.

WYATT, Richard Henry Hartington St Medical Practice, 36-38 Hartington Street, Barrow-in-Furness LA14 5SL; 30 Balmoral Drive, Barrow-in-Furness LA13 0HX — MB BCh Witwatersrand 1990.

WYATT, Robert John The Surgery, Marsh Lane, Misterton, Doncaster DN10 4DL Tel: 01427 890206 Fax: 01427 891311; Heljen House, Caves Lane, Walkeringham, Doncaster DN10 4LS Tel: 01427 891218 — MB ChB Sheff. 1974; MRCP (UK) 1978.

Specialty: Gen. Pract. Prev: Clin. Asst. (Gen. Med. & Endocrinol.) Doncaster Roy. Infirm.

WYATT, Robert Miles Poundwell Meadow Health Centre, Poundwell Meadow, Modbury, Ivybridge PL21 0QL Tel: 01548 830666 Fax: 01548 831085 — MB BS Lond. 1979; DRCOG 1982.

WYATT, Sarah Suzanne Hampton Lodge, Warwick CV35 8QT Tel: 01926 492521 — MB BChir Camb. 1991; MRCP (UK) 1993; FRCA 1997. Regist. (Anaesth.) Soton. Gen. Hosp. Specialty: Anaesth. Prev: SHO (Anaesth.) Soton. Gen. Hosp.; SHO (Anaesth.) Roy. United Hosp. Bath; Regist. (Med.) Chas. Gardiner Hosp. Perth, West. Austral.

WYATT, Susan Elizabeth Paediatric Department, Clarendon Wing, Leeds General Infirmary, Leeds LS2 9NS Tel: 0113 392 2955 Fax: 0113 392 2955 Email: sue.wyatt@leedsth.nhs.uk — MB BS Lond. 1977 (Kings Coll. Hosp. Med. Sch. Lond.) BSc Lond. 1974; DCH Eng. 1979; MRCP (UK) 1981; FRCPCH 1997. Paediatric Rheumatologist, Leeds; Community Paediatrician, Leeds, 1991-2003. Specialty: Paediat. Socs: FRCPCH; BSPAR; BSR. Prev: Sen. Regist. (Community Paediat.) Oxf. RHA; Sen. Regist. (Paediat.) Univ. Coll. Hosp. Lond.; Regist. (Haemat.) Roy. Postgrad. Med. Sch. Lond.

WYATT, Susan Jane St Augustines Medical Practice, 4 Station Road, Keynsham, Bristol BS31 2BN Tel: 0117 986 2343 Fax: 0117 986 1176 — (Univ. Coll. Hosp.) MB BS Lond. 1970; MRCS Eng. LRCP Lond. 1970; DA Eng. 1973; DCH Eng. 1975; MRCGP 1977. Prev: Med. Intern Coney Is. Hosp. New York, USA; SHO (Paediat.) Hull Roy. Infirm.; SHO (Cas.) Edgware Gen. Hosp.

WYATT, Suzanne Ty Fry Farm, Llandow, Cowbridge CF71 7NT — MB BCh Wales 1993; BA Oxon.; FFAEM; MRCP.

WYATT, Thomas Andrew Latham House Medical Practice, Sage Cross Street, Melton Mowbray LE13 1NX Tel: 01664 854949 Fax: 01664 501825 — MB ChB Liverp. 1985; MRCGP 1989; Dip. IMC RCS Ed. 1990. Mem. (Vice-Chairm.) Rutland & Leics. Accid. Care Scehem (Affil. to BASICS); Clin. Asst. (Rheum.) Leicester Gen. Hosp. Specialty: Accid. & Emerg.; Rheumatol. Socs: BASICS; Primary Care Rheum. Soc.

WYBORN, Alison Jane Nerina The Gratton Surgery, Sutton Scotney, Winchester SO21 3LE — BM Soton. 1990; DCH RCP Lond. 1993; DFFP 1994; DRCOG 1994; MRCGP 1995. GP Asst. The Grattan Surg. Hants.; GP Asst. Endless St. Surg. Salisbury. Specialty: Gen. Pract. Prev: Trainee GP Nightingale Surg. Romsey Hants.; SHO (Psychiat.) Salisbury; SHO (O & G) St. Mary's Hosp. Portsmouth.

WYBORN, Mary Vinnien Thomson Ivry Street Medical Practice, 5 Ivry Street, Ipswich IP1 3QW Tel: 01473 254718 Fax: 01473 287790 — MB BS Lond. 1971 (St. Mary's) MRCS Eng. LRCP Lond. 1972; DObst RCOG 1973; DA Eng. 1975. Prev: Clin. Asst. (Anaesth.) Huntingdon Co. Hosp.; Regist. (Anaesth.) Addenbrooke's Hosp. Camb.; Regist. (Anaesth.) & SHO Hillingdon Hosp. Uxbridge.

WYBREW, Maria Elizabeth Wentworth Street Surgery, 15 Wentworth Street, Huddersfield HD1 5LJ Tel: 01484 530834; Brook House Farm, Clough Road, Golcar, Huddersfield HD7 4JX — MB ChB Manch. 1985 (Manchester) BSc (Hons.) Manch. 1982; MB ChB (Hons.) Manch. 1985.

WYBREW, Robin Wilfrid James Wentworth Street Surgery, 15 Wentworth Street, Huddersfield HD1 5LJ Tel: 01484 530834; Brook House Farm, Clough Road, Golcar, Huddersfield HD7 4JX — MB ChB Manch. 1983 (Manchester) MRCGP 1988; Dip. Clin. Hypn. (Distinc.) Sheff. 1991.

WYCHERLEY, Christine Rebecca Sidney Powell Avenue Family Health Centre, Sidney Powell Avenue, Westvale, Kirkby, Liverpool L32 0PL Tel: 0151 546 5103 Fax: 0151 547 2729; 1 Tennyson Drive, Billinge, Wigan WN5 7EJ — MB ChB Liverp. 1977.

WYCHRIJ, Oryst Brook Haven, Princess of Wales Hospital, Stourbridge Road, Bromsgrove B61 0BB Tel: 01527 488284 Fax: 01527 488281 — MB ChB Birm. 1975; MRCPsych 1981. Cons. Psychiat. Elderly BromsGr. & Redditch. Specialty: Geriat. Psychiat.; Gen. Psychiat.

WYCLIFFE-JONES, Keith Culduthel Road Surgery, Ardlarich, 15 Culduthel Road, Inverness IV2 4AG Tel: 01463 712233 — MB ChB Ed. 1983; BSc (Med. Sci) 1981; DRCOG 1986; FRCGP 1994, M 1987.

WYCLIFFE-JONES, Stephen Christopher Ashley (retired) 7 Morven Road, Inverness IV2 4BU Tel: 01463 235880 — MB BS Lond. 1949 (St. Mary's)

WYDENBACH, Kirsty Ann Flat 10, Dorset Court, Dorset Street, London W1U 6QX Tel: 020 7224 0929 Email: kwydenbach@yahoo.co.uk — MB BS Lond. 1998 (Imperial Coll.) BSc Lond. 1995; FRCA Lond. 2003. SpR (Anaesthetics) St. Mary's Hosp. Paddington, London. Specialty: Gen. Surg.

WYER, Anthony Ian — MB BS Lond. 1998 (St Bart. & Roy. Lond. Hosp.) BA (1st cl. Hons.) Oxf. Specialty: Gen. Pract.

WYER, Jonathan Francis 23D Bromell's Road, Clapham, London SW4 0BN Tel: 020 7720 6114 — MB BS Lond. 1990. SHO (Paediat.) Qu. Mary Hosp. Childr. Sutton.

WYER, Simon Richard 19 Westlands, Comberton, Cambridge CB3 7EH — MB BCh Wales 1998.

WYETH, Simon Walter Faversham Health Centre, Bank St., Faversham ME13 8QR Tel: 01795 532192; 27 Abbey Street, Faversham ME13 7BE — MB BS Lond. 1983; DRCOG 1985; DCH RCP Lond. 1986; MRCGP 1987.

WYGANOWSKA, Maria Ewa Teresa 13 Squirrels Heath Avenue, Gidea Park, Romford RM2 6AD — LRCPI & LM, LRSCI & LM 1953; LRCPI & LM, LRCSI & LM 1953.

WYKE, Barry Darrell 25 Boundary Road, London NW8 0JE Tel: 020 7624 0491 — MD Sydney 1965; MB BS (Hons.) 1945. Dir. Neurol. Research Unit RCS Eng.; Sen. Lect. Applied Physiol. Inst. Basic Med. Scs. Univ. Lond.; Mem. Bd. Studies in Physiol. Univ. Lond.; Examr. (Physiol.) Exam. Bd. in Eng. Socs: Brain Research Assn. Internat. Assn. Study Pain.; DHSS Working Gp. Back Pain. Prev: Fell. Rockefeller Foundat. 1948; Beit-Memor. Research Fell. 1949-50; Clin. Research Asst. Nuffield Dept. Surg. Oxf. 1949-50.

WYKE, Margaret Elizabeth Watling Vale Medical Centre, Burchard Crescent, Shenley Church End, Milton Keynes MK5 6EY Tel: 01908 501177 Fax: 01908 504916; 7 Rylstone Close, Heelands, Milton Keynes MK13 7QT Tel: 01908 314227 — MB BS Lond. 1978; MRCS Eng. LRCP Lond. 1978; DRCOG 1982. Prev: Trainee GP Bedford VTS; Ho. Off. (Med.) Wexham Pk. Hosp. Slough; Ho. Off. (Surg.) Burton Gen. Hosp.

WYKE, Peter Leonard (retired) Trefynant Hall, Trefynant Park, Acrefair, Wrexham LL14 3SR Tel: 01978 822867; Trefynant Hall, Trefynant Park, Acrefair, Wrexham LL14 3SR Tel: 01978 822867 — MB BS Lond. 1978 (Camb. & Univ. Coll. Hosp.) FIChemE 1996, M 1994, G 1960; FIMechE 1996, M 1962; C Eng 1965; MA Camb. 1978, BA 1974; MFOM RCP Lond. 1993, A 1987; LLM Wales 1993; Spec. Accredit. Occupat. Med. JCHMT 1995. Prev: Sen. Med. Off. (Toxicol.) Imperial Chem. Indust. Ltd. (Chem. Polymers Ltd.).

WYKE, Richard John The Ipswich Hospital, Heath Road, Ipswich IP4 5PD Tel: 01473 712233 — MB BS Lond. 1972 (St. Geo.) AKC; MRCP UK 1975; MD Lond. 1983; FRCP Lond. 1995. Cons. Phys. & Gastroenterol. Ipswich Hosp. Specialty: Gastroenterol. Prev: Sen. Regist. (Gen. Med.) Walsgrave Hosp. Coventry; Research Fell. Liver Unit King's Coll. Hosp. Lond.; Regist. (Gen. Med.) Leeds Gen. Infirm.

WYKES, Catherine Beatrice 27A Canonbury Square, London N1 2AL — MB BS Lond. 1993.

WYKES, Clare Elizabeth 6 Byng Road, Tunbridge Wells TN4 8EJ Tel: 01892536421 Fax: 01892536421 — MB BS Lond. 1998 (LHMC (University of London)) Specialty: Haematology.

WYKES, Emma Louise Clattwm, Trefnant, Denbigh LL16 5UP — BChir Camb. 1996.

WYKES, Kathryn Jane Liverpool Road Health Centre, 9 Mersey Place, Liverpool Road, Luton LU1 1HH Tel: 01582 31321 — MB ChB Liverp. 1989; MRCGP 1993. Trainee GP Wycombe HA VTS.

WYKES, Peter (retired) Beech House Surgery, Beech House, 69 Vale Street, Denbigh LL16 3AY Tel: 01745 812863 Fax: 01745 816574 — MB BS Lond. 1968 (St. Geo.) Prev: Ho. Phys. St. Geo. Hosp. Lond.

WYKES, Peter Revill (retired) The Spire House, New Square, South Horrington, Wells BA5 3LA — MB BS Lond. 1956 (Westm.) MRCS Eng. LRCP Lond. 1956; DA Eng. 1958. Prev: Ho. Surg. (Gyn.) Westm. Hosp.

WYKES, Mr Philip Robert 23 Avon Road, Hale, Altrincham WA15 0LB — MB ChB Bristol 1993; FRCs 1998. Specialist Regist. Orthop. N. W. Rotat. Specialty: Otorhinolaryngol.

WYKES, Richard James Clattwm, Plas Chambers Road, Denbigh LL16 5UP; 32 Gerald Street, Wrexham LL11 1EL — MB BS Lond. 1993; DRCOG 1996. SHO (Gen. Med.) Wrexham; GP Regist.

Wrexham Area. Specialty: Gen. Med. Prev: SHO (Paediat.) Wrexham; SHO Timam, New Zealand; SHO (O & G) Wrexham.

WYKES, Timothy Robert (retired) c/o Mr A.G. Chard, 31 Fernheath Road, Bournemouth BH11 8SF Mob: 0776 5584842 — MRCS Eng. LRCP Lond. 1967 (TC Dub.) MA Dub.; LMCC 1972. Prev: Surg. Chief Off. Roy. Fleet Auxilliary Serv. (Merchant Navy).

WYKES, Mr William Nicholas Ross Hall Hospital, 221 Crookston Road, Glasgow G52 3NQ Tel: 0141 810 3151; 20 Merrylee Road, Newlands, Glasgow G43 2SH — MB ChB Bristol 1976; DO RCS Eng. 1982; FRCS Eng. (Ophth.) 1983; FRCOphth 1988. Cons. Ophth. & Clin. Dir. South. Gen. Hosp. Glas. Specialty: Ophth. Socs: UKISCRS; BOPA; SOC. Prev: Sen. Regist. Univ. Hosp. Wales Cardiff & St. Woolos Hosp. Newport; Regist. Princess Alexandra Eye Pavil. Edin.; SHO (Ophth.) Northampton Gen. Hosp.

WYLD, Lynda Walker Edge Farm, Walker Edge, Bolsterstone, Sheffield S36 4ZA — MB ChB Sheff. 1990; FRCS Eng. 1994; FRCS Ed. 1994. Specialty: Gen. Surg.

WYLDE, Edith Margaret (retired) St. Katharine's House, Ormond Road, Wantage OX12 8EA — MB ChB St. And. 1950; DObst RCOG 1952; DA Eng. 1955. Prev: MO i/c Matern. & child health,Kuala Lumpur.

WYLDES, Michael Peter Birmingham Heartlands Hospital, Bordesley Green East, Birmingham B9 5SS Tel: 0121 424 2000 Fax: 0121 424 3130 Email: michaelwyldes@heartsol.wmids.nhs.uk — MB ChB Leic. 1983; BA Oxf. 1980; MRCOG 1988; FRCOG 1990; MA Oxf. 1992; DAdvObstUltrasound RCR/RCOG 1993. Cons. Obst. & Gynaecologist; Private Obstet. & Gynat. Practice; Clin. Lead for W. Midlands Congen. Register; Director for Midlands Ultrasound and Med. Servs. Specialty: Obst. & Gyn. Socs: Brit. Med. Ultrasound Soc.; BMFMS; BMUS. Prev: Sen. Regist. Manor Hosp. Walsall; Regist. (O & G) Centr. Birm. & S. Birm. Hosps.; Cons. O & G Birm. Heartlands Hosp.

WYLIE, Alan Scott Room F17, Primary Care Trust, Stobhill Hospital, Glasgow Tel: 0141 531 3231 — MB ChB Aberd. 1985; MRCPsych 1990; Dip. Forens. Med. Glas. 1995. Cons. & Hon. Sen. Lect. (Psychiat.) Glas. Community & Ment. Health Care Trust. Specialty: Gen. Psychiat. Socs: Soc. Study Addic. to Alcohol & Other Drugs. Prev: Sen. Regist. & Hon Lect. (Psychiat.) Glas. HB; Assoc. Psychiat. Lond.; Regist. (Psychiat.) Warlingham Pk. Surrey.

WYLIE, Anne Margaret Hunter Health Centre, Andrew Street, East Kilbride, Glasgow G74 1AD Tel: 01355 906676 Fax: 01355 906676; 9 Moor Road, Eaglesham, Glasgow G76 0BA Tel: 01355 303597 — MB ChB Glas. 1990; DRCOG 1993; MRCGP 1994.

WYLIE, Anne Mary North Bar Surgery, 21 North Bar Without, Beverley HU17 7AQ Tel: 01482 882546 — MB ChB Glas. 1976; DRCOG 1978; MRCGP 1980.

WYLIE, Cecilia Elizabeth Community child health, Maple House East Surrey Hospital, Canada Avenue, Redhill RH1 5RH Tel: 01737 768511 Ext: 6872; 72 Hazelwick Road, Crawley RH10 1NH — MB ChB Dundee 1982; DRCOG 1984. SCMO (Child Health) E. Surrey HA Redhill. Specialty: Community Child Health.

WYLIE, Professor Charles Murray 26 Clarence Way, Horley RH6 9GT Tel: 01293 771038; 1607 Dicken Drive, Ann Arbor MI 48103, USA Tel: 00 1 313 769 2632 — (Glas.) MB ChB Glas. 1947; DrPH John Hopkins 1956; MD Glas. 1957; DTM & H Eng. 1958; FFCM RCP (UK) 1972; FFPHM RCP (UK) 1990. Indep. Pract. (Geriat. Med.) Ann Arbor Michigan, USA; Prof. Emerit. Pub. Health Administ. & Prof. Health Gerontol. Univ. Michigan Sch. Pub. Health, Ann Arbor, USA. Specialty: Care of the Elderly. Socs: Fell. Amer. Pub. Health Assn.; Fell. Amer. Geriat. Soc. Prev: Assoc. Prof. Pub. Health Administ. Johns Hopkins Univ. Sch. Hyg. Baltimore, USA; Lt-Cdr. Med. Corps USN Washington, USA.

WYLIE, David Wright (retired) 11 The Highway, Sutton SM2 5QT — (Glas.) BSc (Hons.) Glas. 1946, PhD 1949, MB ChB 1953. Prev: Chairm. & Pres. Europ. Div. Sterling Drug Inc.

WYLIE, Eric Samuel (retired) Blacmoor Hall, Blackmoor Road, Ormskirk L40 2QE Tel: 01704 822240 — MB ChB Liverp. 1954. Prev: Ho. Phys. Clatterbridge Hosp.

WYLIE, Gordon Leonard 3 Calton Road, Lyncombe Hill, Bath BA2 4PP Tel: 01225 429247 — MB ChB Glas. 1949. Socs: BMA. Prev: Surg. Lt.-Cdr. RN; Ho. Surg. West. Infirm. Glas.; Ho. Phys. Roy. Infirm. Worcester.

WYLIE, Graeme Woodland View Surgery, Woodland View, West Rainton, Houghton-le-Spring DH4 6RQ Tel: 0191 584 3809 Fax: 0191 584 9177; 6 Marsham Close, Cleadon Village, Sunderland SR6 7PP Tel: 0191 536 2702 — MB ChB Sheff. 1983; MB ChB (Hons.) Sheff. 1983; BSc Sheff. 1983; Cert. Family Plann. 1987; MRCGP 1987; DRCOG 1987. Aurthur Hall Gold Medal Path. 1981. Prev: Ho. Phys. (Profess. Med. Unit) North. Gen. Hosp. Sheff.; SHO (Gen. Med. Rotat.) Freeman & Newc. Gen. Hosps. Newc. u. Tyne; Trainee GP Northumbria VTS.

WYLIE, Graham Leatham Parexel Lts, River Court, 50 Oxford Road, Denham,, Uxbridge UB9 4 Tel: 01895 23800 Fax: 01304 618299; Red Tiles, Beauchamps Lane, Nonington, Dover CT15 4EZ — MB BS Lond. 1987 (St. Bart. Hosp. Lond.) BSc Lond. 1982. Med. Dir.- Europe N.sea Region. Specialty: Pharmaceutical Medicine. Socs: BMA- Full Mem.; RCM. Prev: Business & Quality Developm. Manager Pfizer Ltd. Sandwich; Clin. Developm. Operat. Manager Pfizer Ltd. Sandwich; Dir. Pfizer Inc. New York.

WYLIE, Mr Ian Gordon The London Imaging Centre, 11 Wimpole St., London W1M 7AB Tel: 020 7580 5255; 44 Cronks Hill Road, Redhill RH1 6LZ Tel: 01737 245990 — MB BS Lond. 1961 (St. Mary's) MRCS Eng. LRCP Lond. 1961; FRCS Ed. 1968; DMRD Eng. 1970; FFR 1972; FRCR 1975. Cons. Radiol. Roy. Lond. Hosp. Specialty: Radiol. Socs: Eur. Soc. Neuroradiol. & Brit. Soc. Neuroradiols. Prev: Ho. Surg. St. Mary's Hosp. Lond.; Regist. (Gen. Surg.) SE Metrop. RHB; Sen. Regist. (Radiodiag.) Lond. Hosp.

WYLIE, Iris Lorraine 38 Derrycreevy Road, Dungannon BT71 6RZ — MB BCh BAO Belf. 1997.

WYLIE, James Pinson Christie Hospital NHS Trust, Wilmslow Road, Manchester M20 4BX Tel: 0161 446 3341 — MB BS Lond. 1990 (St. Thomas's Hospital, London) FRCR; MRCP (UK) 1993. Cons. (Clin. Oncol.) Christie Hosp. Manch. Socs: Connective Tissue Oncology Soc. (CTOS). Prev: SpR (Clin Onco) Christie Hosp.; Clinical Fellow Princes Margaret Hosp. Toronto, Canada; SHO (Clin. Oncol.) Christie Hosp. Manch.

WYLIE, Jennifer Margaret Great Ayton Health Centre, Rosehill, Great Ayton, Middlesbrough — MB BS Lond. 1988. SHO (Accid & Emerg.) Middlesbrough Gen. Hosp. Specialty: Gen. Pract. Prev: Ho. Off. (Surg.) Harrogate Dist. Hosp.; Ho. Off. (Med.) Derbysh. Roy. Infirm.

WYLIE, John Buchanan 10 Southlands, Holmes Chapel, Crewe CW4 7EU Tel: 01477 35787; 10 Southlands, Holmes Chapel, Crewe CW4 7EU Tel: 01477 35787 — MB ChB Glas. 1963; DObst RCOG 1965; DA Eng. 1968; MRCGP 1972. Specialty: Civil Serv.

WYLIE, Judith Haematology Department, Darlington Memorial Hospital, Holyhurst Road, Darlington DL3 6HX Tel: 01325 380100 — MB BS Newc. 1983; MRCP (UK) 1988. Staff Grade (Haemat.) Darlington Memor. Hosp. Specialty: Haematology. Prev: Sen. Regist. (Genitourin. Med.) Sunderland Dist. Gen. Hosp.; Regist. (Haemat. & Gen. Med.) Sunderland Roy. Infirm.

WYLIE, Kevan Richard Porterbrook Clinic, 75 Osborne Road, Nether Edge, Sheffield S11 9BF Tel: 0114 271 8674 Fax: 0114 271 8693 Email: k.r.wylie@sheffield.ac.uk; Royal Hallamshire Hospital, Glossop Road, Sheffield S10 2JF Tel: 0114 271 3334 — MB ChB Liverp. 1985; FRCPsych 2003, M 1989; MMedSc Leeds 1991; MHSM 1992; DFFP 1993; DTC 1993; DSM 1994; MD 1999. Cons. Psychiat. Sheff.; Cons. (Sexual Med./Urol.) Roy. Hallamsh. Hosp. Sheff. Specialty: Gen. Psychiat.; Psychosexual Med.; Urol. Special Interest: Sexual Med. Socs: Inst. Health Servs. Managem.; Soc. for Scientif. Study of Sexuality; Accred. Mem. BASRT. Prev: Sen. Regist. (Psychiat.) Yorks. RHA; Regist. Rotat. (Psychiat.) Leeds; SHO (A & E) Walton Hosp. Liverp.

WYLIE, Lesley Anne — MB ChB Ed. 1988.

WYLIE, Myra (retired) 11 The Highway, Sutton SM2 5QT — (Glas.) BSc Glas. 1949, MB ChB 1954. Prev: Med. Off. Lond. Boro. Sutton.

WYLIE, Paul Gerard 19 Shalloch Park, Doonfoot, Ayr KA7 4HL — MB ChB Dundee 1981; DRCOG 1983; MRCGP 1985; DA (UK) 1991; FFA RCSI 1993. Cons. AnE.hetist, Ayrsh. & Arran Hosp.s. Specialty: Anaesth.; Intens. Care. Socs: Assn. Anaesth.; Glas. & W. Soc. of AnE.hetists; Scott. Intens. Care Soc. Prev: Sen. Regist. (Anaesth.) N. & Yorks. Region.; Regist. Rotat. (Anaesth.) Vict. Infirm. Glas.; GP Hemel Hempstead.

WYLIE, Philip Arthur Lawson 2 West Walks, Dorchester DT1 1RE — MB ChB Bristol 1984; BSc Bristol 1981; MRCP (UK) 1987; DCH RCP Lond. 1987; DTM & H RCP Lond. 1993. Cons. Paediat. Specialty: Paediat.

WYLIE, Robert Daryll Stewart Camps Bay House, Downderry, Torpoint PL11 3LG — MB ChB Aberd. 1984.

WYLIE, Robert Malcolm Church Lane Surgery, 24 Church Lane, Brighouse HD6 1AS Tel: 01484 714349 Fax: 01484 720479 — MB ChB Leeds 1978; DRCOG 1981; MRCGP 1982. Clin. Asst. (Genitourin. Med.) Huddersfield. Specialty: Genitourinary Medicine. Socs: BMA.

WYLIE, Ronald John (retired) flat 6D, Pollokshields Square, Pollokshields, Glasgow G41 4QT Tel: 0141 423 9713 Fax: 0141 423 9713 Email: ron.wylie@btinternet.com — (Glas.) MB ChB Glas. 1957; DObst RCOG 1961; DA RCPSI 1966.

WYLIE, Sandra (retired) 16 Shorelands, Greenisland, Carrickfergus BT38 8FB Tel: 02890 862072 — MB BCh BAO Belf. 1950; FRCGP 1980. Prev: Res. Med. Off. Roy. Vict. Hosp. Belf.

WYLIE, Stewart — MB ChB Glas. 1993. GP in Dumfries, Scotland.

WYLIE, Susan St Margarets Health Centre, St. Margaret's Drive, Auchterarder PH3 1JH Tel: 01764 662614/662275 Fax: 01764 664178 — MB ChB Ed. 1987; DA (UK) 1989; DCH RCPS Glas. 1992; DRCOG 1992; MRCGP 1994. Prev: Trainee GP Alloa; SHO (Anaesth. & Med.) Ashington Gen. Hosp.

WYLLIE, Professor Andrew David Hamilton Department of Pathology, Tennis Court Road, Cambridge CB2 1QP Tel: 01223 333691 Fax: 01223 339067 Email: ahw21@cam.ac.uk — (Aberd.) PhD Aberd. 1975, BSc 1964; MB ChB Aberd. 1967; MRCP (UK) 1971; FRCPath 1987, M 1975; FRSE 1991; FRCP Ed. 1993; FRS 1995; DSc Aberd. 1998. Prof. of Path. & Head of Dept. of Path. Univ. of Camb. Specialty: Histopath. Socs: Path. Soc.; Amer. Assn. Cancer Research; Found. Mem. Acad. Med. Sci. Prev: Head Dept. Path. & Prof. Experim. Path. Univ. Edin.; Research Fell. Cancer Research Campaign; Lect. (Path.) Edin. Univ.

WYLLIE, Anne Margaret 9 Crawford Crescent, Uddingston, Glasgow G71 7DP Tel: 01698 324377 — MB ChB (Hons.) Aberd. 1960; DO Eng. 1963; FRCS Ed. 1966. Cons. Ophth. Lanarksh. Health Bd. Specialty: Ophth. Socs: Scott. Ophth. Club. Prev: Sen. Regist. (Eye) Aberd. Gen. Gp. Hosps.; Lect. (Ophth.) Univ. Manch.

WYLLIE, Brendan Warren (retired) Lower Wythall, Walford, Ross-on-Wye HR9 5SD Tel: 01989 57755 — MB BCh BAO Dub. 1941; BA, MB BCh BAO Dub. 1941. Prev: Med. Off. Matern. & Child Welf. Clinics Rolvenden & Wittersham.

WYLLIE, Miss Frances Jane 12 Glamis Drive, Dundee DD2 1QL Tel: 01382 668700 — MB ChB Ed. 1975; FRCS Ed. 1979. Med. Off. (Plastic Surg.) Ninewells Hosp., Dundee. Specialty: Plastic Surg. Socs: Profess. Assoc. Brit. Assn. Plastic Surgs.; Assoc. Mem. Brit. Soc. Surg. Hand. Prev: Med. Off. (Plastic Surg.) Dundee Roy. Infirm.; Fell. Louisville Hand Surg. Kentucky, USA; Regist. (Plastic Surg.) Bangour Gen. Hosp.

WYLLIE, George Alexander McHarg (retired) Overbeck, 7 Old Godley Lane, Halifax HX3 6XQ Tel: 01422 359692 — (Glas.) MB ChB Glas. 1961; FRCOG 1980, M 1967. Prev: Cons. (O & G) Halifax Gen. Hosp.

WYLLIE, Professor John Hamilton (retired) 10 Seaview Road, Cummingston, Burghead, Elgin IV30 5YU Tel: 01343 835946 Email: jh.wyllie@btinternet.com — MB ChB (Hon.) Aberd. 1957; MD (Hon.) Aberd. 1961; BSc Aberd. 1954; FRCS Eng. 1964; FRCS Ed. 1964. Emerit. Prof. Surgic. Studies Univ. Coll. Lond. Med. Sch. Prev: Hon. Cons. Gen. Surg. Whittington Hosp. & UCL Hosps.

WYLLIE, Jonathan Peter Department of Neonatology, The James Cook University Hospital, Marton Road, Middlesbrough TS4 3BW Tel: 01642 850850; 42 Langbaurgh Road, Hutton Rudby, Yarm TS15 0HL — FRCP; BSc (Hons.) Experim. Immunol. & Oncol. Manch. 1983, MB ChB 1986. Cons. Neonat. The James Cook University Hospital, Middlesbrough. Specialty: Paediat. Socs: FRCP; FRCPCH.

WYMAN, Mr Andrew Northern General Hospital, Herries Road, Sheffield S5 7AU Tel: 0114 226 6985 Fax: 0114 271 4480 — MB ChB Sheff. 1982; FRCS Eng. 1986; MD Sheff. 1992. Cons. Surg. N. Gen. Hosp. Sheff. Specialty: Gen. Surg. Prev: Sen. Regist. (Surg.) Roy. Hallamsh. Hosp. Sheff.; Vis. Lect. (Surg.) Chinese Univ. Hong Kong; Lect. (Surg.) Univ. Sheff. & North. Gen. Hosp. Sheff.

WYMAN, David Anthony Park Lane Surgery, 8 Park Lane, Broxbourne EN10 7NQ; 22 Graham Avenue, Broxbourne EN10 7DP Tel: 01992 443979 — MB BS Lond. 1974 (Westm.) MRCS Eng. LRCP Lond. 1974; DObst RCOG 1976. Clin. Asst. (Diabetes) Qu. Eliz. II Hosp. Welwyn Gdn. City. Specialty: Gen. Pract. Socs: Roy. Soc. Med.

WYNANDS, Roel Wilhelmus Anna Filey Surgery, Station Avenue, Filey YO14 9AE Tel: 01723 515881 Fax: 01723 515197 — Artsexamen Rotterdam 1988.

WYNCOLL, Duncan Lloyd Andrew St Thomas Hospital, Adult Intensive Care, Lambeth Palace Road, London SE1 7EH Tel: 020 7960 5843 Fax: 020 7960 5842 Email: duncan.wyncoll@gstt.sthames.nhs.uk — MB BS Lond. 1989; FRCA 1994; EDIC 1997; DICM 1998. Cons. (Intens. Care) St. Thomas Hosp. Lond. Specialty: Intens. Care. Special Interest: ARDS; Pancreatitis; Severe Sepsis. Socs: Intens. Care Soc.; Europ. Soc. of Intens. Care Med.; Soc. of Critical Care Med. Prev: SHO (Anaesth.) Guy's Hosp. & Lewisham Trust Hosp.; Sen. Regist. Kings Hosp. Liver Unit, Lond.; Sen. Regist. Dept of Anaesth., Guys Hosp. Lond.

WYNDHAM, Jonathan Gabriel 2 Hill Rise, London NW11 6NA — MB BS Lond. 1973 (Westm.) DCH Eng. 1977; MRCP (UK) 1979. Prev: Ho. Phys. Qu. Mary's Hosp. Roehampton; SHO (Clin. Chem. & Haemat.) Northwick Pk. Hosp. Harrow; SHO (Paediat.) St. Stephen's Hosp. Fulham.

WYNDHAM, Michael Trevor Lane End Medical Group, 25 Edgwarebury lane, Edgware HA8 8LJ Tel: 020 8958 4233 Fax: 020 8905 4657 — MB BS Lond. 1978 (Westm.) MRCS Eng. LRCP Lond. 1978; DRCOG 1980; MRCGP 1983. Course Organiser Barnet MTW Hosp. VTS. Prev: Clin. Asst. (Thoracic) Northwick Pk. Hosp. Harrow.

WYNES, Christopher William (retired) Sutton Hill Medical Practice, Maythorne Close, Sutton Hill, Telford TF7 4DH Tel: 01952 586471 Fax: 01952 588029; Field Lane, Kemberton, Shifnal TF11 9LW Tel: 01952 586471 — MB BS Lond. 1965 (King's Coll. Hosp.) MB BS (Hnrs. Med.) Lond. 1965; MRCS Eng. LRCP Lond. 1965. Staff Grade (Psychiatry). Prev: Med. Off. Internat. Grenfell Assn. N.W. River Labrador.

WYNESS, Phyllis Jane 101 Newark Street, Greenock PA16 7TW — MB ChB Aberd. 1969. SHO Larkfield Hosp. Greenock.

WYNFORD-THOMAS, David Wynford Department of Pathology, University of Wales College of Medicine, Cardiff CF14 4XN Tel: 029 2074 2700 — MB BCh Wales 1978; PhD Wales 1982; MRCPath 1987. Prof. Path. Univ. Wales Coll. Med. Cardiff.

WYNICK, David Department of Medicine, Bristol University, Marlborough St., Bristol BS2 8HW Tel: 0117 928 3396 Fax: 0117 928 3976 Email: d.wynick@bris.ac.uk; 19 Old Sneed Park, Bristol BS9 1RG Tel: 0117 928 3396 Fax: 0117 928 3976 Email: d.wynick@bristol.ac.uk — MB BS Lond. 1983 (Middlx.) MRCP (UK) 1986; BSc (Hons.) Lond. 1980, MD 1994; FRCP 1998; PhD 1998. Sen. Lect. & Hon. Cons. Bristol Roy. Infirm.; Hon. Sen. Lect. RPMS. Specialty: Endocrinol. Prev: MRC Clin. Scientist Roy. Postgrad. Med. Sch.; Regist. Rotat. (Med.) Hammersmith Hosp. Lond.; Wellcome Trust Train. Fell. Roy. Postgrad. Med. Sch. Hammersmith Hosp. Lond.

WYNICK, Sarah Pennina Child & Family Department, Tavistock Clinic, 120 Belsize Lane, London NW3 5BA Tel: 020 7435 7111 — MB BS Lond. 1988; BSc Lond. 1985. Cons. (Child & Adolesc. Psychiat.) Tavistock Clinic Lond. Specialty: Child & Adolesc. Psychiat. Prev: Regist. (Psychiat.) Roy. Free Hosp. Train. Sch.; Sen. Reg. Tavistock Clinic.

WYNN-MACKENZIE, David Michael The Shaftesbury Practice, Abbey View Medical Centre, Salisbury Road, Shaftesbury SP7 8DH Tel: 01747 856700 Fax: 01747 856701 Email: david.wynn-mackenzie@gp-j81026.nhs.uk; Tout Hill House, Tout Hill, Shaftesbury SP7 8LX Tel: 01747 854051 Email: david.wynn-mackenzie@talk21.com — MB BS Lond. 1976 (Middlx.) MRCP (UK) 1978; DCH Eng. 1979; DRCOG 1981; MRCGP 1983. Partner & Trainer, Shaftsbury. Specialty: Gen. Pract. Prev: SHO (Med.) Roy. Free Hosp. Lond.; SHO (Paediat.) Middlx. Hosp. Lond.; SHO (Obst.) Centr. Middlx. Hosp. Lond.

WYNN, Gregory Robert Melford Park Farm, Alpheton, Sudbury CO10 9BN Tel: 01284 828747 — MB BS Lond. 1996; BSc (Neuroanat.) Lond. 1992; MRCS Lond. 2000. SpR (Gen. Surg.) South Thames Deanery (NTN). Specialty: Gen. Surg. Socs: MDU; BMA; ASGBI. Prev: SHO Rotat. Kings Lynn.

WYNN, Jeremy Benet 460 Didsbury Road, Heaton Mersey, Stockport SK4 3BT — MB ChB Manch. 1986.

WYNN, John Stephen 41 The Downs, Altrincham WA14 2QG Tel: 0161 928 0611 Fax: 0161 927 9175; Hill Croft, Chelford Road,

Great Warford, Alderley Edge SK9 7TL Tel: 01625 582553 Fax: 01625 582553 — MB ChB Manch. 1975; DCH Eng. 1979; MRCP (UK) 1981; MRCOG 1981; FRCOG 1996; FRCP 1999. Cons. O & G Wythenshawe Hosp. Manch. Specialty: Obst. & Gyn. Socs: N. Eng. Obst. & Gyn. Soc.; Brit. Soc. Gyn. Endoscopy; Sale Med. & Dent. Soc. Prev: Sen. Regist. (O & G) Freedom Fields Hosp. Plymouth; Sen. Regist. (O & G) Groote Schuur Hosp. Cape Town; Regist. (O & G & Neonat. Med.) St. Mary's Hosp. Manch.

WYNN, Marie Dorothy 113 Newland Park, Hull HU5 2DT Tel: 01482 341410 Fax: 01482 341410 — MB ChB Liverp. 1951; DCH Eng. 1955.

WYNN, Michael (retired) 34 Orrok Park, Edinburgh EH16 5UW Tel: 0131 666 1353 — (Aberd.) MB ChB Aberd. 1964. Med. Manager, Med. Servs., Sema Gp., Edin. Prev: GP Edin.

WYNN, Nwe Nwe Willow House, 23 Grosvenor Road, Aldershot GU11 1DL Tel: 01252 350387; 22 Windermere Walk, Heatherside, Camberley GU15 1RP Tel: 01252 505887 — MB BS Med. Inst. (I) Rangoon 1980; MRCPsych 1995. SCMO Gen. Adult Psychiat. Specialty: Gen. Psychiat.

WYNN, Patrick 28 Aberford Road, Bramham, Wetherby LS23 6QN — MB ChB Manch. 1992.

WYNN, Philip Adrian 6 Heatherstones, Queensgate, Halifax HX3 0DH — MB ChB Aberd. 1990.

WYNN, Robert Francis Royal Manchester Children's Hospital, Hospital Way, Manchester M27 4HA Tel: 0161 727 2172 — MB BChir Camb. 1989; MRCP (UK) 1992; MRCPath 1997. Cons. Paediatric Haematologist Roy. Manch. Childr.s Hosp. Specialty: Haematology.

WYNN, Simon Mostyn Hayden 4 Maris Drive, Burton Joyce, Nottingham NG14 5AJ — BM BS Nottm. 1988; BMedSci 1986; MRCGP 1993; MRCP (UK) 1993; DFFP 1994.

WYNN, Professor Victor 21 Redington Road, Hampstead, London NW3 7QX — MB BS Melbourne 1944; MD Melbourne 1953; FRCPath 1967, M 1964; FRCP Lond. 1974, M 1967. Chairm. Wynn Inst. for Metab. Research; Emerit. Prof. Human Metab. Lond. Univ. Socs: Assn. Phys. & Med. Research Soc.; Assn. Path.; Assn. Clin. Biochem. Prev: Prof. Human Metab. Univ. Lond. at St. Mary's Hosp. Lond.; Civil Cons. (Human Metab. & Endocrinol.) RAF & Med. Serv. Brit. Airways; Dir. Alex. Simpson Laborat. Metab. Research St. Mary's Hosp. Med. Sch. Lond.

WYNN-JONES, Dylan Y Gaer Wen, Cae Meta, Llanrug, Caernarfon LL55 3AY Tel: 01248 671925 — MB BS Lond. 1996 (St George's Hospital Medical School) BSc (Hons.) Lond. 1993; MRCP UK 2000. SpR (Radiology) All Wales Higher Train. Scheme. Specialty: Gen. Med. Prev: SHO (Med.) Princess of Wales Hosp. Bridgend.

WYNN-JONES, John Well Street Surgery, Well Street, Montgomery SY15 6PF Tel: 01686 668217 Fax: 01686 668599; The Lions, Lions Bank, Montgomery SY15 6PT Tel: 01686 668569 Fax: 01686 668569 — MB BS Lond. 1975 (Guy's) BSc (Hons.) Lond. 1972; MRCS Eng. LRCP Lond. 1975; DCH Eng. 1978; DRCOG 1978; MRCGP 1979. Clin. Dir. Team TeleMed. Project Powys; CME Tutor N. Powys; Bd. NHS Staff Coll. Wales. Specialty: Ment. Health. Socs: (Sec.) Montgomery Med. Soc.; RCGP (Comm. Mem. Rural Task Force).

WYNN PARRY, Christopher Berkeley, MBE British Association for Performing Arts Medicine, Totara Park House, 34-36 Grays Inn Road, London WC2 Tel: 0845 602 0235; 51 Nassau Road, London SW13 9QG Tel: 020 8748 6288 — BM BCh Oxf. 1947; MA, DM Oxf. 1954, BA 1947; DPhysMed Eng. 1950; FRCP Lond. 1972, M 1959; FRCS Eng. 1978. Cons. Rheum. Brit. Assn. for Permorming & Med. Specialty: Rehabil. Med.; Rheumatol. Socs: Fell. Roy. Soc. Med.; Brit. Soc. Surg. Hand; Brit Assoc. Reum. Prev: Dir. (Rehabil.) King Edw. VII Hosp. Midhurst & Roy. Nat. Orthop. Hosp. Lond.; Gp. Capt. RAF Med. Br.

WYNN-WILLIAMS, David Llewelyn, SBStJ Roper and Partners, Syston Health Centre, Melton Road, Syston, Leicester LE7 2EQ Tel: 0116 260 9111 Fax: 0116 260 9055; Vine House, Chapel St, Syston, Leicester LE7 1GN Tel: 0116 260 8333 — MB BChir Camb. 1963 (Camb. & King's Coll. Hosp.) BA Camb.; DObst RCOG 1964; MRCGP 1974. Socs: BMA; Leic. Med. Soc. Prev: Cas. Off. King's Coll. Hosp. Lond.; SHO Vict. Childr. Hosp. Hull; Clin. Asst. (Med.) LoughBoro. Gen. Hosp.

WYNNE, Afshan c/o Mr K.S. Wynne, South Tyneside District General Hospital, Harton Lane, South Shields NE34 0PL — MB BS Punjab 1982; MRCOG 1994.

WYNNE, Austen Trevor Health Centre, 407 Main Road, Dovercourt, Harwich CO12 4ET Tel: 01255 201299 — MB BS Lond. 1976 (Roy. Free) MRCS Lond. 1976; FRCP Lond. 1976; FRCS Ed. 1981. GP Princip.; Clin. Asst. Orthapaedics, Colchester Dist. Gen. Hosp. Specialty: Gen. Pract.; Orthop.

WYNNE, Catherine Sophia Department of Paediatrics, St James's University Hosital, Beckett St., Leeds LS9 7TF Tel: 0113 243 3144; 25 Woodlea Garth, Meanwood, Leeds LS6 4SG — MB ChB Leeds 1997. Specialty: Paediat.

WYNNE, David McGregor 18 Fettercairn Gardens, Bishopbriggs, Glasgow G64 1AY — MB ChB Glas. 1998.

WYNNE, Hilary Anne Royal Victoria Infirmary, Queen Victoria Road, Newcastle upon Tyne NE1 4LP Tel: 0191 232 5131 — MB BS Lond. 1980; BA Camb. 1977; MRCP (UK) 1983; MD Newc. 1991; FRCP Lond. 1995. Cons. Phys. (Geriat.) Roy. Vict. Infirm. Newc. u. Tyne. Specialty: Care of the Elderly.

WYNNE, Ian Charles Patterdale Lodge Medical Centre, Legh Street, Newton-le-Willows WA12 9NA Tel: 01925 227111 Fax: 01925 290605; 123 Ashton Road, Newton-le-Willows WA12 0AH — MB ChB Bristol 1976; MRCGP 1986.

WYNNE, Jane Margery Clarendon Wing, Leeds General Infirmary, Leeds LS2 9NS Tel: 0113 292 6106 Fax: 0113 392 6219 — (Leeds) MB ChB Leeds 1969; MRCP (UK) 1973; FRCP Lond. 1992. Cons. Community Paediat. Leeds Gen. Infirm. & Hon. Sen. Lect. (Clin. MLeeds. Specialty: Paediat. Prev: Lect. (Child Health & Community Paediat.) Leeds Univ.; Sen. Regist. (Paediat.) Kings Coll. Hosp. Lond. & Roy. Alexandra Hosp.Sick Childr.; Brighton; Regist. (Paediat.) Nottm. City Hosp. & Childr. Hosp. Nottm.

WYNNE, John Stuart Wellington Medical Centre, Bulford, Wellington TA21 8PW Tel: 01823 663551 Fax: 01823 660650; Headweir, Washford, Watchet TA23 0LB Tel: 01984 640743 — MB ChB Leic. 1983 (Leicester) MRCGP 1988. GP Partner Wellington Med. Centre Wellington; Clin. Asst. (Urol.) MusGr. Pk. Hosp. Taunton Som. Specialty: Gen. Pract. Prev: GP S. Ct. Minehed Som.

WYNNE, Mr Kamil Shameen South Tyneside District Hospital, Harton Lane, South Shields NE34 0PL Tel: 0191 202 4014 Fax: 0191 202 4081; 239 Sunderland Road, South Shields NE34 6AL Tel: 0191 455 9827 — MB BS Punjab 1982 (King Edward Medical College Lahore, Pakistan) FRCS Eng.; FRCS Ed. 1987. Cons. Surg. Specialty: Gen. Surg.

WYNNE, Richard Charles Warren Broughton, 14B Fairlands Road, Stourbridge DY8 2DD Tel: 01384 371999 Fax: 01384 371812 — LMSSA Lond. 1970 (Leeds) BSc St. And. 1961; DObst RCOG 1972; FRCGP 1992, M 1974. Benefits Agency Examg. Med. Pract. Med. Servs., Manc.; Private Homeopathic Doctor. Specialty: Homeop. Med.; Disabil. Med. Socs: Assoc. Mem. Fac. Homoeop. Prev: Trainee GP Ipswich VTS; SHO (O & G) Ipswich Gp. Hosps.; Ho. Phys. & Ho. Surg. Pinderfields Hosp. Wakefield.

WYNNE, Ronan D'Arcy 15 White Furrows Cotgrave, Nottingham NG12 3LD — MB BS Newc. 1972; BSc (Hons. Physiol.) Newc. 1969; Dip. Pharm. Med. RCP (UK) 1982; FFPM RCP (UK) 1992. Cons. Pharmaceutical Phys. Specialty: Pharmacology. Prev: Med. Dir. Fujisawa Pharmaceut. Co Ltd Europ. Clin. Research Centre Lond.; Head of Clin. Pharmacol. Knoll Pharmaceut. Nottm.; Hon. Clin. Asst. (CVS Med.) Univ. Hosp. Nottm.

WYNNE, Sian Philippa Morgan 29 Elm Drive, Wirral CH49 3NP — MB ChB Birm. 1991; BSc Birm. (Pharm.) 1988, MB ChB (Hons.) 1991; MRCP (UK) 1994. Trainee GP/SHO (Med.) Merseyside VTS.

WYNNE-DAVIES, Ruth (retired) 2 Dale Close, St. Ebbe's, Oxford OX1 1TU Tel: 01865 727525 Email: ruth.wynne-davies@doctors.org.uk — MB BS Lond. 1953 (Roy. Free) MA Oxon. 2003; FRCS Eng. 1960; PhD Ed. 1973. Hon. Cons. Med. Genetics Churchill Hosp. Oxf. Prev: Reader (Orthop.) Genetics Research Univ. Edin.

WYNNE EVANS, Barbara Karyn Caeherbert Lane Surgery, Caeherbert Lane, Rhayader LD6 5ED Tel: 01597 810231 Fax: 01597 811080; Bryn Llewenydd, Rhayader LD6 5LT Tel: 01597 810313 — MB ChB Liverp. 1969. Prev: Ho. Phys. & Ho. Surg. Wrexham, Powys & Mawddach Gp. Hosps.; Med. Off. (Gen. Duties) Anglo-Amer. Co. Kitwe, Zambia.

WYNNE-JONES, Geraint Rhoslan Surgery, 4 Pwllycrochan Avenue, Colwyn Bay LL29 7DA Tel: 01492 532125 Fax: 01492 530662 Email: geraint.wynne-jones@gp-w91031.wales.nhs.uk — MB ChB Liverp. 1980 (Liverpool) DRCOG 1984. Specialty: Gen. Pract.

WYNNE-JONES, Guy Alexander Flat 2, 144 Kennington Lane, London SE11 4UZ Email: guy.wynne-jones@virgin.net — MB BS Lond. 1993; PhD Lond. 1990; FRCS 1998.

WYNNE-JONES, Melanie Louise Marple Medical Practice, 50 Stockport Road, Marple, Stockport SK6 6AB Tel: 0161 426 0299 Fax: 0161 427 8112 — MB ChB Manch. 1978; DRCOG 1982; MRCGP 1991. Freelance Med. Jl.ist Chesh.; GP Trainer. Prev: GP Gatley & Runcorn.

WYNNE-ROBERTS, Caroline Rosales Seager Morgan c/o Lloyds Bank, Victoria House, Southampton Row, London WC1B 5HR — MB BS Lond. 1961 (Roy. Free) LMSSA Lond. 1960. Socs: Amer. Rheum. Assn.; New York Acad. Sci. Prev: Assoc. Prof. (Rheum.) South. Illinois Univ. Sch. Med. Springfield; Staff Phys. & Rheumatol. Veterans Admin. Hosp. Pittsburgh; Chief, Electron Microscopy Unit Veterans Admin. Hosp. Pittsburgh.

WYNNE-SIMMONS, Anne Penelope Mary Old Hall, Stiffkey, Wells-next-the-Sea NR23 1QJ Tel: 01328 830161; 148 Harley Street, London W1G 7LG Tel: 020 7935 1207/020 7935 1900 — MB BS Lond. 1971 (Roy. Free) MRCS Eng. LRCP Lond. 1971; DCH Eng. 1973; MRCGP 1979; MFHom RCP Lond. 1985. Homoeop. Phys. Lond. Specialty: Homeop. Med.

WYNNE-WILLIAMS, Hilary Victoria 18 Tyler Court, Shepshed, Loughborough LE12 9SJ — MB BS Lond. 1968; MRCS Eng. LRCP Lond. 1968. Prev: SHO (Obst.) Univ. Coll. Hosp. Lond.

WYNROE, John Christopher Nab Top Farm, Dale Road, Marple, Stockport SK6 6NL — BM Soton. 1994.

WYNROE, Susan Iris Romiley Health Centre, Chichester Road, Romiley, Stockport SK6 4QR Tel: 0161 430 2573 Fax: 0161 406 7237; Nab Top Farm, Dale Road, Marple, Stockport SK6 6NL Tel: 0161 427 6569 — MB ChB Manch. 1966; DObst RCOG 1969; DA Eng. 1970; MRCGP 1978. Socs: BMA. Prev: Regist. (Anaesth.) Crumpsall Hosp. Manch.

WYNTER, Meriel Jennifer Claire Otford Medical Practice, Leonard Avenue, Otford, Sevenoaks TN14 5RB Tel: 01959 524633 Fax: 01959 525086; The Gables, 41 Zion St, Seal, Sevenoaks TN15 0BD — MB ChB Dundee 1988; DCH RCP Lond. 1991; DRCOG 1992. Socs: Med. & Dent. Defence Union Scotl.

WYON, Agnes May (retired) Ford Cottage, Thirlby, Thirsk YO7 2DJ Tel: 01845 597466 — MB ChB Leeds 1937; DObst. RCOG 1938. Prev: Med. Off. (Family Plann. & Child Welf.) N. Yorks. AHA.

WYPER, John Forrester Brown (retired) Stable End, Blackhills, Leochel-Cushnie, Alford AB33 8LQ Tel: 01339 883468 — MB ChB Glas. 1938; BSc. Glas. 1935, MB ChB 1938; FRCOG 1957, M 1942. Prev: Cons. Gynaecol. & Obstetr. Grampian Health Bd.

WYSE, Colin Terris (retired) Seaholme, Chapel Green Road, Earlsferry, Leven KY9 1AD — MB ChB St. And. 1951.

WYSE, Matthew Kevin Walsgrave NHS Trust, Clifford Bridle Road, Coventry CV2 2DX Tel: 024 76 538952 — MB BS Newc. 1990; FRCA 1995. Cons. anaesth. Walsgrave Hosp. Coventry. Specialty: Anaesth. Socs: BASICS.

WYSE, Sheena Dobson Chubbs Farm, Pound Lane, Burley, Ringwood BH24 4EF Tel: 01425 402298 — MB ChB Manch. 1967; FFA RCS Eng. 1972. Specialty: Anaesth. Prev: Cons. Anaesth. Groote Schuur Hosp. Cape Town, S. Afr.; Regist. (Anaesth.) Brompton Hosp. Lond. & Univ. Coll. Hosp. Lond.

WYTHE, Paul County Practice, Barking Road, Needham Market, Ipswich IP6 8EZ Tel: 01449 720666 Fax: 01449 720030 — MB ChB Liverp. 1974; DTM & H Liverp 1994.

WYTHERS, Deborah Jayne 25 St Mary's Road, Tickhill, Doncaster DN11 9NA Tel: 01302 742503 Fax: 01302 752293; 120 Broom Road, Rotherham S60 2SU Tel: 01709 375947 Email: deborah.wythers@virgin.net — BM BS Nottm. 1992; MRCGP 1996.

XAVIER, Alfredo Bruno College Street Surgery, College Street, Southampton SO14 3EJ Tel: 023 8033 3729 Fax: 023 8022 7233; Xaviers, Canada Road, West Wellow, Romsey SO51 6DE — MB ChB Leeds 1970 (Univ. Leeds) BSc (Hons.) Lond. 1963; MRCS Eng. LRCP Lond. 1970. Prev: Regist. (Gen. Med.) Dorset Co. Hosp. Dorchester; SHO St. Mary's Hosp. Leeds; Ho. Off. (Med., Neurol. & Surg.) Chapel Allerton Hosp. Leeds.

XAVIER, Patrick Lloyd Culbert (retired) 24 Cherry Gardens, Billericay CM12 0HA Email: xaps@aol.com — MB BS Lond. 1970 (Westm.) BSc (Physiol., Hons.) Lond. 1967; FRCR 1981. Prev: Cons. Oncol. and Radiother. OldCh. Hosp. Romford.

XAVIER, Richard James Harrison (retired) Birnam Lodge, Nursey Road, Loughton IG10 4EF Tel: 020 8508 1393 — MRCS Eng. LRCP Lond. 1952 (St. Bart. & W. Lond.)

XAVIER, Stephanie Christine Yvonne Sita (retired) 3 Woodland Place, Hemel Hempstead HP1 1RD — MB BS Ceylon 1964 (Colombo) Prev: Clin. Asst. (Histopath.) Hemel Hempstead Gen. Hosp.

XAVIER, Surahi Marisha St Lukes Surgery, Warren Rd, Guildford GU1 3JH Tel: 01483 572364 — MB BS Lond. 1993 (UMDS (United Medical & Dental Schools of Guy's & St. Thomas) DRCOG 1998; DFFP 1998; MRCGP 1999. Three quarter time Princip. in Gen. Pract. Prev: Clin. Asst., Genito-Urin. Med., Farnham Rd Hosp., Guildford, Surrey.

XENITIDIS, Kiriakos Department of Psychological Medicine, Institute of Psychiatry, De Crespigny Park, London SE5 8AF Tel: 020 7740 5287 Fax: 020 7701 9044 — Ptychio Iatrikes Athens 1984; MRCPsych 1993; MSc Univ. Lond. 1995. Cons. Psychiat. Hon. Sen. Lect. Specialty: Gen. Psychiat. Prev: Sen. Regist. Maudsley & Guys NHS Trusts; Regist. & SHO (Psychiat.) Univ. Edin.; Research Fell. & Hon. Sen. Regist. (Psychiat.) Inst. Psychiat. Lond.

XENOPHOU, Xenakis c/o Mr Filshie's Secretary, B Floor East Block, Queen's Medical Centre, Nottingham NG7 2UH — MB BS Adelaide 1986.

XERRI, Salvino Bridge Medical Centre, Wassand Close, Three Bridges Road, Crawley RH10 1LL Tel: 01293 527 114 Fax: 01293 553560; 10 Trinity Close, Pound Hill, Crawley RH10 3TN Tel: 01293 883910 — MD Malta 1976 (Roy. Univ. Malta)

XIFARAS, George Paul 58 Purnells Way, Knowle, Solihull B93 9EE Tel: 0156 453977 — Med. Dipl. Univ. Athens 1961; MRCS Eng. LRCP Lond. 1969; FFA RCS Eng. 1969. Cons. Anaesth. W. Birm. Gp. Hosps. Specialty: Anaesth. Prev: Sen. Regist. Anaesth. Birm. United Hosps. & Birm. RHB; Regist. Anaesth. & SHO Anaesth. Aberd. Teachg. Hosps.

XUEREB, John Henry Division of Molecular Histopathology, Box 231, John Bonnett Clinical Laboratories (Level 3), Addenbrooke's Hospital, Hills Road, Cambridge CB2 2QQ Tel: 01223 762607 Fax: 01223 762610 Email: jhx1000@cam.ac.uk; 1 Capstan Close, Cambridge CB4 1BJ Tel: 01223 522762 — MRCS Eng. LRCP Lond. 1977 (Roy. Univ. Malta) MRCP (UK) 1981; MD Malta 1984; MRCPath 1990; MD Newc. 1990; T(Path) 1991; MA Camb. 1994; FRCPath 1999. Sen. Lect. (Path.) Univ. Camb. & Cons. (Neuropath.) Addenbrooke's Hosp. Camb.; Fell. and Dean St Catharine's Coll. Camb. Specialty: Neuropath. Special Interest: Neurodegenerative Disorders. Socs: Fell. Roy. Soc. of Med.; Brit. NeuroPath. Soc.; Internat. Soc. of Neuropath. Prev: Sen. Regist. (Neuropath.) Addenbrooke's Hosp. Camb.; Regist. (Neuropath. & Neurol.) Region. Neurol. Centre Newc. Gen. Hosp.; Regist. Profess. Med. Unit Manch. Roy. Infirm.

YAAKUB, Roselina 38 Housefield, Willesborough, Ashford TN24 0AF — MB ChB Liverp. 1988.

YACOB, Zuhair Matti Colliers Wood Surgery, 58 High Street Colliers Wood, London SW19 2BY Tel: 020 8540 6303 — MB ChB Baghdad 1972.

YACOUB, Sophie Flat 10, Arundel House, 21 Lawn Road, Portswood, Southampton SO17 2ER — BM Soton. 1998.

YADAV, Anupam 25 Winchester Close, Woolton, Liverpool L25 7YD — MB ChB Manch. 1996.

YADAV, Desh Gaurav Sheffield Road Surgery, 170A Sheffield Road, Barnsley S70 4NW Tel: 01226 293232 Fax: 01226 280432 — MB BS Patna 1960. GP Barnsley, S. Yorks.

YADAV, Hans Raj The Surgery, 192 Tudor Drive, Kingston upon Thames KT2 5QH Tel: 020 85490061 Fax: 020 8549 9488 — MB BS Delhi 1964 (Maulana Azad Med. Coll.) Socs: BMA. Asst. Surg. Grade I Ordnance Factories, India.

YADAV, Jai Kant Earle Road Medical Centre, 131 Earle Road, Liverpool L7 6HD Tel: 0151 733 5538 Fax: 0151 733 6914 — MB BS Ranchi 1975.

YADAV, Mr Shambhu Narayan Lorn & Island District General Hospital, Glengallan Road, Oban PA34 4HH Tel: 01631 567500 Fax: 01631 567133 — MB BS Bihar 1972; MS Bihar 1975; FRCS

Glas. 1980. Cons. Surg. (Gen. Surg.) Lorn & Is.s Dist. Gen. Hosp. Oban. Specialty: Gen. Surg. Socs: Assn. Surg.; W Scotl. Surgs. Assn. Prev: Lect. (Surg.) Univ. Papua, New Guinea.

YADAV, Surinder Singh 5 Britland Close, Barnsley S75 2JP — MB ChB Liverp. 1994.

YADAVA, Rajendra Prasad Merton Surgery, Merton Street, Longton, Stoke-on-Trent ST3 1LG Tel: 01782 322966 Fax: 01782 322914 — MB BS Patna 1964 (P. of Wales Med. Coll.) DTM & H Eng. 1967; DCH RCPS Glas. 1972; MFFP 1995; FRCGP 1997. Specialty: Gen. Pract.; Family Plann. & Reproduc. Health.

YADEGAR, Mr John 2 Linnet Close, Bushey, Watford WD23 1AX — MB BS Lond. 1991; FRCS Eng. 1995; FRCSI 1995. SHO (Transpl. Surg.) Addenbrooke's Hosp. Camb.

YAGER, Robert Stewart (retired) 19 Vicarage Gardens, Scunthorpe DN15 7BA Tel: 01724 856378 — MB BS Durh. 1948.

YAGER, Thomas Andrew Bridge House, Bury Road, Rickinghall, Diss IP22 1EJ Tel: 01379 890233 — MB BS Lond. 1982; DRCOG 1985; MRCGP 1988; MA (Philosophy of Healthcare) Wales 1994.

YAGHAN, Mr Rami Jalal Kalajari 2/2, 16 Blantyre Street, Glasgow G3 8AP — MB BS Jordan 1986; FRCSI 1992.

YAGNIK, Romesh Dayashanker 356 James Reckitt Avenue, Hull HU8 0JA Tel: 01482 796121 — MB BS 1966 (B.J. Medical College Ahmedabad (GUJ) India) FRCS (Ed.) 1970; (ECFMG) USA 1971; MD USA 1971. GP Princip. (full time '74); Vasectomist, Minor Surg,. I/A Pericuticular Surg. (on contract NHS). Prev: Urol. & Vasc. Surg. '72-'74, Ahmedabad (GUJ) India.

YAGOUB, Sobhi Mill View Hospital, Nevill Avenue, Hove BN3 7HZ Tel: 01273 696011 — MB ChB Tanta 1983; DPM Dub. 1997; MSc Lond. 1999; DIC Lond. 1999. Cons. (Psychiat.) Mill View Hosp. Hove. Specialty: Gen. Psychiat.; Geriat. Psychiat.

YAHIA, Abdalla Osman Dorothy Pattison Hospital, Alumwell Close, Walsall WS2 9XH Tel: 01922 858000 Fax: 01922 858085; 415 Birmingham Road, Walsall WS5 3NT Tel: 01922 648456 Fax: 01922 648456 — MB BS Khartoum 1978 (Khartoum University, Sudan) DPM RCPSI 1989; MRCPsych. 1992. Cons. (Psychiat.) Walsall Community Health NHS Trust W. Midl.s. Specialty: Gen. Psychiat.; Geriat. Psychiat. Prev: Sen. Regist. Rotat. NE Thames; Regist. (Psychiat.) St. Matthew's Hosp. Burntwood Walsall; Regist. & SHO (Psychiat.) St. Clement's Hosp. Ipswich.

YAHYA, Anwar Eaglestone Health Centre, Standing Way, Eaglestone, Milton Keynes MK6 5AZ Tel: 01908 679111 Fax: 01908 230601 — MB BS Lucknow 1966.

YAKELEY, Jessica Wood The Maudsley Hospital, Psychotherapy Unit, Denmark Hill, London SE5 8AZ Tel: 020 7919 2385/020 7919 2514 — MB BChir Camb. 1990 (Univ. Camb. Trinity Coll. & Univ. Coll. Middlx. Sch. Med.) MA Camb. 1990; MRCP (UK) 1993; MRCPsych 1996. Specialist Regist. (Psychother.) Maudsley Hosp. Lond.; Assoc. Mem. of Brit. Psychoanalytic Soc. Specialty: Psychother. Prev: Regist. Rotat. (Psychiat.) Maudsley Hosp. Lond.; SHO Rotat. (Psychiat.) Maudsley Hosp. Lond.; SHO Rotat. (Neurol. & Med.) Roy. Free Hosp. Lond.

YAKUBO, Mr Alkassim Dept. of Urol., Burnley General Hospital, Burnley Tel: 01282 474 442 Email: yakubu@aol.com — MB BS Ahmadu Bello U 1981; FMCS (Nig) 1989; FRCS (Edin.) 1991; Dip. Urol. (Lond.) 1997; FRCS Urol. 2001. Cons. Urol., Burnley Gen. Hosp. Specialty: Urol. Special Interest: Oncology. Socs: British medical Association; Brit. Assn. of Urol. Surg. Prev: Specialstist Regist., N.. Irel.; Specialist Regist., Bournemouth Roy.

YALE, Christopher Ipswitch Hospital NHS Trust, Department of Child Health, Hath Road, Ipswich IP4 5PD Tel: 01473 702176 Email: chris.yale@ipsh-tr.anglox.nhs.uk — MB BS Lond. 1985; BA (1st cl. Hons.) Camb. 1982; MRCPCH 1991. Cons. Paediat. Ipswich Hosp. NHS Trust. Specialty: Paediat. Prev: Sen. Regist. (Paediat. Rheum.) Gt. Ormond St. Hosp.; Sen. Regist. (Paediat.) Watford Gen. Hosp.; Regist. (Paediat.) Northwick Pk. Hosp.

YALE, Vijaydev 104 Sudbury Court Road, Harrow HA1 3SQ Tel: 020 8904 2937 — MB BS Bangalore 1974; DLO RCS Eng. 1986. Specialty: Otorhinolaryngol.

YALLOP, Deborah 4 Old Hall Close, Trowse, Norwich NR14 8TB — MB BS Lond. 1998.

YAM, Tat Shing 2 Greenvale, Dunmurry, Belfast BT17 9LR — MB BCh BAO Belf. 1994.

YAMEY, Gavin Mark 56B Market Place, London NW11 6JP — MB BS Lond. 1994.

YAMIN-ALI, Richard Glenn 60 Baronscourt Road, Carryduff, Belfast BT8 8BQ Tel: 01232 814803 — MB BCh BAO Belf. 1992; FFARCSI 1997. Specialty: Anaesth.

YAN, Christopher 216 Widney Manor Road, Solihull B91 3JW — MB ChB Aberd. 1998.

YAN AUNG, Dr 4 Deepdale, Leigh WN7 3EG — MB BS Med. Inst. (I) Rangoon 1972.

YANAH, Mr David Kwame 134 Grove Road, London E17 9BY — MB BS Durh. 1967 (Newc.) FRCS Ed. 1977; FRCS Eng. 1979. Regist. (Gen. Surg.) St. And. Hosp. Lond. Specialty: Gen. Surg. Prev: SHO (Orthop.) Blackburn Roy. Infirm. & Whipps Cross Hosp. Lond.; SHO (Surg.) Hull Roy. Infirm.

YANDELL, Caroline Jane 8 Breach Road, Bristol BS3 2BD — MB ChB Bristol 1997.

YANEZ PEREZ, Leopoldo Manuel (retired) Eldene Health Centre, Eldene, Swindon SN3 3RZ Tel: 01793 22710 — LRCP LRCS Ed. 1961 (W. Lond.)

YANNEY, Michael Peter 32 Fitch Court, Laburnum Road, Mitcham CR4 2ND — MB BS Lond. 1993.

YANNI, Mr Dimitri Hassan c/o Bromely Hospital, Cromwell Hospital, Bromley BR2 9AJ Tel: 0208 687442 — MB BS Lond. 1983 (Guy's) FRCS Ed. 1987; FRCS Eng. 1988; FRCS (Orth.) 1992. Cons. (Orthop. & Hand Surg.) Bromely Hositals NHS Trust. Specialty: Orthop. Socs: Fell. Roy. Soc. Med.; Fell. Brit. Elbow & Shoulder Soc. Prev: Sen. Regist. (Orthop. Surg.) SE Thames Train Progr.; Sen. Regist. Cappagh Orthop. Hosp. Dub.; Fell. (Hand Surg.) Pulvertaft Hand Centre Derbysh. Roy. Infirm.

YANNI, Mr George Armia Wellhouse NHS Trust, Barnet General Hospital, Wellhouse Lane, Barnet EN5 3DJ Tel: 020 8440 5111; 16 Holmstall Avenue, Edgware HA8 5JH Tel: 020 8205 2410 — MB BS Khartoum 1980; FRCS Ed. 1991. Regist. (Surg.) Barnet Gen. Hosp. Herts. Specialty: Gen. Surg. Prev: Regist. (Surg.) Edgware Gen., Univ. Coll. & Middlx. Hosps. Lond.

YANNI, Ghada 55 Avondale Road, Bromley BR1 4HS — MD NUI 1991; MB BCh BAO 1984; LRCPI & LM, LRCSI & LM 1984; MRCPI 1986. Sen. Regist. (Rheum. & Gen. Med.) Guy's Hosp. Lond. Specialty: Gen. Med. Prev: Research Lect. (Rheum.) Univ. Coll. Dub.; Regist. (Rheum. & Gen. Med.) Beaumont Hosp. Dub.; SHO Rotat. (Med.) St. Laurence's Hosp.

YANNI, Mr Omar Nicolas William Harvey Hospital, Ashford TN24 0L — MB BS Lond. 1989; FRCS Ed. 1993.

YANNY, Laila Boshra Lister House, 473 Dunstable Road, Luton LU4 8DG Tel: 01582 571565 Fax: 01582 582074 — MB BCh Cairo 1972.

YANNY, Wasfy Albert St Albans City Hospital, Normandy Road, St Albans AL3 5PN Tel: 01727 866122 Fax: 01582 461210 — MB BCh Cairo 1969 (Kasr EL Aini) DA Ireland 1975; FFARCSI Ireland 1980. p/t Cons. (Anaesth.) W. Herts NHS Trust. Specialty: Anaesth. Special Interest: Intens. Care Med. Socs: Roy. Soc. of Med., Lond.; Roy. Coll. of Anaesthetics, Irel.; B.M. Association/HCSA. Prev: Sen. Regist. (Anaesth.) Qu. Eliz. Hosp. Birm.; Sen. Regist. (Anaesth.) The Middlx. Hosp. Lond.

YAP, Beng Khiong 11 Kerscott Road, Manchester M23 0GD — MB ChB Dundee 1992.

YAP, Mr John Yin Ming Royal Brompton Hospital, Sydney St., London SW3 6NP Tel: 020 7352 8121 — MB ChB Glas. 1986 (Glasgow) FRCS Glas. 1991; MD (Glas) 1999. Specialist Regist. Cardiothoraric Surg., Roy.Brompton Hosp., Lond. Specialty: Cardiothoracic Surg. Socs: BMA; RCSP (Glas.).

YAP, Lok Bin 91 Ravenshaw Street, London NW6 1NP — BM BS Nottm. 1998.

YAP, Peng Lee Edinburgh & SE Scotland Blood Transfusion Service, The New Royal Infirmary of Edinburgh, 51 Little France Crescent, Edinburgh EH16 4SA Tel: 0131 242 7526 Fax: 0131 242 7514 — MB ChB Ed. 1974; BSc (Hons.) Ed. 1971, MB ChB 1974; FRCPath 1993, M 1980; PhD CNAA 1980; FRCP Ed. 1994. Cons. Blood Transfus. & Immunol. Edin. & SE Scotl. Blood Transfus. Centre; Sen. Lect. Univ. Edin. Specialty: Immunol.; Blood Transfus. Prev: Roy. Soc. Med. Foundat. Vis. Prof.; MRC Clin. Research Fell. 1976-79.

YAP, Soong Loy Maypole Health Centre, 10 Sladepool Farm Road, Kings Heath, Birmingham B14 5DJ Tel: 0121 430 2829 Fax: 0121 430 6211; 77 Hay Lane, Shirley, Solihull B90 4TZ Tel: 0121 745 9244 Fax: 0121 745 9244 — MB ChB Dundee 1987. Specialty:

Acupunc.; Diabetes. Prev: Trainee GP/SHO (Gen. Med.) Walsgrave Gen. Hosp. Coventry VTS; Ho. Off. (Gen. Med. & Surg.) & SHO (ENT & Psychiat.) Walsgrave Hosp. Coventry.

YAP, Sue Ching 25 Abbey Road, Beeston, Nottingham NG9 2QF — BM BS Nottm. 1998.

YAP, Yee Guan 36 Fitzroy Crescent, Chiswick Place, Chiswick, London W4 3EL — BM BS Nottm. 1992 (Univ. Nottm. Med. Sch.) BMedSci (Hons.) Nottm. 1990; MRCP (UK) 1996. Brit. Heart Foundat. Research Fell. (Cardiol.) St Geo.'s Hosp. Med. Sch. Lond. Specialty: Cardiol. Socs: Fell. Roy. Soc. Med. Prev: Clin. Research Fell. (Cardiol.) St. Geo. Hosp. Med. Sch. Lond.; SHO (Gen. Med.) St. Geo. Hosp. Lond.; SHO (Neurol.) Atkinson Morley Hosp. Lond.

YAPANIS, Michael 7 Heddon Road, Barnet EN4 9LD — MB ChB Ed. 1991.

YAPP, Julia Anita 3 Snowdrop Valley, Crich, Matlock DE4 5BT — MB BS Lond. 1991; DRCOG 1993.

YAPP, Julie Kencot Lodge, Kencot, Lechlade GL7 3QX; 37 Brook St, Winsor, Brisbane, Queensland 4030, Australia Tel: 07 3861 1585 — MB BCh Wales 1988 (Cardiff) DCH RCP Lond. 1992; DRCOG RCOG 1993; MRCGP RCGP 1995.

YAPP, Paula Anthea 191 Monmouth Road, London N9 0LE; 11 Spellbrooke, Hitchin SG5 2NB Tel: 01462 627788 — MB BS Lond. 1992; DRCOG 1996. Phys. (Drug Safety) Roche Products Welwyn Garden City. Specialty: Gen. Pract. Socs: Med. Sickness Soc. Prev: GP Locum; GP Regist. N. Finchley; SHO (Paediat.) VTS Barnet.

YAPP, Thomas Rowland Princess of Wales Hospital, Coity Road, Bridgend CF31 1RQ Tel: 01656 752487 Fax: 01656 752487 Email: tom.yapp@bromor-tr.wales.nhs.uk — MB BCh Wales 1988 (Cardiff) FRCP (UK). Cons. Gastroenterologist/ GP Princess of Wales Hosp. Bridgend, Wales. Specialty: Gastroenterol. Socs: Brit. Soc. of Gastroenterol.; BMA. Prev: Cons. gastroenterologist / Gen. Phys., Roy. Gwent Hosp. Newport 2000-2003.

YAQOOB, Mohammed Ali 27 Neville Street, Cardiff CF11 6LP — MB BCh Wales 1992.

YAQOOB, Mohmad Eaton Place, 47 White Elme Road, Danbury, Chelmsford CM3 4LR — MB BS Bombay 1973; FRSH 1983.

YAQOOB, Najma 54 Station Road, Birmingham B14 7SR — MB ChB Birm. 1991. SHO (Med.) Dudley HA.

YAQOOB, Rabia GP Direct, 5/7 Welback Road, West Harrow, Harrow HA2 0RH Tel: 020 8515 9300 Fax: 020 8515 9300; 33 Kingsway, Wembly Park, Wembley, London HA9 7QP — MB BS Lond. 1991 (Univ. Coll. & Middlx. Sch. Med. Lond.) DFFP 1994; DCH RCP Lond. 1995; DRCOG 1996; MRCGP 1998. GP Princip. GP Direct. Prev: SHO (O & G) Chase Farm Hosp. Enfield; SHO (Paediat.) Chase Farm Hosp. Trust Enfield; SHO (A & E) WellHo. Trust Barnet Gen. Hosp.

YAQUB, Mohmad The Health Centre, Cliffe Road, Brampton, Barnsley S73 0XP Tel: 01226 753321 Fax: 01226 753321 — MB BS Jammu & Kashmir 1968.

YAQUB, Sami Ullah 18 Malford Grove, London E18 2DX — MB BS Lond. 1990.

YAQUB, Zia Ullah 18 Malford Grove, London E18 2DX — MB BS Lond. 1997.

YAR KHAN, Sayeed Afridi The Rooms, Elemran, Aston Lane Shardlow, Derby DE72 2GX Tel: 01332 792871 Fax: 01332 799946 Email: humkalam@aol.com; Elemran, 5 Aston Lane, Shardlow, Derby DE72 2GX Tel: 01332 792871 Fax: 01332 792871 — MB BS Punjab 1956 (King Edwd. Med. Coll.) BSc Bombay 1949; MS Punjab 1962; DPM Eng. 1972; MRCPsych Eng. 1973; T(Psychiat.) 1991. Indep. Cons. Derby; Unit Med. Represen. to Gen. Managem. Team. Specialty: Forens. Psychiat. Socs: BMA. Prev: Cons. Psychiat. Aston Hall Hosp. Aston-on-Trent; Regist. & SHO (Psychiat.) Severalls Hosp. Colchester; Sen. Regist. Roy. East. Co. Gp. Hosps. Essex.

YARDLEY, Denis Noel Alma Road Surgery, 68 Alma Road, Portswood, Southampton SO14 6UX Tel: 023 8067 2666 Fax: 023 8055 0972 — MB ChB Liverp. 1967. Specialty: Gen. Pract.

YARDLEY, Mr Mark Peter John ENT Department, Royal Hallamshire Hospital, Glossop Road, Sheffield S10 2JF — MB BCh Wales 1984; FRCS Ed. 1989; MPhil Sheff 1996. Cons. (ENT) Roy. Hall Hosp. Sheff.; Cons. (ENT) Sheff. childr.'s Hosp.; Hon. Lect. Univ. Sheff. Specialty: Otolaryngol.

YARDLEY, Michael Hilton Lyngford Park Surgery, Fletcher Close, Taunton TA2 8SQ Tel: 01823 333355 Fax: 01823 257022; 27 Avon Close, Taunton TA1 4SU Tel: 01823 275726 — BM BCh Oxf. 1972 (Oxford) MA Oxf. 1982, BA 1969; MRCGP 1980; DRCOG 1981; DLO RCS Eng. 1982; DFFP 1994. Hon. Med. Off. W. Som. Railway. Specialty: Gen. Pract. Prev: Trainee GP Taunton VTS; SHO (ENT) MusGr. Pk. Hosp. Taunton; Med. Off. St. Lucy's Hosp. Tsolo Transkei.

YARDLEY, Ralph Andrew Castle Mead Medical Centre, Hill Street, Hinckley LE10 1DS Tel: 01455 637659 Fax: 01455 238754; 32 Winchester Drive, Burbage, Hinckley LE10 2BB Tel: 01455 634471 — MB ChB Birm. 1965; DCH Eng. 1968; MRCP (UK) 1973. Prev: Regist. (Paediat.) Leics. AHA (T); SHO Neonat. Paediat. Sorrento Matern. Hosp. Birm.; SHO Med. Groby Rd. Hosp. Leicester.

YARDLEY-JONES, Mr Anthony Chelsea and Westminster Hospital, 369 Fulham Road, London SW10 9NH — MB ChB Liverp. 1975 (Liverpool) Dip. Med. Acupuncture; FRCS Ed. 1979; Cert Av. MoD (Air) & CAA 1980; DIH Soc. Apoth. Lond. 1981; DIH Eng. 1981; FFOM RCP Lond. 1993, MFOM 1984; PhD Surrey 1988. Cons. in Ocupational Med. Chelsea and Westminster Hosp., Lond.; Hon. Consg. Ocupational Toxicologist, Nat. Poisons Inf. Serv., Birm.; Hon. Sen. Clin. Lect. (Occupat. Health) Univ. Birm.; Hon. Cons., King's Coll. Hosp. Occ Health Dept. Specialty: Occupat. Health; Acupunc. Special Interest: Human performance and heart rate variability; Stress. Socs: Soc. Occup. Med.; Regist. Toxicol. Brit. Toxicology Soc.; Fellow Royal Society of Medicine. Prev: Med. Dir., Castrol / B.P.; Chief Med. Adv., Burmah Castrol Trading Ltd, Swindon; Sen. Occupat. Med. Adv. Shell UK Ltd.

YARDUMIAN, Dorothy Anne Department of Haematology, North Middlesex Hospital, Sterling Way, London N18 1QX Tel: 020 8887 2428; Church Farm House, Luffenhall, Walkern, Stevenage SG2 7PX — MD Lond. 1988; MB BS (Hons. Obst. & Gyn. & Path.) 1979; MRCP (UK) 1982; MRCPath 1988; FRCP 1996; FRCPath. 1996. Cons. Haemat. N. Middlx. Hosp. Lond. Specialty: Haematology. Prev: Lect. & Sen. Regist. (Haemat.) Middlx. Hosp. Med. Sch. Lond.

YARDY, Neil David East Kent Hospitals NHS Trust, Dept. Anaesthesia, William Harvey Hospital, Kennington Road, Ashford TN24 0LZ Tel: 01233 633331 Fax: 01233 616118 — MB BS Lond. 1987 (Guy's Hospital Medical School) FRCA 1996. Cons. Anaesth., E. Kent Hosps. NHS Trust. Specialty: Anaesth. Socs: Fell. Roy. Coll. Anaesth.; Assn. Anaesths.; Difficult Airway Soc. Prev: GP Canterbury & Thanet HA.; Specialist Regist. (Anaesth.) N. W. Region.

YARGER, Nishi 101 Ellesmere Road, London NW10 1LH — MB BS Lond. 1994 (University College London) BSc. Regist. (Child & Adolesc. Psychiat.) Northwick Pk. Hosp. Harrow, Middlx. Specialty: Gen. Psychiat.

YARHAM, Dorian David Portcullis Surgery, Portcullis Lane, Ludlow SY8 1GT Tel: 01584 872939 Fax: 01584 876490; Birchlea, Caynham, Ludlow SY8 3BJ Tel: 01584 875423 Fax: 01584 876240 — MB ChB Glas. 1984; DRCOG 1987; MRCGP 1988. Med. Adviser Ludlow Hosp.; Non-Exec. Dir. & Chairm. Shrops. Drs. Co-Op. Socs: BMA; Chir. Soc. Glas. Prev: SHO James Paget Hosp. Gt. Yarmouth VTS; Ho. Off. (Med.) Glas. Roy. Infirm.; Ho. Off. (Surg.) Stobhill Gen. Hosp. Glas.

YARNALL, David John Queen Square Surgery, 2 Queen Square, Lancaster LA1 1RP Tel: 01524 843333 Fax: 01524 847550; 54 High Road, Halton, Lancaster LA2 6PS Tel: 01524 811025 — MB ChB Bristol 1976; DCH Eng. 1979; MRCGP 1980. GP Lancaster; Crowd Doctor Reebok Stadium Bolton Wanderers FC; Course Organiser Lancaster GP VTS. Prev: Med. Off. CECIB Heysham.

YARNALL, Nicholas John, Surg. Cdr. RN, Surg. Lt.-Cdr. RN — MB ChB Leeds 1991; DRCOG 1998; MRCGP UK 1999; MFOM 2004. Specialty: Occupat. Health; Gen. Pract.

YARNELL, John William Gordon Department of Epidemiology & Public Health, Mulhouse Building, Queen's University of Belfast, Grosvenor Road, Belfast BT12 6BJ Tel: 01232 894614 Fax: 01232 231907; 61 Magheralane Road, Randalstown BT41 2NT — MB ChB Manch. 1968; DPH Bristol 1972; MFCM 1979; MD Manch. 1981. Sen. Lect. (Epidemiol.) Qu. Univ. Belf. Specialty: Epidemiol.; Pub. Health Med.; Cardiol. Socs: Soc. Social Med.; Eur. Soc. Cardiol. (Working Gp. Epidemiol. & Preven.); Internat. Soc. & Federat. Cardiol. Prev: Mem. Scientif. Staff, MRC Epidemiol. Unit Cardiff.

YARNLEY, Paul Arthur IMASS LTD, 10 Southway Lane, Roborough, Plymouth PL6 7DH Tel: 01752 782211 Fax: 01752 782299 Email: imass@mass.freeserve.co.uk — MB BS Lond. 1976; AFOM RCP Lond. 1993. Clin. Dir. Indust. Med. & Safety Serv. Ltd. Specialty: Occupat. Health. Socs: Soc. Occupat. Med.

YARNOLD, John Robert 27 Killieser Avenue, London SW2 4NX — MB BS Lond. 1972; MRCP (UK) 1974; FRCR 1977. Professor & Hons. Cons. Inst. Cancer Research & Roy. Marsden Hosp. Specialty: Oncol.

YARR, Julie Elaine 9 Beanstown Road, Lisburn BT28 3QS — MB BCh Belf. 1997.

YARR, Nicholas Tudor North Road Medical Practice, 182 North Road, Cardiff CF14 3XQ Tel: 029 2061 9188 Fax: 029 2061 3484 — MB BCh Wales 1980; MRCGP 1984; DRCOG 1984.

YARR, Susan Nicola 3 Millvale Wood, Hillsborough BT26 6JB — MB BCh BAO Belf. 1990; MRCP (UK) 1993; MRCGP 1995; DRCOG 1996. Specialty: Gen. Pract.

YARRANTON, Helen Thrombosis & Haemostasis Research Unit, University College Hospital London, 98 Chienes Mews, London WC1E 6HX — MB ChB Bristol 1993; MRCP (UK) 1996; MRC Path 2001. Research Regist. Haemat. Specialty: Haematology. Prev: Specialist Regist. (Haemat.) Camb.

YARROW, Andrew David 3 Thistle Hill Court, Thistle Hill, Knaresborough HG5 8LS Tel: 01423 866944 — BM BCh Oxf. 1972; DRCOG 1977.

YARROW, Dudley Ernest (retired) Little Winsford, Woodland Rise, Sevenoaks TN15 0HY Tel: 01732 61817 — MB BChir Camb. 1938 (Camb. & Lond. Hosp.) MRCS Eng. LRCP Lond. 1936; DCH Eng. 1945. Prev: Capt. RAMC.

YARROW, Hal 27B Devonshire Street, London W1N 1RJ Tel: 020 7935 1694; West Green, Preston, Hitchin SG4 7UB — (St. Bart.) MRCS Eng., LRCP Lond. 1935. Med. Dir. Dermal Labs Ltd. Specialty: Dermat. Socs: Fell. RSM; BMA. Prev: Ho. Surg. Gravesend & N. Kent Hosp.; Clin. Asst. St. Johns Skin Hosp. Lond.; Police Surg. & Pub. Vaccinator.

YARROW, Simon Home Farm Cottage, 6 High St., Weston, Towcester NN12 8PU Tel: 01295 760069 — BM BCh Oxf. 1993; DA (UK) 1996; FRCA 1999. Cons. & Specialist Regist. in Anaesth., Oxf., Deaney. Specialty: Anaesth. Prev: SHO (Anaesth. & ITV) Univ. Hosp. Birm.; SHO (Anaest) City Hosp. Birm.

YARWOOD, Gary David Princess Elizabeth Hospital, Guernsey GY4 6UU Tel: 01481 725241 — MB BS Lond. 1985 (St Bart.) FRCA 1990. Cons. Anaesth. & Dir. Intens. Care Qu. Eliz. Hosp. Guernsey. Specialty: Intens. Care; Anaesth. Socs: Assn. of Anaesth.s GB and Irel.; Intens. Care Soc. Prev: Sen. Regist. (Anaesth.) St. Bart. Hosp. Lond.

YARWOOD, Rosemary Manor Park Surgery, Bell Mount Close, Leeds LS13 2UP Tel: 0113 257 9702 Fax: 0113 236 1537 — MB ChB Leeds 1984; MRCGP 1989. Prev: Trainee GP Pinderfields Gen. Hosp. Wakefield VTS; SHO (A & E, Paediat., Obst. & Psychiat.) Pinderfields Gen. Hosp. Wakefield; SHO (Anaesth.), Ho. Phys. & Ho. Surg. Pinderfields Hosp. Wakefield.

YARWOOD SMITH, Colin Hugh Wychbury Medical Centre, 121 Oakfield Road, Wollescote, Stourbridge DY9 9DS Tel: 01562 882277; 12 Cochrane Close, Pedmore, Stourbridge DY9 0ST Tel: 01562 884706 — MB ChB Birm. 1981 (Birmingham) Cert. Family Plann. JCC 1985; MRCGP 1985; DRCOG 1985. Chairm. Dudley LMC; Chairm. Stourbridge PCG. Socs: BMA (Ex-Chairm. Dudley Div.). Prev: Trainee GP Wycombe DHA VTS; Ho. Surg. Kidderminster Dist. Gen. Hosp.; Ho. Phys. Med. Profess. Unit Qu. Eliz. Hosp. Birm.

YASHODA, Punreddy c/o Dr K.R. Reddy, 12 Langholme Close, Wigan WN3 6TT — MB BS Osmania 1967.

YASIN, Khaled Mustafa Brentford Health Centre, Boston Manor Road, Brentford TW8 8DS Tel: 020 8321 3822 Fax: 020 8321 3808; 1 Daver Court, Mount Avenue, London W5 1PL — MB BS Lond. 1982.

YASSA, Janet Ghobrial Sheffield Children's Hospital, Sheffield S10 2TH — MRCS Eng. LRCP Lond. 1970.

YASSEEN, Baheig El Sir Mohamed 36 Streatham Common, London SW16 3BX — MB ChB Ain Shams 1965.

YASSIN, Raouf (retired) Mallards, The Rickyard, Shutford, Banbury OX15 6PR — MB ChB Cairo 1956; LMSSA Lond. 1964. Prev: SHO (Med., Paediat. & Surg.) Horton Gen. Hosp. Banbury.

YATE, Brian Hugh Whitlera, Dryslwyn, Carmarthen SA32 8SJ — MB ChB Manch. 1968.

YATE, Paul Michael London Hospital, Anaesthetics Department, Whitechapel, London E1 1BB — MB BS Lond. 1974 (Lond. Hosp.) FRCA 1979. Cons. Anaesth. Barts & The Lond. NHS Trust. Specialty: Anaesth. Prev: Sen. Lect. & Hon. Cons. (Anaesth.) Lond. Hosp. Med. Coll.

YATES, Andrew Department of Anaesthetics, Queen Alexandra Hospital, Cosham, Portsmouth PO6 3LY Tel: 023 92 286279 Fax: 02392 286681; Rosina Cottage, Church Road, Newtown, Fareham PO17 6LE Tel: 01329 835218 — MB BS Lond. 1975 (St. Thos.) FFA RCS Eng. 1983. Cons. Anaesth. Portsmouth Hosps. NHS Trust; Ass. Clin. Dir. Theatres, Portsmouth Hosp. NHS Trust. Specialty: Anaesth. Socs: Assn. Anaesth.; Soc. Naval Anaesth.; Vice-Pres. AODP. Prev: Cons. Anaesth. Roy. Naval Hosp. Haslar; PMO HMS Ark Roy. & HMY Britannia.

YATES, Andrew John 88 Framingham Road, Sale M33 3RJ — MB ChB Sheff. 1981; MRCPath 1992. Cons. Histopath. Tameside Gen. Hosp. Specialty: Histopath. Prev: Sen. Regist. (Histopath.) N. West. RHA.

YATES, Mr Anthony James (retired) 24 Hawthorn Avenue, Lenzie, Glasgow G66 4RA Tel: 0141 776 4502 — MB ChB Ed. 1966; FRCS Ed. 1971. Prev: Cons. Urol. Surg. Stobhill Gen. Hosp. Glas.

YATES, Brendan Davidson — MB ChB Otago 1979; BA (Hons.) Otago 1984; MPH Glas. 1988; FFPHM 1990. Cons. Pub. Health Med. NHS Exec. S. W. Bristol. Specialty: Pub. Health Med. Prev: Cons. in Pub. Health Med. S. W. RHA; Cons. in Pub. Health Med. Northern and Yorks. RHA; Cons. in Pub. Health Med. Yorks. RHA.

YATES, Bryan Hulme 115 Wingrove Road, Newcastle upon Tyne NE4 9BY — MB BS Newc. 1998.

YATES, Charles Michael (retired) 25 Bloomfield Terrace, London SW1W 8PQ Tel: 020 7730 3650 — MB BChir Camb. 1953 (St. Thos.) MA Camb. 1986, BA (Hons.) 1950, MB BChir 1953. Prev: Med. Cas. & Ho. Surg. St. Thos. Hosp. Lond.

YATES, Mr Christopher John Percy Wellington Health Centre, Chapel Lane, Wellington, Telford TF1 1PZ Tel: 01952 226000; The Mill House, High Ercall, Telford TF6 6BE Tel: 01952 770394 — MB BS Lond. 1971 (St. Bart.) MRCS Eng. LRCP Lond. 1971; FRCS Eng. 1977; DRCOG 1982. Prev: Regist. Rotat. (Surg.) St. Geo. Hosp. Lond.; Research Fell. (Periferal Vasc. Unit) St. Jas. Hosp. Lond.; Regist. (Surg.) Leicester Gen. Hosp.

YATES, Mr Colin Department of Oral & Maxillofacial Surgery, Wexham Park Hospital, Slough SL2 4HL Tel: 01753 634076 Fax: 01753 691343; Squirrels, Hatton Hill, Windlesham GU20 6AD Tel: 01276 472100 — MB ChB Birm. 1972; BDS Birm. 1963; FDS RCS Eng. 1967. Cons. Oral & Maxillofacial Surg. Heatherwood & Wexham Pk. Hosps. Trust; Specialty Tutor E. Berks. RCS (Eng.). Specialty: Oral & Maxillofacial Surg. Socs: Fell. Brit. Assn. Oral & Maxillofacial Surg.; BMA & BDA. Prev: Sen. Regist. (Oral & Maxillofacial Surg.) King's Coll. Hosp. Lond. & Mass. Gen. Hosp. Boston, USA; SHO (Oral Surg.) Hosp. Sick. Childr. Lond.; Ho. Surg. Birm. Accid. Hosp.

YATES, David Anthony University Hospital Birmingham NHS Trust, The Queen Elizabeth Hospital, Department of Neuroradiology, Edgbaston, Birmingham B15 2TH Tel: 0121 472 1311 Fax: 0121 627 2578; The Cottage, 6 Cotton Church Lane, Cotton Hackett, Rednal, Birmingham B45 8PT Tel: 0121 445 1293 — BM BCh Oxf. 1970; BA Oxf. 1968; FRCR 1980. Cons. Radiol. Qu. Eliz. Hosp. Birm.; Hon. Sen. Lect. Univ. Birm. Specialty: Radiol. Socs: Brit. Soc. Neuroradiol.; Sen. Mem. World Federat. of Intervent. & Therap. Neuroradiol.; Fell. RCRadiol.

YATES, David Anthony Hilton Adams Cottage, Bramshott, Liphook GU30 7SJ Tel: 01428 723075 Fax: 01428 723075 — MB BS (Hons.) Lond. 1953 (St. Thos.) FRCP Lond. 1974, M 1957; DPhysMed Eng. 1960; MD Lond. 1963. Emerit. Phys. St. Thos. Hosp. Lond.; Emerit. Rheum. HM Armed Forces. Socs: Fell. Roy. Soc. Med. (Ex-Pres. Rheum. Sect.); (Ex-Pres.) Brit. Soc. Rheum. Prev: Cons. Rheum. King Edwd. VII Hosp. Offs. Lond.; Cons. Phys. St Thomas Hosp. Lond.; Regist. (Thoracic Med.) & Cas. Off. St Thomas Hosp.

YATES, David Beresford Taunton & Somerset Hospital, Musgrove Park, Taunton TA1 5DA Tel: 01823 342132 Fax: 01823 344542; Vexford Court, Higher Vexford, Lydeard St. Lawrence, Taunton TA4 3QF Tel: 01984 656735 Email: dbyates@doctors.org.uk — MB BS Lond. 1967 (King's Coll. Hosp.) MRCS Eng. LRCP Lond. 1967; MRCP (UK) 1970; FRCP Lond. 1983. Cons. Phys. Taunton & Som. Hosp. Specialty: Gen. Med.; Rheumatol. Socs: (Counc.) Brit. Soc. Rheum.; (Pres.) SW Wessex & S. Wales Rheum. Soc.

YATES, David Herbert (retired) Wintergreen, St.. Jidgey, Wadebridge PL27 7RE Tel: 01208 812391 — MB ChB Manch. 1949; DPM Eng. 1960; FRCPsych 1986. Prev: Cons. Psychiat. St. Lawrence Hosp. Bodmin.

YATES, David Owen Jary, Yates and Brown, Well Street Medical Centre, Well Street, Stoke-on-Trent ST10 1EY Tel: 01538 753114 Fax: 01538 751485; Vinewood Farm, Marlpit Lane, Denstone, Uttoxeter ST14 5HH Tel: 01889 591185 Email: dyates@doctors.org.uk — MB ChB Dundee 1976; MRCGP 1981. Clin. Asst. (Elderley Care) Cheadle Hosp.

YATES, David William Kent and Sussex Hospital, Tunbridge Wells TN4 8AT — BM Soton. 1977; FFA RCS Eng. 1982. Cons. Anaesth. & Intens. Care Tunbridge Wells. Specialty: Anaesth. Prev: Lect. Univ., Zimbabwe.

YATES, Professor David William (retired) Hope Hospital, Salford, Manchester Tel: 0161 206 4397 Fax: 0161 206 4345 Email: dyates@fs1.ho.man.ac.uk; 22 Westminster Road, Eccles, Manchester M30 9EB — MB BChir Camb. 1967 (St. Thos.) MD Camb. 1990, MA 1967; FRCS Eng. 1972; MChOrth Liverp. 1975; FRCP 1998. Director of Admissions at Manch. Med. Sch.; Hon. Cons. Emerg. Med. Hope Hosp. Salford; Mem. Scientif. Staff N. West. Injury Research Centre.

YATES, Eric John, DSC (retired) The Weir House, Boat Lane, Welford-on-Avon, Stratford-upon-Avon CV37 8EN Tel: 01789 750546 — MB ChB Manch. 1938. Prev: Ho. Surg. Ancoats Hosp. Manch.

YATES, Francis Alexander (retired) C1 Marine Gate, Marine Drive, Brighton BN2 5TN Tel: 01273 672077 — (King's Coll. Hosp.) MB BS Lond. 1952; MRCS Eng. LRCP Lond. 1952. Prev: Ho. Phys. Bolingbroke Hosp. Lond.

YATES, Frank Wright 1 Rivington Lane, Headless Cross, Anderton, Chorley PR6 9HQ Tel: 01257 483042 Fax: 01257 482642 — MRCS Eng. LRCP Lond. 1960 (Liverp.) LMSSA Lond. 1957. Specialty: Occupat. Health.

YATES, Geoffrey Alan Belmont Farm, Great Harwood, Blackburn BB6 7UY — MB BS Lond. 1991 (St George's) Specialty: Gen. Med.

YATES, Gordon 75 Stoke Road, Shelton, Stoke-on-Trent ST4 2QH Tel: 01782 745325 Fax: 01782 747617; Wyndowne, Bedcraft, Barlaston, Stoke-on-Trent ST12 9AL Tel: 01782 372155 Fax: 01782 747617 — MRCS Eng. LRCP Lond. 1956 (Camb. & Middlx.) MA, MB BChir Camb. 1956; DIH Soc. Apoth. Lond. 1963. Indep. Cons. Occupat. Med. Stoke-on-Trent. Specialty: Occupat. Health. Socs: BMA & N. Staffs. Med. Inst. Prev: Ho. Surg. Middlx. Hosp.; Ho. Phys. N. Middlx. Hosp. Lond.; Nuffield Trav. Fell. 1968.

YATES, Helen Anne Grosvenor Medical Centre, 23 Upper Grosvenor Road, Tunbridge Wells TN1 2DX Tel: 01892 544777 Fax: 01892 511157 — BM Soton. 1989; DRCOG 1993; MRCGP 1995. GP Princip. Prev: Trainee GP Tunbridge Wells VTS.

YATES, Mrs Janette Avril 18 Union Street Surgery, Kirkintilloch, Glasgow G66 1DH Tel: 0141 776 1238; The Ferns, 24 Hawthorn Avenue, Lenzie, Kirkintilloch, Glasgow G66 4RA Tel: 0141 776 4502 — MB ChB Ed. 1966.

YATES, John Benjamin Alexander Wintergreen St Judgey, St Issey, Wadebridge PL27 7RE — MB ChB Glas. 1994.

YATES, Professor John Robert Watson Department of Medical Genetics, Box 134, Addenbrookes Hospital NHS Trust, Hills Road, Cambridge CB2 2QQ Tel: 01223 216446 Fax: 01223 217054 — MB BS Lond. 1977 (Univ. Coll. Hosp.) MA (Physics) Oxf. 1970; MRCP (UK) 1981; FRCP Lond. 1994. Prof. of Med. Genetics, Dept. of Med. Genetics, Univ. of Cambridge; Hon. Cons. In Med. Genetics. Dept. of Med. Genetics, Addenbrooke's Hosp., Cambridge. Specialty: Genetics. Prev: Reader in Med. Genetics, Dept. of Med. Genetics, Univ. of Cambridge.

YATES, Judith Anne Wand Medical Centre, 279 Gooch Street, Highgate, Birmingham B5 7JE Tel: 0121 440 1561 Fax: 0121 440 0060 — MB ChB Birm. 1975; DRCOG 1979. GP Birm.

YATES, Kenneth Philip The Surgery, Mill Hoo, Alderton, Woodbridge IP12 3DA — MB ChB Manch. 1974.

YATES, Mabel 5 St Catherines Walk, Leeds LS8 1SB Tel: 0113 266 8801 — MB ChB Leeds 1956. Med. Panel Mem. of the Appeals Serv. Specialty: Community Child Health. Prev: Princip. Clin. Med. Off. Leeds E. HA; SCMO (Hearing Impairm.) Leeds East. HA; Ho. Phys. Geriat. & Ho. Surg. ENT & Ophth. St. Jas. Hosp. Leeds.

YATES, Mark Timothy Market Harborough Medical Centre, 67 Coventry Road, Market Harborough LE16 96X — BM BS Nottm. 1996. GP Princpal. Specialty: Ophth. Prev: SHO, Orthalmology, W. Norwich Hosp., Norwich.

YATES, Mark William 12 Avon Close, Taunton TA1 4SU Tel: 01823 256512 — MB BS Monash 1986.

YATES, Martin 16 The Sycamores, Bramhope, Leeds LS16 9JR — MB BS Newc. 1985; MRCPsych 1990; MRCP (UK) 1994. Regist. (Gen. Med.) Roy. Gwent Hosp. Newport. Specialty: Gen. Med.

YATES, Mhairi Stewart 15 Lee Fold, Tyldesley, Manchester M29 7FQ — MB ChB Liverp. 1991.

YATES, Michael David The Surgery, 239 Mosley Common Road, Boothstown, Manchester M28 1BZ Tel: 0161 790 2192 Fax: 0161 799 5046 — MB BS Lond. 1967 (Westm.) MRCS Eng. LRCP Lond. 1967. GP Churston Ferrers Brixham. Prev: SHO (O & G) Canad. Red Cross Hosp; Paediat. Westm. Childr. Hosp. Lond.; Ho. Surg. Qu. Mary's Hosp. Roehampton.

YATES, Michael John Frimley Green Medical Centre, 1 Beech Road, Frimley Green, Camberley GU16 6QQ Tel: 01252 835016 Fax: 01252 837908; 156B Frimley Green PD, Camberley GU16 6NA Tel: 01252 835254 — MB BS Lond. 1972 (St. Geo.) BSc Lond. 1969; DObst RCOG 1974; MRCGP 1981. Prev: Ho. Phys. & SHO (O & G) St. Geo.'s Hosp. Tooting; Ho. Surg. Ashford Hosp., Middlx.

YATES, Michael Simon The Pines, 71B Westhall Road, Warlingham CR6 9HG — MB BS Lond. 1987.

YATES, Moira Jean St George's Surgery, 46 a Preston New Rd, Blackburn BB2 6AH Tel: 0125 453791 — MB ChB Ed. 1992; DRCOG 1995; MRCGP 1996; DFFP 1996. Specialty: Gen. Pract. Socs: RCGP (NW Eng. Fac.); BMA; Scott. Family Plann. Assn. Prev: Trainee GP Inverness-sh. VTS.

YATES, Muriel Grace (retired) Bryn Aber, Nantgwynant, Caernarfon LL55 4NW — (Ed.) MB ChB Ed. 1949; DCH Eng. 1951. Prev: Asst. MOH Surrey CC.

YATES, Nicholas The Kintbury Medical Practice, Kintbury Surgery, Newbury Street, Kintbury, Hungerford RG17 9UX Tel: 01488 658294; 5 Halfway, Bath Road, Newbury RG20 8NG Tel: 01488 658092 — MB BS Lond. 1975; BSc (Ophth. Optics) Manch. 1969; MRCGP 1980; DCH Eng. 1980; DRCOG 1980. Prev: Regist. (Paediat.) Ninewells Hosp. Dundee; Ho. Surg. & Ho. Phys. (Paediat.) St. Thos. Hosp. Lond.

YATES, Paul Anthony 118 Doveleys Road, Salford M6 8QW — MB ChB Bristol 1982.

YATES, Peter Albert Academic Unit of Child & Adolescent Psychology, 3rd Floor QEQM, St Mary's Hospital, Norfolk Place, London W2 1PG Email: p.yates@ic.ac.uk — MB ChB Cape Town 1989; MRCPsych 1996. Specialist Regist. Child & Adolesc. Psychiat. Gt. Ormond St Hosp., Lond.; Hon. Clin. Research Fell., Acad. Unit of Child & Adolesc. Psychiat., Imperial Coll. Sch. Of Med. @ St Mary's, Lond. Specialty: Child & Adolesc. Psychiat.

YATES, Philip Blood Transfusion Centre, Aberdeen Royal Infirmary, Foresterhill, Aberdeen AB25 2ZW Tel: 01224 685685 — MB ChB Manch. 1979 (Manch. Univ.) MRCP (UK) 1984; MRCPath 1988; FRCP Ed. 1995; FRCPath 1997. Cons. Transfus. Med. Aberd. & NE Scotl. Blood Transfus. Serv. Aberd. Specialty: Blood Transfus. Prev: Assoc. Specialist (Transfus. Med.) Aberd. & NE Scotl. Blood Transfus. Serv.; Sen. Regist. Rotat. (Haemat.) Bristol Roy. Infirm.; Regist. (Haemat.) West. Gen. Hosp. Edin.

YATES, Philip Andrew Orchard Medical Centre, Macdonald Walk, Kingswood, Bristol BS15 8NJ Tel: 0117 980 5100 Fax: 0117 980 5104 — MB ChB Bristol 1979; DRCOG 1982; MRCGP 1984; DFFP 1996. Chair S. E. Gloucestershire PCG.

YATES, Philip David 2 Ashgill House, Clayton Road, Newcastle upon Tyne NE2 1TL — MB ChB Manch. 1991.

YATES, Rachel Helyn Theresa 65 The Fairway, Saltburn-by-the-Sea TS12 1NG — MB ChB Liverp. 1993.

YATES, Rachel Olwyn Nethergreen Road Surgery, 34-36 Nethergreen Road, Sheffield S11 7EJ Tel: 0114 230 2952 — MB ChB Sheff. 1974; BSc Sheff. 1969.

YATES, Richard William Peel Hilo House, St. Clements Coast Road, St Clement, Jersey JE2 6SA Tel: 01534 22381 — MB BS Lond. 1953 (Guy's) MRCS Eng. LRCP Lond. 1953.

YATES, Robert William Smith Kilmory, 22 Ralston Road, Bearsden, Glasgow G61 3BA — MB ChB Glas. 1977; MRCOG 1984. Lect. Dept. O & G Univ. Liverp. Prev: Regist. Infertil. Clinic

Roy. Infirm. Glas.; Research Regist. Univ. Glas. Dept. O & G Roy. Infirm. Glas.

YATES, Robert Wright Royal Manchester Children's Hospital, Paediatric Intensive Care, Pendlebury, Manchester M27 4HA Tel: 0161 794 4696 Email: robert.yates@cmmc.nhs.uk — MB BS Lond. 1986 (Roy. Free) MRCP (UK) 1990; DA (UK) 1991; MSc Univ. Lond. 1996; FRCPCH 1996. Cons. Paediat. Intens. Care Manch. Childr. Hosps. Specialty: Paediat. Prev: Sen. Regist. (Paediat. Intens. Care) Gt. Ormond St. Hosp. Lond.; Regist. (Paediat.) Chelmsford; Regist. (Anaesth.) Roy. Lond. Hosp.

YATES, Roger Alan Zeneca Pharmaceuticals, Medical Research Department, Macclesfield SK10 4TG Tel: 01625 582828; 3 Racecourse Park, Wilmslow SK9 5LU Tel: 01625 520246 — MB BChir Camb. 1971; MA Camb. 1972; PhD Bristol 1976; MRCP (UK) 1977; MFPM RCP Lond. 1990; FFPM RCP Lond. 1993. Sen. Clin. Pharmacol. Zeneca Pharmaceuts. Div. Alderley Pk. Specialty: Pharmacology. Prev: Clin. Research Asst. (Therap. & Clin. Pharmacol.) Qu. Eliz. Hosp. Birm.; MRC Jun. Research Fell. Dept. Pharmacol. Bristol Univ.

YATES, Rowena Catharine 2 The Horseshoe, York YO24 1LX Tel: 01273 707546 — MB BS Lond. 1965 (Guy's) MRCS Eng. LRCP Lond. 1965. Clin. Asst. (Psychiat.) Clifton Hosp. York. Prev: Regist. Dept. Child Psychiat. St. Jas. Hosp. Leeds; Regist. (Psychiat.) St. John's Hosp. Stone.

YATES, Sarah Mounts Medical Centre, Campbell Street, Northampton NN1 3DS Tel: 01604 631952 Fax: 01604 634139; 39 Aldwell Close, Wootton, Northampton NN4 6AX — MB BS Lond. 1968; MRCS Eng. LRCP Lond. 1968; DFFP 1993. Prev: Lect. Univ. Malta.

YATES, Sarah Catherine Longdon, Shipley Rd, Southwater, Horsham RH13 9BQ — BM Soton. 1997 (Soton) GP Trainee.

YATES, Sarah Catriona 24 Sandy Lane, Lymm WA13 9HQ — MB ChB Liverp. 1991; MB ChB 1991 Liverp.

YATES, Stewart Paul Barnsley District General Hospital, Gawber Road, Barnsley S75 2EP Tel: 01226 730000 — MB ChB Sheff. 1983; BMedSci 1980; FRCR 1990; T(R)(CR) 1991. Cons. Radiol. Barnsley Dist. Gen. Hosp. Specialty: Radiol. Prev: Sen. Regist. (Radiol.) Sheff. HA; Regist. (Med.) Rotherham Dist. Gen. Hosp.

YATES, Sylvia Helen (retired) Gemini, Lanham Lane, Winchester SO22 5JS Tel: 01962 861681 — MB ChB Sheff. 1952; Acad. DPH Univ. Lond. 1956. Prev: SCMO Winchester HA.

YATES, Mrs Victoria Mary Orchard Cottage, 40 Leighton Beck Rd, Beetham, Milnthorpe LA7 7AX Tel: 01539 564129 — MB ChB Sheff. 1974; MRCP (UK) 1976; FRCP Lond. 1993. Cons. Dermatol. Roy. Bolton NHS Trust & Univ. of Manch. Dept. of Dermat. Specialty: Dermat. Prev: Cons. Dermat. Blackburn Roy. Infirm.; Sen. Regist. (Dermat.) Skin Hosp. Manch.; Sen. Regist. & Regist. (Dermat.) Stobhill Hosp.

YATES, Wendy Ann (retired) 3 Racecourse Park, Wilmslow SK9 5LU Tel: 01625 520246 Email: wenyates@yahoo.co.uk — MB BChir Camb. 1971 (Cambridge) MA Camb. 1972, MB BChir 1971; DObst RCOG 1973; DFFP 1996. Prev: Assoc. Specialist (Cytol. & Colposcopy) St. Mary's Manch.

YATES-BELL, Mr Andrew John (retired) King's College Hospital, Denmark Hill, London SE5 9RS; The Oaks, Manor Park, Chislehurst BR7 5QE — MB BChir Camb. 1959 (King's Coll. Hosp.) BA Camb. 1959; FRCS Eng. 1966. Hon. Cons. Urol. King's Health Dist. (T). Prev: Regist. (Surg.) St. Peter's Hosp. Lond.

YAU, Chi Yuen 2A Harvesters Close, Gillingham ME8 8PA — MB BChir Camb. 1992.

YAU, Kar-Man Raymond 76 Rofant Road, Northwood HA6 3BA — BM Soton. 1993.

YAU, King Wai Royal National Orthopaedic Hospital NHS Trust, Brockley Hill, Stanmore HA7 4LP — MB ChB Birm. 1981; FRCA 1986. Specialty: Anaesth.

YAU, Susan Zi May 34 Wonford Street, Exeter EX2 5DL — MB ChB Bristol 1998.

YAU, Wing Him The Surgery, Rough Road, Kirkstanding, Birmingham B44 0UY; 14 Lapworth Drive, New Oscott, Sutton Coldfield B73 6QG — MB ChB Ed. 1980; DCH RCP Glas. 1982; Cert. Family Plann. JCC 1983; DRCOG 1984.

YAU, Yun Yin 10 Barned Court, Maidstone ME16 9EL — MB BS Lond. 1997.

YAXLEY, Katharine Mary Fulwood Clinic, Lytham Road, Preston PR2 4JB Tel: 01772 401300; 6 Beechfield Avenue, Wrea Green, Preston PR4 2NX Tel: 01772 681619 — BM Soton. 1985; DCH RCP Lond. 1990. Staff Grade Practitioner (Community Paediat.), Preston acute Hosp.s NHS Trust. Specialty: Community Child Health. Prev: Staff Grade Pract. (Community Child Health) Norwich Community Health NHS Trust; Clin. Med. Off. (Community Child Health) Norwich Community Health NHS Trust; Ho. Off. (Gen. Med., Cardiol., Urol. & ENT) Norf. & Norwich Hosp.

YAZDANI, Monwar Shariar South West Herts Health Centre, Oxhey Drive, South Oxhey, Watford WD19 7SF Tel: 020 8421 5224.

YAZDANI, Qudsia 10 Ashby Road, Tamworth B79 8AG — MB BS Punjab 1972.

YAZDANI, Ramin 7 Coleridge Walk, London NW11 6AT — MD Teheran 1992; MRCP. Sen. Ho. Off. (Oncol.) Roy. Free Hosp. Lond.

YAZDIAN-TEHRANI, Hamid — MB BS Lond. 1998 (UMDS) SHO (A&E), Conquest Hosp. Hastings. Specialty: Accid. & Emerg. Prev: HO, Sug., Frimley Pk. Hosp.; Ho. Off. Med., Conquest Hosp. Hastings.

YEALLAND, Susan (retired) 9 Clarkson Road, Cambridge CB3 0EH — MB BS Lond. 1949 (Roy. Free) MRCS Eng. LRCP Lond. 1949; DO Eng. 1975.

YEAMAN, William Taylor McKenzie (retired) 22 Jedburgh Road, Dundee DD2 1SR Tel: 01382 668601 — MB ChB St. And. 1955.

YEANG, Yvonne Yee Wan 30 Deansway, East Finchley, London N2 0JF Tel: 020 8883 6951 Fax: 020 8883 6951 — MB ChB Ed. 1971 (Edinburgh University) BSc (Med. Sci.) Ed. 1968, MB ChB 1971; MRCP (UK) 1974; Dip. Pharm. Med. RCP (UK) 1986; FFPM 1995. Dir. Clin. Investig. Pharmaceut. Company. Specialty: Pharmaceutical Medicine.

YEAP, Joo Seng Room 3 Upper Wing, Louise Fleischmann Building, Royal National Orthopaedic Hospital, Brockley Hill, Stanmore HA7 4LP — MB BCh BAO Belf. 1992.

YEAP, May Lynn Bristol Royal Hospital for children, Upper Maudlin Street, Bristol BS2 8BJ Tel: 0117 923 0000 Email: myeap@doctors.org.uk; 2 Priory Road, Clifton, Bristol BS8 1TX — MB ChB Bristol 1995; DCH 1998; MRCPCH 1999. Research Fell. (Endocrinol. & Oncol.) Bristol Roy. Hosp. for Childr. Specialty: Paediat. Socs: Med. Defence Union; BMA; Med. Protec. Soc. Prev: Sen. Ho. Off. (A & E) Roy. Infirm. Leicester; Ho. Off. (Surg.) Bristol Roy. Infirm. & Southmead Hosp.; Ho. Off. (Med.) Bristol Roy. Infirm.

YEARSLEY, Deborah Margaret Marlborough Medical Practice, The Surgery, George Lane, Marlborough SN8 4BY Tel: 01672 512187 Fax: 01672 516809; Fairways, 28 The Thorns, Osbourne Chase, Marlborough SN8 1DY Tel: 01672 516698 — MB BCh Wales 1985; DRCOG 1991. Prev: Trainee GP Ramsbury Wilts.

YEARSLEY, John Kenneth Noel, MC (retired) 46 Middlebridge Street, Romsey SO51 8HL Tel: 01794 522317 — MB BS Lond. 1952 (St. Thos.) DTM & H Liverp. 1954. Prev: GP Ramsgate, Kent.

YEATES, Caroline Elizabeth Swn y Gwynt, Day Hospital, Tir y Dail Lane, Ammanford SA18 3AS Tel: 01269 595473 — MB BS Lond. 1984; DRCOG 1988. Staff Grade Doctor (Psychiat.) Swn y Gwynt Day Hosp. Ammanford. Specialty: Gen. Psychiat.

YEATES, Curtis Bernstein Big J's Supermarket, Lower Harbour St., Falmouth Post Office, Trelawny, Jamaica; 2 St. Lawrence House, Melville Road, Edgbaston, Birmingham B16 9NQ Tel: 0121 454 6840 — MB BS West Indies 1989; BSc (Hons.) New York 1984; MRCP (UK) 1994. Specialty: Nephrol.

YEATES, Francis Alexander The Thorndike Centre, Longley Road, Rochester ME1 2TH Tel: 01634 817217; 27 Beresford Road, Kits Coty, Aylesford ME20 7EP Tel: 01634 861374 — MB BS Lond. 1982; DRCOG 1987.

YEATES, Mr Hugh Alan 2 Inver Park, Holywood BT18 9NF — MB BCh BAO Belf. 1971; FRCS Ed. 1976; FRCS (Orthop.) Ed. 1980. Cons. Orthop. Surg. Musgrave Hosp. Belf.; Cons. Orthop. Surg. Ulster Hosp. Dundonald. Specialty: Orthop.; Trauma & Orthop. Surg. Socs: Brit. Orthop. Assn. & Ulster Med. Soc.

YEATES, Sybil Ruth (retired) 185 Lawrie Park Gardens, London SE26 6XJ Tel: 020 8778 8148 — MB BS Lond. 1947 (Roy. Free) MRCS Eng. LRCP Lond. 1946; FRCPCH 1997. Prev: Cons. Optimum Health Trust Lond.

YEATMAN, Alison West Suffolk Hospital, Hardwick Lane, Bury St Edmunds IP33 2QZ; Caius Cottage, Bardwell Road, Barningham, Bury St Edmunds IP31 1DF — MB BS Lond. 1991.

YEATMAN, Nigel William Johnathan 1C Tredegar Square, Bow, London E3 5AD Tel: 020 8980 4181 — MB BS Lond. 1974 (Lond. Hosp.) BSc Lond. 1972; DRCOG 1976; DCH Eng. 1977; MRCP (UK) 1978. Lect. (Med. & Dent. Educat.) Barts & The Lond. Sch. Med. & Dent. Prev: Lect. (Immunol.) Lond. Hosp.; SHO (Cas.) Whipps Cross Hosp. Lond.; SHO (Paediat.) Lond. Hosp.

YEDLA, Suryaprakash Rao c/o Dr S. Motha, 41 The Sutton, St Leonards-on-Sea TN38 9RA — MB BS Andhra 1975.

YEE, Amah Tyrone Road Surgery, 99 Tyrone Road, Thorpe Bay, Southend-on-Sea SS1 3HD Tel: 01702 582670 Fax: 01702 589146 — MB BS Dacca 1965; MRCS Eng. LRCP Lond. 1983.

YEE, Main Ching 40 Chapel Road, Weldon, Corby NN17 3HP — MB ChB Leic. 1992.

YEE, Mee Lian Flat 1, Trident Court, 3 Gilbertstone Avenue, Birmingham B26 1LD — MB ChB Sheff. 1983.

YEGANEH-ARANI, Erfan Church Grange Surgery, Brambeys Drive, Basingstoke RG21 8QN; 32 Ellenborough Road, London N22 5HA — MB ChB Manch. 1995 (Manchester) DRCOG 1998. SHO (O & G) N. Hants. Hosp.; GP Regist. Ch. Grange Basingstoke Surg. Specialty: Gen. Pract. Socs: Med. Protec. Soc. Prev: SHO (Pub. Health Med.) N. & Mid Hants. Health Auth.; SHO (Psychiat.) Roy. J. Hants Hosp.; SHO (Med.) Burnley Gen. Hosp. Lancs.

YEGHEN, Tullie King's College Hospital, Denmark Hill, Lewisham High St., London SE5 Tel: 020 7737 4000; 20 Stokenchurch Street, London SW6 3TR Tel: 020 7736 8400 — MB BS Lond. 1986; BA Oxf. 1982; MRCP (UK) 1990; DRCPath 1993. Sen. Regist. (Haemat.) King's Coll. Hosp. Lond. Specialty: Haematology. Prev: Sen. Regist. (Haemat.) Lewisham Hosp. NHS Trust Lond.; Research Fell. (Haemat. & Microbiol.) Roy. Free Hosp. Lond.; Regist. (Haemat.) St. Geo. Hosp., Roy. Marsden. Hosp. & Roy. Surrey Co. Hosp.

YEH, James Shue-Min 44A Upcerne Road, London SW10 0SQ Tel: 020 7351 1396 — MB ChB Ed. 1995; BSc Ed. 1993; MRCP (UK) 1998; ALS Cert 1999. Specialist Regist. (Gen. Med.) Hammersmith Hosp. Lond. Specialty: Gen. Med. Socs: BMA; Fell. RSM. Prev: SHO (Gen. Med.) King's Coll. Hosp. Lond.; SHO Oncol. Myertein Inst. of Oncol. Middlx. Hosp. Uni. Coll. Lond. Hosp., Lond.; Ho. Off. (Gen. Surg. & Gen. Med.) Roy. Infirm. Edin.

YEH, Mr John Sho-Ju The Royal London Hospital, Barts & the London NHS Trust, Queen Mary University of London, Department of Neurosurgery, Whitechapel, London E1 1BB Tel: 020 73777000; 71 Plover Way, London SE16 7TS Email: j.s.yeh@doctors.org.uk — MB BChir 1989 (Univ. of Camb.) BA 1987; MA 1991; FRCSEd 1994; FRCSEd (Neuro.Surg) 2001. Sen. Clin. Lect. & Cons. Neurosurg. Specialty: Neurosurg.; Research; Spinal Surgery. Socs: Brit. Cervical Spine Soc.; Fell. Roy. Coll. Surg. Edin.; Soc. of Brit. Neurol. Surgeons. Prev: Research Regist. (Neurosurg.) Midl. Centre for Neuosurg. & Neurol. Birmingham; SHO (Neurosurgery Cardiothorasis Surg. Gen. Surg. Orthopaedics) N. Staffs. Roy. Infirm. Stoke-on-Trent; Ho. Phys. (Gen. Med. & Haemat.) & Ho. Surg. (Urol. & Gen. Surg.) Addenbrooke's Hosp. Camb.

YEH, Peter Shue-Yen 71 Plover Way, London SE16 7TS Tel: 020 7252 3899 Fax: 020 7252 3899 Email: yehpeter@hotmail.com; 15 Kestell Drive, Cardiff CF11 7BF Tel: 029 2066 5931 Fax: 029 2066 5931 Email: yehpeter@hotmail.com — MB BChir Camb. 1992; MA Camb. 1993, BA (Hons.) 1989; DFFP Lond. 1997; MRCOG London 2001. Clin. Research Fell. Fetal Med. Oxf. Radcliffe Hosp. NHS Trust; McLoghlin Schol. RCS Eng. Specialty: Obst. & Gyn. Prev: Regist. (O & G) Hammersmith Hosp. NHS Trust Lond.; Regist. (O & G) Oxf. Radcliffe Hosp. NHS Trust; Ho. Off. (Gen. Med. & Haemat.) Addenbrooke's Hosp. Camb.

YELD, Rophina Owen Southbourno Surgery, 337 Main Road, Southbourne, Emsworth PO10 8JH Tel: 01243 372623 Fax: 01243 379936 Email: rophina.yeld@gp-h82078.nhs.uk — MB BS Lond. 1987 (Charing Cross and Westminster) DRCOG 1993; DFFP 1994. GP at Southbourno Surg. Prev: Trainee GP S.bourne, Hants.; SHO (A & E) St. Richards Hosp. Chichester; SHO (Anaesth.) Poole Gen. Hosp.

YELDHAM, Denise Linda The Lawels, Newton Abbot Hospital, 62 East Steet, Newton Abbot TQ12 4PT Tel: 01626 357335 — MB ChB Leeds 1975; BSc Leeds 1972; MRCPsych 1979. Cons. Psychiat. S. Devon Healthcare Trust. Specialty: Gen. Psychiat.; Psychother. Socs: Assoc. Mem. Brit. Assn. Psychother. Prev: Med. Dir., Cons. Psychiat. & Psychother. Pk.lands Ment. Health Servs. Mid-Surrey HA; Cons. Psychiat. & Psychother Ment. Illness Mid. Surrey HA; Sen. Regist. (Adult Psychiat.) St. Geo. Hosp. Lond.

YELL, Jennifer Anne Hope Hospital, Salford M6 8HD Tel: 0161 206120 Fax: 0161 787 1998 Email: jennifer.yell@srht.nhs.uk — MB ChB Cape Town 1985; MRCP UK 1987; MD Cape Town 1998; FRCP UK 2000. Cons Dermatol Salford Roy. and Trafford. Specialty: Dermat. Socs: Brit. Assn. Dermat.; Brit. Soc. Study VD; BSID. Prev: Cons. Dermat. Wrightington Wigan & Trafford Gen. NHS Trust & Salford Roy. Hosps. Manch.; Sen. Regist. & Regist. (Dermat.) Oxf. Radcliffe Hosp.; Fell. (Dermat.) Univ. N. Carolina Chapel Hill, USA.

YELLAND, Mr Andrew Nigel Porter Breast Unit, Royal Sussex County Hospital, Eastern Road, Brighton BN2 5BE Tel: 01273 696955; 72 Woodland Drive, Hove BN3 6DJ — MB BS Lond. 1986 (St. George's) FRCS Ed. 1993; MS Lond. 1994. Lead Cons. Breast Surg. Roy. Sussex Co. Hosp. Brighton. Specialty: Gen. Surg. Socs: Breast Surgs. Gp.; Roy. Soc. Med.; Assn. Surg. Prev: Regist. Rotat. (Surg.) S. Thames (W.); Research Fell. (Med. Oncol.) Char. Cross & Westm. Med. Sch. Lond.

YELLAND, Elizabeth Sian 51 Drymen Road, Bearsden, Glasgow G61 2RN — MB ChB Glas. 1994. Specialty: Paediat.

YELLIN, Sharon Diana Leeds Health Authority, Blenheim House, West One, Duncombe St., Leeds LS1 4PL; 19 The Avenue, Roundhay, Leeds LS8 1JG — BM BCh Oxf. 1986; MPH Leeds 1992; MFPHM RCP (UK) 1993; MRCGP 1997. Cons. Pub. Health Med. Leeds HA. Specialty: Pub. Health Med.

YELLON, Trevor John 6 The Drive, London NW11 9SR — MB BS Lond. 1998.

YELLOP, Lisa Jane 1 Green Row Fold, Methley, Leeds LS26 9BG Tel: 01977 603671 — BM BS Nottm. 1994; MRCGP.

YELLOWLEES, Alexander John Priory Hospital, 38 Mansion House Road, Glasgow G41 3DW Tel: 0141 636 6116 Fax: 01738 440431 Email: alex.yellowlees@onet.co.uk — MB ChB Ed. 1977; MPhil Ed. 1984, BSc (Med. Sci.) 1974; MRCPsych 1981. Specialty: Gen. Psychiat. Special Interest: Eating Disorders. Socs: Som. Eating Disorder Assn.(Patron). Prev: Cons. Psychiat. Murray Roy. Hosp. Perth; Sen. Regist., Regist. & SHO (Psychiat.) Roy. Edin. Hosp.

YELLOWLEES, Gillian Mary MHET Melburn Lodge, Borders General Hospital, Melrose TD6 9BS Tel: 01896 827105 Fax: 01896 827114 — MB ChB Bristol 1983; MRCPsych 1988. Cons. Psychiat. (Old Age) NHS Borders, Melrose. Specialty: Geriat. Psychiat.; Gen. Psychiat. Prev: Cons. Psychiat. (Old Age) Borders Primary Care Trust Melrose; Sen. Regist. (Psychiat.) Newc.; Sen. Regist. Rotat. (Psychiat.) Bristol.

YELLOWLEES, Sir Henry, KCB (retired) 33 Lea Road, Harpenden AL5 4PQ — (Middlx.) BM BCh Oxf. 1950; MA Oxf. 1950; MRCS Eng. LRCP Lond. 1950; FRCP Lond. 1971, M 1966; FFCM 1972; Hon. FRCPS Glas. 1974; Hon. FRCPsych 1977; FRCS Eng. 1984; FRCP Ed. 1993. Prev: Chief Med. Off. DHSS Educat. Sci. & Home Off.

YELLOWLEES, Ian Henry Kippilaw Mains, Melrose TD6 9HF Tel: 01835 822015 Email: ian.yellowlees@painco.co.uk — MB ChB Bristol 1983; BA (Hons.) Engin Sci. Oxf. 1977; FCAnaesth 1989; MPhil (Engineering) 1990. Cons. & Dir., The Pain Co Ltd.; Med. Dir. Quantics Consulting Ltd. Specialty: Anaesth. Special Interest: Insurance/Legal Assessments; Return-to-work Schemes. Prev: Cons. Anaes. & Pain Manag. Borders Gen Hops. Melrose; Sen. Regist. Rotat. (Anaesth.) Newc.; Regist. (Anaesth.) Bristol.

YELLOWLEES, Walter Walker, MC (retired) The Cottage, Alma Avenue, Aberfeldy PH15 2BW Tel: 01887 820277 Email: w.syellowlees@virgin.net — (Ed.) MB ChB Ed. 1941; FRCGP 1970. Prev: RMO 5th Bn. Qu. Own Cameron Highlanders.

YELLOWLEY, John Crisp (retired) 30 Lumsdaine Drive, Dalgety Bay, Dunfermline KY11 9YU Tel: 01383 824870 — MB ChB Ed. 1952.

YELLOWLEY, Thomas William 106 Edge Hill, Ponteland, Newcastle upon Tyne NE20 9JQ — MB BS Durh. 1961; DObst RCOG 1963.

YELNOORKAR, Kamalakar Galleries Health Centre, Washington Centre, Washington NE38 7NQ Tel: 0191 416 7032 — MB BS Marathwada 1968. GP Washington, Tyne & Wear.

YEN, Mr William 49/50 Leinster Gardens, Bayswater, London W2 3AT — MB BS Lond. 1959; MRCS Eng. LRCP Lond. 1959; FRCS Ed. 1963; FRCS Eng. 1964.

YENTIS, Irvan Lavender Wall, 12 Warren Road, Ickenham, Uxbridge UB10 8AA Tel: 01895 235867 — MB BS Lond. 1947 (Guy's) MD Lond. 1950; FRCP Lond. 1973, M 1951; DMRD Eng. 1953; FFR 1957; FRCR 1975. Specialty: Radiol. Socs: (Ex-Pres.) Windsor & Dist. Med. Soc. Prev: Dist. Clin. Tutor E. Berks. HA; Cons. Radiol. King Edwd. VII Hosp. Windsor & Wexham Pk. Hosp. Slough; Sen. Regist. (X-Ray Diag.) Univ. Coll. Hosp. & Hosp. Sick Childr. Gt. Ormond St. Lond.

YENTIS, Steven Marc Magill Department of Anaesthesia, Chelsea & Westminster Hospital, 369 Fulham Road, London SW10 9NH — MB BS Lond. 1984 (Univ. Coll. Hosp.) FRCA 1989; BSc Lond. 1981, MD 1994. Cons. Anaesth. Chelsea & Westm. Hosp. Lond. Specialty: Anaesth. Prev: Sen. Regist. (Anaesth.) Char. Cross & Westm. Hosps. Lond.; Regist. (Anaesth.) St. Mary's Hosp. Lond.

YEO, David Woon Tjun 412 Park W., London W2 2QT — MB BS Lond. 1998.

YEO, Elaine Ruth Abernethy House, 70 Silver Street, Enfield EN1 3EP Tel: 020 8366 1314 Fax: 020 8364 4176; 9 Glebe Avenue, Enfield EN2 8NZ Tel: 020 8363 1019 — MB ChB Birm. 1972; DObst RCOG 1974; DCH Eng. 1975; MRCGP 1984. GP Course Organiser Enfield VTS. Prev: Ho. Off. (Obst.) & SHO (Paediat.) N. Middlx. Hosp. Lond.

YEO, Hazel Eunice Dorothy Pennells and Partners, Gosport Health Centre, Bury Road, Gosport PO12 3PN Tel: 023 9258 3344 Fax: 023 9260 2704 — MB BS Lond. 1978 (Univ. Coll. Hosp.) BSc Lond. 1975; DRCOG 1980; MRCGP 1982. Prev: GP Guildford; SHO (Paediat. & ENT) Roy. Surrey Co. Hosp. Guildford.

YEO, Jane Elizabeth Tilehurst Surgery, Tylers Place, Pottery Road, Tilehurst, Reading RG30 6BW Tel: 0118 942 7528 Fax: 0118 945 2405; 9 Norman Avenue, Henley-on-Thames RG9 1SG Tel: 01491 577915 — MB BS Lond. 1961; MRCS Eng. LRCP Lond. 1961; MRCGP 1983. Prev: GP Barbados.

YEO, Kok Cheang, CMG (retired) 10 Rowbarns, Battle TN33 0JQ Tel: 01424 772803 — MB BS Hong Kong 1925; DTM & H Eng. 1927; DPH Camb. 1928; MD Hong Kong 1930. Prev: Asst. Psychiat. St. Ebba's Hosp. Epsom.

YEO, Mr Richard Adams Farm, Sandrock Hill, Crowhurst, Battle TN33 9AY Tel: 01424 830255 — MB BChir Camb. 1959 (Westm.) MChir Camb. 1967, MA, MB 1959, BChir 1958; MRCS Eng. LRCP Lond. 1958; FRCS Eng. 1962. Hon. Cons. Gen. Surg. Conquest Hosp. St. Leonards-on-Sea. Specialty: Gen. Surg. Socs: Sec. Brit. Surg. Stapling Gp.; Surg. Vasc. Soc. of Gt. Brit. & Irel. Prev: Cons. Gen. Surg. Roy. E. Sussex & St. Helen's Hosps. Bexhill Hosp. & Rye Hosp.; Res. Surg. Off. Brompton Hosp.; Sen. Regist. (Surg.) King's Coll. Hosp. Lond.

YEO, Richard Castle Hill Hospital, Castle Hill Road, Cottingham HU16 5JQ Tel: 01482 875875; Bank House Farm, Main St, Etton, Beverley HU17 7PQ Tel: 01430 810459 — MB BS Lond. 1968 (St. Geo.) DObst RCOG 1970; FRCOG 1987, M 1973. Cons. O & G E. Yorks. Hosp.s Trust Hull. Specialty: Obst. & Gyn. Socs: Lond. Obst. & Gyn. Soc.; Hull Med. Soc. Prev: Sen. Regist. (O & G) Char. Cross Hosp. Lond.; Regist. (O & G) Pembury Hosp.; SHO (O & G) Princess Margt. Hosp. Swindon.

YEO, Seng Tee 31 Wyncote Court, Jesmond Park Est., Newcastle upon Tyne NE7 7BG — MB BS Newc. 1991.

YEO, Siaw Ing Flat 36, Campania Building, Atlantic Wharf, 1 Jardine Road, London E1 9WE Tel: 020 7790 3180 — MB BS Lond. 1993 (UMDS Guy's and St. Thos. Hosps.) MRCP (UK) 1996. Specialist Regist. (Rheum. & Med.) S. Thames. Specialty: Gen. Med.; Rheumatol. Prev: Clin. Research Fell. (Rheum.) King's Coll. Hosp.; SHO (Rheum.) Lewisham NHS Trust.

YEO, Wilfred Winston Section of Clinical Pharmacology & Therapay, University Department Medicine & Pharmacology, Floor L, Royal Hallamshire Hospital, Glossop Road, Sheffield S10 2JF Tel: 0114 271 3789 Fax: 0114 272 0275 Email: w.w.yeo@sheffield.ac.uk; 7 Glebe View, Barlborough, Chesterfield S43 4WF Tel: 01246 570454 — MB ChB Sheff. 1984; MD 1996, Sheff; BMedSci (Hons.) Sheff. 1983; MRCP (UK) 1987. Sen. Lect. in Med., Clin. Pharmacol. & Thrapeutics; Hon. Cons. Phys., Centr. Sheffeld, Univ. Hosp. Trust. Specialty: Gen. Med. Socs: Brit. Pharm. Soc.; Brit. Hypertens. Soc.; Clin. Sec. BPS. Prev: Sen. Regist. & Lect. (Med. & Pharmacol.) Roy. Hallamsh. Hosp. Sheff.; Research Regist. (Pharmacol. & Therap.) Roy. Hallamsh. Hosp. Sheff.

YEOH, Jo Han Staffordshire General Hospital, Deparrtment of Thoracic Medicine, Weston Road, Stafford ST16 3SA Tel: 01785 230971 Fax: 01785 230980 Email: jo-han.yeoh@msgh-tr.wmids.nhs.uk — MB BCh Wales 1991; MRCP Lond. 1996. Cons. Respirat. Phys. Mid-Staffs. Gen. Hosps. NHS Trust. Specialty: Respirat. Med.; Gen. Med.

YEOH, Mr Lam Hoe Epson & St Helier NHS Trust, Weythe Lane, Carshalton SM5 1AA — MB BS Singapore 1976; DLO Eng. 1979; FRCS (Otol.) Eng. 1982; MSc Manch. 1988. p/t Cons. Phys. (Audiol.) Epsom & St Helier NHS Trust Surrey; Cons. Phys. (Audiol.) Portland Hosp. Lond.; Cons. Phys. (Audiol.), Cromwell Hosp. Lond.; Cons. Phys. (Audiol.), St Anthony's Hosp. Cheam; Cons. Phys. (Audiol.), Ashstead Hosp. Ashstead. Specialty: Audiol. Med. Special Interest: Noise Damage; Tinnitus; Paediatric Audiology. Socs: Brit. Assn. of Audiological Physicians; Internat. Assn. of Physicians in Audiol. Prev: Cons. Phys. (Audiol.) Merton & Sutton HA.; Sen. Regist. (Audiol. Med.) Mersey RHA; Sen. Regist. (Otorhinolaryng.) Mersey RHA.

YEOH, Michael John Department of Anaesthetcis, Salisbury District Hospital, Odstock Road, Salisbury SP2 8BJ — MB BS Melbourne 1991.

YEOMAN, Andrew David The Rectory, Merthyr Mawr Road N., Bridgend CF31 3NH — MB BCh Wales 1998.

YEOMAN, Colin Michael Highpoint, Church Lane, Thropton, Morpeth NE65 7JB — MB ChB Manch. 1994.

YEOMAN, Lindsey Jane Department of Radiology, Barnsley District General Hospital, Gawber Road, Barnsley S75 2EP Tel: 01226 730000 — MB BS Lond. 1983; MRCP (UK) 1986; FRCR 1990; T(R) (CR) 1991. Cons. Radiol. Barnsley Dist. Gen. Hosp. Specialty: Radiol. Prev: Cons. Radiol. City Hosp. Nottm.

YEOMAN, Neil Christopher 14 Meynell Gardens, London E9 7AT — MB BS Lond. 1987.

YEOMAN, Peter David Waterloo Surgery, Thoroton Street, Blyth NE24 1DX Tel: 01670 396560 Fax: 01670 396579 — MB ChB Manch. 1983 (St Andrews & Manchester) BSc St. And. 1980; DRCOG 1986. Bd. Mem. PCG. Prev: SHO (Paediat.) Cumbld. Infirm.; SHO (O & G) Newc. Gen. Hosp.; Ho. Off. (Med.) Lewis Hosp. Stornoway.

YEOMAN, Roger Willow Surgery, Coronation Rd, Downend, Bristol BS16 Tel: 0117 970 9500; 26 West Mall, Clifton, Bristol BS8 4BG Tel: 0117 973 7552 — MB ChB Manch. 1986 (St. Andrews/Manchester) BSc Med. Sci. 1983, St. And; D.A Coll. Anaestetists 1991. Specialty: Gen. Pract. Socs: Cossham Med. Soc.

YEOMANS, Julian David Ian Somerset House, Manor Lane, Shipley BD18 3BP Tel: 01274 531536 Fax: 01274 770779 — MB ChB Manch. 1985; BSc St. And. 1982; MRCPsych 1990; MMedSc Leeds 1992. Cons. Psychiat. (Adult Psychiat.) Bradford Community Health Trust. Specialty: Gen. Psychiat. Prev: Sen. Regist. (Adult Psychiat.) Yorks. Region; Hon. Tutor (Psychiat.) Univ. Leeds.

YEOMANS, Neil Paul 6 Leopold Drive, Bishops Waltham, Southampton SO32 1JU — MB ChB Leeds 1998.

YEOMANS, Steven John 35 The Broadway, Tynemouth, North Shields NE30 2LL — MB BS Lond. 1992 (Guy's Hosp., Lond. Univ.) BA Oxf. 1989; MRCP (UK) 1997. Specialist Regis., (Gen. & Geriat. Med.), Bishop Auckland Hosp.; Cons. Physician/ Geriat. N. Tees Hosp. Specialty: Care of the Elderly. Socs: Brit. Geriat. Soc. Prev: Specialist Regist., S. Cleveland Hosp.; Specialist Regist., Sunderland Roy. Hosp.; Specialist Regis., N. Tees Hosp.

YEONG, Chee Chew Warrington Hospital NHS Trust, Lovely Lane, Warrington WA5 1QG Tel: 01925 662457; 24 Greenway, Appleton, Warrington WA4 3AD Tel: 01925 604899 — MB BCh BAO Dub. 1982; MRCP (UK) 1987; FRCR 1992; T(R) (CR) 1993. Cons. Radiol. Warrington Hosp. NHS Trust. Specialty: Radiol. Prev: Sen. Regist. N. Staffs. Hosp.

YERASSIMOU, Pamela Marcella 15 Belmont Court, 93 Highbury New Park, London N5 2HA — MB BCh Wales 1994.

YERBURY, Christopher Michael Grange Road Surgery, Grange Road, Bishopsworth, Bristol BS13 8LD Tel: 0117 964 4343 Fax: 0117 935 8422 — MB BS 1985 (U.C.H, London) BSc Lond. 1982; DCH RCP Lond. 1988; DRCOG 1992; MRCGP 1993. GP Bristol. Prev: GP VTS, Bath; Med. Off. Kikuyu Hosp. Kenya.; Med. Off. Eshowe Hosp. Zululand.

YERBURY, Grace Margaret (retired) Timber Close, Church Lane, Oakley, Bedford MK43 7RP Tel: 01234 825432 — MB BS Lond.

1954 (Middlx.) FRCPH; DObst RCOG 1956; DCH Eng. 1957; MPhil Cranfield Univ. 1993. Prev: Regist. (Paediat.) Addenbrooke's Hosp. Camb.

YERBURY, Nicholas Olyffe New Court Surgery, Borough Fields, Wootton Bassett, Swindon SN4 7AX Tel: 01793 852302 Fax: 01793 851119 — MB BS Lond. 1972 (Guy's) MRCS Eng. LRCP Lond. 1972; DObst RCOG 1974; MRCGP 1979. Socs: Soc. Apoth. Lond. Prev: Sen. Med. Off. RAF Lyneham; Ho. Off. (Obst.) Roy. Sussex Co. Hosp. Brighton; Ho. Off. (Paediat.) Southmead Hosp. Bristol.

YESUFU, Aminu Omonikhe 279 Katherine Road, London E7 8PP — MB BS Ibadan 1978; MRCOG. Specialty: Obst. & Gyn.; Disabil. Med.; Gen. Pract. Prev: Staff Grade Obst.& Gynae., St Cross Hosp., Rugby,January 1997.

YETTON, William Rex (Surgery), 4 St Peters Place, Brighton BN1 4SA Tel: 01273 606006 Fax: 01273 623896; 49 The Droveway, Hove BN3 6PR Tel: 01273 558274 — MRCS Eng. LRCP Lond. 1973; FFA RCS Eng. 1980. GP Brighton. Specialty: Anaesth. Prev: Regist. (Anaesth.) Roy. Sussex Co. Hosp. Brighton.

YEUNG, Eric Sze Tsun 44 Castle Grove, Portchester, Fareham PO16 9NZ — MB BS Lond. 1996.

YEUNG, John Ngai Man Whittington Hospital, Highgate Hill, London N19 5NF Tel: 020 7272 3070; 108 Clarence Gate Gardens, Glentworth St, London NW1 6AL Tel: 020 7724 1299 — MB ChB Ed. 1988; MBA Warwick 1990; MRCP (UK) 1992. SHO (Paediat.) Whittington Hosp. Lond. Specialty: Paediat. Prev: SHO Rotat. (Med.) Battle & Roy. Berks. Hosps. Reading; Ho. Off. (Med.) Dumfries & Galloway Roy. Infirm.; Ho. Off. (Surg.) West. Gen. Hosp. Edin.

YEUNG, Justin Ming-Chi 11 Hazelmere Grove, Lenton, Nottingham NG7 2EH — BM BS Nottm. 1996.

YEUNG, Shun May Flat 16, 45 Barkston Gardens, London SW5 0ES — MB BS Lond. 1991.

YEUNG, Stephen Roy The General Infirmary at Leeds, Great George Street, Leeds LS1 3EX — MB ChB Leeds 1968; Dip. Pract. Dermat. Wales 1991. Assoc. Specialist Dermat., Leeds Teachg. Hosps. NHS Trust. Prev: Research Clin. Asst. (Neurol.) Leeds Gen. Infirm.; Ho. Phys. Leeds Gen. Infirm.; Ho. Surg. St. Jas. Hosp. Leeds.

YEUNG-WYE-KONG, Mr Chin-Kian Pontefract General Infirmary, (Pinderfields and Pontefract Hospital Trust), Friarwood Lane, Pontefract WF7 7EL; Green Knoll, Pontefract Road, Ackworth, Pontefract WF7 7EL — MB ChB (Hons.) Leeds 1969; FRCS Ed. 1974; FRCS Eng. 1975. Cons. Surg. Pontefract Gen. Infirm. Pinderfields & Pontefract Hosp. Trust. Specialty: Gen. Surg. Prev: Sen. Regist. (Surg.) Leeds & Bradford Health Dists.; Research Fell. Univ. Dept. Surg. Leeds Gen. Infirm.; Surg. Regist. Nottm. AHA (T).

YI, Chung-Yiu Guy's Hospital, St. Thomas St., London SE1 9RT Tel: 020 7955 5000 — MB Camb. 1992; BChir 1991; MA Camb. 1993; MRCP (UK) 1995. SHO (Renal Med.) Guy's Hosp. Lond.

YIALLOUROS, Michael 2 Camlet Way, Barnet EN4 0LH Tel: 020 8440 1628 Fax: 0208 447 1627 — Ptychio Iatrikes Thessalonika 1971. Specialty: Gen. Med.

YIANGOU, Mr Constantinos Queen Alexandra Hospital, Cosham, Portsmouth PO6 3LY Tel: 023 9228 6263 Fax: 023 9228 6547 Email: constantinos.yiangou@porthosp.nhs.uk — MB BS Lond. 1987 (St. Mary's Hosp. Med. Sch.) BSc (Hons.) Lond. 1984; FRCS Eng. 1991; FRCS (Gen Surg.) 1999. Cons. Surg. Qu. Alexandra Hosp., Portsmouth; Hon. Sen. Lect., Univ. of Portsmouth. Specialty: Gen. Surg. Socs: BMA; Brit. Assn. Of Surgic. Oncol.; Assn. of Breast Surg. Prev: Sen. Specialist Regist. (Gen. & Oncol. Surg.) Lister Hosp. Stevenage; Specialist Regist. (Gen. Surg.) Hemel Hempstead Hosp.; Sen. Specialist Regist. (Gen. & Breast Surg.) Char. Cross Hosp. Lond.

YIANGOU, Georgia Grosvenor House, 147 Broadway, West Ealing, London W13 9BE Tel: 020 8567 0165/5172 Fax: 020 8810 0902; 11 St. Michaels Avenue, Wembley HA9 6SJ — MB ChB Manch. 1981; Cert. Family Plann. JCC 1982. Specialty: Gen. Med.

YIANNAKOU, John Yiannakis 10 Raglan Street, Kentish Town, London NW5 3DA — MB ChB Dundee 1986.

YIANNI, John 9 Newman Road, Hayes UB3 3AL Email: john.yianni@physiol.ox.ac.uk — MB BS Lond. 1996.

YICK, David Chee Kong — BM BS Nottm. 1996; BMedSci; MRCP.

YIEND, Margaret Elizabeth (retired) The Jays, Lynwood Road, Lydney GL15 5SG — MB ChB Leeds 1950. Asst. MOH Matern. & Child Welf. Plymouth.

YIH, Jean-Paul Lai Bong 34A Belsize Road, London NW6 4RD — MB BS Lond. 1990; MA Oxf. 1993. SHO Moorfields Eye Hosp. Lond. Prev: SHO (Ophth. & Plastic Surg.) Hosp. Childr. Gt. Ormond St. Lond.; SHO (Neurosurg. & Ophth.) Roy. Lond. Hosp.

YII, Mr Michael Yang Yong Cardiothoracic Surgical Unit, Royal Postgraduate Medical School & Hammersmith Hospital, Du Cane Road, London W12 0HS Tel: 020 8743 2030; 16 Vellacott House, Du Cane Road, London W12 0UQ Tel: 020 8746 0627 — MB BS Melbourne 1990; FRCS Eng. 1994. Research Regist. (Cardiac Surg.) Roy. Postgrad. Med. Sch. & Hammersmith Hosp. Lond. Specialty: Cardiothoracic Surg.

YIN YIN WIN, Dr 6 Burnsall Close, Brackendale, The Droveway, Pendeford, Wolverhampton WV9 5RU; Wall Lane House Young People's Centre, St. Edwards Hospital, Cheddleton, Leek ST13 7EB — MB BS Med. Inst. (I) Rangoon 1979; MRCPsych 1996. Specialty: Child & Adolesc. Psychiat.

YING, Ian Alaistair Ashby Clinic, Collum Lane, Scunthorpe DN16 2SZ Tel: 01724 271877; 135 Moorwell Road, Scunthorpe DN17 2SX Tel: 01724 840742 Fax: 01724 840742 — MB BS Lond. 1963 (St. Bart.) MRCS Eng. LRCP Lond. 1967; MRCOG 1969. Prev: Cons. O & G Geo.town Hosp. Guyana; Regist. (O & G) Beckenham Matern. & Beckenham Gen. Hosps.

YIP, Alex Shing Biu 48 Childebert Road, London SW17 8EX — MB BS Lond. 1981 (St. Bart.) MRCP (UK) 1984. Regist. (Med.) Roy. United Hosp. Bath. Prev: SHO (Cardiol.) Lond. Chest Hosp.; Ho. Phys. Whipps Cross Hosp. Lond.; Ho. Surg. St. Bart. Hosp. Lond.

YIP, Brigitte Hairmyres Hospital ,
Department of Medicine for the Elderly, Eaglesham Road, East Kilbride, Glasgow G75 8RG Tel: 01355 585000 Email: brigitte.yip@lanarkshire.scot.nhs.uk — MB ChB Glas. 1985; FRCP. Cons. (Phys. in Geriat. Med.) Hairmyres Hosp. E. Kilbride. Specialty: Care of the Elderly. Special Interest: Stroke Med.

YIP, Lai-Ching Kathleen 28 Highbury Road, Glasgow G12 9DZ — MB ChB Ed. 1987; MRCGP 1991. Prev: Med. Off. (Community Paediat.) Optimum Health Servs. Lond.; SHO (Obst.) Paisley Matern. Hosp.; Trainee GP Greenlaw Med. Centre Paisley.

YIP, Richard Ying Wai 10 Hancroft Road, Bennetts End, Hemel Hempstead HP3 9LL Tel: 01442 236693 — MB BChir Camb. 1990; MRCGP 1994. Socs: Brit. Med. Acupunct. Soc. Prev: Trainee GP Hemel Hempstead.

YIP, Yee Yan c\o 62 Elmslie Point, Ackroyd Drive, Mile End, London E3 4LD — MB BS Hong Kong 1967; DTM & H Liverp. 1968.

YISA, Mahazu Ajayi 81 Claydon Drive, Beddington, Croydon CR0 4QX — MB BS Ibadan 1976; MRCP (UK) 1984.

YIU, Carolyn Anne Cornerways Surgery, 50 Manor Road, Beckenham BR3 5LG Tel: 020 8650 2444; 56 Barnfield Wood Road, Park Langley, Beckenham BR3 6SU Tel: 020 8658 1739 — MB BS Newc. 1975; MRCGP 1979.

YIU, Mr Chu Yiu Queen Elizabeth Hospital, Stadium Road, Woolwich, London SE18 4QH — MB BS Lond. 1976 (Univ. Coll. Hosp.) FRCS Eng. 1981; BSc (Hons.) Anat. Lond. 1973, MS Lond. 1990. Cons. Surg. Qu. Eliz. Hosp. Woolwich. Specialty: Gen. Surg. Socs: Brit. Assn. Surg. Oncol; Assn. Coloproctol.; St. Mark's Assn. Prev: Regist. (Surg.) Chase Farm Hosp. Enfield Middlx.; Wellcome Lect. (Surg.) Sch. Med. Univ. Coll. Lond.; Sen. Lect. (Surg.) UCL Med. Sch.

YIU, Cynthia Oi San The Hurley Clinic, Ebenezer House, Kennington Lane, London SE11 4HJ Tel: 020 7735 7918 Fax: 020 7587 5296 — MB BS Lond. 1983; DCH RCP Lond. 1991; MRCGP 1995; ILTM 2002.

YIU, Hsiang-Sung, Robert 35 Hendon Avenue, Finchley Central, London N3 1UJ Tel: 020 8349 2360 — MB BS Hong Kong 1955.

YIU, Mr Patrick 26 Woodberry Way, North Finchley, London N12 0HG — MB BS Lond. 1989 (UMDS Guy's & St. Thos.) BSc (Hons.) Lond. 1986; FRCS Eng. 1994. Research Regist. (Surg.) Middlx. & Univ. Coll. Hosps. Lond. Socs: BMA; Roy. Soc. Med.; Roy. Coll. Surg. of Eng. Prev: Regist. (Cardiothoracic) Lond. Chest Hosp.

YODAIKEN, Myer Mark Steppinghill Hospital, Poplar Grove, Stockport SK2 7JE; BMI The Alexandra Hospital, Mill Lane, Cheadle SK8 2PX; BUPA Hospital, Russell Road, Whalley Range, Manchester

M16 8aj Tel: 0161 232 2277 Fax: 0161 232 2255 — MB BCh Witwatersrand 1990; FRCS; FCS (Ophth). Cons. (Ophth.) Steppinghill Hosp. Stockport; Privat. Pract. BMI Alexandra Hosp. Cheadle & BUPA Hosp. Manch. Specialty: Ophth. Special Interest: Cataract & Refractive Surg. Socs: UK Society of Cataract & Refractive Surgeons; America Academy of Ophthamology; European Society of Cataract & Refractive Surgeons.

YOGALINGAM, Muttukumaru 182 Upper Shoreham Road, Shoreham-by-Sea BN43 6BG Tel: 01273 591183 — MB BS Ceylon 1971. Specialty: Rehabil. Med.; Rheumatol.; Care of the Elderly.

YOGANATHAN, Kathirgamanathan 24 Rhydydefaid Drive, Sketty, Swansea SA2 8AJ Tel: 01792 204615 — MB BS Sri Lanka 1981; MRCP (UK) 1988; MRCS Eng. LRCP Lond. 1989; FRCP 1998. Cons. Phys. (Genitourin. Med.) Singleton Hosp. Swansea. Specialty: Genitourinary Medicine. Prev: Sen. Regist. (Genitourin. Med.) King's Coll. Hosp. Lond.

YOGANATHAN, Malarmagal 24 Rhydydefaid Drive, Sketty, Swansea SA2 8AJ Tel: 01792 204615 — MRCS Eng. LRCP Lond. 1988; MRCS Eng LRCP Lond. 1988; DFFP 1995. Clin. Asst., (ENT & Rheum.); GP since Oct. 1999. Specialty: Otolaryngol.; Rheumatol. Prev: Locum Staff Grade Phys. in Elderly Care, Hill Ho. Hosp., Swansea.

YOGARAJAH, Subraya Chettiar Department of Radiology, Milton Keynes General Hospital, Milton Keynes MK6 5LD Tel: 01908 660033 — MB BS Ceylon 1966 (Colombo) DMRD Eng. 1975; FRCR 1976. Cons. Radiol. E. (Glas.) Health Dist.; Hon. Clin. Lect. (Radiodiag.) Univ. Glas. Specialty: Radiol. Socs: Brit. Inst. Radiol. & Brit. Med. Ultra-Sound Soc. Prev: SHO (Med.) Haslemere & Dist. Hosp.; Regist. (Radiol.) & Sen. Regist. (Radiol.) Roy. Infirm. Glas.

YOGARATNAM, Sarojinidevi 3 Churchill Close, Aylestone Hill, Hereford HR1 1DH Tel: 01432 352308 Fax: 01432 276527 — MB BS Sri Lanka 1973. Clin. Asst. Gen. Hosp. Hereford.

YOGASAKARAN, Bhuwaneswari Sivakumarie Dept. of Anaesth., Luton & Dunstable Hospital, Lewsey Road, Luton LU4 0DZ Tel: 01582 497 230 Fax: 01582 497 230 Email: bsyoga@aol.com — MB BS Sri Lanka 1974 (Univ. of Colombo, Sri Lanka) FFA RCS Eng. 1982. Consultant Anaesthetist. Specialty: Anaesth. Special Interest: Chronic Pain. Socs: The Pain Soc. (UK); IASP; Assn. of Anaesthetics. Prev: SMO Grantham Hosp., Hong Kong; Cons. Waikato Hosp., Hamilton. New Zealand.

YOGASAKARAN, Namasivayam Registrar in Anaesthetics, Princess Alexandra Hospital, Harlow CM20 1QX; 38 Sheldon Avenue, Clayhall, Ilford IG5 0UD — MB BS Ceylon 1974; DA Eng. 1981; FFA RCSI 1984. Specialty: Anaesth.

YOGASUNDRAM, Sanath Naresh The Old Bakery, 25 West St, Easton on the Hill, Stafford PE9 3LS Tel: 01780 753898 — MB ChB Leic. 1990; BSc (Hons.) Leic. 1987; MRCGP 1995. Partner GP. Specialty: Gen. Pract. Prev: PeterBoro. VTS; SHO Rotat. (Med.) P'boro. VTS.; SHO Wollongong Hosp. NSW, Austral.

YOGASUNDRAM, Mr Yoganathan 4 Winmarleigh Road, Ashton, Preston PR2 1ET Tel: 01772 726992 — MB BS Ceylon 1958; FRCS Ed. 1964; FRCS Eng. 1965. Assoc. Specialist (Surg.) N. W. RHA. Prev: Tutor in Surg. Univ. Ceylon; Regist. (Orthop.) Gen. Hosp. Colombo.

YOGENDRAN, Logesvaran Global Clinical Safety & Pharmacovigilance, Glaxo SmithKline Research and Development Ltd, Greenford UB6 0HE — MB BS Colombo 1983; MFPM; MSc; MRCP (UK) 1989. Med. Director (Global Clin. Safety & Pharmacovigilance) Glaxo SmithKline Research & Developm. Greenford,Middlx. Specialty: Pharmaceutical Medicine.

YOGESWARAN, Pararajasingham 82 Hillside Road, Northwood HA6 1PZ — BM Soton. 1994.

YONACE, Adrian Harris Bournemouth Nuffield Hospital, 65-67 Lansdowne Road,, Bournemouth BH1 1RW Tel: 01202 291866 — BM BS Nottm. 1975; BMedSci (Hons.) Nottm. 1973; FRCPsych 1994, M 1980. Cons. Psychiat. Private Pract.; Hon. Cons. Roy. Bournemouth and Poole Gen. Hosp.s; JP; Ment. Health Review Tribunal; SOAD Ment. Health Act Commiss. Specialty: Gen. Psychiat. Prev: Cons. Psychiat. St. Ann's Hosp. Poole; Cons. & Hon. Sen. Lect. Frien Hosp. & Roy. Free Hosp. Sch. Med. Lond.; Lect. & Hon. Sen. Regist. Roy. Free Hosp. & Regist. Maudsley Hosp.

YONG, Agnes Siew Mee 28A Benbow Road, London W6 0AG — MB BCh BAO Belf. 1990; MRCP (UK) 1993. Regist. (Haemat.) Hammersmith Hosp. Lond. Specialty: Haematology.

YONG, Audrey Alice 7 Park Drive, Wickford SS12 9DH — MB BS Lond. 1991 (St Bartholomew's) FRCS 1995. Specialty: Radiol.

YONG, Chee Heng Medical Residency, Morriston General Hospital, Heol Maes Eglwys, Cwmrhyceirw, Swansea — MB ChB Ed. 1987.

YONG, Collin Kah Khion 21 Stephenson Close, Leamington Spa CV32 6BS — MB ChB Leic. 1989.

YONG, Diana Elizabeth Jane Department of Paediatrics, Peterborough District Hospital, Midgate, Thorpe Road, Peterborough PE3 6DA Fax: 01733 874326 Email: diana.yong@pbh-tr.nhs.uk — MB ChB Aberd. 1989; MRCP (Paediat.) (UK) 1993. Cons. Paediat. & Neonatol. Specialty: Paediat. Prev: Specialist Regist. (Paediat.) Leicester; Specialist Regist. (paeds) PeterBoro. Dist. Hosp.; Hon. Clin. Lect. Univ. Aberd.

YONG, Kwee Lan Flat 28, Corringham, 13-16 Craven Hill Gardens, London W2 3EH — MB BS Lond. 1984.

YONG, Patrick Foh Khing c/o 11 Brocas Close, London NW3 3LD — MB ChB Bristol 1998.

YONG, Pauline Poh Lin St Mary's Surgery, 1 Johnson Street, Southampton SO14 1LT Tel: 023 8033 3778 Fax: 023 8021 1894 — BM Soton. 1985. SHO (O & G) Dorchester. Socs: BMA. Prev: Ho. Off. Isle of Wight & E. Dorset HA.

YONGE, Geoffrey Pragnell, TD (retired) Foxhollow, Merlewood Drive, Chislehurst BR7 5LQ Tel: 020 8467 6117 — MB BS Lond. 1949 (Middlx.) Prev: Chief Med. Off. Provident Mutual Life Assur. Assn.

YOON, Jeannie Swee Lynn 1 Addison House, Grove End Road, London NW8 9EH — MB BS Lond. 1986.

YOON, Lai Lan 31 Ashleigh Manor, Windsor Avenue, Belfast BT9 6EJ — MB BCh BAO Belf. 1992.

YOONG, Adrian Kah Hean Birmingham Women's Hospital, Department of Histology, 1st Floor Laboratories, Edgbaston, Birmingham B15 2TG Tel: 0121 627 2729 Fax: 0121 607 4721 Email: adeyoong@hotmail.com — MB BChir Camb. 1983 (Cambridge) MA Camb. 1985; MRCPath 1991; T(Path) 1991; FRCPath 1999. Cons. Gyn. Histo/Cytopath. Birm. Wom.'s Hosp.; Hon. Sen. Clin. Lect. Univ. of Birm. Specialty: Histopath.

YOONG, Ann Fui-En Department of Obstetrics & Gynaecology, St. Mary's Hospital, Newport PO30 5TG Tel: 01983 534348 — MB ChB Birm. 1983; MRCOG 1988; MD Birm. 1993; FRCOG 2001. Cons. (O & G) St. Mary's Hosp. I. of Wight. Specialty: Obst. & Gyn. Special Interest: Menstrual Disorders; Pelvic Surgery; Urinary Incontinence. Prev: Lect. O & G St. Mary's Hosp. Manch.

YOONG, Soo Yee Zetland House, Friarage Hospital, Northallerton DL6 1JG; 27 Copperclay Walk, Easingwold, York YO61 3RU — MB ChB Aberd. 1982 (Univ. Aberd.) DCH RCP Lond. 1986; MRCP (Paediat.) Glas. 1992; MMedSc Leeds 1997. Specialty: Community Child Health.

YOONG, Wai Cheong 72 Winchfield Drive, Birmingham B17 8TR — MB BCh BAO Belf. 1987; MRCOG 1995. Clin. Research Fell. Dept. of O & G Roy. Free Hosp. Lond. Specialty: Obst. & Gyn. Prev: Rotat. Regist. (O & G) W. Midl.

YORK, Ann Helen Child & Family Consultation Centre, Richmond Royal, Kew Foot Rd, Richmond TW9 2TE Tel: 020 8355 1984 Fax: 020 8355 1977 — MB BS Lond. 1982 (Roy. Free) MRCPsych 1987. Cons. Child & Adolesc. Psychiat. Child & family consultation Centre, Richmond; Hon. Sen. Lect., Child & Adolesc. Psychiat., St Geo. Hosp. Med. Sch. Lond (P/T). Specialty: Child & Adolesc. Psychiat. Socs: Mem. of Roy. Coll. of Psychiat.s. Prev: Sen. Regist. (Child Psychiat.) St. Geo. Hosp. Lond.; Clin. Asst. (Addic.) Qu. Mary's Hosp. Lond.; Regist. (Child Psychiat.) Ealing Child Guid. Ealing.

YORK, Anthea Hilary The Surgery, Queens Road, Earls Colne, Colchester CO6 2RR Tel: 01787 222641; The Cottages, Lamarsh Road, Bures CO8 5EW Tel: 01787 227490 — MB ChB Birm. 1969.

YORK, Elizabeth Louise 6 Manor Court, South Brent TQ10 9RA Tel: 01364 649 120 — MB ChB Ed. 1996. SHO(Anaesth.) Plymouth Hosps. NHS Trust. Prev: SHO S. E. Scotl.; SHO Med., Frenchay Healthcare NHS Trust.

YORK, James Richard Brynhyfryd Surgery, Brynhyfryd Square, Brynhyfryd, Swansea SA5 9DZ Tel: 01792 655083; 29 Bryn Hedydd, Llangyfelach, Swansea SA6 8BS — BM BS Nottm. 1988; MRCGP 1992. Prev: Trainee GP York VTS.

YORK, Josephine Helen The Cottages, Lamarsh Road, Bures CO8 5EW — MB ChB Sheff. 1998.

YORK, Stephen Arthur Horton Bank Practice, 1220 Great Horton Road, Bradford BD7 4PL Tel: 01274 573696/572573 Fax: 01274 521605; Arrowbutt Lee, Catherine House Lane, Luddenden Dean, Halifax HX2 6XB — MB ChB Leeds 1976.

YORK, Susan Mary 1 Southview Gardens, Ravenshead, Nottingham NG15 9GB — BM BS Nottm. 1976.

YORK-MOORE, David William Litchdon Medical Centre, Landkey Road, Barnstaple EX32 9LL Tel: 01271 23443 Fax: 01271 25979 — MB BS Lond. 1976 (London Hospital) DRCOG 1981; MRCGP 1982. Specialty: Gen. Pract. Prev: Trainee GP N. Devon VTS.

YORKE, Peter Harold (retired) The Old Coach House, Buttery Lane, Teversal Village, Sutton-in-Ashfield NG17 3JN — MB BS Durh. 1958. Med. Off. Notts. Water Bd. & Alan Smith Gp. Nottm. Prev: Dent. Anaesth. for Sch. Dent. Serv.

YORKE, Reginald Angelo (retired) Briardale, 3 Wicks Lane, Formby, Liverpool L37 3JE Tel: 017048 72187 Email: wd71@dial.pipex.com — MB ChB Liverp. 1954; FRCGP 1996, M 1988. Prev: Regist. (Med.), Ho. Surg. & Ho. Phys. Liverp. Roy. Infirm.

YORKE, Ronald James Health Centre, Civic Centre, Ebbw Vale NP23 6EY; Errigal, Bryn Deri Road, Ebbw Vale NP23 6DG — MB BCh BAO Dub. 1947.

YORKE, Sydney Clifford Brookfield Anna Freud Centre, 21 Maresfield Gardens, London NW3 5SD Tel: 020 7794 2313; Fieldings, Paper Mill Lane, South Moreton, Didcot OX11 9AH Tel: 01235 814555 Fax: 01235 814555 — (King's Coll. Hosp.) MRCS Eng. LRCP Lond. 1946; DPM Lond. 1951; FRCPsych 1981, M 1971. Hon. Cons. Psychiat. Anna Freud Centre Lond. Socs: Fell. Roy. Soc. Med.; Brit. Psychoanal Soc. Prev: Cons. Psychotherap. Psychiat. Unit Watford Gen. Hosp.; Cons. Psychotherap. Napsbury Hosp.

YORKSTON, Neil James Stockton Hall Psychiatric Hospital, The Village, Stockton on the Forest, York YO3 9UN — MB BS Sydney 1952; FRACP 1973, M 1956; DTM & H Sydney 1957; DPM Eng. 1962; FRCPsych 1979, M 1971; FRANZCP 1990. Cons. Psychiat., Stockton Hall Psych. Hosp, York; Emerit. Prof. Psychiat. Univ. Brit. Columbia Vancouver, Canada. Specialty: Gen. Psychiat. Socs: Co-Winner, Soc. of Psychother. Research Award. Prev: Cons. Psychiat. S. Durh. Health Care NHS Trust Darlington; Prof. Dept. Psychiat. Univ. Brit. Columbia, Canada; Assoc. Prof. Psychiat. & Med. Univ. Minnesota Minneapolis, USA.

YORSTON, Caroline Mary Didcot Health Centre, Britwell Road, Didcot OX11 7JH Tel: 01235 512288 Fax: 01235 811473; 2 Chestnut Avenue, Radley College, Abingdon OX14 2HS Tel: 01235 520081 — MB ChB Bristol 1988 (Univ. Bristol) DCH RCP Lond. 1991; DFFP 1993; DRCOG 1993; MRCGP 1994. Specialty: Gen. Pract. Prev: Trainee GP Oxf. & Exeter VTS.

YORSTON, Graeme Andrew St. Andrew's Hospital, Billing Road, Northampton NN1 5DG Tel: 01604 616000 Fax: 01604 616015 Email: gyorston@standrew.co.uk — MB BS Lond. 1986 (Westm.) BSc (Hons.) Lond. 1983; MRCPsych 1994; MSc (Forens. Psychiat.) Lond. 2004. Cons. Old Age Psychiat., St. And.Hosp., Northampton. Specialty: Geriat. Psychiat. Socs: Brit. Assn. for Psychopharmacol. Prev: Cons. (Old Age Psychiat.) Lanarksh.; Sen. Regist. (Psychiat.) Oxf.; Regist. (Psychiat.) Fife.

YORSTON, Jessie Campbell (retired) Luibeg, Gardeners Lane, East Wellow, Romsey SO51 6BB — MB ChB Aberd. 1953; MD Aberd. 1956. Prev: Med. Off. (Family Plann.) Hants. AHA.

YORSTON, Malcolm Bruce (retired) Luibeg, Gardeners Lane, East Wellow, Romsey SO51 6BB Tel: 01794 512054 — MB ChB Aberd. 1953; DA Eng. 1955; FFA RCS Eng. 1961. Prev: Cons. Anaesth. Soton. Univ. Hosp. Gp.

YORSTON, Robert Allan (retired) Templehall, Longforgan, Dundee DD2 5HS Tel: 01382 360242 — MB ChB St. And. 1951; DLO Eng. 1960. Prev: Assoc. Specialist (ENT) Ninewells Hosp. Dundee.

YOSEF, Hosney Mohamed Ahmed Ali Beaton Oncology Centre, Western Infirmary, Dumbarton Road, Glasgow G11 6NT — MB BCh Cairo 1965; DMRE Cairo 1968; FRCR 1973. Cons. (Radiother. & Oncol.) Gtr. Glas. Health Bd. Specialty: Oncol.; Radiother.

YOUAKIM, Sherif Samir Fayez 1 Admiral Gardens, Knowle Hill, Kenilworth CV8 2XJ — MB ChB Alexandria 1983; MSc Lond. 1998.

YOUART, Ann Haematology Department, Hartlepool General Hospital, Holdforth Road, Hartlepool TS24 9AH — MB BS Newc. 1975; MRCP (UK) 1978; DMRT Eng. 1980; FRCPath 1996, M 1985. Cons. Haemat. Hartlepool Gen. Hosp. Specialty: Haematology. Prev: Sen. Regist. Haemat. Nottm.

YOUD, David James Brookroyd House Surgery, Cook Lane, Heckmondwike WF16 9JG Tel: 01924 403061 — MB ChB Manch. 1978.

YOUDALE, Dennis Auguste (retired) Oak House, Oak Lane, Minster-in-Sheppey, Sheerness ME12 3QP Tel: 01795 872723 — (Leeds) MB ChB Leeds 1955; DObst RCOG 1957. Prev: SHO (O & G) Fulford & Matern. Hosps. York.

YOUDAN, Michael Eric Northcroft Surgery, Northcroft Lane, Newbury RG14 1BU Tel: 01635 31575 Fax: 01635 551857 — BM BCh Oxf. 1972; MA; MRCGP 1977. Prev: Trainee GP PeterBoro. VTS.

YOUELL, Adrien George (retired) 3 The Lakeside, Blackwater, Camberley GU17 0PQ Tel: 01276 36642 — (TC Dub.) MB BCh BAO Dub. 1970; MA Dub. 1973. Prev: Fell. (Path.) AFIP Washington DC.

YOUELL, Catherine Dorothy 4 Holmer Down, Woolwell, Plymouth PL6 7QW — MB BS Lond. 1980; MRCGP 1985.

YOUENS, John Edward Bentley Bretton Health Centre, Rightwell, Bretton, Peterborough PE3 8DT Tel: 01733 264506 Fax: 01733 266728; 25 The Rookery, Orton Wistow, Peterborough PE2 6YT Tel: 01733 239659 — MB BCh Wales 1979; UMDS Lond.; DCH RCP Lond. 1988; DRCOG 1989; MSc (Grnd. Prac.) 1998. Prev: Regist. (Clin. Biochem.) New Adenbrooke's Hosp. Camb.; Med. Off. Brit. Antartic Survey.

YOUHANA, Mr Aprim Yousif Cardiac Centre, Morriston Hospital, Morriston, Swansea SA6 6LN Tel: 01792 704126 Fax: 01792 704141; 28 Joiners Road, Three Crosses, Swansea SA4 3NY Tel: 01792 875804 — MB ChB Baghdad 1977 (Badhdad) FRCS Ed. 1990; FRCS (Cth.) 1995. Cons. Cardiothoracic Surg. Cardiac Centre Morriston Hosp. Swansea. Specialty: Cardiothoracic Surg. Socs: Soc. Cardiothoracic Surgs. GB and Irel.; Roy. Soc. Med. Prev: Cons. Cardiothoracic Surg. Roy. Hosps NHS Trust. Lond.; Sen. Regist. Roy. Brompton Hosp.; Sen. Regist. Lond. Chest Hosp.

YOUKHANA, Ishow Skharia 4 Fobbing Farm Close, Basildon SS16 5NP Tel: 01268 593638 — MB ChB Mosul 1974; DA (UK) 1991; FRCA 1994. Cons. Anaesth. Basildon Hosp., Basildon, Essex. Specialty: Anaesth. Socs: BMA; MDU; Assn. of Anaesth.s of Gt. Britain & Irel. Prev: Regist. (Anaesth.) Yeovil Dist. Hosp.; Specialist Anaesth 1987-90; Regist. (Anaesth.) Qu.'s Med. Centre Nottm.

YOUL, Bryan Douglas Royal Free Hospital, Pond Street, London NW5 1TU; 50 Lady Somerset Road, London NW5 1TU — MB BS Melbourne 1980; MD; FRCP; FRACP; BMedSc Melbourne 1977. p/t Cons. (Clin. Neurophysiol.) Nat. Hosp. & Roy. Free Hosp. Lond. Specialty: Neurol.

YOULTEN, Lawrence John Francis London Allergy Clinic, 66 New Cavendish Street, London W1G 8TD Tel: 020 76379711 Fax: 020 75809749 Email: l-a-c@lineone.net; Periteau House, High Street, Winchelsea TN36 4EA Tel: 01797 224045 Fax: 01797 222694 Email: lyoulten@aol.com — MB BS Lond. 1961 (Guy's) MRCS Eng. LRCP Lond. 1961; PhD Lond. 1968; FRCP Ed. 1992; FFPHM RCP (UK) 1993. p/t Cons. and Director, Lond. Allergy Clinic; Vis. Cons.. Dep of Allergy & Clin. Immunol., Addenbrookes Hosp., Camb.; Emerit. Cons., Dep of Allergy & Clin. Immunol. Guy's & St. Thomas' Hosps. NHS Trust. Specialty: Allergy. Socs: Brit. Soc. Allergy & Clin. Immunol. (Mem.). Prev: Dir., Clin. Pharmacol. Compliance Smith Kline Beecham Pharmaceuts.; Sen. Lect. (Pharmacol.) Inst. Basic Med. Scs. RCS Eng.; Sen. Lect. (Physiol.) Lond. Hosp. Med. Coll.

YOUNAN, Mr Fekry Hemaya Hazel Oak, 2 Blythewood Close, Knowle, Solihull B91 3HL Tel: 01564 774518 — MB ChB Cairo 1969 (Kasr El Eni) FRCS Eng. 1978. Assoc. Specialist Warwick Hosp. NHS Trust; Cons. Surg. King Faisal Milit. Hosp. Khamis Mushat, Saudi Arabia. Specialty: Gen. Surg. Prev: Asst. Prof. Surg. King Saudi Univ. Abha, Saudi Arabia; N. Eng. Research Soc. Regist. (Surg.) Med. Sch. Univ. Newc.

YOUNG, Adrian Charles (retired) Bletchingdon Road Surgery, Bletchingdon Road, Islip, Kidlington OX5 2TQ Tel: 01865 371666 Fax: 01865 842475; Wirepool Cottage, Oddington, Kidlington OX5 2RA Tel: 01865 331284 — MB BS Lond. 1974 (Char. Cross) BSc Lond. 1971; DRCOG 1977. Prev: Trainee GP Mid-Sussex VTS.

YOUNG, Alan George St Giles Road Surgery, St Giles Road, Watton, Thetford IP25 6XG Tel: 01953 889134/881247 Fax: 01953

885167 — MB BS Lond. 1969 (Univ. Coll. Hosp.) BSc (Anat.) Lond. 1966, MB BS 1969; MRCGP 1974; DObst RCOG 1975. Prev: Ho. Phys. & Ho. Surg. Univ. Coll. Hosp. Lond.

YOUNG, Alasdair Patrick 6 Hills Mews, Florence Road, Ealing, London W5 3RG — MB ChB Glas. 1998.

YOUNG, Alastair Cushnie BUPA Hospital, Russell Road, Whalley Range, Manchester M16 8AJ Tel: 0161 226 0112 Fax: 0161 226 1187; Oakleigh, 3 Euxton Hall Gardens, Euxton, Chorley PR7 6PB — MB ChB Aberd. 1964; MRCP (UK) 1970; FRCP Lond. 1985. Cons. NeUrol. BUPA Private Pract., Manch. Hosp. & 57 Chorley New Rd. Bolton; Private Med. & Medico-Legal Pract., Neurol., Manch. & Bolton. Specialty: Neurol.; Medico Legal. Socs: Fell. Manch. Med. Soc.; Mem. Acad. of Experts. Prev: Cons. Neurol. Salford Roy. & Bolton Roy. NHS Trusts; Sen. Regist. (Neurol.) Oxon HA; Regist. (Med.) Aberd. Gen. Hosps.

YOUNG, Alexander Harley (retired) 22 Eden Park Drive, Batheaston, Bath BA1 7JJ — MRCS Eng. LRCP Lond. 1964 (Roy. Free) BDS Glas. 1955; FDS RCS Eng. 1959; FDS RCS Ed. 1959. Clin. Lect. (Dent. Surg.) Univ. Bristol Dent. Hosp. Prev: Cons. (Oral & Maxillofacial Surg.) Bath Health Dist. & Bristol & Weston Health Dist. (T).

YOUNG, Alexander Muir Morton Alyth Health Centre, New Alyth Road, Alyth, Blairgowrie PH11 8EQ Tel: 01828 632317 Fax: 01828 633272; Boglea House, Alyth, Blairgowrie PH11 8NU Tel: 01828 632442 — MB ChB Dundee 1973; MRCGP 1981. Clin. Asst. (Diabet.) Ninewells Hosp. Dundee. Prev: Trainee GP Dundee VTS.

YOUNG, Professor Allan Hunter School of Neurology, Neurobiology & Psychiatry, Division of Psychiatry, Royal Victoria Infirmary, Newcastle upon Tyne NE1 4LP Tel: 0191 232 5131 Ext: 24258 Fax: 0191 227 5108 Email: a.h.young@ncl.ac.uk — MB ChB Ed. 1984; MRCPsych 1988; MPhil Ed. 1990; PhD Ed. 1996. Prof. of Gen. Psychiat. Univ. Newc. Specialty: Gen. Psychiat. Prev: Research Fell. & Hon. Sen. Regist. (Psychiat.) Univ. Edin.; Clin. Lect. (Psychiat.) Univ. Oxf.

YOUNG, Allan Russell Castlemilk Health Centre, 71 Dougrie Drive, Glasgow G45 9AW Tel: 0141 531 8585 Fax: 0141 531 8596; Allanvilla, 2 Threestanes Road, Strathaven ML10 6DX Tel: 01357 21165 — MB ChB Glas. 1965; DObst RCOG 1972.

YOUNG, Amanda Jane Albion House Surgery, Albion Street, Brierley Hill DY5 3EE Tel: 01384 70220 Fax: 01384 78284 — MB BS Lond. 1987 (University College London) BSc (Hons) Lond. 1984; DRCOG 1989; MRCGP 1991. Specialty: Gen. Pract.

YOUNG, Amber Elizabeth Russel North Bristol NHS Trust, Dept. of Anaesthesia, Frenchay Hospital, Bristol BS16 1LE Tel: 0117 970 2020 Fax: 0117 957 4414 Email: amber.young@dial.pipex.com; Clifton Retreat, Clifton Hill, Clifton, Bristol BS8 1BN Tel: 0117 974 5220 Fax: 0117 957 4414 Email: amber.young@dial.pipex.com — MB ChB Bristol 1987; BSc Bristol 1984; FRCA 1993. Cons. Paediat. Anaestetist, Frenchay Hosp., Bristol; Chairm. Paediatric Standards Comm. Specialty: Anaesth.; Intens. Care. Socs: Paed. Intens. Care Soc.; Intens. Care Soc.; Brit. Burns Assn. Prev: Sen. Regist. (Paediat. Anaesth.) Roy. Childr.'s Hosp. Melbourne, Australia; Research Regist. (Neuro. & Intens. Care) Frenchay Hosp. Bristol; Post Fellowship Regist. (Paediat. Anaesth.) Gt. Ormond St. Hosp. Childr. NHS Trust.

YOUNG, Mr Andrew Buchanan (retired) 46 Darnley Road, Glasgow G41 4NE Tel: 0141 423 6814 — MB ChB Glas. 1950; FRCS Ed. 1959; FRCS Glas. 1979. Prev: Cons. Orthop. Surg. Glas. Roy. Infirm.

YOUNG, Andrew John Silver Springs Medical Practice, Beaufort Road, St Leonards-on-Sea TN37 6PP Tel: 01424 422300/426464 Fax: 01424 436400; High Firs, Silverhill Avenue, St Leonards-on-Sea TN37 7HG Tel: 01424 752640 — MB BS Lond. 1975 (St. Bart.) MRCS Eng. LRCP Lond. 1974; DRCOG 1977; MRCGP (UK) 1981. Prev: GP Trainer, Hastings; SHO (O & G) Northampton Gen. Hosp.; SHO (Paediat.) Qu. Mary's Hosp. Childr. Carshalton.

YOUNG, Andrew Jonathan 15A Morton Way, London N14 7HS — MB BS Lond. 1993.

YOUNG, Angeline Mary Rubislaw Medical Group, 7 Rubislaw Place, Aberdeen AB10 1QB Tel: 01224 641968 — MB ChB Aberd. 1983; DRCOG 1986; MRCGP 1987. GP Principal.

YOUNG, Ann Shona 1 Bagnall Cottages, Cinderhill Road, Bulwell, Nottingham NG6 8SD — MB ChB Ed. 1992. Specialist Regist. (Anaesth.) Qu. Med. Centre Univ. Hosp. Nottm. Specialty: Anaesth.

YOUNG, Anna Catriona Micaela The Surgery, Denmark Street, Darlington DL3 0PD — MB BCh BAO NUI 1989; DRCOG 1992; MRCP 1994. GP Princip.; Clin. Asst. Psychiat. Specialty: Gen. Pract.

YOUNG, Anna-Mary 28 Woodborough Road, London SW15 6PZ — MB BS Lond. 1998.

YOUNG, Anne Elizabeth The Surgery, Doctors Lane, West Meon, Petersfield GU32 1LR Tel: 01730 829333 Fax: 01730 829229; Ann Cottage, Kilmeston, Alresford SO24 0NW Tel: 01962 771472 Fax: 01962 771899 Email: anne.e.young@bigfoot.com — MB ChB Glas. 1974; DRCOG 1985. Gen. Practitioner, Hants.

YOUNG, Anne Hall (retired) 20 Claremont Drive, Hartlepool TS26 9PD Tel: 01429 279446 Email: brian@bguttridge.freeserve.co.uk — MB BS Durh. 1959; DPH Durh. 1964; MFCM 1974. Prev: Dep. MOH & Dep. Princip. Sch. Med. Off. Hartlepool Co. Boro.

YOUNG, Mr Anthony Elliott St Thomas' Hospital, London SE1 7EH Tel: 020 7188 7188 Ext: 82571 Fax: 020 8244 5467 Email: anthony.yung@gstt.sthames.nhs.uk — MB BChir Camb. 1968 (St. Thos.) MChir Camb. 1979, MA 1969; FRCS Eng. 1973. Cons. Surg. St. Thos. Hosp. Lond.; Cons. Surg. King Edwd. VII's Hosp., Lond. Specialty: Gen. Surg. Special Interest: Endocrine and Breast. Socs: Fell. Roy. Soc. Med.; BMA; BASO. Prev: Med. Director, Guy's and St Thomas' Hosp. Trust.

YOUNG, Mr Antony John 2 Berners Mansions, 34-36 Berners Street, London W1T 3LU Email: tony.young@ucl.ac.uk — MB BS Lond. 1994 (UCLMS) FRCS Eng. 1998. Specialist Regist., Urclogy, William Harvey Hosp. Ashford, Trent. Specialty: Urol.

YOUNG, Professor Archie Geriatric Medicine, Department of Clinical and Surgical Sciences, University of Edinburgh, The Chancellors Building, Room SU220, 49 Little France Crescent, Edinburgh EH16 4SB Tel: 0131 242 6481/2 Fax: 0131 242 6370 Email: a.young@ed.ac.uk — MB ChB (Commend.) Glas. 1971; MRCP (UK) 1973; BSc (Hons.) Glas. 1969, MD 1983; FRCP Glas. 1985; FRCP Lond. 1989; FRCP Edin. 1999. Prof. Geriat. Med. Univ. of Edin. Specialty: Rehabil. Med. Socs: Med. Res. Soc. & Europ. Soc. Clin. Investig.; Amer. Coll. Sports Med. Prev: Prof. Geriat. Med. Roy. Free Hosp. Sch. Med.; Clin. Lect. & Hon. Cons. Phys. Univ. Oxf.; Clin. Lect. (Human Metab.) Univ. Coll. Hosp. Med. Sch. Lond.

YOUNG, Mr Austen (retired) Fairways, Ynyslas, Borth SY24 5JX Tel: 01970 871234 — MB ChB Ed. 1937 (Univ. Ed.) FRCS Ed. 1946; FRCS Eng. 1948. Prev: Aural Surg. Roy. Infirm. Sheff. & Childr. Hosp. Sheff.

YOUNG, Barry Philip Medical Centre, Craig Croft, Chelmsley Wood, Birmingham B37 7TR Tel: 0121 770 5656 Fax: 0121 779 5619 — MB ChB Birm. 1983; DCH RCP Lond. 1986. Specialty: Gen. Pract.

YOUNG, Barry Stuart Avondale Surgery, 5 Avondale Road, Chesterfield S40 4TF Tel: 01246 232946 Fax: 01246 556246 — MB ChB Sheff. 1976; DRCOG 1980; MRCGP 1981. GP Chesterfield; Company Doctors Stage Coach Bust Company Med. Therapeutic Research.

YOUNG, Basil (retired) 81 Woolton Hill Road, Liverpool L25 4RE — MRCS Eng. LRCP Lond. 1951 (Liverp.) MRCGP 1968. Prev: Med. Pract. (Dermat.) Newsham Gen. Hosp. Liverp.

YOUNG, Brian Keith Shelley Surgery, 23 Shelley Road, Worthing BN11 4BS Tel: 01903 234844 Fax: 01903 219744; Oliver's Cottage, 141 The St, Patching, Worthing BN13 3XF Tel: 01903 871251 Fax: 01903 871251 — BM BS Nottm. 1980 (Univ. Nottm.) BMedSci Nottm. 1978; DRCOG 1982; DCH RCP Lond. 1984; MRCGP 1984.

YOUNG, Caroline Jayne — MB ChB Birm. 1992 (Birmingham) BPharm (Hons.) Nottm. 1986; DFFP 1996; MRCGP 1998. GP Princip.; Civil. Med. Practitioner RAF Stafford; Occupational Health Phys. Spool Pottories; Occupational Health Phys. Tarmac. Socs: Pharmaceut. Soc. & BMA. Prev: Locum GP UK & New Zealand; SHO (Orthop.) N. Staffs. Hosp. Centre; GP Trainee Hall Gr. Surg. WGC.

YOUNG, Carolyn Anne Walton Centre for Neurology & Neurosurgery, Lower Lane, Fazakerley, Liverpool L9 7LJ Tel: 0151 529 5711 Fax: 0151 529 5512 — MB ChB Bristol 1985; BSc (Hons.) Bristol 1982; MRCP (UK) 1989; Euro. Dipl. Of Rehab. Med, 1994; FRCP 1998; MD 1998. Cons. Neurol. Walton Centre for

Neurol. & Neurosurg. Merseyside; Hon. Sen. Lect. (Neurol.) Univ. of Liverp.; Cons. Neurologist, Rathbone Brain Injury Rehabil. Centre. Specialty: Neurol.; Rehabil. Med. Special Interest: Brain Injury; Motor Neurone Dis.; Multiple Sclerosis. Socs: Assn. Brit. Neurol.; World Federat. Neurol. Sec. Neurol. Rehab. Research Gp.; Brit. Soc. Rehabil. Med. Prev: Sen. Regist. (Neurol. & Rehabil.) & Higher Train. Post Merseyside RHA; Regional Regist. Rotat. Merseyside.

YOUNG, Catharine Janet The Old Vicarage, Llancarfan, Barry CF62 3AJ Tel: 01446 751175 Fax: 01446 750206 Email: janetyoung@doctors.org.uk — MB ChB Manch. 1980; DRCOG 1983; MRCGP 1985. Princip. Forens. Phys. S Wales Police; GP Barry S Wales.

YOUNG, Catherine Margaret Pershore Health Centre, Priest Lane, Pershore WR10 1RD Tel: 01386 502030 Fax: 01386 502058 — MB ChB Leic. 1984; DRCOG 1987. Princip. In Gen. Pract. Socs: Med. Protec. Soc. Prev: Trainee GP Kettering VTS.

YOUNG, Catherine Pamela Rasharkin Health Centre, 10 Moneyleck Road, Rasharkin, Ballymena BT44 8QB Tel: 028 2557 1203 Fax: 028 2557 1709; Windyridge, Finvoy, Ballymoney BT53 7JW Tel: 0126 65 71203 — MB BCh BAO Belf. 1971; MB BCh BAO (Hons.) Belf. 1971; DCH RCPS Glas. 1973; MRCP Glas. 1979. Sessional Med. Off. (Paediat.) Route Hosp. Ballymoney.

YOUNG, Christine Anne Viewpark Health Centre, Burnhead Street, Uddingston, Glasgow G71 5SU Tel: 01698 813753 Fax: 01698 812062 — MB ChB Dundee 1983. Socs: Med. Protec. Soc. Prev: SHO (Med. & Surg.) St. Michael's Hosp. Hayle; SHO (Paediat.) Inverclyde Roy. Hosp. Greenock; SHO (Psychiat.) Ravenscraig & Inverclyde Roy. Hosp. Greenock.

YOUNG, Christopher Donald Central Surgery, Brooksby Drive, Oadby, Leicester LE2 5AA Tel: 0116 271 2175 Fax: 0116 271 4015; 1 Pinetree Gardens, Oadby, Leicester LE2 5UT — MB BS Lond. 1982 (St Mary's Lond.) DRCOG 1984. Princip. GP & Sen. Partner. Socs: Leic. Med. Soc.

YOUNG, Christopher Maugham St Richard's Hospital, Department of Medical Imaging, Spitalfield Lane, Chichester PO19 6SE Tel: 01243 788122 Ext: 3472/01243 831771 Fax: 01243 831452 Email: chris.young@rws-tr.nhs.uk — MB BS Lond. 1975 (Roy. Free) MCRS Eng. LRCP Lond. 1975; FRCS Ed. 1984; FFRad (D)(SA) S. African Coll. of Med. 1992. Cons. (Radiol.) St Richards Hosp. Chichester. Specialty: Radiol. Special Interest: Breast Imaging; GI Radiol.; Interventional Radiol. Socs: BIR; BSIR. Prev: Cons Radiologist Groote Schuur Hosp., Cape Town, S. Africa; Cons. Surg. Groote Schuur Hosp., Cape Town, S. Africa.

YOUNG, Mr Christopher Paul Guys & St Thomas' NHS Foundation Trust, St. Thomas' Hospital, Lambeth Palace Road, London SE1 7EH Tel: 020 7188 1077 Fax: 020 7188 1006 Email: christopher.young@gstt.sthames.nhs.uk — MD Sheff. 1991; MB ChB 1980; FRCS Eng. 1984. Cons. Cardiothoracic Surg. & Hon. Sen. Lect. St. Thos. Hosp. Lond. Specialty: Cardiothoracic Surg. Special Interest: The Aortic Valve; Thoracic Aortic Vascular Disease. Socs: Soc. Cardiothoracic Surgs. GB. & Irel.; Edit. Bd. Soc. Cardiovasc. Surg.; Roy. Soc. of Med. Prev: Sen. Regist. (Cardiothoracic Surg.) Hosp. Sick Childr. Gt. Ormond St. Lond.; BHF Jun. Research Fell. Rayne Inst. St. Thos. Hosp. Lond.

YOUNG, Claire Alexandra 19 Woodbine Road, Gosforth, Newcastle upon Tyne NE3 1DD — MB BCh Wales 1992; MRCP (UK) 1996. Specialty: Gen. Med. Prev: SHO (Gen. Med.) Univ. Hosp. Wales.

YOUNG, Claire Fiona Freeman Hospital, Newcastle upon Tyne NE7 7DN; 13 Haldane Terrace, Jesmond, Newcastle upon Tyne NE2 3AN Tel: 0191 281 7309 — MB ChB Glas. 1995; MRCS (Eng.) 1998. Specialist Regist. (Orthop.) Freeman Hosp. Specialty: Trauma & Orthop. Surg. Prev: SPR (Orthop.) Newc. Gen. Hosp.; SPR (Orthop.) Wansbeck Gen. Hosp.; SPR (Orthop.) Cumbld. INF.

YOUNG, Claire Sutherland Norbury Resource Centre, 2 Crabtree Road, Sheffield S5 7BB Tel: 0114 226 2560 — MB ChB Manch. 1982; MRCPsych 1994. Cons. Old Age Psychiat. Northern Gen. Hosp., Sheffeld. Specialty: Geriat. Psychiat. Prev: Regist. (Psychiat.) Roy. Dundee Liff Hosp.

YOUNG, Colin Mark 249 Holywood Road, Belfast BT4 2EW — MB BCh BAO Belf. 1986.

YOUNG, Mr Cyril John, TD, Deputy Lt. Queen Elizabeth Hospital Trust, Stadium Road, Woolich, London SE18 4QH Tel: 0208 836 4501 Fax: 0208 836 4504; 75 Hornfair Road, London SE7 7BB Tel: 020 8319 2567 — MRCS Eng. LRCP Lond. 1966 (King's Coll. Hosp.) FRCOG 1988, M 1972; MSc Surrey 1977. Cons. O & G Qu. Eliz. Hosp. Woolich; Rep.Dep.Lieut.L.B.Greenwich. Specialty: Obst. & Gyn. Socs: Soc. Apoth.; W Kent M-C Soc. Prev: Cons. O & G Greenwich Dist. Hosp.; Cons. Obst. Brit. Hosp. Mothers & Babies Lond.; Sen. Regist. (O & G) Qu. Charlotte's Hosp. Wom. Lond.

YOUNG, Professor Daniel Greer Department of Paediatric Surgery, RHSC Yorkhill NHS Trust, Glasgow G3 8SJ Tel: 0141 201 0169 Fax: 0141 201 0858; 49 Sherbrooke Avenue, Glasgow G41 4SE Tel: 0141 427 3470 — MB ChB Glas. 1956; DTM & H Liverp. 1959; FRCS Ed. 1962; FRCS Glas. 1975; FRCPCH 1996. Prof. Paediat. Surg. Univ. Glas.; Hon. Cons. Surg. Roy. Hosp. Sick Childr. Glas. Specialty: Paediat. Surg. Socs: (Ex-Pres.) Roy. M-C Soc. Glas.; (ex-Pres.) Brit. Assn. Paediat. Surg.; (Ex-Chairm.) W. of Scot. Surg. Assn. Prev: Sen. Regist. & Resid. Asst. Surg. Hosp. Sick Childr. Gt. Ormond St.; Sen. Lect. (Paediat. Surg.) Inst. Child Health Lond.; Hon. Cons. Surg. Hosp. Sick Childr. Gt. Ormond St. & Qu. Eliz. Hosp. Hackney.

YOUNG, David Alan The Surgery, Bridgemary Medical Centre, 2 Gregson Avenue, Gosport PO13 0HR Tel: 01329 232446 Fax: 01329 282624 — MB ChB Bristol 1974.

YOUNG, David Anthony (retired) Restormel, Penpol, Devoran, Truro TR3 6NW Tel: 01872 865433 — (Middlx.) MB BS Lond. 1957; MRCS Eng. LRCP Lond. 1958; DA Eng. 1959; FFA RCSI 1966; FFA RCS Eng. 1967. Prev: Cons. Anaesth. Bromley HA & Clin. Dir. (Anaesth. & Allied Servs.) Bromley Hosps. NHS Trust.

YOUNG, David John 5 Thingwall Road E., Thingwall, Wirral CH61 3UY — MB ChB Liverp. 1980.

YOUNG, David Robertson Milliken and Young, The Surgery, Castlehill Loan, Stirling FK8 3DZ Tel: 01786 870369 Fax: 01786 870819 — MB ChB Glas. 1983; MRCGP 1987. Prev: GP Cumnock.

YOUNG, David Wallace Laxey Medical Centre, New Road, Laxey IM4 7BF Tel: 01624 781350; Rock Rose, Ballacollister Heights, Laxey — MB ChB Glas. 1973; BSc (Hons. Biochem.) Glas. 1969. Prev: Sen. Med. Off. St. Helena Is., S. Atlantic; GP Broxburn W. Lothian.

YOUNG, David William Young and Partners, The Ryan Medical Centre, St Marys Road, Preston PR5 6JD Tel: 01772 335136 Fax: 01772 626701 — MB ChB Dundee 1975.

YOUNG, David William City Hospital NHS Trust, Birmingham B18 7QH Tel: 0121 554 3801 Fax: 0121 523 6125 — MD Manch. 1983; MB ChB 1963; FRCP Lond. 1982, M 1967; MFCM RCP (UK) 1982. Phys. Birm. City Hosp. NHS Trust; Sen. Clin. Lect. Univ. Birm.; Clin. Adviser Informat. Policy Unit NHS Exec. Specialty: Ophth. Prev: Lect. (Med.) Univ. Birm.; MRC Clin. Research Fell. Qu. Eliz. Med. Centre Birm.; Regist. Qu. Eliz. Hosp. Birm.

YOUNG, Donald James Reid 5 Woodside Gardens, Clarkston, Glasgow G76 7UG — MB ChB Manch. 1998.

YOUNG, Donya Carolyn Denise Wickhampark Surgery, 2 Manor Road, West Wickham BR4 9PS Tel: 020 8777 1293 Fax: 020 8776 1977; 9 Bishops Avenue, Bromley BR1 3ET Email: donyayoung@arsenalfc.net — MB BS Lond. 1985 (King's College Medical School, London) DRCOG 1988; MRCGP 1990; DFFP 1995. Prev: Trainee GP FarnBoro. Hosp. VTS.

***YOUNG, Dudley Paul** The Old House, Mill Lane, Hurstpierpoint, Hassocks BN6 9WL Email: dudleypyoung@hotmail.com — MB BS Lond. 2003; BSc (Hons.). PRHO (Gen. Med. & Care of the Elderly).

YOUNG, Duncan Niel The Health Centre, Dunning Street, Stoke-on-Trent ST6 5BE Tel: 01782 425834 Fax: 01782 577599; The Gables, Alsager, Stoke-on-Trent ST7 2HT — MB ChB Sheff. 1991; BSc Dund 1986; MRCGP 1997. Specialty: Gen. Pract. Prev: GP Regist. Sheff.

YOUNG, Edward 68 Beech Lane, Earley, Reading RG6 5QA — MB BS Lond. 1961 (Guy's) MRCS Eng. LRCP Lond. 1961; DObst RCOG 1963; DA Eng. 1965; FFA RCS Eng. 1969. Cons. Anaesth. W. Berks. Health Dist. Specialty: Anaesth. Prev: Sen. Regist. (Anaesth.) United Oxf. Hosps.; Ho. Phys. Pembury Hosp.; Ho. Surg. New Cross Hosp.

YOUNG, Eileen Barbara Barr (retired) Vectis Lodge, 74 Victoria Road S., Southsea PO5 2BN Tel: 02392 821682 — BM BCh Oxf. 1953 (Oxf. & St. Mary's) MA Oxf. 1957, BM BCh 1953; FRCGP 1981, M 1968. Prev: Princip. GP Portsmouth.

YOUNG, Elaine Anne 75 Higher Lane, Lymm WA13 0BZ — MB ChB Liverp. 1988; MRCP (UK) 1992; FRCR 1998. Specialist Regist.

(Clin. Oncol.) Christie Hosp. Withington. Specialty: Oncol.; Radiother. Prev: Trainee Radiother. Christie Hosp. Withington.

YOUNG, Elizabeth Anne West Barton Farm, Horwood, Bideford EX39 4PB Tel: 01271 858495 — MB ChB Sheff. 1970; DCH RCP Lond. 1972. Sch. Med. Off. N. Devon HA. Prev: Clin. Med. Off. Trafford HA; SHO (Paediat.) Childr. Hosp. Sheff. & Jenny Lind Hosp. Norwich; Ho. Off. (Gen. Med.) North. Gen. Hosp. Sheff.

YOUNG, Eric Thomson (retired) Holly Lodge, Fulbeck, Morpeth NE61 3JT Tel: 01670 512052 — MB ChB Glas. 1959; FRCP Ed. 1975, M 1963; FRCP Glas. 1974, M 1963; FRCP Lond. 1977, M 1964. Cons. Phys. N.d. AHA & Newc. AHA (T). Prev: Sen. Regist. (Med.) Roy. Vict. Infirm. Newc.

YOUNG, Fergus Ian Department of Pathology, Cumberland Infirmary, Newtown Road, Carlisle CA2 7HY Tel: 01228 523444 — MB ChB Dundee 1985. Cons. (Histopath.) Cumbld. Infirm. Carlisle. Specialty: Histopath.

YOUNG, Francesca — MB ChB Manch. 1998.

YOUNG, Francis Louis Dermot (retired) 32 Granville Court, Granville Road, Eastbourne BN20 7EE Tel: 01323 723926 — (Guy's) MRCS Eng. LRCP Lond. 1940; DPM Eng. 1948. Prev: Dir. Psychogeriat. Servs. Nova Scotia Hosp. & Cons. Psychiat. Halifax Co. Regional Rehabil. Centre, Canada.

YOUNG, Frank Maurice (retired) Dormy Cottage, 5 Fortune Hill, Knaresborough HG5 9DG Tel: 01423 862411 — (St. Geo.) MB BS Lond. 1960; MRCS Eng. LRCP Lond. 1960; DObst RCOG 1964. Prev: Ho. Phys. & Cas. Off. St. Geo. Hosp. Lond.

YOUNG, Gail — MB ChB Sheff. 1985; Cert. Family Plann. JCC 1988; DCH RCP Lond. 1988; DRCOG 1989; MRCGP 1990; T(GP) 1991. Specialty: Gen. Pract.

YOUNG, Gavin Leslie Temple Sowerby Medical Practice, Temple Sowerby, Penrith CA10 1RZ Tel: 017683 61232 Fax: 017683 61980 — MB BS Lond. 1975 (Univ. Coll. Hosp.) DRCOG 1979; MA Oxf. 1980; FRCGP 1993, M 1980. Socs: Founder Mem. (Ex-Chairm.) Assn. Community Based Matern. Care; Fell. Roy. Soc. Med.

YOUNG, Gavin Robert Department of Neurology, James Cook University Hospital, Marton Road, Middlesbrough TS4 3BW Tel: 01642 850850 — MB ChB Manch. 1987 (Manchester) MRCP (UK) 1990; MD Manch. 1997; MD Manchester 1997. Cons. Neurol. Middlesbrough Gen. Hosp. Specialty: Neurol.

YOUNG, George Brims Gall Green Health, 979 Stratford Road, Hall Green, Birmingham B28 8BG Tel: 0121 777 3500 Fax: 0121 325 5514 Email: george.young@southbirminghampct.nhs.uk; 7 Norcombe Grove, Cheswick Green, Solihull B90 4PA Tel: 0121 7445 8016 Email: george.young@southbirminghampct.nhs.uk — MB BS Lond. 1980; DRCOG 1983; MRCGP 1984. GP Trainer Birm.; GP Mcmillan Cancer Lead. Birm. PCT; Primary Care Lead Birm. Cancer Network. Socs: Exec. Mem. NHSPCG Alliance (PREV NACGP). Prev: Chairm. Hall Green GP Commissioning Project; GPCA Chest Med. Birm. Chest Clinic; Trainee GP/SHO E. Birm. Hosp. VTS.

YOUNG, Mr George Ivan (retired) 38 Magheralave Road, Lisburn BT28 3BN Tel: 02892 664166 — Cons. Surg. Lagan Valley Hosp. Lisburn; MB BCh BAO Belf. 1949; FRCS Ed. 1956; FRCS Eng. 1956. Prev: Surg. Fell. Lahey Clinic Boston, U.S.A.

YOUNG, Glenda Kaye (retired) 21 Sealand Court, Shorts Reach, The Esplanade, Rochester ME1 1QH Tel: 01634 845834 — (Roy. Free) MB BS Lond. 1961. Prev: Clin. Asst. (Psychother.) Canterbury & Thanet Community Healthcare Trust.

YOUNG, Grace Maria North Staffordshire Hospital Emergency Department, Windsor House, 223 Princes Rd, Hartshill, Stoke-on-Trent ST4 7JW Tel: 01782 554503 Fax: 01782 747179 — MB ChB Birm. 1982. Assoc. Specialist (A & E), N. Staffs Hosp. NHS Trust. Specialty: Accid. & Emerg. Prev: SHO (Anaesth.) E. Birm. Hosp.

YOUNG, Mr Graeme Bruce (retired) 5 Tipperlinn Road, Edinburgh EH10 5ET Tel: 0131 447 7318 — (Ed.) MB ChB Ed. 1939; FRCS Ed. 1947; DMRD Ed. 1961; FFR 1964; FRCR 1975. Prev: CMO Mission Hosp. Jalna Deccan, India.

YOUNG, Graham Kemnay Medical Group, High Street, Kemnay, Inverurie AB51 5NB Tel: 01467 642289 Fax: 01467 643100; 18 Fetternnear View, Kemnay, Inverurie AB51 5JF Tel: 01467 642681 — MB ChB Aberd. 1972 (Aberdeen) DObst RCOG 1976; FRCGP 1992, M 1977. Staff GP Inverurie Hosp. Specialty: Gen. Pract.

YOUNG, Mrs Gwyneth Vivien Wright 63 Lee Road, London SE3 9EN Tel: 020 8852 1921 Fax: 020 8244 5467 — MB BS Lond. 1969 (St. Thos.) DCH Eng. 1971; MRCPCH 1997. Assoc. Specialist (Paediat.) Greenwich Dist. Hosp. & Qu. Eliz. Hosp. Lond. Specialty: Paediat. Socs: Harveian Soc. & Med. Soc.; BACCH & Brit. Paediat. Assn. Prev: SHO (Paediat.) & Ho. Phys. Kingston Hosp.; Ho. Off. (Surg.) St. Thos. Hosp. Lond.

YOUNG, Hamilton Nat (retired) 19 Kingston Road, Bridlington YO15 3NF Tel: 01262 401372 — (Glas.) MB ChB Glas. 1958; DObst RCOG 1960; DA Eng. 1965. Prev: GP (Robt.son Young Mundy and Harris).

YOUNG, Harry Lawrance 15 Blythwood Road, Crouch Hill, London N4 4EU — MB BS Lond. 1952.

YOUNG, Helen Kathryn 6 Cooper Crescent, Enniskillen BT74 6DQ — MB ChB Ed. 1993.

YOUNG, Helen Louise St Andrews, Herbert Road, Chelston, Torquay TQ2 6RW — MB BCh Wales 1998.

YOUNG, Helen Sara Department of Dermatology, Hope Hospital, Stott Lae, Salford, Manchester M6 8HD — MB ChB Manch. 1994 (Manchester University) MRCP 1997. Specialist Regist. Dermat., Hope Hosp., Manch. Specialty: Dermat. Prev: SHO (Dermat.) Hope Hosp., Manch.; SHO Rotat. (Gen. Med.) Hope Hosp. Manch.; SHO (Cardiothoracic Med.) Wythenshawe Hosp. Manch.

YOUNG, Hoi Wah Soon Khow 33 Eriskay Avenue, Newton Mearns, Glasgow G77 6XB; 24 Longpark Place, Eliburn, Livingston EH54 6TU Tel: 01506 419116 Email: soon@skyoung.freeserve.co.uk — MB ChB Glas. 1989; FRCS; FRCR. Specialist Regist. Radiol. Specialty: Radiol.

YOUNG, Howard (retired) 6 Kinfauns Drive, High Salvington, Worthing BN13 3BL; 6 Kinfauns Drive, High Salvington, Worthing BN13 3BL — MB ChB Birm. 1952.

YOUNG, Mr Howard Anthony 24 Albyn Place, Aberdeen AB10 1RW Tel: 01224 595993 Fax: 01224 584797 Email: info@albynhospital.co.uk; 18 Edgehill Road, Aberdeen AB15 5JH Tel: 01224 324554 Email: howlou@lineone.net — MB BS Newc. 1968; FRCS Eng. 1974. p/t Cons. Otolaryngol. & Head & Neck Surg. Grampian Univ. Hosps. NHS Trust Aberd.; Head of Serv. Otolaryn & Head & Neck Surg.; Hon. Sen. Clin. Lect. (Otolaryngol.) Aberd. Univ.; Cons. Otolaryngol & head and neck Surg., at Albyn Hosp., Aberd.; Vis. Otolaryngol. Orkney & Shetland Health Bds. Specialty: Otolaryngol. Special Interest: Paediatric Otolaryngol. Socs: Fell. Roy. Soc. Med. (Mem. Otol. & Laryngol. Sect.); Brit. Assn. Otol. & Head & Neck Surg.; Scott. Otolaryngol. Soc.(Ex-Pres.). Prev: Sen. Regist. (Otolaryngol.) Tayside HB; Regist. (Otolaryngol.), Ho. Surg. & Ho. Phys. Roy. Vict. Infirm. Newc.; Hon. Lect. (Otolaryngol.) Univ. Dundee.

YOUNG, Mr Howard Lewis School of Postgraduate Medical & Dental Education, University of Wales College of Medicine, Cardiff CF14 4XN Tel: 029 2074 4934 Fax: 029 2075 4966 Email: younghl1@cf.ac.uk — MB ChB Dundee 1973 (Univ. Dundee) FRCS Eng. 1978; ChM Dund 1983; MBA Open 1993. Vice Dean Sch. Postgrad. Med. & Dent. Educat. & Hons. Cons. Surg.; Non-Executive Director, Cardiff & Vale NHS Trust. Specialty: Gen. Surg. Socs: Fell. Assn. Surgs.; Surgic. Research Soc.; Assn. Coloproctol. Prev: Sub-Dean & Dep. Dir. Postgrad. Med. Educat. for Wales & Hon. Cons. Surg.; Sen. Lect. & Lect. (Surg.) Univ. Wales Coll. Med. Cardiff; Clin. Research Off. (Surg.) Welsh Nat. Sch. Med. Cardiff.

YOUNG, Hugh Boyd (retired) 22 Broomvale Drive, Newton Mearns, Glasgow G77 5NN — MB ChB Glas. 1942. Prev: Cons. Phys. Lyle Ship Managem. Glas.

YOUNG, Iain McGregor — MB ChB Glas. 1991; FFAEM; Dip FMS; MRCP (UK) 1996. Cons. A&E Roy. Alexandra Hosp. Paisley. Specialty: Accid. & Emerg. Socs: Brit. Assn. Accid. & Emerg. Med.; Fac. Accid. & Emerg. Med. Prev: Specialist Regist. (A & E) W. of Scotl.

YOUNG, Professor Ian Douglas Department of Clinical Genetics, Leicester Royal Infirmary, Leicester LE1 5WW Tel: 0116 258 5736 Fax: 0116 2586 057 Email: iandyoung@hotmail.com — MB BS Lond. 1973; MD Lond. 1981, MSc 1978, BSc (Hons.) 1970; DCH Lond. 1976; MRCP (UK) 1976; FRCP Lond. 1989. Cons. Clin. Genetics & Vis. Prof., Leicester Roy. Infirm. Specialty: Genetics. Socs: Clin. Genetics Soc. & Europ. Soc. Human Genetics. Prev: Sen. Lect. (Clin. Genetics) Univ. Leicester; Sen. Regist. (Med. Genetics) Univ. Hosp. Wales Cardiff; Clin. Fell. Hosp. Sick Childr. Toronto, Canada.

YOUNG, Mr Ian Edward 4/9 South Elixa Place, Edinburgh EH8 7PG Tel: 0131 659 5375 — MB ChB Ed. 1992; FRCS Ed. 1996. Specialty: Gen. Surg.

YOUNG, Ian Malcolm Department Reproductive Physiology, St. Bartholomew's Hospital, 51 Bartholomew Close, London EC1A 7BE — MB BS Lond. 1972.

YOUNG, Professor Ian Stuart Department of Medicine, Mulhouse Building, Royal Victoria Hospital, Belfast BT12 6BJ Tel: 012890 632743 Fax: 012890 235900 Email: i.young@qub.ac.uk — MB BCh BAO Belf. 1985; BSc (1st cl. Hons.) Biochem. Belf. 1982, MD 1994, MB BCh BAO 1985; MRCP (UK) 1988; MRCPath 1992; FRCP Lond. 1998; FRCPath 2000; FRCPI 2002. Prof. of Med., Qu.'s Univ. Belf.; Cons. Clin. Biochem. Roy. Gp. Hosps. Belf. Specialty: Biochem. Special Interest: Nutrit., Micronutrients, Lipids. Prev: Sen. Lect. (Clin. Biochem.) Qu. Univ. Belf.

YOUNG, Mr Ian William (retired) 1 The Beeches, Lydiard Millicent, Swindon SN5 3LT Tel: 01793 770483 — BM BCh Oxf. 1954 (Oxf. & Univ. Coll. Hosp.) MA Oxf. 1954; FRCS Eng. 1962. Prev: Cons. Orthop. & Accid. Surg. Princess Margt. Hosp. Swindon.

YOUNG, Ian Wilson 294/4 Craigcrook Road, Edinburgh EH4 7BA Tel: 0131 336 3604 — MB ChB Ed. 1967. Exam. Med. Pract. Med. Servs. Edin.; Med. Adviser, Recruit Selection Centre, Glencorse Barracks, Penicuik. Specialty: Disabil. Med. Socs: BMA. Prev: Clin. Asst. Haemophilia & Haemostasis Centre Roy. Infirm. Edin.; Princip. GP Folkestone; Sessional Med. Off. Edin. & S. E. Scotl. Blood Transfus. Serv.

YOUNG, Isaac 8 Ashfield Lodge, Palatine Road, Didsbury, Manchester M20 2UD — MB ChB Leeds 1939. Prev: Cas. Off. Stockton & Thornaby Hosp.; Asst. Med. Off. Hollymoor Emerg. Hosp.; Med. Off. RAFVR 1940-46.

YOUNG, Isabella Noble 39 Milcote Road, Smethwick, Smethwick B67 5BN — MB ChB Ed. 1975; DRCOG 1977. Prev: Ho. Surg. (Obst.) Mothers' Hosp. Lond.; Ho. Phys. & Ho. Surg. Law Hosp. Carluke.

YOUNG, Isobel Margaret (retired) 56 Broomwell Gardens, Monikie, Dundee DD5 3QP Tel: 01382 370451 — MB ChB St. And. 1947 (Qu. Coll. St. And.) Prev: Med. Ref. Scott. Home & Health Dept.

YOUNG, James Crawford 49 Ravelston Road, Bearsden, Glasgow G61 1AX — MB ChB Glas. 1971; FRCP Glas. Cons. Phys. (Geriat. Med.) South. Gen. Hosp. Glas. Specialty: Care of the Elderly.

YOUNG, James David Dr Moss and Partners, 28-38 Kings Road, Harrogate HG1 5JP Tel: 01423 560261 Fax: 01423 501099 — MB ChB Sheff. 1977; DRCOG 1980; FRCGP 1991, M 1981. Prev: Trainee GP Harrogate VTS; Ho. Surg. Roy. Hosp. Sheff.; Ho. Phys. St. Geo. Hosp. Lincoln.

YOUNG, Mr James Drummond Harding (retired) South Kinrara, Fairmount Terrace, Perth PH2 7AS Tel: 01738 625343 — MB ChB Liverp. 1964; FRCS Ed. 1970; FRCOphth 1988. Cons. Ophth. Dundee Teach. Hops. NHS Trust. Prev: Cons. Ophth. Tayside HB.

YOUNG, James Graham Watergates, Ashbourne Road, Blackbrook, Belper DE56 2DA — BM BCh Oxf. 1993; FRCS Eng. Specialist Regist. (Urol.), Char. Cross Hosp., Hammersmith, Lond. Specialty: Urol. Prev: SHO (Urol.) Kent & Canterbury Hosp. Canterbury; SHO (Gen. Surg.) Roy. Berks. Hosp. Reading.

YOUNG, James Jack 15 King Street, Paisley PA1 2PR Tel: 0141 889 3144; Creggan, Arthur Road, Paisley PA2 8AZ Tel: 0141 889 9831 — MB ChB Glas. 1956.

YOUNG, James Richard 51 Beech Court, Darras Hall, Ponteland, Newcastle upon Tyne NE20 9NE — MB BS Durh. 1962 (Newc.) DMRD Eng. 1966; FFR 1968. Cons. Radiol. Qu. Eliz. & Freeman Trust Hosps.; Clin. Lect. Radiol. Newc. Univ.; Clin. Dir. Breast Screening & Assessm. Centre Gateshead. Specialty: Radiol. Prev: Cons. Radiol. i/c Radiol. Qu. Eliz. Hosp. Gateshead.

YOUNG, James Richard Keeling Street Doctors Surgery, Keeling Street, North Somercotes, Louth LN11 7QU Tel: 01507 358623 Fax: 01507 358746; 3 Meteor Road, Manby, Louth LN11 8UB Tel: 01507 328784 Fax: 01507 328784 Email: jyoung7234@aol.com — MB BS Lond. 1983 (Roy. Free) DRCOG 1987; DFFP 1995. Specialty: Obst. & Gyn.; Gen. Pract. Socs: Assoc. Mem. RCGP; BMA; Fell. RSM. Prev: Trainee GP Harrogate; SHO (O & G) York Dist. Hosp.; SHO (ENT Surg.) Roy. Gwent Hosp. Newport.

YOUNG, Jane Elizabeth 65 Lethbridge Road, Wells BA5 2FW — MB BS Lond. 1994.

YOUNG, Jane Frances Hampton Medical Centre, Lansdowne, 49a Priory Road, Hampton TW12 2PB Tel: 020 8979 5150 Fax: 020 8941 9068; (branch Surgery) Tangley Medical Centre, 10 Tangley Pk Road, Hampton TW12 3YH — MB BS Lond. 1968 (St. Mary's) MRCS Eng. LRCP Lond. 1966; DObst RCOG 1968; DFFP 1993. Med. Off. Hampton Sch. Middlx. Specialty: Gynaecology; Diabetes.

YOUNG, Janet Cecilia Josephine 37 Nightingale Avenue, Cambridge CB1 8SG — MB BS Lond. 1955; MRCS Eng. LRCP Lond. 1955.

YOUNG, Janet Margaret Seivwright Church Street Surgery, St Mary's Courtyard, Church Street, Ware SG12 9EF Tel: 01920 468941 Fax: 01920 465531 — MB BS Lond. 1976; BSc Lond. 1973, MB BS 1976; MRCP (UK) 1979; MRCGP 1988.

YOUNG, Jean Isobel Lanark Doctors, Health Centre, South Vennel, Lanark ML11 7JT Tel: 01555 665522 Fax: 01555 666857 — MB ChB Aberd. 1972; DObst RCOG 1975; DCH RCP Lond. 1975; MRCGP 1984.

YOUNG, Jean McIver 41 Beechwood Drive, Broomhill, Glasgow G11 7ET Tel: 0141 357 6600 — MB ChB Glas. 1952; LFHom 1997 (Licenciate). Specialty: Homeop. Med. Socs: LFHOM. Prev: Clin. Med. Off. West. Health Dist.; Med. Off. Lanarksh. CC; Ho. Surg. Roy. Hosp. Sick Childr. Glas.

YOUNG, Jean Morrison The North Glasgow University Hospitals NHS Trust, Glasgow G11 0YN; 79 Campsie Gardens, Clarkson, Glasgow G76 7SF — MB ChB Glas. 1983 (Bristol) MRCP (UK) 1986. Specialist Regist. (Gen. Internal Med. & Geriat. Med.) N. Glas. Univ. Hosps. NHS Trust. Specialty: Care of the Elderly; Gen. Med. Socs: Soc. Occupat. Med.; Brit. Geriat. Soc. Prev: Sen. Regist. (Gen. & Geriat.) Longmore Hosp. Edin. Sen. Regist. (Geriat.s) Vict. Infirm. NHS Trust Glas.; Regist. (Geriat.) Lightburn Hosp. Glas.; Regist. (Med. & Neurol.) Inst. Neurol. Sci. South. Gen. Hosp. Glas.

YOUNG, Jennifer Ann University of Birmingham, Department Pathology, Medical School, Birmingham B15 2TT Tel: 0121 414 4002 Fax: 0121 414 4019 Email: 1.a.young@bham.ac.uk; 18 Frederick Road, Edgbaston, Birmingham B15 1JN Tel: 0121 455 7775 — (T.C. Dub.) MA, MD, Dub. 1982, BA; MB BCh BAO Dub. 1961; FFPath RCPI 1985; FRCPath 1998. p/t Cons. Cytopathologist Univ. Hosp. Birm. Socs: Internat. Acad. Cytol. Pathol. Soc. GB & Irel.; Vice-Chairm. Brit. Soc. Clin. Cytol. Prev: Sen. Regist. (Path.) Qu. Eliz. Hosp. Birm.; Research Regist. (Cytol.) Glas. Roy. Infirm.; Edit. Bd. Mem. Cytopath. & Diagn. Cytopath.

YOUNG, Jennifer Margaret Ball Tree Surgery, Western Road North, Sompting, Lancing BN15 9UX Tel: 01903 752200 Fax: 01903 536983; 64 Mill Road, Lancing BN15 0QA — MB ChB Birm. 1973. GP Lancing. Socs: BMA.

YOUNG, Joanna Hilda Grangemead, 1 Hawthylands Rd, Hailsham BN27 1EU Tel: 01323 442144 Fax: 01323 847822 — MB BS Lond. 1985 (St Georges, London) MRCPsych 1992. Staf Psychiat.(Old Age), Eastbourne & Co. Healthcare NHS Trust. Specialty: Geriat. Psychiat.; Gen. Psychiat. Prev: Staff Psychiat. (Forens.) Ashen Hill Hailsham; Staff Psychiat. Eastbourne & Co. Healthcare (NHS Trust).

YOUNG, Joanna Mary 70 South Street, Greenock PA16 8QJ — MB ChB Glas. 1998.

YOUNG, Joanne Community Paediatrics, Borders General Hospital, Melrose TD6 9BS Tel: 01896 826000; Lyme House, 51 Shedden Pk Road, Kelso TD5 7AW Tel: 01573 226107 — MB ChB Glas. 1980; MPhil Glas. 2000. Staff Grade (Child Health) Roxburghsh. Specialty: Community Child Health. Prev: Med. Off. BTS; SHO (Anaesth.) Dudley Rd. Hosp. Birm. & E. Birm. Hosp.; Ho. Off. (Surg.) St. Chad's Hosp. Birm.

YOUNG, John (retired) 21 Furners Mead, Henfield BN5 9JA Tel: 01273 2708 — MB ChB Glas. 1921 (Univs. Glas. & Camb.) DPH Camb. 1922. Prev: MOH Leics. & Rutland Comb. Dists.

YOUNG, John Archibald — MB ChB Aberd. 1973; MRCGP 1977. GP Princip. Alva; Trainer (Gen. Pract.) Alva. Specialty: Gen. Pract. Socs: BMA; Roy. Coll. Gen. Pract. Prev: Trainee GP Aberd. VTS; Resid. Ho. Off. City Hosp. Aberd. & Aberd. Roy. Infirm.

YOUNG, Professor John Braithwaite Department of Medicine for Elderly, St. Luke's Hospital, Bradford BD5 0NA Tel: 01274 734744 — MB BS Lond. 1977; MRCP (UK) 1980; FRCP Lond. 1994; MSc Lond. 1989, MBA (Open Univ.) 1995. Cons. Phys. St. Luke's Hosp. Bradford; Assoc. Prof. Sheff. Inst. for studies on Ageing (SISA); Vis. Prof. Nuffield Inst. for Health, Leeds; Prof. Assoc., Sch. Health Care Studies, Bradford. Specialty: Gen. Med.; Rehabil. Med.

YOUNG, John Charles Norwood Medical Centre, 99 Abbey Road, Barrow-in-Furness LA14 5ES Tel: 01229 822024 Fax: 01229 823949 — MB ChB Dundee 1987; MRCGP.

YOUNG, John Dewar Consett Medical Centre, Station Yard, Consett DH8 5YA Tel: 01207 216116 Fax: 01207 216119; Shortycroft, Stocksfield NE43 7SB — MB BS Newc. 1977; BMedSc 1974; MRCGP 1988.

YOUNG, John Duncan Adult ICU, John Radcliffe Hospital, Headley Way, Oxford OX3 9DU — BM Soton. 1979; FFA RCS Eng. 1984; DM Soton. 1992; FMedSci 2001. Cons. in Anaesth. and Intens. Care, John Radcliffe Hosp., Oxf.; Sen. Clin. Lect., Univ. Oxf. Specialty: Anaesth.; Intens. Care. Prev: Clin. Reader (Anaesth.) Univ. Oxf.

YOUNG, John Hildreth Merck Sharp & Dohme, Hertford Road, Hoddesdon EN11 9BU Tel: 01992 452341 Fax: 01992 479191 Email: john_young@merck.com — MB BS Lond. 1968 (St. Thos.) Dip. Biochem. Lond 1965; MRCP (UK) 1973; FRCPath 1993, M 1982; FFPM 1990; FRCP Lond. 1990. Med. Dir. Merck, Sharp & Dohme Ltd. Specialty: Pharmaceutical Medicine. Socs: Brit. Soc. Rheum. & Brit. Geriat. Soc. Prev: Lect. (Chem. Path.) Univ. Soton.; Regist. (Med.) Northwick Pk. Hosp. Harrow; Regist. (Chem. Path.) Hosp. Sick Childr. Gt. Ormond St. Lond.

YOUNG, John Howard Ball Tree Surgery, Western Road North, Sompting, Lancing BN15 9UX Tel: 01903 752200 Fax: 01903 536983; 64 Mill Road, Lancing BN15 0QA — MB ChB Birm. 1977; FFA RCS Eng. 1977. Specialty: Anaesth.

YOUNG, John Murray, OStJ, Surg. Capt. RN Retd. (retired) 29 Kennedy Crescent, Alverstoke, Gosport PO12 2NL Tel: 023 9258 0168 — MRCS Eng. LRCP Lond. 1956 (Oxf. & St. Mary's) DPhil Oxf. 1971; MFCM 1974; MFOM 1978; FFOM RCP Lond. 1987; MFPHM 1990. Prev: Cons. Occupat. Phys. Gosport.

YOUNG, John Murray Miller (retired) Cairngorm, 20 Lyons Lane, Appleton, Warrington WA4 5JG — MB ChB Glas. 1952; MRCGP 1968.

YOUNG, John Peter Russel High Tide, 11 Kilmuir, By North Kessock, Inverness IV1 3ZG Tel: 01463 731446 — MB BChir Camb. 1963 (St Thos.) MRCP Lond. 1969; MPhil Lond. 1969; MA Camb. 1970; MD Camb. 1971; MRCPsych 1971; FRCPsych 1986; FRCP Lond. 1987. Emerit. Cons. in Psych. Med., Guys & St Thos. NHS Trust. Specialty: Gen. Psychiat.

YOUNG, Mr John Riddington, OStJ, TD Department of Otolaryngology, North Devon District Hospital, Raleigh Park, Barnstaple EX31 4JB Tel: 01271 322736; West Barton Farm, Horwood, Bideford EX39 4PB Tel: 01271 858495 — MB ChB Sheff. 1970; DLO Eng. 1974; FRCS (Otol.) Eng. 1976; MPhil Brussels 2001. Sen. Cons. ENT Surg. N. Devon Hosp. Barnstaple; Col. (Commanding Off.) 211 Wessex Field Hosp. RAMC (V); Area Surg. (N. Devon) St. John Ambul. Brig. Specialty: Otolaryngol. Socs: Mackenzie Soc. Prev: Sen. Regist. (ENT Surg.) Manch. Roy. Infirm.

YOUNG, John Robert Burns 65A Links Lane, Rowlands Castle PO9 6AF Tel: 023 9241 2009 — MB ChB Glas. 1960; DObst RCOG 1962; FFA RCS Eng. 1967. Cons. Anaesth. Portsmouth Gp. Hosps. Specialty: Anaesth.

YOUNG, Jolyon David Chilcoate Surgery Practice, Hampton Avenue, St Marychurch, Torquay TQ1 3LA Tel: 01803 316333 Fax: 01803 316393 — MB ChB Birm 1981.

YOUNG, Juanita Jane, Maj. RAMC Revilo, Maybourne Rise, Mayford, Woking GU22 0SH — MB BS Lond. 1985; DCH RCP Lond. 1988; MRCGP 1990. SHO (Gen Med.) Camb. Milit. Hosp. Aldershot; GP Aldershot VTS. Prev: SHO (Paediat.) Regtl. Med. Off. Army.

YOUNG, Katharine St Paul's Road Medical Centre, 248 St Paul's Road, Islington, London N1 2LJ Tel: 020 7226 6333 — BM BCh Oxf. 1990; DCH RCP Lond. 1992; MA Oxf. 1994; MRCGP 1994.

YOUNG, Katherine Alice (retired) Highfield, Silverdale, Carnforth LA5 0SQ Tel: 01524 701234 Fax: 01524 701234 — MB ChB Ed. 1946.

YOUNG, Katrina Elizabeth Magdalen Medical Practice, Lawson Road, Norwich NR3 4LF Tel: 01603 475555 Fax: 01603 787210; Church Farm, Church Lane, Eaton, Norwich NR4 6NW Tel: 01603 457302 — MB ChB Aberd. 1972.

YOUNG, Katrina Mary St Marys Surgery, 37 St. Mary's Street, Ely CB7 4HF; 81 Downham Road, Ely CB6 3DY Tel: 01353 610870 — MB BS Lond. 1985; DA (UK) 1993. Prev: SHO (ENT & Anaesth.) Cheltenham Gen. Hosp.; Resid. Med. Off. Grafton Cone Hosp., Austral.; Clin. Asst. (Anaesth.) Hinchingbrooke Hosp. Huntingdon.

YOUNG, Keith The Surgery, High Street, Epworth, Doncaster DN9 1EP Tel: 01427 872232 Fax: 01427 874944 — MB ChB Sheff. 1976; DRCOG 1980; MRCGP 1980.

YOUNG, Keith Adam City Hospital, Department of Rheumatology, Waverley Road, St Albans AL3 5PN Tel: 01727 897859 Fax: 01727 897042 Email: adam.young@whht.nhs.uk; 36 Platts Lane, London NW3 7NT — MB BChir Camb. 1972 (Camb. & St. Geo.) MA Camb. 1969; MRCP (UK) 1975; FRCP Lond. 1991. Cons. Rheum. St. Albans & Hemel Hempstead NHS Trust. Specialty: Rheumatol. Socs: Brit. Soc. Rheum.; Roy. Coll. of Physicians. Prev: Sen. Regist. (Rheum.) Middlx. Hosp. Lond.; Regist. (Neurol.) Centr. Middlx. Hosp. Lond.

YOUNG, Keith Evans 52 St Michaels Road, Llandaff, Cardiff CF5 2AQ — MB BCh Wales 1958 (Cardiff) DObst RCOG 1961. Prev: Ho. Phys. Roy. Infirm. Cardiff; Ho. Surg. (Obst.) St. David's Hosp. Cardiff.

YOUNG, Keith Richard Consultant Obstetrician and Gynaecologist, Scunthorpe and Goole NHS Hospitals Trust, Cliff Gardens, Scunthorpe DN15 7BH Tel: 01724 282282 — MB BS Lond. 1973; FRCOG 1993. Cons. O & G Scunthorpe & Goole Hosps. Trust. Specialty: Obst. & Gyn. Socs: Brit. Soc. Colpos. & Cerv. Path.; Brit. Soc. Gyn. Endoscopy. Prev: Cons. O & G RAMC.

YOUNG, Keith Stewart (retired) Chester House, 24 Bell Lane, Kesgrave, Ipswich IP5 1JQ Tel: 01473 624306 — MB BChir Camb. 1962 (Univ. Coll. Hosp.) MA Camb. 1962; DCH Eng. 1964; DObst RCOG 1964. Prev: SHO (Paediat.) & Ho. Surg. (Obst.) Ipswich & E. Suff. Hosp.

YOUNG, Kenneth Herbert McKenzie, OBE, Brigadier late RAMC Retd. (retired) 58 Forest Drive, Theydon Bois, Epping CM16 7EZ Tel: 01992 812337 — MB BCh BAO Dub. 1946 (TC Dub.) DPH NUI 1964; FRCGP 1977, M 1972; DTM & H Eng. 1972. Prev: Director of Army Gen. Pract.

YOUNG, Lesley Jane Department of Geriatric Medicine, Sunderland Royal Hospital, Kayll Road, Sunderland SR4 7TP; Broadbeck, Leazes Villas, Burnopfield, Newcastle upon Tyne NE16 6HW Email: lesleyyoung99@hotmail.com — MB BS Newc. 1989 (Newcastle) Dip. Med. Sci.; MRCP (UK) 1992. Cons. Geriat. Specialty: Gen. Med.; Care of the Elderly. Socs: Brit. Geriat. Soc.

YOUNG, Lesley Rita London Weekend Television, South Bank TV Centre, London SE1 9LT Tel: 020 7261 3132 Fax: 020 7261 3132; 26 Strawberry Hill Road, Twickenham TW1 4PU Tel: 020 8891 0638 — MB BS Lond. 1970 (St. Mary's) MRCS Eng. LRCP Lond. 1970; DObst RCOG 1973. Med. Off. Lond. Weekend Television; Med. Off. P&O Bulk Shipping. Specialty: Occupat. Health. Socs: Soc. Occupat. Med.

YOUNG, Linda Anne 84 Glenview Road, Nab Wood, Shipley BD18 4AR — MB BChir Camb. 1977; MA, MB Camb. 1977, BChir 1976.

YOUNG, Lindsay Fiona — MB BS Lond. 1987.

YOUNG, Lorna Bruce Manchester Eye Hospital, Oxford Road, Manchester M16 8AJ; 8 Winton Road, Bowdon, Altrincham WA14 2PB Tel: 0161 927 7469 — MB ChB Ed. 1975; DO Eng. 1980. Assoc. Specialist. Ophth. Specialty: Ophth. Socs: MRCOphth. Prev: Assoc. Specialist Ophth. Princess Alex. Eye Pavilion Edin.

YOUNG, Malcolm John Bridgeflat, Bridge of Weir PA11 3SJ Tel: 0150 587 2595 — MB ChB St. And. 1970; MRCP (UK) 1973; FRCP Glas. 1985. Cons. Dermat. Argyll & Clyde Health Bd. Specialty: Dermat.

YOUNG, Margaret Anne Rena Orchardton, Garlieston, Newton Stewart DG8 9DE Tel: 01988 600612 — MB ChB Glas. 1980 (Glasgow) MRCGP 1984; BA Open 1996.

YOUNG, Marie Jane 28 Cairn Gardens, Cults, Aberdeen AB15 9TE — MB ChB Aberd. 1989.

YOUNG, Mark Andrew St John's House Surgery, 28 Bromyard Road, Worcester WR2 5BU; 14 Upper Ferry Lane, Callow End, Worcester WR2 4TL Tel: 01905 831218 — MD Manch. 1990 (Manchester) MB ChB 1975; MRCP (UK) 1981. GP Princip. Specialty: Gen. Pract.; Cardiol.; Gen. Med. Socs: Brit. Hypertens. Soc.; Assur. Med. Soc.

YOUNG, Mark Andrew Stapenhill Surgery, Fyfield Road, Stapenhill, Burton-on-Trent DE15 9QD Tel: 01283 565200 Fax: 01283 500617; The Fieldings, 51 Main St, Rosliston, Swadlincote

DE12 8JW — BM BS Nottm. 1984; BMedSci Nottm. 1982, BM BS 1984; Cert. Family Plann. JCC 1988; MRCGP 1989. GP Burton-on-Trent. Prev: SHO (Anaesth.) Leighton Hosp. Crewe.

YOUNG, Martin Paul Alistair Department of Histopathology, St. George's Hospital Medical School, Cranmer Terrace, London SW17 0RE Tel: 020 8725 5265; 3 Charlesworth Place, Eleanor Grove, Barnes, London SW13 0JQ Tel: 020 8392 8611 — MB BS Lond. 1980 (St. Geo.) BSc Lond. 1977; MRCOG 1987; MRCPath 1994. Cons. Histopath. St. Geo. Hosp. Med. Sch. Lond.; Cons. Histopathol. & Cytopathol. St. Geo. Hosp. Lond. Specialty: Histopath. Socs: Assn. Clin. Path.; Path. Soc. Prev: Lect. & Hon. Sen. Regist. Univ. Coll. Lond. Med. Sch.; Regist. (Histopath.) Univ. Coll. Hosp. Lond.; SHO (Path.) Manch. Roy. Infirm.

YOUNG, Matthew James 2 Manor Road, West Wickham BR4 9PS; 9 Bishops Avenue, Bromley BR1 3ET — MB BS Lond. 1986 (Univ. Lond. & Westm.) BSc Lond. 1983; MRCGP 1990; DRCOG 1990. GP Adviser for GP Newspaper Lond. Prev: Trainee GP/SHO Qu. Mary's Hosp. Sidcup VTS; Ho. Surg. Mayday Hosp. Croydon; Ho. Phys. Qu. Mary's Hosp. Lond.

YOUNG, Matthew John Department of Diabetes, Royal Infirmary of Edinburgh, Lauriston Place, Edinburgh EH3 9YW — MB BS Newc. 1985; MRCP (UK) 1989; MD Newc. 1994. Cons. Phys. & Diabetologist Roy. Infirm. Edin. Specialty: Gen. Med. Prev: Sen. Regist. Glas. Roy. Infirm.; Research Fell. Manch. Roy. Infirm.; Regist. North. Gen. Hosp. Sheff.

YOUNG, Maura Fiona 19 Waterfoot Road, Magherafelt BT45 6LF — MB BCh Belf. 1997.

YOUNG, Michael (retired) 21 Sealand Court, Shorts Reach, The Esplanade, Rochester ME1 1QH — MB BS Lond. 1961 (Roy. Free) MRCS Eng. LRCP Lond. 1961; DObst RCOG 1965. Assoc special. (Palliat. Med.) Heart of Kent Hospice Aylesford. Prev: GP Rochester.

YOUNG, Mr Michael Harry (retired) 12 Park Road, Padyr, Cardiff CF15 8DG Tel: 029 2084 2975 — MB ChB (Hons.) Sheff. 1960; MD (Commend.) Sheff. 1964; FRCS Eng. 1966. Prev: Cons. Orthop. Surg. S. Glam. AHA (T).

YOUNG, Michael John Young, Ellis and Overton, 41 David Place, St Helier JE2 4TE Tel: 01534 723318 Fax: 01534 611062; 3 Albermarle, LA Grande Route Des Sablons, Groyville, Jersey JE3 9FP Tel: 01534 851256 Fax: 01534 857642 — MB BS Lond. 1957 (Guy's) MRCS Eng. LRCP Lond. 1956. Socs: MRCGP; Jersey Med. Soc. Prev: SHO (Gen. Med.) Princess Beatrice Hosp. Lond.; Ho. Phys. (Paediat.) & Ho. Surg. Guy's Hosp.

YOUNG, Michael Peter Northlands Wood Surgery, 7 Walnut Park, Haywards Heath RH16 3TG Tel: 01444 458022 Fax: 01444 415960 — MB BChir Camb. 1970 (Univ. of Camb. Univ Coll. Lond.) MRCP (UK) 1973; DCH Eng. 1974; DObst RCOG 1974; MRCGP 1980.

YOUNG, Nathaniel Stuart (retired) 6 Sackville Way, West Bergholt, Colchester CO6 3DZ Tel: 01206 240045 — MB BS Lond. 1964 (Guy's) MRCS Eng. LRCP Lond. 1964.

YOUNG, Neville Widdrington Hilton (retired) 39 Allen House, Allen Street, London W8 6BH Tel: 020 7937 7426 — MB BChir Camb. 1953 (Camb. & Middlx.) MRCS Eng. LRCP Lond. 1950; DRCOG 1956.

YOUNG, Nicholas James Sevenposts Surgery, 326A Prestbury Road, Prestbury, Cheltenham GL52 3DD Tel: 01242 244103; 34 Kings Road, Cheltenham GL52 6BG — MB ChB Birm. 1983; DRCOG 1987.

YOUNG, Nicholas John Holly Lodge, Fulbeck, Morpeth NE61 3JT — BM BS Nottm. 1992.

YOUNG, Nicola Department of Medical Microbiology, The Old Medical School, Leeds General Infirmary, Great George Street, Leeds LS1 3EX Tel: 0113 3926818 — MB ChB Manch. 1992; BSc St. And. 1989; DTM & H, Lond. 1998; MRCPath London 2001. Specialist Regist. (Med. Microbiol.) Roy. Hallamshire Hosp. Sheff. Prev: Regist. (Med. Microbiol.) North. Gen. Hosp. Sheff.; Registrar (Med. Microbiology), Sheffield Teaching Hospitals Trust.

YOUNG, Mr Nigel John Alexander Clementine Churchill Hospital, Harrow HA1 3RX Tel: 020 8422 3464 Email: nigelyoung1@aol.com — MB BS Lond. 1968 (Middlx.) FRCS Eng. 1977; FRCOphth. 1988. Cons. Ophth. Watford Gen. Hosp. Specialty: Ophth. Prev: Cons. Ophth. Centr. Middlx., Northwick Pk. & Mt. Vernon Hosps.; Chief Clin. Asst. Moorfields Eye Hosp. Lond.; Res. Surg. Off. Moorfields Eye Hosp. Lond.

YOUNG, Norman (retired) 71 The Broadway, Walsall WS1 3EZ Tel: 01922 622144 Fax: 01922 622144 Email: youngnorman@lycos.co.uk — MB ChB Glas. 1950; DObst RCOG 1954; MRCGP 1963; LMCC 1969. Prev: Ho. Phys. & Ho. Surg. Stobhill Hosp. Glas.

YOUNG, Pamela Joy (retired) 22 Dumpton Gap Road, Broadstairs CT10 1TA — (Leeds) MB ChB Leeds 1964; DObst RCOG 1967; DPM Eng. 1972.

YOUNG, Pamela Ruth Greyfriars Surgery, 25 St. Nicholas Street, Hereford HR4 0BH Tel: 01432 265717 Fax: 01432 340150 — MB ChB Birm. 1983; DRCOG 1986; MRCGP 1989. Prev: Trainee GP Shrewsbury; SHO (Psychiat.) Tokanwi Hosp. New Zealand; SHO (Paediat. & O & G & Geriat.) & Cas. Off. Roy. Shrewsbury Hosp.

YOUNG, Patricia Margaret NHS Lothian:Women & Children's Directorate, Community Child Health Services, 10 Chalmers Crescent, Edinburgh EH9 1TS Tel: 0131 536 0000 Ext: 20470 Fax: 0131 536 0570 Email: Patricia.Young@luht.scot.nhs.uk; 35 Fox Covert Avenue, Edinburgh EH12 6UQ Tel: 0131 316 4010 Email: pmy@blueyonder.co.uk — MB ChB Dundee 1983; Cert. Family Plann. JCC 1986; DCH RCP Lond. 1986; MRCGP 1987; T(GP) 1991; DFFP 1993. p/t Staff Grade Paediat. Edin. Sick Childr. NHS Trust. Specialty: Community Child Health; Gen. Pract. Socs: Fac. Community Health; Assn. Research in Infant & Child Developm.; Roy. Coll. of Gen. Practitioners. Prev: GP Partner & GP Asst. Hull; SCMO Hull & Holderness Community Health Care Trust; Trainee GP Hull VTS.

YOUNG, Patrick Michael 1 Cardington Drive, Heath Farm Estate, Shrewsbury SY1 3HD — MB BS Lond. 1984.

YOUNG, Peter Frank Little Arowry Cottage, Little Arowry, Hanmer, Whitchurch SY13 3DD — MB ChB Ed. 1984. SHO (O & G) Shrops. HA. Prev: SHO (Med.) Princess Roy. Hosp. Telford.

YOUNG, Peter Frederick Pallion Health Centre, Hylton Road, Sunderland SR4 7XF Tel: 0191 567 4673 — MB BS Durh. 1964 (Newc.) Socs: Sunderland W. End Med. Soc. Prev: SHO (O & G) Sunderland Gen. Hosp. & SHO (ENT) Roy. Vict. Infirm. Newc.; Ho. Phys. Gen. Hosp. Newc.

YOUNG, Peter Jeffrey 17 Branksome Road, Norwich NR4 6SN — MB ChB Ed. 1990.

YOUNG, Peter John William (retired) Boundary House Surgery, Mount Lane, Bracknell RG12 9PG Tel: 01344 483900 Fax: 01344 862203 — MB BChir Camb. 1963 (Middlx.) BA Camb. 1959.

YOUNG, Peter Nesbitt (retired) 112 Linden Avenue, Prestbury, Cheltenham GL52 3DS Tel: 01242 520459 Email: pnyoung@argonet.co.uk — MB BChir Camb. 1964 (Univ. Coll. Hosp.) DObst RCOG 1968; FFA RCS Eng. 1971. Prev: Cons. Anaesth. Cheltenham Gen., Glos. Roy. & Tewkesbury Hosps.

YOUNG, Peter Timothy Hay Lodge Health Centre, Neidpath Road, Peebles EH45 8JG Tel: 01721 720380 Fax: 01721 723430; 19 Morning Hill, Peebles EH45 9JS — MB ChB Glas. 1984; MRCGP 1990. Prev: Trainee GP Glas. VTS.

YOUNG, Peter Westgate Plumstead Health Centre, Tewson Road, Plumstead, London SE18 1BB Tel: 020 8854 1898 Fax: 020 8855 9958 — MB BS Lond. 1975; MRCS Eng. LRCP Lond. 1974; DRCOG 1977.

YOUNG, Philip Charles, Surg. Lt.-Cdr. RN Royal Hospital Haslar, Gosport PO12 2AA Tel: 023 9258 4255 Email: 106225.1276@compuserve.com — MB BS Lond. 1985; FRCA 1995. Cons. Anaesth.; Hon. Cons. (ITU) Oxf. Radcliffe NHS Trust. Specialty: Anaesth.; Intens. Care. Socs: BMA; Assn. Anaesth. Prev: Hon. Sen. Regist. Oxf. Radcliffe NHS Trust.

YOUNG, Rachel Caroline 19 Leigh Hill Road, Cobham KT11 2HS — MB BS Lond. 1990.

YOUNG, Mr Richard Aretas Lewry West Middlesex University Hospital, Twickenham Road, Isleworth TW7 6AF Tel: 020 8565 5768 Fax: 020 8287 2778 Email: youngral@compuserve.com; 26 Strawberry Hill Road, Twickenham TW1 4PU Tel: 020 8891 0638 Fax: 020 8287 2778 — MB BChir Camb. 1968 (Camb. & St. Mary's) MRCS Eng. LRCP Lond. 1967; FRCS Eng. 1972. Cons. Surg. W. Middlx. Univ. Hosp. Lond.; Recognised Teach. Univ. Lond.; Examr. Find MB, BS Lond. Specialty: Gen. Surg. Socs: Fell. Roy. Soc. Med.; Fell. Assn. Surgs.; Vasc. Surgic. Soc. Prev: Sen. Regist. (Surg.) St. Mary's Hosp. Lond.; Bernard Sunley Research Fell. RCS Eng.; Regist. (Surg.) Roy. Free Hosp. Lond.

YOUNG, Mr Richard Charles 1 Broomsleigh St, West Hampstead, London NW6 1QQ — BM BCh Oxf. 1993; MA Camb. 1994; FRCS Eng. 1995. Research Fell., Blond Mcindoe Laboratories, Roy. Free Hosp. Lond. Specialty: Plastic Surg. Prev: SHO (A & E) John Radcliffe Hosp. Oxf.; SHO Rotat. (Surg.) Frenchay Hosp. Bristol; Demonst. (Anat.) Univ. Camb.

YOUNG, Richard Edward 25 Lawmarnock Crescent, Bridge of Weir PA11 3AS — MB ChB Glas. 1971; MRCP (UK) 1977. Cons. Phys. Geriat. Med. Argyl & Clyde HB. Specialty: Care of the Elderly. Prev: Regist. (Med.) West. Infirm. Glas.; Research Asst. Univ. Dept. Med. & SHO (Cardiol.) West. Infirm. Glas.

YOUNG, Richard John Paston Surgery, 9-11 Park Lane, North Walsham NR28 0BQ Tel: 01692 403015 Fax: 01692 500619; Home Farm, Barton Turf, Norwich NR12 8BQ Tel: 01692 536475 — MB BChir Camb. 1989; DRCOG 1992; MRCGP 1993. Hon. Sen. Lect. Sch. of Med. U.E.A. Prev: Course Organiser Norwich VTS.

YOUNG, Robert Alasdair Brims Castle Craig Hospital, Blyth Bridge, West Linton EH46 7DH Tel: 01721 722763 Fax: 01721 752662 Email: al@old-forge.demon.co.uk — MB ChB Glas. 1972; MRCPsych 1976. Cons. Psychiat. & Treatm. Director Castle Craig Hosp. Specialty: Gen. Psychiat.; Alcohol & Substance Misuse. Special Interest: Dual Diag. Prev: Regist. St. Crispin Hosp. Northampton; Hon. Clin. Teach. Soton. Univ. Med. Sch.; Sen. Regist. St. Jas. Hosp. Portsmouth & (Psychiat.) Roy. S. Hants. Hosp. Soton.

YOUNG, Mr Robert Andrew Michael 23 Millvale Road, Hillsborough BT26 6HR Tel: 01846 682387; Department of Urology, Craigavon Area Hospital, Craigavon BT63 5QQ Tel: 01762 334444 — MB BCh BAO Belf. 1983 (Queen's University Belfast) FRCSI 1987; MD Belf. 1993; FRCS (Urol.) 1996. Cons. Urol. Craigavon Area Hosp. Specialty: Urol. Socs: Brit. Assn. Urol. Surg.; BMA & Ulster Med. Soc. Prev: Sen. Regist (Urol.) Belf. City Hosp.; Regist. (Surg.) Roy. Vict. Hosp. Belf.; Research Fell. Roy. Vict. Hosp. Belf.

YOUNG, Robert Douglas (retired) Highfield, Silverdale, Carnforth LA5 0SQ Tel: 01524 701234 Fax: 01524 701234 — (Ed.) MB ChB Ed. 1943; FRCP Ed. 1971, M 1950; MD Ed. 1958. Prev: Cons. Phys. Lancaster & S. Cumbria Health Dists.

YOUNG, Robert Kyle Barr Brunthill Farm, Fenwick, Kilmarnock KA3 6HX Tel: 01560 700242 — MB ChB Glas. 1966; FFA RCS Eng. 1971. Cons. Anaesth. N. Ayrsh. Dist. Gen. Hosp. Specialty: Anaesth. Prev: Sen. Regist., Regist. & SHO (Anaesth.) Glas. Roy. Infirm.

YOUNG, Robert Marryat New House Surgery, 142A South Street, Dorking RH4 2QR; Puffins, Newdigate Road, Beare Green, Dorking RH5 4QN Tel: 01306 711920 — MB BS Lond. 1976 (St. Mary's) MRCS Eng. LRCP Lond. 1975; DRCOG 1978. Specialty: Gen. Pract. Prev: Trainee GP Lond.; SHO (Cas. & O & G) St. Mary's Hosp. Harrow Rd.; SHO (Anaesth.) Worthing Hosp.

YOUNG, Roger Christopher (retired) Yennadon Spinney, Dousland, Yelverton PL20 6NA Tel: 01822 777 — MB BS Lond. 1956 (Middlx.) DObst RCOG 1958; DA Eng. 1960. Prev: Ho. Phys. Warneford Hosp. Leamington Spa.

YOUNG, Ronald (retired) Westfield House, Calow, Chesterfield S44 5AD Tel: 01246 73845 — LMSSA Lond. 1954 (St. Bart.) Prev: Sen. Ho. Off. (Ophth.), Ho. Phys. & Ho. Surg. (Gyn.) Derby Roy.

YOUNG, Rowena 22 Edenpark Drive, Batheaston, Bath BA1 7JJ Tel: 01225 858212 — MB BS Lond. 1966 (Roy. Free) MRCS Eng. LRCP Lond. 1966; DObst RCOG 1968. Assoc. Specialist Roy. United Hosp. Bath. Socs: BMA; Brit. Diabetic Assn. (Med. & Scientif. Sect.). Prev: Ho. Surg. (Obst.) S. Lond. Hosp.; Ho. Phys. W. Kent Gen. Hosp. Maidstone; Ho. Surg. Roy. Free Hosp. Lond.

YOUNG, Russell Andrew c/o Hull Royal Infirmary, Anlaby Road, Hull HU3 2JZ Tel: 07930 193617 Email: winfield19@aol.com; 5 Albert Terrance, Beverley HU17 8JU Tel: 01482 882146 — MB ChB Manch. 1997. SHO (Gen. Surg.) Hull Roy. Infirm. Specialty: Gen. Surg. Prev: Ho. Off. (Gen. Med.) Trafford Gen. Hosp. Manch.; SHO Orthpaedics; SHO (A&E).

YOUNG, Russell Murray Department of Clinical Biochemistry, Queen Alexandra Hospital, Cosham, Portsmouth PO6 3LY Tel: 023 92 286349 Fax: 023 92 286265 Email: russell.young@porthosp.nhs.uk — BM BS Nottm. 1976; BMedSci Nottm. 1974; Dip. Health Managem. Keele 1993; FRCPath 1995. Cons. Chem. Path. Portsmouth Hosps. NHS Trust. Specialty: Chem. Path.; Endocrinol. Special Interest: Fertility. Socs: Hon. Sec. Assn. Clin. Pathol.; Assn. Clin. Biochem. Prev: Sen. Regist., Chem. Path., Yorks. Regional Health Auth., Leeds; Regist., Chem. Path., Leeds Area Health Auth., Leeds.

YOUNG, Ruth Amelia (retired) 5 The Manor House, Upper Green, Tettenhall, Wolverhampton WV6 8QJ Tel: 01902 756168 Email: rayoung@amserve.com — (Univ. Glas.) MB ChB Glas. 1946, DPH 1949. Prev: Gen. Practitioner Wolverhampton.

YOUNG, Samuel Knibb, SBStJ (retired) 39 Newlands Avenue, Bishop Auckland DL14 6AJ Tel: 01388 602495 — (Camb. & St. Thos.) LMSSA Lond. 1954; MA Camb. 1954. Prev: Sen. Partner in Gen. Pract., Bishop Auckland.

YOUNG, Sandra Hurst Holly Lodge, Fulbeck, Morpeth NE61 3JT Tel: 01670 512052 — MB ChB Glas. 1961. Clin. Asst. (Dermat.) Roy. Vict. Infirm. Newc., Tynemouth Vict. Jubilee Infirm. & Northld. AHA. Prev: SHO Dept. Dermat. Vict. Hosp. Glas.; Ho. Off. Ballochmyle Hosp. Mauchline.

YOUNG, Sara Camilla (retired) 19 Kingston Road, Bridlington YO15 3NF Tel: 0126 401372 — (Sheff.) MB ChB Sheff. 1963. Prev: SCMO E. Yorks. Community Healthcare.

YOUNG, Sarah Catherine Russel 30A Kemplay Road, Hampstead, London NW3 1SY Tel: 020 7794 7983 — MB BS Lond. 1991; BSc Lond. 1986. Prev: SHO (O & G) Hammersmith Hosp. Lond.; SHO (Med.) Johannesburg Hosp., SA.

YOUNG, Sarah Louise Doctors Surgery, Forge Close, Hayes, Bromley BR2 7LL Tel: 020 8462 1601 Fax: 020 8462 7410; 13 Beadon Road, Bromley BR2 9AS — MB BS Lond. 1986; MA Oxf. 1983; DCH RCP Lond. 1989; DRCOG 1992. Specialty: Gen. Pract. Socs: BMA.

YOUNG, Sarah Margaret 8 Oxford Road, Teddington TW11 0PZ — BM BS Nottm. 1998.

YOUNG, Sean Patrick New Surgery, Victoria Street, Pontycymer, Bridgend CF32 8NN Tel: 01656 870237 Fax: 01656 870354; Llangeinar House, Bttius Road, Llangeinar, Bridgend CF32 8PH — MB BS Lond. 1989; MRCGP 1994. Prev: Trainee GP/SHO (Psychiat.) M. Glam. VTS.

YOUNG, Sharon Moiran Midgley University Health Service, University of Edinburgh, Richard Verney Health Centre, Edinburgh EH8 9AL Tel: 0131 650 2777 Fax: 0131 662 1813; 8 Succoth Place, Edinburgh EH12 6BL — MB ChB Ed. 1979; DCCH RCP Ed. 1985.

YOUNG, Sheila Haxby & Wigginton Health Centre, The Village, Wigginton, York YO32 2LL Tel: 01904 760125; 6 The Willows, Strensall, York YO32 5YG — MB BS Newc. 1982; DRCOG 1988.

YOUNG, Shina Ann Birchwood Surgery, Birchwood, Arisaig PH39 4NJ Tel: 01687 450258 — MB ChB Aberd. 1967. Prev: Clin. Med. Off. Highland HB; GP Kinlochleven; Resid. Roy. Aberd. Hosp. Sick Childr. & Woodend Hosp. Aberd.

YOUNG, Simon John Brenkley Avenue Health Centre, Brenkley Avenue, Shiremoor, Newcastle upon Tyne NE27 0PR Tel: 0191 251 6682 Fax: 0191 219 5700 — MB ChB Manch. 1989. GP Newc.

YOUNG, Simon Peter — MB ChB Aberd. 1998.

YOUNG, Stephanie Kim 11 Sheridan House, Wincott Street, London SE11 4NY — MB ChB Otago 1992; MRCPsych 2000. Specialty: Gen. Psychiat.

YOUNG, Mr Stephen Kenrick South Warwickshire Hospital, Lakin Road, Warwick CV34 5BW; Sussex Gardens, Grafton Lane, Binton, Stratford-upon-Avon CV37 9TZ — MB BChir Camb. 1979; FRCS Ed. 1983. Cons. Orthop. Surg. S. Warks. Hosp. Specialty: Orthop. Prev: Sen. Regist. (Orthop.) Bristol Roy. Infirm.

YOUNG, Steven Charles 9 Ash Grove, Carnock, Dunfermline KY12 9JT — MB ChB Dundee 1978; MRCPsych 1987. Cons. Psychiat. State Hosp. Carstairs Lanarksh. Specialty: Ment. Health; Forens. Psychiat.

YOUNG, Steven Jackson Oakham Medical Practice, Cold Overton Road, Rutland, Oakham LE15 6NT Tel: 01572 722621; Lyndon View, 12 Church Street, Wing, Rutland, Oakham LE15 8RS — MB ChB Manch. 1979; DRCOG 1987; MRCGP 1988; MSc Sports Med. Nottm. 1994. Clin. Asst. (c/o Elderly & Fract. Clinic) Rutland Memor. Hosp. Oakham. Specialty: Sports Med.

YOUNG, Stuart Shepherdson 9 Longmans Lane, Newgate St., Cottingham HU16 4EA Tel: 01482 876700 — MB ChB Sheff. 1952; MRCS Eng. LRCP Lond. 1952; DObst RCOG 1956; DCH Eng. 1956.

YOUNG, Susan Elizabeth Jean (retired) 51 Wilton Road, London N10 1LX — MB BCh BAO Dub. 1958 (T.C. Dub.) DCH Eng. 1961;

MRCP (UK) 1971; Dip. Bact. Lond 1973. Specialist in Community Med. (Epidemiol.) Communicable Dis.

YOUNG, Susan Forsyth Hunter Health Centre, Andrew Street, East Kilbride, Glasgow G74 1AD Tel: 01355 906611 Fax: 01355 906615 — MB ChB Glas. 1988. Specialty: Obst. & Gyn.

YOUNG, Susan Margaret 301 Westmount Road, Eltham, London SE9 1NR — MB ChB Leic. 1990.

YOUNG, Susan Miranda Department of Genitourinary Medicine, Kings Mill Hospital, Mansfield Road, Sutton-in-Ashfield NG17 4JL Tel: 01623 622515 Ext: 4095 — MB ChB Dundee 1977; Dip. Ven. Liverp. 1984; MRCPI 1988. Specialty: Genitourinary Medicine. Prev: Sen. Regist. (Genitourin. Med.) Leic. Roy. Infirm.; Regist. (Genitourin. Med.) Roy. Liverp. Hosp. & Arrowe Pk. Hosp. Upton.

YOUNG, Thomas Behnam 3A Horn Lane, London W3 9NJ Tel: 020 8993 2313 Mob: 07718 276060 — MB ChB Mosul 1970; FRCS Glas. 1980.

YOUNG, Thomas William Stewart Email: TWSY@doctors.net.uk — MB ChB Leeds 1994. Specialty: Accid. & Emerg.

YOUNG, Timothy Michael — MB BS Lond. 1997 (King's Coll. Hosp.)

YOUNG, Timothy Stuart Staveley Temple Sowerby Medical Practice, Temple Sowerby, Penrith CA10 1RZ Tel: 017683 61232 Fax: 017683 61980 — MB ChB Ed. 1982; DRCOG 1986. Clin. Asst. (Ophth.) Cumberld. Infirm. Carlisle. Prev: Trainee GP Fife Health Bd. VTS.

YOUNG, Torrence Martyn (Tod) (retired) Department of Anaesthetics, Manchester Royal Infirmary, Oxford Road, Manchester M13 9WL Tel: 0161 276 4551 Fax: 0161 273 5685; 64 Stamford Road, Bowdon, Altrincham WA14 2JF Tel: 0161 928 4912 — MB BS Lond. 1950 (Univ. Coll. Hosp.) MRCS Eng. LRCP Lond. 1950; DA Eng. 1954; FFA RCS Eng. 1956. Prev: Hon. Cons. Anaesth. Manch. Centr. Dist.

YOUNG, Venetia Emma Beech Lodge, Carleton Clinic, Carlisle CA1 3SU Tel: 01228 602392; Eden Croft, Temple Sowerby, Penrith CA10 1RZ Tel: 017683 61647 Fax: 017683 61980 Email: youngjckvg@compuserve.com — MB BS Lond. 1975 (Univ. Coll. Hosp.) BSc Lond. 1972; MRCGP 1979; DRCOG 1979. Clin. Asst. (Family Psychother.) Carleton clinic. Carlisle; Dip. Family Ther. Specialty: Psychother.

YOUNG, Mr Vincent Kieran Coleraine Road, Maghera BT46 5HZ; 4 Avondale Lawn, Carysfort Avenue, Blackrock, Dublin, Republic of Ireland Tel: 00 353 1 833420 — MB BCh BAO Dub. 1986; FRCS Eng. 1990; FRCSI 1990. Regist. (Gen. Surg.) Waterford Regional Hosp. Specialty: Gen. Surg.

YOUNG, Violet Boyle (retired) Orphir, Main Road, Rhu, Helensburgh G84 8RB Tel: 01436 820698 — MB ChB Glas. 1941; DA Eng. 1944. Prev: Med. Off. Blood Transfus. Serv. Glas.

YOUNG, William Alister Highpoint House, Bromley, Bexley and Greenwich, Child and Adolescent Mental Health Service, Memorial Hospital Shooters Hill, London SE18 3RZ Tel: 0208 836 6418 Fax: 0208 836 6436 Email: bill.young@oxleas.nhs.uk; 60 Craigerne Road, Blackheath, London SE3 8SN Tel: 020 8853 4863 Email: byoung@dircon.co.uk — MB ChB Manch. 1983; DCH RCP Lond. 1985; MRCP (UK) 1987; MRCPsych 1989; FRCPCH UK 1999. p/t Cons. Child & Adolesc. Psychiat. Bromley, Bexley & Greenwich Child & Adolesc. Ment. Health Serv. Lond.; Cons. Psychiat. Abbeycrest Adolesc. Psychiatric Unit Upper Norwood Lond. Specialty: Child & Adolesc. Psychiat. Special Interest: Health Servs. Managem. Socs: Assn. of Family Ther.; Trustee of Young Minds; Fell. Roy. Coll. of Paediat. and Child Health. Prev: Cons. Adolesc. Psychiat. & Clin. Dir. (Oakview Adolesc. Unit) St Mary Cray, Orpington; Sen. Regist. (Child & Family Psychiat.) Tavistock Clinic Lond.; Regist. (Psychiat.) Maudsley Hosp. Lond.

YOUNG, William Brewitt (retired) Black Charles Barn Cottage, Underriver, Sevenoaks TN15 0RY — MB BChir Camb. 1941 (King's Coll. Hosp.) Prev: Ho. Surg. Mildmay Miss. Hosp. Lond.

YOUNG, William David Viewfield Medical Centre, 3 Viewfield Place, Stirling FK8 1NJ Tel: 01786 472028 Fax: 01786 463388 — MB ChB Glas. 1969; FRCOG 2003. Hosp. Prac. (Genitourin. Med.) Orchard Hse. Health Centre Stirling. Specialty: Gen. Pract. Prev: Regist. (O & G) Stirling Roy. Infirm. & Stobhill Gen. Hosp. Glas.; Regist. (Biochem.) Qu. Mother's Hosp. Glas.

YOUNG, William Hayward 15 Nottington Court, Weymouth DT3 4BL Tel: 01305 812818 — MRCS Eng. LRCP Lond. 1967 (Westm.) BSc Lond. 1961; AKC 1971; DMRT Eng. 1972. Forens. Med. Examr. (Police Physician), Weymouth. Socs: Assn. Palliat. Med. Prev: Assoc. Specialist, Radiother. & Oncol., S. Cleveland Hosp., Middlesborough; Sen. Regist. (Radiother.) Christie Hosp. & Holt Radium Inst. Manch.; Assoc. Specialist Radio Ther. & Oncol. S. Cleveland Hosp. Middlesbrough.

YOUNG, William Morrison Douglas Street Surgery, 1 Douglas Street, Hamilton ML3 0DR Tel: 01698 286262 — MB ChB Aberd. 1980; DRCOG 1983; MRCGP 1984.

YOUNG, Windsor Tudor X Ray Department, Princess of Wales Hospital, Bridgend CF31 1RQ Tel: 01656 752425; Old Cogan Hall, Sully Road, Penarth CF64 2TQ — MB BCh Wales 1980 (Welsh National School Medicine) MRCP (UK) 1983; FRCR 1988; FRCP 1998. Cons. Radiol. Princess Wales Hosp. Bridgend. Specialty: Radiol. Prev: Sen. Regist. (Radiol.) Univ. Hosp. Wales.

YOUNG, Yvonne Maria 40 Mount Road, London SW19 8EW — MB BS Lond. 1983; BSc (Hons.) Lond. 1980; MSc Lond. 1990. Cons. Communicable Dis. Control/Publ. Health Med. Specialty: Pub. Health Med. Prev: Research Regist. (Microbiol.) Westm. Hosp. Lond.; Regist. (Pub. Health Med.) SW Thames RHA.

YOUNG-HARTMAN, Marrigje 5 Fairlands Park, Coventry CV4 7DS Tel: 024 7641 8684 — Artsexamen Amsterdam 1981 (Univ. Amsterdam) Cert. Community Paediat. Warwick 1984; Dip. Community Paediat. Warwick 1986. SCMO (Child Health) Coventry HA. Prev: Occupat. Health Phys. S. Warks. HA; SHO (Paediat.) & Ho. Off. Coventry DHA.

YOUNG MIN, Marie Sandra Department of Haematology, Birmingham Heartlands Hospital, Bordsley Green East, Birmingham B9 5SS; 27 Blackwood Road, Bromsgrove B60 1AN — MB ChB Birm. 1991; BSc (Hons) Birm. 1988; MRCP (UK) 1994. Specialist Regist., Birm. Heartlands Hosp. Specialty: Haematology.

YOUNG MIN, Steven Andrew Newcastle General Hospital, Newcastle upon Tyne NE4 6BE Tel: 0191 273 8811; 172 Osborne Road, Jesmond, Newcastle upon Tyne NE2 3LE Tel: 0191 281 7593 — BM BCh Oxf. 1994; BA (Hons.) Oxf. 1991. SHO (Med.) Newc. Gen. Hosp.

YOUNGE, Paul Andrew Emergency Department, Frenchay Hospital, Bristol BS16 1LE Tel: 0117 959 5112 Email: paul.younge@north-bristol.swest.nhs.uk — BM Soton. 1987; BSc (Hons.) 1981; DA (UK) 1989; MRCP (UK) 1993; FFAEM 1998. Clin. Fell. Paediat. Emerg. Med., Cons. in Emerg. Med.; Clin. Lect. in Child Health; Sen Lect. in Emerg. Med. Prev: Clin. Fell. (Paediat.) ICU, Bris. Childr.'s Hosp.; Specialist Regist. (Emerg. Med.) Bris. Roy. Infirm.

YOUNGER, Jane Mary 7 Ormiston Gardens, Belfast BT5 6JD — MB ChB Liverp. 1998.

YOUNGER, Kirsten Alexandra Tandrup, Hill View Road, Claygate, Esher KT10 0TU — MB BS Lond. 1983 (Lond. Hosp.) BSc (Physiol. with Basic Med. Sci) Lond. 1980; FRCR 1990. Cons. Radiol. Epsom Gen. Hosp. Specialty: Radiol. Prev: Regist. (Radiol.) St. Geo. Hosp. Lond.; SHO Rotat. (Surg.) Roy. Surrey Co. Hosp. Guildford.

YOUNGHUSBAND, Andrea Joan Broadway Medical Group, 164 Great North Road, Gosforth, Newcastle upon Tyne NE3 5JP Tel: 0191 285 2460; Hawthorn Cottage, East Heddon, Newcastle upon Tyne NE15 0HD — MB BS Newc. 1985; MRCGP 1990.

YOUNGMAN, James Robert 15 Corinne Road, London N19 5EZ — MB BS Lond. 1990.

YOUNGMAN, Lisa Margaret 51 Chepstow Road, Leicester LE2 1PB — MB ChB Leic. 1997.

YOUNGMAN, Peter Robert Hamilton Road Surgery, 201 Hamilton Road, Felixstowe IP11 7DT Tel: 01394 283197 Fax: 01394 270304; The Cottage, Thorpe Common, Trimley St Martin, Felixstowe IP11 0RZ Tel: 01394 273688 — MB BS Lond. 1977 (Middlx.) BSc Lond. 1974; DCH Eng. 1980; DRCOG 1981.

YOUNGS, Elizabeth Rosa County Hospital, Microbiology Department, St Anne's Road, Lincoln LN2 5RF Tel: 01522 528607 Fax: 01522 546997 Email: elizabeth.youngs@ulh.nhs.uk — MB ChB Manch. 1977 (St And. & Manch.) BMedSci 1974; DBact. 1982; MRCPath 1984; FRCPath 1995. Cons. Microbiol. Co. Hosp. Lincoln. Specialty: Med. Microbiol.

YOUNGS, Giles Robert Kopsey Cottage, Rattlesden Road, Drinkstone, Bury St Edmunds IP30 9TL — MB BChir (Hons. Path.) Camb. 1966 (Camb. & Lond. Hosp.) FRCP Lond. 1982, M 1969;

MA Camb. 1967, MD 1972. p/t Examg. Med. Practitioner (Disability Analysis) Dept. of Work & Pens. Prev: Cons. Phys. (Med. & Gastroenterol.) Countess of Chester Hosp. Chester.; Sen. Regist. (Med.) Soton. Gen. Hosp.; Ho. Phys. Profess. Med. Unit Lond. Hosp.

YOUNGS, Jane Claire Higherfield, Horrabridge, Yelverton PL20 7RW — MB ChB Birm. 1997.

YOUNGS, Mr Robin Peter Gloucestershire Royal Hospital, Great Western Road, Gloucester GL1 3NN Tel: 01452 394205 — MB BS Lond. 1980 (Westm.) MRCS Eng. LRCP Lond. 1980; FRCS Eng. 1984; MD Lond. 1993. Cons. Otolaryngol. Gloucestershire Royal Hospital; Vis. Lect. Inst. Laryngol. & Otol. Univ. Lond. Specialty: Otolaryngol. Special Interest: Endoscopic Sinus Surg.; Middle Ear Surg. Socs: Fell. Roy. Soc. Med.; British Rhinological Society; European Rhinological Society. Prev: Sen. Regist. (ENT) St. Bart. Hosp. Lond.; Regist. (ENT) St. Mary's Hosp. Lond.; TWJ Research Fell. Univ. Toronto, Canada.

YOUNGS, Sarah-Louise Emma Charlotte Lockwood Springfold, Cherry Tree Road, Rowledge, Farnham GU10 4AB — MB ChB Birm. 1994; DFFP 1998; DRCOG 1999; MRCGP 2000. GP Princip.; Med. Off. Cheltenham Ladies Coll. Specialty: Gen. Pract. Prev: GP Reg. Cheltenham.

YOUNGSON, Elaine Margaret 80 Kidderminster Road, Hagley, Stourbridge DY9 0QL — MB ChB Ed. 1986. GP Princip.; GP Locum Hagley Med. Pract. Specialty: Gen. Pract. Prev: Trainee GP Livingston; SHO (Paediat.) Falkirk Roy. Infirm.; SHO (Psychiat.) Bangour Village W. Lothian.

YOUNGSON, Professor George Gray Royal Aberdeen Children's Hospital, Cornhill Road, Aberdeen AB25 2ZG Tel: 01224 681818 Fax: 01224 550642 Email: ggyrach@abdn.ac.uk; Birken Lodge, Bieldside, Aberdeen AB15 9BQ Tel: 01224 861305 — MB ChB Aberd. 1973; FRCS Ed. 1977; PhD Aberd. 1979. Cons. Paediat. Surg. Grampian Univ. Hosps NHS Trust; Regional Adviser RCS of Edin.; Hon. Prof (Paediat. Surg.) Univ. of Aberd. Specialty: Paediat. Surg. Socs: Assn. Surg.; Brit. Assn. Paediat. Surg. Prev: Lect. (Surg.) Aberd. Univ.; Resid. (Cardiac Surg.) Univ. West. Ontario & Fell. Clin. Surg. Hosp. Sick Childr. Toronto, Ontario, Canada.

YOUNGSON, Robert Murdoch, OStJ, Col. (retired) 26 St Leonard's Avenue, Blandford Forum DT11 7NY Tel: 01258 452465 Email: robert_youngson@compuserve.com — (Aberdeen) MB ChB Aberd. 1951; DTM & H Eng. 1964; DO Eng. 1965; FRCOphth 1988. Full-time Med. & Sci. Writer. Prev: Cons. Ophth. Qu. Eliz. Milit. Hosp. Lond.

YOUNIE, George Grant, TD (retired) 5 Laurelwood Avenue, Aberdeen AB25 3SY Tel: 01224 636491; Balvenie, Linn of Dee Road, Braemar, Ballater AB35 5WT — MB ChB Aberd. 1948.

YOUNIE, Mai Louise Amanda 1 All Saints Road, Thurcaston, Leicester LE7 7JD — MB ChB Bristol 1997. SHO (A&E). Specialty: Accid. & Emerg. Prev: Ho. Off. (Surg.); Ho. Off. (Med.); SHO Orhopaedics.

YOUNIS, Mr Farouk Mustafa (cons. rooms), 129 Harley Street, London W1N 1DJ Tel: 020 7487 4897 Fax: 020 7224 6398 Email: fmyounis@aol.com; 4 Langton Avenue, Whetstone, London N20 9DB Tel: 020 8446 1672 Fax: 020 7224 6398 Email: fmyounis@aol.com — MB ChB Baghdad 1971; FRCS Eng. 1977. Cons. Surg. Princess Grace Hosp. & Hosp. of St John & St Eliz. Specialty: Gen. Surg.; Urol.; Gastroenterol. Socs: Fell. Roy. Soc. Med.; BMA; Fell. Assoc. Surg. GB & Irel. Prev: Cons. Surg. Whittington Hosp (Locum); Regist. (Gen. Surg. & Urol.) Huddersfield Roy. Infirm.; Regist. (Gen. Surg.) Whittington Hosp. Lond.

YOUNIS, Naveed 58 Norton Street, Manchester M16 7GR — MB ChB Manch. 1993.

YOUNIS, Yasmeen 156 Queens Road, Halifax HX1 4LN — MB ChB Dundee 1997.

YOUNUS, Mr Naeem 36 Buckland Road, Leyton, London E10 6QS — MB BS Punjab 1990; FRCS Ed. 1995.

YOUSAF, Rauf 16 Yew Tree Close, Lords Wood, Chatham ME5 8XN Tel: 0973 671151 — MB ChB Dundee 1995.

YOUSEF, Zaheer Raza 25 Pollards Close, Goffs Oak, Cheshunt, Waltham Cross EN7 5JP; Flat, Alpika Court, Saunders Road, London SE18 1NT Tel: 020 8355 7755 Email: zyousef@dircon.co.uk — MB BS Lond. 1992; BSc (Hons.) Lond. 1988, MB BS 1992; MRCP Lond. 1996. Clin. Research Fell. (Cardiol.) Guy's & St. Thos. Hosps. Lond. Specialty: Cardiol.

YOUSIF, Abdul Ridha Salman 14 Bowyer Walk, Ascot SL5 8QS — MB ChB Baghdad 1970.

YOUSIF, Emad Habib Colchester PCT, Heath House, Grange Way, Colchester CO2 8GU Tel: 01206 747781 Email: emad.yousif@newpossibilities.nhs.uk — MB ChB Baghdad 1971; MRCPsych 1985; LD psych 1990; T(Psych) 1991. Cons. Psychiat. (Learning Disabil. Psychiat.) New Possibilities NHS Trust. Specialty: Ment. Health; Gen. Psychiat.

YOUSIF, Sami Yousif 9 Southwold Spur, Slough SL3 8XX — MB ChB Baghdad 1973; MRCPI 1991.

YOUSSEF, Evelyn Elia Birmingham and Midland Eye Centre, Dudley Road, Birmingham B18 7QU Tel: 0121 554 3801; 3 Becontree Drive, Baguley, Manchester M23 9WQ — MB BCh Assiut 1976; FRCSI 1992. Specialty: Ophth.

YOUSSEF, Hanei Mohamed Hosny Ali Princess Mary's Hospital, RAF Akrotiri BFPO 57 Tel: 00 357 2596 5562; 17 The Green, Radyr, Cardiff CF15 8BR Tel: 029 2084 2781 — MB ChB Alexandria 1972; DGO Dub. 1977; FRCOG 1997, MRCOG 1984. Civilian Cons. (O & G) MoD. Specialty: Obst. & Gyn. Special Interest: Infertil. Socs: Brit. Fertil. Soc. & Brit. Menopause Soc. (former). Prev: Cons. (O & G) & Acting Chief (O & G) King Abdul Aziz Hosp. & Oncol. Centre Jeddah Saudi Arabi; Cons. O & G Vict. Sq. Med. Centre P. Albert Canad.; Chief (O & G) Yanbu, Saudi Arabia.

YOUSSEF, Haney 5 Poppyfield Ct, Coventry CV4 7HW — MB ChB Birm. 1997.

YOUSSEF, Mr Magdy Mohamed Kamal Ibrahim 7 Roebuck Close, Ingleby, Barwick, Stockton-on-Tees TS17 0RZ Tel: 01642 762336 — MB BCh Cairo 1979; FRCS Glas. 1989; FRCS Gen. Dub. 2001. Cons. Breast and Gen. Surg. Wansbeck Hosp. Ashington, Northumbria. Specialty: Gen. Surg.

YOUSSEF, Samir Morcos (retired) — MB BCh Ain Shams 1958; DTM & H Ain Shams 1964; DMedRehab Eng. 1978; MRCS Eng. LRCP Lond. 1979. Prev: Regist. (Rehabil.) Raigmore Hosp. Inverness.

YOUSSEF, Youssef Yacoub Lady Close, Warrington Road, Mere, Knutsford WA16 0TE Tel: 01565 830517 — MB ChB Alexandria 1964; FFA RCSI 1973; DA Eng. 1973. Cons. (Anaesth.) N. (Manch.) Health Dist.; Hon. Lect. Univ. Manch. Specialty: Anaesth. Socs: Assn. Anaeth. Gt. Brit. & Irel.; Obst. Anaesth. Assn.; Pain Soc. of G.B. & Irel. Prev: Coll. Tutor.

YOUSU KUNJU, Mohamed Glyn Ebwy Surgery, James Street, Ebbw Vale NP23 6JG Tel: 01495 302716 Fax: 01495 305166; 5 Green Street, Victoria, Ebbw Vale NP23 8WR Tel: 01495 309505 — MB BS Kerala 1974 (Trivandrum Med. Coll.)

YOUSUF, Enver Yunus 35 Sutherland Avenue, London W9 2HE — MB BS Lond. 1994; BSc (Hons.) Lond. 1991.

YOUSUF, Mr Ishrat Muhammad Chesterfield Royal Hospital & NHS Trust, Chesterfield S44 5BL Tel: 01246 277271; 15 Blackthorn Close, Hasland, Chesterfield S41 0DY Tel: 01246 551853 Fax: 01246 551853 Email: ishrat@ishrat.fsnet.co.uk — MB BS Karachi 1983 (DOW Medical College, Karachi) FRCSI 1991. Staff Grade (ENT) Chesterfield Roy. Hosp. Specialty: Otolaryngol. Prev: SHO (ENT) Dudley Rd. Hosp. Birm. & Sunderland Dist. Gen. Hosp.; SHO (Gen. Surg.) Neville Hall Hosp. Abergavenny.; Regist. (ENT) Stoke Mandeville Hosp. Aylesbury.

YOUSUF, Kolothum Thodi 7 Bridle Hey, Nantwich CW5 7QE — MB BS India 1976.

YOUSUFF, Mr Anser Mohammed 27 Laxton Garth, Kirkella, Hull HU10 7NN Email: yousuff@aol.com — MB BS Madras 1986; FRCS Glas. 1991; Dip Urol. Lond. 1994. Staff Grade Urol. Roy. Hull NHS Trust. Specialty: Urol.; Gen. Surg. Prev: Act. Regist. (Urol.) Burton Hosp.; Regist. (Surg.) Stockport/Trafford/Ashton-u-Lyme.

YOUSUFZAI, Noor Mohammad (retired) BUPA Hospital, Little Astor, Sutton Coldfield B74 3HP; 203 Walsall Road, Four Oaks, Sutton Coldfield B74 4QA Tel: 0121 353 0656 Fax: 0121 353 6255 — MB BS Sind 1963 (Liaquat Med. Coll.) DPM Eng. 1970; FRCPsych 1991, M 1973. Cons. Psychiat. BUPA Hosp. Little Astor. Prev: Cons. Psychiat. Dorothy Pattison Hosp. Walsall Burntwood Psychother. Unit Bloxwich Hosp. Walsall.

YOXALL, Charles William Neonatal Intensive Care Unit, Liverpool Womens Hospital, Crown Street, Liverpool L8 7SS Tel: 0151 708 9988 Fax: 0151 702 4082 — BM BS Nottm. 1986; BMedSci Nottm. 1984; MRCP (UK) 1990; MD Liverpool 1998; FRCPCH 1999. Cons. Neonat. Paediat. Liverp. Wom. Hosp.; Paediatric Train. Progr.

Director, Mersey Deanery. Specialty: Neonat. Socs: Eur. Soc. Paediat. Research; Neonat. Soc.; MRCPCH. Prev: Lect. Dept. Child Health, Univ. Liverp.; Clin. Research Fell. (Neonat.) Univ. Liverp.; Regist. (Paediat.) Mersey Region.

YOXALL, James Henry Blackbrook Surgery, Lisieux Way, Taunton TA1 2LB Tel: 01823 259444 Fax: 01823 322715; West Lodge, Pitminster, Taunton TA3 7AZ Tel: 01823 421396 — MB BS Lond. 1977; DRCOG 1980.

YU, Christopher Bing On — MB BS Lond. 1991; FRCOphth 1996; FHKAM 1999.

YU, Dominic Fergus Quok Ching King's College Hospital, Denmark Hill, London SE5 Tel: 020 7346 3331 — MB BS Lond. 1991; MRCPI 1997; FRCR 2001. Specialist Regist. (Diagnostic Radiol.) King's Coll. Hosp. Specialty: Radiol. Prev: SHO (Gen. Med.) Medway Hosp.; SHO (Gen. Med.) Chase Farm Hosp.; SHO (A & E) Watford Gen. Hosp.

YU, Dominic Shu Lok 70 Leybourne Avenue, London W13 9RA — MB BS Lond. 1996.

YU, Koa Hung Green Wrythe Surgery, 411A Green Wrythe Lane, Carshalton SM5 1JF Tel: 020 8648 2022 Fax: 020 8646 6555; 24 The Highway, Sutton SM2 5QT Tel: 020 8661 6242 — MB BS Colombo 1980. GP Surrey. Specialty: Cardiol.; Paediat.; Gen. Med.

YU, Ling Faang Marfleet Group Practice, 350 Preston Road, Hull HU9 5HH Tel: 01482 701834; PO Box 13954, Kota Kinabalu, Sabah 88845, Malaysia Tel: 00 60 88 245088 — MB ChB Glas. 1990; MRCP (UK) 1995; DDSc Wales 1996; MSc Wales 1997. Specialty: Dermat.

YU, Raymond Chi Hung 99 Harley Street, London W1G 6AQ — MB BChir Camb. 1983; MRCP (UK) 1988; MD 1994; FRCP 2000. University College Hospitals NHS Trust. Specialty: Dermat.

YU, Shee Hung 27 Chestnut Close, London N14 4SG Tel: 020 8447 9452 — MB BS Sri Lanka 1975; LRCP MRCS Eng. LRCP Lond. 1979; DRCOG 1984. Specialty: Gen. Med.

YU, Sui Cheung 24 Aspen Close, London W5 4YG — MB ChB Leeds 1992; BSc Leeds 1989. Med. Off. (Anaesth. & Intens. Care) P. of Wales Hosp. Hong Kong; Adjunct Tutor Chinese Univ. Hong Kong. Specialty: Anaesth.

YU HO YAM, Henry Golden Pine, Charles II Place, 77 King's Road, Chelsea, London SW3 4NG Tel: 020 7352 6499 — MB BS Lond. 1966; LMSSA Lond. 1964; FRACS 1973.

YU WAI MAN, Patrick Yee Sem Youn Royal Victoria Infirmary, Eye Department, Queen Victoria Road, Newcastle upon Tyne NE1 4LP — MB BS (Hons.) Newc. 2002; BMedSci (Hons.) Newc. 2001. SHO Opthalmology Roy. Vict. Infirm. Newc.-u-Tyne. Specialty: Ophth. Prev: PRHO, Roy. Vict. Infirm. Newc.-u-Tyne.

YUDKIN, Gillian Diana James Wigg Group Practice, Kentish Town Health Centre, 2 Bartholomew Road, London NW5 BX Tel: 020 7530 4747 Fax: 020 7530 4750; 28 Huddleston Road, London N7 0AG Tel: 020 7607 3855 — MB BChir Camb. 1967 (Camb. & Univ. Coll. Hosp.) DCH Eng. 1971.

YUDKIN, Professor John Stephen 28 Huddleston Road, London N7 0AG Tel: 020 7607 3855 — MB BChir Camb. 1967 (Camb. & Univ. Coll. Hosp.) FRCP Lond. 1988, M (UK) 1971; MD Camb. 1975. Prof. Med. Univ. Coll. Lond. Specialty: Gen. Med. Socs: Med. Res. Soc. & Brit. Diabetic Assn. Prev: Cons. & Sen. Lect. (Gen. Med. & Diabetes) Whittington & Univ. Coll. Hosps. Lond.; Lect. Metab. & Endocrine Unit Lond. Hosp. Med. Coll.; Sen. Lect. Fac. Med. Univ. Dar es Salaam, Tanzania.

YUE, Arthur Man-Hin 41 Kings College Court, 55 Primrose Hill Road, London NW3 3EA — BM BCh Oxf. 1994; MA Oxf. 1996; MRCP (UK) 1997. Specialist Regist. Rotat. (Cardiol.) Wessex & SW Thames. Specialty: Cardiol. Socs: Brit. Echocardiogr. Soc.

YUEN, Alan Wah Cheong 9 Elmwood Park, Gerrards Cross SL9 7EP Email: alan@yuen.freeserve.co.uk — BM BCh Oxf. 1977; MA Camb. 1978; MRCP (UK) 1979; MRCGP 1982; FFPM RCP (UK) 1996. Med. Research Nat. Soc. Epilepsy. Specialty: Pharmaceutical Medicine. Prev: Manager Global Licensing.

YUEN, Albert Kin-Chung 134 Gillespie Road, London N5 1LP — MB BS Lond. 1994.

YUEN, Conrad Hong Wai — MB ChB Liverp. 1994; MRCOphth 1997. SpR (Ophth.) Mersey Region. Specialty: Ophth. Prev: SHO (Ophth.) Southport & Formby NHS Trust Southport Gen. Infirm. (Eye Unit); SHO (Ophth.) St Paul's Eye Unit Roy. Liverp. Univ. Hosp.; SHO (Ophth.) Glas. Roy. Infirm. NHS Trust.

YUGAMBARANATHAN, Kandiah 7 Harefield Close, Enfield EN2 8NQ — MB BS Colombo, Sri Lanka 1978; MRCP (UK) 1993.

YUILL, George Martin (cons. rooms), 16 St John Street, Manchester M3 4EA Tel: 0161 834 2554 — MB ChB Manch. 1965; Cert. Av Med. MoD (Air) & Civil; BSc (Physiol.) Manch. 1962; FRCP Lond. 1982, M 1968; Aviat. Auth. 1979; BA Open 1988. Cons. Neurol. N. Manch. Gen. Hosp.; Lect. Med. Univ. Manch. Specialty: Neurol. Socs: Assn. Brit. Neurols. & N. Eng. Neurol. Assn.

YUILL, Gordon McLellan Flat 2, Tall Trees, Mersey Road, West Didsbury, Manchester M20 2PE Tel: 0161 718 1949 — MB ChB Manch. 1994; BSc (Hons.) Manch. 1991. Specialist Regist. Anaesth., N. W. Rotat. Specialty: Anaesth. Socs: MRCAnaesth.; Assn. Anaesth. Prev: SHO (Anaesth.) Stepping Hill Hosp.; SHO (Anaesth.) Roy. Oldham Hosp.

YUILL, Robert Alexander Border Medical Ltd., 10 Hunters Walk, Canal Street, Chester CH1 4EB — MRCS Eng. LRCP Lond. 1970. Med. Examr. to Civil Aviat. Auth.

YUILLE, Frances Anne Pascoe Western General Hospital, Crème Road, Edinburgh EH4 2XU Tel: 0131 537 1000; Poldrait, Preston Rd, Linlithgow EH49 6QL Tel: 01506 842124 — MB BS Lond. 1987; MRCP (UK) 1990; FRCR 1994. Cons. in Clin. Oncol. Western Gen. Hosp. Eninburgh. Specialty: Oncol.

YUILLE, Pamela Mary Bridgnorth Medical Practices, Northgate House, 7 High Street, Bridgnorth WV16 4BU Tel: 01746 767121 Fax: 01746 765433; Underton Cottage, Underton, Bridgnorth WV16 6TY — MB BS Lond. 1975; MRCP (UK) 1978; DRCOG 1980; MRCGP 1982.

YUILLE, Tom Dalling Glan Clwyd Hospital, Bodelwyddan, Rhyl LL18 JUJ Tel: 01745 334225 Fax: 01745 534194 Email: drtom.yuille@cd-tr.wales.nhs.uk — MB BS Lond. 1969 (Roy. Free) MRCP (U.K.) 1972. Cons. Paediat. Conwy & Denbighsh. NHS Trust. Specialty: Paediat.

YUKSEL, Bulend Barnet and Chase Farm Hospital NHS Trust, The Ridgeway, Enfield EN2 8JL Tel: 020 8366 6600 Fax: 020 8967 5903; 40 Leaside Avenue, Muswell Hill, London N10 3BU Tel: 020 8444 7276 — Tip Doktoru Istanbul 1980; MD Istanbul 1984; DCH RCP Lond. 1990; MRCPI 1994; FRCPI 1997; FRCPCH 1997. Cons. (Paediat. Neonat.) Barnet & Chase Farm Hosp. Enfield; Hon. Teach. Univ. Coll. Lond. Hosps. 1996-; Assoc. Prof. Univ. Istanbul 1993. Specialty: Paediat. Socs: Eur. Respirat. Soc. (Sec., Neonat. & Paediat. Intens. Care Grp.); Amer. Thoracic Soc.; Neonat. Soc. Prev: Clin. Research Fell. & Hon. Sen. Regist. King's Coll. Hosp. Lond.; Specialist (Paediat.) Univ. Istanbul 1984.

YULE, Adrian John Hunters Chase, Rockbourne Road, Coombe Bissett, Salisbury SP5 4LP — MB BCh Wales 1989. SHO (Paediat.) Winchester. Prev: SHO (Ophth.) Cardiff.

YULE, Alexander Graeme St Julians Medical Centre, 13A Stafford Road, Newport NP19 7DQ Tel: 01633 251304 Fax: 01633 221977; 12 Llangorse Drive, Rogerstone, Newport NP10 9HJ — MB BCh Wales 1988. GP Princip.; Clin. Asst. Drugs Project in Newport; Med. Off. Cross IGMS Rugby Club.

YULE, Constance Margaret (retired) 8 Ash Tree Grove, Bolton Le Sands, Carnforth LA5 8BD Tel: 01524 822070 — MB ChB Aberd. 1949.

YULE, Diana Pratt (retired) 3 Abbey Farm, St Bees CA27 0DY Tel: 01946 823155 — MB ChB (Distinc.) St. And. 1945; DObst RCOG 1946. Prev: Assoc. Specialist W. Cumbld. Hosp.

YULE, George William Golder (retired) Orchard Cottage, Little Longstone, Bakewell DE45 1NN Tel: 01629 640414 — (Manch.) MRCS Eng. LRCP Lond. 1953; DObst RCOG 1956; AFOM RCP Lond. 1983. Works Med. Advis. & Appt. Doctor (Lead Regulat.) H.J. Enthoven's Lead Smelter Darley Dale. Prev: Clin. Asst. (Orthop.) Devonsh. Roy. Hosp. Buxton.

YULE, Ian Golder (retired) 14 Malthouse Court, Thornham, Hunstanton PE36 6NW — MB ChB Manch. 1954; DCH Eng. 1960; DPH 1962; FFCM 1973. Prev: Dist. Med. Off. & Dir. Serv. Plann. Aylesbury Vale HA.

YULE, Mr James Herbert Burton (retired) 216 Newton Drive, Blackpool FY3 8JE Tel: 01253 32880 — BM BCh Oxf. 1947 (Guy's) MCh Oxf. 1961, MA BM BCh 1947; FRCS Eng. 1954. Prev: Cons. Surg. Blackpool & Fylde Hosp. Gp.

YULE, Joan Matthewson 17 Mellerstain Road, Kirkcaldy KY2 6UB — MB ChB Aberd. 1995. Specialty: Gen. Pract.

YULE, John Charles Rutherford House, Langley Park, Durham DH7 9XD Tel: 0191 373 1386 Fax: 0191 373 4288 — MB BS Newc. 1970.

YULE, Mr Robert (retired) 4 Copperfield Court, New Street, Altrincham WA14 2QF Tel: 0161 928 5878/01666 510353 — MB ChB Ed. 1949; FRCS Ed. 1956; FRCOG 1974, M 1957. Prev: Cons. Cytopath. Christie Hosp. & Holt Radium Inst. Manch.

YULE, Robert Martin 14 Station Road, Hest Bank, Lancaster LA2 6HP — MB ChB Dundee 1975.

YULE, Steven Murray Eisai Ltd., 3 Shortlands, London W6 8EE; Saffron House, Saffron House, Old Stowmarket Road, Woolpit, Bury St Edmunds IP30 9QS Email: richard.west25@btinternet.com — MB ChB Dundee 1986; BMSc Dund 1983; MRCP (UK) 1989; PhD Newc. 1996. Med. Adviser, Oncol. Specialty: Oncol.; Haematology; Paediat.

YULE, Steven Robert — MB ChB Aberd. 1989; MRCP (UK) 1992; FRCR 1996. Cons. Radiologist, Aberd. Roy. Infirm. Specialty: Radiol. Prev: Regist. (Radiol.) HA Manch.; SHO (Med.) Aberd.

YULE, Susan Frances The Lofts, 24 Ash Lane, Collingtree, Northampton NN4 0ND — MB ChB Leeds 1998.

YULE-SMITH, Annabel Louise Church Street Surgery, Church Street, Hibaldstow, Brigg DN20 9ED Tel: 01652 650580; West Farm, Hunts Lane, Hibaldstow, Brigg DN20 9EH — BM BS Nottm. 1987. Socs: BMA.

YULL, Derek Neil 1 Nightingale Road, Rickmansworth WD3 7DE — MB BS Lond. 1994.

YUNAS, Sohail 2-D Mossfield Road, Birmingham B14 7JB — MB ChB Liverp. 1994.

YUNG, Bernard Man-Chak Basildon & Thurrock Hospital, Department of Respiratory Medicine, Nether Mayne, Basildon SS16 5NL — MB BCh Wales 1988; MRCP (UK) 1991; MD London 2001. Cons. Phys., Basildon Hosp. (Gen. & Resp. Med.). Specialty: Respirat. Med.; Gen. Med. Socs: Brit. Thorac. Soc. Prev: Specialist Regist. (Gen. & Respirat. Med.) Barnet Gen. Hosp.; Clin. Tutor & Research Fell. (Respirat. Med.) Roy. Brompton Hosp. & Nat. Inst. Heart & Lung Dis. Lond.; Clin. Research Fell. (Cystic Fibrosis) Sect. Respirat. Med. Univ. Wales Coll. Lond.

YUNG, Mr Man Wah The Ipswich Hospital, Ear, Nose & Throat Department, Heath Road Wing, Ipswich IP4 5PD Tel: 01473 712233 — MB BS Hong Kong 1978; DLO RCS Eng. 1980; FRCS Ed. 1982; PhD Liverp. 1987. Cons. Otorhinolaryng. Ipswich Hosp. NHS Trust, Ipswich. Specialty: Otorhinolaryngol. Socs: Politzer Soc.; Euro. Acad. In Otol. & Neuro-Otol. Prev: Lect. (Otorhinolaryng.) Univ. Liverp. 1986-1987; Sen. Regist. (ENT Surg.) Roy. Liverp. Hosp.

YUNG, Sui Yin Ruth c/o Mr. S. Tang, 56 Eighth Avenue, Newcastle upon Tyne NE6 5YB — MB BS Newc. 1985.

YUSAF, Baber Stowhealth, Violet Hill House, Violet Hill Road, Stowmarket IP14 1NL Tel: 01449 776000 Fax: 01449 776005 — MB BS Lond. 1982 (The Lond. Hosp.) BSc Lond. 1979; DRCOG 1988. GP Stowmarket.

YUSOF, Alvin Idrishah Rossdale CMHT Resource Centre, 12 Haughburn Road, Pollok, Glasgow G53 6AB; Flat G, 49 Bellshaugh Gardens, Kelvinside, Glasgow G12 0SA — MB ChB Glas. 1994. Rossdale CMHT Resource Centre, Glasgow. Specialty: Gen. Psychiat. Socs: BMA. Prev: SHO Rotat. (Psychiat.) Woodilee Hosp. N. Glas. Train. Scheme.

YUSOFF, Farhanah Crosshouse Hospital, 41 Simpson Street, Kilmarnock KA2 0BE Tel: 01563 21133 — MB ChB Glas. 1993.

YUSUF, Farah Yasmin 228 Killinghall Road, Bradford BD3 7JL — MB ChB Leeds 1987; MRCGP 1992. Specialty: Gen. Pract. Prev: Trainee GP Manch.

YUSUF, Imtiaz Ahmed Maybury Surgery, Alpha Road, Maybury, Woking GU22 8HF Tel: 01483 728757 Fax: 01483 729169; Plymlea, Triggs Lane, Woking GU22 0EH — MB BS Lond. 1984 (Char. Cross) D.Occ.Med. RCP Lond. 1995; AFOM RCP 1997. Occupat. Health Phys. Brit. Airport Auth. Heathrow; GP. Specialty: Occupat. Health. Socs: Soc. Occupat. Med. Prev: Med. Advisor (Occupat. Med.) Roy. Surrey Co. Hosp.; Ho. Surg. Hertford Co. Hosp.; Ho. Phys. Char. Cross Hosp. Lond.

YUSUF, Mr Mohammed Ormskirk & District General Hospital, Wigan Road, Ormskirk L39 2AZ — MB BS Lucknow 1960 (G.S.V.M. Med. Coll. Kanpur) MS (Orthop.) Lucknow 1963; FRCS Ed. 1976. Prev: JHMO Promenade Hosp. Southport; SHO Orthop. & Accid. Dept. N. Staffs. Roy. Infirm. Stoke-on-Trent; SHO Orthop. & Genito-Urin. Unit Wrightington Hosp. Wigan.

YUSUF, Muhammad Najib Richmond Community Healthcare, Hamlet, Kew Foot Road, Richmond TW9 2TE Tel: 020 8940 3331 Fax: 020 8940 2490; 30 Stewart Close, Hampton TW12 3XJ Tel: 020 8941 6059 Fax: 020 8941 6059 — MB BS Sri Lanka 1978; LRCP LRCS Ed. LRCPS Glas. 1985. Assoc. Specialist (Community Paediat.) St Geo. Healthcare NHS Trust. Specialty: Community Child Health. Socs: Roy. Coll. Paediat. & Child Health; MRCPCH. Prev: Sen. Staff Community Paediat. Richmond, Twicknham & Roehampton Healthcare Trust; SCMO Greenwich Healthcare NHS Trust.

YUSUF, Mrs Saadat Ahmed Junaid 60 Kewstoke Road, Willenhall WV12 5DL Tel: 01922 400838 Fax: 01922 445106 — MB BS Punjab 1965 (Fatima Jinnah Med. Coll. Lahore) Specialty: Anaesth.

YUSUF, Sarah Flat 7, Westfield Hall, Hagley Road, Birmingham B16 9LG — MB BS Lond. 1992 (St Geo.) Specialist Regist. (Radiol.). Specialty: Radiol.

YUSUF, Mr Syed Waquar Royal Sussex County Hospital, Eastern Road, Brighton BN2 5BE — MB BS Karachi 1987; FRCS Eng. 1991. Specialty: Gen. Surg. Socs: Assoc. Fell. Amer. Coll. Angiol.; Internat. Soc. Endovasc. Surg.

ZABETAKI, Eleni 46 Fairfield Crescent, Edgware HA8 9AH — Ptychio Iatrikes Patras 1988.

ZABIHI, Mr Tahmoures Department Orthopaedics, South Cleveland Hospital & Middlesbrough General Hosp., Middlesbrough Tel: 01642 850850 Ext: 5914; 5 Welburn Grove, Ormesby, Middlesbrough TS7 9BN Tel: 01642 325937 — MD Tehran 1968; MS (Orthop.), MS (Gen. Surg.) Tehran 1968, MD 1955. Staff Grade Surg. S. Cleveland Hosp. Middlesbrough Gen. Hosp.; Assoc. Specialist S.T.H.A. MiddlesBoro. Gen. Hosp. Specialty: Gen. Surg. Socs: Brit. Orthopaedic Assn.

ZACHARIA, Ajit Yhomas 16 Chedworth Road, Nettleham Park, Lincoln LN2 4SL — MB BS Kerala 1983.

ZACHARIAH, Jolly Central Milton Keynes Medical, 1 North Sixth Street, Saxon Gate West, Milton Keynes MK9 2NR Tel: 01908 605775 Fax: 01908 676752; 16 Haltonchesters, Bancroft, Milton Keynes MK13 0PF — MB BS Mysore 1977 (J.J.M. Med. Coll.) MRCS Eng. LRCP Lond. 1981.

ZACHARIAH, Mr Samuel Raymond Gubbins Lane Surgery, 89 Gubbins Lane, Harold Wood, Romford RM3 0DR Tel: 01708 346666 Fax: 01708 381300; 48 Chelmsford Road, Shenfield, Brentwood CM15 8RJ — MB BS Calcutta 1971; FRCS Eng. 1979.

ZACHARIAH, Shanti Elizabeth 17 Westrick Walk, Wrenside, Prestwood, Great Missenden HP16 0RZ — MB BS Lond. 1968; MRCS Eng. LRCP Lond. 1968; DA Eng. 1975; FFA RCS Eng. 1981. Assoc. Specialist (Anaesth.) Wycombe Gen. Hosp. Bucks. Specialty: Anaesth.

ZACHARIAS, John Trent View Medical Practice, 45 Trent View, Keadby, Scunthorpe DN17 3DR Tel: 01724 782209 Fax: 01724 784472; 7 The Dell, Silica Lodge, Scunthorpe DN17 2XB Tel: 01724 850120 Fax: 01724 850120 — MB BS Bangalore 1967. Prev: SHO (O & G) Fulford Matern. Hosp. York; SHO (Gen. Surg.) & SHO (Gyn.) W. Cumbld. Hosp. Whitehaven.

ZACHARIAS, Peter Lindsay 88 Rodney Street, Liverpool L1 9AR Tel: 07831 886535 — MB ChB Liverp. 1971; MA Cantab. 1970; DIH 1979; MFOM 1982. Independent Occupational Therapist. Specialty: Occupat. Health.

ZACHARY, Anne Rosemary Portman Clinic, 8 Fitzjohn's Avenue, London NW3 5NA Tel: 020 7794 8262 Fax: 020 7447 3748; 13 West Park Road, Kew Gardens, Richmond TW9 4DB Tel: 020 8876 7531 — MB BS Lond. 1975 (Roy. Free) MRCS Eng. LRCP Lond. 1975; DRCOG 1977; MRCPsych 1982; FRCPsych 1998. Cons. Psych. (Psychother.) Portman Clinic Lond. Specialty: Psychother. Socs: Assoc. Mem. Brit. Psychoanalyt. Soc. Prev: Sen. Regist. (Psychother.) Cassel Hosp. Lond.; Regist. (Psychiat.) Roy. Free Hosp. Lond.; Locum Cons. Psychother. Maudsley Hosp. Lond.

ZACHARY, John Bransby Barnsley District General Hospital, Gawber Road, Barnsley S75 2EP Tel: 01226 730000 — BM BCh Oxf. 1973 (Oxf. & Lond. Hosp.) MRCS Eng. LRCP Lond. 1972; BA Oxf. 1967, MA 1973; DObst RCOG 1975; DMRD Eng. 1977; FRCR 1980. Cons. Radiol. Dist. Gen. Hosp. Barnsley. Specialty: Radiol.

ZACHARY JENNINGS, Caroline Michelle 33 Trewince Road, London SW20 8RD — MB BS Lond. 1994.

ZACK, Philip 49 Selby Road, Carshalton SM5 1LE — MB BS Lond. 1993.

ZADEH, Mr Hamid G West Middlesex University Hospital, Twickenham Road, Isleworth TW7 6AF Email: zadeh@zadeh.co.uk — MB BS Lond. 1987 (Guy's) FRCS Eng. 1991; FRCS (Orth) 1997. Cons. Orthop. Surg., W. Middlx. Univ. Hosp. Specialty: Orthop. Socs: Assoc. Mem. BOA; RCS (Eng.). Prev: Specialist Regist. Roy. Nat. Orthop. Hosp. Trust Rotat.

ZADIK, Elena (retired) 131 The Avenue, Leigh WN7 1HR Tel: 01942 673488 — MB ChB Sheff. 1943. Prev: Clin. Asst. (Anaesth.) Wigan & Bolton Health Dists.

ZADIK, Paul Michael 8 Spout Copse, Sheffield S6 6FB — MB BCh Oxf. 1974; MSc (Med. Microbiol.) Lond. 1981; MRCPath 1982. Cons. Microbiol. Pub. Health Laborat. N. Gen. Hosp. Sheff. Specialty: Med. Microbiol.

ZADIK, Sarah Anne Selborne Road Medical Centre, 1 Selborne Road, Sheffield S10 5ND — MB ChB Ed. 1977; BSc (Med. Sci.) Ed. 1974; DCH RCPS Glas. 1979; MRCP (UK) 1981; MRCGP 1987. GP Princip. Sheff. Health.

ZADOO, Kishori Lyndhurst Drive Surgery, 53 Lundhurst Drive, Leyton, London E10 6JB Tel: 020 8539 1663 Fax: 020 8556 1977 — MB BS Jammu & Kashmir 1970; FRCOG London.

ZADOROZNY, Vanda Lorraine 15 Protea Gardens, Titchfield, Fareham PO14 4TJ — MB BS Lond. 1991 (St Bart.) BSc Lond. 1988. Specialty: Gen. Pract.

ZAFAR, Afia 41 Greenburn Park, Lisburn BT27 4LS — MB BS Karachi 1982.

ZAFAR, Muhammad Hanif 9 Lincoln Avenue, London SW19 5JT — Vrach Kuban Med. Inst. 1985.

ZAFAR, Noreen 19 St David's Close, Worksop S81 0RP — MB BS Punjab 1990; MRCOG 1995.

ZAFAR, Syed Ali The Surgery, 192 Charles Road, Small Heath, Birmingham B10 9AB Tel: 0121 772 0398 Fax: 0121 772 4268 — MB BS Bihar 1967 (Darbhanga Med. Sch., Bihar) MRCP (UK) 1976. Hosp. Pract. Diabetic Clin. Birm. Specialty: Diabetes.

ZAFAR, Syed Sibte 25 Oswald Street, Rochdale OL16 2LA — MB BS Pakistan 1984.

ZAFAR, Tahira 30 City Way, Rochester ME1 2AB Tel: 01634 818449; 332A, Lane 4, Peshawar Road, Rawalpindi, Pakistan Tel: 00 92 51 474765 Email: azmalik@hotmail.com — MB BS Punjab 1978 (King Edward Med. Coll. Pakistan) MRCPath 1994. Cons. Haemat. Armed Forces Inst. Path. Rawalpindi, Pakistan. Specialty: Haematology.

ZAFAR, Mr Waheed Uz Macclesfield District General Hospital, Victoria Road, Macclesfield SK10 3BL Tel: 01625 421000 Fax: 01625 663064; 16 Brampton Avenue, Macclesfield SK10 3DY Tel: 01625 265727 Email: waheedzafar@hotmail.com — MB BS Punjab 1983; BSc Islamia 1980; FRCSI 1990. Staff Urol. Macclesfield Dist. Hosp. & Vict. Roy. Hosp. E. Chesh. NHS Trust. Specialty: Urol. Special Interest: Erectile Dysfunction. Socs: Brit. Assn. Urol. Surgs. Prev: Regist. (Urol.) Portsmouth Hosps. NHS Trust; SHO (Urol.) E. Yorks. NHS Trust; SHO (Urol.) Macclesfield Dist. Gen. Hosp.

ZAFER, Ibtsam Mohamed Zaki 9 Horsley Close, Epsom KT19 8HB Tel: 013727 21233 — MB BCh Cairo 1963; DA 1971. Anaesth. E. Surrey & Mid. Surrey HA. Socs: Assn. Anaesth. Gt. Brit. & Irel.

ZAFFAR, Mahmood Ahmad (retired) 7 Lavender Sweep, London SW11 1DY — MB BS Punjab 1954 (King Edwd. Med. Coll.) Locum GP. Prev: SHO Bristol Roy. Infirm.

ZAFFAR, Muzaffar 7 Lavender Sweep, London SW11 1DY Tel: 020 7223 7475 — MB BS Lond. 1996 (Char. Cross & Westm.) BSc (Hons.) Lond. 1993. SHO (GP Train. Scheme) Mayday Univ. Hosp. Lond. Socs: BMA. Prev: Hse. Surg. St. Peter's Hosp. Chertsey; Hse. Phys. Chelsea & Westminster Hosp. Lond.

ZAHANGIR, Mohammed Monkland District General Hospital, Monkscourt Avenue, Airdrie ML6 0JS Tel: 01236 787787 Fax: 01236 760015; 6 North Avenue, Carluke ML8 5TR Tel: 01555 751034 — MB BS Dacca 1966 (S.S. Med. Coll.) DPM Eng. 1974; MRCPsych 1975. Cons. Psychiat. Lanarksh. Health Bd. Specialty: Gen. Psychiat.

ZAHEER, Pervez Cinderford Health Centre, 19 Abbots Road, Cinderford GL14 3BN Tel: 01594 822097 — MB BS Karachi 1964. GP Cinderford, Glos.

ZAHEER, Mr Syed Asghar The Briery, 3 Orchard Place, Rectory Rd, Wokingham RG40 1DW Tel: 0118 979 2902 — MB BS Lucknow 1954; BSc Allahabad 1949; FRCS Ed. 1961; FRCS Eng. 1962. Chief Cons. Surg. & Urol. Igbinedion Hosp. & Med. Research Centre Okada, Nigeria. Specialty: Gen. Surg. Socs: Fell. Internat. Coll. Angiol. (NY) 1967; Fell. Assn. Surgs.; Sen. Mem. Brit. Assn. Urol. Surgs. Prev: Cons. Surg. E. Antrim Gp. Hosps.; Cons. Surg. Merthyr & Aberdare Gp. Hosps.; Regist. (Surg.) SE Kent Gp. Hosps. & Withington Hosp. Manch.

ZAHER, Samir Abd El-Azim Flat 2/01, 91 Greenock Road, Paisley PA3 2LF Tel: 0141 840 1757 — MB BCh Cairo 1965.

ZAHIR, Mr Abol Ghassem 152 Harley Street, London W1G 7LH Tel: 020 7935 2477 Fax: 020 7224 2574; 72 Onslow Gardens, Muswell Hill, London N10 3JX Fax: 020 8883 6027 — MB BS Lond. 1964 (Lond. Hosp.) MRCS Eng. LRCP Lond. 1962; FRCS Eng. 1967; Specialist Accredit (Orthop.) RCS Eng. 1973. Cons. Orthop. Surg. Whipps Cross (Forest Healthcare). Specialty: Orthop. Socs: Fell. Roy. Soc. Med. & BOA. Prev: Cons. Orthop. Tehran Clinic, Iran; Sen. Regist. (Orthop.) Lond. Hosp.

ZAHIR, Keyvan Enfield & Haringey Health Agency, Alexander Place, Lower Park Road, New Southgate, London N11 1ST Tel: 020 8361 7272 Fax: 020 8361 6126; 72 Onslow Gardens, Muswell Hill, London N10 3JX Tel: 020 8365 2430 Fax: 020 8883 6027 — MD Tehran 1967; DPH Lond. 1970; FFCM 1993, M 1985. Dir. (Pub. Health Med.) Enfield & Haringey Health Agency. Specialty: Pub. Health Med. Prev: Dir. Pub. Health New River HA; Specialist (Community Med.) Haringey HA; Sen. Regist. NW Thames RHA.

ZAHIR, Maryam Edgware Community Hospital, Burnt Oak Broadway, Edgware, Edgware HA8 0AD Tel: 020 8732 6566 Fax: 020 8732 6474; 58 Blake Road, London N11 2AH Tel: 020 8368 2990 — MB BS Lond. 1984 (Roy. Lond.) BSc McGill 1979; DCH RCP Lond. 1987; MRCP Paediat. (UK) 1989. Cons. Community Paediat. Barnet Healthcare NHS Trust. Specialty: Paediat. Socs: Roy. Coll. Paediat. & Child Health; Eur. Assn. Childh. Dis. Prev: Lect. (Community Paediat.) Camberwell HA; Regist. (Paediat.) St. Mary's Hosp. Lond.; SHO (Neonat.) Hammersmith Hosp. Lond.

ZAIB, Sajid Ali 3 Whitelands Way, High Wycombe HP12 3EH — MB BS Lond. 1994.

ZAIDI, Mr Abul Abbas District General Hospital, Moorgate Road, Rotherham S60 2UD Tel: 01709 304420/01709 304775 — MB BS Sind 1968 (Liaquat Med. Coll. Hyderabad) DO RCPSI 1971; FRCS Glas. 1978; FCOphth 1989. Cons. (Ophth. Surg.) Dist. Gen. Hosp. Rotherham. Specialty: Ophth. Prev: SHO (Ophth.) Maelor Gen. Hosp. Wrexham; Regist. (Ophth.) Chester Roy. Infirm.; Sen. Regist. Roy. Eye Hosp. Manch.

ZAIDI, Mr Ahsan Zafar c/o Mr. S.M. Rasheed, 13 Dalmeny Crescent, Hounslow TW3 2NT Tel: 020 8847 4210 — MB BS Aligarh 1972; FRCS Eng. 1979; LRCP LRCS Ed. LRCPS Glas. 1980. Prev: Gen. Surg. & Chief Surg. Civil Hosp. Khamees Mushayt Saudi Arabia; Regist. (Gen. Surg.) N. Middlx., Lond. & Roy. Lancs. Infirm.

ZAIDI, Amir Masood 3 The Forge Mews, 501-503 Wilmslow Road, Withington, Manchester M20 4AW — MB ChB Manch. 1989.

ZAIDI, Farhan Husain 28 Bedford Road, South Woodford, London E18 2AQ — MB BS (Hons.) Lond. 1994; FRCS (Gen) Eng. 1997; MRCS (Ophth) Ed. 2001; MRCOPhth 2002. Research Fell. Imperial Coll. Sci., Technol. & Med., The Hammersmith, St Mary's & The West. Eye Hosp. Lond. Socs: Middlx. Hosp. Med. Soc. Prev: SHO (Ent) Roy. Nat. Throat, Nose And Ear Hosp.; SHO (Surg.) UCL Hosps. Lond.; Ho. Phys. N. Middlx. Hosp. Lond.

ZAIDI, Iram — MB BS Lond. 1994.

ZAIDI, Mone Biochemical Medicine, St George's Hospital Medical School, Tooting, London SW17 0RE Tel: 020 8682 3380 Fax: 020 8784 2946; 33 Oakwood Park Road, Southgate, London N14 6QT Tel: 020 8886 8867 — MB BS Lucknow 1984; MRCPath 1990; PhD Lond. 1987, MD 1991; FRCPI 1994, M 1993. Sen. Lect. & Cons. St. Geo. Hosp. Med. Sch. Lond.; Research Worker Physiol. Laborat. Univ. Camb. Specialty: Gen. Med. Socs: Amer. Soc. Bone & Mineral Research & Soc. Endocrinol. UK. Prev: Lect., Sen. Regist., Regist. & Research Schol. Endrocrine Unit Dept. Chem. Path. Roy. Postgrad. Med. Sch. Lond.

ZAIDI, Nerjis Huma 10 Halvis Grove, Manchester M16 0DX — MB ChB Manch. 1994.

ZAIDI, Sarwat Eastwood Surgery, 348 Rayleigh Road, Eastwood, Leigh-on-Sea SS9 5PU Tel: 01702 525289 Fax: 01702 520134; 91 Eastwood Road, Leigh-on-Sea SS9 3AH Tel: 01702 476543 — MB BS Punjab 1962; DRCOG 1976; DFFP 1996. Specialty: Gen. Med.; Family Plann. & Reproduc. Health; Obst. & Gyn.

ZAIDI, Syed Ali Raza 19 Arbour Way, Hornchurch RM12 5BS — MB BS Karachi 1968; FFA RCSI 1975.

ZAIDI, Syed Babar Abbas Head of Healthcare Services, HM Prison, Barrack Square, Gloucester GL1 2JN Tel: 01452 529551 Fax: 01452 310302 — MB BS Dacca 1970; DPM Eng. 1982; Dip. Addic. Behaviour Lond. 1992. Head Health Care Servs. HM Prison Gloucester. Specialty: Alcohol & Substance Misuse. Socs: Med. Protec. Soc. Prev: Clin. Asst. (Psychiat.) E. Dyfed HA.

ZAIDI, Mr Syed Husain Afzal Morriston Hospital, Swansea SA6 6NL — MB BChir Camb. 1990 (Camb. & Guy's Hosp.) MA (Cantab) 1991; FRCS Eng. 1994. Cons. (Cardiothoracic Surg.) Morriston Cardiac Centre. Specialty: Cardiothoracic Surg. Socs: Soc. Cardiothoracic Surg. GB & Irel. Prev: SpR All Wales Rotat. in Cardiothoracic Surg.; Transpl. Research Fell. Papworth Hosp.; Regist. Cardiothoracic St. Bart.'s Hosp. Lond.

ZAIDI, Syed Husain Jamal Department of Obstetrics & Gynaecology, Conquest Hospital, The Ridge, St Leonards-on-Sea TN37 7RD Tel: 01424 755255 Fax: 01424 758086 Email: jamal.zaida@esht.nhs.uk — MB BS Lond. 1987 (King's Coll. Hosp.) MRCOG 1992; MD Lond. 2000; FRCS (Cardiothoracic) 2002. Cons. (O & G) Conquest Hosp., The Ridge, E. Sussex & BUPA Hosp. Hastings. Specialty: Obst. & Gyn. Special Interest: Endoscopic Surgery; Reproductive Medicine; Ultrasound. Socs: Brit. Fertil. Soc.; Internat. Soc. Ultrasound in Obst. & Gyn.; Amer. Soc. for Reproductive Med. Prev: Sen. Regist. (O & G) John Radcliffe Hosp. Oxf.; Regist. (Clin. Research) King's Coll. Hosp. & Lond. Wom. Clinic. Harley St.; Regist. (O & G) King's Coll. Hosp. Lond.

ZAIDI, Syed Ishrat Ali St Nicholas Health Centre, Canterbury Way, Stevenage SG1 4LH Tel: 01438 357411; 54 Dowlands, Stevenage SG2 7BH — MB BS Karachi 1962 (Dow Med. Coll.) DA Eng. 1973. Prev: Med. Off. H.H. Agha Khan Hosp. Mombasa, Kenya; Regist. (Anaesth.) Stafford Gen. Infirm.; SHO (Anaesth.) Roy. Hosp. Wolverhampton.

ZAIDI, Syed Masoodul Hasan Kilmarnock Infirmary, Kilmarnock; Accident & Emergency, Crosshouse Hospital, Kilmarnock KA2 0BE Tel: 01563 521133 — MB BS Karachi 1961. Cons. A & E CrossHo. Hosp. Kilmarnock. Specialty: Accid. & Emerg. Socs: BMA; BAEM.

ZAIDI, Syed Mohammad Nawab 87 Farnham Road, Guildford GU2 7PF Tel: 01483 68715 — MB BS Karachi 1968 (Dow Med. Coll.) DPM Eng. 1971; MRCPsych 1972; DPM Eng. 1982. Cons. Psychiat. Brookwood Hosp. Knaphill. Specialty: Gen. Psychiat.

ZAIDI, Syed Mohammad Zafar 118 Albert Road, Jarrow NE32 3AG Tel: 0191 489 7002 Fax: 0191 428 5640 — MB BS Karachi 1983. GP Jarrow, Tyne & Wear.

ZAIDI, Syed Nayyar Abbas 10 Halvis Grove, Manchester M16 0DX — MB ChB Manch. 1990.

ZAIDI, Syeda Talat Abbas Kent Elms Health Centre, Rayleigh Road, Leigh-on-Sea SS9 5UU Tel: 01702 421888 Fax: 01702 421818; 335 Eastwood Road N., Leigh-on-Sea SS9 4LT Tel: 01702 529817 — MRCS Eng. LRCP Lond. 1978; MB BS 1973.

ZAIDI, Zafar Husain 28 Bedford Road, South Woodford, London E18 2AQ Tel: 020 8989 3090 — MB BS Lucknow 1955 (King Geo. Med. Coll.) DCH Eng. 1960; FRCP Ed. 1980, M 1965; FRCPCH 1994. Cons. (Paediatr.) King Geo. Hosp. Ilford & Oldchurch Hosp. Romford. Specialty: Paediat. Socs: Ilford Med. Soc. (102nd Past Pres.). Prev: Prof. & Head, Dept. Paediat. Univ. Aligarh, India.; Chief Resid. (Paediat.) Univ. Ottawa Gen. Hosp., Canada; Past Clin. Dir. (Paediat.) Barking & Havering Hosp. NHS Trust.

***ZAIN, Amir Azlan** 23 Tattershall Drive, Beeston, Nottingham NG9 2GP; 17 Templemead, Witham CM8 2DF — BM BS Nottm. 1997; BMedSci. (Hons.) Nottm. 1995. Specialty: Gen. Med.

ZAINUDDIN, Ani Amelia 44 Helmsley Road, Sandyford, Newcastle upon Tyne NE2 1DL Tel: 0191 261 8944 Fax: 0191 261 8944 — MB BS Newc. 1996. SHO Dept. O & G Directorate of Wom.'s Servs. Newc.-u-Tyne. Specialty: Obst. & Gyn. Socs: BMA; Med. Protec. Soc. Prev: Surg. Ho. Off. Med. Ho. Off. S. Tyneside Dist. Hosp. Tyne & Wear.

ZAINUDDIN, Idris Abdulkader Flat 21, Gatehill Court, 166 Notting Hill Gate, London W11 3QT Tel: 020 7229 6404 Fax: 020 7221 2691; Maimoon Manzil, 10 The Glebe, Worcester Park KT4 7PF Tel: 020 8335 4051 Fax: 020 8335 4152 — MB BS Punjab 1962; DOMS Vienna 1966. Specialty: Ophth.; Neonat. Socs: BMA. Prev: Clin. Asst. Roy. Eye Hosp. Lond.; SHO (Ophth.) Sunderland Eye Infirm. & Ophth. Hosp. Maidstone.

ZAJICEK, John Peter Department of Neurology, Derriford Hospital, Plymouth PL6 8DH — MB BS Lond. 1984; BA Camb. 1981; MRCP (UK) 1987; PhD Camb. 1993; FRCP 2000. Hon. Cons. Neurol. Derriford Hosp. Plymouth; Hon. Sen. Lect. Univ. of Plymouth; Reader in Neurol., Peninsula Med. Sch. Specialty: Neurol. Prev: Clin. Lect. Addenbrooke's Hosp. Camb.

ZAKANI, Regina Upton Road Surgery, 30 Upton Road, Watford WD18 0JS Tel: 01923 226266 Fax: 01923 222324 — State Exam Med Hamburg 1988. GP Princip. Upton Rd. Surg. Watford. Specialty: Gen. Pract.

ZAKARIA, Abul Kashem Mohd Upper Road Medical Centre, 50 Upper Road, London E13 0DH Tel: 020 8552 2129 Fax: 020 8471 4180 — MB BS Dacca 1969.

ZAKARIA, Faris Benjamin Peter St Peter's Hospital, Chertsey KT16 0PZ Tel: 01932 872000 — MB BS Lond. 1990. Cons. (Obst. & Gyn.) St Peter's Hosp. Chertsey. Specialty: Obst. & Gyn.

ZAKARIA, Ghulam Yusufzai Afghania House, 35 Marlings Park Avenue, Chislehurst BR7 6QN Tel: 020 8850 2779 — MB BS Karachi 1962; BSc Peshawar 1956; DCH RCPS Glas. 1968; MD Jalal-Abad 1975. Managing Sec. Afghania Educat. Trust. Socs: GP Research Gp.; BMA & BDA. Prev: Research Asst. Lennard Hosp. FarnBoro.; Clin. Asst. (Diabetol.) Greenwich Dist. Hosp.; Clin. Asst. (Diabetol.) W.hill Hosp Dartford.

ZAKARIA, Mohamed Yahia Withybush Hospital, Haverfordwest SA61 2PZ — MB BCh Cairo 1980.

ZAKARIA, Mohd Idzam 38 Southbank Road, Manchester M19 1PX — MB ChB Manch. 1998.

ZAKARIA, Nada Abdalla 11 Ruskin Court, 4 Champion Hill, London SE5 8AH Tel: 07881 824914 Fax: 020 7738 6960 Email: nadawho@hotmail.com — MB BS Khartoum, Sudan 1989; MRCP (UK) 1994. Research Regist. (SpR Gastroenterol./GIM) Inst. of Liver Studies, King's Coll. Hosp. Lond. Specialty: Gastroenterol.; Gen. Med. Socs: MRCP (UK); MDU. Prev: SpR Gastroenterol., Liver Unit, King's Coll. Hosp. Lond.; SpR Gastroenterol., Qu. Mary's Hosp. Roehampton; SpR Gastroenterol., Ashford Hosp. Middlx.

ZAKHOUR, Hani Arrowe Park Hospital, Upton, Wirral CH49 5PE — MD Prague 1973 (Charles Univ. Prague) MD Charles Univ. Prague 1973; MRCS Eng. LRCP Lond. 1979; FRCPath 1993, M 1982. Cons. Path. Arrowe Pk. Hosp. Wirral; Director of Training and Educational Standards - Royal Coll. Of Pathologists. Specialty: Histopath. Socs: Internat. Acad. Path.; Assn. Clin. Path.; Past Pres. NW Br. Assn. of Clin. Pathol. Prev: Director of Postgrad. Educat. Wirral Hosp. Trust; Sen. Regist. (Histopath.) North. Gen. Hosp. & Clin. Tutor (Morbid Anat.) Univ. Sheff.; Regist. (Histopath.) Wythenshawe Hosp. Manch.

ZAKI, Aida Said Stechford Health Centre, 393 Station Road, Stechford, Birmingham B33 8PL Tel: 0121 784 8101 Fax: 0121 785 0565 — MB BCh Alexandria 1970; Family Planning Certificate. GP. Prev: GP Since 1988; 1974-1978 Gyn. & Obstetric; 1978-1986 Anaesth.

ZAKI, Mr Graeme Anderson Queen Alexandra Hospital, Maxillofacial Unit, Cosham, Portsmouth PO6 3LY Tel: 023 9228 6466 Fax: 023 9228 6089 — MB BS Lond. 1983; BDS Lond. 1976; FDS RCS Eng. 1986; FRCS Ed. 1988. Cons. Oral & Maxillofacial Surg. Qu. Alexandra Hosp. Portsmouth. Specialty: Oral & Maxillofacial Surg. Socs: Fell. Brit. Assn. Oral & Maxillofacial Surg.; BMA. Prev: Sen. Regist. St. Geo. Hosp. Lond.

ZAKI, Irshad 19 Knightsbridge Crescent, Stirchley, Telford TF3 1BN — BM BS Nottm. 1987; BMedSci (Hons.) Nottm. 1985; MRCP (UK) 1990. Cons. (Dermat.) Solihull & Heartlands Hosp. Specialty: Dermat. Prev: Sen. Regist. (Dermat.) Nottm.

ZAKI, Mohammed Dilnasheen, Pyle Hill, Mayford, Woking GU22 0SR — MB BS Delhi 1969 (Maulana Azad Med. Coll.)

ZAKI, Mona Morad Ramzy Northern Residence, Singleton Hospital, Sketty, Swansea SA2 8QA — MB BCh Cairo 1988; MRCOG 1995.

ZAKI, Shereen 33 Cheam Road, Epsom KT17 1QX — MB BS Lond. 1991. SHO (Cardiol.) Cardiothoracic Centre Liverp. Prev: SHO (Gen. Med.) Joyce Green Hosp. Dartford Kent; SHO (A & E)

Newham Gen. Hosp. Lond.; Ho. Off. (Surg.) Roy. Cornw. Hosp. Treliske.

ZAKI AHMED, Syed Mohammad Malinslee Surgery, Church Road, Malinslee, Telford TF3 2JZ Tel: 01952 501234 Fax: 01952 594555; 19 Knightsbridge Crescent, Stirchley, Telford TF3 1BN — MB BS Osmania 1962 (Gandhi Med. Coll.) DPH Osmania 1967. Specialty: Accid. & Emerg. Socs: BMA & Overseas Doctors Assn.; Small Practs. Assn. Prev: Asst. Prof. Gandhi Med. Coll. Hyderabad, India; Asst. MOH Municip. Corpn. Hyderabad; Asst. Surg. Urban Family Plann. Clinic Hyderabad.

ZAKI-KHALIL, Ihab Ahmed Victoria Hospital, Whinney Heys Road, Blackpool FY3 8NR — MB ChB Cairo 1975; DRCOG 1986; MRCOG 1988. Regist. (O & G) Torbay Hosp. Torquay. Specialty: Obst. & Gyn. Prev: Regist. (O & G) Grimsby Dist. Gen. Hosp.

ZAKLAMA, Magued Sabet, Maj. RAMC (retired) Birch Hill Hospital, Rochdale OL12 9QB Tel: 01706 77777; Amon-Ra, 1 Broadhalgh Road, Bamford, Rochdale OL11 5NJ Tel: 01706 649985 Fax: 08700 547740 Email: mszak@mszak.demon.co.uk — MB BCh Cairo 1970; FRCOG 1992, M 1977. Cons. O & G Rochdale Dist. HA. Prev: Cons. O & G Brit. Milit. Hosp. Hannover, BFPO 33.

ZAKRZEWSKA, Joanna Maria Barts & the London NHS Trust, Oral Medicine, Dental Institute, Turner Street, London E1 2AD Tel: 020 7377 7053 Fax: 020 7377 7627 — MB BChir Camb. 1980; BDS Lond. 1972; FDS RCS Eng. 1980; MD Camb. 1990; FFD RCSI 1991. Sen. Lect. & Hon. Cons. Bart Lond. Dent. Inst. Socs: Fell. Roy. Soc. Med.; Brit. Soc. Oral Med.; Internat. Assn. Study of Pain. Prev: Cons. & Hon. Sen. Lect. (Oral Med.) Eastman Dent. Hosp. & Univ. Coll. Hosps. Camden & Islington NHS Trust; Cons. Camden & Islington Community NHS Trust; Hon. Cons. Nat. Hosp. Neurol. & Neurosurg. Lond.

ZAKRZEWSKI, Henryk John Pendleside Medical Practice, Clitheroe Health Centre, Railway View Road, Clitheroe BB7 2JG Tel: 01200 421888 Fax: 01200 421887 — MB ChB Manch. 1990 (Univ. Manch.) DRCOG 1993; DFFP 1993; MRCGP 1994. GP Princip. Pendleside Med. Pract., Clitheroe Lancs.; GP Trainer. Specialty: Gen. Pract. Socs: (Treas.) Blackburn & Dist. Med. & Dent. Soc. Prev: Asst. GP Pendleside Med. Pract. Clitheroe; Trainee GP Montague Health Centre Blackburn; Trainee GP/SHO Qu. Pk. Hosp. Blackburn VTS.

ZAKRZEWSKI, Kajetan Krzysztof Kasta Clinic, 9 Carlisle Road, Eastbourne BN21 4BT Tel: 0870 240 2370 Fax: 0870 240 2370 — Lekarz Warsaw 1974; Specialist Psychiatrist 1983, Institute of Psychiatry & Neurology Exam. Board Warsaw; MRCPsych 1987. Cons. Anaesth. Roy. Hallamshire Hosp. Specialty: Gen. Psychiat. Socs: BMA; Roy. Coll. Psychiatr. Prev: Cons. Psychiat. Leics. Ment. Health Servs. & Eastbourne Co. NHS Trust; Cons. Psychiat. & Alcoholism, Warsaw, Poland; Specialist Psychiat. Inst. Psychiat. Neurol. Warsaw.

ZAKY, Saroj 17 Doncaster Close, Coventry CV2 1HW — MB BS Rajasthan 1973.

ZALA, Navin Naran Marling Way Surgery, 117 Marling Way, Gravesend DA12 4RQ Tel: 01474 533201; 128 Elaine Avenue, Rochester ME2 2YP — MB BS Poona 1975 (BJ Med. Coll.) DObst 1980. Clin. Asst. (Paediat.) Gravesend & N. Kent Hosp.; Vis. Med. Off. Community Ment. & Handicap Unit Dartford & Gravesham HA. Prev: SHO (Gen. Med.) Gravesend & N. Kent Hosp.; Trainee GP Dartford VTS.

ZALIDIS, Sotirios The Surgery, 52B Well Street, London E9 7PX Tel: 020 8985 2050 Fax: 020 8985 5780; 140 Powerscroft Road, Clapton, London E5 0PR Tel: 020 8986 9479 — Ptychio Iatrikes Athens 1973; MRCP (UK) 1982. Specialty: Gen. Med.; Psychother. Socs: Soc. Psychosomatic Research; Balint Soc.

ZALIN, Anthony Maurice — MB BChir Oxf. 1969; MRCP Lond. 1971; MD Camb. 1976; FRCP 1983. Specialty: Gen. Med. Special Interest: Diabetes and Endocrinol. Prev: Cons. Phys. Dudley Gp. of Hosps. 1976-2002.

ZALIN, Mr Harold (retired) 13 Heathfield Close, Church Road, Potters Bar EN6 1SW Tel: 01707 651522 — MB ChB Liverp. 1937; DLO Eng. 1945; FRCS Ed. 1947. Prev: Cons. Surg. ENT Walton Hosp. Liverp.

ZAMAN, Ahmed Darwen Health Centre, Union Street, Darwen BB3 0DA Tel: 01254 778377 Fax: 01254 778372; 48 Richmond Park, Darwen BB3 0JX Tel: 01254 702319 — MB BS Dacca 1962; BSc Dacca 1955. GP Blackburn; Clin. Asst. (Psychiat.) & Clin. Asst. (Geriat.) Qu.'s Pk. Hosp. Blackburn; Trainer Family Plann. Assn. Socs: Fell. Inst. Psychiat. Prev: SHO (Med.) Maelor Gen. Hosp. Wrexham; Regist. (Infec. Dis. & Geriat.) Ladywell Hosp. Salford; SHO (Chest & Med.) Lodge Moor Hosp. Sheff.

ZAMAN, Anwar Ghaus 132A Barnsley Road, Hemsworth, Pontefract WF9 4PG Tel: 01426 241202 — BM BCh Oxf. 1986; MA Camb. 1987; MRCP (UK) 1989; FRCOphth 1991. Cons. Ophth. Surg., Qu.s Med. Centre Nottm. Specialty: Ophth. Prev: Vitreoretinal Fell. Moorfields Eye Hosp. Lond.; Vitreoretinal Fell. Manch. Roy. Eye Hosp.; Sen. Regist. Ophth., Qu.s Med. Centre.

ZAMAN, Ashrif Cheyenne 85 Vickers Road, Sheffield S5 6WA — MB ChB Sheff. 1995.

ZAMAN, Azfar Ghaus 132A Barnsley Road, Hemsworth, Pontefract WF9 4PG — MB ChB Leeds 1985; BSc Leeds 1982; MRCP (UK) 1988; MD Leeds 1995. Cons. Cardiol., Freeman Hosp., Newcastle-Upon-Tyne.

ZAMAN, Herbert Winthrop River Surgery, 110 London Road, River, Dover CT16 3AB; White Horses, Cliff Road, Kingsdown, Deal CT14 8AJ Tel: 01304 373397 — MB BS W. Indies 1967; ECFMG Cert 1976. Locum GP. Socs: Fell. Roy. Soc. Med. Prev: GP Princip.

ZAMAN, Khalid Holly House, Nunroyd, Heckmondwike WF16 9HB — BM BS Nottm. 1996.

ZAMAN, Maqsuda 15 Sylvandale Avenue, Manchester M19 2FB — MB ChB Liverp. 1992.

ZAMAN, Mohammed Justin Samuel Middlesex Hospital, Mortimer St., London W1T 3AA — MB BS Lond. 1997.

ZAMAN, Nasser Ali Derby Lane Medical Centre, 30 Derby Lane, Derby DE23 8UA Tel: 01332 773243 — MB ChB Manch. 1989.

ZAMAN, Neelofer Yasmin 132A Barnsley Road, Hemsworth, Pontefract WF9 4PG — MB ChB Leeds 1989; BSc (Hons. Path.) 1986; MRCP Ed. 1993. Specialty: Radiol.

ZAMAN, Qaisar HMP Strangeways, Southall Road, Manchester M60 9AH Tel: 0161 834 8626 — MB BS Peshawar, Pakistan 1972. GP HMP Strangeways Manch.

ZAMAN, Rashid Imperial College School of Medicine, Division of Neurosciences & Physiological Medicine, Paterson Centre, 20 South Wharf Road, London W2 1PD Email: r.zaman@ic.ac.uk; 265 Mill Road, Cambridge CB1 3DF Email: rash@peak88.freeserve.co.uk — MB BChir Camb. 1988; BSc (Hons.) St. And. 1980; LMSSA Lond. 1986; DGM RCP Lond. 1989; MRCGP 1991; MRCPsych 1996. Lect. & Hon. Specialist Regist. Div. of Neurosci.s & Physiol. Med. Imperial Coll. Univ. of Lond.; GP Camb.; Psychiat. Research Lond. Specialty: Gen. Psychiat.; Forens. Psychiat. Socs: BMA; Roy. Coll. Psychiatr.; Internat. Soc. Transcranial Stimulation. Prev: Regist. (Psychiat.) Char. Cross Hosp. Lond.; Research Regist. Leavsden Hosp. Herts.; Regist. & SHO (Psychiat.) Char. Cross Hosp. Lond.

ZAMAN, Saira Judith 17 Brentwood Avenue, West Jesmond, Newcastle upon Tyne NE2 3DQ — MB BS Newc. 1996.

ZAMAN, Salman Mohammad Radiology Department, Leighton Hosptial, Middlewich Road, Crewe CW1 4QJ Tel: 01270 612153 Fax: 01270 612156 Email: salman.zaman@virgin.net — MB BS Peshawar 1985 (Khyber Med. Coll. Peshawar) MRCP (UK) 1990; FRCR 1995. Cons. Radiol. Mid. Chesh. Hosps. Trust. Specialty: Radiol. Prev: Sen. Regist. & Regist. Sheff. Radiol. Train. Scheme; SHO Rotat. (Med.) Camb.; SHO Rotat. (Med.) Hull.

ZAMAN, Shamas 114 Spencer Street, Keighley BD21 2QB — MB ChB Leic. 1995.

ZAMAN, Sonya Rownak Green Acre, Brookhouse, Laughton, Sheffield S25 1YA — MB BS Lond. 1998.

ZAMAN, Syed Nuru Southampton General Hospital, Department of Medicine for Older People, Tremona Road, Southampton SO16 6YD Tel: 023 8079 4329 Email: Syed.Zaman@suht.swest.nhs.uk — MB BCh BAO NUI 1988 (Roy. Coll. Surgs. Irel.) Cons. Phys., Med. for Older People, Soton. Gen. Hosp. Specialty: Gen. Med.; Care of the Elderly. Socs: Brit. Geriat. Soc.; Brit. Soc. for Heart Failure; Arrhythmia Alliance. Prev: Sen. Regist. (Med & Geriat.) Wessex; Regist. (Med.) Broomfield Hosp. Chelmsford.

ZAMAN, Tahir Mahmood 596 Bromford Lane, Birmingham B8 2DS — MB ChB Manch. 1990; BSc (Hons.) Manch. 1987.

ZAMAN, Tariq Mahmood 162 Cherrywood Road, Bordesley Grove, Birmingham B9 4UN — MB ChB Dundee 1988.

ZAMAN, Zahur Department of Clinical Chemistry, University Hospitals Leuven, Catholic University of Leuven, Herestraat 49,

Leuven B-3000, Belgium Tel: 00 32 16 343390; 38 Milton Lawns, Chesham Bois, Amersham HP6 6BH Tel: 01494 726110 — MD Louvain 1985; PhD Soton. 1973, BSc (Hons.) Physiol. & Biochem. 1969. Cons. Chem. Path. Univ. Hosps. Leuven, Belgium; Reader Catholic Univ. Leuven, Belgium. Specialty: Chem. Path. Prev: Sen. Regist. (Chem Path.) Centr. Middlx. & St. Mary's Hosps. Lond.; Research Fell. Sc. Research Counc. Univ. Soton.; Sen. Research Fell. Dept. Med. Catholic Univ. Louvain, Belgium.

ZAMANTHANGI, Jadeng Mani Church Road Health Centre, Manor Park, London E12 6AQ Tel: 020 8478 0686 Fax: 020 8478 1666; East Ham Memorial Building, Shrewsbury Road, London E7 8QR — MB BS Gauhati 1966. SHO Emerg., Cas. & Orthop. Dept. E. Ham Memor Hosp. Prev: Ho. Off. Med. Dept. Bruntsfield Hosp. Edin.; SHO Geriat. Dept. East. Gen. Hosp. Edin.

ZAMBANINI, Andrew Department of Clinical Pharmacology, NHLI, Imperial College, St. Mary's Hospital, Praed Street, London W2 1NY Tel: 020 7886 6827 Fax: 020 7886 2207 — MB BS Lond. 1991 (St Geo.) MRCP (UK) 1995; CCST Clin. Pharmacol. & Therap. 2001. Clin. Research Fell. in Clin. Pharmacol. NHLI, Imperial Coll., Lond. Specialty: Pharmacology; Gen. Med.; Vasc. Med. Socs: Roy. Coll. Phys.; Lond. Hypertens. Soc.; Roy. Soc. Med. (Fell.). Prev: Sen. Regist., Clin. Pharmacol., Chelsea & Westm. Hosp. Lond.; Research Fell. (Cardiovasc.) Green La. Hosp., Auckland, New Zealand; Regist. (Gen. Med.) Chelsea & Westminster & Watford Hosp.

ZAMBARAKJI, Mr Hadi Jihad Department of Ophthalmology, Whipps Cross Hospital, London E11 1NR Tel: 020 8539 5522 Fax: 020 8535 6466; 10 Lowndes Square, Flat 20, London SW1X 9HA Tel: 020 7259 6765 Email: hzambarakj@aol.com — MB ChB Dundee 1990; FRCOphth 1995. Specialist Regist. (Ophth.) N. Thames Rotat. Specialty: Ophth. Socs: BMA; MRCOphth.; Med. & Dent. Defence Union Scotl. Prev: Fell. (Diabetic Retina Ophth.) Qu. Med. Centre Nottm.; SHO (Ophth.) Char. Cross Hosp. Lond.; SHO Stirling Roy. Infirm.

ZAMBLERA, Dante University Hospital Lewisham, Lewisham High Street, London SE13 6LH Tel: 020 8333 3065 Fax: 020 8690 1963 — MB BCh BAO NUI 1988; LRCPSI 1988. Cons. (O & G) Univ. Hosp. Lewisham. Specialty: Obst. & Gyn. Prev: Regist. (O & G) Guys & St Thos. Hosp. Lond.

ZAMBON, Maria Caterina Virus Reference Laboratory CPHL, 61 Colindale Avenue, Colindale, London NW9 Tel: 020 8200 4400 Fax: 020 8200 1569 — BM BCh Oxf. 1989; PhD Univ. Lond. 1984; FRCPath Lond. 1996. Cons. Virologist Virus Ref. Laborat. Centr. Pub. Health Lab. Lond. Specialty: Virology. Socs: Soc. Gen. Microbiol.

ZAMIR, Rebecca Jayne 7 Chatsworth Drive, Tutbury, Burton-on-Trent DE13 9NS — BM BS Nottm. 1993.

ZAMIRI, Iraj 225 Lake Road W., Cardiff CF23 5QY Tel: 029 2075 8316 — MB BS Durh. 1964 (Newc.) MRCS Eng. LRCP Lond. 1964; MD Newc. 1973. Sen. Lect. Welsh Nat. Sch. Med. & Hon. Consult. Univ. Hosp. Wales; Hon. Cons. Pub. Health Laborat. Cardiff.

ZAMIRI, Mozheh 27 Lonsdale Terrace, Newcastle upon Tyne NE2 3HQ — MB ChB Ed. 1996.

ZAMIRI, Parisa 31 Alison Road, London W3 6HZ — MB BS Lond. 1991.

ZAMMIT, Stanley George Department of Psychological Medicine, University of Wales College of Medicine, Cardiff CF14 4XN — BM BCh Oxf. 1993.

ZAMMIT, Vincent (Surgery) 50 Church Road, Ashford TW15 2TU Tel: 01784 254041; 10 Sheperds Close, Shepperton TW17 9AL Tel: 01932 243337 — MD Malta 1965; Cert. Family Plann. JCC 1978; MRCGP 1987.

ZAMMIT-MAEMPEL, Ivan Department of Radiology, Freeman Hospital, Newcastle upon Tyne NE7 7DN; 19 Baronswood, Gosforth, Newcastle upon Tyne NE3 3UB — MB ChB Manch. 1982; MRCP (UK) 1985; FRCR 1988. Cons. Radiol. Freeman Hosp. Newc. u. Tyne. Specialty: Radiol. Prev: Sen. Regist. (Radiol.) NW RHA; Regist. (Radiol.) NW RHA; SHO (Med.) Wythenshawe Hosp.

ZAMMIT-MAEMPEL, Joseph George The Meadow Fields Practice, Chellaston Park, Snelsmoor Lane, Chellaston, Derby DE73 1TQ Tel: 01332 700455 Fax: 01332 700628; Longlands Farm, 19 Main St, Findern, Derby DE65 6AG Tel: 01283 703203 — MB ChB Dundee 1984; DCH RCPS Glas. 1986; DRCOG 1987. Specialty: Gen. Pract.

ZAMMIT-TABONA, Michael Victor Lanhael House, 34 High Street, Toft, Cambridge CB3 7RL Tel: 01223 263589 Email: mtabona@aol.com — MB BChir Camb. 1976 (Westm. & Camb.) MA Camb. 1975; MRCP (UK) 1978; Dip. Pharm. Med. RCP (UK) 1986; MFPM 1989. Specialty: Pharmaceutical Medicine; Respirat. Med. Socs: Brit. Thorac. Soc. & Amer. Thorac. Soc. Prev: Med. Dir. & Vice-Pres. Europe, Smithkline Beecham Pharmaceut.; Research Fell. (Respirat. Med.) Univ. Brit. Columbia, Vancouver; Regist. (Med.) Hammersmith Hosp.

ZAMMITT, Nicola Naomi 7 (Flat 1), Glengyle Terrace, Edinburgh EH3 9LL Mob: 07803 619669 Email: nicolazammitt@hotmail.com — MB ChB Ed. 1998; BSc (Med. Sci.); MRCP Ed. 2002. Specialty: Diabetes.

ZAMORA EGUILUZ, Maria Christina Leyton Green Neighbourhood Health Service, 180 Essex Road, Leyton, London E10 6BT Tel: 020 7539 0756 Fax: 020 7556 6902 — MB ChB Birm. 1981.

ZAMORA VICENTE DE VERA, Francisco Javier Colchester General Hospital, Turner Road, Colchester CO4 5JL — LMS U Autonoma Madrid 1990.

ZAMVAR, Mr Vipin Royal Infirmary of Edinburgh, 51 Little France Crescent, Edinburgh EH16 4SU Tel: 0131 536 1000 Fax: 0131 242 3930 Email: vipin.zamvar@luht.scot.nhs.uk; BUPA Murrayfield Hospital, Corstophine Road, Edinburgh EH12 6UD — MB BS Bombay 1988; MS Bombay 1991; FRCS Glas. 1992; FRCS (CTh) Glas. 1998. Cons. Cardiothoracic Surg. Roy. Infirm. Edin.; Cons. Cardiothoracic Surg. BUPA Murrayfield Hosp. Edin.; Ed. Bd. Mem. Heart Surg. Forum. Specialty: Cardiothoracic Surg. Special Interest: Aortic Valve Surg.; Off Pump Coronary Artery Surg.; Total Arterial Revascularisation. Socs: Soc. Cardiothoracic Surg. Gt. Britain & Irel.; Europ. Assn. Cardiothoracic Surg.; Internat. Soc. Minimally Invasive Cardiac Surg.

ZANDER, Karine Marguerite 39 Chestnut Road, London SE27 9EZ — MB ChB Bristol 1993. SHO (Med.) Frenchay Hosp. Bristol.

ZANE, Jeffrey Neil Colne House Surgery, 99A Uxbridge Road, Rickmansworth WD3 7DJ Tel: 01923 776295 Fax: 01923 777744; 16 Dunsmore Way, Bushey, Watford WD23 4FA Tel: 020 8950 6705 Fax: 020 8950 1112 — MB BS Lond. 1972 (Univ. Coll. Hosp.) MRCS Eng. LRCP Lond. 1972; DA Eng. 1974. GP Princip. Specialty: Paediat. Dent.

ZANIEWSKI, Francis Teodor 2 Braemar Mansions, Cornwall Gardens, London SW7 4AF — MB BS Lond. 1973 (St. Thos.) MRCS Eng. LRCP Lond. 1973; DCH Eng. 1975; MRCP (UK) 1976.

ZAPATA, Luis Camilo 31 Riverside Road, Oxford OX2 0HT — MB BS Lond. 1994.

ZAPATA-BRAVO, Enrique 31 Riverside Road, Oxford OX2 0HT Tel: 01865 721933 Fax: 01865 724645 — Medico Cirujano Chile 1964; AFOM RCP Lond. 1983; MSc Oxf. 1984; MRCPsych 1987. Cons. Psychiat. Oxf. RHA; Med. Dir. Milton Keynes Community NHS Trust.; Acad. Tutor RCPsych. Milton Keynes. Specialty: Gen. Psychiat.; Geriat. Psychiat. Prev: Cons. Psychol. Med. Oxf.; Cons. WHO Brazzaville; Dir. Hosp. del Torax Santiago.

ZAPHIROPOULOS, George Constantine Walsgrave Hospitals NHS Trust, Clifford Bridge Road, Coventry CV2 2DX — MB ChB Alexandria 1961; LMSSA Lond. 1967; MRCP Lond. 1969; FRCP Lond. 1985. Cons. Rheum. Coventry & Nuneaton Hosps., Walsgrave Hosps. NHS Trust & Geo. Eliot Hosp. NHS Trust. Specialty: Rheumatol. Socs: Brit. Soc. Rheum.; Midl. Rheum. Soc.; W Midl. Phys. Assn. Prev: Sen. Regist. (Rheum.) Guy's Hosp. Lond. & Roy. Sussex Co. Hosp. Brighton; Regist. (Med.) Roy. Vict. Hosp. Bournemouth.

ZARAGOZA CASARES, Pablo 22 Colston Road, East Sheen, London SW14 7PQ — LMS U Complutense Madrid 1994.

ZARD, Chantal Maurice 2 Chiltern Close, Croydon CR0 5LZ — MB BS Lond. 1989.

ZARDIS, Michalakis Chris Testvale Surgery, 12 Salisbury Road, Totton, Southampton SO40 3PY Tel: 023 8086 6999/6990 Fax: 023 8066 3992; Little Busketts, 184 Woodlands Road, Woodlands, Southampton SO40 7GL — BM Soton. 1984; MRCP (UK) 1987; DRCOG 1989; MRCGP 1990. Prev: SHO (Paediat. Cardiol.) Soton. & SW Hants. HA.

ZAREMBA, Eleanor Lois Stonewold, Hunton Road, Catterick Garrison DL9 3NN — MB BS Lond. 1998.

ZARGAR, Bashir Ahmad 12 Turnbury Close, Branston, Burton-on-Trent DE14 3GZ Tel: 01283 539603 — MB BS Kashmir 1967. Cons. for Older Adults, Lichfield/Tamworth S. Staffs. NHS Trust. Specialty: Gen. Psychiat. Prev: Clin. Med. Off. (Community Health) Blackpool, Wyre & Fylde HA; Clin. Med. Off. (Gen. Psychiat.) Premier Health Trust Burton-on-Trent.

ZARGAR, Ghulam Akbar 18 Langport Close, Fulwood, Preston PR2 9FE — MB BS Sind 1976.

ZARGAR, Ghulam M Druids Heath Surgery, 27 Pound Road, Druids Heath, Birmingham B14 5SB Tel: 0121 430 5461 — MB BS Patna 1967.

ZARIFA, Mr Zuhair Khalil Custom House Surgery, 16 Freemasons Road, London E16 3NA Tel: 020 7476 2255 Fax: 020 7511 8980; 5 Ffordd Hendre, The Ithens, Wrexham LL13 7EZ — MB ChB Ain Shams 1976; FRCS Glas. 1985.

ZARNOSH, Mohammad Royal Eye Unit, Kington Hospital, Galsworthy Road, Kingston upon Thames KT2 7QB; 12 Manor Drive North, New Malden KT3 5PB — MB BS Punjab 1968 (Nishter Med. Coll. Multan) DO Eng. 1975. Clin. Asst. (Ophth.) Kington Hosp. Specialty: Ophth. Prev: SHO (Thoracic Med.) Aintree Hosp. Liverp.

ZARO, Mushtaq Ahmad The Surgery, 6-7 Aspen Court, Belvoir Park Road, Cleethorpes DN35 0SJ Tel: 01472 291977 — MB BS Janu & Kashmir 1969; MD Kasmir Univ. 1977; DCCH Sheff. 1994. GP Med. Off. GTFC. Specialty: Paediat.; Gen. Pract.; Sports Med.

ZAROD, Mr Andrew Peter 14 St John Street, Manchester M3 4AZ Tel: 0161 834 9900; 31B Carrwood Road, Bramhall, Stockport SK7 3LR Tel: 0161 485 3100 — MB ChB Liverp. 1973; FRCS Ed. 1980; FRCS Eng. 1980. Cons. ENT Surg. The Pennine Acute Hosps. NHS Trust & Centr. Manch. and Manch. Childr.'s Univ. Hosps. Specialty: Otorhinolaryngol. Socs: Founder Mem. (Ex-Counc. Mem.) Brit. Assn. Paediat. Otorhinolaryngol.; Roy. Soc. Med. (Vice-Pres. Sect. Laryngol. & Rhinol.). Prev: Lect. (Anat.) Univ. Manch.

ZARYCKYJ, Michael Park Road Medical Centre, 17 Park Road, St. Annes on Sea, Lytham St Annes FY8 1PW Tel: 01253 866978 — MB ChB Manch. 1978. GP St. Anne's on Sea.

ZATMAN, Perry Ty Gwyn, 4 Westfield Road, Newport NP20 4ND Tel: 01633 672416 — MB BS Lond. 1991; BSc Manch. 1986. Gen. Practitioner. Prev: Specialist Regist., Radiol. Uni. Hosp. Of Wales.

ZATMAN, Syeda Tahsin Fatima 13 Fernbank Close, Stalybridge SK15 2RZ — MB BS Lond. 1992.

ZATOUROFF, Michael 145 Harley Street, London W1G 6BJ Tel: 020 7935 4444 Fax: 020 7935 2725 — MB BS Lond. 1961 (Lond. Hosp.) MRCS Eng. LRCP Lond. 1961; DCH Eng. 1964; FRCP Lond. 1982, M 1966. Hon. Sen. Lect. (Med.) Roy. Free Hosp. Lond.; Lect. (Med.) Lond. Foot Hosp.; Examr. Med. Soc. Chiropodists; Examr. Med. ConJt. Bd. Eng. Specialty: Gen. Med. Socs: (Counc.) Med. Soc. Lond.; Sec. Osler Club. Prev: Regist. (Med.) Roy. North. Hosp. Lond.; Regist. Univ. Coll. Hosp. Ibadan; Phys. Kuwait Govt.

ZAVODY, Maria 42 Buckland Avenue, Slough SL3 7PH Tel: 01753 523575 — MD Pecs Hungary 1963. Staff Psychiat. Reading. Specialty: Child & Adolesc. Psychiat. Prev: Staff Psychiat. Huntercombe Manor Hosp. Taplow; Regist. (Psychiat.) Pk. Prewett Hosp. Basingstoke.

ZAW MIN, Mr — MB BS Mandalay Burma 1973; FRCS Ed. 1984; FRCOPhth 1989. Clin. Asst. (Eye Department) Darent Valley Hosp. Dartford Kent; Clin. Asst. (Eye Department) Farnborough Hosp. Farnborough Kent; Clin. Asst. (Eye Department) Qu. Mary's Hosp. Sidcup Kent. Specialty: Ophth. Special Interest: Retina.

ZAW WIN, Dr 53 Taunton Way, Stanmore HA7 1DJ — MB BS Med. Inst. (I) Rangoon 1971. SHO (Anaesth.) ScarBoro. Hosp.

ZAYYAN, Mr Kasimu Sanusi 218 Sandycombe Road, Kew, Richmond TW9 2EQ Tel: 020 8948 7823 — MB BS Nigeria 1983; FRCS Ed. 1990; FRCSI 1990.

ZBAEDA, Matouk Mohamed Ormskirik District General Hospital, Wigan Road, Ormskirk L39 2AZ Tel: 01695 656280 Fax: 01695 656282 Email: m.zbaeda@southportandormskirk.nhs.uk — MB BCh Al Fateh, Libya 1981; FRCPCH; MSc; MMed Sc; DCH; FRCPI; MRCPI 1993. Cons. Paediat. Ormskirk Dist. Gen. Hosp.; Cons. Paediat. Renacres Halll Hosp. Ormskirk. Specialty: Paediat.; Neonat.; Respirat. Med. Socs: Roy. Coll. of Paediat. and Child Health; Roy. Coll. of Physicians of Irel.; Brit. Assn. of Perinatal Med.

ZBRZEZNIAK, Wiktor Stanislaw Caythorpe Surgery, 52-56 High Street, Caythorpe, Grantham NG32 3DN Tel: 01400 272215 Fax: 01400 273608 — MB BS Lond. 1985; BSc (Hons.) Lond. 1982; DCH RCP Lond. 1988; MRCGP 1989. Prev: Trainee GP Lincoln VTS; Ho. Phys. & Ho. Surg. Guy's Hosp. Lond.

ZDZIARSKA, Caroline Anne Child Health Department, Mansfield Community Hospital, Stockwell Gate, Mansfield NG18 5QJ Fax: 01623 424062; 45 Haddon Road, Ravenshead, Nottingham NG15 9EZ — BM BS Nottm. 1988; BMedSci Nottm. 1986; MRCGP 1994. Community Paediat. (Staff Grade) Centr. Healthcare Trust Notts. Socs: BACCH. Prev: GP.

ZEALLEY, Andrew King (retired) Viewfield House, 12 Tipperlinn Road, Edinburgh EH10 5ET Tel: 0131 447 5545 Fax: 0131 447 5545 — MB ChB Ed. 1959; FRCP Ed. 1974, M 1963; DPM Ed. 1966; FRCPsych 1979, M 1971. Chairm., Lothian Research Ethics Comm. Prev: Phys. Superintendent and Med. Director, Lothian Healthcare NHS Trust.

ZEALLEY, Helen Elizabeth, QHP, OBE Lothian Health, Deaconess House, 148 Pleasance, Edinburgh EH8 9RS Tel: 0131 536 9163 Fax: 0131 536 9164; Viewfield House, 12 Tipperlinn Road, Edinburgh EH10 5ET Tel: 0131 447 5545 Fax: 0131 447 5545 — MB ChB Ed. 1964; MD Ed. 1968; Dip. Soc. Med. Ed. 1973; FFPHM 1980, M 1974; DCCH RCP Ed. (Hons) 1982; FRCP Ed. 1987. Chief Admin. Med. Off. & Dir. Pub. Health Lothian HB; Hon. Sen. Lect. Univ. Edin. Specialty: Pub. Health Med. Prev: SCM Lothian HB; Med. Off. Scott. Counc. Postgrad. Med. Educat.; Regist. Regional Virus Laborat. City Hosp. Edin.

ZEALLEY, Ian Alexander Department of Radiology, Ninewells Hospital & Medical School, Ninewells Avenue DD1 9SY Tel: 01382 660111 Email: ian.zealley@tuhr.scot.nhs.uk; 76 Holly Avenue, Jesmond, Newcastle upon Tyne NE2 2QA Tel: 0191 281 3334 — MB ChB Ed. 1991; BSc (Med. Sci.) (Hons.) Ed. 1989; MRCP (UK) 1994; FRCR 1997. Cons. Radiologist, Abdom. & Interventional Radiol., Ninewells Hosp., Dundee. Specialty: Radiol. Special Interest: Abdom. & Interventional Radiol. Socs: (Ex-Jun. Pres.) Roy. Med. Soc. Edin. Prev: SHO Rotat. (Med.) Newc. Teach. Hosps.; Ho. Phys. & Ho. Surg. Roy. Infirm. Edin.; Regist. Rotat. (Radiol.) N. & Yorks. Region.

ZEALLEY, Kirsten Elizabeth 12 Tipperlinn Road, Edinburgh EH10 5ET Tel: 0131 447 5545 Fax: 0131 447 5545 — MB ChB Dundee 1991; DCH RCP Lond. 1994; DFFP 1997; MRCGP 1997. Specialty: Gen. Pract. Prev: GP/Regist. Inch Pk. Surg. Edin.; SHO (Psychiat.) Roy. Edin. Hosp.; SHO (O & G) Gosford Hosp. NSW, Austral.

ZEALLEY, Monica Margaret (retired) The Old Vicarage, Southstoke, Bath BA2 7DU Tel: 01225 832080 — MB ChB Ed. 1946.

ZEB KHAN, Aurang Birch Hill Hospital, Birch Road, Rochdale OL12 9QB Tel: 01706 377777 Fax: 01706 755663; 23 Hawthorn Road, Rochdale OL11 5JQ Tel: 01706 44290 — MB BS Peshawar 1978 (Khyber Med. Coll.) DCH Punjab 1980; MCPS Pakistan 1982; DCH Dub. 1985. Staff Grade (Paediat.) Birch Hill Hosp. Rochdale. Specialty: Paediat. Prev: Regist. (Paediat.) W. Dorset Gen. Hosp., Altanegalvin Area Hosp. N. Irel. & Waterford Regional Hosp. Irel.

ZEBRO, Tadeusz Julian Microprep Pathology Laboratory, Ross House, Church Street, Wistow, Huntingdon PE28 2QE Tel: 01487 823131 Fax: 01487 824484 — Lekarz Krakow 1953; MD 1st Med. Inst. Moscow 1956; FRCPath 1980. Cons. Histopath. Microprep Laborat. Servs. Huntingdon. Specialty: Histopath. Socs: Assn. Clin. Path.; Eur. Soc. Pathol. Prev: Cons. Histopath. Hinchingbrooke Hosp. & Cromwell Clinic Huntingdon; Vis. Prof. & Hon. Cons. Path. King's Coll. Hosp. Med. Sch. Lond.; Vis. Prof. Inst. Path. Giessen Univ. Med. Sch. W. Germany.

ZECKLER, Sharon-Rose The Wall House, Mongewell Park, Wallingford OX10 8DA — MB BS Lond. 1996.

ZEDAN, Mr Abdel-Majeed Anwar 166 Leicester Road, Barnet EN5 5DS Tel: 020 8441 5727 — MB BCh Cairo 1980; FRCS Ed. 1993. Staff Surg. (ENT) Chase Farm Hosp. Enfield.

ZEEGEN, Ronald, OBE Westminster & Chelsea Hospital, 369 Fulham Road, London SW10 9NH Tel: 020 8746 8599 Fax: 020 8392 1607 Email: ron@zeegan.co.uk; 36 Clare Lawn Avenue, East Sheen, London SW14 8BG Tel: 020 8876 4622 — MB BS Lond. 1962 (St. Bart.) DObst RCOG 1964; MRCS Eng. LRCP Lond. 1964; FRCP Lond. 1980, M 1967. p/t Emerit. Cons. Phys. and Gastroenterologist, Chelsea and Westm. NHS Trust, Lond.; Cons. Phys. and Gastroenterologist, Ulster Hosp., Lond. Specialty: Gastroenterol.; Gen. Med. Socs: Med. Soc. of Lond.; Brit. Soc.

Gastroenterol.; Brit. Med. Assn. Prev: Sen. Regist. (Med.) Westm. Hosp. Lond.; Research Fell. & Sen. Regist. (Med.) St. Bart. Hosp. Lond.; Cons. Phys. (Gen. Med. & Gastroenterol.) Westm. & Chelsea Hosp. & The Lister Hosp. Lond.

ZEGLEMAN, Fiona Elizabeth 4 Wester Coates Avenue, Edinburgh EH12 5LS Tel: 0131 337 1900 — MB ChB Ed. 1980; MRCPsych 1985.

ZEIDAN, Marwan Moorfields Eye Hospital, City Road, London EC1V 2PD Tel: 020 7253 3411 — Approbation Leipzig 1971. Specialty: Ophth.

ZEIDAN, Sabri Fadel Princess Alexandra Hospital NHS Trust, Hamstel Road, Harlow CM20 1QX Tel: 01279 827448 Email: sabri.zeidan@pah.nhs.uk — MB ChB Cairo 1975; FRCPCH; MRCP UK; MSc. Cons. Paediat., Princess Alexandra Hosp. Harlow; Cons. Paediat., The Rivers Hosp., Sawbridgeworth. Specialty: Paediat.; Respirat. Med. Socs: Brit. Paediatric Respirat. Soc. Prev: Cons. Paediat., Dhahran Health Centre, Saudi Arabia.

ZEIDER, Mr Paul Alfred The Surgery, 3 Candover Street, London W1W 7DE Tel: 020 7636 4311 — MB ChB Sheff. 1969; MRCOG 1974; FRCS Ed. 1975.

ZEIDERMAN, Mr Michael Richard Southport & Ormskick NHS Trust, Town Lane, Kew, Southport PR8 6NJ Tel: 01704 704252 — MB ChB Liverp. 1978; FRCS Eng. 1982; BSc (Hons.) Liverp. 1975, ChM 1988. Cons. Gastroenterol. & Gen. Surg. Southport & Ormskick NHS Trust; Clin. Lect. (Surg.) Univ. of Liverp. Specialty: Gastroenterol. Prev: Lect. Univ. Dept. Surg. North. Gen. Hosp. Sheff.; Lect. & Hon. Sen. Regist. Sheff. & Chesterfield Hosp.; Research Fell. Leeds Gen. Infirm. 1983-5.

ZEINA, Bassam Milton Keynes Hospital, Dermatology Department, Milton Keynes MK6 5LD Tel: 01908 243852 Fax: 01908 243852 Email: zeinabassam@yahoo.co.uk — MD Damascus 1984. Assoc. Specialist (Dermat.) Milton Keynes Hosp. Specialty: Dermat. Special Interest: PDT; Skin Cancer.

ZEINELDINE, Ahmed Amr 109 Commercial Way, London SE15 6DB Tel: 020 7703 6460 Fax: 020 7701 2266; 99 Great Brownings, College Road, London SE21 7HR Tel: 020 8670 7488 Fax: 020 8488 7872 Email: amr.zeineldine@which.net — MB ChB Alexandria 1975; MRCGP 1989; T(GP) 1994. Specialty: Gen. Pract. Socs: Diplomate Fac. Family Plann. RCOG. Prev: Trainee GP Lond.; GP Riyadh Armed Forces Hosp.

ZEITLIN, Professor Harry UCL, Academic Department of Psychiatry, Wychelm House, Hamstel Road, Harlow CM20 1QX; 3 West Grove, Greenwich, London SE10 8QT Tel: 020 8692 6403 Fax: 020 8691 9477 — MRCS Eng. LRCP Lond. 1962 (Lond. Hosp.) MD Lond. 1983, MPhil 1971, BSc (Hons. Physiol.) 1959; FRCP Lond. 1988, M 1967; FRCPsych 1972, M 1972. Prof. Child & Adolesc. Psychiat. Univ. Coll. Lond.; Hon. Cons. N. E. Essex, Ment. Health. Specialty: Child & Adolesc. Psychiat. Socs: Fell. Roy. Soc. Med. Prev: Reader (Child Psychiat.) Char. Cross & Westm. Med. Sch. Lond.; Sen. Regist. Childr. Dept. Maudsley Hosp. Lond.; Regist. Lond., Maudsley, & Southend Gen. Hosp.

ZEITOUN, Mr Hisham Glan Clwyd Hospital, Bodelwyddan, Rhyl Tel: 01745 534259 Fax: 01745 534160 — MB ChB Alexandria 1984; FRCS Glas. 1993; FRCS (ORL-HNS) 1998. Cons. Otolaryngologist, Head & Neck Surg., NHS Trust, N. Wales. Specialty: Otorhinolaryngol.

ZEITOUNE, Mr Samir Moussa Noble's Ilse of Man Hospital, The Strang, Bradden, Douglas IM4 4RJ — MB ChB Alexandria 1968; FRCS Glas. 1982.

ZEKI, Mr Sabah Mohammed Room 1/110, Gwynedd Hospital, Bangor LL57 4TL — MB ChB Baghdad 1971; DO RCS Eng. 1980; FRCS Glas. 1986; MSc (Med. Sci.) Glas. 1990; FRCOphth 1993. Cons. Ophth. Surg. Gwynedd Hosp.; Cons. Ophth. Surg. N. Wales Med. Centre Llandudno. Specialty: Ophth. Prev: Sen. Regist. Rotat. W. Midl.; Sen. Regist. & Regist. (Ophth.) Tennent Inst. Ophth. Glas.

ZELAYA-MENDIVIL, Gonzalo Felipe (retired) Tigh-Na-Mara, Kirkton, Glenelg, Kyle IV40 8JR Tel: 01599 522272 Fax: 01599 522272 — Medico Cirujano San Andres, Bolivia 1970. Prev: Princip. GP Glenelg.

ZELENKA, Robert Martin Friarage Hospital, Accident & Emergency Department, Northallerton DL6 1JG Tel: 01609 763334; Old School Cottage, Hornby Road, Great Smeaton, Northallerton DL6 2EY Tel: 01609 881357 Email: robzelenka@lineone.net — MB BS Lond. 1988 (Guy's) MA Oxf. 1981; MRCGP 1994; DFFP 1994. Assoc. Specialist in A&E Med., Friargate Hosp., Northallerton, N. Yorks DL6 1JG. Specialty: Accid. & Emerg. Prev: Trainee GP Harrogate VTS; SHO (Orthop.) Friarage Hosp. Northallerton; SHO (Psychiat.) Harrogate Dist. Hosp.

ZELIN, Jill Margot Barts Sexual Health Centre, St Bartholomews Hospital, West Smithfield, London EC1A 7BE Tel: 020 7601 8090 Fax: 020 7601 8601 Email: j.zelin@bartsandthelondon@nhs.uk — MB BCh Wales 1984; MFFP; Dip GU Med. Soc. Apoth. Lond. 1990; MRCOG 1991. Cons. Genitourin. Med. St. Bart. Hosp. Lond. Specialty: Genitourinary Medicine; Family Plann. & Reproduc. Health. Prev: Sen. Regist. (Genitourin. Med.) St. Bart. Hosp. Lond.

ZELISKO, Richard Stephen 1 Edinburgh Drive, Ickenham, Uxbridge UB10 8QY — MB BS Lond. 1975. Specialty: Blood Transfus.

ZEMAN, Adam Zbynek James Western General Hospital, Department of Clinical Neurological Sciences, Edinburgh E44 2XU Tel: 0131 537 1167 Email: adam.zeman@ed.ac.uk — BM BCh Oxf. 1984; BA Oxf 1979; MRCP UK 1987; DM Oxf 1994. Cons. Neurol. West. Gen. Hosp. Edin.; Sen. Lect. Univ. Edin. Specialty: Neurol. Special Interest: Cognitive Neurol.; Sleep disorders. Socs: Brit. Sleep Soc.; Internat. League against Epilepsy; Brit. Neuropsychol. Soc. Prev: Sen. Regist. (Neurol.) Addenbrooke's Hosp. Camb.; Regist. Nat. Hosp. for Neurol. & Neurosurg. Qu. Sq. Lond.; Regist. (Neurol.) Radcliffe Infirm. Oxf.

ZENGEYA, Stanley Tamuka Great Western Hospital, Department of Paediatrics, Marlborough Road, Swindon SN3 6BB — MB ChB Zimbabwe 1982; MRCP UK 1991. Specialty: Paediat.; Neonat.

ZENTLER-MUNRO, Patrick Luke Department of Medicine, Raigmore Hospital, Inverness IV2 3UJ Tel: 01463 704000 Fax: 01463 705460; Brae House, Canonbury Terrace, Fortrose IV10 8TT Tel: 01381 620039 — MB BChir Camb. 1972; MRCP (UK) 1975; MA 1973, MD 1985; FRCP Ed. 1989. Cons. Phys. In Gen. Med. and Gastroenterol., Reigmore Hosp., Inverness; Hon. Clin. Sen. Lect. Univ. Aberd. Med. Sch.; Advisory Council Drug Therap. Bull. Specialty: Gen. Med.; Gastroenterol. Prev: Hon. Clin. Asst. Brompton Hosp. Lond.; Sen. Regist. St. Geo. Hosp. Lond.; Research Fell. St. Geo. Hosp. Med. Sch. Lond.

ZEPEDA, Mr Armando Ramon 323 Skircoat Green Road, Halifax HX3 0NA Tel: 01422 54874 — MD El Salvador 1973.

ZEPPETELLA, Giovambattista Stone Barton, Hastingwood Road, Hastingwood, Harlow CM17 9JX Tel: 01279 773 770 Fax: 01279 773 771 Email: jzepperella@stclare-hospice.co.uk — MB BS Lond. 1985 (Univ. Coll. Hosp.) BSc (Hons.) Lond. 1981; MRCGP 1991. Med. Director St Clare Hospice Essex; Hon. Princess Alexandra NHS Trust Harlow. Specialty: Palliat. Med. Prev: Cons. Palliat. Med. St. Joseph's Hospice Lond.; Hon. Barts and the Lond. NHS Trust.

ZERAATI, Mr Mehdi Bassetlaw District General Hospital, Department of Orthopaedics, Blyth Road, Worksop S81 0BD — MB ChB Sheff. 1981. Specialty: Trauma & Orthop. Surg.

ZERAFA, Raphael Paston Health Centre, Chadburn, Peterborough PE4 7DH Tel: 01733 572584 Fax: 01733 328131 — MD Malta 1967.

ZERMANSKY, Arnold Geoffrey Park Edge Practice, Asket Drive, Leeds LS17 1HX Tel: 0113 295 4650 Fax: 0113 295 4663 Email: arnoldz@easynet.co.uk; 11 Wike Ridge Grove, Leeds LS17 9NW Tel: 0113 268 3802 Email: arnoldz@easynet.co.uk — MB ChB (Hons.) Leeds 1970; DObst RCOG 1972; MRCGP (Distinc.) 1978. p/t Vis. Hon. Sen. Research Fell. Sch. of Healthcare Studies Univ. of Leeds; Tutor (Gen. Pract.) Univ. Leeds; Mem. Leeds LMC. Special Interest: Medicines Managem.; Therapeutic misadventure. Socs: (Ex-Pres.) Leeds Jewish Med. Soc. Prev: Chairm. E. Leeds Primary Care Gp.; Med. Adviser Leeds FHSA; Gp. Mem. Leeds E. Dist. Managem. Bd. & Chairm. Leeds E. Dist. Med. Comm.

ZERMANSKY, William Simon — MB ChB Birm. 1998.

ZEWAWI, Mr Ali Salem Flat A, 43 Rectory Road, Crumpsall, Manchester M8 5EA — MB BS Garyounis, Libya 1976; FRCSI 1990.

ZEYA, Kyaw 6 Burnsall Close, Pendeford, Wolverhampton WV9 5RU Tel: 01902 781096 — MB BS Med. Inst. (I) Rangoon 1979; LRCP LRCS Ed. LRCPS Glas. 1986.

ZEZULKA, Alexander Vratislav Airedale Hospital, Skipton Road, Steeton, Keighley BD20 6TD Tel: 01535 292018 Fax: 01535 292019 — MB BS Lond. 1977 (Westm.) BSc (Physiol.) Lond. 1974; MRCP (UK) 1980; MD Lond. 1993; FRCP 1999. Cons. Cardiol. Airedale Hosp. Steeton W. Yorks. Specialty: Cardiol. Socs: Brit.

Cardiac Soc.; Brit. Cardiac Interven.al Soc.; Brit. Pacing and Electrophysiol. Soc. Prev: Sen. Regist. & Regist. (Cardiol.) Leeds Gen. Infirm.; Sen. Regist. (Med.) Profess. Med. Unit, Leeds Gen. Infirm.

ZIA, Mohammad Imran — MB BS Lond. 1996.

ZIA, Mubashar 48 St Kilda Drive, Jordanhill, Glasgow G14 9LT — MB BS Punjab 1986; FFA RCSI 1993.

ZIA-UL-HASAN, Dr 4 Abbots Way, Westlands, Newcastle ST5 2ET — MB BS Peshawar 1984; MRCP (UK) 1994.

ZICCHIERI, Francesco Luigi Robin Lane Medical Centre, Robin Lane, Pudsey LS28 7DE Tel: 0113 295 1444 Fax: 0113 295 1440; Woodland Villas, 84 Bachelor Lane, Horsforth, Leeds LS18 5NF — MB ChB Leeds 1985; MRCGP 1989. Specialty: Ophth. Prev: SHO (Ophth.) Bradford Roy. Infirm.

ZICKERMAN, Anna Maria 6 Aber Road, Stoneygate, Leicester LE2 2BA Tel: 0116 270 9565 Fax: 0116 270 9565 — MB ChB Leic. 1994; MSc (Sports Med.) Nott. 2001. GP Locum. Specialty: Gen. Med. Prev: SHO Rotat. (Med.) Leicester; VTS Regist. (Rotat.) O & G, Leicester Gen. Hosp.; Flexible Trainee.

ZIDEMAN, David Anthony, QHP, CStJ 31 Moss Lane, Pinner HA5 3BB Email: david@zideman.demon.co.uk — MB BS Lond. 1972 (Lond. Hosp.) BSc (Hons.) Lond. 1969; FFA RCS Eng. 1976; Dip. IMC RCS Ed. 1995; FIMC RCS Ed, 2000. Cons. Anaesth. Hammersmith Hosp. & Hon. Sen. Lect. (Anaesth.) Imperial Coll. Sch. of Med.; Chief of Serv. for Anaesth., Hammersmith Hosps. Trust. Specialty: Anaesth. Socs: Chairm. BASICS; Exec. Comm. Resusc. Counc. (UK); Chairm. Europ. Resusc. Counc. Prev: Sen. Regist. (Anaesth.) Hammersmith Hosp. Roy. Postgrad. Med. Sch.; Fell. (Anaesth.) Hosp. Sick Childr. Toronto, Canada; Regist. (Anaesth.) St. Mary's Hosp. Lond.

ZIEGLER, Emma Samantha Mary 27 Love Lane, Petersfield GU31 4BP — MB ChB Bristol 1988. Specialist Regist. (Occupat. Health) Camb. Specialty: Occupat. Health.

ZIELINSKI, Richard Antoni 3 Fell Grove, Birmingham B21 8JQ — MB ChB Birm. 1993.

ZIERVOGEL, Mark Allan (retired) 2 Robinsfield, Balmore Road, Bardowie, Milngavie, Glasgow G62 6ER Tel: 01360 622268 — MB ChB Glas. 1969; BSc Natal 1959; DMRD Eng. 1972; FFR 1974; FRCR 1975. Prev: Cons. Radiol. Roy. Hosp. Sick Childr. Glas. & Stirling Roy. Infirm.

ZIGMOND, Anthony Stephen Newsham Centre, Seacroft Hospital, York Rd, Leeds LS14 6WB — MB ChB Birm. 1975; MRCPsych 1979. Cons. Psychiat. Leeds Mental Health Trust. Specialty: Gen. Psychiat.

ZIGMOND, David North Aisle Medical Centre, St James Church, Thurland Road, London SE16 4AA Tel: 020 7237 4066 Fax: 020 7740 1031 — MB ChB Birm. 1969; DPM Eng. 1975; MRCGP 1976. Specialty: Psychother. Socs: Inst. Transactional Anal.; Assn. of Gp. and Individual Psychother. Prev: Sen. Lect. NE Lond. Polytechnic; Vis. Tutor Brit. Postgrad. Med. Federat.; Hon. Lect. Roy. Postgrad. Med. Sch. Lond.

ZIKO, Abdulrahman Osman Aly 57 Rectory Lane, Bury BL9 7TA Tel: 0161 797 9528 — MB BCh Ain Shams, Egypt 1980; MRCP (UK) 1994. Assoc. Specialist (Anaesth.) Fairfield Gen. Hosp. Bury.

ZILAHI, Clara Clotilde (retired) 31 Wimbotsham Road, Downham Market PE38 9PE — MB BChir Camb. 1955; FRCS Eng. 1965.

ZILKHA, Kevin Jerome Cromwell Hospital, Cromwell Road, London SW5 0TU Tel: 020 7460 5668 Fax: 020 7460 5669 — MB BS Lond. 1953 (Guy's) MRCS Eng. LRCP Lond. 1953; FRCP Lond. 1970, M 1958; MD Lond. 1962. Emerit. Hon. Neurol. King's Coll. Hosp. Lond.; Emerit. Hon. Phys. Nat. Hosp. Qu. Sq. Lond. Specialty: Neurol. Socs: Fell. Roy. Soc. Med.; Assn. Brit. Neurols. Prev: Hon. Neurol. Army & Roy. Hosp. Lond.; Sub-Dean Inst. Neurol. Qu. Sq. Lond.; Ho. Phys. (Neurol.) Guy's Hosp. Lond.

ZILKHA, Timothy Robert Tarr House, Kingston St Mary, Taunton TA2 8HY — MB BS Lond. 1984 (Guy's) FCAnaesth. 1990. Cons. Anaesth. Taunton & Som. Hosps. Specialty: Anaesth. Socs: Assn. Anaesths. Prev: Sen. Regist. (Anaesth.) & Research Fell. (Pain Relief) King's Coll. Hosp. Lond.; Regist. (Anaesth.) St. Bart. & Southend Gp. Hosps.

ZILLWOOD, Sarah Jane 28 Malling Avenue, Broughton Astley, Leicester LE9 6QS — MB ChB Leic. 1989.

ZILVA, Professor Joan Foster (retired) 30 Lavington Court, 77 Putney Hill, London SW15 3NU Tel: 020 8789 1585 Email: JZilva@aol.com — MB BS Lond. 1951 (Roy. Free) FRCP Lond. 1971, M 1955; BSc (Special Physiol.) Lond. 1947, MD 1958; FRCPath 1974, M 1964. Emerit. Prof. Chem. Path. Univ. Lond.; Hon. Cons. Chem. Path. Riverside HA. Prev: Prof. Chem. Path. Char. Cross & Westm. Med. Sch.

ZIMBLER, Nicoletta 23 Rosebery Crescent, Jesmond, Newcastle upon Tyne NE2 1EU — MB ChB Leic. 1991; MRCP (UK) 1994. SHO (Anaesth.) Sunderland Dist. Gen. Hosp. Prev: SHO (Infec. Dis.) Dundee; SHO (Med.) Nottm.

ZIMBWA, Peter Mark The John Radcliffe, Department of General Medicine, Headley Way, Oxford OX3 9DU — MB ChB Zimbabwe 1992. Specialty: Gen. Med.

ZIMMER, Stanley 29 Burn Road, Darvel KA17 0DB — MB ChB Glas. 1970; FFA RCS Eng. 1974. Cons. Anaesth. NHS Ayrsh. & Arran. Specialty: Anaesth.

ZIMMERN, Ronald Leslie Public Health Genetics Unit, Strangeways Research Laboratory, Worts Causeway, Cambridge CB1 8RN Tel: 01223 740228 Fax: 01223 740200; Hall Farm House, Great Abington, Cambridge CB1 6AE Tel: 01223 891996 — MB BChir Camb. 1972 (Middlx.) MRCP (UK) 1973; MA Camb. 1976; MFCM 1987; FRCP Lond. 1992; FFPHM RCP (UK) 1993. Dir., Pub. Health Genetics Unit; Assoc. Lect. Univ. Camb; Cons. in Pub. Health Med. Specialty: Pub. Health Med. Socs: Brit. Assn. Med. Managers (Bd. Dir.); Roy. Soc. Med. Prev: Cons. Pub. Health Med. Addenbrooke's Hosp. Camb.; Hon. Sen. Regist. (Neurol.) Addenbrooke's Hosp. Camb.; Sen. Regist. (Community Med.) Camb. HA.

ZINCKE, Horst Department of Uro-Oncologic Surgery, Health Care International (Scotland) Ltd., Beardmore St., Clydebank G81 4HX — State Exam Med Frankfurt 1966.

ZINKIN, Pamela Margaret 45 Anson Road, London N7 0AR — MB ChB Leeds 1956; FRCP Lond. 1981.

ZINNA, Rosario Federico 23 Wharfedale Road, Westbourne, Bournemouth BH4 9BT — MD Naples 1948; Dip. Psych. McGill 1960; ECFMG Cert. 1962; Dip. Amer. Bd. Psychiat. & Neurol. 1965; LAH Dub. 1970; MRCPsych 1971. Cons., W. of Eng. Laser Centre, Som. Nuffield Hosp., Taunton. Specialty: Child & Adolesc. Psychiat. Socs: Corresp. Mem. Amer. Med. Psychiat. Assns.; BMA. Prev: Clin. Tutor Duke Univ. Med. Sch., Univ. N. Carolina Med. Sch. & Dartmouth Coll. Med. Sch., U.S.A.

ZINTILIS, Spyros Andrea London Road Surgery, 49 London Road, Canterbury CT2 8SG Tel: 01227 463128 Fax: 01227 786308; 31 Longacre, Chestfield, Whitstable CT5 3PQ Tel: 01227 792452 Fax: 01227 792132 — MD Athens 1973; MRCS Eng. LRCP Lond. 1975.

ZIPRIN, Anna Elisabet 6 The Closes, Haddenham, Aylesbury HP17 8JN — MB ChB Manch. 1992. Specialty: Gen. Pract.

ZIPRIN, Jennifer Hilary 5H Castlebar Park, Ealing, London W4 1DD Tel: 020 8930 1103; 20 Christchurch Road, Malvern WR14 3BE — MB BCh Wales 1993; MRCP Paeds. Specialist Regist. Neonatology Univ. Coll. Hosp. Lond. Specialty: Neonat. Prev: SPR Paediat. Hillingdon Hosp. Lond.

ZIPRIN, Paul 4A Churchfield Road, London W13 9NG Tel: 020 8566 0877 Email: paul@ziprin.freeserve.co.uk — MB BCh Wales 1992; FRCS (Eng) 1996. NW Thames Specialist Regist. Rotat. (Surg.). Specialty: Gen. Surg. Prev: Regist (Gen. Surg.) Roy. Gwent Hosp.; SHO (Gen. Surg.) Cardiff Roy. Infirm.; SHO (Urol.) Cardiff Roy. Infirm.

ZIRK, Maia Helga (retired) 15 Beechwood Close, Leicester LE5 6SY — Med. Dipl. Tartu 1944.

ZIYADA, Nadia Fatima Adnan — MB ChB Baghdad, Iraq 1984.

ZMYSLOWSKI, Andrzej Jerzy 24 Chester Avenue, Southport PR9 7ET — MB BS Newc. 1980; Cert. Family Plann. JCC 1983; DRCOG 1983; MRCGP 1984; DCCH RCGP 1984; Dip.Med.Ac 1997. Med. Exam. for Benefits Agency Med. Serv.; Registered Med. Examr. Gen. Counc. Brit. Shipping; Indep. Acupunc. Pract. Specialty: Gen. Pract.; Acupunc. Socs: Brit. Med. Acupunct. Soc. Prev: Med. Off. P & O Lines; GP Houghton-le-Spring; Indep. Acupunc. Co. Durh.

ZOBAIR, Mike Swan Street Surgery, 35-41 Swan Street, Longtown, Carlisle CA6 5UZ Tel: 01228 791202 Fax: 01228 791942 — MB BS Patna 1968 (P. of Wales Med. Coll.) GP Princip. Single Handed; Civil Med. Pract. MoD Establ. Socs: BMA; SPA. Prev: SHO Gen. Med. Chester-le-St., Durh.; Ho. Off. (Gen. Surg.) Sunderland Gen. Hosp.; SHO (Gen. Med., ENT & Eyes) Patna Med. Coll. Hosp., India.

ZOHA, Mir Moin 24 Queen Elizabeth Drive, London N14 6RD — MB ChB Birm. 1992.

ZOHDY, Mr Gamal West Wales General Hospital, Carmarthen SA31 2AF Tel: 01267 227749 Fax: 01267 227414 Email: zgamal@yahoo.com — MB ChB Alexandria, Egypt 1982; FRCS Ed. 1993. Assoc. Specialist (Ophth.). Specialty: Ophth. Prev: Staff Grade (Ophth.) Shrops. HA; Regist. (Ophth.) W. of Scotl.

ZOLCZER, Laszlo Department of Orthopaedics, Mayday University Hospital, London Road, Croydon CR7 7YE Tel: 020 8401 3000 Fax: 020 8401 3100 — MD Semmelweis, Hungary 1985; Hungarian Trauma & Orthop. Board 1990. Locum Cons. Surg. (Orthop.) Mayday Univ. Hosp. Croyden Surrey. Specialty: Orthop. Socs: Brit. Orthop. Assn.; Hungarian Trauma & Orthop. Assoc. Prev: Sen. Regist. (Orthop.); Staff Surg. (Orthop.).

ZOLESE, Maria Gabriella Springfield University Hospital, Department of General Psychiatry, 61 Glenburnie Road, London SW17 7DJ — State Exam Rome 1980. Specialty: Gen. Psychiat.

ZOLKIPLI, Zarazuela 15B Canonbury Square, London N1 2AL — MB ChB Ed. 1996.

ZOLLINGER-READ, Paul John Mount Chambers Surgery, 92 Coggeshall Road, Braintree CM7 9BY Tel: 01376 553415; 2 Grove Field, Braintree CM7 5NS — MB BS Camb. 1986; MA Camb. 1986; DGM RCP Lond. 1989; DRCOG 1990; DCH RCP Lond. 1991. Specialty: Obst. & Gyn.

ZOLLMAN, Catherine Esther 11 Cliftonwood Crescent, Bristol BS8 4TU Tel: 0117 921 1247 — MB BS Lond. 1989; BA (Physiol. Sci.) Oxf. 1986; MRCP (UK) 1992. Dir. Med. Educat. Servs. Research Counc. for Complementary Med. Lond.; GP Montpelier Health Centre, Bristol. Specialty: Gen. Pract. Prev: GP/Regist. Montpelier Health Centre Bristol; Regist. (Oncol. Med.) Qu. Eliz. Hosp. Birm.; SHO (Paediat. Oncol.) Bristol Childr. Hosp.

ZOLTIE, Mr Nigel Leeds General Infirmary, Accident & Emergency Department, Great George Street, Leeds LS1 3EX Tel: 0113 392 6470 Fax: 0113 392 2810 Email: nigel.zoltie@leedsth.nhs.uk — MB ChB Bristol 1977; FRCS Ed. 1982; FFAEM 1994. Cons. A & E Leeds Gen. Infirm.; Hon. Sen. Clin. Lect. (A & E) Leeds Univ. Specialty: Accid. & Emerg. Prev: Regist. (Plastic Surg.) W. Norwich Hosp.; Sen. Regist. (A & E) Leeds.

ZOLTOWSKI, Mr Janusz Andrzej Highfield Surgery, Holtdale Approach, Leeds LS16 7ST Tel: 0113 230 0108 Fax: 0113 230 1309 — Lekarz Warsaw 1970; FRCS Ed. 1977; MPhil Leeds 1982.

ZOMA, Asad Abood Hairmyres Hospital, Eaglesham Road, East Kilbride, Glasgow G15 8RG Tel: 01355 584821 Email: asad.zoma@laht.scot.nhs.uk — MB ChB Baghdad 1971; MRCP (UK) 1979; FRCP Glas. 1989; FRCP Lond. 1999. Cons. Phys. (Rheum.) Lanarksh. Acute Hosps. Trust Scotl.; Sen. Clin. Lect. Univ. of Glas. Specialty: Gen. Med.; Rheumatol. Special Interest: Inflammatory Jt. Dis.; SLE. Socs: Brit. Soc. Rheum.; Scott. Soc. Rheum. Prev: Sen. Regist. (Gen. Med. & Rheum.) Roy. Infirm. Glas.; Regist. (Gen. Med.) Gartnavel Gen. & West. Infirm. Glas.

ZOMAS, Athanassios Academic Department of Haematology & Cytogenetics, Royal Marsden Hospital, Downs Road, Sutton SM2 5PT Tel: 020 8642 6011; 8 Salisbury House, Bessborough Gardens, Pimlico, London SW1V 2HJ Tel: 020 7821 0350 — Ptychio Iatrikes Thessalonika 1988. Hon. Sen. Regist. (Haemat.) Roy. Marsden Hosp.; Hon. Regist. (Haemat.) St. Geo. Hosp. Med. Sch. Lond. Specialty: Haematology.

ZOOB, Betty Constance (retired) 5 Kenbrook House, Kensington High St., London W14 8NY Tel: 020 7602 3329 — MB BS Lond. 1944 (Lond. Sch. Med. Wom.) Prev: Clin. Asst. Bloomsbury Rheumat. Unit. Arthur Stanley Ho. Lond.

ZOON, Elizabeth 137 Humberston Avenue, Humberston, Grimsby DN36 4ST — Artsexamen Rotterdam 1989.

ZORAB, John Stanley Mornington (retired) Holmray Cottage, Park Street, Iron Acton, Bristol BS37 9UJ Tel: 01454 228757 Fax: 01454 228295 Email: jzorab@compuserve.com — (Guy's) MRCS Eng. LRCP Lond. 1956; DA Eng. 1959; FFA RCS Eng. 1963. Emerit. Cons. Anaesth. Frenchay Hosp. Bristol. Prev: Cons. Anaesth. & Med. Dir. Frenchay Hosp. Bristol.

ZORAB, Walter John (retired) Flat 18, Village Gate, Southampton Hill, Fareham PO14 4BJ Tel: 01327 847351 — (King's Coll. Hosp.) MRCS Eng. LRCP Lond. 1939. Prev: Ho. Phys. (Midw. & Anaesth.) White Lodge Hosp. Newmarket.

ZORIC, Bozena St Peter's Hospital, Guilford Road, Chertsey KT16 0PZ — MD Zagreb 1982; MRCP (UK) 1987; MSc Lond. 1996. Cons. Paediat. Specialty: Paediat. Prev: Sen. Regist. (Paediat.) Soton.; Regist. Nottm. City Hosp.; Research Fell. (Paediat.) MRC Nottm.

ZOSMER, Nurit Ratzoni Samuel 5 Western Avenue, London NW11 9HG — MD Tel Aviv, Israel 1983.

ZOTKIEWICZ, Marek Jozef Bentcliffe, 9 Devonshire Road, Hope, Salford M6 8HY — MB ChB Manch. 1982; BSc (Hons.) Manch. 1979. Dir. of Health Care Servs. HM Prisons Garth & Wymott Leyland, Preston. Specialty: Civil Serv.

ZOUKOS, Ioannis Darent Valley Hospital, Darenth Wood Road, Dartford DA2 8DA — Ptychio Iatrikes Athens 1982. Cons. Neurol. Darent Valley Hosp. Dartfd. Specialty: Neurol.

ZSIGMOND, Andrew Consulting Rooms, 43 Rodney Street, Liverpool L1 9EW Tel: 0151 709 7441 Fax: 0151 708 0526 Email: doctor@zsigmond.co.uk — MRCS Eng. LRCP Lond. 1962 (Liverp.) Cert Av Med MoD (Air) & CAA; Aviat. Auth. 1974; MFOM RCP Lond. 1979. Authorised Med. Examr. Civil Aviat. Auth., Fed. Aviat. Admin. & Civil Aviat. Auth., Canada; Med. Examr. RAF Liverp.; Asbestos Cons. Liverp. Specialty: Occupat. Health; Aviat. Med. Socs: (Ex-Pres.) Liverp. Med. Inst. 1995-96; (Ex-Chairm.) Assn. Aviat. Med. Examrs. 1998-2000. Prev: Ho. Phys. Walton Hosp. Liverp.; Ho. Surg. (Orthop.) Roy. South. Hosp. Liverp.; SHO (Radiother.) Clatterbridge Hosp. Bebington.

ZU SOLMS-BARUTH, Caroline-Mathilde Elisabeth (retired) Barn Cottage, The Green, Bledington, Chipping Norton OX7 6XQ — MB ChB Stellenbosch 1961; MSc Cape Town 1955. Prev: GP Banbury.

ZUBAIRU, Mohammad Bankole The Health Centre, Braithwell Road, Maltby, Rotherham S66 8JE Tel: 01709 798822 — Vrach 1st Leningrad Med. Inst. USSR 1972. Socs: BMA & Soc. Occupat. Med. Prev: Area Sen. Med. Off. S. Yorks. Brit. Coal; Dep. Area Med. Off. S. Midl. Area Nat. Coal Bd.; Regist. (A & E & Orthop.) N. Lincs. HA.

ZUBAIRY, Mr Aamir East Lancashire NHS Trust, Burnley General Hospital, Casterton Avenue, Burnley BB10 2PQ Tel: 01282 475227 Fax: 01282 474848; Abbey Gisburne Park Hospital, Gisburn, Clitheroe BB7 4HX Tel: 01200 445693 — MB BS Karachi 1987; FRCS (Trauma & Orth.); FRCSI. Specialty: Trauma & Orthop. Surg. Special Interest: Foot and ankle Surg. Socs: MDU. Prev: Cons. Orthopaedic Surg. Burnley Gen. Hosp.

ZUBERI, Mohammad Mustafa, CBE 1A Davenham Avenue, Northwood HA6 3HW — MB BS Punjab (Pakistan) 1953 (King Edwd. Med. Coll. Lahore) DPH Lond. 1964; DIH Eng. 1968; FFOM RCP Lond. 1986. Cons. Occupat. Health Medicentres, Lond. Specialty: Occupat. Health. Socs: Soc. Occupat. Med. Prev: Cons. Occupat. Health BUPA Occupat. Health; Med. Adviser Health Policy Health & Safety Exec.; Regional Dir. & Dep. Dir. Med. Servs. Health & Safety Exec.

ZUBERI, Sameer Mustafa Fraser of Allander Neurosciences Unit, Royal Hospital for Sick Children, Yorkhill, Glasgow G3 8SJ Tel: 0141 201 0141 Fax: 0141 201 9270 Email: sameer.zuberi@ntlworld.com/ sameer.zuberi@yorkhill.scot.nhs.uk — MB ChB Ed. 1989; MRCP (UK) 1992; MRCPH 1997. Cons. (Paediat. Neurol.) Roy. Hosp. Sick Childr. Glas.; Hon. Sen. Lect. in Child Health, Univ. of Glas. Specialty: Paediat. Neurol. Socs: Roy. Coll. Phys. Edin.; MRCPCH; Brit. Paediat. Neurol. Assn.

ZUBIER, Mustafa Mohammed — MB BCh Al Fateh 1991. Cons. (Paediat.) Hull Roy. Infirm. Specialty: Paediat.

ZUCK, David (retired) Craigower, St. Andrew's Close, Woodside Avenue, London N12 8BA Tel: 020 8445 4685 Email: n2o@dsl.pipex.com — MB ChB Birm. 1945; FRCA 1988; DA Eng. 1948; FFA RCS Eng. 1953; DHMSA Lond. 1975. Hon. Cons. Anaesth. Enfield Dist. Prev: Capt. RAMC Graded Anaesth.

ZUCKERMAN, Professor Arie Jeremy Royal Free & University College Medical School, Royal Free Campus, Rowland Hill St., London NW3 2PF Tel: 020 7830 2579 Fax: 020 7830 2070 — MB BS (Hons) Lond. 1957 (Roy. Free) MRCS Eng. LRCP Lond. 1957; DObst RCOG 1958; MD Lond. 1963; FRCPath 1977, M 1965; Dip. Bact (Distinc.) 1965; MSc (Genetics.) Birm. 1962, BSc (Hons.) 1953, DSc (Experim. Path.) 1973; FRCP Lond. 1982, M 1978; FMedSci 1998. Prof. Med. Microbiol. Univ. Lond.; Dir. WHO Collaborating Centre for Ref. & Research on Viral Dis.; Edr.-in-Chief Jl. Med. Virol. & Jl. Virol. Methods. Specialty: Med. Microbiol. Socs: Soc. Gen. Microbiol.; Amer. Assn. Study Liver Dis. Prev: Cons. Med. Microbiol.

Roy. Free. Hampstead NHS Trust; Prof. Virol. Univ. Lond.; Dir. Anthony Nolan Bone Marrow Trust.

ZUCKERMAN, Charles Howard Zuckerman, Felderhof and Ali, Northfield Health Centre, 15 St Heliers Road, Birmingham B31 1QT — MB BS Lond. 1971; DObst RCOG 1975; DCH Eng. 1975; FRCGP 1993, M 1976. Sec. Birm. LMC. Prev: Regist. Guy's Hosp. Lond.; Ho. Surg. St. Pancras Hosp. Lond.; Ho. Phys. St. Jas. Hosp. Lond.

ZUCKERMAN, Jane Nicola Royal Free & University College Medical School, London NW3 2PF Tel: 020 7830 2999 Fax: 020 7830 2268 Email: j.zuckerman@rfc.ucl.ac.uk — MB BS Lond. 1987; MD Lond. 1996; MFPM Lond. (Roy. Coll. Phys.) 2000; FFPM Lond. (Roy. Coll. Phys.) 2002; FBiol. 2003; FRCPath 2003. Head & Hon. Cons. Acad. Cent. Travel Med. & Vaccines; Med. Director Clin. Trials Centre, Roy. Free & Univ. Coll. Med.; Dir. Clin. Trials Cent. Roy. Free & Univ. Coll. Med. Sch.; Sen. Lect. & Elective Tutor Roy. Free & Univ. Coll. Med. Sch., Lond.; Med. Dir. The Roy. Free Travel Health Centre. Specialty: Infec. Dis.; Trop. Med.; Pharmaceutical Medicine. Socs: Brit. Assn. Pharmaceut. Med. Res. Soc.; RCP UK Fac. of Pharmaceutical Med.; Brit. Infec. Soc. Prev: Sen. Research Fell. Roy. Free Hosp. Sch. Med. Lond.; Clin. Research Fell. Occupat. Health Unit Roy. Free Hosp. Lond.; Regist. & SHO (A & E & ITU) Roy. Free Hosp. Lond.

ZUCKERMAN, Mark Adam Health Protection Agency, London & London South Specialist Virology Centre, King's College Hospital, King's College School of Medicine & Dentistry, East Dulwich Grove, London SE22 8QF Tel: 020 8693 3005 — MB BS Lond. 1985 (Univ. Coll. Hosp.) MSc (Clin. Microbiol. Lond.) 1990, BSc (1st cl. Hons. Microbiol.) 1980; MRCP (UK) 1989; MRCPath 1993; FRCPath 2001. Cons. Virol. & Hon. Sen. Lect. Dulwich PHL & Med. Microbiol. King's Coll. Sch. of Med. & Dent. Specialty: Virology. Prev: Regist. (Med. Microbiol.) The Lond. Hosp.; SHO (Med.) Ipswich Gen. Hosp.; Ho. Surg. Stoke Mandeville Hosp.

ZUHA, Roslin 3 The Paddock, Hove BN3 6LT — MB BS Lond. 1994.

ZUHRIE, Shadman Riaz Northwick Park & St Mark's NHS Trust, Watford Rd, Harrow HA1 3UJ Tel: 020 8235 4231 Fax: 020 8426 6002 Email: rzuhrie@mds.qmw.ac.uk; 16 Duffield Close, Harrow HA1 2LG Tel: 020 8424 0160 — MB BS Poona 1971 (Armed Forces Med. Coll.) PhD Lond. 1991. MRC Clin. Scientist & Hon. Clin. Assist. Med., Northwich Pk. & St Mark's NHS Trust Middlx. Socs: MBA; BMS (Menopause Soc.); SSM (Social Medium). Prev: MRC Clin. Scientist & Hon Sen. Regist. MRC, Epidemiol. Med. Care Unit. St Bart. Hosp. Lond.; Research Regist. Clin. Immune Defic. Dis. Research Gp., MRC Clin. Research Centre, Northwich Pk. Hosp. Middlx.

ZUK, Ronald Joseph Department of Histopathology, Monklands District General Hospital, Monkscourt Avenue, Airdrie ML6 0JS — MB ChB Dundee 1981; BMSc (Hons.) Dundee 1978; MRCPath 1989.

ZULUETA MADINABEITIA, Luis Sandwell District General Hospital, West Bromwich B71 4HJ Tel: 0121 553 1831; 39 Avern Close, Tipton DY4 7ND Tel: 0121 557 3991 — LMS Basque Provinces 1989. Clin. Asst. (Anaesth.) Sandwell Dist. Gen. Hosp. W. Bromwich. Specialty: Anaesth. Prev: Clin. Asst. Geo. Eliot Hosp. Nuneaton; SHO Sandwell Dist. Gen. Hosp.

ZUMLA, Professor Alimuddin Royal Free University College London Medical School, Centre for Infectious Diseases, Windeyer, Institute Room G41, 46 Cleveland St., London W1T 4JF Tel: 020 7679 9187 Fax: 020 7679 9311 Email: a.zumla@ucl.ac.uk — MB ChB Zambia 1979; BSc Zambia 1976; MSc Lond. 1981; MRCP Lond. 1984; PhD Lond. 1987; FRCP Lond. 1995; FRCP Ed. 1999. Prof. of Infec. Dis. & Int. Health Univ. Coll. Lond., Roy. Free & Univ. Coll. Med. Sch.; Cons. Phys. (Infec. Dis.) Univ. Coll. Lond. Hosps. Trust; Hon. Prof. Inst. of Child Health Lond. Specialty: Infec. Dis.; HIV Med.; Trop. Med. Socs: Internat. Union Against Tuberc. & Lung Dis.; Brit. Soc. Immunol.; Fell. Roy. Soc. Trop. Med. Hyg. Prev: Vis. Prof. & Utzam Dir. Sch. Med. Univ. Zambia; Assoc. Prof. Centre for Infec. Dis. Univ. Texas, Houston, USA; Sen. Regist. (Clin. Immunol. & Rheum.) & Hon. Lect. Roy. Postgrad. Med. Sch.

ZUREK, Andrew Alexander Antoni — MB ChB Ed. 1964; MRCGP 1976. Prev: Hon. Clin. Lect. (Med.) Univ. Liverp.; Sen. Clin. Lect. (Gen. Pract.) Univ. Liverp.

ZUREK, Andrew Maria — MB BChir Camb. 1991; MRCP (UK) 1994. Cons. in Respirat. and Gen. Med., Roy. Berks. and Battle Hosps. NHS Trust, Reading. Specialty: Respirat. Med. Prev: SpR (Respiratory Medicine) S.W. Deanery; Clinical Research Fellow/Hon. Registrar (Respiratory Medicine) Soton. University.

ZURICK, Natasha Jane Weald Cottage, Sheerwater Avenue, Woodham, Addlestone KT15 3DP — MB ChB Bristol 1994; BSc Bristol 1991.

ZURUB, Amer Ahmad Health Centre, High Street, Bedworth, Nuneaton CV12 8NQ Tel: 024 7631 5432 Fax: 024 7631 0038; 17 Chilworth Close, The Poplars, Nuneaton CV11 4XE Tel: 01203 351363 Email: amer@zurub.freeserve.co.uk — MB BCh BAO NUI 1988 (RCSI) LRCPSI 1988. Socs: Med. Protec. Soc.

ZUTSHI, Derek Wyndham 36 Eton Court, Eton Avenue, Hampstead, London NW3 3HJ Tel: 020 7722 6316 — MB ChB Bristol 1957; DObst RCOG 1959; FRCP Lond. 1991, M 1967. Specialty: Rehabil. Med.; Rheumatol. Socs: Fell. Roy. Soc. Med.; Fell. (Ex-Pres.) Hunt. Soc.; Fell (Ex-Counc.) Med. Soc. Lond. Prev: Cons. Phys. Rheum. P. of Wales' & St. Ann's Hosps. Lond.; Sen. Regist. (Rheum.) Lond. Hosp.; Ho. Phys. Profess. Med. Unit Bristol Roy. Infirm.

ZUTSHI, Mr Mohan Krishen 9 Meyricks, Coed Eva, Cwmbran NP44 6TU Tel: 01633 675421 Fax: 01633 675421; 57 Priory Gardens, Ealing, London W5 1DY Tel: 020 8997 4198 — MB BS Agra 1957 (S.N. Med. Coll.) FRCS Glas. 1967 FRCS Ed. 1966; FRCS Eng. 1969; FICS 1973. Specialty: Gen. Surg. Socs: Fell. Roy. Soc. Med.; BMA. Prev: Regist. (Surg.) Gen. Hosp. Burton-on-Trent; Sen. Cons. Surg. & Head (Surg.) Gen. Hosp. Pondicherry, India & St. Martha's Hosp. Bangalore, India.

ZUTSHI, Risheshwar Nath (retired) 40 Villiers Crescent, Eccleston, St Helens WA10 5HR Tel: 01744 27177 — BSc (Allahabad India) 1942; MB BS Lucknow 1948. Prev: GP St. Helens.

ZWAAL, Jacob Willem Kingston Hospital, Department of Anaesthetics, Galsworthy Road, Kingston upon Thames KT2 7QB. Cons. (Anaesth.) Kingston Hosp. Specialty: Anaesth.

ZWARTOUW, Carol Louise Rosser and Partners, Crewkerne Health Centre, Middle Path, Crewkerne TA18 8BX Tel: 01460 72435 Fax: 01460 77957; Little Plot, Silver St, Misterton, Crewkerne TA18 8NG — MB BS Lond. 1978; DRCOG 1981; DA Eng. 1981.

ZWI, Morris — MB BCh Witwatersrand 1982; Hon. FRCPsych; MRCPsych 1989; Diploma in Systematic Reviews Methodology UCL 2000. Cons. Child & Adolesc. Psychiat. S. W. Lond. & St George's Ment. Health NHS Trust Richmond Roy. Hosp. Specialty: Child & Adolesc. Psychiat. Special Interest: Attention deficit hyperactivity disorder; Epidemiol.; Evidence-based Pract. Socs: Centre for Evidence Based Ment. Health; Child Psychiat. Research Soc. Prev: Sen. Regist. Child & Adolesc. Psychiat., N. W. Thames Rotat.; Regist. Psychiat., Barnet Rotat.

ZWINK, Patricia Jessie Swan Woodthorpe, St. Mary's Avenue, London E11 — MB ChB St. And. 1944.

ZWINK, Mr Roger Bryan Accident & Emergency Department, Broomfield Hospital, Chelmsford CM1 7ET Tel: 01245 514601 Fax: 01245 514223 Email: roger.zwink@meht.nhs.uk — MB BCh Wales 1981 (Welsh Nat. Sch. Med.) BDS Wales 1972; FDS RCS Eng. 1976; FRCS Ed. 1987; FFAEM 1994. Cons. (A & E) Broomfield Hosp. Chelmsford; Recognised Clin. Teach. Univ of Camb. Sch. of Clin. Med.; Regional Advis. N. Thames (E.) Fac. of Accid. & Emerg. Med. Specialty: Accid. & Emerg. Prev: Sen. Regist. (A & E) Oldch. Hosp. Romford; Regist. (Oral & Maxillofacial Surg.) Welsh Nat. Sch. of Med. Cardiff.

ZYCH, Zdenek Princess Alexandra Hospital, Harlow CM20 1QX Tel: 01279 444455 — MRCS Eng. LRCP Lond. 1970; DA Eng. 1972; FFA RCS Eng. 1974. Specialty: Anaesth.

ZYGMUNT, Professor Stefan Carol Queen Elizabeth Hospital, Department of Neurosurgery, Queen Elizabeth Medical Centre, Edgbaston, Birmingham B15 2TH — Lakarexamen Linkoping 1977. Cons. Neurosurg. Qu. Eliz. Hosp. Birm. Specialty: Neurosurg.

ZYLSTRA, Heinrich Johan 20 Grange Close, Godalming GU7 1XT — MB ChB Cape Town 1983.

ZZAMAN, Kazi Ansaru Zaman, Marus Bridge Health Centre, Highfield Grange Avenue, Wigan WN3 6SU — MB BS Calcutta 1962.

Index by Postal District: London

Joyce, C
Khan, S A
Lam Kin Teng, L T
Mahendran, S
Manam, A
Moussa, M M H
Munro, M H W
O'Moore, G R
Patel, A
Patel, D
Patel, K I
Patel, Y I
Rafiq, S S
Rashid, Y
Robinson, K A
Ruhi, S O
Sherwood, S M
Sinha, B K
Somorin, A O
Swedan, S K S
Uddin, M M
Vyas, V C
Wood, S A
Yesufu, A O

E8

Ajuied, A
Benn, R S
Cahill, M F A
Caplin, L A
Cooper, S A
Cowley, S J
Darnley, B J M
Fade, P Z
Fontaine, E J
Hendricks, Y J
Heyse-Moore, L H
Highton, R S J
Hopson, A S M
Jackson, K
Jamil, M N
Jarrett, L
Kirton, J L
Marlowe, S N S
Mdingi, G V
Pilkington, A C
Read, J M
Ribeiro, M D C
Sanfey, J J
Senior, R S
Tibrewal, S P
Williams, R D A
Windsor, J P W

E9

Adireddi, V S P
Aitken, M J
Amin, S N
Amos, R J
Aung, S
Balakrishna, J
Bays, S M A
Bhanji, A B
Blanshard, C
Bliss, W H
Boast, N R
Bodenstein, M E
Bothamley, G H
Bower, R C
Britton, M E
Bucknall, J L
Bull, R H
Burns, D A
Charles, H J
Choi, A Y S
Cohen, R M
Costeloe, K L
Cowden, F
Cross, M R
Cullinan, T P
Cumming, I R
Cumming, K J
De Souza, B A
Dean, P J
Dex, E A
Dorman, E K
Elgadi, S M A
Erskine, K J
Fang, S H
Forrester, A
Freedman, P S
Gibson, R J
Green, S C
Guha, M K
Gurtin Zorkun, D
Halfpenny, D M
Hamid, S S
Harrad, J D
Heyman, J
Highton, C R
Holland, M E
Husain, S M
Hutchinson, C J
Jones, P S
Joseph, S
Julian, P A C
Karcher, A M
Kong, K C
Lehmann, A B
Leslie, K S
Lockley, M
McCarthy, D M
Mahir, M S
Mootoo, R V
Mustafa, M
Olusanya, A A A
Parton, S D
Patel, G H
Patel, H G
Payne-James, J J
Peirce, K S
Petterson, L E
Power, L M
Prasad, R
Pugh, G G
Rajakulasingam, K
Ratnam, D S
Rizvi, S P J
Roberts, C H
Roper, J
Salter, M S
Shidrawi, R G
Singer, R
Tang, C P-Y
Taylor, C J A
Tham, L C H
Timmis, P K
Tobias, G J
Tollins, A P
Tunstall Pedoe, D S
Vafaie, K
Van Velsen, C L
Washington, A J
Watson, J D
Yeoman, N C
Zalidis, S

E10

Abora, Y Y
Adams, W
Ali, S M
Allybocus, S A H
Ariff, M H I
Biss, G C
Biswas, A
Bose, K
Casey, D R
Crowe, M B
Das, P K
Das, R
Dhillon, P S
Fernandes, D A
Hafeez, I
Huddart, M J
Kalra, T K K
Kapoor, D
Kapoor, R
Khawaja, S S
Mallick, G
Mallick, K B
Pal, G S
Pandit, S N
Patel, M R
Phillips, S
Radix, J C A
Ramsis, H E
Sen, S K
Singh, J C I
Sun Wai, W Y S
Wey, E Q
Younus, N
Zadoo, K
Zamora Eguiluz, M C

E11

Adam, S A
Adly Habib, N
Ahmed, A U
Aiyegbusi, M
Akin-Olugbade, O
Akramuzzaman, M
Ali, L
Alstead, E M
Amin, M R
Amin, R T
Anderson, C C
Annan, H G
Arulefela, M M
Ashley, E J
Aswani, K
Atando, S W
Aveling, W
Baillie, C T
Balkind, J
Beasley, I F R
Bewley, A P
Bhattacharyya, A K
Bjorndal, E
Bohra, C G
Boruch, L A
Brearley, S
Brent, W M
Bright, C M
Browning, M J
Chalabi, G
Chaudhuri, S
Choudhury, M A H
Cotterill, A M
Crinnion, J N
D'Oyley, D A
Darkwah, J A
Das-Gupta, M
Davies, R J
Davison, R M
Dawda, P
Donnelly, S P
Doshi, S
Doyle, D V
Duncan, B B A
Duthie, A
Ezekwesili, R A
Fagin, L H
Ferdinandus, E L C
Frankel, E
Gadhvi, H M
Gauci, C A
Gibbon, K L
Gilmour, R F
Goldie, B S
Hamilton-Farrell, M R
Hassan, S
Hasslocher, D
Hines, J E W
Hird, K H
Hogan, J C
Holden, S T R
Hollingworth, A A
Hotton, M E
Hunt, M T
Hurley, P D
Hussain, K
Hussain, S A
Hutchings, A
Islam, A K M S
Jacklin, M C
Jacobs, D S
Jain, C
Jestico, J V
Kafetz, K M
Kavanagh, M
Kenyon, G S
Khan, H N
Khan, M A
Khan, M S H
Khan, N
Kiyani, T M
Kolosinska, Z S
Lamba, M S
Lim, S C
Littler, B O
Louis, N
McElligott, G M F
Mansi, E G
Matthews, W C
Meadows, C I S
Melville, R L
Muir-Taylor, J H
Norris, G F
O'Callaghan, E M
O'Carroll, A-M
O'Farrell, J M
Owen, R A
Pahwa, B K
Peters, J L
Prabhu-Palav, S S
Rattan, D S
Ray, N
Reading, N G
Reed, A R
Rees, D G
Roberts, C M
Robinson, S E
Russell, S S
Samuel, M
Sandhu, S S
Savla, N C
Sawyerr, A M
Sharma, P
Siggins, P C
Silas, A M
Singh, R
Singh, T
Sloczynska, C W
Soole, M J
Stables, A B J
Storring, R A
Sudderuddin, A
Taylor, R F H
Thomas, P A
Togobo, A K
Towler, H M A
Tranmer, L S
Travers, W J E
Walshe, M B A
Wijeyekoon, S P
Williams, D V
Willson, L A H
Youssef, H A E F E S
Zambarakji, H J

E12

Alagrajah, P
Ambris, M G
Dalrymple, A
Dhariwal, S K
Ethell, M E
Farnham, F R
Gopakumar, C G
Graham, P
Gunathilagan, G J
Hussain, A A
Jones, P T C
Mridha, K B
Mridha, M S A
Nasralla, A H K
Ojagbemi, F O
Pople, A R
Raina, C P
Ramesh, N
Rees, J E
Sai Sankar, N
Shekar, S
Shetty, M K
Sohi, M S
Staunton, T H F
Sullman, B
Thirumamanivannan, G
Vijaya, V
Zamanthangi, J M

E13

Abbas, K F
Addai, S A
Ahmed, A U
Ahmed, Z
Al-Mudallal, G B
Andrew, C J
Baffour-Kodua, M O A
Basu, I
Basu, S K
Beaver, M R
Bewaji, A F
Bhagrath, M S
Bhatti, H U
Brown, R C M
Bulusu, S
Buscombe, J A
Chaudhuri, B B
De Las Heras Garcia, L
Dolan, T G
Faire, G M
Gelding, S V
George, G H M
Gonsai, R B
Gwynne, M V P
Halberstadt, I
Hallam, P L
Hanmer, O J
Higgins, R G
Kalhoro, S
Ko, M L B
Le Fur, R
Leung, Y-L
Littlejohns, D W
McGhee, T D
Madipalli, S
Maplethorpe, R P
Maynard, A H
Mihaimeed, F M A
Naftalin, A A
O'Shaughnessy, T C
Oliver, J M
Packe, G E
Patel, J
Pauleau, A
Pradhan, V S
Princewill, O M
Rao, M V
Röhricht, F M
Sahin, A
Silverman, L S
Smith, R F A
Suliman, A M H
Tan, K M
Ugochukwu, U O
Umrani, W M
Velupillai, S
Venugopal, R
Vijayaraghavan, S
Wilson, G E
Wisdom, A R
Zakaria, A K M

E14

Absolon, C M
Adusu-Donkor, A
Allred, J E
Atkin, P A
Baker, C J
Bari, N
Barraclough, M A
Belsey, J D
Bennett-Richards, P J
Betteridge, C L M
Boomla, K R F
Chandr-Ruang-Phen, P
Cheeroth, S A
Chok, S L-M
Chong, C F
Cirolli, R G M
Crombie, J L
Daniels, B J
Dobbing, C J
Doig, K M
Douglas, N A
Empeslidis, T
Epstein, L J
Farrand, S R
Fitchett, M J
Fraser, K E
Hall, G J
Harrison, C
John, C R
Kayzakian, A M
Ketley, J B
Khan, Z A
Kinsler, R A
Kirby, D A
Lamb, P M
Lee, S
Linford, S
Livingstone, A E
Lunniss, P J
McAteer, E J
MacGreevy, B M C
Mahajan, V D
Nagrath, K D
Nandy, S K
Owa, A O
Parsons, S L F
Pietroni, T L
Playford, V J
Porter, H
Qureshi, T M
Ray, N L
Richardson, J R
Robson, J P
Sarkar, B
Schilling, C J
Self, J E
Sharma, A
Shukla, A C
Siriwardena, D K
Speldewinde, D C M
Taylor, J R
Thormod, C E
Vickers, A R
Walton, S
Whitley, T B H
Wigmore, T J
Wood, J B

E15

Bhowmik, P R
Brohi, A Q
Chang, M K L
Fleming, M E
Khan, M S J
Lalude, O A
Najam Ud Din, Dr
Ojuro, I V
Pashankar, D S
Pashankar, F D
Qadri, A Q
Rahman, A R
Shah, A M
Stacey, S J
Uzoka, K A O
Verma, U K

E16

Adedeji, E A
Adeyemi, M S
Comyns, M J
De Cocq, D F F
Edginton, S
Jones, J O E
Lwin, T
Ornadel, D
Patel, B P
Quigley, I G
Ryanna, K B W
Saha, M
Sehra, R T
Seneviratne, G N
Seneviratne, K B C
Shore, E M
Siddiqui, N
Zarifa, Z K

E17

Akuffo, E O
Arasaradnam, R P
Arastu, N
Bailey, J
Barnes, N R
Belton, P A
Birrell, W L
Bishop, R A
Coomarasamy, D
Cooney, S
Darko, K
Deva, A
Dhital, R P
Garelick, A I
Gracias, C J L
Gupta, R K
Gupta, U
Horne, A D
Huda, M F
Ibrahim, A
Isaacs, S
Jabbar, F
Jethwa, R N
John, T M
Kariyawasam, H H
Kawar, P M
Khalid, A F A
King, C A J
Lindall, S
Malhotra, A K
Malik, Z I
Monteiro, R F
Omololu, A G
Oraelosi, F N O
Parsons, M A
Payne, H A
Rajput, P B
Ray, J C
Reeve, A C
Rowse, N J
Seedat, N I
Shah, M R
Shah, R B
Shantir, D Y A-R
Sheikh, A Q
Siddiqui, A M
Sinason, M D A
Sowemimo, G M
Stearn, A C
Stearns, E J E
Stolar, M
Subramanian, P B
Sureshkumar, T
Swedan, H I
Tennekoon, M
Yanah, D K

E18

Atun, R A
Barrett, A A
Chard, D T
Collins, J A
Dempsey, C M
Dus, V
Edwards, J G
Elliott, P R
Franklin, J J
Hanley, M L
Hines, K C
Howlett, S F J
Johannsson, H E
Karim, M R
Kulhalli, V

McNeill, J M
Masani, V D
Munjal, S
Nokes, T J C
Penfield, B
Philp, T
Rather, G M
Ryan, J M
Shah, M V
Shaw, S A
Smith, S D
Staley, M
Stapley, M L
Thompson, AV
Webster, F
Wolkind, S N
Yaqub, S U
Yaqub, Z U
Zaidi, F H
Zaidi, Z H

EC1
Abdelaziz, M M
Abdullah, S
Abrams, S M L
Addison, P K F
Amoroso, P
Anderson, J
Anderson, J V
Andrea-Barron, D R
Andreou, P S
Angell-James, J E
Armstrong, P
Arora, A
Assi, A
Baines, P S
Banim, S O
Barton, K
Beaconsfield, M
Bessant, D A R
Bird, A C
Born, G V R
Brelen, H M
Britton, K E
Bruce, T J R
Buchholz, N P
Buckley, R J
Carr, C A
Carter, J L B
Catarino, P A S D R A
Cavenagh, J D
Charteris, D G
Chew, S L
Clark, A J L
Coakley, J H
Coghlan, K M
Coid, J W
Coleman, K A
Cooke, E D
Cooling, R J
Coombes, A G A
Cordeiro, M F
Cottrill, C P
Crake, T
Dambo, K U
Daniel, R D
Dart, J K G
Das, S S
Dauncey, M K
Davies, A J
Davies, N P
Dickinson, C J
Dilkes, M G
Dinan, T G
Domizio, P
Doust, P J
Dowler, J G F
Drake, W M
Driver, H E
Earnshaw, G
Evans, S I R
Farrugia, D C
Ficker, L A
Fielder, A R
Franks, W A
Gallagher, C J
Galton, D J
Gartry, D S
Gattuso, J M
Geoghegan, C J
Ghufoor, K
Glenn, M S
Goldstone, A P
Gormley, F C
Granowska, M
Greenhough, S G
Grossman, A B
Guymer, R H
Hajioff, S
Halliday-Bell, J A
Hardie, R M
Harris-Jones, R D L
Hemming, A E
Hincks, S S M
Hinds, C J
Howell, P R
Hulbert, M F G
Hutchison, I L
Ihenacho, A O
Ionides, A C W
Jacks, A S
James, J A
Jeffries, D J
Jenkins, P J
Jeyarajah, A R
Johnson, C-A
Johnson, G J
Johnston, L B
Jurek, P M P
Kadim, M Y
Kamal, D S
Kelsey, S M
Khaw, P-T
Kon, C H
Kurbaan, A S
Kwan, S L A
Landers, A M
Langford, R M
Larkin, D F
Lehmann, E D
Lehmann, O J
Leslie, R D G
Levene, R
Lightman, S L
Lister, T A
Litchfield, P
Lockwood, C M
Loh, C P L
Lower, A M
Lugone, H A
Luthert, P J
MacCallum, P K
MacGregor, E A
MacIntyre, I
McLaren, D S
McLean, A M
McNeish, A S
Mair, G H M
Menzies, R C
Miller, G J
Miller, N E
Mirakian, R M
Monson, J P
Moodaley, L C M
Moore-Gillon, J C
Mulholland, B
Murdoch, I E
Nagendran, K
Nargund, V H
Neaman, G M
Newell-Price, J D C
Nockler, I B
Nolan, W P
Norton, A J
Nutting, C M
O'Byrne, S R T
Odufuwa-Bolger, T O
Okhravi, N
Oliver, R T D
Ong, K-B
Oza, A M
Parkin, J M
Parmar, D N
Patel, H K B
Patel, P
Patterson, L J
Pearson, R M
Perry, N M
Phillips, C F
Powell, M E B
Pozzilli, P
Prior, P F
Pritchard, N C B
Propper, D J
Quigley, C S M
Rao, K A
Rimmer, B K
Rodriguez Arnao, J
Ruckert, L A L
Rudd, R M
Sauvage, J A M
Savage, M O
Schilling, R J
Schwartz, E C
Sethi, A S
Shah, P
Shamash, J
Sharma, K K
Shepherd, J H
Shingadia, D V
Sigston, P E
Smith, L F F
Steele, J P C
Stevens, J D
Sullivan, P M P
Thexton, P J
Tho, J H
Thomas, G P L
Tuft, S J
Turner, T H
Vasserman, D
Verity, D H
Vinnicombe, S J
Viswalingam, N D
Viswanathan, A C
Wald, N J
Watkiss, J B
Wedzicha, J A
Wells, C A
Wells, P
White, D P
White, D A
White, P D
Whitmore, A V
Wilkins, M R
Wilkinson, D J
Williams, C M
Wilson, P
Wood, A J
Wormald, R P L
Young, I M
Zeidan, M
Zelin, J M

EC2
Bell, P A
Brackenridge, R D C
Brown, S E
Collier, P M
Cowie, C M
Dark, C H
Evans, M R E
Fletcher, C L
Forman, C W
Griffiths, M A
Hanly, J F
Harvey, A M
House, J M
Kelly, D
Landon, J
Lumley, J S P
Lyons, V L
Macaulay, D E S
McRae, S C C
Makings, E A
Morganstein, D
Reid, H L M
Richards, J M
Royan, C N
Roythorne, C
Stacey, A C E
Tay, E S W
Terry, A E
Wallington, D M
Walsh, D I
Wilcox, D T
Wildman, S M C

EC3
Arnison-Newgass, P
Boylan, T M
Chesney, R
Cunningham, G A B
Guider, P J
Lohn, M S
McGrath, J G
Macleod, G A
O'Donoghue, M G
Spier, G W
Thompsell, A A B
Vaile, E
Webb-Wilson, G J

EC4
Agius-Ferrante, M-T
Black, A J M
Campbell, I D
Cooper, J R B
Cunard, M A
Dawood, R M
Ferrante, A M A
Friston, M H
Gill, C R W
Paul, M
Pollock, E M M
Samaratunga, V S
Solomon, F S
Taylor, S W

N1
Addous, A
Addy, N
Adrangi, B
Asteriades, H E
Bain, B J
Banerjea, P
Bannerman-Lloyd, F
Barkham, D W
Barton, A C G
Baumgarten, S
Beaumont, B R
Bethapudy, S R
Bhargava, A
Bhatti, N
Blackwood, N J
Bloor, I A M
Booth, P J
Boyd, N R H
Brooker, C B
Bunt, R J
Candlin, R E
Casson, D H
Cattell, C A
Chan Tun Lun, A-F
Chapman, M J
Chianelli, M
Cikurel, K
Clements, E A F
Cochrane, G A
Cohen, B
Colvin, D R
Connolly, J O
Cranitch, J A
Dacie, J E
Dana, E C
Davies, S
De Couteau, M E
Dean, A D
Deighan, J
Dixon, J A
Duggan, P J
Dunn, J M
Eigener, K F E
Evans, J P M
Evans, R C
Fahey, J D
Fidler, S J
Findley, I L
Fleetwood, M E
Foster, P M M
Fox, B D
Franks, L M
Fuller, J H S
Garway-Heath, D F G
Gillies, L
Gillis, S
Giwa, S O
Goldberg, R G
Gore, J C P
Grandison, A L
Gupta, N
Hagdrup, N A
Hai, S A
Harrison, S M
Hassim, C E
Haughey, S J
Henry, J
Hickling, J A
Hillman, K A
Hodes, D T
Holland, M W
Hollander, R
Hopkins, R J
Hossain, A
Howling, S J
Hunter, J V
Hurwitz, B S
Hutchins, R R
Indapurkar, N R
Jacks, M E
James, I G
Jeffcote, N A
Jenkins, S M
Kavanagh, J
Khazne Charimo, Z
Kouimtsidis, C
Kouvarellis, D S
Laban, C A
Laing, G J
Lambert, C
Liu, R S N
Livingston, J P
Lloyd-Owen, S J
Lloyd, J K
Loud, S G
MacBean, A L
McCartney, P R
McGilligan, J A
McGoldrick, S
McLoughlin, I C
Maheswaran, M
Marley, R T C
Marshall, J S
Meerstadt, P W D
Miflin, G K
Mills, S M
Milner, Q J W
Montemagno, R
Moody, J M
Morgans, M E
Mummery, D F
Narayanan, S
O'Connor, P D H
O'Driscoll, C M
O'Rourke, L E
Pandit, A
Pilston, M J
Pote, A H
Pracy, J P M
Qureshi, R N
Roberts, J V
Rottenberg, G T
Roy, S
Sattar, D A
Scott, L V
Seal, D V
Sennett, K J
Shanson, R L
Shiels, A M
Simon, R D B
Skalicka, A
Skelly, C M
Slater, N D
Smillie, D C
Soldi, D F
Sowdager, A
Spackman, D R
Speight, L
Stacey, C M
Stafford, C J
Stibe, E
Stirland, A M
Summerfield, K E
Sutherland, C J
Taylor, J F
Thompson, P B
Tibble, M J K
Umaria, N
Varley, B Q
Weinbren, H
Wise, D
Wiseman, S M
Wollaston, S L
Wright, J L
Wykes, C B
Young, K

N2
Abrams, A B
Akita, A G M
Anderson, L D
Andrews, S J
Assem, E-S K E-S A
Baker, L D
Bloomer, J M
Braham, A N
Brooks, H R
Camara, B S
Chataway, S J S
Dakin, P K
Davies, G J
Dezateux, C A
Ehigie-Osifo, E
Ellis, H
Fairhead, I A
Fox, M F R
Freaker, W A
Gibeon, S
Goldberg, A A J
Gregson, R S I
Hanouka, A
Ioannou, N
Isenberg, L A
Jacobs, J J
Josephs, I
Kashi, I
Kelly, T
Kreel, L
Leigh, M E M
Levin, P D
Livingston, G A
Lucas, R N
McNicol, F J
Matharu, M S
Mellins, R A
Mouchizadeh, J
Naidoo, R O M
Nathan, N L
Osrin, D
Poncia, J R
Powell, A
Prasad, V
Rabin, N K
Salkind, M R
Samad, E M A-M
Samanta-Laughton, M
Shadwell, R N
Shore, P M
Singarayer, K N
Singer, A
Slesenger, J P
Spencer, M J
Steinberg, S D
Sutton, V E
Tailor, R
Tang, S C
Tarnesby, G M S
Timmis, J B
Tobin, J A
Tong, T
Tong, T
Twena, D M
Ugboma, I A F
Wagner, S D
Wai, A S-Y
Wilcox, T
Wilkinson, A H
Wong Kam-Kee, S
Wong, G J W S
Wood, G

N3
Bangham, C E
Beatus, D
Bejekal, R A
Bradley, J J
Cavendish, J A
Chak, M H G
Chan, A H
Chandrapal, K E
Chowdhury, N I
Christodoulou, A A
Desai, S R
Durden, N P
Dvorkin, L S
Elton, N K
Elton, C
Fernandez, R
Foley, C L
Foley, P E
Giannoulatos, S
Gibbons, E M
Gilbert, A
Gimmack, G
Hague, D E
Hamzah-Sendut, I
Harkin, E J
Hart, C A
Herxheimer, A
Herxheimer, J C G
Ismail, A R
Kazemi, A-R
Keane, P M
Keidan, I J
Khan, S
Kochhar, N
Levin, G E
Mehta, P
Melnick, S C
Meltzer, M L
Mohamed, R
Mooncey, S
Morris, N H
Mumtaz, F H
Mumtaz, T
Nataraju, M R
Okonkwo, N A
Patel, A
Patel, N
Pattni, T A
Perkins, A L
Popat, U R
Prasad, S
Rahman, F A
Ramachandran, M
Rashid, A H
Rathore, C K
Rees, H L
Robinson, A C
Rosswick, R P
Rowlands, A E
Sadana, A
Scott, B D

Scott, K
Shah, L D
Shah, M
Shah, V P
Sperber, G
Stacey, S M
Talwatte, B Y
Talwatte, D B B
Thangaraj, I L
Tonucci, D F M
Varnava, A M D
Vigano, P C
Vyas, D K
Wang, R Z
Watkins, G O
Weyman, C
Winship, A Z
Wong, T-S
Yiu, H-S R

N4
Alam, M S
Ali, M
Amarasena, G A C
Anyamene, N A
Arfeen, Z-U
Ariff, B B
Barbenel, D M
Carver, R T
Chinyama, N C
Davies, D W L
Ekwuru, M O
Haas, J M
Harris, S J A
Hockey, J S
Hotonu, O E O
Hubbard, A D
Hubbard, M
James, E A
Khan, G M
Krisnamurthy, M
Kwok, Q S K
Li Ting Wai, L S
Lipitch, H S
Ma, R M M N
Mack, D J
Masterson, S W
Meghani, S
Morrison, I R
Newman, P J
Nubi, W A O
Panja, A S
Patel, P C
Porte, M E
Ruhul Amin, M A K M
Sanders, F E
Shah, N S
Shier, D L
Teo, S G
Ullah, K M S
Varughese, R T J
Vijayakumar, M
Wolff, A H
Young, H L

N5
Alexander, N
Anand, V
Bataille, V
Bennett, S D
Calder, P R
Caller, H A
Casasus Borrell, T
Challands, J F
Collie, M H S
Crawford, T A
Dervish, H
Dervish, H
Dimmock, S A
Dock, V J
Dutton, J A E
Foord, M L
Gawronski, J G S
Gupta, S P
Hunningher, A
Hussain, S M
Indar, R A
Jacobs, F K S
Kaplan, J
Magnifico, F
Mazrani, W
Morrison, H E
Nicholson, R H
Patel, J D
Perera, S R
Slack, S J
Smirl, J E
Trosser, A
Warren, A K
Whitlock, P R
Yerassimou, P M
Yuen, A K-C

N6
Alberman, E D
Alimo, E B D
Andrews, L H
Baig, L
Bardsley, I M
Bax, M C O
Beardwell, N A
Beaugie, A V
Bernhardt, L W
Briffa, J P J
Broadhurst, E R
Browne, E F
Chan, K K L
Chataway, A M
Cheng, A
Chesshyre, M H
Choudhry, S O
Clemente Meoro, M D C
Collie-Kolibabka, G A
Cooper, C P
Crockard, M C A
Dawid, F E
Dickie, S J
Dukes, S A
Feldman, M M
Ferner, R E
Frank, N J
Frankl, A R
Galton, C J
Galton, J S
Gibbons, R K
Graham, R L
Grover, N
Harbin, L J
Harding, K R
Harding, L
Harrod, S T S-C
Hindley, C P
Hinton, A E
Holtby, V C
Hosie, G P
Howitt, G B
Hudson, H N G
Jacob, S J
James, E C W
Jelenowicz, E
Johal, P S
Keeble, T
Knowlden, M J
Knowlden, P R
Lam, W W-L
Latimer-Sayer, E G
Legg, N J
Levine, D
Lewis, E
Lloyd-Thomas, H G L
Mamaloukas, E
Margulies, H H
Mayer, R D
Meadows, C A
Mikhailidis, A M
Mulvany, S R
Myers, D S
Myerscough, N
Nandi, L R S N
Ng, J C M
Nonoo-Cohen, C
Ong, E G P
Patel, K
Patel, R S
Paterson, M T
Pathmanathan, Y
Pearse, P A E
Pomson, H R
Prudo-Chlebosz, R R Z
Riddell, J D
Robertson, S M
Rockall, T A
Romanos Betran, M T
Rosen, J-P D
Rushman, N R
Rustin, J K
Schmidt, A E
Schon, F E G
Semenov, R A
Shove, D C
Sidhu, S K
Silman, R E
Smith, S M
Smits, M M
Spankie, A C
Stern, G
Thum, A M E
Vicary, F R
Webster, G J M
Woodrow, C J

N7
Amin, D J
Asher, P N
Bantock, H M E
Battle, G N
Bryant, P A
Chow, W C
Coutinho, M L P
Cripwell, M T
D'Arrigo, W L
Davidson, D
Desai, B R
Dockery, F
Dopfmer, U
Eagleton, F M B
Edoman, S
Fertleman, C R
Field, P M
Funnell, M S
Getachew, U
Grender, B C
Gupta, V K
Haigh, D J G
Hall, I S
Hart, J K
Hart, P E
Hau, Y G
Hayes, M E B
Hewitt, J
Ho, S W T
Hopper, A H
Howard, J M
Hunt, S T
Hussein, A A G
John, L H
Joshi, C S
Kinsella, L M J
Krause, U
Krywawych, M N
Marinker, M L
Mpanga, L A Z
Muttunayagam, G M
Nguyen, C T
Oakley, G M
Ogundipe, E M
Patel, A
Patel, R N
Piachaud, M J H
Savage, A W G
Sayer, G L
Sills, M D
Sinclair, S I G
Sitaras, D
Storey, S M
Tarlow, J
Tarlow, S
Tatham, M E
Tounjer, I A
Windsor, J
Yudkin, J S
Zinkin, P M

N8
Adeniran, F G A
Ali, T M M I
Amlot, N
Bardani, I
Beck, E R
Beck, R O
Benson, K J
Berk, C
Blackburn, T D V
Blass, D M
Bolland, E
Brown, J G
Busaidy, F S
Cooper, J A
Cotton, M-A
Datta, D
Dhorajiwala, D
Dolman, W F G
Eccles, N K
El-Kinani, S
Ellerby, M J
Fehler, B M
Fitzgerald, J M
Giotakis, I
Gothard, S C
Greenbury, E
Gueret-Wardle, T
Hassiotou, A
Ishaque, M A
Jefferies, N J
Johns, J
Jolliffe, V M L
Jones, G
Jones, G V
Jootun, N
Kessel, A S
Korner, J
Locke, I
McCartney, S A
Maneksha, S
Marriage, S C
Masters, D
Matsakis, M
Meek, J H
Miles, D W
Moorey, H C
Munro, J M
Nikolopoulos, J
Oli, J M
Onyeabo, B C
Perera, C A M
Photos, E
Raja, A U K
Ramgoolam, N
Rosenthal, A N
Rosenthal, D
Rosenthal, J J
Rosin, R A
Rubra, T D
Sampson, A
Sharma, S
Shashikanth, S
Sher, C
Skogstad, H
Smith, S D C
Stock, D J
Stock, R D
Strycharczyk, K J
Talat, M
Trew, J M
Walker, A
Wood, K A

N9
Anyanwu, A C
Bolcina, A L
Bumrah, R S
Clare, D
Exworthy, T P N
Ghazi, A H
Gill, D P
Gnanandan, J
Herekar, S R
Jones, A S
Jones, A
Jowett, S A
Kattan, G V
Logan, M B
Meltzer, E S
Mistry, C R
Patalay, T
Philippou, G N
Pillai, K O
Pillai, S W
Reshamwalla, D K N
Singer, R V J
Sternberg, S
Warren, J S
Yapp, P A

N10
Abrams, M E
Amlot, P L
Benians, R C
Berzon, D
Betts, J C
Blackstone, V H
Blend, D M
Brecker, N A
Brocklesby, S J
Brown, D W G
Brueton, R N
Chaloner, E J
Christian, P K
Christopher, E
Cohen, C R G
Corridan, B J P
Das, C K
De Silva, H A
Demades, J
Dzumhur, S
Farrow, S C
Finch, R J
Foley, M F
French, S L
Friedmann, B
Funaki, A
Gerrard, T J
Hale, R B
Hatjiosif, R
Healy, R
Hill, J P
Hinton, E A
Isaacson, R
Jaumdally, J-U-D R
Karunaratne, D C P
Kell, P D
Kolocassides, K G
Laverick, S
Lawes, D A
Levine, S
Lewis, S N
MacQuillan, J G
Mantides, G E
Marks, R J
Menzies, E A D
Mootoosamy, I M
Mulkis, H B
Neuling, K F S
O'Donoghue, D M
Putris, S H
Robinson, K J
Rotblat, F
Russell, A G
Safranek, M M S
Salkind, S R
Segal, H M
Sharfuddin, I
Sharma, R C
Shaw, J C L
Sivakumar, T
Solomons, N
Swale, J
Trompeter, S
Van Hagen, T C
Waterhouse, E T
Weatherley, P L
Werth, F
Woolfson, S B

N11
Adamson, E
Albon, L I M
Brooks, J
Corcoran, D
Deshmukh, B A
Dickie, C H
Dimitrakos, M-A
Goraya, A
Govind, A
Haidar, A
Hamilton, S J
Holt, L W J
Khumri, A
Lawal, O
Lewis, R M
Mansfield, J D
Markham, J E R
Maroof, Dr
Miah, S I
Okonkwo, S I
Parmar, S J
Patel, S M
Plunkett, C N
Rifkin, S
Saglani, S
Schamroth, A J
Selwyn, V G
Shah, H R
Shah, S M
Sherman, L M
Siddiqui, G K
Singh, R
Smith, G W T
Thillainathan, S
Twine, M R
Waldron, G
Waldron, H A
Zahir, K

N12
Abdul-Ghani, A K M
Ahmed, A R
Amdurer, M A
Astruc, D M N
Baker, J
Barnes, S J
Barrett, P J
Berkovitz, S R
Besherdas, K
Bezuidenhout, P B
Bhatia, S
Brett, C J S
Brull, D J
Brunner, M D
Buckman, A
Burney, S R M
Chan, K S
Chari, P
Chari, S
Cheung, K Y P
Chong, A Y-L
Corcoran, J S
Daitz, A R
Dardis, P M
Deboutte, D
Docherty, S M
Douglas-Wilson, I
Farooque, P G B
Fish, M
George, B
George, P M
Gilley, J A
Goulden, N J
Goulden, P K
Jarvis, E T
Jennings, S J
Jones, N
Jordan, A J
Klein, A A
Leighton, M H
Mahadeshwar, S S
Ming, H Y
Mohapatra, J R
Mok, H L-H
Momoh, J A
Myttas, N
Ng, B K W
Olaitan, A
Parker, A M
Patel, N R
Patel, R S
Peisach, C M
Raneem, I
Richards, L M E
Riley, C E
Sargent, C S
Sebastianpillai, N J
Singh, A K
Skia, B
Stephens, C A
Strouthos, M
Tang, Y-T K
Tauzeeh, S M
Wee, A A B L
Yiu, P

N13
Achike, D I O
Ahmed, A A S M
Ahmed, A
Ali, K M
Ali, T
Crossley, H
Daitz, H
Dick, A R
El-Oush, T M M
Gibbs, J G
High, J E
Kolman, P C
Kouloumas, G
Leedham, S
Llahi Camp, J M
Malone, T B A
Mavrides, A
Naik, P N
Nandadeva, P G
Nicholaou, T A
O'Mahony, J F
Obiekwe, M N
Osman, R
Patel, M H
Sinha, K M
Szlosarek, P W
Tan, K C B
Warren, L M
Wright, G A K

N14
Abedi, M K A
Aetheris, P S
Ahmad, S N
Ali, S A
Amarasinghe, L M
Amarasinghe, M A
Annaradnam, R J
Ara, B K
Aristodemou, A
Behr, H L
Brener, N D
Broster, G M
Campbell, A C H
Caplan, H
Cattell, H R
Chau, B L
D'Souza, L R
Dancygyer, A M
De, S K
El Ashry, A A

Eldridge, C D
Geffin, B B
George, M J
Hamid, M S M
Ho, N C Y
Ho, V C L
Howell, D C J
Islam, M N
Islam, V
Ismail, H
Ismail, H
Ismail, I H M
Jarvis, K J
Jayaratnam, A S V R
Kaleel, M F
Khan, T B
King, A-M
Kiss, I S
Kooner, P
Lakhani, N N
Lau Lai Lin, L
Lipkin, B D
McClure, J L
Marcus, N J
Moran, E
Muhundhakumar, S
Muhunthakumar, P
Neehall, D J
Ng, P H
Ninis, N
Niranjan, N
Owino, W E J
Patel, P G
Pati, J
Phadnis, S G
Phillips, R L
Prothero, D
Rasiah, N J
Richardson, E J L
Robinson, G M
Seal, A N
Seal, L J
Sebastianpillai, C
Sebastianpillai, F B Y
Shaddick, R A
Shah, D K L
Sheldon, L A
Shergill, S S
Sissou, P
Smith, G D
Sonigra, H K
Synge, J
Thomas, J M
Turk, J L
Van Someren, R N M
Veale, D M W C
Watts, V K
Wray, G M H
Young, A J
Yu, S H
Zoha, M M

N15
Afghan, K
Bateman, A W
Bilginer, H T
Blanchard, M R
Callan, A F
Caplan, R S
Chadwick, J M
Chowdhury, D H
Chowdhury, H
Dickinson, M J
Fenton, K A
Furlong, R C S
Ghosh, A K
Ghosh, D
Hawkes, G I N
Hazelwood, S R
Hoar, A C D
Holmes, D A
Ikwueke, J K
Isaacs, G
Isorna, V
Johnson-Sabine, E C
Kirk, M
Kundu, D K
Lingam, S
Majewski, A A
Mukhopadhyay, D N
Nageswaran, A S
Noktehdan, N
Oji, K N
Pandya, J K
Phimester, M E
Popat, R T
Portsmouth, S D
Rachman, S C
Read, J H M

Rohan, J S
Sabat, A L
Seargeant, J M
Shaw, T B
Sirri, T N
Sivasinmyananthan, K
Smith, W G
Thambapillai, A J
Thiruvudaiyan, P

N16
Ansorge, R
Bench, M T
Bohn, P M
Brandner, B
Browne, N B
Buchin, E M
Carr, J B
Caviston, P M
Chowdhury, F B
Clouter, G
Cross, L C
Dalton, M J T
Davidson, K
Dell, A J
Derrett, C J
England, R
Evans, T K A
Faruhar, M
Fitzpatrick, M J
Foster, C S
Gadhvi, M R
Gadhvi, N M
Gangola, R L
Garner, G M
Goodhart, L C
Green, S G
Gupta, S P
Hindley, M C
Jaffer, N
Kambitsis, N
Kay, P T S
Keene, A D
Kiernan, S J R
Levy, A L
McKie, J M
Madge, S J
Maloney, C
Mann, N G
Marks, C M
Mitchell, H J
Morton, A D
Osen, H E
Ozcan, K
Phelan, D R
Prasad, S N
Qureshi, M A H
Ramanna, M
Rasburn, B
Spitzer, J
Virjee, S
Waldman, L J
Weinstock, S
Wilkinson, J M
Williams, C D
Williams, D S
Williams, J
Withers, D J
Woodgate, M
Wright, F A

N17
Abomeli, D O
Agyeman, K
Amato, G A
Augustt, A G
Barnett, P
Bastianpillai, L S K
Curtin, J T
Dadzie, O E
Dowler, S A
Ebigbo, A P M
Henderson, A M
King, E
Lindsay, M S
Louka, L
Marotta, S
Mazzon, S
Moossun, H
Morrison, C M
Ostle, K
Pereira, J M D S
Pierre, S L
Ranmuthu, A H
Svenne, D
Udenkwo, D
Woollacott, M

N18
Alsford, L J
Alwan, A H
Aziz, M N
Bell-Gam, Dr
Borgstein, R
Chattopadhyay, B
Cohen, M E H
Davies, S A
Deo, S I
Dixon, P J
Drabu, Y J
Evans, F A
Fowlis, G A
Girgis, F L
Hiew, S C C
Husien, A M A
Ithayakumar, E S
Jayasena, S D
Karp, S J
Khan, A
Kumaran, T O
Luckit, J K
McDonald, J A
Makker, H K
Maxwell, P R
Mehtar, S
Millar, A D
Mistry, A D
Onwubalili, J K
Patel, B C
Rees, J A
Sala, C
Schwenk, A
Shah, H R
Sheinman, B D
Silver, M E
Sinclair, H D
Stoker, D L
Sultana, A A
Sundaresan, M L
Thapar, R
Thiagarajah, K A
Tindall, H
Ubogagu, M
Viswanathan, M
Weithers, E C
Woolf, V J
Yardumian, D A

N19
Aarons, S D
Ardeshna, K M
Arnold, A M
Atia, W A
Bacarese-Hamilton, I A
Banerjee, A
Barnes, S D
Beatson, S M
Bebbington, P E
Bernardis, C K
Bielawska, C A
Blake, S M
Blumerg, R M
Brady, R
Brett, B T
Bryan, R L
Buszewicz, M J
Campbell, M F S
Chase, J C C
Chaudhuri, R
Cheung, C M G
Chong Siew Foon, E
Coppola, W G T
Dacre, J E
Dalton, J
Darley, M P
Dennell, L V A
Desai, S A
Desmond, N M
Din, R R
Dufton, K E
Dunstan, M E
Durrant, K J
Ellis, D G
Feeney, J T
Fraser, R J
Gluck, T A
Grande, M J
Grant, D S
Greenhalgh, P M
Hannam, S
Hardman, S M C
Hargreaves, C G
Harkness, A
Haselden, S P
Heaton, G M A
Helman, C G
Heman-Ackah, C A

Henson, G L
Ingham Clark, C L
Inwald, A C M
Jacobs, S R
Jaswon, M S
Jolowicz, K
Jukes, M M R
Kateb, H J
Kelsey, M C
Ko, A H N
Koya, M R
Kraemer, J W S
Kyei-Mensah, A A A
Lock, M R
Lock, S H
Mackinnon, H S
McLure, C E
Makinde, O
Malone-Lee, J G
Martin, J R
Martinez-Alier, N G
Miller, R A
Mitchell, P O
Mitchell, S J
Morgan, A A
Mountford, L
Nesbitt, S J
Olateju, M A O
Panch, G
Parker, N E
Patterson, D L H
Rands, G S J
Restrick, L J
Roberts, J E
Robins, A W
Robinson, I F
Ross, A M
Rossi, M
Saeed, B O
Seckl, M J
Semrau, U
Shah, M R
Shaw, C A
Singer, A
Southgate, L J
Stevens, J P
Sullivan, C M
Suri, D
Swinn, M J
Tan, S-Y
Thomas, M R
Ticktin, S J
Tucker, S K
Vos, A L
Walters, K R
Wills, A J
Wilson, A J
Wonke, B
Wooller, D J A
Worrall, J G
Yeung, J N M
Youngman, J R

N20
Bayreuther, J L
Bray, P M
Callaghan, B D
Chrysopoulo, M T
Davidson, R A
Dyer, N C
Eisen, S M
Epstein, E F
Flynn, F V
Free, D G C
Goldman, M H
Grantley, B
Griffith, J D A-H
Gross, G
Hayward, A E
Hobsley, M
Howells, J
Jankowska, P J
Jeffreys, P A
Kapur, S B
Katz, R E
Lawlor, M G
Lever, C G
Lubin, J R
Lucas, E A
Lumley, K
Maxwell, J R
Milnthorpe, J C
Page, F M L
Patel, T B
Poobalasingam, N
Sampson, R D
Scurr, A J
Scurr, C F
Seevaratnam, N S

Shaikh, N A
Silk, J
Smith, H G
Smith, H R
Viapree, R O
Ward, S L
Whiter, A J
Whiter, G L
Willis, K M
Wood, D R

N21
Abdel Khalek, A I
Ballah, N D
Banim, R H
Bhattacharyya, M R
Chakraborty, A
Edhem, I
Elias, T H
Fletcher, I H
Freeman, M J
Georgallou, M
Golara, M
Gormley, S J
Halil, O
Harris, R D
Herriott, M
Herriott, T D
Hume, R C
Huq, K K
Jash, K
Jenkins, G C
Jenkins, M D
Jesuthasan, M
Jones, H S J
Jones, M O
Karia, N
Krass, I M
Ling, K S L
Maciolek, J S
MacKenzie, G D
MacPhail, M
Makuloluwe, C L K
Masters, A B
Mottalib, E A
Nicola, K P
Nolan, F C
Noor, R
North, J R
Olakanpu, O A
Parbhoo, R
Pathmanandam, H
Perera, W A T E
Samtani, A
Selwood, J E
Sethi, P
Shah, P R
Shah, P
Shah, R C
Sheville, E
Stern, G M
Topiwala, N P
Trathen, D P
Tudberry, R A
Wiggins, L J
Wragg, A

N22
Acharya, R J
Aldulaimi, D M
Bodhinayake, B
Botros, H
Christoforou, C
Clarke, P C
Cleanthis, T M
Connolly, G M M
Dave, M S
Deeney, H N
Eren, E
Graham, N W
Higgins, C J
Hoque, A T M M
Jadeja, A K
Jalloh, S S
Jurangpathy, M F
Kamal Nor, N
Kaya, B
Kaya, E
Koziol, L F S
MacGowan, J R
Man, F W A
Manheim, V H
Matheson, P J
Pantazis, A
Patel, H M
Patel, K L
Patel, M K
Paun, S M
Pelendrides, H

Raza, M
Salek Haddadi, A A
Samarasinghe, L
Scott, A J
Sivananthan, N
Soutter, P G
Steinberg, S
Stekelman, S
Strommer, T R
Sultana, K
Theodorou, M
Visavadia, B G
Windle, M F

NW1
Akinyanju, O O
Al-Adnani, M S
Alcorn, R J
Allinson, R N
Andersen, S L
Antoniades, C G G
Anwar, F S
Arnold, K G
Arnold, N
Assheton, S J
Avery, N R
Awad, W I I
Aziz, M V
Bahl, M R
Baraitser, P
Barker, M A
Barlow, J S
Benaim, S
Bloom, P A
Bradley, E A
Brenman, E
Brockbank, M H
Brogan, P A
Buchanan, A J
Carlton, O H
Castell, F A
Cathcart, S J
Chakrabarty, S
Challoner, T E
Connor, H E
Cook, C A G
Cook, G C
Cooper, C A
Corbett, M C
Corcuera Maza, M A
Coren, A
Cowan, D A
Cowan, G O
Cullum, A R
Darbyshire, J H
Davidson, J
Davis, H J
Davis, R M E
Dinning, W J
Drummond, P M
Duguid, I G M
Dunlop, L J
Eapen, E
Edmunds, L E S
Elphinstone, P E
Faghihi Naraghi, A M
Fairhead, S M
Ferguson, C N
Fikree, M A
Gibb, D M
Giunti, P
Gledhill, R C
Goodstone, A S
Greaves, S
Gregory-Evans, K
Hackett, G H
Hailstone, J D
Harbord, R B
Harris, D N F
Hecker, K V
Hennelly, K J
Herst, E R
Hird, V
Hooper, H J
Hoque, M
Horton, R C
Horwitz, N I
Hoult, J E
Isaacs, A D
Jain, S
Jenkinson, A D
John, L M
Joyce, C M M
Joyston-Bechal, S
Kaleem, N
Kanaan, R A A
Katz, A W
Kemp, K S A
Kerr, I E

Landeck, A
Latchman, M Z
Lawrence, C J
Lawrie, H S L S
Layland, W R
Lieberman, G
Lindsay, K D
Ling, K L C
Luttrell, S R R
McCormack, S M G
McCullagh, G M
McDonald, F M A
Martin, C B
Matthews, S J
Miller, J W
Moore, D A J
Morris, J E
Morrison, R C
Morrison, S C
Nadarajah, S
Nagle, C J
O'Donnell, J G M
Ormston, R M A
Parry, R J
Paul, G A
Peirce, N S
Peters, D
Petrou, P P
Phan, P-A T
Pickard, C A M
Pierides, M
Pollock, R M
Preston, J W P
Puxon, C M
Qamar, A
Ragge, N K
Rao, S K
Ratcliffe, G E
Reid, A S
Renfrew, I
Roques, T W
Roux, B R
Sabeti, H
Sanderson, P J
Sarma, R C
Scarffe, J H
Senanayake, I P
Shaw, K L
Shina, A G
Siddiqi, N I
Siow, W
Skensved, H
Smaje, L H
Smith, E R
Smith, S M
Sohn, L
Southall, T R
Speakman, M J
Strachan, A M J
Svasti-Salee, D
Taylor, R W M
Teoh, S K
Thompson, C M
Vernon, P R
Wander, A P
Wedeles, E H
Weston, T E T
Whitcombe, E M
White, M
Winnett, A R D

NW2

Agranoff, J
Ahuja, A
Ajdukiewicz, K M B
Al Sahlani, U Y A
Allen, R L
Amin, Y K
Andrawis, N F
Appiah, L K
Baghai-Ravary, R
Barter, J A
Bashey, A
Bennett, J A
Biggs, S
Brennan, M T
Bunn, A W
Burch, A M
Burton, C H
Chaudhury, S D
Coates, S M
Cohen, J
Cohen, N A
Craig, A P
Dalsania, A V
Datoo, M M A
Davis, L
De Kare-Silver, N S
Dudley, A F
Elmiyeh, B
Ezquerro Adan, A
Faal, M A
Forbat, S M
Frosh, B J
Ganny, A S
Graham, J J
Halsted, C J
Hassan, M A
Haynes, K G
Heuschkel, R B
Houston, M E
Howard, M R
Husain, S T
Imeson, J
Isaacs, J D
Jeswani, T A
Jolles, M A
Joshua-Amadi, M I
Joslin, J M
Kahtan, S R
Khan, Z
Lepski, G R
Lodhi, M A K
Lyon, A R
McCollum, M P
Marshall, J R
Mehta, K A
Mehta, R K
Mitchley, S E
Najim, Z N
Neerkin, J
Negus, R P M
Neoman, I F Z
Nesa, Q U
Newman, L T
Nissenbaum, H
Nwozo, J C
O'Donovan, M R
Oliver, M T
Onyeador, M I
Osakwe, E A
Patel, M K
Perinpanayagam, R M
Phelan, M S
Potter, J D F
Prempeh, T B
Qureshi, A I
Rahman, F Z
Raja, M A K
Rakshi, J S
Ranade, J U
Rasooly, R
Richman, G
Robinson, A L
Rudge, P J
Samarasinghe, K P B
Sathia, U L
Schelvan, C S K
Shah, U U
Shah, U R
Sheth, J G
Siriwardhana, S A
Skelker, M H
Slome, J J
Sohi, D K
Sorungbe, A O O
Talmud, J C
Taylor, J
Thackray, J E
Thomas, J M
Thursfield, S R
Tilley, J M
Ukachukwu, I
Vanderpump, M P J
Wadhwa, P
Ward, P A
Weisz, G M
White, D M

NW3

Achkar, J C
Adler, M A
Ahmed, S M
Akerele, O F
Akinsola, S A
Al-Damluji, S
Ali, A A
Allum, C A
Altschulova, H J
Ameen, A A
Anderson, C R S
Angel, A M
Angus-Leppan, H
Annis, H M
Anthony, A
Aung Hpyoe, Dr
Babar-Craig, H
Bahri, A K
Bailey, J N R
Baillod, R A
Baker, D M
Balakrishnan, I
Balcombe, J N
Bannister, B A
Bark-Jones, E M H
Barker, D A
Barnes, E J
Bates, A W
Bates, S J
Bayes, A R R
Beary, M D
Beckles, M A
Begent, R H J
Behr, E R
Bell, C L
Belsham, P A
Bendor, A M
Bentley, T J
Berelowitz, M O
Berger, L A
Bevan, K E
Bird, A S
Black, C M
Black, J M
Blakeley, C J
Bonner, C V
Bostock, T S V
Boukalis, A
Bouloux, P-M G
Bourne, S
Bowen, E M
Bowler, J V
Bradley, E F
Bradley, S M O
Brafman, A H
Bridgewater, J A
Brook, J H R
Brough, G M
Brown, G N
Brumfitt, W
Burke, O C A
Burman, A M
Burroughs, A K
Burton, B J L
Buscombe, J R
Butler, P E M
Caplin, M E
Carr-Brion, J M H
Cassell, J A
Caufield, H M
Chan, C S Y
Chan, O
Chan, S S C
Chao, D
Chapman, J T V
Chapman, M V
Chapple, J C
Chee Keng Jin, A
Cheng, G C W
Choi, S P
Claff, H R
Clayton, W J
Cockcroft, A E
Coghlan, J G
Cohen, S
Collee, G G
Copell, J A
Cox, S J
Croft, G A
Cropley, I M
Crow, J C
Crowston, J G
Cummings, G E
Curtis, C J
Cwynarski, K L
Daniel, J R
Danso, M A
Davarashvili, T I
Davenport, A
Davey, C C
Davidson, B R
Davidson, T I
Davies, A E
Davison, H W
De Mare, P B
Denton, C P
Dick, R
Dilworth, J P
Dinner, L
Dirmeik, B F
Djazaeri, B
Djazaeri, B
Dooley, J S
Dorward, N L
Dowd, G S E
Downie, P M
Drake, B E N
Duncan, D D
Dunn, J
Durkin, C A
Dusheiko, G M
Dytham, A J
Eber, T R
Economides, D L
Edwards, S E
Eid, C S
Eid, N H
Eisen, T G Q
Ellis, J M
Epstein, O
Evans, A L
Evans, T R
Fairclough, A D
Fancy, N E
Faraj, K S
Farfan, G A
Fatnani, D T
Feldmann, P J
Fernando, O N
Finlay, S C
Fleischman, A P
Fogarty, A B
Fok, D H S
Foster, J W
Foster, S
Fox, S B
Frankel, T L
Freedman, J
Gabriel, G
Garlick, N I
Gertner, G
Ghosh, J M
Gibb, E L
Gibbs, J M
Gillespie, S H
Ginsberg, L
Goddard, N J
Gracey-Whitman, L J
Grasse, A S M
Griffiths, P D
Grun, L M
Gulati, S
Hakeem, A
Hallgarten, R J
Hamilton, G
Hamilton, M I R
Harbord, M W N
Hargest, E L
Harper, N C
Harris, M J
Harrison-Read, P E
Hawkins, P N
Heaton, J M
Heelan, B T
Henderson, J H
Henryk Gutt, R
Hettiarachchi-Abeya, M
Higgs, B D
Hilson, A J W
Ho, R L-M
Ho, S S M
Hobson, R P
Hodgson, H J F
Hoffbrand, A V
Hoffbrand, S E
Hoffmann, K A
Hood, C
Hood, J R
Horton, J P
Howie, A J
Huang Yun Pui, B
Hutchings, S L
Hymanson, E N
Ijaz, S
Ioannidis, A
Ioannidis, C
Irish, C J
Jackson, D J
Jacobs, M G
Jaffe, R
Jareonsettasin, T
Jarmulowicz, M R
Joels, S L
Johnson, A M
Jolles, S R A
Jones, A L
Jones, C L
Jones, J A
Jones, J M
Jones, M M
Jourdan, I C
Jourdan, M H
Kallberg, M H
Kampfner, F B E
Kasinski, K L J
Kenton-Smith, J
Keshav, S C
Khan, N Q
Khan, S R
Khara, M
Khoo, P C
Kibbler, C C
Kidd, D P C C
Kiely, N M
Killaspy, H T
King, M B
Kingdon, E J
Kinston, M A
Kinston, W J
Kirk, R M
Kleinman, R L
Koh, T N
Kohn, M R
Koso-Thomas, O M
Kreindler, J R
Kurowska, A C
Kurzer, L
Laniado, M E
Laqueur, S R
Laurence, A D J
Laurence, D R
Lawson, J M M
Leddy, K
Lee, C A
Lee, D R
Lee, M A G H
Lefford, F
Leigh, E D
Lewis, A A M
Lewis, P D
Lim, C J
Lim, P S C
Lindsey, C R W
Lipman, M C I
Little, B C
Lloyd, B W
Loo Wing Hing, H
Lord, R H H
Lotzof, K G
Loughridge, F A
Lozewicz, S
Lucas, C
McCarthy, J E
McGuinness, A M
McLean, A G
Maclean, A B
Magos, A L
Majid, S
Majzlisz, A
Mak, T W C
Malek, B
Malhotra, U
Mallett, S V
Martin, M D
Marwaha, S
Mason, H M C
Maurice-Williams, R S
Meer, S
Meeson, A
Meeson, B
Mehta, A
Mehta, A B
Mendonca, L M
Meyer, T
Mikhael Matta, W H
Mikhail, G W I
Mikhailidis, D
Miranda Fernandez, F J
Mollison, P L
Moore, K P
Morgan, M Y
Morgan, S L
Morris, D C
Moss, C H
Muammar, M
Murch, S H
Myint, F P-O
Nahai, S C
Nathan, B E
Nazareth, I
Newby, J C
Newsholme, W A
Ng, R L H
Nonis, C N A
Obholzer, A M
Ogunbiyi, O A
Oguz, C
Okolo, S O
Oon, L L E
Ordman, A J
Orrell, R W
Orteu, C H
Osborn, D P J
Owen, N J
Papadopoulou, A M
Patch, D W M
Patrick, M P H
Payne, N D G
Peachey, T D
Pepys, E O
Pepys, M B
Perry, D J
Pigott, J L
Pigott, K H
Platts, A D
Potter, M N
Pounder, R R E
Powis, S H
Prais, S S
Prelevic, G
Raeburn, J R
Raven, P W
Reed, J R
Rees, L H
Rees, M C
Rees, P H
Regan, J L
Reid, W M N
Renwick, S R
Robinson, P H
Roche, N A
Rolles, K
Rubio Lainez, C R
Sacks, M D
Sandford, J M
Sayer, C S
Schapira, A H V
Scott, E M
Scott, P D C
See Chye Heng, A
Senanayake, L F N
Shamash, A
Sharma, A K
Shaw, E H
Shein, I G
Sheldon, J H
Shenfield, F
Shieff, C L
Shiu, K Y
Siddiqi, A
Sienkowski, I K
Simons, R S
Simpson, K M
Sklar, J
Smeeth, L
Snowdon, B A
Sofi, M A
Speight, R G
Stafford, S
Stanley, C A
Stewart, H
Stoll, L J
Stone, A B
Stone, R M E
Stone, S P
Stratton, R J
Stuart Morrow, C
Stuart-Smith, S J
Stuart, A B D
Suppree, D A
Sutcliffe, A G
Swain, A F
Swain, C P
Sweeten-Smith, B A
Sweny, P
Tam, T C
Tanner, M A
Taylor, A A
Taylor, B
Taylor, C P F
Taylor, D
Temple, N O T
Thomas, J R L
Thomson, M A
Tibballs, J M
Tormey, V J
Toszeghi, A D
Tuck, S M
Van Someren, V H
Vaz, O K
Vizza, E
Wajed, S A
Walker-Smith, J A
Walker, E M
Warbey, V
Warner, T T
Watts, J D
Webber, I T A
Webster, A D B
Weich, S R
Whittaker, S J
Williams, C J S

Williams, S S
Wilson, A D H
Wilson, L A
Winder, A F
Winslet, M C
Wise, M E J
Wiseman, P J T
Wolfe, I J
Wong, J M
Wong, L T
Wootliff, A B
Wu, A
Wynick, S P
Wynn, V
Yong, P F K
Yorke, S C B
Young, S C R
Yue, A M-H
Zachary, A R
Zuckerman, A J
Zuckerman, J N
Zutshi, D W

NW4

Abelman, W
Aggarwal, R K
Al-Dabbagh, Z T N
Alijani, M
Almeida, A Z
Aronica, G F
Aziz, V M
Baker, G
Bashir, F A
Benepal, T S
Benjamin, C A
Benjamin, E D
Chatrath, V M
Cohen, M
Cooper, K S
Cooper, S H
Crosby, C P
Datoo, S A L
Davis, C P
Davis, H
Donegan, J L M
Fernando, B S
Fox, S D
Fraser, K E
Goldman, J H
Gosain, R K
Graham, K E
Hart, P S
Hoffbrand, C R
Holder, B
Ihara, T
Jackson, R A
Jaffe, V
Jaja, D M
Jolic, G
Jones, P E
Joshi, R
Josse, S E
Kark, A E
Katz, G
Khonji, A A
Kielty, V J
Kleinberg, S R
Kohli, B L
Kohli, S K
Kotecha, K M
Kurzer, M N
Lauffer, G L
Lawson, S E
Mailoo, R J
Markiewicz, M
Maxwell, V B
Milofsky, R
Missakian, S K
Musgrave, M S
Okaro, C O
Pambakian, Y E L A
Patel, S A
Peters, E M
Popat, J T
Qureshi, Z
Rahmanie, N
Ray, S
Raymond, G P M
Razzaq, N
Rees, J D S
Rosenberg, J N
Sakkadas, A
Samuel, J L
Samuel, S
Sarma, U C
Schwartz, J S
Shah, R M
Shelat, C C
Sheng, M H-T
Stein, G
Steuer, L R
Sudan, S
Thrower, P A
Toledano, H
Townsley, W
Upadhyay, V A
Uzoka, A A E
Whitton, T
Wilkes, A

NW5

Alnaes-Katjavivi, P H
Amiel, S M
Asen, K M
Ashworth, N P
Blackburn, V M M
Boyce, W J
Bunker, J R
Cleverley, J R
Davis, J C
Davison, M
Dean, J
Dean, Z-U
Dickinson, C M
Dixon, G L J
Dormandy, T L
Dow, A M
Empson, B D
Farmer, M
Fitzpatrick, C M
Fleming, C
Fox, M P
Freedman, B
Freudenberg, S
Gaminara, E J
Gammell, S J
Graham, N
Graham, P J
Graham, S H
Granger-Taylor, C P
Grant, D M
Gyorffy, G
Hajioff, J
Hale, A D
Halford, S E R
Hannan, F M
Hawting, R A
Heath, I C
Hinshelwood, B G
Hughes, D A
Hunt, S J
Ivens, D R
Jegadeva, A N
Jennings, E A L
Keyvan-Fouladi, M
Klouda, A T
Koperski, M T
Leff, A P
Lockett, C J
Lowe, J N
Macdonald, M
Macgregor, D R
McNaught, A S
Malik, M A
Mariotti, P
Matthewman, P J
Mehta, A
Moran, M M
Moyes, B A
Myat, J M
Oddy, M J
Oswald, I H S G
Palmer, S C
Posner, P J
Rahman, S
Ramachandran, S
Rich, E M
Richman, N S
Riddell, A F
Robbins, S A
Roberts, O A
Robinson, K A
Roedling, A S
Rose, C D L
Sackville West, J E
Sayer, M M R
Schneidau, A
Sinclair, N E
Sinha, S
Sinha, S K
Steel, A C
Summerfield, D A
Tendall, J D
Toeg, D
Wakeham, N R
Yiannakou, J Y
Youl, B D
Yudkin, G D

NW6

Abraham, M D
Afridi, S K
Ames, D J
Angeloglou, M
Ansell, E
Asafu-Adjaye, D S
Ashdown, A C
Ballaro, A P C
Barnett, J M
Basir, N
Berry, M G
Binks, M H
Blesovsky, L T
Braude, W
Braunold, G A
Briffa, A C
Britton, R S
Budewig, K
Burgoyne, P W
Burman Roy, S A
Calaminici, M
Cantons, C A
Caparrotta, L
Caplan, A
Carey, P A
Carulli, M T
Chandler, K E
Cohen, S L
Coker, F B A
Cunningham, F L
David, L T
De Zulueta, P C B
Dettori, H L
Di Luca, C
Dietch, D M
Eames, S A
Edmondson, C R
Elliott, S M
Eneli, A C
Esterson, A
Farah, A E T
Fatemi Langroudi, B
Footerman, D S
Ford, C H
Fox, K F
Gill, M W
Gottlieb, I
Gotto, J
Gozali, S
Grant, A J
Griffith, G D W
Gumpel, S M
Halpern, H S
Hammad, M K A H H
Hill, J M
Hinshelwood, L S
Hobdell, R A
Holmes, M J
Howell, A
Iliffe, S R
Kansagra, D M
Keane, F
Keays, R T
Kudrati, M E
Kustow, B
Landau, S C
Lazanakis, M S
Le Roux, P H
Lee, C C-Y
Levy, D M
Levy, M J
Lim, J C M
Lucas, J M
Luksenberg, S R
MacDermot, K D
McGuinness, O E
Magara, G
Mallett, P
Man, K W
Marcus, E
Maxwell, S L
Morris, M G A
Morris, P D
Morton, O
Murphy, E
Murray, E
Nathan, M P
O'Sullivan, E P
Obichere, A
Offer, M
Osrin, I
Patel, C S
Pelekoudas, N
Pelling, M X
Powis, M R
Qubaty, M A-M
Ramsay, S J
Reinald, F N C
Robinson, D J C
Rosenfelder, A F
Sandby-Thomas, M G
Scatchard, K M
Segall, J M
Shah, M V
Shah, N I
Shakokani, A A
Shaw, F M
Sherif, T E B A F
Smith, A M
Smith, D K
Smith, S C
Spencer, L L
Stein, A G
Stratton, M R
Sumption, C A
Tate, A L
Thomson, B J
Tobias, M
Tonnesmann, M E H P
Tooth, B
Trefzer, S
Vijeyasingam, R
Vites, J
Wainhouse, C L
Watson, T P
Wayne, A N
Whitworth, J A G
Wiseman, O
Wongtschowski, K G J
Wood, E F
Wright, D E
Yap, L B
Yih, J-P L B

NW7

Albert, P J R
Antebi, D
Armstrong, A
Aslan, T
Bailey, D A
Bangham, A M
Beynon, H L C
Brown, B E
Claasen, G
Crawford, C E
Cuttell, P J C
Dawson, J D
Dimson, H P
Durojaiye, O M
Fairweather, D V I
Faulkner, P
Fields, P A
Figa, S A
Flower, S P
Fluck, N C
Fluck, S L
Frost, D K
Gandamihardja, T A-K
Goldsmith, E
Gomes, M F A
Greenbaum, A S
Hitchcock, S-C
Imtiaz, F
Joshi, N D
Joshi, N D
Khan, S N
Lagnado, M L J
Lai Chung Fong, P
Levy, J
Lewis, D S
Lineen, P M
Lloyd, M H
McDermott, E
Makanjuola, A O
Maruthainar, K
Maruthainar, N
Moorthy, S S
Murad, J
Nandi, R
Newman, M J
Noori, S N
Oduro-Yeboah, A
Osman, E M
Pei Yaw Liang, G
Pei, K C B
Pei, Y M D
Peter, J L T
Qureshi, I A
Remington, G A
Remington, K N
Reynolds, M A
Reynolds, W H
Robles, A
Rosefield, A R
Sawdayee-Azad, A
Singer, J
Sirisena, U N H
Sood, M K
Tang, Y C
Thwaites, S V
Tobias, A R
Valentine, N J
Wijetilleka, A B S A
Wiseman, A J

NW8

Abadi, D I
Abdel Aal, N M Y
Al-Barjas, H S A
Al-Duri, Z A A A K
Al-Simaani, M T
Alorda Boscana, M M
Amis, S J
Anderson, G
Antoniou, A K
Bakker, A A
Bentley, C R
Beukes, A J
Bhattacharya, K
Bivona, D
Black, P D
Brennan, D J J
Brown, R A
Campbell, M D
Chambers, R F
Chan, E Y-L
Charkin, S M
Chau, G K-O
Cheah, E-G
Cheesman, A D
Conway, J S
Craft, N
Cram, L A
De Fonseka, S E
Dick, J R F
Dunn, C J
El Sayed, T F E B
Elias, D A
Elton, A
Emery, R J H
Forman, R G
Fortune, F
Freedman, L
French, A J
Garfinkel, H A
Gillingham, N S
Glazer, G
Golding, C E M
Graham, J M
Grahame, R
Harris, D W S
Hogewind, G L
Hunt, S R
Jacobson, U
Jarman, B
John, L C H
Kanoria, S
Kauffmann, E A
Kazi, T
Khan, A
Lam, F H T
Lancaster, R
Lavelle, E T
Lever, E G
Levin, A
Lewis, K H
Lister, D A
Love, W E
Lowick, S J
Lyons, J D
Mackay, J A
Mallon, E C
Marston, R A
Masani, J J N
Mason, A A
Mehta, A R
Mintz, H G
Mira, S A
Mitra, A N
Mohammed, I
Mulla, N A
Nancekievill, D G
Nwakakwa, V C
Oldershaw, P J
Pang, A
Panos, G Z
Panos, M Z
Parbhoo, S P
Quinn, D W
Ralph, D J
Ramsbottom, N
Ratnaval, N
Razavi, L M
Rogol, B
Ross, A
Sarner, M
Schuff, G H
Seifert, M H
Shahdadpuri, V D
Sharp, M A
Shellim, M A
Shirlaw, N A
Silove, Y M
Singh, J K
Singh, R
Smith, G M
Snell, W M
Soh, J K
Sonnabend, J A
Sonoda, L I
Soyer, J A
Super, P
Taylor, C J
Vecht, R J
Wasan, B S
Wellwood, J M
Wilkins, R A
Wilton, J F
Wong, T H T
Wyke, B D
Yoon, J S L

NW9

Abdullah, A M
Ahmed, G M S U
Ahmed, S
Alpren, C G
Amakye, C A
Bachelani, A
Burnett, A C
Cahalin, P A
Catchpole, M A
Chandran, V
Chandrasekara, B S D
Chapman, L E
Cheeroth, S R
Chong, I
Cole, C A
Contreras, M
Cookson, B D
Crowcroft, N S
Dave, D V
De Silva, M
Deshpande, H B
Dinshaw, D
Dutta, J
Ehrenstein, J S
Evans, B G
Finlay, B R
Fitzgerald, A M
Fox, A S
Fry, T
Fung-A-Fat, A G E
Furtado, A
Gajjar, A
Gallagher, L M
Gandhi, P
George, R C
Ghani, K R
Gill, O P N
Guhadasan, R
Harpalani, V B
Harrison, J F
Hewitt, P E
Heyse-Moore, J P
Huehns, E R
Hunyi, S J
Irfan, S A
Johnson, P M
Kaul, A
Kearney, J W
Kelsey, W A
Kirkbride, H A
Kumar, P V
Lamba, M K
Lloyd, R V
Madi, M S
Makhecha, R L
Martin Palma, E
Mathew, G
Mathew, N G
Mirza, H
Modi, A J
Mondal, A A
Moore, M C
Morafa, O A
Morgan, D
Mortimer, P P
Newby, R T
Ng Chieng Hin, S M C
Nicoll, A G
O'Brien, S J
Ofoe, V D
Om Prakash, M
Onuoha, O O

Patel, J
Pattani, S K
Pundit, M
Qureshi, N A
Ramaswami, R A
Ramsay, M E B
Ray, S
Raza, N
Regan, A F M
Richards, D
Rowe, B
Selwyn, A
Shah, J
Shah, U
Shah, Y Z
Sim, F M
Smith, P D
Sobti, U K
Stanwell Smith, R E
Steele, S
Tobiansky, R I
Towuaghantse, E
Vadgama, S
Vetpillai, M
Vetpillai, S
Vogel, M
Walford, D M
Warwick, R M
Watson, J M
Whitlingum, G L
Wilkinson, P J

NW10

Abdalla, A H
Abrahams, L N
Agbim, O G
Akinosho, B O
Amerasinghe, C N
Aminu, A K
Amobi, C A E
Armar, N A
Arnold, A E
Ayles, H M
Badiani, D
Bain, G A
Bansel, J K
Beaconsfield, T
Bell, R A
Bose, U
Bowman, P
Boyce, M J
Brook, M G
Bumby, A F
Carne, A J
Cayley, A C D
Cheong-Leen, R
Colaco, C B
Cummings, T A
Dalby, M C D
Davies, D D
De Roeck, N J
Depala, B T
Deshmukh, S B
Dharia, R R
El-Sadig, S E G
Erskine, M K
Eza, D E
Fletcher, M D
Fletcher, S D
Gellert, A R
Gellert, S L
Godward, S
Graham, V A L
Green, D M
Grenfell, A
Habib, M
Hine, A L
Hollingdale, J P
Howells, H V
Hughes, R T
Humphries, P D
Ibrahimi, M-Q
Igboaka, G U A
Irani, G S
Israni, G K
Johnston, F A B
Joseph, J P
Joshi, R
Kapoor, A
Kay, L
Kerslake, S
Kirollos, C T
Kirubaharan, K
Klein, J L
Kong, E K C
Lee, V
Levy, S G
Loftus, J K M
Low, J K
Lubega, S L
McManus, R J M
Mak, V H F
Mallik, D
Manning, E A D N B
Markham, G C
Marks, A J
Marks, M M
Marris, R
Mohammad, T S
Murphy, S
Murugesu, I
Nancarrow, J G
Naorose-Abidi, S M
O'Brien, M S G
Ogakwu, M O
Ogugua, V O
Parkar, H B
Patel, C
Patel, I P
Patel, S B
Pearse, M
Peter, A M
Powell, R B
Prosser, R E
Ramdahen-Gopal, S
Ray Chaudhuri, K
Richardson, A
Riordan, J F
Robayo Castillo, L V
Roberts, A J
Rolfe, L M
Ryan, N M A
Salmasi, A-M
Samuel, J
Schwartz, R H
Shabrokh, P
Shafi, M S
Shah, D
Shapiro-Stern, P R
Shaw, B E
Sherman, D I N
Shields, J
Shorvon, P J
Singh, S P
Sklar, E M
Tachakra, S S
Tan, S
Taylor, P C A
Thompson, S M
Toh, C T
Veiras, M B
Vergnaud, S
Warrington, S J
Wijetunge, A
Woko, E C
Woko, S C
Wong, K K Y
Woolich, J G
Yarger, N

NW11

Adler, J S
Adler, S
Adomakoh, N K P
Ahmad, S
Andrew, M
Angell, C L
Armonis, A
Asaria, R H Y
Atkin, N B
Been, J B
Benjamin, A R
Bentley, J
Bethlehem, A K
Blanchon, B J R
Bloch, L G
Blom, P S
Brenner, B N
Buckman, L
Carlos, A J
Catania Aguero, S
Cavendish, M N
Chalk, B-Z
Cheong, F M
Chow, P Y
Clark, M
Cohen, R J
Cohen, S I
Croft, E
Curwen, J L
Day, B L
De Souza, M V
De Souza, V C
Desai, S J S
Dollery, C T
Donovan, C F
Dubowitz, D J
Dubowitz, G
Dubowitz, L M S
Duckworth-Smith, H C
Dutt, S
Eccleston, S E
Elgar, J D
Evans, A T
Fisher, M
Flores De Laurnaga, B
Foo, I S M
Garrett, K R
Gergel, I P
Gishen, F S
Gledhill, M T
Gold, D B
Goldberg, M
Golden, B J
Goldin, J G
Goodchild, H
Gordon, G
Greenberg, M
Greenstein, A S
Greenstreet, Y L A
Grossmark, K R
Gubbay, A D
Harris, C
Harris, M
Harverd, L B
Heald, S C
Herbert, P J
Hill, J M
Hochhauser, D
Hooper, P A
Ibrahim, F
Jayaweera, R L A
Jayaweera, R D
Kabeli, S
Kates, W E
Kaufman, D
Kaufman, L
Kessel, M S
Khan, I U H
Khwaja, H
Kirklin, D L
Kucheria, R
Kurer, M H J
Kwapong, A O
Kwong, A
Lalvani, M
Laznowski, A
Lindop, P J
Liu, C K L
Long, C W
Mahir, S A
Malhotra, M
Manson, J J
Mathur, A
Meyer, D L
Miller, A C
Miller, D M
Moross, T
Moss-Morris, S B
Nadal, M J
Narvani, A A
Oberman, A S
Ong, C
Page, C M
Parikh, A M
Patel, B C
Patel, M M
Patel, N R
Pepys, M E
Peters, C J
Phillips, C J
Price, E H
Price, L C
Rasheed, S A A
Ratnasabapathy, L
Ray, S
Riaz, S
Roberts, B L
Robinson, P D
Rogers, D J S
Rowbury, C A
Roy, P
Russell, N H
Sanati, M
Sanders, K
Scheuer, P J
Shah, J C
Shah, S N
Shah, S P K
Shanson, D C
Sharman, V L
Shukla, K K
Steiner, J
Steiner, M C
Stern, M
Stoll, B A
Teller, R H M
Thomas, M E M
Townley, A D
Trivedi, S K
Tunkel, S A
Valman, H B
Vandervelde, E M
Varchevker, J A
Vinayagum, S R
Warman, L H
Weber, J
Wengrowe, N E
Wyndham, J G
Yamey, G M
Yellon, T J
Zosmer, N R S

SE1

Abbs, I C
Acharya, B
Adam, A N
Agathonikou, A
Agrawal, M R
Ahmed, A A
Amin, D M
Anderson, D R
Andrews, T C
Andrews, V
Aps, C
Archibong, E I
Atkinson, S H
Bagshaw, Dr
Baker, E J
Bankes, M J K
Barker, J N W N
Barkley, A S J
Barnett, M B
Baron, I D
Barrington, S F
Bateman, N T
Bauer, P
Bbeid, M A M
Beale, R J
Beaney, R P
Beckley, J
Beechey-Newman, N
Bejon, P A
Bennie, M J
Bewley, S J
Beynon, T A
Bialas, I
Bihari, D J
Bingham, J S
Bird, C F
Biswas, G
Black, M M
Blaney, S P A
Blauth-Muszkowski, C I A
Bodani, M
Booton, P
Bosley, C M
Boulton, J E
Bradbeer, C S
Braude, P R
Breathnach, S M
Brennand-Roper, D A
Bridgwood, W G
Briscoe, O V
Brooks, M
Brostoff, J
Brunjes, H O
Bucknall, C A
Burnand, K G
Burney, P G J
Buxton, N J
Calman, F M B
Calver, D M
Carapeti, E A
Carr, R
Carroll, P V J
Catto, G R D
Chambers, J B
Champion, M P
Chan, K
Chappell, L C
Chelliah, J V
Chevretton, E B
Chia, H M Y
Chowdhury, P
Ciclitira, P J
Clark, A G B
Clark, K G A
Clark, T B
Clarke, D G
Clarke, S E M
Clayden, G S
Cochrane, G M
Coltart, D J
Connaughton, M
Connell, P A
Cooke, R A
Cooper, B M S
Corr, L A
Corrigall, R J
Corrigan, C J
Cowling, M G
Cox, A D
Cranston, I C P
Cremona-Barbaro, A
Crook, M A
Crowson, R A
Cunningham, C S
Cunningham, D G
Curry, P V L
Curson, S
D'Cruz, D P
Daniels, J G
Davies, E A
Davies, G M
Davies, T W
Davis, A R
Davison, S E
Dawe, S A
De Ruiter, A
Demetroulis, C
Dervos, H D
Dickson, J P
Djurovic, V
Dobbs, H J
Dodhia, H
Doherty, S J
Donnan, S P B
Dowling, R H
Dratcu, L
Duerden, B I
Dussek, J E
Eady, R A J
Earnshaw, P H
Eckle, I
Elkington, N M
Ellis, P A
Evans, A V
Evans, G
Evans, S M
Farmer, C K T
Fentiman, I S
Ferguson, J S J
Ferro, A
Fisher, M J
Fishlock, D J
Flinter, F A
Fogelman, I
Foley-Comer, A J
Forbes, M J
Fotiadou, M
Fottrell, E M
Fox, E F
Fraser-Andrews, E A
Fraser, H M
Fraser, J S
French, G L
Fry, A H
Fryer, J A
Gadd, E M
Gaind, R
Garnham, I R C
George, M L
Germain, S J
Ghosh, G J
Giannelli, F B
Gibson, K A A
Gill, A D S
Gill, H K
Gleeson, M J
Gnudi, L
Goldsmith, D J A
Graham, E M
Gransden, W R
Gray, D C
Griffiths, M A
Gruden, G
Gulliford, M C
Gunasekara, H L
Haig, J
Hamann, W C
Hamed, H H A
Hampson, N
Haq, M R
Harari, D
Harborow, P W
Harris, A N G
Harris, M B
Harris, S J
Harrison, C N
Hartley, H M
Haworth, F L M
Haycock, G B
Heathcock, R M
Heatley, F W
Herbert, A
Hextall, J M
Hicks, B H
Hilton, R M
Ho, W T V
Hodgkiss, A D
Holloway, J B
Holt, G M
Hopkinson, N S
Hubbard, J G H
Hughes, G R V
Hughes, R A C
Hunt, B J
Hunter, D N
Hussain, K
Islam, M T
Izatt, L P
Jackson, B T
Jackson, G
Janse Van Rensburg, M
Jarvis, D L
Jeannon, J P
Jennings, M P
Jezzard, R G
Johnson, J-A
Joiner, C L
Jones, A J
Justins, D M
Kaiser, A M
Kanabar, D J
Kavalier, F C
Keable-Elliott, D A
Keen, H
Khader, M A B A
Khamashta, M A
Khan, L N
Khan, S S
Khor, T T G
Kinirons, M T M
Kirby, N G
Kmiot, W A
Kobza Black, A
Koffman, C G
Kopelman, M D
Koutroumanidis, M
Kovalic, A J
Kubba, A A
Kulasegaram, R
Lamas, C D C
Lambiase, D P
Landau, D B
Landfester, C
Langford, K S
Lankester, T E
Lawman, S H A
Leach, R M
Lee, C
Lee, S L C
Lee, T H
Lee, Y-C
Leeds, A R
Leese, E J
Lehner, T
Leigh, T H
Leighton, M A
Lekakis, G
Leslie, M D
Levy, S J
Lewis, G H
Lewis, P J
Lewis, R R
Lim, M
Lin, J-P
Linton, R A F
Lipsedge, M S
Lloyd, C P
Lo, R S-K
Lockie, S M C
Lowy, C
Ludgate, S M
Mabey, D M
McAlindon, T E
McCarthy, M M
MacDonald, D M
MacDonald, L M
McGibbon, D H
McGrath, J A
McGregor, J M
McGuinness, C L
McGurk, M
McLuckie, A
MacMahon, E M E
Madan, R
Mahadeva, U
Maisey, M N
Mant, T G K
Mantell, A E

Marber, M S
Markey, A C
Markowe, H L J
Marlowe, K H S
Marshall, S A
Martin, F C
Martin, L J
Maryon-Davis, A R
Mascarenhas, L J
Maslen, T P J
Master, D R
Mathews, J A
Mawer, C
Mayer, E
Maynard, R L
Mehrez, Y G M
Mekawi, L M F
Mellerio, J E
Mellor, S
Midgley, D Y
Milburn, H J
Mills, P R
Milner, A D
Milner, D G G
Mishra, M
Misra, K K
Modarai, B
Mohammed, S N
Morgan, J R
Morley, A P
Morris-Jones, R
Motto, S G A
Muller-Pollard, C S
Mulvey, M J
Naftalin, R J
Nath, B K
Nelson-Piercy, C
Newton, N I
Ng, G Y T
Nunan, T O
Nunn, D
Nyeko, C
O'Brart, D P S
O'Brien, M D
O'Connell, M E A
O'Dell, E
O'Donnell, P J
O'Sullivan, D G M
O'Sullivan, G M
Panayi, G S
Parikh, K S
Parnaby-Price, A
Patel, D
Pattison, J M
Payne, C O
Pearce, A C
Pearson, A D
Pearson, T C
Peel, M R
Penman Splitt, M C
Peters, B S
Pettigrew, R A
Pietroni, R A Y
Pither, C E
Plunkett, T A
Pocock, C F E
Pohl, K R E
Polani, P E
Polychronis, A
Pope, F M
Porter, J S
Poston, R N
Potter, J G
Povlsen, B
Powrie, J K
Powroznyk, A V V
Price, N M
Priest, T D
Pritchard, J
Qureshi, S A
Radclyffe, V G
Rakhit, R D
Ramachandra, S
Ramirez, A J
Ramsay, R L
Randall, S J
Rankin, S C
Rao, M R
Razzaque, M
Reddy, M
Redfearn, A
Redfearn, P M
Redwood, S R
Reed, L J
Rees, P J
Reid, C J D
Reidy, J F
Richards, A
Richards, M A
Ridgway, G L
Ridley, D M
Rigden, S P A
Rissik, J M
Ritter, J M
Robb, S A
Robinson, P D
Robinson, R O
Robson, M G
Rodgers, C A
Rona, R J
Rosen, B K
Roth, C E
Rowlands, E C
Rowsell, A R
Roxburgh, J C
Roy, D H
Rudd, A G
Russell-Jones, R D
Russell, R E K
Rycroft, R J G
Ryle, A
Rymer, J M
Sacks, S H
Salimee, S G
Salisbury, D M
Santos Ramon, A
Saunders, A J S
Saunders, P J
Savidge, G F
Scarisbrick, J J
Schey, S A
Scott-Mackie, P L
Setterfield, J F
Seymour, A-M F
Shaheen, S O
Shanti Raju, K
Sharief, M K
Sharland, G K
Sharp, H R
Shaw, M C
Shennan, A H
Shepherd, P S
Sherry, E N
Shilling, J S
Simcock, R A J
Simpson, J M
Singh, S D
Siva Prakash, P G
Skidmore, F D
Smith, G N
Smith, M J M
Smith, S J
Sonksen, P H
Soo, S S
Spalton, D J
Spector, R G
Spector, T D
Spencer, J D
Staffurth, J N
Steer, S E
Stefan, M D
Stern, C M M
Stock, D G
Stone, I M
Summers, L K M
Sundaresan, V
Tan, K-H
Tate, A T
Taylor, J D
Taylor, P R
Teo, C E-S
Thadani, H
Thoburn, C R
Thompson, A E
Thompson, R P H
Thomson, R D A
Tibby, S M
Tilzey, A J
Timothy, A R
Tiptaft, R C
Tolhurst, D E
Tonge, K A
Torry, R
Treacher, D F
Treasure, J L
Treasure, T
Tungekar, M F M Y
Turnbull, S M
Turner, A
Twitchen, M J
Twort, C H C
Ungar-Sargon, J Y
Van Den Hurk, P J
Vassiliadis, N
Vaughan, J M M
Velazquez Guerra, M D
Venn, G E
Verikiou, K
Vernon, J A
Viberti, G F
Wain, E M
Wale, L W
Walker, S C
Wallis, D N
Walsh, R M
Ward, J
Waring, M
Waterstone, M P M
Watson, M S
Webb-Peploe, M M
Webb, J F W
Webb, M C
Whitmore, B L
Widdicombe, J G
Wierzbicki, A S
Wight, A L
Wilkinson, M L
Williams, A J
Williams, B T
Williams, D G
Williams, E R L
Williams, K N
Williams, R E
Williamson, J B
Williamson, T H
Wolfe, C D A
Wong, A P L
Wong, W
Wood, C H
Wrigley, R A
Wyncoll, D L A
Yi, C-Y
Young, A E
Young, C P
Young, L R

SE2

Al-Zaidy, A K
Anand, P
Cannon, W J
Flynn, A G
Gravestock, S M
Menezes, G R
Milstein, P A
Pulsford, D R
Robinson, S J
Smith, C C M
Todd, V A
Troughton, V A

SE3

Ahmed, S S
Aravinthan, J
Arnold, R W
Bains, J J S
Bassi, S K
Begum, J A
Besson, J A O
Black, P J
Chapman, P
Chesterton, J R
Chowienczyk, P J
Claoue, C M P A
Colvin, L J
Cumberland, A G
Davies, N H
Dhadly, M S
Elliott, R M
Fender, L J
Field, B C T
Gillbard, J
Gregory, F P
Guest, R M
Guppy, A E
Harrison, T A
Hay, J F
Heliotis, M
Holland-Gladwish, J J
Hooper, S E
Houghton, S H
Huang, C P
Huang, D C S
Jackson, P G
Jennings, J M
Jones, H I
Kailey, L K
Kalairajah, Y
Krall, K
Lee, S R
McCarthy, C A
McCullagh, A G
McKee, S N K
McNicholas, F C P
Mahesh, Dr
Manna, V K
Megias Martin, E M L
Mehta, M S M
Melchor Ferrer, C
Mikhail, W I
Montgomery, A C V
Mori, K
Moscuzza, F
Muhammad, L M
Muir-Taylor, D J
Mustapha, A A
O'Connell, B
O'Riordan, J B A
Onyeama, W P J C
Patel, S K
Penney, C C
Petty, L G
Plana Vives, F
Poulton, M B
Powell, M B
Price, T R
Purdy, B
Radcliffe, H
Rahman, S M L
Refsum, E
Roberts, A P
Ross, O C
Rowntree, C
Rowntree, M
Sales, J M
Saunders, K B
Schnepel, B
Senior, D F
Skyrme, A D
Smith, S G T
Songhurst, L Z
Sotiriou, S
Stephenson, M T
Stevenson, K E
Stoker, A P
Stoker, T A M
Stokes, T C
Sutaria, P D
Thilagarajah, M
Thomas, A J
Thomas, D
Thompson, A B R
Thompson, D G
Turner, A J
Ward, D G
Wengraf, C L
Westwick, R J
Whitfield, G P
Williams, A B
Windsor, R E
Wood, W E A
Woollett, R J
Young, G V W

SE4

Alderman, E W R
Asherson, P J E
Bacon, L E
Bolam, M J
Byrne, P R
Cahn, A P
Chan, S Y Y
Davies, M P N
Fellows, E W
Griffiths, M P
Haines, D H
Jiao, L
McCullagh, M M M
McIntyre, D H
Majid, F
Malde, G M
Neal, F R
Parker, J H
Parsons, D L T
Pawlowska, E
Reshi, S H
Sagay, A S
Sobolewski, O A
Springer, S E
Watts, A M
Wiggins, C A T

SE5

Abas, M A
Aclimandos, W A I
Adair, A
Ahmed, A M M
Aitchison, K J
Al-Chalabi, A
Al-Nawab, M D A-D
Al-Sarraj, S T
Alarcon Palomo, G
Alcock, E L
Allin, M P G
Amiel, S A
Amusan, K A
Ashley, E M C
Aylwin, S J B
Bailey, C S
Bailey, P J
Baker, H J W
Balendran, P
Ball, C S
Ball, D M
Banerjee, S S
Barnes, P R J
Barrett, C H R
Begley, E A
Bellingham, A J
Bernard, S H
Berry, H E
Bhatt, G B
Bhugra, D K M L
Bindman, J P
Bindra, R
Binnie, C D
Bird, J
Birtchnell, J A
Bjarnason, I T
Bowden, P M A
Bowles, M J
Bras, P J
Brex, P A
Brown, A S T
Brown, R M
Buchanan, A W
Buchanan, C R
Buckland, M S
Bullock, P R
Buxton-Thomas, M S
Cairns, H S
Cardozo, L D
Cavanagh, J B
Cervilla Ballesteros, J A
Chan, D H Y
Chandler, C L
Chau, N-M
Cheah, E K L
Checkley, S A
Child, F J
Chin, D T-E
Chitkara, N
Chong, M S
Chong, N H V
Choy, C N K
Choy, E H S
Cleare, A J
Clough, C G
Cohen, A T
Cole, E D E J
Compson, J P
Connor, S E J
Conway, J L C
Cottam, S J C
Cotton, H M
Crane, J L
Crayford, T J B
Crick, R P
Critchley, G R
Critchlow, D G
Cross, Z E
Crouchman, M R
Curson, R
Curtis, V A
D'Alba, R
Dare, J R
Davenport, M
David, A S
Davies, R A
Davies, S N
Davison, S C
Dawson, A
Dawson, J M
Dayanandan, R
De Meeus, J-B
De Zulueta, F I S
Deasy, N P
Desai, J B
Desai, S
Devane, S P
Devereux, S
Dickinson, L
Dilley, M D
Dowell, J K
Driver, M V
Durston, R S
Easterbrook, P J
Eben, F
Eddleston, A L W F
Edmonds, P
Edwards, J G
Elkington, H M
Ellis, C M
Elwes, R D C
Evans, J A
Evanson, R L
Fabre, J W
Fahy, T A
Farmer, A E
Farrell, M P
Ferguson, J D
Fife, A J
Finch, E J L
Finnerty, G T
Fisher, A P
Fleminger, S
Forgacs, I C
Gall, N P
Gardner, W N
Garrett, J R
Gayle, C M
Ghufoor, Z
Ginsburg, R
Glucksman, E
Goldberg, D P B
Gonde, J E
Goodman, R N
Goodwill, C J
Granger, A C P
Gray, B J
Green, D W
Greenough, A
Griffin, M
Grime, P R
Groom, A F G
Groves, P A
Gullan, R W
Gunn, J C
Gurm, H S
Ha, Y W M
Hadden, R D M
Hadfield, P J
Hadzic, N
Hakkak, M S
Hanna, M H
Harris, P E
Harrison, P M
Harry, R A
Hart, I J
Harwood, G
Healy, M R
Height, S E
Henderson, R C
Hendry, B M
Hester, J B
Heyman, I
Higgins, E M
Higginson, I J
Homolka, M P P
Honavar, M
Hopkins, D F C
Hopster, D J
Hotopf, M H
Howard, L M
Howard, R J M W
Howells, R B
Howes, O D
Huggon, I C
Hugh-Jones, P
Hughes, M W
Hutchinson, G A
Hutchison, D C S
Ismail, K
Jamieson-Craig, T K
Jenkins, R
Jewitt, D E
Jones, N A E
Joseph, S E O
Juhasz, Y C
Jurkovic, D
Kalra, L
Kelly, A J
Kelly, C P
Kelly, D M C
Kerwin, R W
Khan, M Z
Klein, S
Krasucki, C G
Langdon, J D
Lawton, F G
Layton, D M
Lee, W E
Leech, S C
Lees, C C
Leigh, P N
Limb, S P
Lingford-Hughes, A R
Lloyd, C M
Lo, S K
Lovestone, S H
Lucas, P A
Lucey, J V
Lyons, A J

MacCarthy, P A
MacDonald, B K
McDonald, E M P
McDonnell, N P
Macedo, P
McGinley, E
McGregor, A M
McGuffin, P
McGuire, P K
McInerny, T M
McKenzie, N C
MacKinnon, A G
McManus, T J
Macvicar, A D L
Maden, A
Maiden, H K
Malligiannis, P
Man, W D-C
Manuelpillai, N L
Marks, I M
Marrinan, M T
Marsh, M S
Marshall, E J
Marshall, W J
Massil, H Y
Meeran, H
Meldrum, B S
Melissari, E
Messent, M
Michaelis, C
Mieli Vergani, G
Mills, K R
Misch, P A
Mohamed Rela, S
Moniz, C F
Moorey, S
Moriarty, J
Mortimer, J M P
Morton, M A S
Mostyn, P A
Moxham, J
Muiesan, P
Mulvin, D W
Munro, J C
Murphy, K C
Murphy, S M
Murray, R M
Naidu, V
Nash, R M
Nashef, L
Natucci, M
Ng Hock Oon, P
Ng, V W K
Noble, P J
Noble, P R
O'Brien, A J
O'Brien, I M
O'Connor, B J
O'Dowd, L R
O'Grady, J G M
Olajide, O O
Osborne, S A
Pagliuca, A
Palmer, C
Park, H G J
Parkin, J R
Parmar, H
Parsons, J H
Parton, M J
Patel, A G
Patel, A J
Patel, J V
Peebles, D M
Perez Celorrio, I
Peters, T J
Phillips, S L
Philpot, M P
Philpott-Howard, J N
Picchioni, M M
Pocock, J
Polkey, C E
Polkey, M I
Pollock, L E
Ponte, J C
Portmann, B C
Pouria, S
Prasad, S
Price, J F
Purves, A M
Rahman, S
Rashid, H I
Rees, D C
Reiss, D
Rennie, J M
Rennie, J A
Retzlaw, E
Reynolds, E H
Reynolds, P A
Ridsdale, L L
Rifkin, L
Riordan-Eva, P
Robinson, S
Romilly, C S
Rood, J P
Rose, M R
Rosemen, J J
Rowell, A M
Rushton, D N
Russell, M A H
Rutter, M L
Saha, M
Salisbury, J R
Salman, M S
Samuel, M C
Sangala, A V
Saunders, D E
Savvas, M
Sayal, K S
Scott, D L
Seaman, J A
Sedgwick, J V
Selway, R P
Shah, A M
Sham, P C
Sharland, R J
Shaw, S C
Sheehan, B D
Sheikh, A
Siddique, F H
Sidhu, P S
Simonoff, E A
Sinha, J
Skinner, J A M
Spencer, J P G
Springer, J
Stagkou, A
Stephens, A D
Stewart, R J
Strang, J S
Strong, A J
Subotsky, F E
Sutherby, E K
Tanner, S P
Taylor, A M
Taylor, C B
Taylor, E A
Taylor, R E
Tenant-Flowers, M
Thein, S L
Thomas, J N
Thomas, N W M
Thompson, P M
Thomson, D S
Thornicroft, G J
Tiller, J M
Travis, M J
Trill, A S
Turner, L
Upton, K E
Vergani, D
Virji, A A N
Von Kaisenberg, C S L
Vougas, V
Wade, J J
Wainwright, R J
Waterstone, J J
Watkins, P J
Watson, D-M K
Watts, P M
Webster, P M
Welch, J M
Wendon, J A
Wessely, S C
Wheatley, E A
Whitehead, M I
Wickstead, D H
Wilkinson, M C P
Williams, I L
Williams, I T
Wilson Jones, C F
Wilson, S P
Winston, I
Wolff, G S
Wong, T H G
Wood, B L
Woolley, J B
Wright, I C
Wright, J B
Wyatt, H A
Xenitidis, K
Yakeley, J W

SE6

Abang-Taha, A B
Akinbolue, O S
Akomea-Agyin, C
Allan, P E M
Allen, M C
Alonso Urrutia, A M
Amiruddin, K M
Augustine, A S
Ayeko, M O
Dare, C
Doble, N S
Entwistle, H J
Heathcote, J A
Hughes, E F
Ismail, K
Joseph, M J G
Lasoye, T A
Lee, J F
Macauslan, K M
McCredie, J E
McIntosh, D M
Mangan, C M
Mills, A W
Mireskandari, K
Misselbrook, D P
Nguyen, T D
O'Connor, K B
Pavar, J S
Pektas, T
Ragupathy, M
Shanaz, M
Sharpe, D S
Surridge, N J
Thomas, M R
Twort, R J
Weston, J C
White, P T

SE7

Abel, D C
Barker, K
Browne, D G
Corston, S H
Dickson, E J
King, L A
Palmer, S J
Parkash, V K
Parsons, M S J
Rowlands, R G
Santos, J P D
Sharpe, E E
Skelton, M L

SE8

Batra, B K
Caffrey, E A
Gandhe, A J
Hashmi, K Z
Ikogho, O O
Jain, A K M
Khan, O
Mohamedali, A
Olobia, E V A
Patel, J
Sanghera, S
Singh, S

SE9

Abel, H B
Agarwal, V
Alcalay, M
Baksh, M
Boddy, J L
Brahmbhatt, G A
Campbell, P I
Durve, D V
Edghill, H B
Evans, D P
Field, R
Fortune, D C
Hack, H H A
Hack, M E
Jacobson, R R
Jarrett, P H
Kenny, D A
Khanam, A N
Lal, J
Lazim, T R
Livingstone, J S
McCarthy, K
Mahfuth, Z S
Martin, R K
Massey, R M
Mulvaney, J K
Owen, W A
Pearlgood, M
Pratap, R
Saldanha, G J F
Sandrasagra, V
Sennik, S K
Shahab, K L
Singh, H
Sithamparanathan, T
Sizer, E
Surenthiran, S S
Taylor, R L
Thenuwara, C D
Varma, C
Varma, R B
Wade, C B
Young, S M

SE10

Ahmed, I
Barclay, G A
Bennett, E P T
Brown, A P
Clark, B R
Cochran, G O
Davies, J K
Dyke, T N
George, S P
Haque, Q S M
Harris, A J
Janmohamed, K M I
Lee, J A
Lesnik Oberstein, S Y
Lindsay, I
McCarthy, K H
O'Riordan, S E
Perks, N F
Perry, N D
Phillips, H M
Phillips, P M
Ratnarajan, N
Ratnarajan, S T
Richards, T J L
Ryan, M J
Seymour, W M
Sivagnanam, C
Smith, A D
Stott, R B
Thomas, A L
Tibrewal, S B
Wilkinson, A C H
Wilmshurst, J M
Wright, E S

SE11

Allen, D K
Amin, N K F
Armstrong, D
Ashworth, M
Badger, K M
Barnick, C G W
Bruce, R C H
Campbell, J L
Cantillon, C J P M
Collins, A D
Cutting, C W M
Cutting, H A
Dudley, F L
Falkov, A F
Fitzpatrick, S A
Foley, P T
Fourie, H
Gaspar, H B R
Harker, R J
Harrison, N A
Henwood, N D
Honeyman, A E
Hunt, T M
James, S
Jones, R H
Khorsandi, S E
Latham, J A
Lees, M
Loader, P J
Lorek, A K
Madan, A K
Martin, W N
Mercurio, G G
Murdoch, E
Olayemi, A O
Pelfrene, E
Poole, D
Rossor, E B
Sayour, S
Scrutton, M J L
Shaffer, J
Smyth, J M
Spencer, G T
Summers, P D
Tangang, V N
Theodore, C M
Timms, P W
Tynan, M J
Van Reenen, S
Walsh, D M
Wass, V J
West, H
Wynne-Jones, G A
Yiu, C O S

SE12

Balachandran, S
Bamberger, D C
Bentham, J C P
Byford, S
Ghuran, A V
Helm, E J
John, R I
Kenning, B R
Khanem, N M
Kreeger, C G
McCarthy, H J
MacDonagh, I R J
Malik, Y D
Mian, I
Morgan, D S
Nguyen, D Q A
Oakley, R J
Ong, F G-C
Santhakumar, D
Selvanathan, G A J
Seth, P
Stark, J P
Taylor, K A
Uhama, J N
Whitworth, M
Willis, J H P

SE13

Abraham, D M
Aitken, E M
Al-Janabi, T A J
Alister, M E
Bahri, A H
Bharaj, H S
Birch, D J
Boss, G
Byng, R N
Cochrane, R M
Coogan, J S V S R
Cooney, J M
Daman Willems, C E
Del Amo Valero, J
du Peloux Menagé, H G
Dudley, J M
Dunn, N J
Dykes, E H
Eiser, N M
Evans, R G
Farrington, T
Fathulla, B
Fidler, H M
Garcia Gimeno, I
Garvie, D C
Gibbs, S E M
Goddard, N P
Gore, R V
Gostling, A C
Haines, H M
Harris, T M
Heath, M L
Hill, M D
Holloway, G
Hossain, A T M A
Hossain, Z A
Isaac, M T
Jack, T C L
Jacobs, B R
Jacomb-Hood, J H
Jarrett, P S
Jolaoso, A S
Kabir, A M N
Kabir, J M M
Kennedy, D C M
Kenny, P A
Khalpey, Z I
Khwaja, F A
Kingsley, G H
Lam, J S J
Lanigan, C J M
Leslie, A
Lettington, W C
Lewis, S J
Linsell, J C
Mohammed, S A
Morgan, M B F
Mounty, E J
Nayeem, N
Norton, J
O'Donohue, J W
O'Sullivan, A G
Ogufere, W E
Page, J M
Petriccione Di Vadi, P
Phillips, M G
Pierpoint, S
Plugge, E H
Powell, C M
Prince, M J
Reffitt, D M
Richards, C A
Roberts, A P
Roberts, J M
Roe, C M
Ross, A P
Roulson, C J
Sajjanhar, T
Sakka, S A A
Salama, N Y
Sands, A M
Sarker, P
Seth, R V
Shafik, A M
Shaw, S J
Shelton, D M
Smith, C H
Songo-Williams, R A
Starke, I D
Stroobant, J
Suddle, A R
Uduku, N O-A
Walker, G A
Wellesley, A J
Wilson, E J
Wiseman, M R
Worsley, A P
Zamblera, D

SE14

Almeida, E J J
Almeida, N M
Banks, P A
Blackie, P J
Bruce Ja Ja, D F
Charmantas, M G
Chesterman, L P
Dargan, P I
Dias, S A N
Gordon-Brown, A D
Haire, A R
Himid, K A
Humm, T E
Jenkins, R G
Jeyanathan, S
Jones, A L
Kandavel, R
Karalliedde, S
Karlman, I M
Leonardi, G S
McColl, J L
MacDermott, A J
MacFarlane, A E
Maisey, N R
Martin, P
Murray, V S G
Palin, C
Persaud, R A P
Pickard, S J
Prior, K R E J
Sarder, M O G
Sayyah-Sina, K
Shah, B B
Steele, G J
Tiwary, R N

SE15

Abel, K M
Abeysinghe, A D
Allen, R G
Alyas, F
Amir-Ansari, K
Banjo, A A
Birch, F
Butler, H V S
Chappiti, S S
Coan, K M
Crawshaw, A
Do, M K
Effiong, P
Feazey, A J
Gersten, A E
Graham, J H
Heatley, C J
Hossain, M
Huynh, P S N
Iriyagolle, I M R C
Iu, M
Kumar, S
Lomas, D M
Lupton, M G F
Marks, P
Mathieson, D M
Mehta, P P
Morris, R J C
Pratt, T
Rakowicz, A S
Reyburn, H W

Roe, Y O W
Sales, R C
Seeraj, E C
Seevaratnam, M S
Sekweyama, S G G
Simmons, J
Stolkin, C
Tan, S W
Wall, P R
Watson, F J
Watson, H S
Weeramanthri, T B
Wieland, S S L
Wong, C M
Zeineldine, A A

SE16
Abbasi, K A
Ahmed, S
Beales, P L
Bhatt, J N
Boardman, A P
Chamberlin, A J
Coles, D R
Coyle, F M
Donmall, R C
Easter, R A
Fawibe, O O
Ferguson, J K
Gammon, M
Gangoli, S V
Harding, L D
Hegarty, D D
Holden, P J
Jani, F M
Jani, P
Kadhim, R Y
Kanagalingam, J
Kandiah, N
Kelly, J C
Kent, A S H
Kho, B C
Kirkpatrick, A H
Kirkpatrick, W N A
Li, A M
Lo, S H-S
Magrath, H P
Manam, V R
Marrinan, P J M M
Moses, D V K
Nalla, J
O'Neill, E V
Otty, C J
Patel, S M
Rheem, J Y
Richards, E R
Ringrose, D K
Sandhu, C
Shiv Shanker, V
Stamenkovic, S A
Thomas, M R
Wan, K-M B
Wijetunge, D B
Wong, D C H
Yeh, P S-Y
Zigmond, D

SE17
Abdoolcader, T
Brew-Graves, E H
Brown, J R I
Davenport-Jones, C I
Diffley, F S
Eddy, B A
Evans, B E K
Glasper, A J
Haigh, C S
Herzmark, V J
Higgs, R H
Hodges, J M
Kay, S
Kian, K
Kiernan, E J
Klimek, J V
Lask, B D
Mackay, J E
Maycock, A J
Nixon, S J
Noohu Kannu, A
Page, E A
Pickering, R A
Pryor, A D
Quick, D G C
Rao, N
Robinson, S P
Round, L
Samudri, M F
Sangowawa, O O

Tennent, T D
Thomas, W K

SE18
Agnihotri, S
Ali, M S
Aston, N O F
Baggaley, M R
Banerjee, S
Bragman, S G L
Brox, G A
Burch, J
Cameron, M L
Cetti, N E
Chadha, M S
Char, D N
Chinduluri, C M R
Coakley, P G L
Colvin, S
Dickens, E L
Divall, S E
Edmonds, N R V
Ekpo, E B
Ferraris, G M C
Ghosh, S K
Gibbs, C J
Gupta, S K
Heath, D I
Huggon, A-M
Hughes, R K F
Hussain, S
Ireland, R M
Jenkins, J H
Johnston, J D
Karder, M A
Khan, A
Le Ball, K M
Mackay, A D
McNair, A N B
Markovic, D
Metcalf, S W
Mohamed, A M S
Nagendran, R
Njuki, F I
Oke, O O
Okocha, C
Onyali, K O
Parikh, J
Patel, B K
Pinto, T
Pollock, I
Power, S J
Rached, S T
Raphael, N
Robson, D J
Roden, C E
Saleem, S
Seehra, C S
Seehra, T K
Sen, A
Shah, B A
Siddiqi, M N
Singh, S P
Smith, J R G
Spencer, M E
Sri Krishna, M
Sri Krishna, R
Steadman, P W M
Tanega, K R M
Taylor, M B
Venn-Treloar, J M
Wahba, H F
Watkin, P M
Webb, J R
Yiu, C Y
Young, C J
Young, P W
Young, W A

SE19
Arvin, B
Bolade, I O A
Cheung, B Y Y
Choyce, A
Condon, J R
Deegan, K M
Diver, A O
Elliott, M K
Fakim, A
Gatward, C C
Gray, C J
Heyer, E J
Hickin, L A
Holden, A
Jacobs, B W
James, L E
Khandwala, S
Lams, E J
Lidgey, S I

Luff, R H
Macdonald, I
Mahdi, A M
Ng Cheng Hin, P
Nguyen, C T
Nunn, P A
Patel, R N
Patel, V C
Roditi, E
Sharma, M A
Sinha, S K
Sivathasan, S
Smith, S E
Somalingam, R
Tan Eng Looi, C
Taylor, C L
Trivedi, R S
Virdi, D S
White, P T
Wong Lai Cheng, Dr

SE20
Abraham, J
Davda, K G
Fishtal, A
Hellyar, A G
Manidas, S
Mason, J H
Nalliah, S J
Prasad, P N
Silva, P S
Stoner, S J
Sutton, R B O
Wheeler, D W
Wilson, S E

SE21
Aranki, D A
Aranki, S F I
Assersohn, L C
Athanassiou, S
Baker, S J
Black, J W
Bradbeer, T M
Broughton, S J
Cawson, R A
Chow, C
Cook, J V
Davidson, M J
Di Ceglie, D
Di Ceglie, G R
Doig, R J
Drake, D P
Duff, S E
Edeh, J C T
Evans, T G J R
Fieldhouse, R D
Flower, G P
French, J C
Gupta, R
Hamilton, E B D
Harwin, B G
Hatton, M A
Holden, C A
Howard, K A
Howarth, A E
Howell, C W
Hulf, J A
Jenner, C S
Karalliedde, J L
Katugampola, S M
Kiln, M R
Lams, B E A
Lams, P M
Leonard, R A
Leung, W C D
Lim, J C S
McCaul, J A
Macdonald, A J D
Mahon, C C W
Mann, S N
Miller, S C
Nicolaides, K H
Parris, M P
Pemberton, J
Pemberton, P L
Perry, C M
Pieris, M J A
Polkey, A E
Price, D E
Raeburn, J N
Rohatiner, A Z S
Roseveare, M P
Sandberg, S U T
Siddique, A B M
Sivanandan, M
Smith, J A J
Soni, N C
Starr, D R P

Steger, A C
Taggart, L P
Tamale Ssali, E G
Turvill, J L
Turvill, S B
Wakely, C
Walters, H L
Walters, S J
Whooley, D J

SE22
Abbas, A
Adam, G
Ahmed, M J
Ajayi, R A
Akpobome, G
Alexander, A M
Amir-Ansari, B
Appleby, E L
Barlow, D
Barlow, N P
Barnardo, A T
Barrett, D
Bhatia, A
Blackburn, A M
Breen, C P M
Carucci, P
Chauhan, N
Clark-Jones, A
Cliffe, J M
Close, J C T
Cooper, S R
Corbett, S A
Costello, M C L
Cranston, R D
Curran, I E
Curtis, L D
Dalgliesh, D
Davies, A
Dewji, H
Dimitriou, G
Dowson, A J
Draper, A G
Drobniewski, F A
During, M E
Elston, W J
Evans, J M
Fowler, H M
Fuller, L C
Gallagher, N J
Ghufoor, W N
Graham, H J
Grant, S A
Gulliford, T J G
Gupta, R P
Haq, M I
Hicks, A E
Hill, J P
Hitchins, J E
Holden, N C
Ibrahim, S
Jackson, S H D
Kavadia, V
Kon, S P
Lewis, S J
Luce, P J
Macdougall, I C
MacKeith, J A C
McKenzie, K J
Mallinson, C
Manos, J
Osborn, D M
Parbhoo, I
Parbhoo, K
Pettingale, K W
Pritchard, M J
Pullen, A J
Rhodes, B
Rogers, A D
Rogerson, M E
Round, J E C
Ryan, D J
Saunders, J P
Scoffings, D J
Scorer, R M
Stenhouse, P D
Swift, C G
Tegner, H
Thompson, R J
Wainford, C M
Waller, S C
Ward, S J
Westall, G P
Wistow, T E W
Zuckerman, M A

SE23
Bomford, A B
Bradshaw, C R

Brodie, C
Chow, W C S
Cottrell, C K
Crown, I W
Cudlip, S A
Dein, S L
Dilly, P N
Edwards, M V
Fogazzi, G B
Hickey, M A J
Hu, M T-M
Hyatt, P J
Israel, J
Lamptey, C
Ledger, S
O'Sullivan, N T
Oldershaw, K L
Rosenberg, D A
Rowland, R M
Schroeder, K E M
Slovick, S
Soile, D O
Sykes, A C
Van Cooten, S E
Wheeler, J H

SE24
Ball, S P
Blackburn, T K
Blackman, G M
Bowen, E F
Chieveley-Williams, S A
Chinegwundoh, J O M
Dasan, R
Deasy, H C A
Dhingra, J K
Dick, M C
Dickinson, G
Ellsbury, G F
Evanson, E J
Fenwick, P B C
Finn, A P
Galdos Tobalina, M P
Gleeson, J M
Hampton, A C
Hanna, S J E
Hornsey, J M
Houghton, M A
Hughes, G J
Ish-Horowicz, M R
Joashi, U C
Jones, P R
Kasaka, N
Kemp, R A
Kulkarni, A K
Lamb, S N
Lasserson, E M
Ledger, D H
McClintock, T L
Meares, T M
Morris, M S D
Naraynsingh, P A
Noble, P L
Pallecaros, A S
Papapanagiotou, G
Peakman, M
Pope, M E
Rathbone, R G
Rayner, H C A
Riley, U B G
Robertson, D E
Roth, M G
Ruiz, R G G
Saunders, A P G
Scaravilli, N
Scott, S B C
Shaffi, S
Silverman, A M
Steele, J M B
Stephens, D
Streather, C P
Tovey, D I
Willcox, R
Wright, C J G

SE25
Allan, E M
Ameerally, P J
Arjun, N V L
Attard, A C
Barber, K W
Bhatti, F N K
Critchley, P A
Cutler, N A L
Dhoat, J S
Dhoat, N
Dunnet, R
Emara, M M K

Furnell, P M
Jackson, P M
Jahangir, M T
Khan, A R
O'Hara, S V
Ogedegbe, A J
Pickup, J C
Ranson, R
Shipolini, A R
Sondhi, R
Spicer, J E A
Srivastava, G

SE26
Austin, B M
Batrick, N C
Birch, D M L
Campbell, J E
Chaudhri, B B
Cheal, C
Christie Brown, J S
Christie Brown, M E
Clarke, S D
Cole, R B W
Cordery, R A
Da Fonseca, J M G
Ellington, N C
Evans, A G
Fisher, B H
Gibbs, L M E
Gothard, J W W
Hughes, P L
Kangesan, K
Kok, K W
Liew, C F
Liew, L C H
Lindo, D O N S J
Nesbitt, A
Platman, A M
Raeside, D A
Rakhit, A
Redenham, A J
Robinson, F O
Sikorski, J J
Snowden, S A
Sykes, N P
Thickett, D R
Thomas, S E
Whitworth, G R
Williams, R
Wu, F S-M

SE27
Acton, K J
Ashley, M H
Bruce, A E
Choyce, J
Daynes, T J
Hawxwell, S G
Haxby, E J
Hu, Y J
Mendonca, C O
Rampersad, R F
Sapuay, B C
Vaz, F M
Zander, K M

SE28
Asafu-Adjaye, H B
Chalmers, J A C
Cristofoli, L E
Kennedy, J M
Lewins, P G
Lobley, C F M
Wheeler, D M

SW1
Abdalla, H I
Abdul Aziz, A B Z
Alexander, F M
Amery, J E
Ashe, A G R
Athanassiou, E
Bache, X J S
Bailey, V F A
Barshall, C E
Bates, P F
Bewley, B R
Bewley, T H
Bone, A
Breuning, S G E
Brewer, C L
Brewerton, D A
Broomfield, A A
Brouckaert, S M
Browne, D R G
Brunton, K S
Budden, J M
Bushnell, M G

Carter, J T
Chapman, J
Chaudhry, T A
Cheng, W
Chirgwin, M E
Chiu, C K F
Chong, G W
Cockell, A P
Connan, F H
Copeman, P W M
Corall, I M
Cowen, J
Cox, H E
Craig, R P
Criswell, M I
Cutting, J C
Davidson, M J F
Dicker, A P
Donaldson, L J
Dorrell, W
Dorrington Ward, P
Dow, C
Easmon, C J
Eggleton, D A
Ferguson Smith, J
Fergusson, I L C
Ferris, M M
Fogelman, F
Foot, V H
Foster, D H C L
Fox, L
Furness, M J
Gafar, A H
Garcia-Lozano Gomes, F J
Garcia, S P
Gayner, J R
Goddard, P F
Godfrey, G
Graff, C T
Greenburgh, A L
Hammond, J
Hancock, R P D
Harding, M J H
Harley, J R
Harvey, C J
Hazlewood, J G
Helps, S A F
Herbert, D C
Herman, A M
Hickey, M U
Hsin, M K-Y
Hudson, T G
Hunt, J P H
Ilbert, R C
Ind, J E
Jarvis, L J
Jennings, G A
Jerjian, J C
Joy, A
Kalina, M A
Kapff, P D
Keys, L
King-Lewis, P W
Kingman, C E C
Kirker, J M
Knapman, P A
Kwok, J
Laing-Morton, P A
Langley, C N M
Lee, M R
Levinson, C M
Littlewood, E M
Lloyd-Harris, Q L G
Longfield, M
Ludford, C N
Lyndsay, D M
McAlinney, P G
McDonald, I O
McDonald, J
McKiernan, M J
McLaren, A R H
McOwan, A G
Macpherson, D A
Madan, I
Maniera, D M
Mathias, J C
Mayou, B J
Mayou, S C
Mills, S B
Mitchell, A J
Mostad, H
Muir, J A H
Muir, V R-J
Munday, J E L
Murray Bruce, D J
Murrison, A W
Myers, N J
Negus, D
O'Keeffe, A G
Ogunsanwo, O A O
Okoh, D
Oram, J J
Padfield, N L
Pao, C S-L
Parry, D L
Pattison, J R
Pattison, P B
Payne, J G
Peacock, C
Phillips, B L D
Platt, H S
Poncia, J
Price, G D L
Pryor, J P
Pugh, K E
Raffaelli, P I
Ragoowansi, R H
Rankine, S E
Reed, J L
Reeve, J
Rinsler, M G
Roberts, J R L
Salt, B D
Sandberg, M D A
Saraki, O A A
Sarkar, S P
Scott, J E
Scurr, J H
Shanks, J M
Sieratzki, J H
Sippert, A
Smith, J R
Smith, S C
Sodipo, J O
Somasundaram, V
Sopher, S M
Squires, N F
Stables, P R J
Stone, C M
Studd, J W W
Sweeney, M G
Tao, M
Tayler, E M
Tew, J S T
Thomas, J M
Tiner, R S
Tlusty, P J
Triay, C H
Troop, P A
Van Der Walt, L
Van Tooren, R
Vaskovic, T
Velkes, V L
Vernon, G R P A
Volkers, R C
von Bertele, M J
Wedgwood, J
Wells, J C
Wheeler, P J
Wilks, D M W
Wilson, M S G
Win, M T
Wolman, R I
Woo, K C D
Woodcock, P W
Wren, M E
Wright, B

SW2

Agranoff, D D
Ah-Moye, G R
Andlaw, M R
Arthur, R G
Bennett, D S
Brooks, T A V
Chakrabarti, B K
Chatoo, S B
Chaudhari, S A
Cohen, J R
Cook, M
Davis, L A
Estyn-Jones, H
Eyears, J M
Fairclough, P J
Farrugia, P
Fernandez Panos, M
Freeman, S V
Fuller, M D
Geh, S Y V
Georgiou, M
Giwa-Osagie, O O
Guinane, M J
Hayfron-Benjamin, J M S
Hewes, D K M
Kayes, M I
Kitteringham, L J
Kouriefs, C
Lavender, H A
McCarthy, S P
Mancey-Jones, M S
Mir, N
Moore, N L
Newton, A A T
Patel, V C
Peringer, J E
Pinder, M
Roberts, C D
Ruttley, M-E
Saif, M R
Shannon, C N
Shannon, G M
Slater, M A
Somasundaram, A A
Stannard, C L
Thomas, P B
Tilzey, S E
Vincent, C M A
Webb, S E
Wedgwood, F
Whyte-Venables, M
Wilkie, C E
Winter, L N
Wood, M
Yarnold, J R

SW3

Abd Allah, S A H
Al-Nasiri, N
Alexander, C
Allen, M J
Archer, D J
Balfour-Lynn, I M
Barata, L M
Barnes, P J
Bearn, J G
Benson, C
Beresford, N W
Blake, P R
Boffard, K D
Bolger, A P
Bordat, S P E
Bradfield Stowell, P
Brazil, L C A
Broadley, K E
Burman, J F
Bush, A
Catovsky, D
Celin, G
Cheung, D L C
Chisholm, D G
Chung, K F
Clarke, M J
Cleator, S J
Coats, A J S
Cole, P J
Collins, P
Cordingley, J J
Corrie, L A C
Corrin, B
Cowie, M R
Datnow, A D
Daubeney, P E F
Davey, J B
Davies, S W
De Lorenzo, F F
De Souza, A C
Devchand, D
Douek, M
Du Bois, R M
Durham, S R
Edwards, L
Ellison, C
Evans, T W
Feldman, S
Ffytche, D H
Finney, S J
Fisher, C
Flather, M D
Fogg, K J
Fox, K M
Geddes, D M
Gibson, D G
Gillbe, C E
Goldstraw, P
Gore, M E
Gormley, M A
Graneek, B J
Green, M
Greenwood, C H
Griffiths, M J D
Gui, G P H
Hansel, T T
Hansell, D M
Haq, S E A
Harmer, C L
Harrington, K J
Harris, P A
Haselden, B M
Hawley, K E
Hay, M A
Herford, T
Hickey, H B M
Hilliard, T N
Holesh, S A
Hon, J K F
Hong, A
Hooper, R J L
Horsewood-Lee, S M
Howe, L J
Hussein, J R
Jaggar, S I
Johnston, S R D
Jones, F P
Jungels, A L
Kakkar, S K
Kay, A B
Keogh, B F
Kilner, P J
King, T J
Kontogianni, I
Kozlowska, W J
Ladas, G
Lazari, M A
Lim, S
McDonald, J C
McGuiness, C N
Macrae, D J
Magee, A G
Maini, A
Mainwaring, P N
Mallick, U
Matutes Juan, M E
May, O S
Mbamali, J O
Miller, D E
Mitchell, D N
Mitford-Slade, F D
Moat, N E
Moskovic, E C
Muir, J M H
Newman Taylor, A J
Nicholson, A G
Northridge, G H
Ostermann, M E
Page, N G R
Panting, J R
Parry-Jones, N
Pennell, D J
Pierce, J F
Poole-Wilson, P A
Powell-Brett, C F
Power, J
Purcell, I F
Rakus, M R
Rhys Evans, P H
Rigby, M L
Robarts, W M
Rose, A J
Rosenthal, M
Ross, J R
Russell, J P A
Sachdeva, R
Sacks, N P M
Scallan, M J H
Scoote, M
Scudder, C C
Searle, A E
Sethia, B
Shembekar, M V
Sheppard, M N
Shinebourne, E A
Simonds, A K
Skewes, D G
Slavik, Z
Smith, I E
Snell, N J C
Soulioti, A M A
Southcott, A M
Stevenson, J C
Stevenson, M C
Swanston, J S K
Thomas, D J
Thomas, S R
Till, J A
Trott, P A
Turner, J S
Tutt, A N J
Underwood, S R
Van Zyl, J E
Vandenburg, M J
Vella Bonello, L M
Venables, K M
Viggers, J M
Walden, P A M
Wallace, W M
Watters, K J
Webb-Peploe, K M
Westbury, C B
Wilson, D R
Wilson, N M
Wilson, R
Wilson, V S
Wotherspoon, A C
Wright, J A G
Yap, J Y M
Yu Ho Yam, H

SW4

Aitken, D M
Allt-Graham, J
Ashton, P S
Bailey, E A
Balazs, J R
Ball, R
Bickerstaff, H E
Brain, P D
Burton, C A L
Calder, I
Callaghan, I M
Carey, B J
Cassidy, L
Child, C S
Choudhuri, K
Clark, A
Coffey, D P
Collins, S R
Cotton, M H
Curran, D P M
Cutter, W J
D'Arcy, C A
Davies, N J
Dyer, B J
Edwards, B M F-A
Ferentinos, A
Fraser, S A
Ghosh-Chowdhury, N
Gilham, P A
Glanville, T A
Glasson, C
Gupta-Wright, S R
Hacking, M B
Hanekom, W V H
Hanscheid, T
Harper, J R
Haworth, S G
Haywood, P T
Healy, J C
Heenan, P N
Henderson, H W A
Hughes, K R
Hull, D A
Johnston, I B
Keane, M A R
Keating, A R
Lamuren, T E
Lewis, R J
Low, N M
MacDiarmid, D
McDonagh, M J
McKenzie, R J
McLachlan, A J
Majeed, F A
Marsh, A M
Mathers, D
Munden, A
Neuber, M
Oteng-Ntim, E
Phillips, R J W
Prahalias, A A
Rodgers, M E
Sharif, H
Shelock, C F M
Shepherd, S T
Smith, S M E
Stevens, H P
Sunthankar, G
Todd, J A
Vass, N N
Vogt, J
Waight, C T
Wallat, W
Walsh, R
West, J A
Whittet, S E
Williams, E J
Wilson, G H M
Wolstenholme, V
Wyer, J F

SW5

Al-Haddad, H B
Almeida, A M
Awwad, A M
Batool, M
Bester, P K
Biadene, G
Bricka, C
Brooke Barnett, J W
Cantor, D D
Costello, J
Crock, H V
De Siena, P M
Dewast-Gagneraud, C
El Borai, M R
El-Gamel, A M H M
Faridian, P
Forster, D M C
Glazebrook, W R
Grande, R A
Hamami, N A A J
Harling, J D
Ho, K M T
Howard, E R
Ibrahim, S A H
Keaney, F P S
Khadjeh-Nouri, D
Kulatilake, A E
Ladbrooke, T E
Lancaster, M J
Lewis, C A
Lhopitallier, O M
Lowrey, S
Malik, F R
Mallett, P J
Mansour, F
Martin, V M
Minasian, H
Mooney, V M B
Morris, N F
O'Brien, K M
Odgers, P B
Paterson, F W N
Peries, A
Periyasamy, T
Pickard, B H
Prasad, S
Qureshi, M A
Qureshi, N M
Ramishvili, A
Ramsay, I D
Reid, R W S
Retsas, S
Room, G R W
Rose, G S
Rub, A
Simons, E G
Skeggs, D B L
Tabrizi, S J
Vashisht, R
Wallace, C E
Yeung, S M
Zilkha, K J

SW6

Ahmed, M
Ahrens, G N
Arunasalam, P
Atkinson, J A
Aw Yong, Y M
Baraniecka, V T
Bilagi, P S S K
Blair, G
Bray, J K
Buchanan, G N
Buckley, J F
Burgess, E H
Chan, K A
Chapman, R C
Chaudhry, A N
Cheshire, E R D
Christian, W J
Clegg, J M
Cowper, D M
Daborn, A K
De Sousa, L A S
Deeming, K F
Dellaportas, C
Dove-Edwin, I A
Downs, M H
Draper, H L
Duquesnay, R F
Eccles, S J
Edwards, S C
Elliott, C L
Eltringham, I
Evans, M A L
Fleming, D C
Forster, N J
Frain, J D J
Freeman, G K
Gilchrist, F C
Graham, T L

Gunston, E L
Harper-Wynne, C L
Harris, N A
Harrop-Griffiths, J L
Hicks, J P
Hoban, B L
Holmes, P M
Howsam, S E
Hussain, Z
Jackson, E A
Jelley, A P
Jenkins, R T
Johnston, A K
Jones, A T
Karwatowski, S P
Keown, P J
Klosok, J K
Ladenburg, H I
Lawley, G C
Lawson, R I
Low-Beer, N M
Lyons, F M
McAndrew, F C M
McMichen, H U S
McMichen, I K S
McNicholas, T J
MacSweeney, D A
Mangwana, K L
Mantafounis, A
Martin, A
Mee, S J
Meenan, J K P
Mehrotra, R
Millen, J S
Morgan, N F A D
Mulcahy, A J
Murphy, D M
Muthiah, R N
Nageh, T
O'Farrell, N
O'Shea, D B
Palfrey, A J
Pariente, L
Paris, S T
Patel, A
Patel, S D
Peckett, W R C
Peters, J M
Peters, R M
Pickering, A E
Porter, J D H
Powrie, S E
Pugh, S F
Rahmat Pour Monfared, M
Rezvani, K
Robinson, I E
Roomi, R
Ross, P J
Roylance, R R
Sandison, A
Scriven, A J
Selvarajan, B S
Singhai, S
Stone, A F M
Stroudley, J L
Thomas, K
Trenfield, S M
Vaughan, J R
Vigars, S P
Walker, E J
Warden, M G
Wasfi, F M
Webb, L J
Westcott, M C
Williams, A M
Williams, N M
Wilson, I D
Worsdall, A K

SW7
Al-Khawaja, I M S
Archard, J C
Auden, R R
Bareille, J-P
Baudon, J J
Bayliss, R
Bealing, C L B
Bhagat, K
Boreham, J J C
Boyle, N H
Boyton, R J
Caro, C G
Cela, E
Cheung, B
Cheung, H
Chu, S K
Critchley, J M
Dauncey, J K
Deane, T H W
Edwards, C R W
Ehteshami, S
El-Meliegy, D A N
Freedman, S A
Geraud, C
Ghadimi, H
Good, C D
Hargrove, R C A
Hawawini, A
Hussein, S E
Innes, C A
Jairaj, P
Judge, R
Khater, M S E D
King, H L
Kirkham, A P S
Lau, Y K
Ledingham, S J M
Lefever, R
Levin, A G
Luxen, A A J
MacDermot, J
McKeown, M D
Mahmud, T
Manocha, K F
Marston, J A P
Marston, S
Mina, F S
Murad, J S
Neri, M
Papamichael, D
Perepeczko, B
Rowley, P D
Sabroe, I
Sarker, S K
Sethi, T J
Sharpe, L D
Staight, G B
Stott, C J
Swann, A B
Viegas, M
Watrelot, A
Weinreb, I R
West, J R C
Wood, T A
Zaniewski, F T

SW8
Ala, A J K
Astroulakis, Z M J
Barratt-Johnson, M F R
Beale, D M
Bowker, T J
Branker, M D
Burgess, P A
Chesshire, N J
Cohen, D G
Collins, J D
Costa, D
Dhillon, R S
Down, M W F
Dunne, J
Emberson-Bain, D I
Haase, G
Harrison-Woolrych, M L
Harrison, P J
Hawkins, C E A
Heath, C P M
Hopper, J M
James, D H
Jefferys, D B
Job, S A
Law, J E
Lawrence, A G
Le Fanu, J R
Lee, E H
Logan, P J A
Losa, I E
MacFarlane, D A
MacLennan, I P B
Markey, G S
Matthews, J G
Muhammad, H A
Narayanan, G
Onwuchekwa, W O
Page, M C
Parikh, C
Peacey, J M
Powell, M
Powlson, M
Robinson, M D
Robinson, N M K
Saidin, D
Sedar, M I
Singh, S S
Skuce, A M
Smith, C L
Smith, I W
Speirs, C F
Steen, J S M
Suvarna, J R
Taylor, S J
Thatcher, M J
Tylden, E
Wharram, J
Woodings, D F
Woods, K L

SW9
Abaecheta, H C
Adeoba, S A
Alikhan, R
Atkinson, S A
Azuonye, I O
Beck, N A
Bell, S M
Berlyn, R A D
Boocock, A M
Bradley, L J
Breach, C S
Browne, N D F
Church, R S
Corry, D G
Cresswell, B E
Crocombe, M J
Cruise, A S
Davies, N J
Dunning, V I
Edwards, H G
Fong, J J
Halse, G G
Hitchens, J
Hopkinson, K A
Hutchinson, N A
Jenkins, C J R
Joseph, J V
Konzon, N I
Lee, H K P
McCarthy, D P J
McCoy, R N
McCready-Hall, L P
McGinn, E P
Maxwell, N J
May, S D
Ndegwa, D G
Nwaboku, H C I
O'Flynn, D W
Patel, H J
Patel, S N
Prendergast, K F
Ruben, P E
Rust, P A
Savage, R A
Shaw, A C
Stevens, T G
Toyne, A
Van Den Berk, J C L M
Wallis, R M
Wicks, R M

SW10
Abrahamson, E L
Adekunle, O O
Allen-Mersh, T G
Anderson, J R
Andreyev, H J N
Asboe, D
Ayida, G A
Baird, P R E
Ball, S G
Barton, S E
Basquill, J G
Bedford Russell, A R
Bell, J R G
Benatar-Catillon, J
Biddulph, D R
Bieler, Z A
Bispham, A
Boag, F C
Booth, S J
Bowden-Jones, O
Bower, M D
Bridges, J E
Bridges, N A
Bridgett, C K
Browne, R E
Brueton, M J
Bunker, C B
Burkill, G J C
Carter, A E S
Catalan, J
Cavanagh, J
Cavanagh, P A
Chinn, R J S
Claxton, A P
Collins, J V
Cooper, B J
Costello, C E M
Cox, M L
Cox, S
Dakin, M J
Dinneen, M D
Durbridge, J A
Eckersley, J R T
El-Refaey, H A
Emerson, P A
Emiliani, O
Etchegoyen, A
Evans, S C
Farrar, S E
Feher, M D
Fell, J M E
Fleet, M S
Fox, P A
Garnham, F E
Gazzard, B G
Georgiou, C
Gibberd, F B
Gilleece, Y C
Haddad, M J Y
Hargreaves, P I
Harrison, M C
Hawkins, D A
Holdcroft, A
Hopper, S A
Hulme, A L
Hunter, M R A
Inge, K S-K
Isaacs, A J
Jackman, J G
Johnson, M R
Jones, R M
Joshi, N
Kaddoura, S
Kampers, W T
Katsarma, E
Kaye, S A
Kazim, H A A
Kennedy, A M D
Khan, M M T
Klemperer, F J
Kotak, A
Kovar, I Z
La Paglia, J E
Lant, A F
Lavelle, J R
Lawson, A D
Levin, J
Lowe, J C
McCall, J
McCall, J M
MacCormack, S M
Madden, N P
Mahendran, B
Mallal, G M
Manisali, M
Margarson, M P
Martin, D L
Martin, J P
Meehan, J P
Menon, R R
Miao, Y M
Mitchell, S M
Morgan, D J R
Morris, A K
Napier, K C
Newman, C G H
Nordin, A J
Norman-Taylor, J Q
Nott, D M
O'Connor, K A
Ogden, C W
Padley, S P G
Papayannakos, E
Patel, K
Patterson, A E J
Pelly, M E
Penn, Z J
Penrice, J M
Pozniak, A L
Rafique, F
Rees, T S
Roberts, N E M
Rufford, H J
Schulte, A C
Sedgwick, E
Sender, H
Sender, S N
Shah, P L
Sharpe, B D
Sinclair, E A
Singer, J D
Singh, S
Skinner, R R
Sleigh, G
Smellie, W J B
Smith, C E
Stafford, M K
Stanford, H M
Stanford, M R
Staughton, R C D
Steer, P J
Sweeney, B J G
Theobald, N J A
Thomas, V J E
Thompson, J N
Thomson, G A
Thorpe-Beeston, J G
Voss, S B
Wales, N M
Walsh, J C
Wastell, C
Williams, D J
Windross, P M
Yardley-Jones, A
Yentis, S M
Zeegen, R

SW11
Abokarsh, K
Ahad, N I
Ameke, I N
Artley, M L
Barnes, E S
Bevan, D H
Bourke, S K
Brigden, C E
Brock, J E C
Budd, A J
Butt, R
Carruth, J S
Chittick, D G H
Coker, C B A O
Cramp, H A
Cramp, M E
Creamer, J D
Creamer, K L
Durham, M G
Eden, J C P
El Beze, Y S
Ellin, C
Ellingham, M J
Falworth, M S
Fernando, S B
Finch, D G
Fitzgerald, S F
Flis, C M
Frazer, C K
Freeman, S P
Gazzard, J A
Geary, S C
Ghosh, D B
Gibson, A R
Goldberg, C D S
Gordon, E M
Grannell, J
Grundy, A
Gulati, R K
Haddock, J A A
Hanbury-Webber, R
Hicklin, L-A C
Holmes, P A
Hossain, A B M M
Jayamanne, D G R
Joekes, M
Johnson, E A
Khan, D B A
Kinmonth, R J
Klaye, T O
Lascelles, K P
Le Roux, A E
Levitt, C
Lofts, J A
Lucas, H M
Meacock, W R
Meares, H D D
Mills, R J
Mills, S A
Monahan, A M
Moschat, P
Muttalib, M
Nasiruddin, I J
Nesdale, A D
North, S L P
O'Dwyer, A-M
Owens, D F
Payne, D N R
Penge, D J
Perera, R C
Price, M L
Pugh, H M
Puvinathan, H
Richardson, P G G
Robinson, S C
Rowson, N J
Salim, A
Salim, S H
Savage, R A
Scott-Fleming, M S
Scott, M F
Shah, W A
Shakir, N A
Shaw, S E
Snape, E E
Sporik, R B
Stavron, K J
Surawy, A J
Taghizadeh, A K
Walden, A P
Walsh, E A M
White, L A M
Williams, F M K
Wolff, E P F
Woolf, R L
Wyatt, M E
Zaffar, M

SW12
Ahsan, A N
Akah, F B C
Akbar, N
Antwi, D N K
Baretto, R L
Biswas, D
Blair, A M
Brinkmann, D A
Brosnan, C M
Cartwright, R H
Darowski, A
Djerkovic, G S
Egan, A C
Ferguson, C N
Gillespie, S M
Green, P G
Hamblin, L G
Hamblin, M T
Han, L-Y
Haque, S E
Heriot, J A
Johns, J
Jopson, C J
Kathirgamanathan, K
Keatings, V M
Kirwan, J F
Koh, B C
Lapsley, D H M
Lapsley, M
Leaker, B R
Leung, R S
Lipowsky, R
Lloyd, G W L
Lobo, C E
McLachlan, S
Magnall, R J
Manikon, M I
Mazhar, M
Mazhar, N A
Morgan, A T
Morris, K A
Ng Sui Hing, N Y K
Nicholas, P L
Okusi, D
Parry-Jones, A J D
Patel, K M
Patel, S
Peach, C J D
Qazi, N A
Rahman, M S
Ratcliffe, P W
Reid, K
Ribeiro, C A
Robinson, G E
Salt, N J
Salter, P A
Serajuddin, M
Shah, N C
Shariff, A T
Singh, P
Sreetharan, M
Tan Phoay Lay, C
Thomas, M P
Torossian, F S B
Turner, A W M
Vowles, R E
Wong-Lun-Sang, S

SW13
Bartlett, N A
Beales, P H
Berman, L H
Botting, J P

Browne, G P R
Burnett, L J B
Doherty, P F
Elkington, A G F
Elkington, J R S
Ellman, T J
Fender, G R K
Flood, R J
Gibson, P W
Harries, M
Hassan, T H A
Hockney, E A
Honnor, S E
Johnson, L
Lewis, E A
Main, A M
Makey, A R
Martineau, A R
Mathias, T W
Metaxas, N
Minton, N D
Muntarbhorn, S
Nicholas, S C
Oliver, C D
Olney, S M
Palacci, A E
Plant, M J
Powell, K D
Redstone, D
Reid, S
Rice-Jones, M C
Ross Erro, A-L
Saklatvala, J
Shetty, A K
Tubbs, S C
Waters, H
Watson, J

SW14

Adams, P J
Al-Yassiri, M M H
Barnes, P K
Beard, C A S
Boheimer, K
Brand, A J O
Bullen, C
Bunje, H W
Bush, J L
Castello-Cortes, A H
Clarke, J A
Craighill, A R
Crollick, A J
De Burgh-Thomas, A G
Ellison, M M
Emery, E R J
Geffen, T J B
Grayson, C E A
Gregory, S M
Ismail, F
Jezierski, M R
Kidd, A L
Lambert, H P
Lawrence, R M
Lewis, N U
Mahomed Keshavjee, S N
Mofeez, M A
Moore, F P
Nicholson, J A
Rundle, P K
Sharaf, T F A
Smith, M V
Strickland, P
Thomas, H M
Tomlinson, D R
Warren, C J
Watts, C C W
Weeks, R L
Zaragoza Casares, P

SW15

Aarons, B M
Adam, R
Ahmad, S
Ahmed, Y
Al-Ahmad, S K Y
Al Mahdy, H
Al Mizyen, E
Al-Sager, A H J
Andrews, K
Arthur, R M F
Bailey, C R
Balassa, G
Bale, R J
Ballard, R M
Basarab, T
Bass, C S
Beach, J L
Bearn, V M
Bennett, E D
Bhide, A M
Black, E A
Boultbee, J E
Bowen, P L
Bradley, L J
Bradshaw, A J
Brook, N E
Brown, E M
Bulstrode, N W
Burt, L
Cadogan, F
Calwell, W P K
Chan, J J K
Chau, I T M
Chess, E J
Clement, A
Collins, M N
Collyer, J
Cowie, V A
Cull, A D
Dashti, H
Davies, G I
Day, J M C
De Boer, R F A
Deas, S C
Degorrequer-Griffith, T B H
Dennis, D L
Drzymala, M K
El Dabouni, M A M
Elliott, P M
Estall, R J
Evans, O G
Farrell, T G
Festa, M S
Fitzgerald, A J
Fitzmaurice, M
Georgiannos, S
Gil Rivas, S
Grice, C A
Grimwade, D J
Halileh, S O M
Hammond, R J
Harrison-Hansley, E J
Harrop-Griffiths, A W
Hedayati, B
Heriot, A G
Hickey, J B
Hoveyda, F
Hoveyda, N
Huff, A G
Ilves, P J
Islam, S
Jasani, A F
Kataria, M S
Kelly, D H W
Khadra, A
Khoubehi, B
Kilduff, R C
Kimberley, A P S
Kirkland, A A L
Kleanthous, K L
Kooner, M
Lebus, J C M
Lister, P J
McKee, K J
McKenzie, D J
Major, A
Mallya, B
Manjula, G
Martin, A C
Mathews, C J
Mavalankar, A P
Mendonca, D R
Mireskandari, M
Morton, K E
Naudeer, S F M
Navamani, A S
Ngan, H
Nirmalan, R
North, S M
O'Neill, J M B
O'Reilly, M A R
Pantin, P L
Paulding, E A
Payne, F M
Plumley, S M
Pourgourides, E K
Ratnayake, B C N
Redding, W
Riccio, M
Richardson, H J
Roberts, J M
Robinson, K P
Roet, B C
Rowan, P R
Russell, A L
Ryan, S M
Scarlett, N J D
Shanahan, S E E
Sherriff, E A
Shur, E
Sindall, F M
Sooriakumaran, S
Speirs, J M
Stephens, K
Stilgoe, J R
Suckling, R J
Swierczynski, S
Tan, S-Y
Tattersall, S J
Temple, S E
Theodossi, A
Watters, O F
Wattie, M L
Williams, S L
Wong, C Y
Worth, R W
Wright, G M
Young, A-M

SW16

Addo, J K
Adeboyeku, D U
Afzal, M M
Ah Chong, A K
Akoojee, E
Amin, M
Amure, A O
Ashby, P M
Baker, E H
Barrett, P P
Beranek, M D
Beumelburg, N J
Beyzade, B
Blacklay, H C
Blair, D A
Blankson-Beecham, G
Brett, J M
Calder, F R
Chaudhary, M F
Choukroun, C
Clarke, K
Clarke, S
Climie, R P
Cohen, A C
Cross, T G
Cummings, I G
De Almeida, S T L
Desai, N
Duff-Miller, D B
Duncan, E H
Edwards, R
Eliatamby, S R-K
Foster, T R
Freeman, J
Graham, A S
Graham, M H
Groen, B G S
Gunasuntharam, T
Handa, S K
Hasan, R
Hayes, J
Healey, J
Hoque, K A
Huggins, E M
Kaba, R A
Keane, M F
Lee, S B J-P
MacIver, M
Mackenzie, S J
Madhav, R T
Mahadevan, D
Masterton, J W
Menezes, L J X
Mirza, A H
Mirza, D
Modder, J V J
Mullin, M M
Nadeem, F
Newell, A M B
Nowicki, M T
Nzegwu, G O
Osborne, P P
Otuteye, E T
Pankhurst, M-T A
Parton, E Q
Patel, B R
Patel, C T
Patel, N K
Peck, A B
Phipps, J A
Potter, A N
Raghunath, J V
Raghunath, N J
Rahman, Y
Samarasinghe, A M
Samarasinghe, C R
Samarasinghe, D G
Savage, S J
Sharma, A O
Steele, A P H
Thomson, P G
Towers, J F
Vickers, B A J
Vyas, A
Wallace, E L M
Watt, L L
Weatherup, J
Willsher, T
Wilson, M
Wittek, I H
Worthington, K A
Wright, J P
Yasseen, B E S M

SW17

Abayawardana, R D
Abou Saleh, M T
Adam, E J
Adams, F R A
Ahmad, I
Ahmad, R N
Ahmed, A
Ahmed, M I
Aitken, P H L
Akram, F
Al-Saady, N M M
Ala, A
Alam, S
Alford, P F
Allison, H J
Almeida, B M
Anderson, C J
Anson, K M
Arulkumaran, S
Axford, J S
Bailey, M J
Bain, M D
Ball, J A S
Ball, S E
Barker, D S
Barlow, F M
Belli, A-M
Bennett, M A
Bernal, S J
Bicanic, T A
Bircher, M D
Birthistle, K A J
Bland, J L
Blenkinsopp, P T
Boddy, S-A M
Bolton, J S
Borgstein, B M E
Bose, M
Bourne, T H
Bower, P J
Breathnach, A S
Brecker, S J D
Britton, J A
Brook, H D D
Brown, R W
Buckenham, T M
Burke, A W
Calvert, S A
Camm, A J
Campion, H C R
Capps, S N J
Cappuccio, F P
Carrasco, M P
Carter, P G
Cartledge, A G
Cashman, J N
Chalmers, A G W
Chambers, T J
Chandraharan, E
Chandrasekaran, V
Chang, R W S
Checinski, K M
Chemla, E S
Child, A H
Chow, W M J
Chowdhury, S
Chowns, J C
Christopher, J A
Clifton, A G
Clifton, A
Cloud, G C
Coates, A R M
Colgan, J F
Collier, J G
Collinson, P O
Corbishley, C M
Costa-Michael, M
Courtenay, K P
Crawley-Boevey, E E
Crusz, T A M
Curry, I J
Dalgleish, A G
Damaskinidou, K
Dash, A
Dashwood, C S
Davis, N
Day, A C
De Rooy, L J
De Silva, L S
Dhiman, A
Dimond, C W
Donohue, E P G
Dormandy, J A
Drummond, C R
Drummond, D C
Drummond, L M
Dumonde, D C
Dundas, D D
Eastman, N L G
Eastwood, J B
El-Kholy, A A-K A-F
El-Sayeh, H G S K
Elanchenny, N
Elanchenny, P
Elmslie, F V
Evans, C L
Fahey, C A
Fairbank, A C
Farnsworth, G M
Farrer, K F M
Fegan-Earl, A W
Fernando, M D A K S
Field, C M
Finlayson, C J
Fisher, N R
Fitzpatrick, G S M
Fleming, A N M
Foster, O J F
Franklin, M
Gallagher, M M
Ganeshalingham, R
Garcia Asensio, M D P
Gateley, D R
Gavrielides, I
Ghaem-Maghami Hezaveh, S
Ghodse, A H
Given-Wilson, R M
Goldenberg, S M
Goodwin, C S
Gordon-Smith, E C
Graham, A
Gribbin, N M
Griffin, G E
Griffiths, J R
Grounds, R M
Hall, G M
Ham, J A
Hamilton-Fairley, D
Hamilton, P A
Hampson-Evans, D C
Hanafiah, Z
Hanspal, J S
Hartikainen, J E K
Harvey, F A H
Harvey, I
Hastie, I R
Hawkins, R L
Hay, P E
Heath, P T
Heenan, S D
Hermon-Taylor, J
Heron, C W
Hilson, G R F
Hindley, P A
Hinton, E A
Hodgson, S V
Holliman, R E
Hollins, S C
Holmes, S J K
Holwill, S D J
Hubble, D
Hughes, N C
Hughes, P M
Hughes, P P M
Humphrey, M E D
Hunter, G
Hussain, I R
Hutchinson, L R
Hutchinson, S E
Hwang, D T W
Hyde, N C
Iheanacho, I O
Jarman, C M B
Jazrawi, R P E
Jeffrey, I J M
Jones, K J
Jones, P W
Jordan, G M
Judge, J E
Kadambari, S R
Kanagasabay, R R
Karmani, M S
Keane, C J
Keen, D V
Kenny, S J
Kent, A J
Khan, Q-U-A
Khan, S A
Khaw, K-T
Kidd, M
Kiely, P D W
Killoughery, M P
Kingdon, C C
Kirkland, P M
Kist, P C M
Lacey, J H
Laczko-Schroeder, T J
Larkin, G B R
Last, K
Lau, R K W
Laugharne, R A
Lawal-Rieley, T C
Lee Khet Leong, D
Leicester, R J
Liban, J B
Lofts, F J
Lovell, R A
Macallan, D C
McAnulty, G R
McCoubrie, M
McGowan, M E L
MacGregor, G A
Macmichael, C J
MacPhee, I A M
Madden, B P
Mahroof, H M
Malik, F A
Malik, M H K
Malik, R J A
Mansi, J L
Mansour, S
Manyonda, I T
Marsden, R A
Marsh, H T
Marsh, J C W
Martin, A J
Maxwell, J D
Meagher, P J
Mellor, A J
Melville, D M
Mezey, G C
Midgley, S N
Minattur, D J
Minhas, P S
Mitchell-Heggs, N A
Mitchison, D A
Mitton, S G
Mokbel, K
Morgan, R A
Morgan, S V
Morley, H L
Morris, C M
Mortimer, P S
Moss, A L H
Mughal, M S
Mughal, N J
Mukherjee, R A S
Muralitharan, V
Murdoch, L J
Naqvi, S B
Nduka, C C
Nelson, S R
Nemeth, W
Newton, C R
Nussey, S S
O'Callaghan, P A
O'Flynn, N M
O'Riordan, J A
Oakeley, P S
Oakeshott, P
Obel, O A
Okafor, B E
Oliveira, D B G
Olugbile, A O B
Ostlere, L S
Oyebode, B O
Paine, P A
Panahloo, A A
Parker-Williams, E J
Patel, P C
Patel, S Y
Patel, U
Pathak, S
Pathmabaskaran, S
Patton, M A

Pettengell, R
Philips, B J
Pilcher, J M
Pollok, R C G
Porter, S-A M
Poullis, A P
Powell, B W E M
Prime, K P
Pumphrey, C W
Rahman, M
Rayner, C F J
Razis, P A
Redmill, B S
Rehman, Z
Rhodes, A
Rice, P S
Rich, P A
Riordan, D C
Robertson, S J
Rogers, D J
Rostron, C K
Rowland, E
Ruggier, R
Sagar, S M
Saggar, A K
Saleemi, S A
Saxena, S K
Sayer, R E
Schwartz, M S
Scott, K A
Selvadurai, D K
Shah, F N
Shannon, M S
Sharland, M R
Sharma, A K
Sherman, Y
Shiraz, M
Sibthorpe, R J
Singh, R
Sinha, M K
Sivarajan, K
Skillern, L H
Smith, E E J
Snashall, S E
Soomro, G M
Stanton, A W B
Stark, M M
Starkey, C N
Stern, J S
Stevens, J R D
Strachan, D P
Styles, C J
Sueke, H M
Sultan, M S
Sunil Babu, V
Szolach, M R
Tham, S W
Thomas, V A
Thompson, G M
Thompson, M M
Thurlbeck, S M
Thurlow, A C
Tibbs, C J
Tilley, R C
Toma, A
Tomlinson, M A
Turk, J
Twisleton-Wykeham-Fiennes, A G
Uddin, J M
Ugwumadu, A N
Vallance, P J T
Van Besouw, J-P W G
Varghese, D
Vince, J
Vinestock, M D
Vyvyan, H A L
Walters, D V
Wansbrough-Jones, M H
Warwick, H M C
Westlake, A S
Whincup, P H
White, G J
Wilbraham, D G
Wilkinson, L S
Williams, A R
Williams, A F
Williamson, P A
Willis, F M
Wilson, P O G
Wood, D M
Yip, A S B
Young, M P A
Zaidi, M
Zolese, M G

SW18
Adamson, D L
Aderinto, J B
Afaq, M A
Auty, F T
Bamber, D B
Bamford, N J
Barnard, A E
Barthes-Wilson, E L
Battley, C J
Bavar, G
Bell, P A J
Bickerton, A S T
Bijlani, N
Bobak, S A
Bovill, I P
Bradley, U P
Bradley, W N
Brara, N
Bull, M E
Chapman, E P
Chow, K Y
Christie, C L
Coffey, T A
Cooper, Y
Costales, E L
Cumberland, M A
Davies, B A
Deuchar, A J
Ewen, R A
Gibbons, C R
Gibson, A T
Goddard, J
Gomez, C K R
Gomez, K R
Gordon, D H
Gorman, J J
Hagger, R W
Harris, T J
Hollamby, R G
Horwood, N
Iadevita, G
Jacobs, S
Jones, N
Khan, M-U H
Kidd, G T B
Lawrence, E S
Lynch, B A
McCrone, H E M
Nicholas, A M
O'Connell, J M
O'Neil, R
Olver, R E
Onoche, A O
Patel, L C
Patel, M B
Perraudeau, M K
Perry, N
Phillips, A A
Rashid, M A
Redelinghuys, J
Roberts, L M
Robertshaw, H J
Roche, C J H
Rousseau, N C
Rudzinski, B M
Scott, G M S
Serafini, F
Seymour, H R
Shorten, J B
Siddiqi, S A
Solan, N L
Sullivan, A K
Taylor, H P
Vreede, E
Waite, J C
Ward, E S
Ward, L
Weinstock, N G
Whitehead, S C
Wilcock, F M
Winstock, G B M
Wood, C C

SW19
Ahmad, N
Allen, J M S
Appadurai, I R
Atkins, M J
Ayub, M S
Aziz, N
Baig, M N
Baillie, C J A
Bakowska, A J
Balasingam, V
Balsingham, S
Bending, M R
Bett, N J
Bettridge, R F
Biswas, D
Blegay, R N
Blonstein, L H
Bolton, J G F
Bonar, J A
Booth, T R
Bossowska, I J
Bridle, S H
Bulman, W K
Bunting, R M
Butt, M W
Cadsky, O
Chakrabarti, U
Chakravarty, S K
Chuaqui, P B
Clarke, J T
Cock, S
Coleman, C M
Cooney, V B
Cross, J A
Cundy, P R
Cunningham, A R
Cunningham, S F
Cuthbert, N D
Dadarkar, P
Darke, K F
Darr, A J
Davidson Parker, J J
Davies, D D
Davies, S C
De Souza, N M
De Winter, E
Devan, V R
Dick, G M
Dinsmore, J E
Dirmikis, H
Dooley, D
Drury, A
Dunfield-Prayero, A C
Elstub, J
Emerson, E M
Feilding, E L
Field, A M
Flynn, P E
Forsyth, D S
Freeman, E J K
Frenkiel, A L
Gaillard, B
Gibbs, C F
Gnanapragasam, J
Gnanapragasam, J B
Gnanapragasam, V C
Gomez, G
Gray, T J P
Greenfield, P M
Haq, S H
Hargreaves, M
Harper, I D R
Hearth, M W
Henderson, E R
Heron, T G
Hill, L C
Hollick, E J
Horner, D R M
Howell, D D
Iya, D
Iyer, M G
Jackson, S A
Jajbhay, M
Jamil, M
Jay, B S
Jenkinson, K A
Johnson, M W
Jones, H W
Jones, J R
Jones, T N
Joshi, A K
Joyce, E L
Jupp, S M
Kanapathippillia, R
Kenyon, K L
Kerac, M
Langley, K J C
Leigh, G I
Li, W-Y
Mackie, A
McKinnon, M E
Maguire, M
Maitra, S
Matsuda, T
Message, S D
Mills, F C A
Moloney, E F
Moorthy, I T
Morris, S C
Mosahebi-Mohammadi, A
Mulcahy, R P C
Munsie, A J
Murphy, H C
Murray, A D
Mushin, J S
Nabijee, A H A A
Naha, B
Nandanwar, C
Neil, A F
Nortley, E R W
Ntountas, I
O'Riordan, M D
Ohri, A K
Osborne, A W H
Pagadala, V
Paton, N I J
Paul, J R
Payne, J P
Plimmer, A L
Plimmer, W N
Portas-Dominguez, L-C
Powell, S N
Powles, T J
Provost, G C
Rabbin, D C
Rahman, S G
Rajakariar, R
Ransome (Mrs Heron), J
Ratnasingam, L
Ray, D K
Rees, M
Reynolds, M W
Rhind, T P F
Rippingale, C
Roberts, I F
Robertson, W B
Robson, B E C
Rutter, D A
Sabbat, J K M
Saleem, I
Sanders, G M
Sanders, J
Sanderson, I M
Saville, S
Schiffer, G
Scoble, J E
Scott, O L S
Sharma, V
Sibbel-Linz, A-K
Singh-Ranger, D
Singh-Ranger, G
Sithamparanathan, S
Skull, A J
Smallwood, R I L
Soni, R
Sornalingam, N
Spencer, T M
Stammers, T G
Steven, C M
Sundaralingam, J
Suntharalingam, S
Taussig, D C
Taylor-Roberts, T D
Taylor, C G
Taylor, J
Tennant, R C
Thanga, V
Udwadia, Z
Wake, A M
Wake, M C
Wallat-Vago, S B
Watson, H P
White, G M
Williams, D J
Winpenny, H C
Wong, I K C
Wright, G
Yacob, Z M
Young, Y M
Zafar, M H

SW20
Ahmad, S F
Allum Lai-Fook, J T
Appulingam, K
Ayub, N A
Bell, B A
Bierer-Sharp, D
Borthwick, S D
Burling, M B
Byles, N S
Bynevelt, M
Cairns, L M
Chandi, A
Chegwidden, R J D
Chill, C S
Clarke, J M H
Crook, S J
De Wilde, S J
Dhalla, N H K
Edwards, D R L
Emsden, A E M
Freeman, H M
Gabe, C I
Ghauri, A S K
Gnanaratnam, J
Gonsalves, O J
Gowing, N F C
Grieve, J P
Halden, P J
Hamilton, P G
Harnett, P R
Hartley, I C R
Hashmi, H M
Jacob, S
Jarzembowski, M K
Kingsmill, J C
Kolendo, J
Kozielski, Y M
Lawlor, T
Lawrence, C J
Lemberg, M W
Lewis, A K
McCaffrey, B J
McCaffrey, S
Malhomme De La Roche, H J M
Marshall, J
Mason, G J
Misir, S M
Monahan, E C
Moore, A J
Mulcahy, R E
O'Connor, M D
Patel, D
Penrice, L M
Perkins, R M
Peters, A J
Price, T M D
Raghavan, M
Reddy, K M
Roberts, J A
Rohde, S P
Rozewicz, L M
Senthuran, S
Sheth, P K S
Sivayoham, N
Spanton, I D A
Sri Ganeshan, M
Stapleton, S R S J
Stone, P C
Stroud, C E
Taubel, J
Thevathasan, L J
Thompson, P J
Tulloch, A D
Ubhi, V S
Venkatesan, D
Wait, H J
Webber, L M
Wilson, J N
Woods, A L
Woropay, S J
Wren, D R
Zachary Jennings, C M

W1
Aarons, E J
Abecassis, M
Abood, E A
Abraham, R R
Abramovich, S
Achan, N V
Achan, P
Achan, V
Adams, B G
Adams, P W
Adeniyi-Jones, R O C
Adiseshiah, M
Afshar, F
Ainley, C C
Akle, A
Akle, C A
Al-Ani, H M
Alhejazi, M B R H
Allibone, J B
Almeyda, J J R
Alusi, G
Amakye, J
Ames, P R J
Amin, Z
Andersson, L C
Anthony, S
Appleby, B P
Armstrong, N P I
Ashby, P H
Astley, B A
Atkinson, F G
Aylward, G W
Badenoch, D F
Badrawy, G A
Bailey, C M
Bailey, C S
Baker, H
Baker, L R I
Balcon, R
Baldeweg, S
Balfour-Lynn, L P
Barker, S G E
Barnard, M J
Barretto, J H
Bartram, C I
Baskerville, P A
Basra, D S
Bekir, J S
Bengani, K S
Bentovim, A
Berry, H
Bessant, R
Besser, G M
Betteridge, D J
Beynon, G P J
Bischoff, R E H
Bishop, C C R
Bishop, C
Black, A D
Blackburne, J S
Blackie, R A S
Blair, A A D
Blau, J N
Bleehen, S S
Bloom, S L
Blott, M J
Boag, A G
Bomanji, J
Bond, S A
Booth, H L
Bor, S
Botros, F N
Boulos, P B
Bourke, B E
Bowen, J E
Bowen, M L
Bowerman, J E
Bowler, P J
Bown, S G
Box, J E
Boyde, T R C
Bradbrooke, S A
Brain, C E
Brazier, D J
Breach, N M
Brendel, S C
Brenton, D P
Briggs, P C
Bright, H
Bristow, A S E
Bromley, L L
Brook, C G D
Brookes, G B
Brookes, J A S
Brooks, J H
Brough, M D
Browett, J P
Buckley-Sharp, M D
Bucknill, T M
Bull, T R
Bultitude, M I
Burton-West, K E
Bush, K
Byers, P D
Byrne, M A S
Calnan, C D
Campbell, A M
Campbell, L B
Campos Costa, D
Carnell, D M
Carpenter, R
Carruthers, G B
Carruthers, M E
Carter, S S C
Carver, N
Casburn-Jones, A
Cass, P L
Cassone, A M
Catterall, A
Chamoun, V
Chapman, M
Chapman, R H
Chapman, R
Chase, H D
Chignell, A H
Choong, K S S
Choy, Y-S
Christie Brown, J R W
Clark, M L
Clarke, C R A
Clarke, P D
Clarke, S G
Clein, L J

Clements, R V
Clynick, F E
Cnattingius, J A
Coakes, R L
Cobb, J P
Cockburn, H A C
Cohen, B
Cohen, S
Coleridge Smith, P D
Collin, J R O
Connolly, R C
Conway, G S
Cooper, B S
Cooper, R M
Cory-Pearce, R
Court, S A
Cowan, D B
Coxon, A Y
Craft, I L
Crawley, E M
Cream, J J
Crichton, P
Croft, C B
Crooks, R A J
Crown, S
Croxson, R S
Cullen, N M
D'Silva, R P
D'Souza, R E
Dalrymple, J O
Daniel, R
Dartey, P K W
Das-Gupta, R
Davey, G
Davies, A E
Davies, A E
Davies, D G
Davies, D M
Davies, D W L
Davies, G
Davies, G J
Davies, J E
Davies, R
Davies, T S G
Dawson, J R
Dawson, P
Day, J H
Daya, H
Daya, S M
De Bono, E F C P
Deman, E J
Dervisevic, S
Devlin, J J
Diggory, P L C
Dilke, T F W
Dingle, M L D
Dische, F E
Dixit, B B
Dixon, J
Douch, G
Douek, E
Douek, E E
Dowd, P M
Drewry, H R
du Vivier, A W P
Duchesne, G M
Dunaway, D J
Dutt, T P
Dymond, D S
Dymond, G S
Dyson, P H P
Ebrahim, I O
Edgar, M A
Edmonds, J A T
Edmondson, P C
Edmondson, S J
Edwards, J C W
Ehrenstein, M R
Eisenhandler, S J
El-Sherbini, R M
Elias, J A
Ell, P J
Ellahee, N
Ellingsen, J D
Emberton, M
Empey, D W
England, J P S
Enslin, R C
Erian, A
Eskander, A A
Etherington, G A
Ettlinger, P R A
Evans, C J
Evans, D G
Evans, I M A
Evans, M J
Falcon, M G
Farid, N
Farjo, B K P
Farjo, N P F
Farrag, M Z A E R
Farrar, D
Farthing, A J
Feitelson, Z
Fenton, D A
Ferguson, V M G
Ferrett, C G
ffytche, T J
Field, L H
Fine, J H
Firth, J B
Fison, P N
Fitzgerald O'Connor, A F
Foale, R A
Ford, S P
Forecast, D J
Fowler, P B S
Frank, O S
Frankland, A W
Freeman, H L
French, B T J
Fry, L
Gabriel, S S
Gander, D R
Gant, A R I A
Garson, J A
Gawler, J
Gaya, H
Gaze, M N
George, C F
George, P J M
George, R J D
Gerlis, L S
Ghatak, S K
Ghilchik, M
Ghosh, J C
Gibb, D M F
Gil-Rodriguez, J A
Gilkes, J J H
Gillams, A R
Gillard, M G
Gilmore, O J A
Gilmour, B D
Glenville, B E
Glynne, A
Goldie, L
Goldstone, J C
Goodhardt, L S
Gordon, A B
Goswamy, R K
Graham, D F
Graham, J M
Grant, H R
Gravett, P J
Grayson, M F
Greenberg, M P
Greene, A M
Greenwood, M H
Greer, A J
Greeves, J A
Gregor, Z
Grespi, L
Greville, A C
Griffiths, W A D
Grindle, C F J
Grobbelaar, A O
Gross, M
Grossmann, M E
Grover, R
Groves, R W
Guéret Wardle, D F H
Gurling, H M D
Gyselinck, P
Haacke, N P
Haas, D S
Haddad, F S
Hall-Craggs, M A
Hammond, C R
Harcourt, J P
Harland, S J
Harper, P G
Harrington, K F
Harris Hendriks, J M
Harris, A M
Harris, J R W
Harris, M N E
Harris, M
Harrison, D H
Harrison, M A
Hart, R A
Harvey, P K P
Hassiotis, A
Hatfield, A R W
Hatton, M J
Havard, C W H
Hawley, P R
Hazell, J W P
Healey, N J
Heard, C R
Hend, M F A
Henry, M M
Hensher, R W
Hickey, J D
Hill, A F
Hill, P D
Hilton, P J
Hitchings, R A
Ho, B M L
Hobbs, J T
Holder, D
Honey, M
Hooper, A A
Hosking, G P
Howard, C H
Howell, R J S
Hugh, D J
Hughes, A F R
Hughes, L
Hungerford, J L
Hunt, D M
Hunter, P A
Hurel, S J
Huskisson, E C
Hutton, J N T
Hyatt, D W
Hykin, P G
Ioannides, C
Irvine, D H
Isenberg, D A
Isworth, R A
Jackson, A M
Jacobs, H S
Jacobson, R A (
Jadav, J S
Jadhav, S S
Jagger, J D
Jalili, I K
James, D G
James, D R
James, P L
Janikoun, S G
Jansen, K L R
Jasani, M K
Jelliffe, A M
Jeya-Prakash, A
Johns, M E D
Johnson, I S
Johnson, J R
Johnson, N M
Jones, B M
Jones, O W
Jory, W J
Joseph, H T
Joyce, B
Joyston-Bechal, M P
Kaisary, A V
Kallis, P
Kapadia, L H
Kaplan, B
Katona, C L E
Katz, D R
Katz, M
Kavouni, A
Kay, L A
Keene, M H
Kelada, E
Kelleher, C J
Kellett, M J
Kellow, N H
Kelly, C A
Kendall, S
Kenig, M
Kennedy, K W
Kenney, A
Keshtgar, M R S
Kharbanda, R K
Khwaja, M G
King, J D
Kingdon, A J
Kinnear, P E
Kirby, R S
Kirkham, J S
Kirwan, E O G
Klaber, M R
Knight, M J
Kocjan, G
Kolvekar, S K
Konotey-Ahulu, F I D
Kotowski, K E
Kraft, T
Kratimenos, M L K
Kreeger, L C
Krikler, D M
Kurtz, A B
Kushalappa, C K
Kwok, K D
Lai, L M
Laidlaw, D A H
Lam, S J
Langley, J F A
Laurence, M
Lavy, J A
Lawrence, R E
Laws, I M
Lawson Baker, C J
Layton, C A
Leader, G L
Leathem, A J
Ledermann, J A
Lee, J P
Lee, S M
Lees, W R
Leonard, J N
Leonard, T J K
Levene, S
Levy, I S
Lewis, B
Libby, G W
Lilleyman, J S
Lim, F T K S
Littlewood, R M
Liversedge, R L
Lloyd, G G
Lloyd, G J
Lloyd, U E
Loeffler, F E
Logan, M A J
Lovat, L B
Lowe, D G
Lowe, M D
Lowe, N J
Lucire, Y
Luke, I K
Lunken, C R
McAra, A C
Maccabe, J J
McCoubrey, I A
Macdonald, N-J
Mace, M C
McEwan, J R
McGovern, C F M
McHardy-Young, S
McHugh, J D A
Mackay, I S
McKenna, W J
Mackenzie, P W
Mackie, I A
Mackinnon, D M
Mackinnon, J
Mackintosh, C E
McMillan, D L
McNab Jones, R F
MacSweeney, J E
Magee, P G
Magovern, P M J
Maguire, A
Mahendra, B
Mahmud, T
Mak, I Y H
Mallinson, C N
Mandel, J E
Mann, F B
Mansell, M A
Maratos, J
Marsh, R J
Marwood, R P
Mason, P W
Mason, R R
Mathalone, M B R
Matti, B A
May, M W
Meadows, J C
Meleagros, L
Mellett, P G
Mellon, C F M
Mezey, A G
Michelagnoli, M P
Migdal, C S
Millar, J M
Miller, M H
Millner, W F
Mills, A M
Mills, P G
Milroy, E J G
Mindell, J S
Mirpuri, N G
Misiewicz, J J
Mitchell, H
Mitchell, V S
Moore-Gillon, V L
Moran, J D
Morgan, R J
Morley, T R
Morris, S D
Morris, V H
Morrison, G A J
Morton, C M
Muir, J R
Muirhead-Allwood, S K
Mullins, M M
Mumtaz, H
Mundy, A J
Mundy, A R
Murphy, A M
Murphy, D A
Murphy, H M
Murray-Lyon, I M
Mushin, A S
Mythen, M G
Nag-Chaudhury, S R
Nagasubramanian, S
Nasser, N A
Nauth-Misir, R R
Naylor, C H
Nazeer, S
Neal, A J D
Neild, G H
Nemeth, C H
Newman, J H
Newton, J R
Newton, W K
Ng, N S-H
Nicholls, R J
Nield, D V
Nixon, J E
Noordeen, M H H
O'Brien, J P
O'Connell, J P J
O'Doherty, C S J
O'Donoghue, N
O'Driscoll, P M
O'Neill, G F A
Oakley, N W
Odedun, T O
Ohri, R
Olobo-Lalobo, J H
Oram, D H
Ornstein, M H
Osborne, J L
Osho, O F
Ostberg, J E
Pacifico, M D
Page, J E
Pandey, M
Panting, G P
Pardy, B J
Pariente, D
Parkhouse, H
Parsons, D W
Pattison, C W
Pavlou, C
Pedley, J E
Persoff, D A
Petty, H R
Peyman, M A
Pfeffer, J M
Phelan, M R
Phelan, M B
Phillips, K D
Phillips, W S
Pilcher, R
Pitcher, D C R
Plowman, P N
Pollock, R C
Power, J W
Price, J D
Price, S L
Primavesi, R J
Prinja, A
Prvulovich, E M
Pugh, M A
Quiney, R E
Radcliffe, A
Radcliffe, G J
Rahman, M A A
Rahmathunisa, A A
Raine, G E T
Raji, A M
Ralph, D J
Ransley, P G
Raphael, M J
Ratsey, D H K
Read, F E
Redgment, C J
Rehman, A J
Resek, G E
Reynolds, T J
Rickards, D
Roberts, A H
Roberts, D N
Robertson, M J S
Robertson, M M
Robinson, T W E
Rockall, A G
Rodriguez De La Sierra, L
Rogers, J
Roodyn, L
Rook, G A W
Rosalki, S B
Rose, F C
Rose, G E
Rosen, R C
Ross, D N
Rowbotham, H D
Rowland Payne, C M E
Rubens, M B
Rubin, A P
Rudolf, N M
Russell, R C G
Rustin, M H A
Ryan, P D
Sabetian, M
Sainsbury, J R C
Salah, M W
Salmon, P R
Salt, J C
Samuel, A M
Sanders, R
Sanders, S
Sarkany, I
Saunders, C M
Savin, G E
Sawyer, C N
Schetrumpf, J R
Scholes, G B
Schulenburg, W E
Scott, W A
Sebagh, J-L
Sebastian, J
Sear, M
Selby, L M
Semple, J C
Sergeant, H G S
Setchell, M E
Sevitt, L H
Shah, P J R
Shaikh, A A
Shanahan, W J
Sheaves, R M
Shephard, E
Shephard, E P
Sherwood, M P
Shiers, L G P
Shine, I B
Shipley, M E
Showghi, S
Shuker, M T
Sidaway, M E
Siddins, M T B
Sikora, K
Sillers, B R
Silver, J
Silverstone, A C
Simpkin, P
Sims, C D
Sinclair, L
Singer, M
Slevin, M L
Smith, J H
Solomons, B E R
Somerville, J
Sommerfield, J
Somper, J D
Sood, S C
Speechly-Dick, M E
Spence-Jones, C
Spiro, D M
Spiro, S G
Spittle, M F
Sporton, S C E
Spoudeas, H A
Springall, R G
Spurrell, R A J
Stamp, T C B
Stanek, J J
Stanton, S L R
Starr, M J
Stearns, M P
Steel, A E
Stein, R C
Stephens, J W
Stern, G M
Stewart, A C
Stoker, D J
Stonehill, E
Strigner, A E
Stuttaford, I T
Sullivan, M F
Sutcliffe, J C
Sutton, R
Swanton, R H
Sweetnam, D I S

Swire, N
Syada, M
Tabone-Vassallo, M
Talerman, H J
Tang, D W K
Taor, W S
Tappouni, F R
Tattari, C
Taylor, D S I
Taylor, I
Taylor, J O M
Teasdale, E L
Temperton, H C
Thomas, M G W
Ting, P Y C
Tinker, J
Towers, M K
Townsend, C
Tucker, A K
Tucker, S M
Tufnell, G
Tunio, A M
Turner, S W
Ungar, S C
Unwin, R J
Uppal, R
Van Oldenborgh, H M
Vandendriessche, M A W
Vanhegan, G M
Vesselinova-Jenkins, C K
Vickers, R H
Viel, M
Viel, R
Wade, T H H
Waldman, A D B
Walesby, R K
Walker, P G
Wallace, S A
Walshe, J M
Ward, D E
Ward, K N
Wareing, M J
Warren, R A
Waterhouse, N
Waters, K J
Watkin, B C
Watkin, J E
Watkins, E S
Watson, D M
Watson, N A
Webb, A R
Welldon, E V
Welply, G A C
Weston, M J
Whelan, J S
White, A G
White, H
White, I R
White, S A
Whitelocke, R A F
Whiteson, A L
Whitfield, H N
Whitfield, P J
Wignall, B K
Wilkinson, C L
Williams, A T D
Williams, H P
Williams, R L
Wincewicz, A M
Winspur, I
Witchalls, J R
Witherow, R O N
Witt, J D
Witt, M J
Wolfe, J H N
Wong, S K
Wontumi, J A
Woo, P M M
Woodhouse, C R J (T
Woolfson, G
Wright, J E
Wright, J L W
Wright, M G
Wrong, O M
Wydenbach, K A
Wylie, I G
Yarrow, H
Youlten, L J F
Young, A J
Younis, F M
Yu, R C H
Zahir, A G
Zaman, M J S
Zatouroff, M
Zeider, P A
Zumla, A

W2

Abdalla, S H
Abdullah, H S N
Acha Gandarias, P
Al-Onaizy, Z Y
Alberti, K G M M
Alexander, H P M
Alexander, S M
Ames, D E
Anderson, S T B
Arora, S
Ashworth, S F
Atkinson, S
Aylin, P P
Balakrishnan, J A
Ball, J A
Barghouti, W Y
Beesley, M L S
Bell, S S J
Berlin, A P
Bevan, P J
Beveridge, I G
Bharucha, M-P E
Bilagi, P
Blake, J C
Brooks, M J
Cairns, T D H
Cattell, V
Chalhoub, N M Y
Chambers, W M
Chambler, A F W
Cheshire, N J W
Chew, A-L
Chiotakakou, E
Chong, K K
Clifford, K A
Cobb, E I
Cooper, E S
Corlett, S K
Coulter, C A E
Cowan, D L
Craig, F
Crane, J S
Crawford, M J
Crème, M L
Crofton, M E
Cronje, W H
Cunningham, D A
Damant, H G
Darzi, A W
Davies, D W
Davies, H T
De Munter, C
Deal, J E
Dick, E A
Doo, A K
Duckworth, G J
Easmon, C S F
El-Farhan, M H
Elder, A H
Elkeles, R S
Elliott, P
Epenetos, A A
Epstein, J
Evans, D J
Fairney, A
Faliakos, S
Farmer, S F
Faust, S N
Fielder, M H
Fitzharris, P F
Flitcroft, D I
Fluxman, J D
Forbes, S J
Franks, S
Gadelrab, R R
Gandhi, N D
Gangar, K F
Garralda Hualde, M E
Gautama, S
Ghali, S
Gill, S
Gilling-Smith, C M-T L
Gledhill, J A
Glyn, J H H
Goldin, R D
Gonzalez-Garcia, J
Goon, P K C
Gorchein, A
Gould, D A
Greene, L A
Guy, M A
Habibi, P
Hadjiminas, D
Hakim, N
Hamilton, R D
Hanna, N
Hansell, A L
Hardman, C
Harris, J E
Hart, R
Hartley, S L
Hassan, A H A
Heggessey, L S
Hemingway, H J S
Henebury, R E D
Henry, J A
Hewitt, C A H
Hickey, M
Higham, J M
Hodes, M
Holdsworth, G M C
Holloway, P A H
Hopkins, C E O
Horn, A R
Huang, Y L E
Hughan, I C
Hughes, A D
Hulme, B
Hussain, W
Indar, R
Ismail, A H
Jeffery, K J M
Jepson, A P
Joffe, M
Johnson, M A
Johnston, D G
Johnston, S L
Jones, D M
Jones, R M
Joseph, P L A
Judge, D J
Kadas, T
Kalodiki, E
Kammerling, R M
Kampmann, B
Karimjee, S
Karmi, G
Kessell, M
Khaliq, S A
Khullar, V
Killick, C J
Kitson, J
Kojodjojo, P
Kon, O M
Kong Yao Fah, S K
Kroll, J S
Kwan, J S K
Kywe, H
Lacey, C J N
Lack, G
Lamb, G M
Lamba, H S
Langdon, N
Lee, D M
Lee, W S
Leonard, R C
Leyton, H R
Lishman, E J
Lissauer, T J
Lomax, D M
Lyall, E G H
McElwee, C S E
MacLeod, K G A
Maguire, H C F
Main, J
Maini, S
Markides, V
Marriott, S V L
Maru, L
Mason, J
Mathias, C J
Mayet, J
Mikou, P
Miskry, T S
Mitchell, D M
Mok, M H H
Montgomery, S A
Mowbray, J F
Moyes, S T
Murphy, K W
Musajo, F G
Mussa, M Y
Nadel, S
Narula, A A P
New, H V
Ng, K J
O'Hare, R
O'Sullivan, F E
Oberoi, A
Odgaard, A
Odunuga, B A
Oldfield, W L G
Olufunwa, P B
Ong, J
Openshaw, P J M
Osborne, G E N
Palmer, A B D
Papas, K
Patel, A
Patel, K S
Paterson, C M
Percy, D B
Persad, K
Peters, N S
Philip, G E
Platt, M W
Poulter, N R
Powles, A V
Pursell, N R
Reed, A M
Rees, R G
Regan, L
Rice, A S C
Rivers, R P A
Robinson, S
Roche, S W
Rosin, R D
Sanderson, A L
Saxsena, S P
Schachter, M
Schonfield, S
Scott, S L
Sever, P S
Shahrad, P
Shaw, F E
Shawis, T N
Sheridan, D J
Shortall, T N
Shroff, K J
Shum, W K
Silva, D
Simpson, J E P
Smyth, C L
Smyth, D P L
So, E
Sondheimer, J
Soucek, S
Stanbridge, R L
Stanton, A V
Summerfield, J A
Summerfield, O J
Tabandeh, H
Taub, P-S A
Taylor-Robinson, D
Taylor, G P
Teare, J P
Teoh, T G
Thiru, Y
Thom, S A M
Thomas, H C
Thomas, H J W
Thompson, E M
Thompson, P K
Thursz, M R
Tolley, N S
Touquet, R
Trigg, C J
Tweedy, M H
Vale, J A
Venkat Raman, N
Vine, A M
Vranakis, K
Wakelin, S H
Walker, J G
Walker, M M
Wallace, A L
Walters, M D S
Ward, H
Watkins, R P F
Webb, S A R
Weber, J N
Weir, J G
Wilkinson, D M
Wilson, L F
Wolff-MacDonald, E M
Wright, A R
Yates, P A
Yen, W
Yeo, D W T
Yong, K L
Zaman, R
Zambanini, A

W3

Annadani, S R
Arora, G S
Azzopardi, D
Baber, P M
Bakala, A I
Bayney, R D
Borrows, R J
Bull-Soukeras, S
Burns, A
Cabot, K L
Campbell, B J
Campbell, E
Chambers, M M
Chong, P
Collier, I F
Crawford, C L
Datta, S N
Davies, C D
Dehghani, M
Dhatt, M
Evans, J A
German, K A
Gupta, A N
Hassanaien, M M
Haverty, P F
Ickringill, J C W
Jacobs, E B A
Jeffreys, G E S
Kaur, S
Kazzaz, H J S A
Khan, N Z
Khashaba, A M H
Kolokithas, D
Koziell, S
Laurie, A S
McGovern, U B
McKeigue, S J
Magner, E H
Marden, P F
Martinez, J
Measday, I F
Morrell, J E
Moustafa, W M
Mulchandani, H
Pambakian, N H
Pullaperuma, S P
Reddy, C P
Reynolds, P J
Rimmer, D M D
Rimmer, Y L
Robinska, E M
Saujani, A V
Scully, A G
Shahrabani, R M J
Sinha, B P
Smith, M A
Spencer, S M
Takhar, G S
Taraba, P
Ukra, H A H R
Vowles, J E
Wielogórski, A K
Womersley, B J
Young, T B
Zamiri, P

W4

Al-Benna, S
Anderson, F M
Baker, C B
Barnes, S K M
Bennett, D M
Bennett, N C
Betancor Martinez, M
Bhatt, V B
Burbidge, N V
Bushby, A J R
Butler, S P
Campion, H M R
Chan, S T K
Chandran, B S
Chiu, D C
Chiverton, S G
Choudhuri, D
Cole, A S
Colfor, A M
Connell, R J
Cooper, J E
Czajkowski, M A
Davis, J R
Devine, A R Y
Doulia, E
Dumskyj, M J
Edmonds, E V J
Edwards, K M J
Ezekwe, C K C
Garcia-Praderas, I
Gardiner, C A
Gilvarry, A M
Grover, V P B
Groves, C J
Guntis, E
Hall, S A
Halliday, M W
Harris, M F
Haslehurst, J M
Heinsheimer, R J
Hirst, S L
Holderness, Y M
Hughes, G V
Hunt, S M
James, C E
James, D C O
Jansen, A
Kaplan, M J
Keen, J W
Khalifa, W
Khalique, S
Killeen, M A
Kirtchuk, G H
Konieczko, K M
Lander, D K
Lechler, R I
Levison, A V
Lim, W W D
Lockett, M J
McCormack, M
MacDonald, R S
Matthews, S H M
Mearza, A A
Mendes Da Costa, C J
Milojkovic, D
Moseley, I F
Moussa, R
Munro, A R
Murdoch, I A
O'Brien, K M
Paszkowska, K
Patel, H
Patel, M B
Pattison, J
Pejovic, I
Phelan, M B
Pigott, J D
Polkinghorne, K R
Porto, L O D R
Proner, B D
Reinstein, D Z
Ridgway, E S
Rizvi, N
Rocker, M D
Rogers, C
Rumian, A P
Sacks, G P
Salama, A D
Sargent, A M F
Sethurajan, S
Shah, B R
Shah, S N
Shaw, P J
Smith, I
Soysa, P N
Stableforth, C F
Stevens, L M
Szyszko, J M
Taggart, P I
Taylor, W J
Thakrar, N A
Thompson, P M
Venkatesham, G
Ventresca, G
Vroegop, P G
Walden, S J
Wasan, H S
Wasan, P K
Waygood, A R
Weber, A M
Whiten, C J
Williams, K A
Yap, Y G
Ziprin, J H

W5

Abadir, W F
Abeyasinghe, N I
Al-Saidi, N H M
Ali, S H
Allan, S E
Allen, G M
Aluvihare, V R
Amin, M A
Ashby, D R
Aziz, M R A
Azzopardi, J G
Balasegaram, M V
Balasegaram, U
Baruch, U B H
Beardow, R V
Benierakis, C
Billington, S A M
Bradley, L A
Broomhead, L R
Buxton, P A
Campbell, S
Campbell, T J
Carter, F E
Chalmers-Watson, J I
Charitou, A
Cogill, G O
Crowley, C J

Dalal, R R
Dalal, S R
Das, L
Dave, J
Dave, R
Day, A M
De Rosa, S
Dixon, P J V
Dowling, M
Downer, J P
Duff-Miller, M T
Dundon, E A
Dunkley, A B
Dureja, A
Dybas, B
Engler, C F
Evans, D C M
Farley, K L
Ghosh, G K
Giam, N K L
Gill, J S
Gittins, J C
Greenway, R A C
Grewal, P S
Hamilton, J A
Hanslip, J I
Haque, S J
Harding, C S J E
Harper, E S
Hayman, G R
Hennebry, M C
Higgins, S J
Hiwaizi, F S
Holbrook, D M A
Horner, R
Hunt, K D
Irvine, S M T
Jeffery, R M R
Johnson, D S
Jones, M R
Kaler, S S
Kamalarajah, B
Kamalarajah, S
Karim, Q N
Karthikesalingam, S
Keddilty, J T H
Knox, K L
Kochan, M D
Kohn, A D
Krasucki, R E
Kyriakou, K P
Laskiewicz, B M
Lauder, M M
Lawes, R J
Lewanski, C R
Li, C K-C
Lloyd, D
Logan, B
Lucas, C M
Lydon, C
McLure, H A
Mander, D S
Mastihi, A
Meer, H
Melikian, N
Mendel, D J
Meurer-Laban, M M
Mitko, A Z
Mohamed, G E Y
Nadersepahi, A
Nafie, S A E-A A
Neave, F
O'Callaghan, A C
Owen, M J
Pakarian, B F
Pande, M
Patel, G A A M
Paul, N K
Peatfield, R C
Philp, B M
Picard, J J
Pietroni, R G
Pope, S J
Rampling, M J
Ramsamy, T
Richmond, P J M
Rogers, D A
Rollason, S B
Sapsford, R N
Sarwar, M N
Sharma, S
Sherafat, H
Shnyien, N K
Sikorski, J M
Simpson, A B
Simpson, J C
Stephenson, D T
Sturge, R A
Toale, E
Trivedi, V J
Tung, M-Y
Twomey, J L
Walji, S F
Warren, A J
Whitehead, A P
Whitehead, P T
Whitehurst, A M
Williams, H M
Williams, S R R
Wilson, M B
Wright, C S W
Wright, S D
Young, A P
Yu, S C

W6

Ahmad, M
Alaghband Zadeh, J
Alexander, S
Alusi, S H
Arrigoni, P B
Asplund, O A O
Ault, E A
Azadian, B S
Bagshawe, K D
Baker, C S R
Banati, R B
Banks, L C
Bansi, D S
Barber, N J
Barling, J M
Barrett, S P
Bartels, A R D
Bellringer, J F
Bench, C J
Bennett, P R
Beski, S
Billett, A F
Birtle, A J
Blane, D B
Blunt, S B
Bolton, A
Boolell, M
Brock, C S
Bronstein, A M
Brown, E A
Carby, A E
Choudhury, M A Q
Christmas, T J
Clarke, F
Clarke, P M
Clifford, C P
Colquhoun, I R
Combe, E A
Coomes, E N
Cope, A P
Courtenay-Mayers, B B P
Crimlisk, S N
Cummin, A R C
Dalrymple, S D
David, A L M
Davies, A H
Davies, S E
Davis, A
Dawson, P M
Deacon, M B
Dennis, R T
Di Pasquale, A B
Dutta, R L
Elkington, P T G
Evans, P J D
Falconer, A
Fauvel, N J
Feldmann, M
Fernandes, P F R
Fitzgerald, T J
Fletcher, M
Flood, A J
Foadi, M D
Forester, A J
Fotiadis, R J
Francis, N D
Frank, J W
Franklin, I J
Frazer, A N L
Gaer, J A R
Gibson, A J
Gladdish, S J
Glaser, M G
Glees, J P
Glickman, S
Glover, M
Gopinath, S
Gordon, J S
Grant, W E
Green, A N
Green, R
Greenhalgh, R M
Guiloff, R J
Gupta, V K
Guz, A
Hamblett, C J
Hanham, I W F
Hariri, M A
Harper, F V L
Harrington, D J
Harris, R L
Hart, N
Hayward, M P
Hirsch, S R
Ho, S-A
Howard, J V
Hrouda, D
Hucker, J C
Hughes, R A
Hughes, S P F
Husain, M
Ion, L E
Isaac, D L
Jankowski, S K
Jarvis, S C
Jaye, P D
Johnson, M R
Johnson, P V
Joyce, E M
Joyce, S
Kennard, C
Khalil, N M
Koppel, J I
Lane, R J M
Larché, M J
Lawson, L L
Lee, C P
Letsky, E A
Levy, J B
Lim, C H
Linjawi, S
Lynch, M J
Lynch, V M
McCartie, J D
MacDonald, D H C
McEwan, J A M
MacInnes, L E
McKee, H J
McLaren, S A U
McLean, K A
Maier, M
Maini, R N
Maitra, B
Mak, I Y N
Malik, O
Manson, A J
Maraj, B H
Masoli, M P D
Matthews, T D
Meacher, R L
Mead, S H
Mendoza, N D
Millington, H T
Miskelly, F G
Misra, R R
Mitchell, A W M
Mizen, C S
Mohith, A B
Morley, S J
Naguib, M E N
Nanchahal, J
Newlands, E S
Newson, D H
Norman, B J
Nuthall, T R A
O'Keeffe, C J
Olver, J M
Owens, C M
Palmieri, C
Park, A J
Partridge, M R
Partridge, S E
Patel, M C
Percival, N J
Perkin, G D
Persaud, M C
Pett, S J
Phelan, M C
Phillips, M E
Poor, S H
Porter, F V
Powell, C G B
Pritchard, C A
Proll, S
Ramsay, J W A
Ratcliffe, M J H
Razzak, A H M H W M
Reder, P
Redman, S P
Rees, B W
Rees, H C
Rice-Edwards, J M
Roddie, M E
Roney, S M
Roohanna, R
Rose, F G
Ross, G M
Rudge, S D E
Rugg, S A M
Salooja, N
Salt, P J
Sanderson, J D
Scriven, J E
Shakir, R A W
Shaoul, D D R
Shaoul, E
Sharma, P
Shortt, M W
Shousha, M S M
Simon, D W N
Sinnett, H D
Slater, L B
Smith, J J
Smith, N A
Southcott, B M C
Steiner, T J
Steuer, A
Stewart, J S W
Su, R C W
Svensson, W E
Tan, S V S-M
Taylor, A
Taylor, D G
Taylor, P C
Taylor, S D
Thomssen, H
Tipples, M K
Trendell-Smith, N J
Tyrer, P J
Venables, E M
Wade, J P H
Walton, I G
Ward, P M
Watson, D G A
Wetton, C W N
Wheatley, D P
White, J F
Williams, W
Wilson, J A
Wingfield, D J C
Wood, D A
Wood, S H
Wright, C J E
Yong, A S M
Yule, S M

W7

Baldock, J E
Ballard, J
Bennett, C N
Bennett, D N
Cummings, T M
Derham, R J M
Dhillon, A P
Freeman, A L
Gill, G S
Hallums, A L
Hereward, J M
Hereward, J O
Jackson, A E
Kyrionymou, G
Lees, A R
Lewandowska, A
Light, F W
Naish, R
Pambakian, A L M
Pambakian, H
Pambakian, S
Pinney, S A
Pipon, M L
Rogers, Z J
Sahota, O S
Sivaramalingam, T R
Stapleton, S
Stewart, R C
Thomas, C S
Waldes, R M

W8

Alderson, E H
Bell, M
Bozek, T
Bronsdon, C E
Candelier, C K
Cohen, A S
Cohen, C E M
Cole, M L
Corbett, P C
Dahdal, M T E
De Brito, A J F
Dimitriadis, I
Doidge-Harrison, K J
Ernsting, J
Farnham, C W E
Freeman, R T
Gomersall, C D
Hall, A J
Hamlyn, E M
Hammond, R O
Hashemian, H A
Hayes, J M
Kang, C H
Kaye, G S
Khammar, G S
Kiernan, P J
Kitiyakara, C
Kurtz, Z
Lasa Georgas, A E
Lea, G
Lee, S K
Lopez-Ibor Alcocer, M I
MacGreevy, B I P
Malhas, M H
Malhas, S M
Moore, S P G
Nour-Eldin, F
O'Sullivan, J C
Pawlikowski, T R B
Peterson, D C
Refson, A R
Richardson, P J
Samaan, N M
Sharara, A M
Smith, J B
Smith, M P
Stanowski, M
Tahbaz, A
Tharmaratnam, A K
Thompson, J R
Wong, F-M

W9

Abrams, D J R
Adams, D L
Adshead, J M
Bancroft, R J
Barreto, A
Barry, S M E
Basham, S C
Bearsted, C J
Beetles, C
Berger, A J
Bevington, R L S
Borton, C
Brennand, D J
Bull, D R
Cantrell, P J
Carey Smith, R L
Chan, J P L
Church, S M
Congreve, K A M
Constantinou, J
Contell, F N
Curtis, R N M
Cusano, C
De Silva, P S
Dexter, S L
El-Gazzar, Y A S
Elvin, E J
Fraser, J I C
Fung, Y
Garfield, A M
Garner, J S
Gibson, D J
Giles, M J
Gorham, T J
Hart, S K
Helme, M A
Hepper, F J
Hicks, R A
Hidalgo Simon, M A
Hirsh, A V
Ho-Asjoe, M S K W
Honey, S E
Houghton, J M
Houghton, S L
Ishaque, J S
Johnson, M A
Jones, B A S
Jones, E C A
King, P M
Kitchen, V S
Kopelowitz, L
Lawal, A H
Leader, A R
Lockie, J
McGilligan, J M P
McGilligan, R C
Malone, A A
Meir, N S
Miles, M M
Miles, M V
Moorhead, J F
Nelson, P D
O'Neill, N M D R
Owen-Reece, H
Pallis, D J
Pirie, A
Puttick, M I
Quilliam, R P
Qureshi, M
Ratip, S
Rich, P M
Roeves, A J
Rucklidge, M W M
Rutter, P
Sahota, K K
Sarnicki, M A
Sorour, G A
Stafford, M T
Stormont, F C
Symons, S B V
Taherzadeh, O
Tennant, S J
Toubia, N F
Uppal, R S
Varawalla, N Y
Vogel, M W
Wei, C W
Williams, G J P
Williamson, P D
Wright, H E
Yousuf, E Y

W10

Abbas, W S
Ahmed, N
Alam, R
Anthony-Pillai, R D
Ardern, M H
Bordin, P
Brunner, I C
Burton, R C
Butler, R E
Chang, Y H
Dathi, H H M
De Ruiter, J M
Densham, E P
Doyle, J M
Eagger, S A
Evans, A H
Evans, R M
Gillespie, H M
Gillespie, H R E
Hasford, C
Heydari, A
Higgitt, A C
Jalisi, Q Z H
Jasani, N
Kelso, I J
Lam, T H
Mackney, P H
Melnik, L
Melville, C S A
Michael, T E
Myers, K G
Naysmith, A
Nijhar, A
O'Rawe, M G D
Ormerod, A E
Parsons, E J
Rahman, M L
Rahman, M L
Ramasamy, N
Sadler, G D
Sash, L
Smith, G N
Smith, P C C
Swade, S N
Webb, S C

W11

Alikhani, S
Ansari, S
Bell, R W
Besse, C P
Bloom, C A
Bonwitt, C
Calman, C R
Chapman, J N
Cheng, W C W
Chin, P C C
Chowdhury, S
Chung, M M
Datnow, E L

Dawson, M E
Demetriou, R S
Dias, V O
Dzendrowskyj, P
El-Kabir, D J
Emanuel, R W
Farrimond, J G
Foong, L C
Gillies, E A D
Haughton, N D
Holden, S J
Hooker, R C
Houang, E T
Huber, C P P
Hutt, R S A
Hyde, T A
Jackson, G D M
Jenkins, G R
Kaz-Kaz, H
Kazi, A B
Khan, M A
Kuteesa, W M A
Mansi, M N
Mohamad, J A
Mok, C A K Y
Munns, J
Nayani, T H
Norman, A R F
O'Connell, B A
O'Connor, C M I
Patten, P E M
Pearl, B A
Pettifer, B J
Preziosi, J J
Price, D B
Radcliffe, S A
Ramsden, S S
Reid, P J
Rosenthal, J M
Rutter, T M
Salkeld, S A
Schachter, J
Scurr, M J
Seemungal, B M
Shoenberg, P J
Soboniewska, K M T
Steele, A C
Stride, J S C
Stringer, K R
Viviers, L
Waldron, J P
Wannan, G J
Wassif, W S
Watson, D
Wijaysinghe, D
Zainuddin, I A

W12
Abel, P D
Adam, E C
Ahmad, R A S
Aichinger, G
Ainley, T C
Aitman, T J
Al-Hamali, S A
Al-Nahhas, A M M
Albrecht, T
Allen, A R
Anderson, J R
Anjarwalla, N K A
Apperley, J F
Archer, S E
Bacon, R C
Badat, A A
Bagger, J P
Baldock, G J
Barakat, M T
Basarab, M
Basma, R
Beatt, K J
Bellamy, M F
Bloom, S R
Bogle, R G
Botto, M
Bourdillon, P J
Bratby, M J
Brooks, D J
Bryan, E M
Bulpitt, C J
Burns, A
Camici, P G
Canisius, D S D
Chadha, S
Chapman, V J
Chu, A C
Clutterbuck, E J
Coker, R K
Coleman, D V
Cook, H T
Coombes, R C D S
Cosgrove, D O
Cowan, F M
Cox, P M
Craddock, C F
Cummings, C S
Dalley, C D
Dandapat, R
Das-Gupta, S
Davies, A E M
De La Fuente Pereda, J
Dhanjal, M K
Dokal, I S
Dornhorst, A
Dowdeswell, K A
Drewett, S J
Drury, R E F
Edmonds, D K
Epstein, R J
Feldman, R G
Fermie, P G
Fisk, N M
Frankton, S
Friedland, J S
Fullerton, S A
Fusi, L
Gabra, H
Garg, A
Gaskin, G
Gates, C D
Gbeckor-Kove, D M
Ghosh, S
Gibbs, J S R
Girgis, S I
Goldman, J M
Goodchild, K A
Gothard, P K
Grippaudo, V M
Hammond, S J
Haskard, D O
Hawkins, T E
Hemingway, A P
Hodes, C B
Holmes, M R
Hornick, P I
Howard, J K
Huddy, J M M
Hughes, J M B
Hughes, T P
Impallomeni, M G
Ind, P W
Jackson, J E
Jenkins, I H
Johnson, I B
Jolly, R V
Jones, B
Kakkar, A K
Kanfer, E J
Keyani, J A
Kirby, S A
Kolomainen, D F
Kumar Surendran, S
Laffan, M A
Lalani, E-N M A
Lavery, S A
Lefroy, D C
Lemoine, N R
Lerman, A J
Lighten, A D
Lightstone, E B
Lindsay, J O
Lockwood, G G
Lowe, E M
Lynn, J A
Maalouf, E F
McClure, N A
McIndoe, G A J
Makgoba, M W
Marcus, C
Margara, R A
Martyn-Johns, D
Mason, J C
Meeran, M K
Miller, S
Mills, J K
Modi, N
Morrison, P A
Morrison, R S
Moses, G
Muntoni, F
Naoumova, R P
Nihoyannopoulos, P
Nikolaou, D
O'Donovan, M
O'Gallagher, D M B
Palin, C A
Panay, N
Panoskaltsis, T
Papakostas, P
Paterson-Brown, S
Piccini, P
Pickering, M C
Pitt, A E
Plaat, F S
Puri, B K
Pusey, C D
Rayner, S A
Redfern, D R M
Richardson, R J
Roberts, I A G
Robertson, N J
Robinson, B H
Rogers, T R F
Rose, G L
Ross, E C
Rutherford, M A
Sellu, D P
Sethurajan, A
Shadbolt, C L
Shah, K R
Shaunak, S
Shaw, R J S
Shovlin, C L
Sigurdsson, H H
Smith, D A
Smith, P L C
Soleimani, B
Soutter, W P
Sriskandan, S
Stavri, G T
Stephen, G W
Strickland, N H
Taheri, S
Tait, N P
Tam, F W-K
Taneja, A K
Tateossian, J K
Taylor-Robinson, S D
Taylor, K M
Thillainayagam, A V
Thompson, G R
Thomson, M A
Tierney, J
Trew, G H
Trikas, A
Tuddenham, E G D
Uppal, G S
Uppal, S
Valentine, L
Van Iddekinge, B
Vassiliou, G S
Vernon, C C
Vigushin, D M
Vyse, T J
Walker, E K L
Walport, M J
Walters, J R F
Warrens, A N
Waxman, J H
Webber, L J
Williams, G R
Williamson, C
Williamson, R C N
Williamson, R
Winston, R M L
Yii, M Y Y

W13
Adams, B K
Azoo, N M
Bailey, S M
Baker, W N W
Bassi, S
Bayer, J M
Beitverda, Y
Bernstein, I A
Bhatti, M A
Biel, E M
Blyth, T P
Burna Asefi, M S
Chamberlain, A L
Clarke, D C K
Cominos, M
Coucher, J R
Courrier, M Y
Cowen, D S
Dasoju, R
Dhillon, G
Drepaul, L R M
Duff, M C
Estreich, L
Fuller, J H
Gopal, B
Gordon, A C
Gordon, G
Gordon, H
Harris, J V
Hooftman, L W F
James, S M
Jarosz, J M
Jazrawi, H H
Kitchener, P A
Kosciesza, E
Lau, P H-H
Lazarov, D
Lemoine, L
McPartlin, D W
Majekodunmi, O O
Mankoo, K S
Markham, J J
Marks, N A
Mason, S J
Master, B R
Nazerali, G A
O'Donohue, M B
Osman, Z
Oyediran, M A
Pathansali, R
Phornnarit, J
Porter, E J B
Price, A B
Rai, R S
Randall, D G S
Ridings, P C
Romano, P
Russell, D A
Salam, S
Seneviratne, S
Shah, A K
Stevens, M A
Sukhia, V D
Thomas, D K
Travis, P J
Watrasiewicz, K E
Watson, A C
Wilkin, D J W
Wimalasundera, H H
Yiangou, G
Yu, D S L
Ziprin, P

W14
Adams, C E A
Alexandrou, D
Avrane, J-J
Binysh, J K
Bourke, K A
Bullen, S A
Campion, J E
Carleton, H C S
Carne, S J
Chao, M A
Chappell, B G
Chen, S D M
Clubb, E M F-S
Clubb, R A
Collins, L
Colquhoun, M C E S
Cotter, P A
Davidson, A W
Davison, M M
Dickinson, R
Dornan, V I P
Dua, J S
Edrich, C L
Elliott, C
Fahmy, H
Fennelly, E D
Frenkel, J
Ghazanfar, R
Giles, A J H
Greenhalgh, R
Harris, J S E
Herman, J S
Hood, D J
Horne, A W
Ind, S H
Jackson, G N B
Kanani, M
Khan-Gilbert, H
Kohner, E M
Lau, A W K
Lewis, D J
Low, S W W
Lyon, J A
McCollum, A
McEvedy, C P
Malik, N N
Martinez Campos, E
Metcalfe, A M
Milne, A G
Mitchell, T N
Moir, J G
Morris, A L
Mort, D J
Motazed, R
Nash, G F
Nihal, A
O'Brady, D S
O'Driscoll, M C
O'Hara, L J
Ogunbiyi, T A J
Oon, V J H
Oshodi, M A
Patwardhan, K
Raj, S J
Rao, R M
Salukhe, T V
Sastre Cabrer, J A
Schofield, E M
Scoones, F H
Scuplak, S M
Sercombe, K M
Sims, H
Thompson, W C R
Turner, M S
Vakis, S
Wilson, J H
Wilson, J L
Wilson, P N
Wong Hong Chai, Dr
Woodruff, S A

WC1
Acheson, J F
Adler, M W
Ahmad, S
Albanese, A
Albert, D M
Alibhai, A A
Allam, J
Allam, M
Allason-Jones, E
Allford, S L
Alvarez Parra, G E
Anagnostopoulos, A-V
Ancliff, P J
Andersen, P A
Anderson, R H
Arden, G B
Assi, G
Atherton, D J
Aylett, S E
Aynsley-Green, A
Babu-Narayan, S V
Badia Vallribera, L
Bagary, M S
Bahra, A
Balamurali, T B S
Baranowski, A P
Barnicoat, A J
Barrett, M D A
Bavin, D J
Baxendale, H E
Beale, T J
Beavis, J P
Behrens, R H
Bellingan, G J
Bellman, M H
Benn, P D
Benton, J S
Bernard, T
Biassoni, L
Bingham, R M
Biscoe, T J
Bitner-Glindzicz, M A K
Black, A E
Black, N A
Boralessa, R
Botma, A M
Botwood, N A J
Boyd, S G
Bradley, D J
Brandner, S
Bremner, F D
Brown, A S J M
Brown, J S
Brown, M M
Brown, M
Brown, P
Bryan, S J C
Bull, C
Burch, M
Burmester, M K
Burns, F M
Cadge, B A
Cale, C M
Cameron, F J
Carney, P J E
Casey, A T H
Cass, H D
Chan, D
Chan, M Y
Chaturvedi, N
Chawda, S J
Chessells, J M
Chiodini, P L
Chisholm, J W
Chisholm, J C
Choa, D I
Chong, W K
Chorbachi, M R
Churchyard, A J
Clarke, A E
Clayton, P T
Cohen, H
Cohen, S L
Coleman, M P
Collinge, J
Collins, J E
Collis, I
Colville, C C
Copp, A J
Corbett, E L
Cordery, R J
Cornah, R A
Costello, A M L
Cowan, F M
Crean, V S J
Creighton, S M
Crockard, H A
Croker, J R
Cross, J H
Cruz Arteaga, J C
Cutner, A S
Cutts, F T
D'Sa, S P
Daly, P E
Daniel, S E
Dattani, M T
Davies, J M
Davies, M C
Davies, R C
Davies, R A
Day, V A
De Leval, M R
De Sousa, C M C P
De Swiet, M
Desai, M M
Devile, C J
Dewhirst, K
Dillon, M J
Dinwiddie, R
Dollery, C M
Donald, A K
Donaldson, J A
Duchen, M R
Duffy, P G
Duncan, J S
Eagleton, T M
East, C A
Elliman, D A C
Elliott, A M
Elliott, C A
Elliott, M J
Ellis, D S
Everitt, A D
Facer, E K
Feather, S A
Fine, L G
Fisher, L F
Fisher, P A G
Foreman, J C
Forouhi, N G
Fowler, C J
Fowler, D J
Frackowiak, R S J
French, P D
Fryssira, E
Galloway, M J
Gardiner, R M
Garrard, P
Gavalas, M C
Gibson, E E
Gilbert, C E
Gilbert, R E
Gillett, G T
Gilson, R J C
Giovannoni, G
Glaser, D R
Glover, M T
Glynn, J R
Glynne, P A
Goadsby, P J
Godfrey, M
Godlee, F N
Goldin, J M
Goldman, A J
Goldstone, A H
Goodman, F R
Gordon, I
Gration, J C D
Greenwood, R J
Griffiths, M H

Groves, P
Groves, P H
Hagard, S
Haines, A P
Hall, A J
Hall, C M
Halvorsen, R T L
Hann, I M
Hanson, G A
Harding, B N
Harding, S R G
Harkness, W F J
Harper, J I
Harrop-Griffiths, K
Hart, A J
Hartley, B E J T
Hartley, J C
Hasan, F A
Hasan, R S
Havard, J D J
Hawdon, J M
Hayward, R D
Healy, C M J
Heard, S R
Henrichsen, T A
Hesketh, T M
Hickman, S J
Hill, R A
Hill, S M
Hill, V A
Hinchcliffe, R
Hirsch, N P
Hobart, J C
Hopper, C
Houghton, A M
Houlden, H J
Hourihane, J O B
Houssemayne Du Boulay, E P G
Howard, D J
Howard, R S
Hyett, J A
Inwald, D P
Isaacson, P G
Iyer, K R
Jackson, N R
Jacobs, I J
Jaffe, A
Jalan, R
Jamieson, A
Jarman, P R
Jauniaux, E
Jayaraj, S M
Jeene, H J E
Jennings, N K
Jones, A M
Judah, J D
Kalavrezos, N
Kallappa, K
Kaluba, J B L
Kapila, P
Kapoor, R
Kent, D G
Khan, N L
Kiely, E M S G
Kilby, A M
King, M J
Kinton, L
Kirkham, F J
Kitchen, N D
Klein, N J
Kotecha, B
Kullmann, D M
Küpper, A-L
Lachelin, G C L
Lakhani, S
Lancaster, D L
Land, J M
Langdon, M L
Larsen, C H
Lau, L K S
Lavelle, C
Law, C M
Ledermann, S E
Lee, M J T
Lee, P J
Lees, A J
Leiper, A D
Levinsky, R J
Levitt, G A
Libri, V
Liesner, R J
Lim, D P
Limaye, S V
Limousin, P
Linch, D C
Lindley, K J
Lloyd-Thomas, A R
Lob-Levyt, J P
Lockwood, D N J
Loke, M Y
Lomas, D E
Losseff, N A
Loudon, D R
Lucas, D J
Lund, V J
Lutman, D H
Luxon, L M
Mabey, D C W
Macallister, R J
MacArdle, B M
McCarthy, M J
McElhinney, J M
McEvoy, A W
McGregor, R M V
Machin, S J
McHugh, K
Mackay, J
McKee, C M
McKeigue, P M
McKintosh, E
McManus, I C
McMichael, A J
McNeilly, R A
Macpherson, M M
Mahoney, P F
Maini, M
Malone, M M T
Mansour, M R
Mantoudis, E
Marcovitch, H
Marks, S D
Marmot, M G
Marnane, C N
Martin, J F
Maskey, S P C
Meade, T W
Meeks, M G
Mehta, A K
Mellado Calvo, N
Mercey, D E
Merry, R T G
Michaels, L
Michalski, A J
Milla, P J
Millar, M R
Miller, R F
Miotti, A M
Miotti, F A
Misra, V P E
Miszkiel, K A
Mitchell, H S
Moghissi, A J
Mok, Q Q
Montgomery, H E
Morris, J N
Moss, F M
Mould, T A J
Mundy, P G
Murray, N M F
Naftalin, A P
Naim, T
Nandi, P R
Naoumov, N V
Nathanson, V H
Nazroo, J Y
Neville, B G R
Newman, L
Newton, M C
Ng, C Y
Nicholls, D E
Nischal, K K
Noah, N D
Norman, P M
Novelli, M R
Novelli, V
Nyiri, P J
O'Brien, P A
O'Donoghue, B M
O'Flynn, P E
O'Higgins, P
O'Riordan, S P
Obasi, A I N C
Okonkwo, O O
Omara-Boto, T C A
Paice, E W
Pal, D K
Palaniappan, R
Pandya, P
Parkinson, M C
Patel, A
Patterson, K G
Peckham, C S
Peckham, M J
Pembrey, M E
Pereira, S P
Petros, A J
Petzold, A
Pierro, A
Pigott, N B
Pillaye, J
Pitt, M C
Plant, G T
Playford, E D
Pollock, A M
Porter, J C
Porter, S R
Powell, M P
Prichard, B N C
Pritchard, J
Quinn, N P
Raglan, E M
Rahi, J S
Rahman, S
Raine, R A
Rajput, K M
Ramsay, A D
Redington, A N
Rees, G E
Rees, J H
Rees, L
Rees, P G
Reinhardt, A K
Revesz, T
Richens, J E
Rieberer, G C
Risdon, R A
Roberts, A J
Roberts, I G
Robinson, A J
Rodeck, C H
Ron, M A
Ross, D A
Rossdale, M R
Rosser, E M
Rossor, M N
Roughneen, P T M
Rubin, J R
Rudge, P
Russell-Eggitt, I M
Ryan, J M
Samaratunga, R D
Sander, J W
Sarasola Lopetegui, J A
Sargent, J C
Saridogan, E
Scadding, G K
Scadding, J W
Scaravilli, F
Scher, H
Schindler, M B
Schott, G D
Scott, R J
Scully, C M
Segal, A W
Segal, T Y
Sethi, D
Shaida, A M
Shekerdemian, L S
Shorvon, S D
Shulman, C E
Singh, D
Singh, M B
Sirimanna, K S
Sisodiya, S M
Skolar, P J
Skuse, D H
Smith, M
Smith, S J M
Solanki, G A
Solomon, S M E
Somerville, F
Spitz, L
Spoulou, V
Stanhope, R G
Stanton, A J
Stark, J
Steer, J A
Stephenson, J M
Stevenson, V L
Stewart, G W
Stirling, L C
Sumner, E
Surtees, R A H
Sury, M R J
Swanwick, T
Tatman, M A
Taylor, J F N
Thom, M H
Thomas, D G T
Thomas, J A
Thomas, M L
Thomas, P K
Thompsett, C
Thompson, A J
Thompson, D N P
Thompson, E J
Thrasher, A J
Tinker, A
Tomkins, A M
Tonks, A M
Trimble, M R
Trompeter, R S
Tsam, L
Upton, K M
Urch, C E
Vadgama, B
Vallance-Owen, A J
Van Doorn, C A M
Van Paesschen, W
Van'T Hoff, W G
Vaughan, J P
Vaz Pato, M
Vellodi, A
Veys, P A
Wadley, J P
Wagg, A S
Walker, I A
Walker, J M
Wallis, C E
Walmsley, K M
Ward, A A
Warren, V J
Watkins, L D
Webb, D K H
Webber, R H
Wei, T C M
Werring, D J
Westcott, G F
Wharton, B A
White, S R
Whitehead, B F
Whiteman, J R
Wilkins, A
Wilkinson, P D
Williams, I G
Williams, J O H
Williams, R
Wilson, A P R
Wilson, L C
Wilson, S R
Winyard, P J D
Wood, N W
Woods, S C P D
Woolf, A S
Wray, S L
Wright, A
Wright, S G
Wroe, S J
Wyatt, J C
Wyatt, J S
Wynne-Roberts, C R S M
Yarranton, H

WC2

Aitken, J
Basu, D B
Bavetta, F
Bloom, M
Bolton, J P G
Byrne, M B
Carroll, S R
Chatamra, K
Debuse, M J
Ellis, P S
Ford, P M
Francis, T
Garner, J F
Goodge, A
Hale, A S
Henderson, M
Hilton, J A M
Jones, D S D
Jones, R H
Kelt, J D
Leng, G C
Marrs, T C
Milliken, T D A
Missen, G A K
Mitchell, J L
Ng, T T C
O'Mahony, M C
Okech, M
Ough, R W
Rady, N A
Ratnavel, R
Ross, E M
Sawney, P E
Sinnatamby, C S
Skinner, R K A M
Stidolph, P N
Szarewski, A M
Tacconelli, F
Thomas, R D
Tomlinson, I P M
Toy, J L
Warren, J B
Wedderburn, L R
Whitear, J R
Whitear, S-N
Wright, P H

Index by Town

Murdoch, H B
Murphy, C A
Murphy, E
Murray, A D
Murray, G
Murray, S
Mutch, W J
Needham, G
Newlands, W J
Newnham, D M
Nicholson, A P
Nicoll, K S
Nicolson, M C
O'Kelly, T J
Ogg, F L M
Ogston, K N
Olson, J A
Olson, S
Ormerod, A D
Orr, J D
Orr, M J
Owen, J A
Page, J G
Palin, A N
Park, K G M
Parkin, D E
Parry Davies, M F
Patey, R E
Payne, S N L
Pearson, D W M
Pennington, T H
Perry, M S
Peterkin, G S D
Petrie, M C
Petty, R D
Philip, R A
Philip, W J U
Phull, E A
Phull, P S
Pirie, C M
Pitt, E S
Pratt, M A
Prime, A J
Primrose, W R
Provan, C D
Provan, J
Qadir, A
Quadhir, M J A
Qureshi, A M
Rait, D E
Rashid, M
Ratcliffe, M A
Ray, P K
Read, J R M
Rees, A J
Reid, A
Reid, C
Reid, D M
Reid, J A
Reid, J P
Reid, T M S
Reith, W
Renny, N M C
Renshaw, P R
Repper, J A
Rhind, G B
Rhodes, P M
Richards, D W L
Richardson, F M
Richardson, F
Richardson, J R
Riddell, R E
Ritchie, A M
Ritchie, C W
Robbie, R B
Roberts, S C
Robertson, C
Robertson, E A
Robertson, K
Robinson, A D T
Robinson, J G
Rodger, S J N
Ronald, A L
Ross, A M
Ross, A M
Ross, E T
Ross, I S
Ross, J A S
Rossi, M K
Rowlands, A B
Russell, G
Samuel, L M
Sarwar, M I M
Scotland, J J
Scotland, T R
Scott, C J
Scott, J
Scott, S T
Seddon, R
Seymour, D G
Seymour, R M
Shand, L M
Shanks, M F
Shearer, A F
Shepherd, G A A
Shirreffs, M J
Shirriffs, G G
Short, D S
Sim, A J W
Simpson, J G
Simpson, S A
Simpson, T W
Simpson, W G
Sinclair, C D
Sinclair, P
Smail, P J
Smart, A R T I
Smart, L M
Smith, A P M
Smith, B H
Smith, C C
Smith, F W
Smith, G
Smith, H
Smith, H P
Smith, I
Smith, M G
Smith, N
Smith, N C
Smith, W C S
Snape, P E
Soper, F R C
Spence, F M
Srivastava, P
St. Clair, D M
Stanbridge, J E
Stark, G P
Starr, K J
Stephen, G
Stephen, W T
Stephen, W S Y
Stephenson, R N
Stewart, C
Stewart, M
Stewart, R J G
Steyn, J H
Stockdale, E J N
Stott, S A
Strachan, F M
Strachan, L M
Strachan, P A
Sulaivany, T-I A
Sutherland, A G
Sutherland, B
Sutherland, J G
Sutherland, L M
Swami, K S
Taylor, A J
Taylor, F A
Taylor, R J
Taylor, V E
Taylor, W E
Telfer, J M
Templeton, A
Terris, M
Terry, P B
Thomas, A D
Thompson, A J
Thompson, C A
Thompson, W D
Thomson, A R
Thomson, J S
Thorpe, A P
Tou, S I H
Treliving, L R
Trotter, P M
Turnbull, P J
Turner, A R
Tuttle, S
Valentine, M J
Vickers, M A
Walker, F
Walker, S A
Wallace, E D
Wallace, J D
Wallage, S
Wallis, J F E M
Walshe, E T
Warrender, T
Warrington, J
Watson, A J M
Watson, H G
Watson, M S
Watson, W A
Watt, M J
Watt, R M J
Waugh, N R
Wearden, D J
Webster, J
Webster, J
Wedderburn, S
Weir, J
Weissen, P R
Weston, A N
Whalley, L J
White, J C
White, M I
White, M
Wilkinson, A T
Wilkinson, S P
Williamson, K M
Wilson, G E
Wilson, J G
Wilson, S J
Wintour, D I
Wisely, I C F
Wood, F T
Wright, M E
Yates, P
Young, A M
Young, H A
Young, M J
Youngson, G G

Aberdovey
Davies, T T
Sayes, R M

Aberfeldy
Cox, V A
Dougall, H T
McBride, H M
Pitchforth, A E
Riddell, D I
Wheater, R A
Wright, D S
Wright, H M

Abergavenny
Abdel-Massih, R S
Alfaro Garcia, G M
Babiker, S E D M
Balboa, S
Barton, H W
Beard, H
Bhatia, A G
Birdi, P K
Blackett, R L
Borg, A
Bowden, B G
Bracchi, A L C A M
Bracchi, R C G
Burrows, D J
Carbarns, N J B
Cave, W P
Clements, J M M
Concha, E M
Cross, N C
Das, I
Davies, A B
Davies, D L
Davies, H G
Davies, P L
Dawson, A J
Dawson, K
Dawson, L K
Dennis, C A
Edwards, G J
Edwards, M
Edwards, P W
El-Serafy, N I
Evans, E C
Everest, M P
Falkner, J D
Fone, D L
Frazer, A C
Ghosh, S
Gibbon, G J
Gruffudd-Jones, D M
Habboush, H W
Haboubi, N Y A
Hargest, R
Harrell, M E
Harrell, R
Heneghan, C P H
Hosen, S C
Howell, S
Hulme, C E
Hutchison, S J R
Jenkins, N H
Jennings, J S R
Jones, I E
Jones, I G
Keely, G M J
Kellett, R J
Kerr, M P
Khanna, PB
Killeen, N C J
Kocan, M K
Lavis, M S
Lawson, J M
Lewis, R M L
Linton, S M
Maddocks, J
Mahmood, A
Martin, M J
Meredith, A S
Morris, M B
Nalini, V
Natarajan, D
Nathdwarawala, Y R
Neville, P M
Parker, A
Parker, T F J
Pickford, R B
Plumb, J M
Poddar, S
Proctor, E
Queen, K B
Reed, D H
Reynolds, J H
Rich, D A
Richard, B L
Robins, G
Robinson, G T M
Rolfe, A B
Rolfe, S E
Ruth, P M
Saafan, A A M
Sampson, S R M
Saunders, J
Sinha, A
Skea, G K
Srinivasan, K
Staples, V J
Stewart, B R
Stokes, I M
Stucke, S K
Taylor, D C
Thomas, J
Walker, R W
Warren, S W
Weekes, C A
Weeks, R A
Wheatley, R J
Williams, R M
Williams, T H C

Abergele
Charles, T J
Clarkson, N C
Davies, H O
Dromey, J F
Edge, J M
Edwards, S G
Garnett, A G G
Honeybun, J J
Innes, H E
Jamil, A
McCormack, J G
Smith, I C E
Srinivasan, J
Stockport, J C

Aberlour
Bonnyman, S D
Cammack, A E
Dennis, T
Ellis, S J
Green, H M
Johnston, N M
McDowall, D J
Miller, D J
Purdie, N L

Abertillery
Clatworthy, M R
Dexter, C G
Hossain, N A
Hossain, S A
Narang, S K
Neville, K F
Roy, C H
Thornton, A J
Venn, C S
Venn, S J

Aberystwyth
Atrah, H I A R
Awad, S A M M
Axford, A T
Bonsu, A K
Boswell, G V
Brookes, J-P C M
Burroughes, A M
Colbourn, C
Collingborn, B M
Cornah, P R
Cunningham, D A
Davies, A G
Davies, E J
Davies, G S
Edwards, R B L
Evans, A
Evans, R
Evans, R A
Gerrard, F E
Godfrey-Glynn, P M N
Haddad, S K
Henderson, R M
Hosker, I T
Humphreys, S W
Jackson, D S
Jones, J A
Jones, P D
Khan, A M
Lloyd, H S
Lord, M G
Lotfi, G
Manning, N A
Meredith, A D
Mishra, K P
Morgan, G W
Morus, L C
Muller, R K G
Myles, R W
Narain, M A
Nicholls, H
Price, M A
Rhys, A
Roberts, R S C
Sahni, K
Saleh, A J
Shanmugalingam, S
Slade, K
Smart, F A
Thomas, B I E
Thomas, M
Walters, D D
Williams, J A
Williams, J L
Williams, J W
Williams, S C
Williams, W

Abingdon
Adams, L R
Allan, E A
Auckland, C R
Bell, N J
Beynon, G W
Bryant, J E
Casson, R T
Cave, R J S
Chipperfield, A
Cox, V A
Crossley, N R
Davis, C J F
Dixon, A D
Duffield, J E
Dugdale-Debney, F W
Dyson, E D
Edge, C J
Elwig, N H
Evans, R F
Gibson, C E
Govier, K L
Graves-Stanwick, T R
Hampson, S C
Hart, M H
Hodgson, D C
Hodgson, H J
Hughes, M
Keeling, A L
King, S J
Lambert, B G
Lapwood, S G
Lea, J R
Lynch-Blosse, R H
McMichael, C F
May, D R
Midwinter, K I
Moore, J N B
Moyses, C
Murray, J L
Nowell, T E
Ogg, C S
Otterburn, D M
Parsons, S J
Pathinayake, B D A C
Pedrazzini, S-L
Pembridge, B T
Phillips, D J
Pinches, R S
Pope, M H M
Reynolds, T D R
Robertson, P M
Rockett, M P
Safranek, P M
Schulte, A C
Shepperd, R A
Smeulders, N
Sperry, L M
Stein, F C
Strugnell, M J
Studholme, K M
Tan, P S T
Tate, P H L
Thorne, A
Thorne, R J T
Tilley, J A
Verjee, S A K S
Westwood, L K

Aboyne
Dawson, H
Dunbar, C M
Glass, J
McCance, K J
Robertson, J L
Scott, J K
Starritt, D R
Taylor, J L
Taylor, M B

Accrington
Batra, G S
Bhat, G M
Brown, N
Cunningham, S L
Dixon, J H
Field, V K
Grady, A K
Gupta, R C
Gupta, S K
Hewitt, K M
Hipwell, M C
Joseph, P K
Kapenda, A Y
Karim, N
Karim, S I
Karim, S I-U
Kelly, A M
Krishna Murti, L
Manjooran, F
Manuel, A
Mills, S S
Ojha, R R
Quinn, P W
Seymour, L K
Smith, A C
Swana, A S
Wallworth, R A
Ward, C A
Westwood, G R
Woodcock, D R

Acharacle
Buchanan, M E

Achnasheen
Arnold, P A

Addlestone
Carter, S E
De Netto, M-A K
Denison, D M
Gargan, R E
Godrich, J E
Grob, P R
Harvey, P R
Zurick, N J

Airdrie
Ahmed, A
Alagar, S P
Angus, M M M
Atkinson, J
Beshr, A S M S
Bodane, A K
Brough, G D
Butt, A J M
Cargo, P E
Carlin, G F
Cassie, R
Cook, R J
Crawford, J G
Curle, J M
Darroch, J N
Dobbie, C M
Douglas, W S
Dunn, B P
Dutta, K
Evans, C D

Gardiner, D S
Gibb, F D M
Gopinathan, V
Gray, H G M
Gupta, G
Guse, J V
Halliday, J
Hamilton, A S S
Hammersley, N
Handa, J L
Harrower, A D B
Howatson, S R
Hughes, K
Imrie, J E A
Inglis, M D
Innes, D T
Jardine, S L
Jarvie, F E
Johnston, A
Johnston, S A
Johnstone, P A
Kennedy, N
Laird, B J A
Lees, C T W
Lough, J R M
Lwanda, J L
McAlpine, L G
McAvoy, N C
MacDonald, A
MacInnes, A N
McIntyre, J E
McIntyre, J M
Mackenzie, R E
McKerlie, L C
McKillop, H T
McLaren, I
McLaughlin, M-J
McPhail, N J
Maculloch, S M
Mathew, G
Matthews, D M
Milligan, J
Mills, E E
Mitchell, K M
Monaghan, M T
Murphy, D S
Murphy, J A
Paterson, P
Paulus, U
Pollock, E E
Pollock, J M M
Prach, A T
Reid, V T
Roberts, J E
Ross, C S K
Ross, P M D
Schultz, S S
Scullion, W
Shilliday, I R
Siddiqui, M F
Siddiqui, M F
Strong, A M M
Sugden, C J
Teo, N B
Thompson, J
Todd, W T A
Wainwright, N J
Walker, D
Walker, L
Wallers, K J
Watson, W H
Watt, M
Weerackody, R P
Wilson, K E
Zahangir, M
Zuk, R J

Alcester
Armitage, J P
Bexfield, S M
Bulchand, R
Chaffey, R F
Dencer, D
Embley, C
Haden, R M
Harman, S A
Hutchinson, P J
Nava, P L
Neville, T P
Popplewell, J A
Popplewell, M
PremcHand, V B
Singh, M B
Singh, P D

Aldeburgh
Ball, S C
Barrick, D N
Boswell, A M
McGough, J G
Simmonds, S-J
Standley, T D A

Alderley Edge
Chaudry, I H
Clough, P H
Davidson, J
Gardiner, J S
Gibson, J M
Hall, H E
Hammonds, G
Hammonds, R M
Hirst, G C
Macdonald, D J H
Merchant, S D
Mohindra, S
Moore, P E
Newton, E R
Sambrook, P
Taylor, J A
Thompson, H E
Walton, G M
Williams, J P
Williams, R J

Alderney
Fegan, W G
Mark, J F
Seymour, R N

Aldershot
Anderson, D R
Bartlett, S G A
Brigg, P D
Brooks, C E
Brown, W
Davis, L C
Ebrahim, N
Fahmy, M
Gamble, D S C
Gonçalves-Archer, H C
Gruebel Lee, D M
Head, J E
Hilditch, J
Innes, A C
Kingston, F R A
Lansley, P H
Law, K V
Leopold, C A
MacLeod, M D
O'Callaghan, S E
Pallant, J M
Paterson, R A
Pearson, C A
Riggs, M
Robertson, B
Romaya, B F
Scantlebury, B
Scott, M J
Shalley, M J
Shaw, A J
Sherwood, K E
Stewart, T D S
Whatmough, P M
Whitby-Smith, B J
Wictome, J
Wynn, N N

Alexandria
Al-Khafaji, M N M
Barber, T S
Baxter, A D
Cameron, A E
Campbell, P M
Carmichael, H A
Clark, D P
Clarke, I S
Cox, H
Douglas, G A
Dunn, J A
Dunn, S
Easy, W R
Fabling, M
Flett, S R
Forbes, F
Guthrie, C E
Harper, A S
Hassan, K
Haxton, M J
Herd, G W
Hunter, C A P
Johnson, G
Kenyon, N J
McClure, I M
McCruden, D C
McGlinchey, I
Mackay, N S D
McLachlan, K R
MacRae, M M
Maiden, N L
Mamdani, G H
Manning, N T
Murray, E L
Nassar, A H M
Peacock, J E M
Robertson, E W
Sajid, M
Scullion, M
Series, J J
Shand, J M
Shouler, P J
Sievert, J
Simpson, M P
Towlson, K L
Trust, P M
Tully, A M

Alford, Lincolnshire
Carter, I M
Carter, S
Charlton, K
Ferguson, D W
Spenceley, K R
Woollard, A E

Alfreton
Bingham, M S
Blyth, J M
Broderick, M M
Burstow, A C
Cooper, R E
Duffield, M W
Gruffydd, D R
Gundkalli, A A
Gundkalli, I
Hill, J P
Hills, E S
Holland, D D
Holloway, R
Holtham-Taylor, D A
Jones, T L
Kelman, M B
Lawrence, R A A R
McKay, N P
Meakin, A H
Needham, H M
Noronha, M D
Parkin, T
Pryce, J C
Richmond, G A
Skidmore, J R
Sowerby, H A
Taylor, D W
Tippetts, R
Tipping, P J
Veale, M J

Alloa
Borland, D S
Collins, I P
Dullea, B C A
Green, F R
Greig, J E W
Hood, G J
Kirk, D P
Macgregor, J
MacInnes, P
Patrick, A G
Proctor, S J R
Rasul, S
Sime, L A
Stirling, K W
Walters, W D
Ward, A L
Webster, R W J

Alness
Baxter, P N
Hutton, J F
Jackson, J D
Kelly, S J

Alnwick
Bridge, A J
Brown, C R
Brown, R C A
Davison, D C
Dodd, M J
Dodd, S J
Embleton-Black, C C
Fortune, W A
Fraser, G S
Fraser, J C
Guy, M J
Lishman, S H
McKenna, A M
McKenna, K
Mitford, E
Renner, S L
Robertson, E
Smith, M
Stevenson, C J

Alresford
Baker, W J
Cassidy, S J
Clark, M J
Cribb, R A
Crosse, S M
Fairley, C J
Green, D H
Green, D J
Hall, Z M
Happel, S M
Hill, D M
Isbister, A R
Lowman, A C
Masters, A J
Read, J M
Sandison, A L
Sargent, P M
Seaburne-May, M P
Stebbing, J E
Stokes, P J
Sword, L J
Tanner, S J

Alston
Dawson, M J

Alton
Amery, A H
Bethell, H J N
Burch, P
Collins, C L
De Quincey, M M
Fletcher, V J
Hall, M J
Hamilton, J M I
Hayward, M G
Hopwood, P N
Isaac, P W
Jones, N A
Kelly, L F
Louden, S F
Macnamara, M
Myers, S F
Nonhebel, A C
Over, J M
Rickard, A J
Stubbington, H L
Sword, A J
Terry, K J
Wassef, M A-E
Watters, S R
West, P
White, N J
Willis, J A R
Wozniak, T

Altrincham
Adams, M E
Al-Khaffaf, H S
Al-Safar, J A
Aldean, I M A
Ali, A K M
Allred, J P
Awan, S K
Bailey, P J
Beardsmore, J D
Bee, P
Belloso Uceda, A
Bhatt, A M
Bhatt, M K
Biswas, S
Bowman, R A
Bromley, E J T
Brooks, R D
Brown, I C
Brown, J D K
Buck, P
Burke, D M
Burns, J
Butler, J D
Cameron, P M
Caplan, B
Carroll, K B
Cave, S B
Chan, K T
Cheah, T-S
Cheyne, E H L
Cheyne, L R P L
Chung, A S
Conboy, A O
Condliffe, H A
Davies, C J
Davitt, M C
Davy, R A
De Lacy, S E
Desai, S C
Dover, B
Drabu, G J
Duthie, V J
Edwards, P D
El-Kafrawy, U
Elliott, C E
Estcourt, T
Fitzgerald, C H
Fitzgerald, J J
Frank, T L
Freeman, L B
Furrows, D C
Furrows, S J
Ghaneh, P
Gowrisunkur, J S
Gratwick, L C
Greenwood, B K
Gregory, M W
Hallas, S F
Halpern, I B
Haslam, P G
Haslett, R S
Haslett, R C
Herrington, L M
Heywood, M W
Hilton, R M
Holmes, P
Hoosen, Y
Huddlestone, L
Iglesias Alvarez, M
Ingram, J C
Jackson, A
Jacovelli, J B
Jellinek, D C
Jenkins, S
Johnson, T W
Jolley, S P
Jones, P E
Kelly, J
Kelman, C G
Kiel, J E
King, A T
Klass, H J
Klein, L E
Krysiak, P
Kuna, P
Ladha, S S
Laha, S
Laitt, R D
Landes, C J
Lee, K G
Leech, G
Leggate, J R S
Lennie, M E
Lieberman, I
Lloyd, M J
Lord, N P
Macdonald, B N
McKinnon, K A
Mackrodt, K M
McNab Jones, S E
Mahmood, N
Manns, J J
Marsden, A R
Marshall, B E
Martin, C P
Maybury, H J
Menon, S
Mitchell, G G
Moyo, C
Mrozinski, R A
Myatt, T S
Naik, C S
Newson, L R
Nicholson, D A
Norman, S A
Norris, K J
O'Driscoll, D P
Parks, R J
Patel, M
Pathak, P N
Pearson, D J
Pearson, D
Pengelly, C D R
Phillips, G
Pumphrey, J H
Qureshi, N S
Rahmanou, P
Remington, S A M
Reynolds, S M
Richardson, M J
Rickman, A J
Rimmer, S
Robinson, S P
Roland, J
Rothera, M P
Rowland, G F
Ryley, H E
Saleh, R
Santaniello-Newton, A
Scarsbrook, A F
Shamas-Ud-Din, S
Shaw, J
Shekelton, F A
Sheridan, A J
Shipston, A M
Shipston, J E
Sieff, I
Singh, I P
Smith, B G
Smith, S
Smith, V L
Sommerfield, A J
Southworth, S A
Sutherland, H C
SymcOx, H A
Taylor, A E
Thompson, A M S
Tighe, N J
Tolhurst-Cleaver, C L
Toon, C G E
Trask, M D
Trehan, A
Tytler, J A
Vasa, S A
Vincent, J A
Weighill, P A
Wells, S L A
West, S L
Westwood, C
Wilkins, G S
Will, S C C
Williamson, J C
Woodhead, R J
Woodhead, Z M
Wooldridge, W J
Wooster, S L
Wykes, P R
Wynn, J S

Alva
Abel, G A
Byrne, A J
Clark, J M
Collier, F
Crocket, A
Hay, G I
Hurry, R A
Johnston, F I
Musk, D C

Ambleside
Birket, I J
Bishop, E S
Blackburn, J C
Crossley, D R
Davies, P J
Davis, L R
Earnshaw, D H
Forrester, M B T
Harris, M T M
Jackson, A H
Lawrence, V J
Mathieson, A E T
O'Connell, G
Rimington, J E
Robson, M
Smith, R I
Stanley, J R
Warburton, R A

Amersham
Barnes, R J
Batten, C
Bennett, N J
Brown, A J
Buchanan, G E
Burgess, J M
Burne, B H
Carter, P A
Carter, V L
Cheema, S
Coady, A T
Couch, A L
Curling, O M
Davies, C J W
Davies, D L
Dellow, A C
Enright, S M
Ferguson, D M
Ferraro, A J
Fieldsend, R C
Foote, A A
Forti, A D

George, S A
Gibbs, A E R
Gough, D
Hall, M L
Helps, E P W
Hynes, K A
Jenner, P N
Kanga, S B
Kilgour, J L
Lamont, R F
Laube, S
Lilley, C S
Mace, A D
Morris, E H
Nash, C J
Neal, B L
Orton, D I
Palfreman, T M
Palmer, P A
Pienaar, G F
Sapsford, R A
Sharma, R
Skinner, D V
Slater, A J
Stevens, R J
Summers, L A
Sunderland, R
Thompson, S G
Thorne, S J
Vesely, M J J
Wayte, J A
Weaver, A E
Whittaker, C A
Wilkinson, J D
Wiseman, A
Wood, A

Amlwch
Austin, B N
Griffith, B A
Jones, S T
King, A H
Owen, J P
Thomas, A

Ammanford
Bizby, L J
Capper, W M
Coombe, A D
Edwards, A L
Evans, D A
Griffiths, J S
Griffiths, M J
Jones, G J
Jones, S
Mason, B W
Morris, H D
Morris, P
Murfin, D E
Powell, F I
Rahman, K M
Rowlands, H W D
Salisbury, R D
Smith, D E
Thomas, G
Watkin, A R
Williams, D M
Yeates, C E

Andover
Allan, M J
Armstrong, A J M
Batham, D R
Bond, S
Bowden, T
Bruford, M K
Bryan, T A
Carr, S A
Collins, P A
Cook, A E
Daley, S E
Davies, L A L
Davies, T M
Gailey, D A H
Greig, A D
Griffiths, R J
Harries-Brown, R A
Hickey, S
Hobhouse, S L
Hoole, M
Humphreys, M F
Irwin, W J
Islam, A M
Jackman, J S G
James, T R
Johnston, D
Lambert, R
Lockwood, M J
Loudon, G M
Mann, J N
Matheson, R M
Needham, V H
O'Halloran, P D
Pawley, A F
Perry, I C
Porter, G D
Potter, A R
Rossiter, M A
Shields, R S D
Stone, M
Verity, J C T
Walker, A M
Wallis, C J
Wells, R D W
Wessely, T L
Wilkins, C J
Willson, H J

Anglesey
Roberts, E L
Thomas, G D

Annan
Abd Karim, Z
Baillie, N A
Byers, D L
Coyle, C J
Kelly, N G
Kerr, J S
Kieran, W J G
Lapka, B A
McCallum, E M
Maggiori, T K
Millar, S
Ocansey, J A
Paul, D H
Ross, S D

Anstruther
Brunton, C
Bumbra, L A
Francis, C P
Kyle, A W
McGonigal, J A
Marston, D J W
Mitchell, A V
Ross, P W
Tarvet, F

Antrim
Alderdice, J M
Ashe, R G
Bali, I M
Bill, A
Bittar, W
Black, I H C
Brady, S T
Browne, R J
Carson, J G
Critchlow, S G
Crossan, I
Currie, R E S
Cusick, P B
Daly, J G
Delap, T G
Dripps, K
Duff, Y R
Elliott, T P
Ferguson, J A J
Ford, B N
Galway, J P
Gamble, W
Garstin, W I H
Gregg, W V H
Harbinson, M T
Henry, G
Hogg, W
Howard, P B
Humphreys, W G
Hunter, P
Hutchinson, W D
Jenkins, J G
Kapur, D K
Kearney, M P
Kelly, C B
Kenny, B D
Kyle, E A
Leyden, P E F
Lim Hoe Kee, J
McAloon, J
McBrien, M E
McCabe, R E
McCartney, K N
McCaughey, M
McClelland, C J
McCloskey, M
McGinnity, M G A
McIlroy, G H C
McIlwee, C A
McKeown, P P J
McLarnon, J F
McMillen, R M
McMurray, A H
MacPherson, J E
Mannion, M F
Marriott, C M
Millar, J R
Moss, J E
Nelson, H F J
Nelson, W M
Nicholson, J
O'Gorman, C J
O'Loan, M D
Rainey, D S
Ritchie, W A H
Robb, J J
Stewart, E C A
Todd, G R G
Toner, G G
Trouton, T G
Turk, G N
Turner, M D
Watson, M R
Whiteside, M C R

Appin
McNicol, D
McNicol, I D
Mathieson, D A M

Appleby-in-Westmorland
Box, B
Gill, C R
Leitch, J B
Sharpe, G F
Sharpe, K T

Arbroath
Acheson, A J
Anderson, C J B
Bird, S P G
Boyd, E J S
Cherry, J S
Gray, M W
Hornsby, A H
Inglis, J D A
Kolhatkar, L M
Langlands, J M
Ledson, M A
McKay, C M
Moffat, G L
Muir, G L
Noltie, A C K
Ogilvie, J R
Reid, P J
Smith, W R
Speirs, R B
Sutherland, G M
Taylor, H M
Walker, R J
Ward, A E
Weir, I G C

Ardgay
Carbarns, S A
Crabb, G R
Hamblet, K M
Lumsden, W
Macdonald, P M
Mair, C J
Mair, J M

Ardrossan
Clark, P
Haggerty, G
Johnstone, C P
Merry, A J
Raghavendra, K
Weetman, M G
Weir, G
Whyte, M D R
Wight, A M

Arisaig
Young, S A

Armagh
Allen, J M
Anderson, R
Beckett, E P
Bergin, S P
Canning, U B
Carlile, R M
Cartmill, J L
Cassidy, C E
Colvin, P W B
Corrigan, D B
Dorman, D E
Dorman, R H
Douglas, K M J
Eames, M H A
Edwards, D J
Fearon, E D
Fee, P M
Fitzsimons, O
Gaffney, S S M
Garvin, C C
Gillespie, J F
Jones, M N R
Kellett, P S
Knipe, C W D
Leetch, R J
McAlinden, E S
McAlinden, P M
McBride, S J
McCahon, R A
McClung, J P
McCollum, W R K
McConnell, V P M
McConnell, W B
McConville, J P
McElnay, R E
McEvoy, M P C
McGuinness, J F
McMullan, J E
McNally, M S
Magee, T F
Marshall, K M
Marshall, N C
Mayne, D G
Millar, K J
Morgan, O M
Nicholson, G M
O'Hagan, A H
O'Hagan, F T
O'Reilly, G V
O'Reilly, R
Reaney, E A
Reilly, R P
Robinson, F L
Sam, G J
Smyth, A E
Steed, A J
Telford, A M
Tohani, V K
Turtle, A M
Walsh, J B
Whelan, L M
Wright, T P

Arrochar
Fettes, P H
Troup, D F

Arundel
Eve, R H
Farquhar-Thomson, D R
Foulkes, A
Gibbs, R G J
Jenkins, M E C
Larsen, T A
Levantine, A V
Mott, A N
Peters, D J
Pullan, D S B
Stenson, K
Thompson, K C

Ascot
Afzal, N
Akinsola, M
Al-Chalabi, T
Armstrong, P M C
Bevan, C A
Burgess, N D S
Craze, A L
Davies, R J
Deane, G
Denny, S
Drake, N B
Dyerson, K J
Fanning, A P
Ferrero, T M
Furness, R H S
Gall, R G
Gatha, D N
Grace, K L R
Green, B J
Gunther, H N C
Gunther, M H D
Harding, J W
Harkness, V I K
Hartstone, R E
Hussain, M A
Jones, G D
Khaksar, S J
Lansley, M J
Luck, C A
McDonald, D G
Moore, R K G
Natorff, B L
Norminton, D R H
Rawlinson, J R
Selvey, D M
Sexton, S A
Sheikh, N
Sherley-Dale, A C
Singer, G C
Smith, M J
Sodhi, R K
Spring, J E
Tasker, G D
Walker, D M
Warren, J B
Whitfield, P N
Wilson, G K
Wraight, W J
Yousif, A R S

Ashbourne
Ashworth, J M
Baines, D A
Bridge, M-L T
Dent, K S
Erskine, R J
Fenwick, H C
Fulford, R K
Gage, P R
Geary, R J
Ghadiali, H H
Ghadiali, H N
Hanson, R J
Harvey, J A
Henshall, T D
Joel, C E
Kirtley, P R
Macleod, I S C S
MacLeod, S M
Martin, S J
Mills, C A
Morley, W L
Ogley, R
Richardson, C M
Shepherd, S J
Tattersall, E P
Tomlinson, R C
Tothill, C L
Ward, D R
Wedgwood, J P

Ashby-de-la-Zouch
Addison, J
Clifton, C J
Davies, R A
Foulds, G E
Harrison, P L
Hoffman, J
Matthews, A R
Minhas, R S
Morgan, A J
Patel, S P
Randev, P
Randev, P K
Singh, M P
Spiegler, W J
Tailor, H
Woolgrove, C G

Ashford, Kent
Addison, R L
Al-Maarof, M S M
Al-Shaikh, B Z T
Bafadhel, Z A
Banks, J C
Bates, T
Bernhardt, J R C
Bradley, G W
Bull, P W
Bushnell, T G
Chance, P S G
Chianakwalam, C I
Chissell, S A
Choi, W H
Church, W E
Clark, J E
Coleman, J E
Colledge, R E J
Cooney, J A
Corfield, N S
Coulson, E A M
Cowley, C
Davies, C C A
Davies, J O
Divekar, A B
Dove, S J
Dunnet, W J S
Eggleden, J C
Fairley, J W
Farrell-Roberts, M G J
Freeston, U H
Frohnsdorff, K G E
Gardner, M C
Ghulam, S J
Greaves, B P
Green, C P
Griffiths, N J
Hamer, M S F
Harper, K J
Hensman, E R
Horn, N J
Horn, S H
Hossain, J
Husain, S M S
Insall, R L
Irvine, C
Kamalvand, K
Kazmi, S M A
Klim, E A
Lai, A K T
Lake, J
Lawson, C W
Learmont, J G
Levi, S R
Li, K C
Long, D R
Macdonald, A M
Mackey, C J
Menon, R
Miller - Jones, C M H
Miller, I D C
Mirza, G H
Moffat, W J
Morris, A J R
Morris, J E
Munro, N A R
Nagesh Rao, G
Nuttall, J S
Paciorek, P M
Parker, S L
Phipps, M E
Porter, C A
Pragnell, A A
Price, C A
Ralfs, I G
Rampton, A J
Robinson, P S
Rowden, K W
Ryley, J P
Sands, M J
Seaton, J E V
Sewell, J R
Shah, V N
Shakir, S A W
Shrivastava, R K
Smith, O O
Smith, R A
Smithard, D G
Stossel, C A
Taffinder, N J
Thurrell, W P
Tolba, M A-A
Traill, C G
Ursell, W
Vella, M A
Vogel, M L
Waitt, R H F
Waller, R
Waluube, D D F
Webb, W M
Webster, D J
Wheeler, P C G
White, C P
Williams, C D
Williams, R E T
Williamson, S
Yaakub, R
Yanni, O N
Yardy, N D

Ashford, Middlesex
Adams, A J
Alvi, S A
Aweid, A M S
Bailey, B M W
Balakrishnan, P H
Bellamy, E A
Belstead, S M
Bond, H R
Bramble, B
Dalton, R
Das, A
Dawson, J C

El Ashouri, A R
Ellis, B W
Garner, A
Grossmith, C M
Horner, J
Irani, M S
Kandela, P
Keenan, C E S
Khan, S
Kirk, N R
Kulkarni, R P
Matthew, J
Meekings, E L
Moore, R G W
Newberry, D J
Paul, L
Reiff, D B
Roushdi, H R I M
Sandrasagra, A J R
Sidhu, D S
Skeldon, I
Surtees, H F A
Wilkinson, P R
Zammit, V

Ashington
Amin, S M
Bagott, M J
Beattie, W H
Bell, A D
Bradburn, D M
Carr, M
Cleverley, S J
Conn, A G
Cox, J G C
Crook, P R
D'Souza, R C M
Daniel, C
Derrick, S-A
Dewar, M S
Fraser, G B
Geoghegan, A T
Gilfillan, L J
Gregory, W L
Hatch, T
Higham, P D
Hobbs, J J
Hodgson, J
Innes, A R
Jones, S M G
Lambourn, R J
Lauckner, D I
Laurenson, J A
Lavin, T A
Leitch, J M
McCubbin, A T G
Milne, R K
Neilly, I J
Parkins, D R J
Partington, P F
Plummer, C J
Rasoul, M S
Rennison, C M
Richardson, D A
Roberts, A E
Rushmer, R J
Sellers, J
Senarath Yapa, R S
Sill, P R
Smith, D A
Willoughby, C M
Wotherspoon, W C

Ashtead
Anderson, A M
Boardley, A C
Cobb, A G
Eldridge, S B J
Evans, G M
Hartnoll, G
Inglis, M S
Jones, H W
Lewis, C K
Litman, C L
Lowes, J J
MacTavish, S D
Mavrikios, A
Papadopoulos, A J
Poundall, C E
Robb, G H
Soden, K A
Stephenson, J R
Taylor, E J S
Taylor, R S
Williams, M K
Williams, S D
Wood, J M D

Ashton-under-Lyne
Allan, G
Basnayake, P
Baynes, D B P
Bhachu, H S
Biswas, B
Biswas, C
Boyes, B E
Brammah, T B
Burke, D K
Campbell, C H
Chand, K
Chopra, M P
Clothier, P R
Coates, M
Coote, J H
Creedon, R J
Creighton, F J
Dalal, N
Davies, B C
Dixon, G R
Dunningham, T H
Ebizie, A O
Edge, A N
El Safadi, N
Ellenbogen, S
Freeman, J S
Gandhi, S D
Greenhough, C M
Haque, M E N
Hesten, F J
Husaini, M H
Hutton, A J
Idrees, F
Ilyas, M
Iserloh, H J
Jenkins, L K
Jolobe, O M P
Jude, E B
Kokiet, S J
Kushlick, A
MacCowan, J S R
McDade, G
Massarano, A A
Mistry, K
Munro, D I
Needham, E
Obeid, E M H
Oliver, F
Parham, A L
Parry, E J
Patel, G R
Pena, M A
Porter, S W
Rajendram, S
Rakicka, H
Rhodes, R J
Rubner, J V
Sadik, S M
Shaw, C M
Shoo, E E
Siddiqui, K H
Simpson, J
Smith, P A
Sridhar, J
Stagg, M J
Telfer, I
Tewari, S K
Theophilopoulos, N
Tiwari, K
Unsworth, P F
Wan Ho Hee, H
Watson, A J S
Wells, P A
Whatley, G C A
Williamson, A H M

Askam-in-Furness
Barker, J M
Jain, P R
Lewis-Jain, M

Atherstone
Alam, S Z
Bone, A M
Chant, B W
Chapman, K M
Cheetham, A M
Clemons, M J
Gooding, T N
Hull, J M
Thomson, A S
Weston, D A
Winward, J M

Attleborough
Byrne, H A
Craig, J P
Croot, G M

Howard-Alpe, G M
Leach, B M
Lindner, R H
Main, T J
Martin, A A
Martin, H M
Oxley, C F S
Scase, A E
Thornton, R J

Auchterarder
Burnett, J P
Carter, S J
Crease, G A G
Dickson, J D
Grant, J A
Laird, J C
MacLarty, H J
McLeay, G F
Morton, C A
Paterson, R W
Robertson, A J
Stevenson, P
Watson, A S
Wilson, J W
Wylie, S

Augher
Bingham, M T
Clarke, R C N

Aughnacloy
McCord, W D G

Aviemore
Berkeley, M I K
Checkley, B H B
Garraway, W M
Irvine, G E
Jachacy, G B
Langran, M
MacNeill, A
Patterson, A C
Stewart, K M

Avoch
Anderson, E M
Leslie, S J
Todd, A W

Axbridge
Friend, J P D
Frost, S M
King, R
Nicholl, S

Axminster
Cobley, T D D
Dixon, S M
Evans, D N
Golding, C L
Hodges, S R
Hodges, Y M B
Taylor, P A
Taylor, P J R
Vann, J A

Aylesbury
Adams, J N
Adlard, P
Ahmed, N
Allanson, J
Ammar, M A W
Ashworth, M F
Attwood, A I
Baez Gandia, J A
Bakhshi, K N
Balfour, A J C
Banwell, P E
Baruch, J D R
Beck, G S
Beesley, H S
Benjamin, L
Betmouni, M K
Bhowmick, B
Black, H J
Blackwell, J N
Boakes, A J
Bodley, R N
Booth, A
Bowen, B M
Bransbury, A J
Brown, R S
Burwood, D F S
Butland, H J
Cameron, D F
Campbell, C D
Campling, C
Cann, K J

Chaubal, N D
Cheung, D S-H
Chung, T W H
Clare, T D
Clarke, J
Cloke, A
Collins, P
Coombes, S J
Cooper, S M
Cox, S N
Crabtree, J M
Curtis, M O
Danton, S J
Davis, R D
Derry, F
Desai, S N
Downey, W R H
Durkin, C J
Eagleton, H J
Edmonds, S E
Edwards, P J
Edwards, R S
Evans, B-J
Farouk, M O
Forman, C H
Frankel, H L
Gammon, A P J
Gardner, B P
Gillett, A P
Gordon, J F
Goy, J A
Graham, A
Graham, C T
Hannaford, K L
Haroon, M
Harries, W J L
Harris, N M
Hawken, W J
Henderson, N J
Heywood, A J
Holdich, S Y
Hollis, L J
Howcutt, M T
Ikpeme, O B
Isaac, J S
Jackson, G J
James, C B
Jamous, M A
Johnson, K L
Jones, T L
Karmali, J
Kennedy, N D
Kiff, P S
Kindell, C
King, B R H
Knight, A H
Lamb, C T
Leeper, R Q
Lindsay, M K M
Loosemore, M P
Mackenzie, J F
Mackenzie, J M
McLaskey, S
Mallik, S k
Marr, J
Marshall, J P
Mayers, M M
Melvin, C A
Mitchell, T D
Money-Kyrle, A R W
Moorman, C M
Moreton, P W
Muldoon, C G
Mulholland, M N C
Newton, E K
Ng, C H S
Noone, C
Norton, R C
Nuseibeh, I M
O'Driscoll, J C
O'Hea, A-M
Ochoa Grande, J
Packham, J C
Padel, A F
Panikkar, K K
Parge, F M E
Patterson, D M
Paul, M
Peacock, T G
Peberdy, R J
Plummer, R B
Powell, J A
Pyott, J J
Rainford, D J
RamcHandani, P G
Ratnavel, R C
Record, C
Reed, R A
Reid, M B

Renfrew, A C
Ribes Pastor, P
Richards, A M
Riley, D M
Rizzo-Naudi, J L
Roberts, A H N
Robertson, L J
Robinson, J G
Sadler, J C
Sale, J P
Sames, M P
Savage, P E
Schuman, A N
Scott, G A
Scott, M J L
Segui Real, B
Shaikh, G F
Shanmuganathan, K
Shanmuganathan, M
Sharif, R A M
Shepard, C L
Shield, M J
Smith, C M
Smith, C M
Smith, R G
Smith, R S
Smith, V M
Stott, D G
Stradling, H A
Stradling, P A
Subramaniam, K P
Sullivan, M E
Sutton, J C
Taylor, A R
Tewson, J
Theobald, A J
Thirlwall, M
Thiyagarajan, C A
Thomas, S M
Tinnion, S A
Trower, C S G
Tudway, A J C
Turner, M
Tweedie, J H
Tyler, M P H
Usherwood, M M
Vasi, V
Vogelzang, S A
Wakefield, M A
Walker, S R
Walters, A M
Ward, S J
Watson, A
Watt, A D
Webley, M
Weldon, M J
Whittington, J M
Williams, F C
Williams, G M
Williams, S J
Wilson, R B
Wood, P F
Wool, R J
Ziprin, A E

Aylesford
Baluch, S
Bergmann, M
Bowen, R L
Canavan, J S F
Cantor, T J
Charlesworth, W G
Chesover, D F
Cochrane-Dyet, C E
Forsythe, D T
Humphreys, S
Lissamore, J R
Rana, B S
Ridsdill Smith, R M
Sandifer, Q D
Shakespeare, K M
Swann, R I A

Ayr
Adamson, M W
Afzal, T
Al-Aummran, M E
Alcorn, N J
Alexander, R G
Ashcroft, J L
Bain, R
Balachandran, C
Barvaux, V
Bass, J C
Beattie, N G M
Begg, J A
Berry, I E
Blair, J M
Blair, M

Bowbeer, J
Brown, C J
Brown, H C
Bunting, R W
Carswell, T M
Clark, N M
Craig, A D
Craig, J A
Creaney, K L
Creaney, W J
De Mey, R D
Doherty, J
Douglas, R J
Dowell, R C
Downie, T J
Duncan, G
Duncan, M R
Dunne, B J
Ferguson, A E
Ferguson, J T
Flowerdew, J A
Forsyth, M T
Fraser, M H
Fraser, S
Gaikwad, G A
Gaskell, A
Gemmill, J D
Gibson, D H
Gibson, F M
Gilliland, S J
Glencross, J F
Gow, A C
Grant, E D M J
Grant, P K
Hannah, A C
Hardie, R A
Hartung, S H-J
Hendry, S W
Hodelet, N P
Hollins, G W
Holms, J S M
Huda, A S
Huda, Q
Huda, S S
Hunter, N J F
Hunter, T W
Jackson, R E
Jamdar, S
Jeffries, C A
Johnston, T G
Kennedy, A J C
Kerr, S P J
Kettlewell, S
Kothari, S H
Large, D F
Lawrie, J G
Lennox, B
Linden, D
Linton, C M
Logan, M C
Lumsden, A S
McCabe, C G
McCamily, J
McGee, T C
McHardy, J
Mackie, N F T
McMahon, R
McNally, P
McNally, S J
McNicol, I F
McTaggart, W A
McVeigh, G
Madden, A M
Maharajan, S V
Martin, S W
Meddings, R N
Meiklejohn, B H
Miller, J B
Morrison, A
Morrison, D M
Muir, R F
Muirhead, A G
Muirhead, C S M
Murdoch, J M
Murray, E L A
Murray, J G S
Murray, J L
Niblock, J L
O'Sullivan, B C
Park, K A
Paterson, F C
Paterson, G W H
Paul, J
Pieper, H
Potter, R S
Rae, P S
Reynolds, P M G
Rose, J D R
Russell, T V N

Ryan, D A
Salih, K M
Shah, P
Shearer, P E
Simpson, A C
Smellie, M K R
Sood, R K
Stevens, P G
Stewart, G
Swanson, F M
Taylor, D
Teenan, D W
Watson, J M
Watts, M I
White, A A J
Whymark, C H
Williamson, J
Wilson, C
Wilson, E C
Wong, M M
Woodburn, C
Wylie, P G

Bacup
Greenwood, J D
King, B
Sattar, N
Sharma, Y
Wilkinson, P A
Williams, K V
Williams, P

Badminton
Epps, H
Mitchelmore, A E

Bakewell
Ashton, M G
Bartlett, N C
Bendefy, I M
Birkinshaw, K L
Chadwick, M S
Cohen, A
Griffiths, J A
Harris, G C
Holloway, J
Lockhart, O A
Martys, C R
Newton, J C B
Pickard, R J
Savage, A C
Smith, G H
Stephenson, I
Stuart, O M
Williams, P D

Bala
Davies, R M
Jones-Evans, D H
Jones-Evans, R A
Jones, T
Lazarus, D H
Roberts, I E

Baldock
Cockburn, M K F
Dorrell, C E
Georgiou, G
Hall, H I
Hoffman, M G
Korgaonkar, S V
Macrae, I F
Masood, M R
Moynihan, F D
Nevison, J
Old, S E
Outhoff, K
Parkinson, H
Russell, S C J
Seymour, J E A
Thomas, M M
Trathen, B C
Wong, Y L A

Balerno
Beattie, C M M
Boddy, K
Dickson, M J
Fergusson, N S
Jackson, J E Z
Krauth, G A
Millar, C G
Preston, J E
Rae, S M
Ritchie, C A M
Williams, A J K

Ballachulish
McKenzie, J P M

Ballasalla
Blackman, A M
Hockings, J E
Scott, J A
Taggart, C C

Ballater
Cruickshank, D M
McLeod, E D J

Ballindalloch
Aldridge, O R V
Crowley, D J
Derounian, J N
Whyte, B

Ballycastle
Farnan, C A
Guzhar, A R
Hunter, A M
Killough, E A
McKinley, P M
McLister, M S
McNulty, O M C

Ballyclare
Baird, G V
Baird, H
Baird, S H
Bill, R H
Bill, S M E
Cameron, J D
Clarkson, I P
Craig, M
Crooks, G M
Dawson, C A
Doherty, J F
Gardiner, E W
Ghosh, R M
Green, R G H
Hill, M J
Jefferson, W W
Jenkinson, H A
Laird, J D
Logan, J H C B
Ly, M H
McAteer, C O
MacFarlane, S E
McIlmoyle, C A
McIlrath, J P
Manderson, J E
Minford, E J
Moore, J
Munro, P I
O'Kane, E M
Rea, R D
Robinson, H
Stirling, J A
Thompson, T J
Whitehead, E M
Woodburn, E M A
Wright, T J W A

Ballymena
Agarwala, S
Allen, D J
Allen, G J
Armstrong, H M
Armstrong, K J
Bali, S
Barr, R S
Beckett, M
Black, I M
Black, J H A
Black, M C
Boyce, S A
Bunting, L
Burnside, P
Cameron, D
Carlisle, H A I
Clarkson, L
Cubitt, E D
Davison, L B S
Delargy, K P
Dick, C M
Dick, P T H
Doyle, D C
Dundee, R C
Ferguson, J
Flanagan, P G M
Fox, P J
Gardiner, G D
Gaston, W D M
Gilchrist, A
Glover, B D
Grainger, D J
Harper, J
Heggarty, P C
Henderson, R E

Hogg, J H
Hopkins, D M
Hughes, P G
Hunter, J B
Hutchinson, S P
Johnston, D J
Johnston, R S
Johnston, R E
Kennedy, D M
Kennedy, F D
Kennedy, J P
Kenny, R J
Khanna, S
King, R
Love, H E S
Low, B K
Lowry, J
Lowry, M
MaCartney, C
McCaughern, J
McCleery, M
McCluney, N A
McCollam, M P
McCoy, K J
McCready, D V
McCusker, D P
McFarland, J R L
McGahey, D T
McGavock, E
McKelvey, J
McKelvey, J K
McKelvey, R D
McKillen, J M
McLoughlin, K H
McManus, O B
McMullan, M G
McMullan, N J
McNeill, O A
McQuillan, J D
McSparran, A J M
McSparran, J A
McWilliams, E A
Magowan, M C
Magowan, T D
Mairs, A P
Marshall, M
Maxwell, G J
Mudd, P D
Mullan, J M
Nesbitt, S F
Newell, J
O'Hanlon, S
O'Hara, M G
Patterson, B G
Pothanikat, M G
Purce, E J
Ramsey, T L
Rea, R E
Redmond, M R
Redmond, R A A
Redmond, V A
Reid, J A
Russell, S G
Simms, K C
Simpson, A H
Simpson, J D
Sinclair, C J
Smith, J J
Smyth, N W
Stafford, S J
Stewart, R A
Stockman, A
Swan, K O
Tawia, A
Turtle, F
Vercoe-Rogers, J P
Waldron, G J M
Watson, J D
Willoughby, C E
Wilson, J
Wilson, P C
Wilson, W J C
Wright, G F
Young, C P

Ballymoney
Adams, J R
Boyd, K L
Fannin, E S
Flynn, J G
Gaston, J T
Hardy, T J
Harvey, W R
Johnston, D W H
Johnston, J E
Johnston, R J
Lee, D T
Lynch, B S
McCartney, R N J

McLaughlin, J
Matthews, J G W
Moles, M R
Murdock, O W N
O'Kane, M P
O'Sullivan, B M P
Robb, J D
Robb, J D A
Robinson, I H W
Sterne, A P
Virapen, M P
Wallace, J A

Ballynahinch
Ashton-Jennings, C A
Bailie, A G
Banks, I G
Bassett, J W
Beatty, H G
Christy, M W D
Courtney, A E
Courtney, C H
Ferguson, R W
Gillespie, P H
Gunn, S C
Harrison, R T S
Lowry, J H
McAdam, J G
McGlew, J M
Mills, E M
Nirodi, P
Nirodi, S
Nirodi, V N
O'Duchon, O
O'Gorman, E C
Poland, K M
Ross, R W D
Sands, F M
Scott, R
Smyth, E F
Watson, S J
Watterson, B R

Bamburgh
Hull, C J

Bampton
Harper, E
Landray, R
Mackenzie, R M
Perry, M G
Ward, N A L

Banbridge
Auld, J E
Boyce, C A
Carlisle, R J T
Cassidy, C A
Cocks, G R
Connolly, K S
Cupples, B B
Downey, A C
Graham, K E
Hollinger, M J
Hopkins, J P
Huey, M J
Knight, E D
McCandless, W
McConville, R M
McCreedy, A E
McNiff, C G P
Mallon, J H
Mawhinney, C
Moran, M B
Morrow, B A
Murray, L J
Murray, M A E
Ramsey, J K
Ramsey, P J
Robinson, T J

Banbury
Addison, S L
Aldous, M R
Allison, N Q
Appleton, G V N
Arnold, I R
Atoyebi, O I
Bell, R A F
Bentley, S
Boyle, D S
Budd, B M
Budd, D W G
Campbell, H R
Canty, S H
Chalmers, J S
Chamberlain, S K
Chambers, J C
Copcutt, E G

Cordingley, J L
Cornwall, L J
Crawford, P
D'Souza, M A J
Davenport, C F
Day, C W
Dehalvi, M N
Eatock, E M
Edwards, H A M
Ellis, A J
Elphick, M
Evans, C P
Everatt, J C D C
Everatt, S
Garud, S P
Gate, B
George, G J C
Gillham, N R
Goode, A F
Granne, I E
Greywoode, G I N
Griffiths, C L
Griffiths, H
Hall, C J
Harris, D M
Harris, M A M
Harrison, J M
Haynes, S A
Holt, C S
Hughes, A W
Hunter, M F
Hyslop, D A
Johnson, J
Kemp, S H
Klenka, L H
Large, S H
Laurie, P S
Lehman, R S
MacLaren, D M
Mahy, N J
Mann, C
Mann, R Q
Marshall, R E K
Marshall, T P
Mason, G P H
Miller, S J
Moran, S F
Ng Cheng Hin, H S
Nicholls, J S D
North, C E
O'Donnell, H F
O'Farrell, B D
Paranjothy, S
Parsons, P W
Patton, M K
Pollard, J P
Reid, N G B
Robinson, S L
Rodrick, I W
Rogers, G Y
Rogers, S J
Ruddock, F S
Shafighian, B
Shapley, R
Sheybany, S
Shia, G T-W
Smith, S R
Soden, F B
Spackman, D D
Tasker, J A
Tideswell, D J
West, J D P
Whitehead, T C
Wignell, D J
Willatts, D G
Williams, J A G
Wookey, S L M
Wright, J A

Banchory
Barclay, D G
Bayliss, A P
Bayliss, M A
Brynes, G D
Carroll, A L
Carroll, D S
Donald, K J
Johnston, S J
Kentish, L E
McCrone, M G
Maclean, A F
Mair, F F
Morton, K M
Pearson, M J
Proctor, D W
Secrett, T J
Sudder, J A
Watt, S J
Webster, N R

Banff
Anderson, J E
Bruce, C E
Campbell, R J
Chung, C W
Innes, G D D
Lees, R F B
Mandal, K C
Ross, J B
Smith, M R
Wallace, E A H

Bangor, County Down
Archer, K L
Archer, L J
Bailie, R K
Baird, W J S
Baker, R C
Ball, G M
Ballard, J D
Beckett, N
Bingham, G P
Bleakney, R R
Brooks, S
Brown, A P
Bryans, R
Cairns, P N E
Campbell, G A M
Carroll, R A
Chambers, C A
Christy, J R O
Crawford, G M
Crowe, J A
Crowther, S M
Dinsmore, E A
Doran, G
Douglas, J H E
Drew, J L
Garland, J M
Gault, L D
Gibson, C
Gilmore, C P
Graham, P J K
Guy, D D
Hainsworth, A M
Harbinson, S A
Hardy, C L
Harper, S
Haslett, W H K
Heaney, A E
Hill, C
Hunter, J
Jones, D D
Jordan, N P D
Kennedy, M N
Kerr, H
Killiner, W S
Lavery, H A
Lavery, J T
Lightbody, C J
Loughrey, C M J
Lowry, K J
Lynas, T H
Mcadam, T K
McAuley, W J
McBride, R J
McBride, S T
McClelland, A M
McCoubrey, M A
McGrane, C T
McGrattan, B M
McManus, D K
McMinn, S A
Majury, N T
Mannis, N D
Millar, W J R
Miller, J
Monaghan, D A T
Mulholland, K C
Mulholland, M L E
Murphy, A L
Murray, P D
Nicol, P A
Nixon, J R
Page, A B
Patterson, G J
Patterson, R N
Phipps, B M
Redmill, D A
Reid, R D
Rennie, I M
Rogers, H J
Sharpe, T D E
Slater, R M
Stout, A W
Thompson, K R
Todd, S A
Turner, J

Walford, G A
Wetherall, L M
Wilson, E A
Wilson, L E
Woods, A J

Bangor, Gwynedd
Adams, C J
Baldwin, C D
Barr, G S
Bate, T E
Bates, A B
Benfield, G F A
Birch, P D
Bloodworth, L L O
Bolton, L M
Bowen, E S
Bracewell, R M
Caukwell, J P
Chowdhury, M W R
Crawford, R C
Devakumar, M
Devaraj, K S
Edwards, N I
Elliston, P R A
Fowell, A J
Francis, A F
Gilleece, M H
Harris, T J B
Healy, D T M
Heinersdorff, N R
Hodges, N
Horn, J S M
Hughes, J A
Hughes, R C E
Iqbal, J
Jibani, M
Johnston, J G
Jones, D A
Jones, D P A H
Jones, G L
Jones, I W
Jones, M W
Kassab, S C
Kinahan, P J
Korn, H E T
Kurian, G V
Leeson, S C
Lewis, J A
Lynch, F K
Macfarlane, A W
McMonagle, T M M
McSweeney, L
Maddison, P J
Madkour, M B E-D
Mammen Korulla, B
Mehta, H K
Mehta, M H
Miles, L
Mithan, W J
Mortimer, J A
Nicholas, S G
Nickson, P J
Owen, B C
Owens, D
Pennant-Lewis, R
Poeppinghaus, V J I
Powell, T G
Prichard, D R
Radford, A M
Roberts, D P W
Roberts, E
Roberts, G E W
Roberts, G L W
Roberts, L R
Roberts, M A
Rosser, C
Savage, M C
Seale, J R C
Shambrook, A S J
Singh Josson, K
Sriwardhana, K B
Stuart, N S A
Subash Chandran, R
Tivy-Jones, P
Tyldesley, D B
Walker, A M
Watkin, G T
Wayte, D M
Wenham, S J
Whiteley, G S W
Williams, L G
Williams, M A C
Williams, R M
Williams, R S
Woolley, J L
Zeki, S M

Bangor, North Wales
Johnson, I A T

Banstead
Ahmad, M
Archibald, R M
Arduino, L A
Banerjee, D K
Basu, R
Cartwright, H F
Digby, S T C
Efthymiou, C
Fielder, H C
Gallagher, H
Geer, P L
Kirk, H L
Lancefield, K S
McCurdie, I M
MacRae, R C
Majumder, J L
Nathan, L A
Ngan-Soo, E M-S
Pande, S K
Pearson, P J T
Perlman, F J A
Planche, T D
Powles, R L
Rafi, I
Till, R J W
Tinton, M M
Wray, R M

Banwell
Mee, M S

Bargoed
Baig, M Z
Caesar, E
Caesar, H
Das, N
Majumdar, S K
Prior, G T J
Thomas, A-J
Watkins, N R
Williams, E D G

Barking
Abudu, I A
Ahmad, H
Ahmed, A B J
Akinola, S E
Ali, M M
Baghla, D P S
Barclay, G
Booth, H C
Chopra, A S
Gupta, S N
Harvey, L J
John, A
John, K
Kateck, V H
Mathur, P
Moazzez, K
Moghal, I A
Nguyen, D D H
Parikh, N S
Rahmatullah Khan, Dr
Sainsbury, J
Seth, P V
Sheril, D B
Thomas, G L
Tolia, K J
Tote, S P
Uncle, K A
Watts, C J

Barmouth
Bradley, M C S
Hassan, S P
Haworth, R A
Hickey, M S
Short, S P
Taaffe, P
Whitehead, W H

Barnard Castle
Austin, P G
Cuthbert, C R
Fordy, K
Hamilton, F J
Harrison, C M S
Nainby-Luxmoore, J C
Ross, A M
Ross, I H
Ryan, P M
Smith, A H
Stewart, P D

Welch, F M
White, J J

Barnet
Anchor, S C
Anwar, U S
Arunachalam, S
Baig, K A
Bajekal, N R
Baker, K W
Barnes, A J
Bell, D J
Berger, J
Berney, S I
Bird, R L R
Bloomfield, A E
Bolton, J P
Bradford, A T
Bradley, J C
Breeze, R W
Briggs, T P
Broadbent, J A M
Brown, E G
Bunce, C J
Burke, B J
Burn, M J L
Cartmell, E L
Cooper, S M
Creer, D D
Curran, P M
Dar, V K
David, L S
Davies, A C
El Jabbour, J N
Evans, J
Fage, V A A
Ferris, B D
Fine, W
Fox-Male, P
Fox, D B
Fuller, G
Garland, M H
Goodwin, R W
Greenbaum, R A
Harbinson, P L
Huseyin, T S
Ibrahimi, G S
Johnston, I E
Joseph, L R
Kamath, B S K
Kanabar, S D
Kaplan, G R
Khan, S
Khiroya, D V
Khiroya, V P
Kidson, I G
Kirk, A
Kumar, G
Kurien, J
Lagnado, E A
Lai Chung Fong, P
Laufer, N E
Laurent, S J
Lee, F Y K
Lehovsky, A J
Levy, N A
Lindsey, S K
Livingston, S I
Livingstone, D A
Lodge, P J
Loh, A
Loh, C K
Lupin, L
McGowan, P R
Mackay, K H
Males, S M
Marcus, A J
Margerison, N J
Maudgal, D P
Milaszkiewicz, R
Miles, S J
Minchin, A J
Moman, R B
Monkman, D S
Natkunarajah, S
Natkunarajah, S
Nicholls, M D W
Nikapota, H M V L B
Norris, J C
Painter, A N
Patel, D J
Patel, M K
Patel, S
Patel, S
Pavey, S K
Pearson, A J G
Philippson, M E A
Raman, C
Ranasinghe, D U

Ranasinghe, N
Rean, Y M
Ribet, P W L
Ribet, R P
Rosenbaum, N L
Rossouw, D J
Roth, S C
Russell, R C
Ryan, F M
Sanghani, V V
Savege, P B
Shafi, G
Shah, S S
Shanthakumar, R E
Sharkawi, E
Sheridan, P J
Sireling, L I
Sittampalam, G
St. John Smith, P
Strawbridge, L C
Sturridge, B F
Symons, I E
Tait, D
Tanner, P A S
Tham, N
Thambapillai, R
Troyack, A D
Vellodi, C
Virchis, A E
Watt, S J
Watts, N
Weston, P M
Wiseman, P A
Wolfman, M J
Yanni, G A
Yapanis, M
Yiallouros, M

Barnetby
Grant, B M
Vora, A

Barnoldswick
Dick, D G
Evans, A J
Hare, A C
Holmes, S G T
Huxley, P A

Barnsley
Aboobakar, B
Adebajo, A O
Ahmad, A
Al-Bazzaz, M K I M
Allen, D J
Allen, K W
Alvarez Escurra, M F
Alvarez Iglesias, M
Amonkar, J A
Appelqvist, I P
Athale, D M
Balac, N
Ballingall, D A T
Banerjee, K
Bannister, J J
Baxter, A P
Beck, J M
Bell, A R
Bell, C
Bell, N J
Bennett, R I
Bhartia, R R
Bhaskara Rao, B
Bhaskaran, N C
Birinder, K T
Birkinshaw, R I
Bodhe, M M
Booth, D
Bothwell, J E
Bowns, C M
Bradbury, R A
Brenchley, J
Bridger, C A
Bryant, P A
Bullimore, D W W
Burgin, M I
Burton, S J
Carlin, E M
Chan Lam, J M F D
Chaudhry, T A
Claydon, P J
Coup, A J
Courtney, M E
Crowe, M
Czepulkowski, E C
Darby, D C
Davis-Reynolds, L M R
Dehadray, M G
Eldred, J B

Firth, S H
Franklin, J S Q
Freeborn, C M
Gear, S L
Gill, N P
Goh, G C
Granger, K A
Harban, J
Harrison, K
Heyes, T G
Hicks, D A
Hirst, W S J
Hoda, M Q
Hooson, T K
Hourihane, B
Jain, V K
Johnson, M E
Jones, T H
Kakoty, P C
Kapur, K C
Keini, K S
Kershaw, D A
Khan, G H
Khan, M A
Kini, K K
Krishnaswamy, C K
Lavender, A
Law, C E
Leabeater, B F
Lee, D E
Leese, C W
Leigh, J
Littler, W W
Loh, R Y M
Lotfallah, H N
McDonald, A R
McDonald, K W
McFeely, D F
McNicholas, J L
Marshall, A D R
Matuk, M D
Mehta, B M
Menezes, A R
Metson, J R
Mian, R S
Middleton, F H
Miller, A J
Mitra, S
Myint, Y
Naish, C
Nayyar, N A
Ng Ping Cheung, J-P
North, C
O'Dwyer, P F
O'Reilly, B N
O'Sullivan, D J
Okoko, A E J
Ostrowski, J L
Palmer, N W
Panezai, J U R
Pearson, V
Piper, I H
Pollock, A L
Prasad, Y N
Price, A G
Puttagunta, B
Quincey, C
Ravi, A
Ravi, S
Reed, P D
Rhoden, W E
Richards, F A
Robertson, J G
Rose, D
Roy, R
Ruddlesdin, C
Ruiz Fito, J R
Sagar, J L
Sattar, S A
Sattar, S A
Scargill, M A
Shiwani, M H
Sics, M R
Sillifant, K L
Singh, D
Singh, R P
Smith, A K
Spencer, H D
Sriramulu, V
Stobart, J A H
Swinhoe, A L
Swinhoe, C F
Sykes, L
Tambar, B K
Tyerman, G V
Tyerman, P F
Vaghani, J T
Varley, R
Vinod Kumar, I

Waddington, R T
Wahedna, I
Wakefield, V A
Walker, A
Ward, A S
Way, B G
Weatherill, J
Welchew, K L
Wickham, M H
Wilkerson, J N
Wood, C B
Yadav, D G
Yadav, S S
Yaqub, M
Yates, S P
Yeoman, L J
Zachary, J B

Barnstaple
Alexander, H M
Ashton, M G
Attock, B
Averns, H L
Baker, A W T
Bargery, A
Barker, A J
Barker, J R
Barron, E K
Barwise, K
Bastiaenen, H L R
Beer, R J S
Bigge, T L
Bosley, A R J
Boss, J M
Boucherat, A
Boyle, A H W
Brennan, N
Buchanan, I
Bull, A D
Bunney, R G
Claydon, E J
Coberman, M
Compton, N J
Davies, J H
Dickson, J
Dodds, J M
Eckford, S D
Enoch, B E
Forster, S J
Gillard, J D
Hart Prieto, M C
Harvey, D R
Hawkins, M J
Helsby, J
Holman, R A
Holmes, J A
Hooper, C A
Horman, L M
Howlett, A J
Hubbard, H C
Hunt, S J
Jack, I F M
Kalsi, B S
Kay, M
Laycock, G J A
Le Dieu, H R
Lewin, I G
Loader, B W
McCabe, J G
McCaie, C P
McElderry, E M
Malcolm, B
Markham, N I
Marston, J A
Matthews, H C
Miller, A L
Miller, J E
Miller, T E
Mills, C L
Moore, P C H
Moran, A
Morgan, M R
Myers, S
Nicholson, S D
O'Donovan, N P
Oliver, M H
Osborne, C L E
Peet, J S
Podmore, M D
Quinton-Tulloch, J C
Reynolds, R J
Reynolds, Z M
Richards, D A
Roberts, G A
Roberts, T L
Rutter, M J
Sadek, R I M
Sanderson, A J
Saunders, J M

Sewell, M S
Sinclair, B J
Skinner, L J
Smith, P F
Smithson, J M
Socrates, A
Sowden, G R
Speirs, G E
Steinlechner, C W B
Suresh Shetty, V
Taylor, A D
Taylor, C P
Treble, N J
Treweeke, P S
Turner, J G
Van Buren-Schele, M
Walder, A D
Wheble, A M
White, J C
Whittle, E R
York-Moore, D W
Young, J R

Barrhead
Gemmell, W E
McAleer, M
Mitchell, M B
Morton, I C
Naven, T
Nicholson, A F

Barrow-in-Furness
Allan, D
Allington, M D
Ashcroft, A J
Ashcroft, C N
Askari, S H
Ball, C S
Baqai, A N
Boardman, A J
Brewer, I L
Burden, M F
Cockshott, C U
Coker, D M
Courtman, N H
Crawshaw, P J S
De Clercq, S M
Dieker, A
Egan, J A
Glew, M
Govenden, V
Green, C J
Harrison, R
Hasan, M R-U
Hearn, H J
Hodkinson, J N
Hussein, I Y
Jeelani, G
Joglekar, V M
Jolliffe, G C
Kamalanathan, V
Keating, J J
Knott-Craig, J L
Lee Cheong, L F L
Lindley, J C
Maalawy, M M
MacDonald, B R
McGroarty, V
Macheta, A T
McQuillan, S T
Mangal, A
Mardel, S N
Memon, Y
Mohammed, O E N
Murugappan, N
Nasmyth, D G
Ni Chuileannain, F M
Nugent, E M
Nugent, J J
O'Donovan, I A M
Oldham, T P
Page, A
Pai, K G
Partridge, S M
Patel, M C
Rathi, R K
Robinson, K M
Rogerson, J W
Rogerson, S H
Sayer, N J
Sekhar, R
Sharples, P J
Stoney, P J
Story, T W
Swinglehurst, P A
Taylor, A
Todd, D
Tupper, C H
Wear, I J

Wiejak, A P
Williams, L J
Williams, P S
Wilson, R Y
Wyatt, M G
Wyatt, R H
Young, J C

Barry
Baig, A
Brook, J F
Brown, G G
Bugler, H
Burfitt, E M
Chapman, J R
Coleman, M A T
Coyle, F M
Coyle, J M A
Davies, D
Davies, E J
Davies, G F
Davies, S H
Doherty, E F
Donaghy, C E
Donnison, P E I
Evans, J G
Harfoot, D A
Holgate, S K
Hooper, R A
Hortop, S E
Hughes, A
Jones, S D
Lazarus, G F
Lindsay, S D
Parker, S J
Rhys-Dillon, C C G
Richards, L F
Smith, S J
Sullivan, M A L
Sutton, L J
Tasker, D G
Walton, E E
Weatherup, A
Williams, A J
Williams, A J
Williams, D E
Williams, R D
Witte, K K A

Barton-upon-Humber
Bacon Kinsella, C E
Birtwhistle, T J C
Dickinson, J A
Jaggs-Fowler, R M
Lobacz, R M
Longden, P
Macmillan, F N
Pemberton, J
Rowles, N

Basildon
Agombar, A C
Agrawal, A
Agrawal, R L
Ali, A
Ali, P M
Askwith, J H
Barton, I K
Bell, R J
Biswas, K
Biswas, S K
Catterall, M D
Cavaroli, M E
Chajed, G
Chan, A W C
Chan, T Y K
Colby, R
Collier, D S J
Colliver, D W
Cook, L
Cornforth, B M
Cotta, R G
Coward, L J
David, A C
Denham, A
Eade, P F
Fayad, G
Galea, C
Gendi, N S T
Gertner, D J
Goyal, R L A
Griffin, A B
Gupta, G R
Hastings, L A
Herath, N L B
Hoogsteden, L
Hopcroft, K A
Huwez, F U

Jas, B B
Jeddy, T A
Jenner, G H
Karia, S J
Kerrigan, P J C
Khan, F H
Khan, R
Khorshid, S M
Lafferty, K
Lal, A S
Latif, A
Lefevre, D C
Lehner, K G
Linehan, I P
Lockwood, C A
Lovett, B E
Lowe, D M
Lowe, M R
McFarlane, S H
Malhotra, A E D
Mampilly, J
Marshall, R B
Martin, C J
Martin, P B
Maunder, R F
May, M S
Memon, W M
Millins, S
Mitchell, A J
Morgan, S H
Moulds, A J
Mulcahy, M P E
Murray, A M
Najim, H A
Nimmo, S
Ojutiku, M A
Ozua, P O
Palit, J
Patel, N
Patel, P C
Pereira, C M
Prem Swarup, I J
Pretty, M A
Punchihewa, V G
Pusey, R J
Ramanan, R
Rao, H S
Rawlingson, C J
Rosen, M R
Rylah, L T A
Sage, R J
Salahuddin, A
Saw Myint, Dr
Sharief, N N Y
Sharpe, R A
Sims, M A
Singh, P K
Singhal, H
Smith, R B
Spraggins, D
Targett, J P G
Tarn, M
Taylor, H W R
Utting, H J W
Vohra, A
Vyas, J K
Wakeman, R
Watts, E J
Whitehead, J P
Willert, E J
Woodgate, D J
Yung, B M-C

Basingstoke
Adamson, G
Aertssen, A M G
Allen, J F
Arianayagam, S V
Aronstam, A
Ashworth, J S
Ashworth, M E
Assadourian, R
Aston, D L
Bates, R G
Baxter, P J C
Bell, J W
Bernstein, J J
Birtwistle, S M
Bishop, A J
Blanshard, J D
Booth, L V
Boswell, P A
Bowen, S P
Brain, G R H
Brian, J
Britton, A E M
Britton, J M
Brookes, C I O
Browne, R J S

Burgess, E J
Button, P D
Cameron, A H
Carman, S J
Carnegy, A
Church, J P
Cochrane, T R C
Cole, A T
Coppin, R J
Crone, A M
D'Souza, E
De Mars, C
Dent, C J
Dent, T H S
Dixon, C G
Eden, C G
Eustace, J D
Faithfull-Davies, D N
Farquharson, S M
Fawcett, H A
Fisher, E P
Fraser, N B
Freeman, H J
Fry, R P W
Gall, J
Geach, A R
Gold, D M
Gould, S W T
Gowers, L E
Green, I L
Greenslade, J H
Greenwood, A J
Guy, R J C
Haas, A J
Heald, R J
Hettiaratchy, S W
Heys, M
Hiorns, P E
Hoar, D H M
Hobby, J L
Hogan, A M
Hudson, S W
Hudson, W S
Hullah, G J
Hunter, E M M
Hurley, J E
Iffland, C A
Ilangovan, P B
Ilesley, I C
James, P D
Jamil, S
Jardine-Brown, K
John, T G
Jones, S H
Jones, T J H
Jones, V J I
Keightley, S J
Kerawala, C J
Knight, D K S
Knowles, P M
Knowles, S P
Koch, S
Lee, A C
Levy, T M
Limbrey, R M
Lindsay, J A
Lorge, R E
McGonigal, G
McKinlay, K P
McLay, I A B
Macve, J S
Maltby, J D
Matti, S J
May, A-M
Milne, A E
Mitchell, A T
Mitchell, M I
Morgan, J G
Morrell, R R J
Morsman, C D G
Moss, D
Moss, M L
Mostafid, A H
Munro, D F
Mycock, H D
Myles, B J
O'Neill, H M-J
O'Sullivan, G F M
O'Sullivan, M J B
Ollerhead, K J
Pagdin, J C
Pal, C R
Parker, J C
Parker, R L E
Patel, S
Patterson, G M
Peppercorn, P D
Pimenta, D J
Plant, G R T

Platt, K A
Pleydell-Pearce, J S J
Plyming, A V L
Powell, J J
Preston, H G
Prouse, P J
Radja, N
Ramage, J K
Rathod, S L
Rees, J
Rees, M
Reid, C G
Richards, A B
Richardson, J
Robins, D W
Roy, A
Roy, L
Sacco, D F
Sandy, C J
Sayer, T R
Shawe, D J
Shelley, D F
Simpson, H K
Sorby, N G D
Spencer, G M
Spraggs, P D R
Stebbing, M A
Stephenson, D A
Stranks, G J
Summers, L J
Teall, J G
Thomas, N P
Thomson, K D
Todd, G P A
Tristram, S J
Trueman, R S
Tupper, D J L
Turner, R G
Ubhayakar, G N
Upchurch, S
Vanita, Dr
Vinitharatne, J K P
Walters, R O
Waring, N J
Warren, P A
Wells, J K G
Western, N V B
Wigfield, R E
Wilkins, D F
Willcocks, J A J
Williams, E A
Williams, G A
Williamson, D J
Wilson, P T J
Wright, D J T
Wright, P G Y
Yeganeh-Arani, E

Bath
Abu Zaid, E-H A
Acharya, B
Ahmed, A W
Alabaster, C J
Alexander, A G
Allan, M D
Amos, C
Andersson, M I
Antcliff, R J
Aplin, C G
Archer, P
Ashmore, A M
Aston, S J
Atkinson, P J
Austin, V M A
Avery, A F
Awan, R J
Baer, R M
Bagley, S R V
Baird, M B
Barclay, J A
Bardner, D J
Barton, B J J
Bateman, D E
Bates, T S
Batten, K L
Batterham, I A
Beaven, J T
Bell, R C
Bennett, J M
Bennett, P F
Berrisford, C E
Bevan, C M
Bhalla, A K
Biddlestone, L R
Billson, A L
Binzenhofer, J
Bishay, M S K
Blackmore, J E
Blackstock, J

Blain, C R V
Bliss, P
Bointon, G B H
Booth, P J
Botham, J R W
Bottomley, M B
Boucher, K J
Bovill, B A
Bradbury, N
Britton, D C
Bromwich, H L
Brooks, J D
Brooks, S J
Bruce-Jones, W D A
Bubna-Kasteliz, B
Budd, J S
Cahill, T E
Cairney, P
Calin, A
Canter, R J
Capper, R
Carr, D W R
Carter, A C
Cash, H C
Cashman, J P
Chalmers, A H
Chapman, J A
Charles-Chillcott, R J
Clark, N
Clark, T W
Clarke, A K
Colfox, L S M
Collins, A J
Conway, B M
Cook, S J
Cooper, A M
Cooper, D J
Cooper, S J
Cornish, J M M
Cosgrove, P V F
Cottee, C S
Cottman, S B
Coulter, G G
Craft, T M
Cromby, J W
Crook, A E
Cumpsty, C E
Cumpsty, J R
Darch, G R
Davies, J
Davies, J A
Davies, W R
Davis, M
Deane, L S
Dinwoodie, J M
Divall, P A W
Donovan, A D
Dorman, S
Douglass, S J
Dow, L
Downie, C J C
Dowson, D I
Duignan, M
Dunlop, D A B
Dunlop, D C
Dunn, R B
Dunster, G D
Eavis, P M
Edwards, E A
Ewbank, J A
Fallon, K M
Farrant, J M
Finlay, R D
Fitzgerald, J H
Foley, N M
Fuge, C A
Galimberti, A
Gallegos, C R R
Gibbs, Z K
Giddins, G E B
Gilbert, J H
Gilby, E D
Gillberry, M A
Gillies, F C L
Gillies, R M
Glaser, S
Glew, D
Goddard, D A
Goodwin, A P L
Grabham, R E
Green, P J
Griffiths, J M
Groenhuysen, C
Gupta, K J
Hall, T B
Hallett, A M
Hamling, H M-C
Hamling, J B
Hampton, J

Handel, J M
Hansell, J
Hanson, B E
Hardman, J A R
Harries, J M
Harris, M F
Harris, T J
Harrison, F M
Hartley-Brewer, V F
Hayes, A L
Hayward, S J
Head, A J
Hersch, E
Hersch, E V
Hertlein, R A
Hill, C P
Hill, S L
Hillen, R S
Hills-Wright, P A
Hirschowitz, L
Hodson, R S
Hooper, A I
Horn, C K
Houghton, H J
Howell, G P
Howell, M E
Howlett, D M
Howse, N L
Hubbard, W N
Hudson-Jessop, P
Hughes-Davies, D I
Hughes, J
Humphries, E A M
Irish, W T
Jackson, A C
Jackson, F P
Jackson, H J
Jacobson, S K
Jelley, T M
Jenkinson, T R
Jennings, P J F
Jiggins, M P
Johns, W A
Johnson, M R
Johnson, N
Johnson, T M
Jones, C B
Jones, C D
Jones, D E P
Jones, J P
Jones, N C R
Jones, R
Jones, R W
Jones, S W
Judge, C B
Karanjavala, J D
Kaye, A
Kellas, A R P
Kennaway, C V
Kingston, P
Kitching, P A
Knechtli, C J C
Kocheta, A A J
Korendowych, E
Langdon, I J
Laverty, T A
Leach, C L
Leahy, E P
Lechi, A
Legassick, R A
Lenton, S W
Lim, A B H
Lovell, C R
Luck, J
Lutterloch, M J
Lyons, P R
McCrea, J
MacDougall, M H
McFarlane, J P
McHugh, L A
McHugh, N J
Mackay, G H
McKechnie, E J
McMaster, V J
McNab, M A
McNeir, C
Maddox, P R
Magee, P T
Maguire, K M
Mahto, R S
Maken, S
Malin, A S
Mallet, C M
Malthouse, M E
Malthouse, S R
Mann, J B
Marden, B J
Marjot, R
Mauri Sole, I
Mayor, A H
Medworth, S
Meehan, C J
Meisner, S J
Michael, B
Miller, A M
Millington, C
Milner, P C
Monro, A D
Montgomerie, J
Moore, D C
Morgan, K F H
Morrice, A A G
Morris, A K
Morris, J C
Morrison, M
Morrison, P J M
Mowat, J S S
Muddiman, M J
Mundy, F H
Murison, I C
Murray, S R
Nixon, J
Noakes, M J
Nolan, J P
North, P C
Novak, S A
Nulliah, K
O'Brien, A T J
Orpen, I M
Osborne, J P
Padkin, A J
Parr, M J A
Paterson, M P
Pauli, H M
Pavy, C R
Payton, C D
Pearson, M L
Peden, C J
Pemberton, D P
Perry, N K
Peters, C D
Pizey, N C D
Playfair, J R
Pointing, T D
Pollock, K J
Porter, R J
Potter, R G
Pozo, J L
Prees, K A
Price, L E N
Proffitt, C M
Protheroe, D T
Provan, A B
Radford, S R
Reckless, J P D
Redman, A G O
Reynolds, N J
Richardson, J C
Roberts, B J
Robertson, D A F
Robinson, B L
Rolls, R L
Rooney, N
Rose, D S C
Rose, H J
Ross, A C
Rudd, P T
Rumball, C L
Rye, S
Sammes, H R
Sanchez-Andrade Bolanos, J M
Sandeman, A P
Savine, R
Schnetler, J F C
Schofield, H M
Seagger, R M
Seagger, R A
Seppelt, I H
Sharman, S L
Shaw, L J
Sheppard, C A
Sholapurkar, S L
Simpson, N
Simpson, T J P
Singer, C R J
Singh Ranger, R
Slack, R W T
Smith, A
Smith, J
Smith, J C
Smith, J G
Smith, P K W
Souter, A J
Speed, M A
Spelman, J F
Spurling, S G
Stagg, C E
Standing, B L
Stanton, R A
Stewart, M S
Sykes, P H
Tan, R S-H
Tate, J J T
Teoh, R E
Thomas, C L
Thomas, J
Thomas, R D
Thorley, A P
Tilley, J S
Tonge, H M
Towers, J S
Tuckey, J P
Turnbull, A R
Tyrrell, J C
Umpleby, H C
Usman, F
Valentine, J P
Waldron, J
Walker, D J
Walker, G D
Watson, D P H
Wayte, C
Webber, S M
Wernham, C M
Wexler, S A
Wharton, R L
White, A
Whitfield, B E
Widdowson, E J
Wilde, J M
Wiles, I D
Willars, C M
Williams, C J
Williams, D J
Williamson, M E R
Williamson, T J
Worsdall, G M
Wylie, G L
Young, R

Bathgate
Al-Ubaid, K S
Bader, R
Bell, P C
Bradshaw, Q P
Brady, B M
Brown, K J
Carlaw, W G
Chaudhury, A J
Cook, A J C
Duncan, I D
Easter, H J
Ferguson, A
Ferguson, S R
Hay, D J
Hayward, C D
Ibrahim, M
James, B K D
Kerr, A M
Laird, G W
Lees, J S
Macaulay, D
McCallum, J M
McCollum, D
MacGillivray, D
McKinstry, B H
McKitterick, M J
McNutt, A P W
Merrilees, H F
Milne, S M
Mooney, J K
Phillips, C J
Porter, L J
Ritchie, V
Robertson, C M M
Stewart, C M
Stewart, J H
Thomson, J
Toellner, C B
Tydeman, G S J
Wallace, J A K
Williamson, S M
Wilson, C E
Winter, M D

Batley
Ashraff, Y N
Barker, D R
Bham, A Y
Bham, Y G M
Bottomley, S E
Cowie, I W R
Desai, P M
Elders, M K
Fowers, D E
Ghanchi, F D
Gillson, S T
Glover, P D
Hooper, J M
Houghton, C S
Jones, J F M
Kalla, V K
Lawler, J S
Lawson, S J
Lee, J H
Lidhar, J K
Lidhar, K S
Lobb, B R
Longmore, T B
Lynch, B D
Lynch, M P
Mackereth, A C
Miller, P A
Mullhi, P S
Mulrennan, S
Rajpura, A
Rajpura, A
Scales, M F
Singh, N K
Tarrant, D A
Walker, E C
Wright, J R

Battle
Beal, R J
Belcher, N G
Campbell, D A
Griffith, D G C
Hargreaves, C D
Jardine-Brown, T
Justice, R J
Kemm, I S J
Lloyd-Jones, D
Merrick, C D
Mogan, J E
Rademaker, J W
Rice-Oxley, C P
Rivett, J G
Rivett, P M
Silva, L U
Stern, S R
Underhill, T J
Vale, K E
Wakeford, N A A
Wood, M C
Yeo, R

Beaconsfield
Agbeja, A M
Amin, C L
Balmforth, J R
Bayliss, M A
Blackmore, S J
Brodie, D P
Brown, S P
Bulger, J M
Churn, M J
Coggan, A M
Cox, S A L
Crawford, D S
Crawford, J L
Dalton, J I F
Davies, K E
Dell, R J
Devoy, M A B
Donnelly, R J
Elliott, C
Feegrade, M D
Fletcher, G R L
Gallagher, S K
Glover, J D
Grover, E R
Hagger, A O
Hambly, J F E
Hardy, J
Harris, G
Hart, R A
Hern, E E
Horn, R F H
Jones, R D
Lang, G S
Lomax, S H M
McDermott, H W
McGirr, B P
Mackenzie, V F
McPherson, G A D
McVey, V M
Marsden, D A
Murray, M L
Musaji, M A
Roberts, P D
Sellors, G P
Slater, S D
Smallwood, E H
Stanworth, S J
Stoneham, M D
Thomas, S I
Walker, B J
Widgington, N J
Wilson, J F

Beaminster
Goodhart, R A G
Kettell, J A
Payne, J M V
Robinson, T W
Sinclair, E R

Beauly
Baecker, T E
Forsyth, R S
Fullerton, L A
Habermann, F F
Hawco, M J
Janssens, M
Kane, I A
Kane, T P C
McIntyre, A J
McLardy, J
MacLeod, M
MacVicar, J
Paul, N
Whittle, E J

Beaumaris
Fowell, A
Jones, H W
Jones, R Y
Macvicar, S
Parry, D H
Pringle, M
Richards, G
Vousden, J E
Waite, H C

Beaworthy
Al-Doori, A A A-M
Bowden, L J
Filer Cooper, R
Human, M S
Miller, S W M

Bebington
Haylock, B J
Klenka, H M
Sagar, S
Thomas, J

Beccles
Battye, I R
Berry, P S
Brown, A E
Bubb, A R
Bungay, E K
Cadman, S
Cockshott, A M
Collins, G W
Douglas, K D S
Frears, J F
Harrison, D A
Holly-Archer, F K M
Kinsey, W L
Latoy, J J
McMahon, P J T
Morton, T J
Pitt, J M
Smith, P R
Wells, A L

Beckenham
Abdullah, V
Baker, A J
Barnett, H C
Bearn, J A
Boakes, J P
Broadfield, J B
Bugler, J A
Buttriss, C J
Campbell, A C
Carroll, K P C
Cassar, S D
Daly, H C S
Davidson, S P
Donald, J L
Dunachie, P A
Dyer, K E
Eayrs, P J
Ephson, P M J
Fisher, M F
Fitt, C S
Fitzpatrick, D G
Fowle, A S E
Frimpong, G A A A
Funnell, N J
Gale, R F
Gibson, T J
Gilbert, A M
Glanfield, M D
Glenister, P W
Gnanachelvan, S
Gordon, H L
Harris, L S
Harrison, M C
Holder, S E
Holloway, F
Hoo, C A
Horgan, M M
Horwood, E
Husain, S S-Y
Hutchinson, D B A
Ilo, O A
James, J D
James, P R
Johnson, C
Kamalanathan, F A
Kandavel, R
Kaye, A M
Kazmi, S M N A
Kelleher, K G
Kerawala, J J
Latham, J
Little, C P
Little, V
McColl, C L
McQueen, J
McWilliams, S E
Maini, R
Malhi, G
Manuel, J B
Martin, J R
Medcalf, M S
Mercer, D M
Motahar, M M
Mozley, C R
Naylor, R
Needham-Bennett, H
Norton, M R
Onen, T S
Pandya, D
Paranjape, R N
Pook, J A R
Rajap, T I
Reddy, K P
Sampson, S A
Silver, T
Simmons, I G
Stone, C J
Tempest, J E
Tilsley, D W O
Tinson, R E
Trezies, A J H
Underhill, H C
Vella, R
Wagstyl, J W
Ware, R J
Wells, R A
Williams, D J
Williams, K G D
Wozniak, A P
Wraige, E A
Yiu, C A

Beckermet
Cheetham, R B

Bedale
Ashworth, J
Bell, R E
Collier, C N
Fisken, J M
Thompson, J M
Thompson, M J
Willox, M F

Bedford
Agarwalla, B
Agrawal, A T
Agrawal, M L
Agrawal, P
Agrawal, T
Aldrich, I D
Allingham, J P
Anderson, J M
Arasaratnam, R B S
Attia, F F
Au, K H-K
Aylward, J G
Azher, M
Baker, A S
Baker, P A
Baldwin, H C
Barter, S J
Berman, J W

Besag, F M C
Bhamra, G S
Binns, J C
Blackshaw, A J
Blackshaw, M J
Bogle, G D
Bone, J W
Brookes, N R
Buckingham, C J
Budden, G C
Burtt, G J
Butlin, J A
Callam, M J
Cambridge, G C
Cameron, E A
Clark, E C
Cochrane, J G
Coles, S R
Coombes, A M A
Cooper, I C
Cooper, J P
Cooray, P G
Crawford, B J F
Dalton, A M
Daniels, D G
Davies, R J E
De Groot, W T
Deane, S E
Didier, H P
Done, A R
Dorling, B
Edwards, W J
Egan, A M
Eldin, A M I S
Elliman, A M
Fardell, S J
Farhoud, J S L
Feast, S M
Fenske, M
Ferguson, S A
Fisher, F F
Fitch, L E
Foley, R J E
Fox, J M
Frampton, M C
Fuad, F
Gallivan, R J
Glaze, M E
Gnanakumaran, G
Godbole, V
Godbolt, A K
Gooding, R G
Gordon, E A C
Goulding, J A
Gray, A P
Grice, G C
Griffith, T P
Hadfield, J I H
Hamilton, B H
Haque, S
Harling, R E
Harries, A M
Harvey, R S J
Haywood, R J
Haywood, R M
Hedges, K M
Hicks, I P
Hoare, T J
Hood, J E
Hopper, C
Howard, D J
Howell, A P
Howes, D T
Hughes, S P
Hurst, S L
Hyder, M N
Inskip, T G
Iqbal, M
Jackson, R F
Jaiswal, R S
Jones, B G
Jones, C J
Jones, S R
Jones, T M
Kathane, R H
Kavan, R
Kedward, J F
Khanbhai, A T
Khokher, T H
Kirubakaran, S
Kotecha, N
Kruszewska, J W M
Leigh, M
Leonard, S J
Lessell, C B
Lindo, D G
Lindsay, J I
Ling, H-L
Liu, D W H
Lockley, W J
Lotay, N S
Lowe, S W
Lua, S H
MacInnes, R E
Mackellar, B N
McNamara, P A
Manford, M R A
Markar, H R
Marner, S P
Martin, W A
Mason, R C S H
Mehta, R D
Mody, A S
Monk, B E
Monks, D C
Morris, R H
Morris, S J
Morrish, N J
Moxon, R A
Munno, A
Murphy, J P
Murray, R M B
Mutch, A F
Nagreh, B K
Nawal, H C S
Nayar, V K
Neale, E J
Nel, G
Niblett, D J
Nixon, C J
Noel, M G B
Norris, R
O'Neill, E M
O'Rourke, M H
Oakley, R H
Obara, L G
Ogborn, A D R
Onyekwuluje, C E
Parry Okeden, P C U
Patel, A G
Peacock, B
Pead, M E
Pettman, S B
Pocha, M J
Pope, I M
Prior, M
Rae, S A
Rawlins, R D
Read, N E
Reynolds, S F
Riding, W D
Rimmer, D B
Roberts-Thomson, J H
Rochford, J J
Ross, F M
Rowe, P G
Rupasinghe, E P
Ryan, R P
Sattiarajah, A I
Saunders, J H B
Shah, D K
Shaikh, M I
Shankar, A N
Shankar, S
Shanmugaratnam, K
Sharrock, J K C
Simmonds, M J
Singhal, A
Sivabalan, T
Sizer, J M
Skipper, D
Small, D J
Smith, J J M
Snape, S L
Soni, V K
Southgate, C R W
Sowerby, R F
Stanton, J R
Stow, S L
Suddle, A N
Sydenham, D J
Tatman, P J
Taylor, F R
Thomas, H L
Tisi, P V
Todd, O R
Toovey, A J
Toovey, A R
Tredget, J M
Trounson, W N
Ungaro, A R
Valentine, J C
Wallace, R M
Wallis, M
Walsh, A C
Walters, M
Waterfall, N B
Webster, L K
Wheldon, D B
Wijayaratne, W M T
Wilden, S D
Wilkins, I A
Wilkins, M J E
Wilkinson, P S
Wilson, J J
Wilson, J U

Bedlington
Abbey, H B
Forster, D P
Harris, P J S
Harrison, J
Hobson, J E
Marshall, C M
Munro, E W
Starkey, G
Summers, D J
Tallantyre, P M
Todd, J

Bedworth
Charles, E
Menage, J

Beith
Campbell, L M J
Isbister, G I
McCarroll, S E
McRae, C A
Madsen, S
Morrissey, A F
Peggie, D A

Belfast
Abdo, K R
Abernethy, E V
Abraham, H M
Abram, W P
Adair, I V
Adair, J J
Adair, N S S
Adair, S R
Adams, D A
Adams, G
Adams, H E
Addidle, M
Addley, K
Adgey, A A J
Agnew, L M
Alcorn, J R M
Alderdice, J T
Ali, A
Allen, D C
Allen, G S
Allen, G E
Allen, I V
Allen, J D
Allen, J A
Allen, M J
Anderson, N H
Anderson, R J
Anderson, W J A
Andrews, C T
Armstrong, A M
Armstrong, D L
Armstrong, D K B
Armstrong, F T
Armstrong, R
Atkinson, R J
Atkinson, S
Austin, S J
Bailey, I C
Bailie, K E M
Baird, D J R
Baird, R H
Bakry, M A A
Ball, P A
Bamber, J H
Bamford, K B
Barbour, J V R
Barr, R J
Barros D'Sa, E A
Beattie, D C
Bedi, A
Beirne, P K
Beirne, P A
Bell, A H
Bell, A L
Bell, D J A
Bell, J D
Bell, J M
Bell, P F
Bell, P M
Bell, P
Bentley, A J
Beringer, T R O
Best, B G
Best, R M
Beverland, D E
Bharucha, H
Bhat, K K
Bill, K M
Bingham, E A
Black, A J
Black, C E
Black, E A
Blair, J M
Bolton, P W
Bolton, S D J
Bond, E B
Bonnar, G E
Boreland, G J
Bowden, J B
Bowers, M J
Boyd, D D
Boyd, H G M
Boyd, N A M
Boyd, S A S
Boyd, T H
Boyle, D D
Boyle, D M
Boyle, M M I
Bradley, J A G
Bradley, P
Bradley, T
Breach, J F
Bready, K A
Breene, E R
Brennen, M D
Briggs, G M
Briscoe, M
Brooker, D S
Brotherston, T M
Brown, H M
Brown, H C
Brown, J G
Brown, J H
Brown, J A
Brown, P T K
Brown, S
Brown, T
Brown, W M
Browne, F W A
Browne, G A
Browne, J N
Bruce, I N
Bryson, C A
Buchanan, H K
Buchanan, T A S
Buckley, M R E
Burke, B E
Burns, G E
Burrows, B D
Burrows, D
Busby, R E
Byrnes, C K C
Byrnes, D P
Byrnes, S M A
Byrnes, T J D
Cairns, A P
Cairns, C M
Calderwood, C J
Calderwood, J W
Callaghan, M J
Callender, B E
Cameron, R I
Campbell, D K
Campbell, W I
Campbell, W J
Carabine, U A
Carey, P D
Carnaghan, L E
Carser, J E
Carson, C A
Carson, D J
Carson, F D G
Carton, P F
Casement, M E
Casey, Y A
Cashell, C F
Cashell, M P
Cassidy, E E
Caughley, L M
Chakravarty, B
Chambers, S A
Chambers, S J
Chan, S K
Chan, W S
Chan, W C
Chapman, C J D
Chapman, R C
Cheah, F S
Chee, T O C
Cheng, K E
Cheung, C C
Chew, E-W
Chew, M W
Cheyne, D B
Chidrawar, M M
Chin, T M M
Choudhari, K A
Christie, E M
Cinnamond, M J
Clarke, E W
Clarke, G S E
Clarke, J I M
Clarke, J C
Clarke, K E
Clements, J G
Clements, R A
Clements, W D B
Cochrane, B A
Cochrane, D J
Cole, C M
Cole, T B
Colgan, B J
Colleary, G
Collier, J F
Collins, A J
Collins, C J
Collins, F J
Collins, J P
Collins, K M
Collins, V C A
Colton, F M E
Compton, S A
Conn, P G
Connolly, J D R
Connolly, M J
Connolly, N P
Convery, P N
Conway, K P
Conway, M F
Cooke, E A
Cooke, J-L
Cooke, R S
Cooper, S J
Corbett, J R
Corkey, C L
Corr, J F
Corrie, P R
Cosgrove, A P
Cosgrove, S D
Coulson, S M
Coulter, J E M
Cowie, G H
Coyle, D J
Coyle, J M
Coyle, V M
Craig, B F
Craig, B G
Craig, C L
Craig, J J
Craig, J S
Crane, J
Crawley, U C
Crean, P M
Critchlow, M R
Cromey, G M
Cromey, R S
Cromie, A J
Crone, M D
Crossin, C M
Crossin, J D
Crossin, T C
Crothers, J G
Crowther, G R
Crozier, C L
Cruickshanks, S T
Cullen, B M
Cullen, C M
Cullen, M E
Cullen, M
Cummings, A J
Curran, F P
Curran, H J M
Curran, P S
Currie, W P
Curry, R C
Cuthbert, R J G
D'Arcy, F G
Dallas, A J
Dalzell, G W N
Dargan, C B
Darragh, J H
Darragh, P G
Davis, R I
Dawson, J F
Dean, B E
Dearden, C H
Deasy, D M
Deeney, S
Deignan, E B
Dempsey, S I
Devendra, D
Deyermond, R E
Diamond, A M
Diamond, M C
Diamond, P J
Diamond, T
Dick, A G
Dick, C J
Dinsmore, W W
Dixon, R T
Dobson, G
Doherty, C C
Doherty, G M
Doherty, J K
Doherty, M M
Dolan, J J
Dolan, L M
Dolan, O M
Donaghy, J F
Donaldson, R A
Donnelly, C S
Donnelly, D E
Donnelly, M J
Donnelly, M C
Donnelly, R P
Doran, N F
Dougan, J P
Dowey, K E
Downey, M P
Downing, R R C
Doyle, J
Doyle, S M
Droogan, A G
Duffin, M S
Duffy, C M
Duncan, C G
Dunlop, J M
Dunlop, P A
Dunlop, R
Durkan, V J R
Dynan, C E
Dynan, K B
Eakin, R L
Edgar, J D M
Egan, J
El Agnaf, M R
El-Gaddal, A A H
Elliott, J R M
Elliott, P
Emanuel, M Q
English, B
English, F C
Esmonde, T F G
Essandoh, R S
Eu, T Y
Evans, A E
Evans, J R
Fair, B E
Farling, P A
Farnan, B J
Farnan, E P
Farnan, T B
Farrell, J G
Faulkner, P R
Fee, J P H
Ferguson, C J S
Ferguson, H R
Fetherston, M S
Finch, M B
Finlay, F O
Finlay, S R
Finlay, S S A
Finnegan, J M
Finney, E J
Fisher, R B
Fitch, C M
Fitch, M
Fitzpatrick, C R
Fitzpatrick, K T J
Fitzpatrick, M S
Flannery, D J
Fleming, J C
Flett, R H
Flynn, P A
Fogarty, B J
Fogarty, D G
Fogarty, P P
Fon, L J
Forbes, J M
Foy, C J
Frazer, D G
Frew, N C
Froggatt, P
Fryers, S G
Fullerton, K J
Gallacher, C
Gallagher, A
Gallagher, E J
Gallagher, G M
Gardiner, K R

Gardner, C S
Gaston, C H
Gavin, A T
Gawley, S P
George, K A
Gibson, F M
Gibson, J M
Gibson, R
Giles, C M
Giles, C J
Gillespie, I A
Gillespie, P E
Gilligan, C J
Gilligan, M T
Gilliland, A E W
Gillvray, K E
Gilmer, S O
Gilmore, D H
Gilmore, I R
Gilroy, D G
Glackin, S
Glasgow, A C A
Glasgow, J F T
Gleadhill, D N S
Gleadhill, V F D
Glenfield, J E
Glenn, D R J
Glover, P J
Goldsmith, E C
Gordon, D J
Gordon, D S
Gorman, C C
Gorman, C C
Gormley, G J
Gormley, M J J
Gormley, S M C
Gough, F C
Gough, P J
Gracey, S E
Graham, A C
Graham, A
Graham, C J
Graham, D T
Graham, E A
Graham, E L
Grant, B
Gray, J E
Gray, W J
Green, J N S
Gregory, A L
Grey, A C
Gunning, L M
Guy, R L
Guy, S E
Hadden, D R
Hadden, D S M
Hall, J D I
Hall, J G
Hall, J A
Halliday, C
Halliday, H L
Halliday, J A
Hamilton, E A
Hamilton, I S
Hamilton, M S
Hampton, M A
Handley, J M
Hanna, E V
Hannon, R J
Harley, J M G
Harper, E E
Harper, G K
Harper, K W
Harper, M A
Harper, R
Harris, P G
Hart, D C
Hart, P M A
Harvey, C F
Haslam, L J
Hawthorne, P W
Hay, R J
Heaney, A P
Heaney, L G
Hegan, P D
Henderson, S A
Hendron, J G
Henry, P G
Henry, R W
Herdman, G J
Herity, N A
Herron, B M
Hickey, M C A
Higgins, J A
Higgins, S M
Higginson, J D S
Hill, A E
Hill, D A
Hoey, D P W

Holmes, E J
Holmes, L M R
Holterman, K A
Hood, J M
Horner, G F B
Houghton, J P
Houston, J K
Houston, K E
Houston, R F
Howe, J P
Huda, U
Hughes, D A
Hughes, D M
Hughes, J A F
Hughes, M L
Humphreys, R O
Hunter, C M
Hunter, D C
Hunter, O G
Hunter, S J
Huntley, L E
Hurwitz, D S
Hurwitz, J L
Hutchinson, S J
Hyland, M A
Hyland, P N
Hynes, J M
Irvine, A
Irvine, G J G
Irvine, J J B
Irwin, A W
Irwin, D G
Irwin, E A
Irwin, S T
Jackson, C H D
Jackson, W E
Janes, E S
Jefferson, J A
Jhagroo, R R
Johnson, M J
Johnston, G D
Johnston, J M
Johnston, J R
Johnston, L E
Johnston, L C
Johnston, P B
Johnston, P G
Johnston, P W
Johnston, S D
Jones, F G C
Jones, M
Jones, P
Jong, M
Kealey, W D C
Keane, H M I
Keane, M T
Keane, P F
Keilty, S R
Kelly, B E
Kelly, E R
Kelly, J E
Kelly, J E M
Kelly, L S
Kelly, M M T
Kelly, M G
Kelly, M C
Kelly, R E
Kelly, S A T M
Kendrick, R W
Kennedy, J A
Kennedy, P
Kennedy, P T
Kennedy, T G
Kenny, L M
Kerr, A G
Kerr, A N
Kerr, D N
Kerr, H
Kerr, P P
Kerrigan, B M
Kervick, G N
Kettle, P J
Keys, C M
Khan, K
Khoo, B C H
Khosravi-Nezhad, B
Kidd, A M
Kidwai, B J
Kilbane, M P J K
Kilgore, H J
King, C M
King, S M
King, T C F
Kinney, A M
Kirk, C D
Kirk, G R
Kirk, K S
Kirk, S J
Kirkpatrick, D H

Kitara-Okot, P
Knight, C M
Knox, L M
Kuan, Y C
Kyle, S J
Lai, H K
Lalsingh, I R
Lambe, D E
Lamki, H M N
Lasa Gallego, M A
Laverick, M D
Lavery, A G
Lavery, P E
Lawler, A M
Lawson, J T
Leach, J G
Lee, A L
Lee, D E T
Lee, J T-S
Lee, S M
Leggett, J J
Leggett, P F
Leitch, A J
Lenfesty, J P
Lennox, J D
Leonard, A G
Leonard, N
Lewis, A E
Li, A H-Y
Lim, C T S
Lim, C C
Lim, P L
Lim, Y Y
Lindsay, K G
Little, J M
Little, M A
Livingstone, A F
Loane, B J
Loane, R A
Lockie, P D
Logan, J I
Logan, M-L
Lotery, A J
Loughrey, A C B
Loughrey, C B M
Loughrey, C M
Loughrey, C M
Loughrey, M B
Loughrey, P G
Loughridge, E A
Loughridge, J C H
Loughridge, R J
Loughridge, W G G
Lovell, S L
Lowry, J P S
Lowry, K A
Lowry, K G
Lua, Y C
Lundy, G P P
Lynas, R F A
Lynas, W J
Lynch, G M
Lynch, J V
Lynch, T H
Lyness, R W
Lyons, J D M
Lyons, S M
Lyttle, J A
Lyttle, K D L
McAlea, P M
McAleer, J J A
Mcaleese, J J
McAllister, A S
McAllister, J M
Mcareavey, F E
MaCartney, C A
McAtamney, D G
McAteer, J A
McAteer, M P
McAughey, J M
McAuley, D F
Macauley, D C
McAuley, D M
McAuley, E M J
Mcauley, M R
McBride, M O
McBride, W T
McCabe, N E E
McCaffrey, J E
Mccallion, W A
McCance, D R
McCann, J P
McCarroll, C P
McCarthy, B T
McCarthy, M A
McCarthy, M D
McCartney, M
McCarty, D
McCarty, H A

McCaughan, J F G
Mccaughey, C P J
McCaughey, M
McCauley, A A M
McCay, N M
McClean, M
McCleery, A J
McCleery, M R
McClelland, R
McClelland, W M
McClements, B M
McCloskey, B V
McCloskey, M S
McCloy, M P
McCluggage, J R
McClure, K A
McClure, M C
McClure, N
McCluskey, C
McCluskey, D R
McCollum, J S C
McComb, D W
McConkey, C D
McConkey, M J
McConnell, L A
McConnell, R G C
McConway, J H F
McCormack, S R E
McCourt, K C
Mccoy, E P
McCoy, G F M
McCracken, S R C
McCrea, G W
McCreesh, G A
McCrory, D C
McCullagh, C D
McCullagh, M R
McCullins, M E
McCutcheon, A
McDonald, G H
McDonald, P A
McDonnell, A
McDonnell, G V
McElhenny, B E
McElwaine, A V
McEvoy, M D
McEwen, E A M
McFarland, G L
McFarland, M A
McFarland, R J
McFerran, K
McGarrity, S J
McGarry, C J P
McGarry, P J
McGarvey, L P A
McGeough, P T
McGeown, J G
McGibben, B F
McGinn, C M S
McGinnity, F G
McGlade, K J
McGleenon, B M
McGlennon, D M
McGonigle, R J
McGovern, A E
McGovern, M C
McGovern, S M M
McGovern, T D
McGovern, V M
McGowan, D J
MacGowan, S W
McGrath, K J
McGrogan, P J
McGuffin, K M
McGurk, C T
McHenry, S M
McHugh, C J
McHugh, J O P
McHugh, S J A
Mcllmoyle, E L
Mcllrath, E M
Mcllroy, R L
Mclver, M S
Mclvor, P J
McKaigue, J P
McKane, W R
McKay, A C
McKee, C H W
McKee, G J
McKee, R H
McKeever, G J K
McKelvey, A
McKelvey, S T D
McKenna, D J J
McKenna, G L
McKenna, J F
McKenna, K E
McKenna, M P
McKenna, M P

McKeown, D S P
McKeown, E F
McKeown, P B
McKeown, R P
McKernan, M F
McKie, L D
McKinney, M S
McKinstry, A R
McKinstry, C S
McLaverty, D M
MacLennan, B A
McLorinan, G C
McLoughlin, C M
McLoughlin, C C
McLoughlin, J C
McLoughlin, J S
MacMahon, J
McMahon, N M
McMahon, R
McManus, D T
McManus, J
Macmanus, M P
McManus, T E
McMaster, J I
McMechan, S R
McMillan, J A
McMillan, J C
McMillan, M I
McMillen, H K
McMillin, W P
McMullan, M J
McMullen, E A
McMullin, M F
McNaboe, E J D
McNally, D P G
McNally, J R A
McNamee, D A
McNamee, H M
McNarry, A F
McNeill, J
McNeill, S I
McNicholl, B P G
McNutt, C E
Macpherson, C
Macsorley, M P
MacSorley, P J
McVeigh, G E
McVeigh, L M
McVicker, J M
Magee, A C
Magee, G D
Mageean, A M
Magill, E A
Maginn, P
Maguire, B
Maguire, D F
Maguire, O T
Maini, A K
Mainie, I M L
Maitland, J E
Mallon, P W G
Manderson, L L
Mangan, B G
Mangan, C M
Manoharan, G
Manwell, M K C
Mark, M C
Markey, G M
Marsh, D R
Marshall, B A
Marshall, C A
Marshall, D F
Martin, A C
Martin, D
Martin, G R C
Martin, J B
Martin, M F T
Martin, P S
Masroor, T
Mathews, H M L
Matthews, C F
Maw, R D
Mawhinney, H J D
Maxwell, A P
Maxwell, M
Maxwell, R J
Mee, J D
Meenan, G W
Mercer, C I
Middleton, A M N
Miller, R L
Milligan, K R
Milligan, S
Milliken, J A H
Minford, H D F
Mirakhur, A
Mirakhur, M
Mirakhur, R K
Mitchell, D J

Mitchell, E
Mitchell, R M S
Molloy, M E
Monaghan, C A
Moncrieff, E M
Montgomery, E A
Montgomery, S A
Moohan, V P
Moore, A L
Moore, J E
Moorehead, R J
Morgan, B J F
Morris, T C M
Morrison, P J
Morrison, R L
Morrow, J I
Morrow, V S
Mottiar, N S
Moyes, D A
Moynihan, P
Muldoon, O T
Mulgrew, J A
Mulhern, M F
Mulholland, H C
Mulholland, K C
Mulholland, M G
Mullally, B
Murdock, E M
Murnaghan, M E
Murphy, B G
Murphy, G J J
Murphy, R D
Murphy, T F B
Murray, J M A
Murtagh, E G
Murtagh, J G
Murthy, K
Mustafa, M A B
Neagle, E H
Neeson, C
Neill, A K
Nelson, J K
Nelson, J K
Nelson, K A
Nelson, W E
Nelson, W M
Nethercott, R G
Newlands, L C
Ng, B Y
Ng, C S H
Ng, K S L
Nicholas, J
Nicholas, R M
Nicholls, D P
Nicholson, M J
Noh, M B M
Nolan, C P
Nugent, A M
O'Connor, B G
O'Connor, M G
O'Connor, P J
O'Doherty, A J
O'Donnell, M T
O'Gorman, C
O'Hagan, S J
O'Hara, M D
O'Hare, D M
O'Hare, M P
O'Kane, A E
O'Kane, D J
O'Kane, D
O'Kane, H F G
O'Kane, H O
O'Keeffe, D B
O'Loan, A A
O'Neill, G D
O'Neill, H F
O'Neill, T W
O'Rawe, A M
O'Rourke, D M
O'Sullivan, A K
Odling-Smee, G W
Ogbobi, S E
Oneill, M F
Ong, G M L
Ong, H Y
Ong, Y L
Ong, Y L
Orr, D H
Owens, P J
Owusuansa, N
Park, E J
Park, R M
Parke, R C
Parke, S C
Parks, L
Parks, T G
Passmore, A P
Paterson, A

Patterson, A S
Patterson, C E
Patterson, D G
Patterson, G C
Patterson, J K
Patterson, V H
Patton, L
Patton, W C
Paulin, M N M
Paxton, L D
Pendleton, A
Perrin, M E
Phillips, A S
Pinkerton, R M
Pitt, J B
Porter, G J R
Potts, S R
Power, M J P
Price, J H
Primrose, E D
Purcell, C
Quinn, F M
Quinn, M J
Quinn, S R
Rafferty, C G
Rafferty, M S
Rainey, G J
Rainey, G W
Rainey, N A
Rainey, R S
Ramsay-Baggs, P
Ramsey, H C
Ramsey, J C P
Ranaghan, E A
Rankin, S J A
Raphael, A M
Rea, G R
Refsum, S E
Reid, A J M
Reid, I A C
Reid, J E
Reid, M A
Reid, M M
Reid, P T
Reilly, P
Renfrew, C W
Rethinasamy, E L
Richardson, R J
Richardson, S G
Riddell, G
Riddell, J W
Ritchie, I S D
Roberts, M J D
Roberts, R N
Roberts, S D
Robinson, F E
Robinson, J M
Robinson, K A
Robinson, R K
Rocke, L G
Rodden, N D
Roddie, K A
Rodgers, C
Rodgers, S A
Rodrigues, R J C
Rogan, J T
Rooney, P J
Ross, A M
Ross, R W D
Rowan, I G
Rowan, M G
Rowney, W R
Rudralingam, M
Rudralingam, V
Ruiz Herrero, A L
Rusk, R A
Russell, C F J
Russell, J C
Russell, M F
Rutherford, J R
Ryan, A M
Ryan, R J
Sadler, M A
Salathia, K S
Samuel, M
Sandhu, S K
Savage, D M
Savage, J M
Sawh, B
Sawhney, B B
Scally, M J
Scoffield, J L
Scott, C E
Scott, J N
Scott, K C
Scott, K W
Scott, L C
Scott, T J
Shamoun, O S A M
Shannon, J M
Sharkey, J J M
Sharkey, P J
Sharma, P
Sharp, E
Shaw, R A
Shaw, V J E
Shaw, Y P
Shearer, K
Shearer, R M
Shepherd, D R T
Sherwood, J I
Shields, E G
Shields, M D
Shiels, A M K
Shum, P L
Shyamsundar, S
Silvestri, G
Simpson, D I H
Simpson, R
Singh, S
Sinnott, B S
Skan, D I M
Skelly, R T
Sloan, J M
Sloan, M K
Sloan, S
Sloan, S C
Small, C
Small, F M
Small, J O
Small, R B
Smith, D J
Smith, P
Smyth, E T M
Smyth, F
Smyth, F B
Smyth, J S
Smyth, R
Somerville, J E
Spence, R A J
Spence, S D
Stamm, R G W
Steele, E K
Steele, I C
Steele, W K
Steen, H J
Stevens, A B
Stewart, A H R
Stewart, F J
Stewart, M C
Stewart, P C
Stewart, R C
Stockman, N J T
Stout, R W
Stranex, S
Swain, A
Swain, K B
Swain, W D
Swann, M A
Sweeney, D
Sweeney, L E
Sweet, D G
Taggart, A J
Taggart, C M
Taggart, H M
Tallon, G M
Tan, K S
Tan, M C S
Tate, S
Tay McGarry, G S
Taylor, I C
Taylor, R H
Taylor, T C
Tennet, H M
Tham, T C K
Thompson, A W
Thompson, A M
Thompson, E M
Thompson, E J
Thompson, N S
Thompson, R N J
Thompson, W
Thornbury, G D
Thornbury, K D
Thornton, C M
Thornton, P D
Toal, B J
Todd, D O
Tohill, M P
Toland, J M P
Toner, J G
Tracey, M E
Traub, A I
Trimble, F M
Trimble, W G C
Trinick, T R
Tsang, W C
Tsang, W K
Turner, A J
Twinem, G S
Ullah, R M
Vallely, S R
Vaughan, P K
Wadgaonkar, P S
Walby, A P
Walker, N J P
Walker, S
Walker, S H
Walker, W H A
Wallace, W F M
Walsh, I K
Walsh, M Y
Ward, R P S
Wasson, C
Waterman, M R
Watkins, D C
Watt, M
Watters, J P
Waugh, P K
Weaver, J A
Webb, C H
Webb, S W
Weir, P E
Wells, M D
White, D W
White, D S
White, J A
White, J B
White, S T
Whiteside, R J
Wiggam, M I
Wilde, J C
Wilkinson, A J
Wilkinson, P
Williamson, G F
Williamson, G
Williamson, S K
Willis, C E
Willis, J
Wilson, A E J
Wilson, A G C
Wilson, B G
Wilson, C S
Wilson, C M
Wilson, C M
Wilson, D B
Wilson, G A
Wilson, J M
Wilson, J E
Wilson, J M
Wilson, L
Wilson, P J K
Wilson, P J
Wilson, R H
Wilson, R K
Wilson, S J
Wilson, S D
Wilson, W N
Wilson, Y T
Windrum, P
Winn, J H
Wolsley, K
Wong, G T
Wong, Y W
Woodman, A M
Woodrow, E A
Woods, J P
Woods, J D
Wright, G D
Wright, R E R
Yam, T S
Yamin-Ali, R G
Yarnell, J W G
Yoon, L L
Young, C M
Young, I S
Younger, J M

Belford
Gill, D K
Miller, E C
Miller, S N
Pawson, R H
Williams, P G

Bellshill
Bradshaw, T A
Duncan, E M
Elder, A G
Fletcher, L O A
Kelly, C A
Lindsay, K
McKibbin, C M
Muir, W J
Ritchie, S A

Belper
Atherton, S J
Barkham, M H
Batty, R
Bold, T A W P
Brentnall, C J
Brett, M J E
Bronks, I G
Chapman, M G T
Cooke, D
Fairweather, J E
Giovannelli, M A
Hanson, S A
Leyland, B
Marshall, P M
Moore, R J
Narborough, G C
O'Flanagan, P H
Poll, D J
Rutherford, J M
Stephenson, J D
Stevens, C E
Venables, M G M
Wright, D G
Young, J G

Belvedere
Adagra, M B
Dave, R J
De Waal, F
Kapur, S K
Lyons-Nandra, S S
Mandl, S A
Pattison, D C
Roy, S R
Sehgal, N N
Taylor, E C

Bembridge
Kaula, C V
McComb, P E F
Thomas, D S

Benfleet
Baker, R J N
Beresford, T P
Betts-Brown, A
Bunney, J A
Dhingra, S K
Gardiner, R A
Gill, S S
Gupta, S K
Gutteridge, H J
Hiscock, S C
Leahy, P D
Lemmens, J A
Lester, M J
McGladdery, J A
Mott, H W
Patel, B R
Patel, R M
Pope, J A F
Smith, M J
Smithson, D L
Tan, L A
Timms, R L
Trotter, G G
Waiwaiku, K N
Wessels, H M A H
Wilde, J P

Berkeley
Higgs, S J
James, F E
Longstaff, A J
Ludlow, B P
Walshe, P B
Wilson, P

Berkhamsted
Aitchison, E I
Andrews, C J
Banerji, A K
Chuter, G S J
Cohen, J A
Conway, Z F
Corbin, C J
Currie, C L A
Dalton, R S J
Evans, J B
Evans, S C
Franc, N L
Garner, A J J
Hallan, L A
Manton, H E
Merrett, K D
Nath, A R
Nicholls, M J
Ormiston, I N R
Ponsonby, C E
Ramsay, B
Rennie, I G
Rice-Edwards, S A
Roythorne, J P
Sargaison, J M
Squire, A J
Suchy, K C
Taylor, R A
Thirlwall, A S
Thornber, A J
Walker, R I
Williams, H F
Williams, R A

Berwick-upon-Tweed
Bromly, A C
Cheek, B N
Fisken, J
Knight, R A
Mather, R F
Mitchell, J H
Nesbitt, L E
O'Dwyer, T M
Reavley, P D A
Semple, G A
Smith, B C H
Spink, M
Watson, I F
Watson, J M
Wood, P F A
Wooding, R M S
Wright, H M

Betchworth
Crawshaw, J W A
Jenner, G J
Kober, P H
Mathews, B H
Rawson, L E
Sevenoaks, T A
Webster-Smith, C S
Whiteley, J S

Betws-y-Coed
Metcalfe, R E
Park, A V

Beverley
Ali, S A
Ashley, S D
Bawn, B L
Bestley, J W
Branton, J F
Carruthers, S C
Chapman, R D
Clayton, G L
Clifton, J
Cooper, D D
Dale, S S
Dale, S P
Donnan, R H C
Donohue, J S
Fairfield, G E
Gillespie, J M
Glover, K J
Griffin, S C
Hardisty, P
Harley, A M
Hill, S A
Hogg, D C
Huckvale, B F
Hutchinson, W A
Ikin, P N
Ilangaratne, J B
Jones, P G
Kennan, N M
Kerin, M J
Lee, P W R
Lyons, C L
Mabbott, J L
Mann, S L
Marwah, K S
Menon, M
Milner, A C
Mixer, P R
Morris, P J
Murphy, B A M
Patmore, J E
Phillips, K
Ratnavel, C D
Rowland, G P
Ryan, D H
Shaw, J N
Shearing, L J
Slade, A M
Sowerby, M K J
Stafford, H G
Stafford, N D
Stirling, J G
Stirling, V A
Sugars, K H
Suri, H S
Sutton, R J
Sykes, A J
Underwood, A D
Wade, A
Walters, M I
Weatherill, W F
Weldon, D P
White, A S C
Williams, D F
Williams, G D V
Williams, S B
Williams, T I R
Wilson, J A
Wylie, A M

Bewdley
Bidgood, R A
Cooper, J H
Dyson, J A
Gottschalk, B
Green, C A
Haynes, S V Z
Holloway, B J
Inglis, I M
Kumar, R
Limbrick, R A
McLachlan, C J H
Marriott, R G
Meggy, J M
Montandon, P E
Mulder, F A
Orange, M
Paton, J S H
Prince, C B
Rumley, S J

Bexhill-on-Sea
Al-Ansary, Y
Ashby, S M
Brown, E
Chalkias, I
Craig, G R
Crawford, J A
Dewhurst, P D
Eaton, J C R
Elias, R G
Emmanuel, J H
Gonzalez Polledo, J
Hadley, L A-A
Harrison, K M
Hawley, W L
Hunter, G M
Kinch, H W A
Kramer, S
Kremer, D J
Lacey, E M
Lawton, D J
Ludwig, Z J
Maloney, F E
Maxwell, T G
Myrddin-Evans, T O W
Newell, D N
Plumpton, H P
Radwan, R R M I
Rajanathan, E
Ramachander, C B
Robinson, M K
Scott, L G
Sharma, R
Singh, G
Sitwell, I A H
Southward, S P
Thompson, A J
Thompson, A R
Thomson, A G
Thomson, S R
Waller, J G
Walter, N R
Warden, D J
Watson, D B D

Bexley
Ayto, R M
Banerjee, A
Banerjee, T K
Boomla, R F
Chan, J M W
Cota, A M
Guryel, E H
Hirons, J M
Hoogewerf, M
Malone, S T
Mendonca, S
Owen, S

Pyszora, N M
Raine, G J
Saiz, A M B
Simmons, R L L
Skarsten, A R H
Somasegaram, P D
Srinivas, R K
Sykes, R A
Thavapalan, N D
Thenuwara, C
Virdee, M S
Walter, I M
Wedderspoon, A D

Bexleyheath
Barnett, A M
Berg, S N
Cameron, E A
Chase, P N
Chase, S B
Chowdhury, A M
De Souza, P B
Easwar, M D
Forshaw, H B B
Goddard, C A
Griffin, A E
Hale, J M
Hammatt, M D
Harrison, N S C
Hatfull, D M
Joyner, N
Kumar, S K
Kwan, W K C
Maini, P
Maizels, D W
Malone, A M
Mehta, M M
Nour, H
Perera, D C
Pollock, J A
Quarterman, E A
Rajaratnam, S
Rajshekhar, M S
Shah, H K
Singh, R
Stoate, H G A
Streetly, A
Strevens, M J
Thavapalan, M
Thomas, J C
Tolhurst, J
Whitehead, G A
Williams, R I J

Bicester
Ainsworth, Q P
Anderson, T W D
Attwood, S P
Bailey, R C
Bennett, L S
Bliss, G A S
Brand, J S G
Brooks, A S B
Burgess, S A
Cox, G H
Curry, M J
Ealing, K M
Flintan, B A
Fox, R A
Galuszka, J A
Gibson, A F B
Grimshaw, D R
Halsey, C
Hannon, D G
Holt, J
Horne, C A
Jackman, J R
Jones, J R
Langstaff, R J
McDonald, B
Martin, H P L
Miller, B J
Moncrieff, G C
Murphy, A E H
Ragheb, E A A
Ridley, N T F
Robbins, S E
Rowlands, A
Saunders, L J
Saunders, T H
Stephenson, R H
Talbot, J M
Thompson, N
Tofts, L J
Van Stigt, E S
Wait, C M
Weaver, H P
Williams, T
Windsor, A M

Bideford
Atkinson, E
Belsey, G
Bradbeer, P J
Brown, K P
Brummitt, P J
Buckland, R H
Clayton, M R
Cook, G T J
Cracknell, M M
Daly, G A
David, J C C
Dean, R P
Diamond, A J
Ford, R G
Ford, S G
Henderson, A S
Herriott, S L
Hill, S G
Knight, G
Latham, A
Loka-Saleh, R M
Milburn, D W
Moore, A
Moore, E M
Pritchard, K A
Spencer, G S
Wilson, J G M
Wood, J S
Young, E A

Biggar
Bewsher, M R
Browning, J A
Cameron, F S
Cameron, J A
Carvel, D R
Clerihew, L J
Dobbie, A E
Elder, A M
Galloway, R J
Goldie, A M D
Gourlay, R G
Leitch, J M
Leitch, R G
McGregor, P G
Munro, A M
Rodger, K A
Tiley, M J
Watt, A M

Biggleswade
Butcher, R A
Chowdhary, U M
Dowsett, A O
Evans, C M
Hollington, W A
Low, A C S
Marshall, F T
Mason, R B S
Momen, S A
Murnal, S B
Taylor, A J

Billericay
Afifi, A
Almond, M K
Brown, F M
Butler, S J C
Chatterjee, K L
Chatterjee, S
Clear Hill, B G R
Cockcroft, J H J
Copsey, M D
Das Gupta, A L
Das Gupta, R
Denham, M M
Durani, S K
Fernie, T C
Giles, R M
Gupta, C P
Hayden, P G
Hui, W L
Knight, J S
Kukathasan, P
Kumar, S
Lai, S H-L
Lazell, G J
Lee, S P-C
McGoldrick, A N
Morley, C
Nadarajah, K
Nunn, T
Pain, V M
Pollard, M A
Roberts, J K
Sarfraz, A M
Sarfraz, M-U-H
Shen, R N

Sirotakova, M
Sofoluwe, G O
Thomson, L F
Tin Loi, S F
Ware, S J
Wilkinson, N M R
Williams, A C P
Willoughby, C P

Billingham
Adebayo, A O
Chatterjee, P P K
Clish, D
Elborough, A Y
Fenwick, S
Fordham, J N
Gartner, C P
Geoghegan, H F
Gittens, M J
Goorbarry, M D
Gosalia, N H
Irvine, A J
Joyce, C A
Lockey, K N
Longwill, J M
Murphy, R S
O'Donoghue, J P
Rasool, S
Reynolds, R P
Ritchie, P
Sinclair, J A G
Walton, L J
West, S C

Billingshurst
Balme, G M
Broughton, M D
Crabb, S J
Drummond, J
Dunne, R D C
Jones, N J
Leach, A R
Margetts, G
Meanock, C I
Polwin, P J S
Rouse, D A
Tabb, P A
Williams, A E
Wood, C G M

Bilston
Adma, L
Anandakumar, P
De, S K
Hossain, M
Kumar, S
Lal, C
Morris, T A
Patel, M K
Pope, J D K
Rangel, R L
Sharma, S V
Than, M
Tinsa, J S

Bingley
Andrews, E C
Bairstow, T E
Busby, C R
Claxton, B A
Davies, A B
Dawe, B C E
Duke, F C
Fieldhouse, D C
Findlay, J M
Flockton, E A
Haslam, G H
Hassan, F A
Hattam, S A L
Horsfield, M J
Jeffrey, R F
Jennings, K L
Jones, S E
Jowett, L J
Knappett, P A
Ludlow, E L
Newton, D A G
Price, J J
Pushpangadan, M
Rai, N
Robson, K H
Stewart, P A H
Vesey, J
Vesey, R J
Wallis, G G

Birchington
Eddington, J
Eddington, W A

Fletcher, M W
Freedman, R C
Garland, J K
Hayden, J T D
Jackson, N C
O'Donoghue, E

Birkenhead
Alauddin, K
Amily, G S
Arthur, C P
Austen, J M
Boylan, B G
Brace, C A
Brayley, M
Brodbin, C
Cameron, E F
Caslin, A W
Charles, E J
Cookson, I B
Cookson, N M P
Coombs, D M
Courtney, D B
Cullen, M
Cunningham, J L
Davies, J A
Davies, M G
Dillon, I J
Dixon, T A
Dodd, M D
Dow, J M
Dow, S C
Edwards, E M H
Edwards, R W
Ellis, B R
Fallowfield, R E
Ferguson, R E
Franklin, J
Freeman, M J
Galvani, D W
Grant, P J
Green, D H
Green, M J
Hardaker, E A
Harding, S G
Harris, N L
Hill, D R
Hilton, R C
Holley, J M
Howard, J E
Hughes, P A
Jones, M M
Jones, W W
Karyampudi, P
Kenyon, C M
Kidd, C M T
Leigh, R F
Lewis, A H
Lowe, D C
McKay, J P
Mairs, P P
Malcolm, J E
Mantgani, A B
Massey, K
Mawdsley, J
Melville, J A
Metcalfe, C E
Mohan, D
Munro, M A
Naughton, M D
Noorpuri, R S
Nuttall, P J
Onion, C W R
Oolbekkink, M
Owers, D L
Owers, F M
Patel, R S
Paterson, E A
Raines, R J H
Ratnaike, N D A
Ream, J E
Renwick, J A
Roberts, M L
Romaniuk, D A
Roper, J P
Rowlands, A G
Ryall, C J
Salahuddin, M
Satchithananthan, S
Seager, J
Selvarajah, D T
Seymour, P J
Smethurst, F A
Soe Aung, Dr
Stevens, L E
Stokell, R A
Strang, L
Sturgess, R P
Syed, M F

Tan, A T-L
Taylor, A J
Taylor, B W
Thomas, J G
Thomson, L E
Vaillant, C H
Vangikar, M M
Vogwell, P C
Walker, C V S
Walters, A E
Wardale, J G
Whalley, J T
Williams, D H
Williams, R M
Woodrow, J C
Wu, K H J

Birmingham
Aas, O G B
Abbas, S
Abrol, V
Abudu, A T
Acharya, M P
Acheson, N
Ackroyd, R S
Acland, P R
Adab, P
Adam, D J
Adams, J L
Adlakha, S
Adu, D
Affie, E M
Afnan, A M M
Agwu, S C
Ahamed, H A
Ahamed, M
Ahmad, N
Ahmad, S
Ahmad, S Z
Ahmad, Y
Ahmed, A H
Ahmed, B
Ahmed, I
Ahmed, I
Ahmed, Q W
Ahmed, R
Ahmed, S K
Ahmed, Z
Ainsworth, J R
Aitchison, F A
Ajimal, S K
Akbar, A
Akhtar, A
Akhtar, R
Al-Aaraji, Y M S
Al-Ansari, I K
Al-Kadi, K
Al-Mawali, S H
Alam, M
Aldridge, F R
Ali, A
Ali, A H M S
Ali, Z
Allan, A-M T
Allan, R N
Allaway, E J
Allen, C H
Allen, G M
Allen, M P
Allin, D M
Allington-Smith, P J
Allroggen, H
Alonzo, K H R
Alton, H M
Aluwihare, N P
Ambasht, D P
Amin, U R
Amir, W P
Anees, N W
Anfilogoff, N H
Ansari, M Z R H
Anwar, M
Appiah, S K
Appleford, J K
Archer, V R
Arif, M H
Arif, M R
Arif, S
Arkell, D G
Armitage, L E
Armstrong, F M
Armstrong, H J
Armstrong, L B
Arnold, A J
Arora, G R
Arora, K J
Arora, P P
Ashcroft, M E
Ashton, J

Ashton, W D
Asif, M
Asif, M
Asker, D C
Asquith, J R
Atwal, S S
Aukland, A
Auth, M K-H
Aveyard, P N
Aw, T-C
Aylin, D R
Azam, S
Bache, C E
Bacon, P A
Badawi, H I
Badger, I L R
Baghdadi, S H N
Bagshaw, O N T
Bailey, G M
Bainbridge, E T
Baird, M S
Bajaj, B P S
Bajpai, A C
Bakhshi, S S
Balasubramaniam, R N
Ball, J A
Ball, S T
Ballantyne, S L
Ballesteros Jeronimo, M S
Baloch, K G
Bancroft, G N
Bancroft, J
Bandara, D S P K
Bandopadhyay, S
Bandyopadhyay, B C
Bandyopadhyay, S
Banerjee, D J
Banerjee, S T
Banerjee, S K
Banham, S P
Banks, M J
Bansel, J K
Barber, J M P
Barber, K J
Barber, P J
Barford, D J
Barker, C P G
Barnes, S J
Barnett, A H
Barraclough, C R
Barratt, D J
Barret, C M
Barrett, J S
Barrett, T G
Barron, D J
Barros D'Sa, I J
Barry, J-S
Barry, R J A
Bartlett, M A
Basil, K-T
Batch, A J G
Bate, C
Bates, G D L
Bath, S S
Bathla, V
Batra, S
Batta, K
Baxter, M A
Bayliss, H G
Beach, J R
Beath, S V
Beatson-Hird, J F
Beattie, J M
Beazley, M F
Beedie, M A
Beevers, D G
Begum, H
Beighton, P G
Belhag, M A A
Benbow, J A
Benham, J D
Benham, M
Bennett, J M
Bennett, R J
Bent, J A
Berovic, M N
Berry, K
Betts, T A
Bevan, P G
Beyer, P M
Bhadri, A D
Bhardwaj, M K
Bhaskar, V A P
Bhatia, R K
Bhatt, K B
Bhattacharyya, B
Bhatti, R A
Bhatti, S

Bhimji, Y S
Bhomra, D S
Bhullar, M S
Bickley, P
Bindal, T
Bindman, E
Bion, J F
Birch, L J
Bird, A P
Birkill, R J
Birmingham, J S
Birmingham, L S
Birtle, J
Bishay, E S S
Bissenden, J G
Biswas, S
Biswas, S
Blackford, P
Blaggan, A S
Blake, D H
Bland, N C
Blaney, A
Blows, M
Bluglass, J M K
Bluglass, R S
Blunt, S M
Boden, J M
Boden, J L
Bond, M
Boniface, K J
Bonser, R S
Boorman, D G
Booth, I W
Borg-Bartolo, P P
Bosworth, M R
Botha, R A
Boulter, A R
Bowden, G
Bowden, M I
Bowser, J
Boyce, D E
Bradberry, S M
Bradbury, M J E
Bradby, G V H
Bradford, A P J
Bradish, C F
Bradley, S A
Bradshaw, K A
Bradwell, A R
Bramhall, S R
Brammer, R D
Brawn, C M
Brawn, W J
Brewin, M D
Brierley, A F M
Bright-Thomas, R M
Bright-Thomas, R J
Bright, P
Brinksman, S
Bromley, P N
Brookes-White, P J S
Brookes, S K
Broomhead, M E
Brown, A M S
Brown, G T
Brown, G J
Brown, M
Brown, N P
Brown, R M
Brown, S E
Browne, S D
Brueton, L A
Bruton, L A
Bryan, R T
Bryson, P H R
Buckels, J A C
Buckley, A M
Budh-Raja, V P
Buick, R G
Buller, N P
Burden, A C
Burdon, M A
Burge, A
Burge, P S
Burges, D C E
Burke, S J
Burls, A J E
Butcher, A J
Butler, J A M
Butler, L
Cadbury, N L
Cadigan, P J
Calderwood, D K O D
Calderwood, V S
Cameron, D S A
Cameron, J
Campbell, A J G
Campbell, C M
Campbell, F E
Canham, N L E
Carey, M P
Carlish, S
Carnie, J C
Carroll, A M
Carruthers, D M
Carson, A J B
Carter, S R
Carter, S R
Cartmill, A D
Carver, E D
Cash, H T
Cassam, K
Casson, P A
Caswell, L P
Cathcart, M
Cathcart, V H
Cayton, R M
Chadwick, V L
Chan, K K
Chan, N T-Y
Chan, S Y
Chander, A
Chaparala, B C
Chapman, A L N
Chapman, S
Charon, J-P M
Chaudary, A H
Chaudhary, S M
Cheel, C
Cheema, M N
Cheetham, J N H
Cheng, K K
Cherry, R C
Chetiyawardana, A D
Cheung, G W Y
Cheung, R C-Y
Child, V M
Chilton, A P
Chilvers, J P
Chitnis, A J
Chokshi, N C
Chokshi, U N
Choudry, G A
Chowdhary, S
Christodoulou, C
Chu, W W-C
Chudley, S M
Chukwulobelu, R N
Chunduri, D R
Clarke, C E
Clarke, H G
Clarke, J R
Clarke, P F F
Clarkson, M E
Clay, S N
Cleasby, M J
Clifton, P J M
Clutton-Brock, T H
Cockel, R
Cockerham, R
Cockwell, P
Coddington, T
Coe, T R
Cole, F
Cole, R
Cole, T R P
Coleman, G M
Coleman, N S
Collard, J M
Colley, J J
Collin, M B
Collingham, K E
Collins, P L
Colloby, P S
Commander, M J
Commander, R A D
Condie, R G
Condley, M
Conlon, M H
Conrad, V A
Constantinides, S
Cook, D M
Cook, M A
Cooke, A M
Cooke, M A
Cooner, M K
Cooper, B T
Cooper, G M
Cooper, H M
Cooper, J P
Cooper, M R
Cope, R V
Corfan, E
Corkery, J J
Cormac, I D
Corrie, T
Cotterill, C P
Court, B V
Coward, A D
Coward, C M A
Cox, P A
Craigen, M A C
Crawford, S L
Crocker, C B
Crocker, C
Crombie, C M
Cross, V H
Crowe, P M
Crowley, N L H
Cullen, L
Cullen, M H
Cunliffe, I A
Cunningham, M J I
Curran, R C
D'Silva, M R
D'Urso, P J
Dadheech, H H
Dadheech, V K
Dakin, M C
Dalal, B M
Dale, R C
Daly, A S J
Daly, J E
Daly, P J
Damoa-Siakwan, S A
Daniell, P A
Das, I
Dasgupta, S R
Davies, A J
Davies, A L
Davies, A M
Davies, C M
Davies, J H
Davies, P H
Davies, R R
Davies, S R
Davis, H
Davis, J M
Dawkins, D M
Dawson, D E
Dawson, K G
Daya, P
De Giovanni, J V
De Wildt, G R
Deacon, K R
Deb, S
Debelle, G D
Debenham, S E
Deiry, A A
Del Bene, R
Delaney, B C
Deluz, J E
Derrick, G M
Derry, D D
Desai, M
Deshmukh, S C
Desveaux, J-C
Deuchar, N J
Devarajan, R
Dhaliwal, J S
Dhamija, S K
Dhanji, F Z
Dhariwal, A S
Dibdin, E M
Dicker, B J
Diwan, S P
Dodson, P M
Doe, W F
Doggett, J M
Doherty, A P
Doherty, N J
Dominey, J A
Donaldson, I
Donnelly, H M
Donovan, I A
Dor, R
Doughty, H-A
Dover, M S
Downes, M K
Dowson, L J
Doyle, M A
Doyle, P
Drake-Lee, A B
Drake, S M
Drayson, M T
Drever, W M H
Du Feu, M
Dubash, D H
Duddy, M J
Dudley, P M
Dullehan, R M S
Dunlop, D J
Dunne, F P M
Dunstan, C M
Dunstan, E J
Durbin, G M
Durkin, D J
Durston, G W
Dwarakanath, L S
Dyer, P H
Eagle, C D
Eardley, K S
Ebert, F H
Eccleshall, S C
Eccleston, D B
Edmunds, J P
Edward, M G
Edwards, G J
Edwards, J H
Edwards, S C
Ehtisham, J
Ehtisham, S
Eke, A J
El-Farok, M O
El Mankabady, S F
El-Sheikh, O A-E A
Elcock, S K
Elgon, J J A
Elias, E
Elliott, C I
Elliott, S C
Elliott, T S J
Ellis, C J
Ellis, S C
Ellwood, H L
Ely, J C J
Emens, J M
Emery, D G
Empson, K
England, E J R
Engledow, A H
English, M W
Enriquez Puga, A
Escofet Martinez De Arenzana, X
Evans, H M
Evans, M L
Evans, R C
Evans, R F
Ewer, A K
Exon, D J
Ezikwa, F Z
Faisal, K N M A
Faisal, N A
Farhadian, F
Farmer, A J
Farmer, C M
Farndon, P A
Farrar, D J
Faull, C M
Fawcett, C J
Fedee, J L
Felderhof, J C
Fenton, T W
Ferguson, W J
Fernando, I N
Ferner, R E
Field, S K
Field, S J
Brown, R M
Fisher, E W
Fitzmaurice, D A
Fleming, D M
Fletcher, R I
Flinn, R M
Fogell, M
Foggensteiner, L
Folb, J E
Ford, D R
Forsey, P R
Forster, P M
Foulds, I S
Fownes, H E
Fox, J E
Fox, S J
Fraise, A P
Fraise, M C
Francis, A E
Francis, G H
Franklyn, J A
Franks, S C
Frempong, J
Gaballa, N E
Gabra, G S
Gabriel, S G J
Gallacher, K G
Gallacher, T
Gammage, M D
Gandhi, I K
Gangotra, G
Ganiwalla, T M J
Gannon, M X
Garcia De Vinuesa, C
Gardner-Medwin, J M M
Gardner, G T G
Gaspar, A S
Gaspar, K
Gaspar, L S
Gasson, G B
Gazis, A G
Gearty, J C
Gee, H
Geh, J I
George, M
Gibbons, P J
Gibson, J M
Giddings, P
Gill, J K
Gill, M J
Gill, P S
Gill, S K
Gillies, A J
Girgis, Y S
Gittins, P R
Gittoes, N J L
Gladwell, S R F
Glaholm, J
Glass, A
Glass, R G
Glithero, P R
Goh, J C B
Gohil, N M
Gohil, S
Gold, L M
Goldin, J H
Goldman, M D
Goldstein, A R
Goldstein, A L
Goldstein, J E
Gonsalves, P
Gonzaga, R T
Goode, N J
Goodman, M H
Goodyear, H M
Gordon, C
Gordon, W L
Gospel, R L
Goswami, V P
Gough, A C
Gould, M J
Gourevitch, D
Gowar, J P
Graham, T R
Grainger, C R
Grant, I J M
Green, M A
Green, S H
Greening, J S
Gregg, E M
Gregory, K S
Greig, J M
Griffith, M E
Griffiths, A
Griffiths, F D
Griffiths, K J
Griffiths, M P
Griffiths, R K
Grimer, R J
Grocutt, M S J
Grundy, R G
Guest, P J
Guirguis, H M
Gupta, A
Gupta, J K
Gupta, M
Gupta, T N
Hadley, J W
Hafeez, A
Hafeez, F
Hafeez, U
Hahn, A M
Haider, F S
Haigh, S F
Hakeem, A G
Hales, A D M
Hall, J M
Hall, M G
Hallissey, M T
Hambleton, D
Hamer, A R
Hamilton, P A
Hammersley, R L
Hamnett, E
Handy, S
Hanif, M
Hankin, J E
Haq, I U
Hardie, A D
Harding, L K
Harding, N J
Hardwick, C I
Hardwick, J M
Hardy, R G
Harland, S P
Harley-Mason, G R
Haroon, A M
Harper, L
Harris, D M
Harris, P
Harris, Q
Harrison, G R
Harrison, T M
Hart, D P
Hashmi, M
Hassan, M S U
Hassan, M S U
Hassan, U S
Hawker, C F
Hawker, J I
Hawkey, P M
Hawkins, D J
Hayes, G S
Heafield, M T E
Heath, C M
Heath, C W
Heath, D A
Heitmann, M
Henshall, S M
Heritage, J H
Hero, I
Herodotou, N
Heslop, J M
Hettiaratchy, S P
Hewins, P
Hewitt, M L
Hickman, M D
Hijazi, L
Hill, A C
Hill, F G H
Hill, P R
Hinder, S A J
Hirsch, M V
Hiscock, E
Hobart, A G
Hobbs, F D R
Hocking, M D
Hockley, A D
Hodgson, J
Hofmann, H A
Hollier, K P
Hollingworth, T
Hone, J H
Honeybourne, D
Honeyman, M M
Hooper, C L
Hooper, M B
Hope-Ross, W M
Hopkins, J D
Hopkinson, R B
Horton, G
Horton, V C
Hoth, T
Hourani, A H I
Howes, D M
Hubscher, S G
Huddleston, R E
Huengsberg, M
Huggins, L J
Huggins, N J
Hughes, J M
Hughes, M A
Hughes, S J
Hughes, T J
Hulten, M A
Hulton, S-A
Humphreys, M S
Hunt, D A
Hunt, E
Hussain, A
Hutton, P
Hvidsten, S J
Hyde, C J
Hyde, J A J
Hylton, S M
Hyman, B M
Ievins, F A
Iles, P B
Imlah, N W
Indwar, C
Iqbal, A
Iqbal, J
Ireland, P S
Irgin, S M
Isaac, D T
Isaac, S
Iskander-Gabra, S D
Islam, N
Ismail, A
Itrakjy, A S J M A
Iyengar, P G
Jackowski, A
Jackson, A P F
Jackson, S A

Jaffer, K
Jairaj, M B
Jaitly, V K
Jajoo, J N
Jamaluddin, M
Jameel, S Y
Jameel, T
James, J M
James, N D
James, P J
James, S R N
Jamieson, D G
Janardhan Reddy, S R
Jaron, A E G
Jassel, G S
Jawaheer, G
Jeavons, M P
Jemahl, S
Jenkins, D W
Jenkinson, H C
Jennings, C R
Jeskins, G D
Jessop, H C
Jeys, L M
Jhass, L S
Jheeta, B S
Jhittay, P S
Jobanputra, P
John, P R
Johnson, A P
Johnson, J W E
Johnson, K J
Johnson, S A
Jones, A F
Jones, E L
Jones, E F
Jones, G S
Jones, H H
Jones, M M
Jones, R W A
Jones, R L
Jones, S R
Jones, S E F
Jones, T J J
Jordan, J A
Jordan, P J
Jordan, R H A
Joshi, K
Joshi, M D
Joshi, S M
Jubb, R W
Jukes, D S
Kahn, A
Kandula, V
Kane, K F
Kannan, A J
Kapadia, M K
Kapur, R V
Karamdad, D R
Karim, M B
Karzoun, F K
Kathuria, U C
Kaushal, N A
Kavi, L A
Kay, J
Kayani, J A
Kayente, M L
Kaylan, A S
Keeble, M
Keighley, D M
Keighley, M R B
Kelly, D A M
Kelly, G D
Kelly, L M
Kelly, M M
Kemm, J R
Kendall, M J
Kennedy, J
Kenney-Herbert, J P
Kenyon, B
Keogh, B E
Kersley, J B
Keshri, R
Ketkar, V H
Kett, D W
Khair, O A G B M
Khaira, J S
Khalid, A
Khalid, S
Khalid, U K
Khalil Marzouk, Y F
Khan, A
Khan, I
Khan, M
Khan, M S
Khan, M A
Khan, R
Khanduri, S
Khanna, K A
Khattak, S S
Khattak, S H
Khin-Maung-Zaw, Dr
Kilby, M D
Kinch, D
King, A M
King, B R
King, M J
Kinshuck, D J
Kippax, T P
Kirk, J M W
Kirkby, G R
Knowlden, R P
Knowles, M G
Knowles, P J
Kong, K L
Kong, N
Kordan, M A
Kpiasi, E O
Kulshrestha, M K
Kulshrestha, R P
Kumar, S
Kumble, J R
Kuo, M J-M
Labinjo, K O
Laird, M J
Lamond, I
Lampert, I
Lander, A D
Lane, P J L
Langford, Dr
Langrick, A F
Lanham, J R C
Lanigan, S W
Lashen, H A M A
Latham, T B
Latief, T N
Latif, S A
Latthe, M M
Latthe, M M
Latthe, M A
Lau, E W Y
Lavin, I
Law, D P F
Lawrence, G D
Lawrence, M P
Lawrence, R P
Lawson, S E
Lea, D C J
Lea, R A
Learmonth, D J A
Lee Pek Wan, Dr
Lee, C Y
Lee, J R
Leggetter, P P
Leggott, M J
Leigh, C
Lengua Quijandria, C A
Lester, H E
Lester, J S
Lester, R L
Lester, W A
Levi, N A
Levick, P L
Lewis, H M
Lewis, M
Lewis, M
Lewis, M J V
Lewis, M E
Lidder, P G
Liebling, A J
Liew, C
Liew, L C W
Liley, A
Lilford, R J
Lilley, J-P
Lindsay, J A
Linney, S F
Lip, G Y H
Lip, P L
Lip, P-L
Lipkin, G W
Littler, W A
Lloyd, B E M
Lockley, M R
Loffeld, A
Loftus, C E
Logan, I S
Loizou, E
Lonergan, J G
Lopez Sanchez, C
Loudon, R F
Loughridge, C J
Low, D C
Lowe, A L
Luckas, M J M
Ludman, P F
Luesley, D M
Lumley, L C
Lyon, A K
Mabley, A M
McCafferty, I J
McCollum, D H
McConkey, B
McDonnell, J H
Macerola, G
Macfarlane, D W R
McGrath, C C B
McGuinness, P J N
Machin, P
McHugo, J M
McKechnie, R L
Mackenzie, A A
McKeown, C M E
Mackie, J G
McKiernan, P J
MacLennan, C A
MacLennan, I C M
MacLeod, J
MacLeod, R A L
McLeod, T J
McMaster, P
McMillan, G H G
McMullan, P J V
Macnamara, M A M
McNamara, M J
MacPhail, C V
MacPherson, L K R
McQuillan, E J
McShane, L M
Magee, C M
Magnay, K L
Mahendra, P
Maher, A R
Maher, E R
Maheswaran, V
Mahmood, A
Mahmood, Y
Majevadia, D K
Makin, A J
Malik, A M
Malik, N M
Malik, W
Malins, A F
Mangham, D C
Manji, M
Manley, V C
Mann, A-B
Mann, C H
Mann, J R
Mant, J W F
Manu, M
Manuchehri, K
Manyweathers, V J
Marks, D S
Marns, R S
Marok, I S
Marsden, J R
Marshall, A C
Martin, J P
Martin, K L
Martin, N A J
Martin, U
Masood, M
Matharoo, H
Mathews, E T
Mattar, R G
Matthews, P M
Mattu, G S
Mavi, B S
Mayer, A D
Mayer, P P
Mayor, V
Meakin, L C
Mearns, C A
Mehta, R L
Mehta, R R
Melhuish, L
Melikian, F R
Mendelsohn, R A
Merron, S
Messahel, F M A
Mewar, D
Meyer, C H A
Meyer, H C K
Michael, J
Milford, D V
Millane, T A
Millar, C L
Milledge, D T
Miller, J A L
Miller, K A
Miller, L F
Miller, M R
Miller, P A
Milligan, D W
Millns, J P
Mills, J D
Milo-Turner, G
Mina, M T
Mina, M M M
Mishra, M N
Mishra, P
Miskin, N
Miskin, S J
Misra, P K
Misra, U S
Mistry, T P
Mitchell, A M
Mitchell, R D
Mohan, C B
Moiemen, N S M
Monaghan, A M
Moonga, P S
Moore, J R M
Moore, S J
More, I S
Morgan, D R
Morgan, E J
Morgan, M E I
Morgan, S D
Morland, B J
Morley, R L
Morris, S B
Morrison, I D
Morrison, J M
Morrison, K E
Mortiboy, D E
Mortimer, A T
Mortimer, M J
Morton, D G
Morton, J E V
Mosquera Lopez De Larrinzar, A
Mosquera, D A
Moss, C
Moss, J L M
Moss, M S
Moss, P A H
Mottershead, L M
Moussa, K T
Moy, R J D
Muayed, R M H
Mukherjee, S
Mulcahy, T M
Mulik, R B
Munday, S J
Munden, A C
Munir, S M
Mupanemunda, R H
Murdoch, W
Murphy, M S
Murphy, P D
Murray, A T
Murray, J A
Murray, J A
Murray, P I
Murray, R G
Mushin, S E
Muss, D C
Myskova, I A
Mzimba, Z S
Nagi, H M
Nagle, C J
Nagrani, R
Najada, S F
Najak, B G H
Nall, P T
Nancarrow, J D
Nandi, D K
Narayan, B S
Narhlya, N K
Narhlya, P K
Nathavitharana, C P G
Nattrass, M
Naughton, P E
Nazir, M
Nazki, M T
Negargar, A
Neuberger, J M
Newman, J
Newrith, C R F
Newton, T
Nicholl, P T
Nicholls, A M H
Nicol, D B
Nicum, S
Ninan, T K
Nirdosh, N
Nithiyananthan, R
Niven-Jenkins, N C
Niwa, K
Nixon, H K
Nixon, J R
Noon, A J
Norman, A M
North, J P
Notghi, A
Notghi, L M
Nye, M Y L
Nyholm, E S
O'Brien, C M
O'Brien, D C
O'Brien, P M
O'Connell, J E
O'Connor, B B
O'Dea, J F
O'Donnell, D
O'Driscoll, A M
O'Driscoll, D J
O'Gara, M G
O'Gorman, M E
O'Hara, J N
O'Neill, E C
O'Reilly, P J
O'Shea, J G
Oates, G D
Obeid, M L
Oetiker, U
Ojha, A
Olliff, J F C
Olliff, S P
Oluwole, M O K
Oppenheim, E M
Osman, K H E
Owen, A J
Owen, J J T
Owen, K R
Owen, K C
Oyaide, O M
Oyebode, O A
Page, A J
Pahor, A L
Pal, P
Pal, P K
Palin, S L
Palmer, H E
Palsingh, J
Panagamuwa, C S B
Pandit, S S
Pankhania, R
Panton, S
Papini, R P G
Paramanathan, K
Paramanathan, S
Parashar, K
Pardoe, I S
Parikh, D H
Park, C A
Parkes, J
Parle, H J E
Parle, J V
Parmar, S
Parnaik, V G
Pasupathy, D
Patel, A R A
Patel, A
Patel, C
Patel, H
Patel, J N
Patel, K C
Patel, R R
Patel, S
Paterson, J T
Patodi, S K
Pattni, B L
Paul, A
Paw, R C
Payne, E S
Payne, M L
Payne, R J
Peake, D R
Pearce, D E
Pearman, K
Pears, P E
Pearson, A J
Pearson, G A
Peet, A C
Penfold, S E
Pennington, S J
Pentecost, B L
Perkins, S L
Phelps, S R
Philip, W M
Pillay, D
Piqueras Arenas, A I
Pirie, A M
Pitt, M P I
Plant, P A
Platt, C C
Platt, S G
Plewes, J J L
Pogmore, J R
Pointen, E J
Pollock, G T
Poltock, T L
Pomeroy, R T
Poole, C J
Porter, H P
Porter, K M
Poultney, J M
Pradhan, C B
Prais, L
Prasad, K T
Prasad, P
Prasher, V P
Pratt, D A
Pratt, J D
Prendergast, M
Pretlove, S J
Prime, C F
Pritchard, T R
Proops, D W
Pugh, L J L
Puleston, R L
Raafat, F
Rabb, L M
Radcliffe, K W
Radvanyi, M
Rafiq, M
Raghavan, S
Rahber, M S
Rahim, A
Rahman, A S M M
Rahman, H U
Rahman, I
Rahman, S-A
Rahman, S
Rai, H S
Raichura, V K
Raine-Fenning, N J
Raine, R A
Raj, G R
Raja, J H
Rajesh, P B
Rajput, K S
Rajput, S
Rajput, V K
Ralston, C S
Ralston, G R D
Ramachandram, R S
Ramani, P
Ramarao, M V
Rami Reddy, S
Ramjohn, M A
Rana, K
Rana, T A
Randhawa, V
Rankin, E C C
Rao, J N
Rao, V
Rashid, A
Rati, N
Ratib, K
Raut, S L
Rauz, S
Ravindrababu, G
Ray, S
Rayner, H C
Rayner, I R
Rayner, P H W
Rayton, E L
Raza, K
Rea, D W
Reddy, K S P
Reddy, N S
Redfearn, E
Redman, H K A
Reed, A
Rees, A H
Rees, E N
Rees, G L
Rehmany, K M
Reid, A P
Reid, R E G
Rewhorn, I D
Reynolds, J H
Riaz, A
Rice, P F
Richards, N T
Richards, P W
Richings, C I
Rickards, E H G
Riddell, P L
Riddington, D W
Ridgway, J C
Ridley, C C S
Riordan, F A I
Rippin, J D
Roberts, F E
Roberts, M
Robertson, A S
Robertson, D N
Robertson, P A

Robinson, A L
Robinson, B H B
Robinson, J S
Robinson, S J
Robson, C H
Robson, N J
Rock, I W
Rodgers, R T B
Rodrick, C J
Rodrigues, A J
Rogers, J M
Rogowski, P
Rooney, M J
Roper-Hall, M J
Roper, H P
Roper, P H
Rose, J H
Rose, S J
Ross, A M
Ross, J D C
Rothery, D J
Rouse, A M
Rowe, J
Roy Choudhury, M
Roy, A
Roy, H
Roy, M
Roylance, J
Ruby, A
Rummens, L J
Rummens, S D
Rumsey, J M A
Russell, G S J
Russell, I D
Russell, S H
Ryan, P G
Ryder, C A J
Ryder, R E J
Sabir, N M
Saeed, T
Saeed, Z P
Sagar, C V
Sahay, P K
Saigol, M Y
Saikia-Varman, N
Saikia, S
Saini, M S
Saini, M S
Sakhuja, S B
Saksena, S C
Salama, A A K
Salamat, A A
Saldanha, L J
Saleem, M A
Sales, T S
Salib, S S E
Salim, M
Salim, S N
Salmon, D N
Salt, P J
Samarasinghe, L A
Sambatakakis, A
Sandhu, S S
Sandilands, D W I M
Sandler, D
Sandrasegaran, K
Sanghera, J S
Sangra, R A S
Sarin, S
Sarmah, B D
Sarwar, S
Sashidharan, S P
Saunders, D M
Saunders, E J
Saunders, P B
Savage, C O S
Sawers, R S
Schuppler, P E R
Scott-Cook, H R
Scott, P E
Scott, R A H
Scott, S J
Seaborne, L
Seakins, E C
Searle, S J
Sellarajah, A
Sempa, A V
Sen-Gupta, T
Seth, A
Settatree, R S
Seymour, A H
Sgouros, S
Shafi, M I
Shah, A U
Shah, B M
Shah, F
Shah, J L
Shah, M J
Shah, N K
Shah, P R
Shah, V M
Shah, Z H
Shahmanesh, M
Shahmanesh, M
Sham, S-Y
Shameem, M
Shankernarayan, M G
Shannon, J R
Shannon, N L
Shannon, S W
Shapiro, J A
Shapiro, L R
Sharif, K W S
Sharma, A
Sharma, A
Shastri, M M
Shaw, M J
Shehab, A M A
Sheikh, M A
Shelton, F C
Sheppard, M C
Sherlaw, J A
Sherrington, J M
Sherwood, N A
Shevket, M
Shinkwin, C A
Shinner, G
Shinton, R A
Shipman, P A M
Short, J M
Shumsheruddin, D M
Siddeeq, M U
Sidhom, A T M
Sigurdsson, A S
Sills, J A
Silove, E D
Silverman, S H
Simkiss, D E
Simms, M H
Simon, P D
Simons, D M
Simpson, M
Sims, D G
Sinclair, A S
Singal, A
Singh, B K
Singh, G
Singh, P
Singh, S P
Singh, S
Singh, S
Singh, V K
Singhal, S
Singhal, S
Sinha, M
Sintler, M P
Sipple, M A
Siriwardena, G J A
Skingle, I S
Skinner, A M M
Slater, N A J
Slator, R C
Smart, C J
Smart, S J
Smith, A G
Smith, A
Smith, B S
Smith, E G
Smith, G R
Smith, J E
Smith, K M
Smith, K J
Smith, L J A
Smith, M R
Smith, N A
Smith, P R
Smith, R V
Smith, R N
Smith, S R G
Smith, S A
Sneath, R J S
Snell, A D
Sobti, A K
Solari, J R
Somasundara-Rajah, J
Somasundara-Rajah, K
Somerset, D A
Somerset, R B
Sood, M R
Soon, Y
Southwood, T R
Spanner, R M
Spannuth, F
Sparkes, J M
Spiller, P A
Spray, C H
Srivastava, A S
Stableforth, D E
Stamp, E J
Stanley, D P
Stannard, W A
Stanton, E C R
Stark, E G
Stark, P J
Stedman, J K
Stedman, S R
Steedman, G
Steele, R T
Stern, S
Sterne, A J
Steven, N M
Stevens, A J H
Stevens, M C G
Stevenson, I H
Stewart, P M
Stirling, A J
Stockley, R A
Stoddart, B C
Stokes-Lampard, H J
Stokes, M A
Strange, S W
Stumper, O F W
Subzposh, S Y A
Sud, S K
Suggett, N R
Suleman, S T
Suleman, Z
Sullivan, A L
Sullivan, C A
Sumathipala, S
Sunderland, R
Sungum-Paliwal, S
Super, P A
Surdhar, H S
Sutcliffe, A J
Sutherland, G A
Sutton, G A
Swain, A J
Swain, D G
Swales, N V
Swani, M S
Sweeney, H R
Syed, A B
Syed, N Y
Sykes, J J W
Sylvester, A R
Tabani, A R
Tadros, W S
Takes, H M
Tan, C Y
Tan, L C
Tandon, N K
Tandon, U R
Tattersall, D J
Tavares-Mott, N E
Taylor, A J
Taylor, A P
Taylor, C M
Taylor, C J C
Taylor, D G B
Taylor, E I R
Taylor, F T
Taylor, J M
Taylor, K G
Taylor, M H
Taylor, S A
Taylor, W
Teale, G R
Temple, J G
Temple, R M
Thake, A I S
Thakur, S
Than Than Swe, Dr
Thandi, K S
Thebridge, P J
Then, K Y
Thethy, R S
Thind, I
Thomas, A M C
Thomas, E
Thomas, M K
Thompson, A G
Thompson, A K
Thompson, A P
Thompson, I M
Thompson, R D
Thompson, S M
Thomson, H J
Thorburn, D
Thorne, S A
Thwaites, A J
Tierney, J N
Tillman, R M
Timoney, N
Tinkler, R
Titley, O G
Todd, R S
Toozs-Hobson, P M
Toyn, C E
Tricklebank, B
Trimble, K T
Trivedi, K M
Trotter, S E
Tsakonas, D
Tse, W Y
Tubbs, O N
Tudor, V S
Tudway, D C
Turner, E S
Turner, N O
Turner, P R W
Turpin, P J
Udokang, M J
Ullyatt, K J
Unsworth, J
Uppal, H S
Usher-Somers, N
Usmani, I
Vachhani, M K
Vaile, J C
Vale, J A
Valsalan, U
Van Marle, W
Van Mourik, I D M
Varma, R
Vatish, R K
Vella, A
Venkat, K R
Venkatesan, P
Verma, A N
Verma, A
Verma, S K
Viney, R P C
Virdee, M S
Vora, A K
Waddell, C A
Wadhwa, H K
Wagstyl, S
Wainscott, G R D
Wake, M J C
Waldram, M A
Walford, S
Wali, G
Walji, M-T I
Walker, S L
Walker, W E
Wall, R A
Wallace, D M A
Wallace, P A
Wallis, P J W
Walsh, A R
Walshe, A D
Walt, H J
Walt, R P
Walters, S
Walton, K W W H
Walton, M J
Ward, J P Q
Warfield, A T
Wasserberg, J
Wassmer, E
Waters, R A
Watkins, R A
Watkins, S J D
Watkinson, J C
Watkinson, M
Watson, D N
Watson, E A J
Watson, K A
Watt, J M
Wearn, A M
Weaver, J B
Webb, D R
Webber, J
Webster, K
Weddell, D J
Weeks, M C
Weerasena, L
Weller, M D
Weller, P H
Weller, T M A
Wells, M B
West, N S
West, R J
Wheatley, V J
White, A C
White, D J
White, R J
Whitehouse, S J
Whiteley, J T
Whittaker, C M
Whittington, R M
Whittle, M J
Whyte, J A
Wiggins, M R
Wigley, E J
Wijnberg, A W A
Wilcox, C
Wilcox, R G
Wilcox, R M L
Wild, N J
Wildbore, P M
Wilde, J T
Wildman, M J
Wilkes, M P
Wilkey, A D
Wilkinson, C D
Wilkinson, M J B
Williams, A C
Williams, C R
Williams, D C
Williams, D K
Williams, D P C
Williams, E D
Williams, H J
Williams, J P
Williams, J K
Williams, J
Williams, L R
Williams, M D
Williams, N A
Williams, R C
Williams, S J
Williams, S P
Williamson, E J E
Willis, T A
Willmot, M R
Willson-Lloyd, J M
Wilson, B E
Wilson, F
Wilson, I C
Wilson, M
Wilson, P G
Winer, J B
Wingate, J P
Wingate, V A
Winkley, L M
Winter, H R
Wise, R
Wiseman, E S
Wishart, E H
Wolverson, R L
Wong, A K M
Wong, C H
Wong, P C
Wood, A L
Wood, J K
Wood, P R
Wooding, N J
Woodward, C L
Woollaston, K A H
Woolley, S L
Woolley, S M
Wozniak, I A
Wozniak, J T
Wozniak, S
Wrenn, P A M
Wright, C J
Wright, D
Wright, J M
Wright, J G C
Wright, M J
Wright, P R
Wyldes, M P
Yap, S L
Yaqoob, N
Yates, D A
Yates, J A
Yau, W H
Yee, M L
Yoong, A K H
Yoong, W C
Young Min, M S
Young, B P
Young, D W
Young, G B
Young, J A
Youssef, E E
Yunas, S
Yusuf, S
Zafar, S A
Zaki, A S
Zaman, T M
Zaman, T M
Zargar, G M
Zielinski, R A
Zuckerman, C H
Zygmunt, S C

Bishop Auckland

Airlie, K R
Baliga, K V S
Bateson, M C
Benstead, S E
Bibby, C B
Bolton, G M
Bowron, P
Bremner, I S
Chandrasiri, R B C M
Cottrell, A J
Deytrikh, N
Eccleston, E C
Fairclough, B E
Findlay, S M
Ford, G D
Forge, J A
Fox, J V
Gonsalves, H J B
Hackett, M T C
Harris, D
Hema Kumar, J
Hetherington, A
Hill, A M
Howells, L
Jayasekera, L A G
Johnson, M K
Johnston, A M
Jones, P M
Jones, S R
Khan, S H
Lamb, W H
Langford, D C
Layzell, T
Lewis, A
Lumb, S A
McCulloch, A J
McGregor, G S
Macleod, A H
McManners, R
Mahdi, K S
Mahmoud, M M Y
Mees, G P
Mehrzad, A A
Needham, I C
Nyamugunduru, G
Oghoetuoma, J O
Orr, P K
Pickworth, J C
Pike, B R
Pike, E E
Pindolia, N K
Prentice, M C
Priddy, R J
Pugh, K
Roberts, C
Robertson, I
Said, J R
Sanghera, S K
Sarkar, D
Scott, C M
Sivayokan, P
Smellie, W S A
Smith, H L
Spurr, J I
Stephen, J G
Stock, S E
Vijayaraghavan, S
Vose, H C
Waller, D C E
Ward, M A
Weerasinghe, B D

Bishops Castle

Howell, N C B
Penney, A P S J

Bishop's Stortford

Agarwal, S
Al-Fattal, S M A S
Arafa Ali, K A L
Banatvala, J E
Bhuller, A S
Bradbury, N J L
Carew, R I
Carrick, P A
Chauhan, A
Chisnall, A
Clemans-Gibbon, T M
Crowe, G H
Currey, J
Dain, A V
Davies, R G
Davis, R A
Degun, W J
Dixon, J A
Dolling, M
Donnelly, J S
Dove, P R
Emmett, V E
Fawcett, I M
Fearby, S
Fitness, S J
Gilchrist, I C
Goldspink, M H F

Greenlees, F R
Hardwick, M J
Hardy, J D
Hickman, P J
Jabbar, N K A
Jellis, T S
Jenns, M A
Jordan, A F
Kapadia, Y K
Kent, R V
Lloyd, J E
MacHale, S J
Mand, H S
Moore, P J
Morris, E C
Nutley, P G
Oates, N R
Orton, K A
Orton, P K
Pandor, S B
Raine, J M
Rayner, J M
Rogers, M J
Schofield, J G
Scott, L A
Shaw, K
Tennekoon, M S
Tischkowitz, M D K-E
Todd, R M
Trivedi, K G
Wallace, J T
Watson, A T
Whetstone, S
Wilson, P C
Wilson, S D

Bishopton
Alexander, J O
Bennie, A M
Boyce, J
Bradford, C A
Downie, F B
Gowling, G E
Gray, D G
Gray, J S
Hodgson, M E
Masterton, J G
Miller, J

Blackburn
Agarwal, K N
Ahmad, T U
Ahmed, M M
Al Ani, F S S
Ali, A A
Ali, M O
Amarasinghe, G P W
Amran Bin Marzuki, Dr
Apaloo, F K B
Aravind, S P
Ariyaratnam, S
Ashe, P J
Azfar, S S
Bahia, H I
Balasubramanian, M
Barker, R F
Barrie, J L
Benson, J W T
Benson, R C
Bhattacharjee, G B
Bhojani, I H
Bristow, A I
Buckley, N G E
Burch, K L
Burn, K E
Bux, Z M
Calow, A J
Carter, P S
Chadwick, E
Chang, D
Chattree, S
Cherry, J R
Chorlton, M I
Chowdhury, M R
Clark, C E
Clarke, S J
Clarkson, S
Crowley, B
Datta, M K
Datta, S
Davenport, G A
Davey, R J
Dawson, C R
Dervan, M F
Dugmore, W N
Duong, T V
Earnshaw, D P
Emmott, R S
Evans, D A
Fakhry, H A G
Farooq, H M
Fletcher, L M
Fourie, P G
Fox, D J
Franks, D
Gamble, A R
Gargye, U
Garwood, P J
Gavan, D R
Gavan, J
George, T K
Gilligan, S J
Golding, T M
Goodall, D
Gooder, P D
Goodfellow, P B
Grayson, R P
Green, R M
Grimes, D S
Gunn, S D
Gupta, D
Hamlin, G W
Hancock, S A
Haq, Z
Hardy, C I
Hardy, S C
Hardy, S K
Hartley, R C
Hindle, J
Hodkinson, P S
Horsfield, N
Hossain, M O S M
Islam, N
Jadhav, S D
Jeyaseelan, S
Jones, D A
Jones, G R
Jones, L S
Jones, R P
Jones, R C
Joshi, S V
Karim, T
Kaur, S
Kirkpatrick, H W
Koneru, U S
Kumar, A
Ladlow, M E
Lewis, F W
Lomax, S R
Lowe, S E
Lowrie, I G
Lynch, D A F
McCarthy, M J
McEwan, A B
Maiti, S K
Marlborough, J J C
Maskell, A P
Mene, A R
Minto, G W
Misra, N
Mohammed, T
Moodie, I J
Moosa, H A U
Morar, P
Mousdale, S
Mowbray, C H
Mukherji, D J
Murdoch, A J M
Myers, A
Nagpal, N
Nagpal, S
Nandakumar, E
Nataraj, V
Neilson, D
Nicholson, R W
Nylander, A G E
O'Donovan, P A
Ormerod, L P
Osman, M
Owen, C M
Paley, J D
Paley, M D
Panikkar, J
Paris, J A G
Parry, A K
Patel, Z
Paton, R W
Pearce, S
Perera, G S G S
Phillips, E B
Phillips, J K
Pollock, R S
Premraj, K
Prescott, R J
Privonitz, D M
Rahman, M A
Rahman, M
Rakshit, B C
Randall, J C
Rao, K C
Rashed, N F
Rautray, R C
Rautray, R
Ravat, F E
Reed, P F
Rehman, S A
Roberts, N A
Roberts, T A
Romachney, P
Rosbottom, J M
Rose, D J A
Royle, J D
Rushton, C E
Russo, P
Salaman, R A
Sarodia, U A
Schram, C M H
Searson, J J
Shah, F Z
Sharma, M
Sivagnanam, T
Smith, C P
Smith, D
Smith, N A
Soliman, E S
Srirangam, S J
Stanley, I R
Suleman, M H J
Teh, L-S
Timms, M S
Timson, I
Trafford, P D
Tresadern, J C
Tucker, K P
Upton, S N
Valluri, P
Vijaykumar, A
Virdi, R P S
Walmsley, P N H
Walsh, J
Walter, C M
Watson, R J
Weerakone, R S
Wemyss-Holden, G D
Whyte, I D
Wiggans, S M
Wilkinson, R
Wlodarczyk, K K
Yates, G A
Yates, M J

Blackpool
Abellan-Antolin, F J
Adinkra, J P
Anandappa, A J A
Anderson, W J
Apaloo, E C
Arrowsmith, S
Arthur, I D
Arya, M
Arya, S
Arya, S C
Ashworth, R N
Au, J K K
Aulakh, H S
Awbery, S M
Baloch, A G
Barlow, D J
Bedell, J
Beet, P L
Bell, H J T
Bevis, C R A
Billington, P
Biswas, P K
Boak, M
Boissiere, P F T
Bolton, M
Bonsell, E M
Bottomley, W W
Bowyer, P K
Bury, R W
Byrne, S
Calvert, C A D
Calvert, J S
Campbell, C D
Chamberlain, M E
Chandra, V
Charles, D P
Chattopadhyay, P K
Choudhury, A K
Clarke, C W M
Cookson, A J
Cooper, J D
Cornah, M S
Cowin, S W
Crookenden, D
Cupitt, J M
Curtis, P D
Cushing, S
Dabrowski, M T
Dale, M C
Duncan, A J
Dunne, J A
Duthie, S J
Edwards, V A
Eggington, W R O
Ellis, S K
Evans, C G
Faux, P A L
Fawkes-Palmer, R
Fewster, S D
Finucane, U A
Flanagan, N G
Flegg, P J
Gadallah, E F
Gajawira, N P
Garstang, A R
Gavin, N J
Goode, G K
Green, K L
Greenaway, W E
Greiss, G G
Guirguis, A F A
Guisasola-Gorrochategui, I
Harper, N G
Harrison, D
Harrop, H J
Harrop, S N
Hausser, B I
Haworth, D A
Hayes, B
Hayes, P J
Hayes, S D A
Heath, J C D
Hemmings, S C
Hiles, A
Hinchcliffe, D E
Hindley, C J
Hoadley, G M
Horton, S J R
Hulme, A V
Humber, J C
Humphries, C A
Inmonger, J
Iqbal, M
Ireland, D
Isaacs, P E T
Johnson, A G
Johnson, G W
Kane, T P
Kay, D S G
Kelly, P D
Kelsey, P R
Khawaja, U L
Kitching, C
Knowles, A C
Lake, P J
Lambert, I K
Lau, S C
Leather, K E
Lee, L K
Li Kam Wa, T C
Lippmann, M E M
Liu, S M
Lord, B M
Lowson, T A
Lucking, M T
Lunn, M K
Macbeth, A J
McConachie, I W
McGovern, A J
Macheta, M P
Mackay, J D
McLoughlin, S J
Madan, A K
Madan, K K
Madan, S
Mannion, S J
Martin, M H
Meichen, F W
Miller, H S
Miller, J
Mistry, D D
Mitchell, S L
Molodynski, C J
Montgomery, D P
Morcos, M I
Morgan, R J M
Murray, D G
Naguib, M A E-A A
Nasr, E F
Naylor, G
Neary, P J
Newiss, L P
Nigam, A
Nolan, J A
Nugent, J P
O'Reilly, J F
O'Donnell, M J
Parham, A L S
Parikh, R K
Parker, S P
Parkinson, G F
Parr-Burman, S J
Perricone, V
Pettit, S H
Pollock, J E
Pollock, W S T
Prakash, H
Preskey, M S
Raines, M F
Randall, N P C
Ravi, S
Rees, A N
Riding, G S G
Riding, K J
Robb, A K
Roberts, D H
Rothwell, P J N
Rowlands, A J
Rudnick, L R
Saeed, A M
Salah, I H I
Sampath, S A C
Sarkar, P K
Saunders, M G
Scott, C W
Sedgwick, M
Self, M C
Shanmugasundaram, O
Shearer, S A
Shorrock, C J
Shravat, B P
Smith, S T
Sogliani, F
Srivastava, A
Srivastava, S P
Steel, A
Suriya, A
Thomas, M R
Thompson, S W
Tun, S T
Vardy, P I
Vasudev, K S
Vaughan, S T A
Verma, R K
Vyse-Peacock, A
Walker, M C M
Walshaw, C F
Ward, T W
Wells, R A
Wheatley, R
Wilcox, F L
Williams, M E
Wilson, J M
Wojciuk, J
Zaki-Khalil, I A

Blackwood
Datta, B N
Harris, C
Jacques, R M
Jayadev, A
Khan, B
Lloyd, A L
Miles, O H
Ray, D K
Rogers, J H P
Sahni, P
Shah, I S
Shah, S H
Sweetman, J A
Thompson, W
Waheed, A
Windsor, K

Blaenau Ffestiniog
Boyns, A R
Dafydd, R E
Evans, O W
Jones, H R
Jones, J R K
Morgan, J R
Parry, T

Blaenavon
Buffett, G J G
Grant, D P
Lewis, T L
Lewis, W

Blairgowrie
Buist, A J
Callaway, E J
Dick, J B C
Downie, S E
Faloon, K
Forbes, H F
Gilmour, F B
Greig, G C
Humble, R D
Jack, J F B
Mackay, J M
McNeill, G P
McNeill, K E M
MacVicar, M
Martindale, M M
Mitchell, P E G
Morris, M J
Pyle, R L
Reid, I C
Shaw, J M A
Sim, I J
Slater, W J
Stewart, C T
Williams, J W
Young, A M M

Blandford Forum
Armand Smith, N G
Beadsmoore, E J
Blevins, T C S
Bosworth, P
Burlton, D A
Cade, A N
Cave, W K
Clarke, J J
Clements, J
Creagh-Barry, M J W
Davies, J V
Evans, J M
Ford, M S
French, A M
Gelder, A D
Hillier, E W
Hillier, M J H
Lester, J A
Meyrick Thomas, R H
Oliver, P O
Percival, G N
Pestridge, A D
Prior, R J
Richardson, S M
Scorey, P D
Thomas, A M
Walton, M J
Ward, R F

Blaydon-on-Tyne
Banerji, A
Bolas, R
Duggal, R P
Gibson, A L
Johnson, R M
Khanna, R
Lowery-Leigh, G
McKay, S
Mackie, J H
Matheson, D J
Oldroyd, J C
Robson, S
Williams, P R

Blyth
Allen, J S
Carr, R
Cochran, L
Dodds, W R
Eynon, D M
Fletcher, H J
Ghosh, J K
Gittins, S
Henderson, C A
Hussain, Z
Johri, R
Kimmitt, J
McCollum, R W
McEvedy, P A
Morgan, D C
Murphy, R A
Rawes, G D
Redfearn, A
Sukumaran Nair, C
Turner, J P
Urquhart, A S
Westgarth, D
Yeoman, P D

Boat of Garten
Riach, I C F

Bodmin
Bruce, J D

Buckley-Evans, J D
Coulthard, C W S
Cox, P J R
Eastwood, N J B
Eddy, J H
Evans-Jones, R J
Farrar, D I
Hignell, S P
Hogbin, P A
Koch, B
McCarron-Nash, B K
Maguire, J
Maher, T M
Owen, N T P
Partington, A G
Rouncefield, A M
Stead, M S
Tullberg, H T W
Tyler, J A
Watkins, S J O
Woodfield, M

Bodorgan
Morris, C D
Roberts, J M
Thomas, K J
Wilkinson, D C
Williams, A W
Williams, M

Bognor Regis
Ahmed, E R
Amaladoss, A S P
Bradstock-Smith, M R
Cahill, C
Callaway, P L
Dormer, M J S
Ellis, E A
Esslemont, A
Fox, C M
Fox, M H
Fulton, R
Furlepa, K A
Grainge, C L
Greenway, J H
Hanan, P M
Jackson, R A
Kerr, S A
Kipling, M L
Kirkwood, J L
Lavender, A J
Lean, A T
McLoughlin, J N
Mather, S D
Naylor, A M A
Paterson, F N
Price, J R
Rehman, F U
Ridley, M G
Robinson, G R E
Rogers, W J
Shaw, M M
Sodera, V K
Southgate, H J
Spurrier, P D
Twist, M H C
Wallis, P
Williamson, C M

Boldon Colliery
Aitken, G J
Cole, F R
Hall, W
Nellist, P J
Simpson, J H
Thorniley-Walker, E G A

Bolton
Adam, Y
Ainley-Walker, P F
Allamby, D L
Allan, A E
Ariff, A
Atcha, A W
Atcha, S
Atcha, Z I
Baker, F
Baker, P
Bancroft, K
Banerjee, A
Banerjee, A K
Banks, A J
Benjamin, M S
Berry, S G
Bishop, H M
Bisset, D L
Board, T N
Bolt, J C D
Bora, R
Bowman, F M
Bradford, J M
Bratt, A
Brocklebank, M C
Brown, M C
Brownlee, M R
Bullen, T F
Bunn, D T
Buttoo, S
Caldwell, I D
Canty, S J
Chan, K-K
Chandra, M
Charidemou, C
Chia, K V
Chishti, J M
Chowdhury, M
Cooper, M M
Cooper, R M
Craig, S K L
Crank, A
Curless, E
Dady, I M
Dakshinamurthi, M
Danson, S J
Das, D
Dave, A K
Dave, V K
Davies, A J
Davies, M R P
Dean, J D
Dennard, D L
Dey, M P
Downes, B
Doyle, S J
Dryburgh, P A
Duncalf, H A
Earnshaw, C J
Eminson, D M
Farrand, R J
Farrell, A M
Fasnacht, M
Faulkner, G S
Ferguson, E
Ferguson, G H
Fildes, S L
Fletcher, C L
Fletcher, M S
Flynn, M J
Ford, P M
Garewal, S
Gartside, M W
Gatenby, J
Gent, R N
Glass, S
Godden, D P
Green, J J
Greenhalgh, C B
Greenhalgh, S
Guhathakurta, S
Habashi, F A
Hailwood, R A
Hall, J M
Hall, M J
Hall, S A
Hamer, I E
Hamilton, S L
Hanif, S T
Hanson, I M
Hardman, J L
Hargreaves, S P
Harris, J
Harris, R P
Hartopp, I K
Haslam, D W
Haslam, N
Hassan, I
Healey, H
Hearn, G M
Hearn, K C
Henderson, A A
Henderson, J J
Hendy, C
Higgins, M C
Hobbiss, J H
Hodgson, S P
Hollows, K B
Holly, L J
Hopkins, R E
Hopkinson, J M
Hossain, M
Hunt, R A
Hutchesson, A C J
Iliff, A M
Ingram, G E
Inkster, C F
Isaac, T C
Jackson, R J
Jagannath, P
James, I G V
Jarvis, A M
Jayasekera, A I
Jayasekera, D S
Jip, J
Johnson, J D
Jones, D K
Jones, I N
Jones, J R
Joyce, E A
Kay, A L
Kelly, S P D D
Kent, L N
Kenward, S E
Khan, S H
Khwaja, M S
Kirby, J A L
Korlipara, K R
Kumar, D
Kwartz, J
Lad, R P
Lamb, A K
Lancashire, G S
Langton, J
Leahy, A R
Leaver, N M
Lipscomb, K J
Liratsopulos, G
Litherland, D J
Littlewood, R
Liversedge, S N
Lobo, C J
Loomba, Y
Lowe, J
Lowry, J C
Lynch, T
Lyon, A L
McAuley, D E
McCallum, A S R
McCurdie, M J
McKenna, M A
McKenna, T D
McKenzie, C J
Mackinnon, C J
McLardy, G
Mahindrakar, N H
Mangrolia, R D
Marles, P J
Mathew, S
Maxwell, A J
Mehta, S R
Mercer, C P
Michie, H R
Miller, B M
Mirza, M A
Mitchell, R G
Mobb, G E
Moriarty, K J
Morrison, A M
Moulton, C
Muhammad, J K
Mukherjee, D
Munshi, S A B
Murphy, D J
Naqvi, S M H
Natha, L A
Navaratnam, Y
Needham, J A
Newgrosh, B S
Newman, B M
Nicholson, J A H
Northover, T H
O'Keeffe, L J
Odonga, F
Ogden, G H
Onwudike, M
Ormiston, P J
Ostick, D G
Page, J
Panja, S R
Parr, A M
Parr, P J
Patel, A M
Patel, K J
Patel, R
Patel, R M
Patel, V K
Peacock, J
Pearson, J M
Perkins, B
Perry, E M
Petrie, P J
Phillips, J P K
Pope, I J
Pownall, P J
Poynor, M U
Price, E W
Priest, P J
Quenault, S L
Rae, P J
RamcHandani, M
RamcHandani, P
Raw, J M
Reading, J G
Reilly, S M
Reynard, A J
Roberts, J W
Robinson, A C J
Roddie, A E
Rothwell, N L
Rowe, S D
Rowlands, F M
Ryan, J P
Ryan, W G
Sarkar, S
Sarker, D
Saul, P A
Schofield, C P
Scott, P J
Seabourne, A E
Selvakumari, S
Senior, T P M
Service, E
Settle, P
Shankland, C R
Shaw, S A G
Sheldon, H E
Sheppard, I J
Sidat, I A G M
Siddiqui, T N
Silvert, B D
Simpson, R A
Singh, S
Singh, V M M
Sivalingam, T
Smith, M C
Smith, N J
Smyth, J W
Somerville, D M
Spurr, D
Strong, P M
Tabor, J E
Taulke-Johnson, T D
Taylor, J
Thomas, C F L
Tomkinson, J S
Tun Min, Dr
Umebuani, V C
Varghese, C M
Varker, J A
Varley, S C
Wakefield, C J
Walker, J R A
Walker, P M
Walker, R J
Wall, D A
Wallis, S W J
Walmsley, T A
Ward, P J
Wardman, L E
Warner, J G
Watson, R
Watt, R W
Watts, G M
Wells, S
West, C G H
Wheatley, E C
Whittle, J K
Widaa, A R
Wilkinson, M J S
Winstanley, J H R
Wood, J P
Woods, C J
Wright, A J

Bo'ness
Crichton, A-M
Easton, D V M
Gilmour, M F W
Hitchcock, R H
Onori, K M
Park, D J
Park, J
Paton, J
Proudlove, R
Sargent, T S P

Bonnybridge
Anderson, S C
Colgan, J M
Dick, A N
Dyer, C F
Dyer, R S
McCalister, B
McCalister, P W
Murray, M D
Weir, J A
Wilson, C C S
Wolff, L E

Bonnyrigg
Brown, I D
Clarke, F J
Dickson, G C
Dyson, F M H
Heggie, L J
Innes, R B
Keith, M A
Lamb, S G
Munro, N H
Norton, A M
Rother, P
Sattar, N
Smart, I S M
Thomson, G G J
Watkinson, H L
Wusu, O O H

Bootle
Ali, A
Beck, R A
Chung, K M
Cleugh, P A
Goldberg, D O
Jha, K K
Lalgee, C H
McCormick, C G S
Misra, G K
Murphy, K E
Newman, T A
Osman, J
Rawbone, R G
Roberts, A W
Sinha, N K
Sinha, S K
Srivastava, P K
Stanley, B
Stephenson, S J
Swarbrick, J G
Vinchenzo, A

Bordon
Beaumont, K M
Beech, P A
Binns, H
Egerton, D C
Read, Z H
Rose, J S

Borehamwood
Adeboye, K A O
Bellau, A R
Bennett, P E
Binks, F A
Cremin, P M
Dattani, R T
Drake, A J
Edwards, M R
Elliott, S C
Graham, J W
Harrison, R A
Hirsch, L
Howe, C J
Jacobson, B L
Lewin, J H
Longbourne, J R
Nicholson, C A
Pugh, D A
Rayat, S
Rose, J D
Smith, A L B
Spring, J T
Thomson, S D
Wilson, A T
Wilson, C E
Woolf, J K

Borth
Fish, S E
Williams, J T

Boscastle
Abbott, P R
Garrod, G D
Jarvis, C A N

Boston
Abdel Khalek, M N A
Adeyemi, O A
Allwood, A C L
Allwood, C R L
Andrews, N J
Arayomi, J O
Basu, S N
Batchelor, G N
Bexton, M D R
Bloom, I R B
Boldy, D A R
Boughey, O M S
Britton, I
Brocklehurst, J R
Bull, C S
Burks, C G
Busch, T A H
Chalmers, E P D
Chapman, R
Chatterjee, S C
Cheung, L C B
Clay, J C
Cope, S F
Crawford, M J
Cressey, J M
Dahar, N A
Datta, S
Dawson, P J
Dichmont, E V
Doddrell, A I
Dogra, K S
Durrant, D C S
Ejaz, T
Elwood, C M
Fairman, M J
Garden, G M F
Garg, N
Germer, M D
Germer, S
Gray, P J
Green, D F
Griffiths, C J
Hanumara, S K
Harris, P J
Hartshorn, J
Hassan, H S A
Holmes, P R
Hughes, A S
Hunt, B P
Jones, R
Kelly, C
Kirk-Smith, P R J
Korrapati, V M C
Lamb, W R
Latchem, R W
Layfield, J N
Loudon, K W
Mackin, J R
Malcolm, P N
Mangion, D
Massey, C I
Massey, J M
Matiti, H H
Meacock, D J
Minhas, T-W H A
Mortlock, A J
Norton, A C
Nyman, C R
Olamijulo, Dr
Olczak, S A
Palit, T
Parkin, N D
Pervez, M
Polling, M R
Rahman, A
Rainford, P J
Rance, D B
Ray, K K
Razzak, M S A
Refaat, R F
Rhys-Davies, S T
Sagar, D A
Sankey, E A
Savory, J N
Savory, S J
Shah, S M
Shaheen, A A M
Sobolewski, S
Spittal, M J
Steel, K C M
Taffinder, L D
Thomas, J
Walling, M R
Wallis, J H
Warren, C E J
Watson, J A S
Westmore, G A
Wheatley, S R
Woods, L
Woods, P J
Wookey, B E P

Bourne
Bevan, S F
Beveridge, V L
Briggs, B A
Burgess, P C
Burr, C R

Elder, R A
Halliday-Pegg, S M
Harris, J C
Pace, I G
Patel, R B
Pears, C R
Premkumar, G
Redding, W H
Sneath, P H A
Stitson, R N M
Turnbull, N B
Wallace, D A
Wheatley, I M
Wright, A M

Bourne End
Bentley-Thomas, C A
Biles, J P
Buxton, S H
Church, M R T
Church, S M
Havelock, T P
Hussain, T
Lee, L J
Newman, P W
Slack, R A
Wakatsuki, M
Wheater, M J

Bournemouth
A'Ness, T L
Abdalla, H O
Adams, R C
Alder, T A
Aldwinckle, R J
Allen, S C
Alsadi, M R H
Armitage, M
Bagnall, P J
Barker, P G
Barraclough, A C
Beck, J M
Bellamy, D
Bellamy, S
Bennett, D H
Benson, R A
Beswick, I C
Betts, R J
Bevan Jones, T M
Bidad, K
Bintcliffe, D J L
Blakeway, C
Blaszczyk, A
Brad, L D A
Bramble, F J
Brewer, A
Bridgman, N M
Bridgman, W M
Bromley, P A
Brookes, K R
Brown, G E
Caplin, G
Carter, C J M
Carter, S J
Cavan, D A
Chadwick, H A
Chau, W F
Cheesman, A M
Cook, M C
Cooke, J E
Cowley, N M
Cox, I M
Cox, S N A
Craig, E S
Creasey, D P
Creasy, T S
Crichton, D A
Crockett, C J
Davies, C
Davies, N
Davison, C R N
Dickson, D M
Donnellan, B S
Dorrell, E D
Drury, A E C
Dunkelman, H M
East, K R
Edwards, A J
Edwards, G A
El-Dars, L D
El Dars, M K
El-Dars, N
Etchells, D E
Evans, A J
Evans, P
Eve, L A
Fila, C
Fisher, J A
Flack, S T
Foot, A S
Fozard, J B J
Frank, H J
Freeth, M O
French, E
French, P F
Friedmann, A I
Gannon, I D
Gardiner, A O P
Garside, L J
Gibson, J F J
Goodier, V A
Goodwin, M I
Gordon, I D
Gould, J M
Gregory, D G
Grice, A S
Gunson, O S
Hardie, A W
Harding, J C
Hargreaves, D M
Harling, M E
Hartley, R H
Harvey, J E
Hassan, K M R
Head, J M
Heatley, I H
Heatley, K A
Hughes, M C
Irwin, N C
Jackson, P H
Jenkinson, D F
Jeyatheva, D N
Joshi, J B
Kennedy, J J A
Kernohan, J G
Kerr, D
Kidman, S P
Killick, S B
King, R A
Kingsley, M
Kissen, L H
Knighton, J D
Lawrance, R J
Lesley, B A
Levitt, A M
Lindall, K
Linnard, C A
Loehry, C A E H
McCullen, M A
McGill, N A
Mahmoud, M A-R
Marsh, C S
Martin, M J
Masding, M G
Mecklenburgh, P E
Michel, M Z H
Middleton, R G
Miller, S
Millward, J
Moran, C J
Moreland, B O
Morris, A H C
Nelemans, I
Nicholson, I G
Norris, C D
O'Connor, D
O'Connor, M J C
Ogden, A S
Oscier, D G
Owens, C T
Pampiglione, J S
Panton, N T M
Parham, D M
Parker, S W
Parvin, S D
Patten, M G
Pearson, N D
Penn, M A
Pennell, S C
Perkins, P D
Perry, D
Poulton, D J
Pratt, D R
Price, N C
Pryce, L S
Radvan, J
Ramsay, M W
Raza, T H
Rintoul, D M M
Rogers, B
Rogers, S A
Rozkovec, A
Scales, A H
Schuster Bruce, M J L
Scott, J W
Scrivener, S L
Scull, D A
Sekhar, C J R
Shakespeare, W M
Shaw, A A A
Shaw, M B
Shepherd, D F C
Sheridan, J J
Singh, A
Skene, A I
Sly, J M
Small, J H
Smith, M C
Smith, S
Southgate, J J
Stephens, J P
Surridge, J G
Sylvester, S E
Tawn, D J
Taylor, G G
Taylor, P
Tetley, G
Thomas, S M
Thurston, A M
Timberlake, T
Torquati, F R
Tunstall, N R
Turnbull, P
Turner, J A M
Van Hasselt, G L M
Vartan, C P
Wadams, S J F
Walker-Date, S E
Waters, J M
Watkins, J M
Weaver, R D
Whitwell, J
Widdicombe, N J
Williams, A J
Williams, C J H
Williams, C P R
Williams, D E
Williams, K G
Williams, S E
Willis, K A
Wimbleton, P A
Winwood, P J
Woodhead, J L
Wright, C J
Yonace, A H
Zinna, R F

Bow Street
Rhys, G
Roy, P B

Bowmore
Farrington, R L
Macdonald, M R S
MacDonald, M R

Brackley
Bennett, C L
Chidwick, D A
Cordingly, K A M
Perrott, C S
Quiney, I D
Rathborne, A C
Rundle, J A
Stephens, C A
Stephens, J
Stevens, P J
Turpin, C D
Widdowson, F J M
Wijayawardena, M A S S
Williams, K E

Bracknell
Afolami, S O
Ball, S K
Barrett, J
Bartlett, J M
Beckley, R A
Bell, A R
Briggs, E D
Caird, C J
Crisp, K E
Curry, K M
Emery, P K
Evans, E C
Gennery, B A
Green, R L
Greig, A P M
Hall, A K
Henman, M E
Holmes, D J
Houston, A C
Jady, K
Johnson, O
Kade, C
Kassianos, G
Keeling, T J
Knight, M G S
Koefman, R J
Lapham, G P
Lawrence, J J
Layng, J E
Leather, M S
Macaulay, O O
McBurnie, P R
McDonald, C F
Machray, A J
Mallipeddi, R
Metson, D
Mitchell, A C S
Mitchell, P B
Moriarty, J M A
Murray, J W I
Newton, K J W
Nielsen, K S
Norman, D P
Northover, S C
Orr, J F
Pardhanani, G
Pegrum, H L
Powers, L A
Ranscombe, B J
Ricketts, K J
Rogers, C E
Schiff, A A
Slemp, M C
Smith, M J
Stirling, J S
Tay, K S
Tobin, M J W
Tong, W
Trowbridge, M D
Verma, N
Weir, G

Braddan
Crerand, J
O'Malley, D N

Bradford
Abbas, N F
Abbasi, Z
Ahmad, M
Akhtar, S A
Akhtar, S
Alemi, A A
Alemi, C M
Ali, S M
Amarendra, V
Anderson, B D
Anikin, V A
Ansari, M I
Ashman, L M
Ashurst, N H
Atherton, P J
Atkinson, P L
Atukorala, A W
Ausobsky, J R
Auty, S J
Azam, A
Azam, M
Bargh, J H
Barnes, C A
Barnes, F C
Barodawala, S
Bartle, E O
Baruah, A
Baruch, M R
Basu, A
Batchelor, N G
Bateman, S P
Batman, P A
Baugh, S J
Bavington, A J
Bem, C C
Bembridge, J L
Bembridge, M
Beresford, N M
Bickford Smith, P J
Bindu, A
Blackburn, S D
Bollen, S R
Booth, A C
Bothra, J
Bowring, N A C
Boyden, J E
Bracken, P J
Bradbury, J A
Bradley, C
Bradley, P A
Brierley, E J
Brierley, S A
Bromley, S E
Brooke, M D
Brooksbank, A J
Brown, B J
Brown, G M
Brown, P M
Budd, S T
Busby, M I
Byrne, C
Callaghan, R T
Calvert, R J
Cann, M L
Cavaliere, V
Chatfield, S L
Chin, D
Chitsabesan, S
Chohan, N S
Clark, J A
Clark, R
Cohen, M S
Cole, A J
Cole, H K C
Coley, K
Collins, J B
Collis, K V
Connolly, A L
Connolly, J M
Corry, P C
Cowan, C L
Cramp, P G W
Craske, D A
Crossland, W D
Daley, A G
Dalton, P K
Danby, J
Davidson, R I
Davies, J B
Davies, T J
Dawson, A D G
De Mowbray, S S
Dedrick, S H
Devonport, H
Dewhirst, C J
Dharma Rajah, S
Downey, S E
Dutta, A
El Azab, A E S A
El Eliwi, R A
Elliott, L-A
Ellis, M P J
Emms, J R
Evans, C S
Evans, E C
Fairbrass, M J
Fenwick, I E
Flannigan, G M
Foo, I T H
Gaguine, D S
Gamie, E M K
Gavin, F M
Gilkar, G M
Gill, J C
Ginbey, D W
Goel, A
Gorman, S R
Gouldesbrough, D R
Gowa, S
Green, S D R
Griffith, J P
Griffiths, A O
Gupta, U
Haigh, D
Haile, A
Hall, R S
Hamilton, J B
Hanna, S N
Hansen, A T
Hardaker, J C
Harris, C P
Harrop, F M
Hawthorne, L A
Henderson, A A
Henderson, L J
Hewson, L A
Hill, S R A
Hillary, G M
Horsman, B A
Hossain, M M
Hossain, U
Hughes-Guy, L
Hughes, A
Hunter, S A
Husain-Qureshi, S
Hussain, S
Ihsan, F
Jacob, B K
Jandu, J
Jandu, M K
Jayatilake, N A
Jennings, S J
Jepson, K
Johnston, C A
Jones, J M
Kamill, P G O
Karet, B J
Karunakara, M
Keeler, J F
Kennedy, S
Khan, A
Khan, A A
Khan, A M
Khan, A
Khan, I A
Khan, M H
Khan, M A
Khan, N
Khan, S
Khan, S I
Khara, B R
Khatoon, A
Khwaja, S A I
King, S
Kluge, W H
Lansbury, A J
Latif, A B
Lawson, M
Lealman, G T
Lee, J E
Leedham, W G
Lennard, R F
Lindsay, H S J
Litvin, N P
London, E M
London, K M
McElligott, A J
McEvoy, A W
McEvoy, J F
Macintosh, M C M
McKean, E J G
McLindon, J P
McWhinney, P H M
Maddison, J L
Maddy, A
Mahmood, M
Mahmood, S
Mahmood, T
Mahomed, I
Majid, A
Malhotra, R K
Malik, T H
Mall, K P
Manchester, S G
Manik, K S
Manning, A P
Marcham, C D
Margerison, M R
Margerrison, C D
Marsh, P J
Martin-Hirsch, D P
Masood, A
Masood, M B
Matthew, A M
Mattocks, A N
May, J C
Mayfield, M P
Mearns, A J
Mellors, P A
Melsom, R D
Mewasingh, D
Micallef, C
Michie, C A H
Miciak, J
Mihajlovic, S
Mills, G A
Modi, D S
Moochhala, H S
Moreea, S M
Morley, C A
Morley, M E
Morrison, G W
Moulson, A J
Mughal, M S
Mughal, Z A
Nair, B
Nawaz, R M
Newmark, J C P
Newmark, P A
Newton, L J
Nigam, R
Obiechina, N E
Oke, A O
Okeahialam, M G
Ossei-Gerning, N
Overend, G S
Parapia, L G H
Parkinson, B F
Parnell, C
Passant, W S G
Paterson, C L
Patterson, C J
Patterson, J A

Paul, N
Peacey, S R
Pennington, E R
Philip, J
Pond, M N
Qasim, A
Qureshi, M A
Qureshi, M T
Raine, A
Raine, C H
Ralph, W H
Rand, R J
Rao, K
Rashid, A A W
Rashid, R
Rehman, M J
Rennie, P R
Reynell, P C
Reynolds, S E
Richardson, J
Riley, G A
Roberts, A M
Roberts, J F
Ross, M
Rout, D J
Rowlands, C J
Rushton, A
Russon, L J
Sabir, M S
Saed, E A-H
Sah, A
Sanderson, G D
Sandhu, K S
Schallreuter, K
Shah, S T K
Shanker, J S
Shaper, N J
Shaw, D L
Sheldon, K P
Shepherd, R I
Shoesmith, D J
Sides, A P
Sidra, R S
Sinclair, P M
Singh, B K
Singh, I M
Singh, J P
Singh, V
Sloan, B E
Smith, K T E
Smith, R A
Sood, S
Spiers, M R
Stark, D P H
Stephens, E C P
Stinson, I R
Strachan, C D S
Strachan, D R
Sullivan, J M
Swapp, H G
Taylor, S E
Temperley, C
Terry, H J
Thandi, H S
Thornton, D M
Throssell, J A
Timmons, M J
Todd, F N
Towers, S M
Trikha, S P
Tucker, A G
Tucker, J S
Tuffnell, D J
Turner, S M
Upile, T
Veeravahu, M
Venables, A J
Venkatesh, U R
Venters, N D
Vowden, P
Wade, I R
Wade, M J
Walker, N G
Wallace, S
Warlow, J J
Wason, A-M
Watson, E J
Watters, A T
Webster, J C T
Welford, J R F
Whitecross, S E S
Whitelaw, D C
Wildig, C E
Williams, A T
Wilson, A R
Wilson, V E
Winn, N B
Withers, A W J
Wright, A L
Wright, A J
Wright, J B
Wright, J P
York, S A
Young, J B

Bradford-on-Avon

Batty, S C
Bolt, J M
Carter, V
Catt, V E
Christie, E A
Cox, J A
Gamble, K R
Gough, N A
Heffer, J S
Higgs, C M B
Johnson, E B
Kendrick, C H
Narang, V P S
Needham, P R
O'Reilly, M
Paterson, L C
Patrick, J
Phillips, S M
Snow, A R
Swale, N F H
Wilkins, D C
Wyatt, N V

Braintree

Antcliff, A C
Archer, G K
Bracebridge, S P
Carter, J A
Cowburn, P J
Cutts, A M
Evans, D M
Gibson, C V
Gibson, I G L
Hildrey, A C C
Horobin, S R
Jackson, M D
Jackson, W L M
King, R L
Knapman, F M M
Kyaw Htun, Dr
Littler, W I
Martin, R H
Mayo, R E P
Meakin, R P
Meesters, H J R
Paterson, J R
Pereira, N B M
Purdie, A V
Richardson, J S
Runacres, A S R
Rushton, S C
Shaw, I C
Slater, J E
Soares, A-M R
Summers, S K
Williams, D A
Mya Than Win, J
Zollinger-Read, P J

Brampton

Blakeman, T M
Byers, M
Gray, P J
Hollings, A S J
Low, G D
Nicholson, S
Rodgers, R C
Royle, J
Wagstaff, R J
Weaving, P G

Brandon

Benke, E J
Campman, G H
Daley, T P
Hicks, T M
Khan, C F
Pugh, C J
Walmsley, S R
Warren, A E

Braunton

Bennett, B L
Bradford, H R
Dissevelt, A C E
Francis, A
Howell, J K
Loveden, L M
Moore, D G
Pearse, H A C
Pote, J
Vale, R J

Brechin

Adams, S A
Allison, C W
Buckley, J R
Callaghan, T S
Cowan, M
Donald, L A
Duff, A R
Fernandez, D B
Frost, S A H
Gillanders, I A
Greig, H D
Huda, A H M Q
McInnes, A M
Mahon, I M
Martin, R W Y
Shaw, A M
Tainsh, J A
Valentine, N W
Weekenborg, M-A

Brecon

Bacon, R W
Birch, R J
Cooper, P J
Davies, C D
Davies, J A J
Dimyan, W A
Dunn, A M
Evans, A V
Faulkner, P O
Ford, E M S
Gardner, Z N C
Goodger, V R
Gooding, P S
Griffith, D J O
Griffiths, M J
Heard, J
Heneghan, M B J
Hill, B J
Jackson, A S
Johnson, D B
Jones, E J
Jones, J K
O'Reilly, S
Rees, D G
Snow, P J
Thomas, W H
Vulliamy, C B
Wainwright, A J
Wainwright, D T
Walker, P C
Williams, B W
Williams, R S
Woodman, G J

Brentford

Alves Teixeira, J M
Bowden, A D
Chisholm, J M
Chojnacki, A
Davies, H W
Dignan, F J
Hill, J F
Horton, R J
Jones, D A
Lane, S M
Lawrence, C E
Murphy, A L
Revell, C P
Rowley Jones, D
Ruggles, R M
Ryan, P J J
Stevens, D J C
Sykes, J E
Wellwood, M R
Yasin, K M

Brentwood

Ainsworth, D P
Apps, M C P
Ariyanayagam, I J
Ariyanayagam, S
Battey, G S
Bennett, S M V
Boralessa, H
Bradbury, V D
Brock, D M
Butcher, J H
Butler, N S
Carter, C M W B C
Cervi, P L O
Chaloner, J M
Chatterjee, D S
Clough, L A
Coull, D B
Curtis, J
Davies, A M
Davies, D N
Dima-Okojie, S I
Dryden, M M
Duce, D J
Dunne, F J
Ekanayake, A T
Evans, C A W
Evans, D E W
Evans, J D
Feakins, M J
Fernando, H G
Fife, D G
Garvan, C J
Goodfellow, A E
Gordon, A J
Gorman, A M
Grewal, R
Gupta, R
Hamilton, M A
Handel, C C
Harper, C A
Hildebrand, S C
Hill, J T
Hillman, G W
Holkar, V E
Horti, J M
Jennings, S J
Karunanayake, M G S
Kassab, R D
Kochhar, M S
Lang-Stevenson, A I
Lewis, E R
Lissmann, M R
McKinnon, M D
Martin, N M
Mead, K I
Moncrieff, J M
Murray, J J
Naeem, A A
Navaratnam, S
Neill, S V
Outen, P R
Paffey, M D
Pandit, D R
Patel, B
Perrett, C M
Peskett, S A
Philpott, J M
Puvanendran, K
Ribeiro, B F
Richardson, J C W
Ridpath, J
Sathananthan, Y
Scott-Russell, A M
Sexton, N J
Steddon, S J
Steer, G L
Stephens, J D
Strachan, S R
Swift, J L
Tallack, J A
Taylor, J L
Tuppen, J J
Varma, R
Villiers, C
Walton, S J
Watson, J
Watts, S J
Woolterton, M C

Bridge of Weir

Aitchison, W R C
Arnot, A D W
Binning, A R
Crawford, J M
Findlay, I N
Geddes, C M
Geddes, N K
Goudie, H M
Hunter, C J
Lawson, P M
Leiberman, D P
McBain, R H
Macdonald, J B
McLaren, G I
O'Kane, G
Pollock, J S S
Rentoul, J R
Shepherd, H J
Smith, J L
Tatek, J
Taylor, K A
Van Der Lee, A J
Young, M J
Young, R E

Bridgend

Ali, I M
Anthony, J R
Ashpole, K J
Balfour, R P
Banerji, C
Barr, D B
Barrett, R M
Bhargava, J P
Blackall, D H
Bowyer, F M
Brodie, S W
Burgess, B J
Capel, M M
Chappell, A G
Chivers, S E
Clarke, E J
Cotter, M M G
Coyle, P J
Craven, A
Cuthill, J M
Davies, A I
Davies, H F
Davies, J P
Davies, K M
Davies, R H
Dawkins, J C
Devalia, V
Donagh, J G F
Edwards, C D
Edwards, P D L
Ellis, E M
English, E M
Evans, D A
Evans, L J
Evans, O
Evans, R A
Farrell, S H
Fletcher, P C
Foster, D R
Gataure, P S
Gilmartin, L M D
Goodwin, A
Gwilliam, G M
Hadley, R J
Hambly, P B
Hapgood, A I
Hapgood, G C
Hasan, D
Hashmi, M S
Hedges, A R
Higgs, J M
Hughes, D W
Hughes, J C
Jagger, P T
James, K C B
James, S H
James, W
Janas, M A
Johnson, R C
Jones, A
Jones, C J H
Jones, D C
Jones, D A
Jones, J S
Jones, J P
Jones, M J T
Joseph, F G
Judd, D
Koppel, S M
Lloyd, S M
Lock, A L
Logan, R A
Lord, M M L
McCann, R J
McHugh, R J
Madelin, S K
Manning, A
Mason-Williams, J
Mason, C H
Meredith-Smith, A
Miller, M D
Mohajer, S K P
Morgan, C A
Morgan, D W
Morgan, R O
Morris, J S
Morris, L M
Morris, P G
Morris, R W
O'Connor, I
Obaid, M P
Obaid, S L
Obaidullah, M
Osborne, J A
Owen, P J D
Owen, R E
Parab, S B
Patel, G K
Poulter, S D
Powner, H R
Price, A
Price, G V
Pritchard, G A
Pyves, C A
Raha, S K
Rahman, N A
Raijiwala, N T
Rees, A M
Reilly, T A A
Richards, G L
Richards, T V H
Roberts, C
Roberts, S A
Sarvotham, R
Smillie, J F
Sollis, M E
Srinivasan, U
Stamatakis, J D
Thomas, D J
Thomas, K
Thomas, R I
Tidley, M G
Trimlett, R H J
Tudor, G R
Vasu, V
Ware, D A
Waters, I R
West, S A
Wilkins, W E
Williams, C R
Williams, E J
Williams, G
Williams, J J
Williams, J P R
Williams, M
Williams, M N
Williams, M-C
Williams, M A
Williams, P D R
Williams, P
Williams, R G
Williams, T M
Wintle, M E
Winton, E
Workman, A R
Yapp, T R
Yeoman, A D
Young, S P
Young, W T

Bridgnorth

Blayney, J E
Burke, L P
Carvell, S P
Cotter, J
Downs, A M R
Gibbs, R H
Gillie, C P
Good, V J
Goodall, M S
Groves, R C C
Hammerton, M D
Hammerton, W
Kneen, L C
MacColl, L J
Magill, M J
Martin, S L
Parsonage, W A
Patel, Y A
Reeves, E M
Sandhu, N S
Seeley, A J
Suett, M J
Sykes, T C F
Torkington, A P J
Yuille, P M

Bridgwater

Aird, P M
Airey, N J
Allen, H M
Barnes, J S
Barrington, P M
Bennekers, J E C
Bidmead, N
Bray, E L
Bray, N J
Budd, J D
Cheek, C M
Constable, G D
Cooke, D I
D'Ambrumenil, P L
Davies, D N I
Deakin, H L
Di Mambro, S L M
Douglass, A W R
Dovey, J K
Evans, R L
Fergusson, G M
Gardiner, S
Goldie, A M

Hansford, P K
Hayne, P S
Hynes, D M
Ives, C L
Jago, H M
Johnson, M F
Johnson, R D
Lambert, R J
Lawler, C E
Lee, B E
Lee, R J
Lemmens, G W
Macadam, C F
McEwen, L M
Matthews, D T
Molyneux, A R
Ogle, J L
Osborne, C J
Paisley, A C
Parratt, J
Pepperell, J C T
Reed, A E R
Reed, P D
Roberts, S E K
Rooke, D K
Searle, W H
Slack, W W
Smart, M A
Stevenson, G R
Swindall, H J
Tanner, G P G
Tanner, H
Taylor, T M W
Tilsley, T M
Tottle, J A
Wright, A
Wrout, J D

Bridlington
Barton, E A
Bayne, J B
Bowden, D F
Burridge, D N
Calaghan, N P
Clarke, A J
Farley, K T J
Francis, A C
Gillespie, J R
Harris, P A
Hickson, D E G
Hillman, J G
MacNab, H K
Meldrum, H R P
Memon, M A
Mundy, P
Nasar, M A
Nisbet, A M
Ridley, P D
Robertson, A S
Robertson, A
Robertson, A S
Robertson, M
Sinha, C
Sinha, R S K
Talbot, A W
Wallam, T D
Watson, A J S
Watson, R M
Webster, M R
Wiles, B G R
Wilson, J F
Wilson, P D

Bridport
Beckers, M J J
Beckers, S R
Burt, B M
Carter, R G
Cotton, J M
Crawshaw, E G A
Crook, A
Hollands, J J C
King, J G
Laven, L E D
Lintner, B
Longley, J I
Millar, A B
Napper, A M S
Neame, R L
Platt, I T
Pratt, C L G
Rossiter, S K
Skellern, G
Smithers, D A
Thomson, M
Webb, P G
Wilson, C B

Brierley Hill
Ahmed, N W
Bundred, M A
Clarke, B W
Craggs, A M S
Craggs, I F
Edwards, C R
El-Sayad, A R A H
Faux, D H R
Fernandes, C
Hafiz, A
Jones, T E G
Khasgiwale, A K
Leung, V K Y
Patel, J A
Plant, S J
Reed, I A
Rigler, M S
Russell, J A
Shah, H V
Shah, R M
Sumaria, M K M
Thornton, A J
Young, A J

Brigg
Burscough, J F
Chester, D W
Crompton, B A
Crowe, N A
Edmondson-Jones, M
Guest, R
Hill, A
Iuel, B M
Lloyd, S
Norris, P E
Reid, F M
Sutton, P A
Travers, A F
Whitaker, V S
Yule-Smith, A L

Brighouse
Aparicio Ledesma, J
Brook, A C
Chambers, S J
Farrow, S
Gatecliff, J R
Gay, D A T
Gorman, P J
Grant, J P
Gurr, J M
Jain, N K
Lamming, R E M
Lawson, J H
Martin, S
Mason, A D
Mason, L E
Matischen, G M
O'Carroll, P J A
Quarcoo, S T
Rajjayabun, P H
Savage, V E
Sharma, N K
Wilkinson, J R
Wylie, R M

Brighton
Aawar, O A
Abraham, A J
Adams, N J
Aiton, N R
Allen, C D
Allenby, L M
Altman, K
Ames, W A
Amess, P N
Anderson, K J
Anderson, K J
Appanna, N
Aston, J E
Atkinson, D C
Austera, J
Baldwin, F J
Banieghbal, B
Barley, M G
Bartlett, C I
Beasley, J V
Beesley, C J
Bell, M E
Bentley, M R
Beresford-Jones, P R
Bhermi, A J
Bickler, G J
Bintcliffe, I W L
Bird, N
Bloomfield, D J
Bodkin, J R
Bowie, J E

Bowman, G O
Bowskill, R J
Boyd, J
Boyd, O F
Bradley, R J
Bradshaw, M J
Brittain, G P H
Brooks, M D
Brown, C F
Bryant, C M
Bryant, G D R
Burt, R W
Burwood, R J
Butt, A M
Carter, H R
Casswell, A G
Chaikin, M J
Chamberlain-Webber, J A A S
Chang, Y F
Child, C S B
Churchill, D R
Clarke, J N
Clarke, S A
Clarkson, P J
Clifford, G J
Cockcroft, M
Cohen, J
Combe, A J
Cordingly, M R
Corner, A J
Cottingham, R L
Craigie, I T
Crichton, A R C
Crossman, I G
Cubbon, M D
Culliford, L D
Curtis, A
Darley, C R
Davey, A J
Davidson, A
Davidson, C
Davies, H J
Davy, A R
De Belder, A J
De Souza, R G J
Deady, J M
Denis Le Seve, P A
Derrick, E K
Devlin, P N P
Dew, A E
Dodge, G S
Doshi, M K
Doyle, T N
Drake, H F
Duncan, J R
Eadie, E J
Ebbetts, J H
Eckstein, M B
Edwards, M K R
Elcock, D H
Elcombe, G M
Elvidge, J B
Evans, A H
Farhoumand, N
Fernandes, L
Firth, S M
Fish, A N J
Forsyth, A T
Fry, A
Gainsborough, N
Garewal, C
Garrett, W V
Gentles, H
George, J Y
Gilhooly, G
Gilman, D H
Goldberg, L C
Goyne, R L
Gray, R
Green, D J M
Gumpert, J R W
Habgood, C M
Hacking, R S
Hale, P C
Halford, J
Hallam, L
Harden, A F
Harding, N J
Harper, D R
Harries, M L
Harris, I M
Harris, S
Harrison, J R
Hartley, J P R
Helps, P J
Hermitage, A P
Herold, J
Hildick-Smith, D J R

Hildick-Smith, P M
Holden, D P
Hollis, P R
Holmberg, S R M
Holt, S G
Homer, P M
Howells, M
Hoyle, A N
Hurst, P A E
Hutchesson, E A
Hyams, A B
Iggo, N C
Ing, R P
Ingram, A S
Ireland, A
Iversen, S A
Jackson, M B
Jarvis, K R
Kalidasan, V
Kanal, L
Kanumakala, S
Karnicki, M T
Kaye, S L
Kelleher, D I F
Kenney, I J
Kenny, M W
Kerr, G A
Khan, N A
Khot, A S S
King, C J
King, E J
Kingswood, J C
Kirkham, N
Kirkland, B
Knott, M H
Kuper, M B
Lamah, M
Larcombe, P J
Larner, T R G
Levack, F C
Lewis, C C
Lewis, J
Lipscombe, S L
Livesey, E A
Lulsegged, A
Lyall, R A
McConnell, R
McDonnell, E D
McKinna, F E
McLeod, B K
MacRorie, N D
Mangat, S S
Meade, P F
Mendonca, M J T
Mockett, R J
Montgomery, J C
Mukadam, G A
Mull, A
Mustill, A L
Neilson, F M
Newman, G H
Newman, P L
Nisbet, A P
O'Connor, F A
O'Neal, H
Paisley, J M
Panja, S K
Papasavvas, G K
Parikh, J K
Parish, S P E
Parry, M G
Parsley, J
Patel, N K
Pateman, J A
Patton, N D
Paul, J
Pay, R K
Perez-Avila, C A
Perry, F M
Philip, G
Phillips, D L
Pierce, E L
Price, G J
Price, M L
Pugsley, W B
Pulley, M S
Punja, A N
Ragab, S
Rainey, A J
Ralph, I
Ramadas, R
Ransom, P A
Roberts, C E A
Robinson, R E M
Rockwell, S R
Roderic-Evans, J E
Rosenberg, M A J
Rowan, J
Rubin, G

Rustom, R
Saadah, E S M
Sacks, S L
Sagar, P J
Saunders, N C
Sayani, M I
Seddon, P C
Shah, A C
Shah, R
Shaheen, J S O
Sharp, M J A
Shaw, C D
Simpson, J K
Slattery, M A
Smith, A M
Smith, H E
Sonksen, C J
Spurrell, J R R
Spurrell, P A R
Srinivasan, S
Sripuram, S G
Stalker, M J
Staniforth, P
Stead, C A
Stewart, V R
Strachan, C J L
Street, M J
Studd, C
Supple, D L
Sutcliffe, V A
Sutton, C J
Swaine, C N
Tate, R T
Tayler, D H
Thomas, P J
Thompson, M W B
Thorp, T A S
Titley, R G
Tranter, R M D
Tredgold, B
Trounce, J Q
Twohig, M M
Van Ryssen, J S M W P
Vaughan, N J A
Vickers, S F
Vincent, R
Vokins, C G
Voyce, M E
Walters, M T
Wastie, J C
Waters, A M
Watkins, R C
Watson, C A
Watson, P M
Weighill, J S
Weir, F J
Wells, A A
Whale, W R
White, H A
White, S M
Wilkinson, P R
Williams, C R P
Williams, D I
Williams, R A
Willis, C H
Willison, K A
Winter, R A
Withecomb, J L
Woollaston, M E F
Woollons, A D
Wostenholm, D K
Wright, C M V
Yelland, A
Yetton, W R
Yusuf, S W

Bristol
Abrams, P
Ackroyd, C E
Adams, E J
Adams, K J
Addison, S J
Addleson, D J
Ahmed, M
Al-Mufti, R A W M L
Al Wakeel, G M
Alderson, D
Aleeson, R
Alexander, J I
Alexander, K M M
Ali-Khan, A S
Allen, C S
Allen, P E
Allen, P L
Alonso Madrazo, C
Alsop, K R
Amar, K A K A
Anderson, D N

Anderson, E G
Anderson, R S
Andersson, C S
Andrews, H S
Andrews, J H
Angelini, G D
Ansell, D B
Anstey, E J
Appleton, A S
Archer, C B
Arkell, S M
Armstrong, C P
Armstrong, S J
Arnold, R P
Arul, G S
Aspinall, R L
Atherton, M T
Atherton, W G
Atkins, J L
Atkins, R M
Atkins, S E
Atter, C C
Axson, D M
Aylard, A P
Aylard, P R
Azurmendi Sastre, V
Backhouse, M F
Bacon, J M
Badger, G
Bagshaw, P J
Bailey, C C
Bailey, D J G
Bailey, J S H
Bailey, J A
Bailey, J E
Bailward, T A
Baird, R N
Baker, A R
Bakker, P A G
Baldwin, D L
Baldwin, R J
Bannister, G C
Barber, M J
Barber, R D
Barham, C P
Barkley, A C
Barlow, G M
Barnes, A D
Barnes, H E
Barrett, A J
Barry-Braunthal, J A
Barry, R E
Barwell, J R
Barwell, P J
Barwell, W B A
Bassi, S C
Bates, J H J
Bates, M
Baxter, I T
Bayley, G L
Bayly, G R
Bayly, R A
Bazeley-White, D L
Beale, R J
Beare, N A V
Bell, C J
Ben-Shlomo, Y
Bench, L J
Benger, J R
Bennet, E G
Bennett, E M
Bennett, J A
Bennett, J A
Bennetto, L P
Beresford, R J A
Beringer, R M
Berkley, R J
Bevir, T A
Bingley, P J
Binns, C E
Birch, K
Birchall, J E
Bird, J M
Bird, J M
Bird, S A A
Birkett, P B L
Bishop, N L
Bisson, D L
Black, A M S
Black, S M
Blacker, C V R
Blackwell, M M
Blake, A J
Blazeby, J M
Blewitt, N
Bloss, D E
Blunsum, E A
Blythe, A J
Bobrow, C S

Bodard, S J
Boden, S K
Bolger, C M
Bolt, J L
Bolt, S H
Bolton, J
Bonnet, M S
Boone, D L
Boreham, P A
Borhanzahi, K
Bowden, J E
Bowen, J T
Bowen, R L
Bower, C P R
Bowler, V A
Box, M P
Box, O M
Boycott, A
Boyd, K E
Bradfield, P C
Bradley, B A B
Bradley, S N
Bradshaw, J R
Bragg, J M
Bragonier, R
Brain, S P
Branfoot, K J
Braybrooke, J P
Bredow, M T
Bremner-Smith, A T
Brett, M T
Briggs, J A
Brightley, K M
Brindle, P M
Britten, S
Brokate, A
Bromham, B
Bromley, J
Brosh, S J
Brown, A C
Brown, E M
Brown, J
Brown, J M
Brown, R A
Brown, R P M
Bryan, A J
Buckingham, R A
Buckley, P A
Buhrs, E G J
Bunting, R A
Burd, D A R
Burge, T S
Burke, S P
Burness, J H
Burney, P J
Burnham, W H
Burns-Cox, C J
Burrow, J E
Burton, C J
Butler, A V J
Butler, N R
Byrne, A
Byron, M A
Caddick, J F
Cahill, D J
Caine, S E
Cairns, P A
Callaway, M P
Callow, G
Cameron, M-Y
Campbell, C J
Campbell, C P
Campbell, M J
Candish, C G
Caputo, M
Carey, R J
Carney, L J
Carnie, P W
Carpenter, P K
Carr, R J
Carrington, D
Carson, K G S
Carswell, A M
Carswell, F
Carter, J A
Carter, M
Carter, S E
Case, C P
Cash, I D
Caswell, H J
Catterall, J R
Cawthorn, S J
Cembrowicz, S P
Cervantes, A J
Chadwick, S A
Chambers, J
Chambers, S
Chambers, T L
Chan, K X-H
Chan, S K M
Chandler, R J
Chatakondu, S C
Chatakondu, S
Cheesman, M G
Cheetham, E J
Chesney, D S
Chesser, T J S
Cheung Ming Hon, M
Chidley, K E
Chillistone, D J D
Churchill, A J
Ciulli, F
Clark, A J B
Clark, J B
Clark, M E
Clarke, G J
Clarke, S P
Clavert, K L
Clay, M E
Clayton, T J
Clement, M J
Clifford, J
Cloote, A H
Coakham, H B
Coates, D P
Cobby, M J D
Cobby, T F
Cochrane, B
Cochrane, D F
Codling, B W
Coggins, R P
Cohen, A M
Cohen, M A H
Coleman, P D
Coles, C J
Colley, J R T
Collis, R J
Colman, A R
Combe, G M
Coniam, S W
Connor, A P
Conrad, J M
Constantinides, H
Conway, P J
Cook, S D
Cooke, L B
Cooling, H S
Cooper, S J
Coote, E A
Coppock, W A
Corcoran, M T K
Cordell, A J
Cornes, J S
Cornes, P G S
Corrall, R J M
Coulson, A
Coulson, C
Coulson, C E
Coulson, T J
Cox, C M
Cox, D E
Cox, J W
Craig, J K
Craig, N J
Creamer, P
Crichton, N R
Cripps, T R
Crown, A L
Crowne, E C
Croxson, S C M
Culling, J A
Cunliffe, J L
Cunliffe, P N
Currie, A D M
Currie, L J
Dacombe, C M
Daglish, M R C
Dalton, G R
Daniel, R M
Daniels, K R
Darby, M
Darcy, M K
Darley, E S R
Darvill, D R
Darwent, M
Davey-Smith, G
David, M G J
Davidson, E J
Davidson, R G
Davies, D I
Davies, F J
Davies, I M
Davies, S J C
Davies, V M
Davis, A
Davison, P A
Dawson, N J
Day, P J
Dayan, C M
De Berker, D A R
De Cothi, G A
Deakin, G J
Dean Revington, P J
Dedman, P A
Degens, G C
Delaney, R J
Dennison, M
Denton, K J
Denton, R S
Di Mambro, A J
Diamond, J P
Dibdin, S J
Dick, A D
Dieppe, P A
Difford, F
Dinani, S
Dix, P J
Dixon, A R
Dixon, J C
Dixon, J H
Dixon, N M
Dobbie, J A
Donald, C C
Donald, F A
Doney, I E
Doris, J F
Douek, I F
Douglas, N T E
Dowling, S F O
Down, R C E
Dowse, C T
Dowson, S R
Doyle, M J
Draycott, T J
Dresser, I G
Du Heaume, J C
Duck, J L
Dudderidge, T J
Dudley, C R K
Dudley, J A
Duke, L C
Duke, N C
Duncan, A W
Duncan, K R
Dunnet, J M
Dunnett, I A R
Dunnill, M G S
Dunning, B H
Durdey, P
Dwarika, W M
Dwyer, N A
Eames, P G
Eastaugh-Waring, S J
Eastman, F V
Easty, D L
Eaton, J M
Ebrahim, S B J
Eccles, M J
Eddison, D M
Eddison, R M
Edwards, A G
Egginton, A M
Eldridge, J D J
Eley, E A
Ellis, C
Ellis, J C
Elstow, G A
Eltringham, W K
Emond, A M
Emsley, S P
Entrican, J H
Erskine, K F
Evans, A J
Evans, A E
Evans, E M
Evans, G A
Evans, J C W
Evans, J L
Evans, M J
Evely, R S
Ewen, J M
Ewins, D
Eyers, P S G
Falk, S J
Farey, H K
Farnall, E A
Fearon, H C
Feest, T G
Felce, D W
Feller, R
Fenn, S E
Fenton, J A
Ferguson, I T
Ferguson, J W
Fernandes, F J
Fernandez De Castillo Torras, B
Ferris, J D
Feuchtwang, A C
Fielden-Smith, S A
Fielding, A S
Fields, R
Findlay, A M
Finn, A H R
Finn, H P
Flanagan, P M
Fleming, J O
Fligelstone, J S
Follows, P M
Foot, A B M
Forbes, K
Ford, M R W
Ford, S M
Foreman, P S
Fornear, J E
Forrest, M J
Fosbury, S J F
Foster, D M
Foster, L M
Foubister, W J
Fowler, C A
Fowles, S J
Fox, A B E
Fox, C A
Fox, D P
Frank, J D
Frankel, S J
Franklin, T C
Frewer, J D
Frewin, T
Frost, N A
Furlong, E
Gaal, E
Gale, E A M
Gamble, E A
Ganly, S A
Gardner, I C
Gargan, M F
Garner, J E
Garrett, T
Garrod, T J
George, M J
Gepi-Attee, S
Gething, E
Ghosh, A R
Gibbs, C E
Gibbs, G H R
Gibson, A G F
Gilbert, P S
Gill, A A
Gill, S S
Gillatt, D A
Gilmore, K J
Gingell, J C
Ginn, H E
Gleeson, R E
Glew, C
Glover, D A
Glover, S C
Godfrey, I B
Godfrey, P S A
Godfrey, P F
Goldie, M
Golding, S J
Goldstraw, E J
Goldsworthy, L L
Golledge, J
Gollin, T J
Gompels, M M A
Goodden, G F C
Goodland, D S
Goodman, N W
Goodman, S E
Goodrick, M J
Goram, J B K
Gordon, F H
Gordon, J R
Gordon, U D
Gough, R
Gould, T H
Goyder, N P
Graham, A L
Graham, J D
Granier, S K
Grant, D A
Gray, H C
Gray, J F
Green, A J
Green, M E
Green, P R
Green, R E
Green, S M
Greene, J R T
Greenhalgh, K L
Greenhouse, P R D H
Greenslade, G L
Greenwood, H
Gregory, M
Grenfell-Shaw, J M
Grenfell, P M
Grey, R H B
Grice, G L
Grier, D J
Griffith, N W
Griffiths, C A
Grindey, C A
Gruenewald, P
Grundy, P L
Guest, J
Guest, P G
Guilding, T M
Gumb, J P
Gunnell, D J
Gutteridge, G J
Guy, P R
Haddy, C E L
Haggett, T I
Halford, J M
Hall, C M
Hall, C R
Hamilton, M A
Hammer, B
Hancock, J P
Hanks, G W
Hanmer, R L
Hannon, M A
Harbord, P N
Hardie, R J
Hardiman, G V
Harding, K A
Harding, R J
Hardy, H D
Hardy, J R W
Hare, L
Hargreaves, H M
Harland, R F
Harling, C C
Harlow, E D
Harman, I P
Harper, S J
Harrad, R A
Harries, H J
Harris-Lloyd, C M
Harris, P P
Harrison, E
Harrison, G L
Harrison, L S
Harrison, M D I
Harrison, V M
Hart, J C D
Hartnell, V H
Harvey, J E
Harvey, R F
Hashim, H
Hatton, C E
Havers, A R
Hawley, R M
Haworth, J M
Haworth, J M A
Hayes, A M
Hayes, F M
Hayes, J R
Haynes, R J
Hayter, J D
Heading, C M
Hearn, K P
Heath, R W
Heidelmeyer, C F
Hellier, P A
Hellier, W P L
Hembry, J N
Hemmings, M A
Hepburn, P R
Herborn, A
Herod, S J
Herron, M L
Hetzel, M R
Hewer, R L
Hewes, J C
Hewitt, J A
Heyderman, R S
Heywood, P
Hibbert, V L
Higgins, A S
Higgs, S A
Hill, M E
Hillier, J C
Hills, M W
Hine, C E
Hine, I D
Hinton, R A
Hobbs, C G L
Hockey, B J
Hodges, C
Hoffman, C L
Hoffman, N J
Hoffman, R J
Hogg, D C
Hogg, G P
Hoghton, M A R
Hoh, H B
Holden, N E S
Holdsworth, J E
Holland, D E
Holland, R K
Holland, S M
Holliday, D B
Hollingworth, P
Holmes, K M
Hooper, N R J
Hopwood, J A
Horner, P J
Horrocks, C T
Hosking, E-J
Houghton, K J
House, W
Hovey, T M
Howe, A M
Howe, R A
Hows, J M
Hoysal, N
Hoyte, C A E
Hudson, J G
Hughes, C W
Hughes, D G
Hughes, G
Hughes, J L
Hughes, S
Humphreys, N
Humphries, A B D
Hung, I F-N
Hunt, R J
Hussain, N
Hutchinson, M J
Hutter, J A
Hynam, P
Ibrahim, N B N
Iles, S
Illingworth, S C
Inward, C D
Irvine, C E W
Irvine, G H
Izhar, M
Jackson, M
Jackson, N J
Jackson, S A
Jahfar, S C
James, H A
James, J A
James, J R
James, L
James, S C
Jardine, P E
Jefferson, K P
Jeffrey, D R
Jelfs, J P
Jenkins, G M
Jenkins, I A
Jenkins, J M
Jewell, M D
Jewkes, J
Jobanputra, R
Joels, L A
Johar, M A
John, N G
Johnson, C J H
Johnson, D P
Johnson, D M
Johnson, R S
Johnson, R W
Johnston, S L
Johnstone, C G
Jones, A J
Jones, A M
Jones, C M
Jones, E V
Jones, J V
Jones, J E
Jones, K E
Jones, M S
Jones, M L
Jones, N
Jones, R
Jordan, L M
Joy, V J
Kabala, J E
Kalfayan, P Y
Kane, L A
Kane, N M
Karabatsas, K
Kay, A R
Kaye, J I
Keen, G
Kelland, S A

Kemp, H J
Kemple, T J
Kendall, C E
Kendall, J M
Kenealy, J M
Kennedy, C T C
Kennedy, R P
Kenney, B A K
Kenny, J R
Kent, N J
Kenwright, P
Kerfoot, N E
Kershaw, D M L
Kessler, D S
Khabaza, E
Khan, F
Khan, S
Khong, C H
Khong, S-Y
Kindleysides, A
Kings, G A
Kingston, J M
Kinsella, S M
Kirkpatrick, A J J
Kirkup, M E M
Kirwan, J R
Kitching, D F
Knight, C J
Knights, S E
Koehli, N
Krischer, J M
Kvalsvig, A J
Kyle, M V
Kyle, P M
Lafferty, E M
Laing, J D
Lalla, S C
Lam, P S E
Lambert, P A
Lambert, R G
Lamont, M M
Lamont, P M
Langfield, J A
Langton Hewer, S C
Langton, F A
Laszlo, G
Latham, S G
Lau, D F
Lauder, G R
Laue, B
Laurence, N J I
Laurence, R Q
Lavelle, A B
Lavin, E P
Lawlor, D A
Lawrence, J C
Lawrence, T M
Lawson, R H
Leaf, A A
Leahy, T C
Lear, P A
Learmonth, I D
Leary, P M
Lee, E C
Lee, R C
Leigh, J
Leitch, A
Lesley, S W
Leslie, I J
Levy, A
Lewis, G M
Lewis, H J
Lewis, N L
Lewis, T T
Li, S T B
Lightman, S L
Lim, B K
Lindeck, J F
Linter, S P K
Lismore, J R
Loader, J S
Lockey, D J
Lockyer, J S
Lockyer, M S
Loke, A J
Longhurst, S E
Lopez, A
Lounamaa, R H K
Love, S
Loveday, E J
Lowis, S P
Lowrey, S
Lunt, P W
Lunts, E S
Lupton, H A
Luty, J S
Lyell, V R
Lyons, A F M
Lyons, M

McCafferty, I J
McCaldin, M D
McCarron, P G
McClatchey, A
McCormick, B A
McCulloch, N A
Macdonald, A J R
Macdonald, R D
McEvoy, S C
MacGowan, A P
McGowan, M T
McGraw, M E
Macgregor-Morris, R
Macintyre, A E R
Macipe, M E
Mackenzie Crooks, D J
Mackenzie, E F D
Mackenzie, J C
Mackintosh, M A
McLeod, F N
Macpherson, R I
Macquire-Samson, I M P J
McQuoney, P A
McRobert, M S
McVey, F K
McWatters, V
Madden, A P
Maendl, A C J
Maher, J
Mahyoub Abbas, M A
Main, J A
Main, P G N
Majid, M A
Makins, R J
Malcolm, G P
Male, P P
Malki, A A-E-H G
Mallory, S
Malone, J D
Manara, A R
Mancero, S
Mandeville, J E
Manoharan, P
Mansfield, K B
Mansfield, N C
March, E J
Markham, D H
Markham, R H C
Marks, D I
Marsh, P J J
Marsh, R D
Marshall, D E
Martin, R P
Martin, V C
Martindale, S J
Masacorale, S V
Masheder, S
Maskell, N A
Mason, C F
Mason, E E
Massey, E J R H
Massey, S R
Mather, S J
Mathieson, P W
Mathison, A C
Mathison, D M
Maw, A R
Maxwell, R B H
Mayes, A J
Meadows, P S
Meads, A E
Meehan, S
Melichar, J K
Meller, R H C
Memel, D S
Menke, T
Menson, E N
Mercer, N S G
Metcalf, J V
Mian, I H
Millar, A B
Mills, M S
Milne, J D
Milne, M R
Mital, D
Mitchell, D C
Mitchell, R M
Mitchell, T J F
Mitchell, W B
Mitcheson, J I H
Mobbs, J
Mokete, M
Moncrief, A C
Monk, C R
Monsell, F P
Montague, A P
Montague, H J
Montague, R F

Montgomery, S M
Moon, D J
Moore, A G
Moore, N J
Moore, P J
Moorman, N E
Moralee, P
Moreno Garcia, J
Morgan, H G
Morgan, J A
Morgan, J D T
Morris, E W
Morris, E A J
Morse, M H
Moss, T H
Mostafa, M A A
Mountford, R A
Muir, R M
Mumford, D B
Mungall, S B
Munro, A E B
Munro, E N
Murdoch, J B
Murphy, K P M
Murphy, P J
Murray, J R
Mussett, J M
Mutch, H J
Myers, P P V
Myles, J S
Naish, J M
Nandwani, N
Nash, A P
Nation, C B M
Naughton, C A
Naysmith, M C
Ndirika, A C
Neal, D M
Negus, A G
Nelki, M F H
Nelson, I W
Nereli, B E
Ness, A R
Newbery, F E
Newbury-Ecob, R A
Newell, E L
Newman, C A
Newman, H F V
Newman, J H
Ng, S Y
Nicholas, M
Nicholls, G
Nicholls, K
Nichols, K C
Nicholson, H D
Niven, P A R
Norfolk, G A
Norman, J M
Norman, M L
Norman, M A
Norman, S P
Norman, S
Norton, R H
Norton, S A
Nowers, M P
Nunez, D A
Nutt, D J
Nutt, N R
O'Brien, C M
O'Carroll, M G
O'Connor, S
O'Hara, G V
O'Higgins, F M
O'Leary, A J
O'Mahony, M Y
O'Neill, P J
Oakhill, A
Oakland, C D H
Oakley, G A
Odum, S
Oke, S C
Oliver, E J H
Oliver, S E
Orlando, A
Ormerod, F
Ormerod, I E C
Osborne, N J R
Osborne, S F
Ostins, A W
Otton, S H
Over, D C
Overton, C E
Owen-Jones, J L
Owen, G
Owen, J H
Owen, W I
Oxley, J
Page, F B
Page, S J

Paine, T F
Pamphilon, D H
Pandit, J C
Papacostopoulos, D
Papouchado, M
Parker, J C
Parker, L R C
Parker, M
Parker, S E
Parkinson, J M T
Parmenter, J G
Parnham, A
Parrott, J P S
Parry, A J
Parry, H R
Parry, M O L
Partridge, D R
Passmore, K E
Patel, B P
Patel, P S
Patel, S D
Paterson, C F
Paterson, J P
Paterson, T A
Pattison, H F
Pattison, S H
Paul, I R
Pawade, A M
Paxton, C P C
Payne, C J I
Payne, F B
Payne, N E S
Payne, P A G
Peacock, G F
Pearce, K J
Peel, D J
Pegg, G C
Pemberton, P E
Penning-Rowsell, V W
Pentlow, B D
Pepper, S H
Persad, R A R
Petrie, N C
Pettit, E K
Pheby, D F H
Philipp, R
Phillips, D G
Phillips, S M
Phillips, W R
Pickering, V
Pickett, D A
Pike, A A
Pike, J
Pitman, M A
Pitts Crick, J C
Plummeridge, M J
Pomirska, M B
Pople, I K
Portas, C D
Porteous, D J
Porter, C J
Porter, D G
Porter, I J
Porter, K
Potokar, T S
Pottinger, R F
Potts, M J
Poulsom, W J
Pounsford, J C
Powell, L A
Price, C G A
Price, D M
Price, S P
Primrose, P A
Probert, C S J
Probert, J L
Pryn, S J
Prys-Roberts, C
Przemioslo, R T
Purkiss, R H
Quader, K
Quinn, M J
Raffety, R C
Rahman, M A
Rahman, S N
Randall, M E H
Rasanayagam, S R
Rashid, I
Rawlinson, G V
Rawlinson, J N
Rawlinson, S M
Raynal, A L
Rayter, Z
Read, K G
Reading, C A
Reavley, S B
Record, C A
Redmond, J V
Ree, C J

Rees, C M
Rees, C A
Rees, G J G
Rees, H J
Rees, J R
Rees, J S
Rees, J R E
Rees, R
Reeve, M
Reeves, G E
Reeves, R W K
Reid, C D
Reid, C M
Reid, D L L
Revington, P J
Reynolds, N M
Rice, G A
Rich, M G
Richards, C M
Richardson, S A
Ridler, S L
Ridley, P
Rigby, H S
Riley, K
Ring, N P
Roberts, A S
Roberts, C M
Roberts, C J C
Roberts, C J
Roberts, D G V
Roberts, D M
Roberts, S K
Robertson, R J
Robinson, B
Robinson, D E
Robinson, P J
Rodgman, M E
Roe, A M
Rogers, D G C
Rogers, J E G
Rogers, J C
Ronson, J G
Rooth, J A
Rosengren, H
Ross, A J
Rossdale, M G P
Routledge, T A
Rowley, C
Roy, B F
Royston, V H
Rudge, C J
Russell, E C
Russell, S R
Ryan, A G
Sacks, L J
Sadler, J A
Sage, C H
Sahay, S
Sale, S M
Saleem-Uddin, M A
Salisbury, C J
Salmon, G M
Sampson, M T
Samuels, A
Sandeman, D R
Sanders, A D
Sanders, D J
Sandford, J J
Sandhu, B K
Sandry, S A
Sansom, J E
Sant, A M
Sarangi, P P
Sarma, K P
Sartori, R A
Sasada, M P
Saunders, E S
Saunders, M W
Saunders, P W
Saungsomboon, D
Savage, J R
Savage, P E
Sawford, R W
Sawyerr, C
Scanlon, J M
Schaefer, J A
Schembri Wismayer, F
Schofield, E C
Schulte, J F
Scott-Moncrieff, C M
Scott, A J
Scott, B A
Scott, G L
Scott, M P Y
Scull, T J
Searle, J M
Seddon, J D M
Self, F R
Sellers, S M

Sellick, C S
Sells, H
Senior, C J
Sephton, E A
Sephton, T J
Sergi, C
Seymour-Shove, R
Shah, M J
Shahid, H
Sharp, D J
Sheard, T A B
Sheffield, E A
Shepherd, A M
Shepherd, S G
Shepherdson, D
Sheppard, C J
Shere, M H
Sheridan, R P
Sherriff, R J
Sheshgiri, J B
Shield, J E H
Shield, J P H
Shinde, S
Shlosberg, C B
Short, C A
Shutt, L E
Shyamapant, S
Sias, A
Sibley, G N A
Siddiqui, M M F
Sidebotham, P D
Sieradzan, K A
Silbiger, C A
Silvey, H S
Simmonds, M R
Simons, P S
Simpson, A L
Simpson, P J
Sims Williams, H G
Skelton, D A W
Skew, B L
Skinner, A V
Slack, N F
Slade, R R
Smalldridge, J
Smith, A J
Smith, C S
Smith, D L
Smith, F C T
Smith, J E
Smith, J M
Smith, P J B
Smith, P M
Smith, P A
Smith, R M
Smith, R P P
Smith, S J
Smith, S N
Smith, S M
Smith, T J T
Smithson, J E
Smithson, S F
Smyk, D
Smyth, G T C
Snow, J A
Soar, J
Solomon, L
Soodeen, D E
Soodeen, S J
Soothill, P W
Southwood, T M
Spare, T J
Speller, D C E
Spence, D S
Spence, R W
Spencer, R C
Spicer, R D
Spurling, B M
Stainer, K J
Stambuli, P M
Standen, G R
Stanley, D J P
Stanley, O H
Stannard, C F
Stansbie, D L
Steeds, C E
Steele, T
Steiner, M R
Stephens, A D
Stephenson, C R
Stevens, R J G
Stevenson, B J
Stevenson, J
Steward, C G
Stimpson, G G
Stoddart, H
Stoddart, P A
Stoodley, N G
Struthers, C A

Stuart, A G
Stubbs, P D
Styles, C L
Sullivan, J G
Summerskill, W S M
Sutcliffe, M C
Sutton, E M
Sweerts, M I E
Swingler, R
Swithinbank, D W
Swithinbank, L V
Sylvester, P A
Symes, M O
Tait, C P
Tallis, P M
Tam, B S M
Tan, C
Tan, S Y
Tarleton, D E B
Tate, D W
Tattan, T M G
Tawodzera, P B-C P
Taylor, C
Taylor, J D M
Taylor, J S W
Taylor, M J
Taylor, N W G
Taylor, P A
Taylor, R A
Taylor, R G
Taylor, S D
Telling, J P
Teo, H T H T C
Terry, D M S
Tharmaratnam, D
Thin Kyu, Dr
Thomas, H M
Thomas, J S
Thomas, K A
Thomas, K D
Thomas, M S
Thomas, M G
Thomas, S J
Thomas, T A
Thompson, E A
Thompson, E C M
Thompson, K M
Thompson, M J
Thompson, M H
Thompson, S A
Thornley, P
Thornton, M J
Thornton, P G N
Tierney, P A
Tilley, A J
Timoney, A G M
Titcomb, D R
Tizard, E J
Tobias, J H
Tobin, G W
Todd, E J
Todman, E
Tole, D M
Tometzki, A J P
Tomison, A R
Tomkins, S E
Tomlinson, J M
Tomson, C R V
Tonge, J M A
Totham, A
Townsend, P L G
Treloar, E J
Tremaine, K J
Trenfield, J D S
Tricks, C D
Trinder, J
Truscott, J H
Tsai-Goodman, B
Tuffrey, C
Tulloh, R M R
Tunstall, S R
Turner, R J
Tyler, J E
Umarji, S I M
Underwood, S M
Unsworth, D J
Vahdati-Bolouri, M
Van Asch, P
Vassallo, A A
Verne, J E C W
Vernon, J M
Vickers, J H
Vickery, C J
Vickery, C W
Vickery, I M
Vieten, D
Virjee, J P
Vyas, S K
Waddell, A N
Wakeley, C J
Walford, N Q
Wallace, C A
Wallington, T B
Walsh, D S
Walsh, E M
Walsh, ND
Walters, A S
Walters, F J M
Walters, J H
Ward, A J
Ward, G R
Ward, L L
Wardle, P G
Warin, W A
Warinton, A D
Warner, D L
Warnock, M M
Warr, C A
Warr, E E
Warr, R P
Warren-Browne, C Y
Watkins, C J
Watson, G W
Watt, E M
Watt, F A
Watt, F K
Watts, A R
Watts, D P
Watts, D R
Watts, H R
Weale, A E
Webb, E J
Webb, J C J
Wehner, H E
Weil, D M
Weir, P M
Weller, R M
Welsh, M A
Wensley, S K
West, S H
Whaley, A P
Whallett, D J
Whallett, E J
Wheatley, A M
Wheeler, A
Whipp, E C
Whitaker, N T
White, H
White, M T
White, R J
Whitelaw, A G L
Whiteside, B G
Whittlestone, T H
Whitton, T L
Whitwell, F D
Whone, A L
Wickert, A J
Wickremaratchi, M M
Wigfield, C C
Wight, D J
Wilcock, G K
Wilde, R P H
Wilkins, J
Wilkinson, D A C
Wilkinson, E J
Wilkinson, S A
Willems, P J A
Williams, A B
Williams, B M
Williams, C J
Williams, C E M
Williams, C S
Williams, C J H
Williams, C
Williams, G
Williams, J D
Williams, M P
Williams, N B
Williams, R E M
Williams, R W
Williams, R J W
Williams, T D
Willmott, S L
Wilmshurst, M J
Wilson, A M
Wilson, M P
Wilson, N H
Winson, I G
Winterborn, R J
Winteringham, T
Winters, Z E
Wiszniewska, R H
Witcher, J W
Wong, C K M
Wong, R C W
Wood, C E
Wood, D A
Wood, F A
Wood, J A
Woodhead, A E
Woodward, C M
Worsley, G E
Wrathall, G J
Wright, J S
Wright, M P J
Wright, M E
Wyatt, S J
Wynick, D
Yandell, C J
Yates, P A
Yeap, M L
Yeoman, R
Yerbury, C M
Young, A E R
Younge, P A
Zollman, C E

Brixham

Acheson, E A
Acheson, P
Ansley, D G H
Avery, P J
Bromige, R M
Brown, K R M
Brown, L M M
Brown, R M
John, T C
Johnson, P B
Langley, D C
Langley, P S
Lee, E J
McConnell, M B
Montgomery, R W
Paton, A N
Tapp, M J F
Washington, R J M
Williams, D C
Wood, D N

Broadstairs

Ajayi, J D
Arnold, C S
Bachlani, M M
Bean, J N
Cardwell, M D
Cook, J A M
Cook, R M M
Corti, K D F
Cunard, A J K
Cutting, R J
Davies, M
Gill, R S
Goldberg, S M
Gunn, K P
Hartt, A S
Herron, J T
Hewitson, M W A
Karunadasa, A T R K
Limentani, A E
McAvoy, B J T
Marshall, A
Marshall, D I
Martin, T S
Misgar, B A
Nairac, B L
Pheils, P J
Poole, R G
Sahadevan, S
Shariff, S Y
Soppitt, R W
Stephen, I B M
Tuppen, N M
Wilson, P E
Wilton, H J

Broadstone

Briggs, M W
Cartwright, L N
Davies, H C R
Dinley, R R J
Drake, B E
Dudding, G J
Dutson, M E J
Fleming, P A
Jones, J H A
Lawrence, J S
McCall, C J
Marsh, K E
Nixon, S M
Ortega, L S
Panda, J K
Panda, V P
Pharaoh, J M
Richardson, M I
Saynor, A M N
Shakespeare, R M
Sharp, N S
Timmis, R G
Watkins, A J

Broadway

Bloch-Ashbridge, K M
Bloch, T P S
D'Agapeyeff, A P
Juckes, T R B
Marlborough, M
Mockler, E M
Townshend, N W N
Vincent, E J
Williams, A C

Brockenhurst

Baynes, S C
Benson, R J
Birt, C H
Godfrey, I M
Green, R V
Humby, E M
Jones, N F
Lawrence, K M
Moss, S J
Newbury, L
Thomas, V L

Brodick

Brown, M M
Buchanan, R A
Grassie, A D
Grassie, E H S
Guthrie, E L
Kerr, M M
MacVicar, F T
Sloss, G A
Tinto, B A
Tinto, R G

Bromley

Ahmed, Q Z
Al-Chalabi, N
Allen, P R
Arora, A
Arul, D R
Bassett, D J
Berman, N A
Best, E A
Bhinda, H P
Bird, S F
Birmingham-McDonogh, S M L
Bradley, M D
Breese, E O
Broadhead, J C
Broom, A M
Castell, R
Castles, W J B
Chang, Y-C
Collins, M E
Comper, S J
Coombes, S K
Cornish, E M
Cox, A
Crook, J M
Davies, D S T
Davies, N E
Dawkins, G P C
De Cothi, E M
Dhadly, P P S
Eapen, V
Edmonds, G M
Ellice, R M
Ellul, J P M
Farooqi, F M
Fathulla, B B
Fergusson, D A N
Fernando, E C K
Fisher, E J
Fowler, T J
Franklin, A
Ghali, F A M
Gnanachelvan, K
Gray, P J P
Guckenheim, P D L
Gupta, B N
Gupta, D
Guram, N S
Hadley, E M
Hall, S E
Hamid, S
Hanna, L S
Harvey-Smith, E A
Haughey, N M
Haywood, J M
Hazra, D
Hedley, R M
Higgs, S I L
Hill, N C W
Hunt, J B
Jalajam, M P
Jeanes, A L
Jenkins, A P
Jenkins, V M
Job, M C H
Jones, N C
Kahlon, K S
Kapadia, A P
Kaur, I
Kendall, G
Kenyon, J B
Kharade, M A
King, P B
Leather, A J M
Leather, S C
Lewis, B S
Lumley, P W
Luong, C B
Lyttle, M E A C
MacCann, E
MacKillop, A J J
MacLeod, M J
Mahendrarajah, A
Malekniazi, D
Martin, A
Matthews, M A
Meire, H B
Michael, W F
Midwood, C J
Mullally, J J
Munday, A N
Murphy, J M
Nackasha, E P
Neelamkavil, D P S
Ng, L V-L
Noori, M
Nurse, D E
Osborn, S V
Page, J E
Pallant, E A
Patel, A B
Patel, C R
Payne, N M
Pritchard, E L
Procter, L
Quastel, A S
Quirk, J A
Rajamenon, A
Rakowicz, S P
Ramanathan, J S
Rao, V R K
Rashid, A
Ratneswaren, N
Rault, J P R
Reed, H
Russell, G F M
Ryba, P C J
Samuel, M S
Satkurunath, G
Saunders, R C O
Sehmi, S K
Selby, M R
Selvanathan, E S
Shah, J K R
Shahnawaz, G
Sharma, K K
Sheppey, M C
Shivanathan, S
Singh, H
Singh, N
Sivagnanasundaram, S
Smith, I F
Smith, S M
Spiby, J
Staffurth, J S
Statham, H C
Stein, G S
Surenthiran, S
Swift, M R
Tampiyappa, T N
Tatford, E P W
Tattersfield, H G
Taylor, P A
Tharmaseelan, K
Tseng, E H Y
Vine, P R
Wegstapel, H
Whiteside, W N
Wilkins, A
Willatt, R N
Wing, L G
Wragg, P G
Yanni, D H
Yanni, G
Young, S L

Bromsgrove

Ashton, F
Aust, T R
Bailey, S R
Banerjee, S
Blunt, R J
Byrnes, R
Bywater, B
Chakraverty, R C
Coles, V R
Collins, S J
Cooke, R A
Crooks, M P
Dale, J E
Dowley, S P M
Dowley, W G H
Dykes, P A
Eardley, M L
Evans, A J
Fellowes, M A
Finnegan, J A
Goldman, I G
Gorman, S L
Griffiths, A C
Grove, L H
Hall, F J
Hall, R J
Hallows, M R
Heath, C D
Hotham, D S
Jack, D A
Jack, O P
Jack, R A F
Jackson, J R
James, V H C
Jenkins, R M
Laxton, C J S
Leci, M K
Lee, A J
Leigh, B A
Lewin, J S
Morgan, D W
Morgan, P A P
Morrey, I A
O'Neill, D
Penfold, B M
Pryke, D S E
Radcliffe, M E
Reddie, E M
Schirrmacher, U O E
Sefton-Fiddian, P
Simoyi, T
Souza Faria, F P
Spires, R C S
Swire, H
Wall, L T
White, F M
Whiteford, L J
Wilkinson, R D
Wychrij, O

Bromyard

Barnes, J M
Brockington, I F
Bull, L
Clear, M R
Ganderton, P
Ilsley, J K
Kirrage, D C
Scott, S F O
Spicer, N A A
Tait, I J
Wilmshurst, S L

Brora

Fortune, M H
Main, M M

Broseley

Bhageerutty, J D
Brace, A A

Brough

Allen, S P
Arrowsmith, J S
Bray, J H
Charlson, P B
Dobson, E M
Ferguson, R A
Harper, C L
Hart, W A
Livesey, J P
Macpherson, H
Marshall, S R
Mathew, B G
Partridge, S
Purdy, G M
Richardson, W N
Rosenberg, F G
Searle, S M
Smith, S L

Snell, L R
Spencer, J
Summerton, A M
Tinker, N R
Tod, I A A
Webb, A T

Broughton-in-Furness
Bates, T H
Harvey, S C

Broxbourne
Allen, K H
Blackman, M
Condon, R N H
Dignan, J E P
Hiscock, B M V
Manlow, C J
Mukherjee, A
Sheridan, J S
Watt, N K
Wood, A G
Wyman, D A

Broxburn
Cuthbert, D A
Ferguson, T H
Fowler, G
Heath, L
Kent, B
Lewis, B
Lyons, G L
McRae, F C
Priyadarshi, S
Russell, J C
Santer, P M
Semple, S M
Sives, D A
Wood, N R

Bruton
Genton, H E
Naumann, U
Nicole, T M
Player, M H

Buckfastleigh
Barton, T J
Draper, C A
Dunstan, E R R
Edwards, P D
Hedger, J R
Kealy, M R
Towers, J R

Buckhurst Hill
Adamson, M I
Ah-Moye, M
Allum, T G L
Arif, S
Barnardo, A N
Briggs, A C
Collett, P M R
Daniel, C A
Dhanji, A-F A-A
Dodd, P P
Fiamanya, W K
Fieldman, N R
Heavens, M A C
Hussain, I
Jackson, E R
Leahy, J D
Liao, S
McAuliffe, T B
McMillan, A-M
Melson, L C
Moss, C E
Nunneley, J B
Osborough, F
Ross, G A W
Ruben, S T
Slater, A J
Stuart, R D
Sudarsanam, P
Taylor, G B
Taylor, J S G
Thomas, A M
Thomas, D J B
Tranmer, C
Viniker, D A
Walker, A

Buckie
Arnould, K M
Gallacher, W A
Hood, C M
Jaffrey, W G A
McLintock, M G

Martin, M S
Morrison, R M
Morrison, S G
Pringle, G M
Rennie, J M
Tuckerman, J G
Walker, L
Welsh, B M

Buckingham
Austin, M W
Cash, C J C
Clark, W I C
Dickson, R N
Fairfield, J J
Harrington, R W E
Hens, M
Largent, T
McDonald, N J
McMullan, A D
Mason, M R
Mason, P D
Mathews, S R
Preston, A E
Preston, K E
Pryse, R D
Richardson, D
Robb, E
Robins, A E
Simons, G D
Straker, D M
Stranks, S J
Suddes, K P
Tizzard, S P
Trafford, P J
Wetherill, M H
Whittington, J R
Woodroffe, R W

Buckley
Attree, R C
Barnard, C S
Botham, S A
Chadwick, J M
Clarke, W B
Hoggins, G R
Hopkins, R S
Lucas, R M
Manson, M D
Owen, S J
Speakman, P F
Spencer, C W
Tansley, A G
Tobias, N F

Bude
Batty, C G
Brown, A J
Forrest, A K
Gurd, D E P
Haddon, P W
Hammond-Evans, J M
Morwood, C I
Moss, A Y D
Register, P W
Rowlands, A M
Sweet, D J
Thres, G V

Budleigh Salterton
Davis, T S
Fletcher, S E
Franklin, S
Hughes, S
Lewis, A A G
Mejzner, R H
Reese, J M
Ross, F K
Taylor, G E
Wright, M

Builth Wells
Davies, S D L
Edmondson, C L
Gibbins, R L
Harriss, A R W
Wallace, A R
Walters, R B

Bungay
Emerson, A R
Emerson, R G
Goss, B M
Hand, C H
Kaytar, J
Self, A E
Sethia, K K
Williams, G

Buntingford
Bryant, J G
Handysides, N S P
Lancaster, P A
Partington, M J
Withers, D P

Bures
Cattermole, R W
Magnus, I A
Patey, D G H
Pilgrim, L L
York, J H

Burford
Mackenzie, F M
Moore, J A
Sharpley, O J
Slater, C
Willby, L A

Burgess Hill
Barker, G M
Broadley, C E
Carter, J R
Cheng, M-N
Claiden, M
Eastman, K E
Ebbage, J C
Gankerseer, S A
Gigli, C
Harman, F E M
Harrop, J E
Holwell, I A
Hornby, R C
Longthorne, P N
Lyle, P T W
MacGuire, J D
Mahapatra, K C
Napier, J C
Pepera, T A A
Plant, S H
Rahman, M K
Read, J M
Roche, D F E
Ross, B
Siddiqui, U A
Turton, C W G

Burnham-on-Crouch
Bailey, K L
Harris, S J
Jayasekara, K S
Kamlow, F J
Ketteley, S J
Latif, M H
Phillips, J D

Burnham-on-Sea
Gauld, D A
Green, M J
Holl, S G
Matthews, N K
Sampson, H C R
Thomson, M R
Wildbore, R D

Burnley
Abdul-Nabi, M J
Ahmad, S M
Al-Amin, M
Al-Dawoud, A A F
Ali, S T
Anafi, R F
Arif, N
Ariyaratnam, R
Asghar, N M
Ashworth, F J
Ateaque, A
Bailey, D W
Bailey, S
Barker, T M
Barsby, M R
Bayton, E A
Beech, K J
Berry, C M
Best, R A
Bhattacharyya, S
Biswas, S R N
Brew, J R
Brierley, A J
Brown, I H
Burke, M J
Calow, C E
Chatterjee, A K
Clark, E J
Clarke, F R
Cleasby, S J
Cooke, B E

Corkhill, S E
Coulson, I H
Craig, A E
Craven, N M
Crumbleholme, G K
Dabir, Z M
Daly, B M
Dalziel, E A
Das, R
Das, S
Deegan, S P
Dennison, J M A
Dilraj Gopal, T R
Donald, C J M
Dooldeniya Perera, D
Downes, J
Durkin, M A
Farag, A M
Fishwick, K T
Fraser, D J
Gadsby, J B
Green, A T
Greenwood, A P
Grimley, C E F
Gross, E
Gupta, S N
Hamer, F C
Hanna, M I
Haq, A
Haq, K S
Hartley, P C
Hassan, A
Hebden, S
Horsman, G
Hyatt, R H
Hyder, C K Z
Inglis, T C M
Iqbal, J
Jenkins, A J
Kendra, J R
Khan, L U R
Khan, N A
Khatu, B V
Kirby, J M
Kumar Singh, P K
Langton, S G
Launer, M A
Limaye, P
Limaye, S H
Littley, M D
Lockwood, E
Lotha, L M
McDevitt, M W
Mackenzie, T H M
Mahady, I W
Mahady, V E
Malik, S
Masanjika, J P
Maung, M
Mellody, J
Milne, I L
Mishra, M S
Morris, T
Naha-Biswas, P
Narayana, V
O'Hagan, D P
Ogden, J R
Phillips, G E H
Rahi, M A
Raza, S S
Rhodes, P C
Robertson, J G F
Rusius, C W
Sahu, R C
Saikia, A N
Salman, W D
Sandilands, D G D
Sarin, R
Sarkar, P K
Sayers, C L
Schmitgen, C
Schmitgen, G
Scott, P D
Seavers, J E
Seavers, P
Seeney, B
Shahid, M
Shakir, A A K
Singh, N
Singh, R K
Singh, S K
Singh, S
Sinha, R P
Smith, M V
Sundararajan, P
Swann, A
Swann, I L
Syed, I A
Tan, M M S

Tattersall, N
Taylor, J P
Tripathi, D N
Vohra, S
Walton, M R
Watts, J C
White, D J
Whittaker, K
Wilson, D G
Wong, C K
Wright, D H
Zubairy, A

Burntisland
Bell, M D
Chishti, Z J
Duncan, D
Fleming, L E M
Forbes Smith, P A
Halliday, I M
Lees, S
Macdonald, J H B
Mowbray, A
Stewart, A J

Burntwood
King, J C
Reynolds, C E
Winter, J M

Burry Port
Anderson, P M
Davies, R J
Gower, G E
Hughes, D G
Lodha, L A
Thomas, F J
Williams, J M

Burton-on-Trent
Allen, C
Anderson, J D
Atkinson, M G W
Baldock Grimes, S M
Barrow, A S
Beckett, P A
Benn, J J
Black, A
Bradbury, E L
Bucknall, T E
Butchart, G D
Cartwright, P H
Chawdhary, S
Cleary, J J L
Collier, S L
Corfield, R A
Crosse, J M
Dickson, D E
Doyle, P T
Dutton, D A
Dutton, G C D
El-Khanagry, M F F
Farrar, C D
Free, G
Gent, K S
Ghori, M U
Gompertz, R H K
Green, D M
Green, L C
Greenwood, C M
Gregory, B A
Grey, J M
Gunstone, C C
Gunstone, E M
Hall, C J
Hann, H C L
Harrison, R J
Heal, C M
Heath, A C
Hegde, R T
Hextall, R A
Hill, J D
Hingorani, T V
Holgate, P W
Hollingworth, J
Hopper, J M
Horton, R M
Hughes, M W
Ibrahim, Y G
Jacob Samuel, T
Jenkins, R G
Johns, A M
Jones, P L
Jordan, A D
Kamath, U M
Kasthuri, N
Khan, H A
Khan, M A
Laban, S J

Law, H M
Law, S D
Lee, R E
Lobb, C J
Lockwood, J A F
Long, J M
Luft, G A N
Mager-Jones, J
Manzoor, A
Martin, J W
Masani, H M
Matharu, G S
Millar, S W
Minn Din, Z
Mirfattahi, M M B
Moloney, P G
Murray, C A
Needham, P
Nelson, H M
Newton, M P
Nweke, A J
O'Dwyer, F G J
Oakley, W E
Oates, J
Ong, P S
Pelekouda, E
Pidsley, C G L
Pinhorn, A
Piracha, A
Porter, A J
Rafique, A
Rau, U B N
Rauf, A
Reisner, C
Reynolds, T M
Roberts, A I
Roberts, A D G
Roberts, I
Robinson, P N
Rockley, T J
Rogers, C A
Saweirs, W M
Scheel, T A
Seigel, J F
Sellens, K F
Sheldon, J W S
Shipman, J A J
Singanayagam, J
Skinner, H D
Smith, I B
Smith, K L
Spencer-Jones, J M
Spencer-Jones, R G
Spencer, N M
Staley, F M
Stenhouse, C W
Stevenson, M P
Stokes, M J
Street, M N
Sverrisdottir, A
Tansey, J M
Thomas, D M
Thompson, A C
Tombs, D G
Trelinski, M J
Vickers, R J
Waddy, E M
Walker, N L
Wallace, M E
Watmough, D
Webb, C A
Wellstood-Eason, M J H
White, J A
White, J C
Why, H J F
Willis, A C
Winchurch, S R
Worstmann, T
Young, M A
Zamir, R J
Zargar, B A

Bury
Adamson, C L
Ahmed, S
Anjum, I A
Ashraf, S
Baig, M K
Baig, S
Bansal, A
Bashir, A A
Bene, J
Best, C T
Beveridge, A J
Bhalla, K
Bhatt, P R
Bowers, S L
Bradburn, J C

Brammer, C G
Brandrick, J T
Brewood, A F M
Brigg, D J
Britton, C A
Buchanan, M J
Bugg, G
Chande, C
Cheong, C Y
Chidambaram, V
Cleary, P M
Contractor, N
Cornmell, C A
Cumarasamy, K
Danson, J A
Dawson, N J
De Sousa, B A
De Sousa, E L
De Vial, S R
Deakin, H
Demetriou, A
Devlin, J C
Dockrell, J C
Doyle, J
Duce, C L
Dutt, S
El-Malek, E A A
Ellison, M F
Evans, S A
Finnegan, M J
Fletcher, D P
Fletcher, K L
Fletcher, P F
Frassek, B
Freschini, D L
Gadiyar, V
Garg, N
Gormally, J
Gosall, G S
Grey, M R
Hampson, J R
Harbottle, J A
Harvey, G C
Hashemi, M Z
Haworth, K S
Hayden, B E
Hayden, J
Herd, M E
Hill, A D
Hough, M
Hughes, R D
Hurst, J R
Jackson, J C
Jackson, P A
Jenkins, S A P
Joseph, N
Karwowski, I S
Kataria, K K
Khan, A M
Kirkham, S K
Kotak, P K
Kutiyanawala, M
Kyffin, D N
Lal, D P S S
Leahy, M M P
Lippett, S C
Livingstone, J
Lo, S V
Lyons, A J
McGivney, R C V
McGowan, A K
Mackinnon, A S R
Mackinnon, G
Mamoowala, H E
Mattison, M L
Maudsley, I S
Mirza, S R
Munir, M
Murray, C J
Mutucumarana, C S
Neininger, P D R
Norman, P R
North, P J
O'Callaghan, K M
O'Connor, F
Oates, B C
Pearson, K W
Phillips, B S
Phillips, S D
Prabhu, P U
Pressler, J M
Prudham, R C
Qurashi, I
Ralhan, R
Rowland, A G
Russell, A J
Saab, M
Sankar, V S
Sarkar, D
Sarkar, S K
Savage, M W
Scott, K M
Senarath Yapa, S C
Sethi, P
Shekar, C
Siegler, S A
Sims, A J
Singanayagam, S
Sinha, S K
Sinniah, A R
Smith, A C
Sopher, B J
Standing, P A
Stokes, R A
Stone, F
Stoner, J M
Subbiah, S
Sumner, A H
Suteria, Y
Tan, G D
Thaker, K K
Thornton, S J
Tolan, E L
Turck, W P G
Vaidya, S M
Wadhwa, V K
Wake, C R
Wakefield, R M
Watts, J P
Wheater, A W
Wilson, D C
Woodcock, P J
Ziko, A O A

Bury St Edmunds
Abu-Haneeffa, M
Adams, C N
Adams, P J
Alam, N A
Arjani, K A
August, A C
Aung, T T
Bannon, R P
Barabas, A A
Barnet-Lamb, M
Bedford, A F
Bell, M A C
Blunt, M C
Booth, S A
Bower, E L
Bowling, P I V
Boys, J E
Bradford, H W
Bradley, R K
Brain, A R
Brereton-Smith, G
Broadhurst, A D
Brookes, M T
Brown, S M
Bruton, J A
Buck, J J
Burgess, J
Burns, A M
Cannon, J C
Cantlay, J S
Chow, A E
Clark, J D A
Clements, S L H A
Cooledge, J S
Cooledge, R C
Crickmore, C T
Darley, J S
Darrah, E R A
Davies, J A
Dean, P R
Derbyshire, E V
Dunne, C T P
Edwards, S K
Evans, I E
Evans, P R
Fasler, J J
Field, J M
Finn, P J
Finn, P S
Gibson, J E
Giles, C E
Giles, R W H
Godwin, R J
Gove, J R W
Grace, K R
Grace, T
Graham, H M
Greener, J S
Greener, W A
Grove, L M
Gull, S E
Haider, Z S
Hall, J D
Handfield-Jones, S E
Harpur, N C W
Harrison, P D
Harston, A P B
Hart, C D
Haslewood, S M
Heywood, L J
Hickson, L P
Hodgson, C C
Hopkinson, G P
Hutton, R A
Jones, M R C
Jones, R C
Jordan, K
Kasbarian, A
Keeling, N J
Kelvin, G
Kennedy, C L
Kilner, P B
King, B J
Lamb, R J
Lambert, E L
Langford, R A
Lee, E M
Lewis, G M
Little, W R
Livermore, A L
Lockyer, M J
Love, K D
Lowe, S S
Mabin, D C
McBrien, M P
McDonald, W V
McLoughlin, J
Majeed, J F
Martin, S C
Mason, A M
Masters, J E
Matheson, K H
Mauger, J S
May, S A
Mayer, C N
Mistry, M K
Moffat, J R
Moody, A M
Morrison, C M
Motha, J T
Munglani, R
Newell, J R L W
Nicolson, A
O'Flynn, R R
O'Reilly, D T
O'Riordan, D C
Odegaard, E R
Oliver, S F
Pearson, D A
Penfold, N W
Pike, K C
Porteous, M J L F
Ramsay, A S
Ravisekar, O
Recaldin, S
Reynolds, G A
Riddick, A C P
Ridsdill-Smith, W P
Rix, G H
Robinson, R C
Robling, S-A
Russell, A J
Russell, L K
Rutherford, J
Rycroft, N E
Sach, M
Sauvage, A D P
Sawyer, R J
Sengupta, A
Sharma, P K
Sharpe, C E
Sharpstone, D R
Siklos, P W L
Sjolin, S U
Slade, J M
Slade, J M
Slater, A
Smith, C
Smith, R M L
Soper, R H
Spencer, P J
Stairmand, R A
Starck, A L
Stringer, B M
Stroud, D S
Tasker, W J
Teo, H S
Thompson, A M S
Thompson, J B
Thompson, M G
Tolland, E M
Tremlett, C H
Urquhart, J C
Vassilas, C A
Wallace, E C
Waters, F S
Watson, D H
Watson, L J
Webb, T E
West, R J
Wignall, O J
Wilson, C S
Wilson, H M
Winton, F E
Wood, M K
Wootton, J C
Wright, E D
Yeatman, A

Bushey
Mandalia, P A

Bushmills
Dunlop, M L
Wee, S-C

Buxton
Barrett, P D
Best, E A
Blomfield, S J W
Bradbury, E M
Bridge, A-L
Briggs, A P
Collier, A J
Cox, P J
Culshaw, M C
Doig, C M
Fitzsimmons, C R
Graham, S M
Grimbaldeston, A H
Haddon, J
Hallam, C A
Hardman, M
Hardman, S F
Harry, J D
Hartley, A W
Hockenhull, C H
Hodgkinson, T C
Kay, S M
King, S F
Mark, C T
Martin, P J
Pearson, L A
Reynolds, M A
Short, P R D
Smallbone, D F
Stirling, R J
Swinhoe, D J
Weir, K M
Williams, B R
Wilson, A
Woods, S E

Caernarfon
Bee, R W
Crabtree, P G E
Davies, R H
Evans, G M
Evans, J G
Farquhar, G N
Griffiths, N G
Gutting, P A
Holland, H T
Huws, N O
Jones, J M
Jones, J S
Jones, M W
Jones, W A
Llwyd, E M
McCann, K
Morgan, L G
Morgan, P R
Oddy, A V
Ohri, P N
Owen, M
Owen, M E
Owen, T J
Owens, G W
Parry-Jones, G
Parry, A L
Parry, E E
Parry, M I
Parry, R
Parry, W G W
Pearson, N M
Pierce, E W
Rees, K S
Roberts, H L
Roberts, W O
Thomas, M
Thompson, J C B
Tickle, E K
Turner, S L
Watson, S J
Williams, A G
Williams, E
Williams, I P
Williams, R S
Williams, R W
Wynn-Jones, D

Caerphilly
Abou-Zeid, S M A-H
Ahmad, H B
Allan, D E
Anderson, R A
Bailey, D S
Bashar, N A
Bignall, J A
Chapman, M D
Chidgey, M A
Cox, C J C
Davies, D R
Davis, D H J
Doulah, M A U
El Garib, A E M H
Evans, S E
Ferguson, S D
Goddard, R J
Griffiths, M
Harney, P J
Harper, R J
Hourihan, B M
Jayawickrama, N S
Jenkins, D
Jones, R
Lewis, J W
Morgan, P D
Pathak, P K
Penrose, G L
Reed, M
Reid, A
Salam, S
Shannon, J L
Stacey, C S
Stout, T V
Thevathasan, M
Thomas, A K
Thomas, E W
Watson, H P
Watt, A
West, S M

Caersws
Green, M W
Smith, S M L B
Wallbank, G R

Cairndow
Basu, T K

Callander
Baillie-Hamilton, P F
Gibson, I M
Ingle, G T
Mathewson, K G
Scott, A M-L
Scott, R M
Strang, G D M
Watkins, O

Callington
Bartram, J W
Bleksley, M C
Chaplin, S
Kratky, A P
Steggles, B G
Warren, E J

Calne
Beale, N R
Bishop, D S
Clarke, B P
Dilley, J C
Gough, S L
Hatherley, C C A
Lawson, P R
Leach, R M C
Lovell, A G
Pritchard, S A
Sandford-Hill, A M
Searle, M A
Taudevin, E J
Thornton, A S

Calstock
Bowie, A N
Fitzgerald, M B
Mantle, E M

Camberley
Ahmad, S S
Al Khalaf, S S I
Al-Rawaf, S A A
Alston, W C
Alton, P A
Andrews, D M
Ashbrooke, A B
Bajwa, N P S
Bala, K
Barker, S E
Barrie, E
Bartlett, C I S
Bergman, B P
Beynon, D W G
Blackman, R H
Blackmore, M J
Booth, B P
Bown, R L
Boyd, M J
Brinklow, K A
Brown, K J
Buchan, R N M
Buchanan, P L
Burnham, D A
Chakrabarti, G N
Chissell, H R
Chiswell, R J
Cockburn, J E
Collinson, J R
Corbet Burcher, E A
Coulson, M L
Coulter, S A
Cumberland, N S
Cureton, P C
Cureton, R E
Daoud, R A
Darroch, R C
Davidson, J A
Davies, M L
Davies, M H
De Ferrars, R J M
Debrah, K M
Dempster, D W
Denham, P L
Denton, S E
Dias, D R C
Divan, A M
Donovan, B
Drever, I R
Drury, R R
Edwards, D P
El Mahallawy, M H A A
Embling, K F
Fabricius, P J
Ferguson, B M
Fernando, D S
Fisher, M G P
Galbraith, S N
Garber, S A
Gill, M E C
Goddard, G F
Gordon, E
Grady, K B
Graham, S J
Green, A D
Griffiths, M F P
Gudgeon, A M
Hadley, N S
Hague, N J
Hall, J R W
Harris, J R
Hassan, G A E-S M
Hawthorne, M E
Hearn, D L
Hearn, F J
Henderson, A D
Hern, J D
Hey, G B
Hinton, R M
Hoad, N A
Hodgetts, T J
Hogben, R K F
Holdbrook-Smith, H A
Holden, C E A
Holliman, S M
Holmes-Smith, J G
Howard, F M
Hull, J B
Humphreys, D M
Ineson, N
Ingram, R K
Irish-Tavares, D N
Jakeman, R D
Jennings, C S
Jewitt, J A L
Jonathan, D A
Jones, S R

Joshi, P
Kabil, Y A E-M
Keightley, A M
Kilpatrick, S M
King, S J
Knight, R K
Kumar, R
Leopold, P W
Lillywhite, L P
Lloyd, M E
Lothe, K J
Lowes, T
Lucas, M A
McClenahan, A F
McCombe, A W
Mayall, M N A
Mellor, S G
Millar, W S
Miller, S A S J
Montgomery, B S I
Moorthy, B
Morgan-Jones, D J
Mundy, K I
Nadarajah, R
Naerger, H G A
Neill, F E
Nethercliffe, J M-S
Niemiro, L A K
Noyelle, R M
O'Leary, D A
O'Sullivan, D P D
Oliver, P J R
Ooi, R G B
Orr, J E K
Ottley, V R
Paley, M R
Paterson, I M
Pike, J M
Price, B A
Pugh, P J
Rahman, M K A
Raymond-Jones, J G
Reilly, P A J
Renbourn, E T
Restall, J
Roberts, G D
Robinson, G M
Rust, N E
Rutherford, J
Sakellariou, A
Simpson, R G
Singh, S
Sleator, D J D
Smail, J K
Smart, P C
Smith, C E T
Sreenivasa Rao, P M
Starr, R L
Strudley, M R
Sukumaran Nair, P K
Sukumaran Nair, S
Tandon, M K
Tanner, C C
Taylor, N M
Teale, T E
Tettenborn, M A
Thillaiambalam, N
Tiller, G
Tong, J L
Toplis, P J
Trippe, H R
Turner, C E
Uheba, M A
Upadhyay, A K
Van Den Bosch, C A
Waine, J M
Wang, T W-M
Wells, J M
White, I L
Williams, M
Yates, M J

Camborne
Ahling-Smith, H E M
Barton, S R
Bergin, J R
Blake, I D
Brooks, J W
Collins, W E
Cotton, S A
Dowling, K A
Harvey, R A
Hawker, L B
Henderson, K J
Keech, T P
Lay, E T
McCabe, C R
MacDonald, K E
Perkins, P J
Thomas, J E
Whiting, S L
Whittle, K G

Cambridge
Abad Alejandre, J
Abrahams, P H
Acerini, C L
Addison, P D
Adey, E M
Adlam, D M
Adlam, S A
Adler, A I
Ah-See, S-Y W
Ahluwalia, J S
Ahmad, T
Alderson, M L
Alderson, T S J
Alexander, G J M
Alexander, S J C
Allen, C M C
Allen, L E
Amin, A N
Amure, B O
Anderson, J R
Anderson, M R
Andreasen, M-J
Antoun, N M
Aparicio, S A J R
Appleton, D S
Arends, M J
Arno, J
Arrowsmith, J E
Ashurst, N J
Aslam, A
Atkinson, P R T
Aylott, C L
Baglin, T P
Bailey, A R
Bailey, P A
Baldwin, E C
Baldwin, P J W
Ball, S J A
Ballantine, D M
Bankes-Page Chapman, C A
Baralle, D
Barclay, S I G
Barker, R A
Barnard, S A
Barnes, J L C
Barnes, R J
Barnett, G C
Bartlett, D W
Bass, S P
Bastable, R B
Bateman, A M
Bateman, P J
Battersby, A J
Bavalia, K
Baxter, P J
Bearcroft, P W P
Beardsall, K
Beattie, S L
Behr, S B
Bell, D
Bell, I F
Bennett, A M D
Bennett, C M
Benson, J R
Bentham, P W
Bentley, S
Berrios, G E
Bertram, R C R
Bettinson, H V
Biggs, J S G
Bilton, D
Birks, E I
Bisset, J A
Blaine, F
Blandford, N S
Bleehen, N M
Bobrow, L G
Bobrow, M
Bolland, J L M
Bolton, P F
Booth, S
Borer, E F
Boyle, J R
Bradley, J A
Bradley, J R
Brain, A J L
Brant, J M
Brassett, C
Brayne, C E G
Brecknell, J E
Breeze, A C G
Brennan, L
Brett, M
Brice, J H
Brimblecombe, P R
Brinsden, P R
Britton, P D
Broadley, S A
Brodie, D A
Brodie, G D
Brook, S S
Brown, C K
Brown, C H
Brown, D L
Brown, M J
Brown, N M
Browning, C J
Budd, E O
Bufton, K E
Bukhari, T
Bullmore, E T
Bullock, K N
Burgen, A S V
Burnet, N G
Burrell, C G
Burrows, N P
Burton, G J
Burton, M H
Butcher, A
Butler, A J
Butterworth, J L
Buttery, P C
Calladine, M R H
Calloway, S P
Camilleri-Ferrante, C
Campbell-Hewson, G L
Campbell, G A
Carmichael, A J
Carmichael, J
Carne, C A
Carrell, T W G
Carroll, N R
Cary, N R B
Challen, A D
Chaloner, A B
Chan Lee Gaik, Dr
Chatterjee, V K K
Cheney, G T
Cheow, H K
Cheriyan, J
Chester, S C
Chesworth, T J
Chilvers, E R
Ching, H S
Choksy, S A
Chua, V W T
Clark, A T
Clarke, S C
Clements, A L
Cocheme, M A X
Coleman, N
Coles, A J
Coles, C E
Coles, J P
Collins, V P
Compston, A S
Compston, J E
Condliffe, A M
Conlan, D P
Connan, P D
Constant, C R
Cooper, C M
Cormack, G C
Cornish, F E
Corrie, P G
Cosgrove, M P
Coulden, R A R
Cowley, H C
Cox, E J C
Cox, L J
Cox, T M
Cozzi, E
Craig, J I O
Crawford, I E M
Crawford, R A F
Crisp, A J
Crosbie, A D
Cross, J J L
Crossman, P
Croucher, P E
Culank, L S
Cullum, S-J
Cummings, G E
D'Amore, A
Dalton, K J
Dandy, D J
Dansie, A R
Davies, R G
Davis, J A
Davison, B C C
Dawnay, N A H
Dawson, I H P
De Lacey, P A
De Vries, P J
Deans, C L
Debenham, P J
Dening, T R
Denman, F M C
Desselberger, U
Dinneen, S
Diston, C F
Dixon, A K
Dixon, C M
Donagh, A C
Dowson, J H
Drake, B J
Draper, J
Duff, C H
Dunning, J J
Earl, H M
East, M M
Edgar, A C D
Edwards, D J
Edwards, O M
El Tahir, E F M M
Elliott, M L
Ellis, P D M
Elton, N H
Emerson, C V
Emerson, M S
English, M C
Evans, C A
Evans, K A
Evans, M L
Evans, P M
Ewan, P W
Exley, A R
Farnell, J E
Farrant, C G C
Farrington, M
Fernandes, H M
Fersht, N L
Fertig, A
Ffrench-Constant, C K
Fife, K M
Finer, N
Fingleton, P G
Firth, H V
Firth, J D
Fisher, A F
Fistein, E C
Fitzsimons, J T
Fleming, W R
Flinn, A J
Flint, J E
Flynn, P D
Forouhi, P
Forsyth, D R
Foweraker, J E
Freeman, A H
Freeman, R A V
Froggett, S M
Gair, R W
Gant, R M
Gardner, R
Gaston, C M
Gaston, J S H
Gattens, M
Gaunt, M E
Gelson, A D N
George, S
Georgiou, T
Ghosh, S
Gibbon, C E A
Gibbons, A H
Gibbs, P
Gidwani, F N
Gilbert, L K
Gilder, F J
Giles, A P
Gillard, E S E
Gillard, J H
Gilligan, D
Gilmore, A M C
Gimson, A E S
Girling, D M
Glazebrook, C W
Gleave, J R W
Goh, S-G J
Goldbeck-Wood, S J
Goldsmith, P
Goodyer, I M
Gordon, D N
Gould, J M
Grace, A A
Graeme-Barber, M
Graham, A J
Grant, I
Grant, J W
Gray, R F
Gray, S J
Green, A R
Gregory, C A
Griffin, D R
Griffin, S J
Griffith, F M
Griffiths, W J H
Grimshaw, K M
Grounds, A T
Groves, A M
Groves, R M
Grubb, H E S
Gunning, K E J
Gupta, A K
Gurnell, M
Gwynn, A M
Habib, S B
Habib, S E
Hackett, G A
Haigh, E
Hales, C N
Hall, N R
Hall, P N
Halliday, S E
Harcombe, A A
Hardwick, R H
Hardy, D G
Hardy, I
Harper, J M
Harris, P A
Harrison, N G
Harrison, R L
Harrison, R J
Harten-Ash, V J
Hashim-Iqbal, H
Hassan, J
Hatfield, A D
Hatsiopoulou, O
Haydock, S F
Hayhoe, F G J
Hazleman, B L
Herbert, J
Herrick, M J
Hewlett, J L
Hewlett, T G
Higgins, J N P
Hignett, C L
Hill, D J
Himsworth, R L
Hirschfield, G M
Hitchcock, C T
Hobbiger, S F
Hodges, J R
Hogg, N J
Holland, A J
Holland, T M
Holmes, J R
Holmes, S M
Hopkinson-Woolley, J A
Horn, N M A
Howell, J E
Huang, C L-H
Hugh-Jones, M C
Hughes, D R
Hughes, I A
Hughes, M
Hughes, V C
Humphreys, A J
Hung, C T
Hunt, C R
Hunt, M N S
Hunt, N J
Hunt, T J
Huntbach, J A
Hunter, J O
Hussey, A S
Hutchinson, H C
Hutchinson, P J A
Hyde, J B
Hymas, N F S
Iles, R W
Iregbulem, L M
Irwin, M S
Isherwood, D L
Jackson, J M C
Jaffa, A J
James, D C
Jamieson, N V
Jandziol, A K
Jayawardena, B
Jayne, D R W
Jenkins, D P
Jenks, C E
Jessop, F A
Jones, D H
Jones, J G
Jones, L M
Jones, P B
Jones, S E
Jorgensen, T A
Josse, J D
Kaloo, P D
Karet, F E
Keene, G S
Kelsall, A W R
Kelvin, R G
Kennedy, D J
Kenney, C G
Kent, C J
Kerr- Muir, M G
Kett-White, C E R
Kettle, M A
Keynes, R J
Khaw, K-T
King, A J
King, A
King, D K
King, M S
Kinmonth, A-L
Kirby, D P J
Kirker, S G B
Kirkpatrick, P J
Kirollos, R W M
Klein, J R
Klinck, J R
Knapton, P M
Kneeshaw, J D
Kuczynska, A-M E J
Kuczynska, M J
Kuczynski, A
Kumararatne, D S
Lachmann, H J
Lachmann, P J
Lachmann, R H
Lai, R Y K
Laing, R J C
Lalli, C A
Lam, R W F
Lamberty, B G H
Lamberty, F
Lane, S
Latcham, F
Latimer, J A
Latimer, M D
Lattimore, C R
Lawson, C R
Lawton, C A
Lea-Cox, C M
Leggatt, V J
Lehner, P J
Lennox, G G
Lessan, N G
Lever, A M L
Levick, M P
Levine, G
Lewis, E J
Lillicrap, M S
Lindop, M J
Linehan, G M
Lockett, G A
Lomas, D A
Lomas, D J
Lomas, P E S
London, M
Ludlam, H A
Lum, L C
Macanovic, S
Macartney, F J
McCabe, J A
McClure, R J
McConachie, C F J
McDonald, C J
MacDougall, M J
Macfarlane, M P
Macfarlane, R
MacGibbon, R
Machen, J M
Mackay, J H
McKee, T A
McKenna, P J
McKenna, P J
McKeown, J M I
McKiernan, D C
McLean, A C J
Mahaffey, A M
Maibaum, A
Maimaris, C V
Malata, C M
Males, A G
Males, R
Malik, S N
Mallet, M L
Maloney, E J E
Marcus, N K K
Marcus, R E
Marcus, S F
Marriott, R M
Martin, P J

Mathews, T
Matthewson, M H
Meggitt, B F
Meldrum, D J
Menon, DK
Merricks, M J
Meyer, P A R
Middleton, S J
Miles, B J
Millar, A J W
Miller, R
Mills, A J D
Mills, I H
Milne, C
Milton, P J D
Minshull-Beech, C S
Minto, C L
Mitchell, A L
Mitchell, A U
Mitchell, C S
Mitchell, J N
Mitchinson, M J
Moffat, D A
Moore, A T
Moore, N N
Morrell, N W
Morris, P J
Morris, S A
Moseley, R P
Mowat, C M
Muller, D J
Mulroy, S E
Murphy, P J
Nachev, P C
Naima, S J
Nashef, S A-M
Nasser, S M S
Neal, D E
Neill, A-M
Newman, D K
Newport, M J
Newton, P J
Nicholl, C G
Nicholson, J C
NiemcZuk, P
Nind, N R
Norris, P G
Nussey, A P
O'Donnell, E A
O'Donnell, D R
O'Leary, D A
O'Rahilly, S P
O'Reilly, A J
O'Shaughnessy, K M
O'Sullivan, D M
Oakeshott, S
Oduro-Dominah, A
Offen, D N
Ogilvy-Stuart, A L
Ong, K K L
Ostenfeld, T
Ostor, A J K
Owens, J
Paine, D S
Parameshwar, K J
Park, G R
Park, S-M
Parker, A P J
Parker, I R
Parkes, M
Parkin, I G
Patel, H C
Paterson, J S
Patient, C J
Paw, H G W
Pawley, J J
Paxton, P J
Paykel, E S
Pencheon, D C
Pepke-Zaba, J W
Peppiatt, T N
Perera, S D
Perrin, V L
Perry, J R
Petch, M C
Peters, A M
Peters, D K
Petter, J R
Pharoah, F M
Pharoah, P D P
Pickard, J D
Picken, S
Pinder, S E
Pinnington, J
Polack, C
Polkinhorn, M E
Ponder, B A J
Poole, S B
Popham, P A B
Power, D M
Powles, J W
Praseedom, R K
Prentice, A
Prentice, H G
Purr, J M
Purushotham, A D
Pye, R J
Rabey, G P
Rajalingam, U P
Ralevic, D
Ramana, R
Ranasinghe, R S
Ranasinghe, W A E P
Randall, T M K
Rankin, A
Rankin, J
Rann, S F
Rao, G S
Rashbass, J L
Ray, J L
Ray, N
Raymond, F L
Reading, J M
Redwood, M D
Reed, N J H
Rees, J K H
Reid, E A L
Richards, D A
Richards, S D
Ridsdill Smith, G P
Rigg, E L
Ring, H A
Rintoul, R C
Ritchie, A J
Roberts, C P
Roberts, D S
Roberts, J T
Roberts, M T M
Robinson, A H N
Robinson, F M
Robinson, S M
Robson, J M
Roe, P G
Roper, G P
Ross Russell, R I
Roth, M
Rothwell, S E
Round, C E
Rowland, M G M
Rubenstein, D
Rubery, E D
Rubinsztein, D C
Rubinsztein, J S
Rudd, J H F
Ruddock, J M
Rudolph, J
Rushton, N
Rushton, S M
Russell, S J
Rytina, E R C
Saich, A J
Sale, J E
Salisbury, R S
Salmon, R P
Sanders, C R
Sandford, R N
Sansome, A D
Sapsford, D J
Sarkies, N J C
Sartori, P C E
Satchithananda, D K
Saunders, M T
Save, V E
Sayeed, R A
Schofield, P M
Schramm, C J
Scott, J D
Scott, P M
Seed, M J
Set, P A K
Shah, N C
Shapiro, L M
Sheares, K K K
Shepherd, B C
Sherriff, H M
Shneerson, A
Shneerson, J M
Silverman, B H
Silverman, J D
Simpson, R M
Sinha, S
Sinnatamby, R
Sissons, J G P
Slack, R O
Smailes, C M
Smellie, A S
Smith, A D
Smith, G C S
Smith, I E
Smith, S K
Smith, T A
Snead, M P
Soh, V A L
Soilleux, E J
Somers Heslam, J
Sonnex, C
Soo, K G
Sopwith, A M
Spooner, V J
Stebbing, B
Stein, P E
Stephens, C J
Stephenson, C M E
Sterling, J C
Stevens, J F
Stewart, A J
Stewart, S
Stone, D L
Sule, B A
Suter, C M
Swami, A B
Tan, L T
Tasker, A D
Tasker, R C
Tavare, S M
Tayabali, M
Taylor, A J
Taylor, L K
Tempest, H V
Terlevich, A
Tewson, P J
Thirunavukkarasu, S
Thomas, C M
Thomas, G J
Tidswell, A T
Tiley, C G
Tilley, R E
Toase, P D
Tobin, G B
Todd, P M
Tolley, M E
Tooze, R M
Torpey, N P
Towriss, M H
Traub, M M
Tsui, S S L
Tuckfield, C J
Turner, J M
Turner, M W H
Turner, P S
Tweedale, J L
Valente, J E
Vallance-Owen, J
Varty, K
Verghese, R
Verity, C M
Verney, G I
Vickers, D W
Villagran Moreno, J M
Villar, R N
Vuylsteke, A
Wade, J D
Wagstaff, A E
Walker, M A
Wallace, B A
Wallwork, J
Walsh, C M
Walton, J D
Warburton, E A
Ward, M
Wareham, N J
Warren, A J
Warren, A Y
Warren, A R
Warren, R M L
Waters, A
Waters, F H
Waters, J K
Watson, A B
Watson, C J E
Watson, M E C
Watson, P G
Webster, S G P
Weisblatt, E J L
Weissberg, A
Weissberg, P L
Wells, F C
Werno, A M
West, D J
Whale, R
Wharton, A J
Wheeler, V A
White, C
Whitehead, A L
Whitfield, J J
Whittle, E
Wight, D G D
Wight, N J D
Wight, W J
Wilkinson, G
Wilkinson, I B
Wilkinson, P O
Williams, D M
Williams, E D
Williams, M P L
Williams, M V
Williamson, J R W G
Williamson, L M
Willocks, L J
Wilson, C B J H
Wilson, J M
Wilson, K J
Winter, R J D
Wiseman, J R
Wishart, G C
Wishart, M O
Withers, E J
Wolff, C B
Wong, C C
Wong, J K W
Wong, O Y
Wong, S P Y
Wood, D F
Woodrow, S L
Woods, S E
Woodward, J M
Worrall-Kent, L S
Wraight, S K
Wright, D R
Wright, N L
Wyer, S R
Wyllie, A D H
Xuereb, J H
Yates, J R W
Young, J C J
Zammit-Tabona, M V
Zimmern, R L

Camelford
Garrod, A C
Haddon, J E
Hrynaszkiewicz, A
Richardson, J P S

Campbeltown
Cook, K M
Elder, M R
Hall, M D
Hyndman, A M
Jackson, R N
Lazarus, M
Leask, J T S
Norrie, I A
Wallace, A D

Cannock
Apta, R D
Ballinger, P M
Berriman, T J
Chapman, P
Farr, D R
Gallimore, J R
Gibbins, S R
Hands, S J
Hardwick, N
Holbrook, J A P
Hulme, L V
Lochee Bayne, E M
Murugan, M
Nicklin, S
Patel, D A
Price, T
Sainsbury, J A
Satchwell, V J
Sathia, P J
Sathia, P
Sathia, U
Selvam, A
Singh, P K
Speedie, C A
Thaker, P K
Thompson, A J
Threepuraneni, G
Verma, A
Warburton, A L
Williams, E J
Woo, M P

Canonbie
Mann, P J
Rose, A J
Tinker, M D

Canterbury
Abdool Raman, A C D
Al-Hasani, M K A-K
Ananda Balendran, V
Ananthakopan, S
Andrew, N C
Armstrong, H E
Baker, G R C
Baker, J L
Bamber, R W K
Batty, G M
Beaton, A
Beats, B C
Beaumont, A C
Biggs, P E
Blanco Davila, R
Bland, J D P
Bliss, S M G
Bobba, J R
Bradburn, B G
Brown, S A
Burrowes, P W
Byrom, H
Byrom, K
Byrom, R G
Cameron, A
Carmichael, P
Carpenter, G I
Caswell, S J
Chowdhury, S R
Christodoulou, C C
Coakley, A J
Cocks, E M
Colchester, A C F
Collier, J
Collins, R E C
Coltart, R S
Coopamah, L D
Cornelius, P G
Das, P K
De Cock, R
Di Biasio, N
Dibble, J B
Didehvar, R
Downes, M O
Dowse, S C
Drouot, J E
Eaves, D L
Edwards, R S
Ellis, S B A
Entwisle, K G
Evans, J W H
Eve, M D
Fegent, J A
Field, S
Flynn, M D
Foord, A L
Forsythe, J M
Gable, D R
Garsed, M P
Goddard, K A
Goggin, M J
Greaves, D J
Greaves, S J
Grice, D J P
Heddle, R M
Heller, A J
Herraiz Morillas, R
Hettiarachchi, S P
Hoda, A W
Horton-Szar, D A J
Housden, P L
Hughes, J A
Hughes, W L
Hussain, S A
Irwin, K Z
Jackson, D B
Johnson, A J
Jones, D M
Jones, G L
Kalidindi, S
Kerr, J
Kinnersley, D S
Kittle, D J
Kurstjens, S P
Laing, R T R
Lamb, C J
Lambie, L
Larkin, V J
Lawson, K
Learner, J M
Lilley, J
Little, S R C J
Livesey, P G
Lloyd, R J
Love, E R
Lythall, D A
McCormick, D C
McIvor, J E M
Mackenzie, E C
Mackinnon, J C
Macklin, A V
McWilliams, R N
Mah, M S L
Mahapatra, P K
Manson, G
Maryosh, J A A
Matheson, P
Mikhail, A S I S
Mitchell, D B
Mithal, N P
Moran, N F
Morrison, I D
Moskovits, P E
Muller, A F
Muller, M A
Murray, K H A
Nash, I T
Neales, K E
Newson, T P
Nichols, M J
Noble, T C
Norman, M H
Nosenzo, L
O'Sullivan, C C
Opdam, H I
Owen, A
Padgham, N D
Panday, S
Parks, Y A
Pay, C L
Plummer, W P
Pollock, S S
Potter, J M
Pratt, D G
Puleston, J M
Rafla, M
Rake, M O
Rehling, G H
Richardson, M H
Roberts, B K
Robertson, B R
Royston, R G
Saleh, M I
Sarkhel, R P
Sarkhel, S T
Sawitzky, C
Schlien, M
Shah, B A
Shaw, K A
Simmonds, R
Smedley, H M
Smith, A R
Snow, J T
Sorefan, O M A
Srinivas, S
Stevens, M R C
Stevens, P E
Stewart, K R
Stewart, R M
Stillman, K
Storrs, T J
Sturgess, I
Sutherland, I R
Sykes, P H
Tamimi, N A M
Tasou, A
Toon, P D
Tyler, P A
Walkington, R P E
Way, C F
Weatherley, A
Wells, J A
Wetherell, R G
Wharfe, S M W
Wickham, E A
Wijesurendra, C S
Wijesurendra, I T
Wilkins, P
Wilkinson, P A
Williams, H J H
Williams, Y F S
Wilson, N V
Winter, J B M
Withrington, R H
Workman, I C E
Wright, M
Zintilis, S A

Canvey Island
Aslam, M
Ghauri, J B
Jena, R
Kanapathippillai, S
Levy, A J
Limage, S J
McCarthy, T J
Patel, D S
Rahman, H U
Skeet, W A G
Sughra, G

Swami, P M
Tay Za Aung, Dr
Vavrecka, M J F
Wilson, L E

Cardiff
Abdel-Nabi, A G H A G
Abel, J V
Abel, R J
Abolade, B K
Abouharb, A T
Adams, M
Adisesh, L A
Affley, B T
Aggarwal, O P
Ahmad, A B
Ahmad, S
Ajayi, B A
Al-Jader, L N
Al-Wafi, A A
Al-Samsam, R
Alcolado, J C
Aldridge, C R
Ali, M S A H
Allanby, C W
Alldrick, M D
Allouni, S
Amodeo, P A
Amso, N N J
Anderson, D J W
Andrews, J D
Anwar, A M G E
Ap Gwilym, E R M
Arana Galdos, M A
Archer, H L
Arif, M
Armstrong, T S H
Ashworth, D R
Atkins, M C
Atkins, S J
Attwood, S J
Aubrey, D A
Aylward, M
Aymat Torrente, A
Baban, V
Backer, H
Badminton, M N
Baghomian, A
Bagshaw, M J M
Baker, J H E
Baker, K L
Bako, A M
Barnes, R A
Barr, S M
Barr, V J
Barrett-Lee, P J
Barrett, I T
Barry, A J
Barry, J E S
Barry, J D
Barton, D M
Basheer, A
Batt, M C
Beattie, R B
Bebbington, A
Beck, M
Beck, P
Bedwani, S J
Bellamy, R J
Benedict, C
Bennett, A J
Bensusan, D
Bentley, D P
Bentley, R P
Bentley, R P
Benton, I J
Bevan, M A
Bhal, P S
Bhogal, J
Bisson, J I
Black, J J A
Blake, L-L
Bloomfield, M C
Bolton, C E R
Bondeson, J
Bongilli, J S
Borysiewicz, L K
Bowen, R G
Bragg, E A
Braithwaite, P A
Bratton, M L
Brewster, A E
Brooks, R M
Broughton, J M
Brown, E S
Brown, H M
Brown, N K
Brown, N J
Browning, M R
Bufton, H J S
Bunce, N H
Burnett, A K
Burr, M L
Burrell, C C
Burwell, D R
Butchart, E G
Butler, C C
Byron, M G
Callaghan, R R
Callen, N R
Camara Xardone, P M
Cameron, I R
Camilleri, J P
Campbell, S H
Cantor, R
Capstick, M E L
Cardno, A G
Carter, K M
Carter, R L
Cartlidge, P H T
Casali, G
Casey, R C E
Cattermole, G N
Chandrani, R
Chant, D J
Chapman, J A
Charles, H M J
Chaudhary, S N
Chaudhry, W N
Chawla, J C
Cheang, P P
Chellaram Hathiramani, K G
Chin, S S
Chowdhury, M M U-H
Chubb, H L
Chubb, L V
Chung, T Y
Ciampolini, I
Clarke, A J
Clarke, A J
Clyburn, P A
Coakley, M N
Cochlin, D L
Cockcroft, J R
Cocks, D W N
Coekin, S E
Cole, K E
Coles, E C
Coles, G A
Coles, P F
Colgate, R E T
Collier, G M
Collins, P D
Collins, P W
Collis, R E
Colquhoun, M C
Conlon, F V
Conner, C E
Conroy, M C
Cook, D S
Cook, E A
Cooper, A M
Cooper, H L
Corbett, J
Cotter, M
Cox, D A
Coyle, E F
Craddock, N J
Craig, B R
Crane, J A
Creaby, M M
Cronje, A M L
Crosby, D L
Crosby, G
Crowe, L J
Cunningham, N
Curran, E F
Cuthill, A R
Daniels, A W
Daniels, H F
Daniels, I R
Daoud, Z A-S
Darmani, A A
Das, S
Datta, S N
David, C
David, M Y
Davies, A J P
Davies, C
Davies, C S
Davies, C E
Davies, E G
Davies, H J
Davies, H W
Davies, I H
Davies, J S
Davies, J M
Davies, J S
Davies, M
Davies, M
Davies, M R
Davies, N J
Davies, P R
Davies, S E
Davies, S J
Davies, W T
Davis, N C
Davison, A M
Dayananda, K S S
De Alwis, E
De Lloyd, L J
Dearden, A R
Dexter, A M
Dey, P
Dhaliwal, J K
Dhallu, T
Dhariwal, D K
Dickinson, L
Diez-Rabago Del Barrio, M V
Dimpel, H L
Dingley, L D
Doherty, C B
Dolby, A E
Donovan, K L
Doyle, C
Drage, M P
Drayton, M R
Duff, E J
Dunne, N M
Dyer, J R W G
Edwards, A T
Edwards, E A
Edwards, J
Edwards, P H
Edwards, R P
Edwards, R T M
Edwards, S M
El-Khatieb, M M H
El Mahayni, N M R
El-Shaboury, A-H M
Elder, G H
Elder, S H
Elsarrag, M E
Elwood, P C
Elwyn, G J
England, R C D
Enoch, M D
Evans, A R
Evans, A
Evans, C E
Evans, C G
Evans, C L
Evans, C
Evans, D E N
Evans, D L
Evans, D G
Evans, H O
Evans, J
Evans, K T
Evans, L T I
Evans, M H
Evans, M R
Evans, N A
Evans, P M S
Evans, R E
Evans, R J
Evans, R O N
Evans, R C
Evans, R J
Evans, S A
Evans, S G
Everest, S F
Fagan, D
Fairclough, J A
Fardy, C H
Fardy, M J
Farley-Hills, E M
Farrell, A M
Farrier, J N
Farrow, A K
Fegan, C D
Fenton-May, J M
Feyi-Waboso, A C
Fiander, A N
Fielding, P A
Findlay, C M
Findlay, G P
Finlay of Llandaff, I G
Finlay, A Y
Flackett, L K
Foster, M E
Fox, R
Foy, J G D
Foy, J M
Fraser, A G
Fraser, E D
Fraser, W I
Frayling, I M
Freedman, A R
Frenneaux, M P
Frost, A
Fudge, B J
Fuge, B
Gaffney, C C
Gajraj, M
Gallop-Evans, E M L
Gandhi, P S
Gantley, J M
Garrett, J G
Gibbon, F M
Gibbs, C R
Gilbart, W S
Gildersleve, C D
Gill, J S
Gilmour, J P
Glascoe, S P
Glover, G
Godkin, A J
Gooderham, E P
Goodfellow, J
Goodwin, N
Goodwin, V H
Gordon, T L
Gouldson, R
Graham, G P
Graham, J A
Granger, M E
Gravell, R M
Gray, S R
Green, J M J
Green, M F
Gregory, J W
Grey, J E
Griffin, J D
Griffith, I P
Griffith, T M
Griffiths, B
Griffiths, D F R
Griffiths, E H
Griffiths, G B
Griffiths, J J
Griffiths, K U
Griffiths, M C
Groom, P J
Groves, A H
Groves, N D
Groves, P H
Grundler, S
Grundy, P F
Grzybowska, P H
Gunawardena, S M
Hadjikoutis, S
Hailwood, R L
Hall, J E
Hall, R
Hamilton, S A
Hanif, J
Hanna, C L
Harding, K G
Harding, L J E
Harmer, M
Harper, M
Harper, P S
Harries, I G
Harries, J
Harries, S E M
Harris, B B
Harrison, M D
Harrison, S K
Harry, G
Hart, P R
Hart, S M
Hasan, K
Hatfield, R H
Hauke, A H
Havard, C
Hawthorne, A B
Hawthorne, K
Hayes, G J
Heavens, C
Henson, S E
Henton, N J
Hicks, C E
Higgins, M A G
Hill, S M
Hillier, J
Hilling, G A L
Hocking, J A
Hodzovic, I
Holden, B M
Holland, J W
Holme, S A
Holt, P J A
Hombal, J W R
Hope-Gill, B D M
Hope, D A
Hopkins, C L
Hopkins, S D
Hopkins, T
Hopkinson, I
Hourihan, M D
Houston, H L A
Howard, A J
Howe, T M
Howell, T K
Howells, D
Howells, R M
Howes, J P
Huddart, S N
Hughes, D J
Hughes, J D
Hughes, O D M
Hughes, R C
Hughes, T A T
Humphries, A M
Hunter, J W
Hunter, P J
Hurle, R A
Hutton, K A R
Inman, C G
Ions, E
Isaacs, S L
Ismail, S M
Jackson, P M
Jacob, Dr
Jacobs, R
Jacobson, L D
Jain, S
Jamal, A S
Jamal, Z
James, G R
James, H W H
James, N M
Jamil, N F
Jani, J J
Jasani, B
Jawad, M S M
Jawad, N H
Jefferson, M J
Jenkins, A I R
Jenkins, B J
Jenkins, B J
Jenkins, C
Jenkins, D M
Jenkins, D R L
Jenkins, H R
Jenkins, J R
Jenkins, M W
Jenkins, P L G
Jenkins, S A
Jenkins, T D O
Jenney, M E M
Jewkes, F E M
Johansen, A M
John, A W
John, N E
Johnson, J
Johnson, M L
Johnston, K R
Jones, A R
Jones, A
Jones, A C
Jones, A
Jones, D L
Jones, D L
Jones, D R
Jones, D T
Jones, E C
Jones, G S
Jones, H L
Jones, H W
Jones, J I L
Jones, M R
Jones, M
Jones, N K
Jones, P L
Jones, P W
Jones, R M
Jones, R G
Jones, R D
Jones, S M
Jordan, G J
Judodihardjo, H
Kabeer, U
Kamarylzaman, S B
Kamath, S K
Karseras, A G
Kaye, P D
Keen, M R
Kell, W J
Kellam, A M P
Kemp, A M
Kerby, C
Kerby, I J
Kerkar, N R
Key, S J
Khan, N A
Khan, T
Khatib, H A
Khatib, M J
Kini, U S
Kinnersley, P
Kirby, A H
Kirov, G K
Kite, J E
Klentzeris, L D
Knight, A G
Knight, B H
Knoyle, P A
Krimmer, M H
Krishnamurti, D
Kshetry, L D
Kulatilake, E N P
Kumar, P
Laidlaw, S T
Laidler, P
Lammie, G A
Lane, A G
Lane, C M
Lane, I F
Lane, S J
Latto, I P
Lawrence, M S
Lawrie, B W
Lawton, H L
Lazarus, J H
Lazda, E J
Leadbeatter, S
Lee Hai Leong, Dr
Lee, E S G
Leeson, N A
Lewis, C G E
Lewis, D K
Lewis, G
Lewis, H
Lewis, J E
Lewis, J M
Lewis, M J
Lewis, M E
Lewis, S A R
Lewis, S M
Li, W C W
Lim Su Ping, R
Lim, F K B
Lim, J T K
Lim, K C-K
Lim, P O
Lindsey, H C
Livingstone, M D
Llewellyn, J O
Llewelyn, A A
Llewelyn, M B
Lloyd-Jones, S J
Lloyd, A R
Lloyd, D C F
Lloyd, E
Lloyd, G E
Lloyd, H A
Lloyd, H J
Lloyd, I W
Lloyd, P A R
Lloyd, R H G
Lloyd, S D
Lloyd, T H L
Logan, S W
Longstaffe, J E
Lowe, G L
Lowe, K J
Ludlow, E J
Lukaris, C P
Luscombe, J C
Lush, S G
Lyne, P N D
Lyons, I
McBeth, C
Macbeth, F R
McCann, N
McCarthy, G M T
McConnochie, K A
McCracken, D
McDowell, I F W
McHugh, L J
Mackie, I G
McKirdy, H C
McKirdy, M L
Maclaren, A M
Maclean, A C W
Maclean, A
McLean, M J
McLoughlin, N P T
McPherson, R J E

McQueen, I N F
Maddox, J C
Maheson, M V S
Mannari, N S
Mansel, R E
Manuel, A R G
Manuel, D D
Marks, R
Marsh, H S
Marshall, G E
Martin Oliver, M J
Martin, J C
Martinez, G
Marx, H M
Mason, M D
Mason, S J
Matthews, F J
Matthews, P
Matthews, P N
Maughan, T S
Mayo, H G
Meades, D C
Meghani, D K
Meyrick, R S
Millar-Jones, D J
Milligan, J P
Mills, R G S
Minton, D K
Mischel, E L
Mitchell, S H M
Moffat, D B
Moghal, A M
Mohamed, M Y
Monaghan, S P
Mondal, D
Moore, R H
Morgan, B P
Morgan, C A
Morgan, C E
Morgan, C
Morgan, D L
Morgan, G F
Morgan, J E
Morgan, R M L
Morgan, S M
Morgan, S J
Morley, A R U
Morris, G
Morris, H R
Morris, R L
Morris, S J
Morris, T J
Morse, R E
Moss, L J
Motley, R J
Mott, A M
Mower, J
Mowle, S H
Mudd, S J
Muen, W J
Munro, J A
Murrin, K R
Nam, S
Narang, I
Nayar, R N
Neal, J W
Nelson-Owen, M E C
Ng, W T
Nokes, L D M
Norton, C A
Nowayhio, F A
Nunn, A N
O'Doherty, D P W
O'Donovan, M C
O'Dwyer, H S
O'Sullivan, M
Oelmann, G J
Ogden, J N
Oldham, T A
Ong, J P L
Owen, A M
Owen, D C
Owen, M J
Owens, E P
Owens, R E
Owens, R W
Palmer, D J W
Palmer, S R
Parkinson, D J
Parry-Morton, M
Parsons, A S
Parsons, J M
Parsons, S L
Patel, N D
Pathy, D J G
Payne, E E
Pearce, A V
Pearson, J R
Pegge, N C
Penketh, R J A
Penny, E P
Penny, W J
Peters, J R
Phillips, A O
Phillips, S
Pickersgill, T P
Pierrepoint, M J
Pierry, A A
Pilz, D T
Pippen, C A R
Pitt, D J
Plant, M J
Powell, A
Powell, J R
Poynton, C H
Premawardhana, L D K E
Presley, R
Price, M M
Price, M
Price, M A
Prichard, J E
Pritchard, M H
Procter, A M
Prokop, R
Pugh, C N
Pugh, S C
Puntis, M C A
Purnell, R M
Quarry, D P
Quarry, S J
Rafter, M J
Raghunathan, K
Raghupati, R
Rattigan, S M
Ravine, D
Raybould, A D
Razouqi, B M
Read, M S
Reddy, D P
Rees, A E J
Rees, A
Rees, B M
Rees, B I
Rees, H G
Rees, J A E
Rees, J I S
Reeves, D M
Reid, S A
Rhodes, P
Richards, C J
Richards, S
Richmond, J K
Richmond, P W
Riley, S G
Rishko, A J
Rivron, M J
Roach, H D
Robbe, I J
Roberts, A
Roberts, A W
Roberts, A J
Roberts, B C
Roberts, B N
Robertson, S W
Robinson, B G
Robinson, C J
Robinson, M D
Roblin, D G
Roblin, M W
Rochfort, A M C
Rogers, C
Rogers, M T
Rosen, M
Rothwell, A C
Routledge, P A
Rowe, S M
Roy, W S
Rudge, P
Rudling, J L
Ruttley, M S T
Ryan, A G M J
Ryder, R C
Rye, A D
Saad, M
Sabir, A W
Sabir, A T W
Sadiq, S S Q
Sadler, S J
Saha, T K
Sakel, R
Salmon, R L
Salter, D G
Sampson, J R
Samuels, A J L
Saunders, K
Savage, P M
Scanlon, M F
Scarle, T J B
Scherf, C F
Schofield, S J A
Scholey, J A
Scolding, K J
Scorer, R C
Scott, A K
Scourfield, J
Secker Walker, J
Shah, H V
Sharma, S K
Sharma, S
Sheen, M
Shehadeh, E S
Shelling, D
Shepherd, E H
Sheraton, T E
Shewring, D J
Shewring, J I
Shewring, S A
Shone, G R
Shortland, G J
Shrivastava, S K
Siddall, B L
Sim, K T
Simmons, M D
Simpson, B A
Sinclair, A J
Singh, H B
Singhal, K
Sinha, A K
Skyrme, M L
Skyrme, R J
Smail, S A
Smart, J A
Smith, G C
Smith, J S
Smith, L-A
Smith, P H
Smith, R
Smith, R A
Smithies, M N
Soukias, N
Sparks, R A
Stacey, M R W
Stephens, S D G
Stephenson, T P
Stevenson, A I
Steward, J A
Stewart, J I M
Stone, A M
Stone, R L
Stork, A F
Strachan, A G
Sullivan, B A
Sultana, K
Sultana, R
Sumption, J C
Sumption, N J
Sweetland, H M
Sykes, H E
Syson, A
Tan, K L
Tan, K H-V
Tang, W Y
Tapper-Jones, L M
Taylor, C
Thapar, A
Thomas, A M
Thomas, C E
Thomas, D M
Thomas, D R
Thomas, G A O
Thomas, H O
Thomas, J A
Thomas, J
Thomas, M
Thomas, M J
Thomas, M J E
Thomas, T H
Thompson, J P
Thompson, T H R
Thompson, W M
Tiwari, R
Tjandra, J J
Todd, G B
Todd, S E
Tomlinson, S
Trigg, S E E
Triggs, A J
Tromans, J P
Tufail, A
Tweddel, A C
Vaid, S
Van Der Voort, J H
Van Woerden, H C
Vasanthakumari, S
Vaughan, D L J
Vaughan, R S
Verrier Jones, K
Vetter, N J
Vig, S
Von Oppell, U O
Votruba, M
Vujanic, G
Wainwright, J R
Wakeling, J A
Walker-Baker, L
Waller, J A
Walters, R F
Ward, D A
Ward, D E
Ward, N W
Warner, J T
Wat, D S-C
Watson, M R
Watson, M W
Watts, K A
Watura, R
Weaver, S R
Webb, E V J
Webster, D J T
Webster, V J
Wenham, G A
West, S C
Westall, W G
Westlake, H E
Westlake, J D
Westmoreland, D
Wheeler, R A E
Whiston, R J
Whitaker, G
White, S V
Whittaker, S M
Whitten, M P
Wigley, A M
Wiles, C M
Williams, A J
Williams, B D
Williams, D T
Williams, E V
Williams, E H
Williams, G L
Williams, G T
Williams, H E
Williams, J D
Williams, J E
Williams, L B
Williams, N J
Williams, P E
Williams, P R
Williams, R L
Williams, R G
Williams, R I
Williams, R S
Williams, S M
Williams, S A
Williams, T N
Williamson, D W
Williamson, J B
Willis, B A
Wilson, C
Wilson, I C
Wilson, K M O N
Wiltshire, E J M
Win Ko, Dr
Windhaber, R A J
Wong, C Y
Wong, S Y S
Wood, A M
Wood, S M
Woodhouse, K W
Woodnutt, D J
Woods, K M
Woolf, A M
Woolley, C M
Worwood, G
Wright, P A
Wynford-Thomas, D W
Yaqoob, M A
Yarr, N T
Young, H L
Young, K E
Zamiri, I
Zammit, S G

Cardigan

Cuddigan, A S
David, O J
Fischer, C M
Hemington, A
James, D W
Knight, S N K
Noakes, J P L
Rendle, D E
Russell, B T
Stephens, N G
Thomas, S E M
Thomas, S G

Carlisle

Adam, G P
Allison-Bolger, V Y
Amos, T A S
Anderson, J G
Ashton, H
Ashton, J R
Asquith, C E
Athey, G N
Athey, R J
Baker, C M
Baker, C D
Barber, H M
Barber, L M
Barnsley, R J
Bearn, M A
Beastall, A
Bennett-Jones, D N
Billett, J S
Black, A D F
Bone, J A
Brammah, A L
Briggs, M A
Brignall, C G
Britton, J N
Britton, N R
Brodie, C A
Brookes, C E
Brown, A A
Burke, D A
Calvert, N I R
Cawley, N
Chin, P-L
Clark, D R
Clark, M G
Clough, H A
Corrigan, C
Cowley, M L
Cox, N H
Cumming, J A
Davies, D P
Deeble, J
Depla, D N
Dickson, U K
Dobson, J M
Dodgeon, L M
Dorken, P R
Dunckley, H G
Dyson, P
Edgar, A J
Edge, J M H
Edwards, A D
Evans, A T G
Evans, D R
Ewbank, J A
Faux, J W
Ferrier, G M
Foster, J C
Foxworthy, J V
French, J A
Frost, J C
Furlong, L R
Gardner, D W
George, J
Goold, M F
Gordon, J E
Grainger, I M
Gregson, C A
Harker, C G
Harper, K L
Hasan, S Q
Hay, S R
Hayes, D G
Head, M O C
Herrick, A C
Herrmann, K
Hindle, J M
Hinson, F L
Hipple, L J
Holdsworth, A C
Holmes, K M
Horne, A R
Huggins, C L
Ions, G K
Jackson, J E
Jardine, G W H
Jayawardena, G M U
Jenkins, M
Jennings, P G
John, M R
Jones, D F
Keir, S L
Kennedy, S
Kerss, I M S
Kewley, M A
Kidd, C E
King, A L
King, P H M
Kirke, C N
Knowles, M A
Koussa, F C
Large, D M
Lawley, R
Leesley, D A
Lewis, C K
Lightfoot, R J
Loftus, J
Lord, C
Ludlam, R B
McClay, W J A
McCrea, J D
Macdonald, C E
McDowell, J F
MacFadzean, J A C
Mackay, T I
Mackenzie, G M
McKenzie, Y
McNeill, R H
McStay, K C
Margerison, L N
Mead, P A
Melrose, I C
Mitchell, C P
Morgan, W H
Murrant, N J
Murray, A C
Murray, I H F
Murray, R H
Mustchin, C P
Neal, G
Nicoll, J J
Noblett, J J
Nolan, J A
O'Brien, H A W
Orr, M J
Palmer, J G
Palmer, V F
Paterson, A W
Paterson, W D
Patterson, C
Pattinson, C P
Payne, M R
Paynter, A S
Pearson, S E
Philp, L D
Popple, A W
Putnam, G D
Raimes, S A
Rea, A J
Read, R E
Reay, S
Reed, R C
Reid, F M
Reid, W
Rickerby, E J
Rigby, M F
Rippon, C
Roberts, M H W
Roberts, S A
Robson, A K
Robson, R H
Ross, M G
Sabir, O M E
Salisbury, M S
Saxton, J S
Scott, S W
Scroggie, B M R
Sells, M F L
Sevar, R
Shanks, A B
Shetty, T T
Singh, T M
Sixsmith, M
Smith, K P
Smith, R P S
Stanley, B S
Stitt, G W
Storr, J N P
Storr, T M
Stride, P C
Strover, A R M
Stuart, P
Swain, R A H
Swindells, A
Tait, K F
Tayler, P J
Taylor, M C
Thomson, J C
Tidmarsh, M D
Tiplady, P
Twomey, M P K
Tzabar, Y H
Ward, D B
Wheatley, D S
White, M J

White, P M
Whiteley, J
Wholey, V G
Wicks, R
Wigmore, N P
Williams, M R
Wills, H G
Wolstencroft, P J
Wood, M E
Wright, N F
Young, F I
Young, V E
Zobair, M

Carluke
Arnott, S
Baldwin, S H G
Boyd, J C
Buck, L M
Chaubey, S
Christie, I R
Delahunty, C
Gemmill, S
Guha, S
Gunn, I R
Guthrie, G M
Haque, M S
Hodsman, N B A
Howard, M E
Innes, A C
Jackson, A W
Kaiqobad, R M
Kennedy, G
Lynas, A M
McCallion, J
McCallion, J S
Mackintosh, C L
O'Brien, I A D
Patterson, A A
Redpath, J B S
Scott, J J
Shajahan, P M
Sharma, B D
Stewart, J F N
Teoh, Y P
Workman, A J G
Wright, A D G

Carmarthen
Al-Abdullah, A F I
Arvind, A S R
Battu, V R
Bennett, M
Black, R J
Bloomfield, T H
Brennan, D R
Briggs, G D
Brown, P M
Carter, S H
Chapman, T H
Chatterji, S
Coleman, M C
Cumber, P M
Daniel, O
Davies, D A
Davies, G W M
Davis, B R
Denholm, R B
Dowling, M A
Edwards, H
Eustace, J R
Evans, H A
Evans, K P
Eynon, A M
Gana, B M
Gibbin, P P
Gibby, S A
Goriah, S A
Gravelle, I P
Greenacre, J A
Griffith, M J
Griffiths, S E
Griffiths, W G
Harries, D K
Harrison, G A J
Hasan, M A S
Hooper, C A
James, W M
John, C L
Johnson, S J
Johnson, S R
Jones, C
Jones, C A M
Jones, D W M
Jones, D
Jones, E
Jones, E W
Jones, M H
Jones, S C
Jose, K
Kanapathy Raja, M S
Kinnear, J C
Laxton, A G P
Lewis, A L
Lewis, G H
Lewis, G E
Llewellyn-Jones, C G
Locker, A P
Loyden, C F
McGinley, J F
Magee, T M
Mahon, S V
Masoodi, M N
Mistry, P G
Morgan, N J
Morgan, S
Moyle, C D
Murphy, D L
Murphy, J K
Murphy, R C
O'Riordan, B G M
Owen, G
Potter, H A
Powell, D E B
Prasad, R
Purcell, P M J
Ramadan, A M
Rees, A
Rimell, P J
Rincon Aznar, C
Ritchie, W N
Roberts-Harry, T J
Rowlands, I G
Salam, I
Salinas, J
Sargeant, M P
Saxena, V R
Sheridan, W G J
Stephens, C L
Tan Tong Khee, Dr
Taube, M
Thirunawarkarisu, K S
Thomas, C W
Thomas, D H
Thomas, M A
Thomas, T P L
Thomson, W
Tirunawarkarisu, K P
Turtle, M J
Vamadeva, P
Walapu, M F M
Walker, M
Wan, S K H
Warren, P M
Warren, S
Wilding, H I
Wilkins, M F
Williams, J H
Williams, R G
Wright, R G
Yate, B H
Zohdy, G

Carnforth
Abraham, N J
Bates, P
Beagan, M M
Blewitt, R W
Bryan, S R
Clarke, J M
Crosfill, F M
Docton, R K E
Fleetwood, A L
Fletcher, M M
Fowden, A
Granger, C E
Gray, P F
Hall, P J I
Halsey, J P
Hampson, J L
Hobbs, G A T
Johnson, J A
Kopcke, D H F
Lakeland, D A
Longley, J P
Lowson, K
McConnell, A T
Matchett, A A
Morgan-Capner, K
Morris, J A
Park, W G
Partington, A
Placzek, M M
Robinson, R E
Sewell, R N
Shakespeare, J
Sheals, G
Smith, E A
Sutton, D E
Thomas, D G
Till, C B W
Torkington, M J
Wall, W H J
Wickenden, G H

Carnoustie
Campbell, L
Chalmers, S D
Clark, M F
Crosby, F R G
Easton, A I M
Gallon, M E
Hutcheon, S D
Leslie, H
McKendrick, A D
Morton, L J
Robb, O J
Stubbs, M C
Thornton, P W

Carrickfergus
Addis, S R D
Anderson, M R
Andrews, W J
Baird, T A
Bolton, L H
Bradley, S
Buckley, O M
Calwell, A M I
Calwell, A I J
Campbell, H S
Courtney, D
Crothers, E D
Darragh, P M
Davison, D N
Dixon, N D
Esler, J R D
Ferguson, J R
Ferres, C J
Gordon, D V
Green, D F
Harper, D S
Hunter, K
Hutchinson, A F
Lewis, A
Logan, I D
Mcallister, J G
McCluggage, W G
McCrory, C A W
McDonald, L J
McGrath, J J O
Mahood, K M
Muir, A D
Peoples, S
Rainey, J C A
Robinson, W J E
Russell, C H
Ryans, R I
Shahidullah, B S
Smith, S P
Stone, M P
Turkington, J R A
Vahid Assr, M D
White, J S
Wilson, J P

Carshalton
Akinmade, O
Ali Khan, N F
Andrews, P A
Assinder, F R S C
Atallah, M G
Attard, M T
Baig, S N
Bansal, A S
Barron, J L
Barry, J J G
Behrens, J
Benson, M J
Bird, J
Blewitt, S D
Boardman, D R
Boyd, P J R
Brown, J M
Burren, C P
Byrne, P D
Chesser, J J S
Chong, S K-F
Citron, N D
Clancy, R M
Clarke, M F
Cockbain, J M R
Cooke, D A P
Cooke, N T
Dar, A
Dar, S
Das, S K
Davies, G W
Ditri, A
Doyle, A P
Duke, O L
Estreich, S
Farhat, S Y
Favre, A
Field, R E
Foran, J P M
Forrest, A J
Fouque, C A
Frangoulis, M A
Froley, A
Galloway, A
Ghaznavi, A H
Gilford, H J
Goel, K L
Goel, R K
Halfhide, C P
Harland, C C
Harris, F E
Hastie, A L
Hawkins, S S
Hebrero Matobella, E
Hodson, N J
Howard, P J
Hyer, S L
Jones, C R
Kavanagh, T G
Khan, F
Khong Yang-Sui, M
Knott, P D
Kwan, J T C
Ling, S
Liu, M Y
McWhinney, N A
Madina, T
Makanjuola, A D
Mantell, J
Marsden, M R
Maynard, J P
Mercieca, J E
Mohiud-Din, F
Mohiud-Din, S M
Mojiminiyi, O A
Moncrieff, D P M
Nehra, D
North, E A
Ogilvie, D
Palmer, M K
Patel, S R
Patel, V R
Penna, L K
Pinto, A P R
Pujara, M S
Quinton, C F
Radford, P
Renwick, S J
Ringer, W S
Rodin, D A
Ross, L D
Rudolphij, A J
Samadian, S
Shellim, A J
Shephard, E R
Siala, M-D
Singh, L N
Singh, N
Smith, A R C
Stevens, K L H
Stockwell, M A
Sultan, V
Tayar, R
Taylor, J D
Thomas, P R S
Toosy, T H
Varney, V A
Ward, M C
Warren, M E
Wartan, S W
Wells, M P P
Whaley, K E
Wheildon, M H
Whitlow, B J
Wilcox, A H
Williams, C R
Yeoh, L H
Yu, K H
Zack, P

Carterton
A'Court, C H D
Clough, F C
Jones, N M
Reid, G E

Castel
Balls, J L
Clark, R N W
Gee, I B
Hanna, R G J
Mowbray, E S M J I

Castle Cary
Collins, D P
Ketley, A M D
Roylance, M K

Castle Douglas
Armstrong, W H
Carmichael, I A
Carson, E A
Clarke, M D B
Greeley, N C
Halliday, K C R
Jones, B G
King, M
Livingstone, S E
Neil, S P
Oliver, N M
Purdie, G
Scott, P J
Sproat, L M E
Walker, K R
Wilkinson, A P D

Castlebay
Campbell, M E
Hidson, J M
Savory, J C
Sinclair, A-M

Castlederg
Bailie, R W A
McElroy, R G
McHugh, R
O'Hare, B J
O'Hare, I P

Castleford
Aldridge, G R
Atkinson, R
Bance, H R
Cuttell, E J
Gallagher, P
Godridge, A C
Gopinathan, K K
Harris, L D
Henein, R R
Lloyd, C
McClintock, C B
Minocha, D
Nambiar, S C
Pierechod, B A
Prasad, A
Ravindran, A
Sanzeri, M
Sloan, R E G
Subramanian, S
White, D A

Castletown
Brewis, V T
Harris, S A
Smith, P H
Swainson, S M

Castlewellan
Chestnutt, J A J
Magorrian, M T

Caterham
Bantick, G L
Benn, C L
Brocklebank, A-M N
Cole, B W
Crispin, S A
Defriend, K P
Dodson, H J
Dunnet, E L
Heath, M T
Howard, J V
Hutchinson, A
Irvine, R E
Lazarus, N R
Lewis, J M
McKeran, R O
Miller, A J
O'Brien, F C
Peermahomed, R
Piper, R O J
Roberts, P F
Sinclair, R D
Stead, T L
Walls, N J
Wand, P J
Wright, R E

Catterick Garrison
Anderson, J
Cox, V M
Fulton, G W O
Gillespie, P N
Lord, S R
McManus, F B R
Robertson, D G
Turner, M A
Watt, S E
Williams, D
Zaremba, E L

Chalfont St Giles
Allison, N
Fung, D A
Harmer, D
Hatfield, E C I
Heywood, D
Holton, T S
Sutherland, S C

Chard
Beaven, J H
Bowie, C
Davies, S J
Down, A G
Eales, M J
Evans, J M
Freeston, W
Glanvill, A P
Goddard, C L
Harris, S W
Jones, D R H
Montague, I A
Saintey, P A
Staveley, C D
Tresidder, A P T

Chatham
Ahern, M D
Aslam, T
Badiger, R V
Bellary, S V
Broom, T
Chaudhry, M A
Cohen, J
Dabestani, M
Davis, F C
Gopalji, B T
Hanson, L M H
Hussain, A
Iles, S E
Imlach, A A
Jha, A B
Judge, S
Karim, M M
Khan-Lodhi, N
Khan, M A
Mahapatra, K S
Mahmood, A
Masand, M
Modha, P G
Mohamed, M S H
Morton, V J
Nathan, N
Norris, R W
Padma, K
Panesar, H S
Qureshi, K N
Raval, J K
Raval, P B
Raval, V P
Sethi, C S
Sethi, J K
Shaikh, R A
Sharma, A
Shum, C M
Szwedziuk, P
Talavlikar, P H
Tooby, D J
Tucker, B R
Ukachi-Lois, J O
Verheul, M R
Vibhuti, R
Virdee, B S
Webb, P J
Windmill, M E
Yousaf, R

Chatteris
Herbert, A T
Szekely, J M
Watts, S J

Cheadle
Abdulezer, T R
Adams, J R
Aggarwal, R

Armstrong, M A
Aslam, N F
Atkinson, N H
Bazley, P D
Bennett, C A
Bowman, A H
Boyd, J
Brady, J L
Cahill, A
Carroll, R N P
Chaudhry, A A
Connolly, P T
Cowie, R A
Cumming, W J K
Das, A
Davidson, D G D
Davies, C P
Davison, A J
Day, J F
De Kretser, D M H
Deakin, D P
Dean, K M
Deiraniya, A H K
Delaney, J A
Depares, J
Devakumar, V N
Doherty, C H
Dunlop, P M
Ellis, J
Fuller, A R
Gilbert, D J
Glicher, S R
Goodwin, S H J
Gore, P J
Grant, E M
Green, B H
Hardman, A
Higson, V L
Hopkins, S M
Hudson, G R
Ingleby, I
Isherwood, M J
Jackson, H
Jobling, A J
Johnson, S M
Keenan, J
Kiely, G P
Knox, G M
Lang, D M
Lansbury, J
Lee, S J
Lemon, J G
Lord, G M
Lord, R H
Lund, S T
McFarlane, T
McGirr, P W
McKeown, S P
McLaren, J E
McLauchlan, D G
Maclellan-Smith, I
Mamelok, J P
Markham, D E
Mather, A J
Miller, T C
Milligan, J C
Mirski, T I M
Mishra, K
Moore, S J
Morewood, G A
Mottershead, M S
Naeem, N S
Nassar, W Y
Newbon, S
O'Driscoll, J B
Oldale, M J
Olujohungbe, A B K
Oommen, P K
Patel, S J
Payne, C R
Priest, A V
Priestley, G S
Radcliffe, D
Rowlands, D J
Russell, J R
Sandars, J E
Sanderson, J H
Sassoon, J H
Seabrook, R J
Shalet, S M
Sillince, C
Strachan, A N
Sutton, J K
Swainson, C J
Sykes, J R
Sylvester, B S
Taylor, A K
Testa, H J
Thorne, J A
Turnberg, D
Vaid, V
Weatherby, E D
Webb, A K
Webb, L J
Webster, A P
Weiner, C A
Wensley, R T
Whiteson, S D
Woods, M R
Wright, A T

Cheddar

Davies, T E
Hincks, J R
Thomas, S Y A

Chelmsford

Agarwal, A
Agrawal, A
Ahmad, S
Ahmed, M A
Ahmed, W
Al-Hasani, A J
Al Janabi, K J S
Alexander, W L
Allan, H F
Anderson, C S
Anfield, A C D
Archer, M
Astbury, C
Bagchi, R
Bailey, M C
Bakewell, S M
Barron, E T
Baugh, O H A
Baylis, T M
Bell, M P
Bell, T A G
Bevan, C J
Birn-Jeffery, J
Blainey, A D
Boira Segarra, M B
Boon, C S
Booth, J T
Boyle, R J
Bradbury, P G
Brain, A G C
Brain, H P S
Brann, L R
Bridgman, J C
Bridgman, J F
Brook, V
Brown, M T
Brown, P D
Browne, T F
Bulkeley, J D L
Cacket, N E
Carter, J A
Cass, S
Chad, R K
Clesham, G J
Collins, C J
Cooper, N I
Cormack, J F
Cory, P
Cummins, T A
Cunnah, D T E
Cunniffe, G A
Dann, C F
Davies, P J
Davies, R A
Davis, M E
Dawton, A J
De Meza, P
Dilley, S P
Dodd, H J
Duku, A Y
Durcan, J J
Dyson, A E
Eaton, J E
Edelsten, M
Everett, S C
Fallowfield, M E
Ferguson, J L
Fisher, J M
Flanagan, J
Flemming, A F S
Forbes, D I
Forde, I
Frame, J D
Frost, M W
Garrod, P J
Garvey, J C
Gaskell, W G
Gittos, M J B
Goodfellow, C F
Gopakumar, C K
Grant, F M
Greene, M L
Griffith, D W
Guttikonda, A
Guttikonda, K L
Guttikonda, M
Guy, J
Guy, L M
Hanson, B C
Hariram, P
Harpur, J E
Harverson, A R V
Harverson, G
Harvey, M H
Hashmi, S T A
Hashmi, S Z A
Hatton, C-L
Hattotuwa, K L
Hock Heng Tham, Dr
Hooper, D M
Hopkins, P A
Huddy, N C
Huddy, V J
Hudson, S J
Hunt, N G
Ivermee, S P
Ives, A J
Iwuagwu, F C
Jackson, G M
Jader, S N
Jegede, A A
Jenkins, G W
Johnson, P D
Jonas, M
Kamala, K
Kelly, D A
Kelly, R A
Khin, C C
Klaber, M C V
Klijnsma, M P
Lach, S
Lewi, H J E
Lints, A V
Lipscomb, A P
Little, J C
Lloyd, J
Logan, A
Longhurst, H J
Lyall, H A
McAllister, P D
MacCarthy, P R
McGeachy, D J
Macgregor, M F
McLean, G E
Mahesh Babu, R N
Manickasamy, T A
Mann, S A
Mathai, J T
Maxwell, J F
Mayet, A
Melamed, R
Merritt, J L
Middleton, M I
Monsell, N
Montague-Brown, H J
Morgan, B H
Morley-Jacob, C A
Murphy, E A
Murray, C
Murray, D M
Nadra, A
Nair, A L
Nickol, K H
Niranjan, N S
North, M A
Noury, S A M
Osborne, D R
Pace-Balzan, A
Pain, A N
Palmer, S J
Panagiotopoulos, T
Partington, C K
Passani, S
Pateman, M T
Peck, S
Philpott, G J
Pitt, B M
Pluck, J C
Pratt, P G
Qureshi, A S
Qureshi, S
Ramsay, H V
Randell, R
Rao, V R
Richardson, N G B
Robarts, P J
Roberts, M E
Robson, E J
Ross, A H M
Rushbrook, S M
Russell, S M
Salom De Tord, R
Santhiapillai, D
Sarjudeen, M T
Sauven, P D
Savage, N A
Saverymuttu, S H
Short, A I K
Singh, C B
Sinha, A
Sommerlad, M G
Soria, A
Spence, M R
Spurr, M J
Srinivasan, A M
Stallwood, M I
Stead, C H
Stern, P M
Stevens, S A
Steyn, M P
Su, A P C C
Swallow, E B
Swallow, R A
Tarjuman, M
Taylor, M F S
Teare, E L
Tetstall, A P
Thilagarajah, R
Thoung, M T
Thway, Y
Timmins, A C
Tiwari, A
Tiwari, I
Towers, E M
Towson, N B D
Tucker, S E
Tuite, J D
Utting, J A
Vincent, N R J
Vucevic, R
Wagle, S G
Walker, J E G
Ward-Booth, R P
Whitney, R W
Wickramasinghe, S G M
Williams, D J M
Williams, W W
Wilson, A D
Winton, P E
Wissa, A H
Wood, E C
Wood, M K
Wood, P J C
Wood, S M
Wright, J M
Yaqoob, M
Zwink, R B

Cheltenham

Ackroyd, A
Adams, J F R
Ainscow, D A P
Alcock, P S
Allum, W E
Anderson, J T
Arnott, M S M
Aung Thu, Dr
Bailey, C E
Batten, J H
Bennett, J M
Benstead, K
Bialas, M C
Billings, R A
Blundell, E L
Bohm, Y H
Bond, R
Borley, N R
Bowley, R N
Brampton, W J
Bramwell, J C
Bristol, J B
Brooks, K M
Brown, E F
Buckley, W E G
Bugaighis, A E
Buntwal, N E
Burgess, C C
Burkett, J D
Caesar, R H
Cairns, I L
Campbell, A J
Casey, W F
Chamberlain Webber, R F O
Chan, H Y
Chapman, D C
Chapple, R D
Clarkson, J M
Clarkson, K R
Collyer, S P
Cooper, M A
Cooper, R A
Copp, M V
Copps, C A
Counsell, R
Court, S E
Cowen, C J
Cox, A-M
Cummin, C G
Curtis, K W
Dalton, R J
Davies, P H
Davies, S L
Day, A J
De Courcy, J G
De Moor, M M A
Deering, A H
Delhanty, M H V
Disney, J N
Dye, H M
Dykes, R M
Eaton, D J
Edmondson, S G
Edwards, H E
Elliott, S A
Ellis, M F S
Elyan, S A G
Field, J
Fielding, P D
Fletcher, P J
Flowers, C S
Flynn, J F
Forsyth, H M
Galey, S M
Gazet, A C
Gee, A S
Gibson, J M
Gilbert, H W
Giraldi, D J
Glen, R T
Glover, L A
Goodman, A J
Goodrum, D T
Green, A R
Green, S
Gubbay, N
Hamilton-Ayres, M J J
Hamilton, D C M
Hande, H R S
Hanna, E M
Hardwick, T J
Harrison, J M
Harrod, R R
Haseler, C M
Healy, T J G
Henson, A
Hill, E L
Hiorns, M P
Hollands, J M
Hollands, R D
Holmes, D M
Hyatt Williams, M G
Hyatt Williams, S
James, B G
James, G S E
Jaycock, P D
Jeffrey, D I
Johnston, R L
Jones, R L
Joyce, M
Kerr-Wilson, R H J
Kinchin, C G J
Kinder, R B
Kinder, S M M
Kirkpatrick, J N P
Kloer, J
Kloer, M J
Knights, A L
Lamden, C S J
Lee, S A
Liebert, I J
Llewellyn, T D
Lloyd, D J
Lyburn, I D
Lyle, D W
McCarthy, K P
McDowell, A M
McGrath, J C
McKenzie, I F
Mackinnon, H M
Mackinnon, J G
MacKinnon, M D
Mackintosh, G I S
McMinn, S G E
McNaught, A I
McPherson, I S
McSwiney, M M
Marshall, J A
Marson, D
Martin, A
Martin, D C
Martin, K
Mather, C M P
Mathers, R G
Medforth, L J
Medland, L F
Mehta, C P
Miles, W R
Milroy, S E C
Minett, A R
Mitchell, E A
Mohankumar, S
Moliver, A A
Moliver, S
Moore, J B
Morgan, P D
Morison, N J
Morphew, K J
Morrow, P C
Mortimore, I L
Murphy, E A
Nelson, S A B
Nicholas, M E
Nicolson, B R
O'Conor, H M N
O'Leary, C M
Olver, J D
Ormerod, T P
Owen, J R
Owen, K L
Pearson, J G
Pearson, S E
Penketh, A R L
Penny, E C
Perkins, C S
Philpot, K A
Pillai, M B
Pomeroy, A
Poskitt, K R
Pratt, S F
Price, D G
Price, E D P
Price, N C
Pygott, Y M
Ramsay, I D
Ranger, M
Rawstorne, S
Richards, M J
Ritchie, P A
Robinson-White, C M
Robinson, C P
Robinson, F M
Rooker, G D
Ropner, R J R
Roscoe, P
Ross, A
Rouse, G M
Routh, G S
Rowles, S V
Russell, H C
Ryley, S P
Sanchez-Moyano Lea, J M
Sanderson, P M
Saunders, A
Sawers, J S A
Scanlon, P H
Scott, S J
Shepherd, S F
Sherringham, P E C
Skillman, J M
Slimmings, P G
Sloan, F J
Smellie, V R
Smith, S P
Stedeford, J C
Steele, N A
Sutton, M
Sweet, A J
Thompson, C L
Thomson, R G
Thornett, J A
Timlin, C E
Todd, K H
Toner, P G
Treharne, A E
Tribley, A R
Trueman, M D
Van Rooyen, E
Vernon-Smith, J W
Wand, J S
Watkins, D J
Webb, M R
West, S L
West, S E
Whyman, M R

Wickham, H E H V
Wilson, G M
Wilson, J M
Withers, A F D
Wreford, J
Young, N J

Chepstow
Allison, R J
Berger, C P M
Dallimore, J N
Daly, M H
Davies, H L
Dickson, W A
Edwards, T J
Gibbon, G V
Hancox, D J
Hawkins, P
Jacks, S M
Jacks, T A
Jenkins, K
Jones, N J P E
Jones, P H
Jones, R H
Jovasevic, B
Lougher, L J
Matthews, C N A
May, J E
Merrick, J M
Moore, E J
Morton, P P
Oldham, J C
Pendleton, A P M
Pullen, F J
Roberts, P
Savage, C
Seale, A N
Tayton, K J J
Thompson, P D
Twamley, H W J
Van Buren, A E
Williams, S T B

Chertsey
Aggarwal, R
Bahl, S
Bahmaie, A
Barnes, D
Baxter, M A
Bearn, P E
Bennett, C E
Blewitt, N J
Bowyer, J J
Britton, M G
Brodribb, P F
Butler, B
Canty, M C
Castleton, B A
Chin, K H
Chong, H P
Cole, R S
Cooper, P J F
Crawshaw, P A G
Creagh, M F
Creagh, T M
Davidson, S M
Dawson, K J P
De Ruiter, M J
Dodd, S M
Donaldson, D R
Donaldson, J A
Elias, A H
Evans, J A
Farjad Azad, F
Finch, P J
Fluck, D S
Fowle, A J
Franciosi, P G
Fuzzey, G J J
Gelman, W
Gilani, S S M
Glover, J R
Greaves, K
Grundy, H C
Haddad, D F
Hadley, J M
Hall, G M
Hall, M
Harris, A J
Hennessy, R E
Ho, P P
Hollingsworth, R P
Houlton, P G
Hulme, S-L
Hung, W Y-C
Ibrahim, S K
Joy, M D
Knight, S E
Kumar, K
Kumar, P
Lawn, E M
Long, C A
Manaktala, K J R
Manjubhashini, S
Mann, H M
Mantel-Cooper, N
Martin, P B
Maxfield, H S
Miller, A L C
Nackasha, W L
Neill, S (M
Newman, K J H
Newton, R C F
Nordstrom, M E
North-Coombes, D P
Patil, K P
Pinder, D C
Rafferty, A M
Rana, P S
Rizvi, S S A
Sarris, I
Sebestik, J P
Seehra, K K
Sen Gupta, A K
Sharma, V
Singh, A P
Singh, S
Stuart, F M
Thomas, M H
Thornton, J R
Towie, H G
Vaughan Jones, S A
Vincent-Brown, A M B
Weston, J A B
Wright, J T
Wyatt, M L
Zakaria, F B P
Zoric, B

Chesham
Appleby, M I
Aulaqi, A A M
Baxter, T
Bishop, A P
Boast, P W
Cooper, N C
Dineen, R A
Firth, R M
Flint, P J
Jordan, R A
King, S M
Masters, G L
Morris, A E
Mowat, K J
Norman, M
Paul, M L H
Payne, G P I
Phibbs, P A T
Rashiq, H N
Roberts, J P
Russell, T
Stevens, D C
Verrinder, C J L
Wilkie, J N
Wood, N R

Chessington
Currie, A P
Edgar, F M
Elford, M T
Gray, J E
Jayasekera, N
Khan, K A
Law, P K
Riley, S J
Somanathan, L
Udal, M S
Visva Nathan, S

Chester
Adams, E J
Adams, R M
Al Shamma, F A S
Amin, A W A K
Anderson, L E
Armstrong, S
Arnold, R T
Ashton, A J E
Assheton, D C
Baker, C M
Baker, M A H
Barlow, J M
Battersby, N C
Beckitt, T A
Bender, S
Berry, J
Bertram, A
Billings, A C
Blacklock, N S
Blake, A C
Bland, A K
Bobic, V
Boothroyd, E C
Bourne, M W
Bowles, S A
Bowyer, J D
Boyd, J P
Bradshaw, D J
Braithwaite, I J
Bricker, S R W
Bronnert, N H
Brookes, R
Brown, L G
Bulgen, D Y
Bushell, K E
Butcher, J M
Byam, J E
Cain, J E
Campbell, D
Carter, L
Charles-Jones, J E D
Cheater, L S
Clough, J V
Coghlan, S F E
Cook, M A T
Cope, T M
Cornforth, C M
Cotgrove, A J
Coughlin, L B
Coyle, P R
Craven, B M
Cresswell, A D
Crinyion, I J
Crowe, A V
Curphey, J M
Curtis, J M
Da Gama-Rose, B M
Dalzell, A J C
Danczak, E M
Daniels, I S
Davidson, J S
Davies-Humphreys, J
Davies, R M
Davies, T J
De Cossart, L M
Debray, R
Dennitts, P J
Dhital, S K
Dignon, N M
Dimitri, S K Z
Doyle, G J
Duffin, D N
Duffin, L B
Dunbavand, A
Dunn, H D
Edwards, P R
Elder, J
Ellerby, S E
Evans-Jones, F G
Evans-Jones, J G
Evans-Jones, L G
Ewins, D L
Fantom, E S
Farrall, D L
Fergusson, N V
Finnegan, V L
Finnerty, J P
Fisher, C D
Forbes, A M
Forrest, E T S
Forsyth, M C
Foster, G E
Fowler, A
Franks, A R
Fryar, C P
Galaud, J B
Gardiner, M R
Ghebrehewet, S
Gibbs, J M
Gillies, H C
Gilmore, C
Golder, N D B
Gowers, S G
Gray, K E C
Greensill, V L
Griffith, A W
Griffiths, M D
Guest, V J
Guinan, K T
Hamid, B N A
Hargreaves, W J
Harlin, S J
Harris, N A
Harrison, D A
Harvey, I A
Hawe, J A
Hill, S E
Hodgson, J
Hogan, G M
Holland, J L
Holley, G E
Holme, C-A
Hood, J S
Houghton, J E
Hughes, A C
Hughes, I L
Hunter, P R
Inchley, D C
Jameson, P M
Jayaram, R
Johnson, M A
Johnston, M N
Jones, A J
Jones, R D
Jones, V W
Joyce, P K
Kane, J F
Kaufman, A L
Kaye, S N
Keeping, I M
Kenningham, J A
Kenyon, W E
Khan, R U
Kini, K N
Langrick, H E
Larmour, P F
Lee, E S-H
Lee, R M
Leech, S G
Leggat, H M
Leng, G
Littlejohns, C S
Logan, A S C
Lowrie, M J S
McCaig, R H
McClure, E A
McClure, R H
McCormack, M J
McDonald, P C
Macdonald, S E
McGeorge, D D
Mackinnon, N A
McNutt, A R J
Makower, R M
Malik, S
Manche, M
Mannion, P T
Meachim, S M
Mead, G E
Mendelsohn, S S
Mills, B
Milner, P M
Minshall, I R
Monk, D N
Moon, J K
Morgan, N K
Nelson, R A
Neukom, C R
Nicholson, D G
O'Donnell, J
O'Mahony, C P
Overton, C
Pascall, O J
Peattie, A B
Powell, C S
Powell, D L
Pughe, C T
Ramsdale, J E
Redmond, E J
Reid, P G
Riley, L M
Roaf, R
Robertson, M F
Rogahn, D
Rogers, A J
Rogerson, I M
Rowe, B R
Roylance, P D
Russell, I A
Rutter, M K
Saunders, T P
Scanlan, J
Schofield, C E
Scott, P
Sedgwick, M L
Self, R J
Setty, P H R
Shanahan, A P
Simpson, R J
Sinha, B N
Sissons, C E
Sissons, D A
Sissons, G R J
Sivananthan, A
Skilton, R W H
Skues, M A
Smith, B J
Smith, D F
Somauroo, J D
Sowerby, R G
Spencer, H F
Spencer, M G
Staiano, J J
Stanley, J D
Steele, P R M
Stephens, J M
Stewart, A G
Stewart, R C
Stronach, A J
Swallow, M D
Swanson, M A
Taylor, C J
Temple-Murray, A P
Temple, R H
Thomas, A
Thompson, M W
Thompson, V
Thornton, L
Tighe, S Q M
Tsekouras, A
Tutton, M K
Walker, D J
Waters, M R
Weatherley, R E
Westlake-Guy, C H
White, G B
Whiteoak, K L W
Williams, G
Williams, J H
Willis, R G
Worth, J M
Worth, R C
Worthington, T R
Wright, E A
Yuill, R A

Chester-le-Street
Alexander, K
Bennett, C J
Bowman, S J
Bray, J A
Brockington, J M
Colman, G
Cookey, N C
Crackett, G
Derrick, J P
Douglas, A R H
Duke, A M
Duke, W A
Featherstone, G L
Fletcher, P T
Garcia-Miralles, J R
Gollings, A J
Hall, R S
Herring, D W
Holmes, C J
Hughes, J M
Johnston, T P S
Le Dune, P L
Lilly, R J
Lombard, D C
Mackay, V E
McMichael, J L
Nair, R R
Owen, T D
Portergill, N C
Preston, J G
Rahman, S
Rhys Evans, G
Robinson, A B
Shave, N R
Shirbhate, N C
Sinclair, S
Steele, J W
Sullivan, A
Timmons, M T G
Tyson, A J
Underwood, M C
Vincent, P W
Wheatley, R

Chesterfield
Ahmed, K A
Ahson, A A
Ainsworth, A J
Alam, M M
Aldred, P R
Allen, C C
Allen, T R
Anderson, D I
Andrew, M F
Apaya, J A
Archer, A G
As'Ad, S M
Aziz, N H
Babirecki, M
Bailey, R C
Baker, G C W
Banning, M D
Beauchamp, C G
Bescoby-Chambers, N J C
Bhalla, D
Bhattacharyya, R N
Black, D W
Blagden, M D
Booth, C J
Bose, J C
Boucher, N R
Bourne, J T
Bradley, M A
Brooks, D J
Bullock, J
Cansfield, P J
Carley, J M
Chadwick, D R
Chand, A D
Chawla, V
Chedumbarum Pillay, O D
Chew, D
Church, E J
Clark, D J
Collin, R C L S
Collins, G
Colver, G B
Contardi, P A
Cook, J P
Cook, N J
Cooper, C M
Cooper, C M S
Coup, A
Cresswell, J L
Crooks, S W
Crowther, P S
Cunnane, J G
Dale, J I H
Dastidar, B G
Dave, D
Davies, S J
Day, C D
De Carteret, J R
Dilley, S E
Dods, I M
Dornan, M G
Dowsett, S J
Dowson, C M
Dunphy, N W
Durward, H D
Early, N E
Elmore, D M
Else, C P
Ennis, K A B
Euinton, H A
Eustace, R W
Everett, C F
Everitt, N J
Fairburn, K
Fermer, F E
Fey, C M
Fowler, C S
Fraser, P A
Freeman, W H
Garbutt, D
Gardner, J A
Gedge, A S
Gell, I R
Gillam, S C
Glaves, J
Grant, J S
Green, M A
Groves, J B
Grundman, M J
Gupta, R
Hadfield, J W
Hadfield, S C
Hanwella, J S
Harley, D H
Hawley, C L
Hay, D P
Hehir Strelley, M E
Heston, J P
Holt, S
Howell, E S
Humphries, T A
Ibrahim, I F
Iqbal, P
Jackson, C W P
Jackson, M G
Jackson, P C
Jaiswal, R C
James, M J
Jones, W A K
Kale, N J

Kellock, S L
Kemp, C E
Kimmins, B A G
Knott, D K
Knowles, T K
Krishna Kumar, P
Lambert, K J
Lambert, W G
Langan, S
Lendrum, K
Leveckis, J
Livings, R R
Lloyd, S
Loveday, J H
Lowe, T
Lower, B M
McConnell, T J D
McConville, A E
McDonnell, J M
McKenna, D M
McNab, D A
Madden, C A
Makkison, I
Mann, J R
Markus, K
Mason, S M
Masters, P W
Matthews, A P M
Medcalf, P
Mee, R A
Miller, P E
Mishra, A D
Mitton, D J
Mohamad, K K F
Moon, J A
Murray, S
Murton, M D
Nair, K V
Natt, A L
Neep, R J
Neofytou, S K T
Nissenbaum, S H
Nofal, F M
O'Neill, P
Oluwajana, F M
Palmer, A
Parker, A P
Parnacott, S M
Parratt, J R
Parry, J C
Parthasarathy, P B
Patel, C B B
Payne, J N
Perera, A N R
Pilcher, C J
Preece, P M
Preston, H S
Price, D A
Raby, C
Ray Chaudhuri, R
Ray, S C
Rayner, P R
Rengan, D C
Riches, E
Roberts, I F
Rowlands, R P
Ryan, D
Ryan, J B
Sandler, D A
Scotland, H W F
Searle, J M
Sengupta, S K
Serrell, I R
Sharma, A K
Sharma, G
Shaw, W A
Sheikh, A Z
Shrestha, B K
Simms, J M
Singleton, C D
Sivarajan, V
Smith, A E R
Snee, K
Spencer, M R
Stafanous, S N
Start, R D
Stevens, J D
Stevens, P J
Stewart, R M
Stirland, J D
Talati, V R
Thambirajah, G R
Than, S
Thickett, K M
Thomas, K
Thornton, D M
Thurstan, J W
Tromans, P M
Tsang, G M K
Tupper, R C A
Tyler, R M
Tyler, S S A
Van Der Heijden, L P J
Walton, R D
Webster, J
Whalley, S A
Wilbourn, G
Williams, P M
Wood, S A
Worthington, C A
Wroth, R P
Young, B S
Yousuf, I M

Chichester
Aldridge, J F L
Allen, D R
Allen, S J E
Amesbury, B D W
Ashby, C R
Ashford, N S
Atkins, M
Banuls Pattarelli, M
Barnett, A L
Barratt, F M
Bartle, D G
Beattie, D K
Bell, F J
Berry, P A
Betts, N E
Bevan, P C
Beynon, J L
Birtchnell, S A
Birtley, E J
Bonsey, M M F
Bowyer, R C
Bracewell, M A
Bradbury, P A
Brigden, W D
Britton, J P
Bromley, L M
Buchanan, I Y
Burns, B J
Candy, D C A
Carpenter, J P
Carruthers, L R B
Carter, P G
Cavanagh, S P
Chadwick, K C
Chai, D T C
Challis, R E
Chishick, A R
Clarke, P D
Coburn, P R
Collis, J W
Condon, H C
Conroy, J M
Conyers, A B
Copsey, A
Corke, A R
Covell, T
Crinion, A R
Cripps, N P J
Crossman, R P
Dalgleish, J G
Deavall, T
Dempster, S J
Dennis, S C R
Densham, C A
Dewhurst, A G
Doll, N W
Dunlop, B N B
Edwards, T G
Elliott, B
Fernando, K T M
Fieldhouse, R M A
Findlay, A M T
Fox, P D
Gilbert, M E
Gomez, B K
Gomez, M P G A
Gorrie, G H
Greenwood, M C
Gregory, A B
Greig, M A
Hagen, D L
Haigh, R A
Hammans, S R
Hammond, T J
Hargreaves, J
Harris, G J C
Harris, R
Hartland, S J
Hartree, C J
Harvey, A J
Hester, R F
Hill, R P
Hoare, D M
Holden, F M J
Holman, R A E
Hooker, J G
Hounsome, C E
Howarth, M W
Howlett, R A
Hunniford, Y E
James, S L
Janes, S L
Johnson, P A
Johnstone, C I
Johnstone, T
Jones, C M
Kay, D N
Kelly, G S-B
Kelly, S K
Lacey, M J
Lacey, M L
Lake, A C
Lamont, L S
Lartey, J P A
Laseinde, O O
Lee, G B
Leegood, H M J
Lewis, F J
Low, N M H
Lytton, A
McDonald, P F
McGuinness, C L
McHale, S P
Macpherson, D W
Madden, G J
Mallam, W D C
Matthews, M B
Miller, K A
Missen, J C
Moffitt, V K
Moore, J J
Morrison, I M
Mortimer, K E
Morton, S J
Moss, M C
Mulatero, C W
Mullett, S T H
Murphy, A
Murphy, C F
Murphy, M M
Murray, T G S
Nicholls, D R
Norton, A E
Nott, M R
O'Brien, J I
O'Shea, J K
Orr, M J
Owen-Smith, B D
Paterson, R G
Platts, H A
Poots, G G L
Pratt, P L
Price, J M
Quiney, J R
Quinnell, P M
Reid, C J
Reid, D E B
Revell, E
Rice-Oxley, M
Ross, D J
Rotz, B
Sartory, F B
Shand, D
Shankar, R K
Shapiro, E B A
Shipsey, C M
Simpson, R D
Simson, J N L
Sloley, L J
Smith, C
Solan, K J
Spender, Q W
Stephens, I F D
Stott, J A V
Stross, W P
Stupple, J M G
Tamlyn, G J
Tanner, J A
Taylor, T M
Townend, J R L
Turner, C L
Turner, G A
Van Arenthals, A J S
Vardy, D L
Venn, S N
Walker, F C E
Wallace, A C M
Ward, D J
Ward, S P
Wartnaby, H
Watts, G V
Webb, A J
Whitehouse, R J
Whittaker, B E
Whittaker, P J D
Williams, J L
Williams, L K
Wilson, R J
Winch, T
Witts, E J
Young, C M

Chigwell
Ansari, S A
Beling, G E A
Brandman, S
Celaschi, D A
Chana, J S
Chattopadhyay, U
Chitra, G
Chopra, P S
Dandekar, S S
Dauid, L M
Davies, R M E
Farzaneh-Far, A
Flasz, M H
Hamal, A
Hing, C B
Inayat, Dr
Jackson, J A
Jain, A S
Jain, A K
Jumani, A N
Lall, K S
Lee, R A
Lillywhite, A V
Lillywhite, E K
Memon, M A
Osen, J S
Osen, M A
Qureshi, A H
Rajah, V
Roback, S D
Rushton, G J
Schapira, R C
Strehle, E-M
Weatherstone, R M
Weera, C R W

Chinnor
Ball, K E
Crick, A P
Green, S G
Hood, C A
Hood, C A
Knightley, M J
Pinto, A A
Stamp, S A

Chippenham
Allard, L L
Allen, P
Barter, J A W
Barton, T C
Bools, C N
Bridgens, J P
Brosch, J A
Brown, N H
Brunyate, P H
Cartwright, J
Constantine, S J
Dewland, P M
Firman, M A
Gabriel, R J
Gaunt, R M C
Gilroy, F M
Grandison, I M
Hartington, K
Henry, W S
Holbrook, A G
Jones, M R
Kay, J T M
Keatings, B T
Lashford, A M
McCay, N J P
McCormack, N W
McCune, C A
McKibbin, A R
Meudell, C M
Moore, M T
Morgan, J E
Morley, C E
Muir, R F
Nowlan, W A
Page, C J
Palmer, R B
Patrick, G M
Pickthall, P D
Russell, J G
Seddon, J M
Stanton, E F
Turek, T A
While, R S A
Wilkinson, C E
Williams, I R
Wilson, E
Wright, A T S

Chipping Campden
Brook, W A D
Denning, A M
James, M J
Smith, J A
Wallbank, W A

Chipping Norton
Bayliss, H J
Bond, H E K
Chambers, M D
Edwards, D R
Edwards, J E
Elliott, C A
Goves, J R
Hall, W L
Harbinson, R D
Hebden, A
Keenan, C
Keenan, M F
Matthews, J L
Moore, J G
Moran, P A
Nixon, D P
Pargeter, J M
Paul, E H M
Peniket, A J
Platten, M C
Queenan, M B
Scott, G
Shaw, H J
Somaiya, R S
Walker, J R
Walton, J A
Williams, H M

Chislehurst
Agarwal, P C
Barbary, N S
Becker, W G E
Brander, E A S
Bryant, A J
Carr, D A
Choong, M L O
Datta, V
Deacon, C
Dean, E A
Denvir, L
Gupta, V K
Hamblyn, N C
Hitman, G A
Kamdar, B B
Kotak, D C
Lindley-Jones, M F H
Olley, L M
Parson, A F
Proffitt, D
Qazi, F A
Ratneswaren, S
Rub, H-U
Savine, R E
Shah, A H
Shah, N
Sharma, P
Sivakumar, B
Terry, J
Trueman, G B
Wasty, S W H
Williams, A G
Williamson, K F
Zakaria, G Y

Choppington
MacDonald, W P
Parker, B L
Sanderson, P W
Turner, W

Chorley
Abbott, P
Ainsworth, P
Almond, W R
Baghdjian, R B
Barker, C
Bennett, A M
Bennett, R J C
Blake, P M
Brade, D A
Brown, A K
Burford, S A
Calleja, M A
Clarke, C B
Dare, E K
Desai, H
Edwards, S J
El Halhuli, O A E R S
Evison, M N
Evison, R A
France, M M
Gale, M S J
Gallagley, A
Galletly, S C
George, P P
Hall, I M
Halstead, G A
Hartley, R D
Haslam, K E
Heald, S J
Hilton, S N
Howarth, D E
Hronis, V G
Hunt, A E
Hunter, J T
Hussain, S A
Imam, S H
Khanna, V K
Knapp, J A
Leonard, I J
Letch, R D
Lofthouse, J A
Lord, S R
Lyons, R M
McAllister, D M
Madi, S I
Manji, A K
Manus, N J
Mason, S J
Montero Garcia, J M
Motappashastry, V
Mughal, M M
Mumford, P A
Naqvi, S N H
Ne Win, Dr
O'Donnell, E L
Parker, M R
Pinheiro, N L
Robinson, L J
Ross, D
Ruiz Gonzalez, M
Sambrook, A J
Savage, M E
Scott, J M
Service, M A
Shah, V S
Sharma, S
Sharma, V N
Sloan, M A
Smith, I G
Soe Than Myint, Dr
Spinks, B C
Stockwell, R C
Symes, J E
Symes, S R
Tasker, M
Troop, A C
Vaidya, A
Wallis, S C
Walsh, J M
Watmough, P J
Whalley, J
Whitaker, H J
Wilson, W W
Wood, W M
Wren, P J J
Yates, F W

Christchurch
Archard, G E
Aveyard, S C
Birch, H E W
Blaikley, A B
Boyd, A P M
Boyde, A M
Carey, N F
Collier, J D
Collins, S C P
Coupe, S C
Critchley, E
Dague, J R S
Debenham, E J R
Dunne, K A
Dunnill, R P H
Edwards, K
Fulford, L G
Gamper, M A
Gamper, N H
Gilbertson, R C
Gregson, J P
Halder, S R
Hall, K E
Hamdi, S S

Harris, J D C
Hazell, M
Hickish, A E
Hickish, G W
Hodgson, L E
Hopkinson, N D
Jenkinson, R
Josephs, L K
Kay, T A
Kelly, B J
Klein, G
Lee, J M
Livingstone, M
Lloyd-Thomas, A R
McCarthy, K
Menzies, A R
Ni'Man, M N
Odbert, R M
Pillinger, J E T
Pugh, R J
Rana, B S
Rana, M Z K
Randall, F M
Rangaswamy, V
Reeve, S D
Rhodes, G A
Rogers, D J
Savage, N J
Scott-Jupp, W M
Tallant, N P
Tang, Y Y M
Terry, C M
Thomas, R L
Walden, A
White, J S
Williams, M A
Wood, A W
Wood, M B

Chulmleigh
Beer, M H
Bowman, C R
Brown, B A
Burke, J E T
Fisher, S R
Kemp, N H
Wielink, R C A D

Church Stretton
Beach, J F
Beach, J W
Cook, L R
Griffiths, C C
Howard, J A
Malone, C J
Matthews, W L
Parker, T G
Peer, E J
Riding, S M
Robinson, K A
Rushton, P F
West, C A
West, D R S

Cinderford
Adams, J M
Arthurs, D
Burrows, C D M
Gadsby, I C
Lane, D M
Roberts, R C
Shaw, D G
Zaheer, P

Cirencester
Beales, D M
Beales, D L
Binfield, P M
Cameron, E A
Coleridge, H C C
Drysdale, S W
Dukes, C S
Duncumb, C E
Evans, D J
Evans, M
Evans, P M
Evans, R I
Gale, D G L
Goldie, C J
Gomara, C J B
Grantham, C F
Hawkins, M
Hewett, H E
Hewett, M F
Hutchison, C R
Jacob, M P
Jardine, C V
McInerney, G M
MacKinnon, A D
MacKinnon, J R
Marriott, C M
Miller, J E
Mitchell, D C
Moorhead, P M
Patuck, D
Pawson, R M
Price, P A
Ramsay, J R S
Reynolds, P A
Robson, C E
Sethi, R
Simpson, I J
Tallon, J G J
Thurston, N
Troughton, A H
Waddell, J A
Whittles, S E
Wigfield, M F
Winter, J M

Clackmannan
Bowman, A M
Gray, R D
Jackson, L S
Macphail, D I
Scott, V A
Thomson, I B

Clacton-on-Sea
Barry, M P
Bowsher, F M
Buchanan, L A
Burton, D J
Cochrane, W H
Colquhoun, J H C
Cox, S
Cullen, T J
Faerestrand, H I
Faerestrand, W M
Feldmar, G L
Flood, A G
Garas, S F
Garside, J M
Grange, A R
Guille, J L
Halstead, D E
Howden, P
Hunt, J W
Leach, J N
Letton, D J
Letton, P H J
Lineen, J P P
Littlemore, A J
McCurdy, J F
Mackenzie, A D C
MacMillan, S J
Mann, M
Mathias, R D
Morrison, A J
North, C D
Puvi, N
Sarathchandra, C B
Shiers, C
Slawson, J A
Stedman, A J
Stewart, A G E M
Sweeney, G A
Tan, S
Whippman, S C

Cleator
Thursz, A D
West, N C

Cleckheaton
Brayshaw, S A
Crosbie, E G
Fox, G S
Greenwood, A
Hatfield, S J
Kelly, D
Khan, M S A
Marsh, J M
Midgley, R S-J
Rix, K J B
Stringer, J
Waters, S H
Wood, P J W

Cleethorpes
Ahluwalia, S
Bhaduri, S K
Choudhury, P
Crombie, R N
Dailey, L
David, H
Doldon, J L
Hurst, P
Lavin, R J
Pearse, H A
Purser, P C
Rees, A L
Sarkar, D
Singh, K P
Singh, N P
Sutherland, I A
Williams, F
Zaro, M A

Clevedon
Begley, P J
Bullock, R D
Ford, J J
Green, D
Hime, M C
Horner, G R
Horry, P A
How, G C
Martin, J K
Miller, I S
Nicholas, F E
Parfitt, C J
Patrick, E A S
Pill, S H C
Porter, L
Rukunayake, G N C
Russell, C I F
Stewart, E J

Clitheroe
Bartle, M R
Brown, A M
Burns, J
Bywater, N S
Carter, J A F
Crawford, M J
Cronin, M A
Crowther, A
Eddleston, M P
Flatley, M
Fogg, C J
Franks, K N
Freeman, R A
Harrison, CM
Heaton, W M
Higson, R J
Higson, W A
Holgate, S
Huson, A S
Hutchison, B T N
Hutchison, S J
Ibbotson, I J
McCree, T
Mackean, W G
McKinlay, W J D
McLaughlin, J
McMeekin, N H
Morris, S J
Pearson, S
Porter, C
Porter, J H
Razzaque, M A
Rees, G
Saunders, J
Smith, B
Smith, M M
Tang, D T S
Turner, I M
Zakrzewski, H J

Clydebank
Anderson, M I M
Bell, D R
Clarke, E A
Clegg, B D
Crawford, G M
Doverty, M R
Fletcher, M
Gorrie, S M
Harper, P I
Hollier, L H
Houston, D R
Jaberoo, D W
Johnson, C O
Khogali, K A
Light, J K G
McCall, J M
McDevitt, A G
McKenzie, J
Maclean, N M
Mitchell, E I
Potter, A W
Rahman, A Q M H
Ramayya, P
Ray, D A A
Rogerson, G G
Sardi, A
Sarmiento, A
Simpson, D B
Spence, D G
Sutcliffe, N P
Templeton, L M
Veidenheimer, M C
Wade, A G
Wilding, A M
Wilson, A M
Wilson, R J M
Zincke, H

Coalville
Baker, J
Chawda, N J
Hammond, T M
Hazlehurst, G J
Hepplewhite, E A
Horsburgh, C
Jolleys, J V
Khirwadkar, P M
Lawrence, R W
Lewis, A M
Morgan, L M
Morris, M W
Mutimer, J N
Neville, P G
Newman, D J
Ollerton, J E
Pulman, N R
Robinson, I C
Wittels, P L
Woods, D M

Coatbridge
Agnew, M
Bawa, S S
Bell, D W
Brankin, E
Connolly, S A
Coull, R S
Daisley, S E
Docherty, J V
Feeney, J
Holt, S M
Kilgour, D
McGowan, J D
McMorris, S
Marcuccilli, N S
Morcos Hanna, M Y
Ooi, K H
Park, D J
Picozzi, G L
Picozzi, J
Singh, K B P
Turnbull, E B

Cobham
Allen, R J
Austen, J C
Bailey, C
Bell, J G
Chisham, M
Desor, M I N
Eliopoulos, F B
Hobbs, M D B
Huchzermeyer, P M
Johnston, F G
Kelly, J A
Knudsen, E T
Kumar, S
Lewin, J M
McClure, P S
MacDougall, I S
Meurisse, F L A
Nguyen, D M
Nguyen, H B
Restorick, H M
Small, Y J
Stuart, L M
Trent, M P
Watson, A
Young, R C

Cockermouth
Berrill, W T
Campbell, G C
Campbell, G L
Clarkson, D G
Claxton, A
Cowan, N R L
Desert, S A
Dutta, S K
Edwards, A N
Edwards, P J
Eldred, A E
Eynon, S M
Eyre, T A
Gilchrist, S
Hargreaves, A
Hodson, M J
Horder, E A
Hossain, M A
Hossain, S
Howarth, J P
Lees, D M
Mason, A R
Pearson, A J
Thomson, C
Travis, A
Wandless, R J
Whiteley, J
Wilkinson, J S

Colchester
Ahmad, A
Ahmad, N
Aitken, J M
Al-Dabbagh, M A T
Al-Sad, H M H H
Anderson, E A
Arrindell, A P
Ashok Kumar, T L
Austin, R C T
Ayache, F K
Backhouse, C M
Baldwin, S P
Baloch, K H
Baloch, N
Banna, A
Barkham, J D T
Barnes, L S
Bashir, A
Bateman, D J
Bateman, D J A
Beardmore, C E
Beauchamp, J E
Beckingsale, A B
Bennett, V S
Blaxill, J M
Bodmer, C W
Bohannan, P J
Booth, C M
Boots, M A
Bradley, J A
Brayley, N F
Brayley, S L
Brogan, D P
Brown, J A
Byrne, P A C
Carlyon, L
Carr, P J
Cavenagh, N F
Chambers, C
Chyc, A D
Claridge, P M
Clark, D G C
Clubb, V J
Cockwell, K
Colclough, A B
Collingwood, P D
Conn, P C
Cope, A I
Coulson, R W S
Cowan, R E
Coxhead, M S
Coxhead, N
Cutler, R C
Daunt, S O N
Davidson, A G H
Davies, C F
Davies, G L S
Davies, J L
De Silva, R J
Dixon, N T
Dixon, P E
Dixon, S J
Dixon, S M
Doney, A S F
Dowson, H M P
Doyle, R
Duffy, S M
Eddy, J W
Eldridge, A G
Elrington, G M
Elston, A C
Elston, R A
Emerson, B M
Emery, P J
Evans-Jones, J C
Farnworth, H E
Ferguson, A L
Finch, S A B
Foreman, J T
Forsyth, M C
Fox, V E N
Frampton, M A
Gamble, G E
Gatland, J C
Gay, F W
Gear, P
George, M D
Ghosh, I R
Gibbs, M L
Gilbert, C R
Goodwin, A M
Gould, M
Grant, J
Gray, J D
Griffiths, J J
Grimm, B W
Gunawardena, S A
Hale, J C P
Halfhide, P J A
Hall, C B
Hall, S
Handley, A J
Handley, S A J
Hare, M F
Hargreaves, M J
Henderson, D J
Hickman, M P
Hilton, N J
Hine, K L
Hinshelwood, R D
Hoodboy, S A
Howes, T Q
Huber, J P
Hughes, N J
Hunt, M J N
Irwin, E B
James, H M
Jayaratnam, A V H
Jeffries, J D
Jones, C E B
Justice, A A
Karim, N
Kempster, S J
Khan, A R
Khetarpal, B K
King, W D
Kitchen, P
Konarzewski, W H
Kong, H A
Lakshman, H W D
Landsmeer, R E
Lennard-Jones, A M
Lind, J F
Loeffler, M D
Lothian, A W R
Macallan, C R
McCarthy, M J
MacDonald, L M
MacDonnell, S P J
McFerran, D J
McGinty, M J
McKeever, C S T
Mackenzie, S I P
MacNeill, F A
McRae, R D R
Mahon-Daly, L M E
Marfleet, J C
Marfleet, P
Marsh, S K
Marshall, A S
Marshall, P A
Marshall, W
Matthes, P A
May, A R L
Meanley, J A
Meanley, T H
Menzies, D
Millar, D M
Milne, D R M
Monk, M C
Moore, D J
Moore, K
Moore, M H
Mossop, H E J
Motson, R W
Mukerji, A K
Mukerji, S
Murphy, M J
Murray, B
Murray, P A
O'Callaghan, E G
O'Callaghan, U C
Ogilvie, A J
Owens, J M
Palmer, E G
Parker, G D
Parry, C W K
Parthasaradhi, K
Patel, A C
Patient, P S
Pickering, R S
Pinkey, B

Polak, L
Ponty, R W
Poole, R R G
Pratt, W R
Ramster, D G
Ranasinghe, D N
Ranasinghe, P N I
Ranawat, N S
Rao, M
Rasor, P A
Read, D J
Robinson, A F
Ross-Marrs, R P
Rudge, S D
Rudra, T P
Rushbrook, L A W
Sagar, S A
Salter, H A
Sanderson, D A
Sarathchandra, S F
Seddon, I
Shah, S Z H
Sheldrick, C M
Shuttleworth, D
Sihra, B S
Singh, R K
Singh, S D
Smith, C N
Smith, C M
Smith, J M
Snook, N J
Spooner, L L R
Spowage, P M
St. Joseph, A V
Stannard, E J
Stedman, S L
Steiner, N B M
Stephens, D D
Strowbridge, N F
Symons, J C
Tang, K H
Tarala, C T
Taylor, B O T
Thavabalan, P B
Thibaut, R E
Thomas, C E
Thomas, T L
Thompson, C F D
Thompson, M A
Thomson, S J
Thorogood, A
Tillett, A J
Toms, R M
Treharne, I A L
Tucker, D L
Tucker, K E
Tucker, P M
Tupper-Carey, D A
Turner, N A
Urwin, G
Wakely, J N
Wall, M
Ward, W D
Warrington, J S
Whyte, A P
Wilbraham, K
Willenbrock, P C
Williams, J F
Wilson, M A
Withnall, D
Wood, J A
Wood, M E
Woods, P M
Wright, P L
York, A H
Yousif, E H
Zamora Vicente De Vera, F J

Coldstream
Marynicz, P
Schleypen, P F H M J
Veitch, E M H

Coleford
Cummins, B D
Ford, L I
Longley, R H
Wilkinson, N M

Coleraine
Adams, S M
Alderdice, D K
Beck, A W
Beck, A W
Bell, M A
Bonnar, B C
Brown, J A
Brown, J S
Brown, M G
Burns, R W
Church, A W E
Clarke, L W A
Coleman, E
Connor, B W D
Cooper, A R
Davies, E A
Dixon, L J
Donnelly, M E C
Ellard, M A
Finnegan, O C
Friel, A M
Fyvie, K R J
Ghaie, S S
Glass, R
Hadden, I J
Henderson, W A
Huey, S
Hunter, R F
Irwin, K R
Kapur, K
Kelly, S G
Kernohan, R M
Kerr, A H
Kerr, J B K
Ledwith, M V
Lee, B C
McAuley, R G
McClenahan, M C
McCollum, A S
McConnell, P
McCormack, J P
McGavock, H
McGlade, J F X
McGowan, W A W
McGurk, G M
McMaster, I J
Marshall, B M S
Martin, R P
Matthews, R S
Millar, D
Mitchell, B W
Moore, R H
Mullan, K R
Nevin, L J
Newman, C E
Nicholl, M E
Nutt, D J P
O'Donnell, H E
Orr, D S A
Orr, R D
Pollock, C L
Quiery, A F J
Rollins, M D
Scally, C M
Shannon, E N
Sharieff, S F
Siberry, H M
Stewart, D G T
Stewart, H E
Swinson, B D
Symington, J J M
Telford, K J
Thompson, M K J
Topping, W A
Tracey, T J
Turner, T B
Wali, J
Wallace, S
Walsh, D A
White, T J
Wilson, G S

Colne
Bower, I
Cowpe, T V
Cox, P T
De Vries, H
Jackson, R S
Jackson, S M
Kenny, R
Kerridge, F J
Miller, P G
Mitchell, A D
Northridge, C S
Sahar, M A
Singh, R C P
Spencer-Palmer, C M
Spencer, A E
Sulaiman, S A L
Sulaiman, S M U
Watson, C C
Watson, H D
Woodhead, P M

Colwyn Bay
Algawi, K D M
Armer, M L
Barry, P
Breese, V L
Corkery, P B
Cowell, E W
Crawford, D J
Davies, W R A
Edwards, M
Evans, J D A
Farah, A G
Frost, C S
Gupta, B K
Hindle, C M
Hughes, E P
Humphreys, E W
Jones, G H
Kelly, K J
Kiehn, B
Klimach, V J
Laraman, C
Lloyd, D H O
McIlroy, P W J
Malik, A E D T M
Midgley, J M
Owen, E
Owen, K
Owen, R
Parry-Williams, A W
Powell, M A
Ratcliffe, M J
Reynolds, R
Rouse, R T
Sissons, H M
Thackray, C P
Watkins, S C
Widdowson, D J
Williams, J W
Williams, W R
Wood, D G E
Wynne-Jones, G

Colyton
Askew, M F
Carmichael, D S
Jones, J R
Thomas, D O

Congleton
Atkin, K J
Baker, T H
Bennett, P H
Bromley, P T
Brooks, J B S
Carter, E A
Daly, R C
Dutton, A C
Fray, D
Gokhale, V L
Green, A N F
Hart, T B
Hesketh, M
Highland, A M
Jesudason, E C
Kay, G E
McLean, J H
Norris, M G
Rigby, P J
Rosson, A K
Sivakumaran, S R
Sugden, P E
Taylor, C M
Thomas, S A
Thomson, C M
West, D R

Coniston
Wood, R A B

Consett
Anderson, E J
Astley, D A
Bright, S T
Douglass, U E
Elliott, J C
English, S P J
Flynn, E J
Hamilton, J R
Hasan, S
Iqbal, A
Levick, J F
Levick, S
McKinney, C F
Mountford, J A
Murray, A W
Nave, E W
Petterson, D M
Raine, C
Rao, C S
Sambasiva Rao, G
Shah, P R
Stevenson, W J
Stuart, J M E
Turner, J
Tyerman, K S
Welsh, L
Whitfield, E M
Young, J D

Conwy
Barber, V E
Barnard, R E
Bell-Davies, D E
Crawford, A H
Edwards, P J
Evans, J G
Grout, P
Harrison, E T
Hunter, S G
Jayaram, M
Jones, D A
Kraaijeveld, L M-A
Leask, H J G
Osborne, B V
Parry, D C
Parry, J J
Whitley, L L
Williams, M
Wright, P B

Cookstown
Acharya, K P
Barnes, S A
Black, J H
Black, R G
Burns, F J
Corrigan, J C
Curry, P A
Dalzell, M C
Doonan, J F
Finch, R S
Flanigan, P P J
Gilfillan, R C
Hamilton, R J
Irwin, A I
Irwin, P B
Johnston, T C
McBride, J B
McKeever, G T M
Mullan, R P
O'Kane, J B
Smyth, J E

Corbridge
Caird, J D D
Cowling, B E
Crack, L A
Cunningham, W F
Dykins, R J
Egan, M J
Harle, D G
Kingett, R W J
Manship, J M M
Melrose, T M
Michelmore, K F
Perry, J J
Swaddle, M
Waddell, F M
Walters, P L

Corby
Appleton, C R
Baxter, R D
Beric, V
Bhattacharya, B R
Bowie, I M
Buckingham, P V
Graham, C
Harris, A R
Harris, T J N
Hart, J J
McCahill, J P
Mellor, J G
Misra, S C
O'Neill, A
O'Neill, J D
Palmer, D A
Partington, C T
Rodgers, F M
Sumira, R P
Treharne, I R
Turner, D C
Wade, S
Wadsworth, S M
Whittaker, R N
Wilczynski, P J G
Williams, K R
Yee, M C

Corsham
Allan, E B
Baker, H E
Bullen, J A
Burrell, S J
Cowie, A S
Daniel, P G
Green, D M
Hatherell, M J
Johnson, W D K
Jones, K G
Kelley, S P
Leyden, H E
MacArthur, D J
Starr, L M
Walker, S J

Corwen
Deady, R
Park, K C
Roberts, D G
Williams, I C M

Cottingham
Ahmad Turkistani, I Y
Almond, D J
Avery, G R
Billings, D
Bowden, H F
Cain, T J
Cale, A R J
Caplin, J L
Clark, A L
Clark, J P
Clarke, P D
Cleland, J G F
Cowen, M E
Culbert, B D
Drew, P J
Duthie, G S
Dyet, L E
Elliott, L
Evans, P
Exon, M E
Farnsworth, T A
Finlay, M E
Fox, J N
Gower, S N
Greenstone, M A
Guvendik, L
Hall, C E
Harkness, G J
Harmer, R H
Hart, N B
Hartley, J E
Haworth, C M
Howard, J S
Hussain, S R
Hutchinson, C M
Johnson, G S
Joshi, U Y
Kastelik, J A
Kaye, G C
Kieran, D N
Knox, J
Korab-Karpinski, M R
MacDonald, A W
McGivern, D V
Mahapatra, T K
Michie, E W
Mohiuddin, S A
Mohsen, A M M A
Monson, J R T
Morice, A H
O'Hare, P M
O'Neill, P A
Pearson, L
Pollock, C G
Redington, A E
Reiss, S H
Richmond, I
Robson, J
Shaw, C J
Shields, M L
Thackray, S D R
Thind, J
Tilsed, J V T
Tomlinson, I W
Tsai, H H
Wharton, I P
Whitehead, P
Willson, J C
Yeo, R
Young, S S

Coulsdon
Asirdas, S R N
Boffa, P B J
Brogan, V M
Chitkara, S C
Cruickshank, I D
Goddard, M J
Irfan, M
Iu, P-C
Johnston, M J
Khan, J A
McAllister, W J
MacCallum, R
Murphy, D J
Northfield, J W
Partridge, E D
Ramakrishnan, K P
Sawyer, A N
Silverton, K L
Smith, M L W
Stephenson, V J
Stewart, A D
Takhar, B
Von Backstrom, A G

Coventry
Agarwal, I C
Aggarwal, P
Ahmed, I
Ahmed, Z P
Al-Bayati, A H A R
Al-Chalabi, A N
Aldersley, M A
Aldridge, M J
Ali, S
Ali, T
Allan, P S
Allen, M E
Ansari, M Z A
Anyanwu, A L
Armstrong, L E
Ashley-Smith, A
Atwal, A S
Awonuga, A O
Baguant, N K
Ballantine, R J
Bambridge, P R
Barbieri, M
Barclay, A J G
Barclay, G
Barfield, L J
Barker, P J
Barnett, M M
Barros D'Sa, A A J
Bastow, N M
Batten, J
Bayman, I W
Beamer, J E R
Beaumont, P A
Been, M
Bellamy, E P D
Benning, R
Bera, S K
Berth-Jones, J
Bhandal, M S
Bhattacharya, S
Blacklock, A R E
Blakemore, M E
Bland, J W
Bloor, J M
Boateng, K E
Bodalia, B
Bodalia, R
Bogahalande, S
Booker, J M
Booth, L J
Borman, C A
Borman, E M
Bowman, D M
Brady, P A
Brennan, M E
Briffa, N P
Brown, W F
Calder, I G
Calder, S J
Camm, M J
Carter, Y H
Chaggar, H S
Chandy, J
Charlson, M J
Chaudhry, A Y
Chen, K
Cherry, R J
Chohan, B P S
Choksey, M S
Choudree, A C
Cietak, K A
Cleaver, M H
Clegg, J
Clowes, D P
Coad, N A G
Cockerill, M J
Coe, A W

Cole, B
Cooke, M W
Coole, L
Coolican, M A
Cooper, G M
Coppock, J E
Coppock, J S
Cordle, J E
Cowan, E W H
Cowley, A D
Craggs, L A
Cunnington, P M D
Dadhania, M R
Dale, J R
Dawda, V G
Dawes, D L
De Silva, G E F
De Souza, T J
Dean, F M
Deegan, T F
Dekker, P J
Desai, K M
Dhillon, M S
Dhillon, S K
Dickson, T D
Dilip Kumar, R
Dimitri, P J
Dimitri, W R
Docker, C
Donegan, A M
Dooley, P T
Dosanj, R S
Dosanjh, H S
Douzenis, A
Downing, M E N
Dukes, H M
Duncan, A A
Dunn, M W
Durr, C S
Dutta, R K
Eaden, J A
Ebrahim, D W
Edmunds, M E
Edwards, R B
Elton, R J
Emery, J C
Essex, C
Evans, D R
Evans, H C
Evans, S F
Exon, S M
Ezzat, A A
Feltbower, A R
Ferryman, S R
Fink, C G
Fletcher, S
Foguet Subirana, P R
Francis, K S
Franks, A L
Fraser, I A
Fulford, K W M
Garala, M
Geddes, G B
Ghataore, K S
Gill, H K
Gill, R
Girvan, R B
Gold, M R
Gonzalez Sanz, N
Goodfellow, T
Gough, M W R
Gray, C T
Greenwood, R S
Grieve, R J
Griffin, P J
Griffiths, F E
Guha, T
Halder, S R
Halliday, B L
Hamilton, R J
Harkness, M C H
Harris, J B
Harverson, A D
Hasan, S
Hazarika, P D
Heer, A S
Herd, A M
Higgins, R M
Hill, M N
Hobson, S
Hocking, M L
Holton, K M
Horn, P J
Humber, C E
Hussain, M J
Hutton, R M
Hyare, H K
Igwiloh, C O K
Ilchyshyn, A
Imray, C H E
Irwin, C J R
Jaspal, M S
Jayaratnam, M
Jayaratnasingam, S
Jetty, U
Jones, D G
Jones, R D
Jones, W K
Joshi, R
Judelsohn, F A
Judge, G S
Kakad, K L
Kalloor, G J
Kandaswamy, S
Kanji, H K
Kapwepwe, S
Kashi, S H
Katti, S S
Kavia, S
Keane, C C
Kearney, S E
Kelly, C
Kennedy, C R
Kennedy, N M J
Kenton, A R
Kenyon, P S
Khalifa, Y
Khara, B S
Kirkham, C J
Kisnah, V P
Klocke, R
Kolacki, B M T
Krikler, S J
Kukreja, A S
Kukreja, N
Kukreja, R K
Laird, A N
Lal-Sarin, R R
Lawford, C V P
Lawton, M E
Lea, P M
Lee, M J R
Leigh, E A
Leung, H H-Y
Loft, D E
Long, R J
Louden, J D
Lovatt, W P
Lupton, S C
Lyall, S S
McAleese, G A
Macartney, J C
McCulloch, W J D
Macdonald, I
Macdougall, C F
Mace, C J
McIntosh, J S
Mackie, F D
McLachlan, K P
Macpherson, J H
Madan, H
Madhu, K R
Maheson, A
Majevadia, S K
Mangat, K S
Mann, G S
Margetts, M J
Marsh, R M
Marston, G M
Matyka, K A
Mirza, Z A
Mishra, K
Misra, V K
Mistry, B P
Mistry, D K
Mistry, S H
Mitchell, A D
Morris, R
Morris, R M J
Mulholland, P J
Mulrooney, P
Munday, D F
Murrin, R J A
Murthy, B V R N
Muruganinrajah, S
Mwale, E M Y
Nahl, S S
Navin, W P
Newbold, K M
Norton, R
Nwokolo, C U
O'Brien, J A
O'Brien, P W M
O'Hara, R J
O'Sullivan, J F X
Obaid, S
Oliver, C B D
Ong, W W
Osman, F
Pai, M S
Paige, P G
Pandya, H K
Parfitt, G G
Parker, R W
Parker, S J
Parr, S M
Patel, D
Patel, J M
Patel, K
Patel, M P
Patel, P
Patel, P J
Patel, R
Patel, S J
Pathan, M A
Peile, E B
Perez De Albeniz, A J
Perlik-Kolacki, D B
Pickin, M C
Ponsford, J R
Porter, J M
Purnell-Mullick, S
Quabeck, G
Rahman, A
Rai, H S
Rajput, R S
Ramachandra, R R
Ramsden, K L
Rauchenberg, P M
Rhodes, C A
Richards, P E I
Richards, S M
Richardson, W
Riddoch, D
Robbins, M C O
Robert, P S
Roberts, P N
Robinson, R E
Rosin, M D
Saad, K F G
Sadrani, P J
Saeed-Ahmad, S
Sahota, J K
Sandhu, J S
Sathyanarayana, C N
Selwyn, E M
Shad, A
Shah, V S
Shahabuddin, M
Shanmugalingam, V
Sharma, M
Shatwell, W J
Sheard, S C
Shehu, A
Shergill, N S
Sherlala, K H
Shields, S D
Shillinglaw, D
Shine, D F
Shiu, M F
Short, A K
Sihota, J S
Simmonds, E J
Singer, D R J
Singh, H
Singh, S
Singh, S
Singh, S S
Singh, T
Sitjes Llado, N
Slibi, M
Smith, H M
Smith, J L
Smith, R C
Smithers, A J
Snead, D R J
Snowdon, J C
Sood, T S
Spalding, T J W
Spencer, N J
Spokes, G A
Spokes, R M
Srodon, P D
Stableforth, P J
Stanworth, P A
Stein, A G
Stevens, M
Stewart-Brown, S L
Stirling, H F
Stockdale, A D
Strantzalis, G
Subhani, M
Sullivan, W R
Taggart, C M
Taylor, M T
Taylor, S A
Thacker, S L
Thavasothy, M
Thavasothy, R
Thevendra, S
Thin Thin Aye, Dr
Thomas, G O
Thomson, K T
Thornhill, R J
Thornton, D A
Thornton, S J
Thornton, S
Tilbury, J G
Tran, A T H
Trent, R S
Tsagurnis, I
Turner, S M
Vallet, E A
Venkataraman, M
Viira, D J
Vishwanath, M R
Vlachtsis, H
Vohrah, A R
Wade, A A H
Wade, P J F
Walker, R S
Wallace, M E H
Walton, A M
Ward, I J
Ward, J A
Webster, S J
Wellings, R M
Whatmore, W J
Wheatley, K A
Williams, N
Wills, M I
Wong, L H
Wood, L E P
Wood, M A
Wooding, C D
Wyse, M K
Young-Hartman, M
Youssef, H
Zaky, S
Zaphiropoulos, G C

Cowbridge
Allman, A C J
Armstrong, R L
Bowrey, D J
Broughton, L A
Cohen, D A
Dent, C M
Dowdle, J R
Elliott, S E
Evans, A G
Evans, C E
Evans, S
Fenn, N J
France, J E
Goodfellow, R M
Graham, I M
Houghton, I
Howells, E B
Howells, K L
Hughes, D L
Jenkins, E K
Jones, B S
Jones, D A S
Jones, D I
Jones, R D
Kemble, H R
Lever, J
McDowell, M J
McGovern, D J L
Meller, K E B
Morris, I D
Naysmith, C
Newham, J R T
O'Hanlon, T M
Page, M D
Pardoe, T H
Plummer, S J
Pugh Williams, S
Stuart, T M
Taylor, C L
Taylor, J M
Thomas, A O
Thomas, D G
Thomas, P H
Thomas, T E
Todd, A J
Varma, P N
Watkins, T G L
Webb, D B
Wilkinson, C D
Wilkinson, E J
Woodsford, P V
Wyatt, S

Cowdenbeath
Alcock, J
Choudhury, R
Dunn, A
Johnston, M A
McRobbie, I A
Steele, A H
Wright, J W

Cowes
Bisset, J G V
Chopra, R
Clements, S D
Finch, E A M
Fordham, S E
Freytag, C U
Gardiner, J C
Hinchliffe, J
Noble, H A
Stainer, G
Stainer, M R
Swarbrick, R H

Cradley Heath
Chaggar, J S
Mahon, J P
Muthuveloe, D W
O'Brien, D J

Craigavon
Adams, G F
Adams, J D
Armstrong, V L
Bailie, N A
Barr, J W R
Bell, J A
Best, J A
Best, S J
Black, R J
Black, V E
Bronte, J E
Brown, N A
Budd, S K
Bunting, H E
Burnett, J A
Burnett, R A
Campton, J L
Carl, I L
Carson, G F
Carson, P E R
Chada, N
Chambers, M F
Clarke, M A R
Clarke, S E
Connolly, M
Conran, T M
Craig, S E
Cupples, M E
Damani, N N
Davidson, M E
Davis, R M W
Dillon, J M
Dobson, W
Doyle, M F
Dunseith, P G S
Eakin, J M
Eedy, D J
English, S A
Evans, A J
Geddis, A E
Geddis, T H
Golchin, K
Good, B J
Good, P D
Gormley, J D
Gracey, D G R
Grant, V E
Gray, P L
Hall, S J
Hamilton, A J
Hamilton, R A
Hanratty, B
Hanratty, C G
Heasley, R N
Higazey, M A M
Horan, M A
Houston, S J
Hunter, D M
Hunter, H S
Jamison, C A
Jennings, J E
Landy, S J
Lappin, K J
Lee, R J E
Lemon, S E
Lennon, S P
Livingstone, K
Logan, R A
Lowry, D W
Lowry, D S
McAnallen, C
McAnallen, J G
McAteer, E J
McCaffrey, M J
McCann, E
McCann, G J
McCaughey, W
McCleane, G J
McClure, T C
McConaghy, P M
McConnell, E M
McConnell, J P
McConville, K F
McConville, M T
McCrory, M
McCune, N S C
McDonald, C M
Mackle, C P
Mackle, E J
Mackle, R A
McLoughlin, D C
McMullen, J V
MacSorley, F J
Maguire, S R G
Maguire, S H
Martin, K R G
Mathews, C W
Mathews, J W
Menown, I B A
Miller, V A
Mitchell, D M
Mockford, B J
Mockford, J A
Moriarty, A J
Morton, M R J
Murdock, A M
Murdock, J
Murugan, S P
News, M T
Nicholson, M R
Nugent, A G
O'Brien, A
O'Kane, B M
Orbinson, H M
Orr, D A
Orr, I A
Parker, S J
Patton, D T
Patton, M
Pickering, Z G
Rice, R H
Ritchie, C M
Sabherwal, P
Sami, S A
Sharpe, P C
Sharpe, S W
Shaw, C L
Sheehan, B E
Shepherd, C W
Shields, G L
Sidhu, H K
Southwell, A G
Spence, P J
Stewart, A
Stirling, W J
Tay, T W
Thompson, I P C
Thompson, W B
Tipping, C G
Titterington, M B
Troughton, A M J
Troughton, K E V
Vallely, C T J
Wallace, N S
Wallace, W D
Webster, K
Weir, C D
Wharton, E V
Wilkinson, A M
Williams, M
Wilson, C S
Withers, R J
Woods, J K
Woolsey, S M

Craighouse
Merz, L H

Cramlington
Ahmed, A B M E
Ainsworth, S B
Brown, D M G
Cripps, E J
Davison, E P
Dickinson, G M
Dove, A P
Dunbar, G
Erridge, J F

Fail, M
Ferguson, E M
Foster, L A
Green, P A T
Holding, B E
Khan, M A U
Khan, U Z
Kuruvilla Zachariah, K
Laing, J A
Leith, D
McKenzie, S A
Macmillan, J D R
Maddison, P
Morris, J
Patton, M
Prank, C J
Quayle, S E
Reddy, K S
Thompson, G H
Waddell, J M
Ward, C C
Watson, J P

Cranbrook
Al-Kassim, N
Blundell, R J
Brettingham, L C
Butler, H J
Conry, B G
Crowe, D J
Cubison, T C S
Dale, R F
Dean, S C
Dewing, C R
Digby, R J
Grant, A C
Hefni, M A
Hindmarsh, D J
Jepp, K
Kefford, P J
Kefford, R H
Llewellyn, H
McGlone, K J
Macpherson, D S
Mahadevan, S
Moore, E
Player, P V
Potu, P
Quaife, J
South, L M
South, P J
Van Der Plas, F P
Wood, A M
Wotton, L D
Wratten, J C

Cranleigh
Bratty, C A
Bundy, M J
Christie, D
Clark, M L
Fawkner-Corbett, R
Glover, R E
Hamer, H M
Hart, C J
Hawley, R T
Ingham, J F
Kolind, A L
Lewis, R J W
Lynch, T M
Mitchell, W A L
Myhill, M D H
Price, R N
Read, J M
Stevens, C V
Verdon, J H
Wightman, S J

Craven Arms
Appleby, D J
Bell, J H
Challiner, J
Davidson, J M
Garlick, M J
Gray, J C S
Record, D M
Stanford, C A
Williams, S E
Winter, P R X

Crawley
Abayomi, E M-J
Abdel-Hadi, S E A M
Alexander, P
Alexander, R
Anderson, I P
Armstrong, J E
Atkinson, P I
Bailey, R J
Bennett, G
Bevan, K
Bhargava, A
Birch, J K
Blechynden, J C
Bower, S M
Brayden, P C
Brightwell, C G
Buchan, K R
Burgess, C S
Caldbeck, C R
Carter, S J
Chhaya, B C
Chorley, S J
Clemens, N J
Clifford, A D
Cooper, A L
Craik, J I O B
Croucher, L C
Davies, J M C
De La Mota Nicolas-Correa, M D P
Donnellan, I M
Donnelly, S J
Evans, S A
Foley, H M
Gleeson, C M A
Goodwin, R J
Gossage, A A R
Greengrass, A
Haworth, R N
Hawrych, A B
Hiam, R C
Hicklin, J A
Hill, D A
Hoare, R W
Hopkins, N F G
Hornung, E A
Hunter-Craig, C J
Hurrell, K J
Husain, T
Jackson, N W
Kansagra, B A
Kansagra, I B
Leigh, R K
Leigh, T R
Lewis, I G
Luke, J R
Lyle, D J R
Mabrook, A F
McDonogh, B A
McIntosh, I D
Manjiani, J D
Mohabir, N A
Murray, P V
Myint Thein Khine, Dr
Nandi, A C
Narouz, N
Newman, V J
Oliver, J E
Pallett, J L
Palmer, C R
Pannu, G S
Parker, S M
Phillips, R C
Procter, M S
Rafique, A
Rivers, M D
Rofail, S D
Rose, S E
Roy, A
Royds-Jones, J A
Sattianayagam, A
Schirge, A S
Shah, S
Singh, D R
Sinha, R K
Smith, W C
Spoto, G
Stapley, S A
Stillman, P
Stone, C D P
Storer, N R
Suntharanathan, A
Sutaria, N
Thom, P M
Thomas, G H
Tin, N K
Truter, K W C
Turner, B C
Turner, R
Turner, R C
Vallon, A G
Veerabangsa, M
Vekes, K
Venkataratnam Babu, K
Vinson, P S
Vive, J U
Waldron, M J
Ward, R J
Watson, S V
Wellbelove, P A
Weston-Burt, P M
Weston, J
Wilkinson, A M
Williamson, D J
Wilson, A
Xerri, S

Crediton
Anderson, C
Anderson, J M E
Berridge, P D R
Blackman, S E-A
Davidson, J L
Friend, H M
Hall, A M
Homer, A C
Johnstone, C A P
Kekwick, C A
Kennerley, P C
Kent, C P
Maycock, C H
Murphy, M H
Niklaus, L J
Pearson, K J
Rodd, C D
Selley, P J
Shorney, J S
Shorney, N M
Smith, C F
Stephenson, R E
Westwood, P A
Wright, G C

Crewe
Armatage, R J
Atkins, S L
Bache, J B
Blakebrough, I S
Board, P N
Booth, P A
Brooks, N C
Brough, S J
Brown, R M
Calderhead, R J
Calvey, T A J
Chambers, D K
Clarke, M J
Cooper, J G
Cooper, J
Cooper, M S
Davies, J E
Davies, J M
Deans, J A J
Dingle, A F
Dobson, H S
Dodds, P A
Doherty, A G
Doring-Basso, S
Edwards, B A
Ellison, J A
Evans, M E
Evans, S E
Evennett, P M
Fairey, J
Farrell, A J
Felmeden, D C
Felmingham, J E
Findlay-Domes, E
Freeman, M R
Gay, S P
Gillies, R M
Göpfert, M J
Gould, A A
Gray, J L
Guy, A J
Hall, K H
Hanafy, M E E D
Harris, A J
Hensel, E A
Hodgson, D I
Howard, J C
Hudson, M F
Hufton, B R
Hyde, K R
Hyder, N
Hynes, E F
Irvine, A W
Jackson, A D
Jeyadevan, K S
Jeyadevan, N N
Jones, H W
Jones, K E
Lane, M B
Lawrence, M
Lewis, P
Lloyd, D
Lloyd, J
London, I J
Lovatt, G L
Lovett, J W T
McDonald, A D
McKay, J S
Malins, T J
Mallya, S
Martin, A J
Martin, T J M
Matin, M P
Millward, R G
Milsted, R A V
Mitchyn, M
Moriarty, B J
Moss, S J
Mukhopadhyay, T K
Nahabedian, A M
Neugebauer, M A Z
Nicol, A
O'Donoghue, M A T
O'Driscoll, M
O'Sullivan, G P
Oleshko, C G
Patel, N
Patterson, M J L
Pearce, P A
Pegg, D J
Piggott, A
Pover, A B
Prigg, N J
Pugh, A
Ravindra Kumar, K
Redfern, T R
Rigby-Jones, T
Roberts, S L
Robinson, M P
Sackey, A H
Salusbury-Trelawry, J M
Scally, J
Schofield, K P
Scott, G I
Scott, W G
Selvachandran, S N
Sharma, P
Shridhar, S
Slavin, J P
Smirk, T W
Smith, D G
Smith, T G
Somasunderam, B
Spooner, A L
Stephens, G P
Stuart, F E
Stubington, S R
Tate, S R
Thomas, D G
Thomson, A P J
Thorburn, R A F
Torrens, R L
Trowler, E P
Vickers, G A
Vickers, J C
Walker, J
Watson, J M
Whiston, R J
Willdig, K M
Williams, J E A
Williamson, D P H
Wilson, E M
Wilson, N G M
Wylie, J B
Zaman, S M

Crewkerne
Balian, B H
Bevan-Mogg, K J
Camsey, J M
Field, M W
Gilson, R A J
McInerney, M A
Rosser, J G
Zwartouw, C L

Criccieth
Roberts, G H
Webb, J G

Crickhowell
Bradbury, A G
Braeman, C
Gregory, D W
Kakas, M A
Lewis, R J
Paton, D H H
Porter, T
Price, D A
Stoker, C J
Taylor, M E
Williams, F

Crieff
Bradley, E
Bushby, D R P
Cooper, J A
Crabbie, E M
Don, J B
Ewing, P A
Gaskell, D E
Jeffery, S L A
Johnston, A M
Johnston, J H
Kirkwood, H L S
McLeod, G G
McPhail, L M
Martin, A E
Matthews, A E
Mitchell, D G
Morrison, A
Murray, R H S
Nicol, K M
Randfield, R S
Sales, J D
Savage, G
Sutherland, G
Wishart, I H

Cromarty
Charley, H G
Hussey, S
Matheson, I U

Cromer
Arbuthnot, J H
Becker, F
Ding, C D
Lennox, A M
Lennox, V C
Norman, W A
Oliver, R M
Ripley, P
Symes, M H A

Crook
Banerjee, A K
Banerjee, A K
Banerjee, A K
Barmby, D S
Carney, M R
Catterick, D I
Chadwick, E T
Clarke, J A
Gayer, M A
Holbrook, G D
Middleton, R A
Sarnaik, N B

Crowborough
Ankrett, V O
Bruce, C E J
Clarke, E M
Crosbie, B J
Davies, J O G
Doherty, J E
El-Nagieb, O M
Fox, R M
Gallannaugh, S C
Golton, M J
Hall, D K
Halliday, N P
Loftus, D A
McGillivray, J L
Maciver, C A
Marriott, P J
Morris, J V
O'Connell, M C
Pereira, J A
Price, T W
Sampson, C S
Sinclair, K G A
Spencer, M A
Stokes, C E
Taylor, S J
Thornton, B A
Thornton, V G
Watts, M E

Crowthorne
Adshead, G M J
Basson, J V
Chau, E P W
Cheung, M S-M
Crampton, A
Damania, A
Davies, A G
Doherty, A J
Forshaw, D M
Fox, W T A
Gupta, A J
Hind, E J
Horne, A S
Humphreys, S A
Iles, S A
Johns, A R
McGauley, G A
Meux, C J
Minne, C C M
Mohan, D J
Murray, K J
Oakley, C J
Payne, A J
Smith, G K
Spanswick, R
Spinks, J
Thomas, R S L
Veeramani, R
Vermeulen, J W
Withers, M

Croydon
Abbot, H P
Abbott, A
Abhayaratne, R N
Abili, O B
Abulafi, A-M
Acevedo, I A
Adabie, K H
Adcock, G N
Ahmadani, H
Akanga, J M C
Akbar, S S
Al-Sheikhli, A R J
Amarasekara, R N S
Amonoo-Kuofi, K
Ansari, A R
Aquilina, C
Atayi, M A
Ayliffe, W H R
Bailey, C V
Balendran, N
Barretto, C J
Baruya, M
Barzanji, A J
Baskaran, B
Beal, V E D
Bees, N R
Bernadt, M W
Berry, D W
Booker, M W
Bootes, J A H
Bowen-Wright, H E
Brightwell, P
Burke, D V
Byrne, P J
Cambridge, N A
Canepa-Anson, R
Carter, N J
Chandra, G
Chang, Y L
Charlton, P P
Chaudery, N
Cheema, A A
Clarke, A M
Coppen, M J
Cottrall, K
Courtenay-Evans, R J
Crowe, M J
Cutting, D A
D'Souza, A C
Darko, D A
Darougar, S
Dave, S S
De Alwis, D V
De Silva, N T
Derodra, J K D
Desai, I T
Diggory, P
Doig, A D
Eason, J R
Ebbs, S R
Ede, J N
El Beshty, M M
Elliman, A J
Epie, G M
Fenton, T H M
Fernandes, A T
Ford, N T
Francis, G G
Fyvie, A D
Gardiner, D A
George, S E
Goberdhan, P D
Graham, C R
Griffin, M H
Griffith, D N W

Hanifa, Y
Hart, S M
Hashemi, K
Hayes, M J
Heidari-Khabbaz, N
Henry, R A
Hill, J J
Hoskins, M C
Howell, G E D
Howell, S D
Htay Nyunt Kyi, Dr
Hughes, J E
Hughes, J G
Husbands, S D
Hussain, S
Ikpoh, A C A
Jaganmohan Reddy, G
Jayaratne, B S S
Kansagra, K
Karim, N B
Kashif Al-Ghita, F A A
Kemp, T J
Khan, K A
Khan, S H
Knibb, A A A
Knight, J R
Kooner, H S
Krysa, J
Lam, Y H
Lennard, R H
Lowe, S
McCrea, D W K
Madhavan, B
Madziwa, D
Mahran, R M A
Maitland, J A
Manoharan, S
Marsh, G D J
Marson, B S
Massoud, M S
Mayahi, L
Mendall, M A
Miller, A C
Miranda Palomino, J F
Monks, P S
Mowbray, M A S
Mufti, F H
Murray, C T A
Nath, R
Navaratnarajah, M
Nawrocki, A
Ng, C L L
Nievel, J G
Noronha, H D S
Owen, A M
Palmer, R N
Patel, N
Patel, S R
Patel, Y S
Paul, S N
Pawa, C M
Peebles-Brown, A E
Peiris, L H S
Persaud, R D
Price, R K
Puvanendran, P
Qureshi, M B
Ramasubbu, K
Ramaswamy, A C
Rathwell, C A
Ravetto, M P C
Ravishankar, G
Redvers, A
Reilly, M M
Salama, N S I
Salerno, J O
Salerno, J A
Sand, P R
Saravanan, K
Sarkany, R P E
Sarma, D I
Sathananthan, K
Seward, H C
Shah, P N
Shaikh, S S
Shaikh, S A
Shakir, S A W
Shanks, J E
Shanmugaraju, P G
Sharif, M
Sheen, A J
Shenoy, A N
Siddiqui, A R
Simenacz, M A
Sinclair, A M
Smahliouk, P
Smaldon, D L
Sneary, M A B
Soutter, A P
Stacey, A G
Sultan, A H
Tan, J L
Tarn, A C
Tay, H H
Thakar, B R
Tharmarajah, P
Thatcher, P G
Thawda Win, Dr
Theano, G
Thiagalingam, N
Thomas, S M
Timans, A R
Toosy, A T
Treml, J
Tross, S Z
Vaja, R
Varughese, M A
Velasco, N
Verstraten, L
Waitt, D J
Walker, K P
Wallace, E J
Walton, D P
Ward, G
Warren, S J
Wesson, I M
White, M S
White, S
White, T G E
Whitfield, R J
Wilcock, C J
Williams, M A
Williams, S K
Willis, M P L
Wimalasuria, S B
Yisa, M A
Zard, C M
Zolczer, L

Crumlin
Carey, F M
Gallagher, H J
Gallagher, J P
Gallagher, O T
Hyndman, R W
Larkin, C J
MacCreanor, C M
McDermott, B M L
McLean, T W B
McQuillan, C
O'Neill, C P
Roughton, S A
Thompson, G
Thompson, L E
Thomson, J H
Weir, J M

Cullompton
Ball, L J
Bellamy, J E
Bodger, M A
Couldrick, M W
Davies, J N
Fairrie, A J
Farmer, C E
Harris, H M
Hook, P C G
Jenner, D R
McLintock, D M
Martin, A M
Rew, R J
Rhys-Davies, N
Rushton, N P
Smith, A G
Straughan, S J
Ward, A G
Willson, S A

Cumnock
Adams, R A
Bhatkar, R L
Burley, J A
Chaplin, D A
Christie, I T
Christie, J H
Findlay, C A
Hasan, M T
Latoria, J K
Latoria, R
Lockens, R
Low, K M
Macnair, C F
MacNair, D M B
Macnair, J A
Macnair, J M
Naczk, A
Nandy, D C
Ramsay, I
Smith, B A
Strath, I D

Cupar
Allison, A S
Anderson, L J
Arbuckle, E
Arthur, J
Barlow, H C
Blyth, A C
Booth, D J W
Brown, M M
Cachia, P G
Cardno, G W
Carey, S J
Cavanagh, P J
Cruickshank, A
Dakin, H E
Dickson, W E
Field, M A S
Findlay, A
Gourley, P E M
Graham, D J M
Grant, H S
Gray, A J
Gray, D A
Griffiths, L K
Hargreaves, P N
Hargreaves, V S
Harry, R M
Hendry, C V
Hendry, M D
Hogg, I K
Hyland, J M
Ince, A H
Johnston, S S
Kenny, N M
Kerr, J A
King, W J
Leonard, K A
Macdonald, L M
McFarlane, J A C
McGregor, H M
McKellican, J F
MacManaway, P J
MacPherson, I R J
MacPherson, S A
Melhuish, R O
Melville, E M
Murphy, J
Neilson, D R
Pickard, M A
Pollington, G D
Pryde, A N M
Robertson, L M
Rowling, D E
Scott, E A H
Sherret, I R
Taylor, D L
Thomson, M F
Warner, B G
Wightman, D
Winslow, G S

Currie
Andrews, D
Clinkenbeard, J M
De Lima, V R F
Dennis, G A M
McColl, A D
McGavigan, P P
McGrath, W D
Potter, M A
Scott, E C
Venters, G L
Wallace, W F

Cwmbran
Allen, L M
Baldwin, R J T
Birchley, D W
Busby, H I
Butcher, J L
Davies, R A
Davies, S S
Ensaff, S
Evans, H S
Fok, M E
Hickson, V M
Holgate, G P
Hunter, S
Hussain, R I
Kabeer, A W A
Kabeer, A A K
King, J L
Kinnaird, T D
Law, P J
Lewis, C S
Lohfink, A B
Morgan, N A
Nicell, D T
Nirmal, D L
Nolan, W P
Paramagnanam, N
Purcell, A M
Roberts, G A
Rowlands, P J
Shah, R B
Skitt, R C
Smith, S A
Thear-Graham, M R
Thomas, B E
Thurgood, M C
Vermaak, Z A
Warrington, R
Wharton, E
Whatmore, K S H
Zutshi, M K

Dagenham
Adedeji, A
Asadullah, M
Ashraff, S M M
Baird, S R
Bajpai, S
Bishop, D A
Connell, T E
Ellul, N
Fateh, M
Ghosh, T K
Gosai, P M
Goyal, M
Heinink, P A
Henderson, H J
Hora, S
Hora, S C
Jaiswal, D P
Junaid, K N
Junaid, R A
Kadva, A B
Kalra, R S
Kaulu, K K
Khan, G M A A
Kugapala, G
Kumar, A
Kumar, M
Kumar, S
Mitra, A K
Mittal, A K
Mohan, T C
Quansah, B B
Roy, M
Saxena, D
Wijekoon, J B

Dalbeattie
Cowe, L
Neilson, A M
Neilson, D J C
Pflanz, S
Wilson, O

Dalkeith
Binnie, J A H
Copp, P A J
Court Brown, C M
Glencross, A H
Glidden, J M
Grant, N C R
Ireland, V M E
Kilday, J-P
Marshall, G I
Marshall, W D
Miller, J N
Murray, M E D
Murray, M J
Philpott, H G
Robertson, D
Smart, L
Westwood, D L
Wilson, M S

Dalry
Andrews, I M
Arnott, G L
Kirke, E M
Law, M J A
Stevenson, J
Taylor, J A
Wilson, M T

Dalton-in-Furness
Amos, C E
Johnson, R N
Maguire, J C
O'Donovan, J J

Darlington
Abu-Rajab, R B
Alam, M M
Ali, A S M
Bagshaw, I M M
Barnes, E W
Bawarish, M A
Berenguer Pellus, J V
Berry, J
Biggin, A E
Birnie, T
Bosanquet, H G
Bradey, N
Bradshaw, J
Braid, J
Bray, G P
Broadbent, C
Brookes, J L
Brookstein, R
Brown, C D
Bruggink, E M A
Buckley, S A E
Burdis, B D
Burton, L L
Byrne, W H T
Carnwath, T C M
Carpenter, R F
Carr, P H
Carrick, H J
Carter, F C
Chan, L
Chan, T
Charlton, R S
Chou, C W K
Christie, J S
Connolly, C K
Corner, N B
Dang, M S
Davison, C P
Dillon, E
Dixon, H H
Drummond, R S
Elliot, J W
Enoch, D A
Fenwick, K W H
Finnie, S M
Fuat, A
Gooch, I J
Gunning, K A
Haidon, J L
Handyside, W B
Hargreaves, M J
Hargreaves, R J
Hargroves, D R
Harris, G
Haslam, J D
Henderson, R G
Hindmarsh, J R
Hodgson, J D S
Humphrey, A R
Husain, S A
Izzat, A B
James, R D
Jeavons, D A
Jones, A B
Kukreja, N
Lam Shang Leen, G
Langham, P J
Latimer, J
McIlhinney, S E
Mackenzie, M S
Mallinder, P A
Marshall, A J
Martin, S D
Mather, J S
Maughan, J H
Melrose, D M
Metcalfe, G J G
Michie, A F
Monro, J S C
Montgomery, A
Mowbray, P
Munshi, S
Murphy, J J
Naismith, S M
Neville, A C
Neville, M J
Nicholson, G
Parameswaran, R
Peart, E J
Penney, B F
Pheara, J
Phipps, A J
Potter, G J A
Pugh, E J
Rajah, P A N
Rhodes, M
Ruckley, R W
Russell, D
Saha, D
Saha, S
Sathananthan, D
Satyavadanan, B S
Senanayake, G
Senthilnathan, G
Shaw, A
Sloss, J M
Spark, J I
Stahl, T J
Stevens, R C H
Stone, S A
Strong, D A
Suri, Y P
Talluri, S C
Tan, Y M
Tarelli, S V
Temple, M J
Thakur, I M
Townshend, J M
Trewby, C S
Trewby, P N
Trewhella, M J
Tulloch, C J
Tyre, N W F
Uitenbosch, M
Upshall, R T P
Wade, R
Wade, S J
Waldin, I E G
Walton, D A
Waterworth, S M
Watson, C
Whittaker, A M
Williams, G V
Williams, G B G
Wylie, J
Young, A C M

Dartford
Aburn, S P
Addison, A K L
Alban Davies, H
Anderson, J B
Andrews, V E
Baines, M J
Beazley, P M C
Beer, M D
Bhargava, S
Bhatia, P P K
Brooke, D B M
Browne, S E
Corbett, D J R
Cybulska, E
Dave, S R
Davies-Wragg, C
Davis, A E
Delport, B C
Denholm-Young, H M
Dickinson, I K
Dickinson, K A
Ede, R J
Elazrak, S M H
Enchill-Yawson, M K
Farquhar, C W
Fernandes, N B
Fernando, P H Q
Fitzpatrick, W J F
Fraser, J A
Ghozlan, H K B
Gladman, M A
Grant, C E
Greer, B L
Gunasingham, V
Hamblyn, M J
Harryman, Dr
Hood, J
Hubbard, B M
Hunt, A B
Hunter, F M
Jamall, A
Jeans, V C
Jones, D R
Jones, M H
Kelly, E P
Khakoo, A A
Khan, M M
Kirk, J M E
Koo, C K
Lawrence, D J
Leyshon, A
McCann, M G
MacDermott, R I J
McIrvine, A J
Madill, S A
Mathew, V M
Melia, W M
Mohan, A J S
Mohan, S

Morgan, S A
Nicolson, J A
Parker, M C O
Parrott, J M
Parry, G M
Patel, D C
Patel, H T
Patel, H R
Patel, H
Patel, R A
Patel, T P
Peiris, M L Q
Peppiatt, R
Perry, N
Pimenta, N G
Pimenta, S M
Prendergast, M T A
Protopapas, M
Pugh, H W
Pyle, S J
Rashid, A M F
Ravi, R
Rawcliffe, J F X
Rose, S L
Rowe, V B
Saheed, A H
Sait, M S
Sarkar, J C
Schreiner, A L
Scott, J F
Selvaratnam, M A
Sharma, R
Sharma, T
Shaw, A C
Shora, B S
Short, D H
Short, N L
Sikdar, N
Spensley, C A
Symes, J B L
Thebe, P R
Thomas, G E
Toth, M
West, C H
Wickens, C L
Zoukos, I

Dartmouth
Anderson, A C
Barrell, S R
Ellerby, R
Eynon-Lewis, A J
Giblin, M
Giblin, M M
Gray, J M
Green, J E
Lockerbie, G D
Pearson, C J P
Ross, M P
Shalders, K
Woodroof, G M F

Darvel
Kondol, A J
Rait, E A
Robertson, M A
Sargaison, M F R

Darwen
Ahmed, S
Alam, S K
Andrews, D M
Bolton, A
Butterworth, D J
Dalton, C R
Higab, M G B
Hirst, A M
Jagadesham, P
Memon, M I
Mills, A
Morris, P J
Patel, R
Schofield, I J
Sinclair, A A
Zaman, A

Daventry
Beer, T C
Boulton, D J
Craig, A J
Davies, M G
Gardiner, P S
Harding, T A C
Harvey, R S
Herbert, K C
Jeffers, L M
Kirkham, S E
Lovatt, C J
Middleton, P H

Moser, J B
Redpath, A M
Rookledge, M M
Sewell, J M
Silverman, A J
Sims, R J A
Verso, N E
Voeten, F

Dawlish
Alborough, E A
Brook, G K
Clements, A J P
Diprose, R H
Donovan, W M
Dorkins, C E
James, A J B
Jeffery, D C J
Oxborrow, S M
Pajovic, S
Raby, P R
Whitehead, J R E

Deal
Barron, H L
Bulmer, J N
Dunn, J M E F
Dyer, J K
Heeley, M E
Hoffmann, F
Hollingsbee, E R
Ison, E
Joslin, J E M
Kaduruwane, E N
Lee, M A
Maginn, S
Rawlings, K L
Russell, S A
Rutherford, S J
Ryder, S-A
Scholfield, D P
Sharp, J F
Sharvill, N J
Smith, G M
Sparrow, I R C
Taha, H M
Viney, M T
Walter, M V

Deeside
Barlow, G D
Bos, E G
Cameron, M C
Currie, A E
Curry, J A
Donaldson, M
Dreyer, C P
Dyer, T J
Fells, J F
Gavin, W B J
Harney, M A J
Hughes, T G
Jeffries, M G
Jones, C W
Jones, T M W
Jones, W R S
Markey, B M
Morris, D E
Pritchard, R M
Rathbone, N
Roberts, D F
Roberts, D Y
Salt, A
Skilbeck, B
Stiggelbout, H J

Denbigh
Appleton, F
Banks, R
Davies, C R
Davies, M W
Eve, J L
Giles, M A
Hackett, P L
Heaton, A
Jenkins, S E
Jones, D G
Jones, R H
Jones, R W
Madoc-Jones, J C
Marshall, A G
Owen, G W
Parry, D E
Parry, E
Roberts, B
Roberts, J M
Roberts, R J
Rodgers, B
Rowe, A J S

Salusbury, C A
Sheers, R
Thomas, J C
Trevelyan, T R
Turczanska, E
Watkin, H
Webb, R D
Webb, T B
Williams, G L
Williams, S A
Wilson, C S
Wykes, E L
Wykes, R J

Denny
Blyth, T H
Boyd, M N
Campbell, I K
Craig, I F
Deuchar, R A
Donaldson, S W
Downs, F M
Flynn, F M
Giles, G M
Kay, D H
Kay, P A
McElhinney, A S J
McGettigan, J T
McLean, K F
Ryrie, G E
Slann, H E R
Wilm, A R

Derby
Abrahams, J W
Adamson, E A
Aitchison, P J M
Aiton, C G
Allen, G R
Allen, L J
Allen, R A
Allsop, J R
Ambrose, J S
Ancliff, P M
Anderson, C M
Anderson, T
Archer, S J
Ashby, J H
Askew, A E
Atkin, M P
Bailey, G R
Bainbridge, L C
Bainbridge, M A
Bains, H S
Bakshi, J
Banbury, J E
Barrett, S
Barron, D A
Barron, N M
Basi, S K K
Bates, B J
Bates, B J
Bates, R C E
Bavister, P H
Bawden, M J
Bell, M M
Benjamin, P D
Berrisford, R C
Bhowmik, M M
Binnie, D J
Birch, P C
Birtwell, A J
Black, I L
Blacker, P A
Blackshaw, G L
Blackwall, M C H
Bland, E S
Bland, S A
Bleiker, T O
Blissett, J E
Boddy, P J
Booth, D F
Brewin, J E
Broadbent, C R
Brooks, A J
Brown, A G
Brown, H M
Browne, M N K
Bullock, D W
Bungay, P M
Burn, S
Bush, J A
Butler, G
Byrne, P H
Callum, K G
Calthorpe, D A D
Cameron, S
Cargill, A O
Cartwright, D P

Cartwright, N P
Chakraborti, A
Chakraborti, P K
Chamberlain, S T
Chapman, M A S
Chapman, R L K
Charlton, J A
Chawla, O P
Chen, H C
Chilka, S Y
Chilton, C P
Choonara, I A
Choudhury, A R
Chowdhury, P A H
Chowdhury, S M I
Church, R D
Clark, D I
Clayton, A R
Clulow, C
Coate, C E H
Cole, A T
Cowlishaw, P J
Cox, J R
Cox, J
Cozens, N J A
Crompton, J G
Crossley, A W A
Cust, M P
Dada, T
Daniells, J J
Dann, N
Davidson, G A
Davies, P B
Dawson, J S
Day, H M M
De Nunzio, M C
Derrington, M C
Dew, S E
Dhadda, A S
Disney, D J
Dixon, W G
Docherty, P T C
Dodd, K L
Donnelly, R
Doris, E J
Dua, R
Edyvean, I K
Edyvean, R J F
Eglitis, H M
Eisenberg, J N H
Ellis, S R
Elsherbini, M M
Evans, A G
Evans, D J
Evans, G F
Farmer, D
Farrell, K A
Farrow, R J
Fellick, J M
Ferrer, I R
Fey, R E
Field, S Y
Fieldhouse, M L
Filer, J L
Fisher, S A
Fitton, R P
Fletcher, J D
Fletcher, V L
Fluck, R J
Forde, M E
Forster, M C
Forster, N D
Foskett, L A
Foster, J H
Foster, N J
Fowlie, A
Fraser-Moodie, W A
Freeman, B
Freeman, J R
Fyall, A A
Game, L M
Gardner, I D
Gartside, J M
Gayed, S L
Gembali, M
Gilchrist, A M
Girn, S S
Goddard, A F
Godridge, H
Golding, D J
Golding, P R
Goodwin, J F
Gorman, W P
Gray, J M
Grenville, J S
Guthrie, D
Haddow, A M
Hale, W M
Hall, R I

Hamilton, R J
Hands, B G
Hanna, N P
Harper, R D
Harris, A P
Harrop, A J
Harrop, J S
Harvey, C M
Hay, J M
Hayes, P D
Heappey, M
Henry, A P J
Herberts, P J D
Hewitt, R I
Hill, P A
Ho, B Y M
Hobday, S R
Hocknell, J M L
Hodgkins, J
Hodson, P B
Hogg, J R
Holliday, C M
Holliday, H W
Holloway, S A
Holmes, G K T
Hope, D T
Hopper, I P
Hopton, S S
Horden, P J
Horner, M E A
Horry, P E
Howard, P W
Howarth, N J
Howell, D A
Howell, P J
Howells, D P M
Hudgins, D
Hunt, D J
Hutchinson, J W
Huxley, C A
Ibrahim, F R
Iddon, P W
Iftikhar, S Y
Isherwood, J P
Jack, B A
Jackson, S N J
James, P D
James, R A
Jefferson, R D
Jenkins, H M L
Jibodu, M O
Jibodu, O A
John, T M
Jones, K
Joshi, A A
Kai, J P
Kapila, I
Karim, U H A
Kazmi, F A
Kazmi, M A
Keeley, V L
Keeling, C J
Keeling, M
Kelsey, R E
Kennedy, J L
Keys, S S S
Khalil, N G
Khan, A Q A
Khan, J A
Khosla, S
King, P
Kinsella, H P
Kirupananthan, S
Komocki, E C
Lacey, P G
Langham, B T
Lawson, I J
Leeder, P C
Leveaux, V M
Little, S W
Lloyd, C G
Long, J
Lunn, A J F
McCance, A J
McCance, S L
McFarlane, H W
McGhee, M
McGibbon, I
McGrath, C M P
McIntyre, J W
Mackaness, C R
McKenny, J G
McKernan, A M
McLean, K A
Macleod, G F
Maginnis, C M
Majumdar, B
Malhi, S S
Marak, W K

Marshall, T J
Matthews, H L
Matthews, I W
Matthews, J I
Maung Maung Tun, N
Mayne, S
Millar Craig, J A
Millar-Craig, M W
Miller, M T V
Milner, S A
Minford, J E
Mitchell, D C
Moar, A K
Molloy, K J
Monteiro, J L
Moore, J K
Mordey, P L
Morrissey, J J
Morton, R E
Moss, P J
Muhiddin, K A L
Mukhopadhyay, S
Mulvey, D A
Murphy, M A C
Murray-Leslie, C F V
Mylvahan, N
Nash, J R
Nath, M
Nathan, P A
Navaratnam, R M
Nelson, C S
Newton, R J
Nichols, G J
Nicholson, J
Norton, B
O'Donoghue, A E M A
O'Reilly, M K
O'Reilly, S C
O'Rourke, E J
Oppong, A C K
Orchard, J M
Orr, R L
Otim-Oyet, D
Owen, R T
Panton, S
Parker, D A
Parkes, I R
Patel, K C
Patel, P K
Patel, R C
Pavis, H M
Pavlidis, S
Piotrowicz, A J K
Pitts, C M
Pore, P S
Potter, T B
Pound, N
Pritty, P E
Quarmby, J W
Quinnell, R C
Rahman, F R
Rajakumar, R
Ralph, S J
Ramzan, M
Rao, K
Ratcliffe, A B
Ratcliffe, V A
Ratnayaka, B D M
Rayment, A
Rayner, S S
Redlaff, L
Regan, M R
Reynolds, J R
Rivers, J A
Rixom, J A
Robertshaw, J K
Robertshaw, K A
Robinson, I A
Robinson, J F C
Rogers, P N
Rogerson, D
Rossiter, J M
Rowan-Robinson, M N
Rowles, J M
Ruggins, N R
Salem, H A M
Schroven, I
Scothern, G E
Scott, I V
Scott, T N B
Searle, A E
Semeraro, D
Shand, I R
Sharp, J F
Shaukat, M N
Shaw, R W
Sherman, M A
Sherwood-Jones, D M
Sibbering, D M

Simmons, M H
Singh, D N P
Singh, H P
Singh, K S P N
Sinha, L
Sinha, S
Sisodia, N
Smailes, R A
Smalley, D M
Smith, A D A
Smith, F D
Smith, H J
Smith, K
Smith, K
Smith, M R
Smith, P G L
Smith, S J
Spincer, J
Sreevalsan, s K
Sreevalsan, S K
Staley, P K
Stanley-Smith, S P
Steele, G A
Stephenson, D K
Stevenson, J M
Stoddard, D R
Summers, G D
Summerscales, A
Sumner, K R
Symonds, I M
Tamizian, O
Tangri, C
Tatla, T
Taylor, G J
Terrell, E S
Thacker, S P
Thomas, J A
Thomson, D J
Tindall, M J
Tinklin, T S
Tran, M N
Tresidder, J S
Turnbull, A E
Turner, C B
Turner, G M
Vater, M
Verma, R
Vinayagamoorthy, P
Voice, A
Walsh, J T
Wanger, K M
Ward, C D
Warner, C E J
Watkinson, S E
Weir, N U
Wells, D T
Westbrook, A P
Wharton, P J
Wheatcroft, M S
Whitaker, R
Whitehall, A L
Whitehead, S M
Wicks, M H
Williams, D A
Williams, N R
Williams, R A
Williams, S E
Wilton, T J
Windebank, W J
Wood, P A A
Yar Khan, S A
Zaman, N A
Zammit-Maempel, J G

Dereham
Abell, C A
Bailie, H C
Carroll, R L
Carroll, S M
Clemo, J
Colman, J E R
Cooper, S F
Crampton, S A
Dun, M
Ewing, J M
Grahame-Clarke, C N E
Hibberd, S C
Hodge, A L
Hughes, R J R
Jackson, A O
Jones, E A
Jones, H W
Kreeger, A J
Lavelle, K G
Lee, A J
MacNair, A D
Marczewski, A G
Moore, S C
Rose, C J
Strickland, P J
Taylor, S J
Thorneley, C W
Tracey, C A
Turner, S D
Webb, K R

Devizes
Akhtar, M A
Archer, R D J
Dunbar, P G
Evans, M R W
Featherstone, J M
Flood, J E
Godfrey, J M
Godwin, L C
Gompels, M A B
Hallward, C G
Hallward, G G
Hamid, E A H M
Heaton-Renshaw, J S
Hollway, J C
Kuber, U A
Lindon, R G
Lodge, G J
Madigan, E A
Meredith, S G
Merrick, G D
Miller, J D T
Nash, J C
New, J W
Osborn, H M
Price, S
Pullen, J E
Purcell, B L
Reid, N C
Riley, N P
Sandford-Hill, R C S
Siggers, S H
Spencer Jones, C J
Stevens, D G
Tully, E M K
Twiner, D A N
Vize, C M
Watson-Jones, D L
Watson, C

Dewsbury
Ahmad, M
Ahmad, M
Angus, P D
Ansari, N-U-H
Asmal, Y Y V
Asmar, M A A A
Balasunderam, S
Balasunderam, S
Barnes, S M
Biswas, C K
Booya, N H
Brook, J
Brown, S A
Bullimore, S P
Chapple, M R
Conway, C A
Coore, J R
Cox, N L T
Craig, I R
Crockett, A L
Currie, D C
Dadibhai, E I
Dhir, S
Evans, J M
Farooqui, T M
Ford, G P
Goulden, P
Goyal, A
Gudgeon, P W
Hicks, J
Hildyard, C L
Hordon, L D
Kalli, M
Kemp, T M
Kerner, A M
Khaliq Masood, A
Kumarasena, H A D
Lovegrove, J E
Lyndon, P J
Maarouf, A S M S
Mackay, P M
Maher, O
Medley, S N
Mehrotra, A P
Miles, S M
Myers, N A
Nanabawa, H I
O'Daly, E F
Okereke, C D
Patel, Y V S
Rahman, M F
Rajpura, A I
Rehman, S-U
Robinson, C D
Shah, M
Shea, J G
Smith, P A
Smyllie, J H
Steel, D
Sutcliffe, I M
Taylor, E G
Thimmegowda, H
Trehan, A K
Twist, D C
Wilson, I R

Didcot
Barrett, J M
Batty, B J
Beswick, K B J
Corps, D J
Couldrick, W G R
Deaney, C N
Delfosse, J B
Dickinson, H A
Hawthorne, S E
Jackson, W F
Kemp, H
Kershaw, J A
Lee, A M
Mackenzie, I D
Millar, J M
Nowell, H J
Pritchard, N L
Salzman, N G
Spiro, J G
Starer, R
Tennent, T G
Wagner, A J
Wood, R
Yorston, C M

Dinas Powys
Cherry, A W
Davies, N P
Davies, R
Harvey, J S
Henderson, J E
Jones, J A G
Laurence, K M
Lewis, A G
Liddell, M B
Mackay, K R
Monypenny, I J
Robinson, M E
Sampeys, C S
Seel, E H
Smith, P M
Stears, A J
Thomas, S

Dingwall
Black, D M C
Black, D K M
Davidson, A J L
Eagleson, K W
Hayward, J D
Macdonald, H M
Mack, M B
McKenna, M F
Maclean, H
Macrae, A S
McRorie, J
Millar, J S
Morrison, I A
Rasdale, P
Reid, K J
Ross, C M
Ross, L E
Scott, E R
Steele, S

Diss
Bawden, R H F
Chandler, O J
Clarke, S M
Cooke, T D
Drake, S E
Grogono, R M
Gunaratna, I J
Hassan, A G
Hayward, J M
Hopkins, S M
Hume, I M
Jones, A D
Leftley, P A
Rowan, P A
Twite, M D
Veneto, B
Walsh, J
Wheble, S M

Dolgellau
Bradley, J N
Challen, P D
Edwards, J J
Fisher, J M
Hilton, S M
Hopkins, J P
Lawson, T M
Martin, H M
Ogden, T L
Roberts, I E
Roberts, J G
Thomas, N A

Dollar
Allan, F
Baughan, P M
Borrowman, E H
Galloway, I W Y
Holdsworth, R J
Houston, N M
Jackson, L A
Mok, V S
Morgan, J P
Randfield, H F
Reid, C R G
Risk, W J

Donaghadee
Beckett, H E
Groves, A M
Larkin, J A M
Long, E D
McClelland, J A E
Majury, C W
Miller, J
Rutherford, J H

Doncaster
Abbas, M
Adams, L M
Addey, K M
Ahmad, S
Al-Khatib, M
Al-Najar, M A W A H
Al-Sindi, Z A H A M
Ali-Khan, M V
Anim-Addo, A
Attwood, M D
Baddoo, W A
Baig, M K
Bake, A J
Banga, B S
Banga, R
Barbour, P
Barker, S R
Barrett, V L
Baskar, B
Beal, J A
Benson, P J
Berry, A W
Bittiner, S B
Bloore, C M
Bolton, R P
Bonham, T J
Boon, M R
Booth, S J
Borrill, M A
Bradley, A E
Bradley, J M
Brennan, K
Britten, L D
Brophy, C S
Brown, D J
Brownson, A J
Buckle, R J
Burne, J M
Burroughs, E A
Burton, A C
Carreck, G C
Chadha, D K
Chandler, G P
Chaudhary, R P
Chib, S C
Chikhani, C G A
Clark, A J
Clark, R
Coleman, M C
Connor, G J
Cook, P H E G
Coombes, G B
Cope, M A
Corlett, J R
Crooks, R N
Cubbon, D H
Cunliffe, L F
Cuschieri, R J
Dahanayake, S B M
Dahanayake, W D
Dakin, G H
Das, P D
De Groot, S J
Deere, J J
Desai, S P
Desai, V S
Dexter, A
Dinakaran, S
Doran, K W
Dua, I S
Dua, P
Duffield, J S
Eddison, P F
Emms, N W
Emovon, E
Evans, K J
Everitt, B M
Fagg, P S
Falk, R M
Farmer, S E
Faruqi, M T
Fearns, D C
Fearns, J M
Fearns, S N
Felton, J C
Field, P M
Field, W D
Fitton, D C
Forbes, A L
Gallagher, J M
Gilbert, J
Glaves, P
Godley, H D
Goni, R A
Goodhead, D G
Graham, D
Graves, A C
Griffiths, M A
Hadjikakou, A P
Hall, J L
Hamlin, R A
Haq, M S
Harding, G M
Harris, J J
Hasenfuss, M F
Hattab, M M
Hawkswell, J C
Head, C D
Helm, R H
Heslip, M R
Hezseltine, D
Hill, G M
Hirpara, R H
Ho, A K-M
Hooper, K H
Hosker, J P
Howard, F A
Hoy, C M
Hughes, K B
Hughes, M E
Hughes, T J
Humby, F C
Hurley, P J
Inglis, J
Inglis, S A
Inman, A J
Inman, S R
Islam, G
Jackson, B E
Jackson, J H
Jacob, G
Jadhav, P R
Jagadish, T S
Johnson, A M
Jones, E W
Jones, M G
Jones, R L D
Jones, V E
Jordan, P R
Kayarkar, V V
Kerr, I P
Kesseler, G
Ketchin, G S
Key, C
Khan, A
Khan, A U
Khan, M A
Kilvington, K A
Kingston, M A
Kirby, S
Kolar, K M
Kolli, L R
Kouchouk, A A
Kumar, P N H
Kurien, G
Lambert, J R
Le Vann, A M
Lee, K M S
Leggett, R J E
Leigh, R J
Lockyear, S K
Love, P W
McGrath, H M
Machin, A J
McIlwraith, W
McKenna, B J
Mackenzie, D S
Mackenzie, J
Mackie, A D R
Mackinlay, J Y
McMahon, C
Majumdar, G
Makol, O P
Marsh, V C
Marshall, A J
Martin, P C
Matthews, J G
Middleton, N M
Miller, A M
Milne, B R
Mitchell, D
Moores, W K
Moss, T R
Nelson, J P
O'Horan, P
O'Leary, M
Oakshott, G H L
Orridge, H W
Owen, R P
Owen, R D
Pardoe, R F
Parry, M S
Paskins, J R
Patel, B M
Payne, G E
Phillips, S L
Pilgrim, J A
Pittaway, A J
Platts, K A
Porter, R W
Pounder, F A
Pramanik, P
Prasad Reddy, K
Psaila, J V
Raithatha, H H
Rajathurai, A
Rajathurai, T
Ramgoolam, M
Redden, J F
Rigby, K A
Roberts, J E
Robinson, R J
Rodgers, L J
Rogers, S
Rogers, T K
Saddler, N J
Saha, S K
Salama, N D
Saunders, I M
Savage, D
Sayer, J M
Sellars, N R
Seth, A K
Sewell, P F J
Shannon, P E
Sharp, J E
Sheehan, A L
Sheikh, M E
Shepherd, J B M
Siddiqui, K
Silvester, N W H
Sinclair, N M
Singh, S
Sowden, M C
Stannard, P A
Stewart, D J A
Syed, R U H
Sykes, K B
Sykes, R S
Tahir, S M
Taneja, A
Taylor, M R
Tomlinson, G N
Townend, I R
Train, J J A
Turner, S
Umapathee, P
Urruty, J-P
Ward, C J
Ward, D A
Ward, S
Watson, G M
Watson, M G
Webb, R F
Weeks, I R

Weller, S
Whale, C I
Wilson, A H
Wilson, P D
Wong, C-H
Wood, D J
Wright, A
Wright, C W
Wyatt, R J
Wythers, D J
Young, K

Dorchester
Al-Hilali, M M A
Anscombe, A M
Armitage, P L
Arnall-Culliford, J M
Ball, A J
Ball, S E
Barlow, I W
Barlow, J M
Bawden, S L
Bhide, M
Boardman, C J
Bowering, A R
Bray, L C
Bridger, S
Bruce-Jones, P N E
Cain, D L
Camm, P R
Campion-Smith, C R
Carey, W D H
Cartwright, F S
Chall, D
Chesney, D
Clifford, R D
Coode, W K
Cornaby, A J
Cove, D H
Cove, R D
Crook, S M
De Silva, K P
Dick, D H
Dixon, K
Dobbs, J F R
Dooley, M M P
Doyle, A R
Edwards, T J
El Komy, A A H A
Ellison-Wright, Z R
Fahmy, M E E-D S
Fleet, J C
Flowerdew, S M
Ford, G R
Foxell, R M
Francis, G J
Furse, R M
Gallimore, G R
Gibbens, G L D
Gill, K J
Goonetilleke, C R
Goulden, S E
Graham, M D
Groom, S N
Hall, G
Hankin, R G
Harker, P
Hateboer, N
Hebblethwaite, R P E
Helliwell, M G
Hitchcock, M
Hollis, J N
Hooper, E J
Hopford, R L S
Hopkin, N B
Hovell, C J
Hughes, M P
Iftikhar, M
Ingram, S M
Iparragirre, B
Jeffery, P J
Johnson, A J
Johnson, M G
Kassab, A S M
Knight, H-P F
Krishnamurthy, P
Lagattolla, N R F
Lale, A M
Lamparelli, M J
Lane, S M
Lim, K S
Ling, D
McConnell, W D
Macdonald, A J
Mackay-James, M A
Mackenzie, I F
McNicol, G P
Matthews, M W B
Millner, C B E
Moosa, A H
Murray, E O
Pearce, M Q
Phillips, G D
Porter, G P
Pulletz, M C K
Purvis, R J
Raza, M N
Reck, A C
Riddoch, A J
Robinson, H A
Romanes, G J
Scott, S T
Simpson, S W
Sloan, R H
Smith, N C
Snook, S
Somani, N R
Somani, N
Sowerby, P R
Stanley, S
Tadros, A N
Taylor, J E
Taylor, P N
Thomas, G D
Thomasson, J E R
Tucker, S C
Veasey, D A
Vines, J R
Wakeham, C T
Webb, A J
Weston, C E
Wiley, P F
Williams, E A
Williams, R K T
Winterton, S J
Wright, P F
Wylie, P A L

Dorking
Alloway, R
Arnold, P C
Blockey, G J
Castaldi, P
Chappell, R H
Cornish, G F
Gledhill, R F
Guilder, T F
Guthrie, G M
Gwyther, S J
Hare, A S
Hare, N C
Jeffcoate, S L
Jefferies, S D B
Jepson, G J
Kingsley-Jones, J
Kober, S J
Loveless, S R
Menzies, R D
Monella, S C
Morrow, M
Mulgirigama, L D
O'Donnell, M J
Orr, R G
Pearce, C J
Rasmussen, J G C
Revel, J-C A
Reynard, T J W
Savage, S J
Scott, H J
Stanley-Jones, J K V
Thomas, C W
Thompson, J R
Tomlinson, S J
Venn, R M
Woodcock, J F
Young, R M

Dornoch
Aitchison, K J
Campbell, D E

Douglas
Biggart, M J
Birkin, N J
Blackman, C M
Blankert, M H L
Booth, J B
Bradley, V P
Brownsdon, D J
Bull, D M
Chalmers, D H K
Clague, C P T
Clague, R B
Cretney, J D
Cullen, J P
Currie, J N
Daniels, J K
Evans, G
Evans, P F
Fayle, R J S
Featherstone, R M
Fenton, C M
Garvey, C N
Gavin, N G S
Green, A D L
Hamm, R E D
Hampton, G
Harding, F W
Harris, B D
Harrison, N A
Harrison, P A
Harrop, M C
Hillas, C
Hinds, J C D
Hockings, N F
James, D
Kerruish, T B W
Khan, E G
Khuraijam, G S
Kissack, C M
Levine, W H C
McCrory, J W
Manuja, S L
Moroney, A M
Moroney, L H E
Murray, C R H
Newton, P G
Nicholls, C R
Pilling, A C
Plews, N R
Ritson, R H
Stevens, D B
Thavarajah, V M
Upsdell, S M
Vaughan, A R S
Wardle, J K
Wilkinson, K
Zeitoune, S M

Doune
Cordwell-Smith, C B
Henderson, P M N
Jardine, C K H
McAlpine, J A
Rose, P F
Sawyer, D H

Dover
Anderson, A M
Bahadur, T
Barley, P E
Birks, S F
Bradley, S D
Bundy, A G
Chaudhuri, S
Cloke, D J
Collins, M
Dodd, I H
Flower, K L
Goddard, I M
Hodnett, S F
Jain, S C
Jenkins, D
Jones, M E P
Kelly, B A
Kumi, G O
Lloyd, G L
McSwiggan, G V
Maddaford, K J
Morris, J I J
Mottershead, A C
Naterwalla, R H
Neylon, J J
Premnath, P
Premnath, R
Stellon, A J
Tippu, N I
Torrance, T C
Turner, D J
Ward, K J
Waters, S S
Welch, E F J
Wood, J R
Wright, L M
Zaman, H W

Downham Market
Bungay, A W
Chase, N J
Cvijetic, B P
Garner, P
Gent, T M
MacKichan, A H T
Sconce, J C A
Scott, R D
Sheppard, C T

Downpatrick
Archbold, J A A
Bain, D A
Bell, J C
Boggs, R E
Brown, E
Cheung, H C
Creaney, J
Deeny, A P
Doris, J P
Foy, J M
Foy, W T
Gaffney, B P
Grebbell, F S
Hamill, G
Hamill, J A
Hamill, J P
Hamill, V A
Hanna, B C
Hannah, B A
Harney, A-M
Harney, E J
Hayes, O M
Ingram, R M
Jacob, S
Kelly, M I
Kirk, J E J
Lamberton, M H
MacAleenan, F A
MacAleenan, N A
McDaniel, D
McGill, J U
McGoldrick, H P M
McGrady, B J
McIntosh, H Y
Mollan, R A B
Moore, P R J
Moorehead, C N S
Mulhall, M M
Murphy, M
Napier, E D
Napier, N J
O'Connor, S A
O'Reilly, G M
O'Toole, C E K
Phillips, M R
Sheridan, M C
Small, U R
Stevenson, T H
Stewart, J C M
Storey, R G N
Wain, A A
Watts, A E
Wilkie, A W
Wilson-Davis, M L

Driffield
Anderson, S J
Ascroft, N O
Clarke, A D
Clarkson, G C
Crawford, A N
Crumpton, M
Freeman, R C
Heaton, C H
Kelly, S E
Loqueman, N
Pickering, N
Richardson, P C
Senior, D
Towers, S J
Vincini, C
Walker, Z A
Wigglesworth, D F

Droitwich
Adcock, A V
Blake, A
Bradshaw, T
Brownridge, D S
Clark, A
Cleak, D K
Dykes, C J
Elliott, N M
Ellson, C R
Fernell, D M
Freeman, M J
Gillson, J A
Hamer, J D
Hartwright, D
Horn, A C
Jenkins, N E
Kameen, A F
Keeble, M M
Kelly, A J
Kenyon, A C W
Kerton, I L
Kinsman, R I
Kramer, H
Lancashire, M J
McCloskey, B G
McKie, D J
Newsholme, R G
Pashley, J K
Rawcliffe, P J
Read, L
Rennie, C D
Sawyer, J P C
Smart, J C
Strover, A E
Tarlo, L
Tomlinson, C J
Turner, P J
Vardi, G
Wild, S M
Wilkie, V M
Woof, W R

Dromore
Atchison, E M
Beggs, L H
Cargin, J A
Connery, J A
Corbett, G D A
Cull, M E
Drake, A T
Drake, M B G
Hicks, N C
Hinds, G M E
Humphreys, S R
Kenny, C J
McNeice, R A
Paisley, J A
Patterson, A B
Ruddell, N J
Shannon, G E M
Walsh, S J

Dronfield
Allamby, P R
Barrowcliffe, D G
Bethell, J N
Bull, R E
Davidson, M J
Earl, R C
Foroughi, M
Harvey, G M
Hawley, S K
Park, A J
Parsons, C E M
Spooner, C A

Drybrook
Good, C D
King, P A

Dudley
Acquah, E K
Aggarwal, S P
Al-Ibrahim, J
Al-Rabban, S F
Ali, M S
Anandakumar, P
Ananthanarayanan, V
Andrews, R
Arkell, L J
Banerjee, A K
Bansal, N
Bareford, D
Blackman, A J
Brettell, P B V
Broad, M V J
Butt, M S M
Cartwright, J
Cartwright, S T
Christie, J L
Conlon, D M
Conlon, W P
Craggs, J E
Cullen, P E
Dawes, K R
De Silva, D T
Desai, J
Doherty, M J
Dukes, I K
Elwell, D
Emtage, L A
Farmer, M
Favill, E J
Fiad, T
Fisher, N C
Flahn, G N
Funkel, H
Gee, R W
George, D E
George, N J R
Gnanadurai, T V
Gregan, A C M
Grimley, R P
Gupta, P D
Gupta, R
Gurney, P W V
Haddon, A L
Hall, A D
Hamlyn, A N
Hampson, W T
Harrison, P
Huish, Z K
Husain, R A
Ingle, P R
Ingle, U P
Irani, S
Jain, S K
James, D A
Jayatunga, A P
Jones, B J M
Kevern, A B
Khan, J M
Kitas, Dr
MacAviney, M A M
Mittal, V K
Moors, A H
Morrill, P O
Narad, P K
Norcott, H C
O'Mara, L
Oliver, P S
Oliver, R
Oram, D A
Pall, J
Parkes, A W
Parry, D G
Patel, R
Perera, R K
Poole, C J M
Porter, A M
Potamitis, T
Quinlan, M
Randall, J
Rao, V M K
Reed, I T D
Richardson, S G N
Robertson-Steel, I R S
Rowse, A D
Sangha, S S
Sant, K G
Saunders, W A
Savage, A P
Scriven, P M
Shafquat, S
Shaikh, Z A
Shather, N A
Shave, R M
Shipsey, S J
Smart, V M
Smith, S
Sonksen, J R
Spencer, G
Spiers, R J
Stevenson, M M
Stewart, D G
Stonelake, P S
Swatkins, S
Tye, J C
Warrington, N J
Whallett, A J
White, N C
Whitehurst, P
Wild, S P
Wilson, F
Wolinski, A P
Womersley, D S

Dukinfield
Ali, F S M
Asthana, A
Douglas, C A
Dowling, T I
Kelly, B J
Malik, D
Marr, D H
Procter, J C
Roylance, M H
Seeley, S K
Toyn, J L

Dulverton
Burton, L
Goodwin, F R
Thomson, R G

Dumbarton
Alcorn, T
Barlow, T H
Berry, C
Bidwell, L A M
Braidwood, E A

Byrne, F J
Byrne, J A
Byrne, M A
Cairns, E E
Campbell, E C
Crawford, E G
Doig, A
Downie, J F
Foote, S J
Logan, D R
Lynn, K N
Maciver, S A H
Mackenzie, J A
McMaster, T
McNamee, R N
McNamee, S A
Mason, M R
Mitchelson, A V
Morton, D E
Rainey, V
Renshaw, S B H
Stevenson, J G
Sweeney, J M
Thomas, M M
Wales, R M
Watson, J M

Dumfries
Armstrong, H E
Auld, A R
Auld, C D
Ball, D R
Baptist, G P
Beaumont, C G
Bedford, G J B
Bennie, D B
Bone, F J
Bonn, G
Breen, D A
Brewster, H A
Brown, C A
Buchan, C C
Burton, J W
Carruthers, J W
Cathcart, J B T
Cathcart, R A
Clark, M H
Clayton, P
Clyde, J W
Cowie, I D S
Currie, H D
Currie, R A
Cusworth, E J
D'Ambrogio, M S
Dale, B A S
Dang, R K B
Dewar, C S
Downie, A
Drever, E A
Evans, D A
Falconer, J A G
Fellowes, E C
Ferguson, K M
Flint, E F
Flockhart, D R
Garcia-Baquero Merino, M T
Geals, M F
Gibson, I H
Gibson, J L
Gibson, J C
Gordon, R G
Graham, J M
Grant, C I
Grieve, R M K
Gurney, M F
Gysin, J
Halliday, B W
Halliday, S P
Hassall, J E S
Hay, I F C
Henderson, M A
Holden, R
Holt, M C W
Howie, G M
Hutchison, P G
Irving, M A M
Isles, C G
Isles, R M
Jamieson, C
Johnston, L F E
Jones, D N
Jones, S
Kiely, D G
Lawrence, J R
Leuvennink, J C
Lowry, W S
Lutfy, A M
Lyon, A R
McCreadie, R G
McCullough, A M
McFadzean, J
McGrouther, R I
McKay, D A
McKechnie, J M
Maclean, I H
McMahon, M J
McQueen, K J
Maggiori, L A E
Martin, L C
Meek, R
Mensah, P K A
Metcalfe, S F
Morris, S
Morrison, R
Morton, M L
Muir, I M
Neilson, J
O'Brien, F G M
Park, R W
Perkins, V
Powell, E F
Power-Breen, P A
Power, B J
Power, N R
Rafferty, P
Reid, J M
Rhind, G B
Rizvi, S T M
Robertson, S E
Robson, J E
Rutherford, J S
Saad, K J
Sabur, R Y
Sajid, S A
Sanderson, H
Shearer, M G
Shroufi, S
Simpson, R M
Slinn, R M
Smith, D P
Smith, I G
Spafford, P J D
Stark, A N
Stoddart, M G
Strachan, D A
Tait, G W
Taylor, D D
Taylor, S B
Thomson, A M
Thomson, R B
Tilak-Singh, D
Toolis, F
Unyolo, P M
Waite, A
Walls, A D F
Walter, R D
Waterhouse, J
Watson, N T B
White, J M
Williams, D R
Wilson, M C G
Wilson, W A M
Wisdom, S J
Wood, E R M

Dunbar
Badger, T R
Black, C N
Brewster, A M
Cassells, D A
Gordon, A I
Hare, E H
Horn, C R
McLaren, P J
Rogers, M E

Dunbeath
Usher, N E

Dunblane
Abercrombie, M R
Barnes, J F
Barron, C M
Bengough, E A
Buchan, D A
Butts, S L
Crow, Y J
Gardiner, A J S
Garrett-Cox, R G
Hamilton, B
Herbert, J M
Kerr, A L
King, I
McGarva, J
McNeill, A
McShane, L J
Pollock, A M
Price, F J
Rodger, R A
Roxburgh, D A
Smith, C M
Swan, W G
Trench, A J
Watson, R G
Wood, J M
Wright, F G

Dundee
Abu-Bakra, M A J
Adamson, D J A
Adlakha, H L
Adlakha, S
Agustsson, P
Aird, F K
Al-Dabbagh, A S K
Al-Sanjari, N A G A
Allen, M-E
Allison, R H
Andersen, R M
Anderson, J A
Arblaster, L A
Arthur, I D
Arthur, S J
Avison, G G
Bain, J
Baldacchino, A M
Ballantyne, E S
Banerji, S
Bannister, J
Basra, S
Beale, J P
Beattie, P E
Begg, J D
Belch, J J F
Birrell, A L
Birrell, D H
Blair, R L
Bonnar, S E
Bowen, D T
Bree, S E
Brown, A D
Brown, D W H
Brown, D C
Brown, E H
Bruce, D A
Bruce, J T
Bruce, L E
Bryden, A M
Buchan, A B
Buckney, M N M
Cairns, M
Cameron, F M L
Cameron, R C P
Campbell, K L
Cavanagh, J
Cezanne, H H
Chakraverty, S C
Chan, R H F
Chan, Y Y
Charlett, P J
Che Abdullah, S T
Checketts, M R
Chesters, E M
Chishti, S K K
Chong, Y M
Clarke, R
Clift, B A
Coid, D R
Coleiro, J A
Colvin, B A J
Colvin, J R
Colvin, M A
Connolly, C M N
Constance, N D
Cook, A M
Copland, A M
Cormie, C A
Coull, S L
Coventry, D M
Crighton, A J
Crighton, A D
Curr, E A
Dance, J C
Das, S
Das, S
Dauleh, M I M
Davey, P G
Davidson, H A
Davis, B C
Davis, M H
Dawson, A J
Day, R K
De Zeeuw, F J
Dent, J A
Devereux, S L M
Dewar, J A
Dick, P H
Dillon, J F
Doig, S N
Donaldson, K J
Donaldson, L
Dorling, J S
Dorward, D W T
Dow, E
Dowell, J S
Duffy, M C
Duke, S L
Dunbar, A P
Dunbar, D S
Duncan, I D
Duncan, M R
Dunkley, M P
Dymock, B A
Dymock, T
Edwards, S L
Eljamel, M S
Ellis, E
Ellis, J D
Ellison, L E
Emslie-Smith, A M
Emslie-Smith, K M
Esparon, J A
Evans, A T
Fahey, T P B
Fairlamb, A H
Farquharson, C A J
Fee, M C D
Fellowes, J L
Ferguson, G
Ferguson, J
Fergusson, R A
Findlay, D J
Flavahan, C
Fleming, C J
Fleming, R A
Fletcher, F
Fletcher, J D
Fogarty, M Y
Forbes, J H D
Forrester, A G
Forsyth, J S
Forsyth, J D J
Foster, J
Foubister, G C
Fox, P
France, A J
Franklin, V L
Freeman, C A
Freshwater, K H
Galloway, A J
Gardiner, Q
Gardiner, S
Gelly, K J
Gemmell, D F
Gentleman, D R
George, M J A
George, N D L
Ghosh, U K
Gillespie, L M
Gillespie, N D
Goodman, C M
Gorman, L J
Gorog, D A
Gossip, J M
Goudie, B M
Goudie, D R
Graham, J G I
Grant, K P M
Gray, M
Green, C M
Greene, S A
Griffiths, G D
Grimmer, C
Grimmond, L M C
Guha, P K
Gusa Lavan, S G
Haining, R E B
Hajipour, L
Hall, P A
Hankinson, C A
Hannah, S R
Hanslip, J L
Harden, R M
Harrold, A J
Hartmann, D
Haut, F F A
Hayes, M G
Henderson, L M
Henman, P D
Hew, W-S R
Hewick, S A
Hewitt, P M
Hogg, M C
Hopwood, D
Hopwood, S E
Houston, J G
Huang, D S W
Hulbert, J K M
Hume, R
Hunt, V J
Hunter, S M
Hussain, S S M
Husselbee, K M
Hutchison, G L
Ibbotson, S H
Irwin, J
Jaafar, H M I B
Jain, A S
Jeffers, R F
Johnston, B B
Johnston, D A
Jones, K D
Jones, M C
Jones, P A
Jung, R T
Kastner-Cole, D
Kavi, J
Kazmi, S A-H
Kenicer, K J A
Kennedy, D W
Kennedy, M S
Kerr, L M
Key, B
Kilgallon, B
Kirkpatrick, M R
Kyeremateng, S P K
Lafferty, M E
Laing, D E
Lall, R
Lamb, J S
Lang, S
Leadbitter, H
Leese, G P
Leese, R A
Leiper, J M
Leslie, J R S
Levack, I D
Levin, C A
Levison, D A
Levison, J L
Levison, S E
Lewis-Jones, M S
Lewis, A H O
Lo, M C K
Locke, J W
Locke, R M
Lockwood, P
Lorimer, S
Lowe, E M
Lowe, J G
Lowe, K G
Lowe, L M
Lyall, M H
McAllion, S J
McCarthy, R
McClymont, W
MacConnachie, A A
McConnell, K D
McCormack, D J
MacCormack, J G
MacCowan, H A S
McCowat, L C
McCulloch, A S
McCulloch, J M
McCullough, J B
McDevitt, J M
MacDonald, T
McEwan, M S R
MacEwen, C J
McEwen, J
McEwen, J R
McGlone, L
McGowan, D W
McHarg, A M
MacIntyre, J M
Mackenzie, N
Mackie, J I
Mackinnon, A J
McLean, S M
McLellan, A
McLoughlin, P M
McMurdo, M E T
Macpherson, E S
Macrae, W A
MacWalter, R S
Magro, J J
Main, G
Malcolm, J B
Malcolm, R M
Malik, S
Man, I W-P
Manthri, P R
Maple, C
Martindale, J P
Mathew, P
Mathewson, Z M
Matthews, K
Meikle, J N
Mellish, R W E
Millar, J P
Miller, A S C
Miller, D C
Milne, S E
Mitchell, L H
Moir, C L
Montgomery, A J
Moore, J A
Morley, S M
Morris, A M
Morrison, A
Morrison, W G
Mowle, D H
Muir, A H
Munnoch, D A
Murray, S J
Naasan, A
Naismith, K I
Narsapur, S L
Nassif, M G G
Nathwani, D
Neville, R G
Newton, J R
Newton, R W
Nichol, N M
Nicoll, D
Nicoll, L M
Nicoll, S M
Nimmo, M J
Noaman, L A
O'Donoghue, C R
O'Riordan, J I
Ogilvie, K E
Okhai, A A H
Oliver, T B
Olver, W J
Orange, G V
Owen, L E
Payne, R J
Peart, C L
Pegg, S M
Petrie, R X A
Phillips, M G A
Pippard, M J
Prakash, U
Preece, P E
Pringle, S D
Pringle, T H
Proctor, I
Prodhan, C R
Prophet, L E
Proudfoot, D J
Pullar, T
Purdie, C A
Quinn, K
Rae, G B
Raj, M
Rajendran, S
Ramachandran, N K
Ramage, L
Ramsay, A E
Rankin, E M
Ravikumar, A
Reid, A H
Reid, D C
Reynolds, N
Riad, M M A
Richards, J P
Richmond, J D
Rickhuss, P K
Ritchie, D K
Roberts, R C
Robertson, A J
Robson, C J
Robson, J P
Rorie, D A
Rorrison, H W
Rosbottom, R
Rowley, D I
Rundle, C M
Russell, A G
Russell, D W
Ruta, D A
Ruthven, E
Ruthven, J L
Ryan, M F
Ryder, K O
Sadler, D W
Saggar, K D
Salisbury, J
Sanders, A F
Sanderson, J B
Savage, A J
Scahill, S J

Scanlan, P H
Scott, A
Scott, F M
Scott, K N L
Scott, R F
Scullion, L T
Semple, M M
Senior, P A
Severn, A
Sharma, M M
Sharpe, G D M
Shearer, A J
Shearer, K H
Shepherd, C
Shimi, S M
Simonsen, H
Simpson, N S
Sinclair, B L
Siu, S K L
Slane, P W
Smeaton, N C
Smith, A H W
Smith, D R W
Smith, G D
Smith, R W
Smith, R N
Sohail Sahibzada, A
Spencer, J
Spiers, E M
Spillane, K
Spruce, B A
Staziker, A C
Steele, R J C
Steele, S M
Stewart, C I L
Stewart, D P
Stewart, J
Stoddart, J W A
Stonebridge, P A
Struthers, A D
Summers, G
Suttie, K Y
Swingler, R J
Symon, M A
Taig, C
Taig, D R
Tait, I S
Tarnow-Mordi, W O
Taylor, J H
Taylor, T W
Taylor, W J
Thakore, S B
Thompson, A M
Thomson, A J M
Thomson, E S
Thomson, J M D
Thomson, R
Thurairajah, K
Tiffin, P A C
Timperley, J C
Toller, R A
Townell, N H
Tunstall-Pedoe, H D
Tunstall-Pedoe, O D
Uqlat, L N E
Vaid, M A E
van Twuyver, P V
Veitch, T
Vernon, J P
Vernon, M M
Vincent, D S
Walker, P J
Walker, W F
Wallace, D J
Ward, M C
Watson, A D
Watson, A M
Watson, G D
Watson, G C
Watson, Y M R
Webster, L H
Weir, C J
White, K D
White, P S
Whiteside, C E
Wilcock, M A
Wildsmith, J A W
Wilmshurst, A D
Wilson, S M
Winter, J H
Wood, C R
Wood, C M
Wood, R A B
Woodley, A G
Wyllie, F J

Dunfermline
Adams, W E
Alexander, A C A
Alexander, D
Allan, S J R
Anderson, H E
Anderson, T J
Austin, A E
Birkinshaw, K J
Bray, J C
Briggs, S J
Brown, A G
Brown, T M
Brownlie, R
Burt, G F
Burt, J R
Burt, J R F
Cameron, I A N
Carter, R G
Chan, Y K
Christmas, E R
Claisse, A Z
Conway, N T
Copeland, C L
Cross, W A
Curry, P D
Daniel, T
Dean, B
Downie, F D H
Duncan, R W
Duthie, P C
Emery-Barker, J A
Evan-Wong, L A
Falzon, M
Farrar, S M
Firth, C E
Fleet, M S
Fletcher, G M
Garvie, S J
Gilbert, S S
Gillespie, G D
Gilmore, D R
Gowans, M
Grant, S M T
Hadoke, J K
Hicks, J D
Hill, C
Holligan, E M
Howd, A
Hyde, A J A
Jenkins, D A S
Johnston, B E
Johnston, G
Jones, B J
Jones, D G
Kao, R N P
Keston, R B
Laggan, M J
Langham, M I
Lester, R B
Lyall, J B F
Lyth, D R
Macaulay, K E C
McBride, K D P
McGovern, A W
MacIsaac, A B
Mackay, K M
Mackay, S K
MacLeod, D C
McMinn, C S
Malcolm, W N
Malik, T Y
Marks, R C
Masaud, M K
Mason, I L
Mathie, I H
Mathie, Y M
Milne, A A
Moxey, J E
Moy, J R
Murdoch, G E
Nicholas, M P
Nisbet, R M
Niven, C F
O'Regan, M B
Oliver, C J R
Park, M J
Patel, G J
Peyton, P A
Philipsz, M L
Prentice, L-A
Proudfoot, M C
Reid, S R
Robertson, M I
Russell, S C
Scott, M R
Scott, T M
Scragg, S E
Seaman, F M
Selby, C D
Shah, S K
Shaw, D R
Sinclair, A
Stuart, F M
Sutherland, M S M
Thomas, I G
Thores, O A
Turner, A R
Walker, M W
Walsh, J P
West, A M

Dungannon
Baird, T J
Barbour, P M
Bogues, B E
Brodison, A M
Campbell, R
Casey, F
Coogan, K
Corr, F M
Costello, L M
Cummings, D H
Currie, A A
Donaghy, S M
Gallagher, M E
Gamble, W J
Garvin, J S M
Girvin, F G
Gribben, T M
Hackett, P J
Hagan, P M
Haughey, J P
Herron, A
Herron, M J
Hobson, L A
Hughes, S
Hunter, C F
Jenkinson, W R
Johnston, I H
Johnston, S E
Jones, A M
Kelly, E
Kennedy, H M
Kennedy, M
Logan, J M
Logan, J J
McAliskey, D P
McCammon, L C
McCoy, B G
McGuinness, B
MacHenry, J C R M
McIvor, D E L
McKay, J J
McKenna, P H
McKeown, P F
McMenemy, P L
McNeill, H G
McQuade, E
McShane, A M
McVeigh, J E
Marshall, P
Millar, E J
Nugent, T P J
O'Loughlin, M A
Palmer, J M
Peyton, J W R
Pothanikat, G
Rodgers, A A
Rodgers, D A
Sands, C J
Stinson, P G
Streahorn, D
Symington, S K
Thompson, M R
Tierney, J P
Walker, N W
Watson, M S
Wylie, I L

Dunkeld
Binnie, D S
Brooks, J E
Donnelly, J D
Patel, N B
Silburn, J N
Silburn, M D W
Wright, G A

Dunmow
Castleden, L S
Davies, P G
Griffiths, R L
Hartgill, T W
Healy, D W
Howlett, R W
Hudson, I R B
Hughes, S A
Jackson, J S B
Kellerman, A J
Malone, A H
Miller, R
Nunn, R A
Nunn, T R
Pinchen, C J
Pugh, E C
Pye, M J
Raybould, S A
Slack, M C
Stevens, J A
Tailor, R A
Tayler, M J
Tee, M K
Turner, D R
Vernon, J G

Dunoon
Adamson, D M R
Campbell, P T
Clark, C M
Johnston, D I
Johnston, S M
Lawson, C A
Lilley, I N
Pearce, J M
Raghavaiah, L S
Stewart, A J
Stewart, J G H
Thomson, A W
Turner, A R
Wilkie, W J

Duns
Aitken, W B
Auld, B M
Dobie, V J S
Fingland, I W W
Fowles, R G
Inglis, S A
Macallister, D J
McCann, S R
Mitchell, D L
Ross, E J W
Sim, G

Dunstable
Bell, J R
Benedikt, N A
Berry, J E
Bilton, K
Bodhani, H D
Carter, G B
Carter, M I
Chowdhury, U K
Cro, R J
Curt, N E
Dashore, J P
Day, M J I
Donald, A
Freeman, K A
Fsadni, J
Goutam, P K
Haq, M F
Hassan, P C
Hawking, K M
Jackson, P G
Jones, M R
Long, A C
Mallik, A K
Neal, R C
O'Toole, O B
Pal, U
Perkins, J D A
Peters, J
Prendergast, J M
Quartly, C F
Reyner, L J
Robinson, R C
Shah, C N
Shah, R
Speakman, H M A
Stein, S M
Sullivan Standen, A
Sykes, C M
Towler, J M
Twivy, S B
Weir, W M

Durham
Akindolie, O
Alifieri, E
Allison, D
Anderson, J E
Aye, C C
Bain, I M
Banks, J G
Barnes, A J
Barnes, S E
Beard, J R
Beggs, G C
Bernard, P M
Berry, R B
Birrell, K G
Birrell, V L
Bremner, W G M
Bristow, E A
Brown, H A
Butterworth, G A
Buxton, C S J
Carr, M M
Catty, R H C
Cave, M H
Charters, J W
Cheeseman, S J
Chester, P G
Chuck, A J
Clark, A D
Clark, J A
Clifford, D G
Collings, P A J
Conway, V G
Cook, A I M
Cook, P J
Cooper, R
Cotes, J E
Craddock, S C
Cunliffe, T P
Dabner, S
Darling, B M
De Silva, C
Desai, S M
Docherty, T B
Dowson, S
Dunning, P G
Earnshaw, M A
Ehtisham, M
El-Harari, M B A
English, P J
Erdmann, M W H
Fisher, C J
Flanagan, P A
Gardner, S
Glover, M E
Gorton, R K
Graham, P M A
Green, M R
Green, S E
Greenwell, D G
Gregory, R J H
Gururaj Prasad, K B
Hammond, R J
Hand, R W
Harnor, K J
Harrington, J
Harrison, J H
Harrison, J E
Hawkins, C
Hawthorn, I E
Hazell, M J
Helliwell, G M
Herd, A N
Hickson, G M
Holmes, E J
Horton, A J
Hubbard, M P
Hutchinson, F H
Ibbott, J M
Irons, D W
Irving, H M
Jackson, R M
James, S
Jones, D W
Judson, M L
Keenan, F M
Kemball, H J
Kirkup, W
Lane, M R
Leaver, A A M
Lewthwaite, P W
Lothian, M
McBride, P A
McConnell, F K
Macintyre, A
McLean, A T M
McLean, N R
Maddison, B
Maddison, G M
Mahto, N K
Maini, V
Maloney, D J L
Maloney, G
Mangion, P
Mansfield, S D
Mansour, S H S
Marsden, P J
Martin, S J S
Mattinson, P J B
Maung, S W
Miller, J C
Milne, B E
Milne, J E C
Milne, P
Mitchell, R W D
Moon, A P
Moran, P
Munro, G
Munro, N C
Murray, R W
Nagi, S S
Neely, R D G
Neilson, F M C
Noble, D L
Noel, I
Osborne, K A
Pascall, C M E
Patel, A S
Patel, K M
Pearce, S J
Peel, P H
Petterson, T
Phillips, C E
Prescott, R W G
Quasim, M
Ramakrishna, G M D
Ramarao, P
Randle, M
Ray, P
Rhind, J R
Robertshaw, B A
Rocker, P B
Rodriguez Garcia, F J
Rooney, C M
Roper, N A
Ruffett, D I
Ryan, J M
Sandall, D
Sanders, E
Sanjeeva Rao, V
Selby, N M
Shaw, N J
Sinclair, S A
Siriwardana, N C P
Smart, D W
Smith, D R S
Snashall, P D
Speight, A N P
Spencer, I
Stewart, H V
Sutherland, I A K
Tatham, P C
Terry, G
Thalayasingam, B
Thomas, D G
Thomas, D G
Thompson, C S
Thompson, S J
Tomkinson, J S
Turner, H D
Twite, S J
Underwood, I R
Vallance, J H
Walling, A E
Walton, P R
Walton, S E
Wardropper, A G
Weatherill, D
Welsh, G H
Whalley, F E
White, C
White, D R
Whitfield, S J
Whyte, S D
Wilford, N J
Will, R
Williams, R A-I W
Wilson, D
Wingate-Gray, E
Wolsey, L A F
Wood, D W
Wood, P J
Woods, R
Wright, K U
Wright, P J
Yule, J C

Dursley
Alvis, S J
Bewley, J S
Cole, G J
Curtis Hayward, K S
Frankau, T G
Freeman, M J
Gornall, C B
Kenny, D
Lewis, R M
McDowell, M J
Milson, J A
Opher, S J

Rix, S P
Roberts, J K
Steel, J A P
van't Hoff, H C
Wardell-Yerburgh, T C
Wills, E

Dymock
French, R J

East Boldon
Baines, D L
Benton, K
Board, H R
Clark, D
Cooper, D G
Crabtree, H L
Dhar, R
Fawzi, H W
Howard, T J
O'Dair, G N
O'Dair, J D
Obonna, R
Reed, L

East Cowes
Andrews, C J A
Davies, M L R
Gillan, S A

East Grinstead
Arnstein, P M
Ashworth, C
Aylesbury, H E
Barham, C J
Belcher, H J C R
Bellamy, S J
Berkovitch, A P
Blair, J W
Boorman, J G
Bowley, N B
Brooks, K J
Brown, A E
Brown, J M
Christopher, B W C C
Cullen, K W
Curran, J E
Dheansa, B S
Diba, A
Digges, C N O N
Dunstan, R J R
Enskat, A R D
Erlam, A R
Foulger, V A L
Genevieve, M Y
Gilbert, P M
Harborow, P C
Hoare, G L
Hoe, W K-C
Khilkoff-Choubersky, A
Lavery, K M
Mackenzie, A A J
Martin, A
Moshegov, C N
Parkhouse, N
Pearson, E R
Pickford, M A
Smith, R W
Sneddon, K J
Squires, S J
Sugden, J J
Teo, T-C
Van Gelderen-Swart, A G
Venn, P J
Vevers, J J
Wong, P

East Linton
Cameron, J M W
Guy, D
Hare, K M

East Molesey
Brant, S E
Britton, S E
Collie, I F
Coxon, I D
Gajraj, M K
Gajraj, N M
Galvan De La Hoz, A
Glanville, S B C
Gray, J
Hamill, J S
Jeffcoate, C M
Kapoor, A
Lark, K A
Marks, K A
Paramothayan, B N

Robak, K R
Rowe, T L
Tapping, P J

Eastbourne
Adoki, I I
Adolph, M P N
Ahmed, S A
Al Hajaj, W H
Aldridge, A J
Allan, S M
Anderson, H J
Argent, V P
Argiriu, P
Armitage, A R
Ashby, C P
Barnes, J D
Beeney, M A R
Bell, T J
Bending, J J
Bishai, I A H
Bland, L W
Bloor, G K
Bonnici, A V
Brennan, B P M
Brown, G C
Canagaratnam, N
Canavan, A C
Casey, J M I H
Chowcat, N L
Chui, D K C
Clarke, H J
Cook, J H
Cooke, R P D
Cookey, I P
Coutts, G M
Curry, P S
D'Arcy, J C
Darwent, A
De Muinck Keizer, J W
Deery, R W
Dickens, P R
Dimond, J P
Dugan, U M
Dunk, A A
Durrani, A-R
Edwards, R E
Elliott, D H
Emslie, A J
Evans, G H C
Evans, S K
Evason, M R
Eyre, S J
Fan, Y S
Folwell, G A J
Forster, R A
Francis, K M J
Frisby, P A
Gaffney, M S J
Garlick, D J
George, L
Gietzen, T W
Gilmour, A M
Ginimav, S P
Gover, P A
Grace, R J
Hargreaves, J N
Hobbs, S D
Hughes, D V
Hunt, C B M
Inayat, M
Isibor, F O
Jackson, L V
James, S E
Kamugisha, C K
Kelleher, B J
Kinder, J
King, T A
Kinniburgh, N A
Kisler, J D
Lawrence, W T
Leeson, K E
Liddell, K
Liebenberg, M
Livingston, S
Lofts, J A
Lytton, S T
McGregor, R R
McNally, S A
McNaughton, I C
Malak, T M
Manjaly, G
Marchbank, N D P
Marshall, M F P
Martyr, J W
Masotina, A
Matin-Siddiqi, S A
Maxwell, D L
Miller, W G

Moffat, C J C
Murray, H G S
Murray, M E
Myerson, K R
Mynott, M J
Nahhas, A S
Nash, P J
Nicholls, S
Nicoll, S J B
Noble, G E
Northrop, M M
O'Brien, P J
Parker, A P
Patel, N R
Paterson, I W
Pawley, S E
Plumb, A P
Prosser, J K
Rabuszko, J P
Rajendra, S
Richards, D J
Richardson, T N A
Rimington, P D
Robertson, D E
Ross, K R
Ruffell, E A
Salam, M A
Sallomi, D F
Sasada, K
Saunders, M P
Scarisbrick, P H
Shawcross, J
Sheikh, M A
Shepherd, C D
Shepherd, P R
Simpson, J M W
Squires, M J
Steer, B
Stewart, A N
Stockton, M G
Stone, J M
Stoodley, B J
Sulke, A N
Surtees, S J
Taha, A S A
Thomas, H F
Vickery, K
Waddy, R S
Walmsley, A J
Walter, M
Walton, S M
Warren, G A R
Waters, S J
Watson, G M
Watson, N A
Wearmouth, E M
Westlake, A C
Wilkinson, J R W
Williams, P G
Wojtulewski, J A
Writer, M D L
Zakrzewski, K K

Eastleigh
Aley, M C
Anderson, D F
Arden, C D
Babar, J L
Balachandra, K
Black, G H
Bodagh, I Y O
Brodrick-Webb, C A
Brough, B J
Browning, A C
Burbidge, A A
Carter, R C
Chaplin Rogers, S P
Chojnowska, E I
Clark, L-J
Colmsee, M R
Connolly, E A
Courtney, P M
D'Arcy, A H E
Dakeyne, M A
Das, A
Drabu, R K
Dunger, G T
Egan, J N T
Ezad, L
Ezad, M A
Farmer, I F
Fitchet, M Q
Foote, G A
Forrest, L V
Fowler, K M A
Fox, A D
Frank, T G
Gardner, A C
Gavin, J

Godfrey, P K
Goodbody, R A
Gorrod, E R
Greenhalgh, J H
Gregory, K L
Gupta, M P
Harvey, A R
Hillam, A C
Hood, W A F
Humphries, S A
Jenner, C E
Kell, G
Latham, J M
Lavanchy, O R
Lee, S K M
Liakos, G M
Luff, A J
McAulay, J
McCarthy, M E
Manners, J M
Morgan, A T
Murphy, D P
Murphy, H R
Olson, J J
Patel, P
Peckham, C L
Pickvance, N J
Rickenbach, M A
Rowen, D
Sadler, C J
Sadler, M A
Salmon, A P
Shearer, J R
Tansley, M C
Terry, J M
Turner, A M
Walker, J
Ward, S A P
Weavind, G P
Whyte, S P
Williamson, J F

Ebbw Vale
Alford, G
Davies, S W
Goddard, L
Hunt, L E
Jain, A K
Khan, M R
Mohindru, A C
Morgan, J H
Morgan, W D
Nookaraju, K
Pitman, I J
Rice, K J
Sodhi, S S
Sodhi, S P S
Varshney, G K
Wasim, M
Williams, D W
Yorke, R J
Yousu Kunju, M

Edenbridge
Bayley, T R L
Eclair-Heath, C M
Garrett, T Y
Gillespie, M M
Ilsley, M D
Jones, B R
Kelly, K B
King, L E
Milner, B S
Morrison, S J
Shaw, J H T
Spear, B S
Williams, S A

Edgware
Abenyeka-Nunma, P O K O
Ahluwalia, S M S
Ajitsaria, R
Alam, S K
Amin, S P
Annear, J M
Arora, N
Bard, V
Barnard, M E
Beney, J C
Braham, D L
Briggs, B H J
Chakraborty, C
Challis, D M
Cooklin, M
D'Costa, R A F J
Davies, H J
Davis, S
Dey, A

Fernandes, A L C
Ferris, M
Festenstein, J B
Feuchtwang-Foy, J N H
Gainza, C F A
Ganesh, T
Goldmeier, D
Gondhia, A
Goonawardana, P R
Gordon, H
Gugenheim, P S
Harman, W B
Hommel, L
Hopkins, W B
Hornik, R J
Hossain, S
Huelser, R E
Ikkos, G
Jain, P
Kapacee, D R C
Kapse, A A
Kapse, N A
Kawsar, M
Kearney, T M
Keni, M
Kirpalani, G
Kohll, S J M
Krasner, D H
Kurian, K M
Makanji, H
Malik, A
Manning, A D
Manning, G L
Manzur, K M A
Matin, M W
Maybaum, S W
Mei Yuk Luk, Dr
Miller, H
Moodaley, D
Mtandabari, T M R
Nagpaul, S
Narendran, P
O'Shea, E M A
Pampel, M M
Parsons, G M
Patel, A M
Patel, N R
Patel, S
Patel, S K
Pinto, Z A
Platt, S R
Psiachou-Leonard, E
Rampes, H
Roberts, L L
Rosenberg, D
Rozewicz, E
Saldanha, M B Y
Sanyal, A
Saraf, I M
Sbano, H
Scambler, S M
Schipperheijn, J A M
Shah, J
Shah, K
Shah, K K
Shah, R C
Shamsuddin, A B
Sharman, G
Shelley, S A
Sivasanker, K
Small, N M W
Songra, A K
Stephenson, L K
Susman, R D
Taktak, S G
Tharumaratnam, D B
Trafford, P A
Varughese, P S
Wagman, L
Weinbrenn, G H
Wyndham, M T
Zabetaki, E
Zahir, M

Edinburgh
Abdelkader, M M F
Abernethy, P
Abernethy, P J
Adams, A D
Adams, L J
Affleck, R L
Affolter, J T
Airlie, M A A
Aitken, J
Aitken, R J
Akram, A P
Akroyd, S A
Akyol, A M

Al-Shahi, R
Al-Nafussi, A I A
Aldridge, L M
Aldridge, R D
Alexander, W D
Allan, A G L
Allan, D J M
Allan, J R
Allan, P L P
Allan, S R
Allison, M E
Alston, R P
Anderson, C E
Anderson, E D C
Anderson, K M
Anderson, K D
Anderson, M E
Anderson, N H
Anderson, R A
Andrews, J M
Angus, M M
Annan, F J
Annan, I H
Archibald, F L M
Armstrong, E M
Arnstein, F E
Arthurson, I H
Ashfaq, I
Ashley, R H
Auckland, K J
Avery, B J
Aw, J
Ayles, A C M
Aylward, R L M
Ayub, M
Bailey, L
Bain, D
Bain, E M
Bain, M R S
Baird, D T
Balfour, R F
Ballantyne, A
Bancroft, P J
Bancroft, T P
Barclay, G P T
Barlee, R J
Barnes, C F
Barron, M C
Bartolo, D C C
Bashir, F A
Bashir, W A
Bateman, D N
Bath, L E
Bathgate, A J
Baylis, P J
Beach, C A D
Beal, T A
Beamish, D
Beattie, T F
Becher, J-C
Beedel, A
Beggs, I
Bell, A M R
Bell, J E
Bell, K
Bell, M F J
Bell, N J
Bellamy, C O C
Bennison, J M
Bennison, J M
Benton, E C
Benton, T F
Benzie, S J
Berg, J N
Berger, G E
Bickler, C B
Birkett, E S
Bisset, A F
Bissett, E M
Black, F M
Black, G
Black, R N H
Blackwell, C D
Blackwood, D R
Blaikie, K J
Blair, A S
Blake, S J
Bloomfield, P
Bloomfield, S M
Bodasing, N
Boeing, L
Bolland, W T
Bolton, R E
Bond, A J
Bond, I D
Boon, N A
Boron, I
Bouki, K
Bowler, G M R

Box, S A
Boyd, A C
Boyd, G
Bracewell, A C E
Brackenbury, E T
Bradbury, M D
Bradbury, P
Bremner, A R F
Brettle, R P
Brewster, D H
Briggs, L M
Brittenden, J
Broadbent, M R
Brockington, A R
Bronte-Stewart, C M
Brookman, C A
Brotherston, K G
Brough, M D
Brown, A D G
Brown, C
Brown, D R
Brown, D T
Brown, D C
Brown, J C R
Brown, K J A
Brown, L M
Brown, O J
Brown, S
Brown, T S
Browning, G G P
Bruce, M S
Brush, J P
Bryan, I R J
Brydon, R A
Brydone, G F C
Buchan, A S
Buchan, J A
Buchanan, R B
Buck, S M
Buckley, E G
Bull, M W
Burnett, H M
Burnett, R
Burnett, R C S C
Burns-Brown, I L
Burns, J E
Burns, S M
Burt, A J
Burt, J P
Bury, J K
Busuttil, A
Buttery, R C
Byrne, M P
Caesar, D H
Cairns, D A
Cairns, M J
Calder, A A
Calvert, J M
Calvert, S H S
Cameron, A V
Cameron, D A
Cameron, G
Cameron, H S
Cameron, J M
Cameron, S T
Camidge, D R
Campbell, A S
Campbell, B C
Campbell, C
Campbell, D A
Campbell, F A
Campbell, H
Campbell, J P M
Campbell, W A
Cannon, N
Cantley, P M
Caplin, B D
Carey, F A
Carmichael, G L M
Carruthers, D B
Carter, T A H
Casey, J J
Cash, M P
Cavanagh, J T O
Cay, S E B
Chaddock, M E
Chadwick, A E P
Chalmers-Watson, C E
Chalmers-Watson, T A
Chalmers, J W T
Chalmers, R T A
Chalmers, S R
Chalmers, T M
Chapman, B J
Chapman, J S
Chapman, M E
Chapman, N C
Charnley, N G
Chaudhry, M T
Chawla, H B
Cheesman, C A
Chevassut, T J T
Chew, I S H
Chick, J D
Chin, D M F
Chiswick, D
Choo, C H
Christie, J
Christie, J E
Chui, E-C
Clark, V A
Clive, S
Clouter, M A
Codispoti, M
Cohen, K D J W
Coia, J E
Cole, S K
Colledge, N R
Collie, D A
Collingham, N T
Colver, H M
Colvin, L A
Comiskey, G A
Conlon, C F
Connan, A L
Connolly, K C
Cooper, E J
Cooper, G
Corbett, G T
Cormack, C R H
Cornbleet, M A
Cosgrove, L E
Cowan, C
Cowan, D L
Cowan, J
Cowell, M M
Cowie, V J
Cox, N M
Cozens, A L
Craig, G
Cramond, S A C
Craven, J M
Crawford, C E H
Crawford, D H
Crean, A M
Creed, J J
Cremona, F R
Cresswell, J E
Crichton, A
Crichton, J H M
Crispin, J D
Crispin, J R
Critchley, H O D
Crofts, F M
Crofts, T-J
Crompton, G K
Cronin, H M B
Crookes, D P
Crosbie, P A J
Cross, M D
Crosswaite, A G
Cull, R E
Cullen, A K
Cullen, M J
Cumming, A D
Cunningham, S
Cupples, W A
Currie, C T
Currie, I H
Currie, J R M
Curtis, A
Da Costa, J A G
Dalgleish, J
Dalkin, T J
Dall, G F
Dames, G
Darling, K E A
Davenport, R J
Davidson, A W
Davidson, E D L
Davidson, E M
Davidson, K L
Davidson, K
Davie, E G
Davie, I T
Davies, M J
Davies, P E
Davies, S J
Dawson, L K
De Beaux, A C
De Beaux, I
Deary, I J
Deery, C H
Delvaux, A
Denison, F C
Denison, R S
Dennis, M S
Dennis, R E
Denvir, M A
Devey, L R
Dhall, P
Dhillon, B
Dhillon, V B
Diamond, R L
Dickson, E M
Dickson, J E A
Dickson, M A S
Dickson, R I
Dimigen, M
Din, N A
Dixon, J M J
Dixon, R E J
Dobbie, J W
Dobbin, A E
Dobson, G A
Dodds, A D
Doherty, V R
Donald, A G
Donald, J B
Donald, S M
Donaldson, K
Donat, R
Donnelly, J G
Donnelly, M P
Donnelly, S C
Donovan, W R
Douglas, A J
Douglas, N J
Dow, R J
Dowling, N J
Downie, R G
Doyle, P R
Drake, A J
Drever, J H
Drewitt, D J N
Drewitt, H P
Drummond, D C
Drummond, G B
Duncan, L E
Duncan, M E
Duncan, W
Duncan, W C
Dundas, S
Dunhill, Z M
Dunlop, A
Dunn, J L
Dunn, M J G
Duvall, E
Ebmeier, K P
Edington, J H R
Edmunds, W T
Edwards, H V
Eglinton, D J
El Hag, O A O
El-Khatib, A R R
Elder, A T
Ellis, R A
Elmubarak, M Y
Elswood, R
Emmanuel, F X S
Emond, M W
Ennis, J E
Ennis, J S A
Erridge, S C
Errington, J R
Errington, M L
Eunson, G J
Evans, C D J
Evans, G C
Evans, J I
Evason, S E
Ewart, D W
Ewing, F M E
Ewing, K A
Faccenda, J F
Fair, J F
Fairhurst, K
Fallon, M T
Farah, H H
Farmer, K D
Farquharson, D I M
Fawcett, P G
Fearon, K C H
Fentiman, G J
Fenton, I S
Ferguson, A
Ferguson, C A
Ferguson, M J
Fergusson, R J
Fernandez Dair, N
Fettes, M R
Fineron, P W
Fink, G
Finlayson, N D C
Finnie, L R
Fisher, J A C
Fitzgerald, T
Fitzpatrick, D R
Flapan, A D
Fleck, B W
Fleming, P A
Fleming, S
Foo, I T H
Forbes, F C M
Forbes, G I
Forbes, K
Forbes, W
Fordyce, D T
Forfar, I M L
Forsey, J H
Forsyth, K C
Forsythe, J L R
Foster, C A
Fowkes, F G R
Fox, K A A
Foy, R C
Francis, C M
Francis, R R M
Franks, K L
Fraser, A K
Fraser, D R K
Fraser, S C A
Freeman, C P L
Freeman, J A
Freestone, S
Freshwater, J V
Fried, M J
Frier, B M
Fulford, P E
Galea, G
Gallagher, J M C
Gallivan, P R
Garden, O J
Gardner, D L
Gardner, K M
Garner, J A M
Gaskell, P A
Gatiss, S-J
Gebbie, A E
Gemmell, H M
George, C M
George, F O
Geraghty, J R
Ghaly, A F F
Gibb, A P
Gibson, D A
Gibson, J N A
Gibson, P H
Gibson, R J
Gilchrist, J J
Gillespie, I N
Gillingham, F J
Gillon, J
Gilmour, H M
Glasier, A F
Glaze, R C J
Glen, E M
Glen, J L
Glen, S K
Gold, H J
Gonzalez Prieto, M C
Gordon, A C
Gourlay, K A
Gow, G
Gowans, I D
Graham, L J C
Grant, D J
Grant, I S
Grant, L J C
Grant, N A
Grant, R
Grant, S M
Gray, D A
Gray, H C
Greening, A P
Greer, J R
Gregor, A
Greig, L D
Grieve, D C
Grieve, F J
Griffiths, J M T
Grigor, H
Grigor, J
Grigor, K M
Gronski, M J
Grubb, M A
Gunn, J M
Gunn, W J
Gurmin, V J
Guthrie, B
Gutierrez Rodriguez, A
Habeshaw, M J
Hailey, J A
Hall, A M
Hall, R J P
Hallam, N F
Halloran, E M
Hamer-Hodges, D W
Hamill, A M
Hamilton, H R
Hamilton, J M S
Hamilton, M I
Handyside, R
Hanley, J P
Hannaford, P F
Hannon, P A C
Hanson, M F
Hardie, C L
Hargreave, T B
Harkin, C
Harkness, R A
Harris, P A
Harrison, A R
Harrison, D J
Harrison, N
Harrison, R E
Hart, S P
Harvey, F M K
Haslam, C J
Haughney, M G J
Hawkins, J W
Haydon, G H
Hayes, P C
Hayward, R L
Heidemann, B H
Henderson, C E A
Henderson, K
Henderson, L F
Henderson, R N
Henderson, R E
Hendry, S J
Henriksen, P A
Henry, C N M
Hepburn, T
Hepple, P A
Herbert, I
Hewitt, A N M
Hill, J
Hintjens, K L
Hiremath, K
Hoare, P
Hodgson, M M
Holland, P J P
Hollingdale, E E
Hollis, S
Holloway, A J
Holmes, S-E J
Holton, D W
Holton, F A
Homer, D E
Hook, A C P
Horn, H M
Horne, P M
Hornibrook, S C
Horsburgh, J C
Horsfall, H S C
Hosie, J E
Howard, G C W
Howard, R G
Howie, C R
Howie, G M
Huby, C L
Hughes, D J
Hughes, J E
Hughes, M L
Hughes, R G
Hunter, A J C
Hunter, I
Hunter, J M
Hunter, J A A
Huntly, B J P
Hurst, J R
Hutchison, J K
Hutton, C L
Iliffe, A L
Illingworth, S G M
Imray, E A
Inglis, J H C
Ingram, S M
Innes, E M
Innes, J A
Inwood, J M
Ireland, H M
Ironside, J W
Ironside, J A D
Ironside, M J
Irvine, D S
Irvine, W J
Irving, R J
Jaap, A J
Jack, W J L
Jackson, P D
Jalan, A R
Jamie, G M
Jamieson, N S D
Jamieson, W S
Jamnicky, L
Jellinek, E H
Jenkins, A M
Jenkins, J
Jenkins, M G
Jigajinni, M V
Jodrell, D I
Johnson, G A
Johnson, P R E
Johnstone, E C
Johnstone, F D
Johnstone, M M
Jolliffe, D W
Jones, C W
Jones, R I A
Jordan, L B
Jordan, L J
Kamel, H M H
Kaufman, M H
Kavanagh, G M
Keating, J F
Keel, A M
Keeling, J W
Kellett, R J
Kelly, C A
Kelly, K P
Kelman, J R
Kelman, L
Kelnar, C J H
Kemmett, D
Kent, J A
Kent, V J
Ker, J S
Kerr, A I G
Kerr, I J
Kerr, J M
Kerr, N G D
Khalifa, B E B
Kidd, S L
King, M R G
Kirkup, J R
Kirwan, E V
Knox, K W
Kondracki, S G
Kreitman, N B
Kuenssberg, B V
Kunkler, I H
Kurt-Elli, S L
Labinjoh, C
Laing, I A
Lakhdar, A A
Lam Shang Leen, C
Lamb, D I H
Lamb, K
Lamb, P J
Lambert, C M
Lambie, S H
Lane, O S
Lang, C C E
Lang, F H
Lang, H M
Lang, J A
Langa Ferreira, B A
Latham, T
Laurenson, I F
Lawrie, S M
Lawson, C S
Lawson, G M
Lawson, R A
Lawson, S R
Le Fevre, P D
Learmonth, A C
Leckie, A M
Leckie, S M
Lee, A
Lee, D
Leitch, J E B
Lello, G E
Leonard, P A
Leonard, R C F
Lessells, A M
Lessells, K M
Leung, R C-Y
Levack, P A
Lever, M J
Lewin, C A
Lewis, J
Liddle, R E
Lim, C S
Lim, W C
Lindsay, R S
Liston, W A
Little, F A
Little, K
Littlechild, P
Littlewood, D G
Lloyd, E L
Lodge, A M

Lodge, M C
Logan, M R
Logie, L J
Loh, D L
Lord, H K
Lorenzo Gallego, S
Lorge, M A
Lorimer, S M R
Lossock, F H
Loudon, J A Z
Low, G W Y
Lowry, L M
Ludlam, C A
Lumsden, G R
Luqmani, R A
Lyall, R M
Lyon, A J
Lyon, W M M
McAlister, C A
McAndrew, L J H
McArdle, C S
Macari, A C
Macartney, M M
Macaulay, R A A
McAuslane, S E
McBirnie, J M
McCall-Smith, E D A
McCallum, J R
MacCallum, L R
McClelland, D B L
McClure, J H
McCool, H J
McCord, N
McCowen, E M
McCrae, A F
McCulloch, G J
McCulloch, I M
McCullough, C T
McDermott, R A
McDonald, C F
MacDonald, E R
Macdonald, I D
Macdonald, K
MacDonald, L A
MacDougall, G M
MacDougall, M W J
MacDuff, A
McElearney, N L G
McFadyen, I J
MacFarlane, R M
McFee, L L M
Macfie, J A
McGalloway, B A
MacGilchrist, A J
McGoogan, E
McGregor, A H
McGregor, C J
McGregor, G
McGregor, J C
McGuigan, C C
McGuigan, P S
McHale, S J
MacHale, S M
McHardy, G J R
McIlwaine, G M
McIntosh, A H
Mcintosh, A F
McIntosh, A M
McIntosh, C E
McIntosh, N
MacIntyre, D J
MacIntyre, I M C
McIntyre, M A
Macintyre, S C
McKain, A D
Mackay, A
Mackay, A R
Mackay, G R
McKay, I I
Mackay, T W
Mackean, M J
McKee, I H
Mackenzie, A
McKenzie, A G
Mackenzie, C J R
MacKenzie, C D
Mackenzie, J
MacKenzie, J R
Mackenzie, J E
McKenzie, K J
Mackenzie, P A P
Mackenzie, S B P
Mackenzie, S J
Mackenzie, S
Mackenzie, S
Mackenzie, W C
McKeown, D W
Mackie, C F
Mackie, M J
Mackie, S E R
MacKinlay, G A
Mackinnon, H F
Mackinnon, H L
Mackinnon, R K J
McKnight, J A
MacLachlan, D C
McLaren, D B
MacLaren, F B
McLaren, J A
McLaren, K M
McLaren, R C
McLean, A M
McLean, C M
Maclean, M H
MacLean, M E
McLellan, S A
McLennan, J M
MacLennan, W J
MacLeod, A D
MacLeod, C M
MacLeod, J G
Mcleod, K A
Macleod, M R
Macleod, M A
McLeod, N W
McLeod, C J
MacLullich, A M J
McMillan, A
Macmillan, I M M
McMillan, S A
McMillan, T M
McNamara, N J
MacNee, W
MacNeil, C
McNeill, S A
Macnicol, M F
McNiven, A C
McPartlin, G M
Macpherson, A G H
MacPherson, H D
Macpherson, S G
McPhillips, M A
McQueen, M M
McRorie, E R
McVean, A E
Mahadevan, M M
Main, T D
Maingay, C H
Mander, B J
Manders, D N
Mankad, P S
Manson, T W
Maran, A G
Marsden, A K
Marshall, A F
Marshall, H
Martin, H M
Mason-Apps, S P
Mason, B P
Mason, J K F
Masterton, G
Matheson, G H
Matheson, L M
Matthews, A G
Mattick, A P
Maudsley, I M
Maule, M M
Mayer, N J
Maynard, C A
Mee, B
Melvin, W D
Menon, G
Mepham, S O
Merino, SV
Merricks, E K
Mervyn-Thomas, J W
Metcalf, J
Middleton, A J
Middleton, W G
Midgley, S
Millar, A M
Miller, H C
Miller, K A
Miller, N M
Miller, R J
Milligan, G R
Mills, R P
Millwater, C J
Milne, C A
Milne, J A
Mishra, P
Mitchell, C
Mitchell, D H
Mitchell, I D C
Moffat, I A
Moffat, R C E
Moffoot, A P R
Mohamed, F
Mohan, M
Moir, A T B
Moir, F M
Moir, S B
Mok, J Y Q
Monaghan, H
Moor, S
Moralee, S J
Morgan, K P
Morley, H S
Morris, E J B
Morrison, A G
Morrison, A
Morrison, D P
Morrison, F M
Morrison, M M
Morton, C M
Morton, C P J
Morton, D N
Morton, S L
Moultrie, S J
Mounstephen, A H
Mountain, D A
Moussa, S A
Mukherji, P S
Mumford, C J
Munro, F D
Murchison, J T
Murie, J A
Murphy, T J C
Murray, A W
Murray, H M
Murray, I E L
Murray, J G
Murray, J E
Murray, M
Murray, N S
Murray, S A
Mushtaq, T
Myerscough, P R
Myles, L M
Myskow, L M
Nagle, R S
Neil, J R K
Nelson, F R
Newby, D E
Nicholson, S
Nickerson, C B
Nicol, S G
Nicoll, J A
Nimmo, A F
Nimmo, G R
Nimmo, J
Nimmo, S M
Nimmo, W S
Nixon, D L
Nixon, S J
Noble, K W
Northridge, D B
Norton, B
Nuki, G
Nussey, F E
Nutton, R W
O'Donnell, M
O'Hare, A E
O'Neill, J M
O'Neill, K M
O'Neill, O B
O'Neill, W M
Ogilvie, M M
Ojar, D H
Oliver, C W
Ong, E K
Orr, J A
Orr, J D
Osifodunrin, O O O
Ostrowski, N M J
Oswald, J
Owen, M
Owens, D G C
Oxenham, H C
Paisley, A M
Palmer, K S
Palmer, K R
Papachrysostomou Evgenikos, M
Parker, S S
Parks, R W
Parris, M R
Partridge, J M
Patel, D K B
Paterson-Brown, S P
Paterson-Brown, S
Paterson, A
Paterson, D R
Paterson, I
Paterson, J W
Paterson, R L
Paterson, S M
Patrick, A W
Patterson, W J
Peat, M L
Pedder, C E
Penman, I D
Penny, J M
Pentland, B
Perry, C H
Peters, J A
Peutherer, J F
Phanjoo, A L
Phelps, R G
Philip, L
Phillips, C I
Phillips, H A
Phillips, J
Phillips, J E
Pilkington, A
Piris, M
Plant, W D
Plevris, I
Plews, D E
Polson, H W M
Pope, D G
Porteous, M E M
Porter, D E
Potter, G M
Potts, S G
Pound, S E
Prendergast, A E
Price, A
Price, G M
Price, G C
Price, J F
Prince, K L
Pugh, G C
Pullen, I M
Purdie, D W
Purdue, B N
Quaba, A-A-R A
Quinn, T J
Raczkowski, R M
Rae, H H
Rae, P W H
Rajack, S M
Ralston, S H
Ramkissoon, A M
Ramsay, D A
Ramsay, L J
Ramsay, R G
Rasool, T P
Ray, D C
Ray, R E
Raza, Z
Razzaq, G
Read, H S
Redhead, D N
Redpath, C J
Reeves, I C
Regan, C C
Reid, A G
Reid, A G
Reid, D A
Reid, F M
Reid, W A
Reiss, J E
Reive, A R
Rennie, L M
Rhein, H M
Richardson, J M
Riches, H I
Rigden, J
Rigg, R C
Rimmer, C S
Rimmer, S
Ritchie, C M D
Ritchie, E L
Ritson, E B
Robb, J E
Robbins, A G
Roberts, J
Robertson, G
Robertson, J R
Robertson, J M
Robertson, M J C
Robertson, P J
Robertson, P
Robinson, C M
Robison, C
Robson, M J A
Roddie, P H
Rodgers, A J C
Rodgers, H C
Rodgers, H J
Rogers, C E
Rooney, M M E
Rose, M
Rosie, H A
Ross, F M H
Ross, I R F
Ross, L A
Ross, M T
Ross, P J
Rothwell, P M
Rowney, D A
Royle, H M
Russell, E B A W
Russell, G T
Russell, K A
Russell, L F M
Russell, T
Ruth, M J
Rutledge, M L C
Rutledge, P
Ryan, M F
Rycroft, H D
Sala Tenna, A M
Salem, R J
Sandercock, P A G
Sanders, R
Sanderson, R J
Sangra, M S
Santana Hernandez, D J
Sargent, W
Savill, J S
Savin, J A
Saweirs, W W M
Schneider, V
Schofield, O M V M
Scott, A
Scott, A I F
Scott, C J
Scott, D H T
Scott, E A J
Scott, G J C
Scott, G R
Scott, M
Scott, P M
Scott, R J
Searl, C P
Seaton, A
Seckl, J R
Seiler, E R
Sellar, R J
Seth, S A
Seyfollahi, S
Shand, A G
Sharpe, F M
Sharpe, M C
Sharwood-Smith, G H
Shaw, R J
Shaw, T R D
Sheikh, A
Shepherd, A M
Shepherd, P C A
Shiels, R M
Sim, J S N
Sime, J L
Simmons, C M
Simon, E J
Simpson, A H R W
Simpson, C A
Simpson, D L
Simpson, H
Simpson, K J
Sinclair, A A
Sinclair, C J
Sinclair, F M
Singh, J
Skene, C G
Skinner, F M
Skinner, R
Slater, E M
Slater, E
Slatford, K
Slorach, C A
Small, M J
Smart, G E
Smith, A I
Smith, A D S
Smith, A F
Smith, B J
Smith, G
Smith, J E
Smith, J K
Smith, S J
Smith, T J S
Smithson, N J
Smyth, J F
Sneddon, D J C
Sojitra, N M
Somerville, E M
Song, S H
Soon, S Y
Soutar, C A
Soutar, I
Soutter, F A
Spence, A A
Spens, H J
Spiller, J A
St. John, H E
Stanley, M C
Stansfield, M H
Stark, M J
Starkey, I R
Starr, J M
Starritt, N E
Statham, P F X
Steers, A J W
Stein, K W T
Stenson, B J
Stephenson, R N
Stevenson, A J M
Stevenson, A G
Stevenson, D J D
Stevenson, J E
Stevenson, L V
Stewart, A R
Stewart, A J
Stewart, B J C
Stewart, E A
Stewart, G T
Stewart, I C
Stewart, L H
Stewart, R A L
Stewart, R C
Stewart, W G
Steyn, J P
Stirling, A M
Stone, J
Storey, D
Struthers, R A
Stuart, J C
Stuart, W P
Sudlow, C L M
Sudlow, E M
Sudlow, M F
Sumeray, M S
Sutherland, G R
Sutherland, J K
Sutherland, K A
Sutherland, R W
Swainson, C P
Swarbrick, P J
Sykes, C J
Symmers, W S C
Tait, W A
Tannahill, A J
Tay, C C K
Taylor, D M
Taylor, F
Taylor, J C G W
Taylor, J
Taylor, L M
Taylor, S G
Telfer, A H
Telfer, J R C
Temple, C M
Than Nyunt, M P
Theodosiou, C A
Therapondos, G P
Thomas, A E
Thomas, J S J
Thomas, M J C
Thompson, C I
Thompson, E J
Thompson, J R
Thompson, J M
Thompson, M J
Thomson, A J
Thomson, C M
Thomson, D M
Thomson, D G
Thomson, K J
Thomson, L D G
Thomson, L A
Thomson, P G
Thomson, S A
Thorn, J B
Thyne, D H S
Tidman, J S M
Tidman, M J
Ting, A Y-H
Todd, I C
Todd, J R C
Todd, W G
Toft, A D
Toft, N J
Tolley, D A
Tolley, M S
Torrance, A M E
Torres, M D R C
Tothill, S A
Treasure, W
Tripathi, D
Tripp, J C S

Trotter, S H
Tulloch, D N
Tulloch, L J
Turnbull, C M
Turnbull, L W
Turner, A N
Turner, D
Turner, M L
Turney, T M
Twiddy, P J
Tybulewicz, A T
Underwood, J R
Uren, N G
Uttley, J M C
Uttley, W R
Varma, K B
Varma, M
Varma, S
Venters, B
Virgo, M A
Wadehra, V
Walayat, M
Walker-Kinnear, M H
Walker, B R
Walker, D E
Walker, F C
Walker, G A
Walker, J C
Walker, J
Walker, S W
Wall, L R
Wallace, A M
Wallace, C J
Wallace, G M F
Wallace, I W J
Wallace, N W
Wallace, W H B
Wallis, C B
Walls, E W
Walmsley, F J
Walsh, J S J
Walsh, T S
Walton, H J
Ward, H J T
Wardlaw, J M
Warlow, C P
Warnock, S M
Waterer, S C
Watson, F E
Watson, G M
Watson, M L
Watson, P A
Watson, R A M
Watson, S J W
Watt, G
Watt, K P
Watts, D A
Webb, D J
Weller, R P J B
Welsby, P D
Wenham, V C
Wharton, S B
Whatling, P J
Whimster, J H
White, I R
White, L J
White, P G
Whitley, M W
Whittle, I R
Whittle, J R S
Whitwell, J R
Whitworth, C E
Whitworth, D M
Whyte, H
Widdowson, J
Wight, R M
Wightman, A J A
Wigmore, S J
Wild, S R
Wildgoose, C D
Wilks, D P
Will, D J
Will, R G
Williams, A H
Williams, A R W
Williams, A T
Williams, H J
Williams, L P
Williams, M J
Williams, R J
Williamson, J
Wilson-Storey, D
Wilson, A G
Wilson, D C
Wilson, D M
Wilson, D F
Wilson, E S
Wilson, E G
Wilson, I M
Wilson, J A
Wilson, L M
Winney, R J
Wong, J K F
Wong, N A C S
Wood, B R
Wood, M J
Woodburn, K J
Wright, A F
Wright, D J
Wright, E
Wright, M R
Wyatt, J P
Yap, P L
Young, A
Young, I E
Young, I W
Young, M J
Young, P M
Young, S M M
Yuille, F A P
Zamvar, V Y
Zealley, H E
Zealley, K E
Zegleman, F E
Zeman, A Z J

Egham

Allen, E B
Bethel, R G H
Brand, N S
Burmanroy, S
Elliott, J V
Galazka, L S
Galazka, N M I
Hawk, L J
Kidd, S J
Morris, R O
Nicholson, P J
Pavesi, L A
Priestley, V R
Salmon, R P
Vaughan-Davies, S L
Warwicker, P M
Whiteley, J D

Egremont

Bewick, M
Creed, A L N
Gallacher, R H
Galloway, F D
Goodman, S E
Heijne Den Bak, J
Jakobson, R A
Veitch, J W

Elgin

Albiston, E M
Anderson, D J S
Anderson, D M
Bagnall, R A
Bedford, S J
Bredell, P M
Brown, D F
Brown, K M
Cartwright, B L
Chen, T M C H
Dawson, G A W
Duthie, G M
Evans, D C
Fell, L F
Findlay, P F
Ghanim, S N
Gunn, I G
Harper, I
Hart, C L
Hawkins, J L
Henderson, M G
Hodges, A E
Hornsby, C A
Houliston, M D
Johnston, M I
Lim, M-N
Lowe, R J
MacEachen, M L
McFarlane, C
McFarlane, D E
McIntyre, R
McLauchlan, A J W
McPherson, A
Maitland, H M
Miller, J D B
Milne, G G
Mitchell, F L
Mobbs, J M
Morrison, W M
Morrison, Y A
Nash, C H
Nicol, J W
Pearson, R L
Robertson, J G
Rodger, A B
Simpson, A I
Stewart, R D M
Taylor, G R
Taylor, J C
Tennant, N J
Todd, J O
Trew, J M
Trythall, J
Walker, K J
Wilson, J T

Elland

Bylina, E P
Clarkson, J E
Holroyd, J B M
James, T E
Naz, E M
Naz, F
Parmar, P P
Spencer, S F

Ellesmere

Morgan-Jones, R L
Newton, S J
Richards, P A
Wess, J M

Ellesmere Port

Bowman, S N
Chitty, R N
Dowson, J T
Faulks, G
Judge, A P
Seddon, D J
Stringer, J
Wall, C E
Wall, C M
Warren, F M
Wearne, J P
Wilkinson, J F

Ellon

Bell, R M R
Brown, P J
Burgess, C S
Burnett, R J
Chisholm, R I
Donaldson, A E
Mackay, D I
McKerchar, D J
Morrison, W J
Murphy, P A
Pearson, A R
Penney, G C
Pucci, M J
Simpson, I T
Stephen, H J
Taylor, M
Walker, D M

Ely

Aniskowicz, J S
Baker, I H
Barltrop, A H
Bond, C A
Burnford, R P
Byrne, M M
Coupe, L C
Devereux, J G J
Dober, M H
Douglas, A S
Dunn, A J
England, M
Findlay, S C
George, A M
Green, A J
Harding, S E
Holt, J
Horne, C R
Howard, J E
Hughes, J P
Kenny, P
King, S L
Lindsay, I D
Lynch, V J
McBryde, C W
McCormack, D H P T
McHugh, J
Martin, A P
Mee, S E
Molyneux, A H
Morgan, A M
Norris, K L
O'Connell, C R W
Partha, J
Ragu, H K S
Shackleton, J R
Smith, H L
Tierney, D M
Woods, D G
Young, K M

Emsworth

Allen, P
Atkinson, C L
Baker, N J
Bale, R N
Bateman, J E
Bateman, N D
Bowen, A H
Collings-Wells, J S
Crundwell, N B
Cummins, S J G
Edsell, M E G
Foley, M E M
Gale, C W
Griffiths, W E G
Hertzog, J L
Hollis, M J
Ingram, D L
Kelway, S P
Kirkham, P W
Knight, K E
McDonald, G E
Newman, P M
Richardson, G A
Ryland, J M
Seymour-Jones, J A
Seymour, E J
Shannon, C J
Speed, C A
Sussex, J E
Taylor, S M
Thomas, A L
Thomas, D J
Thomas, P M A
Tibbs, P G
Tilley, E A
Vinnicombe, J
Wright, I A
Yeld, R O

Enfield

Akinkunmi, A
Al Ayoubi, A
Amarin, J O
Amin, N
Andrews, H T T
Appleton, H
Archibald, D A A
Arnold, J A
Attalla, F E
Balachandran, T
Barnes, M A
Barnes, P
Baynes, C
Beeharry, R
Benjamin, L D
Bryant, C A
Bukhari, N A S
Bull, R K
Bull, T M
Carmi, M A M B
Carrick, J C
Chahal, R
Challis, J H
Chan, K H
Chang, C T N
Chatterjee, K
Clark, E
Coffey, M S
Conacher, R S R
Connaughton, J T
Copland, R F P
Craig, A R
Croft, R J
D'Souza, A S
Davies, R H
De Taranto, N E
Devereux, M H
Dissanayake, H R M
Donnelly, P F
Downes, E G R
Duffield, G A
Duignan, I J C M
Eldon, H M
Erkeller-Yuksel, M F
Fajemisin, B A
Farag, M Z M
Fryszman-Fenton, A J
Gardham, J R C
Garland, B
Garner, B J
Gaukroger, M C
Gocman, M C
Gomes, A N V
Gopalakrishnan, G
Grace, D L
Griffin, A J
Habashi, S
Hamilton, L W E
Hampton, N R E
Handa, N
Hare, J M S
Harvey, D C M
Head, J E
Hinchley, G W
Hindley, C B
Hitchings, V
Iqbal, A
Jackson, A E
James, K K
Jayran Nejad, Y
Jenkins, M G
Jepson, C M
Jones, G R B
Kanse, P T
Kaplan, S A
Karvounis, S-S
Kataria, B
Kearns, A
Keating, P G D
Kelland, P
Kember, M J
Kennedy, H G
Khiroya, R C
Knott, L J
Knowles, R L
Larkin, S C
Love, S V
Macartney, N J D
McLay, J S
McQueen, J E
Marks, A S
Mazumder, R
Meek, D B
Menzies, L J
Mier Jedrzejowicz, A K
Mikhail, H M T
Mikhail, S W I
Mok, A W-F
Moosvi, R S
Morcos, M Y
Morganti, K M
Munro, B F
Nduka, S A
Newton, P M
Nicholas-Pillai, A
O'Mahony, P H M
Palaniappan, S
Panjwani, S
Pathan, A H
Pavlou, P T
Pavlou, S
Pollock, I
Postlethwaite, J C
Prout, J R
Rahman, A T M L
Ramanathan, P
Ratnarajah, K
Ravindran, A
Reid, A S
Reid, H A S
Rice, N E
Ridge, A T
Rohan, C F
Rooban, R A
Roux, H J
Rubenstein, I D
Rubenstein, P
Salih, H
Savage, D E
Sawdy, R J
Scurlock, H J
Shah, A R
Shaw, S
Shridhar, S
Sidhu, G S
Sinniah, A T
Spencer, R E
Stanton, M B
Subanandan, P
Subrahmanyam, P C
Syed, A
Taylor, L B
Theivendra, M
Theron, J S
Trieman, N
Tuthill, D P
Valls Ballespi, J
Varatharaj, J
Verma, D K
Waddington, R J
Walgama, S K L
Walker, R E
Ward, M W N
Warren, S J
Watkin, L A
Weinstein, A F
Whittaker, W E
Williams, P S
Withana, K A
Wood, J J
Worswick, J C
Yeo, E R
Yugambaranathan, K
Yuksel, B

Enniskillen

Armstrong, J D
Asghar, M M
Auterson, T N
Blake, P N
Bothwell, J E
Boyd, J D
Brady, M C I
Brady, P J
Caithness, J S
Campbell, M E
Cathcart, M E H
Cody, M W J E
Conneally, P
Connor, E
Cromie, W N
Darling, J R
Day, D E M
Deeny, E D M
Devlin, K F
Dolan, F M
Elliott, M E L
Forster, E M H
Forster, S W H
Gallagher, A B
George, M G
Gilroy, J B
Graham, C W
Groves-Raines, J C
Harrold, P F M
Herdman, C G
Jentsch, T
Keaney, A A M
Kelly, J F
Kiernan, T F
King, L J
Kirby, A M
Kirby, J M
Leary, R T
Long, R M
Lynch, P N
McAleer, B G A
McCaffrey, P E
McCaw, C J
McConville, M E
McCusker, J A
McDermott, B A
McGowan, P J A
McManus, B M
Mallon, M J
Marshall, S G
Mellotte, M
Montague, J J
Moran, N M
Mulligan, G R
O'Dolan, C A
O'Donohoe, J M
O'Hare, C V
O'Hare, R A
O'Reilly, P J D
Pippet, D J
Rahman, M M
Rea, M A
Reidy-Brady, N M
Richey, R E M
Scott, M J
Smyth, M G
Sweeney, C J
Sweeney, K M M
Treacy, P J
Varma, M P S
White, A B
Williams, J R
Young, H K

Epping

Amen, A A A
Ashaye, O A
Ashford, A L
Barker, D A V
Barrie, M A
Bolton, P J
Casaubon Alcaraz, F J
Chapman, R A M
Darcy, J A

Dawkins, R S
Dempsey, E M
Evans, F J H
Fadl, S E D R A
Gold, J-A
Higham, C
Hill, J D
Hynds, W R G
Jenkins, S H
John, C E H
Jones, R M
Lan Keng Lun, K F
Leake, J
Letcher, R G M
Lowry, D M
Mayer, A-P T
Morris, R W
O'Connor, D M E
Peck, M J E
Pradhan, R M
Richards, G J
Roy, B K
Shepherd, D T S
Stanhill, V
Walker, Z
Waller, J F

Epsom
Al-Musawi, D M M
Ardern-Jones, M R
Badami, A J
Baird, J E
Baldwin, M J
Barker, R J
Beadles, W I
Beckaya, A
Bellenger, W S
Bendig, J W A
Bishay, S S
Bottomley, N
Boughton, P R
Brown, J
Bunn, M N
Burton, R H
Canton, L C
Charig, C R
Charlton, R M
Chen, A W Y
Chen, B
Clarke, D J
Cobb, R A
Connolly, F H
Cooper, P J
Coppen, A J
Cowlard, R J
Cunningham, J A
Darlington, L G
Davis, P A
Desborough, J P
Dutta, S
El-Dosoky, A M R A
Ellis, C E G
Elrahman, I H A A
Etherington, J
Ewah, B N
Farooqi, M R
Flower, J F
Ford, P N
Free, A J
George, C D
Goddard, R K
Gould, S R
Gregory, A M
Hammond, P J
Harris, D M
Harun, S
Hay, G C
Haydon, S C
Hayes, M A
Hayward, A J
Hayward, C M M
Henderson, A
Holbrook, J
Hopkins, G O
Howard, C M
Howlett, D C
Hughes, S G
Irvine, A T
Jayasena, K
Jayawardhana, S R
Jones, D W
Kakumani, V
Katesmark, M
Katiyar, A K
Khakhar, M B
Leaver, S
Lim, A G
Liyanage, P P
McCullough, T K

McFarland, R J
Mackay, C J
McKee, N D
Mahadevan, M
Manghat, N E
Markose, G
Markose, V M
Masood, J
Masood, U
Matthews, A J
Miller, A L
Mitchell-Heggs, P F
Mitchell, H J
Mitchell, P A
Mitchell, S C
Mok, D W H
Moore, S
Morrell, D C
Morrell, J M
Morton, E E
Narang, K K
Nicholls, J M
Nightingale, M D
Odemuyiwa, O
Orton, J J
Pais, W A
Parker, B C
Pattinson, C J
Ranasinha, K W
Ranganath, L R
Rangedara, D C
Ransom, W T M
Ravago, E
Raweily, E A A
Rees, J A
Reynolds, J C
Richardson, T
Robb, P J
Roberts, S A
Rollin, A-M
Rollin, H R
Rosbotham, J L
Rundle, S K
Salem, N
Semple, M J
Senhenn, J S A
Sevenoaks, M R
Seymour, A L
Shankar, S
Shanmuganathan, T
Sharpe, A P
Shephard, E A
Sheriff, S
Sheth, T R
Silva, F B
Sneath, P
Sreetharan, M
Steventon, P N
Stott, R A P
Suleman, S K
Sweeney, C M
Temple, L N
Thornton-Smith, A N
Twyman, R S
Walker, J L
Walker, R M H
Waters, F M
Wilson, J H
Wilson, R
Wilson, S G
Wong, F
Wormley, R L
Zafer, I M Z
Zaki, S

Erith
Arnaot, M R Z T
Browning, S M
Dhatariya, R C
Fok, W W F
Franklin, V
Ghosh, M H
Kailey, S S
Le Geyt, J D
McIntyre, M R
Mehrbakhsh, A
Nandra, K S
Nguyen, H
O'Neill-Byrne, K
Patel, V S
Roberts, P J
Sellappah, S

Erskine
Afuakwah, J K
Aikman, M
Griffith, D B
Hanley, T-A
McFadyen, T

McGavigan, M E
Patel, S
Tabony, W M
Tarrant, P D

Esher
Ainslie, D
Al-Jezairy, A I K
Andersen, U H
Baldock, A M
Bates, T D
Breathnach, A S
Bull, B I
Cross, J M
Dance, P J
Dixon, M H N
Evans, J C
Forrester, P C
Franks, Q B
Fyfe, A L A
Gannon, M C
Gavins, P W
Gibson, I D
Goldsack, A M
Hall, C A
Harper, C A
Hendry, J A
Holden, A M
Hoy, A M
Hui, F C
Hutton, M D C
Kamboj, A S
Karim, A
Kearsey, S Y
Leach, J B
Leach, R D
Leary, R M
Low, I H
Lucas, C F
McGinn, O M
Mearing-Smith, T M
Munnelly, J T
Munro, N M
Owen, P J
Pao, D S P
Patel, H F
Radford, M J
Sanchez, M-J
Shine, A M
Sim, H G
Smith, G B
Spooner, J B
Stanbury, R M
Stewart, A
Thorns, A R
Wales, E
Wilkinson, E K
Wright, T S
Younger, K A

Etchingham
Bolton, C F
Burton, K J
Cowey, A J
Gilbert, C P
O'Neill, D F
Packham, B A
Ustianowski, P A
Woodgate, J E

Evesham
Burton, G
Cox, M J
Cross, H M
Cross, R L
D'Arcy, C M R
Doran, J S
Edwardes, J A
Grant, S C
Gregorowski, L F
Henry, I J
Herold, D C
Jackson, N R
Johnson, S J
Jones, D A
Lloyd, J H
Logan, P J
Milner, J C G
Nava, G
Ounsted, C M
Richards, L E J
Serenyi, A G
Shackley, E C
Shore, K M
Smith, I L T
Swindlehurst, A L
Wolfe, J
Wright, J A

Exeter
Abbood, K H
Abdel Rahman, I E
Adcock, C J
Adey, J
Adkins, C T
Allman, K G
Amin, R
Anderson, R J
Arshi, H
Ayres, R C S
Babajews, A V
Bailey, A M
Baines, R
Baker, P J S
Ballard, P K
Barnes, A P
Barnes, S L
Barnett, A M
Bayliss, C R B
Beaman, M
Beck, W A
Berry, C B
Berry, J A
Beynon, R P
Bhalla, N K
Bhatia, N
Black, S E
Blewett, A E
Bliss, P
Boaden, R W
Bogdanovic, M D
Bolden, F M
Booth, R A D
Bradley-Smith, G C
Bradley, M K
Bradley, N C A
Branton, D W
Brightwell, A P
Briscoe, M H
Broad, G J
Brown, A M E
Bunkall, S C
Bunker, T D
Byles, D B
Campbell, W B
Campling, J M
Challenor, J
Chapman, O G
Christie, J M L
Clark, J T M
Clarke, T J
Clarke, W L
Clarkson, R L
Clements, C L
Clunie, J M J
Coleman, J R
Coleman, L J
Coleridge, S D
Colley, N V
Collins, P A
Collinson, A C
Colville, A
Conn, D A
Cooper, M J
Coote, J M
Cowan, A R
Cox, P J A
Crowe, C A S
Curtis, H A
D'Souza, R J
Daly, A J
Daneshmend, T K
Daniel, S
Daniel, V
Daugherty, M O
Dawrant, J M
Dawrant, M L
Day, C J E
Day, D W
De Boer, R C
De Carteret, S L
Devaraj, V S
Dick, C L
Douglas, A M
Drewe, C D
Dudbridge, S B
Dunlop, J L
Dunn, J M
Eggleton, J D P
Elderkin, R A
Elzik, C S
Ernst, E
Eskander, R I
Evans, A
Evans, L J
Evans, P H
Evans, S E
Ewings, S A

Fahmy, F S
Faircloth, H O
Fenwick, G M
Ferguson, A D
Ferguson, B M
Fernando, G C A
Fiorentini, T
Foster, E A
Fredriksson, S T
Freer, T H
Gallwey, P L G
Gandhi, M M
Gardner-Thorpe, C C
Gardner-Thorpe, C
Gardner, N H N
Garth, R J N
Gellett, L R
Gie, G
Gilbert, J
Giles, N C L
Giles, S H
Goodman, A G
Gopal, R
Goulding, T J
Greenwood, B P
Gutowski, N J
Halford, J G
Halpin, D M G
Hamad, S N
Hamilton-Wood, C
Hamilton, W T
Hampshire, M S B
Hanington, S J
Harington, J M
Harries, S R
Harrill, J G M
Harris, A R
Harris, S A C
Harrison, A J
Hart, A M
Hart, J C C
Hattersley, A T
Hayes, P A
Heal, P C
Helliar, N H
Hemsley, A G
Herdman, J
Heron, W C
Hewin, D F
Hill, R F
Hilton, D C W
Hilton, M P
Holding, J
Holme, C O
Honan, W P
Hong, A
Hooper, D C
Hopwood, B C
Howard, I T
Hubble, M J W
Hudson, A J R
Hudson, A J
Hughes, A G
Hulin, S J
Irvin, T T
Jabarin, Z S
Jacob, J S H
Jacoby, R K
James, M A
Jameson Evans, D C
Jefferies, A E
Jeffreys, O M E
Johnson, D S
Jolliffe, P H G
Jones, A M B
Joyner, M V
Kay, P H
Kealey, L E
Keen, C E
Keith, J R
Kent, E M
Kernick, D P
Key, H
Kinsella, D C
Knight, J W H
Knox, A J S
Lawn, E N
Lee, A J
Lee, R W H
Leeder, D S
Leete, R J
Leger, B J
Lewis, V E
Lin Sin Cho, G L
Ling, R S M
Lloyd, J G
Logan, G S
Lowings, E A
McBay, I W

McConville, R J
McCorkindale, R A
McCrindle, D C
McCullagh, P J
Mackenzie, K G P
McKinnel, S R
McLauchlan, C A J
McLean, E K
McLennan, A S
Macleod, K M
McNinch, A W
Malone, T J L
Mann, R S C
Marshall, F P F
Martin, M R
Mason, C H
Meredith, M J
Midgley, A K
Mole, M R
Montgomery, C D
Moody, R H
Moore, G J M
Morgan, G M
Morgan, M S
Morgan, W I C
Mossop, G W E J
Moxon, G W
Munn, J
Mynn Htyn, Dr
Napier, M P
Nelson, T R
Nicholls, A J
Northover, R P
Norton, M R
O'Sullivan, M E
Oades, P J
Onyett, R M
Osborne, P B
Owen, M R
Packer, T F
Pagliero, K M
Palmer, H J G
Palmer, J H
Parker, Y-M A
Parkyn, T M
Pearce, V R
Perkins, J H
Perriss, B W
Piercy, M L
Plummer, H
Pocock, M A J
Pocock, R D
Powis, R A
Ragbir, M
Ragi, E F E
Rains, S G H
Ramell, M D
Reaves, C S
Reaves, E C
Rees, J E G
Regan, J M
Renninson, J N
Renouf, A C D
Richardson, D E M
Richardson, J S
Ridler, B M F
Rinaldi, C A
Riordan, T
Roberts, F L
Robinson, T J
Rogers, A R
Rolfe, M G
Rosser, V C E
Rossiter, A
Round, A P
Rowland, C G
Rudin, C
Russell, D J
Rutter, J A
Saddler, J M
Salzmann, M B
Sandhar, B K
Saunders, E M J
Saxby, P J
Schranz, P J
Scott, A P B
Sharpe, D P
Sharpe, I T
Shaw, D B
Sheehan, D J
Sheldon, C D
Sheldon, J C
Shewell, P K
Simcock, P R
Simpson, R H W
Smallwood, N N
Smith, A E
Smith, L D R
Smith, R C

Spencer, H
Spiers, A S D
Spyer, G
St. Johnston, C F
Stanley, B L G
Stead, J W
Steele, R J F
Stewart, A J
Stone, C A
Stott, M A
Stowell, G M
Sturley, R H
Sweeney, K G
Talbot, N J
Teasdale, A R
Telford, R J
Thomas, K M J
Thomas, R D
Thompson, J F
Thorne, C P
Tillett, R I L
Timperley, A J
Toy, E W
Travers, P R
Tripp, J H
Turner-Warwick, R T
Turner, C
Turner, R J
Turnpenny, P D
Van Nimmen, B
Van Staden, G N
Varian, J A
Vercoe, S
Walker, A C
Walker, J A
Warin, A P
Warin, J M
Watkinson, A F
Watson, M B
Watson, T M
Weatherley, C R
West, J H
West, P G
Wilkie, J R
Wilkins, L K
Williams, A
Wilson, I H
Withers, N J
Withey, J M
Woods, A J
Wormald, P N
Wray, G
Wride, J P
Yau, S Z M

Exmouth
Argent, J D
Beed, M J
De Kretser, A J H
Debenham, T R
Donald, R G
Enright, H M
Fewings, P E
Hepburn, J A C
Hopkins, R J
Hull, M G
Johnson, M J
Johnston, N F A
Kay, S R
Lewis, A P
May, C J
Nicholson, M E J
Nicholson, T F
Pocklington, S L
Price, S R
Quinn, P M
Richmond, G O
Ross, S D J
Sanderson, L
Scott, C L
Spiers, D R
Stubbings, C A
Stubbings, S M
Vasey, S E
Ward, S

Eye
Colley, S P
Cooper, P H
Eckersley, E
Ellis-Jones, M
Goodge, B M
Holmes, S J
Macmillan, F K
Morris, J A C
Partridge, C J
Read, G M
Thirlwell, C
Vaudrey, B

Eyemouth
Dorward, I M
Fenty, M A
Macdonald, J A
Mason, A P
Swan, I L H

Fairford
Benzie, A S
Bingham, C
Frazer, D C
Gardiner, A E
Knights, M J G
Lunney, D C
Sabourin, A C

Fakenham
Bennett, D J N
De Marco, P
Joshi, M
Reinhold, P H
Taylor, A B W

Falkirk
Ainsworth, J H S
Anderson, S W
Ark, S S
Arthur, I S
Barnes, S
Barth, C
Bennett, K M E
Birch, A D J
Borg Grech, V
Briggs, E W W
Broome, I J
Brown, E
Brown, H G
Brzeski, M S
Buchanan, L M
Clafferty, R A
Close, S A
Cordeiro, N J V
Crawford, G
Crichton, F J B
Crookston, A
Crowe, A M
Dodds, G
Duncan, P L
Edwards, G P
Evans, S M
Ewing, R G
Gardner, H W
Gilbert, J
Gillespie, M D
Glen, K A
Grant, K A
Hargreaves, A D
Harris, N W S
Harvey, J M
Haywood, H A
Hogarth, E D A
Holliday, M P
Howland, N J
Hunter, I
Jack, M E
Johnston, V J
Kerr, G D
Khurana, C
Khurana, I K
Krosnar, A
Laurie, G A
Law, R G
Lehany, G P
Leonard, J D
Lim, J A
Lim, P C-K
Lindsay, J R
Luke, W M
McCabe, E M
McCall, A C
McDonald, A
MacFlynn, G M P
McGhee, C
McGlynn, J M
McInnes, G K
McLean, G S
McManners, J
McSorley, P D
Maguire, N M
Merrick, B M
Middlemiss, S A
Millar, E
Miller, W D W
Morrison, D
Morrison, S S
Moses, P C
Multani, S S
Murdoch, P S
Nadeem, R D

Neilson, R F
Nimmo, T W
Ogilvie, C K
Oram, M C H
Orr, K M
Peddie, M M
Peden, N R
Ramsay, D M
Ramsay, K
Reid, J
Robb, H M
Robertson, A A
Robertson, A
Salatian, M
Sankey, S J
Scott, A D
Scougal, I J
Shanks, H A C
Shields, M F
Smith, M F
Smith, R C
Stewart, J D
Stewart, M P D
Sydney, R
Taylor, H
Thomson, R C G
Underwood, G H
Waldron, S M
White, W G
Whitelaw, C A
Wilkie, G
Wright, S C

Falmouth
Blundell, J A T
Burnett, P
Cheetham, C E
Clover, A M
Davis, G W
Dommett, P G
Downey, A
Hichens, S M
Hindley, F
Hobbs, J H
Hyland, J
James, R D G
Jones, H
Lester, A A
Miller, D G
Morris, M
Reeves, M A
Roberts, A B
Roberts, P
Rotheray, A D
Rowe, A J
Sage, F J
Sellwood, K
Siddall, H S C
Simcock, A D
Slater, P D
Stacpoole, H A
Wight, V L

Fareham
Allen, N J
Ashton, R E
Baldock, N E
Barnard, K D
Barr-Taylor, P
Bellenger, R A
Brims, F J H
Chaderton, N H
Chatwin, H C
Christie, I G
Clark, A D
Coleman, H
Coote, A L
Daoud, J B
Delves, G H
Diggens, S E
Dixon, K E
Douglas, T G C
Dover, R W
Du Feu, G J C
Dunbar, D A
Dunton, M J
Durrant, D A E
Evans, S A
Foggitt, A C
Foot, J L
Gill, P K
Gonem, M N H
Gordon, A C
Griffiths, S J
Hahn, H J A
Harley, J E
Harris, F E
Henry, C
Hillam, G H

Hopkins, P N
Howell, R D
Hurren, J S
Jackson, A R
Jonas, M M
Jones, C
Jordan, B L
Kyd, K L
Lambert, F R
Lambert, V M J
Larmer, S D
Larson, A G
Lowe-Ponsford, F L
Lusznat, R-M G
MacAdam, R C A
McCabe, S E T
McLean, A D
Maguire, A C
Moore, A L
Morris, J C
Munden, A J
Mushens, E J
Nagvekar, V
Nelson, R
O'Byrne, J J
O'Grady, J C
Ormsby, J M
Page, K M
Pai, K S
Palmer, B M
Paterson, A J
Pechal, A J
Polson, R G
Potiphar, D W
Prosser, J G S
Prout, W G
Rayner, S A L
Richards, P L
Robins, S J
Ronayne, K L
Roope, R M
Samarajiwa, H K
Schopp, M J
Sewell, N B
Shaw, G D
Shaw, K M
Shepherd, T H
Siggers, B R C
Sims, J S
Sinclair, D J
Sirr, H C R
Smallwood, S H
Sommerville, G P
Sotheran, W J
Southern, K J H
Swanson, N C P
Tandy, J C
Taylor, A V
Taylor, M E
Tenters, M T
Tibble, H C
Toleman, S E
Tottle, S
Tucker, A J
Wade, N R
Wakefield, C J
Walmsley, B H
Walmsley, T
Ward, C T
Ward, T P
Warner, J R
Webster, E M
Wolpe, A P
Yeung, E S T

Faringdon
Bartholomew, G J
Cartwright, S R
Chesterton, L J
Craighead, I B
Douglas, A M R
Erskine, S P E
Heanley, C P
Holdsworth, F E
Last, S E M
Pinches, P J E
Scott-Brown, G
Stenhouse, J N
Vanhegan, R I
Warner, M D
Watters, M P R
Williamson, L

Farnborough
Ahmed, M A
Barnard, S A
Boorman, S R
Caird, G R
Carvalho, A

Cave, A M
Clasper, J C
Curran, A
De Verteuil, J A
Desai, A J
Draper, P D
Eggeling, I T
Fairbairn, O J
Ferguson, N R
Gibbons, A N
Hargreaves, U
Haywood, J
Headley, C A
Heywood, S A
Hughes, N J
Kay, W D
Linton, L S K
Linton, S P
Marshall, C B
Micklethwaite, G
Nejo, T A
Noorani, F
O'Hara, F R
Opie, N J
Poots, D F J
Ramachandran, K
Reid, J E
Sales, N R
Simon, J W
Smyth, M
Stack, M M
Stone, K P
Stuart, I M
Sumner, T L
Sutherland, I A
Tanner, K J
Toms, M E
Vakil, P A
Walczak, J P B
Welch, R A
Whitcher, H W

Farnham
Abbas, T
Ainsworth, R W
Bandara, I S
Beare, B C
Bird, K L
Blagden, S P
Blundell, F J
Bourne, R R A
Boxer, C M
Braithwaite, J M
Brown, D
Burgess, J E
Burton, S L
Byren, J C
Carvill, J M
Chadha, A-N C
Christmas, A R
Clarke, S
Cothay, D M H H
Coull, J T
Davies, S J M
Davies, W G
Dempster, J B
Elliott, A J
Elliott, A J
Evans, C R
Fahmy, A I
Felix, R H
Fisher, N J
Fisher, R L
Fozard, J R
Giles, P R
Gooding, A
Govan, J A A
Guy, M P
Head, F F
Hemsley, C J
Hodgson, M C
Holmes, B J
Holt, D I
Ibrahim, A J
Ibrahim, I K
Inman, S E
Jenkins, S L
Joiner, I M
King, D M
Laidlaw, I J
Lallemand, R C
Luscombe, T D
Lynch, N P
McClay, A O
Macnair, P A
Massouh, H
May, W J
Mehta, M K
Milligan, G M

Moore, J W A
Morris, C B
O'Donnell, H
O'Dowd, C E
Ody, C L M
Palfrey, E L H
Parker, P M
Partridge, R J
Payne, M J
Powell, L J
Price, R D
Pryke, J R
Quaile, A
Quin, M M
Raw, A J A
Regan, K J
Ridley, P J
Rishworth, V C
Roberts, H J M
Robinson, P C
Russell, C J
Scott-Perry, S J
Slater, J C
Spink, M
Standring, A F
Straiton, J M
Sushila, S
Swage, T H
Taylor, A J
Tibbott, C W
Trotter, M I
Way, M
White, D G
Wood, B G
Woollam, V A M
Youngs, S-L E C L

Faversham
Barnes, A D
Chopra, G
Chopra, M S
Corble, G
Curry, R D
Cwynarski, M T
Dawson-Bowling, P R
Everest, N J
Hodgkiss, R V
Kesson, R A
Knowles, P A
Logan, L C
Lynch, C G M
Lynch, M A
Moore, D J
Potter, V J
Reichhelm, T
Scarlett, A J
Taylor, A J
Wood, S
Wyeth, S W

Felixstowe
Beaton, K C
Clarke, B M G
Davenport, R A
De Cleen, M
Feltwell, S R J
Forde, H H
Holloway, G J T
McKee, W B
McMurray, J
Moon, D N L
Moss, C J
Pearce, K W
Powell, K U L
Reed, T J
Rowe, F J
Silovsky, K
Sudell, W A
Tempest, L C
Youngman, P R

Feltham
Amarasinghe, A R
Anderson, I R
Aswani, G T
Ayala Gonzalez, A
Bhullar, B K
Dagg-Heston, R
Dong, B
Ghosh, A K
Gill, P S
Howes, N R
Hussain, T
Kotian, P D
Lynch, C M
McInnes, E G
Mahon, C M
Meagher, M A
Mecci, Z H

Moran, J R
Muzafer, M H
Navani, L
O'Connor, J B
Patel, V N
Ranjithakumar, S
Scopes, I
Sen, S K
Stent, V M
Takeda, S
Winayak, V K

Ferndale
Banerjee, P
Dutta, R
Guhaniyogi, S B
Lloyd, M
Nath, K
Rahman, M
Sengupta, S

Ferndown
Adams, L A
Barcellos, A A
Bennett, S F
Clarke, S V
Davenport, E J
Ferguson, W J
Gillett, M J
Green, R K
Jenkins, N M W
Ladd, J E
Laishley, R F
Luckie, M J
McKinstry, T H
McPhail, A L
Molina Navarro, C
Ottley, G B
Paine, D H D
Pilling, P J
Rees, C R
Sarwar-E-Alam, A K M
Strauss, J P

Ferryhill
Cadigan, P
Drew, S C
Hall, N A
MacDougall, B K
McGlade, D R
Merson, P J
Moore, H E
Oakenfull, A G P
Orlandi, M
Schneeloch, B
Stevenson, G
Tijsseling, A C
Willis, D M

Ferryside
Griffiths, D R
Jenkins, D M G
O'Donnchadha, B P

Filey
Ablett, J J L
Donovan, A G
Garnett, J F P
Hazledine, C
Meeson, M D
Nunn, B R
Shepherd, C M
Skitt, B
Wynands, R W A

Fishguard
Davies, D B
Davies, N G
Evans, H D

Fivemiletown
McKeagney, K E
McKibbin, C
Rutledge, E M

Fleet
Arscott-Barber, J A
Barker, S S
Basher, M J S
Batstone, G F
Beal-Preston, R M C
Billinge, V A
Brasher, P F
Bromley, C L
Clark, N A D
Clarke, S A
Coombe, D H
De Glanville, T B
Fraser, J H
Garsed-Bennet, D J C
Goldring, S T
Hamann, J C H
Hannington-Kiff, J G
Healey, J C
Heffernan, S
Henderson, K
Higgins, C J C
Hoare, J M
Kimber, C J
King, S
McGinty, H J
McOwan, M M
Michel, A B
Murphy, J F D
Prior, A R J
Saxton, T N
Sharp, A L H
Shiells, L A
Speers, A G
Swift, M A
Thomas, M J G
Tilly, H V
Tollett, B J
Townsend, L Z
Waters, R J

Fleetwood
Ali, S M
Aziz, M M
Carpenter, P G
Clark, R J
Fairhead, S
Grenier, H P
Hardwick, J L
Hockings, M
Kirk, S J
Natrajan, K
Page, M J S
Ramesh, C
Rowley, E
Singleton, N J
Smyth, R A C
Spencer, M
Tse Sak Kwun, P C
Whiteside, A
Wilde, S
Wilson, M J

Flint
Barnard, W K H
Daniel, P
Davies, C P
Kapoor, J C
MacKirdy, J E
Mathews, E D
Rehman, Z-U

Fochabers
Ewing, C P
Kennedy, A-M
McNie, H
Pakenham, R W
Scott, C R

Folkestone
Allen, K E
Amin, Y Y
Arulanantham, N Y
Attara, G A
Bailey, A D
Beach, G R
Beckett, M E
Blaxland, N N
Blinston Jones, M P
Calver, G D
Catto, C E
Cox, M C L
Dallin, V J
Deane, A M
Evans, D P
Farebrother, L A
Farrow, D J
Felstead, S J
Fernandes, M A A M
Findlay, G H
Goodman, J L
Goodwin, A M
Goodwin, D P
Govier, E A
Hossain, M A
Inglis, P M
Jackson, D
Jackson, R G M
Jedrzejewski, J A
Jequier, P W
Keown, D
Khine-Smith, M C K
McGregor, B L
McPartlin, J F
Maitra, D K
Malcolm, R G
Marlowe, M J
Maze, S T
Musselwhite, D H
Neild, V S
Roberts, G A
Robertson-Ritchie, H
Sheikh, N A
Sholl, P P
Smith, L S
Sudheer, K
Veenhuizen, P G
Veenhuizen, P A
White, K J

Fordingbridge
Ashby, J B B
Cooke, S S
Downes, P G C
Gannon, M J
Gemmell, I M M
Hensel, C M
Knight, C E
Kuttler, A D S
Mccallum, M
McGee, J A
Morris, H J L
Newstead, S M
Shephard, N W
Smith, S
Staunton, E B
Wallis, T D
Wardley, J R

Forest Row
Baseley, J A
Del Mar, A R
Josephson, J-M
Miller, S A

Forfar
Beveridge, J B
Burt, D P
Davies, F J M M
Dick, P R
Dixon, A
Edmond, H L
Edwards, A I
Erskine, F M
Houghton, A
Houghton, E S
Kerr, F M
MacCallum, K S
MacDonald, A J A
McPhail, I J
McWilliam, L S
Mitchell, L D N
Morris, A H M
Nolan, J A C
Raitt, N
Smith, D M
Smith, W T M
Wake, D J
Woodroffe, G C
Woodroffe, S A

Forres
Anderson, J A
Angel, H R M
Govan, G
Hutchison, S
Johnson, D S
Kennedy, R J
Kerr, D
McMullen, B J
Mead, D E
Renwick, A A
Roy, L K M
Sabiston, M A
Sneddon, D T
Stevenson, D
Stewart, R J
Sutherland, D J
Thomson, A S
Wallace, J
Willetts, S J

Fort Augustus
Farmer, I D
Skeoch, J E

Fort William
Baggallay, A J
Douglas, J D M
Foxley, M E M
Goodall, J A D
Irving, E W
Lachlan, G W
Lachlan, M
Leeson-Payne, C E S
Leeson-Payne, C G
McArthur, C A
MacDonald, E C
McKay, J
Massie, A
Munro, A J
Munro, D J
Robinson, C
Roy, H L
Roy, M
Sedgwick, D M
Shirley, J
Smith, A D
Tangney, D J
Tregaskis, B F

Fortrose
Fraser, U S
Howes, J A
Lloyd, N M
Macdonald, C J
MacGregor, A M

Fowey
Hamilton, M H
Middleton, A
Ross-Mawer, J H R
Waldron, M J

Fraserburgh
Beattie, A G
Bichan, R M
Crockett, C S
Dick, M J W
Duthie, R M
Fowler, H M
Kinnon, J F
Lee-Mason, F V A
McPherson, J R
Murray, R S M
Packham, G B
Smith, A R
Steele, W M
Strachan, G M
Tweedie, D M
Watt, A N
Wisley, A B

Freshwater
Hill, M K
Magee, K J
Marshall, J C
Moffat, W C
Scivier, A
Thomson, G E
White, D H

Frimley
Barnardo, P D
Bartels, U J A
Chaudhary, R
Foster, J M G
Frankel, R J
Gerrard, D J
Hendrickse, A D

Frinton-on-Sea
Davies, J S
Elvin, G H
Exworth, D B
Fludder, V
Harrison, I D
Moore, G S
Stubbs, V M
Wall, M T

Frizington
Donald, C
Jackson, A
Oxby, C L

Frodsham
Ansdell-Smith, M

Frome
Booth, A C
Bungay, D M
Clacey, R P
Ellis, C J
Ellis, J A J
Griffiths, R L
Gumbley, M
Hall, C L
Henderson, V E
Holden, P E
Hunt, M A
Jelly, J R
Kingston, H M
Knight, F J
Mansfield, B G
Merry, T L
Millar, J M
Muscat, S
Rawlins, D C
Scheurmier, N I M
Scotchman, F G V
Taylor, J C
Vose, M A
Whitehead, N F

Gaerwen
Bowden, D F
Davidsson, H J
Fairhurst, B J
MacQuisten, S

Gainsborough
Basu, S K
Bedford, T A
Brown, P C
Carmichael, C M
Clarke, S L
Done, K L
Fickling, K A
Hale, E G
Hockey, J A
Hoggard, N
Hunt, C S
Hyde, P R
Jolly, D A
Kademani, Y
Lannon, P G
Millns Sizer, S A
Morris, M-A M
Padley, R G
Percival, I D
Pollard, M
Procter, G S
Taiwo, C B
Walker, A P
Warnes, G D
Wilkins, R A
Wragg, C M

Gairloch
Marshall, A L
Mitchell, G A
Robertson, R H
Smith, Y

Galashiels
Arbuckle, G M
Brown, M I
Cramond, P M
Cross, R A
Glenfield, J R
Gollock, J M
Greenwood, C A
Johnston, J R
Johnston, R L
Johnstone, A V
Leaver, R J
Lindsay, M K
Maclaine, G N
Megahy, F R C
Miller, I I A
Owen, D J
Rodgers, F R
Smith, R R
Soutter, R I
Timperley, L R
Wright, A K J

Galston
Dean, W M F
McCall, J S
McWhirter, J W
Nicoll, W S
Robertson, A K

Garve
MacLeod, A
Whitteridge, S M

Gateshead
Aird, I A
Antrobus, J N
Ashour, H Y H
Austin, A H
Barer, D H
Bartley, C F M
Beeby, A R
Beesley, J R
Bhaskaran, A R
Bhattacharya, V V
Bird, C M
Bone, D
Bonnington, R M
Bowman, A
Bowman, D E
Brandon, H A
Browell, D A
Browne, B D P
Brumby, P
Bryson, J M
Calvert, S
Cassidy, P D
Chalmers, J E
Cock, C E
Comerci, G
Condie, W H
Congera, G P
Cope, M T
Cox, R A
Cross, P A
Cunliffe, W J
Daniels, S P
Datta, D
Dawson, C J
Dodds, S R
Dorani, B
Dowson, T
Dutta, D K
Errington, D R
Errington, M G
Eseonu, O C
Fairs, R G
Field, S M
Fisher, R J
Galloway, H J
Gardner, C A
Gilbert, P S
Groom, H M
Gupta, D
Haines, R M
Hanson, G H G
Harness, J D
Harrison, D A
Harrison, R W S
Hendrick, A M
Henry, J A
Heycock, C R
Holmes, A
Hood, M P
Horlock, L
Hudson, S J
Hughes, T
Hunt, A J
Ilyas, M
Imam, S M
Jones, K P
Kanu, F C S
Kaura, A
Kaura, V C
Kell, W
Kelly, C A
Kennan, E
Kenny, C
Killen, J W W
Kumar, A
Kunju, M P K
Lambert, K H
Leon, C M
Liston, J E
Lopes, A B
Lunt, L G
Lustman, F
Mcauley, F T
McClintock, I R
McErlane, F E
May, H A
Mercer-Jones, M A
Morris, N A
Mudawi, A M
Muthu Krishnan, N
Naik, R
Naylor, F L
Nutting, L M
Orritt, S G C
Pannu, U S
Parker, C L
Pattekar, B D
Prudhoe, K
Ranu, H K
Razvi, S S
Reveley, C H
Rickards, M
Robson, J C
Rutenberg, S M
Schumm, B A
Scott, A M
Scott, C D
Shankar, N
Sherratt, M

Singh, K J
Singh, R K
Smith, D D
Smith, D A
Smith, L
Stack, W C
Steele, A M
Stevenson, P S
Streit, C E
Suchdev, M S
Tasker, B E
Tate, J
Tetlow, S
Thompson, P
Varghese, M A
Warwick, J S
Williamson, S L H
Wilson, S-A
Wise, C F
Wotherspoon, M

Gatwick
Cooke, J N C
Evans, A D B
Johnston, R V
Schenk, C P

Gerrards Cross
Aldwinckle, T J
Allan, G
Amin, S
Armstrong, J W
Barber, R T
Bartkiewicz, A J
Baxendine, D M
Bell, G S
Bray, S J
Butcher, S J
Chandra, A
Chandra, A K
Churchman, I R
Clayton, P P
Dean, A E
Dhesi, G S
Fiddian, A P
Forsyth, S
Foskett, R A
Foster, K E
Fowler, G R J
Ghouze, A
Grassick, B D M
Grieve, D K
Gristwood, J
Harrison, E L
Hart, A M
Hell, S C
Heywood, R L
Hughes, M J
Irwin, P F
Johal, J S
Kingdom, L G
Leaver, S
Mackinnon, S
Michell, E P G
Moiz, M
Myant, N B
Ogden, W S
Patel, S R
Paul, S S
Pilbrow, L K
Pye, G F
Quiney, M J
Rakhit, M K
Regan, R J
Robertson, S J
Seimon, J W M D J
Shotbolt, J P
Thomas, C C
Townsend, E R
Try, J L
Turner, N S
Webber, A M
Westcott, E D A
Whitwell, G S
Williams, E J
Wilter, P H
Yuen, A W C

Gillingham, Dorset
Fawcett, K J R
Freeland, M S
Groom, M R
Mole, K F
Short, M A

Gillingham, Kent
Addy, N C
Adesida, O A
Adlam, D
Ahmed, A I H
Al-Sinawi, A A H S
Aldouri, M
Andrews, B G
Badrinath, M R
Bassily, A A E
Beattie, A M
Beeby, D I
Beerstecher, H J
Bewicke, R W
Bhatti, S A
Bloor, A J C
Boutros, N W M
Brennen, R G
Bui, T A
Buist, R J
Butler, C M
Corall, J M
Damri, M
Davis, J P
Day, R C
Day, S
Debenham, M J
Dholakia, R P
Diwakar, K N
Ducker, D A
Duckett, J R A
El Kary, S I
Ferrin, L V
Fleetcroft, J P
Frank, M J
Garrard, O N I
Gluckman, P G C
Gupta, J
Hahn, S
Hasan, K
Haworth, K L
Hayward, M J
Hoile, R W
Hoque, H M R
Imam, N
Ismail, S
Jani, B R
Joshi, S
Karim, Y
Karwal, N
Khan, O
Kitchen, P A
Lakshman, J C
Landham, T L
Lindley, R P
Mahmud, S Z
Manuel, P D
Mason, M A
Moore, D M
Morrice, A E
Mufti, G R
Mukherjee, K
Nagmoti, V G
Naseem, M S
Norman, S G
Oliver, R M
Palmer, J H
Parwani, G S
Patel, M G
Penman, D G
Procter, E A
Prothero, J D
Quatan, S M H
Quigley, M C
Qureshi, M-U-D
Qureshi, S M
Randall, B J
Reddy, K
Rucinski, J
Ryan, P J
Sarmotta, J S
Scobie, I N
Selvan, S T
Shaunak, L N
Shetty, A A
Silhi, R B
Simpson, D A
Singh, A K
Singh, B N
Sivathasan, S
Smith, A
Stewart, A G
Stone, P T
Suresh, K
Symonds, R L
Toye, R
Tsang, W-M
Varada Reddy, P S
Velamati, M D
Wahab, M A
Welland, H A
West, A G
Wilcox, A-M C
Williams, P M
Williams, P L
Wilson, T J
Yau, C Y

Girvan
Anderson, D G
Barr, G W
Cowell, G G
McFadyen, E P
Malloch, T
Maxwell, H L
Moore, C D
Smith, T C G
Strachan, G R

Glasgow
Abbas, A
Abedin, K J
Abel, B J
Abu-Seido, H-E-D A A
Adam, J S
Adams-Strump, B J
Adams, B W
Adams, E A P
Adams, F G
Adams, J N
Addis, G M
Addis, G J
Adjei, S S
Adlung, B
Afuakwah, R J
Ahmad, T
Ahmed, R
Ahmed, S I
Ahmed, S
Aitchison, M
Aitken, I C
Akhtar, M
Akhter, R
Akhter, Z
Al-Alousi, L M E
Al-Badran, L
Al-Badran, R H
Al Bahnasawy, L M S
Al-Jilaihawi, A N A
Al-Kadhimi, A R J H
Al-Shamma, M R R
Alam, M F
Alam, T A
Alcock, S R
Alcorn, D L
Alexander-Sefre, F
Alexander, A M
Alexander, C A
Alexander, C I
Alexander, R J T
Alexander, W D
Algie, T A
Alguero, L
Ali, A
Ali, A
Ali, H O M
Ali, S K
Allahabadia, A
Allahabadia, A
Allahabadia, J K
Allam, B F
Allam, S
Allan, D B
Allan, J G
Allen, D K
Allen, J M
Allison, A G
Allister, A
Alves, C B
Alwan, M A R
Amin, V S
Anderson, A A S
Anderson, A S
Anderson, B G
Anderson, D L
Anderson, D E
Anderson, E G
Anderson, H M
Anderson, I W R
Anderson, J M
Anderson, J S
Anderson, J H
Anderson, J R
Anderson, J S
Anwar-Ul-Haq, M
Anwar, M
Apiliga, M T
Appleby, A B
Arbab-Zadeh, A
Archer, S C
Arfan, A
Armour, A A
Armstrong, I A
Asbury, A J
Asghar, B
Ashley, A M
Ashley, E A
Aslam, A
Athavale, D
Auld, M H
Austin, A V
Aylmer, D A
Azmy, A A M F
Baillie, D
Bain, D J
Bain, K E
Baird, C R W
Baird, D R
Baird, J W
Baird, J A
Baird, K S
Baker, M
Balfour, A E
Ballantyne, D
Ballantyne, J P
Ballantyne, J P
Ballantyne, R
Balmain, S
Balmer, S
Bancewicz, D
Banerjee, A K
Banham, S W
Bankowska, U Z
Barber, J M
Barker, J
Barlow, G
Barlow, M
Barlow, P
Barnes, J J
Barnes, J
Barnes, M F L
Barr, M C
Barrett, B G J
Barrett, C F
Barrett, H A
Barrett, K F
Barrett, R
Barrett, S V
Barrie, A A O
Barrie, R
Barton, J
Bashir, A A
Baxter, G M
Baxter, R H
Beardsley, S J
Beattie, A D
Beattie, G J
Beattie, J O
Beattie, R M
Beattie, S C
Beattie, T J
Bedi, C I
Bedi, T S
Beesley, S A
Begg, C J
Behan, C M H
Behan, W M H
Belcher, O P P R
Bell, A M
Bell, C A
Bell, E
Bell, G
Bell, G T
Bell, J M
Benaran, C
Benbow, S J
Bennet, A C
Bennet, G C
Bennett, N L M
Bennie, E H
Berardelli, C E
Berg, G A
Bergin, R L
Berrie, A K
Berry, F
Berry, M M
Best, C J
Best, W A
Beveridge, E J
Beynon, J A
Bhachu, H S
Bhandari, S
Bhatt, A
Bhattacharya, J J
Bhatti, N T
Bhawal, R
Bhopal, A S
Bigrigg, M A
Bilsland, D J
Bingham, B J G
Bissoonauth, S
Black, C J M
Black, E A
Black, M
Black, R A L
Blackwood, D L
Blair, A M
Blair, A J
Blair, D L
Blair, J A S
Blair, S J A
Blatchford, M E
Bleasby, C J F
Blincow, A H
Blyth, M J G
Boag, J W
Boddy, F A
Bolt, J M W
Bond, M R
Bone, I
Bong, J L
Bonnes, T M
Booth, M G
Booth, R H
Borthwick, J M
Bouch, C J K
Boulton-Jones, J M
Boulton-Jones, R V
Bowman, C M
Bowring, S A C
Boyce, S H
Boyd, A L
Boyd, C
Boyd, F F
Boyd, G
Boyd, M A
Boyd, W P
Boyle, D
Boyle, K C
Boyle, K
Boyle, M A
Boyle, S C
Brady, A J B
Branchfield, P J J
Brandon, A-M
Bransby-Zachary, M A P
Brechin, S
Bremner, A D
Brennan, A F
Brennand, J E
Brittliff, J
Brodie, A F
Brodie, D J
Brogan, R T
Brookes, R W
Brooks, S G
Brooksbank, K L
Brown, A J
Brown, D H
Brown, D J G
Brown, D R P
Brown, G J
Brown, G A
Brown, I D M
Brown, I G
Brown, I L
Brown, J H
Brown, K M
Brown, M R
Brown, R C
Brown, R M
Brown, S M R
Brown, S A
Brown, S E
Browne, B H
Browning, G G
Browning, J J
Browning, J P
Browning, J G
Bruce, C L M
Bruce, D J
Bruce, E J
Bruce, S J
Bryce, I G
Bryden, F M
Bryden, H S
Bryden, J S
Brydie, D H
Brydon, C W
Bryson, M S
Buchanan, M E B
Bucknall, C E
Buist, L J
Buksh, K
Bullock, M R R
Burden, A D
Burgoyne, M
Burleigh, E A
Burnett, C
Burnett, E B
Burnett, R A
Burns, H J G
Burns, J W
Burns, J M A
Burrell, H E
Burrow, M A L
Burton, A E
Burton, K A
Bush, A C
Butler, J G
Butler, S J
Butt, A M
Butt, N M
Byford, D M
Byrne, G C
Cadenhead, A L
Cairns, T
Calder, C B
Calder, J F
Calder, N J
Caldwell, J C
Calman, K C
Cameron, A D
Cameron, E
Cameron, H A
Cameron, N M
Campbell, A
Campbell, A T
Campbell, A J
Campbell, A C
Campbell, A M
Campbell, C
Campbell, C W
Campbell, D S
Campbell, F A
Campbell, G J
Campbell, G
Campbell, G A M
Campbell, I C
Campbell, J L
Campbell, J G
Campbell, J M
Campbell, L M
Campbell, M S
Campbell, P C
Campbell, S
Campbell, S E
Canning, G J
Canning, G P
Canning, M
Cannon, I A N
Cannon, R N
Capaldi, A D
Capell, H A
Caplan, R P
Caponigro, F
Carachi, R
Carlile, D
Carmichael, J
Carmichael, R M
Carnon, A G
Carrick, D G
Carroll, G
Cartledge, E A
Cartlidge, I J
Carty, M J
Cassels, M C
Cassidy, M
Castle, E A
Cathcart, A
Caulfield, S F
Cavallo, A V
Caven, E A
Cavoura, C
Chakrabarti, H S
Chalmers, A M
Chalmers, E A
Chalmers, G W
Chan, P K H
Chang, J W
Chapman, R M
Chatfield, M M
Chatfield, W R
Chaudhri, O S
Chaudhry, S R
Chazan, N
Cheah, P Y
Chen, C X
Cheriyan, S
Cherry, L A
Chiah, K S
Chiah, S A
Chiang, C C P
Chisholm, I M
Chita, B S
Chong, D
Chong, P S
Choudhery, V P

Chowaniec, A M
Chowdhury, M M M
Chowdhury, M
Chowdry, A S
Christian, M T
Christie, C A
Christie, J M
Christie, S F
Christison, M K
Chung, D A
Church, A C
Church, J A
Church, M V
Clark, C E
Clark, C J
Clark, C
Clark, D
Clark, H B
Clark, L A
Clark, L J
Clarke, P T
Clegg, S K
Clements, R
Clifford, D J
Climie, P B
Clinton, E
Clokey, G J
Clubb, C
Cobbe, S M
Cochran, D P
Cochran, K M
Cochrane, L M
Cochrane, L M
Cochrane, R A
Cockburn, A F
Cockburn, F
Cohen, H N
Coia, D A
Cole, A T
Coll, L
Collie, S J
Collins, K E
Colquhoun, I W
Colville, D R
Conn, I G
Connaughton, K J
Connell, J M C
Connell, L E
Connell, R A
Connelly, J A
Connolly, C M
Connolly, M A
Connolly, P J
Connor, J M
Connor, J M
Connor, R A C
Conroy, S
Conway, D I
Conway, V A
Cook, G
Cooke, L D
Cooke, T G
Cooper, B
Cooper, S-A
Cooper, S M
Copeland, L E K
Corbett, R H
Corcoran, G D
Cordiner, C M
Cordiner, J W
Corfield, A R
Corrigan, D L
Cossar, D F
Cossar, J H
Cotton, P
Cousland, G
Coutts, J A P
Coutts, S B
Cowan, C A
Cowan, J B
Cowan, M S
Cowan, M D
Cowden, J M
Cowie, F J
Coyle, A C
Coyle, H E
Craig, M B
Cram, L P
Crampsey, V R
Crawford, C M
Crawford, J A
Crawford, L A
Crawford, M
Crawford, R
Cron, A M
Crooks, J E
Crorie, J W
Crosbie, D I
Crowther, J A
Cruickshank, A M
Cruickshank, D M
Cruickshank, M C W
Cuchel, M
Cuddihy, T P
Cuddihy, V
Cullen, M P
Cullen, T J O H
Cumming, S A
Cunning, B W
Cunningham, A A
Cunnington, A-L
Curran, A J
D'Silva, M C
D'Silva, R
Dabydeen, L
Dabydeen, S W Y
Dagg, K D
Dalling, R
Dalton, D J N
Dancer, S J
Danesh, B J
Daniel, M K
Dargie, H J
Dargie, R
Darlow, J M
Das, A C
Das, R
Das, S
Datta, S
Daud, S M
Davda, A N
Davda, N S
Davidson, A J W
Davidson, C B
Davidson, F A
Davidson, H R
Davidson, I T
Davidson, K G
Davidson, M C
Davidson, S M
Davie, A P
Davie, C A
Davie, J W
Davies, G J
Davies, N P G
Davis, J A
Davis, P R
Dawes, P F H
Dawoud, R A
Dawson, M F
Dawson, R D
Day, R E
De Caestecker, L
Deane, R F
Deeny, M
Dell, A E
Dely, C J
Desai, G
Deshpande, N P
Deshpande, P M
Deubel, E L
Devanney, M C
Devers, M C
Devine, B L
Devine, J
Devine, M M
Dhiya, S
Diaper, C J M
Dick, D H
Dick, E S
Dickson, E J
Dinardo, L R B
Doak, W M
Dobson, C C
Dobson, H M
Docherty, D J
Docherty, R C
Dochery, A
Dodds, M
Doherty, A M
Doherty, P A
Doherty, S M
Doig, H P
Doig, W B
Doig, W M
Dominiczak, A F
Dominiczak, M H
Donald, J R
Donaldson, L
Donaldson, M D C
Donnelly, J W
Doraiswamy, N V
Doran, C A
Dorrance, H R
Dougall, H G G
Dougall, H I
Douglas, A M
Douglas, R N C
Dove, P M
Dover, S B
Dow, J S M
Dow, T G B
Dowers, A D
Downey, M G
Downie, A C
Downie, C J
Doyle, A S P
Doyle, D
Drummond, M B
Drummond, M W
Drummond, R S
Drury, J K
Drysdale, R G
Duff, G M
Duffy, M
Duffy, M T
Duke, E M C
Dummett, N J
Dunachie, S J
Duncan, A C
Duncan, C L
Duncan, J R
Duncan, M S
Duncan, R
Duncan, R D D
Dunleavy, M J
Dunn, A J
Dunn, I B
Dunn, J M
Dunn, J J
Dunn, L T
Dunn, R T
Dunn, S G M
Dunnigan, M G
Dunwoodie, W M
Durnin, J V G A
Durward, W F
Duthie, B A M
Duthie, F R
Duthie, N J
Dutta, S
Dyker, G S
Dyker, K E S
Dysart, J G
Eason, S M
Easson, M T
Edgecombe, J F
Edmond, P
Edwards, B A
Edwards, D J
Edwards, G F S L
Edwards, R D
El-Lemki, M A M
Ellahi, R T
Elliott, H L
Ellis, G
Ellison, J
Elms, S T
Esler, D J
Evans, S M
Evans, T J
Evans, T R J
Eves, S C
Ewart, P A
Ewen, G
Ewen, S J
Fadaly, A-H A
Fagan, C
Faichney, A
Fairgrieve, R
Fairley, A
Fairlie, A B
Fairweather, R A
Fakhoury, V A
Fallon, C W
Fallon, H M
Farish, G
Farrell, A M
Farrell, A A
Farrow, J
Fazzi, M
Fazzi, U G
Featherstone, C J
Fegan, P G
Felix, D H
Fell, E
Fell, N
Fellows, K P
Fergie, I
Fergie, N
Fergus, G C
Ferguson, A E
Ferguson, A G
Ferguson, D R
Ferguson, E
Ferguson, J C
Ferguson, R J
Fern, A I
Fernie, C G M
Ferrell, W R
Field, M
Fife, J
Fife, R J A
Finch, A K
Findlay, L
Finlay, E R
Finlay, I G
Finnegan, A A
Finney, A A W
Fisher, B M
Fitch, W
Fitchett, A A
Fitzpatrick, A P
Fitzpatrick, J J
Fitzpatrick, J P
Fitzsimons, E J
Fitzsimons, P A
Flanigan, C M
Flanigan, P G
Fleming, G
Fleming, M
Flowers, A-M
Flynn, E M
Flynn, M-A
Foley, C A
Ford, A D
Ford, J A
Ford, L B
Ford, S J
Forrest, A E M
Forrest, A
Forrest, J A H
Forrest, K M
Forrester, P B
Forsyth, A
Forsyth, A C
Foster, J E
Fouad, A A M M
Foulds, W S
Foulis, A K
Fowlie, J E
Fox, J G
Frame, D W
Frame, M H
Frame, M Y
Frame, W T
Francis, R
Franklin, I M
Fraser, A A
Fraser, C P
Fraser, E M
Fraser, G
Fraser, J
Fraser, L D
Fraser, M H
Fraser, P A
Fredericks, B J
Freer, C B
Fu, Y L
Fullarton, G M
Fyfe, A H B
Gaballa, M A A
Gabri, R A M I
Gaffney, D
Gajree, A K
Galbraith, J
Galbraith, S L
Galbraith, S B
Galea, P F
Gallacher, K A
Gallacher, S J
Gallagher, G A
Gallagher, J
Galloway, D J
Gandhi, R A
Gardee, M R
Gardiner, H M
Gardner, E R
Gardner, F
Garrioch, M A
Garthwaite, M E K
Garvie, A C E
Garwood, E J
Gaudoin, M R
Gavin, M P
Gaw, A
Gaw, N J
Geddes, C C
Geddes, I C
Geddes, K M
Geddes, P M
Geddes, S M
George, M I
Ghosh, K
Ghosh, P
Ghosh, S K
Ghouri, N A
Gibson-Smith, B K
Gibson-Smith, S
Gibson, A J
Gibson, B E S
Gibson, H
Gibson, I W
Gibson, N A
Gihooly, T C
Gilchrist, C-A M
Gilchrist, I N
Giles, M D
Gilhooly, C J
Gillani, N
Gillespie, E
Gillespie, G
Gillespie, G N
Gillespie, J A
Gillies, C
Gillies, G W A
Gillies, M A M
Gillis, C R
Gilmartin, G
Gilmore, M C
Gilmour, D G
Gilmour, H N
Girdwood, R W A
Glasser, A I
Glasser, J M
Glavin, R J
Glen, P
Goddard, M J
Goh Huat Seng, M
Going, J J
Going, S M
Goldberg, D J
Goldberg, J A
Goldie, J G S
Goldie, J
Goldin, E J
Goldthorp, S L
Gooch, C L
Goodfield, N E R
Gordon, D
Gordon, I M H
Gordon, J A
Gordon, J
Gordon, J N
Gordon, J S
Gordon, M W G
Gordon, M M
Gordon, R A
Gordon, S M J
Gorrie, M J
Goudie, S G
Goudie, S E G
Gow, R L
Graham, A M R
Graham, A R
Graham, A S
Graham, D I
Graham, I K
Graham, W M
Granger, J M
Grant, P T
Gray, A J R
Gray, A G
Gray, F M
Gray, G R
Gray, J A
Gray, J K M
Gray, R M
Gray, R F
Gray, T M
Greene, J D W
Greer, A
Greer, I A
Greig, K
Grierson, D J
Grieve, C
Griffiths, H L
Groden, R E
Grom, I A P
Grossart, K W M
Grosset, D G
Grosset, K A
Gruer, L D
Gruszecka, K A T
Gunneberg, N
Gupta, D
Gurbanna, B A
Gurling, S R
Guse, G E W
Gusterson, B A
Guthrie, C I
Guthrie, E
Habeshaw, T
Haddock, G
Haddow, K A R
Hadley, K M
Haggerty, S J
Haggith, A K
Hague, R A
Haigh, J S E
Hair, A
Hajivassiliou, C A
Hall, G L
Halliday, J C
Hamayun, M P
Hamid, S K
Hamilton, G W
Hamilton, G M
Hammer, H M
Hamoudi, A H
Handa, U
Hanlon, P W
Hannah, E G
Hannah, P M
Hannay, J A F
Hanretty, K P
Harchowal-Muir, V S K
Harden, K A
Hardie, M J
Hardie, M R W
Hardman, R J
Harkins, L
Harkins, M
Harley, E C
Harper, A C
Harper, A M
Harper, C M
Harris, F E
Harris, M C
Harris, M I
Harrison, J M
Harrison, P G W
Harrison, S C
Hart, A M
Hart, D M
Harvey, A M R
Harvey, K J
Harvie, A
Hassan, K S
Hathorn, I A
Hatter, T J
Haughney, J A F
Haworth, G
Hawthorn, R J S
Hay, E J
Hay, J H
Hay, L A
Hay, W M
Hay, W I
Hearns, S T
Hems, T E J
Henderson, A P K
Henderson, F
Henderson, J R
Henderson, J J
Henderson, K M
Henderson, L K
Henderson, R
Henderson, S C
Henderson, T F
Henderson, W I F
Hendry, C
Hendry, D S
Henry, G P
Hepburn, M
Hepburn, M E
Hepple, S E
Herbison, J
Herron, J J
Hickey, K M
Hide, T A H
Higgins, A
Higney, M C
Hilditch, W G
Hillan, K J
Hillis, W S
Hinnie, J
Hitiris, N G
Ho, G-T
Ho, J T F
Hodge, W R
Hogg, K-J
Hogg, P
Hogg, R B
Hoh, C S L
Holden, R J
Holden, R M
Holland, B M
Holms, C M
Hood, J
Hood, V D
Hooper, D K B
Hooper, K M
Hopkinson, Z E C

Horgan, M P
Horne, G M
Hosie, G A C
Hosie, J
Hossain, T
Houston, A B
Houston, F M
Houston, V
Howat, C
Howat, T P
Howat, T W
Howatson, A G
Howie, E B
Howie, F M C
Hubbard, K E
Hughes, K S
Hughes, R L
Hughes, V E
Hughson, A V M
Hukin, S L
Hullin, M G
Hume, M A
Hunter, G W G
Hunter, J A
Hunter, M A
Hunter, R
Hussain, N
Hussain, Z
Hutchison, A S
Hutchison, B M
Hutchison, D A
Hutton, I
Ibrahim, F H
Imrie, C W
Imrie, F R
Imrie, G J
Imrie, W L
Ingham, D G
Inglis, A C
Inglis, A I
Ingram, R R
Ip, J C K
Ireland, A J
Ireland, R W
Irshad, N
Irvine, H J
Irvine, R W
Irvine, S A
Irwin, G J
Isa, A Y
Ismail, I S
Jackson, A P
Jackson, D J
Jackson, G A
Jackson, H J
Jackson, J A
Jackson, L E C
Jackson, R
Jackson, S A
Jacobs, L
James, A M
James, E A
James, J M
James, K S
James, W B
Jamieson, D G
Jamieson, H T
Jamieson, M E
Jamieson, M P G
Jamieson, R R
Jandial, S
Jardine, A G
Jarrett, P M
Jarrett, R F
Jarvie, A
Jauhar, P
Jay, J L
Jay, M J H
Jeffrey, J S
Jennett, S M
Jennings, K
Jheeta, J S
Johnmian, C J
Johnpulle, A F S
Johnson, D T
Johnson, M K
Johnston, A N
Johnston, F A
Johnston, R A
Johnstone, C
Johnstone, W A
Jones, B L
Jones, C C
Jones, G C
Jones, I G
Jones, R D
Jones, S
Jordan, M T
Joseph, S
Joss, N M
Juhasz, P L
Junor, B J R
Junor, E J
Jury, C S
Kamat, N D
Kamming, D
Kasem, K F
Kausar, M S
Kausar, S
Kavanagh, D
Kay, A J F
Kean, D M
Keane, J A
Keddie, J
Keeble, W
Keighley, B D
Kell, M R
Kelly, C J G
Kelly, D R
Kelly, G M
Kelly, M D
Kelly, M P
Kelly, M H
Kelly, R C C
Kempsill, G R J
Kennedy, D H M
Kennedy, E M M
Kennedy, I M
Kennedy, J H
Kennedy, J A
Kennedy, P G E
Kennon, B
Kenny, G N C
Kent, F J
Kent, M A
Ker, N D
Kerr, A M
Kerr, I C
Kerr, I F
Kerr, J I
Kerr, K J
Kerr, M H
Kerr, R E I
Kerr, W J
Kershaw, P W
Kesson, C M
Kestin, I G
Khan, A L
Khan, M W A
Khan, S A J
Khand, A
Khand, R
Khanna, R
Kidd, V E
Kiddie, J M
Kim Lin Lim, Dr
Kincaid, R J
Kincaid, W C
King, A E
King, S A
Kingsmore, D B
Kinnear, F B
Kinninmonth, A W G
Kinsella, J
Kirk, A J B
Kirk, D
Kirkland, I B
Kirkness, C M
Kirkpatrick, J J R
Kirkwood, W S
Kleinglass, A H
Knight, D G
Knill-Jones, R P
Koch, J E
Kochar, A
Kohi, Y M
Koppel, D A
Kraszewski, A
Krause, A A
Krishnan, P
Kubba, A K
Kuhan, V
Kyle, K F
Kyle, P M
Lafferty, T G
Laing, M S
Laird, L
Laird, S
Lalloo, D
Lamb, E W B
Lamb, K S R
Lan-Pak-Kee, L Y K
Land, J H
Lang, S C
Lang, W
Langan, C E
Langan, J J
Langridge, S J
Lanigan, D J
Lappin, S J
Larisma, P
Larkin, J G
Larkin, M P
Lau, P F
Laude, A
Lauder, J C
Laurie, A N
Laurie, M
Law, A T
Lawrence, C A
Lawrie, S M
Lawrie, T D V
Lawson, A A
Lawson, R A
Lean, M E J
Leanord, A T
Ledingham, M-A
Lee, A J
Lee, J C L
Lee, K M
Lee, W R
Lees, J T
Lees, J C
Lees, K R
Lees, N W
Leggate, P A
Legge, S
Leitch, J J
Leith, J M
Leman, J A
Leng, J E
Lennox, I M
Leonard, M
Leonard, M J
Leslie, D W
Leslie, M E
Leung, E W-Y
Leven, C F
Lever, R S
Levy, B
Levy, I A
Levy, R D
Lewis, G D
Lewis, J M D
Lewis, M T
Lewis, R F M
Leyland, K G
Li Yim, D F M
Li, K-W K
Liddell, A R
Liew, B S
Lindop, G B M
Lindsay, A C
Lindsay, E L S
Lindsay, G
Lindsay, J M
Lindsay, K W
Lindsay, K A
Lindsay, N J F
Ling, S C
Lingam, S M K
Litherland, J C
Livingston, E
Livingston, M G
Livingstone, E D
Livingstone, H W
Lockhart, G D
Logan, J A
Logue, J A
Love, G H
Lovett, J M
Low, R A L
Lowe, G D O
Lucie, N P
Luck, J F
Lui, G J L
Lukman, H
Lumsden, M A
Lunan, C B
Lunan, H R
Lupton, M F
Lyall, H
Lynas, A H
Lynas, G J
Lynch, B
Lynch, J
Lyon, S C
Lyons, D
Lyons, J C
M'allistev, K F
McAlavey, P S
Macalister, A
McAlpine, A C
McAlpine, C H
McAlpine, H M
MacAndie, C
MacAra, L M
McArdle, P A
McArthur, A A
MacArthur, G E
McArthur, J D
McAulay, E M
Macaulay, L
MacBain, G C
MacBrayne, J
Macbrayne, J F
McBurnie, V A
McCabe, R J R
McCallum, M M
MacCallum, R D
McCallum, S M
McCann, C M
McCann, G
McCann, S J
McCarlie, I
McCarter, D H A
McCartney, D J
McCaul, J A
McClure, K R
McColgan, C C
McColl, K E L
McConnell, J M
McConnell, V A
MacCormick, A S
McCormick, M F
McCreath, B J
McCreath, C M
McCreath, S W
McCruden, E A B
McCubbin, T D
MacCuish, A C
MacCuish, S K
McCulloch, A C
McCurley, J
McDevitt, J
McDevitt, R L
McDonagh, M F
McDonagh, T A
Macdonald, A G
Macdonald, A G
MacDonald, A S
McDonald, C F M
Macdonald, E B
MacDonald, G J
Macdonald, H E
Macdonald, I M
MacDonald, I K G
McDonald, J E
McDonald, J S
McDonald, K J
Macdonald, M E
MacDonald, P D
McDonald, S W
McDougall, A N
McDougall, C
McDougall, J W
McDougall, S J
McDougall, V M
Mace, A T M
McElroy, K
McEntegart, A
McEntegart, M B
McEwan, H P
MacEwan, T H
McFadyen, M B
Macfarlane, D W
MacFarlane, G P
Macfarlane, G N
McFarlane, J H
McFarlane, T
McFatter, F B
McGarrity, J D
McGarrity, M
McGarry, F J
McGarry, G W
McGeoch, P D
McGeorge, A P
McGettrick, S M
McGhee, D P
McGhie, J
McGill, P E
McGinley, A L
McGivern, C
McGlone, G C
McGlone, M C
McGonigal, A
McGowan, M P
McGown, D S
McGrath, A M
McGregor, E A
MacGregor, F B
MacGregor, K E
McGregor, K A
McGregor, M S
Macgregor, S E
McGurk, F M
McGurk, S F
McHenry, P M
McHugh, O C
McIlhenny, C
McIlwaine, L M
Macinnes, B N
McInnes, G T
Macintosh, I D
MacIntyre, D
McIntyre, K J
Mack, D S
Mack, K M
McKane, J P
McKay, A J
Mackay, A J
McKay, C J
McKay, I
Mackay, I M
Mackay, I R
Mackay, I G
Mackay, K J
Mckay, V
McKean, S J C
McKean, W P
McKechan, K F
McKechnie, S A
McKee, A H
McKee, P B
McKee, R F
McKeeve, G
McKenna, E A
McKenna, K J
McKenna, M P
Mackenzie, A G
Mackenzie, A M
Mackenzie, F M
MacKenzie, J A B
Mackenzie, J F
Mackenzie, P C
Mackenzie, P A
Mackenzie, R J
Mackenzie, R A
MacKenzie, S
McKeon, S C
McKeown, A C
McKeown, R C
Mackie, R M
McKillop, A C
McKillop, J H
Mackinnon, A D M
McKinnon, C
MacKinnon, H B
Mackintosh, C J
Mackintosh, L N M
Mackintosh, W A
Mackle, J
Macklin, J P
Macklon, N S
McKnight, D W
McKnight, J M
McLachlan, D D
MacLachlan, J S
McLaren, A D
McLaren, E H
McLaren, J
McLauchlan, J H
McLaughlin, A-M
McLaughlin, E
McLaughlin, I M
McLaughlin, I S
McLaughlin, K J
McLaughlin, M E
McLay, A L C
McLay, W D S
Mclean, A N
McLean, A H
Maclean, G P
MacLean, J A
MacLean, M A
McLearie, S
McLellan, A R
McLellan, D M
McLellan, D R
McLellan, E M
McLennan, C
MacLeod, A
MacLeod, D J
McLeod, F
MacLeod, G A
Macleod, H E
Macleod, I A
Macleod, M C M
McLeod, S A
Macleod, U M
McLintock, T T C
McMahon, A J
Macmillan, A H M
McMillan, A C
McMillan, K
McMillan, L J D
McMillan, M A
McMillan, N C
McMurray, J J V
McNally, A M
McNaught, P L
McNee, A
McNeil, H
McNeil, N
MacNeill, D R
McNeill, R J
McNeish, C I M
McNeish, G
McNicol, A M
McNicol, L R
McNicol, M F
McNicol, R A
McPhaden, A R
MacPhail, A K
Macphee, G J A
McPhee, S G
MacPhee, W P
Macpherson, C M
McPherson, E A
Macpherson, I
MacPherson, M J
Macpherson, S G
McQuaker, I G
McQueen, A
Macrae, C M
Macrae, K A
Macrae, M E
MacRae, W J
MacSween, R N M
MacSween, R M
McTaggart, H
Mactier, H
Mactier, R A
MacVicar, S M
McWilliam, R C
Madhok, R
Madhok, V K
Madi, A M
Maguire, A M
Mahal, P S
Mahmoud, O A R
Mair, R M
Makar, S
Malcolm, M R
Malcolm, R S
Malik, A K
Malik, H Z
Mallinson, A C
Mallon, E A
Mallon, J M
Mamode, N
Manchip, A J
Mandeville, H C
Mandeville, R P
Mani, C
Mann, A C
Mann, T S
Mansouri, M
Mardon, J M
Marney, Y M
Marsden, D M
Marsh, D R G
Marsh, J I
Marshall, A J
Marshall, J W V
Marshall, J M
Martin, A C
Martin, B J
Martin, C L
Martin, D J
Martin, G M
Martin, J I
Martin, L J
Martin, N
Martin, W G
Masterson, E
Mathers, A M
Mathewson, W B
Matthew, T B
Maule, B H
Maule, J H
Maxwell, H
May, B J
May, J A
Mealyea, M T M
Meek, D
Meek, R M D
Meggs, A M
Meighan, D P
Meikle, F S
Mellon, A
Melrose, D
Melrose, H G
Melville, C A

Menzies, G F
Mercer, S W
Metcalfe, R A
Midgley, N M
Midgley, P C
Miles, B M
Millar, A J
Millar, A Y
Millar, B A
Millar, E A
Millar, G
Millar, S
Miller, C D
Miller, G S
Miller, J C
Miller, K J
Miller, S A D
Milligan, J A
Mills, P R
Milne, R
Milroy, R
Minhas, H B
Minnis, H J
Mir, N U
Misra, P C
Misra, S
Mitchell, A
Mitchell, A C
Mitchell, A G
Mitchell, C M
Mitchell, I J
Mitchell, J R
Mitchell, K F
Moffat, K J
Moffett, A W G
Mohammed, N
Mohammed, R
Mohammed, Y
Moir, J S
Molloy, R G
Monaghan, P B
Moncrieff, J
Mone, A J
Mone, J G
Monie, R D H
Moonie, A
Moore, J M
More, I A R
Morgan, A H
Morley, J R
Morley, K D
Morrice, M S
Morris, A R
Morris, A J
Morris, S T W
Morrison, A C M
Morrison, A E
Morrison, C E
Morrison, D A N
Morrison, D S
Morrison, G B
Morrison, H M
Morrison, J D
Morrison, J M
Morrison, J M
Morrison, J L
Morrison, L M
Morrison, M
Morrison, S
Morrissey, M S C
Morrow, H M
Morton, A L
Morton, M J S
Morton, N S
Morton, R
Moschos, M
Moses, A G W
Mosley, A M
Moss, J G
Moss, N M
Mowat, A M
Mowat, C
Mowat, E M
Mowat, W
Moyes, E C
Mucci, B
Muhammad Taib, R H
Muir, A J
Muir, D F
Muir, K W
Mukherjee, M R
Mukherjee, S K
Mulhearn, J F
Mulhearn, N M
Mulholland, G M
Mullin, A M
Munro, C S
Munro, L M
Murch, C R
Murday, V A
Murdoch, D L
Murdoch, D R
Murdoch, F
Murdoch, J R
Murdoch, R M
Murnaghan, C
Murphy, A V
Murphy, D J
Murphy, G A
Murphy, J B
Murphy, L
Murray, C
Murray, C C
Murray, C D
Murray, F
Murray, J B
Murray, L A
Murray, N S
Murray, S B
Murray, T S
Murray, V
Murray, W R
Mutch, S M
Mutch, W M M
Naftalin, L
Nahar, P N
Nairn, L M
Naismith, A J W
Naismith, A J
Nandwani, R
Napier, D E
Napier, E S
Napier, J M
Nasib, A
Neill, H
Neilson, D W
Neilson, E G
Nelson, J K M
Newman, L H
Newman, P M
Newman, W D
Newton, A I
Newton, J
Newton, J M
Newton, W D
Nicoll, J A R
Nicolson, J M
Nightingale, A M
Nijjar, A S
Noble, J S C
Norman, J E
Norris, A
Northcote, R J
Notman, I A
Nzewi, O C
O'Connor, M R
O'Connor, P
O'Donnell, N G
O'Donoghue, F J M
O'Driscoll, D P
O'Dwyer, P J
O'Hare, K J
O'Leary, C P
O'Neill, A S J
O'Neill, G T J
O'Neill, K A
O'Neill, K F
O'Neill, S M
O'Reilly, B F
O'Reilly, C V
O'Reilly, D S J
O'Reilly, P V
O'Rourke, N P
Oates, B D
Oates, J D L
Oates, P D
Oates, V E M
Ockrim, J L
Ogg, E C
Ogilvie, D B
Oglethorpe, R J L
Ohri, C K
Ohri, K M
Oien, K A
Oldroyd, K G
On, F W
Orr, D J
Orr, L A
Orr, R M
Ortega Sipan, A M
Osborne, K N A
Osborne, S C
Osborne, S A
Osbourne, G K
Osman, I
Overell, J R
Overton, J G
Owen, P
Pace, N A
Padgham, K L
Padmanabhan, N
Paice, B J
Pandis, V
Panesar, B S
Papanastassiou, V
Park, H M
Park, R H R
Parke, T R J
Parker, A N
Parker, B
Parkinson, H S
Pate, E G
Patel, K R
Patel, M
Paterson, A M E
Paterson, K R
Paterson, P J
Paterson, R E
Paton, J Y
Patrick, J A
Patrick, W J A
Patterson, R
Paul, D L
Pauleau, N F
Peacock, A J
Pearsall, F J B
Pearsall, R W H
Pell, J P
Pelosi, A J
Pemberton, L S
Pender, J
Penney, S C
Percy-Robb, I W
Perera, M J
Periasamy, P
Perry, C G
Perry, S F
Perry, S C
Peters, S E
Petrie, J R
Pettigrew, A F
Pettigrew, G
Petty, R K H
Peutrell, J M
Pexton, N F
Pezeshgi, D S
Phillips, G M
Phillips, K
Phillips, S H
Pickard, M A D
Pickard, W R
Pickering, C P
Pickett, M E J
Pirret, M F
Pirwany, I R
Pithie, A D
Pitt, W H
Plenderleith, A C H
Plenderleith, J L
Poddar, M L
Pole, I
Pollock, J C S
Pollock, K M
Pomphrey, E O H
Poon, F W
Porru, D
Porter, D R
Porter, M E
Pourghazi, S
Powell, J J
Powell, J C
Power, A
Powls, D A
Prabhu-Khanolkar, S D
Prakash, D
Prasad, V
Price, R J
Priddle, D J
Priest, M
Pringle, S
Pugh, D N
Purdie, A T
Pyone Pyone Myint, Dr
Quasim, I
Quasim, T
Quate, L Z
Quigley, A J
Quin, L M
Quinn, A C
Quinn, E A
Rae, A P
Rae, A J
Rae, C A
Rae, C P
Rae, R
Raeburn, R M
Raeside, J
Rafferty, C V
Raine, P A M
Raine, W J B
Rajar, R M
Ramayya, A
Rampling, R P
Ramsay, C N
Ramsay, I N
Ramsay, J E
Ramsay, L M
Rankin, A C
Rankin, E M
Rankin, M
Rankin, P M
Rashid, R
Ratani, T H
Ray, B C
Ray, K
Raza, A
Reavey, J
Reece, G J
Reed, N S E
Reekie, R M
Rees, D E
Rees, G L
Reeve, W G
Rehana, H A
Reid, A W
Reid, A A
Reid, D M
Reid, E K
Reid, I L
Reid, I M
Reid, J P S
Reid, J L
Reid, J A
Reid, R P
Reid, W
Reilly, D
Reilly, T G
Rejali, S D
Rennie, A L
Rennie, A N
Rennie, A C
Reynolds, G M
Reynolds, K N
Richardson, J P
Riches, S M-T
Richmond, H A N
Richmond, J R
Richmond, M
Riddell, E M
Ridgway, T J
Ritchie, A N
Ritchie, A J
Ritchie, B W
Ritchie, D A W
Ritchie, D M
Ritchie, J
Ritchie, R M
Ritchie, S N
Ritchie, W P
Riyami, B M S
Roan, C A M
Roberts, D T
Roberts, F
Roberts, J C
Roberts, J I
Roberts, M A
Robertson, A W
Robertson, A N
Robertson, A G
Robertson, A
Robertson, D J
Robertson, D K
Robertson, G A
Robertson, H M
Robertson, I W
Robertson, J I S
Robertson, J M
Robertson, K J
Robertson, K W
Robertson, L M
Robertson, M M D
Robertson, N A
Robertson, R A
Robinson, K E
Robinson, P H
Robless, P A
Rodger, C J
Rodger, J
Rodger, J C
Rodger, M W
Rodger, R S C
Rodie, V A
Roditi, G H
Roemmele, B J
Rogers, K M
Rogers, P N
Rollo, A G
Ronghe, M D
Rooney, D P
Rose, K I
Ross, J S
Ross, J J
Ross, L M
Ross, M A
Rouse, M E
Roushdy-Gemie, M
Rowlands, C M
Rowlands, G C
Roxby, E M
Roy, D H
Roy, M S K
Rubin, P
Ruiz, G A
Ruiz, M-C
Rumley, J J
Runcie, C J
Russell, A J C
Russell, D I
Russell, F M
Russell, J M
Russell, K A
Russell, L H F
Russell, R I
Russell, S
Russell, S A
Russell, T J
Ryan, P F
Sabharwal, A J R
Sadiq, H A
Salim, R
Samavedam, S
Sambrook, M G
Sammon, D J
Sanaghan, S A
Sanai, L
Sandford, A E
Sandham, P A
Sands, M G
Sardar, S A
Sarkar, S K
Sarvesvaran, J S
Sattar, N A
Schofield, A D G
Schulz, U C
Scollon, D
Scorgie, I G
Scott, E G
Scott, J L
Scott, J I
Scott, K
Scott, M G B
Scott, N B
Scott, P D R
Scott, P J W
Scott, R N
Scoular, A B
Scullion, H C
Scullion, J C
Scullion, J F
Scullion, R
Seenan, C F
Seltzer, B K
Seltzer, M S
Semple, C G
Semple, L C
Semple, P F
Sengupta, S
Senthil Kumar, C
Senthilkumar, C
Serpell, M G
Sewell, R A
Sewnauth, D K
Sha'Aban, M A J
Shah, I M
Shah, S
Shahriari, S
Shaker, A G
Shakur, J
Shand, J
Sharif, M M
Sharma, P
Sharma, V
Sharp, G L M
Sharp, J M
Sharp, R A
Sharpe, J E
Shaw Dunn, G
Shaw, B G
Shaw, R L
Shaw, R W
Shearer, L M
Sheerin, D F
Sheikh, S H
Sheil, L J
Shemilt, J C
Shepherd, J
Shepherd, M C
Sheridan, M C
Sheridan, P G
Shetty, M A
Shields, S A
Shoaib, T
Short, L M
Shott, C H
Shujaat, R
Siann, T L
Sidiki, S S
Silverdale, M A
Simmons, A L E
Simmons, M
Simmons, W
Simms, C M
Simpson, C C
Simpson, D C
Simpson, H W
Simpson, I G
Simpson, J A
Simpson, J C
Simpson, K R
Simpson, L N
Simpson, N J
Simpson, R G
Sinclair, J
Sinclair, J F
Singer, I O
Singh, B J
Singh, I
Sinha, R N
Skeoch, C H
Skeoch, H M
Slane, F
Slater, A C
Slater, V M A
Slavin, J A
Sloan, J B
Slorach, C C S
Small, M
Smiley, E
Smith, A M
Smith, C A
Smith, D M
Smith, D C
Smith, D
Smith, F M
Smith, G L
Smith, G L F
Smith, G H
Smith, G Y
Smith, I D
Smith, I S
Smith, J F F
Smith, K
Smith, L R N
Smith, M
Smith, M A E
Smith, M B
Smith, M C
Smith, M J
Smith, N C
Smith, R G
Smith, R H
Smyth, M G
Snaith, R J
Snedden, A E
Sockalingam, R R
Somerville, M J
Sommerville, M J
Sommerville, W T
Sonthalia, V B
Sood, A
Sood, L
Soraghan, P G
Sorooshian, K
Soukop, M
Soussi, A C
Soutar, A L D
Soutar, D S
Soutar, R L
Souter, M J
Spence, D F
Spence, G G
Spence, J C
Spencer, M H
Spilg, E G
Spilg, S J
Spowart, K J M
Sproule, M W
Sprunt, E M
Stack, B H R
Stallard, S
Stanley, A J
Stanton, T
Steen, B M
Steinberg, S V

Steingold, H
Stenhouse, P G
Stephen, C M
Stephen, L J
Stephen, M R
Stephens, C S
Stephens, M S
Stephenson, J B P
Steven, J M
Steven, K
Steven, R R
Stevenson, A G M
Stevenson, D J
Stevenson, M J
Stevenson, R D
Stewart, A I
Stewart, A M
Stewart, C J R
Stewart, D A
Stewart, E
Stewart, I
Stewart, I S
Stewart, J F G
Stewart, L B
Stewart, M E
Stewart, M D C
Stewart, M
Stewart, P M
Stirling, J B
Stirling, J L
Stockwell, M C
Stoddart, D G
Stone, D H
Stone, P A
Stother, I G
Stott, D J
Stott, S M
Strain, G B
Strathern, C H C
Struthers, I R
Stuart, B S
Sturrock, A M
Sturrock, M M
Sturrock, R D
Suckle, N E
Sullivan, F M
Summers, W B
Sunderland, G T
Sutherland, A M
Sutherland, C A H
Sutherland, D F
Sutherland, G A
Sutton, A M
Swain, E
Swan, F A
Swan, I R C
Swan, L
Swann, IJ
Sweeney, B
Sweeney, D
Sweeney, K T
Sweenie, A C
Syme, I G
Symington, I S
Syyed, R
Taggart, H F
Taggart, I
Tait, C M
Tait, R C
Tan, K Y
Tang, B Y W
Tansey, P J
Tappin, D M
Targosz, S A
Tavadia, S M B
Taylor, A D
Taylor, D A
Taylor, J L
Taylor, J R
Taylor, M F
Taylor, M
Taylor, S G
Taylor, Y
Teasdale, G M
Teh, L G
Templeton, D J
Tengku Ismail, T S
Teoh, C-M
Teoh, Y Y
Thakker, B
Thampy, R S
Thom, A A
Thomas, M J
Thomas, S R
Thompson, N F
Thompson, T D B
Thomson, A J
Thomson, A M P
Thomson, B F M
Thomson, D F
Thomson, E C
Thomson, G L
Thomson, J K
Thomson, J
Thomson, J E
Thomson, J
Thomson, N C
Thomson, S M
Thomson, W B
Thorburn, P J
Thoris, S
Thorp, J M
Tillman, D M
Tindal, M T
Tobias, E S
Tobias, J A
Todd, A M
Todd, M C
Tolhurst, J E
Tolmie, J L
Tomnay, J
Torley, D
Toshner, D
Tough, A M
Townsley, A
Tran, H N P
Travers, J F
Traynor, J P
Treadgold, N J
Trent, R J
Trollen, R M
Tsang, P
Tullett, W M
Turfrey, D J
Turnbull, A
Turner, J M
Turner, K J
Turner, M S J
Turner, P
Turner, T L
Tweddell, G A
Ullah, M I
Unwin, L G
Ure, D S
Urquhart, C S
Vallance, B D
Vallance, N B
Vallance, R
Vanezis, P
Vardy, J M
Vartikovski, R
Vasey, P A
Venner, R M
Vernham, G A
Vernon, D R H
Vickers, L E
Vilaplana Cannon, J P
Vincent-Smith, L M
Waddell, G A B
Waddell, M M
Wagstaff, A
Walbaum, D W
Walker, A E
Walker, A M Z
Walker, A B
Walker, C R C
Walker, D S
Walker, I D
Walker, J W S
Walker, J M
Walker, K G
Walker, M H
Walker, P I T
Walker, R G
Walker, R S
Wallace, D G
Wallace, I W
Wallace, J B
Wallace, W H
Walsh, E S
Walters, M R
Ward, D M B
Waterson, P G
Watkins, R
Watkinson, G
Watson, D J
Watson, F G
Watson, G C
Watson, M J
Watson, R J
Watt, A J B
Watt, A D
Watt, G C M
Watt, L J
Watt, N
Weaver, L T
Webb, A E
Webster, G D
Webster, M H C
Weiler-Mithoff, E M
Weinhardt, A B
Weir, A I
Weir, C R
Weir, J P
Weir, R J
Weir, R
Welch, G H
West, B A K
West, G P
Westwater, J J
Wheatley, D J
Wheeldon, K
Wheeldon, V C
Wheelwright, E F
Whitby, S
White, A
White, A
White, M P
White, R J
Whitefield, G A
Whiteford, M L
Whitelaw, A S
Whitelaw, S C
Whitham, G T
Whiting, B
Whitmarsh, T E
Whitty, B L
Whyte, L
Whyte, S J
Whyte, S F
Whyte, W G
Wiggins, P S
Wilcox, A
Wilcox, D E
Wilford, J M
Wilkie, S C
Wilkinson, A E R
Wilkinson, J D
Wilkinson, L M
Will, M
Willens, M
Williams, A M H
Williams, B O
Williams, C J
Williams, L
Williams, L
Williams, P J
Williamson Duffy, L M
Williamson, L
Willis, F R
Willison, H J
Willocks, C M
Willox, D G A
Willox, J C
Wilmington, S M
Wilson, A B
Wilson, B N
Wilson, C S
Wilson, C R
Wilson, C A
Wilson, E A
Wilson, E H C
Wilson, F A
Wilson, F W
Wilson, H E
Wilson, J W
Wilson, L L
Wilson, M E
Wilson, M P
Wilson, N
Wilson, N I L
Wilson, P C
Wilson, P M J
Winston, A
Winter, A J
Winter, H L
Winter, J W
Wirth, M A
Wise, A
Witherspoon, P
Witkiewicz, T S
Woldman, S J
Wolfe, R
Womersley, J
Wong, D J
Wong, R A
Wong, S C O
Woo, Y M
Wood, S F
Woodger, B A
Worrall, E P
Wray, D M
Wright, C M
Wright, D M
Wright, F
Wright, L
Wright, L M
Wright, P M
Wu, W C K
Wykes, W N
Wylie, A S
Wylie, A M
Wynne, D M
Yaghan, R J K
Yates, J A
Yates, R W S
Yelland, E S
Yellowlees, A J
Yip, B
Yosef, H M A A
Young, A R
Young, C A
Young, D G
Young, D J R
Young, H W S K
Young, J C
Young, J M
Young, J M
Young, S F
Yusof, A I
Zia, M
Zoma, A A
Zuberi, S M

Glastonbury

Acland-Hood, P L F
Corfield, A R H
Hancock, J M
Helsby, M R
Hughes, R M
Jackson, P A
Jones, D K L
Jones, P A
Macdonald, N D
Molina Sanchez, B
Montagnon, S A
Muir, W J
Sephton, J E
Strawford, I D
Welford, R A
Woolley, A C

Glenrothes

Aitken, C J D
Ball, M E
Ballingall, T A
Bell, J M
Campbell, R G
Carlyle, B E
Carlyle, D L
Carr, W D
Chien, F W
Clayton, M K
Downie, C H
Dunlop, W B
Fawzi, M F F F
Galloway, J P
Gergis, E M F
Gordon, G M
Grant, R M
Hellewell, D R
Howell, R A
Hyndman, N C
Iskander, S Y
Krishnaswamy, B R
McBride, I M
MacDiarmid, N G
Macdonald, W
McElhinney, J H
MacLeod, D S T-Y
Michael, C E
Milne, J A
Paisley, J M
Philipson, G P
Pryde, I
Reglinski, F A
Reid, D I
Robertson, R C G
Russell, F E
Smith, J
Stewart, H
Wallace, E L

Glossop

Adams, R C
Addy, J A
Ansons, A M
Appaji Gowda, M B G
Banerjee, B
Bennett, T
Bhanumathi, K S
Bhatt, S C
Broome, C J
Broome, J D
Daly, J
Dow, A J
Hanna, W J
Kershaw, S W
Oldham, J
Palmer, L A
Parikh, R V
Purnachandra Rao, V
Roberts, G J
Thorley, N J
Thornley, A P
Vuyyuru, S
Westmerland, S P
Woodyer, A B
Worrall, M A C

Gloucester

Adriaans, B M
Allen, P
Artamendi Larranaga, P
Asante, D K
Atine, G I O
Bailey, R C
Bailey, R G
Bailey, S C
Bakewell, S E
Baldwin, R N
Bancroft-Livingston, M K
Banks, R A
Barnes, R J
Barrick, V E
Barrow, J M
Barrow, P M
Basker, E L
Bell, R W
Bennett, D J I
Bennett, I M
Bertone, R
Billington, M T
Birch, P A
Brooke, A E
Brooke, J A
Brown, J L
Brown, J L
Bruce, S A
Buckley, C I W
Buckley, J F
Butland, R J A
Byrne, R J F
Carr, K L
Challenor, V F
Champion, C J
Charles, R
Chaudhuri, A K
Chaudhuri, A K
Chaudhuri, M
Chown, S R
Cobbe, J M
Coker, W J
Conaty, D J
Cook, T A
Cooke, S G
Corrigan, L D
Crabb, I J
Craig, J B
Cranmore, F J
Crawshaw, C C V
Croft, J J
Dale, C
Davidson, J C
Davies, N F
Dawes, R F H
Dicks, A G
Docherty, A D
Dodwell, P J
Donald, I P
Drinkwater, S L
Duffell, E F
Dutton, C S
Earnshaw, J J
Ellis, M S
Elphinstone, L H
Eltringham, R J
Evans, N J R
Fairbairn, G R H
Fairbairn, M L
Falkus, G K J
Fear, C F
Foster, J E
Foster, W H
Fowler, G J
Fuller, G N
Gabbott, D A
Gadsden, P M
Garbutt, N I B
Garcia-Rodriguez, C R
Garstang, J E
Gilbert, N J
Godden, D R P
Gold, C J
Goodwin, F C
Graham-Cumming, A N
Grayling, M
Graystone, S J
Green, C P
Griffiths, P F
Harbottle, T G
Harcourt, W G V
Hardingham, M
Hardy, P A J
Harney, B A
Harrington, A K
Hartrey, R
Hasan, N
Haynes, W D S
Heather, B P
Henderson, M S
Hidson, O J
Hoare Nairne, J E A
Hodges, P
Hodgson, G I
Hollingworth, M
Holmes, K A
Jadresic, L P
James, A J S
Jaques, R D
Jarvis, I S
Jewell, A P
Jewell, F M A
Johnson, G J
Jones, D J
Jones, S E
Joseph, R H
Kapoor, S
Kazi, B M
Kelsey, I G
Laidlaw, J D D
Laite, P A
Lala, A B H
Layzell, J M
Lazar, L K
Leitch, S P
Lewis, D A
Lindsay, D C
Livingstone, J A
Lloyd, G L
Logan, M N
Lucarotti, M E
Lush, P S L
Lynch, A S
McCarthy, J H
McCrum, A
McCrum, J C
McDowall, N A
Mackay, R H
Macleod, I N C
Macnair, D R
McNulty, C A
Macpherson, R
Mahendran, D
Majkowski, R S
Mann, J E
Marchant, M J
Martin, D R
Martin, R J
Mason, J E
Mathers, G C
Matthai, M S
Maxted, D F
Meecham Jones, D J
Miller, H J
Milne, J T
Moate, T J R
Moffitt, D L
Moodie, S F
Moore, P C L
Morris, T J
Mulhall, R M
Munir, A
Munir, M
Murphy, J R
Murphy, S D
Nair, H T
Nair, S
Nicol, A
Noonan, W J
Norwich, R P
Owen, M E
Pack, S F
Padfield, H J
Parfitt, V J
Parnham-Cope, D A
Parsons, C R
Paterson, R J
Paynter, H E
Peniket, J B
Petersen, M E V

Pickett, T M
Pike, W J
Porter, W M
Prior, J G
Pryle, B J
Read, M D
Reid, A N C
Remfry, C J C
Remfry, R M
Richards, R K
Richards, S E
Ritchie, A W S
Roberts, C J
Roberts, D M
Roberts, L A
Ropner, J E
Ross, D E
Ross, Carr
Rouse, M E
Russell, G A
Salter, M W A P
Sammon, A M
Sammon, H M K
Samuel-Gibbon, A G
Sarkar, J
Sarkar, S
Savage, J E
Savidge, M J
Seacome, M P S
Seymour, A
Shaw, I S
Sheehan, G E M
Shepherd, N A
Silva, M T
Sivananthan, N
Skirrow, M B
Smith, D J
Soundy, V C
Spargo, A E
Spargo, P J R
Spencer, E M
Steinhardt, S I
Stevens, D L
Stevens, D W
Sulaiman, M Z C
Tasker, T P B
Taylor, L E
Taylor, N H
Thomas, D M
Thomson, W H F
Thornberry, E A
Thornton, E J
Towle, N D
Uff, J S
Ulahannan, T J
Unwin, J
Valori, R M
Vanner, R G
Vassall-Adams, N I
Vipond, M N
Wagstaff, M H
Wallington, M
Watkins, R M
Watson, K M
Webb, J L
Webb, M S C
Webster, R H
Wheatley, A H
Whitehead, P N
Whittaker, M D
Whittaker, M A
Whittle, R A S
Wilcock, A C
Wilkinson, A R
Williams, B A
Williams, K J
Williams, K D N
Williams, L
Williams, N J
Winterbottom, P M
Youngs, R P
Zaidi, S B A

Godalming
Anderson, C M
Bigos, J E
Bland, H A
Blowers, J F A
Borthwick, A
Bott, S R J
Bray, R L
Brunet, M D
Bryett, A G
Campbell, P M F
Cerullo, A
Childs, K J
Clark, S E
Cook, A S
Craske, S
Davis, M E L
Dooley, J F
Fleetcroft, C T
Flynn, M J
Green, K
Gundry, A C
Hill, G W R
Howe, T V T
Hudson, M G
Hudson, P T P
Jagger, C R
Jameson, J K
Jenkins, M A
John, M
Jones, A K
Kahlenberg, H G
Kershaw, E J
McCluskie, P J A
Murray, L F
O'Donnell, M
O'Donnell, P S R
Overington, F J
Page, R F M
Riley, S J
Russell-Jones, D L
Savundra, J E
Sears, A F
Shah, T M
Simons, S E D
Simpson, E K
Slade, V J
Thomas, K E
Thomas, M
Thorburn, T G
Van Dorp, F A
Van Dorp, M H
Wathen, S J
Whitaker, J A J
Wilks, P R
Woolrych, J M
Zylstra, H J

Godstone
Al-Hilaly, N H D
Egerton, D F
Frost, S M
Glover, M
Howard, C W

Golspie
Begg, A B
Reid, A R
Thomson, K J

Goodwick
Davies, D E
Van Kempen, C E

Goole
Booth, F H
Brews, A J
Brown, D A
Clark, J E
Evison, D
Gogoi, N K
Greenwood, R
Hardy, D G
Harrison, R W
Kumar, B
Kurtis, R E
Moghissi, K
Moran, A G
Mukherji, S
Pinder, J R
Prendergast, B
Price, R B
Rana, A K
Reid, G F
Sim, J W
Smith, J L
Wignall, J R N
Wrightson, L

Gorebridge
Cremona, A
Lithgow, R S
McKeating, S H
Matear, E A
Murray, E M
Russell, J A
Scales, E A
Stoddart, D
Storrie, M P

Gosport
Anderson, J L
Anderson, J T H
Andrews, N P
Asbridge, M S
Bailey, D J W
Banks, V A
Barton, J A
Beasley, P A
Beck, S
Bennett, N J
Black, D H
Blacklock, N J
Brand, J J
Brigg, M J
Brook, S J
Brooks, G J
Brown, D C
Brunning, J
Burlein, G
Buxton, P J
Cavanagh, M C
Chilvers, D M
Coddington, R
Coggon, S
Collins, B G
Coltman, T P
Cook, D E
Coonan, B
Cooper, M P
Crean, D M
Davis, M C
Dean, M R
Edwards, C J A
Edwards, S A
Erskine, D O
Firth, M
Forster, J E
Fox, D J
Garratt, P P
Glover, M A
Golden, F S C
Golding, P L
Grocock, J H
Haddon, R W J
Hajiantonis, N C
Iddles, A J
Jagdish, S
Jones, J
Kershaw, C R
Kilbey, J H
Knapman, A C
Lacey, P A
Lenoir, R J
Lloyd, J P
Lynch, D N
Lynch, S M E
Millar, C W
Morgan, S R E
Morgans, B T
Mutch, C E
North, D
Nwokora, G E
Okhandiar, A
Parrish, M M
Parry, C A
Patrick, K
Pennells, R A
Peters, E J
Peters, N J M
Pingree, B J W
Pipkin, C
Pitkin, A D
Reston, S C
Rickard, R F
Risdall, J E
Scerri, G
Scott-Brown, M M
Sharpley, J G
Shaw, F R
Shawcross, C R
Skinner, T A
Skipper, J J
Swain, D L
Sykes, E M
Traynor, D B
Treharne, P G
Vassallo, D J
Watkins, M J G
Whitbread, T
Whiteoak, R
Whittaker, M A
Williams, M D
Yeo, H E D
Young, D A
Young, P C

Gourock
Adams, J C
Blair, D
Craig, J D
McGarrity, K M
McKinnon, S S
Murray-Lyon, R N
Nelson, E C
Robinson, M
Russell, D D
Russell, M C
Sridhar, S

Grange-over-Sands
Allen, J R
Barton, N V
Birch, A
Boyce, A C L
Irwin, J E
Lovatt, H M
Mason, N
Milligan, S D
Norman, J R
Phizacklea, S
Raymond, T M J R
Ruell, S D
Siddiqi, S C
White, T C

Grangemouth
Anderson, B G
Ballantine, D I
Carlyle, A K
Cruickshank, L J W
Deans, M
Deans, N J
Duggie, J G
Dunsire, M F
Gawn, A V
Hamilton, I R
Hegde, B D
Mohan Adyanthaya, K R R
Morrison, R A
Murdoch, I B
Murray, D R
Nicol, G J C
Selfridge, D I

Grantham
Abdel-Nasser, M R
Akhrass, A
Allsebrook, I
Baker, D J
Bamber, M G
Barker, S J
Birch, C R
Breckenridge, J L
Buck, J C
Caley, R
Campbell, G D
Campbell, J H
Campbell, M A
Camphor, S
Clarke, J D
Coombes, S
Cory, C E
Croft, K F
Crossley, I B
Cruickshank, J A
De Silva, S R
De Silva, S D
Dighe, V C
Dorrington, R F
Doughty, J M
Dunkin, J W
Elder, J B
Favier, J-P M
Fraser-Darling, A
Gallop, D M
Garbutt, F E
Garrick, H D O
Gee, R A
Gibson, P J
Gilmore, S J B
Gonzalez, O
Goru, S S R
Hale, C
Halliday, A E G
Hargreaves, P
Helmy, E L
Higgins, M T C
Hogg, C L
Holderness, D M
Houghton, A R
Husemeyer, R P
Ikhena, E I
Jayamaha, A A S
Kathel, B L
Kerr, J S
McKechnie, A
Manistre, S J
Mawdesley-Thomas, J
Mills, S J
Molave, E R
Moran, D G M
Munday, S A
Nicholson, K M
Nicoll, J M V
Nqumayo, C C
O'Riordan, S M
Onugha, C O
Parkin, M G
Patel, M N
Porter, A D
Porter, F N
Potdar, N P
Rankin, L C G
Rodrigues, C
Roper, D J
Shrouder, R D
Sie, T H
Sneddon, J J
Soni, R K
Southall, J G A
Stafford, E J
Stewart, K R
Surtees, A
Tedbury, M J
Terrill, L M
Tore, V B
Townsend, J S
Valerio, D
Van Lany, P
Vogt, S
Walker, I W
Wallace, K R
Watts, A J
Webster, M H
West, E A
Wiggins, B L
Wijayawardhana, U D
Wilson, J A
Zbrzezniak, W S

Grantown-on-Spey
Burns, F W
Grant, P F
Hamilton, S A
Lennon, R I
Mathers, S B
Peters, S B
Pirie, L K

Gravesend
Ahmad, I
Ali-Khan, G
Bailey, J A
Barker, C E
Bee, A J
Biswas, B K
Board, A P
Boyle, P
Brown, M P
Brown, P E
Carne-Ross, I P
Crawford, I
El-Faramawi, M A A
Fraser, C M
Giles, J H
Haider, S
Haider, Z J
Hall, J
Handy, C F
Harris, A R B
Hopkins, A D
Howie, J H
Jackson-Voyzey, E N
Jerreat, P G
Kent, J E
King, S G
Kooner, T S
Leung, T Y D
Markwick, C P
Martin, L P
Millar, I S
Moran, S G
Morgan, A H
Mounty, J P
Nada, E M E
O'Connor, D C
Ozua, C I
Pahal, G S
Palmer, A P
Patel, J R A
Patel, M M
Payne, D J
Price, L
Rao, G H
Shanks, R
Shergill, S S
Spurgin, H M K
Strens, L H A
Sumner, D J
Taruvinga, M
Taylor, H W
Thomson, A J
Todd, R G
Townsend, J C
Vallely, A J B
Vasudaven, B
Ward, J W
Westbrook, M A
Woodhead, D M J
Woodhead, N J
Zala, N N

Grays
Abeyewardene, A K
Aggarwal, D R
Bansal, A
Bose, A
Byrne, G P
Cameron-Mowat, I C
Colburn, M
D'Mello, J M T
Dambawinna, R
Dunn, G O
Dutta, B
Gunasekara, K V
Gupta, O P
Gupta, S S K
Headon, O T
Hurter, M D
Jayakumar, S
Jolly, G
Jones, S R
Khan, A A
Khan, K M
Khan, R S
Martin, P A B
Masson, H
Masson, K K
Mitchell, A H
Mitra, R K
Mohile, R V
Mohile, V V
Moore, J E A
Motashaw, R D
Newell, B A T
Rahim, M H
Ramachandran, M K
Shah, R
Shaikh, A
Shergill, S S
Sidana, S S
Sirisena, W G
Smith, D G

Great Missenden
Cairns, D W
Cottam, S-L G
Jenkins, C E
Jenkins, L M
Kadirgamar, A G V
Kanji, A A A
Kennedy, P A
Kirton, V
Laybourn, M L
Llewellyn Smith, M
Mair, J H D
Mallard-Smith, R J
Mitchell, M J
Neale, T W
Oliver, L J
Pattinson, J K
Peggs, K S
Pool, C J F
Purnell, N
Rogers, M H
Silver, J R
Smith, M C
Spencer, A J
Thomson, H G
Tingey, W R
Wilson, S J P
Wise, K S H
Zachariah, S E

Great Yarmouth
Absalom, S R
Adams, D E
Ahmad, N
Ahmed, E
Allan, A C
Amanat, L A
Aukland, P
Baker, H A
Betts, A F
Black, P D
Bonner-Morgan, B M
Bonner-Morgan, R P
Branch, K G
Cheema, A M

Cliffe, A M
Cotter, T P
Cowan, F M
Cremades Tudela, E
Crick, M R
Dalton, W T G
Dawson, J T
De Kock, A J
Delany, O J
Dissanayake, M P
Durance, P G
Eastwood, L H
Edelsten, A D
Ekbery, D J
Ellis, D A
Evans, H A
Fanous, N I
Fleetcroft, R C
Flores, M
Forster, P J G
French, A J
Gay, M P
Gerken, A
Gould, J
Gould, N S
Grabau, W J
Greenwood, P A
Hamza Aly, H
Harris, B R
Harrison, P R
Harry, T C
Hathaway, C
Hems, R A
Huston, N R
Ibrahim, G M A E-M A
Inyang, V A
Jarvis, R J T
Jesudason, K
Jewell, C
Jeyam, M
Jones, R N
Koessler, H
Kumar, V
Lal, R
Le Jeune, H J
Liddle, A C
Liddle, G C
Lipp, A C
Livingstone, N M
McIver, N K I
Mallion, J A
Mehta, G U
Mercer, R
Millican, D L
Minns, T
Mitchell, T R
Nagpal, S
Nagpal, S
Neaves, J M
Newstead, M R
Noakes, P C
Notcutt, W G
Novak, A Z S
Oosthuysen, S A V R
Outwin, W R
Oyeleye, A O
Pace, T
Patil, D B
Penn, A
Pereira, J H
Petri, G J
Poole, B J
Premachandra, D J
Qazi, S
Rafique, M
Rumble, M
Safwat, S M M
Sale, A C B
Salvary, I A
Santori, L B
Savage, J S
Schneider, H J
Shaw, I
Shelton, P J
Simpson, A D
Singh, S K
Statter, N R
Stevens, L F
Stewart, G S J A
Stuart, W H
Studley, J G N
Sturzaker, H G
Sudlow, S
Suresh Babu, G
Tadross, A A
Thomas, E A
Trigg, S L
Verma, A K
Verma, R
Vining, R M
Watson, D G
Watson, N J
Watts, M R
Willamune, N B
Win, S S
Wright, M M
Wright, R M

Greenford

Abdel-Hadi, O B A
Ahmad, J
Ahmed, S
Al Asady, M H S
Alles, R M
Anderman, J E F
Barrington, P
Barton, C M
Barton, J
Choudry, A A
Corn, T H
Doherty, B M
Eckland, D J A
Felton, J M
Finn, A M
Garbett, N D
Gayed, E S
Ghataura, S S
Goraya, B S
Goraya, S S
Guha, S
Gunput, M D
Heavey, D J
Hernon, J M
Hunjan, M S
Issac, N E
Jafree, A J
Jenkins, D A
Jenkins, M M
Jeyasingh, N
Jeyasingh, S
Jurges, E S
Kakar, S
Kapoor, K
Keerthi Kumar, S
Kooner, H S
Lewis, R A
Lones, A R W
Malhi, A M
Meehan, R A
Miall-Allen, V M
Moore, R C
Munn, S E
Narang, R S
Nasar, R B
Nizam, M
Patel, H
Patel, K
Quarishi, N A
Rapeport, W G
Ross, I R
Rut, A R
Salahuddin, M J
Sandhu, I K
Segal, N H
Segal, S M
Shackell, M M
Shah, R R
Sharma, S D
Steel, H M
Swords, J
Sykes, J A
Tak, A M
Vanderpuije, J A
Wah, T M
Webster, A
Williams, M L
Williams, P M
Winter, C W M
Yogendran, L

Greenhithe

Langley, S H

Greenock

Ayana, A E
Ayana, G E
Barr, P S
Bartholomew, A J
Biggs, E A C
Blyth, A C
Burton, J N
Campbell, I B
Deveney, G
Dickson, A R
Dilawari, J B
Fisher, S A
Foster, D A
Gallagher, J O
Ganai, N K
Haggerty, K A
Hamilton, E M
Harkins, L H
Henderson, W B
Hillman, A
Hlaing, T T
Hulme, A W
Hyett, E L
Jefferies, G D
Kapasi, M A
Kerr, B A
Kerridge, S C E
Kohlhagen, N
Kurian, O K
Leighton, K M
Lusman, D
McCallum, H S
McCarey, D W
McConnell, A A
McGarrity, G
Macnab, G M
McNeil, W
Majumder, B C
Malloch, A J
Mansfield, D C
Marshall, D A S
Montgomery, J
Morrison, A M
Moultrie, P A
Munro, F J
Murdoch, F A
Orr, F G G
Papaconstantinou, H
Petrie, A J
Pettigrew, A M
Pow, C E L
Rainey, M G
Reidy, J J
Roach, E
Robins, J B
Roy, J
Rutherford, A
Semple, J M
Semple, P A
Seywright, M M
Sharma, D C
Sihra, P K
Sim, Y T
Small, H M M
Sykes, R A D
Tam, W K
Taylor, E W
Thomas, M A
Thompson, J B
Thomson, J E
Tong, G Y K
Valentine, C B
Walker, N P
Ward, R
Watt, I
Welsh, S L
Wright, K C
Wyness, P J
Young, J M

Gretna

Herrick, P R
Kamar, S H
Rigg, A W
Stenhouse, S M

Grimsby

Abourawi, F I
Adhikaree, S N
Adiotomre, J A
Adiotomre, P N A
Ahmad-Salem, M I M A R
Al-Atrakchi, S
Albuquerque, W J
Amin, H H S
Anderson, J
Bagga, P
Bagga, T K
Bain, R J I
Ballantyne, J F
Bandyopadhyay, S
Barton, R O
Belcher, P D
Bellini, M J
Blanco Mayo, F
Bolaji, I I
Bramwell, R G B
Bruning, T J
Bwalya, G M
Calthorpe, W R
Campbell, A E R
Carter, P A
Chalmers, I D S
Chappel, E C
Chauhan, S
Choudhury, K
Collett, K A
Culshaw, T D
Deodhar, B G
Dobson, A H J
Donaldson, L A
East, M R
Elder, D C
Finch, A A
Foulkes, K K
Gough, M D
Gough, M B
Gowribalan, R
Harries, R W J
Harris, P
Heath, P
Hobbes, C J C
Holland-Keen, L B
Hopkins, E N
Hopper, D E
Ingram, I J
James, D W
Jethwa, H
Kelly, J D C
Kershaw, J B
Khan, K U
Kidson, C J
Knight, S J
Koonar, K S
Kotta, S
Kumar, R
Kweka, E L M
Laver, S R
Law, A L C
Lawless, P
Leitch, D G
Lopez Sanchez, J E
Majumder, A K
Matthews, T K
Melton, P J
Moss, S
Mounfield, P A
Nathwani, N
Nicholson, T C
Opie, P M
Overton, R C
Packer, P F
Panigrahi, P
Parrish, F J
Peacock, K
Pearson, H J
Peters, W M
Plotnek, J S
Pool, R W
Potter, J R C
Rajasekhara, K S
Rizvi, I H
Roberts, J A
Saha, A
Salim, G M
Salisbury, A K
Samaan, A A A
Samy, A K E M
Samy, M A E
Sarkar, S K
Seal, R H
Sharma, R P
Shweikh, A M
Sikka, S
Simhachalam, D
Singh, B
Smith, M F
Spalding, A E
Speed, K R
Stergides, A C
Sumbwanyambe, N W
Suresh Babu, P
Tait, T J
Tandon, B
Thrippleton, S A
Tilston, M P
Twomey, C A
Twomey, P A
Vicca, A F
Ward-McQuaid, J M
Wardle, E N
Watkin, J I
Wobi, B
Woosnam, L
Zoon, E

Grouville

Alwitry, A
Blandin, B O
Howard, R D
Philips, F K

Guernsey

Allen, K V
Allen, N H
Allsopp, R H
Andrews, C W
Arduin, M-L
Bacon, H F
Barker, R W F
Biggins, P
Birchall, H M
Bodkin, S E
Boyle, A S
Boyle, A G
Brache, J A
Brand, D S
Brennand Roper, S M
Brereton, M J
Byrom, N P
Chamberlain, M R
Chankun, T S L
Degnen, F H
Downing, M P R
Edirisooriya, A W
England, R A
Erskine, J
Farmer, C J
Ferguson, J
Gibbs, J R
Gibson, H M
Gill, T R
Gomes, P J
Harcus, A W
Haskins, R H
Henry, S L
Heyworth, S P
Hollwey, S J
Johnson, A D
King, N C
Laidlow, E H
Lean, B W
Lee, T R
Lewis-Jones, H J
Longan, J F
Lyons, R A
McCarthy, M D W
McClymont, C
Mellors, S F
Monkhouse, C R
Mowbray, M
Mullen, P J P
Norris, E M
O'Donnell, A J
Oswald, G A
Paluch, N A F
Parkin, B D
Parkin, L
Pearce, J G
Pratt, C I
Pring, D J
Quanten, P P L
Raderschadt, E L
Reilly, G D
Reilly, S J
Rice, J G
Richards, P W
Richards, S J
Simpson, P
Sinnerton, T J
Smith, E J
Stocker, J C
Sutherland, A M
Taberner, C R
Thompson, P J
Tooley, P J H
Turner, J J
Van Der Hauwaert, N
Williams, P G
Wilson, D S M
Wilson, S J V
Wolfe, M J
Wray, S
Yarwood, G D

Guildford

Abood, E A
Ackerley, D
Adams, A E
Al-Khatib, F A H
Arbuckle, J D
Arnold, S J
Arnold, T D
Baerselman, G M
Bailey, M E
Bailey, V E
Barbour, L A A
Barnardo, J N
Basarab, A O
Beaumont, J D
Bedson, C R
Behn, A R
Belshaw, C P
Bevington, W P
Bews, S M M
Blair, R A
Bland, C J H
Blight, A R
Bloomberg, T J
Blundell, R E
Bodgener, S
Boodhoo, M G
Booth, A J
Breimer, L H
Britton, P
Brookshaw, J D
Brown, J G
Butler-Manuel, S A
Cane, P J
Carlyon, A M E T
Carpenter, S
Carr-Bains, S
Carr-White, G S
Carroll, J D
Chambers, S
Chandrasekaran, B
Chapman, P
Chapman, S J
Christopher, A N
Chua, T P
Clarke, J
Coates, C J
Coats, P M
Cook, M G
Cordingley, R A
Couper, D M
Craven, R M
Cross, A P
Crutchley, E
Cummin, A R E
Cunliffe, I F
Curtis, E P P
Daborn, L G
Danford, M H
Das, S N
Daulton, D P H
Davies, A P
Davies, J H
Davies, J H W
Davis, A K
De Lusignan, S
Deacock, S J
Dellow, E L
Demetriadi, F E
Domizio, S A G
Douglas, C N
Douglas, I D C
Drury, S J M D
Dumbreck, L A
Edkins, C L
Elliott, D R
Evans, C M
Evans, J J
Ewart, I C
Eyre-Brook, D G
Fairey, A E
Farmer, R D T
Faulkner, E
Fawcett, W J
Ferns, G A A
Ferreira, I
Fisher, W J
Flannery, M C
Foley, J H
Foley, P W X
Foley, T H
Franks, O H B
Franks, V E
Gabriel, J R T
Gallagher, T M
Gibbons, J W
Gibbs, N M
Gibson, P J
Gilbert, S
Godden, C W
Gordon, C J
Gosal, H S
Gray, R E S
Grisewood, H L
Grisewood, M
Guest, C S
Hadwin, R J
Halfpenny, D V A
Hall, J R
Halliwell, I K
Hampson, S W
Han, C F
Harvey, M P
Hatrick, C M
Helliwell, C J V

Hibbert, J
Hillman, H
Hockey, A J
Holliday, M G
Hornett, G A W
Howard, L C
Humphrys, C M
Hutt, R
Isaac, J
Jackson, E G A
Jackson, P A
James, S E
Jayarajan, V
Jenkins, J G
Jenkins, T P N
Johnson, P A
Jones, S L
Jordan, M J
Jump, A E
Kalu, G U
Karanjia, C R
Karanjia, N D
Keenan, J M
Kemball, G A
Keown, C E
Kissin, C M
Kissin, M W
Knight, C A
Laing, R W
Langley, S E M
Laurence, D T
Lawrenson, R A
Layer, G T
Leatham, E W
Lee, E
Lee, N J
Leigh, J M
Lennox, H R G
Longman, R J
Lopez, A J
Lukaszewicz, C M
McAllister, W A C
Macdonald-Watson, A
MacMillan, D M
McMullan, C A
Magnussen, P A
Marks, C G
Marsh, J E
Mead, A L
Metcalfe, C
Money-Kyrle, J F
Morrison, M C
Moss, S M
Neal, A J
Nichols, J A A
Nickells, J S
Nigam, A K
Norris, J S
O'Connell, M P
Obi, B C
Oh, C J E
Oxenbury, J L
Packham, I N
Paremain, G P
Paremain, T J
Patel, V
Piper, E J
Piper, S
Powell, J H P
Qureshi, T I
Rathnavarma, C V R
Rauh, P B
Rawal, K M
Rayner, C M
Read, M T F
Rees, J D G
Reid, K W
Riaz, N U
Rimmer, A F G
Robbins, G
Rossdale-Smith, G J
Rosson, J W
Rowe-Jones, J M
Rushen, J E
Rushton, K L
Ryalls, M R
Sales, R A
Sarin, U
Saunders, P R
Schweitzer, F A W
Scott, J C R
Sekhawat, B S
Sender, J
Seth, V
Shirley, J A
Shoeb, I H A-H
Sisson, J
Slater, G H
Sleight, S P
Smith, M R
Smith, M G M
Smith, M J
Sockett, G J P
Solomons, N B
Speirs, N I
Stebbing, J F
Stephenson, K A
Stiles, P J
Stoner, K B
Sudderick, R M
Sutton, C J G
Sutton, J A
Swindale, F E
Tahir, S S
Tailor, A J
Tansley, R G
Tarzi, M D
Taylor-Barnes, K
Taylor, J D
Tinkler, A M
Topham, C A
Trend, P S J
Trigg, H A
Tutin, A F
Tutin, A M
Tyrrell, G R
Valentine, P W M
Van Every, T H
Volikas, I
Wachtel, S L
Walker, W J
Walsh, R N
Wan Fook Cheung, W C H
Watson, S J
Weir, N F
Werrett, G C
Whitcroft, S I J
White, W F
Whitehead, A M
Whitelaw, E A
Whiteley, M S
Wilkinson, A B
Willett, C J
Williams, J G
Wong, E
Wong, G E
Worthington, S
Wright, J W
Xavier, S M
Zaidi, S M N

Guisborough
Ashraf, A
Bell, A J
Bergin, A J
Brownlee, M J
Davis, P A
Dobie, F D
Dobson, L P
Garry, R
Gilliat, J M F
Halloway, A J
Hilton, A
Hobkirk, D W
Irving, S A
Kaiser, J P
Katib, J
Lewis, A M
Marr, D C
Newnam, P T F
Phillips, A G
Prince, S
Smith, A J
Todd, R L
Williams, S M

Gullane
Auld, J W
Cusworth, C J
Durie, A W
Eunson, P D
McPhail, P M
Millar, D R
Quigley, M G

Gunnislake
Bowhay, A A
Buxton, N D
Heslop, J V M
Stewart, A P

Haddington
Alexander, G
Baptie, J A
Branwood, A W
Brown, J K
Carrell, M
Fulton, J F
Glendinning, S M R
Hastings, P D
Hogg, V J
Holton, D E
Laidlaw, S C
Langlands, R W D
Lavelle, F M M
Lawson, R J
McInnes, K E
Mercer, G W
Morrison, L
Riddle, W J R
Robertson, P E
Rogers, T D
Sheldon, A J L
Wright, H W

Hailsham
Ahmed, S K
Alston, R H
Baker, G R H
Carson, R G
Croucher, M D
Davison, D A
Doraiswamy, W
Dunphy, P W
Gardner, G A
Griffiths, S S
Grimston, A J
Hall-Smith, R G
Hanraty, D A
Hays, P L
Heap, B J
Holden, J S F
Holmes, P C B
Hope-Gill, M C
Jenkins, A F
Knight, M B
MacLeod, A
Mason, J
Matravers, P J
Monk, F L
Pearce, A J
Savvas, S
Torkington, J
Tourle, C A
Wainwright, C J
Young, J H

Hale
Haslam, R J
Serafi, S

Halesowen
Akufo-Tetteh, H N
Allen, H C
Ayliffe, G A J
Ball, C J
Bathija, A S
Campbell, D J
Coates, S J
Constantine, G
Cutler, D H
Darby, J H
Dervish, O O
Gingell, K H
Gurney, I
Halford, C F
Horsburgh, T B
Hughes, C C M
Jackson, A R
Johnson, B P
Johnson, R A
Khetani, M J
Lennie, J E
Lewis, R A
Little, R M
Lloyd, H
Love, G M
Milsom, P
Mina, A G
Modi, V
Qaiyum, M-U
Saffar, N
Southam, R J
Spychal, R T
Stanton, I D P
Thorns, R

Halesworth
Abbott, A B
Anderson, A J
Baker, S M
Forsythe, D E
Lock, S
Neil, W J
Northover, C S
Peel, D M
Roy, R R
Shapland, J M

Halifax
Aiyappa, K S
Akram, A P
Aldabbagh, A
Alderson, P J
Anand, V K
Anderson, C M S
Aspinall, S R
Awan, A W
Bailie, R
Bain, R B
Bamber, P A
Banerjee, A K
Banerjee, S
Bangar, V
Barnes, G H
Bartholomew, K M
Bazaraa, T A S
Binns, H A
Bolland, H M
Britto, D J J
Brown, R T
Bukunola, B
Burley, D
Carsley, H A
Chadwick, C J
Chandratre, P S
Chandratre, S N
Chater, S N
Chatterjee, J H
Chaudhry, Q
Chiang, M S
Choucri, M C A
Clayton-Stead, A J
Clogher, L
Clowes, M A
D'Ambrogio, V J
Debono, M A
Dunning, T L
Dyson, S J
Edwards, R J
El-Bereir, G M A
Ellahi, T
Ellis, G N
Ellwood, D S
Esmond, J R
Felton, H M
Fernandez, B
Findlay, M J
Flood, B M
Freeman, M N
Galvin, H L
Gardiner, S C
Glencross, I H
Goffe, T R P
Goodall, R J R
Goyal, P
Goyal, S K
Grant, S C D
Green, S R
Gunson, E J
Gupta, J
Gupta, P K
Hamal, P B
Hamilton, S M
Hammond, E L
Hanson, M R
Hardy, R L
Harris, S R
Hasnain, R T-U
Hava, M A S
Highley, M S
Houghton, M W
Howell, J H
Humberstone, P M
Hussain, I
Hussain, I
Hutchinson, C H
Johnson, R V
Jones, D
Kanumilli, N
Kazi, A M M A
Kumar, K V
Lalor, B C
Lesser, P J A
Lockey, A S
McMichael, C M
Maguire, J P
Malenda, A N
Manthy, I
Mayland, F A
Modgill, V K
Moncrieff, A B
Mulder, M
Muscat-Baron, J
Nunn, D
Oade, Y A
Ormerod, I R
Parikh, B K
Parry, C S
Patrick, R K
Pickles, L J
Price, F M
Qureshi, M S A
Ramanathan, C
Rocheteau, M S
Rogawski, K M
Roulson, J-A
Rust, J H
Saadien-Raad, M
Salt, S D
Sawczyn, P G
Scriven, N A
Sen, B
Shakir, I
Shetty, P R
Smith-Moorhouse, G P
Smith, D I H
Somerville, I D
Somerville, J J F
Spencer, J G
Spencer, S R
Steed, A J
Sukumaran, S O
Sutton, L N
Tandon, A P
Taylor, C L
Taylor, D A
Taylor, J V
Taylor, R G
Than Htay, Dr
Thomas, G D H
Thomson, J
Thornber, S
Ullah, H
Vaughan, R
Walker, S M
Wynn, P A
Younis, Y

Halstead
Bainbridge, I M
Bristol, M P
Burton, J H
Duffus, P J
Edwards, N V
Giblin, M E
Healy, M J
Jones, S E
Markham, J E
Morgan, K L
Newhouse, S M
Salmon, N J
Spencer, B J
Symington, A J F

Haltwhistle
Adamson, R J
Baker, M
Ridley, J G
Ridley, P G
Thomson, D A

Hamilton
Baboolal, A W
Barton, P J M
Birney, S M
Black, K M
Braithwaite, C P
Brown, D R
Brown, F L
Brown, R H
Campbell, M-A
Cromie, D T
Curtis, M
Dawson, C A
Dobbie, D T
Duncan, J
Equi, A C
Findlay, S
Fowler, G E
Gaddis, S
Graham, A
Grant, J M
Hamilton, L M
Hannah, J A M
Herbert, M M
Hunter, I P
Hunter, L C
Ide, C W
Irvine, K G
Kohli, H S
Koteswara Rao, M
Lynas, B R
McCorkindale, C M C
McLay, R K
Marshall, L J
Mathie, D S
Miller, J M
Moir, D C
Murray, S A
Naismith, D S
Paterson, M E
Russell, S L
Smyth, S C
Stewart, M H
Tansey, B J
Tansey, M T
Tsang, S W M
Van Beinum, M E
Wallace, D H
Webster, A M
Wedlock, K
White, S M
Wickes, A D
Wilson, I D
Young, W M

Hampton
Baldwin, J M
Bhatia, K S S
Bignall, S
Brenner, E R
Brooks, A A
Carty, P A
Chaku, S K
Clarke, D J A
Cribb, R J
Dave, S D
Davies, D H
Davis, I R
Devaraj, A
Devaraj, S
Dhalla, P
Dighe-Deo, D
Feilberg, K A
Gupta, S
Howard, N M
Irving, C J
Isaac, R G
Kember, S M
Knights, K V
Kurl, D K
Kyriacou, E
Lewis, G J
Mitchell-Heggs, C A W
Morcos, S A G
Nielsen, E
Rieck, J
Rusby, J E
Smith, C A
Subramanyam, P V
Walkden, L
Whyte-Venables, D H
Wile, D B
Williams, R
Wright, A J
Young, J F

Harleston
Compton, J
Frew, P W
Heath, M J
Kemp, A H
Kemp, P W
Valori, A M
Way, B J

Harlow
Abraham, S M
Al-Samarraie, M T K T
Aldous, S
Allen, P W
Anthony, R Y
Arfman, M H J
Ashar, K N
Bachtalia, P
Bailey, K
Bansal, S
Barber, C J
Barker, K F
Bedford, C A
Bellingham, J M
Beshyah, S A
Bishop, C W
Bradpiece, H A
Bulpitt, D C H
Campbell, M
Chan, R H
Chhibber, F A
Chowdhury, N
Clifton, M A
Crossley, D J
Daud, S

Dillon, J A
Dodd, H
Elamin, M E
Elfarra, K
Eschle, M R
Firth, S A
Flaye, D E
Flower, N G
French, R C
George, T H G
Gerlis, R D
Hemming, C E
Higgens, E W
Ingham, E J
Jacobs, M C
Jenkins, S C
Kapasi, F M
Kawa, Z I
Khimji, H M R
Kozdon, A
Krishnamurthy, A K
Lamb, C E M
Leek, C A
Lockwood, J E
Long, M A
Loveday, B J
Loxley, C G W
Lurkins, M D
Mays, C S
Meehan, D M
Mistry, P
Mitchell, A
Morgan, R F
Nairn, D S
Nash, W N C
Orrell, M W
Oxley, V E
Pajwani, K S
Paliwala, A H
Patel, N
Philipson, R S
Phillips, J A J
Phillips, R H
Portelly, J P
Potluri, B S
Preston, D M
Radhakrishnan, T
Rajani, M H
Richards, C H
Roberts, M J
Rogers, S P
Sayer, J W
Sequeira, J M
Shrimpton, S B
Slack, R F Y
Smalley, C
Smalley, D S
Sreeharan, N
Stoner, E A
Stoner, S J
Swainsbury, J S
Taylor, A M
Tharakan, J
Thomas, S E A
Tully, K N
Vanner, A M
Vempali, V M R
Virdi, J S
Visuvanathan, S
Warren, J P
Yogasakaran, N
Zeidan, S F
Zeitlin, H
Zeppetella, G
Zych, Z

Harpenden
Addiscott, C L
Argyle, C M
Bail, H C K K
Balderamos-Price, J M
Barber-Lomax, C A
Bayer, C J
Belderbos, S M
Bell, L E
Bird, D O
Bolger, J P
Cashyap, A
Chafer, A T H
Chatterjee, D
Cole, A B J
Connolly, C N M
Cook, C J
Cranston, D P
Davies, K S
Davis, N J
Eardley, A J N
Evers, A M A
Farrow, C A
Feeney, A J
Feeney, M A
Festenstein, F
Gibbs, R J
Goodwin, T G
Habeshaw, J A
Hall, T
Harris, G E
Hemsi, D N
Henshaw, D J E
Holmes, G M
Horwell, D H
Hughes, G K
Impey, J A
Ingram, S D
Jack, M J E S
Jones, R B
Keir, P M
Kelly, F E
Lamb, K M
Langdon, J A
Lawson, P J
Logan, R F L
Long, E K
Loweth, S M
Mann, K A
Marsden, H L
Miller, R B
Mills, K E
Mitchell, I C
Norbrook, P J
Ostler, P J
Owens, O J D
Phillips, D G L
Pocock, K N J
Quinn, D C
Rajah, A
Reid, P C
Sanderson, G
Smith, S
Stirling, C F M
Stranders, A P O
Tattersfield, J F
Walker, R
Wang, M K
Wright, D J

Harrogate
Aldred, J E
Amaku, E E
Asaad, I
Asaad, L
Atkinson, F M
Baker, R F
Banks, P C
Bannatyne, D F
Bargh, I A
Barnett, A A
Beaini, A Y
Beardsell, I D M
Beeken, S A
Beer, H L
Beer, M J
Bird, A
Boyle, S P
Bradshaw, J H
Bray, M K
Bridge, G W K
Brotheridge, S P
Brothwell, J A
Buxton, E J
Bynoe, A G
Calvert, R M
Campbell, A J
Campbell, J R
Carey, M L
Carradine, S
Chave-Cox, R V
Chetcuti, P A J
Clark, A M
Collier, A M
Conway, K M
Coral, A P
Crouch, G A
Cubitt, K A
Cutler, P G
Da Costa, A A
Day, M S
Dennis, R W
Dias, B P
Dias, J-P
Dodwell, D J
Dyke, G W
Ellis, M
Emms, K J
Falshaw, R L
Fennerty, A G
Foley, S
Fowler, O J W
Frater, R A S
Gammack, A J
Gardiner, S
Gasser, A J
Gillies, D R N
Gilmore, D A
Givans, R J
Gledhill, A
Gohil, S R
Gray, C
Greenwood, S
Hain, B
Halaka, A N A M
Hall, C J
Hall, R S
Hammond, C M
Hammond, P J
Handley, A K
Hardcastle, J E
Harrison, G L
Harrison, J D
Haves, S E
Henderson, E T
Henderson, J E
Houston, M E
Hulse, W
Ikpeme, J O
Jamieson, A E
Jones, P A
Jones, R S
Kaye, P D C
Kaza, M
Kaza, R
Kidd, L C
King-Evans, V M
King, A M
Laird, A M
Larkin, H
Law, H
Lawson, A H
Lawson, D G B
Layton, A M
Leach, M A
Leinhardt, D J
London, N J
McClure, L
McEnery, R S K
McEvoy, M W
McIntosh, I M
McLusky, E G C
McPherson, S J
Mahapatra, S B
Mann, E T
Mark, J P
Metcalfe, S
Metcalfe, T W
Minty, S J
Morgan, C
Moss, H A
Murray, D K
Nehaul, J J
Newman, R J
Nicoll, D A P
North, C E
O'Connor, R D
O'Neill, M S G
Parkin, G
Penman, R A
Perkins, C A
Polito, T C
Poon, P Y A
Prakash, H C
Quartson, J K
Rawson, I A
Richards, C A L
Rider, M A
Riley, J M
Rowell, E R M
Rugg, A J
Russell, E
Ryan, C M
Saagandi, F W
Sarin, G
Sarma, J
Scatchard, M A
Scott-Knox-Gore, C L
Scullion, D A
Sharp, R J
Shepherd, G H
Shire, C M E
Short, L C
Shriman Narayan, R
Smith, D E
Spain, J R
Speight, M B
Spencer, R M
Stanworth, A W
Sullivan, C J
Sultan, H Y
Sweeney, R C
Symon, T
Taylor, D S
Taylor, E
Taylor, N P
Thirlwall, P J
Thompson, A C
Thornton, T J
Toop, M J
Town, V J
Travers, C V
Turner, R D
Umesh, S
Vincenti, G E P
Walsh, C J L
Ward-Campbell, G J
Ward, J P
Warren, J
Waterworth, A M
Webster, R A
Weeks, P J
Whitaker, J J
White, D A
Whiteside, O
Wild, S M
Woods, J C
Young, J D

Harrow
Abrar, S
Adler, L M
Ahluwalia, S
Ahmad, S
Ahmed, A
Ajina, I A A H
Akhtar, N
Akhtar, S
Akinwunmi, J O
Al-Adnani, M
Al-Mousawi, A H F
Al-Mrayat, M A-J K
Alesci, G
Allan, L G
Allard, S
Amin, K M
Andrews, P J
Asante-Siaw, J
Asgari-Jirhandeh, N
Auerbach, R
Barnard, M L
Barrington, A J
Bartlett, M J
Bates, H
Batten, C O
Bentley, P I
Bethell, H W L
Bhagat, A
Bhandari, J
Blair, M E
Blazquez Angulo, J A
Bodani, H
Bodin, M A
Bounds, G A
Boyle, S
Bracey, E E C L
Brady, A F
Brooker, J C
Budgett, R G M
Burke, M
Chadwick, S J D
Chadwick, T S
Chait, I B
Charlton, J S
Chatlani, P T
Chatterji, U
Cherry, P M H
Chidambaram, M
Chua, E S K
Cliff-Patel, S
Cohen, D L
Cohen, R I
Colbeck, R A
Collins, D R
Costello, M M
Cumberworth, V L
Cummins, S M
D'Almada Remedios, D J
Daniels, C C
Darakhshan, A A
Das, P K
Dattani, M
Davey, M E
David, P J
Davidson, R N
de Lacey, G J
De Silva, G U Y
Dean, M R
Devine, M E
Dhillon, R S
Dhillon, S S
Duggal, V
Eddington, M P
Elkabir, J J
Esah, K M
Farooqi, S M A
Feizi, T
Ferguson, H A
Fernandes, C F
Fernandez, S M B
Forbes, A
Frank, A O
Freedman, L S
Fyfe, I S
Gabe, S M
Gallagher, G M
Garrett, C
George, K
Gill, S K
Gleeson, M J
Golden, G A
Goldstein, S Y
Gomes, J A
Goonewardene, T I
Graham, G W S
Grayeff, S B
Green, M C D
Green, R
Greenstein, D
Grigor, C J
Gross, M L P
Gulamali, I H
Gumpel, J M
Gupta, P
Halligan, M S F
Hand, A
Harbin, L
Hardy, A
Harries, M G
Harris, J W
Hart, J J
Hassan, N
Hayat, S
Hegarty, M K
Herath, S N B
Hewlett, A M
Higgens, C S
Hilton, C F
Hinton, J
Hughes, M P
Hunjan, A S
Hussain, F F
Hussain, S T
Hwong, M-T
Hyer, W F
Jacobs, B
Jacyna, M R
Jaffe, R
Jaibaji, M M
Janossy, G
Janossy, K M
Jayesinghe, D C R
Jefferys, P M
Jeganathan, S
Jogarajah, T
Justice, J M
Kamlin, C O F
Kamm, M A
Katz, D E
Kaye, P J
Keat, A C
Kelshiker, A R
Kelshiker, R Y
Kelshiker, S Y
Kessling, A M
Khaja, G
Khan, M R H
Khurjekar, S
Knottenbelt, C M
Knottenbelt, J D
Knottenbelt, R G
Kulasekeram, V
Kulkarni, P R
Kulkarni, S P
Kurzer, A J
Lachman, P I
Lakhanpaul, R S
Lancer, R
Landau, R
Lee Chong, L P F
Lee, J H T
Lee, L C L
Lever, L R
Leverton, T J
Levine, T S
Levy, M L
Lewis, A J
Lloyd, D J
Loughnan, B A
McCloghry, F J
McCullough, C J
McDonald, A H
McDonald, P J
McIntyre, W
Malik, H M
Malnick, S D H
Malone, M J
Mangat, H K
Manickarajah, P
Mannix, P A
Marais, J
Marshall, M M
Marshall, S A
Massoud, A F
Mathur, C P
Mee, A D
Mehta, P C
Mehta, R
Mehta, S P
Mehta, S P
Melhuish, H F
Merali, N R
Michaelson, S
Missula, A S
Mistry, H G
Moore, A F K M
Moriarty, M A
Mukherjee, J
Mullerat, J
Munshi, F R
Naik, S
Nathwani, A
Nathwani, D C
Nicholl, R M
Nithyanandarajah, G A L
Nixon, N L P
Njoku, L I
Northover, J M A
Nurmohamed, A
Oyesanya, O A
Paffenholz, M
Paktsun, L W-P
Pallawela, G D S
Pandya, M D
Paraskeva, P A
Parfitt, J
Parmar, B
Parnell, K E
Pasupathy, A
Pasvol, G
Patel, A
Patel, A G
Patel, D K C
Patel, F
Patel, H B
Patel, J R D
Patel, N P
Patel, P C
Patel, S
Patel, S
Pattani, S M
Paun, S H
Peiris, J G C
Pereira, R S
Peter, L H
Peters, W
Phillips, R K S
Pitcher, M C L
Pitkin, J
Poblete Gribbell, M X
Priddy, A R A
Qureshi, R
Radhakrishnan, S
Ragbir, R
Rajabali, S
Ralleigh, G
Ramachandra, V
Ranganathan, S
Ravikumar, V
Regunathan, P
Renton, S C
Reuben, J R
Rhodes, M T
Robinson, A C
Robinson, C G G
Roden, A T
Rogers, L A
Rozewicz, D P
Rutter, M D
Ryan, R M
Sado, G D
Saifuddin, A
Sala, M J
Saleh, A
Samadi, N
Saravanamuthu, J

Sargeant, C F
Saunders, B P
Savundra, P A
Scambler, P J
Senanayake, H M
Senathirajah, S S
Senior, R
Seyan, S S A S
Shackleton, G E
Shah, A H
Shah, B N
Shah, D
Shah, K P
Shah, R
Shah, S R
Shah, S K
Shaida, W A
Shaikh, S
Sharma, S M
Sharp, P S
Shaw, A J
Shek, F W-T
Sherif, T
Shukla, R B
Silva, O S G
Sinnatamby, S
Sodhi, M S
Sodhi, S M
Solomons, G E
Soutzos, T
Spencer, J A D
Srikantharajah, I
Stephens, N G
Stern, J M
Stevens-King, A
Sufraz, R
Suri, R
Suri, S
Swinburn, J M A
Tadrous, P J
Talbot, I C
Talwar, S
Tam, D
Taor, P J
Taylor, V M
Thakrar, J P
Thanabalasingham, Y
Thiruchelvam, T R
Thirunathan, J
Thomas, R M
Timlin, M A
Topper, R
Turner-Stokes, L F
Vaizey, C J
Vaughan, D J A
Vijayanathan, S
Vohra, A D
Vora, M S
Vyas, J
Walsh, W J
Warren, N P
Wasu, P S
Watkins, S D
Wee, C E L
Weerasinghe, B P
Weerasinghe, P M
Wells, G J
Wignakumar, V
Wijendra, S D
Wijeratne, J J
Williams, G R
Wilson, J A
Wilson, S Y
Windsor, A C J
Wong, C P
Wong, M C-C
Woyka, W J G
Yale, V
Yaqoob, R
Young, N J A
Zuhrie, S R

Hartfield
Bott, M C
Furneaux, P J S
Hancock, P J
Hellmann, K
Tam, N L K

Hartlepool
Adair, A D
Agarwal, A K
Ahmad, M H-U
Alder, J L
Anam, Z
Andelic, S H
Apte, P P
Armstrong, R W W
Awad, A H
Ayre, M A
Bansal, P
Bew, D P
Blandford, A C
Brash, C J H G
Bruce, D W
Burrell, P G
Cacciato, A M
Chaudhury, B K
Cooper, A P
Crow, J
De Miguel Artal, M
Downs, A P
Dunn, N A
Eaton, A H
El Menabawey, M A-A A
Faiyaz, F
Fortune, J M
Frater, J K S
Frost, G
Gallagher, J
George, I R
Gibson, R
Hazle, S K
Heggs, C G
Holmes, A R
Howe, J B
Jani, J
Johnston, F R P
Jwad, A I
Kalmanovitch, D V A
Khan, M C
Kidambi, A V
Kirby, R
Leigh, J M
Leigh, R D
Lennox, C M E
Lennox, J M
Lowcock, J
McGowan, P F
McKinty, M C
McLatchie, G R
McPhee, J J
Milligan, G J
Moncrieff, R
Moody, R G
Naqesh-bandi, H A
Nicholson, O P
Nutt, C J
Oldroyd, D
Oliver, S M
Omer, F
Pagni, P A
Parker, C D
Parker, C S
Quinn, N D
Ray, D K
Reece, D A
Relton, P G S
Richardson, R W
Roberts, S A M
Robinson, B W
Roy, M K
Russell, F R
Shaheen, M A E-K
Simpson, A N
Singh, A K
Smith, M J
Smith, M I
Southward, R D
Stoves, C
Sutton, P P
Symon, D N K
Tang, S C
Tchikhiaeva, T
Thompson, J
Trimming, H M
Trory, G H
Tuma, T A-K
Wajid, M A
Watson, L A
Windram, J D
Wood, C P L
Youart, A

Harwich
Alldrick, A R
Balin, G V
Child, S W
Christie, S W
Ford, G C
Hoskyns, J C
Nightingale, P J
Norman, J C
Rankin, J G
Strachan, J C M
Sullivan, B A
Sullivan, J V
Wilson, R J
Wynne, A T

Haslemere
Ashwood, N
Campbell, C G
Cant, M E
Claridge, M W C
Cornish, J W M
Cowan, N M
Davis, J M E
Elliott, D H
Forsythe, F M
French, J
Hampson, E K
Hanly, D J
Hurst, M
O'Sullivan, W J
Panchaud, M L T
Randall, G R
Ridsdill Smith, P A
Samways, D M
Sharratt, M
Sherriff, R G
Stoneham, J R
Sutcliffe, P J
Taylor, C P
Thomas, A A L
Whitaker, S P
Wilks, M

Hassocks
Bellamy, J D F
Christie, T H
Cook, R I
Deering, R B
Farrands, P A
Haigh, A C
Harper, R H
Heeley, P J M
Jeffery, R N
Juniper, C P
Kemp, R J
Kinane, C F S
Knight, R
MacDermot, V D
McGorry, K M
Moore, A H
Morris, M T
Rawlinson, W A L
Reid, H S
Shearn, C A
Strachan, K A
Tombleson, P M J
Tunnadine, C H J
Warburton, M C
Weppner, G J

Hastings
Bennett, G G
Bray, L M U
Chinery, C G
Chisholm-Batten, R E
Connor, J A
Cooper, C
Cooper, T F M
Das, P
Dhalla, P N
Doe, J C
Driver, N P
Dutchman, D A J
Giles, J A
Henry, J G
Hicks, I R
Higginson, B M
Horsley, I T
Howie, F J T
Hughes, H E
Jones, H B
Jones, L O
King, D
Kumar, R
Meredith, A P E
Nicholson, H P
Paget, S E
Paget, S C
Patel, H C
Pronger, E A
Radia, K
Seal, P L
Sheill, M J
Waller, C M
Whelan, D E
Whincup, G
Wilcox, G E
Wisby, L R
Wray, R

Hatfield
Brooks, R V
Clements, S
Colter, E F
Davies, G S
Durkin, A
Dytham, N K
Elson, D F
Jowett, V C
Kerr, J P
Kipgen, D
Lavelle, R C W
Lewis, G H
Lim, S C
Lock, J A M
McDowall, G K
Oates, P E
Rajaratnam, M
Restell, C A
Roe, M F E
Salmon, A H J
Steward, M R
Tiwari, N V
Wikner, R A
Williams, D J
Willson, T H
Wotton-McTurk, P H

Havant
Allan, T C
Anandan, C W R
Ayling, P J
Ball, N A
Balthazor, D P J
Barrett, D F
Batty, J A
Bedford, F J
Bowley, E C
Cogswell, D F
Cogswell, L K
Cole, C J
Corbin, M J
Dewar, R
Earley, M J
Earley, M A
Geoghegan, J
Grafen, L
Green, A I
Hardy, T J
Hazeldene, M J
Hughes, J R
Kennedy-Cooke, C J
Maclean, M J
McNeill, A I N
Magee, D B
Melville, D H
Morrison, C E
Moss, N H
Naing, S Y
Nash, K L
Neville, C E
Pearson, R N
Robinson, B S
Ryle, C A
Sinclair, J C
Sizer, K A
Summerhays, B G
Sutton, R M
Thakrar, P M
Thomas, T R
Timms, D P
Torode, N B
Warlow, C N
Williams, M G
Willicombe, P R

Haverfordwest
Barnes, A
Bartlett, M
Barton, A D
Bates, C M
Bell, C J
Bryant, J D
Buntwal, V
Burns, R W
Clow, W M
Cooke, D A
Cooke, R A
Cross, R
David, D R
David, R E
Davies, D H
Edwards, E D
Evans, G W L
Forman, S M
Gammon, R S G
Griffiths, R B
Grimshaw, R J
Hamilton, S A
Hesketh, S J
Howells, M R
Hughes, B J
Jafri, M S
James, C M
Jones, G R M
Jones, J N
Jones, R W
Jones, R P
Jowett, N I
McEvoy, R C
Martin, I R
Maxwell, W A
Milewski, P J
Mohanaruban, K
Narayan, V
Neumann, K M
Noott, G G
Nur, O A
Paterson, A M
Perry, M E R
Polacarz, S V
Premkumar, C S
Read, K M
Richards, A D
Richardson, E M
Saleem, A K N
Saleem, M F
Singh, P D N
Sinha, S
Thomas, D A
Thomas, J E
Thomas, S E
Thompson, R W G
Vas Falcao, C M G
Vipulendran, V
Weaver, A J
Weaver, A L B
Williams, L G
Wilson, P
Wort, R L
Zakaria, M Y

Haverhill
Baker, R W
Cornish, C A
Donovan, D H
Katrak, P M
Lawfield, M F M
Mann, N M
Mohan, H B
Patel, A
Selby, J N
Servant, J B
Smith, S T
Stephenson, P S
Tate, P A
Worthington, R C

Hawes
Hamer, J M
West, P K A

Hawick
Bianchi, G
Bishop, J P
Boon, R L
Brogan, E
Bruce, L M
Cameron, W R
Lockie, P
Macdonald, J M
Macmaster, H
Macrae, F
Manson, P G C
Michie, R W
Oliver, C H
Palmer, A A
Rolland, D M
Rolland, M B
Ross, G M J
Wilson, C J F
Woolfenden, E C

Hayes
Ahluwalia, N S
Anand, S
Campbell, H G
Grace, D M
Hamid, M S
Hasan, S A
Iqbal, S
Joshi, V P
Kanthan, P R
Khan, F A
Lauwers, A J
Lucas, B B
Lukmany, M F
Madhavan, T
Malik, N S
Mehta, K
Michaels, R
Nair, S
Nanavati, M K
Nelson-Iye, A C
Patel, H S
Prunty, M J
Quadri, S A
Rahim, M S
Raju, T D
Rashid, A Y
Sembhi, S K
Sethi, K K
Smith, A M J
Stephens, P J
Thomas, B M
Thurlow, S K
Vyas, K H
Wood, D R
Yianni, J

Hayle
Blair, B E
Croft, A M
El Gammal, M M Y
Evans, J N
Fuller, F M
Gibson, N H
Higgs, M J E
Kingshott, B M-M
Maskell, A M
Olds, E M
Parasuram, P
Patrudu, M N
Slater, J
Stevens, D

Hayling Island
Chilcott, R C
Coombs, S E
D'Alton-Harrison, J J
David, S T
Keogh, J M E
Lancaster, T V
McCall, K E
Mossman, A D
Perrin, C E
Prestwood, J M
Stratford, A J
Thomas, R J
Turner, C
Walton, J H
Williams, R H M

Haywards Heath
Abdel Gawad, A A
Adams, H G
Alden, S R
Allen, J C
Alvarez-Ude, J M
Angel, R J
Arundale, N
Barrie, F M M
Barrie, N J
Bashir, T A
Begg, A H
Bellis, D J
Berresford, P A
Berry, J M
Birch, I D
Blundell, J M
Bridger, A D
Chandrasekera, C P
Chappel, W A
Cheal, H J
Clenshaw, J E E
Corbett, C R R
Cox, S R
Creek, I M
Dale, J W
Dawes, B J
Dawson, P J
Denney, R W
Donaldson, P M W
Durrant, C C J
Eastcott, H R
Elkins, A V
Emerson, R M
Fearn, C B A
Firth, P S
Fulford, W G
Ghandi, S
Gunasekera, W S L
Gurner, A C
Harding, A S
Hardingham, J E
Hardwidge, C
Harker, H A

Hart, P C
Harvey, M R
Harvey, R A H
Hayward, P J
Hill, P R
Hine, K R
Holloway, N J
Hoyal, R H A
Hutchinson, M C E
Jannoun, U
Janvrin, S B
Jeffree, M A
Jenkins, E M
Jones, C N O
Jones, I E
Jones, K G
Jones, M A
Jones, R H
Khine, T T
Kini, M D
Kiss, A
Lafreniere, L M
Lambert, R B H
Lavelle, M A
Lawrence, A J
Lawson, E M
Lawson, K M
Liddell, J
Littlejohn, I H
Lynch, M V
McKenzie-Gray, B
McMinn, L
Male, I A
Marshall, C E
Mather, K L
Mather, R J
Metcalfe, J M
Mims, C A
Morris, R P
Morrish, P K
Mort, L E
Moseling, D M
Nagendra, K H V
Nath, J
Nawrocki, J D
Noble, D C
Norris, J S
O'Brien, W
Olney, J S
Parnell, E J
Parnell, N D J
Patterson, M H
Pilkington, S A
Pyle, E J
Rath, S
Read, D H
Ricketts, D M
Rose, P E
Rouse, J M
Smith, C M
Snape, O J
St. John Jones, L S
Stuart, B M
Sumner, M J
Tahzib, F
Taylor, E P
Tildsley, G J
Walter, P H
Ward, P J
Wheatley, T
While, J A
Williams, I R
Wiseman, R A
Young, M P

Heanor

Ahmed, I
Gilbert, A E
Graham, A B
Houlton, S C
Lodge, R
Manley, R
Mellor, S
Noble, J
Tompkinson, J M
Walker, A

Heathfield

Aldridge, M S
Almeida, J H
Blakey, R T
Casares, M E
Dodge, C J
Eggleston, A
Griffin, S
Jeans, A F
Mcconkey, G N
McGowan, J F
Palmer, S
Pertwee, R
Rees, E L
Underhill, Y M
Wadman, S M
Woods, C M

Hebburn

Boll, S
Brady, M
Burns, M
McIntosh, G D
Minchin, A H
Nicholls, K-M
Oliphant, C J
Vinayak, I P
Vinayak, V
Withington, B R

Hebden Bridge

Allcock, H
Blomfield, R G
Child, D
Gooch, J A
Grainger, R L
Hawkes, F A
Lyons, M J
McInnes, S J
Taylor, N G
Wadsworth, J A
Wild, D A

Heckmondwike

Findlay, D J
Khan, K
Laher, J P S
Woodhall, A J
Youd, D J
Zaman, K

Helensburgh

Arneil, G C
Brown, A J
Brown, C A R
Brown, W R H
Burgess, J L
Burgess, R C A
Calder, B D
Campbell, E B
Clarke, S A
Coulter, F
Cox, A L
Doyle, A J
Duncan, M J P
Dunlop, T D
Falconer, A D
Flatman, W L
Kirk, A W
Lee, C W
Linzee-Gordon, P A H
McKelvie, J D
McLachlan, B
Macleod, C
McMenemin, I M
Mascarenhas, R A
Morrison, M E E
Newberry, J
O'Donovan, J P J
O'Regan, M E
Ram, A J
Reay, P L
Reitano, T
Robin, J G
Sharara, F
Smith, M D
Stephen, A J
Storey, N D
Taylor, F G
Underwood, E M L
Woodburn, A G

Helmsdale

Singh, D

Helston

Barton, P A
Coward, N H
Cuff, C M
Davidson, N J
Davies, L A
Dorrell, M G
Duckworth, J
Edgerley, R I
Fremantle, J E
Frisken, I K
Gearing, K E
Harris, P J S
Hawkins, R T J
Hosking, R D
Johnston, R P
Kitson, M M
Lansdowne, J D
Lawton, B
Lord, J M
Old, F T
Oliver, J P
Richards, F J A
Shelley, R A
Smith, R S
Smith, S P
Williams, M S
Wolstencroft, R F
Wood, M

Hemel Hempstead

Ali, A
Allistone, J C
Antscherl, H E
Bailey, D M
Bairoliya, R P
Bakshi, A
Barrison, I G
Bayliss, J F J
Beacon, J P
Benson, G L
Bhamra, R S
Bhatt, S K
Bhatti, T S
Borkett-Jones, H J
Boucher, S L
Bradnock, B R D P
Brazier, J C
Bulger, G V M
Bull, M J
Cairn, J W N C
Carr, A M
Catnach, S M
Chadwick, S L
Collinson, D J
Crane, V R
Darasz, K H
Di Monaco, M
Divers, A R
Drake, M J
Dunphy, K P
Dutta, T
Dyson, L
El Naggar, H M A
Farag, R R
Fernandes, T D
Gallow, R J
Gannon, P F G
Goddard, H C
Gordon, T M
Graham, R S
Grimer, D P
Guirguis, E G R
Guirguis, S A (
Gunawardena, H
Ha, H C Y
Hackett, D R
Hall, J M
Hallan, R I
Harrison, J F M
Heatley, P T
Hill, S F
Hinsley, D E
Hinsley, S C
Hirji, F M
Hislop, J E
Hobbs, R C
Hodge, K
Hogg, S J
Hurst, Z H
Johnston, C L W
Johnston, D F
Kane, J L
Kerry, D B
Khatri, H I
Khattak, M A K
King, A L
King, D S
Lang, J E
Lim, L S
Lucas, S O
McFarlane, K J C
Mapara, R
Martlew, K G
Mazhar, R
Mishra, K M
Monro, J A
Moring, C F
Mugge, L E A
Nicholls, J C
Nodder, J H
O'Reilly, A P
Ormiston, M C E
Pancharatnam, M D
Parry, J I
Phillips, B E
Pigott, T G
Pontefract, C A
Price, R M J
Ratneswaran, D
Raudnitz, L C B
Richardson, A S
Roots, P J
Royston, I M
Rudramoorthy, T
Saunders, A J
Savla, M P
Seetulsingh, P S
Shipley-Rowe, A P
Sofat, A
Stambach, T A
Stier, S
Thacker, J G M
Thomson, C C B
Tipple, B G
Toorawa, D A
White, G Y
Wiener, A J
Wiggins, R J
Wright, J R
Wright, L P
Yip, R Y W

Henfield

Burdsall, J
Cairns, S R
Crawford Clarke, K E
Gibson, A D
Haylett, A C
Horley, J F
Kenney, N C
McLean, M S
Norman, J R
Simpson, V M A
Smyth, G V

Hengoed

Ali, M M
Antao, V R F L F
Greville, W D
Griffiths, H M
Heneghan, S J
Jones, E
Jones, H O
Jorro, M T C A
McCann, K M
Rogers, S
Rosser, C A
Scourfield, A J
Williams, D T
Williams, M L

Henley-on-Thames

Ashby, P A
Bacon, A S
Barrass, B J R
Barton, J H
Bergel, R C
Blagg, S E
Bromilow, J E
Collett, E
Copeland, J A M R
Craik, M C
Dudeney, T P
Easton, C S
Elliott, M J
Friend, K J F
Ganly, N A
Garrett, J
Guest, E L H
Hall, S L
Holt, C M
Jones, H G
Kinsler, V A
Langley, H K
Lukats, V E J
McCullough, S
McEwen, H C
McEwen, L M
McKeogh, M M
McWhirter, J H
Milligan, J M
O'Gorman, W J
Pigott, P V
Pitt, N S
Ratcliffe, C G
Robertson, J
Silver, L R
Snell, B J
Stephens, V J
Sutherland, S D
Sykes, A
Terris, A J M

Henlow

Batchelor, A J
Bird, O J
Broadbridge, R J M
Bruce, D L
Collins, H E
Connor, M P
Cullen, S A
Dave, N P G
Devnani, K C
Dexter, D
Green, N D C
Greenish, T S
Hill, I R
Matthews, R S J

Hereford

Adams, S J
Allen, C J
Allsopp, L E
Ballance, J H W
Ballham, A
Barber, M D
Barling, T C
Bathurst, C E
Beach, B
Bhattacharyya, S
Bracebridge, M C
Brooks, W
Broome, M R
Butterfill, A M
Butterfill, J B
Bywater, N J
Caine, D J
Canavan, R E M
Canning, C L
Carter, R C
Cartledge, W S
Cohn, M R
Collins, K J
Collins, R J
Connor, H
Coombs, E
Corder, A P
Corfield, A P
Cousens, A R
Crossley, A W
Dallimore, J S
Dalziel, J A
Davies, D M
Davies, W H
Day, A C
Deakin, M T
Deutsch, J
Dinnen, J S
Donovan, M J R
Doran, R M L
Dowling, R M B
Duffett, J M
Eggar, R J
Epps, M T
Evans, N-W D
Eyre, A J
Farmer, R E
Ferguson, S
Fraser, N C
Frith, C W
Garlick, P R
Gee, R P
George, L
Glancy, J M
Godbert, K
Goodfellow, D P
Goodfellow, J C
Gray, B
Gray, J A
Grech, P
Griffiths, R L
Grigg, J A
Grocott, E C
Hall, M J
Hanna, G S S
Hargraves, A
Harper, P H
Harris, P
Hasan, S
Hayes, M
Heal, A J
Hearne, M J
Helme, M M
Henderson, R J
Hession, M A
Hirst, R M
Holt, J L
Hutchinson, J D
Jay, P I
Jenkins, C
Jennings, S F
Jobst, K A
Johnson, A S
Johnson, A
Johnson, M L
Jones, A G
Kaye, P M
Kennedy, F L
King, H A
King, R A
King, R E
Kramer, J J
Laird, C J F
Laird, R B
Lattey, N J
Lewis, A M G
Litchfield, J A
McGinty, F
Mackie, V J
Majeed, D
Majeed, L J A
Malins, D M
Marsden, S M
Maslen, M J
Matthews, P J
Maxwell, J M
Mears, T P
Medcalf, K R
Menzies, L J
Millard, K
Montgomery, H R
Moore, W J
Morison, C J
Newcombe, G L
Nicholson Roberts, T C
Orr, A M
Overstall, P W
Pawley, M K
Penney, O J S J
Penney, R M
Pimblett, J H S
Pollard, N A
Pratt, G
Press, J D
Ransford, R A J
Reed, A J
Rendall, J R S
Reynolds, I S R
Richardson, B P
Ridgway, S
Roberts, C C N
Roper, I W M
Rose, N M
Rothwell Hughes, M E
Rowe, G M
Ryan, P J
Ryding, F N
Salmon, N P
Salter, S H
Scotcher, S M
Seal, P V
Seal, P A
Shewell, P C
Shields, D A
Shirazi, J E
Sibly, T F
Singh, R
Sleath, J D
Slee, G C
Smallwood, B H
Smith, M C F
Smith, R B
Sole, G M
Southall, P H
Steven, C A
Subak-Sharpe, R J
Sykes, R A
Symonds, K E
Thomas, C J
Thomas, H R
Thompson, A J
Turnbull, M
Wade-Evans, V J
Wagner, N A G
Walsh, P R
Walter, H P
Warner, R G
Warsap, A J
Waters, M R
Watt, I D
Watts, A C
Weavers, B J
Wheeler, J G
While, A C A
White, C A
Williams, D H
Williams, R B
Williams, R G
Williams, S
Willoughby, S J B
Wilson, J M

Wilson, P R
Wilson, S
Wrench, J R E
Yogaratnam, S
Young, P R

Herne Bay
Barton, D G
Brian, C J
Cleverley, H R
Collier, G M
Davis, S G
Dunn, S J
Gadhia, N
Green, C R
Jenkins, R M H
Manson, H M
Parsloe, J B K
Prince, A W
Ritchie, I W
Senthiraman, V
Sigurdsson, R G
Strutt, M D
Stubgen, S O
Turner, C L
Wheeldon, R
Wilson, R E M

Hertford
Atwill, K N
Black, G C
Bossley, C J
Cembala, J A
Cheesman, C A
Corlett, K J
Craighead, S K
Crossthwaite, D I
Curtin, B G
Daborn, D K R
Darlow, N E
Devine, A J P
Eames, J R
Forshaw, M J
Grabarska-Kreiss, B K
Griffin, L J
Hamilton, P G
Handysides, J M
Harris, S
Horsman, A M
McClure, I R
McLees, D J S
Maiti, H
Mathew, G
Mobley, R J
Murray, N H
Newton, J E
O'Reilly, F E
Oates, A P
Rank, T J
Refson, J S
Roach, R T
Robinson, W
Sloper, C M L
Sloper, P
Stott, C M
Taylor, P J
Titcombe, J L M
Watson, L J
White, A W

Hessle
Abraham, T
Adhami, Y
Arnold, A G
Crafter, P F
Dore, A M
Grout, P
Haines, D R
Kell, B
Locker, I
Lorences Ruiz, C I
McInnes, A J
Mathur, S
Nicholson, A A
Riddle, M A
Robertson, A C
Robinson, G
Sherman, J M
Sinha, S
Whitty, R T

Hexham
Al-Ali, M S M
Ambrose, J A
Anderson, I
Baillie, M
Blades, D S
Bradbeer, E G
Carney, T A
Chippindale, A J
Coleman, S A
Condie, P W
Crick, J M J
Cuthbertson, J E
Devlin, A M
Edmonds, P P F
Ford, S D
Forsey, J P
Gallagher, E J
George, M M
Gholkar, J
Gold, J S
Gray, A L
Harte, B D
Helliwell, C D
Henderson, M T
Hogarth, M C
Johnson, N G
Keep, N K
Longrigg, J N
McCollum, J P K
Macklon, A F
Maddick, G
Middleton, C S H
Morrow, G
Mungall, I J
Nandy, M K
Parry, M R
Patrick, D
Patterson, C A
Petty, D R
Powell, F M N
Quibell, R M
Redpath, A
Rose, K F
Sims, P F
Sutton, R A
Thompson, E G E
Thompson, J J
Thompson, J W
Wainwright, C J-P
Walker, M C
Walsh, W K
Weaver, R M
Wells, N J
Wildmore, J C
Wilson, T M
Wright, A J
Wyatt, P H

Heywood
Adshead, P A
Bailey, S
Bunting, S L
Duffy, C J
Gibson, J A
Hanif, M
Inceman, H
Krysztopik, R J
Marshall, J A
Mooney, E M
Onon, T
Osborne, E S
Parashchak, M R
Plumb, S
Pokinskyj, S K
Rasheed, S
Salkin, C
Saxena, R
Saxena, R
Williams, A
Wood, R A

High Kelling
Chapman, A C
Cooper, J D
Crawley, H B
Franklin, P K
Grove, S J
Latten, A

High Peak
Almond, I D
Austin, D J
Bartholomew, A D
Bullock, R E
Callister, M E J
Caplin, S
Cooper, S P
Crosby, P
Dobbing, J
Edwards, R N
Edwards, S
Ferris, P I
Holderness, J A
Jones, R A
Kumar, B
Lord, W D
Losel, T M
McWilliam, L J
Moore, H L
O'Donoghue, J
Parker, R S
Potts, W A
Riddell, D J
Storm, M
Williams, D E
Wilson, K L

High Wycombe
Afridi, M V K
Aitchison, R G M
Akbar, F A
Al Hillawi, A H S
Allen, D S
Allim, R M
Aly, H E B M
Amin, S
Anderson, D M
Anzak, M
Armitage, F H
Armitstead, J G
Aslam, N
Aslam, N
Attar, G S
Atwell, S A
Bacon, N F
Bath, E M
Baxter, E N
Bdesha, A S
Bennett, A J M
Bennett, A R
Berry, J F
Birch, K E
Blair, Z A
Bonney, G L W
Booth, M I
Bopearachchi, T J P
Bose, P P K
Bowker, M H
Branagan, J P
Bray, E C
Burton, A J
Cadman, P J
Capper, J W R
Carless, J J
Carter, F C
Channon, G M
Chapman, P J V
Charlesworth, C H
Cheetham, C H
Clark, H E
Clarke, T J
Combe, W A D
Corless, D J
Cowland, G N D
Cox, G A
Crittenden, G
Dahiya, S
Delamore, J A
Dexter, T J
Dudley, J
Duvall-Young, J
Earley, A R C
Eley, N A
Erskine, J A
Eustace, D L S
Fawcett, V A T
Fernandez-Martinez, P
Finch, R
Flint, R P
Foord, C D
Fraser, K C B
Gallen, I W
Gamell, A P
Garnham, J C
Gatzen, C
Gilchrist, N
Gorard, D A
Graham, D G
Gray, J C
Haffiz, T
Hameed, A
Hasan, A K H
Hasnain, Y A
Havelock, P B
Herbert, J J F
Homer, J R
Horner, J R
Ilyas, S
Inman, N J
Jackson, M C
James, H C
Johnson, H C
Kapoor, V
Kazer, M
Kelleher, J P
Kelly, C M
Kelly, S J
Kepetzis, M N C
Kettle, S J A
Khan, S N
Khooshabeh -Adeh, R
King, M M K
Kirby, A C
Kuhn, K A
Landon, H M
Lethbridge, K G
Lowe, P J
Luzzi, G A
Lyons, M M
McAllister, R
McCarthy, A L
McCay, D A
McClelland, A J
McIntyre, A S
Malpass, T S
Manchanda, S
Martin, F H
Masters, N J
Matthews, M G
Mawdsley, S K V
Maxmin, J S
Medhurst, A W J
Middleton, S J
Moretto, J C
Morgan, N J
Munro, J H M
Newton, D J
Nice, A M
Northeast, A D R
O'Sullivan, M C
Patten, M J
Payne, J M
Payne, M A
Pearson, D C
Phillips, J N
Potts, D J
Pounder, L
Price, S R
Rahman, F
Rajendran, V
Rastogi, G C
Reidy, R N
Roblin, S
Robson, M S
Rogers, S J
Sawhney, K K
Scott, D M
Shaine, B J
Shaw, D E
Slater, K E
Smith, D G
Spalding, E M
Stapleton, T
Strube, P J
Sumner, D
Tan, K S-W
Taylor, D A
Taylor, E J
Taylor, G J
Thomas, E G
Thompson, A C
Titheridge, R E
Turner, M J
Venning, G R
Waghorn, D J
Wallace, K D
Walter, J A
Wathen, C G
Watson, P J Q
Wayne, C J
Wighton, C J
Wilson, A J
Wise, M P
Woolnough, M J
Worth, C T
Wright, D D
Zaib, S A

Highbridge
Anderson, S J
Barry, P H
Bizon, M J
Clapham, C M
Edwards, M C
Gough, A L
Griffith, R A
James, D M
O'Brien, R A D
Reynolds, C A
Stoddart, P G P
Trowell, G M

Hillsborough
Bell, S M
Bingham, J M M
Burns, D M
Chambers, J M J
Coulter, N C
Cupples, S J
Dorman, L A
Eames, N W A
Eames, R S
Farrar, M
Ferguson, J I
Field, G G
Fitzpatrick, O J
Fleming, J K
Forde, A
Hogan, M M
Hunter, C M
Hunter, I M
Jackson, A C J
Johnston, A J
Kirkpatrick, M H E
Lappin, J M
Lawther, R E
Lee, C E
McBrien, H S
McCreary, R D
McFarland, A R
Mulholland, M G
Owen, T A
Page, W
Patton, H H T
Rogers, P P
Shillington, R K A
Smylie, A
Uprichard, A C G
Urey, M R
Walker, J
Wilson, G M
Wilson, J C
Wright, S A
Yarr, S N
Young, R A M

Hinckley
Alun-Jones, J E
Bowler, H L
Cracknell, I D
Finnegan, J P
Gilberthorpe, C
Harrison, J
Havard, L K
Howes, H K
Johnson, S
Kothari, A K
McCole, L C
Maity, P B
Marlow, K D M
Mason, P S
Muthiah, M
Parkinson, A M
Pearson, J R
Rowe, V L
Ruban, E P
Sacha, B S
Sil, S K
Singh, B
Sladden, C S
Solanki, P
Sood, A K
Sutton, F J
Taylor, R S
Warner, R H L
Willmott, N J
Yardley, R A

Hindhead
Baldock, N J D
Cavannagh, L C
Colyer, E E S
Dunbar, S J
Ford, J M
Hancock, K G
Jenkinson, P M A
Jobson, P H
Sleator, A M G
Tobin, D E
Tomes, J S
Wise, V A

Hitchin
Aldeghather, J T
Anklesaria, R P
Baker-Glenn, E J
Bancroft-Livingston, G H
Barwick, A C
Bhatiani, R
Blackman, J M
Bols, R M-C
Carragher, M S
Clarke, M G
Cooper, F
Cox, J P H
Daniel, K J
Downey, M F
Gilvarry, M C
Golding, J H
Gradwell, D P
Greenish, K B
Griffiths, S J
Haigh, A B
Hallwood, P M
Hillman, R A
Hodgson, M J
Hope, S A
Ingram, R M
James, N K
Kelly, P D
Kendell, N P
Kennerley, P M
Kenny, C J
King, C M P
Lacy, M K
Lawrence, J M
Leaver, A T
Lewis, R S
Lim, M S T
Lincoln, D S
Machen, J
Pickett, L C
Rand, J I
Raymond, F D
Richardson, S M
Ryecart, C N
Seaman, R A J
Shellock, A J
Slattery, M A
Smith, I M
Smith, R N
Stevenson, J L
Tadros, A
Tadros, O I
Taylor-Robinson, K
Tidy, G
Tresman, R L
Vorster, M A
Wandless, S
Watkins, S M
Williams, D P
Woodman, M J

Hockley
Aukett, M A
Bernardo, M V
Cornes, P S
Donnelly, C A
Galvin, E A S
Layzell, S
Rees, T P
Taylor, D S
Thomas, P D
Tullett, D C

Hoddesdon
Adlard, R E
Andrews, M
Baxter, B
Blankfield, C P
Clayton, F G
Davies, A W
Guptha, S
Henderson, F J
Hiscock, I M K
Jolliffe, R J
Parkes, G
Patterson, M S
Record, J L
Roberts, J L
Robinson, P J
Robson, J J
Sandler, M G
Tomiak, R H H
Tyne, H L
Waddington, C
Wenley, M R
Willis, D A
Young, J H

Holmfirth
Harding, J R
Hopkinson, N A
Moffitt, S J

Holmrook
Thornton, A

Holsworthy
Betts, J B
Green-Armytage, G K

Hillebrandt, D K
Human, S J
Kandasamy, R
Page, R J
Price-Thomas, S P
Shaw, R F
Wardle, R M

Holt
Atiomo, P-L
Birt, A J
Brett, S L
Colebrook, R D
Fowle, C S
Freeman, D
Harvey, P T
Jolliffe, M V
Marriott, J M
Norwood, M G A
Paddon, A J

Holyhead
Bertorelli, S W
Bowen, D J
Burnell, S H
Clyde, R J
Davies, R P
English, H L
Ford, G
Francis, S B
Griffith, H B
Harrison, M
Ijaz, Q
Leigh, J A
McCoy, B T
Nicholson, B
O'Toole, J G
Parry, H
Petty, M G D
Roberts, D M
Roberts, J K
Robson, D J
Torbohm, I K-H
Tsang, H K
Walker, C F
Williams, D T
Windall, K M

Holywell
Allsopp, L B
Boiston, P A
Chowdhury, S D
Harper, H M
Jones, G O
Jones, G M
Jones, S
Kapur, Y P
McIntyre, O B
Major, R G
O'Keeffe, V M
Roberts, A
Rowlands, M

Holywood
Adamson, S I G
Arnold, R G
Caddy, G R
Cleland, J A
Cosgrove, C T
Courtney, J R
De Jong, J
Dornan, J C
Eardley, M
Egerton, T J A
Foster, G C
Graham, S M
Greer, H P
Hamilton, K
Hannam, C R
Kane, J R B
Lawson, G T N
Lawson, R G
Lindsay-Miller, A C M
Little, B T
McCall, J R
McCrea, A P
McCreery, J
McGibben, P D
McGimpsey, J M
McGimpsey, W M M
Millar, R
Miller, A R
Morrison, G C
Orr, L E
Ryan, T G F
Sheeran, M R M
Stevens, R F
Strong, J E
Wallace, R G H

Watson, R G P
Williams, M A
Wright, A M
Wright, O L
Yeates, H A

Honiton
Barber, P C
Courtney, P T
De Sousa, B
Donohoe, M E
Forbes, A E
Gibson, J J S
Harvey, N E
Leach, R
Lee, J E
Peat, J M
Penwarden, D B
Poels, P J
Seamark, C J
Seamark, D A
Wallace, O N
Ward, D G
Ward, J A
Webb, P J

Hook
Barns, H C C
Clay, A E
Collins, A J
Cox, J
Davies, A J
Evans, D J
Fernando, A M
Gilbody, J S
Goncalves-Archer, E B
Goold, I J
Heywood, H C F
Hunter, C J
Lieberman, S
Longstaff, S F
Love, D M
Morgan, G N
Page, J M
Rees, J
Rimmer, C J
Shand, C R
Stedman, S A
Weaver, A D

Hope Valley
Adler, T J
Beeley, J M
Bell, J H
Brennan, S R
Burton, J A
Clarke, S E
Dale, S M
De Carteret, A M
Farrell, R W R
Fordham, E J
Glanfield, P A
Gow, W M
Howson, B E
Hutchinson, D I
Hutchinson, S P
Jackson, P H
Jordan, L K A
Morton, E A
Moseley, D J
O'Connor, K R
Read, C A
Ridley, N A
Robinson, A P
Robinson, J
Ross, J J
Simpson, J L
Smith, P D

Horley
Butcher, R M
Chapman, P J C
Conaty, T A
Cook, L A
Courtenay-Evans, P A
D'Costa, E F
Daruwalla, N K
Diack, H J
Dormer, J K
Dyke, T N
Goodwin, S A
Hole, S G
House, J H
Jenkins, E M
Keay, D A
Lightwood, A M
Lightwood, R G
Middleton, K G
Moyle, P L

Olliver, R J
Parkes, C A
Ramanathan, R S
Ring, P A
Rolland, P S
Stanley, R S
Tallent, D N
Townsend, P T
Vethanayagam, S
Wambeek, N D
Williamson, R D C
Wylie, C M

Horncastle
Burman, L
Dalton, J E
Duckham, C M J
Owen, Y E M
Read, S M
Watkins, T

Hornchurch
Aggarwal, A
Ahmad, S
Ahmad, S N
Arasu, P
Asadullah, H
Bell, E
Bhargava, A
Bland, T C
Blewitt, M J
Brodie, K
Caira, J C E
Carruthers, H J
Chopra, B D
Deshpande, A R
Edison, M M
Farrow, S J
Haq, M F
Inglis, S L
Jaiswal, A L
Kendall, K S
Kershaw, P S
Kithulegoda, L M
Kornfeld, A
Kundu, T
Mann, E J
Mannall, J
Matthews, T H J
Moghal, A
Mohan, I C
O'Moore, J C F D
Omoregbee, A I K
Parker, L B
Patel, P M
Rahman, M M
Rawal, J L
Samanta, N
Sethu, P
Seymour, M W
Sharma, A K
Sharma, P
Sivapathasundaram, P
Sloan, D J
Sohal, H
Tilly, A
Tinslay, P I
Tsoi, K C F
Uberoy, V K
Vanniasegaram, I
Zaidi, S A R

Hornsea
Collingwood, P I
Dawber, E E
Hall, J
Sibley-Calder, I C
Walker, J E S

Horsham
Adcock, H M
Ali, H E A
Barker, B M
Binns, T B
Black, T R L
Blackburn, S C F
Brookes, J D
Cameron, G M
Clarke, J E
Clement, J M
Darcy, J F
De Bono, J M
Dean, S J
Deere, H M R
Dubrey, S W
Duncan, A C W
Fisher, E M
Fisher, S R
Gliddon, R P N

Godfrey, V A
Grant, M E
Hall, M
Heath, C J
Heatley, J P
Hillman, G
Hills, N D
Hodson, A C
Hodson, J M
Holwell, D W
Jarratt, W J
Kewley, G D
Khalafpour, T
Latif, M A
Lawson, T K S
Liu, H L
McGregor, A R
McNeil, I D
Madan, N
Marshall, S R
Monro, B B
Morris, J S
Moult, E M
Mountain, B A
Mulvey, J M
Namasivayam, K
Noel-Paton, M K H
Owen, E R T C
Pal, A
Pallister, D H
Palmer, J C
Parkes, R T
Pearse, S B
Pearson, L S
Peters, J J
Piper, S J
Pothecary, I C
Ramsay, F M
Scanlon, F L
Scott, E B M
Shattles, W G
Sheikh, A A
Skipp, D G
Skipp, H J
Smethurst, M E
Smith, P J
Thwaites, I G
Topham, E J
Venables, M T
Vohra, S
Vohra, S L
Walton, N P
Watson, R I
Williams, G J
Williams, S J
Willis, L K
Woods, P M
Yates, S C

Houghton-le-Spring
Ancliff, J E
Barker, J M
Dingle, P R
Goff, D K
Goudie, R A
Hepple, E C
Johnson, A G M
Jones, A I
Laws, D
Lilley, R J
Linnett, P J
McElroy, J H
Mackay, J C S
McLaughlin, C
McVie, J L
Marashi, M T
Mishreki, S K
Muthu, B S
Nicholson, J C
Pappachan, V J
Pepper, H M
Prudhoe, R H
Quinn, M G
Roberts, P R G
Sartoris, A
Sekhar, P R
Shorten, P J
Shrestha, K L
Thalayasingam, M E L
Thomas, E J
Thornton, H L
Turnbull, D M
Wallace, A S
Watkinson, S A P
Watters, J G
Wylie, G

Hounslow
Aladerun, S A

Bajoria, R
Bakshi, J M
Bambawale, A K B
Barringer, J
Baum, G
Baum, M R
Bhalla, R K
Bhardwa, J M
Bharti, H K
Bhatti, T J N
Chambers, R M
Chitnavis, S P
Chowdhury, V
Cliffe, D J
Coll, A J
Copenhagen, H J
Cresswell, G J
Das, A
Dhadwal, A K
Dhillon, H S
Dutta, J
Ganeshananthan, M
Garcha, P S
George, B
Gill, K
Gill, P S
Grewal, H S
Gunjal, D
Hanid, M A
Hanif, R
Hannan, S
Husein, Y A
Hyde, C S
Ikram, S
Irani, B H
Jeer, P J S
Jeynes, A M
Jogia, P L
Kaiser, R A
Kalha, I S
Kalsi, J S
Kanagaratnam, C N
Kanani, S
Kanchan, S
Khan, T I
Khan, Z I
King, W C
Kirk, A E M
Kooner, R K
Kullar, H S
Lamont, J E
Lessing, D N
Loomba, R L
Malhotra, A
Mangat, S K
Mann, A P S
Mannan, M A
Martin, C B
Mayor, S K
Melichar, K B
Mellors, K D
Mendel, P R
Menon, S
Mohindra, R K
Moran, F M
Mughal, A H
Munro, A J
Murray, N A
Nag, S
Nagra, A
Nanda, D
Nijjar, A S
O'Bryan-Tear, C G
Omayer, A S
Osman, M
Pankhania, A C
Patel, B C
Patel, B
Patel, V
Perera, S H B
Prince, C A
Rai, J S
Rajasingam, D
Rajendram, R
Rawll, C C G
Robinson, N D P
Sachar, A
Saini, M
Saini, S R
Sandhu, S S
Sandhu, V
Seddon, L
Sharma, B
Sharma, S
Shenton, P A
Singh, P
Sinha, V N P
Smith, R H
Sood, S

Tan, K H
Thanabalasingham, S T
Thomas, B
Thomas, S
Tripathi, D P
Turner, M R
Vedi, V
Winayak, K
Zaidi, A Z

Hove
Adams, J A
Ahmad, N
Al-Hussaini, A S
Allan, P
Ashton-Key, M
Assin, M
Assin, W D
Badalbit, A
Baker, S C
Barker, C R
Berelowitz, G J
Bodkin, N L
Bound, D S
Brierly, R D
Briggs, M J
Buck, T J
Channing, N A
Chauhan, S K
Clark, A W
Condon, J A
Condon, N I
Court, C S
Daly, P G
Davidson, R A
Deutsch, G P
Dobbs, F B
Donaghy, J B
Donnelly, J P P
Dossetor, R S
Emmanuel, S S
Evans, D J E
Evans, P C
Fergie-Woods, D F
Fielding, R E
Fletcher, M S
Forsdick, P B
Fox, H G
Gayton, P
Gilsenan, K L
Gimbrett, R C
Godber, G N L
Greenwood, C E
Gutjahr, C
Haslam, N P
Hempling, S M
Henderson, E J D
Higson, N
Hindley, M G
Holloway, K A
Hume, D C
Jackson, R N
Janes, J S
Jenkinson, J L
Keep, J W
Kelly, M C
Kocen, J L
Krafft, J M
Laurence, W N
Lean Su-Tseng, I S
Liu, C S C
McMinn, T G
Mak, V Y Y
Mancey-Barratt, W A
Melcher, D H
Mills, S J
Milroy, S J
Morgan, J W
Nurick, S
O'Doherty, C M
Ojo, O A
Osborne, D M
Pilley, C H F
Polmear, A F
Pritchard, H W
Purwar, S
Rabbs, J M
Richter, G
Risk, A M M
Roberts, C
Royle, M G
Rukmani, K S
Saadah, M A
Scott-Smith, W
Sharman, M J
Sharpstone, P
Stearman, A S L
Stewart, D B

Stuart, M H
Sudhakaran, N
Tabor, A S
Tate, A R
Taylor, A D
Taylor, A M C
Treger, A
Turnbull, T J
Turner, K L
Walker, H J
Walley, D R
West, E A
Williams, J H
Wren, E M
Yagoub, S
Zuha, R

Huddersfield
Adam, M J
Aggarwal, A
Aggarwal, S
Aguirre Vila-Coro, A J
Ahmed, M S N
Ahmed, S
Akam, R M
Al-Doori, M I
Al-Egaily, S S
Al-Quisi, N K S
Al-Saigh, G S
Alcide, J M
Anathhanam, J J K
Anderson, D G
Anderson, E J
Angus, R J
Annan, G
Atkinson, S M
Bagchi, S K
Bairstow, J A
Balendran, N
Bamford, N J
Banks, J
Barnwell, D
Barrett, E C
Bashir, S
Benett, S A
Benson, H A
Benster, B
Berry, P W D
Bhabra, K
Bhasin, B B
Bhattacherjee, S
Black, S K
Bottomley, J P
Bower, R L
Bradley, G
Brennan, S A
Brook, M E
Buckle, J
Burnett, I A
Burrows, A W
Butt, M
Buxton, R L
Caligari, A M
Cameron, A J
Cameron, S
Cannon, P D
Care, A E
Case, W G
Cashin, D A
Cassidy, P P
Chakravorty, N K
Chaudhry, F
Cheema, H S
Cheema, S P S
Cheesbrough, M J
Clayden, J R
Clayton, M G G
Cleary, J E
Clogher, C A
Clowes, J R
Cole, G
Cooling, N J
Crossland, R M
Curtis, J M
D'Cruz, P A
Dafalla, B E D A
Das, A K
Das, P
Davey, K G
Deacon, A R
Deane, M E F
Dempsey, H M
Dewhurst, A
Dissanayaka, N
Dunne, K M
Eagland, K G
Eales, G
Effa, N N
Elliott, M
Evans, R P
Exley, A
Farooque, H
Faulkner, P P J
Feeney, A-M R
Ferro, M
Fitton, P H
Forrest, K A T
Fox-Hiley, P J
Fox, J E
Gannon, C D
Gehlhaar, E W
George, A F
Gowa, S H N
Graham, A
Greenhalgh, N M
Guest, T D
Haigh, S J
Hameed, F
Hamid, A R A S
Hamilton, A H
Handa, S M
Hanson, J R
Hargreaves, D C
Hariharan, T
Hasanie, N U H
Hawkswell, J A
Heaton, R W
Higgins, E
Hill, B A
Hindle, D J
Hooper, M D
Hughes, D M
Hussain, A
Irving, C D
Isaac, C F
Islam, M N
Ives, V J
Jabczynski, M R
Jackson, R M
Jameson, R J
Jenkinson, R D
Jennings, F O
Jennison, P R
Jindal, B K
Joffe, J K
Jolly, N C
Jones, S C
Juby, L D
Kaftan, S M H
Kathuria, B S
Kay, S
Kaye, N M
Kazemi-Jovestani, A
Kazemi-Jovestani, M
Khan, A
Kiely, M T
Kucharczyk, W A J
Kumar, A
Landon, C R
Larkin, E
Littlewood, J
Lloyd, D R
Lord, J R
Lucas, L E
Lumsden, G V
Mcallister, J M
McCarthy, F J F
McCormack, K G
Macdonald, R C
MacIver, N
McKenzie, I P
Manning, J E
Mansoor, W
Martin, N
Martin, V H
Martland, C P
Miller, M G
Mitchell, R D
Mohammed, A
Morris, I R
Murphy, A G
Mustafa, S
Naik, K S
Nandakumar, C G
Naylor, J R
Nazareth, H A A
Newbegin, C J R
Newbegin, H E
Nightingale, J A
O'Shaughnessy, C V
Ong, Y E
Ong, Y G
Orme, L J
Pace, H E
Pacynko, M K
Paes, A R
Parker, C R
Parker, H
Parker, J A
Preston, J A H
Priestman, J F W
Ramsden, C S
Rana, P S
Raper, S C
Rawcliffe, D S
Read, S G
Reece, R J
Reed, L
Roberts, C L
Rushton, R J
Salaman, J H
Samanta, K
Samanta, R
Sanderson, A
Sanderson, I A
Schembri, J A
Sebastian, T C
Seeley, D
Shamsee, M Y S
Sharaf, L A M
Sharman, R A
Shenolikar, A
Shortt, A M
Siddiqui, A A
Siddiqui, S A
Siddiqui, U S
Sills, M A
Smelt, G J C
Smith, A J
Smith, G B
Smith, I J
Smith, J M P
Smith, M L
Smith, R E W
Sobala, G M J
Sohail, R
Spencer, H M R S
Spencer, S M
Standring, J N
Stevenson, R N
Steyn, A M
Stiles, M A
Swift, T D
Sykes, D P
Tattersall, A E
Taylor, M J
Taylor, M A
Taylor, M
Tebbit, A
Thornton, P
Tomlinson, J F
Tomlinson, R J
Varma, A
Waddington, D
Wade, K
Wallwork, M A
Wardley, A M
Wattis, J P
Watts, C
Welch, M T C
Welsh, C J P
Wilkinson, A
Wise, D I
Woodhead, R B
Wright, M J
Wybrew, M E
Wybrew, R W J

Hull
Abd-Mariam, N T
Aber, C P
Ahmed, A E
Ahmed, R E
Al-Saleh, A S
Alexander, N
Ali, S L
Allison, T
Armstrong, D J
Arowojolu, A O
Ashworth, I A
Atkin, S L
Awan, R K
Ayyub, M
Azaz, A M A
Bajalan, A A A
Balshaw, J
Balshaw, M
Barnes, D J
Barraclough, M
Bartlett, R J V
Beddis, I R
Best, J G
Bhandari, S
Bhaskara, R G
Blackburn, C W
Blackburn, P A
Blake, S R
Blow, J D
Bolton, T
Bott, M H
Brocklehurst, G
Brown, M J
Burgess, P A
Cafferty, M D A N
Campbell, A P
Campion, P D
Carter, C
Chan, D W-S
Chandy, J
Chapela, J M
Chauhan, G S
Chia, P S
Colman, A W
Cooksey, G
Costello, D F A
Courtney, E D J
Craig, M O
Creighton, S I J
Crick, D L A
Crossley, M C
Cundill, J G
Curran, G J
Dakkak, M
Datta, S K
Davis, P S J
Doherty, S M
Donaldson, M D J
Dore, P C
Drennan, J D
Driver, R K
Drummond, G B
Dunlop, J M
Dunlop, J L
Dunn, S R
Eadington, D W
Early, A S
Earnshaw, J H
Edwards, G M
Ell, S R
Ellwood, R W
Emmott, S M
English, P
Ettles, D F
Fairhurst, C T
Farr, M J
Felgate, M J
Findley, M
Galea, I A
Gandhi, J D
Gee, D G
George, P
Ghosh Ray, G C
Ghosh, P C
Gibson, H G
Goebells, P
Gooding, C R
Goring-Morris, J
Gray, B M
Gray, P A
Green, A M
Green, D A
Green, L C
Greensides, J L
Gurnell, P
Guthrie, K A
Haley, P F
Halstead, K A
Hammersley, C A
Hammersley, K A
Hanna, C M
Hay, D M
Hendow, G T
Henshaw, M E
Hepburn, D A
Hetherington, J W
Heylings, P N K
Hirst, J M
Holmes, M E
Holmquist, J C
Horton, D
Hovell, B C
Howell, F R
Hunter, A I
Hussain, A W
Hussain, S M
Imrie, A H
Innes, A D
Jackson, T R
Jaffe, L
Jaworska-Grajek, M
Jayawardhana, B N M
Jefferson, I G
Johnson, B F
Johnson, K
Jones, E J S
Jones, J J
Jones, P N
Jones, P A H
Jones, T P J
Jorna, F H
Joshi, S U
Kamath, M B
Keczkes, K
Khan, I H
Killick, S R
Kilpatrick, E S
Kings, G L M
Knox, A P
Kundu, P M
Kutte, K J
Lambert, C J
Lawley, D I
Lees, S A
Leng, M D
Levett, I J S
Lewis, C M P
Lewis, J P D
Lindow, S W
Long, E D
Loose, J H
Lorenz, J R
Lovett, M S
Lowery, S D
Luffingham, R L
McAlpin, P G R
McClean, H L
McCollum, P T
McDiarmid, M K
McDonald, N H
McIntyre, G B
Macphie, S
Maguiness, S D
Mahdi, G E D M
Mallik, M K
Mansoor, M A
Mansoor, M R
Markova, I
Martin-Smith, M H A
Massey, R F
Masson, E A
Mather, A A
Mawer, S L
Meigh, J A
Meigh, R E E
Melville, A J
Melville, C R
Miller, J
Mitchell, P C
Mohla, D J
Moody, M E A
Morris, K M
Mortimer, A M
Musil, J
Nandi, S
Naughton-Doe, P E G
Nayar, J K
New, N E
Newman, P F
Nirodi, G N
Noble, S C
Nyunt, A
Ogunlesi, T O O
Oliver, R M
Ong, V H
Pairaudeau, P W
Pande, K
Parker, G T
Parker, J S
Parkin, A E
Patmore, R D
Pepper, A V N
Percival, R
Pestell, A
Platts, C H
Prasad, N
Pratap Varma, M J
Price, J D
Queenan, P J
Rai Choudhury, K
Rangwala, G D
Rasool, H
Rasool, M A
Raut, R
Rawson, M D
Read, J R
Renwick, P M
Richards, K J C
Richardson, J W
Richardson, W T
Riusech Mas, I
Rizk, M S
Rochford, F M M
Rogerson, R
Roper, D J
Rosen, C
Rotherham, J
Rowland Hill, C A
Royston, C M S
Russell, I F
Salvage, D R
Samaan, A
Sande, W G T
Sattari, M
Scarfe, S A
Sedman, P C
Sefton, G K
Sellars, L
Selmi, F
Semeniuk, P
Setiya, M S
Shaikh, M
Sherman, K P
Shields, R H
Shores, J G
Siddiqui, A S
Singh, M N
Smales, C
Smithson, J A J
Snowden, G
Soul, J D
Spokes, J M
Starr, D G
Steel, N R
Stephenson, J T
Stewart, O G
Subramaniam, S
Sutton, P R
Tang, K M
Taylor, A D
Thackray, P
Thomas, M C
Thomas, R C
Thompson, E C
Thomson, F J
Tommins, K S
Trowell, J E
Turner, W H
Turpin, D F
Tyrrell, S N
Ubhi, S
Umerah, F N
Upadhyay, S K
Van Maarseveen, P L
Venugopal, J
Walster, V M J
Walton, S
Warran, P
Weir, J A D
Whitehead, E
Whitley, I
Win, A Z
Withington, B S
Wong, M K
Wright, P J
Wynn, M D
Yagnik, R D
Young, R A
Yousuff, A M
Yu, L F

Hungerford
Bray, J K
Colthurst, J R
Dace, H M
Dunn, R J
Hamilton, R A
Hetherington, P I G
Johal, N S
Montague, C C
Pihlens, H L
Powell, H B
Rice, H M
Symon, R
Williams, C E
Yates, N

Hunstanton
Baluch, M A
Burgess, J E
Charles, I P
Hutfield, D C
Le Masurier, R R
Machin, C

Huntingdon
Aggarwal, A K
Aggarwal, R
Al-Kurdi, M
Allan, R B
Amara, S N
Archer, C C
Babbington, S P
Bacon, N A
Banfield, C C

Baxter, R
Benison, P M
Bermingham, D F
Biram, R W S
Blake, D E
Booth, A J
Booth, J V
Borland, C D R
Bower, P S
Boyle, B E
Boyle, J A
Bray, J D
Brinsden, M D
Brook, J M
Brookes, J M G M
Brooks, A M J H
Brown, S J
Cameron, B A
Carlyle, R F
Caswell, J D
Challener, J
Chan, E W-S
Churms, B K
Collinson, J E
Cook, S L
Cormack, L E
Cox, A J
Cox, D C A
Cracknell, D D
Crockatt, D R
Culloty, S M
Cutress, M L
Das, R K
De Cates, C R
Dean, H C
Diamond, J G
Dickinson, R J
Donnelly, K F
Dumbelton, I B
Fells, J N
Ferreira, F G
Flanagan, D W
Fletcher, P R
Forbes, P B
Forster, S M
Foster, P J
Ghosh, T N
Glover, M W
Goodwin, P R
Greatrex, A F
Gryf-Lowczowski, J V D
Hage, W K
Harding, P J
Harper, A D
Haslam, D A
Haslett, E A
Hoggarth, C E
Holland, H F
Horsnell, J M
Hubbard, C S f
Hunter-Campbell, P
Hunter, D
Irish, N
Irwin, D S S
Jamali, N
Jenaway, A
Jenner, J A
Jennison, K M
Jessop, C H
Jewell, J A
Johnson, A T
Johnson, S A
Jones, J A
Jones, S P
Kakani, S R
King, S M
Lasman, F C A
Latcham, R W
Latham, B V
Latimer, R D
Liggins, A J
Lim, B H
Lund, K A
Lyle, T
McCullough, F W
Mackay, H M
McKay, R J
Macleod, C A
MacLeod, K R
Martin, D J
Matsiko, K S
Mayhew, C A
Miles, R N
Millard, P W
Mills, C A
Moazzam, A
Moor, M J
Mullinger, A V
Nashef, A J
Newby, M R
Ni Bhrolchain, C M
Norden, A G W
Norman, C W
O'Sullivan, F T
Okagbue, C E
Oubridge, J V
Outram, D P
Owen, A
Paraskevaides, E C
Parwaiz, K
Patel, A
Patterson, A
Paul, S C
Pedersen, S W
Perkins, P J
Picts, A C
Pike, J M
Platten, H M J
Pountain, G D
Price, V
Purbick, A
Quek, S L G
Quick, C R G
Randhawa, S S
Rands, C E
Rawlinson, J
Rea, D P
Reed, J B
Reeve, A A
Rege, K P
Rej, E
Rene, C
Reynolds, G C S
Richardson, A J
Roberts, D H G
Rodgers, D J
Rutherford, H J
Saban, P A
Sackin, P A
Salman, M N
Schofield, J P
Searle, P J
Sewell, P F T
Sharp, C
Slack, M C
Small, G
Smerdon, G R
Smith, R J
Southgate, G W
Stanger, R J R
Stenner, J M C
Sugden, J H
Sutcliffe, R C
Sweetenham, I A
Swinscoe, A W
Taggart, S C O
Taylor, N J
Thomas, T M
Tiffin, E J
Tulloch, B C
Turner, J V
Turnill, A
Vaughan-Lane, T
Vickerstaff, K M
Walsh, K J
Walters, S E
Warbrick-Smith, D
Watson, B J
Weyell, R S
Whitelock, D E
Whitton, M W
Wilcock, J M
Williams, I G
Williams, P H
Wilson-Haffenden, C F
Wright, A D
Wright, M H G
Wojclk, A
Zebro, T J

Huntly

Arthur, A L T
Carter, G
Cosgrove, E E
Easton, D A H
Gatenby, R A B
Lockyer, J A
Lyons, K A
McEwen, J
Shirreffs, G C
Sinclair, A G
Troup, J D G
Watt, B

Hyde

Ashworth, W D
Aziz, T Z
Baguneid, M S
Banks, A J
Bellhouse, W
Bhatti, Z B
Bradshaw, F R
Carroll, D H
D'Silva, K
Farrar, S W
Gulati, R K
Gutteridge, L C
Haji-Suhailee, H-A
Harvey, J M
Islam, T
Johnston, E M
Kelly, P A
Kinsey, M A
Lee, S S
Loose, H C
MacGillivray, A
Maclaverty, K G J
Mohd Sani, A K
Moysey, J O
Napier, I G
Patel, R
Peravali, B
Pole, P M
Procter, H M
Proctor, S C
Purves, J D
Reynolds, L J
Roney, D B
Schofield, P F
Shah, M P
Singh, G P
Tanna, V N M
Thornton-Chan, E W C
Wickenden, D H
Williams, J M
Wintle, F C

Hythe

Allen, A P
Bedford, B
Besley, C R G
Briggs, R D
Campbell, D R
Chandrakumaran, K
Davidson, K W
De Caestecker, J P
Foster, I L
Grainge, S M W
Hiscocks, E S
Immelman, R E
Klugman, D J
Lock, M
Martin, F J
Menin, P T
Oakes, J L
Padley, N R
Pitts, J R
Rial, S C
Robertson, A
Stewart, C M
Torrance, A M
Wells, D G
Whitby, M E

Ilford

Abdul-Razak, N A J
Abidogun, K A O
Afzal, M
Ahmad, R
Ahmad, S M A
Ahmed-Shuaib, A
Akhtar, N
Al-Qassab, H K
Ali, M L
Ali, S N
Arawwawala, D P
Ashraf, W
Atalar, A T
Azad, A
Bagg, L R
Bakhai, R P
Bakhsh, N
Balakumar, T
Baloch, A H
Balraj, V
Banerjee, L
Banerjee, N
Banerji, S
Barnardo, A E M
Basra, S S
Bastianpillai, B A
Batheja, M
Beg, M S A
Bellin, U
Bennett, D L
Bettany, G E A
Bhadra, N B
Bishai, K R T
Boctor, S Z
Briggs, J C
Brown, N
Bullon Barrera, F J
Cameron-Mowat, R J
Chatterjee, H
Choudhury, A K
Clarke, F A
Cleary, M P
Cochrane, G W
Colgate, E J
Crabbe, I F
Croker, N
Cronin, B
Dabrera, M G A V
Davison, S C
Deb, N K
Desai, J D
Duffett, R S
Dutta, N N
Ehsan, M
El Hussein, N A
Elias, S A
Enver, M K
Fang, C R
Fiberesima, S L
Gautama, P
Ghosh, M
Goel, A
Goel, R
Grainger, S L
Grant, I R
Green, E M
Greenaway, B J
Haldar, G
Hanna, N J
Harar, R P S
Hargreaves, C A
Harwood, C A
Hervel, G M
Hobson, J G
Hodges, M J
Hollingworth, B A
Hossain, F
Hossain, M
Hossain, M M
Husain, S A
Hussain, K
Hussein, S
Huston, R B
Ip, M
Islam, T M
Iwegbu, C G
Jan, M B
Javed, E B
Jayatillake, S M D
Jethwa, S R
Joshi, N
Kadir, N
Kalebic, B
Kaltsas, D S
Kanagasabai, K
Kanagasundrem, A
Karki, B D
Kashin, M A H
Kerawala, F M
Khan, M Y
Kollipara, P
Kulasegaram, Y
Kulendran, S
Kullar, N S
Kumar, R
Kumarakulasingham, R
Lau, A Y-H
Lester, J F
Levack, B
Levy, R B
Littlejohn, R
McDougall, C M
Mackenzie, G D
McMillan, G J S
Mahendra-Yogam, P
Mahmood, M
Makar, A S
Mandavia, B J
Margo, A M
Martin, D G
Mayer, T C
Mehta, A
Mehta, R C
Mendes, R L
Moss, D
Mughal, R M
Munneke, G J
Munneke, R
Mustfa, G
Naganathar, I
Navaneetharaja, N
Niranjan, K
Nirmalananthan, S
Nischal, V K
Nylander, H H
O'Brien, A E
Ojo, A A
Osei, E
Padmanathan, C
Pandit, V
Pandya, J
Parmar, H R
Patel, G D
Patel, R B
Patel, R S
Paul, E A A
Piyarisi, D L
Purushothman, G
Qayyum, A
Quraishi, M A
Qureshi, M A
Rahim, S
Rainsbury, P A
Rana, D-E-S
Randall, R
Rastogi, R
Ratnakumar, K
Ratnakumar, S
Ray, D
Rizvi, S I H
Robinson, D L
Rodrigues, M J P
Row, K P
Rupal, A
Sadheura, M K
Sadideen, M
Saggu, R S
Saha, A R
Saha, T K
Sahdev, A
Sahu, U N
Sakthibalan, M
Saleh, F A A
Sanghvi, M V
Sclare, H
Seehra, S S
Segal, M P L
Sen, D
Sennik, A K
Shabestary, S M
Shah, A K
Shah, S A
Shan, K
Shanahan, D
Sharif, S
Sharma, K
Sharma, S
Sharma, V K
Shaw, F J
Shergill, B S
Shillito, M
Shirsalkar, A M
Shubhaker, U D
Shubhaker, U
Siddique, Y
Singh, H
Sinha, S K
Sinnathamby, S W
Smith, S J
Snooks, S J
Soares, P O B
Solebo, J O
Solomon, W C A
Soosay, G N
Spencer, J R
Spiteri, H P
Springer, H W
Srinivasan, S
Steinbergs, G G
Subberwal, K
Suri, A C
Tahir, M
Taslimuddin, A S M
Tek, V
Thurairajah, G
Tsang, D T K
Tse, D T K
Uddin, S
Van Der Putt, R P
Vanstraelen, M
Vijaya Ganesh, C
Viswanath, I
Wakeel, R A P
Webster, E A
Wellings, M J
Wickremasinghe, S P
Wickremasinghe, S M
Wijayakoon, A P

Ilfracombe

Bevan, S A
Eames, M R
Fenner, M T
Griffiths, B J
Hunt, S J
Kilner, G F
Mather, M J C
Ross, J D
Wallace, D I R
Womersley, J S B

Ilkeston

Adams, R D
Bagshaw, K J
Bailey, E W E
Binnie, F J F
Brammer, A
Brown, B D
Connell, H E
Crowder, L E
Crowley, G S
Dawson, R D E
Donovan, J A
Downes, N M
Finch, G
Futers, G
Halls, P J
Johnson, T M
Kirk, D A
Lalloo, R D
Langdon, M D
Miller, S J
Parfitt, C J
Portnoy, A E
Portnoy, D
Purnell, S L
Thomson, J
Tierney, G M
Tooley, I R
Travell, P D
Turner, D P J
Varnam, R M
Walton, G M
Webb, C L
Weston Smith, P A

Ilkley

Atkins, F E
Atkins, P
Barron, R
Batool, T
Beard, D J
Bearpark, A D
Beck, I
Bramwell, E R
Brand, I R
Brooke, A
Brown, A C
Chang, B
Clarke, A
Clarkson, A D
Cockshoot, D
Dickson, P
Dickson, S D
Evans, V J
Fox, S E
French, M J R
Goodwin-Jones, R B
Hanson, K E
Hargreaves, R E
Haynes, P A
Hicks, J S
Lewis, M A
McLellan, A E
Martinez, D
Milnes, J P
Murray, H
Neasham, J P
Newby, E A
Newton, E M G
Ogilvy, J E
Pacsoo, T C
Pickles, E J W
Poulier, R A
Powell, A L
Ragunathan, P
Raubitschek, E
Rawling, A H
Rawling, R G
Roberts, S J
Rolfe, H C
Shann, D J
Smith, C A
Srinivasan, T R
Tinker, A J
Valentine, J
Van Terheyden, N J E R

Wales, A C
Weatherill, J R
Williams, E A
Willoughby, B J
Woodford, A

Ilminster
Anton, D J
Austin, A D L
Barber, R N
Boyce, D J
Gayer, S J
Hazlewood, J
Hodges, A E J
Outram, M
Patuck, D F
Patuck, J F
Pearce, S N
Reeves, W G
Schmidt, K E
Sen Gupta, P
Simpson, R C
Wilson, A G M
Wilson, J E

Ingatestone
Acorn, D J
Bolton, M E
Cheung, K-K
Coffin, J P
Emond, R A
Feldman, P M
Hughes, C A
Lightowler, C
Lightowler, J V J
Macpherson, T J
Medford, N C
O'Reilly, R J
Orford, E D
Pal, S K
Rilstone, F W B

Innerleithen
Cumming, R L
Oswald, I
Ward, P M

Insch
Kay, D M
Morrice, G M
Teale, S J

Inveraray
Bijral, H S
Bijral, H S
Bijral, K S
Colley, I H
Colley, J K

Invergordon
Barker, P A
Carr, P D
Hutchison, B S

Inverkeithing
Allan, J J
Duncan, L E
Grant, A R
Jackson, A R
Jalil, M
Jamieson, K A
Ritchie, K B
Slight, R D
Taylor, D M

Inverness
Aitken, A G F
Ashton, M A
Austin, J B
Baijal, E P
Baikie, M L
Ball, J L
Ball, L M
Beasley, R J
Blagden, A K
Boyd, F E
Bramwell, S P
Brown, C A
Caird, L E
Campbell, A F
Campbell, D
Campbell, H O C
Chancellor, C I
Charters, F K
Chesser, R M
Chun, P K
Collier, M K
Convery, K A
Cook, C M
Cormack, J G
Cormack, T G M
Cox, Q G N
Davidson, K E
Davies, I J T
Deans, J
Dempster, S
Docherty, J G
Duncan, J L
Edmonstone, Y G
Ennis, C J
Escott, T E
Farmer, G
Ferguson, I C
Finlayson, D F
Fisher, L R
Gajda, A
Gamblin, A J
Gillies, N W
Gilmour, R J
Glen, A I M
Godden, D J
Goff, D G
Goodlad, J R
Gordon, P M
Graham, A J
Grant, C E
Gray, S A
Griffiths, C A
Guy, R D
Hadley, D C G M
Haggerty, S R
Hamilton, A
Harrison, S B
Harvey, R D
Hay, A G
Hay, A J
Hendry, P J
Herd, D J
Ho-Yen, D O
Hulks, G
Hutchison, S M W
Jack, S A
Jamieson, A D
Jamieson, N F
Jennings, P
Johnston, I G
Johnston, J M
Johnston, R
Jones, C J
Keen, J C
Kelly, S M
Kerr, F
Khaweri, F A
Kiln, P A
Kirkwood, G A
Laing, M R
Lamont, A M
Lees, D A R
Logie, J R C
Lumley, S P
Lush, C J
McBride, E
McClure, S
McClymont, L G
MacDonald, I A R
McFadden, J A V
Mcfarlane, A
Macfarlane, E
McFarlane, E A
McGrath Ross, L
MacGregor, A
MacGregor, C
MacGregor, C M
Machin, J R
McKenna, J G
Mackenzie, I
Mackenzie, M E F
McKerrow, W S
Mackinlay, M G
Mackintosh, G J
Mackintosh, L E
Maclaren, M H S
Maclean, B N
Maclean, M L
MacLellan, L D
MacLeod, A A
MacLeod, A J M
Macleod, A C
Macleod, C L H
Macleod, R S
Macleod, S E
Macleod, S K
MacLean, R
McNamara, H I
Macneil, A
MacPherson, M J P
McPhie, J L
MacRae, J A M
Macrae, M J
MacRury, S M
MacVicar, D
MacVicar, L C
MacVicar, R
Malcolmson, S E
Martin, C M
Martin, J A M
Martin, J R
May, J R
Munro, A
Munro, N A
Murphy, N M
Murray, W
Nicholls, J
Nichols, D M
Oates, K R
Palmer, T J
Palombo, A S
Pearl, S A
Philip, D
Potts, L F
Quinn, K S
Ramsay, J W
Rankin, R
Robertson, D A
Robertson, P
Ross, J
Ross, W A
Rosser, A K D
Russell, I C
Sampson, R P
Scott, I G
Shanks, S D
Shearer, H L
Sim, A J
Skipsey, I G
Smith, A D
Smith, I R
Smith, S L
Snow, A F
Somerville, D W
Soulby, G C
Spenceley, J A
Spenceley, N C
Stark, C R
Steven, M M
Stevenson, A W
Stone, G V
Strachan, H M C
Struthers, A D
Sweenie, J F
Syme, A I C
Taylor, J E
Taylor, T G
Thin, M J
Thomas, R
Thompson, J
Tracey, D M
Traill, E R
Urquhart, C
Vestey, J P
Walker, A
Walsh, P V
Watt, S M
Waudby, H
Whillis, D
Whillis, J E
Whyte, D K
Whyte, I F
Wilkes, P R
Williams, F R
Williams, H
Williams, P
Wilson, J C
Wolf, B
Wrench, J G
Wycliffe-Jones, K
Zentler-Munro, P L

Inverurie
Bainton, R
Beattie, J A G
Black, J E
Brewis, G M
Cannon, A M
Cassidy, K A
Ewen, D M
Fraser, J H E
Harkness, S M
Hawson, D S
Hood, D B
Humphrey, C A
Ingram, S E
Johnston, V W
McDonald, L
Mack, H N
McKay, F M A
Murrison, B L
Oliver, J
Paterson, K E
Rutledge, D G A
Shepherd, J H
Wallace, R M
Watson, C J
Young, G

Ipswich
Abuown, A A
Adair, H M
Adapa, U D
Archer, T J
Badcock, S
Bailey, D M
Ball, R
Bamford, M F M
Barsoum, M Z
Bawden, S E
Bellhouse, J E
Bethell, P A
Bhatia, I L
Bowditch, M G
Broadway, J W
Brown, C M D
Brown, V J
Browne, M J
Buckley, R M
Burn, P W
Bush, P A
Cameron, A E P
Campbell, J M
Carey, J M
Cavanagh, R A
Cave, D R
Chalmers, I M
Chalmers, J A
Chowdhary, Z A
Chung, N A Y
Clark, C J
Clunie, G P R
Coady, T J
Collins, R J
Coode, P E
Cook, C I M
Cook, M H
Coomber, S (E L
Cope, E M
Craggs, R A
Cruickshank, G M
Cupper, N C
Cushen, M J
Cutler, T P
David, P S
Davies, H T
Davies, R A
Day, J L
Deacon, D J
Dineen, S J
Dixon, J M
Dodd, N J
Donaldson, P J
Dubois, S V
Duncan, J N
Edelsten, C
El Gaddal, M E H
Evans, W B
Everitt, C R
Exley, P
Fairhead, M M
Fairweather, J A
Flather, J N
Freestone, M D
Fryer, P J
Garber, S J
Garfield, P
Gazeley, S D
Gibbons, N C
Gibbs, A N
Gibbs, S S S
Glancey, G R
Glason, M S L
Glass, S A
Goble, R R
Goodess, J E
Goodwyn, J R
Gould, J D M
Goyder, E C
Grierson, C A
Grimmer, S F M
Guirguis, R W
Guirguis, W R
Hadden, F M
Hague, J S
Halford, J D
Hall, D R
Hall, S R
Hall, S W
Hallett, J P
Hancock, S P
Hands, D H
Hardman Lea, S J
Harley, S C L
Hartfall, W G
Hartley, K E
Head, L
Helps, C M
Henderson, J C
Henshall, L A H
Hilger, A W
Hirst, S G
Hodgkinson, D W
Holloway, P
Howard-Griffin, J R
Howard-Griffin, R M
Howell, P J
Huddy, S P J
Hudson, I
Hutchinson, J R M
Innes, N J
Irvine, N A
Irwin, P T J
Jackson, E P
James, L M
James, R S
Jarvis, A P
Jennings, P E
Jesuthasan, A J
Jogeesvaran, S
Johal, B
Jones, P H
Jones, S E M
Jupp, E J
Karia, K R
Keeble, B R
Kent, R J
Kiel, A W
King, A M
King, D R
King, K A
Knight, M A
Kong, A S
Laukens, A E P
Lazar, S C
Le Vay, J H
Leather, A T
Lelijveld, H A B M
Lewis, D A A
Lloyd, M
Lockington, T J
Lockwood, T J
Lush, A M
McCullagh, M G
McCurdy, D L
McElhinney, D J
McGrath, D R
McKall, K C
McKay, P W
Mamujee, A M
Mamujee, N V
Manji, H
Mansfield, M D
Marsh, M J
Marsh, T D
Marx, C L
Mehta, K H
Mercer, R E
Midforth, J E
Mills, A M
Mills, J W
Mills, P J
Mindham, M R
Mohamed, M S
Moncrieff, M D S
Mooney, P
Morgan, J S
Mortimer, C J D
Moser, S
Mowles, A J
Nabarro, R M G
Narayanan, S
Nicholl, A D J
O'Neill, K P
Ogden, B E P
Orrell, J M
Palmer, M I
Parry, J R W
Pavitt, J A
Pearce, R J
Peecock, F P M
Penkethman, A J
Peyton, H N
Phillips, N E
Phillips, P A
Picken, G
Pitt, J
Powell, J M
Powell, O J
Rae, D M
Rauniar, A K
Rayman, G
Reader, C E
Reader, F C
Remeh, B S
Renshaw, N D
Richards, G D H
Roberts, S J
Roberts, T J H
Robertson, K J
Rowe, R C G
Roy, P K
Royce, S M
Ruddy, M C P
Rush, E M
Salam, M A M E-H
Schurr, A J V
Scott, I H K
Seaton, D
Seaton, E D
Servant, C T J
Shanahan, M D G
Sharman, A
Sharp, D J
Sharpe, C R
Sheehan, J M
Sheehan, L J
Siddique, A Q
Sinclair, M T
Skinner, J B
Smith, K S
Smith, S L
Smith, S J
Smithson, N
Sonnex, T S
Spencer, C P
Squire, C M
Steiner, R R
Stevens, I
Stevens, M J
Strubbe, P A M J
Tate, R J
Taylor, S J
Thiruchelvam, N
Thomas, D L C
Thomas, G
Thomas, P D
Thompson, E J
Thurairaj, T
Thurtle, O A
Todd, A E
Trowell, J E
Tucker, S R
Turner, D A
Vasey, D P
Wadera, S P
Wankowska, H C
Ward, D M
Ward, T
Warren, M D
Watson, M
Watson, R J
Watts, J P
Webber, J E
Weir, I K
Wellingham, C B
Whale, S A
Whitear, W P
Wilden, J
Wilkinson, A J
Wilkinson, S L
Williams, B E B
Williams, J R
Williams, P F
Williams, S A
Williams, S G J
Wilson, M E S
Wiltshire, S J
Woodley, J M
Wright, K J T
Wright, R
Wyborn, M V T
Wyke, R J
Wythe, P
Yale, C
Yung, M W

Irvine
Adamson, A
Alexander, B K
Barber, J M
Burnett, R R
Campbell, W D
Cunningham, D
David, M C
Doig, M F
Dryden, C M
Godfrey, J B

Graham, K
Hewitt, A P
Irvine, G A
Kerr, P
Luis Ruiz, D
MacDonald, C E
McElhone, J P S
McGlone, P
McGregor, C M
McHugh, C
McKeith, D D
Macleod, I
Macrae, R A
McSherry, G J
Miller, A F
Mullin, L
Nelson, J
Nixon, A A
Park, L M
Paterson, M T
Russell, S G
Sharma, V C
Stirling, A J
Wagner, R M
Wood, I H Y

Isle of Benbecula
Dawson, S K
Senior, A J
Tierney, F

Isle of Colonsay
Currie, J S

Isle of Eigg
Weldon, R H

Isle of Harris
Latham, A C
Naylor, A I

Isle of Islay
Buchanan, E C
Buller, A J
Knowles, J M
Latta, D
Perrons, A J
Wood, R J

Isle of Lewis
Barker, J A
Clark, I
Collacott, R A
Hamilton, R W
Maciver, I
Macleod, M
Marshall, L S
Murray, D R
Nichols, D
Rigby, D J
Roberts, A M
Smith, J
Vishu (Vishwanath), M C

Isle of Mull
Charlier, A R
Douglas, M
Jack, J A
Kennedy, S D

Isle of Skye
Baker, F M
Ball, J R
Banks, T W F
Cheyne, M F
Crichton, C L
Johnston, H M
McCabe, S D
Maclean, M
Pearce, T
Shaw, K J
Tallach, C
Toms, J S M
Turville, S A

Isle of Tiree
Holliday, J D P

Isleworth
Abhaya Kumar, S
Adam, B S
Ahmad, S S
Al-Obaidi, M K
Ali, N T
Allard, S A
Anderson, M G
Andrew, R
Antebi, D L
Archibald, C
Ashley, J S A
Banerjee, B
Basu, S
Beckett, M W
Bhattacharyya, B K
Bhave, N A
Cassar, J
Cheetham, D R
Collins, C E
Craig, R G
Dalton, M E
Daniels, D G
Davis, D M
Doctor, R S
El Khidir, H H
Ezzat, M H
Fox, J S
Girling, J C
Greenwood, T W
Guha, I N
Guru-Murthy, K
Habel, A
Hakeem, V F
Harrison, S J
Ho, K N V
Hughes, R G
Hussain, H K
Idia, T I J
Jogiya, A
Jones, E C
Kaikini, D W W
Kane, S P
Khattar, R S
Kurar, A K
Kyi, M S
Lau, D P-C
Lett, K S
Macedo, C
Mannan, M A
Massoud, M A K
Matson, A M
Miller, C S
Naunton Morgan, T C
Oliver, J R
Owen, E J
Pabari, D
Papasiopoulos, S
Parker, S C
Patel, S N
Peters, T M
Platt, J S
Pusavat, L T
Ramesh, S
Rangasami, J J
Raslan, F
Richmond, C E
Rogers, H S
Sekhar, M
Sensky, T E
Shah, S
Shah, S M A
Shettar, C K
Sodsai Nathan, S M
Thein, M
Thorpe, P A
Venkataraman, G
Walia, S
Warnock, W A
Whitmarsh, S P
Winning, A J
Young, R A L
Zadeh, H G

Iver
Banner, B H
Gilani, N
Gilani, S M N
Jenkins, L K
Nowers, C D
Rigby, G V
Robinson, V P
Shafi, M A
Trythall, D A H
Webster, P J R

Ivybridge
Anderson, R B
Behennah, L M
Bleiker, P F
Broadley, A J M
Burnell-Nugent, H M
Campbell-Smith, T A
Campbell, L J F
Cornock, S J
Day, H C
Evans, L E
Gregory, G
Griffiths, T N
Hamlyn, E C
Harker, R J
Holley, P J
Johnson, A L M
Jones, K A
Langsford, M J
Laurens, C
Martin, J R C
Morris, J R
Ousey, T J
Pinsent, S E M
Price, J N
Price, M J
Richardson, J B
Sheppard, S C
West, D
Willcox, J R
Wyatt, R M

Jarrow
Bedi, A K
Bem, J L
Brewster, N
Cordner, D E S
Davison, M A
Dias, B F
Farrar, M W
Griffiths, K
Lodhi, K A K
Overs, K
Palmer, H M
Radley, J
Zaidi, S M Z

Jedburgh
Booth, T F
Cook, G A
Dorward, C R
Mitchell, R J
Muir, E S

Jersey
Allardice, J T
Bailhache, N A
Balbes, D I
Barrett, M E
Bates, P R
Blampied, A M
Bonn, S M J
Borthwick-Clarke, A
Brown, J R
Brown, R L
Bruce, M P
Buist, W E S
Burke, W M M
Callander, G W R
Cameron, I L
Cameron, Z A
Clifford, R P
Clinton, C
Coates, J A
Coleman, P
Comerford, M B
Connor, T P
Coverley, C T
Curtis, N R
Day, J B
Drew, O E
Earley, M A
Evans, J E M
Evans, S N
Faiz, G F
Fortun, P J
Foster, S J
Frank, D C
Franklin, W H
Georgelin, D J
Gibson, H N
Gibson, M
Ginks, S E
Ginks, W R
Gleeson, M H
Glynn, P J H
Goodson, T C
Goulding, H
Gracey, N G A
Grainger, C R
Halliwell, A C
Hamilton, D G B
Harvey, J D
Hickson, B
Hickson, R M
Higgins, P
Hill, P J
Himayakanthan, S
Holmes, M B
Howell, J B
Hurst, R K
Ilangovan, C K
Ince, D A J
Ince, G J
Ingram, N P
Isham, C
Kellett, B C
Kinross, I
Konstantinov, D T
Krohn, P L
Kumar, A
Labia, J B
Landor, E C
Lane, J R
Lapasset, MMF
Le Bas, P S
Le Cocq, H D
Le Cornu, J
Lea, P A W
Leadbeater, N A G
Lissenden, J P
McBride, M E
MacLachlan, N A
Macmichael, I M
Marson-Smith, R A
Matthews, P J M
Mattock, C
Maxey, J M
Mickhael, N F
Milner, S M
Minihane, N A
Mirvis, L M
Mitchell, A R J
Mourant, P N
Muhlemann, M F
Muscat, I
Naidu, G C P
Nanson, J K
Newell, J R
Norman, A L S
O'Sullivan, D A
Osmont, J M
Pai, K P
Pope, D G
Preston, S D
Prince, G D
Purcell-Jones, G
Raghu, C G
Reid, A C
Reid, J
Richardson, M R
Russell-Weisz, D J
Santos, S R
Selvachandran, P S
Shah, N D
Shenkin, I R
Simmonds, K A
Sinfield, K E
Siodlak, M Z
Slater, E M
Smart, P H
Smylie, C A
Southall, P J
Sparrow, S A
Spratt, H C
Standring, P
Stewart-Jones, J
Swann, J D
Taylor, J J
Taylor, W D
Twiston Davies, C W
Usha, T R
Venn, P M
Watts, N
Webster, N J
Wildy, G S
Williams, A D
Wilson, L
Winspear, M
Yates, R W P

Johnstone
Ahmad, R S
Ahmad, S
Alston, A B
Baxter, M M
Biggart, B S
Bland, R M
Borthwick, M J
Brandon, D J
Campbell, A R
Clark, R R
Coats, A E
Cunning, C A
Dhiya, L H
Dorward, F C
Dunlop, W W
Erwin, L
Fergusson, A J
Fisher, D E
Forrest, G J
Ghaus, P
Gibson, J A
Harris, G K
Innes, M R
Jones, C M
Khanna, D S
McBryan, D D
Matson, I C
Milburn, R A
Mitchell, M M
Ramsay, A L
Raveenthiranathan, C
Renwick, E C
Russell, A M
Scade, T P
Shadbolt, C J
Singh, T N
Storey, M E
Stromberg, P
Todd, J G
Todd, W
Umesh, S
Wallace, J A
Wallace, K A G
Wallace, P G M
Webb, L A
Wills, J F
Wright, A H

Keighley
Adley, R
Al-Muhandis, W M
Alim, S A
Allen, D E
Almond, F A
Appleyard, I
Armstrong, R K
Aspin, A J
Baker, D A
Belsey, R L
Belton, A
Blake, J G
Booth, J A (L
Bostan, A M
Bradburn, H
Bradford, N C
Brash, J H
Britland, A A
Brown, D R
Brown, T S
Brunskill, P J
Burton, J H W
Bushby, M
Cadamy, M E
Chambers, C H
Clark, D
Clements, D G
Clements, E J
Collinson, A
Cooper, A M
Cox, H
Cradick, N H
Crawford, S M
Cruikshank, G M
Cunliffe, G
Cuthbert, A C
Da Costa, P E
Day, S W
Dev, V J
Dewar, E P
Dinnen, R L
Dudley, M J
Dunbar, A M
Duncan, M J
England, J K
England, M A
Faraj, A A M
Ferguson, I G
Fisk, J A
Fontana, J W
Foster, J E
Gabbitas, S M
Gill, J C S
Gopal, D T
Grunshaw, N D
Hakin, B A
Hakin, R N
Harrington, M G
Harrison, A P
Hayes, M L
Haywood, J A
Healey, C J
Helliwell, M F
Hill, R E
Hodgson, G A
Hodgson, J D
Hosker, H S R
Howe, J G
Hoyle, M K
Hudson, R B S
Hughes, M J
Huxley, J C
Ilett, S J
Iskander, N Y
Jagger, J H
Jeyasangar, G
Jones, G M
Kapadia, C R
Kay, P M
Kehoe, R F
Khan, P
Khan, R B N
Kharbanda, Y
Lindsay, K
McCulloch, E E
McGill, R
McLellan, G S M
Middleton, R J
Milbourn, M R
Mohammed, R A
Moore, J A
Nagaraja, E G
Nair, R R
Névin, J A
Nejim, A
O'Dowd, J J
Onafowokan, J A
Opira-Odida, F X
Orgles, C S
Parker, C R
Parry, J H
Partridge, G W
Phillips, R J M
Pickles, J S
Pope, R M
Porter, G G
Pratt, O W
Preshaw, J M
Pue, P
Purvis, M J
Raashed, M
Reisig, V M T
Richardson, S M
Robertson, J A
Samtaney, N T
Savage, B F
Savill, G A
Severs, P H
Shaikh, N A
Silverton, N P
Simpson, F M
Sims, C D P
Skarrott, P H
Smith, N A L
Smith, N R
Smith, P A
Solomons, R E B
Sonanis, S V
Stanton, J M
Starkey, C
Taylor, P
Thorburn, W S
Todd, J A
Tones, B J
Towers, S
Ullah, S
Waite, K E
Walshaw, C A
Ward, K P
Whamond, W N
Wilkinson, K N
Williams, G C
Wilson, N D
Wray, C C
Zaman, S
Zezulka, A V

Keith
Gould, D C
Green, C L
Harrington, J H
Heneghan, T T
Hutchison, K R
Hutchison, R B
Morrison, W M
Shaw, S M
Thomason, J

Kelso
Cutting, R I
Fingland, I G
Fish, M J
Hood, W G
Johnston, C A
Lawley, M A
Millar, J A
Mooney, G
Morris, A R

Nisbet, R
Potter, S F
Sutherland, A S

Kelty
Melville, A W T
Pryde, L A
Sheil, P A

Kendal
Brennan, C
Buckler, J A
Buckler, P W
Chadwick, I G
Coulson, R A
Dean, G
Dolton, W D
Donnelly, J M
Duggan, E J
Duxbury, S C
Edgell, A F
Elliott, M
Finlay, A M
Foster, H E
Gardner, S J N
Gill, A L A
Green, S A
Heaven, W G
Howse, M L P
Howse, M L
Huggett, I M
Ingram, H J
Lee, A K
MacKenzie, A G
Meyrick, M R P
Milnes, R S W
Mingins, C
Mitchell, R W
Mukherji, M J
Obale, B A
Oliver, K J
Ostick, S
Payne, J
Pigott, J E
Reeder, S A
Scott, R W
Shaw, C S
Shaw, C P
Simpson, P D
Sloss, J D G G
Smith, M G
Stokes, C S
Stringer, R M
Thomas, P C
Urquhart, A
Wilkinson, H L
Williams, E C

Kenilworth
Allinson, F
Allsopp, E J
Appleyard, K M
Archibald, E H
Beckford, L C
Birchall, L A
Botherway, A H
Cable, H R
Clayton, K C
Cremonesini, D P
Curley, M
Davies, C L
Davies, R N
Delaney, A J
Dickson, C W
Eaton, T J
Foster, L M
Geddes, J H
Grogan, R J
Harvey, S G
Jones, D A
Jones, H D
Kander, P L
Lewis, M W D-L-H
McCreadie, M A
Mander, A V L
Matthews, G A
Miller, P C
Pai, S M
Prosser, S E
Rapley, D M
Ray, C K
Rudd, A G
Spraggett, D T
Street, K N
Walker, E H
Whelan, R M
Youakim, S S F

Kenley
Carroll, C
Collins, F M
Collomosse, J R W
Jones, G N
Qureshi, S
Ray, G
Stanway, P A
Sturgess, M J

Keston
Child, S C C
Neve, J M
Paddle, J S
Paddle, J J
Singh, K K

Keswick
Atack, J A
Blakemore, R
Bulman, J M
Hadkins, R
Hammond, A
Hodgson, D J
Hooper, T M
Mackay, H J
Moore-Ede, M C
Rennie, S M
White, P M
Woodliff, H J

Kettering
Abdallah, H M H
Abdel-Latif, M M A
Ablett, J C
Aherne, J J A
Al-Sudani, M L
Antcliffe, R D
Aspinall, W P
Bahal, V
Baines, G F
Balloch, C B
Barclay, P
Barrington, R L
Beckett, N S
Betambeau, N
Birring, S S
Biswas, S P
Bland, K M
Bland, R M
Blindt, D M
Branford, W A
Braybrooks, L S
Britton, M J
Bromage, J D
Brown, A R
Bryant, K M
Burnell, J C
Carr, A S
Chambers, J S
Child, R J
Clearkin, R J
Cotterell, S J
Craven, A F
Dancocks, A C
Datta, A K
Davison, O W
Dempster, R K
Fitton, J H K
Glover, S J
Goh, G J M
Gonzalez Santos, R
Gostelow, B E
Graham, L S
Gunasekera, N P R
Hadaway, E G
Harrop, C W
Haughney, R V M
Holden, J M
James, M G
Jones, A E
Jones, J R
Kapur, R K
Kelsey, H C
Khan, K M
Kiddle, M W
Langendijk, J W G
Lawrence, J H
Lee, R J
Leyden, P V
Loo, P S L
Loveday, N F J
Luthman, J A
Macleod, F K
McManus, J B
Matthews, S R
Mattingly, P C
Maye, A J
Maye, M J

Michel, V J-M
Milkins, S R
Mistry, N H
Moody, R A
Moore, J S
Morris, I M
Moss, H
Mukhopadhyay, T
Mukhtar, A I
Nanayakkara, C S
Neill, L G
O'Malley, B P
Parkinson, M S
Patel, J B
Pease, J J
Penney, T M
Perera, G L S
Perkins, A
Perry, D
Peterson, S
Piechowski, L
Pinnell, J R
Pollak, T E
Pratt, C A
Rashed, M D
Reeve, R G
Rose, C F
Ross, S M
Russell, A J B
Samtani, B K
Sansome, J D W
Sanyal, B
Scanlon, J J
Shackleton, C D
Sheppard, J
Sibson, K R
Smith, J S
Smith, R J
Staff, D M
Stephen, A A
Stewart, R D
Stocks, P J
Streeter, H L
Sugunakara Rao, Y V K
Sulch, D A
Taylor, O M
Thamizhavell, R C
Thompson, A J
Tilley, N J
Treharne, L J
Turner, S
Twohey, L C
Vaal, M F
Veasey, K A
Walters, R L
Wildgoose, A D
Williams, J B
Williams, Dr
Wood, P L E

Kidderminster
Ahmed, N
Allen, T M W
Armitstead, P R
Bennett, A J
Blanchard, G F
Bolton, C
Booth, S N
Boyle, H C
Budhani, S J R
Burridge, J M
Butcher, L H
Campion, G R C
Campion, T C
Carter, A G
Cawdery, H M
Chaudoir, P J
Cockrell, N B
Cushley, M J
Dauncey, A C C
Davies, R A
Eeles, E M P
Farraj, D A A
Ferguson, I M C
Frost, G J
Gajjar, A P
Gerrard, J
Ghobrial, E I
Girgis, M S
Gray, S R
Hayward, C J
Herbert, R E
Hill, B D
Holzman, R H A
Ireland, R W
Irlam, C A
Jarvie, N C
Kaushal, P

Kelsey, R J
Labib, M M
Lewis, M L
Lindsay, S-A
Malcomson, D H
Malcomson, E J
Mallen, C D
Mann, P
Marsh, C R
Mendes Da Costa, B
Morgan, F B
Mukoyogo, J M
Murrin, K L
Newrick, P G
Nixon, D
Pathirana, C K
Perry, S R
Phillips, L J
Saverymuttu, T M
Schrieber, V P
Sherwood, B T
Smith, C R
Smith, C M D
Smith, J V
Smith, K L
Smith, S A
Spalding, J P
Stanley, J K
Starkie, D W
Stewart, P A
Summers, A R
Summers, G D
Tallents, C J
Taylor, C L
Tewari, S
Thompson, P
Thorley, C H
Trezise, C A
Tudor, J G
Udeshi, U L
Wadsworth, T M
Wetherall, A P
Wilkie, S
Williams, P W
Wilner, J M

Kidlington
Aitken, A C
Bangham, C R M
Banks, A
Bryceson, W T
Bryson, N H L
Carr, J M
Durrant, I J
Ellis, M L
Evans, D J
Gunasekera, K D
Heaf, J M
Lee, G J
Lehane, J R
Marshall, V E
Newman, W J
Pandher, K S
Parker, I W
Price, H M R
Rogers, P M
Sherwood, W J
Street, S H
Stuart, E A
Stubbings, M A
Tranter, J
Turner, R S L
Wall, I J
Wallace, M J
Watts, A J

Kidwelly
Acharya Baskerville, M
Baskerville, R
Dundrow, J M
Edmunds, E G-H
Hopkins, M P
Standley, C

Kilbirnie
Colquhoun, A B
Ferry, D A
Hillman, R G
Kilpatrick, A
MacInnes, P
Smith, R R

Kilgetty
Jones, R M
Williams, S J T

Killin
Hope, G M
Rough, S A

Syme, D M
Turner, E I

Kilmacolm
Ellis, D L
Fisher, C J
Fyfe, T
Gemmell, J A
Knight, P V
Laurie, H C
McGill, A M
McGinn, G H
McLellan, I S
Morris, G E
Powell, J M
Robertson, J K
Soinne, N
Strathern, H M
Winning, T J
Wootton, R P

Kilmarnock
Adamson, M R
Afzal, M
Allardyce, J G S
Anderson, K
Barr, M E
Beveridge, R D
Black, J P
Boag, D E
Brown, E
Buchanan, I R
Carruthers, J G
Carton, A T M
Chestnut, R J
Courtney, J M
Coy, S E
Crichton, I S
Curran, J D
Currans, J M
Currie, W J R
Currie, W J R
Dean, L H
Dean, R T
Dempster, J H
Diament, R H
Drummond, J W
Duke, J D
Dunlop, P A
Dunn, F J
Dwyer, C M
Erskine, J G
Fallows, R
Foxworthy, M P
Gaffney, P G
Gardner, F M
Gold, I L
Graham, I
Grant, L
Hambly, K N
Henderson, B C
Hills, S
Hislop, W S
Holland, J
Horne, M A M
Howie, P G
Illingworth, D M
Inglis, F G
Innes, A
Irvine, K H
Johnston, C P
Joussef, M M A-M
Kalman, C J
Khaliq, K
Kilpatrick, J M
Kyles, I M
Lang, J A
Lannigan, A M
Lennox, S E
Lipka, A W
Livingston, W S
Lochrie, A S
Lough, M
Mcadam, J A
McAdam, L A E
Mcadam, S R
McAlpine, W A
McBride, J
McClure, J P
MacDonald, A A
McDougall, L
McGeechan, P
McGregor, E M
McGregor, J R
McHardy, C
McIntyre, L A
McMurtrie, F
MacPherson, J N
McTaggart, A

Magee, J R
Marshall, A H
Martin, C S
Masterton, R G
Melrose, E B
Micallef-Eynaud, P D
Michie, A R
Mikhail, W M F
Miller, D E
Miller, L R
Morris, A J
Morrison, C A
Mulugeta, Y
Murphy, J T
Murray, A
Nairn, E R
Osman, M K
Palchaudhuri, M R
Paxton, G C
Paxton, J R
Powell, G J
Pugh, R M
Ralston, G J
Ratnasabapathy, U
Rawlings, D
Richards, I M
Robertson, W S M
Rodriguez Santos, J
Schwigon, S S
Sengupta, U
Shamlaye, C F
Shanks, E M
Shaw, D
Shaw, K C
Short, R M
Sirisena, L A P
Smith, S M
Smyth, M J
Sommerville, J M
Staines, J D
Stewart, W
Sword, L
Syme, B A
Tait, G R
Tellechea Elorriaga, F J
Thompson, S E
Timmons, M J
Walker, E
Wardrop, P J C
Watson, D
Watts, J D
White, R J
Whitford, P
Williamson, A E
Wilson, P A
Wood, M J
Young, R K B
Yusoff, F
Zaidi, S M H

Kilwinning
Allen, D J
Groves, T
Hall, R D
Huggan, D K
McCreadie, S L
McInroy, B
Miller, D J
Scollay, G
Sutherland, F T

Kings Langley
Birdwood, G F B
Brownfield, M O N
Cave, T R C
Cohen, S J
El Borai, C L
Farrow, L J
Kanani, S-A
McLellan, J M
Perahia, D G S
Percy, C M
Popli, S
Reidy, M J
Wallis, E G

King's Lynn
Abdel Gadir, M A
Abdy, S
Abukhalil, S H
Aickin, J C
Al-Taher, H
Allen, G B
Anderson, J A R
Arafat, Q W
Atkinson, L K
Bansal, B
Barber, C G
Barber, J C

Barclay, A J
Barter, D A C
Bartlett, D L
Bhupathi, V
Biran, R K
Black, D M S
Bone, C D M
Brown, J M
Burchett, K R
Burchett, N
Burgess, A S
Butt, Z A
Byatt, C M
Campbell, I K
Chakrabarti, A
Chakrabarti, I U
Chakraborti, S
Chan Seem, C P
Coates, P B
Collett, A
Connolly, C A
Crosby, G L
Crowe, M T I
Cullen, P T
Cunningham, M D
Cupper, G A
Daly, M M
De Silva, K S M
de Whalley, P C S
Denny, N M
Devane, L S
Dhumale, R G
Dootson, G M
Dossetor, J F B
Douds, A C
Duncan, B M
Eames, R A
Eaton, A C
Edris, M A M
Ell, M S F
Elston, C C
Florance, R S K
Galloway, J M
George, E
George, R
Gough, P G
Greatorex, R A
Hambling, C E
Harris, S J
Harrison, E A
Hart, N
Herrod, J J
Ho, L W
Hobbiger, H E
Hopkin, D J
Hotchin, I K
Howard, S H F
Hughes, A L E
Iyengar, M O P
Jacobs, T E
James, M E
Jeffery, J A
Jelfs, B R
Jennings, A M
Johnson, N A
Keidan, A J
Kenny, M T
Kenny, M K
King, A D
Knott, S R G
Kumar, E B
Kurma Rao, B
Lacey, H P
Lake, A K
Lavallee, P J
Lazarus, H I
Li, M N
Luxton, D E A
McGouran, R C M
McGourty, J C
Mack, I J
Maclean, A R
Martin, J D
Martin, J S
Murray, A
Nicholls, E A
Nockolds, C L
Nooh, A M M K
O'Brien, A A
O'Brien, J R
O'Brien, P D
O'Neill, A E
Outred, R
Patel, A R
Pawlowicz, A
Phillips, J R N
Phillips, S
Plumley, M H C
Pryn, R B
Pushpanathan, R J
Ramachandran, V
Redhead, K A
Redman, R C
Redwood, N F W
Richardson, G
Richardson, S J
Rimmer, M J
Robinson, A A
Rubin, S P-A
Russell, J J
Sapey, E
Sasitharan, N
Sconce, F M
Scott, J M
Shaw, N C
Sheppard, L C
Sherwood, A N
Showell, D G L
Singh, S M
Sivakumar, K
Sparks, M J W
Stabler, R J
Suchak, K K
Summers, S R
Tasker, P R W
Thorpe, N C
Tiernan, D G M
Tigchelaar, E F
Venning, S L
Warren, H W
Waterson, I M
Webber, P A
Weli, T D
Wheater, M
White, N
Whiteman, P D
Williams, J D
Wilson, A W
Wilson, M G C
Wright, F G L

Kingsbridge
Baldwin, J R
Boughton, B A
Brett, A D
Carter, N W R
Chopin, K T
Cole, R J
Elliott, D M
Everitt, M T
Game, D S
Hargreaves, S J
Harvey, A J
Holcombe, D R
Jackson, P N
King, J B
McIntosh, C G
Reeve, B J
Smith, M A
Syn, T
Thomson, I G
Trounce, C C
Turner, C L
Williams, S G

Kingston upon Thames
Abayasiriwardana, J M
Al-Wakeel, B A R
Alhadi, B Z R
Allen, W M C
Andrew, L J
Bak, J E
Barker, G H
Barrie, M
Barton, F L
Beare, J D L
Beattie, J C
Betts, J
Bevan, R K
Bloom, I T M
Bowskill, P A
Bowskill, S J
Boxer, J C
Brown, C L
Buchan, M C
Burn, L
Cahill, C J
Chaliha, C
Choudhury, S S A
Chouhan, M A
Christie, P N
Chua, S M
Clark, D L
Clements, D M
Coombs, R R H
Crow, M A B
Culling, W
Curtis, M J
D'Souza, M J
D'Souza, M F
Daly, K E
Davey, P A
Davies, J R
Davis, P K B
Delves, C E
Dick, J A
Dixon, A N
Duckham, J M
Eardley, G R
Fawcett, A
Fernandez, C
Foddy, S E
Gibbons, C E R
Gillespie, I H
Girgis, A J
Goel, R N
Grant, E C G
Gregory, S A
Gupta, N
Hampton, R W D
Hawker, D J L
Hetherington, D J
Heymann, T D
Hickman, N L A
Hilton, S R
Hindmarsh, P C
Hopkins, D M
Horgan, S E
Hughes, A R
Jacobs, L R
Jameson, C F
Jawed, S
Jayne, W H W
Jebb, D N
Jeevaratnam, S
Kane, J A
Katay, E I
Kennaugh, A J
Kenyon, B K M
Knee, G
Knowles, G K
Kreeger, L C R
Lee, A K T
Lee, C N
Li, W-Y
Lourudusamy, S
McAuliffe, R L
McCall, A W
McCarthy, G A
McCrimmon, F E
McHugh, P J F
MacKenzie, D L
Mackie, S
McNabb, W R
Manning, C L
Marwaha, S
Mason, A M
Mathie, A G
Matthews, T J
May, D P L
Moalypour, S-M
Morley, R
Morris, O K
Mullen, M J
Myers, C A
Nandakumar, K N
Neville, L O
Newman, P J
Norris, P M
Omer, S E D M
Parekh, V J
Parrish, J R
Patel, K R
Patient, D N
Pearson, H H
Perera, I M F
Polanska, A I
Pooley, A S
Proctor, M T
Rafferty, P G
Railton, G T
Raimondo, C
Ravalia, A
Ray, A
Ray, S A
Reed, M G
Reynolds, P R
Rhodes, A I
Richardson, A E
Richardson, H D
Rigg, C D
Roberts, S H
Robinson, R A
Rodrigues, C A
Rowe, D J
Rowley, M R
Sabih, M R
Sammut Alessi, C W
Schiess, F J
Shah, D S
Shallal, S A M A-T
Sheikh, H F
Sinton, R I R
Slee, I P
Smith, A T M
Smith, J M A
Smith, P S
Sommerville, G P
Spring, M W
Stacey, R G W
Steer, C G
Strickland, I D
Sykes, H
Thakerar, J G
Thayalan, A S
Thonet, R G N
Todd, C E C
Vines, B H
Wang, M Y E
Ward, C S N A
Ward, D A
Ward, R D
White, M
Whitfield, R L
Whittam, D E
Wijayasinghe, G E S
Willson, P D
Wimalasiri, R W
Wimalasundera, R C
Winrow, A P
Wong, H J
Yadav, H R
Zarnosh, M
Zwaal, J W

Kingswinford
Basheer, M
Bloor, J A
Carr, J F
Cripps, D F
Dawes, P
Foster, H M
Gallimore, D J
Hamza, P
Kendle, G
Keogh, S P
Kiteley, N A
Kuligowski, M
Parnell, S J
Pinfold, T J
Plant, N A
Potter, S J
Rathore, J S
Rowlands, J L
Shekhawat, F S
Skilbeck, A B
Swain, C M
Tweddell, W H
Williams, M D

Kington
Crawshaw, J M
Lias, M
Murphy, B J M
Rannie, G H

Kingussie
Anderson, M E M
Convery, A
Michie, A R
Munro, D G M

Kinlochleven
Headden, G D

Kinross
Aitken, E
Anderson, D P
Campbell, D
Carragher, P J
Ferguson, W M
Gardiner, J
Hogg, D H
Krishnaswamy, D
Lee, M A
Mason, C J
Osborne, C J
Robson, P G
Spens, F J
Thornber, M
Wallace, E D

Kirk Michael
Smith, M E

Kirkby Stephen
Hallam, C S M
Huck, S
MacDonald, A
Merckel, J C

Kirkby-in-Furness
Clayson, H
Hall, N L

Kirkcaldy
Adam, M P
Allen, R A
Anderson, S M
Ballantyne, K C
Barker, G G
Barker, J A
Bee, D E
Beg, M H A
Black, A G
Boyce, S
Brown, G M
Brown, T I S
Buchanan, I J
Buchanan, R C
Buxton, R A
Campbell, I
Chalmers, J
Clark, C A
Cruickshank, G S
Duncan, A D G
Duncan, C
Ferguson, J M
Ferguson, K D
Ferguson, L A
Flynn, A M
Fraser, D M
Galloway, S J
Gergis, M I
Ghosh, D
Gourdie, R W
Greig, G E
Hakim, S M
Hanafiah, S R
Janczak, J J
Karim, S Z
Kelleher, J J R
Kendall, D J
Lafong, A C
Lees, A P
Linnemann, A M
Loudon, M A
McCallum, A E
McCallum, C J
Macdonald, E A
MacGlone, C M J M
McGourty, L J
McGowan, F J
McLeod, L S
McMillan, J F
MacMillan, M G
McTaggart, J
Mahmood, T A
Mair, S J
Meek, J L A
Mitchell, M C
Moonie, L G
Morris, C A
Morris, R L
Mughrabi, M A M
Murray, H A
Oates, W K
Oudeh, B A R M
Paisley, T A
Pal, S
Petrie, G R
Pinion, S B
Priyadharshan, R
Rahilly, M A
Rahman, M A-U
Rebello, G
Redpath, M
Reid, D A
Richardson, T J
Robertson, J D
Robertson, R
Rochow, S B
Rogers, S Y
Russell, S C S
Satyanarayana, P
Scott, R G A
Smith, A G
Smith, D H K
Smith, G F N
Smith, R P
Steel, J M
Steer, C R
Stewart, M E
Stobie, F J
Thrower, M M
Tomlinson, J E M
Urquhart, D R
Wilson, J S
Wilson, J A
Yule, J M

Kirkcudbright
Branson, R R
Dow, R C
Locke, W J
Mack, R H
Morton, J M
Rutherfurd, J A F

Kirkliston
Carson, D P
Douglas, E
Milne, R M
Mitchell, J
Simpson, W S

Kirkwall
Al-Mukhtar, A A M A
Beaven, S R
Borland, C W
Deans, W J D
Dewar, I G
Dohrn, M
Fay, E D J
Fay, P J
Hamilton, L M
Hamilton, W M
Hepburn, B
Konstam, S T
Laird, C
MacInnes, D J
MacInnes, R J N
Nicolson, A L
Van Schayk, M
Wright, T F

Kirriemuir
Farquhar, A M
Gilmour, J R
Guthrie, M F
Learmonth, J C M
Lendrum, A B G
McAdam, N W
Morrison, S L
Ritchie, J M
Watts, M C
Weir, A D
Wilmshurst, A P

Knaresborough
Alpin, H R
Banks, J C D
Burton, J L
Carradine, J S
Corrin, S E
Downes, A J
Hall, J L
Jobling, D I
Keenleside, C L
Keogh, A J
Lee, J N
Mawhinney, R R
Murphy, A M
Newman, C P S J
Norton, P M
Robinson, R M
Roy, S N
Sapherson, D A
Smith, R B
Walton, S F
Ward, J R
Watson, W F
Yarrow, A D

Knebworth
Campbell, P J
Cooper, M E
Daniel, R A
Dent, R G
Edmunds, I G
Faulkner, R E
Kalilani, M J M
Kite, S A
Lawson, A
Peace, S
Salter, J P H
Sinclair, F M
Stratford, M
Turner, J E
Wood, D C

Knighton
Cross, P L

Howcroft, K M
Kiff, M L
Myhill, S B

Knottingley
Atkins, D
Baruah, P C
Berridge, L S
Brahma, P K
Earnshaw, P
Newland, L A
Pinder, C A
Pinder, I F
Rashid, N A

Knutsford
Arthur, D K
Bayliss, L A
Berrisford, M H
Billingham, J W
Caldwell, J
Clements, A C
Conroy, J L
Cowling, H E
Eaton, J D
Evans, P J
Fitzgerald, J D
Gibbons, D R S
Heseltine, J S
Highcock, M P
Holt, A K I
Howarth, K L
Johnson, S M
Kearns, P J
Khan, A T M M H
La Coste, J J
Lawn, J A
Leicester, G
McHugh, F J
Mallon, T J
Morgan, J P
Muston, G C
Muston, G C
O'Shea, S J
Oldham, B
Price, H S
Ramsden, A R
Redfern, E
Reeves, S M
Robertson, C M
Shackleton, D A
Smith, M C
Smith, V J
Stephenson, R J
Stones, R N
Taylor, J I
Wardle, T D
Watters, E A
Youssef, Y Y

Kyle
Hurding, S B
Mackinnon, R E
MacRae, K E A
Morgan, P J P
Tallach, J R

Lairg
Cadamy, A R
Dickson, A
Fitzsimons, B J
Hughes, A J
Macdougall, M
Slator, D A
Vine, R J

Lampeter
Davies, I N
Howley, H M
Jones, E W
Jones, T M L
Mathew, R
Phillips, A M
Sawyer, M N
Seal, M T

Lanark
Anderson, C M
Black, W
Carleton, R L
Christie, A J
Christie, L H
Connaughton, J A
Copland, J
Criggie, W R
Duncan, J M
Grant, A M
Hacking, J
Hill, J G
Islam, Z U
Kane, I M
Kerr, A T
Kerr, S
Lang, A E
MacGregor, F M
McKnight, F E
McMahon, D J
McQueen, D
MacRitchie, D M
MacRitchie, P A
Martin, J
Murie, J
Nunn, T J
Robb, A G
Scott, W S
Steel, E A
Ward, N M
White, T
Young, J I

Lancaster
Abraham, J S
Agababian, A A
Agarwal, M
Ahmed, S I
Ainsworth, P
Allen, J W
Ashworth, L J
Bali, P L
Baraka, M E F M
Bateman, A M
Batty, P D
Beaumont, J M
Bird, T M
Bollard, R C
Breckon, K E
Brigg, J K
Brown, A K
Brown, S M
Bukhari, M
Bulman, C H
Burch, D J
Burnett, J M P
Burr, R H
Byers, E A
Carling, D
Carvill, P T
Caun, K
Chandoo, A H
Coltman, D B
Connell, S J
Cook, N K
Craven, A J
Crawford, A I M
Crighton, I L
Curzon, I L
Dafforn, E M
Dalziel, M
Davies, J R
Dendy, R A
Denver, M D
Dodd, A J
Dodds, W N
Donnelly, J M
Duffy, P M
Durham, S T
Earnshaw, T G
Eckersley, N G
Ellam, M
Elley, C M
Erulkar, J
Feldman, A Y
Flanagan, P M H
Fleet, T W
Foster, N J
Foster, S F
Freeman, P
Gallagher, A R
Gaskell, R K
Gibson, P A G
Gill, R W
Gill, V
Gorst, D W
Guinan, I
Hacking, J E
Hallam, D
Halstead, H C
Harding, S A
Harrison, L E
Harrison, P V
Healy, E T
Heywood, R J
Higham, A D
Hodge, J C
Jackson, R G
Jenkinstone, T M
Johnstone, N A
Jones, K
Kamal, A K M
Khan, D S A
Kingston, M R
Lavelle, J M
Leese, T
Longden, D J
Lunt, T J
McCafferty, J I
McCaldin, A M
McDonnell, D S
McGlone, R G
McGregor, J C
McIllmurray, M B
Mahendran, S M
Marriott, J D
Marshall, P D
Mason, W T M
Mathen, G
Mechie, G L
Milson, J E
Mom, J S
Morgan, W P
Murgatroyd, A B
Murgatroyd, M J
Ness, L M
Nicholls, G C
Nightingale, P B
North, J K
O'Donnell, M
O'Neill, F C
Opdebeeck, G P E M T
Orr, J T
Owen, I T
Parkes, A W
Partington, J R
Paton, A L
Pearson, J D
Peat, M J
Pilling, G M E
Povedano Canizares, C E
Prasad, B K
Pugh, H
Rabbett, H L C
Riley, P M
Roffey, M
Ruscillo, G A
Seddon, T M
Severn, A M
Shepherd, R J
Shukla, Y P
Sidhu, K
Singh, C A
Smith, A F
Smith, D J
Smith, M B
Stacey, D J
Staff, W G
Stewart, H D
Stewart, M
Story, C A
Sullivan, R
Taylor, A
Taylor, E
Telford, D R
Thomas, J M
Toy, A J
Tynan, P F
Vaughan-Jones, N
Vickers, A P
Wales, D A
Walker, B H
Wall, W H J
Walmsley, D
Watt, C S
Watts-Tobin, M E A B
Wedley, J R
Wetherell, S C
Whittaker, R G
Whitton, A D C
Willey, R F
Wilson, P
Wong, K E
Wong, M K Y
Wright, S G
Yarnall, D J
Yule, R M

Lancing
Al-Hasani, L J
Brummitt, P I
Burton, J P
Campbell, A J
Feeney, P J
Hobson, D G
Ilkiw, P S J
King, H A P
O'Sullivan, P J G
Peskett, D J
Starbuck, D P
Tierney, P T F
Tobias, A J
Varty, C P
Woolcock, J A
Young, J M
Young, J H

Langholm
Phillips, H C
Phillips, M L C
Scott, A
Spencer, G R
Williamson, M B

Langport
Balai, R
Bond, A K
Chubb, S
Gibson, D W R
Hussey, O J
Knight, K M
Nightingale, E A E
Nightingale, P J
Pollock, D M
Richards, M L
Shrimpton, H D
Strutte, L J F
Talbot, S
Tyler, C L

Larbert
Barron, J
Boyd, J
Brown, S T C
Cole, R A
Duncan, C M
Ellison, D P
Finegan, W C
Ghobrial, O S
Gibson, G A
Gibson, L M
Hillan, L R
Leeming, J A
Lynch, P P
McNab, M J W
Martin, J H
Massey, J B
Paton, D H
Preshaw, C T
Robinson, J A
Suresh, T
Thomson, C R
Tuddenham, L M

Largs
Auld, A
Brown, H B
Cooper, M I
Ewing, C G
Greenfield, M R
Heaney, S J
Howie, S P
Jamieson, I S
Johnstone, M
Lewis, S G
McClure, J R
MacDonald, A A
McGurk, D A
Park, C M
Shaw, A J
Simpson, J A
Soutter, D A
Turner, S L
Walsh, P F

Larkhall
Baird, S H
Balkrishna, N
Cama, E F
Duncan, D
Fattah, H M
Harvey, G M
Kinniburgh, D E
Martin, A R
Mormesh, N M
Morrison, J D R
Ofili, E A
Parker, C P
Renfrew, D M
Roy, J P
Russell, C R
Sim, N A
Skehan, P F J
Smart, J F
Spence, E
Telfer, C A L
Thompson, A T
Vyas, R B
Wilson, J R

Larne
Bell, J H
Booth, K
Breen, E P
Bridges, J G M
Campbell, G
Chin, A K L
Craig, A M
Crory, G A C
Cullington, S J
Dornan, J O G
Dunn, J B
Ferguson, K
Gray, S B
Heyburn, G
Hopkins, M P
Howie, P K
McCloskey, S M
McIlroy, A
McIlroy, D J
McMinn, D J S
Mitchell, W A
Murphy, E
Shanks, B
Steele, C
Varghese, M
Wasson, L F
Wilson, J R W
Worthington, J M

Lasswade
Chapman, K A
Combe, J R
Jones, N C
Macdonald, D J
MacLeod, W A
Pettigrew, N M E

Lauder
Cormie, P J
Crombie Smith, H J C
Lowles, J M
Macrae, M C

Launceston
Baker, P J
Collier, P T
De Glanville, R G
Felton, J R
Fitzpatrick, E L
Morice, R O
Smith, G T
Stevens, A G
Wells, M L
Wheal, J D

Laurencekirk
Anderson, M J
Anderson, N J
Box, K M
Lyall, A R
Mulcahy, P D
Pirie, K
Wood, J R

Laxey
Mcalister, J
Moran, P J
Mullan, M H
Stone, A K
Wilson, K G
Young, D W

Leamington Spa
Ainsworth, P
Allsopp, G M
Anderson, J H
Ashmore, M W
Baker, D S
Benning, T B
Bickerton, R C
Bonsall, P A
Boothroyd, C M
Campbell, F S
Carter, J C
Chan, E A
Chhina, N
Christopher, P M
Clowes, C T
Collins, R J C
Courtenay, R T
Davis, P J M
El-Gingihy, A S A
Emery, J C
Eykyn, M L
Farrall, L A
Fullbrook, J E
Galbraith, E A
Glass, J M
Gough, A
Green, M J
Greenwood, C R
Hancock, J L
Harban, F M J
Hawkes, G
Higman, D J
Holloway, E H
Holmes, J E
Hortas, C
Hyland, V M E
Janda, A
Johnston, A O B
Khan, S Y
Knell, A J
Knight, T J
Larard, D G
Leigh-Hunt, N J
Lodwick, L M
Lucas, J B
Mactier, F C A
Mann, J
Marshall, J R
Moffatt, C D
Nippani, K J
Oliver, L
Pearson, L C
Pearson, M J
Perks, B M H
Potts, D A
Privett, J T J
Robson, A M
Rohatgi, S
Saluja, R K
Shakespeare, D T
Shenkman, J J
Shipton, P F
Singh, G
Snowdon, C M
Stewart, F E
Sumra, R
Taylor, R A S
Taylor, S
Trevelyan, N C
Trye, C J
Watt, A M
Weinstein, V F
Wilkinson, J J A
Wilmot, J F
Wilne, B D
Wilson, T D P
Yong, C K K

Leatherhead
Anderson, W J
Bailey, C S
Banerjee, A K
Barr, W S R
Belbeck, J S
Bennett, T J
Birtwistle, M L
Blow, C M
Bourne, S J
Buchanan, S R J
Chinn, G L
Claridge, G B
Clark, S J
Close, J B
Cross, J A
Davies, L C
Deane, C J
Degaitas, P
Down, N A C
Draper, R J
English, P M B
Evans, A M
Finnamore, V P
Garnett, R
Gosden, C W
Gray, M S
Harper, D A
Harrington, N J
Hibbert, J
Jarrett, P E M
Johnson, P A
Johnston, P M
Jones, K H
Jones, L J B
King, H M
Lawrenson, A L
Lee, J D
Leung, Y L
Lewis, N R
Littleton, E T
Marazzi, P J M
Martin, C

Martin, E A
Martinez Del Campo, M
Mead, A J
Menzies, R W
Meynen, F G C
Moore, J R
New, L C
O'Connell, M R
Patel, C
Pickin, J H
Pilkington, G A
Powell, S J
Prowse, A D
Rose, J A
Rowe, C J
Speirs, C J
Spurgeon, J
Stephenson, J D
Stewart, P J
Strickland, A D
Thomas, E J
Thompson, C
Thomson, R S
Torode, S A
Upchurch, F C
Vithayathil, K J
Walter, R M
Watson, J U
Williams, A A
Williams, D O
Wong, J S K
Wyatt, C M

Lechlade

Greenwood, R E
Hancock, F B
Stephens, H M A
Thomson, I A
Yapp, J

Ledbury

Conway, K R
Crook, M C
Draper, M R
Greenall, G
Hiley, C D
Hunter, W J
Johnson, R
Ranasinghe, A M
Sandison, R A
Scholefield, R D
Scott, B C
Smith, E N
Smith, M D
Thorp-Jones, D J
Tomlinson, M J

Lee-on-the-Solent

Ashby, G H
Bassett, J H
Beale, E A
Bell, I S
Butler, R E
Craig, J R
Evans, S D
Parsons, M H
Ross, R J
Taylor, C A

Leeds

Abbott, C G
Abbott, C R
Adams, I D
Adams, J
Adams, J M
Adams, R J
Adcock, C A
Addlestone, M B
Addlestone, R I
Ade, C P
Adlard, J W
Adshead, D W
Ahmad, N
Ahmad, R
Ahmed, I
Ahmed, Y S
Aitken, C
Akagi, H
Akhtar, S
Albert, D J
Aldridge, S J
Alexander, C M
Alexander, J M
Alexander, M S
Ali, F S
Ali, S A
Alison, D L
Allen, A W
Allen, F S
Allibone, R O
Allison, E A
Allison, S C
Allman, I G
Alpin, H R
Alvi, N-S F
Ambrose, N S
Amery, C M
Ang Wan-Ming, C
Anthoney, D A
Appleby, M A
Apps, J M
Archer, I A
Armitage, J D
Arnold, R
Arthur, R J
Arundel, P
Ash, D V
Asiedu-Ofei, E S
Atherley, C E
Atkinson, H G
Atkinson, J D
Atter, M
Aumeerally, Z B
Austin, S
Aviv, R I
Axon, A T R
Ayres, J E
Bagnall, W E
Baig, M W
Bailey, C C
Baker, R J
Balen, A H
Ball, R J
Ball, S G
Ball, S A
Balls, M A
Balmford, S E
Bamford, J M
Barclay, I
Barnard, D L
Baron, S E
Barth, J H
Batchelor, A G G
Batra, N
Batra, R K
Baxter, K F
Beacock, D J
Beckwith, L
Beecroft, C L
Belchetz, P E
Belfield, P W
Bell, A P
Bellamy, M C
Bem, M J
Bennett, C P
Bennett, E K A
Bennett, M I
Bennett, R J
Benson, S E
Berkin, K E
Berlet, J K
Berridge, D C
Berridge, J C
Berridge, J M
Berridge, K I
Berridge, M J
Berrill, A J
Best, A C
Bew, N M
Bew, S A
Bhakta, B
Bhandary, L V
Bhandary, U V
Bhartia, B S K
Bhatia, M S
Bhattacharyya, P K
Billsborough, S H
Bingham, S J
Biran, L A
Birchenough, S J
Bird, H A
Birkin, A E
Birnage, K M
Bishop, N
Bishop, R I
Biwer, J E
Black, D A
Black, M A
Black, S J
Blacker, A J R
Blomfield, I A
Bobet Reyes, R M
Bodansky, H J
Boddy, J E
Bolland, H E
Bolton, A J
Bong, J J
Bonsor, G
Bonthron, D T
Boon, A P
Boonin, A S
Botterill, I D
Bottger, S
Bottomley, D M K
Bower, S J
Bowie, P C W
Bowman, C E
Boyd, K L
Boylston, A W
Bradbury, K M
Brady, S K
Branfoot, J T C
Brennan, C L
Brennan, T G
Brew, S
Bridges, L R
Broadhead, T J
Broch, J I
Brogden, P R
Brookes, S D
Brooks, A S
Brown, H
Brown, H B
Brown, J L
Brown, M A
Brown, S J
Browne, J M
Browning, C A
Browning, F S C
Brownjohn, A M
Brownlee, K G
Buch, M H
Budgen, S A B
Burke, B M
Burke, D
Burkill, A D
Burn, W K
Burns, E
Burr, J M
Burr, W A
Burrows, D A
Burton, D J C
Bury, R F
Bush, D J
Bush, S
Butler, G E
Butt, W P
Bynoe, J K
Bywaters, J L
Cade, A
Cahill, B T
Cairncross, R G
Cairns, A
Calder, S J
Caldicott, L D
Calvert, S M
Cameron, A
Cameron, I H
Cameron, S J
Campbell, D J
Campbell, D A
Campbell, F M
Campbell, J A
Campbell, S D
Carder, P J
Carey, B M
Carmichael, D J
Carmody, E A
Carpenter, M J M
Carrington, N C
Carroll, B N
Carswell, N S
Carter, J
Carter, R F
Cartwright, R A
Cassels-Brown, A
Cassidy, J F
Cassie, J A
Catto, A J
Cave, E M
Chalmers, A G
Chalmers, D M
Chamberlain, M A
Chapman, A H
Chapman, R A
Chappelow, S
Chapple, K S
Charlton, J S
Charlton, P N
Chennells, P M
Chesser, S G S
Chester, J D
Child, J A
Childs, A-M
Christian, A S
Christou, T
Christys, A R
Chu, C E
Chu, C H P C
Chung, A K K
Clappison, D P
Clare, C M
Clark, A E
Clark, S M
Clarke, J
Clarke, M D
Clarke, M A
Clarke, P R
Clarkson, K S
Claydon, S M
Clyde, C A
Cohen, A E
Cohen, A P
Cohen, A T
Cohen, A F
Cohen, E M
Cohen, J M
Cohen, M B
Cohen, S A
Cole, P J
Colling, P N
Collinson, M P
Congdon, H M
Conway, S P
Cooke, M L
Cookson, T W
Cooper, L R
Cooper, N A
Cornette, L
Corrado, O J
Cottrell, D J
Cowan, J C
Cowan, P J
Coyle, C A
Crabbe, D C G
Crawshaw, A L
Creaby, G E
Creighton, J E
Crellin, A M
Crew, A D
Critchley, A T
Crofton-Biwer, C J
Crone, A A
Cross, M H
Cross, R J
Crossland, G J
Crowson, J B
Cruickshank, J L
Cruickshank, R H
Cubbon, R M
Culliney, P
Cundall, D B
Cunliffe, W J
Cunningham, J A
Curgenven, A
Curran, S
Dai, C-C A
Dall, B J G
Danks, J F
Darbyshire, P G
Darling, J C
Darnborough, A
Darnborough, S
Darowski, M J
Davey-Quinn, A P
Davidson, L A
Davies, A-M
Davies, J A
Davies, M H
Davies, R M
Davis, F I
Davis, S M
Davison, A M
Davison, S M
Day, A T
De Boer, G M
de Pauw, K W
De Silva, C
De Silva, N A
Deacon, V
Dean, S G
Dear, P R F
Dearden, A M
Dearden, N M
Denton, D V
Denton, M
Denyer, M E
Devaraj, K S
Devaraj, S R
Devaraj, V
Devitt, H J
Dexter, S P L
Dickinson, C J
Dickinson, D F
Dickinson, J R E
Dickson, D E
Dickson, R A
Diekerhof, C
Dintinger, E L
Dixon, J A
Dixon, J J
Dixon, J A
Dixon, M F
Dodman, J D
Doig, R L
Dolben, J
Donaldson-Hugh, M E A
Donnelly, H S
Doughty, C
Douglas, I A C
Dowell, A C
Dowley, A C
Downing, C
Dowson, D G
Dresner, M R
Drife, D E
Drife, J O
Dryhurst, D J
Duffy, S R
Duncan, B
Dunham, R J C
Dunn, E M
Dunphy, R H
Dwyer, A S
Dwyer, N M
Eardley, I
Eastham, D G
Easton, A M E
Eastwood, D S
Eastwood, P G
Eccles, J T
Edwardson, R S
El-Sayed, M E N M
Ellis Emeritus, F R
Ellison, C
Elmslie, A G M
Elton, S M
Emerton, M E
Emery, C
Emery, P
Essom, J M
Evangelou, L
Evans, J
Evennett, H C
Everett, B D
Everett, M P
Everett, S M
Fairfield, J E
Fairley, I R
Fale, A D
Farrell, P
Fatheazam, S
Fatheazam, S L
Fear, J D
Febbraro, S
Feely, M P
Feeney, M T
Feldman, S M
Fellerman, S M
Fenwick, J D
Ferrie, C D
Ferriman, E L
Field, A M
Finan, P J
Firth, D C G
Fisher, R B
Fisher, S E
Fitzgerald, T A
Fitzpatrick, M M
Flannigan, C B
Flynn, C M
Foley-Nolan, N D R
Ford, A C
Ford, H L
Ford, P A
Forrester, D W
Forster, S
Foster, C A
Foster, K
Fowler, R C
Fox, T P
Fraser, A
Frazer, J B
Freeman, C B
Freeman, L
Freeman, M S
Friend, A R
Frieze, M
Frost, S F
Gambles, C S
Garrett, C J
Gbolade, B A
Geraghty, P G M
Gerrard, G E
Gerrard, J W
Gesinde, M O
Ghoneim, A T M
Giannoudis, P
Gibbs, J L
Gibbs, K
Gibson, J S
Gibson, R M
Gilbey, J E
Gilbey, S G
Gilchrist, C M
Gill, A B
Gilliam, A D
Gilmore, M
Gilmore, R D
Gilson, D
Gimeno Sentamans, C M
Glaser, A W
Glass, M R
Gledhill, J E
Glynn, P M
Godfrey, D J
Godfrey, G
Gokhale, J A
Golding, W R
Gooi, H C
Gopakumar, B N
Gough, M J
Gould, M I
Goulding, P J
Gozzard, J G
Grant, P J
Green, A L
Green, J B
Greenway, J
Greenwood, J P
Griffin, N R
Griffith-Jones, M D
Grogan, E
Groves, J
Guckian, D M F
Guillou, P J
Gulliver, S A
Gupta, K K
Guthrie, J A
Hackney, R G
Haigh, L I G
Hainsworth, R
Hall, A S
Hall, G D
Hall, G I
Hall, R D
Hall, S K
Halpe, N L
Halsall, P J
Hamer, D W
Hamilton, S C C
Hammond, C J
Hanson, D R
Haq, R
Haque, M E
Hardo, P
Harkin, P J R
Harkness, K A C
Haroon, M M
Harries, C J
Harris, A M
Harris, C M
Harris, K A
Harris, K M
Harris, N J
Harrison, D F
Harrison, E A
Harrop, G B C
Hassan, T B
Hatcher, S M
Hatton, P
Haward, R A
Hawkhead, J L
Hawkings, M D
Hawkins, A
Hayden, J D
Hayes, S L
Hayward, D M
Haywood, H L
Heal, S J V
Heatley, R V
Heeralall, D
Helliwell, P S
Henry, M T
Heppell, D
Hervey, G R
Hesse, G W A
Heywood, P L
Hibble, C J
Hicks, C A
Hicks, F M

Hickson, J R
Higgins, D G
Higgins, J C
Hillhouse, E W
Hillman, B
Hillman, J S
Hind, S P
Hirschowitz, P M
Hobbs, C J
Hobman, J W
Hodge, D G
Hodgson, A J
Hodgson, R E
Hogan, S K
Holland, P C
Hollyoak, V A
Holman, D S
Holmes, C P
Holmes, J D
Hopkins, P M
Horgan, K
Hornbuckle, J
Horner, J H
Horsley, S
Houghton, A M
Houghton, A L
House, A K
House, A O
Howden, P
Howdle, P D
Howell, S J
Hudson, J
Hudson, P C
Hughes, D
Hull, M A
Hume, M J
Humphreys, A C
Humphris, S D
Hunjin, M S
Hunter, C M
Hurley, M B
Hurwitz, D C
Huston, C
Huston, G J
Hutchinson, K
Hutchinson, S
Igbaseimokumo, U
Iles, P J
Illingworth, K A
Illingworth, R N
Ilsley, D W
Ilyas, M
Ingham, J S
Inweregbu, K O
Irving, H C
Isaacs, J D
Islip, M R
Ivbijaro, G O
Iwantschak, A
Jabeen, S
Jack, A S
Jackson, A P
Jackson, K A
Jackson, T L
Jain, A
James, P N E
Jamieson, D R S
Janik, A J
Jankovic, Z
Janulewicz, M A
Jardine, K L
Jarman, R D
Jarrett, S J
Jarvis, E H
Jayne, D G
Jenkins, G
Jerram, T C
Johnson, E J
Johnson, G S
Johnson, J
Johnson, M H
Johnson, P A
Johnson, R J
Johnston, J
Johnstone, P W
Jones, J M
Jones, R G
Jones, S K
Joyce, A D
Juniper, S E J
Kain, K
Kalu, P U
Kaminopetros, P I
Kaul, P
Kay, P H
Kay, S P J
Kearns, N P
Keeble, R J
Keefe, W J
Keep, M J
Kelly, E J
Kennedy, J E
Kent, P J
Kessel, D O
Khan, A S N
Khan, O D
Khan, S N
Khan, Y Z A
Kibria, S M G
Kiltie, A E
Kinsey, S E
Kirkham, J
Kirkwood, C J
Kitchen, C A
Kite, S M
Knight, L C
Knight, P R
Knight, S L
Koslowsky, N
Kumar, V S P
Kurukulaaratchy, R J
Kwok, M C
Lacey, V J
Lam, B L
Lam, W L
Lam, W
Lamb, J T
Lane, G
Lane, P E
Lane, S A
Lanfear, P C
Langford, R M E
Lansdown, M R J
Larvin, M
Last, H A
Lawrence, S L
Lawrenson, F J
Lawson, C A
Lawton, J O
Lawton, S L
Laybourn, J K
Laybourn, S M
Leach, A M
Leahy, M G
Ledger, S J
Lee, A C H
Lee, C E
Lee, P S
Lee, S G
Leeds, J S
Lees, G A
Lessels, F A
Lestner, R A
Levene, M I
Lewis, H N
Lewis, I J
Lewis, P D
Li, A G K
Liddington, M I
Limb, D L
Lindsay, K A
Lindsay, M A
Lintin, S N
Lipman, G
Liston, J C
Livesey, D J
Livingston, J H
Lloyd, S M
Lodge, J P A
Logan, K L
Logarajah, V
Loizou, M
London, J
Long, D E
Longbottom, G
Losowsky, M S
Lough, C D
Loukota, R A
Lowe, R A
Lowther, J J H
Lubrano Di Scorpaniello, E
Lumb, A B
Luscombe, H C
Lynagh, J
Lynch, L A
Lyons, G R
Lyons, S
McAteer, E M
MacCarthy, J P
McClean, P
MacDermott, S J
McDonagh, F M C
Macdonald, D A
McGoldrick, P J
McGonagle, D G
McGowan, A
McGrath, H J
McHugh, P J M
McIntosh, S J
MacKenzie, A C M
McKenzie, F R
McKibbin, M A
Mackintosh, A F
McKittrick, M
Maclean, C M
McLenachan, J M
Maclennan, K A
MacLennan, S
McMahon, A J
McMahon, M J
McMain, S S
McNeill, E J M
McVerry, B A
Madan, C K
Madan, S
Makura, Z G G
Malhotra, A
Malhotra, P A
Malhotra, P K
Mallett, M I
Mallick, A
Manning, S I
Manock, K J
Mansfield, M W
Manyeula, R T
Markham, A F
Marks, P V
Marriott, R G
Marsden, J H
Marshall, A M
Marshman, R I
Martin, M F R
Martins, C A
Mary, A S G
Mascie-Taylor, B H
Mason, E A
Mason, G C
Maston, J
Mathers, J-A
Mathialahan, T
Matthews, N R
Matthews, S J E
Mavor, C J
Mayers, J N D
Maz, S S
Mbizeni, J M
Meadow, S R
Mehay, R
Mehrotra, P N
Mellor, D J
Menon, R
Mercer, K G
Merchant, W J
Meynell, A
Mezas, L H
Millard, J
Millares Martin, P
Millner, P A
Millner, V A
Mills, C R
Millson, C E
Miloszewski, K J A
Mindham, R H S
Minhas, R B
Minhas, S
Mishra, A K
Mitchell, D P
Molto, A
Mooney, A F
Moore, D G
Morgan, A W
Morgan, P W
Morrell, A J
Morris, E J
Morris, M
Moss, E
Mossad, M G
Mounsey, N L
Mourmouris, N
Moxon, J W D
Moxon, P
Mueller, R F
Muers, M F
Muir-Cochrane, R R
Mulley, G P
Muncer, Z K
Munsch, C M
Murdoch Eaton, D G
Murphy, C E
Murphy, S A
Murray, R A
Murty, J A
Naik, J
Nair, S
Nair, U R
Najmaldin, A
Nawaz, S
Nazir, N
Neal, R D
Nelson, J W
Nelson, M A
Nelson, M
Nelson, S
Nensey, M
Neumann, V C M
Newbound, A D
Newell, D
Newell, S J
Newman, K L
Newman, P P
Newstead, C G
Newton Bishop, J A
Nicholas, A C S
Nicholas, B M
Nix, A L
Nix, P A
Nkonde, P M
Noble, B A
Noden, J B
Norfolk, D R
Norwood, C
Nunn, G F
O'Brien, T P
O'Connor, P J
O'Donovan, P J
O'Loughlin, B A
O'Mahony, J G
O'Neill, D P
O'Shea, T S
Ogden, L M
Okereke, R A
Oldroyd, G J
Oliver, S D
Ollerton, S J A
Olsburgh, J D
Orton, C J
Osman, C H
Ottman, S C
Owen, R G
Owens, D W
Oxborrow, N J
Page, R L
Pai, H U
Panezai, A M
Papagiannopoulos, K
Papworth-Smith, J W
Parkin, G J S
Parkin, R D
Parry, D J
Parsloe, M R J
Patel, A
Patel, J V
Patel, K K
Patel, K
Patel, N K R
Patel, P M
Patel, S
Patel, T B
Paul, A B
Paul, A C
Peacock, S G
Pearson, E M
Pearson, R E
Pearson, S B
Pearson, S G
Pease, C T
Peckham, D G
Peckham, F C
Pedder, S J
Pedley, I D
Penn, N K
Penn, N D
Pepper, C B
Perren, T J
Perrins, E J
Phelan, F J
Philippidis, P
Phillips, N I
Pickering, I F
Pickles, V M
Picton, S V
Pieroni, J E
Pinder, A J
Pittard, A J
Plant, P K
Pollard, S G
Pollock, K D
Porter, K G
Potts, N J
Potts, R K
Pountney, A J
Pouya, A
Power, A P
Power, B E
Powersmith, P S M
Prakash-Babu, P C
Prasad, B
Pratt, D
Prescott, S
Preston, S R
Prestwich, N C
Price, P M
Pritlove, J
Procter, J J
Puntis, J W L
Puri, S C
Quinn, M A
Quirke, P
Raines, J E
Raistrick, D S
Rait, G
Raja, U
Ralph, S G
Ramsden, W H
Randall, M S
Rane, V A
Ranjitkumar, S
Rankine, J J
Raper, J M
Ravenscroft, A J
Ravi, K
Raynor, Y M
Razzaq, I
Read, P E
Reece, A
Reid, J A
Reid, K
Rembacken, B J
Renwick, D S
Renwick, S J K
Reynard, K
Reynolds, A
Reynolds, M T
Reynolds, P D
Rhodes, N D
Richards, E M
Richold, J P
Rickards, A F
Ridgway, D M
Roberts, A B
Roberts, F
Roberts, J H
Roberts, T E
Roberts, T E
Robertson, I R
Robertson, R J H
Robinson, A S A
Robinson, A
Robinson, J E R
Robinson, M B
Robinson, P F
Robinson, P
Robinson, P J A
Robson, D J
Roden, R K
Rooney, C M
Rooney, F J
Rose, D M
Rose, N J
Rosenberg, K
Rothwell, R I
Rowe, C E
Rowell, N R
Rowland, G D
Rudolf, M C J
Ruigrok, A
Russell, J L
Russell, L E
Rutherford, A J
Rutledge, G J
Sadaba, J R
Sadiq, F J
Sadler, R S
Saffer, C M
Sager, J M
Saha, S C
Sainsbury, P A
Samuel, C A
Sandle, G I
Sapsford, R J
Sarvananthan, R
Satur, C M R
Saunders, E J
Saunders, E J
Saxena, I R
Schallamach, S
Schweiger, M S
Scott, B W
Scott, D
Scott, D J
Scott, D J A
Scott, E M
Scott, J N
Scott, N
Seal, A K
Sebag-Montefiore, D J
Sedler, M J
Sefton, S
Selby, P J
Sellors, J E
Selsby, D S
Semple, P
Setia, R
Settle, F C
Seymour, M T
Shah, M V
Shah, T H
Shapiro, H
Share, A I S
Sharma, S
Shaw, J D
Shaw, N H
Shaw, S A
Shaw, S H
Sheard, T S
Sheehan-Dare, R A
Sheerman-Chase, G L
Shelly, M A
Shenderey, K D
Sheridan, M B
Sheridan, P
Sherwood, G J
Shevlin, P V
Shillito, T J A
Short, B
Sillender, M
Silman, H
Simm, J M
Simmons, A V
Simmons, M A
Simpson, K H
Simpson, N A B
Sims, A C P
Sinclair, G
Singh, G P
Singh, J L
Sivananthan, U M
Sixsmith, A M
Skelton, R E
Skinner, J
Slaymaker, A E
Sleightholm, M A
Sloan, J P
Sloan, M C
Smeed, R C K
Smith, D A
Smith, E S
Smith, G E C
Smith, G M
Smith, G M
Smith, I M
Smith, I S
Smith, N A G
Smith, P S
Smith, P H
Smith, R M
Smith, R T
Smith, W E
Smith, W H T
Snell, J A
Sood, R N
Sooltan, A R
Sooltan, M A
Southern, K W
Southern, P B
Souyave, J
Spencer, H A
Spinty, S
Spokes, E G S
Squire, B R
Srivastava, S K
Stables, G I
Stahlschmidt, J
Stakes, A F
Stanley, P J
Stanton, J A
Stanton, M
Stead, H
Stevens, A M H
Stockton, M R
Stone, M H
Storer, D
Storr, E F
Straiton, J A
Stringer, M D
Stuttard, S
Sue-Ling, H M
Sugden, J C
Sutcliffe, R I
Sutton, J B
Sutton, J
Swaby, M J
Swanwick, M V

Swift, S E
Swinburne, M L
Swirsky, D M
Syed, N A
Sykes, N F
Sykes, S J
Szulecka, T K
Tagg, G V
Tan, L-B
Tattersall, R S
Tay, J I-Y
Taylor, C M
Taylor, G B
Taylor, G M
Taylor, H E
Taylor, J M
Taylor, P F
Taylor, P L
Taylor, R M
Taylor, R E
Teale, C
Templeton, P A
Thakur, M C
Than, N
Thistlethwaite, J E
Thomas, A J H
Thomas, D F M
Thomas, H J
Thomas, S J
Thompson, A J
Thompson, D J
Thompson, J C
Thorburn, J S
Thorpe, J A C
Thrower, A J
Timothy, J
Timperley, J
Todd-Pokropek, C J
Todd, N J
Tolan, D J M
Tolley, J M
Tolman, C J
Tompkins, D S
Toogood, G J
Tooley, D A
Townley, A
Townsend, P S
Trigwell, P J
Trumper, A L
Tuggey, J M
Tummala, V R
Turley, J M
Turner, C M I
Turner, G
Turner, J A
Turney, J H
Upadhyaya, G
Uzochukwu, B C
Valeinis, M
Van De Velde, R I
Van Hille, P T
Vardy, E R L C
Varnavides, C K
Vautrey, R M
Veldtman, G R
Verdi, K
Veysi, V T
Vucevic, M
Wachsmuth, R C
Waite, A
Walden, F
Waldenberg-Namrow, C
Walford, L J
Walker, A
Walker, A M
Walker, B E
Walker, J J
Walker, M F
Wall, O R
Wallace, S
Walls, M J
Walls, W K J
Walsh, G
Walsh, M E
Wanklyn, P D K
Warren, E R
Waters, A D
Waterworth, A S
Watkin Jones, A
Watson, C S
Watson, D L
Watson, J P
Watson, T E
Watters, J K
Welch, K A
Welch, R B
Welsh, M C
Wessell, H N
Weston, A L
Weston, M J
Wheeler, M S
Whelan, P
White, S A
Whiteley, S M
Whitmarsh, K A
Wickremasinghe, A S
Wilcox, M H
Wilkinson, D
Wilkinson, N
Wilkinson, S M
Will, E J
Williams, C J C
Williams, D R R
Williams, E M
Williams, G J
Williams, M A T
Williams, S
Williams, S G
Wills, P M
Wilson, A T
Wilson, A R
Wilson, C L
Wilson, I G
Wilson, J D
Wilson, R C
Winyard, G P A
Wong, C L
Wong, C I
Wong, Y F S
Wood, C M
Wood, P M D
Woodhead, C J
Woodley, H E
Woodrow, G
Woods, D R
Worrall-Davies, A E
Wright, A L
Wright, A L
Wright, E M
Wright, F J
Wright, N M J
Wurr, C J
Wyatt, J I
Wyatt, S E
Wynne, C S
Wynne, J M
Yarwood, R
Yates, A P B
Yates, M
Yates, M
Yellin, S D
Yellop, L J
Yeung, S R
Young, N
Zermansky, A G
Zigmond, A S
Zoltie, N
Zoltowski, J A

Leek

Brookes, G S
Carpenter, G R
Elsdon, S J
Evans, D J
Goodwin, S M
Harvey, A M
Hughes, D H
Joseph, C P
Norrie, S D
Piggott, R M
Porcheret, M E P
Rees, A F
Scriven, B E
Shiers, D E
Somerville, S J
Ward, R A
Westaway, C E

Leicester

Abbott, R J
Abbott, S M
Abdul Aziz, F W
Ackerley, R G
Adam, S
Adkinson, R K
Agarwal, V K
Ageed, A B M A
Agrawal, S
Ahmad, S
Ahmed, M-U-D
Akingba, M A
Akowuah, E F
Al-Azzawi, F A L M
Alexander-Williams, J M
Alexander, C C
Ali, N S
Allen, J C
Allen, J N B
Allen, K M
Ambekar, M
Ambus, I A
Amin, A J
Anastasiou, N
Anderson, C S
Anderson, I G
Anderson, P G
Andrade, G G S
Andrew, D C
Andrews, H B
Anwar, M
Anwar, Z R
Appiah, E K
Aram, G E
Archer, C K
Archer, R P
Argiros, G
Ashton, L A
Astles, J G
Au-Yong, R C L
Austin, D J
Austin, M W E
Bahra, R S
Baigent, D F
Bailey, S A
Baker, A K
Baker, K
Baker, R H
Baker, R W
Ball, E L
Ball, K J
Bandesha, G
Bapodra, S V
Baragwanath, P
Barber, B
Barnett, D B
Barrie, W W
Barry, P W
Barton, R P E
Baxendine, C L
Beck, A J
Beck, F
Beddows, M E
Beech, S H
Bell, P R F
Bell, P J R
Benamore, R E
Benghiat, A
Bennetts, R J
Benninger, B L D
Bentley, A J J
Berry, D P
Best, A J
Bhandal, N K
Bhangoo, P
Bhangoo, R S
Bhangoo, S S
Bhate, M S
Bhaumik, S
Bhogadia, H
Bhowal, B
Bhutani, H C
Bibby, K
Bing, R F
Birch, J F
Bland, D G
Blanshard, K S
Bloor, A C
Bohin, S
Bolia, A A
Bolt, S B
Borley, S R
Borrill, L S
Bouch, D C
Bouch, D C
Bourne, C M
Bourne, T M
Bowry, S
Bradding, P
Bramble, N P
Brammar, T J
Braybrooke, J R
Brazil, E V
Bretherton, K F
Brightling, C E
Brittain, R V
Brocksmith, D
Brombacher, J H-P
Brooke, A M
Brooks, H
Brown, A R
Brown, V A
Browne, L E
Browning, M J
Bruce, D I
Bruce, J M
Brugha, T S
Brundell, S M
Brunskill, J
Brunt, K E
Bryant, G M C
Bu'Lock, F A
Buck, K S
Buck, R G
Buckler, M E L
Bukhari, S S
Bunn, H J
Buras, J J
Burd, R M
Burgess, I C
Burke, J G A M
Burnett, M P
Burns, D A
Byer, L D
Byrne, E J H
Cameron, D
Camp, R D R
Campbell, S H
Campling, P M
Canorea, F
Cappin, J M
Cappin, S J
Carey, A-M D
Carr, R M
Carr, S J
Chada, N K
Chadwick, C A
Chaloner, D A
Chan, J C K
Chan, K C
Chapman, C S
Chapple, S-J
Charles, T H S
Chatteris, D J
Chaudhari, I
Chauhan, A
Chauhan, A
Chauhan, B
Chauhan, B
Chauhan, N
Chave, T A
Cherryman, G R
Cheung, E S-K
Chidlow, G
Chillala, S
Chohan, J
Chohan, S S
Church, V A
Churchward, H C V
Clark, C J
Clarke, R
Coakley, F V
Coggins, M M
Cole, A G H
Collett, B J
Conboy, P J
Cook, A G
Cook, E M
Cook, G D
Cooke, S D S
Cooper, J G
Corbett, V
Cottee, C A
Cotton, B R
Craig, D S
Cretney, P N
Critchley, P H S
Crombie, R D
Croom, A J
Crump, B J
Currie, A E
Curwood, V L
Cusack, R J
Dacie, J
Dadge, N G
Daintith, H A M
Dale, A R
Danaher, P J
Daniels, D F
Darlington, B G
Davda, M
Dave, S
Dave, S K
Davenport, P G
Davies, F C W
Davies, M J
Davies, M J
Davies, P
Davies, S
Davison, H K
Davison, I S
Dawson, S L
de Bono, A M
De Caestecker, J S
de Chazal, R C S
De-Melo, A E
Deane, J S
Deans, R F
Dennis, M J S
Dennis, M S
Desai, B N
Desai, S P
Desor, R
Dey, S K
Dhesi, J K
Di Lustro, M J
Dias, J J
Dickinson, F L
Dickinson, L M
Docrat, F
Dogra, N
Doughman Marzouk, T
Downs, P A
Drummond, G A
Duddridge, M
Duggan, F E
Duke, C
Duke, T G
Duncan, C H
Dunkley, M J
Dunn, R A S
Durkan, R M
Dux, A E W
Duxbury, M J
Dyer, M J S
Eastley, R J
Edwards, R G
Elias-Jones, A C
Elliot, C A
Ellis, R
Eltigani, E A H
Elton, C D
Emberton, P
Esler, C N A
Evans, K
Evans, P A
Evennett, J
Everson, N W
Fahy, G T
Fairfield, M C
Falconer Smith, J F
Fallow, S M
Farhan, M M
Farid, B T
Featherstone, S M
Feehally, J
Fell, D
Field-Lucas, A S
Finlay, D B L
Finucane, K A
Firmin, R K
Firth, W R
Fisher, R M
Fishwick, N G
Fisk, P G
Flint, N J
Flynn, C C
Ford, S E
Fotherby, M D
Fox, A J
Frain, I K M
Fraser, M
Fraser, R C
Fraser, S M F
Freeman, R F
Frost, S J
Fry, J M
Fullard, M J
Furlong, C M
Furness, P N
Gajebasia, S S
Gardi, P D
Gardner, F J E
Gardner, J M
Garrido Ferrer, A
Gattoni, F E G
Geelan, S D
Gibbons, C P
Gibbons, G R
Glastonbury, R R
Glover, N A J
Godsiff, S P
Goffin, P S
Goh, G T Y
Gohil, V N L
Golshetti, V G
Goodchild, J
Goodier, J C
Gopal, M N
Gotla, D W
Gould, M J
Goulstine, D B
Goulstine, M B
Graf, R E
Graham-Brown, R A C
Gray, J
Green, M R
Green, T P
Greer, A J
Gregory, R
Greiff, J M C
Griffin, B J
Grigg, J M
Grundy, N J
Habiba, M
Hainsworth, B H A
Hall, A P
Hall, A W
Hall, A S
Halligan, A W F
Hamer, V A
Hamill, J J
Hampson, J M
Hanger, S J
Hanly, T P
Hanning, C D
Hardcastle, S J
Harman, K E
Harris, K P G
Harrison, R E
Harrison, R F
Harrisson, P A
Harvey, N J
Hassan, W
Hastings, A M
Hay, A D
Hay, G C
Hayter, J P
Hayward, N S E
Heer, R
Hellendoorn, J W
Hemingway, D M
Henderson, H P
Hetherington, S L
Hewett, N C
Hewitt, C D
Hickey, M S J
Hickinbotham, P F J
Higgins, H P
Hiley, A L
Hinchliffe, A C
Hirani, A
Hirani, N A
Hirani, S
Hoffler, D E
Holbrook, J D
Hollington, A M
Holton, A F
Hopes, D R
Horst, C
Hoskinson, J
Hoskyns, E W
Houtman, P N
Howlett, T A
Hsu, R T-H
Hubner, P J B
Hubner, R A
Huddy, C L J
Hudson, I
Hudson, N M
Hugh-Jones, S
Humphries, J M
Hunter, A E
Hurwood, R S
Hussey, P G
Hutchinson, C V
Inman, J K
Iqbal, S J
Ireland, D
Ives, D R
Jackett, D M R
Jameson, J S
Jameson, V J
Jankowski, J A Z
Jarvis, A
Jayakumar, K N
Jefferies-Beckley, A L
Jenkins, G
Jennings, T R
Jervis, P N
Jethwa, A A
Jeyapalan, I
Jeyapalan, K
Johnston, G A
Jolliffe, D M
Jones, D M
Jones, G W
Jones, I P
Jones, J M
Jones, M J
Jones, P A
Jones, S D
Joshi, N H

Joshi, R
Jugessur, D
Julian, S L
Kanabar, R C
Karim, K A
Karwatowski, W S S
Kaul, A
Kaul, H K
Kay, D P
Kaye, H J
Keal, R P
Kelly, M J
Kelvin, N B
Kendall, B R
Kendall, C H
Kenrick, J M T
Kerbel, D G
Kerby, C
Kershaw, C J
Kershaw, I F M
Khalid, A M
Khan, N S
Khan, S L
Khandhadia, S D
Khong, T K
Khoo, E Y H
Khoosal, D I
Khunti, K
Khunti, P
Kiana, S
Kilpatrick, J R B
Kilty, B
King, A L
King, C F
King, N W
Kinsella, B W
Kirk, L A
Kirwan, P H
Kishore, K
Knight, A J
Ko, S H
Kockelbergh, R C
Koffman, D
Kong Yao Fah, S-C M-F
Konje, J C
Kotecha, S H
Kovac, J
Krarup, K C
Krishnan, H
Krishnan, R
Kuncewicz, I
Lakhani, D R
Lalji, M K
Lampard, R
Langford, K J
Larkin, E P
Lauder, I
Lawden, M C
Lawrence, I G
Lawrence, N W
Lawrie, I
Lazarus, P A
Leach, R A
Leather, G S J
Lee, D J
Lees, B E
Lennox, A I A
Leslie, N A P
Levene, L S
Leverment, I M G
Lewington, A J P
Lewis, C
Lewis, D G
Lightstone, B L
Lightstone, R J
Lim, V R
Lindesay, J E B
Lloyd-Evans, M
Lloyd-Powis, N
Lloyd, T D R
Lo, N M K
Lo, T C N
Lodhia, B R
Loftus, I M
Loke, S C
Loke, W I
London, N J M
London, S P
Longworth, S
Lucas, B A C
Lucraft, L
Luyt, D K
McAuley, D M
McCarthy, M J
McCaskie, A W
McCullough, J
McGarrity, C
McGrother, C W
Mackay, E H
McKinley, R K
McLaren, I M
McLellan, I
McLoughlin, S J
McNally, P G
McNulty, J M
McParland, P C
Madira, W M
Maharaj, V
Maini, M
Mandalia, I R
Mansingh, S
Marcer, H J
Marchant, J
Maskell, T W
Matharu, G S
Mathers, A
Maxted, S H
May, A E
May, D W F
Mayne, C J
Mead, M K
Mead, M G
Meakin, C J
Medcalf, J F
Mehta, R L
Mengher, L S
Messios, N
Metcalfe, C A
Milner, A R
Milton, J
Milward, T M
Minhas, H S
Miodrag, A
Mistry, A K
Mistry, A D
Mistry, B
Mistry, H R
Mistry, S
Mlynik, A
Mobley, K A
Modhwadia, M M
Modi, B V
Mohamed, M
Moltu, A P
Moncrieff, C J
Monk, P N
Montague, M A
Moody, C M E
Moore, A E J
Moore, K A
Moran, H V
Morar, K K
Morgan, B
Morgan, M D L
Morgan, S J
Moriarty, R J
Morley, C
Mortimer, N J
Muehlbayer, S
Mukadam, H
Mulcahy, K A
Mulla, S C
Muller, S
Murphy, R M
Myint, S H
Naftalin, N J
Nana, A
Naylor, A R
Neale, G
Neilson, J R
Neuberg, K D
Neuberg, R W
Nevitt, G J
Newland, C J
Newley, K P
Newstead, P
Newton, J D
Ng, E W O
Ng, G A
Ng, L L
Ngwu, U O
Nichani, S H
Nichol, F E
Nicholas, R C
Nicholls-Van Vliet, M A T
Nicholson, M L
Nielsen, F
Nightingale, J M D
Nixon, M C
Noble, M D
Nolan, E M
Nour, S A E-R M
O'Brien, R J
O'Callaghan, M
O'Callaghan, P A
O'Carroll, T M
O'Connor, S R
O'Keeffe, D F
O'Reilly, K M
Offer, G J
Okundi, A J A
Oldham, R
Oldring, J K
Oni, O O A
Oppenheimer, C A
Ormiston, I W
Osborn, D E
Osborne, J E
Osborne, N W
Osman, A E M
Ottey, D S
Palin, R D
Panacer, D S
Pancholi, P
Pandya, R P
Panja, K K
Pannu, H S
Panton, I R
Papageorgiou, G L
Pararajasingam, R
Parker, J L
Parkin, A
Parmar, H P
Parry, J S
Partridge, F J
Parwaiz, P
Pasi, K J
Patchett, I D
Patel, B S
Patel, B P
Patel, B D
Patel, D
Patel, G M
Patel, G D
Patel, I G
Patel, J K V
Patel, M
Patel, M
Patel, P
Patel, P C
Patel, R
Patel, R N
Patel, S
Patel, S S
Patel, S S
Patel, V R
Pathak, P
Pathak, P L
Pathmanathan, R K
Pattar, S M
Pavord, I D
Pavord, S R
Peake, M D
Peat, I M
Peek, G J
Pepperman, M L
Peterson, M
Petillon, C M
Pettit, A I
Philpott, C M
Pickard, G A
Pickering, M A
Piper, J A
Pitt, F A
Platts, P
Pohl, D S
Pook, A
Porter, H J
Poskitt, V J
Potter, J F
Power, C A
Power, R A
Prasad, A
Preston-Whyte, M E
Prettyman, R J
Price, C M
Price, R J
Prowse, G D W
Prydal, J I
Pugh, V W
Purdom, D J
Purnell, D
Purohit, S J
Pye, I F
Quinn, M B
Quinton, D N
Rabbitt, C J
Rabey, P G
Raghavjee, I V
Rahman, M
Rai, J
Raitt, D G
Raja, A S
Rajakaruna, C S
Ralli, R A
Ramsay, D W
Range, S P
Ranpura, N
Rashid, A
Ratan, D A
Rathbone, B J
Rathbone, G V
Rayner, J A
Rea, P A
Reddy, P
Redfern, S J
Redzisz, B
Reek, C
Rees, I W J
Rejman, A S M
Reuben, M J
Reveley, M A
Rhodes, A J
Richards, C J
Richardson, T C
Rickett, A B
Riisnaes, A M
Ring, S J
Ritchie, E C
Robertson, G S M
Robinson, L O
Robinson, R J
Robson, F S
Rodgers, M
Rodgers, P M
Roper, P W
Rose, H M
Rosenthal, F D
Ross, C
Rotchford, A P
Rothwell, K
Rowbotham, D J
Rowe, M J
Rowley, H A T
Roy, G A
Rudd, G N
Ruddock, C J
Russell, J A
Russell, W C
Rutter, D P
Rutty, G N
Ryder, J J
Sabri, K
Saldanha, G S
Salkin, D S
Salt, M J
Samani, N J
Samanta, A K
Sandhu, D P S
Sansome, D A W
Sarvananthan, N
Saujani, V K T
Sayed, M A
Sayeed, A
Sayers, R D
Scarborough, N P
Schober, P C
Schofield, J
Scott, A D
Scott, K-A
Scott, S A
Scotton, J E
Scriven, J M
Scriven, S D
Self, J B
Sell, P J
Sellen, E M
Senior, N M
Shaffu, N G
Shafi, S
Shah, B J
Shah, P
Shah, Y B
Shahidullah, H
Shanks, M P
Shannon, R S
Sharma, G K
Sharma, H K
Sharma, N-K
Sharma, R A
Sharma, S K
Sharma, V K O
Shawket, S A J
Sheerin, N S
Sheikh, M N
Sheikh, S A
Sheldon, P J H S
Shepherd, D J
Sher, K S
Sherriff, D
Shikotra, B K
Shrimpton, A R
Shukla, R
Sian, S S
Siddiqui, F
Siddons, E M
Silverman, M
Simpson, K
Singh, H
Singh, K
Singh, P J
Singh, R
Singh, V K
Skehan, J D
Skoyles, J R
Sladden, M J
Slorach, J
Small, M J
Smeeton, R J
Smith, G
Smith, J T
Sosnowski, M A
Spaul, K A J
Sperry, T L H
Spooner, S M
Squire, I
Stanley, A G
Stephens, M F T
Stephens, W J
Stern, M C
Steward, W P
Stewart, C R
Stewart, J A D
Stockley, R A
Stockton, G
Stoddart, P R
Stokes, T N
Stollery, N A
Stotter, A
Stoyle, T F
Straw, R G
Stray, C M
Sturmer, H L
Summer, M
Swales, P P R
Swann, R A
Swift, P G F
Symonds, R P
Szemis, A H
Tagboto, S K
Tajuddin, M
Talwar, S
Tanna, A G
Tanna, R
Tanna, S A
Tansley, P D T
Taylor, D J
Taylor, G A
Taylor, G J S C
Taylor, J A
Taylor, S
Temple, A R
Terry, T R
Tew, R P
Thakor, R S
Thomas, A L
Thomas, E E
Thomas, G D
Thomas, M E
Thomas, N E
Thomas, O
Thomas, P A
Thomas, R G
Thomas, R S A
Thomas, W M
Thompson, J P
Thurston, H
Tighe, K E
Timmins, A J
Tincello, D G
Trayner, J W
Trembath, R C
Trivedi, H V
Trivedi, S H
Trotter, T N
Trower-Greenwood, B G
Tsang, B
Tura, J E
Twigg, L J
Ubhi, S S
Uprichard, W O
Vaghela, H K
Vallance, T R
Valmiki, V H
Vania, A-K
Varma, S K
Vass, A D
Vell, T J
Verma, S S S
Vijayakumar, N
Vindlacheruvu, M
Virdee, D S
Vlachou, P
Vyas, H D
Vyas, J R
Waldrum, C I
Wales, A T
Wales, J M
Walker, C A
Walker, R A
Walker, S R
Walters, G D
Wandless, J G
Ward, A
Ward, D J
Ward, K L
Ward, S C
Warwick, G L
Waspe, S R
Watkin, E M
Watson, H J
Watson, P
Watt, F E
Wells, G R
Wells, J M
Wellstood-Eason, S P
Welsh, K R
West, K P
Weston, P J
Wheatley Price, N
Wheeler, P C
Wicks, A C B
Wildin, C
Williams, B A
Williams, B
Williams, G D
Williams, M A
Williams, O E
Williams, S T
Willmott, A M
Wills, A D
Wilson, A D
Wilson, J I
Wilson, L
Windle, R
Wiselka, M J
Witcomb, A H
Wohl, M A
Wolf, P A
Wong, J Y W
Wong, L S
Wong, M K Y
Woo, D G
Wood, J A
Wood, J K
Woodbridge, S
Woodruff, G H A
Woolford, M C D
Wordsworth, M T
Wright, A J
Wright, J M
Wright, M J
Wyatt, R
Wynn-Williams, D L
Young, C D
Young, I D
Youngman, L M
Younie, M L A
Zickerman, A M
Zillwood, S J

Leigh

Babladi, M N
Bell, M S
Bottomley, J G H
Chan, C K C
Chau, S K H
Cottrill, M R B
Crompton, J L
Dongre, A S
Doublet-Stewart, M P H
Downes, R M
Duper, B
Fletcher, T S
Fox, S
Fulton, P
Geoghegan, S L
Hardcastle, P F
Hilton, R
Hindle, A T
Holbrook, M C
Horne, R J
Jha, B K
Kohen, D D
Lancaster, P S
Lewis, J L
Martin, S M
Molajo, A O
Pickin, J M
RamcHandani, M

Rathod, B K
Richardson, P S
Stewart, E J C
Thomas, A
Tomar, S S
Wardman, A G
Yan Aung, Dr

Leigh-on-Sea
Alawi, M H
Behn, A
Bevan-Jones, A B
Beverton, M J
Bowen, D R V
Bull, L A
Chalmers, J A
Craig, M F
Craig, P J
Dickens, L A
Doshi, H V
Fasey, C N
Gretton, K L
Halls, G J
Hasan, S Y H
Hassaan, A M H
Hayter, A P
Hayter, N P
Hodge, J-C
Idrees, F
Idrees, F
Jayatilaka, G K
Kennedy, H R
Khakhar, A
Kongar, N
Latif-Puri, A A L
Levy, T L
McConnell, J
Malik, S A
Mills, M J
Nagle, L R
Ng, H W K
O'Neill, K S
Peters, G
Porter, J E
Sathanandan, S
Singer, L
Sivaji, C
Sudlow, R A
Watkins, E P H
Wise, L K
Zaidi, S
Zaidi, S T A

Leighton Buzzard
Ana, J E
Bolton, T W
Butteriss, M
Chapman, R G
Cochrane, T J D
Dry, F J
Dunford, G P
Evershed, E Z G
Ewart, J C
Fothergill, S M
Gibby, M J
Hacking, D F
Harding, R A
Henderson, J L
Hesford, S E
Horkan, M C
Kilpatrick, J W M
King, J M
Lane, T M
Lilley, J A
McHugh, F C
Marshall, C D W
Meade, A M
Minney, P C
Palmer, R D
Peel, E M
Povey, M S
Scudamore, J A
Shafi, M M
Srinivasan, R
Taylor, B
Taylor, C L
Thompson, I W
Wallace, I M
Watkins, R P
Watkins, S E
Watts, E T
Wray, D G

Leiston
Hopayian, K
Jobson, D H
Jones, G V
Osler, K

Leominster
Armitstead, M
Bowen, G J
Boyles, D J
Cathcart, C
Davis, M
Dubberley, J
Dubberley, R V
Fisher, C A H
Gaunt, K J
Gray, J D
James, W A
Jeffery, D G
Jenkins, I
Knight, A L
Knight, C J
Mansell, R C
Marshall, P F
Mathias, T G
Ovenden, P A
Pritchard, J A
Rees, M P
Thompson, R M
Voysey, J R

Lerwick
Anderson, Y D
Brew, I F
Clarke, G A
Cooper, A B
Coutts, A G
Cox, F C
Farquhar, G
Freshwater, G T
Johnson, F J
O'Connor, P J
Rarity, R A
Shaw, S N
Veen, H

Letchworth
Aldridge, F J
Aldridge, R P
Ashwood, C G
Bond, A M
Boomers, G W M
Boomers, O W
Brooks, C A
Brugman, M J J
Chand, R
Coker, T P
Day, S L
Graham, R J O
Graham, S M
Hamilton, A L
Heelis, G
Irvine, N S
Jarvis, M A
Jaworski, W F
Judd, M B
Kanakaratnam, G
Kirby, M G
Leigh, M
Lucas, V C
Nevard, R S C
Rahman, J
Ramsbottom, T J
Rodger, A
Strowger, T B C
Tyler, G J
Walsh, J I
Webb, J B

Leven
Ashcroft, L P
Barclay, D A
Bisset, L G M
Bonde, K
Bumbra, J S
Campbell, I W
Christie, L C
Clark, J R
Cruickshank, I N
Cruickshank, R
Delaney, E K
Duncan, J A
Dunn, R
Egerton, P J
Gibson, J H
Heap, A L
Ireland, H C
Keir, R D
Lee, C A
MacIntyre, P A
McLaren, G S
McLean, D F
Martin, L A
Mills, G W
Mukherjee, S

Page, R M
Pattison, R B
Petrie, C J
Pringle, A F
Rodger, S N G
Ross, J D
Sinclair, D M
Skelton, C E
Sloan, R L
Sneddon, A J C
Springer, A L C
Stevens, H M
Thompson, K J
Thrower, S M
Wallace, I
Ward, M J
Woolard, F E

Lewes
Allaway, A J
Arlett, P R
Ashby, P H
Baker, K F
Beasley, M J
Bennett, J
Bjorn, J M
Bridger, P C
Carter, E J
Clarkson, P
Claydon, P E
Collins, C A
Crean, E E
Critchley, M
Dyer, S J
Edmands, D F
Estcourt, P G
Ferns, R A
Fine, E
Forster, E M
Gillams, C L
Hall, R A
Hall, W D
Hargrave, C
Hawke, C I
Heap, D G
Heath, J A
Heath, M J
Hempshall, I N
Hill, J C
Horan, F T
Jensen, J H
Jones, B E
Khan, Y
Lamb, E F
Lamberty, J M
McGibben, L J
Marriott, J C
Merritt, C L
Moore, P N
Norris, E M
Price, H L
Price, J S
Ramsay Smith, S R
Randall, J M
Rees-Jones, A
Robinson, E K
Ross, D
Ross, R A
Rowland, R G
Ryan, A M
Rydon, A H B
Scanlon, T J P
Shiel, J I
Simmons, J A
Stevens, A P
Street, M K
Swaine, C A
Swaine, D J
Szekely, G
Thompson, M A
Thurston, K
Warren, R E
Way, B P J
Welsh, F K S
Williams, O A
Williams, P J

Leyburn
Brown, J M
Dawson, A M
MacIntosh, K C
Palmer, J V
Riley, G A
Walker, G R
Wheatley, B
Wheatley, C J

Leyland
Garg, K K
Mainey, V G

Lichfield
Allan, A
Bird, R H
Blundell, S J
Booth, D J
Bramwell, H M
Bretland, C B
Brown, J R D
Buxton, K M
Causer, M S E
Chung-Faye, G A
Cole, N C S
Cooper, P H
De, D
De, P R
Evans, J
Gregory, P J
Hackett, G I
Hallifax, L J
Harrington, L T
Harris, A R
Henshaw, R W
Herbert, T J
Huisman, G B
James, J D
Jones, B
Khan, M T
Langdown, A J
Le Maistre, S
Lockwood, C M
Millar, E L
Mohanna, K
Morrison, H M
Muller, E J
Newson, D C
O'Leary, C L
Pilkington, C J
Plant, I M
Rockett, J W
Saleem, M
Saleem, T
Sidaway, S F
Skanderowicz, A G
Southall, G J
Tan, W M
Todd, E A
Varadarajan, R
Voice, E A
Webb, T R
Wells, W D E

Lifton
Sparrow, M A

Lightwater
Barnie-Adshead, R T
Lander, S J
McFarlane, S M
Whitfield, A J
Wood, E V
Wood, J V

Limavady
Callaghan, K A
Carson, R L
Day, T K
Devlin, B M
Devlin, D P
Donaldson, D P
Farquharson, I K
Finlay, W P
Fulton, R A
Harkin, D W
Heaney, G L
Henderson, M E
Hutchinson, D R
McCleery, W F
McIlmoyle, N A
McKenny, N V
McLaughlin, J A
McQuillan, B J
Magee, W H K
Mercer-Smith, N
Patton, M S
Ryan, S S
Spratt, J S
White, R J

Lincoln
Abbas, B K
Abbas, E M
Adelman, M I
Ahmed, I
Ajimoko, B A
Al-Ghonaimi, G S

Albuquerque, K V P
Anderson, B L
Andrew, D R
Andrews, R
Ansari, S M
Ash, C E
Asirvatham, R
Atkins, P F
Atkinson, R J
Attrup, M
Backhouse, C A
Bakar, S J
Baker, M
Bali, B
Bali, H S
Barczak, P J N
Barczak, S M
Barker, S G
Barlow, A P
Barton, S J
Batty, C J
Beden, R S
Beer, F D
Bell, S J
Bell, W A
Beswick, P N
Bibby, S R
Binks, S E
Birch, J-A
Birch, P M
Birch, P S J
Bowater, R L
Breeson, A J
Brightman, C A J
Brooks, D S
Broughton, L J
Brown, C A
Campbell, J R C
Carmichael, J R
Carty, M H
Carty, S M
Caruana, A
Catterall, E A
Chaudhary, B A
Chippington, S J
Clark, R
Clarke, D J
Clarke, H J M
Coffey, J F
Craven, J R
Curtis, M D
Delaki, E
Diffey, R F
Drummond, P M
Dyer, I R
Elwood, P Y
Fallon, A M
Fallon, M E
Fathers, E T
Fernley, C A
Firth, S H
Fisk, G G
Freeman, K
Fussey, C E
Ghaharian, K
Gibbs, J C
Glencross, J D
Golding, M J
Goldstein, H
Gough, G W
Graham, F M
Grant, D I
Griffiths, A L
Griffiths, G J
Groggins, R C
Grundy, K N
Gwilliam, N J
Habib, S
Haigh, K M C
Hanson, K B L
Harkness, D G
Hepburn, N C
Hillier, R J
Hinchcliffe, R J
Hindocha, L S
Hindocha, S
Hogg, S G
Hughes, G R
Hui, E H K
Hurst, A
Hutton, I M
Hyde, I D
Inder, G M
Jackson, E
Jenkins, K J
Jones, M E
Jones, M W
Kaar, J D W
Kelly, S J

Kennedy, D H
Khatib, S N
Kucyj, M D
Kutarski, A A
Lacy, I R
Lamb, M P
Lamerton, A J
Lansdall-Welfare, R W
Latham, M J
Layton, S A
Leach, S
Leeper, K C
Lennon, M M
Lewins, I G
Li Wan Po, G L T N
Locker, M
Logendran, M
Loosmore, S J
Lough, T A M
Mcdonald, B J
McGowan, M B
McLoughlin, J G
McManners, T
McRae, A R
Magee, M A
Mahalingam, M
Mallett, S A
Mallett, V A
Manandhar, L D
Mark, I R
Marris, S L
Matusiewicz, S P
Maughan, E H
Mehta, T B S
Mendel, L
Millns, C P
Morris, E W
Nouri-Dariani, E
O'Grady, T J
O'Kelly, R M
Oakford, A C
Ojo, O E
Owen, G O
Pack, M Y A-M
Parker, J L W
Parkin, J L
Parsons, P A
Paterson, I C
Paxton, A G
Pearson, B J
Perry, C A G
Petherbridge, S P
Phillips, D C
Pillay, J G
Pirzada, A F
Pirzada, B-U-I
Pirzada, O M
Pontin, A J
Porter, M C B
Powles, A B
Protheroe, M C
Protheroe, S A
Pyrgos, N
Pyrgos, V
Qureshi, A H
Qureshi, M Z
Ramon, A J
Rawden, A M
Reasbeck, P G
Reeves, D M
Reynolds, A D
Richardson, M
Robbins-Cherry, A M
Sadler, A G
Scammell, A M
Scarisbrick, D A
Scott, B B
Scott, D G
Scott, J A
Scott, R B
Sharpe, G A
Shewan, D M
Singh, J
Siriwardena, A N
Smith, D I A
Smith, R N E
Smith, R P R
Sood, V B
Sowerby, R
Stacey, S
Stonham, J
Stratton, P
Sturton, P R
Suresh-Babu, M V
Tekriwal, A K
Thava, V R
Thompson, A E
Thompson, M E
Thomson, J D R

Thornton, R J
Thorpe, G W
Thurkettle, A J
Tyler, C K G
Velaudapillai, C P
Vellacott, I D
Victoria, B A
Vijayasimhulu, G T
Waller, S L
Wallis, T D
Ware, C C
Watts, T
Webb, A M
Whitlow, W M
Wight, C O
Wilkinson, J M
Wilson, R J
Wilson, R P
Wood, D A
Wood, M J
Woulds, M
Youngs, E R
Zacharia, A Y

Lindfield
Knight, S A
Spensley, K M R
Taylor, E J

Lingfield
Allen, F J
Cliffe, P A H
Francis, I S
Gardner, J E
Noble, S I R
Northen, M E
Robertson, A J
Rose, W J M
Whittaker, D J
Wright, H M E

Linlithgow
Ahmed, M
Boyle, M F
Boyle, N J
Brockway, M S
Cawood, T J
Davie, J M
Fitzgerald, A J
McCallum, C A
McGhee, A R
MacKenzie, K W
McLay, C K A
McNab, J M
Mickel, D R
Millar, E D
Morley, A D
Orr, T A
Payne, E M C
Ramsay, S G
Ratcliffe, H D
Scothorne, A W
Sengupta, F R
Sengupta, T K
Smart, H E
Wardall, G J
Wood, S

Liphook
Barrett, J A
Berry, D J
Bore, J T
Cooper, A S
Hardwick, J C H
Hardwick, R J
Hayes, S A
Jackson, W F M
Landes, A H L
Neville-Towle, A
Ng, J M-Z
Rushton, B E A
Van Der Most, R N

Lisburn
Adair, A I
Anderson, H M
Anderson, N W
Archbold, J A L
Atkinson, A B
Baird, A E
Balnave, K
Baxter, A E
Beers, H T B
Best, J L
Bolleddula, K P
Boydell, L R
Brown, E F
Bryars, J H
Bryars, N E

Bunn, R T N
Cairns, I R
Calvert, G J
Campbell, N S
Carlisle, R P
Carragher, A M
Carson, M P
Chadwick, L
Chapman, N
Clenaghan, S D
Close, M E
Collins, J S A
Cormack, E C
Curry, P M
Daly, O E
Davis, A
Deacon, J M M
Devaney, N M
Doherty, T P
Elder, O P P M
Fleming, B
Gilpin, G N
Gilpin, J L
Gleadhill, I C L
Goodman, A M
Grahame-Smith, H N
Gray, M N
Hamill, D I W
Harrison, L W
Hegarty, J E
Henderson, H J
Henry, J S R L
Hewitt, R S
Hrabovsky, A
Humphrey, C A
Hutchinson, P D
Ireland, B J
Irwin, A G H
Jefferson, H A
Johnston, S R
Johnston, S E
Jose Thampi, C M
Knox, S G
Lawton, N R
Logan, G
Logan, K R
Loughlin, V
Love, A M
McAlister, J C
McAuley, R T
McBrien, J J S
McClean, H J M
McCloskey, E V
McCullough, G W
MacDonald, S F
McFarland, D
McKeown, A J P
McKeown, M E
Magee, N D
Malcomson, C I
Martin, R E
Mawhinney, I N
Milliken, C R
Moore, S
Mulvany, S A
Neagle, W B
Norris, A M
Nutt, A E C
O'Hanlon, J J
O'Neill, M J
O'Neill, S B
Palmer, R M
Patterson, M R
Patterson, S C A
Patterson, W R M
Porter, F J
Press, J R
Primrose, W J
Quigley, C N
Quigley, D G
Richardson, R P
Robb, K H
Rodgers, C J
Ruddell, M A
Russell, C M
Sands, S L
Shorten, W W J
Soye, J A
Spence, G M
Stanfield, S M
Stanley, J C
Stevenson, J H
Stewart, A J
Stewart, H J
Turner, L M
Wales, I F H
Walker, J M
Walker, T S J
Walmsley, A E

Watson, F L
Weir, J M P
White, A J
Wilson, J D
Wilson, R A
Wilson, R R
Yarr, J E
Zafar, A

Liskeard
Auckland, G D
Cater, E V
Coad, W M
Critchley, J
Eardley, R A A
Fagg, C G C
Hargadon, D J
Jefferies, S B
Kneebone, C A
McCartney, M R
Macfarlane, J L
Massey, M R
O'Leary, D R
Piper, A R
Ronchetti, M G
Smalley, A D
Sneyd, F M C
Toms, G R
Ussher, J H
Wood, P H N

Liss
Bevan, J R
Cairns, A W
Edwards, C S
Egelstaff, S J
Hennelly, M F
Mackie, A P
Morris, S J
O'Leary, C F
Panton, D J
Sedgwick, J R
Selby, L M P

Littleborough
Brazier, D T
Chew, R
Frost, S K
Gordon, D
McCarthy, J P
Sen, P K
Sidhu, S S
Thakor, S B
Walton, N

Littlehampton
Atkinson, T D
Bach, C D
Barrett, J W V
Beeching, Y G H
Brown, C K
Burcombe, D R
Bush, P K D
Byars, G K
Chandrarajan, C S
Coulthard, M
Critchfield, T O
Davies, T A
De Silva, V G
Deans, J S
Farrer-Brown, D
Gerard, S W
Greenwood, J
Handley, D J
Harland, M
Harrison, A J
Hart, G R
Hart, S R
Kimber, T J
Liddiard, A M
Liston, M P
Lovell, P
Lovell, R A
McLeod, D W
Miller, M R D
Morgan, W
Morton, J A B
Oliver, J
Palmer, S H
Plagaro Cowee, S
Roberts, R E
Stapleton, G A G
Storey, J L
Taylor-Roberts, M G W
Tilley, E J
Walsh, J M M
Walsh, S J M
Weinbren, H K
Williams, D G

Williams, S
Wiseman, M
Withers, D J
Wright, S J

Liverpool
Abang Mohammed, D K
Abbott, P M
Abdu, S A M
Abernethy, L J
Abraham, V V
Acharya, S P
Adab, N
Adisesh, L T
Agarwal, R P
Agius-Fernandez, A
Ah-Fat, F G
Ah-Weng, A
Ahmad, B
Ahmad, R
Ahmed, I
Ahmed, I
Ahmed, P R
Ainley, N J
Akhter, H
Al-Aloul, M
Al-Janabi, M A M
Alawattegama, A B
Albert, P S
Alexander-White, S
Alexander, J L
Ali, S I
Allmand, C A
Allsup, D J
Alty, M
Amadi, A
Ammir, T F E R
Ananthakrishna Rao, A
Anderson, R J
Angus, R M
Anthony, K
Appleton, E J
Appleton, R E
Armstrong, A M
Armstrong, J
Armstrong, K M
Armstrong, R
Arora, P
Arora, R M
Arunachalam, N
Arya, E C
Arya, R P
Ashok Kumar, J M
Askari, S H
Aspinall, D J
Atherton, L A
Attwood, M
Au, P W H
Avann, H J
Aziz, N F
Azurdia, R M
Backhouse, J E
Baderin, A A
Baig, M A A
Bainbridge, E A
Baines, P B
Baird, M A
Bajaj, R K
Bajaj, R K
Bajaj, V
Baker, A
Bakran, A
Ball, A R
Bamber, M J
Barclay, P M
Barlow, C
Barnes, R C
Barnes, S N
Barnett, R N
Barrett, P J
Barry, M G
Barry, P
Barton-Hanson, N G
Barton, S B
Bass, A
Basu, R
Bates, C M
Bateson, P M
Batra, R P
Batterbury, M
Bayley, T J
Beacon, S
Beattie, C H
Beattie, J K
Bebb, C E
Beckett, P
Beeching, N J
Bell, G M

Bell, H K
Bennett, A J
Bennett, S P
Bentley, J T
Beresford, M W
Bergel, E
Bevan, G P
Bhatnagar, P K
Bhushan, V
Bickerstaffe, W E
Billingham, I S
Billingsley, P
Birch, J C
Birchall, E W
Birchall, M A
Birley, H D L
Birt, C A
Bishop, S E
Blackburn, D J
Blackie, D M
Blackwell, L K
Blakeborough, J L
Bliss, J L
Bode, D
Boggild, M D
Bogle, I G
Bone, J M
Booker, P D
Boon, R L J
Bowden, A N
Bowers, S G
Bowhay, A R
Bowsher, D R
Box, D E O C
Boyars, L
Boyce, R P
Boyd, I M
Boyle, W J
Brabbins, C J
Brabin, B J
Bracey, A P
Bradley, M G
Bradley, P
Bradshaw, H D
Brady, J A
Breakell, A
Brearey, S P
Brennan, J A
Brewster, J A
Brice, D D
Briggs, M C
Briggs, P E
Brindley, A J
Brinksman, H J
Broadbent, D M
Brodbelt, A R
Bromilow, A
Brook, L A
Brookes, M R
Brown, A B
Brown, D J
Brown, J S
Brown, J W
Brown, R E
Brownson, P
Bruce, C E
Bruce, L B
Bruce, N G
Brunton, J N
Bryson, J R
Bucknall, R C
Bundred, P E
Bunn, J E G
Burdett-Smith, P
Burke, A G
Burke, U B
Burnham, P R
Burns, J
Burns, L S
Burns, M S
Burra, V S M
Burrow, C T
Buse, P
Butler, I G
Butterell, H C
Buxton, N
Byrne, E J
Byrne, I M
Byrne, M F
Byrne, W
Caldwell, J
Callaghan, J M
Callaghan, M
Callaghan, T A
Callow, D M
Calverley, P M A
Campbell, F
Campbell, J
Campbell, R S D

Cantarini, M V
Canter, A K
Capewell, S J
Carey, P B
Carlton, E A
Carroll, N S
Carroll, R
Carter, J M
Carter, N J
Cartwright, J L
Cashen, J A
Cashin, R J
Casson, I F
Caswell, M
Cavadino, A
Cave-Bigley, D J
Cavendish, M E
Cawley, J C
Chadwick, D W
Chakrabarti, B
Chan, A T Y
Chan, R K-Y
Chandna, A
Chandrashekhar, M N
Chapman, L J
Chapman, R
Charles, R G
Charters, P
Chaudhury, G B
Chaudhury, M
Chawla, N K
Cheesbrough, M F
Cheng, K Y M
Cheong, B Y C
Chester, M R
Chisnall, D P
Chitkara, D K
Choudhary, P
Chow, T W P
Chu Chi-Mai, P
Chung, K O
Chung, T T
Church, E N
Clague, J E
Clancy, M J
Claria-Olmedo, M J
Clark, A R
Clark, D I
Clark, R E
Clarke, K W
Clarke, M A
Clarke, R W M
Clarkson, J D
Clayton, G S
Clewes, A R
Coady, A M
Coady, D A
Coleman, J M
Coleman, N A
Coleman, N H
Collins, J D
Colville, L J
Connelly, D T
Connolly, C M
Connolly, J K
Connolly, S D
Connolly, S
Conroy, T A
Cook, G R
Cooke, R W I
Corbett, H J
Corcoran, G D
Cornford, P A
Corrighan, G A
Costigan, K J
Coulter, J B S
Couriel, J M
Craig, S V
Cranney, M
Crawford, N P S
Crawford, V H
Cribbin, L J
Crooke, J W
Crooks, D A
Cross, J S
Crowder, S W
Croy, M F
Cuckson, A C
Cullen, S P
Cunliffe, M
Cunliffe, N A
Cunningham, N
Curpen, N C
Currer, M
Cuthbert, J A
Dalton, J R
Dalzell, A M
Damato, B E
Dangerfield, P H

Dar, M A
Darabshaw, G S
Darcy, A E
Darcy, C M
Darcy, P F
Darcy, Y A
Darla, S R
Darroch, C J
Das, A
Das, B
Das, K S V
Daud, A S
Davenport, S A
Davidson, D C
Davidson, E G
Davidson, N C
Davies, E J
Davies, L
Davies, M W
Davies, P D O
Davis, A J M
Davis, A H
Davis, G K
Davis, J
Davis, R J N
De Matas, M
De Souza, J M A
Demnitz, U H
Dempster, I A
Denny, C M
Desai, S K
Desmond, A D
Desmond, M J
Devaney, J Y
Devine, A
Dewhurst, D J
Dhorajiwala, J M
Diab, M A
Diack, A M
Dickinson, P S
Didi, M A
Dihmis, W C
Dilworth, A
Disley, R
Dixon, J L
Dixon, M S
Djabatey, E A
Dobson, C M
Dobson, N U
Dodd, R J
Dominic, M A
Donnell, S C
Doran, C L
Doran, M
Dorgan, J C
Dove, W L
Dover, O
Dowrick, C F
Doyle, A M
Drakeley, A J
Drakeley, M J
Duckenfield, F M
Duerden, M G
Duffy, M F
Earis, J E
Early, K
Eccles, D R
Edirisinghe, D N
Edwards, W M
Edynbry, K D
Ejuoneatse, M O
El-Jassar, R P
El-Sayed, F E H
Eldridge, J A
Eldridge, P R
Ellis, A
Ellis, I H
Ellis, P M
Emmott, M N
Enevoldson, T P
Ensor, J M
Entwistle, A N
Epstein, A C R
Epstein, G A
Ervine, I M
Evans, E M
Evans, F M
Evans, J
Evans, K J
Evans, M D
Evans, R C
Evans, R A
Evans, T R
Exley, D
Fabri, B
Faint, D
Farquharson, R G
Farrington, G A
Fazlani, N A
Feld, M S
Fewins, H E
Finch, L D
Findlay, G
Finlay, I G
Finnegan, D M
Fish, B M
Fisher, M
Fiske, A P
Fitzgerald, B
Flanagan, D M
Flattery, P J
Fletcher, N A
Fook, L J
Forbes, A M W
Ford, C D
Forrest, J M
Forster, A
Forsyth, H G M
Forsyth, L J
Foster, C S
Foster, J E
Fox, M A
Foy, P M
Frais, M M
Franks, R E
Fraser, B J
Fraser, M D
Fraser, W D
Freeman, K B N
Frostick, S P
Fryer, A E
Gabbay, M B
Gadhvi, B
Gadhvi, D
Gaier, S
Gallagher, C
Gallard, S C A
Galloway, S W
Galtrey, A C
Gama, J G
Garden, A S
Gardner, K A
Garner, P A
Gauthier, J-B M
Gaynor, E S
Gaze, B I
George, A
Gerg, R K
Ghose, S L
Gibson, M G
Gibson, N E
Gibson, P J
Gibson, S P
Gilbertson, A A F
Gilbody, J
Gilchrist, I R
Giles, A A
Gill, G V
Gilles, H M J
Gilling-Smith, G L
Gilmore, I T
Gipson, M
Gladman, G
Goddard, M L
Godfrey, J J
Goenka, G
Goenka, N
Goffman, H L
Goldberg, I J L
Goldsmith, D H
Goldstone, J
Gomes Deraniyagala, G B
Gonsalves, J V
Gonzalez-Martin, J A
Goodman, B E
Goodwin, A M
Goonatilleke, M D A P
Gordon, I J
Gore, D M
Gosney, J R
Gould, D A
Goulden, M R
Gradden, C W
Graham, I F M
Graham, J C
Grant, L J
Gray, I C M
Green, G B
Greenfield, P J
Gregg, J E M
Gregson, J M
Grey, P
Griffiths, E M
Griffiths, G E
Griffiths, J M
Griffiths, P M
Griffiths, R D
Grossman, M L
Gunstone, A J
Gupta, P L
Gupta, R L
Gupta, S K
Guy, J M
Hackett, S J
Hadcroft, J
Haddock, A W
Hadji, F
Haines, J R
Haji Misbak, N
Halabi, S
Haley, C J
Halstead, G M
Hamad, S A K M
Hammad, A-E-K S A-E K
Hammond, C
Hanafi, Z
Hankin, T
Hanratty, B
Haqqani, M T
Haque, Q M
Hardie, J E
Harding, M J
Harding, N
Harding, S P
Harding, S
Hargreaves, F T
Harkins, K J
Harley, A
Harley, J S
Harper, N P A L
Harper, S J
Harrington, Y M
Harris, L
Harris, P C
Harris, P L
Harrison, C B
Hart, C A
Hart, G
Hart, I K
Hartley, M N
Harvey, G
Harvey, V A
Hattaway, B M
Hawkes, D J
Hayes, C F
Hayes, S C
Hayward, P B
Head-Rapson, A G
Heaf, D P
Heatley, M K
Hedge, R N
Hehar, S S
Helliwell, T R
Hennessy, E P
Herod, J J O
Herrington, C S
Hershman, M J
Hewitt, J
Hibbert, W K
Higgie, M R
Hill, J W
Hind, C R K
Hiscott, P S
Ho, V W C
Hobbs, W J C
Hodder, R J
Hoddes, J A
Hodgson, C A A
Holcombe, C
Holemans, J A
Holland, M J
Holland, M A J
Hollingsworth, J D K
Holme, V E
Honey, G E
Hornung, R S
Horton, W A
Hossain, M M
Houghton, R P
Howard, C V
Howard, E C
Howard, H L
Howitt, R J
Hoyen-Chung, E G
Hubbard, A J
Hubbert, C M
Hughes, B
Hughes, D A
Hughes, D M
Hughes, D W
Hughes, J H
Hughes, M I
Hughes, M L
Hughes, P J
Humphrey, P R D
Hung, C C
Hunn, M K
Hunt, A L S
Hunukumbure, S B
Hussain, J A
Hussain, S M
Hussain, S
Hussey, J A
Hussey, R M
Ibreck, R F
Idama, T O
Innes, C F
Iqbal, D S
Iqbal, J
Jabeen, Z
Jack, C I A
Jackson, C T
Jackson, S R
Jacobs, V J L
Jaffey, L H
Jagoe, R T
James, D
Jameson, P P M
Jane, M J
Jardine, J V
Jayaram, N
Jayson, S J
Jeanrenaud, P
Jeffreys, R V
Jenkinson, M D
Jepsen, F
Jesudason, G R R
Johnson, C P
Johnson, P P
Johnson, S R
Johnston, B M
Johnstone, M J
Johnstone, S A
Jones, A G H
Jones, A G
Jones, A S
Jones, A S
Jones, A F
Jones, C A
Jones, C A
Jones, N E B
Jones, P L
Jones, R G
Jones, T D
Jones, W A
Joseph, J V
Journeaux, S F
Judd, B A
Judge, B P
Judge, J
Jukka, C M
Kalinsky, S
Kamal, A
Kan, S M
Kapoor, V
Kazi, H A
Kehoe, A
Kelly, J E
Kemp, G J
Kent, M J
Kenyon, R M
Kerr, A R
Kerrigan, D D
Kewn, D
Keyser, A T
Khan, J A
Khan, S
Khera, G
Kidd, B C
Kidd, G M
King, R I
Kingsland, C R
Kingston, R E
Kinloch, T S
Kinn, D R
Kinnersley, A
Kirkman, J L
Kirkpatrick, U J
Kishan Rao, V
Kneen, R
Knowles, I
Koh, C S V
Kothari, H P
Krasner, N
Krasner, N I
Kumar, A
Kumar, S
Kumar, S A
Kumar, V
Kuruvilla, G
Kwok Chai Sum, A
Kyaw Lwin, Dr
Kyle, G M
Lahiri, M
Lakhani, D N
Lalloo, D G
Lamb, G H R
Lamont, G L
Lamplugh, G
Larner, A J
Lawrence, A
Leach, J P
Lecky, B R F
Ledson, J F
Ledson, M J
Lee, Y C
Lemmens, F M
Lennon, K J
Leonard, D
Lesser, T H J
Levy, M L
Levy, M
Lewis-Jones, D I
Lewis-Jones, H G
Lewis, D K
Leyland, M C
Li, D
Lim, K C
Lim, K H
Lister, R K
Littlewood, A H M
Littlewood, C M
Lloyd-Jones, G H
Lloyd-Jones, W
Lloyd, D A
Lloyd, E A
Lo, K W
Lock, J D T
Lombard, M G
Losty, P D
Lowe, P L
Lu, J C Y
Lubman, D I
Luck, S E
Lwin, M K-K
Lye, M D W
Lynch, M C
Lynn, K L
Lythgoe, M W
Maassarani, F
Maassarani, H A
McBrien, A
McCahy, H J
McCormick, M S
McCoy, D G L
McCrossan, P J
McCulloch, P G
McCutcheon, M R
McDowell, D K
McDowell, H P M
McElroy, C A
McFadyen, I R
MacFarlane, I A
McFarlane, X A
McGettigan, C P
McGibbon, C
McGuiness, S P
Machin, D G
Machin, P L
McKay, J A
McKean, C D
Mackean, J M
Mackean, W M
McKendrick, C S
McKendrick, H M
Mackenzie, A J
McKernan, C
Mackie, C R
McLoughlin, G A
McLoughlin, K C
McLoughlin, P L
McLoughlin, R
McMenamin, M
McNamara, P S
McNulty, S J
McQuail, P A
McQuillan, S
Macrae, F M H
McVicar, J T
McVicker, J T
Madanayake, S K
Magee, C J
Magennis, J P M
Maher, B
Maher, S J
Mair, F S
Maitra, S
Majeed, F A A
Malik, D R
Malik, M I A
Mallaiah, S
Mallucci, C L
Malpas, C E
Mangan, S A
Manley, A F
Manley, S M
Manning, E M C
Marsh, D M
Marsh, I B
Marshall, A G
Marson, A G
Martin, L
Martin, R M
Martlew, V J
Masip Oliveras, T
Maskrey, N
Massey, G S
Massey, R R
Mathie, A G
Matthews, T P
Mattison, H
Maudsley, G
Mawson, S L
May, P L
Mediratta, N K
Mehta, M N
Mehta, R K
Meldrum, D
Mendick, M
Menton, J P
Mercer, N P
Merriman, M G
Messing, Z R
Metcalfe, J W
Metcalfe, P
Metcalfe, R M
Middleman, M J
Milford, C D
Miller, A R O
Miller, D H T
Miller, D H
Mills, K G
Mimnagh, A P
Mimnagh, C J
Minn Lwin, Dr
Mintz, B J
Mohanan, K S
Mohteshamzadeh, M
Molokhia, M
Moloney, D T
Moloney, D M
Monk, C J E
Monk, D A
Monk, J P
Montgomery, S C
Mooney, P J
Moore, A P
Moore, E W
Moore, K S
Moores, C
Moots, R J
Moran, B P
Moreton, P
Morgan, S J S
Morris, A I
Morris, J
Morrison, W L
Morriss, R K
Morton, S H
Moss, A C
Mostafa, S M
Mugglestone, S J
Mullen, P F
Mullett, H S
Mullett, S S
Mullin, M S
Mullin, T
Mullins, S D
Muogbo, J C
Murphy, M
Murphy, N D
Murphy, P E
Muruganathan, N
Murugananthan, N
Muthu, S
Muthu, V S
Myerscough, E G
Mytton, J A
Nagpal, I S
Nahser, H-C
Naik, J N
Nash, J R G
Nash, T P
Navaneetharajah, N
Nayagam, S
Nayak, G P
Naylor, K P
Neal, T J
Needham, A D
Neill, M P
Neilson, J P
Nelki, J S

Neoptolemos, J P
Newsham, J A
Newson, M P
Newstone, J
Nicolaides, P
Nielsen, H J
Nirula, R P
Niven, S D
Nolan, J
Noland, D J
Nurmikko, T J
Nye, F J
O'Brien, C G
O'Brien, D J
O'Brien, L S
O'Brien, M J
O'Brien, T G
O'Connell, N M
O'Connor, B D
O'Donnell, J F
O'Donnell, J D
O'Donnell, M J
O'Dowd, G M
O'Grady, E A
O'Hanlon, C
O'Hara, D P
O'Leary, M A
O'Neill, J M
O'Neill, M B E
O'Riordan, J E G
O'Shea, P J
O'Toole, P A
Ochefu, O A
Oelbaum, S
Ogden-Forde, F E
Ogden, D J
Ogilvie, C M
Okhah, M
Ooi, J L
Ooi, K H
Oppenheim, A I
Orlans, D A
Orlans, M
Orme, N J
Osman, H M
Over, K E
Owen, A W M C
Owens, A S
Owens, K E
Owens, P M
Owens, S
Page, R D
Pai, V P
Palejwala, A A
Pande, S K
Pande, S K
Pang, L
Parfrey, H
Parker, C J R
Parkins, K J
Parry, D M
Parry, G R
Parslew, R A G
Parsons, K F
Patel, N M
Patsalides, C T
Patterson, R C
Pearson, M G
Peart, I
Peddi, N C
Peddi, V
Pellegrini, A V
Pembleton, A
Pendleton, N
Pennie, B H
Pereira, A C
Perera, H D P W
Perrin, P F
Perry, R A
Pettitt, A R
Pfeiffer, U
Phillips, B M
Phillips, B J
Phillips, G
Phillips, M F
Philpott, R M
Photiou, S
Pigott, T J D
Pirmohamed, M
Platt, M R
Platt, M J
Playfor, S D
Pollack, J
Pollard, C E
Poole, R G
Poonawala, S S
Poston, G J
Powell, P M
Pozzi, M
Pramanik, K
Prasad Rao, G
Prasad, N
Prasad, T
Preston, E M
Price, G
Prince, G H
Pritchard, D M
Proctor, J L
Proudlove, D A
Pryce, A C W
Pullan, D M
Purewal, T S
Pyatt, J R
Quigley, C
Quinn, M C
Radcliffe, S N
Radha Krishna, L K
Radhakrishna, G
Rai Chowdhury, S L
Rajlawot, G P
Rakowski, J H
Ramadan, M F
Ramamoorthy, S N
Ramsdale, D R
Rao, M S
Rao, P B
Rashid, A
Rastogi, S
Rastogi, T K
Ratcliffe, J M
Ratti, N
Ravey, M
Razvi, S A H
Reade, D W
Reddington, J A
Reddy, A V G
Redmond, P V S
Redmond, S J
Redmond, T K
Rees, B
Rees, M
Reeve, J L
Regan, M M C
Reid, M M
Reilly, P C
Renton, M C B L
Rhodes, J M
Rhodes, L E
Riaz, A
Richards, D E W M
Richardson, D
Richardson, P
Richardson, W R
Richmond, D H
Rickwood, A M K
Rigby, P
Rintala, R J
Robb, C A
Roberts, D
Roberts, J W
Roberts, P J
Roberts, R A
Robertson, J L
Robinson, C J S
Robinson, M L
Robson, W J
Rodgers, I D
Rodrigues, E A
Rodrigues, J
Roe, D A
Roebuck, H
Rogers, J H
Rogers, M G H
Roland, N J
Romer, H C
Rooney, P S
Rosanwo, E O
Rose, A P
Rose, S A
Rosen, M P
Rosenbloom, L
Rosenthal, J M
Rostron, P K M
Rothburn, M M
Roulston, L
Rowlands, J K
Rowlands, M H
Rowlands, P C
Royle, M J
Rushambuza, F G
Rushambuza, R P M
Russell, G N
Ryan, D P M
Ryan, M F
Rylands, A J
Saba, G Y S
Sadik, W B
Sadiq, P M
Saha, A K
Saleem, A
Sanderson, C J
Santer, G J
Sapre, S
Sarginson, R E
Sarker, S
Satchithananthan, N
Saunders, P A
Scarland, M G
Scawn, N D A
Schlecht, B J M
Schmidt, B E
Scott-Samuel, A J R
Scott, I G
Scurr, J R H
Sekhar, K T
Selby, A M
Sells, R A
Semple, A B
Semple, M G
Sen, J
Sendegeya, C
Sephton, V C
Setty, S
Shah, D K
Shamas-Ud-Din, S
Shantha, A L
Sharma, A K
Sharma, A
Sharma, A K
Sharma, P
Sharma, S P
Sharpe, G R
Shatwell, M A
Shaw, C R
Shaw, M D M
Shaw, S D
Sheard, J D H
Shearer, E S
Shears, P
Sheeran, E
Sheeran, P B M
Shenkin, A
Shepherd, A J N
Shiffman, I F
Shiffman, K
Shoker, B S
Short, A D
Short, L J
Siddiqi, M A
Siegler, J
Siller, C S
Sillitoe, A T
Silver, N C
Simpson, G T
Singer, R
Singh, B D N
Singh, H K
Singh, N P
Singh, S
Singh, S
Singh, S B P
Singh, S
Singh, S N
Singh, Y
Singhal, A K
Sinha, B K
Sinha, B K
Sinha, S
Sivabalan, P
Sivori, R E
Skaife, P G P
Smart, H L
Smerdon, A W
Smith, D F
Smith, D J
Smith, M L
Smith, M R
Smith, M J
Smith, M R
Smith, P J
Smith, P A
Smith, P A
Smith, T K
Smyth, R L
Snowdon, R L
Snyder, M
Sobowale, A O
Solomon, T
Soorae, A S
Soulsby, T P
Spofforth, P
Squire, S B
Stables, R H
Stamboultzis, N
Stanaway, S E
Steiger, C A
Steiger, M J
Stephens, E A
Stevenson, H L
Stevenson, I M
Steyn, R S
Stone, A
Strain, W D
Struik, S S
Suares, M
Subhedar, N V
Sudhakar, K
Sulaiman, H M
Sumner, D J
Suri, A K
Sutton, R
Sweeney, M E
Sweeney, M T
Swift, A C
Taggart, T F O
Tagore, N K
Tamin, J S F
Tatam, M E
Taylor-Robinson, D C
Taylor-Robinson, J W
Taylor, A J N
Taylor, A S
Taylor, W
Taylor, W N
Tewari, V K
Thakur, S C
Theophanous, M
Thom, C M H
Thomas, A G
Thomas, B
Thomas, D A
Thomas, D G
Thomas, E E
Thomas, H O
Thomas, J M
Thomas, K J
Thomas, L S
Thomas, P J
Thomas, S D
Thompson, R N
Thong, K F
Thoo, C K
Thornington, R E
Thurston, H A
Tobias, M
Todd, D M
Toh, C H
Toke, E
Topping, J
Townley, S A
Tree, A M
Tseung, K W
Tucker, A K
Tulley, P N
Tunn, E J
Turnbull, L S
Turner, J J
Turnock, R R
Tweedie, I E
Upsdell, M A
Usher, J L
Van Heyningen, C
Van Saene, H K F
Van Velzen, D
Varma, T R K
Vella, I
Verbov, J L
Verma, S K
Verstreken, P
Vickers, M J
Vitty, F P
Volk, H M J
Vora, J P
Voruganti, U R
Waghorn, A J
Wake, P N
Walker, B A
Walker, C R
Walker, P P
Walker, P E
Walkinshaw, S A
Wallbank, I W
Walley, T J
Wallis, H L
Walmsley, P J
Walsh, C
Walsh, H P J
Walters, C M
Warburton, C J
Ward, J B
Warenius, H M
Warnke, P
Watkin, E J
Watkin, F M
Watson, A J M
Wauchob, T D
Webb, A M C
Webster, D
Webster, M
Webster, S W
Weindling, A M
Welby, S B
Welch, G P
Welch, J A
Wells, J C D
Welsh, C D
Wenstone, R
Weston, P J
Whelan, E
Whelan, M J
Whitby, P J
White, F E
White, N P
White, R P
Whitenburgh, M J
Whiteside, C L
Whitley, S
Whittaker, J A
Wieshman, U C
Wilder-Smith, O H G
Wilding, J P H
Wildsmith, P H
Wilkinson, E A J
Wilkinson, M
Williams, C E
Williams, C
Williams, E
Williams, E M I
Williams, I R
Williams, S M
Williamson, B H
Wilson, K C M
Wilson, N J E
Wilson, N L
Winstanley, P A
Winter, J A C
Winterburn, R
Wishart, P K
Wolf, A
Wolfman, L C
Wolfman, S S
Wong Ching Hwai, S Y
Wong, A
Wong, K C
Wong, S C P
Wood, R N A
Woodall, P L
Woodcock, B E
Woods, I M M
Woods, T O
Woodward, J
Woodward, R B
Woolfenden, K A
Woollard, S J
Wright, D J
Wright, E J
Wright, F J
Wright, N B
Wycherley, C R
Yadav, A
Yadav, J K
Young, C A
Yoxall, C W
Zacharias, P L
Zsigmond, A

Liversedge
El Sarraff, M R
Ghafoor, N H
Khan, H
Sarathy, P
Sears, A L
Steward, M A
Thompson, J A

Livingston
Adwani, H P
Anderson, D N
Anderson, W D
Aspin, J D
Backett, S A
Bailey, P S
Bartholomew, R S
Bateman, M J A
Beveridge, C J
Brown, T M
Buchan, I C
Butterworth, M S
Campbell, A M
Chambers, S E
Cooper, T K
Davie, R M
Dewart, P J
Farquhar, D L
Ferguson, J B
Finnie, R M
Forbes, J W
Fothergill, N J
Freeland, P
Gibson, N M
Gourlay, E J
Gribben, S C
Grigor, M J
Handley, J E
Hay, K W
Henderson, D J
Hendry, J D
Hennessey, C M
Hogg, F J
Jacob, A J
Jones, R D G
Koay, P Y P
Lonsdale, M
McCullough, D A
Macdonald, R J M
McEwan, A J
McGowan, N J
McKinnon, M G M
McLauchlan, M A
Macleod, A J
McLeod, I C
Macleod, M F
Martin, E G
Mauchline, R M
Mazza, D J
Mitchell, R
Montgomery, B W
Morrison, L M M
Neal, S M
O'Donnell, A M
Patel, M S A
Pringle, J R
Ramesar, K C R B
Ritchie, J M
Robertson, D A
Robertson, P
Robinson, H J
Roscrow, S E
Russell-Smith, E D
Sim, D W
Skinner, B C
Skinner, L P
Sloan, R D
Smart, L M
Steel, R M
Tripathi, B P
Tybulewicz, S M
Walker, J D
Weir, A M
Wild, K A
Williamson, E C M

Llandeilo
Davies, C M
Davies, T R
George, R I
Leopold, J G
Llewelyn, A D
Nakielny, E A
Thomas, C M J
Thomas, D P

Llandovery
Boulter, M J M
Briscoe, C R
Rees, P J
Richards, J L
Salt, R W

Llandrindod Wells
Arkinstall, G M
Brown, W M R
Buchan, J
Davies, E
Gillett, A S
Hilsden, E I
Jones, S A
Matson, J S
Tattersall, T
Warrick, M J S
Warrick, S M

Llandudno
Akasheh, K
Brigg, W M M
Carri, M P
Davey, R J
Davies, P R C
Emmett, P A
Gilmore, R
Green, J J
Gubay, A
Hampton, E
Hana, A B

Hay, D J
Hindle, J V
Hotston, S J
King, G D
Mitchelson, P A
O'Beirn, D P
Price, V J
Roberts-Puw, E H
Shaw, R R
Simpson, B
Thomas, E L
Thomas, S K
Vaterlaws, A L
Williams, S

Llandysul
Adair, A A
Cule, J H
Evans, M S
Gard, R J
Gordon, K J
Jay, A L
Jefferson, F A
Jeremiah, D S
Jones, D T
Llewelyn, N
MacBean, S M
Reiter, M E K
Roberts, D A T
Taylor, N C
Thomas, I M
Thomas, M S

Llanelli
Ahmed, K
Anthony, E L
Aston, A R
Bajoria, S K
Caiach, S M
Cassidy, L J
Cnudde, P H
Daniel, M A M
Davies, A F-D
Davies, B R
Davies, D M
Davies, H E
Davies, R M
Davies, W F T
Devichand, P
Devonald, R C
Dew, M J
Drummond, R N
Edmunds, E C H
Edmunds, E
Ellis-Williams, G W
Evans, D W
Evans, H J R
Evans, J V
Evans, T N
Evans, T N W
Gravell, D L
Gravell, E W
Green, M T
Griffiths, A W
Gupta, B
Gwynne, B M
Harries, A I
Hill, A A
Holmes, S C
Holt, S D H
Howarth, A J
Huws, R G
Jaidev, V C
John, M H
Jones, G L
Jones, G R
Jones, K E
Jones, M E
Lefebvre, L M
Lewis, R W
Majer, R V
Morris, G C
Nigam, A K
Pease, N J F
Prakash, K G
Prigmore, G T
Rees, J E
Richards, A P
Satarasinghe, K A S
Scourfield, A E
Scourfield, E J
Sharaiha, Y M
Slader, C J
Slader, M I
Thomas, D R
Thomas, D B
Thomas, G
Thomas, J S I
Thomas, J M

Thomas, R W
Thomas, W C T
Treharne, C J
Treharne, E
Vaughan, M O
Vaziri, M
Waghorne, N J
Walters, P M
Williams, A J
Williams, D D W
Williams, I M
Williams, T D M

Llanerchymedd
Masters, R R
Parry-Jones, C E

Llanfairfechan
Cambridge, I J
Carolan, C M
Ellis, A
Flannery, M D
Hughes, C M
Hughes, S
Luithle, E R E
Scott, J M
Summers, D W B
Walker, R M
Williams, N H

Llanfairpwllgwyngyll
Davidsson, G K
Gammon, K
Glyn-Jones, S
Griffiths, A G R
Jamison, M H
Jones, H R
Jones, J
Leyland, M F
McEwan, L M
Pleming, A W
Roberts, G
Williams, J G

Llanfyllin
Evans, H C
Griffiths, K R
Hancorn, M K
Jones, L B P
Jones, P N G
Weston, A H S

Llangefni
Edwards, J I
Griffiths, P H
Hughes, B A
Jones, H I
Morgan, G W
Morgan, J P
Williams, J P

Llangollen
Davies, D R W
Davies, J R A
Downes, A J
Edwards, A E
Evans, A D
Gemmell, L W
Green, J L
Jones, H L
Kalra, L A
Malster, M G
Tanner, R M
Williams, E J
Williams, R E W
Williams, R B

Llanidloes
Jones, N H
Leslie, S M
Scrase, A M
Scrase, E T

Llanon
Staite, P E

Llanrwst
Hughes, A J
Johl, S
Kenrick, R M
Ramsay, R B

Llantrisant
Abdullah, A N
Al-Aslan, S M A K
Alcolado, R
Arnold, J M
Davies, C J
Davies, S G

Griffiths, R H
Hodges, I G C
Lewis, M H
Pugh, D H O
Rhys, R
Rivron, R P
Sandhu, G S
Sewell, J M A
Strang, J I G
Sullivan, S C
Wagle, A U
Woodward, A

Llantwit Major
Ashworth, C S L
Bevington, W R P
Crimmins, G J
Foreman, A J
Harris, J A
Leuchars, K L
Morris, J M
Richards, B F
Summors, R E
White, J P

Llanybydder
Davies, A W
Rowlands, S G

Llanymynech
Poole, G G
Thwaite, D S

Loanhead
Dickson, T C
Henderson, I J M
Herbert, G N
Leslie, A
Moonsawmy, S A
Weir, D J G
West, C P

Lochboisdale
Powell, A P

Lochgelly
Cattanach, S J
Farrell, A A
Garvey, N
Gordon, H J
Goyal, A K
Khan, F
Khan, M A R
Khan, S
Kidd, C A
Lindsay, S M
MacFarlane, J R
McKean, J R
Mistry, C U
Patel, R V
Rahman, M A

Lochgilphead
Brailsford, M M
Corrigan, F M
Fergusson, G M
Guy, P M M
Mackay, A V P
MacKenzie, S D
Mackie, C S
Millar, B-A M
Phillips, J K
Provan, A A
Ranger, A F
Simpson, M J
Thompson, P
Ward, A D
Wells, A D

Lochmaddy
Keiller, P W
Pilkington, B S

Lochwinnoch
Blair, M M R
Dalrymple, J G
McCormick, C V
McCusker, C D
McInnes, J C
Waterston, P F

Lockerbie
Costigan, P S
Frost, D
Hill, J J
Maclean, N
Marr, A W
Norris, J F B
Norris, S C

Ogden, A C
Ogden, E C
Porteous, G A
Powell, H K R
Rigg, N D
Smith, J D
Taylor, D J

Londonderry
Abbott, F A A
Aquino, P J
Ashenhurst, E M
Baird, D S C
Bankhead, K B
Barr, S H
Beirne, J A F
Black, E T J
Boyd, L E
Boyle, N B J
Brennan, N R
Brennan, R J
Brennan, V J
Brown, C M
Brown, D A
Brown, R M
Burns, J A
Byrne, G A
Cadden, I S H
Canavan, H R
Casey, L J
Cavanagh, V J
Chauhan, N D
Chestnutt, W N
Connolly, D F
Cosgrove, J P
Cosgrove, J J
Cosgrove, K J
Cosgrove, P A
Craig, T J M
Dace, J S
Dale, V A
Daly, C A P
De Burca, D I
Deane, D M
Devlin, E G
Devlin, E M
Devlin, M M A
Devlin, P B
Devlin, S B
Dickey, W
Doherty, A M
Doherty, J A
Doherty, P J
Dolan, D M
Downey, N J
Duffy, N K
Dunn, H M
Durand, M D M
Elder, F R
Eyre, D G
Fallon, P T
Fallows, S A S
Flanagan, D J
Foster, S E
Frazer, A F
Gamble, W R
Gardiner, P V
Garvey, A J
Gerber, D G
Gilliland, R
Glynn, G M A
Gordon, I R O
Grace, D
Grant, D J
Gunn, M B
Hamilton, C A
Harper, E J M
Hassett, P D A
Hasson, F P
Healy, M J
Hegarty, J D
Hetherington, C H R
Hill, J M M
Howe, A R
Hughes, A-M T
Hughes, D F
Hughes, S J
Imrie, C B
Jadhav, S T
Johnston, F P D
Johnston, H C
Johnston, J J E
Kane, E P
Kasturi, S
Keegan, D A J
Keenan, G F
Khow, G M
Knowles, E T
Leeson, W P J

Linton, A F
Lynas, A G A
McCallion, N E
McCarron, M O
McCartie, B S J
McCauley, D A
McCauley, W J
McClay, M J
McClean, J R
McCloskey, M E
McCloskey, M A
McCord, F B
McDermott, S M
McEvoy, J D
McEvoy, P J
McGilloway, M M E
McGinley, I G
McIlwaine, J E J
McIvor, P C A
McKelvey, M A
McKinney, L A
McLean, R D W
MacMahon, B M
McNeill, A J
McNicholl, F P
Madden, M G
Magee, S E E
Magnier, M R
Manning, R W
Mariswamy, S B
Martin, A G M
Martin, D H
Mayes, R C D
Millar, J K
Millen, S A
Moles, K W
Molloy, P G
Moohan, J M
Morgan, M M
Morrison, A M
Morrison, C M
Morrow, B C
Mulholland, D A
Mullan, C H
Mullan, J R
Munro, C K
Murphy, C A
Murphy, S M
Murray, A P V
Nairn, R M
Nelson, D E
O'Connor, F A
O'Donnell, J J J
O'Flaherty, K A
O'Hara, A G
O'Kane, C M
O'Kane, D P
O'Kane, J J
O'Kane, M J
O'Kelly, J K
O'Neill, R J
O'Sullivan, M J B
Palin, I S
Panesar, K J S
Parker, M J R
Patterson, D R
Patton, N
Phellas, P
Porter, J M
Purvis, J A
Quinn, K M
Quinn, R J M
Rea, S M
Reidy, J
Reilly, M P
Robertson, I D
Samson, J D
Sharma, N K
Siddiqui, A M
Simpson, J T
Singh, I P
Sinton, J E
Smith, B T M
Smithson, R D
Smyth, H J
Spence, J E
Stafford, M A
Steele, J A
Stewart, D P E
Stewart, G R
Stone, J C
Taylor, M A
Tedders, B
Thompson, R L E
Toland, M
Varadarajan, C R
Vazir, M H
Walpole, G A M
Ward, M J

Warne, S A
Warnock, A M M
Watt, L M J
White, C V
Wilson, C J
Wray, A R

Longfield
Armstrong, C B
Carter, P M
Davies, P R
Davies, Y M
Dott, A G
Faddoul, E
Fraser, M R
Hatrick, J A
Herring, J
Hosny, A A
Kamdar, B A
Luffingham, J N
Moftah, F S
Patel, H T
Patel, S T
Patel, T D
Ramanathan, N
Ramanathan, S
Rebel, D J
Selwood, D P
Singh, K H P E
Smith, P K E
Thompson, F C
Williams, A A

Longniddry
Knight, R S G
Lowe, C H
Lowe, C S
Martin, D L
Wood, P

Looe
Brewer, P J J
Davies, G N
Gates, J C
Horner, J C
Palmer, M J
Roy, I G
Staff, A

Lossiemouth
Barclay, A
Barr, E J
Bishop, L D
Featherstone, C J F
Pleasant, E A
Sabiston, N
White, I H
Williams, D

Lostwithiel
Bowen, H P
Bowen, I R
Denn, P G
Harrison, J M
Howe, R W
Mackinnon, F M

Loughborough
Ahmad, H K
Almassi, M
Aust, W J
Badiani, K N
Bagley, A M
Bal, A S
Barlow, A R
Barlow, C R
Bassi, S K
Benton, J J N
Bhatia, G S
Borsada, S C
Brewis, C
Brocklesby, K J
Campbell, S S
Cannon, P M
Cawdron, B A
Chander, R
Clode-Baker, E G
Cornish, D C
Cox, H
Croker, L R
Cullis, S A
Davis, R J
Dean, A D P
Dipple, H C
Drakes, A H
Duffy, S A
Euden, M
Evans, K J
Eveson, S E

Ferguson, M R
Fossey, S M
Foulds, R A
French, A J
Frisby, J J
Frost, M F
Furber, P J
Furlonger, A J
Gerrie, S E
Ghaly, M S
Gill, H K
Gordon, P D
Graham-Brown, M M R A
Gray, J M
Green, R C
Hale, M C
Hall, E A
Hall, T D
Hall, W B
Hallam, C F
Hanlon, G P
Harding, M L
Harding, R J P
Harries, M J
Harries, S S C
Harrison, M J
Haynes, D I
Hazlewood, J H
Heap, B M
Holt, P R
Hoyle, J T E
Hughes, H J
Hughes, M W
Hunter, M C C
Jasoria, S
Jassal, S S
Jewson, D G
Jivan, S
John, A P K
Jolleys, J C W
Jones, B E
Jones, R T
Kaitiff, N C
Kelly, A T
Khalid, L J
Kingsley, P J
Lakhani, M K
Larsen, J E
Leeson, C P M
McDonald, C I
McHale, J F
MacSween, P J
Mak, F
Matthews, K T A
Matts, S J F
Matts, S G F
Mayer, J H
Middleton, J F
Moir, A A
Moore, N A
Newton, A F
Nicholson, K G
O'Toole, S J
Oliver, K J
Parker, S C
Parrott, C E
Patel, B
Patel, R S
Patel, V
Phillipson, E M
Price, C
Price, R J A
Quinn, A G
Redferne, J H
Riley, V C
Ryan, D P
Saund, N S
Schofield, I R
Shortt, S J
Simpson, A J G
Simpson, N H R
Sivaguru, A
Southwell, K F
Stafford, P J
Stead, B E
Tandon, S
Tatham, P F
Ugoji, U U
Unitt, H M
Vadher, S
Vaghela, N N
Veitch, Y
Volpe, N
Wallis, D E
Ward, B J
Ward, J W
West, K J
Wheeley, M S G
Whymark, A D
Wilde, S M
Wray, H A
Wynne-Williams, H V

Loughton
Bagguley, K A
Banerjee, B
Barnes, S
Batchelor, C M
Baxter, D
Bhagrath, R A S
Chew, R E
De Silva, W M C
Dighton, D H
Dubinski, J
Frootko, N J
Hasan, A
Ide, J E
Kalkat, G S
Kanamia, T
Kari, J A A
Khan, A A
Khan, H U
Lukey, D C
Matthews, S A
Mirchandani, M V
Mitchell, F L
Nath, N K
O'Neill, A P
Pang, H T
Pradhan, A M
Prajapati, D
Ramsey, M C
Ribbens, S C
Runagall, S E
Smith, C J M
Stone, A G H
Tomlins, F G

Louth
Ahmed, M
Birch, J J
Drake, H M
Dwyer, M J A
Gallagher, A J
Grant, C E P
Hanslip, J M
Humberstone, I P
Jain, S K
Jones, D A
Khan, M M R
Khan, M U
King, N H T
Knight, P T
Maity, S
Mowat, A J
Parker, G S
Parkes, N R Q
Pike, L C
Qadir, M
Ramkhalawon, M
Ravindra Nath, A
Reynolds, D J
Ross, G
Staunton, D
Stovin, P H
Taylor, G R
Topham, S P
Vaquas, S M
Westwood, C A
Young, J R

Lowestoft
Ababio, S N
Atkins, J L
Aylward, M J
Berry, R V
Bigg, A R
Bond, R I
Bouch, K
Brabbins, L J
Butt, M S
Calver, R
Cox, S M
Dakin, R
Drane, N R
Duncan, R W
Ehmann, J F
Gunn, K
Halder, D
Hamelijnck, J A
Hartley, E M
Henderson, D R
James, R G
Johnston, D
Kathuria, R L
Kerry, F M R
Krishnaswamy, S
Krishnaswamy, U
Lall, R S
Lawrence, P W
Lockyer, G J S
McLean, C R
Mann, R A M
Mawer, B J M
Mohan, G
Moon, E A C
Moorthie, G A
Morrison, J M
Nadarajan, P
Nettleton, M A
O'Driscoll, F A
O'Regan, M H
Periselneris, S R
Prince, S R
Sanger, J L
Seehra, M S
Truman, L A
Turner, D J
Van Den Broek, A J C M
Van Pelt, H J F
Walker, A G

Ludlow
Attlee, W O
Beswick, T S L
Cook, G P
Cullen, J D
Davies, R D
Farnell, B J
Farnell, N J
Foster, S
Irani, D A
Klein, V H
Lane, J W J
Perks, A
Smith, S D
Snape, S R
Yarham, D D

Luton
Abuhadra, K S
Acellam-Odong, C C
Adams, M E
Adler, B R
Adler, F P
Ahad, M F R
Ahmad, A
Ahmad, Q
Ahmad, Z
Ahmed, N
Alexander, M A
Alexander, M S M
Ali-Khan, A
Amin, M R
Anam, K A K M
Ar-Rikaby, H A
Ashford, A C C
Attais, M
Attias, M
Austwick, D H
Balachandran, T
Balasubramaniam, K
Barhey, M
Bashir, R
Bath, P S
Bietzk, R G
Bissoondatt, R S
Blessing, E
Bright, K J
Brosnan, S G
Burrell, S J
Chan, C-H
Chawla, O P
Cheslyn-Curtis, S
Claramunt Romero, M D C
Clark, E A
Cockerill, K J
Condell, H M
Craske, E
Dand, P A
Day, J J
Deeley, D P
Denis-Smith, D
Dhabuwala, N D
Dorman, A H
Duffy, U M C
Ebrahim, A-R
Elliott, K E
Ellis, C D W
Erotocritou, P P
Farbotko, T A
Fleming, A E
Flora, H K
Foley, M
Ganju, D
Gardner, E S
Griffiths, M
Gupta, M
Gupta, R K
Haider, T
Hall, P L
Hamilton, A J
Harris, C G M
Harris, D J
Harris, F A R
Hey, P A
Hill-Smith, I
Hill, H M
Houghton, D A
Houston, B D
Howard, S V
Hussain, I
Ikeagwu, E O K
Iqbal, T
Jabbar, M A
Jackson, S J
Jain, V K
Jeffs, N G
Johnson, G M
Jutla, G S
Kearney, C E
Khan, M Y
Khanchandani, R
Khanu, D D
Kirubakaran, P
Lewis, P A
MacBrayne, J T
McGill, H L
Mcloone, M B E
Mahadevan, N
Marsden, J K
Martin, S J
Mirza, I A
Mitchell, A M D
Mylvaganam, K
Nafis, M A
Nesaratnam, S
Nicoll, D M
Norman, S G
Novell, J R
O'Malley, J F
Patel, S M
Patroclou, A
Patten, M T
Paul Choudhury, S K
Peterson, D B
Pickles, J M
Pillai, J A
Pinto, R T
Pinto, S C
Pittam, M R
Prakash, O
Rahman, S
Rajapakse, Y S
Ramsay, J R
Rao, Y B J
Rasamuthiah, T
Raut, V V
Ravichandran, D
Rieger, C A
Roberts, M D
Robinson, C A
Roud Mayne, C C A
Rowsell, R B
Russell-Taylor, M A
Safdar, M
Sahdev, A K
Saleh, I
Schembri Wismayer, J
Seery, J A
Semark, D W
Shah, D V
Shah, H M
Shah, S D
Shakoor, A
Shamprasadh, V
Shaper, K R L
Sharma, S
Sherratt, R M
Shokar, N K
Siegler, D I M
Simmonds, N J
Singer, P A
Sinha, R P
Sivakumar, P
Skyers, P A
Soo, S-C
Spears, F D
Spira, M
Stanton, J R
Stodell, M A
Sule, K K
Summers, J A
Swallow, H M
Swan, K M
Tabert, J E K
Talbot, P A J
Tant, D R
Tew, J H
Thiruchelvam, A
Thit Thit, Dr
Thompson, D S
Thompson, M H
Thomson, M
Tolia, J J
Towler, G M
Tsahalina, E
Twigley, A J
Ullah, S
Verghese, A R
Verity, T
Von Arx, D P
Wakefield, P C
Waldock, A
Ward, E M C
Warren, M J
Warriner, S E
Watson, S A
Williams, H J
Williams, N
Williams, P G
Wykes, K J
Yanny, L B
Yogasakaran, B S

Lutterworth
Alexander, C A
Allcock, J N
Bartram, D H
Brown, L J R
Coates, A P M
Dorok, A J
Dowell, C G
Flaxman, P A
Greaves, J M
Guppy, J M
Hampton, R H
Jennings, R S
Khong, C K
Masharani, U B
Masharani, V
Reynolds, J C
Robertson, I K
Warburton, D J R
Watson, D M
Wiggins, W J

Lydbrook
Coates, A J M
Pearce, A F B

Lydney
Bee, A L
Bennett, P J L
Bounds, R J
Chambers, J
Christmas, R
Ellis, D L I
Fellows, P R
Gibbs, M
Hayes, M F
Ibbotson, R B
Jones, R B
Miller, M D
Nancollas, C E
Sharma, S R
Swannack, R

Lyme Regis
Austin, M A
Bowles, R M L
Conway, I M
Eyres, M G
Rajaratnam, D V
Robinson, B J
Ryan, R A

Lymington
Arnold, A J
Badham, D S
Bailey, S G
Birch, S J
Bodley Scott, D D
Collings-Wells, J A
Cracknell, B D
Davies, N J H
Gaunt, S P
Gay, J C C
Green, S N
Hawthorn, E M
Hempsall, V J
Hobson, A R
Humby, M D
Jackson, R K
Johnston, I N L
Johnston, S
Keatinge, J M
Law, C J
Lees, R M
Lloyd, T W
Lowe, N J
Macalister, A M
McCafferty, J D
Macdonald, D M
McEwen, T H
McNaught, J A
Mason, H K
Read, D E
Read, J A J M
Rogers, B J
Rogers, J D
Rowe, P B
Seward, C F
Simon, C A E
Smith, S A C
Spencer, D J
Steadman, A F
Taylor, M C
Turner, G F
Walker, C B
Walker, G D
Wilkie, D J K
Wood, B C

Lymm
Allan, E
Atherton, E A
Bamforth, M A
Beattie, E L K-M
Bell, M H
Carlin, J
Cheetham, E D
Cottrill, P N J
Dodd, F M
Goodall, J R
Green, P M
Haqqani, M F
Harle, C C
Henderson, S J
Johnstone, A H
Kelsall, O M
Lynch, M P
Morgan, K P
Morgan, R J
Morton, A K
Murray, C S
Oxynos, C
Plunkett, S G
Ramsden, G H
Semple, D M
Shard, H M
Swindlehurst, R A
Webster, A L
White, M M S
Williams, B O
Yates, S C
Young, E A

Lympstone
Hayes, C
Ross, R A

Lyndhurst
Allin, A C
Balfour, A M
Balfour, D M
Chinn, S E
Hughes, S R
McAll, F A M
Neil-Dwyer, J S E
Noble, A D
Olliff-Cooper, A K
Smart, J M
Stokes, V V
Struthers, S L
Trickett, J P

Lynton
Allaway, G W
Ferrar, R J
Frankish, J B

Lytham St Annes
Acornley, A J
Atherton, M T C
Bamford, C
Barnsley, C J
Bedford, N A
Bilbey, F
Boardman, A D
Boardman, J

Charles, W J
Connolly, C V
Cooke, F J
Craw, N I
Curzon, R N
Dale, M J
Dempsey, H F M
Duncan, K M
Edwards, T P
Ellwood, S T
Fielding, J D
Fisher, A J
Forrest, L
Foster, K A A
French, P A
Greenwood, K M
Greenwood, S F
Groarke, P
Hall, T M
Hedley, N G T
Hellier, R J
Hough, D J
Irving, A G
Jackson, P J C
Johnson, M C G
Khanna, V K
Laundy, N P
Legg, W J J
Lewis, R N
Lingam, R P
Logan, W F W E
Lowe, N C
Mackey, W T
McLennan, K M
Milner, I G
Molodynski, A C
Moorhouse, P J
Murray, S M
Newman, M
Niman, W
Pitt, S M
Poyner, J G
Reed, R W
Reid, C M B
Reid, S P J
Renvoize, E B
Schofield, C E
Seed, C A
Sloan, M E
Smith, G P
Stevens, R
Stewart, A F S
Tattersall, C W
Thorpe, R J
Vasudev, N S
Wallace, V A
Whitson, A
Williams, R W
Wilmington, A M
Zaryckyj, M

Mablethorpe
Wright, S J

Macclesfield
Aglan, M Y A E A
Akerman, N
Allcock, C
Arnold, B D C
Arnold, C L
Ashley, D L
Auchincloss, J M
Auty, R M
Banner, C V
Bardgett, D M M
Barge, A J
Baskeyfield, H M
Beckett, A K
Beckett, S E
Belliappa, K P
Black, D
Black, S M
Blackledge, G R P
Bowie, J S
Bowie, R A
Bradley, W P L
Branson, K
Braude, W M
Brimelow, A E
Brownhill, A J
Burrows, E J
Calleja, J
Cameron, H A
Carbarns, I R I
Carter, M G
Chalmers, C R
Charlesworth, B R
Choudhury, G
Clack, G I S
Clay, R S
Cochrane, L
Colville, J C
Coope, G A
Coope, M L
Cragg, D K
Dale, R H
Davies, A H
Davies, M
Davison, C E
Dean, S
Drake, R J
Duce, G M
Dunlop, P D M
Earp, A D
Egdell, R M
Entwistle, M P
Fagg, S L
Farrington, A
Finch, E L
Ford-Young, W P D
Forrester, C
Forsythe, B J
Foster, P N
Fox, E M
Galloway, J C R
Garcia-Vargas, J E
Gates, S
Gathercole, N J
Gilbert, J
Gray, A J
Gray, H S J
Hall, V
Handler, K E
Hanson, J R
Harris, R A
Hastings, S C
Heathcote, J A
Heron, R J L
Heyworth, R C F
Higgins, S A
Hodgson, J M
Holden, D
Holden, H M
Hopkins, K J
Hughes, A M
Hughes, M S
Huyton, M C
Iqbal, J
Jackson, C
Jones, D
Kay, M R
Kelly, D F
Kramer, I M E
Link, C G G
Lockton, J A
Loughran, C F
Loughran, M T
McLean, A F F
Macleod, H
Madden, P L
Madhusudan, M G
Marshall, A M
Matheson, D M
Maurice, A R
Maxwell, D A
Meir, A R
Mellor, S
Mina, M A Y
Mines, G P
Minton, N A
Monaghan, K N
Morris, C Q
Morris, D R
Morris, L J
Morris, Y S
Murgatroyd, H K
Nagaraj, H N
Nair, R G
Namasivayam, S
Nuttall, A M
Olverman, G N
Owens, J R
Parkinson, I M
Partridge, E M
Patterson, J S
Pears, J S
Perkins, C M
Pickles, V A
Plant, G D
Powell, C V E
Preece, R M
Quayle, A R
Rajaratnam, A
Rajaratnam, K
Ramsden, V M
Richards, J B
Rimmer, T W
Robinson, S J
Rodgers, E M
Rogers, J M
Rothwell, M P
Rowlands, D
Roycroft, R J
Shackleton, D B
Shribman, A J
Sinclair, P K
Singer, J A
Smith, L K R
Smith, M P
Smith, R A
Snow, H D J
Spencer, A C
Spillman, I D
Stead, R J
Steep, E
Stirling, A W
Strutt, K L
Studds, C J
Tampi, S C
Taylor, M A R
Thomas, H J
Thomasson, D I
Towers, E A
Tucker, S E
Usher, J R
Van Ross, R T G
Waheed, N
Wales, J E J
Walker, D J
Walker, J M
Wallis, N T
Walton, S R
Waring, H L
Weaver, A B
White, H L
Whiteman, I A
Willdig, P J
Williams, A R
Williams, A J
Yates, R A
Zafar, W U

Macduff
Brooker, I P
Hoddinott, P M

Machynlleth
Hayter, R C
Hughes, R M
Morpeth, S J
Tedders, R A
Thapa, T B
Unsworth, F J
Upadhyay, M

Maesteg
Bassett, S D
Davies, W A
Ferguson, B J M
Griffiths, H
Jones, D M
Kirsop, B A
Lewis, R J P
Lodwig, G S
Peregrine, A D
Rogers, A
Rogers, M A
Sharma, A
Smith, G L
Spiller, J E
Stratford, K A
Thomas, K W
Thomas, N B
Walby, C

Maghera
Convery, R P
Harkin, M S
Mullan, B A
Mullan, R N
Murphy, G J
Overend, J S
Scullin, P
Stevenson, M M
Young, V K

Magherafelt
Bailie, J C T
Barker, D
Barton, C M
Charlton, M A
Chaturvedi, R R
Clark, H S G
Doherty, Y E
Doyle, M B
Glancy, B P
Harkin, A J
Harkin, C A
Harkin, K A
Hawe, M J G
Henry, A M
Heron, M O
Hinds, M C
Hunter, E K
Ingram, E R
Keatley, J D
Kuriacose, J K
Lambrechts, H A
Lowry, C G
McCloskey, C L
McConnell, A A M
MacLarnon, P G
McRobert, R
Miller, M F
Mills, H M
Mulholland, B A
Mulholland, J K
Murphy, B
Nesbitt, M E
Noble, I S
O'Kane, A G
O'Neill, C O
O'Neill, M P
Pyper, P C
Rankin, P V
Scullion, D F
Scullion, U M E
Shastri, K D
Shaw, G M
Tohill, M
Walker, L J E
Walls, A T R
Walls, F B
White, C
White, F A
Wilson, C H
Wilson, L L
Wray, R H
Young, M F

Maidenhead
Aldington, D J
Ammar, T
Baillie-Hamilton, A B
Barker, J E
Behrman, R G A
Bezulowsky, V
Birdi, A Z
Blackmore, S C
Boyd, J G
Brealey, D A
Brock, P G
Burnley, S R
Butler, A H
Butler, A J
Butt, T Y
Coleby, M D
Colyer, P E
Cutting, P A
Dhillon, P T S
Easparathasan, V P
Englishby, V L
Fanning, P P
Fletcher, P A
Flew, R
Francis, G C
Gilroy, K J
Grewal, J S
Grewal, N A S
Gutteridge, W H C
Habershon, R J
Harrold, J D
Haslam, D J
Hawkins, F D
Head, C E
Hemmings, P M
Hill, J R
Hutchings, C M
Jobling, S A
Johnson, M V T
Jones, I S
Joshi, G C
Keiller, N P
Khoo, C T-K
Kinder, J A
Kitchin, N R E
Kon, P
Lambton, M
Langdon, C G
Langdon, J A
Lloyd-Williams, D J
Lockhart, S P
Louth, S
Lytton, J M
McIntosh, E D
Mahmoudi, M
Martin, G G
Maudgil, B D
Maudgil, D
Mawson, H N C
Mercer, D R V
Mercer, J C
Milne, A D T
Mitchell-Fox, T M
Mitchell, A J
Montague, G R
Newman, M
Nuvoloni, M C C
Obi, B C
Owens, L A
Parker, J C
Petersen, L A
Pillitteri, A J
Platt, T L C
Pountney, A M
Pratt, S
Ratti, B M
Riley, P J
Roberts, H L
Roberts, J C U
Roberts, P J
Robertson, A M
Rosewall, H L
Rushton, J M
Rutter, P C
Scorer, H J M
Scothorne, C L
Segal, D S
Shaw, P J
Sithirapathy, S
Slater, A M
Smith, R D
Southgate, M J
Spier, S J
Stawarz, M J
Stearnes, G N
Stone, J P
Symons, K W
Symons, R C F
Tattersall, M L
Thomas, H G
Thomas, J A
Toal, M J
Townsend, C L
Valentine, J L
Watson, M W
Wells, L C
Wheeler, J S
Wickramasinghe, S N
Williams, M K
Williams, S L
Wiltshire, R J

Maidstone
Abson, C A
Adjaye, N T
Akhtar, R
Akram Chaudhry, T M
Alexander, H C
Alkass, W A Y
Anderson, H E
Andrews, S M
Aragones Arroyo, M L
Ashton, J B
Barrett, D M
Batley, M A
Bearcroft, R I
Beesley, S H
Belham, M R D
Bhaduri, B R
Bingham, J R M
Bird, G L A
Biswas, M
Bonds, P R
Brice, C H
Brown, E W J
Brunell, C L
Bulmer, P J
Burman, A S
Christmas, S
Cook, G E
Coutts, M A
Cranston, C J
Cross, G D
Czaykowski, A A P
Da'Ood, M S
Dawes, L
Dawes, M
De Zoysa, W S L
Dening-Smitherman, P
Dennison, J A
Derry, C P
Dickenson, J E
Dickie, A R
Dolman, L J
Donaldson, J G
Downing, H M
Dunham, A M
El-Menshawy, H M M
Ellis, S C
Fernando, B V E
Fernando, H M T
Fernando, R L
Fincham, A C
Fish, D E
Gammanpila, S M
Gammanpila, S W
Gardner, R F A
Gaston, J C
Gaule, E W
Geadah, M W
Gerhards, M
Gilmore, R J
Godsmark, C J
Goodman, J D S
Gray, R N M
Gundry, M F
Hagan, G C
Hammond, A
Hancock, D J
Hanrath, P H J
Haque, F
Haque, S Q
Harland, E C
Harland, T G
Harris, C
Hart, R
Henderson, A F
Henry, R C
Hesketh, S C
Hibbert, D J
Hill, M E
Hobday, P J
Holt, P M
Hulse, J A
Iyer, S P S H V
James, R D
Jenkins, C D G
Jenkins, D G
Jessel, C R
Johnson, S R
Jones, A M
Jones, C A
Jones, M C H
Jones, P A
Jones, P V
Jones, S E
Kavi, S
Kemp, L I
Kidd, M N
Laurent, R J
Leech, R C
Lewis, P L
Lilley, J A
Little, L
Little, T M
McAllister, R H
McEwan, G D
MacFarlane, A I
McGavin, D
McIlwraith, G R
McLean, I F
McMillan, P J
McMullen, I D H
Mason, A B
Matin, M A
Meech, S H
Mennie, R H
Milroy, A J
Mirza, I H
Mongalee, M-E-R
Morgan, L V
Morgan, M D
Mortimer, A R
Mosa, M A M
Moss, M L
Mounter, N A
Mya Win, Dr
Navaratne, M
Newman, D A
Oakley, L H
Parkes, K N
Parris-Piper, T W
Pollington, B I
Powell-Jackson, P R
Puffett, A R
Pulham, N L
Rao, A
Rao, I V
Reddy, P J
Reed, A M
Reeves, N A
Renkema, S E
Rex, S D

Reynolds, E M R R
Richards, S K
Rifaat, M
Ritchie, J P
Roberts, I
Sadler, G M
Schofield, J B
Scott, O J
Shahabdeen, M M
Shahrad, B
Shaikh, T R
Shamim, S U
Sheth, H
Siggers, G R
Simmons, H O
Singh, K
Sinha, G C
Sivakumar, K
Slater, R N S
Smith, H J
Soorma, A
Spicer, A J
Sritharan, S
Subash Chandran, S
Summers, J
Taylor, D H
Thom, C H
Thom, R B
Thomas, A J
Thomas, J G
Thornburgh, I L
Timms, C M J
Towner, H D
Tudor De Silva, H P B
Unter, C E M
Van Seenus, T E
Van Wyk, G J
Vaux, R H C
Virden, J C
Wahby, C C T
Walker, A E
Walker, C J
Waters, T C
Whistler, D M
Widd, S E
Wilford, P J
Williams, N J
Williams, R C
Witt, J M
Worden, R J
Yau, Y Y

Maldon
Booker, P
Bozman, E H
Cargill, C L
Carr, M J T
Causton, J A
Chapman, A B C
Cronin, M T
Deasy, J M
Furze, R J
Haeger, M P
Jones, R A
Lim, L
Macdonald, R J M
McDowell, I R
Molife, L R
Morley, S L
O'Connell, M S
Roper, R M
Shirodaria, C V
Smithson, C J
Stylianides, L

Malmesbury
Badcock, K
Barron, G J
Botell, R E
Charles, D L
Crawford, C E J
Graham, V H J
Harrison, J D
Heathcock, J P
Martin, J L
Neale, J S
Owen, C G
Pettit, J G
Pettit, P C
Pickering, N J

Malpas
Davies, L M C
Howarth, A J
Hulbert, C C
Hulbert, G M
London, A A M
Monck-Mason, J M

Price, M L
Smith, A C

Malton
Balmer, R L
Balmer, S L
Campbell, L
Carrie, D R
Diggory, C J
Diggory, T M
Grant, W C
Grove, L
Hobkinson, L M
Lynch, M
Rayne, D
Sleeman, M L
Taylor-Helps, D F
Taylor, H P
Thornton, S M
Umbrich, P

Malvern
Adeney, C G
Allbright, M
Allbright, S E
Barnes, R D
Bates, P A S
Black, J
Brocklebank, D M
Budd, J M
Busher, G L
Edwards, J
Fuller, D J
Gilbert, R F
Grant, M I
Harcup, J W
Henry, G F J
Herriot, B W A
Herriot, S E
Hinchliffe, M
Holland, C R
Houghton, P G
Jarrett, K W
Lambert, R A
Lavin, J B
McCarthy, P H V
McCracken, A L
Mackman, C J
Macleod, I R
Mather, J M
Mayner, P E
Millard, N R H
O'Flynn, M W
Orgee, J M
Palmer, E N E
Pearce, J C
Radley, D J
Richards, J A
Richards, M J
Rogers, P J
Rose, P
Sefton-Fiddian, J
Senior, E L
Tarr, K E
Trueman, T
Tuck, B A
Turner, C E
Vaughan, J A
Vaughan, M M
Walsh, P J F
Ward, B-A
Wight, K C
Williams, G M

Manchester
Abbas, A C
Abboud, S H
Adams, J E
Adamski, J K
Addis, V P
Addison, G M
Ag Hj Mohd Hassan, D H
Agius, R M
Ahluwalia, A
Ahluwalia, A S
Ahluwalia, R S
Ahmad Mohd Zain, Z
Ahmad, M Z
Ahmad, M
Ahmad, M M
Ahmad, Z H
Ahmed, A R
Ahmed, Z
Ainscow, G
Akbar, A
Akhter, S
Al-Abady, A
Al-Asadi, A D

Al-Dabbagh, A K R
Al-Gailani, M A-M A-R
Al-Moomen, A H A
Al-Mulla, A
Alderson, D M
Alexander, G S
Ali, G
Ali, H H H
Ali, N S
Allan, B K
Allaun, D H
Allcock, S
Allen, D J
Allen, D L
Allen, G
Allen, N H P
Allweis, B
Alnuamaani, T M
Alvi, F-U-H
Ammori, B J I
Amos, H T
Anandadas, J A
Anderson, I M
Ang, C W-M
Anshar, F M
Anwer, K
Appachi, E
Appleby, C
Appleby, L
Arnold, M M
Arora, S C
Arrowsmith, J M
Ashford, P
Ashleigh, R J
Ashworth, H M
Ashworth, J L
Aspinall, G R
Atalla, A E
Ataullah, S M
Atrey, A K
Atrey, N
August, P J
Azam, F S
Azam, M
Bahgat, M S
Bahia, S S
Baildam, A D
Baildam, E M
Bailey, E V
Bailey, N
Bailey, S M
Baird, R M
Baker, P N
Bakhat, A A
Balayogi, K K
Ballardie, F W
Ballin, I A
Ballon, M D
Banerjee, S
Banks, R H
Bannister, C L
Bannister, C M
Bannister, P
Baral, S
Barber, N P
Barber, P V
Barker, J M
Barman, D N
Barnard, S J
Barnes, A J
Barnes, D G
Barnes, N L P
Baronos, E
Barooah, K
Barooah, P S
Barr, L
Barrow, J
Barson, A J
Bass, K
Basu, P S
Batchelor, J S
Bates, A C
Baxandall, M L
Baxter, D N
Bayman, D C
Beadsworth, M B J
Beards, S C
Beetles, U M
Begum, S
Behardien, J Y
Behrana, A J
Bellantuono, I
Belli, A
Bellis, A J
Benbow, E W
Benett, I J
Benjamin, S
Bennett, D H
Bentley, A M

Benton, K G F
Berger, S M
Bernstein, R M
Bhatia, T
Bhatti, W A
Bianchi, A M
Bianchi, S M
Birchall, W
Birrell, F N
Birtwistle, I H
Birzgalis, A R
Bishop, P N
Bishop, P W
Bisset, R A L
Black, J E B
Blake, I C
Blakey, A F
Bodey, S A
Boggis, C R M
Bolton, M J
Bonington, A
Bonington, S C
Bonshek, R E
Borg Costanzi, J M
Borrill, J K
Borrill, Z L
Boulton, A J M
Bouskill, J
Bowden, L S
Bowdler, G R
Bowley, C A
Boyce, C T
Boyd, M I
Boyd, R
Bracegirdle, A P
Bradbury, A J
Bradbury, G A
Bradley, A J
Bradley, D S
Braganza, M A
Braine, K
Bramley, R
Brear, S G
Brennan, B M D
Bridgewater, B J M
Brien, P F
Briggs, C H
Bromley, A B
Brooks, D
Brooks, N H
Brosnan, R D
Brough, P J
Brough, R J
Brown, A G
Brown, A A
Brown, A B
Brown, A P T
Brown, G N
Brown, G C S
Brown, H
Brown, J R
Brown, S M
Broxton, J S
Bruce, J
Buchalter, I M
Buchan, I E
Buckley, C H
Budden, P D
Bundred, N J
Bungay, C J
Burgess, H
Burman, A
Burnie, J P
Burns, A S
Burt, P A
Burton, I D
Burton, I E
Bussin, J L
Butler, A S
Butterworth, D M
Byers, R J
Byrne, E J
Byrne, G J
Calderwood, R O D
Callander, M J
Camilleri, A E
Campbell, A A
Campbell, C S
Campbell, I T
Campbell, L H
Campbell, N J
Campbell, R H A
Cant, M M
Canty, D P C
Capek, M E Y
Caplan, G
Caplan, M
Carley, S D
Carlisle, H R

Carpenter, J E
Carpenter, L J
Carrero Cabo, A C
Carrington, B M
Carrington, P A
Carter, N
Cartlidge-Eighan, R E
Cassidy, J M
Cater, E J
Caulfield, H M
Chadwick, I S
Chadwick, P C
Chakravarty, M R
Chalmers, N
Chalmers, R J G
Chan, K P
Chandiok, S
Chandiramani, V A
Chang, J
Chant, H J
Charles-Jones, H D
Charles, S J
Charlesworth, D
Charnley, J
Chaudhuri, H
Chaudry, I A
Chaudury, F R
Checkley, E J
Cheema, R A
Chen, C E
Cheshire, C M
Chew-Graham, C A
Chintapatla, S
Chiswick, M L
Chiu, C T
Chiu, T W
Choi, C F
Choi, D
Choi, P
Chopra, R
Choudhri, A H
Chowdhury, B A
Christmas, R J
Cinkotai, K I
Clark, A F
Clark, A J
Clark, L J
Clark, S J
Clarke, A D
Clarke, B
Clarke, C P C
Clarke, N W
Clayson, A D
Clayton Smith, J
Clayton, A J
Clayton, P E
Cleary, B J
Cleator, P J
Clegg, D S
Clift, A D
Clough, D L
Clutton, H A
Cockayne, L M
Coe, G J
Coles, P K L
Colgan, S M
Colligan, D
Connolly, L P
Conroy, J I
Contractor, A S
Cook, A E
Cooke, C A
Cooke, M J
Cooper, A
Cooper, P N
Corlett, A J
Cornish, E L
Costello, C B
Couper, D M
Court, J E
Cowie, A G
Cox, A E
Coyne, J D
Craig, C V
Crane, M D
Craufurd, D I O
Creed, F H
Crocombe, S J
Crook, I
Crook, S A
Crowther, D
Cruickshank, J K
Cryer, L M
Cumming, A M
Cunningham, M B
Cunningham, S A
Curran, J
Currer, B A
Curzen, N P

D'Souza, S W
Dainton, M C
Dalton, S J
Daly, E L
Danczak, A F
Dangoor, A
Dar, S A
Das, P K
Das, V K
Dass, L
Dass, S
Datta, P
Davenport, P J
Davenport, R
David, T J
Davidson, S E
Davies, D R A
Davies, R R
Davies, R
Davis, J R E
Davis, N
Davison, P
Dawes, N J
Day, J R
Day, J N
Day, J B
De Mello, W F
De Weever, A C A
De, R N
Deakin, J F W
Dean, A
Dean, G L
Dean, N
Dearlove, O R
Deas, J
Decalmer, S A
Decatris, M P
Deighton, J G
Delaney, M J
Dellagrammaticas, D
Denning, D W
Densem, C G
Desai, M S
Desmond, J
Dewsnap, C H
Dhadli, M K
Dickson, A P
Dickson, J
Dinerstein, J
Dixon, N W
Dixon, P A
Dodd, A S
Dodd, C L
Doffman, S R
Dolan, L J
Dolan, M C
Donnai, D
Donnai, P
Doody, P
Doran, H E
Doran, H M
Dornan, C C
Duane, L P
Dube, P
Dubicka, B W
Ducker, G M
Ducksbury, C F J
Duddy, O M
Duffy, D J
Duncan, J E
Duncan, T
Dunkley, M A
Dunkow, P D
Dunn, K W
Durrington, P N
Dymock, I W
Eden, O B
Eden, R I
Eden, S
Edmondson, E D
Edmondson, G M P
Edwards, J D
Eeckelaers, M C W
El Gadi, I A
El-Ghazawy, M A L M A
El-Khashab, T A F
El-Mikatti, N
El Teraifi, H A A
Element, P
Elliot, S D
Ellis, R M
Elsworth, C F
Eltoft, M E
Emmerson, A J B
England, R E
Enoch, B A
Enoch, L C
Etteh, B E

Evans, D G R
Evans, J E C
Everett, J
Ewing, C I
Fallon, J S
Farrington, M R
Farrington, W T
Faza, H N
Fenerty, C H
Ferguson, A M
Ferguson, A P
Ferguson, D A
Fink, P R
Finke, A S
Firoze, A
Firoze, K V
Fitzgerald, Z
Fitzmaurice, R J
Fitzpatrick, A P
Fitzpatrick, H J
Flascher, S M
Fleming, D H
Fletcher, K M
Foex, B A
Ford, J M
Forman, W M
Fortune, P-M
Foster, M E
Fox, D M
Fox, H
France, M W
Frank, P L
Fraser, I S
Fraser, W R
Freed, L
Freedman, F
Freeman, A S
Freeman, S R M
Freemont, A J
Froggatt, P A
Fuller, J E A
Fyans, P G
Fyfe, D W
Gadd, J R
Gage, A J
Gale, A C
Gan, Y C
Gandhi, A
Gangaprasad, G
Ganvir, P L
Garcia Alen Garcia, L
Gardner, R W
Garg, T L
Garrett, H M
Garston, J B
Garvey, T P N
Gatley, M S
Gatoff, H
Gattamaneni, H R
Ghani, R
Ghosh, A K
Gibbs, M G
Gibson, P D
Gilani, S A A
Gill, A K
Gill, L S
Gill, P
Gill, S
Gillespie, J E
Glass, A L
Goel, R P
Golding, J L
Goldstone, J
Goldwater, D E
Goodall, B
Goodman, M A
Goodman, R E
Gordon, D
Gordon, R I
Gore, D
Gore, H
Gough, D C S
Gough, V M
Gow, D P
Graham, S
Green, J M
Green, R
Greenalgh, D
Greenaway, T J
Greenbaum, A R
Greene, A
Greig, D G
Griffiths, A G
Griffiths, M R
Griffiths, P J
Griffiths, R W
Grinter, K R
Groarke, A W
Grotte, G J
Groves, C J
Gudgeon, E A
Gulati, R C
Gunda, A F
Gupta, N K
Guthrie, E A
Guthrie, G E
Guy, R C
Gwinnutt, C L
Hadjiloucas, I
Haider, Y
Haji-Michael, P G
Halder, N
Halder, S L S
Hall, C M
Halstead, L G
Hamdy, R
Hamilton, A J
Hamilton, R M
Hammer, M R
Hamour, A O A A A
Hampson, F G
Hanley, S P
Hannah, J C
Happold, M E
Haque, I-U
Harake, M D J
Hardinge, K
Hardy, C C
Hardy, L A
Hargreaves, F M
Hargreaves, G K
Harper, N J N
Harris, B V
Harris, C P
Harris, H J
Harris, M A
Harris, P L
Harrison, A M
Harrison, B J
Harrison, C J
Harrison, J A
Hart, E A
Hartley, L A
Hasleton, P S
Hassan, I A
Hassoon, A A M
Hawes, S J
Hawgood, E A
Hawkins, K C
Hawkins, R E
Hawnaur, J M
Haworth, D
Haworth, J I
Hay, C R M
Hay, G G
Hayes, M J
Heagerty, A M
Healey, A E
Healy, T E J
Heathcote, I T
Helbert, M R
Hellewell, J S E
Helman, S C
Hennessy, D M
Herbert, E A
Heron, E C
Hershon, E
Hibbert, D L
Hickling, D J
Higgins, G A
Hill, A S
Hill, J
Hill, J M
Hilton, S R
Hindley, D T
Hirsch, P J
Hoad-Reddick, D A
Hobson, S J
Hoddes, C E
Hodson, S A
Holland-Elliott, K
Hollingshead, S
Holloway, J
Holmes, S J
Holt, L P J
Homer, J J
Hooper, T L
Hope, B
Hopgood, P
Hopwood, P
Hore, B D
Horrocks, A W
Horsman, E L
Hosker, H B
Hoskins, A
Hotchkies, I L M
Hotchkies, S A C
Houston, E C
Howard, E M
Howard, R E
Howat, J M T
Howden, M D
Howe, M C
Howell, A
Howell, R J
Howell, S J
Hughes, D G
Hughes, J G
Hughes, M I
Hughes, N R
Hughes, S M
Humphreys, J
Huq, H H
Huq, Z
Hurley, E
Hussain, I
Hussain, Z
Hutchinson, C E
Hutchinson, D J
Hutchison, A J
Hutton, A J F
Hyams, N A
Hyde, S M
Hyman, J G
Hynes, J E
Ibrahim, A F
Iddon, J
Igielman, F I P
Ioannidou, S S
Isaacs, A B
Isaacson, D M
Isalska, B J
Islam, C O F
Islam, M S
Islam, M S
Issa, B G
Ivinson, M H L
Iyengar, E N
Iyengar, M
Jacks, S P
Jackson, A
Jackson, L E
Jacobs, E M
Jafaree, S A H
Jafari, B
Jaffe, S M
Jaffe, W
Jain, P
Jalaluddin, Z
Jamal, W
James, J M
James, P F
Jari, S
Jarratt, J W
Jarvis, R R
Javidi, M
Jayson, D
Jayson, G C
Jayson, M I V
Jeffery, K F K
Jeffries, M
Jeffries, S C
Jenkins, J P R
Jenkins, N P
Jepson, F K
Jilani, S A
John, A B
Johnson, D A W
Johnson, R J
Johnson, R W G
Johnson, R A
Johnston, T A
Jolly, G K
Jolly, S S
Jones, A S
Jones, A M
Jones, C I
Jones, D J
Jones, D L
Jones, K E
Jones, M T
Jones, N P
Jones, S L
Jones, T M
Joseph, S G
Joshi, G D
Joshi, V B
Joyce, P R
Judge, M R
Jukes, R A M
Julien, D R
Juma, N M H
Kaczmarski, E B
Kale, M
Kalim, K
Kamaly-Asl, I D
Kaminski, D J
Kanagasegar, S
Kane, K
Kane, S
Kathirgamanathan, A
Kauffmann, L A D
Kaur, R
Kaur, S
Kaushal, K
Kawafi, K R
Kawonga, R M P
Kay, C L
Kay, M J R
Kaye, A H
Kaye, J E
Keaney, M G L
Kebbie, M M
Keenan, D J M
Kelly, A-M
Kelsall, M E
Kelsey, A
Kenny, N W
Kenrick, D A
Kerns, W
Kerr, M E
Kerr, S J
Kerrane, J
Kerrin, D P
Kerry, A L
Kershaw, P
Keynes, G R E
Khan, A N
Khan, G M
Khan, M A H
Khan, M A
Khan, M H Z
Khan, N S
Khan, S S
Khan, S
Khan, Z A
Khanna, M
Khanna, V
Khiani, R
Khoo, S H
Khurana, K M
Khurana, M
Kidd, C M
Kiff, E S
King, J E
Kingston, H M
Kingston, P A
Kingston, R D
Kinsella, T J
Kirby, A
Kirk, P R
Kirwan, C C
Kissen, G D N
Kitchener, H C
Kitching, W J
Kiwanuka, A I
Kleinberg, J E
Knox, W F
Kok Shun, J L C S
Kolb, C S
Kondratowicz, T
Koria, K
Kotegaonkar, K S
Kotegaonkar, M K
Kujawa, M L
Kukula, M S
Kulkarni, J R
Kulshrestha, R K
Kumar, P
Kumar, S
Kuna, K
Kurdy, N M
Kwok, S
Kwong, H T
Kwong, L J
Kyriakides, C A
Ladusans, E J
Laha, S N
Lai, P
Lalloo, F I
Lancashire, S C J
Lang-Sadler, E
Langley, S J
Lansbury, E S
Lascelles, R G
Lau, Y N
Lavin, M J
Law, J B
Lawrance, J A
Lawton, V
Lea, S
Leach, J M
Leahy, B C
Leahy, M D
Leask, K M
Leatherbarrow, B
Lee, H S
Lee, S H
Lee, W R
Leech, A M
Leitch, D
Lendon, M
Lendrum, J
Lennon, S P
Lennox, B J
Leon, E A
Leschziner, G D
Leveson, C M
Levine, E L
Levy, R D
Levy, R G
Lewis, H M
Lewis, M A
Lewis, M R
Lewis, S W
Liaw, V P
Libbert, D H
Lieberman, B A
Lighton, L L
Lindsay, S D
Linforth, R A
Lissett, C A
Liu Yin, A
Lloyd, H
Lloyd, I C
Lockwood, M
Loncaster, J A
Longson, D
Lorigan, P C
Louca, L L
Love, E M
Lovell, M E
Lowe, H
Lucas, G S
Ludlow, J P
Lumb, P D
Lyons, C A
Ma-Fat, R
McArdle, M T
McCann, R A
McCarthy, D K
McCloy, R F
McCollum, C N
McCorkindale, S
McCrea, R R
MacDiarmaid-Gordon, A R
Macfarlane, L
MacFarlane, N D
Macfoy, D
McGawley, C M
McGonigle, T P
McGrath, B A
McGrath, G J
McGrogan, L P
McGrouther, D A
McIntyre, F J
McKenna, F
McKenna, R
Mackenzie, K R
McKibbin, V P
McKinlay, D M
McKinlay, I A
Mackway-Jones, K C
McLaren, J S
MacLean, I M
McLean, J M
MacLennan, I
McLeod, D
McMahon, R F T
McMenzie, A J
Macnab, W R
McNamara, J F
McNulty, S J
McNulty, S M
McQuillan, O M A
McVey, R J
Madan, M
Magee, B J
Magennis, R F
Mahafza, T A
Mahmood, T
Majid, Z
Makin, D
Makin, G W J
Makin, W P
Malik, A A
Malik, R A
Malik, R A
Mallick, N P
Malloy, N P
Maltby, B
Manchester, D J
Mangar, S A
Mansfield, J D
Marco Molina, M L
Marcus, R L
Marcuson, R W
Maresh, M J A
Margison, F R
Mark, P E
Marshall, C F
Marshall, M N
Marshall, R E
Marsland, A
Martin, C E G
Martin, D F
Martin, R B
Martin, S E
Massie, J A
Matthews, R C
Mattison, A F
Maudar, J A
Maurice, S C
Maw, A E
Mawer, G E
Mayall, F G
Mayall, R M
Maynard, S M
Mazhari, H K
Mead, G S
Meakin, G H
Mehraj, Q R
Mehta, S G
Mene, R
Merrill, K J
Metzger, R E
Meyer, S
Michael, L A
Middlehurst, R J
Miles, J F
Miller, J P
Miller, L J
Milligan, H S
Mills, A E
Mills, K B
Milton, R S
Mistry, N U
Mitchell, J C
Mitchell, S R
Mo, C-N
Modi, N K
Modi, S P
Mohammad, D
Mohammad, W
Mohr, P D
Mokashi, A V
Moloney, A M
Momen, A
Monaghan, S J
Monteiro, B T
Moore, C E G
Moore, M A
Moran, A
Morris, D P
Morris, E M
Mortimer, A J
Morton, R J
Moss, D A
Moyo, P K
Mughal, M Z
Mukherjee, V
Mullin, N H
Mullins, P D
Mumtaz, H M
Munro, K A
Munshi, S B
Murray, S R
Murthy, P
Musgrove, B T
Mutton, K J
Myerscough, A
Naidoo, R K A
Nanavati, B A
Napier-Hemy, R D
Naqui, F A
Nasim, A
Natha, M I
Nayar, R
Naylor, K M T
Needham, D J
Neville, T E
Newbould, M J
Newlove, R M
Newman, W G J
Newton, J S
Newton, R W
Nicholson, S
Nightingale, P
Niven, R M
Noble, J L
Noble, J
Nolan, D M
Noone, J F

Noone, M A
Norburn, P S
Norbury, L P
Noronha, E A
Noronha, M J
Nunez Miret, O
Nunoo-Mensah, J W
Nurennabi, A K M
Nussbaum, T
Nylander, D L
Nysenbaum, A M
Nzelu, E N
O'Brien, K
O'Carroll, D J
O'Connor, A M
O'Connor, J M
O'Connor, L M
O'Connor, M B
O'Donnchadha, E P
O'Donnell, A
O'Donoghue, N B
O'Driscoll, G
O'Driscoll, S C
O'Dwyer, S T P
O'Keeffe, N J
O'Malley, P A
Ocansey, P
Odom, N J
Oram, J C
Orton, C I
Osborne, M A
Osu, B A
Owen, K R
Owen, R A
Painter, G E
Painter, M J
Pal, B
Panagea, S E
Panigrahi, H
Panikker, S
Pantelides, M L
Parihar, P
Parihar, S S
Parrott, N R
Parry, N S
Pasha, M
Patel, D
Patel, L
Patel, R H
Patel, R G
Patel, R R
Pathak, P L
Patrick, M R
Patton, J T
Pattoo, B A
Paul, A S
Payne, S R
Pearson, R C
Pemberton, M N
Pereira, D T M
Pereira, J R
Perera, D M D
Perkins, R J K
Perry, M S
Peters, L A
Petrie, H P
Pettit, W J
Phillips, K A
Picardo, L
Pickering, C A C
Pickering, G
Pickin, C A
Pike, A C
Pilkington, R S
Pitches, D W
Plant, L A
Plant, N D
Plenderleith, M
Pollard, B J
Poller, L
Porczynska, K R
Porritt, A J
Porter, J N
Postlethwaite, R J
Poston, B L
Poynton, A M
Prabhakar, D T C
Prendergast, B D
Prescott, M C
Prestwich, H R
Price, D A
Price, L J
Price, P M
Price, R
Price, R M
Procter, A W
Prodhan, M S
Puddy, V F
Pugh, E W
Pumphrey, R S H
Puri, S
Purohit, N N
Purser, J H
Qasim, F J
Quddus, S F
Quine, D J
Quinnell, A J
Qureshi, K
Qureshi, M I
Radford, J A
Radford, R
Rahim, O
Rahman, J
Rahman, K M
Rahman, T S
Rahuja, S A S
Rajagopal, R
Rakhit, A K
Ralston, A J
Ramesh, C A
Rampling, K
Ramsden, R T
Rana, D N
Rana, S K
Randall, P E
Randhawa, J S
Rankin, W J
Rannan-Eliya, R W D G
Ranote, S R
Ranson, M R
Rao, P J
Rapado Santaolalla, F
Rasheed, F
Ratcliffe, D S
Ratcliffe, J
Rawson, A
Ray, D W
Ray, S G
Rayner, C R
Razzak, A
Razzaq, F
Reddy, Dr
Redmond, A D
Redmond, B
Reisler, R
Renehan, A G
Reynolds, K M M
Riad, H N
Richards, J L
Richardson, J A
Ridgway, A E A
Riley, S F
Rittoo, D B
Rittoo, D
Riza, I M
Rizvi, Q R
Roach, S C
Roberts, D J
Roberts, M E
Roberts, P-J
Roberts, R E I
Roberts, S P
Roberts, S A
Robertson, J D
Robins, N M
Robinson, A J
Robson, G E W
Robson, S A
Roche, M E
Rogers, J E
Rolan, P E
Roland, M O
Ronalds, C M
Rose, G K
Rose, K G
Rosenberg, B
Rosenberg, R B
Ross, C E
Ross, K G M
Rossini, J
Roussak, J B
Roxburgh, R H S R
Rozycki, A A
Ruiz De Arcaute, J
Russell, E
Russell, S A
Rutherford, J D
Rutter, R A
Ryan, B P
Ryan, K E R
Sabar, M A
Sadiq, M
Sadiq, S A
Sadiq, Z A
Saeed, N
Saeed, R
Saeed, S R
Sahni, A S
Sahni, V A S
Saidi, S A
Saleem, A
Saleh, S
Salim, R
Samad, A
Samanta, A K
Sambrook, M A
Sanchez, E G
Sanders, K J
Sanders, P A
Sandhu, S
Sandle, L N
Sandle, L H
Sanehi, O P
Sangha, M S
Sanyal, D
Sarangi, B B
Sarmah, N N
Sastry, S R
Sathi, N
Saunders, M P
Sawyer, R H
Schady, W
Scholes, P E Q
Schroeder, U E
Schryer, J
Schwarzer, A
Sclare, P D
Seehra, H
Seely, M F
Seex, D M
Segar, S L
Selby, L A
Selby, P L
Sell, L A
Sen, D
Sen, S A
Seriki, D M
Seshappa, V
Shah, D K
Shah, S M A
Shaikh, N
Shakespeare, E J
Shanks, J H
Sharma, M M
Sharma, S K
Sharples, A
Shaw, A
Shaw, A L
Shearer, K
Sheehan, P Z
Sheikh, M Y
Shelly, M P
Shepard, G J
Sheppard, G E
Sheridan, E G
Sherlock, D J
Sherman, L H
Sherry, S J
Shlosberg, D
Short, C D
Shortall, D A
Shreeve, D R
Shroff, S
Siddiqui, S
Siew Tu, C-L
Simenoff, C J
Simler, N R
Simon, A S
Simpson, A
Simpson, J C G
Singh, H S G
Singh, H
Singh, K V
Singh, M
Singh, Y S
Singleton, N A
Sinha, A
Sinha, S
Siriwardena, A K
Siviter, G
Slack, C B T
Slade, D A J
Slater, C S
Slater, R M
Slevin, N J
Sloan, G D
Smalldridge, A
Smith, A R B
Smith, E P
Smith, E J
Smith, H R
Smith, J H J
Smith, M G
Smith, N S
Smith, P J
Smith, P H
Smith, R A
Smith, S J
Smith, V J
Smithson, S E
Smyrniou, N N
Smyth, J V W
Snowden, H N
Snowden, P R
Sodipo, J A J
Soman, V B
Soni, S G
Sookur, D
Soothill, J S
Spencer, L G
Spooner, S J
Sproston, A R M
Spyrantis, N
Sreedharan, K
St. John, J M
Stalley, L F
Stanbridge, T N
Stedman, H G B
Steele, C
Steller, P H
Stevens, E D
Stevens, R H
Stewart, A L
Stewart, D
Stewart, W A
Stone, M J
Stone, P A
Storey, A B
Stout, R
Sugarman, P M
Summers, C L
Summers, Y J
Summerton, C B
Super, M
Sutton, E J
Sutton, J F
Sutton, R S
Swan, J W
Syed, O A
Sykes, A J
Sykes, P A
Symmons, D P M
Symons, S J
Szofinska, B
Tait, W F
Talbot, J S
Tallis, R C
Tamin, S K F
Tamkin, E J
Tamkin, W P
Tasker, I T
Tasker, P R S
Tatnall, S K
Taylor, M B
Taylor, M J
Taylor, P A C
Taylor, P M
Taylor, S J
Teale, K F H
Telford, R M
Tench, D W
Tennant, B D
Teo, H-G
Than Kyaw, Dr
Thapar, A K
Thatcher, N
Theodossiadis, A
Thomas, A G
Thomas, C S
Thomas, N B
Thomas, P W V
Thompson, A R T
Thompson, D
Thompson, H F
Thompson, J C
Thompson, J L
Thoms, G M M
Thurnell, C A
Tint, A K
Tobias, C M
Tonge, G M
Torr, B
Torr, J B D
Townend, W J K
Tragen, D J
Trainer, P J
Trehan, V K
Trenholm, P W
Trump, D
Tsolakis, M G
Tuck, J S
Tudor, G J
Tuffin, J R
Tullo, A B
Tumman, J J W
Tunbridge, R D G
Turley, I M
Turner, A J L
Turner, G S
Turner, M A T
Turner, S L
Turner, S J
Turya, E B
Tyrrell, N M
Unwin, M R
Utting, M R
Vadeyar, H J
Valdez, F N
Vallance, H D
Vallance, R L
Valle, J W
Van Ross, E R E
Varma, B N
Vasanth, E C
Vause, S H
Venning, M C
Verma, S G
Vickers, K
Vites, N P
Vohra, A
Vowles, H A
Vu, T Q
Wacks, H
Waddell, N M R
Wadsworth, R
Waite, I
Waldman, S J
Walker, C A
Walker, H A C
Walker, M G
Walker, R W M
Walker, S
Walker, W D
Walkley, J H C
Waller, C J
Walls, J
Walter, D P
Walton, J M
Wan Hussein, H Y
Ward, D
Ward, K
Ward, S J
Warnes, T W
Waterhouse, D G
Webb, F M
Webb, N J A
Webber, M C B
Webster, L
Webster, R C
Weetman, J P
Weighill, F J
Weiner, M
Weinstock, H S
Weir, D C
Welch, I M
Welch, M
Wheatly, R S
Wheeldin, W
Whitaker, D K
Whitaker, M J
Whitby, D J
White, C E
White, C S
Whitehouse, R W
Whiteley, J M
Whiteman, S J
Whiting, M R
Whittaker, J
Whittaker, N A
Whitworth, H E
Whorwell, P J
Wijeyesekera, K G
Wilcock, D J
Wilcock, J
Wiles, P G
Wilkins, E L
Wilkinson, A J
Wilkinson, B A
Will, A M
Williams, B J
Williams, B T J
Williams, M L
Williams, P H
Williams, Y
Williamson, J B
Williamson, R
Wilson, A C
Wilson, C A
Wilson, G E
Wilson, G B
Wilson, M
Wilson, M D
Wilson, S W
Winslow, L
Wisely, N A
Wong, G A E K-C
Wood, A J
Wood, D M
Wood, N J
Woodcock, A A
Woodhead, M A
Woodhead, N J
Woodhouse, C J
Woodman, C B J
Woodman, M
Woodwards, R T M
Worden, T W J
Wraith, J E
Wren, A M
Wright, E A
Wright, N J S
Wright, S A
Wroblewska, M H
Wu, F C-W
Wylie, J P
Wynn, R F
Yap, B K
Yates, M S
Yates, M D
Yates, R W
Young, A C
Young, H S
Young, I
Young, L B
Younis, N
Yuill, G M
Yuill, G M
Zaidi, A M
Zaidi, N H
Zaidi, S N A
Zakaria, M I
Zaman, M
Zaman, Q
Zarod, A P
Zewawi, A S

Manningtree
Bartley, B J
Hoodbhoy, A P
Kelly, J C
Pain, S J
Southgate, C J
Wilkinson, H C
Wilshaw, H A E

Mansfield
Afacan, A S
Ahmad, N
Allfree, A J
Baranauskas, C V
Baugh, S J
Bilas, Z
Booth, A P
Brauer, S E
Brown, C L
Butler, E V
Butler, T J
Carlisle, R D
Creedon, J
Crosby, M E
Dale, J H
Dalton, M J
Dawson, P P
Day, S P
Dornan, J T
Dutt-Gupta, J
Dutt-Gupta, R K
Foster, D M C
Frith, P J B
Genever, R W
Ghosh, B
Hampton, J A L
Haque, M A
Hay, E H
Huggard, S E
Hughes, D W
Joashi, Y C
Jones, G I
Joshi, A R
Kaur, M
Kendall, J B
Krishna, G
Kumar, V
Lim, K L
Linney, P J
Loker, J E
Lucassen, A E A
Macdougall, P W
Macgregor, C J
Maddock, S J R
Mandal, J
Masud, H
Mills, J E

Mulrooney, L
Murphy, J P
Nair, V P R
Ockelford, S J
Park, H L
Peacock, V A
Pearce, V L
Phipps, K N
Pollard, V A
Powell, W M
Quinlan, R M
Rae, D E
Rahman, A B M S
Rahman, A
Rahman, T
Ransford, J
Rasheed, M H
Roberts, D T
Rockett, H E
Sharma, M S
Sheikh, R R
Shrestha, S M
Singh Khanna, H D
Singh, V
Smith, C J
Steiner, E S
Stephan, T F
Sudell, C J
Sudell, R P
Temple, D R
Topley, E M
Tut, T T
Ward, S J
Watkins, M D A
Whitaker, A J
Williams, D A
Zdziarska, C A

Marazion
Hamilton, A B
Killeen, D M
Thacker, S J
Walden, N P M
Weber, B E

March
Bhatia, S-S
Collings, B R
Goswami, T K
Harrison, W N
Hirson, R B
Ley, C C
Sengupta, C
Taylor, M J
Thomas, M G
Walsh, E J
Warrender, T S
Win Maung, Dr
Wyatt, R D

Margate
Abdel-Hadi, A H S A Q
Audah, S A
Badkoubei, S
Belgaumkar, P V
Carrington, B
Carrington, M E
Casha, J N
Ciccone, G K
Cornell, M S
Davies, E H
De Lord, D A
Dickin, P D
Diggens, D
Fajemirokun, E A
Giancola, G L
Gibbs, S A L
Greenhalgh, A M
Gunasekera, J B L
Hameed-Ud-Din, S
Hamour, M A A A
Henry, S I
Joy, G J A
Kazmie, M
Kelsey, R W
Kha, O S
Laing, E M S
Langworthy, J N D
Lattimer, C R
Leak, A M
Lillicrap, S H
McCafferty, H
Martin, C M
Morcos, W E
Morgan, A D
Morgan, M G
Mukherjee, S K
Patterson, W M P

Rahman, M R
Rahman, T
Ramachandra Raju, K
Rfidah, E H I
Rogers, G J
Russell, A I
Ryder, J E
Sarmah, A
Scott, H W
Shaw, L M A
Sivakumar, M
Smith, C W E
Summerfield, B J
Tse, N Y
Tumath, D E F

Market Drayton
Ackroyd, C R
Adams, R J
Bates, C G
Bremner, A
Burns, S C E
Byrne, J
Coleman, G P
Crocombe, J M
Forrest, J F
Garson, S
Green, C J
Green, M B
Halstead, S
Hares, R A
Hixson, R C
Hopkinson, G B
Leno, E M
McCulloch, D A
Mairs, T D
Mehta, J R
Picton-Robinson, I
Raichura, N
Richards, R W
Rodge, S L
Rowe, S C
Simons, A W
Thinn, K
Thorley, H
Tufft, N R
West, D J
Wilkinson, T S
Wilson, A J T
Wood, R G B

Market Harborough
Allen, M J
Ayton, P R S
Bagnall, A J
Barouch, C A
Beadsworth, A J
Bennett, A P
Biggin, M F
Bird, C R
Bishop, F M
Blake, T M
Bowles, A
Briggs, P
Butterworth, P C
Craven, E R
Crawford, A
Crowley, S E
Delargy-Aziz, Y K
Delargy, H J
Eardley, R E
Hadley, S E
Hartopp, R J
Healey, P D
Johnson, A T
Lancaster, J G
Leach, N T
Lyttelton, M P A
Maxwell, J C
Mistry, H K
Moyes, D G
Pirie, L E
Sellers, W F S
Shaw, F A
Twidell, S M B
Van Diepen, H R
Wilkinson, A F R
Wilson, J M
Woods, D J
Yates, M T

Market Rasen
Bee, D M
Eames, M R
Holford, L C
Manners, C E
Maxwell, T M
Nicol, K
Parry, L G

Peacock, T E
Rhodes, M J
Telfer, J R
Tennant, A W
Vessey, W C
Watson, F J
Weeks, R V
Whitbread, R P
Wood, G C

Markfield
Fernandez, H D
Hailstone, T R
O'Connor, D J
Trzcinski, C J

Marlborough
Ballard, T H
Bishop, D
Butters, P B
Chesshire, D G
Chinneck, P J E
Clapp, B R
Colquhoun, A J
Crofts, P K
Cruickshank, E K
Dalziel, N I
Davies, J M
Duke, H N
Faber, V C
Hanson, S M
Hyson, G E
James, C C
King, P A
King, T J
McCleery, W N C
Manchip, S P
Mapstone, J
Maurice, D P
Maurice, N D
Miller, A
Miller, T N
Morris, J
Muller, G S
Nicolle, F V
Owen-Jones, R J F
Paddon, A M
Papenfus, C B
Prout, R
Ramsay, J H
Rayner, J M H
Roberts, J M N
Rosalie, R
Rosedale, J O B
Tulloch, P M B
Williams, J H
Yearsley, D M

Marlow
Addison, R A
Beresford, A P
Black, M J
Burgess, V M
Calwell, H B
Crawford, S P
Davies, G S R
Fearn, S J
Hayter, J M I
Hobbs, A M B
McColm, J A
Mahoney, A
Maxwell, K J
Merritt, J C
Mitchell, G E
Mogg, A J
Mogg, E J
Morrow, T J
Moston, R H
North, C I
Plater, M E
Redgrave, E A
Sprott, M M
Summers, L W
Swietochowski, J P G
Van Den Berghe, R C
Vincent, E C
Walsh, H M
Watkins, S M
Willsdon, H F

Martock
Bailey, M
Beattie, J K
Bridge, A R
Coates, B M (L
Eaton, A T
Majid, M
More, S J
Quayle, A J M

Maryport
Chaudhri, F L
Collins, T M
Longstaff, K
Money, B I
Overend, A J
Roberts, M B R
Thornley, S K

Matlock
Bathgate, J T
Bennett, C A C
Burd, D
Cannings, I R
Chamberlain, C A
Clark, D M
Connolly, B P S
Currie, A T
Curtis, R A P
Dawson, J V
Draisey, J H
Edwards, M S D
El-Farhan, N M M
Emmerson, R C
Fray, N F
Holden, P J P
Hyde, J L
Hyde, T W
Knight, A M
Lindop, A R
Lingard, P S
MacArthur, D G
Macfarlane, C S
MacFarlane, J F
Mayes, N J
Milner, E C R
Pickworth, D C
Rapoport, J
Ritchie, N J
Rudd, S E
Sinnott, A D
Smallman, R I
Steed, J M
Ward, M G
Wilderspin, M P

Mauchline
Campbell, W T
Cleland, J R
Cleland, J
Currie, J M
McMillan, E S
May, J B
Morrison, K M
Ramsay, W
Scott, A L
Walker, A D W

Maybole
Donaldson, B
Duncan, J A L
Lindsay, M M
Paton, G
Scobie, B
Steele, E S

Mayfield
Bell, D M
Coates, A J
Felton, A E
McAuley, D J
Mathams, A J
Tallett, P R

Melksham
Durrant, G M
East, R M
Frankland, S M
Harrison-Smith, M K
Hill, J D H
Howgrave-Graham, T R
Kahane, R M
Kingston, P M
Lennon, C H
Phillips, P J
Rendall, C M S
Rosser, S A

Melrose
Abdel-All, M A H
Ainslie, D
Amin, A I
Arbuckle, P E M
Bazoua, G
Beighton, R C
Bennett, S A
Blake, J L
Braidwood, J M

Broadhurst, P A
Bryce, J A
Burley, L E
Burns, J M
Clowes, C B
Clutterbuck, D J
Cormie, C M
Crichton, J L
Cripps, T P
Cumming, G P
Dennyson, W G
Dunbar, J A
Duncan, R A
Eade, O E
Gordon, A J
Halpin, R M B
Hardwick, D J
Hosny, M A
Houston, K E
Humphries, C P
Kerr, A D
Leary, N P
Leaver, D C
Leslie, P J A
Love, D R
Low, C B
Lowles, I E
McDonagh, N J
McDonald, R D
McGhee, A-M
McRitchie, H A
Magowan, B A
Maguire, P A
Montgomery, C E A
Montgomery, J N
Mordue, A
Morrice, J S
Murray, R I
Norris, C A
O'Neill, J S
Pearson, A J
Reid, J H
Richard, C J
Richmond, R
Rodgers, J
Sadullah, S
Sharp, C W
Shepherd, W F I
Sloan, M G
Syme, P D
Tucker, J
Wilson, G D
Yellowlees, G M
Yellowlees, I H
Young, J

Melton Mowbray
Ackerley, G C
Adams, M J
Ardron, M E
Barnsdale, E R
Barnsdale, P H
Barrow, D A
Bolt, C E
Bousfield, J D
Corvin, D J
Davies, S M
Gallop, A J
Gosling, O E
Harvey, D J
Harvey, J M
Holt, B E
Hooper, G
Howe, P J C
Hykin, J L
Hykin, L R
Johnston, P W F
Kirby, H
Kirkup, B
Logan, F A
Lovett, D M
Martin, G E
Merrill, J F
Nassim, M A
O'Shea, R A
Patel, S P
Phillips, K G
Rathbone, P S
Reeves, J P
Riley, P
Sidwell, R U
Slevin, P G
Smith, T D W
Thew, R J
Wong, M F M C
Wooding, S C
Wyatt, T A

Menai Bridge
Edwards, H A
Farquharson, G C
Hesketh, G M
Iorwerth, A
Lowes, M E
Maxwell, R T
Maxwell, S E L
Morris, O G
Palin, S J
Parry-Jones, A
Parry, E
Roberts, J G
Robinson, G A
Thomas, E O
Tripp, S J

Merthyr Tydfil
Blankson, J M
Cassidy, D M
Chandran, V S
Chillal, B
Choudhary, P C
Choudhury, N
Choudhury, S K
Clements, S A C
Cooze, P H
Davies, D B S
Davies, M J
Drah, M A
Evans, K M
Evans, R W
Evans, W V
Ézsiás, A
Fleming, J F
Gabr, S M
Ganesh, S
Gaugain, J V
Gilchrist, H
Gottumukkala, V R
Hanna, F W F
Hawkes, N D
Hourahane, B E
Hussain, A
Hussein, O T M K
Ismaiel, A H M A
Iyer, B R
Izzidien, A Y
Jayadev, B U
Jayaraman, N
Jones, H
Karpha, S
Kelly, B V
Kennedy, G P
Khan, M I
Kumar, P D
Lalla, M M
Maguire, M J
Maulik, T G
Megharaj, P D M
Menon, L
Mirando, U S
Mukasa, F J
Murdeshwar, S S
Myers, K
O'Dwyer, G A
Owen, A C
Patel, B T
Quirke, R J
Rahim, A
Rangarajan, T
Richards, J P
Saigal, S
Selvananthan, P
Shah, K
Shah, P S
Slyne, D J
Smith, F G M
Srivastava, A K
Steed, E A
Sudhakar, M
Sullivan, G
Tang, S Y
Thomas, D W
Thomas, K R
Vali, A M
Vatsala, C N

Mexborough
Agrawal, D L
Cooper, D N
Lathia, I
Leach, M C
Muthulingaswamy, M
Nagpal, I C
Sarkar, S H
Senaratne, K M J

Middlesbrough
Acquilla, D B
Aitchison, J D
Ajekigbe, O L
Al-Shukri, S J A
Amann, M E
Anderson, J T
Ankcorn, C T
Ashraf, S
Austin, G L R
Avery, B S
Bailey, S M
Baptiste, C E
Barham, N J
Barlow, S S
Barnes, L
Barsoum, M K
Barton, H R
Baxter, S M
Beere, D M
Bilous, R W
Blakey, J
Boggis, A R J
Bonner, S M
Bowes, C H G
Boxall, M C
Bramble, M G
Broughton, D L
Brown, P M
Buckle, S M
Burke, H B
Cann, P A
Canning, J T
Carmichael, A J
Chadwick, D J
Chandler, J E
Chappelow, E M
Chaudhry, B S
Chew, K S
Chilton, S A
Choo-Kang, A T W
Clarke, F
Clarke, F L
Clarke, J R
Coady, M S E
Cole, A W K
Compitus, B A
Cooke, W M
Corbett, B P
Corbett, W A
Cornford, C S
Cornwall, P L
Cruickshank, D J
Cuthbert, A
Dave, S V
Davies, A
Davies, J L
de Belder, M A
Dickinson, G
Dolan, J C
Donovan, D T
Doughty, J
Drury, J
Duggleby, M R
Duncan, T
Dunlop, P R C
Dunn, L E
Durning, P
Easby, J
Edge, C J
El-Naggar, M H R A
Ellerton, C R
Faulkner, M H
Firth, S
Fisher, R R
Flood, L M
Foley, M
Foster, T A
Fraser, W C
Frood, J D L
Garnett, A R
Gash, A J
Gavin, N A
Gedge, J
Gedney, J A
Geiser, P
Geldart, J R
Gjertsen, T A
Graham, S G
Grainger, J
Green, N J
Green, P A
Greenough, C G
Gribbin, H R
Gutteridge, E
Guy, I T
Hall, J A
Hampton, F J
Han, K H
Hardman, P D J
Hargate, G
Harrison, A M
Hartley, R W J
Haslock, D I
Hawthorne, M R
Helbert, D
Herbert, D W
Heywood, P J
Hodgson, G
Holtby, I
Horne, H L
Houldsworth, F J
Hovenden, J L
Howitt, M J
Hughes, J H
Hunter, S
Hunton, J
Hutchison, R S
Iqbal, S
Irvin, P J
Isserlin, B
Jacott, N J
Jawad, M S M
Jones, R A
Jones, S B
Joshi, N R
Kane, P J
Keegan, P E
Kelly, W F
Kendall, S W H
Kerr, R
Kessell, G
Khair, S S
Knox, J W S
Koh, J C H
Kokri, M S
Kon, P Y
Krishnan, R
Kuvelker, G W
Lakeman, J M
Lakin, A R
Lamballe, J
Lamplugh, M
Land, H R
Land, N M
Lau, W L M
Lawler, P G P
Lehmann, G A
Leigh, H
Levie, B B
Linker, N J
Lone, I A
Lucas, P A
McCarty, M
McCormack, P
McGuire, D P
McIlhinney, S W
McKeown, C O
McLean, K A
Main, J M
Majupuria, A
Malden, M A
Mamujee, S A
Marks, S M
Marshall, M
Martin, F W
Masinghe, N R
Masri, Z
Mehta, M
Meikle, R J R
Mian, M S-N
Middleton, L G
Miller, N B
Miller, R J
Milne, S
Mitra, S
Mohammed, H
Montgomery, R J
Morgan, J M
Morgan, T R M
Morrison, W J
Morritt, G N
Morritt, J A
Muckle, D S
Muddappa, Y N
Murdoch, R
Murphy, J G
Mutton, A E
Nagarajan, S
Nagendar, K
Nahhas Oubeid, A G
Naisby, G P
Naismith, L J
Nicolson, A
Noble, S G
Nugent, D
Oatway, H B
Oladipo, J O O
Oo, M
Opaneye, A A
Oswald, N T A
Owens, W A
Palczynski, S H
Park, G E
Park, J D
Parry, A D
Pettit, M
Phellas, A
Phellas, A J
Prasad, R C
Puttick, N
Ramwell, J
Ramzan, A Y
Rathmell, A J
Reaich, D
Reilly, J G
Ribeiro, A
Riddle, I F
Risebury, M J
Ritchie, C
Roberts, J H
Robertson, J D A
Robson, N J
Roth, L J
Rowell, N T
Royal, D M S J
Ryan, S M
Saha, R
Sanders, G L
Sandresegaram, K
Santosh, C G
Sarangapani, K
Scoones, D J
Selby, E M
Senor, C B
Seymour, H M
Shaw, S R
Shehade, S
Shrinath, M
Silcock, J G
Simpson, M D C
Sinclair, C J
Sinclair, D J M
Slade, P H
Smerdon, D L
Smith, R
Srivastava, P K
Starford, H
Stewart, M J
Stothard, J
Strachan, R D
Struthers, G D
Sutherland, M S
Sutton, W E
Symon, M A
Taggart, S
Tawse, S B
Taylor, P J
Taylor, W D
Teece, S C
Thompson, K W
Tiah, H A
Tilley, P J B
Toop, K M
Townend, A M
Ullah, A S
Van Der Voet, J C M
Veitch, D
Viva, C
Wakefield, S E
Wakerley, R L
Wallis, J
Walshe, D K
Ward, C R
Wasson, J F M
Waters, H J
Watson, D J
Webster, D D
West, A
Wetherell, H C
Wheeler, R J
White, C
Whiteway, J E
Wight, R G
Wilkinson, D B
Williams, B R
Williams, H I
Williamson, S F
Willimott, E J
Wilson, J K
Winnard, J A
Winter, A
Wood, A C
Wood, J
Wright, R A
Wyatt, G P
Wylie, J M
Wyllie, J P
Young, G R
Zabihi, T

Middlewich
Atherton, J B
Clifton, M R
Conrad, J J A
Curbishley, P G
Ford, D L
Jones, N L
Ratcliffe, B L

Midhurst
Brownlee, W C
Davis, E P
Dolin, S J
Forshall, S W
Foster, C J
Gabe, I T
Guthrie, T
Halfacre, J A
Hemming, J C
Hill, T J
Hopkirk, J A C
Horne, J H M
Hudson, A
Kelly, J B
MacCallum, A G
MacCallum, S K
Marien, B J
Masding, J E
Older, M W J
Power, N A
Sherrington, J M
Wilkinson, J C

Milford Haven
Evans, D L
Evans, P J
Garrett, C A
George, W T
Gunning, M P
Hickson, M J
Jones, T T
Lynch, W M G
Mackintosh, J F
Mathias, H C
Meagher, E M
Picton, J M
Sheikh, T B N
Warlow, A L
Williams, A D
Wright, C M

Millom
Cook, G
Johnson, E A
Matheson, I C C
Patchett, P A
Pogrel, G P
Walker, R C M
Walters, P J

Millport
Bryson, E A
Bryson, J A M

Milltimber
Al-Sayer, H M
Chabert, C C
Chithila, C J M
Denholm, M J
Downie, A J
Eagles, J I
Hogenboom Van Den Eijnden, M G E
McLauchlan, J
Morton, M A
Noble, C
Patterson, J E

Milnthorpe
Black, S L
Bonwick, H E
Calvert, F R
Cleary, P R
Darby, C T
Gorrigan, J H
Grocott, M P W
Irving, J A
Jackson, S F
Lomax, R J
Orton, C M
Parker, P J
Pearson, E J
Perham, E
Warren, M R
Wilson, S R
Yates, V M

Milton Keynes
Abbas, D
Allsopp, A
Anaman, S S
Anderson, F M
Anderson, N M
Araez Guarch, R
Assaf, A A-R S
Barker, G J
Barker, R W
Bates, R A
Bedford, C
Berger, A B
Berkin, P L
Bradley, C J
Bradley, J H
Bramley, M J
Brandon, E L
Bridgman, K A
Brown, P M
Bunting, N G
Butterworth, R J
Carson, N P S
Carter, R C
Cassidy, M P
Chambers, K H
Chambers, P H
Chowdary, K V
Clerkin, P M M
Clewett, V
Cowen, M J
Craggs, M E
Crankson, S J
De Gorter, J-J
Dewji, M R M
Dhanoa, S K
Douse, N A
Drouet, F H
Dua, J A
Dun, A F
Edwards, S
Evans, P A M
Fernandes, V
Fisher, C W S
Garai, G
Goodman, J C
Grinyer, S A
Gunn, R S
Hadi, Q M A
Hadida, A
Hanna, G F B
Haq, A-U
Hardingham, C R
Hassan, A O
Havard, A C
Hawkins, J M C
Haynes, J W
Haynes, P J
Herman, C R
Hickman, R J
Hildick-Smith, B A
Hilmy, H H
Hilmy, N M H
Hilton-Jones, D
Ho-Yen, R G
Holford, C P
Holowka, K A
Houston, J D A
Howard, E A
Huish, E F
Jaderberg, E M
Jawaid, H
Jeevananthan, V
Jenkins, E A
Jeyaratnam, D
Jeyaratnam, R
Johannes, S G
Jones, A P
Joss, D V
Kadom, A H M
Karia, A V
Katumba-Lunyenya, J N
Kempster, A
Khurana, P
King, B A
Kingston, A H
Labrum, A S
Lakhani, P K
Lambley, J C G
Lanzon-Miller, S
Latham, P J
Liesching, R A
Logan, C J L
Logsdail, S J
Lourie, J A
Lwin, K Y
Lynch, C B
McBride, D D
McCune, G S
McIlwain, L I M C
Mackenzie, L E
McWhinnie, D L
Madhotra, R
Mahendran, M
Mallick, D K
Marshall, A J
Mead, J L
Miles, P D
Miller, E J
Miller, G F
Mitchell, A
Mohammed, K I
Moore, P L
Morrison, D J
Moyle, J T B
Muir, J W
Mulligan, I P
Mwansambo, C C V
Nasiri, A Z
Nayani, G R
Nicolaou, A C
Nicolls, D B
Nott, J G H
O'Malley, S P
Odedra, N
Pai, E S
Patel, B B
Patel, R H
Paterson, R A H
Paton, R C
Petrides, S P
Philbin, J C
Philbin, K H
Pitkin, L J
Platford, J
Porter, J
Prisk, A J
Punch, D M
Reddy, J
Reddy, V L N
Robinson, G B
Rog, D J
Rogers, M J
Rohlfing, R F
Rose, E D
Roy, M
Sadiq, M N M
Sagoe, K B
Satchitananda, M
Schmidt, A C
Scott, S J
Shah, M R
Shapero, J S
Sharda, A D
Sharma, A
Shubsachs, A P W
Smith, N L
Smith, R W
Smith, T S
Sorrell, J E
Souter, R G
Staten, P
Suleman, A
Teago, P J
Thakker, Y
Thalakottur, J M
Thomas, P C
Toff, W D
Ullah, H
Walker, E M
Wanigaratne, D S
Watson, A
Weatherhead, S M
Wedgbrow, C S
White, A P
White, D M
Wolfendale, M R
Wyke, M E
Yahya, A
Yogarajah, S C
Zachariah, J
Zeina, B

Minehead
Currie, A L
Currie, M A
Davies, R
Earle, A M
Higgie, J M M
Hunt, C F
Jones, A M M
Kelham, I
Lamacraft, G
Mackie, C M

Nelson, A R
Neville, P S
Paine, Dr
Slade, P J B
Thomas, E A
Thomas, H G
Vale, S S

Mirfield
Bedford, M R
Best, M E
Clarke, J H
Cowan, D
Davison, M J
Dyson, G D
Eabry, E S
Gooding, J H
Grason, H G
Hall, P J
Hamilton, C M
Lukic, M
Mahmood, T
Panter, S J
Parker, R
Ridge, J A F
Warner, S T

Mitcham
Adjepong, K
Akinfenwa, O O
Akoo, M S
Butt, A
Chana, N S
Cochrane, M E M
Cohen, A R
Colborn, R P
De Silva, J V
Dewsnap, P A
Emmanuel, J J
Foster, H D
Freeman-Wang, T B R
Furey, A H
Ghodse, B
Gough, J S
Gunatilleke, A
Hannah, M C
Hill, K P
Hollier, G P
Kirupanantham, P
Lasserson, J A
Mangaleswaran, S
Mansfield, P A
Otley, A J
Patel, S S
Patel, S J
Rang, E H
Ravetto, S
Saxena, M K
Schapira, H
Shah, M A A
Strangeways, J E M
Syed, S B
Thet Tun, Dr
Thomas, A T
Vivekananthan, M
Von Fraunhofer, N A
Whitehead, P J
Yanney, M P

Mitcheldean
Martin, R E
Rodgett, A F
Weiss, P D

Moffat
Crosby, R R
Gillies, R
Gillies, S R
Graham, J A
MacEwen, G L
Robertson, J A
Sharkey, A S
Sloan, L M

Mold
Ali, M A
Banerjee, S
Baron, C E
Beckett, E I
Bickerton, D A M
Crossland, J S
Davies, A P
Graham, C M
Jones, R A
Muckle-Jones, D E
Mwambingu, F A L T
Payne, S A
Ranole, A-L G
Salib, Z R

Saunders, F M
Selman, R M
Shillito, R N
Shillito, W E
Woodward, S

Monmouth
Alliott, R J
Bagwell, A D
Blease, S C
Booker, D F
Calland, A L
Galbraith, J
Griffiths, A R
Harries, B D J
Jennings, J P
Jones, A H
Jones, C
Kelly, M-C M
Kindy, G R
Loffhagen, R J
Marsden-Williams, J
Matharu, M S
Matharu, N M
Messing, H J
Morris, C R
Payne, J H R
Phillips, A E M
Seymour, J
Shaw, S H D
Shute, J C
Steiner, D A
Visser, M J

Montgomery
Currin, S
Davies, R M
Lindsay, P H
Reid, A
Wynn-Jones, J

Montrose
Begg, A G
Calder, J G
Clunie, F S
Craig, D L
Cranswick, R C
Diack, P P
Diack, W G H
Drayson, A M
Forbes, W
Gammie, S C
Gavin, A J
Goode, H
Griffith, H E
Griffith, J M
Grove-White, I G
Hillyear, M E
Ireland, M
Kramer, G A
Logie, S A
Noble, J E
Orr, A W
Peden, K I
Rice, P M
Rodriguez Castello, C
Voice, S-A M
Walker, D R
Wilson, P M

Morden
Ali, S S
Anandarajah, T
Arulrajah, S
Day, C I
Frempong, R Y
Hariharan, S
Hawkins, P
Ho, G S W
Ikomi, A E A
Jephcott, J J
Jethwa, N K
Lawrence, E R
Lee, W P
Parameswaran, U
Perera, S T B
Piyasena, C
Sivagnanavel, S
Smith, A L N
Smith, N J
Soyemi, A O
Vivekananda, C
Wardle, N S

Morecambe
Bell, D T S
Brear, S E
Dillon, R
Ellis, J A T

Evans, C D
Forsyth, A S
Gartside, T
Grealy, M G
Grealy, S E
Greenwood, A M
Herd, G M
Ingham, W G
Ingram, D J
Kapur, H L
Khan, M I
Knapper, D O
McKinney, N H M
Macleod, A J
Maher, S P
Pidd, S A
Routledge, R
Seville, M H
Simm, F
Smith, F
Sykes, R A
Thomas, H R
Townley, P A
Williams, S J
Wilson, S M
Wimborne, J M
Winfield, P J W
Wood, G M

Moreton-in-Marsh
Barling, R G
Birts, R J
Bloxham, R E
Dastgir, M B
Every, M
Eyre, D H
Lutter, P S
Morton, C C
Towler, A

Morpeth
Anderson, P
Armstrong, H A
Barker, D C
Baylis, S M
Blair, A S
Bradley, P G
Cameron, A G
Cassie, G J
Cavill, G
Colver, A F
Colver, P A
Conn, J S
Craft, I
Craig, L J
Creighton, P A
Day, K A
De, D
Dower, F H
Dunstan, A
Edmondson, L
Edwards, S B V
Elphick, S J
Familton, H
Farndale, J A
Finch, K R
Flood-Page, P T
Fraser, A R
Gordon, S
Grant, W N M
Greaves, J D
Greenaway, M E
Griffiths, H W
Guest, J
Gunn, A
Gunn, M C
Hankinson, J
Harris, C L
Hatch, A L
Healicon, J E
Heggie, N M
Holland, H-C
Hopson, P R
Horner, M S
Howe, J W
Howells, K A
Hughes, A C
Hunt, P G
Jobling, S
Joyce, J P
Kerr, D M
Lothian, J L E
Lyons, G J
McElhinney, I P M
McLaren, A T
McParlin, M J
Marr, C
Menage, C M
Mitford, P

Morton, S T
Myers, J M
O'Driscoll, F H
Perini, A F
Pettifer, M W
Phipps, C K L
Power, J A S
Proctor, S E
Quinn, J S
Ridley, D C
Russell, J K
Sanderson, J
Savage, R
Scott, T B
Seager, M C
Sher, J L
Singleton, S J
Soundararajan, P C
Steel, C S
Stonelake, A V
Sykes, E
Tallantyre, H M
Thompson, K J
Thomson, G D
Tinegate, H N
Toop, R L
Turnbull, G H
Watkins, G D
Watson-Jones, E M C
Watson, H M S
Wilkes, S
Wilkinson, M E
Williams, L S
Winslow, N R
Wubetu, T
Yeoman, C M
Young, N J
Young, S H

Motherwell
Ashraf, M
Bell, L
Blake, K
Callaghan, M
Campbell, R J
Child, N J
Cross, T W
Cumming, A J
Fleming, M-C
Forrest, E F
Goudie, A W
Hamilton, R M
Henderson, J N
Hogan, L A
Hogg, W J
Hughes, N
Keegans, P
Keenan, J
Kerr, E C
Lando, J K
Liddle, R D S
Lochhead, J
Logan, A
Logie, B R
McBride, D F
McGill, B W
McGrane, S
MacInnes, D C
McKenzie, H J
Menon, K V K
Mishra, A N
Robertson, J F R
Robison, J M
Rose, G D
Russell, R J
Shah, M
Short, L C
Siddiquie, S
Sturgeon, J L
Thomas, E M
Tilley, M M E

Mountain Ash
Krishnamurthy, R S S
Kulkarni, S R
Manjunath, M
Morgan, D M T
Patel, M R
Putta Gowda, H M
Rajapaksa, R A M
Sanghani, J V
Sanghani, N
Sanghani, R
Skaria, J

Much Hadham
Brookbanks, C F G
Fiddler, G I
French, J L H

Haimes, P F
Mayson, R L
Milne, J R

Much Wenlock
Benbow, R J
Gainer, A J
Goodall, R C

Muir of Ord
Laing, M
MacDougall, D A
McKenna, M J
Pearson, S J

Munlochy
Fettes, C D
McNeill, L A
Watson, D A

Musselburgh
Binns, C A
Blaymires, K L
Blyth, A B
Carr, K
Clark, I M
Clubb, A S
Cochrane, M A
Duncan, S E
Fisken, M N
Frew, J M
George, R E J
Goh, D E
Hind, J
Johnston, I S
Jones, M E
Langsley, N
MacDonald, H L
Macdonald, P A G G
Maguire, E S
Marshall, I J
Miller, L M
Pearson, S L
Shaw, J
Walker, E C
Weeple, J A

Nairn
Adam, A
Adam, M G
Barrington-Ward, B
Bremner, H A
Cox, J B
Hogg, J Q G T
Macaulay, C Z
MacLennan, A
Noble, A L
Noble, J L
Scott, C H R
Scott, J M
Simpson, K
Stanfield, A C
Worthington, J

Nantwich
Alexander, R K
Appleton, R A
Barron, A A
Basu, R K
Blanchard, H C
Booth, N P
Brady, D W G
Brighten, K A
Cherry, T
Clowes, N W B
Coupe, A S
Davenport, G J
Deans, A J
Edgecombe, S J
Emery, F M
Fitzpatrick, C
Galiot Garcia, F
Hadrill, K C V
Harris, J P
Harrison, M O
Heal, M R
Holdsworth, S
Hollowood, A D
Hulme, S A
Hunter, P A
Johnston, R H
Jones, D M
Jones, R
Jones, V P
King, B A
King, N A
Knapman, J H
Mahmoud, A M A
Mayor, P E

Monaghan, S D
Moorhouse, P R
Morgan, J M
Okell, R W
Payne, J
Pugh, R E
Raeburn, A L
Rawsthorne, A M
Rawsthorne, G B
Roberts, K N
Schur, T
Smith, C D
Smith, M S
Spargo, J R
Walsh, S J
Warren, E
Winson, M D
Yousuf, K T

Narberth
Allen, P K
Cadbury, R C
Davies, A R
Edwards, F
Ghosh, A L
Harries, E W
Jones, D I
Mackintosh, M
Palit, A
Rees, D G
Rees, J E P
Vasfalcao, I I
Wood, S J

Neath
Ayers, R J
Bask, N T
Bennett, A C
Bowen, A C
Cook, B T
Copp, L
Davies, A S
Davies, D P
Davies, J P
Devichand, P
Driemel, S J
Dryden, P R
El Shazly, A H A
Elias, J
Evans, G V
Evans, W E
Gupta, M L
Hardie, D M
Harris, A A G
Herdman, G
Higgs, D S
Howe, A D
James, K E
Jenkins, D M
Jeremiah, G M
John, R B
Jones, R M
Jones, S L
Kahan, G K S
Kahan, R O
Kelly, D R
Khan, S
Khosa, N S
Langston, A
Langston, L
Lethbridge, J
Lewis, D
Lewis, R H
Li, M L
Lilley, A J
McMillan, A E
Madhavan, P
Mercurius-Taylor, L A
Morgan, D K
Morgan, H
Morris, H L
Muir, A M
Page, G C T
Pawar, J E
Phillips, S E
Potter, H C
Pradhan, K T
Pusey, C
Richardson, J
Roberts, M
Rogers, J H
Roper, B W
Rosser, C A
Rule, J
Schwarz, P A
Sheehan, B D
Skidmore, R B D
Sobhi, N H
Thomas, G R

Thomas, J
Ware, C-L
Westwood, P R
Wilkes, H F
Williams, E M

Nelson
Ashworth, I R
Aziz, S
Baldwin, K A
Banaszkiewicz, P A
Carr, J
Dodds, A A
Fleming, D R M
Golding, S K
Gude, S J
Guha, P K
Haque, F J B
Haque, M A
Haworth, J L
Ions, W M
Iwuagwu, C O
Jehangir, Q M
Lumb, M A
McDowell, D P
Marsden, N
Marshall, A R
Middleton, C M
Naheed, Y
Palmowski, B M
Pearson, J M
Pickens, S
Qazi, R A
Qureshi, Z A
Sarwar, N
Sarwar, S
Summers, J A
Thornton, S J
Webborn, D J

Neston
Meyer, G
Mitchell, S L M

New Malden
Acharya, D D
Acharya, J
Al-Yaqubi, N N
Arullendran, P
Austen, J C
Bailey, P E M
Balendran, R
Barrie, D
Berkinshaw-Smith, E M I
Bhattacharyya, S
Bindi, F
Brown, S E
Chang, S L-L
Chapman, C M
Chodera, J D
Choudhury, Z N
Crawford, P
Dale, C P
Denis Le Seve, P T
Dhond, G R
Dhond, M R
Fordham, G T
Garewal, D S
Gayed, H W
Ghosh, M
Ghosh, P K
Goel, G S
Goel, M
Grimmett, B M S
Gunasekera, A D
Gupta, B K A
Harris, J N
Harris, S M
Hassanally, D A
Insole, J
Iqbal, N
Jaitly, S
Jivani, A K
Jivani, N A
Lamb, F J
Levak, V
Lewis, S A
Luckett, J P
McAuley, C
McDonald, A M
Modarres Sadeghi, H R
Morgan, H M
Murphy, J B
Nathan, T
Nay Win, Dr
O'Connor, M P
Patel, H J
Patel, M B R
Phelan, A E
Phillips, S R
Qureshi, A M
Rahman, M
Reeve, S
Reid, B R
Sadiq, S T
Saeed, M
Samarasinghe, N
Samarasinghe, P C
Satkurunathan, S
Seddon, B M
Sharples, P E
Sheldon, N H
Sherski, L A
South, J R
Subesinghe, N
Syed, G M
Thursby-Pelham, A K
Thursby-Pelham, F W V
Wiessler, R E

New Milton
Bargh, D M
Barker, A S
Bentley, K D
Brewer, P
Campbell, P J
Clark, R M
Dathan, J R E
Davies, G A
Davies, J F
Davies, J W H
Ferguson, D J
Jenkins, D
Kent, J T
Lam, J Y C
Lambden, P M
McLeod, J B
Maule, L C
Parker, D J
Rutherford, A N
Thacker, M P
Thurston, T J
Watson, N F
Watts, B L
Willard, C J C

New Quay
O'Connor, L D
Rees, Y
Williams, D

New Romney
Cochrane, P T
Deane, J F
Swoffer, S J

Newark
Andrews, C A
Ashton, M B
Ayre, A N
Barber, P
Barker, J A
Bennett, J D
Bird, D I
Britt, R G
Britton, D E R
Busson, M
Campbell, L A
Chalmers, R M
Charlesworth, J P
Clayton, C P L
Compton, E H
Cosslett, A K
Coupland, R E
Davies, I W
De Gay, A
de Gay, N R
De Silva, P C
Dennis, P J
Donohue, S M
Durnin, C A
Finch, K M
Finch, M E
Gains, J E
Garrow, A D
Goodyear, P W A
Hardwick, E
Head, S
Healy, J M
Hind, R E
Ho, T H
Hogg, M J
Hull, R E
Hunter, M
Hutton, D A
Ilett, R J
Innes, C G
Jensen, P M
Johnson, J
Johnston, A J
Jones, P D
Keegan, N J
Kharkongor, S K
Knight-Jones, D
Lawrence, L K
Lawrenson, C J
Layfield, D J
Leach, V
Lennox, B R
Loudon, M F
McGill, J G
Machell, R K
Maung, S W
Mile, D J
Nelson, F G
Parkin, A J
Porter, J D
Prasai, J K
Pringle, M A L
Pullinger, S
Ramalingam, Dr
Reeves, P O
Reid, D A
Richards, R G
Ripley, M I
Roffe, T H
Ross, I N
Schlicht, J
Seivewright, H E
Selwyn, J E
Shearstone-Walker, C G
Smith, J M
Stenson, S L
Sullivan, C J
Sullivan, F D
Tweed, C R
Vohrah, R C
Waller, J M
Ward, H E
Ward, S M
Wathen, D J
West, T P
Wright, A C

Newbiggin-by-the-Sea
Imam, S B
Stephenson, T

Newbridge
Pandolfi, A L

Newbury
Agnew, N M
Anees, W M
Arnold, P D
Batagol, D M
Beverley, E A
Bingham, E
Bishop, M A
Bond, S E L
Britz, M
Brooke, P N R
Burman, R E M
Cave, J A H
Chapman, S
Chapman, S J
Choudhuri, S K
Clarke, B B
Collins, O D G
Davies, C E
Davies, D J
Donaldson, M J
Dyson, M
Ellis, E J
Elvin, B C
Endersby, K
Goodyear, K
Goulden, A D
Harrison, G M
Hughes, G M
Hunter, A E
Hyde, M F
James, S E
Johnson, I C
Jones, J R
Jones, J A
Jones, T J
Letham, B B
Lovegrove, S C
Lowenthal, L M
McManus, B N
Millard, P M R
Mitchell, I D
Morgan, P G
Muir, A M
Murdoch, C H
Nickson, J
Norman, M G
Norwell, N P
Penny, L A
Rendel, S E H
Ribeiro, N M
Robertson, P M
Rowe, J A
Sharpe, C M
Shillam, G N
Sievers, P F
Smyth, P J E
Steare, A L
Stiff, G H
Sullivan, A J
Tapper, R J
Taylor, M J
Thomas, J M
Thomas, K E
Thomas, M L
Titcomb, M L
Totten, E
Totten, J W
Treadgold, U A
Walker, S B
Walter, T N
Watson, R D
Weller, R J G
West, C J
Willis, C J
Wilson, B E
Wotherspoon, M G
Youdan, M E

Newcastle, County Down
Boyd, M W J
Bready, W D
Colgan, S J
Cox, G A
Cunningham, J
Denvir, C M O
Donnelly, M
Farrell, S
Flynn, M E C
Gallagher, F J
Gibson, J C
Graham, D M
Gray, O M
Hanna, G G
Hyland, S C
Keown, A P
Leggett, C D
Macauley, M R
McBride, D I
McCammon, W J
McCormick, J K
MacPherson, E S
O'Connor, N F
O'Neill, P M
Rafferty, C M
Ringland, R A
Sherrard, K E
Smith, A L
Torney, J J
Walker, R A
Walshe, K G

Newcastle, Staffordshire
Aber, G M
Agarwal, K K
Agarwal, S
Agarwal, S
Ashford, R P
Au, B T
Bell, G S
Bellingham, K M
Bhuvanendran, V
Bould, M D
Bowcock, L
Brooks, A R
Brown, A J
Butler, M J
Campbell, E D
Carmichael, I W D
Carson, P H M
Chadalavada, U B
Chitrapu, R K
Common, J D A
Cooper, W J
Cox, P W
Dias, P S
Dilly, S A
Dudson, C M
Dukes, S
Durber, C
Elliott, M D
Farrell, A J
Franklin, P J
Fraser, D G W
French, M E
Ganapathy, D H
Gardner, G I
Garnish, R P
Gray, J G
Green, R J
Griffiths, E A
Hapuarachchi, J S A
Heron, J R
Hollinshead, J F V
Hussain, F K
Hussain, S K
Jeyaratnam, P
Khan, M A
Khanam, S
Kirby, R M
Kulkarni, B N
Kulkarni, S B
Lauckner, M E
Lee, K W
Levine, A J
Little, S A
Lloyd, M E
McGowan, S W
McRobie, E R
Manudhane, V V
Martin, L M
Mellor, S J
Millson, D S
Morgans, G P
Naeem, A
Obhrai, M S
Pasi, K C
Patel, R D
Peasegood, J A
Prowse, K
Pugsley, A D
Ravichandran, S S
Rotondetto, S
Seddon, S J
Shah, S S
Sharma, S C
Shaw, P A
Shenton, K C
Shufflebotham, J Q
Skinner, M D
Thacker, B V
Tommey, M F
Tsang, W C
Tubbs, D B
Turner, N B
Tyler, P V
Wallbank, N J
Walters, F J
Williams, N D
Withers, P A
Zia-Ul-Hasan, Dr

Newcastle Emlyn
Brook, M T
Cole, D R
Davies, R J
Fitzwilliams, B C A L
Jones, H P
Lindsay, A O

Newcastle upon Tyne
Aal, B
Adams, B R
Adams, D M
Adams, E M S
Adams, P C
Adkin, D E
Advani, A
Agarwal, K
Aggarwal, M L
Ah-Kine, D
Ahmad, I
Ahmad, S
Ahmad, Y A
Ahmed, H S
Al-Barjas, M
Al-Harbi, O M A M
Alcorn, A S
Alexander, E M
Alexander, F W
Ali, A A
Ali, H M M D A
Allcock, L M
Allcock, R J
Almond, J A
Anand, Dr
Anand, A
Ancliff, H M
Anderson, C C P
Anderson, S N
Andrews, R M
Ansari, I A
Antoun, P C
Anumba, D O C
Appleby, M A S
Archbold, R A
Archer, K
Armstrong, J E
Armstrong, S E
Arya, A
Ashby, C B
Ashley, B K
Atkinson, R S
Awadh, M
Bach, S P
Bachh, Z J
Back, C P N
Badman, M
Baines, L A
Baker, L C
Baker, S F
Ball, S G
Ballard, C G
Banerjee, B
Barber, R
Barbour, J A
Barker, C
Barker, W A
Barnard, S P
Barnes, M P
Barnes, M P
Barrett, A M
Barrow, P M
Bartlett, S
Bassendine, M F
Batchelor, A M
Bates, C L
Bates, D
Bates, G H N
Baudouin, C J
Baudouin, S V
Baylis, P H
Bayly, P J M
Beacham, K J
Bell, D R
Bell, R
Bell, S J
Bell, S M
Benn, D K
Bennett, M K
Bennett, R P
Bethell, M J
Bethune, C A
Bevan, J D
Bexon, M F
Bexton, R S
Bhala, N
Bhaskaran, A M
Bhate, V S
Bhojani, M A
Biggin, C S
Binmore, T K
Bint, A J
Bint, A H
Birch, M K
Black, D A
Black, N M I
Black, S M
Blades, S M
Blain, P G
Blair, E L
Blessed, G
Bliss, R D
Blundell, M D
Bolton, D T
Bolton, J R
Bond, M E
Bone, M
Boobis, L H
Boonham, J C
Borthwick, M A
Bosanquet, R C
Bose, A K
Bourke, J P
Bourke, S C
Bourke, S J
Bower, S
Bowmer, R G
Boyce, R C L
Boyd, K T
Boyle, K R
Bozzino, J M
Bragg, P M
Branson, A N
Bratch, J S
Bray, R J

Brennan, P
Brettell, F R
Brewster, N T
Briggs, P J
Brittlebank, A D
Brock, J A
Bromly, J C
Brookes, P H
Brougham, C A
Browell, J A
Brown, A L
Brown, A S
Brown, J E
Brown, K
Bryson, M R
Bubb, S C
Buchanan, J M
Buchanan, J
Buchanan, R
Bullock, R E
Bunn, M R
Burden, P L
Burdon, A C J
Burn, D J
Burn, J
Burnett-Hall, C F
Burns, K M
Burridge, A
Burt, A D
Burton, C H
Bushby, K M D
Bythell, V E
Calder, C E
Callanan, K W R
Caller, P J
Calvert, A H
Cameron, D S
Campbell Hewson, Q D
Campbell, A T
Campbell, F C
Cant, A J
Carding, K A
Cardno, N
Carey, G R
Carmichael, J
Carr, W M
Carrie, S
Carrington, P M
Cartlidge, M E
Cattell, E L
Cavet, J
Chalmers, A J
Chalmers, G
Chamley, M
Chandler, B J
Channon, M E
Chaplin, D A
Chapman, C E
Charlewood, A M
Charlton, B G
Charlton, F G
Charlton, J
Charnley, R M
Chater, N C
Chatterjee, M
Chaudhri, S M B
Cheetham, T D
Chinnery, P F
Chipchase, B B
Chishti, A D
Chishti, S
Chopra, R
Choyce, M Q
Church, C J
Clark, A K
Clark, J E
Clark, S R
Clark, S C
Clark, S
Clarke, J
Clarke, L C
Clarke, M J
Clarke, M P
Clarke, T N S
Clasper, S
Cleghorn, N J
Clement-Jones, M T
Coapes, C M
Coates, L E
Codd, A A
Cogan, B D M
Cogswell, C C
Coipel, P M
Colbridge, M J
Cole, A J
Collins, A K
Collins, N S
Comaish, J S
Comiskey, M C
Conlan, B R
Connolly, J A
Conrad, K W
Cook, S
Cooke, R J
Cookey, H G
Cooper, E
Cooper, H B
Cooper, J C E
Cooper, K
Cooper, P D
Cooper, P N
Cope, M R
Cornelissen, P L
Corris, P A
Cosgrove, J F
Cottrell, D G
Coulthard, M G
Court, S
Cowell, H
Cowen, D
Cowlam, S R
Cox, J E M
Coyne, H M
Coyne, P M
Craft, A W
Craig, A M S
Crawford, D C
Crawford, P J
Cray, S H
Cree, N V
Cree, R T J
Crisp, A J
Croft, R J
Crompton, D E
Crooks, B N
Crossman, J E
Crossman, L C
Cruickshank, S G H
Cumberlidge, D F
Cummings, R A
Currie, A
Curry, K M
Curtis, H J
D'Silva, G C J
Dahabra, S
Dahl, M G C
Dalal, D K
Dalby, K V
Dalton, S J
Danjoux, G R
Dark, J H
Darling, C H
Datta, H K
Datta, K J
Davenport, R J
Davey, P
Davidson, E M
Davidson, N C
Davies, J B
Davies, M J
Davis, M
Davison, J
Davison, J M
Davison, S
Day, C P
Dayan, M R
De La Hunt, M N
De Soyza, A G
Deane, M
Deegan, J
Deehan, D J
Dexter, C S
Dhariwal, M
Dharmapriya, N S K
Diamond, C
Dias, C J
Dickinson, A J
Dickinson, W M
Diddee, R K
Dignum, H M
Dixon, J
Dixon, J H
Docton, A J M
Dodds, P A
Donkin, I
Donne, A J
Douglas, G
Douglas, R
Dowden, N
Drake, G P
Dresner, S M
Drinkwater, C K
Drought, T K
Dunleavy, D L F
Dunlop, W
Dye, R K
Dyer, H E G
Dyer, M P
Earl, C F
Eastham, E J
Eccleston, D W
Eccleston, D
Edmondson, R J
Edmunds, R B
Elliott, S T
Ellison, D W
Eltringham, M T
Embleton, N D
Emmerson, C I
Engeset, A-M
Evans, J A
Evans, S M
Evemy, K L
Eyre, K E
Fagan, J M
Fairbairn, A F
Falope, Z F
Fanibunda, H
Farley, A J
Farr, P M
Fawcett, P R W
Fay, A C M
Fay, F J
Feggetter, J G W
Fender, D
Fenton, A C
Ferrand, R
Ferrier, V
Field, A B
Findlay, N G
Finn, K L
Fisher, S
Fitzgerald, J M
Fletcher, I R
Fletcher, R M
Flett, M E
Flint, R A
Flohr, C
Flood, M K
Foo, C K
Ford, G A
Forrest, I A
Forsyth, R J
Forty, J
Foster, H E
Fowler, C E L
Fox, P S
Francis, A J
Francis, R M
Fraser, C J
Fraser, K A
Freake, D
Fulton, B
Furniss, S S
Fyfe, N C M
Gall, S A
Gallagher, H J
Galloway, A
Garner, P J
Garner, R E
Garrood, P V A
Gascoigne, A D
Gaur, A S
Gedney, J
Gee, M N
Gennery, A R
George, A M
George, M
Gerrand, C H
Gholkar, A R
Ghura, P S
Gibb, R C
Gibbons, C T
Gibson, G J
Gibson, M T
Gibson, M J
Gillett, T P
Gillie, R F
Gilvarry, E
Girling, D K
Gnanapragasam, V J
Gold, R G
Golden, L A M
Golightly, K L
Goode, P N
Goodship, J A
Goonetilleke, U K D A
Gordon, L R
Gould, F K
Gowda, R
Grace, J B
Graham, J Y
Graham, J C
Graham, L A
Grainger, D N
Gray, C
Gray, R J
Green, S M
Gregory, D A
Gregory, J
Greveson, G C
Gribbin, G M
Griffin, S M
Griffiths, A B
Griffiths, I D
Griffiths, J
Grime, I D
Groom, P I
Grubin, D H
Guellard, P S
Gumbrielle, T P M
Hainsworth, P J
Hale, J P
Hall, A G
Hall, K
Hall, R R
Hall, V A
Hamdalla, H H M
Hamilton, I J
Hamilton, J R L
Hamilton, S J
Hampton, P J
Hanley, N A
Hanley, S A
Hanratty, C M R
Hanratty, J G
Hanson, J M
Harding, S L
Hargrave, S A
Hargreaves, J N S
Hargreaves, K
Harpin, R P
Harris, A M
Harris, F P
Harrison, J W K
Harrison, M S
Harvey, J R
Hasan, S T
Haslam, N
Haslam, P J
Hassan, M S
Hawley, V
Hawthorne, G C
Hayes, N
Haynes, S R
Hayward, D
Healicon, R M
Healy, E P
Heap, R
Heardman, M J
Hearn, A J
Heaviside, D W
Heaviside, V A
Henderson, L M
Hendrick, D J
Henshall, A L
Herrema, I H
Hewitt, V A
Heycock, L J
Hide, I G
Hierons, A M
Higgins, B G
Higgins, E M
Hill, J
Hill, P M
Hilton, C J
Hilton, P
Hingorani, K
Hnyda, B I
Hodges, S
Hodgkinson, P D
Hodgson, J
Hogg, D W B
Holland, J P
Holland, J J
Hollingworth, R
Hollinrake, P U
Holloway, J S
Holtham, S J
Home, P D
Horgan, A F
Horn, J A
Horn, P A
Hornby, R
Horne, C H W
Horne, M
Hornung, T S
Howarth, D J
Hubbard, G H
Hudgson, M J
Hudson, J C
Hudson, M
Hudson, R M
Hughes, A N
Hughes, D G
Hughes, J C
Hughes, S C
Hunt, S J
Hunter, A S
Hunter, J
Hutchinson, D R
Insley, C A
Irvine, E M
Irvine, S T
Jackson, C R
Jackson, G H
Jackson, I D
Jackson, J M H
Jackson, M J
Jackson, R W
Jaffray, B
Jaiswal, A
Jalpota, S P
James, H
James, O F W
Jarvis, S N
Jenkins, A J
Jessen, E C
Jewitt, C B
Johnson, I J M
Johnson, S J
Johnston, I G
Jokelson, D R
Jones, C T A
Jones, D E J
Jones, D W
Jones, E A
Jones, F E
Jones, H E
Jones, M H
Jones, M S
Jones, N A G
Jones, P M
Jones, R B
Joseph, S A
Joughin, B M
Kanagasundaram, N S
Kandasamy, R
Kaplan, C A
Karat, D
Katory, M
Kaura, V
Kay, A J N
Kay, D W K
Kay, L J
Kaye, B
Kearns, P R
Keavney, B D
Keenlyside, R M
Kelliher, J
Kelly, C G
Kendal, R Y
Kennair, P
Kenny, M A
Kenny, R A M
Kent, R M
Kerr, C M
Khan, A L
Khanum, K
Khattab, A A E N H
Kilburn, J R
Kilner, A J
Kirk, C R
Kirk, S F
Knight, N F
Kong, S C
Kor, H S
Kumar, N
Kumarendran, M
Ladbrooke, K J
Lai, H M
Laidler, C W
Laker, M F
Lakha, S H
Lamballe, P
Lambert, D
Lambert, H J
Lambert, K E
Lane, A S
Lawrence, C M
Laws, D P
Lawson, A
Lawson, C N
Lawson, J E
Le Couteur, A S
Lee, A F C
Lee, I C
Lee, K S Y
Leech, N J
Leech, S N
Leeder, A
Lees, T A
Lees, Y C
Legg, J
Leigh, S
Lennard, A L
Lennard, T W J
Leonard, N
Leontsinis, T G
Lester, S E
Leung, H Y
Lewis, J
Liddle, A L
Lim, K L H
Lindley, A M
Linford, D V
Lingam, R Y
Lipman, D T
Liston, A M
Lloyd-Jones, N D
Lockett, A E
Lombard, L
Lonsdale-Eccles, A A
Loose, H W C
Loraine, C D
Lord, S W
Lovedale, C
Lovedale, I L
Lovell, P R
Lowes, S C
Lowry, S C
Lucey, R
Lucraft, H H
Lunn, B S
Lunney, R W
Lustman, A J
McAllister-Williams, R H
McAllister, V L
McArdle, P A
Macaulay, A
McCahy, P J
McClure, D
McClure, S J
McComb, J M
McCombie, C
McConnell, H D S
McConnell, T F
McCormick, K P B
McDonagh, J E
Macdonald, D W R
McDonald, F E
McDowell, G A
Mace, M
McInerny, D A
McIntyre, E A
Mackay, D C
McKay, G A
McKay, N D
McKeith, I G
MacKenzie, N T
McKenzie, T M
Macklin, H R
McKnight, C K
McLean, L M
McLelland, J
Macleod, S R
McMahon, C C
McMenemie, F M E
McNamara, C M
McNamara, P J G
McNulty, J F
Macphail, S
Macritchie, K A N
Maguire, A A
Mann, J
Mannix, K A
Mansfield, J C
Mansour, D J A
Marshall, C
Marshall, H F
Marshall, J R
Marshall, S M
Martis, P D
Marwaha, S S
Massey, C J
Masson, L J
Matthews, P R
Matthewson, K
Mattinson, A B
May, C D
Mears, C
Medhi, A C
Meggitt, S J
Mehra, P
Meikle, D
Mendelow, A D
Mensah, E
Menzies, R J
Metcalfe, S M
Michael, E M
Millar, M A
Miller, J S G

Milligan, D W A
Milne, D D
Milne, E M G
Milner, R H
Mitchell, L E
Mitchell, L
Moate, B J R
Moghal, N E
Mohammad, S
Mohammed, P D
Moore, A R
Moore, J M
Moorghen, M
Moorhead, S R J
Moran, G D
Morch-Siddall, J
Morgan, P
Morris, D
Morris, P T
Morrison, R P
Morrison, R H
Mulvenna, P M
Munir, A
Murchner, M P
Murdoch, A P
Murphy, C L
Murphy, O M
Murray, S A
Murrell, H M
Mushet, G L
Musson, J C
Myers, R E
Nanson, P
Nargolwala, V S
Nath, S
Needham, G K
Needham, H J
Nerurkar, M
Netts, P H
Newby, V J
Newton, J L
Nice, C A
Nichol, I E
Nicolle, A L
Nielsen, K C
Nissen, J J
Noble, G M
Noble, J M
Noronha, D T
Nyholm, R E
O'Brien, B S
O'Brien, C J
O'Brien, J T
O'Brien, S G
O'Connell, O
O'Hara, L A
O'Neill, K R
O'Reilly, M F
O'Shea, D D P
Oddie, S J R
Oliver, G
Olley, P W
Ong, L C E
Ong, T K
Orr, K E
Osborne, W L
Osei-Bonsu, M A
Owen, T C
Owens, J
Paes, P V
Page, K I
Page, V J
Pandit, R J
Panikkar, A
Parkin, J
Parkins, J
Parks, S
Parry, G
Parry, S W
Patel, H R H
Paterson, H R
Pattman, M G
Payling, S M
Payne, T C
Peakman, D J
Pearce, S H S
Pearson, A D J
Pearson, G L
Pearson, R C A
Pearson, T J
Pearston, G J
Peatman, S J
Pedler, S J
Pelham, A
Pemberton, J A
Pennington, S E
Perriss, R W
Perros, P
Perry, R H
Pettit, K E O
Peverley, M C
Phillips, E M G
Pickard, R S
Pickering, F C
Pickering, W G
Pilkington, G S
Pinder, I M
Pinnington, S
Platt, P N
Plummer, E R
Plusa, S M
Podd, T J
Poole, J
Pooley, J
Posner, N C
Postlethwaite, K R
Potter, J
Potter, S M
Potterton, A J
Potts, M
Powell, H
Powell, P H
Prentice, W M
Preston, M R
Price, S M
Price, T R H
Prince, M I
Procter, C N
Proctor, A J
Proctor, S J
Purves, I N
Quattainah, M A
Quigley, M P
Quinby, J M
Quinton, R
Qureshi, K N
Rahman, S A
Rainey, L
Rainford, P A
Raj, S K
Ramachandrappa, G
Ramesh, V
Ramli, N
Ramsden, A J
Ramsden, P D
Ramshaw, A L
Ranasinghe, H
Rangecroft, L
Rangecroft, M E H
Record, C O
Redfern, N
Reece, A T C
Rees, J L
Rees, R M
Regnard, C F B
Reid Milligan, D A W
Reid, C A
Reid, D S
Reid, M
Reid, M M
Reissmann, G F
Reynolds, N J
Rich, A J
Rich, G F
Richards, C G M
Richards, H C M
Richards, J E
Richardson, A
Richardson, C A
Richardson, D L
Richmond, S W J
Ringrose, T R
Rix, D A
Roberts, D R D
Roberts, J T
Roberts, M
Robertson, L M
Robinson, C A
Robinson, D P
Robinson, D C
Robinson, I S
Robinson, L A
Robinson, S J
Robson, D J
Robson, P
Robson, S C
Robson, V-A
Rodgers, A
Rodgers, H
Rooney, D
Rose, J D G
Rose, P G
Ross, D G
Ross, E
Ross, W E
Routledge, D J
Rowe, P W
Roysam, C S
Ruddle, J E
Ruff, S J
Rutt, G A
Ryan, D W
Ryan, J D V
Ryder, C
Rye, G P
Rylance, G W
Ryman, A E
Saigal, R H
Salih, I
Salkeld, D V
Salkeld, J V
Sammut, M S
Sanders, J H L
Sankar, K
Sarang, K
Saravanamuttu, K M
Sarma, T C
Saunders, P W G
Scarlett, C E
Schlesinger, A J
Schmid, M L
Schofield, I S
Scott, D J
Scott, M E
Scott, S J
Sein, E P
Self, C H
Sen, A
Sen, B
Sengupta, R P
Shabde, I
Shah, P J
Shah, S H
Shah, S G
Shakoor, S
Shamsah, M A
Sharma, P
Sharma, V
Sharp, C
Sharples, P M
Shaw-Binns, S
Shaw, F E
Shaw, J A M
Shaw, J P T
Shaw, P J
Shenfine, J
Shenfine, S D
Shiells, G M
Shinnawi, A K
Shipsey, D
Siddique, N
Siddiqui, F N
Silva, K G
Silver, A J
Simpson, K L
Simpson, N
Simpson, N B
Singh, M M
Skinner, J S
Skinner, R
Slatter, M A
Slorach, M
Slowie, D F
Smith, A J
Smith, D M
Smith, G A
Smith, J E
Smith, J E
Smith, J H
Smith, J P
Smith, K L
Smith, M J
Smith, M A
Smith, M R
Snell, C J H
Snow, M H
Snowden, C P
Sobo, A O
Solomon, S N
Somner, J
Sooltan, Y
Soward, K M
Sparey, C
Speight, E L
Spencer, B T
Spencer, D A
Spencer, I
Spencer, J A
Spickett, G P
Sprake, C M
Srinivasa Murthy, L N
Stafford, F W
Stafford, I
Stafford, M A
Stainsby, D
Stamp, P J
Standart, S
Stanley, J S
Stannard, K P
Stansby, G P
Stansfield, R E
Steckler, T H W
Steel, M D
Steel, S
Steiner, H
Stenton, S C
Stephenson, T
Stevenson, G
Stewart, J A
Stewart, M W
Stoddart, J C
Strick, M J
Strong, N P
Stuart, P R
Stuart, S
Sturgiss, S N
Sudarshan, G
Summers, S P
Sunter, J P
Sutton, D N
Swann, A G
Swanson, L
Sweeney, J E
Szeki, I K
Tacchi, M J
Talbot, D
Tansey, P A H
Tapson, J S
Tay, H L
Taylor, A E M
Taylor, P R A
Taylor, P J S
Taylor, R
Taylor, S C
Taylor, W B
Tharakan, P M
Thein Thein Wynn, Dr
Thick, A P
Thomas, A J
Thomas, D J
Thomas, J E
Thomas, P
Thomas, S H L
Thompson, A P
Thompson, M D
Thompson, N P
Thomson, P J
Thomson, R G
Thoppil, J P
Thornton, D
Tickle, C
Tiffin, P A
Todd, K P
Todd, N V
Tough, S L
Townshend, D N
Turkington, D
Turley, J F
Turley, S A
Turnbull, D M
Turner, A J
Turner, J M
Turner, S L
Turner, S M
Tweddle, D A
Twelves, N
Tyrer, S P
Tyrie, C M
U-King-Im, J M K S
Unwin, N C
Vallis, C J
Van Miert, M M
Van Zwanenberg, T D
Varma, J S
Veeder, A S
Velangi, M R
Venkata Rama Sastry, K
Vijayaratnam, D D
Villaquiran Uribe, J A
Vincent, A
Wadge, V A
Wagstaff, T I
Wake, P J
Wakeling, Z C
Waldron, A C H
Walker, D J
Walker, D R
Walker, J H
Walker, M
Walker, P A
Walker, R A
Wallis, J P
Walls, M Y
Walls, T J
Walters, F M
Walwyn, J L
Ward Platt, M P
Ward, J C R
Ward, K L
Ward, L E
Ward, M K
Wariyar, U K V
Warnell, I H
Warrington, S
Wastell, H J
Waterman, D
Waterston, A J R
Waterston, E
Watson, B G
Watson, D S
Watson, P G
Watson, S
Waugh, M
Weaver, J U
Weaver, M K
Weaver, N F
Weeks, P A
Weir, D J
Weithaus, N
Welbury, R R
Welch, A R
Weldon, J R
Weldon, O G W
Weller, C S
Wells, A W
Wells, C W
Welsh, J L
White, M J R
Whiteman, H R
Whitfield, K J
Whitford, D L
Whitley, S P
Whitney, P G
Whitty, P M
Wigglesworth, M D
Wild, N J
Wilkes, G
Wilkes, J A
Wilkins, D E M
Wilkinson, B J
Wilkinson, S A
Williams, C D
Williams, D O
Williams, J R
Williams, N
Williams, T L
Williams, V L
Wills, S J
Wilson, E M J
Wilson, J A
Wilson, K M
Wilson, N J
Winburn, P E I
Windebank, K P
Winter, E
Winterton, I S
Winterton, S
Wollaston, J F
Wood, M E
Wood, P C
Woodford, H J
Woodhouse, J
Woolfall, P
Woolhouse, I S
Woolley, M J
Worthy, S A
Wren, C
Wressell, S E
Wright, A J
Wright, C
Wright, M J
Wright, S E
Wyatt, M G
Wynne, H A
Yates, B H
Yates, P D
Yellowley, T W
Yeo, S T
Young Min, S A
Young, A H
Young, C A
Young, C F
Young, J R
Young, S J
Younghusband, A J
Yu Wai Man, P Y S Y
Yung, S Y R
Zainuddin, A A
Zaman, S J
Zamiri, M
Zammit-Maempel, I
Zimbler, N

Newcastle-under-Lyme
Bydder, M
Hay, E M
Hill, P
Hollins, M P
McBride, D J
Panayiotou, B N
Swan, C H J

Newcastleton
Blair, J F
Blair, M I
Kennedy, H W

Newent
Anns, J P
Bick, E E
Brooks, M E
Drewett, K A
Leigh-Smith, S J
Malkan, D H
Sillince, D N
Williams, D G
Wright, P H

Newhaven
Argent, L B
Barker, A M
Bradbury, A
Daintree, R A
Figgins, R
Kavanagh, M J P
Sharp, D J

Newmarket
Abel, M E
Alberts, J C J
Andrews, F
Arthur, N S
Bailey, T R S
Baxter, L A L
Bright, E A
Calvert, J W
Clifton-Brown, A F
Ellis, K A
Fawcett, C M
Gumpert, E J W
Kass, T L
Lloyd-Jones, K J
Lloyd-Jones, P M
Lomas, J A
Longman, R J
McLaren, J A
Magnusson, A
Polkinhorn, J S
Shaw-Smith, C J
Silverston, P P
Slowe, M R I
Sriskandan, K
Virgo, F E
Wace, M
Wace, R O
White, A J S
White, W L

Newmilns
Leslie, G J
Mackenzie, P M

Newnham
Bhageerutty, R V
Hutchison, J K
Nobbs, W M A
Parsons, C J
Reader, C A

Newport, Dyfed
Ennis, O W
Evans, H I
Lyon, T
Rees, D A
Revill, S I

Newport, Gwent
Al-Mitwalli, K A H I
Al-Mitwally, Q A H
Alderman, P M
Ambegaokar, S
Anstey, A V
Arnold, R C
Arsanious, N H N
Bassi, R
Bates, C A
Beech, C J
Bernard, M S
Blackmore, M G
Blyth, C P J
Bonn, W A

Bose, M K
Bowen, M E
Bright, J C
Brook, F M A
Brown, J W
Brown, J V
Brown, P
Browne, S E M
Burton, A J
Buss, P W
Callander, C C
Capper, R H A
Carr, A W R
Chandrasekaran, T V
Clark, G S
Clason Thomas, D H
Clayton, M I
Cole-King, A
Costello, J P
Cranfield, F R
Cribb, P E
Crocker, P D
Crosbie, J P
Curtis, J T
Dale, P J
Daniel, D G
Das, R P
Davies, D
Davies, E A
Davies, E G L
Davies, G J
Davies, G P
Davies, J
Davies, R
Davies, R W
Dennis, B D
Diggle, J H
Draper, T J
Dumont, S W
Dye, D J
Edmonds, J E
Edwards, W H
Evans, D R
Evans, V M
Faheem, F G
Farley, C A
Feltham, E R
Freeman, E A
Gateley, C A
Gibby, O M
Glynn, R P
Golden, M P
Gonsalves, R
Goodman, B
Goodman, K
Gower, R L
Gray, A R
Greenway, I P C
Griffith, G H
Hallikeri, C G
Hamilton Kirkwood, L J
Hanna, B W
Hannaford-Youngs, S J
Harding, J R
Hart, J K
Hasan, F
Hayat, M
Hayes, C
Hayes, M F
Haynes, T K
Hicks, J A
Holgate, N J
Holland, P A
Houghton, S J
Hughes, D S
Hughes, J M
Ingrams, D R
Jackson, D M A
Jackson, H A
James, T E
Jenkins, D A
John, C D
John, D W
John, R A
Jones, D G
Jones, G D
Jones, P A
Jones, P E
Jones, R N
Jones, R H
Jones, R G
Jones, S A
Jones, S N
Khan-Singh, J
Khonji, N I
Kilsby, A B
Kruger, M
Kubiak, E M
Kuzel, J J
Lalla, O V
Leitch, L M
Lewis, A J
Lewis, H
Lewis, J C
Lewis, P M
Lewis, W G
Llewelyn, J
Llewelyn, J G
McCarthy, G J
McCarthy, P M
McKenzie, J
Maguire, S A
Matthias, S
Mian, T M
Michael, R F
Mills, C M
Mintowt-Czyz, W J
Mishra, M D
Misir, A
Moffat, E H
Mohamed, H E A M
Monelle, T J
Morgan, D M
Morgan, W J
Morrison, M L
Moses, K W
Nichols, P K T
O'Duffy, D
Osmond, D F
Penney, M D
Perrin, S M
Petheram, C D
Phillips, D L
Phillips, S E
Powell, L J
Price, C J
Rackham, J P
Rampa, B R
Rawlinson, A
Rees, S
Rees, W H R
Richardson, F J
Riley, A J
Roberts, J E
Robson, D A
Rosehill, S
Russell, G K
Ryan, H S S
Sage, M
Saleem, H
Salvaji, A
Salvaji, C S
Sanikop, S B
Savage, R
Saxena, R N
Scholey, G M
Scholler, I W
Shandall, A A A E F
Shankar, Y P
Sheppard, T J H
Sherif, A S A
Shooter, M S
Sinha, J
Sinnett, K J
Sivagamasundari, U
Small, H J
Smith, T D
Srivastava, E D
Staniforth, J
Steiner, J
Stephenson, B M
Stewart, C G
Stone, A L
Stone, M
Stone, N M
Sturdy, D E
Sykes, P J
Tejura, H
Telang, S M
Thomas, A E
Thomas, A G
Thomas, D L
Thomas, S J
Thompson, S D
Toner, J M
Tonkin, L V
Trivedi, J
Tyers, R N S
Vellacott, K D
Venkataramanan, P R
Waheed, W
Wake, A M
Walpole, R H
Watkins, D W
Weerakkody, C S
Whittaker, A J
Wiener, J J
Williams, D H
Williams, D I
Williams, E R
Williams, J C
Williams, L M
Williams, P I
Williams, R S
Williamson, I J
Williamson, K
Wilson, G B
Wintle, C J
Wintle, J M

Newport, Isle of Wight

Alleyne, P J E
Baksi, A K
Basten, J E
Bateman, B J
Beisly, N L
Berrange, E J
Bingham, P
Brooks, M R
Budihal, S S
Cardew, S M
Cave, A P D
Chapman, S T
Chulakadabba, A
Close, P J
Demissie, A
Dick, C A
Elsmore, S
Ewell, E J
Gove, A R
Greenwood, N
Grimaldi, P M G B
Guthrie, A
Hakim, E A
Halder, S
Harwood, D M J
Hill, P J
Hobbs, N J
Jilani, M G-U-S
Johnson, I S
Knight, R J
Landon, K
Lindefors-Harris, B-M
McEwen, A W
Makunde, J T
Marsh, B A H
Mehmet, V
Mikel, J J
Mobbs, C N A
Murphy, D
Nasra, S E
Newson-Smith, J G B
Parsons, B E A
Premsekar, R
Pugh, M T
Routledge, N G
Russell, H J
Salih, M A
Saxena, S
Sherpa, T P
Shinkfield, M N F
Smith, J
Tobey, I
Watson, A H
Wellington, P E
Whelan, T R
Wilks, M
Wills, P C
Yoong, A F-E

Newport, Shropshire

Allan, T W B
Bayliss, L
Collier, S G
Davies, J
Dennis, J M
Egleston, A A
Fitzgerald Frazer, J S
Henderson, R J
Hopgood, E L
James, V U G
Jones, L A
Large, J
Lisk, C H
Mercer, D S
Patterson, R D
Rosevear, C
Saran, S
Sharan, K
Tindall, N J

Newport, South Wales

Ashraf, M T H
Webber, S K

Newport Pagnell

Beaver, D J F
Carter, I S
Greig, A V H
Hickson, C K R
Lees-Millais, J V H
Paton, A C
Skinner, P J
Slavin, B M

Newport-on-Tay

Adam, K P
Alexander, V A L
Clark, A D
Curran, J S M
Duncan, H S C
Gallagher, P M
Gray, I G
Hepworth, D M
Hundal, L M
Ingledew, M E
Johnston, M A
Kenicer, M B
Kilpatrick, A D
Mackintosh, N J
McQueen, F
McWhinnie, A J
Merrylees, N
Morton, I P B
Nixon, J M
Ricketts, N E M
Shepherd, B M
Von Goetz, T C B
Walton, L M

Newquay

Blackford, K E M
Boulton, J V W
Buscombe, P
Cornah, L J
Ettling, T M
Hunter, C B J
Ingle, J H
Irvine, W N
Judd, O F
Kersh, L G
Macready, D
Rigby, J M
Sleep, T J
Woolterton, S J

Newry

Ajam, G S
Allen, J A D
Allen, T P
Beattie, G C
Blundell, J
Brown, J R
Brown, R J
Byrne, T P
Campbell, C I
Campbell, R L
Carroll, A M
Conlan, E F
Connolly, N B
Corkey, C W B
Craig, J T
Cranley, B
Cunningham, A M
Cunningham, C
Cunningham, M J J
Curran, A M
Daly, C
Deane, M G
Devlin, B A
Devlin, J E
Digney, J M G
Dillon, B A
Donnelly, P M
Dooley, A P
Farrell, W J A
Fearon, M J
Fearon, P V
Fegan, M
Finnegan, D P
Finnerty, M
Flood, R B
Flood, R D
Flynn, C
Forshaw, S E A
Foster, J H
Gaskin, P M
Gaw, D H
Gilpin, D A
Goss, K C W
Hanna, W J
Harty, J C
Heaney, H A
Hughes, J
Kearney, A B
Kelly, M
Lambe, M B
Larkin, M P
McAlinden, J M F
McAreavy, J
McAteer, H M
McAteer, J
McBreen, G M M
McCaffrey, P M
McCann, B H G
McCann, J J
McCann, M C
McCormick, M T
McDonnell, O L
McDowell, H M
McEvoy, P M
McGivern, A
McGivern, A M
McGivern, J
McKeown, R M E
McKinney, K A
Mackle, M G E
McKnight, M
McLaughlin, A B
McLaughlin, H
McVerry, I T B
McVerry, M M J
McVerry, M G
McVerry, R G
Magee, D J
Maguire, B M
Maguire, P B
Maguire, S M
Mathew, P M
Mercer, J M
Morgan, L C M
Mulholland, A O
Mulligan, P M
Mulvaney, D G
Mulvaney, G P
Mulvaney, G A
Murphy, M J
Murray, L E
Nash, D T L
O'Brien, C J
O'Donoghue, D B
O'Donoghue, P
O'Hanlon, D T J
O'Hare, A G M
O'Hare, M
O'Hare, M F
O'Leary, T
O'Loughlin, A M
O'Neill, M M
O'Reilly, D M M
O'Reilly, N
O'Rourke, F M
O'Shaughnessy, D M K
Poots, S A
Quigley, P J G
Quinn, F M
Quinn, M M
Quinn, M F
Quinn, R P
Radcliffe, J C
Ratnavel, K K
Reynolds, J M
Rice, E A
Ryan, P F M
Sadler, E
Shannon, E G M
Shields, M O
Shortall, M T
Sim, D A J
Simpson, J A
Sloan, R
Smyth, A
Stokes, M A
Sweeney, C M
Synnott, M E
Treanor, O T
Vettiankal, G G
Walshe-Brennan, K S
Ward, P J
Watters, B V
Woods, W G
Wright, J M
Wright, P J

Newton Abbot

Al-Ashbal, S
Al Fulaij, S
Almond, A J
Arain, A M
Arthur, P J D
Ashworth, R N
Avery, C M
Bates, K J
Beable, R A
Beck, J-K W
Beddoe, V K
Bellamy, P
Bellis, F
Bennett, J R
Bloom, V R
Bowen, J M
Branson, H I
Brown, E A
Brown, K A
Brown, N P R
Bryant, R N
Campbell, B M
Clarvis, M C
Clegg, A J
Cooksley, R
Crawford, S G W
Curtice, M J R
D'Arcy, N J
Densham, P R
Doidge, N H
Dommett, R M
Dudgeon, T A
Dunn, A R
Dunn, J W
Dunn, W K
Dyer, S J
Ellis, D J S
Every, H M
Galli, P R
Gordon, C
Greatorex, D G
Hale, A
Hammersley, A G
Harber, M A
Hatton-Ellis, G W
Hay, D S
Heather, J D
Henwood, B P
Hickey, S A
Hoffman, M M D
Hopkins, R J
Houghton, P W J
Howell, J R
Howes, D E L
Hughes, A S
Hunter, N O
Kelly, D J
Kennaird, D L
Kinsey, V E
Lee, M J C
McDermott, M E
Marsh, S G
Martinus, P M
Melluish, V S-A
Milburn, D
Millar, J P
Morris, T A W
Munk, M E V
Murphy, C A
Orr, R B F
Orton, D A
Parke, R J G
Parker, F A
Parker, P W M
Pearce, D N
Phemister, J C
Ranjit, R
Richards, M J
Roberts, N I
Robinson, A J
Robinson, S T
Rowe, E
Rushton, S R L
Sharp, B T
Smout, S M
Stackhouse, J R
Stanley, P H
Stride, A
Wade, C G B
Wade, R G H
Watkins, N A
Weeden, A C
Wildgoose, N W
Wills, R E
Wollaston, S
Wood, P T
Wright, K J
Yeldham, D L

Newton Aycliffe

Apps, A J L
Bamford, M R

Clarke, A S
Ferguson, G
Jones, M G
Luder, H J
Martin, H
Pounder, R
Qidwai, A
Ramsay, P D
Scott, C W D
Sheldon, D M
Shenton, A F
Sudarshan, C D
Walker, G R

Newton Stewart
Baird, D M
Bremner, B-J
Clark, K
Conner, A M
Ducker, C J
Grove, R A E
Jones, T A
McClintock, C P
McLean, I C
McNab, D S
Marshall, M
Miscampbell, N T
Murphie, R W
Roe, J
Sutherland, S J

Newton-le-Willows
Arya, R
Bentley, J I
Brierley, J
Crotch-Harvey, M A
Foster, R N
James, A
Lim, H H
Lowe, S H
Mahajan, H R
Malham, P A
Pitalia, A K
Pitalia, P L
Raza, M
Shetty, N V
Smith, C
Whittaker, J A T
Wynne, I C

Newtonmore
Fraser, D R M
Kirk, A M
Martin, E P

Newtown
Griffiths, D L
Harries, J D
Hayes, H J
Hughes, G J
James, S P
Lewis, K A
McVey, T J
Nevill, C G
O'Brien, M B
Porter, A
Schaefer, W
Selly, E W
Swan, A J
Wilson, M S G K

Newtownabbey
Abdul Rahim, S
Allen, J S D
Archbold, G P R
Armstrong, D J
Bailey, M C
Balmer, G J
Beattie, I J
Bell, R E
Bennett, E V
Boston, B K
Boyd, K
Brolly, T B
Brown, G L
Buchanan, I S
Buchanan, S B
Byrne, E P
Charlwood, A P
Condron, C K
Corrigan, M M
Crosbie, P J
Darrah, A J J
Davies, P L
Davies, R C S
Davison, P M
Devine, P M
Doggart, E R
Donaghy, P F
Duke, D F
Evans, S A
Ewart, K E
Fair, E A
Flynn, P G
Gamble, J A S
Gibson, J A
Gilmore, J E
Gould, C H G
Gray, J G
Harbinson, M E E
Hart, D J
Hegan, M C
Hendron, M P
Herron, N M
Hill, G
Houston, J R
Ingram, P J
Jenkins, L E
Jennings, R K
Kane, R
Kennedy, R J
Kyle, C J
Lyons, P
McCloskey, A M
McConkey, K
McCullough, A I
McCusker, T M M
McGimpsey, W D
McGowan, C M
McGrath, J S
McKenna, U M
McKenzie, R J
McKeown, D F G
McSorley, F A
Meenagh, C P
Meenagh, G K
Montgomery, D A
Neary, D M
Neary, J G
O'Connor, B S
O'Hare, J
Oakey, H M
Page, B E
Patterson, A J
Poh, C H
Rendall, J C
Seymour, S C
Sloan, S A
Small, L L
Smyth, W R
Spence, C S
Stewart, E J
Toland, W J
Whiteside, M L
Wright, D G

Newtownards
Anderson, J
Armstrong, M F J
Bailie, L M
Bamford, L C
Beattie, C K
Bissett, J
Boston, V E
Bradley, M L
Brown, S J
Bryson, J M
Buchanan, S
Bunn, R J
Calvert, C H
Campbell, H
Cathcart, J-M B
Clarke, P
Clements, W I
Cobain, T G
Compton, D M
Coulter, R S
Davidson, K E
Donaghy, U M
Donaldson, D J
Duke, F J
Elwood, S L
Ferguson, W P
Ferris, J H N
Foster, W F
Gibson, D R
Gilbert, J H
Gilbert, J K
Glennie, A C
Green, J F
Groves, D H M
Harbinson, H J
Henry, I B G
Hicks, E M
Higgins, D A
Hinds, O
Houston, D G
Hughes, D F
Hughes, P L
Jack, C M
Johnston, N J
Kennedy, G D
Kennedy, R D
Kirk, K T K
Lees, E J
Leonard, E J
Lowry, R C
McAuley, D J
McCance, J M
McClements, P G
McClure, P T
McElheron, M L
McGaughey, D G
McIlfatrick, S D
McIlwaine, W J
McKeown, M E
Mageean, R J
Marsh, W G
Martin, P S
Mathison, C D
Mitchell, M A
Mitchell, P J
Moffatt, W R
Moffett, G S J
Moles, G I D
Moorehead, R A
Newell, K A
Noble, J R
Park, J M W
Peacock, D
Petherick, C S
Poulter, A E
Price, G F W
Quaite, T J
Reid, G D
Riley, M S
Savage, D M
Scott, A
Scott, L I
Semple, D K
Shanks, N R
Smith, M R
Smyth, R J
Steele, H D
Steele, M A
Stelfox, D E
Stronge, K A
Trinder, T J
Winter, J K J

Normanton
Aruna Prasad, G
Barber, E A
Bazin, M L F
Clift, J L
Dewhirst, P
Ellis, J
Gupta, R P
Hunter, I A
Shaw, C Q
Wunna, R

North Berwick
Boardman, A E
Boylan, B P
Crawford, M E L
Flynn, M W
Jones, N D
McEwan, P N
Mulrine, A T
Petrie, A M
Pretsell, A O
Salucci, G U

North Ferriby
Alexander, P J
Barchard, M C
Beardsworth, S F
Bennett, S R
Carter, D A
Clarke, R G
Dealey, R A
Griffith, R J
Holwell, A D
Hood, E A
Hunter, P J
Innes, J R
Klakus, J A
Koul, K K
Maguet, H
Mitchell, R G
Naylor, U V P
Rogers, M A
Rutherford, S
Saleh, A H S
Siuda, Z E
Speck, E H
Tuck, S P
Walton, C
Ward, A E
Welch, C J

North Shields
Akak, A M
Anderson, K N
Baird, M E
Bale, C J
Barton, J R
Bates, A M
Benjamin, C M
Bennett, S M A
Bertram, R W
Bolton, A R
Carter, L J
Cassidy, J V
Chatterjee, A K
Chinyandura, M N
Clark, J A
Cobden, I
Cox, J E
Curless, R H
Derry, J A
Doig, J C
Drury, C A
Earl, D S
Eaton, S E M
Emam-Shooshtari, M
Evans, D A
Firth, R J
Freeman, H C
Freeman, L J
Gandy, A S
Gayner, A D
Genever, A V
Ghazal Aswad, S
Goring, C C
Goulbourne, I A
Greenwell, S K
Grove, M L
Harrigan, P
Horgan, L F M
Houlsby, W T
Hughes, J C
Hussain, S
Jackson, J M
Jaiyesimi, R A K
Jelley, D M
Johri, S
Jones, A I
Kasaraneni, R
Kelly, S B
Knox, J C
Lambert, M W
Lawrence, M R
Lewis-Barned, N J
Livingston, M M
Lowry, R J
McCallum, J E
McKenna, P
McManners, M M
Majumdar, A
Mason, C A
Megson, K
O'Hanlon, S
Parkinson, D R
Parkinson, G
Patterson, H
Peel, E T
Pollard, R
Prasad, M G
Ramachandra, C R S
Reed, M R
Riordan, D M
Roberts, J B
Roberts, S H
Robertson, J
Rodgers, A D
Safe, G
Sedgwick, P A
Shabde, N
Slater, B J
Smith, S E
Spink, C E A
Stainthorp, D H
Tapsfield, W G
Taylor, A J
Tennant, D
Tiwari, R K
Tomson, D P C
Van Kampen, M
Walker, R W
Walker, S E
Welare-Smith, J M
Westgarth, T J
White, L F
Woodhams, A M

North Walsham
Davidson, S L
Dunn, W T P
England, M H
Everden, P R
Pickersgill, D E
Pickersgill, H B
Price, G A R
Robinson, D T
Ryan, C E
Strivens, E
Tyrynis Thomas, S A
Vavasour, S M A
Whitfield, F
Young, R J

Northallerton
Allan, J M
Allen, L-C
Allerton, K E G
Allison, C E
Benford, S C
Berens, J
Bhatt, B M
Bosman, D A
Brereton, A G
Browning, M E
Browning, N M
Bryce, F C
Burton, L J
Butterworth, K
Caramello, A J
Carpenter, M R
Cummings, T F
Curry, A W
Das, K
Dickson, D J
Eames, A M
Edon, P J
Enevoldson, H J
Erena Minguez, C
Essex-Cater, A
Fenwick, M J
Fisken, R A
Foster, S
Gough, A
Hannon, C
Hebblethwaite, N
Henderson, D C
Herbert, A P
Hilborne, J
Jackson, D G
Jackson, G D
James, J R
James, R
Jayasuriya, T G
Kabuubi, J B L
Kane, G G
Leigh-Howarth, M
Liow, R Y L
Lough, M J
McNeela, H E
Miers, S W P
Mountain, D
Mumford, J D
Oates, C G
Prasad, K V
Puranik, I
Ramsden, P A
Roberts, A P
Samarage, S U
Sarathy, S
Simpson, C J
Smith, W M V
Thompson, M C
Todd, C L
Tune, G S
Van Hoogstraten, J W A P
Waldron, J H
Walters, A
Walton, M R
Walton, R S
Ward, D C
Weightman, N C
Wilson, A E
Wolfe, S S
Yoong, S Y
Zelenka, R M

Northampton
Abbatt, R J
Abbott, V J
Absoud, E M
Ackland, F M
Aitcheson, P E
Al-Hamed, M H
Aldrich, C J
Alston, D J
Anthony, J P
Arnold, P D
Astbury, P
Atkinson, A J
Bailey, R D
Bainton, V C
Barritt, S A
Barrowclough, M D
Bassett, L C
Beeson, M
Bell, C R W
Berry, A R
Bhala, A
Birch, N C L
Bird, N J
Birkhead, J S
Bissessar, E A
Blackman, C P
Blanshard, C G
Bolland, J A
Bond, M L
Bonthala, C M
Boon, J E
Bowen, A L
Bridges, M J
Brown, E M
Brown, H J
Brunt, N J
Buck, D C
Buckler, D G W
Budge, T S
Burston, D J
Button, M R
Byrne, P K
Cain, P T
Caldwell, N E
Cazes, C I W
Chandarana, V C
Cherry, J E
Chipchase, J G A
Chmielewski, A T
Clark, A R B
Clarke, J
Cleal, D J
Coghill, H M
Coghill, S B
Collinson, J G
Coneys, T D D
Coombs, M C
Cowper, R A
Cradduck, G W
Crawford, T E
Crawfurd, E J P
Crowhurst, E C
Damle, A D
Davey, P P
Davies, E S
Davies, R E
Davis, T C
Dawson, J W
De Brauw, D F R
Donald, E A
Donald, J F
Duggan, L M
Duncan, A R
Duncan, C F
Dwivedi, K N
Eagland, J M
Edwards, A T J
Ellam, K S
Ellis, D Y
Fairlie, N C
Fearnley, I R
Fenton, J
Ferguson, H C
Ferguson, J S
Fletcher, J K
Fogarty, A C
Fox, C J V
French, C M
Frerk, C M
Gardner, R R
Ghobrial, L A I
Gibbons, K J
Gidden, D J
Gidden, F A
Gill, T J
Gillam, D M
Gillam, M L
Gilmore, A
Gleeson, C M A
Goldsmith, M J
Goodwin, M W P
Gordon, A C H
Gordon, C A
Goulding, S R
Gower, S G
Gralton, E J F
Greening, S L

Gregory, A L
Gregory, S D
Griffin, J M
Gurr, P A
Haines, M E
Hallas, C L
Halstead, H E
Halstead, P J
Hamer, D B
Hancock, A
Hancock, R J
Hare, J D
Harisha, J
Haw, C M
Heaney, D C
Heaney, P C
Hein, N
Hellen, E A
Hewertson, J
Hewitt, C S
Hewitt, N D
Hicks, R C J
Hill, J H W
Hill, K E
Hillier, A R
Ho, M
Hollway, M C
Hopkisson, J F
Horsnell, S P
Hunt, I J
Hunt, J A
Hunter, D C
Ireland, J P
Islam, S
Jain, A K
Jayasuriya, H
Jeffrey, A A
Jeffreys, D G F
Johnson, J M
Johnstone, E D
Kay, N H
Kay, V J
Kaye, P M
Kendrick, R G M
Kerr, G R
Khalil, K H
Kilvert, J A
King, J E
Kirkbride, D A
Kirresh, Z O I
Kirwan, M
Krishna Rao, C
Kunkler, R B
Kyriazis, M
Lad, N
Lakha, A A
Lamba, K S
Leroy, A E
Leyden, K M
Lindenbaum, K M
Lindenbaum, R J E
Littlewood, P B
Lloyd, C P
Lloyd, K
McCracken, M
McCullough, W L
McFarlane, J O
McKenzie, J
Macmillan, C H
McNicholas, J J K
McQuillan, W J
Mahood, J M
Makhani, F A
Makwana, N V
Mann, C M
Marsh, R H K
Marshall, C I
Mason, F L
Mason, F M
Mather, D C
Mathew, R
Mattingly, S
Mead, H M B
Meara, J R
Meeking, D R
Miller, D W J
Miller, M A W
Minassian, M A N
Moffat, B
Molla, A L
Molyneux, A J
Moore, C J F
Moore, F C
Morgan, P R F
Morgan, R J
Morrant, B L
Moss, C
Moss, F L S
Mudaliar, R K
Mukherji, C S
Murali Krishnan, M
Natarajan, R
Nawaz, M
Nevison-Andrews, D G
Norton, K J
Nottingham, J F
Nuttall, J B
O'Callaghan, D P
O'Connor, M
O'Donnell, J G
Ogilvie, A L
Orr, M W
Oswald, T F B
Otto, A D
Paine, D L S
Patel, S R
Penfold, H A
Perez, A
Perryer, C J
Pickering, A J-M C
Povey, J R
Poyner, F E
Price, S M
Pyke, M R
Pyke, R
Quinn, L A
Raouf, A H
Raphael, J A G
Ratliff, D A
Reddy, G
Reeder, J A
Reynolds, T H
Ribbans, W J
Rickerby, J
Rigden, B R
Roberts, J
Robinson, K N
Rogers, S M
Rose, M J
Ross, J R Y
Sankar, S
Saqib, M N-U
Saynor, C E
Sebugwawo, S
Sefton, D
Seiger, D G
Shaxted, E J
Sherwood, P V
Shmueli, E
Shribman, J H
Shribman, S J
Smart, D J
Smith, S J E
Smith, W P
Soloff, N
Sood, K K
Southcott, M R
Spencer, H J
Sprigings, D C
Staley, C J
Stevens, G C
Stewart, J A
Stockley, A T
Stockton, E F
Stubbs, R P
Sugarman, P A
Surendra Kumar, D
Sutton, A
Sutton, T M
Swaroop, M
Swart, S S
Tahghighi, J P
Tanqueray, J F
Tapsell, S H J
Taylor, J C
Taylor, J B
Thomas, D
Thomas, V
Thompson, F J
Thompson, S A
Thompson, S
Thornton, D J
Tickle, S A
Timmins, B C
Toseland, O R
Tough, H G
Tripney, R E S
Tunnicliff, M
Twigg, A I
Twigg, S F
Vann, A M
Vince, A S
Von Widekind, C H E
Wacogne, I D
Wade, D C
Wadley, M S
Walker, C A
Walker, G J
Walsma, P
Walton, J L
Ward, A R G
Warwick, H M
Webster, R E
West, R C
Wharton, R Q
Wheeler, J M D
White, J B
White, R R
White, T J
Wilkinson, M B
Williams, A N
Williams, A J
Williams, R F
Willis, A W
Willis, E M
Willows, M A
Willows, R I R
Wilson, B A
Wilson, C R M
Wolverson, K
Wood-Allum, C A
Wood, I R
Wood, P
Woodhams, L J
Yates, S
Yorston, G A
Yule, S F

Northolt

Ali, S O
Azra, S
Balachandran, G
Bell, L C
Bhatt, R K
Campbell, D J
Hopkins, C T
Hui, K W
Hundal, K S
Hussain, M
James, A K
Joshi, B V
Kassam, S G
Khanna, M
Knight, D G
Koupparis, L S
Lewis, A D
Nwachuku, O M
Pal, D
Pal, M
Patel, C B
Patel, D
Prashar, S
Quadri, F R
Sarna, N R
Seimon, J W M S C
Seimon, J W M J B
Wogu, G U E

Northwich

Adams, A S
Anthwal, V M
Ashworth, M
Barratt, C J
Bartlett, G V
Beastall, R H
Bill, E J
Brennan, A L
Brettell, A
Brown, S J
Buckley, P W
Cade, D
Cawthray, P A
Chapman, R O
Cranmer-Gordon, C R
Cronin, P A C
Curran, A L M
Daniels, M S
Dentschuk, A
Dickinson, M A J
Eastaway, A T
Entwistle, G D
Flippance, P D A
Forsyth, W J
Fox, E E
Gurnani, H M
Haeney, L K
Hambidge, D M
Hammond, J H
Harding, V
Hignett, R
Hollinrake, M S B
Hughes, R J
Jackson, S R
Jefferson, M F
Jenkins, J E
Jennings, A C M
Kerslake, J C
Kilby, F K
Langworthy, G W
Llewellyn, M B
McGregor-Smith, F A
McIntosh, R E
Morris, C M
Murphy, R J
Norman, A S
O'Byrne, E K
O'Donoghue, A
O'Sullivan, J J M
Oldfield, P D
Patrick, J M
Rickard, S P L
Rossall, A M
Royle, R A
Rushton, A M
Russell, N A
Saunders, G J
Slaney, C J
Smith, T A
Strefford, T I
Taberner, D A
Torrance, J M
Westwood, S L
Whittaker, W A
Wilkinson, G M

Northwood

Abrahams, Y
Amos, C F
Ansari, M A
Apthorp, G H
Apthorp, H D
Ashford, R F U
Ataullah, I J
Atkins, J-A L
Ayoub, A-W A A
Baddeley, H
Basden, R D E
Bell, G T
Bleehen, I S
Brodrick, P M
Brown, M J C
Bucknill, A T
Burcombe, R J
Carr, D H
Chalmers, A J
Chatoo, M H B
Coleman, J D
Collins, K M
Cussons, P D
Dawrant, M J
Denton, A S
Dhupelia, I R
Dische, S
Duncan, M H
Eykelbosch, G
Fermont, D C
Gajjar, B
Gandhi, A G
Gardiner, G T
Gault, D T
Geary, P M
Giora, A R
Glover, G W
Glynne-Jones, R G T
Goh, V J-L
Goodman, H
Goodwin, P R
Goolamali, S K
Greenhow, D S
Grenville-Mathers, A
Grewal, R S
Haider, S I
Hall, M R
Hammond, T M
Haring, S J
Hoskin, P J
Hughes, P A
James, E B
Jeetle, G S
Jeffery, L A
Kang-Budialam, N V
Kant, S R
Karia, K
Khan, J
Khaw, K S
Kingsley, S M
Lab, D M
Lamb, J K
Lemon, C
Liebeschuetz, S B
Lyn, B E
Machesney, M R
McKeating, J B
Maddox, A J
Maher, E J
Majid, A
Makepeace, A R
Makris, A
Mansoubi, H
Melia, H C
Melia, N P
Mellor, S J
Mills, D C
Mitchell, M H
Mitchell, R
Mitchenere, P
Murtuza, B
Murugesh-Waran, S
Nathoo, Y
Navapurkar, V U
Nawarski, B J
Nicholas, N S
Obadiah, R
Padhani, A R
Phillips, J B
Potts, J J
Rees, G F M
Rivlin, R S
Rustin, G J S
Sarin, S
Saunders, M I
Sayeed-Uz-Zafar, Dr
Scadding, F H
Scott, F R
Sellaturay, R
Sellaturay, S
Shackman, S G
Shapiro, S M
Sharih, S
Smith, P J
Solomon, T A
Stewart, H C
Story, P
Thakkar, D H
Thakkar, I D
Thakrar, D N
Thomas, P M
Thompson, E A
Thompson, F D
Walford, C S
Wong, S J
Yau, K-M R
Yogeswaran, P
Zuberi, M M

Norwich

Abbott, R T
Ahmed, N
Ainsworth, L F
Alawattegama, H D B
Albert, J S
Alden, D J
Allan, A
Allanson, N K
Allen, R W H
Applegate, J M
Arie, T H D
Armon, M P
Ashby, L M
Ashford, N P N
Astbury, N J
Atkinson, A G
Atkinson, L
Auger, B M
Aylott, C E W
Baako, B N
Bailey, J R
Baker, R S
Ball, H N
Ball, R Y
Bamber, S C
Bangham, C H
Barclay, H
Barclay, R P
Barden, S D
Bardsley, A F
Bardsley, V
Barker, G L
Barker, P
Barker, T H W
Barkley, A M
Barltrop, I
Barnard, P B
Barratt, J
Barrett, A
Barrie, P M
Barrie, R E
Bastable, G J G
Baxter, L D
Bayliss-Brown, P J
Beach, R C
Beales, I L P
Beales, M S
Beeby, M J
Beezhold, J N
Bennett, E R L
Bennett, J C
Berry, P J
Beton McCulloch, M L
Bhadrinath, B R
Birks, K A
Blackburn, A L
Blundell, C M
Blyth, J A
Bracher, D
Braithwaite, J E G
Brambleby, P J
Branson, E
Brantigan, P D
Brisley, G D
Brito Ramos, J M
Brittain, D R
Brooks, R
Brooksby, I A B
Brown, S W
Bryce, D K
Buckton, C
Bulman, A S
Bulto Chirivella, M D M
Burgess, N A
Burns, S A
Burrell, M A
Burrows, P J
Bush, A P
Butt, S J
Cahir, J G
Calder, D A
Campbell, C R D
Cant, B
Carlyle, D N
Carver, P H
Cator, S E
Chapman, P G
Charfare, G H G M
Cheesbrough, A J M
Cheetham, A C
Chitale, S V
Chojnowski, A J
Chuah, T P
Clark, G S
Clark, J R
Clark, W A
Clarke, E D
Clarke, J M F
Clarke, P
Clayton, C L
Clayton, G M
Coathup, P A
Cole, B S
Coleman, C J
Conway, S
Copson, S G
Coupland, C R
Cox, K A
Craig, J C
Craig, K D
Crawford, R J
Crook, W S
Crowle, V J
Curtin, J J
Dalrymple, J S O
Dalrymple, P A
Datta, V
Davies, P D
Davies, R E
Dawson, B G
Daykin, S M
de Boer, F C
Deane, A M
Del Rio Basterrechea, I
Delvin, D G
Denton, E R E
Devine, E A
Devine, R
Devonshire, R E
Dhatariya, K K
Dhesi, A S
Dick, D J
Donell, S T
Double, D B
Downs, S M
Dryhurst, K M
Duncan, I
Dyke, M P
Echebarrieta, J M
Edmonds, S M
Eke, T
Ellis, M C
Elsby, K P
Elvy, B L
Evans, A M
Evans, J K
Evans, P J

Evison, P R H
Fairclough, A A
Farman, R D C
Farquharson, S
Fellows, I W
Ferrari, M R
Few, A S
Fielden, A L M
Finney, J M
Fisher, J M
Fiske, S J
Fletcher, H C
Fletcher, S J
Forsythe-Yorke, W E I
Fox, J J
Fox, S A
Francis, C R T
Francis, R N
Fraser, C S
Fraser, D I
Freeman, L J
Frost, J S
Fry, T M
Fryers, G R
Fulcher, R A
Furniss, P
Gaffney, J K
Gair, J D
Gall, A R
Gallagher, E G
Garioch, J J
Gaskin, M A
George, A
George, J D
Gibson, A G
Gibson, I S
Gilbert, R F T
Gillings, M J
Gilson, J M
Girling, A C
Girling, S D
Glasgow, M M S
Glenn, A M
Glennon, P E
Godfrey, A W H
Goldser, D S
Gow, I A
Grattan, C E H
Gray, A J G
Green, C A
Green, M B
Green, N A
Greenwood, R H
Griffiths, T R L
Grove, A J
Guy, A D
Guy, D J
Hall, R J C
Hameed, M B
Hamilton, D V
Hamlin, P J
Hampsheir, R P
Hancock, G D
Harley, D W
Harper, P C W L
Harris-Hall, J J
Harris, J R
Harris, P R
Harris, P R
Harrison, B D W
Harrison, F D
Harrison, K R
Harston, P J R
Hart, A R
Harvey, I M
Harwood, J M
Hatoum, A F
Hattersley, T S
Hawthorn, S J
Haydn, K F
Hayward, A P
Head, F A
Heaton, A
Heaton, K
Henley, P A
Herrero Diaz, M
Heyburn, P J
Hillam, J C
Hillen, H A
Hodgson, S
Hoey, T E
Holland, S J
Holt, S P
Holtom, N C
Hood, D H J
Househam, E A
Howe, A C
Howe, D C
Howe, R J
Hudspith, M J
Hughes, L O
Hughes, W C
Hunter, L C
Hurst, G R
Hutchings, P J G
Hutchinson, C T
Innes, A J
Innes, H E
Ireland, N J
Iver, E B A
Jackson, A W
James, P M L
Jathanna, S D
Jenkins, J R
Jenkins, P F
Jones, C N
Jones, D V
Jones, R D
Jones, S M
Kaszubowski, H A
Kelly, B K
Kennedy, H J
Kerr, L I
Kestin, K J
Kitchener, P G
Kitson, M C
Knights, R C
Lambert, M A
Latham, J B
Laurence, M D
Lawson, P R
Leadbeater, M J
Leaman, A M S
Leary, T S
Ledward, D J
Leeming, D J
Legg, N G M
Leinster, S J
Leney, P M
Lesley, C A
Levell, N J
Lewis, M P N
Ling, D A
Lipp, A K
Lister, A J
Lister, G E
Lloyd, A H
Lock, P T
Lockett, S R
Logan, A M
Loke, Y K
Lonsdale, R N
Luck, J D
McCann, B G
McCarthy, J J
McCartney, I M
McDonald, N G
McEvett, F C
McFerran, D H
McGlashan, K A
McGovern, D O
McIntyre, J D
McIntyre, K E
Mackay, J E
Macrae, S E
Macris, S
McShane, R
Mair, J U
Maisey, D N
Malcolm, J P
Mallinson, R H
Malpas, C A
Malpas, L C
Mann, C J V D
Mansfield, T G R
Manson-Bahr, P G P
Marshall, A T
Marshall, T J
Martin, S
Martin, W M C
Mathur, A B
Maxwell, J R
May, H M
May, S R
Meaden, J D
Merry, P
Meyer, F J
Meyer, M
Miller, J E
Miller, M P
Mirza, W J
Mitchell, I R
Moreton, C A
Morgan-Hughes, G J
Morgan, J H
Morgan, W S
Morris, C H
Morris, E P
Morris, M-A C
Morris, N M
Morrow, D R
Morton, I N
Mosedale, B M
Mould, J
Munson, D J
Murphy, H J
Naguib, M F
Nash, C M
Naunton, W J
Newman, R J
Nicol, A
Nieto Velillas, J J
Nisbet-Smith, C
Noble, M J
Nolan, D F L
Nolan, J E
Nolan, J F
Norman-Taylor, F H
O'Neill, H B
O'Neill, T J
O'Shea, J R
Ogden, J S M
Okoro, J O
Olive, J E
Oliver, L E
Ostrowski, M J
Overy, R D
Page, A J F
Palframan, A
Pannett, R N
Parikh, A
Parry, G W
Patel, A
Payne, B V
Payne, J F
Pearce, C P
Pennell, A M
Percival, G O
Perez-Morales, M M
Perry, G L
Pfang, J A
Pickworth, F E
Pilch, D J F
Pilling, J B
Pilling, J R
Pinching, N J
Pinder, N R
Plunkett, T G
Poliakoff, L J
Pope, L E R
Porter, G E
Poulton, B B
Powell, J S
Pratt, N J
Press, A M
Preston, J T
Preston, P G
Preston, W E B
Price, C P J
Price, D B
Price, F M
Price, M E
Prinsley, P R
Prior, A
Pugh, C R
Pyne, J R
Pyper, A J
Raggoo, M D R
Rai, A S
Raithatha, N
Ralphs, D N L
Ramsay, C F
Ranger, I
Rannan-Eliya, Y F
Rao, B R S
Rash, G J E
Rattner, G J
Reading, R F
Rees, J H
Rees, R T
Reynolds, C M
Rhodes, M
Richards, A E
Richards, J
Ridley, S A
Rigby, A J
Rippy, E E
Rivett, J F
Rix, T E
Roberts, M D
Roberts, P F
Robinson, C R
Roche, M T
Rolls, N P
Ross, C N
Rowe, S
Rowe, W L
Rumball, D
Saada, J
Sabanathan, K
Sambandan, S
Sampson, J S
Sampson, M J
Sams, V R
Sanson, J R
Sassoon, E M
Sattar, M
Scherzinger, S H
Scott-Barrett, S
Scott, D G I
Scott, J D
Scott, S D
Scouller, F E
Senarath, V L
Shaw, C
Shaw, M S
Shaw, T J
Shepherd, P D W
Shields, S A
Shinh, N
Shutes, J C B
Sides, J R
Signy, C M
Simmons, H
Simpson, R J
Skipper, C
Smith-Howell, M A
Smith, S J
Solomka, B T
Spalding, D R C
Speakman, C T M
Spencer, S P
Stanley, A K
Stanley, K P
Staufenberg, E F A
Stebbings, W S L
Steel, N
Steel, S F M
Steele, R G
Stone, R
Stuttard, C A
Summors, A C
Sutton, I J
Tarbuck, A F
Temple, R C
Tewson, G R
Thalange, N K S
Thirkell, C E
Thomas, J M
Thompson, K O
Thompson, R S
Thorn, D R
Thorpe, R S
Thurlow, J
Tighe, M R
Tilford, M P
Timms, R F
Tolley, I P
Tomlinson, D
Toms, A P
Torrens, J D
Tsang, T T M
Tucker, J K
Turner, G E
Twentyman, O P
Tyler, X M
Upton, C J
Valentine, J M J
Valentine, L
Varvel, D A
Vaughan, D A
Vaughan, R
Vaughan, S J
Verma, N K
Verma, R
Viale, N J
Wadsley, J C
Wales, R M
Wallace, M C
Walsh, S J
Warren, R C
Waterhouse, C
Watkin, S W
Watkins, D
Watkins, J
Watkins, R J
Watson, D C T
Watson, M A
Watt-Smyrk, C W
Wayman, J
Welton, T
Went, E L
White, P M B
Whitehead, T R S W
Wickstead, M
Wilkinson, K A
Wilkinson, L M
Wilkinson, M J
Williams, H M S
Williamson, K S
Willis, M D F
Willits, D G
Wilson-Nunn, D L
Wilson, A M
Wilson, J R M
Wilson, P A J
Wimperis, J Z
Wong, N C-K
Wood, P M
Woodall, N M
Woodhouse, P R
Woods, A D
Woollam, C H M
Wright, C J
Yallop, D
Young, K E
Young, P J

Nottingham

Abbott, M D
Abdul-Hamid, S
Abdul, S
Abell, J D
Abercrombie, C A
Abercrombie, J F
Adams, A D
Aderogba, A
Aderogba, K O
Aghel, M M
Ahmed-Jushuf, I H
Ahmed, S I
Ahrens, C L
Ahsan, A J
Aitkenhead, A R
Alagesan, K
Ali, A R
Ali, S I
Allan, A N
Allen, B R
Allfree, J M
Allison, S P
Amar, S S
Ambler, J J S
Amin, J
Amin, S
Amirchetty Rao, S R
Ammar, K M
Amoaku, W M K
Ancliff, N B
Anderson, E R
Ankenbauer, M R
Ansell, I D
Anwar, A E
Arandhara, K K
Arden-Jones, J R
Armitage, F E
Armitage, N C M
Armstrong, R S
Arya, T
Ashpole, R D
Ashworth, A J
Aslam, T M
Aston, I R
Atherley, D B
Atherton, J C
Atkinson, M J
Au, L
Auger, M J
Austin, A S
Aveline, A J D
Aveline, M O
Avery, A J
Bain, C N
Bajek, G
Baker, T M
Baldwin, D R
Baldwin, P M
Balfour, C E
Ballin, N C
Banks, D C
Banner, R W
Barkataki, H C
Barrett, P J
Barrett, S M L
Barry, B P
Bassi, N S
Bassi, S R
Basu, K K
Bates, C P
Bath, P M W
Batt, M E
Baxendale, B R
Beale, L J
Beatty, J H
Becker, G W
Beckingham, I J
Bedforth, K J
Bedforth, N M
Bedi, N K
Beggs, F D
Bell, C H
Bendall, M J
Bennett, J W
Bennett, J A
Bennett, M W R
Bentley, S C
Berman, P
Bertenshaw, C J
Bessell, E M
Bhandal, S K
Bhanji, N P
Bharmal, S
Bhatia, A A
Bhojani, T K
Bhojwani, S C
Bignell, C J
Bignell, J A
Bilkhu, J S
Birchall, A D
Birchall, J P
Bishop, L J
Bishop, M C
Bisson, M A
Biswas, A C
Biswas, A
Bittiner, P
Black, D G
Bladon, Y M
Blake, M J
Blakeman, J M
Blamey, R W
Blumhardt, L D
Blundell, A G
Bogod, D G
Bolarum, S R
Bolsher, S J
Bond, S J
Booth, R
Boswell, T C J
Bourke, J B
Bourke, S L
Bowering, K
Bowler, C
Bowley, C J
Bowling, T E
Bowman, C A
Bradley, P J
Bradley, S J
Braithwaite, B D
Bramley, M D
Bratt, K G
Bratty, J R
Brewin, J S
Bridgewater, A L
Brittain, A H
Britton, J R
Broderick, N J
Brookes, C E
Brown, C M
Brown, K P H
Brown, L M
Brown, M M
Brown, M E
Brown, S F
Brown, T P L H
Browne, N C
Bruce, B I
Bruce, J E F
Buck, S
Buckell, N A
Budge, H J
Bulmer, N J
Bunnage, S J
Burden, R P
Burns, R A
Burns, S M
Burr, R W
Burrell, H C
Burton, G A
Burwell, R G
Butler, T K H
Byrne, J L
Byrne, P O
Bywater, K H
Caffery, I L
Calder, G R
Calder, J
Campbell, F A
Campbell, I W
Cantwell, R
Caplin, S A
Capra, M L
Carberry, P J
Carmichael, J

Carolan, B A
Carr, M E
Cartmill, M
Cartwright, J E
Cassidy, M J D
Cawthron, P A
Chahal, P S
Challen, K B
Chamberlain, M H
Chan, C Y-Y
Chan, K L
Chan, Y T S
Chapman, J E
Chapman, L
Chapman, N D
Charlton, C P J
Chaudhri, Q
Chaudri, M B
Chaudri, M B
Cheeseman, S L
Chester, D L
Cheung, K L
Chishti, R S
Chua, W L
Churchill, R D
Clamp, M
Clark, C T
Clarke, J L
Clayton, J A
Clifford, W A
Cockburn, A P
Cockrill, J
Coffey, F M
Cole, O J
Coleman, T J
Coles, R R A
Colley, M S V
Collinson, B
Colton, C L
Comaish, I F
Connery, T P
Cooper, J E
Coppens, M
Copping, J R
Corcoran, M E
Corcoran, R
Cornforth, B M
Coutts, F
Coutts, S R J
Cox, G M
Cox, G J
Cox, S A
Crighton, I M
Crosby, V L
Cross, B W
Culverwell, N J C
Curnock, D A
Curran, F M
Curran, J P J
Cutajar, P
Cwynar, B U
D'Mello, B J
D'Mello, K A
D'Mello, M T
Dalton, C M
Daly, J C
Davidson, I R
Davies, B W
Davies, D
Davies, G J
Davies, G R
Davies, M G
Davis, C J
Davis, G R
Davis, M E
Davis, T R C
Dawson, A
Day, J S
De Silva, E S
De Sousa, C G
Deane, M
Deighton, C M
Denley, H E
Denny, P A
Desai, K
Devadason, M J N
Dewar, J R
Dexter, P J
Dhar, S
Dickenson, A J
Dixon, H
Dixon, K
Dodd, S L
Doddy, J A
Doherty, M
Dolan, G
Donald, F E
Donnan, A B
Doran, J
Dornan, J D
Doshi, B
Dove, A F
Dowell, J D
Dowell, K
Dowling, F M
Downes, R N
Downing, N D
Dua, H S
Duffy, A M
Duffy, J P
Duggan, A E
Duggins, R A
Dunderdale, M A
Dunn, F A
Dunn, M
Dunstan, S P
Durcan, S F
Durrant, J M
Dyson, A
Earnshaw, S A
Earwicker, H M
Earwicker, S C
Edington, P T
Elliott, R H
Elliott, S
Ellis, I O
Ellis, J A
Elston, C W
Emerson, F-M
Emery, J G B
Emmerson, A M
Engler, J H W
English, J S C
Esberger, D A
Evans, A J
Evans, J H C
Everton, M J
Exley, P M
Fagan, D G
Farquhar, F J
Farquhar, I K
Felstead, A
Feneley, M R
Ferguson, B G
Fillmore, E J
Filshie, G M
Finch, R G
Finn, D L
Finnegan, G F
Firth, J L
Fisher, K M
Fitz-Henry, J K
Flambert, H M
Fletcher, A J P
Flewitt, A P
Flowerdew, G D
Foot, V M
Ford, A R
Ford, S A
Forman, K
Forster, I W
Foss, A J E
Foulds, A M J
Foweraker, K L
Fowler, R
Fowlie, S M
Fradd, S O
Fraser, N
Freeman, N J
Freij, R M
Friedman, T
Fullerton, D G
Gale, C P
Gale, R P
Gallagher, C
Galloway, N R
Galloway, S C
Game, F L
Gan, K B
Ganatra, R H
Garcia-Orad Carles, C
Gard, P D
Gavrilovic, A
Gaywood, I C
Gee, T M
Geh, E
George, K J
Geutjens, G
Ghattaora, A S
Ghattaora, R S
Gibbin, K P
Gibbs, E R
Gibson, S M
Giddins, J C
Gill, D C
Gilmore, N M S
Girdher, A R
Gladman, J R F
Glencross, S J
Gnanalingham, G M
Goddard, A J P
Goddard, W P
Godfrey, P A L
Gokhale, N S
Gokhale, S L
Goldsbrough, J
Gorbutt, N
Gordon, E B
Gordon, J C
Gormley, P D
Gould, N V
Grant De Longueuil, M C
Grant, J
Gray, D
Greaves, R J
Green, A
Green, D J
Green, R H
Gregson, E D
Gregson, R M C
Gregson, R H S
Grevitt, M P
Gribbin, C M
Griffiths, I L
Griffiths, J P
Guha Ray, P K
Guion, A J
Gulati, R
Gunther, A L
Guyler, C J L
Hage, M D
Hahn, D M
Hall, E J
Hall, I P
Hall, L
Hall, T J
Halliday, K E
Halstead, P
Hama, T M
Hama, Z A
Hambleton, K L
Hamilton, J B
Hammersley, B W
Hammond, R H
Hampson, M E
Hampton, J L
Hampton, J R
Hancock, S M
Hannah, D W
Hapgood, D S
Hapgood, R W
Haq, S-U
Hardcastle, J D
Harden, J C
Hargreaves, E L
Harris, J P
Harris, S J
Harrison, A M
Harrison, A T
Harrison, D J
Harriss, D R
Harte, J H
Hartley, S
Hartman, J A
Harwood, R H
Haskew, E E
Hatfield, P
Hathway, K L
Hatton, M
Hawkey, C J
Haworth, S M
Haycock, J C
Hayes, L J
Haynes, R J
Hayward, A C
Hazlewood, E B
Headley, B M
Heaton, M J
Hedley, R N
Heeps, J M M
Heining, M P D
Henderson Smith, R
Henderson, R A
Henfrey, L J
Henley, M
Henley, M J
Henry, D J
Henry, J K
Henry, R I F
Henshaw, R C
Hepden, M
Hewitt, M
Hewitt, M J
Hewitt, S M
Higton, C R
Hildyard, K J
Hippisley-Cox, J
Hobbs, G J
Hodgkinson, V
Hogarth, T B
Holbrook, M R
Holden, N L
Holdsworth, U J
Hollis, C P
Hollis, H R
Holt, J C
Hopkinson, B R
Hopkinson, G R
Hopkinson, H E
Hopton, C
Horn, E H
Hornbuckle, J
Horsfield, P W
Horton, J L
Horton, T C
Hosking, D J
Houghton, B L
Howard, J R
Howard, M A
Howell, C J
Howell, L M
Howell, S J
Howman, E M
Huang, D Y-H
Hubbard, R B
Huggins, D A P
Hughes, S A
Huissoon, A P
Hull, D
Hulman, G
Humberstone, M R
Hunter, J B
Hunter, R
Hussain, F N
Hussain, S A
Hussain, T
Hutchinson, A
Hutchinson, N J
Hutchinson, R
Hutson, M A
Hutter, C D D
Ibrahim, P
Ilyas, N
Ingram, G R
Irving, W L
Jacklin, P J
Jackson, B R
Jackson, D J
Jackson, R J
Jain, S
James, C A
James, D K
James, J J
James, L
James, P D
James, P J
Jan, I A
Jaram, I
Jardine, A D
Jarrett, L N
Jaspan, T
Jayakumar, Y
Jayamaha, J E L
Jeelani, N U O
Jeffcoate, W J
Jelpke, M F D
Jenkinson, D
Jobling, J C
Johnson, C
Johnson, I R
Johnson, M E
Johnson, S R
Johnston, D I
Johnston, I D A
Johnston, M N
Jones, A C
Jones, A M C
Jones, J E
Jones, J A
Jones, J A
Jones, M C
Jones, N S
Jones, P A
Jones, P A E
Jones, S A
Jones, T D
Jones, W L
Jowett, A
Junaid, O
Kachroo, M K
Kalsheker, N A
Kandola, L H K
Karim, R S
Karim, R
Karney, V M
Kaur, K
Kayan, A
Kazem, R
Kean, L H
Keavney, P J
Kendall, D J
Kendrick, D
Kennedy, C M
Kerslake, R W
Kesari, V
Khalique, A
Khalique, P
Khan Madni, M M
Khan, M S
Khan, Z
Kiani, S H
Kime, R
King, R L
Kingdon, S J
Kinnear, W J M
Kirwan, M M
Kitchin, S E
Kleimanis-Taylor, N S
Klonin, H
Knight-Jones, E
Knight, D J W
Knights, D T
Knights, S G
Knox, A J
Kolowski, S J
Kumar, R
Kupfer, R M
Kuruvatti, C C
Kyriakides, J P
Kyriakides, K
Lakhani, M
Lakhanpaul, M
Lakshminarayana, C
Lam, K S
Lamb, J M
Lambourne, J E
Landman, R S
Lane, P W F
Large, G A
Largey, P M
Lata, A
Latief, K H
Latimer, R K
Lau, Y S
Lavelle, P
Lawton, P A
Leach, I H
Leake, V F
Leask, S J
Ledger, C H
Lee, A S
Lee, M
Lee, S J
Leibowitz, R H
Leiper, C A
Leman, P C M
Lemberger, R J
Lennon, K H
Lester, T D
Leuty, G M
Levitt, M J
Levy, D M
Lewis, C
Lewis, M
Liau, F O
Lichtarowicz, E J
Lim, A K P
Lim, K K J
Lim, K T C
Lioumi, D
Lipman, A
Lipp, C
Littlewood, S M
Liu Tek-Yung, D
Livesey, O M
Livesey, R M
Lloyd Jones, J K
Lloyd, J A
Lo, S D C
Loch, A B
Logan, R F A
Logan, R P H
Long, R G
Lonsdale, R E
Lott, C M
Lott, D J
Low, H L
Low, K-W
Lowe, J S
Lowe, J R
Lowe, S J
Luxton, M C
Macarthur, D C
McCall, J
McCauley, P M J
McConachie, N S
McCracken, F M
McCulloch, A E
McCulloch, I W L
McDermott, D M
McDermott, E M
Macdonald, J A
Macfarlane, J T
McGlashan, J A
McHale, N P
McHugh, T M A
McKean, M C
McKinlay, R G
McLachlan, A N
McLachlan, R E
McLaren, A J
MacLean, J C R
McLean, P C
McLoughlin, E T M
McMillan, A K
McNulty, I C
Macpherson, M B A
Macsweeney, S T R
McVicar, E H
McVicar, I H
Maddock, E F
Madeley, J R
Madeley, R J
Magnago, T S I
Maguire, M F
Mahajan, R P
Mahida, Y R
Maile, L J
Maini, D
Majid, N A
Malik, I A
Mann, G S
Manning, P A
Mansell, P I
Manson, C M
Marder, E
Marenah, C B
Marks, P J
Marlow, N
Marsden, K J
Marsh, A J
Marsh, L F
Marshall, A H
Marshall, R H
Martin, G D R
Martin, P H
Mascari, R J
Maskery, J J
Masud, T
Mather, G I
Matthew, J L
Matthews, A J
Mattick, J A
Maxwell-Armstrong, C A
May, T
Medley, I R
Mehat, B S
Mehdian, M H
Mellor, D V
Mellor, L J
Mellor, M
Michel, C A
Middleton, H C
Milburn, J
Miles, H C
Millard, L G
Miller, P J
Milligan, L J
Mills, T A
Minhas, A K
Miranda, S M
Mitchell, I M
Mmono, X M K
Montgomerie, S D
Moorby, T J
Moppett, I K
Moran, C G
Morewood, J H M
Morgan, A G
Morgan, D A L
Morgan, L J
Morgan, N M J
Morgan, S A
Morgan, W E
Morley, J
Morrant, J D
Morris, A J
Morris, G K
Morris, R O
Moulds, J
Moulton, A
Moxon, J

Mueller, K-M
Mukherjee, S K
Murad, M J R
Murthy, A A
Myers, B
Myers, D
Naidoo, A S
Narnor, F W D
Nash, D L
Nathan, A R
Nathanson, M H
Naylor, E L
Neal, K R
Nelson, J S
Nessim Morcos, I
Neumann, L
Neville, A J
Ng, Y K
Nguyen-Van-Tam, J S
Nickalls, R W D
Nowicki, R W A
Nunns, D
O'Donoghue, G M
O'Donovan, T J
O'Dowd, J K
O'Mahony, J B
O'Neil, H A
O'Neil, M J
O'Shea, R M
Oates, M R
Oliver, P A D
Oni, J
Ovenden, L A
Oza, N
Oza, P
Pabla, H S
Packham, C J
Padfield, C J H
Padmasri, P
Page, K E
Page, L J
Page, N P F
Page, R C L
Page, S R
Pallan, A
Pallan, J P
Palmer, N I
Pande, I
Pang, K-K
Park, S B G
Parken, H F
Parken, P N S
Parker, S J
Parmar, S C
Parsons, B L
Parsons, S L
Patel, H
Patel, R R
Patel, S R
Paterson, M A
Pathak, B K
Pathak, C A
Patmore, S J H
Patrick, P R
Pegg, C A S
Percival, H J
Perez Teruel, M I
Perkins, W
Perks, A G B
Perry, J J
Petty, D J
Phillips, J W
Phillips, N N V
Phillips, N V-K
Pickering, S A W
Pillai, C N
Pinner, G T
Place, G F
Pollock, J G
Polnay, L
Poon, J H-W
Porter, J F H
Powell, M C
Powell, R J
Pradeep Kumar, N
Preston, B J
Prince, H G
Pullan, C R
Punt, J A G
Pushparajah, S
Queiroz, J E
Quenby, S M
Qureshi, I F
Qureshi, N
Qureshi, S M
Radford, P J
Raeburn, J A
Raj, D
Rajbhandari, S M
Rajendra, B
Rakhit, T
Ramsay, M M
Randall, P J
Randerson, J M
Rangwani, P M
Raniwalla, J
Rao, A R
Rao, M J
Rao, Y V V S
Raoof, A
Ravenscroft, J C
Rawcliffe, J A
Rayner, P M C
Redfern, M A
Redwood, R
Rees, A M
Rees, J A
Rees, S
Reid, A R
Reid, J A
Reid, M F
Resnick, J V
Reynolds, N J
Rezaul-Karim, S M
Rhoden, F M
Rhodes, J E
Rhodes, K E
Richards, C W
Richens, D
Ridley, D
Rigg, K M
Riley, B
Riley, S P
Ripley, G S
Rizk, S N M
Roberts, E M
Roberts, L
Robertson, I J A
Robinson, M H E
Robson, D K
Rodrigues, K F
Roe, S D
Rogers, R T N
Roith, E
Rose, D H
Rosser, R L
Rotherham, M J
Rotherham, N E
Roughton, H C
Rowlands, B J
Rowson, J E
Roy, S P
Royle, D J
Rubin, P C
Ruddell, M C
Rudham, S J
Rudrashetty, S
Russell, A S
Rutter, N
Rutter, S M
Ruzicka, J M V
Ryan, C J
Ryder, S D
Sabir, S
Sagar, S D
Sahota, O S
Salama, F D
Sama, A
Sammons, H M
Samuels, L S
Sandher, D S
Sanjeev, D
Saunders, A C
Saunders, P
Saunders, P C
Sawle, G V
Sayers, J D
Scaffardi, R A
Scammell, B E
Scholefield, J H
Scott, A R
Scott, A R
Sears, R T
Seddon, D J
Seevaratnam, D M
Selwood, A
Sewell, H F
Shackley, T R
Sham, J K W
Sham, T
Shanley, M J
Shanmuganathan, V A
Sharma, K
Sharma, N K
Sharma, O P
Shaw, H M
Shaw, J M
Sheik Hossain, S M
Shephard, R H
Shepherd, J M
Sherman, R W
Shetty, A
Shields, P A
Shore, I
Siddiqi, A G
Silcocks, P B S
Sills, R O
Simms, M S
Simpson, J D
Simpson, J
Singh Bachra, P
Singh, P J
Singh, S P
Siva, R
Skelton, J B
Sklar, I D
Slack, R C B
Small, P G
Smart, P J E
Smeeton, F J
Smereka, A K
Smethurst, D P
Smith, E M
Smith, J G E
Smith, J C
Smith, J D
Smith, N J
Smith, N K G
Smith, S J
Smith, S A
Smyth, A R
Soar, N M
Somers, J M
Sommers, A J
Sommers, S M
Soo, S-S
Sood, H C
Sood, N C
Soomro, I N
Sparrow, I M
Sparrow, N J
Sparrow, R A
Spencer, C M
Spiller, R C
Sprackling, P D
Stack, W A
Staines, J A
Statham, R
Stebbings, N E
Stephen, A B
Stevens, M A J
Stewart, I D
Stewart, P J
Stryjakiewicz, E G
Sturrock, N D C
Sturrock, S M
Suffield, M J
Sugden, B D
Sullivan, C F
Sully, L
Sunman, W
Swamy, M S
Swinscoe, B D
Symonds, E M
Szabadi, E
Szypryt, E P
Tambyraja, A L
Tan, K C E
Tangri, A K
Tarrant, C J
Tattersfield, A E
Tavernor, R M E
Tavernor, S J
Taylor, A J
Taylor, A M
Taylor, H D
Taylor, H J
Taylor, S M
Teahon, C
Tedstone, I K
Teed, A R
Teh, C P L
Temple, J D
Tennant, W G
Thelwell, C M
Thew, D C N
Thew, M E
Thomas, A E
Thomas, D A
Thomas, D G
Thomas, H J M
Thomas, W A
Thompson, A
Thompson, G M
Thornhill, J D
Thornton, P J
Thornton, S J
Tinsley, M J
Tiong, H Y
Tiwari, P P
Tiwari, S R
Toft, K C
Tomlinson, J D
Tomlinson, P A
Toms, D A
Toms, E S
Topham, L A
Tredgett, M W
Trimble, I M G
Trueman, A M
Tse, Y H A
Turner, B P
Turner, P C T
Turner, R J
Twining, P
Twomey, J M
Ubhi, C S
Udenze, C C
Underwood, F S H
Vaghela, H M
Van Schaick, S H
Varma, R
Varma, S
Varnam, M A
Vassiliadis, H S
Venning, H E
Verma, M S
Vernon, S A
Vettraino, M D
Village, A L
Vindla, M
Vohra, J P S
Vyas, H G
Waite, J
Wake, S L
Wale, M C J
Walker, D A
Walker, J D S
Walker, S L
Wallace, W A
Walsh, D A
Walsh, M M T
Walsh, R J
Walton, S A
Ward, J E H
Ward, L M
Wardle, S P
Warner, J A
Warren, C A
Warsop, A D
Watkin, S L
Watson, A R
Watts, S J
Wayman, M J C
Webb, J K H
Webster, J
Webster, V L
Weir, A
Welch, N T
Wenham, P W
Werchola, L O
West, J
Weston, V C
Whitaker, S C
White, A
White, B D
White, K K
White, L R
Whitehouse, A M
Whitehouse, W P A
Whiteley, A M
Whiteley, P
Wiecek, M R
Wilcock, A
Wilcox, R G
Wilde, S M J J
Wilkinson, E J
Williams, C B
Williams, H C
Williams, L
Williamson, K M
Wills, C J
Wills, J S
Wilson, A R M
Wilson, D I
Wilson, D N
Wilson, R J
Wilson, S H
Wilson, S L
Winter, R J
Wolff, A
Wood, A M
Woods, A H
Woods, L A
Woods, M J
Woodward, E A
Woolrich, L H
Worsey, C J
Worth, K V
Wright, S R
Wynn, S M H
Wynne, R A
Xenophou, X
Yap, S C
Yeung, J M-C
York, S M
Young, A S

Nuneaton
Abdul Wahab, M A-R
Agrawal, V K
Allen, S J
Apakama, I G
Arora, M K
Batchelor, Y K
Beadman, A M
Beckles, D-E P T
Bee, H W
Benton, P J
Binyon, S E
Bluck, G M
Brown, L A
Bruck, P E
Bullen, A W
Burnett, M G
Castells, V
Chapman, P J
Charles, D P J
Chaudhuri, A K
Clamp, I J
Cossey, A J
Crosby, P S
Crutchlow, E J
David, L M
Drage, M W
Fagan, J M
Fear, C R
Gadsby, R
Ganapathi, E N
Garala, K
George, M
Giles, A
Gill, R S
Godfrey, A J
Gorringe, H R
Gossain, R N
Graham, C N
Grant, H M B
Groves, A R
Groves, C F
Guest, M
Gummery, R M
Gupta, A
Haider, Y
Hajat, C
Handslip, P D J
Haynes, I G
Henderson, B L C
Hickson, P J
Hodges, E J
Howarth, N J
Howl, M
Hyslop, R N
Ingrams, G J
Jacob, J
Jones, K L
Jones, S H
Jones, T A
Kachhia, B G
Kenyon, V G
Khan, K
Kisku, W
Law, D G
Lillo Torregrosa, J J
Lim, P V H
Manek, N
Marson, S
Matthews, R N
Mentor, J M
Meystre, C J N
Morrissey, J R
Moshakis, V
Muthiah, C Y T
Nangalia, R
Narayanan, M N
Nasser, Z A-A I
Navaneetham, N
O'Brien, C
Parkianathan, V
Patel, A R
Patel, C R
Patel, R J
Perera, H M G
Perera, W N R
Phelps, S V
Phipps, J H
Prasad, K K
Quadri, S A
Quarcoopome, W N S
Quasim, M
Reddy, M A
Redfern, A C
Reily, C M
Sabih, I
Sayed, S
Sharif, D
Shenoy, K K
Shirazi, H A
Sidhu, B S
Singh, H
Sinha, S
Smith, A M B
Smith, J E
Srivastava, S
Steingold, R F
Summers, M W
Taggart, P C M
Thankey, K L
Thomas, M P
Thompson, A
Todd, J L
Toone, R P D
Topham, P S
Upponi, S S
Upponi, S K
Vaidya, G A
Vallance, K A
Venkatesh, M N
Walzman, M
Whitehouse, A B
Willett, M
Williams, J G
Wilson, H J A
Woo, M T C
Wood, G M
Zurub, A A

Oakham
Baker, J W
Barrow, M
Bennison, D P
Cheverton, S G
Clitheroe, E G
Clitheroe, M B
Crosthwaite, J D
Dighe, S V
Drye, E R
Eaves, M
Fenby Taylor, J W
Fox, H J
Gallimore, C H
Gavins, E N
Goraya, J
Guthrie, A E
Inman, S M
Jones, E G
Jones, J P
Ker, D A J
Lennard, N S
McCormack, G E
Martin, M K
Martin, S G
May, D R
May, S A
Newman, M R B
Nunn, N K
O'Hare, D J
Phillimore, C E
Rees, H E G
Richards, C A
Scotney, A J
Selmes, S E
Seymour, N R
Shewry, S M
Tring, J P
Venn, M G P
Ward-Booth, S
Webster, S E
Whitelaw, J
Woolford, D J
Young, S J

Oban
Adams, K J
Ambrose, L J
Cameron, A T
Cameron, M E
Campbell, N M A
Grant, D F
Hannah, G D
Henderson, A F
Henderson, A K
Jespersen, E
Lane, P J

Lennox, I B
Loynds, P A
Lyon, J M
Macdowall, P
Milne, E J B
Murchison, A G
Murray, A M
Robertson, C Y B
Robertson, M A H
Scobie, D J
Shand, J D
Taylor, S
Walker, J S
Wilson, C M
Wilson, E M
Yadav, S N

Okehampton
Bell, T R D
Box, D C
Carter, A P
Cox, A L
Downie, M C
Gandy, P J
Gundry, D R T
Hart, H M
Ledger, J A
Macklin, S C
Nielson, P C
Padfield, N N W
Rowe, A
Stainer-Smith, A M
Twomey, J C
Vile, K S M
Warre, J H
Watkins, S A

Oldbury
Andreou, B A
Blewitt, L A
Chan, J L M
Collier, S J
Dau, H S
Demajumdar, R
Finch, J
Garfield, M J
Granville, C M
Griggs, N J
Hanna, H S F
Holtom, K
Indwar, A C
Jasim, W A L
Jenkins, P J
Jones, F W
Kamal, L
Kaur, S
Khan, M M
Kharaud, B S
Naeem, A
Nagra, A S
Patel, B
Quli, X H
Rothwell, B P
Springall, C J
Sykes, I R
Tarin, M K
Thacker, A J
Tyler, J E

Oldham
Aboel Saad, A B
Ahmad, J J
Ahmad, N
Ahmed, Z
Al Saidi, T K J
Alam, S
Alexander, A
Allen, G
Amin, B C
Anderton, L C
Ashraf, D
Aslam, M
Asumu, T O
Atherton, D A
Atkinson, M W
Aziz, N L
Bailey, J S
Baker, R P
Bakht, T
Baldwin, E S
Bandara, D J
Bari, M A
Barrie, J R
Bayman, R L
Bhan, G L
Bhatnagar, D
Boden, M G
Braddock, A
Brady, M C
Brett, I
Brocklehurst, I C
Brown, A I
Buch, K A
Buckley, K G
Callow, P J
Capuano, A
Carswell, W
Chakrabarti, A
Chowdhury, M
Clegg, S
Clough, T M
Cogan, F M
Collin, P G
Conroy, D P J
Cook, L B
Cook, P R
Cooper, F
Cope, A
Coupe, M O
Daud, L R
Davies, T L
Derbyshire, S A
Devaraja, V C
Dhanawade, S
Dixon, S E
Dunbar, E M
Dyson, K
Edozien, L C
Emslie, B
Faulkner, M A
Ferguson, M E
Fischel, J D
Fleming, D I
Foster, M E
Fox, A M
Friedman, E H I
Garside, S H
Gibbons, A M
Goodall, K L
Green, J E
Green, N D
Gregory, M A
Gupta, P
Hackett, L
Hadfield, M B
Hall, S E
Hampson, R M
Heyes, P
Hulton, N R
Hutton, S J
Inston, N G
Isaacs, V R
Jackson, N A
Jacobs, L G H
Jain, S R
Jayakumar, L
Jeeves, R S
Jethani, P R
Jeyagopal, N
Jojo, K A J
Kamar, Z
Kapur, J K
Keba, S
Kelso, J W
Kenworthy, J W
Kenyon, S J
Kershaw, S A
Khan, M T
Khan, R S H
Khan, S
Khiroya, R
Khurana, A
Khurana, J C
Khurana, R
Khwaja, N
Klimiuk, P S
Knowles, W P
Kobbekaduwe, A E R
Kohli, R
Lester-Smith, D
Lewis, B
Lipton, J R
Logan, S H M
Luthra, P K
Lynch, B M
McArthur, A
McCoye, A J
McEwan, K L
McGeachie, J F
McGee, H M J
McInnes, R
McIntosh, C A
McIntosh, I H R
Mackenzie, I J
Mehra, S K
Melling, P R
Menzies, D A
Milnes, I
Milton, M H
Mirza, S
Mistry, N T
Mkandawire, E A
Mohanty, A
Mokate, T
Ncube, W
Northfield, M
Nwokolo, C F
Nye, A D
O'Brien, T D
O'Malley, H A
O'Malley, M
Odeka, E B O
Oshodi, T O
Owens, H S
Page, F C
Pal, S K
Panigrahi, K
Patel, K R
Patel, R K
Patrick, J F
Paulley, J S
Pedley, D K
Puddy, B R
Radcliffe, G
Rajasansir, J G S
Ramachandran, K
Rate, A J
Ravishankar, R
Reid, P V
Richards, D M
Rivera De Zea, A
Robinson, J E
Saha, N K
Salah, M M R M
Samji, F
Saraf, R
Schofield, E C
Schofield, L P
Scott, C G
Shackley, D C
Shah, I K C
Sharma, V L
Shepheard, B G F
Shipp, P A
Shoaib, A
Sidra, L M
Sikander, N
Smith, D E
Sobhani, S
Solomon, S A
South, A L
Speden, D J
Spikker, A C W
Sturgess, H
Suharwardy, J M A
Suresh, C G K
Suryanarayan Setty, R S
Sydney, J P M
Syed, S H
Taylor, A W
Taylor, M
Thomas, W
Thompson, J
Trewinnard, P J
Umeh, C F
Vedi, K K
Walsh, P A
Watson, I P M
Watt, T C
Whitley, I G
Wilkinson, J
Wilkinson, J
Wright, J M
Wright, P N

Olney
Bartlett, D R
Beal, S E
Bentley, G
Cockings, J G L
Curtin, M J
Hall, J P
Partridge, B E
Reed, P A
Scott, E A
Short, S D
Snashall, D C
Swallow, P N
Winter, M E

Omagh
Allen, A J
Anand, K
Bindal, K K
Blair, A L T
Bownes, I T
Bradley, P B
Brannigan, R
Breen, H A
Brogan, K B M
Cockburn, I R
Connolly, D F
Connolly, T P
Corry, M J
Courtney, P A
Curran, M P
Davis, W S
Deehan, J A
Deeny, C K M
Dillon, D A
Donnelly, A M
Downey, D G
Fox, D P
Gallagher, P M
Garrett, P J
Gervais, T G
Gormley, D G
Haigney, S A
Hassan, I-U
Hendly, A J
Hodkinson, E H
Irwin, J M A
Jackson, H G
Kaluskar, S K
Kelly, B P
Kemp, M T A
Lalsingh, R R
Law, K P
Loughrey, G J
McBain, C A
McCallion, W
McCann, J J
McCavert, M
McColgan, B J
McDermott, M A
McDermott, M G
McDonald, B T
McGirr, G P
McGlinchey, P G
McGrath, C
McMullan, E A
McSorley, J D
Magfhogartaigh, L G M
Maginness, J M F
Manley, P A
Martin, H
Meehan, D D
Miller, G A B
Mitchell, C J H
Monaghan, K F
Morris, P
O'Boyle, C P
O'Neill, C A
Pinto, D J D T
Pollock, N C
Quinn, P H M
Robinson, F P
Russell, C J M
Russell, J E
Rutledge, M R
Scully, P G
Scully, P J
Smith, R A
Stewart, G E
Strain, A G
Sweeney, B E
Thompson, D R P
Toal, P A
Tracey, N G T
Vishweshwar Rao, V
Watson, I R G

Ongar
Dickinson, M C
Leach, P M
Lloyd, A R N
Menon, N K
Munro, R D
Rix, B D
Rogers, D A
Taylor, H F
Waters, S D
Winter, C D

Orkney
Broadhurst, R J D
Brooke, J V
Buchan, J
Haunschmidt, S M
Hazlehurst, R V
Johnstone, D D
Kemp, C A
Kemp, S
Kettle, P R
Le-Mar, C A
Lester, M H
Linklater, M
Logan, E S
Malhotra, V B
Trevett, A J
Woodbridge, K F

Ormskirk
Adam, R F
Adejumo, S W A
Allan, J M
Andrews, S J
Ash, G M
Atkinson, R B
Baldwin, A C
Barker, D L C
Bhatti, S S
Bishop-Cornet, H R L
Biswas, S
Boocock, G R
Bradbury, C M
Bradley, J J
Burford, P A
Cervoni, E
Cook, F
Coppock, L A
Corke, R T
Cottam, D C
Crilly, M A
Cunnington, A J
Darley, S N
Devine, W C
Dobson, S
Edwards, J W L
Edwards, R P
Forrer, J A
Fowler, J
Frampton, S P
Gardiner, A J
Gray, M P
Greenhow, T J
Gupta, J K
Hammond, J S
Hawkes, B L
Hawkes, R A
Hendy-Ibbs, P M
Holden, A M
Horsley, J R
Hughes, P L
Hurst, P L
Jones, S V
Juste, R N
Kakati, B
Kaye, L C
Kewley, I S
Kiire, C
Kingsley, D M
Kippax, A G
Kirby, I J
Knowles, M
Kumar, A S
Kumar, A
Kumar, P
Lamden, K H
Ledson, H
Lee, T G
McCormick, P J
MacIver, M
McKenzie, M H
Mader, U C
Makepeace, D J
Marshall, S R
Matich, M D
Meehan, S E
Mellor, M S
Mellor, N W M
Memon, A A
Menon, R J
Menon, T J
Navan Eetha Rajah, P
Navaneetharajah, B M J
Naylor, G M
O'Brien, B W
O'Brien, D V
Oelbaum, R S
Orrell, J C
Park, P M B
Parker, J C
Porteous, M R H
Price, E
Randall, C
Ratoff, J C
Redfern, L
Reston, P J J
Rosbotham-Williams, G M
Sammon, P M
Saunders, H J
Sechiari, G P
Shaha, M R
Simpson, C H
Sinha, G
Smith, D J
Smith, H R
Smyth, C C A
Smyth, C M
Stanley, J C
Stanley, J K
Statham, A M
Stubley, M W
Suraliwala, K H
Suri, S
Suri, S
Taggart-Jeeva, S
Tong, N A
Travis, C D
Underwood, B
Vian, A S
Watson, H M
Weerakoon, B S
Weldon, B D
Wickham, T A
Williams, C J
Yusuf, M
Zbaeda, M M

Orpington
Abdullah, A J J
Abumahlula, M A
Acquaah, V L
Adeoye, O A
Ahmad, A M
Ahmed, M
Al-Salihi, O N
Allan, G D L
Arulambalam, K J
Asante, M A
Aung Myint Kyaw, Dr
Bailey, I R
Bailey, J H L
Baldwin, R W M
Barker, G R
Barker, P R
Barnass, S J
Barrett, J F
Bastian, N
Bates, R E
Begum, M J
Bell, J-A
Bhan, A
Bicknell, C D
Bindra, A P S
Black, J
Botfield, C H
Bradley, L
Brennan, J W
Brierley, E-J
Brown, K G E
Brown, R N
Caldwell, C
Carver, R A
Cheung, S T H
Choong, B H
Clement, M
Cook, M A
Coonjobeeharry, K R
Coumbe, A
Crosland, S J
Crowell, E M L
Da Costa, N P
Dalal, P U
Daniell, S J N
De Lord, C F M
De Silva, M
Dennis, K S
Dhanji, A-R A-A
Dyer, A A
Edmondson, R A
Edwards, E J
Erian, J
Fernando, R A M
Fleming, A
Foo, P S L
Ford-Adams, M E
Forton, J T M
Fraser, C M B
Gancke, A E
Gardner, R L
Girija, N
Golding-Wood, D G
Gupta, R M
Harris, P W R
Hennigan, T W
Hildick-Smith, K W R
Hobbins, S M
Hones, H J

Hou, D
Jaisri, S S P
Jenson, C M
Jessop, M E
Kensit, J G
Kessel, B L
Kong, K F
Lamb, J L H
Langford, E J
Lanigan, L P F
Leggett, J C M
Lester, P K
Livesley, V A
Lock, B A
Lokulo-Sodipe, O A
Long, A M
Luckhurst, S P
McAllister, J C R
Mackenzie, C I
Maheswaran, S
Mansi, A R E
Menon, V N
Mercer, J D
Moosvi, S R
Motto, J E
Napier, A C
Neville, L A
Nicholls, M J
Ogunremi, A O
Orphanides, D
Palin, J A
Panesar, R S
Parker, V L
Pearce, D A
Perera, A D
Perera, P H M A
Perera, P
Pitt, P I
Powell, C R
Purwar, R
Pushparajah, C R
Radford, R C
Rajasundaram, S
Ranasinghe, D P
Rand, C
Reid, P J
Rhodes, K M
Riches, M C
Ring, K P
Roberts, H S A
Roberts, M E
Roe, S E
Ross, J A
Rush, J M
Sahi, M K
Sarfraz, M A
Sauve, P S
Sawczenko, A B J
Sawicka, E H
Selvarangan, R
Selway, J R
Sharif, J
Sharples, E J
Sharr, M M
Singh, S
Steel, G
Steer, C V
Stell, I M
Tavabie, A
Tavabie, J A
Terry, R M
Thomas, A M K
Thompson, R T
Timberlake, C M
Toner, C C
Trew, D R
Tritton, B A
Trotter, G A
Tsui, J C S
Udoeyop, U W
Vidgeon, S D
Walker, G A
Walton, J C
Waters, M B
Wells, D L
Wharton, C F P
White, J P
White, R J
Wijayawardhana, P
Wiles, J
Wilkinson, A L
Williams, D L
Williams, J
Wootton, O R

Ossett
Booth, J E
Cokill, B M
Furness, F
Jones, C S
Putman, H R
Reed, S M
Senior, J E

Oswestry
Alageli, N A
Alcock, R J
Barling, P S L
Barling, R
Beeston, K M
Braddock, L
Breese, H T R
Bromley, C L G
Butler, R C
Cassar-Pullicino, V N
Davie, M W J
Dixey, J
Dyke, W A
Eden, S
Eisenstein, S M
El Deeb, B B E D
El-Masry, W S
Emmett, C P
Evans, C R
Evans, G A
Evans, L S
Ford, D J
Glatzel, T G
Gregson, P A
Hadden, N D
Hamade, P M
Harris, D
Hay, S M
Hill, S O
Hodnett, H T
Hutchison, A G
Jaffray, D C
James, M P
James, M W
Johnson, M D
Jones, R S
Jones, S M
Kendall, J G
Kiely, N T
Leather, J
Lewer Allen, C M
Lloyd, C R
Lloyd, E A
Llywarch, B V
Loveday, D J
McCall, I W
Mackereth, A I
McMurray, R G
Makin, M K
Martin, N P
Middleton, P I
Morgan, B A
Newey, M L
Northmore-Ball, MD
Osman, A E-T F
Pabbineedi, R
Park, A E
Pfeifer, P M
Quinlivan, R C M
Rees, D
Rees, H M
Richardson, J B
Roberts, A P
Roberts, S N J
Rummens, I F
Scott-Knight, V C E
Short, D J
Smith, A L
Taylor, A S J
Thomas, A J
Treasure, R A R
Walker, A N
White, S H
Whittingham, F G
Willows, H

Otley
Allen, N J
Bearpark, A
Gogna, C J
Hide, E M
Knott, S
Leung, P M
Lloyd, G M
Lund, J A
Middleton, C H
Monte, S L
Montgomery, H D
Morgan, H E G
O'Hara, S D N
Protheroe, A S
Richmond, J B
Robinson, S D
Shaw, C E
Spencer, P
Stanley, A M
Stanley, S E A
Sykes, O M
Whitehead, S A

Ottery St Mary
Ackroyd, J T
Baker, D M
Brown, J M
Cox, T J
Cullen, M
De Sousa, N A
Dilley, C J
Gurney, K J
Hatfield, P A
Kerr, S J
King, M R
Rose, C M
Stone, B C
Tibble, R K

Oxford
Abrahams, A H
Adams, C B T
Adams, R F
Adcock, J E
Addy, E V
Adwani, S S
Agulnik, P L
Ahmad, T
Ahmed, S
Akinola, M O
Akiwumi, B O
Al-Barazi, S A
Alcock, C J
Alderson, P R
Ali, M T
Allport, T D
Alp, N J
Altmann, P N S
Amery, J M
Anand, S
Anderson, K L
Anderson, K J
Andrews, T M
Angus, B J
Anscombe, M K
Anslow, P L
Anthony, M Y
Armitage, J M
Armstrong, R C
Aronson, J K
Ashworth, G J
Aspel, J L
Atenstaedt, R L
Athanasou, N A
Atkins, B L
Attenburrow, M E J
Babb, A G
Bagnall, M J C
Baigent, C N
Bailey, A J
Banks, E
Banning, A P
Bannon, M J
Barlow, D H
Barnes, P D
Barnett, R J
Barrios Martinez, P
Barter, K L
Bartlett, G E
Bartlett, R A L
Bashir, Y
Bass, C M
Bateman, K L
Bates, G J E M
Bates, N P
Beasley, N J P
Beazer, R
Becher, H H H
Beer, S
Bell, R M H
Bender-Bacher, H F F R
Benham, S W
Bennett, C C
Bennett, D H
Benson, A A
Benson, C A
Benson, M K
Benson, M K A
Beral, V
Berg, B E M
Berg, S J
Bernau, F L
Bethell, D B
Betts, T R
Bevan, A
Bhattacharya, S
Binney, L E
Birch, A G
Black, J J M
Black, R S
Blair, E M
Blakeley, A J
Blazewicz, L W
Blesing, C H
Blogg, C E
Boardman, P
Bodmer, H C
Bogdanor, J E
Bottrill, I D
Bowker, C M
Bowler, I C J W
Bowyer, R L
Boyd, C A R
Boyd, P A
Bradley, K J
Bradley, O P
Brady, S
Brewster, S F
Briggs, M
Briggs, R A
Brink, A K
Britton, B J
Brocklehurst, P
Brodie, J-A B
Bron, A J
Brown, G K
Brown, M A
Brown, M C
Brown, R C
Brown, S
Browne, J S
Brownlow, H C
Brownrigg-Gleeson, J A J
Bryan, P L D
Brylewski, J E
Buckley, C D
Budden, M L
Bullard, H
Bullock, D B
Bulstrode, C J K
Bunch, C
Burge, P D
Burge, S M
Burgess, S E P
Burgner, D P
Burke, G
Burke, P D
Burne, S R
Burns, E C
Burns, T P
Burt, G
Burtenshaw, F G R
Burton, E A
Burton, M J
Butler, R M
Byren, I V
Byrne, J V
Cadoux-Hudson, T A D
Caldicott, F
Calvert, J K
Campbell, A J
Campbell, F J
Campbell, L A
Cantwell, B
Carapiet, D A
Carney, G E
Carr, A J
Carré, E A B
Cassell, O C S
Cerundolo, V
Chadwick, J D H
Chalmers, I G
Chamberlain, P F J
Chan, S M H
Channon, K M
Chapel, H M
Chapman, D E
Chapman, G P
Chapman, R W G
Charnock, F M L
Cheetham, M
Cheng, H
Chivers, C A
Christopher, A V
Clampitt, L B
Clarke, N R A
Clarke, R J
Clelland, C A
Clemmey, W R L
Clubb, J M
Cocuzza, C E A
Coghlan, M C
Cole, D J
Coleman, D J
Collin, J
Collins, R E
Conlon, C P
Cook, P J
Cooke, P H
Cookson, W O C
Corfield, L F
Costello, C H
Cowan, F J
Cowan, N C
Cowen, P J
Cox, G J
Craig, S W
Cranshaw, J H
Cranston, D W
Craze, J L
Crofts, B J
Cronan, W S
Crow, T J
Crowther, R L
Cunliffe, D R
Cunliffe, R N
Curtis, S P
Darby, C R
Davey, A F
David, A F
David, J B
Davidson, L E U
Davies, D R
Davies, R J O
Davison, P S
Dawber, R P R
Day, N P J
De Newtown, R K
Dean, G S
Dendy, P R
Denman, M S
Dennis, P D
Dickson, H A
Dike, A E
Dimech, J
Dobson, M B
Dodd, C A F
Doll, R
Donaghy, M J
Dorkins, H R
Dorling, D M
Dorrell, L
Dorrington, K L
Drage, S M
Drury, N
Du Toit, J E
Dubowitz, M N
Duley, L M M
Duncan, E L
Duong Wust, N T H
Duthie, R B
Duxbury, F R C G
Dwight, J F S J
Dyar, O J
Eastwood, I Q
Edge, J A
Edwards, A
Edwards, J H
El-Kabir, D R
Elithorn, A
Elston, J S
Emery, J D
English, R E
Epstein, A
Erin, R J
Esiri, F O U
Esiri, M M
Evans, J M
Evans, R D
Fairburn, C J A G
Fairley, A
Fairweather, D S A
Farmery, A D
Faust, G E S
Fazel, M S
Fazel, S B
Feldman, E J
Fell, P J
Fennell, D A
Fenton, M J
Ferguson, D E J
Ferris, R J
Fillenz, M
Finnigan, A E
Firoozan, S
Fisher, A
Fleming, K A
Fleminger, M
Fletcher, E C
Flint, J
Flower, T D
Foex, P
Foord, T F
Forfar, J C
Forrest, G C
Forsyth, K D
Fowler, G H
Franklin, S L
Frankum, S C
Fraser, G R
Frayn, E H
Freeland, A P
Freeman, S D
Friend, P J
Frith, P A
Gaba, M D
Gabriel, S L
Galloway, P D
Gancz, G
Ganesan, T S
Gardner, L
Garner, P
Garrard, C S
Gatter, K C
Geddes, J R
George, B D
Giangrande, P L F
Gibbons, C L M H
Gibbons, R J
Gilchrist, J T
Gillmer, M D G
Gilmour, N C
Gleeson, F V
Glynn, C J
Godfrey, A M
Godlee, C J
Godsland, J
Goldacre, M J
Golding, S J
Goldman, D L
Goodacre, T E E
Goodfellow, J W
Goodman, T R
Goodwin, G M
Gould, S J
Govier, J L
Graham, R D
Grange, C S
Grant, H W
Gray, D W R
Gray, J A M
Gray, W
Grebenik, C R
Green, J M
Green, L R
Green, R A
Greenall, M J
Greenhall, E A
Greenhall, R C D
Greenwood, C E L
Gregg-Smith, S J
Gregory, D R
Gribble, F M
Gundle, R
Haeney, J A
Hafizi, S
Hague, S
Hall, G W
Hall, M A
Hall, R M
Halliday, B L
Hambleton, S
Hammersley, H N
Hammersley, M S
Hammond, N A
Handa, A I
Handley, R C
Hands, L J
Harden, P N
Harding, N G L
Hardinge, F M
Harnden, A R
Harris, A L
Harris, E
Harrison, P J
Hart, Y M
Hatton, C S R
Hawton, K E
Hayles, S
Haywood, K M
Heatley, M I
Hempson Brown, J
Herbert, M A
Herdman, P
Hicks, L J
Hicks, N R
Higgs, D R
Higham, H E
Hildebrand, G D
Hill, A V S

Hill, A M
Hill, P F
Ho, L-P
Hobbs, M J D
Hodge, M G
Holburn, A M
Hollinghurst, D
Holman, R R
Hook, P J
Hope, R A
Hormbrey, E L
Hormbrey, P J
Hornby, C J
Horne, S T
Houghton-Clemmey, R S A
Hoult, S L
Howarth, L J
Howie, K L
Hrouda, D
Huckstep, M R
Hughes, C M
Hughes, K A
Hull, J
Humzah, M D
Hurley, P A
Hurst, J A
Impey, L W M
Ioannides, A
Isaac, P
Ives, N K
Jack, T M
Jackson, S R
Jacoby, R J
James, A C D
James, D V
Jarrett, M E D
Jayawant, S S
Jefferson, T O
Jenkins, E L
Jessop, E
Jewell, D P
Johnson, D
Johnson, H J
Johnson, M A
Johnson, P
Johnson, P R V
Jones, A C
Jones, A M
Jones, D P H
Jones, L A
Jones, N
Jones, P H
Julier, M
Junger, D
Kaklamanis, L
Kambouroglou, G
Karamichalis, I M
Karpe, P F
Kay, J D S
Kearley, K E
Kearns, C F
Keeling, D M
Keenan, J
Kemp, E F
Kennedy, J E
Kennedy, M M
Kennedy, S H
Kennett, R P
Kenworthy-Browne, J M
Kenyon, C M
Keoghane, S R
Kerr, D J
Kerr, R S C
Keys, R I
King, S J A
Klenerman, P
Knight, M
Knight, T H
Knox, J M
Kurwa, H A
Kwiatkowski, D P
Lalvani, A
Lancaster, T R
Lane, D J
Lavery, B A
Law, S
Leach, A
Leaver, L B
Leonard, J V
Lessing, M P A
Levitt, N C
Levy, J C
Lewis, P J
Lewis, P S
Licence, K A M
Liebling, R E
Lindsell, D R M
Lintott, P N T
Littlewood, T J
Livesley, B
Llopis Miro, R
Lloyd, J W
Lo, Y-M D
Loach, A B
Loh, L
Lortan, J E
Lyn, C W
McBeath, H A
McCarthy, M I
McCleery, J M
McCloskey, R M H L
McDonnell, C T
Macfarlane, J A
McGee, J O D
MacIntosh, C M A
Mackenzie, D N
MacKenzie, I Z
McKenzie, P J
McLardy Smith, P D
MacLennan, D N
Maclennan, S A
McManus, E M
McMichael, A J
McNab, I S H
McNally, E G
McNally, M A
McPherson, A
Macpherson, G G
McQuay, H J
McQuay, T A I
McShane, M A
McShane, R H
McTavish, S F B
Maddison, A D
Magill, P J
Malladi, R K
Malmberg, A K
Mandelbrote, B M
Manek, S
Manji, H H
Mann, M S
Manning, A N
Mant, D C A
Marsden, A P
Marsden, R B
Martin, C B
Martin, S V
Martinez Devesa, P
Mason, D G
Mason, D Y
Mather, R J
Matthews, D R
Matthews, P M
Maynard, N D
Mayon-White, R T
Mayou, R A
Mehta, P S
Mendes Ribeiro, H K
Merriman, H M
Meston, N
Middleton, M R
Milford, C A
Millar, D E
Millard, P R
Millard, T P
Miller, D S
Miller, D M
Milner, A A
Minton, M J
Misbah, S A
Mitchell, C D
Mitchell, S A
Moher, M G
Molyneux, A J
Moncrieff, M W
Moore, E J
Moore, N R
Moore, P J
Morgan, B L
Morgan, J R
Morris, J E
Morris, J F
Morris, M J
Morris, P J
Morrison, J D
Morrison, S D
Mortensen, J A
Mortensen, N J M
Moser, S C
Moss, K H
Mould, T L
Moxon, E R
Mufti, W-I-S
Murphy, M F G
Murphy, M F
Murray, B J
Murray, D W
Myerson, S G
Nadlacan, L M
Nairne, A A
Neale, I A
Neil, H A W
Nemeth, A H
Newsom-Davis, J M
Newton, J N
Newton, P N
Newton, R E
Nicholson-Lailey, T J F
Nicholson, R S
Noble, J G
O'Brien, T S
O'Byrne, K J
O'Donoghue, M F
Ogg, G S
Oliver, D W
Oppenheimer, C V R P
Orme, R M E
Ormerod, O J M
Ostlere, S J G
Outhwaite, J M
Owen, A C
Owen, J E
Pakenham-Walsh, N M
Palace, J A
Pandit, J J
Park, R J
Parker, C E
Parker, J D
Parry, A M M
Parry, C M
Parsons, D S
Patel, C K
Patsios, D A
Patterson, J A
Pawson, R
Peacock, S J
Pearce, M-J
Peedell, C
Peereboom, J M
Pendlebury, S T
Percival, H G
Pereira, M L
Periappuram, M
Perkins, J M T
Perkins, M J
Perry, R J
Perryer, S E
Perumalpillai, R G
Peto, T E A
Phillips-Hughes, J
Phillips, A J
Phillips, C M
Phillips, R E
Phizackerley, P J R
Pigott, A E
Pike, M G
Piris, J
Plint, S J
Pluck, N D
Pointon, A D
Pollard, A J
Pollard, R C
Poole, E W
Porter, B H
Porter, D
Poulton, J
Powell, A S
Powell, S M
Price, A J
Price, E M
Price, J D
Price, J R
Prior, N G
Pugh, C W
Punt, L
Puvanendran-Thomas, R
Qizilbash, N
Quaghebeur, G M-M
Quested, D J
Quinlan, M J
Rahemtulla, A
Raine, N M N
Rajagopalan, B
Rajakulendran, T
Randall, A A S
Randhawa, B
Rannan-Eliya, S V
Ratcliffe, P J
Ratnatunga, C P
Rawcliffe, P M
Redman, C W G
Rees, C M P
Reynolds, D J M
Reynolds, S M
Richards, P G
Riddle, P J
Robbins, P A
Roberton, M
Roberts, C
Roberts, D J
Roberts, I S D
Robertson, C M
Robins, D P
Robinson, A J
Robinson, E T
Robinson, M
Robinson, S P
Roblin, J
Roblin, P H
Robson, G M W
Robson, M J
Robson, P J
Roddie, A M S
Rogers, R
Rook, C D
Rose, N D B
Rose, S
Rosen, P H
Roskell, D E
Ross, B D
Rowell, N P
Rowland-Jones, S L
Runciman, D M I
Russell, R M
Rutter, H R
Rutter, L E
Sacks, G E
Sadler, G P
Sainsbury, M C
Saleem, S
Salisbury, A J
Salmon, J F
Samra, J S
Sanderson, F
Sargent, P A
Saunders, P M
Scarfe, D R
Schofield, N M
Screaton, G R
Screaton, N J
Sear, J W
Selkon, J B
Series, H G
Shakespeare, J M
Sharma, R
Shawcross, D L
Shefler, A G
Shennan, J C
Shepherd, J E E
Shepstone, B J
Sherrard, J S
Sherrington, L J
Shewan, D B
Shine, B S F
Shlugman, D
Shuker, J P
Sichel, J H S
Side, L E
Sidebottom, P
Silvester, R D
Simon, S D
Sinclair, M E
Sington, J D
Slack, M P E
Slade, M G
Slater, A
Slater, J D E
Slater, J N
Slavotinek, A M
Sleight, P
Small, D G
Smarason, A K
Smith, B J
Smith, K A
Smith, R
Smith, S C
Solomon, R A
Spalding, J M K
Spilling, R A E
Spivey, R S
Squier, M V
Stanton, A P
Stearn, M R
Steel, H C
Stein, A L
Stein, J A
Stein, J F
Stein, T R
Steiner, J A
Stephenson, C J
Stern, D M
Stevens, J E
Stevens, R M
Stewart, A
Stewart, H S
Stirzaker, L
Stoneham, M D
Stores, G
Stradling, J R
Sugden, E M
Sullivan, P B
Swan, M C
Swarup, N
Tagg, C E
Taggart, D P P
Talbot, D C
Talbot, K A
Taylor, A
Taylor, K A
Taylor, M J O
Teddy, P J
Teh, J L Z
Teschke, C J
Thakker, R V
Theodoulou, M T
Theologis, T
Thomas, M G
Thomas, S J
Thomson, A M
Thomson, A H
Threlfall, A K
Tilleard-Cole, R R R
Todd, B S
Toff, P R
Townsend, A R M
Traill, Z C
Travis, S P L
Trowell, J M
Turberfield, L M
Turner, N C
Turner, R J
Tuson, J R D
Uberoi, R
Uden, J A
Underwood, P M
Unia, C
Usiskin, S I
Vallis, K A
Vassallo, C M
Vaughan Williams, E M
Vaux, D J T
Venables, P A
Venning, V A
Vessey, M P
Viale, J P
Vincent, A C
Viney, D B
Virr, A J
Von Eichstorff, P D G
Vyas, P
Wade, D T
Wain, E C E
Wainscoat, J S
Wainwright, A M
Walker, N P J
Wallace, T M
Waller, D J
Walton, R T
Ward, M E
Ware, L M
Warner, N J
Warner, O J
Warrell, D A
Warrell, M J
Warren, B F
Warwick, J P
Wass, J A H
Watkin, N A
Watt Smith, S R
Weaver, A
Webster, P N
Wee, B L
Welding, R N
Weston-Davies, W H
Wheatley, S-A
Wheeler, A J
Wheeler, K A H
Whitaker, P J
White, A C
White, P M
Whybrew, K J
Wiesemann, P
Wilde, G P
Wilkie, A O M
Wilkinson, A R
Wilkinson, D A
Wilkinson, M
Wilkinson, P B
Willatt, J M
Willcox, H N A
Willett, K M
Williams, D L
Williams, E M
Williams, L P
Williams, P R
Williams, S M
Williamson, D
Williamson, K N B
Wilson-MacDonald, J
Wilson, A S P
Wilson, D J
Wilson, J
Wilson, R P E
Wilson, S J
Wilson, S R
Winearls, C G
Winner, S J
Winnifrith, T J A
Wojnarowska, F T
Wood, M J A
Wood, S
Woodman, J R
Woods, K A
Wordsworth, B P
Worlock, P H
Wright, E C
Wright, J A
Young, J D
Zapata, L C
Zimbwa, P M

Oxted

Burns, D
Campbell, A J
Caplan, B A
Everington, T F
Griffiths, R J
Haig, S D
Hill, D J
Hills, S J
Ince, J W
MacLean, K S
Marsh, C K
Morley, P K
Morris, A J
Myers, M J
Pinder, C G
Skellett, S C C
Spiller, R W
Teasdale, K J
Thomas, D C
Williams, J S
Williams, R M J

Padstow

Emrys-Jones, G J H
McKelvey, I A
Priest, M S

Paignton

Ackers, J W L
Alcroft, J E
Austin, M L
Avery, D A
Ballance, P G
Banks, A A
Batstone, J H
Bishop, H
Bridge, J R
Bullen, J G
Cottrell, M A
Coxon, J P
Deakin, J P
Deakin, V E
Dibble, L
Eggleton, M L
Foreman, L P
Green, P A
Hardy, E A
Howitt, W P F
Kuur, C R
Lansdown, S R P
Lowes, A J
MacLoughlin, P J
Masters, R C
Mills, D C
Norley, I
Phare, A J
Pletts, R C
Richards, G A
Richards, I M
Richardson, A P
Roberts, J D V
Slomka, H
Smith, N P
Somerfield, D J
Southall, E
Spicer, N A J K
Steele, Y E
Straiton, N

Thompson, M G
Walden, A F D
Watt, W M
Williams, D L
Wright, M

Paisley
Ahmed, S U
Al-Janabi, S
Allister, C A
Anderson, J M
Anderson, M A J
Anderson, W G
Arokianathan, M C
Baxter, W P
Bell, D
Blatchford, O M W
Bloomer, J
Boag, J C
Bonham, D A
Brown, C W
Brown, R C
Buchanan, A
Byrne, K E
Campbell, I H
Candlish, W
Canning, J C
Chapman, K M
Chaudhri, S
Chawla, J C
Chee, L C
Cheriyan, K E
Chitnis, S L
Clark, K
Crampsey, F M
Cuddihy, A M
Dahill, S W
Davidson, D C
Davies, M-L
Dinnett, E M
Dolan, G P A
Dorward, A J
Downie, A R
Ejaz, S
El-Fallah, M E-M
Evans, C J
Feeney, L A
Fitzpatrick, D
Fitzsimons, C P
Frew, W A
Ganguly, D K
Ganly, I
Gibson, S E G
Gravil, J H
Gruer, N E M
Hamilton, G J
Hamilton, I J D
Hanlon, L C S
Hardie, K G
Hardy, I G
Harkin, H M
Hay, I C
Hay, R E
Herron, C A
Hislop, J M
Hislop, L J
Hislop, W S
Hodgson, C W L
Innes, C Y
Ireland, T
Jenkins, J T
Johnstone, C J M
Jones, A M
Jones, R W
Kinniburgh, A J
Knox, A D
Leighton, J L
Leonard, J F
Livingston, H M
Lowe, K
McAlpine, D M
McArthur, D R
McArthur, S M
McCormick, S
McCourtney, J S
Macdonald Speirs, N A H
MacDonald, C M
McDonald, L A B
McIntyre, M
MacIntyre, P D
McKay, P J
MacKenzie, J C
McKirdy, M J
Maclennan, A C
McLoone, J
McMahon, C P
McMillan, R M
McNaughton, G W
McPeake, J R
Macpherson, T D
Mahmood, A
Makin, M G
Marr, S A P
Marr, S T P
Mason, I S
Meehan, C
Miller, S M
Mitchell, K G
Monaghan, S C
Murray, C M
Negrette, J J
Orr, J E
Pennycook, J A
Porteous, C
Quinn, A J
Ramsay, A
Reay, L M
Reid, C B
Richmond, R M
Rimmer, E M
Roberts, G C
Robertson, M R I
Robson, B J
Scorgie, B M
Scott, B J
Scott, W
Scullion, D M
Selim, A M H
Sengupta, P
Shepherd, R C
Sim, J C
Simpson, G K
Simpson, R B
Smith, L A
Steel, G F
Stewart, G
Stothers, J
Strang, I
Struthers, L J
Sutherland, C G G
Thom, D E
Thomson, A J
Thomson, J E
Unni, A G
Vinson, M C
Waclawski, E R
Wallace, A D
Walsh, J E
Watson, G M
Watson, M A
Weir, J B V
Weir, W I
White, A
Wilkie, L M
Williams, C L C
Williamson, B W A
Winton, D B
Wright, L
Young, J J
Zaher, S A E-A

Par
Gullam, J E
Hannett, B F
Haskins, N
Molyneux, N R
Monk, P E
Nash, S R
Overshott, R A
Rowe, J G
Tempest, P K
Towell, J D

Pathhead
Dummer, D S
Sanderson, E P
Wilson, C M

Peacehaven
Byrne, L G
Curtis, A J
Etherton, J E
Gupta, V K
Gurtler, C J
Jefford, H A
Mandal, L B
Milne, G J
Patel, B A
Patel, C J
Schapira, D J
Starling, A J

Peebles
Bacon, M M C
Baird, D
Clyde, E M S
Duncan, M E
Hegarty, D M
Hunt, K A
Love, D R
McDonald, I A
McEwan, M A
McIntosh, G E
Moore, C S
Morrish, C
Noyes, K J
Pyatt, R N
Simpson, K E
Watt, J V
Young, P T

Peel
Christian, R P
Gray, O S M
Hanks, R J
Hannan, M C
Hudson, A B
Jones, K J
Shaw, D M
Shepherd, R T

Pembroke
Cox, M O
Cuff, B E
Davies, J V
Hannaford, R W
Lewis, S J G
Nagaraj, C B
Naik, D R
Power, F J
Roberts, J G
Scadden, J E
Thomas, M D
Windsor, A C M
Windsor, P A

Pembroke Dock
Bury, R N
Cooper, M M
Evans, A N
Goodson, P
Helliwell, J R
Tobin, F A

Penarth
Al-Sabah, A
Attanoos, R L
Back, I N
Barnes, P M
Bates, J L
Bayer, A J
Baylis, E A H
Bell, S M
Bleehen, R E
Bowler, I
Buchalter, M B
Campbell, I A
Care, E A
Chilcott, J L
Clarke, V
Cobley, M
Cornish, C J
Crane, M D
Creese, K H
Danielsen, M S
Davies, A E J
Davies, B H
Davies, C E
Davies, G
Davies, H L S
Davies, M C
Davies, R P
Edwards, S A
El-Gaylani, N
Erin, E M
Evans, A S
Evans, J G
Ferguson, C J
Frost, P J
Gelder, C M
George, L D
Gibbs, A R
Gough, J
Green, J T
Griffith, E F
Griffiths, T L
Hain, R D W
Halpin, S F S
Hasan, M
Hebden, M W
Hubbard, R E
Jasper, A L
Kafetzakis, E
Lari, J
Lewis, K E
Lewis, P R W
Lindsay, P C
Lloyd, A
Long, C C
Major, V
Matthews, S B
Meek, J C
Mehta, A
Morris, J E
Morris, S
O'Mahony, M S
Owens, D R
Parker, C R
Parry, D E
Peet, E J R
Prickett, F M E
Quoraishi, A H M A H
Radcliffe, A G
Ribeiro, C D
Robinson, T A
Shah, N S
Sim, M F V
Stephens, R C M
Stone, M D
Sutton, D A O
Swift, G L
Thomas, H D
Thomas, J G
Thomas, R H
Tinker, G M
Turton, J
Vafidis, J A
Walker, N A
Warren, C A
Williams, D M
Williams, S R
Wilson, E A
Wright, E M

Penicuik
Begg, A D
Begg, D M
Bell, J K
Carluke, I
Collins, R M
Cooney, M K
Fraser, I M
Gillespie, D H
Griffin, T M J
Hider, C F
Johnston, N M
Levstein, C
Livingstone, A G
Macdonald, S T
McKay, K M
MacLean, J
McLintock, L A
McRorie, A
Marchant, A E
Marwick, T J
Murray, C M
Reid, H A H
Smith, C C
Wood, A P

Penrhyndeudraeth
Clarke, J H
Daplyn, I R
Endaf, A I
Jones, D P M
Prichard, O M
Thomas, A J

Penrith
Barr, J E
Barr, R
Booth, D
Boulter, P S
Brock, P A C
Bruce, E M
Cama, L S D
Davidson, F
Dunlop, J
Dunlop, M S
Dunning, H A
Eckersall, A C
Ellerton, J A
Frost-Smith, B M
Goulding, P G R
Hall, R W
Hallewell, C L
Hanley, M T
Hearsey, J A
Hodkin, J P G
Hutchinson, P M
Johnson, C A
Jupp, C M L
Kirk, J M
Lawler, W
Long, H A
Mans, M
Matheson, A
Metcalfe, D H H
Mills, S L
Pritchard, I P
Purdy, V L
Reed, A
Smith, J K L
Thompson, J A
Tiffin, N J
Unwin, D E J
Wells, C A
Weston, T P
Young, G L
Young, T S S

Penryn
Beckett, R J
Bourne, A J
Brown, I M C
Burns, H
Ellis, M F
Green, B G J
Katz, J
Paxton, M J
Seddon, A J
Sutherland, C J
Upton, P M
White, E M
Wood, R M T

Pentraeth
Starczewski, A R

Pentre
Bihari, K
Choudhary, B P
Choudhary, H N
Choudhary, M
McCrystal, D J
Medlicott, S A
Morgan, R D
Sami, S Z A
Stephenson, C
Stone, A R
Tomkinson, A

Penzance
Armstrong, W N
Bonnar, A J
Carruthers, D M
Cormie, P J
Cox, P J
Currie, I D C
Ellery, A
Fletcher, N J
Freeman, M K
Freeman, Z R L
Griffiths, F J
Halls, G A
Harker, R
Harvey, J R
Hicks, P M M
Hunter, C J K
Jones, M R
Lack, J J
Levine, D F
Long, M H
Mackenzie, M
Manser, R F
Martin, F J
Mulholland, S N P
Paterson, A G
Peller, S E
Pring, J E
Purchas, S F
Rutherfurd, S F
Ryan, J F
Senior, R E
Sproson, J C
Turner, J S
Wearne, S
Williams, S J
Wilson, P P
Wilson, S J S

Perranporth
Hallworth, N A
Jones, C A
Lenz, R J
Merrin, P K
Murdoch, K A
Partington, S I
Sidebotham, C F
Turfitt, M E

Pershore
Atkinson, A C
Barber, K
Borchardt, F J
Carter, J J
Chui, S L
Cluley, S
Edwards, K M R
Hird, J M
Johnstone, G E
Keating, P J S
O'Loghlen, N A
Ooi, Y W
Perks, C E
Pitts-Tucker, T J
Preston, M J
Ralphs, G J G
Rankin, J S
Richards, V J
Thomas, K P
Thompson, P J M
Weatherup, C H
Wunsch, C M
Young, C M

Perth
Allan, Y D
Allen, R E
Angus, S L
Balfour, R O
Bates, D
Beale, N J
Bell, M
Birch, R
Blaikie, A J
Boyd, A T
Brewster, J H
Brown, P H
Bulcraig, A R
Burnett, L D
Cameron, H M
Capper, M E
Carey, D T
Carlin, D D
Carter, G E
Cavanagh, E M
Cockburn, E A
Coe, P A
Coe, S M
Colquhoun, H A
Compson, L J
Connacher, A A
Connelly, P J
Cowie, A J H
Crichton, J A
Currie, F R J
Dewhurst, N G
Dolan, L C
Donald, I M
Dowse, S M
Dutton, A H
Easton, L J C
Eccleston, A D
El-Miligy, M Y M
English, J B
Eriksen, C A
Espley, A J
Falconer, A F
Flinn, J
Fok, P J
Forbes, D W
Forster, L F
Forster, M R
Forster, R E
Foster, D S
Fowler, K G
Franks, D M
Fyfe, J
Gamble, P
Garton, M J
Georgeson, E J
Gordon, A F
Gordon, G J
Gourley, A A
Gray, E C
Hadden, W A
Halliday, P
Hamilton, J R
Hewitt, S J
Ho-A-Yun, J E F
Islam, H R U
Kirk, H
Kirk, J
Kirkwood, D W
Klaassen, B
Kynaston, J H F
Lambie, A M
Lamont, D C
Law, S A T
Lawson, D D A
Lendrum, S
Little, C L

Lowdon, N M
Lyon, R L
Lyons, E
MacCall, C A
Mcclelland, S M
McClure, I J
McFarlane, A G
MacGregor, D F
McGuire, B E
MacKay, R M
Maclean, C M
MacLean, J G B
McLeod, N A
Magahy, F D
Mayland, C R
Mellor, I
Melrose, G A
Melville, R H D
Menzies, E M
Meyers, R M
Murdoch, R W G
Murray, W J G
Napper, A J
Norris, A
Page, C S
Pearson, R H
Peebles, M K
Peek, B
Phillips, W D P
Prentice, N P
Priestley, M B
Pritchard, G
Protheroe, D E
Pugh, C E
Qureshi, S A
Raschkes, B J
Ratcliff, A J
Reay, B A
Reid, G S
Reid, J H
Reid, R P
Reilly, B M A
Renfrew, M A
Richard, K W
Ripley, C S
Ripley, J S
Ritchie, E D
Romotowski, L I
Ross, N
Rowland, L J
Roxburgh, C M C
Roxburgh, S T D
Shackles, D A
Shennan, W J S
Shepherd, A N
Shepherd, N I
Sinclair, J I
Sinclair, S
Singer, B R
Stewart, C D
Tait, D H H
Watson, E T
Watson, J I
Will, M B
Williams, S
Winship, S M
Wood, S M
Wright, D W

Peterborough

Abdul Karim, A P S S M S
Agbasi, N N
Aladin, A
Anand, J K
Anderson, A A
Arnold, S J
Asplin, E J
Baker, P M
Banner, A V
Barrett, M
Basi, R S
Beeton, J R
Bhari, J K
Bhat, N A
Bhullar, T P S
Bishop, M C
Blackford, H N
Blake, D C S
Blatchford, H L
Blundell, J W
Bond, A J
Briggs, F A
Brown, C M
Burley, T K
Cartmel, R M
Cawood, R H
Chambers, G M
Chopra, N B
Choy, L S A
Clarke, J W
Clayton, D A
Cole, D R
Cooper, A M C
Cope, A R
Coxon, T C
Cradwick, J C
Dalal, M M
Damany, D S
Das, P A
Davies, T M
Dawson, C
Dennis, B
Dennis, P M
Denton, M J
Devonald, M A J
Dilley, C M
Dodwell, D J F
Doran, J F
Dryburgh, E H
Du Plessis, J V B
Dugdale, C M
Eadie, K M
Edey, M M J
Eldred, K F
Evans, G E
Ewing, A Y
Ewing, G
Famoriyo, A A A
Farrell, M C
Feggetter, G S
Fitt, A W D
Fletcher, N J
Flores, F R
Fowler, L
Frow, R W
Gall, A J
Gardiner, L J
Gardiner, S E
Gemmell, J H
Gerada, A
Gibbons, A J
Glavina, H M
Glavina, M J
Gleeson, C M
Gormly, L M G
Grant, C M
Grant, S J
Greaves, I
Gregg, A K
Griffiths, R
Guy, R J
Hackman, B W
Hammersley, D
Haque, S T A
Harris, M D
Hartropp, P
Hemmaway, C J
Henchy, M C N
Hipwell, P M
Hobbis, J M
Holmes, J T
Hoole, K
Horrocks, C L
Howlin, S G
Hughes, S P
Hunt, E R
Hutchings, P T
Iyer, V K S
Jachuck, M S J
Jackson, M A
Jackson, N R
Jacobs, L
Jelen, I
Johns, D L
Johnston, P L
Joshi, K M
Kapila, H
Kauser, A
Kent, J
Kerr, D N S
Khan, J A
Kilgallen, C J
Kitson, R M
Knights, A J
Krijgsman, B
Langley, B C E
Laundy, T J
Leung, D P Y
Lewis, S L
Lumb, M R
McAdam, K F
McKeown, B J
Maddula, M R
Mahmoud, N A H
Malki, D S
Mallett, R B
Marshall, N W
Maxey, A M
Mazumdar, R K
Mbanu, A
Mehta, M J
Menzies, S J
Merrill, S B
Mistry, C D
Mitchell, B
Mitchell, C A
Mitchell, D W
Modha, J D
Modha, N J
Morgan, N K
Moshy, R E
Moss, C E
Mungall, I P F
Murthy, V
Myszka, Z J
Nair, P
Nally, R E
Navamani, S
Nnochiri, C C P
Norcliffe, P J
Norman, A W
O'Donnell, P A
O'Reilly, V H
Okonkwo, O J
Okubadejo, A A T
Outar, K P
Panday, S
Parker, M J
Patel, R C
Paterson, B A
Petangoda, G
Pfleiderer, A G
Phipps, J S K
Pryor, G A
Purcell, R T
Rajiv, K
Randall, J M
Rankin, S M
Rao, T L N
Rawdon Smith, H S
Reed, P N
Richards, S D
Rigg, K S
Rimmer, T J
Robertson, J M
Rogers, S D
Roland, J M
Rowlands, D B
Sadler, M G
Sagovsky, R
Salameh, Y M M H
Sampson, K
Samrai, P S
Sanders, N P
Satya Prasad, K
Sayegh, H F
Scarisbrick, C D
Scott, C G
Scott, R M
Senior, A
Shah, M L
Shair, A B E
Sharma, S D
Sheehan, N J
Shilliday, P F
Shoban, B K
Short, S M
Simhadri, N
Sivakumaran, M
Smith, H S
Squire, J K
Sriemevan, A
Stanton-King, K D
Steel, S A
Stovin, O J
Stuart, H C
Takhar, A P S
Thakker, P
Thein, M
Thillaivasan, K
Thomas, J A
Thompson, J S
Thorpe, J
Thorpe, J W
Trounce, R F
Tuck, G
Tuck, S J
Turner, A G
Tweedie, R J
Urwin, S C
Van Den Bent, P J
Vardy, S J
Varley, G W
Walker, R T
Walker, S E
Watson, S J
Watts-Russell, J V A
Wilmot, R A
Wilson, N S
Winfrey, P M
Wishart, K C
Withers, R A
Womack, C
Woodcock, M G L
Woolf, D A
Wozencroft, D W
Yong, D E J
Youens, J E B
Zerafa, R

Peterculter

Harris, D C M
Lawson, C
McHardy, F E
Millar, D G
Skerrow, B A
Stewart, L J

Peterhead

Armstrong, P
Bruce, G M
Campbell, D G D
Donaldson, P H
Fenwick, D K F
Ferguson, G G
Gauld, A R
Gauld, H M G
Kennedy, D J G
Lacey, E J
Lawrie, D
Lawrie, R F
Leslie, M A
McInnes, R
Mackay, J R
Millar, J
Nicol, D R H
Pollock, M R
Ritchie, L D
Robertson, J B
Sandeman, J M
Small, I R
Stephen, R S
Stout, J C
Strachan, B T
Strachan, K A B
Tait, J
Taylor, J M
Watt, G M C
Webster, D

Peterlee

Abbott, R G
Anderson, D G
Barlow, P
Burleigh, A R S
Chandy, J
Choudhary, S R
Gallagher, P G
Hays, K J
Pearson, G
Popov, A
Ramakrishna Gupta, M D
Russell, I S
Sil, A K
Thomas, A H
Thompson, I
Willson, G

Petersfield

Abercrombie, G F
Angell, M P
Bartlett, C V
Bates, T M
Buckley, S J
Bulmer-Van Vliet, J
Bush, C J D
Christie, C
Christie, J S
Coni, H J A
Cox, C M
De Halpert, P A
Ellis, B G
Francis-Lang, A M
Griffin, E L
Holden, A F H
Holden, S J
Lewis, C E
Litchfield, M A
MacKeown, I L
Mileham, P A
Perry, R K K
Renton, N J
Ryan, N C
Sinclair, C C R
Tyler, A K
Welch, C B
Young, A E
Ziegler, E S M

Petworth

Bonsall, J L
Boothby, H A
Clarke, R G
Dally, P J
Howard, P
Lyons, G M
Morgan, R
Pett, S
Quiney, N F
Roehr, S P
Shaw, S L
Simpson, S A
Smith, R C
Waugh, P J

Pevensey

Baig, M I
Bansel, A
Briggs, J A
Darwent, J P
Hewett-Clarke, A H R
Vandenwijngaerden, S

Pewsey

Davis, A E
Green, I
Grundy Wheeler, N J
Heaton, J C
Hewartson, R M
Hutson, A J
Jenkins, P D
McGee, P J
Mahroof, M R
Phillips, S W
Ring, J P G
Shirehampton, T A
Vickers, P J

Pickering

Blacklee, M E
Capes, D E
Cottingham, D
Duddington, M
Thornton, T J

Pinner

Ahmad, N
Allen, J A
Baum, A S
Benattar, K D
Brewerton, J M
Byers, A H
Catto, J W F
Chang, L P-Y
Chang, S H-P
Collins, M R
Cumberbatch, G L
Curran, L A
Dastur, N B
Dawood, R B
Dove, N A R
Doyle, M
Edwards, A
Edwards, D M
Farooqui, O A
Fishman, D
Fong, K J
Groom, R V
Hardman, A
Hazell, N W R
Homapour, B
Hudd, C A M
Hughes, G
Inada-Kim, M
Jamil, F W
Jayabalan, S N
Jenner, C S
Kapembwa, M S
Kelshiker, A S
Kirmani, S S
Kodilinye, H C
Laurence, B E
Liberman, D
Lubel, D D
Majus, R
Markanday, A
Marks, J E R
Mediwake, R G
Miller, D L
Mistry, K
Nicholls, A J S
O'Toole, G A
Paul, K
Payne, C E
Rajani, K K
Reid, C D L
Rizki, S
Rookledge, M A
Rudd, B C
Rudolph, J K
Saville, S D
Schiller, G I
Shah, S Z
Sidhu, J S
Sittampalam, L W
Sofat, N
Stevenson, J F
Sundaresan, R
Thakur, M
Tomic, D A
Tran, T L
Uszycka, B S A
Walton, K R
Weller, I V D
Zideman, D A

Pitlochry

Campbell, A J
Cruikshank, D A
Davis, A G
Dreghorn, J
Faulds, M M
Finlay, K C
Kennedy, D S
Leaver, D P
McCrory, G W
MacHugh, J I R
Simmons, R E

Plockton

Knox, K D
Mackenzie, A

Plymouth

Acharya, U R
Ackford, H G
Adams, J A
Adams, W M
Alderson, J W
Alexander, I
Alexander, J J D
Anderson, G H
Anderson, S R
Andrews, C J H
Archer-Koranteng, E
Arkle, J H
Ashley, S
Aughey, T T
Awan, M Y
Ayling, R M
Bailey, J V
Bailey, N J
Bakheit, A M O
Balmer, H G R
Basterfield, J E
Baumer, J H
Baxter, L A
Beasley, A J
Beckley, S L
Bell, S P
Benjafield, R G
Bennett, M J
Bennett, S G
Benton, J I
Beresford, J K
Bertie, T M
Biggs, J E
Binchy, J M E
Blackstone, H B
Bligh, J G
Booth, A P
Bouhaimed, M M
Bowler, S K
Boyhan, C R
Breddy, P N
Brenton, J E
Bridger, M W M
Britten, C M
Brodribb, A J M
Brooks, P R
Brown, C
Brown, E L
Brownlie, G S J
Bryson, P J V
Budge, A
Budge, C J
Burdett, N G
Burdon, M S
Burge, A J S
Burgess, A J
Burrell, C J
Burridge, M G

Butcher, J L
Butler, J R
Calder, A D
Campbell, H M
Campbell, J C
Campbell, J K
Campbell, P G
Carlson, J N R
Carr, A S
Cassidy, S A
Chakraverty, A C
Challenor, R M
Chapman, J M
Charnley, G J
Chiappe, N P
Chowdhury, M S H
Chowdhury, R Y
Coard, K C M
Coates, M B
Coates, P J B
Coghill, J C
Coleman, M G
Copper, J R
Copplestone, J A
Corkill, R J
Cormack, A J R
Cornish, J F
Couch, J C
Courtney, D J
Cox, R R
Craig, A J
Cronin, A J
Cronshaw, S J
Crook, P A
Cunningham, R
Cunningham, S J
Dalrymple-Hay, M J R
Dance, D A B
Daniel, F N F
Daniels, J P
Dashfield, A K
David, H G
Davidson, H E
Davies, P R F
De Mendonca, P M S
Dean, J D
Deardon, D J
Defriend, D E
Dickinson, A J
Dobbs, F F
Donaldson, C A
Downes, C M
Drabble, E H
Drury, R A B
Dubbins, P A
Dudleston, K E
Duff, P W
Eadie, G B
Eason, J D
Elphinstone, M G
Embleton, M A
Esson, W R
Evans, D A
Evans, J
Evans, N M
Evans, P E L
Evans, R E
Falconer, A D
Farrington, W
Fearon, J
Feddo, F K
Ferguson, S S
Fisher, D W
Fletcher, C P
Ford, R A
Ford, R L
Fox, B M T
Franklin, J R
Frappell, J M
Freegard, T J
Freeman, J
Freeman, R M
Freeman, S J
French, A E
Fuller, J R
Fullilove, S M
Fulton, J D
Gale, J E S
Galloway, P H
Ganapathy, M
Gasim, A
Gaunt, P N
Gerwat, J
Gibson, J D
Gillespie, K
Glew, P A
Golding-Cook, A N
Gorham, P F
Grant, I C
Grayson, M J
Greene, K R
Greenway, B A
Griffiths, H M
Guly, H R
Gurry, B H
Gutteridge, C M
Habib, N E N
Halawa, M
Hambly, J
Hammonds, J C
Hampshire, J E
Hardy, P H
Harnett, C L
Harold, R S J
Harris, D L
Harry, A J
Harvey, P B
Hasan, S
Haslam, E C
Hateley, S J
Hayfron-Benjamin, T R M
Hayward, C M
Haywood, G A
Heath, R M
Hickling, P
Hill, G A
Hill, W T
Hilton, D A
Hirst, R S
Hobbs, S J F
Hodgins, I R
Hofinger, E
Hopkins, M J L
Hosie, K B
Hughes, C H
Hughes, G W
Hughes, P D
Hunter, K R
Hutton, C W
Jackson, S A
James, H D
Johnston, C G
Jones, A C
Jones, A M H
Jones, G M
Jones, P A
Jones, P
Jones, R W A
Jones, R C M
Jones, S J
Kaminski, E R
Kapila, R
Keddie, F S
Kelly, S A
Kersey, P J W
Khan, N A S
Kingsnorth, A N
Kingsnorth, J M
Kirby, J
Kirkham, M J
Kitson, M P
Knight, W A
Knights, D L
Kuo, J H U
Lambert, A W
Lambert, P M
Lambert, S H
Langton, J A
Lawrence, A J
Lawrence, P K
Lenden, G J
Lenden, P M
Lewis, C T
Lloyd, C J F
Lloyd, C E F
Lochhead, J
Longhurst, M J
Longworth, J L
Loopstra, E M
Lovett, J J
Lowe, C H
Loxdale, P H
Luyt, K
Lynch, P
Lytle, J
McArdle, P J
Macartney, S I
McBride, K
McCormick, C S F
McEwing, D J
McGavin, C R
McGill, R M
McInerney, J L
McInerney, P D
MacLeod, P M
MacNaughton, P D
Madar, R J
Mahmood, N
Mahony, J
Makin, J S
Malaree, S L F
Mantoura, O A
Marchbank, A J
Marshall, A J
Matheson, A J
Mears, J E
Melhuish, J E
Mildmay-White, A A
Millard, S W
Monaghan Addy, D J
Moorcroft, J V
Moorman, D J E
Morgan, N V
Morris, D J
Morris, R J
Morrison, G D
Morsman, J M
Motwani, J G
Mugridge, A R
Murphy, F M
Murphy, M
Murphy, W J C
Murray, A E
Murray, S J
Nagabhyru, A
Nagabhyru, A
Natale, S
Neve, H A
Nichols, E A
Nimmo, S B
Norrie, D M
O'Neill, R C O H
Ohlsson, V
Oldman, M J
Oliver, P D
Olsen, N D L
Oppong, F C
Osborn, F A
Overal, S G
Owen, M H
Padley, T J
Page, R M
Pai, R U
Palin, D J
Palmer, J D
Payne, S D
Pearson, S A
Perham, T G M
Perks, J M
Perry, J N
Pickard, J G
Pinch, E T
Pitman, J
Pobereskin, L H
Pollard, B J
Pollitt, Y
Poplar, C C E
Potter, A B
Prance, S E
Price, DK
Prior, R C
Protheroe, C K
Quinton, A A G
Rahamim, Y
Rai, K D
Rance, J M
Rawlings, E
Rawlings, I D
Read, A C
Reilly, E P
Riden, D K
Ring, A E
Ring, N J
Riou, P J
Robbins, J A B
Roberson, F E D
Roberts, S R
Robinson, S J
Rogers, A K J
Rogers, K
Romilly, S A
Roobottom, C A
Ross, J W B
Rossiter, N D
Rowe, P A
Rowland, P G
Rowlands, T K
Rule, S A J
Sair, M
Salz, M
Scott, D J
Scott, N W
Shales, C A
Sharples, A
Shaw, J F L
Sherwood, A J
Shewring, P M
Shrestha, R
Sims, D E
Smith, M E F
Snelson, M G
Sneyd, J R
Soul, A R
Stayte, W M
Steeden, A L
Steel, J R
Stephens, L C R
Stevens, R J
Stevens, R J
Stewart, A E
Stewart, I P
Stitson, D J
Stocker, M E
Storrow, K J
Story, T S
Streets, C A
Strobel, S
Taams, K O
Tai, G K L
Tatham, R H B
Tayler, D J
Taylor, P A
Thom, W F
Thomas, A J
Thomas, H C
Thomas, H A
Thomas, S
Thornberry, D J
Thorpe, S S
Thrush, D C
Thurstan, N D A
Thurston, B J
Tomlinson, G C
Tooke, J E
Torabi, K
Toynton, N J
Toynton, S C
Tuckley, J M
Turner, M S
Tyrrell, C J
Vital, M F
Walker, A J
Walker, M B
Walker, S
Walsh, G J
Ward, P S
Warlow, P F M
Warrell, R J
Warren, S J
Watkins, R M
Watts, M A
Webb, J K G
Westhead, M J
Weston-Baker, E J
Westwood, C N
White, A R
Wilkin, T J
Wilkins, D C
Wilkinson, S P
Williams, M P
Williams, P
Wilson, C E
Windle-Taylor, P C
Wood, A C
Woods, J M
Woods, R R
Wright, H P
Wrigley, S R
Yarnley, P A
Youell, C D
Zajicek, J P

Polegate
Adcock, R J
Bedford-Turner, C M
Birks, D A
Brierley, R P
Brown, R D
Desmond, H
Dickson, S R
Felce, J M
Hammett, A I
Holme, S B
Johnston, P
Lawrence, E F
Sharp, M P
Simpson, M B
Suleman, M I

Pontefract
Abbott, V P
Acuyo Pastor, L
Allen, C L O
Bazaz, M L
Belk, W J
Binns, M S
Bonney, G
Brooksby, W P
Broughton, A C
Brown, J G
Buckley, R
Butler, S E
Caddy, J M
Chakraborty, S K
Chandy, J
Cording, V L
Crabtree, J
Crawley, L C
Davenport, G J
De Dombal, E
Diggle, D P
Dodman, B A
Dunphy, R A
Eastwood, J M
Eccles, D
Evans, A E
Fox, P A
Galvin, H P
Ganorkar, V D
George, E M
Gordon, P G
Grove, A M
Hanney, I P G
Harvey, A R
Hashmi, A A
Hassoon, M M
Hawkins, A E
Horsfall, H O
Huggett, A M
Johnson, A O C
Johnson, M T
Jones, G
Jordan, P D
Joyner, S R
Kamal, L R M
Kanani, R R
Kaul, V
Kupelian, S M
Lannon, M G
Lewis, R V
McClintock, J E
McClintock, J H N
Macdonald Hull, S P
Macdonald, I W C
Martin, A M E
Meulendijk, H N
Mistry, D B K
Montgomery, J S
Moulton, E A
Needham, K L
Nugent, A
Okine, E A
Osselton, M
Perkins, A
Playforth, M J
Prasad, V
Quartley, R G S
Riley, D
Roberts, D G
Roche, R E
Sanderson, K J
Shahi, A
Shutkever, M P
Singh, R K
Singh, S P
Sinha, S K
Slack, G B
Smith, G D
Soar, B A
Stone, K E
Strike, P C
Sweeney, A N
Syam, V
Sykes, A
Tanna, A D
Taylor, J M
Thompson, R M
Thorp, J K
Tobin, C P
Uzoigwe, A O
Viswanathan, P
Wakefield, D A
Waring, J R
Watson, D B
White, C
Wilson, G S L
Wright, D
Yeung-Wye-Kong, C-K
Zaman, A G
Zaman, N Y

Pontyclun
Anness, V R
Bayoumi, M
Benjamin, J A
Bunston, M J
Champ, C S
Cremin, D D
Davies, P S
Davies, T D
Davies, W W
De Alwis, C
Dewar, R I
Duffin-Jones, A
Duggan, M A K
Gower-Thomas, K L
Havard, T
Hawksworth, N R
Hopkin, M
Hughes, R J
Hutton, R D
Jerrett, C S
Jones, R M
Latif, A H A
Majumdar, R K
Millar-Jones, L
Mills, L M
Moody-Jones, W D T
Moorcraft, J
Morgan, C J L
Morgan, R J H
Morris, I B
Parker, V A
Pemberton, D J
Pembridge, J M
Perry, H M
Robinson, D J
Sami, A S A E H
Singh, K R
Singh, T H
Smith, J M
Tanner, J G
Thomas, J P
Thomas, O R
Tudball, P
Wardhaugh, A D
White, D G
Williams, F G
Williams, H O L
Winter, R K

Pontypool
Ahmad, N
Aitken, S J
Anthony, N J
Bapuji Rao, V
Bevan, R A
Brown, P D
Clewer, G J
Cormack, A S
Cormack, H S
Cottam, D J
Cunningham-Davis, P G
Dare, D R
Davies, K
Davies, P A
Davis, J P
Devlin, O P
Edwards, D M
Graham, G I
Grant, K T
Grantham, C E D
Harries, J M
Hobbs, D J
Hughes, A
Hughes, T M
Jeffs, S A
Jilani, M M
Jones, D G H
Jones, D F
Joshi, H P
Khan, A K M S
Layzell, J C M
Machado, F R D S
Mars, P H
Nutt, M R
O'Sullivan, D P
Palmer, J E
Patel, S C
Prabhakaran, U P
Pugh, A C
Rahman, A
Smart, K
Taylor, J
Temple, J M F
Thomas, M P
Williams, D G

Pontypridd
Ackerman, S
Allim, A S
Appanna, T C

Billington, K
Blair, A D
Bristow, G D
Brooks, P T
Brown, M A
Burkhardt, K I
Clarke, J P J
Clee, W B
Darwish, A K
Davies, D H
Davies, G E
Davies, T J
El Naamani, B
Elwood, N F
Evans, G R L
Evely, C L
Gasson, J N
Harris, W H
Hasan, M
Heatley, M K
Heywood, W
Howarth, P J
James, D S B
Jones, A H
Jones, C D V
Jones, D R
Jones, K A
Khalil, D S
Lewis, A S
Lewis, M
Lewis, P S
Li, C Y A
Lloyd-Williams, C B A
Menon, R G
Mogford, N J
Morgan, I G
Morris-Stiff, G J
Mukhopadhyay, A K
O'Leary, T P
Ozdemir, J
Pascoe, K F
Perry, A
Pierrepoint, S E
Pinkham, K L
Prabhu, P S A
Purbey, B N
Randell, D T H
Rees, D R
Rees, W E L
Richards, J D
Robinson, N A
Samuel, M J
Sengupta, P S
Sherwood, H
Slade, D E
Taylor, C E
Thomas, J
Thomas, N M
Tipping, T R
Varde, K
Vijaya Bhaskar, P
White, D G
Williams, D H
Williams, R J L
Willis, L G F
Wu, K-C

Poole
Ainley, E J
Al-Khazraji, M R A H
Alam, M A
Alner, M R
Arnold, E J
Ashton, W B
Atkinson, P H
Atkinson, S R
Ballinger, F C
Barnett, M A
Battcock, T M
Bayley, K L
Begley, J P
Bell, A J
Black, M M
Blakeway, A C
Boyd, C M
Brady, S
Brailsford, J A D
Bray, G M
Britton, N
Bruce, D L
Burn, J P S
Campbell-Ede, S C
Cheng, K
Cheng, Z
Choudry, N
Clein, G P
Cole, C C
Collinson, J D
Cope, D
Coppen, R J
Cousins, C G
Cowley, N
Cox, H J
Crellin, R P
Crick, M D P
Crowther, S D
Cuthbert, C J
Darke, S G
Davies, J B
Day, R W B
Deacon, R J L
Dean, S E
Dent, P
Dewar, A L
Dormon, F M
Edwards, J N T
Ellis, C J K
Ellis, K D
Fairhurst, H E
Farrar, M J
Farrier, C D
Fawkner, K J
Fiddian, N J
Flanagan, P G
Forbes, P J
Frymann, S J
Fullerton, I S
Gadd, C M
Gankande, A U H
Garland, S J
Gatling, W
Goode, T D
Goodworth, D J
Graham, D A
Griffith, A H
Griffiths, S J
Hadley, J L
Hall, R L
Hanna, A R Y
Hardwick, P J
Harries-Jones, R
Harrington, J G
Hatch, G R
Hattersley, R W
Hayward, M J
Henry, R J W
Herbetko, J
Herring, J P
Hext, J E
Heyworth, T
Hickey, J R
Hill, R A
Hill, R M F
Hill, R D
Hill, S F
Hillard, T C
Hillier, C E M
Hitchings, N B
Holmes, D M
Hosking, S W
Howe, A H
Howell, M E
Howell, M-C
Huebner, R
Hussein, K A
Hussey, M H
Ilankovan, V
Jack, F R
Jallali, N
Jankelowitz, G S
Jones, C M
Jones, S N
Jowett, A J L
Kelsall, J E
Kidd, K R
Kirkham, S R
Laurence, V M
Levitt, R J
Lewis, V
Liddiard, G S
Liddiard, G S
Linley-Adams, A C
Litchfield, M
Lockey, B F
Lomax, G P
Lovejoy, J J
Lucas, C
Lyons, F M
McAulay, A H
McCann, D F
McLeod, A A
Maiden, A
Malik, N A
Matthews, D C
Maycock, R R
Millar, J W
Miller, J
Milligan, N S
Milligan, N M
Molyneux, H M
Morris, A E
Morris, S
Moy-Thomas, J M
Moyse, G A
Muir, D P R
Murcott, C A
Myatt, J K
Mynors-Wallis, L M
Neave, S M
Nelms, M T
Newman, A J
Newth, J B
Nicholas, A P
Nicholas, D S
O'Connor, J E
O'Connor, J C
Osborne, R J
Ould, G A
Owen, J C
Packham, R N
Pain, J A
Pandher, G K
Parkin, B T
Peters, C J
Pettit, D R
Playfair, C J
Ponton, A W G
Pouramini, M
Powell, C E
Power, K J
Pratt, E J
Price, S M
Pridgeon, J M
Primavesi, S M
Prossor, J E
Rao, K R
Rastogi, S C
Ray, J A
Redpath, S
Reichl, M
Rein, H I
Richards, S C M
Richardson, D P
Rigby, C M
Roberts, G W
Robson, N K
Rogers, A M
Rowe-Jones, D C
Rundle, J S H
Rushen, D J
Rutland, A F K
Sakhrani, L
Scott, C M
Scott, J S C
Scott, P M J
Seal, P J
Searle, G F
Sharer, N M
Sharma, R C
Shearman, A J
Sheehan, A J
Shelley, F C
Sheridan, E A
Shortland, D B
Sinha, S K
Smith, G D
Smith, R N
Smith, T
Snook, J A
Sorapure, J B
Stanley, G E
Stephens, C J M
Stewart, A B
Street, S Q I
Stuart, A L G
Surridge, J M
Sutherland, J
Talbot, R W
Tarver, D S
Thomas, M
Thomas, S M
Thompson, P W
Tidswell, A T H
Tsamis, M
Upton, C E
Ventham, P A
Villar, M T A
Vithana, T
Walder, G P
Walkden, S B
Ward, A M V
Warlow, S
Wayne, H L
Webb, J N
Wee, M Y K
Wegner, M-P
Wenzerul, A M
Whalen, S H
Wilkins, M C
Wilkinson, C P
Willcocks, L C
Williams, D J
Williams, E J
Williams, S R
Wise, H J
Wood, A D G
Worsley, A M
Wulff, C H

Port Erin
Brocklehurst, M Y
Conlon, D E G
Conlon, M B
Gupta, N
Mousley, N
Wignall, D C

Port Glasgow
Farrell, J P
Holms, L F
McCartney, M
McKay, D J
Manasses, E
O'Rourke, B
Ramanathan, RG
Smith, M H
Wilkie, D J
Wootton, A C

Port Isaac
Barker, J M B
Budd, W E R
Davison, S D K
Larkin, J M G
Lunny, J J
Partington, E P
Sainsbury, A D
Scovell, E E

Port Talbot
Ames, S J
Barnes, J C
Burridge, J W
Clark, S H
Cobbledick, M
Davies, H J
Davies, V G
Dossa, M S
Gibbons, B J
Goodwin, M J
Griffiths, H
Hunt, K P
Isopescu, G A
Jones, P D
Llewellyn, M H
Lodwig, T S
Mouyen, G J M
Patel, Y A
Penney, R J
Roach, D L
Roberts, E M
Rohman, S O
Subbu, V S
Townsend, P
Trott, L I
Tyler, R J

Portadown
Armstrong, C J
Hewitt, G R
Hunter, I W E
Murphy, P P

Porth
Bali, V P
Bali, V
Benjamin, A
Bishara, S A
Carne, M S
Choudhury, G S
Das, S
Duffin-Jones, L
Kaushal, V L
Lawthom, C
Lloyd, G A
Narayan, R D
Powar, M R
Williams, H
Williams, K M
Wilton, A

Porthcawl
Bond, S E
Eales, T D
Evans, J R
Feltham, A M
Ghose, R R
Guest, S
Jenkins, R G
Kirkby, J A
Longley, M A
Mackey, P M
Mohajer, C J
Moore, R P
Overton, M J
Parry, H D
Parry, J G
Parry, P A
Pearson, O R
Rees, G B
Shinkwin, M P
Smith, G S
Thomas, K S
Thomas, R J
Tinkler, G G
Tracy, P M
Williams, C A

Porthmadog
Edwards, J M
Niesser, A J
Niesser, A A
Williams, M W

Portland
Allsop, E J T
Brook, M I
Goodman, S
Hargrave, D B
Mason, P J
Ninham, M C
Sami, N
Whisker, R B

Portree
Crichton, C M
Finlayson, J A D
Macdonald, A N
Macrae, C A
Macrae, C O

Portrush
Anand, K
Bailie, J S
Bresland, M K
Edmundson, H F
Finlay, L
Finlay, S
Gardiner, M C
Logue, C P
McMillan, R L
Murphy, E M
Rea, O H

Portsmouth
Abdul Aziz, L A S
Absolom, M E
Al-Safi, W S A
Allan, A J
Allcock, A C
Arkanath, M
Ashton, M R
Atchison, D G
Atchley, J T M
Bagshaw, H A
Barker, D P
Baylis, R J H
Bayon, J
Beaumont, J M
Beech, L D
Bevan-Thomas, M-A M
Beynon, J H
Boase, D L
Boote, D J
Bowker, C H
Brindle, R J
Brockman, B J
Buchanan, J D
Buckley, H K
Burby, N G
Burden, R J
Cahill, C J
Campkin, N T A
Carss, G A
Castle, N A
Catterall, G A
Charlton, B
Chaudhary, R
Clark, R J
Clarke, H J
Cockcroft, P M
Colin-Jones, D G
Collins, E
Connor, D J
Cook, L J
Cox, J S
Cranfield, T G
Cree, I A
Crisp, M D
Cummings, M H
Dakin, S M
Davies, D W
Dhundee, J
Dickson, R J
Doherty, R P
Domjan, J M
Dowd, A B
Dubois, J D
Duncan, H D
Edmondson-Jones, J P
Eldridge, A J
Ellis, R D
Evans, A R
Ewen, S P
Exton, L C
Farnworth, D
Fellows, E J
Flynn, N A K
Foley, C A
Foley, S E
Franklin, L L
Franks, S H
Freeman, A E L
Gabb, J H
Galloway, A M
Ganczakowski, M E
Gaught, F J
Giddens, J E
Gill, R J
Gillmore, R J
Glasgow, M C
Goggin, P M
Green, B A
Green, P J
Green, W T
Grindrod, R M
Grover, M L
Guirgis, R R
Harindra, V
Harper, G D
Hatfield, A G
Haworth, A E
Haydon, J R
Hedger, N A
Higginson, A P
Hirri, H M
Hodkinson, S L
Hogan, J P R
Hogston, P
Holmes, S A V
Homer-Ward, M D
Howell, M A
Hughes, B R
Hughes, R M
Hull, R G
Isasa Fino, I
Jarrett, D R J
Jeffrey, M J
Jeffrey, M N
Jones, R A
Kalra, P R
Keohane, S G
Khan, T
Khin, M H
Khoury, G G S
King, F M
Lalor, A J M
Langham-Brown, J J
Lawson, A
Leach, T D
Ledingham, J M
Lee, A G
Lee, G
Lewis-Russell, J M
Lewis, C H
Lewis, J E
Lewis, R J
Littledale, E J
Logan, R F
Longbottom, D N
Loxton, J E
McArthur, C J G
MacConnell, L E S
McCormick, D A
McCrae, F C
MacGuire, M H
McKenning, S T
McLaughlin, N P
Maclean, A H
Maclennan, I R
McLeod, A D M
McQuillan, P J
Marley, N J E
Mason, J C

Medbak, S H
Mellor, T K
Merton, W L
Milligan, W L
Millroy, S J
Mitchell, S W
More, R S
Morgan, D L
Moss, F S
Mustafa, M S
Nessim, A A
Neville, E
Nilssen, E L K
O'Callaghan, A M
O'Rourke, N P
Okonkwo, A C O
Old, P J
Olford, C A
Oram, D C
Palmer, R J
Pemberton, R M
Peters, S A
Phillips, S A
Plenty, D R
Poller, D N
Poulton, S E
Pringle, M B
Quine, M A
Randall, S
Randall, V R
Randle, M P
Raw, D S
Reid, R I
Resouly, A
Richards, R H
Richardson, A M E
Riley, A P
Robinson, G J
Rogers, D C
Rogers, P D
Rooke, H W P
Russell, B N
Sadek, S A
Sadler, P J
Sanderson, R A
Saunders, M L
Scott-Brown, A W
Senapati, A
Severs, M P
Shrivastva, D P
Smart, D J G
Smith, G B
Snow, R E
Solomon, L
Somers, S S
Spedding, A V
Stevens, J M
Stevenson, K M
Stewart, A D
Summerton, D J
Sweatman, C M
Thompson, J A
Thompson, M R
Thornber, D R
Thornton, J N D
Thwaites, R J
Tobin, J M
Tollast, A R
Tuckey, J E
Tudor, J C
Tweeddale, M G
Underhill, G S
Vardon, V M
Venkat-Raman, G
Vieweg, R
Wace, J R
Walker, J M
Walters, A M
Ward, S C
Watkins, J
Watson, K J
Watt-Smith, J A
Weaver, P C
Wernick, S P
West, P D B
Wilcockson, A Q
Wilkins, A C
Wilkinson, T J
Williams, A I
Williams, M
Williams, P L
Williamson, K M
Wilson, M S
Wise, M
Witham, F M
Wood, M L B
Woolas, R P
Wotherspoon, F
Wozniak, E R
Yates, A
Yiangou, C
Young, R M
Zaki, G A

Portstewart
Boyd, H K
Carlin, P G M
Corrigan, N P
Dick, C R
Donnelly, E E
Elliott, N W A
Gilmore, P
Harley, J B
Higgins, P M
Hughes, C M
Jack, H M
McCartney, M D
Magee, S K
Morrison, C C M
O'Loan, P R
Tracey, F
Wright, T R

Potters Bar
Abo Abood, N
Barnard, M M E
Carter, P J
Ciezak, R F
Dain, C J
Davies, R P L
Duncombe, C L
Edwards, S R
Elder, R J
Ferris, A R
Forman, J D
Grafton, A J
Henderson, A
Mizan, J
Montegriffo, V M E
Munro, C M
Nicol, A E L
Norris, R M
Patel, A
Ramsell, N J
Ramsell, S E
Ritchie, A F
Salkin, B D
Simmons, A J
Somerset, A M
Stewart, M J
Stone, M C
Tanner, M
Thomson, P J
Traue, D C
Trevor, S
Trowell, J A
Woods, B T

Poulton-le-Fylde
Atkinson, P A
Au, G T
Beswick, S J
Brooks, A
Brown, S
Burnett, W
Byrd, L M
Cook, M C
Costello, F T
Davies, S J
Dempsey, V J
Didsbury, C L
Evans, M J
Furniss, A E
Isherwood, D
Kirkham, I C
Lewin, J P
Lockhart, A S
Lynch, S
Morrison, W D
Murphy, R
Noblett, A K
Qualtrough, J E
Rayner, T A
Rhodes, R R
Simmons, G
Sissons, M C J
Sissons, P J
Smith, P C
Walker, A K
Watt, J N
Whiteley, G L

Prenton
Elhibir, E I
Ho, K W K
Karyampudi, R S

Prescot
Abrams, J
Allen, K D
Amegavie, F L
Andrews, F J
Atherton, D P L
Atherton, S T
Aung, T M
Ball, J B
Baskett, D W
Bolton-Maggs, B G
Breeze, C
Brindley, L J
Brown, A S
Brown, T D
Buchanan, G K
Buckley, R M
Capewell, A E
Cawdell, G M
Chana, L V
Chaudhuri, P S
Choudhury, A
Choudhury, A
Church, S E
Clayton, M R
Conway, P G
Corless, J A
Cramp, J C
Crook, V A
Curley, R K
Denton, J S
Desmond, J M A
Dissont, A D
Dutta, A
Dutta, A
Edrich, P J
El Badri, A M
Falder, L S
Feldberg, L E J
Gana, H B-Y
Giles, V A
Gilligan, R E
Gordon, H L
Graham, C S
Graham, D R
Green, A R
Griffiths, S C
Hamed, H M
Hancock, K
Hardy, K J
Hasan, N U
Hasan, Y H
Hendry, J
Hiranandani, M
Howard, R P
Ince, C S
James, M I
Karunaharan, P
Kelly, S A
Kirby, A J
Kumar, P
Leong, K S
Mcauley, P A
McIlwain, J C
Macmillan, R R
McNeilly, P
Maitra, D
Manning, M P R A
Massey, J A
Meek, D R
Mehra, R K
Moore, G R
Morton, J D
Mukembo, S M
Mylvaganam, A
Nandapalan, V
Nee, P A M
Nelson, V M
Ng, D P-K
Nwosu, E C
O'Donnell, K M
O'Ryan, M F N
Padmakumar, K
Pontefract, D R
Prabhu, U A
Raftery, S M
Raghupati Raju, A S
Rahman, M K
Rahman, N N
Ramstead, K D
Ray, A
Ridyard, J B
Sachdev, A P S
Sachdev, R S
Sanderson, C J
Sandland, R M
Sarkozy, V E
Satchithananthan, G
Scott, M H
Sharma, V
Silke, C M
Sills, J A
Soren, D
Stilwell, J H
Teanby, D N
Varma, M R
Vinod Kumar, P A
Watt, S G
Wide, J M
Williams, L
Wilson, R N
Woodhall, C R

Prestatyn
Braun, M S
Campbell, F
Davies, R L
Dogra, R S
Faulkner, A J
Gozzard, A
Howes, P T
Hughes-Roberts, H E
Jessup, E D
Jones, H G
Jones, H
Jones, L M
Kamaluddin, S M
Kerfoot, J A
Lewis, J
Mahad, D J
Mahadanaarachchi, J C
Mesure, J G
Miller, F B
Morrison, C L
Neville, A E
Neville, W P
Phillips, P R
Roberts, S
Scriven, W A
Sixsmith, D J I
Swinburne, A
Wares, A N
Wickramasekera, D
Williams, P H

Presteigne
Goodall-Copestake, J
Martin, J D C
Schofield, W N
Spring, R D L
Whitfield, C T
Williams, W D C

Preston
Abou Shanab, K S
Addada, J E
Adhikary, H
Adhikary, M
Aggett, P J
Ahad, G W
Ahmad, A
Ahmad, Q
Ali, M M
Allister, A H
Allsup, S J
Almond, S L
Alvarez, E V
Armour, A
Ashcroft, M M
Ashton, K L
Atherton, E N
Atkin, G K
Atkinson, D
Bailey, E A
Bale, R S
Ball, D R
Barkby, G D
Barnes, C
Barnes, R K
Baroudi, G
Basnyet, D B
Battye, R
Berends-Sheriff, P J
Beswick, D
Bewlay, M A
Bird, E E
Biswas, A
Biswas, S
Blades, R A
Blue, A C
Boon, F J
Boothman, B R
Boothman, J
Bourne, M J
Bowker, S G
Bowman, A
Boyle, S
Bradley, S M
Bradshaw, F L
Brearley, J M
Brooks, B V
Brooks, D A L
Brown, J C M
Brown, P M
Bruce, I A
Buckley, A M
Buckley, E I J
Bunting, P
Burnett, H L
Burton, A L
Cain, A C M
Cairns, A J
Cairns, J P
Cairns, S A
Callaghan, L C
Campbell, A N
Carew-McColl, M
Carter, F
Carter, J H P
Cassels, H T
Chaloner, J H
Chand, T G
Chattha, E A
Chattopadhyay, P K
Chaudhri, K
Cheesbrough, J S
Chesworth, R J H
Chikhalikar, G T
Chikhalikar, G
Choudhary, B
Clarke, J
Clarke, J
Clelland, I A
Coaker, M J
Cooper, M J
Corkill, R G
Cornah, J
Cottam, S N
Coughlin, P A
Coughlin, S P
Courtney, E
Coutinho, M C A
Coward, R A
Craig, M
Crispin, Z L
Croft, J A
Cross, W R
Curley, J W A
Curtis, P R
Daley, A J
Daniels, C J
Das Gupta, R
Das, B T
Davis, C H G
Dawson, T P
Deacon, R H
Deakin, D P W
Dickson, C J
Dix, F P
Dixon, N J
Donaldson, I C
Duff, C G
Duff, D A
Duncan, P W
Ebdy, M J
Eccles, J C
Edge, D M
Edwards, J M
Everiss, J
Eves, M J
Eyre, J A
Fairhurst, R J
Farrington, J L
Faux, J C
Feaks, R J
Ferrie, R
Finlay, B M
Flaherty, T A
Fletcher, D J
Foley, A L
Forbes, A S
Forrester, I R
Fowler, S J
Francis, C Y
Fryer, J M
Garg, A
Gask, L
Gater, R A
Gaze, N R
Gee, S D
Ghori, S S
Gibbon, S P
Giencke, K
Giles, E A
Giles, M B
Glenn, M P
Gonzalez, V G
Goodfellow, R C
Graham, F
Greening, A P
Greenwood, S T
Gregson, J
Grenfell, R C
Griffin, S J
Griffiths, J O
Gulati, V
Gurusinghe, N T
Hacking, N M
Hamad, G M E-S A
Hanson, J M
Hardwick, S A
Harrison, C J
Harrison, G
Hart, R O
Hart, R J
Hartley, C
Harwood, P J
Haslam, G M
Hassan, A I
Hatton, D J
Haward, E C
Hawcroft, J
Hayton, M J
Hearn, A R
Heath, S T
Hendy, M S
Hicks, A P
Hill, J C
Hindley, A C
Hirst, S N
Hodskinson, R
Hogg, M S
Holden, C A
Holden, D W
Hothersall, E L
Howat, A J
Howcroft, A J
Howell, S A
Hudson, D M
Hudson, J M
Hughes, R
Hunt, J L
Hunt, N
Hussain, F I
Hynes, C J
Irvine, M S
Isherwood, C N
Jackson, P L
Jamdar, R P
James, M R
Jandu, M S
Jefferies, E M
Jha, J N
Jhooti, T K
John, M E
Johnson, J A
Johnson, T
Jolley, C J
Jones, D S
Jones, G N
Jones, I P
Jones, M J
Kapadia, M
Karri, B
Kelly, A J
Kelly, D R
Kennedy, S
Khan, S
Khanna, A
Kilgour, A J
King, H R
Kirby, A P
Kitching, G T
Laitung, J G
Lambert, M E
Lancaster, C J
Latiff, A
Laurence, A S
Lee, P F S
Leelakumari, T
Leigh, N F
Lekwuwa, U G
Letheren, M J R
Lewis, S E
Linn, P K K
Lonie, D S
Loudonsack, J R
Lowe, R
Lowrie, A
Lupton, M E
Lusk, J A R
Luthra, R
McCann, J F
McCann, P
McCraith, N S

McGaahan, C
McGrath, P J
McKenna, J T
Mackie, J
McKiernan, E P
McMeekin, B A
McWilliam, C
Mahadun, P
Mahawish, L
Mahmood, D A
Majeed, T
Mallam, K M
Marrott, S
Marshall, A J
Martlew, R A
Massey, L J
Matanhelia, S S
Mawson, A C
Mayor, A C
Michel, J M
Millns, D
Minshall, C
Mitchell, J D
Moir, C C
Molloy, R H
Moore, D R
Moreland, N J
Moss, S D
Mulla, H M
Muttucumaru, N J
Naik, R K
Nawrooz, N M J
Newton, P J
Nirula, N
Nixon, P
Noble, A M
Noble, J G
O'Donnell, E I
O'Donnell, V A
Orduna Moncusi, M
Ormerod, P S
Parker, G
Parker, J
Parry, H S
Parry, R T
Parson, A M Y
Patel, A N
Patel, A R
Patel, D
Patel, H P
Patel, K B
Patel, K
Patel, M
Patel, V H
Pavey, I S J
Pavey, K M F G
Pennington, S H
Perez-Cajaraville, J J
Phillips, A B
Phipps, K
Pidgeon, N D
Pitt, M A
Prasad, R K
Pritchett, A H J
Pusey, J M
Rambihar, B V
Read, G
Reddy, G A N
Rees, P
Reid, A D
Riley, A J
Robb, A
Robb, G A
Roberts, N
Roberts, R E P
Robertshaw, M F
Robertson, A
Robinson, P W
Robson, A E
Rodriguez, J M
Rossall, C J
Rowlandson, G
Saha, N G
Saikia, B
Sathananthan, N
Senathirajah, D
Seth, A
Shah, J K
Shahid, S Z
Shaw, J J
Shaw, S J
Shaw, S J
Shek, R J
Siddiqui, H
Silva, E P C
Simpson, D
Singh, A
Singh, B
Singh, H
Singh, J K
Singh, M
Skailes, G E P
Slater, A
Slater, C
Small, M L
Small, M
Smith, E M
Smith, R B
Solomon, L R
Southern, L P
Stevenson, W T J
Stewart, D J
Stivaros, S M
Stringfellow, H F
Sule, H D
Sule, S H
Sundaralingam, S
Susnerwala, S S
Talbot, E M
Tandon, K
Taylor, L A
Tedd, R J
Tew, E
Tew, J A
Thakur, B
Thomas, P T
Thompson, D F J
Thomson, G J L
Tidswell, P
Todman, R H
Tomlin, P I
Townsend, N W H
Tree, D A
Tuck, J J H
Tunstall, S
Turner, M A B
Vakil, S D
Vice, P A
Vijayadurai, P
Walsh, I
Walsh, M F
Walton, S M
Warburton, R
Ward, S T
Warner, K L
Watson, J B
Watson, M E
Watson, V F
Webster, M
Whalley, J A
Wharton, L H
Wharton, M R
White, C C
White, H D
White, S R
Whittaker, J D
Wignall, J B W
Wijethilleke, G G K
Williams, J G
Williams, N
Wilson, C M
Wilson, L J
Wood, G C
Woodroffe, J B
Woollard, A J
Woollard, C M
Wright, D M
Wright, P A
Yaxley, K M
Yogasundram, Y
Young, D W
Zargar, G A

Prestonpans

Blake, R A
Bremner, D
Brown, D G
McNeill, I S
Menzies, S E
Pollock, W
Reeks, J L
Scott, G R H
Simmonte, M G
Turvill, J W

Prestwick

Anderson, D G
Barrie, P J
Cattanach, D J
Cornelius, J M
Forster, A L
Glen, S B
Hardie, R
Lambert, B A
Leslie, C J
Lindsay, J E
McCall, J G
Martin, L M
Park, W D
Percival, R
Roy, D C
Sillars, J
Smith, A E C
Smollett, M A
Taylor, I N
Watson, A
White, G J
Wilson, C S

Princes Risborough

Appleton, P N J
Appleton, S G
Barden, R K
Breese, C W
Cahill, J F B
Cooney, J A
Durban, J
Forbes, A M
Griffiths, J R
Hodder, R W
Jones, M H
McKenzie, R A
Maisey, A R
Partridge, C R-A
Rainbow, J R
Sheerin, S M
Weir, J S L

Prudhoe

Anderson, L M
Berney, T P
Egan, A
Haywood, S C
Jennings, C E
Quilliam, S J
Richardson, A G
Wright, J C

Pudsey

Antrobus, R D
Ball, N S
Belderson, L
Broom, C
Cook, J N
Daly, R
Darlington, S
Darnborough, D C
Devereux, T A
Follows, D M
Follows, G A
Galloway, S J
Groarke, M I
Guerrero, K L
Hall, J F
Hearnshaw, C A S
Kripal, K
Lee, A V
Lee, S M
Lindsay, P J
McGechaen, K W
Maddy, P J
Mason, C M
Mason, J B
Minhas, E-U-M
Minhas, H L
Minhas, H A
Ross, R J
Senior, M A
Steward, K A
Tawse, B M
Watson, K J
Waugh, M A
Woodhead, R
Zicchieri, F L

Pulborough

Bailey, J E
Bartlett, J S W
Brooks, A Y
Clarke, R A
Collyer, T C
Cooper, M
Cooper, M F
Couchman, D R
Diver, J P
Duncan, P A
Ellis, L M
Evans, C A
Ferrie, J I
Fitzpatrick, S C B
Fooks, T J C
Gibbon, E A A
Hanbury-Aggs, C A
Hard, P L S
Herbertson, R A
Jeffery, M P
Kalaher, M E
Kilpatrick, F R
King, C P M
King, C J
MacWhirter, G I
Morson, B C
Page, B M
Poole, K K
Shillingford, M J
Tse, B S-W
Turner, Y J
Vickerstaff, H J
Whitehead, D M

Purley

Bandyopadhyay, U
Basu, C
Blake, H M
Blake, J
Carlisle, J M
Cohen, H C
Counsell, B R A
Dhesi, R K
Gayford, J J
Grasso, P
Hawker, H J
Hopkins Jones, K M
Johnson, J M
Karani, J B
Keyes-Evans, O D
Lawther, P J
Linney, J G
Lloyd, M S
McKenzie, C H
Martin, J C
Newlands, P W
Overton, R D C
Pandita-Gunawardena, N D
Peatfield, B J D
Phillips, P C
Pollard, C M
Premachandran, S
Rogers, D A L
Rourke, A
Rudolphy, S M
Samarawickrama, P G
Shobowale, F O
Shore, H R
Sivaloganathan, M
Sivaloganathan, S
Sivaloganathan, S
Stechman, M J
Terriere, E C
Theva, R
Thin Thin Saing, Dr
Wright, E C

Pwllheli

Chapman, J A
Davies, H M
Harris, K
Jones-Edwards, G
Jones, B G
Jones, R E
Langley, P R
Lawrence, E
Lawrence, I J
Liddle Davies, H L
Ogilvie, P J
Ogilvie, P N
Owen, G T
Parry-Smith, H J
Pritchard, H R O
Pritchard, R I
Robyns-Owen, D
Thomas, D G H
Williams, A
Williams, D K
Williams, R I

Radlett

Bevan, G
Bowen, D A L
Clark, M P A
Cooray, G M
Cooray, S E
Croft, M D
Deeny, J E
Donne, R L
Drake, D A
Farewell, J G
FitzGerald, G M
Fitzgerald, S B
Freedman, W
Glover, D H
Gold, I D
Gray, K E
Griffiths, D C
Handelsman, S M
Herod, J E
Hulin, S J
Ingram, M J
Jackson, N
Lancer, K L
Lawton, G
Leaback, R D
Leung, A W
Lynn, A H
McDermott, P J C
Marriott, S E
Maxwell, C W
Miller, R M
Mitchell, S E H
Moses, M A
Murray, J M
Ogden, E M
Pegg, M S
Rasaratnam, R
Ruston, J J S
Ruston, M A
Sweeney, P M
Taylor, F C
Verdin, S M
Walton, B
Watters, P T
Wildman, M A

Radstock

Hartley, J D
Jackson, G E
Musgrove, H E

Raglan

Davies, E
Downing, J A
Holt-Wilson, A D
Lillywhite, A R
Pantlin, A W
Pook, C W

Rainham

Adur, R M
Awan, B
Evans, J E
Kemp, P S
Mills, J N
Mushtaq, I
Ogbuehi, N J
Stiff, J H
Subramanian, K A
Toni, E E
Wani, M A

Ramsey

Allinson, A J
Armour, J K
Brownsdon, J K
Chan, M S
Clarke, H M
Cowley, L C
Jones, E J
Kelsey, A S C
Parry, A C
Revill, H
Teare, H C
Walsh, W R
Wilson, G M

Ramsgate

Afridi, K W
Attwood, P R A
Banerjee, S
Beale, J D
Charley, A R
Crosfield, C E
Gajjar, G S
Hancock, M-C
Hardaker, J M
Harries, D G
Johnstone, J R
Kitchener, A D
Law, V A
Leeming, C A
Macpherson, A M
Miller, R J
Morcom, R C
Neden, C A
Neden, J W D
O'Brien, D A
Ratnasingham, P
Reeves, M T
Rickenbach, C A M
Sadler, R O
Semple, W J
Stuart, G W
Tigg, A
Timmins, S F
Ward, N C

Rayleigh

Anglin, M
Binns, G
Dayson, C C
Glover, P
Kittle, G P
Kulkarni, P
Nicholls, J E
Pinkerton, A L
Soppet, P E R
Swinburne, R M
Thorp, J S
Walton, A W J
Wier, J

Reading

Abdulla, A J
Abid, F
Abid, M
Agathangelou, C O
Aiono, S
Aitken, F J
Akhtar, J
Allott, H A
Anderson, P M D
Anderson, R G W
Andrew, S L
Attwood, K
Bacon, A S
Badie, F Y
Baker, J P
Bal, H S
Balkwill, J M
Barker, E A
Barker, L C
Barrow, I
Battram, J W R
Baxter, S A C
Beacham, W D
Bell, J A
Benham, C L
Bhasin, R
Billington, B M
Bindra, H S
Bird, C W H
Bird, J E
Bird, S
Birks, M E
Blackburn, B S
Blackwell, B
Blowers, D A
Bohn, G L
Boon, A W
Boon, J E
Booth, C J
Booth, J C L
Borthwick, R M
Boulos, G B
Bowley, C L
Boyle, M D
Bradlow, A
Brain, A I J
Brand, A D
Brar, S
Bray, J E C
Brito-Babapulle, F M C
Brock, N J
Brown, A L
Brown, R S
Brown, S G E
Bruce, D G
Bruce, E
Brunt, E L
Bucher, J
Buckle, D J
Buckley, J B
Budd, A K
Burden, P
Burke, R A
Burnett, G A M
Busby, M F
Busfield, G D
Bywater, J R
Bywater, J E
Cabrera-Abreu, J C
Campbell, M
Campion, K M
Chadha, R K
Chadwick, H N
Chadwick, J M
Chapman, A J
Chapman, J A
Charlton, C D A
Chua, C N
Churchill, D A
Ciecierski, A J K
Clayton, D J
Clayton, J M
Clements, M J

Clouting, E M
Colenso, S M
Collett, R W C
Collett, S M
Collin, C F
Colquhoun Flannery, W
Connor, J H
Constable, P H
Cook, I J
Coomber, A S
Copeland, S A
Corbridge, R J
Corstorphine, W J
Cottrell, J S
Courtney, S P
Cox, I D
Cracknell, M G
Crawford, J F
Crawley, H S
Creed, M E
Croft, R P
Crystal, A M
Cuningham, P M
D'Cruz, G L
D'Cruz, J E M
Dallas, N L
Davies, C W H
Davies, J B
Davies, M G
Dawson, W G
De Silva, G E
Dean, L J
Dehn, T C B
Delany, G M
Derbyshire, N D J
Dill-Russell, P C
Dils, R C
Dixon, J C
Dodds, R D A
Dodson, M J
Drake, E J
Dudek, M K
Edees, S
Edwards-Moss, D J
Edwards, A M
Eggleton, S M
Elson, E M
Emerson, K M
Ewart, M C
Faber, R G
Fane, S K
Farrugia, P D
Faulkner, A-M
Fawcett, D P
Fearfield, L A
Felton, J R
Fergusson, C M
Fitzherbert Jones, R C
Fleischer, C C
Flint, S K
Foley, S J
Fraser, D J
Freebairn, A J E
French, G S
Frodsham, P F
Froud, E B
Fulford, C J
Galland, R B
Gargav, A
Gargav, A K
Garside, P J
George, H M S
Ghorashian, S
Gibson, M R
Gilbert, M J
Gildersleve, J Q
Gold, A
Gonzalez Garcia, L V
Goode, A G
Gordon, A F
Goring, J A
Gosney, M A
Grantham, V A M
Gray, P
Grech, H
Grecj, H
Green, C E
Greenhalf, J O
Greenhalgh, L J
Greenland, J H
Gregory, R P
Grice, D M
Griffiths, B J
Grover, N
Hagger, D C
Hague, G F
Haigh, R
Hall, R M
Hamilton, R W
Hamilton, V H
Hampton, J N S
Hardman, S C
Hardwick, C E
Harris, P D
Harrold, M
Hayes, L J
Haynes, P D
Headon, M P
Hegarty, H M M
Hennessy, A M
Heppell, A C H
Herdman, R C D
Hickson, M S
Higgins, C R
Hislop, R M
Holcombe, E L
Holden, W A
Holt, E M
Hookway, K M
Horne, D K
Horton, L W L
Houston, J P
Howlett, C R
Hudson, G
Hussain, A
Hussain, S
Hussey, J S
Hyman, N M
Inglis, G S
Irvine, A T
Jackson, E G
Jacobs, I R M
Jacobs, M A
James, C
James, J M
James, M P
Jarman, S J
Jarvis, E J
Jefferson, R J
Johnson, P P
Johnston, E M
Jolly, P N
Kamel, K M
Kapila, A
Karim, A H M H
Kaur, S
Kemp, I C
Khan, R J K
Kinnell, H G
Kitching, M R
Knott, F A
Knowles, L J
Kumar, P
Lade, J C
Lancaster, J
Lander, D A
Latchford, N C
Lawrance, C A
Lee, H A
Lees, W C
Lennox, J S H
Leslie, F M
Levy, O
Lewis, N J
Leyland, M D
Lister, B A
Locham, J
Longfield, J C
Longhurst, N
Luxton, K D
Lyall, J R W
Lynch-Farmery, E M
McAllister, V D M
McCann, F J
McCormick, C J
McDonald, B
MacLachlan, K G
McMullan, T F W
McNally, J D
Macrae, A J
Madgwick, S A
Magee, T R
Makowska, M T
Malcolm, S J
Malik, A S
Malone, P R
Mann, N P
Mansell, N J
Markham, D C
Marks, A M
Marks, N J
Markwell, D C
Marshall, J C W
Marshall, P J
Marshall, R W
Martin-Bates, C R
Mary Das, T A
Mascarenhas, R F
May, A J
Mee, A S
Mellors, B E
Middleton, I A
Middleton, S B
Mikhail, M M S
Millar, J M
Miller, J M
Miller, S M
Milligan, D D
Mittal, R K
Mobey, L J
Modi, K
Modi, S K
Moens, V R T
Moffitt, J A
Mohan, N
Moore, J
Morando, S J
Morgan, N J
Morris, S A R
Morrison, C P
Morrison, H P
Murphy, W A
Myszor, M F
Naik, R B
Nanu Kandiyil, V
Naran, K B
Narayan, R
Nash, J M
Nehring, J V
Newman, C L
Newrith, S F
Noone, O P
Nugent, I M
O'Connell, N J
O'Hanlon, S G
Oppenheimer, M M G
Ormonde, S E
Orr, W P
Paige, G J
Paige, H
Pailthorpe, C A
Pandher, B S
Parke, T J
Patel, N G
Patel, S M
Patel, S
Patey, G L T M
Pemberton, D J
Perry, R J
Pick, S
Pickup, A J
Pimm, J T
Pizura, V A
Podichetty, M
Pollitzer, M
Potter, S M
Powell, A R
Powell, H M
Powell, J V
Powell, M P
Puddy, M R
Purcell, P F
Quilty, B M
Rahim, N S
Ralfe, S W
Raman, A
Raman, V
Ranson, S A
Razak, Dr
Read, P R
Reeves, E R J
Requena Duran, M D M
Richards, A B
Richards, D
Richards, J G
Richards, S A
Richardson, T I L
Richmond, H S
Riddell, N J
Riley, D A
Rimmer, M E
Ritzema-Carter, J L T
Roberts, V M
Robertson, R S C
Rock, C L
Rogers, P B
Ronay, S A
Rose, A F
Ross, A E
Ross, J K
Rout, J P
Roy, R
Ruffle, S P
Rushton, S C
Saad, I E D B
Salim, A
San, S M
Sandercott, A M
Sanders, L R
Selinger, M
Sharma, R P
Sharp, R J
Sharpe, R C
Shaw, M B
Sheppard, H W
Siddal, J N
Sidery, J C
Simmons, J D
Simmons, P A
Sinclair, G W
Sinclair, M
Six, S
Slater, C B
Smith, M D
Smith, R A R
Smith, R A
Soysa, S M
Spensley, P J
Stacey, A R
Stansfield, J M
Stickland, J K
Stoppard, E R
Strang, C J B
Street, P
Sumitra, J V
Sutton, L J
Swami, M L
Swami, S
Swan, S E
Taghipour, J
Tait, C R S
Talbot, A J
Talbot, R M
Tang, A L F
Tanner, V
Themen, A E G
Thilo, J B
Thomas, H L
Thomas, P L
Thomson, M A
Thurston, J S
Tinto, E I
Tomboline, D S
Tomlins, C D C
Torrie, E P H
Townsend, R M
Tremlett, J C
Tulley, M M
Turnbull, H E
Umeh, H N
Underwood, T A
Van Wyk, A L
Vega Escamilla, I
Verghese, C
Vivian, C T B
Waldmann, C S
Walker, C P
Walker, J W
Walker, T M
Wallis, S M
Walton, P K H
Warwick, N G
Weeks, R M
Weinstein, C
Welbourn, R B
Welham, R A N
Wells, T A
Westcar, P D
Westermann, W B
Weston, D M
Whalley, M J
Whitwell, D J
Wildman, G M
Williams, D L
Williams, F A B
Williams, G W
Williams, M L L
Williams, R A M
Williams, R M
Williams, S E
Willis, B M
Willoughby, R A G E
Wilton, A Y
Winchester, J P
Yeo, J E
Young, E

Redcar

Ashcroft, D A
Bailey, P
Barker, K M
Barron, R M
Bentley, J
Coleclough, G
Cowser, J
Davidson, R C
Doherty, J C
Elliott, P A
Fairbairn, I P
Ingledew, D C
Jones, C S
Kakkar, A
Kumar, N
Lal, B K
Lal, K R
Lyle, J H
Machender, K
Michie, M H
Moore, D R
Moore, W P F
O'Flanagan, W J D
Orlandi, J R
Rudd, C
Smith, F C
Smith, R
Stocking, A J H
Summers, E J
Thomas, A B
Thompson, A C
White, J S
Whitehouse, D H
Williamson, M R
Woolder, S L

Redditch

Ackroyd, D F W
Ahmad, F
Al-Ali, S H A
Ananthram, S
Arafa, M A M
Ashworth, B M
Awaad, M O M A
Battin, D G J
Bell, K M
Birrell, L N
Boon, H M
Booth, F
Borastero, E W
Caranci, G A
Cassidy, J J
Chandler, S I J
Clarke, G R
Close, G C
Cochrane, J D
Cooper, G R
Cowburn, J E
Da Rocha-Afodu, O
Das, B N
Davenport, R W
Davey, J W
Dawes, N C
Deller, J G
Dior, A R
Doherty, N P
Dow, J D C
Eckersley, P J
El Dosoky, M E
Elias-Jones, J H
Fischer, H B J
Ford, R N
Franklin, S M
Fraser, B E
Geddy, P M
Greaves, D N J
Grier, L M
Grieve, A M
Gupta, D R
Hakeem, J A
Hall, M F R
Hanna, W E M
Haqqani, M R
Haque, S
Harris, G P M
Hill, C A L
Holland, P
Hopkins, D W J
Hudson, D R
Jenkins, F H
Jenkins, S J
Jenkinson, S D
Johnstone, C M
Kai, P
Karagevrekis, C
Keogh, B P
Kerr, K M
King, J R
Kirby, C P
Kondratowicz, G M
Leach, T A
Lister, E S
Locke, P R
Lowe, K S
Lowry, P J
McGregor, C H
Macpherson, G H
McPherson, J J
Mann, M C
Millard, R C
Mosieri, C N
Munir, M
Nathavitharana, K A
Nithianantham, V T
Obeid, D
Ojukwu, C I
Ounsted, J M
Overton, D J
Parkinson, S J
Phillips, C J
Pike, S H
Porter, S M
Price, A J
Pryke, G R
Purser, N J
Ranganathan, S
Reading, A D
Reavley, C M
Roberts, F P
Robinson, A J
Sankey, R J
Seyler, I B F
Sidford, K I
Singhal, S N
Sivapragasam, S
Smallman, L A
Smith, B E
Smith, T C
Tha, Z
Tonge, M F R
Tucker, W F G
Vathenen, S
Velineni, V E
Wells, J J
Williams, A J
Wong, P A
Wosornu Abban, D

Redhill

Abayawickrama, P C K J
Ainley, N C W
Ameen, M
Ansell, R W
Arnold, C J
Aslett, D J
Bajorek, P K M
Bale, C G
Ball, A B S
Barrow, K
Bhaduri, S
Bray, B M
Bullock, D L E
Butler, J A
Butler, W H
Ceccherini, A F A
Chopdar, A
Cowley, N C
Dasan, S
Davies, U M
De Zoysa, S
Dissanayake, M A
Doyle, J C
Drabu, K J
El-Hariry, A A W M
Ferguson, A E
Ferguson, A J
Foster, K J
Gaitonde, A M
Gaynor, P A
Giallombardo, E
Gordge, K
Gordon-Wright, A P
Gordon-Wright, H M
Green, M A
Griffith, S M
Guess, H M
Hale, J E
Hieatt, M S
Hildreth, V A
Hill, B M
Hughes, A J
Hughes, C A
Hughes, D J
Jackson, R S
Jenkins, P
Jesudason, T A
Kanagarajah, D
Kar, S S
Kimber, J R E
King, M O
Lambden, P W
Long, M G
Loosemore, T M

McAvinchey, R P
McDonald, F A
McIntosh, C S
Matthey, F
Maurice, H D
Miller, P D
Momjian, L L B
Mukasa, D H K
Nkanza, K M
O'Sullivan, M F
Onugha, E N
Pangayatselvan, T
Perera, B S F
Phongsathorn, V
Piper, P C
Prajapati, C L
Puzey, S H
Sage, F J
Sambrook, J H
Schierenberg, T S F
Sethugavalar, C
Shinewi, F F
Skeats, C J
Smith, C D
Sneddon, J F
Spolton, M W
Stacey-Clear, A
Stapley, A M
Stern, S C M
Stewart, B A
Tite, L J
Tomei, L D
Tompkin, D M B
Twaij, M H A R A
Walbrook, E E
Warrington, G
Watkins, M E
Wells, A J
Williams, M E M
Wilson, J R
Wilson, R S
Wylie, C E

Redruth
Badve, M I
Baker, T J S
Blake, C E
Blight, S
Carter, A J
Charnaud, A B
Davies, J E
Davies, W A
Edmunds, T C
English, C L
English, J D
Evers, J A
Foster, J S
Gethin, I P
Hayes, P M
Holland, C E
Hollingworth, H C
Hughes, G B
Jones, H M
Jones, P B T
Kinder, C
Knowles, S R F
Lindsey, M P
Lusty, W J
McDermott, C A
McGuinness, J A
MacMahon, D G
Naylor, J M
Naylor, S R
Philpott, D N
Roger, M D
Rogers, T A
Ruscoe, M N J
Scott, J P D
Smith, J M
Spittle, M C
Swithinbank, I M
Trevail, P R
Wilkinson, A M
Wilson, C W

Reigate
Basha, M A
Bragg, A J D
Casson, A J
Curry, P H
Evans, C S
Fahy, H
Forsyth, C J
Guinness, E A
Guinness, L F
Haynes, L E R
Hubert, H M
Jackson, J P
Jackson, P
Kaiser, T
Kerr, P D
Killick, V
Knight, D
Lambourne, P
Lekh, S K
Lindley, C B
Lyons, J P
McKee, C N
Makomaska, B M A
Middleton, G W
Neeson, L E
Nicholls, R D
Pattinson, K T S
Pipe, N G J
Pritchard, J M
Sussman, H S
Wadzisz, F J
Whitfield, G A

Renfrew
Anderson, A M R
Davidson, S L
Ellis, E L
Lyons, K G B
McCall, J
McQuoney, Q J
Ramage, A E
Seath, G L
Shapiro, B W
Sunderland, A

Retford
Abdulla, H R
Anderson, A R
Atkinson, J F D
Badcock, R J
Bendall, P
Brodie, V A
Brown, A L
Brown, R L
Chapman, J E
Cherrill, G
Clark, C R
Cochran, D S
Corbett, C L
Cordess, C C
De Silva, G B D N
Emmerson, J
Foster, P
Gahir, M S
Gilbert, I J
Hardman, P R J
Herbert, J M
Herbert, P M
Ho, T P
Jiwa, M
Johnston, S J
Keitch, I A P
Langley, R E
Milne, E A
Mundy, E M
Murphy, F B
Nwulu, B N
Pearson, C H
Prabhu, M A
Radhakrishnan, G
Roberts, J
Rowell, S R
Sawires, M A A
Scott, H M
Sivridis, A
Slingsby, A J
Souflas, P
Tonge, J
Travers, R F
Vardy, S B
Waas, M J H B
Walker, J M

Rhayader
Hamer-Davies, E A
Joy, P W
Wynne Evans, B K

Rhyl
Alexander, M J
Anderson, S H
Archard, N P
Baig, M F A
Balaji, V
Banfield, P J
Bastawros, S S
Beirouti, Z A Y
Bell, C F
Bellamy, C M
Bellamy, J L
Bickerton, N J
Bishop, J M
Bracewell, B F
Byrne, R A
Cairn, A M
Cartlidge, D
Champion, A E
Chohan, Z L
Clay, N R
Coulton, E R
Craig, A D A
Dalton, A D A
Daniel, C E
Davies, C J
Davies, G
Davies, N S
Davies, P L
Denman, G
Dobson, S J
Edwards, J A
Fayaz, M
Finnie, I A
Frost, N
Ganeshram, K N
Gollins, S W
Goodwin, G W
Gozzard, D I
Green, G J
Greenway, M W
Hammad, Z
Hardway, J M
Hoyle, C F
Jones, C
Jones, E G
Jones, J
Jones, L W
Jones, M O
Khalil, A A
Khalil, K I
Klimach, O E
Lake, A P J
Lanceley, C P
Landon, R A
Leatt, P B
Lister, R F
Looker, D N
Macaulay, M E
McConnell, C A
Nethersell, A B W
O'Donnell, M A
Osborne, J E
Parry, D L
Penfold, C N
Phillips, J G
Pierce-Williams, G
Pritchard, H M
Seager, S J
Shah, M K
Sinha, A
Srinivasan, V
Stuart-Smith, K
Stutchfield, P R
Tehan, B E
Thomas, D J
Vedpathak, V S
Waters, B
Whyler, D K
Williams, A J
Williams, E G N
Williams, F E
Yuille, T D
Zeitoun, H

Rhymney
Jones, S D
Potts, T M
Roberts, J D

Richmond, North Yorkshire
Barker, E V
Dootson, J C
Dunkley, C P
Dykes, L K
Enevoldson, N S P
Fernandes, T J
Hall, M C S
Heaton, N R
Heron, F J
Hodges, C B
Keavney, M J
Lacamp, C J
Lake, B
Lawson, R M
Minns, J P
Morrison, J F B
Mowbray, M
Paterson, A G
Richmond, C S A
Robertson, J D
Swan, T F

Richmond, Surrey
Akhtar, S A A
Anderson, L J
Andrews, L J M
Attard, H W
Bainbridge, A D
Ball, R A
Barker, S J
Barnard, J A
Bartlett, T P
Bates, F M
Bayne, M C
Bell, L D
Bitensky, L
Blake James, J W
Bocking, L J
Boyle, O H C
Boyle, R M
Burman, R H
Burrows, R
Calder, J D F
Carnegie, C M D
Casimir, C L
Chapman, M H
Chiesa, M C
Chung, G J-H
Collis, C H
Cornell, M N P
D'Netto, P E
Davies, H W
Donaldson, R J
Drew, C D M
Engineer, M P
Farmer, R
Feldschreiber, P
Fox, W
Frater, A J
Gaster, R A
Gawlinska, M H
Gowan, A S O
Greenland, A D
Griffiths, A P
Hanief, M R
Hargreaves, C
Harris, R W
Hawkins, S F S C
Healy, K J
Jacobs, B P
Jayawardene, S A
Kenn, C W
Kingston, C A
Kirkbride, A V
Knight, R J
Levin, J M
Levinson, A M R
Lewis, R O
Lorch, C U
McQuattie, A
Maher, J
Montford, H
Morgan, J F
Napier, J A
Natas, S A
Norton, A M
Norton, M L S
Nunes, M D A
O'Donovan, C P
Ooi, M M
Parker, R H
Pattinson, B
Penrose, R J J
Philip, V J
Pilkington, T R E
Raffle, J A
Richter, A G
Rosling, L E A
Ryder, T S
Samson, G J
Savy, L E
Sellwood, M W
Sinclair, T A L
Skogstad, W H
Smith, V C
Solman, N
Stubbs, P J
Symons, G V
Walker, M J
Ward, M M
Ward, W A
Ward, W D
Weir, R E P
Weston, S J
Wheatley, C H
Wiersema, U F
Witherow, H
York, A H
Yusuf, M N
Zayyan, K S

Rickmansworth
Airey, T P
Amess, J A L
Amess, R M
Angel, J H
Auplish, R N
Auplish, S
Aurora, M
Bennett, F
Brew, D S J
Broome, P C
Bycroft, J A
Carswell, J W
Cary, A J
Cole, C J
Colford, C A
Cooke, G S
Cooke, R T R
Corp, N
Dale, G C
Dane, V J
Davies, E R
Davies, K D
De Souza, E L
Diaz-Guijarro Hayes, J
Dunlop, L S
Farago, S A S
Fenton, F M
Fernando, A G R
Flude, I D
Foreman, N E
Foster, G R
Fountain, S W
Fox, J P
Fox, R H
Friston, K J
Golin, M R
Goodwin, A T
Grundy, E M
Haddad, P F
Hernandez, P M
Hilmi, O J
Iacoponi, E
Jones, R W
Kemp, D M
King, D J
King, S K F
Lakasing, E
Larkworthy, A J
Macdonald, K M
McNeil, M S
Mahmood, B
Messer, C P
Middleton, F R I
Miller, D C
Mitchell, K I
Moon, A J
Murray, A X
Nathwani, A C
Pollock, B J
Pollock, D J
Rajani, B
Rajani, V
Sandler, L M
Savani, A C K
Savani, N Y
Sharih, G
Shaw, A P L
Shaw, D G
Shaw, K N
Sheikh, I
Shepherd, D A
Thomas, R E
Topping, A P
Toy, M J
Toy, R
Whisker, L J
Yull, D N
Zane, J N

Riding Mill
Harle, J

Ringwood
Ansell, G L
Boogert, T H W
Bowry, J
Brigstocke, T W O
Cary, M T A
De Silva, A N
Denman, Y L
Fautley, M
Gayer, A H
Gemmell, R J
Goodwin, P G
Hatrick, R I
Henshelwood, J A
Hughes, D C C
Laband, K M
Langford, D P
Lewis, D
Mason, J D
Mathews, C A
Mavor, W O
North, J
Reed, N L
Shaw, C H
Shield, N B
Sizmur, F M
Spark, E D
Taylor, S J
Thompson, S P
Wilson, E A
Wyse, S D

Ripley
Aspinall, J W
Elliott, L M
Gillatt, D C
Horsfield, M F A
Jones, M D
Newport, S M
Nightingale, S L
Williams, P A
Wordley, A R

Ripon
Abbott, G R
Akester, H A
Bennett, C J
Bigham, R L O
Burton, H V
Davies, W M
Dickson, P J L
Fletcher, C H
Fletcher, J V
Gardner, J M
Grenfell, R C
Harford-Cross, E S
Harford-Cross, M
Higson, R H
Ingram, A J
Jeary, D
Ledger, J L
Lightowler, C D R
Livingstone, A M
Livingstone, P R
McDowall, M S
McEvoy, C W R
McEvoy, P A E
MacTaggart, M R
Mansfield, R J R
Martindale, A D
Methuen, C D
Moss, S L
Richardson, J O
Roberts, G R
Robinson, J F
Saunders, I G G
Saunders, M
Thwaites, R
Webb, C B

Robertsbridge
Ben-Eliezer, E J
Clark, J S
Comer, U
Elliot-Pyle, E M
Land, R C
Mills, M
Munro, J L C
Raven, S C
Shalhoub, J T

Rochdale
Abdelatti, M O
Adler, K M
Akhtar, K
Anglin, J T
Ansari, A S
Archibald, L J
Ariyawansa, I
Aslam, R
Babar, I K
Barnes, B W
Beard, M J
Birkett, J A
Blumenthal, I
Bodner, A
Bowden, A P
Bowker, D M
Bradgate, M G
Bradley, R S D
Budhoo, M R
Caldwell, B M
Cartmill, T D I
Chakrabarti, B
Choudary, V R

Clinton, S T
Cohen, P R
Collighan, S J
Conlong, P J M
Crook, A J
Datta, S
Dawes, S A
De Silva, S
Dhanawade, V
Doshi, M R
Doyle, J S
Eastwood, A S
Edmond, N L
Elliott, J T
Emerson, C E
Etherington, J G
Firstbrook, K J
Fletcher, M F
Flook, D J
Forman, M L
Forman, P C B
Foster, D N
Fraser, A M A
Ghafoor, M B
Ghosh, N
Gibson, A
Gillighan, J C V
Godbole, S
Goodman, M J
Greenwood, E
Guest, K L
Gunn, A C
Haines, L J
Halstead, J C
Hampson, L A
Haq, M I-U
Harris, V J
Hartley, R H
Higgs, E L
Hilmi, F G
Horrocks, J E
Hossack, G F W
Hudson, D J
Ibbotson, G P
Irfan, A
Jones, P E
Kasperowicz, R E
Keighley, J
Kelly, J S
Khan, A
Khan, K M
Kidd, R J G
Knight, M T N
Kourah, M A E A K A
Lacey, H B
Lewis, B
Lomax, P M
McCallum, S J
McFarlane, A R T
Mamman, P S
Mansfield, D J
Martin, J E
Mather, J M
Mawdsley, M D
Mazumder, J K
Meagher, V M C
Morley, T L
Morris, A P
Nelson, J J
Nrialike, P O
O'Doherty, M-A
O'Reilly, M A
Osborne, D C
Pandey, V A
Parton, A B
Paska, L M
Patterson, L J
Payne, D A
Platts, H F M
Platts, T S
Porter, R H
Pradhan, S
Prakash, N G
Quinn, S J
Raja, R S
Ransome, J A
Rauf, A
Reynolds, D
Rhodes, S M
Rimmer, D R
Roberts, A P
Rose, J A
Rothery, S P
Rowlands, P
Saeed, A
Salman, S M
Sankar, D
Sarginson, J
Sarkar, U
Sermin, N H
Singh, S
Slack, C J
Smith, E E
Smithard, D J
Solomon, B
Solomon, P
Speed-Andrews, S C
Stratton, F J
Sundar, M S
Swamy, G N
Taraphdar, S
Taylor, D A
Taylor, G S E
Taylor, K J
Thomas, K T
Thomason, F W
Threlfall, A E
Tierney, E
Tierney, P B
Travis, S E
Turner, W D W
Tutton, E V M
Verity, L J
Verity, R H
Vidyavathi, M
Walton, K
Warrington, S
Winarso, P
Worsell, K E
Zafar, S S
Zeb Khan, A

Rochester

Abbott, M A S
Agarwal, G C
Agarwal, V
Armstrong, C A
Avasthi, A
Baht, H S
Balachander, C S
Bannar-Martin, B R
Bhatia, V K
Birdi, J S
Broadbent, J V
Brophy, J V
Carman, D H
Chakrabarti, B
Clarke, J D
Colbert, T S
De Jong, N S
Dhindsa, A S
Elman, H A
Etheridge, H E
Fargher, G
Fitzwater, R E
Fitzwater, T A
Gandhi, N S
Gandhi, S S
Gee, S
Gilbert, P H
Green, P H
Hand, K W
Hart, I J
Harte, M R
Hothi, D K
Hubbard, D C
Hull, S E
Indrasenan, N
James, B J
Johnson, H S
Kunasingam, V
Ladd, H C
Lee, K W
Liem, D B
Lobo, V J E D
Loftus, R C
Lonsdale, J K
Machin, V G
McKeever, G
Malladi, K S
Mara, H K-M
Martin, G
Minhas, R
Munasinghe, D W S
Murtagh, F E M
Oliver, D J
Osman, A E A A E M
Parkes, N M
Parnell, C J
Pattanayak, K
Phillips, J V
Phillips, L J
Pile, N R
Pimm, J
Pimm, J
Premaratne, R V
Rahman, M S
Rao, V P
Ray, J N
Redman, J H
Sahota, M
Salter, A G
Sastry, M R
Shamshad, S
Siddiqi, M A
Spinks, J T W
Stewart, A J
Story, P S
Tanday, J S
Tandon, S L
Weeks, J H
Wheeler, A K
Yeates, F A
Zafar, T

Rochford

Alcock, G S
Birt, R C
Black, A K
Bone, A R
Boylan, M D
Cordess, W S C
Edwards, A
Langan, B C
Puzey, A J
Saville, M J
Singh, B
Tanqueray, A B
Timmins, D J G

Romford

Abbas, A M A
Acheson, D C
Adams, G G W
Adeotoye, O A
Adhami, Z N
Ahmad, F B S
Ahmad, M
Ahmed, S
Akramul Haq, A K M
Al-Okati, D A K A G
Al-Sabti, A H A-R
Al-Saffar, A A
Ali, M M
Ashworth, K L
Aspoas, A R
Baldry, S J
Bampoe, S A
Banan, H
Barua, I
Barua, J M
Bass, D J
Bavetta, S
Bawa, G P S
Beddoe, R J
Beheshti, B
Bell, T
Benjamin, J C
Bhatt, S M
Bond, S L
Boralessa, H
Brownell, A I
Burack, R J
Burke, S J
Carabott, F
Chakravarty, K K
Chawla, J S
Cheatle, T R
Clarke, G R
Coker, A A
Colvin, D A
Coyle, P J
D'Souza, B
De Silva, R N
Douglas, M M
El-Hihi, M A
Elian, M
Ellis, N
Ellis, P C
Enwo, O N
Fahal, I H
Falconer, D T
Farrow, R E
Feldman, M R
Findley, L J
Fowler, R W
Fuks, K
Gademsetty, S R
Gamble, H P
Gershuny, A R
Gibbs, S J
Gilbert, I
Gill, D S
Gill, K S
Goonetilleke, U K D A
Grant, R W
Gujral, S S
Gunasekara, R D
Gupta, N K
Halim, A
Hamilton-Smith, J A
Hamilton, D M
Harris, E
Hartley, S J M
Haskell, K J
Haskell, S J
Hawkes, C H
Hawkes, M
Hawkins, E
Hepworth, C C
Heylen, V F M
Hollanders, F D
Hossain, M N
Howard, T E
Hughes, A S B
Irtiza-Ali, A S
Ismail, W W M
Jabbar, A
Jayapal, P
Jeevan, S K
Jibrin, U F
Johnston, D H
Jones, A C N
Kadr, H H
Kakad, J C
Keefe, J V
Kelsey, C R
Khoo, D E S A
King, A P
Knowlson, H A
Kuchhai, N A
Kumar, S
Lauchlan, M
Leahy, M J
Lecamwasam, D A G
Lee, J
Leigh-Collyer, N
Liu, S H
Lord, C J
McClean, S J
McDonald, A R
McDonald, H F
MacLellan, G E
Mahmood, K
Marks, C T C
Marshall, A K
Martin, E E V
Masud, P F
Mazumdar, S
Mehta, K J
Mehta, R M
Mikhael, M S H
Moffat, M
Myers, P C
Nair, I
Namnyak, S S
Newell, S J
Newton, M
Nigam, S C
O'Doherty, C A
O'Donovan, D G
Ola, A O
Oldfield, R H
Palit, S
Patel, A N
Patel, A M
Patel, H D
Patel, L M
Patel, S H
Patel, V J
Patel, V M
Pathak, M L
Pathak, S K
Pemberton, N C
Plaha, H S
Poologanathan, S
Prasad, J
Prasad, R S
Purdie, H R M
Rabindra-Anandh, K
Roy, K K
Saeed, I T
Saharay, M
Saheecha, B S
Saini, G S
Salisbury, J A
Sathananandan, S-M
Saunderson, E M
Schwartz, M
Scowen, B
Selvarajan, M
Shah, R S
Shami, S K
Shamil, A S A R
Sharma, A
Sharma, S S
Sims, E C
Singh, R R
Sircar, M
Smith, M A
Soneye-Vaughan, F T
Spencer, G M
Srivatsa, S S
Storey, V C
Subramanian, G
Syed, I A
Syedah, N A
Szollar, J
Taghizadeh, A
Tang, C Y K
Tang, K H
Tanna, K
Tate, P A
Teckham, P N S
Teotia, N P S
Thompson, R J
To, M S
Toms, G C
Udo, E A
Umo-Etuk, J M-E
Wajid, A
Wickramasinghe, L
Wickramasinghe, L S P
Wyganowska, M E T
Zachariah, S R

Romney Marsh

Codlin, R M S
Cullen, R F
Downie, P L
Hatcher, A
Kanegaonkar, V G
Robinson, A A

Romsey

Abbott, R M
Akerman, F M
Akerman, H F
Allen, S M
Bamford, S L
Barratt, J A
Burge, D M
Burn, A J
Burrows, C J
Burrows, P J
Charlton, G A
Chinn, J D
Colthurst, S E
Davis, A J M
Dempster, J G
Edwards, A E
Fallowfield, J A
Ferguson, H J
Fitzgerald, J A W
Friedmann, P S
Gamba, E
Glanville, J D
Herbertson, M J
Iles, D J B
Johnson, A D S
Johnson, C E M
Keightley, M A
Keith, I A
Kelly, S R
Kenyon, J B
Kirby, C M
Lalonde, A K
Lambert, E J
Lawrence, M
Lowndes, K E
Lowndes, S A
McCarthy, A H S
Mitchell, M L
Mooney, A
Patel, J
Peace, R H
Pearson, C F
Peebles, C R
Platt, M R
Prosser, Y I J
Roberts, L J
Russell-Smith, R
Rutter, D V
Steer, H W
Still, M A
Thomas, C P
Tippett, S A
Varney, P R
Warner, G
Warner, K J
Wedderburn, A W
White, P J
Williams, M T
Winn, C R
Wright, I C

Roslin

Chambers, M
Craig, R J
Grubb, N R
Hunter, A R A
McDonald, J M
McIntosh, L G

Ross-on-Wye

Beach-Thomas, J M
Clark, A S G
Clayton, P F
Cook, J M
Cook, R J
Crosland, S J
D'Arcy, B L
Davis, E T
Downey, P F
Fletcher, J L M
Hartshorn, C R
Hayward, R J
Janis, N B
Jardine, M A
Jones, G A
Leeman, A J
Marlowe, G T S
Mellor, R J
Part, M
Richards, J L
Rogers, A J
Silver, S N
Townsend, A J

Rossendale

Ainsworth, C J
Babicki, J W
Berrisford, S B
Bunting, J
Choudhry, T W
Coates, M J
Darlington, J M
Deacon, R E
Doherty, D M
Gill, M S
Grover, M
Hardie, C J
Hinchliffe, W S
Karoo, R O S
Lee, J B
Moustafa, A E-F M
Power, M P
Ramsden, A
Reddy, V
Rishton, P
Sellens, G S
Smith, V H
Smurthwaite, G J

Rotherham

Abbas, A M A
Abbey, S J
Abdul, K A C
Abed, R T
Ahmed, T M
Ainsworth, G
Akram, A
Alexander, M C
Allaqaband, G Q
Amos, M W
Aravindakshan, K K
Avery, G C
Bader, M S
Baker, J L
Balch, K J
Bardhan, K D
Barker, H F
Barker, W E
Barragry, L F
Basran, G S
Bassuini, M M A
Beck-Samuels, P R
Beck, S
Bhamra, M
Bhimpuria, Y R
Brynes, R M
Bulugahapitiya, D T D
Bulugahapitiya, D S
Burns, S B
Casapieri, M
Chakrabarti, I
Chambers, G
Charity, R M
Chattopadhyay, S
Clark, M C
Clark, T J
Clarke, P J
Cleminson, K D
Coates, J W
Cobb, J J

Cole, A J
Collinson, R C A
Cooper, C A
Cooper, J C
Cronly, J P
Crosher, R F
Crowley, G E
Dibb, S
Dudani, P V
Durkan, A M
Dziemidko, H E
Essmaili Shad, J
Everett, B J
Faruq, A
Fawthrop, F W
Fearnside, J E
Ford, J B
Fulbrook, R D
Ganguli, A
Gashut, A M
Ghosh, M K
Goel, P K
Goni, A-U-H
Gopinath, M K
Grant, J
Green, N T W
Griffith, P C
Grover, S R L
Haddad, A Q
Harkness, P A
Harris, J C
Harrison, C J
Harvey-Dodds, L M
Harvey, L
Haste, A R
Hayes, G D
Heyes, F L P
Hinchliffe, R F C
Holt, M E
Hood, H L
Hulley, C M
Husain, M H
Hutson, C A
Islam, K
Islam, M B
Jabir, M A
Jacob, L
Jarjis, H A
Jarvis, H
Jayaswal, B N
Jayaswal, R
Jespersen, S B
Jolley, R M
Jones, B A
Jones, C M
Jones, R B
Jubb, A S
Kacker, R
Kapur, B
Kapur, R
Kear, C S J
Keith, A J
Kesseler, M E
Khan, Z A
Kitlowski, J A
Kitto, W D
Lai, D
Lambertz, M M
Lancer, J M
Lee, J A
Lee, S D
Leese, G J
Littlewood, A J
Luker, B C H
Lyle, H M
McCrea, P H
MacFarlane, P I
McWhinnie, R N
Mahadevan, S
Majumdar, P
Manson, P R
Martin, P L
Matthews, P J
Mellor, A D
Mendelson, E F
Miller, M
Mirza, B B
Mohammed Ismail Kadar Sha, S H
Mohsini, A A
Mondal, B K
Moore, T
Mosharaf, A
Muirhead, R J
Mukhopadhyay, T K
Muncaster, A E
Muthusamy, R
Myers, C P
Nemeth, G
Nesha, M
Newby, D M
Ogden, A D
Okwera, J M
Oliver, P P
Palmer, D H
Parys, B T
Patel, N A
Peckitt, G B
Peckitt, K
Phillips, S
Plews, D J
Polkinghorn, D G
Price, R E
Proctor, J C C
Qureshi, H
Qureshi, N
Rabbani, A A M Z
Raha, H D
Ralph, I F
Reddy, S V
Redgrave, A P
Rees, A J S
Reid, H C
Rosenberg, B C
Salim, F
Sanders, J A
Sayed, Z
Sen, S R
Shankar, D
Shrivastava, O P
Shrivastava, R
Simpson, E W
Sinha, A K
Spencer, P A S
Spooner, S F
Stacey, R K
Stott, D R
Suckling, R J
Suri, S S
Swallow, M B
Tan Hark Hong, K
Taylor, E A S
Taylor, P C
Thakkar, B C
Thambirajah, S
Thomas, P G
Thompson, J S
Thornton, R J
Trend, U
Vatish, M
Velamail, V
Venables, M
Venkatraman, T B
Venkiteswaran, N T
Viswesvaraiah, M
Wallis, C B
Warren, G C
Willemse, P J A
Wilson, D H
Wood, M L
Wright, S R
Zaidi, A A
Zubairu, M B

Rothesay
Berrich, A S
Clark, R D
Herriot, D T
Jerome, J M C
Mackenzie, A R
Morton, J S

Rowlands Castle
Bacon, M T
Boswell, C M
Harrison, J R
Neal-Derks, J A M
Pounder, D
Sissons, J P
Williams, M
Wilson, C J
Wren, S M E
Young, J R B

Rowlands Gill
Armstrong, P A
Blair, S
Clarke, A J
Dawson, R T
Imlah, M
Jones, S B
Liddle, A B G
Malley, R
Quigley, P J L
Smith, G J
Stroud, C R
Turner, P

Rowley Regis
Gold, D V
Riley, J P M

Royston
Bambrick, M
Barnett, S J
Beadsmoore, C J
Brand, A J
Brownrigg, M R
Cairns, N J W
Clubb, T C
Coladangelo, R C
Cox, R A F
Dancey, F M L
Dancey, G S
Foster, J E
Freedman, D J
Gough, P
Greatrex, S J
Hacon, D S
Handcock, L J
Hay, R N
Hedges, J R
Holding, T A
Hone, M P
Inman, R D
Langdale-Brown, M E
Leighton, T J
Lilley, M E
Linnett, P J
Longwill, S L S L
Mann, T A N
Maxim, R E G
Piccinelli, K J
Polge, C M
Riddell, A J
Rigney, A T
Rodda, L C
Taylor, J C
Upward, J W
Van Terheyden, K M R
Watkins, G D
Wickens, L C
Williams, O A
Wright, J F

Rugby
Abdel-Mageed, A
Ahluwalia, J S
Atwal, T S
Aulakh, J M S
Balasubramaniam, T S
Balcombe, N R
Barhey, J S
Barhey, N K
Bartram, G F
Bedi, S S
Bemand, B V
Berridge, E M
Biggs, P I
Black, D
Branscombe, F M
Bridgeman, K
Brittain, R D
Brown, S L
Bryant, R M
Canale-Parola, A
Carne, D R
Clemons, K R
Cook, N J
Corbey, M T
Cotterill, J W
Cumming, E J
Czerniewski, I W D
D'Mello, M S
Dahmash, F H
De Veer, G E
Deliyannis, S N
Derrick, J C A
Dhillon, D P
Douse, H E
Douse, J E
Draper, I B
Ducharme, A L
Ducharme, W A
Duckitt, K
Edgar, K J
Edmunds, E V
Eedle, E K
Fielding, W J
Gallagher, B
Gammell, H J B
Gaunt, R M
Goddard, J A
Griffiths, R L M
Harvey, A J
Hodges, L M-C
Holcroft, P J
Holdsworth, R K
Hooke, R L
Houghton, M P
Ingram, D A
Jacoby, M N J
Jones, D A
Kavuri, S B
Khan, S
Kilvert, P J
Koria, A P
Leach, K J
Menon, M R G
Miarkowski, R F
Mistry, D K
Mohamed, W N A E-R
Morris, P
Moule, I
Nethisinghe, S
Nethisinghe, S K N
O'Hare, J P
Parmar, K B
Parsons, A D
Patel, J N
Raj, S
Rao, P C
Ray-Chaudhuri, D S
Ray-Chaudhuri, S B
Reynolds, K M
Ribeiro, A A
Richards, D A
Richards, S M
Roberts, E J
Rowe, R L
Rye, K A
Saeed, I
Seaman, T F
Shields, G G
Shore, D J
Sinha, R K
Sivapathasuntharam, L
Tassadaq, T
Tyagi, D C
Veysey, S L
West, C A
Williams, J M
Willis, S A

Rugeley
Ansell, G J
Bevan, K W
Boyce, K E
Crawford, C D
Davies, N A
Deb, K
Deb, S
Garden, T B
Ibrahim, I H
James, R L
Light, L
Longbotham, R C
MacMonagle, P J
Milestone, A N
Mirsadgady, S Y
O'Hara, H
Rastogi, N C
Sivanesan, V N
Sorrell, J A
Stokes, M J

Ruislip
Ahmad, F S A
Ahmed, S
Ansari, R
Aurora, R P
Baines, J D
Bhattacharya, M
Brunner, P C
Chandok, H S
Chandok, R S
Coe, D F
Conn, G E
Connell, S E
Dangoor, H E L
Duncan, R J
Feast, M J
Feuer, D J
Garg, R
Hobbs, J R
Hobbs, W G R
Howells, B J
Jaggi, S K
Jayakumar, R
Joseph, P F
Karim, A
King, M N R
Lama, A K
Latif, M A
Liberman, M
Livingstone, J A
McDermott, I D
Marriott, A M
Mashru, M K
Modi, N
Newbery, S R
Patel, P B
Pocock, D I G
Price-Williams, R D
Raj, L
Raj, N
Siddiqui, M L R
Sojka, Y J F
Solomon, C M
Solomon, J I
Timmis, C G
Whitten, S M

Runcorn
Abbott, P M
Allen, C M
Barendt, A B
Bell, B T
Bladen, C
Bohra, P K
Bohra, U
Canfield, C J
Chapelhow, S J
Colin-Thome, D G
Conway, J D
Corrado, K M
Cottier, F M
Davies, H M
Ewing, R
Fearon, H P
Findlay, C D
Fountain, M A
Frith, A G B
Frood, R A W
Gibson, J
Green, M H P
Harris, S E
Jenkins, R J
Johnson, J N
Jowett, S L
Kearney, M J
Khaleeli, A A
La Frenais, W S L
Lawrence, S K
McDermott, D
Mallya, R K
Mirski, E B
Morgan, G J
Mottram, S A
Moulana, N
Murphy, G J
Murphy, M G
Newey, J A
Orpin, M M
Otiv, S
Perumainar, M
Pollet, J E
Pollet, S M
Richards, C G
Rose, E L
Saksena, M K
Sandhu, H S
Savin, P T
Shehu, T
Skinner, J M
Smyth, M D L
Staples, B
Thorpe, M J L
Trevor, A J
Ugwu, C N
Watson, C A
Wild, A-M
Williams, J G
Williamson, J C
Wilson, D H
Wreglesworth, J K

Rushden
Barber, V E
Branford, M
Burch, A J
Clifford, P D
Duncan, A M
Fairweather, N J
Findlay, J B
Hanspaul, A S
Hogg, S J
Kelly, J J
Reading, J H
Richards, D J
Subramaniam, M K
Thomas, T
Wali, J D
Williams, D G
Wingfield, S N

Ruthin
Barrie, A R
Barrie, N
Birkin, P J
Evans, C E J
Higgitt, A
Prys-Jones, O E
Roberts, G H
Roberts, L G R
Seddon, J G W
Tudor, N L

Ryde
Arthure, J E
Atine-Okello, M L
Beable, A E
Boyd, N A
Brown, R E
Burton, G E W
Byron, A J
Cooney, K D
De Belder, M J K
Denman-Johnson, M
Edsall, K C
Fullerton, J R
Goodwin, P E
Green, A J
Griffiths, S C
Hazell, Y E
Hughes, E J
Lammiman, D A
Legg, M D
McNeal, A D
Majumdar, B
Majumdar, K
Manning, C J F
Martin, A
Meltzer, J E
Osman, B E D I A E M
Partridge, J
Pradhan, N S
Rees, B S J
Rezk, R N
Ridout, S M
Rogers, J M C
Shah, B K
Sim, P G
Sim, R J
Symes, J M
Vijaya Kumar, M N
Williams, R C

Rye
Carroll, J
Chishick, H B J
Dyson, A J
Ferguson, N J
Griffin, A L
Halpin, K D
James, L P
James, P M
Jeelani, M S W
Jeelani, R A
Neale, D V
Neilson, W R
Rae, S J

Ryton
Bosman, D L
Brown, S J
Chapman, S W
Doshi, A
Greenough, K R
Hilton, S M
Johnson, M A
Kneale, B N
Phillips, M K
Priestley, A C
Purvis, J

Saffron Walden
Alsos, B
Bassett, J H D
Brand, F J
Brown, C
Brown, J D
Clayton Payne, C D
Cowley, C
Dixon, R M
Duke, C J B
Eaton, C J
Ellis, J C
Fox, T D C
Gande, A R
Handley, J A
Huey, K A
Lort, D J
Lort, E A
O'Donnell, P N S

Pagano, K
Paul, C C
Rockley, P A
Rumsey, S
Shires, S E
Sills, P R
Smith, A E R
Stevens, M N
Walter, F M
Warner, M W
Weir, J J
West, J R

Salcombe
Barnicoat, K T N
McLarty, E W
McLarty, E
Saxby, N V
Stanley, H W

Sale
Abraham, A P
Al-Hakim, A H A
Armshaw, K L
Banait, G S
Berry, J P
Bradley, B L
Braganza, D M R
Broadfield, E-J C
Broomfield, D J
Brotherton, M J
Buckley, P
Burdett-Smith, C B
Burke, Y L
Chakrabarty, K H
Chandraker, A K
Chattopadhyay, T K
Cherian, A
Clare, R G
Curtis, M D
Datta, J
Davies, L A
Devine, J C
Drake, D J
Edmondson, D L
Edwards, D L
Evans, J D
Frier, S R
Gasiorowski, E R
Gayen, A K
Geggie, D A R
Grace, P M
Gray, P A
Greenbaum, J D
Grice, J A
Griffith, J L M
Gwanmesia, I L
Hall, C N
Hall, P J
Hargreaves, S J
Hockenhull, N J
Holloway, M J
Jackson, N D
Jackson, P A
Jamal, A F
Jarvis, M A
Jones, P H
Jones, R G G
Joseph, A
Kim, J B
Kirk, S R
Knowlson, G T G
Kocialkowski, A
Labarre, S M
Larkin, B A
Lavin, J M
Leyland, H E
Lupton, E W
MacDermott, N J G
McKaigue, O J
McMahon, C
Macmillan, F T
Marchi, C J B
Mazeika, P K
Millman, G C
Moley, F M
Mughal, M S
Musgrave, S R
Neary, W D
Needham, S B
Ngan, C Y
O'Connor, M M
O'Malley, G
Olojugba, O H
Palmer, A R
Pattrick, M G
Platt, G
Pole, D M
Porter, S

Ramamurthy, L
Raynor, M K
Regan, D M
Riley, D J
Riley, L
Royle, J S
Saad, E S M
Sarangi, K K
Schofield, R P
Sehat, K R
Shaath, N M
Shackcloth, M J
Simpson, P M A
Skrzypiec-Allen, A I
Smart, D K A
Smith, C J
Smithurst, H J
Stewart, A P
Stokes, J M
Sutton, K J
Swain, D R
Taylor, C R
Taylor, N R
Tebb, J B T
Tierney, N M
Tunney, P J
Waldman, E I
Welsh, P J
Wilson, R G
Yates, A J

Salford
Addlestone, L S
Allan, M W B
Allonby-Neve, C L
Amr, M A Y
Anderson, I D
Andrew, J G
Andrew, S M
Ardern, K D
Armstrong, G R
Atkins, M R
Attwood, S E A
Austin, M A
Babbs, C
Bacall, L
Baishnab, R M
Bancewicz, J
Barnes, P C
Basu, S
Boland, G P
Bowles, B J M
Brooke, R C C
Brookes, C N
Buckler, H M
Campbell, M S
Carlson, G L
Chadwick, P R
Chetty, M S
Chew, L-C
Chisholm, R A
Chowdhury, H R
Cohen, D L
Collier, P A
Cooper, R G
Crossland, J A
Das, D N
Dass, B K
Davis, W S
De Silva, A K L
Dick, J P R
Dieh, A P T
Dornan, T L
Earlam, C M
El Mahmoudi, B K A
Ferguson, J E
Finegan, N A
Finlay, M
Fitchet, A
Fitzgerald, D A
Forbes, W S C
Formela, L J
Freed, D L J
Garson, M
Gavin, C M
Geraghty, I F
Ghosh, P R
Girvent Montllor, M
Gonsalkorale, M
Goodman, K L
Goorney, B P
Griffiths, C E M
Haber, S
Haddad, P M
Haeney, M R
Hague, M E
Harris, J N
Harris, L S D
Hasan, A

Heald, A H
Herrick, A L
Hilton, R C
Houghton, J B
Hughes, D G
Hurri, H O
Jackson, S J
Jeet, I
Jeffree, J S
Jesudason, P J
Jones, A K P
Jones, I H
Joseph, L A
Kallis, P F
Kalra, P A
Kassam, N N
Kelly, M C J
Kelly, T
Kochhar, P K
Lakshmi, V
Larah, D G
Lear, J T
Lecky, F E
Levenson, S
Leventhall, P A
Lewis-Parmar, H J
Lloyd, R E
Lopian, N H
Lowenson, L F C
McElroy, H
McLaughlin, J T
Majid, I
Marsh, M N
Maxwell, H A
Million, R
Mitchell, S J
Morgan, R J
Moss, G E
Muir, L T S W
Munjal, R S
Muston, H L
Neary, D
O'Brien, D P
O'Donoghue, D J
O'Driscoll, B R C
O'Driscoll, D
Owen, W A
Palmer, J H M
Parkar, W
Parsons, V J
Pira, A
Polson, D W
Pramanik, A
Protheroe, R T
Quantrill, S J
Quinn, V P
Railton, A
Raj, V B
Randall, S C
Rees, W D W
Reeve, R S
Rehman, S-U
Robinson, J A
Robinson, J
Robinson, M J
Rodgers, M E
Rogers, C M
Rosenberg, S E
Ross, E R S
Routledge, R C
Rudenski, A
Saleh, N
Salim, A
Saxby, K M
Scott, N A
Shaffer, J L
Shaw, E A
Sherrington, C R
Simon, S
Slade, R J
Soni, S
Spanswick, C C
Staniland, J R
Stewart, M F
Stout, I H
Strickland, P L
Sultan, M
Sussman, J D
Talbot, P R
Tankel, J W
Telfer, N R
Thomas, A N
Thompson, D G
Turkington, P M
Turnbull, I W
Tyrrell, P J
Victoratos, G
Waldek, S
Watt, J W G

Willatt, D J
Williams, J D L
Wright, J R
Yates, P A
Yell, J A
Zotkiewicz, M J

Salisbury
Adams, H C
Adams, R A
Adams, R K
Adams, T S T
Annis, J A D
Armstrong, W L
Baker, C C
Barclay, I H
Barnes, L M
Barnsley, R
Barrett, R F
Barrow, G I
Barter, P P
Beaumont, A R
Bentley, B
Beswick, R W
Biggart, S A W S
Boddy, N
Bond, H R L
Borrelli, P B
Bottomley, E L
Box, C J
Boyle, J A
Brockbank, M J
Brooks, T J G
Brown, R M
Buchanan, P
Burrows, L J
Burrows, N C
Cadier, M A M
Calvert, S L
Carter, L D G
Carty, N J
Carvell, J E
Chapple, D C L
Clark, K A
Claydon, P J O
Coats, N L B
Cockroft, S
Cole, R P
Collier, J M
Collier, R G
Collins, M M
Collyer-Powell, R G
Cook, M J
Cooke, T J C
Corlett, J C R
Cotterill, S L
Crabbe, R W
Crane, R G
Cullis, J O
Dalton, J R
Darlow, H M
Davies, P C
Davies, T G
Dean, I A M
Docherty, P W
Downie, I P
Duggal, J A
Eastman, S V
Easton, J A
Edgington, P J
Ellis, R M
English, J M
Evans, S A
Finnegan, T P
Finnis, D
Flood, T R
Flowerdew, A D S
Fountain, S A
French, R B
Frost, R A
Fuller, C E
Gailey, M D H
Garrett, W R
Geddes, J D
Glanville, H J
Glaysher, C M R
Gotham, C R
Gray, M I H
Gready, E M
Green, M J
Griffiths, G W
Griffiths, M A
Grummitt, W M
Grundy, D J
Guy, P J
Haggis, J F
Hall, A
Healey, F B
Hegarty, S E

Helyer, K A-L
Hewetson, R P
Higgins, C S
Hobby, J A E
Horlock, N M
Howgrave-Graham, A J
Hudson, J D P
Humphry, R C
Jack, I L
Jagger, G M H
Janmohamed, S G
Jewson, T E
Johnson, K A
Jonas, D R C
Jones, A L
Jones, S M
Jowett, R
Kerr, J S
Khan, S M
Kidman, L V
King, J V
King, R A
Lacey, O J
Laidlaw, F C
Lewis, S J
Lightfoot, N F
Lintin, D J
McArthur, P
McCallum, M I D
McDowall, R A W
McGee, S G G
McIntosh, G S
McKenna, D M
McKinley, N P
McKinley, P E
McNee, P A J
McNeill, D C
Macready, L
Mann, R G
Marigold, J H
Markey, T E
Martin, H S
Mash, K M
Maslin, P S
Meader, H L
Mein, D C
Millar, K N A
Mitchell, D M
Moore, M V
Morgan, D R
Morgan, M C
Morris, A D P
Morris, M R
Morse, G R
Mullan, D P
Murray, D P
Myint, C M
Nazeer, A F
Nettle, C J
Newton Dunn, A R
Nodder, E M
O'Connell, N M
O'Connor, K M
Orchard, J A
Owers, R C
Parry, H F
Parry, R M
Payne, R F
Peach, F J
Pelly, H J W
Podkolinski, M T
Pope, J B
Powell, G A
Powell, M J
Ranaboldo, C J
Ray, M
Ray, R J
Reeve, A P M
Reid, R A
Rice, P
Richardson, A J
Richardson, W W
Ridley, N H L
Roberts, M J
Robertson, J C
Robertson, M E
Rose, M A
Ross Russell, F M
Rossi, L F A
Rushforth, G F
Russell, A M
Rustom, J W
Scott-Jupp, R H
Scott, C A
Scott, R P F
Seal, S H
Sears, C A N
Sears, E F

Shashidharan, M
Shaw, E J
Shergill, C S
Short, P A
Simpson, C L
Smith, M R
Smithies, A
Soopramanien, A
Stanger, E L
Stanger, N R Y
Stevens, M T
Stone, J A S
Stratton, D
Strelitz, N S
Swayne, P
Thomas, M A
Thomas, S D
Thompson, C S
Thompson, P J
Thorne, B M
Tibbitts, A R
Todd, G B
Tromans, A M
Tyers, A G
Tyers, R C B
Viney, P L
Vyas, S K
Vyrnwy-Jones, P
Walters, D P
Warley, A R H
Waters, E A
Weaver, S A
Webb, E M
West, P S
Whetham, J M
Whittingham, H W
Whitworth, I H
Wilde, J A
Williams, E M
Willis, R J
Witts, H M
Wood, C D
Wright, G D S
Wright, J V
Yeoh, M J

Saltash
Booth, C W
Bowes, P J
Bredemeyer, A
Broadhead, A D
Brown, C
Charlton, S C
Cook, R C
Cundy, A L
Davies, P S
Devonport, N J
Erith, M J
Farrant, S J
Fisher, N G
Fox, C L
Fullalove, S
Gegg, J M
Gronow, H J
Hopper, M A
Hughes, B D
Jackson, S
Kneen, R C B
Mercer, R F
Moore, J R A
Parrish, J
Parrish, R W
Potter, H L Z
Sissons, M P
Smith, D K
Stableforth, W D
Thomas, W G
Webster-Harrison, P J

Saltburn-by-the-Sea
Armitage, A
Betterton, M J
Brownlee, N H
Clements, B W
Connolly, H M F
Costello, B
Dall'Ara, R G
Fish, K P F
Glasby, M S
Greaves, S H L
Harris, E E
Harvie, A K
Johnson, S A
Lavelle, P H
Milner, M L
Palumbo, L
Parkin, R A
Saxton, J C R
Shepherd, D J

Strang Wood, S
Waite, C J
Yates, R H T

Saltcoats
Briggs, E J
Cameron, K J
Hales, D S M
McKinlay, J J
Norton, J C G
Robertson, D I S
Timmons, J A

Sandbach
Armitage, A J
Armitage, J D
Baker, D L
Baxter, R T
Broadbent, P J
Brown, S R
Evennett, A J
Hassall, H
Kinder, A J
Mercer, J D
Olver, M J
Rao, K S
Robinson, M
Tate, M J
Tebby, S J

Sandhurst
Azurdia, M R
Brown, S N
Davies, I Z
Halliwell, R P
Kanjaria, N J
Pidgeon, C A
Routledge, H C
Shivayogi, M
Thing, J R
Vakil, A

Sandown
Botell, L T
Brand, J V
Brand, P
Gent, N R E
Griffiths, A
McMullen, D J
Moore, J S
Randall, P G
Summerhayes, P J
Trowell, H M

Sandwich
Allen, M J
Berti, C A
Birchall, C E
Browning, R C
Carnegie, A M
Carnegie, M R
Child, B G
Colquhoun, K B M
Davies, M J
Davis, A E
Edwards, M R
Ellis, A J
Geewater, D M J
Han, S W
Harris, G
Healy, C J
Hughes, J D
Marchant, B G
Milligan, P M
Mridha, K A
Nurbhai, S
Osterloh, I H
Power, A C
Roblin, D
Wismayer, E C

Sandy
Baker, M R
Baxter, J A
Bourke, B E
Drake, L K
Fowler, S E
Gledhill, P D
Green, C A
Greig, M M
Heslop, D A
Howes, P J W
Kapur, A K
Karamé, M M A
Momen, M
O'Brien, M J
Patel, A M
Reddy, A N
Summers, G D

Taine, D L
Tansey, M J B

Sanquhar
Baker, I R
Burton, C D

Saundersfoot
Allan, R C
Canton, D E
Davies, H E
Fleming, V A
O'Doherty, K
Thomas, G C

Sawbridgeworth
Aldam, C H
Gonzalez Contreras, R B
Gunetilleke, L
Hartwell, R
Hempel, A C A
Jones, K A
Kearns, D M
Keller, P H
Miller, C H
Perry, J E
Pontin, A R
Webb, A R
Wilkinson, M I P

Saxmundham
Backhouse, K M
Buchanan, J
Dunn, H J
Hallam, P J B
Havard, J S
Parks, C J
Tesh, A E C

Scarborough
Abrines, M J
Adams, T J
Adamson, J
Adamson, S J
Akar, P E
Allan, B J
Ames, D S
Andrews, C M
Arundale, D E
Bacon, P J
Bakeer, G M
Baker, J G D
Barron, L
Beardsley, F J
Bradley-Stevenson, C L
Bradley, J G
Brame, K G
Brentnall, A L P
Broadhurst, C
Brown, P M
Brown, S J
Buckley, P M
Cappleman, T A
Carnegie-Smith, K
Cheetham, C M
Chow, W M
Clark, R S
Coppack, J J
Crowson, J D
Davidson, A J
Davies, D R L
Dawes, J A
De Pont, S A M T
Dewar, D H
Dewar, D J
Dewar, M E
Drake, J M
Dyer, J D
El Barghouty, N M N
El Tahir, M A
Fettes, I F
Ford, D J
Fraser, N C
Gill, P M
Glaves, I
Greenan, J
Halloran, K M
Hamp, I R
Hark, A J
Hawkyard, S J
Hayes, G
Holland, I M
Hollins, B J
Hopkirk, T J
Hughes, P J
Humphriss, D B
Jackson, A M
Jacques, A M

Johnson, M J
Jones, D F
Jones, M E
Kaye, H H
Kinch, A P J
Knowelden, D J
Kok, R H C
Lahoud, G Y G
Laljee, R M
Laws, M G
Lister, A H
Livesey, S H
Macfie, J
Mahadeva, S
Marimon Ortiz De Zarate, M
Marshall, N E V
Mason, R A
Matteucci, P L
Meiwald, J M
Mensah, J A
Missen, M R
Mitchell, C J
Moederle-Lumb, D A
Morgan, D R
Morton, R N
Mumby, P S
Nicholson, R D
Noble, E P
Noble, M C B
Normandale, J P
North, A D
O'Sullivan, K M
Oldroyd, D A
Penfold, J J
Percival, S P B
Perry, E P
Phillips, P D
Pitts, I D
Poole, D R
Pretorius, M
Reay, J M R
Redmond, R M
Richardson, S
Rigg, P
Robinson, D W
Robinson, P
Robinson, P J
Saffman, C M
Said, W A D K
Saunders, C
Scarborough, M A
Scarborough, S A B
Schaefer, A M
Scott, C J
Sheikh, A A
Stanley, W E
Stoker, J A
Svoboda, D
Taylor, J A
Thompson, G L
Thompson, R M
Tring, I C
Turner, M A
Volans, A P
Walker, A
Walker, J M
Ward, R W
Western, J M
Whelan, N H
Whitby, E B
Williams, A C
Williams, B J
Williams, R J
Worters, J R

Scunthorpe
Ahmad, S M
Akande, O
Al-Adwani, A A
Aye, O
Baker, F G
Balasanthiran, S
Barbier, B F
Barrantes Gallego, R
Basu, D K
Beer, S F
Bowman, R J
Brown, J A
Butler, M A
Caley, G L
Chaudhary, A K
Chaudhary, D
Coe, A J
Dean, R
Devlin, J
Dhawan, J
Dwyer, M J
El Rakshy, M M B E D

Fernando, I A P N
Fraser, A J
Ghosh, A
Ghosh, A
Goldthorpe, S B
Gordhandas, A M
Grattage, T J
Hall, C J
Hamad, A A M
Hayes, G J
Hockey, M S
Hunt, C M
Isaacs, J A
Jalihal, S S
Jedrzejczyk, A
Jha, R R
Kapil, G P
Kar, A K
Kenny, R H
Kerss, A S
Kulkarni, V A
Kumar, S
Lee, A W
Lees, A M
McCormack, P
McGlasham, G
McNeil, I A
Maharaj, A K
Maitra, T K
Maitra, T B
Mallik, T K
Maslin, S C
Mawhinney, E O
Melrose, J R
Mohamed, A R A A
Molitor, P J A
Molloy, I
Moore, P J
Nasr, I S I M
Newman, C G
Odukoya, A O
Oliver, E M
Pais, V
Pemberton, J M
Penston, J G M
Phillips, E P K
Raha, A K
Rai, N
Rajkumar, S
Ranasinghe, S
Rashid, K
Riley, P B
Roberts, L J
Ryan, E P M
Sabharwal, S
Saleh, B T
Sanderson, M L
Sewell, W A C
Shafqat, S O
Sharara, K E-S H
Sharkey, D
Shekhar, S
Stanford, M F
Stewart, N
Summerton, N
Taylor, A P
Taylor, J W
Terreros Berruete, O
Thant, M
Thompson, J F W
Tindall, S F
Trueman, C J
Vijayakumar, K
Walshaw, R J
Walter, J C
Walton, T J
Webster, P A
Weeks, A D
White, D E
Widders, J
Wilken, B J
Woollands, I G
Worah, R
Ying, I A
Young, K R
Zacharias, J

Seaford
Austin, M J
Barnes, M H
Bayles, I
Bayles, J M
Bayne, G M
Blenkarn, R N
Brown, C S
Cockburn, J M
Dunbar, P A
Foster, S J
Fuller, S

Harvey, C L
Harvey, R W
Jones, J G
Lewis, C J
Light, D C
Lloyd, M M
McGhee, K J
Macleod, T H R
Mellor, C S
Morris, M J
Pickering, B J
Sharman, M A
Shears, M-R B
Turner, C J

Seaham
Angus, G
Appanna, B
Barkataki, N
Bresnen, D
Dusad, R K
George, M E
Gustafsson, J V
Kapoor, A L
Kapoor, K R
Muscat, S M
Napier, D C
Rawling, K G
Reddy, C N
Reddy, K V
Stancliffe, J B

Seascale
Adkins, G G
Carhart, P A
Curry, I P
Jay, S A
Longworth, A E
Lowrey, G E
McAndrew, I W
Macgregor, D H
Maguire, B G
Sowton, T J
Stevenson, M D
Walker, B

Seaton
Bastin, C J
Bramley, R J
Coop, J A
Daniels, R J
Farrell, P J S
Fox, M R
Hurst, J R
Pitt, G H
Rolls, A
Slater, L K
Stewart, D H
Webb, P S
Wickins, M C

Seaview
Cahill, A B
Hounsfield, V
Loach, R S

Sedbergh
Lumb, W J
Newson, E R A
Orr, P A
Orr, W G
Syred, J R
Thomas, T S

Selby
Bilcliffe, E M
Bond, G
Chau, H N
Dalby, R J
Davis, P R
Docherty, C
Docherty, P F
Edwards, D W
Haworth, S R
Hepworth, D
Hildore, L M
Hills, R C
House, E V
Jackson, N
Kaufman, R B
Lewis, I A
Lord, E R
McGrann, P J
Pearson, T E
Reid, J D
Robson, A
Scott, E J
Shardlow, D L
Stanford, A J

Taylor, A R
Wakefield, R J
Williams, M E

Selkirk
Cullen, J G
Davies, S R
Fiddes, W F G
Gillies, E M
Gillies, J C M
Glen, S E
Love, E M
Ross, C C
Sharpe, C J
Wheelans, J C
Wilson, J F

Settle
Birkett, C I
Hall, W W
Lewis, J M
Littlejohn, C I
Longhorn, P D
Longhorn, R K
Moakes, H
Renwick, C J
Sandoe, J A T
Ward, E

Sevenoaks
Arnott, N D
Ashworth, H L
Barker, P G
Barnaby, J
Barnes, J
Bates, C J
Best, M H
Botha, M E
Brignall, K A
Brook, R
Broomby, R C W
Clark, F J
Clarke, N A H
Cook, G E
Cox, J A
Creagh, T M
Creed, H S
Daniel, A C M
Dibble, A M
Dowling, O M T
Dowrick, S E
Dunn, R P
Evans, D K
Farraway, N J
Farthing, C P
Forbes, N J
Ford, M A
Fry, R W
Furness, S J
Giffin, N J
Giorgi, L
Grant, N M
Harris, J W S
Haworth, G M
Haworth, S C
Holder, P D
Horne, P W
Hosseini, M
Hull, K E
Husband, R G
Irvine, T E
Jariwalla, A
John, G
Johnson, F R
Keenor, C
Khakoo, S I
Kotting, S C
Landy, P B
Larchet, P K
Lay, C J
Legg, J R
Lesseps, A
Lindsay, Y
Linnett, D A
Lockhart, N S
Lynam, A M
McCusker, F E M
MacDonnell, A J R
Martin, M S
Moosvi, S K
Morgan, S C
Morton, S V
Parker, N J
Parkes, J D
Patel, V
Pearse, H R
Porter, E
Razzell, P J
Rissik, K M

Rodway, A E P
Ross, F A
Roxburgh, A C
Shairp, B E
Shannon, S E
Sillitoe, C
Solan, C L
Stubbs, E J
Taggart, G E
Taggart, M
Taor, L P M
Taylor, A J
Thomas, D G
Thomas, D M
Tonge, A R
Toothill, S V
Turner, L M
Unwin, P W
Walker, K J
Watson, J N
Whitlock, J A
Winbow, A J
Wright, J J
Wynter, M J C

Shaftesbury
Appleyard, D S
Daddy, S
Dodson, J W
Easterbrooke, S J
Emms, R J
Hewetson, C T
Horner, S S
Jackson, R A
Patterson, D D L
Tapper, G W
Weir, A W
Wynn-Mackenzie, D M

Shanklin
Frame, A G
Gent, G M
Ghurye, R S
Rivers, J W
Stone, B E
Willetts, J M

Sheerness
Armstrong, F J
Brew, M D
Clune, F A M
Cook, L
Dhillon, J S
Ellis, D J
Fahmy, M M E-S
Ramu, V K
Rowe, M P
Tadros-Caudle, M E
Uppal, H K
Whiting, B H

Sheffield
Abell, D J
Ackroyd, R
Adamo, S J
Adams, M
Adams, M G
Adshead, S-L
Afzal, A
Ahmad, J
Ahmedzai, S H
Ainger, M C
Ainscow, C B
Akil, M
Al-Wali, W I A
Alderson, J D
Alison, L H
Allsopp, E S
Amin, S N
Amin, S N O
Amos, R S
Anagnostou, E
Anderson, A J
Anderson, J B
Anderson, J E
Anderson, P B
Anderton, M
Andrzejowski, A Z
Andrzejowski, A R M
Andrzejowski, J C
Angel, C A
Ansons, C
Appleyard, T N
Aratari, C
Arcelus Alonso, J
Asghar, R B
Ashby, A F
Ashmore, G T
Aswani, N M

Atkin, C E
Atkin, M
Atkins, C J
Atkinson, A M
Atkinson, J
Atkinson, R E
Atun, A R
Austin, C A
Ayling, L A
Azmy, I A F
Bailey, H
Baird, A M
Baker, E
Baker, R H
Ball, S E
Balsitis, M
Bandekar, M S
Barclay, C S
Barclay, J H
Bardsley, P A
Barik, S
Barker, I
Barley, J A
Barnes, R J
Baron, D E
Baron, S
Barrington, N A
Bates, C J
Battersby, R D E
Battye, J E
Bax, D E
Bax, N D S
Baxter, A J
Baxter, P S
Beahan, J
Beard, J D
Beaumont, D G
Beckett, J P
Bedford, M
Beechey, A P G
Beetham, M D
Belfield, J C
Bell, M J
Bell, S J
Bellamy, D C
Benjamin, J G
Bennett, A N
Bennett, V R
Benns, J S
Bentley, C C
Bergvall, U E G
Bernard, J
Berthoud, M C
Bethell, J
Bhan, A
Bickerstaff, D R
Birch, J L
Bird, S I D
Birkby, E A
Birks, D M P
Birks, D V
Birks, R J S
Birtwhistle, M B
Bishop, H E
Bishop, J M
Bishop, N J
Blakeborough, A
Bleakley, C J
Blockey, P
Boldy, J A
Boston, P F
Bottomley, D R W
Bowers, J C
Bowes, R J
Bowman, S J
Bowry, A
Bowry, V A
Boyd, V
Boyle, M S
Bracewell, M A
Bradbury, C E
Bradbury, P A
Bradley, A R
Bradley, K E
Braidley, P C
Brammar, D K
Brand, A E
Brand, C S
Brar, A S
Brawn, L A
Breen, D P
Bremner, J A G
Brennan, P O B
Bridgewater, C H
Brimacombe, M C
Brinkley, A M E
Brinkley, D C
Broadley, P S
Brockbank, J E

Brodie, D B
Brook, P N
Brookes, L D
Brown, A
Brown, C B
Brown, J N
Brown, K E
Brown, M B
Brown, P M
Brown, P G
Brown, P W G
Brown, S R
Brown, V A
Brown, W H
Bruce, A S W
Bryan, B A
Bryant, R C
Bryant, R J
Bryson, P N
Buckingham, K L
Buffin, J T
Bull, M J
Bull, P D
Bullas, B H
Burke, J P
Burns, B J
Burton, J
Bush, J M
Bustani, P C
Butler, G
Butler, J M
Butler, U G
Byrne, J W
Caddick, S L
Caddy, C M
Caldon, L J M
Caley, M J
Calladine, C
Cameron, I C
Campbell, A M
Campbell, N M
Campbell, P
Campbell, S
Cannon, J S
Carey, P E
Carlile, W W
Carr, A J
Carter, G S
Carter, M J
Caunt, J A
Chadha, P
Chalmers, J L
Chambers, G
Chan, D T Y
Chan, P
Chan, R
Chan, T K J
Chandrasekharan, S
Channer, K S
Chantry, A D
Chaplais, J Z
Chapman, C L
Chapman, D F
Chapman, J E
Chapple, C R
Charles, B M
Charlton, H M
Chatterjee, D K
Christie, J P
Chua, I C-I
Clark, G P M
Clark, J C
Clark, J D F
Clark, J R
Clark, P J
Clark, S J
Clement, F M
Cleveland, T J
Clout, C
Clowes, J A
Coad, N R
Coan, A C
Cobb, J A
Cockayne, S E
Cohen, G L
Coker, A E O
Cole, A A
Coleman, R E
Coley, S C
Collins, G D
Collins, J S
Collins, M A
Collins, M C
Collins, R K
Colver, D C B
Colver, S E
Connell, H
Connelly, H R
Connolly, S A

Connor, M E
Conway, J V
Cook, J A
Cooke, H M G
Coombs, R C
Cooper, G J
Cooper, J R
Cooper, J E M
Cooper, M W
Cooper, M J
Cooper, M T
Cooper, S M
Cooper, W G
Cork, M J
Cornell, S J
Cort, J M
Cowey, R V
Cox, R M
Cracknell, P
Craig, J M
Craven, P J
Crawford, S E
Creagh, F M
Crehan, P
Cressey, D M
Crimlisk, H L
Critchlow, J I
Croot, L M
Crosby, A C
Cross, S S
Crossland, D S
Crossman, D C
Cullen, D R
Cullen, R J
Cumberland, J E
Cummins, E M
Currie, Z I
Czauderna, J M
D'Mello, B M T
Da Costa, D F
Da Silva, C K
Dalal, S
Dallas, F
Daly, R F
Danskin, J M
Darby, A C
Darling, S P
Das, A
Dass, M
Datta, D
Davidson, A J
Davidson, I W
Davies-Jones, G A B
Davies, A
Davies, A G
Davies, B M
Davies, D P
Davies, G P
Davies, H A
Davies, J G
Davies, J R
Davies, N P
Davis, C J
Davis, K J
Dawson, D J
De Mortimer-Griffin, C A E
De Noronha, R J
Deakin, P J
Dennis, A R
Dey, S K
Dibble, T L
Dilke-Wing, G M
Dobbs, P
Dobson, P M S
Dodd, P D F
Doddridge, N J
Doidge, C L
Donnelly, M T
Dorman, T
Douglas, D L
Downie, W A
Driscoll, P H
Dube, A K
Duckworth, T
Duff, G W
Dujon, D G
Duncan, M E
Dunn, K S
Durling, M E
Eastell, R
Edbrooke, D L
Edenborough, F P
Edney, P
Edwards, M P
Edwards, N D
Ee, H L
Egner, W
Eilbeck, S C

El-Shazly, M M E-D K
Elliott, S J
Ellis, J D
Ellis, S J
Elphinstone, C D
Emerson, S
Emerson, V J
Englert, L J
Eskin, F
Evans, C A
Evans, H P
Evans, M
Evans, R S
Everard, M L
Everson, G S
Ezzat, V A
Fairbrother, J M
Fairlie, F M
Fardon, N J M
Farkas, A G
Farrell, M B
Faulkner, R D
Fenton, P A
Ferguson, C A
Fernandes, N O J
Field, N J
Fieldsend, G A
Fieldsend, R L H
Filby, H J
Fisher, P M
Fisher, P C
Fisher, V M
Fishwick, D
Fitzgerald, D M
Fitzgerald, G
Flann, P-J A
Fletcher, A K
Flowers, M J
Flynn, M E S
Foran, B H
Forrest, A R W
Forrester, A M
Forster, G
Fothergill, D J
Fowler, A J
Fowler, I A
Fox, A M
Fox, M
Fox, S
France, M J
Francis, K L
Francis, T A
Franks, S E
Fraser, R B
Freedlander, E
Freeman, C
Freeman, R
French, N M
Furber, A S
Furniss, D L S
Gajjar, P D
Gallagher, D
Gallagher, D F
Gallaher, J M
Gamsu, M J
Ganapathy, T S
Ganley, P D
Gardner, J M
Gaubert, R A P
Gawkrodger, D J
Geh, L C J
Gelipter, D
Gent, A M
Gentle, S M
George, R R
Gerrard, M P
Gerrish, S P
Getty, C J M
Gholkar, S A
Giannoukas, A
Gibson, R J B M
Gilchrist, J A
Giles, J
Gili, N L
Gill, P V
Gillett, M
Gillott, J H
Gillott, T J
Gleave, C R
Gleeson, D C
Glover, S C
Goddard, J M
Goepel, J R
Goh, K K
Goldberg, K A
Gonzalez, D M
Goodacre, S W
Goodall, H J
Gordon, J E

Gordon, R M
Gossiel, R
Gott, E J
Gowlett, S J
Grainger, R G
Grant, I C
Grantham, G H
Gray, J T
Gray, T A
Greaves, C W K H
Greaves, J A H
Greaves, W E
Green, D T
Green, M
Green, M A
Green, N E
Green, S T
Green, T
Greengrass, S R
Greenstreet, D
Greenwell, T J
Greenwood, L J
Griffin, J J
Griffiths, P D
Griffiths, R W
Grimshaw, M S
Grimshaw, S L
Grover, A
Groves, E R
Grunewald, R A
Gunn, J P G
Hackney, J S
Hackney, M A
Haddock, R
Hadjivassiliou, M
Hafiz, R M
Hall, C M
Hall, D M B
Hall, J
Hall, N A M
Hall, S M
Hamdy, F C
Hamdy, N A T C
Hamer, A J
Hamer, D J
Hamilton, M
Hampton, K K
Hancock, B W
Hancock, S W
Hannay, D R
Haq, I U
Harding, M J
Hardisty, C A
Hardy, P J
Hardy, P G
Harker, T G
Harpin, V A
Harrington, C I
Harris, H J
Harris, J L
Harris, R M
Harrison, B J
Harrison, D A
Harrison, N
Harvey, P R
Harvey, P J
Hasan, J R
Hastie, K J
Hatcher, I S
Hatton, C T
Hatton, E R
Hatton, M Q F
Hayes-Allen, M C
Heap, M J
Heathcote, J A
Heathcote, P R M
Heatley, C T
Heller, S R
Hempseed, G D
Hen, B Y
Hendra, D A
Hendra, T J
Henry, L
Hepple, S
Herdman, C P
Herrera Vega, L
Hettiarachchi, C D
Hickman, L
Hicks, A G
Higenbottam, T W
Higgins, K S
Hill, C
Hillman, B
Hird, C J
Hoare, R J
Hobden, M A
Hobson, N A
Hodgson, T J
Holden, V A

Hollingworth, K M
Holmes, P C
Holt, G M
Hood, G
Hope, A M
Hopkins, B J
Hopkins, J
Hopkinson, D N
Hopper, A D
Hopwood, B
Horner, O J
Hough, R E
Houghton, A M
Howard, A Q
Howard, A C
Howard, K
Howard, P
Howell, S J L
Hudson, A J
Hughes, D E
Humphrey, J A
Hunsley, J E
Hunter, J I
Hunter, S J S
Hutchcroft, B J
Hutchinson, A
Hutchison, G
Huws, R W
Illingworth, C M
Ince, P G
Inch, H M
Ireland, S J
Irwin, K
Islam, B
Jaafar, A S
Jaafar, F
Jackson, B J
Jackson, B C
Jackson, P R
Jakubowski, J
James, A F
James, M D
James, V
Jarratt, J A
Jarvis, C P
Jayasinghe, D S
Jeavons, P
Jellinek, D A
Jenkins, S B
Jenner, F A
Jennings, M
Jewes, L A
Jivraj, S S
Joesbury, H E
John, R E
Johns, R G
Johnson, D A N
Jokhi, R P
Jones, D A
Jones, M L
Jones, M A C
Jones, P
Jones, S J
Jordan, C N
Jordan, N
Joshi, K
Kacker, P P
Kacker, S
Kacker, S
Kandler, R H
Kang, S
Kanis, J A
Karim, M S
Kavanagh, J
Kay, A J
Kay, N R M
Kearsley, N J
Keating, D A
Keegan, S
Keel, J D
Keen, J A
Kell, C
Kelly, C L
Kemeny, A
Kemp, R C
Kemp, R T
Kemplen, A M
Kendall, K M
Kendall, T J G
Kennedy, R M
Kennedy, R
Kenny, C
Kerr, K
Kerry, R M
Kershaw, J D
Ketchell, R I
Khan, A M
Kilding, R F
Killey, S H

King, B C A
King, H
King, J A
King, M
King, P J
Kinghorn, G R
Kirkbride, P
Kirkbride, V
Kitlowski, A J
Knowles, P R
Kudesia, G
Kumar, D
Kurpiel, A J
Kwarko, K A
Lane, V J M
Lang, I M
Lankshear, W M
Latham, C A
Laugharne, J D E
Lawson-Matthew, P J
Laycock, C L
Lazner, M R
Ledger, W L
Ledingham, R G
Ledingham, S N
Lee, C H
Lee, F K T
Lee, V
Leicester, S
Leigh, G
Leigh, V F
Lenthall, J
Leonard, D A
Lethem, K R
Levy, D P
Liddell, A M
Liddle, B J
Lightfoot, D M
Liljendahl, S
Lin, K W
Lindley, R M
Lindop, D J
Linnard, G
Littlewood, C
Livesey, D S J
Lloyd, F E
Lobo, A J
Locke, T J
Lockwood, C S
Lockwood, S E
Loescher, A R
Long, G
Longan, M A
Longfield, S R W
Longshaw, C L
Longshaw, M S
Longstaff, S
Lonsdale, R J
Lord, R C C
Lorenz, E
Lucas, K
Lumb, S E H
Lunt, R L
Lupton, S D
Luscombe, M D
Lyons, V H
McAlindon, M E
McAll, G L G
McAllister, D P
MacAskill, N D
McAvoy, J
MacCallum, E A
McCarthy, S
McCormick, S R
McCullough, H C
McDermott, C J
McDonagh, A J G
McDonough, H M
MacDowell, A D
McElwaine, J G
McFarlane, A
McGorrigan, J L L R
McGraw, S J
McIntyre, H
McKendrick, M W
McKenna, J F
McKenna, M M
McKenzie, A I
Mackenzie, C A
Mackenzie, F A
MacKeown, S T
McKevitt, F M
Mackinnon, A E
Macleod, I C
McMillen, G V
McNaught, R
MacNeill, A
McTavish, K
Magennis, J K

Maheswaran, C M
Maheswaran, R
Majeed, A W
Makris, M
Manley, C A
Mann, M
Manning, L V
Mark, J S
Marples, M
Marr, J E
Marshall, A S
Marshall, T L
Martin Delgado, R
Martin, A G
Marven, S S
Marvin, C M
Massey, N J A
Mathers, N J
Mathers, P M A
Matthews, S
Mayers, G P
Mehrotra, P
Mehrotra, V B
Mehrotra, V N
Mehta, S
Messenger, A G
Metcalf, H M
Metcalfe, B C
Mezilis, N
Michael, S
Michaels, J A
Miller, J G
Mills, C A
Mills, G H
Milner, N A
Milroy, C M
Mirza, M
Mitchell, C A
Mohammed Fauzi, A R
Moll, J M H
Monaghan, D
Mooney, P N
Moore, C A
Moore, K T H
Moorhead, P J
Moorhead, S P
Moran, D G
Morgan, J E F
Morgan, J P
Morgan, J M
Morgan, S A
Morgan, S M
Morley, A F
Morris, F P
Morris, H D
Morris, H J
Morton, L A
Moss, G D
Moss, L S
Moss, P J
Moulsher, P J
Moxon, D
Muggleton, R J
Mundy, J V B
Munro, J F
Murphy, I J
Murray, P
Murray, R J
Myers, A M
Nabi, D W
Nadkarni, S
Nahami, G R
Naik, D R
Naik, R
Nakielny, R A
Nandasoma, U C
Narayanan, A N
Narodden, M N
Nassef, A H K
Nawaz, S
Nawaz, S
Neal, L M
Neal, M R
Nehring, S J
Nelson, K W
Nelson, M E
Nerurkar, I D J
Newman, C M H
Nieder, M
Noble, D A
Noble, T W
Nohr, K
Norman, P
Norris, M J
Norris, S H
North, G N
North, R A
Norton, P G
Nutt, M N

O'Connell, J P
O'Connor, F P
O'Connor, S P J
O'Dwyer, J M E
O'Rourke, A J
Oakes, S M
Oakley, G D G
Oakley, N
Oates, C S
Oates, D E R
Ogden, J
Okorie, N M
Oliver, R
Omokanye, S A
Ong, A C M
Orme, S
Orth, A
Osborne, M A
Otten, K A
Outtrim, J E N
Ow, K K H
Owens, E J C
Padfield, A
Page, H
Page, K B
Page, R E
Palmer, C D
Panarese, A
Panniker, R M
Papageorghiou, A T
Parker, A J
Parker, D A
Parker, G
Parker, M J
Parkes, A M
Parsons, H K
Parsons, M A
Partington, R J
Pascoe, R J M
Patel, G U
Patel, N H
Patel, P S
Patel, R V
Patel, V R
Paterson, M M F
Paterson, M E L
Payne, A J
Peace, J M
Peacock, J E
Pearse, R G
Peat, C C
Peat, J
Peck, R J
Peel, N F A
Peers, L A
Peet, M
Pereira, N H
Perrett, K
Peters, S
Pettinger, G
Pettinger, R
Phillips, A F
Phillips, J K
Phillips, W S
Phillpots, S
Philp, I
Phythian-Adams, J M
Pickin, D M
Pinches, C E
Platt, J
Pledge, S D
Porteous, M
Porter, A J
Potter, D
Powell, B P
Poyser, J
Prakasam, S F R
Pressley, K J
Preston, F E
Primhak, R A
Procter, A E
Prosser, L J
Purcell, W
Purdy, R H
Pycock, J E
Qamar-Uz-Zaman, S
Quarrell, O W J
Quiyum, S A
Qureshi, I
Radford, J M C
Radley, H M
Radley, S C
Radstone, D J
Rafferty, R
Raftery, A T
Rahman, S U
Rahman, Z
Rainford, A
Ralston, D R

Ramakrishnan, S
Ramsay, H M
Ramsay, L E
Rana, T
Rangi, P S
Rashid, S
Ravichandran, G
Rawlin, M E
Rawson, A
Read, N W
Read, R C
Redding, H L
Reed, M W R
Reid, J J
Reilly, C S
Reilly, J T
Rennie, I G
Revill, J
Rhodes, M J
Richards, M
Richardson, C D
Rickards, D F
Rickman, M S
Ridgway, B A
Ridgway, E J
Riley, S A
Rimmer, A
Ringrose, C S
Rittey, C D C
Rivett, K A
Rivlin, I
Roberts, A J
Roberts, J P
Robertson, B J
Robertson, N J
Robinson, C J
Robinson, M H
Robinson, R T C E
Rochester, J R
Roddick, J N
Roden, D
Rogers, M S S
Rogers, N K
Rogstad, K E
Romanowski, C A J
Roper, E C
Rosario, A J
Roscoe, T J
Ross, R J M
Rosted, P
Rowbotham, C
Rowland, M
Rowland, S J
Rowlands, D A
Rowling, J T
Ruck, M J Y
Ruck, S E
Rughani, A N
Ruiz, K
Rundle, P A
Russell, M A G
Russell, R G G
Ryan, C J
Ryan, F P
Rybinski, E A
Rybinski, P
Sadler, K M
Safe, A F
Sagar, H J
Saha, J R
Saleem, M
Salfield, N J
Samarage, L H
Samuel, R C
Sanders, A J
Sanders, D S
Sandhu, A S
Sandler, G
Sandys, R M
Sarwar, N
Saunders, N J S G
Saunders, S J
Savage, D A
Savani, R K
Savani, U K
Saxena, S C
Saxena, S
Say, D T
Schatzberger, P M
Scheele, K H
Scholefield, J H
Schrecker, G M K
Scorah, P J
Scott, G R
Scrimgeour, K M A
Sedler, P A S L
Seeley, D W
Selby, K F
Seth, C

Seth, P C
Seymour, J
Shackley, F M
Shaikh, A M
Sharma, A
Sharma, S S
Sharma, S
Sharp, D J
Sharp, F
Sharpe, M S
Sharrard, M J
Shaw, A J
Shaw, I C
Shaw, T J I
Shaw, W A
Shawcross, C J
Shawcross, C S
Shawis, R N S
Sheard, R M
Shenton, G A
Shepherd, D B
Sherry, K M
Sherry, S
Shickle, D A
Shiell, K A
Shirley, R A
Shirt, D J W
Shore, S L
Shorrock, K
Short, J A
Shorthouse, A J
Shrestha, B M
Shum, K W
Shurmer, D M
Siddiqui, S
Simms, R J
Simpson, K L
Singh, A P
Singh, T S
Sinuff, S H
Sivarajan, S
Skan, J P
Skidmore, D J
Skinner, P P
Skull, J D
Slater, D N
Slater, R
Sloan, L M
Sloan, M E
Sloan, S B
Smailes, J
Smallwood, D M
Smethurst, M
Smith, A H L
Smith, A T
Smith, C M L
Smith, C E
Smith, H N
Smith, H J
Smith, J A R
Smith, J H F
Smith, M E
Smith, M F
Smith, N W P
Smith, R L
Smith, R H
Smith, S N
Smith, T W D
Snelson, E J
Sooklall, C R S
Sorsbie, L
Souper, K
Spear, F G
Spencer, H L
Spinks, M J
Spooner, L
Sprigg, A
Sprigg, N
Sprigg, S J
Spyriounis, P
Squirrell, D M
St. Leger, S A
Stack, C G
Stanley, C K
Stanley, D
Starbuck, M J
Starr, P L
Start, S A
Steel, E A
Steiner, H R
Stenton, K J
Stephenson, J A
Stephenson, P M
Stephenson, T J
Stewart, A-M
Stewart, K
Stewart, P
Stierle, C
Stirling, S C

Stockley, I
Stoodley, K J
Stow, R E
Strachan, K J
Strode, P A
Strong, E P
Studholme, T J
Sugden, J S
Suhail, M
Suliman, M E G R
Sundar Eswar, Dr
Sutcliffe, M K
Sutherland, J A
Sutton, P M
Suvarna, S K
Swales, V S
Swarbrick, M J
Swinden, S J
Sykes, D
Tait, N K
Talbot, H
Talbot, J F
Talbot, M D
Tan, S
Tanner, M S
Tantam, D J H
Tatton, P
Taussig, J-A
Tay, P Y S
Tayler, D I
Taylor, A J
Taylor, C J
Taylor, C J
Taylor, M S
Taylor, N M
Taylor, P R P
Taylor, R
Teasdale, K
Tesfaye, S
Tesfayohannes, B
Thewles, M J
Thomas, D G
Thomas, S E
Thomas, S M
Thomas, S N
Thomas, W E G
Thompson, D
Thompson, M C
Thompson, R
Thorman, N A
Till, S H
Ting, S C H
Tinker, R M
Tooth, D R
Tooth, J A
Tophill, P R
Treacy, P J
Tsintis, P A
Tungland, O P
Tupper, N A
Turner, B A
Turner, D C
Turner, E C
Tweed, C S
Tweney, J C S H
Udejiofo, S F
Underwood, J C E
Usher, A S G
Van Geene, P
Vandenberghe, E A M
Variend, S
Varkey, A T
Varkey, S
Veall, G R Q
Venables, G S
Verity, R G
Vlissides, D N
Vohra, S
Von Schreiber, S K
Vora, A J
Wales, J K H
Walewska, R J
Walker, A H
Walker, C J
Walker, D J
Walker, D A J
Walker, G T
Walker, J
Wallace, W A H
Wallbridge, C M
Waller, R E
Wallis, E J
Walsh, J S
Walsh, M P
Walton, C E
Walton, J J
Ward, A M
Ward, C J
Ward, D L
Ward, S E
Wardrope, J
Wareham, C A
Warner, R W
Warren, C W
Warren, W E
Washington, S E J
Watkinson, P J
Watson, N
Watt, V B
Watton, R J
Watts, C
Webber, S J
Webster, J
Webster, R E
Weetman, A P
Weir, R D
Welch, J C
Welch, R A
Welchew, E A
Wells, G E
Wells, M
Welsh, C L
Wembridge, K R
Wenham, T N
West, J
West, J N W
West, J A
Westin, T A B
Wharton, S P
Wheeldon, N M
Whelehan, I M
White, B M
White, D J K
White, J C
White, R W
White, S A
White, T O
Whitehurst, L M
Whiteside, R S
Whiting, P C
Whittaker, S J
Whyte, M K B
Wight, J P
Wilbush, J
Wilfin, A H
Wilkie, M E
Wilkinson, D J
Wilkinson, G A L
Wilkinson, J M
Williams, D G
Williams, J L
Williams, N H
Willoughby, S J
Wilson, A G
Wilson, L M
Winder, S
Winfield, D A
Winfield, J
Witana, J S
Withers, M R
Woll, P J
Wong, T I
Wood, G E
Wood, N S
Wood, N I
Wood, R J
Woodcock, P J
Woodruff, M J
Woodruff, P W R
Woods, H F
Woodward, D K
Wren, M C
Wrench, I J
Wright, A M
Wright, F W
Wyld, L
Wylie, K R
Wyman, A
Yardley, M P J
Yassa, J G
Yates, R O
Yeo, W W
Young, C S
Zadik, P M
Zadik, S A
Zaman, A C
Zaman, S R

Shefford
Baldock, C A R
Baxter, M J
Bietzk, J E
Cakebread, S R
Clough, S C
Davy, K J
Griffith, S K W
Hooper, B K
Moffitt, S J
Morgan-Gray, K J
Puritz, R
Radford, R

Shepperton
Andrews, J D B
Atkin, C M
Bates, C C
Bates, P G
Bellamy, S J
Candappa, N J C
Carty, S J
Choat, D J M
Dash, P K
Dowdell, J W
Floyer, C E
Norman, J L
Rogers, F A L
Walters, J N
Watson, G C
Wilson, S A

Shepton Mallet
Bourke, M P
Cottle, A G
Cotton, J
Cudmore, J K
Howes, C M
Kenyon, R C
Lindsay, J D I
Llewellyn, I E
Norris, C S
Sharp, G M
Sleap, A G
Stronkhorst, C H
Swayne, J M D
Walker, T R W
Waters, H M

Sherborne
Armstrong, P
Bartlett, I A C
Burke, L J
Byfield, D M
Cave, S G F
Childs, R A
Collins, R E
Ellis, C M
Elsworth, C P
Fazakerley, N W
Forward, R F M
Foster, C A
Gaymer, A R
Gledhill, J M
Griffiths, C S
Hearnden, A J
Hinton, J M
Huins, H F
Jackman, C C
Loud, B W
Maxted, M J
Miles, G
Morris, S R S
Mottram, S N
Pittman, J A L
Purcell, G R G
Robinson, M S
Schofield, L E
Sherwin, N J P
Stronach-Hardy, S
Thomas, J
Townsend, D W
Tuke, J U

Sheringham
May, R G
Roebuck, P D
Sampson, P W
Smith, I C

Shetland
Aquilina, M P M
Baird, J L
Begg, C M
Bowie, S J
Brown, A E
Cleminson, F B
Coutts, E H A
Henry, E B
Hunter, M D
MacFarlane, D
Malcolm, D
Marshall, B
Teunisse, F
Ward, H M

Shifnal
Anderson, E
Brinkley, M A
Leigh, P J
MacWhannell, A
Robson, J-A
Serhan, J T
Whiting, S W

Shildon
Baliga, S K
Bhagat, A K
Evans, B
Grimes, L K
Walton, I T

Shipley
Alexander, S A
Allard, S A
Antrum, R M
Armitage, C M
Baker, A M
Baker, M R
Besrest-Butler, C R
Bibby, J A
Bradley, M C
Brooke, C M
Carr, M H
Chadwick, S P
Chitsabesan, P
Chitsabesan, P
Clayton, S D
Craig, J G
Cuthbert, M M
Dawson, R J
Driscoll, P A
Driver, N J
Edwards, P R
Eisner, M C
Elliott, H
Ellison, J A
Fay, M R
Gallagher, L B S
Gaunt, M L
Goldman, L H
Gomersall, P M
Halloran, J
Harrison, L J
Henderson, P A L
Hickey, K
Hodgson, J D
Holt, A A
Hopker, S W
Humphrey, S H
Keating, E F
Kernohan, E E M
Khan, F N
Livingstone, H J
Livingstone, R I
Lynch, C
Marfell, K
Matthews, S
Metcalfe, J
Narang, S K
Passant, C C
Pearson, N R
Petty, J
Rajaratnam, G
Rewilak, A T
Roberts, H E
Roberts, S E
Ruffe, S H
Rutter, I P
Ship, R H
Slinger, B C
Stead, G W
Tedd, C B
Tonks, W S
Turner, S R
Urwin, S
Van Heel, D A
Webb, S
Yeomans, J D I
Young, L A

Shipston-on-Stour
Gilder, J E
Hance, J R
Morgan, D L
Nixon, C M
Schofield, T P C
Scrivens, J W
Thorogood, C
Wemyss-Holden, S A
Whiteley, A M
Williams, G P

Shoreham-by-Sea
Aboutalebi, S
Bagley, G
Banerji, K
Baskar, N
Beardmore, H J
Bisset, A J
Clark, D W
Daneshmand, L
Dias, A M
Dighe, A M
Fellingham, W H
Floyd, M J
Foley, C M
Gordon, D N
Howard, S A
Jha, P K
Lyons, N S
MacLintock, R M
Nines, R J
O'Dwyer, J P
Raiman, A C
Ratnarajah, C R
Selvadurai, V
Smith, A D
Stevenson, T R T
Tucker, G P
Turner, P
Walker, T
White, M-E
Yogalingam, M

Shotts
Galloway, C F
Kasem, H
MacFarlane, C P
MacFarlane, V A
Milliken, S W G
Myatt, P S
Novosel, S
Walimbe, S

Shrewsbury
Agrawal, R K
Allen, S
Allsop, C J
Archer, A D
Awwad, S T
Baguley, I
Bailey, J J
Ballantyne, J H
Barritt, P W
Bartlett, J I C
Beacock, C J M
Bell, D L
Benady, D R
Bennett, J M
Bennett, P S
Bentick, B
Beresford, P M
Bevington, D J
Biddulph, J C
Bing, A J F
Blomfield, P I
Breese, S J
Brice, J E H
Bright, J
Brunner, H E
Buckett, W M
Bunting, C
Cameron, A M
Campbell, D C
Campbell, P L
Carr, R J
Carter, E J
Chapple, S A
Clarke, H M
Clements, G M
Clesham, D J
Clover, A J P
Clowes, P
Cockill, S
Collins, A J
Coppinger, S W V
Corfield, A J
Coventry, P J
Craig, E A
Cramp, C E
Cribb, G L
Critchley, M A
Crow, P G
Dapling, R B
Darvell, F J
Das, A K
Davies, G T
Davies, R J
Davis, J A
Davis, L K
Deahl, M P
Dean, F K
Dean, M R E
Deshpande, S A
Dobrashian, R D
Dobrashian, R M
Downes, V B
Eden, B W
Eden, J E
Edmunds, S J
Edwards, S C
Elliott, A J
Everett, P S
Fallon, M J
Farrow, J S
Feather, S D W
Fenton, C J V
Fielding, J A
Fletcher, K D
Fox, A D
Fraser, R A
Fry, D J
Fryer, M E
Gill, D B E C
Glover, N M
Good, S I
Gould, T J
Gowans, W J
Green, N J
Griffith, V J
Griffith, W F
Griffiths, T C
Hallatt, S E
Harnden, C E
Harnett, S J O
Hatts, R
Hawkridge, H
Hay, A M
Heaversedge, J T
Hill, L F
Hill, S N
Hill, T R G
Hilton, C M
Hinwood, D C
Hollings, N P
Houghton, A D
Houghton, A L
Hudson, C F E
Hughes, R K G
Humber, S A
Hunt, T M
Hurlow, R A
Hussein, R S A
Jones-Perrott, S E
Jones, J I W
Jones, S G
Joscelyne, J C
Kadiani, M R
Katti, S M
Kelly, C P
Kelly, S E
Kendall, C N
Kent, S E
King, D H
King, N J
Lacey, B W
Lancaster, K L
Lane, J
Latto, D M B
Leaman, C A
Leedham, P W
Lewis, D C
Linford, S M J
Llewellyn, R E
Lovett, M C
Lowdon, D G R
Lowe, M D
Lowe, P P
Lucas, P L M
McCarthy, M U
McCloud, J M
McGeoch, C M
Macleod, A F
Malcolm, A J
Matthias, J E
Maurice, C D J
Mike, N N H
Miller, M W
Molodecki, C A
Moorcroft, A J
Morris, J M
Morris, P
Mott, P A E
Muir, J N
Murphy, C J
Murphy, S M
Myers, D H
Neale, A J
Nehaul, L K
Neil, W F
Newell, R A
Nicholls, P E
Nicholson, A B
Nightingale, S R
Norman, W J

O'Connor, N T J
O'Dowd, R L
O'Neill, P M
O'Shea, M J
Oates, S E
Oldroyd, R E
Olley, S F
Orme, R I
Otter, A E
Otter, M I
Page, M J
Palmer, R M
Park, R
Parry, J M
Patrick, J H
Pattison, A
Penman, E H G
Pepper, J M
Perks, W H
Pickard-Michels, P M H
Pickard, S J
Povey, J M
Povey, J D
Prescott, M V
Prichard, A J N
Pringle, R G
Quayle, J B
Quinton, P J
Redford, D H A
Rees, R J
Reeves, S E
Reid, F
Reid, S C
Robinson, D
Rooney, S J
Rousseau, M J
Russell, J R
Russell, K
Russell, N C
Sansom, H E
Savage, A P
Schofield, A D R
Scott, A R
Shaikh, G
Shipstone, D P
Simmons, M E
Singh, A B
Skinner, D W
Slocombe, G W
Smith-Stanleigh, P
Smith, J A
Smith, M S H
Smith, R G M
Smith, Y L O
Somervaille, T C P
Stapleton, E M
Stringer, J K
Stringer, J R
Tann, C J
Tapp, A J S
Taylor, N J
Taylor, P D
Taylor, W R J
Thevathasan, P A
Thomas, C D
Thompson, A
Thompson, G R
Thompson, R H
Thorne, A K
Thorne, W I J
Tiley, S J
Tomlinson, C J
Toms, A D
Trethowan, W N
Tully, W M M
Tyrrell, C G
Ullegaddi, A F
Ullegaddi, R
Underwood, T J
Waite, A J
Walker, P M
Wallbridge, D R
Walton, W J
Warren, R E
Watson, H R
Watson, T R
Watt, J B
Wedgwood, D L
Welch, R J
West, N E J
West, T E T
Westwell, D F
White, J F
Whittingham, W P
Whitworth, N H
Williams, I
Williams, S J
Williamson, J M
Wilmshurst, P T
Wilson, R S E
Woodford, C P
Wright, I P
Young, P M

Sidcup

Aboel-Sood, A A M A
Ahluwalia, M S
Amin, R
Bamji, A N
Barry, W C W
Bhattad, H L
Bhogal, H S
Black, D A
Bokhari, S A J
Bowcock, S J
Chavda, D
Cheung Chun Wah, N T
Chopra, M
Cooper, J E
Crinall, F J
Das Gupta, P
Davies, T W
Davis, M I M
Davis, T P
Donnelly, J E
Donnelly, W J
Durcan, T G
El-Radhi, A S
Elsey, T A
Evans, C D
Geraghty, R J
Gibbens, M V
Gill, P
Goligher, J E
Gould, B A
Guite, H F
Harding, D R
Hassan, M H
Hemlock, A
Hill, M D
Housley, R C E
Hugkulstone, C E
Jha, A K
Jones, E M
Joyce, J J
Kagalwala, A R
Karunakaran, V
Kerwat, R
Keshavarz-Kermani, H
Khawaja, H
Khoo, C K
Kingston, J M
Laganowski, H C
Lancaster-Smith, M J
Lang, A C
Leary, S M
Maaita, M E K
McKinnon, J
Mani, G V
Mascarenhas, F J
Mason, N C
Medhurst, J
Mehmet, S
Millard, E M
Milne, D
Money, R P
Neal, C J
Nichols, R W T
Nikolaou, C M
Nosseir, M N A H
O'Gorman, A J
Oliver, B J
Pain, A K
Parchure, N
Patel, H
Patel, I S
Patel, K C
Patel, N
Patel, O T S
Pervaiz, K
Prior, C A
Rajayogeswaran, S
Rajvanshi, R
Rao, S G
Rassam, S M B
Ritchie, K A
Roberts, E J
Schuller, I
Scott, S E
Sharif, A T
Shee, C D
Shepherd, T P
Smart, C C
Smith, R N J
Sweet, P R
Tanna, V
Taylor, C J
Ward, S M
Whitaker, D C
White, A M
Whitefield, L A
Wickramasuriya, B P N
Woodward, J W
Woolfson, J

Sidmouth

Anderson, J C
Carless, C A
Hailey, S R
Hall, D P
Kinder, J J
Matthews, C E
Morris, E N
Naylor, P F D
Nelson, S C
Pepper, G J
Read, N J
Ridler, A H
Slot, M J W
Spence, J S

Sittingbourne

Brown, C J
Cantor, F M
Cotton, J P
Cousins, P
Crawford, I C
Cusworth, R J
Dias, A S
Else, O F
Farquharson, M J
Garousha, S A
Gill, J M
Gray, P
Hall, A P
Hickman, R C
Hickman, S J
Hipkins, K C
Hudsmith, J G
Jones, D G
Kumar, R B
Kyle, D W
Marsh, C M
Morrish, C H F
Norris, M C
Philpott, M J
Ponnampalam, J S
Puranik, A
Rees, R J
Saha, B K
Selby, K
Sikdar, A N
Staker, P
Thompson, I G
Valli, P
Wilcox, K E
Witts, S J

Skegness

Archer, G A
Chaggar, J S
Chester, S K
Cotton, P A
Dewar, D D
Garg, S
Ghani, U
Good, W R
Lawson, S A
Mitchell, P D V
Najmi, S M A
Rudrappa, C
Seal, R L
Sykes, S A G

Skelmersdale

Bisarya, A K
Bisarya, A
Brennan, D J M
Chang, D S K
Faza, M K
Flood, G
Gerval, M-O
Gouda, M A-H M
Harrower, J E
Hicks, A J
Hopkins, C
Littler, A D
Minchom, A M
Modha, J S
Orr, G A
Qamruddin, A O
Qamruddin, M
Ryder, P G
Saxena, S
Sharma, A
Sibery, A J
Singh, B B
Singh, U
Sur, S K
Tekle, I
Watras, G J
Wilkinson, S L
Williams, L R

Skelmorlie

Balmer, F
Balmer, F J
Balmer, I M
Di Paola, M P
Dunn, H M
McColl, C M
McColl, D J
Seenan, P J
Tam, P G E

Skipton

Allen, J P
Baker, J R
Bostock, E A
Bransfield, J J
Bundock, A D
Callin, S E
Churcher, S J
Clarke, J
Cotter, D H G
Crabtree, N A
Craig, C J
Daggett, H R
Davies, A
Fisher, G B R
Gazzard, A M
Goodall, J R
Gregory, P A
Hamman, M
Harrison, C R
Hassey, Dr
Hill, R
Holmes, B M
Imrie, J M
Jackson, A J
Keppie, W
Kidd, J L
Kinnish, I K
Kleyn, C E
Pearson, D J
Pilkington, C E
Powell, J O J
Roper, J P
Smulders, T C
Sumnall, A G
Thomas, J A
Thomas, K E
Webber, R J
White, T M
Whitehead, P S
Wilkinson, H S
Woodhouse, B A
Woods, S M

Sleaford

Aldaya Lorenzo, J M
Aslam, M
Aslam, N-S
Carlyle, A E
Cartwright, M A
Collinge, J D
Denton, G
Gamble, W G H
Hackney, J H
Hill, K E
Humphry, N J C
Lorimer, A H
Mukherjee, T
Murphy, D A
Parry, J E
Pinchbeck, F W
Price, P T
Radomski, J W
Timperley, A C
Varah, S
Walsham, A C
Webster, J A
White, P N G
Wiseman, E C

Slough

A-Ali, N
Adam, N S-E
Aggarwal, M
Ahmad, R S
Al-Basri, I A I
Ali, R S
Allen, S M
Allum, R L
Andraka, D
Armstrong, A P
Arora, S K
Ashby, M
Badr, A A G M
Bahia, S O
Bailey, C F
Bain, R R
Bambridge, E J C
Bantick, R A
Barakat, K
Barnes, S F
Barrett, A R
Barrett, D
Bartman, M
Baxter, S T
Benedict, C B
Bhargava, R
Bienz, N
Birman, P
Blackwood, R A
Bleach, N R
Bradley, S G
Brockless, J B P
Bukht, M D G
Burden, G J
Burfoot, C
Burkitt, R T
Campbell, E J
Cassell, P G
Charig, M J
Chaudhry, S H
Chawla, K K
Cheese, N E
Chinn, R E
Christophi, G
Chung, H E
Chung, H M
Clark, C I M
Clark, R L
Clarke, E D
Clifford, E M
Coleman, N S
Cook, I S
Cowen, J M
D'Souza, E R
Daily, S D J
Dalton, A N
Davies, G R
Davies, S
Dawson, G H
Dawson, S G
Dega, R K
Depani, A J
Desai, A L
Dhatt, M S
Dickinson, J C
Dimitry, E S
Dogra, V K
Draper, P W
Duggal, A
Edwards, J N
Evans, S M
Evans, W M I
Eyers, J G
Fairbank, J
Farooq, N
Fell, R H
Fernandes, J R
Fernandes, P
Forrest-Hay, A
Foster, D F
Fryer, H A
Gibson, M
Gilbert, J M
Gilfeather, L B C
Gordon, N
Green, B J
Green, R W
Green, S J
Grewal, P D
Gunawardene, K A
Hamid, A W
Havelock, C M
Hayward, S A
Hear, G S
Heath, P K
Hemantha Kumar, M L R
Holdstock, G E
Hussain, M
Irvine, M C G
Iyer, R V
Jack, R D
Jamal, F
Jamil, M T
Jefferis, A F
Jones, C A
Jones, R A K
Kanski, J J
Karim, O M A
Khan, A
Khan, N
Khan, Q A
King, A
Kochhar, A
Kumar, H
Kumar, S
Kumar, S
Lakhan, A K
Lane, R E
Larcombe, C
Lenox-Smith, A J
Levi, S
Lewis, C
Lewis, N L
Lewis, Y K
Litchfield, J C
Llewellyn, M J
Lloyd Parry, J M
Lorch, D M
Loughlin, S L
Loveland, R C
Lunn, J A
Lynch, S M
McDonnell, M P
McIlroy, D I
McIntyre, M P J
MacMahon, M T
Maidment, C G H
Malik, K Z
Mann, S S
Masood, T
Matheson, A C W
Mayadunne, G A Y V
Mehta, R
Mickiewcz, A J
Mohan, V
Moreau, A P M
Motiwala, H G
Mountford, T H
Muneer, A
Nabi, I M
Neale, R J H
Newson-Smith, G R
O'Dowd, J G M
Ostle, K E
Overton, M R
Parameswaran, S S
Parbhoo, P H
Paul, M
Peck, B W
Perry, L J
Peter, T
Pickering, A H
Pope, R T
Pumford, N A
Purvis, D J
Rahul, C
Raj, I
Rajapaksa, T J
Reece, A H M
Reed, J M
Reginald, P W
Rehman, H
Robinson, M V
Rodgers, D M
Rosenberg, R M
Sadhra, K S
Salmon, J G D
Sandhu, G S
Sawant, N H
Shayo, S D
Singh, K M
Skelly, W J
Smith, B L
Sohal, M
Spelina, K R
Stapleton, C
Steare, S E
Strawford, J
Sudbury, P R
Sulh, J S
Sumanasuriya, R C
Sutlieff, P A
Tansey, S P
Telford, M E
Tewari, R M
Thompson, J N
Thomson, H A
Thyveetil, M D
Trivedi, J
Tyagi, A K
Umapathy, A
Vinayak, B C
Walkden, V M
Walker, J A B L
Watson, L

Watts, M B
Wiggins, J
Wild, R N
Wood, C B
Wood, S J
Wright, K D
Yates, C
Yousif, S Y
Zavody, M

Smethwick
Chawla, H S
Chawla, S
Child, D L
Choudhary, B P
Clark, D
Dhillon, A S
Etti, O R
Grant, S E A
Grubb, H R
Hale, M C
Jackson, A A
Joseph, A P
Kang, L S
Loader, A C
Loader, S M
Loveless, R A
Mann, M S
Matharu, S S
Middleton, J D
Palmer, A E S
Parmar, T S
Rahman, A K M R
Ridley, J
Sam, R C
Sharma, D
Towers, D G
Wanke, M E A
Wright, S L

Snodland
Fahmy, G E I F
Khehar, S
Terrell, H M

Solihull
Abdou, M S
Ainsworth, A F C
Ali, N
Anfilogoff, R
Annetts, S E
Arbuthnot, J E
Aston, W J S
Bagga, T R
Ball, C M
Ball, E F
Banerjee, A K
Bannourrah, F E A
Barkell, E M
Barraclough, J E
Barsoum, G H G
Baxter, JGB
Beale, D J
Beaumont, H E
Begum, Z
Benson, M T
Bhatti, M E
Bieker, M
Bleby, M J
Boyce, A
Bramley, R H
Bramley, S
Bray, A J
Brigstocke, S-J
Brooks, S
Brown, N S
Bsat, R A-G
Byrne, P G
Cameron, P S
Campbell, J B
Canning, W C
Challens, A S
Charlton, R C
Chitnis, J-G
Chopra, R
Clapham, M C C
Clarke, J P
Cogbill, P G
Congdon, A M
Congdon, R M
Cooper, R F
Cowles, S M
Cox, J R
Crichton, B E
Croft, J A
Darling, S G
Davenport, J A
Davies, C M
Davies, P M
Dedicoat, M J
Delaney, M P
Dennison, P H
Deval, S
Dharmaratnam, R
Dobson, H R
Dunn, K R
Dwyer, S D N
Dyas, A C
Edwards, E
Edwards, S
Ellis, C V
Ellis, M
Evans, G A
Evans, K R L
Farag, S F S
Farmer, G S
Farmer, P R
Fear, R C
Feehan, C J
Finch, T M
Fisher, L J
Fletcher, C J
Font Olive, M D M
Forster, E N
Fox, J
Francis, A
Gandhi, B R
Gay, M A
Geddes, A M
Georgy, M S
Ghannam, I M T
Gibbs, R A
Gray, J W
Green, K N
Green, S L
Greenwood, N K
Grewal, G K
Grillage, M G
Gupta, V
Hagon, J A
Hall, S W
Halloran, C M
Harrison, L J
Harrower, R F
Harrower, S I
Hattotuwa, K A G
Heagerty, A H
Hill, E B
Hill, M R
Hogan, D J
Hoggart, B
Holland, C J
Holt, J A
Holweger, W I
Hope, J I
Houghton, A S
Howarth, G F
Hughes, H M
Hukin, A J
Innes, J A
Inwood, J L
Jackson, B R
Jacobs, P
Jago, D G T
Jarrett, G R
Jenkinson, D M
John, R S
Jones, E
Joshi, R K
Kadow, K W
Kale, V R
Kale, V
Kandula, P
Keenan, R D
Kershaw, M J R
King, B A
Kinning, E
Knickenberg, C J
Kondratowicz, E A
Kotecha, S B
Lawley, J L
Lee, L K
Leese, J
Lewis, C A
Lewis, G A
Leyton, E
Liegeois, H M
Liley, H T
Little, J A
Longson, P J
Love, P S
Lupoli, A
Lynch, W A
McCarthy, B E
McDarmaid, E J
McDermott, A-L
Maceachern, D A
McNabb, S J
McRoberts, M T
Maskill, J M
Melrose, P A
Ment, J L
Milan, P A
Milligan, W M
Milner, G L
Moore, V J
Moppett, J P
Morgan, I D P
Morgan, R H
Morgan, T A
Moss, S A
Mukherjee, S
Nagra, I S
Nakhla, V
Naylor, C R
Nicol, B J
Nicol, G L J
Nicol, M J M
Nicol, R E
Nicum, R
Orakwe, S I
Paget, R I J
Palmer, R G
Parkes, S J
Patel, E D
Patkar, A A
Pearson, M J
Perry, D W
Peters, M J
Peters, S E
Phillips, W J
Pickering, A M
Pilling, K J
Playfor, B E
Polson, R J
Portsmouth, O H D
Powis, M D
Pratt, G E D
Price, P H
Priestley, K A
Prosser, G H
Qureshi, S
Ray, E H
Rayner, C R W
Reddy, V A P
Reid, J
Reuben, A D
Robson, J L
Rowbotham, C J F
Rowlands, S C
Rulewski, N J
Ryder, I G
Sandler, M
Satchell, S C
Sengupta, D
Seymour Mead, R
Sharma, N
Sheikh, A J
Shilling, R S
Shinton, N K
Shortland-Webb, S C
Skinner, G R B
Sloan, P J M
Smith, C A
Smith, C D
Smith, R R
Sothi, S
Stacey, L
Stanton, A S
Stenhouse, T
Sterry, M J G
Stevenson, L
Stewart, A M
Stokes, E L
Stores, O P R
Stuart, I R
Sturdee, D W
Sutton, J F
Tadros, F F
Taylor, C M
Teare, L J
Thorp, S L
Tibbatts, L M
Tincombe, M R
Tomkins, M J
Travis, P J
Upton, W S
Vanhouse, S H
Vijh, M
Waddell, A M
Waddell, J E
Waddell, N J H
Walker, R A
Wallis, A J
Ward, E G
Watts, S G T
Weale, A R
Wears, R
West, C A
Weston, C G
Wijayawickrama, A
Wilkes, D
Wilkinson, J P D
Willshaw, H E
Winter, S C A
Xifaras, G P
Younan, F H

Somerton
Barnett, J M
Bonnington, S P A
Griffiths, R E
Sleap, P G F
Smith, R A
Steele-Perkins, A P
Wolton, A D

South Brent
Busfield, A
Halliday, J J
Hart, M T W
Hill, J D
Kelly, A S
Vorster, D S
York, E L

South Croydon
Ablett, J G
Adegoke, A O
Ahmed, S
Baverstock, R A
Burrin, E M
Campbell, P
Cashman, M E
Chadha, A
Clementson, M R
Cockell, J L B
Danbury, R
Deane, A M
Dempsey, O P
Ferguson, R
Found, S M
Gajjar, S
Gallagher, V A
Garratt, P M
George, M S
Georgekutty, K K A
Gillgrass, J W
Gnani, S
Green, E E
Haq, A I
Heal, K
Jasper, W M
Kanagasundaram, M
Khan, M A A
Kurwa, B R
Lawlor, K M
Lyell, D A
McEwan, A
McEwan, G J
Malhotra, D K
Malik, I S
Matthews, G G
Meeran, M H M
Mitchiner, M B
Ohuiginn, P
Patel, N
Perera, P G A A
Perera, P S A
Sachdev, B
Sanderson, R D S
Sathananthan, R
Sathananthan, S
Smart, L K
Snelling, T H
Sornalingam, C
Southcott, R D C
Stiby, E K
Strymowicz, C
Sugumar, K
Towner, C H
Trompetas, A
Urquhart, J F
Wallace, W J
Woolf, S

South Molton
Biss, T T
Darling, J C
Doddington, R A
Gibb, C A
Hadfield, C S L
Hawkins, C J
Morris, D
Shelley, J R
Sherlock, W
Westcott, R H

South Ockendon
Bellworthy, S V
Davies, A M
Haque, M A
Horgan, J T C
Jayakumar, C S
Khraishi, D M M S
Lafferty, P M
Leighton, L F A
Okunola, O O
Williams, M

South Petherton
Buckle, J R

South Queensferry
Ashworth, A J
Cackette, C G
Carson, A J
Creber, C J
Gilchrist, A M
Hart, W M
Leckie, G J M
Love, C D B
Robertson, J F
Stewart, L
Stirrat, F W
Stuart, J D
Williamson, E J

South Shields
Al-Durrah, F M I
Alfakih, K M A
Andrews, J I
Ansari, S H
Armitage, T G
Arthur, J B
Bennett, R J
Bhalla, R
Bhalla, R
Blair, T T
Bone, M F
Bora, A U
Bradshaw, C
Bryson, L G
Chander, S
Cope, L H
Craig, M S
Cronin, S M
Curtis, R J
Daya, S G
Duncan, L E
Eggleston, J M
Evans, M
Fairbairn, D
Gallagher, J E
Gallagher, M
Gandhi, H B
Haque, M A
Haque, M A
Hargreaves, C S
Holmes, R I
Jackson, A
Jana, K
Jay, R H
Jenkinson, J R
Jones, N K
Joypaul, B V
Karandikar, N
Kulkarni, D J
Lambert, M F
Lishman, A H
Lochan, R
Lockman, H
McClure, A M
McManus, W H
Macmillan, M
Madhok, R
Malik, B A
Massam, M
Miller, S G
Minty, I L
Muchall, A J
Mullea, M S
Muncaster, J W
Naroz, N A
Nasser, A
Nwabineli, N J
Okugbeni, G I
Olajide, V F
Owen, T
Parr, J H
Pattekar, J B
Pattison, I
Perrins, J K
Pervaiz Khan, N
Pollard, K P
Proctor, G
Reece, V A C
Rees, C J
Roy, S C
Roy, S P
Roysam, G S
Sarkar, M
Scott, S
Setty, G R
Seymour, K
Singh, R S
Spencer, H S
Swai, E A
Tose, J
Vis-Nathan, S
Watson, D M
Wilson, C N
Wynne, A
Wynne, K S

South Wirral
Awan, M T S
Barber, N C
Barr, A D B
Birch, A D
Brocki, J L
Cassidy, R V
Cowan, B B
Darling, R A
Dickinson, J E
Dupont, M M B
Flattery, H B
Fraser, F
Graham, P J
Guest, N D
Harvey, D J
Hayle, G B
Hoyles, R K
Jackson, R A
Jellicoe, P A
Jones, L E
Kennedy, M R
Klafkowski, G
Knowles, K
Knowles, P A
Lockwood, A J
Lockyer, M W
Macdonald, C J
McGuigan, J R
Mills, R D
Mills, S J
Mitra, S
Mohiuddin, R J
Morrison, I A
Murphy, J
Murphy, P N
O'Shea, M
Owen, S W
Perkins, J M M
Reilly, E I
Riley, K J
Roberts, J
Roohi, S
Shaw, S A
Smith, N
Snook, R N
Steere, C E
Stuart, R A
Thorneloe, M H
Tolley, P F R
Townson, P J
Washington, M I
Willan, A L
Willcox, R
Wood, N

Southall
Aali, S A
Abrahamson, G M
Acland, K M
Adrian, N S
Aggarwal, A K
Amor, T J
Anderson, D J
Anyaegbuna, N T
Armstrong, G H
Arnold, J D
Ash, S A
Ashraf, M
Aujla, K S
Barnes, T R E
Baxter, R D
Baylis, C A
Beverly, M C
Bharal, I
Birring, R K
Botros, A M
Bracey, B J

Bradshaw, E G
Bullock, T
Cummins, M C
Dabas, V K
Davis, A J
De Sica, A
Dent, J A
Dhandee, I S
Dhesi, S S
Eggleston, J
Falzon, M R
Fellow-Smith, E A
Gautam, S K
Gerulakos, G
Gowrie Mohan, S
Hayat, F
Hee, M
Hegde, U M
Hinds, N P
Hogarth, M B
Hoxey, K L A
Hutchins, K J
Iyer, S K K
Jagdev, D S
Jagdev, S P K
Jhooty, H K
Johal, K K
Johal, S S
Johl, R
Kahtan, N
Karagounis, A
Khin Thet Maw, Dr
Kohli, V K
Korpal, K
Kyaw Htin, M
Lack, S J
Lahon, K
Laishley, R S
Lally, S S
Lambert, M T
Lock, M P A W
McNeil, N I
Malik, A H
Mangat, H K
Mangat, N S
Mann, B S
Martindale, B V
Mather, H M
Mathur, R
Mendel, D
Michie, C A
Nathwani, D K
Naughton, M A
Papadakis, A
Patel, P R
Payne, S D W
Petch, E W A
Philpott, N J
Qadan, H M A
Qureshi, S A
Radhakrishnan, S
Rahman, F K
Rai, J S
Randhawa, R S
Richman, S
Rosen, S D
Rosenbaum, T P
Rudolf, M
Saluja, R S
Samra, G S
Sandhu, P J S
Schmulian, C
Scott, J C
Sehdev, R S
Seiden, Z A S
Shakir, N A
Sharma, A K
Sharma, K
Sharma, V
Singh, K
Sivanesan, R
Sloper, K S
Soljak, M A
Stanford, M E
Taw, H
Taylor, R H
Thexton, R
Tolmac, J
Toor, K S
Treasaden, I H
Verma, S
Walker, A E
Waller, K G
Walsh, P M J
Wesby, R D
Westman, A J
Whitehead, E M
Williams, D O
Wong, A K M W
Woodbridge, K

Southam

Coker, T C
Madan, L S
O'Mahony, G A M
Pannell, B M B

Southampton

Addis, B J
Adey, D F W
Ahmed, E B
Ahmed, S
Aihie Sayer, A P
Ajaz, M A
Allen, T E
Alveyn, C G
Anderson, H H
Angus, W H N
Annas, E G
Appleton, P J
Arden, N K
Armstrong, R D
Arney, N P
Arthur, M J P
Arulrajan, A E
As, A K
Ashburn, A E A
Ashton-Key, M R
Asopa, V
Atkinson, A C
Austen, B L
Ayres, C M
Baber, F R
Bailey, I S
Bailey, R L
Bainbridge, B M
Baird, J
Bajwa, S
Baker, A K
Baker, S S
Bakowski, M T
Balkwill, P H
Bamforth, J
Barber, Z E
Barker, C S
Barker, D J P
Barker, R M
Barnes, K
Barnes, R M
Barnfield, M
Barrett, D S
Bartens, A
Bartlet, L B
Basarab, A
Bass, P S
Bateman, A C
Batty, V B
Bauchop, A
Bayley, E K
Bayly, R A
Benning, A S
Bentley, I S
Betts, M T
Betts, P R
Bevin, S V
Bhatt, H B
Bhatt, S J
Biddle, A
Billington, T R M
Bingham, M A
Birch, B R P
Birch, S
Birch, S J
Blandy, S E
Blaquière, R M
Blount, A M
Blunden, J
Boddington, H J
Boeree, N R
Bolt, S A
Bosman, J J
Boulton, F E
Bowyer, G W
Boyd, U B
Brading, L S
Bramley, K W
Brearley, R L
Breen, D J
Brewster, A L
Briggs, R S J
Brighouse, D H
Briley, M
Britt, J R
Brock, S J
Brooke, M J
Brown, A S
Brown, E M
Brown, I
Brown, J A
Buchanan, R B
Buis, C
Burns, A C R
Burrows, S
Burton, J
Bush, J T
Bute, K J
Butler, D A
Butler, J A
Butler, P J
Byrne, C D T
Callahan, H M
Calver, A L
Cameron, D J S
Cameron, I T
Campbell, D
Canning, C R
Carey, J A
Carlisle, A J
Carr, N J
Carroll, M J
Carruth, J A S
Carter, M R
Cates, C A
Cawley, M I D
Chadwick, B D
Chapman-Sheath, P J
Chaudry, Z R
Chesterfield, M P
Chisholm, I H
Choksi, S M D
Clancy, M J
Clarke, N M P
Clarke, P J
Clayton, B E
Cleak, V E
Clearkin, P M
Clough, J B
Clouter, C A
Clover, J A
Coggon, D N M
Cole, A M
Coleman, G P
Coleman, M A G
Connett, G J
Constable, G L
Cookson, S F
Cooper, A F A P
Cooper, C
Cooper, E K
Coppin, B D
Coppola, A M T
Corfe, S E
Correa, J B
Corser, R B
Costa, S
Coutts, J F
Crawford, S C
Crawford, V A
Crook, T L
Crosse, M M
Crutchley, D G
Culora, G A
Cumming, J
Cunliffe, J
Cunningham, L M
Damms, J C
Darch, M H
Das, P
Dave, B-R P
Davidson, B K S
Davidson, P H
Davies, C J
Davies, E M
Davies, M S
Davies, S D T
Davis, D
Dawkins, K D
Dawson, J A
Dawson, P R
Day, I N M
Day, L R A
Dayson, D F
Delany, D J
Dennis, N R
Dennis, S T
Dennison, E M
Dennison, M L
Detsios, C L
Devane, M J D
Dewbury, K C
Dibben, C R M
Dickson, N K
Dinapala, P L
Diprose, P
Dixon, C J
Djukanovic, R V
Douglas, M F
Dracass, J F
Du Boulay, C E H
Duffill, J
Dulay, J S
Duncombe, A S
Dunlop, D G
Dunn, N R
Dyer, M J
Eccles, D M
Eccles, L M
Edwards, C J
Edwards, J G
Egleston, C V
Elliott, E J
Entwisle, I D
Evans, B T
Evans, G B
Evans, N A A
Evans, P W G
Eynon, C A
Faarup, C L
Fairhurst, J J
Fall, C H D
Fennell, J M B
Fernando, S M
Field, J
Fine, D R
Fisher, M S
Fitzpatrick, W J
Fleming, W S
Foster, C R M
Foulds, N C
Fowler, A V
Fowler, S P
Frankel, J P
Fraser, S D S
Frew, A J
Frost, E V
Fugleholm, K
Fung, P J
Gabbay, F J
Gabbay, J
Gallagher, J M
Gallagher, P J
Gandhi, N
Garman, W M
Gaston, H
Gawne Cain, M L
Geldart, T R
George, S L
Gibb, W R G
Gibbs, P J
Gibson, D J K
Gill, C P
Gill, P S
Gillibrand, A
Gillibrand, P N
Gillibrand, S
Girgis, M M R
Glasspool, J A
Gnana Pragasam, J J
Gnanapragasam, J P
Godber, C
Goddard, J M
Godfrey, K M
Godfrey, S J
Godwin, D S
Goodall, H N
Goode, S J
Goodison, S J F
Gordon, A D G
Gorrod, W D
Gotzaridis, E
Gove, R I
Graham, J
Graham, K A
Gray, B A
Gray, H H
Gray, P J
Gray, W P
Greaves, F H
Greenberg, N
Gregoire, A J P
Gregory, P H
Gregory, R K
Griffiths, D M
Griffiths, M
Grimble, S A J
Grimshaw, J S
Grover, A L
Gulliford, C J
Guly, J K
Gupta, R
Guyer, C H
Habib, M J
Hackett, C L
Hacking, C N
Hadfield, A A
Hadfield, H W
Haig, P S
Haji Abdul Hamid, M
Hall, I S
Hall, M A
Hall, N F
Hamilton, A C E
Hamilton, C R
Hamilton, J C
Harden, S P
Hardie, C J W
Hargreaves, D G
Harley, J M
Harman, A N
Harris, C J
Harris, J K
Harvey, J R
Hatchwell, E
Haw, M P
Hawa, L
Hayes, M C
Hayes, N R
Hayes, S F
Hazelgrove, J F
Heafield, R J
Heal, S W P
Heames, R M
Heath, C M
Hemming, C S
Hemming, P A
Henderson, C A
Hennayake, S P
Hervey, V E J
Hettiaratchy, P D J
Heyes, C B
Heyworth, J R C
Hicks, K A
Hill-Cousins, J L
Hill, A W
Hill, C M
Hill, S A
Hillier, E R
Hillier, S J
Hitchcock, A
Hoang, T M
Hockey, P M
Hodgkins, P
Hodgson, A K
Hogg, J I C
Hogg, P S
Hoghton, G B S
Holgate, S T
Hollands, M D
Hook, J L
Howard, J C
Howarth, P H
Howden, P E
Howe, D T
Hudson, S J
Hughes, A H
Hughes, M D
Hunter, B J
Hunter, S C
Hunter, S L
Hunter, S
Hutchin, A K M
Hutchings, C J
Hutchinson, D
Hutchinson, R C
Hwang, C-Y
Ibbitson, D J
Illidge, T M
Ingamells, S
Iqbal, Z
Iredale, J P
Ironton, R
Iveson, T J
Jackson, C L
James, C J
James, R
Jariwala, S
Javaid, M K
Jeffery, I T A
Jellicoe, J A
Johnson, C D
Johnson, P W M
Johnson, W J
Johnston, A
Jolly, C B
Jones, A
Jones, D S
Joughin, N A
Judd, M J M
Kadri, A Z
Kakkar, S
Kakkar, V V
Karran, S J
Katifi, H A
Keefe, M
Keeton, B R
Kelly, J M
Kelly, R W
Kelpie, A G
Kendrick, A R
Kennedy, P
Kent-Johnston, C A
Kidsley, S G
King, A T
King, H
King, L J
Kingdon, D G
Kinsman, F M
Knight, A O C
Knight, J W
Kohler, J A
Kolli, S V
Krentz, A J
Kulkarni, S K
Kumar, S
Kurukchi, E F
Lachlan, K L
Laing, H C
Lall, D G
Lambert, G M
Lambourne, V A
Lang, D A
Lang, I J
Last, A T J
Lawes, E G
Lawrence, C
Lawrence, I S
Lawton, N F
Laycock, J R D
Le Besque, S E M
Leaper, V A
Ledger, M A
Lee, J A
Lee, M T W
Lee, R D
Lees, P D
Legg, J P
Lennon, A J
Leonard, E M
Leppard, B J
Lewis, M
Lewis, M N
Lewith, G T
Lim, S H B
Little, P S
Littlejohns, P A
Lockyer, C R W
Lowes, J A
Lucassen, A M
Luckens, C J
Lyons, J P
McAndrew, H F
McCaughey, E S
McDonald, D S
McElwaine-John, H A
McFarlane, A T
McFarlane, V J
McGill, J I
McGinn, F P
McGrigor, V S
McKay, A
Mackie, E J
McLaren, M I
Maclean, D A
Maclean, J K
Macleod, D B
McQuitty, A F
Mairs, M L
Malone, P S J
Mandair, I S
Manners, R
Mansbridge, B J
Mansell, A J
Marsden, R
Marsh, M J
Marshall, B G
Marshall, C A
Marshall, G S
Marshall, R P
Martin, I G
Martin, L M
Martin, R M
Martinez Saenz, J A
Martyn, C N
Matthews, H P
Mavridou, D
Mavroleon, G
May, J M
May, P G R
Mayers, A J
Mayo, L K
Mead, G M
Meadows, A J
Meadows, A E R

Meakins, P G W
Metcalf, K S
Mettam, I M
Midwinter, M J
Miell, S J
Miles, J C
Miles, R
Miles, S C
Millar, J S
Miller, J M
Millman, A M
Milln, J E M
Milln, P T S
Mills, P M
Mills, R G
Millward-Sadler, G H
Milne, R I G
Mitchell, S J
Mitchell, T E
Monkhouse, M
Monro, J L
Moore, T W
Moors, A
Morfey, D H
Morgan, C J
Morgan, D J
Morgan, J M
Morris, G E
Morris, P N
Morris, R J
Mortimore, A J
Mostyn, A A R
Mountfield, S J
Mountford, J J
Mowbray, A G H
Mufti, S T
Muller, G W
Munro-Davies, L E
Munro, M R
Munro, N P
Murdoch, S R
Murphy, C R C
Murphy, F R
Nasr, M S A
Nasrallah, D F K
Naylor, J S
Neil-Dwyer, G
Neil-Dwyer, J G
Nevin, M
Newman, C J
Newsom, R S B
Nichols, P H
Nielsen, M S
Nightingale, J H
Nixon, C V C
Nixon, J R
Nolan, C M
Northover, J R
Norwood, F L M
Nugent, K P
Nurse, J M
Nutton, M
O'Callaghan, F J K
O'Sullivan, B M
Obin, O M
Odurny, A
Oeppen, R S
Ogilvie, B C
Ohri, S K
Onslow, J M
Orchard, K H
Ord-Hume, G C
Osborne, A H
Osgood, V M
Ottensmeier, C H H
Padday, R
Page, A R W
Pal, R
Pallett, A P
Palmer, E A
Palmer, K T
Panakis, N
Pappin, C J E
Parry, K T
Patankar, R S V
Patel, J P
Patel, S
Patten, T J
Paynton, D J
Pearce, C B
Pearce, N W
Pearce, S
Pearson, G C
Peek, W H
Peoples, J A
Pepe, G
Percival, R E
Perry, R J
Pettifer, C F
Peveler, R C
Phillips, C P
Phillips, D I W
Phillips, M J
Pierce, J M T
Pinder, A
Pitt, I
Plenderleith, S J
Pockney, P G
Polkinghorn, C L H
Porter, P J
Press, C M
Prevett, M C
Price, N S
Price, S E
Primrose, J N
Pringle, J J A
Prinsen, A K E
Putnam, E A
Radcliffe, M J
Railton, K L
Rajapaksa, P N
Randall, C J
Rani, R
Ratan, H L
Rees-Jones, S V
Reid, J M
Rew, D A
Reynolds, K V
Reynolds, R M
Richards, S T M
Richardson, D S
Roberts, C J
Roberts, H C
Roberts, P R
Robinson, N A S
Robinson, S J
Roche, J
Roche, W R P
Roderick, P J
Rogerson, M E
Rolles, C J
Rolles, T F
Rosell, P A E
Rosenberg, W M C
Rosenvinge, H P
Roseveare, C D
Rowden, J D
Royle, G T
Rubin, C M E
Russell, C
Russell, M M A
Salmon, G L
Salmon, G B
Sampson, M A
Sandeman, D D
Sanderson, H F
Sansome, A J T
Sargeant, R J
Saunders, D A
Savill, P J
Schofield, S P
Scott, E R
Scott, J A
Scott, R J
Sealey, S L
Sedgwick, J E C
Selley, C A
Sewell, A C
Shand, G
Sharpe, G
Shaw, D A S
Shaw, K I
Shearman, C P
Shelly, R W
Shephard, J N
Shepherd, H A
Shepherd, N J
Sheron, N C
Shillinglaw, C L
Shore, D F
Short, G P
Short, P M
Shrubb, V A
Simmonds, P D
Simmons, M R L
Simpson, I A
Simpson, R L
Simpson, R M
Singh, G K
Singh, J P
Singha, H S K
Skeates, S J
Skidmore, J R
Slaney, M
Smalley, C A
Smallwood, J A
Smart, C J
Smedley, J C
Smith, A G
Smith, C L
Smith, D C
Smith, P J
Smithies, J M A
Solomon, C L
Somerville, J M
Spargo, P M
Sparrow, O C
Spencer-Smith, M
Spencer, J E
Stacey, B S F
Steadman, K E
Steer, J M
Steinbrecher, H A
Stephens, C R
Stephens, F R
Sterling, N
Stevenson, P G
Stobbs, I P
Stones, R W
Stredder, D H
Stride, J D
Stringfellow, M J
Stroud, M A
Stuart Taylor, M E
Subramanyam, M
Sunak, Y
Sutherland, P D
Sutton, D N
Sutton, G L J
Swales, H A
Swann, C M
Synek, M
Tang, A T-M
Tanna, M
Tate, G H A
Tayler, T M
Taylor, I R
Taylor, J K E
Temple, I K
Terry, P M S Q
Thaker, C S
Theaker, J M
Thomas, C A
Thomas, D
Thomas, E J
Thomas, N H
Thomas, P L
Thomerson, M C R
Thompson, C M
Thompson, C L
Thompson, M J J
Thornett, A M
Threlfall, A L
Tice, J W S
Tolcher, R A
Tomson, C M C
Townsend, S J
Trewinnard, B F
Trewinnard, K R
Trotter, C A
Tung, K T
Turner, J J
Uglow, M G
Ursell, C E
Van Der Star, R J
Vance, G H S
Varney, A D
Varsani, G B
Vettukattil, J J
Vulpe, A-M
Vyas, D R
Waddington, G E
Waddington, S J
Wade-West, S C
Wainwright, A C
Waite, N R
Wakeling, H G
Walbridge, D G
Waldron, M
Walker-Bone, K E
Walker, F
Walker, V
Walsh, J L
Walters, A D
Walton, R J
Ward, C P
Ward, I R
Warner, J O
Warwick, D J
Watson, R
Watson, T E
Webster, A R
Weddell, C R
Weeden, D F N
Weidmann, P J C
Wellesley, D G
Westensee, W
Wheeler, R A
Whitaker, S G
White, P J
Whitehead, R H B S
Whitehorn, M
Whitehouse, C
Whitehouse, P A
Wield, C E
Wild, S H
Wilkins, B S
Wilkins, D C
Wilkinson, D G
Williamson, I G
Willmott, F E
Wilson, A W
Wilson, D
Wilson, H N
Wong, Y K
Wood, R M
Wood, T A
Woodbury-Smith, M R
Woodcock, T E
Woodward, R M
Woolner, C A
Wrigley, K
Xavier, A B
Yacoub, S
Yardley, D N
Yeomans, N P
Yong, P P L
Zaman, S N
Zardis, M C

Southend-on-Sea
Aggarwal, N K
Aggarwal, V P
Agha, Dr
Back, G W
Baqai, A
Bavishi, R K
Beales, S J
Boston, D A
Bowring, A R W
Browne, G R
Chauhan, C
Clappen, J A
Coull, A B
Davison, A G
Dhanapala, R P I
Fairbrass, S P
Fearnley, G
Fowler, E F
Gent, C B
George, V K
Goodchild, C A V
Grant, D L
Grant, J T
Greenwood, E J
Greig, A J
Gupta, R
Heath, M
Henderson, S M
Hutter, U C
Jack, M E W
Jupp, K
Khan, F
Khokhar, A A
Kinnear, J A
Kirkpatrick, R A
Kolli, S
Latif, M K
Liebeschuetz, H M
Mackay, J
Martin, A J L
Moss, P N B
Mountain, A J C
Nerminathan, V
Nicol, M E
O'Sullivan, M G
Odd, D E
Osborne, C E
Pearmain, B M P
Pearson, R V
Pelta, D E
Pocock, T J
Rigby, D
Roberts, P
Ross, G G
Rothnie, R J D
Samak, M A R
Seath, K R
Sen, A K
Sen, G
Shah, B D
Shah, M N
Shah, N K
Shanker, J
Shrivastava, A
Siddique, H A
Sills, D W
Singh, D G
Sowerby, E L
Stuart, M H
Swinburn, H M
Vashisht, S L
Verghese, G S
Ware, C C
Weeks, W T
Weston, M D
Woodham, M J
Yee, A

Southminster
Barclay, A G
Bowton, P A
McGeachy, J E
Southey, T J

Southport
Abdul-Jabbar, T V A
Ajayi, J F
Akingbehin, A
Ali, M A-S
Allan, G M
Amer, K J
Anderson, R J L
Artioukh, D Y
Bannock, A E A
Benjamin, E J S
Bennett, S
Bhatnagar, M
Binymin, K A
Boardman, K
Bolton, C J
Bond, A M
Bond, M D I
Bonnet, S J
Bowley, J A
Brown, M A
Burns, S H
Butcher, G P
Butterfield, J S
Carden, D G
Charway, C L
Coackley, A
Coney, S
Corder, C E
Cornwell, M
Cowling, R J
Currie, F
Dawson, R E
Dey, N G
Donnellan, J
Dundas, S A C
Ellis-Jones, W B E
Entwistle, P B
Equizi, F
Evans, A F
Evans, V A
Eyre, O
Farley, T M
Fearns, G M
Firth, G M
Fletcher, G
Foat, G
Forshaw, M A
Fox, J A
Fox, J P
Gardner, S E
Garston, H N
Giannelli, P B L
Gibb, A M
Gokul, K
Grenyer, D R
Groves, K E
Hancox, D
Harrison, I D
Hedley, G S
Hewitt, W E
Higgins, M R
Howard, N
Hughes, I M
Hussain, E S
Iskander, L S F
Iskander, M N
Islam, S
Izmeth, B
Izmeth, M G A
Janardhanan, K C
Jayson, D W H
Jolly, I M
Jones, D R
Jones, J E
Kilshaw, I M
Koram, K O
Lang, P W
Leonard, N J
Levy, A M
Lewis, C R
Lowe, J
McCormack, M P
McNally, S R
Mansoor, I C
Mansour, P
Marriott, K N
Mason, P F
Milligan, H P
Mon Mon, G
Naidoo, G R
Naidoo, K R
Naidoo, R S
Nelson, C E
Nishith, S
Nugent, C M
O'Donnell, L V
Orford, C E
Parry, R L
Patel, R R
Pati, U M
Popely, C S
Pozzoni, L S
Ramamurthy, A B
Rao, P J
Ratcliffe, C A
Richman, A V
Rigby, J C
Rigg, J H
Ronson, J A
Rostron, E A
Russell, R M
Ryan, A J
Samuels, B
Scott, C C
Searson, J D
Serlin, M J
Sett, P
Sharma, N K
Sharma, S D
Sharpe, G H M
Simmonds, J P
Simmons, S
Singh, G
Slater, L K
Smith, P
Smyth, J H
Soni, B M
Stubbens, G
Sutcliffe, J R
Swift, E F
Sykes, H R
Szczesniak, L A
Thomas, K
Thompson, T J
Tobin, S D M
Tomlinson, R J R
Treasure, J
Trivedi, D V
Trivedi, V A
Turner, J G
Turner, P M
Twist, A M
Vaidyanathan, S
Venkateswarlu, V
Vesey, S G
Watson, A P
Watt, J W H
Wesson, M L
Wilson, C F
Wray, J R E
Zeiderman, M R
Zmyslowski, A J

Southsea
Arnold, T J M
Barron, G R
Bedford, A D
Bennett, J B
Berney, D M
Caiger, B N
Caiger, M
Cannon, L B
Causer, C A
Collins, L S
Dale, B J
Darlow, S J
Dee, G
Emerson, A C
Fleming, P M
Foord, R D
Golland, I M
Gorham, D J
Hilton, D D
Lake, R S
Malbon, K M
Masheter, S N
Minay, I F
Mitchell, B D

Moore, N H
Norman, A M
Ostler, K J
Parkin, G T
Pearson, D G R
Peel, S
Preston, A P
Price, J P D
Robinson, M
Rollins, J W
Schofield, S A
Sowden, L M
Sparkes, D J
Spolton, E M
Sprott, V M A
Taylor, A
Trapiella, B
Tutte, K P
Tyrrell, R F
Uppal, M S
Varma, A
Vernon, K G
Vincent, J C
Viner, C R
Wallace, F
Watkins, S C
White, A J
Williams, C V
Wilson, M R
Winfield, J

Southwell
Ali, N J
Ashcroft, D G
Byrne, A J
Clarke, V J
Cottell, H C
Danby, P R
Duffy, M S
Duffy, M R
Duffy, N C
Leach, A J
Macmillan, R D
Norris, A M
O'Nunain, S S
Platts, B W
Reeves, S D
Sym, R A
Vidhani, K
Ward, K L
Worth, A J J

Southwold
Baylis, J H
Butt, S A
Castle, C R
Church, R E
Eastaugh, A N
Marshall, C G

Sowerby Bridge
Acharya, S R
Bradley, C M
Catlow, S I
Higham, A
Hinds, R O
Hinton, C A
Hinton, P J
Knowles, M L
Littlewood, C R
Pickersgill, D E
Pool, R W
Rogerson, L J
Sarker, M A K
Whisker, W B
Whitaker, B
Wyatt, B T

Spalding
Bell, A I
Booth, C C
Brookes, R H
Burgess, D A
Cole, C R
Corlett, D J
Cowell, J M
Hamblin, C A
Hewat-Jaboor, D F
Jacklin, J B
Jamieson, E C
Lennon, C P B
Low, N J
McCall, A
McCombie, P
Morris, E S
Nathu, A
Peter, M W
Price, M
Rance, B H
Rayner, S
Richardson, B D
Riley, D J
Rodgers, P F E
Scott, C A
Stone, A D R
Sykes, A
Thorpe, R W
Wheatley, G
Wiscombe, K A R

Spean Bridge
Godfrey, J F
Tregaskis, M

Spennymoor
Henderson, A J
Ibbott, N E
Kotwall, F B
Long, A J
Patel, S K
Roy, D V
Sanderson, A A F
Sensier, A E
Staines, J E
van den Brul, K A
Wood, M R D

Spilsby
Caranza, R A
Cartwright, D E
Latto, R J
Morgan, M S
Mowat, A M
O'Kelly, N I
Wain, M O

St Agnes
Bradshaw, H J
Fussell, I J
Guttridge, B
Henderson, N D
Julian, J T
McNeill, E
Newton, C E
Thompson, H M
Thorley, J N
Whitworth, C M

St Albans
Akroyd, I H
Al-Jassim, A H H
Allen, M W
Allistone, A C
Alloway, L J
Anderson, A L
Aram, J A
Atkinson, C V
Avis, R C
Bacchus, R A
Bartlett, J A
Bell, A D
Bevis, M A
Bishop, J F
Blake, K H
Bonnet, J M
Boodhun, R
Bowman, R M
Bremner, A J
Broadwith, E A
Buckley, B E
Burke, S A
Burnett, F E
Butterworth, P M
Cabot, R
Cannell, M C S
Carruthers, G J
Clegg, J P
Conlan, P
Coombs, G A
Corbett, T J
Corlett, H M
Covell, B R
Davies, A A
Davies, A H
Day, L M
Dean, B C
Dearing, N C
Dexter, K E
Douglas, T J
Dow, I A M
Dowling, S E
Elstow, S M
Evans, H
Fairbairn, I M
Ferguson, J W
Franks, D M
Freedman, J E
Gilham, D
Godlee, J R L
Gorton, J D
Griffin, P L
Haider, R U
Halpin, J E
Hamilton, I A
Harrison, G D
Hart, G M
Haseler, A R
Hatch, K M S
Heller, M D A
Hoole, S M
Hynes, M C
Ingram, K L
Irwin, A S
Jaiswal, I
James, L
Jameson, D M
John, J
Johnson, N S
Jones, J E
Jordache, S M
Karunapala, L G H
Kedia, K
Kedia, N
Kedia, P
Kennedy, R C
Khalid, A R
Khan, I H
Kulkarni, S S
Lee, M H M
Lees, M P
Lewis, B
Livesey, P M
Lofthouse, S
McDonnell, J J
Mainwaring, P J
Margereson, A E
Martin, H A D
Matthews, G V
Maurice, P D L
Mitchell, J D
Moore, P R
Mummery, J
Murray, M J
Nathan, J M
Nicholls, H A
O'Sullivan, G H
Olin, R H
Pace, J E
Parfitt, M D
Parsons, L M
Paul, P K
Pearce, J A
Pearse, R M
Penney, D J
Peters, M J
Pinkerton, S M
Platts, A J
Putterill, J S
Puxley, D M
Queen, J K
Ramdeo, A
Ramsay, R
Raymond, S P
Sage, R E M
Sagor, G R
Saleh, M S A D A H
Sasitharan, T
Saunders, S M F
Sawyer, P E L
Schofield, J K
Sebaratnam, N P
Sepai, T M
Sherif, A H M
Singh, S
Sinha, G
Sirker, A A
Sivakumar, R
Skelton, P E
Small, C M
Smith, H
Stephens, J
Strain, H A
Sullivan, N
Sumners, D G
Sutton, R H
Taylor, R D
Tayob, Y
Terry, D A
Thomson, A R
Thurston, A V
Tominey, D P
Usher, S M
Vinayagamoorthy, C
Wajed, M A
White, S K
Whitworth, J C
Wickramasinghe, K M S S
Wilkin, P M R
Williams, R L
Willis, M H G
Woodwark, C
Yanny, W A
Young, K A

St Andrews, Fife
Arnott, J M
Backhouse, S S
Bindon, C I
Bowman, A
Cobb, C J
Cunningham, G L W
Cuschieri, A
Davidson, C M
Delaney, J W
Donald, M J
Duncan, P S
Gifford, J
Lawrie, D M
Lobban, W D
McDonald, J M
MacMillan, C S A
McTavish, J C
Mathewson, I B
Mills, J A
Neil, J M
Orr, V A
Qureshi, T R
Reid, D H S
Reid, M
Rutherford, D
Seddon, P J
Sinclair, D W
Sinclair, M A
Smyth, G P
Sommerville, J A
Steel, C M
Stewart, J E
Sullivan, D B
Swift, P A
Tait, H A
Thomas, D B
Tweedie-Stodart, N M
Weekes, R D M

St Asaph
Arnold, J P
Barnsley, T M
Bhowmick, A K
Cameron, J
Davies, J E
Duffy, J E
Lloyd Williams, M A
Morton, C E
Nagendran, S
Ng, C S
Osei-Frimpong, S
Puvanachandra, K
Saunders, D C
Wainwright, J R
Williams, D

St Austell
Atcha, Z
Banerjee, S S
Blackwell-Smyth, P
Burke, F E
Cecil, J R
Chapel, H
Charman, C R
Corbett, E J L
Davis, A
Dibb, A
Dowling, M F
Forsdick, S J
Foster, P B
Hargreaves, P N
Hereward, A C
Hotton, T H E
Iles, R E
James, A M
Jenkin, D R
Kitson, N I
Lang, D V A
Leigh, J R O
Mackrell, D R
Mather, E P
Mather, R H
Miles, D P B
Mitchell, M M
Nasruddin, I N
O'Brien, B
Penfold, G K
Phillips, P G
Robinson, C D
Robinson, M G
Schenk, P M
Sharp, G T
Travis, P
Wakeford, T D
Whitehouse, A R

St Bees
Greene, K J
Greene, M K

St Columb
Turfitt, E N

St Helens
Abernethy, V E
Atiba, O E
Bainbridge, B A
Baines, J H E
Banat, J J
Beeby, K
Birchall, D
Boyd, C E
Chadha, J C
Corner, T R J
Cox, S J
Crabtree, C
Cunningham, A S
D'Arcy, J R
Denno, H M
Desmond, M
Dilworth, P A
Ellison, J
Ferguson, N J
Ferguson, P W
Filletti, P
Finnegan, B C
Finney, S M
Gaffney, M P
Ghaffar, A R K
Gillanders, V T
Glover, T F
Green, S
Gregan, A C F
Gregan, M J
Gregan, P
Gupta, P
Hanrahan, J M
Hargreaves, S A
Harrison, R J
Hart, N J
Higgins, J
Hindley, J S
Houghton, J I
Hughes, J E
Hunt, E J
Hyde, S W
Johnson, S
Joyce, P W
Junaid, O H
Kilroy, I M
Kurzeja, J A
Liptrot, S
Long, A A
McCourt, B A
McGrath, A E
McManus, C J
Macrae, E M R
MacRae, R A D
Maini, R
Mansoor, S
Markey, P G
Mason, K
Mather, J M
Memon, M S
Mercer, L A
Middleton, J B
Mikhail, K H T
Mooney, P
Morris, J L
Moss, S
Nathan, R N
O'Brien, M
O'Donnell, J J
Paul, P J
Pitalia, S
Pogue, L J J
Rahil, H M
Richmond, J P
Rimmer, M G
Roberts, I
Sagar, P
Sathe, S B
Schofield, J
Shah, M
Smith, A
Smith, G L
Sutton, J M
Taylor, M A
Taylor, R B
Thomas, N F
Thomas, R S
Tolan, S P
Topping, S
Tunstall, P J
Van Dessel, M G
Vaughan, P H
Webb, P
Webster, J
White, G
Whitmore, J M
Whittaker, A
Williams, S E
Wilson, P E
Wotherspoon, J
Wright, R W

St Helier
Bellamy, M J
Carpenter, M
Ellis, B D
Fullerton, M E N
Guillochon, M A H
Hugh, J E
Jackson, J D
King, S C
Le Gresley, J S
Marks, M F
Overton, M A
Parris, R
Porcherot, R C
Robertson, B C
Rosser, M J
Slaffer, S N
Stevens, N B
Thacker, R H
Vincent, A P
Wilson, M G
Young, M J

St Ives
Currie, S
Freegard, S P
Harris, A E
Hayes, B J
Hosking, L A
Jewell, W E
Johnson, H D
Lakic, J
Manley, R
Marshall, R J
May, C M I
Moran, S A
Pardoe, T S
Philip, C J
Royston, A M
Sanderson, M R
Sell, J N
Wilkins, A N J

St Leonards-on-Sea
Al-Saleem, M A W
Apthorp, L A
Auld, B J
Baer, S T
Banfield, J M
Barker, J P
Barnes, W S F
Beard, J
Board, R H
Boxer, M E
Bruce, S A
Bryden, P J
Buchanan, J A F
Bullen, E K
Butler-Manuel, P A
Cameron, D J
Chowdhury, M R
Clee, M D
Consterdine, E
Dennison, J
Doig, A S
Foord, K D
Freeman, M P
Furley Smith, E A
Gorsuch, A N
Gregory, P T S
Guy, R L
Hawley, I C
Henderson, E B
Hinves, B L
Jones, D E
Kaliniecki, J P J
Khoury, G A
Kinloch, D R
Leach, A B
Lee, J V
Lethbridge, J R

Lyttle, J A
M'Munoru, M M
MacCarthy, N E
McIntyre, H F
Mehta, P A
Motha, S
Mutiboko, I K
Nasar, M A
Parker, L S
Pitts, J E
Plail, R O
Rahmani, M J H
Rai, S K
Rajbee, F T
Rajbee, T Y
Rashbrook, P S
Sandison, A J P
Sapper, M E
Scott, D J
Searson, J W
Segar, E P
Sengupta, G
Serrano Garcia, J A
Shah, C H
Shepherd, M A W
Sinha, P
Smith, S G W
Stewart, J G
Stock, J G L
Strouthidis, T
Sudhakar Rao, S
Taubman, R L
Vethanayagam, S V
Walker, D M
Ward, T J
Whitehead, S M
Wright, E P
Yedla, S R
Young, A J
Zaidi, S H J

St Mary's
Davis, A J G
Drake, M R
Gale, J
Gleadle, R I
Jeffries, D J

Stafford
Aggarwal, A K
Aggarwal, S K
Ahmed, S A
Albright, E J
Allbeson, M
Allen, D B
Ander, P G M
Archer, J D
Baichoo, S
Barnes, C N
Bates, A S
Beal, R M
Bee, E M
Bhoora, I G
Bishop, D G
Blanchard, D S
Bland, J M
Brackley, P T H
Bramley, C
Broader, J H
Burra, F F R
Byrne, F
Calhaem, M N
Campbell, T M
Carr, D M
Carrasco, C D P
Chakraborty, S K
Clifford, G N
Coates, P A A
Collier, J D
Connellan, S J
Cooner, B S
Cooper, C J
Crisp, J A
Daggett, P R
Daniels, R J
Dapaah, V
Davenport, S M
David, V C
Davies, J A
Davies, W A D
de Boer, C H
De Murtinho-Braga Ossa, J J
Deane, A G
Dixon, J E
Duggal, H V V P
Dunn, C K
Durrans, D
El-Fakhry, T T
Elizabeth, J E
Eqbal, Z S
Eva, L J
Evans, K
Evans, R M
Fairfax, A J
Finn, T L
Gallimore, J
Gandham, S R
Gee, B C
Geller, R J
Gendy, R K
Gibson, J A
Glennon, P
Gordon-Nesbitt, D C
Grewal, M S
Griffin, N V
Grocott, A E
Gwynn, B R
Haig-Ferguson, D R
Hannigan, J P
Harper, N N
Harris, S C
Hawkins, W J
Hearing, S D
Hearn, J S
Hiley, P E
Hiley, S M
Hodgkinson, B R
Houlder, A R
Howell, J V
Hoyle, M D
Hughes, R G M
Husselbee, A J
Hutchinson, R
Iddenden, D A
Iqbal, Z
Jankowski, S L
Jones, L M
Jones, M C
Joshi, V
Kathuria, V
Kawecki, J Z
Kelly, S E
Khan, A A
Khan, A
Knight, S J
Knight, S M
Lamb, A S T
Lamb, A B
Lambah, P
Lambah, P A
Leong, Y H
Liss, M R
Lloyd, R S
Lockhat, M D
Logan, A J
Lotz, J C
Loynes, R D
Loynes, R P
Luck, B M
McGeehan, D F
Macleod, A M
Markos, A R M
Martin, H M
Mateu-Lopez, E
Merriott, D E
Miller, C L
Muir, A
Munslow, D J
Nanavati, B T
Nanavati, C B
Nock, I D
O'Connell, E P
Oliver, M D
Palmer, D J L
Palmer, K S
Panis, E A H
Patel, P
Postings, S J
Prasad, N
Pringle, K
Quader, S E
Raby, M B
Rawle, M S
Reddy, T N
Revell, P G
Richard, H W
Roberts, S F
Roddy, E
Ross, C D
Salwey, M G
Schofield, S F
Sellwood, W G
Singh, P
Skilton, G H S
Skilton, J A
Smith, P D F
Sofoluwe, G O
Spiers, J M
Steele, N J
Steventon, D M
Stewart, A I
Suarez, V
Summers, B A
Swinson, D E B
Szafranski, J S
Talbot, J L
Taylor, R C H
Thambirajah, M S
Thomas, A
Thomas, E
Thuraisingam, A I
Travlos, J
Turner, I M
Turner, P E M
Vaggers, S D
Vidyasagar, H N
Vishwabhan, S P
Wagner, H
Wall, M K
Walsworth-Bell, J P
Watts, M
Watwood, K
Westwood, T L
Wiley, C A
Wilson, I
Woodmansey, P A
Yeoh, J H

Staines
Bansal, R
Basra, S K
Blackburn, J R C
Bridger, D H
Curtis Jenkins, G H
Curtis, H S
Dawson, S J
Hughes, P J
Irani, M R
Jurado, R
Martin, J R J
Martin, M E
Menzies-Gow, A N
Mills, C D
Owen, D A
Pittard, J B
Poots, S J
Quraishy, M M
Salahuddin, M
Salaria, D A
Silver, D M
Stephens, H E
Tarzi, N
Thapar, V
Wallis, M G
Wells, J M
Williams, M G
Wilson, F M

Stalybridge
Ahmed, S
Ansari, J K
Asthana, J C
Athwal, S S
Barber, N A
Bircher, J
Bircher, R
Bowers, P J
Haider, M
Hasan, M Q
Hershon, A L N H
Howarth, V S
Howorth, P
Johnson, A E
Kakade, M
McNeil, A F
McNeil, N C H
Matin, M A
Peters, J G
Rao, J
Rashid, S M
Reeves, S J
Syed, S N
Tapley, M P
Urmila-Rao, N
Walsh, R
Ward, T
Zatman, S T F

Stamford
Ahmed, I
Anandan, N A
Armstrong, V J
Babbs, D J
Briggs, A C
Callow, N
Delaney, J A
Donnelly, N P
Dronfield, M W
Fairham, S A
Fields, J R
Gleeson, H K
Glynn, B G
Gobbett, A M
Gregory, G A
Hall, J H
Hall, S J
Hudson, P M
Hume, N S
Hunt, P C W
Kelly, G E
Kent, S J S
Khan, M A J
Knight, E
Lankester, K J
Ley, R J
Livingstone, R K
Lowry, S R
McInerney, L J
Mann, A L
Mason, S A
Mitchell, J V
Noble, K L
Pring, C M
Reiss, S B
Riley, R E
Smith, A L
Spencer, S A
Stafford, H M
Sutcliffe, M L
Warner, A A
Watt, M J
Weisz, M T
Wells, A D
Williams, J P
Williams, N E

Stanford-le-Hope
Chatterjee, L M
Hanson, K J
Holder, E H
Kotecha, M G
Makhdum, R
Mull, P J
O'Doherty, A
Patel, B N
Pattara, A J
Pusey, J M
Tresidder, N J
Waraich, M K

Stanley
Astell, S L
Bhattacharya, K F
Bidwell, C M
Clasper, P
Cronin, M S
Dhuny, A R
Douglas, S
Gallwey, B A
Gomathinayagam, A
Harbinson, M J
Hijab, A R A
Knowles, G M
Lambert, B
Mackay, J A
Nath, P U
Nath, P V
Pandey, S K
Parthasarathy, D
Parthasarathy, M
Rahman, M M
Ramesh, C N
Walker, A
Watson, P J

Stanmore
Abood, Y A
Agyare, K
Barcroft, J P
Basu, P
Bates, P D
Bayley, I J L
Benn, J M
Berkowitz, J L
Berman, J S
Bhatiani, W
Bhudia, S K
Birch, R
Brealey, S
Briggs, T W R
Cannon, S R
Carlstedt, P T
Colvin, I B
Cowan, J M A
Curry, S H
D'Souza, S A
Dalah, M
De Souza, D S M
Eastwood, D M
Edge, P G
Elwerfalli, M M
Falk, H C
Fox, R S R
Frankel, A H
Gad-El Rab, R R
Gall, A
Garcia, S H
Gerrard, J
Goldhill, D R
Gould, A M
Gould, L N
Green, R A R
Harrison, D J
Hashemi-Nejad, A
Henry, D B
Herman, S S
Hetreed, M A
Highman, V N
Ismail, F F
Jeffery, R C S
Keen, R W
Kumar, K
Lalwani, K
Lam, K H F
Lambert, S M
Lehovsky, J
Lewis, J G
Lokugamage, A U
Madeley, N J
Mandalia, H N
Marks, L J
Maruthappu, J
Mehta, R A
Michael, G M
Miller, G
Mistlin, A
Moss, K E
Mownah, A
Nagpaul, C
Nash, J T
Noori, Z F A S
O'Sullivan, N N V
Patel, J I
Patel, S
Pearse, D J
Prasad, R
Pringle, J A S
Ravikumar, R
Rose, P A
Sassoon, S M H
Seingry, D R J
Shah, D P
Shah, N K
Shukla, C J
Silver, G A
Singh, D
Somaratne, D A
Spier, A
Sumners, S M
Syed, S B
Taylor, B A
Trouli, C
Veldtman, U M
Vijayan, K P
Wieselberg, H M
Wilkes, N
Williams, A M
Wolman, R L
Yau, K W
Yeap, J S
Zaw Win, Dr

Stansted
Dove, S E
Ferns, M
Hamilton, B A
Jones, P G
Jones, S E

Stevenage
Ahmed, O A
Al-Shafi, K M K
Al-Shihabi, B A
Babinskyj, R M
Baird-Smith, S V
Banerjee, Dr
Baxani, R
Bhardwaj, S K
Binder, A
Borthwick, L J
Brooke, A J
Brooks, P T
Catterall, A P
Chilvers, M R
Chin, S C-P
Coreira, M C
Coxall, S J
Croft, R D
Dalla Valle, G M
Davies, S A
Delany, M G
Dickson, M G
Dorrell, J H
Duggan, M J
Ellis, S I
Fahmy, S
Farrington, K
Frosh, A C
Gale, S A
George, D W R
Gillam, S J
Gogbashian, C A
Greenwood, R N
Gregory, M M
Grimsell, C H
Hanbury, D C
Holme, T C
Hope, P G
Hyde, J C
Irvine, S A-M
Jani, K
Jothilingam, S
Kenyon, A P
Kerr, P S S
Khan, S A
Kostick, A R
Lacey, S J
Lalor, J M
Lambourne, P J
Lee, H M
McNicholas, T A
Mahaffey, P J
Meer, J A
Mochloulis, G
Ninan, M
O'Donoghue, P
Ogilvie, D M H
Oo, M M
Osborn, G R
Osindero, A O
Palmer, B V
Powell, C E
Powles, D P
Prendergast, C M
Reid, P M
Reiser, J
Richardson, D A
Rickford, W J K
Rouse, B R
Salvesen, D R
San Thein, Dr
Sargeant, I R
Sarkar, J S
Saunders, C J
Selvadurai, M A
Selvakumar, S
Sengupta, P
Shareef, S H
Singfield, C J
Singh, M
Sockalingham, I
Sowah, A
Tew, C J
Thiagarajan, J
Thompson, H H
Uthayakumar, S
Wahab, M A
Wallis, M O
Warner-Smith, J D
Wilson, A J
Zaidi, S I A

Stevenston
Martin, C J

Steyning
Annan, M H
Davey, N B
Frank, A J M
Goldsmith, C S
Noren, C E
Parr, D C
Pembrey, R L
Schofield, P C H
Shrimpton, G R
Wetson, R E

Stirling
Abel, R A
Allatt, J M
Baddon, A C J
Balendra, P R
Balnave, S E

Beattie, M T
Berry, P D
Beyer, M S
Bishop-Miller, J
Booth, D B
Bramley, P N
Bridges, A B
Briggs, R D
Brown, R J H
Bryan-Jones, J C
Bryce, R P
Cathcart, I R
Clarke, D N
Clayton, D L
Coles, R J
Connor, W C
Cooper, G L
Crawford, G A
Cunningham, C
Cunningham, H E
Davidson, G G K
Denovan, J
Doherty, A M
Dunsmore, H
Evans, T W
Fairley, R
Ferguson, E J
Fisher, W G
Forsyth, D E
Foster, G R
Gallacher, J H
Gillen, J
Glen, D A
Green, F C
Greenshaw, C
Grewal, G K
Haddow, L J
Hamilton, N W
Hanley, R I
Harrington, D S
Hehir, M
Hendry, W S
Higgins, M T
Hill, D J
Hosking, A G F
Howie, A D
Huggan, J D
Jabbar, A A
Johnston, S M E
Johnstone, F M
Kasthala, R P
Kelt, C H
Kennedy, B W
Kennedy, S M
Kennie, D C
Kerr, T S
Kilgour, S W L
King, D B M
Kippen, D J
Lenton, R J
Leonard, M L T
Lindsay, A
Lindsay, R S R
Logan, J M
Longmate, A G
Loudon, J B
Lyle, F E
McArthur, J G
MacDonald, A J
Macdonald, J K
McEwen, J P J
MacFadyen, U M
McGavigan, J
MacGregor, D B
McIntosh, I B
Mackay, G M
McKenzie, A K
McKinlay, R G C
Mackintosh, J
McLeod, M E
McMullen, K W
McWhirter, M
Maddox, B R A
Mair, C J
Mair, W B
Michie, B A
Milliken, N K C
Morrice, D J
Morrison, A B
Morrison, F K
Morton, K D
Muir, A R
Mullen, C C
Murdoch, G J
Oto Llorens, M
Paterson, H M
Pettigrew, A M
Pollok, W M
Prabhu, M R
Rankin, J N E
Renwick, C J C
Richardson, I R
Riley, A
Ritchie, I K
Ritchie, J M R
Roberts, J J K
Roberts, J L B
Robertson, J U
Ross, D J
Ross, J R
Ruddell, W S J
Saboor, T
Schulga, A
Schulga, J
Scott, J A
Semple, A J
Sharp, G R
Simpson, D S
Simpson, G D
Sinclair, A M R
Smith, A
Smith, J F B
Smith, M W
Sprunt, D C C
Stenhouse, E J
Steven, J D
Stewart, F K
Stewart, K S
Stewart, S L
Stuart, A B
Stuart, C A
Tweedle, J R
Walford, S A
Ward, S M
Watters, J
Webster, A
Webster, J A
Weir, I R J
Whiteley, M C W
Worsley, M H
Young, D R
Young, W D

Stockbridge

Adams, M S
Austin, G R
Bates, A T
Burnfield, A J
Duffy, J N
Durnford, S J
Evans, G
Hodgkinson, C R
Mackintosh, L A
Mackintosh, N B
Mackintosh, T F P
Manchett, P
Rooms, M A
Simpson, D C
Townsend, A P
Vincent, P J

Stockport

Abadjian, M
Adair, M G M
Adenwala, Y T
Adhya, G
Ahluwalia, N K
Ahmed, B A
Alam, M
Ali, A A
Ali, J
Alladi, V R
Allan, P J
Allister, J W
Anderson, C
Ansell, K S
Archer, G J
Arepalli, N
Armstrong, M H
Arora, A
Arora, N
Arrandale, L A
Ash, H C
Ashworth, J
Aswani, D
Atkinson, C J
Ayres, J
Ayub, A
Azeem, T
Azmy, H H
Baillie, N M
Bain, H M
Bakaya, R
Ballin, M S
Bamford, D J
Banerjee, B
Bardsley, S J
Baron, R L
Beardsell, R S
Benjamin, S J
Bennett, P W
Benson, J P
Berry, P M
Bhargava, J S
Bilbey, H
Billington, T N
Bills, G
Birch, J S
Black, G C M
Black, L D
Bolton, B
Booty, J
Bostock, D
Boyd, T H
Bradshaw, S J
Briggs, R S
Broadbent, P A
Brochwicz-Lewinski, M J
Brodie, G
Brooman, P J C
Brough, W A
Brown, S C W
Buckley, A
Buckley, M
Burns, H J
Burrows, G C
Butler, M L
Butterworth, D I
Byrne, J P
Byrne, R L
Capper, S J
Carmody, M C
Carr, H M H
Carroll, C D C
Carter, G J
Chambers, B J
Chanda, M
Chang, J M
Channing, G M
Cheadle, B
Checkland, K H
Cherry, E M
Chopra, P
Choudhuri, A M
Chung, P W-M
Clarke, S
Cockersole, G M
Coghlan, B P
Cole, S J A
Coley, A N
Coley, J C
Collins, G N
Collyer, I T
Condliffe, R A
Cook, G A
Cooper, R A
Cottrell, K A
Critchlow, B M
Crook, G C
Cryer, R J
Curley, J
Curran, F J M
Curran, N C
Cutts, M W J
Dada, D N
Dalal, R B
Datta-Chaudhuri, M
Dawson, D L
Day, C A
De Courcy Grylls, S C
Deans, G T
Derbyshire, N
Devine, N J
Dickie, I W
Dickson, R D
Dillon, J A
Donnan, I G
Douglas, J K
Downton, J H
Drake, C N
Dymock, S M
Ead, R D
Eadsforth, P
Edwards, R
Eeckelaers, E A
El Tayeb, H T
Elbeih, N M K I
Ellis, D J
Ellis, R A
Eyong, E
Fahmy, N R M
Fallowfield, J M
Farrell, D M
Feinmann, R
Fisher, A S
Fountain, A N
Fowler, E
Francis, J N
French, J A
Garner, M R
Geary, J A
Ghafoor, A
Ghosh, B N
Gill, R S
Gillespie, A
Gilman, A R
Gilmour, S A D
Gilmour, S K
Glass, S E
Goddard, C J R
Gor, M
Gradwell, M W
Graham, W B
Greenhough, S G
Gringras, M
Haboubi, N Y
Hale, P J
Hale, R J
Hall, J D
Hall, L M
Hamlet, G
Hammersley, S E
Hanley, M
Haque, M A
Hardie, L
Hardman, R G
Harrison, R
Harrison, R K
Harrison, T J R
Hawkes, D J
Hayward, L
Heald, J
Heath, R M
Hedley, P J
Helliwell, W E
Herbert, D L
Hercules, B L
Herd, J
Hernon, C A
Heyworth, T L
Hick, A G
Hick, P G
Higginbotham-Jones, K J
Hill, H F
Hingorani, A D
Hope, S M
Hopkinson, J R
Horsfall, A T
Housley, L E
Hughes, N
Hull, C A
Hume, D D
Hunt, C R
Hussain, A
Hussain, N
Huthart, P A
Ikram, K
Isherwood, I
Jacques, H E
Jain, A K
Jameson, R A
Jenkins, S M
Johari, S
Johnson, D S
Jones, D M
Jones, M M
Jones, N F
Jorasz, B M
Kaklugin, V I
Kalra, S K
Keeling-Roberts, C S
Keenleyside, G H
Kenyon, N
Khan, M A
Kilmartin, E J
Kilroy, D A
Kirwan, J M J
Knowles, D
Kumar, J S
Lalloo, N C
Lapsia, J
Lapsia, S K
Laughton, J M
Laxminarasimhaiah, T H
Lee, J W K
Leitch, C R
Lennox, R A
Levy, S F
Lewis, C J
Lewis, P S
Lightowler, B K W
Lindon, E F
Lipshen, G S
Logue, J
Lowe, J
Lundy, M T
McArdle, C-A
McCarthy, B P R
McCarthy, J F
McCluskey, A
McDermott, R P
McEnroe, G
McGregor, A E
MacKinnon, R J
Maguire, A M P
Maguire, D
Maher, T V
Mallikarjun, T S
Manton, J R
Marks, J S
Marshall, J S
Marshall, K C
Martin, B W
Martin, C J
Martin, M A
Mason, C J
Mathewson, R C L
Maxwell, S
Maxwell, W O
Meadows, D P
Meadows, T H
Mehta, R S
Mehta, S C
Mehta, S
Melzer, M
Menzies, D G
Midgley, M
Miller, J E
Miller, P F W
Miller, P I
Milnes, J E
Milson, J E
Mishra, A M
Misra, H N
Mitchell, H A
Mohamed, Q A
Moola, M I
Moore, A W
Moore, S A L
Morgan, I D F
Morgan, K G
Morgan, L H
Moriarty, A P
Morris, M A
Morrison, J E
Mortimer, J S
Moss, J
Muddu, V
Mukherjee, S K
Murthy, A P
Murugan, G
Nankhonya, J M
Nathoo, V
Nayar, A
Nazir, T Y
Needham, M J
Nelson, J M
Ng Man Kwong, G
Nuttall, I D
O'Flynn, K J
O'Neill, S S
O'Reilly, P H
Oldham, J R
Oldham, R A
Owen, J R B
Owen, P A
Pal, S
Parikh, R A
Parker, G
Parker, M R
Parker, T J
Parkinson, H M
Parkinson, M J
Partridge, C A
Patel, A M
Patel, L S
Paul, C A
Paul, N R
Pease, E H E
Phillips, M E
Pickersgill, A
Pocklington, A G
Pollard, A J
Pontefract, L
Pritchard, G M
Quinlan, M H
Quraishy, E
Radcliffe, M H
Raftery, P
Rains, K M
Rao, S
Rash, A
Rees, G A
Reeve, H A
Reeve, N L
Roberts, M J
Rodman, R
Rogers, W A
Roland, J
Roll, M J S
Rooney, M J
Rose, D H
Rowlands, M
Royle, D T
Royle, S G
Saeed, N R
Saeed, N R
Sahal, A K
Sarmah, A
Sayeed, I A
Schnieden, V
Semple, I C
Sethi, G
Sharma, A
Sharma, P D
Sharma, T
Sharma, Y D
Shelley, K E
Shepherd, A D
Sim, D M
Simpson, R
Singer, H G
Sinha, V
Sitlani, P K
Smith, J A
Smith, J U A
Smith, M C G
Spence, I P W
Spreckley, D E
Sridharan, G V
Stanley, C H
Start, N J
Stewart, I D M
Stone, M D
Stones, N A
Strelau-Sowinska, J
Sturgess, D A
Sutton, A G
Sykes, R
Tait, A C
Tait, W
Tandon, D K
Taylor, M E
Taylor, S L
Theodosiou, L J
Thomas, D R
Tinsley, H M
Tipping, K E
Todd, B D
Travenen, M J
Turner, P G
Tweedle, I S
Vasanthi-Sreenivasan, P
Vasey, R O
Vause, M H
Vickers, D M
Von Fraunhofer, M A
Walker, E H
Walker, J
Warburton, I R
Ward, S C
Watkins, S J
Watt, C M
Watt, G J
Weeks, A K
Wells, K
Wild, A F
Wilde, N T
Wilkes, J M
Wilkins, H M
Wilkinson, P M
Wilks, D
Wilson, M C
Wolfendale, K D
Woodhouse, M N
Wynn, J B
Wynne-Jones, M L
Wynroe, J C
Wynroe, S I
Yodaiken, M M

Stocksfield

Corbett, L
Eastwood, J R
Feeney, D P
Hall, J R
Hawkesford, B
L'Anson, M-J
McFetrich, A J
McKechnie, E P

Mansour, M S A
Pike, J L
Robson, J D
Said, W Q

Stockton-on-Tees
Adams, R N
Adamson, K A
Adamson, R M
Ahmad, M A
Anderson, D J
Anderson, R L
Andrew, L
Ashley, B D
Attalla, Y A
Barber, T M
Barlow, A P
Bayliss, N C
Berry, J
Bonavia, I C
Boylan, J J B
Broadway, P J
Brown, K J
Buchan, A
Budge, E M
Burrows, P S
Butler, M
Cameron, M J
Carr, D
Cattermole, T J
Chappel, D B
Chaudhry, S
Contractor, B R
Contractor, H B
Cook, A P
Craven, R M
Cresswell, P A
Davidson, G E
Davies, A L
Daynes, G K
De Burca, T T
Devlin, B
Dias, P J
Dias, R C
Dickens, D
Dobson, J A
Douglass, R A
Duckett, S P
Duval, C M
Dwarakanath, A D
Dyson, C
Ellenger, K
Elliot-Smith, A
Emerton, D G C
English, C J
Entwistle, W
Farooqi, A U
Frain, J P J
Fry, E N S
Gaskarth, M T G
Gill, P T
Gilliland, E L
Gordon, R D
Hall, K G
Hannigan, B F
Hardwick, J C
Harley, J J
Harrington, F M
Harrison, R N
Hatem, M
Hazelton, D C
Hearmon, C J
Hennessy, C
Herd, B M
Hinman, M M
Hoque, M H
Horne, R A
Howorth, P W
Hungin, A S
Jhawar, K
Jones, P R M
Kamlana, S H
Kenyon, S E
Khan, Z
Kiberu, S W
Kingscote, A D
Kingscote, J M
Kirkbride, I R
Krishna Kumar, V
Krishna, M
Kwan, T C O
Larcombe, J H
Lawson, A J
Leaper, D J
Leech, D L
Leitch, D N
Levan, D
Levan, S M
Litster, R Y
Lowe, J W
Lowerson, B
McBride, J E
McCarthy, T J
McGowan, P J
McGuinness, P D
McGuire, J
McInally, J
McKenna, A
Mackenzie, C
Maheshwaran, S S
Maheswaran, S
Makwana, R D
Mann, B M
Massey, K B
Monaghan, C M
Monkhouse, D
Montgomery, J E
Montrose, M K
Mounter, P J
Mulgrew, C J
Naisby, M G
Needham, S J
Nicholas, J R
Norrie, M S
O'Byrne, K P
O'Neill, C P
Oliver, G
Parrott, R J
Patel, R B
Peel, A L G
Phillips, M A T
Phyu Phyu, Dr
Poyner, T F
Pratt, R K
Quasim, M N I
Rai, S S
Ramaswamy, A
Ramphul, N
Rettman, C
Rigby, C J
Ritchie, A F
Roberts, L H
Roberts, R F
Robinson, N
Roddam, P A
Rosenberg, I L
Royal, V M
Royle, P
Scaife, B
Scane, A C
Scarth, J C
Scott, B
Shaw, D G M
Shaw, J
Shyam Sundar, A
Sidney, J A
Sinha, R N
Smith, R H
Snowden, K A V
Stephen, G W
Stephenson, C J
Stockley, S N
Stubbs, L A
Sudhakar, J E
Swords, P J K
Sylvester, S H H
Tabaqchali, M A
Tanner, A R
Thompson, A C
Thompson, W D
Thornham, J R
Tunio, F
Turner, A M
Turner, L A
Turner, R V
Upton, M N
Van Loo, G
Ventress, M A
Verber, I G
Walton, S M
Webb, L A
White, D H
Wignarajah, N
Wilkinson, J R
Williams, S R
Woodhouse, P
Youssef, M M K I

Stoke-on-Trent
Abdu, T A M
Abraheem, A
Adjogatse, J K
Ahmed, S
Aitken, C M
Aldridge, N A
Allen, M B
Allt, J E
Angris, S
Arshad, S H
Ashraf, M
Ashworth, J
Badcock, L J
Bagchi, D N
Bailey, I S
Bailey, N A
Bajwa, S
Baker, C E
Bamford, W M
Barakat, N
Barber, J M
Barker, C L
Barnes, S J
Barnes, S B
Barrett, K
Barrie, B T
Barrow, K E
Bartlam, A S
Bashford, J N R
Bedson, J
Bennett, A G
Bennett, J D C
Bloor, R N
Boddie, H G
Bolia, S
Bourne, H C
Bradbury, S M
Braithwaite, M
Bridgman, S A
Bridgwood, P S
Brind, A M
Bromley, J S
Brookfield, D S K
Brown, L S
Brown, M F
Brown, M A I
Brown, R D
Brunt, A M
Brydon, H L
Burton, K M
Butcher, A B
Campbell, C A
Carlin, N E
Carlin, W V
Carpenter, E H
Carr, D M
Carter, A J
Cartwright, D J
Casement, J R
Chadalavada, R
Chadalavada, V S R
Chamakuri, V
Chambers, R M
Chan, S C Y
Chand, G T
Chandler, P A
Chatterjee, A
Chehata, J C G
Child, H F
Clarke, M
Clayton, R N
Cook, A M
Cooper, J C
Cooper, V
Corcoran, H M
Courteney-Harris, R G
Cowan, K A
Cox, J L
Creamer, J E
Crisp, W J
Croft, P R
Crome, I B
Crome, P
Cunningham, N J
Dallow, P C
Davidson, J
Davies, M B
Davies, S J
Davis, J A S
Davison, P M
Dawes, P T
De Takats, D L P
Deakin, M
Dent, A R
Donoghue, C A
Dos Remedios, I D M
Dove, J
Dover, S J
Dowell, I S
Duffy, T J
Dunn, A T
Dwyer, J S J M
Eardley, R C
Edgley, J N
Edmends, S
Egginton, J A
Elder, J B
Elliot, I R
Ellis, S J
Emery, D F G
Evans, D M
Fernando, L R T A
Fisher, C J
Forrest-Hay, I
Foster, C E
French, T A
Garnham, P A R
Gerry, Z L
Ghosh, D C
Ghosh, J
Gilby, J A
Gillow, J T J
Gohil, K B
Golik, P
Gopalan, V
Graetz, K P
Graetz, P A
Gray, C A M
Gray, J
Green, J C
Green, J R B
Griffiths, D
Grime, P D
Hall, C
Hancock, M R
Hand, M F
Harbidge, C J
Harris, A
Harrison, N J
Hartland, A J
Hassan, M K
Hawkins, K A
Heath, P D
Henshaw, C A
Hickson, A F
Hill, E W
Hobson, C M
Hobson, J A
Hodgson, R E
Holland, J
Hopcroft, J D
Hopkins, C S
Hopkins, S E
Hopwood, M E F
Howell, C J
Howis, A
Hughes, G M
Hully, R
Hurley, D
Hurlstone, D P
Hussain, K
Jafri, A
Jafri, S A
Jafri, S K A
Jain, N K
Jary, S R
Jheeta, A S
Jones, A
Jones, C M
Jones, D H
Jones, R G
Jordan, T L
Keates, M D
Keating, G W
Kerr, C A
Khan, A H
Khunger, A C
Kilding, J-A
King, J M
King, S E
Knapper, S
Knight, C L
Kundu, S
Lam, F Y
Lata, P S
Lawrence, A D M
Lear, G A
Lee, S W
Leese, I D
Lenney, W
Lightfoot, P J
Lithgow, P A
Little, J T
Liu, S
Loughney, D G M
Lovett, L M L
Lyons, E L P
McCarthy, J J
McCarthy, M E F
McCartie, K M
McConnell, J R L
McGowan, J M
McMaster, P
McVerry, D N
Maffulli, N
Magnay, A R
Male, C G
Malgwa, A
Malgwa, P R
Mali, M
Mallepaddi, N R
Manning, G L
Manudhane, V S
Masson, G
Matthews, N C
Mawby, N C
Mayland, P A
Meaton, M L
Mehta, K K
Menon, B K V
Merali, N A
Merifield, W K
Millinship, J
Mirza, S M
Mohajer, M P
Morgan, R H
Morris, P T
Morrison, P J
Mottershead, N J
Mucklow, J C
Naeem, M
Nayar, O K
Nayeemuddin, F A
Neary, R H
Negrycz, R J
O'Brien, A P
O'Brien, P M S
Oakley, P A
Oxtoby, J W
Oxtoby, J D
Page, R J
Pantin, C F A
Parikh, H S
Park, A J
Parkinson, K
Parkinson, R J
Parmar, J M
Patel, B D
Patel, C V
Patel, K P
Patel, S V
Patterson, J A
Pearson, R A
Pedrazzini, A E
Perry, M J
Phillips, C J
Phillips, D W
Pilpel, J M
Pilpel, P J
Plunkett, M C
Prabhakaran, N
Pratap, B R
Price, D J
Przyslo, F R
Pullan, A D
Rabie, S M M
Raffeeq, P M
Ramachandran, S
Rao, S Y P C P
Rathi, A K
Reddy, G V
Redman, C W E
Reeves, H L
Reynolds, E R
Reynolds, K A
Rice, C P
Richards, P J
Richardson, B
Rickards, N P
Rizvi, F H
Roberts, J O
Rogerson, M E
Rohatgi, M K
Rohatgi, S
Roy, T K
Russell, G I
Ryan, M M B
Saklatvala, J
Salpekar, S D
Salt, M J
Samal, K
Samuels, M P
Sanghera, P
Sankaran, M
Saxby, M F
Scarpello, J H
Scheepers, B D M
Schur, P E
Scoble, J E
Scott, C A
Scragg, G M
Seth, K N
Sethi, K B S
Sgouros, X
Shadforth, M F
Shah, P H
Shah, S S
Shaikh, M S
Shamsi, S A
Sharaf-Ud-Din, S
Sharaf, A
Shaw, H M A
Shaw, P H
Sheikh-Sajjad, A R
Sheppard, D A
Shevlin, B A
Sieber, F A
Singh, G
Singh, J
Sinha, A K
Sinha, R N
Sivapalan, S
Sivardeen, G M F
Sivardeen, K A Z
Smallpeice, C J
Smith, A G
Smith, B A C
Smith, I
Smith, P J
Smith, S D
Soliman, M O A M
Solis Reyes, C
Spencer, S A
Stafford, D M
Standage, K F
Stephens, M
Stocker, D I
Sule Suso, J
Suxena, S R
Synnott, M B
Talpur, H A
Tan, B B
Tattum, C M
Tattum, K T
Taylor, K M
Thomas, G R W
Thomas, M P S
Thomas, P B M
Tomlinson, A A
Tomlinson, I M
Tooth, J S
Topple, N A
Turner, P J
Turner, S E
Turner, W W
Vaghmaria, A
Van Der Linden, H H E M
Vaze, B C
Verborg, S A
Verma, H L
Verma, R K
Verma, R K
Wakley, G M
Walker, A B
Walsh, A K M
Ward, A B
Watson, R A
Watts, D J
Weatherby, S J
Webster, A P
Webster, V G
Weeder, R G
Wells, R D
Welton, M D M
Wilcock, D J
Wilkins, C J
Williamson, A D
Willmott, P A
Wood, A F
Woodcock, C J
Wright, N J
Yadava, R P
Yates, D O
Yates, G
Young, D N
Young, G M

Stoke-sub-Hamdon
Blaydes, K E
Bulley, R J
Collins, H F
Scott, P J

Stone
Acey, G
Anderson, I V
Atkins, C S
Ballinger, J P
Campbell, C F L
Challiner, R A
Clark, R M
Clubb, A W
Crump, A A S C W
Eames, J K

Hamilton, E C
Hamilton, P G
Hand, S E
Hart, C N
Hassell, A B
Holden, S W
Ibbotson, R M
Johnson, A M
Kadam, U T
Kimber, V R
Lamb, A J
MacSharry, M J
Murphy, F
Powers, D S
Secker, C J
Stafford, A J
Taylor, I A
Templeton, J
Wooding, S J

Stonehaven
Chan, T T B
Cordiner, D S
Dossett, A G
Fisher, P M
Herd, J M R
Hopper, N B
Houghton, E J
Howard, D M
Innes, I
Johnson, B
MacCuish, A
McIntosh, G H
Mackenzie, I S
Mackenzie, L M
McLay, K A
Maclean, V M
Macleod, F
McLeod, I
Morgan, A H
N'Dow, K E
O'Hara, A W
Patience, L A
Reary, S
Stewart, A L
Stewart, A D
Thomson, J M G
Weir, M J

Stonehouse, Gloucestershire
Anslow, S R F
Cartwright, K A V
Lake, L A
Latter, M J
Sivyer, J E
Wenham, J A
Woodland, J

Stornoway
Cunningham, G K
Davis, J N
Dickie, A M
Dickie, R J
Ferguson, M
Gray, G L
Hothersall, A P
Maclean, D A
MacLennan, C R
Macleod, M M
Michie, A B
Murray, D J
Raff, P F
Scott, L
Sim, A J W
Walker, M J

Stourbridge
Allen, E K
Allen, S M
Allison, E C
Andrew, T A
Ashton, C T
Bache, J C
Barrett, E C A
Barrett, S R
Baxter-Smith, D C
Beardsmore, D M
Berwick, S J M
Bracka, A
Brindley, R J
Browning, D J C
Burbridge, B J
Bury, J P
Butler, A C
Callender, R
Carter, M P
Chaloner, J D
Chandra, E
Clark, A L
Clymo, A B
Cooke, M J
Coope, B J
Cooper, T A
Czapla, K
Davies, S J
Davis, R E
De Silva, M S
Delamere, J P
Digger, T J
Dingwall, I M
Donovan, R M
Drury, V W M
Dudley, B G
Dunn, R M
Edwards, T R
Evans, L C
Farley, P S
Feghali, E
Firth, J
Fisher, G C
Flint, E J
Ghose, A
Gittins, N S
Grainger, M F
Griffiths, C A
Hale, M
Healy, M D
Heywood, T R
Higgins, R P
Hobson, M I
Homer, L M
Hunton, M
Hyde, J N
Hyne, S J
Innes, P A
Iqbal, A
Irfan, F A
Issitt, J S
Jabar, M F
Jenkins, K L
Joy, T K
Kelly, A N
Kelly, S D E
Khalid, N
Killalea, S E
Killin, W P
Krick, R C B
Labib, M H Z
Lewis, G J
Leyland, F C
Lim, S
Louca, O A B
McKenzie, M A
McMinn, D J W
McMinn, M J
Mangat, T K
Mann, S J
Mazey, N S
Meer, L C
Megyesi-Schwartz, F C
Merotra, S K
Mifsud, R
Mitchell, T D
Mohite, A S
Moleele, G T
Moore, E C
Mucklow, J T
Mudgal, R
Orange-Lohn, B
Partridge, S J
Patodi, M
Pennock, H C
Perry, K A
Phillips, A F
Porter, W A B
Powell, D F
Powell, D J S
Price, M
Raafat, L
Rees, D A
Renny, F H B
Reshamwala, N K
Richards, D S
Richards, J E H
Riley, K P
Roberts, G A
Rose, M N
Sajid, M
Sarhadi, N S
Shah, N H
Shaw, J L
Smith, R S
Sockalingam, M
Speakman, J K
Steven, R E
Stone, M J
Tai, Y M A
Tanner, M T
Taylor, V R
Tebbutt, N C
Thomas, S S
Thompson, S D
Tzifa, C
Walker, M A
Walmsley, R S
Warwick, A P
Watkins, B J
Watson, R S
Watt, A J M
Watton, D
Weyham, C J
Wild, A G
Wilkinson, S D
Wilson, G R
Yarwood Smith, C H

Stourport-on-Severn
Al-Khayat, M A R M
Batty, P F
Brohan, E
Franklin, M E
Gait, A J
Goodman, J S
Hickman, L J
Horton, R J
Kanas, R P
Kingston, W E
Parsons, G J
Rumley, S L P
Ward, R A

Stowmarket
Campbell, D M T
Clapp, R M M
Egan, D J
Fenning, A H
Fielder, J P S
Gill, J R
Grundy, R E
Hall, R M
Head, P H
Helliwell, M C J
Herman, J M
Jenkins, I A R
Jennings, T B
Kubis, V M
Macpherson, H M
Muir, J E
Reti, S R
Rudland, S V
Shenton, M I
Tuke, J W
Wankowski, A F
Yusaf, B

Strabane
Carey, S A
Cavanagh, P J
Diamond, P M
Donnelly, D M
Duffy, M P
Friel, F C
Fullerton, A T
Gallagher, J
Gillespie, J G
Harron, J C
Harron, M E
Kerr, E G
Leahy, B J P
McCarron, S B
McCluggage, H L
McCrea, K J
McGuinness, A P
McHale, J G A J
Mullen, S M
O'Donnell, J S
O'Flaherty, G M
O'Neill, M P O M
Patton, S N
Quigley, B M
Rawdon, C M
Robinson, D P
Stewart, S D
Watson, G H V

Stranraer
Adams, A R
Balmer, J N W
Calvert, J A
Donnelly, C M
Gall, J F
Gordon, J J
Lee, J
Lennon, E M
McDougall, F M
McTaggart, J C
Narain, B
Reid, S C T
Ritchie, I M
Spicer, R J
Vaughan, D A
White, R J
Wooff, D J

Stratford-upon-Avon
Adam, I J
Alliston, J E
Allwood, I J
Batt, E M
Bothwell, P W
Brace, W D
Buckley, D M
Carrington, I M
Carus, A M
Chambers, S J
Clarke, K L
Coulthard, R A
Craddock, D J
Crook, T G
Crowfoot, J
Dalton, J D
Derbyshire, D R
Fitchford, R J
Fitchford, W J
Gabathuler, H
Garratt, D M
Gowans, J
Henderson, R M
Hodson, J P A
Jones, J A
King, K J
Kinoulty, M
Kitchen, H J
Lindahl, A J
McMorran, J P
McMorran, S H
Madagan, N G
Mingo, R M
Morgan, A J A
Peer, R M
Phalp, C G A
Rudge, J W
Schofield, A M
Supple, N T
Sykes, G W
Thorne, R J
Winstanley, A M
Winstanley, C S
Wood, N C
Woodward, M N

Strathaven
Campbell, C M C
Campbell, W M
Dow, R E
Fulton, J M
Godley, C C
Hackett, J S
Hassall, C M
Hynes, P C
McGowan, J H
Pepperell, J
Porte, A M
Shapiro, F N
Sharma, D
Sharma, S
Sharma, U C
Smith, S M
Whitelaw, F M

Strathcarron
Cargill, J M
Murray, D B

Strathdon
Craig, M S
Dudley, H A F
Fitton, J L

Strathpeffer
Gate, H B
Macpherson, T S
Wood, A J

Street
Clark, H M
Elkin, T
Last, R D
Merrick, J
Merry, E J
Monro, A J
Owen, R J
Rushford, C A
Seymour, B J
Singhal, V K
Wolfe, C S

Stromness
Diament, M L
Pyle, W D
Rae, C K
Trickett, A R

Stroud
Allan, M
Babor, B E
Baddeley, P G
Barraclough, K
Bayly, J R
Blatchley, C
Boddam-Whetham, A H C
Booker, N J
Bouzyk, P C A
Bridger, C
Brown, C M
Brown, P F
Bye, I M
Campbell, M M F
Croser, D H
Crouch, T
Davie, R C
Dickson, A F L W
Driscoll, R C
Du Toit, J A
Evans, K L
Evans, M R
Fairgrieve, H
Haffenden, D K
Hall, G D
Holmes, R P H
Hutter, A
Isaac, D C
Isaac, G J
James, M E
Jansen, C A M
Jones, N D H
Jorro, B S C
Keating, V J
Kelly, P G
Lake, I D
Latham, A M
Lavis, R A
Lewis, E D
Livingstone, D N
Lucas, A J
McKie, N I P
Marlow, A-M
Meikle, V M
Mills, S J
Morgan, C E
Pearson, P
Perry-Keene, G H
Poole, R A
Porter, M C M
Pouncey, D A C G
Quekett, J T S
Reed, A
Richards, H
Ridge, A L
Sackett, K M
Salter, J C
Savage, M J
Shepherd, C B
Simpson, A P F
Slim, J M
Smith, D A
Staniforth, C
Stephenson, R H
Stirland, E
Swindell, P J
Tann, O R
Thomas, D M
Thomas, S
Thompson, D R
Van Zyl, M E
Vestey, S B
Waldon, R D
Walters, J C
Weir, S
Wood, R
Woods, C J

Studley
Ash, J V
Buckley, M P
Cartledge, J D
Edwards, D A
Harris, P J
Wade, R J
Walsh, R C

Sturminster Newton
Burton, E C
Casson, E J
Clayton, S J
Cripps, M G
Hopkins, K I
Perkins, K M
Robinson, J P J
Sparrow, G E A
Vardill, D
Wilson, W G

Sudbury
Adams, E B
Barker, M J M
Bevan, D C P
Bone, A D W
Chambers, M E W
Chase, R P
Crouch, A D K
De Pass, J P C
Deb, A K
Donnelly, R
Feneck, R O
Garrett-Moore, T R
Goodliffe, C D
Hawkins, J A
Hayhow, B
Haythornthwaite, G E
Heller, K B
Hughes, R A
Jetha, S K
Kemp, A R
Lesser, G F
McClellan, E
MacDiarmid, F M
Norris, T C M
Sarda, K
Side, C D
Sills, S C J
Stewart, A D
Stewart, J A B
Swampillai, J S
Taylor, D L
Taylor, M E
Williamson, S S
Wynn, G R

Sunbury-on-Thames
Al-Ani, S-A A
Ali, M
Baker, P D
Barnett, R
Bhular, J S
Byrne, B
Chapman, G B
Elvin, V
Hodson, S E
Maclaurin, J R C
Martin, A M
Pearce, J J
Pearce, N R
Saunders, A P
Van Rhijn, M

Sunderland
Abu-Harb, M
Adedeji, O A
Ahmed, N
Al-Khalidi, B G O
Ali, S S
Allchin, R W
Allen, E D
Anjum, S
Arrowsmith, A E
Atchison, R K
Bagchi, S P
Banjeree, G
Banks, D C F
Bansal, S K
Barton, J W
Basu, A P
Bell, G D
Bell, R W D
Bendelow, K
Bernardi, R E
Bhate, S M
Bignardi, G E
Birnie, A J M
Bolel, S B
Bose, A A K
Brigham, J D
Brown, A M D
Brown, C J
Brown, M J
Burton, R L
Buswell, W A
Button, C
Cameron, H M

Carey, P J
Cassidy, T P
Cervenak, R F E
Chapman, A J
Chapman, F M
Chay, S T S
Chhabra, D R
Chiquito-Lopez, P E
Clague, H W
Clark, L
Cleland, P G
Cloak, B J
Cochrane, H R
Connor, J A
Corson, R J
Crone, N M
Cronin, P M
Cross, A T
Crummie, A J M
Dalton, M E
Danjoux, J-P
Datta, P S
Davies, A J
Daymond, T J
Deady, J P
Deshpande, M K
Devapal, D
Dhar, R L
Dhariwal, N K
Dillon, R D S
Donaldson, K I
Donoghue, R E
Dowd, H D
Dulson, K
Dunlop, P
El-Faki, A E H M A
El Mekkawy, E E-D A-K
El Safy, A M I E
Ela, M A A
Emmerson, C M
Featherstone, T
Fernandes, C
Fetherston, T J
Fletcher, R D M
Ford, R N
Forester, N D
Fraser, K M
Fraser, S G
Furness, J C
Galloway, M J
Gautam, S
Ghosh, A
Gill, P J
Glass, L G
Glatt, D
Glatt, H S
Goldsmith, P V
Golledge, P
Gough, D G
Grant, J A
Gray, C S
Green, J D
Gupta, S D
Hall, S J
Hallikeri, S G
Hamad, A H
Harvey, G T
Heard, A M B
Heaton, J M
Henderson, D P
Heycock, E G
Heycock, R W
Hind, J M
Hinshaw, K
Holland, C D
Hunsley, D
Hyder, M T
Inglesby, D V
Irwin, L R
Johnson, R
Jones, A J
Jones, R E
Joshi, N A
Junejo, S
Kanta, K
Karn, K P
Kaul, O
Keaney, N P
Kelly, J M
Kennedy, R L
Kew, F M
Kilgour, T C
Kirchin, V S
Lahiri, B
Lahiri, S
Langtry, J A A
Lawrie, A W
Lawson, G R
Lee, J
Leeks, A D
Lefley, P J
Leigh, R J
Levy, B
Liang Lung Chong, M E K
Lobo, F X
Lyndon, S
McBride, G P
McDonald, J W
Mackay, L J
Mackee, I W
Mackrell, J R
MacNab, G
Maidment, G
Mair, J A
Malik, M M A
Maredia, M N
Marsh, R L
Martin, A M
Martin, E R
Martin, I C
Mellon, A F
Miller, P D
Milne, D S
Mitchison, H C
Mitchison, S
Morgan, E
Morgan, S J
Motwani, C A
Mukherjee, S P
Murphy, A-M
Murray, B J
Murray, R B
Muwanga, C
Natarajan, S
Nepali, P K
O'Connell, J E
Oakley, H
Owen, N M
Parker, A J
Partington, J S
Patnaik, S
Patnaik, S N
Patterson, P R N
Pawaroo, L
Phelan, P S
Pickworth, R W
Pilapitiya, R B
Pillai, S S
Place, M
Powell, S L
Price, K A
Pugh, S E
Raman, T S
Raphael, G A J
Raphael, M
Rashid, S
Razvi, F M
Reddy, G M
Reid, C J
Richardson, J
Richardson, W A W
Roy, A I
Rubin, G P
Rutherford, R G
Saharia, E
Samuel, P R
Sandbach, C S
Sarma, K M
Sarson, D
Sein Win, L C H
Settle, C D
Sharma, K N
Shepherd, R B
Shetty, B K K
Singh, H C
Singh, L
Small, P K
Smith, J J
Smithson, S R
Spagnoli, E A
Steel, A M
Steel, D H W
Steele, S C
Stephenson, K
Stirrat, A N
Stone, A W
Sultana, A M U
Surtees, P
Tayal, S A
Taylor, I K
Thomas, J B
Thorpe, A C
Velangi, S S
Waine, C
Walker, M J
Walton, C J
Ward, G C
Watson, A J
Watson, I D
Watters, M M
Weatherhead, M P
Weaver, K N J
Welbury, J
Wetherall, M R B
Whiting, K A
Widdrington, I H
Wilkinson, R
Wilson, I J
Wong, L H
Wong, N C
Wortley, P M
Wright, W
Young, L J
Young, P F

Surbiton

Agrawal, K
Agrawal, R K
Aldous, C A
Barlin, C A
Bartlett, D
Baruch, A L H
Benney, S A J
Boullin, J P
Bowey, O
Byramji, N K
Campbell, N G
Cassell, D M C
Cockburn, J J
Collini, P J
Crawley, S J
D'Souza, J C H
Dalzell, J
Dhir, K S
Edwards, J M
Gaya, D S
Gentle, S C
Ging, J E
Gordon, D J
Haddo, O
Hindle, K S
Hinsley, A M
Holdsworth, W G
Holton, A R
Hulse, M G
Kalsi, M S
Kelly, J
Kodikara, M
Langridge, P
Lee, R K L
Luke, J J
Mansour, N S N
Martin, E C
Maxwell, M J
Milton, R S
Mitra, S
Mohan, T C
Montgomery, D H
Moore, P D
Moutoussis, M
Munby, J S
Munby, J C A
O'Driscoll, M J
Oshea, C P
Pall, A A
Peter, J
Prentice, M G
Prentice, P A
Punter, J
Rafique, M A
Rajani, R
Rathakrishnan, R
Roberts, D L
Saha, B N
Somers, L J
Spotswood, V J
Syed, A A
Syed, J A
Thaman, R
Thurairaja, R
Topp, J M
Turner, C L S
Waters, M J
Weeks, P H
Whitlock, N J
Wilding, G
Wilding, L J
Wolfson, M S

Sutton

Aboud, M A
Akberali, A F
Akram, N S
Ali Khan, M F S
Allum, W H
Amin, S M
Arendse, S D
Atra, A A A
Baird, R D
Barrett, J J
Barsey, H
Barsey, L
Benyamin, F
Bhattachan, C L
Bhoyrul, S
Bignell, M D
Bingle, K C
Blackwell, M J
Bloom, H S
Brada, M
Brennan, C A M
Bristow, M F
Brown, G
Brown, J H
Bryan-Brown, A B E
Canepa-Anson, A C M
Carter, T R G
Chana, P
Chana, T
Chilvers, A S
Churchill, M A
Coldrey, D A
Cook, G J R
Cooling, R A
Craig, J O M C
Croucher, J J
Cunningham, D
Cunningham, D
Curtis, J R
Dark, G G
Davies, C E
Davies, K A
De Silva, P V
Dearden, C E
Dearnaley, D P
Dearnaley, J M M
Dinnick, S E
Doyle, E X P
Eeles, R A
Eisinger, A J
Elliott, C J
Elliott, S D C
Evans, R A
Evans, S A
Fernandez, M D
Filshie, J
Fish, D G H
Fleet, H J
Ford, H E R
Free, A J
Free, M C
Gardner, M W
Ghosh, M K
Gossain, S R
Gough, P M
Govender, S
Greer, H S
Grice, S J
Hall, J G
Hardy, J R
Hargrave, D R
Harris, C B
Havelock, J M
Henk, J M
Hji Yiannakis, P
Hobbs, A R
Hogg, H A
Horwich, A
Houlston, R S
Howell, M L
Howell, S E
Huddart, R A
Hudson, B
Husband, J E S
Jelly, L M E
John, A C
Jolley, A W
Jones, D B D
Jones, V A
Joseph, S P
Judson, I R
Kalmus, E J
Kanthan, K K
Karunasekera, I K
Kathirgamakanthan, S
Kattan, M M
Kay, D M
Kaye, S B
Kazmi, M S
King, M M
Kothari, J J
Kuppusami, T N
Kurwa, A R
Lall, R P
Latham, D
Latifi, Q A
Latifi, S Q
Lee, M S
Leghari, J A K
Leitch, R J
Likeman, M J
Linnell, A E T
Lodge, J W
Longley, J M
McCready, V R
McElvanney, A M
McInnes, P B
McIntosh, C S
Macleod, A T
Magauran, D M
Mason, R H
Mathers, C B B
Mehra, M
Merritt, L G
Middleton, S
Mirnezami, A H F
Morgan, B J
Morgan, G J
Mugglestone, C J
Mullane, M C
Nash, A G
Neville, K M
Neylan, C M M A
Norton, K R W
O'Brien, J T
O'Brien, M E R
O'Donnell, P J
O'Sullivan, C J
Ogeah, Dr
Orchard, R T
Oshowo, A O
Palmier, B M
Paramothayan, N S
Patroni, B
Pearson, I C
Pembrey, J S
Perkin, M R
Perry, A R
Pinkerton, C R
Popat, S B
Pourgourides, C K
Pritchard-Jones, K
Quek, F M
Querci Della Rovere, G
Quigley, M M
Rabindra, B
Ramsey, J M
Ramsey, P M
Rathod, R C
Redwood, D R
Richards, M A
Roberts-Shephard, A
Rodin, M J
Rostom, A Y
Rubio Rodriguez, M D C
Ruse, G A
Said, A
Said, A J
Saluja, T R
Samuel, D P
Sarin, R
Scully, M A
Seyan, R S A S
Shah, S M
Sharma, A
Shedden, R G
Shepherd, J C
Shiew, C M
Shiew, M M F
Singhai, S
Smit, I D
Smith, I D
Smith, J N
Smith, R E
Sohaib, S A A
Soomal, R S
Soon, C C Y
Souberbielle, B E
Spring, L C
Stern, R S
Stinson, D M
Sumpter, K A
Swerdlow, A J
Tait, D M
Thethravusamy, J A
Thomas, D V P
Thompson, A M
Tinkler, J M
Tonge, A E
Treleaven, J G
Tylee, A T
Tyler, M J
Tyrrell, J M
Ursell, P G
Vernon, J E
Vijayakulasingam, V
Wadhwani, G H
Warren, A P
Whitaker, S J
Whitlow, C M
Williamson, A D B
Wills, G T
Wood, E J (D
Wright, J C
Wurm, R E
Zomas, A

Sutton Coldfield

Abbas, S
Abd-El-Massih, G K
Abdalla, M A-E H M
Abdo, O A
Abdul Cader, A H M
Al-Salihi, T
Alam, M
Albright, S W
Allan, L M
Ananta, M P P
Archer, D F J
Bains, J
Baker, A C
Banerjea, B L
Baxter, R J
Beaumont, A L
Bennett Britton, S
Benyon, S L
Bhatt, P I
Bhatt, R I
Bickley, C M
Bleasdale, J P
Blight, A P
Bond, A R
Booth, K R
Brake, R C
Brennan, A P
Briscoe, J J D
Broomhead, C R M
Brown, J H
Browse, D J
Burton, C C
Burton, P W
Cartmill, R S V
Cassam, S
Cave, N S
Chapman, J P O
Cheetham, P J
Chiam, T K
Churchill, D
Clarke, M P
Collier, I P
Collier, J B
Constable, T J
Constantine, G
Cope, S J
Coutts, A S
Crawford, W S
Cuthbert, A J
Damerau, N B L E
Darby, S E
Davies, A C
De Wit, A
Deshpande, A H
Deshpande, V A
Divall, J M
Dodds, S R
Dolman, M J
Down, S K
Dugas, M J
Duggal, R
Dunbar, M R
East, D M
Eddy, J D
Edwards, J G
Elliot, J M
Elmardi, A A A
Evans, S C
Farooqi, I S
Finn, C B
Flacks, R M
Fletcher, T J
Forshaw, M L
Fortes Mayer, K D
Foster, M C
Francis, D A
Gent, R J
Ghosh, C
Ghosh, K
Gibbins, S J
Goel, V K
Gonzalez Naranjo, D S
Goodwin, I D

Gordon, S A
Gossain, S
Grant, P H
Griffin, M J W
Gupta, K K
Hamilton, M S
Harris, A W
Hassam, Z
Hayward, P J
Hill, S A
Hodgson, R J
Humpherson, C E
Hunter, M D
Ingham, B
Ingham, P J
Iszatt, M E
Iyer, S J
Jarratt, R M
Jeetley, P S
Jeeva Raj, M V
Jeffery, D M
Jewkes, A J
Jobanputra, S M
Johnston, P
Jones, B G
Jones, S L
Joseph, R
Kanagaratnam, P
Kapur, P
Kaul, S
Kaul, S
Khaira, G K
Khaira, H S
Khanna, R
Lai, W K
Langley, A M
Laycock, R J
Lee, T J
Lenton, C D
Lesshafft, C S
Lester, H D E
Leung, A Y-T
Leyva-Leon, F A
Light, A M
Lumley, M A
McCabe, E J
McDonald, A J
Mackay, A D
Martin, S C
Messih, M N A E
Metwally, A M
Miller, I M
Milles, J J
Mirza, M
Moloney, M D
Moorjani, N
Moorjani, R
Moreton, E I J
Mortimer, H J
Mundy, P J
Murray, P F
Narayan, P L
Natalwala, S
Nelson, C A
Oakley, J R
Owens, J
Pai, S H
Pal, B R
Parkin, J W
Parnell, A P
Patel, A E
Pennington, J M
Perris, T M
Petty, M J
Phillips, L A
Platt, R
Price, R A
Rajeshwar, M
Ramnarine, V D
Rastogi, A
Rawal, P
Ray, L C
Reddy, E
Rees, T W
Reynolds, J H
Richardson, D
Rimmer, J M
Roberts, N G
Robinson, W H
Rogers, V J
Rolland, P A
Ruiz Martin, M
Sagoo, V S
Sahota, B S
Sawar, M O
Seehra, M
Sen, A
Shearer, A C I
Sheldrake, J H
Sheldrake, L J
Shepherd, A J
Sherlaw, S R
Simons, M A P
Singh, H B
Singh, S
Slominski, H B
Smith, R E A
Solari, T J
Soorae, S S
Speak, N J
Spiers, D P
Spooner, D
Storer, J I
Strachan, R A
Surendra Kumar, R
Surendrakumar, S M
Tamma, S
Taylor, J G
Thirumala Krishna, M
Thomas, C P
Thomas, D I
Thomas, D R
Thomas, L J
Thompson, A R
Thompson, R J W
Thrush, S
Upthegrove, R A
Valsalan, V C
Vanner, T F M
Walker, E J
Walker, S A
Wall, D W
Walsh, G D
Walsh, L J
Webster, M A
Whitehouse, D R
Whitticase, J E
Willis, A P D
Wulff, D E

Sutton-in-Ashfield

Abbott, L P
Ali, S
Alker, M
Allen, S M
Barrett, P
Bishton, I M
Bliss, D F
Bond, D W
Bull, P T
Chandran, Q
Chandran, T R
Cooke, G A
Ewbank, G S A
Fairbrother, B J
Finn, G P
Greasley, L A
Hambidge, J E
Harris, R F
Hastings, A G
Hill, K J
Hill, K J
Hook, R A
Idris, I R
Jenkins, J R F
Jones, S G
Lacey, A J
Lloyd-Mostyn, R H
Logan, E C M
McInerney, B A
Mason, J S
Mathew, T K
Meats, P S
Mowbray, M J
Needoff, M
Nigam, K
Nithianandan, P
Nithianandan, S
Panto, P N
Pickles, C J
Rahman, M
Robertson, N M
Ross, M T
Rowley, J M
Salter, E J
Sands, K A
Smith, P G
Stein, G
Subramaniam, S
Subramanian, T
Taylor, M C
Temple, P I
Thomson, G A
Ulliott, E E J
Ward, M J
Ward, S J
Williamson, J R
Worsley, A P
Young, S M

Swadlincote

Buckler, E C
Clegg, A
Corbett, E A
Davidson, A S
Davies, G P
Field, M
Follows, R L
Gravestock, N
Hannon, M C
Hignett, A W
Jamison, R W
Kenny, T M
Khalid, T
Kirk, J S
Robinson, J
Stack, M M
Starey, N H L
Taleb, S M
Trotter, R F
Vaughan, J M
Von Fragstein, M F F
Walker, J D

Swaffham

Barton, D I
Dorling, R F
Draper, N E
Haczewski, I
Hatfield, J M R
Hendrie, O R S
Holmes, M J G
Holmes, N K
Musson, R I
Rayner, R A
Sorensen-Pound, D J
Willy, D M M

Swanage

Baker, R W
Caruana, M P
Clark, J C D
Clark, P M R
Elfes, C J
Freeman Welham, S
Haines, D A
Heard, W E
Karlowski, T A
Knott, D
Lane, H L
Leigh, P R
Lodge, J A
Munday, J N R
Murphy, K M
Petri, M P
Rowland, A G

Swanley

Brooman, I C
Burrows, L M
Gregson, S N
Lynch, V J
Muthappan, A K
Pomeroy, W S
Ramphal, P S
Rizwan, M M
Rumfeld, W R

Swansea

Adams, L J
Adams, R
Agarwal, N K
Aird, D W
Aird, I A
Al-Ismail, S A D A R
Albuquerque, S R J
Allen, H
Anani, A R A
Anderson, M H
Annear, R O D
Antao, A J O
Apsitis, B
Arthurs, Y M C
Askill, C S
Asscher, A W
Austin, M W
Avery, J G
Avery, P G
Baines, P I B
Baker, R H
Bamber, C S
Banks, J
Barrow, T V
Barton, C R
Baxter, J N
Baxter, P W
Beddall, A C
Beese, E N A
Bell, J P
Bennett, D G
Benton, M A
Bevan, C J
Bevan, J C
Beynon, J
Beynon, P
Biswas, S
Blackford, S L W
Blackwell, A L
Blair, J M
Boladz, W P
Bourne, S J
Bowen-Simpkins, P
Bowen, A
Bowen, H G
Bowen, H J
Bowen, I
Bowen, I E
Bradley, P A
Bradley, S J
Bradley, W A
Brady, T L
Brick, S J
Brown, T H
Browning, H
Browning, S T
Buck, M E
Burrow, S
Buxton, T S
Byrne, A J
Calvert, J P
Campbell, A E
Carr-Hill, S M M
Carr, N D
Catling, S J
Ch'ng, C L
Chamberlain, G V P
Chamberlain, J O P
Chare, M J B
Clement, D A
Clements, D M
Closs, S P
Cobbold, S S
Collinson, M A
Coombs, I P
Cooper, M A C S
Cosgrove, M
Costello, C
Craven, S
Cray, E B
Cribb, C T
Crossland, P E
Cummings, P
Daniel, C J
Danino, C E
Danino, S M
Davies, A W
Davies, D E
Davies, D H
Davies, D H
Davies, E G
Davies, I
Davies, J L
Davies, J O C
Davies, J S S
Davies, J H
Davies, L
Davies, M
Davies, M M R
Davies, M J
Davies, O M
Davies, P J
Davies, R S
Davies, R N
Davies, S E
Davies, S P
Davies, T M
Davis, P L
Dawkins, C J
Dawson, A
De Arce Seuba, C D
Delahunty, A M
Devichand, N
Dinsdale, C L
Donnelly, P
Donnelly, P D
Downes, E M
Downing, H A
Drew, P J
Duane, P D
Dwyer, R E
Dyer, D F
Eales, M C
Ebden, P
Edwards, A G K
Edwards, P A
El-Sharkawi, A M M
Elkholy, M E S M
Emery, S J
Eshun, J A
Evans, A D
Evans, D H
Evans, D R
Evans, H J
Evans, J E
Evans, J E
Evans, K E
Evans, M L
Evans, M J
Evans, M J
Evans, R J
Evans, R M
Evans, R B
Evans, S L
Evans, S E
Evans, T I
Factor, D C
Fareedi, M A
Fareedi, S
Ferguson, M M
Fielder, C P
Fligelstone, L J
Flowers, C I
Flynn, P M
Foulkes, A L
Gajek, A
Gajek, W R
Ganeshanantham, S
Ghosh, S
Ghuman, B S
Gibbons, C P
Gibbs, M D
Gilbey, A G
Giltinan, W M
Goni Sarriguren, A
Gowda, S
Gray, H M
Griffiths, C J M
Griffiths, R D
Grimes, C J
Gunneberg, A
Gwynne Hughes, L A
Hammond, T J
Hancock, C
Harding, A M
Harkness, J M
Harrigan, M J
Harris, E E L
Harris, J A
Harris, L A
Harris, P
Harris, R C
Harris, W
Harrison, N K
Harry, C R
Harry, L E
Harvey, D J
Hawkins, A K I
Hayes, S L
Helan, S A
Hennessy, A I
Henwood, M
Hill, J A
Hill, R J
Hilliard, J J
Hilliard, J S
Hockridge, K S
Hodder, S C
Hoddinott, H C
Hopkin, J M
Hopkins, C L
Hopkins, M K
Horsman, D C
Howells, G
Howells, M L
Hudson, A J R
Hudson, C N
Hughes, D P
Hughes, E
Hughes, K
Hughes, R I
Hutson, H S F
Huws, A M
Ingram, W A
Irvine, R J M
James-Ellison, M Y
James, E T R
Jenkins, C I
Jenkins, C
Jenkins, G H
Jenkins, K L
Jenkins, S P
Jerwood, D C
Joannides, T
Johns, C J C
Johns, P F
Johns, S R
Jones, A
Jones, A W
Jones, B G
Jones, C E
Jones, D A
Jones, D M
Jones, E W L
Jones, E G
Jones, G O
Jones, G H
Jones, H M
Jones, I T
Jones, J
Jones, L E L
Jones, M
Jones, M K
Jones, R R
Jones, S R
Jones, T R
Jones, T A
Jones, W H L
Joynson, D H M
Keveligham, E
Khan, M A L
Kumari, A V B
Laing, J H E
Lake, D N W
Lathbridge, A B
Lawrence, M R
Laws, D E
Leary, J A
Lennox, S D
Leopold, J D
Levy, B
Lewis, A M
Lewis, A M
Lewis, H B
Lewis, M
Lewis, M S
Leyshon, R L
Littlepage, B N C
Llewellyn-Jones, S A
Llewelyn, R W
Lloyd Jones, F R
Lloyd, A P
Lloyd, B W
Lloyd, D R
Lloyd, K R
Lloyd, R C
Long, D H
Long, H R
Lucas, M G
Lyons, R A
McCabe, M J
McCarry, M E
McCarthy, M E
McDonald, J
McFadzean, W A
McGill, F J
McGregor, A D
McKenzie, R J
Maddock, H
Maddocks, J A
Maganas Aguilera, I
Maggs, A G
Maggs, R G
Major, E
Major, H G
Mamiso, J A
Mangat, P S
Mansell-Watkins, T
Manson, E F
Manson, J M
Mason, R A
Masoud, R
Matthes, J W A
Matthews, P C
Matthews, P L
Meecham Jones, S M
Mellor, C H
Meredith, E L
Milling, M A P
Millington, I M
Moore, D
Morgan, A G L
Morgan, A R
Morgan, B
Morgan, C R
Morgan, G
Morgan, I L
Morgan, J R
Morgan, J E
Morgan, J E
Morgan, L B
Morgan, L G
Morgan, M
Morgan, P G

Morgan, R N W
Morgan, S M
Morris, A D
Mortimer, R J
Murison, M S C
Najib, R A M
Nash, P E
Nesling, P M
Newington, D P
Newman, F
Noone, B E M
Norris, P
Norton, A
Nowak, J J R
O'Brien, C J
O'Kane, M J
O'Malley, H F
Oldham, M M
Olliffe, D J
Oppel, A B L G
Owen, D
Parker, J L
Patel, B
Patel, G M
Patel, N
Perkins, P P
Phillipps, J J
Phillips, G B
Phillips, S J
Pickering, A
Pickering, E E
Pincott, R G
Piskorowskyj, N
Pogson, D G
Potter, R J
Poulden, M A
Powell, N
Power, A L
Prasad, P M
Price, D E
Price, N
Pritchard, A
Pritchard, S R
Raichoudhury, B S
Ramsey, M W
Rayani, A P
Raynsford, A D
Redfern, R M
Rees-Jones, E C
Rees, A D
Rees, A M
Rees, H G
Rees, J W
Rees, L J
Rees, S D R
Rees, S O
Regan, F M
Richards, A M
Richards, D G
Richards, K
Richardson, C E
Rickards, C
Rickards, M
Ridgewell, M C
Riordan, T P
Roberts, D L L
Roberts, D E
Roberts, S M
Rogers, D W
Roman, R M
Rose, M B
Rosser, B
Rowley, K H M
Rushworth, F H
Russell, I D
Sadler, M J
Sait, C L
Salter, K E U
Samuel, C
Samuel, T W
Sansbury, M A
Sartori, J E
Sartori, N
Sawhney, I M S
Schreuder, F B
Scott, G
Seager, M J
Sharaf, U I
Shenolikar, V
Shuttleworth, G N
Silvester, K C
Simpkins, H G
Sinha, A K
Sinha, S
Sivakumaran, V
Slowey, H F
Stanton, J A
Staple, G
Statham, B N
Steene, L
Stefanutto, T B
Stevenson, A D
Stubbs, P G
Sullivan, C L
Sullivan, M J
Sullivan, H J
Sweetman, B J
Talbot, J S
Talukder, S B
Tarr, G
Thomas, A
Thomas, D W
Thomas, D C
Thomas, I R J
Thomas, J S
Thomas, L A
Thomas, M A
Thomas, P
Thomas, R
Thomas, S D
Thomas, W I
Thomas, W R G
Thorpe, C M
Todd, C
Tofazzal, N
Tomos, H W
Treseder, A S
Truman, K H
Tudor-Jones, T
Upton, N
Vaughton, K C
Wagstaff, J
Wall, T J
Wani, M A
Watkeys, J E M
Weatherill, B A
Webster, P P
Weiser, R
Werner, D J S
West, A P
Westerholm, R
Weston, C F M
Weston, S N
White, C P
White, M
White, N M L
Whitehead, M J
Whittet, H B
Wilkins, E A
Williams, A J
Williams, B
Williams, D D R
Williams, D J
Williams, D W
Williams, J G
Williams, J G
Williams, J C
Williams, M E
Williams, N W
Williams, N S
Williams, P A M
Williams, S
Yoganathan, K
Yoganathan, M
Yong, C H
York, J R
Youhana, A Y
Zaidi, S H A
Zaki, M M R

Swindon
Achar, U
Adams, S
Ahilan, R
Ahmad, S L
Amies, P L
Armstrong, J S
Arya, R
Aslam, H B H
Aslam, M N
Austin-Pugh, C K W
Babington, P C B
Bahia, S S
Baker, A R M
Barnard, H
Barnes, M D
Barnes, P A
Barry, C N
Batten, D A
Beale, A M
Beeby, C P
Bentley, J
Best, N R
Bestwick, J R
Bhambra, M K
Birley, D A H
Blesing, N E
Bliss, W A
Bond, A P
Brooke, S R M
Buck, J W
Bullock, R A
Burgess, P
Campbell, D N C
Campbell, H J
Cannon, C H
Carroll, N J
Carron, R I
Chalstrey, S E
Chandler, H A
Chippendale, S M
Clements, P J
Cluett, B E
Colley, C M
Collins, C A M
Collins, D A
Crossley, N A
Crouch, P A
Cullimore, J E
Currie, I G
Dale, A
Davies, A G
Day, J R
De Silva, L W
Deo, S D
Dhanulshan, P
Eastgate, J W
Elliman, J C
Entwistle, M D
Evans, G J
Eyre, R
Fan, S F
Ferguson, D R
Finch, D R A
Finch, D J
Flew, J P
Fogg, A J B
Foy, M A
Freakley, G C H
Frost, J A
Galea, M H
Gent, P M
Gilbert, C J
Gill, J
Glass, R E
Glover, J R
Godfray, D M
Graham, F C
Grain, L A T
Gray, A G
Green, D E
Green, E S
Griffiths, D J
Guilding, R C
Gupta, H M
Hall, C A B
Hanson, P J V
Hardy, R P
Hassan, S N
Heaton, D C
Hellier, J M
Hellier, M D
Hibbert, G A
Hicks, S C
Hillman, R
Hilton, J W
Hocken, D B
Holden, C G
Holden, R E M
Holliday, E
Holmes, R J L
Howard, D J
Hunt, N G
Iacovou, J W
Ivory, E A
Ivory, J P
Jackson, D M
Jackson, L K
Jackson, P D
James, B H E
James, C M
Janson, W R
Jephson, C G
John, D D
Jones, A M M
Jones, H E
Jones, R M
Juniper, M C
Kandiah, A
Kelly, A R M
Kendall, I G
Kidney, E M
Kilaru, N P P
Killick, F M
King, J M
Kowalczyk, A M
Kumar, R
Lal, A
Lavelle, S E
Lawrence, R N
Le Coyte, T S J
Lee, M J
Leonard, A J
Leung, J O S
Ling, E A
Lloyd, C R
Lowdon, I M R
McCrea, W A
Maciejewska, E M
Macintyre, A R
Mack, P R
McKemey, M J
Mackinlay, C I
Macoustra, S A
Maitland-Ward, K
Mann, R J
Mansour, J T
Marshall, J M H
Mayes, P J
Mearns, E A
Mercer, J H
Metcalfe, J A
Milner, S L
Mukherjee, D
Myatt, I W
Narayan, H
Nath, R
Newell, A G
Newton, A S
Newton, H
Nixon, R G
O'Brien, M K
O'Brien, T P
O'Connell, P J
O'Connor, M
O'Keeffe, P T A
O'Kelly, S W
Oliver, E
Owen-Jones, J M S
Parks, R G
Pickworth, A J
Pierzchniak, P
Pigott, S C
Price, E J
Price, H L
Ramananandan, A
Rawlins, D B
Rhodes, S
Robbins, J C
Robinson, D K
Rooney, G J
Schlesinger, P E
Scholes, K T
Scott, T E
Scurr, J A
Sewell, S P
Shad, I A
Sleggs, J H
Smith, A M L
Smith, I D
Smith, P T
Speller, C J
Stagles, M J
Stean, M L
Steptoe, A M
Strong, A M
Swinyard, P W
Ta, T C
Tang, C W M
Tattersall, M P
Taylor, E J
Taylor, S J
Tew, D N
Thavaraj, M
Thilakawardhana, W D P
Thomas, H G
To, S S
Turbin, D R
Valentine, M J
Van Hamel, J C M
White, J H
Whitworth, A G
Williams, P M G
Williamson, D M
Winfield, D
Woodhouse, W J
Woods, D A
Woodworth, A E
Wooller, D M
Wright, F A
Wright, J F
Yerbury, N O
Zengeya, S T

Tadcaster
Cronin, H F
Dryburgh, W A
Hayes, M
Haynes, J C
Inglis, A E
James, D
Lee, T W R
Parsons, J M
Peel, A J
Reeves, W J
Turton, C L
Turton, E P L
Willis, D
Woodhouse, J C

Tadley
Adler, V
Bhanot, S D
Brough, P R
Caren, C A
Castle, S L
Colley, S J
Finch, J M
Hawken, R M A
Kenshole, D H
Knowles, C
Perkins, A M Y
Peters, J
Ridsdale, P A
Waddingham, R

Tadworth
Adams, R E
Ahmad, N
Battinson, A N
Bowen-Davies, P E
Brown, E A
Cantopher, T G A
Carpenter, S F
Croft, R S
Day, B P
Dua, L G S
Fielding, A
Goodger, N M
Gordon, S J
Graham, A E
Hargreaves, R M
Harris, S A
Haywood, S
Hermon, G A
Hudson, S L
Jenkins, P A
Juchniewicz, H J
Krapez, J R
Kumar, D
Kumar, K A
Lam, K-P
Malik, A
Moorthy, V
Orme-Smith, E A
Pawulski, Y M
Phillips, C E W
Pitsiaeli, A P
Rowlands, M W D
Singh, S A
Stephenson, C A
Stott, P C
Symes, D M
Verity, H J
Webb, J

Tain
Colvin, I G
Gordon, S R
Graham, P D
Grant, G
Greenwood, J P
Macdonald, M
Macleod, I C
Runcie, J
Savage, K J
Skinner, J A

Tamworth
Ballard, P
Barker, G M
Beecham, K
Benkert, S T
Bird, S C
Boss, D P
Boss, V C
Bowen, Y M
Bruce, G J C
Carlisle, T A
Chambers, J S
Clamp, H
Clayson, M C
Cooke, L H
Crofts, K H M
Cutting, D L
Dabestani, E
Davis, M S K
Deshpande, A A
Edwards, A M
Fitzgerald, H M
Foist, J M E
Gordon, G
Griffiths, H M
Gummery, A R
Halpin, D C
Harrison, P S
Hawkes, R A
Hawkins, J B
Jawed, S H
Jones, C J
Jones, S P
Khan, L A
Killeen, P D
King, J M
King, M I
Lawrence, D R
Mair, B M
Martin, C A
Moosa, A S
Moroney, M M
Odber, E A
Pascoe, K L
Patel, R M
Popple, M D
Rajput, R A
Rajput, V K
Rastall, S J
Richardson, W L
Samson, H C
Sherlock, J D
Smith, J W
Spenceley, S R
Sreehari Rao, S
Stabler, J M
Turfrey, D M
Vaughan, P J
Wood, P M
Yazdani, Q

Tarbert
Gourlay, N J
Graham, F M
Howat, I M G
Maitland, J
Stewart, H V A

Tarporley
Bashford, S E
Black, H E W
Caesar, S R
Campbell, P A
Cartwright, A J
Chantler, S
Chappell, G M
Crockford, T K
Durrant, M A
Etherington, R J
Gething, J
Gleek, R N H
Grant, R H E
Griffin, J M
Halstead, N A
Hoy, A N
Hutchinson, K F C
Jones, M B
Mann, P M
Meekins, J W
O'Callaghan, N G
Phillipson, A P
Rowland, K
Stowe, H E
Taylor, K V
Vickers, J P

Taunton
Abdullah, S H
Ahmed, W
Anderson, E J
Ashworth, S L
Ballance, R J
Ball, J E
Barlow, H V L
Barrett, N K
Bates, A K
Beecher, H M
Bell, J M
Berry, M A
Bett, C J
Bevis, M J
Bhattacherjee, J W
Bhattacherjee, S
Bidgood, K A

Bilbrough, M
Bird, D F
Bird, R J
Black, P R M
Bolt, H L
Boyle, J
Brocksom, L A
Brook, R
Brown, T R
Browne, B L
Bryce, G M
Bulloch, C
Burton, H L
Cadman, D H
Cairns, S R M
Chadwick, R M
Chester, J F
Claridge, K G
Clarke, A M
Clear, J D
Close, C F
Cockett, A D
Collins, C D
Collins, S J
Cooper, S C
Cottrell, P W A
Crabb, K A
Crabtree, B J
Crabtree, R E
Davidson, J E
Davidson, M J C
Davies, S V
Dayani, A
Daykin, A P
Dean, D C
Desborough, R C
Devine, M D
Downs, D J
Drysdale, A J
Dunn, E J
Duthie, Y L
Edmondson, D B
Ellwood, M G
Evans, M
Eyre-Brook, I A
Fathers, E E
Fernando, A M R
FitzGerald, M R
Fletcher, M H
Forster, H
Fox, R
Frazer, S J
French, T J
Gardner, R J
Gauntlett, I S
Geraghty, E M
Geraghty, J M
Gillen, C D
Gorman, M S
Gormley, H K J
Gover, D E
Gover, S M
Gray, R H
Hakin, K N
Halfyard, A E A
Halliday, N J
Hamilton, S G
Hamlyn, J F
Hammerton, S P
Hanson, S D
Hanspal, R
Harris, N M C
Harrison, S R B
Hart, R J
Hesford, A C
Hickman, J
Highley, D A
Hinds, P J
Hobbs, R J
Howes, T R J
Husband, A D
James, M A
Jenkins, C
Johnson, C A
Johnson, S A N
Jones, C
Jowett, A E
Kelly, A J
Kelly, S E J
Kennedy, N J
Kilbey, R S
Klidjian, A M
Lane, P J
Laversuch, C J
Linder, A M
London, R J
Louis, J L
Lucas, J G
MacConnell, T J
MacDonagh, R P
MacGregor, R J
MacIver, D H
Mackenzie, N C
Mann, C J
Mann, R J
Manning, H P
Marsh, H
May, T F
Meads, J E D
Moore, J C
Moyse, B C
Needham, P J
Newell Price, R J
Nicholls, B J
O'Connell, S M
Ogilvie, C
Ostler, E G
Parkin, S G
Pascall, C R
Pascall, E J
Paul, M N
Pearson, N J
Pendered, L F
Penny, P T
Perry, A J
Pfeifer, C Z
Pollock, L M
Poole, A J
Powers, M J
Price, A N C
Pryce, D W
Pugh, S
Pullin, J A
Rainey, H A
Ramus, N I
Ravenscroft, P J
Rees, J L
Reilly, S J
Richardson, J A
Rivett, A
Rivett, R S
Robinson, B F
Rosser, M A
Rostron, M G
Roy, L C
Ruell, J A
Savage, R H
Scanlon, J G
Scott, G J
Sells, R W B
Siddique, M F
Sidwell, I P
Silsby, J F
Skinner, P J
Slack, A J
Sladden, J M
Smith, K
Smith, M P
Smith, M D
Smith, S C
Snell, R O L
Solanki, T G
Speakman, M J
Squire, P L B
Stone, R A
Swinburn, C R
Symons, L C
Tandy, A D
Thomas, H G
Thomas, P D
Thompson, C C
Thompson, E H
Thorpe, P L P J
Tighe, M
Till, K
Tipping, J P
Tolliday, J D
Trotter, P A
Turner, D R
Twomey, J M
Upton, J J M
Vipond, A J
Ward, T M G
Webster, M H
Welbourn, C R B
Wells, R
Wells, S K
Wells, S C
Williams, M H
Wrede, C D H
Yardley, M H
Yates, D B
Yates, M W
Yoxall, J H
Zilkha, T R

Tavistock

Allenby, W J
Barker, C S
Barrand, K G
Bertram, J
Craig, S M
Cullen, M S
Cummings, G C
Davies, I L
Evans, J A L
Evans, V L
Farr, A P
Gibbs, D S
Gude, R A
Jayarajah, J M
Kelsey, A M
Kersey, J P W
Liggins, S J
Lorenzi, A R
MacRostie, J A
Metcalf, E P
Nicholls, C S
Norgren, P M
Ostler, A M
Porterfield, P N
Rea, W E
Ridout, S S
Roberts, M A
Rodgers, P J
Speller, J C
Stokkereit, C
Vicarage, P H
Williams, H C
Wilson, R J

Taynuilt

Armstrong, K M D
Davies, A M

Tayport

Baxter, A G
Mires, G J
Simpson, H A
Torrance, W N

Teddington

Blake, C H
Bradley, J A
Brockbank, J
Brougham, P A
Brown, A M
Childs, A J
Cobb, J P
De Bruyne, V
Hempenstall, K
Johnson, T W
Kendall, A M
Mindlin, M J
Nicholas, R J
Pace, R F E
Patel, V
Patton, A
Ryle, D M
Scriminger, M W
Sinnott, C R
Wilson, J E H
Young, S M

Teignmouth

Best, F W
Billyard, J J C
Cooling, R M
Cullen, D
Finneran, N K
Halford, M
Halford, M G
Henley, A J
Karakusevic, C A
King, M H
McCormick, A J A
McGrath, P D P
Melluish, P G
Peirce, C R
Powell, E A
Randalls, P B
Rowbury, J L
Squires, J P
Tuck, S C
Venton, T J
Warland, J C

Telford

Ackroyd, P L
Ahmad, M
Ali, S F N
Awty, M W
Balasubramaniam, C
Bandak, R
Bartlett, M H
Barua, A R
Bateman, J M
Beck, G P
Blackmore, J
Brahmachari, A K
Brown, C I W
Calvert, J
Campbell, R R
Capps, E G S
Capps, N E
Carley, R H
Christmas, D
Chuter, P J
Clevenger, E O
Corser, G C
Coventry, C L
Crichlow, T P K R
Dawson, M J
De Klerk, C J
Diggory, R T
Donnellan, I M
Douglas, T A
Duffield, R G M
Frain, S P T
Freeman, C J
Goode, T B
Hailey, R W
Hastings, L I
Heber, M E
Herd, E J
Hickmott, K C
Hinde, F R J
Hinton, C E
Hinton, C P
Hogg, J S
Hoque, M S
Hugh, S E J
Hughes, D S
Hughes, T J H
Inglis, A R
Ingram, L C
Innes, M A
Jacobson, G A
Joy, R M
Kallan, B
Keohane, K M
Kirby, P J
Lane, M W
Leaman, A M
Lees, D A
Lewis, C J
McDonnell, T C
Manns, R A
Marray, P J
May, P C
Mell, A K
Metcalfe, E M
Mishra, S K
Mohamed, A O
Moudgil, H
Newman, P F
Nolan, E M
Northern, D G F
O'Gorman, D
Pandya, L
Park, D P
Parrish, D J
Pearson, C A R
Pelton, C I
Phillips, G H
Picard, L
Pringle, A J
Pritchard, S J
Rathbone, A R
Rathbone, E
Richards, G P
Richards, N C G
Richardson, J P A
Sanghera, S S
Shaw, P Q
Siddiqui, R
Singh, J
Spencer, K P
Summers, B N
Swallow, J W
Taylor, T L O
Thompson, G D
Usman, T
Visick, J
Wainwright, G A
Walsh, M T J
Ward, L S
Williams, M R
Williams, T D
Wright, D J
Yates, C J P
Zaki Ahmed, S M
Zaki, I

Templecombe

Beach, F X M
Courtenay, T M A
Reid, M J
Speight, J M

Tenbury Wells

Brereton, W J
Chesshire, J S I A
Eames, S M
Foster, N J
Goddard, S
Hardiman, J M A
Hardiman, M C
Hunter, J L
Lear, R J A
Mocroft, A P
Tinkler, R F W
Wright, A M

Tenby

Bowen, E J
Bowen, J M
Bowen, J R
Griffiths, A J
Hughes, W E
Riley, S E
Roberts, H G

Tenterden

Alaily, A B E
Charlesworth, D N
Clothier, J G
Cox, S P
Dodds, D H H
Dowling, J M
Ingle-Finch, F M
Lloyd-Smith, A R
Lloyds, D
Oliver, M C
Rowlands, D M

Tetbury

Kirby, A K
Leonard, L
Walsh, A
Wardell-Yerburgh, S J

Tewkesbury

Ashbridge, K
Atwick, D L
Buckley, R G
Carver, C H
Crossley, I R
Crowther, A N
Crowther, M A A
Cunningham, A C E
Davis, R W
Dore-Green, F
Dunlop, E M
Gormley, K M
Hutchison, S R
Johnson, J V
Lewis, M F
Lewis, M H
Macmorland, L A
Macmorland, T D L
Milliams, S L
Mitchell, M D
Mulrenan, M J
Renfrew, C C
Rigby, A N
Shervey, C S J
Stone, T D
Tuck, A W
Williams, K
Williams, R

Thame

Burch, K W
Chubb, C H T
Farmer, A J
Fisher, J D
Geaney, D P
Gleadle, J M
Green, S B J
Harrington, R V M
Jackson, T J
Jobson, T M
Keeley, D J
Markus, A C
Markus, P J M
Millo, J L B
Mistry, A
Neal, D A J
Paul, H-J
Taylor, H E A
Turner, S D
Vaughan, M S

Thames Ditton

Barnes, G M
Bezant, F J
Bullen, S
Cason, A P E
Gardner, C M
Glasgow, L V M
Griffiths, P K
Jebb, G A
Keating, F S J
Magrill, L H
Matthews, D J
Miller, A J
Mills, F
Mitchell, T J
Munn, O M A
Roberts, C A

Thatcham

Bahia, B S
Barrett, V J M
Caddy, A J
Harris, P
Hayward, J M
Mackinnon, A-L
Morgan, M W M
Nimmagadda, S R
Porter, K A
Rice, E D
Rixon, R A
Robertson, E A
Robertson, G A
Rudgley, R J
Smith, C C
Tayton, R G
Thompson, T M
Vevers, G W G
Williams, V N

Thetford

Ball, S M
Belsham, M P
Bryson, J L
De Bass, F W J
Gibbs, T J
Gray, P S L
Gregson, D
Hadley Brown, M
Hahn, I R
Henderson, W B
Hughes, M J M
Hunter, D M
Leventhorpe, J R B
Mahatme, D A S
Martin, S A
Nisbet, I G
Overy, M K D
Riddell, C W
Sagar, G A
Schram, J E
Smith, G R
Taylor, J
Williams, R J
Young, A G

Thirsk

Casey, P A
Cook, E J
Donald, J
Frith, M-D S
Garside, J H
Harrison, M T
Hiles, R J
Lyth, N A
Parker, C M
Pooley, S F
Potts, M A
Redman, J W
Shaw, C J
Spence, D P S
Trzeciak, A W
Wight, G R
Williamson, D K

Thornhill

Brodie, R
Brown, I M
Kennedy, J C B S
Robertson, E
Vernon, F H
Woolrych, R S

Thornton Heath

Bakare, R O
Dosaj, A K
Gooneratne, H
Holt, S N
Johnson, P H
Lumley, H S

Mehta, A J
Newland, R A
Newman-Sanders, A P G
Patel, C R
Ramsbotham, S E
Reardon, J A
Rodrigues, N F B
Suganthi, D P
Tarrant, K N
Whitehead, M A
Wilson, E B

Thornton-Cleveleys
Ahmed, R Y
Azurza Sorrondegui, K M
Boissiere, J A
Broadley, R M
Brown, H G
Cartmell, N V
Cooper-Smith, J H
Cowpe, J
Ford, W L
Forster, D M
Hendrickse, M T
Horsfield, P
Kitchen, S P
Llewellyn, D J
Matthews, J J
Naughton, A
Page, M E
Palin, P H
Pananghat, T P
Pilling, D J
Powell, M F
Rowland, B J
Sundar Rao, P
Turner, B A
Walford, D H H
Whittle, A D

Thurso
Brooks, A G
Burnett, G R M
Deans, J P
Findlay, S R
Fraser, M E
Irons, G S
Kelly, D J
Lee, J A W
Lee, R J
Mackay, N
Macleod, W J J
McNeill, D
McNeill, W
Morris, G J A
Morrison, J D
Page, J P A
Robertson, A H A

Tidworth
Harley, O J H
King, B M
Kuber, A
Piper, M E

Tighnabruaich
Carle, G
Irvine, J I

Tilbury
Archer, R
Lake, C G
Malvankar, G K J
Saha, P K
Sundaresan, T

Tillicoultry
Basquill, M P
Brodie, J E
Clark, G P
Edmunds, N J
Galloway, L
Harrower, N A
King, J A
Seaman, F M

Tintagel
Richardson, R

Tipton
Bradley, K M
Browne, C J
Dayani, L N
Leadbeater, C M
Loryman, B J L
Patel, H D L
Robinson, A J
Solomon, G
Sullivan, R P
Swiestowski, I
Walton, I J

Tiverton
Backhouse, P J
Batth, M S
Bloom, J N A
Bull, P M
Clark, C E
Coulter, M E
Davies, J R L
Davies, M C
Grieve, D I
Johnson-Ferguson, S J
Leach, A L M
Maltby, S D
Marcus, P
Mew, C J
Miller, A J
Miller, P M
Monahan, J
Mounsey, R M
O'Kelly, F P
Peters, G K
Revolta, A D
Rumble, P B
Seymour, M T J
Seymour, S-J
Sheridan, J H

Todmorden
Cormack, A S
Davey, N P
Dearden, V A
Ehrhardt, P O G
Grewal, A P S
Harrison, A J
Ketley, S J
Lofthouse, R A
Ransome, P J
Ryland, D A
Sacco, J
Williams, G

Tonbridge
Anderson, I R M
Anderson, J S N
Baker, J W
Baldwin, A
Bench, P D
Blewett, K A
Borley, N C
Bowman, C M
Brookes, E J
Castro, K A
Cheales, N A
Christophers, J
Coles, S R D
Cowan, N A
Davies, M C
Dawson, M J
Devenport, C E
England, J M
Evans, K G C
Evans, N J
Ford, J M T
Fraser, I M M
Gibbins, N E
Gildeh, P B
Goodridge, D M G
Goozee, P R
Hayden, J T
Howitt, A J
Ironmonger, M R
Jenner, M J R
Jutting, I G C
Kelynack, J B
Kirby, G
Law, E M J
Legg, O C
Lloyd Davies, S H
Love, M E
McCarthy, L S L
Mahadevan, J
Manifold, D K
Manifold, N J
Marshall, M A B
Minett, N P
Moore, J P
Morgan, J E
Morris, M J
Nida, A M
O'Carroll, A A
Palmer, T A
Potter, N D M
Potterton, K L
Quinlan, J M
Reynolds, M M
Ripley, L H
Roberts, J M
Russell, E C
Sanders, F L
Sleight, C L
Smale, S J
Smith-Laing, G
Stuart-Buttle, C D G
Taylor, A F
Thomas, K J
Warner, C M
Watson, J V
Whillier, D E
Whitehead, E J
Wilson, J A
Woodhouse, P A

Tonypandy
Baron, R T
Barr, R S G
Edwards, D A
Jenkins, M A
Jones, D S
Lees, A P
Llewellyn, R
Morgans, D L
Rahman, M A
Rahman, S
Tirupathi-Rao, M

Torpoint
Bristow, A H
Crook, J C
Davis, A J
Davis, M P
Fraser, V G
Gask, J
Jolly, R T
Kehoe, J E
McEleny, P C
Mallett, B L
Mattholie, K M
O'Leary, T D
Pollard, J G
Scaglioni, F G
Stewart, M W
Woffenden, L R
Wylie, R D S

Torquay
Ackford, C
Adams, S J
Alderson, D J
Allen, K P
Alston, A K
Anderson, L
Ashworth, M J
Athow-Frost, T A M
Bailey, N P
Barrington, J W
Barton, P M B
Birdsall, P D
Bosley, P V
Bradbrook, R A
Broomhall, J
Brown, M R
Buley, I D
Burke, N J
Campbell, N N
Cannizzaro, S
Carey, C M U
Chadwick, R G
Cole, M D
Crocker, K L
Currie, I C
Da Cruz, D J Z
Daniels, C H L
De Friend, D J
Douglas, P S
Dyer, R G
Edwards, D
Elliott, H A
Ellis, A W
Fearnley, R H
Fearnley, S-J
Field, K J
Fisher, N
Fitchett, L
Fitter, A C
Fletcher, T G
Fordyce, A M
Forward, P J
Foster, R N
Fothergill, G
Foulkes, J E B
Fox, L C
Fox, M
Gardner, G C E
Gardner, G J
Gardner, S J
Ghazi, A
Gillespie, C M
Goldman, J M
Gould, S M
Graham, C M
Greenwell, D G
Hamad, Z M S
Hearn, M
Horner, J E
Horvath, R S
Houghton, K
Huckle, J A
Hughes, R G
Hunt, P G
Hutchinson, P F
Hutchison, J D
Imong, S M
Irvine, G B
Isaacs, J L
Jacobs, A G
James, C R H
Jones, G
Judge, B P P
Keeling, P J
Kember, P G
Kendall, G P N
Kuyyamudi, C U
Ladwa, V G
Lambourn, J
Law, D J
Lewis, P
Livesey, S J
Lowes, J R
Lydon, A P M
McCarthy, D A
McCarthy, R J
MacDermott, J P A
Maceachern, A G
Mackay, N N S
McKay, R E
Mahy, I R J
Malherbe, C J
Marshall, J H
Martin, A C
Mason, M
Mew, I P
Mihssin, N K
Mitchell, S J
Molan, C J
Montgomery, J E
Moore, P L
Morrell, I R
Morris, E
Morris, S C
Natusch, D I
Nofal, M A-E M S
Paisey, R B
Paley, H
Pappin, J C
Perry, J F
Pullan, R D
Roberts, P J
Rovira, P A
Ryley, N G
Sadler, A P
Sainsbury, C P Q
Scanlan, C M
Scott, C A
Seymour, R
Shute, P A
Sinclair, D G
Sleight, P J
Smith, K J
Smith, S R
Smith, S J
Snow, D J
Speake, J G
Spear, D W
Stainforth, J N
Stannard, P J
Swart, M L
Tackley, R M
Takyi, A
Teague, R H
Thomas, E A
Thorn, V M
Tresidder, I R
Tucker, A J
Tucker, H S
Tucker, S C
Tudor, G P
Turner, D L
Urquhart, G W
Varvinsky, A M
Watts, E C
White, P G
Williams, C A K
Williams, D A W
Willmer, J M
Wilson, P G
Womersley, H C
Young, H L
Young, J D

Torrington
Armstrong, B D J
Armstrong, T
Bangay, A P D
Berger, D W
Bremner, A E
Lamb, N C
Martineau, J G
Patterson, M D
Thomas, R A N

Totnes
Barratt, D K
Benatt, J
Benzies, R A O
Blackshaw, R E
Born, A J
Buckingham, S J
Burston, J
Cooper, N A
Crickmay, J R
Crowe, S P
Curtin, D M
Feloy, J M L
Frankland, A W
Franklin, J A C
Greene, W J W
Hall, G F M
Hanrott, S F
Harrison, S L
Hayne, D
Hendy, S C
Hubregtse, G
Hunt, M S
Ingham, J N
Ingoldsby, B J
Leney, B V
Lewendon, G
Lewis, A D
Lewis, R J
Loverock, M
Manser, T I
O'Brien, J A
Oxtoby, S J
Pettinger, A J
Peyton-Jones, B
Richi, M N M
Somerville, M
Tatham, P H
Teague, G
Thompson, E M
Thould, G R
Todd, N B

Towcester
Campion, J C
Davies, A J
Greenhalgh, J E
Greenhalgh, M G
Gwilt, D J
Hamer, S A
Hooker, A N
Sayers, I G
Stoddart, P E B
Sunderland, J R
Supple, M A
Wallace, R B
Ward, N J
Yarrow, S

Tranent
Cameron, C
Crawford, Y E B
Donaldson, I D
Driscoll, P J
Halliday-Pegg, J C
Ingham, L J
Lange, P J
MacNair, J D
Macrae, A M
Morrison, J
Reid, A I
Russell, K J
Salter, D M

Tredegar
Baker, D
Davies, H J
Hla Bu, Dr
Lamerton, R C
Payne, S A
Pritchard, M G
Singh, A
Sinha, S

Tregaron
Gealy, S E
Heneghan, F A
James, J A
Langley, R C
Thomas, K L

Treharris
Batuwitage, B T
Das, D
Dharmasiri, A H C
Morgan, N S
Nath, M L
Phadke, A S
Rees, J L
Williams, A J

Treorchy
Gopala Krishna, P
Obaji, A K K
Sarnobat, M S
Sarnobat, S R
Singh, H

Trimdon Station
Carter, J M
Robinson, D E
Saunders, F C
Srirangalingam, S
Srirangalingam, T S S

Tring
Baxter, R M
Cannon, H L
Gupta, A
Hall-Jones, A H
Higginson, A G
Lane, R S
Livingston, G
Livingston, S J M
Ogden, D J
Roberts, R N F
Thallon, D F E
Tomlinson, P
Wainwright, A J R
Woodward, A J

Troon
Auld, C M
Baird, C H
Baird, P J
Beatson, J M
Brown, J
Crumlish, P
Elliott, M E
Hamilton, R M
Hildebrand, P J
Hill, A M O
Lawrie, S C
Lloyd, H J
McGregor, A J
McHattie, A G
Mackay, D H W
Macpherson, J M
Miller, T D
Mohammed, E P
Morran, C G
Morrison, A D
O'Neill, D M
Pittam, J K
Potts, H E
Scott, M E
Sugden, B A
Thomson, P H G
Whyte, R B
Williams, G R

Trowbridge
Baker, Z C
Bimbh, K S
Bryant, G
Clark, S J A
Collins, R A
Cookson, T W S
Duckworth, M J B
Foggett, C
Gracias, S A
Harris, A
Hole, J G
Jay, G E
Jones, R N
Locke, S M
Lodge, L J
Munro, M E
Nelson, G S
Nye, B M

Parr, L S
Rope, T C
Rowlands, S C
Slack, J E
Smales, K A
Swan, I R
Thompson, L V

Truro
Adams, E F M
Adcock, S D
Al-Rawi, S J A
Asplin, C M
Ball, H J
Ballam, J M D
Barnes, J N
Barton, S J
Battle, M O
Bendall, R P
Bishieri, S Y G
Bishop, L S
Black, M P
Boissonade, J
Bolton, J A R
Bourne, R
Bowers, P W
Bracey, D J
Bridger, V J
Bridges, V J
Bryson, P R C
Caldicott, M L
Callen, P J
Campbell, G F
Campbell, S M
Carruthers, W A F
Casey, S F
Chambers, J C
Christensen, D M C L
Conrad, G J
Cook, P G
Coutts, I I
Cox, R
Cran, J S
Creagh, M D
Crouse, M W
Dalal, H M
Dalton, H R
Dalziel, K L
Daniels, M V
Davies, J N
Davies, M T
Dingwall, A E
Dodenhoff, R M
Edwards, G P L
Evans, C D
Evans, S J
Evers, J-A G
Fairman, H D
Falkner, M J
Farmer, K D
Fern, E D
Ffrench-Constant, E P S
Follett, O J
Foote, J W
Galbraith, D
Gilbertson, N J
Godbehere, P R
Gray, N I D B
Gray, S J
Graymore, R I
Griffiths, D P G
Gripper, M B
Gripper, S M
Grundy, G V
Grundy, J R B
Gunn, K L
Hambly, A T
Hancock, J H O
Harper, S H
Harvey, A J N
Harvey, W R
Hasan, S S
Hawkins, S J
Hayes, D F G
Hellyar, E A
Hobbs, A J
Hocking, M A
Hood, D A
Howarth, P A W
Howarth, S M R B
Hussaini, S H
Hutchins, P M
Hyslop, J S
Jakt, L M
James, K M
Jervis, M J
Johnston, P A
Johnston, R T
Jones, K R
Joseph, E
Julian, C G
Keane, F E A
Laing, C M
Lansley, C V
Lee, A S
Lester, J E
Lichy, R J
Liddicoat, A J
Lloyd-Davies, E R V
McIntosh, S P
McKendrick, M N
McLean, B N
Maling, D J
Maskell, G F
Mathew, J
May, A J
Metcalfe, M W
Mitchell, M D
Mohammed, S
Moon, C A L
Morgan, G A R
Morgan, J
Mourant, A J
Munyard, P F
Murrell, J S
Murrell, S J
Myers, E
Myers, J D
Newman, R M
Noble, R S
Nyman, V A
O'Rourke, J S
O'Shea, S B
Parsons, S W
Peace, P K
Perrett, J M
Pettit, B
Pinching, A J
Pitcher, R W
Pitman, R H
Portch, H R
Powell, J F
Price, A S
Proctor, M C D
Radford, I S
Raj, A A
Raj, S P
Rayner, N
Redding, G A
Redington, A N
Rickford, C R K
Rotheray, C F
Round, K W
Rowe, P R
Rozario, J A C
Schofield, C M
Scott, T D
Short, P
Siddig, M A N
Simpson, L
Sinclair, J R
Slade, A K B
Smith, G D P
Smith, I M
Smith, W H
Stepp-Schuh, K
Stockwell, A J
Stone, D R
Sullivan, M
Taylor, G P
Telfer Brunton, W A
Thacker, E J
Theophilus, M N
Thompson, A B
Thorogood, S V
Tisdale, J B
Vaidya, D V
Veal, C T
Vowles, S C
Walker, A K Y
Warner, A P
Wheatley, D A
White, C R
Whiteley, W N
Widdison, A L
Wilde, A D
Willis, R G
Wilson-Holt, N J
Winterton, E A
Winterton, M C
Wood, K A
Woodward, W M
Woolf, A D

Tunbridge Wells
Aron, U
Asprey, J C
Bamford, P N
Banks, P
Banks, R A
Barnaby, H J
Barnes, D J
Bell, J A
Bentley, P G
Bergin, P M D
Boles, P R
Bolger, P G
Bolsover, W J
Bolton, J M H
Bolton, V J
Bowden, A S
Bowden, P C
Bowes, R J
Bradshaw, N J M
Bruce, J M
Buckland, A G
Bull, A R
Cameron, A J
Charlwood, G P
Charlwood, G J
Chase, A J
Chellappah, M
Christopher, J B
Chung, R A
Cooke, J B
Cordell, R J
Costain, D W
Cottrell, P R
Cripps, J R
Crosby, Z V
Cynk, M S
Davie, W J A
Day, P
Delaney, D M
Dismorr, K J
Dodman, S
Doyle, Y G
Edwards, A R
Edwards, D M
Ellwood, N H
Engleback, M
Everest, M S
Finlay, K D
Firth, D A
Flanagan, J J
Fleming, I M G
Flute, D F
Flynn, G M
Ford, T F
Fordyce, M J F
Gabbott, M C
Galliford, J W
Garrett, J P
Garrioch, D B
Garthwaite, S E
Gibb, P A
Gillett, D S
Gladstone, D I
Green, D J
Grieve, A J
Hall, S A
Hangartner, J R W
Hardie, T J
Harrington, D W M
Harris, A W
Hassan, H M G E D
Hedley, K R
Hicks, G E
Hirst, C I
Hughes, J A
Hurlow, D
Hutchinson, H T
Ignotus, P I
Ironside, J G
Jacques, S L
James, S
Jenner, M R
Jones, A C
Jones, D I
Kendall, C
Kilcoyne, M T
Kirwan, M C
Kirwan, S E M
Knight, D M A
Kwong Hong Tsang, P H H
Langrish, C J
Lawes, M R
Lawson, C S
Lewis, J L
Lewis, S G
Liebmann, R D
Lloyd Davies, S K
Loke, H T R
Loveday, R
McAllister, T W J
Macdonald-Brown, A J
MacDonald, J C
Mace, P J E
McEvedy, M B
MacFarlane, D G
McPherson, J S
Maling, J A
Mancais, P A
Marshall, J K
Martin, P J
Matthews, M P
Maw, D S J
Mills, P M M
Mills, P M
Mueller, M F F
Nicholl, J E
Pearson, J M
Pedlow, P L
Pyne, A
Raju, K S
Reeves, K E G
Reynolds, P J
Robards, M F
Roberts, L A
Robson, E
Rodwell, N A
Roome, J K
Roome, P C
Rorke, S
Rose, C E
Russell, G A
Sachdeva, L
Sachdeva, S K
Sawyer, C J
Schellander, F G
Sergeant, R J
Shakoor, S
Sharma, N
Shotton, J C
Sikorski, A D A
Sinclair, R M
Sinden, M P
Skerry, C A
Skinner, P W
Smith, D E
Somerville, D R
Soon, S Y
Stone, N
Streeten, N C
Tanner, N S B
Taylor, A L J
Taylor, C G
Tharakaram, S
Topa, G N F
Tuckwell, G D
Turrell, C M
Tuson, K W R
Twydell, H J
Tyrrell, M R
Wakankar, H M
Walmsley, G L
Warr, O C
Welch, N M
Whichello, K J
Wilcox, M A
Williams, I
Williams, S J
Williams, T G
Wilski-Jaloszynski, A
Winceslaus, S J
Wolfle, A D
Woolgar, M J
Worthley, P
Wykes, C E
Yates, D W
Yates, H A

Turriff
Connell, D G
Duthie, K E S
Fraser, K G
Fraser, R B I
Graham, K
Guthrie, P N
Henderson, S C
Liddell, R W
Milne, M H
Robertson, A G C
Robertson, S B
Smith, A P W
Watson, C

Twickenham
Adams, A M
Alexander, D J
Andrews, J L
Badgett, W J L
Bird, J H
Boohan, T L
Cash, M E
Cawrse, N H
Chapman, C M
Christie, B A
Cook, V A M
Davey, L F
Dhillon, P J
Edmonds, J
Elliott, D S
Gallagher, L M G
Gardner, M L
Goldwyn, C R L
Gonzalez Carvajal, J R
Hall, A J M
Hameed, S A
Harper, M N
Holmes, S C
Hotson, P A
Johal, B S
Kanchan, B S
Kemp, S P T
Khan, S
Kumaran, J
Kumaran, V E
Loughridge, L W
McCarthy, M R
McCarthy, T
Mathew, M C F
Mehta, M H
Moore, K J
Mullan, E M
Ng, W S
Nicholas, R S J
O'Flynn, K G
Payan, J
Pearson, J G H
Pugh, J K
Raheja, S K
Rees, J P M
Rigby, S P
Robertson, A G
Rowlands, G P
Salih, A R M M
Sandler, M
Sardesai, B S
Sardesai, S H
Savage, P
Sebaratnam, N R
Sharma, R
Shenton, F G A
Smith, C J
Somani, R
Sood, A
Sowden, P A
Stevenson, C W
Teodorczuk, A M
Thomas, F M
To, T H
Todd, D B
Trayner, I A M
Turvey, J S
Unadkat, M D
Unadkat, M M
Vaziri, K
Walawender, A J
Warren, E S L
Whittingham, C G N
Wilson, C L

Tycroes
Williams, O M

Tyn-y-Gongl
Jones, C A C
Lewis, J D
Lupton, D J
Williams, D L

Tywyn
Bishton, R B B
Church, D S
Coward, J
Farrell, D L
Lycett, N A
Taylor, T A

Uckfield
Argyrou, N A
Brown, C L
Clare, C A
Fabre, C D
Gent, P N C
Giles, J W
Gurney, M J T
Jephcott, C G A
Johnson Smith, E J
Mayo, K M
Meikle, C J P
Merritt, R A
Nicholl, J L
Oliver, J
Petit, C G C
Phillips, M C R
Rogers, M C
Sawcer, D
Sewell, E
Skinner, C P R
Sly, I L C
Wright, D S

Ullapool
Diack, G A M
Dumughn, D B
Hartley, I M
McDougall, C
Peebles, M A C
Stewart, A
Watmough, G I

Ulverston
Bottrill, D
Brady, D
Brice, J A R
Butler, A S
Callingham, R F
Cooper, M A
Elliott, S A
Forbes, R D
Graham, J P
Horsley, S D
Hubbard, I H
Johnstone, I C
Lyness, A L
Maguire, G R
Milne-Redhead, B
Moore, G J
Parnell, C E
Rayner, L
Redman, P J
Savage, M
Schmidt, J
Sherwin, J R A
Sherwin, K E
Unnikrishnan, M
Wilson, L A

Umberleigh
Hambley, A B
Harper, G D
Mair, A
Payne, C E
Payne, M J

Upminster
Anfilogoff, M E
Anthony, J R
Baig, M M
Baig, S S
Beaton, A
Brooks, W V
Chakravarty, P
Chopra, P K
Dahs, C
Daniel, D
Foley, E P
Haider, S S
Haider, S I
Hails, A J
Hollowbread, A
Maitra, K
Menon, N P
Rix, R D
Sangar, S K
Sudha, I K
Werry, C A

Upton
Anderson, J A
Ferguson, R
George, E
Hennessy, M S
Rittoo, D

Usk
Allison, M C
Bodley Scott, R
Botting, J R
Brown, G M
Brown, M J K M
Fairweather, S J
Frampton, C
Hartley, R B
Howells, R J
Huckle, P L
Jarrett, A G
Jarrett, S A
King, M R
Nandy, D

Parry, A
Perry, A
Perry, D R A
Preece, J M
Robinson, D A
Watkins, J

Uttoxeter
Aldridge, R V H
Barron, O P
Bennett, J
Brookfield, C D R
Burlinson, A A
Burton, R C
Dalton, T M
Holroyd, B
Johnson, A F
Jones, S G W
McCosh, C
Magapu, V
Pashby, N L
Sicha, M A
Trewin, P J H
Wainwright, C T
Webster, N C H

Uxbridge
Ackland, G L
Ahmad, S
Amrani, M
Armstrong, F M
Arthur, I H
Asher, R
Assaf, A K
Atrah, S G K
Banerjee, R
Bangham, L C
Banner, N R
Barbir, M
Barker, F G
Barrett, S T
Begg, N T
Bhatia, R
Bodey, W N
Boscoe, M J
Buchdahl, R M
Burke, M M E
Cain, P A
Chana, G S
Charig, E M
Chatrath, V K
Chetty, M N
Cleary, K J
Collier, S D
Connell, P A
Conway, A S
Copland, D R
Cruwys, M J
Daily - Jones, H R
Das, S K
Dodhy, B M A
Doherty, J M
Dollow, S C
Dovey, P
Edwards, B D
Finlay, M N
Franklin, R C G
Garsin, M D
Geraint, M
Gill, R G
Gonzalez Gracia, I M
Grocott-Mason, R M
Gupta, N K
Hagan, G W E
Hall, A V
Hall, D C
Hanspal, R S
Herbert, J R
Hillson, R M
Hogarth, A M
Hughes, J R
Ilsley, C D J
Jackson, N V
Jaffe, P
Janmohamed, R M I
Jassal, B S
Jawad, A N
Jones, C A
Jouhargy, W Y I
Kantor, R J
Kaplan, V
Kelion, A D
Kelley, C J
Kerin, P J M
Khaghani, A
Khakoo, G A
Kircher, M
Kubie, A
Lal, P
Lam-Po-Tang, K L M
Lasker, S S
Lavis, L S
Lazem, F J
Le Fevre, E J W
Lee, N B
Lees, J M
Leong Mook Seng, C C K
Loveless, P M
McBeath, J I
McDade, H B
McEwen, M
Maclean, A M
Madhok, M
Marshall, M J
Mason, M J
Mehta, A
Mehta, A
Millington, M
Mitchell, A G
Mitchell, J B
Mohsen, Y M A
Mort, S J A
Muhairez, M A-Q
Murphy, J P
Musawwir Ali, M
Namjoshi, S
Nel, M R
Oliver, A N
Paes, T R F
Palmer, J C
Parry, A C
Partridge, J B
Patel, K P
Phillips, T
Pope, A J
Price, J
Price, S H M
Radley Smith, R C
Rahmaan, G
Rajagopal Arokiadass, S M
Rawal, B K
Raza, K
Rigby, J P V
Robertson, J M
Robinson, C A
Round, P M
Saunders, Y
Serra Mestres, J
Shad, S K
Shawe, E A
Shears, D J
Shirley, I M
Siddiqui, A S
Singh, I
Singh, K N
Singh, K
Snowise, N G
Stonelake, P A
Stratton, J D
Studdy, P R
Sweatman, M C M
Takhar, K
Tonge, K A
Turnbull, M J
Usmani, I A
Usmani, M P
Vaughan-Smith, S
Walker, C P R
Watson, N R
Weinbren, J
Williamson, J M S
Wills, P J
Wood, J R
Woodham, S E
Wright, I G
Wylie, G L
Zelisko, R S

Ventnor
Alleyne, H M A
Coleman, P A
Doggett, S J
Harding, I J
Hicks, N J
Hossenbocus, A
Kitt, R
Lock, M W
Oakley, E H N
Porter, S M
Tippett, R J
Turner, D P
Walsh, T H

Verwood
Brammer, P A
Chamberlain, A S E
Devereux, H J
Layman, P R
O'Driscoll, M
Polkinghorn, A
Sandy, N K
Segal, J M L

Virginia Water
Barrett, E L
Carratt, S L
Dhenin, G H
Hargreaves, G F
Kalinkiewicz, M C
Lock, D J
Loxton, P M
Pawsey, S D
Rice, A J
Walker, K A

Wadebridge
Blatch, M J
Brooke, E M
Foster, J A
Griffiths, F V
Hewitt, C M B
Johnson, P M
Morphew, J A
Saitch, C D
Spencer, C G C
Venner, E A
Watkins, K P
Yates, J B A

Wadhurst
Bishop, J M
Blackburn, A M T
Burdett, H J
Busuttil, W
Collis, A J
Etkin, H
Goodman, K A
Hill, E A
Lewis, W G
Macdonald, A
Macdonald, A
Mills, C S
Offord, C M
Pickering, M E A C
Pipe, R A
Roche, D
Ronder, J T
Sugg, D J
Turnbull, G J

Wakefield
Abbott, C F
Ahmed, K
Ahmed, K
Ahmed, M
Al Ani, K I J
Alcock, K M
Ali, S
Anand, U
Azmy, M A L
Baker, E J
Balen, F G
Ballesteros Jimenez, J A
Barker, H E
Barker, P N
Barodawala, K
Basu, H
Bates-Kreuger, J G
Batin, P D
Becker, S J
Belk, D S
Bell, G J
Berry, A D I
Bird, G G
Birkinshaw, S E P
Blakemore, L T
Bloye, D J
Boon, S J
Bottomley, J M
Brain, G A
Brown-Doblhoff-Dier, D
Bryant, V M
Burns, L J
Butterfield, J K
Carmichael, R D G
Carpenter, M A
Carpenter, S E
Carroll, A-M
Ch'Ng, K T
Clark, N H
Clarkson, A G
Collins, P J
Cooper, A L
Cosimini, A J
Crabbe, S J
Crawford, K P
Cruickshank, C A
Cruickshank, H E
Curley, P J
Daniel, A C
Darling, C
De Silva, T
De Souza, C C A
De, K R
Dean, T A G
Dick, S M
Donnan, J S
Donner, C M
Dourado, J R
Dublon, G P N
Dublon, V E
Dunne, C L
Dunwoody, G W
Edmonds, J P F
Edwards, A S
Ellingham, J H M
Elliott, N
Ellis, J R C
Evans, A
Farooq Dar, M
Farrar, H E
Fenton, O M
Fletcher, S J
Fodden, D I
Foo, R P
Fowler-Dixon, R H
Fyfe, D R
Gair, T
Gairin Deulofeu, I
Gajjar, J G
Galvin, M C
Garthwaite, E A
Gaunt, J
Ghali, N N
Gilbert, R J
Gill, S S
Glass, E J D
Gollapudi, S
Gray, N R
Green, N J
Gupta, R C
Hall, C J
Hall, D J G
Hallott, D E
Hancocks, G H J
Hanif, S
Harrison, S C W
Haskayne, L F
Hatfield, A C
Higgins, J A
Hillmen, P
Hossain, J F M M
Humphry, R J
Irvine, C D
Ismail, A A
Ismail, Y
Jackson, A M
Jackson, K A
Jardine, M Y
Jeffery, D M
Jepson, A M
Johns, H V
Jones, R
Jones, S T
Judkins, K C
Kakroo, S
Kent, J H
Khan, I A
Khondaker, E H
Kidd, A J
King, L H S
Kirk, G E
Kirkbright, A
Kulanthaivelu, A R S
Kulanthaivelu, M
Lawn, J P J
Leading, A D
Lee, J D
Limb, C A
Littlewood, M S
Lowe, J A
Lowe, R
McDonald, M
Macfaul, R
McIver, S
McKee, D H
Maclean, A B
Maclean, N
Macrow, P J
Mahanty, S K
Mantell, A J
Mathew, E
Maynard, D G
Merson, A T
Mieszkowski, J
Millar, E M
Mitchell, D A
Mitchell, D A
Mitchell, G F B
Mone, A D
Morgan, I
Murphy, F M
Musa, S A
Mushtaq, N
Myers, C E
Nagar, M P
Nagdee, K A
Nagi, D K
Najm Al-Din, A S
Naseem, M
Nhemachena, C M
North, A C
Oo, M K
Owen-Smith, R J
Palmer, M A
Patel, D P
Paton, R H
Pattison, A C
Phipps, A R
Pinder, G A
Platt, A J
Pollock, C T S
Potts, E D A
Powell, S M J
Prasad, P
Prasad, S N
Prasad, U K
Qarshi, A A
Rainey, A E S
Rajan, G
Ram, S
Ramnani, S M
Rao, V R
Rashid, S A
Rashid, S T
Rawes, M L
Robinson, M
Rogers, M J
Roy, S L
Samaranayake, B M
Samaranayake, J J
Schindler, J L
Schofield, P J
Scott, J E
Scott, M E
Sharma, R K
Sharma, S B
Shaw, M B K
Sheppard, A P
Shields, M D
Shinn, C P
Siddiqui, N A
Silva, L F A
Singh, A
Singh, M
Slater, G D
Smith, A N
Smith, D A
Smith, S N
Sohal, A S
Souter, K M
Stanners, A J
Stewart, R G
Stickley, E A
Stockill, R A
Sutton, G C
Switalski, B J
Tabner, J A
Tabner, S A
Tan, K-S
Tawfik, R F
Taylor, C M
Taylor, M L
Tobin, M V
Tosh, J
Tree-Booker, D A
Turner, P J
Twomey, J A
Ufodiama, B E
Upadhyay, B B
Vaughan, M
Vellenoweth, S M
Walls, J B
Walls, W D
Wass, A R
Weston, P M T
Whitaker, W
White, A J
Williams, S E
Wilson-Sharp, R C
Wilson, J I
Winrow, A M
Womack, N R
Woodrow, J M
Wroe, S J

Wallasey
Amendy, U
Boydell, J S
Bradley, N A
Broadbelt, R P
Caine, J M
Cargill, A F
Coulson, A
Dunne, W T
Effingham, W H
Fegan, K J
Gardner, D
Gibbons, J J P
Goyal, A L
Hargreaves, T H
Hayes, M G
Hickey, J J M
Hollmann, M G
Hopewell, R E
Johnson, P H
Kingsland, J P
Lehane, F M
Lodh, M K
McCormack, P M
Magennis, S P M
Moulton, L C
Mukherjee, A
Mukherjee, S K
Nagesh, K
Patel, H R
Patel, R G
Peters, H
Quinn, B N E
Roberts, A
Roberts, G C S
Rudnick, S P
Shah, S C
Smye, R A
Stevenson, P A
Swift, N D
Tandon, P K
Tandon, R
Taylor, S K
Thomas, C M
Wainwright, E A
Wilkes, R G
Wright, L A

Wallingford
Agass, M J B
Anderson, J A
Collett, P R G
Cornell, J M
Crisp, S R C
Da Roza Davis, J M
Duggleby, J E
Helling, J W
Hughes, C P
Huins, T J
Ingham, F E
Jarman, D M
Jones, A
Jones, C A
Jones, S B
Ledger, S
Newnham, C T
Parker, D L
Ramage, V M
Rogers, G
Rose, P W
Sanders, M N
Sansom, A E A
Shaw, H E
Stinchcombe, C E
Thompson, C J
Trower, K J
Turberville, S M
Vernon, A R
Vickers, J R
Wilson, D T R
Zeckler, S-R

Wallington
Asirwatham, J S
Barnwal, A
Basu, S
Bilston, A E
Boulis-Wassif, S
Dimmock, D P
Erskine, M E
Fagbohun, M
Ghoorbin, V B
Golding, S J J
Halder, T K

Jones, D R E
Joseph, A E A
Kaura, D
Lal, M M
Lasrado, M F
Lewis, B P
Lings, H R
Meller, M T
Montgomery, V J
Munden, J E
Petrie, R A N
Phelan, L K
Pogson, C J
Radford, N M
Ratcliffe, R M H
Smith, R G
Sutton, S G
Thorpe, E J
Wadey, L P
Wilson, I M

Wallsend
Abraham, P
Bell, J P
Blair, S E
Broad, A J
Carrie, L A
Coles, J S
Coomber, S J S
Dewan, V
Evans, R L
Fawcett, C E
Fitzgerald, J O
Foxen, P
Griffiths, V A M
Kelly, D M
Kenny, B J
Lloyd, A J
McColl, A W
Malik, M N
Matthews, J D
Ng, J L
Oakley, T N
Page, J M
Potts, L A
Riddle, F J
Soulsby, N W
Stoves, J
Sweetman, A C
Thomas, S A
Thornton, R D
Tinkler, S D
Vaughan, G J
Westwood, M A
Wright, M

Walsall
Agrawal, B G
Agrawal, K G
Agrawal, V K
Al-Allaf, A A K
Allan, E R
Allen, C A
Alo, G O
Anand, H
Anand, M S
Antani, M R
Antani, R D
Arteen, P B
Arumainayagam, J T
Ashraf, A S
Babatola, F D O
Bagchi, I
Baig, M M A
Balachandar, C
Balagopal, V P
Banerjee, K
Banerjee, S P
Barry, T N
Basu, B J
Basu, D B
Batra, H C
Bevan, W J
Bromwich, P D
Brooks, R W S
Browne, H M R
Browne, M J
Buch, A N
Buch, M H
Butler, L M
Carter, P F B
Chandramani, S
Chattopadhyay, A K
Chhaya, S C
Coleman, T D
Conod, K C
Cooper, M H
Cotterhill, A T
Crowther, M F
Cunnington, A R
Das Gupta, S
Datta Gupta, R
Davies, M K
Davis, B W
De, S
Dean, S
Denihan, C
Dent, T F
Devasia, N D
Dewada, C
Din, K M A U
Drew, D
Dugas, M N
Durrell, N G
Ellis, L
Elves, A W S
Fehilly, B
Ferrie, B G
Galvin, G P
Gatrad, A H M
Gatrad, A R
Ghaffar, A
Ghatge, R
Ghosh, P
Giles, P D
Gray, A J
Green, S T
Hadfield, G T
Haire, A K
Harrison, J M
Harrison, K
Harvey, R A
Head, A C
Hock, Y L
Hodgins, P S
Hoskisson, D M
Houlahan, D P J
Hudecek, I P
Hunday, D S
Iqbal, M J
Ismail, S
Janes, J L
Jarrams, R G
Javeed, M
Johnson, D C
Katragadda, U
Kaul, P L
Kehler, L M
Kelly, R N
Khan, A
Khan, R
Khattak, T M
Klair, P S
Kukathasan, G
Kundu, S K
Kushwaha, A P S
Langton, G M
Latthe, R B
Lloyd, C E
Lochee Bayne, W A
Lockwood, G M
McMillan, E J
Malik, N J
Mallick, S H
Mallik, S
Manjunatha, S
Marshall, C
Mayne, A J
Min, A
Minhas, S S
Misra, G S
Mo-Szu-Ti, M S Y
Monnington Howe, M-A A
Moore, A J
Muscroft, T J
Nambisan, L S
Neeves, Z W
Newson, C D
Newton, A W
Nicholls, J E
Nixon, K
Norton, M H
Norwood, J M
Nuruzzaman, M
Okubadejo, A A
Owen, S J
Page, M M
Pansari, N G
Patel, A B
Patel, P K
Patel, S
Pathak, N D
Paw, J D
Peacock, K E
Pedder, G H
Pitkeathly, W T N
Qureshi, M U
Qureshi, M A
Rai, H
Rajeshwar, K
Rao, V D
Rashid, N Z
Ray, K C
Reddy, R M
Rifat-Ghaffar, Dr
Rolston, E T
Roy, D K
Rozario, E L
Ryatt, K S
Sadique, T
Sahu, S P
Sameja, S
Sandhu, R S
Sayaji Rao, K
Sehjpal, A
Sen, S C
Shek, K-C
Siddiq, M A
Siddiqui, M A J
Sikka, J S
Singal, A K
Singal, A K
Singh, G
Sinha, G P
Sinha, M
Sinha, S
Stanton, R J
Stewart, J
Sulaiman, S K
Suri, A S
Tewary, A K
Thiru, N
Thomas, A R
Thomas, R E
Thuse, M G
Toshniwal, M H
Tozer, A J
Trivedi, M
Turner, J P
Washbrook, R A H
Watkins, S L
Webb, A R
Wharton, J G
White, J D
Wilson, E
Wright, A D
Yahia, A O

Waltham Abbey
Berry, B B
Engineer, S R
Galbraith, S M
Garkal, A
Lakha, A G N
Morris, A G
Pymont, F E

Waltham Cross
Baker, A W
Baldas, A
Bhar, G C
Conway, J C
Galaal, K A
Goodwin, A M
Hasan, M
Hodge, R J
King, I J
Misra, K
Nagpal, K K
Naqvi, A T
Neville, W T
Pasapula, C S
Roberts, D R A
Roberts, N
Sahni, D R
Sengupta, N
Southerton, J
Spinoza, M H
Stanton, S M
Wakefield, S M
Watson, S C
Weadick, P R
Wood, D F
Yousef, Z R

Walton on the Naze
Beardmore, C L M
Frost, I
Geldard, J A F
Roper, N D K
Thompson, J H

Walton-on-Thames
Andrews, S J
Arnold, P F
Banham, M J
Bennett, R J J
Britton, G V
Clark, L A
Cooper, J E S
Edwards, A
Emerson, C A
Fahmi, F M R
Ferriday, U T
Gladman, L M
Holdsworth, J A
Kangesu, E
Lewis, G E
Littlewood, E R
MacVicar, C V
Malde, K
Meechan, P O
Noon, C C
Pirrie, A J
Ratcliffe, D M
Redfern, R
Ribera Cortada, I
Rice, K M
Salih, J E
Sekhon, S S
Shrimpton, S P
Sillick, J M
Warrington, B M V
Warrington, R
Wijnberg, J P
Williams, E C
Woodward, P J

Wantage
Allen, A W D
Ambler, P J
Banwell, M E
Baverstock, A M
Blake, E R
Dinnis, G A
Drury, V M
Dunning, M T
Gillibrand, R
Godlee, R J P
Herd, G J C
Howard, J
Kaye, S M
Kyle, P D
Kyle, S D
Lister Cheese, I A F
Robinson, J C
Shackleton, S C
Sharp, R J
Teare, C M L
Thrippleton, L K
Triffitt, D J
Uridge, C F
Whipple, S J B
Wise, D G D

Ware
Baverstock, M W J
Bridges, I H
Davies, M W
Gibson, S H
Gilbert, D J
Hans, S F
Harris, S C
Law, N W
Lennox, S C
McCreadie, J E
Maddams, D J
Merwaha, N
Morgan, R E
Peters, J L
Preston, P
Rundell, T R
Watson, J C
Young, J M S

Wareham
Bennett, C E
Bennett, J R
Brown, A M
Brown, T S
Cox, J S
Greenfield, R M
Harley, T G
Irwin, C S
Lesna, M
Lesny, J
Lyons, C
Lyons, N T
Ross, P A
Rumbold, C A
Salter, A L
Salter, T C M
Ward, A H
Williams, M G

Warley
Ahuja, D K
Ahuja, J
Bathija, S H
Binks, C
Bloxham, S T
Collier, D J F
Cornish, V M
Desai, P M
Gibson, P L
Hamilton, D G
Harrington, D A
Harris, E
Iqbal, Y
Jhanjee, V K
Kalsi, G S
Khan, F A
Ladha, K
McCathie, N J
Nutbeam, H M
Pall, N K
Pinto, S M
Price, W R
Rahman, K A
Roberts, K E
Ryan, H T
Sharp, J
Srivastava, K K
Vaughan, K F
Willetts, I E
Wong, P T Y

Warlingham
Allenby, F
Beckitt, D
Boorman, P A
Bown, M J
Cruthers, J P
Hinkes, D A
Parry, D M
Ramage, P C V
Stimmler, L
Turner, M J
Yates, M S

Warminster
Arathoon, D A
Asbridge, G
Beach, P G
Bell, J M
Braithwaite, M G
Browne, C H
Church, E
Collyns, T A
Corey, O I M
Fishwick, J J
Goedkoop, L C
Greenhalgh, M C S
Greenwood, A
Houghton, S R A
Lawton, G S
Little, D J
McBride, E
McBride, K N
Moore, J M F
Payne, J S
Price, W J P
Stevens, V J R
Thorpe, M A
Titley, J V
Tremlett, P D
Williams, K L
Wingfield, C A
Woolgar, J D

Warrington
Abbott, J B
Abdullah, A
Adair, R J
Adair, T
Agnew, E M
Agnew, M N
Al-Jafari, M S
Al-Maskari, S M
Alam, M S
Anis, A B
Asamoah, D K
Aslam, M
Awan, T T
Baines, A G
Bannon, J J E
Bansal, V K
Banyard, P J
Barton, P G
Basma, L
Bates, A J
Beare-Winter, A N
Bentley, S J
Bokhari, A A
Bokhari, S A
Boot, D A
Booth, J A
Bradley, G C
Brady, D W J
Brassill, J W
Brett, M C A
Briggs, J R
Brook, N M
Brook, R
Brooker, G E M
Brown, G J
Brown, Z
Burke, B M
Burke, P L
Burke, S L
Burke, W
Burthem, J
Butler, A J
Cann, P C
Cantrell, P
Caplan, M P
Carmichael, D N
Carr, D J
Chetter, I C
Choudhury, A
Clarke, J N
Clayton, W G
Cockburn, K J
Coleman-Smith, I
Colquhoun, R G
Connell, J E
Copeland, G P
Coughlin, M
Cox, D A
Cribb, J S
Croton (Mrs Entwistle), J L L
Das, R
Davies, G J
Davis, A M
Davis, P A
Dennis, M W
Dhir, K
Dixon, A M
Dixon, S P
Doherty, M B
Downey, P
Durkin, C M
Edwards, C V S
Edwards, D W
Edwards, I G
Estlin, E J
Fallon, K M
Fazackerley, E J
Ferran Cabeza, J M
Filobbos, R
Flanagan, S M
Francis, E P
Freeman, C A M
Garvey, R J P
Gerber, S
Ghaffar, A A
Ghazawy, S
Glennon, C M
Gomes, A J
Goodwin, T
Hadland, M D
Haigh, P M
Hall, S J
Halliwell, M C
Hanumanthu, V R
Harney, J M V
Hebbar, G K
Higgs, A G
Hobin, D A
Holland, E F N
Hope, J A
Horton, V M
Hunter, J D
Hussein, A M M K
Hutchinson, G H
Hyland, C
Iceton, N M
Iles, E A
Inman, C D C
Jagadeesh, S V
Jamieson, P A
Jarvis, P D
Jarvis, S J F
John, B
Johnson, E M
Johnson, M
Johnson, R T
Joshi, H
Kanagavel, N
Kelleher, P C
Kerr, M A
Khalil, A L

Kishan, B
Knight, S R
Knill, R
Kowalska, K A
Kozman, E L L
Krishna Reddy, T V
Kumaraswamy, S P
Laycock, A N
Leach, J M
Leigh, A J
Leneghan, J E
Letchumanan, V
Levy, M
Lewis, S J
Linaker, B D
Lloyd, C C
Lynch, S C
McCaig, J
McClean, M
McCormack, J R S
Mackay, M M
Mackin, E A
McNicholas, M J
Malik, Z I
Malkhandi, A D
Malpica, M G
Manning, G F
Manning, G M
Martin, B A
Miall, F M
Miller, W G
Mills, G N
Mills, J K
Milroy, P J M
Moody, A P
Mukhopadhyay, P S
Mundell, R H
Myles, J M
Nalla, R R
Napier, J E
Neary, W J
Nixon, S J
Norgain, H R
O'Colmain, B P
O'Connor, A P
O'Flanagan, J O
O'Flanagan, P M
O'Loan, J
O'Shea, M J
Oglesby, S D
Oldfield, J A
Osborne, A W
Palmer, G R
Paranjothy, C
Park, R
Parkins, A C
Parkinson, D W
Parry, R G
Patel, V
Patiniott, A K
Patiniott, F J
Peckar, C O
Penni, A N
Pepper, J M
Platts, A S G
Plumb, E A
Pomfret, S M
Porter, B J
Priestley, C T
Rahim, M A
Rahman, M B
Rahman, S M S
Ranasinghe, H A N
Rao, S V
Ratchford, A M
Rathe, M
Redfearn, S W
Rees, M
Reynolds, P A
Rimmer, A J
Ritter, A C
Robertson, D E
Robertson, R M P
Robinson, A E
Ross, S M
Rowlands, M
Royle, D A
Salib, E
Salih, A R M
Sathiyaseelan, S
Seddon, J A
Shahbazi, S S A H
Shaw, L C
Sheikh, I H
Sherry, P G
Shome, C
Sillah, A K
Skinner, A C
Slovak, A J M
Smith, A T
Smith, C E
Smith, G D
Smith, S P
Sokhi, J S
Sowden, H
Sowinska, E
Spedding, R L
Stanway, T L
Stewart, G D
Storrar, D A
Stott, J E
Tailby, C H
Tandon, H P
Taylor, B A
Ternent, T
Thomas, M D
Thorburn, R J
Tighe, M J
Tourish, P G
Trotter, C
Turner, H J
Tyrer, M
Umnus, L
Veeravahu, R
Vivekanandamurty, K
Wadsworth, M R
Wales, E L
Wales, E K
Walkden, D
Walkden, J A D
Walton, D J
Ward, B
Watson, I N
Webb, C J
Whitcroft, I A
Wild, N J
Williams, A
Wilson, I S
Winter, S M
Wishart, M S
Wood, R S
Yeong, C C

Warwick
Acharya, A B
Allen, A J
Allim, J S S
Anduvan, S
Anthony, A
Antrobus, J H L
Badwan, D A H
Bates, J
Batra, N
Bedlow, A J
Begg, H B
Beniston, M A
Bhandal, T S
Bishop, J M
Blacklay, P F
Box, M J
Campbell, C A
Carr, R A
Casey, M D
Chamberlain, S J
Charles-Holmes, R
Chell, P B
Clark, H L M
Clarke, D P
Clarkson, S G
Coleman, H E
Cross, T J
Dallaway, C M
Darby, D O D
Davids, E
Davis, L A
Dawkins, C J
Desai, H
Desborough, S H
Dowell, J R
Dumughn, C
Dunn, R M W
Finney, M E
Fraser, I D L
Ghose, A R
Ghose, B
Gopinathan, K P
Gray, D J
Grewal, R
Gunton, H J
Hall, L K
Harries, S A
Hatton, J A
Hawker, P C
Hayward, C J
Hill, L S
Horrocks, P M
Hughes, M
Hughes, T B J
Humphreys, F
Inchley, S J
Jackson, R
Jones, J M R
Jones, R
Joshi, A A
Kapma, J A A
Kennedy, A G
Killeen, I P
Laird, S
Le Tocq, M C L
Lewis, D C
Leyland, G R
Leyland, M J
Lindsey, M W
Long, T M W
Mahmood, A
Marguerie, C P
Martin, S J
Mather, S P
Meaden, R W
Meadows, H
Melton, R P
Menage, J L
Miles, J
Millard, F C
Milner, M A
Mohamed, H H
Morris, I H
Murphy, P D
Nancarrow, J
Natin, D J M
Ngeh, J K T
Nwachukwu, I A
O'Driscoll, A M
Osborne, M J
Panting, K
Parsons, A
Penter, G
Perthen, K S
Phillips, D E
Pinder, S J
Quinn, A C
Ray, P K
Robertson, T D
Robinson, D A
Rogers, J N
Rose, P E
Sansom, D T
Sewell, R C T
Shearman, J D
Silvester, K M
Slowther, C M
Smeyatsky, N R
Smith, F A
Strachan, J R
Struthers, G R
Tait, J S
Tarpey, J J
Templeton, A M
Thurley, P A
Tweedie, D G
Usselmann, B M
Vaz, F G
Viswan, A K
Wells, L G
White, H G
Whitehouse, A J
Whitewood, C N
Whitewood, F J
Wilkinson, C E
Wilkinson, J E M
Williams, P H
Wilmot, E F
Wilson, E M
Wyatt, S S
Young, S K

Washington
Benn, H M
Bhatt, N J
Brandes, E A
Burke, M F
Carney, S M
Cowie, S
Dennison, K C
Dixit, C M
Gollan, J
Heaney, R I
Hegde, A K K
Kulkarni, D R
Lawther, I W
McCabe, M M E
McCabe, M G
Mazarelo, J O
Nanavati, N A
Nanda, N
Nanda, U C
Pegman, A J
Ray, N K
Rutland, R F K
Saravanamattu, K
Sen, I
Shah, T H
Stephenson, G
Thomas, K M
Vakharia, B R
Wong, H S
Yelnoorkar, K

Watchet
Rush, M
Wilson, M L
Wilson, P A

Waterlooville
Bartlett, D
Bateman, A M S
Batten, S F
Blakeley, S L
Bligh, M D
Bowerman, R D
Boyle, P D
Brownlie, H A
Burtenshaw, A J
Burton, K L
Chada, K
Churcher-Brown, C J
Clarke-Williams, J E
Cohen, A E
Croker, G H
Daniel, R J E
Gibbons, P M
Gould, R A
Goulder, T J
Gregori, M
Griffiths, D G
Hanson, R G
Hargreaves, C M
Hargreaves, M D
Hume, A M
Jenkins, S C
Johns, M
Jones, D H
Kenny, T D
King, A P U
McErlean, P
Mann, R D
May Mya Nwe, Dr
Millard, M-L
Millard, R V
Millen, N J
Milne, P S
Moate, R D C
Morey, P-J
Morison, S R
Penfold, H M
Plane, A R
Pringle, J K
Pryce, D P
Roberts, N J
Rowling, A J
Ruddle, A C
Ryan, J A
Ryan, P B
Saville, M A
Shaltot, M A A
Shutte, H A N
Spreadbury, P L
Spruell, D A
Stanley, S P
Walters, H M
Warwick-Brown, J M
Warwick, J R
White, M J

Watford
Ainsley, J
Al-Barazanchi, A J H
Allen, S T
Anthony-Pillai, I
Apple, M F A
Aron, P M
Aslam, S
Atkin, H S
Awad, R W I
Babu-Narayan, R K
Baker, G M
Bankole, C A
Belderbos, R
Belham, G J
Bintcliffe, B J
Blackwell, V C
Bolitho-Jones, A
Bolitho-Jones, P V
Borkett-Jones, S E
Boxer, D I
Boyd, T J
Brent, K A
Brown, N J
Buist, M
Bulman, W H
Cameron, E A B
Cameron, J D H
Cates, C J
Chakrabarti, N
Chaudary, M A
Chesterfield, H M
Chipperfield, R A
Chung, E M K
Clark, E J
Clements, M R
Cohn, A S
Coleman, R M
Collas, D M
Connor, A J M
Cooper, R C
Courtney, R M
Cox, S J
Crisp, J C
Davis, P J
Daya, J
Devine, M A
Dhadwal, K K
Dobney, S
Dodoo, E A
Duckworth, A J
Dullforce, E J
Dyson, A L M B
Eliad, R A
Essam, M A
Fertleman, M B
Fuchs-Goldfarb, S
Furbank, I D J
Galan, Y S
Gale, A N
Gavilan, J
Gelister, J S K
Glover, J I
Gordon, A D
Grice, K
Griffin, D R
Gujral, M K
Hammad, G E-D M
Hart, S M
Hassan-Ali, R
Heckmatt, J Z
Heller, E
Hemmens, S A
Hodes, S
Hussain, F M
Hussain, Z-U
Ineson, N R
Irvine, L M
Isweran, P S
Jackson, A P
Jaffe, M
Jagajeevanram, D
Jessop, J H
Joshi, B P
Kamya, D
Karunasekara, N R
Kat, H S
Keen, M J
Khamzina, E I
Khan, P S
King, J A
Knight, E J
Kodati, S M R
Lazzerini, V R
Leahy, A J
Lee, T L
Leigh, Y
Levison, W B
Lewis, D M
Lim, S C
Livingstone, J I
Loney, E L
McCann, S J
Macfarlane, B J
Mackell, K A
Mackenney, R P
McKitterick, E C
McMurtry, I A
McNally, S A
Markeson, V E
May, A J
Meager, P W D
Meyrick Thomas, J
Mir, R S
Mir, S A
Mital, R K
Moore, P F
Moss, D P
Moulsdale, M T
Mowbray, C K
Mullan, H M
Munday, P E
Murdoch, M E
Murray, M D
Nelstrop, G A
Novak, T V
Nyman, L E
O'Connor, P F M
Oren, C L
Padwick, M L
Pandit, A N
Pandit, N A
Parker, R K H
Parry, H M
Patel, D K K
Patel, S C
Purbrick, S
Rackham, A J
Rae, H E
Raithatha, M M
Rajamanoharan, S
Rajasekaran, J
Ramachandran, N
Ratnavel, T
Raychaudhuri, S
Razzaq, Q M
Reader, P M
Redman, D R O
Reissis, N
Reubin, R D
Richards, B A
Richards, J D M
Rieu, E C
Rizvi, S A H
Robertson, S C
Robinson, E A E
Robson, T W
Rotman, C M H
Rubin, A
Rudran, V
Sa'adu, A
Sainsbury, W A
Saksena, J
Sanusi, F A
Sarva Isweran, M
Scholes, C F
Scott, J M
Searle, C H
Shanmuganathan, C
Shears, D
Sheikh, N F
Shepherd, J S
Sheridan, R J
Simmons, K L
Singleton, C D
Sinha, J K
Slater, M S
Somerville, K W
Somerville, W
Soskin, M A
Starer, F
Steele, C A
Stimmler, A
Supramaniam, G
Tan, S H
Taylor, G D
Thacker, B G
Tso, M T B Y
Uzoho, R
Vyramuthu, N
Walker, J A
Wallace, M H
Wallis, H
Watkinson, D S
Watson, M E J
Webb, R J
Weidmann, S J
Williams, M J H
Wilson, M A
Yadegar, J
Yazdani, M S
Zakani, R

Watlington
Gordon, A C
Gregory, N A P
Miller, T R
Stillwell, J M

Wedmore
Drage, S A C
Howard, J C
Watt, D S
West, A J

Wednesbury
Abedin, M Z
Ahmed, S A
Bhadauria, B S
Buckley, M P

Carr, V A
Huey, D M
Lavender, J P
Morris, C D E
Patel, K K
Pearce, G
Rahman, A-U
Rana, S
Saini, A S
Shah, J
Sikka, C S
Taylor, M B
Tayyebi, G A
Vaid, S J

Welling
Anto, M K
Baruah, A C
Chahal, J K
Colaco, T D C
Cotter, W A
De Souza, R A
Dhital, A P
Fish, P D
Gupta, C L
Hanner, I E
McEwan, J
Martin, J L
Nwamarah, D E
Oxford, P C J
Patel, M
Raoof, H Y
Ryder, J C
Shah, N
Sylvester, G M
Wijayatilake, N

Wellingborough
Alexander, Z
Barton, L M
Bent, J E
Bevan, J M
Box, W D
Byles, L E
Chung, K Y K
Coulson, W J
Cox, J K
Craig, J H
Dent, C C
Dibble, T F C
Dwivedi, A
Ellis, C J
English, J
Evans, A G
Geeves, N P
Gordon, P J
Graves, P B
Harry, M L G P
Hunt, W J
Inns, P
Iriso, N
Jollyman, T M
Kapre, M L
King, G R
Kownacki, S
Lambert, A M
Lawrence, D K
McGarity, K L
McGibbon, A F
Masih, H
Mistry, V K
Nalinasegaren, G
Nandakumar, K
Nayani, S
Neame, R L
Nicholas, I H
Palfreeman, A J
Pepperman, M A
Perry, R M
Purdy, D R
Robertson, A P
Shah, J S
Spencer, M C
Titheridge, K L
Upton, P G
Wainwright, A T
Wall, I F
Whittington, T J

Wellington
Bevan, P W
Bridgman, S J
Cole, J H
Fairbairn, S E A
Frier, J A
Leahy, A C
McCann, D J
Michaels, M
Newmarch, B
Peters, H G
Rickard, A M
Thomson, P J
Waterhouse, P
Wynne, J S

Wells
Ancill, P K
Ashman, R
Barnes, J C
Bench, J J
Bridson, C M
Crawley, H E
Gatrill, R B
Gillen, D P
Goddard, R H
Gould, J C G K
Marshall, D L
Martin, T J
Norman, A S
Pinching, J
Pryer, A A
Young, J E

Wells-next-the-Sea
Ebrill, C S T
Lahbib, F J
Wynne-Simmons, A P M

Welshpool
Brownbill, C L
Evans, A V
Hutchinson, E A
Jones, E L
Jones, J M
Jones, M E
Jones, R M
Lambert, S K
Lewis, M R
Milne, L G
Novick, S M
Riley, M
Ryan, T D
Solomon, A L
Townsend, C S
Williams, J A

Welwyn
Abrahams, R C
Almeyda, J S
Crane, W P
Cropp, J E
Dansie, N B
Derola, T
Drew, A
Goetz, S C
Hammond, T A G
Harrison, S J
Moye, A R
Nandy, A M
Napier, H B
Pardoe, C A
Reed, A
Robbins, G M
Roden, M
Small, B J
Stallard, M C
Stallard, N C
Tobin, M D
Tobin, T A
Trevarthen, F D
Turner, K J
Vaquas, S
Wilson, H O
Wood, S J

Welwyn Garden City
Al-Izzi, M S S
Aldridge, M C
Angwin, H V
Atalla, R K
Axon, J M C
Bakhru, M N
Barathan, I
Bayoumi, A-H M M
Boyce, T H
Brewis, R P
Campbell, S H
Charlwood, L M U
Clarke, R
Conroy, S J
Corser, A J
Cranfield, F M
Creak, D R
Crilly, D
Dallas, J D A
Dasgupta, J
Davies, R P
Davis, H P
Dover, C J
Drew, N C
Duggal, S
Dunster, R J
Egbase, P E
Evison, J G
Fattah, A M N
Feizi, O
Fineberg, N A
Fox, M H
Gautam, V
Goldberg, P L
Greenfield, S M
Griffin, J P
Hanak, B A
Harding, M J
Harvey, D M
Haslam, R G E
Hawley, C J
Hayman, M R
Higgins, S
Hilditch, R J
Hirst, J R
Holden, A A
Holt, P M
Hubbard, A P
Husain, H M
Iafelice, E D
Iqbal, Z
Jenkins, C M
Katz, J R
Khan, S S
Kingsbury, S J
Kirkpatrick, C T
Kitson, J L
Lennox, M S
Lok, S S
Lund, C D
McCallum, A K
McCue, J L
McGettiga, H
McGhee, A G
McIntyre, P B
McLintock, D G
Mercy, L C
Mithra, S D
Moxon, M A
Munshi, N J
Newman, M J
Parmar, H
Phiri, D E D
Pugh, G
Quartey, P K
Raffles, A K M
Roberts, A G
Robson, R A
Rogerson, R E
Rule, M J
Saetta, J P
Samarasinghe, W
Sandhu, B S
Shah, Z P
Sharma, R
Shaw, C A
Sheela Sridhar, K
Sherman, J A
Turner, S J S
Voke, J M
Waldron, M N
Walker, T J
Waller, S M
Wat, C K Y
Waterfield, A H
Watkins, M E
Winocour, P H
Wood, H A

Wembley
Abeysiri, P
Ahmed, A
Amin, M B
Andrade, E J Y
Apley, M S
Ashour, F A A E-M
Azzam, Y M A
Bajaj, S
Balachandran, N
Banerjee, C
Banerjee, S
Bayer, M M
Bernstein, J F
Bhardwaj, R
Bhattacharyya, M
Brent, P G
Clark, M O
Dabas, R
Drage, S M
Dutton, D
Ellis, P F
Estment, P D
Fox, A T
Gandhi, V
Goodchild, L P
Gor, A S
Gor, M S
Greenham, R M
Griffin, C M
Hales, S
Hami, F
Haque, I
Hira, J R
Hunter, C
Hyman, V C
Islamullah, M
Jagadambe, P R
Jegatheesvaran, M
Kaleem, T
Kearns, W E
Khan, A A
Kirmani, T H
Kotecha, M B
Krotosky, L A
Kumar, A S B
Kunapuli, V S
Lee, C H
Lewis, C J
Lovett, P C A
McGovern, H
Maheswaran, W T
Makhija, S K
Malde, N S
Mamtora, M P
Mass, M E
Mehta, S M
Merchant, R
Milik, N S
Mills, J
Murugiah, S
Nandhabalan, K
Naylor, D H R
Negandhi, D B
O'Neill, E M
O'Riordan, D K
Obeng, F
Obeyesekera, S L
Odutola, T A A
Patel, A R
Patel, B B
Patel, B
Patel, H
Patel, J I
Patel, J S
Patel, P B
Radia, D H R
Raichura, M M
Rangr, P
Rapp, D A
Rashid, B U
Ross, J
Saad, A
Sabharwal, C K
Sabharwal, N N
Sabharwal, N K
Salame, M Y
Salinsky, J V
Salker, D M
Scrine, M
Shah, K A
Shah, S
Shah, S M
Shaikh, A
Sheikh, S A
Sheth, G P
Singarayer, C
Singh, I
Singh, T G
Strang, R A
Syed, R
Syed, S U
Tahir, H I S
Tailor, V G
Tansley, E J
Tayal, N
Taylor-Smith, R G
Teelock, B
Thirumavalavan, V S
Thurairajah, A
Twomey, A F J
Ugboma, K J
Vijh, V
Vyas, S
Weeks, V C
Wijayaratna, L O
Wijeratne, W K
Wills, C I

Wemyss Bay
Grabs, A J
McKay, L A
McKechnie, S
Shirazi, T

West Bromwich
Agarwal, M D
Agarwal, N K
Agrawal, G K
Agwu, J C
Ahmed, A H S
Armstrong, J
Bajaj, S
Banerjee, R
Banerjee, S K
Bardha, H S
Bassan, T S
Bellin, J M
Bhatt, R C V
Blissitt, L C
Bose, R C
Brook, F B
Carter, N P
Cave, K L
Chalkley, M J
Chand, D
Clothier, J C
Cobb, C A
Connolly, D L
Crampton, G M
Crowther, C A
Crump, M S
Dar, S
Davis, R C
Daya, V H
Dexter, B H
Doerry, U G
Edwards, S
El-Gohary, T M T
El-Hilu, S
El Shazly, M A M
El-Safty, M M
Ellis, D J
Evans, A R M
Fletcher, J S
Gabbitas, D G
Gilbert, J E
Grindulis, H
Grindulis, K A
Gudi, P V
Hallan, P S
Harb, M M
Harte, N M
Hughes, E A
Jayatunga, R
Jones, MA
Kabukoba, J J
Kaplan, N M F
Karandikar, R V
Kathirgamakarthigeyan, T
Khanna, A
Leahy, J F
Leeming-Latham, L
Macaulay, D D R
McClement, B J
McLeod, D T
Mallya, J U
Mattar, M H
Mehta, B S
Mlele, T J J
Page, N G
Panikker, N R
Parvatham, K
Patel, D R
Patel, R M
Pathak, S K
Perera, B L
Porter, J M
Prasad, K
Rayatt, S S
Robertson, D A
Rose, M
Sajnani, D K
Saunders, D J
Shakeel, M H
Shaw, A S
Singh, C D P
Singh, I
Smith, R K
Sreekanta, G
Tahir, M Z
Tutton, G R
Vairavan, M
Van Den Dwey, K
Verow, P G
Wheatley, K E
Wijewardene, P A
Zulueta Madinabeitia, L

West Byfleet
Bennett, P M J
Cara, D M
Churchill, M P
Cowan, P J
Crossley, J N
Dickson, D G
Dunstan, C J D
Horgan, J L
Hughes, J
Hyzler, A H
Jones, B M
Ker, D B
Lynch, M T
McEvoy, H M
Manuel, H
Meechan, H T
Shepheard, A C

West Calder
Barclay, K
Brook, C M
Campbell, A M
Campbell, C M
Gilkison, J N
Haigh, S J
Hewitt, M J
Robertson, J L
Valentine, D E

West Drayton
Abe, P J A
Andrews, L M
Andrews, P
Byrne, N J
Chandra, L
Dowdall, N P
Eraneva, K A
Grewal, A
Hikmet, S A
McCarthy, T P
McCulloch, W J
Mian, F U R
Montgomery, J
Mooney, S E
Morris, M M
Paramanathan, V
Picton, C E
Ponnappa, M A
Wilkinson, E S

West Kilbride
Arumugam, C
Caskie, J P
Chisholm, L J
Colburn, D D
Davies, F W
Fegan, K G
Graham, H C
Kelly, B M J
Porteous, E M E
Porteous, G S

West Linton
Adamson, P M
Halcrow, J S
McCann, M A
Pollock, A C
Pollock, M W
Young, R A B

West Malling
Barnhoorn, A M
Burland, J G H
Cassim, S D M
Crutchfield, L A
Eggleton, S P H
Hirons, R M
Keane, M A
Musgrave, R J
Newell, R J
Pinder, D K
Rushton, M J
Sadik, S R
Scott, A J
Tomkins, C M

West Molesey
Buchan, I C
Kumar, S

West Wickham
Allen, S D
Amin, S
Arif, M S
Carter, S M

Cheetham, M A
Dilley, R J
Dunlop, A J
Hammill, R M
Holloway, J A C
Jhally, S
Kirby, R N
Langtry, A B
Purwar, V
Ramani, R M
Robertson, S H
Sithamparapillai, S
Standfield, N J
Strathdee, G M
Van Woerkom, A E
Venison, T D
Whittaker, I D
Young, D C D
Young, M J

Westbury
Beale, D A
Edwards, R M
Grier, I W
Hibbert, R S
Kostelnik, J R
Powell, D H T
Siggers, D J

Westcliff on Sea
Adey, A J
Adey, C
Aggarwal, R K
Ahlquist, J A O
Al-Shammari, A A
Ansari, S
Atkinson, P
Babar, I U
Bain, L A
Ball, A J
Boardman, J P
Bowles, J N
Bray, G P
Buckley, J H M
Bullock, A E
Callaghan, S M
Carmichael, D J S
Carr, T W
Chappell, M E
Chaturvedi, K K
Chisnell, P T
Collings, A D
Dasgupta, B
Davies, B S
Diddee, A S
Diddee, S D
Donald, D
Dworkin, M J
Eden, A G Z
Eden, H H A
El-Kasaby, H T
Eraut, C D
Ewart, I A
Franklin, J S
Gabrielczyk, M R
Garofalides, B
Gatland, D J
Ghani, P N
Gordon, T E
Gray, A E
Grover, S P
Gul, J
Halliday, R M
Hamblin, J J
Harter, C
Hewazy, A- H
Higgins, D J
Hollywood, P G
Hughes, S F
Ibrahim, M N
Jakeways, M S R
Jennings, D A
Kalan, A M H
Kelly, P A
Kent, M B
Khan, A
Khan, M R
Khazim, R
Lamont, A
Lane, G F
Leonard, P C
Lewars, M D
Lewis, C P M
Liew, S-H
Lim, K B
Lubel, J S
McKechnie, J
Maher, H A
Majdneya, E
Mellor, J A
Metcalfe, K A
Misbahuddin, A
Mullane, D M
Myers, M
O'Brien, A A J
O'Brien, J D
Packer, G J
Park, D M
Perera, S D
Perera, S J
Prejbisz, J W
Ramdin, L S
Robinson, A C R
Rokan Al-Mallak, H
Rothnie, N D
Roy, S
Rumble, J A
Salter, M C P
Schuster, R
Shah, S S
Shaw, A J
Siani, N M
Sinha, A K
Slovick, D I
Sooriakumaran, V
Spitzer, R J
Spivey, C J
Subasinghe, S Z A
Tosh, G C
Trask, C W L
Tsokodryi, C
Ward, J K
Ward, S
Warwick-Brown, N P
Watters, G W R
Weller, P J
White, A E T
Whybrow, T R
Wisely, J
Wong, W M

Westerham
Carson, S J
Dowling, G C V
Gramsma, A
Ismaili, J A
Ismaili, N
Kapadia, A
Kenwright, K A
Knox, V E
Lord, J A D
Lyttle, T W
Molyneux, P D
Parker, J R
Pearson, C M G
Pinchin, R M E
Pugh, R J
Pullen, M D
Richardson, R G
Sargeant, I D
Singh, K
Singh, S
Skinner, A J
Spivey, M H

Westgate-on-Sea
Abrokwah, J
Dean, A J P
Lall, A
Lall, A
Lewis, M
Meakin, D R
Moore, E L
Standeven, P A H
Turtle, J A

Westhill
Allan, C G
Brownhill, J E
Brownie, E C
Bruce, A W
Burnett, J C D
Cauchi, P
Dean, J H S
Ellis, G G
Harris, C C
Hunter, C M
Hutchison, J D
Jibril, J A
Ritchie, R D

Weston Super Mare
Afifi, R A E M M
Ainsworth, M K
Alam, M M
Bailey, S J
Barff, D M
Bartlett, P G
Bevan, C D
Bhakri, H L
Birkett, J F
Bosson, S
Bowering, R J B
Bradley, A
Britchford, R E
Case, R D
Chitty, J R
Cilasun, O
Clarke, C W
Cockeram, J
Collett, C A
Corcos, C D
Croucher, C L
Daly, R S
Danker, K O
Darling, R M
Davies, H C
Day, A P
Derrington, P M
Devitt, N M
Dixon, J
Easton, P J
England, C M
Evans, D J
Fitzpatrick, R C
Foxton, T M
Foy, G
Frost, C E A
Gallegos, N C
Gamlin, C G
Garvey, G N
Giannoulis, K
Gillis, C V
Gosden, P E
Gould, G A
Hasham, N I
Hinchliffe, A
Horgan, C H
Hugh, D
Johnson, M R
Krekorian, H A W
Lakin, N P
Langkamer, V G
Latif, M M A
Leonard, M J
Lott, M F
Lumb, P G
MaksimcZyk, P
Milnthorpe, P D
Molesworth, T
Murdin, P G
Mussell, F M R
Newton, A P
Osman, M A
Papworth, J E J
Parker, D R
Parker, J
Patel, N D
Paterson, D A
Pearse-Danker, S C
Petty, W H
Pimm, M H J
Piotrowski, A G
Preston, C W
Preston, R C
Pye, G
Roberts, R D
Saunders, J H
Saw Lwin Aung, Dr
Smith, A J
Smith, P R
Stallworthy, E G
Stebbings, S M
Steggall, E A
Todd, I M
Tomblin, M P M
Tomlinson, M J
Vaze, N R
Waring, I S
Watkinson, P M
Wilson, E D
Wilson, P B
Winterton, H M
Woodhead, P J
Wyatt, M T

Wetherby
Atkins, M L
Beard, A D
Blair, I H
Bradley, A M
Brady, M D
Brooke, B M
Browning, B S
Browning, S J
Crabbe, R M G
Dillon, S
Drayson, R W
Durham, N P
Edwards, S
Finch, P J C
Fraser, S E
Hall, R
Hopton, B P
Ireland, A P
Jarvis, G J
Jeffery, J R
Knight, J
Lavalette, D P
Lovisetto, S G
McArdle, J M
Marley, J L
Mate, J D
Mawson, A
Morrell, H B
Moxon, J W A
Murphy, P G
Norman, A T
O'Meara, M E
Pearlman, J A
Rose, T
Roussounis, S H
Smith, A
Staples, E J
Stocks, D A
Taylor, J M
Thom, M V
Walker, A H
Wynn, P

Weybridge
Aylett, M R
Barwell, J G
Bateman, S G
Blackman, J A
Boyle, A M
Brown, I E
Burgess, H K
Burns, A M E
Butler, M
Carr, R J
Cocker, D P
Comber, E
Davidson, S M
Denning, Z P
Desor, D
Dovell, T M
Econs, A
Fozard, L A
Fraser, J M
Glaser, L H
Green, A M
Hinds, R M
Howard, J S
Jakubowski, K A
Jenner, M W
Krol, J E
Lawrence, L M
Lee, B T M
Lewis, A F
Lilliott, M M
McLaren, R D
Marjot, D H
Menzies-Gow, L C
Oh, S Y A
Peachey, G R
Prince, W T
Raymakers, K L M
Russell, M H
Sacoor, M H A
Seiger, C P
Sharma, R
Sharpe, K E
Shefras, J
Sott, A H
Staunton, N J
Stedman, A E
Suryavanshi, V S
Vandeberg, C R E
Vrionides, Y
Walker, C R
White, E A
Wilson, T A H

Weymouth
Baird, P W
Bick, S A
Blease, D J
Blunt, A J
Bowditch, W B
Boyd, D C
Brown, C A
Burgess, D K
Chapman, I
Cheung, S C-K
Chopra, S
Cox, J
Da Costa, I M V N
Davies, F M
De Kretser, J
Dickinson, A G W
Down, P F
Evans, D M
Fernandez, G N
Fowler, N H
Gibbins, P A
Grogono, K
Hall, I R
Hendricks, M A
Hewett, P J
Hodder, S E
Houston, K C
Hull, P J
Hutchinson, W F
Killoch, M M
Kirkham, K V
Knight, W R
Laird, A J
Laird, G D
Llewellyn, H D
Lopez Longas, J F
McEleny, K R
Man, A
Mann, J H
Mitchell, P J
Naylor, K J
Orrell, J M
Page, N E
Pouncey, C M G
Priestley, C J F
Priestley, H S
Puckett, M A
Roberts, A P
Robinson, G J
Savage, R A
Simpson, D S
Slater, D R
Smithson, E F
Stalley, N J
Stewart, J A
Stradling, A J
Talbot, S
Temple, A J
Thacker, C R
Thornton, A
Townsend, J M
Townsend, M
Turberville Smith, R J
Waldron, R W
Ward, A J
Ward, R D
Webb, K I
Woodall, N A
Young, W H

Whitby
Baird, A M
Campbell, G B B
Chadwick, W J
Croft, G
Cunion, D
Davies, W G
De Silva, P N
Emad, F
Fisher, C J
Franklin, R B
Harrison, M M
Holt, T A
Jackson, M
Johnson, P C
Lomas, A C
McAuley, J J
McCormack, T
Metcalfe, P W
Mian, A H
Moore, N
Newman, R R
Nicol, N T
Pearce, R E
Priest, O H
Rippon, D
Smart, A L
Suckling, I G
Vasey, D
Ward, N
Ward, P J
Ward, T A
Wheldon, G R
Williams, B P

Whitchurch, Hampshire
Card, T R
Croft, H D R
Johnson, M H

Whitchurch, Shropshire
Barker, E
Carter, G S E
Clayton, J S
Clayton, R
Flewett, W E
Giles, S N
McCarter, J D
Pritchard Jones, R O
Roberts, P J
Senior, F L
Short, W R
Teather, S J
Terry, R E
Thompson, R J
Vale, P T
Wilson, P F
Young, P F

Whitehaven
Bagshaw, S A
Battistessa, S A
Bober, M J
Bober, S A
Boyle, C E L
Carter, P E
Cartwright, P D
Christie, M C
Cristaldi, M
Davies, K H
Dhebar, M I
Dickson, J M
Dixon, E M
Elasha, H M S
Eldred, J M
Forbat, L N
Godden, M J
Greiss, M E
Griffith, T P
Huntley, L S
Iranzo, J
Ironside, F C
Ironside, G J
Jayatilaka, M N D P
Lamont, D A
Lee, D A
Local, F K
Markandoo, P
Moss, B
Park, P W
Precious, S H
Richards, D G
Rocha Janeiro, M M
Rogers, D J
Rudman, J D
Russell, N J
Saudi, M N S A R
Sellar, P W
Sharp, A S
Stafford, J
Stevenson, N J
Sullivan, V J
Sydney, M A
Timney, A P
Tranter, R
Umar, A
Varghese, S
Verinder, D G R
Walker, M A
Watson, D M
Westhead, J N
Willmer, K A
Woffindin, J

Whitland
Anthony, C J J D L
Griffiths, A E
Griffiths, I J
Jenkins, H C
Jenkins, R T D
McNeil, B D
Maguire, D M

Whitley Bay
Barker, J S
Barnes, P R
Beaumont, D M
Bridgewater, R A M
Buchanan, K J
Burrell, C M
Carlile, A K
Carr, C M E
Cockburn, R A
Corbitt, N E
Coundon, H
Craxford, P A
Cresswell, S M
Crilley, P F

Critchlow, B W
Cross, K A
Dale, G
Emamy, H F
Falconer, I L
Ferriman, J H
French, J J
Glennie, R
Gower, A
Hildreth, K A
Hinds, P R
Huntley, S
Inglis, E
Ingram, A T
Jackson, A W
Johns, G
Kilgour, H A
Lee, C J
Lunn, J S
Lunn, T
McDaid, P
MacLennan, D J
McManners, A J
Mayes, D E
Muir, I G
Murray, D
Olsburgh, B
Piper, M P P
Pridie, A K
Rae, G
Reay, K A
Richardson, S A
Ridley, A E
Robson, C W
Sabourn, P W
Sayers, S J
Srivastava, S P
Swann, K J
Tose, J M
Westgarth, S E
Wills, J C

Whitstable
Birch, S M
Chandler, S J
Cuming, T
Jardine, M A
Johnson, L F
Kanagasooriam, G M H
Lupton, P M H T
Mridha, E U
Pinnock, H J
Puckett, J R
Ribchester, J M
Shar, M B
Stefani, T A
Turner, M E C
Turner, R J C
Wain, M L

Whyteleafe
Collyer, G B
Roberts, A
Slater, A M
Tun, V

Wick
Cheesman, B P
Cobb, E J
Datta, P K
Farquhar, I H
Fisher, P W
Gunn, J
Haughey, F A
Inkster, T J
Johnston, I
Millard, E R
Mowat, J
Olorunda, H L O
Pearson, M R
Shallcross, T M
Stanley, R A

Wickford
Agbaje, O A
Brown, A A
Brown, J C
Chandra Reddy, P
Fernando, M Y D
Harriott, J C
Laker, M K
Maynard, J R
Moore, T M C
Persaud, J
Prem, A G
Reddy, S
Richards, P
Seewoonarain, K S K
Wildin, H M
Yong, A A

Widnes
Biggs, C J
Boggiano, P
Breeden, J S
Brindle, M J
Collinson, J A
Crabbe, S A
Creely, S J
Derham, C J
Edwards, S J
Evans, P J
Fletcher, S N
Gyawali, P
Hallam, C P
Holmes, G P
Howes, A J
Imison, C L
Kumar, S
Kumar, S
Lakshminarayana, M
McKenna, G W
McLaughlin, A G
McMaster, D S
Manning, D R P
Mottershead, J P
Perritt, S J
Saleemi, M H
Schofield, C I
Simmons, D J
Smith, S
Stockton, P A
Tandy, G G
Tierney, C J
Woodforde, C S J

Wigan
Agyeman, A
Ah-Weng, F
Ahuja, A S
Ahuja, R
Ahuja, S K
Alamin, M I
Angior, P G
Arthur, N A
Ashworth, M R
Azmi, A H
Bajkowski, A
Banerjee, D K
Basu, M K
Bateman, A P
Benjamin, U B
Best, A G
Bezzina, C L
Bhadoria, R S
Bhalerao, V R
Bhavnani, M
Blower, A L
Bose, L M J
Braben, P S
Bradshaw, J H
Brodie, D G
Browne, A O J
Burkinshaw, P R
Burza, N A
Chandler, C J
Chattopadhyay, C B
Chattopadhyay, H
Clark, M D A
Clayton, C
Clift, D L
Cooper, C D
Corkan, E J
Coxon, N R
Crook, H E S
D'Arifat, P F D
Dalal, A
Darvill, S P
Davies, J A
Dawson, J K
Dey, N C
Dhesi, I S
Dinnepati, S R
Doherty, R
Donaldson, K
Donnelly, D
Earnshaw, S M
Ellis, A J
Elton, P J
Eshiett, M U-A
Fairhurst-Winstanley, A J
Fairhurst, D A
Fallon, K J
Farrier, M P
Flatt, N W
Fraser, J M K
Fraser, J A
Frayne, J M
Gambhir, A K
Garner, J P
Ghalayini, M
Ghaly, R G
Ghosh, A K
Girgis, M H
Godby, C
Gradwell, E
Graham, A R P
Graham, R C P
Greenwood, A P
Grennan, D M
Hacking, N
Haines, J F
Hall, J S
Harborne, D J
Harland, R N L
Hart, S A
Hassan, C N
Heaton, S G
Heaven, C J
Herbert, J C
Higgins, S P
Hodgkinson, J P
Hogan, R A J
Holden, J D
Holme, A D L
Holme, C A
Holme, J D L
Holme, V J
Hopcroft, P W
Hopcroft, R W
Hughes, J R
Ibrahim, T S
Ishaque, M
Izzat, M
Jacks, R D
Jamdar, S
Jameel, M M M
Jehan, R
Jingree, M
Johnson, F
Jones, F B
Jones, I W
Jones, R J
Kapoor, P D
Kay, P R
Kelsall, R A
Khattab, B
Khattab, H P
Kirk, R S
Knowles, E W
Kofokotsios, A
Koppada, V R
Koussa, F F
Kreppel, P R
Kumar, B N
Lane, A D
Ledson, T A
Levine, H
Livingstone, B N
Llewelyn, J M
Lord, C P
Loudon, J R
Lowe, D B
McCarthy, J P
McCulloch, A B
McDonnell, J G
MacFaul, J P
Mackenzie, N A
Mann, T J
Marcovic, L
Marples, J
Mars, J S
Marsh, D J
Martin, R H
Marwick, T P
Mather, C E
Mellor, S C
Mills, J S
Misra, S N
Mohammed, A
Moore, V J
Morris, P R
Mughal, S
Mukherjee, A
Mukherjee, S
Mulinga, J D
Mullen, D J
Munro, C J
Murali, S R
Murnan, A
Murphy, D
Nagrani, P
Nandi, S R
Naqvi, N
Natha, S
Nayak, B N
Nsamba, C
O'Connell, I P M
O'Connor, R C
Ollerton, A
Owen, I G
Patel, M K
Peach, I D
Peck, R M
Pendry, K
Pinto, A L P
Pitalia, S K
Pollard, M
Poon, C L
Porter, M L
Prabhu, S
Pugh, M D
Purbach, B
Queenborough, R
Raut, V V
Ray, A C
Rayner, C A
Robertson, T C
Rodgers, P
Ross, K
Russell, B S
Rutter, J M
Sanghi, P K
Sathyan, N
Seabrook, J D
Seddon, T A
Shackleton, S E
Shaw, S J
Sheals, D G
Siddiqui, S V A
Sinclair, C M
Smith, M C
Southern, P J
Speakman, A R
Spence, M T
Stansfield, D A
Stewart, J S S
Suntha, S
Sutton, A N
Sweeney, J N
Temperley, D E
Thomas, A L
Thomas, B E
Thompson, A
Thomson, C
Thomson, R M
Thwaite, E L
Titoria, M
Trace, J P I
Trail, I A
Trivedi, A D
Trivedi, D
Turnbull, A D
Twist, W A
Twomey, M J
Tymms, D J
Ugargol, C P
Unwin, H M
Valentine, D T
Van Spelde, J F P
Vasudeva Kamath, S
Vickers, J E
Watson, S D
Watters, J
Welding, I J
White, D A
Whittington, M J
Wilson, L
Wolstenholme, R J
Wood, P L R
Wright, C R
Wroblewski, B M
Yashoda, P
Zzaman, K A

Wigston
Chamberlain, M N
Dauncey, S M
Dayah, A R
Mannan, V
Polak, G J A
Prideaux, C P
Ravat, S
Sharp, A J H
Shaw, J F
Sutton, C D

Wigton
Ajai-Ajagbe, E K O
Brown, G W
Cox, J
Hewson, M J
Higgins, D A
Holdsworth, J D
Honeyman, J P
Howe, J L
Johnston, M B
Jones, R M
Knox, C J
Robinson, D B
Roderick, E M
Russell, C J
Shand, J E G
Spencer, P M
Swan, E A
Swindells, R F C
Townend, M
Turnbull, A T M
Ungar, A

Willenhall
Abdalla, S Z
Badh, C S
Harris, M L
Johal, S S
Lall, G S
Necati, G
Patel, R M
Pendlington, M
Platt, C L
Prasad, A K
Sandhu, R K
Shah, A R
Sharma, N K
Shaw, M J
Shires, K M
Singh-Nijjer, B
Spurlock, C J
Varkey, T A
Vasudevan Nair, D C
Yusuf, S A J

Wilmslow
Ainsworth, J H
Allsager, C M
Anthony, E W
Bedi, K S R
Bedi, M S V
Bell, V A
Bird, J R
Bray, C L
Brennan, M
Bundred, S M
Caprio, L
Carne, P R
Case, K M T
Chatterjee, P C
Chatterjee, S S
Choudhry, H K
Connell, P G
Cope, V
Cowan, R A
Damani, Z B
Darroch, R A
Davies, E T L
Doran, T N H
Fraser, N C
Gain, R T G
Ghosh, A K
Goodger, A R
Gorman, A P
Gregg, R C
Hague, J N
Hindusa, K
Hirst, P
Hore, I D B
Horton, C A
Huddart, J E
Hutchinson, T R
Ismail, A M
Johnson, R H
Johnston, H A
Jones, A D N
Jones, M H
Jones, S T M
Kerr, D F
Khafagy, R S
Khafagy, R T
King, J M
Kingston, T P
Lam, A C W
Lea, R A C
Levy, A H
Levy, L P
Lewis, S E
Longson, J
McDonald, J P
McIntyre, I G
Mamtora, H
Manning, G A K
Maxwell, S R
Moss, R M H
Myers, A E
Nadarajah, M
Neal, B R
Newhouse, R E
Newton, M L
O'Driscoll, B J
O'Sullivan, K A
Patterson, E J
Percival, E J
Pope, V
Powell, K Y
Ramsay, T M
Rawal, S B
Ream, J A
Ring, N M
Rushton, A
Sanville, P R
Scott, G
Scott, M A
Sheikh, J Y
Silverman, S R
Spencely, M
Stockdale, A V K
Stockley, W D
Struthers, J K
Sukumar, P
Torry, M J W
Walker, A M
Walthew, R I
Wasson, C M A
Wasson, S J
Welchman, C L

Wimborne
Adlington, P
Adlington, R J
Ahmed, M A
Allen, R L
Aquilina, R J
Baldwin, H L
Chambers, N
Craigmyle, D
Davidson, C M
Dawson, A J
De Freitas, A J S
Deverell, M H
Dickins, P J N
Edwards, T J
Elder, A M
Francis, J R
Garrard, A C
Gee, A A
Greenway, N D
Harrocks, D R
Hayden, A
Holt, M F
Horgan, J E M
Howard, T R G
Howard, W R G
Lanham, P R W
Lawrence, S J
Lear, B L
Leggett, J M
Leschen, A D
Levinson, A R
Linley-Adams, M J
McKevitt, N L
Maiden, L P
Malpas, S M
Moondi, P P S
Morgan, D F
Nicholas, A S
Pharaoh, A M
Pope, D C
Purandare, A S
Sanders, E M
Sankson, H
Scott, N C
Slade, D E M
Smyth, P R F
Stephens, J R D
Swan, M J
Tan, J B L
Taylor, M S
Trivedi, K L
Tulloch, J G
Walden, T A
Williams, J P
Wilson-Croome, J
Woollard, B P
Wright, N R

Wincanton
Elcomb, A M N
Farrant, C F
Fellows, M J
Gribble, R J N
Phillips, I G
Robertson, G D
Woodland, J M

Winchelsea
Alexander, C A
Doherty, W G
Homi, J

Winchester
Abbott, D F
Acres, D J
Adams, J P
Adamson, A S
Al-Badri, A M T
Antoniou, A G
Arnold, R C
Ashcroft, M W
Ashcroft, P B
Ashken, J V
Aston, C E
Baker, R A
Bavister, A E
Beaumont, S
Bedford, J
Benjamin, E
Bolwell, A G
Bonsall, A M
Bould, E-J
Boyle, D S
Brockway, B D J
Brooke, D J
Brooks, A P
Buchanan, N M M
Buckingham, M S
Burlinson, R A
Burrows, F D C
Burrows, J
Burton, P J
Button, R I
Calogeras, A
Chan-Pensley, E
Chapman, C M
Cheetham, J E
Corkill, R A
Corlett, R J
Cotton, T G
Cox, N L
Craggs, D A
Crawford, A D
Curson, J A
D'Alfonso, A A L
Davies, J C
Davies, S L
Davis, A V H
Deacock, S J C
Dewbury, C E
Diaper, M D
Dreaper, R E
Dryden, M S
Du Boulay, P M H
Eddy, T
Edelsten, M A
Elford, J
England, P G
Evans, M R W
Fairris, G M
Fayers, K E
Firebrace, D A J
Fitzgerald-Barron, A W J
Fon, P J
Foote, K D
Forster, I D
Foster, B J
Fowler, J L
Fox, H J
Gabb, R J E
Gartell, P C
Goldsmith, A L
Gordon, H M
Grant, L J
Grant, S J
Green, B
Grummitt, C C
Guerrier, T H
Hall, V L
Hamer, J E
Hanna, H M
Harrison, E M
Harrison, G S M
Heard, M J
Hemsley, Z M
Henderson, F H M
Hesketh, K T
Hobbs, A
Hook, W E
Howells, C J
Hume-Smith, H V
Hunt, B J
James, C M
Jessop, E G
Jones, D H
Jordan, K M
Kay, E M
Kelly, J E
Keough, A D
Kerkhoff, R V
Khan, H H
King, A W
Kingswell, R S
Knight, H M L
Laidlow, J M
Lambert, M G B
Lane, R H S
Laws, S A M
Lee, P J
Lees, S J
Lewis, A
Lippiett, P V
Lock, D J
Louden, K A
Loughran, J
McGrand, J C
Macleod, J D A
Mahon, D
Mainwaring, C J M J
Mann, K S
Marquis, A M M
Marsh, A J
Marsh, D F
Mears, H J
Miles, A J G
Mitchell, M C
Moitra, R K
Moore, H L
Moore, M G
Morgan, J
Morgan, K
Morris, K E A
Morton, J R C
Mulcock, H
Myers, J H
Nair, S B
Nancekievill, M L
Nicholson, S M
Nicpon, K J
Norman-Nott, A G
Normand, I C S
O'Sullivan, J L
Olliver, M E
Owen, D K
Padgham, M R J C
Page, A C
Paget, T D
Papastathis, D
Paramanathan, N
Parfitt, J C
Pathmadeva, C
Pathmadeva, T W
Pearson, S
Pell, J B
Percival, I M
Phillips, C G H
Pitman, M C
Plant, I D
Powell-Jackson, J D
Powell-Jackson, M A
Rains, A J H
Rainsbury, R M
Rall, M H
Read, J A P
Roberts, J A
Roberts, J M
Roberts, K E
Rose, J W P
Rowe, K A
Rowland, R G
Samuel, A W
Samuel, M
Saunders, W A
Selman, J C
Slack, M H
Slack, S E
Slapak, G I
Slapak, M
Smith, F R
Smith, H R
Smith, J A E
Soekarjo, D D
Spencer-Silver, P H
Spice, C L
Stannard, T J
Stevens, L C
Steventon, N B
Stewart, A J
Stewart, K O
Stewart, R I
Strange, J W N
Summerfield, R J
Sylvester, N C
Thomas, M F
Thomas, R C
Thompson, J A
Toff, N J
Tomlinson, J M
Toone, P C
Trimmings, N P
Van De Pette, J E W
Voisey, S C
Wakefield, C H
Watt, P A
Watt, P J
Watts, J A
Weller, R O
Wethered, O J C
Wheeler, T
White, D
White, L A
White, W D
Wills, D R
Wills, F A
Wilson, A S
Wilson, N M
Woodcock, K R
Wright, H G
Wright, N
Wright, N J
Wyborn, A J N

Windermere
Burns, P
Coleman, K E
Gulliford, P
Hawson, J P
Hynes, J M
Oakden, E W R
Pearson, B C
Roberts, J H
Swan, M
Watson, S M
White, G P
Winter-Barker, J P

Windlesham
Armstrong, K A
Buxton, F A M
Handley, S M
Hatty, S R
Keohane, P P
Lledo Macau, A
Peck, R W
Roberts, E W
Simmons, V E
Simpson, A
Walmsley, A M

Windsor
Alden, C P
Almeyda, R V
Atkins, M
Bacon, D H
Barrett, G S
Barua, B K
Bloomfield, M D
Brudney, J K
Butcher, C B
Cheongvee, E S L
Chukwuemeka, S O
Crossley, R A
Denny, M R L
Denny, M F
Duncan, D
Evans, D E
Evans, D M
Felstead, M
Flower, D J C
Gibbings, C R
Goulds, R K
Hales, D A
Hameed, R S A
Harvey-Hills, N
Hawk, J L M
Holliday, J J C
Horan, S
Howells, J B
Hussain, S A
Inward, J M
Jones, J R
Kinnear, F C
Lelli, N M
Lewis, E S
Lewis, G M
Lewis, M J
Lewis, S I
Liyanage, I S
Liyanage, S P
Luck, R J
Lund, J
McAllister, J A
Macaulay, A J
Mackenzie, J W
Mackie, P H
McKiernan-Krieg, W S
Mills, A P G
Moloney, S J
Morgan, N H
Morrish, L W
Mower, I M
Mower, M T C
Packard, R B S
Patterson, J V M
Pethen, S
Power, R J
Rajagopal, R V
Rao, S K
Roberts, A
Robertshaw, C J
Roddy, R J
Roles, W
Saad, M N
Sammut, D P
Sawhney, S
Scott, R D M
Shin, C Y-M
Smart, R G
Smith-Walker, M T
Song, F M
Stone, J P W
Stoppard, M
Swann, M
Thomas, M
Tillott, R C
Trickey, N R A
Unwin, A J
Van Der Meulen, J J N M
Walsh, J K
Wellington, C M
Wilkins, A J
Williams, S A

Wingate
Fairlamb, C P
Morle, I J F
Simpson, A M
Sinha, P
Stephenson, R
Van Buuren, C M D

Winscombe
Hasham, S
Jackson, J C
John, D H
Newton, J C
Roberts, P H
Ruddell, K B L
Shouls, J C
Smith, I M A

Winsford
Achurch, S M
Bratt, H J
Bundle, A
Fallon, M P M
Gilmour, J E
Green, J H
Hyder, S
Kelly, P D
Loke, E S I
Mozumdar, S K
Price, J-A
Rasaiah, S
Roy, S K
Shuaib, M
Smith, C G
Talukder, R
Thomas, N R

Wirral
Agbamu, D A
Agrawal, G S
Ahmed, W
Airey, C L
Alderman, B
Alderson, M L
Ali, A
Alman, R J
Anthony, K L
Arista, V A
Ashton, P C B
Atherton, A M J
Atherton, J
Avery, M J
Ball, A R
Banks, D S
Bansal, O P
Barnard, P D
Barrett, J A
Baruah, A K
Bates, J W
Berstock, D A
Bhati, R
Bird, H C
Blacklin, J
Blair, S D
Booth, F J
Bousfield, P F
Bousfield, S K
Boyd, A H
Brace, J V
Breckenridge, R A
Brennan, S M
Brewis, J E
Brock, J E S
Brown, A G
Bryson, T H L
Burgess, M B
Bush, K J
Bussey, T J
Byrne, A E
Calderbank, S J
Calow, S A
Campbell, I R
Camphor, I A
Carroll, N
Carter, A J
Carter, H
Carter, P B
Causer, J P
Cervetto, P
Chadwick, C
Chadwick, M A
Chalmers, W D
Chambers, J J
Chapman, R J
Charlwood, C A
Chesters, S A
Chong, W C C
Clark, A H
Clark, J H
Clark, P I
Clarke, E T
Clarke, S P
Clearkin, L G
Cliff, A M
Conway, M
Cooke, K C
Coppock, P J
Cottier, B
Cowie, F A
Coy, A A C
Crosthwaite, O S
Currie, P
Cuthbertson, F M
D'Souza, S P
Dalby, M D
Darwish, D H
Dawson, J
Deeble, T J
Deeks, A J
Delaney, H L
Delaney, J C
Dennis, M W
Devlin, J C
Dixon, L A
Dolan, S-A
Donnachie, N J
Downs, H E
Downward, D C
Doyle, P M
Drury, J H
Dufton, P A
Dunham, W R
Earl, M J
Edwards, G M
Edwards, K E
Edwards, K B
El Boghdadly, S A E-K M
Elkington, J S
Ellis, A M
Emms, H A
Entwistle, I R
Errington, R D
Evans, J C
Evered, C J
Eyes, B E
Faizallah, R
Fletcher, M E
Foggin, W K
Fordham, M V P
Foster, V J
Francis, G G
Gannon, J P
Garrett, A M G
Garrett, M
Geary, N P J
Ghosh, A K
Gibbs, T J
Gidlow, D A
Gillett, M B
Gokhale, G
Gollins, W J F
Good, A M T
Goonesinghe, N S
Grant, K A
Gray, G A
Greaney, M G
Green, A R T
Green, J M
Green, J A
Green, R M
Griffith, C J
Guratsky, B P
Haggett, M J
Hamilton, S E
Harding, J A
Hardman, G
Hargreaves, S J
Harkins, F
Harrison, J C
Harty, S M
Harvey, R A
Hawthornthwaite, E M
Hayes, J C
Hayhurst, V
Healy, A P
Heaton, A J
Hennessy, T D
Hlaing, T
Hodgson, L M
Holmes, J J
Howard, C
Hughes, A P
Hughes, J M
Hulme, G
Hulme, I S
Hunter, J M
Husband, D J
Hussain, A
Hutchinson, S
Jackson, E J
Jackson, S P
Jacobs, E F
Janikiewicz, S M J S
Jayaraman, S
Jefferies, G
Jip, H
Johnson, R
Johnson, T B W
Johnston, A R
Johnstone, R G
Jones, C M
Jones, D C
Jones, D H
Jones, I R
Jones, P O
Jones, S K
Joynson, C P
Katchburian, M V
Kaye, J C
Keetarut, S
Kennedy, T D
Kenny, S E
Kershaw, D
Khalil, H R
Kidd, S A
Killeen, D M
King, D
Kingston, S P
Klenka, Z R
Konig, P C W C
Kutarski, P W
Lacy, D E
Lancaster, J L
Lane, C J
Lang, D M
Lannigan, B G
Larkin, P S
Lawrence, D S
Lawrence, E J
Lecky, J M F
Leigh, T J
Leith, S E
Lenfestey, P M
Levycky, H M
Lewis-Jones, C M
Lipton, M E
Little, A D
Littler, J A H
Lorains, J W
Lynes, J
McAlavey, A J
McClelland, P
McCrone, J W
McGuinness, A J
McKay, S J

Mackenzie, C P
Macleod, A J
McWatt, P J
McWilliams, M J
McWilliams, R G
Madden, M P
Magennis, J
Maguire, J
Mahai, A P K
Makin, C A
Mamman, I
Manning, D J
Marrow, J
Marshall, E
Marshall, M A
Martin Hierro, M E
Martin, H C
Masters, A
Mawby, N E
Maxwell, M J
Meara, R J
Mellors, A S
Moloney, A
Moore, J K
Morris, A D
Murray, A
Murray, A E
Murray, R
Neil, T
Neithercut, W D
Newall, N
Newbury, A L
Newland, A D
Nicholas, K S
Noglik, A M
O'Connor, J
O'Hagan, J E
O'Hanlon, D P
O'Hanlon, K C
O'Reilly, S M M
Oates, J G
Ohiorenoya, B
Oliver, K
Omari, A A A
Owens, J L
Owens, V B
Painter, D J
Parkinson, R W
Parr, N J
Parry, C R
Parry, D G
Parton, M J
Partridge, T M
Patwala, D Y
Payne, J H
Pennycook, A G
Pereira, A A L
Perkins, J A
Phillips, R P
Pickin, R B
Pickles, R L
Pigott, S J
Pilling, D W
Pillow, S J
Pinder, C A F
Pleasance, C M
Porteous, M A
Porter, G C
Potter, A W
Potter, F A
Powell, A P
Prasad, S
Price, A R
Price, D J
Pritchard-Howarth, M R
Quest, L J
Rae, J L
Rafiq, S
Ramdenee, R
Rao, A M
Raraty, C C
Raraty, M G T
Rawlinson, J K M
Raymond, C J
Reid, A G
Reilly, D T
Reuben, S F
Reynolds, J J
Rhodes, E G H
Rich, P N
Richmond, E E
Richmond, I M
Richmond, M S
Roberts, E
Roberts, J R
Robertson, S H
Robin, N M
Robinson, J S
Robinson, L Q
Robson, P W
Romaniuk, C S
Rowlands, D J
Ruddy, J P
Rule, E M
Russell, J
Ryan, S W
Ryan, T D R
Sagar, A
Sangster, G
Sansom, C D
Scott, A K
Setna, F J
Shah, N
Sharma, V
Sharples, R H
Shennan, J M
Sherman, I W
Shiralkar, V M
Sida, E C
Sidky, K H I
Silas, J H
Simison, A J M
Singh, K
Slater, A J
Sloka, R A
Smethurst, M E
Smith, A B
Smith, D B
Smith, D N
Smith, D A
Smith, M W
Snowden, A E A
Sprigge, J S
Stanley, C A M
Stevens, K D
Stevens, R W
Stewart, A B
Stokoe, D
Swales, C L
Sweeney, E
Syndikus, I M
Tansey, D J
Tansley, A P
Tarr, T J
Thaker, D
Thomas, T G
Thompson, J A R
Thompson, S K
Thomson, A J M
Thorp, N J M L
Timmins, D J
Timms, M A J
Todd, P J
Tomlinson, A P
Tomlinson, S D
Townsend, C J
Tracy, H J
Turnbull, C J
Usborne, C M
Vine, D J
Wade, R H
Waller, D P E
Walsh, C J
Walshaw, M J
Walton, H A S
Warren, V J
Watts, M T
Weaver, H
Welch, C R
Wells, S M
Welsh, S H
Weston, N C
White, P C
White, S I
Whiteside, M W
Whitfield, A M
Wight, J A
Wilkins, H M
Wilkinson, C E
Wilkinson, H C
Williams, I A
Williams, R D
Williams, S H
Williamson, V C
Winston, M P
Winston, S R
Wong, S H D
Wood, J G
Woodcock, B M
Woollons, M J
Wort, S J
Wright, A R
Wright, J E M
Wright, J A
Wright, P K
Wynne, S P M
Young, D J
Zakhour, H

Wisbech

Al-Bitar, M Z
Blundell, A C
Chandler, A
Clark, L
Clarke, E J
Doran, K M
Earle, R C
Ferriday, C E R
Fester, J S
Forster, D B
Grant, L A
Hattersley, D A
Hudson, B
Karunaratne, W M
Khetani, B N J
Lees, J M
Lines, J
Mason, I H
Millard, S P
Moffat, G M
Neary, J M
Nelson, S E
Patel, N R
Pryer, M P L
Richardson, M J
Rosier, N C I
Shippey, B J
Somerville, E T
Walker, M P
Webb, R T
Williams, N C
Williams, P R
Wong, Q K K
Wood, C J M
Wordsworth, A D

Wishaw

Ahmed, O N
Al-Kureishi, T
Allan, T L
Allen, I C
Begg, L
Bell, A
Ben-Younes, A H
Callaghan, M W
Campbell, H
Cannon, J D
Clark, C M
Clark, F C E
Connelly, A
Cooper, L A H
Crossan, E M
Curran, J E
Dear, N P M
Dobbie, S
Eatock, C R
Falconer, J S
Gibb, D B
Helenglass, G
Hendry, A
Hotchkiss, C M
Hung Kwok Choi, M J A
Kolhatkar, R K
Lannigan, A K
Lees, C M
Lennox, C E
Logan, A R
McClung, A R
McCoach, A
McConnell, S M
McCrum, D
McGuire, L C
McKay, K E H
Macpherson, B C M
MacSween, W A
Majumdar, A A W
Mann, B S
Milne, A J
Murphy, E A
Murphy, J W
Naismith, J H
O'Dowd, J J M
Ofili, G U
Parker, I
Pickard, R G
Reddy, S S
Reid, D B
Reynolds, M F
Sagoo, R S
Scott, H R
Stewart, D W
Thom, W R
Thomson, J B
Walsh, J M
Westbrook, F
Wilson, T K

Witham

Baqai, A
Baqai, M A
Beatty, D E
Bridgman, G C
Carroll, G D
Courtman, S P
Crane, T P
Davies, D F
Dekker, B J
Fernando, M L P
Foster, W
Gough, B R
Grew, R C
Hawkins, R M
Hopcroft, J P
Hore, A T
Irwin, D J
Karki, C B
Krishnamurthy, K
Krishnamurthy, M R
Millership, S E
Murtaza, L N
Netscher, M M
Parry-Jones, N O
Phillips, P K
Shroff, R
Sizer, B F
Summers, R T
Teverson, E
Watson, P S
Wright, C J

Withernsea

Fouracre, R D
French, R S
Heaton, G D
Herbert, P E
Khoury, F

Witney

Ali, A N
Bacon, N C M
Bailey, J
Baker, F A
Brylewski, S
Caddick, A N
Chakraverty, R K
Chalmers, C A
Chapman, K
Coffey, P P
Connor, P P
Derry, J L
Diacon, M J
Douglas, A
Evans, H W
Graham-Jones, S
Grainger, L
Green, B G
Grimwade, P R
Hale, D J
Hallett, S
Haslam, L
Herries, J W
Hickman, T M
Hyde, B J
Jackson, P C
James, M D
Jarvis, J R
Jones, R J
Kay, P G
Lawrence, M A
Lole-Harris, C A
Manning, C J
Mather, R A L
Maxwell, J M
Morris, C E
Naidoo, N K
Nelson, G L
Peterson, D J M
Prosser, P D
Smith, S M V
Spence, J R
Stanger, M J
Stephenson, P B O
Stewart, B J A
Theodorou, S
Thorley, R A
Walton, S E
Watson, P A

Woking

Ambler, L C
Ambrose, G C
Andrews, G
Armstrong, L J
Atkins, M C
Ayers, A B
Aziz, K A
Aziz, W A
Baker, A W
Barker, N J
Bates, P C
Baughan, C A
Beilby, J O W
Bingham, E M
Bird, M M
Bishop, Y M
Blakey, L
Bourke, M J
Branagan, G W
Brockway, C M
Brown, P A
Buchanan, R M
Cameron, E G M
Chan, S W
Chisholm, E M
Christie, A-M
Christopherson, T A P
Clarke, V A
Cleary, C V
Close, A R
Close, L P
Coe, S M
Collins, T M
Collins, Y D
Condon, R W
Coope, A M
Cummin, A L
Cummin, P J C
Dawkins, J L
De Courcy, S A
Deans, A C
Dear, N J
Dennison, M G
Edmunds, C J
Essa, N I S
Evans, B T
Evans, R P
Eyton, S M A
Foote, J A J
Garrett Ryan, F J
Gillham, A B
Glover, J M
Grieve, N W T
Grove, C E
Hadfield, G
Halepota, M A
Hall, A M
Handousah, S M E
Harding, T M
Harris, K P
Hendry, A E
Hennell, P A
Hindley, D J
Howitt Wilson, M B
Imrie, M M
Jarzabek, J B
Johnson, D
Jones, A F
Keane, R
Kelly, C A
Khan, N H Z
Kirthisingha, V A
Knights, H D
Kruchek, D G L
Kuzmin, P J
Lance, N S
Lander, R M
Leach, J R
Leno, S M
Lewis, S E
Lock, K J
Lucas, E G
Lyle, N J
Lynn, W A
Lytton, G J
McIntosh, S L
Mahmood, A
Manners, B T B
Margary, J J
Mellor, J P
Michelmore, S K
Miller, H B
Miller, J A
Mirza, M R
Morgan, J A
Morgan, J
Morley, N J
Munro, F M E
Murray, S I
Newbold, S M
Newman, H
O'Neill, A-M
O'Neill, V M
Ogden, A B
Panhwar, G-M
Pankhania, B
Parveen, S S
Perera, D D T
Pontin, M J
Pool, R J
Pool, R D
Prior, T
Ratcliffe, N A
Rauf, K G
Riddle, A F
Roberts, L C
Rogers, B A
Rooney, B A
Rudman, T J
Rumball, B J
Ryan, N P
Saunders, M I
Scott, J A G
Sellars, N H L
Sellick, B C
Sheikh, A
Shiel, D A
Simonis, R B
Sinnerton, R J
Smith, P J R
South, J
Spencer, T S
Sreedaran, E
Steele, K
Tennant, F D
Thomas, D H V
Thompson, J M
Thompson, N J
Unwin, T A E
Walker, M C
Wall, A R J
Walsh, M
Ward, P
Wilson Jones, A C R
Wilson Jones, N A H J
Wong, A S-Q
Wright, T G
Young, J J
Yusuf, I A
Zaki, M

Wokingham

Allsopp, M R
Arnold, S M
Beard, G A
Beer, P A
Black, J E B
Butler, K
Carter, K T
Corfield, M H
Darlison, M T
Day, A H
Doran, J R
Dunnet, S C
Edwards, R C
Emmerson, R W
Evans, R J
Evans, S D
Fawke, J A
Foley, G P
Gallagher, C J
Goodwin, L G
Goodwin, M D
Griffith, S
Guyer, B M
Hadfield, K A M
Haslam, M B
Helm, S M
Herman, M J G
Hession, P T
Houghton, D C
Hutchison, J B
Kerr, J D
Kitson, G E
Latham, R A
Lee, M C
McCall, P D
MacDougall, M E
Marwick, S M
Mellows, R J
Mitra Thakur, G G
Moreno Beteta, A
Morton, N B M
Moudiotis, C R
Murphy, A L
O'Donnell, C A-M
O'Donnell, D R
Purchas, M A
Reakes, R E M
Reece-Smith, H
Richards Affonso, N
Ross, P S

Saba, H P
Smyly, P A J
Sowter, E M
Stangroom, C D
Walker, A
Ward, M L
Wardill, L F
Watson, E A
Weeks, N J
Weir, K A J
Win Hlaing, Dr
Zaheer, S A

Wolverhampton
Adeghe, A J-H
Agrawal, L
Agrawal, S
Aiton-MacBean, D R
Anand, S
Anderson, J M
Anees, N N
Annesley-Williams, D J
Asthana, K
Aung, T S
Axon, E J
Babiker, S K
Bagary, D S
Balaggan, K S
Ball, E S
Barnes, P
Barry, K J
Benbow, S M
Bhatia, M M
Bhikha, A
Bilas, R
Black, T J
Blayney, M R
Boddy, R S
Bose, R K
Bould, M
Bradley, J
Bright, J J
Browning, A J F
Bryan, L H
Bulmer, N J
Burrell, J T
Bush, D M
Cameron, H A C
Catchpole, C R
Chohan, M M
Cleeland, J A
Clews, J W
Cockburn, T R
Collins, M A
Cooke, P W
Cooper, M A
Copeman, A J
Coppolo, M
Corridan, P G J
Corston, R N
Coward, J I G
Cox, C W F M
Creed, T J
Cross, T J S
Crossley, D R
Crossley, T M
Curran, F T
Currie, S J
D'Costa, D F
Davies, J E
Davies, M
De Rosa, D
Deacon, C S
Derso, A
Dexter, E L S
Dhillon, G S
Dhingra, H S
Diba, V C
Dison, P J
Djan, N
Dobie, D A
Dobie, D K
Dukes, I T
Duncan, P J
Dunn, S M
Elcock, M
Fairlamb, C A W
Fairlamb, D J
Fan, V T W
Fenner, S G
Fitzgerald, R
Fletcher, A M
Forrest, G A
Foster, C J
Fotherby, K J
Fowler, J M
Freeth, M G
Fuggle, W J
Gama, R M
Gardecki, T I M
Gee, P
Ghosh, A
Gill, A S
Glover, H F B
Gnanasegaram, D
Gnanenthiran, S
Gogna, S C
Goldie, A M
Gonzalez, E
Goodyear, G M
Graff, D J C
Grandhi, V
Green, D I
Grew, N R
Griffiths, J J
Grinsted, R
Grosvenor, L J
Guest, E H
Gupta, A
Gupta, E
Gurney, J
Hadley, C R
Hadlington, K J
Halepota, A A
Hall, H N
Hamad, H A
Handa, S I
Handa, S I
Handley, A F
Hartill, S A
Hassan, H M J
Hibbs, H M
Hickman, P
Higgins, C M
Hogg, R A
Hollands, R A
Hommers, C E
Hooper, C R B
Horton, R C
Hughes, R C
Ilyas, N
Inglis, J A
Isbister, E S
Jackson, M A
Jackson, T N
Jacob, A
Jeewa, M A I
Jenkins, R
Johnson, A
Jolley, D J
Jones, F C
Jones, H E
Jones, L
Jones, P N
Joy, H A
Julka, S K
Kainth, M S
Kalra, D S
Kanodia, S K
Kapadia, S A
Kassim, Z
Kaur, H R
Kelleher, H C
Kemsley, S
Kew, J M D
Khan, A H
Khan, M I
Konu, G K
Krishan, K S
Kumararatne, B
Lantos, H W G
Larkin, E B
Larkin, J M
Lee, E F-Y
Leung, H H
Linnemann, M P
Luis, J L C
MacCarthy, B
McCarthy, S W
McCreadie, D W J
Macdonald, D R
McKenzie, J
Mackie, G
McLaren, R
McNamee, G G
Mahay, G R
Maheru, A K
Maidment, P R
Maji, S
Manley, M E P
Mann, J S
Mantle, M
Mathews, J
Maung, Dr
Mehan, R
Mehmi, M
Meredith, H E
Micklewright, R J
Millar, B G
Mittal, S
Molony, N C
Moran, M
Morgan, I S
Morgans, J P
Mudie, L L
Murray, G S
Naren, M
Nehikhare, F O
Nguyen, A L
Nguyen, M L
Nightingale, P D
Noble, B S
O'Connell, D M
O'Dowd, S
Odum, J
Oliwiecki, S
Pahwa, M K
Parkes, A J
Parkes, J D
Passi, M M L
Passi, U
Passi, V
Patel, K A
Peacock, S R
Pearson, D J
Perry, M R
Peters, C G
Phillips, A W
Phillips, A J
Phillips, M
Philp, N H
Pickavance, G
Plant, A
Pooni, J S
Poornan, A M
Porczynska, W I
Prasad, R
Price, N J
Qureshi, A S
Rahman, M A
Rahman, M H
Rai, J
Ratra, S S
Ravindran, T S
Rayner, R J
Read, C A
Richardson, H B M
Richmond, D J H
Roberts, R N
Rowlands, D C
Rushton, P J
Russon, M J
Ryan, G
Rylance, P B
Rylance, W S
Samra, J S
Samra, M K
Sandramouli, S
Sarkar, A
Sarkar, P K
Sarkar, P K
Scott, K W M
Scotton, S J
Seedhouse, J K
Sehdev, G
Serhan, E
Shah, I A
Shah, N K
Shah, S
Shaikh, M G
Share, A
Sharma, B K
Shortridge, R T J
Shun-Shin, G A
Sidebotham, E L
Simon, G R
Simon, R I
Singh, B M
Singh, B B
Singh, M
Singh, S P
Smith, J K
Smith, J L
Smith, M H
Smith, N I
Snape, S L
Staite, M E
Stoves, R
Strain, G J
Stuttard, G L
Talbot, M S
Tandon, R K
Tandon, S C
Taylor, C
Taylor, D R
Taylor, S A
Tayyab, M
Thet Win, Dr
Thomas, A P
Thomas, R J
Tomlinson, J H
Tovey, G F
Turner, A
Varadharajan, S
Vishwanath, L S
Vishwanath, M S
Wagstaff, P J
Wake, M
Walker, C
Walker, P J
Walton, R S
Wanas, T M
Watson, A M
Waymont, B
White, J F M
Williams, A
Williams, A E
Williams, J G
Williams, J T
Willis, M J
Willis, P
Wilson, M
Wiseman, J
Wrigley, E T
Yin Yin Win, Dr
Zeya, K

Woodbridge
Alden, A E
Allen, R T
Archer, C A
Ball, S P
Bartlett, K L H
Bartlett, M H
Boyd, K D
Brierly, E K
Byrne, A J
Byrne, W F
Crowther, K A
Deliss, L J
Dillon, F C
Driver, I K
Edwards, N J
Elson, C W
Fairweather, D A
Glaister, A M
Goble, O A
Haigh, J W
Hamilton, T J
Healey, D G
James, M R
Jones, J G
Jones, K M
Lewis, R E
Lynch, J P W
McGlennon, M
Mackay, S G
Moffatt, R J
Norton, S C
Odlum, H R
Parkinson, M J
Perkins, S
Rivers, N
Rowell, G H R
Rufford, B D
Simmonds, A J
Slater, C J
Smith, M G
Tate, A C
Taylor, G H F
Verrill, R P
Wright, C E
Yates, K P

Woodford Green
Arora, A K
Barfoot, L C
Baura, G K
Beavis, A K
Bosch, G
Brill, G
Brill, S E
Brohi, A H K
Chatterjee, M
Das, C K
Dasgupta, R
Deo, H D
Devereux, E-J
Divakaran, K
Gandhi, M M
Graham, J D
Green, B
Gutmann, J H
Honey, C M
Innes, W G
Ireland, J
Joiner, C E
Jones, R H
Lawrence, P L
Luthra, P N
Lyons, A G
Mohamed, M A M
Mulligan, M J C
Okosun, O H
Price, R V
Rajakumar, R
Ray, A K
Ray, D
Ryatt, L K
Sahu, D N
Samsami, S M
Sheikh, I S
Sika, M
Smith, I A
Smith, J
Taylor, G A W
Tranmer, F M
Webb, A A C
Whitaker, J W

Woodhall Spa
Butter, K C
Campbell, C S
Malcolm, J M
Murray, M C

Woodstock
Barrington-Ward, D
Billing, J S
Cook, S A
Coombs, H M C
Henville, J D
Hope, S L
Leck, I M
Martin, A J
Orchard, T R
Van Oss, H G
Winterbottom, P M

Wooler
Craig, R
Dean, C R
Spoor, K M

Woolwich
Carr, J V L
Evans, A N W
Ketley, N J
Robertson, S M
Shakespeare, C F
Teall, A J

Worcester
Abudu, T O
Agoston, S A
Aldis, J S
Ali, B
Allen, D J
Allen, P A
Armitstead, C P
Ashton, C E
Austin, D I
Ayshford, C A
Back, D L
Barnard, N A
Barrell, J P
Bellamy, W
Belt, P J
Bennett, S J
Blake, A E
Bond, T P
Bowley, D M G
Breakwell, J
Brookes, P T
Brotherwood, A P
Brown, J F
Brown, L M
Brown, M T
Brown, R
Bryant, M G H
Butler, J
Bywater, A J
Cairns, D
Campbell, I M
Castling, D P
Chapman, T W L
Charny, M C
Chen, T F
Chikwe, J
Childs, F E M
Christys, A G
Clark, J M C
Clear, D B
Cockeram-Paranavitana, M N S
Cockeram, S F
Collett, L A
Collins, R J
Collis, A T G
Colwill, R C
Constantine, C E
Cook, P J
Cope, P G
Corlett, M P
Cottell, K M
Crookall, P R
Cross, S J
Crossman, K J
Cullen, M G
Cutts, S
Dale, J M
Davies, J S
Davies, M C
Davies, T E P
Davis, I J
Davis, M J
Davis, P J C
Day, N J
De Cothi, A J
De Silva, Y
Deighan, M J
Dennis, E A
Dickens, J J
Doward, W A
Downing, R
Dunn, P J S
Dye, P C
Earl, P D
Ellis, W R
England, D W
Everitt, S M A
Ferguson, T A
Fielding, E M P
Fielding, J W L
Franklin, T S M
Gallagher, A C
Georgiou, G A
Glennie, H R
Goldsmith, C
Gommersall, L M
Gonzalez Elosegui, A M
Goodman, J F M
Griffiths, W D
Hak, C
Hamilton, M J
Hardwick, M
Harvey, L
Havercroft, A R
Haynes, S J L
Hickey, N C
Hickling, E J
Higginson, R
Holding, R
Holehouse, G D T
Huppertz, R C M
Hussain, M A
Jackson, P
Jefferson-Loveday, J W
Jenkins, D
Johnson, R A
Jones, C P
Jones, I R
Jones, J C
Jones, T J D
Kerton, J J
King, S G
Laidlaw, A J
Laidlaw, K A M
Lake, S P
Lavin, S J
Lee, B J
Lewis, A M
Lewis, F M
Lewis, R A
Lord, P W
Lowe, S J
Mackichan, R I
Maddison, T J R
Marshall, A E
Mason, B
Mills, A F
Mitchell, P A
Monkley, C R
Morgan, M G G
Morrison, C A
Morrison, R D
Mulira, A J E L
Munro, A J
Murray, D S
Nazare, J C F

Neil, D
Neillie, J L
New, A C
Newey, S F
Norton, W D
O'Driscoll, J P
O'Dwyer, K J
O'Hickey, S P
Osborn, J A
Osborn, N A
Osborne, J
Owen, R D
Paton, R S
Peet, A S
Pennock, P F L
Perkins, S M
Phillips, D M
Philpott, R G E
Pickerell, L M W
Pickrell, M D
Pickworth, M J W
Pinnock, C A
Pitcher, D W
Popert, J
Popert, S J
Popovic, S
Porter, M J
Pratley, J
Procter, R S
Prosser, E J
Prosser, J A
Pugh, W A
Pycock, C J
Radley, J R
Rai, A
Ratcliffe, P J
Reichenberg, F P
Richards, E
Richardson, A J
Rigby, M C
Robertson, C L
Robertson, C S
Robinson, D D
Romer, C
Roscoe, B
Roscoe, E J
Roscoe, S A
Rosewarne, H C
Rosewarne, M D
Rouholamin, E
Rowe, I F
Ruparelia, B A
Sanmuganathan, P S
Sawers, A H
Scanlon, J E M
Selvakumar, S P
Short, A
Simpson, A N B
Slaney, G
Slaney, P L
Smart, R A
Smith, C H
Smith, D M
Smith, G T
Smith, J E
Smith, R M H
Solesbury, K A
Sorensen, M H
South, D
Spencer, S J W
Stedman, Y F
Stockley, J M
Tarry, J E
Teague, I
Thomas, R J
Thompson, J A
Timberlake, A H
Treadwell, E A
Trevett, M C
Tunnicliffe, W S
Turner, A F
Tweddell, A L
Vaughan-Jones, R H
Vella, V M P S
Walker, M
Walker, S C
Ward, R S
Watson, S P A
Watts, J F
Webberley, M J
Webster, C D
Webster, D A
Webster, G M
Whitby, R M
White, R E B
Whitmore, I R
Wilkes, M C T
Williams, H D
Williams, H T
Wilson, G M
Woof, A M
Young, M A

Worcester Park

Aerts, S L F
Al-Khudhairi, M S M
Antonio, S E
Blowers, H V
Bowen-Perkins, H H
Brady, C T M
Chung Hung Tseung, C Y C
Coffey, A J D
D'Souza, G R A
De Silva, E B R
Dosani, S
Fatnani, S T
Greene, W J
Ho, C H-K
Hollings, A M
Jasani, V
Kalsi, B S
Patel, R
Pathmanathan, I K
Riley, P A
Samarasinghe, S R
Solanki, D A
Tran, A D
Vara, R

Workington

Bater, E J
Butler, A C
Crosby, P
Goodwin, R M
Gourlay, M V
Howarth, P
Jay, V C B
Jones, C E
Joy, K R
Kingsbury, Q D
Law, J K
Macbeth, M
McGreevy, N G
Morgan, A J
Mort, M J L
Mujahed, M A
Naylor, H A
Palmer, E M
Proudfoot, R T
Rao, P B
Rudman, R J
Scott, A V
Shaw, N A
Slater, C A
Spencer, J V
Steel, G M
Trafford, R M
Ulyett, I
Walker, R D
Wilmot, J D C

Worksop

Allen, J M
Alloub, M I A
Alwail, A N
Anathhanam, A J
Avill, R
Bickerton, G S
Bodden, S J
Cashmore, R J
Clegg, R T
Collins, D J
Collins, L A
Corbett, M G
Crate, I D
Crossman, H M
Cyriac, J E A
Davies, I F
Davies, M B
Davies, S C
Delaney, W M M
Dixon, A M
Drown, G K M
El Hag, S H
Elson, R A
Emery, M C
Exposito Coll, P
Finbow, J M
Finbow, J A H
Fulton, J A
Goel, R K
Guirguis, M W
Guirguis, M
Haldar, G
Hall, I M
Harris, R W
Harrow, A
Hashmi, S S J
Hepburn, J M
Hobson, P J
Howard, J
Hussain, S M A
Kar-Purkayastha, S K
Kell, S W
Khan, I A
Lazarowicz, H P
Lokubalasuriya, D E A
Mammo, M A R
Mannan, M A
Mellows, H J
Merrill, C R
Merriman, L A
Michel, M Z
Millar, L J
Moxon, P J
Mulenga, H P S
Omokanye, A M
Patel, S C
Paul, B
Renshaw, A J N
Rice-Oxley, J M
Riddell, W S
Robinson, K R
Rossi, C A M
Rossi, S
Salamani, M M H
Saqib, N U
Scarrow, P
Sharmacharja, G
Sharmacharja, N R
Shata, M M H
Sinha Roy, A N
Smith, P
Solomonsz, F A
Stanley, C P
Stillwell, M D
Teasdale, D E
Warner, S N B
Williams, L H P
Zafar, N
Zeraati, M

Worthing

Anderson, J G F
Anderson, S K
Appleton, M A C
Bamigbade, T A
Bates, J
Beard, R C
Beney, J R
Bennett, D G
Blows, L J H
Bull, H J M
Bull, J J
Cairns, A J
Caldwell, G
Cameron, E A B
Campbell, N M
Campbell, P J
Carr, P
Carter, D Y
Chalmers, R M
Chard, M D
Child, J A
Chinoy, V J
Chouhan, A K
Clarke, D S
Clifford-Jones, R E
Coldwell, S
Collier, J A B
Congdon, R G
Congleton, J E
Cook, B A
Craig, D M
Daniels, D W
Daniels, P S
Das, A N
Dean, P J
Dearing, J
Dickson, G H
Drown, E M
Duckering, J
Duddy, J R
Edge, A J
Edwards, I M E
Edwards, R
English, J D
English, M M
Epsom, M
Escobar Jimenez, A M
Evans, J A
Funnell, A R
Galea, A P R
Garg, A K
Garner, D P
Giddins, E A
Gnananandha, C
Grant, J J H
Grasset-Molloy, G J M
Grellier, L F L
Grocutt, M P
Gupta, S K
Hall, D G
Hancock, K J
Hardwick, B R
Hill, C A M
Hills, R K
Hinchcliffe, M G
Holmes, A M W
Hopkins, D R
Howell, M
Hutchings, G M
Imms, J M
Jackson, M E
Jarvis, A C M
Jenkins, C S
Johnson, C A
Juer, L D F
Kelley, S T
Khin Maung Nyunt, Dr
King, I D H
Kneale, B J
Lavies, N G
Lermitte, J G C
Liston, T G
Longmore, J M
Lyons, M A
McCarthy, N R
McClumpha, A I
McCutchan, J D S
Mackinnon, A L
Mannings, D J
Mathew, A
Michaelis, J R
Miles, W F A
Montgomery, J
Moore, E J
Moriarty, G K
Nelson, S A
Newnham, J A
Nicholls, F A J
Nicholls, S W
Niyadurupola, T
O'Driscoll, A M
Orpin, R P I
Pastor, T
Patel, K E
Pathmanaban, P
Pickworth, S A M
Pike, S C
Poulsen, H
Pyper, R J D
Randall, K
Rassam, S M B
Raval, M M
Reardon, M F
Richards, A J
Rist, C L
Riveros Huckstadt, M D P
Roberts, K M
Rockall, L J
Rolph, M J W
Roques, A W W
Roques, C J
Ruoss, C F
Ryan, W J
Rymer, M J
Sargen, F E
Saunders, E S
Sayers, R D
Searle-Barnes, P G
Sethi, P C
Sharma, K K
Shipsey, M R
Shute, P E
Signy, M
Singh, K K
Smith, R A
Smith, S M
Smith, T
Spence, D J
Spence, R N F
Spring, C
Suntharalingam, G
Sweet, P T
Teimory, M
Thiagarajah, S
Thompson, A M
Topham, J H
Tozer, R D
Tree, A L
Trounce, N D
Uncles, D R
Von Biel, T A
Wainstead, H
Waters, H R
Watton, E
Webb, M A H
Weber, S
Willard, H L
Williams, A C
Williams, B W
Wiseman, C E
Woodhams, S D
Woods, W G A
Woodward-Court, R I
Woolley, B
Woollons, A
Wrightson, F M
Young, B K

Wotton-under-Edge

Bailey, A R
Burns-Cox, N
Burrows, W J
Green, S M
Hampson, R S
Joslin, C C
Kabler, J J
McCarthy, M B
Margerison, J C L
Pritchard, P L J
Stokes, M J
Thompson, C L
Twomey, P J
Watt, A J

Wrexham

Ahmad, T
Ahmed, S
Alstead, J A
Alstead, P
Arijon Barazal, M C
Arthurs, G J
Ashworth, I N
Atkin, P D
Atkinson, D
Baker, A
Baker, J T
Banerjee, S M
Barton, P C
Bates, G J
Benjamin, A
Billings, P J
Botham, L
Bottomley, A M
Bradshaw, D M
Braid, N W
Breese, S C
Burdge, A H
Cefai, C
Chandra Mohan, A R
Child, D F
Chowdhury, E A H
Cliffe, R J
Cluett, D
Cochrane, R A
Collins, M M A
Cotter, J A
Coward, A E B
Cowell, R P W
Crumplin, K H
Cummins, M C
Da Silva, A E C F
Davies, D A
Davies, D M
Davies, H R F
Davies, K S
Davies, P I
De Bolla, A R
De Soysa, D L D
Deas, E D
Denkema, J F
Duguid, J K M
Earlam, A D
Edmondson, W C
Edwards, C M
Edwards, D M
Evans, E J S
Ewah, P O
Fernando, M U
Fleming, J S M
Gareh, M D
Graham, B
Greaves, R C
Greensmith, M G E
Halpin, K G
Harborne, G C
Harrington, B E J
Harvey, J N R
Hill, G M
Horrocks, F A
Hughes, H
Husain, A
Hussain, Z
Irvine, C P C
Jackson, S L
Jamieson, A M
Jamieson, J R
Jeffreys, T E
Jones, C C
Jones, D G
Jones, D M
Jones, D
Jones, J S
Jones, S W
Kanagaratnam, T
Kaushik, N C
Kelly, P S
Kelly, S J
Kendall, N D
Khalifa, M S E
Khan, G M
Laine, C H
Laing, P W
Lancashire, B J
Latif, F
Littler, C
McAndrew, N A
McCaddon, A
McDonald, K A
McNeill, J M
Mahdi, S
Makwana, N K
Mason, A
Mercer, J H M
Minchom, P E
Minchom, S E
Moore, C
Murray, G M
Myres, M P
Nadra, A M
Nadra, A
Nankani, A J
Nankani, J N
Navaratnam, M
Nirula, H C
O'Sullivan, M M
Olawo, A O
Oliver, C A V
Owen, G
Owens, G G
Pack, H M
Parker, D A
Perera, C N
Phillips, E A
Pickles, R M
Prathibha, B V
Prendergast, M C
Prussia, C M
Pye, J K
Race, J H
Roberts, M J
Roberts, R C
Roberts, T G
Robinson, S H
Roseblade, C K
Ross, A
Rutherford, P A
Saul, P D
Scriven, M W
Sen, A
Seward, W P
Shaw, C D
Silverstone, E J
Smith, R M C
Sowden, J M
Taffinder, A P
Taffinder, G A
Talkhani, I S
Tanti, G J
Tattersall, H J
Tattersall, J
Thomas, A M
Tinckler, L F
Toon, P G
Turkie, P V
Underhill, S
Upadhyay, R N
Uppala, R G
Vellacott, M N
Vennam, R B
Vlies, M J
Vlies, P R
Wainwright, J E
Walsh, J E
Walters, P E
Watson, D K
Welham, J
White, A D
Williams, C P
Williams, D G

Williams, O E
Williams, T E J
Wood, H M
Wood, H M
Wood, K M
Wootton, J R
Wright, B K

Wylam
Aitchison, E A M
Bartram, S A
Brough, W
Donaldson, R W
Knapton, J
Miller, S M
Porteous, L A
Power, J S F
Roberts, C J
Sprague, N B
Vincent, M L

Wymondham
Calne, J A
Cooper, L C G
Groom, C E
Groom, N H
Groom, T M
Howell, T J
Seaton, D G F
Slocombe, R L
Thorman, C A L
Thurston, S C

Y Felinheli
White, P W

Yarm
Aitken, R H
Berg, I
Bonavia, A
Bryson, D D
Clarke, D
Clifford, K M A
Cooper, D W
Crawford, D
Crawshaw, S M
Curry, R C
Davies, B H
Dodds, C
Dodds, E A
Duncan, T J
Gowland, S N
Graham, K A
Khan, K J
Kibirige, J I
Kyi Kyi Tin-Myint, Dr
Lack, L J
Myers, S M
Neoh, L C
Orr, W S M
Padmore, S J
Paterson, A D
Pollard, S M
Prentice, I J
Prior, K M
Rao, S
Rawlinson, A J
Reynolds, N G
Ryall, D M
Targett, K L
Williams, M S
Wilson, R G
Wright, J G
Wright, S G

Yarmouth
Walker, G M

Yateley
Allison, J
Aulakh, R
Bhatia, N
Bird, S M
Bonnevie, J E
France, R
Hancock, A L
Lister, D
Masoumi-Ravandi, M
Palmer, M A
Rogerson, C A
Sant, K E
Teo, A C W
Viner, M A
Walker, N D
Wang, G K P
Wareham, K P
Williams, P G N G

Yelverton
Ames, J A
Bailey, C L
Baker, J A
Bannon, C F
Beckly, D E
Beckly, J B
Campbell, C J
Chiappe, K N
Cowie, J
Davies, M G
Drennan, P C
Farnham, N G J
Finnigan, A G K
Guest, J E
Harmsworth, N J
Huggett, R J
Leverton, W E J
Longdon, D N
Luscombe, F E
Mallaband, E
Murphy, P M
Nichols, M E
Shephard, J A
Smith, P G D
Soul, J O
Stocker, C A
Stoecker, H
Stokes, J M
Taylor, M B
Tipple, R W
Wells, I P
Youngs, J C

Yeovil
Agnew, I
Allen, A J
Ancill, B R
Ariaratnam, G
Azaz, S Y
Baker, K M
Baldwin, J E
Ball, M J
Bathurst, N C G
Brigden, G S
Brooks, S C
Burrell, N L
Camprodon Gazulla, R
Carr, R G
Cawood, J R
Cheale, S M
Collins, M J M
Cornish, G R L
Cornish, M
Cox, J P
Crowley, G P
Daum, R E O
Davey, H M
Davies, A J
Day, H E
Dearlove, J C
Dennis, S E W
Devonshire, H W
Duffy, L J
Eaton, M J
Evans, A G R
Fawcett, I W
Fisher, C J
Gajraj, H
Gore, S
Gower, J D G
Gregory, A J
Hacking, J C
Hall, F G
Hart, J F
Hay, M
Hayman, J J
Heaton, P A J
Hepple, J N
Hogben, R M
Holmes, M J
Howes, L J
Huins, S J
Hunter, S J
Kennedy, R H
Kipling, R M
Knight, A C
Latimer, S
McCormick, R N
Maleki-Tabrizi, A
Minogue, M J O B
Moore, R I
More, R E A
Nadin, J C K
Naravi, M K
Niayesh, M H
Nott-Bower, W G
Oberthur, E P A
Omran, H T I

Palferman, T G
Parker, C J
Pattison, G T R
Payne, G S
Priaulx, L-R
Qadiri, M R R
Rashed, K A M
Richards, M J
Royle, C A J P
Saywell, W R
Scull, J J
Sheffield, J P
Simmonds, A J
Skeath, T H
Smibert, J G
Smith, L F P
Smith, M J
Summers, A
Summers, S H
Taylor, D R
Tricker, J A
Trower, T P
Umoren, D M
Warner, N J
Wootton, M A
Wright, B Y

York
Adams, R D
Alcock, D G
Alexander, D J
Anakwe, G N
Anderson, A D G
Anderson, A W
Anderson, P I
Anderson, S P
Anderton, C J
Andrew, A C
Ashford, R U
Atkinson, A D
Bagnall, J J
Baines, R J
Ball, R J
Banhatti, R G
Barr, C A
Barradell, R
Barry, G P
Barry, M R F
Basu, S
Bates, C
Batman, D C
Belbin, D J
Bell-Syer, J W
Bennett, D A
Berry, C A
Berry, M I
Beverley, D W
Bill, K A
Black, J J
Blake James, R B
Blakeborough, A J
Blakeborough, J
Blenkiron, P
Boffa, J A
Bolter, P J
Border, D J
Bottom, S F E
Bowker, A M B
Boyd, L M
Bradley, E M
Britton, S A
Brobbel, N J
Bromley, B J
Brooke, J P
Brooks, S G
Brown, D P
Brown, H A
Brown, L M
Brown, R F
Burgess, P J
Burnett, P R
Bush, J K
Buswell, C K
Calder, A S C
Campbell, P
Carpenter, R M
Carter, J J
Cass, M A
Chang Kit, H L
Chaplin, J V
Child, D A
Chubb, S E M
Clarke, A M T
Clarke, P R R
Clarke, S E
Cleary, M M
Coatesworth, A P
Coe, K I
Coleman, R L

Collinson, D G
Cook, H L
Cookson, J B
Coop, D J
Corlett, A J
Cox, E M
Crane, S D
Craven, K W E
Crawford, P M
Crompton, J W
Crook, J R
Cross, D A
De Boer, P G
Dell, R E
Dent, A J
Devlin, M
Donaldson, T J
Donnellan, C F
Downing, N P D
Duncan, A F
Dunham, J M
Dux, M S
Easby, B
Ellingham, R B
Evans, A A
Evans, J C H
Evans, M W
Fair, D S
Faller, P F
Fenwick, H J
Field, A F
Finan, C M
Fisher, R H
Fleat, G
Forde, S C O
Forrester, A M
Foster, G P
Foster, K J
Fowler, E V
Galbraith, D J
Garry, A C
Garthwaite, E
Geddes, D R
Gibson, G C
Gibson, M F
Gilbody, S M
Gill, N J
Gilleghan, S B
Girling, P J E
Glennon, V
Godfrey, J L R
Gopalaswamy, A K
Grace, A R H
Green, A S
Griffith, K E
Griffiths, C J
Grummitt, R M
Guest, P A
Habgood, L C
Haddock, G K
Haleem, M A
Hall, P A
Hall, W J
Hamilton, J C
Hammond, D J
Hardy, R G
Harran, M J
Harris, A L
Hartley, D C
Hasan, S S
Haselden, J B
Hayes, S J
Haynes, J
Hayward, D
Hayward, J M
Heald, A
Henderson, C A
Heseltine, D
Heslop, A J
Hewitson, J D
Highet, A S
Hildebrand, A E C
Hirst, J
Holman, C J
Honnappa, H
Hopkin, J M
Howard, M R
Hrycaiczuk, W
Hughes, T R J
Hunter, A M
Hunter, A J
Hutchinson, B R G
Iredale, J L
Isherwood, J
Iveson, J M I
Iveson, R Y
Jackson, D P
Jackson, G B
Jackson, I J B

Jacobs, P M
Jamal, A A
James, D A
Jenkins, C N J
Jennings, P E
Johnson, R C
Johnstone, N A
Jones, J M
Jones, M H
Jones, P R
Jones, R D
Julian, T R
Kelly, A M
Kelly, S M
Kemp, D S
Kennedy, J M
Kennedy, P F
Kerr, M A
Ketting, K P
Kimuli, M
King, D G
Klar, H-M
Lacy-Colson, J C H
Laing, J H W
Lakin, A J
Lakin, H M
Laughey, W F
Lazenby, R M
Leathem, W E
Lethem, J A
Leveson, S H
Lightwing, D S B
Looker, H C
Love, C A
Lubben-Dinkelaar, M M
Lund, J N
Lyall, I M
Lyon, C C
McBride, P M C
McCall, J
McCleary, A J
MacDermott, K J
McDougle, M D R
Macfie, A J
McHenry, C J
Mackenzie, S E
McLaren, A A A
McLaren, C A N
Macleod, J
McPherson, B
Madej, T H
Madsen, K E
Malik, F
Maloney, J D
Mancey-Jones, J B
Mandour, O E M A
Mannion, R A J
Markham, M V
Markham, R J O S
Marsden, J D
Marson, J M
Matheson, A M
Mattock, E J
May, K J
Maycock, T P
Meakins, S J
Mechie, K
Megarry, S G
Meldrum, J M
Merritt, S M
Miller, G V
Millman, A G
Mitchell, N A
Mitchell, S F
Mitchell, S N
Moger, P W
Moncur, P H
Moore, J R
Moran, N
Moroney, J D
Morrison, J
Morrison, R E
Moss, P J
Moulson, A M
Muhammed, S
Mujeeb-Ur-Rahman, Dr
Munnelly, N
Murdoch, S D
Murphy, K A
Murray, A C
Myatt, A E
Myers, K W
Neary, B R
Newcombe, C P
Newland, T M
Nicholson, S
Nixon, R J
Noble, T J

Oglesby, A I
Old, S
Ormston, B J
Orr, G D
Parker, D
Pathmanathan, S
Patterson, D H
Peel, R K
Pegg, D E
Perez, L A
Phin, N F
Pierce, A A
Pope, S P
Porter, G R
Porter, S M
Potrykus, M
Powley, E
Price, K G
Pring, D W
Procter, D
Pye, M A M
Rea, V
Reaney, S M
Reed, J P
Reeder, M K
Rees, H M
Reid, I N
Reilly, P G
Reilly, S P
Reilly, T M
Richardson, G J R
Riley, J E
Rishworth, R H
Ristic, C D
Rix, S M
Roberts, S A
Robertson, N C
Roman, M V
Ruston, R
Samuel, M S
Saunders, G P
Saxty, P
Schofield, S J
Scott, A K
Scott, E A
Scott, J W
Seaton, J M A
Sedano Bocos, A
Seeni, K
Sen, S K
Shaw, S P
Sheikh, Z I
Shujja-Ud-Din, O S
Siddique, T B
Sigsworth, E R C
Simpson, J O
Simpson, J E
Simpson, R N R
Sinanan, R D K
Smales, J R
Smith, D P
Smith, M R
Smith, P S
Smith, R A
Smith, W M
Smithson, W H
Smythies, J R
Snape, C J
Spenceley, J E
Stainforth, J M
Stamp, M P
Stephenson, C J
Stockdale, W T
Stone, P G
Stower, M J
Sultan, M K
Sutton, A G C
Sweeney, A M
Tait, S K
Tams, J
Taylor, J
Taylor, P J
Taylor, R H
Thompson, R C F
Thomson, R J
Thorne, P M
Thow, J C
Ticehurst, P R
Tilston, S J
Toomey, P J
Torlesse, R M
Towler, G M
Traynor, C P
Trudgill, M J A
Tulloch, J S
Turner-Parry, A J
Ubhi, B S
Urwin, G H
Waise, A

Wakerley, M B
Waldron, F M
Walker, J E
Walker, M M
Walker, R G
Walsh, D A
Walsh, S
Walters, N S
Ward, K J
Warnock, N G
Watson, A B
Watson, G D
Watson, S P
Watson, T O
Watt, I S
Wearne, S M
Webb, B J
Webster, R W
Wedgwood, J J
Welch, L J
Westerman, R
Whicher, J T
Whitaker, I M
Whitcher, D M
White, J E S
White, L A
Whitfield, P H
Wickrema, F R S
Wilkinson, B A
Wilkinson, D J
Wilkinson, S M
Williams, H R
Williamson, J
Wilson, J R
Wilson, M A
Wilson, N J
Wilson, R J T
Wong, W Z
Wood, S M
Woodford, D
Woodrow, S P
Woods, I
Worth, D P
Worth, P J
Wright, H
Wright, J B D
Yates, R C
Yorkston, N J
Young, S

Ystrad Meurig

Rhys, W J S E-G

The Medical Directory 2005

Part Two

Healthcare Organisations in the UK

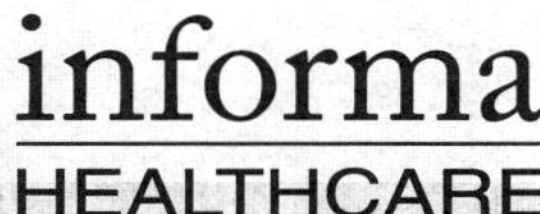

NHS Trusts and NHS Hospitals

England

Adur, Arun and Worthing Primary Care Trust

The Causeway, Goring-by-Sea, Worthing BN12 6BT
Tel: 01903 708400 Fax: 01903 700981
Email: enquiries@aaw.nhs.uk
Website: www.healthinaaw.nhs.uk
(Surrey and Sussex Strategic Health Authority)

Chair Margaret Bamford
Chief Executive Steve Phoenix

Zachary Merton Hospital

Glenville Road, Rustington, Littlehampton BN16 2EA
Tel: 01903 858100 Fax: 01903 858101
Total Beds: 36

Aintree Hospitals NHS Trust

Aintree House, University Hospital Aintree, Longmoor Lane, Liverpool L9 7AL
Tel: 0151 525 5980 Fax: 0151 525 6086
Email: info@aht.nwest.nhs.uk
Website: www.aintreehospitals.nhs.uk
(Cheshire and Merseyside Strategic Health Authority)

Chair John Dray
Chief Executive James Birrell

University Hospital Aintree

Longmoor Lane, Liverpool L9 7AL
Tel: 0151 525 5980 Fax: 0151 529 3286
Total Beds: 938

Accident and Emergency A M Armstrong, J Hollingsworth, R Jones, J Newstone, P Simms, C Stevenson

Anaesthetics S P Acharya, M Bamber, D Brice, H Butterfield, P Charters, L Colville, M Conway, T Cope, J R Dalton, G Dempsey, M Dupont, I F M Graham, D Gray, P Groom, A Guha, M Halligan, J Harrison, M P Hawkins, C Hodgson, W A Horton, E C Howard, R Kandasamy, E Lacasia-Purroy, J Lynes, N P Mercer, D T Moloney, S Nagarajah, J Rodrigues, S A Rogers, S Shaw, E Shearer, G Thind, I Tweedie, B Weldon, C Whitehead, J R Wiles, E Wright

Cardiology A Amadi, K Clarke, G Davis, R Hornung, E Rodrigues, P S C Wong

Care of the Elderly A Aly, J E Clague, D McDowell, A K Sharma, M Siddiqi, J Turner

Chest Disease/Thoracic R Angus, P Calverley, L Davies, P D O Davies, J E Earis, T Jago, J F O'Reilly, M Pearson, C Warburton

Endocrinology S Benbow, I Casson, G V Gill, I MacFarlane, J Pinkney, J Wilding

ENT M Birchall, A S Daud, S Jackson, T Jones, T Lesser, V Nandapalan, M F Ramadan, N Roland, A C Swift

Gastroenterology K Bodger, S Hood, N Krasner, P O'Toole, S Sarkar, R E Sturgess

General Surgery D J Cave-Bigley, J M Dhorajiwala, J Joseph, D Kerrigan, C R Mackie, L Martin, P Skaife, I M Stevenson, R G Ward, A Wu

Haematology R Dasgupta, A Olujohungbe, B Woodcock

Nephrology K A Abraham, C W Gradden

Oncology J Cottier, P Errington, A Flavin, J Litter, D Smith

Ophthalmology D I Clark, A Kamal, G Kyle, I B Marsh

Oral and Maxillofacial Surgery M Boyle, J S Brown, J C Cooper, D C Jones, D Richardson, S N Rogers, E D Vaughan

Orthodontics T Morris

Orthopaedics N Barton-Hanson, A A Bass, C Butcher, R A Evans, S C Montgomery, B Pennie, S Scott, M H Thorneloe

Palliative Medicine G Corcoran

Pathology C T Burrow, M Haqqani, A Khan, J D H Sheard, V Tagore, W Taylor, C Van-Heyningen

Radiology A Ap-Thomas, J Curtis, B E Eyes, R Hanlon, P A H Jones, H Lewis-Jones, J Makowska-Webb, E O'Grady, V Pellegrini, A Smethurst, E Thwaite, J Tuson, D White

Rheumatology and Rehabilitation M Anderson, C Estrach-Roig, N Goodson, R J Moots, K Selverajah, R Thompson, E Williams

Urology D Machin, D O'Sullivan, M Williamson

Walton Hospital

Rice Lane, Liverpool L9 1AE
Tel: 0151 525 5111
Total Beds: 64

Airedale NHS Trust

Trust Headquarters, Airedale General Hospital, Skipton Road, Steeton, Keighley BD20 6TD
Tel: 01535 652511 Fax: 01535 655129
Email: firstname.lastname@anhst.nhs.uk
Website: www.airedale-trust.nhs.uk
(North and East Yorkshire and Northern Lincolnshire Strategic Health Authority; West Yorkshire Strategic Health Authority)

Chair Brian Jewell
Chief Executive Robert Allen

Airedale General Hospital

Skipton Road, Steeton, Keighley BD20 6TD
Tel: 01535 652511 Fax: 01535 655129
Total Beds: 533

Accident and Emergency P Cryer, M J Dudley

Anaesthetics R Adley, S J Almond, J R Baker, J Burns, P M Kay, J Scriven, J M Stanton, C Starkey, K E Waite

Cardiology N P Silverton, A V Zezulka

Care of the Elderly D E Allen, M G Harrington, J P Milnes, J A Onafowokan

Dental Surgery S F Worrall

Dermatology A L Wright

ENT C H Raine, D R Strachan

General Medicine D G Clements, C J Healey, H S R Hosker, S Mawer, C R Parker, R M Pope, M Raashed, R Roberts

General Surgery E P Dewar, I F Hutchinson, C R Kapadia, R B N Khan, A H Nejim

Haematology A C Cuthbert

Neurology J G Howe

Obstetrics and Gynaecology J H Brash, P J Brunskill, K M Graham, N Samtaney

Oncology S M Crawford

Ophthalmology A D Atkins, P L Atkinson, J Bradbury, F D Ghanchi, J N James, A Reynolds

Orthodontics L Mitchell, C E Young

Orthopaedics D J Beard, A A Faraj, S Ravindran, D T S Tang, C C Wray

Paediatrics A A Britland, S J Ilett, R Muthukumar, G A Savill, K P Ward, K N Wilkinson

Palliative Medicine M J Hughes

Pathology N C Bradford, P E da Costa, P G R Godwin, J J O'Dowd

Plastic Surgery M J Timmons

Radiology S G Blake, I R Brand, K A Lindsay, C S Orgles, G G Porter

Radiotherapy and Oncology C J Orton

Urology I Appleyard, N A Shaikh

Airedale General Hospital - Day Hospital for Elderly

Skipton Road, Steeton, Keighley BD20 6TD
Tel: 01535 652511 Ext: 2701 Fax: 01535 655129
Website: www.airdale-trust.nhs.uk

Bingley Day Hospital for the Elderly

Fernbank Drive, Bingley BD16 4HD
Tel: 01274 563438 Fax: 01274 510565

Bingley Hospital

Fernbank Drive, Bingley BD16 4HD
Tel: 01274 563438 Fax: 01274 510565

Care of the Elderly D E Allen

Castleberg Day Hospital for the Elderly

Raines Road, Giggleswick, Settle BD24 0BN
Tel: 01729 823515 Fax: 01729 823082

Castleberg Hospital

Raines Road, Giggleswick, Settle BD24 0BN
Tel: 01729 823515 Fax: 01729 823082
Total Beds: 15

Care of the Elderly M G Harrington

Ilkley Coronation Day Hospital for the Elderly

Springs Lane, Ilkley LS29 8TG
Tel: 01934 609666 Fax: 01943 816129

Ilkley Coronation Hospital (Outpatient and Minor Injuries)

Springs Lane, Ilkley LS29 8TG
Tel: 01943 609666 Fax: 01943 816129

Skipton General Day Hospital for the Elderly

Keighley Road, Skipton BD23 2RJ
Tel: 01756 792233 Fax: 01756 700485

Skipton General Hospital

Keighley Road, Skipton BD23 2RJ
Tel: 01756 792233 Fax: 01756 700485

Care of the Elderly D E Allen, M G Harrington, J P Milnes, J A Onofowokan

General Medicine H S R Hosker, R M Pope

General Surgery E P Dewar, I F Hutchinson, C R Kapadia, A H Nejim

Neurology J G Howe

Obstetrics and Gynaecology N Samtaney

Ophthalmology J N James

Orthopaedics D J Beard, A A Faraj, D T S Tang, C C Wray

Paediatrics K P Ward

Urology I Appleyard, N A Shaikh

Airedale Primary Care Trust

Airedale House, 21A Mornington Street, Keighley BD2 2EA
Tel: 01535 690416 Fax: 01535 672639
Website: www.airedale-pct.nhs.uk
(West Yorkshire Strategic Health Authority)

Chair Elizabeth Wolstenholme
Chief Executive Lyn Wilkinson

Amber Valley Primary Care Trust

Meadow Suite, Babington Hospital, Derby Road, Belper, Derby DE56 1WH
Tel: 01773 525099 Fax: 01773 820318
Website: www.ambervalley-pct.nhs.uk
(Trent Strategic Health Authority)

Chair Adrian Evans
Chief Executive Wendy Lawrence

Babington Hospital

Pennine and Baron Wards, Derby Road, Belper DE56 1WH
Tel: 01773 824171 Fax: 01773 824155
Total Beds: 64

Heanor Memorial Hospital

Ilkeston Road, Heanor, Derby DE75 7EA
Tel: 01773 710711 Fax: 01773 716686
Total Beds: 24

Ripley Community Hospital

Sandham Lane, Ripley, Derby DE5 3HE
Tel: 01773 743456 Fax: 01773 512021
Total Beds: 23

Ashfield Primary Care Trust

Integrated management with Mansfield District Primary Care Trust.

Ransom Hall, Ransomwood Business Park, Southwell Road West, Mansfield NG21 0ER
Tel: 01623 414114 Fax: 01623 653527
Email: info@ashfield-pct.nhs.uk
Website: www.ashfield-pct.nhs.uk
(Trent Strategic Health Authority)

Chair David Kirkham
Chief Executive Eleri de Gilbert
Consultants Greg Finn

Ashfield Community Hospital

Portland Street, Kirkby-in-Ashfield, Nottingham NG17 7AE
Total Beds: 94

Ashford and St Peter's Hospitals NHS Trust

St Peter's Hospital, Guildford Road, Chertsey KT16 0PZ
Tel: 01932 872000 Fax: 01932 723532
Email: forename.surname@asth.nhs.uk
Website: www.ashfordstpeters.nhs.uk
(Surrey and Sussex Strategic Health Authority)

Chair Clive Thompson
Chief Executive Glenn Douglas
Consultants Sue Bateman

Ashford Hospital

London Road, Ashford TW15 3AA
Tel: 01784 884488 Fax: 01784 884017
Total Beds: 327

Accident and Emergency J S Belstead, Mr Kumar

Anaesthetics P H Balakrishnan, J C Dawson, D Holden, A Khadiwal, G Vora, J E J Yates

Care of the Elderly H N C Gunther

Chest Disease A J Winning

Dermatology S Parker

ENT J Hadley, A Robinson

General Medicine P W Adams, D Newberry, J Thornton, P R Wilkinson

General Surgery W N W Baker, N Browning, J Horner, S Shotria

Neurology R Lane

Obstetrics and Gynaecology A Elias, K Gangar, D W Hyatt

Ophthalmology A Gupta, M Rahman

Oral and Maxillofacial Surgery B M W Bailey, R J Carr

Orthodontics C Hepworth, L Jones

Orthopaedics M Bloomfield, H Roushdi, K A Walker

Paediatrics A Hadad, R C F Newton, S Zoritch

Pathology B Bramble, S Ibrahim, C E S Keenan, N R Kirk, A Laurie

Plastic Surgery D Davies

Radiology E A Bellamy, S M Davidson, R Davies, S R Patel, D Reiff

Radiotherapy and Oncology M Gaze

Rheumatology M S Irani

Urology B W Ellis, R Kulkarni

St Peter's Hospital

Guildford Road, Chertsey KT16 0PZ
Tel: 01932 872000 Fax: 01932 874757
Total Beds: 396

Accident and Emergency V O'Neill, P S J Rana

Anaesthetics J Cooper, G J J Fuzzey, P Houlton, M M Imrie, M Jordan, F Lloyd Jones, J J Margary, M H Russell, B C Sellick

Cardiology D Fluck, M D Joy

Care of the Elderly B A Castleton, C Long, E McInnes

Chemical Pathology H G M Freeman, M Knapp

Chest Disease M G Britton

Child Psychiatry Y Parker, J Sebestik

Dermatology S V Jones, J A Miller, S Neill

Diabetes M A Baxter

ENT P Chapman, N Solomons, P Sudderick

Gastroenterology P Finch

General Medicine M G Britton, P Finch, M D Joy

General Surgery E Chisholm, D R Donaldson, G Layer, H Scott, M Thomas

Genitourinary Medicine J Pritchard

Haematology A L Miller, D O'Shaugnessy

Histopathology M Hall, N A Ratcliffe, T Reagh

Medical Microbiology H C Grundy

Neurology D Barnes

Obstetrics and Gynaecology S Bateman, M Bell, S Newbold, T Spencer, J T Wright

Ophthalmology M G Boodhoo, R W Condon

Oral and Maxillofacial Surgery R A Peebles

Orthopaedics D Elliott, R P Hollingsworth, K Newman, R D Pool, C Schofield, R B Simonis

Paediatrics J J Bowyer, P Crawshaw, P Martin, W Nackasha, R C F Newton

Pathology H G M Freeman, H C Grundy, M Hall, M Knapp, A L C Miller, D O'Shaughnessy, D A Ratcliffe

Plastic Surgery R Martin

Radiology C E Bennett, M Creagh, B S Donnellan, J Glover, P P Ho

Rheumatology G Hall, R Hughes

Thoracic Surgery E E J Smith

Urology R Cole, N H Hills

Vascular Surgery K Dawson

Ashford Primary Care Trust

Templar House, Tannery Lane, Ashford TN23 1PL
Tel: 01233 618330 Fax: 01233 618378
Email: ashfordpct.enquiries@ekentha.nhs.uk
Website: www.kentandmedway.nhs.uk
(Kent and Medway Strategic Health Authority)

Chair Peter Smallridge
Chief Executive Marion Dinwoodie

Ashton, Leigh and Wigan Primary Care Trust

Bryan House, 61 Standishgate, Wigan WN1 1AH
Tel: 01942 772711 Fax: 01942 772850
Email: public.enquiries@alwpct.nhs.uk
Website: www.alwpct.nhs.uk
(Greater Manchester Strategic Health Authority)

Chair Lynne Liptrot
Chief Executive Peter Rowe

Avon Ambulance Service NHS Trust

Marybush Lane, Bristol BS2 0AT
Tel: 0117 927 7046 Fax: 0117 925 1419
Email: post@avonambulance.nhs.uk
Website: www.avonamb.nhs.uk
(Avon, Gloucestershire and Wiltshire Strategic Health Authority)

Chair Louis Victory
Chief Executive Kevin Hogarty

Avon and Wiltshire Mental Health Partnership NHS Trust

Bath NHS House, Newbridge Hill, Bath BA1 3QE
Tel: 01225 731731 Fax: 01225 731732
Website: www.awp.nhs.uk
(Avon, Gloucestershire and Wiltshire Strategic Health Authority)

Chair Christine Reid
Chief Executive Roger Pedley
Consultants Christine Vize

Barrow Hospital

Barrow Gurney, Bristol BS19 3SG
Tel: 01275 392811 Fax: 01275 394277
Total Beds: 161

General Psychiatry S Britten, R P M Brown, N Moore, D Mumford, S Oke, J Parker, B Robinson, A J Smith

Blackberry Hill Hospital

Manor Road, Fishponds, Bristol BS16 2EW
Tel: 0117 965 6061 Fax: 0117 925 4832

Forensic Psychiatry J E Smith, A Tomison

Fountain Way Hospital

Wilton Road, Salisbury SP2 7EP
Tel: 01722 336262 Fax: 01722 320313
Total Beds: 80

Green Lane Hospital

Devizes SN10 5DS
Tel: 01380 731200 Fax: 01380 731308
Total Beds: 60

General Psychiatry D Stevens, R Thorpe, C Vize

Long Fox Unit

Weston General Hospital, Grange Road, Uphill, Weston Super Mare BS23 4TQ
Tel: 01934 647069 Fax: 01934 643061
Total Beds: 48

St Martin's Hospital

Midford Road, Bath BA2 5RP
Tel: 01225 832383
Total Beds: 46

Sandalwood Court

Highgrove Road, Swindon SN3 4WF
Tel: 01793 836800 Fax: 01793 836801
Total Beds: 56

Victoria Hospital

Okus Road, Swindon SN1 4HZ
Tel: 01793 481182 Fax: 01793 437636
Total Beds: 46

Barking and Dagenham Primary Care Trust

The Clock House, East Street, Barking IG11 8EY
Tel: 020 8591 9595 Fax: 020 8532 6201
Website: www.barkinghaveringhealth.nhs.uk
(North East London Strategic Health Authority)

Chair Ray Parkin
Chief Executive Hilary Ayerst

Barking, Havering and Redbridge Hospitals NHS Trust

Harold Wood Hospital, Gubbins Lane, Romford RM3 0BE
Tel: 01708 345533 Fax: 01708 708099
Website: www.bhrhospitals.nhs.uk
(North East London Strategic Health Authority)

Chair Ian Kirkpatrick
Chief Executive Mark Rees

Barking Hospital

Upney Lane, Barking IG11 9LX
Tel: 020 8983 8000 Fax: 020 8924 6199
Total Beds: 110

Harold Wood Hospital

Gubbins Lane, Harold Wood, Romford RM3 0BE
Tel: 01708 345533 Fax: 01708 708099
Total Beds: 384

Anaesthetics A Akramul-Haq, S Burke, G Chitra, D De Villiers, S Kapoor, B Robinson

Care of the Elderly M A Smith, L Wickramasinghe

Dermatology A Avermaete, F Carabott, S Matthews

ENT B Chopra, C R Chowdhury, H Kaddour, B Kotecha

General Medicine R Pearson

General Surgery W Ismail, C Muldoon, A Ogedegbe

Haematology A Hughes

Histopathology D Al-Okati, A Goonetilleke, K Mahmood, I Saeed, S Subbuswamy

Medical Microbiology Z Adhami, S Namnyak, A Yaneza

Neurology L J Findley

Obstetrics and Gynaecology P Bolton, Y Coker, E Hawkins, A R Jeyarajah, C Otigbah, U Rao, M Sathanandan, I Tebbutt, A Weekes

Ophthalmology C Claoué, S T Ruben

Paediatrics R S Prasad, J Rawal, G Subramanian

Radiology M Alsewan, I Cameron-Mowat, R Grant

Rheumatology and Rehabilitation K Chakravarty, G Clarke

Urology J Barua, S Gujral, J Hill, M Vandal

King George Hospital

Barley Lane, Goodmayes, Ilford IG3 8YB
Tel: 020 8983 8000 Fax: 020 8970 8001
Total Beds: 555

Accident and Emergency Y Gupta, I Viswanath, S J Ward

Anaesthetics B Bastianpillai, P Dodd, C Gauci, N Hadi, K Hirani, F Igielman, A Khalil, M Khan, D Martin, K Naqushbandi, O Odejinmi

Cardiology A Deaner, C Knight

Care of the Elderly N Ahmad, A Y O Ahonkhai, H Al-Qassab, K Niranjan, V Wijesuriya

Dermatology S Chopra, S Davison

General Medicine W Ashraf, L Bagg, G E A Bettany, S Grainger, K Nikookam, V Sharman, R Storring

General Surgery A Bhargava, J Coker, S Jacob, G Lauffer, A Ojo, S J Snooks

Genitourinary Medicine Y Hooi

Haematology N Akhtar, I Grant

Histopathology P Ashrafzadeh, G Soosay, P Tanner

Medical Microbiology S Lacey, M Melzer

Neurology J Jestico, J McAuley

Obstetrics and Gynaecology S Burgess, G W Cochrane, C Hargreaves, R Howard, P J Kollipara, I Opemuyi, E Osei, J Swinhoe

Ophthalmology S Bryan, H Towler

Orthopaedics C G Iwegbu, S Iyer, D Kaltsas, B Levack

Paediatrics M Ahmed, N Braithwaite, M Hameed, M Keane, D Robinson, A Shirsalkar

Radiology T Jeyakumar, R Obaro, C Padmanathan, M Tahir, S Thenabadu

Rheumatology and Rehabilitation M Dabrera

Urology S Bhanot, P Shridharan

Oldchurch Hospital
Waterloo Road, Romford RM7 0BE
Tel: 01708 746090 Fax: 01708 708137
Total Beds: 565

Accident and Emergency O Abe, T Bell, A Idowu, S Jeevan, A Vasireddy

Anaesthetics M Ather, M Bassilious, G Bawa, H Boralessa, M Gallagher, E Jones, M Mikhael, I Nair, K Raveendran, E Smithers, J Umo-Etuk, P Walker, S Yoganathan

Cardiology T Koh, J Stephens

Care of the Elderly O Adeotoye, R Fowler, J Mannakkara, A Misra

Clinical Genetics S Kumar

ENT A Owa

General Medicine M Ahmed, M Apps, W R Burnham, I Fahal, F Hollanders, A Jubber, H Kadr, E Marouf, M Smith, G Spencer, R Weatherstone

General Surgery T Cheatle, C Hepworth, W Ismail, D Johnston, D Khoo, A Ogedegbe, A Rateme, M Saharay, S Shami, M Wain

Genitourinary Medicine S Ariyanayagam

Haematology A Brownell, D Lewis

Histopathology A King

Neurology S Catania, R N de Silva, L J Findley, C N Hawkes, N Muhammed

Neurosurgery A Aspoas, S Bavetta, J C Benjamin, K David, J Pollock

Oral and Maxillofacial Surgery N Evans, D T Falconer

Orthodontics A Howat, G Howe

Orthopaedics A Ahmad, A Al-Sabti, A Ali, H Banan, A Khan, G E MacLellan, A Makar, H Plaha, K Ratnakumar, J White

Paediatrics J Szoller

Radiology S K Banyikidde, P Butler, S Chawda, A Dabbaghian, R de Kluck, M Farrugia, S R Gademsetty, J Gutman, J Laurila, M Pfeiffer, M Ruch

Radiotherapy and Oncology A R Gershuny, S Gibbs, R Gunasekera, E le Stancbrueziere, M Quigley, E Sims, S Slater

Rheumatology and Rehabilitation C Kelsey

Barnet and Chase Farm Hospitals NHS Trust

Chase Farm Hospital, The Ridgeway, Enfield EN2 8JL
Tel: 0845 111 4000 Fax: 020 8366 1361
Email: firstname.surname@bcf.nhs.uk
Website: www.bcf.nhs.uk
(North Central London Strategic Health Authority)

Chair Peter Brokenshire
Chief Executive Averil Dongworth
Consultants M Al-Dubaisi, H Angus-Leppan, N Bajekal, J Barkder, A J Barnes, J Berger, S Berney, L Bernhardt, R Bird, J Bradley, T Briggs, A Broadbent, S Brocklesby, C Bunce, K J Burke, P E M Butler, D Challis, A Davies, E El-Jabbour, C Elton, J Evans, H Fadl, B Ferris, J B Festenstein, N Feuchtwang, M Gaukroger, J Gelister, T Gluck, R Glynne-Jones, K E Gray, R Greenbaum, P Harbinson, Richard Harrison, G Hinckley, E James, A Jennings, S Johnson, E Jungman, B S K Kamath, G R Kaplan, G Katz, D Khadjeh-Nouri, S Khan, P Lai Chung Fong, S Laurent, T Leslie, D Levy, A Loh, M Maiwand, A Marcus, Sandra McBride, P McGowan, Milaszkiewicz, I Mitchell, P Mitra, E Nevrkla, A E Nicol, V L Nikapota, H Nwaboku, Cate Orteu, P Ostler, Deven Patel, A J Pearson, L Riley, A Rodin, J Rosenberg, D Rossouw, S Roth, Malcolm Rustin, S Shah, R Shanthakumar, B Shravat, D Singh, B Smith, Caroline Smith, H Stevens, I Symons, J Teng, A Virchis, S Watt, M Weir, N Whitelaw, T Wilson, P Wiseman, A Wolff, M Zahir

Barnet Hospital
Wellhouse Lane, Barnet EN5 3DJ
Tel: 020 8216 4000
Total Beds: 459

Chase Farm Hospital
The Ridgeway, Enfield EN2 8JL
Tel: 020 8366 6600 Fax: 020 8366 1361
Total Beds: 469

Barnet, Enfield and Haringey Mental Health NHS Trust

Trust Headquarters, Avon Villa, Chase Farm Hospital, The Ridgeway, Enfield EN2 8JL
Tel: 020 8375 1167 Fax: 020 8366 9166
Email: forename.surname@beh-mht.nhs.uk
Website: www.beh-mht.nhs.uk
(North Central London Strategic Health Authority)

Chair Carl Lammy
Chief Executive John Newbury-Helps

Chase Farm Hospital Site
The Ridgeway, Enfield EN2 8JL
Tel: 020 8366 6600 Fax: 020 8366 9166
Total Beds: 359

Care of the Elderly R A Jackson, A Mahmood, A Weinstein

Child and Adolescent Psychiatry G Broster, G Broster

Community Child Health R Vijeratnam

Forensic Psychiatry A Akikumni, L Hamilton, D James, Dr Kearns, H Kennedy

General Psychiatry C Capstick, M Cody, M Kember, V Watts

Psychiatry of Old Age J Carrick, J Garner

Colindale Hospital
Colindale Avenue, London NW9 5GH
Tel: 020 8200 1555 Fax: 020 8205 6062
Total Beds: 152

Care of the Elderly S Arunachalam, M H Garland, A Homer, L Wilson

Edgware Community Hospital
Burnt Oak Broadway, Edgware HA8 0AD
Tel: 020 8952 2381 Fax: 020 8732 6807

St Ann's Hospital
St Ann's Road, South Tottenham, London N15 3TH
Tel: 020 8442 6000 Fax: 020 8442 6354

Total Beds: 386

Care of the Elderly R Luder, P Ranmuthu, W Woothipoom

Child and Adolescent Psychiatry T M Naidoo, G Stern

General Psychiatry A Bateman, C Burford, R C S Furlong, A Hoar, G S Ibrahimi, E C Johnson-Sabine, R Lucas, W G Smith, M Weller, A Wijeyekoon

Learning Disabilities M Dickenson

Barnet Primary Care Trust

Hyde House, The Hyde, Edgware Road, London NW9 6QQ
Tel: 020 8201 4700 Fax: 020 8201 4701
Website: www.beh.nhs.uk/barnetpct/
(North Central London Strategic Health Authority)

Chair Sally Malin
Chief Executive Charles Hollway

Finchley Memorial Day Hospital

Granville Road, North Finchley, London NW9 5HG
Tel: 020 8349 3121 Fax: 020 8346 6043
Total Beds: 76

Barnsley Hospital NHS Foundation Trust

Established as a Foundation Trust 01/01/2005
Gawber Road, Barnsley S75 2EP
Tel: 01226 730000 Fax: 01226 202859
Website: www.bhnft.nhs.uk
(South Yorkshire Strategic Health Authority)

Chair Gordon Firth
Chief Executive Jan Sobieraj

Barnsley District General Hospital

Gawber Road, Barnsley S75 2EP
Tel: 01226 730000 Fax: 01226 202859
Total Beds: 633

Accident and Emergency M J Bodhe, J Brenchley, D Hughes

Anaesthetics S Abernethy, A Bowry, P Claydon, H J Filby, N P Gill, M A Longan, J Maskill, V F Metias, Y Myint, R Paton, D Roman, A Swinhoe, C F Swinhoe

Care of the Elderly M Al-Bazzaz, A El-Trafi, S Gariballa, S Orme, S Parker

Chemical Pathology A Straffen

Paediatrics M Al-Malik, E A Gouta, R Gupta, D P Kerrin, M Moussa, A Ravi

Dental Surgery J D Price

Dermatology J E Bothwell, R Sabroe, G Sobey, S E Thomas

ENT C Gnanandha, M Nussbaumar, N Siddiqui, M H Wickham

General Medicine M K Al-Bazzaz, D Bullimore, D T Dimov, S Gariballa, T Jones, K Kapur, P Moorhead, T Noble, S Orme, S G Parker, W E Rhoden, B T Saeed, A S G Soliman

General Surgery S Anwar, J J Bannister, P Cutinha, J Hall, J Kenogbon, T Offori, D Rosario, M Shiwani, D Smith

Genitourinary Medicine S Bates, G M Dilke-Wing

Haematology D Chan Lam, J P Ng

Obstetrics and Gynaecology N Khanem, B F Leabeater, R K Raychaudhuri, R Watson, S J Whittaker

Ophthalmology M S Attia, A Ibraheim, Mr Moyardi

Orthodontics J D Holmgren, N Parkin, K Prendergast, A Smith

Orthopaedics A Al-Dadah, P A Bryant, A Ismaiel, M Z G Khan, C Ruddlesdin

Pathology A J Coup, M S Osman, J Ostrowski, C Quincey, A M Straffen

Plastic Surgery R Griffiths

Radiology D Darby, S Gelep, P McAndrew, S Yates, L Yeoman, J Zachary

Rheumatology and Rehabilitation A O Adebajo

Barnsley Primary Care Trust

Kendray Hospital, Doncaster Road, Barnsley S70 3RD
Tel: 01226 730000 Fax: 01226 730054
Website: www.barnsleypct.nhs.uk
(South Yorkshire Strategic Health Authority)

Chair Tom Sheard
Chief Executive Ailsa Claire

Kendray Hospital

Doncaster Road, Kendray, Barnsley S70 3RD
Tel: 01226 777810 Fax: 01226 201435
Total Beds: 77

Alcohol and Substance Abuse B Mehta

Mount Vernon Hospital

Mount Vernon Road, Barnsley S70 4DP
Tel: 01226 777835 Fax: 01226 777836
Total Beds: 74

Manager J Bowser

Care of the Elderly Dr Al-Douri, Dr Baruam, Dr Franklin

Barts and The London NHS Trust

The Royal London Hospital, Whitechapel Road, Whitechapel, London E1 1BB
Tel: 020 7377 7000 Fax: 020 7601 7102
Email: firstname.surname@bartsandthelondon.nhs.uk
Website: www.bartsandthelondon.org.uk
(North East London Strategic Health Authority)

Chair John Ashworth
Chief Executive Paul White

The London Chest Hospital

Bonner Road, London E2 9JX
Tel: 020 7377 7000
Total Beds: 92

Anaesthetics M Messent, S Stacey, K Wark

Cardiology R Balcon, G Clesham, A Deaner, P Kelly, C Knight, P Mills, M Rotham, A Timmis

Cardiothoracic Surgery P Magee, R Uppal, W Weir, K Wong, A Wood

General Medicine N Barnes

Histopathology I Scheimberg

Respiratory Medicine L Kuitert, S Lozewicz, J Wedicha

The Royal London Hospital

Whitechapel Road, London E1 1BB
Tel: 020 7377 7000 Fax: 020 7377 7401
Total Beds: 764

Accident and Emergency T Coats, H Cugnoni, F Davies, G Davies, K Henderson, S Miles, A Wilson

Anaesthetics J Anderson, C Broomhead, J Challands, P Colvin, J Cotter, P Flynn, D Goldhill, S Harrod, M Healy, E Mcateer, J McNeil,

P Monks, A Mulcahy, H Owen-Reece, M Razzaque, C Sadler, G Samra, R Sashidharan, L Struin, A Visram, S Withington, G Wray, P Yate

Dentistry V Booth, M Calvert, M Collins, S Djemal, P Farthing, J Fearne, J Hardie, F Hughes, R Lee, M Thornhill, D Williams, F Wong, P Wright

Dermatology A Quinn (Head), V Bataille, R Cerio, I Leigh, J McGregor

Diabetes S Coppack, G Hitman, P Kopelman

Endocrinology D Wood

Gastroenterology M Glynn, P Kumar, D Rampton, P Swain

General Surgery S Bhattacharya, F Cross, S Dorudi, A W Goode, R Ham, M Sheikh-Sobeh, Mr Siddiqui, M Walsh, N Williams

Genitourinary Medicine G Forster, B T Goh, T McManus, R Shen, C Skinner

Gynaecology P Armstrong, T Beedham, C Davis, G Grudzinskas, V Sivapathasundaram

Haematology B Colvin, F Cotter, C Gutteridge, A Newland, D Proven, P Telfer

Histopathology S Baithun, D Berney, J Martin, M Sheaff

Infection and Immunity G Baily

Medical Microbiology A Mifsud, E Price, A Sefton

Neonatology M Hird, S Kempley, P Mannix

Nephrology Z Chawdhery, J Conningham, F Marsh, M Raftery, C Rudge, R Thuraisingham, M Yaqoob

Neurology P Bradbury, G Elrington, J Fearnley, J Gawler, D Park, M Swash, R Walker

Neuropathology J Geddes

Neurosurgery F Afshar, P Hamlyn, I Sabin, J Sutcliffe

Nuclear Medicine H Jan

Ophthalmology A Mushin

Oral and Maxillofacial Surgery A Aitken, J Carter, K Coghlan, I Hutchison

Orthopaedics C Natali, M Paterson, G Scott

Orthopaedics and Trauma S Ang, M Barry, T Bucknill, D Goodier, W Grange

Paediatrics S Carr, I C Chikanza, C Cord-Udy, V Foster, R Harris, J Kingston, V Larcher, J Lilleyman, S McKenzie, A Martinez, D Misra, D Paige, M Powis, P Rees, V Saha, A Shankar, C Walker

Palliative Medicine D Feuer

Plastic Surgery N Carver, G Moir, M Shibu

Radiology C Blakeney, A Brooks, P Butler, O Chan, M Easty, E Evanson, E Friedman, N Garvie, J Murfitt, A Sharma, C Thakkar

Respiratory Medicine D Empey

Rheumatology and Rehabilitation D Perry (Head), A Jawad, B Kidd, R Stratton

Urology C Fowler, A Paris

Virology C Aitken, J Jeffries

St Bartholomew's Hospital

West Smithfield, London EC1A 7BE
Tel: 020 7377 7000
Total Beds: 407

Anaesthetics P Amoroso, M Ashby, A Bristow, V Carr, J Coakley, C Ferguson, H Hackett, A Hemming, C Hinds, P Howell, N Kellow, J Krapez, R Langford, R Marks, P Saunders, L Tham, B Varley, J Watson, S White, D Wilkinson, L Worthington

Breast Services R Carpenter

Cardiology A Nathan (Head), S Banim, T Crake, R Dawson, D Dymond, S Gupta, J Hogan, O Kurbaan, J Sayer, R Spurrell, J Stephens, D Tunstall-Pedoe

Cardiothoracic Surgery A Wood (Head), S Edmondson, A Lister, P Peters, A Shipolini

Clinical Neurophysiology D Ingram

Clinical Oncology C Cottrill, S Gibbs, G Mair, N Plowman, M Powell, P Wells

Clinical Pharmacology S Abrams

Endocrinology S L Chew (Head), J Anderson, A Clark, A Grossman, P Jenkins, J Monson

ENT M Dilkes (Head), M Keene, J Rubin

Gastroenterology P Fairclough (Head), E Alstead, A Ballinger, P Kumar, G Libby

General Surgery J Lumley, S Purkiss

Genitourinary Medicine C Escourt, P Mayura Nathan, R Melville, J M Zelin

Gynaecology T Al-Shawaf, O Djahanbakhch, G Grudzinskas, I Jacobs, A Jayarajah, A Lower, D Oram, N Perks

Haematology J Amess, J Cavenagh, P MacCallum, A Rohatiner

Histopathology M Calamanici, P Domizio, D Lowe, A Norton, N Singh, C Wells

Immunology M Murphy, A Pinching

Immunopathology J Parkin

Infection and Immunity J Anderson, M Herlbert

Medical Microbiology S Das, M Prentice

Medical Oncology C Gallagher, T Oliver, D Propper, R Rudd, J Shamash, M Slevin

Diabetes P Freedman, D Galton, D Leslie

Neurological Physiology K Nagendran

Neurosurgery P Hamlyn

Nuclear Medicine K Britton

Obstetrics and Gynaecology J Aquilina

Occupational Health D D'Auria

Ophthalmology J Hungerford, R Whitelocke

Paediatric Gastroenterology I Suanderson

Paediatric Medicine N Meadows, M Savage

Pain Management J Foster, J Gallagher

Palliative Medicine D Feuer, C Phillips, T Tate

Radiology P Armstrong, P Cannon, A McLean, M Matson, I Nockler, N Perry, R Reznek, S Vinnicombe, J Webb

Respiratory Medicine J Moore-Gillon

Urology Mr Al Sundani, F Chinegwundoh, V Nargund

Virology D Jeffries

Basildon and Thurrock University Hospitals NHS Foundation Trust

Established as a Foundation Trust 01/04/2004.

Basildon Hospital, Nethermayne, Basildon SS16 5NL
Tel: 01268 533911
Website: www.basildonandthurrock.nhs.uk
(Essex Strategic Health Authority)

Chair David Hooper
Chief Executive Alan Whittle

Basildon Hospital

Nether Mayne, Basildon SS16 5NL
Tel: 01268 533911 Fax: 01268 593757
Total Beds: 321

Anaesthetics H Alhameed, A David, M K Gademesetty, L Hoogsteden, R Jones, D M Lowe, M S May, A M Murray, V G Punchihewa, L T Rylah, M Sun Wai, S J Thomson, S F Tinloi, H J W Utting, J P Whitehead, I Youkhana

Cardiology R Aggarwal, S Iyer, W Serino

Cellular Pathology A Abdulla, N Alsanjari, K Osayi, P Ozua

Dermatology M D Catterall, S M Khorshid

ENT G Fayad, A Latif, B O'Reilly, A P Su

Elderly Medicine C Chan, R Huwez, G H Jenner, A Jubber, D Mullane

Endocrinology R Khan, M Mulcahy

Gastroenterology D J Gertner, J M Subhani, C P Willoughby

Haematology P Cervi, E J Watts

Imaging M Alsewan, T Chan, T Cory, A Hails, A Salahuddin

Internal Medicine E Osman

Microbiology R J Sage

Neurology R Capildeo, A Malaspina

Obstetrics and Gynaecology A R Haloob, A Ikomi, D Ojutiku, R Varma, C C Welch

Oral Medicine J McKechnie, D K Madan, P Weller

Orthopaedics R Grewel, N B Ker, I Lennox, T Peckham, R J Pusey, K J Reddy, J Targett, R Wakeman

Paediatrics J Askwith, K Khalefa, R Ramanan, N Sharief, S J Ware

Palliative Care G Tosh

Renal Medicine I Barton, A Lal, S Morgan

Respiratory Medicine D K Muckherjee, B Yung

Rheumatology N Gendi, J Palit

General Surgery D S J Collier, T Jeddy, F Khan, K Lafferty, I P Linehan, B Lovett, B F Ribeiro, H Taylor

Urology P Ewah, D R Osborne

Orsett Hospital

Grays RM16 3EU
Tel: 01268 533911 Fax: 01268 592227
Total Beds: 200

Anaesthetics M K Gademesetty, D M Lowe, A M Murray, V G Punchihewa, L T Rylah, S J Thomson, S F Tinloi, H J W Utting, J P Whitehead

Care of the Elderly C Cook, A J D Farquarson, G H Jenner, A Jubber, D Mullane

Dermatology M D Catterall

ENT D G Fife, A A Latif, B O'Reilly, A P C Su

Gastroenterology D J Gertner, C P Willoughby

General Medicine J F Bridgman

General Surgery K Lafferty, I P Linehan, H G Naylor, B F Ribeiro

Haematology P Cervi, E J Watts

Histopathology N Aqel, J Leake, E E Peters, S G Subbuswamy

Medical Microbiology R J Sage

Nephrology S Morgan

Neurology R Capildeo

Obstetrics and Gynaecology A R Haloob, M R Martin, R Varma, C C Welch

Oral Surgery J McKechnie, D K Madan, P Weller

Orthopaedics N B Ker, I Lennox, C D R Lightowler, T Peckham, R J Pusey, J Tagett, R Wakeman

Paediatrics D M Easton, R Ramanan, N Sharief, S J Ware

Pathology P W N Gordon

Radiology T Chan, P Cory, R Hails, A Salahuddin, D T Thompson

Rheumatology and Rehabilitation N Gendi, J Palit

Urology D R Osborne

Basildon Primary Care Trust

Phoenix Court, Christopher Martin Road, Basildon SS14 3GH
Tel: 01268 705000 Fax: 01268 705100
Email: info@basildon-pct.nhs.uk
Website: www.basildon-pct.nhs.uk
(Essex Strategic Health Authority)

Chair Alwyn Hollins
Chief Executive Mary-Ann Munford

Bassetlaw Primary Care Trust

Retford Hospital, North Road, Retford DN22 7XF
Tel: 01777 274400 Fax: 01777 274455
Website: www.bassetlaw-pct.nhs.uk
(Trent Strategic Health Authority)

Chair St John Deakin
Chief Executive Louise Newcombe

Bath and North East Somerset Primary Care Trust

St Martins Hospital, Midford Road, Bath BA2 5RP
Tel: 01225 831800 Fax: 01225 840407
Email: info@banes-pct.nhs.uk
Website: www.banes-pct.nhs.uk
(Avon, Gloucestershire and Wiltshire Strategic Health Authority)

Chair Malcolm Hanney
Chief Executive Rhona MacDonald

Paulton Memorial Hospital

Salisbury Road, Paulton, Bristol BS18 5SB
Tel: 01761 412315 Fax: 01761 412315
Total Beds: 28

Manager Dot Mitchard

St Martin's Hospital

Midford Road, Bath BA2 5RP
Tel: 01225 831500
Total Beds: 152

Bebington and West Wirral Primary Care Trust

3 Port Causeway, Bromborough, Wirral CH2 4NH
Tel: 0151 643 5300 Fax: 0151 643 5301
Email: bww@bwwpct.nhs.uk
Website: www.bwwpct.nhs.uk
(Cheshire and Merseyside Strategic Health Authority)

Chair Norman Pursglove
Chief Executive Allison Cooke

Bedford Hospital NHS Trust

Kempston Road, Bedford MK42 9DJ
Tel: 01234 355122 Fax: 01234 218106
Website: www.bedfordhospital.nhs.uk
(Bedfordshire and Hertfordshire Strategic Health Authority)

Chair Helen Nellis
Chief Executive Andrew Reed

Bedford Hospital

Kempston Road, Bedford MK42 9DJ
Tel: 01234 355122 Fax: 01234 218106
Total Beds: 475

Accident and Emergency D Small (Head), S Shankar

Anaesthetics J Sizer (Head), B Fahmy, J E Hughes, J Hurst, R Kavan, D Liu, S Lua, J T McNamara, A S Mody, D J Niblett, S L Snape, J U Wilson

Cardiology I C Cooper, J Cooper

Care of the Elderly I Kamal, K L Nandi, N Thangarajah, W N Trounson

Dermatology E Burova, B E Monk

ENT R Arasaratnam, M C Frampton, T J Hoare

General Medicine M Azher, R S J Harvey, P A McNamara, A Melvin, N J Morrish, J H B Saunders, E Thomas

General Surgery M J Callam, A Eldin, R J E Foley, I Husain, O Omotoso, A Palffy, D Skipper, P Tisi, N B Waterfall

Genitourinary Medicine K Shanmugaratnam

Haematology D T Howes

Neurology M Manford

Obstetrics and Gynaecology G C Budden, E J Neale, D Patel, S F Reynolds, R M Wallace

Oncology V Bulusu, R Thomas

Ophthalmology F F Fisher, D Newman, S J P Pieris, A Sharma

Oral and Maxillofacial Surgery G H Chan, M T Simpson

Orthodontics A B Hewitt

Orthopaedics P A J Edge, C Handley, G Nel, R D Rawlins, J Scott

Paediatrics O Kwapong, M Leigh, R D Mehta, M J Pocha, S Rehman

Pathology A J Blackshaw, D T Howes, F Mutch, D B Rimmer, W S Wassif, M J E Wilkins

Plastic Surgery P J Mahaffey

Radiology I P Hicks (Head), S J Barter, A M Egan, R A Moxon, R H Oakley, C Onyelzwuluje, M I Shaikh

Rheumatology and Rehabilitation S A Rae

Bedford Primary Care Trust

Gilbert Hitchcock House, 21 Kimbolton Road, Bedford MK40 2AW
Tel: 01234 795714 Fax: 01234 342028
Email: information@bedford-pct.nhs.uk
Website: www.bedford-pct.nhs.uk
(Bedfordshire and Hertfordshire Strategic Health Authority)

Chair Alan Loynes
Chief Executive Margaret Stockham

Bedfordshire and Hertfordshire Ambulance and Paramedic Service NHS Trust

Ambulance Headquarters, Hammond Road, Bedford MK41 0RG
Tel: 01234 408999 Fax: 01234 270480
Email: info@bhamb.nhs.uk
Website: www.bhamb.nhs.uk
(Bedfordshire and Hertfordshire Strategic Health Authority)

Chair Maria Ball
Chief Executive Anne Walker

Bedfordshire and Luton Mental Health and Social Care Partnership NHS Trust

Formerly Bedfordshire and Luton Community NHS Trust.

Charter House, Alma Street, Luton LU1 2PL
Tel: 01582 700171 Fax: 01582 700151
Website: www.blct.nhs.uk
(Bedfordshire and Hertfordshire Strategic Health Authority)

Chair Alison Davis
Chief Executive Paul Mullin
Consultants K Bala, F Besag, P Brown, U K Chowdhury, A Fleming, V Frances, A Hussain, M Iqbal, R H Kathane, R MacInnes, H R Makar, K J Morgan Gray, J Muthiah, M O'Rourke, A Patel, T J Phillips, J A Pillai, R Pinto, Y J Rao, A V Roberts, C Royston, J Stein, S M Stein, M Suleiman, R Zaman

Acute Mental Health (North)

Clinical Director Ashok Patel

The Lodge, Twinwoods
Milton Road, Clapham, Bedford MK41 6AT
Tel: 01234 310555 Fax: 01234 310556

Meadow Lodge
Steppingley Hospital, Ampthill Road, Steppingley, Bedford MK45 1AB
Tel: 01525 758400 Fax: 01525 758417
Email: meadow.lodge@sbchc-tr.anglox.nhs.uk

Manager Moira Lawrence

Spring House
Biggleswade Hospital, Potton Road, Biggleswade SG18 0EL
Tel: 01767 224922 Fax: 01767 224921

Manager Jane Kilgour

10a Goldington Road
10a Goldington Road, Bedford MK40 3NE
Tel: 01234 408423 Fax: 01234 408425
Email: goldington@sbchc-tr.anglox.nhs.uk

Manager Phillip Chudley

Weller Wing, Bronte Ward
South Wing Hospital, Ampthill Road, Bedford MK42 9DJ
Tel: 01234 299962 Fax: 01234 299901
Email: bronte.ward@sbchc-tr.anglox.nhs.uk

Manager Mike Jackson

Weller Wing, Keats Ward
South Wing Hospital, Ampthill Road, Bedford MK42 9DJ
Tel: 01234 299955 Fax: 01234 299957
Email: keats.ward@sbchc-tr.anglox.nhs.uk

Manager Bhisma Teeluk

Acute Mental Health (South)

Clinical Director Robin Pinto

Beacon House
5 Regent Street, Dunstable LU6 1LP
Tel: 01582 709200 Fax: 01582 709201
Email: beacon.house@sbchc-tr.anglox.nhs.uk

Manager Jay Nair

Calnwood Court, Inpatient Unit
Calnwood Road, Luton LU4 0LU
Tel: 01582 707563 Fax: 01582 707561

Manager Mega Chetty

Calnwood Court, Outpatients
Calnwood Road, Luton LU4 0LU
Tel: 01582 709150 Fax: 01582 709151

Manager Visu Suppiah

Crombie House
36 Hockliffe Street, Leighton Buzzard LU7 1HJ
Tel: 01525 751133 Fax: 01525 751134
Email: crombie.house@sbchc-tr.anglox.nhs.uk

Manager Pam Skinner

Oakley Court
Angel Close, Off Addington Way, Luton LU4 9WT
Tel: 01582 707596 Fax: 01582 709179
Email: oakley.court@sbchc-tr.anglox.nhs.uk

Manager Harry Sookraj

Townsend Court
Mayer Way, Houghton Regis, Dunstable LU5 5BF
Tel: 01582 707596 Fax: 01582 707599
Email: townsend.court@sbchc-tr.anglox.nhs.uk

Manager Mega Chetty

Mental Health for Older People (North) (MHOP)

Clinical Director Claire Royston

Fountains Court
3 Kimbolton Road, Bedford MK40 2NU
Tel: 01234 310798 Fax: 01234 310128
Email: fountains.court@sbchc-tr.anglox.nhs.uk

Manager Jason Chung

The Lawns (Day Resource)
The Baulk, Biggleswade SG18 0PT
Tel: 01767 224181 Fax: 01767 224180
Email: lawns.mentalhealth@sbchc-tr.anglox.nhs.uk

Manager Sue Inskip

Sheridan Day Hospital
South Wing Hospital, Ampthill Road, Bedford MK42 9DJ
Tel: 01234 299970 Fax: 01234 299901

Manager Kay Stokes

Weller Wing, Chaucer Ward
South Wing Hospital, Ampthill Road, Bedford MK42 9DJ
Tel: 01234 299966 Fax: 01234 299901
Email: chaucer.ward@sbchc-tr.anglox.nhs.uk

Manager Jenny Arden

Weller Wing, Milton Ward
South Wing Hospital, Ampthill Road, Bedford MK42 9DJ
Tel: 01234 299946 Fax: 01234 299901
Email: milton.ward@sbchc-tr.anglox.nhs.uk

Manager Christina Beukes

Mental Health for Older People (North Herts) (MHOP)

Clinical Director Claire Royston

Elizabeth Court
Graveley Road, Stevenage SG1 4YS
Tel: 01438 218141 Fax: 01438 218140

Manager Sue Lomas

Victoria Court
Graveley Road, Stevenage SG1 4YS
Tel: 01438 224005 Fax: 01438 224010

Manager Sue Lomas

Mental Health for Older People (South) (MHOP)

Farley Hill Day Hospital
Whipperley Ring, Farley Hill, Luton LU1 5QY
Tel: 01582 708222 Fax: 01582 708223
Email: farley.hill@sbchc-tr.anglox.nhs.uk

Lime Trees
Calnwood Road, Luton LU4 0DZ
Tel: 01582 707555 Fax: 01582 707554

Manager Louise Trainor

The Poplars
Mayer Way, Off Houghton Road, Houghton Regis, Dunstable LU5 5BF
Tel: 01582 657588
Email: poplarsrv700befordshireandluton@sbchc-tr.anglox.nhs.uk

Manager Elizabeth Langley

Rehabilitation (North)

Clinical Director Ashok Patel

Day Resource Centre
3 Kimbolton Road, Bedford MK40 2NU
Tel: 01234 310044 Fax: 01234 310043

Manager Jo Prior

John Bunyon House
3 Kimbolton Road, Bedford MK40 2NU
Tel: 01234 310330 Fax: 01234 310331
Email: johnbunyan.house@sbchc-tr.anglox.nhs.uk

Manager Tracey Tebbutt

Progress House
36-38 Kimbolton Road, Bedford MK40 2NU
Tel: 01234 310251 Fax: 01234 310252
Email: progress.house@sbchc-tr.anglox.nhs.uk

Manager Brenda Queeley

Rehabilitation (North Herts)

Clinical Director Robin Pinto

Gainsford House
Foxholes, Pirton Road, Hitchin SG5 2EN
Tel: 01462 633680 Fax: 01462 633681
Email: gainsford.house@sbchc-tr.anglox.nhs.uk

Manager Joe Caruana

Hampden House
Elmside Walk, Bedford Road, Hitchin SG5 1HB
Tel: 01462 633666 Fax: 01462 633660
Email: hampden.house@sbchc-tr.anglox.nhs.uk

Manager Laura Rowley

Rehabilitation (South)

Clinical Director Robin Pinto

ACE Enterprises
Oakley House, 60-64 Collingdon Street, Luton LU1 1RX
Tel: 01582 708200 Fax: 01582 708201
Email: ace.enterprises@sbchc-tr.anglox.nhs.uk

Manager Kay Sookun

Biscot House
75 Biscot Road, Luton LU3 1AH
Tel: 01582 707460 Fax: 01582 707459
Email: biscot.house@sbchc-tr.anglox.nhs.uk

Manager Sue Ahiekpor

Leagrave Lodge
Leagrave High Street, Leagrave, Luton LU4 9JU
Tel: 01582 708205 Fax: 01582 708206
Email: leagrave.lodge@sbchc-tr.anglox.nhs.uk

Manager Paul Bates

105 London Road
105 London Road, Luton LU1 3RG
Tel: 01582 708900 Fax: 01582 708901
Email: londonrd@sbchc-tr.anglox.nhs.uk

Manager Mala Curpen

Whichello's Wharf
The Elms, Stoke Road, Linslade, Leighton Buzzard LU7 2TD
Tel: 01525 751170 Fax: 01525 751171
Email: whichellos.wharf@sbchc-tr.anglox.nhs.uk

Manager Sarah Adansi

Secure

Clinical Director Robin Pinto

Orchard Unit
Orchard Unit, Calnwood Road, Luton LU4 0FB
Tel: 01582 657500 Fax: 01582 657501
Total Beds: 32

Manager Maureen Simmons

Services for People who have a Learning Disability (SPLD)

Clinical Director M O'Rourke

Askern House
Manor Road, Kempston Hardwick MK43 9NP
Tel: 01234 853011 Fax: 01234 853566
Email: askern.house@sbchc-tr.anglox.nhs.uk

Manager Chris Cowan

Beech Close Resource Centre
Beech Close, Dunstable LU6 3SD
Tel: 01582 538250 Fax: 01582 538251

Manager Sue Phillips

Carlton House
55 The Causeway, Carlton, Bedford MK43 7LU
Tel: 01234 720737 Fax: 01234 721842

Manager Mike Ullah

Cedar Lodge
9 Sundon Road, Streatley, Luton LU3 3PL
Tel: 01582 883354 Fax: 01582 881916
Email: cedar.lodge@sbchc-tr.anglox.nhs.uk

Manager Deborah Skeldon

Conifers
10 Newbury Lane, Silsoe, Bedford MK45 4ET
Tel: 01525 860495 Fax: 01525 862697
Email: conifers.silsoe@sbchc-tr.anglox.nhs.uk

Manager May McKnight

Country Bungalow
21 Potton Road, Everton, Sandy SG19 2LD
Tel: 01767 692001 Fax: 01767 692759
Email: contry.bungalow@sbchc-tr.anglox.nhs.uk

Manager Gillian Hudson

Crossways
4 High Street, Oakley, Bedford MK43 7RG
Tel: 01234 826056 Fax: 01234 823854
Email: high.street@sbchc-tr.anglox.nhs.uk

Manager Pam Mills

4 Beech Close
4 Beech Close, Dunstable LU6 3SD
Tel: 01582 757660 Fax: 01582 757661
Email: beech.close4@sbchc-tr.anglox.nhs.uk

Manager Gillian Hudson

Little Paddock
30 Hookhams Lane, Renhold, Bedford MK41 0JT
Tel: 01234 772481 Fax: 01234 772930
Email: littlle.paddocks@sbchc-tr.anglox.nhs.uk

Manager Jeanette Franklin

1 Beech Close
1 Beech Close, Dunstable LU6 3SD
Tel: 01582 757645 Fax: 01582 757646
Email: beech.close1@sbchc-tr.anglox.nhs.uk

Manager Naguib Fuzarally

1 The Glade
1 The Glade, Bromham, Bedford MK43 8HJ
Tel: 01234 310730 Fax: 01234 310731

Manager Marion Gant

Orchard Cottage
Church Road, Lower Sundon, Luton LU3 3PB
Tel: 01525 872530 Fax: 01525 877963

Manager Josie Sutton

Overstones
Bowling Green Lane, Luton LU2 7HR
Tel: 01582 876239 Fax: 01582 749201
Email: overstones.luton@sbchc-tr.anglox.nhs.uk

Manager Mark Bailey

Red House Farm
148 Cotton End Drive, Wilstead, Bedford MK45 3DP
Tel: 01234 743225 Fax: 01234 743116
Email: redhouse.farm@sbchc-tr.anglox.nhs.uk

Manager Jan West

Respite Unit
18-20 Calverton Road, Luton LU23 2SX
Tel: 01582 757640 Fax: 01582 757641
Total Beds: 5

Manager Tim Martin

Sharnbrook House
30 Mill Road, Sharnbrook, Bedford MK44 1NX
Tel: 01234 782796 Fax: 01234 783018

Manager Jeremy Jones

The Spinney
31 Luton Road, Wilstead, Bedford MK45 3ER
Tel: 01234 310716 Fax: 01234 310719
Email: the.spinney@sbchc-tr.anglox.nhs.uk

Manager Beverley Martin

3 Beech Close
3 Beech Close, Dunstable LU6 3SD

Tel: 01582 757655 Fax: 01582 757656
Email: beech.close3@sbchc-tr.anglox.nhs.uk

Manager Lucy Gyau-Ampofo

3 The Glade
3 The Glade, Bromham, Bedford MK43 8HJ
Tel: 01234 310740 Fax: 01234 310741

Manager Sandra Parkin

Twinwoods
Milton Road, Clapham, Bedford MK41 6AT
Tel: 01234 310569

2 Beech Close
2 Beech Close, Dunstable LU6 3SD
Tel: 01582 757650 Fax: 01582 757651
Email: beech.close2@sbchc-tr.anglox.nhs.uk

Manager Gladys Quinn

2 The Glade
2 The Glade, Bromham, Bedford MK43 8HJ
Tel: 01234 310735 Fax: 01234 310736

Manager Adrian Henson

Tyndale House
15 Merton Road, Bedford MK40 3AF
Tel: 01234 310725 Fax: 01234 310875
Email: tyndale.house@sbchc-tr.anglox.nhs.uk

Manager Rosa Mactoom

Vincent House
West End Road, Box End, Kempston, Bedford MK43 8RT
Tel: 01234 853443 Fax: 01234 856148
Email: vincent.house@sbchc-tr.anglox.nhs.uk

Manager Lynne Mynard

Washbrook House
50 Washbrook Close, Barton-Le-Clay, Bedford MK45 4LF
Tel: 01582 708326 Fax: 01582 708327
Email: washbrook.house@sbchc-tr.anglox.nhs.uk

Manager Liz Costello

The Willows
4 The Glade, Northampton Road, Bromham, Bedford MK43 8HJ
Tel: 01234 310745 Fax: 01234 310726

Manager Sandra Hukin

Wood Lea Clinic
5 The Glade, Northampton Road, Bromham, Bedford MK43 8HJ
Tel: 01234 310750 Fax: 01234 310751

Manager Steve Burridge

Woodlands
Leamington Road, Luton LU3 3XF
Tel: 01234 310745 Fax: 01582 708325
Email: woodlands.barton@sbchc-tr.anglox.nhs.uk

Manager Simon Tringham

Substance Misuse and Alcohol

Clinical Director Ashok Patel, Robin Pinto

Health Link
26-28 Bromham Road, Bedford MK40 2QD
Tel: 01234 270123 Fax: 01234 365160

Manager Stuart Sage

Maple Lodge
Studley Road, Luton LU3 1BB
Tel: 01582 709100 Fax: 01582 709106

Manager Matthew Johnson

SoBeDAS
15-17 Cardiff Road, Luton LU1 1PP
Tel: 01582 528880 Fax: 01582 528881

Manager S R Manoharan

Bedfordshire Heartlands Primary Care Trust

1-2 Doolittle Mill, Froghall Road, Ampthill, Bedford MK45 2NX
Tel: 01525 631153 Fax: 01525 631168
Email: firstname.lastname@bedsheartlandspct.nhs.uk
Website: www.bedsheartlandspct.nhs.uk
(Bedfordshire and Hertfordshire Strategic Health Authority)

Chair Leslie Watts
Chief Executive Anne Walker
Consultants Sue Gregory, Rachel Joyce

Berkshire Healthcare NHS Trust

Church Hill House, 51-52 Turing Drive, Bracknell RG12 7FR
Tel: 01344 422722 Fax: 01344 867990
Website: www.berkshire.nhs.uk
(Thames Valley Strategic Health Authority)

Chair Lorna Roberts
Chief Executive Philippa Slinger

Heatherwood Hospital (EMI & AMI Units)
London Road, Ascot SL5 8AA
Tel: 01344 623333 Fax: 01344 874340

King Edward VII Hospital (EMI Unit)
St Leonards Road, Windsor
Tel: 01753 860441 Fax: 01753 636107

Newbury Community Hospital (EMI Day Hospital)
Andover Road, Newbury RG14 6LS
Tel: 01628 632012 Fax: 01635 580610

Prospect Park Hospital
Honey End Lane, Titlehurst, Reading RG30 4EJ
Tel: 0118 960 5000
Total Beds: 203

Psychology A Keddie

St Mark's Hospital (EMI Day Hospital)
St Marks Road, Maidenhead SL6 6DU
Tel: 01628 632012 Fax: 01628 635050

Upton Hospital (EMI Unit)
Albert Street, Slough SL2 4HL
Tel: 01753 821441 Fax: 01753 635050

Wexham Park Hospital (EMI & AMI Units)
Wexham Street, Slough SL2 4HL
Tel: 01753 633000 Fax: 01753 634825

Bexhill and Rother Primary Care Trust

Bexhill Hospital, Holliers Hill, Bexhill-on-Sea TN40 2DZ
Tel: 01424 735600 Fax: 01424 735601
Email: surname.firstname@bar-pct.sthames-nhs.uk
Website: www.bexhillandrotherpct.nhs.uk
(Surrey and Sussex Strategic Health Authority)

Chair John Barnes
Chief Executive Rick Stern

Bexley Care Trust

221 Erith Road, Bexleyheath DA7 6HZ
Tel: 020 8298 6000 Fax: 020 8298 6241
Email: contactus@bexley.nhs.uk
Website: www.bexley.nhs.uk
(South East London Strategic Health Authority)

Chair Kathy Balcombe
Chief Executive Ian Leftley

Billericay, Brentwood and Wickford Primary Care Trust

High Wood Hospital, Geary Drive, Brentwood CM15 9DY
Tel: 01277 302516 Fax: 01277 302512
Email: firstname.surname@bbw-pct.nhs.uk
Website: www.bbw-pct.nhs.uk
(Essex Strategic Health Authority)

Chair Angela Bloomfield
Chief Executive Howard Perry

Brentwood Community Hospital

Crescent Drive, Shenfield, Brentwood CM15 8DR
Tel: 01277 302893 Fax: 01277 302870

Manager Sister Phillpot

High Wood Hospital

Geary Drive, Brentwood CM15 9DY
Tel: 01277 302516 Fax: 01277 302512
Total Beds: 50

Manager Jane Evans

Care of the Elderly Dr Wicks

Mayflower House

Blunts Wall Road, Tye Common Road, Billericay CM12 9SA
Tel: 01277 621130 (In-patients), 01277 621140 (Day patients)
Total Beds: 38

Birkenhead and Wallasey Primary Care Trust

Admin Block, St Catherine's Hospital, Church Road, Birkenhead CH42 0LQ
Tel: 0151 651 0011 Fax: 0151 652 2668
Email: birkwallpct@exchange.wirral-ha.nwest.nhs.uk
Website: www.bkwpct.nhs.uk
(Cheshire and Merseyside Strategic Health Authority)

Chair Frances Street
Chief Executive Kathy Doran

Birmingham and Solihull Mental Health NHS Trust

Uffculme Special School, 52 Queensbridge Road, Moseley, Birmingham B13 8QD
Tel: 0121 678 2000
Email: info.comments@bsmht.nhs.uk
Website: www.bsmht.nhs.uk
(Birmingham and the Black Country Strategic Health Authority)

Chair Jonathan Shapiro
Chief Executive Sue Turner

Birmingham Children's Hospital NHS Trust

Birmingham Children's Hospital is one of the largest providers of acute services in the West Midlands specialising in the provision of an integrated child health service.

Diana, Princess of Wales Children's Hospital, Steelhouse Lane, Birmingham B4 6NH
Tel: 0121 333 9999 Fax: 0121 333 9998
Email: child.infoctr@bhanchildrens.wmids.nhs.uk
Website: www.bch.org.uk
(Birmingham and the Black Country Strategic Health Authority)

Chair Joanna Davis
Chief Executive J Sandy Bradbrook

Birmingham Children's Hospital

Steelhouse Lane, Birmingham B4 6NH
Tel: 0121 333 9999 Fax: 0121 333 9998
Total Beds: 295

Accident and Emergency K Berry, B Wilson

Anaesthetics O Bagshaw, A Cranston, S E F Jones, A Liley, A Moriarty, C R Ralston, N J Robson, M Stokes, A Tatman

Cardiac Surgery D Barron, W J Brawn

Cardiology J de Giovanni, R Dhillon, P Miller, O Stumper, J G C Wright

Clinical Chemistry A Green (Head)

Dental Surgery L Shaw

Dermatology C Moss (Head)

Endocrinology N Shaw (Head), T Barrett, J Kirk

Gastroenterology S Protheroe (Head), I W Booth, S Murphy

General Psychiatry G Bates, L Cullen, R El Sharief, F Farook, P Forster, S Handy, D Kat, S Narayan, S Paliwall, D Rothery, D Simmons, L Winkley

Genetics P A Farndon

Haematology P J Darbyshire, F G Hill, S Lawson, M D Williams

Hepatology S Beath, J de Ville de Goyet, D Kelly, I Van Monrik

Intensive Care K Morris, G Morrison, G Pearson, F Reynolds

Medical Microbiology J Gray

Nephrology S A Hulton, D Milford, Dr Stevens, C M Taylor

Neurology S H Green, S Philips

Neurophysiology L Henderson, S Seri

Neurosurgery A D Hockley, S Sgouros, R Walsh

Oncology M English, R Grundy, H Jenkinson, B Morland

Ophthalmology J R Ainsworth, K Butler, H C Willshaw

Oral and Maxillofacial Surgery M Wake

Orthopaedics C F Bradish, P Gibbons, P Glithero, D Marks, J O'Hara

Otolaryngology A Drake-Lee, R Irving, M Kuo, J McRac-Moore, K Pearman, D W Proops, A Reid

Paediatric Surgery R Buick, H Chandran, S Donnell, P Gornall, G Jawaheer, T Lander, K Parashar, D Parikh

Paediatrics G D Belle, V Diwoker, A Goldstein, N McLellan, R Sunderland

Pathology R Brown

Plastic Surgery R Lester, H Nikashawa, R Slater, R Waters, Y Wilson

Radiology H Alton, S Chapman, F Haigh, K Johnson, L McPherson

Radiotherapy and Oncology D Spooner

Respiratory Medicine J Clarke, P Weller

Rheumatology and Rehabilitation C Ryder (Head), J McDonagh, T R Southwood

Thoracic Surgery A Lander, D Parikh

Birmingham Women's Health Care NHS Trust

Birmingham Women's Hospital, Metchley Park Road, Edgbaston, Birmingham B15 2TG
Tel: 0121 472 1377 Fax: 0121 627 2602
Website: www.bwhct.nhs.uk
(Birmingham and the Black Country Strategic Health Authority)

Chair Ann Owen
Chief Executive Caroline Wigley

Birmingham Women's Hospital

Edgbaston, Birmingham B15 2TG
Tel: 0121 472 1377 Fax: 0121 627 2602
Total Beds: 207

Anaesthetics R A Bond, T Bowden, G Cooper, L H Grove, M Lewis, A Malins, P J Millns, A D Wilkey

Clinical Chemistry D Worthington

Cytology A Yoong

Genetics T Cole, P A Farndon, C McKeown, E Maher, J Morton, A Norman

Haematology M Williams

Histopathology S Lee, C Platt, T Rollason

Medical Microbiology J Gray

Obstetrics and Gynaecology M Afnan, S Blunt, K K Chan, J M Emens, H Gee, M Kilby, J R Newton, H O Nicholson, J Pogmore, R S Sawers, M Shati, J Weaver, M Whittle

Paediatrics G M Durbin, M Hocking, I Morgan

Pathology S Lee, T P Rollason, D I Rushton

Radiology J M McHugo, J Mould

Blackburn with Darwen Primary Care Trust

Guide Business Centre, School Lane, Guide, Blackburn BB1 2QH
Tel: 01254 267000 Fax: 01254 267009
Website: www.bwdpct.nhs.uk
(Cumbria and Lancashire Strategic Health Authority)

Chair Nick Kennedy
Chief Executive Vivien Aspey

Blackpool, Fylde and Wyre Hospitals NHS Trust

Blackpool Victoria Hospital, Whinney Heys Road, Blackpool FY3 8NR
Tel: 01253 300000 Fax: 01253 306873
Email: communications@bfwhospitals.nhs.uk
Website: www.bfwhospitals.nhs.uk
(Cumbria and Lancashire Strategic Health Authority)

Chair Beverly Lester
Chief Executive Roy Male

Bispham Hospital Rehabilitation Unit

Ryscar Way, Bispham, Blackpool FY2 0FN
Tel: 01253 655901 Fax: 01253 655903
Email: communications@bfwhospitals.nhs.uk
Website: www.bfwhospitals.nhs.uk/hospitals/bispham
Total Beds: 40

Manager Joanna Beith

Clifton Hospital

Pershore Road, Off Clifton Drive, Lytham St Annes FY8 1PB
Tel: 01253 306204 Fax: 01253 306214
Email: communications@bfwhospitals.nhs.uk
Website: www.bfwhospitals.nhs.uk/hospitals/clifton
Total Beds: 101

Manager Joanna Beith

Care of the Elderly R Gajendragadkar, M E I Khateeb, M J O'Donnell

Devonshire Road Hospital

Devonshire Road, Blackpool FY3 8AZ
Tel: 01253 303364 Fax: 01253 303386
Email: communications@bfwhospitals.nhs.uk
Website: www.bfwhospitals.nhs.uk/hospitals/devonshire
Total Beds: 10

Manager Joanna Beith

Dermatology W W Bottomley, J K Kellett

General Psychiatry C A D Calvert, W J Charles, D S G Kay, C J Molodynski

Fleetwood Hospital

Pharos Street, Fleetwood FY7 6BE
Tel: 01253 306000 Fax: 01253 306029
Email: communications@bfwhospitals.nhs.uk
Website: www.bfwhospitals.nhs.uk/hospitals/fleetwood
Total Beds: 27

Manager Pat Shingleton

Colposcopy A Saeed

Dermatology W Bottomley

Rheumatology I Stewart

Urology N Rothwell

Lytham Hospital

Warton Street, Lytham St Annes FY8 5EE
Tel: 01253 303953
Email: communications@bfwhospitals.nhs.uk
Website: www.bfwhospitals.nhs.uk/hospitals/lytham
Total Beds: 30

Manager Pat Shingleton

Dermatology J K Kellett

Orthopaedics M S Cornah, S McLoughlin

Paediatrics S Byrne

Rheumatology S Jones

Urology C R A Bevis, N Rothwell

Rossall Hospital

Westway, Rossall, Fleetwood FY7 8JH
Tel: 01253 655102 Fax: 01253 655107
Email: communications@bfwhospitals.nhs.uk
Website: www.bfwhospitals.nhs.uk/hospitals/rossall
Total Beds: 40

Manager Joanna Beith

Care of the Elderly R S Gulati

South Shore Hospital
Stony Hill Avenue, Blackpool FY4 1HX
Tel: 01253 306106 Fax: 01253 306101
Email: communications@bfwhospitals.nhs.uk
Website: www.bfwhospitals.nhs.uk/hospitals/south_shore
Total Beds: 101

Manager Kevin Clarkson

Care of the Elderly R S Gulati

Rheumatology S Jones, I Stewart

Victoria Hospital
Whinney Heys Road, Blackpool FY3 8NR
Tel: 01253 300000 Fax: 01253 306873
Email: communications@bfwhospitals.nhs.uk
Website: www.bfwhospitals.nhs.uk/hospitals/victoria
Total Beds: 778

Accident and Emergency S N Harrop, N Kidner, M Sedgwick

Anaesthetics M E Chamberlain, C Clarke, S Corsan, R Cross, J Cuppitt, C Dunkley, N J Gavin, C Harle, N Harper, M Hartley, D Hume, C Humphries, G Johnson, D R Kelly, A Knowles, A S Lockhart, B M Lord, S Mills, R Morgan, A Ramirez-Rodriguez, N P Randall, C Rozario, S Vaughan

Cardiology M Brack, A Chauhan, Dr Eccleshall, G Goode, Dr More, D H Roberts, Dr Waktare

Cardiothoracic Surgery J Au, A Duncan, R Millner, Mr Sogliani, A Tang, J Zacharias

Dermatology W Bottomley, J K Kellett

ENT W Aucott, N Kazmi, A O Keith, A Nigam

General Medicine P Kelsey (Head), A Ahmed, M El-Khateeb, P Flegg, R Gulati, P J Hayes, M Hendrickse, M S Hendy, P E T Isaacs, T Karthikeyan, T C Li Kam Wa, J D Mackay, J McIlmoyle, A Mirakhur, Dr O'Donnell, M Paracha, Y Seth, C J Shorrock, S Talab

General Surgery J Heath, M Khurshid, M E Lambert, H Osman, S Pettit, S Rajan, S Ravi

Genitourinary Medicine A M Saeed, J Sweeney

Neurosurgery B Boothman, C Davis, N T Gurusinghe, T Nixon

Obstetrics and Gynaecology I Arthur, N A Bedford, S J Duthie, M R Steel, F L Wilcox

Oncology Dr Hindley

Ophthalmology J A Dunne, G Naylor, W Pollock, M Raines

Oral and Maxillofacial Surgery J Cornah

Orthodontics Mr Akhtar

Orthopaedics K P Boardman, S D Fewster, I Guisasola, A Javed, S Mannion, S McLoughlin, S Sampath

Paediatrics P Curtis, M E Johnson, N Laycock, R Stevens, M Thomas, R Verma, R Wheatley

Pathology R Duthie, J Johnson, P R Kelsey, M P Macheta, M C J Sissons, K S Vasudev

Plastic Surgery N R Gaze

Radiology P K Bowyer, R W Bury, L Hacking, T P Kane, F Lo Ying Ping, D Montgomery, C Walshaw

Rheumatology S Jones, I Stewart

Urology C R A Bevis, N R Rothwell

Wesham Hospital Rehabilitation Unit
Mowbreck Lane, Wesham, Lytham St Annes PR4 3HA
Tel: 01253 655401 Fax: 01253 655403
Email: communications@bfwhospitals.nhs.uk
Website: www.bfwhospitals.nhs.uk/hospitals/wesham
Total Beds: 40

Manager Joanna Beith

Blackpool Primary Care Trust

Trust Offices (NHS), Derby Road, Wesham, Preston PR4 3AL
Tel: 01253 303211 Fax: 01253 303197
Website: www.blackpoolpct.nhs.uk
(Cumbria and Lancashire Strategic Health Authority)

Chair Tony Shaw
Chief Executive Wendy Swift
Consultants N Gajawira, Saeed, J Sweeney, J Tiley

Blackwater Valley and Hart Primary Care Trust

Winchfield Lodge, Old Potbridge Road, Winchfield, Hook RG27 8BT
Tel: 01252 849000 Fax: 01252 849001
Website: www.bvhpct.nhs.uk
(Hampshire and Isle of Wight Strategic Health Authority)

Chair John Parker
Chief Executive Debbie Glenn

Cranleigh Village Community Hospital
6 High Street, Cranleigh GU6 8AE
Tel: 01483 782400 Fax: 01483 782499
Total Beds: 14

Care of the Elderly H Powell, V Seth

ENT N W Weir

General Medicine T H Foley

General Surgery A E Giddings, N D Karanjia, M W Kissin, C G Marks

Obstetrics and Gynaecology P M Coats, K Morton

Paediatrics P J Gibson

Farnham Community Hospital
Hale Road, Farnham GU9 9QL
Tel: 01483 782000 Fax: 01483 782015
Total Beds: 73

Care of the Elderly K Debrait, I Ibrahim, K Mundy

Dermatology Dr Crone, R H Felix, Dr Woollam

ENT Mr Jonathon, R Kumar, A McCombe, Mr Sudderick

General Medicine Mr Amery, R L Bown, M J Boyd, R J Frankel, Mr Laidlaw, Mr Leopold, Mr Paterson, Mr Rutter

General Psychiatry Mr Hassan

General Surgery M Laidlan, M Leopold, M Singh

Haematology Dr Shirley, J E W Van de Pette

Neurology Dr Trend

Obstetrics and Gynaecology Mr Coates, S E Inman, Mr Riddle, P J Toplis

Oncology Mr Laing

Ophthalmology Mr Elliott, J A Govan, Mr Hashim, M K Tandon

Orthopaedics Miss Ashbrooke, S Davies, D Dempster, Mr Harrison, Mr Magnussen, Mr Pike, Dr Syed

Paediatrics Dr Howard, Dr Maltby, C Sena

Rheumatology and Rehabilitation J H P Cuddigan, Dr Reilly

Thoracic Medicine R K Knight

Urology Mr Kutarski, Mr Notley, Mr Palfrey

Fleet Community Hospital
Church Road, Fleet GU13 8LB
Tel: 01483 782700 Fax: 01483 782799
Total Beds: 31

Haslemere and District Community Hospital
Church Lane, Haslemere GU27 2BJ
Tel: 01483 782300 Fax: 01483 782398
Total Beds: 31

Audiological Medicine V Jayarajan, S E Snashall

Care of the Elderly H J Powell, V Seth

Chest Medicine W A C McAllister

Dermatology E Wong

ENT D McMillan, D Wright

General Medicine T H Foley, M G M Smith, M J Smith

General Psychiatry H Boothby

General Surgery M E Bailey, A E B Giddings, N D Karanjia, M Kissin, C Marks

Neurology P S Trend

Obstetrics and Gynaecology E P Curtis, K Morton, C J G Sutton

Ophthalmology A Gilvarry, S W Hampson

Orthopaedics C J Coates, M C Flannery

Paediatrics P J Gibson, M Ryalls

Plastic Surgery B Powell

Radiology B J Loveday

Rheumatology A R Behn, R E S Gray

Urology J H Davis, F A W Schweitzer

Bolton Hospitals NHS Trust

Royal Bolton Hospital, Minerva Road, Farnworth, Bolton BL4 0JR
Tel: 01204 390390 Fax: 01204 390936
Website: www.boltonhospitals.nhs.uk
(Greater Manchester Strategic Health Authority)

Chair Peter Liptrott
Chief Executive John Brunt

Belmont Day Hospital
Minverva Road, Farnworth, Bolton BL4 0JR
Tel: 01204 390390

Fall Birch Hospital
Lostock, Bolton BL6 4LQ
Tel: 01204 695714
Total Beds: 35

Hulton Day Hospital
Hulton Lane, Bolton BL3 4JZ

Hulton Hospital
Hulton Lane, Bolton BL3 4JZ
Tel: 01204 390262
Total Beds: 42

Minerva Day Hospital
Minerva Road, Farnworth, Bolton BL4 0JR

Rivington Day Hospital
Minerva Road, Farnworth, Bolton BL4 0JR

Royal Bolton Hospital
Farnworth, Bolton BL4 0JR
Tel: 01204 390390 Fax: 01204 390794
Total Beds: 968

Accident and Emergency J C Adams, C Moulton

Anaesthetics J N Aspbury, S Deegan, M J Flynn, J P Ryan, Y Sivalingham, N J Smith

Care of the Elderly K R H Adams, P Baker, A K Banerjee

Dental Surgery D Lewis

Dermatology M H Beck, R J S Chalmers, M Judge

ENT J Mason, L O'Keefe

General Medicine H Bharaj, B J Bradley, J D Dean, K C Hearn, K Moriarty, P J Scott, D Spurr

General Psychiatry M Brownlee, W Dougal, K Mahadeven, M E Taylor

General Surgery G H Ferguson, J H Hobbiss, H Michie, D G Ostick, R J Salem, M J S Wilkinson

Genitourinary Medicine E Curless

Neurology P W Cooper, A C Young

Obstetrics and Gynaecology P Chia, M W Gartside, R E Hopkins, M Tasker

Ophthalmology S P Kelly, J Kwartz, A M Morrison, S J Wallis

Oral Surgery J C Lowry, M R Morton

Orthopaedics A J Banks, A A Henderson, J J Henderson, S P Hodgson, W Ryan

Paediatrics F Bowman, J L Burn, J E Ellis, D M Eminson, T H Northover, P Powell, R W Wall

Pathology D L Bisset, R J Farrand, A M Hawks, A J C Hutchesson, J Jip, J M Pearson, S Wells

Radiology M Gowland, I Hassan, P J Lane, A J Maxwell, P Strong, J S Tuck

Rheumatology R C Hilton

Thoracic Surgery N Odom

Urology M E Mobb, M I Pantelides

Bolton Primary Care Trust

St Peters House, Silverwell Street, Bolton BL1 1PP
Tel: 01204 377000 Fax: 01204 377004
Website: www.bolton.nhs.uk
(Greater Manchester Strategic Health Authority)

Chair Pamela Senior
Chief Executive Kevin Snee

Bolton, Salford and Trafford Mental Health NHS Trust

Bury New Road, Prestwich, Manchester M25 3BL
Tel: 0161 773 9121 Fax: 0161 772 3639
(Greater Manchester Strategic Health Authority)

Chair Julia Chapman-Barker
Chief Executive Lezli Boswell

Prestwich Site
Bury New Road, Prestwich, Manchester M25 3BL
Tel: 0161 773 9121
Total Beds: 349

General Psychiatry S M Bailey, A A Campbell, S Colgan, K J Merrill, E P Owens, P R Snowden, S D Soni

Psychiatry of Old Age G E Moss, I H Stout

Psychotherapy K Hyde

Bournemouth Teaching Primary Care Trust

11 Shelley Road, Bournemouth BH1 4JQ
Tel: 01202 443700 Fax: 01202 434063
Email: firstname.lastname@bournemouth-pct.nhs.uk
Website: www.bournemouth-pct.nhs.uk
(Dorset and Somerset Strategic Health Authority)

Chair Rex Symons
Chief Executive Debbie Fleming

Bracknell Forest Primary Care Trust

Church Hill House, 51-52 Turing Drive, Bracknell RG12 7FR
Tel: 01344 823250 Fax: 01344 823204
Email: bracknell-forest.pct@berkshire.nhs.uk
Website: www.berkshire.nhs.uk/bracknell
(Thames Valley Strategic Health Authority)

Chair Paul Adams
Chief Executive Diane Hedges

Bradford City Teaching Primary Care Trust

Joseph Brennan House, Sunbridge Road, Bradford BD1 2SY
Tel: 01274 424780 Fax: 01274 424781
Email: citypct@bradford.nhs.uk
Website: www.bradfordcity-pct.nhs.uk
(West Yorkshire Strategic Health Authority)

Chair Mohammed Ajeeb
Chief Executive Lynnette Throp

Bradford District Care Trust

Trust Headquarters, New Mill, Victoria Road, Shipley BD18 3LD
Tel: 01274 366007 Fax: 01274 366060
Website: www.bdct.nhs.uk
(West Yorkshire Strategic Health Authority)

Chair John Chuter
Chief Executive Con Egan

Daisy Bank
109 Duckworth Lane, Bradford BD9 6RL
Tel: 01274 494194
Total Beds: 18

General Psychiatry J Throssell

Daisy Hill House
Heights Lane, Bradford BD9 6DP
Tel: 01274 363839 Fax: 01274 363827
Total Beds: 68

Psychiatry of Old Age K Bhatnagar, M Cohen

Leeds Road Hospital
Maudsley Street, Bradford BD3 9LH
Tel: 01274 494194 Fax: 01274 725652
Total Beds: 18

Lynfield Mount Hospital
Heights Lane, Bradford BD9 6DP
Tel: 01274 494194 Fax: 01274 483494
Total Beds: 210

General Psychiatry S J Baugh, K Bhatnager, P Bracken, L Cann, M Cohen, H Daudjee, M Ellis, F Harrop, L Hewson, S Hopker, P Thomas, J Throssell, A Venables, J C T Webster

Rosebery House
40 Rosebery Road, Bradford BD9 7QB
Tel: 01274 547518
Total Beds: 10

Stoney Ridge Hospital
Stoney Ridge Road, Cottingley, Bingley BD16 1UL
Tel: 01274 495737 Fax: 01274 227923
Total Beds: 18

Westwood House
Cooper Lane, Bradford BD6 3NL
Tel: 01274 882001 Fax: 01274 883469
Total Beds: 26

Learning Disabilities T U K Nasir

Bradford South and West Primary Care Trust

Bryan-Sutherland House, Off Dunnock Avenue, Clayton Heights, Bradford BD6 3XH
Tel: 01274 321800 Fax: 01274 321805
Email: enquiries@bradford-ha.nhs.uk
Website: www.bradfordsouthwest-pct.nhs.uk
(West Yorkshire Strategic Health Authority)

Chair Sarah Warner
Chief Executive Barbara Hakin

Bradford Teaching Hospitals NHS Foundation Trust

Established as a Foundation Trust 01/04/2004.

Bradford Royal Infirmary, Duckworth Lane, Bradford BD9 6RJ
Tel: 01274 364788 Fax: 01274 364786
Website: www.bradfordhospitals.nhs.uk
(West Yorkshire Strategic Health Authority)

Chair John Ryan
Chief Executive David Jackson

Bradford Royal Infirmary
Duckworth Lane, Bradford BD9 6RJ
Tel: 01274 542200 Fax: 01274 364026
Total Beds: 882

Accident and Emergency A F Shenton (Head), P Bradley, R Halstead, F N Todd

Anaesthetics P G W Cramp (Head), N H Ashurst (Head), J L Bembridge, M Bembridge, P J Bickford-Smith, R Bowie, A Brennan, S Cheema, B Claxton, D Craske, R I Davidson, A D G Dawson, C S Evans, M J Fairbrass, S J Fletcher, L B S Gallagher, S Gupta, A Hatfield, L A Hawthorne, P A L Henderson, J Horne, A Hughes, M Jones, J Keeler, P A Knappett, K Kyriakides, M E Ladlow, J B Noden, G Oldroyd, J Richardson, C A Sides, R T Smith, A B Swanepoel, P Taylor, M J Wade

Biochemistry M Bosomworth, T J Davies

Breast Services W Case, S Downey

Cardiology S J Lindsay, C A Morley, G W Morrison

Care of the Elderly E G White (Head), S Barodawala, E Brierley, A R Brown, C J Patterson, M Pushpangadan, G B Smith, H J Terry

Diabetes S Peacey, D Whitelaw

ENT C H Raine (Head), C C Bem, I Smith, S Sood, D R Strachan, A G Tucker

Gastroenterology A P Manning (Head), C G Beckett, S Jowett, L Juby, S Morea, P D Reynolds

General Surgery R M Antrum, J R Ausobsky, W Case, J Davies, S Downey, J Gokhale, J Griffith, J C May, M Stewart, D Wilkinson

Haematology L Newton, L A Parapia, A T Williams

Histopathology P Batman, R J Calvert, D R Goldsborough, B Naylor, S O Tijani

Infectious Diseases and Sexual Health P M H McWhinney, P Stanley

Intensive Care P G W Cramp, R I Davidson, S J Fletcher, A Hughes

Medical Microbiology L Campbell, P J Marsh

Medical Oncology C Bradley, S Cheeseman, D Stark, C Twelves

Obstetrics and Gynaecology I Beck (Head), V A Beckett, S M Calvert, S E Jones, N Myerson, P J O'Donovan, C M Ramage, D J Tuffnell, J B Wright

Ophthalmology P L Atkinson (Head), J N James (Head), A D Atkins, J Bradbury, F D Ghanchi, N P Litvin, I Mohamed, A Reynolds

Oral and Maxillofacial Surgery M J Carroll (Head), D N Sutton, S Worrall

Orthopaedics S R Bollen (Head), R S Boome, W De Jager, K Jepson, W H Kluge, C Mann, G Radcliffe, E Schilders, J Shanker, P K Sharma, D L Shaw, T Taggart, A T Watters

Paediatric Surgery D Crabbe

Paediatrics C Day (Head), R Baidgett, S Chatfield, D Ginbey, S Gorman, D Haigh, G T Lealman, A M B Minford, E Moya, S Oddie, S Seal

Pain Management S Gupta, K Kyriakides, J Richardson, A B Swanepoel, P Taylor

Palliative Medicine B Batten, A Daley, L J Russon

Plastic Surgery I T H Foo (Head), D T Sharpe, M J Timmons, D Watt

Radiology R A Lowe (Head), C L Kay (Head), J M Barber, L Elliot, O J W Fowler, T D Gopichandran, C Groves, M Kon, R A Smith, A M Wason, S Whitecross

Respiratory Medicine B K Jacob, D A G Newton, D Saralaya

Thoracic Surgery V Anikin, A J Mearns

Urology G M Flannigan, R Puri, T Shah

Vascular Surgery K Mercer, N J Shaper, P Vowden, D Wilkinson

St Luke's Hospital

Little Horton Lane, Bradford BD5 0NA
Tel: 01274 734744
Total Beds: 192

Breast Services J J Price (Head), W Case, S Downey

Care of the Elderly E G White (Head), S Barodawala, E Brierley, A R Brown, C J Patterson, M Pushpangadan, G B Smith, H J Terry

Child Development Centre P C Corry, E A Mason, C E Wildig, S Yoong

Community Child Care N J H Symons, S Yeung

Dermatology A L Wright

Gastroenterology A P Manning (Head), C G Beckett, S Jowett, L Juby, S Morea, P D Reynolds

Infectious Diseases and Sexual Health P McWhinney, P Stanley

Neurology M I Busby, A J Lanzbury

Neurophysiology J A Twomey

Oral and Maxillofacial Surgery M J Carroll (Head), V K Joshi, D N Sutton, S Worrall

Orthodontics S J Littlewood, L Mitchell, C E Young

Radiology C L Kay (Head), R A Lowe (Head), J M Barber, L Elliot, O J W Fowler, T D Gopichandran, C Grove, M Kon, R A Smith, A M Wason, S Whitecross

Renal Medicine H Akbani, R Jeffrey, R Roberts, J Stoves

Rheumatology P S Helliwell, R A Melsom

Brent Teaching Primary Care Trust

Wembley Centre for Health and Care, 116 Chaplin Road, Wembley HA0 4UZ
Tel: 020 8795 6000 Fax: 020 8795 6018
Website: www.brentpct.nhs.uk
(North West London Strategic Health Authority)

Chair Jean Gaffin
Chief Executive Lise Llewellyn

Brighton and Hove City Teaching Primary Care Trust

6th Floor, Vantage Point, New England Road, Brighton BN1 4GW
Tel: 01273 295490 Fax: 01273 295461
Email: forename.surname@bhcpct.nhs.uk
Website: www.brightonhovecitypct.nhs.uk
(Surrey and Sussex Strategic Health Authority)

Chair Jean Spray
Chief Executive Gary Needle
Consultants Angela Iverson, Rachel Jole, Tom Scanlon, Peter Wilkinson

Brighton and Sussex University Hospitals NHS Trust

Royal Sussex County Hospital, Eastern Road, Brighton BN2 5BE
Tel: 01273 696955 Fax: 01273 626653
Website: www.brighton-healthcare.nhs.uk
(Surrey and Sussex Strategic Health Authority)

Chair Glynn Jones
Chief Executive Peter Coles
Consultants Neil Aiton, Diana Bellis, Rowley Cottingham, Anne Davidson, Chris Davidson, Elizabeth Derrcik, Graham Dodge, Paul Donaldson, Mike Eckstein, Andrew Fish, Nicki Gainsborough, Laurence Goldberg, Peter Hale, Carl Hardwidge, Karen Henderson, Jim Herold, Des Holden, Paul Hurst, Mark B Jackson, Varadarajan Kalidasan, Geoff Newman, Christine Newsome, George Papasavvas, Martin Street, Phil Thomas, Bob Tranter, Nick Vaughan, Chris Williams

Brighton General Hospital

Elm Grove, Brighton BN2 3EW
Tel: 01273 696955 Fax: 01273 626653

Hurstwood Park Neurological Centre

Haywards Heath RH16 4EX
Tel: 01444 441881 Fax: 01444 417995
Total Beds: 53

Anaesthetics R H A Hoyal, W A L Rawlinson, D H Read, J M Rouse, P B Wemyss-Gorman

Neurology R E Clifford-Jones, C Hardwidge, J E Rees

Neuropathology P E Rose

Neurophysiology C P Chandrasekera

Neurosurgery P H Walter, P J Ward

Radiology R S Dossetor, J S Olney

Princess Royal Hospital (East Wing)
Lewes Road, Haywards Heath RH16 4EX
Tel: 01444 441881 Fax: 01444 414174
Total Beds: 286

Accident and Emergency D J Harborne

Anaesthetics H Adams, D Bellis, R H A Hoyal, W A L Rawlinson, D H Read, J M Rouse, P B Wemyss-Gorman

Dermatology D M France

ENT H W Elcock, R Tranter

General Medicine K R Hine, J Metcalfe, J R R Spurrell, T Wheatley

General Psychiatry A Abraham

General Surgery C R R Corbett, M A Lavelle, D J Reid

Haematology P R Hill

Histopathology P A Berresford

Neurology J E Rees

Neurosurgery P H Walter, P Ward

Obstetrics and Gynaecology T Bashir, G D Kerr, B McKenzie-Gray

Orthopaedics C B d Fearn, E Parnell, M H Patterson

Radiology J M Berry, I J Runcie

Rheumatology and Rehabilitation H I Keith

Royal Alexandra Hospital for Sick Children
Dyke Road, Brighton BN1 3JN
Tel: 01273 328145 Fax: 01273 736685
Total Beds: 65

Manager Barry Harmer

Community Child Health E A Livesay

General Medicine N Evans, P Hildick-Smith, P Seddon, J Trounce

Oncology A Davidson

Orthodontics I G Crossman

Paediatric Surgery A Allaway, V Kalidasan, A Van Der Avoirt

Royal Sussex County Hospital
Eastern Road, Brighton BN2 5BE
Tel: 01273 696955 Fax: 01273 626653
Total Beds: 414

Accident and Emergency G Bryant, C Perez-Avila

Anaesthetics E N Armitage, C S B Child, A J Davey, H F Drake, N G S Fisher, A C L Fraser, J M Lamberty, B R P Murray, M K Street, C N Swaine, D Taylor, M Twohig, J H Williams, P A D Williams

Breast Services R Gumpert, G Rubin, A Yelland

Cardiac Surgery A Forsyth, W Pugsley, U Trivedi

Cardiology C Davidson, A De Belder, S Holmberg, S O'Dunain, R Vincent

Haematology J Duncan, M Kenny

Endocrinology J Quin, N Vaughan

Gastroenterology S Cairns, A Ireland

Genitourinary Medicine M Fisher, S Panja, D Williams

Intensive Care O Boyd, M Street

Medical Physics J Lutkin

Neonatology N Alton, F Weir

Neurology P Hughes, P Morrish, A Nisbet

Neurosurgery C Hardwidge, P Walter, P Ward

Nuclear Medicine R Burwood, P Robinson

Oncology D Bloomfield, G Deutsch, D Geoff, N Hudson, J Simpson, M Wilkins

Oral and Maxillofacial Surgery K Altman, J Herold

Private Patients P Austin, D Brett

Public Health Medicine M Cubbon, J Paul

Renal Medicine M Bewick, L Goldberg, N Iggo, C Kingswood, A MacDiarmid-Gordon, P Sharpstone

Thoracic Surgery (Outpatients) J Dussek

Sussex Eye Hospital
Eastern Road, Brighton BN2 5BF
Tel: 01273 606126 Fax: 01273 693674
Total Beds: 22

Ophthalmology P Brittain, A J Casswell, S Vickers

Bristol North Primary Care Trust

King's Square House, 26-27 King Square, Bristol BS2 8EE
Tel: 0117 900 2400 Fax: 0117 900 2677
Email: info@bristolnorth-pct.nhs.uk
Website: www.bristolnorthpct.nhs.uk
(Avon, Gloucestershire and Wiltshire Strategic Health Authority)

Chair Arthur Keefe
Chief Executive Chris Born

Bristol South and West Primary Care Trust

King Square House, King House, Bristol BS2 8EE
Tel: 0117 976 6600 Fax: 0117 900 2548
Email: info@bristolswpct.nhs.uk
Website: www.bristolswpct.nhs.uk
(Avon, Gloucestershire and Wiltshire Strategic Health Authority)

Chair Tom Dowell
Chief Executive Deborah Evans

Broadland Primary Care Trust

St Andrews House, Thorpe St Andrew, Norwich NR7 0HT
Tel: 01603 307000
Email: nicky.jarmain@broadland-pcg.nhs.uk
Website: www.broadland-pct.nhs.uk
(Norfolk, Suffolk and Cambridgeshire Strategic Health Authority)

Chair Nigel Dixon
Chief Executive Mark Taylor

St Michael's Hospital
Cawston Road, Aylsham, Norwich NR11 6NA
Tel: 01263 732341 Fax: 01263 738417
Total Beds: 67

Bromley Hospitals NHS Trust

The Princess Royal University Hospital, Farnborough Common, Orpington BR6 8ND
Tel: 01689 863000
Email: generalenquiry@bromleyhospitals.nhs.uk
Website: www.bromleyhospitals.nhs.uk
(South East London Strategic Health Authority)

Chair Anthony Levy
Chief Executive John Watkinson
Consultants Aza Jamal Jalal Abdulla, M Agrawal, Munir Ahmed, Riaz Ahmed, Paul Allen, Kamalini Arulambalam, Maxwell Asante, Ian Bailey, Edward Baker, Stella Barnass, Claire Botfield, Richard Brown, Carole Caldwell, Frances Calman, Peter Carey, Richard Carver, Michele Clement, Adam Coumbe, Ann Crawshaw, Simon Daniell, Guy Dawkins, Corinne De Lord, Menaka de Silva, Anil Desai, Pat Dhadly, Caroline Dimian, Jane Dobbs, Shamsi El-Hasani, Joseph Ellul, Carl Erhardt, John Erian, Anthony Fleming, Martha Ford-Adams, Alfred Franklin, Claire Fraser, Rosemary Gardner, David Golding-Wood, Shahid Hamid, Christopher Hammond, Russell Hedley, Tom Hennigan, Kathleen Hildick Smith, Nicholas Hill, Susan Hobbins, Massoud Hosseini, Elaine Hughes, John Hunt, Heather Jackson, Anthony Jenkins, Nicholas Jones, Stefan Karwatowski, Belinda Kessel, Peter King, Anil Lakhani, Edward Langford, Lumina Lanigan, Martin Leslie, Bridget Lock, Andrew Long, Adriene Martin, John Maynard, Jack McAllister, Alan McGregor, John McQueen, Derek Mercer, William Michael, Richard Moray, Mark Morgan, Catherine Mummery, Stephanie Munn, Stephen Nash, Diane Nurse, Angela Orunta, Andrew Paix, Ishwara Pathmanathan, Drusilla Pearce, Andrew Pembroke, Roberta Pinchin, Pauline Pitt, Andrew Prior, Alistair Purves, Jennifer Quirk, Rita Radford, Christopher Rand, Kenneth Rhodes, Robert Richards, Honor Roberts, Elzbieta Sawicka, Zaheer Sherazi, Prakash Sinha, Frank Smedley, Richard Stanhope, Christopher Steer, Ian Stell, Katherine Stevenson, Roland Terry, Adrian Thomas, Nigel Thomas, Caroline Timberlake, David Trew, Andrew Turvey, Bipin Vadher, Pauline Vine, Jonathan Walczak, Colin Wallis, Shaun Walter, John Wiles, Dimitri Yanni, Angelika Zang

Beckenham Hospital
379 Croydon Road, Beckenham BR3 3QL
Tel: 01689 863000

Orpington Hospital
Sevenoaks Road, Orpington BR6 9JU
Tel: 01689 863000
Total Beds: 44

The Princess Royal University Hospital
Farnborough Common, Orpington BR6 8ND
Tel: 01689 863000
Total Beds: 525

Bromley Primary Care Trust

Bassetts House, Broadwater Gardens, Farnborough BR6 7UA
Tel: 01689 853339 Fax: 01689 855662
Website: www.bromley.nhs.uk
(South East London Strategic Health Authority)

Chair Adrian Eddleston
Chief Executive Bridget Riches

Broxtowe and Hucknall Primary Care Trust

Trust Headquarters, Priory Court, Derby Road, Nottingham NG9 2TA
Tel: 0115 875 4900 Fax: 0115 875 4910
Email: administration@broxtowehucknall-pct.nhs.uk, firstname.surname@broxtowehucknall-pct.nhs.uk
Website: www.broxtowehucknall-pct.nhs.uk
(Trent Strategic Health Authority)

Chair Mel Hatto
Chief Executive Elizabeth McGuirk

Buckinghamshire Hospitals NHS Trust

Amersham Hospital, Whielden Street, Amersham HP7 0JD
Tel: 01429 526161 Fax: 01494 734753
Email: buckshospitals.info@smh.nhs.uk
Website: www.buckshospitals.nhs.uk
(Thames Valley Strategic Health Authority)

Chair David Croisdale-Appleby
Chief Executive Ruth Harrison

Amersham Hospital
Whielden Street, Amersham HP7 0JD
Tel: 01494 526161 Fax: 01494 734718
Total Beds: 57

Manager W Nartin

Anaesthetics R Allim, N Allison, J Anderson, G Biswas, A Dark, T Dexter, L Graham, A Mahoney, D Overton, C Pal-Soo, P J Strube, E Taylor, J Watson

Care of the Elderly H Al Hillawi

Dental Surgery D Cunliffe, M McKnight

Dermatology S George (Head), M Ali, S A Grabczynska, J Hughes, D Orton, R Ratnavel, J D Wilkinson

ENT J W R Capper, H Thompson

General Medicine I Gallen, D Gorard, M Jackson, B Lavery, A McIntyre, L Sandler, C G Wathen, A Weaver

General Surgery A Bdesha, C Gatzen, J Greenland, J L Grogono, G A D McPherson, A Northeast

Obstetrics and Gynaecology Y Akinsola, D Eustace, M Robson, D Sumner, C Wayne

Ophthalmology N Cox, J Duvall-Young, R Khooshabeh

Orthopaedics G M Channon, A Fernandes, G Matthews, G Taylor, K S H Wise

Pathology R Aitchison, D Bailey, Y Chia, S J Kelly, M Lyons, J Pattinson, S Price, M Turner, D Waghorn

Radiology P Cadman, C Charlesworth, K Hasan, R Horwitz, M Musaji

Rheumatology A Kirk, R Stevens

Urology J P Kelleher

Stoke Mandeville Hospital
Mandeville Road, Aylesbury HP21 8AL
Tel: 01296 315000 Fax: 01296 316604
Total Beds: 520

Anaesthetics Dr Bakhshi

Cardiology Dr Money-Kyrle, Dr Ramrakha

Care of the Elderly Dr Durkin, Dr Yau

Dermatology R Ratnaval

Diabetes Dr Gardner, Dr Knight

Endocrinology Dr Gardner, Dr Knight

ENT G Bates, I Bottrill, G Cox

Gastroenterology Dr Blackwell, Dr Weldon

General Medicine J Blackwell, C J Durkin, M J Weldon, Dr Yau

General Surgery Mr Farouk, Mr Lintott, Mr McLaren, A Northeast, Mr Sharif, A R Taylor, J H Tweedie

Haematology Dr Eagleton, Dr O'Hea, Dr Watson

Neurology D Bridley, Dr Chamoun

Neurophysiology Dr Virgincar

Obstetrics and Gynaecology F Ashworth, I Currie, Mr Dada, Miss Hall, Mr Kemball, M M Usherwood

Oncology C Alcock, N Bates, Dr Salisbury, Dr Warner

Ophthalmology R A Bates, L Benjamin, B James, N Khooshebeh, Mr Manucherhri, Miss Moorman, R G Smith

Oral Surgery Mr Currie, Mr Hodge

Orthodontics Mr Kidner, Mr Manderson

Orthopaedics M E Guindi, H Henderson, D Johnston, B McElroy, Mr Ruiz

Paediatrics P Adlard, R S Brown, Dr Krishnan, C Noone

Plastic Surgery P G Budny, Mr Ghosh, T Heywood, Mr Richards, Mr Tyler

Rheumatology S Edmonds, M Webley

Spinal Injuries Mr Derry, B P Gardner, Dr Graham, Dr Kluger, I Nuseibeh

Thoracic Medicine Dr Williams

Urology Mr Greenland, Mr Raynard

Wycombe Hospital

Queen Alexandra Road, High Wycombe HP11 2TT
Tel: 01494 526161 Fax: 01494 425339
Total Beds: 438

Anaesthetics S Zachariah

Cardiology P Ramrakha

Care of the Elderly H Hillawi, S Manchanda, A Walshe

Dermatology S George (Head), M Ali, S A Grabczynska, J Hughes, D Orton, R Ratnavel, J D Wilkinson

ENT J Capper, H Thomson, S Wood

General Medicine N Ahmadouk, P Clifford, S Firoozan, I Gallen, D Gorard, H Hillawi, S Manchanda, A McIntyre, S Price, L Sandler, D Taylor, A Walshe, C G Wathen

General Surgery W Akinwale, S Appleton, G Cunnick, A Elzayat, C Gatzen, P Lintott, A McLaren, G A D McPherson, A Northeast

Genitourinary Medicine G Luzzi

Haematology R Aitchison, C Barton, S Kelly, J Pattinson

Neurology M Jackson

Obstetrics and Gynaecology Y Akinsola, D Eustace, M Robson, D Sumner, C Wayne

Ophthalmology N Cox, J Duvall-Young, R Khooshabeh

Oral Surgery J Knight, N Saeed

Orthopaedics G M Channon, A Fernandes, G Matthews, G Taylor, K S Wise

Paediatrics R Finch, G Rastogi, M Russell-Taylor, S Salgia, K Sawhney

Plastic Surgery P Budny, C Khoo

Rheumatology A Kirk, R Stevens

Trauma and Orthopaedics S Akram, S Blagg, G Channon, A Fernandes, A Graham, Mr Matthews, A Othman, M Swann, G Taylor, K Wise

Urology A Bdesha, J Greenland, J P Kelleher

Buckinghamshire Mental Health NHS Trust

Manor House, Bierton Road, Aylesbury HP20 1EG
Tel: 01296 393363 Fax: 01296 392606
(Thames Valley Strategic Health Authority)

Chair Shirley Williams
Chief Executive Julie Waldron

Buckingham Hospital

High Street, Buckingham MK18 1NU
Tel: 01280 813243 Fax: 01280 824966
Total Beds: 17

Harlow House

Harlow Road, High Wycombe HP13 6AA
Tel: 01494 436393
Total Beds: 40

Manor House

Bierton Road, Aylesbury HP20 1EG
Tel: 01296 393363
Total Beds: 187

General Psychiatry J Baruch

Learning Disabilities G Barton

Paediatrics M Wakefield

Burnley, Pendle and Rossendale Primary Care Trust

31-33 Kenyon Road, Lomeshaye Estate, Nelson BB9 5SZ
Tel: 01282 619909 Fax: 01282 610223
Website: www.bprpct.nhs.uk
(Cumbria and Lancashire Strategic Health Authority)

Chair James Heyes
Chief Executive David Peat

Burntwood, Lichfield and Tamworth Primary Care Trust

Merlin House, Etchell Road, Lichfield WS13 6JB
Tel: 01543 410020 Fax: 01543 440848
Email: firstname.lastname@blt-pct.nhs.uk
Website: www.bltpct.nhs.uk
(Shropshire and Staffordshire Strategic Health Authority)

Chair Susan Durrant
Chief Executive Alan Snuggs

Hammerwich Hospital

Hospital Road, Burntwood, Walsall WS7 0EH
Tel: 01543 686224
Total Beds: 20

St Michael's Hospital

Trent Valley Road, Lichfield WS13 6EF
Tel: 01543 441400 Fax: 01543 441430

Sir Robert Peel Hospital

Plantation Road, Mile Oak, Tamworth B78 3NG
Tel: 01827 263800 Fax: 01827 263803

Victoria Hospital

Friary Road, Lichfield WS13 6QN
Tel: 01543 442000 Fax: 01543 416729
Total Beds: 32

Burton Hospitals NHS Trust

Queen's Hospital, Belvedere Road, Burton-on-Trent DE13 0RB
Tel: 01283 566333 Fax: 01283 593032
Website: www.burtonhospital.com
(Shropshire and Staffordshire Strategic Health Authority)

Chair Henry Every
Chief Executive Jo Cubbon

Queen's Hospital

Belvedere Road, Burton-on-Trent DE13 0RB
Tel: 01283 566333 Ext: 5557 Fax: 01283 593032
Total Beds: 459

Accident and Emergency F O'Dwyer, E O'Forka

Anaesthetics P Allsop, J D Anderson, M J W Eason, C M Heal, R T Hedge, P Holgate, U Kamath, S W Millar, C Stenhouse, C Webb

Care of the Elderly G S Matharu, C Reisner

Chemical Pathology T M Reynolds

Dermatology P Cartwright, H Nelson

ENT P De, J Oates, T J Rockley, A C Thompson

General Medicine J J Benn, J D Hill, J W S Sheldon, D Watmough, H Why

General Surgery T E Bucknall, R J K Gompertz, R Lee, C A Rogers

Genitourinary Medicine C A Murray

Haematology A G Smith

Histopathology D M Green, N Kasthuri, P Ong

Medical Microbiology J H Paton

Obstetrics and Gynaecology K Anwar, J K Artley, J Hollingworth, Y G Ibrahim, W Oakley, A D G Roberts

Ophthalmology S Chawdhary, R Harrison, A Rauf, T Worstmann

Oral and Maxillofacial Surgery D J Spary

Orthodontics D J Spary

Orthopaedics F Bindi, M R Hamlet, S Khemka, M Wallace

Paediatrics A Choules, T Jacob-Samuel, A Manzoor, M M B Mirfattahi

Radiology N Barraclough, K Nanda, J Singanayagam, A Zafar

Rheumatology M Nisar

Urology R A Corfield, D M Thomas

Bury Primary Care Trust

21 Silver Street, Bury BL9 0EN
Tel: 0161 762 3100 Fax: 0161 764 5042
Website: www.burypct.nhs.uk
(Greater Manchester Strategic Health Authority)

Chair Hilda Harvey
Chief Executive Evan Boucher

Bealey Community Hospital

Dumers Lane, Radcliffe, Manchester M26 9QD
Tel: 0161 723 2371
Total Beds: 16

Manager Mr Clements

Calderdale and Huddersfield NHS Trust

Trust Offices, The Royal Infirmary, Acre Street, Lindley HD3 3EA
Tel: 01484 342000 Fax: 01484 342253
Email: forename.surname@cht.nhs.uk
Website: www.cht.nhs.uk
(West Yorkshire Strategic Health Authority)

Chair Gordon McLean
Chief Executive Diane Whittingham

Calderdale Royal Hospital

Salterhebble, Halifax HX3 0PW
Tel: 01422 357171 Fax: 01422 380357
Total Beds: 517

Accident and Emergency A Lockey, A Mohammed, P Singh

Anaesthetics R Bailie, P A Bamber, K Bartholomew, S N Chater, P Hutchings, R Johnson, N Karandikar, P Knight, P R Knight, P J Lesser, D R Lloyd, H Newbegin, H E Newbegin, G Reah, S A Siddiqui, I D Somerville, F W Than-Htay, J Thomson

Care of the Elderly S N Chandratre, J L Sarin, I Shakir

Child and Adolescent Psychiatry P M Chapman

Dermatology I Barbar, H Galvin, H Hempel, J Holder

Elderly Medicine T A Bazaraa, S Chandratre, K Goodman, I A Manthy, J Sarin, I Shakir

ENT D Boyd, C Ramanathan

General Medicine V Bangar, T Bloomer, S Grant, B C Lalor, M S A Qureshi, N Scriven, A P Tandon, R G Taylor, S Thomas, A Verma

General Surgery S Akhtar, R J R Goodall, P Gupta, D Ilsley, A Mahomed, V K Modgill, N Sharma, A Subramanian

Genitourinary Medicine C Knowles, L Short

Haematology W Simmons, A Steed

Neurology S El-Sadig, A Grueger

Obstetrics and Gynaecology R Aboleyah, M D Bono, C Choy, J Gupta, S Hamilton, S Jamali, D Jones, T Naeem

Ophthalmology M Clowes, C Hutchinson, T James, O Owuru, R Rahman, S Rehman, S Spencer

Oral and Maxillofacial Surgery J Jones

Orthopaedics C Chadwick, A Chapman, B Flood, S C Halder, K Muralikuttan, E Rutten, A R Zepeda

Paediatrics L J Clogher, V Kumar, A Muhammed, Y Oade, G Sharpe

Palliative Medicine S Salt

Pathology D Birkinhead, I Burnett, P Hamal, R Marks, A Padwell, B A Takyi, G Thomas, A Vodovnik

Plastic Surgery I Foo

Radiology N K Jain, M Lintula, H D Montgomery, L N Sutton, M Van Meer

Rheumatology D McGonagle

Urology K Rogawski, J J F Somerville

Holme Valley Memorial Hospital

Huddersfield Road, Holmfirth HD9 3TS
Tel: 01484 681711 Fax: 01484 482357

Huddersfield Royal Infirmary

Lindley, Huddersfield HD3 3EA
Tel: 01484 342000 Fax: 01484 342888
Total Beds: 428

Accident and Emergency R Birkenshaw, M G G Clayton

Anaesthetics N K S Al-Quisi, J J K Anathhanam, J Esmond, B S Ghoorun, P Hall, R M Jackson, F O Jennings, C Lok, C G Nandakumar, J Nunez, J O'Riordan, S N Raizada, M A Salam

Cardiology R Stevenson, C P Welsh

Care of the Elderly M Ahmed, J R Naylor, P Rana, E Silwo

Child and Adolescent Psychiatry I McKenzie

Dermatology M J Cheesbrough, D Cowan

ENT B Doubleday, D Martin-Hirsh, C J R Newbegin, G J C Smelt

Forensic Psychiatry S Bhattacherjee, D Hargreaves

General Medicine A W Burrows, A Graham, R W Heaton, S Jones, O Mandour, G Sobala

General Surgery M I Aldoori, B Dobbins, P J Holdsworth, S Iqbal, M K Jovestani, M Khan, R C Macdonald, I Morris, J Salaman

Genitourinary Medicine S S Al-Egaily, A Kazi, C Knowles

Haematology W Simmons

Immunology D Misbah

Neurology B E D Dafalla, S Z Tun

Neurophysiology K Spillane

Obstetrics and Gynaecology K Bharbra, J M Campbell, S Kaufmann, B Onyeka, M Prafullatha

Oncology B Crosse, J Dent, J K Joffe, M Sen

Ophthalmology N Anand, K E Davey, R Rahman, S Rehman

Orthodontics R Y Shuff

Orthopaedics S Ankarath, G Chakrabarty, A George, A Shenolikar, E Tolessa, D I Wise

Paediatrics C Clogher, E Crosbie, A H Hamilton, M G Miller, G Parry, K Schwarz, M A Sills, V Thiyagesh

Palliative Medicine M Klely

Pathology M Aslam, H Griffiths

Plastic Surgery D T Sharp

Radiology S Gurney, B O Hammond, H Horsfall, A R Paes, K Roberts, F Roman

Rheumatology R Reece

Urology M A Ferro, J Harney

St Luke's Hospital

Blackmoorfoot Road, Crosland Moor, Huddersfield HD4 5RQ
Tel: 01484 343000 Fax: 01484 482409

Calderdale Primary Care Trust

School House, 56 Hopwood Lane, Halifax HX1 5ER
Tel: 01422 397300 Fax: 01422 397301
Website: www.calderdale-pct.nhs.uk
(West Yorkshire Strategic Health Authority)

Chair Joyce Catterick
Chief Executive Martyn Pritchard

Calderstones NHS Trust

Mitton Road, Whalley, Clitheroe BB7 9PE
Tel: 01254 822121 Fax: 01254 823023
Website: www.cstone-tr.nwest.nhs.uk
(Cumbria and Lancashire Strategic Health Authority)

Chair Graham Parr
Chief Executive Russ Pearce

Calderstones

Mitton Road, Whalley, Clitheroe BB7 9PE
Tel: 01254 822121
Total Beds: 230

General Psychiatry A Adewunmi, B Brown, M Ferguson, S Ghosh, A Kumar, M A Razzaque

Cambridge City Primary Care Trust

Heron Court (Block 23), Ida Darwin, Fulbourn, Cambridge CB1 5EE
Tel: 01223 884008 Fax: 01223 885728
Website: www.cambcity-pct.nhs.uk/
(Norfolk, Suffolk and Cambridgeshire Strategic Health Authority)

Chair Evelyn Knowles
Chief Executive Chris Humphris
Consultants Suan Goh, Dorothy Gregson, Tony Luxton, Margaret Sanders

Cambridge University Hospitals NHS Foundation Trust

Formerly Addenbrooke's NHS Trust. Established as a Foundation Trust 01/07/2004.

Hills Road, Cambridge CB2 2QQ
Tel: 01223 245151 Fax: 01223 216520
Website: www.addenbrookes.org.uk
(Norfolk, Suffolk and Cambridgeshire Strategic Health Authority)

Chair Mary Archer
Chief Executive Malcolm Stamp

Addenbrooke's Hospital

Hills Road, Cambridge CB2 2QQ
Tel: 01223 245151 Fax: 01223 216520
Total Beds: 1269

Accident and Emergency G Campbell-Hewson, C Maimaris, S M Robinson, H M Sherriff

Anaesthetics A Bailey, J Bamber, S P Bass, L J Brennan, R Campbell, C Duffy, W A R Erskine, J Fisher, C W Glazebrook, L S Godsiff, K E J Gunning, A K Gupta, M J Herrick, D R Hughes, R M Jones, D J Kennedy, J R Klinck, R D Latimer, M J Lindop, I M J McKenzie, B F Matta, D K Menon, P J Morris, I T Munday, V U Navapurkar, J P Newell, G R Park, J A Pickett, P G Roe, D J Sapsford, N J Scurrah, H L Smith, A B Swami, D N Tew, J M Turner

Blood Transfusion C Beatty, W H Ouwehande, L M Williamson

Cardiology M R Bennett, D P Dutka, A A Grace, M C Petch, P H Schofield, L H Shapiro

Cardiothoracic Surgery S R Large, S S L Tsui, J Wallwork, F C Wells

Care of the Elderly G A Campbell, D R Forsythe, K-T Khaw, C G Nicholl, E A Warburton, K J Wilson

Clinical Biochemistry L S Culank, C N Hales

Clinical Immunology and Allergy P W Ewan, P W Ewan, S M S Nasser

Clinical Microbiology N Brown, U Desselberger, N Farrington, J E Foweraker, A Gerken, H A Ludlam

Clinical Pharmacology and Therapeutics J Brown, M J Brown, S F Haydock, K H O'Shaughnessy, J P Schofield, I B Wilkinson

Dermatology N Flanagan, P G Norris, R J Pye, J C Sterling, P M Todd

Endocrinology V K Chatterjee, S F Dinneen, O M Edwards, M Evans, S P O'Rahilly

ENT P Axon, R F Gray, P Jani, D A Moffat

Gastroenterology M E D Allison, A E S Gimson, J O Hunter, S Middleton, M Parkes

General Medicine A J Carmichael, T M Cox, P B Deegan, D T Fearon, P J Lehner, A M L Lever, M J Newport, D Rubenstein, J G P Sissons

Genetics M Bobraw, C K Ffrench-Constant, H V Firth, J Rankin, F L Raymond, D C Rubinsztein, R N Sandford, D Trump, J R U Yates, R L Zimmern

Genitourinary Medicine C A Carne, C Sonnex

Haematology T P Baglin, J I O Craig, A R Green, R E Marcus, S A J Warren

Histopathology M Arends, L G Bobrow, G Callagy, N Coleman, V P Collins, B Cottrell, S E Davies, A F Dean, J W Grant, F A Jessop, A W Marker, R P Moseley, D G O'Donovan, M L O'Donovan, J L Rashbass, E Rytina, V E Save, S Stewart, S Thiru, A Whitehead, A D H Wyllie, J H Xuereb

Immunology D S Kumararatne

Metabolic Medicine J E Compston, J Reeve

Neurology C M C Allen, R A Barker, D A S Compston, G G Lennox, M R A Manford, J B Pilling, J W Thorpe, S J Wroe

Neurosurgery P J Kirkpatrick, R W Kirollos, R J C Laing, R Macfarlane, J D Pickard, A Waters

Obstetrics and Gynaecology J R Allsop, K J Dalton, G A Hackett, J A Latimer, C Lees, M J MacDougall, P J D Milton, A Prentice, G C S Smith, S K Smith, J R W Williamson

Occupational Health P J Baxter

Oncology A Ahmad, R Benson, S Booth, J Brenton, N Burnet, C Caldas, P Corrie, J Craig, M Daly, H Earl, K Fife, H Ford, D Gilligan, A R Green, S J Jeffries, R Marcus, K McAdam, M Moody, S Old, H Patterson, B A J Ponder, S Russel, L T Tan, R Thomas, A J Warren, J V Watson, M V Williams, C B Wilson

Ophthalmology L Allen, Dr Flanagan, J Keast-Butler, M G Kerr-Nuir, P A R Meyer, D K Newman, C Rene, N J C Sarkies, M P Snead

Oral and Maxillofacial Surgery D N Adlam

Orthodontics R J Rimes

Orthopaedic Surgery D P Conlan, C R Constant, D J Dandy, D J Edwards, P R Hamilton, G Keene, N H Matthewson, P J Owen, A Robinson, N Rushton, R N Villar, A S Wojick

Paediatric Surgery A Aslam, A J L Brain, M P L Williams

Paediatrics C Acerini, J S Ahluwalia, J Challener, D Dunger, I Hughes, R W Iles, A W Kelsall, R J McClure, A L Ogilvy-Stuart, U Ramaswami, R I Ross-Russell, R C Tasker

Palliative Medicine S Booth

Plastic Surgery G C Cormack, P N Hall, M S Irwin, B G H Lamberty, C Malata

Psychiatry G E Berrios, F A M Blake, E Bullmore, S P Calloway, J H Dowson, P C Fletcher, N J Hunt, N F S Hymas, G Isaacs, P B Jones, M London, P J McKenna, R Ramana, J Shapleske, M Stefan, C Walsh

Public Health Medicine P D P Pharoah, N J Wareham, J Whittaker

Radiology N M Antoun, D S Appleton, P W P Bearcroft, L H Berman, P D Britton, N R Carroll, R A R Coulden, C Cousins, J Cross, A K Dixon, A H Freeman, J H Gillard, J N P Higgins, D J Lomas, T Massoud, C Ng, N Sceaton, P A K Set, R Simmatamby, A Tasker, H L Taylor, R M L Warren

Renal Medicine M S Ell, J D Firth, D R W Jayne, F E Karet, D K Peters, K G C Smith, P F Williams

Respiratory Medicine E R Chilvers, E R Condliffe, D A Lomas, K D McNeil, R Mahadeva, N W Morreil, R J D Winter

Rheumatology and Rehabilitation A J Crisp, J S H Gaston, J R Jenner, S G B Kirker, C A Speed

Urology K N Bullock, A Doble, W Turner

Rosie Hospital

Robinson Way, Cambridge CB2 2SW
Tel: 01223 245151
Total Beds: 122

Manager Olive Evans

Anaesthetics A Bailey, C W Glazebrook, D J Kennedy

Obstetrics and Gynaecology R A F Crawford, K J Dalton, G A Hackett, J Latimer, C Lees, M J MacDougall, A Prentice, S K Smith, J R W Williamson

Paediatrics J S Ahluwalia, I Hughes, R W Iles, A W Kelsall, A L Ogilvy-Stuart, R I R Russell, R C Tasker, D M Williams

Radiology P A K Set

Cambridgeshire and Peterborough Mental Health Partnership NHS Trust

Headquarters, Kingfisher House, Kingfisher Way, Hinchingbrook Business Park, Huntingdon PE29 6FH
Tel: 01480 398500 Fax: 01480 398501
Website: www.cambsmh.nhs.uk
(Norfolk, Suffolk and Cambridgeshire Strategic Health Authority)

Chair Owen Ingram
Chief Executive Richard Taylor

Camden and Islington Mental Health and Social Care Trust

2nd Floor East Wing, St Pancras Hospital, 4 St Pancras Way, London NW1 0PE
Tel: 020 7530 3500 Fax: 020 7530 3083
Website: www.cimhscaretrust.nhs.uk
(North Central London Strategic Health Authority)

Chair David Taylor
Chief Executive Erville Millar

Camden Mews Day Hospital

5 Camden Mews, London NW1 9DB
Tel: 020 7530 4780 Fax: 020 7530 4788

Felix Brown Day Hospital

Royal Free Hospital, Pond Street, London NW3 2QG
Tel: 020 7794 0500 Fax: 020 7830 2468

Fordwych Road Day Hospital

85-87 Fordwych Road, London NW2 3TL
Tel: 020 8208 1612 Fax: 020 8208 0889

Jules Thorn Day Hospital

St Pancras Hospital, 4 St Pancras Way, London NW1 0PE
Tel: 020 7530 3391 Fax: 020 7530 3421

Piercey Day Hospital

23 East Heath Road, London NW3 1DU
Tel: 020 7435 7668 Fax: 020 7435 7668

St Luke's Hospital

Woodside Avenue, Muswell Hill, London N10 3HU
Tel: 020 8219 1800 Fax: 020 8219 1801
Total Beds: 72

General Psychiatry E Chesser, I Collis, O Hill, S Stansfield

Camden Primary Care Trust

St Pancras Hospital, 4 St Pancras Way, London NW1 0PE
Tel: 020 7530 3500 Fax: 020 7530 3104
Website: www.camdenpct.nhs.uk
(North Central London Strategic Health Authority)

Chair John Carrier
Chief Executive Rob Larkman

St Pancras Hospital
4 St Pancras Way, London NW1 0PE
Tel: 020 7530 3500 Fax: 020 7530 3510
Total Beds: 105

Care of the Elderly K Arnold, J Croker, J Malone-Lee

Psychiatry of Old Age T Katz

Cannock Chase Primary Care Trust

Block D, Beecroft Court, off Beecroft Road, Cannock WS111JP
Tel: 01543 465100 Fax: 01543 465110
Website: www.cannockchase-pct.nhs.uk
(Shropshire and Staffordshire Strategic Health Authority)

Chair David Littlemore
Chief Executive Jean-Pierre Parsons

Canterbury and Coastal Primary Care Trust

Chestfield Medical Centre, Reeves Way, Chestfield, Whitstable CT5 3QU
Tel: 01227 795008 Fax: 01227 794973
Email: canterbury&coastal.pcg@ekent-ha.nhs.uk
Website: www.canterburyandcoastalpct.nhs.uk
(Kent and Medway Strategic Health Authority)

Chair John Butler
Chief Executive Wilf Williams

Faversham Cottage Hospital
Stone Street, Faversham ME13 8PS
Tel: 01795 562000
Total Beds: 33

Queen Victoria Memorial Hospital
King Edward Avenue, Herne Bay CT6 6EB
Tel: 01227 594700
Total Beds: 24

Whitstable and Tankerton Hospital
174-176 Northwood Road, Tankerton, Whitstable CT5 2HN
Tel: 01227 594400
Total Beds: 50

The Cardiothoracic Centre Liverpool NHS Trust

Thomas Drive, Liverpool L14 3PE
Tel: 0151 228 1616 Fax: 0151 220 8573
Email: forename.surname@ctc.nhs.uk
Website: www.ctc.nhs.uk
(Cheshire and Merseyside Strategic Health Authority)

Chair Mark Fitzsimmons
Chief Executive Michael Bone
Consultants S Behl, Martyn Carr, John Chalmers, P D O Davies, M J Desmond, Walid Dihmis, Michael John Drakeley, Brian Fabri, H Fewins, M A Fox, Elaine Griffiths, P Hardy, J Holemans, J Kendall, M Ledson, Neeraj Mediratta, K Mills, John Morris, William Morrison, J Murphy, A Oo, Richard Page, S H Pennefather, Raphael Perry, Mark Pullan, David Ramsdale, Abbas Rashid, T Ridgway, G N Russell, N Scawn, Ajaib Soorae, Rod Stables, S D Thomas, Derick Todd, Martin Walshaw, R Williams, Jay Wright

Carlisle and District Primary Care Trust

Trust Headquarters, 4 Wavell Drive, Rosehill, Carlisle CA1 2SE
Tel: 01228 603500 Fax: 01228 603612
Website: www.northcumbriahealth.nhs.uk
(Cumbria and Lancashire Strategic Health Authority)

Chair Carole Ferguson
Chief Executive Nigel Woodcock

Wigton Hospital
Cross Lane, Wigton CA7 9DD
Tel: 01697 366600 Fax: 01697 366602
Total Beds: 35

Care of the Elderly J George

General Practice G Brown, J Honeyman, C Russell, R Swindells

Castle Point and Rochford Primary Care Trust

12 Castle Road, Rayleigh SS6 7QF
Tel: 01268 464500 Fax: 01268 464501
Email: info@cpr-pct.nhs.uk
Website: www.castleroch-pct.nhs.uk
(Essex Strategic Health Authority)

Chair Brian Dawbarn
Chief Executive Malcolm McCann

Central and North West London Mental Health NHS Trust

30 Eastbourne Terrace, London W2 6LA
Tel: 020 8237 2000 Fax: 020 8746 8978
Email: forename.surname@cnwl.nhs.uk
Website: www.cnwl.org
(North West London Strategic Health Authority)

Chair Ruth Runciman
Chief Executive Peter Carter
Consultants Philip Joseph

Collingham Gardens
4-5 Collingham Gardens, London SW5 0HR
Tel: 020 8846 6644 Fax: 020 8846 6641
Total Beds: 12

Gordon Hospital
Bloomburg Street, London SW1V 2RH
Tel: 020 8746 5505 Fax: 020 8746 8711
Total Beds: 90

General Psychiatry C Flannigan, O S Frank

Psychiatry of Old Age R Menon

Central Cheshire Primary Care Trust

Barony Hospital, Barony Road, Nantwich CW5 5QU
Tel: 01270 415300, 01270 627469
Email: information@ccpct.nhs.uk
Website: www.ccpct.nhs.uk
(Cheshire and Merseyside Strategic Health Authority)

Chair Pauline Ong
Chief Executive Mike Pyrah

Central Cornwall Primary Care Trust

John Keay House, Tregonissey Road, St Austell PL25 4NQ
Tel: 01726 77777 Fax: 01726 71777
Website: www.cornwall.nhs.uk/centralpct/
(South West Peninsula Strategic Health Authority)

Chair Peter Davies
Chief Executive Lyn Manuell

Falmouth Hospital
Trescobeas Road, Falmouth TR11 2JA
Tel: 01326 434700 Fax: 01326 434769
Total Beds: 34

Fowey and District Hospital
Green Lane, Fowey PL23 1EE
Tel: 01726 832241
Total Beds: 14

Newquay and District Hospital
St Thomas' Road, Newquay TR7 1RQ
Tel: 01637 893600
Total Beds: 22

St Austell Community Hospital
Porthpean Road, St Austell PL26 6AD
Tel: 01726 291120
Total Beds: 66

Central Derby Primary Care Trust

Top Floor, Derwent Court, 1 Stuart Street, Derby DE1 2FZ
Tel: 01332 203102 Fax: 01332 203206
Website: www.centralderby-pct.nhs.uk
(Trent Strategic Health Authority)

Chair John Beswarick
Chief Executive Prem Singh

Central Liverpool Primary Care Trust

Hartington Road Clinic, Hartington Road, Toxteth, Liverpool L8 0SG
Tel: 0151 285 2800 Fax: 0151 733 9213
Email: enquiries@centralliverpoolpct.nhs.uk
Website: www.centralliverpoolpct.nhs.uk
(Cheshire and Merseyside Strategic Health Authority)

Chair Gideon Ben-Tovim
Chief Executive Derek Campbell

Sir Alfred Jones Memorial Hospital
Church Road, Garston, Liverpool L19 2LP
Tel: 0151 250 3000

Central Manchester and Manchester Children's University Hospitals NHS Trust

Manchester Royal Infirmary, Cobbett House, Oxford Road, Manchester M13 9WL
Tel: 0161 276 1234 Fax: 0161 273 6211
Website: www.cmmc.nhs.uk
(Greater Manchester Strategic Health Authority)

Chair Peter Mount
Chief Executive Mike Deegan

Booth Hall Children's Hospital
Charlestown Road, Blackley, Manchester M9 7AA
Tel: 0161 795 7000 Fax: 0161 220 5387

Accident and Emergency S Derbyshire, L Duane

Anaesthetics P Ashford, H L Goldwater, A Griffiths, W D Lord, T Montague, R Perkins, A Razak, Y Y Youssef

Child and Adolescent Psychiatry D Firth, J M Green, A L Trumper

Dermatology T J David, C Ewing, L Patel

ENT Mrs Jaffari, A P Zarod

Gastroenterology S Davidson, V Miller, A Thomas

General Medicine M Bone, T J David, G Hambleton, D A Price, E Wraith

General Surgery J Bowen, A P Dickson, C M Doig

Intensive Care K Hawkins, S Kerr, D Stewart, R Yates

Nephrology M Lewis, N Webb

Neurology M A Clarke, I Hughes, T Martland, R W Newton

Ophthalmology J L Noble

Oral and Maxillofacial Surgery P R White

Orthodontics D Bearn, D Heggarty

Orthopaedics J B Day, T Meadows

Paediatrics E Baildam, M Bone, J M Couriel, T J David, S Davidson, C Ewing, H Jacques, V Miller, L Patel, A Thomas

Paediatrics E M Baildam, M Bone, S Davidson, C I Ewing, H Jacques

Pathology G Addison, C Cullinane, A Milford, M Newbould, R Sanyal, A Will

Plastic Surgery P J Davenport, K Dunn, D J Whitby

Radiology B Barry, C Broome, U Hughes, B P M Wilson

Rheumatology E Baildam, P J L Holt

Manchester Royal Eye Hospital
Oxford Road, Manchester M13 9WH
Tel: 0161 276 5526 Fax: 0161 273 2028
Total Beds: 35

Anaesthetics D Barman, A J Charlton, D G D Davidson, E L Horsman, P W Jackson, A A Khan, I C Lloyd, A K Morton, J Shaw, M E Simpson, R M Slater

Ophthalmology A M Ansons, C L Dodd, N P Jones, M J Lavin, B Leatherbarrow, C Lloyd, D McLeod, K B Mills, J L Noble, E O'Donoghue, A E A Ridgway, A Tullo, G S Turner

Manchester Royal Infirmary
Corbbett House, Oxford Road, Manchester M13 9WL
Tel: 0161 276 1234 Fax: 0161 273 6211
Website: www.cmmc.nhs.uk
Total Beds: 519

Accident and Emergency K Mackway-Jones, R Morton, B Phillips

Anaesthetics J M Anderton, D Barman, R A Bowman, I T Campbell, A K Charlton, D G D Davidson, B R H Doran, L Doyle, J M Eddleston, R Fletcher, S Greenhough, N J N Harper, E J Healey, E L Horsman, A A Khan, A K Morton, N O'Keefe, B J Pollard, J Shaw, M E Simpson, R Slater, T Strang, S Varley, A Vohra, D Whitaker

Audiological Medicine V K Das, V Newton

Cardiology B Clarke, L Cotter, A Fitzpatrick, D J Rowlands

Cardiothoracic Surgery G J Grotte, R Hasen, D J M Keenan, N Odom

Care of the Elderly P Bannister, C M Cheshire, M J Connolly

Chemical Pathology M France

Dermatology R J G Chalmers, H Muston

Diabetes A J M Boulton, R Davies, S Tomlinson

Endocrinology J R E Davies, F Wu

Gastroenterology J M Braganza, T W Warnes

General Medicine M Davies, P Durrington, C C Hardy, A M Heagerty, P Selby, R D G Tunbridge, M A Woodhead

General Psychiatry I Anderson, R C Baldwin, S M Benbow, S Benjamin, D Crauford, F H Creed, J F W Deakin, E Guthrie, J Harrison, D Hughes, G McGrath, F R Margison, A Poynton, A Proctor, N J Simpson, P R Snowden, A G Sutton, L Webster

General Surgery J Hill, R W G Johnson, R F McCloy, I MacLennan, N R Parrott, R C Pearson

Genitourinary Medicine M N Bhattacharyya, T K Chatterjee, B Goorney

Haematology J G Chang, C R M Hay, E M Love, G Lucas, C Shiech, S Shwe, J A L Yin

Immunology J P Burnie, R C Matthews, R S H Pumphrey, J K Struthers

Infectious Diseases B K Mandal

Intensive Care B Doran

Medical Microbiology J P Burnie, R C Mathews, J K Struthers

Nephrology F W Ballardie, R Gokal, A Hutchinson, R W G Johnson, N P Mallick, N R Parrott, R C Pearson, H Riad, L D Short

Neurology J Dick, N McDermott, G Mawer, D Neary, W Schady, P Talbot

Neurosurgery R H Lye, P L Richardson, F A Strang

Nuclear Medicine M C Prescott, H J Testa

Orthopaedics P Hirst, N Kenny, B Maltby, A Paul

Otolaryngology A Birzgalis, P Canty, W T Farrington, R T Ramsden

Pathology A J Barson, E W Benbow, R E Bonshek, C H Buckley, A J Freemont, S Lee, J McClure, R F T McMahon, L Moore, R V Persad, H Reid, C Stanbridge

Plastic Surgery A Brain

Radiology J E Adams, N Chalmers, R A Fawcitt, J E Gillespie, A Jackson, J P R Jenkins, S Lee, S Rimmer, S A Russell, P M Taylor, N A Watson, R W Whitehouse

Rheumatology and Rehabilitation R M Bernstein, P J L Holt, E R E Ross, A Silman

Urology R N P Carroll, J Harney, S Payne

Vascular Surgery R Marcuson, M Walker

Virology A Turner

Royal Manchester Children's Hospital

Hospital Road, Pendlebury, Manchester M27 4HA
Tel: 0161 794 4696 Fax: 0161 727 2364
Total Beds: 182

Anaesthetics O R Dearlove, T Howell, G Meakin, D Patel, D N Robinson, R Walker

Cardiac Surgery G Gladman, E J Ladusans, R G Patel

Chemical Pathology G M Addison

Child and Adolescent Psychiatry R Harrington, M Kelsall, L Kroll, H Lloyd

Clinical Genetics B Kerr, M Super

Developmental Medicine I McKinlay

Endocrinology P E Clayton, D A Price

ENT M P Rothera, D J Willatt

Haematology A Will, R Wynn

Intensive Care K Hawkins, D Stewart, R Yates

Nephrology M Bradbury, M Lewis, R Postlethwaite, N Webb

Neurology M Clarke, I Hughes, T Martland, R Newton

Neurosurgery C Bannister, R A Cowie, J R S Leggate, A Sofat, G Victoratos, C G H West

Oncology B Brennan, T Eden, L Lashford

Oral Surgery I Campbell, R Lloyd

Orthopaedics C S B Galasko, A Henry, E Ross, J Spilsbury, B Williamson

Paediatric Surgery A Bianchi, J Bowen, J Bruce

Paediatrics P Clayton, M Cleary, D A Price, H C Smith, A Thomas, J Walter, J E Wraith

Pathology C Cullinane, A M Kelsey, M Newbould, R Sanyal

Radiology B Barry, B P M Wilson

Respiratory Medicine G Hambleton

Rheumatology E Baildam, A Herrick

Thoracic Surgery R A M Lawson

Transplant Surgery R Stevens, A Will

Urology J Bruce, D C S Gough, U Hughes, K O'Flynn

St Mary's Hospital for Women and Children

Whitworth Park, Manchester M13 0JH
Tel: 0161 276 1234 Fax: 0161 276 6107
Total Beds: 200

Anaesthetics J M Anderton, A J Charlton, D G D Davidson, S Greenhough, N J N Harper, E L Horsman, A A Khan, A K Morton, B J Pollard, J Shaw, M E Simpson, W D Smith, D Whittaker

Cardiology G Gladman, E Ladusans

Genetics J Clayton-Smith, D I O Crawford, D Donnai, G Evans, R Harris, H Kingston

Immunology R S H Pumphrey

Obstetrics and Gynaecology P Buck, P Donnai, T Johnston, H Kitchener, B A Lieberman, M J A Maresh, K Reynolds, M Seif, A R B Smith

Paediatric Surgery A Bianchi, A P Dickson, C M Doig

Paediatrics M L Chiswick, I Doughty, S W D'Souza, A Emmerson, M Z Mughal, D G Sims

Pathology A J Barson, C H Buckley, S Lee, C M Stanbridge

Radiology S Rimmer, S A Russell

University Dental Hospital of Manchester

Higher Cambridge Street, Manchester M15 6FH
Tel: 0161 275 6666 Fax: 0161 275 6776
Total Beds: 14

Dentistry A Mellor, A Shearer

Oral and Maxillofacial Surgery R Middlehurst, B Musgrove

Radiology K Horner

Restorative Dentistry D J Eldridge, J R Heath, P S Hull, J D Lilley, J F McCord, G A Smith, M Wilson, N H F Wilson

Central Manchester Primary Care Trust

Mauldeth House, Mauldeth Road West, Chorlton, Manchester M21 7RL

Tel: 0161 958 4000 Fax: 0161 861 7191
Website: www.centralmanchesterpct.nhs.uk
(Greater Manchester Strategic Health Authority)

Chair Evelyn Asante-Mensah
Chief Executive Sue Assar

Central Suffolk Primary Care Trust

Stow Lodge Centre, Chilton Way, Stowmarket IP14 1SZ
Tel: 01449 616346 Fax: 01449 616340
Website: www.centralsuffolk-pct.nhs.uk
(Norfolk, Suffolk and Cambridgeshire Strategic Health Authority)

Chair Brian Parrott
Chief Executive Carol Taylor-Brown

Charnwood and North West Leicestershire Primary Care Trust

Woodgate, Loughborough LE11 2TZ
Tel: 01509 567700 Fax: 01509 567723
Website: www.cnwlpct.nhs.uk
(Leicestershire, Northamptonshire and Rutland Strategic Health Authority)

Chair Michael Wells
Chief Executive Andrew Clarke

Chelmsford Primary Care Trust

Kestrel House, Hedge Row Business Park, Chelmsford CM2 5PF
Tel: 01245 398770 Fax: 01245 398712
Email: kim.wilks@chelmsford-pct.nhs.uk
(Essex Strategic Health Authority)

Chair Pamela Joughin
Chief Executive Paul Zollinger-Read

Chelsea and Westminster Healthcare NHS Trust

Chelsea and Westminster Hospital, 369 Fulham Road, Chelsea, London SW10 9NH
Tel: 020 8746 8000 Fax: 020 8846 6539
Website: www.chelwest.nhs.uk
(North West London Strategic Health Authority)

Chair Sudahakar Pandit
Chief Executive Heather Lawrence

Chelsea and Westminster Hospital

369 Fulham Road, Chelsea, London SW10 9NH
Tel: 020 8746 8000 Fax: 020 8846 6539
Total Beds: 497

Accident and Emergency P Longstaff (Head), J Booth, P Roberts

Anaesthetics R Keays (Head), P K Barnes, M Bloch, J Chandy, M Cox, S Cox, D Dob, J Durbridge, N Fauvel, K Haire, M Hayes, A Holdcroft, T Kirwan, A Lawson, M Naze, A Rice, J Robotham, N C Soni, V J E Thomas, G Towlerton, M Weston, S Yentis

Cardiology S Kaddoura (Head), S Davies, R Sutton

Care of the Elderly I Bovill, P Kroker, D J R Morgan, M D Pelly

Chest Medicine D Lai (Head), T Evans, P Shah, S Singh

Clinical Pharmacology and Therapeutics M Feher (Head)

Cytology N Livni

Dental Surgery K Barnard, J Smallridge

Dermatology N Roberts (Head), K Agnew, T Basarab, C Bunker, J Cream, S C Mayou, R C D Staughton

Diabetes M Feher (Head), C McIntosh, K Shotliff

ENT P Clarke (Head), J Harcourt, I Mackay

Gastroenterology D Westaby (Head), M Anderson, J Andreyev, J Andreyev, B Gazzard, J Martin, T Vlavianos

General Surgery C Ogden (Head), T Allen-Mersh, M Henry, M Jenkins, D Nott, J Smellie

Genitourinary Medicine D Asboe, S Barton, F Boag, D Hawkins, S McCormack, K Mclean, A McOwan, S Mitchell, M Nelson, A Posniak, N Smith

Haematology C Costello (Head), E Kanfer

Medical Microbiology B Azadian, D J M Wright

Neurology R Guiloff (Head), A Kennedy, I Mak

Obstetrics and Gynaecology G Ayida (Head), S Abdullah, A Bispham, J Bridges, C Gilling-Smith, M Johnson, E Jones, R Marwood, M E Pawson, Z Penn, R Richardson, C D Sims, R Smith, M Stafford, P Steer, J Studd, C Sutton, G Thorpe-Beeston, N Wales, M Williams

Ophthalmology S Mitchell (Head), N Davies, N Joshi, P Kinnear

Oral and Maxillofacial Surgery N Perceval, N Waterhouse, G Wilson

Orthopaedics W Radford (Head), P R E Baird, S Evans, C Gibbons, A Hulme, V Lavelle, A Williams

Paediatrics E Abrahamson, I Balfour-Lynne, A Bedford-Russell, K Bernard, N Bridges, M Brueton, D Caluwe, S Carthigesan, N Cavanagh, B Cooper, M Elsawi, J Fell, S Fernandes, W Grant, M Haddad, J Harcourt, P Hargreaves, G Hartnoll, A Hulme, A Kingi, I Kovar, J Lowe, H Lyall, N Madden, N Madi, M Markiewicz, S Mayou, P O'Driscoll, E Ogundipe, J Penrice, D Piers, N Roberts, A Robin, G Sandhu, J Smallridge, N Waterhouse

Plastic Surgery R Eckersley (Head), G Bantick, A Bremner-Smith, L Ion, E Katsarama, D Martin, S Myers, G Williams, G Wilson

Radiology S Padley (Head), Z Amin, R Chinn, J Healy, J Hiller, D M King, J McCall, L Moore, J Newton, M Phelan, R Pope

Rheumatology A Brand (Head), M Callan, C Mackworth Young

Urology C Ogden (Head), M Dineen, J Ramsay

Cheltenham and Tewkesbury Primary Care Trust

Unit 43, Central Way, Arle Road, Cheltenham GL51 8LX
Tel: 01242 548800 Fax: 01242 548801
Website: www.chelttewkpct.org.uk
(Avon, Gloucestershire and Wiltshire Strategic Health Authority)

Chair Ruth FitzJohn
Chief Executive Caroline Fowles

Cherwell Vale Primary Care Trust

Oxford Road, Banbury OX16 9GE
Tel: 01295 819500 Fax: 01295 819555
Email: firstname.surname@cherwellvale-pct.nhs.uk
Website: www.cherwellvale-pct.nhs.uk
(Thames Valley Strategic Health Authority)

Chair Anita Higham
Chief Executive Barry Thomas

Chipping Norton Community Hospital
Chipping Norton OX7 5AJ
Tel: 01608 628000 Fax: 01608 628011
Total Beds: 20

Cheshire and Wirral Partnership NHS Trust

West Cheshire Hospital, Liverpool Road, Chester CH2 1BQ
Tel: 01244 364368 Fax: 01244 364340
Email: forename.surname@cwpnt.nhs.uk
Website: www.cwpnt.nhs.uk
(Cheshire and Merseyside Strategic Health Authority)

Chair David Eva
Chief Executive Stephen Eames

Ashton House
26 Village Road, Oxton, Birkenhead CH43 5SR
Tel: 0151 653 9660 Fax: 0151 670 9772
Total Beds: 18

Learning Disabilities M T Hand, S Singhal

Elmwood Day Hospital
Liverpool Road, Chester CH2 1BQ
Tel: 01244 364122 Fax: 01244 364027

Ingersley and Millbrook Unit Psychiatric Day Hospital
West Park, Macclesfield District General Hospital, Victoria Road, Macclesfield SK10 3BL
Tel: 01625 663403 Fax: 01625 661118
Total Beds: 127

Psychiatry D Black, A Blakey, J Bowie, W Braude, J Galloway, L Jenkins, H Waring, J Weetman

Kelsall Day Hospital
Liverpool Road, Chester CH2 1BQ
Tel: 01244 364559 Fax: 01244 364561

Leighton Hospital Mental Health Unit
Middlewich Road, Crewe CW1 4QJ

St Catherine's Hospital
Church Road, Tranmere, Birkenhead CH42 0LQ
Tel: 0151 678 7272 Fax: 0151 652 8764
Total Beds: 42

West Cheshire
Liverpool Road, Chester CH2 1UL
Tel: 01244 365000 Fax: 01244 364194

Cheshire West Primary Care Trust

1829 Building, Countess of Chester Health Park, Liverpool Road, Chester CH2 1DU
Tel: 01244 650300 Fax: 01244 650301
Email: ged.taylor@messa.scheshire-ha.nwest.nhs.uk
Website: www.scheshire-ha.nwest.nhs.uk
(Cheshire and Merseyside Strategic Health Authority)

Chair Robert Hodson
Chief Executive Ged Taylor

Chesterfield Primary Care Trust

Scarsdale, Newbold Road, Chesterfield S41 7PF
Tel: 01246 206672, 01246 231255
Website: www.chesterfieldpct.nhs.uk
(Trent Strategic Health Authority)

Chair Tricia Foster
Chief Executive Paul Badger

Ash Green Learning Disabilities Centre
Ashgate Road, Ashgate, Chesterfield S42 7JE
Tel: 01246 565000 Fax: 01246 565014

Walton Hospital
Whitecotes Lane, Chesterfield S40 3HW
Tel: 01246 277271 Fax: 01246 558747
Total Beds: 200

Care of the Elderly D Chew, P Iqbal, P Medcalf, M Reza, P K Sinha

Dermatology G B Colver

Orthopaedics T R Allen, C G Beauchamp, A G Davies, K A Ennis

Psychiatry of Old Age J R Sykes, V M Whittingham

Chesterfield Royal Hospital NHS Foundation Trust

Formerly Chesterfield and North Derbyshire Royal Hospital NHS Trust. Established as a Foundation Trust 01/01/2005.
Calow, Chesterfield S44 5BL
Tel: 01246 277271 Fax: 01246 512737
Email: forename.surname@chesterfieldroyal.nhs.uk
Website: www.chesterfieldroyal.nhs.uk
(Trent Strategic Health Authority)

Chair Michael Wall
Chief Executive Eric Morton

Chesterfield and North Derbyshire Royal Hospital
Calow, Chesterfield S44 5BL
Tel: 01246 277271 Fax: 01246 276955
Total Beds: 570

Accident and Emergency M M Alam, N H Aziz, R C Bailey, K Lendrum

Anaesthetics I R Gell (Head), A E Aziz, S Beavis, C M S Cooper, J M Cort, S J Dale, Y Day, I M Dods, R W Eustace, D Farquharson, J B Groves, E S Howell, G Hutchinson, H Knifton-Smith, I Makkison, J S Mark, R J Murray, A North, P R Rayner, T J I Shaw, C S N Spittle, R P Wroth

Care of the Elderly D Chew, M W Cooper, P Iqbal, P Medcalf, M Reza

Child and Adolescent Psychiatry S Blomfield, J de Cartaret, J Edmondson, E Girgis, J Wilkinson

Dermatology G B Colver, R Murphy

ENT F M Nofal, V R Talati

General Medicine J W Hadfield (Head), A G Archer, M G Ashton, J T Bourne, D J Brooks, C J Cooke, S W Crooks, K L E Dear, K Fairburn, M J Grundman, S M Parnacott, R Robinson, D A Sandler

General Surgery N R Boucher (Head), D Bardsley, D R Chadwick, N J Everitt, J Hall, S Holt, M J James, P K Kumar, W G Lambert

Genitourinary Medicine P A Fraser, K Rogstad

Haematology R C Colin, R M Stewart

Histopathology D Mckenna, K Ramsden, R D Start

Microbiology K Thomas

Obstetrics and Gynaecology G Collins (Head), J L Cresswell, D P Hey, S C Smith, P M Tromans, S Vindla

Ophthalmology C Brand, D Chand, K K F Mohamad, S Stafanous

Oral and Maxillofacial Surgery S J Davies, P T Doyle, P McCloughlin, P J Sandler

Orthopaedics P Williams (Head), S M As'ad, C G Beauchamp, M J Bryant, G Davies, M S d Edwards, K A Ennis, I R Scott, S Shahane, P M Williams

Paediatrics G Collins (Head), K Holt, P M Preece, M Reynolds, I F Roberts, R M Tyler

Radiology A Cohen (Head), P de vos Meiring, J Glaves, K V Nair, M Shaw, P W Sheppard

Chiltern and South Bucks Primary Care Trust

2 & 3 Lacemaker Court, London Road, Old Amersham, Amersham HP7 0HS
Tel: 01494 606606 Fax: 01494 606613
Email: firstname.surname@chiltern-pct.nhs.uk
Website: www.csbpct.nhs.uk
(Thames Valley Strategic Health Authority)

Chair Richard Worrall
Chief Executive Bart Johnson
Consultants Clare Strong

Chorley and South Ribble Primary Care Trust

Jubilee House, Lancashire Business Park, Centurion Way, Leyland PR26 6TR
Tel: 01772 644400 Fax: 01772 227022
Email: enquiries@chorley-pct.nhs.uk
Website: www.chorley-pct.nhs.uk
(Cumbria and Lancashire Strategic Health Authority)

Chair Dennis Benson
Chief Executive Judith Faux

Christie Hospital NHS Trust

Wilmslow Road, Withington, Manchester M20 4BX
Tel: 0161 446 3000 Fax: 0161 446 3977
Email: enquiries@christie-tr.nwest.nhs.uk
Website: www.christie.nhs.uk
(Greater Manchester Strategic Health Authority)

Chair Joan Higgins
Chief Executive Joanna Wallace

Christie Hospital

Wilmslow Road, Withington, Manchester M20 4BX
Tel: 0845 226 3000 Fax: 0161 446 3977
Total Beds: 300

Chest Medicine P V Barber

Clinical Oncology E Allan, P Burt, R Cowan, S E Davidson, D P Deakin, C Faivre-Finn, M Harris, R D Hunter, E Levine, J Livsey, J Logue, B Magee, M Saunders, N Slevin, A L Stewart, R Stout, A J Sykes, R Welch, J Wylie, B Yap

Clinical Pharmacology and Therapeutics P M Wilkinson

Endocrinology S M Shalet, P Trainer

ENT A Birzgalis

Epidemiology A Moran, C Woodman

Haematology R Chopra

Medical Genetics G Evans

Medical Oncology H Anderson, R Hawkins, A Howell, G Jayson, J A Radford, M Ranson, N Thatcher, J Valle, Dr Wardley

Obstetrics and Gynaecology M Kitchener, K Reynolds, R J Slade

Occupational Health R Lennox (Head)

Paediatric Oncology B Brennan, O B Eden, H R Gattamaneni

Paediatric Histopathology A Kelsey

Palliative Care W P Makin

Pathology S S Banerjee, L Menasce, J Shanks

Plastic Surgery A Brain

Psychological Medicine P Hopwood

Radiology R Bramley, B Carrington, P Hulse, R J Johnson, J Lawrance, B Taylor

Surgery A Baildam, N Bundred, S O'Dwyer

Urology N Clarke, M Wilson

City and Hackney Teaching Primary Care Trust

St Leonard's, Nuttall Street, London N1 5LZ
Tel: 020 7301 3000 Fax: 020 7739 8455
Email: barbara.landey@chpct.nhs.uk
Website: www.chpct.nhs.uk
(North East London Strategic Health Authority)

Chair Jane Winder
Chief Executive Laura Sharpe
Consultants Tom Allport, Del Howard, Susan Kermond

City Hospitals Sunderland NHS Foundation Trust

Established as a Foundation Trust 01/07/2004.

Kayll Road, Sunderland SR4 7TP
Tel: 0191 565 6256 Fax: 0191 514 0220
Website: www.sunderland.nhs.uk/chs
(Northumberland, Tyne and Wear Strategic Health Authority)

Chair David Graham
Chief Executive Ken Bremner

Ryhope General Hospital

Ryhope, Sunderland SR2 0LY
Tel: 0191 585 6256
Total Beds: 306

Care of the Elderly S Bansal, S K Basu, J Baxter, T Cassidy, A Davies, S D Gupta, D Hambleton, N Majmudar, A D Mitchell, L J Young

Sunderland Eye Infirmary

Queen Alexandra Road, Sunderland SR2 9HP
Tel: 0191 528 3616
Total Beds: 60

Ophthalmology R W Allchin, E D Allen, R D Bell, F Chapman, J P Danjoux, J P Deady, T J Fetherston, S G Fraser, D V Inglesby, S J Morgan, P S Phelan, D H W Steel, P A C Tiffin

Sunderland Royal Hospital

Kayll Road, Sunderland SR4 7TP
Tel: 0191 565 6256 Fax: 0191 514 0220
Total Beds: 947

Accident and Emergency C L Muwanga (Head), H Dowd, M Jones, K Lambert, M Potts

Anaesthetics Z Arfeen, H Bhaskar, C M E Carr, A K Choudhry, P Cudworth, N Dhariwal, A Dodds, M P Down, B Lal, D Laws, G Lear, A R Mahroo, P McAndrew, M Millar, U Misra, A Morrison, C Richmond, E Rodger, A Roy, L Sekhar, Q Smith, A Taylor, S Varma

Care of the Elderly S Bansal, S K Basu, J Baxter, T Cassidy, A Davies, S D Gupta, D Hambleton, N Majmudar, A D Mitchell, L J Young

General Medicine J Chapman, H Clague, M Farrer, D Hobday, S Junejo, N Keaney, J Langtry, H A A Mansy, M McHugh, H Mitchison, R Natarajan, D Nylander, P Pai, J Painter, S Pugh, K Sridharan, I Taylor

General Surgery A Adedeji, L Boobis, A Brown, J Corson, P Dunlop, M Grey, A J Rich, P Surtees, S Vetrivel

Head and Neck J Ryan (Head), C Hartley, J M Heaton, T Leontsinis, L Lindsey, I Martin, M Morgan, I Shaw

Obstetrics and Gynaecology H Cameron, M E Dalton, K Hinshaw, G Macnab, B J Murray, S Rashid, K M Saravanamuttu, C Steele

Orthopaedics J M Buchanan, A T Cross, G P De Kiewiet, P Dixon, P Gill, L Irwin, A Nanu, S O'Brien, G Roysam, A Stirrat, I Talkhani

Paediatrics M Abu-Harb, P Baines, S Bruce, G Lawson, A Mellon, S W J Richmond, E Saharia, J Welbury, K Whiting

Pathology A Berrington, G E Bignardi, P Carey, H Cochrane, R D S Dhillon, M Galloway, D K Goff, A Hendrick, R Koerner, J McElroy, D Milne, M O'Donnell, C Settle, M Wetherall

Radiology G Bunea, J Connor, S T England, T Featherstone, R L Marsh, S Mukhtar, U Schierle, N Shirbhate, C White

Radiotherapy and Oncology U Mallick, I Pedley

Rheumatology and Rehabilitation T J Daymond, C D Holland, C E Kidd, D Wright

Urology D Greene (Head), P Johnson

Clatterbridge Centre for Oncology NHS Trust

Clatterbridge Road, Bebington, Wirral CH63 4JY
Tel: 0151 334 1155 Fax: 0151 482 7675
Email: info@ccotrust.co.uk
Website: www.ccotrust.nhs.uk
(Cheshire and Merseyside Strategic Health Authority)

Chair Alan White
Chief Executive Tony Halsall
Consultants Peter Clark, A Coackley, Cottier, R D Errington, C Eswas, A Flavin, J A Green, K Hayat, Dave Husband, M Iqbal, A Jhenoy, A Jones, J A H Littler, J Maguire, E Marshall, S Myint, S O'Reilly, C Romaniuk, A J Slater, I Syndikus, N Thorpe

Colchester Primary Care Trust

Health Offices, Turner Road, Colchester CO4 5JR
Tel: 01206 288500 Fax: 01206 288501
Website: www.colchester-pct.nhs.uk
(Essex Strategic Health Authority)

Chair Maggie Shackell
Chief Executive Brendan Osborne

Spencer Close
4 Spencer Close, The Plain, Epping CM16 6TU
Tel: 01279 827303 Fax: 01279 827472

Cornwall Partnership NHS Trust

Porthpean Road, St Austell PL26 6AD
Tel: 01726 291000 Fax: 01726 291080
Email: enquiries@cpt.cornwall.nhs.uk
Website: www.cornwall.nhs.uk
(South West Peninsula Strategic Health Authority)

Chair Sandra Benjamin
Chief Executive Tony Gardner

Bodmin Hospital (Mental Health Unit)
Westheath Avenue, Bodmin PL31 2QT
Tel: 01208 251300 Fax: 01208 251512
Total Beds: 96

Manager Anthea Hancock

Longreach House
Camborne/Redruth Community Hospital Site, Barncoose Terrace, Redruth TR15 3ER
Tel: 01209 881900 Fax: 01209 881920
Total Beds: 67

Manager Juliette Hostick

Lower Cardrew (Mental Health Unit)
North Street, Redruth TR15 1HJ
Tel: 01209 881831 Fax: 01209 881838
Total Beds: 10

Manager David McAuley

Roseveor - Budock Hospital
Union Road, Falmouth TR11 4LQ
Tel: 01326 437600 Fax: 01326 437613
Total Beds: 18

Manager Chris Line

Selwood House (Mental Health Unit)
60 Alexandra Road, St Austell PL25 4QN
Tel: 01726 291250 Fax: 01726 291251
Total Beds: 10

Manager Dave McAuley

Westheath House (Learning Disabilities)
Corporation Road, Bodmin PL31 1QH
Tel: 01208 256250 Fax: 01208 256253
Total Beds: 6

Manager Chris Line

Cotswold and Vale Primary Care Trust

Trust Headquarters, Cirencester Hospital, Tetbury Road, Cirencester GL7 1UX
Tel: 01285 884694 Fax: 01285 884652
Website: www.cotsvalepct.org.uk
(Avon, Gloucestershire and Wiltshire Strategic Health Authority)

Chair Elizabeth Law
Chief Executive Richard James

Berkeley Hospital
Berkeley GL13 9AB
Tel: 01453 562000 Fax: 01453 562001
Total Beds: 20

Manager Barbara Ruthers

Cirencester Hospital
Tetbury Road, Cirencester GL7 1RR
Tel: 01285 655711
Total Beds: 94

Manager Barbara Ruthers

Fairford Cottage Hospital
Fairford GL7 4BB
Tel: 01285 712212
Total Beds: 15

Moore Cottage Hospital
Moore Road, Bourton-on-the-Water, Cheltenham GL54 2AZ
Tel: 01451 820228
Total Beds: 34

Moreton District Hospital
Hospital Road, Moreton-in-Marsh GL56 0BS
Tel: 01608 650456 Fax: 01608 651599
Total Beds: 30

Stroud General Hospital
Stroud GL5 2HY
Tel: 01453 562200 Fax: 01453 562201
Total Beds: 61

Manager Barbara Ruthers

Stroud Maternity Hospital
Field Road, Stroud GL5 2JB
Tel: 01453 562140 Fax: 01453 562141
Total Beds: 9

Manager Michelle Poole

Countess of Chester Hospital NHS Foundation Trust

Established as a Foundation Trust 01/04/2004.

Countess of Chester Health Park, Liverpool Road, Chester CH2 1UL
Tel: 01244 365000 Fax: 01244 365292
Website: www.coch.org
(Cheshire and Merseyside Strategic Health Authority)

Chair Susan Sellers
Chief Executive Peter Herring
Consultants John Cawood, Stephen Chadwick, Linda de Cossart, Sanjiv Dhital, William Fitzroy Smith, Ewen Forrest, Ian Harvey, Neil MacKinnon, Detlev Rogahn, Mark Skues, Sean Tighe, H Waters

Countess of Chester Hospital
Liverpool Road, Chester CH2 1UL
Tel: 01244 365000 Fax: 01244 365292
Total Beds: 591

Accident and Emergency R S Moore, J P Sloan, M Waters

Anaesthetics E T S Forrest (Head), S Q M Tighe (Head), S R W Bricker, N J Campbell, D Childs, N V Fergusson, S E Hill, P M Jameson, A S Logan, P M Mullen, R A Nelson, N M Robin, S Singh, M A Skues, A M Troy

Care of the Elderly S L Choudhury, W D F Fitzroy Smith, K N Ganeshram, B B Spencer

Dermatology A R Franks, S S Mendelsohn

ENT N A MacKinnon (Head), M G Spencer, R H Temple

General Medicine D L Ewins, J P Finnerty, R A Harris, I M Keeping, P G Reid, M A Rutter, M L Sedgwick, J D Somauroo, T D Wardle, R C Worth

General Surgery L de Cossart, S K Z Dimitri, P R Edwards, G E Foster, C E Harding-Mackean, M A Johnson, D N Monk, E J Redmond

Genitourinary Medicine C P O'Mahony

Haematology V J Clough, E S Lee, H M Leggat

Nephrology A Crowe

Neurology M Boggild, A N Bowden, N Fletcher

Neurosurgery T R K Varma

Obstetrics and Gynaecology J Davies-Humphreys, N G Haddad, J A Hawe, S Kirkwood, M J McCormack, A B Peattie, J H Williams

Ophthalmology S Armstrong, J M Butcher, M K Tutton

Oral and Maxillofacial Surgery J I Cawood, D Richardson

Orthodontics S Chadwick, C A Melrose

Orthopaedics I A Harvey (Head), J M Anderton, I J Braithwaite, D Campbell, A P Phillipson, J Rao

Paediatrics L G Evans Jones, J Gibbs, C M V Jones, H Joshi, N P Murphy, D Rogahn

Pathology S A Bowles, J Elder, S A Hales, B N A Hamid, W E Kenyon, R U Khan, P T Mannion

Plastic Surgery S K Dhital (Head), F S Fahmy, A M H Juma

Radiology G T Abbot, G J Doyle, R J Etherington, J E Houghton, W J Pilbrow, G R J Sissons, R A Sloka, E A Wright

Rheumatology and Rehabilitation D Y Bulgen, K E Over

Thoracic Surgery M J Drakely

Urology B A Pettersson, C S Powell

County Durham and Darlington Acute Hospitals NHS Trust

University Hospital of North Durham, North Road, Durham DH1 5TW
Tel: 0191 333 2333 Fax: 0191 333 2699
Website: www.cddah.nhs.uk
(County Durham and Tees Valley Strategic Health Authority)

Chair Angela Ballatti
Chief Executive John Saxby
Consultants J Banks, S Green

Bishop Auckland General Hospital
Cockton Hill Road, Bishop Auckland DL14 6AD
Tel: 01388 455000 Fax: 01388 455127
Total Beds: 354

Accident and Emergency O O Afolabi, H Gonsalves, P Muthu

Anaesthetics Z Daoud, M Johnson, U Saleh, P Sivayokan

Care of the Elderly A Mehrzad, R Prescott

Dermatology M Carr

ENT J Carlin, M Oluwole, R W Ruckley, C Watson

General Medicine R Abbasi, M Bateson, A McCulloch, M Y Mahmoud, A Stewart, G Terry

General Surgery H Hashimi, A Hassn, T Layzell, J Stephen

Genitourinary Medicine C White

Neurology J Young

Neurosurgery J Sinar

Obstetrics and Gynaecology C Lim, J Oghoetuoma, R Wood

Ophthalmology M S Dang, C Dees, J Haslam, R Stirling

Oral and Maxillofacial Surgery C Edge

Orthodontics D McConnell

Orthopaedics N Gandhi, K S Mahdi, M Stewart

Paediatrics A Cottrell, A Johnson, P Jones, W H Lamb, G Nyamugunuru, H Smith

Pathology C Bloxham, T Senadhira, S Smellie

Plastic Surgery P Baguley

Radiology H Jongschaap, P Orr

Rheumatology and Rehabilitation M Sattar

Urology C Roberts

Darlington Memorial Hospital
Hollyhurst Road, Darlington DL3 6HX
Tel: 01325 380100 Fax: 01325 743622
Total Beds: 465

Accident and Emergency H Gonzales, P Muthu, A West

Anaesthetics P Bresland, R S Drummond, D Hamilton, R Hargreaves, R Hixson, H Khalil, C Kotur, P Mallinder, M A Quader, D Saha

Care of the Elderly P H Carr, G V Williams

Dermatology W D Taylor

ENT J Carlin, M Oluwole, R W Ruckley, C Watson

General Medicine E W Barnes, S Mitchell, J J Murphy, P N Trewby

General Surgery R Brookstein, N Corner, S Debrah, K Gunning

Genitourinary Medicine P A Rajah

Neurology P J B Tilley

Obstetrics and Gynaecology R H Aitken, M Ali, D J R Hutchon, J H Macdonald

Ophthalmology S Buckley, M S Dang, C Dees, J D Haslam, R Stirling

Oral and Maxillofacial Surgery C Edge, Mr McConnell

Orthodontics D McConnell

Orthopaedics A Bawarish, M Khan, V Mahendran, T J Stahl

Paediatrics R Ahmed, M Alam, R Carpenter, N On-Tin, I M Thakur

Pathology U Earl, J Sloss, P Williamson

Plastic Surgery P Baguley

Radiology J S Anderson, I Curzon, E Dillon, G Heath, R Henderson

Rheumatology and Rehabilitation M A Sattar

Urology S Fulford, S Vadanan, Mrs Whiteway

Homelands Hospital
Helmington Row, Crook DL15 0SD
Tel: 01388 762339 Fax: 01388 767457
Total Beds: 20

Maiden Law Hospital
Maiden Law, Lanchester, Durham DH1 0QN
Tel: 0191 333 6262

Shotley Bridge Community Hospital
Shotley Bridge Hospital, Consett DH8 0NB
Tel: 01207 583583 Fax: 01207 586003
Total Beds: 336

Anaesthetics D I MacNair, M Sekar

Cardiothoracic Medicine G N Morritt

Community Child Health S K Pandey

Dermatology F A Ive

ENT D S Cameron

General Medicine A P Mukherjee, P Robson

General Psychiatry J M Brockington, K B Gururaj-Prasad, K Hurren, P E Watson

General Surgery J R Mason

Haematology D Stainsby

Obstetrics and Gynaecology B Johnston

Ophthalmology R C Bosanquet, R F Gillie

Oral and Maxillofacial Surgery J M Ryan

Orthodontics I A Shaw

Orthopaedics V S Nargolwala

Paediatrics B Thalayasingam

Pathology D Allison, C M Dobson

Plastic Surgery B Berry, J H James, G S Rao

Radiology J Gholkar, R A Robson, G Timmons

Radiotherapy and Oncology R C B Evans

South Moor Hospital
South Moor, Stanley DH9 6DS
Tel: 0191 333 6262
Total Beds: 20

University Hospital of North Durham
North Road, Durham DH1 5TW
Tel: 0191 333 2333 Fax: 0191 333 2685
Total Beds: 427

Accident and Emergency J G Banks, R Harden, C E Phillips

Anaesthetics H Brar, W G M Bremner, G W Brown, S Dabner, S Dowson, C R D Laird, M Lothian, P A McBride, R W D Mitchell, P Mowbray, A W Murray, I Spencer, D G Thomas, J Watson, D Weatherill, R Will, P J Wood

Care of the Elderly H A Brown, P M Earnshaw, A Gatnash, I Wandless

Chest Disease P Cook, N C Munro, S J Pearce

Dermatology M M Carr, J Langtry, S Natarajan, S Sinclair, S Velangi

ENT T G Leontsinis, L Lindsey, P R Samuel

General Medicine M H Cave, W R Ellis, A F Macklon, E Sanders, J Y Yiannakou

General Surgery I Bain, A I M Cook, P J Cullen, P J English, S Green, I E Hawthorn, D W Herring

Genitourinary Medicine A Wardropper, C White

Haematology A Iqbal, F M Keenan

Obstetrics and Gynaecology D Irons, F H Lloyd, P Marsden, G E Morgan, S Shanmugalingham

Ophthalmology S J Morgan, P Tiffin

Oral and Maxillofacial Surgery I C Martin

Orthodontics I Shaw

Orthopaedics H P Epstein, R J H Gregory, D V Heath, A Jennings, N Shaw, K U Wright

Paediatrics T G Omoregie, D R S Smith, A N P Speight, H V Stewart

Pathology D Allison, P D Barrett, Mrs Day, P Gray, G Horne, D J L Maloney

Plastic Surgery M Erdmann, R B Perry, S Rao

Radiology P Cadigan, S M Desai, S N E Marsden, I Minty

Radiotherapy and Oncology C G Kelly, W B Taylor

Rheumatology A J Chuck, S Hailwood, P Mangion

Urology P Richmond, C Roberts

County Durham and Darlington Priority Services NHS Trust

Earls House, Lanchester Road, Durham DH1 5RD
Tel: 0191 333 6262 Fax: 0191 333 6363
Website: www.cddps.nhs.uk
(County Durham and Tees Valley Strategic Health Authority)

Chair Jo Turnbull
Chief Executive Sandy Taylor

Auckland Park Hospital
Westfield Road, Bishop Auckland DL14 6AE
Total Beds: 52

Bowes Lyon Unit
Lanchester Road, Durham DH1 5RD
Total Beds: 30

County Hospital, Durham
North Road, Durham DH1 4ST
Tel: 0191 333 6262 Fax: 0191 333 3400
Total Beds: 58

General Psychiatry M Appleton, E Jones, K Linsley, S Martin, J Tomkinson

Derwent Clinic
Shotley Bridge Hospital, Shotley Bridge, Consett DH8 0NB
Tel: 01207 583583 Fax: 01207 586049
Total Beds: 40

Earls House
Lanchester Road, Durham DH1 5RD
Total Beds: 93

The Gables
Sedgefield, Stockton-on-Tees TS21 3EJ
Tel: 01740 620521 Fax: 01740 624288
Total Beds: 36

The Goodall Centre
The Goodall Centre, Bishop Auckland DL14 6QW
Tel: 01388 603161
Total Beds: 11

Pierremont Unit and Beaumont
Hollyhurst Road, Darlington
Tel: 01325 743564 Fax: 01325 743588
Total Beds: 95

West Park Hospital
West Park, Darlington
Total Beds: 116

Coventry and Warwickshire Ambulance NHS Trust

Dale Street, Leamington Spa CV32 5HH
Tel: 01926 881331 Fax: 01926 488409
(West Midlands South Strategic Health Authority)

Chair Michael Langman
Chief Executive Malcolm Hazell

Coventry Teaching Primary Care Trust

Christchurch House, Greyfriars Lane, Coventry CV1 2GQ
Tel: 024 7655 2225 Fax: 024 7622 6280
Email: contactus@coventrypct.nhs.uk
Website: www.coventrypct.nhs.uk
(West Midlands South Strategic Health Authority)

Chair Alison Gingell
Chief Executive Laurence Tennant

Caludon Centre
Clifford Bridge Road, Walsgrave, Coventry CV2 2TE
Tel: 024 7660 2020 Fax: 024 7653 8920
Total Beds: 130

General Psychiatry A Ashley-Smith, F A Judelsohn, L G Meesey, E T Rolston, A N Singh, R Thavasothy

Psychiatry of Old Age A Malik, C D Wooding

River House Day Centre
Gulson Road, Coventry CV1 2HR
Tel: 024 76 553344

Tamar Day Unit
Walsgrave Campus, Clifford Bridge Road, Coventry CV2 2TE
Tel: 024 76 602020 Fax: 024 76 538920

Craven, Harrogate and Rural District Primary Care Trust

The Hamlet, Hornbeam Park, Harrogate HG2 8RE
Tel: 01423 815150 Fax: 01423 859600
Website: www.chrd-pct.nhs.uk
(North and East Yorkshire and Northern Lincolnshire Strategic Health Authority)

Chair Johnny Wardle
Chief Executive Penny Jones

Crawley Primary Care Trust

5th Floor Overline House, Station Way, Crawley RH10 1JA
Tel: 01293 572100 Fax: 01293 572172
Email: enquiries@crawleypct.nhs.uk
Website: www.crawleypct.nhs.uk
(Surrey and Sussex Strategic Health Authority)

Chair Malcolm Liles
Chief Executive Lynne Regent

Croydon Primary Care Trust

Knollys House, 17 Addiscombe Road, Croydon CR0 6SR
Tel: 020 8274 6000 Fax: 020 8680 2418
Website: www.croydon.nhs.uk
(South West London Strategic Health Authority)

Chair Toni Letts
Chief Executive Caroline Taylor

Cumbria Ambulance Service NHS Trust

Ambulance Headquarters, Salkeld Hall, Infirmary Street, Carlisle CA2 7AN
Tel: 01228 596909 Fax: 01228 403027
Email: info@cas.nhs.uk
Website: www.cas.nhs.uk
(Cumbria and Lancashire Strategic Health Authority)

Chair Brian Clayton
Chief Executive Tim Lynch

Dacorum Primary Care Trust

The Isbister Centre, Chaulden House Gardens, Off Chaulden Lane, Hemel Hempstead HP1 2BW

Tel: 01442 840950 Fax: 01442 840951
Email: general@dacorum-pct.nhs.uk
Website: www.dacorum-pct.nhs.uk
(Bedfordshire and Hertfordshire Strategic Health Authority)

Chair Mary Pedlow
Chief Executive Falicity Cox

Darlington Primary Care Trust

Dr Piper House, King Street, Darlington DL3 6JL
Tel: 01325 364271 Fax: 01325 746112
Email: info@darlingtonpct.nhs.uk
Website: www.darlington-pct.nhs.uk
(County Durham and Tees Valley Strategic Health Authority)

Chair Sandra Pollard
Chief Executive Colin Morris

Dartford and Gravesham NHS Trust

Darent Valley Hospital, Darenth Wood Road, Dartford DA2 8DA
Tel: 01322 428100 Fax: 01322 428259
Website: www.kentandmedway.nhs.uk
(Kent and Medway Strategic Health Authority)

Chair Sarah Dunnett
Chief Executive Sue Jennings

Darent Valley Hospital

Darenth Wood Road, Dartford DA2 8DA
Tel: 01322 428100 Fax: 01322 428259

Accident and Emergency J Thurston (Head), G R Kerur

Anaesthetics R J C Evans (Head), M A S Abbott, G Disanayake, E P Kelly, B Lobo, R Madan, H T Patel, M Protopapas, J Smith

Care of the Elderly W J Fitzpatrick, S Hussein, W Jayawardena

Dental Surgery Mr Lavery, P Scanlon

Dermatology C Grech

General Medicine H Alban Davies, V Andrews, D Brennand-Roper, R Ede, M Kazmi, W Melia, M Mushtaq, A Tavakkoli, I Vadasz, I Zoukos

General Surgery A J McIrvine (Head), M C Parker, M Stewart, P Strauss, G Thomas

Genitourinary Medicine P Key

Nephrology I McDonald

Obstetrics and Gynaecology A Lesseps (Head), M Jones, R MacDermott, A Schreiner

Oncology M Leslie, M O'Connell, J Prendiville, A Visioli

Ophthalmology M Gibbens, R Goel, L Whitefield

Orthopaedics A K Addison (Head), B A Kamdar, A Leyshon, F Moftah, S Sait

Paediatrics H R Patel (Head), M D'Costa, D Leung

Pathology C Farquhar (Head), V E Andrews, M Kasmi, M Z Khan, A T Rashid, A Shaw, P Thebe

Plastic Surgery R W Smith

Radiology B Al-Murrani, D Allen, J Kirk, C K Koo, N Sathananthan

Respiratory Medicine M Mushtaq, A Tavakkoli

Rheumatology I Vadasz

Urology J K Dickinson, R Ravi

Gravesend and North Kent Hospital

Bath Street, Gravesend DA11 0DG
Tel: 01474 564333 Fax: 01474 574018
Total Beds: 104

Dartford, Gravesham and Swanley Primary Care Trust

Livingstone Hospital, 1st Floor, East Hill, Dartford DA1 1SA
Tel: 01322 622222 Fax: 01322 622384
Email: tricia.bailey@dgspct.nhs.uk
Website: www.dartfordgraveshamswanleypct.nhs.uk
(Kent and Medway Strategic Health Authority)

Chair Martin Henwood
Chief Executive Stephanie Stanwick

Livingstone Hospital

East Hill, Dartford DA1 1SA
Tel: 01322 622222
Total Beds: 38

Daventry and South Northamptonshire Primary Care Trust

Danetre Hospital, London Road, Daventry NN11 4DY
Tel: 01327 705610 Fax: 01327 877058
Website: www.northamptonshire.nhs.uk
(Leicestershire, Northamptonshire and Rutland Strategic Health Authority)

Chair Simon Schanschieff
Chief Executive Kevin Herbert

Danetre Hospital

London Road, Daventry NN11 4DY
Tel: 01327 702113 Fax: 01327 300509
Total Beds: 28

Manager Rita Reeves

Derby Hospitals NHS Foundation Trust

Formerly Southern Derbyshire Acute Hospitals NHS Trust. Established as a Foundation Trust 01/07/2004.

Derby City General Hospital, Uttoxeter Road, Derby DE22 3NE
Tel: 01332 340131 Fax: 01332 625566
Email: jo.yeaman@derbyhospitals.nhs.uk
Website: www.derbyhospitals.nhs.uk
(Trent Strategic Health Authority)

Chair Brenda Remington
Chief Executive Julie Acred

Derby City General Hospital

Uttoxeter Road, Derby DE22 3NE
Tel: 01332 340131
Total Beds: 470

Anaesthetics D P Cartwright, A W A Crossley, W L Dann, G F McLeod, S Piggott, D Rogerson, M Vater, R Verma

Care of the Elderly A J Birtwell, K A Muhiddin, M Mylvahan

General Medicine J R M Bateman, J Bennett, A J Birtwell, J G Freeman, A McCance, N Mylvahan

General Surgery R I Hall, H W Holliday, M Larvin, B McIlroy, J R Reynolds, D M Sibbering, Y Wahedna

Nephrology R Fluck, C McIntyre

Obstetrics and Gynaecology R L K Chapman, M Cust, J F Darne, A Fowlie, H M L Jenkins, I V Scott

Paediatrics K L Dodd, R E Morton, C S Nelson, N Ruggins

Radiology J Minford, J G Pallan, A Turnbull, G M Turner

Rehabilitation Medicine C D Ward

Urology C P Chilton, A M Peracha, S A Thomas, J H Williams

Derbyshire Children's Hospital

Uttoxeter Road, Derby DE22 3NE
Tel: 01332 340131 Fax: 01332 200857
Total Beds: 86

Anaesthetics A Boyd, D P Cartwright, A W A Crossley, G F Macleod, S Piggott, D Rogerson, M Vater, R Verma

Paediatric Surgery P T C Docherty, A P J Henry, R Holden, H Holliday, P W Howard, P Korczak, B Majumdar, J McIntyre, S Mortimore, D Parker, J Reynolds, H A M Salem, J Sharp

Paediatrics T Bleiker, I Choonara, K L Dodd, R E Morton, C S Nelson, N R Ruggins, H Shahidullah, T S Tinklin

Derbyshire Royal Infirmary

London Road, Derby DE1 2QY
Tel: 01332 347141 Fax: 01332 295652
Total Beds: 610

Accident and Emergency A Fraser-Moodie, S M Hewitt, N Howarth, P E Pritty

Anaesthetics M M Ankutse, P H Bavister, A H Boyd, D P Cartwright, A W A Crossley, R Dua, R H Elliott, R J Erskin, P H P Harris, B Hudson, S Kethar-Thas, B T Langham, G F MacLeod, D A Mulvey, S Piggott, S Ralph, D Rogerson, A E Searle, M Vater, R Verma

Cardiology S Burn, A McCance, M W Millar-Craig

Care of the Elderly W P Gorman, R Skelly

Chemical Pathology J S Harrop, P G Hill

Dermatology T Bleiker, J M Gartside, H Shahidullah

ENT M Johnston, B Majumdar, S Mortimore, D A Parker, J Sharp

General Medicine R Donnelly, W P Gorman, G K T Holmes, P King, M W Millar-Craig, B Norton, A R Scott

General Surgery K G Callum, S Y Ifikhar, K Lingham, B McIlroy, J R Nash, J R Reynolds

Genitourinary Medicine R Rajakumar

Haematology A McKernan, S Mayne, D C Mitchell

Histopathology C S Holgate, I P Hopper, I Robinson, D Semeraro

Medical Microbiology D W Bullock

Neurology N Bajaj, D Jefferson, A J Wills

Neurosurgery P O Byrne, T Hope

Ophthalmology H Chen, P T C Docherty, I D Gardner, R Holden, H A M Salem, L Stevenson

Oral and Maxillofacial Surgery A Baker, K Jones, P Korczak

Orthodontics A Murray, O O'Keefe

Orthopaedics D Calthorpe, A O Cargill, D I Clark, G Geutjens, A P J Henry, P W Howard, J W Hutchinson, P G Lunn, D McDermott, R C Quinnell, J M Rowles, T J Wilton

Palliative Medicine J M L Hocknell, V L Keeley, M Swanwick

Plastic Surgery M Henley

Radiology M Cohen, N Cozens, N Dann, M De Nunzio, S Elliot, G Narborough, J Pallam, A Turnbull

Radiotherapy and Oncology P Chakraborti, R Kulkarni, D Otim-Oyet, M Persic, P Woodings

Respiratory Medicine J Bennett

Rheumatology and Rehabilitation L J Badcock, C F Murray-Leslie, S O'Reilly, M R Regan, G D Summers, R A Williams

Nightingale Macmillan Continuing Care Unit

117A London Road, Derby DE1 2RA
Tel: 01332 254900
Total Beds: 19

Derbyshire Dales and South Derbyshire Primary Care Trust

Park Hill, Hilton Road, Eggington, Derby DE65 6SH
Tel: 01283 731300 Fax: 01283 731301
Website: www.southernderbyshire.nhs.uk/dalesandsouth-pct
(Trent Strategic Health Authority)

Chair Peter Purnell
Chief Executive Nina Ennis

Derbyshire Mental Health Services NHS Trust

Kingsway Hospital, Kingsway, Derby DE22 3LZ
Tel: 01332 362221
Website: www.derbyshirementalhealthservices.nhs.uk
(Trent Strategic Health Authority)

Chair Judith Forrest
Chief Executive Mike Shewan
Consultants M A Bhulyan, A T Cole, R Holden, J Kennedy, F Rahman, Peter Stuart, M Wheatcroft, L Whitney

Babington Hospital

Chevin Ward, Derby Road, Belper DE56 1WH
Tel: 01773 824171 Fax: 01773 824155
Total Beds: 10

Derby City General Hospital (Mental Health)

Uttoxeter Road, Derby DE22 3NE
Tel: 01332 340131 Fax: 01332 624587
Total Beds: 173

General Psychiatry M A Bihiliyn, A Clayton, C Clulow, A Cook, R S H Denny, M T Duggan, B Fowler, J Hay, S McCane, R T Owen, K P Rao, M A Sherman, N Sisodia, R Stocking-Korzen

Psychiatry of Old Age P Balakrishnan, J A Hartman, E Komocki, S Pore, S Thacker

Derbyshire Royal Infirmary (Mental Health)

London Road, Derby DE1 2QY
Tel: 01332 347141 Fax: 01332 295652
Total Beds: 33

Psychiatry of Old Age P Balakrishnan, J Hartman, E Komocki, S Pore, S Thacker

Dovedale Day Hospital (Elderly Services)

London Road, Derby DE1 2XX
Tel: 01332 254886

Ilkeston Community Hospital

Woodside Ward, Heanor Road, Ilkeston DE7 8LN
Tel: 0115 930 5522 Fax: 0115 944 1800
Total Beds: 15

Psychiatry of Old Age Dr Komocki

Kingsway Hospital
Kingsway, Derby DE22 3LZ
Tel: 01332 362221 Fax: 01332 331254
Total Beds: 217

General Psychiatry M A Bhuiyan, A Clayton, C Clulow, A Cook, R Denny, M Duggan, D Fowler, J M Hay, S McCance, R T Owen, K P Rao, M Sherman, N Sisodia, R Stocking-Korzen

Psychiatry of Old Age Dr Balakrishnan, J Hartman, E Komocki, S Pore, S Thacker

Resource Centre Day Hospital
Mental Health Resource Centre, London Road, Derby DE1 2QY
Tel: 01332 254818 Fax: 01332 254936

St Oswald's Hospital
Belle Vue Road, Ashbourne DE6 1AU
Tel: 01335 342121 Fax: 01335 300599
Total Beds: 40

Derwentside Primary Care Trust

Headquarters, Shotley Bridge Community Hospital, Consett DH8 0NB
Tel: 01207 594458 Fax: 01207 594438
Email: info@derwentsidepct.nhs.uk
Website: www.derwentside-pct.nhs.uk
(County Durham and Tees Valley Strategic Health Authority)

Chair Peter Innes
Chief Executive Wynn Griffiths

Devon Partnership NHS Trust

Wonford House Hospital, Dryden Road, Exeter EX2 5AF
Tel: 01392 403433 Fax: 01392 208663
Website: www.devonpartnership.nhs.uk
(South West Peninsula Strategic Health Authority)

Chair Keith Portlock
Chief Executive Iain Tulley
Consultants Andrew Blewett, David Jeffrey, Matthew Sewell, David Somerfield

Franklyn Hospital
Franklyn Drive, St Thomas, Exeter EX2 9HF
Tel: 01392 208400 Fax: 01392 208420
Total Beds: 35

Langdon Hospital
Exeter Road, Dawlish EX7 0NR
Tel: 01626 888372
Total Beds: 70

Forensic Psychiatry C E Dorkins, A James

Wonford House Hospital
Dryden Road, Exeter EX2 5AF
Tel: 01392 403433 Fax: 01392 403477
Total Beds: 103

General Psychiatry M Briscoe, R Hill, T Packer, R I L Tillett

Doncaster and Bassetlaw Hospitals NHS Foundation Trust

Established as a Foundation Trust 01/04/2004.

Doncaster Royal Infirmary, Armthorpe Road, Doncaster DN2 5LT
Tel: 01302 366666 Fax: 01302 320098
Website: www.dbh.nhs.uk
(South Yorkshire Strategic Health Authority)

Chair Margaret Cox
Chief Executive Nigel Clifton

Bassetlaw District General Hospital
Blyth Road, Worksop S81 0BD
Tel: 01909 500990 Fax: 01909 502246
Total Beds: 356

Manager Mary Mitchell

Accident and Emergency A Wright (Head), L El-Hag, M El-Salamani

Anaesthetics A M Dixon, R Harris, A J N Renshaw, A Salim, N U Saqib, P Smith

Dermatology B Bittiner (Head)

ENT K Hughes (Head), J Dugar, M Watson

General Medicine M Al-Khoffash, A Alwail, P Chaturvedi, C L Corbett, S Kar-Purkayastha, M M Muthiah

General Surgery R Avill, I Crate, K M Kolar, J Muen

Haematology B Paul

Obstetrics and Gynaecology H Gergis (Head), M Alloub, M Mammo, H J Mellows, M Michel, Mr Solomonsz

Ophthalmology L R Kolli, A Mishra

Orthopaedics M J Farhan, A Mubashir, J U R Panezai, K Shahi, M Zeraati

Paediatrics S J Bodden, H S Mulenga, L H P Williams

Pathology A Anathhanam, A Moffatt, B Paul

Radiology R K Goel, J Howard, C R Merrill

Rheumatology R Amos, A Khoffash

Doncaster Royal Infirmary
Armthorpe Road, Doncaster DN2 5LT
Tel: 01302 366666 Fax: 01302 320098
Total Beds: 800

Accident and Emergency J R Paskins (Head), A Wright

Anaesthetics D Wood (Head), D Graham, T J Hughes, J Jessop, W Karunaratne, G Kesseler, T Kirkpatrick, B R Milne, M Neal, D Northwood, C D Palmer, I Raghavjee, D Raithatha, P Shannon, A Strachan, J A Train

Cardiothoracic Medicine J A Thorpe

Chemical Pathology C E Wilde

Child Psychiatry M Kurian (Head), M Dix

Dental Surgery K Hughes (Head), A Holmes, R K L Lee, J P Simpson

Dermatology S B Bittiner (Head), S B Bittiner, H C McGrath

Elderly Care R Bolton (Head), D K Chadha, A J Oates, A Rajathurai

ENT K B Hughes (Head), J M Dugar, P Harkness, M Watson

General Medicine R Bolton (Head), E W Jones (Head), Z Alsindi, M W Baig, D Chadha, M Highcock, J Hosker, G James, S Kang, J R Lambert, R J E Leggett, A Oates, G Payne, A Rajathurai, T Rogers, J Sayer

General Surgery J Bagley (Head), J Coker, G B Coombes, R J Cuschieri, J K Darrad, G Jacob, N Kazzazi, K Khamis, J Leveckis, J V Psaila, S Singh

Genitourinary Medicine T Moss (Head)

Haematology R Bolton (Head), J Joseph, G Majumdar

Histopathology S Beck (Head), G Kurian, S Rogers, A Sheehan, L Sheehan, A Verghese

Medical Microbiology R Bolton (Head), L A Jewes

Neurology R Bolton (Head), S Howell

Obstetrics and Gynaecology H Gergis (Head), M Alloub, G P Chandler, E Emovon, P Iqbal, W K Moores, P Pisal

Ophthalmology K B Hughes (Head), S P Desai, G Jayamanne, V Kayarkar, L R Kolli, P J Noble

Orthodontics K B Hughes (Head), A Holmes, J P Simpson

Orthopaedics P Fagg (Head), M Al-Khatib, R Helm, J G Matthews, M Pickin, J F Redden, T S F Tadross

Paediatrics M Kurian (Head), S Ahmad, W A Arrowsmith, V Desai, P Field, J Inglis, D Keene, M Madlom

Radiology P Stannard (Head), N Dugar, J Y Mackinlay, P C Martin, D Monaghan, A Sinanan, D G Williams, Q Yamani

Rheumatology and Rehabilitation J Lambert (Head)

Vascular Surgery R Cuschieri (Head), J V Psaila, S Singh, P Tan

Plastic Surgery T M Brotherston

Urology J Leveckis, K Siddiqui, I Townend

Montagu Hospital

Adwick Road, Mexborough S64 0AZ
Tel: 01709 585171 Fax: 01709 571689
Total Beds: 115

Manager Roy Tyson

Anaesthetics M C Hudson, T Kirkpatrick, D Northwood, H H Raithatha

ENT M Watson

General Medicine D N Cooper (Head), R J Leigh (Head), E W Jones

General Surgery R J Cuschieri, J V Psaila

Obstetrics and Gynaecology W K Moores

Ophthalmology P J Noble

Orthopaedics P S Fagg, R Helm

Paediatrics J Inglis

Pathology S Beck, L A Jewes

Radiology J Y Mackinlay, P C Martin, D Monaghan, U Patel, P Stannard, D A Ward

Retford Hospital

North Road, Retford DN22 7XF
Tel: 01777 705261 Fax: 01777 710535

Paediatrics S J Bodden, H S Mulenga, L H P Williams

Pathology B Paul

Radiology Dr Goel, J Howard, C R Merrill

Tickhill Road Hospital

Doncaster DN4 8QL
Tel: 01302 796000 Fax: 01302 796066
Total Beds: 110

Manager Chris Ellingsworth

Elderly Rehabilitation Service D K Chadha (Head), A J Oates, A Rajathurai

Doncaster and South Humber Healthcare NHS Trust

St Catherine's House, St Catherine's, Tickhill Road, Balby, Doncaster DN4 8QN
Tel: 01302 796000 Fax: 01302 796161
Website: www.dash.nhs.uk
(North and East Yorkshire and Northern Lincolnshire Strategic Health Authority; South Yorkshire Strategic Health Authority)

Chair Madeleine Keyworth
Chief Executive Gillian Fairfield

Diana Princess of Wales Hospital

Scartho Road and Dudley Street, Grimsby DN33 2BA
Tel: 01472 874111
Total Beds: 58

Doncaster Gate Hospital

Doncaster Gate, Rotherham S65 1DW
Tel: 01709 820000 ext: 3320 Fax: 01709 304890

Child and Adolescent Psychiatry I Cariapa, M G Thomas

Doncaster Royal Infirmary (Psychiatric Unit)

Armthorpe Road, Doncaster DN2 5LT
Tel: 01302 366666
Total Beds: 82

Loversall Hospital

Weston Road, Balby, Doncaster DN4 8NX
Tel: 01302 796000 Fax: 01302 796066
Total Beds: 127

Rehabilitation Medicine M O'Leary

Rotherham General Hospital Mental Health Unit

Rotherham S60 2UD

St Catherine's

Tickhill Road, Doncaster DN4 8QN
Tel: 01302 796000 Fax: 01302 796066
Total Beds: 87

General Psychiatry J Roberts, N W H Silvester

St John's Hospice

Weston Road, Doncaster DN4 8QL
Tel: 01302 311611 Fax: 01302 796660

Scunthorpe General Hospital (Ward 18)

Cliff Gardens, Scunthorpe DN15 7BH
Tel: 01724 282282 Ext: 2651
Total Beds: 29

General Psychiatry A Chaudhary, B Saleh

Tickhill Road Hospital

Tickhill Road, Balby, Doncaster DN4 8QN
Tel: 01302 796000

Care of the Elderly D K Chandha, A J Oates, A Rajathurai

Elderly Mentally Ill M Broughton, K Wildgoose

Doncaster Central Primary Care Trust

White Rose House, Ten Pound Walk, Doncaster DN4 5DJ
Tel: 01302 320111 Fax: 01302 730362
Email: enquiries@doncastercentralpct.nhs.uk
Website: www.doncastercentralpct.nhs.uk
(South Yorkshire Strategic Health Authority)

Chair Roni Chapman
Chief Executive Simon Morritt

Doncaster East Primary Care Trust

White Rose House, Ten Pound Walk, Doncaster DN4 5DJ
Tel: 01302 320111 Fax: 01302 365234
Website: www.doncastereastpct.nhs.uk
(South Yorkshire Strategic Health Authority)

Chair Roger Greenwood
Chief Executive Christine Boswell

Doncaster West Primary Care Trust

West Lodge, St Catherine's Hospital, Tickhill Road, Doncaster DN4 8QN
Tel: 01302 796796 Fax: 01302 796801
Email: enquiries@doncasterwestpct.nhs.uk
Website: www.doncasterwestpct.nhs.uk
(South Yorkshire Strategic Health Authority)

Chair Ian Olsson
Chief Executive Michael Potts
Consultants Liz Burroughs, Anthony Wilkinson

Dorset Ambulance NHS Trust

Ringwood Road, St Leonards, Ringwood BH24 2SP
Tel: 01202 851640 Fax: 01202 851675
Email: chief.exec@dorsetambulance.nhs.uk
Website: www.dorset.swest.nhs.uk/ambulance/
(Dorset and Somerset Strategic Health Authority)

Chair Trevor Jones
Chief Executive Ken Wenman

Dorset HealthCare NHS Trust

11 Shelley Road, Boscombe, Bournemouth BH1 4JQ
Tel: 01202 303400 Fax: 01202 301798
Email: enquiries@dorsethc-tr.swest.nhs.uk
Website: www.dorsethealthcare.nhs.uk
(Dorset and Somerset Strategic Health Authority)

Chair Michael Parkinson
Chief Executive Roger Browning

Alderney Hospital

Ringwood Road, Poole BH12 4NB
Tel: 01202 735537 Fax: 01202 730657
Total Beds: 103

Mental Health D Cope (Head), M Ford (Head), D Cope, Dr Mynors-Wallis, S Pearson, P Rogers, S Sinha, J Smithers, A Wenzerul

Rehabilitation M Thomas (Head)

Flaghead Unit

Fairmile House, Tasman Close, Jumpers Road, Christchurch BH23 2JT
Tel: 01202 484250 Fax: 01202 496117
Total Beds: 10

Rehabilitation N Choudry (Head)

Hahnemann House

Hahnemann Road, West Cliff, Bournemouth BH2 5JW
Tel: 01202 584400 Fax: 01202 584416

Manager Rebecca Jones

Acute Day Hospital R Allen (Head)

Rehabilitation S Rastogi

Kings Park Hospital

Gloucester Road, Boscombe, Bournemouth BH7 6JE
Tel: 01202 303757 Fax: 01202 395738
Total Beds: 54

Manager Dianne Robinson

Elderly Mentally Ill G Brown (Head), J Hewitt, N Pearson

Learning Disabilities S Ghosh (Head), D Scull

Nightingale House/Nightingale Court

Alumhurst Road, Westbourne, Bournemouth BH4 8EW
Tel: 01202 584300 Fax: 01202 584311
Total Beds: 37

Forensic S Beer (Head)

Rehabilitation S Rastogi (Head)

Oakley House

15 Oakley Lane, Canford Magna, Wimborne BH21 1SF
Tel: 01202 849031 Fax: 01202 849031
Total Beds: 19

Elderly Mentally Ill S Kerwick (Head)

St Ann's Hospital

69 Haven Road, Canford Cliffs, Poole BH13 7LN
Tel: 01202 708881 Fax: 01202 707628
Total Beds: 145

Manager Anna Lewis

Alcohol and Substance Abuse N Choudry (Head)

Elderly Mentally Ill D Cope (Head), G Brown, J Hewitt, N Pearson, J Smithies

Forensic Psychiatry S Beer (Head)

General Psychiatry M Ford (Head), J Bonello, J Bray, L Mynors-Wallis, S Pearson, S Rastogi, G Searle, A Wenzerul

Springbourne House

22 Tower Road, Boscombe, Bournemouth BH1 4LB
Tel: 01202 300024 Fax: 01202 396844
Total Beds: 17

Elderly Mentally Ill J Smithies (Head)

Dudley Beacon and Castle Primary Care Trust

St John's House, Union Street, Dudley DY2 8PP
Tel: 01384 366111 Fax: 01384 366110
Website: www.dudley.nhs.uk
(Birmingham and the Black Country Strategic Health Authority)

Chair Rachel Harris
Chief Executive Robert Bacon

Bushey Fields Hospital

Russells Hall, Dudley DY1 2LZ
Tel: 01384 457373
Total Beds: 168

Ridge Hill Mental Handicap Unit

Stourbridge DY8 5ST
Tel: 01384 457373
Total Beds: 71

General Psychiatry A C Butler

Paediatrics A Sharma

Dudley Group of Hospitals NHS Trust

C Block, Pensnett Road, Russells Hall Hospital, Dudley DY1 2HQ
Tel: 01384 456111 Fax: 01384 244051
Website: www.dgoh.nhs.uk
(Birmingham and the Black Country Strategic Health Authority)

Chair Alfred Edwards
Chief Executive Paul Farenden

Corbett Hospital
Stourbridge DY8 4JB
Tel: 01384 456111
Total Beds: 150

Anaesthetics K Arunsalam, T V Gnanadurai, P M Scriven

Cardiology C Barr, E J Flint, P Forsey

Care of the Elderly A K Banerjee, W A Saunders

Chest Disease M J Cushley, M Doherty

Dermatology Dr Basheer

Gastroenterology A N Hamlyn, B Jones

General Medicine R S Smith, A M Zalin

General Surgery R P Grimley, A P Jayatunga

Neurology R N Corston

Orthodontics M Hammond

Orthopaedics M S Ali, M Butt, R Mifsud

Radiology L Arkell, F H B Renny, A P Wolinski

Urology A D Rowse

Guest Hospital
Tipton Road, Dudley DY1 4SE
Tel: 01384 456111

Anaesthetics T V Gnanadurai

Dermatology Dr Basheer

Genitourinary Medicine Dr El-Dalil, S Oojoo

Ophthalmology S V Aggarwal, J Al-Ibrahim

Rheumatology J P Delamere

Russells Hall Hospital
Dudley DY1 2HQ
Tel: 01384 456111 Fax: 01384 244051
Total Beds: 435

Accident and Emergency R Blayney, I K Dukes, A Mukherjee, C Read

Anaesthetics P Whitehurst

Cardiology C Barr, E J Flint, P Forsey

Dermatology A Basheer

General Medicine S Sivakumar, R S Smith, J Stellmjan

General Surgery R Blunt, R P Grimley, A P Jayatunga, R Patel, A P Savage, K F Yoong

Obstetrics and Gynaecology R Callender, N Fiz-Gibbons, G J Lewis, L Meer, E Watson

Orthodontics M Hammond

Paediatrics Z Ibrahim, Dr Mohite, R Mudgal, A Sharma

Plastic Surgery M Ali, A Bracka, S Sarhadi

Radiology L Arkell, J El-Ibrahim, F H B Renny, A P Wolinski

Rheumatology J P Delamere, G Kitas, A Whallett

Urology L Emtage, A D Rowse

Wordsley Hospital
Stourbridge DY8 5QX
Tel: 01384 456111 Fax: 01384 244395
Total Beds: 368

Anaesthetics E Acquah, K Arunsalam, L Burke, J Danks, T J Digger, H Funkel, T V Gnanadurai, A Moors, P Scriven, J Tye, P Whitehurst

Cardiology M Banks, C Barr, E Flint, P Forsey

Care of the Elderly A Banerjee, S Mandel, J Stellman

Dental Surgery N Grew, N Whear

ENT N C Molony, R T J Shortridge, F Wilson

General Medicine M J Cushley, M Doherty, T Fiad, N Fisher, A N Hamlyn, M Healey, B Jones

General Surgery R Blunt, R Patel, A P Savage

Neurology R N Corston, R Etti

Ophthalmology S P Aggarwal, J Al-Ibrahim, M Quinian, S Shafquat

Oral and Maxillofacial Surgery N M Whear

Orthopaedics M Ahmed, M S Ali, R Mifsud, Dr Subzposh, K Sulaiman

Pathology S Ghosh, P Harrison, M Labib, J Neilson, E Rees, J M Symonds, Dr Wasfi

Radiology L Arkell, A Gregan, P Oliver, F H B Renny, R Shave, A P Wolinski

Radiotherapy and Oncology R Allerton

Dudley South Primary Care Trust

Trust Headquarters, Ridgehill, Brierley Hill Road, Stourbridge DY8 5ST
Tel: 01384 457373 Fax: 01384 400217
Website: www.dudley.nhs.uk
(Birmingham and the Black Country Strategic Health Authority)

Chair David Ibbs
Chief Executive Chris Potter

Durham and Chester-le-Street Primary Care Trust

John Snow House, Durham University Science Park, Durham DH1 3YG
Tel: 0191 301 1328 Fax: 0191 301 1427
Website: www.durhamcls-pct.nhs.uk
(County Durham and Tees Valley Strategic Health Authority)

Chair Ann Calman
Chief Executive Andrew Young

Durham Dales Primary Care Trust

16 Tenters Street, Bishop Auckland DL14 7AD
Tel: 01388 458835 Fax: 01388 458905
Website: www.durhamdales-pct.co.uk
(County Durham and Tees Valley Strategic Health Authority)

Chair Anne Beeton
Chief Executive Andrew Kenworthy
Consultants David Landes, Jean Mather, Jonny Skinner

Ealing Hospital NHS Trust

Ealing Hospital, Uxbridge Road, Southall UB1 3HW
Tel: 020 8967 5000 Fax: 020 8967 5630
Email: firstname.surname@eht.nhs.uk
Website: www.ealinghospital.org.uk
(North West London Strategic Health Authority)

Chair Tony Caplin
Chief Executive Fiona Wise

Ealing Hospital
Uxbridge Road, Southall UB1 3HW
Tel: 020 8967 5000 Fax: 020 8967 5630
Total Beds: 361

Accident and Emergency S Payne (Head), J Redhead

Anaesthetics B J Bracey, E Bradshaw, R Laishley, M Meurer-Laban, M Renna, C Schmulian, R Skinner, E Whitehead

Chemical Pathology P Holloway (Head)

Chest Disease R Mathur (Head), R Mathur, M Rudolf

Dermatology A Chu (Head), K Acland, R Russell-Jones

ENT N Tolley (Head), K Patel

General Medicine J D Arnold (Head), J Kooner, N I McNeil, H M Mather, S Rosen

General Surgery D Sellu (Head), P Abel, P Forouhi, G Geroulakis, A Isla, T Rosenbaum

Genitourinary Medicine B Lynn (Head)

Haematology U Hegde (Head), G Abrahamson, N Phillpott

Infectious Diseases S Ash (Head), W Lynn

Neurology H Jenkins

Obstetrics and Gynaecology Y Abrahams (Head), L Fusi, A Gordon, A D Haeri, N Mahadevan

Orthopaedics M Beverley (Head), M J Evans, R Thomas

Paediatrics M Cummins (Head), N Hasson, C Michie, K Sloper

Radiology W Svensson (Head), Professor Lavender, P R Patel, Dr Stroudley, T Tran

Radiotherapy and Oncology C Lewanski (Head), P Price, S Stewart

Rheumatology and Rehabilitation M Hogarth (Head), M Naughton

Ealing Primary Care Trust

1 Armstrong Way, Southall UB2 4SA
Tel: 020 8893 0303 Fax: 020 8893 0398
Website: www.ealingpct.nhs.uk
(North West London Strategic Health Authority)

Chair Marion Saunders
Chief Executive Robert Creighton

Clayponds Hospital
Sterling Place, London W5 4RN
Tel: 020 8560 4011
Total Beds: 66

Ealing Day Treatment Centre
Britton Drive, Southall UB1 2SH
Tel: 020 8571 1143 Fax: 020 8574 6510

Easington Primary Care Trust

Health Partnership Centre, Unit 2 Fern Court, Bracken Hill Business Park, Easington, Peterlee SR8 2RR
Tel: 0191 587 4800 Fax: 0191 587 4878
Email: info@easingtonpct.nhs.uk
Website: www.easington-pct.nhs.uk
(County Durham and Tees Valley Strategic Health Authority)

Chair Ken Greenfield
Chief Executive Roger Bolas

East and North Hertfordshire NHS Trust

Lister Hospital, Coleys Mill Lane, Stevenage SG1 4AB
Tel: 01438 314333
Website: www.enherts-tr.nhs.uk
(Bedfordshire and Hertfordshire Strategic Health Authority)

Chair Richard Beazley
Chief Executive Nick Carver

Ascots Day Hospital
Howlands, Welwyn Garden City AL7 4HQ

Danesbury
Welwyn AL6 9PW
Tel: 01438 840692
Total Beds: 30

Elderly Care Day Hospital, Lister Hospital
Strathmore Wing, Lister Hospital, Stevenage SG1 4AB
Tel: 01438 314333 Fax: 01438 781449

Hertford County Hospital
North Road, Hertford SG14 1LP

Hitchin Hospital
Oughtonhead Way, Hitchin SG5 2LH
Tel: 01462 422444
Total Beds: 44

Lister Hospital
Coreys Mill Lane, Stevenage SG1 4AB
Tel: 01438 314333 Fax: 01438 781442
Total Beds: 630

Accident and Emergency P D Kelly, P M Reid

Anaesthetics O W Boomers, M R Chilvers, S J Eckersall, G Gowrie-Mohan, K Jani, S Jothilingam, J M Lalor, P Patel, W J K Rickford, P Sengupta, I Sockalingham, J Thiagarajan, L Wickremasinghe

Audiological Medicine B Al-Shihabi

Cardiology C D J Illesley, M Lynch, V Paul

Cardiothoracic Surgery A Rees

Care of the Elderly M Ehsanullah, P Ghosh, S Khan

Chest Disease N N Stanley

Dermatology C A Green

ENT A Frosh, G Mochloulis, S J Quinn

Gastroenterology A Catterall, S Greenfield, I Sargeant

General Medicine L J Borthwick

General Surgery T C Holme, A Mahomed, B V Palmer, S Selvakumar, H H Thompson

Genitourinary Medicine H Maiti, S Uthayakumar

Nephrology K Farrington, R N Greenwood, P Warwicker

Neurology J M Gibbs, T T Warner

Obstetrics and Gynaecology Dr Banerjee, D R Salvesen, R S Sattin, W Tenuwara, J B Webb

Oral and Maxillofacial Surgery A D Giles, M T Simpson

Orthodontics A B Hewitt

Orthopaedics J H Dorrell, P G Hope, P S Kerr, D P Powles, S Wickremsinghe

Paediatrics O A Ahmed, R D Croft, S A Davies, J C Hyde, J Reiser

Pathology A MacDonald, D J Madders, A Rainey, C J Tew, L L Yong

Plastic Surgery M G Dickson, N K James, P J Mahaffey

Radiology N D Amerasekera, J S M Beales, P T Brooks, C M P King, H M Lee, C M Prendergast

Radiotherapy and Oncology B E Lyn, A R Makepeace

Restorative Dentistry A J McCullock

Rheumatology and Rehabilitation A I Binder

Urology G Boustead, D Hanbury, T A McNicholas

Queen Elizabeth II Hospital

Howlands, Welwyn Garden City AL7 4HQ
Tel: 01707 328111
Total Beds: 550

Accident and Emergency V Gautam, Y Saetta

Anaesthetics S Bates, M Fox, P Goldberg, A Maye, M A Moxon, Z P Shah, S Susay, T Walker

Care of the Elderly O Feizi, M Seeveratnam

Dermatology A H Bayoumi, C J O'Doherty

General Medicine A Catterall, R G Dent, S Greenfield, P M Keir, P McIntyre, P Winocour

General Surgery M Aldridge, P Crane, M Dickson, M S Lennox, S Lok, J L McCue

Neurology D Kidd, R W Orrell

Obstetrics and Gynaecology R Atalla, N C Drew, M Hemaya, D G McLintock

Oncology C Coulter, B E Lynn, A Makepeace

Ophthalmology S Campbell, T Coker, B S Sandhu, M Toma

Orthopaedics T Kitson, H V Parmar, M C Stallard, A Waterfield

Paediatrics J Chiyende, A K M Raffles, S Shukia, A M L Shurz

Pathology M Al-Izzi, H P Davis, A Fattah, N Fernando, M Fyffe, J Voke

Radiology B E Hartley, H I Jory, S Khan, A H Lynn, C Ropel

Rheumatology J Axon

Urology J Vanwaevenbergh

Queen Victoria Memorial Hospital

Welwyn AL6 9PW
Tel: 01438 714488
Total Beds: 40

Care of the Elderly M Seevaratnam

Western House Hospital

Collett Road, Ware SG12 7LZ
Tel: 01920 68954
Total Beds: 30

Care of the Elderly O Feizi, M Seeveratnam

East Anglian Ambulance NHS Trust

Hospital Lane, Hellesdon, Norwich NR6 5NA
Tel: 01603 424255 Fax: 01603 418667
Website: www.eastanglianambulance.com
(Norfolk, Suffolk and Cambridgeshire Strategic Health Authority)

Chair Andrew Egerton-Smith
Chief Executive Chris Carney

East Cambridgeshire and Fenland Primary Care Trust

Fenland View, Alexandra Road, Wisbech PE13 1HQ
Tel: 01945 469400 Fax: 01945 469401
Website: www.eastcambsandfenland-pct.nhs.uk
(Norfolk, Suffolk and Cambridgeshire Strategic Health Authority)

Chair Allyson Broadhurst
Chief Executive Audrey Bradford

Doddington Community Hospital

Benwick Road, Doddington, March PE15 0UG
Tel: 01634 585781

North Cambridgeshire Hospital

The Park, Wisbech PE13 3AB
Tel: 01945 585781 Fax: 01945 584316

The Princess of Wales Hospital

Lynn Road, Ely CB6 1DN
Tel: 01353 652000 Fax: 01353 652003
Total Beds: 34

East Cheshire NHS Trust

Macclesfield District General Hospital, Victoria Road, Macclesfield SK10 3BL
Tel: 01625 421000 Fax: 01625 661644
Website: www.echeshire-tr.nwest.nhs.uk
(Cheshire and Merseyside Strategic Health Authority)

Chair Kathy Cowell
Chief Executive John Wilbraham

Congleton and District War Memorial Hospital

Canal Road, Congleton CW12 3AR
Tel: 01260 294800 Fax: 01260 294827
Total Beds: 28

Manager Chris Jervis

Cardiology A Cubukcu

Dermatology Dr Griffiths, T Kingston

ENT J A J Deans

General Medicine C Davison, P N Foster

General Surgery W A Brough, N J Gathercole, D M Matheson

Minor Operations N J Gathercole

Obstetrics and Gynaecology P Dunlop

Ophthalmology L B Freeman

Orthopaedics G W Keys, M G Norris

Paediatrics I E Losa

Radiology C Loughran

Rheumatology S Knight, D Symmons

Urology D Holden

Knutsford and District Community Hospital
Bexton Road, Knutsford WA16 0ED
Tel: 01565 632112 Fax: 01565 632544
Total Beds: 18

Manager Chris Jervis

Cardiology R Egdell

Chest Disease R J Stead

Dermatology T Kingston

Diabetes S Srivastava

ENT J E Davies

General Medicine J Walker

General Surgery D M Matheson

Obstetrics and Gynaecology V Hall

Orthopaedics G W Keys

Paediatrics K Marinaki

Rheumatology S M Knight

Urology D Holden

Macclesfield District General Hospital
Victoria Road, Macclesfield SK10 3BL
Tel: 01625 663306 Fax: 01625 663963
Total Beds: 366

Accident and Emergency N J Gathercole, M Nicol, A Robertson

Anaesthetics P B Backx, D Banks, A P Gorman, J Hunter, S B Rawal, M Rothwell, A J Shribman

Community Paediatrics L Batchelor

Dental Surgery D Eldridge, M Patel

Dermatology T Griffiths, T Kingston

ENT J E Davies, J A Deans

General Medicine M Babores, P N Foster, J V E Roche, R J Stead, D J Walker

General Surgery Dr Brough, D M Matheson, A R Quayle, C Roshanlall

Genitourinary Medicine M H Khan, Dr Morgan

Nephrology M C Venning

Neurology N J MacDermott

Neurosurgery P L Richardson

Obstetrics and Gynaecology S Dean, P Dunlop, V Hall, V A Lether, S Mellor

Oncology S Davidson

Ophthalmology A Hubbard, A Needham, M A Neugebauer

Orthodontics R T P Thompson

Orthopaedics K Barnes, G W Keys, M G Norris, M Waseem

Paediatrics J Gilbert, Dr Laudsans, I E Losia, K Marinaki, J R Owens, I Spillman

Palliative Medicine T Rimmer

Pathology C Burrows, J G Hudson, A R Williams, A Wills

Radiology A D Baxter, J Coffey, Dr Crotch-Harvey, C F Loughran, E Partridge, R Sill

Rheumatology S M Knight, D Symmons

Urology D Holden, S Namasivayam

East Devon Primary Care Trust

Dean Clarke House, Southernhay East, Exeter EX1 1PQ
Tel: 01392 207521 Fax: 01392 270910
Website: www.eastdevon-pct.nhs.uk
(South West Peninsula Strategic Health Authority)

Chair Lynda Price
Chief Executive Hugh Groves

Axminster Hospital
Chard Road, Axminster EX13 5DU
Tel: 01297 32071
Total Beds: 43

Manager Lily Chapman

Budleigh Salterton Hospital
Budleigh Salterton EX9 6HF
Tel: 01395 442020
Total Beds: 20

Manager Les Hickman

Exmouth Hospital
Claremount Grove, Exmouth EX8 2JN
Tel: 01395 279684
Total Beds: 43

Manager Les Hickman

Honiton Hospital
Marlpits Lane, Honiton EX14 2DE
Tel: 01404 540540 Fax: 01404 540550
Total Beds: 32

Manager Paul Boult

Ottery St Mary Hospital
Keegan Close, Ottery St Mary EX11 1DN
Tel: 01404 816000 Fax: 01404 816030
Total Beds: 25

Manager Paul Boult

Seaton and District Community Hospital
Valley View, Scalwell Lane, Seaton EX12 2DU
Tel: 01297 23901 Fax: 01297 24252
Total Beds: 28

Manager Lily Chapman

Sidmouth Hospital
All Saints Road, Sidmouth EX10 8EW
Tel: 01395 512482
Total Beds: 34

Manager Paul Boult

Victoria Cottage Hospital
Sidmouth EX10 8EW
Tel: 01395 512482 Fax: 01395 579326
Total Beds: 34

East Elmbridge and Mid Surrey Primary Care Trust

Cedar Court, Guilford Road, Fetcham, Leatherhead KT22 9RX
Tel: 01372 227300 Fax: 01372 732595
Website: www.eastsurreyhealth.nhs.uk
(Surrey and Sussex Strategic Health Authority)

Chair Jackie Bell
Chief Executive Alan Kennedy

Caterham Dene Hospital
Church Road, Caterham CR3 5RA
Tel: 01883 349324 Fax: 01883 346978
Total Beds: 20

Manager Mark Ogden

Care of the Elderly V Phongsathorn

ENT G Warrington

General Medicine K J Foster

Obstetrics and Gynaecology P Townsend

Ophthalmology S Chatterjee

Orthopaedics H Maurice

Paediatrics M Jawad

Urology P Miller

Dorking Community Hospital
Horsham Road, Dorking RH4 2AA
Tel: 01737 768511 Fax: 01306 741635
Total Beds: 28

Molesey Hospital
High Street, West Molesey KT8 2LU
Tel: 020 8941 4481 Fax: 020 8941 8056
Total Beds: 26

East Hampshire Primary Care Trust

Raebarn House, 3rd Floor, Hulbert Road, Waterlooville PO7 7GP
Tel: 023 9224 8800 Fax: 023 9224 8810
Website: www.easthampshirepct.nhs.uk
(Hampshire and Isle of Wight Strategic Health Authority)

Chair Margaret Scott
Chief Executive John Wilderspin

Havant War Memorial Hospital
59 Crossway, Havant PO9 1NG
Tel: 023 9248 4256
Total Beds: 23

Petersfield Community Hospital
Swan Street, Petersfield GU32 3LB
Tel: 01730 263221
Total Beds: 54

Victoria Cottage Hospital
8 North Street, Emsworth PO10 7DD
Tel: 01243 376041
Total Beds: 15

East Kent Coastal Teaching Primary Care Trust

Protea House, New Bridge, Marine Parade, Dover CT17 9HQ
Tel: 01304 227227 Fax: 01304 225775
Email: ekcpct.enquiries@ekentha.nhs.uk
Website: www.eastkentcoastalpct.nhs.uk
(Kent and Medway Strategic Health Authority)

Chair Jan Askew
Chief Executive Darren Grayson

East Kent Hospitals NHS Trust

Kent and Canterbury Hospital, Ethelbert Road, Canterbury CT1 3NG
Tel: 01227 766877 Fax: 01227 864135
Email: general.enquiries@ekht.nhs.uk
Website: www.kentandmedway.nhs.uk
(Kent and Medway Strategic Health Authority)

Chair George Jenkins
Chief Executive David Astley

Buckland Hospital
Coombe Valley Road, Buckland, Dover CT14 0HD
Tel: 01304 201624 Fax: 01304 214371
Total Beds: 71

Manager Stewart Nisbet

Anaesthetics H G C Bradfield, J N Bulmer, J E Morris

Care of the Elderly M A Vella

Dermatology V Neild

ENT P Robinson

General Medicine G W Bradley, S Kenwright, A J R Morris, P G Wheeler

General Psychiatry M F S Abdurahman

General Surgery T Bates, A M Deane, C D Derry, N J Griffiths, D Keown, J F McPartlin

Haematology D G Wells

Neurology A C F Colchester

Obstetrics and Gynaecology C M Stewart, W Ursell

Orthopaedics M Lock, R Wetherell

Paediatrics C A Porter, S Williamson

Pathology C W Lawson, N R Padley

Radiology D Nadarajah, P Paciorek, A Santhakumaran, R H F Waitt, W H Webb

Radiotherapy and Oncology R Coltart, H M Smedley

Rheumatology and Rehabilitation P W Bull, J R Sewell

Kent and Canterbury Hospital
Ethelbert Road, Canterbury CT1 3NG
Tel: 01227 766877 Fax: 01227 864120
Total Beds: 382

Manager Teo Vogiatzis

Anaesthetics A C Beaumont, B G Bradburn, J Coupe, H Dent, G R Hollister, Dr Jovanovic, C J Lamb, J MacKinnon, Dr Mayall, P Moskovits

Chest Disease A J Johnson

Child Health D Long

Dermatology D Goldin

ENT N Padgham (Head), D Mitchell

General Medicine D I Prosser, M O Rake, C I Roberts

General Surgery R E C Collins, R M Heddle, D B Jackson

Head and Neck A Diabiase

Health Case of Older People G Batty, A J Heller, S O'Riodan, A Owen, J M Potter, I Sturgess

Neurology J D P Bland, Professor Colchester, Dr Moran

Neurophysiology J D P Bland

Nuclear Medicine S Moorhouse, M J O'Doherty

Obstetrics and Gynaecology M P Milligan, K Neales, N M Rafla, L M Shaw

Ophthalmology N C Andrew, R De Cock, R S Edwards, W K Poon

Pathology J B M Winter

Radiology M O Downes, P G Elton, K G Entwisle, I Morrison

Radiotherapy and Oncology R S Coltart, N Mithal, H M Smedley

Renal Medicine Dr Abbas, Dr Delaney, Dr Farmer, Dr John, P Stevens, Dr Webb

Rheumatology R H Withrington

Trauma and Orthopaedics N Blackburn, P Housden, L Loulette

Urology H Evans, K H A Murray, N Shrotri

Queen Elizabeth The Queen Mother Hospital

St Peters Road, Margate CT9 4AN
Tel: 01843 225544 Fax: 01843 220048
Total Beds: 514

Manager Stewart Nisbet

Anaesthetics Dr Adegoke, Dr Ashfaque, Dr Ciccone, E Davies, C Guest, W E Morcos, G Perera, Dr Senashinghe, P Teli, B C Tofte, H J Wilton

Care of the Elderly Y Challiner, M L Jenkinson, S K Mukherjee

Chest Disease N Goldstack

Child Health E Abdelmagid, M Malik, E Rfidah, E Rfidah

Dental Surgery E G Asquith, T J Storrs

Dermatology D Goldin, M Hudson-Peacock

General Medicine J B Cocking, A Marshall, A D Morgan

General Surgery S Gibbs, D Marzout

Genitourinary Medicine C S Wijesurendra

Obstetrics and Gynaecology P V Belgaumkar, A Nordin, Mr Rafla, L M A Shaw, J Shervington

Radiology A H Abdel-Hadi, G Giancola, A M Greenhalgh

Rheumatology and Rehabilitation D DeLord, A Leak

Thoracic Surgery O J Lau

Trauma and Orthopaedics J Casha, M Cornell, S Jain, D Saran

Urology J H Evans, K H A Murray

Royal Victoria Hospital

Radnor Park Avenue, Folkestone CT19 5BN
Tel: 01303 850202 Fax: 01303 854433
Total Beds: 25

Manager Pat Watts

ENT J Fairley, C Howson, G S Kanegaonkar

Ophthalmology R S Edwards, J McConnell

Oral and Maxillofacial Surgery C Hendy

William Harvey Hospital

Kennington Road, Willesborough, Ashford TN24 0LZ
Tel: 01233 633331 Fax: 01233 616008
Total Beds: 573

Manager Pat Watts

Anaesthetics B Al-Shaikh, J Banks, R Bhadresha, H G C Bradfield, J Bulmer, J N Bulmer, T Bushnell, C Davies, S Dolenska, M Gardner, M Hamer, M Jones, A Macdonald, J Morris, A J Rampton, C Toner, A Vroemen-Cermakova, J Vroemen, N Yardy

ENT N Padgham (Head), J Fairley, G S Kanegaonkar, C Robinson, H R Sharp

Haematology V S Ratnayake

Ophthalmology M Fouladi, B Greaves, M Heravi

Oral and Maxillofacial Surgery F Coutts

Orthodontics F Coutts

Paediatrics Dr Birks, Dr Chandola, C Green, Dr Martin, Dr Newsom, Dr Rahman, Dr Saleh, V Shah, O Smith

Pathology A Abdulkadir, S Koslowski, B Maguire, R Oommen, P N Padley, M Pdrenyei, S Szakacs

Radiology Rand David, K Lashkari, P Paciorek, A Santhakumaran, W M Webb

Rheumatology and Rehabilitation P Bull, J Sewell

East Kent NHS and Social Care Partnership Trust

Trust Headquarters, Littlebourne Road, Canterbury CT1 1AZ
Tel: 01227 459371 Fax: 01227 812268
Email: val.woodin@ekentmht.nhs.uk
Website: www.ekct.nhs.uk
(Kent and Medway Strategic Health Authority)

Chair Mary Crittenden
Chief Executive Sue Hunt

St Martin's Hospital

Littlebourne Road, Canterbury CT1 1TD
Tel: 01227 459584 Fax: 01227 812268
Total Beds: 120

General Psychiatry S Anathakopan, B Beats, C Cook, S Wood

Psychology S Hewson

Thanet Mental Health Unit

164 Ramsgate Road, Margate
Tel: 01843 225544
Total Beds: 60

General Psychiatry M Hamour, T Helm, J Kaladini, G Rehling

Western Avenue Day Hospital

Ashford Hospital, Western Avenue, Ashford TN23 1LX
Tel: 01233 623321

East Lancashire Hospitals NHS Trust

Burnley General Hospital, Casterton Avenue, Burnley BB10 2PQ
Tel: 01282 425071 Fax: 01282 474444
Website: www.hospitalsineastlancs.nhs.uk
(Cumbria and Lancashire Strategic Health Authority)

Chair Christine Kirk
Chief Executive John Thomas

Blackburn Royal Infirmary

Bolton Road, Blackburn BB2 3LR
Tel: 01254 263555 Fax: 01254 294572
Total Beds: 322

Accident and Emergency T K George

Anaesthetics W G Hamlin

Cardiology A Myers

Chest Disease N Horsfield, L P Ormerod

Dental Surgery J C Lowry, M E Morton

Dermatology B M Daly

ENT A Abou-El-Farag, J R Cherry, P D Gooder, P Morar, M S Timms

General Medicine G Banait, D S Grimes, G R Jones, D A F Lynch, A Myers, S Ramtoola, L R Solomon

General Surgery D Chang, D A Evans, S C Hardy, R W Nicholson, J C Tresadern, R J Watson

Genitourinary Medicine S L Gayed

Neurology S Shaunak, P Tidswell

Ophthalmology M Abdul-Nabi, M Mohan, A G E Nylander, J P Roper, A Vijaykumar

Orthodontics G C S Cousin, M E Morton, G A Smith

Orthopaedics J L Barrie, J Leito, I G Lowrie, R Mohan, R W Paton, V B Shah, M S Srinivasan

Pathology D A Newsome

Plastic Surgery R P Jones

Rheumatology P J Smith, L S Teh

Urology D A Jones, D Neilson, G D Wymss-Holden

Burnley General Hospital
Casterton Avenue, Burnley BB10 2PQ
Tel: 01282 425071 Fax: 01282 474444
Total Beds: 622

Accident and Emergency S Bhattacharyya

Anaesthetics A Shakir, J C Watts

Cardiology R A Best, G Gladman

Dermatology I H Coulson, N Craven, B M Daly

ENT J R Cherry, A Farag, P D Gooder, M S Timms

General Medicine M N Goorah, A T Green, C E F Grimley, M D Littley, L J Patterson, S Pickens, S Sharma

General Surgery H Al-Khaffaf, T R Dilraj-Gopal, E Gross, A Rahi, D G D Sandilands, P D Scott

Neurology J D Mitchell

Neurosurgery A Golash

Obstetrics and Gynaecology F R Clarke, J M Cruickshank, F C Hamer, T C M Inglis, I W Mahady, H M Ribbans

Ophthalmology M J Abdul-Nabi, M Mohan, A G E Nylander, J P Roper, A Vijaykumar, G Wright

Oral Surgery G C S Cousin, A E Green, S G Langton

Orthodontics P A Banks

Orthopaedics L Markovic, H A J Marynissen, A N Saikia, R Sarin, G Schmitgen

Paediatrics P Ehrhardt, J Iqbal, I L Swann

Pathology J R Kendra

Plastic Surgery J K G Laitung

Rheumatology and Rehabilitation R Ariyaratnan, M J Burke

Urology A McGeorge, M Pillai, A Yakubu

Pendle Community Hospital
Leeds Road, Nelson BB9 9TF
Tel: 01282 474900 Fax: 01282 474980
Total Beds: 72

Queen's Park Hospital
Haslingden Road, Blackburn BB2 3HH
Tel: 01254 263555 Fax: 01254 293803
Total Beds: 414

Care of the Elderly N A Roberts, I Singh, E S Soliman

Obstetrics and Gynaecology N Ahmed, B Debroy, D Goodall, S R Hill, E A Martindale, S K Najia, P A O'Donovan, C H M Schram

Paediatrics J W T Benson, M Lama, K Rakshi, C P Smith

Rossendale Hospital
Haslingden Road, Rawtenstall, Rossendale BB4 6NE
Tel: 01706 215151 Fax: 01706 233210
Total Beds: 29

East Leeds Primary Care Trust

Oaktree House, 408 Oakwood Lane, Leeds LS8 3LG
Tel: 0113 305 9521 Fax: 0113 305 9523
Website: www.eastleeds-pct.nhs.uk
(West Yorkshire Strategic Health Authority)

Chair Linda Phipps
Chief Executive Liam Hughes

East Lincolnshire Primary Care Trust

East Lindsey Locality Office, c/o Louth County Hospital, High Holme Road, North Somercotes, Louth LN11 0EU
Tel: 01507 608342 Fax: 01507 354957
Website: www.eastlincs-pct.nhs.uk
(Trent Strategic Health Authority)

Chair Brian Wookey
Chief Executive Jane Froggatt

Johnson Hospital
Priory Road, Spalding PE11 2XD
Tel: 01775 722386
Total Beds: 28

Manager Andrea Bennett

Skegness and District Hospital
Dorothy Avenue, Skegness PE25 2BS
Tel: 01754 762401 Fax: 01754 760132
Total Beds: 39

Manager Andrea Bennett

Welland Hospital
Roman Bank, Spalding PE11 2HW
Tel: 01775 766800
Total Beds: 28

East London and The City Mental Health NHS Trust

St Clements Hospital, 2A Bow Road, London E3 4LL
Tel: 020 8880 6296 Fax: 020 8880 6250
Website: www.elcmht.nhs.uk
(North East London Strategic Health Authority)

Chair Roger Daily-Hunt
Chief Executive Sheila Foley

East Midlands Ambulance Service NHS Trust

Trust Headquarters, Beechdale Road, Bilborough, Nottingham NG8 3LL
Tel: 0115 929 6151 Fax: 0115 962 7727
Email: forename.sursame@emas.nhs.uk
Website: www.emas.nhs.uk
(Trent Strategic Health Authority)

Chair Chris Faircliffe
Chief Executive Paul Phillips

East Somerset NHS Trust

Yeovil District Hospital, Higher Kingston, Yeovil BA21 4AT
Tel: 01935 475122 Fax: 01935 426850
Email: ask@est.nhs.uk
Website: www.yeovilhospital.nhs.uk
(Dorset and Somerset Strategic Health Authority)

Chair Angela Dupont
Chief Executive James Scott

Yeovil District Hospital

Higher Kingston, Yeovil BA21 4AT
Tel: 01935 475122 Fax: 01935 426850
Total Beds: 354

Accident and Emergency P Ancill

Anaesthetics M Cornish, R Daum, C P Elsworth, S J Hunter, J Kerr, R M Kipling, G R G Purcell, T Scull, M Wootton

Dermatology J Boyle, Dr Downs, D Pryce

ENT G Ford, N B Hopkin, M O'Donnell

General Medicine F X M Beach, G S Brigden, G Chung, I W Fawcett, S Gore, J Grotto, Z H Khan, T Palferman, M Qadiri, K A Rashed, R Sinha

General Surgery H Gajraj, R Kennedy, M Niayesh, J Okrim, C Parker, T Porter, C Royle

Genitourinary Medicine M Fitzgerald

Haematology S Bolam, S Davies, S A N Johnson

Neurology E Farthers, D Foottit, P Heywood

Obstetrics and Gynaecology A J Davies, J Giles, O Osoba, M Zakaria

Ophthalmology L Bray, T Pathmanathan, A N Tadros

Oral and Maxillofacial Surgery M Davidson, J Hamlyn

Orthodontics Miss Atack, C N T Mitchell

Orthopaedics A Chambler, A Chambler, M J Maxted, N Naube, P Porter, D Shardlow, G Smibert, J A Tricker

Paediatrics J C Dearlove, M Eaton, P Heaton, J Higman, M J Smith

Pathology E Cooper, C Fisher, J Heaton, S Knowles

Plastic Surgery Mr Orlando, Mr Tiernan

Radiology J Baldwin, N C G Bathurst, J Hacking, M Hay, C Hopkins, W Saywell

Radiotherapy and Oncology S Falk, S Goodman

East Staffordshire Primary Care Trust

Edwin House, Second Avenue, Centrum 100, Burton-on-Trent DE14 2WF
Tel: 01283 507100 Fax: 01283 507200
Email: heather.evans@es-pct.nhs.uk
Website: www.eaststaffspct.nhs.uk
(Shropshire and Staffordshire Strategic Health Authority)

Chair Alex Fox
Chief Executive Kieron Murphy

East Surrey Primary Care Trust

St John's Court, 51 St John's Road, Redhill RH1 6DS
Tel: 01737 780209 Fax: 01737 767373
Email: enquiries@eastsurrey-pct.nhs.uk
Website: www.eastsurrey-pct.nhs.uk
(Surrey and Sussex Strategic Health Authority)

Chair Martin Kitchen
Chief Executive Elaine Best

East Sussex County Healthcare NHS Trust

Joint management team with West Sussex Health and Social Care NHS Trust.

Bowhill, The Drive, Hellingly, Hailsham BN27 4EP
Tel: 01323 440022 Fax: 01323 842868
Website: www.eastsussexcounty.nhs.uk
(Surrey and Sussex Strategic Health Authority)

Chair Dawn Burnett-Hitchcock
Chief Executive Lisa Rodrigues
Consultants S K Ahmed, P Argiriu, R Bowskill, R Canagaratnan, John Doe, Ros Foulds, J Hargreaves, Ze'ev Levita, Laurence McGibben, Patricia Rashbrook, Noel Swanson

Amberstone Mental Health Unit

Carters Corner, Hailsham BN27 4HG
Fax: 01323 844676
Total Beds: 24

Ashen Hill, Forensic Psychiatry Unit

The Drive, Hellingly, Hailsham BN27 4ER
Total Beds: 15

Roborough Day Hospital

Princess Alice Hospital, Carew Road, Eastbourne BN21 2AX
Tel: 01323 638972

Seaford Day Hospital

Sutton Road, Seaford BN25 2AX
Tel: 01323 490989

Southview Challenging Behaviour Unit

The Drive, Hellingly, Hailsham BN27 4ER
Tel: 01323 440022
Total Beds: 20

East Sussex Hospitals NHS Trust

Eastbourne District General Hospital, King's Drive, Eastbourne BN21 2UD
Tel: 01323 417400 Fax: 01323 417966
Website: www.esht.nhs.uk
(Surrey and Sussex Strategic Health Authority)

Chair John Lewis
Chief Executive Annette Sergeant

Bexhill Hospital

Holliers Hill, Bexhill-on-Sea TN40 2DZ
Tel: 01424 755255 Fax: 01424 213250
Total Beds: 50

Anaesthetics T Arnold, W G Doherty, I Hicks, A B Leach, J R Lethbridge, N McNeillis, M Parsloe, I Reeve, A Slater, J Stock, A Stoddart

Cardiology D Walker, R Wray

Care of the Elderly S A Bruce, J Dennison, H McIntyre, J Rahmani

Chest Disease M Clee, A J Dyson

Dermatology J Vanderwerth

ENT S Baer, A Meredith

General Medicine A Gorsuch, M Whtehead

General Surgery P Callaghan, G A Khoury, J A Lyttle, R Plail, A Sandison, S Whitehead

Obstetrics and Gynaecology A Alaily, J Zaidi

Ophthalmology P T S Gregory, C D Merrick

Orthopaedics H Apthorp, P A Butler-Manuel, B Hinves

Paediatrics S Mansy, D J Scott

Radiology L Apthorp

Rheumatology E Henderson

Conquest Hospital

The Ridge, St Leonards-on-Sea TN37 7RD
Tel: 01424 755255 Fax: 01424 758025
Total Beds: 455

Manager Shirley Whiteway

Accident and Emergency P Cornelius, T Underhill

Anaesthetics T Arnold, W Doherty, I Hicks, A Leach, J Lethbridge, N McNeillis, M Parsloe, I Reeve, A Slater, J Stock, A Stoddart, A R Thompson

Cardiology D Walker, R Wray

Care of the Elderly S A Bruce, J Dennison, M McIntyre, J Rahmani

Chest Disease M Clee, A J Dyson

ENT S Baer, A Meredith

General Medicine K Ahmed, A Gorsuch, J Rademaker, M Whitehead

General Surgery G Khoury, J Lyttle, A Sandison, S Whitehead

Neurology M Chowdhury

Obstetrics and Gynaecology A Alaily, B Auld, P Sinha, J Zaidi

Ophthalmology P Gregory, D Lloyd-Jones, C Merrick

Orthodontics D Vasey

Orthopaedics H Apthorp, J Buchanan, A Butler-Manuel, B Hinves, J Shepperd

Paediatrics L Bray, S Mansy, M Nasar, D Scott, T Ward, G Whincup

Pathology W S Barnes, J Beard, M Boxer, I Hawley, S Weston-Smith, E P Wright

Radiology L Apthorp, K Foord, J Giles, R Guy, R Joarder

Rheumatology E Henderson

Urology P Callaghan, R Plail

Eastbourne District General Hospital

King's Drive, Eastbourne BN21 2UD
Tel: 01323 417400 Fax: 01323 414930
Total Beds: 480

Manager Graham Griffiths

Anaesthetics J Andrews, A Canavan, J H Cook, J Dimond, R Edwards, T King, M Lonsdale, R McGregor, J McGowan, K Myerson, P J Nash, S Nicoll, P O'Dwyer, B Steer, A J Walmsley, N Watson

Dermatology K Liddell (Head)

ENT G Manjaly

General Medicine J J Bending, A A Dunk, T Higgins, G Lloyd, W Macleod, D Maxwell, N Patel, A Pool, A Smith, N Sulke, J Wilkinson

General Surgery A Aldridge, S Allan, G Evans, P H Rowe, M Saunders

Neurology W N Macleod (Head)

Obstetrics and Gynaecology V Argent, K Ayers, D Chui, M Malak, P Rafferty, A Soyemi

Ophthalmology D J Garlick, J Hickman-Casey, I Wearne

Orthodontics J Herold (Head)

Orthopaedics K R Ross (Head), A Bonnici, S E James, A McNally

Paediatrics J Kinder, M Liebenberg, J Mitchell, E Wearmouth

Pathology S K Bangert, P A Gover, R Grace, G Martin, J Mercer, C Moffat, K Ramesar, S Umasankar

Radiology H Anderson, D Howlett, D V Hughes, N Marchbank, E Ruffell, D Sallani, G Watson

Rheumatology A Pool

Urology W T Lawrence (Head), P Rimington, G Watson

East Yorkshire Primary Care Trust

Health House, Grange Park Lane, Willerby, Hull HU10 6DT
Tel: 01482 650700 Fax: 01482 672172
(North and East Yorkshire and Northern Lincolnshire Strategic Health Authority)

Chair Helen Varey
Chief Executive Andrew Williams

Eastbourne Downs Primary Care Trust

1 St Anne's Road, Eastbourne BN21 3UN
Tel: 01323 417714 Fax: 01323 747701
Email: edpct@eastbournedownspct.nhs.uk
Website: www.eastbournedownspct.nhs.uk
(Surrey and Sussex Strategic Health Authority)

Chair Mary Colato
Chief Executive Gina Brocklehurst

Eastern Birmingham Primary Care Trust

Suite 20, Waterlinks House, Richard Street, Birmingham B7 4AA
Tel: 0121 333 4113 Fax: 0121 333 5382
Email: info@easternbirminghampct.nhs.uk
Website: www.easternbirminghampct.nhs.uk
(Birmingham and the Black Country Strategic Health Authority)

Chair Paul Sabapathy
Chief Executive Sophia Christie

Eastern Cheshire Primary Care Trust

Winterton House, Winterton Way, Macclesfield SK11 0LP
Tel: 01625 508300 Fax: 01625 508301
Email: enquiries@echeshire-pct.nhs.uk
Website: www.ecpct.nhs.uk
(Cheshire and Merseyside Strategic Health Authority)

Chair Christine Greenhalgh
Chief Executive Peter Cubbon

Eastern Hull Primary Care Trust

Netherhall, Wawne Road, Hull HU7 4YG
Tel: 01482 335400 Fax: 01482 335446
(North and East Yorkshire and Northern Lincolnshire Strategic Health Authority)

Chair Malcolm Snow
Chief Executive Iain McInnes

Eastern Leicester Primary Care Trust

Mansion House, 1st Floor, 41 Guildhall Lane, Leicester LE1 5FR
Tel: 0116 295 1400 Fax: 0116 295 1464
(Leicestershire, Northamptonshire and Rutland Strategic Health Authority)

Chair Philip Parkinson
Chief Executive Carolyn Clifton

Eastern Wakefield Primary Care Trust

Castleford, Normanton and District Hospital, Lumley Street, High Town, Castleford WF10 5LT
Tel: 01977 605500 Fax: 01977 605501
Email: gisela.clark@ewpct.nhs.uk
Website: www.easternwake-pct.nhs.uk
(West Yorkshire Strategic Health Authority)

Chair Roy Widdowson
Chief Executive Mike Grady

Eastleigh and Test Valley South Primary Care Trust

The Mount Hospital, Church Road, Bishopstoke, Eastleigh SO50 6ZB
Tel: 023 8067 3673 Fax: 023 8067 3674
Email: firstname.lastname@etvs-pct.nhs.uk
Website: www.eastleighandtvspct.nhs.uk
(Hampshire and Isle of Wight Strategic Health Authority)

Chair Lynne Lockyer
Chief Executive John Richards

Eden Valley Primary Care Trust

8 Tynefield Drive, Penrith CA11 8JA
Tel: 01768 245317 Fax: 01768 245318
Website: www.northcumbriahealth.nhs.uk
(Cumbria and Lancashire Strategic Health Authority)

Chair Beth Furneaux
Chief Executive Nigel Woodcock

Brampton War Memorial Community Hospital
Brampton CA8 1TX
Tel: 01697 72534 Fax: 01697 741607
Total Beds: 15

Manager Brenda Wright

Mary Hewetson Community Hospital
Keswick CA12 5PH
Tel: 01768 767000 Fax: 01768 767007
Total Beds: 27

Manager Elizabeth Bateman

General Practice J Atack, M J Hamilton, J D Mitchell, P H White

Ophthalmology M Bearn

Orthopaedics H M Barber

Rheumatology I D L Brewis

Urology J A Cumming

Penrith and Eden Community Hospital
Bridge Lane, Penrith CA11 8HX
Tel: 01768 245300 Fax: 01768 245302
Total Beds: 60

Manager Linda Littleton

Care of the Elderly J S Billett, P L Chin

Dermatology N H Cox, W D Patterson

General Medicine P Mustchin

General Psychiatry C Tyrie

General Surgery J G Palmer

Obstetrics and Gynaecology A A Brown, R G Rangecroft, W Reid

Ophthalmology M Hasan

Orthopaedics C G Brignall, G H H Broome, A N Edwards

Paediatrics J M P Storr

Rheumatology and Rehabilitation I Brewis

Urology R G Willis

Ruth Lancaster James Community Hospital
Alston CA9 3QX
Tel: 01434 381218 Fax: 01434 382134
Total Beds: 12

Manager Sheila Richardson

General Practice M T Hanley, S L Mills

Ellesmere Port and Neston Primary Care Trust

7-9 Civic Way, Ellesmere Port CH65 0AX
Tel: 0151 373 4900 Fax: 0151 356 7403
Email: forename.surname@epnpct.nhs.uk
Website: www.epnpct.nhs.uk
(Cheshire and Merseyside Strategic Health Authority)

Chair Michael Darby
Chief Executive Jacqui Harvey

Ellesmere Port Hospital
Whitby Road, Ellesmere Port CH65 6FQ
Tel: 01244 365000 Fax: 01244 362922
Total Beds: 92

Enfield Primary Care Trust

Trust Headquarters, Holbrook House, Cockfosters Road, Barnet EN4 0DR
Tel: 020 8272 5500 Fax: 020 8272 5700
Email: firstname.lastname@enfield.nhs.uk
Website: www.enfield.nhs.uk
(North Central London Strategic Health Authority)

Chair Carolyn Berkeley
Chief Executive Sally Johnson

Epping Forest Primary Care Trust

Birchwood House, St Margaret's Hospital, The Plain, Epping CM16 6TN
Tel: 01902 902010 Fax: 01902 827847
Email: mail@epping-pct.nhs.uk
Website: www.efpct.nhs.uk
(Essex Strategic Health Authority)

Chair Di Collins
Chief Executive Aidan Thomas

Epsom and St Helier University Hospitals NHS Trust

St Helier Hospital, Wrythe Lane, Carshalton SM5 1AA
Tel: 020 8296 2000 Fax: 020 8641 4546
Email: enquiries@epsom-sthelier.nhs.uk
Website: www.epsom-sthelier.nhs.uk
(South West London Strategic Health Authority)

Chair Michael Doherty
Chief Executive Lorraine Clifton
Consultants Felicity Anderson, Pete Andrews, Serge Bajada, Amolak Bansal, Jeffrey Barron, Sachu Battacharya, Judith Behrens, J Keith Bell, Justin Bendig, Mike R Bending, Marina P Benedict, Martin Benson, Nick Bett, Peter T Blenkinsopp, Sandra Blewitt, Ronald Brandt, Stephen Breathnach, Stephen J D Brecker, Christine Burren, Paul Byrne, Steve Capps, Clive Charig, Muhammed Chawdhery, Sonny Chong, Mark Churchill, Neil Citron, A Clarke, Mary F Clarke, Sandeep Cliff, Val Cook, Nigel T Cooke, David Cunningham, L G Darlington, Joan Desborough, Cheryl Ellis, Steve Estreich, Bernadette Ewah, Richard E Field, Meda A Frangoulis, Julian A Gaer, Martin Gardner, David Gateley, Chris George, H Jane Gilford, Brian M Gompels, Peter Gough, Andrew Gregory, Alison Halliday, Khalid N Haque, Chris C Harland, Simon S Hawkins, M Henk, Hindmarsh, S J Keith Holmes, Philip J Howard, Anwar Hussein, Stanislaw Jankowski, A Chris John, Chris R Jones, Lydia Jones, Viji Kakumani, Mike Katesmark, Manil Katugampola, T Gerry Kavanagh, Michael Keane, Jan Klosok, Jonathan Kwan, Gabrielle Lamb, Bill Landells, John Langdon, Michael Lapsley, Bosena Laskiewicz, R Jane Leitch, Guam Lim, Will A Lindsay, Stanley Ling, Anne Linnell, Bob McFarland, Marion McGowan, C John MacKay, David Male, Janet Mantell, Tina Matthews, Simon T Meller, Jane Mercieca, Daniel Mok, Deborah Moncrieff, Murday, Dhiren Nehra, E Nicholls, Elizabeth A North, John O'Connell, Sola Odemuyiwa, Benedicta Ogeah, Robin T Orchard, Sharon Orton-Gibbs, Winston Pais, Mike K Palmer, Maxine Partridge, Sanjeev Patel, Chris M Perry, Charles W Pumphrey, Patrick Radford, Kinsgsley W Ranasinha, Don C Rangedera, Geoffrey Robb, Peter Robb, Andrew Rodin, A Maria Rollin, Leslie D Ross, Samad Samadian, Stephen Sampson, Margaret Semple, Sanjay Shah, Elizabeth Sherriff, Linda N Singh, Ian Smith, Susan Snashell, Paula Sneath, Sugi Somanathan, Andrew Stewart, Martin A Stockwell, Kathy Stoner, Rene Tayar, L Temple, A Thayalan, A Thurston, Paul Toomey, Veronica Varney, Nestor Velasco, Michael C Ward, Mary Warren, A Hervey Wilcox, Clare R Williams, Peter Williamson, Geoff Wilson, Stephen Wilson, Richard Worth, Robin L Yeoh, Kirsten Younger

Epsom General Hospital

Dorking Road, Epsom KT18 7EG
Tel: 020 8296 2000 Fax: 020 8641 4546
Total Beds: 418

Anaesthetics J K Bell, S Bhattacharya, Dr Desborough, B Ewah, C J Mackay, W A Pais, Dr Pathmabaskaran, A M Rollin

Cardiology S Odemuyiwa

Chemical Pathology Dr Lapsley

Dermatology S Breathnach

ENT B M Laskiewicz, P Robb

General Medicine L G Darlington, Dr Lim, P F Mitchell-Heggs, Dr Rahman, K W Ranasinha, D C Rangedera, G H Robb

General Surgery W Allum, Dr Almusawi, A Halliday, R McFarland, Mr Raj, Dr Toomey

Haematology L Jones, M Semple

Histopathology T Matthews, L Temple

Medical Microbiology J Bendig, S Chambers

Neurology S G Wilson

Obstetrics and Gynaecology C Ellis, V Kakumani, M Katesmark, R W Worth

Occupational Health A Thayalan

Oncology D Cunningham, M Henk

Ophthalmology P Fison, M Frangoulis, Dr Leitch, A Linnell, Dr Shah

Oral Surgery J Langdon, M Partridge

Orthopaedics Dr Cobb (Head), Dr Chockalingam, D Mok, R Twyman

Paediatrics Dr Nicholls (Head), Dr Charlton, Dr Garcia, M Katugampola, J O'Connell, P Sneath

Radiology C George, B M Gompels, A M Gregory, Dr Lamb, K Stoner, K A Younger

Urology M J Bailey, C Charig, Dr Walker

Nelson Hospital

Kingston Road, Merton, London SW20 8DB
Tel: 020 8296 2000
Total Beds: 10

Queen Mary's Hospital for Children

St. Helier Hospital, Carshalton SM5 1AA
Tel: 020 8296 2000
Total Beds: 36

St Helier Hospital

Wrythe Lane, Carshalton SM5 1AA
Total Beds: 600

Anaesthetics M Gardner, S Hawkins, Dr Hussein, S Ling, D Male, P Radford, S Renwick, Dr Said, S Somanathan, C M Steven, Dr Turner, C Williams

Audiological Medicine R Yeoh (Head), Dr Snashall, R Yeoh

Cardiology Dr Brecker, Dr Pumphrey

Care of the Elderly S Samadian, M Ward

Dental Surgery P Blenkinsopp, Dr Brandt, Dr Jones, Dr Orton-Gibbs, Dr Stewart

Dermatology Dr Harland, C A Holden

ENT A C John, Dr Laskiewicz, Dr Williamson

General Medicine M R Bending, Dr Benson, N T Cooke, Dr Duke, P Howard, R Orchard, Dr Rodin, Dr Varney

General Surgery N J Bett, A Chilvers, Dr Nehru, Dr Raja, Dr Thomas, Dr Zaidi

Genitourinary Medicine S Estreich, J Mantell

Nephrology Dr Eisinger (Head), Dr Andrews, M R Bending, Dr Makanjoula, Dr Velasco

Neurology R O McKeran

Obstetrics and Gynaecology Dr Croucher, P Gough, D Moncrieff, Dr Penru, Dr Perry, L D Ross, Dr Shehata, Dr Sherriff

Orthopaedics Dr Chockalingam, M Churchill, N Citron, Dr Field, T G Kavanagh, J Klosok, Dr Patel

Paediatrics Dr Blewitt, Dr Burren, Dr Chong, K Haque, Dr Holmes, Dr McGowan, Dr Ogeah, Dr Rosenthal, Dr Shepherd

Pathology Dr Anderson, Dr Bansal, J L Barron, J Behrens, M Clarke, W Landells, Dr Lapsley, Dr Mercleca, L N Singh, A H Wilcox

Radiology P Byrne, Dr Cook, J Gilford, Dr Keane, E A North, E M O'Sullivan, M K Palmer, R Tayar, Dr Warren

Rheumatology and Rehabilitation O Duke

Urology Dr Boyd (Head), Dr Walker, Dr Watkin

Sutton Hospital
Cotswold Road, Sutton SM2 5NF
Tel: 020 8296 2000
Total Beds: 32

Erewash Primary Care Trust

Ilkeston Health Centre, South Street, Ilkeston DE7 5PZ
Tel: 0115 951 2300 Fax: 0115 951 2350
Website: www.erewash-pct.nhs.uk
(Trent Strategic Health Authority)

Chair Anthea Thompson
Chief Executive Paula Clark

Ilkeston Community Hospital
Heanor Road, Ilkeston DE7 8LN
Tel: 0115 930 5522
Total Beds: 90

Essex Ambulance Service NHS Trust

Broomfield, Chelmsford CM1 7WS
Tel: 01245 443344 Fax: 01245 442920
Email: forename.surname@essexamb.nhs.uk
Website: www.essamb.co.uk
(Essex Strategic Health Authority)

Chair Richard Bourne
Chief Executive Anthony March

Essex Rivers Healthcare NHS Trust

Trust Headquarters, Colchester General Hospital, Turner Road, Colchester CO4 5JL
Tel: 01206 747474 Fax: 01206 742324
Email: firstname.lastname@essexrivers.nhs.uk
Website: www.essexrivers.nhs.uk
(Essex Strategic Health Authority)

Chair Michael Salmon
Chief Executive Peter Murphy

Colchester General Hospital
Turner Road, Colchester CO4 5JL
Tel: 01206 747474 Fax: 01206 742324
Total Beds: 558

Essex County Hospital
Lexden Road, Colchester CO3 3NB
Tel: 01206 747474 Fax: 01206 744572
Total Beds: 56

Halstead Hospital
78 Hedingham Road, Halstead CO9 2DL
Tel: 01787 291010 Fax: 01787 291023
Total Beds: 20

Exeter Primary Care Trust

Dean Clarke House, Southernhay East, Exeter EX1 1PQ
Tel: 01392 207513 Fax: 01392 494726
Website: www.exeter-pct.nhs.uk
(South West Peninsula Strategic Health Authority)

Chair Mary Nisbett
Chief Executive Jill Smith

Whipton Hospital
Whipton Lane, Exeter EX1 3RB
Tel: 01392 208333 Fax: 01392 208307
Total Beds: 33

Fareham and Gosport Primary Care Trust

Unit 180, 166 Fareham Road, Gosport PO13 0FW
Tel: 01329 233447 Fax: 01329 234984
Email: firstname.lastname@ports.nhs.uk
Website: www.farehamandgosportpct.nhs.uk
(Hampshire and Isle of Wight Strategic Health Authority)

Chair Lucy Docherty
Chief Executive Ian Piper

Gosport War Memorial Hospital
Bury Road, Gosport PO12 3PW
Tel: 023 9252 4611 Fax: 023 9258 0360

St Christopher's Hospital
Wickham Road, Fareham PO16 7DJ
Tel: 01329 286321 Fax: 01329 281173
Total Beds: 73

5 Boroughs Partnership NHS Trust

Hollins Park House, Hollins Lane, Winwick, Warrington WA2 8WA
Tel: 01925 664000 Fax: 01925 664052
Email: forename.surname@5boroughspartnership.nhs.uk
Website: www.5boroughspartnership.nhs.uk
(Greater Manchester Strategic Health Authority; Cheshire and Merseyside Strategic Health Authority)

Chair John Gartside
Chief Executive Judith Holbrey

Avenue Day Hospital
Leigh Infirmary, The Avenue, Leigh WN7 1HS
Tel: 01942 264577 Fax: 01942 264576

Manager Alan Slater

Beacon Day Hospital
Billinge Hospital, Upholland Road, Billinge, Wigan WN5 7ET
Tel: 01695 626034 Fax: 01695 626371

Brooker Centre, Halton General Hospital
Hospital Way, Runcorn WA7 2DA
Tel: 01928 753926 Fax: 01928 753219
Total Beds: 73

Fourways
127 Twiss Green Lane, Culcheth, Warrington WA3 4DJ
Tel: 01925 765986
Total Beds: 7

Hollins Park
Hollins Lane, Winwick, Warrington WA2 8WA
Tel: 01925 664000 Fax: 01925 664086
Total Beds: 156

Leigh Infirmary
The Avenue, Leigh WN7 1HS
Tel: 01742 672333 Fax: 01742 264388
Total Beds: 138

Oakdene
Oakdene Unit, Jibcroft Lane, off Twiss Green Lane, Culcheth, Warrington WA3 4TH

Tel: 01925 763764/765335 Fax: 01925 766914
Total Beds: 36

Peasley Cross
Peasley Cross Wing, St Helens Hospital, Marshalls Cross Road, St Helens WA9 3DA
Tel: 01744 458459 Fax: 01744 458522
Total Beds: 49

St Bartholomew's Day Hospital
Station Road, Roby, Liverpool L36 4HU
Tel: 0151 489 6241 Fax: 0151 480 5482

St John's Centre
Alforde Street, Widnes WA8 7QA
Tel: 0151 422 6800 Fax: 0151 420 8351
Total Beds: 10

Sherdley Unit, Whiston Hospital
Whiston, Prescot L35 5DR
Total Beds: 107

Stewart Day Hospital
Peasley Cross Wing, St Helens Hospital, Marshalls Cross Road, St Helens WA9 3DA
Tel: 01744 458393 Fax: 01744 458461

Wexford Unit
Delph Park Specialist Care Centre, Townfield Lane, Winwick, Warrington WA2 8TR
Tel: 01925 575771 Fax: 01925 574589
Total Beds: 8

Frimley Park Hospital NHS Foundation Trust

Established as a Foundation Trust 01/04/2005.

Portsmouth Road, Frimley, Camberley GU16 7UJ
Tel: 01276 604604
Email: firstname.lastname@fph-tr.nhs.uk
Website: www.frimleypark.org.uk
(Surrey and Sussex Strategic Health Authority)

Chair Jane Cooke
Chief Executive Andrew Morris

Frimley Park Hospital
Portsmouth Road, Frimley, Camberley GU16 7UJ
Tel: 01276 604604
Total Beds: 700

Accident and Emergency R Partridge

Anaesthetics Dr Bernardo, Dr Carroll, M H Davies, G F Goddard, Dr Gudgeon, P Joshi, Dr Keeling, S M Kilpatrick, K Markham, Dr Pepall, Dr Shaikh, Dr Slade, Dr Taylor, Dr Walsh, D G White

Care of the Elderly Dr Debrah, I K Ibrahim, K I Mundy

Dermatology Dr Boxer, R H Felix

ENT D Jonathan (Head), Lt Col Hosni, R Kumar, Dr McCombe

General Medicine R L Bown, M J Boyd, R J Frankel

General Surgery Dr Daoud, Dr Gerrard, A M Gudgeon, I Laidlaw, P Leopold, Dr Mellor, I Paterson, Dr Singh

Neurology D Wren

Obstetrics and Gynaecology Dr Bartells, Dr Beynon, J Cockburn, Dr Deans, A Riddle, P J Toplis

Ophthalmology A Elliott, J A Govan, C M Griffiths, M K Tandon

Oral and Maxillofacial Surgery Dr Danford, P Johnson

Orthopaedics A Ashbrooke, Dr Chissell, S Davies, D Dempster, D Harrison, Dr Hull, Dr Pike, Dr Quaile, Dr Sakellariou

Paediatrics F M Howard, P E Walker

Pathology Dr Alton, N Cumberland, P Denham, Dr Elmahallany, J E W Pette, C E T Smith, Dr Wang, M Williams

Plastic Surgery D Martin

Radiology F J Hearn (Head), Dr Ahmad, J Hall, Dr Hatrick, A Keightley, H Massouh

Radiotherapy R Laing

Rheumatology and Rehabilitation Dr Lloyd, P Reilly

Urology B Montgomery, Dr Naeger, E Palfrey

Fylde Primary Care Trust

Derby Road, Wesham, Preston PR4 3AL
Tel: 01253 306305 Fax: 01253 306374
Website: www.fyldepct.nhs.uk
(Cumbria and Lancashire Strategic Health Authority)

Chair Bert Waddington
Chief Executive Julie Goulding

Gateshead Health NHS Trust

Established as a Foundation Trust 05/01/2005.

Queen Elizabeth Hospital, Sheriff Hill, Gateshead NE9 6SX
Tel: 0191 482 0000 Fax: 0191 482 6001
Website: www.gatesheadhealth.nhs.uk
(Northumberland, Tyne and Wear Strategic Health Authority)

Chair Peter Smith
Chief Executive Christopher Reed

Bensham Hospital
Saltwell Road, Gateshead NE8 4YL
Tel: 0191 482 0000 Fax: 0191 478 3357
Total Beds: 151

Care of the Elderly D Barer, D M Beaumont, M Davies

Radiology J Hall, P Lord, R Uberoi

Rheumatology C Heycock, C Kelly

Dryden Road Day Hospital
134 Dryden Road, Gateshead NE9 5BY
Tel: 0191 403 6600 Fax: 0191 403 6601

Dunston Hill Day Unit
Whickham Highway, Dunston, Gateshead NE11 9QT
Tel: 0191 403 6474 Fax: 0191 403 6505

Dunston Hill Hospital
Whickham Highway, Dunston, Gateshead NE11 9QT
Tel: 0191 482 0000 Fax: 0191 403 6408
Total Beds: 70

Queen Elizabeth Hospital
Sheriff Hill, Gateshead NE9 6SX
Tel: 0191 482 0000 Fax: 0191 491 1823
Total Beds: 537

Accident and Emergency B Dorani

Anaesthetics A McHutchon, H May

Child and Adolescent Psychiatry L Barrett, D Bone, J McDonald

Dermatology M C G Dahl

General Medicine N Bailey, D Barer, J Barker, D M Beaumont, M Davies, C T A Jones, C Kelly, L G Lunt, J Mansfield, D J Peakman, T Petterson, C Scott, J U Weaver, L A Webb, J R Young

General Surgery D A Browell, S M Chandhry, W J Cunliffe, M J Higgs

Obstetrics and Gynaecology A Beeby, M Das, S M Field

Oncology N Bailey, T d Lopes, J M Monaghan, D P Sinha

Orthopaedics J A Antrobus, J Pooley

Otology D B Mathias, A R Welch, J Wilson

Paediatrics J R Beesley, S Hodges, A Steele

Pathology M Abela, P Cross, M J Egan, S Hudson, J P Sunter

Radiology J Hall, P Lord

Rheumatology and Rehabilitation C Heycock, C Kelly

Urology H A Ashour, A M M Mudawi

Tranwell Unit
Windy Nook Road, Gateshead NE10 9RW
Tel: 0191 482 0000 Fax: 0191 402 6221
Total Beds: 127

Gateshead Primary Care Trust

Team View, Fifth Avenue Business Park, Team Valley Trading Estate, Gateshead NE11 0NB
Tel: 0191 491 5713 Fax: 0191 491 5727
Email: gatesheadpct@ghpct.nhs.uk
Website: www.gatesheadpct.nhs.uk
(Northumberland, Tyne and Wear Strategic Health Authority)

Chair Alan Baty
Chief Executive Bob Smith

Gedling Primary Care Trust

Headquarters, Byron Court, Brookfield Road, Arnold, Nottingham NG5 7ER
Tel: 0115 993 1444 Fax: 0115 993 1466
Email: gpct@gedling-pct.nhs.uk
Website: www.nottingham.nhs.uk
(Trent Strategic Health Authority)

Chair Derek Stewart
Chief Executive Lynne Winstanley

George Eliot Hospital NHS Trust

Lewes House, College Street, Nuneaton CV10 7DJ
Tel: 024 7635 1351 Fax: 024 7686 5058
Email: enquiries@geh.nhs.uk
Website: www.geh.nhs.uk

Chair Frank McCarney
Chief Executive Duncan Phimister

George Eliot Hospital
College Street, Nuneaton CV10 7DJ
Tel: 024 7635 1351 Fax: 024 7686 5058
Total Beds: 404

Accident and Emergency D Foroughi, G Gordon

Anaesthetics P Taggart (Head), J A Dako, D G Heap, N S Kaduskar, R I Miller, S Nithianandan, S Shawket, P C M Tagg

Biochemistry B Cockrill

Cardiology Y Haider, A Venkataraman

General Surgery I Haynes, S Lele, G Mathew

Genitourinary Medicine L M David, M Walzman

Haematology A Abdul-Cader, M Narayanan

Histopathology N Bajallan, J Nottingham

Microbiology A Manek, R Parn

Oral and Maxillofacial Surgery J Fagan

Orthopaedics A Aboel-Salam, D Sharif, R Steingold

Paediatrics R C de Boer, R C de Boer, M Venkataraman

Palliative Medicine C Meystre

Radiology R Patel, S Sinha, K Vallance

Radiotherapy and Oncology R N Das

Urology K K Prasad

Gloucestershire Ambulance Services NHS Trust

Gloucestershire TriService Emergency Centre, Waterwells Drive, Waterwells Business Park, Quedgeley, Gloucester GL2 2BA
Tel: 01452 753030 Fax: 01452 753031
Website: www.glosamb.org.uk
(Avon, Gloucestershire and Wiltshire Strategic Health Authority)

Chair Carolyn Elwes
Chief Executive Richard Davis

Gloucestershire Hospitals NHS Foundation Trust

Established as a Foundation Trust 01/07/2004.

1 College Lawn, Cheltenham GL53 7AN
Tel: 08454 222222 Fax: 01242 221214
Email: firstname.surname@egnhst.org.uk
Website: www.gloshospitals.org.uk
(Avon, Gloucestershire and Wiltshire Strategic Health Authority)

Chair Janet Trotter
Chief Executive Paul Lilley

Cheltenham General Hospital
Sandford Road, Cheltenham GL53 7AN
Tel: 08454 222222 Fax: 01242 273516
Total Beds: 521

Accident and Emergency P Davies, P Wilson

Anaesthetics W J Brampton, A N Burlingham, M Copp, J G d Courcy, J Francis, D T Goodrum, S Karadia, M McSwiney, C Mather, M Parmar, T Rees, M J Richards, P A Ritchie, G S Routh, S Smith, S West, P N Young

Cardiology V Challenor, R Chamberlain-Webber

Dermatology J Milne

General Medicine S Al-Ahbar, M Bialas, V Challener, I Crossley, A Deering, P Fletcher, I Mortimore, A Penketh

General Surgery N Borlay, J Bristol, H Chan, H Gilbert, A Goodman, R Kinder, K Poskitt, M Whyman

Nephrology A Williams

Neurology G Fuller, R Martin, M Silva

Obstetrics and Gynaecology Dr Holmes, R H J Kerr-Wilson, A McCrum, M Pilllai, M Sutton

Ophthalmology J Ferris, R Johnston, J Kirkpatrick, G Macintosh, A McNaught, J Naime, N C Price

Oral and Maxillofacial Surgery D Godden, J Harrison

Orthodontics J Dickson, L Macey-Dare

Orthopaedics D A P Ainscow, J Field, H Gosal, G Holt, J G McKinnon, G Rooker, J S Wand

Paediatrics S Ackroyd, M Hamilton-Ayres, S Kinder, K Martin

Palliative Medicine D Jeffrey

Pathology E Blundell, S Chown, J Christie-Brown, S G Edmondson, R Jackson, P A Laite, R Lush, V Peterson, A Rye, N Shepherd, P Toner, J Utt

Radiology M Brock, P F Brown, C Bulloch, M Gibson, J Green, R Hopkins, G McGann, C P Robinson

Radiotherapy and Oncology K Benstead, A Cook, R Counsell, S Elyan, D Farrugia, P Jenkins, R Owen, S Shepherd

Respiratory Medicine I Mortimore, A Penketh

Rheumatology D Collins, G Coombes, J Woodland

Urology H Gilbert, R Kinder

Gloucestershire Royal Hospital

Great Western Road, Gloucester GL1 3NN
Tel: 08454 222222 Fax: 01452 310737
Total Beds: 614

Accident and Emergency S McCabe

Anaesthetics Dr Bakewell, J Brown, Dr Clarke, Dr Cooper, Dr Crabb, M A Durkin, R J Eltringham, D Gabbott, Dr Garcia-Rodriguez, C Green, P Hardy, Dr Khor, A McCrirrick, Dr Pryle, C Roberts, P Sanderson, Dr Savidge, E Spencer, A Thornberry, R Vanner, J Waters, N Williams, P N Young

Dermatology Dr Adriaans, J Milne, W Porter

ENT J W Hamilton, M Hardingham, P M Thomas, A M Wheatley, R P Youngs

General Medicine R Banks, Dr Brown, R Butland, D Lindsay, Dr Meecham-Jones, M Peterson, Dr Pickett, J Prior, Dr Ulahannan, R Valori, A J Williams, J Woodland

General Surgery H Barr, Dr Cook, M Gilbert, B P Heather, D Jones, M Lucarotti, A Ritchie, Dr Sammon, W H F Thomson, M Vipond

Genitourinary Medicine D Sulaiman

Neurology G Fuller, Dr Martin, Dr Silva

Obstetrics and Gynaecology Dr James, Dr Mahendran, E Smith, G Swingler, Dr Whittaker

Ophthalmology B Harney, G Mackintosh, J Naime

Oral Surgery Dr Godden, J M Harrison

Orthodontics J Dickson, Dr Macey-Dare

Orthopaedics D Asante, Dr Close, C C Crawshaw, C Curwen, W Harcourt, M Henderson, C Knudsen, R Majkowski, T B Tasker

Paediatrics L Jadresic, Dr Pandya, Dr Rushforth, D W Stevens, M H Wagstaff, M S C Webb

Pathology Dr Chown, Dr Christie-Brown, P A Laite, A Lees, M Logan, K McCarthy, C A McNulty, J E Ropner, N Shepherd, P Toner, J S Uff

Radiology P Birch, E F Brown, S Cooke, R Hopkins, Dr Jelly, F Jewell, S E Jones, A Tottle, Dr Wallace, D Wallace, J B Witcombe

Rehabilitation Services Dr Asghar, M Bannerjee, I Blackman, D Dutta, R Welding

Rheumatology Dr Coombes, J Woodland

Moore Cottage Hospital

Bourton-on-the-Water, Moore Road, Cheltenham GL54 2AZ
Tel: 01451 820228 Fax: 01451 810817
Total Beds: 34

General Medicine J Anderson, V Challenor, I Crossley, A Deering, I Mortimore

General Surgery K Poskitt

Obstetrics and Gynaecology R Kerr-Wilson

Ophthalmology N Kirkpatrick, A McNaught

Orthopaedics G Holt, J G MacKinnon

Paediatrics R S Ackroyd

Rheumatology D Collins

Standish Hospital

Stonehouse GL10 3DB
Tel: 01453 822481
Total Beds: 118

Chest Disease R Butland, J Prior

Orthopaedics D Asante, C C Crawshaw, R A C Davies, C Knudsen, B D A Morris, T P B Tasker

Rheumatology J Woodland

Tewkesbury Hospital

Barton Road, Tewkesbury GL20 5QN
Tel: 01684 293303 Fax: 01684 285887
Total Beds: 50

Manager Rita Holmes

Cardiology V Challenor

Care of the Elderly P Fletcher

Chest Disease I Mortimore

ENT D Thomas

General Medicine V Challenor, P Fletcher, S Sawyers

General Psychiatry M Clarke, M Whyman

General Surgery S Haynes

Obstetrics and Gynaecology D Holmes

Ophthalmology A McNaught

Orthopaedics D A P Ainscow, J Field, J G Mackinnon

Paediatrics R S Ackroyd, A Day, M Hamilton-Ayres, S Kinder

Rheumatology J Woodland

Urology R Kinder

Winchcombe District Hospital

Winchcombe, Cheltenham GL54 5NQ
Tel: 01242 602341 Fax: 01242 604024
Total Beds: 22

General Medicine J Anderson, I Crossley, P Fletcher

General Surgery S Haynes

Obstetrics and Gynaecology M Sutton

Orthopaedics D Ainscow

Paediatrics M Hamilton-Ayres

Urology R Kinder

Gloucestershire Partnership NHS Trust

Rikenel, Montpellier, Gloucester GL1 1LY
Tel: 01452 891000 Fax: 01452 891105
Email: firstname.surname@glos.nhs.uk
Website: www.partnershiptrust.org.uk
(Avon, Gloucestershire and Wiltshire Strategic Health Authority)

Chair Robert Maxwell
Chief Executive Jeff James

Consultants N Ardagh-Walter, S Arnott, B Arredondo, N Buntwal, O Davies, M Dharmendra, C Fear, G Hodgson, J Laidlaw, G Lloyd, M Lowe, R MacPherson, Manju, T Moate, A Moliver, I Pennell, H Richards, R Richards, S Roberts, C Robson, R Ropner, K Sackett, M Scheepers, J Stratford, G Undrill, Sarah Welch, K Williams, K D Williams, P Winterbottom

Charlton Lane Centre
Charlton Lane, Leckhampton, Cheltenham GL53 9DZ
Tel: 01242 272181 Fax: 01242 272105
Total Beds: 80

Manager Marieanne Bubb-McGhee

Consultants M Dharnendra, A Moliver

Denmark Road Day Hospital
18 Denmark Road, Gloucester GL1 3HZ
Tel: 01452 891220 Fax: 01452 891221

Holly House
West Lodge Drive, Coney Hill, Gloucester
Tel: 01452 891380 Fax: 01452 891381
Total Beds: 25

Care of the Elderly N Ardagh-Walter

Stroud Road Unit
136 Stroud Road, Stroud
Tel: 01452 891200 Fax: 01452 891201

Wotton Lawn Hospital
Wotton Lawn, Gloucester GL1 3WL
Tel: 01452 891500 Fax: 01452 891501
Total Beds: 73

Manager Allan Metherall

Consultants N J R Evans, C Fear, G Hodgson, J Laidlaw, J Lugg, R McPherson, K Williams

Good Hope Hospital NHS Trust

Rectory Road, Sutton Coldfield B75 7RR
Tel: 0121 378 2211 Fax: 0121 311 1074
Website: www.goodhope.org.uk
(Birmingham and the Black Country Strategic Health Authority)

Chair Graham Comfort
Chief Executive Anne Heast

Good Hope Hospital
Rectory Road, Sutton Coldfield B75 7RR
Tel: 0121 378 2211 Fax: 0121 311 1074
Total Beds: 550

Accident and Emergency K Gupta, A Tabani

Anaesthetics J Elliott, J Hull, P Johnston, M N A Messih, F Murray, J H Sheldrake, D Siggins, D Thomas

Biochemistry R A Hall

Care of the Elderly J Atiea, A A Farooqi, L Lambert, M P Skander

Child and Adolescent Psychiatry A A E Sorour-El Sharief

Dermatology I S Foulds

ENT E Fisher, A Johnson, D Morgan

General Medicine J Atiea, T Fletcher, P Hillenbrand, L Lambert, A Mackay, J J Milles, M V J Raj, S Singh, M P Skander, R Smith

General Surgery A Allan, P Bearn, M Crowson, M Foster, A Jewkes, B Jones, D R Thomas

Haematology S M Jobanputra, M S Hamilton

Neurology D J Jamieson

Obstetrics and Gynaecology R Cartmill, D Churchill, G Constantine, C Finn, M D Moloney

Oncology T N Latief

Ophthalmology P Lin Lip, M H Ross, P Shah, G A Sutton

Orthodontics S Weerakone

Orthopaedics B Banerjee, G J Benke, G Krishnamusthy, I M Miller, K Wahab

Paediatrics A Baxi, S Bennett Britton, T J Lee, J Meran

Pathology N Aluwihare, A M Light, D Mortiboy, J Tucker, R S Whittaker

Plastic Surgery J H Goldin

Radiology C Bickley, E Millar, C Nelson, A Parnell

Rheumatology T Price, T Sheeran

Urology M C Foster, D R Thomas

Great Ormond Street Hospital for Children NHS Trust

Great Ormond Street, London WC1N 3JH
Tel: 020 7405 9200 Fax: 020 7829 8643
Email: info@gosh.nhs.uk
Website: www.gosh.nhs.uk
(North Central London Strategic Health Authority)

Chair Cyril Chantler
Chief Executive Jane Collins
Consultants P Aurora, Angela Barnicoat, L Biassoni, Maria Bitner-Glindzicz, P Bonhoeffer, Kate Brown, Mandy Bryon, M Burch, Catherine Cale, K Chong, T Cox, D Cubitt, Rose De Bruyn, M de Leval, J Deanfield, G Derrick, R Dinwiddie, Gwynnneth Down, M Elliott, Y Foo, D Glaser, J Goldin, A Goldman, I Gordon, Vivienne Gross, Sarah Gustavus Jones, Christine Hall, B Harding, J Hartley, Daniela Hearst, Isobel Heyman, P Hill, Melanie Hiorns, Jill Hodges, Adam Jaffe, I James, M Kellett, I Kenney, M Kenney, R Liesner, J Mackay, Sue Macqueen, Jenne Magagna, R Maharoon, Marian Malone, K McHugh, Q Mok, D Nicholls, Catherine Owens, M Peters, A Petros, Christine Pierce, N Pigott, Rosemary Radley-Smith, A Ramsay, P Rees, A Reynolds, A Risdon, D Roebuck, Elisabeth Rosser, Margrid Schindler, D Skuse, J Soothill, I Sullivan, Wendy Taylor, V Tsang, C Wallis, Louise Wilson, R Winter, R Yates

Great Ormond Street Hospital for Children
Great Ormond Street, London WC1N 3JH
Tel: 020 7405 9200 Fax: 020 7829 8643
Total Beds: 335

Great Yarmouth Primary Care Trust

Astley Cooper House, Estcourt Road, Great Yarmouth NR30 4JH
Tel: 01493 856156 Fax: 01493 856005
(Norfolk, Suffolk and Cambridgeshire Strategic Health Authority)

Chair Bernard Williamson
Chief Executive Michael Stonard

Greater Derby Primary Care Trust

Derwent Court, 1 Stuart Street, Derby DE1 2FZ
Tel: 01332 224000 Fax: 01332 342881
Email: mail@greaterderby-pct.nhs.uk
Website: www.greaterderby-pct.nhs.uk
(Trent Strategic Health Authority)

Chair Syed Ali Naqwi
Chief Executive Prem Singh

Greater Manchester Ambulance Service NHS Trust

156-158 Bury Old Road, Whitefield, Manchester M45 6AQ
Tel: 0161 796 7222 Fax: 0161 796 0435
(Greater Manchester Strategic Health Authority)

Chair Alan Stephenson
Chief Executive John Burnside

Greenwich Teaching Primary Care Trust

31-37 Greenwich Park Street, Greenwich, London SE10 9LR
Tel: 020 8293 6700 Fax: 020 8269 0787
Email: firstname.surname@greenwichpct.nhs.uk
Website: www.greenwichpct.nhs.uk
(South East London Strategic Health Authority)

Chair Michael Chuter
Chief Executive Jane Schofield

Guildford and Waverley Primary Care Trust

Broadmead House, Farnham Business Park, Weydon Lane, Farnham GU9 8QT
Tel: 01252 305700 Fax: 01252 305701
Website: www.gwpct.nhs.uk
(Surrey and Sussex Strategic Health Authority)

Chair Christopher Grimes
Chief Executive Liz Slinn

Guy's and St Thomas' NHS Foundation Trust

Established as a Foundation Trust 01/07/2004.

St Thomas' Hospital, Lambeth Palace Road, London SE1 7EH
Tel: 020 7188 7188
Email: communications@gstt.sthomas.nhs.uk
Website: www.guysandstthomas.nhs.uk
(South East London Strategic Health Authority)

Chair Patricia Moberly
Chief Executive Jonathan Michael

Grove Park Hospital
Marvels Lane, London SE12 9PD
Tel: 020 8857 1191
Total Beds: 168

Guy's Hospital
St Thomas Street, London SE1 9RT
Tel: 020 7955 5000 Fax: 020 7955 8803
Website: www.hospital.org.uk
Total Beds: 553

Accident and Emergency L Stimmler, D Watson

Alcohol and Substance Abuse M Allen

Anaesthetics M Thompson (Head), M B Barnett, W Coutinho, H D Dervos, J G Diamond, J Hellewell, N Newton, A Pearce, C Wood

Biochemistry R Swaminathan

Cardiology C Bucknall, J Chambers, P V L Curry, G Jackson, G E Sowton

Cardiothoracic Medicine D Anderson, C Blauth, P D Deverall, J Dussek

Care of the Elderly R Lewis, W McNabb

Child and Adolescent Psychiatry A Cox, H Davies, D R Glaser, R J Jezzard, M Wiseman

Cytology N Fagg, I Filipe, B Hartley, D Levison, P Wilson

Dental Surgery F P Ashley, A Banner, S J Challacombe, R Edler, S Farrant, N Fisher, T P Ford, D H Gibb, E Kidd, T Lehner, P Likeman, P Longhurst, M McGurk, M Meikle, J Metclaf, P Morgan, R I Nairn, R Palmer, D Pool, D J Ramsay, G J Roberts, P Robinson, R Savavanamuttu, A M Skelly, B G N Smith, B J Smith, A Thom, L A Usiskin, J D Walter, T L P Watts, E Whaites

Dermatology J N W Baker, R J Hay, D M MacDonald

Diabetes S A Amiel, N Finer, G C Viberti

Endocrinology S A Amiel, S Clarke, I Fogelman, B Hicks, M Maisey, P Winter

ENT E Chevretton, E Douek, M Gleeson, J Hibbert

Forensic Medicine Dr Shepherd, I E West

Gastroenterology R H Dowling, G E Sladen, M Wilkinson

General Medicine G M Cochrane, C J Corrigan, A W Frankland, T Gibson, J Henry, B H Hicks, R K Knight, T Lee, R R Lewis, R McNabb, P J Rees, J Ritter, G Volans, L J F Youlten

General Psychiatry M Dunn, M Lipsedge, A McCarthy, D Master, M Rafferty, A J Ramierez

General Surgery M Jourdan, T L McColl, R Mason, P Taylor

Genetics A C Berry, M Bobrow, S V Hodgson

Genitourinary Medicine S Tovey

Haematology K G A Clark, S Schey, G Smith

Histopathology L Bobrow

Medical Microbiology G French

Neurology A Colchester, R A C Hughes, B Moffat, M D O'Brien

Neurophysiology J Payan

Neurosurgery C Polkey, A J Strong

Nuclear Medicine S Clarke, I Fogelman, P M N Maisey

Obstetrics and Gynaecology S Bewley, M Chapman, T M Coltart, R Forman, K Harding, C Lloyd, D Maxwell, E D Morris, J Rymer, M Thom

Ophthalmology D Calver

Oral and Maxillofacial Surgery P M O'Driscoll

Orthopaedics P Allen, M Laurence, D Nunn, M S Watson

Paediatrics M Agrawal, L Allen, G Baird, E Baker, D M Calver, C Chantler, A G B Clarke, P Evans, G Haycock, M Joyce, M Lynch, I Murdoch, S Qureshi, S Rigden, S Robb, L Stimmler, M Tynan

Palliative Medicine T Bozek

Periodontology M N Naylor, D J Neill, H W Preiskel

Radiology A Adam, T Cox, S Rankin, J Reidy, M R Salari, A J S Saunders

Radiotherapy and Oncology M Chaudary, P Harper, E Macdonald, A Raminez, M A Richards, R D Rubens, S A Schey, D Tong

Renal Medicine J S Cameron, G Koffman, S Sacks, D G Williams

Rheumatology T J Gibson, R Grahame, G S Panayi

Toxicology Mr Edwards, J A Henry, V Murray, G N Volans, B Widdop

Urology J F Flannery, M L Joyce, A R Mundy

St Thomas' Hospital

Lambeth Palace Road, London SE1 7EH
Tel: 020 7928 9292 Fax: 020 7633 9292
Website: www.hospital.org.uk
Total Beds: 813

Accident and Emergency D J Williams

Alcohol and Substance Abuse T S Onen

Anaesthetics C Aps, A J Clement, T Hunt, D M Justins, M Lim, R A F Linton, J A Mathias, G H O'Sullivan, C E Pither, F Reynolds, G T Spencer, K Williams, R P Wise

Cardiology D J Coltart

Cardiothoracic Surgery J Dussek, G E Venn, C P Young

Care of the Elderly A H Hopper, F Martin, A Rudd

Chemical Pathology I S Menzies, B Slavin

Child and Adolescent Psychiatry P Loader, H F Roberts, H Swadi

Clinical Physiology R D Bradley, D F Treacher

Cytology N W Derias

Dermatology D J Atherton, A K Black, M M Black, B M Breathnach, A D M Bryceson, R O R Camp, R A J Eady, M W Greaves, W A D Griffiths, J L M Hawk, R J Hay, R R Jones, G M Levene, P McGibbon, R J G Rycroft, N P Smith, M F Spittle, N P J Walker, I White

Endocrinology R H Jones, C Low, I S Menzies, B Slavin, P H Sonksen, A E Young

ENT E B Chevreton, J N G Evans, A F F O'Connor

Forensic Psychiatry D Murphy

Gastroenterology P J Ciclitera, R J Ede, R P H Thompson

General Medicine N T Bateman, I R Cameron, D J Coltart, P J Hilton, B S Jenkins, F C Martin, O Nunan, R P H Thompson, C H C Twort, M M Webb-Peploe

General Practice F Gelder, M Goyal, G Hillman, R Jones, W S Marson, B Olding, D J Sharp, L I Zander

General Psychiatry Professor Craig, M Samuel

General Surgery N L Browse, K J Burnand, B T Jackson, C W Jamieson, M Jourdan, A E Young

Genitourinary Medicine D Barlow, J S Bingham, C Bradbeer, E M Graham, R N Thin

Haematology R Carr, B Hunt, T C Pearson, G F Savidge, N P Slater

Histopathology C P M Fletcher, P H McKee, H Pambakian

Immunology D C Dumonde, A S Hamblin

Medical Microbiology S J Eykyn, I Phillips

Medical Oncology M A Richards

Neonatology A M Kaiser, A D Milner

Nephrology P Hilton, A J Wing

Neurology R Howard, I C E Ormerod, R W R Russell

Neurophysiology C Panayiotopoulos

Nuclear Medicine D N Croft, T Nunan, H J O'Doherty

Obstetrics and Gynaecology P Braudie, I L C Fergusson, R X Goswamy, A Kubba, K S Raju, E Versi

Occupational Health C Dow, D Snashall

Ophthalmology A H Chignell, M J Falcon, T J ffytche, E Graham, M K Muir, G T Plant, R W Ross-Russell, J S Shilling, D J Spalton

Orthopaedics R N Brueton, F W Heatley, D A Reynolds, M A Smith

Paediatric Surgery H Ward

Paediatrics G S Clayden, G Dumont, G D Haycock, A J Hulse, M L R Lima, C M M Stern

Palliative Medicine D Justins, C Pither

Plastic Surgery P K B Davis, B J Mayou, D Mercer

Proctology B T Jackson, R J Nicholls

Psychiatry of Old Age E Fottrell

Psychology Z Atakan, J A G Besson, H D Kopelman, H F Oakeley, D Roy, J P R Young

Psychotherapy K Dustan

Public Health Medicine W W Holland, R J Rona

Radiology A B Ayers, L M MacDonald, J Pemberton, K A Tonge

Radiotherapy and Oncology T D Bates, R P Beaney, F Calman, H J Dobbs, M F Spittle, A R Timothy

Rheumatology G R V Hughes, J A Mathews, D A H Yates

Thoracic Medicine B Lams, H Milburn, I M O'Brien, G Santis, D F Treacher, C H C Twort

Thoracic Surgery J E Dussek

Urology M I Bultitude, R W L Davies, R Tiptaft

Vascular Surgery N L Browse, K G Burnand, C W Jamieson

Virology J E Banatvala

Halton Primary Care Trust

Victoria House, The Holloway, Runcorn WA7 4TH
Tel: 01928 593672 Fax: 01928 590594
Email: enquiries@halton-pct.nhs.uk
Website: www.halton-health.nhs.uk
(Cheshire and Merseyside Strategic Health Authority)

Chair Jim Wilson
Chief Executive Stephen Parry

Hambleton and Richmondshire Primary Care Trust

Headquarters, Station Road Business Park, Station Road, Thirsk YO7 1PZ
Tel: 01845 573800 Fax: 01845 573805
Email: enquiries@hambrichpct.nhs.uk
Website: www.hambrichpct.org.uk
(North and East Yorkshire and Northern Lincolnshire Strategic Health Authority)

Chair Sue Young
Chief Executive Simon Kirk

Lambert Memorial Hospital

Chapel Street, Thirsk YO7 1LU
Total Beds: 22

Richmond Victoria Hospital

Queens Road, Richmond DL10 4AJ
Tel: 01748 822109
Total Beds: 18

The Rutson HospitaL

Northallerton DL7 8EN
Tel: 01609 779911

Hammersmith and Fulham Primary Care Trust

5-7 Parsons Green, London SW6 4UL
Tel: 020 8846 6767 Fax: 020 8846 6779
Email: name@hf-pct.nhs.uk
Website: www.hf-pct.nhs.uk
(North West London Strategic Health Authority)

Chair Adrian Norridge
Chief Executive Chris Butler

Hammersmith Hospitals NHS Trust

Hammersmith Hospital, Du Cane Road, London W12 0HS
Tel: 020 8383 1000 Fax: 020 8383 4343
Website: www.hhnt.org
(North West London Strategic Health Authority)

Chair Thomas Legg
Chief Executive Derek Smith

Charing Cross Hospital

Fulham Palace Road, London W6 8RF
Tel: 020 8383 0000 Fax: 020 8846 1133
Website: www.nurseslisten.com
Total Beds: 450

Accident and Emergency H T Millington, F P Moore

Anaesthetics P J D Evans, J V Howard, J P Keiller, M P Margarson, M G A Palazzo, J C Salt

Audiological Medicine M A Hariri

Care of the Elderly I G Walton

Dermatology J J Cream

ENT P M Clarke, W E Grant, I S Mackay, H Saleh

General Medicine C S R Baker, A R C Cummin, K F Fox, A H Frankel, M K Meeran, I M Murray-Lyon, W A Seed, S J G Semple, D A Wood

General Psychiatry J S Barrett, S R Hirsch, F J Kelly, M C Phelan

General Surgery A H Davies, R M Greenhalgh, H D Sinnett, R G Springall, N A Theodorou

Haematology D H C McDonald

Histopathology P D Lewis, F J Paradinas

Medical Microbiology S P Barrett

Metabolic Medicine A Domhorst

Nephrology E A Brown, J B Levy, M E Phillips

Neurology P G Bain, S B Blunt, A M Bronstein, R J Guiloff, S H B Hawke, C Kennard, R K B Pearce, R C Peatfield, G D Perkin, R A W Shakir, J P H Wade

Neurophysiology N M Khalil

Neurosurgery N D Mendoza, K S O'Neil, D C Peterson, J M Rice-Edwards, J R van Dellen

Nuclear Medicine J W Frank

Oncology R C D Coombes, M G Glaser, C R Lewanski, C P Lowdell, E S Newlands, R H Phillips, S Retsas, B M Southcott

Ophthalmology W J Dinning, P E Kinnear

Orthopaedics R R H Coombs, K B Desai, M J Evans, D M Fahy, A J Forester, J C Hucker, S P F Hughes, J E Nixon, M Pearse, R K Strachan, A L Wallace

Plastic Surgery O A O Asplund, D M Davies, J Nanchahal, N J Percival, M G Royle, A E Searle, S H Wood

Radiology B K Wignall

Rheumatology A S C Keat, C G Mackworth-Young, R N Maini, P J W Venables

Urology P D Abel, J F Bellringer, S St-C Carter, T J Christmas, D Hrouda, J W A Ramsay

Hammersmith Hospital

Du Cane Road, London W12 0HS
Tel: 020 8383 1000 Fax: 020 8383 3169
Total Beds: 450

Cardiology J P Bagger, P G Camici, G J Davies, J S R Gibbs, D C Lefroy, P Nihoyannopoulos

Cardiothoracic Surgery J R Anderson, P Punjabi, P L C Smith, K M Taylor

Care of the Elderly C J Bulpitt, M Impallomeni, G M Wright

Chemical Pathology S I Girgis

Chest Disease E F Bowen, R K Coker, P W Ind, N B Pride, R J S Shaw, C L Shovlin

Dermatology A C Chu

General Medicine T J Aitman, J Calam, A Dornhorst, S Franks, S Ghosh, R I Lechler, R J Playford, C Rajkumar, A V Thillainayagam, G R Thompson, J R F Walters, G R Williams

General Surgery N A Habib, A K Kakkar, J A Lynn, R C N Williamson

Haematology J M Goldman, E J Kanfer, M A Laffan, A Rahemtulla, E G D Tuddenham

Histopathology N R Lemoine, J M Polak, G W H Stamp

Nephrology E J Clutterbuck, A Darling, G Gaskin, P Hatfield, E B Lightstone, P H Maxwell, C D Pusey, A N Warrens

Neurology D J Brooks, P Piccini, R J S Wise

Obstetrics and Gynaecology P R Bennett, A J Farthing, R A Margara, S Paterson-Brown, W P Soutter, G H Trew, R M L Winston

Oncology H S Wasan, J H Waxman

Paediatrics D Azzopardi, F M Cowan, B Dubowitz, A D Edwards, D R Harvey, A Y Manzur, N K Modi, F Muntoni, N J Robertson, M A Thomson

Radiology D J Allison, G M Bydder, J E Jackson

Rheumatology M F C Callan, D O Haskard, T J Vyse, M J Walport

Urology S K Agarwal, G Williams

Queen Charlotte's and Chelsea Hospital

Goldhawk Road, London W6 0XG
Tel: 020 8383 1111
Total Beds: 120

Anaesthetics G M Stocks

General Medicine M de Swiet

Obstetrics and Gynaecology D K Edmonds, N M Fisk, J C Girling, A L McCarthy, N Panay, G L Rose

Paediatrics D Azzopardi, H M Gardiner

Ravenscourt Park Hospital

Ravenscourt Park, London W6 0TN
Tel: 020 8846 7777
Total Beds: 24

Manager Joe Smyth

Hampshire Ambulance Service NHS Trust

Highcroft, Romsey Road, Winchester SO22 5DH

Tel: 01962 892600 Fax: 01962 842156
Website: www.hampshireambulance.nhs.uk
(Hampshire and Isle of Wight Strategic Health Authority)

Chair Anthony Barron
Chief Executive Claire Severgnini

Hampshire Partnership NHS Trust

Maples Building, Tatchbury Mount, Calmore, Southampton SO40 2RZ
Tel: 023 8087 4300 Fax: 023 8087 4301
Website: www.wht.nhs.uk
(Hampshire and Isle of Wight Strategic Health Authority)

Chair Maureen Robinson
Chief Executive Martin Barkley

Alcohol Advisory Day Hospital
63 Romsey Road, Winchester SO22 5DG
Tel: 01962 825071 Fax: 01962 824247

The Becton Centre
The Fairway, Barton On Sea, New Milton BH25 7AE
Tel: 01425 623802 Fax: 01425 627803

Community Mental Health Team and Day Hospital
Connaught House, 63B Romsey Road, Winchester SO22 5DE
Tel: 01962 825128 Fax: 01962 825280

Crane Ward
Old Manor Hospital, Wilton Road, Salisbury SP2 7EP
Tel: 01722 336262 Ext: 3143 Fax: 01722 425165

The Croft
Badger Farm Road, Winchester SO22 4JG
Tel: 01962 863511 Ext: 404
Total Beds: 8

Leigh House Hospital
Cuckoo Bushes Lane, Chandlers Ford, Eastleigh SO53 1JY
Tel: 023 8025 2418 Fax: 023 8027 0733
Total Beds: 15

Melbury Lodge
Royal Hampshire County Hospital, Romsey Road, Winchester SO22 5DG
Tel: 01962 825507 Fax: 01962 825512

Ravenswood House
Medium Secure Unit, Knowle, Fareham PO17 5NA
Tel: 01329 836000 Fax: 01329 834780

Royal South Hants Hospital, Department of Psychiatry
Brintons Terrace, Off St Mary's Road, Southampton SO14 0YG
Tel: 023 8063 4288 Fax: 023 8023 3189

St James' Hospital
Locksway Road, Milton, Portsmouth PO4 8LD
Tel: 023 9282 2444 Fax: 023 9229 3437
Total Beds: 244

General Psychiatry P M Fleming, N Renton, J Sinclair, C A Trotter

St Waleric (Psychogeriatric Day Hospital)
Park Road, Winchester SO23 7BE
Tel: 01962 841941 Fax: 01962 841590

War Memorial Community Hospital, Day Hospital and Day Surgery Unit
Charlton Road, Andover SP10 3LB
Tel: 01264 835273 Fax: 01264 351424
Total Beds: 10

Weyhill Road Mental Handicap Unit
4 Weyhill Road, Andover SP10 3AA
Tel: 01264 53433
Total Beds: 8

Wolversdene Road
8 Wolversdene Road, Andover SP10 2AX
Tel: 01264 58631
Total Beds: 8

Haringey Teaching Primary Care Trust

St Ann's Hospital, St Ann's Road, London N15 3TH
Tel: 020 8442 6000 Fax: 020 8442 6567
Email: firstname.lastname@haringey.nhs.uk
Website: www.haringeypct.nhs.uk
(North Central London Strategic Health Authority)

Chair Richard Sumray
Chief Executive Tracey Baldwin

Harlow Primary Care Trust

Level 16 Terminus House, Terminus Street, Harlow CM20 1XE
Tel: 01279 694747 Fax: 01279 694741
Website: www.harlowpct.nhs.uk
(Essex Strategic Health Authority)

Chair Tom Farr
Chief Executive Pam Court

Harrogate and District NHS Foundation Trust

Established as a Foundation Trust 01/01/2005.

Strayside Wing, Harrogate District Hospital, Lancaster Park Road, Harrogate HG2 7SX
Tel: 01423 885959 Fax: 01423 555791, 01423 555806
Email: forename.surname@hhc-tr.northy.nhs.uk
Website: www.hdft.nhs.uk
(North and East Yorkshire and Northern Lincolnshire Strategic Health Authority)

Chair Albert Day
Chief Executive Miles Scott

Harrogate District Hospital
Lancaster Park Road, Harrogate HG2 7SX
Tel: 01423 885959 Fax: 01423 555353
Total Beds: 427

Accident and Emergency B Hulse

Anaesthetics J Campbell, J Charlton, P Cutler, M Dakin, R Frater, J Gasser, G Parkin, A Poon, M Siminacz, M Thompson

Cardiology M Appleby, H Larkin

Care of the Elderly A Bennett, S Brotheridge, U Sharan, J Whitaker

Dermatology A Layton

Diabetes and Endocrinology S Ray, S Ray

ENT M Benamer, A Coatesworth, A Nicolaides, P Reilly

Gastroenterology J Ridpath

General Medicine G Davies, A Fennerty, P Hammmond, H Larkin

General Surgery G Dyke, J Harrison, R Knox, D Leinhardt

Genitourinary Medicine C Lacy

Neurology P J Goulding, B Henderson

Obstetrics and Gynaecology A Barnett, S Henalla, L Kidd

Oncology D Dodwell, D Jackson

Ophthalmology T Metcalfe, G Walters

Oral and Maxillofacial Surgery M Telfer, p Whitfield

Orthodontics J Kindelan

Orthopaedics A Collier, N London, J Mitchell, R Newman, G Sefton

Paediatrics S Rahman, D Smith

Pathology A Gledhill, C Gray, J Krishna, L Ragunathan, D Scott, M Toop

Radiology S Carradine, A Coral, R Mawhinney, D Sapherson, D Scullion

Respiratory Medicine A Fennerty

Rheumatology and Rehabilitation A Gough

Urology A Lawson, P Singh

Harrow Primary Care Trust

Grace House, Harrovian Business Village, Bessborough Road, Harrow HA1 3EX
Tel: 020 8422 6644 Fax: 020 8426 8646
Website: www.harrowpct.nhs.uk
(North West London Strategic Health Authority)

Chair Geoffrey Rose
Chief Executive Andrew Morgan

Hartlepool Primary Care Trust

3rd Floor, Mandale House, Harbour Walk, The Marina, Hartlepool TS24 0UX
Tel: 01429 285079 Fax: 01429 286944
Website: www.hartlepoolpct.nhs.uk
(County Durham and Tees Valley Strategic Health Authority)

Chair Gerald Wistow
Chief Executive Angela Hawkes

Hastings and St Leonards Primary Care Trust

PO Box 124, St Leonards-on-Sea TN38 9WH
Tel: 01424 457100 Fax: 01424 457145
Email: enquiries@hs-pct.nhs.uk
Website: www.hastingsandstleonardspct.nhs.uk
(Surrey and Sussex Strategic Health Authority)

Chair Marie Casey
Chief Executive Toni Wilkinson

Havering Primary Care Trust

Bentley Suite, St George's Hospital, 117 Suttons Lane, Hornchurch RM12 6RS
Tel: 01708 465000 Fax: 01708 465300
Website: www.haveringpct.nhs.uk
(North East London Strategic Health Authority)

Chair Leonard Smith
Chief Executive Ralph McCormack

St George's Hospital

117 Suttons Lane, Hornchurch RM12 6RS

Heart of Birmingham Teaching Primary Care Trust

Bartholomew House, 142 Hagley Road, Edgbaston, Birmingham B16 9PA
Tel: 0121 224 4600 Fax: 0121 224 4601
Email: info@hobtpct.nhs.uk
Website: www.hobtpct.nhs.uk
(Birmingham and the Black Country Strategic Health Authority)

Chair Ranjit Sondhi
Chief Executive Antony Sumara

Heart of England NHS Foundation Trust

Formerly Birmingham Heartlands and Solihull (Teaching) NHS Trust. Established as a Foundation Trust 01/04/2005.
Birmingham Heartlands Hospital, Bordesley Green East, Birmingham B9 5SS
Tel: 0121 424 2000 Fax: 0121 424 2200
Website: www.heartsol.nhs.uk
(Birmingham and the Black Country Strategic Health Authority)

Chair Clive Wilkinson
Chief Executive Mark Goldman

Birmingham Heartlands Hospital

Bordesley Green East, Birmingham B9 5SS
Tel: 0121 424 2000 Fax: 0121 424 2200
Total Beds: 950

Accident and Emergency C Park (Head), A Bleetman, E F Jones, A Macnamara, M J Shalley

Anaesthetics J C Carnie (Head), S S Fayek, F Gao, D J Hawkins, R B Hopkinson, J M James, T McLeod, B O'Connor, M J Rooney, A H Seymour, M H Taylor

Cardiology R G Murray (Head), J M Beattie, P J Lowry, P Ludman

Care of the Elderly R M Kamalarajan (Head), D Sandler, R A Shinton, D G Swain, P J W Wallis

Dental Surgery B A Hoyle, C J Meryon

Diabetes A H Barnett (Head), S Bain, P M Dodson, S Gough, S Kumar

ENT J B Campbell (Head), Mr Fisher, M Macnamara, D W Morgan, K Pearman

Gastroenterology I M Chesner (Head), R P Walt

General Medicine R Kamalarajan, S Kumar, M J Leyland, H C Rayner

General Surgery M X Gannon, M D Goldman, D Mosquera, J L Taylor, H J Thomson

Genitourinary Medicine S M Drake, D J White

Haematology D W Milligan (Head), C Fegan

Immunology R A Thompson

Infectious Diseases C J Ellis (Head), A M Geddes, J A Innes

Nephrology H C Rayner, S A Smith, R M Temple

Neurology J M Anderson (Head)

Obstetrics and Gynaecology W E Mackenzie (Head), S W Hall, E Payne, S Sadek, M P Wyldes

Oncology N James

Ophthalmology I Cuncliffe (Head), J R Ainsworth, M T Benson, P Dodson, J M Gibson

Orthopaedics H Rahman, A Sambatakakis, M Shrivastava

Paediatrics S J Rose (Head), H Goodyear, R Mulik, R H Mupaneamunda, T Ninan, L M Rabb, F A I Riordan, H Roper, M J Tarlow, M Venkataraman, M Watkinson, J Williams

Pathology A F Jones (Head), F B Brook, J Crocker, C W Edwards, I D Farrell, M A Hulten, K A James, J Newman, K J Nye, D Pillay, E G Smith, A Warfield

Radiology J H Reynolds (Head), A K Banerjee, J R Ferrando, M J Henderson, G S Jones, S Sangrasegran, D C Tudway

Respiratory Medicine P S Burge (Head), J G Ayres, R M Cayton, D E Stableforth

Rheumatology S Bowman, Dr Faizal, M Pugh

Thoracic Surgery F J Collins (Head), J Khalil-Marzouk, P Rajesh

Urology B D Sarmah (Head)

Solihull Hospital

Lode Lane, Solihull B91 2JL
Tel: 0121 424 2000 Fax: 0121 424 5496
Total Beds: 350

Accident and Emergency T Bagga

Anaesthetics F E Bannourah, B Hoggart, S Parr, R Shilling, C G Weston

Cardiology R G Murray (Head)

Dermatology A Heaggerty

ENT J Campbell (Head), D Morgan, K Pearman

General Medicine R G Murray, S O'Hickey, R Palmer, R J Polson, K Priestley, M Sandler, S Tan, R Wears, R J Wilson

General Surgery G Barsoum, D Burkitt, A Klidjian, G S Sokhi

Neurology M Anderson (Head)

Obstetrics and Gynaecology P Needham, C J F Rowbotham, R S Settatree, D W Sturdee

Oncology A Stockdale

Ophthalmology G Meeson

Orthodontics B Hoyle

Orthopaedics S Brooks (Head), S Bryan, A Murray

Radiology K B Bhatt, N A Chaudhry, C J Fletcher, G Stewart

Heatherwood and Wexham Park Hospitals NHS Trust

Wexham Park Hospital, Wexham, Slough SL2 4HL
Tel: 01753 633000 Fax: 01753 634825
Email: firstname.lastname@hwph-tr.nhs.uk
Website: www.hwph-tr.org.uk
(Thames Valley Strategic Health Authority)

Chair Ruth Watts Davies
Chief Executive Andrew Way

Heatherwood Hospital

London Road, Ascot SL5 8AA
Tel: 01344 623333 Fax: 01344 874340
Total Beds: 244

Anaesthetics J Restall, K Spelina, W J Wraight

ENT A F Jefferis

General Medicine L Hart, R D M Scott, M Smith

General Psychiatry M S L de Silva, R G Gall, W Lang, A J Wilkins

General Surgery G S Barrett, C Desai

Elderly Care R G A Behrman, S K Rao

Neurology M Johnson

Obstetrics and Gynaecology J Fairbank, J Spring

Oral and Maxillofacial Surgery C Yates

Orthodontics D Slattery

Orthopaedics R Allum, G Deane, J Jones, G Singer, M Thomas, A Unwin

Paediatrics J Pearce

Plastic Surgery J Dickinson, C T Khoo

Radiology I Liyanage, C Luck, C Rodgers

Rheumatology and Rehabilitation S P Liyanage

Urology C Hudd, O Karim, H Mottiwala

King Edward VII Hospital

Windsor SL4 3DP
Tel: 01753 860441 Fax: 01753 636107
Total Beds: 20

Care of the Elderly J Harding, S K Rao

Dermatology A Roberts, V Walkden

Diabetes R D M Scott

ENT N Bleach, A F Jefferis

Gastroenterology S Levi

General Psychiatry G Gall, L D Silva

General Surgery G S Barrett

Neurology D J Thomas

Obstetrics and Gynaecology P Reginald, J Spring

Ophthalmology J J Kanski, J A McAllister, R B S Packard

Oral Surgery C Yates

Orthodontics D Slattery

Orthopaedics G Deane, J Jones, M Swann

Paediatrics J Cowan

Plastic Surgery D Crawford

Radiology S Colenso, S Ghiacy

Radiotherapy H Thomas

Rheumatology S P Liyanage

Thoracic Surgery E R Townsend

Urology C Hudd, O Karim

Vascular Medicine P Rutter

St Mark's Hospital

St Mark's Road, Maidenhead SL6 6DU
Tel: 01628 632012 Fax: 01753 638569
Total Beds: 106

Care of the Elderly R Behrman, J Harding

Dermatology A Roberts, J Wilkinson

ENT M Wallace

Gastroenterology M MacMahon

General Medicine R Blackwood

General Psychiatry M Atkins, P D Maddocks

General Surgery A Gordon, P Rutter

Neurology D J Thomas

Obstetrics and Gynaecology S Dinitry, P Reginald

Ophthalmology R Packard

Oral Surgery M Issa

Orthopaedics R Allum, M Thomas

Paediatrics J Connell, J L Pearce

Plastic Surgery C Khoo

Rheumatology S P Liyanage

Urology D Fawcett, C Hudd, O Karim

Upton Hospital

Albert Street, Slough SL1 2BJ
Tel: 01753 821441 Fax: 01753 635050
Total Beds: 105

Care of the Elderly R Behrman, R Chauhan, A Darowski, S K Rao

Chest Medicine M Smith, J Wiggins

Child and Adolescent Psychiatry J Brockless, K Friend, M Kingswood

Genitourinary Medicine S Dawson

Paediatrics M Colbey

Psychiatry of Old Age G Dawson

Wexham Park Hospital

Slough SL2 4HL
Tel: 01753 633000 Fax: 01753 684825
Total Beds: 557

Accident and Emergency J C Litchfield, A C W Matheson

Anaesthetics M D G Bukht, S Davies, R Fernandes, R D Jack, L Leibler, R C Loveland, A May, J Pattison, J Rangasami, T S Silva, B Smallman, B L Smith, K Spelina, E Umerah, R Woolf

Dermatology V Walkden

Elderly Care D Chauhan

ENT C Aldren, N Bleach, A F Jefferis

General Medicine D Dove, S Levi, G Maidment, C Missouris, J Wiggins

General Psychiatry J Brockless, R E Chinn, E Clifford, G Dawson, E D'Souza, J W Harding, W Lang, A McCauley, S Parameswaran, P Sudbury

General Surgery A Desai, J Gilbert, A Gordon, S E Knight, P Rutter

Neurology J Wade

Obstetrics and Gynaecology S Dimitri, P Reginald

Ophthalmology Mr Kanski, Mr Packard

Oral Surgery M Issa, Mr Slattery, C Yates

Orthopaedics R Allum, G Deane, R Dega, J Jones, G Singer, M Swann, M Thomas

Paediatrics J A Connell, J Cowen, Z Huma, R Jones, J L Pearce, P Sebire

Pathology M Ali, N Bienz, H Chapel, C Havelock, A Lessing, M MacIntyre, P H Mackie, Dr Sharif, I Walker

Plastic Surgery Dr Armstrong, Dr Crawford, J Dickinson, CT K Khoo

Radiology Dr Charig, S Colenso, D K Grieve, M Moreland

Radiotherapy and Oncology R Ashford

Rheumatology and Rehabilitation A Hall, Dr Steuer

Urology C Hudd, O Karim, H Mottiwala

Hereford and Worcester Ambulance Service NHS Trust

Bransford, Worcester WR6 5JD
Tel: 01886 834200 Fax: 01886 834210
Website: www.worcestershirehealth.nhs.uk
(West Midlands South Strategic Health Authority)

Chair Joanna Newton
Chief Executive Russell Hamilton

Hereford Hospitals NHS Trust

County Hospital, Union Walk, Hereford HR1 2ER
Tel: 01432 355444 Fax: 01432 354310
Email: forename.surname@hhtr.nhs.uk
Website: www.herefordshire.nhs.uk
(West Midlands South Strategic Health Authority)

Chair Cessa Moore
Chief Executive David Rose

Hereford County Hospital

Stonebow Road, Hereford HR1 2ER
Tel: 01432 355444 Fax: 01432 354310
Total Beds: 340

Anaesthetics J H W Ballance, C A Day, R M B Dowling, I P Hine, J D Hutchinson, W Moore, N P Salmon, W Williams

Care of the Elderly J A Dalziel, C Jenkins, P Overstall

Dental Surgery K Ashley, D Evans

Dermatology J R S Rendall

ENT G Hanna

General Medicine A Blake, H Connor, J Glancy, M Hall, D W Pitcher, P Ryan, J A Spillane

General Surgery A P Corder, E Grocott, P H Harper, G Sole

Obstetrics and Gynaecology M Cohn, R B Smith, R Subak-Sharpe

Paediatrics R Adelman, A M Butterfill, N C Fraser

Palliative Medicine J Sykes

Pathology T J Coleman, J S Dinnen, M Hayes, F McGinty

Plastic Surgery D S Murray

Radiology P Grech, G M Rowe, P Wilson

Radiotherapy and Oncology Dr Elyan, C Roch-Berry

Rheumatology D Rees, R B Williams

Urology A Jha

Hereford General Hospital

Nelson Street, Hereford HR1 2PA
Tel: 01432 355444 Fax: 01432 340425
Total Beds: 106

Accident and Emergency A Ballham

Anaesthetics J H W Ballance, C Day, R M B Dowling, I P Hine, J D Hutchinson, W Moore, N P Salmon, W Williams

Care of the Elderly J A Dalziel, C Jenkins, P W Overstall

Orthopaedics I R S Reynolds, P V Seal, P Shewell, T F Sibly, D Williams

Radiology P Grech, G M Rowe, P Wilson

Victoria Eye Hospital
149-153 Eign Street, Hereford HR4 0AN
Tel: 01432 355444 Fax: 01432 279917
Total Beds: 12

Herefordshire Primary Care Trust

Belmont Abbey, Belmont, Hereford HR2 9RP
Tel: 01432 344344 Fax: 01432 363900
(West Midlands South Strategic Health Authority)

Chair Ted Willmott
Chief Executive Paul Bates

Leominster Community Hospital
South Street, Leominster HR6 8JH
Tel: 01568 614211
Total Beds: 34

Care of the Elderly J A Dalziel, P Overstall

Psychiatry of Old Age R Eggar, V Staples

Ross Community Hospital
Alton Street, Ross-on-Wye HR9 5LQ
Tel: 01989 562100
Total Beds: 32

Stonebow Unit County Hospital
Hereford HR1 2ER
Tel: 01432 355444
Total Beds: 56

Manager Mark Hemming

General Psychiatry P Allman, K Godbert, C Thomas

Psychiatry of Old Age R Eggar, V Staples

Hertfordshire Partnership NHS Trust

99 Waverley Road, St Albans AL3 5TL
Tel: 01727 811888 Fax: 01727 857900
Website: www.hpt.nhs.uk
(Bedfordshire and Hertfordshire Strategic Health Authority)

Chair Hattie Llewelyn-Davies
Chief Executive Bill Macintyre

Hertsmere Primary Care Trust

Barry House, 69-71 High Street, Potters Bar EN6 5AS
Tel: 01707 647586 Fax: 01707 647594
Email: firstname.surname@hertsmere-pct.nhs.uk
Website: www.hertsmere-pct.nhs.uk
(Bedfordshire and Hertfordshire Strategic Health Authority)

Chair Stuart Bloom
Chief Executive Jacqueline Clark

Potters Bar Hospital
Mutton Lane, Potters Bar EN6 2PB
Tel: 01707 53286
Total Beds: 45

Heywood and Middleton Primary Care Trust

London House, Oldham Road, Middleton, Manchester M24 1AZ
Tel: 0161 643 6900 Fax: 0161 655 1548
Email: firstname.surname@hmpct.nhs.uk
(Greater Manchester Strategic Health Authority)

Chair David Edwards
Chief Executive Keith Surgeon

High Peak and Dales Primary Care Trust

Newholme Hospital, Baslow Road, Bakewell DE45 1AD
Tel: 01629 812525 Fax: 01629 817890
Website: www.highpeakanddalespct.nhs.uk
(Trent Strategic Health Authority)

Chair Dianne Jeffrey
Chief Executive Neil Swanwick

Buxton Hospital
London Road, Buxton SK17 9NJ
Tel: 01298 214000
Total Beds: 34

Anaesthetics K O Sullivan

Child Health Dr Preece, M R Reynolds

Chiropody and Podiatry B T Brown

Dermatology J B O'Driscoll

ENT L Ramamurthy

General Medicine N Kong

General Surgery F J Curran, P Gallagher, Mr Heggarty

Obstetrics and Gynaecology A Pickersgill, D Swinhoe

Radiology J Glaves, M R P Shaw

Urology Mr Brough

Cavendish Hospital
Manchester Road, Buxton SK17 6TE
Tel: 01298 79236 Fax: 01298 72054
Total Beds: 48

Care of the Elderly J Catania

Psychiatry of Old Age J Galloway

Newholme Hospital
Bakewell DE45 1AD
Tel: 01629 812525 Fax: 01629 813479
Total Beds: 46

Whitworth Hospital
330 Bakewell Road, Matlock DE4 2JD
Tel: 01629 580211 Fax: 01629 583037
Total Beds: 54

Care of the Elderly D Chew

Dermatology G B Colver

ENT F M Nofal

General Medicine D G Ashton, J W Hadfield

General Surgery D Bardsley, S Holt, W Lambert, J M Sims

Learning Disabilities R Madina

Obstetrics and Gynaecology D Fothergill, J M McDonnell

Ophthalmology K Mohamad

Paediatrics M R Reynolds

Rheumatology J Bourne

The Hillingdon Hospital NHS Trust

Pield Heath Road, Uxbridge UB8 3NN
Tel: 01895 238282 Fax: 01895 811687
Email: forename.surname@thh.nhs.uk, info@thh.nhs.uk
Website: www.thh.nhs.uk
(North West London Strategic Health Authority)

Chair Anthony Woodbridge
Chief Executive David McVittie

Hillingdon Hospital

Hillingdon, Pield Heath Road, Uxbridge UB8 3NN
Tel: 01895 238282 Fax: 01895 811687
Total Beds: 666

Anaesthetics J P Downer (Head), J Anandanesan, A Knight, C Messer, Dr Smith, A Thorniley, S Vashist, Dr Weinbren

Care of the Elderly S J L Brooy, A Parry, Dr Sweetman, Dr Vowles

Dental Surgery Dr Crow, G T Gardiner

Dermatology Dr Hughes

ENT Dr Mareuis, Dr Ryan

General Medicine Dr Dubney, Dr Grocott-Mason, Dr Hilal, R Hillson, G E Holdstock, L H Sevitt, D J Thomas, Dr Tonge, Dr Weedham, Dr Wills

General Psychiatry C Coghlan, Dr Conway, Dr Gouhargy, Dr Hadler, Dr Kincher, B Lucas, Dr Nathan, J Palmer, R W Reid

General Surgery Dr Das, P Mitchenere, Dr Mohsen, T Paes, B A Shorey

Genitourinary Medicine Dr Schroeder, S Waldron

Learning Disabilities I Singh

Neurology Dr Malik

Obstetrics and Gynaecology Dr Jackson, N Nicholas, J Price, N Watson, C S Wright

Ophthalmology P Bloom, Professor Fielder, N Lee

Orthopaedics K M Atrah, W N Bodey, J F Dooley, Dr Kamereri, R Langstaff, Dr Singh

Paediatrics R Buchdahl, M Cruwys, H Hamid, P Jaffe, G Khakoo

Palliative Medicine L Bangham, Dr Lemon, J Maher, G Ruskin

Pathology F Barker, R Jan-Mohamed, R Kaczmarski, D M Rimmer, J Williamson

Psychiatry of Old Age A Conway, J Palmer

Radiology N Chetty, R Devakumar, R J Kantor, Dr Raza, I M Shirley, Dr Whittle

Radiotherapy and Oncology E J Maher

Rheumatology and Rehabilitation R S Hanspal

Thoracic Surgery E R Townsend

Urology Dr Ng, A Pope

Hillingdon Primary Care Trust

Kirk House, 97-109 High Street, Yiewsley, West Drayton UB7 7HJ
Tel: 01895 452000 Fax: 01895 452108
Website: www.hillingdon.nhs.uk
(North West London Strategic Health Authority)

Chair Sarah Pond
Chief Executive Graeme Betts

Northwood and Pinner Cottage Hospital

Pinner Road, Northwood HA6 1DE
Tel: 01923 824182
Total Beds: 24

Hinchingbrooke Health Care NHS Trust

Hinchingbrooke Park, Huntingdon PE29 6NT
Tel: 01480 416416 Fax: 01480 416561
Email: info@hinchingbrooke.nhs.uk
Website: www.hinchingbrooke.org.uk
(Norfolk, Suffolk and Cambridgeshire Strategic Health Authority)

Chair Susan Smith
Chief Executive Douglas Pattisson

Hinchingbrooke Hospital

Hinchingbrooke Park, Huntingdon PE18 8NT
Tel: 01480 416416
Total Beds: 396

Accident and Emergency R K Das

Anaesthetics P M Benison, A J M Brooks, P R Fletcher, I Hardy, M R-U Hasan, B V Latham, K R Macleod, V Price

Care of the Elderly C D R Borland, K J Walsh

Chest Medicine D Bilton, D A Promnitz

Child and Adolescent Psychiatry P W Millard, S W Pedersen

Dermatology C C Banfield

ENT R F Gray, P Jani, P S L Leong

General Medicine C D R Borland, R J Dickinson, R G Henderson, K S Matsiko, M A A Matthews, P J Roberts, K J Walsh

General Psychiatry D Badiani, D F Bermingham, A Jenaway, R W Latcham, M C Royston

General Surgery B A A Bekdash, J R Benson, J V Gryf-Lowczowski, C R G Quick, J B Reed

Genitourinary Medicine S M Forster

Haematology C E Hoggarth, K P Rege

Obstetrics and Gynaecology M Alkurdi, S Bissoonauth, P B Forbes, B H Lim, R S Mathur, H A H Rahman, M C Slack

Ophthalmology D W Flanagan, C Rene, N J Sarkies, C G Stephenson, A Tufail

Orthopaedics S N Amara, D P Conlan, A D Patel, P F T Sewell, G W Southgate, T Vaughan-Lane, A S Wojcik

Paediatrics B D M Algawi, M G Becker, J Challener, L E Cormack, C R de Cates, H Dixon, F Latcham, R N Miles, C M Ni Bhrolchain

Plastic Surgery G C Cormack, M S Irwin

Radiology C S F Hubbard, H L Taylor, A A Warner

Radiotherapy and Oncology D Gilligan, T Li-Tee

Rheumatology and Rehabilitation G D Pountain

Urology K N Bullock

Hinckley and Bosworth Primary Care Trust

Swan House Business Centre, The Park, Market Bosworth, Nuneaton CV13 0LJ
Tel: 01455 293200 Fax: 01455 290700
Website: www.hinckleyboswortpct.nhs.uk
(Leicestershire, Northamptonshire and Rutland Strategic Health Authority)

Chair Ernest White
Chief Executive Colin Blackler

Hinckley and District Hospital
Mount Road, Hinckley LE10 1AG
Tel: 01455 441800 Fax: 01455 441888

Sunnyside Hospital
Ashby Road, Hinckley LE10 3DA
Tel: 01455 251188
Total Beds: 18

Homerton University Hospital NHS Foundation Trust

Established as a Foundation Trust 01/04/2004.
Homerton Row, London E9 6SR
Tel: 020 8510 5555 Fax: 020 8510 7608
Email: enquiries@homerton.nhs.uk
Website: www.homerton.nhs.uk
(North East London Strategic Health Authority)

Chair Andrew Windross
Chief Executive Nancy Hallett

Homerton University Hospital
Homerton Row, London E9 6SR
Tel: 020 8510 5555 Fax: 020 8510 7608
Total Beds: 485

Accident and Emergency H Cugnoni, L Gant, K Henderson, S Miles

Anaesthetics P Amoroso, M W Ashby, V Carr, J Coakley, L Davis, W Gallagher, D Guerin, G H Hackett, D Halfpenny, S Harrod, C J Hinds, P R Howell, Dr Okunso, Dr Tham, J D Watson, D J Wilkinson, Dr Wong, G Wray

Cardiology A Kurbaan, D S Tunstall-Pedoe

Care of the Elderly M Britton, Dr Elegbe, A B Lehmann, K O'Sullivan

Clinical Pharmacology and Therapeutics S M L Abrams

Dermatology R Bull, P Goldsmith

Diabetes J V Anderson, P Freedman

Gastroenterology C Blanshard, P J Kumar, R Shidrawi

General Medicine S M L Abrams, J V Anderson, Dr Blanstard, G Bothamley, Dr Elegbe, P Freedman, A Lehmann, R Mootoo, R Rajakulasingam, D S Tunstall Pedoe

General Surgery S Kadirkamanathan, P Lunnis, M Mahir, Dr Ravikumar, D Shanahan

Genitourinary Medicine J Anderson, S El Gadi, P Mayurahathan

Haematology R J Amos, M Evans

Medical Microbiology A Kärcher, B Macrae

Neurology R J Greenwood, P Jarman

Obstetrics and Gynaecology D Akinfenwa, C Barnick, E Dorman, K Erskine, K Harrington, R J S Howell, C Roberts, C Stacey, N C Wathen, J Yoon

Ophthalmology Dr Daniel

Oral Surgery I L Hutchison

Orthopaedics K C Kong, D M McCarthy, C Mbubaegbu

Paediatrics J Bucknall, K Costeloe, S Fang, Dr Goddard, D Hodes, S Husain, E Maolouf, R Sood, A Washington

Palliative Medicine D Fewer

Radiology S Amin, P M Cannon, K Patel, A Sahdev

Rehabilitation Medicine R J Greenwood

Respiratory Medicine G Bothamley, R Rajakulasingam

Rheumatology A Bhanj, R Mootoo

Urology V Nargund

Horsham and Chanctonbury Primary Care Trust

New Park House, North Street, Horsham RM12 1RL
Tel: 01403 215129 Fax: 01403 215128
Email: info@hcpct.nhs.uk
Website: www.hcpct.nhs.uk
(Surrey and Sussex Strategic Health Authority)

Chair Barbara Wilkins
Chief Executive Angela Ugur

Horsham Hospital
Hurst Road, Horsham RH12 2DR
Tel: 01403 227000 Fax: 01403 227030
Total Beds: 86

Manager Barbara Pink

Care of the Elderly R J Bailey, F Ramsay, A G Vallon

Hounslow Primary Care Trust

Phoenix Court, 531 Staines Road, Hounslow TW4 5DP
Tel: 020 8321 2211 Fax: 020 8321 2249
Website: www.hounslowpct.nhs.uk
(North West London Strategic Health Authority)

Chair Christine Hay
Chief Executive John James

Huddersfield Central Primary Care Trust

Trust Headquarters, St Luke's House, Blackmoorfoot Road, Crosland Moor, Huddersfield HD4 5RH
Tel: 01484 466000 Fax: 01484 466111
Website: www.huddersfieldcentral-pct.nhs.uk
(West Yorkshire Strategic Health Authority)

Chair Rob Napier
Chief Executive Kevin Holder

Hull and East Yorkshire Hospitals NHS Trust

Anlaby Road, Hull HU3 2JZ
Tel: 01482 328541 Fax: 01482 674196
Email: forename.surname@hey.nhs.uk
Website: www.hey.nhs.uk
(North and East Yorkshire and Northern Lincolnshire Strategic Health Authority)

Chair Scilla Smith
Chief Executive Stephen Greep

Beverley Westwood Hospital
Woodlands, Beverley HU17 8BU
Tel: 01482 875875 Fax: 01482 866194

Castle Hill Hospital
Castle Road, Cottingham HU16 5JQ
Tel: 01482 875875 Fax: 01482 623209
Total Beds: 576

Anaesthetics A Saaman (Head), S Bennett, A Coe, A Culbert, P Evans, M Felgate, S Gower, D R Haines, V Hong, B Mikl, Dr Pollock, A H S Saleh, J Thind, F Umerah, R T Whitty, T I R Williams

Cardiology F Alamgir (Head), M F Alamgir, A Clark, J Cleland, G C Kaye, N J Linker

Cardiothoracic Medicine L Guvendik (Head), A Cale, M E Cowen, S Griffin

Care of the Elderly S F Beardsworth, A Farnsworth, J Knox

Gastroenterology M Dakkak (Head), H H Tsai

General Medicine A G Arnold (Head), M A Greenstone, D V McGivern

General Surgery J R T Monson (Head), G S Duthie, J N Fox, J Gunn, J Hartley, T Mahapatra, P McManus, J Tilsed, K R Wedgwood

Infectious Diseases H Thaker (Head), G Barlow, P Moss

Obstetrics and Gynaecology R Yeo (Head), J Gandhi, W Noble, K Phillips, D Poole

Orthopaedics V Johnson (Head), M R Korab-Karpinski, A Mohsen, A Nihal, C J Shaw

Pathology I Richmond (Head), J Meigh, R E E Meigh

Plastic Surgery A Platt (Head), N B Hart, M Riaz, P W R Stanley

Radiology G R Avery (Head), J Cast, A E Hubbard, N Kennan, S L Mann

Rheumatology and Rehabilitation I Tomlinson (Head), B N M Jayawardhana, J W Tomlinson

Surgical Oncology J Monson (Head), P Drew

Thoracic Medicine A G Arnold (Head), M A Greenstone, D V McGivern, A Morice

Urology J Hetherington (Head), D Almond, G Cooksey, S Krauss

Hull Royal Infirmary

Anlaby Road, Hull HU3 2JZ
Tel: 01482 328541 Fax: 01482 674196
Total Beds: 680

Accident and Emergency J Osman (Head), M Higson, T R Jackson, M D C Simpson, W Townend, H Vixseboxse

Anaesthetics A Samaan (Head), G M Bwalya, P Cain, A Coe, M D J Donaldson, M Felgate, B M Gray, P A Gray, C Hibbert, P N Ikin, M R Kamath, A Kuttappa, I Locker, C Melville, R Owen-Smith, G M Purdy, Z Rafique, S Ram, S Ram, C D Rigg, S Roberts, I F Russell, C Smales, I M Smith, F Umerah, J Waterland, B Withington

Cardiology F Alamgir (Head), J L Caplin, M Nasir, R Oliver, A C Tweddle

Care of the Elderly F Thomson (Head), A R Abdul-Hamid, T Aung, M R Mansoor, N R Steel

Dental Surgery A Baxter, C W Blackburn, M R Cope, G F Gregory, D G Starr

Diabetes C Walton (Head), B J Allan, D A Hepburn, E A Masson, J Patmore

ENT S L Smith (Head), S R Ell, R J England, M J Rogers, N D Stafford

Gastroenterology M Dakkak (Head), T Diggory, M H Gaiffer, Dr Khulusi, S Shaji, L Sinha, J Smithson

General Medicine D Bhatia (Head), V K Anand, G G Anderson, S L Atkin, D Bhandari, H Gaili

General Surgery B F Johnson, C O'Boyle, P M Renwick, C M S Royston, P C Sedman

Haematology R Patmore (Head), S Awad Ali, C Carter, M L Shields

Nephrology A T Webb (Head), H Collinson, D W Eadington, D M Lewis, L Sellars

Neurology F Ahmed (Head), P Cariga, H H M Hamdalla, A Ming

Neurophysiology A A A Bajalan

Neurosurgery D O'Brien (Head), P Fewings, B G Mathew, K M Morris, G O'Reilly, J Tarafder

Obstetrics and Gynaecology R Yeo (Head), F Bieruelt, R Jha, S R Killick, P Lesney, S W Lindow, S D Maguiness, E H Speck, S N Tyrell

Ophthalmic Surgery J Innes (Head), M Zaman

Ophthalmology J R Innes (Head), A Babar, S K Datta, A K Mathur, O Stewart, C Vize

Orthodontics J W Coope, P Cove, J J D Neal

Orthopaedics V Johnson (Head), T J Cain, H Cattermole, F R Howell, G V Johnson, M R K Karpinski, G L M Kings, K P Sherman

Paediatric Surgery I Beddis (Head), S Besarovic, R Daniel

Paediatrics I R Beddis (Head), A A A Azaz, M Barraclough, M El-Habbal, A Habeb, H Klonin, R F Massey, V Matthew, P W Pairaudeau, C M Wood, M M Zubier

Pathology I Richmond (Head), D Allsup, P A Burgess, A P Campbell, P C Dore, I Hanning, J Heald, L Karsai, E S Kilpatrick, R P Kumar, E D Long, A W Macdonald, S L Mawer, N E New, J R Read, M Rodrigues, J A Wilson

Radiology G Avery (Head), R J V Bartlett, A M Coady, J F Dyet, A S Early, D Ettles, C Hauff, C R Hill, D Horton, D Nag, A J Paddon, A Razak, G R Robinson, D R Salvage, P Scott, A D Taylor, L W Turnbull

Rheumatology I Tomlinson (Head), E Baguley, S M Doherty, Y I Patel

Vascular Surgery P Renwick (Head), A Akomolafe, P McCollum

The Princess Royal Hospital

Saltshouse Road, Hull HU8 9HE
Tel: 01482 701151 Fax: 01482 676737
Total Beds: 50

Dermatology N Alexander, P Gowda, S Walton

Radiotherapy and Oncology R Patmore (Head), R Barton, A Chaturvedi, A Dealey, S Dixit, C Hamilton, M E Holmes, M Lind, P Mack, A Maraveyas, D Sharp

Humber Mental Health Teaching NHS Trust

Formerly Hull and East Riding Community Health NHS Trust.

Trust Headquarters, Willerby Hill, Willerby HU10 6ED
Tel: 01482 389100 Fax: 01482 303900
(North and East Yorkshire and Northern Lincolnshire Strategic Health Authority)

Chair Ros Taylor
Chief Executive Linda Glasby
Consultants Said Ali, John Astill, Mary Barraclough, John Bestley, Denise Brown, Douglas Gee, Anna Green, Otto Grubl, Graham Harkness, Janine Adelle Henderson, Tarique Hussain, Vinod Iyer, Susan Joseph, Neel Kamal, David Lawley, Mairead Lobban, Jennifer Mabbot, Stella Mahajuodeen, Ivana Markova, Bernadette McInerney, Jan Mead, Stella Morris, Anne Mortimer, Ayung Nyunt, Alison Pierce, Steve Powell, N Prasad, Hufrish Rasool, Mike Reid, David Ryan, Sharaf Salem, Sajja Srikanth, Andy Talbot, Francis Umerah, Simon Wood

Coltman Street Day Hospital and Community Support Teams

Coltman Street, Hull HU3 2SG
Tel: 01482 328807 Fax: 01482 223643

Huntingdonshire Primary Care Trust

The Priory, Priory Road, St Ives, Huntingdon PE27 5BB
Tel: 01480 308222 Fax: 01480 308234
Email: firstname.lastname@hunts-pct.nhs.uk
Website: www.hunts-pct.nhs.uk
(Norfolk, Suffolk and Cambridgeshire Strategic Health Authority)

Chair Michael Lynch
Chief Executive Karen Bell
Consultants Caroline de Cates

Hyndburn and Ribble Valley Primary Care Trust

Red Rose Court, Clayton Business Park, Clayton-le-Moors, Accrington BB5 5JR
Tel: 01254 380400 Fax: 01254 392585
Website: www.hrvpct.nhs.uk
(Cumbria and Lancashire Strategic Health Authority)

Chair Martin Hill
Chief Executive Mark Wilkinson

Accrington Victoria Community Hospital
Haywood Road, Accrington BB5 6AS
Tel: 01254 263555 Fax: 01254 687367
Total Beds: 20

Manager E Dean

Clitheroe Community Hospital
Chatburn Road, Clitheroe BB7 4JX
Tel: 01200 427311 Fax: 01200 442966
Total Beds: 63

Manager Christine Ski

The Ipswich Hospital NHS Trust

Heath Road, Ipswich IP4 5PD
Tel: 01473 712233 Fax: 01473 703400
Email: forename.surname@ipswichhospital.nhs.uk
Website: www.ipswichhospital.org.uk
(Norfolk, Suffolk and Cambridgeshire Strategic Health Authority)

Chair Christine Smart
Chief Executive Andrew Reed

Ipswich Hospital
Heath Road, Ipswich IP4 5PD
Tel: 01473 712233 Fax: 01473 703400
Total Beds: 795

Accident and Emergency A Bose, D Hodgkinson, D Lewis

Anaesthetics D M Bailey, A Bose, J Broadway, J Brown, W F Byrne, P Carroll, I K Driver, M Garfield, I Hatcher, R M Howard-Griffin, P Howell, A P Jarvis, A Kong, N Lillywhite, M D Mansfield, P J Mills, A D J Nicholl, E M Rush, J B Skinner, M G Smith, J Stevens, S J Wiltshire

Cardiology S Chakrabarty, R Chatoor, N A Irvine, R Oliver

Cardiothoracic Surgery D Watson

Care of the Elderly T J Lockington (Head), S F M Grimmer, P A Phillips, L J Sheehan, N Trepte

Clinical Psychology V Potter

Dermatology T P Cutler, S Gibbs

ENT Mr Arasaratum, A Hilger, M Salam, M W Yung

General Medicine R Chatoor, J L Day, D R Hall, N Innes, N A Irvine, Y Miao, R M Oliver, R G Rayman, D Seaton, S G W Williams, R J Wyke

General Surgery H M Adair, T J Archer, A E P Cameron, S P J Huddy, C Mortimer, I Osman, J Pitt, I H K Scott

Haematology J A Ademokun, I Chalmers, N J Dodd

Histopathology J Chapman, D Kamel, J Orrell, R C G Rowe

Nephrology G R Glancey, P F Williams

Neurology H Manji, S J Wroe

Obstetrics and Gynaecology B Johal, A T Leather, P Mooney, T Omara-Boto, G Sellars, R Sharma, M Sule, D P Vasey

Occupational Health S Coomber

Oncology J H Le Vay, J S Morgan, T Podd, C Scrase, K E Sherwin, P Wilkins

Ophthalmology C Edlesten, R Goble, S Hardman-Lea, A Kiel, R E Lewis

Oral and Maxillofacial Surgery H T Davies, T I Davies, R J Tate

Orthopaedics R Baxandall, M A Bowditch, J P Hallett, J Hopkinson-Wooley, I Hudson, C Marx, J M Powell, D G Shanahan, D J Sharp

Paediatrics M F M Bamford, J D M Gould, M James, K Murtagh, K P O'Neill, C Yale

Pathology J Orrell (Head), J Chapman, P Jones

Plastic Surgery A F Bardsley, A M Logan, T J O'Neill

Radiology S Garber, P Jennings, K R Karia, R C Nightingale, G Picken, S Smith, A d C Tate, W P Whitear

Rheumatology and Rehabilitation G Clunie, S Lane, R A Watts

Sexual Health R Noussa, H Wankowska

Thoracic Surgery M Van Levven

Urology S Banerjee, P Donaldson, M Habib, J Parry

Ipswich Primary Care Trust

Trust HQ, 2nd Floor - Trimley, St Clements Main Building, Foxhall Road, Ipswich IP3 8LS
Tel: 01473 329500 Fax: 01473 329050
Email: enquiries@ipswich-pct.nhs.uk
Website: www.ipswich-pct.nhs.uk
(Norfolk, Suffolk and Cambridgeshire Strategic Health Authority)

Chair Peter Gardiner
Chief Executive Carole Taylor-Brown

Isle of Wight Healthcare NHS Trust

St Mary's Hospital, Newport PO30 5TG
Tel: 01983 524081 Fax: 01983 822569
Email: forename.surname@iow.nhs.uk, general@iow.nhs.uk
Website: www.iowht.org.uk
(Hampshire and Isle of Wight Strategic Health Authority)

Chair Rodney Ireland
Chief Executive Graham Elderfield

Frank James Community Hospital
Adelaide Grove, East Cowes PO32 6BZ
Tel: 01983 280700 Fax: 01983 280757
Total Beds: 24

Laidlaw Day Hospital
St Mary's Hospital, Newport
Tel: 01983 524081

St Mary's Hospital
Parkhurst Road, Newport PO30 5TG
Tel: 01983 524081 Fax: 01983 822569
Total Beds: 413

Accident and Emergency P Wellington

Adult Psychiatry A Guthrie, J Newson Smith

Anaesthetics P E Goodwin, H Hay, A Hof, K Landon, A McEwan, H Noble, G Taylor, C Wareham

Child and Adolescent Psychiatry S Parslow

Dermatology M Hazell

ENT P M G Grimaldi

General Medicine H Arshad, A K Baksi, M Connaughton, A Demissie, E A Hakim, A Hossenbocus, D Murphy

General Surgery S Elsmore, V Mehmet, M Shinkfield, J M Symes, T H Walsh

Haematology R Joshi

Histopathology N Greenwood, J Mikel

Metabolic Medicine J Smith

Microbiology S T Chapman

Obstetrics and Gynaecology A D McNeal, D Ridley, A F E Yoong

Old Age Psychiatry D Harwood

Ophthalmology D Dhingra, M Rhatigan

Oral and Maxillofacial Surgery M C Hetherington, T Mellor

Orthodontics S Robinson

Orthopaedics J Gardiner, N Hobbs, S Nagra, K Rahall

Paediatrics P R Cooke, P H Rowlandson, A H Watson

Palliative Care I Johnson

Pathology S Chapman, N Greenwood, R Joshi, J Smith

Radiology APD Cave, P Close, S Voigt

Rheumatology and Rehabilitation M T Pugh

Urology J Makunde

Staplers Road Assessment and Treatment Unit
52 & 52A Staplers Road, Newport PO30 2DE
Tel: 01983 524805
Total Beds: 10

Isle of Wight Primary Care Trust

Whitecroft, Sandy Lane, Newport PO30 3ED
Tel: 01983 535455 Fax: 01983 822142
Website: www.iow.nhs.uk/pct
(Hampshire and Isle of Wight Strategic Health Authority)

Chair Valerie Anderson
Chief Executive Graham Elderfield

Islington Primary Care Trust

110 Hampstead Road, London NW1 2LJ
Tel: 020 7853 5353 Fax: 020 7853 5355
Website: www.islingtonpct.nhs.uk
(North Central London Strategic Health Authority)

Chair Paula Kahn
Chief Executive Rachel Tyndall

Bloomsbury Day Hospital
4 St Pancras Way, London NW1 0PE
Tel: 020 7530 3353

James Paget Healthcare NHS Trust

Lowestoft Road, Gorleston, Great Yarmouth NR31 6LA
Tel: 01493 452452 Fax: 01493 452078
Email: david.hill@jpaget.nhs.uk
Website: www.jpaget.co.uk
(Norfolk, Suffolk and Cambridgeshire Strategic Health Authority)

Chair John Hemming
Chief Executive David Hill

James Paget Hospital
Lowestoft Road, Gorleston, Great Yarmouth NR31 6LA
Tel: 01493 452452 Fax: 01493 452078
Total Beds: 564

Accident and Emergency R Franklin (Head), A Franklin, V Inuang, D Peacock

Anaesthetics H Stuart (Head), Dr Blossfeldt, P Bothma, A Brodbeck, A Engel, S Ganepola, M Gay, J R Jenkins, H Koessler, M Lundberg, R A M Mann, D McKendrick, D Millican, W G Notcutt, S Oosthuysen, S Rhodes, D Tupper-Carey, S Wilson, M Wright

Care of the Elderly P Harrison (Head), M Al-Khafaji, B Brett, T Cotter, A De-Kock, A de Silva, D A Ellis, P J G Forster, A George, W J Grabau, N Huston, K Jesudason, D Vautier, M Williams

Chemical Pathology S Absalom (Head)

Dermatology R M Graham (Head), I Salvary

ENT D J Premachandra (Head), P Prinsley

General Medicine M Al-Khafaji, B Brett, T Cotter, A De-Kock, A de Silva, D A Ellis, P J G Forster, A George, W J Grabau, P Harrison, N Huston, K Jesudason, G Vantier, M Williams

General Surgery Mr Chitre, J Pereira, J R Sansom, Mr Schneider, J Studley, H G Sturzaker

Genitourinary Medicine T C Harry (Head)

Haematology S Sadullah (Head), J Braithwaite

Medical Microbiology A Heggarty (Head)

Nephrology Dr Ross (Head)

Neurology D J Dick, J B Pilling, Dr Woodward

Obstetrics and Gynaecology J Preston (Head), P Greenwood, M Hassanaien, N Oligbo, A Pozyczka, M Rashid

Ophthalmology A Amanat, K Belfer, P Black, Mrs Mulholland, N Watson

Oral and Maxillofacial Surgery S Hadinnapola (Head), S Prince

Orthodontics D Tewson (Head)

Orthopaedics R Jones (Head), C Johnson-Nurse, P Nadarajan, J Petri

Paediatrics R Stocks (Head), J Chapman, A Edelsten, A Goodwin, S Nirmal, R Srueks, A Verma

Radiology V Kumar (Head), F Holly-Archer, A L Laubsher, P W Lawrence, E Thomas

Radiotherapy and Oncology A Bulman, C Martin, M J Ostrowski

Urology G Suresh (Head), A Simpson, G Swell

Lowestoft Hospital
Tennyson Road, Lowestoft NR32 1PT
Tel: 01502 587311 Fax: 01502 589510
Total Beds: 62

Manager Fran O'Driscoll

Child and Adolescent Psychiatry O J Delany

Dermatology R M Graham

General Medicine P Harrison

General Surgery H Schneider

Paediatrics H Goodwin

Northgate Hospital
Northgate Street, Great Yarmouth NR30 1BU
Tel: 01493 337600 Fax: 01493 852753
Total Beds: 36
Manager Andrew Fox

Care of the Elderly P Harrison

Dermatology Dr Salvary

General Medicine Dr Cotter, Dr Forster, W J Grabau

Paediatrics A D Edelsten, R J Stocks

Northgate Therapy Centre
Nothgate Hospital, Northgate Street, Great Yarmouth NR30 1BU
Tel: 01493 337600 Fax: 01493 852753

Kennet and North Wiltshire Primary Care Trust

Southgate House, Pans Lane, Devizes SN10 5EQ
Tel: 01380 733823 Fax: 01380 733729
Email: enquiry@kennetandnwilt-pct.nhs.uk
Website: www.kennetandnwiltspct.nhs.uk
(Avon, Gloucestershire and Wiltshire Strategic Health Authority)

Chair Ron Crook
Chief Executive Carole Clarke

Chippenham Community Hospital
Rowden Hill, Chippenham SN15 2AJ
Tel: 01249 447100 Fax: 01249 444511
Total Beds: 131

Devizes Community Hospital
Devizes SN10 1EF
Tel: 01380 723511 Fax: 01380 726456
Total Beds: 46

Malmesbury Community Hospital
Burton Hill, Malmesbury SN16 0EQ
Tel: 01666 823358 Fax: 01666 825026
Total Beds: 27

Savernake Hospital
Marlborough SN8 3HL
Tel: 01672 514571 Fax: 01672 514021
Total Beds: 36

Kensington and Chelsea Primary Care Trust

Courtfield House, St Charles Hospital, Exmoor Street, London W10 6DZ
Tel: 020 8962 4692 Fax: 020 8962 4690
Website: www.kc-pct.nhs.uk
(North West London Strategic Health Authority)

Chair Terry Banford
Chief Executive Paul Haigh

Princess Louise Hospital
St Quintin Avenue, London W10 6DL
Tel: 020 8969 0133 Fax: 020 8962 4172
Total Beds: 56

St Charles' Hospital
Exmoor Street, London W10 6DZ
Tel: 020 8969 2488 Fax: 020 8962 4041
Total Beds: 97

Care of the Elderly C Pulford, S Roche, S C Webb

Neurology J Ball

Kent Ambulance NHS Trust

Headquarters, Heath Road, Coxheath, Maidstone ME17 4BG
Tel: 01622 747010 Fax: 01622 744167
Email: enquiries@kentamb.nhs.uk
Website: www.kentandmedway.nhs.uk
(Kent and Medway Strategic Health Authority)

Chair Brian Buchanan
Chief Executive Hayden Newton

Kettering General Hospital NHS Trust

Kettering General Hospital, Rothwell Road, Kettering NN16 8UZ
Tel: 01536 492000 Fax: 01536 492295
Email: forename.surname@kgh.nhs.uk
Website: www.northamptonshire.nhs.uk
(Leicestershire, Northamptonshire and Rutland Strategic Health Authority)

Chair Brian Silk
Chief Executive Julia Squire

Kettering General Hospital
Rothwell Road, Kettering NN16 8UZ
Tel: 01536 492000 Fax: 01536 492599, 01536 493767
Total Beds: 560

Accident and Emergency A Dancocks, R Thamizhavell

Anaesthetics S Agarwal, A Bilolikar, D Bland, J C Burnell, R Dravid, R N Enraght-Moony, J Freeman, E G Hadaway, L Hollos, J Luthman, R Moody, N Roberts, M Siddiqui, J Szafranski, L Twohey

Dermatology W A Branford, A Vorster

ENT M A Latif, R J Lee, A Tewary

General Medicine K Ayes, A Chilton, R Clearkin, G Clifford, J Cullen, I Hubbard, A Hussain, B P O'Malley, K Rizvi, N Shavkat, A Steel

General Surgery S Al-Hamali, V Bahal, A Brar, S El-Rabaa, M Rashed, R D Stewart, M Taylor

Neurology R Abbatt, M C Lawden, Y Rajabally

Obstetrics and Gynaecology S Doshi, R Haughney, R Iqbal, M R B Newman, D J W Wilkin, P L Wood

Ophthalmology D Banarjee, P Baranyovits, T Blamires, K El-Ghazali

Oral Surgery C Harrop

Orthodontics J R S O'Neill

Orthopaedics R L Barrington, S P Biswas, J D Bromage, P Latham, D Menon, B Shah

Paediatrics T Acharya, H Bilolikar, T Biswas, C Nanayakkara, P Rao

Pathology B E Gostelow, H Kelsey, M Lyttleton, G McCreanor, S R Milkins, P Stocks, J Uraiby, I Wilson-Morkeh

Plastic Surgery D Ward

Radiology C Clark, G Goh, S Hamid, S Peterson, R G Reeve, A J Thompson, D Walter, D J Woods

Radiotherapy and Oncology C MacMillan, R Mathew

Rheumatology and Rehabilitation G Kallarackal, P C Mattingly, I M Morris

Urology M Al Sudani, O W Davison

King's College Hospital NHS Trust

King's College Hospital, Denmark Hill, London SE5 9RS
Tel: 020 7737 4000 Fax: 020 7346 3445
Email: info@kingsch.nhs.uk
Website: www.kingsch.nhs.uk
(South East London Strategic Health Authority)

Chair Michael Parker
Chief Executive Malcolm Lowe-Lauri

King's College Hospital

Denmark Hill, London SE5 9RS
Tel: 020 7737 4000 Fax: 020 7346 3445
Total Beds: 712

Accident and Emergency R Brown, E E Glucksman, G Little

Anaesthetics J B Broadfield, I M Corall, S Cottam, T D W Davies, F D'Costa, A P Fisher, M F Fisher, T Ginsberg, D Green, M Hanna, C W Howell, P I E Jones, S Peat, J C Ponte, D Potter, R J Ware

Audiological Medicine J V R Sastry

Biochemistry W Marshall, T J Peters

Cardiology D E Jewitt, P Richardson, R Wainwright

Cardiothoracic Surgery J Desai, A T Forsyth, Mr Marrinan

Care of the Elderly A Blackburn, J Close, D J Evans, S Jackson, K Pettingale, C Swift

Chemical Pathology W Marshall, C Moniz, Professor Peters

Child and Adolescent Psychiatry J Dare, F Nikapoka, F Subotsky, L Wheelan

Dental Surgery S N Bhatia, B M Eley, P S Ellisdon, I D Gainsford, J R Garrett, J D Harrison, R D Howard, A T Inglis, M G D Kelleher, J D Langdon, K Marshall, B H Miller, B C O'Riordan, G Parker, C K Schrieber, N J D Smith, P B Smith, R M Watson, S M Wright

Dermatology C Fuller, A C Pembroke, A W P Vivier

Diabetes S Amiel, M Edmunds, S Thomas

ENT W G Edwards, J N Thomas

Forensic Medicine I West

General Medicine J F Costello, A L W Eddleston, I Forgacs, W Gardner, A M McGregor, J Moxham, K W Pettingale, P J Watkins

General Psychiatry L Campbell, G Davies, F Holloway, A D Isaacs, E G Lucas, D McLean, J R Morgan, P Robinson, M Silverman, K Sivakumar, D Somekh, N O T Temple, B K Toone

General Surgery P A Baskerville, I V Benjamin, J Rennie

Genitourinary Medicine A Brooke, P East, T J McManus, C Taylor, J Welch

Haematology D Devereaux, D M Layton, G Mufti, A Pagliuca

Histopathology S Humphreys, B C Portmann

Immunology D E H Tee, D Vergani

Medical Microbiology J N Philpott-Howard, J Wade

Nephrology H Cairns, B Hendry

Neurology P N Leigh, J D Parkes, J Payan, E H Reynolds, D N Rushton, M P Sheehy, K J Zilkha

Neurosurgery P Bullock, C Chandler, R Gullen, J McCabe, C E Polkey, M Sharp, A Strong

Nuclear Medicine M Buxton-Thomas

Obstetrics and Gynaecology S Campbell, L Cardozo, W Collins, D Gibb, F Lawton, J M McEwan, K Nicolaides, J Parsons, M Whitehead

Ophthalmology W A I Aclimandos, R Coakes, P A Hunter

Orthopaedics G Groom, S Phillips, J Sixla

Paediatrics A Baker, C Ball, D Candy, M Crouchman, J Dare, S Devane, H R Gamsu, A Greenough, G Mieli-Vergani, A P Mowat, J F Price, E M Ross, K C Tan

Pathology F E Dische, M Driver, S Humphreys, P J O'Donnell, B Portmann, J Salisbury, I E West, W F Whimster

Public Health Medicine G Bickler, Y Doyle, N Noah

Radiology P Gishen, J Karani, H B Meire, M Michell, N J D Smith, H Walters

Radiotherapy and Oncology F Calman, H Dobbs, A W B Nethersell

Rheumatology and Rehabilitation H Berry, D Choy, C J Goodwill, R Luff, D Scott

Urology P Thompson

Virology S Sutherland, A H C Uttley

Kingston Hospital NHS Trust

Galsworthy Road, Kingston upon Thames KT2 7QB
Tel: 020 8546 7711
Email: forename.surname@kingstonhospital.nhs.uk
Website: www.kingstonhospital.nhs.uk
(South West London Strategic Health Authority)

Chair Christine Swabey
Chief Executive Carole Heatly

Kingston Hospital

Galsworthy Road, Kingston upon Thames KT2 7QB
Tel: 020 8546 7711 Ext: 2814 Fax: 020 8547 2182
Total Beds: 642

Accident and Emergency M Lynch (Head), H Draper, R Goel, M Lynch, S M Moalypour

Anaesthetics S Howsam (Head), A Ravalia (Head), M Alsahaf, L Andrew, F L Barton, A Blyth, B Buxton, A Curtis, R Graham, S Howsam, A Landes, J P Maynard, K Paramesh, S Puranik, B Ratnayake, A Ravalia, G Samsoon, I Sinton, G Smith, C Stableforth, R Stacey, K Stringer, A Volger, J W Zwaal

Care of the Elderly H Lo (Head), C Lee, H Lo, W McNabb, A Neil, C Rodrigues

Dermatology C Fletcher, K J Misch

ENT A E Hinton, T Mugliston, Mr Toma

General Medicine W Culling, T Heymann, G K Knowles, M Oldfield, R Roberts, M Spring, I D Strickland, A Vasudeva

General Surgery J Cahill (Head), P Willson (Head), I T Bloom, J Cahill, R Cummins, P E M Jarrett, R D Leach, S Ray, P Willson

Genitourinary Medicine G McCarthy (Head), A Beardall, G McCarthy, S McMorrow

Neurology H Lo (Head), A Al-Memar, S Omer, J Von Oertzan

Obstetrics and Gynaecology H Anderson (Head), H Anderson, R Bevan, M Davis, O Morris, K Panter, A Pooley, J Wilson

Ophthalmology I Gillespie (Head), J Beare, I Gillespie, S Horgan, C Roberts

Oral and Maxillofacial Surgery P Blenkinsopp (Head), A Jones (Head), B Bailey, P Blenkinsopp, H Chana, R Edler, A Jones, A Stewart

Orthopaedics G Railton (Head), J Bell, R Chapman, M J Curtis, P Davey, R Hampton, S Kendall, M Proctor, G Railton, D Ward

Paediatrics A Winrow (Head), S Al-Jawad, S Al-Wahab, W I Anshasi, T Ayeni, P Christie, E Jurges, D Lindo, I Ojo, R G Wilson, A Winrow

Pathology S Martin (Head), Z Abboudi, S Gothraie Gharaie, C Jameson, G Knee, A Kothari, J B Leach, P McHugh, S Martin, L Neville, M Rowley, D Simms, H V Sykes, H J Wong

Plastic Surgery M Soldin

Radiology C E Todd (Head), S A Evans, P Frank, A Mathie, E O'Sullivan, R H Pearson, A Rhodes, H Richardson, P Scott-Mackie, A S Thornton, C E Todd, C Ward, M M White

Rheumatology and Rehabilitation H Lo (Head), J Foley, S Jawad, H Jones

Urology J A Dick (Head), J A Dick, R Morley, A Thompson

Kingston Primary Care Trust

Hollyfield House, 22 Hollyfield Road, Surbiton KT5 9AL
Tel: 020 8339 8000 Fax: 020 8339 8100
Website: www.kingstonpct.nhs.uk
(South West London Strategic Health Authority)

Chair Neslyn Watson-Druée
Chief Executive Chris Butler

Surbiton General Hospital

Ewell Road, Surbiton KT6 6EZ
Tel: 020 8399 7111 Fax: 020 8390 9920
Total Beds: 44

Knowsley Primary Care Trust

Health and Social Care HQ, Nutgrove Villa, PO Box 23, Westmoreland Road , Huyton L36 6GA
Tel: 0151 443 4900 Fax: 0151 443 4901
Website: www.sthkhealth.nhs.uk
(Cheshire and Merseyside Strategic Health Authority)

Chair Rosemary Hawley
Chief Executive Anita Marsland

Lambeth Primary Care Trust

1 Lower Marsh, London SE1 7NT
Tel: 020 7716 7100 Fax: 020 7716 7103
Website: www.lambethpct.nhs.uk
(South East London Strategic Health Authority)

Chair Jane Ramsey
Chief Executive Kevin Barton

Lancashire Ambulance Service NHS Trust

Broughton House, 449-451 Garstang Road, Preston PR3 5LN
Tel: 01772 862666 Fax: 01772 861003
Email: john.calderbank@las-tr.nwest.nhs.uk
Website: www.lancashireambulance.com
(Cumbria and Lancashire Strategic Health Authority)

Chair Ruth Winterbottom
Chief Executive David Hill

Lancashire Care NHS Trust

Sceptre Point, Sceptre Way, Walton Summit, Bamber Bridge, Preston PR5 6AW
Tel: 01772 695300 Fax: 01772 227080
Email: enquiries@lancashirecare.nhs.uk
Website: www.lancashirecare.nhs.uk
(Cumbria and Lancashire Strategic Health Authority)

Chair Vourneen (Jo) Darbyshire
Chief Executive Finlay Robertson

Avondale Unit

Royal Preston Hospital, Sharoe Green Lane North, Fulwood, Preston PR2 9HT
Tel: 01772 773464, 01772 773466, 01772 773470
Total Beds: 49

Manager Janet Clark

General Psychiatry R Gater, R Morgan, M Robson, A Summers, G Wood

Burnley General Hospital

Casterton Avenue, Burnley BB10 2PQ
Tel: 01282 425071 Fax: 01282 474444
Total Beds: 85

General Psychiatry T Han, M Javeed, S Quraishi

Chorley and South Ribble District General Hospital

Preston Road, Chorley PR7 1PP
Tel: 01257 261222 Fax: 01257 245309
Total Beds: 51

General Psychiatry Dr Ashfaq, Dr Aung, Dr Kala Kala, Dr Patel, Dr Shrevat, Dr Tourish

EMI Unit (Hillview) Day Hospital

Queens Park Hospital, Haslingden Road, Blackburn BB2 3HH
Tel: 01254 263555 Fax: 01254 294572
Total Beds: 20

General Psychiatry S N Waghray

Fleetwood Hospital

Pharos Street, Fleetwood FY7 6BE
Tel: 01253 306029
Total Beds: 40

General Psychiatry G P Opdebeeck

Lytham Hospital

Warton Street, Lytham St Annes FY8 5EE
Tel: 01253 303953 Fax: 01253 303972
Total Beds: 20

General Psychiatry W J Charles, C J Molodynski, E B Renvoize

Ormskirk and District General Hospital

Ormskirk & District General Hospital, Wigan Road, Ormskirk L39 2JW
Tel: 01695 598281 Fax: 01695 598229
Total Beds: 50

Manager Patrick Sullivan

General Psychiatry G Ash, P Cocker, N Fatima, A Gallegley, M McKenzie

Parkwood Psychiatric Unit

East Park Drive, Blackpool FY3 8PW
Tel: 01253 306980 Fax: 01253 306961
Total Beds: 94

Manager Nigel Roberts

General Psychiatry L A Le-Roux (Head), D Kay, J Mequita, Dr Prince, Dr Smith

Pendleview

Queen's Park Hospital, Haslingden Road, Blackburn BB2 3HH
Tel: 01254 263555 Fax: 01254 293406
Total Beds: 68

Manager G Chadwick

General Psychiatry Dr Deo (Head), Dr Adelekan, Dr Ahmad, Dr Chattree, Dr Gossall, Dr Gupta, Dr Husain, P Reed, Dr Saleem, Dr Swana, S N Waghray, Dr Waheep

Ribbleton Hospital

Miller Road, Preston PR2 6LS
Tel: 01772 401600 Fax: 01772 653799
Total Beds: 40

Manager Sue Rowe

General Psychiatry Dr Chattree, Dr MacWilliam

Lancashire Teaching Hospitals NHS Foundation Trust

Established as a Foundation Trust 01/04/2005.

Royal Preston Hospital, Sharoe Green Lane, Fulwood, Preston PR2 9HT
Tel: 01772 716565 Fax: 01722 526565
Website: www.lancsteachinghospitals.nhs.uk
(Cumbria and Lancashire Strategic Health Authority)

Chief Executive Tony Curtis

Chorley and South Ribble District General Hospital

Preston Road, Chorley PR7 1PP
Tel: 01257 261222 Fax: 01257 245309
Total Beds: 400

Accident and Emergency R J Fairhurst

Anaesthetics O E Akinpelu, M A Calleja, J Jayasuriya, C F Loyden

Chest Disease B E Taylor

Dermatology N K Saikia

ENT J Curley, T B Duff, M Small

General Medicine R A Coward, I Drake, R C Gupta, S Madi, S N H Naqvi, S C Wallis, D A L Watt

General Surgery M M Mughal

Neurology P Tomlin

Obstetrics and Gynaecology J F B Clarke, I G Robertson, S K Shah, J D Wright

Oncology R A Cowan

Ophthalmology H P Adhikary, E M Talbot

Oral and Maxillofacial Surgery J Cornah, J Trenouth

Orthopaedics S Ehrendorfer, A I Hassan, A Mohammed, M J Shaw, R B Smith

Paediatrics A N Campbell, S A Clark, D A Mahmood

Pathology P Wright

Radiology S C Galletly, B C Spinks, R Stockwell

Urology S S Matanhelia, R G N Thomson

Royal Preston Hospital

Sharoe Green Lane North, Fulwood, Preston PR2 4QF
Tel: 01772 716565 Fax: 01772 710162
Total Beds: 608

Accident and Emergency J M Hanson, M James, M C McColl

Anaesthetics P Bunting, F DeSilva, P W Duncan, J M Fryer, A J Gosling, J O Griffiths, C Isherwood, G N Jones, S J Keens, A S Lawrence, P F S Lee, A Lowrie, E P McKiernan, R A Martlew, W A Noble, I Selby, A Seth, G K Vanner, J G Williams

Care of the Elderly J McCann, P McDonald, M Waqar Uddin

Dermatology A Butt, J K Kellet, N K Saikia

ENT J d Carpentier, J W A Curley, B Jafari, M Small

General Medicine A L Burton, S A Cairns, R A Coward, A Lakhdar, L Solomon, B E Taylor, J M Temperley, P A Vice

General Surgery A R Hearn, R Hughes, D J Stewart, G Thomson

Genitourinary Medicine A Saeed

Neurology I Bangash, B Boothman, T Majeed, J D Mitchell, P Tidswell, S D Vakil

Neurosurgery C H Davis, N S Gurusinghe, A J Keogh

Oncology A Biswas, A Hindley, G Read, G Skailes, S Susnerwala

Ophthalmology H P Adhikary, A T Ekdawy, G Griffith, E M Talbot

Oral and Maxillofacial Surgery J Cornah

Orthodontics M J Trenouth

Orthopaedics R S Bale, J C Faux, V Shah, S J Shaw, R M Smith, M R Wharton

Paediatrics A N Campbell, S A Clark, D Mahmood, J R Owen, P I Tomlin

Pathology A Armour, T A Flaherty, A J Howat, P G Lynch, C M Nicholson, M A Pitt, F Rugman, N Williamson, P Wright

Plastic Surgery N R Gaze, A J Howcroft, R P Jones, J G Laitung

Radiology J P Bradley, J M Brown, C Coutinho, M Dobson, S D'Souza, W J Gunawardena, I Harris, J C Hill

Thoracic Medicine R W J Millner

Urology B Elem, S Matanhelia, M E Watson

Sharoe Green Hospital

Sharoe Green Lane South, Fulwood, Preston PR2 4DU
Tel: 01772 716565 Fax: 01772 710622
Total Beds: 263

Care of the Elderly J McCann, M Waqar-Uddin

General Medicine A L Burton, B E Taylor, P A Vice

Obstetrics and Gynaecology J F B Clarke, S Hughes, I G Robertson, S K Shah, J D Wright

Orthopaedics R S Bale, J C Faux, V Shah, S J Shaw, R M Smith, M R Wharton

Paediatrics A N Campbell, S A Clark, D Mahmood, J R Owen, P A Tomlin

Langbaurgh Primary Care Trust

Langbaurgh House, Bow Street, Guisborough TS14 7AA
Tel: 01287 284400 Fax: 01287 284401
Website: www.langbaurghpct.nhs.uk
(County Durham and Tees Valley Strategic Health Authority)

Chair David Becker
Chief Executive Jon Chadwick

Leeds Mental Health Teaching NHS Trust

Meanwood Park, Tongue Lane, Leeds LS6 4QB

Tel: 0113 295 2800 Fax: 0113 295 2889
Email: communications@leedsmh.nhs.uk
Website: www.leedsmentalhealth.nhs.uk
(West Yorkshire Strategic Health Authority)

Chair Ian Hughes
Chief Executive Chris Butler

Aire Court Community Unit
Aire Court, Lingwell Grove, Leeds LS10 4RE
Tel: 0113 277 4861 Fax: 0113 277 4895

Aire Court Hospital
Lingwell Grove, Middleton, Leeds LS10 3RE
Tel: 0113 277 4861 Fax: 0113 277 4895
Total Beds: 30

Asket Croft Day Hospital
2 Asket Place, Seacroft, Leeds LS14 1PP
Tel: 0113 305 7000

Crooked Acres
Spen Lane, Leeds LS5 3SJ
Tel: 0113 295 3590 Fax: 0113 295 3288

Learning Disabilities B Easby, S G Read

Hawthorn Day Hospital
St Mary's Hospital, Greenhill Road, Leeds LS13
Tel: 0113 279 0121 ext: 4315

Linden Day Hospital
St Mary's Hospital, Greenhill Road, Leeds LS13
Tel: 0113 279 0121 Ext: 4321

Malham House Day Hospital
25 Hyde Terrace, Leeds LS2 9ON
Tel: 0113 292 6716 Fax: 0113 292 6718

Millfield House
Kirk Lane, Yeadon, Leeds LS19 7LX
Tel: 0113 250 7117 Fax: 0113 250 6751

The Mount
44 Hyde Terrace, Leeds LS2 1JN

Oak Day Hospital
St Mary's Hospital, Greenhill Road, Leeds LS13
Tel: 0113 279 0121 Ext: 4213

St Mary's Hospital
Greenhill Road, Leeds LS12 3QE
Tel: 0113 279 0121 Fax: 0113 231 0185
Total Beds: 63

General Psychiatry A S Zigmond

Psychiatry of Old Age P Bowie, D Deardon

Towngate House Day Hospital
Towngate House, 1 Towngate Close, Guiseley LS20 9LA
Tel: 01943 472000 Fax: 01943 472001

Tuke House
60 Sholebrook Avenue, Leeds LS7 3HB
Tel: 0113 295 2790 Fax: 0113 295 2791

Leeds North East Primary Care Trust

Sycamore Lodge, 7A Woodhouse Cliff, Leeds LS6 2HP
Tel: 0113 305 9763 Fax: 0113 305 9880
Email: forename.surname@leedsnortheast-pct.nhs.uk
Website: www.leedsnortheast-pct.nhs.uk
(West Yorkshire Strategic Health Authority)

Chair Brian Marsden
Chief Executive Thea Stein

Leeds North West Primary Care Trust

Mill House, Troy Road, Horsforth, Leeds LS18 5TN
Tel: 0113 305 7120 Fax: 0113 305 7121
Website: www.leedsnorthwest-pct.nhs.uk
(West Yorkshire Strategic Health Authority)

Chair Martin Drury
Chief Executive Lesley Smith

Leeds Teaching Hospitals NHS Trust

Trust Headquarters, St James' University Hospital, Beckett Street, Leeds LS9 7TF
Tel: 0113 243 3144 Fax: 0113 242 6496
Email: hilda.hardwick@leedsth.nhs.uk
Website: www.leedsth.nhs.uk
(West Yorkshire Strategic Health Authority)

Chair Martin Buckley
Chief Executive Neil McKay

Chapel Allerton Hospital
Harehills Lane, Leeds LS7 4SA
Tel: 0113 262 3404
Total Beds: 259

Anaesthetics M V Shah, J C Sugden

Breast Services K Horgan

Care of the Elderly K I Donaldson

Rehabilitation M A Chamberlain, V Neuman

Rheumatology C T Pease

Cookridge Hospital
Hospital Lane, Cookridge, Leeds LS16 6QB
Tel: 0113 267 3411
Total Beds: 96

Anaesthetics M R Moore

Clinical and Medical Oncology D A Anthoney, D Ash, M G Bond, D Bottomley, C Coyle, A Crellin, D Dodwell, G Gerrard, D Gilson, S Kumar, C Loughrey, J Orton, F Roberts, I Rothwell, D Sebag-Montefiore, M Seymour, M Snee, R Taylor

ENT Z Makura

Leeds Dental Institute
The Worsley Building, Clarendon Way, Leeds LS2 9LU
Tel: 0113 244 0111

Manager William Hume

Anaesthetics E Moss

Dental and Orthodontics M W-Y Chan, P A Cook, M Duggal, S Fayle, A S High, W Hume, M Kellett, F Luther, D M Martin, B Nattress, J P Ralph, A Speirs, C J Watson, C C Youngson

Oral and Maxillofacial Surgery S E Fisher, R Loukota, T K Ong, J Pedlar, J Russell

Leeds General Infirmary

Great George Street, Leeds LS1 3EX
Tel: 0113 243 2799
Total Beds: 1345

Accident and Emergency D W Hamer, T B Hassan, J P Sloan, N Zoltie

Anaesthetics M Arana, S Balaji, M D D Bell, M J Bem, J C Berridge, S Bew, A K Bliss, A R Bodenham, M K G Boylan, R W Brown, N C Bugg, P N Charlton, R R Chatrath, P J Cole, M H Cross, M J Dakin, M E F Deane, N M Dearden, D J R Duthie, A D Fale, J M Freeman, F M C Gamlin, L G Gardner, J S Gibson, H J Gorton, E A Harrison, P T Haywood, W Hinton, J V Howard, Z Jankovic, P Janzen, J I L Jones, S N Lintin, J B Luntley, G R Lyons, E M McAteer, A Mallick, P J McHugh, M H McKeague, H A McLure, D J Mellor, R J Mills, M R Moore, E Moss, S D Murdoch, P G Murphy, J Neasham, G F Nunn, A J Pittard, A C Quinn, R J Roche, D S Selsby, M V Shah, J A Short, S N Smith, N J Snook, J C Sugden, M Vucevic, E R Warren, E J Watkins, K R Welsh, S Williams, A T Wilson

Breast Services A M Bello, K Horgan

Cardiac Surgery P Kaul, P Kay, J McGoldrick, C Munsch, U R Nair, D J O'Regan, K G Watterson, N Weerasena

Cardiology J C Cowan, C J Dickinson, J M McLenachan, C B Pepper, E J Perrins, G Reynolds, U M Sivanathan, L B Tan, G Williams

Care of the Elderly P W Belfield, E Burns, A Cameron, A Catto, O J Corrado, P Wanklyn

Clinical and Medical Oncology D Gilson, I Rothwell, M Snee, R Taylor

Community Paediatrics S Lee, D Murdoch-Eaton, R Skelton, S E Wyatt

Dermatology M J D Goodfield, V Goulden, R A Sheehan-Dare, G Stables, S M Wilkinson

Endocrinology and Diabetes C M Amery, P E Belchetz, H J Bodansky, P Grant, S M Orme

ENT J D Fenwick, D R Hanson, G Kelly, L C Knight, J London, Z Makura, C J Woodhead

Gastro-intestinal Medicine A T Axon, D M Chalmers

Gastro-intestinal Surgery D Burke, S Dexter, P J Finan, M McMahon, P M Sagar, H Sue-Ling

Genitourinary Medicine J Clarke, E F Monteiro, M A Waugh, J D Wilson

Haematology D R Norfolk, G M Smith, D M Swirsky

Histopathology J E Boddy, P Harnden, A S Jack, S Miller, P Quirke, J Sutton

Immunology T E Roberts, P Wood

Neonatology L Cornette, A B Gill, J W L Puntis

Neurology S Jamieson, S E Omer, E G S Spokes

Neurophysiology I S Smith

Neurosurgery P Chumas, P V Marks, N I Phillips, S Ross, G Towns, P T van Hille

Obstetrics and Gynaecology J O Drife, E L Ferriman, M R Glass, C R Landon, G C Mason, N A B Simpson, C Sparey, J Tay

Ophthalmology O Backhouse, B Chang, R M L Doran, M Menage, B A Noble, D O'Neill, H Woon

Orthopaedics S Calder, J L Cruickshank, M E Emerton, R Hackney, N Harris, J O Lawton, M H Stone, P Templeton

Paediatric Cardiology M E Blackburn, D F Dickinson, J L Gibbs, J M Parsons

Paediatric Cystic Fibrosis and Respiratory Medicine P Chetcuti

Paediatric Dermatology S Clark

Paediatric Endocrinology N Alvi, G E Butler

Paediatric Neurology A M Childs, C Ferrie, J Livingstone

Paediatric Neurosurgery A K Tiagi

Paediatric Surgery D C G Crabbe, I Sugarman

Paediatrics Dr Cleary, P C Holland, Dr Williams

Pain Management Dr Dickson

Palliative Care S Kite

Plastic Surgery C Fenn

Radiology R J Arthur, R F Bury, A G Chalmers, P M Chennells, B J G Dall, R J Dunham, R C Fowler, S Macpherson, D Martinez, H Moss, G J S Parkin

Rehabilitation Professor Chamberlain

Renal Services A M Brownjohn, J H Turney, G Woodrow, M J Wright

Reproductive Medicine A Balen, A Rutherford

Respiratory Medicine M Henry, M F Muers, S B Pearson, J Watson

Rheumatology H A Bird, P Conaghan, P Emery, A D Fraser

Thoracic Surgery K Papagiannopoulos, J A Thorpe

Urology A D Joyce, A Paul, S Prescott

Vascular Surgery M J Gough, S Homer-Vanniasikham, A I D Mavor

St James's University Hospital

Beckett Street, Leeds LS9 7TF
Tel: 0113 243 3144 Fax: 0113 242 6496
Total Beds: 1166

Accident and Emergency R N Illingworth, G Johnson, A McGowan, K Reynard, R K Roden

Anaesthetics M C Bellamy, A J Berrill, L D Caldicott, R H Cruickshank, S G Dean, M R Dresner, B Duncan, J E Fairfield, H Klein, S Lloyd, A B Lumb, G R Lyons, P Semple, H A Spencer, A F Stakes, S M Whiteley, I G Wilson, R C Wilson, A P B Yates

Breast Services T G Brennan, M Lansdown

Cardiology E Berkin, A S Hall, A F Mackintosh

Care of the Elderly J Dolben, N J Dudley, J T Eccles, S Mcintosh, G P Mulley, N Penn

Clinical and Medical Oncology D Alison, G D Hall, M Leahy, P Patel, T Perren, P Selby

Clinical Genetics R Mueller (Head), C P Bennett, Y J Crow, J A Dobbie, E Sheridan, C G Woods

Community Paediatrics D Cundall, A J Thomas

Dermatology J A Newton-Bishop, C L Wilson

Diabetes S Gilbey, M Mansfield

Gastro-intestinal Medicine M E Denyer, R V Heatley, P D Howdle, M A Hull, G I Sandle

Gastro-intestinal Surgery N S Ambrose, I Botterill, P J Guillou, D Jayne

Haematology G Cook, R Johnson, S E Kinsey, B A McVerry

Histopathology A P Boon, P J Carder, P Harnden, K A MacLellan, A Roy, C S Verbeke, N Wilkinson, J I Wyatt

Immunology H C Gooi

Infectious Diseases J Minton, P Stanley

Neonatology P F Dear, M Levene, S J Newell, S J Thomas

Neurology J M Bamford, M I Busby, H Ford, P J Goulding, M H Johnson

Neurophysiology A A Da Costa

Obstetrics and Gynaecology T J Broadhead, E J Buxton, D J Campbell, S Duffy, B A Gbolade, M D Griffith-Jones, R C Hutson, G Lane, L Rogerson, A Thein, J J Walker

Ophthalmology A Cassells-Brown, T R Dabbs, M McKibbin, A J Morrell, I Simmons

Orthopaedics I A Archer, S Britten, D A Campbell, R A Dickson, R Dunsmuir, R Farnell, P Giannoudis, D L Limb, D Macdonald, S J Matthews, P Millner, A Rao, B W Scott

Paediatric Cystic Fibrosis and Respiratory Medicine K G Brownlee, S P Conway

Paediatric Gastroenterology, Hepatology and Nutrition S M Davison, P McClean

Paediatric Oncology A Glaser, I Lewis, S V Picton, E M Richards

Paediatric Surgery A Najmaldin, B R Squire, M D Stringer, R Subramaniam, D F M Thomas

Paediatrics F Campbell, J Darling, C J Hobbs, P C Holland, Dr Richards, M Rudolph, C Williams

Palliative Care F Hicks

Plastic Surgery S P J Kay, S L Knight, H Liddington, W Saeed

Radiology D Barron, A H Chapman, A Grainger, J A Guthrie, H C Irving, D Kessel, P O'Connor, J V Patel, W H Ramsden, J Rankine, P Robinson, M B Sheridan, J A Spencer, S E Swift, M J Weston, H E Woodley

Renal Services R J Baker, A F Mooney, C G Newstead, E J Will

Reproductive Medicine V Sharma

Respiratory Medicine M W Elliott, R L Page, P K Plant

Rheumatology M F Martin

Urology J Cartledge, I Eardley, S N Lloyd, A Paul, S Prescott, P Whelan

Vascular Surgery D C Berridge, P J Kent, D J A Scott

Seacroft Hospital

York Road, Leeds LS14 6UH
Tel: 0113 264 8164 Fax: 0113 260 2528
Total Beds: 256

Adult Cystic Fibrosis S P Conway, D G Peckham

Care of the Elderly V Aylett, M Sleightholm, C Teale

Gastro-intestinal Medicine M E Denyer

Radiology L I G Haigh, J Liston

Respiratory Medicine D G Peckham

Wharfedale General Hospital

Newall Carr Road, Otley LS21 2LY
Tel: 01943 465522
Total Beds: 95

Anaesthetics M R Moore, Q L A Robinson

Care of the Elderly M Bradley, I D Thompson

Gastro-intestinal Surgery A W Owen

Leeds West Primary Care Trust

Bremner House, Gelderd Business Park, John Charles Way (off Gelderd Road), Leeds LS12 6QD
Tel: 0113 305 9400 Fax: 0113 305 9481
Website: www.leedswest-pct.nhs.uk
(West Yorkshire Strategic Health Authority)

Chair Kuldip Bharj
Chief Executive Chris Reid

Leicester City West Primary Care Trust

Mansion House, 41 Guildhall Lane, Leicester LE1 5FR
Tel: 0116 295 1100 Fax: 0116 295 1111
(Leicestershire, Northamptonshire and Rutland Strategic Health Authority)

Chair Bernard Greaves
Chief Executive Rob McMahon

Leicestershire Partnership NHS Trust

George Hine House, Gipsy Lane, Leicester LE5 0TD
Tel: 0116 225 6000 Fax: 0116 225 3684
Website: www.leicspt.nhs.uk
(Leicestershire, Northamptonshire and Rutland Strategic Health Authority)

Chair Wendy Hickling
Chief Executive Maggie Cork

Bradgate Unit

Glenfield Hospital, Groby Road, Leicester E3 9QF
Total Beds: 104

The Lewisham Hospital NHS Trust

University Hospital Lewisham, High Street, Lewisham, London SE13 6LH
Tel: 020 8333 3000 Fax: 020 8333 3333
Email: enquiries@uhl.nhs.uk
Website: www.lewisham.nhs.uk
(South East London Strategic Health Authority)

Chair Bala Gnanapragasam
Chief Executive Claire Perry

The Lewisham Hospital

University Hospital Lewisham, High Street, Lewisham, London SE13 6LH
Tel: 020 8333 3000 Fax: 020 8333 3333
Total Beds: 600

Accident and Emergency N Nayeem, W Smallman

Anaesthetics M Albin, R Arnold, N Dasey, P Di-Vadi, W Hamann, M Heath, N V Heerden, C Lanigan, G Lawton, A Marsh, J Pook, C Roulson

Biochemistry P Eldridge

Cardiology J Gill, P G Jackson, S Lewis

Care of the Elderly P Gunawardena, P Luce, I Starke

Chest Disease N M Eiser, P Luce, L Youlten

Cytology C Keen, G Phillip

Dental Surgery S Bhinda

Dermatology H du P-Menarge, J J Ross, C Smith

Diabetes A Worsley

Endocrinology J Miell

ENT D A Bowdler, T Harris, J Rubin, N Salama

General Medicine N Eiser, P G Jackson, P Luce, J Miell, G Sladen, I Starke, R Stott, A Worsley

General Surgery B Edmondson, A Gotlieb, H Hamed, J Linsell, W Owen, N Slater, A Steger, P Taylor

Genitourinary Medicine J Bingham

Haematology Dr Nahheed-Mir, L Tillyer

Histopathology C Keen, C Philip

Medical Microbiology G Rao

Neurology R Chaudhuri

Nuclear Medicine S Clarke

Obstetrics and Gynaecology V Abdo-Nasri, A Jolaoso, P Knott, F Lawton, A Shafik, D Zamblera

Ophthalmology W Acclimandos, D McHugh

Oral Surgery V Rajayogeswaran, P Robinson

Orthodontics D Ramsay

Orthopaedics P Earnshaw, R Gore, B Povlsen

Paediatrics M Agrawal, C Daman-Willems, E Dykes, R Evans, D Garvie, A Lorek, M McCullagh, J Maynard, J Stroobant, H Ward

Palliative Medicine D Bozek

Pathology G Smith

Radiology C Bradshaw, J Jacomb-Hood, C Kennedy, D McIver, M R Salari, R Toye

Radiotherapy A Timothy

Rheumatology G Kingsley, G Yanni

Thoracic Medicine N Eiser, P Luce, D Shelton

Urology J Buckley, R Popert

Lewisham Primary Care Trust

Elizabeth Blackwell House, Wardalls Grove, Avonley Road, New Cross, London SE14 5ER
Tel: 020 7635 5555 Fax: 020 7771 5115
Website: www.lewishampct.nhs.uk
(South East London Strategic Health Authority)

Chair Brian Lymbery
Chief Executive Lucy Hadfield

Lincolnshire Ambulance and Health Transport Service NHS Trust

Cross O'Cliff Court, Bracebridge Heath, Lincoln LN4 2HL
Tel: 01522 545171 Fax: 01522 546834
Email: enquiries@lincsambulance.nhs.uk
(Trent Strategic Health Authority)

Chair Linda Honey
Chief Executive Margaret Serna

Lincolnshire Partnership NHS Trust

Cross O'Cliff, Bracebridge Heath, Lincoln LN4 2HN
Tel: 01522 513355 Fax: 01522 515372
Website: www.lpt.nhs.uk
(Trent Strategic Health Authority)

Chair Alison Healey
Chief Executive Chris Slavin

Ash Villa
Willoughby Road, South Rauceby, Sleaford NG34 8QA
Tel: 01529 488061 Fax: 01529 488239
Total Beds: 12

Manager Tina King

Ashley House
Beaconfield Site, Sandon Road, Grantham NG31 9DR
Tel: 01476 573986
Total Beds: 10

Beckside CMHT
472 Newark Road, Lincoln LN6 8RZ
Tel: 01522 501266 Fax: 01522 696473

Carholme Court
Long Leys Road, Lincoln LN1 1FS
Tel: 01522 577052 Fax: 01522 577225
Total Beds: 30

Elm Resource Centre
Sandon Road, Grantham NG31 9DR
Tel: 01476 584015 Fax: 01476 578210
Total Beds: 10

Maple Lodge
Toot Lane, Fishtoft, Boston PE21 0AX
Tel: 01205 354900 Fax: 01205 354837
Total Beds: 10

Manager Kevin Brooks

Moore House
10/11 Lindum Terrace, Lincoln LN2 5RT
Tel: 01522 513875 Fax: 01522 513405

Manager Jayne Wheway

Rochford Day Hospital
Department of Psychiatry, Pilgrim Hospital, Sibsey Road, Boston PE21 9QS
Tel: 01205 364801
Total Beds: 10

Manager John Steer

Sycamore Assessment Unit
Beaconfield Site, Sandon Road, Grantham NG31 9DF
Tel: 01476 579707 Fax: 01476 579799
Total Beds: 15

Witham Court
Fen Lane, North Hykeham, Lincoln
Tel: 01522 500690 Fax: 01522 500883

Lincolnshire South West Teaching Primary Care Trust

Orchard House, South Rauceby, Sleaford NG34 8PP
Tel: 01529 416000 Fax: 01529 416092
(Trent Strategic Health Authority)

Chair Melanie Hawes
Chief Executive Derek Bray
Consultants Isabel Perez

Liverpool Women's Hospital NHS Foundation Trust

Established as a Foundation Trust 01/04/2005.

Crown Street, Liverpool L8 7SS
Tel: 0151 708 9988 Fax: 0151 702 4028
Website: www.lwh.org.uk

(Cheshire and Merseyside Strategic Health Authority)

Chair Rosemary Cooper
Chief Executive Louise Shepherd

Liverpool Women's Hospital

Crown Street, Liverpool L8 7SS
Tel: 0151 708 9988 Fax: 0151 702 4028
Total Beds: 271

Anaesthetics P Barclay, E Djabatey, S Malliah, G Meadows, B J Phillips, T D Wauchob, R G Wilkes

Genetics I Ellis, A E Fryer, E Greenhalgh, E Sweeney

Obstetrics and Gynaecology E J Adams, N Aziz, P Bousefield, L Bricker, A S Garden, J Herod, M Johnstone, G M Kidd, C R Kingsland, J J Kirwan, D I Lewis-Jones, J P Neilson, D Parkinson, S Quenby, D Roberts, G Rowland, H Scholefield, G Shaw, J Sutherst, C M H Thom, J Topping, S A Walkinshaw

Paediatrics R W I Cooke, N Subhedar, A M Weindling, W Yoxall

Radiology S J King, G H Whitehouse

London Ambulance Service NHS Trust

220 Waterloo Road, London SE1 8SD
Tel: 020 7921 5100 Fax: 020 7921 5129
Website: www.londonambulance.nhs.uk
(South West London Strategic Health Authority)

Chair Sigurd Reinton
Chief Executive Peter Bradley

Luton and Dunstable Hospital NHS Trust

Lewsey Road, Luton LU4 0DZ
Tel: 01582 491122 Fax: 01582 598990
Email: firstname.lastname@ldh-tr.anglox.nhs.uk
Website: www.ldh.nhs.uk
(Bedfordshire and Hertfordshire Strategic Health Authority)

Chair Soraya Dhillon
Chief Executive Stephen Ramsden

Luton and Dunstable Hospital

Lewsey Road, Luton LU4 0DZ
Tel: 01582 491122 Fax: 01582 598990
Total Beds: 600

Accident and Emergency M B Kotecha, M A Nafis

Anaesthetics M A Alexander, S G Brosnan, M I Carter, H M Hill, T V Isitt, N G Jeffs, E M Lang, S Logarajah, M T Patten, CC A Roud Mayne, F D Spears, I D Srikantharajah, A J Twigley, B S Yogasakaran

Cardiology C M Travill

Chemical Pathology D B Freedman

Clinical Oncology K Goodchild, P Hoskin, A Makris, M I Saunders

Dermatology A F Swain

ENT O P Chawla, M C Frampton, D F Johnston, J M Pickles

General Medicine N Finer, D Fishman, A E Griffiths, S R Jain, D B Peterson, D I M Siegler, N J Simmonds, S C Soo, M A Stodell

General Surgery S Cheslyn-Curtis, V K Jain, J R Novell, M R Pittam, J M Towler

Genitourinary Medicine T Balachandran

Haematology H Flora, D S Thompson, J Voke

Histopathology J W Dove, D A S Lawrence, Y Maria-Nayagam

Medical Microbiology R J Mulla

Elderly Care J J Day, K Mandaleson, K Mylvaganam, S Puthrasingam

Neurology A N Gale

Neurophysiology R M Sherratt

Obstetrics and Gynaecology S J Burrell, M Griffiths, D H Horwell, M O Lobb, O J D Owens, P C Reid

Occupational Health P Lewthwaite

Oncology A Makris

Ophthalmology N Anand, J D Heath, A Parnaby-Price, M P Snead, J J Tolia, A Waldock

Oral and Maxillofacial Surgery Mr Chan, D P Von Arx

Oral Surgery A D Giles, M G Gilhooly

Orthodontics L R O Hale

Orthopaedics D H Austwick, P A J Edge, R Pandit, C J Read, J S Sarkar, J M Scott

Paediatrics B R Adler, M J Chapple, D B Houston, P Sivakumar, M H Thompson

Plastic Surgery A O Grobbelaar, R Sanders

Radiology M S M Alexander, S A Allen, S J Barter, G S Jutla, M J Warren, R J Warwick, D J Wright

Radiotherapy and Oncology P J Hoskin, M I Saunders

Rehabilitation Medicine S Mullick

Rheumatology D Fishman

Urology A M Alam

St Mary's Day Hospital

Dunstable Road, Luton
Tel: 01582 721621

Luton Teaching Primary Care Trust

Nightingale House, 94 Inkerman Street, Luton LU1 1JD
Tel: 01582 528840 Fax: 01585 528841
Email: enquiries@lutonpct.nhs.uk
Website: www.lutonpct.nhs.uk
(Bedfordshire and Hertfordshire Strategic Health Authority)

Chair Gurch Randhawa
Chief Executive Regina Shakespeare

Maidstone and Tunbridge Wells NHS Trust

Trust Headquarters, Beech House, Pembury Hospital, Tonbridge Road, Pembury, Tunbridge Wells TN2 4QJ
Tel: 01892 823535 Fax: 01892 825468
Website: www.mtwnhstrust.nhs.uk
(Kent and Medway Strategic Health Authority)

Chair James Lee
Chief Executive Rose Gibb

Kent and Sussex Hospital

Mount Ephraim, Tunbridge Wells TN4 8AT
Tel: 01892 526111 Fax: 01892 528381
Total Beds: 226

Accident and Emergency J M Walker

Anaesthetics J Appleby, L Baldwin, R Chung, H T Hutchinson, R Loveday, T Ludgrove, A J Porterfield, A Pyne, D W Yates

Child and Adolescent Psychiatry R I Bearcroft

ENT R J Sergeant, J Shotton

General Medicine R A Banks, D Barnes, A Harris, J A Hughes, C S Lawson

General Surgery P G Bentley, A J Cook, T F Ford, J L Lewis, M R Tyrrell, T G Williams

Genitourinary Medicine S Winceslaus

Medical Microbiology D I Gladstone

Neurology T J Fowler

Ophthalmology J A Bell, N Rowson

Orthodontics A R Thom

Orthopaedics N J Fordyce, P A Gibb, P W Skinner, K W R Tuson

Paediatrics W J Bolsover, P Day, M F Robards

Radiology B G Conry, J J Flanagan, P Garrett, P R Tallett, C W Whetton

Radiotherapy and Oncology D M Barrett

Maidstone Hospital

Hermitage Lane, Maidstone ME16 9QQ
Tel: 01622 729000 Fax: 01622 224124
Total Beds: 381

Accident and Emergency G Cook, A Soorma

Anaesthetics M Biswas, J Dickenson, S W Gammanpila, D Iyer, A Jappie, S Sritharan, W S L Zoysa

General Medicine G Bird, A Hammond, D J Hibbert, P Holt, G R McIlwraith, P R Powell-Jackson, C Thom

General Surgery P A Jones, L M South, G Trotter

Haematology H J H Williams

Obstetrics and Gynaecology A Dunham, J D S Goodman, R H Kefford

Orthopaedics S Ellis, R N S Slater, C A Stossel, C J Walker

Paediatrics B Badhuri, J A Hulse, C E M Unter

Radiology J Donaldson, P McMillan

Radiotherapy and Oncology M Hill, R Jones, M O'Brien, N Powell, G M Sadler, J Summers

Thoracic Surgery O J Lau

Urology P Reddy

Pembury Hospital

Pembury, Tunbridge Wells TN2 4QJ
Tel: 01892 823535 Fax: 01892 824267
Total Beds: 206

Anaesthetics J Appleby, L Baldwin, R Chung, H T Hutchinson, R Loveday, T Ludgrove, A J Porterfield, A Pyne, D W Yates

Care of the Elderly M Chellappah, P Reynolds, P Tsang

Dermatology S Tharakaram (Head)

General Medicine R A Banks, A Harris, J A Hughes, C S Lawson

General Surgery P G Bentley, A J Cook, T F Ford, J L Lewis, M R Tyrrell, T G Williams

Haematology D S Gillett, C G Taylor

Histopathology R N Basu

Neurology T J Fowler

Obstetrics and Gynaecology P N Bamford, O Chappatte, D B Garrioch

Paediatrics W Bolsover, P Day, M F Robards

Radiology B G Conry, J J Flanagan, P Garrett, P R Tallett, C W Whetton

Maidstone Weald Primary Care Trust

Forstal, Preston Hall, Aylesford ME20 7NJ
Tel: 01622 225750 Fax: 01622 255770
Email: firstname.surname@maidstonewealdpct.nhs.uk
Website: www.kentandmedway.nhs.uk
(Kent and Medway Strategic Health Authority)

Chair Rosanne Corben
Chief Executive Nigel Howells

Hawkhurst Cottage Hospital

High Street, Hawkhurst, Cranbrook TN18 4PU
Tel: 01580 753345 Fax: 01580 754466
Total Beds: 15

Manager Sue Brown

Maldon and South Chelmsford Primary Care Trust

Administration Block, St Peter's Hospital, 32A Spital Road, Maldon CM9 6EG
Tel: 01621 727300 Fax: 01621 727301
Website: www.maldon-pct.nhs.uk
(Essex Strategic Health Authority)

Chair Tony Plumridge
Chief Executive Mike Harrison

Manchester Mental Health and Social Care Trust

Chorlton House, 70 Manchester Road, Chorlton-cum-Hardy, Manchester M21 9UN
Tel: 0161 882 1100 Fax: 0161 882 1001
Website: www.mmhsc.org.uk
(Greater Manchester Strategic Health Authority)

Chair Wyn Dignan
Chief Executive Laura Roberts
Consultants Al-Abbadey, Anderson, Davies, Garvey, R Godsall, J Harrison, Higgo, R Hopkins, J Jones, P Mbaya, A Pavillon, A Poynton, E Pugh, A Theodossiadis, C Thomas, A Wieck

Mansfield District Primary Care Trust

Integrated management with Ashfield Primary Care Trust.

Ransom Hall, Ransom Wood Business Park, Southwell Road West, Mansfield NG21 0ER
Tel: 01623 414114 Fax: 01623 653527
Website: www.mansfielddist-pct.org.uk
(Trent Strategic Health Authority)

Chair Tony Hughes
Chief Executive Eleri de Gilbert

Mayday Healthcare NHS Trust

530 London Road, Croydon CR7 7YE
Tel: 020 8401 3000 Fax: 020 8665 1974
Email: forename.surname@mayday.nhs.uk
Website: www.maydayhospital.org.uk

(South West London Strategic Health Authority)

Chair Sue Eardley
Chief Executive Vanessa Wood

Mayday University Hospital

London Road, Croydon CR7 7YE
Tel: 020 8401 3000 Fax: 020 8665 1974
Total Beds: 750

Accident and Emergency C Blakeley, K Hashemi

Anaesthetics K Amir-Ansari, M Baruya, N Chitkara, D G Cohen, J Collyer, J Heriot, A Knibb, G Menon, Dr Moghal, V Muralitharan, M Navaratnarajah, T Waddell, P Walton

Cardiology R Canepa-Anson, J Orford, P Stubbs

Care of the Elderly P Diggory, D Griffith, V Jones, E Lawrence, A Mehta, P O O'Mahoney

Chemical Pathology A Tarn

Colorectal Surgery M Abulafi

Dermatology E Mallon

ENT L Hicklin, J R Knight, S Mady

Gastroenterology M Mendall, A Theodossi, S M Thomas

General Medicine N L Essex, P Johnson, A C Miller, M Prentice, M Prentice, N Velasco

General Surgery J Derodra, S Ebbs, P Hurley, M Meagher, I Swift

Genitourinary Medicine A Newell, M Rodgers

Haematology J Lumley, J Maitland, C Pollard

Histopathology A Arnaout, E Rawelly, S M Thomas

Microbiology M Sahathevan

Neonatology J Chang, A Kumar

Neurology H Modarres, F Schon

Obstetrics and Gynaecology M Booker, P Clarkson, R Hamid, P Shah, A Sultan, R Thakar, G Ward

Ophthalmology W Ayliffe, D De Alwis, T Richardson, H Seward

Oral and Maxillofacial Surgery N Hyde, M Manisali

Orthodontics A J Banner

Orthopaedics G Howell, A Iossifidis, F Kashif, G Marsh, M A S Mowbray, V Naidu

Orthopaedics and Trauma B Hughes

Paediatrics K Cottrall, T Fenton, S Hart, H Underhill

Palliative Care D E Swann

Pathology M Coppen

Radiology N Bees, H N Blake, R Evans, M C Hoskins, Dr Jeyadevan, S Lowe, S Maheshwaren, A Newman-Sanders, Mr Raju (Shamugaraju)

Restorative Dentistry G Gilmour

Rheumatology and Rehabilitation J A Reardon, R Sathananthan

Urology G Das

Vascular Surgery M Williams

Purley and District War Memorial Hospital

856 Brighton Road, Purley CR2 2YL
Tel: 020 8401 3000
Total Beds: 42

Care of the Elderly D Griffith

Medway NHS Trust

Medway Hospital, Windmill Road, Gillingham ME7 5NY
Tel: 01634 830000 Fax: 01634 825290
Website: www.medwaynhstrust.nhs.uk
(Kent and Medway Strategic Health Authority)

Chair Janardan Sofat
Chief Executive Andrew Horne

Medway Maritime Hospital

Windmill Road, Gillingham ME7 5NY
Tel: 01634 830000 Fax: 01634 815811
Total Beds: 633

Manager Jane Sutherland

Accident and Emergency A Morrice (Head), M Mason, V Sethkumar

Anaesthetics R Buist, G Cross, S Day, N Divekaaar, B Oyesola, C Parnell, M Pick, D Simpson, N Venkat, S Vishnubala, T Wilson

Care of the Elderly M Hayward, B Kundu, A Mamud, P Talavlikar

Chemical Pathology Dr Springbett, R Workman

Dermatology M Boss (Head), C Grech, S Halpern, L Shall, A Shanks

ENT J Davis (Head), P Gluckman, R Henry, V Lobo, M Oyarzabal

General Medicine R Day, A Gough, I O'Brien, I Scobie, A Stewart, D Thompson

General Surgery R Haile (Head), B Andrews, D Beeby, C Butler, O Khan, P Webb, H Westgapel

Haematology R Baker (Head), M Aldouri, J Hayes

Medical Microbiology R Springbett, R Workman

Neonatology D Ducker (Head), B Jani, A Soe

Neurology C Hughes (Head), S Chong, K Cikurel

Nuclear Medicine P Ryan (Head)

Obstetrics and Gynaecology A Ahmed, J Ducket, M Hanson, D Houghton, D Moore, S Norman, D Penman

Occupational Health J Wood

Ophthalmology C Jenkins, A MacFarlane, R Sampath

Oral and Maxillofacial Surgery K Lavery

Orthopaedics J Fleetcroft (Head), K Borowsky, A Hammer

Paediatrics P Manuel (Head), T Little, R Merwaha, P Williams

Pathology L V K De Silva, R Lindley, B Randall

Plastic Surgery H Belcher, P Gilbert

Radiology K Reddy (Head), P Mills, P Reddy, K Segaran, S Sivathasan, M Velamati

Rheumatology and Rehabilitation G George, P Williams

Urology J Palmer (Head), G Mufti

Medway Teaching Primary Care Trust

7-8 Ambley Green, Bailey Drive, Gillingham Business Park, Gillingham ME8 0NJ
Tel: 01634 382777 Fax: 01634 382700
Website: www.kentandmedway.nhs.uk
(Kent and Medway Strategic Health Authority)

Chair Eddie Anderson
Chief Executive Bill Gillespie

Melton, Rutland and Harborough Primary Care Trust

Pera Innovation Park, Nottingham Road, Melton Mowbray LE13 0RH
Tel: 01664 855000 Fax: 01664 855001
Website: www.mrh.nhs.uk/xform.asp
(Leicestershire, Northamptonshire and Rutland Strategic Health Authority)

Chair John Grant
Chief Executive Wendy Saviour

Mendip Primary Care Trust

Priory Health Park, Glastonbury Road, Wells BA5 1XL
Tel: 01749 836500 Fax: 01749 836699
Email: headquarters@mendip-pct.nhs.uk
Website: www.mendippct.org.uk
(Dorset and Somerset Strategic Health Authority)

Chair Stephen Harrison
Chief Executive Robin Smith

Butleigh Hospital
Kingsweston Road, Butleigh, Glastonbury BA6 8TF
Tel: 01458 850237 Fax: 01458 850228
Total Beds: 17

Manager Janet Wright

Shepton Mallet Community Hospital
Old Wells Road, Shepton Mallet BA4 4PG
Tel: 01749 342931 Fax: 01749 330045
Total Beds: 21

Manager Karen Thomas

Victoria Hospital
Park Road, Frome BA11 1EY
Tel: 01373 463591 Fax: 01373 456627
Total Beds: 26

Manager Kay Kittermaster

Wells and District Hospital
Bath Road, Wells BA5 2XL
Tel: 01749 683200 Fax: 01749 683223
Total Beds: 19

Manager Heather Pruett

Mersey Care NHS Trust

Rathbone Hospital, Mill Lane, Liverpool L9 7JP
Tel: 0151 250 3000 Fax: 0151 473 2863
Email: communications@merseycare.nhs.uk
Website: www.merseycare.nhs.uk
(Cumbria and Lancashire Strategic Health Authority)

Chair Stephen Hawkins
Chief Executive Alan Yates

Ashworth Hospital
Parkbourn, Maghull, Liverpool L31 1HW
Tel: 0151 473 0303 Fax: 0151 526 6603
Total Beds: 572

Broadoak Mental Health Unit
Thomas Drive, Liverpool L14 3PJ
Tel: 0151 250 3000 Fax: 0151 250 2325 250 2325 250 2325
Total Beds: 88

Consultants R Higgo, R McCutcheon, M Munro, C O'Brien, G Segarjasingham, E Windgassen

Mossley Hill Hospital
Park Avenue, Mossley Hill, Liverpool L18 8BU
Tel: 0151 250 6127 Fax: 0151 250 6015
Total Beds: 65

Consultants D Anderson, P Metcalf, R Philpott, D Selverajah

Rathbone Hospital
Mill Lane, Liverpool L13 4AW
Tel: 0151 250 3000 Fax: 0151 220 4291
Total Beds: 88

Wavertree Lodge/Wavertree Bungalow
Old Mill Lane, Wavertree, Liverpool L15 8LW
Tel: 0151 250 3000
Total Beds: 12

Windsor House
40 Upper Parliament Street, Liverpool L8 7LF
Tel: 0151 250 5305 Fax: 0151 250 5339
Total Beds: 24

Manager Sue Molyneux

Mersey Regional Ambulance Service NHS Trust

Elm House, Belmont Grove, Liverpool L6 4EG
Tel: 0151 260 5220 Fax: 0151 260 7441
Website: www.merseyambulance.nhs.uk
(Cheshire and Merseyside Strategic Health Authority)

Chair Ken Hoskisson
Chief Executive Janet Davies

Mid Cheshire Hospitals NHS Trust

Leighton Hospital, Middlewich Road, Crewe CW1 4QJ
Tel: 01270 255141 Fax: 01270 587696
Website: www.mcht.nhs.uk
(Cheshire and Merseyside Strategic Health Authority)

Chair Robin Farmer, Simon Yates
Chief Executive Simon Yates

Leighton Hospital
Middlewich Road, Crewe CW1 4QJ
Tel: 01270 255141 Fax: 01270 587696
Total Beds: 700

Accident and Emergency J B Bache

Anaesthetics P Board, M Brown, F M Emery, C S Hopkins, K E Jones, P Lewis, A Martin, R W Okell

Care of the Elderly H W Jones

Dental Surgery J I Cawood

Dermatology P J August, A Harris

ENT J E Davies, J Deans, A Dingle

General Medicine P Dodds, R Kedia, J Lloyd, I Londor, J S McKay, M D Winson

General Surgery D Cade, A Guy, M Hanafi, J Slavin

Genitourinary Medicine M H Khan

Obstetrics and Gynaecology J E Felmingham, M Luckas, G Scott

Ophthalmology L B Freeman, J Hubbard, B Moriarty, M A Neugebauer

Orthodontics C Melrose

Orthopaedics R Gillies, N Hyder, R Krishnan, D Pegg, T R Redfern

Paediatrics J Ellison, R E Pugh, H Sackey, A P J Thomson

Pathology N Cooper, S Mallya, A Nicol, M O'Donoghue, M Patterson, J Stafford

Radiology S Evans, P Mayor, P R Moorhouse, J Scally, A Troop, S Zaman

Urology P Irwin, P Javle, S Stubington

Victoria Infirmary
Northwich CW8 1AW
Tel: 01606 74331 Fax: 01606 74331 ext: 4020
Total Beds: 34

Accident and Emergency J B Bache

Care of the Elderly H W Jones, V Lakshmi

Dermatology P J August

ENT J E Davies

General Medicine J S McKay, M D Winson

General Surgery A Guy, J Slavin

Obstetrics and Gynaecology J E Felmingham, G Scott

Ophthalmology L B Freeman

Orthopaedics D Pegg, T R Redfern

Paediatrics R Pugh

Radiology S Evans

Urology P Irwin

Mid Devon Primary Care Trust

Newcourt House, Old Rydon Lane, Exeter EX2 7JU
Tel: 01392 449864
Website: www.middevon-pct.nhs.uk
(South West Peninsula Strategic Health Authority)

Chair Bud Wendover
Chief Executive Lesley Dunaway

Castle Hospital
1 Castle Walk, Okehampton EX20 1HY
Tel: 01837 52411 Fax: 01837 55507
Total Beds: 35

Crediton Community Hospital
Western Road, Crediton EX17 3NH
Tel: 01363 775588 Fax: 01363 777919
Total Beds: 24

Moretonhampstead Hospital
Ford Street, Moretonhampstead, Newton Abbot TQ13 8LN
Tel: 01647 440217

Okehampton and District Hospital
East Street, Okehampton EX20 1PN
Total Beds: 19

Tiverton and District Hospital
Kennedy Way, Tiverton EX16 6NT
Tel: 01884 235400 Fax: 01884 235545
Total Beds: 47

Mid Essex Hospital Services NHS Trust

Broomfield Hospital, Court Road, Broomfield, Chelmsford CM1 7ET
Tel: 01245 440761 Fax: 01245 514675
Email: enquiries@meht.nhs.uk
Website: www.meht.nhs.uk
(Essex Strategic Health Authority)

Chair David Bullock
Chief Executive Andrew Pike

Broomfield Hospital
Court Road, Broomfield, Chelmsford CM1 7ET
Tel: 01245 440761 Fax: 01245 514166
Total Beds: 800

Accident and Emergency A Mariathas, R B Zwink

Anaesthetics J Alexander-Collins, M Alexander-Williams, J Carter, M Davis, J J Durcan, B Emerson, A Hassani, N Huddy, D Kelly, K Kiff, J Lloyd, C McCartney, C McCartney, L Ooi, S Pal, D Peck, G Philpott, I Seggie, D J M Williams

Burns/Plastic Surgery P Dziewulski, D Elliott, A F S Flemming, T Loshan Kangesu, N Niranjan

Care of the Elderly R K Puri, A Qureshi, V Umachandran

Chest Disease A Blainey, J A Utting

Dermatology A Harrison, M R Klaber

General Medicine G Clesham, D Cunnah, J Fletcher, C Khin, S H Saverymuttu, D R Turner, M J Weston

General Surgery T Browne, M Harvey, Y Panayiotdpoulos, N Richardson, A H M Ross, P Sauven

Neurology P G Bradbury

Ophthalmology T A G Bell, A Sinha, M T Thoung

Orthopaedics J K Dowell, H Lyall, M Pereira, M Taylor, J Tuite, W Williams

Paediatrics A Agrawal, A P Lipscomb

Pathology M A Ahmed, S Al-Sam, K J Al Janabi, O H A Baugh, V Chowdhury, Y Thway

Radiology G Harverson, P H Lee, P G Pratt, H D Punnyadasa, K S Rao, R Whitney, P Wou

Radiotherapy and Oncology N Davidson, T A Lister, S Tahir

Rheumatology and Rehabilitation P G Davies, A Srinivasan

Urology H J E Lewi, T Tassadq

St John's Hospital
Wood Street, Chelmsford CM2 9BG
Tel: 01245 440761 Fax: 01245 513671
Total Beds: 172

Anaesthetics J Carter, M Davis, J J Durcan, J L Handy, A Hassani, N Huddy, D Kelly, C McCartney

Care of the Elderly R K Puri, V Umachandran

ENT D G Fife, A Pace-Balzan, C B Singh

Obstetrics and Gynaecology C F Goodfellow, C J Partington, D J Robarts

Orthodontics G Howe

Paediatrics A Agrawal, G Bridgman, G Kugan, A P Lipscomb, R N Mahesh Babu, L Murtaza

Pathology M A Ahmed, A Al-Sam, K J Al Janabai, O H A Baugh, V Chowdhury, Y Thway

Radiology G Harverson, P H Lee, P G Pratt, H D Punnyadasa, K S Rao, R Whitney, P Wou

St Michael's Hospital
142 Rayne Road, Braintree CM7 2QJ
Tel: 01245 440761 Fax: 01376 558538

Care of the Elderly A Qureshi, V Umachandran

Dermatology A Harrison

ENT C B Singh

General Medicine A Blainey, D Cunnah, S H Saverymuttu

General Surgery Y Panayiotopoulos

Ophthalmology M T Thoung

Paediatrics A Agrawal, G C Bridgman, A P Lipscomb, R N Mahesh Babu

Rheumatology and Rehabilitation P G Davies

St Peter's Hospital
Spital Road, Maldon CM9 6EG
Tel: 01376 551221
Total Beds: 75

Care of the Elderly R K Puri, V Umachandran

Dermatology M R Klaber

General Medicine J Utting, M J Weston

General Surgery P Sauven

Obstetrics and Gynaecology C K Partington

Ophthalmology T A G Bell, A Sinha, M T Thoung

Orthopaedics K Cheah

Paediatrics A P Lipscomb

Pathology M A Ahmed, S Al-Sam, O H A Baugh, Y Thway

Rheumatology and Rehabilitation A Srinivasan

William Julien Courtauld Hospital
London Road, Braintree CM7 2LJ
Tel: 01245 440761 Fax: 01376 552531
Total Beds: 38

Obstetrics and Gynaecology C Goodfellow, J Onwude, C Partington, P J Robarts

Mid-Hampshire Primary Care Trust

Unit 3, Tidbury Farm, Bullington Cross, Sutton Scotney, Winchester SO21 3QQ
Tel: 01962 763940 Fax: 01962 763941
Website: www.midhampshirepct.nhs.uk
(Hampshire and Isle of Wight Strategic Health Authority)

Chair Bridget Phelps
Chief Executive Chris Evennett

Mid Staffordshire General Hospitals NHS Trust

Staffordshire General Hospital, Weston Road, Stafford ST16 3SA
Tel: 01785 257731 Fax: 01785 230538
Website: www.midstaffs.nhs.uk
(Shropshire and Staffordshire Strategic Health Authority)

Chair Tony Brisby
Chief Executive David O'Neill

Cannock Chase Hospital
Brunswick Road, Cannock WS11 2XY
Tel: 01543 572757, 01785 257888
Total Beds: 166

Staffordshire General Hospital
Weston Road, Stafford ST16 3SA
Tel: 01785 257731 Fax: 01785 245211
Total Beds: 410

Accident and Emergency D F McGeehan

Anaesthetics G Earnshaw, M Grewal, W J Hawkins, R W G Johns, A S T Lamb, D A McCulloch, Y M Salib, C Secker, W G Sellwood, A Taylor

Care of the Elderly J Elizabeth, G Jacob, A Oke

Dermatology N Hardwick, A G Smith, K A Ward

ENT V C David, T N Reddy

General Medicine P Coates, P R Daggett, A J Fairfax, J A Gibson, P Singh, P Woodmansey, J Yeoh

General Surgery W Crisp, D Durrans, R Gendy, B Gwynn, R Hutchinson, R Kumar

Genitourinary Medicine A R Markos

Haematology Dr Amos, P G Revell

Histopathology S C Harris, V Suarez

Medical Microbiology E Olson, M L Yee

Neurology B Summers

Obstetrics and Gynaecology K Chin, V Dapaah, J Dixon, A Elmardi, K Powell

Ophthalmology M P Headon, J Price

Oral and Maxillofacial Surgery T Malins

Orthodontics A M Bond, J D Muir

Orthopaedics I Bhoora, T El-Fakhri, M Hoyle, V Kathuria, J Travlos

Paediatrics A Gupta, C Melville, T Randall

Radiology A M MacLeod, S Patel, D Steventon, R Suarez, Dr Willard

Radiotherapy and Oncology A M Brunt, J E Scoble

Rheumatology D Mulherin, T Price, T Sheeran

Mid Sussex Primary Care Trust

Kleinwort, Haywards Heath Hospital, Butlers Green Road, Haywards Heath RH16 4BE
Tel: 01444 475700 Fax: 01444 475757
Email: info@mspct.nhs.uk
Website: www.mspct.nhs.uk
(Surrey and Sussex Strategic Health Authority)

Chair Christine Barwell
Chief Executive Michael Wood

Mid Yorkshire Hospitals NHS Trust

Trust Headquarters, Pinderfields General Hospital, Rowan House, Aberford Road, Wakefield WF1 4DG
Tel: 01924 213850 Fax: 01924 814929
Email: forename.surname@panp-tr.northy.nhs.uk
Website: www.midyorks.nhs.uk
(West Yorkshire Strategic Health Authority)

Chair Malcolm Batty
Chief Executive John Parkes

Castleford, Normanton and District Hospital
Lumley Street, Castleford WF10 5LT
Tel: 01977 605500

Clayton Hospital
Northgate, Wakefield WF1 3JS
Tel: 01924 201688

Dewsbury and District Hospital
Halifax Road, Dewsbury WF13 4HS
Tel: 01924 512000, 01924 816116 Fax: 01924 816192
Email: emma.newsome@dhc-tr.northy.nhs.uk
Total Beds: 514

Manager Angela Watson

Accident and Emergency P K Ancill, S M Barnes, Dr Kerner, Dr Okereke

Anaesthetics S A Brayshaw, J Brook, N Dwyer, P Goulden, K Ismail, O A Maher, J Perfettini, Dr Queneshi, S A Quereshi, Dr Reddy, Dr Riad, P Smith, M A Thickett, Dr Wilson

Cardiology Dr Smyllie

Care of the Elderly C K Biswas, Dr Cox, I Craig

Child and Adolescent Psychiatry Dr Edwards

Dental Surgery Dr Mitchell

Dermatology G Ford, M Shah, G Taylor

Elderly Mentally Ill Dr Booya

ENT Dr Hassan, L C Knight, Dr London, C J Woodhead

General Medicine Dr Chidambra, D C Currie, Dr Fitzpatrick, T M Kemp, B Sivaramakrishnan, Dr Sutcliffe

General Surgery W Case, J Lovegrove, P J Lyndon, C M White

Genitourinary Medicine P A D Silva

Learning Disabilities Dr Galaprathie

Obstetrics and Gynaecology T Aslam-Tariq, K Fishwick, A Trehan

Oncology M Bond, C Coyle, Dr Orton

Ophthalmology A Cassells-Brown, N George, D O'Neill

Orthodontics R Y Shuff

Orthopaedics P D Angus, A Maroof, J Ridge, J G Shea

Paediatrics Dr Allaboa, P Gorham, P MacKay, A M A Soulioti, G M Wilson

Palliative Medicine R Lane

Pathology Dr Cadman, M R Chappell, P W Gudgeon, A Jackson, M M Raj

Plastic Surgery Dr Fenton, Dr Southern

Radiology P L N Ah-Fat, Dr Altikaiti, E Cave, P James, M Vaidya

Rheumatology L Hordon, S Miles

Pinderfields General Hospital
Rowan House, Aberford Road, Wakefield WF1 4EE
Tel: 01924 213850 Fax: 01924 814929
Total Beds: 560

Manager Gordon Walker

General Medicine W A Burr, S E Williams

Medical Microbiology A S Sohal

Neurology A S N Al-Din, L A Loizou

Neurophysiology J A Twomey

Neuroradiology G Bonsor, M Nelson, J Straiton

Ophthalmology K S Toor

Oral and Maxillofacial Surgery D A Mitchell (Head), R A Loukota, K D Mizen

Orthopaedics P Deacon, N N Ghali, A E S Rainey

Paediatrics E Glass, S T Jones, R MacFaul, P Tawfik

Palliative Medicine P Gajjar

Pathology M C Galvin, P B Hamal

Plastic Surgery O M Fenton, L Fourie, K Judkins, A Phipps

Radiology S K Jain, J B Walls, C Wilson-Sharp

Restorative Dentistry V K Joshi

Urology S Harrsion, P Weston

Pontefract General Infirmary
Friarwood Lane, Pontefract WF8 1PL
Tel: 01977 600600 Fax: 01977 606852
Total Beds: 383

General Medicine A K Ghosh, M Gundroo, R V Lewis, M D Peake, M V Tobin, C White

Genitourinary Medicine J Clarke, P A D Silva

Neurology A Burt, L A Loizou

Obstetrics and Gynaecology A Forbes, P D Howe, G Hunter

Ophthalmology K S Toor

Orthopaedics M S Binns, S M Gollapudi, R A Nicholson, D Riley

Paediatrics J M T Alexander, M M Hasson, D Rutter

Pathology M M Aslam, J Haynes, I W C Macdonald

Plastic Surgery L Fouri

Radiology J H M Ellingham, V D Ganorkar, G S Jutlla

Radiotherapy and Oncology A Crellin, R I Rothwell

Urology M R G Robinson

Middlesbrough Primary Care Trust

Riverside House, 18 High Force Road, Riverside Park, Middlesbrough TS2 1RH
Tel: 01642 352370 Fax: 01642 352380
Email: public-affairs@middlesbroughpct.co.uk
Website: www.middlesbroughpct.co.uk
(County Durham and Tees Valley Strategic Health Authority)

Chair Ann O'Hanlon
Chief Executive Colin McLeod

Carter Bequest Hospital
Cambridge Road, Middlesbrough TS5 5NH
Tel: 01642 850911 Fax: 01642 816140

Manager Allison Welsh

Milton Keynes General Hospital NHS Trust

Standing Way, Eaglestone, Milton Keynes MK6 5LD
Tel: 01908 660033 Fax: 01908 669348
Email: mail@mkgeneral.nhs.uk
Website: www.mkgeneral.nhs.uk
(Thames Valley Strategic Health Authority)

Chair Mike Rowlands
Chief Executive Jill Rodney

Milton Keynes General Hospital
Standing Way, Eaglestone, Milton Keynes MK6 5LD
Tel: 01908 660033 Fax: 01908 669348
Total Beds: 410

Accident and Emergency K Kumar, P Thomas

Anaesthetics P H Chambers, J Cooney, M J Cowen, F E Evans, J P Hall, H Howells, V Jeevananthan, H Mangi, J T B Moyle, J Porter, P A Reed, B Slavin, A P White

Dermatology P Duhra

ENT P Brown, P Gurr, S T O'Malley

Gastroenterology S Lanzon-Miller, R Madhotra

General Medicine C W S Fisher, D Gwilt, P Medhi, I Mulligan, R C Paton

General Surgery P C Holford, D Mcwhinnie, K Mainprize, A Mitchell, R G Souter, E M Walker

Neurology R Butterworth, D Hilton-Jones

Obstetrics and Gynaecology R D Fawdry, P Haynes, C B Lynch, G S McCune, A Stock

Ophthalmology A Assaf, R Bates, A Kadom, B Kumar

Orthodontics D G M Greig

Orthopaedics A Floyd, R S Gunn, G F Miller, D Wallace, M Wetherill

Paediatrics V Joss, P K Lakhani, P Latham

Pathology B C Das, T R Gamlen, S S Jalloh, K Y Lwin, E Miller, D J Moir, D White

Radiology Dr Choji, P Evans, O P Fitzgerald-Finch, N Graham, C Hardingham, A Havard, Y Manu, A Ul Haq, S Yogarajah

Urology I Anjum, E Walker

Milton Keynes Primary Care Trust

Hospital Campus, Eaglestone, Milton Keynes MK6 5NG
Tel: 01908 243933 Fax: 01908 694919
Email: mail@mkpct.org.uk
Website: www.mkpct.org.uk
(Thames Valley Strategic Health Authority)

Chair Malcolm Brighton
Chief Executive Barbara Kennedy

Bletchley Community Hospital

Whalley Drive, Bletchley, Milton Keynes MK3 6EN
Tel: 01908 376415
Total Beds: 24

Fraser Day Hospital

Pagnell Grange, Westbury Lane, Newport Pagnell, Milton Keynes MK16 8JA
Tel: 01908 210344 Fax: 01908 218172

Linford Day Hospital

Wolverton Health Centre, Gloucester Road, Wolverton, Milton Keynes
Tel: 01908 316633 Ext: 240

Moorfields Eye Hospital NHS Foundation Trust

Established as a Foundation Trust 01/04/2004.

City Road, London EC1V 2PD
Tel: 020 7253 3411 Fax: 020 7253 4696
Email: info@moorfields.org.uk
Website: www.moorfields.org.uk
(North Central London Strategic Health Authority)

Chair Thomas Boyd-Carpenter
Chief Executive Ian Balmer

Moorfields Eye Hospital

City Road, London EC1V 2PD
Tel: 020 7253 3411 Fax: 020 7253 4696
Total Beds: 80

Anaesthetics C A Carr (Head), S Bailey, A J Budd, N Catteruccia, A Coren, M Kadim, B Logan, R L McAuliffe, C Mathur, C M Moore, S Powrie

General Medicine D J Galton, B T Goh, G Plant

Ophthalmology J Acheson, G W Adams, B Allen, G W Aylward, K Barton, M Beaconsfield, A C Bird, J Brookes, D Charteris, R Collin, C Cunningham, L da Cruz, R D Daniel, J K Dart, A Davis, P Desai, J Dowler, C Egan, E Ezra, L Ficker, P Foster, W Franks, D S Gartry, D F Garway-Heath, Z Gregor, R A Hitchings, S Horgan, J Hungerford, P Hykin, A Ionides, P T Khaw, F Larkin, J P Lee, S Lightman, V Maurino, M H Miller, A T Moore, I Murdoch, N Okhravi, M Papadopolous, C Pavesio, G Plant, G E Rose, C K Rostron, A Salt, D Saunders, J J Sloper, J Stevens, P Sullivan, G Thompson, A Tufail, S Tuft, J Uddin, D H Verity, S Verma, A Viswanathan, A Webster, M Westcott, R Wormald

Paediatrics J Lee, A Salt

Radiology I F Moseley (Head)

Morecambe Bay Hospitals NHS Trust

Westmorland General Hospital, Burton Road, Kendal LA9 7RG
Tel: 01539 795366 Fax: 01539 795313
Website: www.mbht.nhs.uk
(Cumbria and Lancashire Strategic Health Authority)

Chair E Idris Williams
Chief Executive Ian Cumming

Furness General Hospital

Dalton Lane, Barrow-in-Furness LA14 4LF
Tel: 01229 870870 Fax: 01229 871182
Total Beds: 400

Accident and Emergency F McMillan

Anaesthetics S N Costigan, A Dawood, M Haddara, A D Haughton, J N Hodkinson, K Torn, L J Williams

Dental Surgery P V Dyer, V J Hadden, O Keith

Dermatology P V Harrison

ENT P J Stoney, B C S Whitfield

General Medicine A Barton, G Cook, Dr Ghamri, J Keating, W S Mitchell, I Owen, R Sekhar

General Surgery C S Ball, D G Nasmyth, P Patel

Nephrology S Gibson

Neurology K Rauvala

Obstetrics and Gynaecology V Bamigboye, I Y Hussein, P K Misra, V Sharan

Oncology M B McIllmurray

Ophthalmology E Khadem, A L Lyness, B Moate

Oral Surgery P V Dyer

Orthopaedics A N Baqai, N H Courtman, R J Michaud, A Smith

Paediatrics A Olabi, P T Ward

Palliative Medicine N J Sayer

Pathology V M Joglekar, A T Macheta, Dr Spartridge, A Taylor

Radiology P J S Crawshaw

Rheumatology W S Mitchell

Urology K Madhra, R Y Wilson

Queen Victoria Hospital
Thornton Road, Morecambe LA4 5NN
Tel: 01524 411661
Total Beds: 48

Royal Lancaster Infirmary
Ashton Road, Lancaster LA1 4RP
Tel: 01524 65944 Fax: 01524 846346
Total Beds: 437

Accident and Emergency R G McGlone, S Schneidermann

Anaesthetics T M Bird, J R Davies, C Granger, S Harding, Dr Marcham, A Minchom, T Oldham, W G Park, S Richmond, A M Severn, G Siviter, A F Smith, M B Smith, C B Till, A P Vickers

Dental Surgery P V Dyer, V J Hadden, O Keith

ENT M E M Baraka, C H Bulman

General Medicine A Brodison, C M Brown, P B M Clarkson, A D Higham, D McGowan, A B Murgatroyd, I Owen, P Smith, D Walmsley, R F Willey

General Surgery J S Abraham, Mr Bhukari, R C Bollard, J Bonnema, C Bronder, J Calvey, I Crighton, W P Morgan, Mr Tomlinson, M Wilkinson, Mr Wilson

Immunology N Williamson

Medical Oncology M B McIllmurray

Obstetrics and Gynaecology D J Burch, R Ghani, K Granger, K Jones, R J Shepherd

Ophthalmology R K Khanna, G E Ozuzu

Oral and Maxillofacial Surgery P V Dyer

Orthodontics J G McCracken

Orthopaedics Y A Feldman, S K Gary, P Marshall, S N Radcliffe, B Rhodes, H D Stewart

Paediatrics S Cade, P A G Gibson, S Ireland, C Peckham, M M Placzek, J Sandhu

Pathology R W Blewitt, S Dealer, D W Gorst, C L Kozlowski, N Mapstone, J A Morris, R Neary, M Stewart, D R Telford

Plastic Surgery A Howcroft

Radiology P M Flanagan, J M Lavelle, J McGregor, L M Ness, D Sheals, W Stevenson, A K M Taylor, W H J Wall

Rheumatology W N Dodds, J P Halsey

Urology P Duffy, C Rowbotham

Ulverston Hospital
Stanley Street, Ulverston LA12 7BT
Tel: 01229 583635 Fax: 01229 580803
Total Beds: 46

Westmorland General Hospital
Burton Road, Kendal LA9 7RG
Tel: 01539 732288 Fax: 01539 740852
Total Beds: 234

Accident and Emergency R McGlone, S Schneidermann

Anaesthetics T M Bird, J R Davies, C Granger, S Harding, A Highley, Dr Markham, A Minchom, T Oldham, W Park, S Richmond, A M Severn, G Siviter, A F Smith, M Smith, C B Till, A Vickers

Care of the Elderly I Chadwick, I M Huggett

Dental Surgery P V Dyer, V J Hadden, O Keith

Dermatology P V Harrison

ENT C H Bulman, P Stoney, B Whitfield

General Medicine A Brodison, C Brown, A D Higham, P B M Mclarkson, I Owen, P Smith, D Walmsley, R F Willey

General Surgery J Abraham, Mr Bhukari, R C Bollard, J Bonnema, C Bronder, J Calvey, I Crighton, W P Morgan, Mr Tomlinson, M Wilkinson, P Wilson

Obstetrics and Gynaecology D J Burch, R Ghani, K Granger, K Jones, R J Shepherd

Oncology M B McIllmurray

Ophthalmology E Khadem, R K Khanna, A L Lyness, B Moate, G E Ozuzu

Orthodontics J G McCracken

Orthopaedics Y A Feldman, S K Garg, P Marshall, S N Radcliffe, B Rhodes, H D Stewart

Paediatrics S Cade, P A Gibson, S Ireland, C Peckham, M M Placzek, J Sandhu

Pathology R W Blewitt, S Dealer, D Gorst, C L Kozlowski, N Mapstone, J A Morris, R Neary, M Stewart, D R Telford

Radiology P M Flanagan, J M Lavelle, J McGregor, L M Ness, D Sheals, W Stevenson, W H J Wall

Rheumatology and Rehabilitation W Dodds, J P Halsey

Urology P Duffy, C Rowbotham, R Y Wilson

Morecambe Bay Primary Care Trust

Tenterfield, Brigsteer Road, Kendal LA9 5EA
Tel: 01539 797800 Fax: 01539 726687
Website: www.mbpct.nhs.uk
(Cumbria and Lancashire Strategic Health Authority)

Chair Kathy Lubelska
Chief Executive Leigh Griffin

Ridge Lea Hospital
Quernmore Road, Lancaster LA1 3JR
Tel: 01524 586200

New Forest Primary Care Trust

8 Sterne Road, Tatchbury Mount, Calmore, Southampton SO40 2RZ
Tel: 023 8087 4270 Fax: 023 8087 4275
Email: enquiries@nfpct.nhs.uk
Website: www.newforestpct.nhs.uk
(Hampshire and Isle of Wight Strategic Health Authority)

Chair Alex Lander
Chief Executive Angela Jeffrey

Fenwick Day Hospital
Pikes Hill, Lyndhurst, Southampton SO43 7NG
Tel: 023 8028 2782 Fax: 023 8028 2161
Total Beds: 22

Fenwick Hospital
Pikes Hill, Lyndhurst, Southampton
Tel: 023 8028 2782 Fax: 023 8028 2161
Total Beds: 22

Hythe Day Hospital
Beaulieu Road, Hythe, Southampton SO45 7NG
Tel: 023 8084 6046

Hythe Hospital
Beaulieu Road, Dibden Purlieu Hythe, Southampton SO45 5ZB
Tel: 023 8084 6046 Fax: 023 8020 7285
Total Beds: 24

Lymington Day Hospital
East Hill, Lymington SO41 9ZJ
Tel: 01590 676085 Fax: 01590 670749

Lymington Hospital
Southampton Road, Lymington SO41 9ZH
Tel: 01590 677011 Fax: 01590 671787
Total Beds: 93

Lymington Infirmary
East Hill, Lymington SO41 9ZJ
Tel: 01590 676081 Fax: 01590 670749
Total Beds: 37

Milford-on-Sea Day Hospital
Sea Road, Milford on Sea, Lymington SO41 0PG
Tel: 023 8064 3016

Milford-on-Sea War Memorial Hospital
Sea Road, Milford-on-Sea, Lymington SO41 0PG
Tel: 01590 643016 Fax: 01590 645939
Total Beds: 19

Newark and Sherwood Primary Care Trust

65 Northgate, Newark NG24 1HD
Tel: 01636 700238 Fax: 01636 700246
Website: www.newarkandsherwood-pct.nhs.uk
(Trent Strategic Health Authority)

Chair Bonnie Jones
Chief Executive David Sharp

Newbury and Community Primary Care Trust

Headquarters, Avonbank House, Northcroft Wing, West Street, Newbury RG14 1BZ
Tel: 01635 42400
Website: www.berkshire.nhs.uk/newbury/
(Thames Valley Strategic Health Authority)

Chair Bruce Laurie
Chief Executive Sheila Hayes

West Berkshire Community Hospital
Benham Hill, London Road, Thatcham RG18 3AS
Tel: 01635 273300 Fax: 01635 273306

Newcastle, North Tyneside and Northumberland Mental Health NHS Trust

St George's Hospital, Morpeth NE61 2NU
Tel: 01670 512121 Fax: 01670 511637
Website: www.nnt.nhs.uk/mh
(Northumberland, Tyne and Wear Strategic Health Authority)

Chair Sue Whittaker
Chief Executive Alan Hall

St George's Hospital
Morpeth NE61 2NU
Tel: 01670 512121 Fax: 01670 511637
Email: carol.banks@nmht.org.uk
Total Beds: 302

General Psychiatry D Benn, A Brittlebank, W Grant, H Griffiths, C Luke, D L P Marshall, T O'Dwyer, M Parry, S E Proctor, E Sein, A M Walsh, P Yappa

St Nicholas Hospital
Gosforth, Newcastle upon Tyne NE3 3XT
Tel: 0191 213 0151 Fax: 0191 213 0821
Total Beds: 501

General Psychiatry B R Adams, W Barker, S Bhate, M Campbell, R Cawthra, A Cole, D Dunleavy, A F Fairbairn, R G Farquharson, I N Ferrier, E Gilvarry, H Griffiths, F Hassanyeh, S Joseph, T A Kerr, C A Lund, I McKeith, J L Scott, P Tayler, D Turkington

Newcastle Primary Care Trust

Benfield Road, Walkergate, Newcastle upon Tyne NE6 4PF
Tel: 0191 219 6000 Fax: 0191 219 6066
Email: suggestionbox@newcastle-pct.nhs.uk
Website: www.newcastlepct.nhs.uk
(Northumberland, Tyne and Wear Strategic Health Authority)

Chair Gina Tiller
Chief Executive Andrew Gibson

Newcastle-under-Lyme Primary Care Trust

Bradwell Hospital, Talke Road, Chesterton, Newcastle ST5 7NJ
Tel: 01782 425440 Fax: 01782 425445
Email: office@newcastle-ul-pct.nhs.uk
Website: www.newcastlepct.co.uk
(Shropshire and Staffordshire Strategic Health Authority)

Chair Ian Ashbolt
Chief Executive Ian Rogerson

Newcastle upon Tyne Hospitals NHS Trust

Freeman Hospital, Freeman Road, High Heaton, Newcastle upon Tyne NE7 7DN
Tel: 0191 284 3111 Fax: 0191 213 1968
Website: www.newcastle-hospitals.nhs.uk
(Northumberland, Tyne and Wear Strategic Health Authority)

Chair Miles Irving
Chief Executive Leonard Fenwick

Freeman Hospital
Freeman Road, High Heaton, Newcastle upon Tyne NE7 7DN
Tel: 0191 233 6161 Fax: 0191 213 1968
Total Beds: 810

Accident and Emergency J A P Connelly, N J Fox, P N Goode, B Sev, G M Strachan, G F Sweeney, J Wright

Anaesthetics P M Barrow, P J M Bayly, K J Beacham, K R Bell, D T Bolton, M C Burn, T N S Clarke, I D Conacher, D C Crawford, S G H Cruickshank, J A Evans, B Fulton, J Halshaw, S A Hargrave, R P Harpin, S R Haynes, D W Heaviside, N M Heggie, J J Holland, D G Hughes, M S Jones, A J Kilner, C K McKnight, G D McIntosh, D F O'Brien, M L Paes, L R Pardeshi, H Powell, K A Price, A K Pridie, D R D Roberts, C S Roysam, D W Ryan, M S Sammut, S A Scully, I H Shaw, J H Smith, C P Snowden, M Staunton, D A Timon, I H Warnell, O G W Weldon, J A Wilkes, P R Wilkinson, P M C Wright

Biochemistry H K Datta, M F Laker, D McClure, R D G Neely, C H Self, H J Wastell

Cardiology P C Adams, J M Ahmed, R S Bexton, J P Bourke, K L Evemy, S S Furniss, M A Kerry, J M McComb, J J O'Sullivan, L F Purcell, D O Williams, C Wren, A G Zaman

Cardiothoracic Surgery S C Clark, J H Dark, J Forty, J R L Hamilton, A Hasan, C J Hilton, S J M Ledingham, T M Pillay, S Schueler, K Tocewicz

Care of the Elderly E J Brierley, R M France

Chest Medicine P A Corris, G J Gibson, B G Higgins, S C Stenton, A C Ward

ENT D S Cameron, S Carrie, J Hill, I J M Johnson, D Meikle, F W Stafford, A R Welch

General Medicine M F Bassendine, C P Day, A G Dyker, R M Francis, P D Home, M Hudson, O F W James, D E J Jones, R A Kenny, S J Louw, S H S Pearce, M D Rawlins, C O Record, J A M Shaw, S H L thomas, N P Thompson, M Walker, H J Wastell

General Psychiatry M T Campbell, C Cole, D Turkington

General Surgery R D Bliss, R M Charnely, S M Griffin, P J Hainsworth, A F Horgan, B C Jacques, N A G Jones, D Lambert, T A Lees, D M Manas, S M Plusa, S R Preston, G P Stansby, D Talbot, J S Varma, M G Wyatt

Haematology P J L Kesteven

Histopathology A D Burt, N Leonard, S J Needham, M O'Donnell, D M Rassi, M C Robinson, D J Scott, V Wadehra, C Wright

Medical Microbiology M R Barer, A J Bint, R Freeman, A K Galloway, F K Gould, A M Krause, K E Orr, S Pedler, A Turner

Nephrology A L Brown, J S Tapson, R Wilkinson

Neurology M J Jackson, H Rodgers

Neurosurgery P J Crawford, A D Mendelow, R P Sengupta, N W Todd

Obstetrics and Gynaecology K Brown, P Hilton, D J A Mansour, A S McIntosh, A P Murdoch

Oncology P J Atherton, A H Calvert, W Dobrowsky, U K Mallick, I D Pedley

Ophthalmology F C Figueiredo, C C E Neoh, K P Stannard

Oral and Maxillofacial Surgery I D Grime, C Hayward, P J Thomson

Orthopaedics N J Brewster, P J Briggs, D J Deehan, C H Gerrand, M J Gibson, P D Henman, J P Holland, A W Mccaskie, S A Murray, J M Quinby, P L Sanderson, M S Siddique, P R Stuart, D J Weir, J R Williams

Paediatrics J E Clark, M G Coulthard, A M Devlin, M T Gibson, J P Hale, D S F Matthews, D A Spencer

Radiology C J Baudouin, A J Crisp, S T Elliott, A R Gholkar, R W Jackson, B Kaye, R E J Lee, H W C Loose, M M P McElroy, L M McLean, L Mitchell, J D G Richardson, J D G Rose, I Zammit-Maempel

Rehabilitation Medicine N C M Fyfe

Rheumatology B Griffiths, I D Griffiths, S C Isaacs, L J Kay, P N Platt, D J Walker

Urology H Y Leung, P H Powell, P D Ramsden, D A Rix, N A Soomro, D J Thomas, A C Thorpe

Newcastle General Hospital

Westgate Road, Newcastle upon Tyne NE4 6BE
Tel: 0191 233 6161 Fax: 0191 219 5037
Total Beds: 467

Accident and Emergency P N Goode

Anaesthetics R E Bullock, D C Crawford, B Fulton, D G Hughes, I H Shaw, J S Stanley, J A Wilkes

Child and Adolescent Psychiatry S R Bhate, C A Kaplan, D A Ward

General Medicine S J Bourke, G C Hawthorne, D J Hendrick, E L C Ong, M H Snow

General Psychiatry R C G Briel, F M Dunne, S A Joseph, B S Lund, B J Wilkinson

General Surgery S M Griffin

Genitourinary Medicine R S Pattman

Haematology P W G Saunders

Immunology A C Fay, G V Spickett

Neurology D J Burn, U K Goonetilleke, T D Griffiths, T J Walls

Oncology A N Branson, C G Kelly, H H Lucraft, P M Mulvenna, J T Roberts, W B Taylor, M S Verrill

Oral and Maxillofacial Surgery K L Posthlewaite

Paediatrics M M Abinun, F W Alexander, A J Cant, J A Eyre, T J Flood, R J Forsyth, V Ramesh

Plastic Surgery R H Milner

Psychiatry of Old Age A F Fairbairn, E Mukaetova-Ladinska, A G Swann

Radiology K Hall

Newcastle upon Tyne Dental Hospital

Richardson Road, Newcastle upon Tyne NE2 4AZ
Tel: 0191 233 6161 Fax: 0191 219 5037

Oral and Maxillofacial Surgery G S Blair, K B Fanibunda, J E Hawkesford, D J Lovelock

Orthodontics N E Carter, P H Gordon

Pathology J V Soames

Periodontology D G Smith

Royal Victoria Infirmary

Queen Victoria Road, Newcastle upon Tyne NE1 4LP
Tel: 0191 233 6161 Fax: 0191 201 0155
Total Beds: 806

Anaesthetics R J Bray, M R Bryson, V E Bythell, J E Charlton, G R Enever, I R Fletcher, A R Garforth, J D Greaves, I H Herrema, N Redfern, C J Vallis

Cardiology P C Adams, K L Evemy, I U Haq

Care of the Elderly R H Jay, J L Newton, H A Wynne

Dermatology J McLelland, A E M Taylor

General Medicine S V Baudouin, P H Baylis, P G Blain, S J Bourke, D J Hendrick, P D Home, R A James, R A M Kenny, J C Mansfield, S M Marshall, K Matthewson, E L C Ong, R Quinton, C O Record, R Taylor, M Walker, M K Ward, H A Wynne

General Surgery H J Gallagher, C D M Griffith, A B Griffiths, N Hayes, D Karat, T W J Lennard

Genetics J Burn, S A Lynch, M J Wright

Haematology G H Jackson, A L Lennard, S J Proctor, P W G Saunders

Histopathology B Angus, M K Bennett, J N Bulmer, A D Burt, P N Cooper, S J Johnson, D J Scott, J J Shrimankar

Immunology A C Fay, G P Spickett

Medical Microbiology A J Bint, A Galloway, S J Pedler

Neonatology A C Fenton, D W A Milligan, M P Ward-Platt

Nephrology T H J Goodship

Neurology M P Barnes, D Bates, D J Burn, N E F Cartlidge, P J Dorman, P R W Fawcett, D M Turnbull, T L Williams

Neuropathology R H Perry

Obstetrics and Gynaecology M J Blott, J M Davison, A D Loughney, S Macphail, S McPhail, E M Michael, M Roberts, S C Robson, J A Stewart, S N Sturgiss

Oncology B N J Cantwell, P J D Dawes

Ophthalmology M K Birch, R C Bosanquet, M P Clarke, D G Cottrell, M R Dayan, A J Dickinson, F C D Figueiredo, P G Griffiths, C C E Neoh, R J Pandit, N Raychaudhuri, A E Shafiq, K P Stannard, N P Strong, S J Talks

Paediatric Surgery A M Barrett, M N de la Hunt, M S Fleet, B Jaffray, A Lawson, L Rangecroft

Paediatrics M Abinum, F W Alexander, A J Cant, T D Cheetham, M G Coulthard, Simon Court, A W Craft, E J Eastham, J A Eyre, T J Flood, S Hodges, H J Lambert, N E Moghal, C J O'Brien, A D J Pearson, C G M Richards, R Skinner, K P Windebank

Pathology A D Burt, M F Laker, C Wright

Plastic Surgery M J M Black, P D Hodgkinson, N R McLean, S A Pape, C A Reid, N Williams

Radiology A Burridge, A J Chippindale, J P Owen, A J Potterton, J B Wilsdon, S A Worthy

Rheumatology and Rehabilitation H E Foster, S P Tyrer

Walkergate Hospital

Benfield Road, Newcastle upon Tyne NE6 4GQ
Tel: 0191 233 6161 Fax: 0191 213 1968
Total Beds: 325

Care of the Elderly R G Cooper, G A Ford, R M Francis, P Harrigan, O F W James

Newham Primary Care Trust

Plaistow Hospital, Samson Street, London E13 9EH
Tel: 020 8586 6200 Fax: 020 8586 6382
Website: www.newhampct.nhs.uk
(North East London Strategic Health Authority)

Chair Marie Gabrielle
Chief Executive David Stout

The Appleby Centre

63 Appleby Road, London E16 1LQ
Tel: 020 7474 5666 Fax: 020 7445 7008

General Psychiatry D Abrahamson, J Feldman, D Lefevre, R Zimmer

East Ham Memorial Hospital

Shrewsbury Road, Forest Gate, London E7 8QR
Tel: 020 8586 5000 Fax: 020 8586 5099
Total Beds: 83

Plaistow Day Hospital

Plaistow Hospital, Samson Street, Plaistow, London E13 9EH
Tel: 020 8586 6225 Fax: 020 8586 6204

Plaistow Hospital

Samson Street, London E13 9EH
Tel: 020 7472 7001 Fax: 020 8586 6204
Total Beds: 90

Sally Sherman Nursing Home

Albert Dock Hospital Site, Alnwick Road, London E16 3EZ
Tel: 020 7473 4386
Total Beds: 28

Newham University Hospital NHS Trust

Formerly Newham Healthcare NHS Trust

Newham General Hospital, Glen Road, Plaistow, London E13 8SL
Tel: 020 7476 4000 Fax: 020 7363 8181
Website: www.newham-healthcare.org
(North East London Strategic Health Authority)

Chair Mike Smith
Chief Executive Kathy Watkins

Newham General Hospital

Glen Road, Plaistow, London E13 8SL
Tel: 020 7476 4000 Fax: 020 7363 8181
Total Beds: 350

Accident and Emergency J M Oliver

Anaesthetics V S Pradhan, N A Watt

Cardiology K Ranjadayalan

Care of the Elderly M W Gill, S K Lightowlers, C F W Pratt

Chest Disease T O'Shaghnessy, G E Wilson

Dermatology D Fenton, M Glover, F Lawlor

ENT A M Shaida

General Medicine C M Gayle, S V Gelding, V Kulhalli, D Littlejohns, A D Sonibare, G C Toms

General Surgery N R Fieldman, R Le Fur, F M A Mihaimeed, B J Pardy

HIV/Genitourinary Medicine T J McManus, M B Poulton

Obstetrics and Gynaecology J M Boulton, O Djahanbakhch, A R Jeyarajah, R Maplethorpe, A A Naftalin, M Raveenaran

Oncology C J Gallagher

Orthopaedics L de las Heras Garcia, T G Dolan, M Y S El-Zebdeh, R R Gad El Rab

Paediatrics J Allgrove, E S Cooper, V Gopinathan, O J Hanmer, M L Ko, S Mathew

Palliative Medicine C F Phillips

Pathology S Bulusu

Rheumatology and Rehabilitation A S Burney

Urology N P Buchholz, F I Chinegwundoh, I Junaid

St Andrew's Hospital

Devas Road, Bow, London E3 3NT
Tel: 020 7476 4000
Total Beds: 71

Norfolk and Norwich University Hospital NHS Trust

Norfolk and Norwich University Hospital, Colney Lane, Norwich NR4 7UY
Tel: 01603 286286 Fax: 01603 287547
Email: firstname.lastname@nnuh.nhs.uk
Website: www.nnuh.nhs.uk
(Norfolk, Suffolk and Cambridgeshire Strategic Health Authority)

Chair David Prior
Chief Executive Paul Forden

Cromer Hospital

Mill Road, Cromer NR27 0BQ
Tel: 01263 513571 Fax: 01263 514764
Total Beds: 37

Cardiology T Wistow

General Medicine R Greenwood, H Kennedy, M Philips, R Tighe

General Surgery J Clarke, C Speakman

Medicine for the Elderly Y P Chan

Nephrology A Heaton

Neurology J Cochius

Obstetrics and Gynaecology E Morris

Oncology H Baillie-Johnson

Ophthalmology T Burton, T Eke, C Illingworth, C Jones

Orthopaedics D Calder, M Glasgow, P Hallam, C Mann, J Nolan, A Rai

Paediatrics N Thalange

Respiratory Medicine P Grunstein, M Pasteur

Rheumatology K Gaffney, D Scott

Thoracic Surgery W Parry

Urology K Sethia, R Webb

Norfolk and Norwich University Hospital

Colney Lane, Norwich NR4 7UY
Tel: 01603 286286 Fax: 01603 287547
Total Beds: 989

Accident and Emergency T J Daynes, B Finlayson, M A Lambert, K Walters

Anaesthetics G L Barker, L Barker, P Barker, S Brown, D Browne, M Dixon, B Fleming, S J Fletcher, R Garforth, A J G Gray, R Harwood, P E Hodgson, P J G Hutchings, L I Kerr, M J Leadbeater, T Leary, A Lipp, B McGrath, M Naik, D O'Hare, J F Payne, P D Phillips, B Poulton, S A Ridley, W L Rowe, M Sanders, C Sharpe, D Spackman, K A Wilkinson, D Wilson-Nunn, M Wolmarans, N M Woodall, C H M Woollam

Cardiology I A B Brooksby, L Freeman, R Hall, L Hughes, A J F Page, T Whistow

Chemical Pathology G John, T Tickner

Clinical Epidemiology I Harvey

Dermatology J Garioch, C Grattan, N Levell

Emergency Medicine P Jenkins, R Mallinson

ENT A Bath, J Fitzgerald, A J Innes, P Montgomery, D Premachandra, P Prinsley, M Wickstead

Family Planning Clinic C Nash

General Medicine I Beales, D Bell, K Dhatariya, N Dozio, I Fellows, R Greenwood, A Hart, P Heyburn, C Jamieson, H Kennedy, M Phillips, A Prior, M Sampson, R Temple, R Tighe

General Surgery M Armon, J M F Clarke, J F Colin, M Hussein, Sandee Kapur, M Lewis, F Meyer, S Pain, D N L Ralphs, M Rhodes, Leinis Sam, C T M Speakman, W S L Stebbings, S Wemyss-Holden, R Wharton, Y Wilson

Genitourinary Medicine N David, J K Evans, J D Meaden

Haematology M Auger, J Parker, G E Turner, J Wimperis, H Yarranton

Histopathology R Y Ball, V Bardsley, T H W Barker, A Girling, L Igali, W Kinsey, R Lonsdale, B G McCann, D Peat, P F Roberts, V R Sams, X Tyler, M van der Walt, M Wilkinson

Medical Microbiology J Richards, E Rizkalla, S Schelenz, M Sillis, P White, H Williams

Medicine for the Elderly L Bowker, Y P Chan, R A Fulcher, D Maisey, H May, K Metcalf, M Naguib, B Payne, K Sabanathan, P Woodhouse

Nephrology M Andrews, D Hamilton, A Heaton, C Ross

Neurology J Blake, J Cochius, D J Dick, M Lee, J B Pilling, T Staunton, P Worth

Obstetrics and Gynaecology S G Crocker, F de Boer, D I Fraser, F Harlow, E Morris, S Mukhopadhyay, J Nieto, K P Stanley, R C Warren

Occupational Health R Farman, R McCaig

Oncology H Baillie-Johnson, A Barrett, A Bulman, D Epurescu, A Harnett, W M C Martin, M J Ostrowski, T Roques, H Stubbings

Ophthalmology N Astbury, B Beigi, D Broadway, E Burton, T Eke, A Glenn, C Illingworth, C Jones, B Mulholland

Oral and Maxillofacial Surgery S Hadinnapola, S Prince, R Rees

Orthodontics A Slaney, D Tewson

Orthopaedics J S Albert, D Calder, P G Chapman, A Chojnowski, R J Crawford, S Donell, M M S Glasgow, P Hallam, C Mann, J F Nolan, A Patel, H Phillips, A S Raj, J K Tucker, N Walton, J Wimhurst

Paediatric Surgery M Kulkarni, A B Mathur, T T M Tsang

Paediatrics K Armon, R C Beach, V Datta, M Dyke, M-A Morris, M Ni Chroinin, R Proops, R Reading, N Thalange, C J Upton, S Zeitlin

Pain Relief M Hudspith, G Porter, J Valentine

Plastic Surgery A Bardsley, A Logan, M Meyer, T O'Neill, E Sassoon

Radiology C Beadsmoore, M Bennie, J Cockburn, J J Curtin, E Denton, S D Girling, G R Hurst, P G Kitchener, J B Latham, D MacIver, P Malcolm, T Marshall, P E Pickworth, J R Pilling, P G Preston, J Rehman, J Saada, S Scott-Barrett, M Shaw, A Toms, S Williams, P A J Wilson

Respiratory Medicine P Grunstein, B D W Harrison, M Pasteur, C Ramsay, O P Twentyman, S Watkin

Rheumatology and Rehabilitation J K Gaffney, A Macgregor, T Marshall, P Merry, B Ramakrishna, D G I Scott

Thoracic Surgery W Parry, M Van Leuven

Urology N A Burgess, E Ho, S Irving, R Mills, K K Sethia, R J Webb

Norfolk and Waveney Mental Health Partnership NHS Trust

Formerly Norfolk Mental Health Care NHS Trust.

Hellesdon Hospital, Drayton High Road, Norwich NR6 5BE
Tel: 01603 421421 Fax: 01603 421440
Email: info@nwmhp.nhs.uk
Website: www.nwmhp.nhs.uk
(Norfolk, Suffolk and Cambridgeshire Strategic Health Authority)

Chair Maggie Wheeler
Chief Executive Pat Holman

Child and Adolescent Mental Health Service

Mary Chapman House, Hotblack Road, Norwich NR2 4HN
Tel: 01603 421421 Fax: 01603 421990

Manager J Green

General Psychiatry L Ashby, B R Badrinath, X Coll, O Delaney, D Harrison, M Hoogkamer, S Jones, K Sillifant

Hellesdon Hospital

Drayton High Road, Norwich NR6 5BE
Tel: 01603 421421 Fax: 01603 421342
Total Beds: 137

Manager A Bailey, P Thompson, I Young

General Psychiatry J N Beezhold, J Bufton, L Callinan, J S Coogan, K Craig, W Crook, D Double, J Gardner, D Harsh, R L Horne, F Ikhlas, D Jones, M Kitson, I Macmillan, A Nichol, C Reynolds, D Rumball, A C Wagle, R Wales, N Willamune, J Wilson

The Julian Hospital

Bowthorpe Road, Norwich NR2 3TD
Tel: 01603 421421 Fax: 01603 421831
Total Beds: 100

Elderly Mentally Ill N Beezhold, J Bufton, L Callinan, J S Coogan, K Craig, W Crook, D Double, J Gardner, D Harsh, R L Horne, F Ikhlas, D Jones, M Kitson, I Macmillan, A Nichol, C Reynolds, D Rumball, A C Wagle, R Wales, N Willamune, J Wilson

Northgate Hospital
Northgate Street, Great Yarmouth NR30 1BY
Tel: 01493 330054 Fax: 01493 852753
Total Beds: 71

Manager K Chapman

Elderly Mentally Ill H De Waal, J Hillam, C Morris, A Tarbuck, S Wagle, R Wesby

North and East Cornwall Primary Care Trust

Lamellion Hospital, Station Road, Liskeard PL14 4DG
Tel: 01579 335341 Fax: 01579 335343
Website: www.cornwall.nhs.uk/necornwall/
(South West Peninsula Strategic Health Authority)

Chair Mike Matcham
Chief Executive Ian Williams

Bodmin Hospital
Bodmin PL31 2QT
Tel: 01208 251300

Launceston General Hospital
Link Road, Launceston PL15 9JD
Tel: 01566 765650 Fax: 01566 765680
Total Beds: 20

Liskeard Community Hospital
Clemo Road, Liskeard PL14 3XA
Tel: 01579 335600
Total Beds: 52

St Barnabas' Hospital
Higher Porth View, Saltash PL12 4BU
Tel: 01752 857400 Fax: 01752 857429
Total Beds: 17

Stratton Hospital
Hospital Road, Stratton, Bude EX23 9BR
Tel: 01288 287700 Fax: 01288 287729
Total Beds: 17

North Birmingham Primary Care Trust

Blakelands House, 400 Aldridge Road, Birmingham B44 8BH
Tel: 0121 332 1900 Fax: 0121 332 1901
Email: info@northbirminghampct.nhs.uk
Website: www.nbpct.nhs.uk
(Birmingham and the Black Country Strategic Health Authority)

Chair Anne Underwood
Chief Executive Paul Jennings

Sutton Cottage Hospital
Birmingham Road, Sutton Coldfield B72 1QH

North Bradford Primary Care Trust

Level 4, New Mill, Saltaire, Shipley, Bradford BD18 3LD
Tel: 01274 366266 Fax: 01274 366273
Email: nbpct@bradford.nhs.uk
Website: www.northbradford-pct.nhs.uk
(West Yorkshire Strategic Health Authority)

Chair Norman Roper
Chief Executive Ian Rutter

North Bristol NHS Trust

Trust Headquarters, Frenchay Hospital, Blackpool Road, Bristol BS16 1JE
Tel: 0117 970 1212
Website: www.northbristol.nhs.uk
(Avon, Gloucestershire and Wiltshire Strategic Health Authority)

Chair Nicholas Godden
Chief Executive Sonia Mills

Blackberry Hill Hospital
Manor Road, Fishponds, Bristol BS16 2EW
Tel: 0117 965 6061 Fax: 0117 975 4832
Total Beds: 118

Burden Neurological Institute
Frenchay Hospital, Frenchay Park Road, Bristol BS16 1JE
Tel: 0117 956 7444 Fax: 0117 965 4141
Total Beds: 18

General Psychiatry J M Bird, D G C Rogers

Cossham Memorial Hospital
Lodge Road, Kingswood, Bristol BS15 1LF
Tel: 0117 967 1661 Fax: 0117 961 8421

Frenchay Hospital
Frenchay Park Road, Bristol BS16 1LE
Tel: 0117 970 1212 Fax: 0117 956 3880
Total Beds: 548

Accident and Emergency K Jones, C Oakland

Anaesthetics W Blancke, J A Carter, S Coniam, N Dunne, J Dunnet, G L Greenslade, M Gregory, D Harris, C Jewkes, D Lockey, A R Manara, J Mendham, M Milne, J Olday, D Ouer, R J A Pettifer, S Plastow, K Quader, J Rogers, S Shinde, P J Simpson, C Stannard, K Thornton, F J M Walters, T Whitton, G Wrathall, A Young, P Younge

Cardiology M Papouchado

Care of the Elderly R Barber, L Dow, J Pounsford, Professor Wilcock

Chemical Pathology C E Dawkins

Child and Adolescent Psychiatry D L Bazeley-White, J Crooks, I Skeldon

ENT D L Baldwin, M A Birchall

Gastroenterology R F Harvey

General Medicine L Dow, R F Harvey, V Kyle, R J White

General Surgery C P Armstrong, A Baker, S J Cawthorn, A Dixon

Haematology P J Whitehead

Histopathology N B N Ibrahim, H S Rigby

Medical Microbiology E M Brown

Neurology J Bird, N Kane, D Rogers

Neuropathology S Love, T H Moss

Neurosurgery C Bolger, H B Coakham, B H Cummins, S S Gill, R Nelson, I Pople, D R Sandeman

Obstetrics and Gynaecology F N McLeod, P Savage

Orthodontics I S Hathorn

Orthopaedics N Blewitt, I Nelson, A J Ward

Paediatrics H Hargreaves, G Roberts, J Schulte

Plastic Surgery J M Kenealy, N S Mercer, C Reid, L Sacks, P L G Townsend

Radiology J R Bradshaw, M J Cobby, T T Lewis, A J Longstaff, M H Morse, N Slack, R Watura

Rheumatology and Rehabilitation V Kyle

Orchard View Intermediate Care Unit

Pill, Bristol BS20 0HW
Tel: 01275 372661
Total Beds: 21

Southmead Hospital

Westbury-on-Trym, Bristol BS10 5NB
Tel: 0117 950 5050 Fax: 0117 959 0902
Total Beds: 701

Accident and Emergency A Montague

Anaesthetics A Brederode, H Bromhead, D Campbell, M Dirnhuber, F Donald, C Fouque, N Goodman, N Griffith, C R Hall, K Holder, D H Holland, C Johnson, N Koehli, J Leigh, F McVey, A P Madden, Y Marney, G Morris, S Robinson, J Soar, E M Walsh

Care of the Elderly C Chan, M G Cheesman, L Potts

Clinical Chemistry D J Goldie

Clinical Pathology P A Burton

Community Child Health S Clements, A Elmond, H Hargreaves, J Price, G Roberts, J Schulte, O H Stanley

Dermatology C T C Kennedy

ENT D Baldwin, M Birchall, P Robinson

General Medicine J Dwight, E A M Gale, S C Glover, J Harvey, S Hughes, A Johnson, P R Walker

General Psychiatry R Eastley, R M Hawley, R H C Meller, I H Mian, F E Newbery, J Truscott, F D Whitwell

General Surgery P A Lear, D Mitchell, B D Pentlow, A Roe, M H Thomson

Genitourinary Medicine M W Price

Haematology R Evely, R R Slade

Immunology T B Wallington

Medical Microbiology A P MacGowan, D S Reeves

Nephrology C Dudley, T Feest, S Harper, C R V Tomson

Neurology I T Ferguson

Obstetrics and Gynaecology D Bisson, F N McLeod, J Murdoch, P E Savage, P A Smith, S Vyas

Ophthalmology R H C Markham, M Potts

Oral and Maxillofacial Surgery H G Irvine

Orthopaedics C Ackroyd, G C Bannister, E J Smith, I G Winson

Paediatrics T L Chambers, A A Leaf, M E McGraw, B D Speidel, H M Thomas

Pathology P J Berry, P A Burton, J D Davies, I D Fraser, D J Goldie, E MacKenzie, A McIver, D S Reeves, H White

Radiology M Darby

Radiotherapy and Oncology E J Chambers

Rheumatology P Hollingworth

Urology P Abrams, D Gillatt, J C Gingell, A G Timoney

Thornbury Hospital

Thornbury, Bristol BS12 1DN
Tel: 01454 412636 Fax: 01454 281364
Total Beds: 38

North Cheshire Hospitals NHS Trust

Warrington Hospital, Lovely Lane, Warrington WA5 1QG
Tel: 01925 635911 Fax: 01925 662099
Website: www.northcheshirehospitals.nhs.uk
(Cheshire and Merseyside Strategic Health Authority)

Chair Alan Massey
Chief Executive Ian Dalton

Halton General Hospital

Hospital Way, Runcorn WA7 2DA
Tel: 01928 714567 Fax: 01928 753104
Total Beds: 231

Anaesthetics M G D Salem, R K Strahan

Care of the Elderly A Moloney

Dental Surgery S Rudge

Dermatology M M Molokhia

ENT S Kent, K Reddy

Gastroenterology B D Linaker

General Medicine S Church, A Khaleeli, B D Linaker, R Mallya, E Rose, C N Ugwu, J Williams

General Psychiatry M Bamforth, P Decalmer, B Green, M Green, J A Marks, S Pollet

General Surgery G H Hutchinson, J N Johnson, J E Pollet

Genitourinary Medicine M Veeravahu

Neurology Dr Enevoldson

Obstetrics and Gynaecology J Davies-Humphreys, J Langton

Oncology D Errington

Ophthalmology Dr Matthew

Oral Surgery D Richardson

Orthodontics S J Rudge

Orthopaedics D A Boot, P Sherry, G J Stewart

Paediatrics C Bedford, J R Briggs, Dr Mir, N Wild

Radiology J D Conway, F Fraser, T Houghton, G Murphy

Urology R Ewing

Warrington Hospital

Lovely Lane, Warrington WA5 1QG
Tel: 01925 635911 Fax: 01925 662099
Total Beds: 655

Accident and Emergency A Robinson, A J Saleh

Anaesthetics M G Abdel-Salam, P J Barrett, S W Crowder, E J Fazakerley, S V Jagadesh, P Jarvis, A K Malaiya, A Morrison, D K Mwanje, R E Park, C E Smith, J A Tytler

Care of the Elderly G Barton, A A Ghaffir

Dermatology M M Molokhia, M Molokjia

ENT S E Kent, K T V Reddy

General Medicine S J Bentley, J M Jefferson, B D Linaker, S Owen, D Pearson, S J S Virk

General Psychiatry S A Bokhari, N M Brooks, B Soma

General Surgery M Brett, G C Copeland, A P Moody, B A Taylor, P N Wake

Genitourinary Medicine R Rani, M Veeravahu

Neurology A M Dean, T P Easvoldson

Obstetrics and Gynaecology G D Entwistle, H B Griffiths, E F N Holland, E L Kozman, G Ramsden

Ophthalmology P Palimar, C O Peckar, M S Wishart

Oral Surgery J Brown

Orthodontics J W Jones

Orthopaedics D A Boot, H Casserley, M B Jones, I Shackleford, P G Sherry, G Stewart

Paediatric Cardiology K P Walsh

Paediatrics C D Bedford, J R Briggs, N A Mir, N J Wild

Pathology M S Al-Jafari, A Davis, K Dhir, R J P Garvey, N Hasan, D S Shareef

Plastic Surgery P V Kumar

Radiology D K Asamoah, P Cantrell, M P Caplan, J M Desmond, A J Sheridan, R E Wild, C C Yeong

Radiotherapy and Oncology P Clark, B Cottier

Rheumatology A Salih

Thoracic Surgery R Page

Urology L Q Robinson

North Cumbria Acute Hospitals NHS Trust

West Cumberland Hospital, Hensingham, Whitehaven CA28 8JG
Tel: 01946 693181
Website: www.northcumbriahealth.nhs.uk/acute
(Cumbria and Lancashire Strategic Health Authority)

Chair Eric Urquhart
Chief Executive Marie Burnham

Cumberland Infirmary

Newtown Road, Carlisle CA2 7HY
Tel: 01228 523444 Fax: 01228 591889
Total Beds: 442

Accident and Emergency J V Foxworthy

Anaesthetics J Harrison, D F Jones, S Kennedy, A Linsley, M R Payne, R C Rodgers, A Shanks, P C Stride, M D Tidmarsh, Y H Tzabar, M White

Bacteriology M A Knowles

Biochemistry C Lord

Care of the Elderly J S Billett, D P Davies, J George, J M Orgee

Chemical Pathology C Lord

Clinical Genetics J Goodship

Dermatology N H Cox, W D Paterson

General Medicine D Burke, M L Cowley, D M Large, C E McDonald, C P Mustchin, R H Robson

General Surgery F L Hinson, J D Holdsworth, J G Palmer, S Raimes, J E G Shand, M R Williams

Genitourinary Medicine B Stanley

Haematology H A W O'Brien

Histopathology A W Popple, F I Young

Medical Immunology G Spickett, A Todd

Medical Physics W I Keyes

Nephrology D N Bennett-Jones, P Mead

Neurology D Bates, M Jackson

Neurosurgery P Crawford, N Todd

Obstetrics and Gynaecology R Lawley, S E Pearson, W Reid

Ophthalmology M Bearn, D N Depla, M Hasan, R P S Smith

Oral and Maxillofacial Surgery A W Patterson, G D Putnam

Orthodontics R Tyrrell

Orthopaedics C G Brignall, G H Broome, A N Edwards, G Ferrier, G K Ions, M Orr

Otolaryngology D R Clark, N J Murrant, A K Robson

Paediatric Oncology A Craft

Paediatrics J M P Storr, C A Stuart, P Whitehead

Palliative Medicine G Dunkley

Plastic Surgery P Hodgkinson, N R McLean, A C Reid

Radiology G N Athey, J Edge, J Jackson, P Jennings, I Khechane, R McNeill

Radiotherapy and Oncology P Dyson, J Nicoll

Rehabilitation Medicine M H W Roberts

Rheumatology and Rehabilitation I D L Brewis, C E Kidd

Thoracic Medicine M H Holden, G M Moritt

Urology J A Cumming, R G Willis

West Cumberland Hospital

Hensingham, Whitehaven CA28 8JG
Tel: 01946 693181 Fax: 01946 523513
Total Beds: 447

Accident and Emergency M K Greene (Head), C Brett

Anaesthetics R S Frazer (Head), F Graham, M Hodson, Q Kingsbury, M Saudi, A Slaymaker, I Ulyett, G A Van Mourik, N Watkinson, D M Watson

Care of the Elderly F K Local (Head), E Haworth, E O Orugun, N J Russell

General Medicine W T Berrill (Head), L Forbat, J D McCrea, K Willmer

General Psychiatry C Scholefield (Head), A Lamont, G Morley

General Surgery M Walker (Head), S El Rabaa, N Nik Abdulla, D G Richards, A Sowinski

Learning Disabilities A Bassam

Obstetrics and Gynaecology S A Bober (Head), J Eldred, M Jayatilika, M Matar, J Stafford

Ophthalmology P Sellar (Head), S Verghese, M Zaheen

Orthopaedics M I Dhebar (Head), M Greiss, N S Rao, D Verinder

Paediatrics P Carter (Head), M Ben-Hamida, I Boles, D Lee, S Precious

Palliative Medicine E Palmer (Head)

Pathology N C West (Head), S Mathews, C Ozo, S Richards

Psychiatry of Old Age M Bober (Head), P D Benjamin

Radiology T A Eyre (Head), N Huntley, B G Maguire, B Mucci

Rehabilitation Medicine M Roberts

North Cumbria Mental Health and Learning Disabilities NHS Trust

The Carleton Clinic, Carlisle CA1 3SX
Tel: 01228 602000 Fax: 01228 602470
Email: firstname.lastname@ncumbria.nhs.uk
(Cumbria and Lancashire Strategic Health Authority)

Chair Bryan Betterton
Chief Executive Stephen Dalton
Consultants M Bober, J Hankin, C Harvey, M Jefferson, I Joubert, A Lamont, B Laszlo, G Morley, A Muller, D Prosser, D Reynolds, M Rigby, S Scott, P Tayler, S Turner, N Wright

The Carleton Clinic
Cumwhinton Drive, Carlisle CA1 3SX
Tel: 01228 602000

Orton Lea
Orton Road, Carlisle CA9 3QX
Total Beds: 6

Windermere Day Hospital (EMI)
West Cumberland Hospital, Whitehaven CA28 8JG
Tel: 01946 693181 Fax: 01946 523513

North Devon Primary Care Trust

Crown Yealm House, Pathfields Business Park, South Molton EX36 3LH
Tel: 01769 575100 Fax: 01769 373740
Website: www.northdevonhealth.nhs.uk
(South West Peninsula Strategic Health Authority)

Chair Sam Jones
Chief Executive Jacqueline Kelly

Bideford and Torridgeside Hospital
Bideford EX39 3AG
Tel: 01237 472692 Fax: 01237 471408
Total Beds: 68

Care of the Elderly M Dent, G Harper

General Medicine I Lewin, A Moran, M H Oliver, T Roberts

General Psychiatry M V Buren

General Surgery J R Barker, D R Harvey

Learning Disabilities A Boucherat

Obstetrics and Gynaecology A H L Boyle, S Eckford

Ophthalmology R A Gibson

Oral and Maxillofacial Surgery I Buchanan

Orthopaedics V Giles, C Mills, V Treble, P Van Der Wal

Paediatrics A Arend, A J Bosley

Rheumatology H Averns

Urology S Agrawal

Holsworthy Community Hospital
Dobles Lane, Holsworthy EX22 6JG
Tel: 01409 253424 Fax: 01409 254963
Total Beds: 28

Care of the Elderly M Dent

General Medicine A Marshall

General Psychiatry M V Buren

General Surgery M Markham

Orthopaedics M Halawa

Paediatrics A Bosley, M Hughes

Rheumatology Mr Hutton

Urology S Agrawala

Ilfracombe and District Tyrrell Hospital
St Brannock's Park Road, Ilfracombe EX34 8JP
Tel: 01271 863448 Fax: 01271 867813
Total Beds: 14

Care of the Elderly G Harper

ENT J Riddington-Young

General Medicine T Roberts

General Surgery R Bourne

Obstetrics and Gynaecology S Bennett, N Giles

Orthopaedics C Mills, N Treble, P Van Der Wall

Paediatrics M Hughes

Psychiatry M Sewell

Rheumatology H Ferris

Urology S Agrawal

South Molton Community Hospital
Widgery Drive, South Molton EX36 4DP
Tel: 01769 572164 Fax: 01769 574271
Total Beds: 28

Elderly Mentally Ill S Barber

General Psychiatry M Sewell

Obstetrics and Gynaecology S Eckford

Orthopaedics N Giles, C Mills, N Treble, P Van der Watt

Paediatrics J Cox

Rheumatology H Averns

Torrington Cottage Hospital
Calf Street, Great Torrington, Torrington EX38 7BJ
Tel: 01805 622208 Fax: 01805 625108
Total Beds: 14

Care of the Elderly S Barber

ENT J Riddington-Young

General Surgery D R Harvey

Obstetrics and Gynaecology S Bennett

North Dorset Primary Care Trust

Forston Clinic, Herrison Centre, Dorchester DT2 9TB
Tel: 01305 361300 Fax: 01305 361330
Email: email.us@northdorset-pct.nhs.uk
Website: www.northdorset-pct.nhs.uk
(Dorset and Somerset Strategic Health Authority)

Chair Mary Penfold
Chief Executive Andrew Casey

Blandford Hospital
Milldown Road, Blandford Forum DT11 7DD
Tel: 01258 456541 Fax: 01258 450786
Manager Steve Cole

Westminster Memorial Hospital
Abbey Walk, Shaftesbury SP7 8BD
Tel: 01747 851535 Fax: 01747 850152
Total Beds: 33

Manager Vicki Mainprize

Yeatman Hospital
Hospital Lane, Sherborne DT9 3JU
Tel: 01935 813991
Total Beds: 40

Manager Beth Shapland

North East Ambulance Service NHS Trust

Scotswood House, Amethyst Road, Newcastle Business Park, Newcastle upon Tyne NE4 7YL

Tel: 0191 273 1212 Fax: 0191 273 7070
Email: publicrelations@neas.northy.nhs.uk
Website: www.neambulance.nhs.uk
(Northumberland, Tyne and Wear Strategic Health Authority; County Durham and Tees Valley Strategic Health Authority)

Chair Tony Dell
Chief Executive Simon Featherstone

North East Lincolnshire Primary Care Trust

No.1 Prince Albert Gardens, Grimsby DN31 3HT
Tel: 01472 302800
Website: www.nelpct.nhs.uk
(North and East Yorkshire and Northern Lincolnshire Strategic Health Authority)

Chair Valerie Waterhouse
Chief Executive Jane Lewington

North East London Mental Health NHS Trust

Trust Head Office, Tantallon House, Goodmayes Hospital Campus, Barley Lane, Ilford IG3 8XJ
Tel: 020 8590 6060 Fax: 020 8970 8424
Website: www.nelmht.nhs.uk
(North East London Strategic Health Authority)

Chair Jane Atkinson
Chief Executive Paul Gocke
Consultants Emmanuel Akuffo, Jill Chaloner

Chapters House

Goodmayes Hospital Campus, Barley Lane, Goodmayes, Ilford IG3 8XJ
Tel: 0208 590 6060 Fax: 020 8970 8170
Total Beds: 70

General Psychiatry P Caveston, M Cleany, R Duffett, A El-Hadi, M Jones, A Lau, R Littlejohn, M Magner, A M Margo, S Pereira

Mascalls Park

Mascalls Lane, Warley, Brentwood CM14 5HQ
Tel: 01277 302600 Fax: 01277 302602

General Psychiatry J Chaloner, F Dunne, M Frampton, A Majid, S Mathur, A C Purches, S Srikumour, J Taylor

Nasebury Court

2 Merriam Close, London E4 9JQ
Tel: 020 8531 0744 Fax: 020 8531 1851
Total Beds: 40

Manager J J O'Connor

Stonlea

Langthorne Road, London E11 4HJ
Tel: 020 8535 6477 Fax: 020 8535 6530
Total Beds: 29

Woodbury Unit

Whipps Cross Hospital, Samuel Boyce Lodge, 178 James Lane, London E11 1NU
Tel: 020 8538 6475 Fax: 020 8535 6829
Total Beds: 42

Manager Theo Sackey-Addo

North East Oxfordshire Primary Care Trust

Astral House, Granville Way, Bicester OX26 4JT
Tel: 01869 604040 Fax: 01869 604044
Email: firstname.surname@neoxon-pct.nhs.uk
Website: www.neoxon-pct.nhs.uk
(Thames Valley Strategic Health Authority)

Chair Ian Inshaw
Chief Executive Mike Williams

Bicester Community Hospital

King's End, Bicester OX6 7DU
Tel: 01869 244881 Fax: 01869 323302
Total Beds: 12

North Eastern Derbyshire Primary Care Trust

St Mary's Court, St Mary's Gate, Chesterfield S41 7TD
Tel: 01246 551158 Fax: 01246 544620
Website: www.northeasternderbyshirepct.nhs.uk
(Trent Strategic Health Authority)

Chair Ian Mather
Chief Executive Martin McShane

Bolsover Local Hospital

Welbeck Road, Bolsover, Chesterfield S44 6DH
Tel: 01246 827901 Fax: 01246 240373
Total Beds: 72

Clay Cross Hospital

Market Street, Clay Cross, Chesterfield S45 9NZ
Tel: 01246 863031 Fax: 01246 861602

North Essex Mental Health Partnership NHS Trust

Homelands Retail Park, Cuton Hall Lane, Springfield, Chelmsford CM2 5PX
Tel: 01245 318400 Fax: 01245 318401
Email: enquiries@nemhpt.nhs.uk
Website: www.nemhpt.nhs.uk
(Essex Strategic Health Authority)

Chair Mary St Aubyn
Chief Executive Richard Coleman

Chelmsford and Essex Day Unit

New London Road, Chelmsford CM2 9QU
Tel: 01245 318600 Fax: 01245 318601

The Gables Day Hospital

17 Bocking End, Braintree CM7 9AE
Tel: 01376 555700 Fax: 01376 555705

Harwich Day Hospital

419 Main Road, Dovercourt, Harwich CO12 4EX
Tel: 01255 207400 Fax: 01255 207417

Linden Centre

Woodland Way, Broomfield, Chelmsford CM1 5LF
Tel: 01245 318802 Fax: 01245 318801
Total Beds: 55

Longview Adolescent Unit
216 Turner Road, Colchester CO4 5JR
Tel: 01206 228745
Total Beds: 10

Martello Court Day Hospital
Clacton Hospital, Tower Road, Clacton-on-Sea CO15 1LH
Tel: 01255 253540 Fax: 01255 222352

Mayfield Centre (Day Hospital)
93 Station Road, Clacton-on-Sea CO15 1TX
Tel: 01255 207040 Fax: 01255 207044

Rannoch Lodge
146 Broomfield Road, Chelmsford CM1 1RN
Tel: 01245 544869 Fax: 01245 544888

St Margaret's Hospital
The Plain, Epping CM16 6TN
Tel: 01992 561666
Total Beds: 62

Care of the Elderly G Ambepitiya

General Psychiatry S El-Fadl, W Lang, P Robotis, Z Walker

Severalls House
2 Boxted Road, Colchester CO4 4HG
Tel: 01206 228630 Fax: 01206 228660
Total Beds: 21

Stanwell House
Stanwell Street, Colchester CO2 7DL
Tel: 01206 287321 Fax: 01206 287320

White Lodge Day Unit
21 Coggeshall Road, Braintree CM7 6DB
Tel: 01376 308250 Fax: 01376 308251

Willow House
2 Boxted Road, Colchester CO4 5HG
Tel: 01206 228691

Wych Elm House
Hamstel Road, Harlow CM20 1QR
Tel: 01279 692300 Fax: 01279 692323

North Hampshire Hospitals NHS Trust

Aldermaston Road, Basingstoke RG24 9NA
Tel: 01256 473202 Fax: 01256 313098
Email: Laura.Cullum@bas.swest.nhs.uk
Website: www.northhampshire.nhs.uk
(Hampshire and Isle of Wight Strategic Health Authority)

Chair David Emmerson
Chief Executive Mary Edwards

North Hampshire Hospital
Basingstoke RG24 9NA
Tel: 01256 473302 Fax: 01256 313098
Total Beds: 450

Accident and Emergency B C Elvin, J Kitching, H Simpson

Anaesthetics S Ali, P J C Baxter, P Creagh-Barry, A C Haigh, J E Hurley, D W Robins, M A Rose, K Thomas, J K G Wells, P Wilson

Care of the Elderly S Arianaliagam, J Bernstein, J Mallya

Dermatology M Crone, H A Fawcett, Dr Powell

ENT J Blanshard, P Spraggs

General Medicine A Bishop, C Brookes, R J C Guy, K McKinlay, J Ramage, T Yek

General Surgery C Eden, D Gold, T John, B Moran, M Rees, A B Richards, A S Ward

Genitourinary Medicine D H Jackson

Neurology N Lawton, M Prevett

Obstetrics and Gynaecology R Bates, B O'Sullivan, T Sayer

Ophthalmology S Keightley, D Morseman, C Sandy

Oral and Maxillofacial Surgery C Kerawala

Orthodontics R T Reed

Orthopaedics J Benfield, J Britton, J Hobby, G Stranks, N P Thomas

Paediatrics P Llangoyan, A Mitchell, J Pleydon-Pearle, R O Walters, R Wigfield

Pathology D L Aston, J M Finch, E M Husband, A Milne, H S Platt

Radiology I Green, H O'Neill, J C Parker, G R T Plant, D F Shelley

Radiotherapy and Oncology G Sharpe, S Tinkler

Rheumatology C Batten, P Prouse, D Shane

North Hampshire Primary Care Trust

Harness House, Aldermaston Road, Basingstoke RG24 9NB
Tel: 01256 332288 Fax: 01256 312299
Email: firstname.lastname@nhpct.nhs.uk
Website: www.northhampshire.nhs.uk
(Hampshire and Isle of Wight Strategic Health Authority)

Chair Tony Ludlow
Chief Executive Debbie Glenn

Alton Community Hospital
Chawton Park Road, Alton GU34 1RJ
Tel: 01420 82811 Fax: 01420 592884

Chase Community Hospital
Conde Way, Bordon GU35 0YZ
Tel: 01420 488801 Fax: 01420 478720

North Hertfordshire and Stevenage Primary Care Trust

Solutions House, Dunhams Lane, Letchworth SG6 1BE
Tel: 01462 708470 Fax: 01462 708472
Email: firstname.surname@nhst-pct.nhs.uk
Website: www.nhst-pct.nhs.uk
(Bedfordshire and Hertfordshire Strategic Health Authority)

Chair Rachel Fox
Chief Executive Jill Peters

North Kirklees Primary Care Trust

Beckside Court, Bradford Road, Batley WF17 5PW
Tel: 01924 351600 Fax: 01924 475212
Website: www.northkirklees-pct.nhs.uk
(West Yorkshire Strategic Health Authority)

Chair Barry Seal
Chief Executive Philip Sands

North Lincolnshire Primary Care Trust

Health Place, Wrawby Road, Brigg DN20 8GS
Tel: 01652 659659 Fax: 01652 601160
Email: firstname.lastname@nlpct.nhs.uk
Website: www.nlpct.nhs.uk
(North and East Yorkshire and Northern Lincolnshire Strategic Health Authority)

Chair John Mason
Chief Executive Cathy Waters

North Liverpool Primary Care Trust

Cottage No 2, Newhall Campus, Longmoor Lane, Liverpool L10 1LD
Tel: 0151 234 5056 Fax: 0151 284 7517
Website: www.northliverpoolpct.nhs.uk
(Cheshire and Merseyside Strategic Health Authority)

Chair Lily Hopkins
Chief Executive Joanne Forrest

North Manchester Primary Care Trust

2nd Floor, Newton Silk Mill, Holyoak Street, Newton Heath, Manchester M40 1HA
Tel: 0161 219 9400 Fax: 0161 219 9430
Email: catherine.regan@northpct.manchester.nwest.nhs.uk
Website: www.northmanchesterpct.nhs.uk
(Greater Manchester Strategic Health Authority)

Chair Tim Presswood
Chief Executive David King

North Middlesex University Hospital NHS Trust

Sterling Way, London N18 1QX
Tel: 020 8887 2000 Fax: 020 8887 4219
Email: maxine.malpas@nmh.nhs.uk
Website: www.northmid.nhs.uk
(North Central London Strategic Health Authority)

Chair Clive Lawton
Chief Executive Clare Panniker

North Middlesex Hospital
Sterling Way, Edmonton, London N18 1QX
Tel: 020 8887 2000 Fax: 020 8887 4219
Total Beds: 400

Accident and Emergency E Weithers (Head), A E Rajarajan

Anaesthetics I N Rao (Head), A Chan, M Jesuthasan, P Patel, N Poobalasingam, A Ramachandran, D Shah, S Siriwardhana

Cardiology S O Banim (Head), T Crake

Chemical Pathology P West

Chest Disease S Lozewicz (Head), H Makker

Clinical Oncology N Davidson (Head), S A Davies, S J Karp, P Leone, F F Neave

Dermatology J J R Almeyda (Head), T A Mann

Diabetes H Tindall

General Medicine J Ainsworth, A Millar, J Onwubalili, M Vanderpump

General Surgery R J Croft, D M Melville, D L Stoker, J J Wood

Haematology T O Kumaran, J K Luckit, D A Yardumian

Histopathology K J Jarvis, M Sundaresan

Infectious Diseases Y M Yong

Medical Microbiology Y N Drabu, P Lee

Neurology J Gawler

Obstetrics and Gynaecology F Evans, P Hardiman, S Okolo

Ophthalmology G Palexus, R M Phillips, S Shah, E Taylor, K A Thiagarajah

Orthodontics P S G Perera

Orthopaedics J H Challis, M Kurer, Mr Trakru, V Woolf

Paediatrics L Alsford, M Meates, M A Rossiter, A R Shah

Radiology R L Borgstein, A Dinath-Seedat, A Husien, S Pathmanandam, M R Sebastianpillai, J Stroudley

Radiotherapy and Oncology N Davidson, S A Davies, S J Karp, F F Neave

Rheumatology and Rehabilitation M F Grayson, H D Sinclair

Urology G Fowlis, J A McDonald

North Norfolk Primary Care Trust

Trust Headquarters, Kelling Hospital, Cromer Road, Holt NR25 6QA
Tel: 01263 710611 Fax: 01263 710645
Website: www.nnpct.nhs.uk
(Norfolk, Suffolk and Cambridgeshire Strategic Health Authority)

Chair Bruce Barrell
Chief Executive Diana Clarke

Kelling Hospital
Kelling, Holt NR25 6QA
Tel: 01263 713333 Fax: 01263 712000
Total Beds: 57

Manager Sue Kenyon

Care of the Elderly B V Payne

Neurology J Brown

Rheumatology E Arie

North Walsham War Memorial Cottage Hospital
Yarmouth Road, North Walsham NR28 9AP
Tel: 01692 500560 Fax: 01692 407688
Total Beds: 23

Wells and District Cottage Hospital
Mill Road, Wells-next-the-Sea NR23 1RF
Tel: 01328 710218 Fax: 01328 711865
Total Beds: 15

North Peterborough Primary Care Trust

Works with South Peterborough Primary Care Trust and the Adult Social Care Department of Peterborough City Council as Greater Peterborough Primary Care Partnership.

2nd Floor, Town Hall, Peterborough PE1 1FA
Tel: 01733 758500 Fax: 01733 758555
Website: www.greaterpboropcp.nhs.uk
(Norfolk, Suffolk and Cambridgeshire Strategic Health Authority)

Chair Mohammed Choudhary
Chief Executive Chris Town

North Sheffield Primary Care Trust

Welfare House, North Quadrant, Firth Park, Sheffield S5 6NU
Tel: 0114 226 4031 Fax: 0114 226 4030
Website: www.northsheffield-pct.nhs.uk
(South Yorkshire Strategic Health Authority)

Chair Robert Bailey
Chief Executive Andy Buck

North Somerset Primary Care Trust

Waverley House, Old Church Road, Clevedon BS21 6NN
Tel: 01275 546770 Fax: 01275 546769
Email: contact@nsomerset-pct.nhs.uk
Website: www.northsomerset.nhs.uk
(Avon, Gloucestershire and Wiltshire Strategic Health Authority)

Chair Christina Baron
Chief Executive Ray Beale-Pratt

North Staffordshire Combined Healthcare NHS Trust

Bucknall Hospital, Eaves Lane, Bucknall, Stoke-on-Trent ST2 8LD
Tel: 01782 273510 Fax: 01782 275116
Email: enquiries@nsch-tr.wmids.nhs.uk
Website: www.nsch-tr.wmids.nhs.uk
(Shropshire and Staffordshire Strategic Health Authority)

Chair Eddie Slade
Chief Executive Christopher Buttanshaw

Boulton Ward, Haywood Hospital
High Lane, Burslem, Stoke-on-Trent ST6 7AQ
Tel: 01782 425795
Total Beds: 25

General Medicine R C Hayter

Bradwell Hospital
Talke Road, Chesterton, Stoke-on-Trent
Tel: 01782 425400 Fax: 01782 425408
Total Beds: 74

General Medicine P Crome

General Psychiatry M Davies

Bucknall Hospital
Eaves Lane, Bucknall, Stoke-on-Trent ST2 8LD
Tel: 01782 273510 Fax: 01782 275116
Total Beds: 123

Manager Lynn Turner

General Medicine M Browne, R C Hayter, K P Patel, S Sangeelee

Cheadle Hospital
Royal Walk, Cheadle, Stoke-on-Trent ST10 1NS
Tel: 01538 487500 Fax: 01538 487538
Total Beds: 81

General Medicine M Browne

City General Hospital
Elderly Care Unit, 578 Newcastle Road, Stoke-on-Trent ST4 6QG
Total Beds: 84

General Medicine M Browne, P Crome, R C Hayter, K P Patel, C Roffe

Greenfield Centre
Mental Resource Centre, Furlong Road (behind Furlong Medical Centre), Tunstall, Stoke-on-Trent ST6 5UD
Tel: 01782 425740 Fax: 01782 425741
Total Beds: 8

Leek Moorlands Hospital
Ashbourne Road, Leek ST13 5BQ
Tel: 01538 487100 Fax: 01538 487138
Total Beds: 66

General Medicine Dr Paul

Roundwell Place Day Hospital
Roundwell Street, Tunstall, Stoke-on-Trent ST6 5JJ
Tel: 01782 425732

Manager Dr Sivridis

Westcliffe Hospital
Turnhurst Road, Chell, Stoke-on-Trent ST6 6LA
Tel: 01782 425860 Fax: 91782 425878
Total Beds: 68

Care of the Elderly Dr Patel

North Stoke Primary Care Trust

1-6 Whittle Court, Town Road, Hanley, Stoke-on-Trent ST1 2QE
Tel: 01782 227715 Fax: 01782 285293
Website: www.northstokepct.com
(Shropshire and Staffordshire Strategic Health Authority)

Chair Paul Warsop
Chief Executive David Lingwood

North Surrey Primary Care Trust

Bournewood House, Guilford Road, Chertsey KT16 0QA
Tel: 01932 872010 Fax: 01932 875346
Website: www.nsurreypct.nhs.uk
(Surrey and Sussex Strategic Health Authority)

Chair Douglas Robertson
Chief Executive Nick Yeo

North Tees and Hartlepool NHS Trust

University Hospital of Hartlepool, Holdforth Road, Hartlepool TS24 9AH
Tel: 01429 266654 Fax: 01429 235389
Website: www.northteesandhartlepool.nhs.uk
(County Durham and Tees Valley Strategic Health Authority)

Chair Bryan Hanson
Chief Executive Joan Rogers

Peterlee Community Hospital
O'Neill Drive, North Blunts, Peterlee SR8 5TZ
Tel: 0191 586 3474 Fax: 0191 586 6562

University Hospital of Hartlepool
Holdforth Road, Hartlepool TS24 9AH
Tel: 01429 266654 Fax: 01429 235389
Total Beds: 300

Accident and Emergency J Clancy, A Simpson, D Southward

Anaesthetics V L Gupta, H Mohan, D Morle, J J Rao, M K Roy, K Uddin, G Vadnai

Dermatology S Shehade

ENT M Hawthorne

General Surgery H Bandi, R Kirby, R Thomson

Genitourinary Medicine S Tayal

General Medicine D W Bruce, B K Chaudhury, B F Hannigan, A Khan, P P Sutton, C R Ward

Obstetrics and Gynaecology M A El-Menabawey, C Emmerson, A A Robertson, S R Tosson

Occupational Health C J English

Oral Surgery B Avery

Orthodontics N A Fox

Orthopaedics A Rangan, M A Shaheen, A Shetty, S C Tang

Paediatrics S Gupta, J C Jani, D N Symon

Pathology J K S Frater, M O Mohamdee, S Pollard, A Youart

Radiology D Hide, A A Jwad, A V Kidambi, H Kidambi

University Hospital of North Tees

Hardwick, Stockton-on-Tees TS19 8PE
Tel: 01642 617617
Total Beds: 439

Accident and Emergency P Stamp, S Wadhwani

Anaesthetics H Contractor, S Gooneratne, J E Hall, G Harris, P Ritchie, P Royle, V Sarma

Dermatology A Carmichael, A Milligan, W Taylor

General Surgery L Gillland, C Hennessy, A Peel, D Rosenberg, L Rosenberg, M A Tabaqchali, Mr Yassin

General Medicine D Carr, A W Dellipiani, D Dwarakanath, R Harrison, B Herd, A Shyam-Sundar, R Smith, P Snashall, D Spence, D Wright

Obstetrics and Gynaecology E V Gouk, H M Hatem, J Macaulay, I C Macleod, S Walton

Occupational Health C J English

Orthopaedics N Bayliss, M Krishna, S Maheswaran, C Tulloch

Paediatrics R Dias, C I Harikumar, C McCowen, B McLain, M Oo, I Verber

Pathology R Finney, J Hoffman, Z T Maung, C Rettman

Radiology S L Chawla, T Hughes, J Latimer, P Tait, W Thompson, M J Trewhella

North Tees Primary Care Trust

Tower House, Teesdale South, Thornaby Place, Thornaby TS17 6SF
Tel: 01642 352297 Fax: 01642 351644
Email: ntpct@nhs.net
Website: www.northteespct.nhs.uk
(County Durham and Tees Valley Strategic Health Authority)

Chair Graham Prest
Chief Executive Christine Willis

North Tyneside Primary Care Trust

Equinox House, Silver Fox Way, Cobalt Business Park, Newcastle upon Tyne NE27 0EJ
Tel: 0191 291 9292 Fax: 0191 291 9293
Website: www.northtynesidepct.nhs.uk
(Northumberland, Tyne and Wear Strategic Health Authority)

Chair David Luke
Chief Executive Pam McDougall

North Warwickshire Primary Care Trust

139 Earls Road, Nuneaton CV11 5HP
Tel: 024 7664 2200 Fax: 024 7635 1434
Email: general.enquiries@nw-pct.nhs.uk
Website: www.nw-pct.nhs.uk
(West Midlands South Strategic Health Authority)

Chair Chris Bain
Chief Executive Anne Heckels

Bramcote Hospital

Lutterworth Road, Nuneaton CV11 6QL
Tel: 024 7638 8200 Fax: 024 7635 0616
Total Beds: 44

Care of the Elderly A W Bullen, A B Whitehouse

Child and Adolescent Psychiatry S Thavasothy

Brooklands Hospital

Brooklands Way, Coleshill Road, Marston Green, Birmingham B37 7HL
Tel: 0121 779 6981 Fax: 0121 779 4695
Total Beds: 122

General Psychiatry M Baxter, A Roy

Lea Castle Hospital

Wolverley, Kidderminster DY10 3PP
Tel: 01562 850461
Total Beds: 40

Manor Hospital

Manor Court Avenue, Nuneaton CV11 5SP
Tel: 024 7637 4434

North West London Hospitals NHS Trust

Northwick Park Hospital, Watford Road, Harrow HA1 3UJ
Tel: 020 8864 3232 Fax: 020 8869 2009
Email: trust@nwlh.nhs.uk
Website: www.nwlh.nhs.uk
(North West London Strategic Health Authority)

Chair Alastair McDonald
Chief Executive John Pope

Central Middlesex Hospital

Acton Lane, Park Royal, London NW10 7NS
Tel: 020 8965 5733 Fax: 020 8453 2327
Total Beds: 240

Accident and Emergency J Hayes, A Sivakumar, S S Tachakra

Anaesthetics G Abbondati, M A Ali, I F Collier, D Davies, R Griffin, P L Pantin, S Wijegitilleka, M Wrigley

Audiological Medicine D A Bumby

Cardiology T Bowker, C M Dancy, D W Davies

Care of the Elderly C Cayley, B Kaufman, D McCrea

Chemical Pathology P Frost

Dermatology A Powles

ENT S Abramovich, R Ryan, P C A Taylor

Gastroenterology A Raimundo, D Sherman, D B A Silk

General Medicine D Brown, A Grenfell, W M Kong, S Mc Hardy Young, A Palmer

General Surgery M Ghilchick, W Kmiot, N Menzies-Gow

Genitourinary Medicine G Brook, S Murphy

Haematology Z Abboudi, S Davies, K Ryan

Histopathology M Al-Adnani, C N Amerasinghe

Medical Microbiology Dr Rahman, M S Shafi

Neurology R Shakir

Neurophysiology M Elian, N Khalil

Obstetrics and Gynaecology N Armar, S Kerslake, E Manning, N Morris

Occupational Health S Miller

Ophthalmology T Fallon, J Joseph, C Nimalasena, G Vafidis

Oral and Maxillofacial Surgery D J Archer, H Thuau

Orthodontics T Davies

Orthopaedics A Forester, J Goodall, J Hollingdale, M Pearse

Paediatrics H Davies, R Franklin, J Loftus, R H Schwartz, M Scrine, A Sharma

Plastic Surgery J Nanchahal

Radiology C Allen, D Dutton, A Hine, I Nochler, P Shorvon

Radiotherapy C Vernon

Rheumatology B Colaco, Dr Yuksel

Thoracic Medicine V Graham, V Mak, F Moss, D Ornadel

Urology M Gleeson, E Rogers, H Whitfield

Edgware Community Hospital

Burnt Oak Broadway, Edgware HA8 0AD
Tel: 020 8952 2381 Fax: 020 8732 6807

Elderly Medicine P Wiseman

Paediatrics D Challis, N Feuchtwang, E Nevrkla

Northwick Park Hospital

Watford Road, Harrow HA1 3UJ
Tel: 020 8864 3232 Fax: 020 8869 2009
Total Beds: 800

Cardiology H Bethell, N Stevens

Endocrinology P Sharp

Gastroenterology M Pitcher

General Medicine D Cohen

General Surgery L Barker, M Burke, D Greenstein, R Philips, S Renton

Genetics C Garrett

Genitourinary Medicine A Shaw

Immunology A Denman

Infectious Diseases R Davidson

Medical Microbiology P Neilsen

Neurology C Mummery

Obstetrics and Gynaecology A Priddy, J Spencer

Paediatrics A Massoud, R Thomas

Rheumatology C Higgens

St Mark's Hospital

Watford Road, Harrow HA1 3UJ
Tel: 020 8235 4000 Fax: 020 8235 4001
Website: www.stmarkshospital.org.uk
Total Beds: 74

Epidemiology W Atkin

General Medicine A Emmanuel, A Forbes, S Gabe, M Jacyna, M A Kamm, M Pitcher, B Saunders, C B Williams

General Psychiatry J Stern

General Surgery S J D Chadwick, C R G Cohen, P McDonald, R J Nicholls, J M A Northover, R K S Phillips, A C J Windsor

Nuclear Medicine K E Britton, M Granowska

Pathology A Price, I C Talbot

Radiology C I Bartram, S Halligan, M Marshall

Wembley Hospital

116 Chaplin Road, Wembley HA0 4UX
Tel: 020 8903 1323 Fax: 020 8962 4051
Total Beds: 53

General Medicine S M Young

General Surgery M Menzies-Gow

Obstetrics and Gynaecology E Manning

Orthopaedics J Hollingdale

Pathology C N Amerasinghe

Radiology D Dutton

Radiotherapy and Oncology C Vernon

Willesden Hospital

Harlesden Road, London NW10 3RY
Tel: 020 8451 8017 Fax: 020 8451 8030
Total Beds: 76

Care of the Elderly B Kaufman

Chest Disease V A L Graham, V Mak

Oral and Maxillofacial Surgery D J Archer

Pathology C N Amerasinghe

Radiology D Dutton

Rheumatology B Colaco

Thoracic Medicine V Graham, V Mak

North West Surrey Mental Health Partnership NHS Trust

From 04/2005 merging with Surrey Hampshire Borders NHS Trust and Surrey Oaklands NHS Trust to form Surrey and Borders Partnership NHS Trust.

Abraham Cowley Unit, Holloway Hill, Lyne, Chertsey KT16 0AE
Tel: 01932 872010 Fax: 01932 875128
(Surrey and Sussex Strategic Health Authority)

Chair David Rye
Chief Executive Lorraine Reid
Consultants Elaine Alves, Elspeth Bawtree, Paola Franciosi

Abraham Cowley Unit

Holloway Hill, Lyne, Chertsey KT16 0AE
Tel: 01932 872010 Fax: 01932 875128
Total Beds: 82

Ashford Mental Health Services

London Road, Ashford TW15 3AA
Tel: 01784 884488

Hayworth House

Guildford Road, Chertsey KT16 0QA
Tel: 01932 872010
Total Beds: 16

Walton Community Hospital (Mental Health Beds)

Burwood, Rodney Road, Walton-on-Thames KT12 3LB
Tel: 01932 220060 Fax: 01932 253674
Total Beds: 13

Weybridge Hospital

Church Street, Weybridge KT13 8DY
Tel: 01932 852931 Fax: 01932 821966
Total Beds: 30

Care of the Elderly B Castleton

Palliative Medicine C Lucas

Woking Community Hospital (Mental Health Services)

The Willows, Heathside Road, Woking GU22 7HS
Tel: 01483 715911 Fax: 01483 766195
Total Beds: 17

Northampton General Hospital NHS Trust

Cliftonville, Northampton NN1 5BD
Tel: 01604 634700 Fax: 01604 545890
Website: www.northamptonshire.nhs.uk
(Leicestershire, Northamptonshire and Rutland Strategic Health Authority)

Chair Bronwen Curtis
Chief Executive Andrew Riley, David Wilson

Northampton General Hospital

Cliftonville, Northampton NN1 5BD
Tel: 01604 634700 Fax: 01604 545980
Email: teresa.wilkins@ngh.nhs.uk
Total Beds: 748

Accident and Emergency V Holloway, S Moore, F Poyner

Anaesthetics A Chmielewski, J Cressey, A Dash, R Evans, C Frerk, C P O Garrett, M Goodwin, K Gupta, J D Hare, P Jameson, P Kadodkar, N H Kay, C Leng, K Leyden, R H K Marsh, M Murall-Krishnan, K N Robinson, R Webster, J B White, M Wilkinson

Biochemistry J O'Donnell

Care of the Elderly L Brawn, Dr Khan, B Morgan, R Morgan

Clinical Microbiology A H Bentley, M Minassian

Dermatology J Clarke, J Mahood

ENT D J Commins, P Gurr, P Jervis, Mr O'Malley

General Medicine J S Birkhead, C J Fox, A Jeffrey, A Kilvert, Dr MacDonald, A Ogilvie, J Ojoo, Dr Richardson, P Sherwood, E Shmueli, U Shmueli, D Sprigings

General Surgery A Berry, J Dawson, J Harisha, R Hicks, D C Hunter, K Khalil, G Libertiny, D Ratliff

Genitourinary Medicine L Riddell

Haematology A L Bowen, M E Haines, J R Y Ross, S Swart

Histopathology/Cellular Pathology S B Coghill, A Krajewski, A J Molyneux, J F Nottingham, S Swart

Neurology T Beer, P Davies, H Ho, C J F Pursdon-Davis, J Taylor

Neurophysiology A Bissessar

Obstetrics and Gynaecology C Aldrich, J Anthony, J G Bibby, W A R Davies, A R Duncan, W L McCullough, E Shaxted, C von Widekind

Ophthalmology I Fearnley, F Irvine, A Kerr, D Mather, G Reddy

Oral and Maxillofacial Surgery D M Grieg, C Harup, W Smith

Orthodontics D M Greig

Orthopaedics E Crawford, D Gidden, G Kerr, R Natarajn, W J Ribbans, D Stock, A Vince

Paediatrics F M Ackland, J G Collinson, N K Griffin, J Hewertson, S Shribman, A Smith, F Thompson

Plastic Surgery A Heywood, A M Richards

Radiology A Bisset, N Fairlie, R Jones, V Kay, R G M Kendrick, K H Lakin, F L S Moss, C Pal, S Shakhapur

Radiotherapy and Oncology C Elwell, A L Houghton, C Macmillan, R Mathews, J Stewart

Rheumatology and Rehabilitation T C Beer, P Davies, C Fursdon-Davis, M Ho, J Taylor

Urology C Bell, J Potter

Northampton Primary Care Trust

Highfield, Cliftonville Road, Northampton NN1 5DN
Tel: 01604 615000 Fax: 01604 615010
Website: www.northamptonshire.nhs.uk
(Leicestershire, Northamptonshire and Rutland Strategic Health Authority)

Chair John Toby
Chief Executive Mary Burrows

Northamptonshire Healthcare NHS Trust

Provides mental health, learning disability and some specialist services across Northamptonshire.

York House, Isebrook Hospital, Irthlingborough Road, Wellingborough NN8 1LP
Tel: 01993 440099
Website: www.northamptonshire.nhs.uk
(Leicestershire, Northamptonshire and Rutland Strategic Health Authority)

Chair Andrew Scarborough
Chief Executive Ron Shields

Adams Day Hospital

Weedon Road, Upton, Northampton NN5 6UH
Tel: 01604 752323

Psychiatry of Old Age M Bonthala, R Mudalier

Haddon House Day Hospital

Danetre Hospital, London Road, Daventry NN11 4DY
Tel: 01327 872610

General Psychiatry C M Bonthala, A O'Neill-Kerr

Kettering General Hospital (Addington Ward)

Rothwell Road, Kettering NN16 8UZ
Tel: 01536 492000 Ext: 2037
Total Beds: 26

General Psychiatry M Chawla

Princess Marina Hospital

Weedon Road, Upton, Northampton NN5 6UH
Tel: 01604 752323 Fax: 01604 592880
Total Beds: 249

General Psychiatry C M Bonthala, H Masih, R K Mudaliar

Rushden Hospital

Wymington Road, Rushden NN10 9JS
Tel: 01933 440666 Fax: 01933 410754

Total Beds: 42

Psychiatry of Old Age M Branford

St Mary's Hospital
London Road, Kettering NN15 7PW
Tel: 01536 410141 Fax: 01536 493242
Total Beds: 112

Psychiatry of Old Age M Branford, T A Christian

Upton House Day Hospital
31 Billing Road, Northampton NN1 5DQ
Tel: 01604 32958

Northamptonshire Heartlands Primary Care Trust

Nene House, Isebrook Hospital, Irthlingborough Road, Wellingborough NN8 1LP
Tel: 01933 440099 Fax: 01536 494228
Website: www.northamptonshire.nhs.uk/heartlands
(Leicestershire, Northamptonshire and Rutland Strategic Health Authority)

Chair Susan Hills
Chief Executive Richard Alsop

Corby Community Hospital
Cottingham Road, Corby NN17 2UN
Tel: 01536 400070
Total Beds: 19

General Medicine N P R Gunasekera, A Steel, R L Walters

Isebrook Hospital
Irthlingborough Road, Wellingborough NN8 1LP
Tel: 01933 440099
Total Beds: 49

Adult Rehabilitation V Comp, Dr Matthews

Care of the Elderly A Hussein, A Steel

Northern Devon Healthcare NHS Trust

North Devon District Hospital, Raleigh Park, Barnstaple EX31 4JB
Tel: 01271 322577 Fax: 01271 311541
Email: firstname.surname@ndevon.swest.nhs.uk
Website: www.northdevonhealth.nhs.uk
(South West Peninsula Strategic Health Authority)

Chair Ro Day
Chief Executive John Rom

North Devon District General Hospital
Raleigh Park, Barnstaple EX31 4JB
Tel: 01271 322577 Fax: 01271 311541
Email: firstname.surname@ndevon.swest.nhs.uk
Total Beds: 354

Accident and Emergency M Roberts (Head), M Roberts, H Shenavar

Anaesthetics T Cobby (Head), E Barron, H R Bastiaenen, C Colville, S Forster, G Henry, D Hurrell, A Laycock, B Loader, N P O'Donovan, G Rousseau, G R Sowden, A Walder, H Williams

Cardiothoracic Surgery Mr Berrisford

Care of the Elderly A Moran (Head), M Dent, G Harper

Endoscopy A Latham

ENT J Riddington-Young

Family Planning V Nyman

General Medicine A Moran (Head), A Davies, I Lewin, M H Oliver, T Roberts, A Taylor

General Surgery N Markham (Head), J Groome, D R Harvey, N Markham, M Menon

Genitourinary Medicine E Claydon (Head)

Haematology G Speirs (Head), B Attock, R Frewin

Histopathology G Speirs (Head), A Bull, J Davies, N Ward

Medical Microbiology G Speirs (Head), D Richards

Medical Oncology M Napier, Dr Sheehan

Nephrology Dr D'Souza

Neurology D Footit, W Honan

Obstetrics and Gynaecology A Boyle (Head), S Bennett, S Eckford, A M Wheble

Ophthalmology B E Enoch, R A Gibson, K Whittaker

Oral and Maxillofacial Surgery A McLennan (Head), M Moore

Orthopaedics C Mills (Head), M Podmore, N Treble, P Van Der Walt

Paediatrics A Arend (Head), A J Bosley, J Cox

Plastic Surgery Mr Inglefield

Radiology A Sanderson (Head), J MacPherson, J Rhymer, P Treweeke

Rheumatology H Averns (Head)

Thoracic Medicine M H Oliver

Urology J Barker (Head), S Agrawal, M Crundwell, H Syed

Northern Lincolnshire and Goole Hospitals NHS Trust

Diana Princess of Wales Hospital, Scartho Road, Grimsby DN33 2BA
Tel: 01472 874111 Fax: 01472 875357
Email: enquiries@nlg.nhs.uk
Website: www.nlg.nhs.uk
(North and East Yorkshire and Northern Lincolnshire Strategic Health Authority)

Chair Ade Brooks
Chief Executive Andrew North

Diana Princess of Wales Hospital
Scartho Road, Grimsby DN33 2BA
Tel: 01472 874111 Fax: 01472 875392
Email: simon.rigg@ne.lincs-trent.nhs
Total Beds: 650

Accident and Emergency A Shweikh

Anaesthetics A Asumang, R Bramwell, F M Ghandour, M B Gough, R Khan, A A Samaan, B Tandon, J M C Ward-McQuaid

Care of the Elderly S N Adhikaree, J Adiotomre, L Woosnam

ENT H Amin, B Singh

General Medicine R J I Bain, D A Jones, S Moss, A Naqvi, M Walters

General Psychiatry Dr Konar, T V Mohan, L K Roy

General Surgery L A Donaldson, H J Pearson, A Samy, H Souka, M Tilston, C A Westwood

Genitourinary Medicine P C Gupta

Obstetrics and Gynaecology I Bolaji, W Mueller, A Saha

Ophthalmology P Bagga, K Bhattacharya, S Kotta

Orthodontics B Holmes

Orthopaedics T K Bagga, C Grant, J A Roberts, D Stoffelen

Paediatrics P Adiotomre, J M Davies, A Fan, S M Herber, B M Reynolds

Pathology M Ashton, A Borggrech, A Heppleston, J B Kershaw, P Parsons, W M Peters, K R Speed, A Vicca

Radiology R W T Harries, E Kweka, P F Packer, I Rizvi, N W Sumbwanyambe

Radiotherapy and Oncology P Mack

Rheumatology and Rehabilitation T Gillott, D W James, T Tait

Goole and District Hospital

Woodland Avenue, Goole DN14 6RX
Tel: 01405 720720 Fax: 01405 768993
Total Beds: 82

Care of the Elderly P K Dasgupta, A Roy

Dermatology S Walton

ENT P K Bose

General Medicine S Beer, J Dhawan, D G Leitch, J R A Perumal, S Reynolds

General Surgery A Kar, P J Moore

Haematology S Jalihal

Obstetrics and Gynaecology K Young

Ophthalmology Y R Mankad, M D Parekh

Oral and Maxillofacial Surgery A O M Perriman

Orthopaedics P Molitor

Paediatrics J Devlin, I Evans, M E M Wing

Pathology D Kennedy

Radiology M C Fernando, S Maslin, T N Mehrotra, G T Vijay

Radiotherapy and Oncology T Sreeni

Urology M R G Robinson

Scunthorpe General Hospital

Cliff Gardens, Scunthorpe DN15 7BH
Tel: 01724 282282
Total Beds: 504

Accident and Emergency M Hockey

Anaesthetics A Coe, H El-Rakshy, S Goulding, J Jayamaha, C Moore, R Sharawi, J F W Thompson

Cardiothoracic Surgery M Cowen, K K Nair

Care of the Elderly P K D Gupta, A Roy

Chemical Pathology D D Kennedy

Dermatology S Walton

ENT P N Agarwal, P K Bose

General Medicine S Beer, J Dhawan, D G Leitch, J R A Perumal, S Reynolds

General Surgery S M Ahmad, A K Kar, P J Moore, S F Tindall, B J Wilken

Genitourinary Medicine P C Gupta

Haematology S Jalihal

Neurology M D Rawson

Obstetrics and Gynaecology B F Heywood, L Roberts, S Sabharwal, K Young

Ophthalmology Y R Mankad, M D Parekh

Oral Surgery A Perriman

Orthodontics D M Penketh

Orthopaedics P Molitor, S Shafqat, A P Walker

Paediatrics J Devlin, I Evans, Dr Shekhar

Pathology C Hunt, D Kennedy

Radiology M C Fernando, S C Maslin, T N Mehrotra

Radiotherapy and Oncology T Sreeni

Northgate and Prudhoe NHS Trust

Northgate Hospital, Morpeth NE61 3BP
Tel: 01670 394000 Fax: 01670 394002
Website: www.nap.nhs.uk
(Northumberland, Tyne and Wear Strategic Health Authority)

Chair Patrick Lavery
Chief Executive Joe Kewin
Consultants T Field, Graham, Joyce, Prendergast, Punstan, Rayan, Rippon, S Seager, Tyrer

Northgate Hospital

Morpeth NE61 3BP
Tel: 01670 394000 Fax: 01670 394002
Total Beds: 294

General Psychiatry J Joyce, E Milne, G O'Brien, A F Perini, J Radley, P C Rajan

Prudhoe Hospital

Prudhoe NE42 5NT
Tel: 01670 394000 Fax: 01661 514590
Total Beds: 192

General Psychiatry T Berney, M Prendergast, S P Tyrer, S Wilkinson

Northumberland Care Trust

Merley Croft, Loansdean, Morpeth NE61 2DL
Tel: 01670 394400 Fax: 01670 394501
Website: www.northumberlandcaretrust.nhs.uk
(Northumberland, Tyne and Wear Strategic Health Authority)

Chair Richard Holden
Chief Executive Jim Mackey

Northumbria Health Care NHS Trust

North Tyneside General Hospital, Rake Lane, North Shields NE29 8NH
Tel: 0191 259 6660 Fax: 0191 293 2745
Website: www.northumbria-healthcare.nhs.uk
(Northumberland, Tyne and Wear Strategic Health Authority)

Chair Brian Flood
Chief Executive James Mackey, Sue Page

Alnwick Infirmary

Alnwick NE66 2NS
Tel: 01665 626700 Fax: 01665 626761
Total Beds: 60

Manager Jackie Christer

Chest Disease P J E Brown

Dermatology N Simpson

ENT A Welch

General Medicine J C G Cox

General Psychiatry S E Proctor

General Surgery M Griffin

Obstetrics and Gynaecology T A Lavin

Ophthalmology N P Strong

Orthopaedics A Innes, J L Sher

Radiology K Howells

Rheumatology and Rehabilitation P R Crook

Urology J G W Feggetter

Berwick Infirmary

Berwick upon Tweed TD15 1LT
Tel: 01289 356600 Fax: 01289 355665
Total Beds: 74

Manager Jackie Christer

Chest Disease P J E Brown

Dermatology N Simpson

General Psychiatry S E Proctor

General Surgery M Bradburn, A B Griffiths, R F Mather, G R Proud

Obstetrics and Gynaecology P Franks

Orthodontics T G Bennett

Orthopaedics J M Leitch

Radiology K Howells

Rheumatology and Rehabilitation P R Crook

Urology J G W Feggetter

Blyth Community Hospital

Thoroton Street, Blyth NE24 1DX
Tel: 01670 396400 Fax: 01670 396492
Total Beds: 78

Manager Jackie Christer

General Medicine R S S Yapa

Coquetdale Cottage Hospital

Rothbury, Morpeth NE65 7TT
Tel: 01669 620555 Fax: 01669 621527
Total Beds: 17

Manager Jackie Christer

Orthopaedics Mr Partington

Haltwhistle War Memorial Hospital

Westgate, Haltwhistle NE49 9AJ
Tel: 01434 320225
Total Beds: 19

Manager Jackie Christer

Hexham General Hospital

Corbridge Road, Hexham NE46 1QJ
Tel: 01434 655655 Fax: 01434 607920
Total Beds: 98

Manager Bruce Skilbeck

Anaesthetics I Anderson, D Laffey, A Redpath

Dermatology P Farr

General Medicine K Matthewson, A J Wright

General Surgery R M Weaver

Obstetrics and Gynaecology J P Forsey, P F Sims

Ophthalmology R E W Ridley, Mr Strong

Oral and Maxillofacial Surgery J E Hawkesford

Orthopaedics R Sutton, W K Walsh

Otolaryngology C Diamond

Pathology P W Condie

Radiology J B Douglas, E B Garner

Radiotherapy and Oncology H H Lucraft

Morpeth Cottage Hospital

South Road, Morpeth NE61 8UW
Tel: 01670 395600 Fax: 01670 395657
Total Beds: 86

Manager Jackie Christer

General Medicine R S Yeppa

North Tyneside General Hospital

Rake Lane, North Shields NE29 8NH
Tel: 0191 259 6660 Fax: 0191 293 2745
Total Beds: 546

Manager Jim Mackey

Accident and Emergency C C Goring

Anaesthetics P Cooper

Chemical Pathology P McKenna

General Medicine O A Afolabi, I Cobden, C Doig, E T Peel

General Surgery Mr Goulbourne, F J Holmes, S Kelly, R Pollard

Haematology H Tinegate

Histopathology P Birch, S Johri, A D Rodgers

Medical Microbiology R Stansfield

Obstetrics and Gynaecology D A Evans

Orthopaedics S Asaad, J M Caullay, A D Gaynor, D Kramer

Paediatrics W T Houlsby

Psychiatry of Old Age R Adams, M Livingston, G Ramsey

Radiology D Tennant

Sir G B Hunter Memorial Hospital

The Green, Wallsend NE28 7PB
Tel: 0191 262 4403

Manager Jackie Christer

Wansbeck General Hospital

Woodhorn Lane, Ashington NE63 9JJ
Tel: 01670 521212 Fax: 01670 529047
Total Beds: 405

Manager Les Morgan

Norwich Primary Care Trust

St Andrew's House, Northside, St Andrew's Business Park, Thorpe St Andrews, Norwich NR7 0HT
Tel: 01603 307320 Fax: 01603 307421
Email: ann.filby@norwich-pct.nhs.uk
Website: www.norwichpct.nhs.uk
(Norfolk, Suffolk and Cambridgeshire Strategic Health Authority)

Chair Susan Gale
Chief Executive Alastair Roy
Consultants Kate McGlashan, Veena Rodrigues

Colman Hospital

Unthank Road, Norwich NR2 2PJ
Tel: 01603 286286

Little Plumstead Hospital

Hospital Road, Little Plumstead, Norwich NR13 5EW
Tel: 01603 711227 Fax: 01603 711212

Total Beds: 200

General Psychiatry S Brown, V Krishnan, N Verma

Norwich Community Hospital

Bowthorpe Road, Norwich NR2 3TU
Tel: 01603 776776

Nottingham City Hospital NHS Trust

Nottingham City Hospital, Hucknall Road, Nottingham NG5 1PB
Tel: 0115 969 1169 Fax: 0115 962 7788
Email: contact@ncht.trent.nhs.uk
Website: www.ncht.org.uk
(Trent Strategic Health Authority)

Chair Christine Bowering
Chief Executive Gerry McSorley

Nottingham City Hospital

Hucknall Road, Nottingham NG5 1PB
Tel: 0115 969 1169 Fax: 0115 962 7788
Total Beds: 1116

Manager Gerry McSorley

Anaesthetics C Abercrombie, A Aitkenhead, K Alagesan, A Biswas, D G Bogod, C J Bowley, A Byrne, J P J Curran, J Fitzhenry, A J P Fletcher, D E Griffiths, M P D Heining, V Hodgkinson, S Hussain, S Z Hussain, C Hutter, A Jardine, J E L Jayamaha, D T Knights, M J Levitt, R P Mahajan, A Matthews, J Nicholl, R W D Nickalls, N A Okonkwo, A Ravenscroft, M S Shajar, H J Skinner, J R Skoyles, P E Tatham, J M Vernon, J A Warner, L A Woods

Breast and General Surgery R W Blamey, K L Cheung, D Macmillan, J F R Robertson

Cardiology A J Ahsan, M Baig, R A Henderson, G K Morris

Clinical Chemistry C Marenah

Clinical Genetics C Gardiner, T Parkin, J A Raeburn, M Suri

Gastroenterology C M Teahon

General Medicine P Berman, D L Cohen, A W G English, P H Fentem, S M Fowlie, N P Kumar, T Masud, S K Mukherjee, A M Trueman

General Surgery R Blamey, K Cheung, D MacMillan, K Rigg, J Roberstson, U Ubhi, N T Welch

Haematology J L Byrne, S Donohue, A Hayes, P A E Jones, A K McMillan, N H Russell

Histopathology I D Ansell, Z Chaudry, H Denley, I O Ellis, C W Elston, J Johnson, A H S Lee, T A McCulloch, S R O'Connor, Dr Pinder, I N Soomro

Infectious Diseases R G Finch, B J Thomson, P Venkatesan

Integrated Medicine P Berman, S Fowlie, FL Game, W Goddard, DJ Hosking, R Hubbard, WJ Jeffcoate, R Long, T Masud, R O Morris, R C L Page, N Smith, N K G Smith, N D C Sturrock, W Sunman, A Tattersfield, A M Trueman

Microbiology T Boswell, F Donald, S Pugh, S Soo, V Weston

Neurology P M W Bath

Obstetrics and Gynaecology C N Bain, J E F Bruce, T N Fay, I R Johnson, L H Kean, D T Y Liu, S Watkin, K Williamson

Oncology E Bessell, J Carmichael, S Chan, D Fyfe, D Morgan, S Morgan, M Sokal, P Woll

Oral and Maxillofacial Surgery J Rowson

Orthopaedics A P Broodryk, S Dhar, M Hatton, C J Howell, L Neumann, B E Scammell, P D Triffitt, W A Wallace

Paediatrics G Croaker, D Curnock, J Evans, R Gregson, E B Knight-Jones, N Marlow, D Mellor, C Rance, N Rutter, C Smith, A R Smyth, A Watson

Palliative Medicine R Corcoran, V L Crosby, A Wilcock

Plastic Surgery J C Daly, M Henley, A G B Perks, I F Starley, D I Wilson

Radiology N J Broderick, H C Burrell, E J Cornford, A J Evans, K J Fairbairn, D J Green, J James, J C Jobling, J C Jobling, K H Latief, A R Manhire, K S Pointon, D H Rose, J M Somers, A R M Wilson

Renal Medicine R P Burden, M J D Cassidy, S D Roe, M Shehata

Respiratory Medicine D R Baldwin, J R Britton, T Harrison, A J Knox

Rheumatology C M Deighton, M Doherty, A C Jones, J F Mchale, I R A Pande, D Walsh

Sexual Health I Ahmed, C J Bignell, C A Bowman, E M Carlin

Thoracic/Cardiac Surgery F D Beggs, J P Duffy, I Mitchell, W E Morgan, S Nalk, D Richens

Transplantation K M Rigg, M Shehata

Urology M Bishop, M C Bishop, M Dunn, D R Harriss, R J Lemberger, M Taylor

Nottingham City Primary Care Trust

1 Standard Court, Park Row, Nottingham NG1 6GN
Tel: 0115 845 4545 Fax: 0115 912 3300
Email: chiefexec.office@nottinghamcity-pct-nhs.uk
Website: www.nottingham.nhs.uk
(Trent Strategic Health Authority)

Chair David Atkinson
Chief Executive Samantha Milbank

Nottinghamshire Healthcare NHS Trust

Duncan Macmillan House, Porchester Road, Mapperley NG3 6AA
Tel: 0115 969 1300 Fax: 0115 993 4546
Website: www.nottinghamshirehealthcare.nhs.uk
(Trent Strategic Health Authority)

Chair Brian Edwards
Chief Executive Jeremy Taylor

Nuffield Orthopaedic Centre NHS Trust

Windmill Road, Headington, Oxford OX3 7LD
Tel: 01865 741155 Fax: 01865 742348
Email: enquiries@noc.org.uk
Website: www.noc.org.uk
(Thames Valley Strategic Health Authority)

Chair Joanna Foster
Chief Executive Ed Macalister-Smith
Consultants Nicholas Athanasou, Michael Benson, Tony Berendt, Gavin Bowden, Paul Bowness, Matthew Brown, Christopher Bulstrode, Peter Burge, Andrew Car, Paul Cooke, Joel David, Christopher Dodd, Sally Edmonds, Jeremy Fairbank, Max Gibbons, Henk Giele, John Goodfellow, Roger Gundle, John Kenwright, Udo Kischka, Peter McLardy-Smith, Ian McNab, Eugene McNally, Martin A McNally, J Dougall Morrison, Alistair Mowat, David Murray, Simon Ostlere, John Outhwaite, Clare Robertson, Graham Russell, Roger Smith, John Spivey, James Teh, Rajesh Thakker, Tim

Theologis, Derick Wade, John Wass, James Wilson-MacDonald, David Wilson, Colin Woods, Paul Wordsworth

Oldbury and Smethwick Primary Care Trust

Kingston House, 438-450 High Street, West Bromwich B70 9LD
Tel: 0121 500 1500 Fax: 0121 500 1501
Website: www.os-pct.nhs.uk
(Birmingham and the Black Country Strategic Health Authority)

Chair Richard Nugent
Chief Executive Gill Combes

Oldham Primary Care Trust

Primary Care Support Centre, Ellen House, Waddington Street, Oldham OL9 6EE
Tel: 0161 622 6500 Fax: 0161 622 6512
Website: www.oldham.nhs.uk
(Greater Manchester Strategic Health Authority)

Chair Riaz Ahmad
Chief Executive Gail Richards
Consultants Bhatti, John Billsborough, Colette Bridgeman, Chris Howard, Jane Rossini

Oxford City Primary Care Trust

Richards Building, Old Road, Headington, Oxford OX3 7LG
Tel: 01865 226900 Fax: 01865 226970
Email: firstname.surname@oxfordcity-pct.nhs.uk
Website: www.oxfordcity-pct.nhs.uk
(Thames Valley Strategic Health Authority)

Chair Malcom Fearn
Chief Executive Andrea Young

Oxford Community Hospital

Churchill Hospital, Old Road, Headington, Oxford OX3 7LJ
Tel: 01865 225501 Fax: 01865 225506
Total Beds: 30

Oxford Radcliffe Hospitals NHS Trust

The John Radcliffe, Headley Way, Headington, Oxford OX3 9DU
Tel: 01865 741166 Fax: 01865 741408
Website: www.oxfordradcliffe.nhs.uk
(Thames Valley Strategic Health Authority)

Chair William Stubbs
Chief Executive Trevor Campbell Davis

The Churchill

Old Road, Headington, Oxford OX3 7LJ
Tel: 01865 741841 Fax: 01865 225011
Total Beds: 350

Anaesthetics C J A Glynn, T M Jack, H J McQuay

Clinical Genetics E M Blair, G K Brown, J A Hurst, S M Huson, H S Stewart, I P M Tomlinson, A O M Wilkie

Clinical Oncology C J Alcock, N P Bates, C H Blesing, D J Cole, A C Jones, B A Lavery, A J Salisbury, E M Sugden, N J Warner, A Weaver

Dermatology S M Burge, R P R Dawber, S A George, H A Kurwa, J J Powell, S M Powell, R C Ratnavel, R J Turner, V A Venning, F T Wojnarowska

General Surgery C R Darby, D J Deardon, P J Friend, D W R Gray

Haematology P L F Giangrande, D M Keeling, S N Wickramsinghe

Immunopathology H M Chapel, S A Misbah

Infectious Diseases A R Berendt, C P Conlon, P Klenerman, S J McConkey, T E A Peto, S L Rowland-Jones

Medical Oncology T S Ganesan, A L Harris, M R Middleton, A Protheroe, D C Talbot

Mental Health A K Malmberg

Nephrology P Altman, P D Mason, C G Winearls

Paediatrics E C Burns, C M Robertson, J A Shaw

Palliative Medicine J Chamberlain, M G Miller, M J Minton, R G Twycross

Radiology R F Adams, N C Cowan, R E English, F V Gleeson

Rheumatology K R Mackay

Thoracic Medicine L S Bennett, M K Benson, R J O Davies, F Hardinge, M G Slade, J R Stradling

Urology S F Brewster, D W Cranston, J P Crew, J G Noble, J M Reynard

Horton Hospital

Oxford Road, Banbury OX16 9AL
Tel: 01295 275500 Fax: 01295 229055
Total Beds: 200

Accident and Emergency G C George

Anaesthetics J E R Beamer, S K Chamberlain, J Everatt, P S Laurie, A E Richards, M A Sicinski, B A Thornley, C M Wait, D G Willatts

General Medicine I R Arnold, A J Ellis, T M Pathrose, S R (R Smith, A V G Taylor

General Surgery G V N Appleton, M N (N Dehalvi, C L Griffiths, R E K Marshall

Haematology O I Atoyebi

Histopathology G I N Greywoode, N J Mahy

Medical Microbiology C J Hall

Obstetrics and Gynaecology S H Canty, E R Laird, H G Naoum, J S Nicholls

Orthopaedics N R Gillham, A Hughes, J P Pollard, B Shafighian

Paediatrics R I Ahmed, R A F Bell, M F Hunter, E E Matthews, B J A Stewart

Radiology B P Barry, M D Bindal, H F D'Costa, P J Haggett, F K Macleod

The John Radcliffe

Headley Way, Oxford OX3 9DU
Tel: 01865 741166 Fax: 01865 741408
Total Beds: 650

Accident and Emergency J J M Black, P J Hormbrey, R A Pullinger, D V Skinner

Anaesthetics E V Addy, Q P Ainsworth, M T Ali, S J Berg, H S Bridge, G Burt, M B Dobson, K L Dorrington, O J Dyar, J M Evans, R D Evans, A D Farmery, P J A Foex, F A M Gibson, C S Grange, C R Grebenik, P R Hambly, J D Henville, H E Higham, C F Kearns, J R Lehane, A B Loach, L Loh, C McGuinness, P J McKenzie, M S Mann, D G Mason, J M Millar, J J Pandit, T M Parry, D W Pigott, R C Pollard, M T Popat, M J Quinlan, F M Ratcliffe, R Rogers, R M Russell, S V Rutter, M C Sainsbury, N M Schofield, J W Sear, D Shlugman, M E Sinclair, J E Stevens, M D Stoneham, M E Ward, O J Warner, J P Warwick, J L Westbrook, S A Wheatley, D A Wilkinson, E M Williams, J D Young

Blood Transfusion M F Murphy

Cardiology A P Banning, Y Bashir, H H H Becher, S Bhattacharya, B Casadei, K M Channon, J C Forfar, D C Lindsay, I P Mulligan, S Neubauer, O J M Ormerod, H Watkins

Cardiothoracic Surgery S H Armistead, R G Perumal Pillai, C P Ratnatunga, D P Taggart, S Westaby

Chemical Pathology A K Abraha, P A H Holloway, J D S Kay, J Keenan, B S F Shine

Clinical Genetics S M Price

Clinical Immunology J E Lortan

Clinical Pharmacology and Therapeutics J K Aronson

Clinical Physiology B Rajagopolan

Gastroenterology R Aga, R W G Chapman, D P Jewell, S P L Travis, J M Trowell

General Medicine B J Angus, J I Bell, C Bunch, V Cerundolo, J D Collier, J S J Dwight, R J Gibbons, M S Hammersley, A Lalvani, A J McMichael, R E Phillips, C W Pugh, P J Ratcliffe, D J M Reynolds, G R Screaton, P Sleight, R V Thakker, A R M Townsend, D A Warrell, N J White, P M Zimbwa

General Surgery B J Britton, P J Clarke, J Collin, C Cunningham, B D George, M J Greenall, A I Handa, L J Hands, N D Maynard, P J Morris, N J M Mortensen, J M T Perkins, G P Sadler

Haematology G W Hall, C R S Hatton, D R Higgs, S J Kelly, T J Littlewood, D Y Mason, R Pawson, P Vyas, J S Wainscoat

Histopathology I D Buley, C A Clelland, D R Davies, K A Fleming, S B Fox, K C Gatter, W Gray, K Hollowood, M Ilyas, S Manek, P R Millard, F Pezzella, J Piris, I S D Roberts, D E Roskell, K A Shah, B F Warren

Immunopathology A C Vincent, H Waldmann

Infectious Diseases N P J Day, A V S Hill, T G Tudor-Williams

Intensive Therapy S W Benham, J Chantler, C S Garrard, N M McGuire

Medical Microbiology B L Atkins, I C J Bowler, K J Cann, D W M Crook, S J Peacock, M P E Slack

Nephrology R J Cornall

Oral Surgery F R Carls, D R Cunliffe, M G Hodge, S R Watt-Smith

Orthodontics G Kidner, M M McKnight, F G Nixon

Orthopaedics W G Bowden, C J Bulstrode, P D Burge, A J Carr, J C T Fairbank, D R Griffin, R C Handley, G Kambouroglou, R I Keyes, I S H McNab, M A McNally, T N Theologis, G P Wilde, K M Willett, J Wilson-MacDonald, P H Worlock

Paediatric Cardiology S S Adwani, L N J Archer, I Ostman Smith, R C Radley-Smith, D M I Runciman

Paediatric Neurology M A McShane, M G Pike

Paediatric Surgery H W Grant, R J I Hitchcock, P R V Johnson, K K Lakhoo

Paediatrics F M Ackland, S J Allen, J L Craze, D B Dunger, J A Edge, M C English, P J R Goulder, J Hull, Z Huma, M A Johnson, C J Killick, D P Kwiatkowski, C D Mitchell, E R Moxon, J Panisello, A J Pollard, J Poulton, A G Shefler, P B Sullivan, A H Thomson, W G Van't Hoff, J T Warner, K A H Wheeler, T N Williams

Radiology P Boardman, S J Golding, T R Goodman, D R M Lindsell, E McNally, H K Mendes Riberio, N R Moore, S J G Ostlere, J Phillips-Hughes, B J Shepstone, Z C Traill, D J Wilson

Rheumatology P Bowness, M A Brown, M F C Callan, M A Hall, B P Wordsworth

Virology C Roberts

Women's Centre M Y Anthony, D H Barlow, C M Bowker, P G Chamberlain, J E Cullimore, M D G Gilmer, S J Gould, P A Hurley, L W M Impey, N K Ives, N V Jackson, S R Jackson, P Johnson, S H Kennedy, I Z MacKenzie, J E McVeigh, P J Magill, E A Opute, Professor Redman, A R Wilkinson

Radcliffe Infirmary

Oxford OX2 6HE
Tel: 01865 311188 Fax: 01865 224566
Total Beds: 250

Chemical Pathology K Evans

Clinical Neurology E A Bissessar, R P Kennett, A Virgincar, Z Zaiwalla

Diabetes A J Farmer, R R Holman, P F Karpe, J C Levy, D R Matthews, H A W Neil, W M G Tunbridge, H E Turner, J A H Wass

Genitourinary Medicine I D V Byren, A Edwards, G A Luzzi, G Rooney, J S Sherrard

Geriatric Medicine P J Cook, A Darowski, J G Evans, D S Fairweather, H W Jones, N A R Stewart, S J Winner

Medical Oncology D J Kerr

Neurology J E Adcock, D Briley, C J F Davis, M J Donaghy, G Ebers, P B C Fenwick, P T Grant-Davies, R C D Greenhall, R P Gregory, Y Hart, D Hilton-Jones, N M Hyman, M C Jackson, P M Matthews, P J M Newsom-Davis, J M Oxbury, J A Palace, P M Rothwell, K A Talbot

Neuropathology M M Esiri, B McDonald, J H Morris, M V Squier

Neurosurgery C B T Adams, T Z Aziz, R S C Kerr, P G Richards, R J Stacey, P J Teddy

Ophthalmology A J Bron, H Cheng, S M Downes, J S Elston, P A Frith, S Hague, P J McCormack, C K (C Patel, P H Rosen, J F Salmon

Otolaryngology G J E Bates, I Bottrill, M J Burton, R J Corbridge, G Cox, A P Freeland, C A Milford

Plastic Surgery O C S Cassell, C R Charles, D J Coleman, H Giele, T E E Goodacre, M D Humzah, C J Inglefield, A Platt, S A Wall

Radiology P L Anslow, J V Byrne, A J Molyneux, G M Quaghebeur

Oxfordshire Ambulance NHS Trust

Churchill Drive, Old Road, Headington, Oxford OX3 7LH
Tel: 01865 740100 Fax: 01865 741974
Email: office@oxamb.nhs.uk
(Thames Valley Strategic Health Authority)

Chair John Goddard
Chief Executive John Nichols

Oxfordshire Learning Disability NHS Trust

Slade House, Horspath Driftway, Headington, Oxford OX3 7JH
Tel: 01865 747455 Fax: 01865 228182
Email: enquiries@oldt.org.uk
Website: www.oldt.org.uk
(Thames Valley Strategic Health Authority)

Chair Helen Baker
Chief Executive Yvonne Cox
Consultants Tim Andrews, Mark Lewis, John Morgan, K Qureshi, Matthew Stephenson

Oxfordshire Mental Healthcare NHS Trust

Warneford Hospital, Warneford Lane, Headington, Oxford OX3 7JX

Tel: 01865 778911 Fax: 01865 223078
Email: enquiries@oxmhc-tr.nhs.uk
Website: www.oxfordshirementalhealth.nhs.uk
(Thames Valley Strategic Health Authority)

Chair Janet Godden
Chief Executive Julie Waldron

Fiennes Centre
Horton General Hospital, Oxford Road, Banbury

Fulbrook Centre
Churchill Hospital, Old Road, Headington, Oxford OX3 7LE

Littlemore Mental Health Centre
Sandford Road, Littlemore, Oxford OX4 4XN
Tel: 01865 778911
Total Beds: 272

Moorview
2-8 Moorland Road, Witney OX28 6LF
Tel: 01993 202100

Park Hospital for Children
Old Road, Headington, Oxford OX3 7LQ
Tel: 01865 741717
Total Beds: 25

Child and Adolescent Psychiatry G C Forrest, D P H Jones, M Purkis, R Shepperd, A L Stein, G Stores, E Walters

Neurology Z Zaiwalla

Warneford Hospital
Warneford Lane, Headington, Oxford OX3 7JX
Tel: 01865 741717
Total Beds: 81

Child and Adolescent Psychiatry A C D James

General Psychiatry D Chalmers, C Davison, M Elphick, C J A Fairburn, D P Geaney, S Hampson, K E Hawton, R A Mayou, D O'Leary, C Oppenheimer, N Rose

Psychotherapy M J D Hobbs, A S Powell

Oxleas NHS Trust

Pinewood House, Pinewood Place, Dartford DA2 7WG
Tel: 01322 625700 Fax: 01322 555491
Website: www.oxleas.nhs.uk
(South East London Strategic Health Authority)

Chair Dave Mellish
Chief Executive Stephen Firn

Bracton Centre
Medium Secure Unit, Forensic Mental Health, Bracton Lane, off Leyton Cross Road, Dartford DA2 7AP
Tel: 01322 294300 Fax: 01322 293595
Total Beds: 80

Green Parks House
Farnborough Hospital, Farnborough Common, Orpington BR6 8NY
Tel: 01689 880000 Fax: 01689 851211
Total Beds: 88

Manager Kate Thompson

Woodlands
Queen Mary's Hospital, Frognal Avenue, Sidcup DA14 6LT
Tel: 020 8308 3100
Total Beds: 66

Manager Jack Yan

Papworth Hospital NHS Foundation Trust

Specialist cardiothoracic centre. Established as a Foundation Trust 01/07/2004.

Papworth Everard, Cambridge CB3 8RE
Tel: 01480 830541 Fax: 01480 831315
Website: www.papworth.hospital.org.uk
(Norfolk, Suffolk and Cambridgeshire Strategic Health Authority)

Chair John Beadsmoore
Chief Executive Stephen Bridge

Papworth Hospital
Papworth Everard, Cambridge CB3 8RE
Tel: 01480 830541 Fax: 01480 831315
Total Beds: 220

Anaesthetics J Arrowsmith, F Falter, S Ghosh, S Gray, R Hall, R Hall, I Hardy, A Klein, J D Kneeshaw, R D Latimer, J Mackay, A Oduro, A Vuylsteke

Cardiology S Clarke, A Grace, F Murgatroyd, M C Petch, P Schofield, L M Shapiro, D L Stone

Cardiothoracic Surgery D Jenkins, S Large, S A M Nashef, A Ritchie, B Rosengard, S Tsui, J Wallwork, F C Wells

Histopathology M Goddard, D Rassel, S Stewart

Medical Microbiology J Foweraker, A Karas

Oncology D Gilligan

Palliative Medicine M Saunders

Radiology D S Appleton, R Coulden, N Screton, A Tasker

Thoracic Medicine D Bilton, C Haworth, J Peke-Zaba, J N Shneerson, P Sirasothy, I Smith, J Wong

The Pennine Acute Hospitals NHS Trust

Westhulme Avenue, Oldham OL1 2PN
Tel: 0161 624 0420 Fax: 0161 627 3130
Email: enquiries@pat.nhs.uk
Website: www.pat.nhs.uk
(Greater Manchester Strategic Health Authority)

Chair Steven Price
Chief Executive Chris Appleby

Birch Hill Hospital
Rochdale OL12 9QB
Tel: 01706 377777 Fax: 01706 754108
Total Beds: 293

Anaesthetics O Abdelatti, S Drake, A Eskander, J Kini, R Shaikh, A Swayampraksam

Care of the Elderly Dr Buan (Head), R Namushi, R K Sharma

ENT J T Brandrick, D Gordon, D Sheppard

General Medicine M Finaly (Head), T Akintewe, M F Fletcher, D N Foster, R George, M Hargreaves, S Jegarajah, D J Smithard

Neurosurgery Mr King

Ophthalmology N Jacobs, S Kafle, K N Khan, I H Qureshi

Paediatrics E Odeka (Head), S DeSilva, O P Oluwole

Pathology M G Bradgate, Dr Brammer, R Fitzmaurice, Dr Grey

Radiology J Mather, Mr Shah, D P Winarso

Rheumatology and Rehabilitation A Bowden, E E Smith, K Walton

Fairfield General Hospital

Rochdale Old Road, Jericho, Bury BL9 7TD
Tel: 0161 764 6081 Fax: 0161 705 3656
Total Beds: 577

Anaesthetics Dr Gadiyar, K Kataria, P Kotak, Dr Madhavan, Dr Marthi, A H M Mollah, Dr Pandya, N M Tierney

Cardiothoracic Surgery Dr Jones

Care of the Elderly Dr Bowden, Dr Finnegan, Dr Goodman, Dr Haslam, Dr Kouta, Dr Mushahwar, A Narayan, Dr Prudham, Dr Savage, P Sethi, Dr Sinniah, Dr Smith, Dr Smithurst, U N Wadhwa

Dental Surgery A E Green, S G Langton

Dermatology D Fitzgerald (Head), Dr Judge

ENT Dr Bhatnagar, J T Brandrick, D Gordon, Dr Sheppard

General Psychiatry Dr Paul, Dr Prasad, Dr Sagar, K T Thomas, Dr Vaidya

General Surgery Dr de Souza, Dr Kutiyanawala, Dr Sharif

Genitourinary Medicine Dr Lacey

Neurology Dr Mohr

Obstetrics and Gynaecology B Hayden, A Patrick, M Preston, C Rice, A J Russell, C R Wake

Ophthalmology Dr Hashmi, Dr Jacobs, Dr Khan, Dr Qureshi

Orthodontics P A Banks

Orthopaedics A F M Brewood, J Doyle, A I Hegab, Dr Ilango, R McGivney

Paediatrics Dr Bose-Haider, R Levy, E Odeka, P U Prabhu, V S Sankar, R M Wakefield

Radiology S Singanayagam

Radiotherapy and Oncology Dr Slevin

North Manchester General Hospital

Delaunays Road, Manchester M8 5RB
Tel: 0161 795 4567 Fax: 0161 740 4450
Total Beds: 898

Accident and Emergency Dr Derbyshire, L Duane, P E Randall, M J Stuart

Anaesthetics R Bhishma, G S C Brown, I S Chadwick, I K Hartopp, Dr Jones, V Kapoor, P Kirk, I D Macartney, R Mayall, H V Petts, G E W Robson, P H Steller, H D Vallance, H A C Walker, Y Y Youssef

Cardiology P Atkinson, J Swan

Care of the Elderly Dr Ahmed, P Gibson, V Khanna, M Yates

ENT Dr Murphy, Z P Shehab, A P Zarod

General Medicine D C Weir (Head), S P Hanley, H J Klass, Dr Mcfarlane, M G Pattrick

General Surgery J M T Howat, M Madan, D J Sherlock, W F Tait, Dr Vadeyar, Dr Walls, G T Williams

Genitourinary Medicine S P Higgins

Haematology Dr Robertson, M Rowlands

Histopathology D M Butterworth, D M H de Kretser

Infectious Diseases A Bonington, E G L Wilkins

Neurophysiology I H Bangash

Obstetrics and Gynaecology V Osmak (Head), D Adegbibe, A S Jones, D Macfoy, J Patrick, C Rice, C F Rice

Occupational Medicine T Persad

Ophthalmology S J Charles

Oral and Maxillofacial Surgery A G Addy, Dr Bhatti, Dr Boyd, M E Foster, P R White, R T M Wodwards

Orthopaedics A D Clayson, T M Meadows, P Rae, D Sochart, B S Sylvester

Pathology Dr Butterworth, Dr de Kretser, M Hammer, H Panigrahi, Dr Robertson, Dr Rowlands

Radiology M R C Aird, Y S Al-Khattab, R A L Bissett, C Jones, A N Khan, N B Thomas, I W Turnbull, Dr Walker

Restorative Dentistry T Boyd

Rheumatology and Rehabilitation Dr Harrison, N Snowden

Urology D Barnes, W M Chow, C B Costello

Rochdale Infirmary

Whitehall Street, Rochdale OL12 0NB
Tel: 01706 377777 Fax: 01706 655474
Total Beds: 272

Anaesthetics O Abdelatti, R Drake, A Eskander, I Kini, R Shaikh, A Swayampraksam

Cardiology M Hargreaves

Cardiothoracic Medicine J G Grotte

Care of the Elderly M Finlay, R Namushi, R K Sharma

Dermatology R D Ead

General Medicine M Finlay (Head), T Akintewe, M F Fletcher, D N Foster, R George, D J Smithard

General Surgery S Afify, K Akhtar

Genitourinary Medicine H Lacey

Obstetrics and Gynaecology A Atalla, M Dickson, S A F Ghobrial, J Patrick, C Rice, M S Zaklama

Oral Surgery P R White

Orthopaedics S Alcock, M A Ali, V Devadoss, E R Jago

Paediatrics M A Ariyawansa, R Smith

Pathology M G Bradgate, D T I Cartmill, R Fitzmaurice, F J Stratton

Plastic Surgery D J Whitby

Radiology J Mather, R S Raja, K Shah, D P Winarso

Radiotherapy and Oncology Mr Wylie

Rheumatology and Rehabilitation A Bowden, E E Smith

Urology M Kourah

The Royal Oldham Hospital

Rochdale Road, Oldham OL1 2JH
Tel: 0161 624 0420 Fax: 0161 627 3130
Total Beds: 835

Accident and Emergency P S Kumar, P K Luthra, R Sohaie, M Zahir

Anaesthetics J Barrie, M Boyd, L B Cook, P R Cook, M A Gregory, J Kenworthy, A Krishnan, J F McGeachie, J K Orton, B R Puddy, A L Richards, D B Rittoo, H Stewart, T C Watt

Audiology I J MacKenzie

Cardiothoracic Surgery T Hooper

Chemical Pathology D Bhatnaghar

Child and Adolescent Psychiatry L R Daud

Dental Surgery A G Addy, M E Foster

Dermatology R D Ead

ENT N K Saha, V L Sharma

General Medicine B Bajaj, J Barclay, G L Bhan, D Conlong, M O Coupe, P Haynes, P S Klimiuk, B Rameh, A Robinson, S A Solomon, G V Sridharan, W Thomas, J Vassallo, K K Vedi

General Surgery D Flook, M Hadfield, N R Hulton, I H McIntosh, T Oshodi, A Rahe, D Richards

Genetics H M Kingston

Haematology V Sen

Histopathology A Padwell

Medical Microbiology B S Perera

Nephrology P A Kalra

Neurology L E L Sayed

Neurosurgery G Victoratos

Obstetrics and Gynaecology S Ali, O Amu, Z Anjun, N Aziz, A Boulos, J Patrick, J Patrick, C Rice

Occupational Therapy N Clayton, S Logan, F Page, S Turner

Ophthalmology J B Garston, K Goodall, J Suharwardy

Orthopaedics T Asumu, K A Buch, C F Elsworth, L G H Jacobs, M S Sundar

Paediatrics I Blumenthal, E B Odeka, B Padmakumar, N G Prakash

Plastic Surgery V Rees

Radiology N Jeyagopal, M Kumar, L K L Lee Cheong, M Nadarajah, P Solomon, C Swainson

Radiotherapy and Oncology C F Finn, R Stout, R Welch

Rehabilitation Medicine K Walton

Restorative Dentistry S Bhatti, T Boyd

Urology S D Chowdhury, N Sharma

Pennine Care NHS Trust

Tameside General Hospital, Fountain Street, Ashton-under-Lyne OL6 9RW
Tel: 0161 331 5151 Fax: 0161 331 5007
Website: www.penninecare.nhs.uk
(Greater Manchester Strategic Health Authority)

Chair Terence McCabe
Chief Executive John Archer

Birch Hill Hospital

Rochdale OL12 9QB
Tel: 01706 377777 Fax: 01706 754376

Fairfield General Hospital

Rochdale Old Road, Bury BL9 7TD
Tel: 0161 764 6081 Fax: 0161 778 3762

Hyde Hospital

Grange Road South, Hyde SK14 5NY
Tel: 0161 366 8833 Fax: 0161 368 2834
Total Beds: 32

General Psychiatry F Oliver

Orchard House Day Hospital

Milton Street, Royton, Oldham OL2 6QX
Tel: 0161 633 6219

The Royal Oldham Hospital

Rochdale Road, Oldham OL1 2JH
Tel: 0161 624 0420 Fax: 0161 627 8669

Sycamores Day Hospital

Rochdale Road, Oldham OL1 2JH
Tel: 0161 627 8101

Tameside General Hospital

Fountain Street, Ashton-under-Lyne OL6 9RW
Tel: 0161 331 5151 Fax: 0161 331 5007
Total Beds: 128

Mental Health B Baynes, P Bowers, F Creighton, S Darvill, Dr Gonrisvnkar, C E Jagus, A Kushlick, Dr McDade, Dr Shaw, Dr Tait, I Telfer, Dr Theofilepoulos, C Watson

Wood's Hospital

Park Crescent, Glossop SK13 9BQ
Tel: 01457 860783 Fax: 01457 868704
Total Beds: 24

General Psychiatry F Oliver

Peterborough and Stamford Hospitals NHS Foundation Trust

Established as a Foundation Trust 01/04/2004.

Edith Cavell Hospital, Bretton Gate, Peterborough PE3 9GZ
Tel: 01733 874000 Fax: 01733 874001
Website: www.peterboroughandstamford.co.uk
(Norfolk, Suffolk and Cambridgeshire Strategic Health Authority)

Chair Clive Morton
Chief Executive Chris Banks

Edith Cavell Hospital

Bretton Gate, Peterborough PE3 9GZ
Tel: 01733 874000 Fax: 01733 875001
Total Beds: 250

Anaesthetics B Appadu, P Baker, D Blake, A M Cooper, P Das, M Farrell, M Glavina, R Griffiths, S G Howlin, P C Hunt, R F Jeevaratnam, P L Johnston, S B Merrill, A Naunton, P Reed, R Robertshaw, M Saleh, S Short, H Smith, D Smyth, M Weisz

Care of the Elderly H Kapila, R Mittra, D Okubadejo, P Owusu-Aguei

ENT N Bhatt, P Leong, A G Pfleiderer

General Medicine C Mistry, J M Roland, D B Rowlands, S Sahi

General Surgery F Bajwa, E Duggan, J T Holmes, S J Kent

Neurology C M Allen, J Thorpe

Orthopaedics T Bhullar, G M Chambers, A Doran, B K Dutta, S Lewis, G Pryor, I Sargent, M L Sutcliffe, G Varley

Radiology C M Brown, B McKeown, B F Millet, R E Moshy

Rheumatology N J Sheehan, N Williams

Urology H N Blackford, C Dawson, S Sharma, A G Turner

MDHU Peterborough

Thorpe Road, Peterborough PE3 6DA
Tel: 01733 874984

Peterborough District Hospital

Thorpe Road, Peterborough PE3 6DA
Tel: 01733 874000 Fax: 01733 874001
Total Beds: 500

Accident and Emergency A Cope

Anaesthetics B Appadu, P Baker, A M C Cooper, P Das, M C Farrell, M J Glavina, S Howlin, P C W Hunt, R Jeevaratham, P Johnston, S Merrill, A Naunton, P N Reed, R Robertshaw, S Short, H S Smith, D Smyth

Care of the Elderly H Kapila, K M Myint, D Okubadejo, P Owusu-Agyei

Chemical Pathology J F Doran

Dermatology P M Hudson, R Mallett

General Medicine M W Dronfield, C Hunter, T Laundy, C Mistry, I P F Mungall, P Nair, J Roland, D B Rowlands, S Sahi

General Surgery J T Holmes, S J S Kent, R T Walker, A Wells

Genitourinary Medicine A Palfreeman

Haematology S A Fairham, M Sivakumaran

Histopathology P M Dennis, M Gertenbach, C Womack

Medical Microbiology A Hellyar, A J Mifsud

Obstetrics and Gynaecology I Jelen, M Lumb, B Ramsay, J Randall, M Slack, A Sriemevan, S Steel

Ophthalmology A Hashim, T Rimmer, S Vardy

Oral and Maxillofacial Surgery W T Lamb, J M Robertson, R Shepherd

Orthopaedics T Bhullar, G M Chambers, A Doran, B K Dutta, S Lewis, G Pryor, M L Sutcliffe, G Varley

Paediatrics S Babikar, V Reddy, M Richardson, A Sumner, S J Tuck, D Woolf, D Yong

Plastic Surgery P Hall

Radiology A E W Dux, B McKeown, B F Millet, R E Moshy

Radiotherapy and Oncology R Benson, K Fife, K McAdam, - Tan

Thoracic Surgery J Dunning, F Wells

Stamford and Rutland Hospital

Ryhall Road, Stamford PE9 1UA
Tel: 01780 764151 Fax: 01780 763385
Total Beds: 90

Manager Paula Gorst

Plymouth Hospitals NHS Trust

Derriford Hospital, Derriford Road, Plymouth PL6 8DH
Tel: 01752 777111 Fax: 01752 768976
Email: info@plymouthhospitals.org.uk
Website: www.plymouthhospitals.org.uk
(South West Peninsula Strategic Health Authority)

Chair John Bull
Chief Executive Paul Roberts

Derriford Hospital

Derriford Road, Plymouth PL6 8DH
Tel: 01752 777111

Mount Gould Hospital

Mount Gould Road, Plymouth PL4 7QD
Tel: 01752 268011 Fax: 01752 672971
Total Beds: 5

Child and Adolescent Psychiatry S Walker

Royal Eye Infirmary

Apsley Road, Plymouth PL4 6PL
Tel: 01752 662078
Total Beds: 27

General Surgery N M Evans, T Freegard, M Ganapathy, N Habib, V T Thaller

Ophthalmology N Evans, T Freegard, N Habib, V Thaller

Scott Hospital

Beacon Park Road, North Prospect, Plymouth PL2 2PQ
Tel: 01752 550741 Fax: 01752 606958

Paediatrics A J Cronin, R Evans

Plymouth Teaching Primary Care Trust

Derriford Business Park, Building 1, Brest Road, Derriford, Plymouth PL6 5QZ
Tel: 01752 315315 Fax: 01752 315321
Email: enquiries@pcs-tr.swest.nhs.uk
Website: www.plymouth-pct.nhs.uk
(South West Peninsula Strategic Health Authority)

Chair David Connelly
Chief Executive Ann James

Plympton Hospital

Market Road, Plympton, Plymouth PL7 1QR
Tel: 01752 314500 Fax: 01752 314501
Total Beds: 121

Poole Hospitals NHS Trust

Poole Hospital, Longfleet Road, Poole BH15 2JB
Tel: 01202 665511 Fax: 01202 442562
Email: firstname.surname@poole.nhs.uk
Website: www.poolehos.org
(Dorset and Somerset Strategic Health Authority)

Chair Peter Harvey
Chief Executive Roger Packham

Poole General Hospital

Longfleet Road, Poole BH15 2JB
Tel: 01202 665511
Email: firstname.surname@poole.nhs.uk
Total Beds: 798

Manager Roger Packham

Accident and Emergency G Cumberbatch, M Reichl

Anaesthetics R Aquilina, W Ashton, H Brownlow, T Dodd, F Dorman, J Holloway, P R W Lanham, A McCormick, B Newman, R N Packham, K Power, P Smyth, B Sweeney, G M L Van Hasselt, P Ventham, M Wee

Care of the Elderly T Battcock, R Day, P Fade, R Harries-Jones, S Ragab, M Thomas, T Villar

Dermatology M Hazell, C J M Stephens

ENT H Cox, D G John, S Rhys Williams, P Scott

General Medicine D Bruce, D Coppini, S D Crowther, W Gatling, K Greaves, A McLeod, J W Millar, N Sharer, J Snook, E Williams

General Surgery A Clarke, J Edwards, A Evans, J Evans, R Henry, T Hillard, S W Hosking, G Nash, J Pain, J Scott, R Talbot

Neurology J P S Burn, J Cole, C J K Ellis, C Hiller, N M Milligan, C H Wulff

Obstetrics and Gynaecology J N T Edwards, R Henry, T Hillard, R Sawdy, J W Scott

Oncology N Cowley, P Crellin, S E Dean, T D Goode, T Hickish, V Lawrence, R Osborne

Oral Surgery V Ilankovan, A F Markus, W J N Peters

Orthopaedics M Farrar, N J Fiddian, D O'Connor

Paediatrics M M Black, R Coppen, A Dewar, J Kelsall, A H McAuley, S Morris, R Rao, J Renshaw, J Sandell, D B Shortland

Palliative Medicine S Kirkham

Pathology J Alexander, J Begley, A J Bell, C M Boyd, P Flanagan, S Hill, K Hussein, F Jack, D Nicholas, A Worsley

Radiology J A D Brailsford, M Creagh-Barry, J Herbetko, M Ismail, J Jones, C Lee-Elliott, A Maibaum, N K Robson, J Stutley, D Tarver, S B Walkden, A Wood

Radiotherapy N Cowley, P Crellin, S Dean, T D Goode, T Hickish, V Lawrence, R Osborne

Rheumatology and Rehabilitation S Richards, P Thompson

Poole Primary Care Trust

Westover House, West Quay Road, Poole BH14 1JF
Tel: 01202 688880 Fax: 01202 668131
Email: poole.admin@poole-pct.nhs.uk
Website: www.poolepct.nhs.uk
(Dorset and Somerset Strategic Health Authority)

Chair Jim Wilson
Chief Executive Andrew Morris

Portsmouth City Teaching Primary Care Trust

Trust Central Office, St James' Hospital, Locksway Road, Portsmouth PO4 8LD
Tel: 023 9283 8340 Fax: 023 9273 3292
Email: firstname.surname@ports.nhs.uk
Website: www.portspct.nhs.uk
(Hampshire and Isle of Wight Strategic Health Authority)

Chair Zenna Atkins
Chief Executive Sheila Clark

Portsmouth Hospitals NHS Trust

De La Court House, Queen Alexandra Hospital, Southwick Hill Road, Cosham, Portsmouth PO6 3LY
Tel: 023 9228 6000 Fax: 023 9228 6073
Website: www.portshosp.org.uk
(Hampshire and Isle of Wight Strategic Health Authority)

Chair Michael Waterland
Chief Executive Ursula Ward

Queen Alexandra Hospital

Southwick Hill Road, Cosham, Portsmouth PO6 3LY
Tel: 023 9228 6000 Fax: 023 9228 6012
Total Beds: 595

Accident and Emergency C J Cahill, G A Carss, S Mullett

Anaesthetics N W Barnes, R J Burden, N T A Campkin, N Chaderton, G Craig, D A B Desgrand, A J Eldridge, S M Elliott, M Ghurye, G Graig, J Harrison, P J Heath, P Jeyabalam, F King, D F Marsh, P J McQuillan, J J Nightingale, R J Palmer, S Pilkington, D Pounder, P D Rogers, G B Smith, B L Taylor, K Torlot, J C Vincent, J R Wace, J A Watt-Smith, M L B Wood, A Yates

Audiological Medicine P West

Dental Surgery J D W Barnard, H Beckett, G Zaki

Dermatology L J Cook, A Haworth, B Hughes, S Keohane

ENT W S Al Safi, A E Davis, C I Johnstone, G Madden, E Nilssen, M Pringle, A Resouly, P West

General Medicine R J Clark, D C Colin-Jones, M Cummins, H Duncan, R Ellis, P M Goggin, N Hedger, A W Matthews, K M Shaw

General Surgery K Abusin, N Digard, J M Kelly, S Payne, M Pemberton, P M Perry, W G Prout, S A Sadek, A Sanapati, S Somers, G L Sutton, M R Thompson, S Toh, A Walters, P C Weaver, M H Wise, C Yiangou

Genitourinary Medicine V Harindra

Intensive Care G Craig, J Knighton, P McQuillan, G B Smith, B L Taylor, G Tweeddale

Microbiology R J Brindle, P M Crockcroft, G S Underhill

Occupational Health D Shand

Ophthalmology D L Boase, A R Evans, D Farnworth, W Green, M N Jeffrey, H Maclean

Orthodontics D Barnard, H Beckett, D J Birnie, H Hilling, S N Robinson, G Zaki

Orthopaedics H J Clarke, N A Flynn, M Grover, S Hodkinson, J G Hussell, I T Jeffery, D M Longbottom, M McLaren, A S Mansour, R H Richards

Palliative Medicine H Jones

Pathology T Cranfield, J Dhundee, S Di Palma, M Ganczakowski, H Hirri, M J Jeffrey, D A McCormick, N J E Marley, D Poller, A Spedding, R M Young

Radiology J Atchley, J Domjan, M N H Gonem, P Gordon, R Harrison, R G Hull, A R Jackson, J J Langham-Brown, E A Tilley, S P Ward, F Witham

Rheumatology R G Hull, J Ledingham, F McCrae, R Shaban, A L Thomas

Royal Hospital Haslar

Gosport PO12 2AA
Tel: 023 9258 4255
Total Beds: 210

St Mary's Hospital

Milton Road, Portsmouth PO3 6AD
Tel: 023 9228 6000 Fax: 023 9286 6413
Total Beds: 551

Care of the Elderly A D Dowd, J A H Grunstein, D R Jarrett, R F Logan, A Lord, M P Severs, J C Tandy

Dermatology D F Barrett, L J Cook, B Hughes

General Medicine S Evans, T G Farrell, R J Lewis, J G B Millar, E Neville, J Stevens, J Watkins

Genitourinary Medicine V Harindra, J M Tobin

Nephrology R Lewis, J C Mason, S A Sadek, J Stevens, G Venkat Venkat-Raman, A Walters, M Wise

Neurology W Gibb, A M Turner

Neurophysiology W L Merton

Obstetrics and Gynaecology J R Bevan, A D Clark, D W Davies, I Golland, R R Guirgis, P Hogston, V Osgood

Paediatrics M Ashton, M J Hardman, S Peters, R Thwaites, J M Walker, E R Wozniak

Pathology R Brindle, R Buchanan, P M Cockroft, J Dhundee, P J Green, N J Marley, J Mikes, G Underhill

Radiology I M Fairley, T V Lancaster, M H MacGuire, M A A Shaltot

Radiotherapy and Oncology D J Boote, J D Dubois, P F Golding, G G Khoury, E M Low

Rehabilitation Medicine M Homer-Ward

Urology S J Chiverton, S Holmes, B H Walmsley

Preston Primary Care Trust

Preston Business Centre, Watling Street Road, Fulwood, Preston PR2 8DY
Tel: 01772 645500 Fax: 01772 220285
Email: enquiries@prestonpct.nhs.uk
Website: www.prestonpct.nhs.uk
(Cumbria and Lancashire Strategic Health Authority)

Chair Wendy Hogg
Chief Executive Jan Hewitt

Ribchester Community Hospital
Ribchester, Preston PR3 3XD
Tel: 01772 782216
Total Beds: 15

The Princess Alexandra Hospital NHS Trust

Princess Alexandra Hospital, Hamstel Road, Harlow CM20 1QX
Tel: 01279 444455 Fax: 01279 429371
Website: www.pah.nhs.uk
(Essex Strategic Health Authority)

Chair Robert Powell
Chief Executive John Gilham

Princess Alexandra Hospital
Hamstel Road, Harlow CM20 1QX
Tel: 01279 444455 Fax: 01279 429371
Total Beds: 451

Accident and Emergency K Harvey, A Saha

Anaesthetics O Akinniranye, R Cattermole, J Crossley, D Dutta, L N Iskander, A Krishnamurthy, M Michail, N Patel, J Phillips, G Raine, R Rajendram, Z Zych

Care of the Elderly A Dain, R Morgan, J Tharakan

Chest Disease J Waller, J Warren

Dermatology H Dodd

Diabetes S Beshyah

ENT A A Amen, N Flower

General Medicine J R Milne, D Preston, J Sayer, E Stoner

General Surgery H Bradpiece, M A Clifton, J Peters, J Refson

Microbiology S Visuvanathan

Neurology O Cockerell, P Martin, R Walker

Obstetrics and Gynaecology M Al-Samarrai, K El-Farra, R Hartwell, P Kumaranayakan

Oncology J Singer

Ophthalmology I Fawcett, D Flaye, V Vempali

Oral and Maxillofacial Surgery J Carter, K Coghlan, F J Evans

Orthodontics N Hay

Orthopaedics C H Aldam, P Allen, A Amini, R Hill, A Hussein, D S Nairn

Paediatrics M Ali, V Amadi, V Chakravarti, T Hla, K Nimalraj, E Thambapillai, S F Zeidan

Pathology K Agarwal, F Al-Rafaie, S Jader, J Leake, R G M Letcher, J McKenzie, V Oxley, S Thomas

Radiology C Barber, A Chauhan, S Dimmock, B Lan, J Lockwood, M Long, S Redla, T Sikdar

Rheumatology and Rehabilitation K Ahmed, J Currey

Sexual Health G Crowe

Urology B Potluri, J S Virdi

Queen Elizabeth Hospital King's Lynn NHS Trust

Formerly King's Lynn and Wisbech Hospitals NHS Trust.

Queen Elizabeth Hospital, Gayton Road, King's Lynn PE30 4ET
Tel: 01553 613613 Fax: 01553 613700
Website: www.qehkl.nhs.uk
(Norfolk, Suffolk and Cambridgeshire Strategic Health Authority)

Chair Jeffrey Prosser
Chief Executive Tony Andrews

Queen Elizabeth Hospital
Gayton Road, King's Lynn PE30 4ET
Tel: 01553 613613 Fax: 01553 613700
Total Beds: 580

Accident and Emergency N Burchett, R Florance

Anaesthetics J G Allen, A J Barclay, M Blunt, K R Burchett, N M Denny, N H Duncan, R N Francis, S J Harris, Dr Hobbiger, M Miller, M Plumley, B Watson

Care of the Elderly M S Ell, J C McGourty, J Phillips

Chemical Pathology C P C Seem

Dermatology J A R Anderson, G Dootson

ENT B P Cvijetic, P A Webber

General Medicine A Douds, E George, A M Jennings, E Kumar, K Lingam, R C McGouran, A Pawlowicz

General Psychiatry L Ho, G Isaacs, A Ogilvie, A Wagle

General Surgery P T Cullen, P Gough, R A Greatorex, N Redwood, S M Singh, H Warren

Genitourinary Medicine K Sivakumar

Haematology P B Coates, J Keidan

Histopathology R A Eames

Medical Microbiology M A Hegarty

Neurology J Brown

Obstetrics and Gynaecology S H Abukhalil, C D M Bone, S Monaghan, H M A Taher, A B W Taylor

Ophthalmology Z Butt, C Jakeman, N A Johnson, P J Pushpanathan

Oral and Maxillofacial Surgery E A Flower

Orthodontics J Bottomley

Orthopaedics N Coleman, M Gadir, J Jeffrey, A Murray, N P Packer

Paediatrics D A C Barter, J F B Dossetor, S P Rubin, M Wheatley

Radiology Q Arafat, M Crowe, G R Hunnam, M J Rimmer, M J Sparks, J Stabler, M Sultan

Radiotherapy and Oncology A Ahmad, M Daly

Rheumatology J D Williams

Urology A C Eaton

Queen Elizabeth Hospital NHS Trust

Queen Elizabeth Hospital, Stadium Road, London SE18 4QH
Tel: 020 8836 6000
Website: www.qehospital.com
(South East London Strategic Health Authority)

Chair Colin Campbell
Chief Executive John Pelly

Queen Elizabeth Hospital
Stadium Road, Woolwich, London SE18 4QH
Tel: 020 8836 6000

Accident and Emergency A-M Huggon, S Metcalf

Anaesthetics R G H Baxter, H Bretschneider, D Markovic, S Missouri, M Pannell, S J Power, S Ratnakumar, P Ravindran, S M Robertson, V Vijayakulasin, I Wijesurendra

Cardiology C Shakespeare

Dermatology P Bannerjee, A Barkley, D McGibbons

General Medicine M Ali, E Ekpo, T P George, C Gibbs, K Leball, P Marsden, A McNair, V Saxena, W Seymour, T Stokes, D Sulch, J Tremble, J Webb

General Surgery N Aston, D Heath, A Montgomery, O Oke, G Rather, M Siddiqui, K Thakur, C-Y Yiu

Genitourinary Medicine S Mitchell, J Russell

Haematology R Ireland, N Ketley

Histopathology G Menon, J M Munro, T Pinto

Obstetrics and Gynaecology S Ali, J Burch, J V L Carr, C Leitch, R MacDonald, V Palaniappan, N Perks

Orthopaedics M Eskander, F Khan, A Kumar, W Scott, S Tibrewal

Paediatrics B Al-Rubeyi, A Evans, H Issler, J Lord, K Ogbureke, G Young

Radiology N Edmonds, D Naik, S Surenthiran, Dr Wafula

Radiotherapy and Oncology B Bryant, F Calman, S Harris, Dr Landau

Renal Medicine H Cairns

Rheumatology G Coakley, L Dolan, R Price

Urology N Cetti, R Niekrash, N Sarangi

Queen Mary's Sidcup NHS Trust

Queen Mary's Hospital, Frognal Avenue, Sidcup DA14 6LT
Tel: 020 8302 2678 Fax: 020 8308 3074
(South East London Strategic Health Authority)

Chair Elizabeth Butler
Chief Executive Helen Moffatt

Erith and District Hospital

Park Crescent, Erith DA8 3EE
Tel: 020 8302 2678 Fax: 020 8308 3074

Queen Mary's Hospital

Frognal Avenue, Sidcup DA14 6LT
Tel: 020 8302 2678 Fax: 020 8308 3074
Total Beds: 430

Accident and Emergency H Hassan, K Pervaiz

Anaesthetics E Chandrad, Dr Chavda, T P Davis, T Durcan, M Fisher, Dr Ganeshan, D Harding, Dr Kumar, Dr Lee, Dr Palin, W S Rao, E Roberts, Dr Statham, Dr Sweet

Care of the Elderly Dr Abrahim, Dr Bowcock, Dr Curtis, Dr Das Gupta, R Geraghty, Dr Gould, J Kelleher, Dr Lan Smith, Dr Mehmet, Dr Parchure, Dr Rassam, S Roe, C D Shee

Dental Surgery Mr Hossein, Mr Young

Dermatology A Kagawala

ENT Dr Beg, D Golding-Wood

General Medicine D Black, I Cranston, Dr Curtis, B A Gould, Dr Ibrahim, M J Lancaster-Smith, Dr Mehmet, W N Seymour, C D Shee

General Surgery T Davies, Mr Kerwat, H Khawaja, J G Payne, Mr Reyes, T Walters

Haematology S Bowcock, S Rassam, S Ward

Medical Microbiology J Kensit

Neurology T Britton

Obstetrics and Gynaecology A Abbas, L S Hanna, Mr Irvine, Mr Seif, R Smith, Mr Waterstone, J Woolfson

Ophthalmology M Gibbens, Dr Goel, C Hugkulstone, H C Laganowski, L Lanigan, J S Shilling, L Whitefield, T Williamson

Oral Surgery K Hussain

Orthodontics D Young

Orthopaedics P Gill, T Mani, S Rao, M Rowntree, C Smart

Paediatrics W Barry, S A Bokhari, A S El-Radhi, J Sahi, I Schuller

Pathology E J A Aps, S Bowcock, J Cooper, J G Kensit, M K Khan, S Rassam

Radiology I Abdelhadi, A U Ahmed, J E Goligher, M Gotlieb, I Morgan, C G Pinder

Rheumatology and Rehabilitation A N Bamji, C Nap

Queen Victoria Hospital NHS Foundation Trust

The Queen Victoria Hospital is the regional centre for plastic surgery and burns, maxillofacial surgery and corneal surgery. Established as a Foundation Trust 01/07/2004.

Holtye Road, East Grinstead RH19 3DZ
Tel: 01342 414000 Fax: 01342 414414
Email: information@qvh.nhs.uk
Website: www.qvh.nhs.uk
(Surrey and Sussex Strategic Health Authority)

Chair Hugh Ure
Chief Executive Jan Bergman

Queen Victoria Hospital

Holtye Road, East Grinstead RH19 3DZ
Tel: 01342 410210 Fax: 01342 317907
Total Beds: 110

Anaesthetics S Fenlon (Head), C J Barham, J Curran, A Diba, J Giles, P Jones, S Krone, Y M Lam, C Lawrence, C Patel, J Sanders, K Sim, S J Squires, P Venn, N Vorster, G Wearne

Care of the Elderly T Martin (Head)

Corneo-Plastic / Oculo-Plastic Surgery S Daya (Head), R Malhotra

Dermatology S Tharakaram

ENT R V Lloyd, R J Sergeant

General Medicine R A Banks, M Kearney, R Makadsi

General Surgery A Stacey-Clear, T Williams

Histopathology J Allen (Head)

Microbiology D Lyon, B Stewart

Obstetrics and Gynaecology M Long

Ophthalmology S Daya (Head), R Malhortra

Oral and Maxillofacial Surgery A E Brown (Head), K Lavery, K Sneddon, J Tighe, P Ward-Booth

Orthodontics B Smith, A R Thom, L Winchester

Orthopaedics E J Parnell

Paediatrics C Greenaway, K Greenaway, I Lewis

Plastic Surgery P Arnstein, H R Belcher, J W Blair, J G Boorman, K W Cullen, J A Davison, B S Dheansa, P Gilbert, A R Khandwala, N Parkhouse, J Pereira, M Pickford, F Schönauer, R Smith, T C Teo

Psychiatry A Begg, A Shetty

Radiology N Anderson, N B Bowley

Rheumatology R Makadsi

Queen's Medical Centre, Nottingham University Hospital NHS Trust

Derby Road, Nottingham NG7 2UH
Tel: 0115 924 9924 Fax: 0115 970 9196
Email: forename.surname@qmc.nhs.uk
Website: www.qmc.nhs.uk
(Trent Strategic Health Authority)

Chair Ted Cantle
Chief Executive John MacDonald

University Hospital

Queen's Medical Centre, Nottingham NG7 2UH
Tel: 0115 924 9924 Fax: 0115 970 9196
Total Beds: 1366

Accident and Emergency F Coffey, R Dar, A F Dove, D A Esberger, L N Jarrett, S Smith, D Vickery, L Williams

Anaesthetics C A Abercrombie, A R Aitkenhead, P Bachra, B Baxendale, N Bedforth, M Bennet, M Brown, A J Byrne, I M Creighton, J Eastwood, J Emery, K George, C Gornall, S Hancock, J Hardman, J Harris, J C Haycock, G Hobbs, A Hutchinson, A D Jardine, J M Lamb, D J Layfield, D Levy, M C Luxton, S Markham, P Martin, A J Matthews, M H Nathanson, L Neale, J M Nicoll, A Norris, R Nowicki, N I Palmer, H Parekh, M F Reid, P A Tomlinson, P Veale, J E H Ward, P M Yeoman

Care of the Elderly C Gaynor, J R F Gladman, N P Kumar, R M Kupfer, J D Morrant, O Sahota, D Seddon

Child Health M Hewitt, N Marlow, L Polnay, J Punt, N Rutter, T J Stephenson, M Vloeberghs

Dermatology J L Bong, J S C English, S M Littlewood, L G Millard, W Perkins, J Ravenscroft, E M Saihan, S Varma, H C Williams

ENT N Beasley, J P Birchall, P J Bradley, K P Gibbin, N S Jones, J A McGlashan, T Meehan, G M O'Donoghue, A Sama

General Medicine G Aithal, J Atherton, T Bowling, J Corne, M Culshaw, C Fraser-Moodie, A Gazis, T Gray, I P Hall, A Harcombe, C J Hawkey, A Jawhari, S Johnson, I D A Johnston, R Kennedy, W J M Kinnear, P C Lanyon, R F A Logan, Y R Mahida, P I Mansell, S R Page, R J Powell, K Raghunath, P Rubin, S D Ryder, R C Spiller, A Staniforth, T J Walsh, S Wharton, R G Wilcox

General Surgery J F Abercrombie, N C M Armitage, T W Balfour, I J Beckingham, J B Bourke, B D Braithwaite, S N Chandrasekar, J Doran, D Lobo, M S T MacSweeney, C Maxwell-Armstrong, M H Robinson, B J Rowlands, J Scholefield, W G Tennant, P W Wenham, J P Williams

Haematology G Dolan, K Forman, A Macmillan, D Myers

Histopathology R Alliborne, P D James, P V Kaye, K Kulkarni, I H Leach, S J Lee, J S Lowe, D O'Neill, C J H Padfield, D K Robson, A M Zaitoun

Immunology E M C Dermott, R J Powell, H F Sewell

Medical Microbiology O Ala' Aldeen, T Boswell, F Donald, W Irving, P J Jenks, R Madeley, S F Pugh, R C B Slack, S Soo, D Turner, V C Weston

Neurology N Bajaj, C Constantinescu, M Himberstone, P Madison, M F O'Donaghue, A M Whiteley, A Wills

Neuropathology J S Lowe, K Robson

Neurophysiology P Choudhary, N J Smith

Neurosurgery R Ashpole, P O Byrne, M Cartmill, D T Hope, D Macarthur, I J A Robertson, M Vloeberghs, B D White

Obstetrics and Gynaecology W Atiomo, P T Edington, G M Filshie, J Gardosi, R H Hammond, J F Hopkinson, D K James, I R Johnson, R Kazem, O A I Kuran, M B A Macpherson, M C Powell, M Ramsay, J Rutherford

Occupational Health F Curran, D J Fox

Ophthalmology L C Abercrombie, W M K Amoaku, H S Dua, A J Foss, R M Gregson, A King, C S Lim, G M Orr, S A Vernon, A G Zaman

Oral and Maxillofacial Surgery S A Clark, P Hollows, I McVicar, R R Nashed, J E Rowson, A Sidebottom

Orthodontics R R Nashed

Orthopaedics M Batt, J Chell, T R C Davis, S Dhar, N Downing, I W Forster, D Hahn, K Hassan, B J Holdsworth, C J Howell, J B Hunter, P James, A R J Manktelow, P Manning, C G Moran, J Oni, P J Radford, B Scammell, E P Szypryt, A Taylor, W Wallis

Paediatric Surgery B Davies, C H Rance, M Shenoy, R Singh, R J Stewart

Paediatrics C P J Charlton, J Grant, M Hewitt, D I Johnson, D Mellor, D Thomas, H Vyas

Pathology J Gomez, P Prinsloo

Radiology S S Amar, N Broderick, S Dawson, W Dunn, R H S Gregson, K Halliday, I M Holland, T Jaspan, Dr Kersake, Dr Ludman, Dr McConachie, A Moody, B J Preston, J Somers, P Twining, M L Wastie, Dr Whitaker

Reading Primary Care Trust

57-59 Bath Road, Reading RG30 2BA
Tel: 0118 950 3094 Fax: 0118 982 2914
Email: toni.lock@berkshire.nhs.uk
Website: www.berkshire.nhs.uk/reading
(Thames Valley Strategic Health Authority)

Chair Colin Pincombe
Chief Executive Janet Fitzgerald

Dellwood Community Hospital

22 Liebenrood Road, Reading RG30 2DX
Tel: 0118 958 9195 Fax: 0118 959 1217
Total Beds: 43

Redbridge Primary Care Trust

Beckett House, 2-14 Ilford Hill, Ilford IG1 2QX
Tel: 020 8478 5151 Fax: 020 8926 5001
Email: info@redbridge-pct.nhs.uk
Website: www.redbridgepct.nhs.uk
(North East London Strategic Health Authority)

Chair Edwin Doyle
Chief Executive Heather O'Meara

Redditch and Bromsgrove Primary Care Trust

Crossgate House, Crossgate Road, Park Farm Industrial Estate, Redditch B98 7SN
Tel: 01527 507040 Fax: 01527 507041
Email: pct@redditchbromsgrove-pct.nhs.uk
Website: www.randb-pct.nhs.uk
(West Midlands South Strategic Health Authority)

Chair Graham Vickery
Chief Executive Eamonn Kelly

Princess of Wales Community Hospital

Stourbridge Road, Bromsgrove B61 0BB
Tel: 01527 488000 Fax: 01527 488035

Richmond and Twickenham Primary Care Trust

Thames House, 180 High Street, Teddington TW11 8HU
Tel: 020 8973 3000 Fax: 020 8973 3001
Email: firstname.surname@rtpct.nhs.uk
Website: www.richmondandtwickenham.nhs.uk
(South West London Strategic Health Authority)

Chair Sian Bates
Chief Executive Joan Mager

Teddington Memorial Hospital

Hampton Road, Teddington TW11 0JL
Tel: 020 8408 8210 Fax: 020 8408 8213
Total Beds: 50

Manager Jill Downey

Robert Jones and Agnes Hunt Orthopaedic and District Hospital NHS Trust

Gobowen, Oswestry SY10 7AG
Tel: 01691 404000 Fax: 01691 404066
Website: www.rjah.nhs.uk
(Shropshire and Staffordshire Strategic Health Authority)

Chair Michael Bolderston
Chief Executive Jackie Daniel

Robert Jones and Agnes Hunt Orthopaedic Hospital

Oswestry SY10 7AG
Tel: 01691 404000 Fax: 01691 404050
Total Beds: 227

Anaesthetics R Alcock (Head), C Emmett, B Morgan, P M Pfeifer, S Ray

Care of the Elderly Dr Shu Ho

General Medicine M Davie, L Hill, S Hill

General Surgery A Fox, A Schofield

Gynaecology D Redford, S Robinson, A Tapp

Histopathology D C Mangham, J McClure

Neurology G Cole, S Ellis, C Hawkins

Neurophysiology T G Staunton

Orthopaedics P Cool, S Eisenstein, W El Masry, G A Evans, D Ford, P Gregson, S Hay, M J S Hubbard, D C Jaffray, A Jamieson, C Kelly, P Laing, K Lewis, N Makwana, C M McGeoch, J H Patrick, D Rees, J Richardson, A Roberts, S Roberts, D Short, R Spencer-Jones, S White, D H Williams

Paediatrics G A Evans, J Patrick, R Quinlivan, A Roberts

Plastic Surgery J Roberts

Radiology I W McCall, V Pullicino, P Tyrell

Respiratory Medicine R Wilson

Rheumatology R G Butler, J J Dixey

Rochdale Primary Care Trust

164-166 Yorkshire Street, Rochdale OL16 2DL
Tel: 01706 652430 Fax: 01706 632153
Email: firstname.lastname@rochdale.pct.nhs.uk
(Greater Manchester Strategic Health Authority)

Chair Debbie Abrahams
Chief Executive Trevor Purt

Rotherham General Hospitals NHS Trust

Rotherham District General Hospital, Moorgate Road, Oakwood, Rotherham S60 2UD
Tel: 01709 820000 Fax: 01709 304200
Website: www.rotherhamhospital.trent.nhs.uk
(South Yorkshire Strategic Health Authority)

Chair Margaret Oldfield
Chief Executive Paul Nesbitt

Rotherham District General Hospital

Moorgate Road, Rotherham S60 2UD
Tel: 01709 820000 Fax: 01709 304303
Total Beds: 860

Accident and Emergency N Chopra, F L P Heyes

Anaesthetics I Allyon, A Blackburn, V Boyd, A E Cooper, P Dobbs, I C Grant, P J Matthews, M Miller, D M Newby, K Ruiz, R K Stacey, E Taylor, D Warling, M Withey

Care of the Elderly Dr Al-Modarus, M K Ghosh, J O Kwera, B K Mondal

Dermatology M E Kessler, A Muncaster, M L Wood

ENT L Durham, P Harkness, J M Lancer

General Medicine K D Bardhan, P A Bardsley, G S Basran, G Knight, R Muthusamy, S Muzuw, M Prasad, N Qureshi, Dr Soo, P Willemse

General Surgery M Bassuini, J C Cooper, R B Jones, M Lambertz, J Rochester

Genitourinary Medicine T Kyi, A Wright

Obstetrics and Gynaecology D W Fenton, A Kumar, K Lingham, D Patel, C Ramsden, S F Spooner

Occupational Health B Platts

Ophthalmology R Croasier, MR El-Bably, A Gashut, Mr Gerges, Mr Husain, M Jabir, A Mishra, A A Zaidi

Oral and Maxillofacial Surgery P G McAndrew

Orthodontics W L Yap

Orthopaedics M Bhamra, I Chakrabartii, K Ratnakumar, A J S Rees, M J Robson, M M Zaman

Paediatrics S El-Refee, C Harrison, P I MacFarlane, J Mahajan, S Suri

Pathology H Barker, L Harvey, J Lee, R Lord, T Marshall, P C Taylor

Radiology Dr Chua, P Spencer, S Varkey

Rheumatology and Rehabilitation F Fawthres, M E Holt, G Smith

Thoracic Surgery J A C Thorpe

Urology A Ehattack, B T Paeys

Rotherham General Hospital Day Surgery Centre

Moorgate Road, Rotherham S60 3AJ
Tel: 01709 820000 ext: 4560/4565/5906 Fax: 01709 304563

Rotherham Primary Care Trust

Oak House, Moorhead Way, Bramley, Rotherham S66 1YY
Tel: 01709 302000 Fax: 01709 302002
Email: health.enquiries@rotherhampct.nhs.uk
Website: www.rotherhampct.nhs.uk
(South Yorkshire Strategic Health Authority)

Chair Alan Tolhurst
Chief Executive John McIvor

Doncaster Gate Hospital
Doncaster Gate, Rotherham S65 1DW
Tel: 01709 304802

Rowley Regis and Tipton Primary Care Trust

Kingston House, 438-450 High Street, West Bromwich B70 9LD
Tel: 0121 500 1500 Fax: 0121 500 1501
Website: www.rrt-pct.org.uk
(Birmingham and the Black Country Strategic Health Authority)

Chair Doug Round
Chief Executive Geraint Griffiths

Royal Berkshire Ambulance NHS Trust

44 Finchampstead Road, Wokingham RG40 2NN
Tel: 0118 936 5500 Fax: 0118 977 3923
Website: www.rbat.com
(Thames Valley Strategic Health Authority)

Chair Keith Kerr
Chief Executive Ian Ferguson

Royal Berkshire and Battle Hospitals NHS Trust

Royal Berkshire Hospital, London Road, Reading RG1 5AN
Tel: 0118 987 5111 Fax: 0118 987 8042
Email: forename.surname@rbbh-tr.nhs.uk
Website: www.rbbh.nhs.uk
(Thames Valley Strategic Health Authority)

Chair Colin Maclean
Chief Executive Anne Sheen

Battle Hospital
Oxford Road, Reading RG3 1AG
Tel: 0118 987 5111
Total Beds: 274

Care of the Elderly M W Pearson, A Van Wyk

General Medicine J A Bell, N Spyrou

Neurology R Gregory, N Hyman

Paediatrics H A Curtis, S M Wallis

Rehabilitation Medicine C Collin

Respiratory Medicine C Davies, J Thomas

Rheumatology A Bradlow, J D McNally

Prince Charles Eye Unit
King Edward VII Hospital, St Leonard's Road, Windsor SL4 3DP
Tel: 01753 860441

Royal Berkshire Hospital
London Road, Reading RG1 5AN
Tel: 0118 987 5111
Total Beds: 508

Accident and Emergency M Dudek, P Farrugia, S Soysa

Anaesthetics S C Allen, K J Bird, J Collie, C M Danbury, P C Dill-Russel, M C Ewart, J Fielden, R M Hall, F Idrees, R H Jago, R Jones, A Kapila, A J Kitching, K E Krzeminska, K Machlachlan, J W MacKenzie, T Parke, M Rimmer, C Verghese, C S Waldmann, L Worthington

Biochemistry G Challand, G Lester, D Williams

Chemical Pathology D L Williams

Clinical Oncology J M Barrett, C D C Charlton, A Freehairn, J Q Gildersleve, P Rogers

Dermatology C Higgins, J Holder, M P James

ENT W Colquhoun-Flannery, R Herdman, N J Mansell, N J Marks

General Medicine J Booth, M F El Shieikh, A S Mee, M Myszor, R B Naik, J D Simmons, H C R Simpson

General Surgery S P Courtney, T C B Dehn, R G Faber, R Farouk, R B Galland, T R Magee, S B Middleton, H Reece-Smith, H N Umeh

Genitourinary Medicine S Rajamanoharan, A Tang

Haematology F Brito-Babapulle, H Grech, G R Morganstern

Histopathology L W L Horton, C J McCormick, R A Menai Williams, T Saleem

Obstetrics and Gynaecology H A Allott, A M Crystal, J O Greenhalf, E M Holt, M Selinger, J Siddall-Allum, K M Smith, P Street, R M Williams

Occupational Health A Ross

Ophthalmology A S Bacon, B M Billington, P Constable, M Leyland, A R Pearson, V Tanner

Oral Surgery M F Patel, C D C Tomlins

Orthodontics D Bryan, C R Harper

Orthopaedics S A Copeland, R D A Dodds, C M Fergusson, O Levy, R W Marshall, I M Nugent, S T O'Leary, C A Pailthorpe, S Tavares, A E G Themen

Paediatrics A W Boon, M J Clements, S Edees, A Gordon, A J Macrae, N P Mann, C L Newman

Radiology A Brown, N D J Derbyshire, E Elson, M Gibson, C I Meanock, N S Rahim, R S C Robertson, E P H Torrie, T M Walker

Urology D Fawcett, P Malone, H N Whitfield

The Royal Bournemouth and Christchurch Hospitals NHS Foundation Trust

Established as a Foundation Trust 01/04/2005.

Royal Bournemouth Hospital, Castle Lane East, Bournemouth BH7 7DW
Tel: 01202 303626 Fax: 01202 704077
Website: www.rbh.org.uk
(Dorset and Somerset Strategic Health Authority)

Chair Sheila Collins
Chief Executive Tony Spotswood

Christchurch Hospital
Christchurch BH23 2JX
Tel: 01202 486361 Fax: 01202 705225
Total Beds: 210

Manager S Edington

Care of the Elderly S C Allen, K Amar, D Jenkinson, Z Rana

Dermatology P G Goodwin, M Hazell

Palliative Medicine F M Randall

Radiology M Andreas, R Bull, T S Creasy, B Donnellan, A Drury, S N Jones, D F C Shepherd, J Sheridan, J Small, J D Stevenson, D J Tawn

Rheumatology and Rehabilitation C Dunne, N D Hopkinson, K Mounce, B Quilty

Royal Bournemouth Hospital

Castle Lane East, Bournemouth BH7 7DW
Tel: 01202 303626 Fax: 01202 704077
Total Beds: 694

Accident and Emergency G Cumberbatch, K Hassan, A Lelo

Anaesthetics D M Dickson, R P H Dunnill, D M Hargreaves, P Lanham, M Michel, N S Milligan, J K Myatt, M P Rafferty, M Schuster-Bruce, A D Scott, M J Whittle

Dermatology P G Goodwin, M Hazel

General Medicine S C Allen, K Amar, M Armitage, D A Cavan, D Jenkinson, D Kerr, J Radvan, Z Rana, A Rozkovec, J Turner, A J Williams, P Winwood

General Surgery D Bennett, S G Darke, N Davies, J B F Fozard, R J Lawrance, S D Parvin, A I Skene, L Wijesinghe

Genitourinary Medicine A H de Silva, M J Hayward, B Herieka

Obstetrics and Gynaecology A J Evans, R J Henry, J S Pampiglione

Ophthalmology C R Davison, A M Denning, D E Etchells, H J Franks, C S Marsh, B N Matthews, A H Morris, B T Parkin, S A Rowley

Oral and Maxillofacial Surgery A F Markus, W J N Peters

Orthodontics J F Hodgkins, S Power, M Short

Pathology T J Hamblin, M Lesna, D G Oscier, D M C Parham

Radiology M Andress, R Bull, T S Creasey, B Donnellan, A Drury, S N Jones, D F C Shepherd, J Sheridan, J Small, J D Stevenson, D J Tawn

Rheumatology and Rehabilitation N D Hopkinson

Urology F J Bramble, C J Carter, J S Rundle, A Wedderburn

Royal Brompton and Harefield NHS Trust

Sydney Street, London SW3 6NP
Tel: 020 7352 8121 Fax: 020 7351 8473
Website: www.rbh.nthames.nhs.uk
(North West London Strategic Health Authority)

Chair Lord Newton of Braintree
Chief Executive Gareth Goodier

Harefield Hospital

Harefield, Uxbridge UB9 6JH
Tel: 01895 823737 Fax: 01895 822870
Total Beds: 184

Manager Robert Craig

Anaesthetics M J Boscoe, J Farrimond, S George, S Kamath, J Mitchell, D Royston, C Walker, C Wall, G Wright

Cardiology N Banner, M Barbir, M Dubowitz, R Grocott-Mason, C Ilsley, M Mason, A Mitchell, W Wallis

Cardiothoracic Surgery M Amrani, G Dreyfus, W Fountain, J Gaer, A Khaghani, O Maiwand, S Tadjkarimi, E Townend

Chest Medicine D Evans, A Nath, P Studdy

Nephrology F D Thompson

Paediatrics R D G Franklin, R C Radley-Smith

Palliative Medicine L Bangham

Pathology M Burke, D Cummins, A Hall

Radiology A Kelion, T Mittal, J Partridge

Thoracic Surgery S W Fountain, O Maiwand, E R Townsend

Royal Brompton Hospital

Sydney Street, London SW3 6NP
Tel: 020 7352 8121 Fax: 020 7351 8473
Total Beds: 300

Manager Patrick Mitchell

Anaesthetics J Cordingly, T Evans, K Fogg, C Gillbe, J W W Gothard, M Griffiths, E Haxby, D Hunter, S Jagger, A Kelleher, B Keogh, C J Morgan, M J Scallan, R Stenz

Cardiology A Bishop, C Brookes, J Clague, A Coats, P Collins, M Cowie, S Davies, M Flather, K M Fox, M Gatzoulis, M Henein, S Kaddoura, M Mullen, P J Oldershaw, P Poole-Wilson, A F Rickards, R Sutton

Cardiothoracic Surgery A De Souza, M Dusmet, P Goldstraw, G Ladas, N Moat, J R Pepper, P Sarkar, D Shore

ENT I S Mackay

Intensive Care R Peters

Paediatrics I Balfour-Lynn, Dr Buchdahl, M Burmeister, A Bush, J Carvalho, Dr Daubeney, J Davies, H Gardiner, L Gerlis, H La Rovere, J Larovere, D Macrae, A Magee, M L Rigby, M Rosenthal, Z Salvik, B Sethia, E A Shinebourne, J Till

Pathology J Burman, R J L Hooper, J Kerr, A Nicholson, M Sheppard

Radiology C Anagnostopoulos, D Carr, D M Hansell, P Kilner, Dr Mohiaddin, V Naidoo, D Pennell, M B Rubens, S R Underwood, A Van Aswegan

Respiratory Medicine E Alton, P Barnes, R D Bois, K F Chung, J V Collins, T Cullinan, S Durham, T Evans, D M Geddes, M Green, M Hodson, A B Kay, D N Mitchell, A J Newman-Taylor, J Pfeffer, M Polkey, D Robinson, P Shah, A Simonds, M Stern, A Wells, R Wilson

Royal Cornwall Hospitals NHS Trust

Royal Cornwall Hospital (Treliske), Bedruthen House, Truro TR1 3LJ
Tel: 01872 250000 Fax: 01872 252708
Website: www.cornwall.nhs.uk/rcht
(South West Peninsula Strategic Health Authority)

Chair Angela Alderman
Chief Executive Brian Milstead

Royal Cornwall Hospital

Truro TR1 3LJ
Tel: 01872 250000 Fax: 01872 252708
Total Beds: 1020

Accident and Emergency S Barron, M A Hocking, P A W Howarth, J P Wyatt

Anaesthetics J A Boyden, S Currie, M V Daniels, A E Dingwall, W H Fish, M K Freeman, F J Griffiths, R A Harrison, C R Harvey, W R Harvey, A J Hobbs, P Hopton, L M Jakt, W E Jewell, R J Mawer, M D Mitchell, A More, G A R Morgan, R J E Page, A M Pickford, J F Powell, J E Pring, C J Ralph, P A Rich, G M Saville, J R Sinclair, T A Skinner, P M Upton, A K Y Walker, P Waterhouse, A M Weiss, W M Woodward, S D Wragg

Cardiology M R D Belham, S J Evans, R T Johnston, A J Mourant, P Owens, A K B Slade

Care of the Elderly M Battle, R Bland, F Boyd, J A Evers, D G MacMahon, S Renwick, I Swithinbank

Dermatology P W Boweres, T A Chave, K Dalziel, T W Lucke, S Woodrow

General Medicine C M Asplin, J N Barnes, I I Coutts, H R Dalton, J W Foote, L Hosking, S H Hussaini, P A Johnston, D F Levine, J D Myers, R G Parry, J Stratton

General Surgery R Bourne, J N Davies, H U Desmarowitz, E R V Lloyd-Davies, P M Peyser, C R K Rickford, A L Widdison, K R Woodburn

Neurology B N McLean, S Smith, J Stewart

Obstetrics and Gynaecology S A Bates, D L Byrne, P J Callen, S R Grant, R P Holmes, K R Jones, J Lord, A Oladipo

Ophthalmology W A F Carruthers, S Kumaravel, A J Stockwell, W H Westlake, N J Wilson-Holt

Oral and Maxillofacial Surgery S D Adcock, C Lansley

Orthopaedics D J Bracey, J Dainton, E D Fern, P M Hutchins, R J Kincaid, A S Lee, M R Norton, S W Parsons, M W Regan, T D Scott, S Smith, J H Wilson

Otolaryngology P M Flanagan, I M Smith, D J Whinney, A D Wilde

Paediatrics S Daud, N Gilbertson, S M Harris, Y Kumar, Y P Kumar, J P Lewis, P F Munyard, A T Prendiville, R Spork, G R Taylor, J M Topley, M A Wooldridge

Palliative Medicine S P Ife

Pathology M D Creagh, S J Fleming, M Jenkins, H Jones, R J Marshall, J Matthew, R W Pitcher, Y Sivathondan

Plastic Surgery R J Morris

Radiology H E Belcher, P G Cook, A Edwards, K Farmer, R Farrow, J H O Hancock, N D Hollings, J S Hyslop, C M Ivory, G F Maskell, S Mohammed, J Pollock, W H Smith, W H Smith, T V Sulkin, S Sutton, S V Thorogood, S J Travis

Rheumatology and Rehabilitation M J Davis, D Hutchinson, J Morgan, A D Woolf

Urology R Cox, J S O'Rourke, R G Willis

St Michael's Hospital

Trelissick Road, Hayle TR27 4JA
Tel: 01736 753234 Fax: 01736 753344
Total Beds: 69

West Cornwall Hospital

Clare Street, Penzance TR18 2PF
Tel: 01736 874000 Fax: 01736 874081
Total Beds: 110

General Medicine M C Abban, C M Asplin, D Levine

General Surgery P J Cox, M MacKenzie, A G Paterson, K R Woodburn

Royal Devon and Exeter NHS Foundation Trust

Established as a Foundation Trust 01/04/2004.
Barrack Road, Exeter EX2 5DW
Tel: 01392 411611
Website: www.rdehospital.nhs.uk
(South West Peninsula Strategic Health Authority)

Chair Ruth Hawker
Chief Executive Angela Pedder

Royal Devon and Exeter Hospital

Barrack Road, Exeter EX2 5DW
Tel: 01392 411611 Fax: 01392 402067
Total Beds: 850

Accident and Emergency A R Harris (Head), C McLauchlan

Anaesthetics K Allman, P K Ballard, C Berry, R W Boaden, D A Conn, M Daugherty, C Day, A Dow, E Hammond, E Hartsilver, P MacIntyre, F P F Marshall, J Munn, J Pittman, J Purday, F L Roberts, J M Saddler, D Sanders, B K Sandhar, A Teasdale, R J Telford, P Thomas, I H Wilson

Cardiology L D Smith (Head), J Dean, M Gandhi, C Rinaldi

Care of the Elderly S Harris, M James, M Jeffries, V R Pearce

Chemical Pathology M Salzman

Clinical Genetics C Brewer, J Rankin

Clinical Oncology P Bliss, A Goodman, A Hong, C G Rowland, D Sheehan, E Toy

Dermatology C Bower, A P Warin

Emergency Medicine A Harris (Head), C McLauchan

General Medicine R Ayres, M Beaman, J Christie, M Daly, T K Daneshmend, R D'Souza, A Hattersley, K Macleod, A J Nicholls

General Surgery B Campbell, M J Cooper, A Cowan, J Dunn, A Gie, T T Irvin, A J S Knox, J F Thompson

Genitourinary Medicine I Alexander, G D Morrison

Haematology M V Joyner, R Lee, M Pocock, C Rudin

Medical Microbiology A Colville, M Morgan, T Riordan

Medical Oncology M Napier

Neurological Rehabilitation D Footitt

Neurology C Gardner-Thorpe, N J Gutowski, W P Honan

Neurophysiology E Ragi

Obstetrics and Gynaecology J West (Head), N Colley, N Liversedge, J Renninson, R Sturley

Occupational Medicine A Rossiter

Ophthalmology D Byles, J S H Jacob, A Quinn, P R Simcock, G Sturrock

Oral Surgery A V Babajews, A McLennan

Orthodontics M Moore (Head), K M Postlewaite

Orthopaedics T D Bunker, D Chan, P Cox, K Eyres, G A Gie, N Giles, M Hubble, C D Jefferiss, P Schranz, I Sharpe, J Timperley, C R Weatherley

Otolaryngology R Garth (Head), A Brightwell, M Hilton, G Werier

Paediatrics A Collinson, C Hayes, C Holme, S Imong, V Lewis, A McNinch, P Oades, M W Quinn, R Smith, J H Tripp

Palliative Medicine J F Gilbert, M Ryan

Pathology T Clarke, N Cope, C Day, C Keen, C Mason, P MuCullagh, P Sarsfield, R H W Simpson

Plastic Surgery V Devaraj, C J Palmer, P J Saxby, C Stone

Radiology C R B Bayliss, J Coote, L Gellett, C Hamilton-Wood, J Harington, S Harries, D C Kinsella, C Pinder, D Silver, A Spiers, M R Thomas, A Watkinson

Respiratory Medicine D Halpin, C Sheldon, N Withers

Rheumatology R Haigh, R Jacoby

Thoracic Surgery R Berrisford

Urology M Crundwell, R D Pocock, M A Stott

Royal Free Hampstead NHS Trust

Pond Street, London NW3 2QG
Tel: 020 7794 0500 Fax: 020 7830 2468
Email: forename.surname@royalfree.nhs.uk
Website: www.royalfree.nhs.uk
(North Central London Strategic Health Authority)

Chair Pamela Chesters
Chief Executive Martin Else

Queen Mary's House
124 Heath Street, Hampstead, London NW3 1DU
Tel: 020 7431 4111 Fax: 020 7830 2020
Total Beds: 101

Royal Free Hospital
Pond Street, London NW3 2QG
Tel: 020 7794 0500 Fax: 020 7830 2468
Total Beds: 950

Manager Martin Else
Accident and Emergency P Belsham, A Fogarty, A Martin, K Whitwell
Anaesthetics S Shaw (Head), B Agarwal, C Beard, P Berry, I Calder, S Charlton, G Collee, J Cooper, L Dinner, A England, A Evans, R Fernando, T Gruning, S Harrison, B D Higgs, J Howard, D Jackson, S Mallett, W Marchant, R Marks, A J Ordman, T Peachey, M S Pegg, P Pemberton, N Randhawa, S Renwick, J Robinson, J Ruddock, J Ruston, R Simons, L Vella, J Watts

Cardiology G Coghlan, J Davar, T R Evans, D Lipkin

Cardiothoracic Surgery R Walesby

Child and Adolescent Psychiatry M Berelowitz

Child and Family Development A Stein

Clinical Biochemistry D Mikhailidis, D Nair

Dermatology F Child, S McBride, C Orteu, M H A Rustin

ENT H M Caulfield, R Quiney, G Radcliffe, M Stearns

General Medicine S Al-Damluji, M Beckles, P-M Bouloux, A K Burroughs, M Caplin, J S Dooley, G Dusheiko, O Epstein, L Fine, M Hamilton, M Harbord, P N Hawkins, M Hennessy, H Hodgson, I James, M Johnson, S Keshav, M Lipman, N McIntyre, K Moore, M Y Morgan, D Patch, M Pepys, R Pounder, M Press, G Prevelic, M Vanderpump

General Psychiatry A S Bird, M Blanchard, L Caparroita, S Jeffreys, M King, G Lloyd, A McNaught, P Raven, P Robinson

General Surgery D M Baker, B Davidson, T Davidson, O Fafemi, B Fernando, G Hamilton, A A M Lewis, R Lord, F P Myint, G Ogunbiyi, S P Parbhoo, N Roche, K Rolles, D Wheeler, M Winslet

Genitourinary Medicine G Gabriel, D Ivens, A Nageswaran

Haematology S Brown, A Fielding, C Lee, S Mackinnon, A B Mehta, G Miflin, D Perry, C Taylor

Elderly Care A Davies, D Lee, J Morris, S Stone, A Wu

Histopathology J C Crow

Immunology P Amlot, G Janossy, L Poulter, D Webster

Infectious Diseases B Bannister, S Bhagani, I Cropley

Medical Microbiology S H Gillespie

Medical Physics J Agnew

Nephrology A Burns, J Cross, A Davenport, H S Powis, P Sweny, D Wheeler

Neurology H Angus-Leppan, J V Bowler, R E Brenner, C A Davie, A N Gale, J Gibbs, L Ginsberg, D P C Kidd, R W Orrell, L M Parsons, A H V Schapira, T T Warner, P M Watts, L A Wilson, R J S Wise

Neurophysiology M Al-Khayatt, R M Sherratt, B D Youl

Neurosurgery R Bradford, N L Dorward, R S Maurice-Williams, C L Shieff

Nuclear Medicine J R Buscombe, A Hilson

Obstetrics and Gynaecology D L Economides, H Evans, P J J-Hardiman, R Kadir, A B MacLean, A L Magos, S Radhakrishnan, W M N Reid, E M Scott, S M Tuck, P G Walker

Occupational Medicine S Williams

Ophthalmology J D Brazier, C C Davey, J E Forbes, M Harris, J D Jagger, J M M Lawson, B C Little, B Mulholland

Orthopaedics P M Ahrens, G S E Dowd, D M Eastwood, N I Garlick, N J Goddard

Paediatrics D V M Acolet, M W Greenberg, R B Heuschkel, A Lloyd-Evans, B W Lloyd, S H Murch, A G Sutcliffe, B W Taylor, V H van Someren

Palliative Medicine A J Tookman

Pathology M Thomas, D Webster

Plastic Surgery M D Brough, P E M Butler, D C Floyd, P L Malucci, S J Withey

Radiology J R G Bell, L A Berger, J R Cleverley, N H Davies, S Edwards, J A Haddock, J Hinton, B J Holloway, A D Platts, L E Savy, J M Tibballs, A R Valentine, T Wilhelm

Rheumatology H L C Beynon, C M Black, C P Denton, P N Hawkins

Thoracic Medicine M A Beckles, J P Dilworth, M Johnson, M C I Lipman

Urology M Al-Akraa, A V Kaisary, R J Morgan

Virology P D Griffiths

Royal National Throat, Nose and Ear Hospital
Gray's Inn Road, London WC1X 8DA
Tel: 020 7915 1300 Fax: 020 7833 5518
Total Beds: 51

Manager Rob Smith

Allergy G Scadding

Anaesthetics P Bailey, D H Enderby, C Ferguson, A Fowler, B O'Donoghue, A Patel, N Randhawa, J Ruddock

Audiological Medicine R Alles, K Harrop-Griffiths, D Lim, D Lucas, B MacArdle, R Palaniapan

ENT L Badia, G B Brookes, D Choa, C East, J Graham, H Grant, D Howard, T Joseph, B Kotecha, J Lary, V Lund, P O'Flynn, J Rubin, A Shaidar, A Wright

General Psychiatry M Greenberg

Paediatrics M Bellman

Radiology L Savy

Royal Liverpool and Broadgreen University Hospitals NHS Trust

Prescot Street, Liverpool L7 8XP
Tel: 0151 706 2000 Fax: 0151 706 5806
Email: forename.surname@rlbuht-tr.nwest.nhs.uk
Website: www.rlbuht.nhs.uk
(Cheshire and Merseyside Strategic Health Authority)

Chair Roger James
Chief Executive Maggie Boyle

Broadgreen Hospital
Thomas Drive, Liverpool L14 3LB
Tel: 0151 706 2000

Total Beds: 310

Anaesthetics G Bardosi, D D Brice, R Dodd, L Fahy, B G Murthy, A Roitberg-Henry

Biochemistry A Stott

Care of the Elderly N Carroll, G Phillips, J R Playfer

Dermatology R Azurdia, C King, R Parslew, G R Sharpe, N Wilson

Gastroenterology A Ellis, H Smart

General Medicine R C Bucknall, P C Deegan, T Dixon, M Fisher, D Glynne-Thomas, I Hart, J Hobbs, M Walshaw

General Surgery P Carter, M N Hartley, W Lloyd-Jones

Orthopaedics W A Jones, D H Miller, A Taylor, C R Walker

Pathology P Chu

Radiology D A Gould, C Ryall

Urology A D Desmond, M Fordham

Royal Liverpool University Dental Hospital

Pembroke Place, Liverpool L3 5PS
Tel: 0151 706 2000

Anaesthetics D D Brice, P Jarvis, G Lamplugh

Medical Microbiology M V Martin

Oral and Maxillofacial Surgery P Hardy, E D Vaughan

Oral Medicine E A Field

Oral Pathology J Scott, J Woolgar

Oral Surgery J S Brown, G T R Lee, D R Llewelyn, O A Pospisil, D Richardson, J Scott

Orthodontics N Pender, S J Rudge, J Warren-Jones

Plastic Surgery A R Green, L A Holbrook

Radiology J B Hutton

Restorative Dentistry D Adams, J Cunningham, R A Howell, K S Last, M Lennon, L P Longman, T Nisbet, A Watts

Royal Liverpool University Hospital

Prescot Street, Liverpool L7 8XP
Tel: 0151 706 2000
Total Beds: 911

Accident and Emergency P Burdett-Smith, L H Jaffey

Anaesthetics E J T Allsop, L Bardosi, M W Davies, S J Harper, J M Hunter, A G Jones, A Leach, S Mallaiah, G J Masterson, P L Misra, S M Mostafa, B V S Murthy, C Parker, B J Phillips, T D R Ryan, T Sajjad, R Wenstone, R G Wilkes

Care of the Elderly N Carroll, C I A Jack, G Phillips, J R Playfer

Chemical Pathology W D Fraser, G J Kemp, E M C Manning, A Shenkin

Dermatology C M King, G R Sharpe

Endocrinology J P Vora

General Medicine G M Bell, J M Bone, R C Bucknall, T A Dixon, J E Ellershaw, A J Ellis, I H Ellis, C C Evans, A Fryer, C F Gilks, I T Gilmore, M Hommel, M G Lombard, M Molyneux, A I Morris, M Pirmohamed, T S Purewal, J Rhodes, S S Saltissi, J M Skinner, H L Smart, D H Smith, S B Squire, E J Tunn, M J Walshaw, H M Warenius, T Whalley, E Williams, P S Williams, P A Winstanley

General Surgery A Bakran, J A Brennan, G L Gilling-Smith, P L Harris, M N Hartley, M J Hershman, C Holcombe, W Lloyd-Jones, J P Neoptolemos, G J Poston, P S Rooney, R A Sells, R Sutton, J H R Winstanley

Genitourinary Medicine A B Alawattegama, H D L Birley, P B Carey, D J Timmins

Haematology J C Cawley, P Chu, R E Clark, V J Martlew, C H T Toh

Histopathology V Aachi, J R Gosney, T R Helliwell, P Hiscott, P Johnson, J Nash, P A Smith

Medical Microbiology C A Hart, G W Smith, C Y W Tong, D Van Saene, T H Williets

Nephrology R Ahmed, G M Bell, J M Bone, P S Williams

Neurophysiology K A Pang

Nuclear Medicine M L Smith

Ophthalmology M C Briggs, A Chandna, B E Damato, C P Groenewald, S P Harding, S B Kaye, P Whishart, D Wong

Orthopaedics S P Frostick, W A Jones, M C Lynch, S Nayagam, D S O'Donoghue, S K Thompson, C R Walker

Otolaryngology A Jones, M S McCormick

Pathology F Campbell, C S Foster, J R Gosney, D M Guerin, T R Helliwell, C P Johnson, J R G Nash, J P Sloane, L S Turnbull

Radiology A T Carty, C J Garvey, D A Gould, J A Holemans, E Hurley, G H R Lamb, R G McWilliams, K A Meakin, D A Ritchie, P Rowlands, C J Ryall, C Sampson, F E White

Radiotherapy and Oncology J E S Brock, R D Errington, S Myint, A J Slater, I Syndikus

Transplant Surgery (Renal) A Bakran, M W Brown, R A Sells

Urology A D Desmond, M V Fordham, K F Parsons, K A Woolfenden

Royal Liverpool Children's NHS Trust

Alder Hey, Eaton Road, West Derby, Liverpool L12 2AP
Tel: 0151 228 4811 Fax: 0151 288 0328
Website: www.alderhey.com
(Cheshire and Merseyside Strategic Health Authority)

Chair Angela Jones
Chief Executive Tony Bell

Alder Hey Children's Hospital

Eaton Road, West Derby, Liverpool L12 2AP
Tel: 0151 228 4811
Total Beds: 330

Accident and Emergency R Massey, W J Robson

Anaesthetics I S Billingham, P D Booker, A Bowhay, I M Boyd, M Cunliffe, R E Sarginson, R E Thornington

Child and Adolescent Psychiatry J Hill

Dental Surgery J C Cooper, D R Llewelyn, B B J Lovius

Dermatology P Friedman, J L Verbov

ENT J H Rogers, S D Singh

General Psychiatry J S Nelki, A Oppenheim, F E Stewart

General Surgery G Lamont, D A Lloyd, P L May, R Rintala, R Turnock

Immunology T A Dixon, J A Wilson

Neuroradiology N R Clitherow, E T S Smith

Ophthalmology A Chanda, S Kaye

Orthopaedics J C Dorgan, J F Taylor, J Walsh

Paediatrics R Arnold, R W I Cooke, D C Davidson, D P Heaf, J Martin, L Rosenbloom, J A Sills, C S Smith, A Thomson

Pathology P Bolton-Maggs, D Isherwood, G Kokai, H K F Saene

Plastic Surgery J R Bryson, M Gipson, A R Green, G Hancock, J H Stilwell

Radiology L J Abernethy, A E Boothroyd, D W Pilling, A Sprigg

Radiotherapy and Oncology D W Pilling, A Sprigg

Tropical Medicine J B S Coulter

Urology A M K Rickwood

The Royal Marsden NHS Foundation Trust

Established as a Foundation Trust 01/04/2004.

Fulham Road, London SW3 6JJ
Tel: 020 7352 8171 Fax: 020 7808 2094
Email: forename.surname@rmh.nhs.uk
Website: www.royalmarsden.org.uk
(North West London Strategic Health Authority; South West London Strategic Health Authority)

Chair Tessa Green
Chief Executive Cally Palmer
Consultants Desmond Barton, Mike Brada, Caroline Brain, Jane Bridges, Gina Brown, David Chisholm, Mitch Dowsett, Stephen Ebbs, Ros Eeles, Tim Eisen, Cyril Fisher, John Glees, Martin Gore, Gerald Gui, Cive Harmer, J M Henk, Michael Henry, Mark Hill, R A Huddart, Thomas Ind, Stephen Johnston, Ian Judson, Stan Kaye, V Khoo, M E Matutes Juan, Eleanor Moskovic, N Nasiri, Eric Nicholls, Eric Nicholls, Chris Nutting, Mary O'Brien, Cathy Pritchard-Jones, G Querci della Rovere, U Riley, Gill Ross, Assam Rostom, Nigel Sacks, John Shepherd, Diana Tait, J Meririon Thomas, Jeremy Thompson, J G Treleaven, A C Wotherspoon, John Yarnold

The Royal Marsden Hospital (Chelsea)

Fulham Road, London SW3 6JJ
Tel: 020 7352 8171 Fax: 020 7808 2094
Total Beds: 152

The Royal Marsden Hospital (Sutton)

Downs Road, Sutton SM2 5PT
Tel: 020 8642 6011 Fax: 020 8770 9297
Total Beds: 168

Anaesthetics J M Edwards, J Filshie, J J Kothari, D Skewes

Chemical Pathology C R Tillyer

Dermatology P S Mortimer

General Surgery A Nash, P Rhys-Evans, J Shepherd, J M Thomas

Haematology M J S Dyer, G J Morgan

Histopathology C Fisher, P A Trott

Medical Oncology D Cunningham, M Gore, I Judson, I E Smith

Microbiology N Mackenzie

Nuclear Medicine V R McCready

Ophthalmology P J Holmes-Sellors, R Whitelocke

Oral and Maxillofacial Surgery D J Archer

Paediatrics S Meller, K Pritchard-Jones

Radiology J C Husband, D M King, D MacVicar, E C Moskovic

Radiotherapy P R Blake, M Brada, D Dearnaley, H T Ford, J P Glees, C L Harmer, J M Henk, A Horwich, D Tait, J R Yarnold

Royal National Hospital for Rheumatic Diseases NHS Foundation Trust

Established as a Foundation Trust 01/04/2005.

Upper Borough Walls, Bath BA1 1RL
Tel: 01225 465941 Fax: 01225 421202
Email: info@rnhrd-tr.swest.nhs.uk
Website: www.rnhrd.nhs.uk
(Avon, Gloucestershire and Wiltshire Strategic Health Authority)

Chair Kate Lyon
Chief Executive Nicola Carmichael

Royal National Hospital for Rheumatic Diseases

Upper Borough Walls, Bath BA1 1RL
Tel: 01225 465941 Fax: 01225 421202
Total Beds: 85

Manager Nicola Carmichael

Rheumatology and Rehabilitation A K Bhalla, D Blake, A K Clarke, T Jenkinson, N McHugh, E Okirie, M Stone

Royal National Orthopaedic Hospital NHS Trust

Brockley Hill, Stanmore HA7 4LP
Tel: 020 8954 2300 Fax: 020 8954 9133
Email: enquiries@rnoh.nhs.uk
Website: www.rnoh.nhs.uk
(North Central London Strategic Health Authority)

Chair Donald Hoodless
Chief Executive Andrew Woodhead

Royal National Orthopaedic Hospital

Brockley Hill, Stanmore HA7 4LP
Tel: 020 8954 2300 Fax: 020 8954 6933
Total Beds: 239

Anaesthetics K Agyare, J P Barcroft, J S Berman, M Chandra, G M Edge, M E Fennelly, R Fox, R R Gadelrab, D R Goldhill, E M Grundy, M A Hetreed, A P Rubin, F Salim, D R J Seingry, V M Taylor, K W Yau

General Psychiatry G Ikkos, H M Weiselburg

Histopathology A M Flanagan

Neurology G D Schott

Neurosurgery A T C Casey

Orthopaedics J B Allibone, I J L Bayley, R Birch, T W R Briggs, S R Cannon, P T Carlstedt, R W J Carrington, A T C Casey, D M Eastwood, D J Harrison, A Hashemi-Nejad, S M Lambert, J Lehovsky, S K Muirhead-Allwood, M H H Noordeen, J Shah, D Singh, J Skinner, B A Taylor, S K Tucker, L F Wilson

Paediatrics D M Eastwood, A Hashemi-Nejad, S S Herman, B Jacobs, C L Oren

Radiology R A R Green, R Mitchell, P G O'Donnell, A Saifuddin

Rehabilitation Medicine J M A Cowan, A Gall, F R I Middleton

Rheumatology R W Keen, J T Nash, R L Wolman

Royal Orthopaedic Hospital NHS Trust

Bristol Road South, Northfield, Birmingham B31 2AP
Tel: 0121 685 4000 Fax: 0121 685 4100
Email: info@roh.nhs.uk
Website: www.roh.nhs.uk
(Birmingham and the Black Country Strategic Health Authority)

Chair Les Lawrence
Chief Executive Christine Miles

Royal Orthopaedic Hospital
Bristol Road South, Northfield, Birmingham B31 2AP
Tel: 0121 685 4000 Fax: 0121 627 8211
Total Beds: 171

Anaesthetics C Bhimarasetty, V Girgis, D Hawes, B Kumar, T Neal, O Owen-Smith, P Riddell, G Shinner, J Watt

Histopathology D Hughes, V P Sumathi

Orthopaedics A T Abudu, C E Bache, K G Baloch, C F Bradish, S R Carter, G S Chana, M A C Craigen, S C Deshmukh, D J Dunlop, P J Gibbons, P R Glithero, M F Grainger, M A Green, R J Grimer, M L Herron, A Jackowski, D J Learmonth, D S Marks, S Massoud, J N O'Hara, J L Plewes, V Rajaratnam, J B Spilsbury, A J Stirling, A M C Thomas, R M Tillman, R B C Treacy, M A Waldram

Radiology A M Davies, N S Evans, R Popuri

Rheumatology P Jobanputra

Sports Medicine G Brown, R C Chakraverty

Royal Surrey County Hospital NHS Trust

Royal Surrey County Hospital, Egerton Road, Guildford GU2 7XX
Tel: 01483 571122 Fax: 01483 537747
Website: www.royalsurrey.nhs.uk
(Surrey and Sussex Strategic Health Authority)

Chair Alan Howarth
Chief Executive Mathew Swindells

Royal Surrey County Hospital
Egerton Road, Guildford GU2 7XX
Tel: 01483 571122
Total Beds: 520

Accident and Emergency B Brooks, A Wan

Anaesthetics G Dhond, W Fawcett, J R Fozard, T M Gallagher, H B A Griffiths, J G Jenkins, E J Kershaw, M Payne, N F Quiney, P R Saunders, M Scott, J R Stoneham

Audiological Medicine V Jayarajan

Cardiology T P Chua, E Leatham

Cardiothoracic Surgery R E Sayer, E E J Smith

Care of the Elderly A Blight, H Khoshnaw, H Powell, V Seth

Dermatology E Wong

ENT P Chapman, J Rowe-Jones, N Solomons, R Sudderick, N F Weir

General Medicine R Jones, W A C McAllister, M G M Smith

General Surgery M E Bailey, M Karanjia, M W Kissin, C G Marks, J Stebbing, M Whiteley

Neurology P S Trend

Neurophysiology M Sheehy

Obstetrics and Gynaecology E P Curtis, R Hutt, A Kent, K E Morton, C J G Sutton, S Whitcroft

Ophthalmology G Boodhoo, R Condon, A Gilvarry, J Keenan, C McClean

Oral and Maxillofacial Surgery M Damford, P Haers, P Johnson

Orthodontics N Taylor

Orthopaedics C Coates, M Flannery, M Helliwell, P Magnussen, G Paremain, J W Rossen

Paediatrics S Chapman, M Evans, J H Foley, C Godden, M Ryalls

Pathology R L Carter, M G Cook, L Daborn, S De Sanctis, S Deacock, I D C Douglas, G Ferns, P Jackson, E Mannion, G Robbins

Radiology C J Bland, T J Bloomberg, J C Cooke, A Lopez, W J Walker

Radiotherapy and Oncology S Houston, M Illsley, R Laing, G Middleton, A Neal, H Thomas, C Topham, S Whittaker

Rheumatology and Rehabilitation A R Behn, R E J Gray

Urology J Davies, S Langley, A Nigam

Royal United Hospital Bath NHS Trust

Royal United Hospital, Combe Park, Bath BA1 3NG
Tel: 01225 428331
Website: www.ruh-bath.swest.nhs.uk
(Avon, Gloucestershire and Wiltshire Strategic Health Authority)

Chair Mike Roy
Chief Executive Mark Davies

Royal United Hospital
Combe Park, Bath BA1 3NG
Tel: 01225 428331 Fax: 01225 824395
Email: info@ruh-bath.swest.nhs.uk
Total Beds: 566

Accident and Emergency S Meek

Anaesthetics A F Avery, M Baird, T Cook, A P L Goodwin, K Gupta, J M Handel, P Hersch, S L Hill, L Jordan, P McAteer, P Magee, R Marjot, V C Martin, A H Mayor, J Nolan, A Padkin, C Peden, R Seagger, T Simpson, A Souter, J Tuckey

Biochemistry A Taylor

Cardiology R D Thomas

Chest Disease A Alexander

Clinical Genetics R Newbury-Ecob

Dermatology C R Lovell (Head)

Diabetes J P Reckless (Head), E L Higgs, T Robinson

ENT R J Canter, A Jardine, R Slack

Gastroenterology M Davis, M Farrant

General Medicine D E Bateman, T Bennett, M Davis, K Dawson, C L Hall, W N Hubbard, P Lyons, J P D Reckless, D A F Robertson, R D Thomas, R Young

General Surgery D C Britton, M Horrocks, P R Maddox, J J Tate, H C Umpleby, M Williamson

Gynaecology G D Dunster, N Johnson, R J Porter, N C Sharp, T M Tonge

Haematology C Singer, J G Smith

Neurology D E Bateman, K Dawson

Obstetrics and Gynaecology G Dunster, R Holmes, N Johnson, M Tonge, D Walker

Ophthalmology R Antcliff, R Baer, J Boulton, S Webber

Oral and Maxillofacial Surgery J Schnetler

Oral Surgery J Schnetler

Orthodontics A Ireland, H Knight

Orthopaedics M Bishay, N Bradbury, M Burwell, G Giddins, S Gregg-Smith, S Pope, J L Pozo, A C Ross

Paediatrics A Billson, S Jones, J P Osborne

Pathology L Biddlestone, L Hirschowitz, P Kitching, C Meehan, N Rooney, S Rose

Pharmacology P N Bennett

Radiology A H Chalmers, D A B Dunlop, D Glew, D Goddard, J Hardman, M J Noakes, M O'Driscoll, A Phillips, L Robinson, A Sandeman

Radiotherapy and Oncology H F V Newman, G J G Rees

Respiratory Medicine A Alexander, N Foley, A Malin

Urology T Bates, C Gallegos, G Howell

The Royal West Sussex NHS Trust

St Richard's Hospital, Spitalfield Lane, Chichester PO19 6SE
Tel: 01243 788122 Fax: 01243 531269
Email: firstname.lastname@rws-tr.org.uk
Website: www.rwst.org.uk
(Surrey and Sussex Strategic Health Authority)

Chair David Taylor
Chief Executive Robert Lapraik

St Richard's Hospital

Spitalfield Lane, Chichester PO19 4SE
Tel: 01243 788122 Fax: 01243 531269
Total Beds: 405

Anaesthetics A S Carter, A B Conyers, J G Dalgleish, A P Kendall, P F McDonald, S P McHale, M R Nott, C Smith, G A Turner

Audiological Medicine P D West

Chemical Pathology J R Quiney

Dermatology P R Coburn, A V Levantine

ENT A E Davis, C I Johnstone

General Medicine A G Dewhurst, R A Haigh, R A E Holman, G B Lee, I M Morrison, C J Reid, R D Simpson

General Surgery D R Allen, R C Bowyer, R A P Scott, J N L Simson

Genitourinary Medicine M P G Gomez

Haematology P C Bevan, W P Stross, T Umar

Histopathology J Conroy, B French, J P O'Sullivan

Medical Microbiology M Greig

Neurology S R Hammans

Neurophysiology R J van der Star

Obstetrics and Gynaecology J L Beynon, J G Hooker, Z H Z Ibrahim

Ophthalmology P D Fox, T Niyadurupola, M Teimory

Oral and Maxillofacial Surgery D W MacPherson, C J Poate, C A Pratt, J R L Townend, J L Williams, A Wilson

Orthodontics A M Hall

Orthopaedics S Cavanagh, M C Moss, L J Taylor

Paediatrics M A Bracewell, D C A Candy, L S Lamont, T M Taylor, A C M Wallace

Palliative Medicine S J Dolin

Radiology N S Ashford, B J Burns, A M Guilding, D N Kay

Radiotherapy and Oncology G G S Khoury

Restorative Dentistry P D Cheshire

Rheumatology and Rehabilitation M G Ridley

Urology J P Britton, P G Carter

Royal Wolverhampton Hospitals NHS Trust

Trust Management Offices, Hollybush House, New Cross Hospital, Wednesfield Road, Wolverhampton WV10 0QP
Tel: 01902 307999 Fax: 01902 643173
Website: www.royalwolverhamptonhospitals.nhs.uk
(Birmingham and the Black Country Strategic Health Authority)

Chief Executive David Loughton

New Cross Hospital

Wednesfield Road, Wolverhampton WV10 0QP
Tel: 01902 307999 Fax: 01902 642810

Accident and Emergency R Khanna, D W J McCreadie, I Robertson-Steel

Anaesthetics S G Fenner, R J Micklewright, R D Patel, D J H Richmond

Cardiology R C Horton, M S Norell, J W Pidgeon

Care of the Elderly D L Leung

Chemical Pathology R M Gama

Dermatology S Oliwieki, D R Taylor

ENT R J Cullen, L P Glossop, R T J Shortridge, F Wilson

General Medicine D F d'Costa, M A Jackson, S A Kapadia, R Lodwick, J S Mann, J Odum, P B Rylance, B M Singh, E T Swarbrick, A M Veitch

General Surgery I L R Badger, L D Coen, M P M Cristobal, F T Curran, T I M Gardecki, A W Garnham, B Isgar, J G Williams

Haematology A MacWhannel, A M Patel, N A Smith

Medical Microbiology M A Cooper

Neurology R N Corston

Obstetrics and Gynaecology A J F Browning, C W F Cox, S D Jenkinson, D J Little, D J Murphy, J S Samra, H J Sullivan

Oral and Maxillofacial Surgery E B Larkin, B G Millar

Orthopaedics S Chugh, A M Fraser, E S Isbister, R K Tandon, A P Thomas, R J Thomas, A Turner

Paediatrics J M Anderson, P J Dison, D S Kalra, B Kumararatne, C A Moore

Pathology N P Aluwihare, K W M Scott

Radiology C S Deacon, R Fitzgerald, M Hale, G Mackie, Y Osafo-Agyare

Radiotherapy and Oncology R Allerton, C V Brammer, M J Chum, D J Fairlamb, D R Ferry, R C Mehra, A Samanci

Rheumatology H A Ali, P Netwon

Urology J A Inglis, N H Philp, B Waymont

Wolverhampton and Midland Counties Eye Infirmary

Compton Road, Wolverhampton WV3 9QR
Tel: 01902 307999 Fax: 01902 645019
Total Beds: 25

Ophthalmology P Caruana, Y C Chan, C K S Chew, P G J Corridan, M P Headon, N J Price, S Sandramouli, G A Shun-Shin

Royston, Buntingford and Bishop's Stortford Primary Care Trust

Herts and Essex Community Hospital, Cavell Drive, off Haymeads Lane, Bishop's Stortford CM23 5JH

Tel: 01279 827228 Fax: 01279 465873
Email: firstname.lastname@rbbs-pct.nhs.uk
Website: www.rbbs-pct.nhs.uk
(Bedfordshire and Hertfordshire Strategic Health Authority)

Chair Mavis Garner
Chief Executive Gareth Jones

Herts and Essex Community Hospital

Haymeads Lane, Bishop's Stortford CM23 5JH
Tel: 01279 827228
Total Beds: 44

Royston and District Hospital

London Road, Royston SG8 9EN
Tel: 01763 242134
Total Beds: 24

Manager Anne Richmond

Rugby Primary Care Trust

Swift Park, Old Leicester Road, Rugby CV21 1DZ
Tel: 01788 550860 Fax: 01788 513000
Website: www.rugby-pct.nhs.uk
(West Midlands South Strategic Health Authority)

Chair Philip Blundell
Chief Executive Peter Maddock

Rushcliffe Primary Care Trust

Easthorpe House, 165 Loughborough Road, Ruddington, Nottingham NG11 6LQ
Tel: 0115 956 0300 Fax: 0115 956 0302
Email: rcpt@rushcliffe-pct.nhs.uk
Website: www.nottingham.nhs.uk
(Trent Strategic Health Authority)

Chair Martin Suthers
Chief Executive Mark Morgan

Highbury Hospital

Highbury Road, Bulwell, Nottingham NG6 9DR
Tel: 0115 977 0000

Lings Bar Hospital

Beckside, Gamston, Nottingham NG2 6PR
Tel: 0115 945 5577

St Albans and Harpenden Primary Care Trust

99 Waverley Road, St Albans AL3 5TL
Tel: 01727 831219 Fax: 01727 812686
Website: www.stalbansharp-pct.nhs.uk
(Bedfordshire and Hertfordshire Strategic Health Authority)

Chair John Bennett
Chief Executive Jacqueline Clark

Harpenden Memorial Hospital

Carlton Way, Harpenden AL5 4TA
Tel: 01582 760196

Runcie Unit

St Albans City Hospital, Waverley Road, St Albans AL3 5PN
Tel: 01727 897618

St George's Healthcare NHS Trust

Blackshaw Road, Tooting, London SW17 0QT
Tel: 020 8672 1255 Fax: 020 8672 5304
Email: general.enquiries@stgeorges.nhs.uk
Website: www.st-georges.org.uk
(South West London Strategic Health Authority)

Chair Naaz Coker
Chief Executive Peter Homa

Bolingbroke Hospital

Wandsworth Common, London SW11 6HN
Tel: 020 7223 7411 Fax: 020 7223 5865
Total Beds: 78

Care of the Elderly J Coles, M A Cottee, I Hastie, J J Oram, S Samadian

St George's Hospital

Blackshaw Road, London SW17 0QT
Tel: 020 8672 1255 Fax: 020 8672 5304
Total Beds: 979

Accident and Emergency M Lynch, D Wallis, D Wijetunge

Anaesthetics J Allt-Graham, J D Boyd, R W Brown, J N Cashman, J T Clarke, G Farnsworth, I L Findley, R M Grounds, M G Hulse, S E Hutchinson, M Kraayenbrink, J B Liban, L J Murdoch, P J Newman, J A O'Riordan, P A Razis, P A Rich, B J Stanford, B A Sutton, A C Thurlow, J P Van Besouw

Anaesthetics - Atkinson Morley Wing G Hall, T E Hollway, M A Kraayenbrink, P Razis, A C Thurlow

Audiological Medicine E M Raglan, S E Snashall

Cardiology S J D Brecker, A J Camm, W McKenna, C W Pumphrey, D E Ward

Cardiothoracic Surgery A J Murday, R E Sayer, E J Smith, T Treasure

Care of the Elderly J A Coles, M A Cottee, I R Hastie, J J Oram, S Samadian

Chemical Pathology P Collinson, G E Levin

Clinical Genetics V A Murday, M A Patton

Dermatology R A Marsden, P S Mortimer, L S Ostlere

General Medicine J Eastwood, P W Jones, J D Maxwell, C R Newton, S S Nussey, A Panahloo, C F J Rayner

General Surgery J A Dormandy, A Fiennes, A Halliday, M J Knight, D Kumar, R J Leicester, T Loosemore, R McFarland, D Melville, A Sharma

Genitourinary Medicine E A F Davidson, P E Hay, R Lau, J Mantell

Haematology S E Ball, D H Bevan, E Gordon-Smith, J C W Marsh

Histopathology J Chow, C M Corbishley, T Creagh, C J Finlayson, I J M Jeffrey, V A Thomas, P Wilson, M P A Young

Infectious Diseases G E Griffin, M H Wansbrough-Jones

Medical Microbiology A Breathnach

Nephrology M Bewick, R W S Chang, J B J Eastwood, S R Nelson, D Oliveira, C Streather

Neurology D M Barnes, O J F Foster, Y M Hart, H R Modarres-Sadeghi, F Schon, M Schwartz, S G Wilson, D Wren

Neuroradiology J Britton, A Clifton

Neurosurgery B A Bell, F G Johnston, H T Marsh, A Moore, S R Stapleton, P E Wilkins

Nuclear Medicine A E A Joseph

Obstetrics and Gynaecology D Barton, T H Bourne, S Campbell, P Carter, I T Manyonda, G Nargund, S L Stanton, B Thilaganathan, T R Varma

Occupational Health N A Mitchell-Heggs

Ophthalmology W Aylward, C K Rostron, G M Thompson

Oral and Maxillofacial Surgery M Danford, M Manisali

Orthodontics S J Powell

Orthopaedics M D Bircher, S H Bridle, P T Calvert, A Day, A C Fairbank, A M Jackson, R H Vickers

Otolaryngology A E Hinton, V L Moore Gillon

Paediatrics M D Bain, A R Bedford-Russell, S M Boddy, C Brain, S A Calvert, S N J Capps, J A Christopher, E G Davies, D A C Elliman, S J Fonseca, P A Hamilton, S J K Holmes, S Mitton, P J Rye, M Sharland, T T N Sim, S M Thurlbeck

Plastic Surgery D Gateley, A L H Moss, J O'Donoghue, B W Powell

Radiology E J Adam, R A Allan, A M Belli, T M Buckenham, D D Dundas, R M Given-Wilson, A Grundy, H L Hale, C W Heron, A E Joseph, K T Khaw, U Patel, A G Wilson

Radiotherapy and Oncology A Dalgleish, J P Glees, C L Harmer, F Lofts, J L Mansi, R Pettengell

Rehabilitation Medicine B E Bourke, F E Bruckner, P Kiely

Restorative Dentistry P F A Briggs

Rheumatology J Axford, B E Bourke, F E Bruckner, P Kiely

Urology K Anson, M Bailey, R S Kirby

Wolfson Neuro-Rehabilitation Centre

Regional Neurosciences Centre, Atkinson Morley's Hospital, Copse Hill, Wimbledon, London SW20 0NQ
Tel: 020 8725 4764 Fax: 020 8944 9927
Total Beds: 27

Rehabilitation Medicine D G Jenkins

St Helens and Knowsley Hospitals NHS Trust

Whiston Hospital, Warrington Road, Prescot L35 5DR
Tel: 0151 426 1600 Fax: 0151 430 1425
Email: enquiries@sthkhealth.nhs.uk
Website: www.sthkhealth.nhs.uk
(Cheshire and Merseyside Strategic Health Authority)

Chair Mavis Wareham
Chief Executive Ann Marr

Newton Community Hospital

Bradlegh Road, Newton-le-Willows WA12 8RB
Tel: 01925 222731
Total Beds: 30

Care of the Elderly J Abrams

Dermatology R K Curley

ENT J C McIlwain

General Medicine A M G Cochrane

General Psychiatry B John

General Surgery M Scott

Obstetrics and Gynaecology G Buchanan, M Hamed

Ophthalmology J Villada

Orthopaedics M E Cavendish, I M Shackleferd

Paediatrics L Amegavie, E L Badri, C R Woodhall

St Helens Hospital

Marshalls Cross Road, St Helens WA9 3EA
Tel: 01744 26633 Fax: 01744 451321
Total Beds: 211

Anaesthetics G M Edwards, R P Howard, J A Nash

General Surgery R A Audisio, L S Chagla, I M Khan, R S Kiff, C J Sanderson, M H Scott

Ophthalmology N R Cota, M Hiranandani

Orthopaedics B Bolton-Maggs, M B Carsi, J S Denton, V M Kothari, M P R Manning, P J Mobbs, D N Teanby, G Thomas

Pathology G Satchithananthan

Radiology A F Evans

Rheumatology V E Abernethy

Urology J A Massey

Whiston Hospital

Whiston, Prescot L35 5DR
Tel: 0151 426 1600 Fax: 0151 430 1425
Total Beds: 795

Accident and Emergency C S Graham, E F Worthington

Anaesthetics G M Edwards, R P Howard, C S Ince, J A Nash, S M Raftery, A C Skinner

Care of the Elderly J Abrams, A E Capewell

ENT V Nandapalan

General Medicine J B Ball, S E Church, J A Corless, C Y Francis, J P McLindon, S J McNulty, J B Ridyard

General Psychiatry M Al-Nufoury, S A Bokhari, A Dutta, F M Ibitoye

General Surgery R A Audisio, L S Chagla, I M Khan, R S Kiff, D Maitra, C J Sanderson, M H Scott

Medical Microbiology K D Allen

Neurology P Ray

Obstetrics and Gynaecology G M Cawdell, H M Hamed, T O Idama, J Langton, P R Morgan, E C Nwosu

Ophthalmology J Ghosh, P Joyce

Orthopaedics J S Denton, M P R Manning, P J Mobbs

Paediatrics J A Sills

Palliative Care C M Littlewood

Pathology M A M Al-Jubouri, N U Hasan, G Satchithananthan, J A Tappin

Plastic Surgery A R Green, K Hancock, V Kumar

Radiology J M A Desmond, C R Thind

Rheumatology M P Lynch

Urology H B Gana, J A Massey

St Helens Primary Care Trust

Cowley Hill Lane, St Helens WA10 2AP
Tel: 01744 733722 Fax: 01744 453085
Email: info.sthelenspct@sthkhealth.nhs.uk
Website: www.sthkhealth.nhs.uk
(Cheshire and Merseyside Strategic Health Authority)

Chair Nora Giubertoni
Chief Executive Morag Day

St Mary's NHS Trust

Praed Street, London W2 1NY
Tel: 020 7886 6666 Fax: 020 7886 6200
Email: switchboard@st-marys.nhs.uk
Website: www.st-marys.nhs.uk
(North West London Strategic Health Authority)

Chair Joan Hanham
Chief Executive Julian Nettel

St Mary's Hospital

Praed Street, London W2 1NY
Tel: 020 7725 6666 Fax: 020 7886 1017
Total Beds: 700

Accident and Emergency R Brown, J Henry, I Maconochie, J Redhead, R Touquet, P Ward

Anaesthetics A J Hartle, J A Jones, F M Nicholls, M Platt, J E Shepherd, J B Smith

Asthma/Allergy A Croom

Cardiology D W Davies, R A Foale, N Peters, D Sheridan

Cardiothoracic Surgery B Glenville, R Stanbridge

Care of the Elderly D Ames, C Pulford, S Roche, S C Webb

Chest Disease S Johnston, D M Mitchell, Dr Onn Min Kon, P Openshaw

Dermatology F Child, C Hardman, J Leonard, A V Powles, S Wakelin

Diabetes R S Elkeles, A Fairney, D G Johnston, S Robinson

ENT S Abramovich, R Gad, A A Narula, K Patel, S Soucek, J Suri, N Tolley

Gastroenterology J S Summerfield, J Teare, H Thomas, M Thursz

General Medicine R Lancaster, J Main

General Surgery A Darzi, M W Ghilchik, G Glazer, B E Glenville, R D Rosin

Genitourinary Medicine M Byrne, D Goldmeier, L Greene, N Hanna, J R W Harris, G Scullard, G Taylor, G Tudor-Williams, S Walters

Haematology S H Abdalla, B J Bain, A Shlebak, S M Wickramasinghe

Immunology P Kelleher, S Marshall

Neurology J Ball, J Chataway, S Farmer, M N Rossor, D J Thomas

Obstetrics and Gynaecology K A Clifford, C Coulter, A Farthing, S Franks, J Higham, V Khullar, P Mason, K Murphy, C M Paterson, L Regan, J Smith, T G Teoh

Oncology C A Coulter, S Stewart

Orthopaedics J R T Eckersley, R Emery, D Hunt, J Johnson, R Marston, A Odgaard

Paediatric Surgery M Haddad, N Madden

Paediatrics S Bignall, M Coren, C de Munter, J Deal, M Garralda, K Ghaus, P Habibi, M Hodes, M Howard, S Kroll, G Lack, M Levin, T Lissauer, S Nadel, R Rivers, R Schwartz, D Smyth, G Tudor-Williams, S Walters, M Watson

Pharmacology N Poulter, P S Sever, S Thom

Radiology S Burnett, M Clark, M Cowling, M E Crofton, D A Cunningham, W Gedroyc, M Pelling, J M Stevens, A Wright

Renal and Transplant Unit T Cairns, J Contis, N Hakim, A Palmer, D Taube

Rheumatology R G Rees, M H Seifert

Urology A Patel, J A Vale, R O Witherow

Vascular Surgery N Cheshire, M Jenkins, J H N Wolfe

Western Eye Hospital

Marylebone Road, London NW1 6YE
Tel: 020 7402 4211
Total Beds: 20

Ophthalmology P A Bloom, M Corbett, I G M Duguid, S Farmer, V M G Ferguson, A Fielder, A Gorchein, N B Lee, C S Migdal, J Olver, W E Schulenburg, U Vogt

Salford Primary Care Trust

2nd Floor, St James House, Pendleton Way, Salford M6 5FW
Tel: 0161 212 4800 Fax: 0161 212 4801
Email: firstname.surname@salford-pct.nhs.uk
Website: www.salford-pct.nhs.uk
(Greater Manchester Strategic Health Authority)

Chair Eileen Fairhurst
Chief Executive Mike Burrows

Salford Royal Hospitals NHS Trust

Hope Hospital, Stott Lane, Salford M6 8HD
Tel: 0161 789 7373 Fax: 0161 787 5974
Email: enquiries@srht.nhs.uk
Website: www.srht.nhs.uk
(Greater Manchester Strategic Health Authority)

Chair Margaret Morris
Chief Executive David Dalton

Hope Hospital

Stott Lane, Salford M6 8WH
Tel: 0161 789 7373 Fax: 0161 787 5974
Total Beds: 800

Accident and Emergency P A Driscoll, D W Yates

Anaesthetics M W B Allan, B J M Bowles, C Earlam, I Geraghty, C L Gwinnutt, T W Johnson, R Kishen, C M Rogers, C Spanswick, M D Trask

Care of the Elderly M Gonsalkorale, A K M Karim, R C Tallis

Chemical Pathology M F Stewart, C Weinkove

Dental Surgery I D Campbell, R E Lloyd

Dermatology P J August, C E M Griffiths

ENT M P Rothera, D J Willatt

General Medicine P C Barnes, H Buckler, T L Dornan, R O'Donoghue, R O'Driscoll, W D Rees, Dr Sandle, J Shaffer, D G Thompson, S Waldek, R J Young

General Surgery J Bancewicz, N Scott

Genitourinary Medicine B P Goorney

Haematology P Carrington, J B Houghton, R C Routledge

Histopathology G R Armstrong, R H McDonald, R S Reeve

Immunology M R Haeney

Medical Microbiology L A Joseph, M G L Keaney

Nephrology D O'Donoghue, S Waldek

Neurology P D Mohr, A C Young

Neurosurgery R A Cowie, R A C Jones, G G H West

Obstetrics and Gynaecology G F Falconer, G G Mitchell, D Poulson, A Railton

Oncology D Crowther, J H Scarffe

Oral and Maxillofacial Surgery I D Campbell, R E Lloyd

Orthodontics J Brady

Orthopaedics G Andrew, C S B Galasko, J Noble, E R S Ross, J B Williamson

Paediatrics G Hambleton, M J Robinson

Plastic Surgery C I Orton, J S Watson

Radiology J D K Brown, R A Chisholm, W S C Forbes, S G Gupta, D Hughes, H Mamtora, D Nicholson

Rheumatology and Rehabilitation A Herrick, A K P Jones

Urology N Clarke

Ladywell Hospital

Eccles New Road, Salford M5 2AA
Tel: 0161 789 7373
Total Beds: 246

Care of the Elderly M Gonsalkorale, R C Tallis

Haematology J B Houghton, R C Routledge

Medical Microbiology L A Joseph, M G L Keaney

Neurology P D Mohr, A C Young

Radiology J D K Brown, S Thurairajasingam

Rheumatology and Rehabilitation R C Hilton, A K P Jones

Salisbury Health Care NHS Trust

Salisbury District Hospital, Salisbury SP2 8BJ
Tel: 01722 336262 Fax: 01722 330221
Website: www.salisburyhealthcare.org
(Avon, Gloucestershire and Wiltshire Strategic Health Authority)

Chair Luke March
Chief Executive Frank Harsent

Fordingbridge Hospital

Bartons Road, Fordingbridge SP6 1JD
Tel: 01425 652255 Fax: 01425 654705
Total Beds: 40

General Medicine J H Marigold

Salisbury District Hospital

Salisbury SP2 8BJ
Tel: 01722 336262 Fax: 01722 330221
Total Beds: 550

Accident and Emergency N C Burrows, N Robinson

Anaesthetics S Abbas, R F Barrett, S L Calvert, S Cockroft, C Cox, K N Duggal, W Garrett, D J Lintin, M I D McCallum, D P Murray, J Onslow, R J Ray, R P F Scott, P Swayne, I Wright

Burns E Tiernan

Care of the Elderly J H Marigold, D Walters

Child and Adolescent Psychiatry M A Griffiths, M I Vereker

Dermatology R H Meyrick-Thomas, D Mitchell

ENT M J Brockbank, M Collins

General Medicine S Biggart, A Jones, J Marigold, C Page, M Smith, A Tanner, C Thompson, S Vyas, A R H Warley

General Surgery A Aertssen, A Campbell, N J Carty, H Chave, T J C Cooke, D Finnis, C Ranaboldo

Genitourinary Medicine M S A Nasr

Obstetrics and Gynaecology P W Docherty, S A Fountain, D M McKenna, J A Wilde

Oncology R Gregory, T Iveson

Ophthalmology R G Collyer-Powell, R C Humphry, A G Tyers

Oral and Maxillofacial Surgery I Downie, T R Flood, D L Shinn

Orthopaedics A R Beaumont, N Chapple, D R Cox, P Ralih, G F Rushforth, G Shergill

Paediatrics M M M Lwin, A McGeechan, R H Scott-Jupp, D Stratton

Palliative Medicine J Overton, C D Wood

Pathology S Burroughs, J Cullis, C E Fuller-Watson, M Khan, H F Parry, C A Scott

Plastic Surgery M Cadier, R P Cole, J A E Hobby, R A W McDowall, L F A Rossi, E Tiernan, I Whitworth

Radiology J A D Annis, B Bentley, R A Frost, S Hegarty, J Hollway, K Johnson, S G McGee, A D P Morris

Rheumatology and Rehabilitation S Batram, R M Ellis, J C Robertson

Spinal Injuries A Soopramanian, A M Tromans

Sandwell and West Birmingham Hospitals NHS Trust

City Hospital, Dudley Road, Birmingham B18 7QH
Tel: 0121 554 3801 Fax: 0121 507 5636
Email: firstname.lastname@swbh.nhs.uk
Website: www.swbh.nhs.uk
(Birmingham and the Black Country Strategic Health Authority)

Chair Najma Hafeez
Chief Executive John Adler

City Hospital

Dudley Road, Birmingham B18 7QH
Tel: 0121 554 3801 Fax: 0121 523 0951
Website: www.cityhospital.org.uk
Total Beds: 690

Accident and Emergency M Ansari, P John, D Moore, O Okunribido

Anaesthetics J Bleasdale, R A Botha, A Brake, J Chilvers, J Clift, R Dabas, H Ellwood, H Garston, A Hahn, L Homer, A Kabeer, S Kannan, Dr Khan, K L Kong, A McKenzie, A Mosquera, H Nagi, D Newbould, M Patel, R Rasanayagam, A Rayen, P L Riddell, N Sherwood, A Thwaites, S B Vohra

Cardiology G Lip, R MacFayden, T Millane, C Varma, R D S Watson

Dermatology A Abdullah, I S Foulds, S Lanigan, M Ogboli, J Paul, K S Ryatt, C Y Tan

ENT A Batch, T K Bhattacharyya, J O'Connell, M Oluwole, A Sinha

General Medicine A Basu, A C Burden, B T Cooper, P De, R E Ferner, S Hutchinson, P B Iles, T Iqbal, S Kausar, O Khair, N Langford, B Lee, M Lewis, A Raghuram, A Ritch, R E J Ryder, P Sarkar, M A Simons, J A Vale, P Wilson

General Surgery S Bhalerao, H Brown, I A Donovan, F Hoar, P Nicholl, M L Obeid, S H Silverman, R Spychal, L Vishwanath, R L Wolverson

Haematology R Murrin, C Wright

Immunology J North

Medical Microbiology A Fraise, T Weller

Neurology D Nicholl, S G Sturman

Nuclear Medicine A Notghi

Obstetrics and Gynaecology A S Arunkalaivanan, S Baghdadi, S Bakour, N Bhatti, G Downey, L Dwarakanath

Occupational Health J Halliday-Bell

Oncology J Glaholm, C Poole, D Rea, D Spooner

Ophthalmology J Ainsworth, M Benson, M Burden, L Butler, I Cuniliffe, S Elsherbiny, J M Gibson, M Hope-Ross, A Jacks, G R Kirkby, P L Lip, P McDonnell, T Matthews, A Murray, E O'Neill, T Reuser, R Scott, P Shah, S Shah, P Stavrou, V Sung, G Sutton, M Tsaloumas, H Willshaw

Oral Surgery S J Liggins, B Speculand

Paediatrics A Akbar, D Armstrong, A Aukett, J G Bissenden, V Ganesan, J Nycyk, M Plunkett, H M Robertson, N Shaw, P H Weller

Pathology S Y Chan, J C Gearty, M Maheshwari, U Zanetto

Plastic Surgery M S Fatah, G Sterne

Radiology F A Aitchison, J Benham, J Clarke, M Davies, D M Dawkins, K Lee, M J McMinn, M Moss, H-G Teo, S Vydianath, S L Walker, J Wingate

Rheumatology D Carruthers, D Situnayake

Trauma and Orthopaedics S Deshmukh, W Herron, Mr Lin, S Parekh, B K Singh, M S Vishwanath

Urology R Devarajan, P G Ryan, T Sami

Rowley Regis Hospital

Moor Lane, Rowley Regis, Warley B65 8DA
Tel: 0121 607 3465
Total Beds: 76

Sandwell District General Hospital

Lyndon, West Bromwich B71 4HJ
Tel: 0121 553 1831 Fax: 0121 607 3117
Total Beds: 562

Accident and Emergency C J Holburn, S Ishaq, K Murali, J Rizkalla

Anaesthetics J M Bellin, V Bulso, N P Carter, H Daya, D H Dubash, I F Duncan, A Jansen van Vuuren, S Kanari, E Leno, D D R Macaulay, L Murali, A Patel, D Poole, M C Suchak

Cardiology R Ahmad, P Cadigan, D Connolly, R Davis

Care of the Elderly C Crowther, R Dutta, M Hussain, N Page

Gastroenterology C Cobb, S Singhal, N Trudgill

General Medicine I Ahmed, G V H Bradby, P Davies, H Ibrahim, D T McLeod, D A Robertson, L Walsh

General Surgery A Aukland, E T Bainbridge, N Cruickshank, D J Ellis, M Vairavan, K Wheatley

Genitourinary Medicine T Ray

Haematology Y Hasan, P Stableforth

Histopathology S Banerjee, F Brook, S Muzaffar, C Nandini, U Pandey, J Simon

Microbiology A Davies, N Williams

Neurology A Sivaguru

Obstetrics and Gynaecology I Abukhalil, J Kabukoba, R Manivasagam, M Mattar, R K Smith

Occupational Medicine P Verow

Ophthalmology S P Aggarwal, J Al-Ibrahim, M Quinlan, A Tyagi

Orthopaedic Surgery S Kulkarni

Paediatrics C Agwu, H Grindulis, R Jayatunga, D C Low, A J Mayne, H Nachi, M Wallis

Pathology E Hughes

Plastic Surgery A Khanna, J M Porter

Radiology A H S Ahmed, R C Bhatt, D Chand, R M Donovan, A R M Evans, J F Leahy, S Yusuf

Rheumatology K Grindulis, F Khattak

Trauma and Orthopaedics J C Clothier, M M El-Safty, S S Geeranavar

Urology M A Jones, K Kadow

Sandwell Mental Health NHS and Social Care Trust

48 Lodge Road, West Bromwich B70 8NY
Tel: 0121 553 7676 Fax: 0121 607 3290
Email: enquiries@smhsct.nhs.uk
Website: www.smhsct.nhs.uk
(Birmingham and the Black Country Strategic Health Authority)

Chair William Thomas
Chief Executive Karen Dowman

Edward Street Hospital and Day Unit

Edward Street, West Bromwich B70 8NU
Tel: 0121 553 7676 Fax: 0121 607 3576
Total Beds: 96

Psychiatry of Old Age S Edwards

Hallam Street Hospital

Hallam Street, West Bromwich B71 4NH
Tel: 0121 607 3900 Fax: 0121 607 3901
Total Beds: 72

Manager E Quaynor

Heath Lane Hospital

Heath Lane, West Bromwich B71 2BG
Tel: 0121 553 7676 Fax: 0121 607 3070
Total Beds: 35

Manager L Arlidge

Scarborough and North East Yorkshire Health Care NHS Trust

Scarborough Hospital, Woodlands Drive, Scarborough YO12 6QL
Tel: 01723 368111 Fax: 01723 342581
Website: www.scarborough-trust.nhs.uk
(North and East Yorkshire and Northern Lincolnshire Strategic Health Authority)

Chair Richard Grunwell
Chief Executive Alison Guy

Bridlington and District Hospital

Bessingby Road, Bridlington YO16 4QP
Tel: 01262 606666
Total Beds: 164

Manager Sue Wellington

Accident and Emergency A P Volans

Cardiology M A Memon

ENT J G D Baker

General Medicine D B Humphriss, M N Pond

Neurophysiology S M H Al-Ani

Obstetrics and Gynaecology R Yeo

Ophthalmology P J Bacon

Rheumatology I W Tomlinson

Urology K G Brame

Haworth Unit
Scarborough Hospital, Woodlands Drive, Scarborough YO12 6QL
Tel: 01723 342278 Fax: 01723 342244

Manager Dawn Whelan

Malton, Norton and District Hospital
Middlecave Road, Malton YO17 0NG
Tel: 01653 693041 Fax: 01653 600589
Total Beds: 62

Manager Mary Stevens

Ophthalmology P J Bacon
Orthopaedics J G Bradley

Scarborough Hospital
Woodlands Drive, Scarborough YO12 6QL
Tel: 01723 368111 Fax: 01723 344244
Total Beds: 373

Manager Jackie Morton, Lorraine Naylor

Accident and Emergency A P Volans

Anaesthetics D F Jones, I C Tring, M A Turner

Cardiology R S Clark, M A Memon

Care of the Elderly S K Chatterjee, W N R Perera

Dermatology A S Highet

ENT J G D Baker, E B Whitby

General Medicine Z S A Al-Saffar, D B Humphriss, C J Mitchell, J Paterson

General Surgery B Balasubramanian, P J Carleton, N M N El-Barghouty, J Macfie, E P Perry

Neurology A Ming, J Tarafder

Obstetrics and Gynaecology A D Booth, M C B Noble, D R Poole, D W Robinson

Ophthalmology P J Bacon, R M Redmond, J van der Hoek

Orthopaedics C M Andrews, J G Bradley, A Lavender, J P Livesey, A D North

Paediatrics A R Falconer, M A R Quneibi, I M Rawashdeh, U R Venkatesh

Urology K G Brame, S J Hawkyard, A S Robertson

Whitby Hospital
Spring Hill, Whitby YO21 1DP
Tel: 01947 604851 Fax: 01947 820568
Total Beds: 96

Manager Maggie Stevens

Scarborough, Whitby and Ryedale Primary Care Trust

13 Yorkersgate, Malton YO17 7AA
Tel: 01653 602900 Fax: 01653 690804
Email: firstname.surname@swrpct.nhs.uk
Website: www.swr-pcg.nhs.uk
(North and East Yorkshire and Northern Lincolnshire Strategic Health Authority)

Chair Colin Barnes
Chief Executive Michael Whitworth

Malton Community Hospital
Middlecave Road, Malton YO17 7NQ
Tel: 01653 693041

Whitby Community Hospital
Springhill, Whitby YO21 1EE

Sedgefield Primary Care Trust

Merrington House, Merrington Lane, Spennymoor DL16 7UT
Tel: 0191 301 3820 Fax: 0191 301 3821
Email: info@sedgefieldpct.nhs.uk
Website: www.sedgefield-pct.nhs.uk
(County Durham and Tees Valley Strategic Health Authority)

Chair Gloria Wills
Chief Executive Nigel Porter

Selby and York Primary Care Trust

Sovereign House, Kettlestring Lane, Clifton Moor, York YO30 4GQ
Tel: 01904 825110 Fax: 01904 825125
Email: firstname.surname@sypct.nhs.uk
Website: www.sypct.nhs.uk
(North and East Yorkshire and Northern Lincolnshire Strategic Health Authority)

Chair Wendy Bundy
Chief Executive Jeremy Clough

Bootham Park Hospital
Bootham, York YO30 7BY
Tel: 01904 610777 Fax: 01904 726849
Total Beds: 120

Manager A Weerakoon

General Psychiatry R D Adams (Head), P Blenkiron, L M Brown, J Clarke, A J Gopalaswamy, J Holland, J Isherwood, C A Kirk, C Marchant, S P Reilly, S P Shaw

St Monica's Hospital
Long Street, Easingwold, York YO61 3JD
Tel: 01347 821214
Total Beds: 11

Selby War Memorial Hospital
Doncaster Road, Selby YO8 9BX
Tel: 01757 702664 Fax: 01757 213783
Total Beds: 40

Sheffield Care Trust

Fulwood House, Old Fulwood Road, Sheffield S10 3TH
Tel: 0114 271 6310 Fax: 0114 271 6734
Email: firstname.surname@sct.nhs.uk
Website: www.sct.nhs.uk
(South Yorkshire Strategic Health Authority)

Chair Alan Walker
Chief Executive Kevan Taylor

Beighton Hospital
Sevenaires Road, Beighton, Sheffield S19 6NZ
Tel: 0114 271 6572

Forest Lodge
5 Forest Lodge Close, Sheffield S30 3JW
Tel: 0114 271 6081

Grenoside Grange
Saltbox Lane, Sheffield S30 3QS
Tel: 0114 271 6131
Total Beds: 10

Nether Edge Hospital
Cavendish Ward 1, Osbourne Road, Sheffield S11 9EL
Tel: 0114 271 6787
Total Beds: 25

Shirle Hill Day Hospital
St Andrews Road, Nether Edge, Sheffield S11 9AA
Tel: 0114 271 6383 Fax: 0114 271 6382

Shirle Hill Hospital
Cherry Tree Road, Sheffield S11 9AA
Tel: 0114 271 6863
Total Beds: 6

Sheffield Children's NHS Trust

Western Bank, Sheffield S10 2TH
Tel: 0114 271 7000 Fax: 0114 272 3418
Email: sheffield.childrenshospital@sch.nhs.uk
Website: www.sheffieldchildrens.com
(South Yorkshire Strategic Health Authority)

Chair Lynn Hagger
Chief Executive Chris Sharratt

Sheffield Children's Hospital
Western Bank, Sheffield S10 2TH
Tel: 0114 271 7000 Fax: 0114 272 3418
Total Beds: 159

Accident and Emergency P O B Brennan, D Burke, B Tesfayohannes, J Yassa

Anaesthetics I Barker, N R Bennett, T Dorman, J M Goddard, R John, C Kirton, N H Pereira, C Stack

Audiological Medicine O P Tungland

Cardiology D Dickenson, J Gibbs, J Parsons

Chemical Pathology J Bohnam

Dental Surgery L Davidson

Dermatology M J Cork, A G Messenger

ENT P D Bull

General Psychiatry S Hughes, R Waller

Genetics J Cook, O Quarrell

Haematology A Vora

Medical Education H Davies

Medical Microbiology D Harris, L Ridgeway

Ophthalmology D Brosnahan, J Burke

Oral and Maxillofacial Surgery P P Robinson, S E Ward

Orthopaedics M J Bell, A G Davis, D L Douglas, M J Flowers, A C Howard, M Saleh, T W D Smith

Paediatric Surgery A E Mackinnon, J Roberts, R Shawis, J Walker

Paediatrics L H Allison, J dez Chaplais, M Everard, M P Gerrard, C A MacKenzie, G Moss, K Price, R Primhak, S Tanner, C J Taylor, J K H Wales

Pathology S Variend

Plastic Surgery T M Brotherston, E Freedlander, R W Griffiths, J G Miller, R E Page

Radiology P S Broadley, P Griffiths, I Lang, G Long, A Sprigg

Rheumatology R Amos

Sheffield South West Primary Care Trust

5 Old Fulwood Road, Fulwood, Sheffield S10 3TG
Tel: 0114 271 1100 Fax: 0114 271 1101
Website: www.sheffield.nhs.uk/southwestpct
(South Yorkshire Strategic Health Authority)

Chair Ann Le Sage
Chief Executive Janet Soo-Chung

Sheffield Teaching Hospitals NHS Foundation Trust

Established as a Foundation Trust 01/07/2004.

8 Beech Hill Road, Sheffield S10 2SB
Tel: 0114 226 1000 Fax: 0114 226 1001
Website: www.sth.org.uk
(South Yorkshire Strategic Health Authority)

Chair David Stone
Chief Executive Andrew Cash

Charles Clifford Dental Hospital
Wellesley Road, Sheffield S10 2SZ
Tel: 0114 271 7800 Fax: 0114 271 7836

Child Dental Health P Benson, A H Brook, L E Davidson, M Stern, D R Willmot

Oral and Maxillofacial Surgery I M Brook, A R Loescher, P P Robinson, A T Smith, S Ward, C M Yeoman

Oral Pathology G T Craig, C D Franklin, C J Smith

Restorative Dentistry I R Harris, R I Joshi, D J Lamb, A Rawlinson, T F Walsh, R B Winstanley, P F Wragg

Jessop Wing Women's Hospital
Tree Root Walk, Sheffield S10 2SF
Tel: 0114 271 1900 Fax: 0114 271 1901
Total Beds: 119

Northern General Hospital
Herries Road, Sheffield S5 7AU
Tel: 0114 243 4343 Fax: 0114 256 0472
Total Beds: 1200

Accident and Emergency S M Mason

Anaesthetics J D Alderson, T N Appleyard, A P G Beechey, C L Harper, N Harrison, P R Knowles, C A Moore, N J Morgan-Hughes, D J K White, A M Wilson

Cardiology R J Bowes, S Campbell, D C Crossman, J P G Gunn, C M H Newman, G D G Oakley, J Sahu, N M Wheeldon

Cardiothoracic Surgery P C Braidley, G J Cooper, D N Hopkinson, T J Locke, M Matuszewski, G Rocco, P K Sarkar, R Vaughan, G A L Wilkinson

Care of the Elderly D F da Costa, T J Hendra, M Jennings, P J Lawson-Matthew

General Medicine A Al-Mohammad, P B Anderson, C A Austin, W M Bennet, S R Brennan, F M Creagh, M T Donnelly, G W Duff, F P Edenborough, C A Hardisty, S R Heller, J M Hill, B J Hutchcroft, B J Liddle, A D R Mackie, J D C Newell-Price, S A Riley, R J M Ross, J Webster, A P Weetman

General Surgery S N O Amin, S R Brown, P S F Chan, V Chidambaram, P D F Dodd, A Giannoukas, B J Harrison, L M Hunt, M S Karim, R J Lonsdale, J A Michaels, R Nair, A H K Nassef, A T Raftery, B M Shrestha, J A R Smith, A Wyman

Nephrology C B Brown, A M El Nahas, N J M Fardon, W S McKane, A C M Ong, D Throssell, M E Wilkie

Orthopaedics M J Bell, C M Blundell, S H Bostock, J N Brown, S C Buckley, N Chiverton, M G Dennison, D L Douglas, C J M Getty, R J B Gibson, A J Hamer, A C Howard, R M Kerry, S H Norris, D Potter, S L Royston, M Saleh, T W D Smith, D Stanley, I Stockley, P M Sutton

Palliative Medicine P D Gajjar, T W Noble

Pathology T A Gray, S K Suvarna

Plastic Surgery T M Brotherston, C M Caddy, D G Dujon, E Freedlander, R W Griffiths, M I Hobson, J G Miller, R E Page, D R Ralston

Radiology N A Barrington, P W G Brown, M J Bull, H A Euinton, P A Gaines, S Matthews, D J Moore, S M Thomas, C S Tweed

Rheumatology and Rehabilitation D Datta, M R McClelland, N F A Peel, S H Till

Urology P R Tophill

Royal Hallamshire Hospital

Glossop Road, Sheffield S10 2JF
Tel: 0114 271 1900 Fax: 0114 271 1901
Total Beds: 750

Anaesthetics S Ahmedzai, J C Andrzejowski, D F Appleton, R E Atkinson, M Berthoud, R J Birks, D P Breen, A J Davidson, D F Doyle, D L Edbrooke, G A Francis, R Freeman, S P Gerrish, E Groves, J V B Mundy, P Murray, J E Peacock, M Pullman, M N Richmond, D B Shepherd, G R Veall, P A Wilkinson, I J Wrench

Cardiology K S Channer, D Oakley, J N West

Dermatology M J Cork, D J Gawkrodger, C I Harrington, N C Hepburn, A J McDonagh, A G Messenger

Diabetes S L Caddick, M W Savage, S Tesfaye

Endocrinology D R Cullen, G T Gillett, T H Jones, R Ross, J Webster

ENT P D Bull, D F Chapman, A J Parker, O P Tungland, T J Woolford, M P Yardley

Gastroenterology D C Gleeson, A Lobo, M E McAlindon

General Surgery A G Johnson, S R Kohlhardt, A W Majeed, M W R Reed, A J Shorthouse, C J Stoddard, W E G Thomas

Genitourinary Medicine G M Dilke-Wing, P A Fraser, D A Hicks, G R Kinghorn, K E Rogstad, M D Talbot, A M Wright

Haematology K K Hampton, M Makris, F E Preston, D C Rees, J T Reilly, E A M Vandenberghe, D A Winfield

Infection and Tropical Medicine S T Green, M W McKendrick, R C Read

Ophthalmology J Burke, J Chan, S Longstaff, M Nelson, I Rennie, P Rundle, J Talbot, J West, S Winder

Pathology C A Angel, S S Cross, A K Dube, J R Goepel, P G Ince, J A Lee, M A Parsons, A Sherif, D N Slater, J H F Smith, T J Stephenson, W R Timperley, J C E Underwood, C W Warren, M Wells

Pharmacology N D S Bax, P R Jackson, L E Ramsay, H F Woods, W W Yeo

Respiratory Medicine D Fishwick, T W Higenbottam, R Lawson, M K Whyte

Rheumatology M A Akil, R S Amos, D E Bax, C J M Getty, J G Miller, M L Snaith, D Stanley, S H Till, A G Wilson, J Winfield

Stroke Medicine A J Anderson, T J Hendra

Urology J B Anderson, C R Chapple, F C Hamdy, K J Hastie, N Oakley, D J Smith

Weston Park Hospital

Whitham Road, Sheffield S10 2SJ
Tel: 0114 226 5000 Fax: 0114 226 5555
Total Beds: 109

Oncology K S Dunn, P Fisher, B W Hancock, M Q Hatton, P Kirkbride, D P Levy, P C Lorigan, I H Manifold, B Orr, S D Pledge, O P Purohit, D J Radstone, S Ramakrishnan, M H Robinson

Sheffield West Primary Care Trust

West Court, Hillsborough Barracks, Langsett Road, Sheffield S6 2LR
Tel: 0114 226 4600 Fax: 0114 226 4601
Website: www.sheffield.nhs.uk/westpct/
(South Yorkshire Strategic Health Authority)

Chair Louise White
Chief Executive Simon Gilby

Shepway Primary Care Trust

8 Radnor Park Avenue, Folkestone CT19 5BN
Tel: 01303 222481 Fax: 01303 222487
Website: www.shepwaypct.nhs.uk
(Kent and Medway Strategic Health Authority)

Chief Executive Ann Sutton

Sherwood Forest Hospitals NHS Trust

Mansfield Road, Sutton-in-Ashfield NG17 4JL
Tel: 01623 622515 Fax: 01623 621770
Website: www.sherwoodforesthospitals.nhs.uk
(Trent Strategic Health Authority)

Chair Brian Meakin
Chief Executive Jeffrey Worrall

Ashfield Community Hospital

Portland Street, Kirkby-in-Ashfield, Nottingham NG17 7AE
Tel: 01623 785050

King's Mill Hospital

Mansfield Road, Sutton-in-Ashfield NG17 4JL
Tel: 01623 622515 Fax: 01683 621770
Total Beds: 635

Anaesthetics J A Anderson, P Barrett, I Bishton, P T Bull, A Dyson, T Keane, J S Mason, M Mowbray, P J Randall, M T Ross, A Voice, A J Whitaker

Dermatology S M Littlewood, E M Saihan

ENT S Ali, W D McNicoll, - Osiname

General Medicine N Ali, R H Lloyd Mostyn, M Mahmoud, S O'Nunain, J Rowley, K A Sands, J Snape, M Vassallo, M Ward

General Surgery J R S Blake, B J Fairbrother, G H Greatrex, F R Jackaman, D Reid

Haematology M Auger, E C Logan

Medical Microbiology M Rahman

Obstetrics and Gynaecology R Dixon, C A Gie, P Makepeace, C J Pickles, G Shrestha

Occupational Health B W Platts

Ophthalmology T Arulampalam, P Nithianandan, A S Rubasingham

Oral and Maxillofacial Surgery P G Watts

Orthodontics D G Nashed

Orthopaedics J Hambidge, P J Livesley, A Moulton, M Needoff, H G Prince, V M Srivastava

Paediatrics S A Beningfield, R F Harris, D I Johnston, V Noble, A P Worsley

Pathology F M Dowling, G Hulman, P J Stocks

Plastic Surgery F B Baillie, M Deane

Radiology S E Brauer, C C A Butcher, E J Cornford, P Ghosh, P N Panto, S Stinchcombe

Radiotherapy E M Bessell

Rheumatology and Rehabilitation K Lim

Urology R J Lemberger, M C Taylor

Mansfield Community Hospital

Stockwell Gate, Mansfield NG18 5QJ
Tel: 01623 785050 Fax: 01623 635357
Total Beds: 112

Care of the Elderly A Akbar, A B M Rahman, J Snape

Radiology S E Brauer, C Butcher, P N Panto, D Svenne

Newark Hospital

Boundary Road, Newark NG24 4DE
Tel: 01636 681681 Fax: 01636 685971
Total Beds: 101

Anaesthetics F D Sullivan

Chest Disease J MacFarlane

Dermatology S M Littlewood

ENT K P Gibbin

General Medicine C R Birch, R S Chowhan, I N Ross

General Psychiatry D A James

General Surgery V S Maheson, C Ubhi, J L Wilkins

Obstetrics and Gynaecology C Gie, R P Husemeyer, R Spencer-Gregson

Ophthalmology T Arulampalam, D Knight-Jones, A S Rubasingham

Orthopaedics J S Hopkins

Paediatrics C S Nanyakkara

Pathology A Lawrence

Radiology S J Bradley

Radiotherapy and Oncology S Chan

Urology J Dunn

The Shrewsbury and Telford Hospital NHS Trust

Royal Shrewsbury Hospital, Mytton Oak Road, Shrewsbury SY3 8XQ
Tel: 01743 261000 Fax: 01743 261489
Website: www.sath.nhs.uk
(Shropshire and Staffordshire Strategic Health Authority)

Chair Phil Homer
Chief Executive Andrew Pritchard

Princess Royal Hospital

Apley Castle, Telford TF6 6TF
Tel: 01952 641222 Fax: 01952 242817
Website: www.prh-telford.org.uk
Total Beds: 344

Manager Neil Taylor

Accident and Emergency V P Alfonsi, A Leaman

Anaesthetics R H Carley, P D Cartwright, D Christmas, G C Corser, K C Hickmott, G H Phillips, S Sanghera, N Tufft

Chemical Pathology N E Capps

Dermatology S Kelly

General Medicine J Bateman, R R Campbell, M Heber, M E Heber, R Jones, N Mike, H Mollogil, D O'Gorman, G Townson, T E T West

General Surgery R G M Duffield, C P Hinton, J B Quayle

Genitourinary Medicine S V Devendra

Haematology G W Slocombe

Histopathology J M Grainger

Medical Microbiology P O'Neil

Neurology P Newman

Orthodontics D C Tidy

Orthopaedics T P K Crichlow, R Dodenhoff, P May, R D Perkins, B Summers

Paediatrics S Abdu, F Hinde, L Ingram, N Vrahimis

Radiology P Lowe, R A Manns, M T J Walsh

Urology C J M Beacock, S Coppinger, A Hay

Royal Shrewsbury Hospital

Mytton Oak Road, Shrewsbury SY3 8XQ
Tel: 01743 261000 Fax: 01743 261006
Total Beds: 520

Anaesthetics I Baguley, H Brunner, M E Fryer, R Hatts, D H King, C T Major, J E Marshall, M Mehta, G R Thompson, I Williams

Bacteriology N J Mitchell, P M O'Neill, R E Warren

Care of the Elderly S N Agnihotri, S N Hill, Dr Ho

Dental Surgery S F Olley, D Wedgwood

Dermatology S Kelly

General Medicine R C Butler, S P Davies, L F Hill, A F Macleod, D Maxton, W H Perks, M S H Smith, P T Wilmshurst, R S E Wilson

General Surgery A Houghton, T Hunt, R A Hurlow, A Schofield

Genitourinary Medicine S U Devendra

Neurology S Nightingale

Obstetrics and Gynaecology B B Bentick, J Lane, M Mohajer, S Oates, D H A Redford, N N Reed, A S J Tapp

Orthodontics J C Chadwick

Orthopaedics D J Ford, S Hay, C Kelly, C M McGeoch, J Patrick, R Spencer-Jones, S White

Paediatrics J E H Brice, S Deshpande, R C M Quinlivan, J Watt, R Welch

Pathology R A Fraser, J M Grainger, N Green, C E Hinton, T J Jones, P D Leedham, P Murphy, P E Nicholls, N O'Connor, M I Otter, G W Slocombe

Plastic Surgery P Davison

Radiology S M Aldridge, M R E Dean, J A Fielding, W J Norman, R I Orme, H R Watson

Radiotherapy and Oncology A Agrawal, S Awwad

Urology C Beacock, S V Coppinger, A M Hay

Shropshire County Primary Care Trust

William Farr House, Mytton Oak Road, Shrewsbury SY3 8XL
Tel: 01743 261300 Fax: 01743 261303
Website: www.shropshirepct.nhs.uk
(Shropshire and Staffordshire Strategic Health Authority)

Chair Liz Owen
Chief Executive Julie Grant

Bishops Castle Community Hospital
Bishops Castle SY9 5AJ
Tel: 01588 638220 Fax: 01588 638756
Total Beds: 24

Bridgnorth Hospital
Bridgnorth WV16 4EU
Tel: 01746 762641 Fax: 01746 766172
Total Beds: 25

Ludlow Hospital
Gravel Hill, Ludlow SY8 1QX
Tel: 01584 872201 Fax: 01584 877908
Total Beds: 63

Shelton Hospital
Bicton Heath, Shrewsbury SY3 8DN
Tel: 01743 261000 Fax: 01743 261279
Total Beds: 238

West Bank Hospital
300 Holyhead Road, Wellington, Telford TF1 2FF
Tel: 01952 243482 Fax: 01952 641953
Total Beds: 12

Whitchurch Hospital
Claypit Street, Deermoss, Whitchurch SY13 1QS
Tel: 01948 666292
Total Beds: 56

Slough Primary Care Trust

Trust Headquarters, Upton Hospital, Albert Street, Slough SL1 2BJ
Tel: 01753 821441 Fax: 01753 635047
Website: www.berkshire.nhs.uk/slough/
(Thames Valley Strategic Health Authority)

Chair Geoff Cutting
Chief Executive Mike Attwood

Upton Hospital
Albert Street, Slough SL1 2BJ
Tel: 01753 821441
Total Beds: 105

Solihull Primary Care Trust

20 Union Road, Solihull B91 3EF
Tel: 0121 712 8300 Fax: 0121 711 7212
Website: www.solihull.nhs.uk
(Birmingham and the Black Country Strategic Health Authority)

Chair Anne Dorow
Consultants Cathy Feehan, Steve Hinder, Richard Soppitt

Somerset Coast Primary Care Trust

2nd Floor, Mallard Court, Express Park, Bristol Road, Bridgwater TA6 4RN
Tel: 01278 432000 Fax: 01278 432099
Email: somcoast@somcoastpct.nhs.uk
Website: www.somersetcoastpct.nhs.uk
(Dorset and Somerset Strategic Health Authority)

Chair Christine Dore
Chief Executive Alan Carpenter

Bridgwater Community Hospital
Salmon Parade, Bridgwater TA6 5AH
Tel: 01278 451501 Fax: 01278 444896
Total Beds: 66

Manager Sian Teal

Burnham-on-Sea War Memorial Hospital
Love Lane, Burnham-on-Sea TA8 1ED
Tel: 01934 773100 Fax: 01278 793367
Total Beds: 23

Manager Sian Teal

Minehead and West Somerset Hospital
The Avenue, Minehead TA24 5LY
Tel: 01643 707251 Fax: 01643 707251
Total Beds: 33

Manager Jane Fitzgerald

Williton and District Hospital
Williton, Taunton TA4 4RA
Tel: 01984 635600 Fax: 01984 633026
Total Beds: 45

Manager Jane Fitzgerald

Somerset Partnership NHS and Social Care Trust

Broadway House, Broadway Park, Barclay Street, Bridgwater TA6 5YA
Tel: 01278 720200 Fax: 01278 720201
Email: ask@sompar.nhs.uk
Website: www.somerset-health.org.uk
(Dorset and Somerset Strategic Health Authority)

Chair Linda Nash
Chief Executive John Haines
Consultants C M Absolon, Waqar Ahmed, N J Airey, N M Bailey, J S Barnes, Jon Barnes, J Barnett, R Brook, R P Clacey, A D Cockett, D R Davies, S Dobson, M J Eales, S Frazer, Jason Hepple, A Hoar, C Johnson, J Kenny, A Knight, S Koslowski, G Lemmens, David Marshall, C Mortimore, E Ostler, J Rossiter, Steve Rossiter, M Spencer, T Trower, M Upton, A Wolton

Barnfield House
Selbourne Place, Minehead TA24 5TY
Tel: 01643 706999 Fax: 01643 707291
Total Beds: 16

Beech Court
Southgate Park, Taunton Road, Bridgwater TA6 3LS
Tel: 01278 444737 Fax: 01278 446717
Total Beds: 23

Cedar House
Cedar Lodge, Holly Court, Summerlands, Yeovil BA20 2BN
Tel: 01935 428420 Fax: 01935 411612

College House
Broadway Park, Barclay Street, Bridgwater TA6 5YA
Tel: 01278 446149

Cranleigh House
Broadway Park, Barclay Street, Bridgwater TA6 5YA
Tel: 01278 446165 Fax: 01278 446154
Total Beds: 18

Hadspen Wood and Ridley Day Hospital
Verrington Hospital, Dancing Lane, Wincanton BA9 9DQ
Tel: 01963 32006 Fax: 01963 34708
Total Beds: 6

Little Court
2 Pinnockscroft, Burnham-on-Sea TA8 2NF
Tel: 01278 786876 Fax: 01278 795290
Total Beds: 16

Orchard Lodge Young People's Unit
Cotford St Luke, Taunton TA4 1DB
Tel: 01823 432211 Fax: 01823 432541
Total Beds: 14

General Psychiatry A D Cockett

Rosebank
Priory Park, Glastonbury Road, Wells BA5 1TH
Tel: 01749 683320 Fax: 01749 683380
Total Beds: 18

Rydon House
Cheddon Road, Taunton TA2 7AZ
Tel: 01823 333438 Fax: 01823 333287
Total Beds: 32

South and East Dorset Primary Care Trust

Victoria House, Princes Road, Ferndown BH22 9JR
Tel: 01202 850600 Fax: 01202 850601
Email: enquiries@ferndown.sedorset-pct.nhs.uk
Website: www.southandeastdorsetpct.nhs.uk
(Dorset and Somerset Strategic Health Authority)

Chair Ruth Bussey
Chief Executive Andrew Cawthron

St Leonard's Hospital
241 Ringwood Road, Ringwood BH24 2RR
Tel: 01202 871165 Fax: 01202 895945
Total Beds: 52

Manager Terry Pickernell

Swanage Hospital
Queen's Road, Swanage BH19 2ES
Tel: 01929 422282 Fax: 01929 423872
Total Beds: 15

Manager Cath Granger

Wareham Hospital
Streche Road, Wareham BH20 4QQ
Tel: 01929 552433 Fax: 01929 550170
Total Beds: 32

Manager Ruth McEwen

Wimborne Hospital
Victoria Road, Wimborne BH21 1ER
Tel: 01202 858200 Fax: 01202 849516
Total Beds: 42

Manager Teresa North

South Birmingham Primary Care Trust

Trust Headquarters, Moseley Hall Hospital, Alcester Road, Moseley, Birmingham B13 8JL
Tel: 0121 442 5600 Fax: 0121 442 5648
Email: info@southbirminghampct.nhs.uk
Website: www.southbirminghampct.nhs.uk
(Birmingham and the Black Country Strategic Health Authority)

Chair David Cox
Chief Executive Graham Urwin
Consultants Rick Roberts

Birmingham Dental Hospital
St Chad's, Queensway, Birmingham B4 6NN
Tel: 0121 236 8611 Fax: 0121 237 2750

Anaesthetics T Bowden, M D Brewin, G Dickson, M Ghoris, R Hibbert, S Hylton, M King, A Malins, J M Watt

Oral Medicine J Hamburger

Oral Surgery J W Frame, W R Roberts

Orthodontics J W Ferguson, R R Pinson, W P Rock

Paediatric Dentistry L Shaw

Public Health R J Anderson

Radiology J Rout

Restorative Dentistry I Chapple, J C Davenport, W R E Laird, P J Lumley, E A McLaughlin, M S Saxby, M J Shaw, A C C Shortall, A D Walmsley, K Warren

Moseley Hall Hospital
Alcester Road, Birmingham B13 8JL
Tel: 0121 442 4321 Fax: 0121 442 3556
Total Beds: 126

Care of the Elderly P P Mayer, J Rowe, A Sinclair

West Heath Hospital
Rednal Road, Birmingham B38 8HR
Tel: 0121 627 1627 Fax: 0121 627 8228
Total Beds: 138

Care of the Elderly E J Dunstan, M Goodman, A Main, J Rowe

South Cambridgeshire Primary Care Trust

Heron Court, Block 23, Ida Darwin, Fulbourn, Cambridge CB1 5EE
Tel: 01223 885880 Fax: 01223 855705
Website: www.southcambs-pct.nhs.uk
(Norfolk, Suffolk and Cambridgeshire Strategic Health Authority)

Chair Ruth Rogers
Chief Executive Sally Hind
Consultants Fahma Janjug, David Kanka, Elaine Lewis, Alison Samsome, David Vickers

South Devon Healthcare NHS Trust

Hengrave House, Torbay Hospital, Lawes Bridge, Torquay TQ2 7AA
Tel: 01803 614567 Fax: 01803 616334
Email: chiefexecutive.sdhct@nhs.net
Website: www.sdhct.nhs.uk
(South West Peninsula Strategic Health Authority)

Chair David Hudson
Chief Executive Tony Parr

Torbay Hospital
Lawes Bridge, Torquay TQ2 7AA
Tel: 01803 614567 Fax: 01803 616334
Email: chiefexecutive.sdhct@nhs.net
Website: www.sdhct.nhs.uk
Total Beds: 500

Accident and Emergency S Cope, J N T Egan, G Gardner, J Horner, M Sach

Anaesthetics J Ackers, A Bainton, P G Ballance, N Campbell, J Carlisle, S J Fearnley, M Hearn, K Houghton, M Human, J Ingham, A Magides, A Matthews, M Mercer, J Montgomery, D Natusch, I

Norley, J Norman, J C Pappin, D Snow, M Swart, R Tackley, J L Thorn, A Varvinsky

Care of the Elderly G P Kendall, P J Sleight

Child and Adolescent Psychiatry I MacLeod

Dermatology J Adams, T Frost

ENT D Alderson, S A Hickey, F P Houlihan, J D Hutchison

General Medicine C Carey, G Cribbin, L Dobson, R Dyer, C Edwards, K George, J Goldman, P Keeling, J Lowes, I R Mahy, R B Paisey, D Sinclair, J Smith, R H Teague

General Surgery I Currie, P Donnelly, D D Friend, P Houghton, R G Hughes, N Johnson, Mr Kirollos, P Lewis, S MacDermott, R Mason, S Mitchell, R Pullan

Genitourinary Medicine J R Willcox

Haematology P Roberts, N Rymes, S Smith, D Turner

Microbiology T Maggs, P Turner

Neurology M Beaman, S Edwards, J D Gibson, J Hobart, R McGonigle, M Sadler

Obstetrics and Gynaecology J Barrington, M Leggott, G Pandher, R Ranjit, P J Stannard

Oncology D Bailey

Ophthalmology M Cole, A Frost, C M Graham, C R H James, S J Livesey, Y Osoba, T Sleep

Oral and Maxillofacial Surgery D Cunliffe, P Douglas

Orthodontics R Robinson, A J Smith

Orthopaedics M Ashworth, P Birdsall, V Conboy, J Davis, M Hockings, G B Irvine, K Kamesh, R Lofthouse, A G MacEachern, J Marshall

Paediatrics J Broomhall, L Dibble, B Fraser, S Imong, C P Sainsbury, B Singh

Palliative Medicine R Scheffer, J Sykes

Pathology J Bridger, D Farrell, C Garrido, N Ryley

Plastic Surgery P Saxby, C Stone

Radiology D Buckley, R Heafield, S Higgins, S Horton, J Isaacs, P Kember, E Morris, M Puckett, R Seymour, G W Urquhart, P White

Radiotherapy and Oncology A Goodman, A Lydon

Restorative Dentistry S Ellis

Rheumatology N Viner

South Downs Health NHS Trust

Brighton General Hospital, Elm Grove, Brighton BN2 3EW
Tel: 01273 696011 Fax: 01273 242215 (Trust HQ)
Email: enquiry@southdowns.nhs.uk
Website: www.southdowns.nhs.uk
(Surrey and Sussex Strategic Health Authority)

Chair Quintin Barry
Chief Executive Michael Rosenberg

Aldrington Day Hospital

35 New Church Road, Hove BN3 4AG
Tel: 01273 778383 Fax: 01273 738407

Manager Cheryl Richards

Brighton General Hospital

Elm Grove, Brighton BN2 3EW
Tel: 01273 696011 Fax: 01273 242215
Total Beds: 465

Care of the Elderly H O'Neal

General Psychiatry C Aldridge, N Farhoumand, K Shamash, R Whale

Radiology P Gordon, J Jeyakumar, G J Price

Rehabilitation Medicine A Kawajah, S Novak

Chailey Heritage

Clinical Services, Beggars Wood Road, North Chailey, Lewes BN8 4EF
Tel: 01825 722112 Fax: 01825 721063
Total Beds: 5

Paediatrics J Bjorn, C Fairhurst, E Green, Y Khan, R Lipowsky

MacKeith Centre

c/o Royal Alexander Childrens Hospital, Dyke Road, Brighton BN1 3JN
Tel: 01273 328145 Ext: 2139 Fax: 01273 202312

Mill View Hospital

Nevill Avenue, Hove BN3 7HY
Tel: 01273 696011 Fax: 01273 242046
Total Beds: 89

General Psychiatry M Assin, S Baker, L Culliford, R Gimbrett, R Ing, T Ojo, M Rosenberg, J Sanders, H Williams

Nevill Hospital

Laburnum Avenue, Hove BN3 7JW
Tel: 01273 821680 Fax: 01273 265553
Total Beds: 40

Newhaven Downs

Church Hill, Newhaven BN9 9WH
Tel: 01273 513441 Fax: 01273 612134
Total Beds: 40

Care of the Elderly C Aldridge, H O'Neal

Southlands Hospital

Upper Shoreham Road, Shoreham-by-Sea BN43 6TQ
Tel: 01273 455622 Fax: 01273 446061
Total Beds: 35

Victoria Hospital

Nevill Road, Lewes BN7 1PF
Tel: 01273 474153 Fax: 01273 473362
Total Beds: 39

Cardiology C Davidson

Chest Disease M B Jackson, C W Turton

Dermatology C Darley

Gastroenterology S Cairns, A Ireland

General Psychiatry C Aldridge

General Surgery M Brooks, P Hale, P Hurst

Obstetrics and Gynaecology K Boos, D Holden

Orthopaedics R Turner, C Williams

Radiology C Sonksen

Rheumatology B Stuart

Urology N Harrison, P Thomas

Victoria Hospital Day Surgery Unit

Nevill Road, Lewes BN7 1PF
Tel: 01273 474153 Fax: 01273 473362
Total Beds: 38

South East Hertfordshire Primary Care Trust

1-4 Limes Court, Conduit Lane, Hoddesdon EN11 8EP
Tel: 01992 706120 Fax: 01992 706121
Email: general@seherts-pct.nhs.uk
Website: www.seherts-pct.nhs.uk
(Bedfordshire and Hertfordshire Strategic Health Authority)

Chair Lynda Tarpey
Chief Executive Vince McCabe

Cheshunt Community Hospital
King Arthur Court, Crossbrook Street, Cheshunt, Waltham Cross EN8 8XN
Tel: 01992 622157 Fax: 01992 629595

South East Oxfordshire Primary Care Trust

Wallingford Community Hospital, Reading Road, Wallingford OX10 9DU
Tel: 01491 208570 Fax: 01491 208580
Website: www.seoxon-pct.nhs.uk
(Thames Valley Strategic Health Authority)

Chair Tony Williamson
Chief Executive Mary Wicks

Townlands Hospital
York Road, Henley-on-Thames RG9 2EB
Tel: 01491 637400 Fax: 01491 410452
Total Beds: 39

Wallingford Community Hospital
Reading Road, Wallingford OX10 9DU
Tel: 01491 208500
Total Beds: 33

South East Sheffield Primary Care Trust

9 Orgreave Road, Handsworth, Sheffield S13 9LQ
Tel: 0114 226 4050 Fax: 0114 226 4051
Website: www.sheffield-ha.nhs.uk
(South Yorkshire Strategic Health Authority)

Chair Adebola Fatogun
Chief Executive Helen Fentimen

South Essex Partnership NHS Trust

Head Office, Dunton Court, Aston Road, Laindon, Basildon SS15 6NX
Tel: 01375 364650 Fax: 01268 492856
Email: communications@southessex-trust.nhs.uk
Website: www.southessex-trust.nhs.uk
(Essex Strategic Health Authority)

Chair Jai Tout
Chief Executive Patrick Geoghegan

Mayfield Unit, Thurrock Community Hospital, Grays, Essex
Long Lane, Grays RM16 2PX
Tel: 01375 364576 Fax: 01375 394970
Total Beds: 24

Mental Health Unit, Basildon Hospital, Essex
Basildon Hospital, Nethermayne, Basildon SS16 5NL
Tel: 01268 533911
Total Beds: 111

Mountnessing Court
240 Mountnessing Road, Billericay CM12 0EH
Tel: 01268 366054, 01277 634711 Fax: 01277 634684
Total Beds: 28
Manager Frances Kay

Rochford Hospital
Union Lane, Rochford SS4 1RB
Tel: 01702 578000 Fax: 01702 549542

Runwell Hospital
Runwell Hospital, Runwell Chase, Wickford SS11 7XX
Tel: 01268 366054 Fax: 01268 366076
Email: teresa.compton@southessex-trust.nhs.uk
Total Beds: 206

Consultants B Canagasabey

South Gloucestershire Primary Care Trust

1 Monarch Court, Emerald Park, Emerson's Green, Bristol BS16 7FH
Tel: 0117 330 2400 Fax: 0117 330 2401
Email: firstname.lastname@sglos-pct.nhs.uk
Website: www.sglos-pct.nhs.uk
(Avon, Gloucestershire and Wiltshire Strategic Health Authority)

Chair Brian Goodson
Chief Executive Penny Harris

South Hams and West Devon Primary Care Trust

The Lescaze Offices, Shinners Bridge, Dartington, Totnes TQ9 6JE
Tel: 01803 866665 Fax: 01803 867679
Email: enquiries@shandwd-pct.nhs.uk
Website: www.shandwd-pct.nhs.uk
(South West Peninsula Strategic Health Authority)

Chair Sally Foxhall
Chief Executive Alan Tibbenham

Dartmouth and Kingswear Hospital
Mansion House Street, Dartmouth TQ6 9BD
Tel: 01803 832255 Fax: 01803 833693
Total Beds: 16

South Hams Hospital
Plymouth Road, Kingsbridge TQ7 1AT
Tel: 01548 852349 Fax: 01548 857727
Total Beds: 20

Tavistock Hospital
Spring Hill, Tavistock PL19 8LD
Tel: 01822 612233 Fax: 01822 610025
Total Beds: 20

Totnes Community Hospital
Coronation Road, Totnes TQ9 5GH
Tel: 01803 862622 Fax: 01803 868349
Total Beds: 20

South Huddersfield Primary Care Trust

St Luke's House, Blackmoorfoot Road, Crosland Moore, Huddersfield HD4 5RH
Tel: 01484 466013 Fax: 01484 466139
Website: www.southhuddersfield-pct.nhs.uk
(West Yorkshire Strategic Health Authority)

Chair Margaret Dale
Chief Executive Kevin Holder

South Leeds Primary Care Trust

1st Floor, Navigation House, 8 George Mann Road, Quayside Business Park, Leeds LS10 1DJ
Tel: 0113 305 9666 Fax: 0113 295 1677
Website: www.leedssouth-pct.nhs.uk
(West Yorkshire Strategic Health Authority)

Chair Robert Seymour
Chief Executive George McIntyre

South Leicestershire Primary Care Trust

The Rosings, Forest Road, Narborough, Leicester LE19 3EG
Tel: 0116 286 3178 Fax: 0116 286 3787
Email: viv.merry@slpct.nhs.uk
(Leicestershire, Northamptonshire and Rutland Strategic Health Authority)

Chair David England
Chief Executive Julie Wood

South Liverpool Primary Care Trust

Pavilion Six, The Matchworks, Speke Road, Garston, Liverpool L19 2PH
Tel: 0151 234 1000 Fax: 0151 234 1001
Website: www.southliverpoolpct.nhs.uk
(Cheshire and Merseyside Strategic Health Authority)

Chair Beatrice Fraenkel
Chief Executive Aerek Campbell

South London and Maudsley NHS Trust

The trust has over 100 sites covering the boroughs of Croydon, Lambeth, Lewisham and Southwark, and specialist services for Bromley, Bexley and Greenwich. Some services are also provided nationally.

Trust Headquarters, 9th Floor, The Tower Building, 11 York Road, London SE1 7NX
Fax: 020 7919 2171, 020 8777 6611
Email: forename.surname@slam.nhs.uk
Website: www.slam.nhs.uk
(South East London Strategic Health Authority; South West London Strategic Health Authority)

Chair Madeliene Long
Chief Executive Stuart Bell

South Manchester Primary Care Trust

1st Floor, Home 4, Withington Hospital, Nell Lane, West Didsbury, Manchester M20 2LR
Tel: 0161 611 3300 Fax: 0161 611 3900
Website: www.southmanchesterpct.nhs.uk
(Greater Manchester Strategic Health Authority)

Chair Mike Green
Chief Executive Adrian Mercer

South Manchester University Hospitals NHS Trust

First Floor, Tower Block, Wythenshawe Hospital, Southmoor Road, Manchester M23 9LT
Tel: 0161 998 7070 Fax: 0161 291 2603
Website: www.smuht.nwest.nhs.uk
(Greater Manchester Strategic Health Authority)

Chair Jeff Wilner
Chief Executive Peter Morris

Adult Psychiatry Day Hospital
Withington Hospital, Nell Lane, West Didsbury, Manchester M20 8LR
Tel: 0161 447 4367 Fax: 0161 447 4441
Total Beds: 151

Atu Day Hospital
Nell Lane, West Didsbury, Manchester M20 8LR
Tel: 0161 447 4312 Fax: 0161 447 4441

Burton House Day Hospital
Nell Lane, West Didsbury, Manchester M20 8LR
Tel: 0161 447 4509 Fax: 0161 447 3785

Duchess of York Children's Hospital
Withington Hospital, Nell Lane, West Didsbury, Manchester M20 8LE
Tel: 0161 291 4620 Fax: 0161 291 3056
Total Beds: 33

Anaesthetics R Lawton

Cardiology R Patel

Neurology I Hughes

Orthopaedics J G Lemon, F J Weighill

Paediatrics A J Bradbury, A Dickson, D C S Gough, S A Roberts, A Robinson

Plastic Surgery C I Orton

Radiology I Lang

Old Age Psychiatry Day Hospital
Withington Hospital, Nell Lane, West Didsbury, Manchester M20 8LR
Tel: 0161 447 4910

Withington Hospital
Nell Lane, West Didsbury, Manchester M20 8LR
Tel: 0161 445 8111 Fax: 0161 445 5631

Accident and Emergency S Hawes

Anaesthetics S Beards, M Bellman, I T Campbell, M Columb, N El-Mikatti, D Greig, J Hargreaves, A Luthra, M McKavney, H Michael, P Nightingale, D M Nolan, M Osbourne, S P Roberts, M P Shelly, C L Tolhurst-Cleaver

Care of the Elderly A K Bancrjee, N J Linker, P A O'Neill, J M Robinson, V Srinivas

Dermatology J Ashworth, P J August, J Ferguson

ENT A E Camilleri, P H Jones

General Medicine J D Edwards, A M Heagerty, J P Miller, T Roberts, S M Shalet, P J Whorwell

General Psychiatry J L J Appleby, A Burns, J Byrne, B D Hore, C Hyde, S Lennon, S Lewis, C Thomas, L Webster, A Wieck

General Surgery A D Baildam, L Barr, N J Bundred, D Charlesworth, E S Kiff, C N McCollum, S T O'Dwyer, D E F Tweedle

Genitourinary Medicine S Chandiok, P D Woolley

Medical Oncology A Howells

Nephrology P Ackrill, M C Venning

Neurology J Dick

Obstetrics and Gynaecology D J Hickling, P J Hirsch

Oral and Maxillofacial Surgery D J Eldridge, C B Tattersall, J R Tuffin

Orthodontics R P J Thompson

Orthopaedics E M Holt, D M Lang, J G Lemon, F J Weighill

Paediatrics A J Bradbury, S A Roberts, A Robinson

Pathology I Burton, J Coyne, J Craske, N Y Haboubi, E B Kaczmarski, A M Kelly, W F Knox, L McWilliam, B Oppenheim, D A Taberner

Plastic Surgery A N Brain, P J Davenport, K W Dunn, V Lees, C Orton, J S Watson, D J Whitby

Radiology D L Asbury, R J Ashleigh, C R M Boggis, R England, D Martin, S Reaney, S Sukumar, M Wilson

Rheumatology and Rehabilitation B Pal, E R E Ross, P A Sanders

Urology R J Barnard, N J R George, E W Lupton, P N Rao

Wythenshawe Hospital

Southmoor Road, Wythenshawe, Manchester M23 9LT
Tel: 0161 998 7070 Fax: 0161 291 2037
Total Beds: 895

Accident and Emergency B Ryan

Anaesthetics N Braude, P T Conroy, F Dodd, K Grady, D Greenhalgh, H S J Grey, P J Hall, K G Lee, A J Mortimer, P Nightingale, M R Patrick, G Phillips, W A Thomas, M A Tobias, S Wheatly, W Wooldridge

Cardiology D Bennett, C L Bray, N Brooks, R D Levy, S G Ray, C Ward

Chest Disease P V Barber, K B Carroll, J J Egan, C A C Pickering, A K Webb, A Woodcock

Dental Surgery M Patel, K Sanders

Dermatology H L Muston

ENT A R Birzgalis, A E Camilleri, P H Jones

General Medicine S G Brear, J R Crampton, P E Jones, J J Manns

General Psychiatry P Mbaya

General Surgery C N Hall, B D Hancock, D Jones

Medical Oncology H Anderson, N Thatcher

Nephrology P Ackrill

Neurology J Dick

Obstetrics and Gynaecology M Fouracres, D J Hickling, P J Hirsch, G A Morewood, J S Wynn

Ophthalmology G S Turner

Oral and Maxillofacial Surgery M Patel, K Sanders, W Simpson

Orthodontics R P J Thompson

Paediatrics A J Bradbury, D C S Gough, R G Patel, S A Roberts, A Robinson

Pathology P Bishop, H Doran, P S Hasleton, T N Stanbridge

Radiology R Ashley, G Economou, R England, A W Horrocks, A E Mattison, R Sawyer

Rheumatology H N Misra, B Pal

Thoracic Surgery B J Bridgewater, C S Campbell, H K Deiraniya, T L Hooper, M T Jones, R A M Lawson, A Rahman

South of Tyne and Wearside Mental Health NHS Trust

Cherry Knowle Hospital, Ryhope, Sunderland SR2 0NB
Tel: 0191 565 6256 Fax: 0191 569 9455
Website: www.sunderland.nhs.uk/stw
(Northumberland, Tyne and Wear Strategic Health Authority)

Chair Cynthia Rickitt
Chief Executive Yasmin Chaudhry

Cherry Knowle Hospital

Ryhope, Sunderland SR2 0NB
Tel: 0191 565 6256 Fax: 0191 569 9455
Total Beds: 308

General Psychiatry H R Board, I Cameron, P O Miller, S Mitchison, J L C Perera, S Rastogi, K L Shrestha

Psychiatry of Old Age A Cooper, P Cronin, G Harvey, D Hunsley

Monkwearmouth Hospital

Newcastle Road, Sunderland SR5 1NB
Tel: 0191 565 6256 Fax: 0191 569 9248
Total Beds: 52

Queen Elizabeth Hospital (Tranwell Unit)

Sheriff Hill, Gateshead NE9 6SX
Tel: 0191 482 0000 Fax: 0191 491 1823

South Tyneside District Hospital (Bede Wing)

Harton Lane, South Shields NE34 0PL
Tel: 0191 454 8888 Fax: 0191 427 9908
Total Beds: 121

South Peterborough Primary Care Trust

Works with North Peterborough Primary Care Trust and the Adult Social Care Department of Peterborough City Council as Greater Peterborough Primary Care Partnership.

2nd Floor, Town Hall, Peterborough PE1 1FA
Tel: 01733 758500 Fax: 01733 758555
Website: www.greaterpboropcp.nhs.uk
(Norfolk, Suffolk and Cambridgeshire Strategic Health Authority)

Chair Marco Cereste
Chief Executive Chris Town

South Sefton Primary Care Trust

Burlington House, Crosby Road North, Waterloo, Liverpool L22 0QB
Tel: 0151 920 5056 Fax: 0151 920 1035
Email: enquiries@southsefton-pct.nhs.uk
Website: www.southseftonpct.nhs.uk
(Cheshire and Merseyside Strategic Health Authority)

Chair Ken Morris
Chief Executive Ian Williamson

South Somerset Primary Care Trust

Chataway House, Chard Business Park, Leach Road, Chard TA20 1FR
Tel: 01460 238600 Fax: 01460 238699
Email: ask@southsomersetpct.nhs.uk
Website: www.southsomersetpct.nhs.uk
(Dorset and Somerset Strategic Health Authority)

Chair Norman Campbell
Chief Executive Virginia Pearson

Chard and District Hospital
Crewkerne Road, Chard TA20 1NF
Tel: 01460 63175 Fax: 01460 68172
Total Beds: 35

Crewkerne Hospital
Middle Path, Crewkerne TA18 8BG
Tel: 01460 72491 Fax: 01460 75423
Total Beds: 20

South Petherton Hospital
South Petherton TA18 5AR
Tel: 01460 240333 Fax: 01460 242292
Total Beds: 44

Verrington Hospital
Dancing Lane, Wincanton BA9 9DQ
Tel: 01963 32006 Fax: 01963 31898
Total Beds: 50

South Staffordshire Healthcare NHS Trust

St George's Hospital, Corporation Street, Stafford ST16 3AG
Tel: 01785 257888 Fax: 01785 258969
Email: mike.cooke@ssh-tr.nhs.uk
Website: www.southstaffshealthcare.nhs.uk
(Shropshire and Staffordshire Strategic Health Authority)

Chair Andrew Millward
Chief Executive Mike Cooke

The George Bryan Centre
Sir Robert Peel Hospital, Plantation Lane, Mile Oak, Tamworth B79 3NG
Tel: 01827 285598
Total Beds: 29

Margaret Stanhope Centre
Outwoods Site, Burton District Hospital, Belvedere Road, Burton-on-Trent
Tel: 01283 505300
Total Beds: 26

St George's Hospital
Corporation Street, Stafford ST16 3AG
Total Beds: 148

South Stoke Teaching Primary Care Trust

Heron House, 120 Grove Road, Fenton, Stoke-on-Trent ST4 4LX
Tel: 01782 298000
Website: www.southstokepct.nhs.uk
(Shropshire and Staffordshire Strategic Health Authority)

Chair Michael Tappin
Chief Executive Tony McGovern

Longton Cottage Hospital
Upper Belgrave Road, Longton, Stoke-on-Trent ST3 4QX
Tel: 01782 425600 Fax: 01782 425656
Total Beds: 43

Care of the Elderly Dr Patel

South Tees Hospitals NHS Trust

The James Cook University Hospital, Marton Road, Middlesbrough TS4 3BW
Tel: 01642 850850 Fax: 01642 854943
Website: www.southtees.nhs.uk
(County Durham and Tees Valley Strategic Health Authority)

Chair Glenys Marriott
Chief Executive Simon Pleydell

Friarage Hospital
Northallerton DL6 1JG
Tel: 01609 779911 Fax: 01609 777144
Total Beds: 236

Manager John Gibb

Anaesthetics J Berens, D G Jackson, M Thompson, M Walton

Dermatology A Senkeran, S Shehade

ENT J Carlin, R W Ruckley, S P Singh

General Medicine M Connolly, R Fisken, U Somasundram, D Spence

General Surgery R Bryan, M H Edwards, D C Ward

Neurology D Jay

Obstetrics and Gynaecology F Bryce, N Hebblethwaite, Dr Kumarendram

Ophthalmology H S Dang, J D Haslam, G S Willets

Oral and Maxillofacial Surgery A Smyth

Orthodontics E May

Orthopaedics K Allerton, L Van Vumren, A C Weeber

Paediatrics D Dammann, A Essex-Cater, J James

Pathology N M Browning, D C Henderson, K V Prasad, A Waise, N Weightman

Plastic Surgery M Coady, C Vivakanathan

Radiotherapy and Oncology V Der Voet

Rheumatology A Isdale

Guisborough General Hospital (Maternity Services)
Guisborough TS14 6HZ
Tel: 01287 633542

The James Cook University Hospital
Marton Road, Middlesbrough TS4 3BW
Tel: 01642 850850 Fax: 01642 854636
Total Beds: 964

Cardiology A Davies, M A De-Belder, J A Hall

Cardiothoracic Surgery G Morritt, J Wallis

Care of the Elderly A Ashraf, A Bergin, D L Broughton, R Murdoch

General Medicine M G Bramble, P A Cann, J R Cove-Smith, H R Gribbin, J Main, R Murdoch, A D Paterson, D J M Sinclair

General Surgery J R Bell, D Clarke, I A E Clason, W M Cooke, W A Corbett, P Durning, A H Tooley, R G Wilson

Haematology J E Chandler, G P Sommerfield

Nephrology J R Cove-Smith, J Main, A D Paterson, D Reaich

Obstetrics and Gynaecology S Bailey, J A Cosbie-Ross, D J Cruickshank, R Garry, R S Hutchison, P J Taylor, K M Toop

Occupational Health D P McGuire

Paediatrics R C Dias, M S Kibirige, P Morrell, S Sinha, G P Wyatt, J Wyllie

Radiology A S S Ahmed, R S C Campbell, K M A Clifford, R W J Hartley, G L S Leen, M McCarty, G Naisby

Radiotherapy and Oncology S L Chawla, P R C Dunlop, P D J Hardman, A J Rathmell

Rheumatology J N Fordham, I Haslock

Thoracic Medicine H R Gribbin, D J M Sinclair

Urology D Chadwick, J R Hindmarsh, J E Whiteway

South Tyneside NHS Foundation Trust

Formerly South Tyneside Health Care NHS Trust. Established as a Foundation Trust 01/01/2005.

Harton Wing, South Tyneside District Hospital, Harton Lane, South Shields NE34 0PL
Tel: 0191 454 8888 Fax: 0191 427 2197
Email: lorraine.lambert@sthct.nhs.uk
Website: www.sthct.nhs.uk
(Northumberland, Tyne and Wear Strategic Health Authority)

Chair Peter Davidson
Chief Executive Lorraine Lambert

Charles Palmer Day Hospital

Palmer Community Hospital, Wear Street, Jarrow NE32 3UX
Tel: 0191 489 7777 Fax: 0191 428 1072

Monkton Hall Hospital

Monkton Lane, Jarrow NE32 5HN
Tel: 0191 489 4111
Total Beds: 56

Moorlands Day Hospital

South Tyneside District Hospital, Harton Lane, South Shields NE34 0PL
Tel: 0191 454 8888

Palmer Community Hospital

Wear Street, Jarrow NE32 3UX
Tel: 0191 451 6000
Total Beds: 82

Primrose Hill Hospital

Primrose Terrace, Jarrow NE32 5HA
Tel: 0191 451 6375
Total Beds: 16

South Tyneside District Hospital

Harton Lane, South Shields NE34 0PL
Tel: 0191 454 8888 Fax: 0191 427 9908
Total Beds: 538

Accident and Emergency A Reece

Anaesthetics S Deshpande, C Muench, J Mullenheim, Dr Polteneri

Care of the Elderly K Liang, A Rodgers, J Scott

Clinical Psychology A McClure

Dermatology J A A Langtry, J McLelland, S Natarajan

ENT P R Samuel, F W Stafford

General Medicine M F Bone, L G Bryson, K Liang, A Lishman, A Nasser, S Panter, J H Parr, C Rees, S Soo

General Surgery H Gehling, B V Joypaul, C Pritchett, B Weber, K Wynne

Genitourinary Medicine S Rashid

Haematology M Galloway

Medical Microbiology R Ellis

Neurology P G Cleland, A Goonetilleke, R E Jones

Obstetrics V Esen, N Fawzi, A J Jones, N J Nwabineli, S Orife

Obstetrics and Gynaecology U Esen, Mr Hani-Fawzi, A J Jones, N J Nwabinelli, S O Orife

Ophthalmology D Bell, T J Fetherston, P S Phelan, D Steel, P Tiffin

Orthodontics M Smith

Orthopaedics J Fraser, H Fuchs, I A Hugh

Paediatrics N Brewster, S Cronin, M Massam, G I Okugbeni

Pathology K Pollard

Plastic Surgery G S S Rao

Psychiatry M J Akhtar, J M T Damas-Mora, D Neil, Dr Roy

Psychiatry (Child and Family) A McCure, C Nourse

Radiology R Cooper, L H Cope, M Farrer

Urology T Armitage

South Tyneside Primary Care Trust

Ingham House, Horsley Hill Road, South Shields NE33 3DP
Tel: 0191 401 4500 Fax: 0191 401 4590
Email: enquiries@stpct.nhs.uk
Website: www.stpct.nhs.uk
(Northumberland, Tyne and Wear Strategic Health Authority)

Chair Stephen Clark
Chief Executive Roy McLachlan
Consultants Faisal Al-Durrah

South Warwickshire General Hospitals NHS Trust

Warwick Hospital, Lakin Road, Warwick CV34 5BW
Tel: 01926 495321 Fax: 01926 482603
Email: enquiries@swh.nhs.uk
Website: www.warwickhospital.nhs.uk
(West Midlands South Strategic Health Authority)

Chair Roger Thompson
Chief Executive Janet Monkman

Stratford-upon-Avon Hospital

Arden Street, Stratford-upon-Avon CV37 6NX
Tel: 01926 495321
Total Beds: 28

Care of the Elderly H N Desai, F G Vaz, A K Viswan

Warwick Hospital

Lakin Road, Warwick CV34 5BW
Tel: 01926 495321 Fax: 01926 482603
Total Beds: 446

Accident and Emergency M Dunn, J Harrison, J Nancarrow

Anaesthetics J H Antrobus, J M S Aulakh, S Crighton, I A Hall, T M W Long, S P Mather, J Richardson, D A Robinson, E White

Cardiology N R Qureshi

Dermatology A Bedlow, R Charles-Holmes, F Humphreys

ENT R C Bickerton, H R Cable, D E Phillips

General Medicine S Boardman, H N Desai, P C Hawker, L S Hill, P M Horrocks, C Marguerie, S Rigby, J H Shearman, F G Vaz, A K Viswan

General Surgery I D L Fraser, S Harries, P Murphy, M Osborne

Genitourinary Medicine D J Natin

Obstetrics and Gynaecology R Jackson, J Nippani, K S J Olah, M J Pearson

Ophthalmology D David, G P Misson, A M O'Driscoll

Orthopaedics P Binfield, I A Nwachukwu, D T Shakespeare, S K Young

Paediatrics A Acharya, J Davies

Pathology S Basu, R Carr, N Chachlani, A R Ghose, J Kavi, P E Rose, O Stores

Radiology D P Clarke, M Hughes, F C Millard, G D Stewart, P H Williams

Urology D C Lewis, J R Strachan

South Warwickshire Primary Care Trust

Westgate House, Market Street, Warwick CV34 4DE
Tel: 01926 493491 Fax: 01926 495074
Email: general.office@swarkpct.nhs.uk
Website: www.swarkpct.nhs.uk
(West Midlands South Strategic Health Authority)

Chair David Ashton
Chief Executive Catherine Griffiths

Alcester Hospital
Kinwarton Road, Alcester
Tel: 01789 762470 Fax: 01789 764363
Total Beds: 22

Manager Sue Price-Gough

Ellen Badger Hospital
Shipston-on-Stour CV36 4AX
Tel: 01608 661410 Fax: 01608 663373
Total Beds: 35

Manager Penny Whitesmith

Royal Leamington Spa Rehabilitation Hospital
Heathcote Lane, Heathcote, Warwick
Tel: 01926 317700 Fax: 01926 317710
Total Beds: 112

Manager Norma Whittall

St Michael's Hospital
St Michael's Road, Warwick CV34 5QW
Tel: 01926 406789, 01926 496241 Fax: 01926 406700
Total Beds: 90

Manager Maria Fennell

South West Dorset Primary Care Trust

Hillfort House, Poundbury Road, Dorchester DT1 2PN
Tel: 01305 368900 Fax: 01305 368947
Email: email@southwestdorset-pct.nhs.uk
Website: www.swdorset-pct.nhs.uk
(Dorset and Somerset Strategic Health Authority)

Chair Anne Thomas
Chief Executive Peter Mankin

Bridport Community Hospital
Hospital Lane, North Allington, Bridport DT6 5DR
Tel: 01308 422371

Manager Sue Snowdon

Portland Community Hospital
Castledown Road, Portland DT5 1AX
Tel: 01305 820341
Total Beds: 16

Manager Joy Warren

Westhaven Hospital
Radipole Lane, Weymouth DT4 0QE
Tel: 01305 786116
Total Beds: 24

Manager Joy Warren

Weymouth Community Hospital
Melcombe Avenue, Weymouth DT6 5DR
Tel: 01305 760022
Total Beds: 53

Manager Joy Warren

South West Kent Primary Care Trust

Sevenoaks Hospital, Hospital Road, Sevenoaks TN13 3PQ
Tel: 01732 470200 Fax: 01732 470201
Email: enquiries@swkentpct.nhs.uk
Website: www.swkentpct.nhs.uk
(Kent and Medway Strategic Health Authority)

Chair Nigel Branson
Chief Executive Steve Ford

Edenbridge and District War Memorial Hospital
Edenbridge TN8 5DA
Tel: 01732 863164
Total Beds: 23

Sevenoaks Hospital
Hospital Road, Sevenoaks TN13 3PG
Tel: 01732 470200
Total Beds: 47

Tonbridge Cottage Hospital
Vauxhall Lane, Tonbridge TN11 0NE
Tel: 01732 353653
Total Beds: 27

South West London and St George's Mental Health NHS Trust

Springfield University Hospital, 61 Glenburnie Road, London SW17 7DJ
Tel: 020 8672 9911
Website: www.swlstg-tr.nhs.uk
(South West London Strategic Health Authority)

Chair John Rafferty
Chief Executive Nigel Fisher

Barnes Hospital
South Worple Way, London SW14 8SU
Tel: 020 8878 4981 Fax: 020 8876 5471

Henderson Hospital
2 Homeland Drive, Sutton SM2 5LT
Tel: 020 8661 1611 Fax: 020 8770 3676

Nelson Hospital
Kingston Hospital, London SW20 8BD
Tel: 020 8544 9799 Fax: 020 8544 9033

Richmond Royal Hospital
Kew Foot Road, Richmond TW9 2TE
Tel: 020 8940 3331

Springfield University Hospital
61 Glenburnie Road, London SW17 7DJ
Tel: 020 8672 9911 Fax: 020 8682 6703
Total Beds: 449

General Psychiatry J S Bolton, T P Burns, J Colgan, L Drummond, N L G Eastman, N Fisher, H Ghodse, P Hughes, G Mezey, P Moodley, D Oyebode, M Potter, S J Robertson, R S Stern, M G Zolese

Sutton Hospital
Cotswold Road, Sutton SM2 5NF
Tel: 020 8652 7900 Fax: 020 8652 7908

Tolworth Hospital
Red Lion Road, Tolworth, Surbiton KT6 7QU
Tel: 020 8390 0102 Fax: 020 8390 1236
Total Beds: 189

South West Oxfordshire Primary Care Trust

Executive Office, Wallingford Community Hospital, Reading Road, Wallingford OX10 9DU
Tel: 01491 208570 Fax: 01491 208580
Website: www.swoxon-pct.nhs.uk
(Thames Valley Strategic Health Authority)

Chair Fred Hucker
Chief Executive Mary Wicks

Abingdon Community Hospital
Marcham Road, Abingdon OX14 1AG
Tel: 01235 205700
Total Beds: 54

Manager Debbie Brewer

Didcot Community Hospital
Wantage Road, Didcot OX11 0AG
Tel: 01235 205860
Total Beds: 30

Manager Sandra Allen

Wantage Community Hospital
Garston Lane, Wantage OX12 7AS
Tel: 01235 205801
Total Beds: 23

Manager Jill Beckhelling

Witney Community Hospital
Welch Way, Witney OX28 6JJ
Tel: 01993 209400
Total Beds: 61

Manager Penny Joy

South West Yorkshire Mental Health NHS Trust

Fieldhead, Ouchthorpe Lane, Wakefield WF1 3SP
Tel: 01924 327000 Fax: 01924 327021
Email: enquiries@swyt.nhs.uk
Website: www.southwestyorkshire.nhs.uk
(West Yorkshire Strategic Health Authority)

Chair Sukhdev Sharma
Chief Executive Judith Young

Aberford Centre for Psychiatry
Ouchthorpe Lane, Wakefield WF1 3SP
Total Beds: 82

General Psychiatry C A Cruickshank

Castleford, Normanton and District Hospital
Lumley Street, Castleford WF10 5LT
Tel: 01977 605500 Fax: 01977 605501
Total Beds: 24

Child and Adolescent Psychiatry M Kay

Psychiatry of Old Age I Hammad

Public Health Medicine R S Thiagarajah

Fieldhead Hospital
Ouchthorpe Lane, Wakefield WF1 3SP
Tel: 01924 327000 Fax: 01924 327021

Learning Disabilities L F A Silva

Holme Valley Memorial Hospital
Huddersfield Road, Holmfirth HD9 3TS
Tel: 01484 681711 Fax: 01484 482357

Pontefract General Infirmary
Friarwood Lane, Pontefract WF8 1PL
Tel: 01977 600600

St Luke's Hospital
Blackmoorfoot Road, Crosland Moor, Huddersfield HD4 5RQ
Tel: 01484 654711 Fax: 01484 482409

Southmoor Hospital
Southmoor Road, Hemsworth, Pontefract WF9 4LU
Tel: 01977 610661

Stanley Royd Hospital
Aberford Road, Wakefield WF1 4DQ
Tel: 01924 201688

South Western Staffordshire Primary Care Trust

Mellor House, Corporation Street, Stafford ST16 3SR
Tel: 01785 220004 Fax: 01785 221251
Website: www.sws-pct.nhs.uk
(Shropshire and Staffordshire Strategic Health Authority)

Chair Jenny Cornes
Chief Executive William Price

South Wiltshire Primary Care Trust

42-44 Chipper Lane, Salisbury SP1 1BG
Tel: 01722 341319 Fax: 01722 326768
Website: www.southwiltshirepct.nhs.uk
(Avon, Gloucestershire and Wiltshire Strategic Health Authority)

Chair Victor Prior
Chief Executive Jan Stubbings

South Worcestershire Primary Care Trust

Unit 19, Isaac Maddox House, Shrub Hill Industrial Estate, Worcester WR4 9RW
Tel: 01905 760000 Fax: 01905 760002
Website: www.worcestershirehealth.nhs.uk/swpct
(West Midlands South Strategic Health Authority)

Chair David Barlow
Chief Executive Mike Ridley

Evesham Community Hospital
Waterside, Evesham WR11 1JT
Tel: 01386 502345 Fax: 01386 502344
Total Beds: 97

Manager Susan Barker

Anaesthetics J J Lee, D Overton

Care of the Elderly C Ashton, H R Glennie, C Pycock

Dermatology Dr Lewis, W Tucker

ENT H Cable, M Porter

General Medicine R Lewis, S O'Hickey

General Surgery M Corlett, S Lake

Obstetrics and Gynaecology P Moran, M D Pickrell, Y Stedman

Ophthalmology N Price

Oral and Maxillofacial Surgery N Barnard

Orthopaedics K O'Dwyer, L Read, A Reading, E Rouholamin, A Salam, Dr Selvey

Paediatrics A P Cole, M Hanlon, A Mills, J Scanlon

Urology T F Chen, M Lancashire

Vascular Surgery I Nyameckye

Malvern Community Hospital
Lansdowne Crescent, Malvern WR14 2AW
Tel: 01684 612600
Total Beds: 18

Manager Marie McCurry

Care of the Elderly H R Glennie

General Medicine S O'Hickey, C Pycock

General Surgery N C Hickey, C Robertson

Obstetrics and Gynaecology B A Ruparelia, J Watts

Orthopaedics J S Davies, M Trevitt

Paediatrics Dr Childs, A Gallagher, J Scanlon

Pershore Cottage Hospital
Defford Road, Pershore WR10 1HZ
Tel: 01386 502070 Fax: 01386 502082
Total Beds: 19

Manager K L Young

Tenbury District Hospital
Tenbury Wells WR15 8AT
Tel: 01584 810643 Fax: 01584 829987
Total Beds: 16

Manager Marie McCurry

South Yorkshire Ambulance Service NHS Trust

Ambulance Service Headquarters, Fairfield, Moorgate Road, Rotherham S60 2BQ
Tel: 01709 820520 Fax: 01709 827839
Email: info@syas.nhs.uk
Website: www.syas.nhs.uk
(South Yorkshire Strategic Health Authority)

Chair Stephen Hunter
Chief Executive Ray Shannon

Southampton City Primary Care Trust

Western Community Hospital, William Macleod Way, Southampton SO16 4XE
Tel: 023 8090 6904 Fax: 023 8090 6960
Website: www.southamptonhealth.nhs.uk
(Hampshire and Isle of Wight Strategic Health Authority)

Chair Pauline Quan Arrow
Chief Executive Brian Skinner

Harefield Day Hospital
Moorgreen Hospital, Botley Road, West End, Southampton SO30 3JB

Inroads Day Hospital
Western Community Hospital, Walnut Grove, Millbrook, Southampton SO16 4XE
Tel: 023 8047 5401 Fax: 023 8047 5402

Moorgreen Day Hospital
Botley Road, West End, Southampton SO30 3JB
Tel: 023 8047 6233 Fax: 023 8046 3176

Moorgreen Hospital
Botley Road, West End, Southampton SO30 3JB
Tel: 023 8047 5400 Fax: 023 8046 5385
Total Beds: 190

Ravenswood House
Medium Secure Unit, Knowle, Fareham PO17 5NA
Tel: 01329 836000
Total Beds: 58

Romsey Hospital
Mile Hill, Winchester Road, Romsey SO51 8ZA
Tel: 01794 512343 Fax: 01794 524465
Total Beds: 24

Western Community Hospital
Walnut Grove, Millbrook, Southampton SO16 4XE
Tel: 023 8047 5401

Southampton University Hospitals NHS Trust

Trust Management Offices, Southampton General Hospital, Tremona Road, Southampton SO16 6YD

Tel: 023 8079 6172 Fax: 023 8079 4715
Website: www.suht.nhs.uk
(Hampshire and Isle of Wight Strategic Health Authority)

Chair Richard Keightley
Chief Executive Mark Hackett

Countess Mountbatten House

Moorgreen Hospital, Botley Road, West End, Southampton SO30 3JB
Tel: 023 8047 7414 Fax: 023 8047 3501
Total Beds: 25

Princess Anne Hospital

Coxford Road, Southampton SO16 5YA
Tel: 023 8077 7222 Fax: 023 8079 4143
Total Beds: 183

Royal South Hants Hospital

Graham Road, Southampton SO14 0YG
Tel: 023 8063 4288 Fax: 023 8082 5206
Total Beds: 138

Southampton General Hospital

Tremona Road, Southampton SO16 6YD
Tel: 023 8077 7222 Fax: 023 8079 4153
Total Beds: 1065

Cancer Care C A Baughan, H Bush, D A Butler, C L Davis, E Goggin, R K Gregory, V L Hall, C R Hamilton, C M Heath, T Illidge, T Iveson, P Johnson, H Kirk, A T J Last, G M Mead, N Murray, C Ottensmeier, J Overton, G Sharpe, P D Simmonds, S D Tinkler

Cardiothoracic Medicine K Almer, C W Barlow, A Calver, N P Curzen, K D Dawkins, J Gnanapr, H H Gray, M P Haw, B R Keeton, S M Langley, S Livesey, P Lowburn, B Moorthy, J M Morgan, S K Ohri, P R Roberts, A P Salmon, A Sayavan, I A Simpson, G M Tsang, G R Veldtman, J Vettukattil, D F N Weeden

Child Health R M Beattie, P R Betts, D M Burge, B Castle, S Charmer, A L Collins, G J Connett, P V Deshpande, A Dhawan, D M Eccles, N Foulds, R D Gilbert, M A Hall, J Hourihane, A Jackson, C Kennedy, F J Kirkham, J A Kohler, T A Leahy, J P Legg, A Lucassen, E Mackie, P S J Malone, M Morgan, A I A O'Donnell, P Puddy, M Radford, H A Steinbrecher, N H Thomas, N Trevelyn, J Warner, R A Wheeler

Clinical Development H Boddington, C Deal, J Hazelgrove, J Lyon-Maris, J McGill, D St George, N Saunders, J Stubbing, R Weller

Consultants J Gabbay, S L George, R Milne, P J Roderick

Critical Care J Ambler, P J Appleton, K Boyle, D H Brighouse, P J Butler, G A Charlton, M J Clancy, A M Cone, R A Cope, S Cottrel, M M Crosse, N J H Davies, P Dawson, C Deakin, S Dunn, J Fennell, B Flavin, A Gande, C Gill, R S Gill, J M Goddard, S Hallford, J Harris, R Hartrey, J Hazelgrove, J A Hell, M J Herbertson, D Hett, J R C Heyworth, S A Hill, D Hulbert, J A Jellicoe, S C Jenkins, M M Jonas, E G Lawes, E G Lawes, J R D Laycock, M Leiva, I Macintosh, M J Marsh, C A Marshall, N S Maskery, I M Mettam, L Monnery, L Nel, M S Nielson, K M Nolan, J V Pappachan, J M Pierce, M R Platt, C M Price, E A Putnam, O C Ross, D V Rutter, A J T Sansome, D A Saunders, P M Spargo, M Stuart-Taylor, J Stubbing, P D Sutherland, D N Sutton, S Tanser, V L Thomas, A C Wainwright, C Weidmann, L A White, A Wilkins, P Witson, C E Wood, T E Woodcock

General Surgery J A Smallwood, C J Smart, H W Steer

Human Resources I Brown, D N M Coggon, A Kendrick, K T Palmer, J C Smedley

Medicine and Elderly Care J H Adams, A P Aihie-Sayer, F H Anderson, N Arden, R D Armstrong, M J P Arthur, R Briggs, D Browne, A Calogeras, N Carrabina, M Carroll, N Coleman, C Cooper, P Crawford, J R E Dathan, B Davidson, N R Dennis, J S Dulay, G Durward, C Edwards, D R Fine, E Foley, A J Frew, P Friedman, K M Godfrey, R I Gove, A Harper, E Healy, C Henderson, D Hilton, P Hockey, R I G Holt, Dr Howarth, C J Hutchings, M Keefe, A J Krentz, B A Leatherdale, B J Leppard, N Malik, B Marshall, D L McLelland, K Palmer, J A Pascual, P Patel, P A Pees, Dr Phillips, M Plater, B Pradeep, H C Roberts, M E Rogerson, C Roseveare, D Rowen, D D Sandeman, N Sheron, B Stacey, G M Sterling, I J N Sterling, M A Stroud, R C Sunanasuriya, D G Waller, F E Willmott, S N Zaman

Neurosciences N J Baker, N S R Brooke, I P Downie, J Duffil, B T Evans, C A Eynon, J P Frankel, W R Gibb, W P Gray, H Katifi, P Kennedy, A Kurian, D A Lang, N F Lawton, M C Prevett, A Prnto, N R Smith, O C Sparrow, R Van Der Star, A A Webb

Obstetrics and Gynaecology K Brackley, I T Cameron, M A G Coleman, S C Crawford, P Donaldson, D T Howe, S Ingamell, G Masson, K S Metcalf, A K Monga, A Moors, S J Mountfield, N Saunders, R W Stones, T Wheeler, P White

Ophthalmology D F Anderson, C R Canning, I H Chisholm, H Gaston, P R Hodgkins, A J Luff, J I McGill, R M Manners, R J Morris, R S Newsom

Orthopaedics D Barret, N R Boeree, G W Bowyer, P Chapman-Smith, N M P Clarke, A S Cole, E Davies, D G Dunlop, D O Eni-Olotu, E Gent, D G Hargreaves, J M Harley, J M Latham, G R Taylor, W Tice, M G Uglow, D J Warwick

Pathology E O Abu, B J Addis, F Aeinle, M R Ashton-Key, A Basarab, P S Bass, A C Bateman, N Carr, C E H Du Boulay, A S Duncombe, V Foria, P J Gallagher, R J Howitt, G R Jones, S Kazmi, P M Kemp, J A Lowes, G H Millward-Sadler, I E Moore, N Nagaraj, I Nazanti, K H Orchard, D O'Shaughn, A P Pallett, D S Richardson, W R Roche, N Singh, A G Smith, J M Theaker, B Vadgaria, V Walker

Radiology J Argent, C S Barker, V B Batty, S J Birch, R M Blaquiere, D J Breen, M Briley, I W Brown, D J Delaney, K C Dewbury, A Ditchfield, J J Fairhurst, M L Gawne Cain, M Griffiths, C N Hacking, C D Houghton, L J King, G P Michaels, J S Millar, A Odurny, C R Peebles, C M Rubin, M A Sampson, J Smart, K T Tung

Surgery A Adamson, I S Bailey, S Baxter, N E Beck, B R P Birch, J Byrne, J Cumming, P Harries, M C Hayes, W Hellier, R House, C D Johnson, J Mella, Dr Miles, T Mitchell, G E Morris, P H Nichols, K Nugent, N Patel, M Phillips, J N Primrose, R Ramchan, C Randall, D A Rew, J G Rice, G T Royle, C Shearman, J Smallwood, C Smith, H Steer, I Whitworth, N M Wilson

Southend Hospital NHS Trust

Southend Hospital, Prittlewell Chase, Westcliff on Sea SS0 0RY
Tel: 01702 435555 Fax: 01702 221300
Website: www.southend-hospital.co.uk
(Essex Strategic Health Authority)

Chair John Bruce
Chief Executive David Brackenbury

Southend Hospital

Prittlewell Chase, Westcliff on Sea SS0 0RY
Tel: 01702 435555 Fax: 01792 221300
Total Beds: 800

Accident and Emergency B Burgess, S Dima-Okojie, R Ritchie, H Rokan

Anaesthetics R Ali Khan, D Barwell, B Boira, U Bopitiya, C Buckore, N Cocker, I Ewart, M Gabrielczyk, D Higgins, P G Hollywood, D King, J Kinnear, H C Naylor, M Nicol, D Ringrose, E Sompson, A Stone, S J Ward, M J Woodham

Cardiology P Kelly, A Kokhar

Care of the Elderly P Aghoram, H Al-Sardar, A Collings, C Gent, A O'Brien, D Slovick

Dermatology A Banerjee, R Cooper

ENT D J Gatland, N P Warwick-Brown, G Watters

General Medicine J Ahlquist, M Almond, S Ansari, G Bray, D Carmichael, A Davison, D Eraut, K Metcalfe, J F Moro-Azuela, J O'Brien

General Surgery A Brown, M Dworkin, E Gray, M Jakeaways, B V R Praveen, N Rothnie, M C P Salter

Genitourinary Medicine D Evans, H Jaleel

Medical Microbiology S Clark

Neurosurgery J Benjamin, J Kellerman

Neurology H Hewazy, M Mavra, D M Park

Neurophysiology A Gordon, N Muhammed

Obstetrics and Gynaecology V Aggarwai, P Hagan, D Jennings, C Lee, K B Lim, T J Pocock, N Tripathi

Ophthalmology R Aggarwal, W L Alexander, S Kasaby, R Pearson, Z Subasinghe

Oral and Maxillofacial Surgery D Madan, J Makechnie, P Weller

Orthodontics S Nute, A Singh

Orthopaedics D A Boston, C Chauhan, R Kazim, G J Packer, S Raza, S Sarkar, R A Sudlow, A White

Paediatrics F R Awadalla, A Khan, I Margarson, V Nerminathan, A Shrivastava, S Sriskandan

Palliative Medicine C O'Doherty, M Piggott, G Tosh

Pathology P Atkinson, M Chappell, A Eden, H Eden, E F Fowler, M J Mills, S Payne, K Wolfe

Plastic Surgery D Elliott, L Kangesu

Radiology M Aslam, M N Ibrahim, M Lewars, S D Perera, B Shah, A B Tanqueray, T Toma

Radiotherapy and Oncology O Koriech, A Lamont, P Leonard, A Robinson, C C Trask, J Whelan

Rheumatology and Rehabilitation B Dasgupta, T Gordon, W Main Wong

Urology A Ball, T Carr, R Lodge

Southend-on-Sea Primary Care Trust

Harcourt House, Harcourt Avenue, Southend-on-Sea SS2 6HE
Tel: 01702 224600 Fax: 01702 224601
Email: information@southend-pct.nhs.uk
Website: www.southend-pct.nhs.uk
(Essex Strategic Health Authority)

Chair Katherine Kirk
Chief Executive Julie Garbutt

Southern Norfolk Primary Care Trust

The Courtyard, Ketteringham Hall, Ketteringham, Norwich NR18 9RS
Tel: 01603 813820 Fax: 01603 813865
Website: www.southernnorfolk-pct.nhs.uk
(Norfolk, Suffolk and Cambridgeshire Strategic Health Authority)

Chair Helen Wilson
Chief Executive Chris Humphris

Dereham Hospital

Northgate, Dereham NR19 2EX
Tel: 01362 692391 Fax: 01362 695457
Total Beds: 68

Thetford Cottage Hospital

Earls Road, Thetford IP24 2AD
Tel: 01842 752499 Fax: 01842 762035

Southport and Formby Primary Care Trust

5 Curzon Road, Southport PR8 6LW
Tel: 01704 530940 Fax: 01704 536072
Website: www.southportandformbypct.nhs.uk
(Cheshire and Merseyside Strategic Health Authority)

Chair Mark Winstanley
Chief Executive Gill Dolan

Southport and Ormskirk Hospital NHS Trust

Blundell House, Ormskirk District General Hospital, Wigan Road, Ormskirk L39 2AZ
Tel: 01704 547471 Fax: 01704 704541
Website: www.southportandormskirk.nhs.uk
(Cheshire and Merseyside Strategic Health Authority)

Chair Andrew Johnson
Chief Executive Jonathan Parry

Christiana Hartley Maternity Unit

Town Lane, Kew, Southport PR8 6PN
Tel: 01704 547471
Total Beds: 35

Obstetrics and Gynaecology G Foat, M N Iskander, S Sharma

Ormskirk and District General Hospital

Wigan Road, Ormskirk L39 2AZ
Tel: 01695 577111 Fax: 01695 583028

Accident and Emergency V Dhayalan, T Odedon

Anaesthetics S W Adejumo, W Bickerstaffe, K Crockford, J W Crooke, J Hammond, M Vangikar

Care of the Elderly M Ahmed, N G Dey

Chemical Pathology C V Heyningen

Chest Disease M J Serlin

Haematology D O'Brian

Dermatology A A Memon

ENT N J Roland

General Medicine J Horsley, C Kire, M MacIver, P Mennim, R Oelbaum

General Surgery R Anderson, S Jmor, N Matar, S Meehan

Genitourinary Medicine J Forrer

Medical Microbiology J A Bowley

Obstetrics and Gynaecology M Davies, R Edwards, S Jones

Ophthalmology N O'Donnell

Oral and Maxillofacial Surgery T Morris, O A Pospisil

Orthodontics N Trenouth

Orthopaedics T J Menon (Head), R F Adam, K Surallwala

Paediatrics G Boocock (Head), S O'Halloran

Pathology J A Bowley, S Clarke, P Mansour

Radiology P Reston (Head), J Fowler, Q Hague

Rheumatology and Rehabilitation H Sykes, E Williams

Urology M M Gammal (Head)

Ruffwood House

Ormskirk & District Hospital, Wigan Road, Ormskirk L39 2AZ

Southport and Formby District General Hospital

Town Lane, Kew, Southport PR8 6PN
Tel: 01704 547471 Fax: 01704 548229

Accident and Emergency C C Scott

Anaesthetics C L Charway, A Head-Rapson, D Jayson, J Jones, A P Kent, J Kirby, I Wallbank, J W H Watt

Clinical Oncology S Sun Myint

Dermatology A A Memom

ENT L Lesser, A C Swift

General Medicine K Binymin, G Butcher, N Dey, J Fox, M J Serlin, J P Simmonds, H Sykes

General Surgery M R Zeiderman (Head), D Artioukh, D Jones, P F Mason

Maxillofacial Surgery C Balmer, M Boyle

Medical Oncology D Smith, I Syndikus

Orthopaedics M Ali, D E.Carden, A G Hayes

Plastic Surgery A R Green

Spinal Injuries B Sett, P Sett

Urology S Vesey

Southport General Infirmary

Scarisbrick New Road, Southport PR8 6PN
Tel: 01704 547471

Care of the Elderly M Ahmed, N G Dey

ENT T Lesser, A Swift

Obstetrics and Gynaecology G Foat, M N Iskandar, S Sharma

Pathology D Dundas

Southwark Primary Care Trust

Mabel Goldwin House, 49 Grange Walk, London SE1 3DY
Tel: 020 7525 0400
Website: www.southwarkpct.nhs.uk
(South East London Strategic Health Authority)

Chair Mee Ling Ng
Chief Executive Chris Bull
Consultants Alan Maryon Davis, Ajay Sharma

Staffordshire Ambulance Service NHS Trust

70 Stone Road, Stafford ST16 2TQ
Tel: 01785 253521 Fax: 01785 246238
Email: enquiries@staffsas-tr.wmids.nhs.uk
Website: www.staffsamb.nhs.uk
(Shropshire and Staffordshire Strategic Health Authority)

Chair William Gourlay
Chief Executive Roger Thayne

Staffordshire Moorlands Primary Care Trust

Moorlands House, Stockwell Street, Leek ST13 6HQ
Tel: 01538 487234 Fax: 01538 487255
Email: moorlands.enquiries@northstaffs.nhs.uk
Website: www.moorlands-pct.nhs.uk
(Shropshire and Staffordshire Strategic Health Authority)

Chair George Wiskin
Chief Executive Tony Bruce

Stockport NHS Foundation Trust

Established as a Foundation Trust 01/04/2004.

Stepping Hill Hospital, Oak House, Poplar Grove, Stockport SK2 7JE
Tel: 0161 483 1010 Fax: 0161 419 5411
Website: www.stockport.nhs.uk
(Greater Manchester Strategic Health Authority)

Chair Robina Shah
Chief Executive Chris Burke
Consultants N K Ahluwalia, Gordon James Archer, John Ashworth, M Ballin, Gillian Burrows, Susie Caldwell, Claire Chandelier, Connell, Cooper, Finlay James McConnachy Curran, Rakesh Dalal, Debasis Das, David Deakin, J Dowdall, Effi Eyong, Patrick Gallagher, Alistair John Gray, Peter John Hale, R J Hale, Heal, Brian Hercules, Jeremy Holland, Simon Marcus Horner, Houston, David Johnson, Simon Jowitt, Nicholas Kay, Navpieet Kumar Ahluwalia, Philip Stuart Lewis, M Liddle, R Lindsay, Michael Anthony Martin, Sarah Maxwell, Tom McFarlane, D Meadows, Mecrow, Donald Menzies, Miller, K G Morgan, Laurence Morgan, Anthony Moriarty, M A Morris, Joseph Nankhanya, Ian Nuttall, J B O'Driscoll, Kevin O'Sullivan, Manu Patel, Andy Pickersgill, Timothy Ramsey, Ranamurthy, S Remington, Jonathan D Rigg, D H Rose, Mohammed Saeed, Antonio Sanchez-Capuchino, Siddiqi, Johnathan Christian Gerard Simpson, S A Southworth, N Sutcliffe, P R Talbot, Gordon Taylor Deans, Robert Thompson, Bob Tuffin, Michael Venning, D M Vickers, E L Wilkins, Mark Yodaiken, Zubairu

Stepping Hill Hospital

Poplar Grove, Stockport SK2 7JE
Tel: 0161 483 1010 Fax: 0161 419 5003
Total Beds: 750

Anaesthetics J A Bourne, J W Dowdall, M Liddle, R G Lindsay, A McCluskey, C Mason, D Meadows, R G Mitchell, K O'Sullivan, C J Pemberton, S Remington, J Rigg, T Tramsey

Care of the Elderly G P Choudary, M L Dattachoudary, J Downton, G K Duckett

Dental Surgery R P J Thompson

Dermatology Dr Ashworth, Dr O'Driscoll

General Medicine N Ahluwalia, G J Archer, R J Cryer, I W Dymock, R Feinmann, P J Hale, P S Lewis, M A Martin

General Surgery W Brough, M Davies, G Deans, P E England, P Gallagher

Obstetrics and Gynaecology J C Depares, E Eyong, T McFarlane, I D Nuttall

Ophthalmology R Brown, B L Hercules, L M Morgan

Orthopaedics D Bamford, N Fahmy, J M Laughton, M Morris, B Todd, P G Turner

Pathology R Hale, P J Martin, S Maxwell, K Morgan, N L Reeve, D M Vickers

Radiology R D Dickson, W T Easson, T L Heyworth, C S Keeling-Roberts, N Lynch, S Mehta, A J Pollard, P Sanville

Thoracic Surgery A K Deiraniya

Urology P J Brooman, S Brown, G Collins, P H O'Reilly

Stockport Primary Care Trust

8th Floor Regent House, Heaton Lane, Stockport SK4 1BS
Tel: 0161 426 5000 Fax: 0161 426 5999
Email: enquiries@stockport-pct.nhs.uk
Website: www.stockport.nhs.uk/pct
(Greater Manchester Strategic Health Authority)

Chair Sam Moore
Chief Executive Richard Popplewell

Suffolk Coastal Primary Care Trust

Bartlet Hospital Annexe, Undercliff Road East, Felixstowe IP11 7LT
Tel: 01394 458900 Fax: 01394 458901
Email: office@suffolkcoastal-pct.nhs.uk
Website: www.suffolkcoastal-pct.nhs.uk
(Norfolk, Suffolk and Cambridgeshire Strategic Health Authority)

Chair Tony Robinson
Chief Executive Carole Taylor-Brown

Aldeburgh and District Community Hospital
Park Road, Aldeburgh IP15 3ES
Tel: 01728 452778 Fax: 01728 454056
Total Beds: 36

Bartlet Hospital
Undercliff Road East, Felixstowe IP11 7LT
Tel: 01394 284292 Fax: 01394 671384
Total Beds: 56

Felixstowe General Hospital
Constable Road, Felixstowe IP11 7HJ
Tel: 01394 282214 Fax: 01394 671384

Suffolk Mental Health Partnership NHS Trust

Formerly Local Health Partnerships NHS Trust.

Trust Headquarters, Suffolk House, St Clement's Hospital, Foxhall Road, Ipswich IP3 8NN
Tel: 01473 329600 Fax: 01473 329019
Email: firstname.lastname@smhp.nhs.uk
Website: www.lhp.nhs.uk
(Norfolk, Suffolk and Cambridgeshire Strategic Health Authority)

Chair Hugh Davies
Chief Executive Mark Halladay

Hartismere Hospital
Eye IP23 7BH
Tel: 01379 870543 Fax: 01379 870340
Total Beds: 86

Care of the Elderly P Philips

Hillcrest and Phoenix Day Hospital
Hospital Road, Bury St Edmunds IP33 3NR
Tel: 01284 725333 ext: 2384

Minsmere House
Heath Road, Ipswich IP4 5PD
Tel: 01473 704200 Fax: 01473 704227
Total Beds: 35

General Psychiatry M Barsoum, L Head, A Siddique

St Clements Hospital
Foxhall Road, Ipswich IP3 8LS
Tel: 01473 715111 Fax: 01473 276558
Total Beds: 231

General Psychiatry M Barsoum, A J Byrne, R Caracciolo, D Dodwell, M Gaddal, Dr Siddique, M J Stevens

Southwold and District Hospital
Field Stile Road, Southwold IP18 6LD
Tel: 01502 723333 Fax: 01502 782 4216
Total Beds: 17

ENT D J Premachandra

General Surgery P Aukland

Ophthalmology P Black

Orthopaedics R Jones, P Nadarajan

Stow Lodge Day Hospital
Chilton Way, Stowmarket IP14 1DF
Tel: 01449 614024 Fax: 01449 615829

Violet Hill Day Hospital
Violet Hill Road, Stowmarket IP14 1JS
Tel: 01449 673872 Fax: 01449 673872

Whitwell House Day Hospital
Saxon Road, Saxmundham IP17 1EE
Tel: 01728 605652

Suffolk West Primary Care Trust

Thingoe House, Cotton Lane, Bury St Edmunds IP33 1YJ
Tel: 01284 829600 Fax: 01284 829657
Email: linda.davey@suffolkwest-pct.nhs.uk
Website: www.suffolkwest-pct.nhs.uk
(Norfolk, Suffolk and Cambridgeshire Strategic Health Authority)

Chair Colin Muge
Chief Executive Tony Ranzetta

Newmarket Community Hospital
Exning Road, Newmarket CB8 7JG
Tel: 01638 564000 Fax: 01638 564068

St Leonard's Hospital
Newton Road, Sudbury CO10 6RQ
Tel: 01787 371341 Fax: 01787 313977

Walnuttree Hospital
Walnuttree Lane, Sudbury CO10 6BE
Tel: 01787 371404 Fax: 01787 372339
Total Beds: 97

Care of the Elderly J Fasler, J S Greener, M G F Troup

Sunderland Teaching Primary Care Trust

Pemberton House, Colima Avenue, Sunderland Enterprise Park, Sunderland SR5 3XB
Tel: 0191 529 7000 Fax: 0191 529 7001
Website: www.sunderland.nhs.uk/teachingpct
(Northumberland, Tyne and Wear Strategic Health Authority)

Chair Susan Winfield
Chief Executive Karen Straughair

Surrey Ambulance Service NHS Trust

The Horseshoe, Bolters Lane, Banstead SM7 2AS

Tel: 01737 353333 Fax: 01737 370868
Email: lac@surram.org.uk
Website: www.surrey-ambulance.nhs.uk
(Surrey and Sussex Strategic Health Authority)

Chair Brian Smith
Chief Executive Paul Grant

Surrey and Borders Partnership NHS Trust

Formed 01/04/2005 from the merger of North West Surrey Mental Health Partnership NHS Trust, Surrey Hampshire Borders NHS Trust and Surrey Oaklands NHS Trust. Further details not available at time of going to press.

Website: www.sabp.nhs.uk
(Surrey and Sussex Strategic Health Authority)

Chair Graham Cawsey
Chief Executive Fiona Edwards

Surrey and Sussex Healthcare NHS Trust

East Surrey Hospital, Canada Avenue, Redhill RH1 5RH
Tel: 01737 768511 Fax: 01737 231769
Website: www.surreyandsussex.nhs.uk
(Surrey and Sussex Strategic Health Authority)

Chair Adrian Brown
Chief Executive Ken Cunningham

Crawley Hospital

West Green Drive, Crawley RH11 7DH
Tel: 01293 600300 Fax: 01293 600341
Total Beds: 251

Accident and Emergency A Mabrook

Anaesthetics W Chappell, L S J Jones, D J R Lyle, J Manjiani, V Newman

Cardiothoracic Medicine P Jenkins

Care of the Elderly R J Bailey, F Ramsay, A G Vallon

Dermatology S Cliff, N Cowley, A Farrell

ENT K Bevan, J D Brookes, G Warrington

General Medicine D Acharya, A Gossage, W Shattles, J Sneddon

General Surgery A Ball, A Donnellan, N F Gowland-Hopkins, E R T Owen

Genitourinary Medicine N Narouz

Haematology A C Nandi

Microbiology K Knox

Obstetrics and Gynaecology D M Abayomi, S Vethanayagam

Oncology C Topham

Ophthalmology M Spolton

Orthopaedics A J Campbell, C D P Stone

Paediatrics P A Ahtonen, P I Atkinson, C Greenaway, I G Lewis

Pathology C Hunter-Craig, J Weston

Radiology J M C Davies, A B Hawrych, Dr Pascaline, J Vive

East Surrey Hospital

Canada Avenue, Redhill RH1 5RH
Tel: 01737 768511
Total Beds: 419

Accident and Emergency S Akbar, S Dasan, A Mabrook

Anaesthetics S.M. Ali, P Bajorek, B M Bray, M Green, G Kar, F Lamb, F Sage, P Williams

Care of the Elderly T A Jesudason, V Phongasthorn, C Prajapati

Dermatology S Cliff-Patel, N Cowley, A Farrell

General Medicine R J Allen, U Davies, Dr Eisenger, K J Foster, P Jenkins, J P Lyons, E M Phillips

General Surgery M.A. Dissanayake, J Grabham, Dr Jennings, R G Lightwood, T Loosemore, P Miller, A Stacey-Clear

Genitourinary Medicine F Guiness, N Narouz

Haematology F Matthey, S Stern

Microbiology B Stewart

Neurology J Kimber

Obstetrics and Gynaecology Mr Butler-Manuel, A Gordon-Wright, M Long, J Penny, J Pipe, P Townsend

Ophthalmology A Chopdar, F O'Sullivan, M Spolton, R S Wilson

Oral and Maxillofacial Surgery R Siva, P Ward-Booth

Orthodontics A Banner

Orthopaedics A J Campbell, K Drabu, H D Maurice, G Selentakis, T J Selvan

Paediatrics N H Al-Hilaly, Dr Das, C Greenaway, M Jawad, M Williams

Pathology M Ameen, D Fish, B M Hill, R Jackson

Radiology B Anastasi, N Anderson, A Ceccherini, D Eliras, S Gwyther, R McAvinchey, D Mukasa, N Sellars

Radiotherapy and Oncology M Illsley, J Money-Kirle

Reproductive Health Dr Shinewi

Rheumatology S Griffiths

Thoracic Surgery R E Sayer

Urology P Miller, Dr Rane

Harrowlands Rehabilitation Unit

Harrowlands Park, South Terrace, Dorking RH4 2RA
Tel: 01306 740449 Fax: 01306 743190
Total Beds: 20

Manager Alistair Bradley

Surrey Hampshire Borders NHS Trust

From 04/2005 merging with North West Surrey Mental Health Partnership NHS Trust and Surrey Oaklands NHS Trust to form Surrey and Borders Partnership NHS Trust.

The Ridgewood Centre, Old Bisley Road, Camberley GU16 5QE
Tel: 01276 692919 Fax: 01276 605599
(Surrey and Sussex Strategic Health Authority)

Chair Mary Sennett
Chief Executive Fiona Green

Farnham Road Hospital

Farnham Road, Guildford GU2 5LX
Tel: 01483 443535 Fax: 01483 443502
Total Beds: 80

Manager Graham Wilkin

General Psychiatry S Ahmad, J Mugisha, I H Shoeb, S J Watson

Psychiatry for Older People Dr Hall, Dr Zaidi, Dr Zaidi

Ridgewood Centre

Old Bisley Road, Frimley, Camberley GU16 5QE
Tel: 01276 692919 Fax: 01276 605360
Total Beds: 64

Manager Liz McGill

General Psychiatry G Andrews, A Chakrabarti, M Hawthorne, H Jameel, S Khalaf, S Lieberman

Surrey Heath and Woking Primary Care Trust

West Byfleet Health Centre, Madeira Road, West Byfleet KT14 6DH
Tel: 01932 356830 Fax: 01932 358640
Email: name.surname@shawpct.nhs.uk
Website: www.shawpct.nhs.uk
(Surrey and Sussex Strategic Health Authority)

Chair Laurie Doust
Chief Executive Jane Dale

Woking Community Hospital

The Willows, Heathside Road, Woking GU22 7HS
Total Beds: 40

Surrey Oaklands NHS Trust

From 04/2005 merging with North West Surrey Mental Health NHS Partnership Trust and Surrey Hampshire Borders NHS Trust to form Surrey and Borders Partnership NHS Trust.

Oaklands House, Coulsdon Road, Caterham CR3 5YA
Tel: 01883 383838 Fax: 01883 383522
Email: forename.surname@surreyoaklands.nhs.uk
Website: surreyoaklands.nhs.uk
(Surrey and Sussex Strategic Health Authority)

Chair Cathy Rollinson
Chief Executive Maggie Somekh

Sussex Ambulance Service NHS Trust

Ambulance Headquarters, 40-42 Friars Walk, Lewes BN7 2XW
Tel: 01273 489444 Fax: 01273 489445
Email: info@sussamb.nhs.uk
Website: www.sussamb.co.uk
(Surrey and Sussex Strategic Health Authority)

Chair Roger Purchase
Chief Executive Paul Sutton

Sussex Downs and Weald Primary Care Trust

36-38 Friars Walk, Lewes BN7 2PB
Tel: 01273 485300 Fax: 01273 485400
Website: www.sussexdownsandwealdpct.nhs.uk
(Surrey and Sussex Strategic Health Authority)

Chair Beryl Hobson
Chief Executive Fiona Henniker

Crowborough War Memorial Hospital

South View Road, Crowborough TN6 1HB
Tel: 01892 603110 Fax: 01892 603119
Total Beds: 32

Uckfield Community Hospital

Framfield Road, Uckfield TN22 5AW
Tel: 01825 769999 Fax: 01825 745020
Total Beds: 47

Victoria Hospital

Nevill Road, Lewes BN7 1PF
Tel: 01273 474153 Fax: 01273 473362

Sutton and Merton Primary Care Trust

Nelson Hospital, Hamilton Wing, Kingston Road, Raynes Park, London SW20 8DB
Tel: 020 8251 1111 Fax: 020 8715 2770
Website: www.suttonandmerton-pct.nhs.uk
(South West London Strategic Health Authority)

Chair Kay Sonneborn
Chief Executive Ian Ayres

Carshalton War Memorial Hospital

The Park, Carshalton SM5 3DB
Tel: 020 8647 5534 Fax: 020 8773 4980
Total Beds: 90

Consultants S K Das, M Ward

Swale Primary Care Trust

Unit 200, Kent Science Park, Winch Road, Sittingbourne ME9 8EF
Tel: 01795 416800 Fax: 01795 416801
Email: info@swalepct.nhs.uk
Website: www.swalepct.nhs.uk
(Kent and Medway Strategic Health Authority)

Chair John McCrae
Chief Executive John Mangan

Sheppey Community Hospital

Plover Road, Minster on Sea, Sheerness ME12 3LT
Tel: 01795 879100 Fax: 01795 416801
Total Beds: 48

Swindon and Marlborough NHS Trust

The Great Western Hospital, Marlborough Road, Swindon SN3 6BB
Tel: 01793 604020 Fax: 01793 604021
Email: forename.surname@swindon-marlborough.nhs.uk
Website: www.swindon-marlborough.nhs.uk
(Avon, Gloucestershire and Wiltshire Strategic Health Authority)

Chair Patsy Newton
Chief Executive Lyn Hill-Tout

The Great Western Hospital

Marlborough Road, Swindon SN3 6BB
Tel: 01793 604020 Fax: 01793 604021
Total Beds: 604

Accident and Emergency I Kendall (Head), B Aslam, I Kendall

Anaesthetics C P Beeby, A Bullough, D N Campbell, R Craig, A Dale, M D Entwistle, J Griffiths, D M Jackson, H E Jones, N Jones, B Maxwell, M O'Connor, S O'Kelly, A J Pickworth, I Smith, J Stone, C Van Hamel, M Watters

Cardiology E Barnes, M J Hayes, W McCrea

Care of the Elderly E Giallombardo, D J Howard, D Mukherjee, H Newton

Child and Adolescent Psychiatry J W Eastgate, R Eyre, W Woodhouse

Dermatology D Buckley, R J Mann, L Whittam

ENT S Chalstrey, J P Donnelly, D Gupta, A Waddell

Gastroenterology P J V Hanson, M D Hellier, J Maltby

General Medicine S Ahmed, E Barnes, P J V Hanson, M J Hayes, M D Hellier, M Juniper, A Leonard, J Maltby, W A McCrea, C McKinley, P A Price

General Surgery R O Beck, P Burgess, D R A Finch, M Galea, R E Glass, D Hocken, J Iacovou, R N Lawrence

Genitourinary Medicine G Rooney

Neurology S Wimalaratna

Obstetrics and Gynaecology A P Bond, W Clifford, J E Cullimore, P A Forbes-Smith, D Griffiths, K Jones, D N Majumdar, H Narayan

Ophthalmology S E P Burgess, P McCormack, J H Ramsay, T Yasen

Oral Surgery C R Charles

Orthopaedics A Brooks, S Deo, A J B Fogg, M A Foy, J Ivory, I M R London, M Rigby, D M Williamson, D Woods

Paediatrics R Chinthapalli, L Grain, J M King, P T O'Keefe, H Price, S T Zengeya

Pathology J Armstrong, N Blesing, C M Colley, S Dawson, A G Gray, E S Green, D Lazic, M Radojkovic, J A Scurr, F Thomas, P Tidbury

Plastic Surgery D J Coleman

Radiology A Beale, J Cook, T Cousins, J Henson, L K Jackson, A Jones, N Ridley, S J Taylor, A Troughton

Radiotherapy D J Cole

Rheumatology and Rehabilitation D A Collins, E Price, L Williamson

Urology R O Beck, J W Iacovou

Swindon Primary Care Trust

North Swindon District Centre, Thamesdown Drive, Swindon SN25 4AN
Tel: 01793 708700 Fax: 01793 708701
Website: www.swindonpct.nhs.uk
(Avon, Gloucestershire and Wiltshire Strategic Health Authority)

Chair Michelle Howard
Chief Executive Jan Stubbings

Tameside and Glossop Acute Services NHS Trust

Tameside General Hospital, Fountain Street, Ashton-under-Lyne OL6 9RW
Tel: 0161 331 6000
Website: www.tamesidehospital.nhs.uk
(Greater Manchester Strategic Health Authority)

Chair Kevin Corscadden
Chief Executive Christine Green

Shire Hill Hospital

Bute Street, Glossop SK13 9PZ
Tel: 01457 866021 Fax: 01457 857519
Total Beds: 54

Tameside General Hospital

Fountain Street, Ashton-under-Lyne OL6 9RW
Tel: 0161 331 5151 Fax: 0161 331 5007
Total Beds: 676

Accident and Emergency MR Kollimada, Y Sharma

Anaesthetics U Deulkar, Dr Gandhi, Dr Hockman, N Jena, A Kulkarni, J K Mazumder, B Ousta, Dr Prasana, H Rehman, K Sultan

Dental Surgery M E Foster, N Mandell, C McDade

Dermatology E Gilmore, E Parry

ENT A E R Kobbe, P D Sharma

General Medicine S Ahmed, B E Boyes, M P Chopra, A Hameed, E Jude, A Khan, N M O'Mullane, C R Payne, S Puri, H Rakicka, R Sinharay, G Whatley

General Surgery P Clothier, M Cooper-Wilson, Mrs Ellenbogen, K H Siddiqui, Mr Welch, A B Woodyer

Genitourinary Medicine M R Girgis

Neurology C Sherrington

Neurosurgery A Sofat

Obstetrics and Gynaecology S Ali, J Foden-Schroff, A I Kiwanuka, T Mahmood, A Watson

Ophthalmology K Goodall, J Lipton, D Sturgess, J Suharwardy

Orthodontics N Mandell, C McDade

Orthopaedics T H Dunningham, A O Ebizie, B N Muddu, E M H Obeid, M Pena, D F Tandon

Pathology W Hood, P F Unsworth, A Yates

Radiology B Bannerjee, I Brett

Radiotherapy and Oncology Mr Sykes

Rheumatology T Brammah

Urology S Brown

Tameside and Glossop Primary Care Trust

New Century House, Progress Way, Windmill Lane, Denton, Manchester M34 2GP
Tel: 0161 304 5300 Fax: 0161 304 5401
Website: www.tamesideandglossop.nhs.uk
(Greater Manchester Strategic Health Authority)

Chair Ian McCrae
Chief Executive Julian Hartley

Taunton and Somerset NHS Trust

Taunton and Somerset Hospital, Musgrove Park, Taunton TA1 5DA
Tel: 01823 333444 Fax: 01823 336877
Website: www.somerset-health.org.uk
(Dorset and Somerset Strategic Health Authority)

Chair Brian Tanner
Chief Executive Nick Chapman

Taunton and Somerset Hospital

Musgrove Park, Taunton TA1 5DA
Tel: 01823 333444 Fax: 01823 336877
Total Beds: 776

Accident and Emergency G Bryce, C Mann

Anaesthetics B Browne, T M Bull, A Daykin, R C Desborough, I Gauntlett, J Lucas, B Nichols, V J Prior, P J Ravenscroft

Cardiology M James, D MacIver

Care of the Elderly S Cooper, M Evans, T Solanki

Chest Disease C R Swinburn

Dermatology J Boyle, D Pryce

ENT S C Wells, Dr Yates

General Medicine D MacIver, C Swinburn, D B Yates

General Surgery J F Chester, C D Collins, I A Eyre-Brook, S M Jones, I N Ramus

Genitourinary Medicine M Fitzgerald

Infectious Diseases C R Swinburn

Medical Microbiology J W Jones, M Smith

Obstetrics and Gynaecology K Bidgood, H Marsh

Ophthalmology K Bates, J M Twomey

Oral and Maxillofacial Surgery M Davidson

Orthopaedics A Clarke, C M Marsh, C Ogilvie, P Webb

Paediatrics R Mann, A Tandy, M Webster

Pathology S A N Johnson, S C Smith

Radiology J M Bell, P M Cavanagh, D Cooke, H Thomas, S K Wells, S A Willson

Radiotherapy and Oncology J Bullimore

Urology M J Speakman

Vascular Surgery J F Chester

Taunton Deane Primary Care Trust

Wellsprings Road, Taunton TA2 7PQ
Tel: 01823 333491 Fax: 01823 272710
Website: www.tauntondeanepct.nhs.uk
(Dorset and Somerset Strategic Health Authority)

Chair Alan Hopper
Chief Executive Edward Colgan

Dene Barton Community Unit

Dene Road, Cotford St Luke, Taunton TA4 1DD
Tel: 01823 433540 Fax: 01823 433423
Total Beds: 40

Taunton Community Hospital

Musgrove Park, Taunton TA1 5DA
Tel: 01823 343756

Wellington and District Cottage Hospital

South Street, Wellington TA21 8QQ
Tel: 01823 662663
Total Beds: 11

Care of the Elderly M Evans

General Psychiatry D W Ahmed

General Surgery N I Ramus

Obstetrics and Gynaecology J A Richardson

Orthopaedics C H Marsh

Urology P J O'Boyle

Tavistock and Portman NHS Trust

Tavistock Centre, 120 Belsize Lane, London NW3 5BA
Tel: 020 7435 7111 Fax: 020 7447 3709
Email: ntemple@tavi-port.nhs.uk
Website: www.tavi-port.org
(North Central London Strategic Health Authority)

Chair Maggie Wakelin-Saint
Chief Executive Nicholas Temple

Monroe Young Family Centre

33A Daleham Gardens, London NW3 5BU
Tel: 020 7431 5138 Fax: 020 7794 0603
Email: myfc@tavi-port.org

Child and Adolescent Psychiatry H Browne

Portman Clinic

8 Fitzjohn's Avenue, London NW3 5NA
Tel: 020 7794 8262 Fax: 020 7447 3748
Email: portman@tavi-port.nhs.uk

Psychotherapy J Freedman, R Hale, C Minne, M Von Der Tann, J Yakely, A Zachary

Tavistock Clinic

Tavistock Centre, 120 Belsize Lane, London NW3 5BA
Tel: 020 7435 7111 Fax: 020 7447 3709
Email: mrustin@tavi-port.nhs.uk

Child and Adolescent Psychiatry R Anderson, E Bradley, O Burke, D Di Ceglie, R Graham, E Kennedy, C Lindsey, J Pigott, R Senior, D Simpson, J Trowell, A Wiener

Primary Care S Blake, J Launer

Psychotherapy D Bell, A Garelick, E Gibb, P Hobson, M Patrick, J Stubley, D Taylor, N Temple, N Whyte

The Tavistock Mulberry Bush Day Unit

33 Daleham Gardens, London NW3 5BU
Tel: 020 7794 3353 Fax: 020 7794 3354
Email: sanfu@tavi-port.nhs.uk

Child and Adolescent Psychiatry K Kasinski

Tees and North East Yorkshire NHS Trust

Flatts Lane Centre, Flatts Lane, Normanby, Middlesbrough TS6 0SZ
Tel: 01642 288288 Fax: 01642 516460
Website: www.peoplelikeus.nhs.uk
(County Durham and Tees Valley Strategic Health Authority; North and East Yorkshire and Northern Lincolnshire Strategic Health Authority)

Chair Eileen Grace
Chief Executive Moira Britton

St Luke's Hospital

Marton Road, Middlesbrough TS4 3AF
Tel: 01642 850850 Fax: 01642 821810
Total Beds: 226

University Hospital of Hartlepool Mental Health Unit

Holdforth Road, Hartlepool TS24 9AH

University Hospital of North Tees Mental Health Unit

Hardwick, Stockton-on-Tees TS19 8PE

Tees East and North Yorkshire Ambulance Service NHS Trust

Fairfields, Shipton Road, York YO30 1XW
Tel: 01904 666000 Fax: 01904 666050
Email: infoline@tenyas.nhs.uk
Website: www.tenyas.org.uk

(North and East Yorkshire and Northern Lincolnshire Strategic Health Authority; County Durham and Tees Valley Strategic Health Authority)

Chair Nicholas Varey
Chief Executive Jayne Barnes

Teignbridge Primary Care Trust

Bridge House, Collett Way, Brunel Industrial Estate, Newton Abbot TQ12 4PH
Tel: 01626 357000 Fax: 01626 357002
Email: enquiries@teignbridge-pct.nhs.uk
Website: www.teignbridge-pct.nhs.uk
(South West Peninsula Strategic Health Authority)

Chair Christine Cribb
Chief Executive Pam Smith

Ashburton and Buckfastleigh Hospital
Eastern Road, Ashburton, Newton Abbot TQ13 7AP
Tel: 01364 652203 Fax: 01364 653676

Bovey Tracey Hospital
Furzeleigh Lane, Bovey Tracey, Newton Abbot TQ13 9HJ
Tel: 01626 832279 Fax: 01626 835818

Dawlish Hospital
Stockton Hill, Dawlish EX7 9LW
Tel: 01626 868500 Fax: 01626 868543

Newton Abbot Hospital
64 East Street, Newton Abbot TQ12 4PT
Tel: 01626 354321

Teignmouth Hospital
Mill Lane, Teignmouth TQ14 9BQ
Tel: 01626 772161 Fax: 01626 771121

Telford and Wrekin Primary Care Trust

Sommerfeld House, Sommerfeld Road, Trench Lock, Telford TF1 5RY
Tel: 01952 222322 Fax: 01952 265197
Website: www.telfordpct.nhs.uk
(Shropshire and Staffordshire Strategic Health Authority)

Chair Sue Davis
Chief Executive Simon Conolly

Tendring Primary Care Trust

Carnarvon House, Carnarvon Road, Clacton-on-Sea CO15 6QD
Tel: 01255 206060 Fax: 01255 206061
Website: www.tendringpct.co.uk
(Essex Strategic Health Authority)

Chair David Rex
Chief Executive Paul Unsworth

Harwich and District Hospital
Main Road, Dovercourt, Harwich CO12 4EX
Tel: 01255 201200 Fax: 01255 552335
Total Beds: 37

Care of the Elderly V Paramsothy, T Rudra

ENT P Kitchen

General Medicine J M Aitken, C Bodmer, N Chanarin, R E Cowan, T Howes

General Surgery C Backhouse, D Menzies, J Strachan

Obstetrics and Gynaecology D Sanderson

Oncology P Murray

Ophthalmology A Beckingsale

Orthopaedics J Bradley, R C Todd

Paediatrics S Mukerji

Rheumatology P Byrne

Thurrock Primary Care Trust

PO Box 83, Civic Offices, New Road, Grays RM17 6FD
Tel: 01375 406400 Fax: 01375 406401
Email: info@thurrock-pct.nhs.uk
Website: www.thurrock-pct.nhs.uk
(Essex Strategic Health Authority)

Chair Valerie Liddiard
Chief Executive Janet Hunter

Thurrock Community Hospital
Long Lane, Grays RM16 2PX

Torbay Primary Care Trust

Rainbow House, Avenue Road, Torquay TQ2 5LS
Tel: 01803 210910 Fax: 01803 292975
Email: enquiries@torbay-pct.nhs.uk
Website: www.torbay-pct.nhs.uk
(South West Peninsula Strategic Health Authority)

Chair Terry Nicholls
Chief Executive Peter Colclough

Brixham Hospital
Greenswood Road, Brixham TQ5 9HW
Tel: 01803 882153 Fax: 01803 856099

Paignton Hospital
Church Street, Paignton TQ3 3AG
Tel: 01803 557425 Fax: 01803 665245

Tower Hamlets Primary Care Trust

Trust Offices, Mile End Hospital, Bancroft Road, London E1 4DG
Tel: 020 8223 8900 Fax: 020 8223 8907
Email: enquiries@thpct.nhs.uk
Website: www.thpct.nhs.uk
(North East London Strategic Health Authority)

Chair Richard Gee
Chief Executive Alwen Williams

Mile End Hospital
Bancroft Road, London E1 4DG
Tel: 020 7377 7920 Fax: 020 7377 7931
Total Beds: 200

Trafford Healthcare NHS Trust

Trafford General Hospital, Moorside Road, Urmston, Manchester M41 5SL
Tel: 0161 748 4022 Fax: 0161 746 7214
Email: info@trafford.nhs.uk
Website: www.trafford.nhs.uk
(Greater Manchester Strategic Health Authority)

Chair Helen Busteed
Chief Executive David Cain

Altrincham General Hospital
Market Street, Altrincham WA14 1PE
Tel: 0161 928 6111 Fax: 0161 928 5657
Total Beds: 41

Anaesthetics B K Greenwood

Care of the Elderly J A Anandadas, T Kondratowicz, S R Musgrave

Child Health H M Lewis

Dermatology H L Muston

General Medicine B C Leahy, F McKenna, S R Musgrove, W P Stephens, C B Summerton

General Surgery I M Aldean

Obstetrics and Gynaecology A M Nysenbaum

Ophthalmology M J Lavin, G S Turner

Orthopaedics A Fitzgerald, M Ismail, M C B Webber

Paediatrics R H A Campbell, H M Lewis

Pathology D M Alderson, L N Sandle

Radiology Dr Mortimer, P S Norburn

Urology P N Rao

St Anne's Hospital
Woodville Road, Bowdon, Altrincham WA14 2AQ
Tel: 0161 928 5851
Total Beds: 20

Care of the Elderly J A Anandadas

ENT A El-Kholy, E Jaffari

General Medicine F McKenna

Stretford Memorial Hospital
226 Seymour Grove, Stretford, Manchester M16 0DE
Tel: 0161 881 5353
Total Beds: 12

Anaesthetics T J Kinsella

Care of the Elderly T Kondratowicz, S R Musgrave

ENT A El-Kholy

General Medicine B C Leahy, W P Stephens, C B Summerton

General Surgery F X Marazerlo

Obstetrics and Gynaecology G Ainscow, R J Howell

Ophthalmology M J Lavin, G S Turner

Orthopaedics M C B Webber

Trafford General Hospital
Moorside Road, Davyhulme, Urmston, Manchester M41 5SL
Tel: 0161 748 4022 Fax: 0161 746 8556
Total Beds: 537

Accident and Emergency M Ahmad, C L Summers

Anaesthetics M Eltoft, B K Greenwood, T J Kinsella, R T Longbottom, A G Pocklington, A Shaw, C Van Oldenbeek

Audiological Medicine P Kuna
Cardiology P Woolfson

Care of the Elderly J A Anandadas, T Kondratowicz, S R Musgrave

Child Health A A A Bagadi, R H A Campbell, D Jayson, A B John, P Kuna, H M Lewis, E B Turya

Dermatology H L Muston

ENT A El-Kholy

Gastroenterology C Summerton

General Medicine B Leahy, F McKenna, W P Stephens, C B Summerton, S C O Taggart

General Surgery I M Aldean, F Mazarelo

Genitourinary Medicine E Curless

Neurology W Schady

Obstetrics and Gynaecology G Ainscow, Dr Hotchkies, R J Howell, A M Nysenbaum

Occupational Health A Adisesh

Ophthalmology M Lavin, G S Turner

Oral and Maxillofacial Surgery T Boyd, S Caldwell, R E Lloyd

Orthopaedics A Fitzgerald, R P Goel, M Ismail, M C B Webber

Paediatrics R H A Campbell, A B John, H Lewis, E B Turya

Pathology D M Alderson, P A Carrington, J Croall, L N Sandle, M Y Sheikh

Radiology U M Beetles, M D Howden, A Mortimer, P S Norburn

Restorative Dentistry T Boyd

Urology P Downey, P N Rao

Trafford North Primary Care Trust

Integrated management with Trafford South Primary Care Trust.

Oakland House, 2nd Floor, Talbot Road, Old Trafford, Manchester M16 0PQ
Tel: 0161 873 9500 Fax: 0161 873 9501
Email: mail@trafford-pcts.nhs.uk
Website: www.trafford-pcts.nhs.uk
(Greater Manchester Strategic Health Authority)

Chair Fay Selvin
Chief Executive Tim Riley

Trafford South Primary Care Trust

Integrated management with Trafford North Primary Care Trust.

1st Floor, Oaklands House, 34 Washway Road, Sale M33 6FS
Tel: 0161 968 3700 Fax: 0161 968 3701
Website: www.trafford-pcts.nhs.uk
(Greater Manchester Strategic Health Authority)

Chair Leslie Robinson
Chief Executive Tim Riley

Two Shires Ambulance NHS Trust

The Trust provides ambulance services primarily to the 1.3 million people in Northamptonshire and Buckinghamshire with some patient transport and logistics work also carried out in parts of Cambridgeshire.

The Hunters, Buckingham Road, Deanshanger, Milton Keynes MK19 6HL
Tel: 01908 262422 Fax: 01908 265014
(Leicestershire, Northamptonshire and Rutland Strategic Health Authority; Thames Valley Strategic Health Authority)

Chair Ken Cooper
Chief Executive Paul Martin

United Bristol Healthcare NHS Trust

Trust Headquarters, Marlborough Street, Bristol BS1 3NU

Tel: 0117 929 0666 Fax: 0117 928 2588
Email: ubht@ubht.swest.nhs.uk
Website: www.ubht.nhs.uk
(Avon, Gloucestershire and Wiltshire Strategic Health Authority)

Chair Philip Gregory
Chief Executive Ron Kerr

Bristol Eye Hospital

Lower Maudlin Street, Bristol BS1 2LX
Tel: 0117 923 0060 Fax: 0117 928 4686
Website: www.ubht.nhs.uk/eye
Total Beds: 46

Manager Y Quincey

Ophthalmology C Bailey, A Churchill, S Cook, M Creaney, J Diamond, A Dick, D L Easty, R H B Grey, R Harrad, R Haynes, R H Markham, M Potts, J Sparrow, D Tole, C Williams

Bristol General Hospital

Guinea Street, Bristol BS1 6SY
Tel: 0117 926 5001 Fax: 0117 928 6245
Total Beds: 97

Care of the Elderly G W Tobin (Head), S C M Croxson, M MacMahon, P Murphy, G W Tobin

Bristol Haematology and Oncology Centre

Horfield Road, Bristol BS2 8ED
Tel: 0117 923 0000 Fax: 0117 928 2498
Total Beds: 45

Manager Cathy Meredith

Clinical Haematology R S Evely, N J Goulden, J M Hows, J A James, S H Otton, D H Pamphilon, G L Scott, G R Standen

Clinical Oncology A Bahl, V Barley, J A Bullimore, E J Chambers, P G Cornes, S J Falk, S Goodman, J D Graham, K I Hopkins, H Newman, G Rees, P Riddle, E C Whipp

Palliative Medicine Dr Adler, K Forbes, G W Hanks, Dr Hawkins

Bristol Homoeopathic Hospital

Cotham Hill, Cotham, Bristol BS6 6JU
Tel: 0117 973 1231 Fax: 0117 923 8759
Website: www.ubht.nhs.uk/homoeopathy

Manager L Quincey

Homoeopathy D S Spence (Head), D N Anderson, G C How, D S Spence, E A Thompson, R A Welford

Bristol Royal Hospital for Children

Upper Maudlin Street, Bristol BS2 8BJ
Tel: 0117 927 6998 Fax: 0117 928 5820
Website: www.ubht.nhs.uk/bch
Total Beds: 124

Manager I Barrington

Cardiac Surgery A J Parry, A Pawade

Child and Adolescent Psychiatry H E Barnes, S Brassington, J Culling, D Indoe, C Lewin, M Rawlinson, J Smith

Clinical Genetics P Lunt, A McDonald, R Newbury-Ecob, S F Smithson

Orthopaedics P G Allen, J D Eldridge, M Gargan, I W Nelson, F Norman-Taylor, N M Portinaro, P J Witherow

Paediatric Clinical Haematology N J Goulden

Paediatric Nephrology J A Dudley, C D Inward, M E McGraw, M A Saleem, G J Tizzard

Paediatric Surgery E Cusick, J D Frank, L Huskisson, J McNally, G Nicholls, R Spicer

Paediatrics M T Bedow, P Cairns, F Carswell, T Chambers, E C Crowne, A Finn, P J Fleming, A B M Foot, L Goldsworthy, J Hamilton-Shield, A M Hayes, J Henderson, P Jardine, S Langton-Hener, S P Lowis, D Marks, R Martin, M G Mott, A Oakhill, T E Richens, M E Rodgman, G A B Russell, B Sandhu, P M Sharples, A G Stuart, M Thoresen, A J Tometzi, A Whitelaw

Pathology M T Ashworth, P J Berry, H J Porter

Bristol Royal Infirmary

Marlborough Street, Bristol BS2 8HW
Tel: 0117 923 0000 Fax: 0117 928 3413
Total Beds: 481

Manager L Kelly

Accident and Emergency I O'Sullivan, N Rawlinson, A H Swain

Anaesthetics J I Alexander, A M S Black, D Coates, A H Cohen, I M Davies, F C Forrest, T H Gould, D G Hughes, I Jenkins, R W Johnson, S Kinsella, S G Lauder, S P K Linter, S Masey, S J Mather, C Monk, P J Murphy, M Nevin, V Penning-Rowsell, S J Pryn, I G Ryder, L E Shutt, P A Stoddart, D Terry, P G N Thornton, S Underwood, P M Weir, A R Wolf

Cardiology A Baumbach, T Cripps, J V Jones, K R Karsch, J C Pitts-Crick, A G Stuart

Cardiothoracic Surgery K M Amer, G D Angelini, R Ascione, A J Bryan, F Cuilli, C Forester-Wood, J A Morgan, M J Underwood

Care of the Elderly S E Caine, S C M Croxson, M MacMahon, P Murphy, G Tobin

Chemical Pathology C R Boyly, P Richardson, D Stansbie

Clinical Pharmacology and Therapeutics C J C Roberts

Dermatology C G Aplin, C B Archer, D d Berker, G Dunnill, S J Hunt, C T C Kennedy, J Sansom

Endocrinology R Corrall, C Dayan

Gastroenterology D Alderson, P Barham, R E Barry, P Durdey, K W Heaton, R A Mountford, C J Probert, M Thomas

General Medicine R E Barry, J R Catterall, E Gamble, F H Gordon, S D Hearing, K W Heaton, M R Hetzel, R S Hyderman, A Levy, S L Lightman, R A Mountford, C J Probert, C J C Roberts

Genitourinary Medicine P J Horner, A J Scott

Histopathology C J Calder, C M P Collins, N Moorghan, J Pawade, E A Sheffield

Medical Microbiology R C Spencer

Nephrology T G Feest, S Harper

Neurology P H Heywood, S D Lhatoo, I E C Ormerod, K A Sieradzan, G D Wright

Neuropathology T H Moss

Occupational Health C C Harling, R Phillip

Orthopaedics R M Atkins, J D Eldridge, M Gargan, M Jackson, I Learmouth, I J Leslie, J Livingstone, J H Newman, F H Norman Taylor, P Sarangi, A G Weale

Pathology C M P Collins, C A Pennock, H J Porter, D Stansbie

Pharmacology C J C Roberts

Radiology H Andrews, A M Baird, J E Basten, D J Crier, A Duncan, P Goddard, A J Jones, J Kabala, E Kutt, P Murphy, M Rees, J Virjee, C J Wakeley, I Watt, R P Wilde

Respiratory Medicine J R Catterall, M R Hetzel, G Laszlo

Rheumatology A M Al-Saidi, F J Cowen, J R Kirwan, L P Robertson, J Tobias

Thoracic Medicine J R Catterall, M R Hetzel, G Laszlo

Urology M Persad, K Ramasubbu, G Sibley, P J B Smith, M P Wright

Keynsham Hospital
Keynsham, Bristol BS18 1AG
Tel: 0117 986 2356 Fax: 0117 986 2356 ext: 256
Total Beds: 61

Manager L Williams

Care of the Elderly F Bigwood, M Cameron, R G Davidson, N R Nutt

St Michael's Hospital
Southwell Street, Bristol BS2 8EG
Tel: 0117 921 5411 Fax: 0117 928 5842
Total Beds: 270

Manager L Salmon

ENT P G Bicknell, M Birchell, M V Griffiths, A R Maw, M W Saunders

Obstetrics and Gynaecology R S Anderson, D Cahill, N Dwyer, S Glew, U Gordon, J Jenkins, P Kyle, M S Mills, J B Murdoch, P A R Niven, S M Sellers, P Soothill, B Strachan

University of Bristol Dental Hospital and School
Lower Maudlin Street, Bristol BS1 2LY
Tel: 0117 923 0050 Fax: 0117 928 4443

Manager C Donoghue

Consultants M Addy, J G Cowpe, P Crawford, J Eveson, D L Franklin, M J Griffiths, P Guest, N W Harradine, A Harrison, I S Hathorn, I S Hathorn, A Ireland, G Irvine, D C Jagger, P King, H Knight, N Meredith, J Moran, G Pell, S Prime, J Rees, J Sandy, S J Thomas, C M Woodhead

United Lincolnshire Hospitals NHS Trust

Trust Headquarters, Grantham and District Hospital, 101 Manthorpe Road, Grantham NG31 8DG
Tel: 01476 565232 Fax: 01476 567358
Website: www.ulh.nhs.uk
(Trent Strategic Health Authority)

Chair Jenny Green
Chief Executive Roger Paffard

County Hospital, Louth
High Holme Road, Louth LN11 OEU
Tel: 01507 600100 Fax: 01507 609290
Total Beds: 117

Manager Sarah Jane Mills

Anaesthetics H Myint, M Serajuddin

Diabetes M Rehman

General Medicine C Cook, M Teli

General Surgery P Reasbeck

Orthopaedics R Nayak

Grantham and District Hospital
101 Manthorpe Road, Grantham NG31 8DG
Tel: 01476 565232
Total Beds: 198

Manager Dominic Cox

Accident and Emergency H D Garrick

Anaesthetics J L Breckenridge, C E Cory, S Jayamaha, C Onugha, N Platt, T P Shepherd, Dr Tore, Dr Udom

General Medicine C R Birch, J H Campbell, U D Wijayawardhana

General Surgery J G McAdam, D Mathur, D Valerio

Haematology V M Tringham

Histopathology D M Clark

Microbiology J Francis

Obstetrics and Gynaecology R P Husemeyer, S Vogt

Orthodontics J Kotyla

Orthopaedics A E Halliday, W A Niezywinski, S M O'Riordan, Mr Singhavia

Radiology S J Bradley, P J Gibson

Lincoln County Hospital
Greetwell Road, Lincoln LN2 5QY
Tel: 01522 512512 Fax: 01522 573419
Total Beds: 625

Accident and Emergency J G Pillay, N Pyrgos

Anaesthetics J Craggs, J Donnelly, A E Feerick, R Francis, A M Liddle, L Mendel, C A O'Dwyer, D C Phillips, A B Powles, A D Reynolds, R B Scott, J Stonham, R J Thornton, C K G Tyler, A B Victoria, A Webb, N Williams, A S Wolverson

Care of the Elderly A Kamal, D M Stokoe

ENT A Connolly, A R McRae, G Owen

General Medicine S Ahmed, R Andrews, J R C Bowen, Dr Davies-Jones, N C Hepburn, E Hui, H Hussain, S Kelly, S Leach, B MacDonald, A Mandal, S P Matusiewicz, W E Morgan, N S Mytheen, J L W Parker, I C Paterson, R S Prasad, B B Scott, B Sharrack, G Spencer

General Surgery D R Andrew, A P Barlow, P K Basu, P Dunning, O Eremin, H Henderson, J A Jibril, A J Lamerton, I Mark, T Milward, S K Varma, D J Ward

Haematology M I Adelman, A Hepplestone, A Hunter, D R Prangnell, K Speed, C Williams

Medical Microbiology C A J Brightman, E R Youngs

Nephrology J Little, Dr Warwick

Obstetrics and Gynaecology A J Breeson, G W Gough, R Husemeyer, M P Lamb, O E Oteri, I D Vellacott, S Vogt

Ophthalmology A A Castillo, P M Drummond, E G Hale, B Redmill

Oral Surgery M A Coupland, S A Layton, A G Sadler

Orthopaedics R Asirvatham, M Feeney, D Gale, I D Hyde, C Lee, M Maqsood, E W Morris, S M O'Riordan, J M Wilkinson

Paediatrics J Baxter, R C Groggins, M J Lewins, C P Millns, A Scammell, Dr Suresh Babu

Pathology G Cowley, J A Harvey, J M F McClemont, W M Peters

Radiology A L Griffiths, S G Hogg, M Kamal, C I Rothwell, S Stinchcombe, V Thava, G W Thorpe, G Vijayashimhulu, D Wheatley

Radiotherapy and Oncology K Baria, J M Eremin, E C Murray, T M Sheehan, T Sreenivasan

Rheumatology J E Carty, B P Hunt

Pilgrim Hospital
Sibsey Road, Boston PE21 9QS
Tel: 01205 364801 Fax: 01205 354395
Total Beds: 520

Accident and Emergency H Hassan

Anaesthetics A Abbas, B Bakalar, G Batchelor, M D R Bexton, Dr Blazkova, M W Butt, R Caranza, E P D Chalmers, E Dichmont, A I Hagar, L Hruban, N Joachim, R Knight, J M Massey, A C Norton, S Panjwani, D A Sagar, G Samra, M Spittal, L Spooner, A Syed

Care of the Elderly F Ihama, D Mangion, D J Meacock

Dental Surgery D E H Glendinning

Dermatology C Quartey-Papafio

ENT M Chaurasia, J Chelladurai, A Izzat

Gastroenterology M Perry

General Medicine D A R Boldy, M J Fairman, S K Jain, C R Nyman, S A Olczak

General Surgery P K Agarwal, N J Andrews, K Jeyapaul, R Jones, M Khan, J Mohan, P Murphy, D Puthu, A Rashed

Haematology S Sobolewski, V M Tringham

Nephrology J Little

Neurology G Sawle

Obstetrics and Gynaecology D A Adeyemi, S Ikhena, S Magd, J Olamijulo, A Shaheen

Ophthalmology S Ahmed, M Gupta, Mr Nanno, A Rahman

Orthodontics F J Calvert

Orthopaedics D Achary, C Ahrens, - Bismil, R Deshmukh, R J Latto, T H Minhas, W Qadir, A Shaikh, J Watson, J A S Watson

Paediatrics Z Ahmed, M J Crawford, S Germer, S K Hanumara, E Ikhena, M Pervez, B Setty

Plastic Surgery E O'Broin

Radiology M Aslam, I Britton, M Butt, R Haddow, R Jones, P T King, A Kukula, J Maskova

Respiratory Medicine D Clifton, A J Morley-Davis

Rheumatology and Rehabilitation J E Carty, B P Hunt

Thoracic Surgery J Duffy

Urology N A Dahar, P Daruwala, D T L Turner

University College London Hospitals NHS Foundation Trust

Established as a Foundation Trust 01/07/2004.

Trust Headquarters, John Astor House, 16 Foley Street, London W1W 6DN
Tel: 020 7387 9300 Fax: 020 7380 9963
Website: www.uclh.org
(North Central London Strategic Health Authority)

Chair Peter Dixon
Chief Executive Robert Naylor

The Eastman Dental Hospital

256 Gray's Inn Road, London WC1X 8LD
Tel: 020 7915 1000 Fax: 020 7915 1012
Total Beds: 12

Dental Conservation D Setchell (Head), K Gulabivala, K Hemmings, A McCullock, A McDonald, J Wickens

Oral and Maxillofacial Surgery B Aghabeigi, R Davies, N Evans, C Feinmann, B Henderson, C Hopper, S Meghji, S Nair, L Newman, J Stewart

Oral Medicine S Porter, C Scully

Oral Pathology B Barrett, P Speight

Orthodontics S Cochrane, E Horrocks, N Hunt, S Jones, H Moseley, J Noar

Paediatric Dentistry J Goodman, C Mason, G Roberts

Periodontology U Darbar, E Giedrys-Leper, G Griffiths, M Tonetti

Prosthetic Dentisty D Cheshire, B Griffiths, J Hobkirk, J Howlett, R Welfare

The Elizabeth Garrett Anderson Hospital and Obstetric Hospital

Huntley Street, London WCIE 6DH
Tel: 020 7387 9300 Fax: 020 7383 3415
Total Beds: 20

Anaesthetics T Newton-John

Obstetrics G Bahadur, J Iskaros, E R M Jauniaux, M Katz, T Mould, J L Osborne, P Pandya, E Saridogan, A C Silverstone

The Heart Hospital

Westmoreland Street, London W1G 8PH
Tel: 020 7573 8888

Cardiology S Cullen, D Holdright, J McEwan, R H Swanton, J M Walker

The Hospital for Tropical Diseases

Mortimer Market, Capper Street, London WC1E 6JD
Tel: 020 7387 9300 Fax: 020 7388 7645
Total Beds: 22

Leprosy D N J Lockwood

Ophthalmology T J ffytche

Parasitology P L Chiodini

Travel Medicine R H Behrens

Tropical Medicine P L Chiodini, A Costello, T Doherty, P Godfrey-Faussett, A Grant, D C W Mabey, A M Tomkins, S G Wright

The Middlesex Hospital

Mortimer Street, London W1T 3AA
Tel: 020 7636 8333
Total Beds: 454

Anaesthetics B Astley, W Aveling, A Baranowski, J Barcroft, M J Barnard, R Bell, L M Bromley, C Bullen, D W L Davies, R J Frossard, C Goldsack, J C Goldstone, A C Greville, E M Grundy, C Hamilton Davies, J A Hulf, J Lockie, A C McAra, V S Mitchell, M G Mythen, D S Woods, S J Wright

Cancer Services G Blackman, A M Cassoni, C A E Coulter, M N Gaze, S Harland, J Ledermann, S M Lee, H Payne, M F Spittle, R Stein, J S Tobias, J Whelan

Cardiothoracic Surgery P Kallis, S Kolvekar, C Pattison, V Tsang, R Walesby

Care of the Elderly J R Croker, S Luttrell

Chemical Pathology M D Buckley-Sharp, D A Gardner, J Honour, G Rumsby, C Samuell

Dermatology P Dowd, R Groves, F Vega-Lopez, R Yu

Gastroenterology S L Bloom, S G Bown, A R W Hatfield, R Jalan, L Lovat, S McCartney, N V Naounov, S Pereira, R Williams

General Medicine D J Betteridge, H Booth, J Brookes, S L Cohen, J R Croker, S Edwards, L G Fine, J George, S Hurel, P Lee, R MacAllister, J Malone-Lee, J Martin, R Miller, A W Segal, M Singer, S G Spiro, G W Stewart, P Vallance, A Webb, I Williams, A Zumla

General Surgery M Adiseshiah, S Barker, C C R Bishop, P B Boulos, P Coleridge-Smith, M Keshtgar, T Kurzawinski, R C G Russell, R Sainsbury, J H Scurr, I Taylor, C Vaizey

Imaging J Brooks, A R Gillams, M A Hall-Craggs, C Hare, M J Kellett, W R Lees, R R Mason, C M Parks, M J Raphael, D Rickards, A Scheneidau, K M Walmsley

Neurology G Gillett, A J Lees

Nuclear Medicine J Bomanji, D Campos-Costa, P J Ell, E Prvulovich

Ophthalmology J Brazier, P A Frith, M Harris, J Lawson

Oral and Maxillofacial Surgery N Kalavrezos

Orthopaedics J P Cobb, B Cohen, M A Edgar, F Haddad, D Jones, L Williams, J Witt

Paediatrics A M Kilby, M Preece, H Spoudeas, R Stanhope, R Viner, V Wright

Pathology N Brink, R S Tedder, K Ward

Rheumatology and Rehabilitation C Chamberlain, A Ebringer, J C W Edwards, M Ehrenstein, H Fitz-Clarence, R Grahame, D A Isenburg, R Keen, J McDonagh, V Morris, K Murray, A Rahman, M E Shipley, P Woo

Thoracic Medicine H L Booth, P J M George, H K Makker, D Mitchell, S G Spiro

Urology P Cuckow, M Emberton, M Mansell, A Mundy, S Nathan, R Nauth-Misir, G Nield, E O'Donoghue, D Ralph, P Shah, R Unwin, H Whitfield, C R J Woodhouse, R Woolfson

The National Hospital for Neurology and Neurosurgery

Queen Square, London WC1N 3BG
Tel: 020 7837 3611 Fax: 020 7829 8720
Total Beds: 244

Anaesthetics A Baranowski, B Brandner, I Calder, M Chapman, N P Hirsch, P R Nandi, M C Newton, M Smith, S R Wilson

Chemical Pathology J M Land, E J Thompson

General Psychiatry R J Dolan, M M Robertson, M A Ron, M R Trimble

Imaging T C S Cox, R Jäger, K A Miszkiel, J M Stevens, W J Taylor

Neurology K Bhatia, D J Brooks, M M Brown, P Brown, L Cipolotti, C R A Clarke, J S Duncan, S Farmer, R S Frackowiak, G Giovannoni, P J Goadsby, R J Greenwood, M Hanna, R S Howard, P Jarman, R Kapoor, H Kaube, D M Kullmann, A J Lees, N Losseff, H Manji, C J Mathias, D H Miller, E D Playford, N P Quinn, J Rees, M M Reilly, M N Rossor, P Rudge, L Sander, J W Scadding, A H V Shapira, S P Shorvon, S Sisodya, N W Wood

Neuropathology A Briddon, S Heales, J L Holton, G Keir, J Land, D N Landon, P Patsalos, T Revesz, F Scaravilli, M Thorn

Neurophysiology D R Fish, S J Jones, P Misra, N M F Murray, S J M Smith, B D Youl

Neurosurgery A T H Casey, H A Crockard, W F J Harkness, R D Hayward, N D Kitchen, M P Powell, D Thomas, L Watkins

Ophthalmology J F Acheson, E M Graham, G T Plant

Otology A Bronstein, G B Brookes, A D Cheesman, R A Davies, L M Luxon

Paediatrics P Lee

Rehabilitation Medicine A J Thompson

Urology C J Fowler, F Thompson

Royal London Homoeopathic Hospital

Greenwell Street, London W1W 5BP
Tel: 020 7391 8833
Total Beds: 6

University College Hospital

Grafton Way, London WC1E 3DB
Tel: 020 7387 9300 Fax: 020 7380 9104
Website: www.uclh.org.
Total Beds: 898

Accident and Emergency M Gavalas, A M McGuinness, J M Ryan, C L Walford

Anaesthetics B Astley, W Aveling, J P Barcroft, M J Barnard, R Bell, G Bellingham, L M Bromley, C Bullen, D W L Davies, R J Frossard, C Goldsack, J C Goldstone, A C Greville, E M Grundy, C Hamilton-Davies, J A Hulf, J Lockie, A C McAra, V S Mitchell, M G Mythen, C M H Ramage, S D Woods

Cancer Services G Blackman, A M Cassoni, C A E Coulter, M N Gaze, S Harland, S M Lee, H Payne, M F Spittle, R Stein, J S Tobias, J Whelan

Care of the Elderly J R Croker

General Medicine D J Betteridge, H Booth, J Brookes, J Cartledge, S L Cohen, J R Croker, M de Swiet, L G Fine, J George, S Hurel, R MacAllister, J Malone-Lee, J F Martin, A W Segal, M Singer, S G Spiro, G W Stewart, P Vallance

General Surgery M Adiseshiah, S Barker, C C R Bishop, P Coleridge-Smith, J H Scurr

Haematology H Cohen, A H Goldstone, A Khwaja, D C Linch, R Luesber, S J Machin, S Mackinnon, A Nathwani, K G Patterson, J B Porter, K Yong

Imaging J Brooks, A R Gillams, C Hare, M J Kellett, W R Lees, C M Parks, A Scheneidau, P J Shaw

Neurology A J Lees

Obstetrics E Christopher, S M Creighton, A S Cutner, M C Davies, J Guillebaud, H Mitchell, P O'Brien, D Peebles, C H Rodeck, F Shenfield

Paediatric Surgery V M Wright

Paediatrics C Brain, E M K Chung, R M Gardiner, S Harding, J M Hawdon, P C Hindmarsh, A M Kilby, M Michelagnoli, A M O'Rawe, M Sellwood, H Spoudeas, R Stanhope, R M Viner, V Wright, J S Wyatt

Pathology E Benjamin, P Chiodini, J Delhanty, A Dogan, M Falzon, A Flanagan, V Gant, M H Griffiths, P G Isaacson, G Kocjan, S R Lakhani, M Novelli, M C Parkinson, G L Ridgway, G Scott, R Scott, N Shetty, P Wilson

Plastic Surgery M D Brough, P Mallucci, D A McGrouther

University Hospital Birmingham NHS Foundation Trust

Established as a Foundation Trust 01/07/2004.

Trust Headquarters, PO Box 9551, Main Drive, Queen Elizabeth Medical Centre, Edgbaston, Birmingham B15 2PR
Tel: 0121 432 3232 Fax: 0121 627 2834
Website: www.uhb.nhs.uk
(Birmingham and the Black Country Strategic Health Authority)

Chair John Charlton
Chief Executive Siobvon Heasivile
Consultants T Elliott, M Gill, D Mortiboy

Queen Elizabeth Hospital

Queen Elizabeth Medical Centre, Birmingham B15 2TH
Tel: 0121 472 1311
Total Beds: 550

Anaesthetics J F Bion, L Blaney, C Bonnici, M I Bowden, M D Brewin, M Clapham, T H Clutton-Brock, G M Cooper, G Dickson, I F Duncan, M H Faroqui, J Freeman, T Gallagher, D Green, G R Harrison, K Hasan, A C Hill, T Hoth, N Huggins, P Hutton, J Isaac, A P F Jackson, G Jeskins, M J King, M Knowles, M Lewis, J P Lilley, A D Malins, N Murphy, A Patel, S Riddington, R Riddle, D M Rosser, S H Russel, M Suchak, A J Sutcliffe, L Tasker, J Tong, P Townsend, D Turfrey, S Walia, J M Watt, A Whitehouse, M Wilkes, A D Wilkey, M Wilson, P R Wood

Bacteriology T J Elliott, M Gill, D Mortiboy

Cardiology R A Bonser, N Buller, P Clift, M D Gammage, T Graham, M Griffith, W Littler, P Ludman, H Marshall, D Sagar, R Steeds, S Thorne, J N Townend, I C Wilson

Cardiothoracic Surgery R S Bonser, J G Mascaro, D Pagano, S Rooney

Care of the Elderly E Dunstan, A Main, P P Mayer, J Treml, P Turnbull

Dental Surgery A M Brown, M S Dover, A Monaghan, S Parmar, I Sharp

General Medicine D Adams, R N Allan, E Elias, A J Franklyn, J Goh, S Gompertz, M Kendall, U Martin, D Mutimer, J Neuberger, S Pathmakanthan, M C Sheppard, P Stewart, R A Stockley, R Thompson

General Surgery J A C Buckels, L J Buist, M Clarke, D England, J W Fielding, A Francis, D Goureuitch, M Hallisey, T Ismail, C Keh, M Keighley, A D Mayer, D Mirza, D G Morton, A Ready, K Subramonian, L C Tan

Genitourinary Medicine M Huengsberg, J Ross, M Shahmanesh

Haematology M Cooke, C Craddock, T N Latief, J Wilde

Immunology I C M McLennon

Nephrology D Adu, S T Ball, P Cockwell, C Ferro, L Foggensteiner, G W Lipkin, C Savage

Neurology C Barraclough, R N Corston, N Davies, D A Francis, T Heaffield, P J McDonnell, R Mitchell, A P Mocroft, K Morrison, S Nightingale, H Pall, J A Spillane, E Sturman, A Williams, J Winer

Neurophysiology J E Fox, A P Mocroft, D E Rao, M L Villagrasa

Neurosurgery G Cruikshank, G Flint, S Harland, A Kay, C H Meyer, R Mitchell, A R Walsh, J Wasserberg, S C Zygmunt

Otolaryngology A B Drake-Lee, R M Irving, C Jennings, A Johnson, D W Proops, J Watkinson

Pathology P Barber, R Cramb, N Deshmukh, R Harrison, A J Howie, S G Hubscher, E L Jones, S Sanders, A Warfield, J Young

Radiology G M Allen, P Guest, J Hopkins, I McCafferty, B Mahon, K Mangat, B Ogunremi, J Ollif, S Ollif, A J Page, P I Riley, E B Rolfe, C L Sanchez, D J Tattersall, D A Yates

Radiotherapy and Oncology A Chetiya-Wadarna, M Cullen, I Fernando, I Geh, J Glaholm, N James, T N Latief, D R Pearce, D C Poole, D Spooner, A Stevens

Rheumatology S Bowman, C Gordon

Urology Y Z Almallah, A J Arnold, A Doherty, M A Hughes, D M A Wallace

Selly Oak Hospital

Raddlebarn Road, Birmingham B29 6JD
Tel: 0121 627 1627 Fax: 0121 627 8214
Total Beds: 450

Anaesthetics M Arif, C V Bonnici, M I Bowden, S Burnley, P J M Clifton, G Dickson, K England, M Ghoris, A P Jackson, M J King, F A Levins, A Malins, M Manji, J P Millns, J Ralph, J E M Smith, A D Wilkey, P R Wood

Cardiology M H Davies

Care of the Elderly E J Dunstan, A N H Main, P P Mayer

Dental Surgery K Webster

Dermatology H Lewis, J Marsden, D F Shah, D J Stewart

General Medicine S K Banerjee, R Boulton, P Doyle, F Dunne, D Gorman, K Kane, A Kayani, M Miller, H Morrison, M Natrass, S Pathmakanthan, J Webber

General Surgery A Edwards, T Ismail, M H Simms, S Smith, R K Vohra, K Webster

Haematology J A Murray

Occupational Health A Robertson

Ophthalmology M Burdon, A Jacks, G R Kirkby, T D Matthews, P J McDonell, H Palmer, R Scott, M Tsaloumus

Orthopaedics K Baloch, J P Cooper, M Craigen, M Green, K M Porter, I Sargeant, A Thomas, M Waldram

Otolaryngology I Donaldson, J R M Moore, P Pracey, A P Reid

Plastic Surgery C C Kat, L H Lap, N Moiemen, D Murray, J D Nancarrow, R Papini, F Peart, S Thomas, G Titley, V Vijh, R Waters, Y Wilson

Radiology S Bradley, J Clarke, A Davies, M J Duddy, N Evans, V R Kale, D Tattersall, C P Walker

Rheumatology S Bradley, P Jobanputra, R W Jubb, E Rankin

University Hospital of North Staffordshire NHS Trust

Trust Headquarters, North Staffordshire Royal Infirmary, Princes Road, Stoke-on-Trent ST4 7LN
Tel: 01782 715444 Fax: 01782 552001
Website: www.nsht.nhs.uk
(Shropshire and Staffordshire Strategic Health Authority)

Chair Calum Paton
Chief Executive David Crowley

North Staffordshire Hospital

Trust Headquarters, North Staffordshire Royal Infirmary, Princes Road, Stoke-on-Trent ST4 7LN
Tel: 01782 715444 Fax: 01782 555202
Total Beds: 1386

Anaesthetics Dr Akhtar, S A Araffin, J Ashworth, Dr Baker, B Carr, N W B Clowes, N A Coleman, S Edmends, S J Foster, D Frechini, J C Hindmarsh, C Howell, P Jeyaratam, C L Knight, F Y Lamm, M E Lauckner, Dr Lennon, C G Male, N C Matthews, Dr Mills, P Morrison, P Oakley, Dr Payne, C P Rice, S J Seddon, B Smith, I Smith, A I Stewart, A A Tomlinson, J Wilkins, V Williams

Cardiology M Clarke, J Creamer, J A S Davis, J Nolan, P O'Gorman

Cardiothoracic Surgery A J Levine, J Nolan, J M Parmar, P Ridley

Clinical Pharmacology and Therapeutics J C Mucklow

Community Medicine J Davidson, P Lithgow, K Reynolds, S Williams

Dermatology J P H Byrne, A G Smith, B B Tan

ENT M V Carlin, Mr Courteney-Harris, J T Little, P Wilson

Emergency Medicine C Gray, I Phair

Endocrinology R Clayton, J H B Scarpello, A Walker

General Surgery Dr Adjogatse, M Deakin, T J Duffy, J B Elder, J F Forrest, C Hall, G Hopkinson, R Kirby, R Morgan, A Walsh

Genitourinary Medicine G Singh, S Sivapalan

Nephrology S Davies, P N Harden, P Naish, G I Russell

Neurology H G Boddie, S J Ellis, C Hawkins

Neurophysiology P Heath

Neurosurgery H Brydon, P Dias, J Singh

Obstetrics and Gynaecology J Cooper, J D Gough, G Masson, B K V Menon, M Obhrai, P O'Brien, C Redman

Oncology F A Adab, A M Brunt, A Cook, J E Scobie

Ophthalmology R D Brown, J D A Common, T Gillow, P A Shaw

Oral Surgery Mr Grime, T Mallins, Mr Perry

Orthodontics J D Muir

Orthopaedics E N Ahmed, M Brown, I Dos Remedios, J Dove, J Dwyer, D Griffiths, D McBride, N Neale, J Templeton, P Thomas, C H Wynn Jones

Paediatrics D Brookfield, C Campbell, W Lenney, B Ley, A Magnay, A A Melville, K Palmer, P M Rafeeq, M Samuels, P Smith, D Southall, S A Spencer

Pathology R C Chasty, P M Chipping, G Douce, M C Garrido, J Gray, R M Ibbotson, C Musgrove, R H Neary, M Rogerson, V Smith, M Stephens, N D Williams

Plastic Surgery P Davison, Mr Prinsloo, J O Roberts

Radiology S Bajwa, D Bakalinova, M Braithwaite, N Haq, J Oxtoby, P Richards, J Saklatvala, M D Skinner, S Tebby, N A Watson, D West, D Wilcock

Rehabilitation Medicine A B Ward

Respiratory Medicine M Allen, C F A Pantin, K Prowse, M A Spiteri

Rheumatology P T Dawes, A B Hassell, E Hay, T E Hothersall, M F Shadforth

Urology M French, S Liu, M Saxby

University Hospitals Coventry and Warwickshire NHS Trust

Waslgrave Hospital, Clifford Briage Road, Waslgrave, Coventry CV2 2DX
Tel: 024 7660 2020 Fax: 024 7662 2197
Email: info@uhcw.nhs.uk
Website: www.uhcw.nhs.uk
(West Midlands South Strategic Health Authority)

Chair Bryan Stoten
Chief Executive David Roberts

Coventry and Warwickshire Hospital

Stoney Stanton Road, Coventry CV1 4FH
Tel: 024 7622 4055 Fax: 024 7622 1655
Total Beds: 250

Accident and Emergency A Alchalabi, S Vlachtsis

Biochemistry H Griffiths

Chest Disease C V P Lawford

Genitourinary Medicine A A H Wade

Haematology R I Harris, M J Strevens

Medical Microbiology R M Hutton

Neurosurgery A Saxena, P Stanworth, W Whatmore

Ophthalmology N E Brown, L Butler, I G Calder, A J Chadwick, T J Fetherston, M Handscombe, R D Kumar, T Vythilingham

Oral and Maxillofacial Surgery J M Fagan, I Moule

Orthodontics C P Briggs, N A E Robertson

Orthopaedics M J Aldridge, M E Blakemore, J Clegg, W F Merriam, P Roberts, S Turner, P Wade, P E H Wilson

Plastic Surgery A R Groves, R N Matthews

Coventry Maternity Hospital

Walsgrave, Coventry CV2 2DX
Tel: 024 7660 2020
Total Beds: 231

Obstetrics and Gynaecology L J S Cassia, K A Cietak, C R Kennedy, M F Reed

Paediatrics S M Brown, J G Davies, E E Jones, S McNamara

Hospital of St Cross

Barby Road, Rugby CV22 5PX
Tel: 01788 572831 Fax: 01788 545141
Total Beds: 180

Anaesthetics S Nethisinghe

Cardiology M Been

Cardiothoracic Surgery R Norton

Dental Surgery I Moule

ENT A Curry, P L Kander

General Medicine A K Basu

General Psychiatry S Thavasothy

General Surgery A A J D'Sa

Haematology A Abdul-Cader

Neurology J R Ponsford

Obstetrics and Gynaecology A D Parsons

Orthodontics N A Robertson

Plastic Surgery A Groves, R N Matthews

Radiology D M Alexander, J Chandy, N Hadid

Radiotherapy and Oncology R J Grieve

Rheumatology G R Struthers

Walsgrave Hospital

Clifford Bridge Road, Walsgrave, Coventry CV2 2DX
Tel: 024 7660 2020 Fax: 024 7662 2197
Total Beds: 1015

Anaesthetics N Bhasin, M D Boobyer, E Borman, F Choksey, K C Clayton, R Elton, G Evans, K Evans, A Frost, R A Johnson, W McCulloch, M Mead, C Mendonca, P Mulrooney, A Phillips, S Radhakrisna, A Scase, J Sherwin, A Singh, E A Taylor, A Thacker, M Wyse

Breast Surgery B Ackroyd, A Al-Dabbagh, S Habib, T A Waterworth

Cardiology M Been, R K Mattu, M F Shiu, H Singh

Cardiothoracic Surgery N Briffa, W R Dimitri, R Norton, R Patel, M D Rosin

Chest Disease R Bell

Colorectal Surgery N Williams

Dermatology J Berth-Jones, B Dharmagunawarden, A Ilchyshyn

ENT A P Bath, P Kander, P Patel

Gastroenterology M Aldersley, D Loft, C Nwokolo

General Medicine N R Balcombe, R Bell, P I Biggs, L J Booth, A Chaudhry, D P Dhillon, E Hillhouse, I D Khan, M Khan, P Lawford, J R Lismore, A J Sinclair, F P Vince

General Surgery A R E Blacklock, K Desai, I Fraser, D Higman, C Imray, S H Kashi, F T Lam, A Rhodes, P N Roberts, M Wills

Haematology R I Harris, N Jackson, M J Strevens

Histopathology K Chen, S Ferryman, T Guha, J Macartney, P Matthews, M Newbold, T Rollason, J Snead

Intensive Care S Evans, S Jayaratnasingam, B Murphy, I Tsagurnis, D Watson

Medical Microbiology M Weinbren

Nephrology D C Dukes, M Edmunds, R Higgins, S Kashi

Neurology A Grubneac, J R Ponsford, A Shehu

Neurophysiology R Paul

Neurosurgery M Choksey, M Christie, P Stanworth

Obstetrics and Gynaecology A Anyanwu, K A Cietak, L Farrall, K Goswami, S Keay, C Kennedy, S Thornton, P Vanderkerckhove, L J Wood

Oncology I Bown, R Das, R Grieve, M Hocking, C Irwin, D Jones, S Sothi, A Stockdale

Orthopaedics I Dunn

Paediatrics M Al-Moudaris, K Blake, N G Coad, A Coe, E Simmonds, H Stirling

Palliative Medicine M Barnett, A Franks, R Walker

Pathology K Chen, T Guha

Radiology T T Aye, D J Beale, S K Bera, J Chandy, A Duncan, D Durrani, T Goodfellow, C Oliver, M P Patel, P D Phelps, R Rattenhali, W Shatwell, K Sherlala, A Vohrah, R Wellings

Radiotherapy and Oncology R N Das, R J Grieve, D A Jones, A Stockdale

Renal Medicine M Edmunds, S Fletcher, R Higgins, A Stein

Rheumatology and Rehabilitation M Allen, J S Coppock, P Perkins, G R Struthers

Urology A R E Blacklock, K M Desai, M Wills

University Hospitals of Leicester NHS Trust

Headquarters, Gwendolen House, Gwendolen Road, Leicester LE5 4QF
Tel: 0116 249 0490 Fax: 0116 258 4666
Email: public.relations@uhl-tr.nhs.uk
Website: www.uhl-tr.nhs.uk
(Leicestershire, Northamptonshire and Rutland Strategic Health Authority)

Chair Philip Hammersley
Chief Executive Peter Reading

Glenfield Hospital

Groby Road, Leicester LE3 9QP
Tel: 0116 287 1471 Fax: 0116 258 3950
Total Beds: 520

Anaesthetics A G H Cole, M J Jones, D G Lewis, E S Lin, I McLellan, K A Mobley, N A Moore, H Rousseau, T N Trotter, K J West, R Wyatt

Cardiology A H Gershlick, P J Hubner, N J Samani, D J Skehan

Cardiothoracic Surgery R K Firmin, M S J Hickey, J N Leverment, A Sosnowski, T J Spyt

Care of the Elderly R F Bing, J S de Caestecker, M D Fotherby, J F Potter

General Surgery A W Hall, A D N Scott, A Stotter, R Windle

Integrated Medicine R F Bing, J de Caestecker, G J Fancourt, M D Fotherby, J F Potter, J W Ward

Orthodontics R F Deans, T G Leggatt, F A Mackay, R Samuels

Orthopaedics J J Dias, W M Harper, O Oni, R A Power, G Taylor

Paediatric Cardiology R Leanage

Paediatrics R Leanage, S Nichani

Radiology A Crozier, H Daintith, K Jeyapalan, R Keal

Respiratory Medicine M D Morgan, J M Wales

Restorative Dentistry R F Deans, T G Leggat, F A Mackay, R H A Samuels

Leicester General Hospital

Gwendolen Road, Leicester LE5 4PW
Tel: 0116 249 0490 Fax: 0116 258 4666
Total Beds: 680

Anaesthetics S Coley, J M Hampson, C D Hanning, D E Hoffler, I Jeyapalan, D G Lewis, P Rabey, D G Raitt, P Spiers, C M Stray, O Williams

Care of the Elderly D M R Jackett, N Lo, R J Shepherd, T R Vallance

General Medicine P Critchley, R Gregory, J F Mayberry, R Oldham, A C B Wicks

General Surgery W W Barrie, M Dennis, A Dennison, M J Kelly, M Nicholson, P S Veitch

Nephrology S Carr, J Feehally, K Harris, G Warwick

Obstetrics and Gynaecology P Kirwan, C Mayne

Orthopaedics M Allen, R N Chan, Q Cox, T Green, M L Harding, J Hoskinson, J M Jones, C Kershaw, P Sell

Paediatrics A Elias-Jones, E W Hoskyns

Pathology P Furness, R Iqbal, E H Mackay, K O'Reilly

Radiology D Bruce, P Emberton, K A Mulcahy, C Newland, Y Rees

Rehabilitation Medicine P Critchley

Rheumatology R Oldham

Urology D E Osborn, D Sandhu, T R Terry

The Leicester Royal Infirmary

Infirmary Square, Leicester LE1 5WW
Tel: 0116 254 1414 Fax: 0116 258 5631
Total Beds: 1107

Accident and Emergency G G Bodiwala

Anaesthetics R Atcheson, B J Collett, B R Cotton, A E De Melo, R J Eastley, D Fell, M R Ferguson, R H James, G W Jones, R L J Kohn, I McLaren, A E May, M Mushambi, T M O'Carroll, M L Pepperman, D J Rowbotham, W Russell, T A Samuels, G Smith, J Thompson, K Tighe, D A B Turner, J G Wandless

Care of the Elderly M Ardron, D R Ives, A Miodrag

Chemical Pathology S J Iqbal, J Lunec, W M Madira, F Smith

Clinical Pharmacology and Therapeutics D B Barnett, L L Ng

Dermatology R D R Camp, R A C Graham-Brown, P E Hutchinson

ENT J Cook, T A Jones, A A Moir, G Murty, R S A Thomas

Gastroenterology J Nightingale, B J Rathbone

General Medicine M Davies, T A Howlett, P McNally, H Thurston, B Williams

General Surgery P R F Bell, N W Everson, D Hemmingway, D Lloyd, N London, R Naylor, S Nour

Genetics M Barrow, R C Trembath

Genitourinary Medicine P G Fisk, V C Riley, P C Schober

Haematology C S Chapman, V E Mitchell

Histopathology D C Bouch, L J Brown, A Fletcher, C Kendall, P A McKeever, S Muller, P A V Shaw, R A Walker, K P West

Immunology M Browning

Infectious Diseases K G Nicolson, K Wiselka

Medical Microbiology R A Swann

Neurology R J Abbott, M Lawden, I F Pye

Obstetrics and Gynaecology A Azzawi, R C S Chazal, A Davidson, A Halligan, D Ireland, N J Naftalin, R W Neuberg, C Oppenhiemer

Ophthalmology D J Austin, K Bibby, D B Goustine, W Karwatowski, P P Ray-Chaudhuri, G H A Woodruff

Oral Surgery J Hayter

Orthopaedics C Kershaw

Paediatrics S Bohin, E Carter, D P Field, M Green, P Houtman, D K Luyt, S Nichani, C O'Callaghan, R S Shannon, M Silverman, P G F Swift

Plastic Surgery H P Henderson, T Milward, S K Varma, D Ward

Radiology A A Bolia, G R Cherryman, D B L Finlay, K C Krarup, A Liddicoat, N Messios, A Rickett, L Robinson, P M Rodgers

Radiotherapy J K O'Byrne, W Steward, S Vasanthan

Rheumatology and Rehabilitation F E Nichol, A Samanta, P Sheldon

Uttlesford Primary Care Trust

The Old Mill, Hasler's Lane, Dunmow CM6 1XS
Tel: 01371 767007 Fax: 01371 767008
Website: www.uttlesford-pct.nhs.uk
(Essex Strategic Health Authority)

Chair David Barron
Chief Executive Melanie Walker

Saffron Walden Community Hospital

Radwinter Road, Saffron Walden CB11 3YH
Tel: 01799 562900 Fax: 01799 562901
Total Beds: 27

Vale of Aylesbury Primary Care Trust

Verney House, Gatehouse Road, Aylesbury HP19 8ET
Tel: 01296 310000 Fax: 01296 318666
Email: firstname.lastname@voa-pct.nhs.uk
(Thames Valley Strategic Health Authority)

Chair Avril Davis
Chief Executive Shaun Brogan

Thame Community Hospital

East Street, Thame OX9 3JT
Tel: 01844 212727 Fax: 01844 260721
Total Beds: 18

Wakefield West Primary Care Trust

White Rose House, West Parade, Wakefield WF1 1LT
Tel: 01924 213050 Fax: 01924 213157
Email: enquiries@wwpct.nhs.uk
(West Yorkshire Strategic Health Authority)

Chair William Barker
Chief Executive Alastair Geldart

Walsall Hospitals NHS Trust

Manor Hospital, Moat Road, Walsall WS2 9PS
Tel: 01922 721172 Fax: 01922 656621
Email: contactus@walsallhospitals.nhs.uk
Website: www.walsall.wmids.nhs.uk
(Birmingham and the Black Country Strategic Health Authority)

Chair Ben Reid
Chief Executive Susan James

Goscote Hospital

Goscote Lane, Walsall WS3 1SJ
Tel: 01922 710710 Fax: 01922 712195
Total Beds: 103

Care of the Elderly R W S Brookes, S Panayiotou, S K Sinha, M N Zaman

Manor Hospital

Walsall WS2 9PS
Tel: 01922 721172 Fax: 01922 656621
Total Beds: 607

Accident and Emergency D Bowden, N Rashid

Anaesthetics N Akinwale, F D Babatola, B Freitag, I P Hudecek, C Newson, S A Nortcliffe, H Sinha, H Yanny, M S Youssef

Care of the Elderly R W S Brooks, S A M Saeed, V S Senthil, P Waraich

Dental Surgery Dr Larkin

Dermatology K S Ryatt

ENT D M East, S Minhas, N Turner

General Medicine I Ahmad, A Al-allaf, V P Balagopal, T J Constable, M Cox, A R Cunnington, S Dean, T C Harvey, M Matonhodge, A Palejwala, M Payne, D Raskausklene, A Wright

General Surgery K M C Abrew, B Ferrie, M Heitmann, A Khan, S R Konery, G Little, K D F Mayer, T Muscroft, S Odogwu, J Stewart

Genitourinary Medicine Dr Joseph

Haematology G Galvin

Neurology D A Francis

Obstetrics and Gynaecology C Balachandar, M J Browne, A C Head, E J McMillan, S Panda, J Pepper, R Reddy

Ophthalmology P G J Corridan, Dr Sandromouli, S Shin, Dr Yang

Orthodontics J W Ferguson

Orthopaedics G Alo, M A A Khan, T Sadique, Dr Shoaib

Paediatrics I Bagchi, U M Chidrawar, D Drew, A R Gatrad, B J Muhammad, B Sahsh, G P Sinha

Pathology C Allen, G P Galvin, P D Giles, A Hartland, Z A Hassam, Y L Hock

Radiology C L Holland, H Rai, D Ramaema, M G Thuse

Radiotherapy and Oncology A D Chetiyawardana, I Fernando

Walsall Teaching Primary Care Trust

Jubilee House, Bloxwich Lane, Walsall WS2 7JL
Tel: 01922 618388 Fax: 01922 618360
Email: info@walsall.nhs.uk
Website: www.walsall.wmids.nhs.uk/pct/
(Birmingham and the Black Country Strategic Health Authority)

Chair Jindy Khera
Chief Executive Alistair Howie

Bloxwich Hospital

Reeves Street, Bloxwich, Walsall WS3 3JJ
Tel: 01922 858600 Fax: 01922 858639
Total Beds: 40

Manager Fiona McGill

Dorothy Pattison Hospital

Alumwell Close, Walsall WS2 9XH
Tel: 01922 858000 Fax: 01922 858085
Total Beds: 86

Manager Steve Foster

Kings Hill Day Hospital

School Street, Wednesbury WS10 9JB
Tel: 0121 526 4405

Manager Maxine Woodward

Mossley Day Hospital

Sneyd Lane, Bloxwich, Walsall WS3 2LW
Tel: 01922 858680

Waltham Forest Primary Care Trust

Hurst Road Health Centre, Hurst Road, Walthamstow, London E17 3BL

Tel: 020 8928 2300 Fax: 020 8928 2307
Website: www.walthamforest-pct.nhs.uk
(North East London Strategic Health Authority)

Chair Joan Saddler
Chief Executive Sally Gorham

Walton Centre for Neurology and Neurosurgery NHS Trust

Lower Lane, Fazakerley, Liverpool L9 7LJ
Tel: 0151 525 3611 Fax: 0151 529 5500
Email: enquiries@wcnn-tr.nwest.nhs.uk
Website: www.thewaltoncentre.co.uk
(Cheshire and Merseyside Strategic Health Authority)

Chair Joyce Brittain
Chief Executive Bev Humphries
Consultants R Appleton, G Baker, M Bamber, Boggild, A N Bowden, J Broome, N Buxton, D W Chadwick, L Collville, J Dalton, K Das, M Doran, P Eldridge, T P Enevoldson, G F G Findlay, N A Fletcher, A Forster, P M Foy, E Ghadiali, I Graham, A Guha, I Hart, N Hinds, Peter Humfries, Peter Humphrey, A Larner, B R F Lecky, C Mallucci, A Marson, P May, D McCoy, A P Moore, P Murphy, H Nahser, T Nash, S Niven, T Nixon, T Nurmikko, T Pigott, R Pillay, C Pinder, N Rainov, S Shaw, D Smith, E T Smith, M Steiger, B Tedman, I Tweedie, T R K Varma, P Waring, P Warnke, B Weldon, R White, C Whitehead, U Wieshman, J R Wiles, E Wright, C A Young

Wandsworth Primary Care Trust

2nd Floor, Teak Tower, Main Building, Springfield University Hospital, 61 Glenburnie Road, London SW17 7DJ
Tel: 020 8682 6170 Fax: 020 8682 5846
Email: comms@swlondon.nhs.uk
Website: www.wandsworth-pct.nhs.uk
(South West London Strategic Health Authority)

Chair Melba Wilson
Chief Executive Helen Walley

Queen Mary's Hospital

Roehampton Lane, Roehampton, London SW15 5PN
Tel: 020 8789 6611 Fax: 020 8780 1089
Total Beds: 70

Warrington Primary Care Trust

930-932 Birchwood Boulevard, Millennium Park, Birchwood, Warrington WA3 7QN
Tel: 01925 843600 Fax: 01925 843601
Email: hq@warrington-pct.nhs.uk
Website: www.warrington-health.nhs.uk
(Cheshire and Merseyside Strategic Health Authority)

Chair Robin Brown
Chief Executive Allison Cooke

Watford and Three Rivers Primary Care Trust

1A High Street, Rickmansworth WD3 1ET
Tel: 01923 713050 Fax: 01923 718921
Email: enquiries@watford3r-pct.nhs.uk
Website: www.watford3r-pct.nhs.uk
(Bedfordshire and Hertfordshire Strategic Health Authority)

Chair Pam Handley
Chief Executive Felicity Cox

Waveney Primary Care Trust

6 Regent Road, Lowestoft NR32 1PA
Tel: 01502 533733 Fax: 01502 512772
Website: www.waveney-pct.nhs.uk
(Norfolk, Suffolk and Cambridgeshire Strategic Health Authority)

Chair Jane Leighton
Chief Executive Andy Evans

Beccles and District War Memorial Hospital

St Mary's Road, Beccles NR34 9NQ
Tel: 01502 712164 Fax: 01502 714696
Total Beds: 48

General Surgery P Aukland

Oncology J Ostrowski

Orthopaedics G H Moore

Patrick Stead Hospital

Bungay Road, Halesworth IP19 8HP
Tel: 01986 872124 Fax: 01986 874838
Total Beds: 20

General Medicine D Seaton

Orthopaedics R Jones, P Nadarajan

Wednesbury and West Bromwich Primary Care Trust

Kingston House, 438-450 High Street, West Bromwich B70 9LD
Tel: 0121 500 1500 Fax: 0121 500 1501
(Birmingham and the Black Country Strategic Health Authority)

Chair John Crawley
Chief Executive Graham Wallis

Welwyn Hatfield Primary Care Trust

Charter House, Parkway, Welwyn Garden City AL8 6JL
Tel: 01707 361204 Fax: 01707 361286
Email: general@welhat-pct.nhs.uk
Website: www.welwyn-hatfield-pct.nhs.uk
(Bedfordshire and Hertfordshire Strategic Health Authority)

Chair Carol Sherriff
Chief Executive Peter Horbury

West Cumbria Primary Care Trust

The Old Town Hall, Oxford Street, Workington CA14 2RS
Tel: 01900 324220 Fax: 01900 324221
Email: westpct.reception@ncumbria.nhs.uk
(Cumbria and Lancashire Strategic Health Authority)

Chair Bernard Kirk
Chief Executive Nigel Woodcock

Cockermouth Hospital

Isel Road, Cockermouth CA13 9HT
Tel: 01900 822226 Fax: 01900 828698
Total Beds: 16

Millom Community Hospital

Lapstone Road, Millom LA18 4BY
Tel: 01229 772631 Fax: 01229 771121
Total Beds: 14

Victoria Community Hospital
Ewanrigg Road, Maryport CA15 8EJ
Tel: 01900 812634

Workington Infirmary
Workington CA14 2UF
Tel: 01900 602244 Fax: 01946 523053
Total Beds: 21

West Dorset General Hospitals NHS Trust

Dorset County Hospital, Williams Avenue, Dorchester DT1 2JY
Tel: 01305 251150 Fax: 01305 254155
Email: headquarters@wdgh.nhs.uk
Website: www.dch.org.uk
(Dorset and Somerset Strategic Health Authority)

Chair Robin SeQueira
Chief Executive Nick Cox

Dorset County Hospital
Williams Avenue, Dorchester DT1 2JY
Tel: 01305 251150 Fax: 01305 254155
Total Beds: 563

Accident and Emergency D Cain

Intensive Care D S Andrew, Dr Ball, T Doyle, R Foxell, K J Gill, R Hebblethwaite, M Hitchcock, N Hollis, M Hough, J Wilson

Cardiology T Edwards, S Winterton

Care of the Elderly A Blake, Dr Bruce-Jones, A Webb, R Williams

Clinical Chemistry K Wakelin

Clinical Neurophysiology C Wulff

Dermatology S Tucker

ENT H Cox, G Ford, N Hopkin

General Medicine Dr Cove, P Down, C Hovell, A Macklin, G Philips

Genitourinary Medicine C Priestly

Haematology M Al-Hilali, Dr Moosa

Histopathology A M Anscombe, D Parums

Microbiology S Crook, S Groom

Nephrology N Hateboer, C Weston

Obstetrics and Gynaecology M Dooley, M Iftikhar

Ophthalmology L Bray, T Pathmanathan, G Porter, A Reck, A Tadros

Oral Surgery V Ilankovan

Orthodontics H Bellis, D Shinn, M Short

Orthopaedics I Barlow, N Fernandez, G Hall, C Thacker

Paediatrics J Doherty

Radiology P Camm, A Johnson, J Lesny, C Orgles, S Scott, N Smith, P N Taylor

Renal Medicine J Taylor

Rheumatology M Helliwell

Surgery A Flowerdew, C Gosling, M Graham, P Jeffery, N Lagatolla

Urology A Cornaby

West Gloucestershire Primary Care Trust

Units 14-15, Highnam Business Park, Newent Road, Highnam, Gloucester GL2 8DN
Tel: 01452 389400 Fax: 01452 389429
Email: mail.us@wglospct.nhs.uk
Website: www.westglospct.org.uk
(Avon, Gloucestershire and Wiltshire Strategic Health Authority)

Chair Liz Boait
Chief Executive Stephen Golledge

Dilke Memorial Hospital
Cinderford GL14 3HX
Tel: 01594 598100 Fax: 01594 598101
Total Beds: 36

Manager Jeanette Giles

Lydney and District Hospital
Grove Road, Lydney GL15 5JF
Tel: 01594 598220 Fax: 01594 598221
Total Beds: 27

Manager Jeanette Giles

West Hertfordshire Hospitals NHS Trust

Watford General Hospital, 60 Vicarage Road, Watford WD1 0HB
Tel: 01923 244366
Website: www.westhertshospitals.nhs.uk
(Bedfordshire and Hertfordshire Strategic Health Authority)

Chair Rosie Sanderson

Hemel Hempstead General Hospital
Hillfield Road, Hemel Hempstead HP2 4AD
Tel: 01442 213141
Total Beds: 387

Accident and Emergency A Marchon

Anaesthetics M T T Bryant, F J Griffiths, M E Pickering-Pick, W Yanny

Care of the Elderly R R Farag

Dermatology P D E Maurice

ENT H K K Bail, J A Harding

General Medicine I G Barrison, J F J Bayliss, C Johnston

General Surgery J C Nicholls, M Ormiston

Neurology J Gibbs

Obstetrics and Gynaecology J L Kane, D A Rosenberg, Y Tayob

Ophthalmology R N Auplish

Orthodontics L R O Hale

Orthopaedics J P Beacon, G M Hart, D Hirschowitz

Paediatrics B K Lee, H e Naggar

Pathology Dr Gaminara, A P O'Reilly

Radiology B V Clegg, A R Divers, D P Grimer, D S Shetty

Radiotherapy and Oncology E J Grosch

Rheumatology and Rehabilitation M A Wajed

Thoracic Medicine A R Nath

Mount Vernon Hospital
Rickmansworth Road, Northwood HA6 2RN
Tel: 01923 826111 Fax: 01923 844460

Total Beds: 144

Manager Mrs Bowser

Anaesthetics A Arnold, J Binns, P M Brodrick, K Collins, A Hayward, D Mills, D K Patel, E Stielow

Care of the Elderly Dr Al-Douri, Dr Baruam, Dr Franklin

General Medicine T J Goodwin, R Hillson, G E Holdstock, D W B Thomas, D Thomson

General Surgery P Mitchenere, T Paes, J E L Sales

Neurology R Peatfield

Oral and Maxillofacial Surgery G Bounds, G T Gardiner, M Issa

Orthodontics J Noar

Orthopaedics G Belham, W N Bodey, J Dooley, N Reissis

Palliative Medicine I Trotman

Pathology D J Allan, S Amin, W K Blenkinsopp, A Coady, D Cummins, P Mahendra, P I Richman, R Smith

Plastic Surgery P Cussons, D Gault, A Grobelaar, D H Harrison, B D G Morgan, R Sanders, P J Smith

Radiology A W Ayoub, H Baddeley, N Damani, P Dovey, W Wong

Radiotherapy and Oncology B E Lyn, R F U Ashford, D C Fermont, R Glynne-Jones, E J Grosch, P Hoskin, P Lawton, J Maher, A Makepeace, G Rustin, M Saunders

Urology M A Ruston

St Albans City Hospital

Normandy Road, St Albans AL3 5PN
Tel: 01727 866122
Total Beds: 187

Anaesthetics M T T Bryant, D U S Pathirana, W A Yanny

Care of the Elderly Dr Farag

Dermatology P D L Maurice

ENT H K K Bail

General Medicine I G Barrison, J F J Bayliss, C Johnston, I P Williams

General Surgery M C Ormiston, G R Sagor

Genitourinary Medicine J John

Neurology J M Gibbs

Obstetrics and Gynaecology J L Kane, D A Rosenberg, Y Tayob

Ophthalmology J F Tattersfield, M K Wang

Orthopaedics J P Beacon, D Hirschowitz

Paediatrics C M Gabriel

Pathology R L Abeyesundere, E J Gaminara, S F Hill

Plastic Surgery P J Smith

Radiology B V Clegg, D P Grimer, B E Hartley, D S Shetty, E Sheville

Radiotherapy and Oncology E Grosch

Rheumatology and Rehabilitation M A Wajed, K A Young

Watford General Hospital

Vicarage Road, Watford WD18 0HB
Tel: 01923 244366 Fax: 01923 217440
Total Beds: 383

Accident and Emergency H J Borkett-Jones, J Oliver

Anaesthetics G Baker, C P Lung, V Page, H M Parry, D R O Redman

Care of the Elderly M L Cox, A Sa'adu, W Somerville

Dermatology M E Murdoch, F Tatnall

ENT R Auerbach, R Dhillon, R England

General Medicine M R Clements, E J Knight, B Macfarlane, G A Nelstrop, P R Studdy

General Surgery R W Awad, J I Livingstone, S Sarin, J M Thomas

Genitourinary Medicine P E Munday

Neurology G D Schott

Obstetrics and Gynaecology B E Bean, D R Griffin, L Irvine, B V Lewis, M Padwick, R Sheridan

Ophthalmology S Kodati, D Owen, N Young

Oral and Maxillofacial Surgery G Bounds

Orthopaedics J Jessop, R P Mackenney

Paediatrics E Douek, G Supramaniam, M J H Williams

Pathology A McMillan, M T Moulsdale, A Rubin

Radiology D Boxer, B Gajjar, S Pathmanathan, T F E Sayed

Radiotherapy and Oncology R F U Ashford

Rheumatology and Rehabilitation N A Pandit

Urology J C Crisp

West Hull Primary Care Trust

Brunswick House, Strand Close, Beverley Road, Hull HU2 9DB
Tel: 01482 303500 Fax: 01482 303501
Email: info.web@whpct.nhs.uk
Website: www.westhullpct.nhs.uk
(North and East Yorkshire and Northern Lincolnshire Strategic Health Authority)

Chair Kathryn Lavery
Chief Executive Christopher Long

West Kent NHS and Social Care Trust

35 Kings Hill Avenue, Kings Hill, West Malling ME19 4AX
Tel: 01732 520400 Fax: 01732 520401
Website: www.wknhssct.nhs.uk
(Kent and Medway Strategic Health Authority)

Chair Ward Griffiths
Chief Executive Jon Wilkes

Archery House

Bow Arrow Lane, Dartford DA2 6PB
Tel: 01322 227211
Total Beds: 59

General Psychiatry E Clarke, V Gunasingham, Dr Sadik

Highlands House

10 Calverley Park Gardens, Tunbridge Wells TN2 2JN
Tel: 01732 455155
Total Beds: 35

Little Brook Hospital

Bow Arrow Lane, Dartford
Tel: 01322 622222
Total Beds: 52

Medway Maritime Hospital

Adult Mental Health Unit, Windmill Road, Gillingham ME7 5NY
Tel: 01634 830000 Fax: 01634 829470
Total Beds: 65

Pembury Hospital (Psychiatric Services)
Pembury, Tunbridge Wells TN2 4QJ
Tel: 01892 823535 Fax: 01892 823545

Priority House
Hermitage Lane, Maidstone ME16 9PH
Tel: 01662 725000 Fax: 01662 723200
Total Beds: 57

Sittingbourne Memorial Hospital
Bell Road, Sittingbourne ME10 4DT
Tel: 01795 418300 Fax: 01795 418301
Total Beds: 48

Manager G Sainsbury

General Psychiatry S Feeney

Stone House
Dartford DA2 6AU
Tel: 01322 622222
Total Beds: 104

Manager Karen Dorey

General Psychiatry V Matthew, Dr Osmay, R R Sharma

West Lancashire Primary Care Trust

Ormskirk and District General Hospital, Wigan Road, Ormskirk L39 2JW
Tel: 01695 598084 Fax: 01695 598104
Email: feedback@westlancspct.nhs.uk
Website: www.westlancspct.nhs.uk
(Cumbria and Lancashire Strategic Health Authority)

Chair Jim Barton
Chief Executive Jane Thompson

Cockermouth Cottage Hospital
Isel Road, Cockermouth CA13 9HT
Tel: 01900 822226
Total Beds: 17

Ophthalmology S Verghese

Millom Hospital
Lapstone Road, Millom LA18 4BY
Tel: 01229 772631
Total Beds: 14

General Medicine W T Berrill, C Thomson

Obstetrics and Gynaecology M J Bober

Orthopaedics M Greiss

Paediatrics P Carter, S Precious

Psychiatry of Old Age M J Bober

Victoria Cottage Hospital
Ewanrigg Road, Maryport CA15 8EJ
Tel: 01900 812634
Total Beds: 22

General Surgery M Walker

Obstetrics and Gynaecology J Stafford

Workington Infirmary
Infirmary Road, Workington CA14 2UN
Tel: 01900 602244
Total Beds: 91

Care of the Elderly F K Local, N J Russell

Chest Disease W T Berrill

Dermatology J Cox, W D Paterson

ENT J T Taylor

General Medicine C Thomson

General Psychiatry M J Bober

General Surgery D G Richards

Learning Disabilities A Bassam

Obstetrics and Gynaecology S A Bober, J Eldred, M Matar, J Stafford

Ophthalmology P Sellar, S Verghese

Oral and Maxillofacial Surgery S C Banerjee

Orthodontics R Tyrrell

Orthopaedics M I Dhebar, M Greiss, N S Rao

Paediatrics P Carter, S Precious

Radiology T A Eyre, B G Maguire, B Mucci

Rheumatology and Rehabilitation J D McRea

West Lincolnshire Primary Care Trust

Cross O'Cliff, Bracebridge Heath, Lincoln LN4 2HN
Tel: 01522 513355 Fax: 01522 540706
Email: communications@westlincs-pct.nhs.uk
Website: www.westlincspct.nhs.uk
(Trent Strategic Health Authority)

Chair Stanley Keyte
Chief Executive Tim Rideout

John Coupland Hospital
Ropery Road, Gainsborough DN21 2TJ
Tel: 01427 816500 Fax: 01427 816512
Total Beds: 21

West London Mental Health NHS Trust

Trust Headquarters, St Bernards Hospital, Uxbridge Road, Southall UB1 3EU
Tel: 020 8354 8354 Fax: 020 8354 8002
Email: enquiries@wlmht.nhs.uk
Website: www.wlmht.nhs.uk
(North West London Strategic Health Authority)

Chair Louis Smidt
Chief Executive Simon Crawford

Broadmoor Hospital
Crowthorne RG45 7EG
Tel: 01344 773111 Fax: 01334 754388, 01334 773327
Total Beds: 483

Cassell Hospital
1 Ham Common, Richmond TW10 7JF
Tel: 020 8940 8181 Fax: 020 8237 2937

John Conolly Wing
Uxbridge Road, Southall, London UB1 3EU
Tel: 020 8354 8354

Penny Sangam Day Hospital
Osterley Park Road, Southall UB2 4BH
Tel: 020 8571 9676 Fax: 020 8571 2089

Three Bridges Regional Secure Unit
Uxbridge Road, Southall UB1 3EU
Total Beds: 124

West Middlesex University Hospital NHS Trust

Twickenham Road, Isleworth TW7 6AF
Tel: 020 8560 2121 Fax: 020 7631 0102
Email: corporate.affairs@wmuh-tr.nthames.nhs.uk
Website: www.west-middlesex-hospital.nhs.uk
(North West London Strategic Health Authority)

Chair Sue Ellen
Chief Executive Gail Wannell

West Middlesex University Hospital
Twickenham Road, Isleworth TW7 6AF
Tel: 020 8560 2121 Fax: 020 8321 5562
Total Beds: 360

Accident and Emergency M W Beckett (Head), M W Beckett, Z Mirza

Cardiology T Greenwood (Head), T Greenwood

Care of the Elderly B K Bhattacharyya, J Platt

Chest Disease A Winning (Head), A Winning

Dermatology M Pope (Head), S Parker, M Pope

ENT V Cumberworth, N Daly, A Robinson

General Medicine S Allard (Head), S Allard, M Anderson, C Collins, T W Greenwood, S P Kane, A Winning

General Surgery R A L Young (Head), R A L Young (Head), J Ramsay, H Rogers, J Smith, R Vashist, R A L Young

Genitourinary Medicine D Asboe, D Daniels

Nephrology E Brown, C Collins, S Kane

Neurology R Pearce

Obstetrics and Gynaecology J M Baldwin, J Girling, E Owen

Oral Surgery R J Carr (Head), R G D Burr, R J Carr

Orthopaedics K Desai, N Nathan, F W N Paterson, H Zadeh

Paediatrics D Hafiz, V Hakeem, J Rangasami, D Ratnasinghe

Pathology R S Fink (Head), R S Fink, R G Hughes, S Karim, M Kyi, M Sekhar, P A Thorpe

Plastic Surgery G Bantick (Head)

Radiology T Naunton-Morgan (Head), F Aref-Adib, C Miller, T Naunton-Morgan, M Owen, C Ramsay, M Watson

Radiotherapy and Oncology M Spittle

Rheumatology S A Allard (Head), S A Allard

Thoracic Surgery W J Fountain

Urology J Ramsay

West Midlands Ambulance Service NHS Trust

Millennium Point, Waterfront Business Park, Brierley Hill, Dudley DY5 1LX
Tel: 01384 215555 Fax: 01384 451677
Email: enquiries@wmas.nhs.uk
Website: www.wmas.nhs.uk
(Birmingham and the Black Country Strategic Health Authority)

Chair Doug Jinks
Chief Executive Barry Johns

West Norfolk Primary Care Trust

St James', Exton's Road, King's Lynn PE30 5NU
Tel: 01553 816200 Fax: 01553 761104
Email: enquiries@westnorfolk-pct.nhs.uk
Website: www.westnorfolk-pct.nhs.uk
(Norfolk, Suffolk and Cambridgeshire Strategic Health Authority)

Chair Sheila Childerhouse
Chief Executive Hilary Daniels

Swaffham Community Hospital
Sporle Road, Swaffham PE37 7HL
Tel: 01760 721363 Fax: 01760 720613
Total Beds: 18

West of Cornwall Primary Care Trust

Head Office, Foundry Road, Camborne TR14 8DS
Tel: 01209 888222 Fax: 01209 886572
Email: name@westprimcare.cornwall.nhs.uk
Website: www.cornwall.nhs.uk/wocpct
(South West Peninsula Strategic Health Authority)

Chair Ed Ferrett
Chief Executive Antek Lejk

Camborne/Redruth Community Hospital
Barncoose Terrace, Redruth TR15 3ER
Tel: 01209 881688 Fax: 01209 881713
Total Beds: 75

Manager Linda Day

Edward Hain Memorial Hospital
Albany Terrace, St Ives TR26 2BS
Tel: 01736 576100 Fax: 01736 576118
Total Beds: 14

Manager Linda Day

Helston Community Hospital
Meneage Road, Helston TR13 8DR
Tel: 01326 435800 Fax: 01326 435859
Total Beds: 24

Manager Linda Day

Poltair Hospital
Heamoor, Penzance TR20 8SR
Tel: 01736 575570 Fax: 01736 575580
Total Beds: 23

Manager Gordon Pickett

St Mary's Hospital
Hugh Town, St Mary's TR21 0HE
Tel: 01720 422392 Fax: 01720 423134
Total Beds: 14

Manager Linda Day

West Suffolk Hospitals NHS Trust

Hardwick Lane, Bury St Edmunds IP33 2QZ
Tel: 01284 713000 Fax: 01284 701993
Website: www.wsufftrust.org.uk
(Norfolk, Suffolk and Cambridgeshire Strategic Health Authority)

Chair Veronica Worrall
Chief Executive Chris Bown

West Suffolk Hospital

Hardwick Lane, Bury St Edmunds IP33 2QZ
Tel: 01284 71300
Website: www.wsufftst.org.uk
Total Beds: 630

Accident and Emergency A Giles, A Haig, A Sauvage

Anaesthetics N Adams, J Boys, A Burns, J Cardy, P Chrispin, A Christensen, C Duke, J Field, J Hall, S Lowe, A Majeed, J Mauger, D Meldrum, R Munglani, M Palmer, N Penfold, J Slade, J Urquhart, K Williams

Cardiology E Lee, D Stone

Care of the Elderly J Fasler, A Nicholson, M Troup

Dermatology S Handfield-Jones, R Jenkins

Diabetes J Clark, A Wijineike

ENT P Axon, F Fahmy, B Fish, D McKiernan, R Skibsted

General Medicine and Elderly Services A Azim, I Aziz, C Beatty, D Chitnavis, J Clarke, S Edwards, J Fasler, H Ford, E Gurnell, S Handfield-Jones, R Jenkins, P Johansen, C Laroche, P Lawrence, E Lee, J Majeed, A Moody, A Nicholson, D O'Reilly, D Sharpstone, P Siklos, S Sinha, D Stone, W Thomas, M Troup, S Whalley, A Wijenaike, C Woodward

General Surgery J Alberts, Mr Boyle, A Canal, E Coveny, Mr Gaunt, T Justin, N Keeling, D Lawrence, D O'Riordan, O Ravisekar

Genitourinary Medicine S Edwards

Haematology C Beatty

Histopathology R Brais, K Love

Neurology F Crawley, E Harper, G Lennox, P Molyneux

Obstetrics and Gynaecology R Giles, S Gull, P Harris, M Judd, D Ross, P J Spencer

Ophthalmology K Jordan, R J Lamb, A Ramsay, A Vivian

Oral and Maxillofacial Surgery H Davies, R Tate

Orthodontics T I Davies

Orthopaedics A C August, A F Bedford, S Deakin, Mr Dunn, P Nicolai, M Porteous, W Schenk, S Sjolin, M Wood

Paediatrics G L Briars, J Buck, M Clements, I Evans, R Lakshman, M Noone, H M Scott, S Thompson

Pathology R Braise, B Cottrell, K Love, S Martin, S Purdy, C Tremlett, E Wright

Radiology R Darrah, R J Godwin, J Guy, M MacFarlane, L Watson

Radiotherapy and Oncology H Ford, M Moody

Respiratory Medicine I Aziz, C Laroche

Rheumatology Dr Johansen, D O'Reilly

Urology J Allan, C L Kennedy, J McLoughlin

West Sussex Health and Social Care NHS Trust

Joint management team with East Sussex County Healthcare NHS Trust.
Swandean, Arundel Road, Worthing BN13 3EP
Tel: 01903 843000 Fax: 01903 843001
Email: firstname.lastname@wshsc.nhs.uk
Website: www.wshsc.nhs.uk
(Surrey and Sussex Strategic Health Authority)

Chair Neil Matthewson
Chief Executive Lisa Rodrigues

Centurion Mental Health Centre

Graylingwell Drive, Chichester PO19 6FX
Tel: 01243 791898 (Orion Ward), 01243 791919 (Mercury Ward), 01243 791930
Total Beds: 38

Chapel Street Clinic

Chapel Street, Chichester PO19 1BX
Tel: 01243 623300

Colwood Hospital

Haywards Heath RH16 4EX
Tel: 01444 441881

Conolly House

Conolly Way, Chichester PO19 6WD
Tel: 01243 791804 Fax: 01243 791819
Total Beds: 15

Dove Day Hospital

Crawley Hospital, West Green Drive, Crawley RH10 7DH
Tel: 01293 600300 Ext: 3640 Fax: 01293 600414

Horsham Hospital

Hurst Road, Horsham RH12 2DR
Tel: 01403 227000 Fax: 01403 227018
Total Beds: 80

Jupiter House

Graylingwell Drive, Chichester PO19 6WD
Tel: 01243 791924
Total Beds: 10

Meadowfield

Arundel Road, Worthing BN13 3EF
Tel: 01903 843200 Fax: 01903 843201
Total Beds: 48

Ridings Southlands Hospital

Shoreham-by-Sea BN43 6TQ
Tel: 01273 446037 Fax: 01273 446042
Total Beds: 23

Salvington Lodge

Salvington Hill, Off Arundel Road, Worthing BN13 3EP
Tel: 01903 266399 Fax: 01903 266388
Total Beds: 66

Villa Ward, Downsview and Martlet Lodge

Princess Royal Hospital, Lewes Road, Haywards Heath RH16 4EX
Tel: 01444 441881 Fax: 01444 441528

The Weald Day Hospital

West Green Drive, Crawley RH10 7DH
Tel: 01293 600300

West Wiltshire Primary Care Trust

Unit B, Valentines, Epsom Square, White Horse Business Park, Trowbridge BA14 0XG
Tel: 01225 754453 Fax: 01225 754648
Email: wwpct@westwiltshire-pct.nhs.uk
Website: www.westwiltshirepct.nhs.uk
(Avon, Gloucestershire and Wiltshire Strategic Health Authority)

Chair Shiena Bowen
Chief Executive Carol Clarke

Bradford-on-Avon Community Hospital

Berryfields, Bradford-on-Avon BA15 1TA
Tel: 01225 862975 Fax: 01225 867488
Total Beds: 15

Melksham Community Hospital
Spa Road, Melksham SN15 3AL
Tel: 01225 703088 Fax: 01225 708301, 01225 764334
Total Beds: 24

Trowbridge Community Hospital
Adcroft Road, Trowbridge BA14 8PH
Tel: 01225 752558 Fax: 01225 764334
Total Beds: 45

Warminster Community Hospital
The Close, Warminster BA12 8QS
Tel: 01985 212076 Fax: 01985 846286
Total Beds: 24

Consultants B Bubna-Kasteliz

Westbury Community Hospital
Hospital Road, The Butts, Westbury BA13 3EL
Tel: 01373 823616 Fax: 01373 827414
Total Beds: 24

West Yorkshire Metropolitan Ambulance Service NHS Trust

Wakefield 41 Business Park, Brindley Way, Wakefield WF2 0XQ
Tel: 01274 707070 Fax: 01274 707071
Website: www.wymas.co.uk
(West Yorkshire Strategic Health Authority)

Chair Ralph Berry
Chief Executive Kevin Ellis

Westcountry Ambulance Services NHS Trust

Trust Headquarters, Unit 4 Abbey Court, Sowton Industrial Estate, Exeter EX2 7HY
Tel: 01392 261500 Fax: 01392 261510
Email: enquiries@wcas-tr.swest.nhs.uk
Website: www.wcas.nhs.uk
(South West Peninsula Strategic Health Authority)

Chair Heather Strawbridge
Chief Executive Michael Willis

Western Sussex Primary Care Trust

The Bramber Building, 9 College Lane, Chichester PO19 6FX
Tel: 01243 770770 Fax: 01243 770799
Email: enquiries@wsx-pct.nhs.uk
Website: www.westernsussex.nhs.uk
(Surrey and Sussex Strategic Health Authority)

Chair Susan Pyper
Chief Executive Claire Holloway

Arundel and District Hospital
Chichester Road, Arundel BN18 0AB
Tel: 01903 882543

Bognor Regis War Memorial Hospital
Shripney Road, Bognor Regis PO22 9PP
Tel: 01243 865418 Fax: 01243 827125
Total Beds: 61

Midhurst Community Hospital
Dodsley Road, Easebourne, Midhurst GU29 9AW
Tel: 01730 819100
Total Beds: 12

Westminster Primary Care Trust

15 Marylebone Road, London NW1 5JD
Tel: 020 7150 8000 Fax: 020 7150 8241
Email: firstname.lastname@westminster-pct.nhs.uk
Website: www.westminster-pct.nhs.uk
(North West London Strategic Health Authority)

Chair Joe Hegarty
Chief Executive Lynda Hamlyn

Weston Area Health NHS Trust

Weston General Hospital, Grange Road, Uphill, Weston Super Mare BS23 4TQ
Tel: 01934 636363 Fax: 01934 647176
Email: executive@waht.swest.nhs.uk
(Avon, Gloucestershire and Wiltshire Strategic Health Authority)

Chair Ron Ballantine
Chief Executive Mark Gritten

Weston General Hospital
Grange Road, Uphill, Weston Super Mare BS23 4TQ
Tel: 01934 636363 Fax: 01934 647029
Total Beds: 358

Accident and Emergency A Newton (Head)

Anaesthetics J Friend (Head), J Dixon, M Elias, P Slew, A Smith

Dental Surgery J W Ross

Dermatology C B Archer (Head)

ENT D Baldwin, Mr Nunez, Mr Tierney

General Medicine H Bhakri, G Gould, D Parker, D Singhal, R M Srivosrava, D Wright

General Surgery Mr Dickerson, Mr Gallegos, Mr Gillatt, A L Gough, T John, G Pye, M Schuijvlot

Histopathology M Lott, D Paterson

Maxillofacial Surgery Professor Cowpe, G Irvine

Neurology I Ormerod, Dr Sieradazan

Obstetrics and Gynaecology R Afifi, C Bevan, N Dwyer

Ophthalmology S Cook, R H B Grey, I Harrad, D Tole

Orthopaedics M Bould, R Case, J Dixon, V G Langkamer, A Mahajan, M Shannon, R F Spencer

Paediatrics D Barff

Pathology M Lott, D Paterson

Radiology C Cook, C Croucher, E Kutt, J O'Brien, P G P Stoddart, P Woodhead

Radiotherapy and Oncology C Price, M Tomlinson, C J Williams

Rheumatology S Clarke, S Stebbings

Urology Mr Dickerson, D Gillatt, J Probert, H Schwaibold

Whipps Cross University Hospital NHS Trust

Trust Headquarters, Whipps Cross University Hospital, Whipps Cross Road, Leytonstone, London E11 1NR
Tel: 020 8535 6800 Fax: 020 8535 6439
Email: info@whippsx.nhs.uk
Website: www.whippsx.nhs.uk
(North East London Strategic Health Authority)

Chair Stephen Jacobs
Chief Executive Lucy Moore

Chingford Hospital
Larkshall Road, London E4 6UN

Wanstead Hospital
Makepeace Road, London E11 1UU

Whipps Cross University Hospital
Whipps Cross Road, Leytonstone, London E11 1NR
Tel: 020 8539 5522 Fax: 020 8558 8115
Website: www.whippsx.nhs.uk
Total Beds: 784

The Whittington Hospital NHS Trust

Highgate Hill, London N19 5NF
Tel: 020 7272 3070 Fax: 020 7288 5550
Email: deborah.goodhart@whittington.nhs.uk
Website: www.whittington.nhs.uk
(North Central London Strategic Health Authority)

Chair Narendra Makanji
Chief Executive David Sloman

Whittington Hospital
Highgate Hill, London N19 5NF
Tel: 020 7272 3070 Fax: 020 7288 5550
Total Beds: 470

Accident and Emergency G M A Heaton, R Landau

Anaesthetics M E Dunstan, B El-Behesy, S Gillis, S M C Hargreaves, N Harper, A S Ishaq, G H Lim, O Makinde, G Panch, J G Powney, C Shaw, S Walker

Care of the Elderly C A Bielawska, R Gray, S C M Mitchell, G S Rai

Chest Disease N M Johnson, S Lock, R Lyall, L Restrick, M Stern

Child and Adolescent Psychiatry S Kraemer, J Roberts

Dermatology R Wakeel

ENT D I Choa, H Grant, T Joseph

General Medicine M L Barnard, D J Brull, J R Davies, S M C Hardman, J G Malone-Lee, S McHardy-Young, D L H Patterson, M Rossi, D Suri, F R Vicary, J S Yudkin

General Surgery C C R Bishop, M D Brough, M Hashemi, C L Ingham Clark, M R Lock, H Mukhtar, A O Oshowo, J R C Sainsbury, Professor Taylor, A J Wilson

Haematology B Davis, N E Parker

Histopathology D C Brown, R L Bryan, N Khan, S O'Byrne, S Ramachandra, B O Saeed

Medical Microbiology M C Kelsey

Neurology N A Losseff, E D Playford

Obstetrics and Gynaecology T P Dutt, F Eben, T B R Freeman-Wang, G L Henson, A Kye-Mensah, A Lokugamange, C F M Mellon, H Morgan, C P Paul, M E Setchell, A Singer, C Spence-Jones, D E Swiet

Ophthalmology C C Davey, B C Little, B Mulhollan

Orthopaedics D I S Sweetnam (Head), I A Bacarese-Hamilton, C Charambides, S Muirhead-Allwood, P Thomas

Paediatrics R M Blumberg, E R Broadhurst, M S Jaswon, H S MacKinnon, J Raine, A W Robins

Palliative Medicine A C Kurowska

Radiology C A Allum, R Chaudhari, J C Davis, D S Grant, S J Howling, J Kumaradevan, D Murray, J B Timmis, J Young

Rheumatology and Rehabilitation J Dacre, I Wamuo, J Worrall

Urology R A Miller, S Nathan

Wiltshire Ambulance Service NHS Trust

Greenways Centre, Malmesbury Road, Chippenham SN15 5LN
Tel: 01249 443939 Fax: 01249 443217
Email: exec.office@wiltsamb-tr.swest.nhs.uk
Website: www.wiltsamb.nhs.uk
(Avon, Gloucestershire and Wiltshire Strategic Health Authority)

Chair James Carine
Chief Executive Tim Skelton

Winchester and Eastleigh Healthcare NHS Trust

Royal Hampshire County Hospital, Romsey Road, Winchester SO22 5DG
Tel: 01962 863535 Fax: 01962 825190
Website: www.wehct.nhs.uk
(Hampshire and Isle of Wight Strategic Health Authority)

Chair Barbara North
Chief Executive Chris Evennett

Andover War Memorial Community Hospital
Charlton Road, Andover SP10 3LB
Tel: 01264 358811
Total Beds: 100

Mount Day Hospital
Bishopstoke, Eastleigh SO50 6ZB
Tel: 023 8061 2335 Fax: 023 8065 0954

Royal Hampshire County Hospital
Romsey Road, Winchester SO22 5DG
Tel: 01962 863535 Fax: 01962 824826
Total Beds: 530

Anaesthetics J C Criswell, S J Deacock, P M du Boulay, C Fairley, A Goldsmith, R Hutchinson, K Morris, M L Nancekievill, R J Summerfield, G Watson, W D White

Care of the Elderly C J Gordon, K O Stewart

Dental Surgery T H Redpath

Dermatology G M Fairris, D H Jones

ENT P B Ashcroft

General Medicine A P Brooks, M S Hammersley, J D Powell-Jackson, J A Roberts, H A Shepherd

General Psychiatry C Bellenis, E Chan-Pensley, P Courtney, P D Hettiaratchy, S Olivieri, I Plant, C Platz, R I Stewart

General Psychiatry P Courtney

General Surgery P C Gartell, R H S Lane, A Miles, R M Rainsbury, N M Wilson

Genitourinary Medicine K Woodcock

Learning Disabilities A Hobbs

Medical Microbiology M Dryden

Neurology P Kennedy

Obstetrics and Gynaecology M S Buckingham, M J Heard, K A Louden, A D Noble

Ophthalmology A Macleod, R J Morris, J Watts

Oral and Maxillofacial Surgery N Baker

Orthodontics S C Cole

Orthopaedics J L Fowler, H Fox, W E Hook, A W Samuel, N P Trimmings

Paediatrics A G Antoniou, K D Foote, T F Mackintosh, D Schapiro

Pathology R K Al-Talib, B Green, C James

Radiology J Cheetham, J Hogg, J M Laidlow, A C Page, O J C Wethered

Rheumatology and Rehabilitation N Buchanan, N L Cox

Urology A Adamson, G S Harrison

Winchester Day Hospital

Royal Hampshire County Hospital, 8 St Paul's Hill, Winchester SO22 5DG
Tel: 01962 863535 Fax: 01962 824826

Windsor, Ascot and Maidenhead Primary Care Trust

King Edward VII Hospital, St Leonard's Road, Windsor SL4 3DP
Tel: 01753 636801 Fax: 01753 636828
Email: wampct@berkshire.nhs.uk
Website: www.berkshire.nhs.uk/wam
(Thames Valley Strategic Health Authority)

Chair Sally Kemp
Chief Executive Philip Burgess
Consultants Philip Brooks

King Edward VII Hospital

St Leonard's Road, Windsor SL4 3DP
Tel: 01753 636801

St Mark's Hospital

St Mark's Road, Maidenhead SL6 6DU
Tel: 01628 632012

Wirral Hospital NHS Trust

Arrowe Park Hospital, Arrowe Park Road, Upton, Wirral CH49 5PE
Tel: 0151 678 5111 Fax: 0151 604 7148
Email: wirral.enq@whnt.nhs.uk
Website: www.wirralhealth.org.uk
(Cheshire and Merseyside Strategic Health Authority)

Chair Eryl Hoskins
Chief Executive Frank Burns

Arrowe Park Hospital

Arrowe Park Road, Upton, Wirral L49 5PE
Tel: 0151 678 5111
Total Beds: 886

Accident and Emergency C Doherty, A Good, B Ohiorenoya, A G Pennycook

Anaesthetics A Atherton, B Bapat, J J Chambers, C Cowan, J C Devlin, D Eastwood, M Frias-Jimenez, J P Gannon, B P Guratsky, B Hedayati, G Jefferies, S Leith, R Mehra, E W Moore, J K Moore, S Ralston, A Rao, N Scawn, M W Smith, J S Sprigge, K Stevens, R W Stevens, J E Sweeney, T J Tarr, M Van Miert, P Williams

Care of the Elderly J A Barrett, D King, R Morgan, M Pritchard-Howard, J Russell, G Sangster, A Scott, B Spencer, C J Turnbull

Chemical Pathology W D Neithercut

Dermatology S K Jones, S I White

ENT D G O'Sullivan, I W Sherman, V Srinivasan

General Medicine J Corless, P Currie, J Dawson, R Faizallah, R Ferguson, D B Jones, I R Jones, D S Lawrence, J Lorains, D Rittou, J H Silas, K Son Leong, Z K Wahbi

General Surgery J Anderson, D Berstock, S D Blair, R Chandrasekar, M G Greaney, M S Javed, C A Makin, A Masters, D T Reilly, S Sagar, F Swe, C Walsh

Genitourinary Medicine A K Ghosh

Haematology T J Deeble, D Galvani

Histopathology D Agbamu, A H Clark, J Elder, M B Gillett, A R T Green, K Gumparthy, R Seneviratne, K C Sidky, H D Zakhour

Medical Microbiology J Cunniffe, A E Murray

Nephrology A Crowe, P McClelland

Obstetrics and Gynaecology B Alderman, P M Doyle, P Green, N Gul, D J Rowlands, C R Welch, I A Williams

Ophthalmology L G Clearkin, P Pennefather, S Prasad, M Watts

Oral Surgery D Jones, G D Wood

Orthodontics G R P Barry

Orthopaedics N Donnachie, N P J Geary, R A Harvey, M Hennesey, J C Kaye, A D Morris, R W Parkinson, A J M Simison, J Stamer, T G Thomas

Paediatrics C N Bhrolchain, E M J Breen, J Fellick, A Hughes, D E Lacy, D J Manning, P J Seymour, P J Todd

Palliative Medicine C M Lewis-Jones

Radiology P J Evans, A M Garrett, D H Green, D Hughes, U M Hughes, D M Killeen, Z R Klenka, S G Lea, M E Lipton, J Magennis, V C Williamson

Rheumatology and Rehabilitation R Chowdhury, E George, S Keetarut, C Pinder

Urology A M Cliff, P Kutarski, N J Parr, R N Stephenson

Clatterbridge Hospital

Bebington, Wirral CH63 4JY
Tel: 0151 334 4000
Total Beds: 245

Anaesthetics A Atherton, B Bapat, J J Chambers, C Cowan, J C Devlin, D Eastwood, M Frias-Jimenez, J P Gannon, B P Guratsky, B Hedayati, G Jefferies, S Leith, R Mehra, E W Moore, J K Moore, S Ralston, A Rao, N Scawn, M W Smith, J S Sprigge, K D Stevens, R W Stevens, J E Sweeney, T J Tarr, M Van Miert, P Williams

Care of the Elderly J A Barrett, D King, R Morgan, M Pritchard-Howard, J Russell, G Sangster, A Scott, B Spencer, C J Turnbull

Chemical Pathology W D Neithercut

Dermatology S K Jones, D King, S I White

General Surgery J Anderson, D A Berstock, S D Blair, R Chandrasekar, M G Greaney, M S Javed, C A Makin, A Masters, D T Reilly, S Sagar, F Swe, C Walsh

Haematology T J Deeble, D Galvani

Histopathology D Agbamu, A H Clark, J Elder, M B Gillett, A R T Green, K Gumparthy, R Seneviratne, K C Sidky, H D Zakhour

Medical Microbiology A E Murray

Orthopaedics N Donnachie, N P J Geary, R A Harvey, M Hennesey, J C Kaye, A D Morris, R W Parkinson, A J M Simison, J Stamer, T G Thomas

Palliative Medicine C M Lewis-Jones

Radiology P J Evans, A M Garrett, D H Green, D Hughes, U M Hughes, D M Killeen, Z Klenka, S G Lea, M E Lipton, J Magennis, V C Williamson

Rheumatology and Rehabilitation R Chowdhury, E George, S Keetarut, C Pinder

Urology A M Cliff, P Kutarski, N J Parr, R N Stephenson

Victoria Central Hospital
Mill Lane, Wallasey CH44 5UF
Tel: 0151 678 5111 Fax: 0151 639 2478
Total Beds: 52

Witham, Braintree and Halstead Care Trust

Warwick House, Market Place, Braintree CM7 3HQ
Tel: 01376 331549 Fax: 01376 331556
Email: firstname.surname@braintreecaretrust.nhs.uk
Website: www.braintreecaretrust.nhs.uk
(Essex Strategic Health Authority)

Chair Marion Williams
Chief Executive Paul Zollinger-Read

Wokingham Primary Care Trust

Wokingham Community Hospital, Barkham Road, Wokingham RG41 2RE
Tel: 0118 949 5000 Fax: 0118 949 2949
Website: www.berkshire.nhs.uk/wokingham
(Thames Valley Strategic Health Authority)

Chair Alan Penn
Chief Executive Sue Heatherington

Wokingham Community Hospital
Wokingham RG41 2RE
Tel: 0118 949 5000 Fax: 0118 977 5880
Total Beds: 28

Wolverhampton City Primary Care Trust

Coniston House, Chapel Ash, Wolverhampton WV3 0XE
Tel: 01902 444888 Fax: 01902 444877
Website: www.wolverhamptonhealth.nhs.uk/wha/
(Birmingham and the Black Country Strategic Health Authority)

Chair Terence MacKriel
Chief Executive Jon Crockett
Consultants E Arsany, T S Aung, S Benlow, T Black, V Coley, C Dean, S Derasari, A Derso, S Dixey, C Higgins, R Jenkins, D Jolley, F Nehikhare, P Singh, S N Verma

Groves Day Hospital
Penn Hospital, Penn Road, Wolverhampton WV4 5HN
Tel: 01902 444130
Total Beds: 22

Manager Heidi Cater

Learning Disability Service
44 Pond Lane, Wolverhampton WV2 1HG
Tel: 01902 444002
Email: annette.shakespeare@whc-tr.nhs.uk
Total Beds: 19

General Psychiatry Dr Coley

Penn Hospital
Penn Road, Wolverhampton WV4 5HN
Tel: 01902 444141
Total Beds: 40

Manager Heidi Cater

Elderly Mentally Ill S Benbow, S Dixey, R Jenkins, D Jolley

West Park Rehabilitation Hospital
Park Road West, Wolverhampton WV1 4PW
Tel: 01902 444000 Fax: 01902 444085
Total Beds: 109

Manager S Holmes

Care of the Elderly T S Aung, F O Nehikhare, S N Verma

Worcestershire Acute Hospitals NHS Trust

Worcestershire Royal Hospital, Charles Hastings Way, Worcester WR5 1DD
Tel: 01905 763333 Fax: 01905 760555
Website: www.worcestershirehealth.nhs.uk
(West Midlands South Strategic Health Authority)

Chair Michael O'Riordan
Chief Executive John Rostill

Alexandra Hospital
Woodrow Drive, Redditch B98 7UB
Tel: 01527 503030 Fax: 01527 517432
Total Beds: 340

Accident and Emergency M A Ansari

Anaesthetics H B J Fischer, R M Haden, J J McPherson, C Mosieri, C A Pinnock, P V Scott, Dr Smith

Cardiology D W Abban

Care of the Elderly S N Singhal

Dental Surgery A W Harris

Dermatology W F G Tucker

ENT P J E Johnson, J R M Moore

General Medicine D J Carter, L J Libman, P J Lowry, S Singhal, G D Summers, A Vathenen

General Surgery R Brown, J H Burman, Mr Jenkes, C D Rennie, R G Tudor

Haematology D Obeid

Histopathology L Brown, G M Kondratowicz, J Stone

Medical Microbiology H M Cawdery

Neurology C R Barraclough

Obstetrics and Gynaecology J H Elias-Jones, S D Jenkinson, G H Macpherson

Ophthalmology B Das, M J Freeman, S M D Porter, P A Thomas

Orthodontics C Gait

Orthopaedics M A M Arafa, J Bell, O S J Costa, A J Price, L Read

Paediatrics G C Close, C I Fraser, R J Sankey

Pathology P P Brown

Radiology C Dale, J M Elliott, P Holland, F H Jenkins, J L Morgan, C Phillips, S R J Reddy

Radiotherapy A D Stockdale

Urology M J Lancashire

Kidderminster Hospital
Bewdley Road, Kidderminster DY11 6RJ
Tel: 01562 823424 Fax: 01562 825685
Total Beds: 24

Worcestershire Royal Hospital
Charles Hastings Way, Worcester WR5 1DD
Tel: 01905 763333
Total Beds: 550

Accident and Emergency R Johnson, A J E Mulira

Anaesthetics R Alexander, I Davis, M Hardwick, N Jones, J Lee, P W Lord, C Maile, D M Philips, J A Prosser, B Roscoe, N M Rose, C Studd, H Williams

Cardiology D Pitcher

Care of the Elderly C Ashton, R Glennie, C Pycock

Chemical Pathology A J Munro

Chest Disease R A Lewis

Dermatology F Lewis

ENT J E D MacLaren, M Porter

General Medicine N H Dyer, D Jenkins, R A Lewis, S Spencer, S Spencer, M J Webberley

General Psychiatry D Battin, J Doran, G Knowles, E H Richards, J Tarry, J Vaughan, R White

General Surgery J Black, M Corlett, R Downing, N Hickey, S Lake, C Robertson, H T Williams

Genitourinary Medicine A J R Crooks

Haematology A H Sawers, R J Stockley

Medical Microbiology C Constantine, J Webberley

Neurology J A Spillane

Neurophysiology A E Blake, A Munro

Obstetrics and Gynaecology B Ruparelia

Ophthalmology R Hall

Oral Surgery N A Barnard, P Earl

Orthodontics D Evans

Orthopaedics J S Davies, K O'Dwyer, P Ratcliffe, D Robinson, E Rouholamin, M Trevett

Paediatrics A P Cole, M Hanlon, B Mason, A S Mills, J E Scanlon

Pathology P J S Dunn, L Smallman, G Smith

Plastic Surgery D S Murray

Psychiatry of Old Age D G J Battin, J E Tarry

Radiology S Bailey, M Brown, J Mould, D Rosewarne, D South, R S Ward

Radiotherapy and Oncology J J Mould

Rheumatology A Rai, I F Rowe

Thoracic Surgery F J Collins

Urology T Chen

Worcestershire Mental Health Partnership NHS Trust

Isaac Maddox House, Shrub Hill Road, Worcester WR4 9RW
Tel: 01905 681511 Fax: 01905 681515
Website: www.worcestershirehealth.nhs.uk
(West Midlands South Strategic Health Authority)

Chair John Calvert
Chief Executive Sue Hunt, Ros Keeton
Consultants Richard Crellin, William Monteiro, Oryst Wychrij

Brook Haven Mental Health Unit
Stourbridge Road, Bromsgrove B61 0BB
Tel: 01527 488279
Total Beds: 18

Manager Hugh McGlinchey

Hill Crest
Quinneys Lane, Redditch B98 7WG
Tel: 01527 500575 Fax: 01527 500519
Total Beds: 25

Manager Nick Bushell

Princess of Wales Community Hospital
Stourbridge Road, Bromsgrove B61 0BB
Tel: 01527 488027 Fax: 01527 574857
Total Beds: 20

Rowan Day Hospital
Smallwood House, Church Green West, Redditch B97 4BD
Tel: 01527 488620

Worthing and Southlands Hospitals NHS Trust

Worthing Hospital, Lyndhurst Road, Worthing BN11 2DH
Tel: 01903 205111 Fax: 01903 285045
Email: firstname.surname@wash.nhs.uk
Website: www.worthinghospital.nhs.uk
(Surrey and Sussex Strategic Health Authority)

Chair Stuart Heatherington
Chief Executive Stephen Cass

Southlands Hospital
Upper Shoreham Road, Shoreham-by-Sea BN43 6TQ
Tel: 01273 455622 Fax: 01273 446042
Website: www.worthinghospital.nhs.uk
Total Beds: 150

Dermatology P Coburn (Head), J Hextall, A Woollons

Genitourinary Medicine A T Nayagam (Head)

Neurophysiology C P Chandrasekera

Orthopaedics D Clark, J Edge, A C Jarvis, J Lewis, D Llewellyn-Clark, K Narang, S Palmer, S Palmer

Rheumatology and Rehabilitation M D Chard, S Mpofu

Worthing Hospital
Lyndhurst Road, Worthing BN11 2DH
Tel: 01903 205111 Fax: 01903 285045
Website: www.worthinghospital.nhs.uk
Total Beds: 460

Accident and Emergency M Grocutt (Head), S Brady, M Jackson

Anaesthetics R Albertyn, S Anderson, E Chojnowska, R Edwards, W Hauf, C Jenkins, N Lavies, J O'Dwyer, S Panayiotou, C Spring, P Sweet, D Uncles, R Venn, H Wakeling, R Waters, S Weber, A C Williams

Care of the Elderly J Kelly, H O'Neal, R Tozer, A-L Yeo

ENT M Harries, J H Topham, J Weighill

Gastroenterology J Bull, L Grellier, A Sinha, P Thatcher, K Thompson

General Medicine M Signy (Head), H J M Bull, G Caldwell, P Carr, J Congleton, J A Evans, L Forni, L Grellier, B Kneale, S Mpofu, N Pegge, A Sinha, K Steele, K Thompson, K Webb-Peploe, U Weis

General Surgery M Baig, R C Beard, A Johri, T Liston, A Miles, A Salman, M Sayegh, K Singh, S Woodhams, W Woods

Neurology R Chalmers, R Clifford-Jones

Obstetrics and Gynaecology J English, F Pakarian, R Pyper, M Rymer

Ophthalmology P D Fox, C H Kon, T Niyadurupola, S Rassam, M Teimory

Oral and Maxillofacial Surgery C Pratt (Head), J Clark, D W Macpherson, J R L Vincent-Townend, A Wilson

Orthodontics J Clarke, A M Hall

Paediatrics S Nicholls (Head), S Coldwell, A Garg, A Mathew, J Rabbs, P Shute

Pathology M Appleton, J Bates, J Child, J Grant, A O'Driscoll, C L Rist, K M Roberts, A W W Roques, J Southgate

Radiology N Davies, D G Hall, M Hinchcliffe, A McKinnon, M Murray, L Rockall, H Seymour, D Withers

Radiotherapy and Oncology G Newman (Head), D Bloomfield, S Mitra, A Webb

Rheumatology and Rehabilitation M D Chard, S Mpofu

Urology R Beard (Head), T Liston, S Woodhams

Wrightington, Wigan and Leigh NHS Trust

The Elms, Royal Albert Edward Infirmary, Wigan Lane, Wigan WN1 2NN
Tel: 01942 244000 Fax: 01942 822042
Email: firstname.surname@wiganlhs-tr.nwest.nhs.uk
Website: www.wwl.nhs.uk
(Greater Manchester Strategic Health Authority; Cumbria and Lancashire Strategic Health Authority)

Chair Brian Strett
Chief Executive Sheena Cumiskey

Leigh Infirmary

The Avenue, Leigh WN7 1HS
Tel: 01942 672333 Fax: 01942 264388
Total Beds: 87

Anaesthetics D J Allan, J Aslam, P G Coloner, G Field, N W Flatt, P Ford, R Foster, R G Ghaly, V Jaitly, I W Jones, F Koussa, R Saad, P Venkataraman

Care of the Elderly A N Khan, A Kumar, S R Nandi

Dental Surgery I D Campbell, R E Lloyd

Dermatology E Stewart, J Yell

ENT S K Banerjee, D Murphy, C Nsamba

General Medicine D Lewis, V Mani, A O Molajo, N Naqvi, A G Wardman

General Surgery M C Holbrook, J Mosley, W D Richmond

Neurology S Duncan

Obstetrics and Gynaecology C J Chandler, R M El Gawley, C P Harris, R H Martin

Ophthalmology D Banerjee, J S Chawla, S Mars

Orthopaedics M S Bell, A O Browne, P W Hopcroft, B Livingstone

Paediatrics A S Ahuja, R Downes

Pathology D Barker, M Bhavnani, C Faris, U Hatimy, J Marples, J Marples, S Mills, R Nelson, K Pendry

Psychiatry N Bano, M Chowdhury, D Kohen, A A Malik, S Malik, B P Maragakis, B K Rathod, D Sena, J G Thomas

Radiology S Augustine, E J Corkan, S Desai, T Houghton, C L Poon, S Ramachadran, P Rodgers, D Temperley, S D Watson

Rheumatology D R Swinson

Urology W D Richmond

Royal Albert Edward Infirmary

Wigan Lane, Wigan WN1 2NN
Tel: 01942 244000 Fax: 01942 822042
Total Beds: 438

Manager Brian Moore

Accident and Emergency D Harbourne, A Pinto

Anaesthetics D J Allan, J Alsam, P G Coloner, G Field, NW Flatt, R Foster, P J Galea, V Jaitty, I W Jones, F Koussa, R Saad, P Venkataraman

Dental Surgery I D Campbell

Dermatology E Stewart, J Yell

ENT M S Izzat, B N Kumar, V B Pothula

General Medicine C M Bate, D Lewis, V Mani, A Molajo, N Naqvi, D J Tymms, A G Wardman, R J Wolstenholme

General Psychiatry A A Malik, B P Maragakis, B K Rathod, G Thomas

General Surgery A Blower, C Campbell, R Gupta, R N Harland, M C Holbrook, M Jamel, N McKenzie, J Mosley

Genitourinary Medicine J A Forrer

Neurology J Susman

Neurosurgery R A Cowie, J Leggate, C West

Obstetrics and Gynaecology A Bellis, C J Chandler, R M El Gawley, C P Harris, P A Lewis, R H Martin

Occupational Health S Kumar

Ophthalmology D Banerjee, C Heaven, S Mars, S Natha, A Siddiqui

Oral Surgery I D Campbell, R Middlehurst

Orthodontics J Brady

Orthopaedics A Gambhir, T Gough, J Mehta, P Rae, B Taura

Paediatrics A S Ahuja, R S Bhadoria, R Downes, J A Fraser, R Greenham, R B McGucken, P Simpson

Pathology D Barker, M Bhavnani, C Faris, U Hatimy, J Marples, J Marples, S Mills, R Nelson, K Pendry

Radiology E J Corkan, S Desai, D Houghton, C L Poon, S Ramachandran, P Rodgers, D Temperley, S D Watson

Radiotherapy E Allen

Rheumatology D R Swinson

Whelley Hospital

Bradshaw Street, Whelley, Wigan WN1 3XD
Tel: 01942 244000 Fax: 01942 822630
Total Beds: 100

Care of the Elderly S Nandi

Occupational Health S Kumar

Rehabilitation Medicine M Eshiett

Wrightington Hospital

Hall Lane, Appley Bridge, Wigan WN6 9EP
Tel: 01257 252211 Fax: 01257 253809
Total Beds: 165

Anaesthetics U Benjamin, J M Frayne, M Jingree, V Koppada, C Martin, M Tittoria

Orthopaedics A Browne, P Burbacks, J F Haines, M J Hayton, J Hodgkinson, A Mohammed, S R Murali, M L Porter, V Raut, J K Stanley, J H Stilwell, I A Trail, P L R Wood

Pathology D Barker, M Bheunani, C Faris, U Hatimy, J Marples, S Mills, R Nelson, K Penrdy

Radiology S Augustine, J Corkan, S Desai, T Houghton, C L Poon, S Ramachandran, P Rogers, D Temperley, S D Watson

Rheumatology C Chattopadhyay, J Davidson, D M Grennan, A Hassan

Wycombe Primary Care Trust

Rapid House, 40 Oxford Road, High Wycombe HP11 2EE
Tel: 01494 552200 Fax: 01494 522046
Email: enquiries@wycombe-pct.nhs.uk
Website: www.wycombe-pct.nhs.uk
(Thames Valley Strategic Health Authority)

Chair Stewart George
Chief Executive Paul Bennett

Wyre Forest Primary Care Trust

7th Floor, Brook House, Kidderminster Hospital, Bewdley Road, Kidderminster DY11 6RJ
Tel: 01562 826329 Fax: 01562 862767
Email: wyreforest.pct@wyreforest-pct.nhs.uk
Website: www.worcestershirehealth.nhs.uk/WFPCT/
(West Midlands South Strategic Health Authority)

Chair David Priestnall
Chief Executive Eamonn Kelly

Wyre Primary Care Trust

Derby Road, Wesham, Preston PR4 3AL
Tel: 01253 306302 Fax: 01253 306306
Website: www.wyrepct.org.uk
(Cumbria and Lancashire Strategic Health Authority)

Chair Ray Pigott
Chief Executive Doug Soper

York Hospitals NHS Trust

York Hospital, Wigginton Road, York YO31 8HE
Tel: 01904 631313
Email: tracey.dixon@york.nhs.uk
Website: www.yorkhospitals.nhs.uk
(North and East Yorkshire and Northern Lincolnshire Strategic Health Authority)

Chair Alan K Maynard
Chief Executive Jim Easton

St Helens Nelson Court

1A Nelson Lane, Tadcaster Road, York YO24 1HD
Tel: 01904 700651

White Cross Court

Wilson Drive, Huntington Road, York YO31 8FT
Tel: 01904 641464

York District Hospital

Wigginton Road, York YO31 8HE
Tel: 01904 631313
Total Beds: 824

Accident and Emergency M J Williams (Head), S Crane, M F Gibson, G Kitching, M J Williams

Anaesthetics P Hall (Head), J Jackson (Head), T Madej (Head), G Priestley (Head), C Barr, G Cundill, S Forde, R M Grummitt, P Hall, R C Johnson, S Old, H Paw, M K Reeder, R W H Skilton, P Stone, P Toomey, W Watson, B Williams, J Wilson, I Woods

Care of the Elderly A Corlett, J Coyle, D Heseltine, D Kasavan, A McEvoy

Dermatology A Highett (Head), C Henderson, A S Highet, C Lyon, A Myatt, J M Stainforth

ENT A R Grace, A Nicolaides, P G Reilly

General Medicine A Turnbull (Head), R M Boyle, R Crook, A M Hunter, P Jennings, C Jones, S Kelly, S Megarry, M Pye, J C Thow, J Turvill, J E White

General Surgery S G Brooks, S H Leveson, J B Mancey-Jones, A McCleary, G V Miller, S Nicholson

Genitourinary Medicine I Fairley, S Ralph

Neurophysiology H K C Laljee

Neurosciences P Duffy (Head), P M Crawford, P O Duffey, A Heald

Obstetrics and Gynaecology R W Hunter, E J Mattock, S Mitchell, D W Pring, C S Tuck

Ophthalmology J M Haywood (Head), R Taylor (Head), R Ellingham, P J Jacobs, T D Manners, R Taylor

Oral and Maxillofacial Surgery M Telfer (Head), A Coatesworth, J Taylor, P Whitfield

Orthodontics P M Jenkins (Head)

Orthopaedics P G d Boer, P Campbell, A J Gibbon, C A N McLaren, H R Williams

Otolaryngology M Benamer, A Nicolaides, Mr Reilly

Paediatrics R Ball, D W Beverley, M J Harran, A M Kelly, D Smith

Pathology A W Anderson (Head), C Bates (Head), L Bond (Head), A Clarke (Head), A M T Clarke, M R Howard, P R Maheswaran, I N Reid, N Todd

Radiology A Murphy (Head), J Cooper, J Hazelden, C N J Jenkins, D J King, K Kingston, R Mannion, M E Porte

Rheumatology and Rehabilitation M Iveson (Head), J M Iveson

Urology G Urwin (Head), K Seenivasgam, M J Stower, G H Urwin

Women's Health J Dwyer, A Evans, R W Hunter, E J Mattock, S Mitchell, D W Pring

Yorkshire Wolds and Coast Primary Care Trust

Health House, Grange Park Lane, Willerby, Hull HU10 6DT
Tel: 01482 650700 Fax: 01482 672176
Email: emma.jones@ywcpct.nhs.uk
(North and East Yorkshire and Northern Lincolnshire Strategic Health Authority)

Chair Karen Knapron
Chief Executive Adrian Smith
Consultants Delyth Wyn-Jones

Alfred Bean Hospital

Bridlington Road, Driffield YO25 7JR
Tel: 01377 241124
Total Beds: 20

Care of the Elderly M A Nasar

Dermatology Dr Stainforth

ENT Dr Baker, S L Smith

General Medicine P M Brown, Dr Pond

General Psychiatry D Armstrong, A Talbot

General Surgery Dr Duthie, J N Fox, K Wedgewood

Obstetrics and Gynaecology R Yeo

Ophthalmology S K Datta, B K De, S Setty

Orthopaedics Dr Bryant, A D North

Paediatrics J L Nicholas, Dr Skelton, Dr Venkatesh

Radiotherapy and Oncology M Holmes

Rheumatology W Tomlinson

Urology K Brame

Hornsea Cottage Hospital
Eastgate, Hornsea HU18 1PL
Tel: 01964 533146, 01964 535563 Fax: 01964 534273
Total Beds: 22

Withernsea Community Hospital
Queen's Street, Withernsea HU19 2PZ
Tel: 01964 614666 Fax: 01964 615238
Total Beds: 22

Scotland

NHS Argyll and Clyde, Acute Services Division

Formerly Argyll and Clyde Acute Hospitals NHS Trust.

c/o NHS Argyll and Clyde, Ross House, Hawkhead Road, Paisley PA2 7BN
Tel: 0141 842 7200 Fax: 0141 848 1414
(NHS Argyll and Clyde)

Inverclyde Royal Hospital
Larkfield Road, Greenock PA16 0XN
Tel: 01475 633777 Fax: 01475 636753
Total Beds: 368

Anaesthetics A Ahmed, O P Maini, F Munro, M Simmons, M C Thomas, D Thomson, T J Winning

Biochemistry A McConnell

Dermatology C Fitzsimons, M Young

ENT R J McGuinness, I C Paton

General Medicine G Curry, J B Dilawari, A Mackay, D A S Marshall, H Papaconstaninou, P Semple, J E Thomson

General Surgery G Bell, J J Morrice, G Orr, J Reidy, I Watt

Genitourinary Medicine R Nandwani

Haematology D L Ellis, G Rainey

Medical Microbiology A E Biggs

Neurology R Petty

Obstetrics and Gynaecology G S Anthony, L Cassidy, J Robins

Ophthalmology S R Gupta, D Mansfield

Orthodontics B D Collin

Orthopaedics S Barnes, M Di Paola, T K Ghosh, G McGarrity, R Venner

Paediatrics G Hunt, O Kurian, R C Shepherd

Pathology M Seywright, M A Thomas

Plastic Surgery M Webster

Radiology F P Kelly, A Ramsay, R Shaw, P F Walsh

Lorn and Islands District General Hospital
Glengallan Road, Oban PA34 4HH
Tel: 01631 567500 Fax: 01631 567134
Total Beds: 138

Anaesthetics A Murchison, J Walker, C Wilson

Care of the Elderly G G Garabet

General Medicine A F Henderson, A K Henderson

General Surgery D Scobie, S N Yadav

Royal Alexandra Hospital
Corsebar Road, Paisley PA2 9PN
Tel: 0141 887 9111 Fax: 0141 887 6701
Email: Karen.Murray@rah.scot.nhs.uk
Website: www.show.scot.nhs.uk/rah
Total Beds: 596

Accident and Emergency C Allister, L Hislop, G McNaughton, R Marshall, F Russell

Adult Medicine A Dorward, I Findlay, J Gravil, J Hinnie, W Hislop, S Hood, P Macintyre

Anaesthetics H Aitken, J J Canning, S Chaudhri, F Davies, J Dickson, G Fletcher, T Goudie, T Ireland, E James, R L McDevitt, S Madsen, J E Orr, B M Scorgie, R Simpson, M Smith

Biochemistry P Stromberg

Care of the Elderly C Leslie, D Mack, G Simpson, A Uni, C Wilkieson

Dermatology C P Fitzsimons, I Hay, M J Young

ENT R J McGuinness, C Murray, I C Paton, A White

General Medicine A J Dorward, I Findlay, B M Fisher, J Gravil, W S Hislop, P McIntyre, J McPeake

General Surgery J McCourtney, A J McEwan, M McKirdy, K G Mitchell, C Porteous, B W A Williamson

Haematology P McKay, M Robertson

Medical Microbiology A Eastaway

Obstetrics and Gynaecology J A Gemmell, K C Muir, A Quinn, G Sarkar, A Thomson

Ophthalmology H Bennett, L Esakowitz, S B Murray, L Webb

Orthodontics K H Moore

Orthopaedics D A R Aaron, I J Cartlidge, S Chitnis, C Kumar, N Kumar, S Smith

Paediatrics G Hunt, L Nairn, M Ray, R C Shepherd, G Stewart

Pathology W Candlish, S Dahill, C Sutherland

Radiology C Adams, C Alexander, L P Cram, M L Davies, J Negrette, L Semple, M Stevenson, A Wallace

Urology L Morton

Vale of Leven Hospital
Main Street, Alexandria G83 0UA
Tel: 01389 754121 Fax: 01389 755948
Total Beds: 255

Anaesthetics T Barber, A E Cameron, G Douglas, W R Easy, A M Tully

Cardiology M N Al-Khafaji

Clinical Biochemistry J Series

Cytopathology H Scullion

Dermatology J Thomson

ENT L Cooke, D G Garrick

General Medicine M Al-Khafaji, H Al-Shamma, H A Carmichael, D McCruden

General Psychiatry M Al-Mousawi, F Coulter, I McClure, I McIvor, K Towlson

General Surgery P Finn, E W Taylor

Haematology P Clarke

Medical Microbiology S Dancer

Obstetrics and Gynaecology A S Clark, M J Haxton, N Kenyon

Paediatrics M Ray, G Stewart

Pathology F Forbes, E L Murray, M Reid

Radiology J McGlinchey

NHS Argyll and Clyde, Lomond and Argyll Community Services Division

Formerly Lomond and Argyll Primary Care NHS Trust.

c/o NHS Argyll and Clyde, Ross House, Hawkhead Road, Paisley PA2 7BN
Tel: 0141 842 7200 Fax: 0141 848 1414
(NHS Argyll and Clyde)

Chair I Miller
Chief Executive K Murray

Argyll and Bute Hospital
Blarbuie Road, Lochgilphead PA31 8LD
Tel: 01546 602323
Total Beds: 181

General Psychiatry F M Corrigan, G M Fergusson, A V P Mackay, R Sandler, P Thompson

Campbeltown Hospital
Ralston Road, Campbeltown PA28 6LE
Tel: 01586 552224 Fax: 01586 554966
Total Beds: 62

Dumbarton Cottage Hospital
Towned Road, Dumbarton G82
Tel: 01389 763151

Dumbarton Joint Hospital
Cardross Road, Dumbarton G82 5JA
Tel: 01389 762317 Fax: 01389 764677
Total Beds: 42

Dunaros Hospital
Salen, Aros, Isle of Mull PA72 6JF
Tel: 01680 300392

Dunoon General Hospital
Sandbank Road, Dunoon PA23 7RL
Tel: 01369 704341 Fax: 01369 702192
Total Beds: 84

Manager S Munro

Islay Hospital
Gortonvoggie Road, Bowmore PA43 7JD
Tel: 01496 810219 Fax: 01496 810754
Total Beds: 26

Lorn and Islands District General Hospital
Glengallen Road, Oban PA34 4HH
Tel: 01631 567500

Mid-Argyll Hospital
Blarbuie Road, Lochgilphead PA31 8JZ
Tel: 01546 602952 Fax: 01546 606500
Total Beds: 47

Vale of Leven District General Hospital
Main Street, Alexandria G83 0UA
Tel: 01389 754121

Victoria Hospital, Isle of Bute
High Street, Rothesay PA20 9JJ
Tel: 01700 503938 Fax: 01700 502865
Total Beds: 24

Victoria Hospital Annexe
High Street, Rothesay PA20 9JH
Tel: 01700 502943 Fax: 01700 505147
Total Beds: 31

Care of the Elderly P Lawson

Victoria Infirmary
93 East King Street, Helensburgh G84 7BU
Tel: 01436 672158 Fax: 01436 672159
Total Beds: 36

Care of the Elderly N T Manning

NHS Argyll and Clyde, Renfrewshire and Inverclyde Community Services Division

Formerly Renfrewshire and Inverclyde Primary Care NHS Trust.

c/o NHS Argyll and Clyde, Ross House, Hawkhead Road, Paisley PA2 7BN
Tel: 0141 842 7200
(NHS Argyll and Clyde)

Chair G Harcus
Chief Executive A Stafford

Dykebar Hospital
Grahamston Road, Paisley PA2 7DE
Tel: 0141 884 5122 Fax: 0141 884 5425
Total Beds: 332

General Psychiatry D A Bonham, J M Dingwall, J Gallacher, A Jones, S Miller, A J Naismith, M Smith, J Thompson

Psychiatry of Old Age A Hughes, H Livingston, K Philips

Hawkhead Hospital
Hawkhead Road, Paisley PA2 7BL
Tel: 0141 889 8151 Fax: 0141 848 7372
Total Beds: 96

Child and Adolescent Psychiatry N Speirs

General Psychiatry A Hughes

Johnstone Hospital
Bridge of Weir Road, Johnstone PA5 8YX
Tel: 01505 331471 Fax: 01505 336497
Total Beds: 104

Care of the Elderly D Mack, G K Simpson, C Wilkieson

General Psychiatry A Hughes

Merchiston Hospital
Brookfield, Johnstone PA5 8TY
Tel: 01505 328261 Fax: 01505 335803
Total Beds: 176

General Psychiatry A Deering, S Groves, R A D Sykes

Ravenscraig Hospital
Inverkip Road, Greenock PA16 9HA
Tel: 01475 733777 Fax: 01475 721547

Total Beds: 230

Care of the Elderly P Lawson, R E Young

Royal Alexandra Hospital (Care of the Elderly)
Corsebar Road, Paisley PA2 9PN
Tel: 0141 887 9111 Fax: 0141 887 6701
Total Beds: 130

General Psychiatry A Deering, S Groves, H Small, R A D Sykes

NHS Ayrshire and Arran, Community Health Division

Formerly Ayrshire and Arran Primary Care NHS Trust.

c/o NHS Ayrshire and Arran, Boswell House, 10 Arthur Street, Ayr KA7 1QJ
Tel: 01292 611040 Fax: 01292 286762
(NHS Ayrshire and Arran)

Chair Gordon Wilson
Chief Executive Allan Gunning

Ailsa Hospital
Dalmellington Road, Ayr KA6 6AB
Tel: 01292 610556 Fax: 01292 513027
Total Beds: 280

General Psychiatry C Aryiku, E Bennie, J Berry, W Creaney, R De Mey, J A Flowerdew, N Hoderet, T Johnston, C Lind, B Martin, J Stewart

Arran War Memorial Hospital
Lamlash, Brodick KA27 8LE
Tel: 01770 600777 Fax: 01770 600445
Total Beds: 22

Ayrshire Central Hospital (Psychiatric Unit)
Kilwinning Road, Irvine KA12 8SS
Tel: 01294 274191 Fax: 01294 278680
Total Beds: 36

General Psychiatry J Barbour, D Gallagher, S McNulty

Brooksby House Hospital
Greenock Road, Largs KA30 8NE
Tel: 01475 672285 Fax: 01475 672439
Total Beds: 18

Crosshouse Hospital (Psychiatric Unit)
Kilmarnock Road, Kilmarnock KA2 0BE
Tel: 01563 521133
Total Beds: 58

Davidson Cottage Hospital
Girvan KA26 9DS
Tel: 01465 712571 Fax: 01465 714382
Total Beds: 26

Manager Neil Mellon

East Ayrshire Community Hospital
Ayr Road, Cumnock KA18 1EF
Tel: 01290 429429
Total Beds: 74

Manager Janet Shankland

Garnock Day Hospital
Ayrshire Central Hospital, Irvine KA12 8SS
Tel: 01294 323050 Fax: 01294 311747

Holmhead Hospital
Cumnock KA18 1RR
Tel: 01290 422220 Fax: 01290 423589
Total Beds: 56

Kirklandside Hospital
Kilmarnock KA1 5LH
Tel: 01563 525172 Fax: 01563 575408
Total Beds: 85

Lady Margaret Hospital
College Street, Millport KA28 0HF
Tel: 01475 530307 Fax: 01475 530117
Total Beds: 14

Maybole Day Hospital
Maybole KA19 7BY
Tel: 01655 882211 Fax: 01655 889698

NHS Ayrshire and Arran, General Hospitals Division

Formerly Ayrshire and Arran Acute Hospitals NHS Trust.

c/o NHS Ayrshire and Arran, Boswell House, 10 Arthur Street, Ayr KA7 1QJ
Tel: 01292 611040 Fax: 01292 286762
(NHS Ayrshire and Arran)

Chair Martin Cheyne
Chief Executive Jim Currie

Ayr Hospital
Dalmellington Road, Ayr KA6 6DX
Tel: 01292 610555 Fax: 01292 288952
Total Beds: 348

Accident and Emergency F Gibson, T Hand

Anaesthetics D Ryan (Head), L Fell, R Jackson, I MacDiarmid, K MacKenzie, R McMahon, B Meiklejohn, I Taylor, P Wylie

Biochemistry M Lough

Care of the Elderly J M Blair, G Nicol, A G Watt

Dermatology R A Hardie

General Medicine A Collier, M Duncan, J A Elliott, J D Gemmill, P M G Reynolds, J D R Rose, S Woldman

General Surgery S Boom, A L Forster, C J Simpson, G Stewart, D Wallace, C Wilson

Haematology P Eynaud, P Vosylius

Ophthalmology A Gaskell, I T Hanna, B Hutchison, S Maharajan, S S Sidiki, A Singh, D Teenan

Oral Surgery A Carton, S Hislop

Orthodontics J R Pilley

Orthopaedics D Large, A Muirhead, H E Potts, P S Rae, K Young

Paediatrics M Blair, S Kinmond, J P McClure, C Morrison

Radiology K N A Osborne

Rheumatology M R Duncan, P Reynolds

Urology N Al-Saffar, M Gurun, G Hollins, R Meddings

Ayrshire Central Hospital
Kilwinning Road, Irvine KA12 8SS
Tel: 01294 274191 Fax: 01294 278680
Total Beds: 252

Care of the Elderly G Duncan, J B W Godfrey, H McMillan

Obstetrics and Gynaecology C H Baird, H G Dobbie, D H Gibson, G Irvine, D H W McKay, E B Melrose, S M M Prigg, T V N Russell

Paediatrics S Kinmond, J Staines

Rehabilitation Medicine P Mattison

Biggart Hospital

Biggart Road, Prestwick KA9 2HQ
Tel: 01292 470611 Fax: 01292 614546
Total Beds: 165

Care of the Elderly J M Blair, V Nicol, A Watt

Crosshouse Hospital

Crosshouse, Kilmarnock KA2 0BE
Tel: 01563 521133 Fax: 01563 572496
Total Beds: 540

Accident and Emergency A Lannigan, J Stevenson

Anaesthetics A R Michie (Head), J Chestnut, A Devine, C Hawksworth, P J Hildebrand, P Korsah, C S Lawrie, C Martin, T D Miller, S Morris, H Neill, M K Shaw, R J White, P A Wilson, R K B Young, S Zimmer

Biochemistry D Boag, M Lough

Care of the Elderly G Duncan, J B W Godfrey, H McMillan, M Palchaudhur

Dermatology J A Craig, C Dwyer, R A Hardie

ENT J H Dempster, A Murray, E M Shanks, P Wardrop

General Medicine A Taha (Head), A Taha (Head), K Anderson, S Ferguson, H Hartung, A Innes, M MacGregor, I G Mackay, J N MacPherson, D O'Neill, A Shah, N Velasco, G R Williams

General Surgery R H Diament, J R McGregor, C G Morran, A Newland, M Osman, B A Sugden, P Whitford

Haematology J G Erskine, P Eynaud, M McColl, P Vosylius

Medical Microbiology G W Downie, R Hardie, A MacDonald

Oral Surgery W J R Currie, W S Hislop

Orthodontics D Morrant, J R Pilley

Orthopaedics G R Tait (Head), B Fitzgerald, M I Foxworthy, I Mackay, C MacLeod, R Short, B Syme

Paediatrics M Blair, Dr Kinmond, J P McClure, Dr Staines

Pathology N E Cunningham (Head), M R Adamson, I Graham, J Lang, A Milne, E R Nairn, E Walker

Radiology M A H McMillan (Head), N Corrigan, P Crumlish, W M F Dean, E Lindsay, G McLaughlan, D Rawlings

NHS Borders, General Hospital Division

Formerly Borders General Hospital NHS Trust.

c/o NHS Borders, Newstead, Melrose TD6 9DB
Tel: 01896 825500 Fax: 01896 825580
(NHS Borders)

Borders General Hospital

Melrose TD6 9BD
Tel: 01896 826000 Fax: 01896 823476
Website: www.show.scot.nhs.uk/bgh
Total Beds: 322

Accident and Emergency J E Phillips

Anaesthetics R C Beighton, J M Braidwood, T C Cripps, N P Leary, D Love, J N Montgomery, C Richard, I Yellowlees

Cardiology P Neary

Care of the Elderly P A Maguire, C A Norris, P D Syme

Child and Adolescent Psychiatry S Davies, S Glen

Dermatology C Benton, D Kemmet

ENT M Armstrong, S Moralee

General Medicine F Bollert, O E Eade, J Fletcher, J Gaddie, P J Leslie

General Surgery J M Gollock, R Halpin, M Hosny, J S O'Neill

Haematology K Gelly, A Hung, J Tucker

Obstetrics and Gynaecology R Campbell, A J Gordon, J E Lowles, B Magowan

Ophthalmology R I Murray, W F I Shepherd

Oral Surgery M Ross

Orthodontics M Ross

Orthopaedics C B Clowes, W G Dennyson, J E Phillips, G H Tiemessen

Paediatrics A Duncan, A C F Margerison, J C Stephens

Palliative Medicine J Rodgers

Pathology S Bennett

Radiology D Hardwick, H McRitchie, A J Pearson, J Reid

Urology I Mitchell

Borders Geriatric Day Hospital

Borders General Hospital, Melrose TD6 9BS
Tel: 01896 754333 Ext: 1222 Fax: 01896 823476
Website: www.show.scot.nhs.uk/bgh

NHS Borders, Primary Care Division

Formerly Borders Primary Care NHS Trust.

c/o NHS Borders, Newstead, Melrose TD6 9DB
Tel: 01896 825500 Fax: 01896 825580
(NHS Borders)

Coldstream Cottage Hospital

Kelso Road, Coldstream TD12 4LQ
Tel: 01890 882417 Fax: 01890 883954
Total Beds: 14

Eyemouth Day Hospital (Geriatric)

Houndlaw Park, Eyemouth TD14 5DA
Tel: 01890 751101

Firholm Day Unit (Elderly with Dementia)

Innerleithen Road, Peebles EH45 8BD
Tel: 01721 720544 Fax: 01721 724063

Gala Day Unit (Elderly with Dementia)

10 Sime Place, Galashiels TD1 1ST
Tel: 01896 754669 Fax: 01896 754669

Hawick Cottage Hospital

Buccleuch Road, Hawick TD9 0EJ
Tel: 01450 372162 Fax: 01450 373935
Total Beds: 24

Hawick Day Hospital (Geriatric)

Buccleuch Road, Hawick TD9 0EJ
Tel: 01450 370000

Haylodge Day Hospital (Geriatric)
Neidpath Road, Peebles EH45 8JG
Tel: 01721 722080

Haylodge Hospital
Neidpath Road, Peebles EH45 8JG
Tel: 01721 722080
Total Beds: 46

Kelso Day Hospital (Geriatric)
Inch Road, Kelso TD5 7JP
Tel: 01573 225779

Kelso Hospital
Inch Road, Kelso TD5 7JP
Tel: 01573 223441 Fax: 01573 225321
Total Beds: 35

Knoll Day Hospital (Geriatric)
Station Road, Duns TD11 3EL
Tel: 01361 883373

Knoll Hospital
Station Road, Duns TD11 3EL
Tel: 01361 883373 Fax: 01361 882186
Total Beds: 27

Princes Street Day Unit (Adult Mental Illness)
Princes Street, Hawick TD9 7EJ
Tel: 01450 377515 Fax: 01450 373425

Priorsford Day Unit (Adult Mental Illness)
Tweed Green, Peebles EH45 8AR
Tel: 01721 723701 Fax: 01721 724052

Sister Margaret Cottage Hospital
Castlegate, Jedburgh TD8 6QD
Tel: 01835 863212 Fax: 01835 864917
Total Beds: 9

West Port Day Unit (Elderly with Dementia)
Drumlanrig Square, Hawick TD9 OBG
Tel: 01450 378028 Fax: 01450 373482

NHS Dumfries and Galloway

See also separate entry under Health Authorities and Boards.

Crichton Hall, Bankend Road, Dumfries DG1 4TG
Tel: 01387 246246 Fax: 01387 252375
(NHS Dumfries and Galloway)

Chair John Ross
Chief Executive John Burns

Allanbank
Bankend Road, Dumfries
Tel: 01387 249935
Email: euan.macleod@allanbank.force9.co.uk
Total Beds: 48

Manager Euan MacLeod

Annan Day Hospital
Stapleton Road, Annan DG12 6NQ
Tel: 01461 202017 Fax: 01461 201581

Manager C Brockie

Annan Hospital
Stapleton Road, Annan DG12 6NQ
Tel: 01461 203425 Fax: 01461 201581
Total Beds: 24

Manager C Brockie

Castle Douglas Day Hospital
Academy Street, Castle Douglas DG7 1EF
Tel: 01556 502333 Fax: 01556 502370
Total Beds: 8

Manager Elma Hogg

Castle Douglas Hospital
Academy Street, Castle Douglas DG7 1EF
Tel: 01556 502333 Fax: 01556 502370
Total Beds: 21

Manager Elma Hogg

Crichton Royal Hospital
Crichton Hall, Bankend Road, Dumfries DG1 4TG
Tel: 01387 244000 Fax: 01381 247706
Total Beds: 371

General Psychiatry J Graham, D Hall, J Leuvenninic, R McCreadie, A McFadyen, J Mackie, G Morrison, E Powell, R M Slinn, J Waterhouse, E R M Wood

Dalrymple Day Hospital
Dalrymple Street, Stranraer DG9 7DQ
Tel: 01776 706900 Fax: 01776 706918
Total Beds: 10

Manager Gwen McGowan

Dalrymple Hospital
Stranraer DG9 7DQ
Tel: 01776 702323 Fax: 01776 706918
Total Beds: 26

Manager Gwen McGowan

Dumfries and Galloway Royal Infirmary
Bankend Road, Dumfries DG1 4AP
Tel: 01387 246246 Fax: 01387 241639
Total Beds: 392

Accident and Emergency J W Burton (Head)

Anaesthetics D R Ball, D B Bennie, H A Brewster, R Meek, J Palmer, V Perkins, J Rutherford, N T B Watson, D Williams

Bacteriology F J Bone, B S Dale

Biochemistry J R Paterson

Care of the Elderly I Hay, G Rhind

Dental Surgery Mr Aird (Head)

Dermatology J F B Norris (Head), J F B Norris

ENT E Flint, B Joshi, S Metcalfe

General Medicine S Cross, F Green, C G Isles, G Jones, M McMahon, P Rafferty, G W Tait

General Surgery C Auld, I M Muir, A D F Walls

Haematology A Stark (Head), A Stark, F Toolis

Obstetrics and Gynaecology Dr Saha (Head), H Currie, Dr Hallifa, A McCullough, P K A Mensah, Dr Saha, S J Wisdom

Ophthalmology G J Bedford, B J Power

Orthodontics J C Aird

Orthopaedics P Costigan, I McLean, G Nimon, A C Ogden, A Ratnam, K Saad

Paediatrics A Chapman, M Higgs, R M Simpson, R B Thomson

Palliative Medicine L Martin

Pathology W Candlish, I Gibson, A M Lutfy

Radiology D Hill, D N Jones, P Kelly, P Law

Radiotherapy and Oncology I H Kunkler

Rehabilitation Medicine R Holden

Rheumatology M J McMahon

Urology M Shearer

Garrick Hospital
Edinburgh Road, Stranraer DG9 7HQ
Tel: 01776 702323

Kirkcudbright Hospital
Kirkcudbright DG6 4BE
Tel: 01557 330549 Fax: 01557 331825
Total Beds: 14

Manager Elma Hogg

Lochmaben Day Hospital
Lochmaben, Lockerbie DG11 1RQ
Tel: 01387 810255 Fax: 01387 810613
Total Beds: 6

Manager Graham Haining

Lochmaben Hospital
Lochmaben, Lockerbie DG11 1RQ
Tel: 01387 810255 Fax: 01387 810613
Total Beds: 16

Manager Graham Haining

Care of the Elderly M Ullah

Moffat Day Hospital
Moffat DG10 9JY
Tel: 01683 220031 Fax: 01683 220539
Total Beds: 20

Manager Liz Shannon

Moffat Hospital
Moffat DG10 9JY
Tel: 01683 220031 Fax: 1683 220539
Total Beds: 12

Newton Stewart Day Hospital
Newton Stewart DG8 6LZ
Tel: 01671 402015 Fax: 01671 402855
Total Beds: 10

Newton Stewart Hospital
Newton Stewart DG8 6LZ
Tel: 01671 402015 Fax: 01671 402855
Total Beds: 22

Thomas Hope Hospital
Market Square, Langholm DG13 0JX
Tel: 01387 380417 Fax: 01387 381428
Total Beds: 12

Manager David Potter

Thornhill Day Hospital
Thornhill DG3 5AA
Tel: 01848 302505
Total Beds: 12

Manager Elspeth Rae

Thornhill Hospital
Thornhill DG3 5AA
Tel: 01848 330205 Fax: 01848 331931
Total Beds: 13

Manager Elspeth Rae

NHS Fife, Acute Hospitals Division

Formerly Fife Acute Hospitals NHS Trust.

c/o NHS Fife, Hayfield House, Hayfield Road, Kirkcaldy KY2 5AH
Tel: 01592 643355 Fax: 01592 648142
(NHS Fife)

Chair David Stewart
Chief Executive John Wilson

Forth Park Maternity Hospital
30 Bennochy Road, Kirkcaldy KY2 5RA
Tel: 01592 643355 Fax: 01592 642376
Total Beds: 106

Queen Margaret Hospital
Whitefield Road, Dunfermline KY12 0SU
Tel: 01383 623623 Fax: 01383 624156
Total Beds: 401

Victoria Hospital
Hayfield Road, Kirkcaldy KY2 5AH
Tel: 01592 643355 Fax: 01592 643355
Total Beds: 366

NHS Fife, Primary Care Division

Formerly Fife Primary Care NHS Trust.

c/o NHS Fife, Hayfield House, Hayfield Road, Kirkcaldy KY2 5AH
Tel: 01592 643355 Fax: 01592 648142
(NHS Fife)

Chair Doreen Bell
Chief Executive Frances Elliot

Adamson Hospital
Bank Street, Cupar KY15 4JG
Tel: 01334 652901
Total Beds: 39

Manager Eleanor Balsillie

Care of the Elderly D Ghosh

General Surgery K Ballantyne

Obstetrics and Gynaecology D Urquhart

Orthopaedics I Weir

Cameron Hospital
Cameron Bridge, Windygates, Leven KY8 5RR
Tel: 01592 712472 Fax: 01592 716442
Total Beds: 128

Rehabilitation Medicine L Sloan (Head)

Rheumatology J Gibson (Head)

Forth Park Hospital
30 Bennochy Road, Kirkcaldy KY2 5RA

Manager Isobel Wood

Care of the Elderly Dr Zaida (Head)

Glenrothes Day Hospital
1 Lodge Rise, Forresters Lodge, Glenrothes KY7 5QT
Tel: 01592 743505 Fax: 01592 753655
Total Beds: 20

Glenrothes Hospital
Lodge Rise, Glenrothes KY7 5TG
Tel: 01592 743505 Fax: 01592 743655
Total Beds: 62

Care of the Elderly R Shenoy

Rehabilitation Medicine L Sloan

Lynebank Hospital
Halbeath Road, Dunfermline KY11 4UW
Tel: 01383 623623 Fax: 01383 621955
Total Beds: 100

Manager Patricia Colville

Learning Disabilities R Logan (Head), F Rodgers

Netherlea Hospital
65 West Road, Newport-on-Tay DD6 8HR
Tel: 01382 543233
Total Beds: 10

Randolph Wemyss Day Hospital
Wellesley Road, Donbeath, Buckhaven, Leven KY8 1HU
Tel: 01592 712427 Fax: 01592 716267
Total Beds: 20

Manager Anne Callaghan

Randolph Wemyss Memorial Hospital
Wellesley Road, Buckhaven, Leven KY8 1HU
Tel: 01592 712427 Fax: 01592 716267
Total Beds: 54

Manager Anne Callaghan

Care of the Elderly A K Datta (Head)

General Medicine I Campbell (Head), D Bhattacharyya, R Cargill, J Chalmers, M Francis, G Petrie, S Rochow, J Wilson

St Andrews Memorial Hospital
Abbey Walk, St Andrews KY16 9LG
Tel: 01334 472327
Total Beds: 34

Orthopaedics R Buxton

Urology J McFarlane

Stratheden Hospital
Cupar KY15 5RR
Tel: 01334 652611 Fax: 01334 656560
Total Beds: 311

Child and Adolescent Psychiatry D Taylor (Head), R Sime

General Psychiatry S Carey, W Dickson, J Murphy, D Neilson, G Stevenson

Weston Day Hospital
West Port, Cupar KY15
Tel: 01334 652163
Total Beds: 30

Whyteman's Brae Day Hospital
Whyteman's Brae, Kirkcaldy KY1 2ND
Tel: 01592 643355 Fax: 01592 640159
Total Beds: 80

Whyteman's Brae Hospital
Whyteman's Brae, Kirkcaldy KY1 2LA
Tel: 01592 643355 Fax: 01592 640159
Total Beds: 108

Care of the Elderly A K Datta, R Shenoy, Dr Ziada

General Medicine S Clark, J Curran, M Falzon, T Glen, D Reid, M Roll, M Stewart

NHS Forth Valley, Acute Operating Division

Formerly Forth Valley Acute Hospitals NHS Trust.

c/o NHS Forth Valley, 33 Spittal Street, Stirling FK8 1DX
Tel: 01786 463031 Fax: 01786 471337
(NHS Forth Valley)

Chair Campbell Christie
Chief Executive Margaret Duffy

Falkirk and District Royal Infirmary
Westburn Avenue, Falkirk FK1 5QE
Tel: 01324 624000 Fax: 01324 617421
Total Beds: 379

Anaesthetics I Broom, R G Law, A McDonald, H Robb, A J Semple, D S Simpson, W J Thomson

Care of the Elderly A C Grant, R J Lenton, E Millar, P Murdoch, I Scougall, J Taylor

Chemical Pathology M Holliday

Dermatology D C Dick, C Morton

ENT D G Keay, J McGarva, A M Pettigrew, N Tin

General Medicine L Buchanan, D Doig, A Hargreaves, P D McSorley, D Morrison, N R Peden, W S J Ruddell, S C Wright

General Surgery A Al-Asadi, N W S Harris, R C Smith

Genitourinary Medicine J N Harvey

Geriatric Medicine A Grant, R J Lenton, E Millar, P S Murdoch, I Scougal

Haematology A D J Birch

Medical Microbiology I King, J McGavigan

Obstetrics and Gynaecology R A Cole, F Crichton, K A Grant, D McQueen, Dr Prabhu

Ophthalmology Dr Gaboor, J D Huggan, Dr Scott

Oral and Maxillofacial Surgery I Holland, J McManners

Orthodontics C M Wood

Orthopaedics J De Leeuw, F Dewolf, J R Lindsay, B Murray

Paediatrics I Abu-Arafeh, Dr Al-Hourani, J Schulga

Pathology K D Morton

Radiology A J Byrne, D Roxburgh, L Stewart

Radiotherapy and Oncology J Cassidy, L MacMillan, J M Russell

Rheumatology and Rehabilitation M Brzeski

Urology M Hehir, M Smith, J Tweedle

Stirling Royal Infirmary
Livilands, Stirling FK8 2AU
Tel: 01786 434000 Fax: 01786 540588
Total Beds: 469

Anaesthetics C R G Crawford, W Mair, C R G Reid, W Richards, A J Trench

Cardiology Dr Bridges

Care of the Elderly P Beausang, Dr Bishop-Miller, D C Kennie, A McKenzie

Chemical Pathology G F Follett

Child and Adolescent Psychiatry C Greenshaw, B Norten, M E N O'Gorman

Cytology D Sprunt

Dermatology D C Dick, C Morton

ENT S Date, D G Keay, J McGarva, A M Pettigrew, N Tin

General Medicine D N Clarke, S Glen, A D Howie, S B M Reith

General Psychiatry R J McIlwaine, D A Pemberton

General Surgery D B Booth, W H S Henry, Mr Jabaar, A Smith

Genitourinary Medicine J N Harvey

Haematology A D J Birch

Medical Microbiology J McGavigan

Neurology C Hall, R Prempeh

Obstetrics and Gynaecology P Holmes, K S McLellan, K McMullen, R Morriston, J D Steven

Ophthalmology J D Huggan, T Saboor, D Scott

Oral and Maxillofacial Surgery I Holland, Mr McManners

Orthodontics R Fowler, P Rimmer

Orthopaedics R D Briggs, G Mackay, I Ritchie, D J Ross

Paediatrics Dr Abu-Arafeh, Dr Al-Doori, Dr Al-Hoorani, Dr Crocket, U MacFadyen, J Schulga

Pathology K D Morton

Radiology H E Cunningham, P McDermot

Radiotherapy and Oncology E J Junor

Urology M Hehir, M Smith, J Tweedle

NHS Forth Valley, Primary Care Operating Division

Formerly Forth Valley Primary Care NHS Trust.

c/o NHS Forth Valley, 33 Spittal Street, Stirling FK8 1DX
Tel: 01786 463031 Fax: 01786 471337
(NHS Forth Valley)

Chair Marlene Anderson
Chief Executive Anne Hawkins

Bannockburn Hospital
Bannockburn, Stirling FK7 8AH
Tel: 01786 813016 Fax: 01786 812071
Total Beds: 114

Care of the Elderly D C Kennie

Old Age Psychiatry R J Coles, Dr Kidd

Bellsdyke Hospital
Bellsdyke Road, Larbert FK5 4SF
Tel: 01324 570700 Fax: 01324 562367
Total Beds: 102

General Psychiatry Dr Brown, Dr McFlynn, Dr Morrison

Bo'ness Hospital
Dean Road, Bo'ness EH51 0DH
Tel: 01506 823032 Fax: 01506 822680
Total Beds: 40

Care of the Elderly R Lenton, Dr McKean

Bonnybridge Hospital
Falkirk Road, Bonnybridge FK4 1BD
Tel: 01324 814685 Fax: 01324 815652
Total Beds: 90

General Medicine P Murdoch, Dr Scougall

Psychiatry of Old Age G McLean, Dr Woolf

Clackmannan County Day Hospital
Clackmannan County Hospital, Ashley Terrace, Alloa FK10 2BE
Tel: 01259 723840
Total Beds: 20

Clackmannan County Hospital
Ashley Terrace, Alloa FK10 2BE
Tel: 01259 723840 Fax: 01259 724740
Total Beds: 32

General Psychiatry Dr Collins, C Crawford

Psychiatry of Old Age D R Coles

Dunrowan Day Hospital
Maggie Woods Loan, Falkirk
Tel: 01324 639009
Total Beds: 20

Kildean Day Hospital
Drip Road, Stirling FK8 1RW
Tel: 01786 446114
Total Beds: 20

Kildean Hospital
Drip Road, Stirling FK8 1RW
Tel: 01786 446114 Fax: 01786 458605
Total Beds: 30

Care of the Elderly A Mackenie

Psychiatry of Old Age R J Coles

Orchard House Day Hospital
Union Street, Stirling FK8 1PA
Tel: 01786 474161 Fax: 01786 447430
Total Beds: 25

Princes Street Day Hospital
5 Princes Street, Stirling FK8 1HQ
Tel: 01786 474230
Total Beds: 20

Royal Scottish National Hospital
Old Denny Road, Larbert FK5 4EH
Tel: 01324 570700 Fax: 01324 558382
Total Beds: 140

General Psychiatry Dr McVicker

Sauchie Hospital
Sunnyside, Alloa FK10 3BW
Tel: 01259 722060 Fax: 01259 720474
Total Beds: 30

Care of the Elderly J Bishop-Miller

Westbank Day Hospital
West Bridge Street, Falkirk FK1 5RT
Tel: 01324 624111
Total Beds: 20

NHS Grampian, Acute Services Division

Formerly Grampian University Hospitals NHS Trust.

c/o NHS Grampian, Summerfield House, 2 Eday Road, Aberdeen AB15 6RE
Tel: 0845 456 6000
(NHS Grampian)

Aberdeen Maternity Hospital
Cornhill Road, Aberdeen AB25 2ZL
Tel: 01224 681818 Fax: 01224 684880
Total Beds: 144

Anaesthetics A Campbell, F M Knox, A W Sheikh

Neonatology P Booth, P Duffty, D J Lloyd

Obstetrics D R Abramovich, P M Fisher, M H Hall, G D Lang, D E Parkin, N C Smith, A A Templeton, P B Terry

Aberdeen Royal Infirmary

Foresterhill, Aberdeen AB25 2ZN
Tel: 01224 681818
Total Beds: 1100

Accident and Emergency Dr Cooper, Dr Ferguson, Dr Hiscox, J G Page

Anaesthetics G D Adey, J S Blaiklock, G Byers, A Campbell, W R Casson, W Chambers, R W Davidson-Lamb, K Ferguson, G M Johnston, B R Kennedy, F M Knox, H J McFarlane, J D Mckenzie, D M Macleod, M S P Macnab, D Noble, R Patey, G Ramayya, E A Robertson, G S Robertson, D G Ross, A W Sheikh, G Smith, I Smith

Cardiology K Jennings

Dermatology A D Ormerod, L Stankler, M I White

ENT K A McLay, W J Newlands, D J Veitch, L C Wills, H A Young

General Medicine N B Bennett, J S Bevan, P W Brunt, A S Douglas, N Edward, N B Haites, D J King, K C McHardy, A W McKinley, A M MacLeod, N A G Mowat, D Ogston, D W M Pearson, J C Petrie, S Ralston, J M Rowless, T S Sinclair, A H Watt, S J Watt, M J Williams

General Surgery A K Ah-See, G Cooper, J Engeset, O Eremin, S Heys, R A Keenan, P King, N M Koruth, Z H Krukowski, S S Miller, G G Youngson

Genitourinary Medicine A J Downie

Haematology A A Dawson, R R Khaund, P J King

Neurology R J Coleman

Neurosurgery D G Currie

Ophthalmology H R Atta, W H Church, W B M Donaldson, J V Forrester, F D Green, C H Hutchinson, A G R Rennie

Oral and Maxillofacial Surgery N Renny

Orthopaedics J McLauchlan, T R Scotland, J M Scott, P A Slater, D Wardlaw

Plastic Surgery Dr Davies, J D Holmes, P S Kolhe

Thoracic Surgery J S Cockburn, R Jeffrey, S Prasad

Urology S McClinton, L E F Moffat

Dr Gray's Hospital (Acute)

Elgin IV30 1SN
Tel: 01343 543131 Fax: 01343 558504
Website: www.show.scot.nhs.uk/guh
Total Beds: 190

Anaesthetics A Bruce, G M Duthie, C McFarlane

General Medicine R Harvey, R D M MacLeod, D Williams

General Surgery A G Coutts, I G Gunn, R McIntyre, J D B Miller

Medical Paediatrics A Attenburrow, H Stander

Obstetrics and Gynaecology Dr Evans, S Navani

Ophthalmology J Wallace

Orthopaedics D Anderson, G Kilian, M Roos

Foresterhill Hospital

Foresterhill, Aberdeen AB9 8AQ
Tel: 01224 681818 Fax: 01224 840597
Total Beds: 1093

Royal Aberdeen Children's Hospital

Cornhill Road, Aberdeen AB25 2ZG
Tel: 01224 681818 Fax: 01224 840704
Website: www.show.scot.nhs.uk/guh
Total Beds: 113

Anaesthetics G Byers, A Campbell, G Johnstone, G S Robertson, A Sheikh, G Smith

Dermatology A D Ormerod, L Stankler, M I White

ENT K A McLay, W J Newlands, D Veitch, L C Wills, H A Young

General Medicine I A Auchterlonie, P Booth, G F Cole, P Duffty, A D Kindley, D J Lloyd, G Russell, P J Smail

General Psychiatry M Brown, D D Chisholm, C Reed

General Surgery G G Youngson

Neurosurgery C T Blaiklock, D G Currie

Ophthalmology H R Atta, W H Church, W B M Donaldson, J V Forrester, F D Green, C H Hutchinson, A G R Rennie

Oral and Maxillofacial Surgery N W Kerr

Orthodontics S Hewage, G Wright

Orthopaedics P H Gibson, J McLauchlan, T R Scotland

Plastic Surgery J Holmes, P Kohle

Tor-Na-Dee Hospital

Milltimber, Aberdeen
Tel: 01224 867307 Fax: 01224 840771
Website: www.show.scot.nhs.uk/guh
Total Beds: 71

Woodend Hospital

Eday Road, Woodend, Aberdeen AB15 6XS
Tel: 01224 663131 Fax: 01224 404179
Website: www.show.scot.nhs.uk/gov
Total Beds: 332

Anaesthetics G R Dundas

Care of the Elderly P C Gautam, S J C Hamilton, M D MacArthur, D Newnham, W R Primrose, C J Scott, G Seymour, S Wilkinson

Orthopaedics G P Ashcroft, R Battacharya, R B Chesney, P H Gibson, J Hutchison, D Knight, W Ledingham, J McLauchlan, N Maffulli, T Scotland, D Wardlaw

Rehabilitation Medicine J A Cozens, S J C Hamilton, C J Scott, R Seymour

NHS Grampian, Primary Care Division

Formerly Grampian Primary Care NHS Trust.

c/o NHS Grampian, Summerfield House, 2 Eday Road, Aberdeen AB15 6RE
Tel: 0845 456 6000
(NHS Grampian)

Aberdeen City Hospital

Urquhart Road, Aberdeen AB24 5AN
Tel: 01224 663131
Total Beds: 115

Care of the Elderly P C Gautam, D Newnham, J Scott

General Psychiatry M Shanks

Aboyne Hospital

Aboyne AB34 5HQ
Tel: 01339 886433 Fax: 01339 885373
Total Beds: 48

Campbell Hospital

Park Crescent, Portsoy, Banff AB45 2TR
Tel: 01261 842202 ext: 201 Fax: 01261 843971
Total Beds: 26

Chalmers Hospital
Clunie Street, Banff AB45 1JA
Tel: 01261 812567 ext: 71168 Fax: 01261 818074
Total Beds: 58

General Psychiatry D Fowlik

Dr Gray's Hospital (Mental and Community)
Elgin IV30 1SN
Tel: 01343 543131 Fax: 01343 558504

Fleming Hospital
Aberlour AB38 9PR
Tel: 01340 871464 Fax: 01340 871814
Total Beds: 15

Fraserburgh Hospital
Lochpots Road, Fraserburgh AB43 5NF
Tel: 01346 513151 Fax: 01346 514548
Total Beds: 66

General Psychiatry D Fowlik

Glen O'Dee Hospital
Banchory AB31 3SA
Tel: 01330 822233 Fax: 01330 825718
Total Beds: 60

Insch and District War Memorial Hospital
Rannes Street, Insch AB52 6JJ
Tel: 01464 820213 Fax: 01464 820233
Total Beds: 15

Inverurie Hospital
Upperboat Road, Inverurie AB51 3UL
Tel: 01467 620454 Ext: 51723 Fax: 01467 624023
Total Beds: 69

General Psychiatry E Alexander

Jubilee Hospital
Bleachfield Street, Huntly AB54 5EX
Tel: 01224 663131, 01466 792114 ext: 51302 Fax: 01466 794544
Total Beds: 51

Kincardine Community Hospital
Stonehaven AB39 2NH
Tel: 01569 792000 Fax: 01569 792020
Total Beds: 49

General Psychiatry P Olley

Kincardine O'Neil War Memorial Hospital
St Marnan Road, Torphins, Banchory AB31 7JQ
Tel: 01339 882302 Fax: 01339 882580
Total Beds: 11

Ladysbridge Hospital
Whitehills, Banff AB45 2JS
Tel: 01261 861361 Fax: 01261 861779
Total Beds: 165

Leanchoil Hospital
Forres IV36 0RF
Tel: 01309 672284 Fax: 01309 673935
Total Beds: 35

Maud Hospital
Maud Hospital, Bank Road, Maud AB42 5NR
Tel: 01771 604236
Total Beds: 50

General Psychiatry D Fowlik

Peterhead Community Hospital
21 Links Terrace, Peterhead AB42 6XB
Tel: 01779 478234 Fax: 01779 478111
Total Beds: 35

General Psychiatry D Fowlik

Royal Cornhill Hospital
26 Cornhill Road, Aberdeen AB25 2ZH
Tel: 01224 557433 Fax: 01224 403407
Total Beds: 505

General Psychiatry E R Alexander, M Bremner, S Calder, J S Callender, J M Eagles, L M Emslie, D G Fowlie, R Hamilton, D LePoidevin, J Lolley, L A McCrone, I McIlwain, H Millar, M Muir, P Ollem, A G Oswald, A Palin, A D T Robinson, D St Clair, P D Sclare, M Shanks, P Trotter, J Warrington, L Whalley, G E Wilson, Professor Wischik

Seafield Hospital
Buckie AB56 1EJ
Tel: 01542 832081 Fax: 01542 834254
Total Beds: 66

Spynie Hospital
Elgin IV30 2PW
Tel: 01343 53131 Fax: 01343 552185
Total Beds: 66

Stephen Hospital
Dufftown, Keith AB55 4BH
Tel: 01340 820215 Fax: 01340 820593
Total Beds: 21

Turner Memorial Hospital
Turner Street, Keith AB55 5DJ
Tel: 01542 882526 Fax: 01542 882317
Total Beds: 27

Turriff Community Hospital
Balmellie Road, Turriff AB53 4SR
Tel: 01888 563293 Fax: 01888 562431
Total Beds: 19

Ugie Hospital
Ugie Road, Peterhead AB42 6LZ
Tel: 01779 72011 Fax: 01779 471109
Total Beds: 44

General Psychiatry D Fowlik

Woodlands Hospital
Craigton Road, Cults, Aberdeen AB15 9PR
Tel: 01224 663131 Fax: 01224 404018
Total Beds: 64

Learning Disabilities R D Drummond, K McKay

NHS Greater Glasgow, North Glasgow University Hospitals Division

Formerly North Glasgow University Hospitals NHS Trust.

Division Headquarters, 300 Balgrayhill Road, Glasgow G31 2UR
Tel: 0141 211 4200 Fax: 0141 211 4202
Email: forename.surname@northglasgow.scot.nhs.uk
Website: www.ngt.org.uk
(NHS Greater Glasgow)

Chair Ronnie Cleland
Chief Executive Tim Davison

Beatson Oncology Centre
Dumbarton Road, Glasgow G11 6NT
Tel: 0141 211 2000
Total Beds: 135

Palliative Medicine J Edgecombe, A Mitchell, J Welsh

Radiotherapy and Oncology N S E Reed, A A Armour, P Canney, J Cassidy, F J Cowie, D Dodds, D Dunlop, T Evans, G Fraser, R Jones, C H Kodikara, A MacDonald, N Mohammed, N O'Rourke, R P Rampling, D Ritchie, A G Robertson, J M Russell, P Vasey, H M A Yosef

Blawarthill Hospital
129 Holehouse Drive, Blawarthill, Glasgow G13 3TG
Tel: 0141 954 9547
Total Beds: 90

Drumchapel Hospital
129 Drumchapel Road, Glasgow G15 6PX
Tel: 0141 211 6000
Total Beds: 120

Gartnavel General Hospital
1053 Great Western Road, Glasgow G12 0NY
Tel: 0141 211 3000 Fax: 0141 211 3466
Total Beds: 465

Manager Rosie Cherry

Anaesthetics A J Asbury, K M Rogers

Care of the Elderly W J Gilchrist, E G Spilg, B O Williams, J M Young

General Medicine J G Allan, S B Dover, K E L McColl, J B MacDonald, P R Mills, K R Patel, M Small, N C Thomson

General Surgery D S Byrne, G M Fullarton, D J Galloway, A J McKay, R G Molloy, P N Rogers

Ophthalmology T Barrie, G N Dutton, H M Hammer, J L Jay, E G Kemp, C M Kirkness, R M McFadzean

Orthopaedics W J Leach, A T C Reece

Otolaryngology D G Carrick, L D Cooke, N K Geddes, F B MacGregor, M S C Morrissey

Radiology J G Moss

Urology M Aitchison, D Kirk, M A Palmer

Glasgow Dental Hospital and School
378 Sauchiehall Street, Glasgow G2 3JZ
Tel: 0141 211 9600

Oral and Maxillofacial Surgery H A Critchlow, D A McGowan, K F Moos, D I Russell, D Stenhouse, G A Wood

Glasgow Homoeopathic Hospital
1053 Great Western Road, Glasgow G12 0XG
Tel: 0141 211 1600 Fax: 0141 211 1610
Total Beds: 20

Glasgow Royal Infirmary
84 Castle Street, Glasgow G4 0SF
Tel: 0141 211 4000 Fax: 0141 211 4889
Total Beds: 1077

Manager Mark Gordon

Accident and Emergency R Crawford, A Ireland, I J Swann

Anaesthetics M H Basler, M G Booth, W Fitch, M J Higgins, G N C Kenny, B H Maule, E M McGrady, M J McNeil, C J Murdoch, M R Parris, A Patrick, D L Paul, F J B Pearshall, P C Stuart, G A Sutherland, S Tan

Biochemistry R Fleming, N Sattar

Cardiology A J B Brady, H Eteiba, W S Hills, P W Macfarlane, T A McDonagh, J V McMurray, A P Rae, A C Rankin

Cardiothoracic Surgery I W Colquhoun, S R Craig, K G Davidson, A Faichney, A J Murray, S Niak, U U Nkere, J C S Pollock, D J Wheatley

Care of the Elderly J Burns, B L Devine, P V Knight, P Langhorne, D Stott

Dermatology C Clark, A A Forsyth, S C Holmes

ENT A Kishore, K McKenzie, L Swan

General Medicine M M Cotton, C Deighan, B M Fisher, J G Fox, H W Gray, D H Lawson, M E J Lean, G D O Lowe, J F Mackenzie, R A Mactier, J H McKillop, A J Morris, J B Neilly, K R Paterson, R I Russell, H K L Simpson, A J Stanley, R D Sturrock, J Taylor

General Surgery J H Anderson, C R Carter, T G Cooke, I G Finlay, D G Gilmour, P G Horgan, C W Imrie, C J Mckay, R F Mckee, W R Murray, D J Orr, R C Stuart, R P Teenan

Haematology R C Tait, I D Walker

Obstetrics and Gynaecology I A Greer, J H Kennedy, C B Lunan, H Lyall, A Mathers, J Norman, M Rodger, R W S Yates

Oncology A C McDonald, M Soukop, H M A Yosef

Ophthalmology B Browne, M P Gavin, D M I Montgomery

Orthopaedics M J G Blyth, R R Ingram, I G Kelly, A W G Kinninmonth, L A Rymaszewski, S Senthilkumar, R G Simpson, I G Stother, E F Wheelwright

Palliative Medicine P Keeley

Pathology P J Galloway, A R McPhaden, D O'Reilly, J E Tolhurst

Radiology A W Reid, G H Roditi

Urology A C Buck, G E Jones, P J Paterson

Lightburn Hospital
966 Carntyne Road, Glasgow G32 6ND
Tel: 0141 211 1500
Total Beds: 120

Princess Royal Maternity Unit
Glasgow Royal Infirmary, Alexander Parade, Glasgow G31 2ER
Tel: 0141 211 5400
Total Beds: 140

Obstetrics and Gynaecology I A Greer, M Hepburn, J H Kennedy, C B Lunan, H Lyall, A Mathers, M Rodger, R W S Yates

Stobhill Hospital
130 Balonock Road, Glasgow G21 3UT
Tel: 0141 201 3000 Fax: 0141 201 3887
Total Beds: 650

Manager Ian Crawford

Anaesthetics R L Hughes, K Lamb, A H McKee, J B M McKellar, C D Miller, C J Murdoch, D K Sewnauth, P J Slater

Biochemistry N A Siddiqui

Cardiology F G Dunn, N E R Goodfield, K J Hogg

Care of the Elderly A-L Cunnington, J W Davie, P Fraser, C McAlpine, L Simpson

General Medicine B J Danesh, J A H Forrest, J G Fox, D Gordon, E H McLaren, R A Mactier

General Psychiatry J McKnight

General Surgery D T Hansell, A McMahon, M Moschos, K W Robertson, J S Smith

Haematology R L C Cumming, M T J Leach

Obstetrics and Gynaecology J A Davis, M Deeny, C A Forrest, R A L Low, F Mackenzie, P Owen

Ophthalmology T Barrie, B Browne, D M I Montgomery, J R Murdoch

Orthopaedics A W G Kinninmonth, L Rymaszewski, E F Wheelwright

Pathology R B Hogg, G D Smith

Radiology F Bryden, S Ingram, I A Macleod, J Shand, R Stevens

Radiotherapy and Oncology J A Davis, A L H Honeyman, P Symonds

Respiratory Medicine C E Bucknall, R Milroy

Urology J Crooks, M Fraser

Western Infirmary

Dumbarton Road, Glasgow G11 6NT
Tel: 0141 211 2000 Fax: 0141 211 1920
Total Beds: 493

Manager Ronnie Clinton

Anaesthetics J H Brown, C Brydon, K M S Dewar, J R I Dougall, J J Henderson, A Hope, H Howie, I Kestin, T D McCubbin, A D McLaren, I McMenemin, N O'Donnell, N Pace, J L Plenderleith, K M Rogers, C Runcie, L Sanai, M Serpell, P Stone, J G Todd, P G M Wallace

Cardiology H J Dargie, A P Dsvie, I N Findlay, J J V McMurray, K G Oldroyd

Cardiothoracic Surgery G Berg, J G Butler, A Faichney, A J B Kirk, K J D McArthur, V Pathi

Chest Disease K R Patel, A J Peacock, N C Thomson

Dermatology A D Burden, R M Herd, P McHenry, R MacKie, D Tillman

General Medicine M J Brodie, J M C Connell, C C Geddes, W S Hillis, A Jardine, B J R Junor, K R Lees, K E L McColl, E A McGregor, A R McLellan, M McMillan, J Reid, R S C Roger, P Semple

General Surgery J C Doughty, D J Galloway, W D George, R G Molloy, P J O'Dwyer

Obstetrics and Gynaecology J Brennand, A D Cameron, W R Chatfield, J W Cordiner, K P Hanretty, M Lumsden

Orthopaedics P Chatzigrigoris, J F Crossan, U Fazzi, A Gray, M J Jane, M P Kelly, W Leach, J S Moir, A Reece

Pathology W M H Behan, I L Brown, R A Burnett, M Fallowfield, T MacLeod, R N M MacSween, I A R More, R Soutar

Radiology F G Adams, G Baxter, M D Cowan, R Edwards, W Kincaid, N C McMillan, J Moss, N Raby, G Stenhouse, R Vallance, L Wilkinson

NHS Greater Glasgow, Primary Care Division

Formerly Greater Glasgow Primary Care NHS Trust.

Division Headquarters, Gartnavel Royal Hospital, 1055 Great Western Road, Glasgow G12 0XH
Tel: 0141 211 3600
(NHS Greater Glasgow)

Chair Andrew Robertson

Acorn Street Day Hospital

23 Acorn Street, Glasgow G40
Tel: 0141 556 4789
Total Beds: 30

General Psychiatry P C Misra

Campbell House Day Hospital

Gartnavel Royal Hospital, 1055 Great Western Road, Glasgow G12 0XH
Tel: 0141 211 3600 Fax: 0141 334 2408

Denmark Street Day Hospital

101 Denmark Street, Glasgow G22 5EU
Tel: 0141 531 9300 Fax: 0141 531 9304

Easterhouse Day Hospital

Auchinlea House, 11 Auchinlea Road, Glasgow G34 9PA
Tel: 0141 771 3441 Fax: 0141 781 0328

Florence Street Day Hospital

26 Florence Street, Glasgow G5 0YX
Tel: 0141 429 2878 Fax: 0141 420 3464

Gartnavel Royal Hospital

1055 Great Western Road, Glasgow G12 0XH
Tel: 0141 211 3600
Total Beds: 210

General Psychiatry J Bouch, D Brown, R N Herrington, R Hunter, M Kemp, P Kershaw, M Livingston, Dr McCabe, A Nightingale, J Reid, D Scott, I D Smith, J Woods

Hillview Day Hospital

Stobhill General Hospital, 133 Balornock Road, Glasgow G21 3UW
Tel: 0141 201 3918 Fax: 0141 558 1575

Leverndale Hospital

510 Crookston Road, Glasgow G53 7TU
Tel: 0141 211 6400 Fax: 0141 882 8086
Total Beds: 397

General Psychiatry J Baird, D A Coia, C Flanigan, A A Fraser, J Gray, T Henderson, A V M Hughson, G Jackson, D Lyons, J P McKane, A Mitchell, D Palmer, G Shaw-Dunn, J Summers, J Taylor, S Whyte

MacKinnon House

Stobhill Hospital, 133 Balornock Road, Glasgow G21 3UZ
Tel: 0141 531 3100 Fax: 0141 531 3236
Total Beds: 66

Manager Calum MacLeod

General Psychiatry D Ball, D Brown, G Byrne, J McKnight, D Patience, M Taylor, M Turner

The Orchards

153 Panmure Street, Glasgow G20
Tel: 0141 531 5900 Fax: 0141 945 3851

Parkhead Day Hospital

81 Salamanca Street, Glasgow G31 5ES
Tel: 0141 211 8331 Fax: 0141 211 8370

Parkhead Hospital

81 Salamanca Street, Glasgow G31 5ES
Tel: 0141 211 8300 Fax: 0141 211 8312

General Psychiatry E H Bennie, D Brodie, C Flanigan, P Jauhar, Dr Mason, P C Misra, Dr Moore, M M Walker, Dr White, P J Williams

Shettleston Day Hospital

150 Wellshot Street, Glasgow G32
Tel: 0141 778 8381

Southern General Hospital

Psychiatric Unit, 1345 Govan Road, Glasgow G51 4TF
Tel: 0141 201 1100 Fax: 0141 201 1920

Manager Stephen Kerr

General Psychiatry Dr Burley, R Caplan, Dr Crean, A Fraser, A Graham, A Kerr, Dr Livingston, M Malcolm, R McGilp

Woodlands Day Hospital

15-17 Waterloo Close, Kirkintilloch, Glasgow G66 2HL
Tel: 0141 775 3664 Fax: 0141 775 0646

NHS Greater Glasgow, South Glasgow University Hospitals Division

Formerly South Glasgow University Hospitals NHS Trust.

Division Headquarters, 1345 Govan Road, Glasgow G51 4TF
Tel: 0141 201 1100 Fax: 0141 201 2999
Email: forename.surname@sgh.scot.nhs.uk
(NHS Greater Glasgow)

Chair Elinor Smith
Chief Executive Robert Calderwood

Mansionhouse Unit

100 Mansion House Road, Langside, Glasgow G41 3DX
Tel: 0141 201 6161 Fax: 0141 201 6159
Total Beds: 244

Care of the Elderly K Beard, I Lennox, J Potter, M A Roberts, D Stewart

Mearnskirk House

Newton Mearns, Glasgow G77 5RZ
Tel: 0141 616 3742
Total Beds: 72

Care of the Elderly K Beard, I M Lennox, J Potter, M Roberts, D Stewart

Southern General Hospital

1345 Govan Road, Glasgow G51 4TF
Tel: 0141 201 1100 Fax: 0141 201 2999
Total Beds: 965

Accident and Emergency I W R Anderson, D Ritchie

Anaesthetics A Brown, B Cowan, J A Davidson, A Dell, J A Gillespie, G W A Gillies, R Glavin, G Gordon, J C Howie, R L Marshall, J H Maule, J Oates, J Purdie, D Singh, B S Stuart, D F Thomson

Bacteriology G Lindsay (Head), R Lewis, P Redding

Biochemistry H McAlpine, R Northcote

Care of the Elderly K Beard, I Lennox, J Potter, M A Roberts, D Stewart

Chest Disease D McIntyre, D R H Vernon

Dermatology D Bilsland, C Munro, D Roberts

ENT B Bingham, J Crowther, E A Osborne

General Medicine D Ballantyne, K M Cochran, C M Kesson, J Larkin, H MacAlpine, D MacIntyre, R Northcote, D Rooney, S D Slater, D R H Vernon

General Surgery J Drury, G Gillespie, G R Gray, I Pickford, D C Smith, I S Smith

Haematology P J Tansey (Head)

Neurology J P Ballantyne, I Bone, A Chaudhuri, R Duncan, W F Durward, J Greene, D Grosset, P G E Kennedy, A C Mann, R Metcalfe, A Myfanwy Thomas, C O'Leary, R K H Petty, A J Russell, A I Weir, H J Wilson

Obstetrics and Gynaecology S Bjornsson, A Kraszewski, D S Mack, A N McDougall

Ophthalmology W M Doig, P Kyle, J Williamson, W N Wykes

Orthopaedics D R Allan, E R Gardner, T Hems, C Mainds, P D R Scott

Pathology D R McLellan (Head), I Gibson, E A Mallon, W G S Spilg

Radiology J Calder, S E G Goudie, J Lauder, G McInnes, G Millar, W R Pickard

Urology B J Abel, I G Conn

Victoria Infirmary

Langside, Glasgow G42 9TY
Tel: 0141 201 6000 Fax: 0141 201 5206
Total Beds: 420

Accident and Emergency I W R Anderson, D Ritchie

Anaesthetics A Brown, B Cowan, J A Davidson, A Dell, J A Gillespie, G W A Gillies, R Glavin, G Gordon, J C Howie, R L Marshall, J H Maule, J Oates, J Purdie, D Singh, B S Stuart, D F Thomson

Bacteriology G Lindsay (Head), R F M Lewis, P Redding

Biochemistry A Hutchinson (Head), A Glen

Cardiology H McAlpine, R Northcote

Care of the Elderly K Beard, I Lennox, J Potter, M A Roberts, D Stewart

Chest Disease D McIntyre, D R H Vernon

Dermatology D Bilsland, C Munro, D Roberts

ENT B Bingham, J Crowther, E A Osborne

General Medicine D Ballantyne, K M Cochran, C M Kesson, J Larkin, H MacAlpine, D MacIntyre, R Northcote, D Rooney, S D Slater, D R H Vernon

General Surgery J Drury, G Gillespie, G R Gray, I Pickford, D C Smith, I S Smith

Haematology P J Tansey (Head)

Obstetrics and Gynaecology S Bjornsson, A Kraszewski, A N McDougall, D S Mack

Ophthalmology W M Doig, P Kyle, J Williamson, W N Wykes

Orthopaedics D Allan, E R Gardner, T Hems, C Mainds, P D R Scott

Pathology D McLellan (Head), I Gibson, E A Mallon, W G S Spilg

Radiology J Calder, S E G Goudie, J Lauder, G McInnes, M A Millar, W R Pickard

Urology B J Abel, I G Conn

NHS Greater Glasgow, Yorkhill Division

Formerly The Yorkhill NHS Trust.

Division Headquarters, Royal Hospital for Sick Children, Dalnair Street, Glasgow G3 8SJ
Tel: 0141 201 0000 Fax: 0141 201 0836
Email: forename.surname@yorkhill.scot.nhs.uk
(NHS Greater Glasgow)

Chair Sally Kuenssberg
Chief Executive Jonathan Best

The Queen Mother's Hospital

Yorkhill, Glasgow G3 8SH
Tel: 0141 201 0550 Fax: 0141 201 0836
Total Beds: 70

Anaesthetics C S Cairns, J Reid, J Thorburn

Obstetrics and Gynaecology A D Cameron, W R Chatfield, J W Cordiner, K Hanretty, M A Lumsden, L Macara

Paediatrics J Coutts, B Holland, T L Turner

Royal Hospital for Sick Children
Yorkhill, Glasgow G3 8SJ
Tel: 0141 201 0000 Fax: 0141 201 0836
Total Beds: 266

Accident and Emergency J O Beattie, N V Doraiswamy

Anaesthetics G Bell, C Best, P Bolton, P Copples, P Cullen, D Hallworth, R A Lawson, L R McNicol, N S Morton, J Peutrell, J F Sinclair

Biochemistry J M Connor

Cardiology A B Houston, J M McLeod, N Wilson

Cardiothoracic Surgery K McArthur, J Pollock

Child Psychiatry J Barton, R Lindsay, M Morton, J C Shemilt, A Sneddon

Community Child Health S Evans, J Herbison, K Leyland, K McKay, D Stone, A Sutton, D Tappin

Dental Surgery H A Critchlow, D Fung, A Wray

Dermatology D Burden, R Lever, P McHendry

ENT N K Geddes, F McGregor, S Morrisey, H Sadiq

Genetics J M Conner, H R Davidson, J Tolmie, M Whiteford, P Wilcox

Haematology E Chalmers, N Cole, B S Gibson

Neurology R McWilliam, M O Regan, S Zobari

Obstetrics and Gynaecology A Cameron, R Chatfield, J Cordiner, K Hanretty, M Lumsden, L Macara

Ophthalmology J Dudgeon, G T Dutton

Oral and Maxillofacial Surgery J G McLennan

Orthopaedics G C Bennett, R Duncan, D Sammon, D S Sherlock, N H Wilson

Paediatric Surgery A A F Azmy, R Carachi, C Davis, A H B Fyfe, G Haddock, C Hajioassiliou, S O'Toole, P A M Raine

Paediatrics F Ahmed, L Alroomi, J Beattie, D Cochran, J Coutts, M Donaldson, J A Ford, P Galea, N Gibson, R Hague, B Holland, H Maxwell, A V Murphy, J Y Paton, K J Robertson, P H Robinson, C H Skeoch, T L Turner, L T Weaver, M P White

Pathology A G Howatson

Radiology A MacLennan, S Maroo, A Watt, A G Wilkinson

NHS Highland, Acute Hospitals

Formerly Highland Acute Hospitals NHS Trust.

c/o NHS Highland, Assynt House, Beechwood Park, Inverness IV2 3HG
Tel: 01463 717123 Fax: 01463 235189
(NHS Highland)

Belford Hospital
Belford Road, Fort William PH33 6BS
Tel: 01397 702481 Fax: 01397 702772
Total Beds: 49

Manager J Russell-Roberts

Caithness General Hospital
Cliff Road, Caithness, Wick KW1 5NQ
Tel: 01955 605050 Fax: 01955 604606
Total Beds: 96

Manager Sheena Craig

Raigmore Hospital
Perth Road, Inverness IV2 3UJ
Tel: 01463 704000 Fax: 01463 711322
Total Beds: 577

Accident and Emergency N Murphy (Head)

Anaesthetics J Howes (Head)

Bacteriology A Hay (Head)

Care of the Elderly V Sood (Head)

Dermatology J Vestey (Head)

ENT S Denholm (Head)

General Medicine R Harvey (Head)

General Surgery P V Walsh (Head)

Haematology W Murray (Head)

Medical Physics D Crippen (Head)

Obstetrics and Gynaecology L Caird (Head)

Occupational Therapy C Wood (Head)

Ophthalmology C Barras (Head)

Oral Surgery D Macintyre (Head)

Orthopaedics K Baird (Head)

Paediatrics G Farmer (Head)

Pathology J McPhie (Head)

Pharmacy J Cromarty (Head)

Physiotherapy D Sim (Head)

Radiology G Aitken (Head)

Radiotherapy and Oncology D Whillis (Head)

Rehabilitation Medicine L Fisher (Head)

Urology P Walsh (Head)

NHS Highland, Primary Care

Formerly Highland Primary Care NHS Trust.

c/o NHS Highland, Assynt House, Beechwood Park, Inverness IV2 3HG
Tel: 01463 717123 Fax: 01463 235189
(NHS Highland)

Belhaven Ward, Belford Hospital
Belford Road, Fort William PH33 6BS
Tel: 01397 702481 Fax: 01397 702772
Total Beds: 23

County Hospital, Invergordon
Invergordon IV18 0JR
Tel: 01349 852496 Fax: 01349 854328
Total Beds: 44

Dr Mackinnon Memorial Hospital
Broadford, Isle of Skye
Tel: 01471 822491 Fax: 01471 822298
Total Beds: 25

General Surgery J R Ball

Dunbar Hospital
Thurso KW14 7XE
Tel: 01847 893263 Fax: 01847 892263
Total Beds: 16

Gesto Hospital
Edinbane, Portree, Isle of Skye
Tel: 01470 582262 Fax: 01470 582360
Total Beds: 16

Glencoe Hospital
Glencoe, Ballachulish
Tel: 01855 811254
Total Beds: 25

Ian Charles Hospital
Castle Road East, Grantown-on-Spey PH26 3HR
Tel: 01479 872528
Total Beds: 18

Invergordon County Hospital
Invergordon IV18 0JR
Tel: 01349 852496 Fax: 01349 852328
Total Beds: 44

Care of the Elderly P K Srivastava

Lawson Memorial Hospital
Station Road, Golspie KW10 6SS
Tel: 01408 633157 Fax: 01408 633947
Total Beds: 15

Anaesthetics K A Abraham, V Gadiyar, R Nanda Kumar

General Surgery P Fisher, W G Johnston

Lawson Memorial Hospital (Surgical Services) (Cambusavie)
Station Road, Golspie KW10 6SS
Tel: 01408 633157 Fax: 01408 633947
Total Beds: 30

Migdale Hospital
Bonar Bridge, Ardgay IV24 3AP
Tel: 01863 766211 Fax: 01863 766623
Total Beds: 34

Nairn Town and County Hospital
Cawdor Road, Nairn IV12 5EE
Tel: 01667 452101
Total Beds: 19

New Craigs
Inverness IV3 6JU
Tel: 01463 242860 Fax: 01463 236154
Total Beds: 223

Manager Pamela Booth, Mike Perera

General Psychiatry Dr Baeker, K Blagden, J Deans, Y Edmonstone, D Gordon, A Hay, G Jones, A MacGregor

Portree Hospital
Portree, Isle of Skye
Tel: 01478 613200 Fax: 01478 613526
Total Beds: 13

Ross House Day Hospital
Inverness
Tel: 01463 718302 Fax: 01463 718303

Ross Memorial Hospital
Ferry Road, Dingwall IV15 9QT
Tel: 01349 863313 Fax: 01349 865852
Total Beds: 31

Royal Northern Infirmary
Inverness IV3 5SS
Tel: 01463 242860 Fax: 01463 713884
Total Beds: 30

Care of the Elderly V P Sood, P K Srivastava

St Vincent's Hospital
Gynack Road, Kingussie PH21 1EX
Tel: 01540 661219 Fax: 01540 661035
Total Beds: 39

Town and County Hospital
Wick KW1 5NQ
Tel: 01955 604025 Fax: 01955 604606
Total Beds: 20

York Day Hospital
Ness Walk, Royal Northern Infirmary, Inverness IV3 5SF
Tel: 01463 242860 Fax: 01463 713884

NHS Lanarkshire, Acute Services Division

Formerly Lanarkshire Acute Hospitals Division.

Division Headquarters, Strathclyde Hospital, Airbles Road, Motherwell ML1 3BW
Tel: 01698 245000 Fax: 01698 245009
Website: www.show.scot.nhs.uk/laht
(NHS Lanarkshire)

Chief Executive Ian Ross

Hairmyres Hospital
Eaglesham Road, East Kilbride, Glasgow G75 8RG
Tel: 01355 585000 Fax: 01355 584473
Total Beds: 446

Manager David Hume

Accident and Emergency P O'Connor

Anaesthetics J W Burns, G W Davidson, J M Glasser, J V Lees, W A McCulloch, F C McGroarty, G A Weetch

Biochemistry K Cunningham

Care of the Elderly G Cunning, B Martin, M E Stewart, B Yip

Chest Disease C J Clark, M D Clee

Dermatology F Campbell, C Evans, S O Neil, A Strong

ENT J L Handa, G L Picozzi, P S White

General Medicine C J Clark, H N Cohen, K Oldroyd, B D Vallance

General Surgery J R Goldring, D Knight, D F Miller, J R Richards, W O Thomson

Haematology A Roetaf, S Shahriari

Medical Microbiology D Baird

Obstetrics and Gynaecology H Gordon, J M Grant, G K Osbourne, K Spowart

Ophthalmology I Syme

Orthopaedics A Goresori, P J John, W D Newton, J T Watson

Pathology H Kamel, A McLay

Radiology R Connor, R H Corbett, S Millar, R Weir

Rheumatology A A Zoma

Thoracic Surgery A N Al-Jilaihawi, D Prakash

Urology P S Orr, B S Satye Vedanan, L Walker

Monklands Hospital
Monkscourt Avenue, Airdrie ML6 0JS
Tel: 01236 748748 Fax: 01236 760015
Total Beds: 498

Manager Rosemary Lyness

Accident and Emergency M T Brookes, I McLaren, M Watt

Anaesthetics D Clough, T Dunn, M D Inglis, R Mackenzie, S MacVicar, S Marshall, V Muir, A J W Naismith, P Paterson, V Reid, J M Thorp

Biochemistry K J M Cunningham

Cytology S Gardiner, J E A Imrie

Dermatology W S Douglas, C D Evans, A M M Strong, N Wainwright

ENT N Balagji, J Handa, A Johnston, G Picozzi, E Stewart

General Medicine A Gardiner, T Gilbert, M Hand, A D B Harrower, R J Holden, N Kennedy, L McAlpine, D Mathews, A Pell, A Prach, A Raeside, J C Rodger, W J G Smith, W T A Todd

General Surgery Mr Brookes, A McDonald, Mr Mackenzie, Mr Mackenzie, D Murphy, Mr Scott

Gynaecology R Cassie, D Conway, T G B Dow, V Harper

Haematology G Cook, J Murphy, W H Watson

Histopathology R J Zuk

Infectious Diseases N Kennedy, W T A Todd

Maxillofacial Surgery N Hammersley

Neurology D Grosset, R Petty

Ophthalmology A Wylie

Orthodontics M C Easton

Orthopaedics Mr Braidwood, D Bramley, A Campbell, Mr Singh

Paediatrics M Loudon

Radiology J Guse, R M Holden, K Hughes, W Mowat, R Railton, K J Wallers

Urology P S Orr, L Walker

Wishaw General Hospital

50 Netherton Street, Wishaw ML2 0DP
Tel: 01698 361100 Fax: 01698 376671
Total Beds: 633

Manager J Hope

NHS Lanarkshire, Primary Care Division

Formerly Lanarkshire Primary Care NHS Trust.

Division Headquarters, Strathclyde Hospital, Airbles Road, Motherwell ML1 3BW
Tel: 01698 245000 Fax: 01698 245009
Website: www.show.scot.nhs.uk/laht
(NHS Lanarkshire)

Chief Executive Martin Hill

Alexander Hospital

Blair Road, Coatbridge ML5 2EP
Tel: 01698 422661
Total Beds: 20

Birkwood Hospital

Lesmahagow, Lanark ML11 1JP
Tel: 01555 892382 Fax: 01555 894860
Total Beds: 168

Caird House

Caird Street, Hamilton ML3 0AL
Tel: 01698 540182
Total Beds: 10

Cleland Hospital

Bellside Road, Cleland, Motherwell ML1 5MR
Tel: 01698 860293 Fax: 01698 862453
Total Beds: 124

Care of the Elderly J McCallion, R W Pettersson

General Practice Dr McInnes

General Psychiatry A Sinclair

Coathill Hospital

Hospital Street, Coatbridge ML5 4DN
Tel: 01236 421266 Fax: 01236 431252
Total Beds: 86

Care of the Elderly G P Canning, L R Schmulian

Pathology S R Howatson

Hartwood Hospital

Hartwood, Shotts ML7 4LA
Tel: 01501 823366
Total Beds: 223

Kello Hospital

Biggar ML12 6AF
Tel: 01899 220077
Total Beds: 22

General Medicine R H Baxter

General Practice Dr Bewsher

General Surgery J Cannon

Kirklands Hospital

Fallside Road, Bothwell, Glasgow G71 8BB
Tel: 01698 245000 Fax: 01698 852340
Total Beds: 179

General Psychiatry A Langa, C Mani

Lady Home Hospital

Douglas, Lanark ML11 0RE
Tel: 01555 851210
Total Beds: 22

General Medicine M Drah

General Practice Dr Scott

General Surgery J Cannon

Red Deer Day Hospital

Alberta Avenue, Westwood, East Kilbride, Glasgow G74 8N8
Tel: 01355 244254

Roadmeetings Hospital

Goremire Road, Carluke ML8 4PS
Tel: 01555 752242 Fax: 01555 752328
Total Beds: 58

Care of the Elderly J McCallion, R W Pettersson

Strathclyde Hospital

Airbles Road, Motherwell ML1 3BW
Tel: 01698 258800
Total Beds: 70

Manager Craig Cunningham

Udston Hospital

Farm Road, Burnbank, Hamilton ML3 9LA
Tel: 01698 723200 Fax: 01698 710700
Total Beds: 134

Care of the Elderly B Mishra, Dr Semple, M E Stewart

Victoria Cottage Hospital
Glasgow Road, Kilsyth, Glasgow G65 9AG
Tel: 01236 822172
Total Beds: 17

General Practice Dr Walker

Wester Moffat Hospital
Towers Road, Airdrie ML6 8LW
Tel: 01236 763377 Fax: 01236 759913
Total Beds: 60

NHS Lothian, Primary and Community Division

Formerly Lothian Primary Care NHS Trust.

Division Headquarters, St Roque, Astley Ainslie Hospital, 133 Grange Loan, Edinburgh EH9 2HL
Tel: 0131 537 9000 Fax: 0131 537 9500
Email: firstname.surname@lpct.scot.nhs.uk
Website: www.show.scot.nhs.uk/lpct
(NHS Lothian)

Chair Garth Morrison
Chief Executive Murray Duncanson

Astley Ainslie Hospital
133 Grange Loan, Edinburgh EH9 2HL
Tel: 0131 537 9000 Fax: 0131 537 9222
Total Beds: 247

Manager Robert Aitken

Care of the Elderly C T Currie

Rehabilitation Medicine S Donald, J D Hunter, B Pentland, S Smith, I Todd

Belhaven Hospital
Beveridge Row, Dunbar EH42 1TR
Tel: 01368 862246
Total Beds: 40

Care of the Elderly A Jamieson (Head)

Cambridge Street Day Hospital
5-7 Cambridge Street, Edinburgh EH1 2DY
Tel: 0131 229 9581

Corstorphine Hospital
136 Corstorphine Road, Edinburgh EH12 6TT
Tel: 0131 332 2566 Fax: 0131 334 0537
Total Beds: 90

Manager Cecily Henderson

Eastern General Hospital
Seafield Street, Edinburgh EH6 7LN
Tel: 0131 536 7000 Fax: 0131 536 7474
Total Beds: 153

Manager Robert Aitken, Ceciley Henderson

Edenhall Day Hospital
Pinkieburn, Musselburgh EH21 7TZ
Tel: 0131 536 8000 Fax: 0131 536 8152, 0131 536 8153
Total Beds: 39

Elderly Mentally Ill C Rodgers

Edington Cottage Hospital
54 St Baldred's Road, North Berwick EH39 4PU
Tel: 01620 897040
Total Beds: 9

Herdmanflat Hospital
Aberlady Road, Haddington EH41 3BU
Tel: 0131 536 8300 Fax: 0131 536 8500
Total Beds: 97

General Psychiatry G Mercer, W Riddle, C R Rodger, T D Rogers

Loanhead Hospital
Hunter Avenue, Loanhead EH20 9SW
Tel: 0131 440 0174
Total Beds: 40

Princess Margaret Rose Hospital
41-43 Frogston Road West, Fairmilehead, Edinburgh EH10 7ED
Tel: 0131 536 4721

Roodlands Day Hospital
Hospital Road, Haddington EH41 3PF
Tel: 0131 536 8300 Fax: 0131 536 8399, 0131 536 8400
Total Beds: 75

Care of the Elderly A Jamieson, L Morrison

Rosslynlee Day Hospital
Roslin EH25 9QE
Tel: 0131 536 7600 Fax: 0131 536 7637
Total Beds: 108

Consultants J Craig, D Garbutt, A P R Moffoot

Royal Edinburgh Hospital
Morningside Terrace, Edinburgh EH9 1RJ
Tel: 0131 537 6000 Fax: 0131 537 6109
Total Beds: 455

Manager Debbie Jackson

Alcohol J Chick, F Watson

Brain Injury A Carson

Child and Adolescent Psychiatry R Glaze, R MacCabe

Consultants P Hoare, E Johnston, P Lefevre, D Owens

Forensic D Chiswick, J Crichton, A Wells

General Psychiatry D Blackwood, J Christie, T Dalkin, E Ebmeier, C Freeman, E Hare, E Johnson, P LeFerve, A Lodge, P McConville, A L McConville, D Morrison, D Mountain, T Murphy, M Nuttall, D Owens, A Scott, K Slateford, T Welldon, A Wells

Learning Disabilities R Lyall, S Macdonald, P Robertson, J Russell, T Sanderson

Old Age Psychiatry N Anderson, E Holloway, P Morrison

NHS Lothian, University Hospitals Division

Formerly Lothian University Hospitals NHS Trust.

Division Headquarters, Royal Infirmary of Edinburgh, 51 Little France Crescent, Old Dalkeith Road, Edinburgh EH16 4SA
Tel: 0131 536 1000 Fax: 0131 536 1001
Website: www.show.scot.nhs.uk/luht
(NHS Lothian)

Chair Stuart Smith
Chief Executive David Bolton

Chalmers Hospital
55 Lauriston Place, Edinburgh EH3 9HQ
Tel: 0131 536 1000
Total Beds: 60

Liberton Hospital

113 Lasswade Road, Edinburgh EH16 6UB
Tel: 0131 536 7800

Princess Alexandra Eye Pavilion

45 Chalmers Street, Edinburgh EH3 9HA
Tel: 0131 536 1000
Total Beds: 24

Ophthalmology A D Adams, R S Bartholomew, H B Chawla, B Dhillon, B W Fleck, P P Kearns, J Singh

Royal Hospital for Sick Children

9 Sciennes Road, Edinburgh EH9 1LF
Tel: 0131 536 0000 Fax: 0131 536 0001
Total Beds: 151

Accident and Emergency T Beattie

Anaesthetics L Aldridge, E Doyle, J Freeman, I Hudson, J McFadzean, M Rose, D Simpson, C Young

Audiological Medicine D L Cowan, A I G Kerr

Biochemistry J Kirk

General Psychiatry F Forbes, P Hoare, B Norton

Haematology A E Thomas, H Wallace

Orthopaedics M McNicol

Paediatric Surgery G MacKinlay, F Munro, J Orr, D Wilson-Storey

Paediatrics D Brown, J K Brown, J E Burns, J Burt, W A M Cutting, A T Edmunds, P Evenson, M Godman, C Kelnar, N Macintosh, T Marshall, R A Minns, G Stark, W S Uttley, H Wallace, D C Wilson

Pathology J Keeling, K MacKenzie

Plastic Surgery J D Watson

Radiology G M A Hendry, S MacKenzie, M McPhillips, A Wilkinson

Royal Infirmary of Edinburgh

51 Little France Crescent, Old Dalkeith Road, Edinburgh EH16 4SA
Tel: 0131 536 1000 Fax: 0131 536 1001
Total Beds: 766

Accident and Emergency C Robertson, D Steedman

Anaesthetics R P Alston, I H Annan, I Armstrong, F Arnstein, D Beamish, G Bowler, D T Brown, A S Buchan, J Campbell, V Clark, I A Davidson, A Delvaux, M Dickson, J Donnelly, G B Drummond, J N A Gibson, C Howie, J Jenkins, G Keenan, G Lawson, A Lee, D G Littlewood, M R Logan, J H McClure, A Mackenzie, S MacKenzie, D W McKeown, M F Macnicol, A Macrae, N A Malcolm-Smith, N Maran, J McBirnie, M McMaster, J Milne, C Moores, C Morton, A Nimmo, S Nimmo, R Nutton, R Park, A T Pollock, G Pugh, D Ray, J Robb, D H T Scott, D Semple, G H Sharwood-Smith, E Simon, C J Sinclair, A A Spence, H Spens, D Swann, T Walsh, J Wang, D Watson, D Weir

Biochemistry S W Walker

Cardiac Surgery E Brackenbury, E W J Cameron, C Campanella, P S Mankad, S Prasad, W S Walker

Cardiology P Bloomfield, N Boon, A Flapan, K A A Fox, H C Miller, N Uran

Care of the Elderly B J Chapman, N Colledge, C T Currie, D Grant, C Stewart, J Whitwell

Dermatology R D Aldridge, E Benton, D K Buxton, G M Cavanagh, V Doherty, J A A Hunter, G Kavanash, D Kemmett, J Rees, J A Savin, O M Schofield, M J Tidman

ENT D Cowan, W E Grant, A I G Kerr, G Macdougall, R Mills

Gastroenterology N D C Findlayson, P Hayes, R C Heading, A J McGilchrist, J Plevris, K Simpson

General Medicine D Bell, B Chapman, B Frier, R C Heading, E Housley, C Kelly, T Mackay, A Patrick, C Stewart, A Toft, M Uren, J Walker, M L Watson, C Whitworth, M Young

General Surgery D C C Bartolo, T J Crofts, A de Beaux, K C H Fearon, J L Forsythe, S Fraser, O J Garden, D Lee, K K Madhaven, S Paterson-Brown

Genitourinary Medicine A McMillan, G R Scott, C Thomson

Medical Microbiology S Burns, D H Crawford, F Emmanuel, N Hallam, R S Miles, M M Ogilvie, P Simmons, S Sutherland, D M Weir

Metabolic Medicine B Frier, A Patrick, A Toft, J Walker, M Young

Nephrology A D Cumming, R G Phelps, C P Swainson, N Turner, C Whitworth, R J Winney

Neurology C Leueck, C Mumford

Obstetrics and Gynaecology R Anderson, D T Baird, K Boddy, A Brown, A D G Brown, C Busby-Earle, A A Calder, E S Cooper, H O D Critchley, K Dundas, D I M Farquharson, R Hughes, D S Irvine, F D Johnstone, S Lawson, M M Lees, W A Liston, H McPherson, J A Milne, G E Smart, C Tay, C P West

Orthopaedics J Christie, C M Court-Brown, J F Keating, M M M McQueen, C W Oliver, C M Robinson, A Simpson

Paediatrics I Laing, A Lyon, G Menon, B Stenson

Pathology A I Al-Nafusssi, J Bell, A Busuttil, E Cowan, E Duvall, P Fineron, S Fleming, H M Gilmour, K M Grigor, D J Harrison, H Kamel, A Lammie, E McGoogan, K M McLaren, M O'Sullivan, J Piris, B Purdue, W A Reid, D M Salter, A R W Williams, A H Wyllie

Psychology S Machale, G Masterton, S G Potts

Radiology P L Allan, I Beggs, S E Chambers, I N Gillespie, S Ingram, K McBride, G McKillop, S Monssa, S Moussa, J Murchison, D Patel, I M Prossor, D N Redhead, R Sellar, J Walker, J Walsh, A J A Wightman

Respiratory Medicine S Donnelly, N Douglas, C Haslet, A Hill, W MacNee, T Makay, T J Sethi, J Simpson

Rheumatology J Campbell

Thoracic Surgery E W J Cameron, W Walker

Vascular Surgery A Bradbury, R Chalmers, A M Jenkins, D Kitts, J A Murie

Virology M M Ogilvie, S Sutherland

Royal Victoria Hospital

13 Craigleith Road, Edinburgh EH4 2DN
Tel: 0131 537 5000 Fax: 0131 537 5140
Total Beds: 200

General Medicine R Lindley, E MacDonald, R G Smith, J Starr

General Psychiatry E McLennan, A Stewart

Western General Hospital

Crewe Road, Edinburgh EH4 2XU
Tel: 0131 537 1000 Fax: 0131 537 1001
Total Beds: 604

Anaesthetics P Andrews, T Aziz, C Brookman, B Cook, M Cullen, I Foo, J Freshwater, I S Grant, G Jones, K P Kelly, S Mackenzie, S Midgley, M Rutledge, A Stewart, R B Sutherland, C B Wallis, J J Wedgewood, D J Wright

Bacteriology J E Coia, M F Hanson, R G Masterton

Biochemistry J P Ashby, P Rae, P R Wenham

Cardiology M Denvir, D B Northridge, T R D Shaw, I R Starkey, G R Sutherland

Chest Disease A P Greening, J A Innes

Endocrinology R Brown, R L Kennedy, J McKnight, P L Padfield, J S Seckl, B Walker, D J Webb

ENT D L Cowan, W Singh

Gastroenterology S Ghosh, K P Palmer

General Medicine M S Dennis, P L Padfield, W H Price, J S Seckl, D J Webb

General Psychiatry K Slatford, W A Tait

General Surgery E Anderson, U Chetty, M Dixon, M Dunlop, D W H Hodges, C McArdle, I M C McIntyre, S J Nixon, R G Wilson

Genetics D Fitzpatrick, M Porteus, A Wright

Haematology J Davies, M J Mackie

Neurology R Davenport, R Grant, R Knight, C Mumford, P A G Sandercock, G Stewart, C Warlow, B Weller, R Will, A Z J Zeman

Neuropathology J E Bell, J Ironside, G A Lammie, R Will

Neurophysiology R Cull

Neurosurgery P Andrews, G L M Carmichael, D Child, J L Jenkinson

Oncology D Jodrell, J F Smyth

Pathology T J Anderson, J Bell, K M Grigor, J Ironside, G Lammie, A M Lessells, M A McIntyre, P Rae, J S J Thomas, J N Webb

Radiology J P Brush, M Chapman, D Collie, R J Gibson, D C Grieve, R J Sellar, A J Stevenson, C M Turnbull, J Wardlaw, A R Wright, W Young

Radiotherapy and Oncology V Cowie, A Gregor, G W Howard, L H Kunkler, R H MacDougall

Rheumatology N Hurst, R Luqmani, G Nuki

Urology P Boilina, T B Hargreaves, A McNeill, S Moussa, G Smith, L H Stewart, D Tolley, D Tulloch

NHS Lothian, West Lothian Healthcare Division

Formerly West Lothian Healthcare NHS Trust.

Division Headquarters, St John's Hospital, Howden Road West, Livingston EH54 6PP
Tel: 01506 419666 Fax: 01506 416484
Website: www.show.scot.nhs.uk/wlt
(NHS Lothian)

Chair Robert Anderson
Chief Executive Peter Gabbitas

Bangour Village Hospital

Broxburn EH52 6LW
Tel: 01506 419666 Fax: 01506 811727
Total Beds: 56

General Psychiatry S Gilfillan, S Roscrow

St John's Hospital at Howden

Howden, Livingston EH54 6PP
Tel: 01506 419666 Fax: 01506 416484
Total Beds: 479

Accident and Emergency J Fothergill, P Freeland

Anaesthetics P Armstrong, M S Brockway, D Burke, L Carragher, S Edgar, M Fried, D Galloway, D J Henderson, E Martin, L M M Morison, S Neal, J Pahl, S Rowbottom, K G Stewart, J Thomas, K Watson

Bacteriology E Williamson

Care of the Elderly D Farquhar, C Goddard, S Ramsay, J O Walker, A Williams, J A Wilson

Clinical Chemistry D A McCullough

Dermatology V Docherty, O Schofield

ENT R J Sanderson, D W Sim, G A Vernham

General Medicine R S Gray, A J Jacob, W G Middleton

General Psychiatry S A Backett, S Gilfillan, J D Hendry, S Hume, M Mcleod, B Norton, S Roscrow, R Steel

General Surgery D Anderson, G G P Browning

Haematology R Jones, R Shepherd

Hand Surgery G Hooper

Neurology R Malhotra

Obstetrics and Gynaecology G Beattie, T K Cooper, P Dewart, A Macleod, S Nicholson, P G Thomson

Ophthalmology P Koay, A Mulvihull, M Wright

Oral and Maxillofacial Surgery G Lello, J McManners, K Stewart

Orthopaedics R Burnett, A Gibson, G Keenan, G Lawson, R J M Macdonald

Paediatrics A J Burt, H F Hammond, F Munroe, J O Orr, D Theodosiou, D Valentine, D Wilson-Storey

Palliative Care J Spiller

Pathology R M Davie

Plastic Surgery M Butterworth, J C McGregor, A A Quaba, J D Watson

Radiology P Bailey, C Beveridge, S Chambers, I Parker

Radiotherapy G Howard, H Phillips, F Yuille

Rheumatology V B Dhillon, E McRorie

St Michael's Hospital

Linlithgow EH49 6QS
Tel: 01506 842053 Fax: 01506 845746
Total Beds: 30

Care of the Elderly S E Ramsay

Tippethill Hospital

Whitburn by Armdale, Bathgate EH48 3BQ
Tel: 01501 745917 Fax: 01501 745031
Total Beds: 46

Care of the Elderly D Farquhar, J A Wilson

NHS Tayside, Acute Services Division

Formerly Tayside University Hospitals NHS Trust.

c/o NHS Tayside, King's Cross, Clepington Road, Dundee DD3 8EA
Tel: 01382 818479 Fax: 01382 424003
(NHS Tayside)

Chair Murray Petrie
Chief Executive Gerry Marr

Dundee Dental Hospital and School

2 Park Place, Dundee DD1 4HR
Tel: 01382 660111 Fax: 01382 635998
Total Beds: 96

Dentistry C J Allan, E Connor, A J Crighton, S Manton, A Shearer

Ninewells Hospital

Dundee DD1 9SY
Tel: 01382 660111 Fax: 01382 660445
Total Beds: 876

Accident and Emergency M A Johnston, W G Morrison, N M Nichol

Anaesthetics R H Allison, J Bannister, F M L Cameron, M R Checketts, S J Cole, J R Colvin, C Connolly, D M Coventry, S L

Crofts, L Duncan, G L Hutchison, P Johnston, P A Lacoux, I D Levack, N Mackenzie, C S A MacMillan, P A Manthri, W McClymont, B McGuire, G A McLeod, F A Millar, J K Nanson, G E Rodney, A J Shearer, A C Staziker, M F Thomson, E Wilson

Biochemistry E Dow

Cardiology G P McNeill, S D Pringle, T H Pringle

Clinical Radiology J Brunton, R C P Cameron, S Chakraverty, R I Doull, J G Houston, G Main, A S McCulloch, D F McLean, M J Nimmo, B Oliver, D G Sheppard, T Taylor, C M Walker, I Zeally

Cytology S Nicoll

Dermatology J Ferguson, C J Fleming, C M Green, S Lewis-Jones, J G Lowe, S M Morley

ENT R L Blair, B C Davis, Q Gardiner, S Hussain, J Irwin, R E Mountain, M M A Riad, P S White

General Medicine J B C Dick, J F Dillon, D Farmakis, A France, D A Johnston, M Jones, R T Jung, G Leese, R S MacWater, K D Morley, C Mowat, D Nathwani, T Pullar, R P Smith, J H Winter

General Surgery D A Black, D C Brown, K L Campbell, J C Forrester, G D Griffiths, M Lavelle-Jones, D M Smith, P A Stonebridge, R A B Wood

Genetics D R Goudie

Genitourinary Medicine A Ghaly

Haematology P Cachia, D J Meiklejohn

Maxillofacial Surgery P McLoughlin

Medical Microbiology L J Gorman, M Lockhart, P G McIntyre, G V Orange, G M A Phillips

Medical Physics J Davidson

Nephrology M J Andrews, I S Henderson, A Pall, A Severn

Neurosciences E S Ballantyne, M S Eljamel, D Hartmann, W A MacRae, D Mowle, J O'Riordan, K M Spillane, R Swingler, K White

Obstetrics and Gynaecology P Agustsson, E Cato, P Chein, A J Harrold, C McKenzie, N Patel, M Rajkhowa, M A R Thomson

Ophthalmology P S Baines, J A Coleiro, J Ellis, N George, C J MacEwen, S T D Roxburgh

Orthopaedics B Clift, G Foubister, A Jain, M G Naffif, M M Sharma

Paediatrics F Drimmie, J S Forsyth, M Kirkpatrick, W G Manson, R A Wilkie

Pathology F A Carey, A T Evans, A Gilmour, S Lang, J B McCullough, C A Purdie, A J Robertson, S Walsh

Plastic Surgery A Naasan, J H Stevenson, A Wilmshurst

Radiotherapy and Oncology R J Casasola, S Das, J A Dewar, F Scott, P M Windsor

Urology K Baxby, D Byrne, C M Goodman

Perth Royal Infirmary

Jeanfield Road, Perth PH1 1NX
Tel: 01738 623311 Fax: 01738 473206
Total Beds: 232

Accident and Emergency B Klaassen

Anaesthetics C Barthram, M Bell, P Coe, A Davis, W Elsden, D W Forbes, M Forster, F D Magahy, A Ratcliff, E Ritchie, S Winship

Clinical Radiology J Flinn, K Fowler, P Gamble, S McClelland, R H S Murray, R Pearson

Dentistry R Fowler

General Medicine P H Brown, A Connacher, P Currie, N Dewhurst, M Garton

General Surgery A Boyd, E H M El-Seedawy, C Eriksen, P J Fok, R W G Murdoch, W J G Murray

Medical Diagnostics A Shepherd

Obstetrics and Gynaecology R Allen, A Gordon, P Lynch, W D P Phillips

Oral and Maxillofacial Surgery I McClure

Orthodontics J D Clark

Orthopaedics A J Espley, W A Hadden, J G B MacLean, G G McLeod, B Singer

Paediatrics P W Fowlie, D F MacGregor, D Protheroe

Urology P Halliday

Stracathro Hospital

Brechin DD9 7QA
Tel: 01356 647291 Fax: 01356 648163
Total Beds: 53

Anaesthetics C W Allison, I Grove-White, A Houghton

Clinical Radiology J A Tainsh

General Medicine G Brennan, T S Callaghan, N Reynolds

Orthopaedics J R Buckley, P Rickhuss, J E Scullion, N W Valentine

Urology N H Townell

NHS Tayside, Primary Care Division

Formerly Tayside Primary Care NHS Trust.

c/o NHS Tayside, King's Cross, Clepington Road, Dundee DD3 8EA
Tel: 01382 818479 Fax: 01382 424003
(NHS Tayside)

Aberfeldy Cottage Hospital

Aberfeldy PH15 2DH
Tel: 01887 820314 Fax: 01887 829604, 01887 829664
Total Beds: 25

Care of the Elderly I M Lightbody

General Medicine A N Shepherd

General Surgery P J Fok

Arbroath Infirmary

Arbroath DD11 2AT
Tel: 01241 872584 Fax: 01241 872584
Total Beds: 55

Child and Adolescent Psychiatry I C Menzies

Dermatology J G Lowe

ENT B C Davis

General Medicine T S Callaghan, K D Morley, J S A Sawers

General Psychiatry K M G Keddie

Obstetrics and Gynaecology G B James, A A Thomson

Ophthalmology C McEwen

Orthopaedics J E Scullion

Paediatrics J S Forsyth, S A Greene

Radiology W J A Gibson, J A Tainsh

Ashludie Day Hospital

Ashludie Hospital, Monifieth, Dundee DD5 4HQ
Tel: 01382 527830

Ashludie Hospital

Monifieth, Dundee DD5 4HQ
Tel: 01382 423000 Fax: 01382 527849
Total Beds: 215

Care of the Elderly M McMurdo, R S McWalter, W J Mutch, J M Watson

General Psychiatry D J Findlay, A McHarg

Birch Avenue Day Hospital
55 Birch Aveune, Scone, Perth PH2 6LE
Tel: 01738 553920

Learning Disabilities C B Ballinger

Blairgowrie Cottage Hospital
Blairgowrie PH10 6EE
Tel: 01250 874466 Fax: 01250 876194
Total Beds: 62

Care of the Elderly I M Lightbody

Brechin Infirmary
Infirmary Street, Brechin DD9 7AW
Tel: 01356 622291 Fax: 01356 666075
Total Beds: 54

Care of the Elderly J D Fulton

Consultants J Mills

ENT B C Davis

General Medicine T S Callaghan

General Psychiatry A M Drayson

General Surgery A D Irving, N H Townell

Orthopaedics R Buckley

Crieff Hospital
King Street, Crieff PH7 3HR
Tel: 01764 653173 Fax: 01764 654051
Total Beds: 60

Care of the Elderly I M Lightbody

General Medicine N Dewhurst, M Garton

General Surgery R W G Murdoch

Obstetrics and Gynaecology R Allen

Forfar Infirmary
Forfar DD8 2HS
Tel: 01307 464551 Fax: 01307 465129
Total Beds: 50

Consultants R Smith

ENT R P Mills

General Medicine T S Callaghan

General Psychiatry A M Drayson

General Surgery A D Irving

Orthopaedics J E Scullion

Radiology W J A Gibson, J A Tainsh

Glaxo Day Hospital
Ashludie Hospital, Victoria Street, Monifieth, Dundee DD5 4HQ
Tel: 01382 423000 Fax: 01382 527852

Hawkhill Day Hospital
Peddie Street, Dundee DD1 5LB
Tel: 01382 423000

Irvine Memorial Hospital
Pitlochry PH16 5HP
Tel: 01796 472052 Fax: 01796 474279
Total Beds: 27

Care of the Elderly I M Lightbody

General Medicine P Brown, A Connacher

General Surgery P J Fok

Little Cairnie Hospital
Cairnie Road, Arbroath DD11 3RA
Tel: 01241 872584 Fax: 01241 872584
Total Beds: 57

Care of the Elderly J D Fulton, I Gillanders

Montrose Royal Infirmary
Montrose DD10 8AJ
Tel: 01674 830361 Fax: 01674 830361
Total Beds: 44

Care of the Elderly J D Fulton

ENT R P Mills

General Surgery A D Irving, N H Townell

Obstetrics and Gynaecology P W Howie, D J Taylor

Ophthalmology P S Baines

Orthopaedics R Buckley

Murray Royal Hospital
Perth PH2 7BH
Tel: 01738 621151, 01738 621158 Fax: 01738 442630
Total Beds: 340

General Psychiatry P J Connelly, M A Field, H E Kirk, D Mowat, K Richard, D H Tait

Orleans Day Hospital
Orleans Place, Menzieshill, Dundee DD2 4BH
Tel: 01382 667322

General Psychiatry A H Ried, M M Semple

Rosemount Day Hospital
Rosemount Road, Arbroath DD11 2AY
Tel: 01241 72584, 01241 872584

General Psychiatry K M G Keddie

Royal Dundee Liff Hospital
Liff, Dundee DD2 5NF
Tel: 01382 423000 Fax: 01382 423055
Total Beds: 337

General Psychiatry P H Dick, J L Fellows, D J Findlay, A M McHarg, I C Reid, M M Semple, B M Shepherd, A H W Smith

Royal Victoria Day Hospital
Jedburgh Road, Dundee DD2 1SP
Tel: 01382 423000 Fax: 01382 423122

Royal Victoria Hospital
Jedburgh Road, Dundee DD2 1SP
Tel: 01382 423000 Fax: 01382 423122
Total Beds: 180

Care of the Elderly M McMurdo, R S McWalter, W J Mutch, J M Watson

Clinical Radiology J D Begg

General Medicine D Gentleman

Palliative Medicine M Leiper

St Margaret's Hospital
Auchterarder PH3 1JH
Tel: 01764 662246 Fax: 01764 664084
Total Beds: 16

General Medicine P Brown, A Connacher

General Surgery P J Fok

Orthopaedics W Hadden

Strathmartine Hospital
Dundee DD3 0PG
Tel: 01382 423000 Fax: 01382 528027

Consultants C B Ballinger, A H Reid, A H W Smith, P J Walker
Paediatrics E M Merry, K Naismith

Sunnyside Royal Hospital
Montrose DD10 9JP
Tel: 01674 830361 Fax: 01674 830361
Total Beds: 195

General Psychiatry A M Drayson, S Logie, P Rice

Threshold Day Hospital
2-3 Dudhope Terrace, Dundee DD3 6HG
Tel: 01382 423000 Fax: 01382 202585

General Psychiatry P H Dick

Whitehills Hospital
Forfar DD8 3DY
Tel: 01307 464551 Fax: 01307 465129
Total Beds: 38

Care of the Elderly J D Fulton, I Gillanders

Orkney Islands

(NHS Orkney)

Balfour Hospital
Kirkwall KW15 1BH
Tel: 01856 885400 Fax: 01856 885411
Total Beds: 94

Anaesthetics C Borland, J Scott

General Surgery A Al-Mukhtar, M Dohrn

St Magnus Day Hospital
Balfour Hospital, Kirkwall KW15 1BH
Total Beds: 6

Shetland Islands

(NHS Shetland)

Gilbert Bain Hospital
South Road, Lerwick ZE1 0TB
Tel: 01595 743000 Fax: 01595 696608
Total Beds: 70

Anaesthetics P O'Connor, R Rarity

Gastroenterology Z Jussa

General Medicine F Johnson, N D R Laidlay

General Psychiatry D Senior

General Surgery J Brost, H Veen

Montfield Hospital
Burgh Road, Lerwick ZE1 0LA
Tel: 01595 743000
Total Beds: 20

Western Isles

(NHS Western Isles)

St Brendans Hospital
Castlebay HS9 5XE
Tel: 01871 810465
Total Beds: 5

Uist and Barra Hospital
Balivanich, Isle of Benbecula HS7 5LA
Tel: 01870 603603 Fax: 01870 603636
Total Beds: 29

Western Isles Hospital
MacAulay Road, Stornoway HS1 2AF
Tel: 01851 704704
Total Beds: 212

Anaesthetics A P Hothersall

General Medicine J A D Goodall

General Psychiatry I Clark

General Surgery D A MacLean

Obstetrics and Gynaecology D J Herd

Radiology I C F Riach

Wales

Bro Morgannwg NHS Trust

Provides a comprehensive range of integrated services to a population of approximately 300,000. Covers Bridgend, Neath, Port Talbot and Western Vale of Glamorgan localities.

Trust Headquarters, 71 Quarella Road, Bridgend CF31 1YE
Tel: 01656 752752 Fax: 01656 665377
Website: www.bromor-tr.wales.nhs.uk
(Mid and West Wales)

Chair Russell Hopkins
Chief Executive Paul Williams

Cimla Hospital
Cimla, Neath SA11 3SU
Tel: 01639 641161
Total Beds: 40

Croeso Centre
Highland Avenue, Bryncethin, Bridgend CF32 9YL
Tel: 01656 726900
Total Beds: 28

Glanrhyd Hospital
Tondu Road, Bridgend CF31 4LN
Tel: 01656 752752
Total Beds: 105

Groeswen Hospital
Margam Road, Port Talbot SA13 2LA
Tel: 01639 641161
Total Beds: 40

Maesteg Community Hospital
Neath Road, Maesteg, Bridgend CF34 9PW
Tel: 01656 732732
Total Beds: 47

Manager Tracey Rimmer

Neath Port Talbot Hospital
Baglan Way, Port Talbot SA12 7BX
Tel: 01639 862000 Fax: 01639 862583
Total Beds: 270

Manager Karl Murray

Princess of Wales Hospital
Coity Road, Bridgend CF31 1RQ
Tel: 01656 752752
Total Beds: 570

Manager Gaenor Shaw

Tonna Hospital
Tonna, Uchaf, Neath SA11 3LX
Tel: 01639 635404 Fax: 01639 641312
Total Beds: 70

Cardiff and Vale NHS Trust

Cardigan House, Heath Park, Cardiff CF14 4XW
Tel: 029 2074 7747 Fax: 029 2074 2968
Email: enquiries@cardiffandvale.wales.nhs.uk
Website: www.cardiffandvale.wales.nhs.uk
(South East Wales)

Chair Simon Jones
Chief Executive Hugh Ross

The Barry Hospital
Colcot Road, Barry CF62 8HE
Tel: 01446 704000 Fax: 01446 704103
Total Beds: 81

Cardiff Royal Infirmary - West Wing
Newport Road, Cardiff CF24 0SZ
Tel: 029 2049 2233 Fax: 029 2048 39683
Total Beds: 113

Genitourinary Medicine R A Sparks

Geriatric Medicine J E Grey

Lansdowne Hospital
Sanitorium Road, Canton, Cardiff CF11 8PL
Tel: 029 2037 2451
Total Beds: 110

Llandough Hospital
Llandough Hospital, Penlan Road, Llandough, Penarth CF64 2XX
Tel: 029 2071 1711 Fax: 029 2070 8973
Total Beds: 511

Anaesthetics I Bowler, N D Groves, J E Hall, M W Hebden, A Mehta, S Morris, M R W Stacey, C Taylor, A Turley, E M Wright

Chemical Pathology S B Matthews

Community Paediatrics A M Kemp, J M R Morgan, J R Sibert

Dermatology C C Long

General Medicine P Beck, B H Davies, J T Green, J H Lazarus, D R Owens, P A Routledge, G L Swift, J P Thompson

General Surgery J S Harvey, I J Monypenny, A G Radcliffe

Geriatric Medicine M S O'Mahony, M F V Sim, M D Stone, K W Woodhouse

Haematology A I M Al-Sabah

Histopathology R L Attanoos, N S Dallimore, A R Gibbs, R Olafsdottir

Obstetrics and Gynaecology J Evans, P C Lindsay, A E J Rees, A Roberts

Orthopaedics P R Davies, C M Dent, J A Fairclough, G P Graham, S S Hemmadi, J P Howes, A W John, M V S Maheson, R L Morgan-Jones, D P W O'Doherty, D J Shewring, D P Thomas, R L Williams, C A Wilson

Paediatric Oncology R D W Hain, M E M Jenney

Paediatrics and Neonatology M A Alfaham, D P Tuthill

Radiology H Adams, R E Bleehen, M D Crane

Respiratory Medicine I A Campbell, T L Griffiths, D J Shale

Rookwood Hospital
Fairwater Road, Llandaff, Cardiff CF5 2YN
Tel: 029 2041 5415 Fax: 029 2056 4065
Total Beds: 81

Rehabilitation - Spinal Injuries T A T Hughes, C G Inman

St David's Hospital
Cowbridge Road East, Cardiff CF11 9XB
Tel: 029 2053 6666
Total Beds: 100

University Dental Hospital
Heath Park, Cardiff CF14 4XY
Tel: 029 2074 7747 Fax: 029 2074 2421

Dentistry I Chestnutt, S J Crean, M L Hunter, J Knox, E T Treasure

Oral Surgery E G Absi, M J Fardy, C M Hill, J P Shepherd, D W Thomas

Orthodontics P Durning, M L Jones, R G Oliver, S Richmond

Paediatric Dentistry B L Chadwick, B Hunter

Pathology M A O Lewis, A J C Potts

Restorative Dentistry P M H Dummer, D H Edmunds, A S M Gilmour, P H Jacobsen, R G Jagger, R McAndrew, W S McLaughlin

University Hospital of Wales
Heath Park, Cardiff CF14 4XW
Tel: 029 2074 7747 Fax: 020 2074 3838
Total Beds: 970

Accident and Emergency R C Evans, R J Evans, P W Richmond

Anaesthetics R J Abel, I M Aguilera, I R Appadurai, T S H Armstrong, J Azami, J E S Barry, P A Clyburn, M Cobley, R E Collis, T S Dhallu, M P Drage, J A Dunne, J M Foy, C D Gildersleve, S Grundler, M Harmer, R C Hughes, R M Jones, I P Latto, S W Logan, C McBeth, N McCann, P Morgan, K R Murrin, D G Place, S J Plummer, S C Pugh, M S Read, N J Stallard, C N H Tan, G A Wenham, L J Wheeler, M P Whitten, P C Wiener, B A Willis

Cardiology M B Buchalter, J R Cockroft, A G Fraser, P H Groves, N D Masani, P A O'Callaghan, W J Penny, A M Shah, M R Stephens

Cardiothoracic Surgery A A Azzu, E G Butchart, E N P Kulatilake, P A O'Keefe, U O Von Oppell

Chemical Pathology M N Badminton, I F W McDowell, B P Morgan, P E Williams

Clinical Genetics A J Clarke, S J Davies, P S Harper, D T Pilz, F M Pope, D Ravine, M T Rogers, J R Sampson

Dermatology M M U Chowdhury, A M Farrell, A Y Finlay, P J A Holt, R J Motley

ENT G R Shone, S D G Stephens, A Tomkinson, R G Williams

General Medicine J S Davies, A R Freedman, C M Gelder, A J Godkin, A B Hawthorne, M J Lewis, M B Llewellyn, J R Peters, J A E Rees, M F Scanlon, G A O Thomas

General Surgery A Asderakis, W J Byrne, R E Chavez Cartaya, G W B Clark, W T Davies, K G Harding, I F Lane, R E Mansel, M C A Puntis, B I Rees, H M Sweetland, H L Young

Geriatric Medicine A M Johansen, R E Morse, J A Pascual, B S D Sastry, H G M Shetty

Haematology A K Burnett, P W Collins, A P Goringe, C H Poynton, K M O Wilson

Histopathology A M Davison, S Dojcinov, A G Douglas-Jones, D F R Griffiths, D S James, B Jasani, P Laidler, E J Lazda, S Leadbetter, M Varma, G M Vujanic, G T Williams, D Wynford-Thomas

Intensive Care G P Findlay, M N Smithies

Medical Microbiology R A Barnes, B I Duerden, K A N Hosein, A J Howard, J A Munro, C D Ribeiro, D Westmoreland

Nephrology K Baboolal, K L Donovan, R H Moore, D M Thomas, J D Williams

Neurology J P Heath, I N F McQueen, N P Robertson, A E Rosser, P E M Smith, C M Wiles

Neuropathology G A Lammie, J W Neal

Neurosurgery R H Hatfield, B A Simpson, G C Stephenson, J A Vafidis

Obstetrics and Gynaecology N N Amso, R B Beattie, N J Davies, A S Evans, R J A Penketh

Ophthalmology R A Cheema, C Gorman, C M Lane, R J E McPherson, J E Morgan, K N Rajkumar, R F Walters, P O Watts

Orthopaedics P R Davies, C M Dent, J A Fairclough, G P Graham, S S Hemmadi, J P Howes, A W John, M V S Maheson, R L Morgan-Jones, D P W O'Doherty, D J Shewring, D P Thomas, R L Williams, C A Wilson

Paediatric Cardiology O Onuzo, O Uzun, D G Wilson

Paediatric Intensive Care R H Al-Samsam, C H Fardy, M Gajraj, A D Pryor

Paediatric Nephrology G C Smith, K Verrier-Jones

Paediatric Neurology F M Gibbon, S S Jayawant

Paediatric Surgery S N Huddart, K A R Hutton, R H Surana

Paediatrics and Neonatology P H T Cartlidge, D P Davies, C B Doherty, I J M Doull, M R Drayton, H R Jenkins, C V E Powell, G J Shortland

Radiology M W Bourne, D L Cochlin, C Evans, A C Gordon, T M Griffith, S F S Halpin, K Hammer, S K Harrison, M D Hourihan, A Jones, B W Lawrie, D C F Lloyd, K Lyons, S J Morris, J I S Rees, S A Roberts, N G Stoodley, A M Wood

Rheumatology J P Camilleri, S M Jones, M P Pritchard, B D Williams

Transplant Surgery A Asderakis, R E Chavez Cartaya, W A Jurewicz

Urology S N Datta, B J Jenkins, P N Matthews

Women, Children and Community Care M Drayton

Whitchurch Hospital

Park Poad, Whitchurch, Cardiff CF4 7XB
Tel: 029 2069 3191 Fax: 029 2033 6339
Total Beds: 331

General Psychiatry M D Alldrick, J I Bisson, H L Chubb, M M Creaby, G Davies, P D Halford, J Hillier, H P Holmes, S S M Jawad, R G Jones, A M P Kellam, A Korszun, J E Lewis, G Martinez, J Morgan, M J Owen, R Pates, G Phillips, D A Ridley-Siegert, A T Sabir, R C Scorer, S J Smith, A Thapar, C Twining, A J Williams, P A Williams

Carmarthenshire NHS Trust

Mynydd Mawr Hospital, Llannon Road, Upper Tumble, Llanelli SA14 6BU
Tel: 01269 832343 Fax: 01269 832913
Email: forename.surname@carmathern.wales.nhs.uk
Website: www.carmarthen.wales.nhs.uk
(Mid and West Wales)

Chair Margaret Price
Chief Executive Paul Barnett

Amman Valley Hospital

Glanamman, Ammanford SA18 2BQ
Tel: 01269 822226 Fax: 01269 826953
Total Beds: 28

Care of the Elderly G C Morris (Head)

General Surgery H J R Evans (Head), S Rowley, M Taube

Haematology R V Major (Head)

Obstetrics and Gynaecology T H Bloomfield (Head), D N Beruah

Ophthalmology T J Roberts-Harry (Head), D Jones

Bryntirion Hospital

Llanelli SA15 3DX
Tel: 01554 756567

Care of the Elderly T P L Thomas (Head)

General Psychiatry A C Owen (Head)

Llandovery Hospital

Llandovery SA20 0LA
Tel: 01550 720322 Fax: 01550 721270
Total Beds: 18

Manager E Williams

Mynydd Mawr Hospital

Tumble, Llanelli SA14 6BU
Tel: 01269 841343 Fax: 01269 832681
Total Beds: 33

Care of the Elderly G C Morris (Head)

Haematology R V Majer (Head)

Prince Philip Hospital

Bryngwynmawr, Dafen, Llanelli SA14 8QF
Tel: 01554 756567 Fax: 01554 772271
Total Beds: 237

Accident and Emergency M Vaziri (Head), M E Jones

Anaesthetics M Esmail, R Kotian, M Martin, A K Nigam, D C Richards, F Schuetz

Chemical Pathology N A A Haboubi (Head)

Dermatology S L W Blackford (Head)

ENT S Browning, B R Davies, H B Whittet

General Medicine P Avery (Head), Dr Dev, M J Dew, E Edmunds, K Lewis, C Llewelyn-Jones, G C Morris, A Raybould, T P L Thomas, T D M Williams

General Surgery H J R Evans, S D Holt, S Rowley, D Shanahan, U I Sharaf

Haematology R V Majers (Head), S Lewis

Medical Microbiology G Harrison (Head)

Obstetrics and Gynaecology T H Bloomfield, G McSweeney, N Piskorowski

Ophthalmology T J Roberts-Harry (Head), D Jones

Orthodontics D J Howells (Head)

Orthopaedics S Caiach, P Cnuddle, H Fanarof, R S Johnson, H Richards

Paediatrics M Cosgrove, C Sullivan, S Warren

Pathology Dr Major (Head), L A Murray

Radiology J Al-Koteesh, T N W Evans, A Richards

Radiotherapy and Oncology C S Askill (Head), T Joannides

Rheumatology D H Smith (Head), B J Sweetman

Priory Day Hospital
West Wales General Hospital, Carmarthen SA31 2AF
Tel: 01267 227384 Fax: 01267 237662

West Wales General Hospital
Glangwili, Carmarthen SA31 2AF
Tel: 01267 235151 Fax: 01267 227715
Total Beds: 362

Accident and Emergency J H Williams (Head), M E Jones

Anaesthetics A G P Laxton, C F Loyden, V S Mahon, R O'Donohoe, R Prasad, P J Rimell, W Thompson, M J Turtle, B H Yate

ENT B R Davies (Head), N J Morgan, D Stephens, M A Thomas, M Thomes

General Medicine P G Avery (Head)

General Surgery A Locker (Head), M R Nutt, B M O'Riordan, W G Sheridan

Haematology V R Cumber (Head), S Lewis

Neurology C Rickards (Head)

Obstetrics and Gynaecology T H Bloomfield, K G P McSweeney, N Piskorowskyj

Oncology A M El-Sharkawi (Head), M Wilkins

Ophthalmology J Roberts-Harry (Head), P M Brown, D Jones

Oral and Maxillofacial Surgery S C Hodder (Head), K C Silvester

Orthodontics S J James (Head)

Orthopaedics R J Black, S Chatterji, H Fanarof, S R Johnson, H Richards

Paediatrics M Cosgrove, I Doul, J Gregory, M Jenny, G Owen, V R Saxena, C Sullivan, H Traunecker, Dr Vandervoort, J T Waner, S Warren, C White, D Wilson

Palliative Medicine P M Purcell (Head)

Pathology D Major (Head), R B Denholm, N A A Haboubi, J Murphy

Plastic Surgery M A C Cooper (Head)

Public Health Medicine G A J Harrison (Head)

Radiology D I Khechane, S C Nandi, C C Ngoma

Radiotherapy A M M El-Sharkawi (Head)

Sexual Health A Cattell (Head)

Urology B M Gana, M Moosa, M Taube

Ceredigion and Mid Wales NHS Trust

Bronglais General Hospital, Caradog Road, Aberystwyth SY23 1ER
Tel: 01970 623131 Fax: 01970 635923
Email: firstname.surname@ceredigion-tr.wales.nhs.uk
Website: www.ceredigion-tr.wales.nhs.uk
(Mid and West Wales)

Chair Eleri Ebenezer
Chief Executive Allison Williams

Aberaeron Cottage Hospital
Aberaeron SA46 0JJ
Tel: 01545 570225 Fax: 01545 570953

Bronglais General Hospital
Aberystwyth SY23 1ER
Tel: 01970 623131 Fax: 01970 635923
Total Beds: 170

Anaesthetics M Collingborne (Head), G Bonsu, B Campbell, R M Henderson, K P Mishra

Care of the Elderly G V Boswell, P Jones

General Medicine A T Axford, G Boswell, A G Davies

General Surgery D Jackson (Head), J L Edwards, R Visvanathan

Haematology H I Atrah

Obstetrics and Gynaecology Mrs Hammon, Mrs Nan

Ophthalmology Mr Shan

Orthopaedics A D Meredith, W Spaeth, Mr Tandon

Paediatrics D D Walters (Head), A Khan, J Williams

Pathology C G B Simpson (Head), C G B Simpson

Radiology P Cornah

Cardigan and District Memorial Hospital
Cardigan SA43 1DP
Tel: 01239 612214 Fax: 01239 621394
Total Beds: 25

Manager Judith Pitkin

Tregaron Hospital
Tregaron SY25 6JP
Tel: 01974 298203 Fax: 01974 298024
Total Beds: 29

Manager Angela Lloyd-Jones

Conwy and Denbighshire NHS Trust

Glan Clwyd Hospital, Sarn Lane, Rhyl LL18 5UJ
Tel: 01745 583910 Fax: 01745 583143
Email: mail@cd-tr.wales.nhs.uk
Website: www.conwy-denbighshire-nhs.org.uk
(North Wales)

Chair Hilary Stevens
Chief Executive Gren Kershaw

Abergele Hospital
Abergele LL22
Tel: 01745 832295
Total Beds: 71

Manager Kay Hemsley

Chest Disease T J Charles, K Taylor

Orthopaedics S Bastawrous, N R Clay, A O'Kelly, A Sinna

Rheumatology W R Williams

Colwyn Bay Community Hospital
Hesketh Road, Colwyn Bay LL29 8AY
Tel: 01492 515218 Fax: 01492 518103
Total Beds: 42

Manager Jane Trowman

Denbigh Community Hospital
Ruthin Road, Denbigh LL16 3ES
Tel: 01745 812624 Fax: 01745 815851
Total Beds: 49

Manager Eva Edwards

Glan Clwyd District General Hospital

Bodelwyddan, Rhyl LL18 5UJ
Tel: 01745 583910
Total Beds: 683

Accident and Emergency D Cartlidge, S Gandham

Anaesthetics C F Bell, G Davies, A J P Lake, S J Seager, B Tehan, B Waters, T B Webb, E G N Williams

Care of the Elderly B K Bhowmick, M W Greenway, R J Meara, J D D Wood

Dermatology R E A Williams

ENT Z Hammad, J E Osborne

General Medicine T J Charles, G J Green, R Sheers

General Surgery J Clark, C J Davies, C M Evans, D J Hay, O E Klimach, V Srinivasan

Genitourinary Medicine O E Williams

Neurosurgery R V Jeffreys, M T M Shaw

Obstetrics and Gynaecology P Banfield, N Bickerton, J A Edwards, D J Thomas

Oral Surgery C N Penfold, J G Phillips

Orthodontics R C Parkhouse

Orthopaedics N R Clay, M J S Hubbard, J Lewis

Paediatrics P D Cameron, P R Stutchfield

Pathology A D A Dalton, D R Edwards, D I Gozzard, D N Looker, B Rodgers

Radiology N P Archard, R A Byrne, S J Hotson, C A McConnell, E Moss, H G Row, D J Widdowson, J Williams, C H Wright

Rheumatology W R Williams

HM Stanley Hospital

St Asaph LL17 0RS
Tel: 01745 583275
Total Beds: 16

Manager Kay Hemsley

Ophthalmology R Haslett

Llangollen Community Hospital

Abby Road, Llangollen LL20 8SP
Tel: 01978 860226 Fax: 01978 861047
Total Beds: 18

Manager Eva Edwards

General Medicine M D Gareh

Prestatyn Community Hospital

49 The Avenue, Woodlands Park, Prestatyn LL19 9RD
Tel: 01745 853487 Fax: 01745 887479
Total Beds: 12

Manager Jane Trowman

Royal Alexandra Hospital

Marine Drive, Rhyl LL18 3AS
Tel: 01745 343188 Fax: 01745 344574
Total Beds: 54

Manager Jane Trowman

Care of the Elderly B K Bhowmick

General Medicine H Jones

Ruthin Hospital

Llanrhydd Street, Ruthin LL15 1PS
Tel: 01824 702692 Fax: 01824 704719
Total Beds: 48

Manager Eva Edwards

General Medicine J D G Williams

Gwent Healthcare NHS Trust

Grange House, Llanfrechfa Grange, Cwmbran NP44 8YN
Tel: 01633 623623 Fax: 01633 623836
Website: www.gwent-tr.wales.nhs.uk
(South East Wales)

Chair Brian Willott
Chief Executive Martin Turner

Aberbargoed and District Hospital

Commercial Street, Aberbargoed, Bargoed CF81 9BU
Tel: 01443 828728
Total Beds: 28

Manager Sian Millar

Abertillery and District Hospital

Pendarren Road, Aberbeeg, Abertillery NP13 2XA
Tel: 01495 214123
Total Beds: 52

Manager Sian Millar

Blaenavon Hospital

Church Street, Blaenavon NP4 9AS
Tel: 01495 790236
Total Beds: 9

Manager Sian Millar

Blaina and District Hospital

Hospital Road, Blaina NP23 4LY
Tel: 01495 293250
Total Beds: 49

Manager Sian Millar

Caerphilly and District Miners' Hospital

St Martins Road, Caerphilly CF83 2WW
Tel: 029 2085 1811
Total Beds: 111

Manager Sue Rodway

Care of the Elderly M Hasan, M Joglekar

General Medicine D R Davies, L D George, L D K Premawardhana

Obstetrics and Gynaecology M Ashraf, G J Edwards, R Goddard

Chepstow Community Hospital

Tempest Way, Chepstow NP16 5YX
Tel: 01291 636636
Total Beds: 84

Manager Sian Millar

County Hospital

Coed-y-Gric Road, Griffithstown, Pontypool NP4 5YA
Tel: 01495 768768
Total Beds: 97

Manager Sian Millar

Ebbw Vale Hospital

Hillside, Ebbw Vale NP23 5YA
Tel: 01495 356956
Total Beds: 23

Manager Sian Millar

Llanfrechfa Grange Hospital
Llanfrechfa, Cwmbran NP44 8YN
Tel: 01633 623623
Total Beds: 79

Manager Andrew Hopkins

Community Dentistry S Boyce

Community Gynaecology and Sexual Health C Fleming, T McCarthy

Learning Disabilities P V Ramachandran, U Suvagamasundari

Paediatrics Z Vermaak

Maindiff Court Hospital
Ross Road, Abergavenny NP7 8NF
Tel: 01873 735500
Total Beds: 62

Manager Rhiannon Davies, Paul Sussex

Alcohol and Substance Abuse M Rowlands

General Psychiatry I Jones

Psychiatry of Old Age V B Bapujirao, R M L Lewis, P Ruth

Monmouth Hospital
15 Hereford Road, Monmouth NP25 3HG
Tel: 01600 713522
Total Beds: 25

Manager Sian Millar

Nevill Hall Hospital
Beacon Road, Abergavenny NP7 7EG
Tel: 01873 732732
Total Beds: 107

Manager Sian Martin

Accident and Emergency N H Jenkins

Anaesthetics S Bhanumurthy, W P Cave, C Harrison, C Heneghan, D J Hoad, J Howes, M K Kocan, M J Martin, R M Rouse, J A Russell, A C Summors

Care of the Elderly M Edwards, N Y Haboubi, P B Khanna

Child and Adolescent Psychiatry M Shooter

General Medicine E Boyd, A B Davies, S Hutchison, P M Neville, B V Prathibha, J Saunders, J Thomas

General Surgery R L Blackett, C J Bransom, R J Delicata, S Ghosh, R Hargest, D R B Jones

Haematology H Habboush, G Robinson

Medical Microbiology N Carbarns

Neurology F Thomas

Obstetrics and Gynaecology A Dawson, W D Jackson, I M Stokes

Orthodontics H Taylor

Orthopaedics H Davies, I Mackie, A M Nada, Y Nathdwarawala, R Rice, R Walker

Paediatrics A Allman, A M Naughton, M Pierrepoint, T H C Williams

Pathology G B Evans, S Howell, R J Kellett

Radiology N Cross, R B Pickford, D H Reed, D A Robinson, S Wan, F Williams

Rheumatology A Borg, S M Linton, U Srinivasan

Urology K Queen

Oakdale Hospital
Penrhiw Terrace, Oakdale, Blackwood NP12 0JH
Tel: 01495 225207 Fax: 01495 230072
Total Beds: 20

Manager Sian Millar

Redwood Memorial Hospital
The Terrace, Rhymney NP22 5LY
Tel: 01685 840314 Fax: 01685 844928
Total Beds: 21

Manager Lindsey Davies

Royal Gwent Hospital
Cardiff Road, Newport NP20 2UB
Tel: 01633 234234 Fax: 01663 221217
Total Beds: 774

Manager Glyn Griffiths

Accident and Emergency S Jones, F Richardson, A Vaghela

Anaesthetics J Butler, C Callander, A B Carling, G S Clark, J T Curtis, S W Dumont, D J Dye, J Gough, I P C Greenway, J J Griffiths, L Harding, T Haynes, I Hodzovic, K Hoods, D J Hughes, T M Ivanova-Stoilova, J L Janes, D I Jones, H M Jones, S Martan, T Mian, I B Morris, P Nicholls, H S O'Dwyer, M Sage, D L Thomas, R Walpole, S Watson

Dermatology A V Anstey, R Goodwin, C Mills, N Stone

ENT M J K Brown, M I Clayton, D R Ingrams, J M Preece

General Medicine M Allison, N Brown, S E M Browne, J Davies, O M Gibby, M Hack, S Ikram, M Llewelyn, H J Lloyd, H Saleem, E D Srivastava, J Toner, I Williamson, T Yapp

General Surgery C A Gateley, P Holland, W G Lewis, A A Shandall, K Shute, B M Stephenson, K Vellacott, I Williams

Genitourinary Medicine R Das

Haematology C Hewlett, H Jackson, E Moffatt

Nephrology A O Phillips

Neurology J G Llewelyn

Obstetrics and Gynaecology R Gonsalves, M Stone, A N A Weerakkody, J J Wiener, A Wright

Ophthalmology C Blyth, A Feyi-Waboso, D Hughes, M Y Khan, D O'Duffy, S Webber

Oral and Maxillofacial Surgery M Gregory, J Llewelyn

Orthodontics S Wigglesworth

Orthopaedic Medicine S Hannaford-Youngs

Orthopaedics P M Alderman, W J M Czyz, A Grant, K Hariharan, D G Jones, R Kulkarni, P Roberts, R Savage, K J J Tayton

Paediatrics M Barber, J Barton, I Bowler, P Buss, P Dale, S D Ferguson, H Lewis, A Rawlinson, M Schmidt

Pathology E Kubiak, E W Owen, M D Penney, A M Rashid, I W Thompson

Radiology M Bernard, F Brook, R Clements, N Evans, J Harding, D Jackson, A Jones, P Stamper, B Sullivan, G Thomas, A Wake

Rheumatology J Bondeson, P I Williams

Urology C Bates, R L Gower

St Cadoc's Hospital
Lodge Road, Caerleon, Newport NP18 3XQ
Tel: 01633 436700
Total Beds: 94

Manager I Thomas

Child and Adolescent Psychiatry W Barber, E Kapp, D Williams, R J Williams

Psychiatry of Old Age M Reynolds

St Woolos Hospital

131 Stow Hill, Newport NP20 4SZ
Tel: 01633 234234
Total Beds: 191

Manager Sian Millar

Care of the Elderly E A Freeman, D A Sykes, A Whittaker

Occupational Health A Misir

Tredegar General Hospital

Park Row, Tredegar NP22 3XP
Tel: 01495 722271
Total Beds: 58

Manager Sian Millar

Ysbyty'r Tri Chwm

Ystrad Mynach Hospital, Caerphilly Road, Ystrad Mynach, Hengoed CF82 7XA
Tel: 01443 811411
Total Beds: 36

Manager Kevin Wood

Ystrad Mynach Hospital

Caerphilly Road, Ystrad Mynach, Hengoed CF82 7XU
Tel: 01443 811411
Total Beds: 84

Manager Sian Millar

Paediatrics V Antao, H Payne

North East Wales NHS Trust

Wrexham Maelor Hospital, Croesnewydd Road, Wrexham LL13 7TD
Tel: 01978 291100 Fax: 01978 310326
Email: firstname.surname@new-tr.wales.nhs.uk
(North Wales)

Chair Lloyd FitzHugh
Chief Executive Hilary Pepler

Chirk Community Hospital

Off St John's Street, Chirk, Wrexham LL14 5LN
Tel: 01691 772430 Fax: 01691 772342
Total Beds: 31

Manager Carol Davies

Deeside Community Hospital

Plough Lane, Higher Shotton, Deeside CH5 1XS
Tel: 01244 830461 Fax: 01244 836323
Total Beds: 31

Manager Dee Begbie

Dobshill Hospital

Chester Road, Dobshill, Deeside CH5 3LZ
Tel: 01244 550233 Fax: 01244 547872
Total Beds: 46

Manager Myra Allison

Flint Community Hospital

Cornist Road, Flint CH6 5HG
Tel: 01352 732215 Fax: 01352 730494
Total Beds: 18

Manager Dee Begbie

Holywell Community Hospital

Pen-y Maes Road, Holywell CH8 7UH
Tel: 01352 713003 Fax: 01352 715395
Total Beds: 18

Manager Shan Warburton

Lluesty Hospital

Old Chester Road, Holywell CH8 7SA
Tel: 01352 710581 Fax: 01745 534073
Total Beds: 30
Manager Mike Prew

Meadowslea Hospital

Vounog Hill, Penyffordd, Chester CH4 0EA
Tel: 01978 760412 Fax: 01978 762871
Total Beds: 43

Manager Jane Jones

Mold Community Hospital

Ash Grove, Mold CH7 1XG
Tel: 01352 758744 Fax: 01352 750469
Total Beds: 40

Manager Shan Warburton

Penley Hospital

Whitchurch Road, Penley, Wrexham LL14 0LH
Tel: 01948 832070 Fax: 01948 832071
Total Beds: 12

Manager Sheila Felton

Trevalyn Hospital

Chester Road, Rossett, Wrexham LL12 0HL
Tel: 01244 570446 Fax: 01244 571481
Total Beds: 32

Manager Sheila Felton

Wrexham Maelor Hospital

Croesnewydd Road, Wrexham LL13 7TD
Tel: 01978 291100 Fax: 01978 310326
Total Beds: 714

Accident and Emergency M A T Cook (Head), M A T Cook, A Sen

Anaesthetics L W Gemmell (Head), N M Agnew, G J Arthurs, S Coughlan, S J Counsell, C Dowling, C Edmundson, L W Gemmell, J R Jamieson, R A Jones, C Littler, V Scott-Knight, D A Southern, S Underhill, C A Wadon

Cardiology R Cowell (Head), R Cowell, R J Trent

Dermatology J M Sowden (Head), R Lister, J M Sowden

ENT J F Coakley (Head), A R Chandra-Mohan, J F Coakley, D G Snow

General Medicine J Harvey (Head), P J T Drew, J Harvey, S Kelly, N McAndrew, M O'Sullivan, A Ross, P Rutherford, S Stanaway, O Williams

General Psychiatry G C Harborne (Head), H R Cattell, A Cole-King, D R Crossley, T Dyer, C Edwards, G C Harborne, J H Race, R Viswanathan, J Walsh, T Woods

General Surgery J K Pye (Head), P Billings, R A Cochrane, A E da Silva, P Marsh, J K Pye, M Scriven

Genetics A Proctor (Head), A Proctor

Genitourinary Medicine O Williams (Head), O Williams

Medicine for the Elderly I U Shah (Head), M U Fernando, I U Shah, A White

Obstetrics and Gynaecology P R Vlies (Head), C Rosenblade, W Taylor, P G Toon, P R Vlies

Occupational Health P Zacharias (Head), P Zacharias

Oncology A Champion (Head), Dr Al-Samarrie, A Champion, S Gollins

Ophthalmology N C Kaushik (Head), N C Kaushik

Oral and Maxillofacial Surgery C Penfold (Head), C Penfold

Orthodontics J G Heyes (Head), J G Heyes

Orthopaedics K Lewis (Head), N Graham, P Laing, K Lewis, N K Makwana, S Roberts, A L Smith, J Wooton

Paediatrics G G Owens (Head), B Harrington, P E Minchom, N Nehlans, G G Owens

Paediatrics (Community) E G Bos, C Graham, A M Kelly, S Minchom, C Moore

Palliative Medicine M Makin (Head), M Makin

Pathology D K Watson (Head), A H Burdge, C Cefai, J Duguid, D K Watson, C P Williams, R B Williams

Radiology M G E Greensmith (Head), M G E Greensmith, V W Jones, C H Laine, S Meecham-Jones, G M Murray, D A Parker

Restorative Dentistry T Nisbet (Head), T Nisbet

Urology A R Bolla (Head), P S Anandaram, A R Bolla

North Glamorgan NHS Trust

Prince Charles Hospital, Merthyr Tydfil CF47 9DT
Tel: 01685 721721 Fax: 01865 723228
Website: www.nglam-tr.wales.nhs.uk
(South East Wales)

Chair Jill Penn
Chief Executive Jim Hayburn

Aberdare Hospital

Aberdare CF44 0RF
Tel: 01685 872411 Fax: 01685 882741
Total Beds: 89

Manager Keith Powell

Care of the Elderly I B Davies

General Medicine I B Davies, M Drah, B E Griffiths, S Hand, F W F Hanna, T J Morris

General Surgery P A Braithwaite, P N Haray, A Y Izzidien, A G Masoud

Orthopaedics A Hussain, Mr Khalifeh, G C Zaphiropoulos

Paediatrics J M Blankson, R W Evans, M J Maguire

Radiology R A Davies, R M Ginwalla, D W Gregory

Mountain Ash Hospital

Mountain Ash CF45 4DE
Tel: 01685 872411 Fax: 01685 882741
Total Beds: 35

Prince Charles Hospital

Merthyr Tydfil CF47 9DT
Tel: 01685 721721 Fax: 01685 388001
Total Beds: 434

Accident and Emergency G W L Evans, M Obiako, C Tovey

Anaesthetics F Mukasa, D Muthuswamy, S B Sanikop, A Scott, N Un

Care of the Elderly I B Davies, M Direkze

ENT P Johnson, A H Jones, M R P Rivron, V Singh, H O L Williams

General Medicine I B Davies, M Direkze, M Drah, K Giebally, B E Griffiths, S Hand, F W F Hanna, N Hawkes, T J Morris, A H E Shaboury

General Psychiatry P C Choudhury, B Gupta, A Owen, G Sullivan, M Winston

General Surgery P A Braithwaite, P N Haray, A Y Izzidien, A G Masoud

Obstetrics and Gynaecology H R Elliott, A Hamon, T G Maulik, S Mirando

Oral and Maxillofacial Surgery A Ezsias, C S Holland, E S Nash, P T Nicholson, P Stephenson

Orthopaedics A Hussain, K Karras, Mr Khalifeh, G Zafiropolous

Paediatrics J M Blankson, R W Evans, M J Maguire, H Okuonghae, T Rangarajan

Pathology S Kiberu, W A F Mumar-Bashi, K Myers, M I Sweerts, R Tustin

Radiology R A Davies, R M Ginwalla, D W Gregory, O T Hussein, A M Vali

Rheumatology and Rehabilitation C Rhys-Dillon

Urology S Datta, D Jones

St Tydfil's Day Hospital (Medicine)

Upper Thomas Street, Merthyr Tydfil CF47 0SJ
Tel: 01685 723244 Fax: 01685 385171

St Tydfil's Hospital (Mental Health)

Merthyr Tydfil CF47 0SJ
Tel: 01685 723244 Fax: 01685 385171
Total Beds: 162

Care of the Elderly I B Davies, M Direkze

Seymour Berry Community Mental Health Team

Victoria Street, Dowlais, Merthyr Tydfil
Tel: 01685 721671

North West Wales NHS Trust

Ysbyty Gwynedd, Penrhosgarnedd, Bangor LL57 2PW
Tel: 01248 384384 Fax: 01248 370629
Website: www.northwestwales.org
(North Wales)

Chair R Hefin Davies
Chief Executive Keith Thomson
Consultants D C Crawford, N Curzen, A El-Sheikha, J V Hindle, M Jamison, R Kanvinde, L Kaye-Wilson, N Khan, H S Mohammed, D O'Beirn, D R Prichard, H Roberts, K J Thomas, A L Vaterlaws, S Wenham

Bron y Garth Hospital

Penrhyndeudraeth LL48 6HE
Tel: 01766 770310 Fax: 01766 772142
Total Beds: 31

Bryn Beryl Hospital

Caernarfon Road, Pwllheli LL53 6TT
Tel: 01758 701122 Fax: 01758 701295
Total Beds: 32

Care of the Elderly P N Ohri, D R Prichard

General Medicine D R Prichard

Bryn Seiont Hospital

Pant Road, Caernarfon LL55 2YU
Tel: 01286 673371 Fax: 01286 678228

Bryn-y-Neuadd Hospital

Aber Road, Llanfairfechan LL33 0HH
Tel: 01248 682682 Fax: 01248 681832

Total Beds: 113

General Psychiatry F Drouet, L Vati

Psychiatry of Old Age M Devakumar

Carreg Fawr Bed Support Unit at Bryn y Neuadd Hospital
Llanfairfechan LL33 0HH
Tel: 01248 682304
Total Beds: 8

Cefni Hospital
Llangefni LL77 7PP
Tel: 01248 750117 Fax: 01248 753124
Total Beds: 35

Care of the Elderly A R Starczewski

Coed Lys
Llangefni
Tel: 01248 724318
Total Beds: 8

Deiniol Day Hospital
Ysbyty Gwynedd, Penrhosgarnedd, Bangor LL57 2PW
Tel: 01248 384068 Fax: 01248 370629

Dolgellau and Barmouth District Hospital
Dolgellau LL40 1NT
Tel: 01341 422479 Fax: 01341 423684
Total Beds: 33

Care of the Elderly J V Hindle, D P O'Beirn

Dryll y Carr Unit
Llanaber, Barmouth LL42 1YY
Tel: 01341 281049 Fax: 01341 281049
Total Beds: 8

Eryri Hospital
The Park, Caernarfon LL55 2YE
Tel: 01268 672481 Fax: 01286 674380
Total Beds: 36

Care of the Elderly P N Ohri, D R Prichard, A R Starczewski, R Subashchandran

Ffestiniog Memorial Hospital
Wynne Road, Blaenau Ffestiniog LL41 3DW
Tel: 01766 831281 Fax: 01766 830584
Total Beds: 17

Llandudno General Hospital
Llandudno LL30 1LB
Tel: 01492 860066 Fax: 01492 871668
Total Beds: 112

Care of the Elderly J V Hindle, D P O'Beirn

General Medicine J Cunningham, A L Vaterlaws

General Surgery E K N Ahiaku, D J Crawford, L R Jenkinson, G T Watkin, G Whiteley

Mental Health Acute Unit
Hergest Unit, Ysbyty Gwynedd, Penrhosgarnedd Road, Bangor LL57 2PW
Tel: 01248 384384
Total Beds: 60

Minfordd Hospital
Hendrewen Road, Bangor LL57 4DR
Tel: 01248 352308 Fax: 01248 371005

Elderly Mentally Ill M Devakumar

Ty Llywelyn (Medium Secure Unit) at Bryn y Neuadd Hospital
Llanfairfechan LL33 0HH
Tel: 01248 682132
Total Beds: 25

Tywyn and District War Memorial Hospital
Bryn Hyfryd Road, Tywyn LL36 9HH
Tel: 01654 710411 Fax: 01654 712206
Total Beds: 24

Ysbyty Gwynedd
Penrhosgarnedd, Bangor LL57 2PW
Tel: 01248 384384 Fax: 01248 370629
Total Beds: 508

Accident and Emergency P Cutting

Anaesthetics P Barry, C Eickmann, E M Farley-Hills, T J B Harris, W James, I Johnson, R P Lewis, K Mottart, W O Roberts, A Shambrook, S Smith, C H Thorpe, A Valijan

Cardiology S Talwar

Care of the Elderly J V Hindle, D P O'Beirn, D R Prichard, A R Starczewski

Clinical Oncology N S A Stuart

Dermatology A W MacFarlane

ENT G S Barr, M B Madkour, A Sheka

General Medicine W Ahmed, G F A Benfield, L L O Bloodworth, N G Hodges, M Jibani, N Khan, H S Mohammed, D Owens, A Wilton

General Surgery N Abdullah, D J Crawford, W V Humphreys, M H Jamison, L Jenkinson, G T Watkin, G Whiteley

Genitourinary Medicine U Andrady

Haematology D H Parry, J R C Seale

Neurology N Fletcher, B R F Lecky

Neurosurgery P R Eldridge

Obstetrics and Gynaecology L Bolton, S C Leeson, P Tivy-Jones

Occupational Health B C Owen

Oncology N S A Stuart

Ophthalmology K D Al-Gawi, S Amjad, L Kaye-Wilson, P J Kinahan, G Robinson, S M Zeki

Oral and Maxillofacial Surgery C Lloyd

Orthodontics W J Parry

Orthopaedics G A Attara, S G Hunter, M Jones, R Kanvinde, L McSweeney

Paediatrics M J Cronin, R H Davies, B Elnazir, J S M Horn, T G Powell, H Roberts

Palliative Medicine A Fowell

Pathology A W Caslin, K D Griffiths, A M Walker

Radiology C Adams, N C Barwick, P D Birch, R C Crawford, A J Gash, H Godfrey, J Jones, R Y Jones, S Wenham, J G Williams

Rheumatology P J Maddison

Urology E K N Ahiaku, K Thomas

Ysbyty Penrhos Stanley
Holyhead LL65 2QA
Tel: 01407 766000 Fax: 01407 766091
Total Beds: 53

Care of the Elderly K Riniotis

Psychiatry of Old Age M Devakumar

Pembrokeshire and Derwen NHS Trust

Withybush General Hospital, Fishguard Road, Haverfordwest SA61 2PZ
Tel: 01437 764545 Fax: 01437 773353
Email: admin@pdt-tr.wales.nhs.uk
Website: www.pdt-tr.wales.nhs.uk
(Mid and West Wales)

Chair Lynette George
Chief Executive Frank O'Sullivan

Bro Cerwyn Psychiatric Day Hospital
Fishguard Road, Haverfordwest SA61 2PZ
Tel: 01437 773157 Fax: 01437 773057

Bronglais General Hospital
Penglais Hill, Aberystwyth SY23 1ER
Tel: 01970 623131

Brynhaul Day Hospital
Bryntirion Hospital, Swansea Road, Llanelli SA15 3DX
Tel: 01554 756567 Fax: 01554 753519

Brynmair Day Hospital
Brynmair Clinic, 11 Goring Road, Llanelli SA15 3HH
Tel: 01554 772768

Bryntirion Hospital
Swansea Road, Llanelli SA15 2DX
Tel: 01554 756567
Total Beds: 20

Gorwelion Day Hospital
Llanbadarn Road, Aberystwyth SY23 1HB
Tel: 01970 615448

Haven Way Day Hospital
Fort Road, Pembroke Dock SA72 6SX

St Brynach's Day Hospital
Fishguard Road, Haverfordwest SA61 2PZ
Tel: 01437 764545

Manager Hassen Joomraty

St David's Hospital
Carmarthen SA31 3HB
Tel: 01267 237481 Fax: 01267 221895
Total Beds: 154

General Psychiatry R Atkinson, M S Elameer, N Evans, S Girucharanam, C A Hooper, T Magee, H Matthews, C Moyle, E Richardson, M P Sargeant, B Thompson, R Wilson

South Pembrokeshire Hospital
Fort Road, Pembroke Dock SA72 6SX
Tel: 01646 682114 Fax: 01646 774114
Total Beds: 35

Manager Pauline Morrissey

Swn-y-Gwynt Day Hospital
Tir-Y-Dail Lane, Glanamman, Ammanford SA18 3AS
Tel: 01269 595473 Fax: 01269 597518

Manager Sue Richards

Tenby Cottage Hospital
Trafalgar Road, Tenby SA70 7EE
Tel: 01834 842040 Fax: 01834 844097
Total Beds: 13

Manager Pauline Morrissey

Wellfield Day Hospital
Wellfield Road, Carmarthen SA31 1DS
Tel: 01267 236017 Fax: 01267 238506

Withybush General Hospital
Fishguard Road, Haverfordwest SA61 2PZ
Tel: 01437 764545 Fax: 01437 773353
Total Beds: 331

Anaesthetics D Bryant, R A Cooke, R Cross, R B Griffiths, D A Thomas, M J Wort

Biochemistry R G Roberts

General Surgery W Maxwell, P J Milewski

Haematology H Grubb

Integrated Medicine C M James, N I Jowett, K Mohanaruban, A Vaishnavi

Microbiology M Sheppard

Obstetrics and Gynaecology W M Clow, M R Howells, C Overton

Occupational Health R Wort

Oncology S M U Haq

Orthopaedics P Kanse, G Phillips

Paediatrics V Narayan, G Vas Falcao, V Vipulendran

Pathology G R Melville-Jones, S Polacarz

Radiology K Bradshaw, I Martin

Y Delyn Day Hospital
Canolfan Gwenog, West Wales General Hospital, Carmarthen SA31 2AF
Tel: 01267 235151 Fax: 01267 237662

Manager Sue Richards

Pontypridd and Rhondda NHS Trust

Trust Management Offices, Dewi Sant Hospital, Albert Road, Pontypridd CF37 1LB
Tel: 01443 486222 Fax: 01443 443842
Website: www.pr-tr.wales.nhs.uk
(South East Wales)

Chair Ian Kelsall
Chief Executive Margaret Foster

Dewi Sant Hospital
Albert Road, Pontypridd CF37 1LB
Tel: 01443 486222 Fax: 01443 403268
Total Beds: 108

Manager A J Jones

General Medicine R Alcolado, S M A Aslan, P S Davies, R Dewer, J R Dowdle, R T M Edwards, G Ellis, N Evans, P Evans, F L Li Saw Hee, M D Page, G Strang, J White

East Glamorgan Hospital Mental Health Unit
Mental Health Unit, Royal Glamorgan Hospital, Ynysmaerdy, Llantrisant CF72 8XR
Total Beds: 70

Manager A J Jones

Mental Health H Griffiths, R Hailwood, W A Henderson, J Smith, C Staff, Z Summers, S Watkins

Llwynypia Hospital
Llwynypia, Tonypandy CF40 2LX
Tel: 01443 440440 Fax: 01443 431611
Total Beds: 139

Manager A J Jones

Accident and Emergency W D T Moody-Jones

ENT P Johnson, A H Jones, R P Rivron, V Singh, H Williams

General Medicine R Alcolado, S M A Aslan, P S Davies, R Dewer, J R Dowdle, R T M Edwards, G Ellis, P Evans, F L Li Saw Hee, M D Page, A Pandit, G Strang, J White

General Psychiatry R Hailwood, W A Henderson, J Smith, J Smith, C Staff, Z Summers, S Watkins

General Surgery M E Foster, T Havard, M H Lewis, E Williams, R J L Williams, A Woodward

Obstetrics and Gynaecology J M Arnold, J Pembridge, D H O Pugh, S A K Roberts

Oncology R J L Williams (Head), I Kerby

Ophthalmology N Hawksworth, N U Nabi, R Raghu-Ram, S C Sullivan

Orthopaedics J Davies, P D Evans, A I R Jenkins, J M Murray, T Owen, D Pemberton

Paediatrics I Z Z al-Muzaffar, I C G Hodges, L Miller-Jones, J Moorcraft, R J H Morgan

Pathology C Champ, C DeAlwis, D Hullin, J Shannon, D Stock, D White

Radiology C J Davies, G Davies, S G Davies, K Gower Thomas, E Hicks, R Rhys, R Winter

Rheumatology J Martin (Head), C R Dillon, R Goodfellow

Urology D R Jones (Head), J French

Royal Glamorgan General Hospital
Ynys Maerdy, Llantrisant CF72 8XR
Tel: 01443 443443 Fax: 01443 217213
Total Beds: 489

Manager A J Jones

Accident and Emergency A Kamal, W D T Moody Jones

Anaesthetics S Ackerman, M Bayoumi, D Cremin, R Davies, P FitzGerald, T Saleh, J Sewell, T R Tipping, A Wagle, T G L Watkins, P V Woodsford

Child and Adolescent Psychiatry M Hasan (Head), C Bell, A K Darwish, R Duthie, R Potter

Dermatology R A Logan, C Long

Elderly Medicine S M A Aslan, R I Dewar, R T M Edwards

ENT P Johnson, A H Jones, R Rivron, V Singh, H Williams

General Medicine R Alcolado, S M A Aslan, P S Davies, R I Dewar, J R Dowdle, R M T Edwards, G Ellis, N Evans, F L Li Saw Hee, M D Page, A Pandit, G Strang, J White

General Surgery M E Foster, T Havard, M H Lewis, E Williams, R J Williams, A Woodward

Genitourinary Medicine A N Abdullah, A R G Manuel

Neurology I N F McQueen

Obstetrics and Gynaecology J M Arnold, J Pembridge, D H O Pugh, S A K Roberts

Ophthalmology N Hawkesworth, N U Nabi, A R RaghuRam, S C Sullivan

Orthopaedics J Davies, P Evans, A Jenkins, J M Murray, T Owen, D Pemberton

Paediatrics I Z Z al-Muzaffar, I C G Hodges, L Miller-Jones, J Moorcraft, R J H Morgan

Pathology C D Alwis, C Champ, D Hullin, D Stock, D White

Radiology C J Davies, G Davies, S G Davies, K L Gower-Thomas, E Hicks, R Rhys, R Winter

Rheumatology and Rehabilitation J Martin (Head), C R Dillon, R Goodfellow

Urology D Jones (Head), J French

Ysbyty George Thomas
Mattie Collins Way, Treorchy CF42 6YG
Tel: 01443 440440 Fax: 01443 775042
Total Beds: 100

Manager David Jones

Powys Local Health Board

See also separate entry under Health Authorities and Boards.

Mansion House, Bronllys, Brecon LD3 0LS
Tel: 01874 711661 Fax: 01874 711601
Website: www.powyslhb.wales.nhs.uk
(Mid and West Wales)

Chair Chris Mann
Chief Executive Andy Williams

Breconshire War Memorial Hospital
Cerrigcochion Road, Brecon LD3 7NS
Tel: 01874 622443 Fax: 01874 625752

Manager Roseanee Lyles

Care of the Elderly A Pinhorn

Bro Ddyfi Community Hospital Machynlleth
Newtown Road, Machynlleth SY20 8AD
Tel: 01654 702266 Fax: 01654 703795
Total Beds: 43

Manager Delyth Waters

Care of the Elderly R Hayter

General Medicine A T Axford, Dr Davies, Dr Pandya

Obstetrics and Gynaecology Dr Hamon

Bronllys Hospital
Bronllys, Brecon LD3 0LS
Tel: 01874 711255 Fax: 01874 712447
Total Beds: 93

Care of the Elderly A M Dunn

Haematology Dr Haboush

Rheumatology Dr Rees

Builth Wells Cottage Hospital
Hospital Road, Builth Wells LD2 3HE
Tel: 01982 552221 Fax: 01982 554353
Total Beds: 23

Manager Elinor Pennington

Cardiology A Davies, S Huttison

Care of the Elderly A M Dunn

General Medicine R Blackett, J Saunders

Obstetrics and Gynaecology Dr Garwood, P Grech, G Rowe, R Subak-Sharpe, P Wilson

Rheumatology D Rees

Knighton Hospital
Ffrydd Road, Knighton LD7 1DF
Tel: 01547 528633 Fax: 01547 520522

Total Beds: 15

Manager Chrissie Owens

Care of the Elderly A M Dunn

Llandrindod Wells County War Memorial Hospital
Temple Street, Llandrindod Wells LD1 5HF
Tel: 01597 822951 Fax: 01597 828764
Total Beds: 70

Manager Cahterine Davies

Llanidloes and District War Memorial Hospital
Eastgate Street, Llanidloes SY18 6HF
Tel: 01686 412121 Fax: 01686 412999
Total Beds: 36

Manager Mitch Woodcock

Care of the Elderly G Boswell

Montgomery County Infirmary
Llanfair Road, Newtown SY16 2DW
Tel: 01686 617200 Fax: 01686 617249
Total Beds: 48

Manager Dawn Lewis

Care of the Elderly G Boswell

Victoria Memorial Hospital
Salop Road, Welshpool SY21 7DU
Tel: 01938 553133 Fax: 01938 558093
Total Beds: 45

Manager Lorna Luter

Ystradgynlais Community Hospital
Glanrhyd Road, Ystradgynlais, Swansea SA9 1AE
Tel: 01639 844777 Fax: 01639 846479
Total Beds: 46

Manager Graham Powell

Care of the Elderly J Hill, A Pinhorn

Swansea NHS Trust

Central Clinic, Trinity Buildings, 21 Orchard Street, Swansea SA1 5AT
Tel: 01792 651501 Fax: 01792 517018
Website: www.swansea-tr.wales.nhs.uk
(Mid and West Wales)

Chair D Hugh Thomas
Chief Executive Jane Perrin

Cefn Coed Hospital
Waunarlwydd Road, Cockett, Swansea SA2 0GH
Tel: 01792 561155 Fax: 01792 580740
Total Beds: 231

Child and Adolescent Psychiatry S Ames, G Salmon, J S Talbot

General Psychiatry S Davies, P Donnelly, M D Gibbs, A Wooding

Old Age Psychiatry S Albuquerque, M Ellis, D D R William

Clydach War Memorial Hospital
Clydach, Swansea SA6 5DT
Tel: 01792 841447
Total Beds: 20

Fairwood Hospital
Upper Killay, 794 Gower Road, Swansea SA2 7HQ
Tel: 01792 203192
Total Beds: 28

Manager Sarah Knight

Garngoch Hospital
Gorseinon, Swansea SA4 4LH
Tel: 01792 222911
Total Beds: 40

General Psychiatry M D Gibbs (Head), Dr Aiwanczyk, S Davies, P Donnelly, M D Gibbs, A Wooding

Old Age Psychiatry S Albuquerque, E Clarke-Smith, T Crownshaw, M Ellis, D D R William

Gellinudd Hospital
Pontardawe, Swansea SA8 3DX
Tel: 01792 862221
Total Beds: 30

Gorseinon Hospital
Gorseinon, Swansea SA4 2LH
Tel: 01792 897837
Total Beds: 66

Consultants D J Leopold, M Wani

Hill House Hospital
Sketty, Swansea SA2 0FB
Tel: 01792 203551
Total Beds: 86

Morriston Hospital
Morriston, Swansea SA6 6NL
Tel: 01792 702222 Fax: 01792 703499
Total Beds: 850

Accident and Emergency H Allen

Anaesthetics Dr Beese, E P Bennett, J Bowes, A J Byrne, M Davies, J Dingley, S D N Dwyer, M L Evans, D Hope, J A Hughes, L A G Hughes, D C Jerwood, R C King, J Leary, D H Long, W A McFadzean, H W Maddock, S Mahon, E Major, P S Mangat, P C Matthews, J R Morgan, W A Rogers, P A Schwartz, H Speedy, D W Thomas, T J Wall

Cardiology M Anderson, K E Evans, G H Jenkins, M N Ramsey

Cardiothoracic Surgery V Argano, S Ashraf, A Y Youhana

Care of the Elderly D J Leopold, A S Treseder, M Wani

Chemical Pathology A Gunneberg

Chest Medicine K Harrison

Diabetes D E Price

Gastroenterology P Duane, J G Williams

General Surgery J Baxter, T Brown, M Chare, C Ferguson, L Fligelstone, C P Gibbons

Haematology S Al-Ismail, A C Beddall

Histopathology A Dawson, P Griffiths, C J O'Brien, N Toffazzal

Medical Microbiology A Lewis, P D Thomas

Neurology C Rickards, I Sawhney

Neurosurgery J Buxton, J Martin, R Redfern

Occupational Health D Bell

Oral and Maxillofacial Surgery K Bishop, S Hodder, D J Howells, J Knox, K Silvester, A W Sugar

Orthopaedics D A Clement, E M Downes, H C Hoddinott, M Holt, E T R James, R L Leyshon, D Newington, N Price, D J Woodnutt

Palliative Medicine S Closs, H Taylor

Plastic Surgery M A C Cooper, W A Dickson, P S Drew, J H Laing, A D McGregor, M A P Milling, M S C Murison

Radiology A J Davies, J H Davies, R S Davies, R M Evans, S E Evans, C I Flowers, E W Jones, D Markham, N Powell, D G Richards, D E Roberts, P G White

Renal Medicine A J Antao

Rheumatology and Rehabilitation A I Hennessy, D H Smith, B J Sweetman

Urology P Bose, N J Fenn, M G Lucas, K C Vaughton

Singleton Hospital

Sketty Lane, Sketty, Swansea SA2 8QA
Tel: 01792 205666 Fax: 01792 208647
Total Beds: 539

Anaesthetics S Davies (Head), S J Catling, J S S Davies, M Evans, R Falconer, R A Mason, R N W Morgan, A L Murphy, P Nesling, H Slowey, P A Steane, J S Thomas, M J Whitehead, A R Williams

Child and Adolescent Psychiatry S Ames, G Salmon, J Talbot

Community Paediatrics S Jones, A Maddox, J Watkens

Dermatology D L Roberts (Head), S Blackford, I Ralfs, D L Roberts, B Statham

ENT J J Phillips (Head), D W Aird, S Browning, C P Fielder, J J Phillips, H B Whittet

General Medicine J Banks, W Harris, J Hopkin, C Hudson, M K Jones, J G C Kingham, L Thomas, C Weston

General Surgery M C Mason (Head), J Beynon, N D Carr, J Manson, M C Mason, A R Morgan

Genitourinary Medicine V Battue, A L Blackwell, K Yoganathan

Haematology K Rowley (Head), S Al-Ismail, A Beddall, A Benton

Obstetrics and Gynaecology M Bonduelle, P B Bowen-Simpkins, J P Calvert, M Dossa, S Emery, O Freites, J Gasson, E Kevelighan, R Llewellyn, M Morgan

Ophthalmology M W Austin, E G Davies, R J Hill, D E Laws, A Pickering, G Shuttleworth

Paediatrics M Cosgrove, D R Evans, M James-Ellison, G Morris, M O'Hagan, C L Sullivan, C White

Pathology V Shah, P D Thomas, N Tofazzal, D W Williams, N Williams, S Williams

Psychiatry S Ames, G Salmon, J Talbot

Radiology B Patel, A L Power, M White

Radiotherapy K H M Rowley (Head), C S Askill, G Bertelli, A M M El-Sharkawi, W R Gajek, T Joannides, R Leonard, K H M Rowley, Prof Wagstaff

Ty-Einon Day Hospital

Princess Street, Gorseinon, Swansea SA4 2US
Tel: 01792 898078

Velindre NHS Trust

Trust Headquarters, 2 Charnwood Court, Parc Natgarw, Cardiff CF15 7QZ
Tel: 029 2061 5888
Website: www.velindre-tr.wales.nhs.uk
(South East Wales)

Chair Tony Hazell

Velindre Hospital

Whitchurch, Cardiff CF4 2TL
Tel: 029 2061 5888 Fax: 029 2052 2694
Total Beds: 69

Palliative Medicine I F Finlay

Radiotherapy and Oncology M Adams, J Barber, P Barrett-Lee, A Brewster, T Crosby, C C Gaffney, I J Kerby, F Macbeth, M D Mason, T S Maughan, D Mort, I C M Paterson, P Savage, O Tilsley

Welsh Ambulance Services NHS Trust

HM Stanley Hospital, Upper Denbigh Road, St Asaph LL17 0WA
Tel: 01745 532900 Fax: 01745 532901
Website: www.was-tr.wales.nhs.uk
(North Wales)

Chair Roy Norris
Chief Executive Don Page

Northern Ireland

Altnagelvin Area Hospitals HSS Trust

Altnagelvin Area Hospital, Glenshane Road, Londonderry BT47 6SB
Tel: 028 7134 5171 Fax: 028 7131 1020
Website: www.altnagelvin.n-i.nhs.uk
(Western Health and Social Services Board)

Chair Gerard Guckian
Chief Executive Stella Burnside
Consultants P Baylis, L A McKinney, J Steele

Altnagelvin Area Hospital

Glenshane Road, Londonderry BT47 6SB
Tel: 028 7134 5171 Fax: 028 7161 1222
Total Beds: 488

Accident and Emergency L A McKinney (Head), L A McKinney, J Steele

Anaesthetics G Furness (Head), W N Chestnutt, E G Devlin, G Di Mascio, R Franklin, G Furness, D Grace, J N Hamilton, A P Jain, P McSorley, B C Morrow, G A Nesbitt, C O'Hare, M Sheridan, P Stewart

Care of the Elderly J A F Beirne, J G McElroy, D Urquhart

Dermatology R A Fulton, P Podmore

ENT J R Cullen, G McBride

General Medicine J A F Beirne, J G Daly, W Dickey, H M Dunn, P V Gardiner, A Garvey, J G McElroy, A J McNeil, M McCarron, K W Moles, F A O'Connor, J A Purvis, R Sharkey, D Urquhart

General Surgery P G Bateson, S Dace, R J Gilliland, K J S Panesar, R L E Thompson

Genitourinary Medicine W W Dinsmore

Obstetrics and Gynaecology Dr Fallows, S E E Magee, D H Martin, J Moohan, M J Parker

Ophthalmology R Brennan, P Hassett, S Kalamarajah, D Mulholland, N K Sharma, J Sinton

Oral Surgery R C Boyd, M Ryan

Orthodontics R McMullan

Orthopaedics D Acton, A P Charlwood, M J McCormack, H McGee, N S Simpson, J Wong, A R Wray

Otolaryngology J R Cullen, G McBride

Paediatrics D A Brown, N P Corrigan, C Imrie, F B McCord, R J M Quinn

Pathology A M Adas, G M Glynn, J Hamilton, D F Hughes, M Madden, M J O'Kane, M H Vazir

Radiology P B Devlin, C S Elliott, P R Jackson, C C Morrison, M P Reilly, N A Sharkey

Urology C K Mulholland, F Schattka

Ward 5, Waterside Hospital
16 Gransha Park, Londonderry
Total Beds: 18

Manager D Brennan

Armagh and Dungannon HSS Trust

St Luke's Hospital, Loughgall Road, Armagh BT61 7NG
Tel: 028 3741 2446 (Textphone), 028 3752 2381
Fax: 028 3752 6302
Email: info@adhsst.n-i.nhs.uk
Website: www.adhsst.n-i.nhs.uk
(Southern Health and Social Services Board)

Chair Deirdre Dorman
Chief Executive Pauline Stanley

Armagh Community Hospital
Tower Hill, Armagh BT61 9DR
Tel: 028 3752 2381

Manager R Duffy

Audiological Medicine S Hall (Head)

Dermatology K W Scott

ENT R K Hingorani

General Medicine T J Baird, K Balnave

General Psychiatry M McCourt

General Surgery R Campbell, J J O'Neill, J W R Peyton

Obstetrics and Gynaecology R N Heasley, J C R MacHenry

Ophthalmology D G Fraser, C Ware

Orthopaedics J R M Elliot

Paediatrics C Shepherd

Radiology S Hall, R A J Todd

Longstone Hospital
Loughall Road, Armagh BT61 7PR
Tel: 028 3752 2381
Total Beds: 155

Manager Tony Doran

General Psychiatry N Keenan, J F McGuinness

Mullinure Hospital
Loughgall Road, Armagh
Tel: 028 3752 2381
Total Beds: 36

Manager Cathal Doyle

Care of the Elderly B McGleenan

St Luke's Hospital
Loughgall Road, Armagh BT61 7NQ
Tel: 028 3752 2381 Fax: 028 3741 4548
Total Beds: 165

Manager Lucy McManus

Anaesthetics I Samuels

General Psychiatry S Best, C Cassidy, N Chada, M McCourt, C Monaghan, E Saddler

Belfast City Hospital HSS Trust

Belfast City Hospital, 51 Lisburn Road, Belfast BT9 7AB
Tel: 028 9032 9241 Fax: 028 9032 6614
(Eastern Health and Social Services Board)

Chair Joan Ruddock
Chief Executive Quentin Coey
Consultants D C Allen, Grace Allen, Judith Allen, G P R Archbold, R J Atkinson, A Bell, Chitra Bharucha, J W Calderwood, P Declan Carey, Marie E Casement, Eng-Wooi Chew, John Connolly, S J Cooper, Roger Corbett, B F Craig, John J Craig, Z Desai, M J Dinnamond, Stephen P Dobbs, M Doherty, Olivia M Dolan, Richard A Donaldson, J F Douglas, Kathryn Dowey, A G Droogan, Martin Eatock, J D Edgar, J S Elborn, H Elliott, J R M Elliott, R L A Erskine, T F Esmonde, W P Ferguson, K T J Fitzpatrick, Damian G Fogarty, J H Foster, J A S Gamble, Kadayath A George, J M Gibson, I Gillespie, I Gleadhill, Arthur C Gray, Patricia Hart, John Harty, J R Hayes, J E Hegarty, R W Henry, Niall A Herity, J P Howe, D S Hurwitz, S T Irwin, J P Jamison, George D Johnson, L C Johnston, P G Johnston, S R Johnston, Francis G C Jones, P F Keane, J Andrew Kennedy, J G Kennedy, N T Kenny, R M Kernohan, J T Lawson, Bernard Lee, W B Loan, J I Logan, Victor Loughlin, Anne Loughrey, William Loughridge, Thomas H Lynch, R W Lyness, J MacMahon, A P Maxwell, G J McCarthy, Henry R McClelland, Robert J McClelland, William M McClelland, J McCollum, G F McCoy, Gavin McDonnell, Peter McFaul, A McKay, Cormac C McLoughlin, Kieran G McManus, J C McMillan, P T McNamee, K R Milligan, Treen Morris, James I Morrow, H B Murtagh, J G Murtagh, W E Nelson, Ethna C O'Gorman, D B O'Keeffe, M J G O'Reilly, Kiang A Pang, Anthony P Passmore, V H Patterson, K G Porter, J H Price, John C Ramsey, Irene M Rea, S G Richardson, J G Riddell, L Rodgers, B Sawhney, J N Scott, James A Sharkey, B Silke, R A J Spence, F J Stewart, Robert G N Storey, Robert W Stout, Stephen Stranex, J E Strong, T W Swinson, Allister J Taggart, Hugh Taggart, Joseph G Toner, N G Tracey, Anthony P Walby, W F M Wallace, Maureen Y Walsh

Belfast City Hospital
Lisburn Road, Belfast BT9 7AB
Tel: 028 9032 9241 Fax: 028 9032 6614
Total Beds: 708

Accident and Emergency K E Dowey, R B Fisher

Anaesthetics R W Allen, P F Bell, M Brady, G A Browne, J D R Connolly, P Convery, K T J Fitzpatrick, J A S Gamble, K A George, I A Gillespie, J E Hegarty, J P Howe, D S Hurwitz, M C Kelly, N T Kenny, C Kerr, G J McCarthy, J S C McCollum, A C McKay, C C McLoughlin, K R Milligan, O T Muldoon, J E Strong, G Turner, P S Weir, C S Wilson

Anatomy and Physiology J A Allen, W F M Wallace

Bacteriology C Goldsmith, P Rooney

Cardiology E W Chew, N Herity, J G Murtagh, D B O'Keeffe, S G Richardson, M E Scott

Cardiothoracic Surgery J Cleland, D J Gladstone, H O J O'Kane

Care of the Elderly C Foy, K J Fullerton, A P Passmore, I M Rea, R W Stout, H M Taggart

Chemical Pathology G P R Archbold, C Loughrey

Clinical Genetics P J Morrison, F J Stewart

Cytology H Elliott

Dental Surgery N Cambell

Dermatology J R Corbett, J F Dawson, J Handley, J C McKenna, J C McMillan

ENT M J Cinnamond, S Hampton, T J Stewart, J G Toner, A P Walby

General Medicine J S Elborn, J R Hayes, R W Henry, G D Johnson, S D Johnston, J I Logan, G E McVeigh, K G Porter, J G Riddell

General Psychiatry S J Cooper, M Doherty, R Ingram, C B Kelly, R J McClelland, J N Scott

General Surgery P D Carey, A Carragher, R J Hannon, K Khan, B Lee, K G McManus, M J G O'Reilly, S Refsum, C V Soong, R A J Spence, A J Wilkinson

Haematology H D Alexander, R Cuthbert, P Kettle, G M Markey, T C M Morris

Histopathology D C Allen, H Elliot, T F Lioe, R W Lyness, P D McGibben, D T McManus, D M O'Rourke, M Y Walsh

Nephrology C C Doherty, J F Douglas, P T McNamee, A P Maxwell, W E Nelson, J D Woods

Neurology Dr Droogan, T Esmonde, J M Gibson, S Hawkins, J I Morrow, K A Pang, V H Patterson, B Sawhney, M Watt

Obstetrics and Gynaecology M Casement, S Dobbs, H R McClelland, P McFaul, J H Price, S Tharma

Occupational Medicine L Rodgers

Oncology W P Abram, R J Atkinson, J Clarke, B Corcoran, R Davidson, R L Eatkin, M Eatock, R J A Harte, P G Henry, R F Houston, P G Johnston, S Kelly, C M J Loughrey, JJ A McAleer, K P Moore, A J Patterson, D Stewart, S Stranex, R H Wilson

Ophthalmology P M Harte, SJ A Rankin, J A Sharkey

Osteoporosis H Taggart

Pathology N Anderson, L Caughley

Pharmacology G D Johnston, J G Riddell

Plastic Surgery K Khan

Psychology R Davidson

Radiology C Boyd, J G Crothers, L C Johnston, J T Lawson, W Loan, J P Lowry, J McAllister, A M Shiels, N G Tracey, S R Vallely

Radiotherapy and Oncology RJ Atkinson, PG Johnston

Restorative Dentistry J G Kennedy

Rheumatology A L Bell, A J Taggart

Transplant Surgery J K Connelly

Transplant Surgery J Connolly

Urology R A Donaldson, S R Johnston, P F Keane, R M Kernohan, W G G Loughridge, T H Lynch, I K Walsh

Belvoir Park Hospital

Hospital Road, Belfast BT8 8JR
Tel: 028 9069 9069
Total Beds: 208

Causeway HSS Trust

Trust Headquarters, 8E Coleraine Road, Ballymoney BT53 6BP
Tel: 028 2766 6600 Fax: 028 2766 1200
Email: info@chsst.n-i.nhs.uk
Website: www.chsst.n-i.nhs.uk
(Northern Health and Social Services Board)

Chair Jean Jefferson
Chief Executive Brian Dorman

Causeway Hospital

4 Newbridge Road, Coleraine BT52 1HS
Tel: 028 7032 7032
Total Beds: 240

Accident and Emergency A Stewart

Anaesthetics A R Cooper, W A W McGowan, K Pillow, M J Symington, C Watters, D G Wright

Chemical Pathology M Ryan

ENT C Scally

General Medicine O C Finnegan, P Gilmore, D G Sinnamon, F Tracey, A Varghese

General Psychiatry M E C Donnelly, S Kirk, T Leeman, Dr McHugh, M F Walsh

General Surgery M G Brown, F Mullan

Genitourinary Medicine W Dinsmore

Haematology P Burnside

Medical Microbiology E A Davies

Neurology S Hawkins

Obstetrics and Gynaecology W R Harvey, B M S Marshall, S McNeil, J A Wallace

Ophthalmology Miss Hanna

Oral and Maxillofacial Surgery R C Boyd

Orthodontics R McMullan

Orthopaedics A Yeates

Paediatric Cardiology B Craig

Paediatric Neurology E M Hicks

Paediatrics M V Ledwith, M D Rollins, D A Walsh

Radiology M de Jode, D H Kirkpatrick, N McKenzie

Rheumatology E M Whitehead

Urology R Kernohan

Dalriada Hospital

Coleraine Road, Ballycastle BT54 6BA
Tel: 028 2076 2666
Total Beds: 28

Robinson Memorial Hospital

Ballymoney BT53 6HH
Tel: 028 2766 0322
Total Beds: 24

Ross Thomson Unit

Causeway Hospital, 4 Newbridge Road, Coleraine BT52 1TP
Tel: 028 7032 7032
Total Beds: 34

Craigavon and Banbridge Community HSS Trust

Bannvale House, 10 Moyallan Road, Gilford, Craigavon BT63 5JX
Tel: 028 3883 1983 Fax: 028 3883 1993
Website: www.cbct.n-i.nhs.uk
(Southern Health and Social Services Board)

Chair Graham Martin
Chief Executive Glenn Houston

Craigavon Psychiatric Unit

68 Lurgan Road, Portadown, Craigavon BT63 5QQ
Tel: 028 3833 4444
Total Beds: 80

Craigavon Area Hospital Group HSS Trust

68 Lurgan Road, Portadown, Craigavon BT63 5QQ
Tel: 028 3833 4444 Fax: 028 3835 0068
Website: www.n-i.nhs.uk/cahgt
(Southern Health and Social Services Board)

Chair Elizabeth McClurg
Chief Executive John Templeton

Banbridge Polyclinic
11 Ballygowan Road, Banbridge BT32 3QX
Tel: 028 4062 2222

Manager Bernie Kerr

Craigavon Area Hospital
68 Lurgan Road, Portadown, Craigavon BT63 5QQ
Tel: 028 3833 4444 Fax: 028 3835 0068
Total Beds: 414

Accident and Emergency C R A Fee, P P Kerr, H Nicholl, S O'Reilly

Anaesthetics H E Bunting (Head), C Clarke, D Lowry, P McConaghy, M Morrow, D Orr, I Orr, S Oyindola, M Rea, N Rutherfoord-Jones, D Scullion, D Streahorn

Cardiology D T Flannery, C Hanratty, D McEneaney, I Menown

Care of the Elderly P M McCaffrey (Head), A Jones, B McGleenon

Dermatology D J Eedy (Head), A O'Hagen

ENT S J Hall (Head), P Leyden, E McNaboe, K P Singh

General Medicine P Murphy (Head), J Baird, R Convery, M Gibbons, R J E Lee, C M Ritchie

General Surgery E J Mackle (Head), R Campbell, M Epanomeritakis, G Hewitt, R Peyton, W J I Stirling, C Weir

Pathology G J M McCusker (Head), C Armstrong, K Boyd, N N Damani, D Hull, P C Sharpe

Neurology R B Forbes

Obstetrics and Gynaecology R N Heasley, I Hunter, D S Lowry, C MacHenry, H Sidhu, R J Wallace

Orthodontics I Connolly

Paediatrics M M Hogan (Head), B A Bell, C Shepherd, M Smith, S Thompson

Palliative Care O Morris

Radiology C A Carson, M Fawzy, S R Hall, M McClure, E J McAteer, P Rice, J Walker

Urology M Young (Head), A O'Brien

Lurgan Hospital
Sloan Street, Lurgan, Craigavon BT66 8NX
Tel: 028 3832 3262 Fax: 028 3832 9483
Total Beds: 96

Manager Lorna Dilworth

South Tyrone Hospital
Carland Road, Dungannon BT71 4AU
Tel: 028 8772 2821
Total Beds: 41

Manager Mary McGeough

Down Lisburn HSS Trust

Trust Headquarters, Level 5, Lisburn Health Centre, 25 Linenhall Street, Lisburn BT28 1LU
Tel: 028 9266 5181 Fax: 028 9266 5179
Email: enquiries@dltrust.n-i.nhs.uk
Website: www.dlt.n-i.nhs.uk
(Eastern Health and Social Services Board)

Chair Denise Fitzsimons
Chief Executive John Compton

Downe Hospital
9A Pound Lane, Downpatrick BT30 6JA
Tel: 028 4461 3311 Fax: 028 4461 5699
Email: frances_donovan@dltrust.n-i.nhs.uk
Total Beds: 81

Manager Frances Donovan

Accident and Emergency J Martin (Head)

Anaesthetics M Milhench (Head), P Convery, C Hawthorne, C Kerr

Care of the Elderly C M Jack (Head)

Dermatology J Handley

ENT S Hampton, W Harris

General Medicine C M Jack (Head), H Whitehead

General Surgery A Archbold (Head), M Ismail (Head), J Bell

Obstetrics and Gynaecology L Erskine, R G Storey

Ophthalmology O Early

Orthopaedics G McAlinden, D Warnock

Paediatrics P Jackson, L Martel, A Reid, A Thompson

Physicians C M Jack, G Jacob, R R T Shepherd, H Whitehead

Radiology M Thompson

Rheumatology A J Taggart

Vascular Surgery J M Hood

Downshire Hospital
Ardglass Road, Downpatrick BT30 6RA
Tel: 028 4461 3311 Fax: 028 4461 2444
Email: desi_bannon@dltrust.n-i.nhs.uk
Total Beds: 172

Manager Desi Bannon

General Psychiatry B Fleming (Head), M McCleery, P Moynihan, D Shields, A Watts

Lagan Valley Hospital
39 Hillsborough Road, Lisburn BT28 1JP
Tel: 028 9266 5141 Fax: 028 9260 3899
Email: karen_mcilveen@dltrust.n-i.nhs.uk
Total Beds: 159

Manager Karen McIlveen

Accident and Emergency B Low, A McKelvey

Anaesthetics G McCleane (Head), T Beers, M Fassmann, L W Harrison, A Kursurkar, D Potti, N Soomro, G Thompson

Care of the Elderly S P Gawley, R Kelly, H Munro

Dermatology J Dawson

ENT G McKee, W Primrose

General Medicine S Au, J Fyvie, I Gleadhill, T Harding

General Surgery A M Carragher (Head), S Z Hussain, A Kennedy, V Loughlin, Mr Phyu

Obstetrics and Gynaecology L Crooks, A Love, N E E McCabe, A Ramez, S Shahid

Ophthalmology J More, S Rankin

Orthopaedics J G Brown

Otolaryngology G McKee, W J Primrose

Paediatrics P Jackson, D Jones

Psychiatry O Daly, B Fleming, B Kerrigan, N Quigley

Radiology J McNulty (Head), S Ogbobi

Thompson House Hospital
19/21 Magherlave Road, Lisburn BT28 3BJ
Tel: 028 9266 5646 Fax: 028 9266 7681
Email: garry_hyde@dltrust.n-i.nhs.uk
Total Beds: 33

Manager Garry Hyde

Neurology J Morrow

Foyle Health and Social Services Trust

Riverview House, Abercorn Road, Londonderry BT48 6SB
Tel: 028 7126 6111 Fax: 028 7126 0806
Email: madonna.mcginley@foyletrust.n-i.nhs.uk
Website: www.foyletrust.org
(Western Health and Social Services Board)

Chair Anthony Jackson
Chief Executive Joe Lusby
Consultants Burges, Curran, Eyre, S Hutton, C M McDonnell, McGlennon, A Murray, S M Rea, I D Robertson

Gransha Hospital
Clooney Road, Londonderry BT47 1TF
Tel: 028 7186 0261
Total Beds: 138

General Psychiatry C McDonnell, D McGlennon, A Murray, A O'Hara, S M Rea, I Robertson

Stradreagh Hospital
Gransha Park, Clooney Road, Londonderry BT47 1TF
Tel: 028 7186 0261 Fax: 028 7186 0356
Total Beds: 68

Manager Mary Ralphs

General Psychiatry M G Curran, D G Eyre

Waterside Hospital
Gransha Park, Clooney Road, Londonderry
Tel: 028 7186 0007
Total Beds: 55

Manager Pauline Casey

Care of the Elderly J A F Beirne, J G McElroy

Green Park Healthcare HSS Trust

Musgrave Park Hospital, 20 Stockman's Lane, Belfast BT9 7JB
Tel: 028 9066 9501 Fax: 028 9038 2008
Website: www.greenpark.n-i.nhs.uk
(Eastern Health and Social Services Board)

Chair Jim Stewart
Chief Executive Hilary Boyd

Forster Green Hospital
110 Saintfield Road, Belfast BT8 4HD
Tel: 028 9094 4444 Fax: 028 9094 4400
Total Beds: 83

Care of the Elderly T O Beringer, J G McConnell, I Taylor

Child Psychiatry L Cassidy, A Haller

Neurology J McCann, V H Patterson

Joss Cardwell Centre
401 Holywood Road, Belfast BT4 2LS
Tel: 028 9076 8878 Fax: 028 9076 0313

Musgrave Park Hospital
Stockmans Lane, Belfast BT9 7JB
Tel: 028 9090 2000 Fax: 028 9090 2222
Total Beds: 348

Anaesthetics R Allen, P Bell, J P H Fee, J A S Gamble, I Gillespie, J E Hegarthy, D S Hurwitz, N T Kenny, J S C McCollum, A C McKay, C McLoughlin, R Martin, K R Milligan, Dr Muldoon, E Stiby, J E Strong, Dr Turner, Dr Weir, Dr Wilson

Care of the Elderly S P Gawley, D Gilmore, M Gilmore, I Steele, I Wiggan

Orthopaedics I V Adair, Mr Andrews, Mr Barr, D E Beverland, J G Brown, J W Calderwood, J Corry, Mr Cosgrove, G H Cowie, G R Dilworth, J R M Elliott, A Hamilton, S Henderson, H Laverick, C J McClelland, G F McCoy, Mr Maginn, Professor Marsh, H J D Mawhinney, Mr Mobbs, R A B Mollan, R Nicholas, J R Nixon, Mr Nolan, Mr Swain, T C Taylor, R G Wallace, H A Yeates

Radiology M D Crone, Dr Grey, H B Murtagh

Rehabilitation Medicine J P McCann

Rheumatology A Bell, M Finch, Dr Rooney, Dr Wright

Sports Medicine M Cullen

Homefirst Community HSS Trust

The Cottage, 5 Greenmount Avenue, Ballymena BT43 6DA
Tel: 028 2563 3700 Fax: 028 2563 3733
Website: www.homefirst.n-i.nhs.uk
(Northern Health and Social Services Board)

Chair Robert Ferguson
Chief Executive Norma Evans

Holywell Hospital
60 Steeple Road, Antrim BT41 2RJ
Tel: 028 9446 5211 Fax: 028 9446 1803
Total Beds: 220

General Psychiatry A Collins, S Critchlow, J Daly, A Davis, F Duke, T P Elliott, J Finlay, P Gallagher, W Gregg, H Henderson, G Henry, U Huda, C Kennedy, Dr Livingstone, G Lynch, E MacFarland, M Mannion, C Mulholland, J O'Neill, K Troughton, R Wilson

Mater Hospital HSS Trust

45-51 Crumlin Road, Belfast BT14 6AB
Tel: 028 9074 1211 Fax: 028 9074 1342
Email: info@mater.n-i.nhs.uk
Website: www.n-i.nhs.uk/mater
(Eastern Health and Social Services Board)

Chair Anne McCollum
Chief Executive Sean Donaghy

Alexandra Gardens Day Hospital
Old See House, 603 Antrim Road, Belfast BT15 3LJ
Tel: 028 9077 3311 Fax: 028 9077 3311

Mater Infirmorum Hospital
47-51 Crumlin Road, Belfast BT14 6AB
Tel: 028 9074 1211 Fax: 028 9074 1342
Total Beds: 216

Accident and Emergency P Curran (Head), G Lane

Anaesthetics H Matthews (Head), S Austin, P Gormlay, J O'Hanlon, E Thompson

Cardiology B McClements (Head)

Chest Disease S Guy (Head)

ENT F G D'Arcy (Head)

General Medicine M J J Gormley (Head), S Guy, P Lim, B McClements, J C McLoughlin

General Psychiatry A O'Neill (Head), D M Brennan, G McDonald, A McDonnell, E A Montgomery, M O'Kane

General Surgery B Wilson (Head), T Diamond, C F Harvey

Neonatology R Tubman (Head)

Obstetrics and Gynaecology P Weir (Head), R White

Ophthalmology G Kervick (Head), O Earley, B Lacey

Radiology J S McLoughlin (Head), V Bhandari, A Norris

Newry and Mourne HSS Trust

5 Downshire Place, Downshire Road, Newry BT34 1DZ
Tel: 028 3026 0505 Fax: 028 3026 9064
Email: lynda.king@dhh.n-i.nhs.uk
Website: www.newryandmournetrust.n-i.nhs.uk
(Southern Health and Social Services Board)

Chair Sean Hogan
Chief Executive Eric Bowyer
Consultants B Aljarad, J Barr, J G Boyle, R J Brown, C Campbell, C W B Corkney, J Craig, B Cranley, R De Courcey-Wheeler, J E Devlin, D J Eedy, D Gilpin, M Hollinger, J Hughes, Hull, Leonard, P Leydon, C J McClelland, H M McDowell, K McKinney, K McManus, E J McNaboe, C J O'Brien, M F O'Hare, A Page, P Ramsay-Baggs, E Sadler, D Sim, John Simpson, R A J Todd, R Wallace, J Wright

Daisy Hill Hospital

5 Hospital Road, Newry BT35 8DR
Tel: 028 3083 5000 Fax: 028 3025 0624
Email: lynda.king@dhh.n-i.nhs.uk
Website: www.newryandmournetrust.n-i.nhs.uk
Total Beds: 297

Anaesthetics R J Carlisle, P G Loughran, J Wright, P Wright

Dermatology D J Eedy

ENT P Leyden, E J McNaboe

General Medicine J E Devlin, H M McDowell, C J O'Brien

General Psychiatry C Campbell, J Cotter, E Sadler, J Simpson

General Surgery G Blake, R J Brown, B Cranley, D Gilpin

Obstetrics and Gynaecology R De Courcy-Wheeler, K McKinney, M F O'Hare, D Sim

Ophthalmology Y Canavan, A Page

Oral Surgery P Ramsey-Baggs

Orthopaedics J Barr, C J McClelland, R Wallace

Paediatrics B Aljarad, C W B Corkey, J Hughes

Plastic Surgery Mr Leonard, K McManus

Radiology J G Boyle, R A J Todd

Thoracic Surgery K McManus

Mourne Hospital

Newry Street, Kilkeel, Newry BT34 4DP
Tel: 028 4116 2235 Fax: 028 4176 9770

General Medicine H McDowell

General Surgery R J Brown, B Cranley

Obstetrics and Gynaecology R De Courcy-Wheeler, K McKinney

North and West Belfast HSS Trust

Glendinning House, 6 Murray Street, Belfast BT1 6DP
Tel: 028 9032 7156 Fax: 028 9082 1285
Email: info@nwb.n-i.nhs.uk
Website: www.nwb.n-i.nhs.uk/mah
(Eastern Health and Social Services Board)

Chair Patrick McCartan
Chief Executive Richard Black

Muckamore Abbey Hospital

1 Abbey Road, Muckamore, Antrim BT41 4SH
Tel: 028 9446 3333 Fax: 028 9446 7730
Total Beds: 497

General Psychiatry J Galway, D Hughes, J MacPherson, K N McCartney, M McGinnity, C Milliken

Northern Ireland Ambulance Service HSS Trust

Headquarters, Site 30, Knackbracken Healthcare Park, Saintfield Road, Belfast BT8 8SG
Tel: 028 9040 0999 Fax: 028 9040 0900
Website: www.niamb.co.uk
(Eastern Health and Social Services Board)

Chair Douglas Smyth
Chief Executive Liam McIvor

Royal Group of Hospitals and Dental Hospital HSS Trust

Royal Victoria Hospital, Grosvenor Road, Belfast BT12 6BA
Tel: 028 9024 0503 Fax: 028 9024 0899
Website: www.royalhospitals.org
(Eastern Health and Social Services Board)

Chair Anne Balmer
Chief Executive William S McKee

Royal Belfast Hospital for Sick Children

180 Falls Road, Belfast BT12 6BE
Tel: 028 9024 0503 Fax: 028 9023 5340
Total Beds: 129

Anaesthetics P M Crean, T M Gallagher, S R Keilty, R H Taylor

Cardiac Surgery J Cleland, D J Gladstone

Cardiology B G Craig, H C Mulholland

Child and Adolescent Psychiatry M T Kennedy, R R McAuley

Dental Surgery I D F Saunders

Dermatology E A Bingham, D Burrows, J R Corbett

Genetics N C Nevin

Haematology S I Dempsey

Orthopaedics T C Taylor

Otolaryngology D A Adams, M J Cinnamond, R Gibson, A P Walby

Paediatric Surgery V E Boston, S Brown, S R Potts

Paediatrics D J Carson, J F T Glasgow, H L Halliday, E M Hicks, A E Hill, P Jackson, B G McClure, A O B Redmond, M M Reid, J M Savage, M D Shields

Plastic Surgery M D Brennan, A G Leonard, R Millar

Radiology L E Sweeney, P S Thomas

Royal Maternity Hospital
Grosvenor Road, Belfast BT12 6BB
Tel: 028 9089 4656 Fax: 028 9023 6203
Total Beds: 79

Anaesthetics S Atkinson, W Carabine, M A Lewis, K McGrath, D B Wilson

Cardiology B G Craig, H C Mulholland

Genetics N C Nevin

Obstetrics and Gynaecology D D Boyle, J C Dornan, M A Harper, H Lamki, P McFaul, M Reid, W Thompson, A I Traub

Paediatrics H L Halliday, B G McClure, M M Reid

Radiology L E Sweeney, P S Thomas

Royal Victoria Hospital
Grosvenor Road, Belfast BT12 6BA
Tel: 028 9024 0503 Fax: 028 9024 0899
Total Beds: 750

Accident and Emergency C H Dearden, J Martin, L Rocke

Anaesthetics S Atkinson, K M Bill, I W Carson, D L Coppel, H J L Craig, P Elliott, P A Farling, J P H Fee, F M Gibson, K W Harper, H M L Johnston, J R Johnston, G G Lavery, M A Lewis, W B Loan, K G Lowry, S M Lyons, R J McBride, G McCarthy, T J McMurray, R K Mirakhur, T D E Sharpe, J C Stanley, R H Taylor, V K N Unni, D B Wilson

Bacteriology K M Bamford, J G Barr, E T M Smyth, C H Webb

Cardiac Surgery G Campalani, J Cleland, D J Gladstone, H O J O'Kane, M Sarsam

Cardiology J Adgey, N P S Campbell, B G Craig, G W W Dalzell, M M Khan, D MacBoyle, H C Mulholland, S W Webb, C M Wilson

Care of the Elderly T R O Beringer, D H Gilmore

Cytology J Willis

Dental Surgery I C Benington, T Clifford, C G Cowan, D L Hussey, R W Kendrick, D C Kernohan, M J Kinirons, P J Lamey, G J Linden, J G McGimpsey, P Ramsay-Beggs, I D F Saunders, J M Sheridan, T W Swinson

Dermatology G E Allen, E A Bingham, D Burrows, J R Corbett

ENT D A Adams, D S Brooker, J E T Byrne, M J Cinnamond, F G D'Arcy, R Gibson, A G Kerr, W J Primrose, A P Walby

General Medicine A B Atkinson, P M Bell, K D Buchanan, M E Callender, J S A Collins, D R Hadden, A H G Love, D R McCance, D P Nicholls, S D Roberts, C F Stanford, R G P Watson

General Psychiatry A Kerr, G McDonald, P McGarry, W A Norris

General Surgery A A B D'Sa, J M Hood, G W Johnston, R J Maxwell, G W Odling-Smee, B J Rowlands, C J F Russell, A J Wilkinson

Genetics N C Nevin

Genitourinary Medicine W W Dinsmore, D M McBride, R D Maw

Haematology J M Bridges, S I Dempsey, F G C Jones, W M McClelland, E E Mayne

Histopathology H Bharucha, L M Caughley, M Mirakhur, M D O'Hara, M Y Walsh

Immunology D R McCluskey, T A McNeill

Medical Microbiology T A McNeill, D I H Simpson

Nephrology C C Doherty, J F Douglas, P T McNamee, W E Nelson

Neurology J M Gibson, S A Hawkins, J A Lyttle, J I Morrow, V H Patterson

Neuropathology I V Allen, M Mirakhur

Neurophysiology B B Sawhney

Neurosurgery I C Bailey, D P Byrnes, T F Fannin, W J Gray

Obstetrics and Gynaecology D D Boyle, J C Dornan, H Lamki, W Thompson, A I Traub

Ophthalmology D B Archer, J H Bryars, T A S Buchanan, O E Early, D G Frazer, P B Johnston, G McGinnity, C J F Maguire, A B Page

Orthodontics A Richardson

Orthopaedics I V Adair, J Brown, J W Calderwood, C J McClelland, G F McCoy, H J D Mawhinney, R A B Mollan

Paediatrics V Boston

Pathology C Meban, P D A Owens, J M Sloan, P G Toner, E R Trimble

Periodontology G J Linden

Pharmacology G D Johnston, J G Riddell

Plastic Surgery G Ashall, M D Brennen, A G Leonard, R Millar, J O Small

Public Health Medicine P M Darragh, A E Evans, M J Scott

Radiology K E Bell, M D Crone, J G Crothers, J D Laird, M McGovern, E M McIlrath, C S McKinstry, A McNeill, J E McNulty, J O M Mills, A J O'Doherty, L E Sweeney, P S Thomas, A M Thompson

Radiotherapy and Oncology W P Abram, B D Burrows, W S B Lowry

Rheumatology A L Bell, M B Finch, J P McCann

Thoracic Surgery J M McGuigan, K McManus

Urology S R Johnston, J A Kennedy

Virology P V Coyle

South and East Belfast HSS Trust

Knockbracken Healthcare Park, Saintfield Road, Belfast BT8 8BH
Tel: 028 9056 5555 Fax: 028 9056 5813
Email: consumer.relations@sebt.n-i.nhs.uk
Website: www.sebt.n-i.nhs.uk
(Eastern Health and Social Services Board)

Chair Robin Harris
Chief Executive Patricia Gordon

Albertbridge Road Day Hospital
225 Albertbridge Road, Belfast BT5 4PX

Sperrin Lakeland Health and Social Care Trust

Strathdene House, Tyrone and Fermanagh Hospital, Omagh BT79 0NS
Tel: 028 8283 5285 Fax: 028 8283 5286
Website: www.sperrin-lakeland.org
(Western Health and Social Services Board)

Chair Harry Mullan
Chief Executive Hugh Mills

Erne Hospital
Cornagrade Road, Enniskillen BT74 6AY
Tel: 028 6632 4711
Total Beds: 232

Anaesthetics C A Armstrong, T Auterson, M W Cody, W Holmes

Care of the Elderly J F Kelly

Dental Surgery R Parfitt

Dermatology P Podmore

ENT S K Kaluskar, K P Law

General Medicine M P S Varma, J R Williams

General Surgery A Kibbin, Mr Marshall, J Strahan

Haematology Dr Cuthebert

Neurology V Patterson

Obstetrics and Gynaecology S Cheah

Oncology J Clarke

Ophthalmology D Mulholland

Orthodontics R McMillan

Orthopaedics D Beverland, H Cowie, G McCoy

Paediatrics M O'Donahoe

Radiology P Conneally, G Loughey

Rheumatology Dr Gardiner

Tyrone and Fermanagh Hospital

1 Donaghanie Road, Omagh BT79 0NS
Tel: 028 8224 5211
Total Beds: 182

Forensic Psychiatry I T Bownes

General Psychiatry K K Bindal, D D Cody, T Foster, K Gillespie, M A McDermott, P J Mannion

Tyrone County Hospital

Hospital Road, Omagh BT79 0AP
Tel: 028 8224 5211 Fax: 028 8224 6293
Total Beds: 161

Anaesthetics K Anand, R R Lalsingh, J M F Maginnis, F P Robinson

Care of the Elderly E Hodkinson

Dermatology R A Fulton, P Podmore

ENT Mr Babu, S K Kaluskar, K P Law

General Medicine E Bergin, A L T Blair, P Garrett, C J Russell

General Psychiatry P J Mannion

General Surgery G A B Miller, D J D Pinto

Nephrology E Bergin, P Garrett

Neurology V Patterson

Obstetrics and Gynaecology M Anderson, M Cheah

Ophthalmology P Hassett

Oral Surgery Mr El-Atter

Orthodontics R McMullan

Orthopaedics A R Wray

Paediatrics D Halakoohoon, D O'Donahoe, S Simpson

Radiology G J Loughrey

Radiotherapy R F Houston

Rheumatology P V Gardiner

Ulster Community and Hospitals Trust

Health and Care Centre, 39 Regent Street, Newtownards BT23 4AD
Tel: 028 9181 6666 Fax: 028 9182 0140
Email: public.relations@ucht.n-i.nhs.uk
Website: www.n-i.nhs.uk/ucht
(Eastern Health and Social Services Board)

Chair Eileen Grant
Chief Executive Jim McCall

Ards Community Hospital

Church Street, Newtownards BT23 4AS
Tel: 028 9101 2661 Fax: 028 9151 0111
Total Beds: 20

Anaesthetics T H Boyd, D Carson, D Coyle, C Hickey, J K Lilburn, K Lindsay, D M McAuley, C M Wilson

Cardiology J D S Higginson, S R McMechan

Care of the Elderly J Mathai

Day Procedure Unit M J Allen, B G Best, W Calvert, W J Campbell, S J Dolan, S J Kirk, R J Moorehead

Dermatology J F Dawson

ENT T J Stewart

General Medicine R Harper, W J McIlwaine, B MacLennon, T Trinick

General Psychiatry J Anderson, J K Gilbert, J Green, H Harbinson, D J MacFarlane, A Scott

General Surgery M J Allen, B G Best, S Dolan

Haematology M R El-Agnaf

Ophthalmology T A S Buchanan

Orthopaedics G R Dilworth

Pathology M Agnaff, J Hunter, T Trinick

Radiology P D Hanley

Bangor Community Hospital

Castle Street, Bangor BT20 4TA
Tel: 028 9147 5120, 028 9147 5140 Fax: 028 9147 5153
Total Beds: 40

Cardiology D Cochrane

Care of the Elderly J Mathai

Dermatology J Handley

ENT J Toner

General Medicine W J McIlwaine, T Trinick

General Surgery M J Allen, C H Calvert, R J Moorehead

Haematology K Bailie

Obstetrics and Gynaecology P Fogarty, J M W Park

Ophthalmology T A S Buchanan

Radiology R E Wright

Mental Health Day Hospital

Mental Health Directorate, Ards Community Hospital, Newtownards BT23 4AS
Tel: 028 9181 2661 Fax: 028 9151 0111

The Ulster Hospital

Upper Newtownards Road, Dundonald, Belfast BT16 1RH
Tel: 028 9048 4511 Fax: 028 9048 1753
Total Beds: 576

Accident and Emergency S McGovern, J B Martin, C J Martyn

Anaesthetics P Bell, T Boyd, W I Campbell, D Carson, J R Darling, A M Hainsworth, W H K Haslett, D A Hill, C Hinkley, D Hugh, K Lilburn, K G Lindsay, D M McAuley, M S McKenney, N McLeord, M V S Rao, M Reid, C Renfrew, J T Trinder, C M Wilson

Biochemistry T R Trinick

Cardiology D Cochrane, J D S Higginson, S R McMechan

Care of the Elderly J G McConnell, J Mathai, M J P Power, I C Taylor

Child and Adolescent Psychiatry G Walford

Dermatology J F Dawson, J Handley, K McKenna

ENT T J Stewart, J G Toner

General Medicine D M Boyle, B G Craig, R Harder, D Higginson, R J McFarland, W J McIlwaine, W R McKane, B MacLennan, C Mulholand, J K Nelson, Dr Salathia, T Tham

General Psychiatry J Anderson, J K Gilbert, J Green, H Harbinson, D McFarlane, A Scott

General Surgery M J Allen, B G Best, C H Calvert, W J Campbell, S Dolan, S J Kirk, R J Moorehead

Genitourinary Medicine R D Maw

Medical Microbiology A Loughrey

Obstetrics and Gynaecology E B Bond, J M Dunlop, P Fogarty, J M W Park, R N Roberts

Ophthalmology P B Johnston

Oral and Maxillofacial Surgery T A Gregg, R W Kendrick, P Ramsay-Baggs, S M Sheridan

Orthopaedics J G Brown, G R Dilworth, J A Halliday, G McAlinden, P Maginn, R G H Wallace, A Yeates

Paediatric Surgery V E Boston, S Brown, W McCallion, S R Potts

Paediatrics A Bell, E A Black, T Brown, C Gaston, V Gleadhill, J Major, L Martell, D Primrose

Pathology K Bailie, M El-Agnaff, J Hunter, A Moore, T R Trinick

Plastic Surgery M D Brennan, D J Gordon, K J Herbert, A G Leonard, J S Sinclair

Radiology P D Hanley, M Hyland, C Loughrey, J M McAllister, J R A McNally, C W Majury, N R Pathirana, H K Wilson, R E R Wright

Radiotherapy and Oncology W P Abram, J Clarke

United Hospitals HSS Trust

Bush House, Antrim BT41 2QB
Tel: 028 9442 4655 Fax: 028 9442 4654
(Northern Health and Social Services Board)

Chair R Milnes
Chief Executive J Bernard Mitchell

Antrim Hospital

Antrim BT41 2RL
Tel: 028 9442 4000 Fax: 028 9442 4293
Total Beds: 370

Anaesthetics I M Bali, I H C Black, R Ghosh, D J Grainger, P Leyden, H N McLeod

Cardiology T Trouton, C Wilson

Care of the Elderly P G Flanagan, A K Sarkar

ENT R P Agarwala, J H A Black, G Gallagher, C Scally

General Medicine J B McConnell, B A Sims, G R G Todd, M Varghese

General Surgery W I H Garstin, W G Humphreys, A H McMurray, D G Mudd

Obstetrics and Gynaecology R G Ashe, R M McMillen, W A H Ritchie, P Smith

Orthodontics N M Stratford

Orthopaedics W I H Garstin, D N S Gleadhill, W G Humphreys, A H McMurray, D G Mudd

Paediatrics J Jenkins, J H K Lim, J McAloon, C MacLeod, J Nicholson

Pathology J M Alderdice, P Burnside, J G Carson, E A Davies, M P Kearney, B D Kenny, A Kyle, P D McGibben, M Ryan

Radiology S T Brady, J C Clarke, P M Higgins, J P Lowry, C J Sinclair

Renal Medicine H Brown

Rheumatology E M Whitehead

Braid Valley Hospital

Cushendall Road, Ballymena BT43 6HH
Tel: 028 2565 5200 Fax: 028 2563 5385
Total Beds: 75

Care of the Elderly P G Flanagan, A K Sarkar

Mid-Ulster Hospital

59 Hospital Road, Magherafelt BT45 5EX
Tel: 028 7963 1031 Fax: 028 7963 4078
Total Beds: 191

Anaesthetics M O'Neill, A C Scott

Dental Surgery R W Kendrick

Dermatology R S Matthews

General Medicine N C Chatervedi, E K Hunter, L J E Walker

General Surgery M J G Hawe, P Pyper

Haematology P Burnside

Obstetrics and Gynaecology H C Aitken, H Clarke

Ophthalmology M Sharma

Orthodontics J A Scott, N Stratford

Orthopaedics P Dolan

Paediatrics J H K Lim, C MacLeod

Radiology C J Sinclair

Moyle Hospital

Gloucester Avenue, Larne BT40 1RP
Tel: 028 2827 5431 Fax: 028 2827 5346
Total Beds: 45

Dermatology H A Jenkinson

General Medicine G R G Todd, M Varghese

General Psychiatry G Henry

General Surgery I Garston, A H McMurray

Neurology J Morrow

Obstetrics and Gynaecology R McMillen

Ophthalmology J H Bryars

Orthopaedics J R Nixon

Radiology S T Brady

Whiteabbey Hospital

Doagh Road, Newtownabbey BT37 9RH
Tel: 028 9086 5181 Fax: 028 9036 5083
Total Beds: 171

Accident and Emergency R Wylie

Anaesthetics C J Ferres, K Seetha

Cardiology P Crowe

Care of the Elderly E Byrne, J E Gilmore

Chest Disease G Todd

Dermatology H A Jenkinson, R W D Ross

ENT G Gallagher

General Medicine W J Andrews, P F Crowe, J E Gilmore

General Psychiatry J R Noble, P E Potter

General Surgery D Gilroy, D C McCrory

Haematology A Kyle

Obstetrics and Gynaecology R M McMillen, P Smith

Radiology A Hrabovsky, N Pathnana

Channel Islands

Castel Hospital
Neuve Rue, Castel, Guernsey GY5 7NJ
Tel: 01481 725241 Fax: 01481 252099
Total Beds: 100

Manager K Sirett

Jersey General Hospital
Gloucester Street, St Helier, Jersey JE2 3QS
Tel: 01534 622000 Fax: 01534 622886
Email: health@gov.je
Website: www.health.gov.je
Total Beds: 300

Accident and Emergency A Brett (Head), C Clinton

Anaesthetics G Purcell-Jones (Head), P Coleman, G D Prince, C Taylor

Dental Surgery M Belligoi, M Cassidy, B Skinner

Dermatology M F Muhlemann

ENT N Shah, M Siodlak

General Medicine H Gibson (Head), P Bates, M Gleeson, K Hearn, A Kumar, M Richardson

General Psychiatry G W Blackwood, C Coverley, J Sharkey, L Wilson

General Surgery N Ingram (Head), J Allardice

Obstetrics and Gynaecology J B Day, N Maclachlan

Ophthalmology R Downes (Head), B McNeela

Orthopaedics R P Clifford, C Twiston-Davies

Paediatrics T Malpas (Head), C Spratt, P Thiagarajan

Pathology C Mattock (Head), H Goulding, I Muscat, P Southall

Radiology A P Nisbet (Head), A Borthwick-Clarke, N Scott

King Edward VII Hospital Guernsey
Sanitarium Lane, Castel, Guernsey GY5 7NU
Tel: 01481 725241 Fax: 01481 253135
Total Beds: 100

Rehabilitation J Briggs, S Evans, G Turner

Mental Health Services
Queens House, La Route De La Hougue Bie, Jersey JE2 7UW
Tel: 01534 623220 Fax: 01534 623430
Email: advetnh@jerseymail.co.uk
Total Beds: 122

Manager Ian Dyer

Mignot Memorial Hospital
Crabby, Alderney, Guernsey GY9 3XY
Tel: 01481 824415 Fax: 01481 823087
Total Beds: 24

Manager Marc Sumner

Overdale Hospital
Westmount Road, St Helier, Jersey JE1 3UH
Tel: 01534 623000
Total Beds: 120

Manager Richard Jouault

Care of the Elderly M Richardson

Neurology H Gibson

Psychiatry of Old Age L Wilson

Princess Elizabeth Hospital
St Martins, Guernsey GY4 6UU
Tel: 01481 725241 Fax: 01481 710182
Total Beds: 161

Anaesthetics G N Beck, A S Boyle, C McClymont, C I Pratt, N A Van Heerden, M J Wolfe, G D Yarwood

General Medicine W Anees, N P Byrom, F Degnen, S N Evans, P J Gomes, J Green, P J Mullen, G A Oswald

General Psychiatry H Birchall, R Browne, M Costen, L Macey, G McKeough, P B Turner

General Surgery N H Allen, R H Allsopp, D G Beaumont, J Ferguson, D J Pring, J G Rice, M Van den Bossche, N Van der Hauwaert, R H Vowles

Obstetrics and Gynaecology R H Haskins, F J Hopkins, C E Jensen, H Reed

Ophthalmology H F Bacon, S E Dorey, L Kleanthous

Paediatrics S M Eckhardt, B W Lean, P Standring

Pathology C Chinayama

Public Health D Jeffs

Radiology A Edirisooriya, M L Gaunt, B C O'Dwyer

William Knott Day Hospital
Westmount Road, St Helier, Jersey JE2 3LP
Tel: 01534 623062 Fax: 01534 623098

Manager Millie Horman

Isle of Man

Isle of Man

(Department of Health and Social Security, Health Services Division)

Ballamona Hospital
Braddan Road, Strang, Douglas IM4 4RF
Tel: 01624 642642
Total Beds: 188

General Psychiatry D Balakrishna, E Chinn, M N Elias, D N O'Malley, M O'Sullivan

Noble's Isle of Man Hospital
The Strang, Bradden, Douglas IM4 4RJ
Tel: 01624 650000
Total Beds: 314

Manager Paul Shields

Consultants Dr Anwar, N J Birkin, J Brownsdon, Dr Cheema, Mr Cho, M B Clague, R B Clague, J Crerand, M Divers, R J Fayle, R Godfrey, A D Green, Mr Hancock, N A Harrison, N F Hockings, Mr Iskander, E Khan, G S Khuraijam, A Kurien, S L Manuja, A M Moroney, C R H Murray, Mr Page, S E Stock, J P Travers, S M Upsdell, S M Zeitoune

Ramsey and District Cottage Hospital
Cumberland Road, Ramsey IM8 3RH
Tel: 01624 811811 Fax: 01624 811818
Email: ramsey.cottage@dhss.gov.im
Total Beds: 48

General Medicine A Allinson, J K Armour, J K Brownsdon, M S Chan, H Clark, A S C Kelsey, M Maska, G M Wilson

GP Surgeries and Walk-in Centres

England

Abbots Langley

Abbots Wood Medical Centre
12 Katherine Place, College Road, Abbots Langley WD5 0BT
Tel: 01923 673060 Fax: 01923 681643
(Watford and Three Rivers Primary Care Trust)
Patient List Size: 4000

Practice Manager Rehana Khan

GP Zafar HAMID, Abdul Mashkoor KHAN

High Street Surgery
87 High Street, Abbots Langley WD5 0AL
Tel: 01923 262363 Fax: 01923 267374
(Watford and Three Rivers Primary Care Trust)

Practice Manager Richard Jarman

GP Roger Harvey NEIGHBOUR, Elizabeth Jane EVANS, Patricia GRAY, Ian Charles Osborne ISAAC, Peter Michael SIMMONS, Timothy SWANWICK, Susan Ebsworth WILLIAMS

Abingdon

The Abingdon Surgery
65 Stert Street, Abingdon OX14 3LB
Tel: 01235 523126 Fax: 01235 550625
Email: practice@gp-K84054.nhs.uk
(South West Oxfordshire Primary Care Trust)
Patient List Size: 10000

Practice Manager Teresa Young

GP Neil Roderick CROSSLEY, Prit S BUTTAR, John P HAYDEN, Janet Lilias MURRAY, James R VICKERS

Long Furlong Medical Centre
45 Loyd Close, Abingdon OX14 1XR
Tel: 01235 522379
(South West Oxfordshire Primary Care Trust)

Practice Manager Paul Snook

GP Elspeth Anne ALLAN, Nicholas Henry ELWIG, Anne Louise KEELING, Julian Nigel Blinkhorn MOORE, Theresa Eve NOWELL

Lynch-Blosse and Bradley
The Surgery, Watery Lane, Clifton Hampden, Abingdon OX14 3EJ
Tel: 01865 407888 Fax: 01865 407946
Email: practice@cliff-hanger.oxongps.co.uk
(South West Oxfordshire Primary Care Trust)
Patient List Size: 4000

Practice Manager Taz Evans

GP Richard Hely LYNCH-BLOSSE, Nicholas Julian BELL, Sarah Jane BRADLEY

The Malthouse Surgery
The Charter, Abingdon OX14 3JY
Tel: 01235 524001 Fax: 01235 532197
(South West Oxfordshire Primary Care Trust)

Practice Manager Peter Abery

GP Dr BRACE, Frank Warrner DUGDALE-DEBNEY, Hilary Jane HODGSON, Mary HUGHES, Dr KHAN, Elizabeth Heather Thompson LUMSDEN, David Richard MAY, David Michael OTTERBURN, Timothy David Richard REYNOLDS, Dr TAYLOR

Marcham Health Centre
Marcham Road, Abingdon OX14 1BT
Tel: 01235 522602
(South West Oxfordshire Primary Care Trust)

Practice Manager D Williams

GP Jacqueline Elizabeth BRYANT, Bette Theresa PEMBRIDGE, Mary Halcyon Meredith POPE, Patrick Michael ROBERTSON, Patrick TAN SWEE TEONG, Peter Howard Lovel TATE, Dorothy Jane WILLIAMS

Steventon Road Surgery
39 Steventon Road, Drayton, Abingdon OX14 4JX
Tel: 01235 531322 Fax: 01235 559385
(South West Oxfordshire Primary Care Trust)

Practice Manager Richard Trench Casson

GP Richard Trench CASSON

Accrington

Abbey Street Surgery
60 Abbey Street, Accrington BB5 1EE
Tel: 01254 382224
(Hyndburn and Ribble Valley Primary Care Trust)
Patient List Size: 1650

Practice Manager Marie Mootooneeren

GP Alec Yolomoni KAPENDA

Blackburn Road Surgery
257 Blackburn Road, Accrington BB5 0AL
Tel: 01254 233048
(Hyndburn and Ribble Valley Primary Care Trust)

Practice Manager Sue Maynard

GP Philip Wyndham QUINN, Biswa Nath KUNDU, Dr MOTTUPALLI

The Clayton Medical Centre
Wellington Street, Clayton le Moors, Accrington BB5 5HU
Tel: 01254 383131 Fax: 01254 392261
(Hyndburn and Ribble Valley Primary Care Trust)

Practice Manager Michelle Armstrong

GP Christopher Albert WARD, Kathleen Mary HEWITT

Dill Hall Lane Surgery
158 Dill Hall Lane, Church, Accrington BB5 4DS
Tel: 01254 398350 Fax: 01254 386283
(Hyndburn and Ribble Valley Primary Care Trust)
Patient List Size: 2600

Practice Manager Kath Robinson

GP Paramundayil Kuruvilla JOSEPH

The Eagle Street Surgery
119 Blackburn Road, Accrington BB5 5JT
Tel: 01254 384590
Email: amanda.sullivan@gp-P81779.nhs.uk
(Hyndburn and Ribble Valley Primary Care Trust)
Patient List Size: 850

GP Suryanarayana MURTHY

King Street Medical Centre
43 King Street, Accrington BB5 1QE
Tel: 01254 232435 Fax: 01254 394955
(Hyndburn and Ribble Valley Primary Care Trust)
Patient List Size: 1865

Practice Manager Amanda Sullivan

GP Ramesh Chander GUPTA, Sudesh Kumari GUPTA

Kusum Medical Centre
274 Union Road, Oswaldtwistle, Accrington BB5 3JB
Tel: 01254 232351 Fax: 01254 396253
(Hyndburn and Ribble Valley Primary Care Trust)
Patient List Size: 3495

Practice Manager Rita Neil

GP Rekha Rani OJHA

Myrtle House
154 Blackburn Road, Accrington BB5 0AE
Tel: 01254 233651 Fax: 01254 391965
(Hyndburn and Ribble Valley Primary Care Trust)
Patient List Size: 6771

Practice Manager H Instone

GP John Howard DIXON, Arthur MANUEL

Oswald Medical Centre
296 Union Road, Oswaldtwistle, Accrington BB5 3JD
Tel: 01254 356110 Fax: 01254 356113
Website: www.oswaldmedicalcentre.co.uk
(Hyndburn and Ribble Valley Primary Care Trust)
Patient List Size: 9600

Practice Manager Rita Naylor

GP Thomas MANJOORAN, Devinder GUPTA, Shashi Prabha GUPTA

Peel House Medical Centre
Avenue Parade, Accrington BB5 6RD
Tel: 01254 237231 Fax: 01254 389525
(Hyndburn and Ribble Valley Primary Care Trust)
Patient List Size: 15500

Practice Manager Carole Pilkington

GP Michael Carl HIPWELL, Jane ECCLES, Jane KIRBY, Clara Elizabeth MURPHY, Roy Allen WALLWORTH, Gavin Ralph WESTWOOD, David Roy WOODCOCK

Richmond Medical Centre
Brown Street, Accrington BB5 0RS
Tel: 01254 232832 Fax: 01254 393325
(Hyndburn and Ribble Valley Primary Care Trust)

Practice Manager R F Hints

GP Navin KARIM, Syed Irfan-Ul KARIM

Stone Bridge House
Higher Heys Surgery, Heys Lane, Oswaldtwistle, Accrington BB5 3BP
Tel: 01254 396265 Fax: 01254 392453
(Hyndburn and Ribble Valley Primary Care Trust)
Patient List Size: 2200

Practice Manager M P Hyatt

GP Ghullam Mohammad BHAT

Addlestone

Crouch Oak Family Practice
45 Station Road, Addlestone KT15 2BH
Tel: 01932 840123 Fax: 01932 821589
(North Surrey Primary Care Trust)

GP Elizabeth Antonia WHITE, Rosemary Elizabeth GARGAN, Julian HANCOCK, Peter Russell HARVEY, Mohan KANAGASUNDARAM, Maria-Jose SANCHEZ, Neville John STAUNTON

Alcester

Arrow Lodge Medical Centre
Kinwarton Road, Alcester B49 5QY
Tel: 01789 763293 Fax: 01789 764380
Website: www.arrowlodgemedicalcentre.co.uk
(South Warwickshire Primary Care Trust)

GP Mohan Bhadoor SINGH, Rukmani BULCHAND, Richard LAMBERT

Health Centre
Priory Road, Alcester B49 5DZ
Tel: 01789 763060 Fax: 01789 766574
Email: LINDACOOK@PRIORYROAD.NHS.UK
(South Warwickshire Primary Care Trust)
Patient List Size: 6000

Practice Manager Linda Cook

GP Andrew WALLIS, Anthony BURMAN, Mary Ethel HARRISSON, Emma VICKERS

The Health Centre
High Street, Bidford-on-Avon, Alcester B50 4BQ
Tel: 01789 773372 Fax: 01789 490380
(South Warwickshire Primary Care Trust)

Practice Manager Jane Griffiths

GP Peter Michael ROBINSON, Deborah Margaret EDWARDS, Peter Linton NAVA, Timothy Richard SHACKLEY

Aldeburgh

Church Farm Surgery
Victoria Road, Aldeburgh IP15 5EB
Tel: 01728 452027 Fax: 01728 452041
Website: www.aldesurg.co.uk
(Suffolk Coastal Primary Care Trust)
Patient List Size: 4150

Practice Manager P Illingworth

GP J McGOUGH, Dr BALL, Dr CROWTHER

Alderley Edge

George Street Surgery
16 George Street, Alderley Edge SK9 7EP
Tel: 01625 584545/6
(Eastern Cheshire Primary Care Trust)

GP Stuart Douglas MERCHANT, Christine L ARNOLD, Helen Elizabeth HALL, Douglas John Hector MACDONALD, Harry Edwin THOMPSON, Michelle C VAUGHAN

Aldershot

Aldershot Health Centre
Wellington Avenue, Aldershot GU11 1PA
Tel: 01252 324577 Fax: 01252 324861
(Blackwater Valley and Hart Primary Care Trust)

GP Murdo Donald MACLEOD, Janice HAYWARD, Gita NAIR, Christopher Almack PEARSON, Anne-Marie TINKLER

Alexandra Surgery
2 Wellington Avenue, Aldershot GU11 1SD
Tel: 01252 332210 Fax: 01252 312490
Website: www.surgeriesonline.com/alexandrasurgery
(Blackwater Valley and Hart Primary Care Trust)
Patient List Size: 6006

Practice Manager Elaine Beverley

GP Mary RIGGS, Christina Anne LEOPOLD, Julia Madeleine PALLANT, Louise PAYNE, Barbara SCANTLEBURY

The Border Practice
38 North Lane, Aldershot GU12 4QQ
Tel: 01252 344434/332431 Fax: 01252 319100
(Blackwater Valley and Hart Primary Care Trust)
Patient List Size: 8600

Practice Manager Maxine Price

GP Samina AHMED, Narinder BAJUA, Roger Aston LAWRENCE, Basil Francis ROMAYA

Southlea Surgery
276 Lower Farnham, Aldershot GU11 3RB
Tel: 01252 344868 Fax: 01252 342596

(Blackwater Valley and Hart Primary Care Trust)
Patient List Size: 14000

GP Jeffrey WICTOME, Peter BRIGG, Claire Elizabeth BROOKS, Maurice FAHMY, Julie HILDITCH, Alison LENNOX, Sarah Elizabeth O'CALLAGHAN, Stephen SCOTT-PERRY

The Victoria Practice
Aldershot Health Centre, Wellington Avenue, Aldershot GU11 1PA
Tel: 01252 324577 Fax: 01252 324812
Email: mail@victoriapractice.co.uk
Website: www.victoriapractice.co.uk
(Blackwater Valley and Hart Primary Care Trust)
Patient List Size: 7080

Practice Manager Wendy North

GP Murdo Donald MACLEOD, Janice HAYWOOD, Katie LAW, Gita NAIR, Christopher Almack PEARSON, Anne-Marie TINKLER

Alford, Lincolnshire

Merton Lodge Surgery
West Street, Alford LN13 9HT
Tel: 01507 463262 Fax: 01507 466447
(East Lincolnshire Primary Care Trust)

GP Kenneth Reid SPENCELEY, Keith CHARLTON, Keith Edward DUNNETT, Ann Elizabeth WOOLLARD

Alfreton

Birchwood Lane Medical Centre
2 Birchwood Lane, South Normanton, Alfreton DE55 3DA
Tel: 01773 862907 Fax: 01773 510572
(North Eastern Derbyshire Primary Care Trust)
Patient List Size: 3100

Practice Manager Mina Mistry

GP Pushpam VINAYAGAMOORTHY

Blackwell Medical Practice
Gloves Lane, Blackwell, Alfreton DE55 5JJ
Tel: 01773 510065 Fax: 01773 583086
Email: david.holland@gp-C81661.nhs.uk
(North Eastern Derbyshire Primary Care Trust)
Patient List Size: 2365

Practice Manager Rita Holland

GP David HOLLAND, Nick CAUFMEN

Jessop Medical Practice
24 Pennine Avenue, Riddings, Alfreton DE55 4AE
Tel: 01773 602707/742991 Fax: 01773 602706
(Amber Valley Primary Care Trust)

Practice Manager Glynis Blyth

GP Alan Henry MEAKIN, Joanna Marie BLYTH, David Edward HAWORTH, Tania MAY, Saddeck SHEIKHOSSAIN, Nan Yuin TSE, Michael Joseph VEALE

Leabrooks Medical Centre
27 Swanwick Road, Leabrooks, Alfreton DE55 1LJ
Tel: 01773 602746 Fax: 01773 602746
(Amber Valley Primary Care Trust)

Practice Manager Jennifer Wise

GP Terence Livingstone JONES, Colin CLAYTON

Limes Medical Centre
Limes Avenue, Alfreton DE55 7DW
Tel: 01773 833133 Fax: 01773 836099
(Amber Valley Primary Care Trust)
Patient List Size: 7600

Practice Manager A Moody

GP John Michael ORCHARD, Niall McKAY, Andrew MOTT, Timothy PARKIN, D PONTEFRACT, Joanna SOUTHCOTT

Somercotes Medical Centre
22 Nottingham Road, Somercotes, Alfreton DE55 4JJ
Tel: 01773 602141/601700 Fax: 01773 601704
(Amber Valley Primary Care Trust)
Patient List Size: 6800

Practice Manager Elaine Sheldon

GP James Renshaw HOGG, Antony DOWD, John Joseph HAMBLEY, Nicola HAMBLEY, Christopher Mason HOLLIDAY, Heather HOLLIDAY

Staffa Health Centre
189 Birkinstyle Lane, Stonebroom, Alfreton DE55 6LD
Tel: 01773 873557 Fax: 01773 875700
(North Eastern Derbyshire Primary Care Trust)
Patient List Size: 13500

GP Michael William DUFFIELD, Ruth Elizabeth COOPER, Paul GADSDEN, Dewi R GRUFFYDD, A P PARKER, Timothy Nigel Bradshaw SCOTT, Howard Anthony SOWERBY

The Surgery
Limes Avenue, Alfreton DE55 7DW
Tel: 01773 832749/832525 Fax: 01773 832921
(Amber Valley Primary Care Trust)
Patient List Size: 8350

Practice Manager Janet Elliott

GP James Richard SKIDMORE, Dr McARTHUR, John Charles PRYCE

Alnwick

The Bondgate Practice
Bondgate Surgery, Infirmary Close, Alnwick NE66 2NL
Tel: 01665 510888 Fax: 01665 510581
Email: bondgate-surgery.demon.co.uk
(Northumberland Care Trust)

Practice Manager Jeannette Watt

GP Colin Richard BROWN, Gary Smith FRASER, Jane Clare FRASER, Michael John GUY, Adam HENRY, Alison Mary McKENNA, Graham SYERS

Infirmary Drive Medical Group
Consulting Rooms, Infirmary Drive, Alnwick NE66 2NR
Tel: 01665 602388 Fax: 01665 604712
(Northumberland Care Trust)
Patient List Size: 8700

Practice Manager Michael Ainsley

GP Michael John DODD, David Charles DAVISON, Susan Jean DODD, Caroline Clair EMBLETON-BLACK, Katy LAMB, Christopher John STEVENSON, Janneke WOLTHUIS

Alresford

Alresford Surgery
Station Road, Alresford SO24 9JL
Tel: 01962 732345 Fax: 01962 736034
(Mid-Hampshire Primary Care Trust)

Practice Manager Richard Hannay

GP David John GREEN, Sheila Jean CASSIDY, Richard Alan CRIBB, Ann Catherine LOWMAN, Peter John STOKES, Susan WRIGHT

Watercress Medical Group
Dean Surgery, Ropley, Alresford SO24 0BQ
Tel: 01962 772340 Fax: 01962 772551
(Mid-Hampshire Primary Care Trust)

Practice Manager Clive Davis

GP Stephen CROSSE, Susan HAPPEL, Andrew ISBISTER, Amanda MASTERS, C MOWAT, Lindsay SWORD, Sean WATTERS

Alton

Alton Health Centre
Anstey Road, Alton GU34 2QX
Tel: 01420 542542 Fax: 01420 549466
(North Hampshire Primary Care Trust)

Practice Manager Margaret Lockett

GP George Terence CUBITT, M M DE QUINCEY, Jacqueline Mary OVER, Andrew James SWORD, Nicola Janine WHITE

Alton Health Centre
Anstey Road, Alton GU34 2QX
Tel: 01420 541166 Fax: 01420 542975
(North Hampshire Primary Care Trust)

Practice Manager Margarett Lockett

GP James Alexander Ratcliffe WILLIS, Philip Neil HOPWOOD

Boundaries Surgery
17 Winchester Road, Four Marks, Alton GU34 5HG
Tel: 01420 562153 Fax: 01420 546172
Email: margaret.hall@boundaries-surgery.com
Website: www.boundaries-surgery.com
(North Hampshire Primary Care Trust)
Patient List Size: 2520

Practice Manager Peter Hall

GP M J HALL

The Wilson Practice
Alton Health Centre, Anstey Road, Alton GU34 2QX
Tel: 01420 84676 Fax: 01420 543430
(North Hampshire Primary Care Trust)

Practice Manager Marioin Voller

GP Michael George HAYWARD, S DOBBIE, A W FELLOWS, P HOPWOOD, S F LOUDEN, Jane Sandra PECKHAM, Alison Jill RICKARD, R SWART

Altrincham

Altrincham Medical Practice
Normans Place, Altrincham WA14 2AB
Tel: 0161 928 2424
(Trafford South Primary Care Trust)
Patient List Size: 7400

Practice Manager Louise Beech

GP Kate JENNINGS, Mary ADAMS, Robin Adrian DAVY

Barrington Medical Centre
68 Barrington Road, Altrincham WA14 1JB
Tel: 0161 928 9621 Fax: 0161 926 9317
(Trafford South Primary Care Trust)
Patient List Size: 6000

Practice Manager Suzanne Foskett

GP Brian Nicholas MACDONALD, Rebecca I HEANEY, Sikhander LADHA, Nicola J TIGHE

The Family Surgery
94 Navigation Road, Altrincham WA14 1LL
Tel: 0161 929 9300 Fax: 0161 928 2434
(Trafford South Primary Care Trust)
Patient List Size: 1800

Practice Manager Joan Powell

GP Anoop Kumar SAHAL

The Lindens
Barrington Road, Altrincham WA14 1HZ
Tel: 0161 928 6160 Fax: 0161 929 5348
(Trafford South Primary Care Trust)
Patient List Size: 2725

Practice Manager Sylvia Saleh

GP Roy LIE, Brenda Elizabeth MARSHALL

Park Medical Practice
119 Park Road, Timperley, Altrincham WA15 6QQ
Tel: 0161 973 3485 Fax: 0161 973 3088
(Trafford South Primary Care Trust)

GP Stephanie BARLOW-HITCHEN, Nigel GUEST, May Elizabeth LENNIE, Stephen OWEN

Riddings Road Surgery
34 Riddings Road, Timperley, Altrincham WA15 6BP
Tel: 0161 962 9662
(Trafford South Primary Care Trust)

Practice Manager Margaret Holland

GP John KELLY

Shay Lane Medical Centre
Shay Lane, Hale, Altrincham WA15 8NZ
Tel: 0161 980 3835 Fax: 0161 980 9215
Website: www.shaylane.org
(Trafford South Primary Care Trust)
Patient List Size: 6500

GP Colin George KELMAN, Heather CAULFIELD, John CRANSTON, Liz NAYLOR

Shay Lane Medical Centre
Shay Lane, Hale Barns, Altrincham WA15 8NZ
Tel: 0161 980 3835 Fax: 0161 903 9848
(Trafford South Primary Care Trust)

GP Richard Anthony CALDWELL, Mahendra PATEL, Helen Ann SYMCOX

St Johns Medical Centre
St Johns Road, Altrincham WA14 2NW
Tel: 0161 928 8727 Fax: 0161 929 8550
(Trafford South Primary Care Trust)

Practice Manager Rita Shearn

GP Christopher John DAVIES

St Johns Medical Centre
St Johns Road, Altrincham WA14 2NW
Tel: 0161 928 8727 Fax: 0161 929 8550
(Trafford South Primary Care Trust)

GP Lindsay Margaret HERRINGTON, Deborah Jane MARSH

Timperley Health Centre
169 Grove Lane, Timperley, Altrincham WA15 6PH
Tel: 0161 980 2172 Fax: 0161 904 8573
(Trafford South Primary Care Trust)

Practice Manager Sandra George

GP Bernard CAPLAN

Timperley Health Centre
169 Grove Lane, Timperley, Altrincham WA15 6PH

GP Anthony Brian GALLAGHER

Timperley Health Centre
169 Grove Lane, Timperley, Altrincham WA15 6PH
(Trafford South Primary Care Trust)

GP Brendon Glenn SMITH

Timperley Health Centre
169 Grove Lane, Timperley, Altrincham WA15 6PH
Tel: 0161 980 3751 Fax: 0161 904 9678
(Trafford South Primary Care Trust)
Patient List Size: 3500

Practice Manager Sarah Westwood

GP Colin WESTWOOD

West Timperley Medical Centre
21 Dawson Road, Altrincham WA14 5PF
Tel: 0161 929 1515 Fax: 0161 941 6500
Website: www.westtimperleymedicalcentre.co.uk
(Trafford South Primary Care Trust)
Patient List Size: 6515

Practice Manager Amanda Kirk

GP Katharine Joanne NORRIS, Michael William GREGORY, S J ROBINSON, John Anthony VINCENT

Ambleside

Ambleside Health Centre
Rydal Road, Ambleside LA22 9BP
Tel: 01539 432693 Fax: 01539 432520
Email: helen.havnagold@gp-a82005.nhs.uk
(Morecambe Bay Primary Care Trust)

GP Ian James BIRKET, Andrea BAQAI, Paul John DAVIES, Alan Howard JACKSON, John G SLOSS

Old Forge Surgery
Red Lion Yard, Hawkshead, Ambleside LA22 0NU
Tel: 01539 436246
(Morecambe Bay Primary Care Trust)
Patient List Size: 1150

GP John Christopher BLACKBURN

Amersham

Amersham Health Centre
Chiltern Avenue, Amersham HP6 5AY
Tel: 0870 890 2513 Fax: 0870 890 2514
(Chiltern and South Bucks Primary Care Trust)

Practice Manager J Hayes

GP Alan Charles DELLOW, Nicola Jane BENNETT, Clare GABE, Sarah MARSHALL, Simon Gower THOMPSON, Andrea WOOD

Little Chalfont Surgery
200 White Lion Road, Little Chalfont, Amersham HP7 9NU
Tel: 01494 762323 Fax: 01494 765973
(Chiltern and South Bucks Primary Care Trust)
Patient List Size: 4200

Practice Manager Antoinette Ferraro

GP Rajbir BAJWA, Ash AGGARWAL

Rectory Meadow Surgery
School Lane, Amersham HP7 0HG
Tel: 01494 727711 Fax: 01494 431790
Email: nicola.rouse@nhs.net
(Chiltern and South Bucks Primary Care Trust)
Patient List Size: 9300

Practice Manager Nicola Rouse

GP Brynmor Lloyd NEAL, Vivien Lesley CARTER, David Muir FERGUSON, Agnethe Ann FOOTE, Robert Andrew SAPSFORD, Stephane WATTERUX

Andover

Adelaide Medical Centre
36 Adelaide Road, Andover SP10 1HA
Tel: 01264 351144 Fax: 01264 358639
(Mid-Hampshire Primary Care Trust)
Patient List Size: 9850

Practice Manager Trevor Vidler

GP Roderick Macrae MATHESON, Peter Francis ACRES, Susan BOND, Sylvia HICKEY, Marged JENKINS

Andover Health Centre
Charlton Road, Andover SP10 3LD
Tel: 01264 350270 Fax: 01264 336701
(Mid-Hampshire Primary Care Trust)

GP Donald Richard BATHAM, P COLLINS, R GRIFFITHS, R HARRIES-BROWN, A HOUSTON, T JAMES, P O'HALLORAN, C WALLIS

Bourne Valley Practice
10-12 High Street, Ludgershall, Andover SP11 9PZ
Tel: 01264 400300 Fax: 01264 400310
(Kennet and North Wiltshire Primary Care Trust)
Patient List Size: 1901

Practice Manager Maryanne Leish

GP A GREIG, Andrea CLARK

The Castle Practice
Health Centre, Central Street, Ludgershall, Andover SP11 9RA
Tel: 01264 790356 Fax: 01264 791256
(Kennet and North Wiltshire Primary Care Trust)

Practice Manager Paul Bessant

GP Richard WELLS, Alex ARMSTRONG, Toby DAVIES, Michael ROSSITER, Jennifer VERITY

Charlton Hill Surgery
Charlton Road, Andover SP10 3JY
Tel: 01264 337979 Fax: 01264 334251
(Mid-Hampshire Primary Care Trust)
Patient List Size: 9408

Practice Manager Paul Kelly

GP Vernon Harold NEEDHAM, Llewellyn Alan Lewis DAVIES, Henry Robin Clinton FORD, T Michael JACKSON, Daphne JOHNSTON

Derry Down Clinic
St Mary Bourne, Andover SP11 6BS
Tel: 01264 738368 Fax: 01264 738003
(Mid-Hampshire Primary Care Trust)
Patient List Size: 1900

GP Patricia BASSETT, Jerome RIDENT, James ROSE

New Street Medical Centre
130 New Street, Andover SP10 1DR
Tel: 01264 335999 Fax: 01264 334331
(Mid-Hampshire Primary Care Trust)

Practice Manager Carol Ward

GP Jeremy JACKMAN

Shepherds Spring Medical Centre
Cricketers Way, Andover SP10 5DE
Tel: 01264 361126 Fax: 01264 350138
(Mid-Hampshire Primary Care Trust)
Patient List Size: 9150

Practice Manager K Jenkins

GP Peter BEANLANDS, Alan John HAMILTON, Philip Mark HOOLE, Ann Frances PAWLEY, Heather Jane WILLSON

St Mary's Surgery
Church Close, Andover SP10 1DP
Tel: 01264 341424 Fax: 01264 336792
(Mid-Hampshire Primary Care Trust)
Patient List Size: 9100

Practice Manager Sharon Bicknell

GP John BYRNE, Matthew FERRIS, Elaine PRITCHARD, Malcolm STONE, A WALKER

Appleby-in-Westmorland

Appleby Health Centre
Low Wiend, Appleby-in-Westmorland CA16 6QP
Tel: 01768 351584 Fax: 01768 353375
(Eden Valley Primary Care Trust)
Patient List Size: 4800

Practice Manager Rose Smith

GP James Burrell LEITCH, Christine ECKERSALL, Geoffrey Frank SHARPE, Karen Tacye SHARPE

Arundel

The Arundel Surgery
Green Lane Close, Arundel BN18 9HG
Tel: 01903 882517/882191 Fax: 01903 884326
(Western Sussex Primary Care Trust)

Patient List Size: 6500

Practice Manager Julie Palmer

GP Roger Harry EVE, Marco CAVAROLI, Michael Eric Charles JENKINS, Andrew Norman MOTT

Yew Tree Surgery
Yew Tree House, North End Road, Yapton, Arundel BN18 0DU
Tel: 01243 551321 Fax: 01243 555101
(Western Sussex Primary Care Trust)

GP Andrew FOULKES, Thomas Andrew LARSEN, Peter George SPEER, J TAYLOR

Ascot

Green Meadows Surgery
Winkfield Road, Ascot SL5 7LS
Tel: 01344 621628 Fax: 01344 875136
(Windsor, Ascot and Maidenhead Primary Care Trust)
Patient List Size: 10800

Practice Manager Margaret Little

GP Andrew Patrick FANNING, Lucy GARDNER, Barry John GREEN, Jamie MARTIN, Amanda May ROBERTSON

Kings Corner Surgery
Kings Road, Ascot SL5 0AE
Tel: 01344 623181 Fax: 01344 875129
Website: www.sunninghilldoctor.co.uk
(Windsor, Ascot and Maidenhead Primary Care Trust)
Patient List Size: 7600

Practice Manager Clare McAteer

GP David Roger Harold NORMINTON, Amanda CHOUDRY, Jacqueline McGLYNN, Paul Nicholas WHITFIELD

Magnolia House Practice
Magnolia House, Station Road, Ascot SL5 0QJ
Tel: 01344 637800 Fax: 01344 637823
(Windsor, Ascot and Maidenhead Primary Care Trust)

GP Robert Harvey Scott FURNESS, Andrew Leslie CRAZE, Andrew Charles SHERLEY-DALE, Gillian Dallas TASKER

Radnor House Practice
25 London Road, Ascot SL5 7EN
Tel: 01344 874011 Fax: 01344 628868
(Windsor, Ascot and Maidenhead Primary Care Trust)
Patient List Size: 3030

Practice Manager F Ramsay

GP John Robert RAWLINSON, Katie SIMPSON

Ashbourne

Ashbourne Health Centre
Compton, Ashbourne DE6 1DA
(Derbyshire Dales and South Derbyshire Primary Care Trust)

Brailsford Medical Centre
The Green, Church Lane, Brailsford, Ashbourne DE6 3BX
Tel: 01335 360328 Fax: 01335 361095
(Derbyshire Dales and South Derbyshire Primary Care Trust)
Patient List Size: 5700

GP Paul Richard GAGE, Brenda Jean BATES, Rachel WARD, John Philip WEDGWOOD

Compton Health Centre
Compton, Ashbourne DE6 1DA
Tel: 01335 300588
(Derbyshire Dales and South Derbyshire Primary Care Trust)

Practice Manager Jenny Roebuck

GP Paul Richard KIRTLEY, Andrew Michael BROOM, David Ralph WARD, Christine Elizabeth WESTAWAY

Compton Health Centre
Compton, Ashbourne DE6 1DA
Tel: 01335 343784 Fax: 01335 300782
(Derbyshire Dales and South Derbyshire Primary Care Trust)
Patient List Size: 7300

Practice Manager Lindsey O'Brien

GP Christopher Edwin JOEL, John Anthony CURRY, Ian St. Clair Scott MACLEOD, Sheona Mary MACLEOD

Dove River Practice
Gibb Lane, Sudbury, Ashbourne DE6 5HY
Tel: 01283 812455 Fax: 01283 815187
(East Staffordshire Primary Care Trust)

Practice Manager Tracey Burt

GP Carole A MAGUIRE, Jennifer Mary ASHWORTH, Richard K FULFORD, A Martin GILCHRIST, Louise HANDLEY, Edward Paul TATTERSALL

Ashby-de-la-Zouch

Mansion House Health Centre
The Mansion House, 26 Kilwardby Street, Ashby-de-la-Zouch LE65 2FQ
(Charnwood and North West Leicestershire Primary Care Trust)

GP Orest Peter MULKA

North Street Health Centre
North Street, Ashby-de-la-Zouch LE65 1HU
Tel: 01530 414131 Fax: 01530 560732
(Charnwood and North West Leicestershire Primary Care Trust)
Patient List Size: 12700

Practice Manager J Mansfield

GP John ADDISON, Richard Arthur DAVIES, Geoffrey Eric FOULDS, Clare HALLAS, Jeffrey HOFFMAN, Caroline SPENCER, Harshad TAILOR

Ashford, Kent

Charing Surgery
Charing, Ashford TN27 0HZ
Tel: 01233 714141 Fax: 01233 713782
(Ashford Primary Care Trust)
Patient List Size: 7350

Practice Manager Gillian Magson

GP Terence Paul LISTER, Sara Pamela BUTLER-GALLIE, Neil David POPLETT, William Henry Edwin WARRILOW, M WINDMILL

Dr A Thomas
10 Singleton Court, Ashford TN23 5GR
Tel: 01233 639298 Fax: 01233 639298
(Ashford Primary Care Trust)
Patient List Size: 7200

GP Achamma THOMAS

Hamstreet Surgery
Ruckinge Road, Hamstreet, Ashford TN26 2NJ
Tel: 01233 732262 Fax: 01233 733097
(Ashford Primary Care Trust)
Patient List Size: 6200

Practice Manager Marian C Pullen

GP Julian David COLLEDGE, Ruth COLLEDGE, Anthony Ka Tung LAI, Matthew TIMMS

Hollington Surgery
Blue Line Lane, Ashford TN24 8UN
Tel: 01233 622361/624916 Fax: 01233 647621
(Ashford Primary Care Trust)
Patient List Size: 3200

Practice Manager Sue Goodman

GP William John DAVIES, Anthony PRAGNELL

The Medical Centre
Beaver Road, Ashford TN23 7SP
Tel: 01233 625527/624917 Fax: 01233 661227
(Ashford Primary Care Trust)
Patient List Size: 5000

Practice Manager Carol Duggan

GP Victor ALLEN, Simon GRAINEE, Borhan ZAHI

New Hayesbank Surgery
Cemetery Lane, Kennington, Ashford TN24 9JZ
Tel: 01233 624642 Fax: 01233 637304
(Ashford Primary Care Trust)
Patient List Size: 12500

Practice Manager Barbara Williams

GP Resham Singh DIU, Christopher Duncan POWELL, Mary Gerardine BUCKENHAM, W LLOYD-SMITH, Caroline Denise RUAUX, Trevor Mark STANLEY

North Street Surgery
28 North Street, Ashford TN24 8JR
Tel: 01233 661133 Fax: 01233 662727
(Ashford Primary Care Trust)
Patient List Size: 2600

Practice Manager Alyson Pinnock

GP Roger Graham PINNOCK

St Stephens Health Centre
St Stephens Walk, Ashford TN23 5AQ
Tel: 01233 622474 Fax: 01233 611664
(Ashford Primary Care Trust)
Patient List Size: 4000

Practice Manager Lynne Clumpus

GP Abi ABRAHAM, A COULSON, John DUTTON, A LINGAM

Stanhope Surgery
85 Kilndown Close, Stanhope, Ashford TN23 5SU
Tel: 01233 637125/636816 Fax: 01233 662188
(Ashford Primary Care Trust)
Patient List Size: 3500

Practice Manager P Plester

GP Matta Venkataramanaiah S. SETTY

The Surgery
Sydenham House, Mill Court, Ashford TN24 8DN
Tel: 01233 645851 Fax: 01233 638281
(Ashford Primary Care Trust)
Patient List Size: 10700

Practice Manager Pat McDonnell

GP Christopher Paul WHITE, Kim GARDNER, Kenneth HARPER, Edward Andrew KLIM, Rajeev MENON, Charles Gordon TRAILL

The Surgery
Main Road, Sellindge, Ashford TN25 6JX
Tel: 01303 812180 Fax: 01303 814069
Email: name@gp-g82658.nhs.uk
(Ashford Primary Care Trust)
Patient List Size: 3600

Practice Manager Christine Downey

GP Richard George MOREY, Guiseppina DEL BIANCO, Clare Helen EVANS

The Surgery
Front Road, Woodchurch, Ashford TN26 3SF
Tel: 01233 860236 Fax: 01233 861373
(Ashford Primary Care Trust)
Patient List Size: 3500

Practice Manager Paula Francis

GP Charles Martin Anthony BUSK

The Surgery
Clerk's Field, Headcorn, Ashford TN27 9QL
Tel: 01622 890294 Fax: 01622 891754
(Maidstone Weald Primary Care Trust)
Patient List Size: 6900

Practice Manager E Farbrace

GP Paul Richard SCAYSBROOK, John Granville DUTTON, Penelope June KEFFORD, Timothy WINCH

Willesborough Health Centre
Bentley Road, Willesborough, Ashford TN24 0HZ
Tel: 01233 621626 Fax: 01233 622930
(Ashford Primary Care Trust)
Patient List Size: 12000

Practice Manager Gillian Bushell

GP Norman Stanley CORFIELD, Jane Erskine CLARK, Joseph Arthur COONEY, Stuart James DOVE, Amir NAKY, Michael WEIMAR

Wye Surgery
67 Oxenturn Road, Wye, Ashford TN25 5AY
Tel: 01233 812419 Fax: 01233 813236
(Ashford Primary Care Trust)
Patient List Size: 8500

Practice Manager Jo Shepherd

GP Rosalind WALLER, Nick DI BIASIO, Allan Robert FOX, Jolyon Peter MILES

Ashford, Middlesex

Feltham Hill Road Surgery
107 Feltham Hill Road, Ashford TW15 1HH
Tel: 01784 252027 Fax: 01784 469145
(North Surrey Primary Care Trust)

GP Peter KANDELA

Fordbridge Medical Centre
4 Fordbridge Road, Ashford TW15 2SQ
Tel: 01784 242251
(North Surrey Primary Care Trust)

GP Asu Tosh DAS, Abdel ASHOURI, Sujata DAS, Peter William DRAPER

Stanwell Road Surgery
95 Stanwell Road, Ashford TW15 3EA
Tel: 01784 253565 Fax: 01784 244145
(North Surrey Primary Care Trust)
Patient List Size: 7100

Practice Manager Mary Ponsford

GP Michael Charles Nicholas CARTER, Sumita BURMAN-ROY, Ian Stephen FARMER, Philip John TURNER

Studholme Medical Centre
50 Church Road, Ashford TW15 2TU
Tel: 01784 420700 Fax: 01784 424503
(North Surrey Primary Care Trust)
Patient List Size: 15400

Practice Manager T J Simpson

GP John Roderick COUCH, Samir ALUI, Susan Margaret BELSTEAD, Sohail BUTT, Gill McFARLANE, Richard George Waldron MOORE, H C M RICHARDS, Khye Seng TANG

Ashington

Laburnum Medical Group
14 Laburnum Terrace, Ashington NE63 0XX
Tel: 01670 813376 Fax: 01670 854346
(Northumberland Care Trust)
Patient List Size: 2013

Practice Manager Joanne Hodge

GP Mustafa Salim RASOUL

Lintonville Medical Group
Old Lane, Ashington NE63 9UT
Tel: 01670 812772 Fax: 01670 521573

(Northumberland Care Trust)
Patient List Size: 14700

Practice Manager E L Walker

GP Sarah Jane CLEVERLEY, Andrew David BELL, Rakesh CHOPRA, Dr GEDLEY, Lindsay John GILFILLAN

Nursery Park Medical Group
Nursery Park Primary Care Centre, Nursery Park, Ashington NE63 0HP
Tel: 01670 528100 Fax: 01670 557948
(Northumberland Care Trust)

Practice Manager Philip Saddler

GP Channarayapatna Nanjappa RAMESH, Syed Bizaat IMAN, Jane LOTHIAN, Anne E ROBERTS, Helen RYAN

Seaton Hirst Primary Care Centre
Norham Road, Ashington NE63 0NG
Tel: 01670 813167 Fax: 01670 842019
Email: admin@gp-A84028.nhs.uk
(Northumberland Care Trust)

Practice Manager Pat Stevenson

GP John Maxwell CAMPBELL, Timothy HATCH, Robert John LAMBOURN, Richard Melville QUINBY, Valerie Susan WILLIAMS, Anna Louise HATCH, Alan Thomas Grant McCUBBIN, Dorothy Ruth WARRINGTON

Ashtead

St Stephens House
102 Woodfield Lane, Ashtead KT21 2DP
Tel: 01372 272069 Fax: 01372 279123
(East Elmbridge and Mid Surrey Primary Care Trust)
Patient List Size: 6300

Practice Manager Tracey Crickett

GP Philip John COOPER, Lidia Anna KOSTUCH-BUSH, Murray John STREET

Ashton-under-Lyne

Albion Medical Practice
1 Albion Street, Ashton-under-Lyne OL6 6HF
Tel: 0161 214 8710 Fax: 0161 214 8715
Website: www.albionmedicalpractice.co.uk
(Tameside and Glossop Primary Care Trust)

Practice Manager Tracy Wilson

GP Elizabeth NEEDHAM, Antony Norman EDGE, Foozia IDREES, Janette LOCKHART, Martin James STAGG

Bedford House Medical Centre
Glebe Street, Ashton-under-Lyne OL6 6HD
Tel: 0161 330 9880 Fax: 0161 330 9393
(Tameside and Glossop Primary Care Trust)
Patient List Size: 7400

Practice Manager Christine M Russell

GP Thomas OGDEN, Stefan John KOKIET, Stuart Raymond MURRAY

Chapel Street Medical Centre
Chapel Street, Ashton-under-Lyne OL6 6EW
Tel: 0161 339 9292 Fax: 0161 339 7808
(Tameside and Glossop Primary Care Trust)

GP Jean Sutherland Russell MacCOWAN, Andrew John HUTTON, Susan Jane HUTTON, Richard Andrew STRINGER

Market Place Health Centre
Market Place, Mossley, Ashton-under-Lyne OL5 0HE
Tel: 01457 832561 Fax: 0161 330 6266
(Tameside and Glossop Primary Care Trust)

Practice Manager Sheila Alison McConnell

GP Mohammad Ehtesham Nasirul HAQUE, Fiona Jane HESTEN, Latha JAYAKUMAR, Philip Andrew WELLS

Mossley Medical Practice
187 Manchester Road, Mossley, Ashton-under-Lyne OL5 9AB
Tel: 01457 833315 Fax: 01457 834496
(Tameside and Glossop Primary Care Trust)
Patient List Size: 2040

Practice Manager Claire Davanzo

GP Christina Mary GREENHOUGH, Dr SPALDING

Pennine Medical Centre
193 Manchester Road, Mossley, Ashton-under-Lyne OL5 9AJ
Tel: 01457 832590 Fax: 01457 836083
(Tameside and Glossop Primary Care Trust)
Patient List Size: 10951

Practice Manager D Buckley

GP Ann H M ATHERTON, Catherine Hamilton CAMPBELL, Anthony CAPUANO, Peter Timothy MORRIS, Ann Helena Mary WILLIAMSON

Stamford House
Stamford Street, Ashton-under-Lyne OL6 6QH
Tel: 0161 344 0803 Fax: 0161 339 8243
(Tameside and Glossop Primary Care Trust)

GP Kailash CHAND

Stockport Road Surgery
156 Stockport Road, Ashton-under-Lyne OL7 0NW
Tel: 0161 330 2440 Fax: 0161 330 2440
(Tameside and Glossop Primary Care Trust)

GP Simon KEBA, Govindbhai PATEL

Trafalger Square Surgery
1 Trafalger Square, Ashton-under-Lyne OL7 0LN
Tel: 0161 330 2131 Fax: 0161 339 5749
(Tameside and Glossop Primary Care Trust)

GP Bharat U PATEL

Waterloo Medical Centre
1 Dunkerley Street, Ashton-under-Lyne OL7 9EJ
Tel: 0161 330 7087 Fax: 0161 308 2788
(Tameside and Glossop Primary Care Trust)
Patient List Size: 2300

Practice Manager Janette Sadik

GP Samir Monir SADIK

West End Medical Centre
102 Stockport Road, Ashton-under-Lyne OL7 0LH
Tel: 0161 339 5488 Fax: 0161 330 0945
(Tameside and Glossop Primary Care Trust)
Patient List Size: 7000

Practice Manager John Gilmore

GP Harjinder Singh BHACHU, Patrick Arthur DOODY, Andrew Leonard PARHAM

Askam-in-Furness

The Surgery
2 Parklands Drive, Askam-in-Furness LA16 7JP
Tel: 01229 462464 Fax: 0709 235 6823
Email: prakash@jain.net
Website: www.jain.org.uk
(Morecambe Bay Primary Care Trust)

GP Prakash JAIN

Atherstone

The Atherstone Surgery
1 Ratcliffe Road, Atherstone CV9 1EU
Tel: 01827 713664 Fax: 01827 713666
(North Warwickshire Primary Care Trust)
Patient List Size: 14500

Practice Manager Karen Clark

GP Michael Patrick MAHER, Andrea Mary BONE, Trevor Nigel GOODING, Upma KARIA, Samir PURNELL-MULLICK, Andrew Scott THOMSON, David Andrew WESTON, John McGregor WINWARD

Station Road Surgery
45 Station Road, Atherstone CV9 1DB
Tel: 01827 718631 Fax: 01827 712944
(North Warwickshire Primary Care Trust)

GP Shah Zafar ALAM

Attleborough

Attleborough Surgeries (Station Road)
Station Road, Attleborough NR17 2AS
Tel: 01953 452394 Fax: 01953 453569
Website: www.attleboroughsurgeries.com
(Southern Norfolk Primary Care Trust)
Patient List Size: 16500

Practice Manager Michael Barnes

GP Charles Falcon Sterry OXLEY, Hilary BYRNE, Leslie Charles George COOPER, Jonathan Paul CRAIG, Tom FRY, Brian Montague LEACH, Richard Hunter LINDNER, Alistair Anderson MARTIN

Axbridge

Houlgate Way Surgery
Houlgate Way, Axbridge BS26 2BJ
Tel: 01934 732464 Fax: 01934 733488
Email: surgery@axbridgewedmoredoctors.co.uk
Website: www.axbridgewedmoredoctors.co.uk
(Somerset Coast Primary Care Trust)
Patient List Size: 7800

Practice Manager John Hinchliffe

GP Rosamond KING, J W COX, Matthew John DOLMAN, Ewart JACKSON-VOYZEY, G M MILES

Axminster

Axminster Medical Practice
St Thomas Court, Church Street, Axminster EX13 5AG
Tel: 01297 32126 Fax: 01297 35759
(East Devon Primary Care Trust)
Patient List Size: 10160

Practice Manager Shelah Martin

GP David Norman EVANS, Jonathan Mark ALLEN, Sarah Anne ELLIS, Jonathan Grovenor HALFORD, Simon Richard HODGES, B N McKENNA, Philip James Ralph TAYLOR, James Anthony VANN

Aylesbury

Aston Clinton Surgery
136 London Road, Aston Clinton, Aylesbury HP22 5LB
Tel: 01296 630241 Fax: 01296 630033
Website: www.westgrove.com
(Vale of Aylesbury Primary Care Trust)
Patient List Size: 5500

GP Edward Basil PEILE, Emma GARDENER, N SOLAN, Craig Steven WHITE, Gwen WILLIAMS

Bedgrove Surgery
Brentwood Way, Aylesbury HP21 7TL
Tel: 01296 330330 Fax: 01296 399179
(Vale of Aylesbury Primary Care Trust)
Patient List Size: 9500

GP Martin PAUL, Duncan Frederick Strathdee BURWOOD, Andrew John THEOBALD, Audrey Marguerite WALTERS

Brill Surgery
Surgery in the Square, Brill, Aylesbury HP18 9ST
Tel: 01844 238284
(Vale of Aylesbury Primary Care Trust)

Broughton House Surgery
241 Tring Road, Aylesbury HP20 1PH
Tel: 01296 425858 Fax: 01296 393398
(Vale of Aylesbury Primary Care Trust)
Patient List Size: 3890

Practice Manager Paula Martin

GP Helen Sarah BEESLEY, Christine CAMPLING, Helen TAYLOR

Elmhurst Surgery
Elmhurst Road, Aylesbury HP20 2AH
Tel: 01296 484054 Fax: 01296 397016
(Vale of Aylesbury Primary Care Trust)
Patient List Size: 15200

Practice Manager C Watkinson

GP Valerie Mary SMITH, Micheal John ALEXANDER, Gillian S. BECK, Sanjay DAHIYA, Penelope Margaret HOBHOUSE, C KENNEDY, Kevin Paul SUDDES, A THOMSON, Paul VOGWELL

The Health Centre
Banks Road, Haddenham, Aylesbury HP17 8EE
Tel: 01844 291874 Fax: 01844 292344
(Vale of Aylesbury Primary Care Trust)
Patient List Size: 7600

Practice Manager Pam Bright

GP Jonathan Calvert SADLER, Mark HOWCUTT, Hugh Alan STRADLING, Cathy WADE

Mandeville Surgery
Walton Court, Hannon Road, Aylesbury HP21 8TR
Tel: 01296 431515
(Vale of Aylesbury Primary Care Trust)

Meadowcroft Surgery
Jackson Road, Aylesbury HP19 9EX
Tel: 01296 425775 Fax: 01296 330324
(Vale of Aylesbury Primary Care Trust)
Patient List Size: 11270

Practice Manager Jill Blackburn

GP Michael THIRLWALL, Catherine Helen FORMAN, Timothy Guy PEACOCK, John Graham ROBINSON, Christopher Michael SMITH, Shirley Anne TINNION

Mitchell and Partners
New Chapel Surgery, High Street, Long Crendon, Aylesbury HP18 9AF
Tel: 01844 208228 Fax: 01844 201906
(Vale of Aylesbury Primary Care Trust)
Patient List Size: 9900

Practice Manager Diane Marshall

GP Timothy David MITCHELL, Anna FURLONGER, Stuart LOGAN, Catherine Anne SCOTT, Gillian Anne SCOTT, John MacRae WHITTINGTON

Oakfield Surgery
Oakfield Road, Aylesbury HP20 1LJ
Tel: 01296 423797 Fax: 01296 399246
Email: stella.collins@nhs.net
(Vale of Aylesbury Primary Care Trust)
Patient List Size: 5500

Practice Manager Stella Collins

GP C CANTONS, Sally Yvonne HOLDICH, S Y ZAIB

Poplar Grove Surgery
Meadow Way, Aylesbury HP20 1XB
Tel: 01296 482554 Fax: 01296 398771
Website: www.poplar-grove.com
(Vale of Aylesbury Primary Care Trust)
Patient List Size: 11413

Practice Manager Gareth Collings

GP Martin James WAKEFORD, Claire Veronica BONNER, Karen Lesley JOHNSON, Elizabeth Hilary MUIR, S PILLAI, Juliet Clare SUTTON, Christopher Simon Geoffrey TROWER

Waddesdon Surgery
Goss Avenue, Waddesdon, Aylesbury HP18 0LY
Tel: 01296 658585 Fax: 01296 658467
(Vale of Aylesbury Primary Care Trust)
Patient List Size: 5065

Practice Manager Jenny Mansbridge

GP Alan Douglas WATT, Jan KARMALI

Wendover Health Centre
Aylesbury Road, Wendover, Aylesbury HP22 6LD
Tel: 01296 623452
(Vale of Aylesbury Primary Care Trust)

Practice Manager John Batler, M C Downie, Sue Outtrim

GP Richard Quinn LEEPER, Michael Paul LOOSEMORE, Jonathan Paul MARSHALL, Philippa Wren MORETON, Roderick Alan REED

Whitchurch Surgery
49 Oving Road, Whitchurch, Aylesbury HP22 4JF
Tel: 01296 641203 Fax: 01296 640021
(Vale of Aylesbury Primary Care Trust)
Patient List Size: 4100

Practice Manager Rachel Brice

GP Joseph Louis RIZZO-NAUDI, Hazel BUTLAND, Catherine ELPHINSTONE

Whitehill Surgery
Whitehill Lane, Oxford Road, Aylesbury HP19 3EN
Tel: 01296 432742 Fax: 01296 398774
(Vale of Aylesbury Primary Care Trust)
Patient List Size: 10000

Practice Manager Max Washington

GP Nigel Damien KENNEDY, Tina BEARDSWORTH, Susan Jane DANTON, Helen Catherine FLEMING, Graham John JACKSON, Christopher KINDELL, Dr MARTIN

Aylesford

Aylesford Medical Centre
Admiral Moore Drive, Royal British Legion Village, Aylesford ME20 7SE
Tel: 01622 717389 Fax: 01622 790436
(Maidstone Weald Primary Care Trust)
Patient List Size: 6000

Practice Manager Margaret Parry

GP Robert Llewellyn BOWEN, Karen Maud SHAKESPEARE, Helen Denise TOWNER

Thornhills Medical Group
732 London Road, Larkfield, Aylesford ME20 6BQ
Tel: 01732 843900 Fax: 01732 872633
(Maidstone Weald Primary Care Trust)
Patient List Size: 12400

GP Timothy Jefferson CANTOR, David Frederick CHESOVER, Claire Elizabeth COCHRANE-DYET, Andre A D'COSTA, Robert J GILMORE, D T LE

Bacup

Bacup Health Centre
Yorkshire Street, Bacup OL13 9AL
Tel: 01706 876922 Fax: 01706 877037
(Burnley, Pendle and Rossendale Primary Care Trust)
Patient List Size: 5500

Practice Manager Shirley A Brown

GP Fakhree Fakhruddin AZAD, Shivanand Sakharam BONDRE

Bacup Health Centre
Bacup OL13 9AL
Tel: 01706 876644 Fax: 01706 876769
(Burnley, Pendle and Rossendale Primary Care Trust)
Patient List Size: 5631

Practice Manager Olive Doyle

GP Peter WILLIAMS, John O'MALLEY

Stacksteads Surgery
20 Fareholme Lane, Stacksteads, Bacup OL13 0EJ
Tel: 01706 873122 Fax: 01706 874152
(Burnley, Pendle and Rossendale Primary Care Trust)
Patient List Size: 2500

Practice Manager David Taylor

GP Jeremy Devine GREENWOOD, Hilary Jane WAIT, Patricia Ann WILKINSON

Bagshot

Millside Surgery
Church Road, Bagshot GU19 5EQ
Tel: 01276 452025
(Surrey Heath and Woking Primary Care Trust)

Practice Manager Girija Vadi

GP V K HANDA

Park House Surgery
Park Street, Bagshot GU19 5AQ
Tel: 01276 476333 Fax: 01276 479231
(Surrey Heath and Woking Primary Care Trust)

Practice Manager Pam Roberts

GP Maria Elizabeth SHOTTON, T C JOHNSON

Bakewell

Ashenfell Surgery
Church Lane, Baslow, Bakewell DE45 1SP
Tel: 01246 582216 Fax: 01246 583867
(High Peak and Dales Primary Care Trust)
Patient List Size: 4600

Practice Manager P Edmonstone

GP Michael Sinclair CHADWICK, Louise K A JORDAN, Julian Charles Barker NEWTON

Baldock

Ashwell Surgery
Lawyers Close, Gardiners Lane, Ashwell, Baldock SG7 5PY
Tel: 01462 742230 Fax: 01462 742764
(North Hertfordshire and Stevenage Primary Care Trust)
Patient List Size: 7600

Practice Manager D Stapleton

GP S R BLAKE, M G HOFFMAN, M C JARVIS, C RUSSELL

The Surgery
Astonia House, High Street, Baldock SG7 6BP
Tel: 01462 892458 Fax: 01462 490821
(North Hertfordshire and Stevenage Primary Care Trust)
Patient List Size: 11800

Practice Manager G Gee

GP Margaret Marsh THOMAS, Matthew Keith Francis COCKBURN, George GEORGIOU, John GOLDRING, Claire HAYWARD, Helen PARKINSON, Richard Stephen Grant STANLEY

Bampton

Bampton Surgery
Landells, Bampton OX18 2LJ
Tel: 01993 850257
(South West Oxfordshire Primary Care Trust)

Practice Manager Sue Gooding

GP Ronald Mackinnon MACKENZIE, Matthew Giles PERRY, John Anthony UDEN, Nicholas Alexander Lawton WARD

Banbury

Cropredy Surgery
Claydon Road, Cropredy, Banbury OX17 1FB
Tel: 01295 758372 Fax: 01295 750435
(Cherwell Vale Primary Care Trust)
Patient List Size: 3373

Practice Manager B Ware

GP Judith Anne WRIGHT, Christopher William DAY

Deddington Health Centre
Earls Lane, Deddington, Banbury OX15 0TQ
Tel: 01869 338611 Fax: 01869 37009
(Cherwell Vale Primary Care Trust)
Patient List Size: 8600

Practice Manager Sue Wilkins

GP Hugh Francis O'DONNELL, James MILAUGHLIN, Fiona Sue RUDDOCK, Richard RUSH

Godswell Lodge
Church Street, Bloxham, Banbury OX15 4ES
Tel: 01295 720347
(Cherwell Vale Primary Care Trust)

Practice Manager Gill Cook

GP Martin Andrew Michael HARRIS, Hilary Anne Mallett EDWARDS, Timothy Joseph Anthony HURST

Horse Fair Surgery
12 Horse Fair, Banbury OX16 0AJ
Tel: 01295 259484 Fax: 01295 279293
(Cherwell Vale Primary Care Trust)
Patient List Size: 15800

Practice Manager Sue Nottingham

GP Stephen Helliwell LARGE, Timothy John Sipling CHERRY, Hugh Graham GILLIES, Jonathan Lee MOBEY, Deborah Michelle NEVILLE, Nigel George Bruce REID, Jonathan Adam Galloway WILLIAMS

Lehman and Partners
Hightown Surgery, Hightown Gardens, Banbury OX16 9DB
Tel: 01295 270722 Fax: 01295 263000
Email: practice.manager@gp-k84059.nhs.uk
(Cherwell Vale Primary Care Trust)
Patient List Size: 9400

Practice Manager Jean Glasspool

GP Richard Stephen LEHMAN, Douglas Stuart BOYLE, Louise Jane CORNWALL, Pauline CRAWFORD, Harold Sinkwee NG CHENG HIN, Vipul G PATEL

Orchard Surgery
Cope Road, Banbury OX16 2EJ
Tel: 01295 256201 Fax: 01295 277783
(Cherwell Vale Primary Care Trust)
Patient List Size: 7400

Practice Manager H Nulty

GP George Peter Hugh MASON, Nicholas Quentin ALLISON, Claire Elizabeth NORTH, Giles REED

Sibford Surgery
Sibford Gower, Banbury OX15 5RQ
Tel: 01295 780213 Fax: 01295 788280
(Cherwell Vale Primary Care Trust)
Patient List Size: 2600

Practice Manager Susannah Thomas

GP David Derek SPACKMAN, Emma HASKEW

West Bar Surgery
1 West Bar Street, Banbury OX16 9SF
Tel: 01295 256261 Fax: 01295 756848
(Cherwell Vale Primary Care Trust)

Practice Manager Lorraine Pengilley

GP John William David BAUGH, J T CURTIN, Stephen Anthony HAYNES, Brendan David O'FARRELL, Melanie Kay PATTON, G Y ROGERS, Anne SANDERS, John Anthony TASKER, Barry TUCKER, Sarah Lucy Mary WOOKEY

Windrush Surgery
21 West Bar Street, Banbury OX16 9SA
Tel: 01295 251491 Fax: 01295 277706
(Cherwell Vale Primary Care Trust)

Practice Manager Pamela Dove

GP Debra Joan WIGNELL, Simon BENTLEY, Carl Phillip EVANS, Ramjdindredath Singh NANDOE

Banstead

Longcroft Clinic
5 Woodmansterne Lane, Banstead SM7 3HH
Tel: 01737 359332 Fax: 01737 370835
(East Elmbridge and Mid Surrey Primary Care Trust)
Patient List Size: 12200

Practice Manager Barbara Thwaites

GP Laurence Andrew NATHAN, E FULLER, S GODDARD, Sandeep Kumar PANDE, Patrick Joseph Thomas PEARSON, Imran RAFI, N RAY

Nork Clinic
63 Nork Way, Banstead SM7 1HL
Tel: 01737 362211 Fax: 01737 362980
Website: www.norkclinicbanstead.co.uk
(East Elmbridge and Mid Surrey Primary Care Trust)
Patient List Size: 5600

Practice Manager Valerie Shurvell

GP Masood AHMAD, Nuzhat AHMAD, Sally HUDSON, Dr KANTILAL, Victoria MOORTHY, G PATEL

Barking

Barking Medical Group Practice
130 Upney Lane, Barking IG11 9LT
Tel: 020 8594 4353/5709 Fax: 020 8591 4686
(Barking and Dagenham Primary Care Trust)
Patient List Size: 10600

Practice Manager June McGillicuddy

GP Humayun AHMAD, Amarjit Singh CHOPRA, Sulbha Ashok DESHPANDE, Yousef RASHID, Kusum Jagdish TOLIA

Cavendish Gardens Surgery
The Green House, 37 Cavendish Gardens, Barking IG11 9DU
Tel: 020 8594 4700 Fax: 020 8507 1390
(Barking and Dagenham Primary Care Trust)
Patient List Size: 4500

Practice Manager K Leah

GP Victor Henry KATECK, Binal Kumar SHARMA

King Edward Surgery
1 King Edwards Road, Barking IG11 7TB
Tel: 020 8594 2988 Fax: 020 8594 2184
(Barking and Dagenham Primary Care Trust)

GP Aleyamma JOHN, Kochummen JOHN

Ripple Road Surgery
343 Ripple Road, Barking IG11 7RJ
Tel: 020 8594 2770 Fax: 020 8594 3528
(Barking and Dagenham Primary Care Trust)

Practice Manager Tracey Livings

GP Ashfaq Ahmed ANSARI, Shaheen ANSARI

Salisbury Avenue Surgery
7 Salisbury Avenue, Barking IG11 9XQ
Tel: 020 8594 2023 Fax: 020 8594 1132
(Barking and Dagenham Primary Care Trust)

Patient List Size: 3000

Practice Manager Elizabeth Ransom

GP Suraj Narain GUPTA, Ravisha CHIBBER

The Surgery
188 Ripple Road, Barking IG11 7PR
Tel: 020 8594 0212 Fax: 020 8594 2438
(Barking and Dagenham Primary Care Trust)

GP Israr Ahmed MOGHAL, Adel Mohsin ABDULLAH, Nripendra Krishna DEB

The Surgery
51 Upney Lane, Barking IG11 9LP
Tel: 020 8594 3667 Fax: 020 8471 9920
(Barking and Dagenham Primary Care Trust)
Patient List Size: 3400

GP P PRASAD

The Surgery
1 Harpour Road, Barking IG11 8RJ
Tel: 020 8594 1158 Fax: 020 8594 2660
(Barking and Dagenham Primary Care Trust)

Practice Manager M F Haq

GP Mohammed Fazle HAQ, Mohammad Malik RATYAL

The Surgery
60 Victoria Road, Barking IG11 8PY
Tel: 020 8553 5111 Fax: 020 8553 1090
(Barking and Dagenham Primary Care Trust)

GP Virendra Kumar CHAWLA

Thames View Health Centre
Bastable Avenue, Barking IG11 0LG
Tel: 020 8594 1061 Fax: 020 8507 2184
(Barking and Dagenham Primary Care Trust)

Practice Manager Kamal Kalkat

GP Gurkirit Singh KALKAT, Kanika RAI, Dolly SAXENE

Thams View Health Centre
Bastable Avenue, Barking IG11 0LG
Tel: 020 8594 1061 Fax: 020 8594 2184
(Barking and Dagenham Primary Care Trust)

GP Kochummen JOHN, Aleyamma JOHN

Victoria Health Centre
1 Queens Road, Barking IG11 8GD
Tel: 0870 417 3987 Fax: 020 8594 1816
(Barking and Dagenham Primary Care Trust)
Patient List Size: 2500

Practice Manager Azra Ahmed, Wendy Behn

GP Pratibha MATHUR

Barnard Castle

Barnard Castle Surgery
Victoria Road, Barnard Castle DL12 8HT
Tel: 01833 690707 Fax: 01833 690840
(Durham Dales Primary Care Trust)
Patient List Size: 10500

Practice Manager Margaret Taube Brown

GP John Jackson WHITE, Robert Gregson CARTER, Colin Robert CUTHBERT, Fiona Jane HAMILTON, David Alaistair ROBERTSON, Steven J. ROWAN, Flora Mary WELCH

The Surgery
Hill Terrace, Middleton-in-Teesdale, Barnard Castle DL12 0QE
Tel: 01833 640217 Fax: 01833 640961
Email: middletoninteesdalesurgery@gp-a83043.nhs.uk
(Durham Dales Primary Care Trust)
Patient List Size: 3000

Practice Manager Jane Dickson

GP Peter Graham AUSTIN, Jonathan Chave NAINBY-LUXMOORE

Barnet

Addington Medical Centre
46 Station Road, New Barnet, Barnet EN5 1QH
Tel: 020 8441 4425 Fax: 020 8441 4957/4425
(Barnet Primary Care Trust)
Patient List Size: 8000

Practice Manager Soo Kelly

GP Andrew Neil PAINTER, Ayo O AWE, Gareth DEE, Minoti Kalpesh PATEL

Bicknoller
59 Bells Hill, Barnet EN5 2SG
Tel: 020 8449 3514 Fax: 020 8440 1463
(Barnet Primary Care Trust)
Patient List Size: 1900

Practice Manager Mandy Waddon

GP Divya Vinod KHIROYA

Church House Surgery
3 Church Passage, Barnet EN5 4BW
Tel: 020 8449 9622
(Barnet Primary Care Trust)

GP Nalini RANASINGHE, Don Upali RANASINGHE

East Barnet Health Centre
149 East Barnet Road, Barnet EN4 8QZ
Tel: 020 8440 7417 Fax: 020 8447 0126
(Barnet Primary Care Trust)
Patient List Size: 2242

GP Anthony David TROYACK

East Barnet Health Centre
149 East Barnet Road, Barnet EN4 8QZ
Tel: 020 8440 7417 Fax: 020 8447 0126
(Barnet Primary Care Trust)
Patient List Size: 2738

Practice Manager Jackie McGarry

GP David Simon MONKMAN

East Barnet Health Centre
149 East Barnet Road, Barnet EN4 8QZ
Tel: 020 8440 7417 Fax: 020 8447 0126
(Barnet Primary Care Trust)
Patient List Size: 3333

Practice Manager J McGarry

GP Penelope Mary WESTON, Rosalind LANDAU

East Barnet Health Centre
149 East Barnet Road, Barnet EN4 8QZ
Tel: 020 8440 7417 Fax: 020 8447 0126
(Barnet Primary Care Trust)
Patient List Size: 2485

Practice Manager J McGarry

GP Suresh Chand PATNI

East Barnet Road Surgery
113 East Barnet Road, New Barnet, Barnet EN4 8RF
Tel: 020 8449 6443 Fax: 020 8441 5760
(Barnet Primary Care Trust)
Patient List Size: 4100

Practice Manager J Ward

GP Jeremiah McELLIGOTT, Simon John MILES

Holly Park Clinic
Holly Park Road, Friern, Barnet N11 3HB
Tel: 020 8368 7626
(Barnet Primary Care Trust)

Practice Manager Enid Grimes, Smita Raithatha

GP R RAITHATHA

Longrove Surgery
70 Union Street, Barnet EN5 4HT
Tel: 020 8441 9440/9563 Fax: 020 8441 4037
(Barnet Primary Care Trust)
Patient List Size: 10500

Practice Manager Claire Shea

GP Philippa Mary CURRAN, Steven Irving LIVINGSTON, Dr NAIDOO, Margaret Elizabeth Anne PHILIPPSON, Carole Ann SOLOMONS

Old Court House Surgery
27 Wood Street, Barnet EN5 4BB
Tel: 020 8449 2388
(Barnet Primary Care Trust)
Patient List Size: 7985

Practice Manager B Stephens

GP Philippe William Lartigue RIBET, Prashant DESAI, Roisin Patricia RIBET

Station Road Surgery
33b Station Road, New Barnet, Barnet EN5 1PH
Tel: 020 8440 2912 Fax: 020 8441 8711
(Barnet Primary Care Trust)
Patient List Size: 2204

Practice Manager Joan Jackson

GP Roshanali Bhanji MOMAN

Barnetby

The Medical Centre
34 Victoria Road, Barnetby DN38 6HZ
Tel: 01652 688203 Fax: 01652 680841
(North Lincolnshire Primary Care Trust)
Patient List Size: 2000

GP Ajaykumar VORA

Barnoldswick

Edward Street Surgery
Edward Street, Earby, Barnoldswick BB18 6QT
Tel: 01282 843407 Fax: 01282 844886
(Burnley, Pendle and Rossendale Primary Care Trust)
Patient List Size: 7300

Practice Manager Pat Chippendale

GP Alison EVANS, Mike HORSFIELD, Phillip Alexander HUXLEY, Ian David SANGSTER, Esther Grace SMITH

Barnsley

Caxton House Surgery
53 High Street, Grimethorne, Barnsley S72 7BB
Tel: 01226 711228
(Barnsley Primary Care Trust)
Patient List Size: 1600

GP I R SAXENA

Church Drive Surgery
Church Drive, Brierley, Barnsley S72 9HZ
Tel: 01226 711435 Fax: 01226 711625
(Barnsley Primary Care Trust)
Patient List Size: 2000

GP M SHRIVASTAVA

Cope Street Surgery
2A Cope Street, Barnsley S70 4HY
Tel: 01226 244476 Fax: 01226 767349
(Barnsley Primary Care Trust)
Patient List Size: 3000

GP S RAVI

Craven and Czepulkowski
48 High Street, Royston, Barnsley S71 4RF
Tel: 01226 722314 Fax: 01226 728996
(Barnsley Primary Care Trust)
Patient List Size: 6400

Practice Manager Mary Peacock

GP Phillip John CRAVEN, Edward Christopher CZEPULKOWSKI

Darton Health Centre
Church Street, Darton, Barnsley S75 5HQ
Tel: 01226 382420 Fax: 01226 213892
(Barnsley Primary Care Trust)
Patient List Size: 2670

Practice Manager Jane Jones

GP G EKO, Thomas George HEYES

Dr A R Bell
77 Park Street, Wombwell, Barnsley S73 0HL
Tel: 01226 752161
(Barnsley Primary Care Trust)

GP Alan Richard BELL

Dr AL Pollock and Partners
94 Park Grove, Barnsley S70 1QE
Tel: 01226 282345 Fax: 01226 785228
(Barnsley Primary Care Trust)
Patient List Size: 8900

Practice Manager Keith Lyman

GP Anthony Louis POLLOCK, Christopher Alan BRIDGER, Nigel William PALMER, Balaji PUTTAGUNTA

Dr G H Khan
Galtee More, 2 Doncaster Road, Barnsley S70 1UD
Tel: 01226 282555 Fax: 01226 282555
(Barnsley Primary Care Trust)
Patient List Size: 2400

Practice Manager Christine Key

GP Gulzar Hussain KHAN

Dr M Yaqub
Cliffe Road, Brampton, Barnsley S73 0XP
Tel: 01226 753321 Fax: 01226 753321
(Barnsley Primary Care Trust)

GP Mohmad YAQUB

Gold Street Surgery
1A Gold Street, Barnsley S70 1TT
Tel: 01226 205339 Fax: 01226 247932
(Barnsley Primary Care Trust)
Patient List Size: 5450

Practice Manager J Beardshall

GP N BASU, K S DESAI, Satyendu MITRA

Grimethorpe Surgery
Dorbren House, Cemetery Road, Grimethorpe, Barnsley S72 7JB
Tel: 01226 716809 Fax: 01226 712999
(Barnsley Primary Care Trust)
Patient List Size: 4400

Practice Manager Diana Wells

GP Venkataramanappa SRIRAMULU

The Health Centre
2 Duke Street, Hoyland, Barnsley S74 9QS
Tel: 01226 748719 Fax: 01226 360162
(Barnsley Primary Care Trust)
Patient List Size: 4200

Practice Manager Sue Wildsmith

GP Ramakant Ramgopal BHARTIA, J BARUAH

The Health Centre
High Street, Dodworth, Barnsley S75 3RF
Tel: 01226 203881

(Barnsley Primary Care Trust)
Patient List Size: 6300

Practice Manager Ros Mills

GP Raj Pal SINGH, Betty ABOOBAKAR, John Gordon ROBERTSON, Magdi SELIM, Jethalal Tapubhai VAGHANI

The Health Centre
Duke Street, Hoyland, Barnsley S74 9QS
Tel: 01226 743208 Fax: 01226 742557
(Barnsley Primary Care Trust)

Practice Manager Carol Armitage

GP Antony David Roy MARSHALL, M Z MAHMOOD, J D WOOD

The Health Centre
Rose Tree Avenue, Cudworth, Barnsley S72 8UA
Tel: 01226 710326 Fax: 01226 780627
(Barnsley Primary Care Trust)
Patient List Size: 9500

GP Rafi Saleem MIAN, Dinor Madhusudan ATHALE, Catherine M FREEBORN, Martyn Cedric HARVEY, Mohammad Ayub KHAN

The Health Centre
Duke Street, Hoyland, Barnsley S74 9QS
Tel: 01226 742915 Fax: 01226 745585
(Barnsley Primary Care Trust)
Patient List Size: 2300

Practice Manager Jackie Carr

GP A WALKER

Hill Brow Surgery
Long Croft, Mapplewell, Barnsley S75 6FH
Tel: 01226 383131 Fax: 01226 380100
(Barnsley Primary Care Trust)
Patient List Size: 10200

Practice Manager J H Gledhill

GP Arun Kumar AGGARWAL, Christopher NORTH, D W PORTER, Fiona Ann RICHARDS, David ROSE

Huddersfield Road Surgery
6 Huddersfield Road, Barnsley S70 2LT
Tel: 01226 287589 Fax: 01226 731245
(Barnsley Primary Care Trust)
Patient List Size: 10300

Practice Manager Margaret Snell

GP Kenneth Walter McDONALD, Ivan Patrick APPELQVIST, Catherine Elizabeth LAW, Nicholas Dominic Richard LUSCOMBE, Frances Heather MIDDLETON, James Andrew Harley STOBART

Kelvin Grove Surgery
Kelvin Grove, Wombwell, Barnsley S73 0DL
Tel: 01226 752361 Fax: 01226 341577
Email: practice.manager@gp-85012.nhs.uk
(Barnsley Primary Care Trust)
Patient List Size: 7000

Practice Manager V Beaumont

GP Yadu Nandan PRASAD, J A AMONKAR, A MISTRY

Lundwood Medical Centre
Pontefract Road, Lundwood, Barnsley S71 5PN
Tel: 01226 201737 Fax: 01226 731055
(Barnsley Primary Care Trust)

Practice Manager P Taylor

GP Nasima AHMED, John HARBAN

Main Surgery
170 Sheffield Road, Barnsley S70 4NW
Tel: 01226 203190 Fax: 01226 203190
(Barnsley Primary Care Trust)

GP Prakash Chandra KAKOTY, Dr HAKEEM

Mapplewell Health Centre
276 Darton Lane, Mapplewell, Barnsley S75 6AJ
Tel: 01226 233777 Fax: 01226 233773
(Barnsley Primary Care Trust)

Practice Manager Marilyn Bottomley

GP Nikola BALAC, Fernando ALVAREZ ESCURRA

Monk Bretton Health Centre
High Street, Barnsley S71 2EQ
Tel: 01226 771707 Fax: 01226 779874
(Barnsley Primary Care Trust)
Patient List Size: 2400

Practice Manager Marie Sykes

GP Colette Winifred LEESE

Park Grove Surgery
124-126 Park Grove, Barnsley S70 1QE
Tel: 01226 282140 Fax: 01226 213279 (Call before faxing)
(Barnsley Primary Care Trust)
Patient List Size: 3500

Practice Manager Asha Singh

GP Davendra SINGH

Rotherham Road Medical Centre
100 Rotherham Road, Barnsley S71 1UT
Tel: 01226 282587 Fax: 01226 291900
(Barnsley Primary Care Trust)
Patient List Size: 5200

Practice Manager Mike Robinson

GP Gillian Veronica TYERMAN, Mark Innes BURGIN, Monica DUGGAL, Peter Frank TYERMAN

Sheffield Road Surgery
170A Sheffield Road, Barnsley S70 4NW
Tel: 01226 293232 Fax: 01226 280432
(Barnsley Primary Care Trust)
Patient List Size: 2650

Practice Manager Sandra Nicholson

GP Desh Gaurav YADAV

The Surgery
91 Dodworth Road, Barnsley S70 6ED
Tel: 01226 282535 Fax: 01226 241448
(Barnsley Primary Care Trust)

Practice Manager P Hardstaff

GP Stephen James BURTON, Peter Francis O'DWYER, D M SMALLWOOD

Surgery
65D Midland Road, Royston, Barnsley S71 4QW
Tel: 01226 722418 Fax: 01226 700648
(Barnsley Primary Care Trust)
Patient List Size: 9127

Practice Manager Julie Wilson

GP Michael Stanley LITTLEWOOD, Kenneth Paul CRAWFORD, Clare NAISH, Sarah SAKHAMURI

The Surgery
35 Barnsley Road, Goldthorpe, Barnsley S63 9LT
Tel: 01709 880977 Fax: 01709 891457
(Barnsley Primary Care Trust)
Patient List Size: 2000

GP Chelliah Konar KRISHNASWAMY

The Surgery
430 Doncaster Road, Barnsley S70 3RJ
Tel: 01226 216000 Fax: 01226 216002
(Barnsley Primary Care Trust)

GP Armando Rodolfo MENEZES, M E JOHNSON, P F LANE, V PEARSON, M A SCARGILL, C B WOOD

Victoria Medical Centre
7 Victoria Crescent West, Barnsley S75 2AE
Tel: 01226 282758 Fax: 01226 729800
(Barnsley Primary Care Trust)
Patient List Size: 6700

Practice Manager Denise Wilkinson

GP John Noel WILKERSON, Adrienne Margaret RENNICK, Mark Thomas SMITH, Clare TAYLOR, Andrea WALLACE

Wadlerslade Surgery
Walderslade, 194 King Street, Hoyland, Barnsley S74 9LJ
Tel: 01226 743221 Fax: 01226 741100
(Barnsley Primary Care Trust)
Patient List Size: 11000

Practice Manager Judith Pattison

GP R T FARMER, R TAYLOR, Andrea Susan WARD, Rebecca Jane WASTLING, Kathleen Lois WELCHEW

Wombwell Medical Centre
George Street, Wombwell, Barnsley S73 0DD
Tel: 01226 752363 Fax: 01226 270828
(Barnsley Primary Care Trust)

Practice Manager Christina Carroll

GP Christopher Mark BOWNS, Carolyn Jayne DALES, Brian HOURIHANE, Daniel John O'SULLIVAN

Worsbrough Health Centre
Oakdale, Worsbrough Dale, Barnsley S70 5EG
Tel: 01226 204090 Fax: 01226 771966
(Barnsley Primary Care Trust)
Patient List Size: 5100

Practice Manager Angela Adams

GP James Anthony WALKER, Gareth SUTTON, Linda SYKES

Barnstaple

Boutport Medical Practice
110 Boutport Street, Barnstaple EX31 1TD
Tel: 01271 324106 Fax: 01271 347150
(North Devon Primary Care Trust)
Patient List Size: 5300

Practice Manager Sheila Beeney

GP Patrick Christopher Henry MOORE, Annere DISSEVEZT, Stephen MYERS, Daryl PEARCE

Brannams Medical Centre
Brannams Square, Kiln Lane, Barnstaple EX32 8GP
Tel: 01271 329004 Fax: 01271 346785
(North Devon Primary Care Trust)
Patient List Size: 12900

Practice Manager C Ford

GP Thomas Leslie BIGGE, Ian Ferguson Munro JACK, Iain STWEART, Andrew BARGERY, Robert George BUNNEY, John Anthony MARSTON, Charlotte Pelham McCAIE, Zsuzanna Maria REYNOLDS, Charles Peter TAYLOR

Litchdon Medical Centre
Landkey Road, Barnstaple EX32 9LL
Tel: 01271 23443 Fax: 01271 25979
(North Devon Primary Care Trust)

GP Richard John Shapland BEER, Sally Jane HUNT, Brian MALCOLM, Elisabeth Mary McELDERRY, John Ellis MILLER, Penelope Frances SMITH, Julian Geoffrey TURNER, Mark Bailey WOOD, David William YORK-MOORE

The Medical Centre
Beards Farm, Fremington, Barnstaple EX31 2PG
Tel: 01271 376655 Fax: 01271 321006
(North Devon Primary Care Trust)
Patient List Size: 5767

Practice Manager Jenny Gifford

GP Andrew LATHAM, Alan HOWLETT, Bruce HUGHES, Alison LATHAM, John Quinton TULLOCK

Queens Medical Centre
6/7 Queen Street, Barnstaple EX32 8HY
Tel: 01271 372672 Fax: 01271 341902
(North Devon Primary Care Trust)
Patient List Size: 7458

Practice Manager Sheila Beeney

GP Nigel BRENNAN, Miranda COBEMAN, Richard Anthony HOLMAN, Catherine Ann HOOPER, Baljit Singh KALSI

Barrow-in-Furness

Atkinson Health Centre
Market Street, Barrow-in-Furness LA14 2LR
Tel: 01229 821556 Fax: 01229 827171
(Morecambe Bay Primary Care Trust)

Practice Manager Irene Riley

GP Amarnauth MANGAL

Atkinson Health Centre
Market Street, Barrow-in-Furness LA14 2LR
Tel: 01229 821669 Fax: 01229 877185
(Morecambe Bay Primary Care Trust)

Practice Manager Malathi Pai

GP Kasturi Ganejh PAI

Atkinson Health Centre
Market Street, Barrow-in-Furness LA14 2LR
Tel: 01229 821030 Fax: 01229 827171
(Morecambe Bay Primary Care Trust)

Practice Manager Ann Alexander

GP Rajendra Kumar RATHI

Atkinson Health Centre
Market Street, Barrow-in-Furness LA14 2LR
Tel: 01229 822205 Fax: 01229 832938
(Morecambe Bay Primary Care Trust)

GP Antoni Peter WIEJAK, C G COTTAM

Bridgegate Medical Centre
Winchester Street, Barrow-in-Furness LA13 9SH
Tel: 01229 820304 Fax: 01229 836984
Email: diane.clark@gp-982009.nhs.uk
Website: bridgegatemedicalcentre.co.uk
(Morecambe Bay Primary Care Trust)
Patient List Size: 6400

Practice Manager Diane Clark

GP Penelope Susan WILLIAMS, John Paul CULLING, Arthur PETER, Duncan ROCHE, David Philip WAIND

Burnett Edgar Medical Centre
Central Drive, Walney Island, Barrow-in-Furness LA14 3HY
Tel: 01229 474526 Fax: 01229 475282
(Morecambe Bay Primary Care Trust)

Practice Manager Shabina Jeelani

GP Yahya MEMON, Ghulam JEELANI

Dr Nugent and Partners
243 Abbey Road, Barrow-in-Furness LA14 5JY
Tel: 01229 821599 Fax: 01229 821599
(Morecambe Bay Primary Care Trust)
Patient List Size: 7000

Practice Manager Patricia Marshall

GP John Joseph NUGENT, Duncan HAMBLY, Hilary Jean HEARN, Elizabeth Mary NUGENT

Duke Street Surgery
4 Duke Street, Barrow-in-Furness LA14 1LF
Tel: 01229 820068 Fax: 01229 813840
(Morecambe Bay Primary Care Trust)

Patient List Size: 9500

Practice Manager Sheila Lawson

GP Philip James SHARPLES, K BRISTOL, N HUSSAIN, Bruce Robertson MACDONALD, Ian Joseph WEAR

Hartington Street Medical Practice
36-38 Hartington Street, Barrow-in-Furness LA14 5SL
Tel: 01229 820554 Fax: 01229 813718
(Morecambe Bay Primary Care Trust)
Patient List Size: 2873

Practice Manager Rebecca McGlown

GP David Darragh KNOX, Richard Henry WYATT

Hartington Street Surgery
26 Hartington Street, Barrow-in-Furness LA14 5SL
Tel: 01229 820250
(Morecambe Bay Primary Care Trust)
Patient List Size: 2500

Practice Manager Patricia Aguirre

GP Osman El Nur MOHAMMED

Hartington Street Surgery
28-30 Hartington Street, Barrow-in-Furness LA14 5SL
Tel: 01229 870170 Fax: 01229 834677
(Morecambe Bay Primary Care Trust)

Practice Manager Julie Noone

GP Mahendra Kumar Chimanbai PATEL, Julia Margaret BARKER

Liverpool House Surgery
69 Risedale Road, Barrow-in-Furness LA13 9QY
Tel: 01229 832232 Fax: 01229 432156
Website: www.liverpoolhouse.com
(Morecambe Bay Primary Care Trust)
Patient List Size: 5281

Practice Manager Lynda Lowes

GP Christopher John GREEN, Simon Charles HARVEY, Kathryn Margaret ROBINSON

Norwood Medical Centre
99 Abbey Road, Barrow-in-Furness LA14 5ES
Tel: 01229 822024 Fax: 01229 823949
(Morecambe Bay Primary Care Trust)
Patient List Size: 10200

Practice Manager Caroline Lee

GP Amanda Jane BOARDMAN, Michael Fabian BURDEN, Steven Trevor McQUILLAN, Amanda PUGH, Simon ROGERSON, John Charles YOUNG

Rawlinson Street Surgery
128 Rawlinson Street, Barrow-in-Furness LA14 2DG
Tel: 01229 820221 Fax: 01229 824948
(Morecambe Bay Primary Care Trust)

Practice Manager Beryl Pickthall

GP Mikhail Maalway MAALAWY

Risedale Surgery
2-4 Gloucester Street, Barrow-in-Furness LA13 9RX
Tel: 01229 822332 Fax: 01229 433636
(Morecambe Bay Primary Care Trust)
Patient List Size: 2800

Practice Manager Maxine Baron

GP Geoffrey Charles JOLLIFFE, Isabel Mary O'DONOVAN

Barton-upon-Humber

Central Surgery
King Street, Barton-upon-Humber DN18 5ER
Tel: 01652 635435 Fax: 01652 636122
(North Lincolnshire Primary Care Trust)

Practice Manager Nancy Devine

GP Timothy John Charles BIRTWHISTLE, Charles David CHAPMAN, Robert Mark JAGGS-FOWLER, Clare Elaine LAVERY, Paul LONGDEN, Fergus Noel MACMILLAN, Dean WELLINGS

West Town Surgery
80 High Street, Barton-upon-Humber DN18 5PU
Tel: 01652 660041 Fax: 01652 636005
(North Lincolnshire Primary Care Trust)

Practice Manager C Muralee

GP Dr MURALEE

Basildon

Ballards Walk Surgery
49 Ballards Walk, Basildon SS15 5HL
Tel: 01268 542901 Fax: 01268 491246
(Basildon Primary Care Trust)
Patient List Size: 7000

Practice Manager Jackie Mellia

GP Alexander John MITCHELL, Wequar AHMAD, Arun KUMAR

Clay Hill Medical Practice
Southview Road, Vange, Basildon SS16 4HD
Tel: 01268 533151 Fax: 01268 282059
(Basildon Primary Care Trust)
Patient List Size: 8000

Practice Manager Susan Hemmings

GP Robert COLBY, Nihal Lalendra Bandara HERATH, Francisca OGUNBIYI

Dipple Medical Centre
South Wing, Wickford Avenue, Pitsea, Basildon SS13 3HQ
Tel: 01268 556231 Fax: 01268 556231
(Basildon Primary Care Trust)

Practice Manager Sandra Bell

GP Madeline Ann PRETTY, Dave Gobin SINGH

Dipple Medical Centre, West Wing
Wickford Avenue, Pitsea, Basildon SS13 3HQ
Tel: 01268 555115 Fax: 01268 559935
(Basildon Primary Care Trust)
Patient List Size: 9203

Practice Manager D Halliday

GP Robin Joseph BELL, Adekunle ADEOSUN, Joseph Oladeinde ARAYOMI, Michael Andrew SIMS

Dr R J Bell and Partners
Wickford Avenue, Pitsea, Basildon SS13 3HQ
Tel: 01268 555115/555225 Fax: 01268 559935
Email: robin.bell@nhs.net
(Basildon Primary Care Trust)
Patient List Size: 8500

Practice Manager Dee Halliday

GP Robin Joseph BELL, Adekunie ADEOSUN, Joseph Oladeide ARAYOMI, Michael Andrew SIMS

Fryerns Medical Centre
Peterborough Way, Basildon SS14 3SS
Tel: 01268 532344 Fax: 01268 287641
(Basildon Primary Care Trust)

GP Pradeep Kumar SINGH

The Health Centre
Laindon, Basildon SS15 5TR
Tel: 01268 546411 Fax: 01268 493804
(Basildon Primary Care Trust)

Practice Manager Sheila McLean

GP Patrick Joseph Charles KERRIGAN, Robert MAUNDY, Alistair MOULDS

The Health Centre
Laindon, Basildon SS15 5TR
Tel: 01268 546411 Fax: 01268 491248
(Basildon Primary Care Trust)
Patient List Size: 12000

Practice Manager Sheila McLean

GP Robert Francis MAUNDER, Claire LOCKWOOD, Celina Maria PEREIRA, Debra SPRAGGINS

Kingswood Medical Centre
Clayhill Road, Basildon SS16 5AD
Tel: 01268 533727/280514 Fax: 01268 520513
(Basildon Primary Care Trust)

Practice Manager Lorraine Smith

GP Wali Mohammad MEMON, Gautam Champlal CHAJED, Faris J GHANNAM

The Knares Surgery
Great Berry Surgery, Nightingales, Langdon Hills, Basildon SS16 6SA
Tel: 01268 418200/542866 Fax: 01268 417502/491381
(Basildon Primary Care Trust)
Patient List Size: 10400

Practice Manager G Johnson

GP Brenda Mary CORNFORTH, T ADENAIKE, Wynne Janine DEGUN, Mary Clare KLABER, Olatunde MACAULAY, B SALAKO

Knights Surgery
32 Knights, Basildon SS15 5LE
Tel: 01268 415888 Fax: 01268 491318
(Basildon Primary Care Trust)

Practice Manager Patricia Mulcahy

GP Andrew HOLMAN

Laindon Health Centre
Laindon, Basildon SS15 5TR
Tel: 01268 546411 Fax: 01268 491248
(Basildon Primary Care Trust)

Practice Manager Sheila McLean

GP Alistair John MOULDS, Keith Antony HOPCROFT, Ruth Bronia MARSHALL, Christopher John MARTIN, Stewart Hamish McFARLANE, Jane Elizabeth Anne MOORE

Mampilly
Felmores Centre, Felmores, Basildon SS13 1PN
Tel: 01268 728142 Fax: 01268 726567
(Basildon Primary Care Trust)
Patient List Size: 2800

Practice Manager Maria Mampilly, Janet Pape

GP Jojo MAMPILLY

Matching Green Surgery
Matching Green, Basildon SS14 2PB
Tel: 01268 533928 Fax: 01268 289415
(Basildon Primary Care Trust)
Patient List Size: 3300

Practice Manager Shirley Brookes

GP Barid Baran JAS, K JAS

Noak Bridge Medical Centre
Bridge Street, Noak Bridge, Basildon SS15 4EZ
Tel: 01268 284285 Fax: 01268 289324
Email: brij.prasad@gp-F81666.nhs.uk
(Basildon Primary Care Trust)
Patient List Size: 3045

Practice Manager Uma Prasad

GP Brij Kishore PRASAD

Rectory Park Drive Surgery
6 Rectory Park Drive, Pitsea, Basildon SS13 3DW
Tel: 01268 552999 Fax: 01268 559986
(Basildon Primary Care Trust)

Practice Manager Margaret McCarthy

GP Manjula Tribhovandas PATEL, Prafulchandra Chunibhai PATEL

Rectory Road Surgery
201 Rectory Road, Pitsea, Basildon SS13 1AJ
Tel: 01268 727736 Fax: 01268 727045
(Basildon Primary Care Trust)

Practice Manager Janet Smith

GP Krupavathi BISWAS, Dr ASLAM, Susanta Kumar BISWAS

Southview Park Surgery
Southview Park, London Road, Vange, Basildon SS16 4QX
Tel: 01268 553292 Fax: 01268 559805
(Basildon Primary Care Trust)
Patient List Size: 3616

Practice Manager S Hopkins

GP Ratan Lal AGRAWAL, S KHANNA

The Surgery
Felmores Centre, Felmores, Basildon SS13 1PN
Tel: 01268 728108 Fax: 01268 726870
(Basildon Primary Care Trust)

Practice Manager Mary Abraham

GP Kallaracka L ABRAHAM

The Surgery
53 Eastbrooks Place, Chalvedon, Basildon SS13 3QS
Tel: 01268 553455 Fax: 01268 556809
Email: ratan703@yahoo.com
(Basildon Primary Care Trust)
Patient List Size: 2600

Practice Manager Irene Pollock

GP Ratan Lal Agrawal GOYAL, Arjun PRAJAPATI

The Surgery
312 Falstones, Basildon SS15 5DT
Tel: 01268 273436 Fax: 01268 544089
(Basildon Primary Care Trust)

GP Satya Prakash Lal DAS

The Surgery
Wickford Avenue, Pitsea, Basildon SS13 3HQ
Tel: 01268 583288 Fax: 01268 581586
(Basildon Primary Care Trust)

Practice Manager Suman Hindnavis

GP Hindnavis Sudhakar RAO

Whitmore Way Surgery
Aegis Medical Centre, Felmores Centre, Basildon SS13 1PN
Tel: 01268 520641 Fax: 01268 271057
(Basildon Primary Care Trust)

Practice Manager Brenda Birdsey

GP Anil CHOPRA, Nigel Gareth NEWPORT

Basingstoke

Bermuda Practice
Shakespeare house Health Centre, Shakespeare Road, Popley, Basingstoke RG24 9DT
Tel: 01256 454151 Fax: 01256 489270
(North Hampshire Primary Care Trust)
Patient List Size: 4670

Practice Manager Julia Williamson

GP Dr COTTERILL, M SADHEURA, T L WICKRAMASINGHE

Bramblys Grange Health Centre
Bramblys Drive, Basingstoke RG21 8UW
Tel: 01256 467778 Fax: 01256 842131
Email: bgch@lineone.net
(North Hampshire Primary Care Trust)
Patient List Size: 20700

Practice Manager Carole Ellery

GP Gordon Robert Henry BRAIN, Catherine DE MARS, Joanna FOLEY, Philip Edward HIORNS, Shehla JAMIL, Ian Alexander Bruce McLAY, Heather Dawn MYCOCK, Keith John OLLERHEAD, Tania PHILLIPS, Sunil RATHOD

Chineham Lodge
59 Reading Road, Chineham, Basingstoke RG24 0NS
Tel: 01256 466565 Fax: 01256 355234
(North Hampshire Primary Care Trust)

Practice Manager Susan Terry

GP N S BABA

Church Grange Health Centre
Bramblys Drive, Basingstoke RG21 8QN
Tel: 01256 329021 Fax: 01256 817466
(North Hampshire Primary Care Trust)
Patient List Size: 22000

Practice Manager Yolande Newton

GP Richard TURNER, Gemma ADAMSON, Maureen Elizabeth ASHWORTH, Thomas Robert Cedric COCHRANE, Andrew COLE, Dawn COXHEAD, Graham John HULLAH, David Kenneth Sawyer KNIGHT, Ahmed OBAIDI, Judith Claire PAGDIN, Annabelle PLYMING, Rachel QUEW, Richard Simon TRUEMAN

East Barn Surgery
Great Binfield Road, Lychpit, Basingstoke RG24 8TF
Tel: 01256 841654 Fax: 01256 843788
Email: sandie.evans@gp-j82647.nhs.uk
(North Hampshire Primary Care Trust)

Practice Manager Sandie Evans

GP A M MAY, L A JAMES

Gillies and Overbridge Medical Partnership
Brighton Hill, Sullivan Road, Basingstoke RG22 4EH
Tel: 01256 479747 Fax: 01256 320627
Email: enquiries@gilliesandoverbridge.co.uk
Website: www.gilliesandoverbridge.co.uk
(North Hampshire Primary Care Trust)
Patient List Size: 20000

Practice Manager D McCarthy

GP John Spencer ASHWORTH, Tracey BOWDEN, Angus CARNEGY, Christopher George DIXON, Catherine Susan HUYTON, Pamela Mary KNOWLES, Lucy Jane SUMMERS, Nicholas John WARING, Elizabeth Ann WILLIAMS, David James Thomas WRIGHT

Hackwood Partnership
Essex House, Essex Road, Basingstoke RG21 8SU
Tel: 01256 470464 Fax: 01256 357289
(North Hampshire Primary Care Trust)
Patient List Size: 12500

Practice Manager Patricia Bray

GP James RICHARDSON, Susan Patricia BOWEN, Amanda Elizabeth Mary BRITTON, Andrew Hamish CAMERON, Hugh John FREEMAN, Peter George Yardley WRIGHT

Marlowe Partnership
Shakespeare House health Centre, Shakespeare Road, Basingstoke RG24 9DS
Tel: 01256 328860 Fax: 01256 351911
(North Hampshire Primary Care Trust)
Patient List Size: 7000

Practice Manager Karen Wood

GP Vivien Jane Ione JONES, Bee Nah HOBSON, Myint THEIN, Susan UPCHURCH

Oakley and Overton Partnership
Overton Surgery, Station Road, Overton, Basingstoke RG25 3DU
Tel: 01256 770212 Fax: 01256 771581
(North Hampshire Primary Care Trust)
Patient List Size: 10700

Practice Manager Frances Turner

GP Robert Eliot LORGE, D BARTLETT, Susan Mary BIRTWISTLE, Richard John COPPIN, Julia HOPKINS, Judith Anne LINDSAY

South Ham House
96 Paddock Road, Basingstoke RG22 6RL
Tel: 01256 324666 Fax: 01256 810849
(North Hampshire Primary Care Trust)
Patient List Size: 11000

Practice Manager Neil Wright

GP Stephen William HUDSON, Colin MEEKING, Richard Lewis Edward PARKER, Swati PATEL, Patricia Anne RIDSDALE, Nicholas Vernon Blair WESTERN

Stanford Medical Centre
Stanford Road, Brighton Hill, Basingstoke RG22 4LQ
Tel: 01256 469340 Fax: 01256 334115
(North Hampshire Primary Care Trust)

GP K S RAJU

Bath

Bath University
Medical Centre, Quarry House North Road, Bath BA2 7AY
Tel: 01225 462395 Fax: 01225 826489/386489
Email: medicalcentre@bath.ac.uk
(Bath and North East Somerset Primary Care Trust)
Patient List Size: 7800

Practice Manager Frances Ansell

GP Jennifer Mary BENNETT, Andrew LLOYD, Victoria Jane McMASTER, C M REID

Batheaston Medical Centre
Batheaston Medical Centre, Coalpit Road, Batheaston, Bath BA1 7NP
Tel: 01225 858686 Fax: 01225 852521
Email: bmc.docs@mcmail.com
(Bath and North East Somerset Primary Care Trust)
Patient List Size: 5450

Practice Manager Heather du Plessis

GP Paul Francis BENNETT, Karen Adele PREES, Catherine Mary WERNHAM, Alan John YOUNG

Catherine Cottage Surgery
21 Catharine Place, Bath BA1 2PS
Tel: 01225 421034 Fax: 01225 422756
(Bath and North East Somerset Primary Care Trust)
Patient List Size: 2100

Practice Manager Andrew Pearce

GP Catherine Louise LEACH

Combe Down Surgery
Combe Down House, Combe Down, Bath BA2 5EG
Tel: 01225 832226 Fax: 01225 840757
(Bath and North East Somerset Primary Care Trust)
Patient List Size: 7900

Practice Manager Karen Slade

GP Imogen Ann BATTERHAM, S ROBINSON, A SMITH, Julian Stephen TREADWALL

Dr C M Bevan and Partners
Tyning Lane, Camden Road, Bath BA1 6EA
Tel: 01225 331616/480007
(Bath and North East Somerset Primary Care Trust)
Patient List Size: 9760

Practice Manager R C F Craven

GP Christopher Martin BEVAN, John Mark DINWOODIE, Jeremy Heathcote GILBERT, Carole GROENHUYSEN, Helen Marie-Claire HAMLING

Dr P K W Smith and Partners
Waterford Park, Radstock, Bath BA3 3UJ
Tel: 01761 463333

(Bath and North East Somerset Primary Care Trust)

GP James BLACKSTOCK, Paul Kirkel Woodwiss SMITH, Guy Mark WORDSALL

Dr W D Randell and Partners

Radstock, Bath BA3 3PL
Tel: 01761 432121/432540 Fax: 01761 420193
(Bath and North East Somerset Primary Care Trust)

GP Wendy Denise RANDELL, Julian Richard CUMPSTY, Simon Jonathan DOUGLASS, Michael Frank HARRIS

Grosvenor Place Surgery

26 Grosvenor Place, Bath BA1 6BA
Tel: 01225 484748 Fax: 01225 789022
(Bath and North East Somerset Primary Care Trust)
Patient List Size: 3000

Practice Manager Rachael Eade

GP Jane DAVIDSON, Nicole HOWSE

Hillcrest Surgery

Wellow Lane, Peasedown St John, Bath BA2 8JQ
(Bath and North East Somerset Primary Care Trust)

Practice Manager Neil G Mackay

GP D I FIELD

Mendip Country Practice

Church Street, Coleford, Bath BA3 5NQ
Tel: 01373 812244 Fax: 01373 813390
Patient List Size: 5060

GP J SMITH, Bill IRISH, Piers JENNINGS, H MUSGROVE

Newbridge Surgery

129 Newbridge Hill, Bath BA1 3PT
Tel: 01225 425807 Fax: 01225 447776
(Bath and North East Somerset Primary Care Trust)
Patient List Size: 7500

Practice Manager Richard Terry

GP Brian Martin CONWAY, Richard Lloyd WHARTON, Susan Jill COOPER, Ruth Elisabeth GRABHAM

Number 18 Surgery

18 Upper Oldfield Park, Bath BA2 3JZ
Tel: 01225 427402 Fax: 01225 484627
Email: helen.harris@gp-l81049.nhs.uk
(Bath and North East Somerset Primary Care Trust)

Practice Manager Helen Harris

GP Paul Jonathan BOOTH, Charles Edward BERRISFORD, Linda Ann McHUGH, Samuel MEDWORTH, Margaret Joy MUDDIMAN, Christopher WAYTE

Oldfield Surgery

45 Upper Oldfield Park, Bath BA2 3HT
Tel: 01225 421137 Fax: 01225 337808
Email: mail@oldfield-surgery.demon.uk
Website: www.oldfield-surgery.demon.co.uk
(Bath and North East Somerset Primary Care Trust)
Patient List Size: 10200

Practice Manager Pauline Fleming

GP T J HARRIS, A COMBE, P EAVIS, J HAMLING, T JOHSON, J SAVAGE

Pulteney Practice

35 Great Pulteney Street, Bath BA2 4BY
Tel: 01225 464187 Fax: 01225 465622
Email: pulteney@gp-l81068.nhs.uk
Website: www.pulteney.co.uk
(Bath and North East Somerset Primary Care Trust)
Patient List Size: 11500

Practice Manager Stuart Cowper

GP Roger Lewis ROLLS, Stephanie ANDELL, Jon BRUNSKILL, Pippa GREEN, Caroline Elizabeth STAGG, Beth Louise STANDING, John Stewart TILLEY, Ian Derek WILES

Somerton House Surgery

79A North Road, Midsomer Norton, Bath BA3 2QE
Tel: 01761 412141 Fax: 01761 410944
(Bath and North East Somerset Primary Care Trust)
Patient List Size: 5951

Practice Manager Caron Standerwick

GP Alan McLean MILLER, Katherine Mary FALLON, Robert Samuel HILLEN, Joanna Claudia SMITH

St James's Surgery

Northampton Buildings, Bath BA1 2SR
Tel: 01225 422911 Fax: 01225 428398
(Bath and North East Somerset Primary Care Trust)
Patient List Size: 11000

GP J R PLAYFAIR, S L GILLINGS, I MORPEN, J F SPELMAN

St Marys Surgery

St Marys Close, Timsbury, Bath BA2 0HX
Tel: 01761 470880 Fax: 01761 472492
(Bath and North East Somerset Primary Care Trust)
Patient List Size: 4700

Practice Manager J Yates

GP M E HOWELL

St Michaels Surgery

Walwyn Close, Twerton-on-Avon, Bath BA2 1ER
Tel: 01225 428277 Fax: 01225 338484
(Bath and North East Somerset Primary Care Trust)
Patient List Size: 7300

GP James HAMPTON, Dr McNAB, Ian Wyndham PARKER, Dr PAULI, Catherine Mary PROFFITT

The Surgery

8 Queens Parade, Bath BA1 2NJ
Tel: 01225 424460 Fax: 01225 310738
(Bath and North East Somerset Primary Care Trust)
Patient List Size: 3500

Practice Manager P Giles

GP David Martin WALKER

The Surgery

Pondsmead, Oakhill, Bath BA3 5AL
(Mendip Primary Care Trust)

GP P HUTCHINSON

Weston Surgery

36 Combe Park, Bath BA1 3NR
Tel: 01225 446089 Fax: 01225 827639
Email: Val.Hartley-Brewer@gp-L81644.nhs.uk
(Bath and North East Somerset Primary Care Trust)
Patient List Size: 4600

Practice Manager Rosie Murton

GP Valerie Forbes HARTLEY-BREWER, Christina Susannah COTTEE

Widcombe Surgery

3-4 Widcombe Parade, Bath BA2 4JT
Tel: 01225 310883 Fax: 01225 421600
(Bath and North East Somerset Primary Care Trust)
Patient List Size: 6229

Practice Manager Linda Newman

GP Jonathan Andrew CHAPMAN, Francis Peter JACKSON, Rebecca Stacey HODSON, Mary Allison SPEED

Batley

Blackburn Road Medical Centre

Blackburn Road, Birstall, Batley WF17 9PL
Tel: 01924 478265 Fax: 01924 476317
(North Kirklees Primary Care Trust)
Patient List Size: 9900

Practice Manager Y Kernon

GP David Edward FOWERS, Brian Robert LOBB, Timothy Brian LONGMORE, Pauline Ann MILLER

Broughton House Surgery
20 New Way, Batley WF17 5QT
Tel: 01924 420244 Fax: 01924 422490
(North Kirklees Primary Care Trust)

Practice Manager W Loney

GP S CAMERON, J GOGNA

Cherry Tree Surgery
132 Upper Commercial Street, Batley WF17 5DH
Tel: 01924 471115/473221 Fax: 01924 473221
(North Kirklees Primary Care Trust)
Patient List Size: 2450

Practice Manager Margaret Brearley

GP R K SOOD

Grove House Surgery
Soothill, Batley WF17 5SS
Tel: 01924 474674 Fax: 01924 474119
(North Kirklees Primary Care Trust)
Patient List Size: 10000

Practice Manager Dianne Fox, Duncan P Millar

GP Paul Singh MULLHI, Ian Watson Ramsay COWIE, Brian Dermot LYNCH, Maura Paidraigin LYNCH

The Health Centre
130 Upper Commercial Street, Batley WF17 5ED
Tel: 01924 474646 Fax: 01924 474070
(North Kirklees Primary Care Trust)
Patient List Size: 4800

Practice Manager Ann Mitchell

GP Kundan Singh LIDHAR, Jaswant Kaur LIDHAR

Kirkgate Surgery
3 Kirkgate, Birstall, Batley WF17 9HE
Tel: 01924 420242 Fax: 01924 423327
(North Kirklees Primary Care Trust)
Patient List Size: 4000

Practice Manager Amina Priestley

GP Christopher Stephen HOUGHTON, Mohammed ARIF

Undercliffe Surgery
273 Healey Lane, Batley WF17 8DQ
Tel: 01924 403406 Fax: 01924 412890
(North Kirklees Primary Care Trust)
Patient List Size: 8600

Practice Manager Margaret Clarke

GP James Hamilton LEE, Paul David GLOVER, Antony Myles GOODWIN

Wellington House Surgery
Henrietta Street, Batley WF17 5DN
Tel: 01924 470333 Fax: 01924 420981
(North Kirklees Primary Care Trust)
Patient List Size: 9200

Practice Manager Elizabeth Mullins

GP David Rodney BARKER, Sarah Louise HARDING, Sallie J LAWLER, Stuart James LAWSON, Michael Frank SCALES, Deborah Anne TARRANT

Battle

Dr Rice-Oxley and Partners
36 High Street, Battle TN33 0EA
Tel: 01424 772263/772060 Fax: 01424 775569
(Bexhill and Rother Primary Care Trust)

Practice Manager Anne Edmead

GP Charles Patrick RICE-OXLEY, Richard Christopher CLARKE, John Edward MOGAN, John Graham RIVETT

The Surgery
Brede Lane, Sedlescombe, Battle TN33 0PW
Tel: 01424 870225 Fax: 01424 870912
(Bexhill and Rother Primary Care Trust)
Patient List Size: 6100

Practice Manager Judith Collins

GP Timothy JARDINE-BROWN, Caroline Diana HARGREAVES, Steven Richard STERN

The Surgery
High Street, Ninfield, Battle TN33 9JP
Tel: 01424 892569 Fax: 01424 893233
(Bexhill and Rother Primary Care Trust)
Patient List Size: 1933

Practice Manager Julia Scotcher

GP Ian St John KEMM

Beaconsfield

Millbarn Medical Centre
34 London End, Beaconsfield HP9 2JH
Tel: 01494 675303 Fax: 01494 680214
Website: gp-82011.nhs.uk
(Chiltern and South Bucks Primary Care Trust)
Patient List Size: 7500

Practice Manager Margaret Wallace

GP Michael David STONEHAM, Stephen Paul BROWN, Rosemarie Ann HART, John Frederick WILSON

The Simpson Health Centre
70 Gregories Road, Beaconsfield HP9 1PS
Tel: 01494 671571 Fax: 01494 680219
(Chiltern and South Bucks Primary Care Trust)
Patient List Size: 15000

Practice Manager F Denyer

GP Steven Alan Lissant COX, Alison Mary COGGAN, Graeme Robert Lawrence FLETCHER, Simon Harold Michael LOMAX, Hilary Winifred McDERMOTT, Brian Patrick McGIRR, Vivienne Margaret McVEY, Nicola Jane WIDGINGTON

Beaminster

Barton House Surgery
Barton House, Beaminster DT8 3EQ
Tel: 01308 862233 Fax: 01308 863785
(South West Dorset Primary Care Trust)
Patient List Size: 5730

Practice Manager John Skinner

GP Robert Anthony Gordon GOODHART, John Martin Victor PAYNE, Timothy William ROBINSON

Tunnel Road Surgery
24 Tunnel Road, Beaminster DT8 3BN
Tel: 01308 862225 Fax: 01308 863781
Email: postmaster@gp-J81076.nhs.uk
(South West Dorset Primary Care Trust)

Practice Manager S A McConnell

GP P F WILEY, Jonathan Alexander KETTELL, Elizabeth Romana SINCLAIR

Beaworthy

Beech House Surgery
Beech House, Shebbear, Beaworthy EX21 5RU
Tel: 01409 281221 Fax: 01409 281894
Email: stephen.miller@gp-l8312.nhs.uk
(North Devon Primary Care Trust)
Patient List Size: 1850

Practice Manager Stephanie Stacey

GP Stephen William Macdonald MILLER

Blake House Surgery
Black Torrington, Beaworthy EX21 5QE
Tel: 01409 23340 Fax: 01403 231350
(North Devon Primary Care Trust)
Patient List Size: 2300

Practice Manager Tina Dunn

GP Asaad Abed Al-Muhsin AL-DOORI, Dave BERGER, Fiona KEMP

Beccles

Beccles Medical Centre
7-9 St Marys Road, St Marys Road, Beccles NR34 9NQ
Tel: 01502 712662 Fax: 01502 712906
Website: www.beccles.org.uk
(Waveney Primary Care Trust)
Patient List Size: 20000

Practice Manager P Wolton

GP Anthony Roger BUBB, Ian Richmond BATTYE, Paul Stanley BERRY, Elisabeth Kate BUNGAY, Glenn William COLLINS, Keith David Speedie DOUGLAS, Renee L KATHURIA, Timothy John MORTON, Philip Russell SMITH

Beckenham

Cornerways Surgery
50 Manor Road, Beckenham BR3 5LG
Tel: 020 8650 2444
(Bromley Primary Care Trust)
Patient List Size: 8500

Practice Manager Pamela Collison

GP Carolyn Anne YIU, Chu Hing YIU, Nerina Alison BERMAN, Mark Richard NORTON

Eden Park Surgery
194 Croydon Road, Beckenham BR3 4DQ
Tel: 020 8650 9729
(Bromley Primary Care Trust)

GP Janet Mair NEVE, J L DONALD, Rajiv PURWAR

Elm House Surgery
29 Beckenham Road, Beckenham BR3 4PR
Tel: 020 8650 0173 Fax: 020 8663 3911
Email: admin@gp-G84027.nhs.uk
Website: www.elmhousesurgery.com
(Bromley Primary Care Trust)
Patient List Size: 13750

Practice Manager Susan Reeves

GP Michael Charles HARRISON, Andrew AKIRI, Kevin Patrick Charles CARROLL, Angela Mary KAYE, Andreas LINSENMAIER, Kamireddy Prema REDDY, Roger Augustus WELLS

St James's Practice
138 Croydon Road, Beckenham BR3 4DG
Tel: 020 8650 0568 Fax: 020 8650 4172
Email: st.james@gp-G8404.nhs.uk
(Bromley Primary Care Trust)

Practice Manager Celia Gaze

GP Paul Alan DUNACHIE, Kate Elizabeth DYER, Lynda Susanne HARRIS, Jan Wendel WAGSTYL

The Surgery
14 Manor Road, Beckenham BR3 5LE
Tel: 020 8650 0957 Fax: 020 8663 6070
Email: practice.manager@gp-g84008.nhs.uk
(Bromley Primary Care Trust)
Patient List Size: 6548

Practice Manager Pauline McCarthy

GP Ray VELLA, Andrew AGUN, Janet Elizabeth TEMPEST

Bedale

Glebe House Surgery
19 Firby Road, Bedale DL8 2AT
Tel: 01677 422616 Fax: 01677 424596
(Hambleton and Richmondshire Primary Care Trust)

Practice Manager Gill Teasdale

GP Charles Nicholas COLLIER, Dr BELLAS, Dr THOMPSON, Michael Joseph THOMPSON, Stephen James WILKINSON

Bedford

Ampthill Road Medical Centre
178 Ampthill Road, Bedford MK42 9PU
Tel: 01234 266242 Fax: 01234 266242
Email: s.s.basra@aol.com
(Bedford Primary Care Trust)
Patient List Size: 2490

Practice Manager Bubli Basra

GP Satwinder Singh BASRA, Hari NAWAL

Ashburnham Road
8 Ashburnham Road, Bedford MK40 1DS
Tel: 01234 358411 Fax: 01234 273202
Email: m.agrawal@doctors.net.uk
Website: www.agrawalsurgery.co.uk
(Bedford Primary Care Trust)
Patient List Size: 3100

Practice Manager Colin McClean

GP M L AGRAWAL, P AGRAWAL

Bushmead Avenue Medical Centre
21 Bushmead Avenue, Bedford MK40 3QJ
Tel: 01234 267797 Fax: 01234 269649
(Bedford Primary Care Trust)
Patient List Size: 2133

Practice Manager Susan Napper

GP Michael PRIOR

Bushmead Avenue Surgery
21 Bushmead Avenue, Bedford MK40 3QJ
Tel: 01234 349191 Fax: 01234 269649
(Bedford Primary Care Trust)
Patient List Size: 2177

Practice Manager S Napper

GP Roy Francis JACKSON

Carlisle Road Surgery
23C Carlisle Road, Queens Park, Bedford MK40 4HR
Tel: 01234 351661 Fax: 01234 364884
(Bedford Primary Care Trust)
Patient List Size: 8000

Practice Manager Jennie Ingle

GP Narwinder Singh LOTAY, Rihan BASHIR, Michael Olabode FAYEYE, Tariq Hussain KHOKHER, Emily Joy THOMPSON

Cater Street Surgery
1 Cater Street, Kempston, Bedford MK42 8DR
Tel: 01234 853461 Fax: 01234 840536
(Bedford Primary Care Trust)
Patient List Size: 6500

Practice Manager Alison Bampton

GP Alan Roger DONE, A ALI, Simon Peter MARNER

De Parys Medical Centre
23 De Parys Avenue, Bedford MK40 2TX
Tel: 01234 350022 Fax: 01234 213402
(Bedford Primary Care Trust)

Practice Manager Maggie Gardner

GP Christopher John JONES, Penelope Ann BAKER, Penelope Jayne BARTLETT, Nigel Richard BROOKES, Anu GEORGE, John Alexander

GOULDING, Christine HOPPER, Simon Wyndham LOWE, Jason REDDY, Morgan WALTERS

Dr Sydenham and Partners
The Surgery, Hexton Road, Barton-le-Clay, Bedford MK45 4TA
Tel: 01582 528701/528700 Fax: 01582 528714
(Bedfordshire Heartlands Primary Care Trust)

Practice Manager Donna Lopez

GP Margaret Elizabeth GLAZE, Simon Porteous HUGHES, David John SYDENHAM, Frank Richard TAYLOR, Simon Derek WILDEN

Dr Toovey and Partners
2 Goldington Road, Bedford MK40 3NG
Tel: 01234 351341 Fax: 01234 341464
(Bedford Primary Care Trust)
Patient List Size: 11400

Practice Manager Janice Potter

GP Janet Ann BUTLIN, Dankwart Christopher FENSKE, Mary FENSKE, Adri HOFMEISTER, John MURPHY, Amra PACUKA, Angela Joy TOOVEY, Anthony Rupert TOOVEY

Flitwick Surgery
The Highlands, Flitwick, Bedford MK45 1DZ
Tel: 01525 712171 Fax: 01525 718756
(Bedfordshire Heartlands Primary Care Trust)
Patient List Size: 15750

Practice Manager Sandra Hedges

GP Hee-Liong LING, Rajeet BHARTI, William Thys de GROOT, Rebecca Juliet HAYWOOD, Talib MERZA, Sarah J MORRIS

Goldington Avenue Surgery
85 Goldington Avenue, Bedford MK40 3DB
Tel: 01234 349531 Fax: 01234 267455
Email: goldingtonavdrs@nhs.net
(Bedford Primary Care Trust)
Patient List Size: 8045

Practice Manager Sue Adams

GP Timothy Patrick GRIFFITH, Richard James GALLIVAN, Peter John TATMAN, Silkie VAMAR-MATIAR, Vinod VARGHESE

Goldington Road Surgery
12 Goldington Road, Bedford MK40 3NE
Tel: 01234 352493 Fax: 01234 270901
(Bedford Primary Care Trust)
Patient List Size: 3713

Practice Manager V Das

GP V DAS

Greensand Surgery
57 Oliver Street, Ampthill, Bedford MK45 2SB
Tel: 01525 631390 Fax: 01525 631393
(Bedfordshire Heartlands Primary Care Trust)
Patient List Size: 5300

Practice Manager Gill Day

GP Peter George ROWE, Jadwiga Waleria Mary KRUSZEWSKA, Fabienne SMITH

Harrold Medical Practice
Peach's Close, Harrold, Bedford MK43 7DX
Tel: 01234 720225 Fax: 01234 720603
(Bedford Primary Care Trust)
Patient List Size: 5746

Practice Manager Caroline Rigg

GP Frances Mary ROSS, Giles LIMOND, Gert SLAGHUIS

High Street Surgery
137 High Street, Cranfield, Bedford MK43 0HZ
Tel: 01234 750234 Fax: 01234 750588
(Bedfordshire Heartlands Primary Care Trust)
Patient List Size: 7000

Practice Manager Sue Meadows

GP Regina REDDY, Marcus J THOMAS

Houghton Close Surgery
1 Houghton Close, Ampthill, Bedford MK45 2TG
Tel: 01525 402641 Fax: 01525 841107
(Bedfordshire Heartlands Primary Care Trust)
Patient List Size: 9900

Practice Manager P Hillyer-Thake

GP James Gerard AYLWARD, Carol FREEMAN, Peter Jonathan HASLETT, Michelle SAINT, Nicola Mary SCOTT, Helen SMITH

King Street Surgery
273 Bedford Road, Kempston, Bedford MK42 8QD
Tel: 01234 852222 Fax: 01234 843558
(Bedford Primary Care Trust)
Patient List Size: 11450

Practice Manager Ann Lewis

GP Abitalib Tayabali KHANBHAI, Sudha ELANGOVEN, Jacquelyn Susan Lambart FARHOUD, Jane KOCEN, Antonio MUNNO, Nancy MURRAY, Vijay Krishan NAYAR, Annette OCHOLA-KUIPER, Anna PASSMORE, Peter Stephen WILKINSON, Belinda WORSFOLD

Lansdowne Road Surgery
6 Lansdowne Road, Bedford MK40 2BU
Tel: 01234 270170 Fax: 01234 214033
(Bedford Primary Care Trust)
Patient List Size: 7300

Practice Manager L Robson

GP R NORRIS, Dr CORTES-MARTIN, Dr HAYES, Dr INSKIP, Dr THOMAS

Lansdowne Road Surgery
6 Lansdowne Road, Bedford MK40 2BU
Tel: 01234 270170 Fax: 01234 214033
(Bedford Primary Care Trust)
Patient List Size: 7300

Practice Manager L Robson

GP Richard NORRIS, Ruben CORTES-MARTIN, Alison HAYES, Thomas Greville INSKIP, Tom THOMAS

Lathia and Partner
46 Clapham Road, Bedford MK41 7PW
Tel: 01234 357143 Fax: 01234 345902
(Bedford Primary Care Trust)

Practice Manager Pat Huckle

GP Parshottam Naranbhai LATHIA, Muhammad SHAD

Linden Road Surgery
13 Linden Road, Bedford MK40 2DQ
Tel: 01234 273272 Fax: 01234 340339
(Bedford Primary Care Trust)
Patient List Size: 3800

Practice Manager Carole Pope

GP S KANUNGO, Anna Dominique O'BRIEN

London Road Practice
The Health Centre, 84-86 London Road, Bedford MK42 0NT
Tel: 01234 266851 Fax: 01234 363998
(Bedford Primary Care Trust)
Patient List Size: 11000

Practice Manager Gail Dawson

GP Mohammed Nisar HYDER, John Clive BINNS, Naeem-Ur-Rashid CHOUDHRY, John Francis KEDWARD, Padmavathi KIRUBAKARAN, Jaison MATTHEW, Chandu PRESANNAN

Morris and Partners
93 Queens Drive, Bedford MK41 9JE
Tel: 01234 319992 Fax: 01234 319994
(Bedford Primary Care Trust)
Patient List Size: 11300

Practice Manager Richard White

GP Ian David ALDRICH, Roland Howard MORRIS, Rupert Gordon BANKART, Richard COLLINS, Malcom DYER, Stephen Robert JONES, Christopher NIXON, Emmanuel OCHOLA, Jennifer Jane WILSON

Pemberley Avenue Surgery
32 Pemberley Avenue, Bedford MK40 2LA
Tel: 01234 351051 Fax: 01234 349246
(Bedford Primary Care Trust)

Practice Manager Marylyn O'Connar

GP Peter Christopher Uvedale PARRY-OKEDEN, Lindsay HEMY, David Jonathan HOWARD, Julian LANE, Simon ROGERS, Subbiah TAMILARASI

Priory Medical Practice
48 Bromham Road, Bedford MK40 2QD
Tel: 01234 262040 Fax: 01234 219288
(Bedford Primary Care Trust)
Patient List Size: 4410

Practice Manager David White

GP Kam KIRKBRIDE-JAMU, Janet Mair TREDGET

Rothesay Place Health Centre
14 Rothesay Place, Bedford MK40 3PX

GP Martin John SIMMONDS

Rothesay Surgery
14 Rothesay Place, Bedford MK40 3PX
Tel: 01234 271800 Fax: 01234 353722
(Bedford Primary Care Trust)

Practice Manager Penny Hood

GP John Edwin HOOD

Shakespeare Road Surgery
17 Shakespeare Road, Bedford MK40 2DZ
Tel: 01234 330336 Fax: 01234 327710
(Bedford Primary Care Trust)
Patient List Size: 3400

Practice Manager Jo Cordell

GP Anna Rita UNGARO

Silver Street Surgery
26 Silver Street, Great Barford, Bedford MK44 3HX
Tel: 01234 870325 Fax: 01234 871323
(Bedford Primary Care Trust)
Patient List Size: 4600

Practice Manager Sandza Mabbott

GP Brian James Findlay CRAWFORD, Brian PEACOCK, Jonathan WALI

St Johns Street Surgery
16 St. Johns Street, Kempston, Bedford MK42 8EP
Tel: 01234 851323 Fax: 01234 843293
(Bedford Primary Care Trust)

Practice Manager Gill Rees

GP Michael WALLIS, Kevin How-Kok AU

Templars Way Surgery
Templars Way, Sharnbrook, Bedford MK44 1PZ
Tel: 01234 781392 Fax: 01234 781468
Email: sSharnbrook.surgery@nhs.net
(Bedford Primary Care Trust)
Patient List Size: 5600

Practice Manager L Walters

GP Kenneth Mark HEDGES, V J HOWES, John James ROCHFORD

Bedlington

Bedlington Medical Group
Glebe Road, Bedlington NE22 6JX
Tel: 01670 822695 Fax: 01670 531860
(Northumberland Care Trust)

GP Ernest Wilfrid MUNRO, Gary ALFORD, Philippa Jane Scott HARRIS, Katherin Gisela STARKEY, John TODD

The Gables Health Centre
26 St. Johns Road, Bedlington NE22 7DU
Tel: 01670 829889 Fax: 01670 820841
(Northumberland Care Trust)
Patient List Size: 6500

Practice Manager Paul Mitford

GP John HARRISON, Patricia Margaret TALLANTYRE

Bedworth

Drs Jennings and Menage
Bulkington Surgery, School Road, Bulkington, Bedworth CV12 9JB
Tel: 024 7673 3020 Fax: 024 7673 3033
(North Warwickshire Primary Care Trust)
Patient List Size: 4300

GP Janet MENAGE, Roderick Stanley JENNINGS

Belford

Belford Medical Practice
The Belford Health Centre, Croftfield, Belford NE70 7ER
Tel: 01668 213738 Fax: 01668 213072
Email: name@gp-A84008.nhs.uk
(Northumberland Care Trust)
Patient List Size: 4400

Practice Manager Peter Bainbridge

GP David Kirtland GILL, Emma Christina MILLER, Saul Nicholas MILLER, Sebastian MOSS

Belper

Green Lane Surgery
2 Green Lane, Belper DE56 1BZ
Tel: 01773 823521 Fax: 01773 821954
(Amber Valley Primary Care Trust)
Patient List Size: 12300

Practice Manager S Hasiam

GP James John MORRISSEY, Marie-Lou BRIDGE, Michael John DONALDSON, Dr GUEST, Heather Patricia KINSELLA, R C MURRAY, Derek Geoffrey WRIGHT

Riversdale Surgery
59 Bridge Street, Belper DE56 1AY
Tel: 01773 822386 Fax: 01773 829938
(Amber Valley Primary Care Trust)

GP Derek COOKE, Michael John Edwin BRETT, Dominic Bernard Vaughan HEWITT, S E KING, David James POLL, Dr SHEPHERD

Belvedere

Bedonwell Medical Centre
15 Albert Road, Belvedere DA17 5LQ
Tel: 01322 446700 Fax: 01322 446001
(Bexley Care Trust)

GP Varun BHALLA

Cairngall Medical Practice
2 Erith Road, Belvedere DA17 6EZ
Tel: 01322 432315 Fax: 01322 440948
(Bexley Care Trust)
Patient List Size: 9000

Practice Manager Joan Hooper

GP John Frederick BARRETT, Rashmikant Jagannath DAVE, Shirin Rashimikant DAVE, Adrian Piers ROSS

The Surgery
44 Nuxley Road, Belvedere DA17 5JG
Tel: 01322 439707 Fax: 020 8311 5651
(Bexley Care Trust)
Patient List Size: 2709

GP Minocher Bahadur ADAGRA

Benfleet

Belle Vue Medical Practice
271 Rayleigh Road, Thundersley, Benfleet SS7 3XF
Tel: 01702 553140 Fax: 01702 556539
(Castle Point and Rochford Primary Care Trust)

Practice Manager Margaret Waterman

GP Roger Alec GARDINER

Benfleet Surgery
12 Constitution Hill, Benfleet SS7 1ED
Tel: 01268 566400
(Castle Point and Rochford Primary Care Trust)

GP Dr GILL

Essex Way Surgery
34 Essex Way, Benfleet SS7 1LT
Tel: 01268 792203 Fax: 01268 759495
(Castle Point and Rochford Primary Care Trust)
Patient List Size: 8100

Practice Manager Janet Letts

GP Heiltje Wilhelmina MOTT, Syed Manazic KHALIL, Anil Kumar SRIVASTAVA

Hart Road
85 Hart Road, Thundersley, Benfleet SS7 3PR
Tel: 01268 757981 Fax: 01268 795605
(Castle Point and Rochford Primary Care Trust)
Patient List Size: 3400

Practice Manager Jacky Hills

GP Piyush PATEL

High Road Family Doctors
119 High Road, Benfleet SS7 3LA
Tel: 01268 753591 Fax: 01268 794585
(Castle Point and Rochford Primary Care Trust)
Patient List Size: 2750

Practice Manager Adrian Whybrew

GP Kokulo Nyanpee WAIWAIKU

Kents Hill Road Family Doctors
411 Kenshill Road North, Benfleet SS7 4AD
(Castle Point and Rochford Primary Care Trust)

Rectory Road Surgery
41 Rectory Road, Hadleigh, Benfleet SS7 2NA
Tel: 01702 558147
(Castle Point and Rochford Primary Care Trust)

Practice Manager David Baxter

GP John Arthur McGLADDERY, Johannes Antonius LEMMENS, Marcus John LESTER, Dr PETERS, Lan Aik TAN

Rushbottom Lane Surgery
91 Rushbottom Lane, Benfleet SS7 4EA
Tel: 01268 754311 Fax: 01268 795150
(Castle Point and Rochford Primary Care Trust)
Patient List Size: 6088

Practice Manager Claire Sanson

GP Ramnik Mathurbhai PATEL, Richard John Nicholas BAKER, Asha L SWAMY

Rushbottom Lane Surgery
91 Rushbottom Lane, Benfleet SS7 4EA
Tel: 0870 417 3124 Fax: 01268 795150
(Castle Point and Rochford Primary Care Trust)
Patient List Size: 16000

GP Geoffrey Gerald TROTTER, Mon Mon GALE, Sunil K GUPTA, Stephen C HISCOCK, Mohammed R KHAN, Mee Mee ZIN

Berkeley

Marybrook Medical Centre
Marybrook Street, Berkeley GL13 9BL
Tel: 01453 810228 Fax: 01453 511778
(Cotswold and Vale Primary Care Trust)

Practice Manager Sharron Norman

GP Paul WILSON, Simon John HIGGS, Peadar Bernard WALSHE

Berkhamsted

Boxwell Road Surgery
1 Boxwell Road, Berkhamsted HP4 3EU
Tel: 01442 863119/864448 Fax: 01442 879909
(Dacorum Primary Care Trust)
Patient List Size: 5800

Practice Manager Marilyn Wilkinson

GP Andrew John PRIDE, Theresa FINN, Andrea LEVER, Timothy B C STROWGER

The Manor Street Surgery
Manor Street, Berkhamsted HP4 2DL
Tel: 01442 875935
(Dacorum Primary Care Trust)

GP Christine Elizabeth PONSONBY, William John Francis BADO, Lesley Annette HALLAN, Helen Elizabeth MANTON, Richard Irving WALKER

Milton House Surgery
Doctors Commons Road, Berkhamsted HP4 3BY
Tel: 01442 874784 Fax: 01442 877694
(Dacorum Primary Care Trust)
Patient List Size: 8000

Practice Manager P Swatman

GP Edda Inge AITCHISON, Jean Rachel BUNKER, Christopher John CORBIN, Sarah EVANS, Ian Nigel Robert ORMISTON, Judith Patricia ROYTHORNE

Red and White House Surgery
Suite 6, 113-115 High Street, Berkhamsted HP4 2DJ
Tel: 01442 866148
(Dacorum Primary Care Trust)

GP Colin J ANDREWS

Betchworth

The Surgery
Tanners Meadow, Brockham, Betchworth RH3 7NJ
Tel: 01737 843259 Fax: 01737 845184
(East Elmbridge and Mid Surrey Primary Care Trust)
Patient List Size: 8000

Practice Manager Karen Boxall

GP Peter Howard KOBER, Graeme James JENNER, Lucy Elisabeth RAWSON, Jonathan David RICHARDS, Tamsin SEVENOAKS

Beverley

Beverley and Molescroft Surgery
30 Lockwood Road, Molescroft, Beverley HU17 9GQ
Tel: 01482 888690 Fax: 01482 888689
Website: www.molescroftsurgery.co.uk
(East Yorkshire Primary Care Trust)
Patient List Size: 2700

GP Guy Lawrence CLAYTON, D WILLIAMS

The Health Centre
Manor Road, Beverley HU17 7BZ
Tel: 01482 862733 Fax: 01482 864958
(East Yorkshire Primary Care Trust)
Patient List Size: 11500

Practice Manager Barbara Coombes

GP Peter Guy JONES, Elisabeth ALTON, Julie CAVILL, Julia CLIFTON, Stephen Alan HILL, Jeremy Nicholas SHAW, Alan David UNDERWOOD

North Bar Surgery
21 North Bar Without, Beverley HU17 7AQ
Tel: 01482 882546
(East Yorkshire Primary Care Trust)
Patient List Size: 5180

Practice Manager V J Fox

GP Bertha Fiona HUCKVALE, Russell J MARTIN, Anne WYLIE

Old Fire Station
Albert Terrace, Beverley HU17 8JW
Tel: 01482 862236 Fax: 01482 861863
(East Yorkshire Primary Care Trust)
Patient List Size: 11500

Practice Manager Ian Walford

GP Philip Rowland MIXER, Simon Charles CARRUTHERS, Dr DODD, Paul HARDISTY, Dominic Alexander NORGATE, Dr PALUMBO, Gareth David Vaughan WILLIAMS

The Surgery
Samman Road, Beverley HU17 0BS
Tel: 01482 862474
(East Yorkshire Primary Care Trust)
Patient List Size: 1051

GP Bridget Lesley BAWN, Alan Robert Mitchell KELLY

The Surgery
25 Greenwood Avenue, Beverley HU17 0HB
Tel: 01482 881517 Fax: 01482 887022
(East Yorkshire Primary Care Trust)
Patient List Size: 5555

Practice Manager Tina Kettleborough

GP Harminder Singh SURI, Karamjit Singh MARWAH, Heather Gay STAFFORD

The Surgery
29 High Stile, Leven, Beverley HU17 5NL
Tel: 01964 542155 Fax: 01964 543954
(Yorkshire Wolds and Coast Primary Care Trust)
Patient List Size: 10100

Practice Manager Gail Courtney

GP Alan John SYKES, R CHAPMAN, M McMDIARMID, Anthony MILNER, Mary Kathleen Jane SOWERBY, J VERMEIJDEN

Walkergate Surgery
117-119 Walkergate, Beverley HU17 9BP
Tel: 01482 881298 Fax: 01482 861791
(East Yorkshire Primary Care Trust)
Patient List Size: 3600

Practice Manager Josephine Mant

GP Angela Mary HARLEY, L PALUMBO, Dr THORNTON

Bewdley

Bewdley Medical Centre
Dog Lane, Bewdley DY12 2EG
Tel: 01299 402157 Fax: 01299 404364
Email: practicem81057@gp-M81057.nhs.uk
(Wyre Forest Primary Care Trust)
Patient List Size: 14400

Practice Manager Richard Gunn

GP Christopher James Henderson McLACHLAN, Simon GATES, Christine Anne GREEN, Iain Moir INGLIS, Robert George MARRIOTT, Fiona Esther McDOUGALL, Penny MONTANDON, Clive Benjamin PRINCE

Park Attwood Clinic
Trimpley, Bewdley DY12 1RE
Tel: 01299 861444 Fax: 01299 861375
Email: parkattwood@btinternet.com

Practice Manager Shelagh Hart

GP Astrid LINDEBERG, Frank A MULDER, Maurice ORANGE

Bexhill-on-Sea

Collington Surgery
23 Terminus Road, Bexhill-on-Sea TN39 3LR
Tel: 01424 217465/216675 Fax: 01424 216675
(Bexhill and Rother Primary Care Trust)
Patient List Size: 4252

Practice Manager Jean Welling

GP David John WARDEN, Gurcharan SINGH

Old Town Surgery
13 De la Warr Road, Bexhill-on-Sea TN40 2HG
Tel: 01424 219323 Fax: 01424 733940
(Bexhill and Rother Primary Care Trust)
Patient List Size: 6369

Practice Manager Tricia Busbridge

GP Javier GONZALEZ POLLEDO, Lindsay Amy-Anne HADLEY, William Lawrence HAWLEY, Alastair Grant THOMSON

Sea Road Surgery
39-41 Sea Road, Bexhill-on-Sea TN40 1JJ
Tel: 01424 211616 Fax: 01424 733950
(Bexhill and Rother Primary Care Trust)

Practice Manager Kay Davey

GP Roger Garrett ELIAS, Elisabeth Hermine Maria GRUND, Rajiv SHARMA, Stephen Paul SOUTHWARD

Sitwell and Partners
Little Common Surgery, 82 Cooden Sea Road, Bexhill-on-Sea TN39 4SP
Tel: 01424 845477 Fax: 01424 848225
(Bexhill and Rother Primary Care Trust)
Patient List Size: 7400

Practice Manager Judy Coates

GP Isla Ashley Hurt SITWELL, Peter Duncan DEWHURST, Nicola A HAMMOND, Sarah Renata THOMSON

The Surgery
24 Albert Road, Bexhill-on-Sea TN40 1DG
Tel: 01424 730456/734430 Fax: 01424 225615
(Bexhill and Rother Primary Care Trust)

Practice Manager Carole Early

GP David James LAWTON, Sheena Mary ASHBY, C J DIXON, John Callard Robert EATON, Henry William Antti KINCH, Daniel John KREMER, Martha MAKARATZI, David Nicholas NEWELL, Helen Patricia PLUMPTON, Nigel Richard WALTER

The Surgery
7 Buckhurst Road, Bexhill-on-Sea TN40 1QF
Tel: 01424 214757 Fax: 01424 733811
(Bexhill and Rother Primary Care Trust)

Practice Manager Brenda Sammuel

GP Yahya AL-ANSARY

Bexley

Hurst Place Surgery
294A Hurst Road, Bexley DA5 3LH
Tel: 020 8300 2826 Fax: 020 8309 0661

(Bexley Care Trust)
Patient List Size: 6100

Practice Manager Jan Matthews

GP Simona Tanja MALONE, Maria BUTLER, Dan IELAMO

Joydens Wood Medical Centre
111 Summerhouse Drive, Joydens Wood, Bexley DA5 2ER
Tel: 01322 524239 Fax: 01322 529613
(Dartford, Gravesham and Swanley Primary Care Trust)
Patient List Size: 2000

Practice Manager S Cuthbertson

GP R P ARORA

Plas Meddgy Surgery
40 Parkhill Road, Bexley DA5 1HU
Tel: 01322 522056 Fax: 01322 521345
(Bexley Care Trust)
Patient List Size: 5000

Practice Manager Karen Baskett

GP Rachel Anne SYKES, Richard Peter McCARTHY, Ralf SCHMALHORST

Bexleyheath

Albion Surgery
6 Pincott Road, Bexleyheath DA6 7LP
Tel: 020 8304 8334 Fax: 020 8298 0408
Website: www.albionsurgery.com
(Bexley Care Trust)
Patient List Size: 13989

Practice Manager Martin Evans

GP Mukundrai Mulshanker MEHTA, Julian Andrew ARSCOTT-BARBER, Nelun ELPHICK, Nicholas JOYNER, Anna Marie MALONE, S SHAH, Howard Geoffrey Alvan STOATE, Karen Elizabeth UPTON

Bursted Wood Surgery
219 Erith Road, Bexleyheath DA7 6HZ
Tel: 020 8303 5027 Fax: 020 8298 7735
(Bexley Care Trust)
Patient List Size: 5000

Practice Manager V Butler

GP David Warren MAIZELS, Steven Norman BERG, Miren DAVIES

Crook Log Surgery
19 Crook Log, Bexleyheath DA6 8DZ
Tel: 020 8304 3025 Fax: 020 8298 7739
(Bexley Care Trust)
Patient List Size: 8479

Practice Manager Bev McDermott

GP Winnie Kwun Chee KWAN, Philip Benjamin DE SOUZA, Christina MELCHOR, Sunil Kanti ROY, Jacqueline TOLHURST

Mayfair Medical Centre
8 Normanhurst Avenue, Bexleyheath DA7 4TT
Tel: 020 8304 0786
(Bexley Care Trust)
Patient List Size: 3018

GP Meda Dasanna EASWAR

The Medical Centre
41 Lyndhurst Road, Barnehurst, Bexleyheath DA7 6DL
Tel: 01322 525000/01322 558085 Fax: 01322 523123
Email: julia.weal@gp-G83049.nhs.uk
(Bexley Care Trust)
Patient List Size: 8650

GP Edward Lyn MALPASS, Elizabeth Ann CAMERON, Nicholas Stanley Charles HARRISON, Simon John PYLE

The Surgery
58 Cumberland Drive, Bexleyheath DA7 5LB
Tel: 020 8310 5764 Fax: 020 8310 5377
(Bexley Care Trust)
Patient List Size: 1800

GP Samarendra Kumar KUMAR

The Surgery
208 Parkside Avenue, Barnehurst, Bexleyheath DA7 6NW
Tel: 01322 521184 Fax: 01322 525281
(Bexley Care Trust)

GP Neil John SANTAMARIA, Shanti MENDONCA

Thavapalan and Partners
55 Little Heath Road, Bexleyheath DA7 5HL
Tel: 01322 430129 Fax: 01322 440949
(Bexley Care Trust)

Practice Manager Pamela Clark

GP Muruganandan THAVAPALAN, Devi Chandra PERERA

Bicester

Bicester Health Centre
Coker Close, Bicester OX26 6AT
Tel: 01869 249333 Fax: 01869 320314
Email: richard.stephenson@bicesterhc.oxongps.co.uk
(North East Oxfordshire Primary Care Trust)
Patient List Size: 10956

Practice Manager Brian Gallagher

GP John Michael TALBOT, Stephen Paul ATTWOOD, Bernadette Anne FLINTAN, Robin FOX, George Craven MONCRIEFF, Helen WEAVER

Langford Medical Practice
9 Nightingale Place, Bicester OX26 6XX
Tel: 01869 245665
(North East Oxfordshire Primary Care Trust)

Practice Manager Elizabeth Judge

GP Thomas Walter Dalziel ANDERSON, David Richard GRIMSHAW, John Robert JACKMAN, John Richard JONES, Elisabeth Saskia VAN STIGT

Montgomery House Surgery
Piggy Lane, Bicester OX26 6HT
Tel: 01869 249222 Fax: 01869 322433
(North East Oxfordshire Primary Care Trust)
Patient List Size: 12287

Practice Manager Sarah Arnall

GP Michael John CURRY, Stuart BRAND, Alistair Eugene Harvey MURPHY, Aled ROWLANDS, Christine SLOWTHER, Nicholas THOMPSON, Tania WILLIAMS

North Bicester Surgery
Bure Park, Bicester OX26 3HA
Tel: 01869 323600 Fax: 01869 323300
(North East Oxfordshire Primary Care Trust)

Practice Manager V Davies

GP Andrew Forbes Butler GIBSON, Brendan MCDONALD

Victoria House Surgery
Victoria Road, Bicester OX26 6PB
Tel: 01869 248585
(North East Oxfordshire Primary Care Trust)

Practice Manager Sue Burnage

GP John Andrew GALUSZKA, Damian Gerard HANNON, Jill M LEDDY

Bideford

Bideford Medical Centre
Abbotsham Road, Bideford EX39 3AF
Tel: 01237 476363 Fax: 01237 423351
Website: www.bideford-medical-centre.co.uk
(North Devon Primary Care Trust)
Patient List Size: 14250

Practice Manager Olivia Bassett

GP Michael Maurice CRACKNELL, Duncan James BARDNER, Kevin Peter BROWN, Mark Ramsay CLAYTON, Richard Graham FORD, Glenys KNIGHT, Ragai Moris LOKA-SALEH, Kathryn Amelia PRITCHARD, Geoffrey Stuart SPENCER, Alison Mary STAPLEY

Northam Surgery
Bayview Road, Northam, Bideford EX39 1AZ
Tel: 01237 474994
(North Devon Primary Care Trust)

Practice Manager Jane Clark

GP Anthony MOORE, Robin Harold BUCKLAND, Alison Jane DIAMOND, Adrian Scott HENDERSON, Mathew G PIETERSE

Square Surgery
66 The Square, Hartland, Bideford EX39 6BL
Tel: 01237 441200
(North Devon Primary Care Trust)

GP Graham Thomas John COOK, Jonathan Stuart WOOD

The Wooda Surgery
Clarence Wharf, Barnstaple Street, Bideford EX39 4AU
Tel: 01237 471071 Fax: 01237 471059
(North Devon Primary Care Trust)
Patient List Size: 8040

Practice Manager Jane Clark

GP Peter James BRUMMITT, Steven John CHAVASSE, Gillian Anne DALY, Samantha GARDNER, Sara Lucy HERRIOTT, David William MILBURN, John Greer McTurk WILSON

Biggleswade

Biggleswade Health Centre
Saffron Road, Biggleswade SG18 8DJ
Tel: 01767 313647 Fax: 01767 312568
(Bedfordshire Heartlands Primary Care Trust)

Practice Manager Jenny Jessett

GP Samuel Bhaskar MURNAL, Michael Eric CURTIN, Dr EVANS, Stephen Michael FEAST, Jonathan Andrew KIRKHAM, Dr TAYLOR

The Ivel Medical Centre
35-39 The Baulk, Biggleswade SG18 0PX
Tel: 01767 312441 Fax: 01767 603707
(Bedfordshire Heartlands Primary Care Trust)
Patient List Size: 10047

Practice Manager Christina Ward

GP Robert Anthony BUTCHER, Jane Fiona HARTREE, William Alexander HOLLINGTON, Margaret KALILANI, Nigel Peter David SMITH, Anna Barbara Wanda ZAHORSKI

Billericay

Billericay Health Centre
Stock Road, Billericay CM12 0BJ
Tel: 01277 658071 Fax: 01277 631892
(Billericay, Brentwood and Wickford Primary Care Trust)
Patient List Size: 12000

Practice Manager R McDonald

GP Bridget Gytha Rose CLEAR HILL, Usman BUHARI, Michaela CARMACIN, John Henry James COCKCROFT, Tracy FERNIE, Elaine ORFORD, Grahame Oluwole SOFOLUWE, Simon WOOD

Chapel Street Surgery
93 Chapel Street, Billericay CM12 9LR
Tel: 01277 622940/655134 Fax: 01277 631893
(Billericay, Brentwood and Wickford Primary Care Trust)
Patient List Size: 5123

Practice Manager Pat Crew

GP M SAEED, Alyn Christopher Prior WILLIAMS

The New Surgery
27 Stock Road, Billericay CM12 0AH
Tel: 01277 633144 Fax: 01277 633374
(Billericay, Brentwood and Wickford Primary Care Trust)

Practice Manager Maya Gupta

GP Chandra Prakash GUPTA

Queens Park Surgery
24 The Pantiles, Billericay CM12 0UA
Tel: 01277 626446 Fax: 01277 630623
Email: practice.managerf81222@nhs.net
(Billericay, Brentwood and Wickford Primary Care Trust)

Practice Manager Elaine Hemmings

GP Ananda Lal DAS GUPTA, Rita DAS GUPTA

South Green Surgery
14-18 Grange Road, Billericay CM11 2RE
Tel: 01277 651702 Fax: 01277 631894
(Billericay, Brentwood and Wickford Primary Care Trust)
Patient List Size: 3500

Practice Manager D Elam

GP Manzur-Ul-Hassan SARFRAZ

The Surgery
Laindon Road, Billericay CM12 9LD
Tel: 01277 658877 Fax: 01277 631895
(Billericay, Brentwood and Wickford Primary Care Trust)

Practice Manager D E Garrard

GP H U DIN

Western Road Surgery
41 Western Road, Billericay CM12 9DX
Tel: 01277 658117 Fax: 01277 658119
(Billericay, Brentwood and Wickford Primary Care Trust)
Patient List Size: 9500

Practice Manager G Wilks

GP Asadullah AFIFI, Simon James Cawood BUTLER, A M PATEL, Arun PERUMPALLIL, Maria Ann POLLARD, Sheela RAVI

Billingham

The Health Centre
Queensway, Billingham TS23 2LA
Tel: 01642 552700/552151 Fax: 01642 532908
(North Tees Primary Care Trust)
Patient List Size: 7100

Practice Manager Catherine Milburn

GP Hugh Francis GEOGHEGAN, Aileen Yvonne ELBOROUGH, Claire L JACKSON, Suzanne C WEST

The Health Centre
Queensway, Billingham TS23 2LA
Tel: 01642 360033 Fax: 01642 552892
(North Tees Primary Care Trust)

GP Alistair John IRVINE

The Health Centre
Queensway, Billingham TS23 2LA
Tel: 01642 532003 Fax: 01642 557456
(North Tees Primary Care Trust)

GP M CHOUDHURY

The Health Centre
Queensway, Billingham TS23 2LA
Tel: 01642 553389 Fax: 01642 557396
(North Tees Primary Care Trust)

GP William ENTWISTLE, M HAZARIKA

Kingsway Medical Centre
Kingsway, Billingham TS23 2LS
Tel: 01642 553738 Fax: 01642 533011

(North Tees Primary Care Trust)

Practice Manager J E Parker

GP Clive Paul GARTNER, Malcolm James GITTENS, Joyce Maud LONGWILL, C SCHMIDT

Marsh House Medical Centre
254 Marsh House Avenue, Billingham TS23 3EN
Tel: 01642 561282/565068 Fax: 01642 565982
(North Tees Primary Care Trust)
Patient List Size: 8291

Practice Manager Eileen Collingwood

GP J DATTA, Ralf LAMA, Helen MURRAY, John Patrick O'DONOGHUE

Melrose Avenue Surgery
38 Melrose Avenue, Billingham TS23 2JW
Tel: 01642 553055 Fax: 01642 365906
(North Tees Primary Care Trust)

GP A I AWAD, A A G SAAD

Billingshurst

Loxwood Medical Practice
Farm Close, Loxwood, Billingshurst RH14 0UT
Tel: 01403 752246 Fax: 01403 752916
(Western Sussex Primary Care Trust)
Patient List Size: 5501

Practice Manager Philip Slaymaker

GP Andrew Ronald LEACH, Brian Michael GOSS, Christine Ann HOULTON, Emma Mary WOODCOCK

The Surgery
Roman Way, Billingshurst RH14 9QZ
Tel: 01403 782931 Fax: 01403 785505
(Western Sussex Primary Care Trust)
Patient List Size: 10900

GP Charles Geoffrey Millard WOOD, George Maxwell BALME, Michael David BROUGHTON, Rebecca DUNNE, Philip John Stephen POLWIN, Sarah RAVENSCROFT

Bilston

Bayer Hall Clinic
Bayer Street, Bilston WV14 9DS
Tel: 01902 673899
(Dudley Beacon and Castle Primary Care Trust)
Patient List Size: 2100

GP Iqbal Sulemanji ARSIWALA

Bilston Health Centre
Prouds Lane, Bilston WV14 6PW
Tel: 01902 490100 Fax: 01902 445376
Email: indunrn@yahoo.co.uk
(Wolverhampton City Primary Care Trust)

Practice Manager Indu Mudigonda

GP Dr MUDIGONDA

Bilston Health Centre
Prouds Lane, Bilston WV14 6PW
Tel: 01902 492268
(Wolverhampton City Primary Care Trust)

GP Dr RAHMAN

Bradley Community Centre
Wallace Road, Bradley, Bilston WV14 8BP
(Wolverhampton City Primary Care Trust)

GP A KYI

Bradley Medical Centre
83-84 Hallgreen Street, Bradley, Bilston WV14 8TH
Tel: 01902 491323 Fax: 01902 402247
(Wolverhampton City Primary Care Trust)
Patient List Size: 3500

Practice Manager John Guest

GP Chaman LAL

Caerleon Surgery
Dover Street, Bilston WV14 6AL
Tel: 01902 493426 Fax: 01902 490096
(Wolverhampton City Primary Care Trust)
Patient List Size: 4000

Practice Manager Pauline Jones

GP Richard Lawrence RANGEL, Aung KYI

Church Street Surgery
62-64 Church Street, Bilston WV14 0AX
Tel: 01902 496065 Fax: 01902 496384
(Wolverhampton City Primary Care Trust)

GP Dr MAUNG, Min THAN

Clifton Street Surgery
Hurst Hill, Bilston WV14 9EY
Tel: 01902 882170
(Dudley Beacon and Castle Primary Care Trust)

GP S K JAIN

Coseley Medical Centre
32-34 Avenue Road, Coseley, Bilston WV14 9DJ
Tel: 01902 882070
(Dudley Beacon and Castle Primary Care Trust)

GP Perumal ANANDAKUMAR, Sabuj Kanti DE, S PARAMAMATHAM

Shale Street Surgery
1 Shale Street, Bilston WV14 0HF
Tel: 01902 491888
(Wolverhampton City Primary Care Trust)

GP Shyam Kumar KANCHAN

The Surgery
Hill Street, Bradley, Bilston WV14 8SB
Tel: 01902 491659
(Wolverhampton City Primary Care Trust)

Practice Manager Janet Pitt

GP Mosharraf HOSSAIN

Wellington Road Surgery
67 Wellington Road, Bilston WV14 6AQ
Tel: 01902 494464
(Wolverhampton City Primary Care Trust)
Patient List Size: 2048

GP P K MOTWANI

Woodcross Health Centre
Woodcross Lane, Coseley, Bilston WV14 9BX
(Wolverhampton City Primary Care Trust)

GP Dr NOVICK

Bingley

Bingley Health Centre
Myrtle Place, Bingley BD16 2TL
Tel: 01274 562760 Fax: 01274 772345
(Airedale Primary Care Trust)
Patient List Size: 3100

Practice Manager Susan Hardy

GP Kathryn Lesley JENNINGS, Keith Henry ROBSON

Bingley Health Centre
Myrtle Place, Bingley BD16 2TL
Tel: 01274 566617 Fax: 01274 772354
(Airedale Primary Care Trust)

GP Nalini RAI, Frances Carolyn DUKE

Priestthorpe Medical Centre
2 Priestthorpe Lane, Bingley BD16 4ED
Tel: 01274 568383 Fax: 01274 510788
(Airedale Primary Care Trust)

Practice Manager Christine Bennett, Connie M Whitehead

GP N J GREEN, Georgina Helen HASLAM, Richard Charles LAMBERT

Rai and Duke
Bingley Health Centre, Myrtle Place, Bingley BD16 2TL
Tel: 01274 566617 Fax: 01274 772345
(Airedale Primary Care Trust)

Practice Manager Christine Midgley

GP Nalini RAI, Frances Carolyn DUKE

Springfield Surgery
Park Road, Bingley BD16 4LR
Tel: 01274 567991 Fax: 01274 566865
(Airedale Primary Care Trust)
Patient List Size: 5450

Practice Manager John Hutchinson

GP Richard John VESEY, Simon GAZELEY, Jennifer VESEY

Birchington

Birchington Medical Centre
Minnis Road, Birchington CT7 9HQ
Tel: 01843 841384 Fax: 01843 848609
Website: www.birchingtonmedicalcentre.nhs.uk
(East Kent Coastal Teaching Primary Care Trust)
Patient List Size: 9500

Practice Manager Sarah Price

GP Roger KELSEY, Joseph EDDINGTON, John GARLAND, Amer GHAZI, Peter GRAY, Anne MARTIN

Birkenhead

Cavendish Medical Centre
214 Park Road North, Birkenhead CH41 8BU
Tel: 0151 652 1955
(Birkenhead and Wallasey Primary Care Trust)
Patient List Size: 5000

Practice Manager Joyce S Stowe

GP Charles Harry VAILLANT, Christopher S DAVIES, Janet Adrienne MELVILLE

Claughton Medical Centre
161 Park Road North, Birkenhead CH41 0DD
Tel: 0151 652 1688 Fax: 0151 670 0565
(Birkenhead and Wallasey Primary Care Trust)

Practice Manager Barbara Edwards

GP Jill Andrae RENWICK, Charles Peter ARTHUR, Ann CULUMBINE, Bruce Weir TAYLOR

Commonfield Road Surgery
156 Commonfield Road, Woodchurch, Birkenhead CH49 7LP
Tel: 0151 677 0016
(Birkenhead and Wallasey Primary Care Trust)

Practice Manager J Morris

GP Patricia Anne HUGHES, Cornelius BRODBIN, Kathryn MASSEY, Nimal Dushyantha Anthony RATNAIKE

Devaney Medical Centre
40 Balls Road, Oxton, Birkenhead CH43 5RE
Tel: 0151 652 4281 Fax: 0151 670 0445
(Birkenhead and Wallasey Primary Care Trust)
Patient List Size: 8014

Practice Manager J A Elliott

GP Christine Ann BRACE, James William BATES, Peter Julian NUTTALL, David Jeremy STOKOE

Fender Way Health Centre
Fender Way, Birkenhead CH43 9QS
Tel: 0151 677 9103 Fax: 0151 604 0392
(Birkenhead and Wallasey Primary Care Trust)

Practice Manager Debra Fleetwood

GP Janette Gibb WARDALE, Janet Elizabeth REAM

Gladstone Medical Centre
241 Old Chester Road, Lower Tranmere, Birkenhead CH42 3TD
Tel: 0151 645 2306 Fax: 0151 643 1734
(Birkenhead and Wallasey Primary Care Trust)

Practice Manager Debbie Portbury

GP Mohammad SALAHUDDIN, Abel Kehinde ADEGOKE, Khalida ALAUDDIN

Greenway Road Surgery
Greenway Road, Birkenhead CH42 7LX
Tel: 0151 643 6700 Fax: 0151 643 6709
(Birkenhead and Wallasey Primary Care Trust)

Practice Manager Rosemary Stirrup

GP Sally DOW, Julie HARRAND, Peter James HEDGES, Mark John RICHARDS

Holmlands Medical Centre
16-20 Holmlands Drive, Oxton, Birkenhead CH43 0TX
Tel: 0151 608 7750 Fax: 0151 608 0989
Website: www.wirralpcgs.com/holmland
(Birkenhead and Wallasey Primary Care Trust)
Patient List Size: 3410

Practice Manager Pamela Davies

GP R S PATEL, A JONES, V K JOSHI

Miriam Medical Centre
Laird Street, Birkenhead CH41 7AL
Tel: 0151 652 6077 Fax: 0151 651 0018
(Birkenhead and Wallasey Primary Care Trust)

Practice Manager Klazina Brearley

GP Abhinandan Bhupalrao MANTGANI, Debra Ruth HILL

Riverside Surgery
525 New Chester Road, Rockferry, Birkenhead CH42 2AG
Tel: 0151 645 3464 Fax: 0151 643 1676
(Birkenhead and Wallasey Primary Care Trust)
Patient List Size: 7500

Practice Manager Margaret Sinnott

GP Richard Michael WILLIAMS, Robert George JOHNSTONE, Deirdre Annamaria ROMANIUK, Robin Leslie SELBY, Julie WHERE

Victoria Park Health Centre
Bedford Avenue, Birkenhead CH42 4QJ
Tel: 0151 645 8384 Fax: 0151 644 9561
(Birkenhead and Wallasey Primary Care Trust)
Patient List Size: 7500

GP Murray John FREEMAN, David Mark COOMBS, Jane MAWDSLEY, Richard Alexander STOKELL

Villa Medical Centre
Roman Road, Birkenhead CH43 3DB
Tel: 0151 608 4702 Fax: 0151 609 0067
(Birkenhead and Wallasey Primary Care Trust)
Patient List Size: 6200

Practice Manager C Brennan

GP Colin Michael KENYON, Neil Mathew Peacock COOKSON, Marian Morris JONES, Jennifer PERKINS

Vittoria Health Centre
Vittoria Street, Birkenhead CH41 3RH
Tel: 0151 650 1098 Fax: 0151 650 0942
(Birkenhead and Wallasey Primary Care Trust)

GP K S MURTY

Vittoria Health Centre
Vittoria Street, Birkenhead CH41 3RH
Tel: 0151 650 1098 Fax: 0151 650 0942
(Birkenhead and Wallasey Primary Care Trust)

GP K S MURTY

Vittoria Medical Centre
Vittoria Street, Birkenhead CH41 3RH
Tel: 0151 647 7321 Fax: 0151 650 0942
(Birkenhead and Wallasey Primary Care Trust)

Practice Manager Anita Swift

GP Peter Julian GRANT, Robert Wyn EDWARDS, Janet Maria GREEN

Wallasey Village Group Practice
50 Wallasey Village, Wallasey, Birkenhead CH45 3NL
Tel: 0151 691 2088 Fax: 0151 637 0146
(Birkenhead and Wallasey Primary Care Trust)
Patient List Size: 4500

Practice Manager Pat Thorneycroft

GP Ewan Fergusson CAMERON, Kathryn Jane FEGAN, Judith Mary HOLLEY

Wallasey Village Surgery
50 Wallasey Village, Wallasey, Birkenhead CH45 3NL
Tel: 0151 691 2088 Fax: 0151 637-0146
(Birkenhead and Wallasey Primary Care Trust)

GP Ewan Ferguson CAMERON, Dr FEGAN, Dr HOLLY

Whetstone Lane Health Centre
44 Whetstone Lane, Birkenhead CH41 2TF
Tel: 0151 647 9613 Fax: 0151 650 0875
(Birkenhead and Wallasey Primary Care Trust)
Patient List Size: 10024

Practice Manager Anita Jones

GP Clive Martin PLEASANCE, C L AIREY, M LOCKYER, N SHAH, Linda Eileen STEVENS, Amanda Jane TAYLOR

Woodchurch Road Surgery
270 Woodchurch Road, Prenton, Birkenhead CH43 5UU
Tel: 0151 608 3475 Fax: 0151 608 9535
(Birkenhead and Wallasey Primary Care Trust)

Practice Manager Elaine Evans

GP Diana Bowyer COURTNEY, Richard Edward FALLOWFIELD, Jane Elizabeth HOWARD, Andrew LEE

Birmingham

Abbas
Clifford Coombs Health Centre, 70 Tangmere Drive, Castle Vale, Birmingham B35 7QX
Tel: 0121 747 4633 Fax: 0121 747 1587
(Eastern Birmingham Primary Care Trust)
Patient List Size: 5000

Practice Manager Julie Wallis

GP Saeed ABBAS

Abdel-Malek and Matta
Sparkbrook Health Centre, 32 Farm Road, Sparkbrook, Birmingham B11 1LS
Tel: 0121 753 0615
(Heart of Birmingham Teaching Primary Care Trust)
Patient List Size: 5000

Practice Manager Mandy Dance

GP George Talaat ABDEL-MALEK, Inas Y MATTA

Aberdeen Medical Centre
Aberdeen Street, Winson Green, Birmingham B18 7DL
Tel: 0121 554 7311
(Heart of Birmingham Teaching Primary Care Trust)
Patient List Size: 1733

Practice Manager S K Kulshrestha

GP Rajendra Prakash KULSHRESTHA, Sheena KULSHRESTHA

Acocks Green Medical Centre
999 Warwick Road, Acocks Green, Birmingham B27 6QJ
Tel: 0121 706 0501
(Eastern Birmingham Primary Care Trust)
Patient List Size: 3500

Practice Manager Catherine Sen-Gupta

GP Tapan SEN-GUPTA

Al-Shafa Medical Centre
5-7 Little Oaks Road, Aston, Birmingham B6 6JY
Tel: 0121 328 1977 Fax: 0121 327 3755
(Heart of Birmingham Teaching Primary Care Trust)
Patient List Size: 7000

Practice Manager Sameena Akhtar

GP D R KARAMDAD, Zafar ALI

All Saints Medical Centre
1 Vicarage Road, Kings Heath, Birmingham B14 7QA
Tel: 0121 444 2005 Fax: 0121 441 4331
(South Birmingham Primary Care Trust)
Patient List Size: 6000

Practice Manager Cynthia Sutherland

GP Kochu-Teresa BASIL, A OJHA, G VARSANI

Alum Rock Medical Centre
27-29 Highfield Road, Alum Rock, Birmingham B8 3QD
Tel: 0121 328 9579 Fax: 0121 328 7495
(Eastern Birmingham Primary Care Trust)
Patient List Size: 4500

Practice Manager Mohammed Altaf

GP Aleem AKHTAR

Apollo Surgery
619 Kings Road, Great Barr, Birmingham B44 9HW
Tel: 0121 360 8668
(North Birmingham Primary Care Trust)
Patient List Size: 3200

GP Milton MICHALOS, M PRASAD

Ashtree Medical Centre
1536 Pershore Road, Stirchley, Birmingham B30 2NP
Tel: 0121 458 1031 Fax: 0121 459 1182
(South Birmingham Primary Care Trust)
Patient List Size: 3500

Practice Manager Erica Watkins

GP Stephen Denis BROWNE, Margaret Beryl HOOPER

Aston Health Centre
175 Trinity Road, Aston, Birmingham B6 6JA
Tel: 0121 328 3597 Fax: 0121 327 8814
(Heart of Birmingham Teaching Primary Care Trust)
Patient List Size: 2850

GP Mahmudai Rahman KHAN

Baldwin Lane Surgery
265 Baldwin Lane, Hall Green, Birmingham B28 0RF
Tel: 0121 744 1290 Fax: 0121 745 1126
(South Birmingham Primary Care Trust)
Patient List Size: 4000

Practice Manager Sue Sheldon

GP Wagih Shoukry ABDOU, F H YOUNAN

Barnt Green Surgery
82 Hewell Road, Barnt Green, Birmingham B45 8NF
Tel: 0121 445 1704 Fax: 0121 445 7310
(Redditch and Bromsgrove Primary Care Trust)
Patient List Size: 6400

Practice Manager Claire Humpage

GP Frank Thomas TAYLOR, Stuart Robert JONES, Susan Joan SCOTT

Bartley Green Health Centre
Romsley Road, Bartley Green, Birmingham B32 3PS
Tel: 0121 477 4300
(South Birmingham Primary Care Trust)

GP Christine CHEEL, Nuton Ahmed FAISAL, Stephen James David WATKINS

Bellevue Medical Group Practice
6 Bellevue, Edgbaston, Birmingham B5 7LX
Tel: 0121 446 2000 Fax: 0121 446 2015
Website: www.bellevuemedical.co.uk
(South Birmingham Primary Care Trust)
Patient List Size: 6150

GP Frederick David Richard HOBBS, Andrew James Benner CARSON, Stephen John FIELD, Mark Vincent HIRSCH, Patricia HOULSTON, Rekha RAJESH, Sukhdev SINGH, Derek WILLIS

Birmingham Heartlands Surgery
Gray Street, Bordesley Village, Birmingham B9 4LS
Tel: 0121 772 2020
(Heart of Birmingham Teaching Primary Care Trust)

Practice Manager G Kaur

GP Mathew Koduvathrail THOMAS, Vanmala THOMAS

Blakesley Surgery
39 Blakesley Road, Yardley, Birmingham B25 8XU
Tel: 0121 783 4224 Fax: 0121 785 0423
(Eastern Birmingham Primary Care Trust)
Patient List Size: 2000

Practice Manager Hilary Najak

GP Bahadurali Gulam Hussein NAJAK

Bloomsbury Health Centre
63 Rupert Street, Nechells, Birmingham B7 5DT
Tel: 0121 678 3932 Fax: 0121 678 3925
Email: sbbloomsbury@yahoo.com
(Heart of Birmingham Teaching Primary Care Trust)
Patient List Size: 1981

GP Subhashini BATRA

Bloomsbury Health Centre
63 Rupert Street, Nechells, Birmingham B7 5DT
Tel: 0121 678 3932 Fax: 0121 678 3925
(Heart of Birmingham Teaching Primary Care Trust)
Patient List Size: 2300

Practice Manager Rashoa Shanaz

GP Peter Robert HILL

Bordesley Green Surgery
143-145 Bordesley Green, Bordesley Green, Birmingham B9 5EG
Tel: 0121 773 2170
(Heart of Birmingham Teaching Primary Care Trust)
Patient List Size: 5200

Practice Manager Sheila Greeves

GP Minesh Jayantilal SHAH, Varsha Minesh SHAH

Bosworth Medical Centre
16 Crabtree Drive, Chelmsley Wood, Birmingham B37 5BU
Tel: 0121 770 4484 Fax: 0121 779 6818
(Solihull Primary Care Trust)

Practice Manager D Coffey

GP James Ivan STORER, R L CLOWES, S C JERROM, S LOWE, William John PHILLIPS

Bournbrook and Varsity Medical Practice
480 Bristol Road, Selly Oak, Birmingham B29 6BD
Tel: 0121 472 0129 Fax: 0121 472 3775
(South Birmingham Primary Care Trust)
Patient List Size: 6200

GP Victor Herbert CROSS, Christina ALLEN, K ATTWOOD, K POURGOURIDES

Bournville Surgery
41B Sycamore Road, Bournville, Birmingham B30 2AA
Tel: 0121 472 7231 Fax: 0121 472 7231
(South Birmingham Primary Care Trust)
Patient List Size: 2083

Practice Manager Janet Williams

GP Aamer KHAN

Broadmeadow Clinic
Keynell Covert, Kings Norton, Birmingham B30 3QT
Tel: 0121 458 1340 Fax: 0121 459 4459
(South Birmingham Primary Care Trust)
Patient List Size: 2667

Practice Manager Sandra Jackson

GP William Edward WALKER

Broadway Health Centre
Cope Street, Ladywood, Birmingham B18 7BA
Tel: 0121 454 3426
(Heart of Birmingham Teaching Primary Care Trust)

GP Kenneth McNeil BARTLEY, Peter Chike GINI

Bromford Medical Centre
1 Warstone Tower, Bromford Drive, Bromford, Birmingham B36 8TU
Tel: 0121 747 9161 Fax: 0121 749 2676
(Eastern Birmingham Primary Care Trust)
Patient List Size: 1563

Practice Manager J M Heaney

GP Nita SAIKIA-VARMAN, Irene LAVIN

Carnegie Institute
Hunters Road, Hockley, Birmingham B19 1DR
Tel: 0121 554 9920 Fax: 0121 456 5874
(Heart of Birmingham Teaching Primary Care Trust)
Patient List Size: 1600

Practice Manager Rita Radvanyi

GP (Miklos) Nicholas RADVANYI

Castle Practice
2 Hawthorne Road, Castle Bromwich, Birmingham B36 0HH
Tel: 0121 747 2422 Fax: 0121 749 1196
(Solihull Primary Care Trust)
Patient List Size: 8400

Practice Manager Sheila Elliot

GP Anand John CHITNIS, Paul Anthony WALLACE, Kalpana JOSHI, Vanessa Julie MANYWEATHERS, Aryan NEGARGAR

Castle Vale Health Centre
Tangmere Drive, Castle Vale, Birmingham B35 7QX
Tel: 0121 748 8200 Fax: 0121 748 8210
(Eastern Birmingham Primary Care Trust)
Patient List Size: 5953

Practice Manager Linda Aberdeen

GP Francis Henry COLE, Patricia Gillian BEIGHTON, Richard Mathew EDWARDS, Douglas Edward WULFF

Cavendish Medical Practice
2A Cavendish Road, Edgbaston, Birmingham B16 0HZ
Tel: 0121 454 1702 Fax: 0121 455 8084
(Heart of Birmingham Teaching Primary Care Trust)
Patient List Size: 2700

Practice Manager Hari Madhavan

GP P MADHAVAN

Church Lane Medical Centre
111 Church Lane, Stechford, Birmingham B33 9EJ
Tel: 0121 783 2567 Fax: 0121 789 7991
(Eastern Birmingham Primary Care Trust)
Patient List Size: 3803

Practice Manager J M Heaney

GP Nita SAIKIA VARMAN, Irene LANIN

Churchill Medical Centre
191/193 Birchfield Road, Ferry Barr, Birmingham B19 1LL
Tel: 0121 523 3833
Email: prema.iyengar@hobtpct.nhs.uk
(Heart of Birmingham Teaching Primary Care Trust)
Patient List Size: 2600

Practice Manager A Asthana

GP Prema Gopal IYENGAR

City Health Centre
449 City Road, Edgbaston, Birmingham B17 8LG
Tel: 0121 420 2384 Fax: 0121 434 3931
(Heart of Birmingham Teaching Primary Care Trust)
Patient List Size: 2150

Practice Manager Ravinder Kaur

GP Umesh Chandra KATHURIA

City Road Medical Centre
5 City Road, Edgbaston, Birmingham B16 0HH
Tel: 0121 454 8998
(Heart of Birmingham Teaching Primary Care Trust)
Patient List Size: 2300

Practice Manager M Gani

GP Vijayakar ABROL

Cofton Medical Centre
2 Robinsfield Drive, Off Longbridge Lane, West Heath, Birmingham B31 4TU
Tel: 0121 693 5777 Fax: 0121 693 4414
(South Birmingham Primary Care Trust)
Patient List Size: 6700

Practice Manager Julie Walker

GP Dorothy Margaret KEIGHLEY, Nicholas Harry ANFILOGOFF, Kirsten BLACKFORD, James Pangbourne EDMUNDS, Mary Claire FRAISE

College Road Surgery
158 College Road, Moseley, Birmingham B13 9LH
Tel: 0121 777 4040 Fax: 0121 778 6683
(Heart of Birmingham Teaching Primary Care Trust)
Patient List Size: 4000

Practice Manager Deborah Browning

GP Abdul HAFEEZ, Farhat HAFEEZ

Collingwood Family Practice
Collingwood Drive, Great Barr, Birmingham B43 7NF
Tel: 0121 480 5900 Fax: 0121 480 5902
(Walsall Teaching Primary Care Trust)

Practice Manager Alison Phipps

GP Denise Margaret LOMAS, Jagdeesh Singh DHALIWAL, Sukhdev SINGH-SANGHA

Colston Health Centre
10 Bath Row, Lee Bank, Birmingham B15 1LZ
Tel: 0121 622 1446 Fax: 0121 622 6709
(Heart of Birmingham Teaching Primary Care Trust)
Patient List Size: 1900

GP Barry Martin HYMAN

Coventry Road Medical Centre
448 Coventry Road, Small Heath, Birmingham B10 0UG
Tel: 0121 773 5390 Fax: 0121 771 2703
(Heart of Birmingham Teaching Primary Care Trust)
Patient List Size: 4700

Practice Manager Leo O' Toole

GP Yasmin AHMAD, Sajjad AHMAD

Dr Fleming and Partners
Northfield Health Centre, 15 St. Heliers Road, Northfield, Birmingham B31 1QT
Tel: 0121 478 1850 Fax: 0121 476 0931
(South Birmingham Primary Care Trust)
Patient List Size: 10171

Practice Manager Bill Clements

GP Douglas Munro FLEMING, Derek John BARFORD, Judith Margaret HESLOP, Denise KINCH, Barbara Ruth KING, Andrew Munro ROSS, Virginia Sarah TUDOR

Dr MTI WALJI
Balsall Heath Health Centre, 43 Edward Road, Balsall Heath, Birmingham B12 9LP
Tel: 0121 446 2400 Fax: 0121 440 5861
Email: mohammed.walji@hobpct.nhs.uk
Website: www.surgeriesonline.com/balsallheath
(Heart of Birmingham Teaching Primary Care Trust)
Patient List Size: 4131

Practice Manager Renu Sinha

GP Mohamed Taki Ismail WALJI, C BRAWN, S CASSAM, M RASHID

Dr P M Dudley
6 Dyas Road, Great Barr, Birmingham B44 8SF
Tel: 0121 384 4848
(North Birmingham Primary Care Trust)
Patient List Size: 2100

Practice Manager A Chew

GP Paul Maurice DUDLEY

Druids Heath Surgery
27 Pound Road, Druids Heath, Birmingham B14 5SB
Tel: 0121 430 5461 Fax: 0121 436 5669
(South Birmingham Primary Care Trust)

Practice Manager Anne Skidmore

GP Gitanath WALI, Ghulam Mohiuddin ZARGAR, Paramjeet DHILLON

Dudley Park Medical Centre
28 Dudley Park Road, Acocks Green, Birmingham B27 6QR
Tel: 0121 764 7800 Fax: 0121 707 0418
(South Birmingham Primary Care Trust)
Patient List Size: 7300

Practice Manager Karen Carroll

GP Jayshree Narrendra PATEL, Stephen Grant Julian GABRIEL, Mark Alexander KORDAN, J E WADDELL

Eastgate
Gillott Road, Edgbaston, Birmingham B16 0EU
Tel: 0121 454 1712 Fax: 0121 4565174
Email: kandasami.venkat@hobpct.nhs.uk
(Heart of Birmingham Teaching Primary Care Trust)
Patient List Size: 2300

Practice Manager P K Pillai

GP Kandasami Ramaswamy VENKAT

Eaton Wood Medical Centre
1128 Tyburn Road, Erdington, Birmingham B24 0SY
Tel: 0121 373 0959 Fax: 0121 350 2719
(Eastern Birmingham Primary Care Trust)
Patient List Size: 10000

Practice Manager Jan Wilby

GP Sarah Louise PERKINS, J A BALL, A H CHAUDARY, Christopher Marc DAVIES, Hilda Catherine JESSOP, Giuseppe MACEROLA

Ejaz Medical Centre
276 Dudley Road, Winson Green, Birmingham B18 4HL
Tel: 0121 455 6170 Fax: 0121 454 8862
(Heart of Birmingham Teaching Primary Care Trust)
Patient List Size: 3400

Practice Manager Parreen Afzal

GP Fazal AHMED, Aisha RUBY

Erdington Medical Centre
103 Wood End Road, Erdington, Birmingham B24 8NT
Tel: 0121 373 0085 Fax: 0121 386 1768
(Eastern Birmingham Primary Care Trust)

Practice Manager Jenny Quinney

GP Patrick Desmond MURPHY, Samuel Kwasi APPIAH, Robert Luigi MORLEY, Nicholas USHER-SOMERS

Fairway Surgery
475 Bordesley Green East, Yardley, Birmingham B33 8PP
Tel: 0121 783 2125 Fax: 0121 785 0416
(Eastern Birmingham Primary Care Trust)
Patient List Size: 3890

Practice Manager Sue Tustin

GP Meenu BROWN

Fernbank Medical Centre
508-516 Alumrock Road, Birmingham B8 3HX
Tel: 0121 678 3800 Fax: 0121 678 3810
(Eastern Birmingham Primary Care Trust)
Patient List Size: 4350

Practice Manager N Bangash, M A Bowen, S Khan

GP Nawaz H BANGASH, Annie BANGASH

Firs Surgery
87 Kempson Road, Birmingham B36 8LR
Tel: 0121 747 3586 Fax: 0121 749 2070
(Eastern Birmingham Primary Care Trust)

Practice Manager Lisa Hunt

GP Imran Ul HAQ, Mohan Annasahed LATTHE

Frankley Health Centre
125 New Street, Rubery, Birmingham B45 0EU
Tel: 0121 453 8211 Fax: 0121 457 9690
(South Birmingham Primary Care Trust)
Patient List Size: 6000

GP Mukesh Kumar BHARDWAJ, B KALLAN, G SINHA

Gate Medical Centre
120 Washwood Heath Road, Saltley, Birmingham B8 1RE
Tel: 0121 327 4427 Fax: 0121 327 8638
(Eastern Birmingham Primary Care Trust)
Patient List Size: 3200

Practice Manager Margaret Ryder

GP Rai Ahmad Sadiq SANGRA

Goodrest Croft Surgery
1 Goodrest Croft, Yardley Wood, Birmingham B14 4JU
Tel: 0121 474 2059 Fax: 0121 436 7260
Website: www.goodrest@org.uk
(South Birmingham Primary Care Trust)
Patient List Size: 6500

Practice Manager Sue Siddorn

GP Gillian Mary BAILEY, Debby CONDY, Peter GIDDINGS, Jonathan Richard Charles LANHAM, Victoria Jane MOORE

Granton Medical Centre
114 Middleton Hall Road, Kings Norton, Birmingham B30 1DH
Tel: 0121 459 9117 Fax: 0121 486 2889
(South Birmingham Primary Care Trust)
Patient List Size: 8600

Practice Manager Joan Barton

GP Maureen Anne BARTLETT, Susan Elizabeth DEBENHAM, Robert Everett HUDDLESTON, Philip WESTERN

Great Barr Group Practice
912 Walsall Road, Great Barr, Birmingham B42 1TG
Tel: 0121 357 1250 Fax: 0121 358 4857
(Wednesbury and West Bromwich Primary Care Trust)

Practice Manager J M Bennett, A Bhadri, J A McCulloch

GP Aravina Damodar BHADRI, A S KANDOLA, Chandrakant PATEL, Gail STEEDMAN, Kiran Mayee TRIVEDI

Green Lane Surgery
67 Green Lane, Castle Bromwich, Birmingham B36 0AY
Tel: 0121 747 6467 Fax: 0121 749 3613
(Solihull Primary Care Trust)
Patient List Size: 4000

Practice Manager Margaret Webster

GP Ved Prakash BUDH-RAJA, Savita BUDH-RAJA

Green Ridge Surgery
713 Yardley Wood Road, Billesley, Birmingham B13 0PT
Tel: 0121 444 3597 Fax: 0121 441 5839
(South Birmingham Primary Care Trust)
Patient List Size: 5800

Practice Manager Fay Staff

GP Louise Claire LUMLEY, K DEACON, Amanda Claire GOUGH, L S JHASS, R J McMANUS

Griffins Brook Medical Centre
119 Griffins Brook Lane, Bournville, Birmingham B30 1QN
Tel: 0121 476 2441 Fax: 0121 475 0073
(South Birmingham Primary Care Trust)
Patient List Size: 3000

Practice Manager Judith Heath

GP David Gordon EMERY, Julien Helen KHAN

Group Practice Surgery
33 Newton Road, Great Barr, Birmingham B43 6AA
Tel: 0121 357 1690 Fax: 0121 357 4253
(Wednesbury and West Bromwich Primary Care Trust)

Practice Manager Ann Lloyd

GP Paragprasun PAL, Pravinchandra DAYA

Hall Green Health
979 Stratford Road, Hall Green, Birmingham B28 8BG
Tel: 0121 777 3500 Fax: 0121 325 5515
(South Birmingham Primary Care Trust)

Practice Manager Chris Jenkins

GP Diane Claire ASKER, Ann Dolores CARTMILL, Emily Marianne DIBDIN, Peter Thomas NALL, Mosood NAZIR, Eric PENNINGTON, Sheila Jane PENNINGTON, Ajay SINGAL, Stephen William STRANGE, Harminderjeet Singh SURDHAR, Aamir Bakhtiar SYED, Nola Jean WEBSTER, George Brims YOUNG

Handsworth Medical Centre
143 Albert Road, Handsworth, Birmingham B21 9LE
Tel: 0121 554 0980 Fax: 0121 554 3025
Email: vb2326@gp89.birminghamha.wmids.nhs.uk
(Heart of Birmingham Teaching Primary Care Trust)
Patient List Size: 4000

Practice Manager A Bathla

GP Vijay BATHLA

Handsworth Medical Practice
4 Trafalgar Road, Handsworth, Birmingham B21 9NH
(Heart of Birmingham Teaching Primary Care Trust)

GP A SHARMA

Handsworth Wood Medical Centre
110-12 Church Lane, Handsworth Wood, Birmingham B20 2ES
Tel: 0121 523 7117 Fax: 0121 554 2406
Email: philip.hamilton@hobtpct.nhs.uk
(Heart of Birmingham Teaching Primary Care Trust)
Patient List Size: 6100

GP Philip Alexander HAMILTON, Karen BLAKELY, Simon BUTLER, David Baron ECCLESTON, Nicholas HARDING, K MUSTAFA, K M RAILEY

Harborne Medical Practice
4 York Street, Harborne, Birmingham B17 0HG
Tel: 0121 427 5246 Fax: 0121 427 3087
(South Birmingham Primary Care Trust)
Patient List Size: 7500

Practice Manager Sue Smith

GP Michael Lawrence PAYNE, Julia Jane BARNHAM, C ELLIOTT, Peter Malcolm Lloyd GRIFFITHS

The Harlequin Surgery
160 Shard End Crescent, Shard End, Birmingham B34 7BP
Tel: 0121 747 8291 Fax: 0121 749 5497
(Eastern Birmingham Primary Care Trust)

Practice Manager P R Toon

GP Anthony Francis Curtin AINSWORTH, Judith Helen HERITAGE, Rajesh PANKHANIA, S SHAH, Glenys Ann SUTHERLAND, Martin John Brian WILKINSON

Hawkesley Health Centre
375 Shannon Road, Kings Norton, Birmingham B38 9TJ
Tel: 0121 486 4200 Fax: 0121 486 4201
Website: www.hawkesleymedicalpractice.co.uk
(South Birmingham Primary Care Trust)
Patient List Size: 5360

Practice Manager Rhona Woosey

GP Paul Adrian Marc SHIPMAN, D A EDWARDS

Hazelwood Group Practice
27 Parkfield Road, Coleshill, Birmingham B46 3LD
Tel: 01675 463165 Fax: 01675 466253
(North Warwickshire Primary Care Trust)
Patient List Size: 9400

Practice Manager D M Smith

GP David Thomas MILLEDGE, Peter PEARS, Donald POWELL-TUCK, Sarah SHANNON, Patricia WILDBORE, Peter WILDBORE

High Street Surgery
26 High Street, Erdington, Birmingham B23 6RN
Tel: 0121 373 0086 Fax: 0121 373 2041
(Eastern Birmingham Primary Care Trust)
Patient List Size: 6000

Practice Manager Elaine Makinson

GP Carl DUNFORD, F ARMSTRONG, R BAGCHI, A McCOLLUM

High Trees
124 Walsall Road, Perry Barr, Birmingham B42 1SG
Tel: 0121 356 4239 Fax: 0121 356 8914
Email: bhanu.bhattacharyya@pc.birmingham.ha.wmids.nhs.uk
(North Birmingham Primary Care Trust)
Patient List Size: 2752

GP Bhanu BHATTACHARYYA

Highfield Lane Medical Centre
88 Highfield Lane, Woodgate Valley, Birmingham B32 1QX
Tel: 0121 422 0770 Fax: 0121 421 2537
(South Birmingham Primary Care Trust)
Patient List Size: 1250

Practice Manager K Rowlands

GP Inayat ALI

Highfield Surgery
95 Highfield Road, Alum Rock, Birmingham B8 3QE
Tel: 0121 327 4939 Fax: 0121 328 0939
(Eastern Birmingham Primary Care Trust)
Patient List Size: 3220

Practice Manager Hashmat Shaikh

GP Abdul G HAKEEM

Highgate Medical Centre
1 Brinklow Tower, Upper Highgate Street, Highgate, Birmingham B12 0XT
Tel: 0121 440 3605 Fax: 0121 440 5063
(Heart of Birmingham Teaching Primary Care Trust)
Patient List Size: 3838

Practice Manager Dawood

GP Sharad Shripadrao PANDIT

Hilltop Surgery
991 Bristol Road South, Northfield, Birmingham B31 2QT
Tel: 0121 476 9191
(South Birmingham Primary Care Trust)

GP Nicholas Alfred LEVI, Andrew David HARDIE, Linda Mary MOTTERSHEAD

Hockley Medical Practice
247 South Road, Hockley, Birmingham B18 5JS
Tel: 0121 554 1757 Fax: 0121 554 1757
(Heart of Birmingham Teaching Primary Care Trust)

Practice Manager Deborah Pogorzelski

GP Earl Fitzroy O'BRIEN

Hollyoaks Medical Centre
229 Station Road, Wythall, Birmingham B47 6ET
Tel: 01564 823182 Fax: 01564 824127
Email: practice.M81083@gp-M81083.nhs.uk
(Redditch and Bromsgrove Primary Care Trust)
Patient List Size: 5200

Practice Manager David Greenaway

GP Christine M WHITTAKER

Holyhead Primary Health Care Centre
1 St James Road, Handsworth, Birmingham B21 0HL
Tel: 0121 554 8516 Fax: 0121 523 5306
(Heart of Birmingham Teaching Primary Care Trust)
Patient List Size: 3400

Practice Manager Shanti Penduffin

GP Bharaati C CHAPARALA

Jiggins Lane Surgery
17 Jiggins Lane, Bartley Green, Birmingham B32 3LE
Tel: 0121 477 7272 Fax: 0121 478 4319
Website: www.jigginslane.org.uk
(South Birmingham Primary Care Trust)
Patient List Size: 6476

Practice Manager Jackie Shan

GP Sylvia Marion CHUDLEY, Russell Charles CHERRY, Gilles Robert de WILDT, Esther OPPENHEIM, Hilary Jane Elizabeth PARLE

Joshi and Reddy
Aston Health Centre, 175 Trinity Road, Aston, Birmingham B6 6JA
Tel: 0121 327 0144 Fax: 0121 326 9784
(Heart of Birmingham Teaching Primary Care Trust)
Patient List Size: 4300

Practice Manager Suraiya Khan

GP Sharada M JOSHI, Kokkonda Suryaprakash REDDY

The Karis Medical Centre
Waterworks Road, Edgbaston, Birmingham B16 9AL
Tel: 0121 454 0661 Fax: 0121 454 9104
Website: www.karismedicalcentre.uk
(South Birmingham Primary Care Trust)
Patient List Size: 12000

GP Patrick Harold Ross BRYSON, Joanna Elizabeth DALY, Graeme FLEMING, Michael FORREST, Carol GORDON, Gillian Ruth HARLEY-MASON, Malcolm James LAIRD, Aiya SCHOEN, Hendricka Margaret TAKES, Paul Robert Wilson TURNER

Keynell Covert Surgery
33 Keynell Covert, Kings Norton, Birmingham B30 3QT
Tel: 0121 458 2619 Fax: 0121 459 9640
(South Birmingham Primary Care Trust)
Patient List Size: 1700

Practice Manager Janet Weaver

GP Sanat Kumar PATODI

Khyber Surgery
38 Havelock Road, Saltley, Birmingham B8 1RT
Tel: 0121 328 1174 Fax: 0121 328 5340
(Eastern Birmingham Primary Care Trust)

Practice Manager S Millington

GP Atta Ullah SHAH

King's Norton Surgery
66 Redditch Road, Kings Norton, Birmingham B38 8QS
Tel: 0121 458 2550 Fax: 0121 459 2770
(South Birmingham Primary Care Trust)

Practice Manager Gail Fergus

GP Andrew David COWARD, Catherine Margaret Anne COWARD, Damian WILLIAMS

Kingsfield Medical Centre
146 Alcester Road South, Kings Heath, Birmingham B14 6AA
Tel: 0121 444 2054 Fax: 0121 443 5856
(South Birmingham Primary Care Trust)
Patient List Size: 7100

Practice Manager Emma Dent

GP Janusz Tadeusz WOZNIAK, Ursula OETIKER, Helen REDMAN, Frank SPANNUTH, Joyce Kathleen WILLIAMS

Kingshurst Medical Practice
40 Gilson Way, Kingshurst, Birmingham B37 6BE
Tel: 0121 788 8674
(Solihull Primary Care Trust)
Patient List Size: 9000

Practice Manager Jane Nock

GP Rajeshkumar Lalji MEHTA, Geoffrey Neil BANCROFT, Swayam Jyothi IYER

Kingstanding Surgery
26 Rough Road, Kingstanding, Birmingham B44 0UY
Tel: 0121 354 4560 Fax: 0121 354 8981
(North Birmingham Primary Care Trust)
Patient List Size: 5400

GP Khalid CASSAM, Balbir Singh SAHOTA

Kirpal Medical Practice
Soho Health Centre, Louise Road, Handsworth, Birmingham B21 0RY
Tel: 0121 554 0033
(Heart of Birmingham Teaching Primary Care Trust)

GP Ravi Kumar VATISH, P MADHAVAN

Ladywood Surgery
35 Morville Street, Ladywood, Birmingham B16 8BU
Tel: 0121 454 3774 Fax: 0121 456 5713
(Heart of Birmingham Teaching Primary Care Trust)

GP Atef Tawfik Mikhail SIDHOM

The Laurie Pike Health Centre
95 Birchfield Road, Handsworth, Birmingham B19 1LH
Tel: 0121 5540621/5238111 Fax: 0121 554 6163
Website: phc.co.uk
(Heart of Birmingham Teaching Primary Care Trust)
Patient List Size: 10134

Practice Manager Rose Gwillym

GP Margaret Frances BEAZLEY, Brendan Clifford DELANEY, Benjamin David EMPSON, Gwyn Peter HARRIS, William MURDOCH, Naresh RATI, Joanne Louise SHAYLOR

Lea Village Medical Centre
98 Lea Village, Kitts Green, Birmingham B33 9SD
Tel: 0121 789 9565
(Eastern Birmingham Primary Care Trust)

GP Satish Kumar DHAMIJA

Leach Heath Medical Centre
Leach Heath Lane, Rubery, Birmingham B45 9BU
Tel: 0121 453 3516 Fax: 0121 457 9256
(South Birmingham Primary Care Trust)

Practice Manager Katie Howell

GP Nadeem AHMED, Simon Richard CARTER, Kathryn Ann KHANNA, Peter Francis RICE

Lee Bank Group Practice
Colston Health Centre, 10 Bath Row, Lee Bank, Birmingham B15 1LZ
Tel: 0121 622 4846 Fax: 0121 622 7105
(Heart of Birmingham Teaching Primary Care Trust)
Patient List Size: 7400

Practice Manager Joy Fletcher

GP David Ronald MORGAN, Babus AHMED, Sarah BALL, Paul Joseph D'URSO, Amjad IQBAL, Philippa Margaret MATTHEWS, Rheena RAHMAN

Ley Hill Surgery
65 Holloway, Northfield, Birmingham B31 1TR
Tel: 0121 475 1422
(South Birmingham Primary Care Trust)
Patient List Size: 3000

Practice Manager Wendy Loveridge

GP Brian John DICKER, Susan Caryl EDWARDS

Limes Medical Centre
Cooksey Road, Small Heath, Birmingham B10 0BS
Tel: 0121 772 0067
(Heart of Birmingham Teaching Primary Care Trust)
Patient List Size: 5300

Practice Manager Jessica Campbell

GP Vinod Kumar DADHEECH, Hima H. DADHEECH

Lordswood House
54 Lordswood Road, Harborne, Birmingham B17 9DB
Tel: 0121 426 2030 Fax: 0121 428 2658
(South Birmingham Primary Care Trust)

Practice Manager J Marriott

GP Malcolm Greig EDWARD, Ewan HAMNETT, Roisin Helen Anne JORDAN, T M MULCAHY, Gavin Robert Duthie RALSTON, Marion SIMPSON, William VANMARLE, Joanne Tracey WHITELEY

Mabarak Health Centre
8-12 Cannon Hill Road, Balsall Heath, Birmingham B12 9NN
Tel: 0121 440 4666 Fax: 0121 446 5986
(Heart of Birmingham Teaching Primary Care Trust)

Practice Manager M Issaq, I Khan

GP Syed Z AHMAD, Mohammad Bazlay KARIM, Mohammad Shahabuddin RAHBER

Maypole Health Centre
10 Sladepool Farm Road, Kings Heath, Birmingham B14 5DJ
Tel: 0121 430 2829 Fax: 0121 430 6080
(South Birmingham Primary Care Trust)

Practice Manager Mike Pealing

GP Soong Loy YAP, Philipp Andreaus CONRADI, Jacqueline Mary HUGHES

Maypole Health Centre
10 Sladepool Farm Road, Kings Heath, Birmingham B14 5DJ
Tel: 0121 430 5551 Fax: 0121 430 6156
(South Birmingham Primary Care Trust)

Practice Manager Kumud Acharya

GP M P ACHARYA

Medical Centre
Craig Croft, Chelmsley Wood, Birmingham B37 7TR
Tel: 0121 770 5656 Fax: 0121 779 5619
(Solihull Primary Care Trust)

Practice Manager G Davies

GP Dennis Martin ALLIN, Jennifer Ann BENT, M R BOSWORTH, Suriyakumaran DHARMARATNAM, Alison Dorothy Margaret HALES, Richard Thomas POMEROY, Barry Philip YOUNG

Millennium Medical Centre
121 Weoley Castle Road, Weoley Castle, Birmingham B29 5QD
Tel: 0121 427 5201 Fax: 0121 427 5052
Email: mmcentre@lineone.net

(South Birmingham Primary Care Trust)
Patient List Size: 7500

Practice Manager Karen Woodley

GP Peter Paul BORG-BARTOLO, M BOSE, S GOHIL, H RIGBY, Elizabeth Janet WIGLEY

Mirfield Surgery

Scholars Gate, Lea Village, Birmingham B33 0DL
Tel: 0121 785 0795
(Eastern Birmingham Primary Care Trust)
Patient List Size: 3000

Practice Manager Martin Saunders

GP Andrew Leslie GOLDSTEIN

Mirfield Surgery

Scholars Gate, Lea Village, Birmingham B33 0DL
Tel: 0121 789 7607 Fax: 0121 686 4542
(Eastern Birmingham Primary Care Trust)
Patient List Size: 2000

GP Prakash Kumar SAHAY

Misra

Soho Health Centre, Louise Road, Handsworth, Birmingham B21 0RY
Tel: 0121 554 9929 Fax: 0121 507 1527
(Heart of Birmingham Teaching Primary Care Trust)
Patient List Size: 3000

Practice Manager M Misra

GP Unnati Sundri MISRA, Jattinder KUMAR

Moonga

726 Coventry Road, Small Heath, Birmingham B10 0TU
Tel: 0121 773 2094 Fax: 0121 753 0334
(Heart of Birmingham Teaching Primary Care Trust)
Patient List Size: 2800

Practice Manager P K Moonga

GP Paramjit Singh MOONGA

Moor Green Lane Medical Centre

339 Moor Green Lane, Moseley, Birmingham B13 8QS
Tel: 0121 472 6959 Fax: 0121 415 4533
Website: www.surgeriesonline.com/moorgreenlane.mc
(Heart of Birmingham Teaching Primary Care Trust)
Patient List Size: 3374

Practice Manager Jenny Brisroc

GP Raja Segar RAMACHANDRAM, Geeti RAJ, Saima SALIM

Moseley Medical Centre

21 Salisbury Road, Moseley, Birmingham B13 8JS
Tel: 0121 449 0122 Fax: 0121 449 6262
(South Birmingham Primary Care Trust)

GP Jegatheswary SOMASUNDARA-RAJAH, Kandiah SOMASUNDARA-RAJAH

New Road Surgery

104-106 New Road, Rubery, Birmingham B45 9HY
Tel: 0121 453 3584 Fax: 0121 4578443
(Redditch and Bromsgrove Primary Care Trust)

Practice Manager Ann Blackburn

GP J M BODEN, J N H CHEETHAM, M R COOPER

New St Clement's Surgery

56 Nechells Park Road, Nechells, Birmingham B7 5PR
Tel: 0121 327 0147
(Heart of Birmingham Teaching Primary Care Trust)
Patient List Size: 4500

Practice Manager Angela Hargun

GP A S GASPAR, I COX, B JONES

Newtown Health Centre

171 Melbourne Avenue, Newtown, Birmingham B19 2JA
Tel: 0121 554 7541 Fax: 0121 515 4447
(Heart of Birmingham Teaching Primary Care Trust)

Practice Manager Seeta Mahi

GP Subrata RAY, Sarah Victoria Ann BENN, Pramod Kumar MISRA, Samar MUKHERJEE, Rajaiyengar MURALIDHAR

Northwood Medical Centre

10/12 Middleton Hall Road, Kings Norton, Birmingham B30 1BY
Tel: 0121 458 1342 Fax: 0121 458 6921
(South Birmingham Primary Care Trust)

Practice Manager Kirstie York

GP Christopher Jeremy SMART, Matthew Charles DAKIN, Philip Arthur Peter MORGAN, Christopher Michael POTTER, Naila Yasmin SYED

The Oaks Medical Centre

669 Kings Road, Great Barr, Birmingham B44 9HU
Tel: 0121 360 7360
(North Birmingham Primary Care Trust)

Practice Manager Carol Claridge

GP Gertrud Ingeborg Maria BUERSTEDDE, Tow Kwung CHIAM, Richard John DENNING, Gurpreet Kaur KHAIRA, Rajasundram S KUMAR, Sonia L LLOYD, Jawahir Ratilal NAIK

The Old Mill Surgery

22 Speedwell Road, Edgbaston, Birmingham B5 7QA
Tel: 0121 440 4215 Fax: 0121 446 4302
Email: badri.narayan@hobpct.nhs.uk
(Heart of Birmingham Teaching Primary Care Trust)
Patient List Size: 2400

Practice Manager Shabnam Khan

GP Badri Singh NARAYAN, D CROWE

The Old Priory Surgery

319 Vicarage Road, Kings Heath, Birmingham B14 7NN
Tel: 0121 444 1120 Fax: 0121 683 8485
(South Birmingham Primary Care Trust)

Practice Manager Brian Elliott

GP Timothy John HUGHES, Mark St. John GROCUTT, Karen A WATSON

Parkes

Nechells Green Health Centre, 64 Denby Close, Nechells, Birmingham B7 4PF
Tel: 0121 359 2046 Fax: 0121 333 6493
(Heart of Birmingham Teaching Primary Care Trust)

GP Stephen John PARKES

Parkview

Moseley Hall Hospital, Alcester Road, Moseley, Birmingham B13 8JL
Tel: 0121 449 4999 Fax: 0121 442 5635
(South Birmingham Primary Care Trust)

Perry Park Surgery

291 Walsall Road, Perry Barr, Birmingham B42 1TY
Tel: 0121 356 4131
(North Birmingham Primary Care Trust)

GP Kamal Jeet ARORA, Parmjit Singh ARORA

Philip Clarke Medical Centre

1026 Alcester Road South, Kings Heath, Birmingham B14 5NG
Tel: 0121 430 5150 Fax: 0121 436 7274
(South Birmingham Primary Care Trust)
Patient List Size: 2500

Practice Manager Usha Velineni

GP J HARI GOPAL, P SAMRAJYA-LAKSHMI

Poplars Surgery

17 Holly Lane, Erdington, Birmingham B24 9JN
Tel: 0121 373 4216 Fax: 0121 382 9576
(North Birmingham Primary Care Trust)
Patient List Size: 9800

Practice Manager H A Newey

GP Robert Clive BRAKE, Simon Nicholas CLAY, Clive Simeon CROCKER, Adam ISMAIL, Misha VOLKMANSKY, Amantha WALKER

Prasad, Blackford, Commander and Ormiunu
6 Dyas Road, Great Barr, Birmingham B44 8SF
Tel: 0121 373 1885/373 0916 Fax: 0121 382 4907/350 4658
(Eastern Birmingham Primary Care Trust)
Patient List Size: 6700

Practice Manager V Edwards

GP Kumar Tripurari PRASAD, Patrick BLACKFORD, Richard Anthony Dorian COMMANDER, Wilson ORMIUNU

Quinbourne Medical Practice
71 Fellows Lane, Harborne, Birmingham B17 9TX
Tel: 0121 427 1273
(South Birmingham Primary Care Trust)

Practice Manager Diane Payne

GP Shanti Parkash DIWAN, S BANHAM, A DALY, A PERRY

Quinton Family Practice
406 Quinton Road West, Quinton, Birmingham B32 1QG
Tel: 0121 421 6011 Fax: 0121 423 3089
(South Birmingham Primary Care Trust)
Patient List Size: 2260

Practice Manager Sandra Evans

GP John Charles RIDGWAY, Verity A WINGATE

Ramarao
Sparkbrook Health Centre, 32 Farm Road, Sparkbrook, Birmingham B11 1LS
Tel: 0121 773 2104
Email: mvramarao@aol.com
(Heart of Birmingham Teaching Primary Care Trust)
Patient List Size: 2989

Practice Manager Gillian Escott

GP Mallela Venkata RAMARAO

Ridgacre House Surgery
83 Ridgacre Road, Quinton, Birmingham B32 2TJ
Tel: 0121 422 3111
(South Birmingham Primary Care Trust)

Practice Manager L Houghton

GP Stephen BRINKSMAN, Maurice Hugh CONLON, Vanessa Claire MANLEY, Philip Bernard SAUNDERS

River Brook Medical Centre
3 River Brook Drive, Stirchley, Birmingham B30 2SH
Tel: 0121 451 2525 Fax: 0121 433 3214
(South Birmingham Primary Care Trust)
Patient List Size: 4610

Practice Manager Diane Moseley

GP Naresh CHAUHAN, Lisa SEABORNE, Linda Rae SHAPIRO, Elizabeth Jane STAMP

Rotton Park Medical Centre
264 Rotton Park Road, Edgbaston, Birmingham B16 0LU
Tel: 0121 429 2683
(Heart of Birmingham Teaching Primary Care Trust)

Practice Manager M Power

GP Inderjit Singh MAROK

Rotton Park Medical Centre
264 Rotton Park Road, Edgbaston, Birmingham B16 0LU
Tel: 0121 429 1543
(Heart of Birmingham Teaching Primary Care Trust)
Patient List Size: 1500

Practice Manager Margaret Power

GP I MAROK, Dr GILL, R HOPKINS

Roychoudhury
Nechells Green Health Centre, 64 Denby Close, Nechells, Birmingham B7 4PF
Tel: 0121 359 2046 Fax: 0121 333 6493
(Heart of Birmingham Teaching Primary Care Trust)

GP Manik ROYCHOUDHURY

Saltley Centre for Health
Cradock Road, Saltley, Birmingham B8 1RZ
(Eastern Birmingham Primary Care Trust)

GP M G SHANKERNARAYAN, P SHANKERNARAYAN

Saltley Centre for Health Care
Craddock Road, Saltley, Birmingham B8 1RZ
Tel: 0121 327 6444 Fax: 0121 327 2413
(Eastern Birmingham Primary Care Trust)

GP Anup Chandra BAJPAI, Samarendra L SENGUPTA

Saltley Centre for Health Care
Craddock Road, Saltley, Birmingham B8 1RZ
Tel: 0121 327 3321
(Eastern Birmingham Primary Care Trust)

GP Munuswamy Govindarjula SHANKERNARAYAN, Padmaja SHANKER NARAYAN

Satis House
10 Birmingham Road, Water Orton, Birmingham B46 1TH
Tel: 0121 776 7572
(North Warwickshire Primary Care Trust)

GP Mark Nicholas STREET

Selly Oak Health Centre
Katie Road, Selly Oak, Birmingham B29 6JG
Tel: 0121 472 0016 Fax: 0121 472 4912
Website: www.wmids.nhs.uk
(South Birmingham Primary Care Trust)
Patient List Size: 4743

Practice Manager Christine Perks

GP Taufeeq Ahmad SALAR, Dr BECKER

Selly Park Surgery
2 Reaview Drive, Pershore Road, Stirchley, Birmingham B29 7NT
Tel: 0121 472 0187 Fax: 0121 472 0187
(South Birmingham Primary Care Trust)
Patient List Size: 4500

Practice Manager Diane Morgan

GP Patrick Sidney IRELAND, Henry DAVIS, Sarah Gillian PLATT, Laura RUMMENS, Emma SAUNDERS

Severn House Surgery
96 Albert Road, Stechford, Birmingham B33 8AG
Tel: 0121 784 0208 Fax: 0121 789 7351
(Eastern Birmingham Primary Care Trust)

GP Juggit Singh SANGHERA

Severn House Surgery
96 Albert Road, Stechford, Birmingham B33 8AG
Tel: 0121 783 2893 Fax: 0121 785 0914
Email: drwatson@dtn.ntl.com
(Eastern Birmingham Primary Care Trust)
Patient List Size: 1950

GP David Norman WATSON

Shenley Green Surgery
22 Shenley Green, Selly Oak, Birmingham B29 4HH
Tel: 0121 475 7997 Fax: 0121 475 9239
(South Birmingham Primary Care Trust)
Patient List Size: 5707

Practice Manager A Bradshaw, Vicki Chambers, Lynn Goodyear

GP Mayank Mahendraprasad SHASTRI, Andres ENRIQUEZ-PUGA, Katerina GASPAR, Amanda Susan SINCLAIR

Sherwood House Medical Practice
9 Sandon Road, Edgbaston, Birmingham B17 8DP
Tel: 0121 420 0100 Fax: 0121 420 0107
(Oldbury and Smethwick Primary Care Trust)

Practice Manager Karen Woodley

GP Marek Jerzy MORTIMER, Hiltrud Agnes HOFMANN, Ann Elizabeth Gieszczykiewicz JARON, James KAY, James KAY, A J LAM, Lawrence Francis MILLER

Shilpa Medical Centre
1C Ashfield Avenue, Kings Heath, Birmingham B14 7AT
Tel: 0121 444 2668 Fax: 0121 441 1092
(South Birmingham Primary Care Trust)
Patient List Size: 3900

Practice Manager Susan Whitehouse

GP Saroj ADLAKHA

Small Health Medical Practice
2 Great Wood Road, Small Heath, Birmingham B10 9QE
Tel: 0121 766 8828 Fax: 0121 772 0097
(Eastern Birmingham Primary Care Trust)

Practice Manager Julie Patrick

GP James Antony MURRAY, M G O'GARA, Paul Howard ROPER, Helen Ruth SWEENEY

Soho Health Centre
Louise Road, Handsworth, Birmingham B21 0RY
Tel: 0121 523 2343 Fax: 0121 507 1607
Email: mohan.sainil@pc.birmingham.wmids.nhs.uk
(Heart of Birmingham Teaching Primary Care Trust)
Patient List Size: 2300

Practice Manager Lorna Dooley-Lynch

GP Mohan Singh SAINI

Soho Health Centre
Louise Road, Handsworth, Birmingham B21 0RY
Tel: 0121 554 4200
(Heart of Birmingham Teaching Primary Care Trust)

GP Mushtaque E AHMAD

Soho Health Centre
Louise Road, Handsworth, Birmingham B21 0RY
(Heart of Birmingham Teaching Primary Care Trust)

GP A P THOMPSON

Southgate Surgery
11 Bournbrook Road, Selly Oak, Birmingham B29 7BL
Tel: 0121 415 5237 Fax: 0121 472 5414
Website: www.southgatesurgery.net
(South Birmingham Primary Care Trust)
Patient List Size: 1487

Practice Manager Julie Billington

GP Rashmi Rohit MEHTA

Springfield Medical Practice
739-741 Stratford Road, Springfield, Birmingham B11 4DG
Tel: 0121 778 4422 Fax: 0121 702 2662
(Heart of Birmingham Teaching Primary Care Trust)

GP Satpal RAJPUT, Vijay Kumar RAJPUT

Sreerangaiah
St James Medical Centre, 85 Crocketts Road, Handsworth, Birmingham B21 0HR
Tel: 0121 523 6333 Fax: 0121 551 2099
(Heart of Birmingham Teaching Primary Care Trust)
Patient List Size: 2200

Practice Manager Mary Nunn

GP Thiriveedula SREERANGAIAH

St James Medical Centre
85 Crocketts Road, Handsworth, Birmingham B21 0HR
Tel: 0121 554 2980 Fax: 0121 553 9373
(Heart of Birmingham Teaching Primary Care Trust)
Patient List Size: 2498

Practice Manager Santina Deng

GP Zakariah Bol DENG

Stechford Health Centre
393 Station Road, Stechford, Birmingham B33 8PL
Tel: 0121 784 8101 Fax: 0121 785 0565
Email: aida.zaki@pc.birminghamha.wmids.nhs.uk
(Eastern Birmingham Primary Care Trust)
Patient List Size: 2400

Practice Manager Sonia Messih

GP Aida Said ZAKI

Stetchford Health Centre
393 Station Road, Stechford, Birmingham B33 8PL
Tel: 0121 783 2109 Fax: 0121 785 0619
(Eastern Birmingham Primary Care Trust)
Patient List Size: 1400

Practice Manager E Miller

GP M ATTALL

Stockland Green Health Centre
192 Reservoir Road, Erdington, Birmingham B23 6DJ
Tel: 0121 384 8244 Fax: 0121 377 6199
(Eastern Birmingham Primary Care Trust)

Practice Manager Joan Micah-Jones

GP Jaiker Rao KUMBLE

Stockland Green Health Centre
192 Reservoir Road, Erdington, Birmingham B23 6DJ
Tel: 0121 373 5405 Fax: 0121 386 4909
(Eastern Birmingham Primary Care Trust)

Practice Manager J Smith, Judith Williams

GP Mohamed Tariq NAZKI, Mark Mitchell Stirrat WARDLAW

Strensham Road Surgery
4 Strensham Road, Balsall Heath, Birmingham B12 9RR
Tel: 0121 440 3720 Fax: 0121 440 0591
(Heart of Birmingham Teaching Primary Care Trust)
Patient List Size: 3000

Practice Manager Sylvia Salmon

GP Omar Abd-El Aziz EL-SHEIKH, Ahmed ISSA

The Surgery
691 Coventry Road, Small Heath, Birmingham B10 0JL
Tel: 0121 773 4931 Fax: 0121 753 2210
(Heart of Birmingham Teaching Primary Care Trust)
Patient List Size: 7300

Practice Manager Jenny Hall

GP Jonathan Nicholas ALLCOCK, Jeremy Martin John CHAMBERS, Fatin Saleh HAIDER, Amjid RIAZ

The Surgery
192 Charles Road, Small Heath, Birmingham B10 9AB
Tel: 0121 772 0398 Fax: 0121 772 4268
(Heart of Birmingham Teaching Primary Care Trust)
Patient List Size: 4500

Practice Manager Y Husain

GP Santosh Kumar VERMA, Syed Ali ZAFAR

The Surgery
58 Benton Road, Sparkbrook, Birmingham B11 1TX
Tel: 0121 773 4622 Fax: 0121 766 7248
(Heart of Birmingham Teaching Primary Care Trust)

Practice Manager M Y Butt

GP Saima Sajjad KHATTAK, Sajjad Hussain KHATTAK

The Surgery
220 Warwick Road, Sparkhill, Birmingham B11 2NB
Tel: 0121 766 6113
(Heart of Birmingham Teaching Primary Care Trust)
Patient List Size: 3750

Practice Manager R Agarwal

GP Murli Dhar AGARWAL

The Surgery
578 Stratford Road, Sparkhill, Birmingham B11 4AN
Tel: 0121 772 0392 Fax: 0121 766 7509
(Heart of Birmingham Teaching Primary Care Trust)
Patient List Size: 6500

GP Martin Graham HALL, Govinder Singh JASSEL, Balwinder Singh MAVI

The Surgery
Fernley Medical Centre, 560 Stratford Road, Sparkhill, Birmingham B11 4AN
Tel: 0121 772 0284 Fax: 0121 766 5102
(Heart of Birmingham Teaching Primary Care Trust)
Patient List Size: 5500

Practice Manager Nora Grosvenor

GP Syed Yousef SHAH, A B MANN, T L POLTOCK

The Surgery
26 Oakwood Road, Sparkhill, Birmingham B11 4HA
Tel: 0121 777 3082
(Heart of Birmingham Teaching Primary Care Trust)
Patient List Size: 5806

Practice Manager Josephine Shah

GP Farouk K KARZOUN, Shahid Khurshid GILL, Shamim SONDAY

The Surgery
23 Showell Green Lane, Sparkhill, Birmingham B11 4NP
Tel: 0121 766 8447 Fax: 0121 753 0543
(Heart of Birmingham Teaching Primary Care Trust)

Practice Manager H Shirazi

GP Helmy Morcos GUIRGUIS

The Surgery
234 Stoney Lane, Sparkhill, Birmingham B12 8AW
Tel: 0121 449 9685
(Heart of Birmingham Teaching Primary Care Trust)

GP Bashir AHMED

The Surgery
158 Alcester Road South, Kings Heath, Birmingham B14 6AA
Tel: 0121 444 1186 Fax: 0121 444 1094
(South Birmingham Primary Care Trust)
Patient List Size: 2200

Practice Manager Andrea Mitchell

GP Mubashar Ahmad SALEEM

The Surgery
302 Vicarage Road, Kings Heath, Birmingham B14 7NH
Tel: 0121 444 5959 Fax: 0121 441 5040
(South Birmingham Primary Care Trust)

Practice Manager Sushila Verma

GP Amar Nath VERMA

The Surgery
13 Lozells Street, Lozells, Birmingham B19 2AU
Tel: 0121 554 3386 Fax: 0121 523 8439
(Heart of Birmingham Teaching Primary Care Trust)
Patient List Size: 3085

Practice Manager Hafiza Petkar

GP Riyaz AHMED

The Surgery
139 Hamstead Road, Handsworth, Birmingham B20 2BT
Tel: 0121 551 1062 Fax: 0121 551 1618
(Heart of Birmingham Teaching Primary Care Trust)

Practice Manager J T Abhyankar

GP Uday Sadashiv ABHYANKAR

The Surgery
2 The Slieve, Handsworth Wood, Birmingham B20 2NR
Tel: 0121 554 1812 Fax: 0121 554 6830
(Heart of Birmingham Teaching Primary Care Trust)

GP Christopher James FAWCETT, Karl Hilario Reloj ALONZO

The Surgery
190 Aston Lane, Handsworth, Birmingham B20 3HE
Tel: 0121 356 4669 Fax: 0121 356 7020
(Heart of Birmingham Teaching Primary Care Trust)
Patient List Size: 4500

Practice Manager J Shannon

GP Philip BICKLEY, Douglas Neil SALMON

The Surgery
122 Sutton Road, Erdington, Birmingham B23 5TJ
Tel: 0121 373 0056 Fax: 0121 382 3212
(Eastern Birmingham Primary Care Trust)

Practice Manager Sharma Shariff

GP Umadevi VALSALAN, Mehboob Elahi BHATTI

The Surgery
157-159 Reservoir Road, Erdington, Birmingham B23 6DN
Tel: 0121 373 0601 Fax: 0121 373 3263
(Eastern Birmingham Primary Care Trust)

Practice Manager E Archer-Richards

GP John Andrew SHERLAW, Glyn Wedmore DURSTON, Turaabali Mohamedali Jivanjee GANIWALLA, Shirley Rachel SHERLAW

The Surgery
160 Streetly Road, Erdington, Birmingham B23 7BD
Tel: 0121 350 2323 Fax: 0121 382 0169
(Eastern Birmingham Primary Care Trust)

Practice Manager Paul Glover

GP Edward HISCOCK, S HEATH, Joanne Mary KING, Rodney Julian Wesley THOMPSON, Mary Beverley WELLS

The Surgery
115 Humberstone Road, Erdington, Birmingham B24 0PY
Tel: 0121 351 3321 Fax: 0121 313 0919
(Eastern Birmingham Primary Care Trust)

Practice Manager Rosemary Chapman

GP Ariaratnam SELLARAJAH

The Surgery
1222 Coventry Road, Hay Mills, Birmingham B25 8BY
Tel: 0121 772 1898 Fax: 0121 608 1222
(Eastern Birmingham Primary Care Trust)

Practice Manager V B Pattni

GP Bhikhu Ladhabhai PATTNI

The Surgery
15 Rowlands Road, Yardley, Birmingham B26 1AT
Tel: 0121 706 6623 Fax: 0121 706 9888
(Eastern Birmingham Primary Care Trust)

Practice Manager N Peddi

GP Dr PEDDI, Vasundhara KANDULA

The Surgery
172 Garretts Green Lane, Sheldon, Birmingham B26 2SB
Tel: 0121 743 3003
(Eastern Birmingham Primary Care Trust)

GP Raksha CHOPRA

The Surgery
1 Manor House Lane, Yardley, Birmingham B26 1PE
Tel: 0121 743 2273 Fax: 0121 722 2037
(Solihull Primary Care Trust)
Patient List Size: 7800

Practice Manager S P Wilson

GP V SAGOO, M BUTT, F HARDY, R SYED

The Surgery
191 Barrows Lane, Yardley, Birmingham B26 1QS
Tel: 0121 783 2719

(Eastern Birmingham Primary Care Trust)
Patient List Size: 2600

Practice Manager G Wadhwa

GP Harish Kumar WADHWA

The Surgery

315 Sheldon Heath Road, Sheldon, Birmingham B26 2TY
Tel: 0121 743 2626 Fax: 0121 244 8383
(Eastern Birmingham Primary Care Trust)
Patient List Size: 3166

Practice Manager John Pegg

GP Naguib Edward GABALLA

The Surgery

2314 Coventry Road, Sheldon, Birmingham B26 3JS
Tel: 0121 743 2154 Fax: 0121 743 9970
(Solihull Primary Care Trust)
Patient List Size: 4500

GP Nicola Judith GOODE, Richard Franklyn HARROWER, Susan Irene HARROWER

The Surgery

25 Cranes Park Road, Sheldon, Birmingham B26 3SE
Tel: 0121 743 2018 Fax: 0121 743 7688
(Eastern Birmingham Primary Care Trust)
Patient List Size: 2400

GP Mokhlis Mina Mikhail MINA, Mary Talaat MINA

The Surgery

169-171 Church Road, Sheldon, Birmingham B26 3TT
Tel: 0121 743 5511 Fax: 0121 693 9797
(Eastern Birmingham Primary Care Trust)
Patient List Size: 2000

Practice Manager Parmjit Jheetha

GP Bhinder Singh JHEETA

The Surgery

189 Shirley Road, Acocks Green, Birmingham B27 7NP
Tel: 0121 706 5131 Fax: 0121 706 7593
(South Birmingham Primary Care Trust)
Patient List Size: 3150

Practice Manager Sarah Florey

GP Terence Rodney PRITCHARD, C B CROCKER

The Surgery

179 Alvechurch Road, West Heath, Birmingham B31 3PN
Tel: 0121 475 1550
(South Birmingham Primary Care Trust)

GP Gulshan Rai ARORA, Padma ARORA

The Surgery

Selcroft Avenue, Quinton, Birmingham B32 2BX
Tel: 0121 428 2880
(South Birmingham Primary Care Trust)

GP Anthony St John DALY, Mary Patricia GREENE

The Surgery

113 Church Lane, Stechford, Birmingham B33 9EJ
Tel: 0121 783 2861 Fax: 0121 785 0585
Email: linda.hanos@pc.birminghamha.wmids.nhs.uk
(Eastern Birmingham Primary Care Trust)
Patient List Size: 3100

Practice Manager Linda Hanos

GP Hosne Ara AHAMED, I KHAN

The Surgery

36 Bucklands End Lane, Castle Bromwich, Birmingham B34 6BP
Tel: 0121 747 2160 Fax: 0121 747 3425
(Eastern Birmingham Primary Care Trust)

Practice Manager Barbara Wilkins

GP Madhavi Mohan LATTHE, Ramchandra KESHRI

The Surgery

2 Schoolacre Road, Shard End, Birmingham B34 6RB
Tel: 0121 747 2911 Fax: 0121 730 3006
(Eastern Birmingham Primary Care Trust)

Practice Manager S D Bailey

GP Maureen Elizabeth BROOMHEAD, Daniel John HOGAN

The Surgery

140 Coleshill Road, Hodge Hill, Birmingham B36 8AD
Tel: 0121 776 6444 Fax: 0121 688 4544
(Eastern Birmingham Primary Care Trust)
Patient List Size: 2370

Practice Manager Sabitha Pai

GP Srinivas Hemachandra PAI

The Surgery

Aston University, The Aston Traingle, Birmingham B4 7ET
Tel: 0121 359 3611 Fax: 0121 333 6023
Website: astonuniversityhealthcentre.co.uk
(Heart of Birmingham Teaching Primary Care Trust)
Patient List Size: 7281

Practice Manager Angela Hegan

GP Matthew Yau Leung NYE, Nishpal KANG, Prasanna NARAYAN

The Surgery

134 Newton Road, Great Barr, Birmingham B43 6BT
Tel: 0121 357 3309
(Wednesbury and West Bromwich Primary Care Trust)

Practice Manager Lisa Astbury

GP Dinesh Prasad AMBASHT

The Surgery

Sundial Lane, Great Barr, Birmingham B43 6PA
Tel: 0121 358 0082
(Wednesbury and West Bromwich Primary Care Trust)

Practice Manager Elaine Woakes

GP Abu Saleh Mohammad Matinur RAHMAN, Sally-Anne RAHMAN

The Surgery

522 Queslett Road, Great Barr, Birmingham B43 7DY
Tel: 0121 360 8560 Fax: 0121 360 6833
(Walsall Teaching Primary Care Trust)
Patient List Size: 1682

Practice Manager S V Reddy

GP Sanampudi RAMI REDDY

The Surgery

Aylesbury House, Warren Farm Road, Kingstanding, Birmingham B44 0DX
Tel: 0121 373 1078
(North Birmingham Primary Care Trust)

GP Deedar Singh BHOMRA

The Surgery

352 College Road, Erdington, Birmingham B44 0HH
Tel: 0121 373 1244
(North Birmingham Primary Care Trust)
Patient List Size: 8300

GP Graeme HORTON, John Martin COLLARD, Sarah Mary LONG, Sanjeev SARIN

The Surgery

Kingsmount, 444 Kingstanding Road, Kingstanding, Birmingham B44 9SA
Tel: 0121 373 1734 Fax: 0121 377 8292
(North Birmingham Primary Care Trust)

Practice Manager Sandra Green

GP John Andrew SENIOR, Michael Kevin DOWNES, Ian Stewart SKINGLE

The Surgery
65 New Road, Rubery, Birmingham B45 9JT
Tel: 0121 453 3591 Fax: 0121 457 7217
(South Birmingham Primary Care Trust)
Patient List Size: 4150

Practice Manager Angela Styring

GP David Mark FERNELL, Andrew William Alberic WIJNBERG

The Surgery
28 Church Road, Aston, Birmingham B6 5UP
Tel: 0121 327 2348
(Heart of Birmingham Teaching Primary Care Trust)
Patient List Size: 4300

Practice Manager A Care

GP Murari Nand MISHRA, Mukesh SINHA

The Surgery
91 Little Oaks Road, Aston, Birmingham B6 6JX
Tel: 0121 327 0327
(Heart of Birmingham Teaching Primary Care Trust)

GP Harinder Jit SINGH

The Surgery
30 Bloomsbury Street, Nechells, Birmingham B7 5BS
Tel: 0121 359 1539
(Heart of Birmingham Teaching Primary Care Trust)

GP Eamon Joseph McQUILLAN

The Surgery
75-77 Cotterills Lane, Alum Rock, Birmingham B8 3RZ
Tel: 0121 327 5111 Fax: 0121 327 5111
(Eastern Birmingham Primary Care Trust)
Patient List Size: 1258

Practice Manager Linda Edwards

GP Muhammad Younus SAIGOL

The Surgery
183A Woodlands Road, Sparkhill, Birmingham B11 4ER
Tel: 0121 778 5439 Fax: 0121 777 0205
Website: springfieldsurgery.com
(Heart of Birmingham Teaching Primary Care Trust)

Practice Manager Janice Williams

GP Pamela Mary BEYER, Andrew MELCHOIR

The Surgery
1 Newport Road, Balsall Heath, Birmingham B12 8QE
Tel: 0121 449 1327 Fax: 0121 449 5540
(Heart of Birmingham Teaching Primary Care Trust)
Patient List Size: 6280

GP Bashir AHMED, Agha Mohammad HAROON

The Surgery
157-159 Rotton Park Road, Edgbaston, Birmingham B16 0LJ
Tel: 0121 454 0508
(Heart of Birmingham Teaching Primary Care Trust)
Patient List Size: 1500

Practice Manager Catherine Walters

GP Mohammad SALIM

The Surgery
153 Grove Lane, Handsworth, Birmingham B20 2HE
Tel: 0121 554 2493
(Heart of Birmingham Teaching Primary Care Trust)

GP Jerbinder Kaur BANSEL

The Surgery
93 Crompton Road, Handsworth, Birmingham B20 3QP
Tel: 0121 523 0427
(Heart of Birmingham Teaching Primary Care Trust)
Patient List Size: 3000

Practice Manager Surjit Mall

GP Mujeeb Ahmed KHAN

The Surgery
38 Radnor Road, Handsworth, Birmingham B20 3SR
Tel: 0121 554 0070
(Heart of Birmingham Teaching Primary Care Trust)

GP John William Edward JOHNSON

The Surgery
133 Heathfield Road, Handsworth, Birmingham B19 1HL
Tel: 0121 255 4400
(Heart of Birmingham Teaching Primary Care Trust)
Patient List Size: 3262

GP Shiverdorayi RAGHAVAN

The Surgery
174 Rookery Road, Handsworth, Birmingham B21 9NN
Tel: 0121 554 0921
(Heart of Birmingham Teaching Primary Care Trust)

GP Anil Kumar ADAK, Andrew Paul THOMPSON

The Surgery
273 Kingsbury Road, Erdington, Birmingham B24 8RD
Tel: 0121 382 7539 Fax: 0121 386 2482
(Eastern Birmingham Primary Care Trust)

Practice Manager Linda Jeffs

GP Prem Singh JHITTAY

The Surgery
1 Wash Lane, Yardley, Birmingham B25 8SB
Tel: 0121 783 2603
(Eastern Birmingham Primary Care Trust)

GP Bernard Arthur JUBY

The Surgery
194 Sheldon Heath Road, Sheldon, Birmingham B26 2DR
Tel: 0121 743 4444 Fax: 0121 7222044
(Eastern Birmingham Primary Care Trust)

Practice Manager Nindi Sandhu

GP Jagjit Singh SANDHU, Z AMJAD, Vijay BHASKAR, A BHATTACHARYYA

The Surgery
90 Church Road, Sheldon, Birmingham B26 3TP
Tel: 0121 743 3409 Fax: 0121 742 5939
(Eastern Birmingham Primary Care Trust)
Patient List Size: 10651

Practice Manager Christina Machs

GP Paul MACHIN, A BHATT, Jacqueline Ann DOMINEY, Gerwyn James EDWARDS, Richard Charles EVANS

The Surgery
108 Banbury Road, Northfield, Birmingham B31 2DN
Tel: 0121 475 1050 Fax: 0121 476 5847
(South Birmingham Primary Care Trust)

Practice Manager Tina Sham

GP Nasinder BARHEY, L KANG, Sui-Yuen SHAM

The Surgery
263 Tile Cross Road, Tile Cross, Birmingham B33 0NA
Tel: 0121 779 7333 Fax: 0121 770 8432
(Eastern Birmingham Primary Care Trust)

GP Hedathale V ANANTHARAMAN

The Surgery
37-39 Glebe Farm Road, Stechford, Birmingham B33 9LY
Tel: 0121 783 3803
(Eastern Birmingham Primary Care Trust)

GP Aquila KHAN, N AHMAD

The Surgery
119 Sheldon Heath Road, Sheldon, Birmingham B26 2DP
Tel: 0121 784 5465 Fax: 0121 789 6707
(Solihull Primary Care Trust)

Practice Manager L Walsh

GP Patrick Dorairaj SIMON, S K SURYANI

The Surgery
406c Chester Road, Castle Bromwich, Birmingham B36 0LF
Tel: 0121 770 3035 Fax: 0121 779 7109
(Solihull Primary Care Trust)
Patient List Size: 3100

Practice Manager Karen Bense

GP Peter Edward SCOTT

The Surgery
117 Brockhurst Road, Ward End, Birmingham B36 8JE
Tel: 0121 783 2642
(Eastern Birmingham Primary Care Trust)

GP Renu RASTOGI

The Surgery
95 Tamar Drive, Chelmsley Wood, Birmingham B36 0SY
Tel: 0121 749 1313 Fax: 0121 749 3420
Email: tartam.isaac@nhs.uk
(Solihull Primary Care Trust)
Patient List Size: 2400

Practice Manager Prema Pillai

GP Dulichand T ISAAC, Stella ISAAC

The Surgery
107 Warren Road, Kingstanding, Birmingham B44 8QL
Tel: 0121 373 1511
(North Birmingham Primary Care Trust)
Patient List Size: 1200

Practice Manager Adele Morrison Jolley

GP Masud AHAMED

The Surgery
432 Kingstanding Road, Kingstanding, Birmingham B44 9SA
Tel: 0121 377 8244 Fax: 0121 350 0150
(North Birmingham Primary Care Trust)

Practice Manager Margaret Power

GP Patrick GONSALVES

The Surgery
2048 Bristol Road, Rubery, Birmingham B45 9JL
Tel: 0121 457 7966
(South Birmingham Primary Care Trust)

GP David John WEDDELL

The Surgery
229 Victoria Road, Aston, Birmingham B6 5HP
Tel: 0121 327 5421
(Heart of Birmingham Teaching Primary Care Trust)

GP H J SINGH

The Surgery
119 Alum Rock Road, Saltley, Birmingham B8 1ND
Tel: 0121 327 0735
(Eastern Birmingham Primary Care Trust)

Practice Manager K Deathridge

GP Sheik A LATIF

The Surgery
13-15 Washwood Heath Road, Saltley, Birmingham B8 1SH
Tel: 0121 327 3926
(Eastern Birmingham Primary Care Trust)

GP Rashid Ahmed BHATTI

The Surgery
32-34 Naseby Road, Saltley, Birmingham B8 3HE
Tel: 0121 327 1878
(Eastern Birmingham Primary Care Trust)

GP Meraj Din SHEIK

The Surgery
170 Coventry Road, South Yardley, Birmingham B26 1DT
Tel: 0121 743 3003
(Eastern Birmingham Primary Care Trust)

GP K CHOPRA

The Surgery
82 Sandhurst Avenue, Hodge Hill, Birmingham B36 8EJ
Tel: 0121 255 4218 Fax: 0121 255 4222
(Eastern Birmingham Primary Care Trust)

The Surgery
168 Hamstead Road, Handsworth, Birmingham B20 2QR
(Heart of Birmingham Teaching Primary Care Trust)

GP R B CHITRE

The Swan Medical Centre
4 Willard Road, Yardley, Birmingham B25 8AA
Tel: 0121 706 0216 Fax: 0121 707 3105
(Eastern Birmingham Primary Care Trust)

GP David Raymond AYLIN, Karen Geraldine GALLACHER, Denys Bewdley NICOL, Barry TRICKLEBANK

Swanswell Medical Centre
370 Gospel Lane, Acocks Green, Birmingham B27 7AL
Tel: 0121 706 5676 Fax: 0121 765 0160
(Eastern Birmingham Primary Care Trust)
Patient List Size: 6700

Practice Manager Emma Dent

GP Martin Michael JONES, Julie BANCROFT, Philip Ernest Reinhardt SCHUPPLER

Tower Hill Medical Centre
25 Tower Hill, Great Barr, Birmingham B42 1LG
Tel: 0121 357 1077
(North Birmingham Primary Care Trust)

Practice Manager Adele Russon

GP David Kells O'Donel CALDERWOOD, Sirjit Singh BATH, Vivien Sandra CALDERWOOD, Debal K NANDI

University Medical Practice
University Medical Centre, 5 Pritchatts Road, Edgbaston, Birmingham B15 2QU
Tel: 0121 687 3055 Fax: 0121 687 3054
Email: pamela.brazier@pc.birminghamha.wmids.nhs.uk
Website: www.theump.co.uk
(South Birmingham Primary Care Trust)
Patient List Size: 20500

Practice Manager Susan Durbridge

GP S BASRA, Ann Rachel BOULTER, Esme Victoria Ann Pickernell HADFIELD, Vinay Hemant KETKAR, Victoria Alice LILFORD, Simon David RUMMENS

Victoria Road Surgery
21 Victoria Road, Acocks Green, Birmingham B27 7XZ
Tel: 0121 706 1129 Fax: 0121 765 4927
(Eastern Birmingham Primary Care Trust)

GP John CAMERON, Mary Elizabeth O'GORMAN

Wake Green Surgery
7 Wake Green Road, Moseley, Birmingham B13 9HD
Tel: 0121 449 0300 Fax: 0121 442 4057
(South Birmingham Primary Care Trust)
Patient List Size: 10800

Practice Manager Andrea Fray

GP David William KETT, Michael Spencer BAIRD, Catriona Margaret CROMBIE, Philippa Ann DANIELL, Vanessa Clare HORTON, Declan O'DONNELL

Walji
Balsall Heath Health Centre, 43 Edward Road, Balsall Heath, Birmingham B12 9LP
Tel: 0121 446 2500 Fax: 0121 440 5861

(Heart of Birmingham Teaching Primary Care Trust)
Patient List Size: 4200

Practice Manager F Doherty

GP Mohamed-Taki Ismail WALJI

Wand Medical Centre
279 Gooch Street, Highgate, Birmingham B5 7JE
Tel: 0121 440 1561 Fax: 0121 440 0060
(Heart of Birmingham Teaching Primary Care Trust)
Patient List Size: 7500

Practice Manager D M Mann

GP Kanji Harji VAJA, Fay WILSON, Alison Mary CARROLL, Judith Anne YATES

Ward End Medical Centre
794A Washwood Heath Road, Ward End, Birmingham B8 2JN
Tel: 0121 327 1049 Fax: 0121 327 0964
(Eastern Birmingham Primary Care Trust)

Practice Manager Pauline Thorne

GP Julia Marion TAYLOR, Ian David GOODWIN, John HODGSON, Roger John PAYNE, Mohamed Ally RAMJOHN

Weatheroak Medical Practice
35 Warwick Road, Sparkhill, Birmingham B11 4RA
Tel: 0121 772 0352
(Heart of Birmingham Teaching Primary Care Trust)
Patient List Size: 3200

GP Mohammad Nasrullah CHEEMA

Weoley Park Surgery
112 Weoley Park Road, Selly Oak, Birmingham B29 5HA
Tel: 0121 472 1965 Fax: 0121 415 5671
(South Birmingham Primary Care Trust)

Practice Manager Sue Hansard

GP R C ORMOND, A SINGH, M J UDOKANG

West Heath Surgery
196 West Heath Road, Northfield, Birmingham B31 3HB
Tel: 0121 476 1135 Fax: 0121 476 1138
(South Birmingham Primary Care Trust)
Patient List Size: 3330

Practice Manager Nirmal Vora

GP Ashok Kumar VORA

Woodgate Valley Practice
61 Stevens Avenue, Woodgate Valley, Birmingham B32 3SD
Tel: 0121 427 6174 Fax: 0121 428 4146
(South Birmingham Primary Care Trust)
Patient List Size: 4500

Practice Manager K Edwards

GP John Philip Quarrier WARD, Sarah WOZNIAK

Woodlands Road Surgery
57 Woodlands Road, Northfield, Birmingham B31 2HZ
Tel: 0121 475 1065 Fax: 0121 475 6179
(South Birmingham Primary Care Trust)
Patient List Size: 5065

Practice Manager Jenny Clark

GP Martin Paul ALLEN, Mehmet SHEVKET, David Geoffrey Barrie TAYLOR

Wychall Lane Surgery
11 Wychall Lane, Kings Norton, Birmingham B38 8TE
Tel: 0121 628 2345 Fax: 0121 628 8282
(South Birmingham Primary Care Trust)
Patient List Size: 9500

GP Christopher LEIGH, Jean-Claude DESVEAUX, Joanna Hilary McDONNELL, Guy St John RUSSELL, J SHERRINGTON, Richard Merlyn Laurence WILCOX

Wythall Health Centre
May Lane, Hollywood, Birmingham B47 5PD
Tel: 01564 822642 Fax: 01564 829319
Email: martin.chauhan@gp-m81064.nhs.uk
(Redditch and Bromsgrove Primary Care Trust)

Practice Manager Martin Chauhan

GP Anne Elizabeth FRANCIS, Stephen John MISKIN, Sarah Jo MOORE, Anthony Adeniyi OMO-DARE

Yardley Green Medical Centre
73 Yardley Green Road, Bordesley Green, Birmingham B9 5PU
Tel: 0121 773 3838 Fax: 0121 506 2005
Email: rachel.pardoe@ygmc.net
Website: www.ygmc.net
(Eastern Birmingham Primary Care Trust)
Patient List Size: 8300

Practice Manager Rachel Pardoe

GP Neil Peter BROWN, Katherine MARTIN, Elizabeth Shannon NYHOLM, Hunaid RASHIQ, Peter Jonathan THEBRIDGE, Helen WALT

Yardley Green Medical Centre
75 Yardley Green Road, Bordesley Green, Birmingham B9 5PU
Tel: 0121 773 3737
(Eastern Birmingham Primary Care Trust)
Patient List Size: 11700

Practice Manager Linda Parsons

GP Margaret LEWIS, Niall Aidan John MARTIN, Andrew STORER, Philip John TURPIN, Nicholas John Hamilton WADDELL, Kevin Alan Harold WOOLLASTON

Yardley Wood Health Centre
401 Highfield Road, Yardley Wood, Birmingham B14 4DU
Tel: 0121 474 5186 Fax: 0121 436 7648
(South Birmingham Primary Care Trust)
Patient List Size: 10000

Practice Manager Vicky Royston

GP Peter Frederick Franz CLARKE, Sandra Tina BANERJEE, Colin David EAGLE, Christopher John HOLLAND, M KELLY

Zuckerman, Felderhof and Ali
Northfield Health Centre, 15 St Heliers Road, Northfield, Birmingham B31 1QT
Tel: 0121 478 0220 Fax: 0121 476 0931
(South Birmingham Primary Care Trust)
Patient List Size: 5747

Practice Manager Bill Clements

GP Charles Howard ZUCKERMAN, Abad ALI, Jennifer Crawford FELDERHOF

Bishop Auckland

Auckland Medical Group
54 Cockton Hill Road, Bishop Auckland DL14 6BB
Tel: 01388 602728 Fax: 01388 607546
(Durham Dales Primary Care Trust)
Patient List Size: 12500

Practice Manager Susan Atkinson

GP Angus Hugh MACLEOD, Kenneth Russell AIRLIE, Gillian FORD, Catherine Maria Sarah HARRISON, Robert McMANNERS, Mark PRITCHARD, Mark Alistair WARD

Bishopgate Medical Centre
178 Newgate Street, Bishop Auckland DL14 7EJ
Tel: 01388 603983 Fax: 01388 607782
(Durham Dales Primary Care Trust)
Patient List Size: 13000

Practice Manager Philip Jackson

GP Brian Richard PIKE, Susan Elizabeth BENSTEAD, Paul BOWRON, Ian Sherwood BREMNER, Stewart Macpherson FINDLAY, Gordon Strachan McGREGOR

Charlton House
Rear High Street, Ton Law, Bishop Auckland DL13 4DH
Tel: 01388 730251
(Durham and Chester-le-Street Primary Care Trust)

GP Ellen-Ann FINNIGHAN

Pinfold Lane Surgery
Butterknowle, Bishop Auckland DL13 5NU
Tel: 01388 718230 Fax: 01388 718808
(Durham Dales Primary Care Trust)

Practice Manager F Currie

GP Julia Christine PICKWORTH, Richard PICKWORTH

South View Surgery
5 South View, Evenwood, Bishop Auckland DL14 9QS
Tel: 01388 832236 Fax: 01388 833479
(Durham Dales Primary Care Trust)
Patient List Size: 2100

Practice Manager Karen Thompson

GP Joseph Raymond SAID

Stanhope Health Centre
Dales Street, Stanhope, Bishop Auckland DL13 2XD
Tel: 01388 528555 Fax: 01388 526122
(Durham Dales Primary Care Trust)
Patient List Size: 7500

Practice Manager Toni Dickens

GP S BADYAL, Nicholas DEYTRIKH, Matthew Thomas Christian HACKETT, Stephen Andrew LUMB

Station View Medical Centre
29A Escomb Road, Bishop Auckland DL14 6AB
Tel: 01388 663539 Fax: 01388 601847
(Durham Dales Primary Care Trust)
Patient List Size: 10200

Practice Manager John Worrall

GP Ian ROBERTSON, Gordon Mackenzie BOLTON, Elizabeth Clare ECCLESTON, Andrew HETHERINGTON, Narendra Kumar PINDOLIA

The Surgery
Cockfield, Bishop Auckland DL13 5AF
Tel: 01388 718202 Fax: 01388 710600
(Durham Dales Primary Care Trust)
Patient List Size: 2550

Practice Manager A Futter

GP Dilys Claire Elizabeth WALLER, Anne Caroline NEVILLE

Bishops Castle

School House Lane Surgery
School House Lane, Bishops Castle SY9 5BP
Tel: 01588 632285
(Shropshire County Primary Care Trust)

GP Nicholas Charles Blake HOWELL, John Patrick CAMPBELL, Adrian Peter St John PENNEY

Bishop's Stortford

Bishops Park Health Centre
Lancaster Way, Bishop's Stortford CM23 4DA
Tel: 01279 755057
(Royston, Buntingford and Bishop's Stortford Primary Care Trust)

GP Peter Graham NUTLEY, Amrish Sukhadevbhai GOR

Church Street Partnership
30A Church Street, Bishop's Stortford CM23 2LY
Tel: 01279 657636 Fax: 01279 505464
(Royston, Buntingford and Bishop's Stortford Primary Care Trust)
Patient List Size: 15800

Practice Manager Irene Jackson

GP Michael John HARDWICK, Radu BURTAN, Gail DAVIDSON, Rosemary Anne DAVIS, Mark Clifford PENWILL, Martyn John ROGERS, Sarah WHETSTONE

Elsenham Surgery
Station Road, Elsenham, Bishop's Stortford CM22 6LA
Tel: 01279 814730 Fax: 01279 647342
(Uttlesford Primary Care Trust)
Patient List Size: 4342

Practice Manager Jenny walsh

GP J G SCHOFIELD, R A NUNN, J M RAYNER

Hatfield Health Surgery
Broomfields, Hatfield Heath, Bishop's Stortford CM22 7EH
Tel: 01279 730616 Fax: 01279 730408
(Uttlesford Primary Care Trust)
Patient List Size: 7200

Practice Manager Lesley Linford

GP Ian Cameron GILCHRIST, Saadet LAUBLE, K A ORTON, Judith Catherine PLUCK, Raz RASHID

Parsonage Surgery
1A Snowley Parade, Bishop's Stortford CM23 5EP
Tel: 01279 657684 Fax: 01279 506686
(Royston, Buntingford and Bishop's Stortford Primary Care Trust)
Patient List Size: 2800

Practice Manager L Lynn

GP Peter James HICKMAN, Oge AUSTIN-CHUKWU

South Street Surgery
83 South Street, Bishop's Stortford CM23 3AP
Tel: 01279 710800 Fax: 01279 710801
(Royston, Buntingford and Bishop's Stortford Primary Care Trust)
Patient List Size: 198000

Practice Manager Jane Ramshead

GP Mark Andrew JENNS, Roisin BROWN, Paresh DAWDA, S J DIXON, Stuart John FITNESS, Alison Faith JORDAN, Sarah M MACHALE, N S SHUKUR, Milinda Satyajith TENNEKOON

Blackburn

Accrington Road Surgery
85-91 Accrington Road, Blackburn BB1 2AF
Tel: 01254 52002 Fax: 01254 265803
(Blackburn with Darwen Primary Care Trust)
Patient List Size: 2900

GP Gaur Bhusan BHATTACHARJEE

Audley Health Centre
Longton Close, Blackburn BB1 1XA
Tel: 01254 264016 Fax: 01254 696402
(Blackburn with Darwen Primary Care Trust)
Patient List Size: 4600

Practice Manager B Singleton

GP Mridul Kumar DATTA, Saroj DATTA

Bangor Street Health Centre
Bangor Street, Blackburn BB1 6DY
Tel: 01254 674277 Fax: 01254 278573
(Blackburn with Darwen Primary Care Trust)
Patient List Size: 2800

Practice Manager Johanne Shorrock

GP Issak BHOJANI

Bolton Road Surgery
431-433 Bolton Road, Ewood, Blackburn BB2 4HY
Tel: 01254 679781 Fax: 01254 693031
(Blackburn with Darwen Primary Care Trust)
Patient List Size: 5000

Practice Manager Barbara Clare

GP Vasudevan NATARAJ, Shivaji Devrao JADHAV

Brookhouse Medical Centre
Whalley Range, Blackburn BB1 6EA
Tel: 01254 673887 Fax: 01254 697770
(Blackburn with Darwen Primary Care Trust)
Patient List Size: 5900

Practice Manager Jackie Wilson

GP Zuber Mohammed BUX, Mohammed Ibrahim PATEL, H McKEATING

Brownhill Surgery
788-790 Whalley New Road, Blackburn BB1 9BA
Tel: 01254 247477 Fax: 01254 245446
(Blackburn with Darwen Primary Care Trust)

Practice Manager Sue Carr

GP Thomas Llewelyn PHILLIPS, Richard Charles SAMOUELLE

The Cabin Surgery
High Street, Rishton, Blackburn BB1 4LA
Tel: 01254 884217 Fax: 01254 882899
(Hyndburn and Ribble Valley Primary Care Trust)

Practice Manager N Baker

GP Susan Amanda HANCOCK, Dr CHORLTON

The Fargly Practice
Montague Health Centre, Oakenhurst Road, Blackburn BA2 1PP
Tel: 01254 268410 Fax: 01254 268450
(Blackburn with Darwen Primary Care Trust)
Patient List Size: 2310

GP S CLARKSON

Feniscowles Surgery
696 Preston Old Road, Feniscowles, Blackburn BB2 5EP
Tel: 01254 208197 Fax: 01254 200183
(Blackburn with Darwen Primary Care Trust)
Patient List Size: 1490

Practice Manager Anne Geldeard

GP Miraj-Ud DIN

Great Harwood Health Centre
Water Street, Great Harwood, Blackburn BB6 7QR
Tel: 01254 885764 Fax: 01254 877360
Email: susan.upton@gp-p81730.nhs.uk
(Hyndburn and Ribble Valley Primary Care Trust)
Patient List Size: 3300

Practice Manager Judith Smith

GP David SMITH, Susan UPTON

Great Harwood Health Centre
Water Street, Great Harwood, Blackburn BB6 7QR
Tel: 01254 886400 Fax: 01254 877360
(Hyndburn and Ribble Valley Primary Care Trust)

Practice Manager Vicky Hothersall

GP Mohamed Altafur RAHMAN

Great Harwood Health Centre
Water Street, Great Harwood, Blackburn BB6 7QR
Tel: 01254 884295
(Hyndburn and Ribble Valley Primary Care Trust)

Practice Manager Gillian Bull

GP John Dinnis ROYLE

Gunn, Roberts, Fourie and Cooper
Witton Medical Centre, 29-31 Preston Old Road, Blackburn BB2 2SU
Tel: 01254 262123 Fax: 01254 695759
(Blackburn with Darwen Primary Care Trust)
Patient List Size: 11100

Practice Manager Carolynn Leak

GP Paul Gerard FOURIE, Stephen David GUNN, Teresa Agnes ROBERTS

High Street Surgery
87-89 High Street, Rishton, Blackburn BB1 4LD
Tel: 01254 884424 Fax: 01254 884424
(Hyndburn and Ribble Valley Primary Care Trust)

GP Kailash Narain AGARWAL

Infirmary Street Practice
106 Infirmary Street, Blackburn BB2 3SF
Tel: 01254 674665 Fax: 01254 696252
(Blackburn with Darwen Primary Care Trust)

GP Devinder GUPTA

King Street Surgery
King Street, Whalley, Blackburn BB7 9SL
Tel: 01254 823273 Fax: 01254 824891
Email: whalley.surgery@gp-p81017.nhs.uk
Website: www.whalley.surgery.co.uk
(Hyndburn and Ribble Valley Primary Care Trust)
Patient List Size: 10900

GP Geoffrey Alan CARTER, C BROWN, C FOGG, Timothy Michael GOLDING, Ian David WHYTE, Krzysztof Kazimierz WLODARCZYK

Kings Road Surgery
133 Kings Road, Blackburn BB2 4PY
Tel: 01254 201269 Fax: 01254 200717
(Blackburn with Darwen Primary Care Trust)
Patient List Size: 2500

Practice Manager N Rakshit

GP Bhim Chandra RAKSHIT

Larkhill Health Centre
Mount Pleasant, Blackburn BB1 5BJ
Tel: 01254 263611 Fax: 01254 680042
(Blackburn with Darwen Primary Care Trust)

GP Shridhar Vinayak JOSHI, Ramesh Chandra RAUTRAY, Reena RAUTRAY

Little Harwood Health Centre
Plane Tree Road, Blackburn BB1 6PH
Tel: 01254 580931 Fax: 01254 695794
(Blackburn with Darwen Primary Care Trust)
Patient List Size: 11500

Practice Manager Christine Turner

GP Andrew Ian BRISTOW, Maire Frances DERVAN, Christopher Henry MOWBRAY, Dorothea Magdalena PRIVONITZ, Kevan Paul TUCKER

Lower Bank Surgery
54 Preston New Road, Blackburn BB2 6BG
Tel: 01254 262121 Fax: 01254 265969
(Blackburn with Darwen Primary Care Trust)

GP Neville BALL

The Medical Centre
32 High Street, Rishton, Blackburn BB1 4LA
Tel: 01254 884226 Fax: 01254 726190
(Hyndburn and Ribble Valley Primary Care Trust)

Practice Manager Kath Farriday

GP Parthasarathy VALLURI

Montague Health Centre
Oakenhurst Road, Blackburn BB2 1PP
Tel: 01254 268416 Fax: 01254 268450
(Blackburn with Darwen Primary Care Trust)
Patient List Size: 2789

GP Rajiv Pritpal Singh VIRDI

Montague Health Centre
Oakenhurst Road, Blackburn BB2 1PP
Tel: 01254 268436 Fax: 01254 268440
(Blackburn with Darwen Primary Care Trust)
Patient List Size: 7400

Practice Manager Sheila Moss

GP Gill BUTTERWORTH, Jacqueline GAVAN, Ian James MOODIE, John Charles RANDALL, Neil Andrew SMITH

Montague Health Centre
Oakenhurst Road, Blackburn BB2 1PP
Tel: 01254 268425 Fax: 01254 268450
(Blackburn with Darwen Primary Care Trust)

Practice Manager Barbara Tattersall

GP John James Ciaran MARLBOROUGH, M L HARRINGTON

Montague Health Centre
Oakenhurst Road, Blackburn BB2 1PP
Tel: 01254 268456 Fax: 01254 268450
(Blackburn with Darwen Primary Care Trust)
Patient List Size: 2000

Practice Manager Ann Harwood

GP Francis Kwasi Beeby APALOO

Preston New Road Surgery
293-295 Preston New Road, Blackburn BB2 6PL
Tel: 01254 682672 Fax: 01254 696928
(Blackburn with Darwen Primary Care Trust)
Patient List Size: 4000

Practice Manager Shirley Collier

GP Hereward BROWN, Katherine Elizabeth BURN, David Gerard GEBBIE

Primrose Bank Medical Centre
Blackburn BB1 5ER
Tel: 01254 672132 Fax: 01254 699189
(Blackburn with Darwen Primary Care Trust)
Patient List Size: 5200

Practice Manager Zakira Bangue, Helen Lang

GP Ramesh Chandra RAUTRAY, Reena RAUTRAY

Pringle Street Surgery
216-218 Pringle Street, Blackburn BB1 1SB
Tel: 01254 56612 Fax: 01254 681630
(Blackburn with Darwen Primary Care Trust)
Patient List Size: 2113

Practice Manager Liz Collinson

GP Thiet Van DUONG

Pritchard Street Surgery
1A Pritchard Street, Blackburn BB2 3PF
Tel: 01254 56262 Fax: 01254 662835
(Hyndburn and Ribble Valley Primary Care Trust)

Practice Manager R Naylor

GP Thomas MARJOORAN, D GUPTA, S P GUPTA

Redlam Surgery
62-64 Redlam, Blackburn BB2 1UW
Tel: 01254 260051 Fax: 01254 691937
(Blackburn with Darwen Primary Care Trust)
Patient List Size: 6000

Practice Manager L Marsh

GP Sikandar Siraj AZFAR, Alan John CALOW, Anthony DEVINE

Roe Lee Surgery
367 Whalley New Road, Blackburn BB1 9SR
Tel: 01254 680075 Fax: 01254 695477
(Blackburn with Darwen Primary Care Trust)

Practice Manager Ethel Vickers

GP Ian TIMSON, J A SALERNO, Irfan Mahmood ZAFAR

Roman Road Health Centre
Fishmoor Drive, Blackburn BB2 3UY
Tel: 01254 664832 Fax: 01254 695904
(Blackburn with Darwen Primary Care Trust)
Patient List Size: 3000

Practice Manager Marilyn Fox

GP Malcolm RIDGWAY, Claire Ellen Mary Rita RUSHTON

St Georges Surgery
46A Preston New Road, Blackburn BB2 6AH
Tel: 01254 53791 Fax: 01254 697221
(Blackburn with Darwen Primary Care Trust)

Practice Manager Margaret Baines

GP Richard Sayles POLLOCK, Philip John ASHE, Nicholas Godfrey Edmund BUCKLEY, Jane Margaret ROSBOTTOM

St Huberts Road Surgery
153-155 St Huberts Road, Great Harwood, Blackburn BB6 7ED
Tel: 01254 889376 Fax: 01254 877413
(Hyndburn and Ribble Valley Primary Care Trust)
Patient List Size: 2570

Practice Manager Patricia Ahmed

GP Mamdouh Mohamed AHMED

William Hopwood Street Surgery
William Hopwood Street, Audley, Blackburn BB1 1LX
Tel: 01254 52522 Fax: 01254 696086
Email: nirmalanagpal@gp-P81707.nhs.uk
Website: www.surgeriesonline.com
(Blackburn with Darwen Primary Care Trust)
Patient List Size: 4500

Practice Manager Jolene Gregory

GP Nirmala NAGPAL, Amira AL-ABADI, Sisir MUKHERJEE, Satish NAGPAL

Woodlands Surgery
Woodlands, Shadsworth Road, Blackburn BB1 2HR
Tel: 01254 665664 Fax: 01254 695883
(Blackburn with Darwen Primary Care Trust)
Patient List Size: 6500

Practice Manager Liz Bradley

GP Alastair John Macdonald MURDOCH, Angela Karen PARRY, Samantha Jane PROUT, Michael Graham SMITH

Blackpool

Abbey-Dale Medical Centre
50 Common Edge Road, Blackpool FY4 5AU
Tel: 01253 696696 Fax: 01253 691691
(Blackpool Primary Care Trust)
Patient List Size: 2681

Practice Manager D E Hunter

GP Ghulam ABBAS, John POYNER

Adelaide Street Surgery
118 Adelaide Street, Blackpool FY1 4LN
Tel: 01253 620725 Fax: 01253 290765
(Blackpool Primary Care Trust)

Practice Manager Carol Tweedy

GP William James ANDERSON, Edward Cuthbert APALOO, Harnam Singh AULAKH, Paul LYNCH

Arnold Medical Centre
204 St. Annes Road, Blackpool FY4 2EF
Tel: 01253 346351 Fax: 01253 400244
(Blackpool Primary Care Trust)
Patient List Size: 4300

Practice Manager Tracey Swift

GP Suresh Prasad SRIVASTAVA, Anjuli SRIVASTAVA

Ashfield Road Surgery
70 Ashfield Road, Blackpool FY2 0DJ
Tel: 01253 357739 Fax: 01253 596161
(Blackpool Primary Care Trust)

Practice Manager S Wigham

GP Rajesh Kantilal PARIKH

Bispham Road Surgery
154 Bispham Road, Blackpool FY2 0NG
Tel: 01253 352066 Fax: 01253 596083
(Blackpool Primary Care Trust)
Patient List Size: 3600

GP Michael J EVANS, Douglas G MURRAY

Bloomfield Medical Centre
118-120 Bloomfield Road, Blackpool FY1 6JW
Tel: 01253 344123 Fax: 01253 349696
(Blackpool Primary Care Trust)

GP David Chadwick COTTAM, Amanda Mary DOYLE, Janet Elizabeth POLLOCK, Ibrahim Hussein Ibrahim SALAH, Peter Campbell SMITH

Buchanan Medical Centre
73-75 Buckhanan Street, Blackpool FY1 3BN
Tel: 01253 752475 Fax: 01253 752519
(Blackpool Primary Care Trust)

Practice Manager Sue Bird

GP Syed Irfan AHMED

Chain Lane Surgery
26a Chain Lane, Staining, Blackpool FY3 0DD
Tel: 01253 890510 Fax: 01253 885592
(Blackpool Primary Care Trust)

GP Goksel CELIKKOL

Devonshire Road Surgery
467 Devonshire Road, Blackpool FY2 0JP
Tel: 01253 352233 Fax: 01203 590007
Website: www.devonshireroadsurgery-nhs.co.uk
(Blackpool Primary Care Trust)
Patient List Size: 12800

Practice Manager Moira Hall

GP Simon Andrew SHEARER, Karen Lesley GREEN, Janet Anne NOLAN, John Patrick NUGENT, Michael Francis POWELL, William James WARD

Dinmore Avenue Surgery
Grange Park, Blackpool FY3 7RW
Tel: 01253 302794
(Blackpool Primary Care Trust)

Practice Manager Mavis Poracegirdle

GP Goksel CELIKKOL

Dr D Ireland
165 Red Bank Road, Bispham, Blackpool FY2 9EA
Tel: 01253 352780 Fax: 01253 595126
(Blackpool Primary Care Trust)

GP David IRELAND

Elizabeth Street Surgery
61 Elizabeth Street, Blackpool FY1 3JG
Tel: 01253 28949 Fax: 01253 290526
(Blackpool Primary Care Trust)
Patient List Size: 6000

Practice Manager Jacqueline Bainbridge

GP Jagadis Prasad CHATTERJEE, John CLARKE

Harrowside Medical Centre
72 Harrowside, Blackpool FY4 1LR
Tel: 01253 341793 Fax: 01253 346969
(Blackpool Primary Care Trust)

GP David Peter CHARLES, Aruna SINGH

Highfield Surgery
Garton Avenue, Southshore, Blackpool FY4 2LD
Tel: 01253 345328 Fax: 01253 407801
(Blackpool Primary Care Trust)

Practice Manager Jeanette Millward

GP Stuart Edward PRIESTLEY, Stephen HALL, John INMONGER, Paul David KELLY, Michelle MARTIN, Anne McGUIRE

Layton Medical Centre
200 Kingscote Drive, Blackpool FY3 7EN
Tel: 01253 392403 Fax: 01253 304597
(Blackpool Primary Care Trust)
Patient List Size: 7200

Practice Manager Lynn Jones

GP David Alan HAWORTH, Henry James Taylor BELL, Sukumar DAS

Lytham Road Surgery
352 Lytham Road, Blackpool FY4 1DW
Tel: 01253 402800 Fax: 01253 402994
(Blackpool Primary Care Trust)
Patient List Size: 4441

Practice Manager Pauline O'Rourke

GP Dahyu Dullabhbhai MISTRY, Paul STAFFORD

Lytham Road Surgery
352 Lytham Road, Blackpool FY4 1DW
Tel: 01253 402546 Fax: 01253 349637
(Blackpool Primary Care Trust)
Patient List Size: 5800

Practice Manager Susan Smith

GP Graeme Francis PARKINSON, Nish KARUNASKARA, Mark Christopher Michael WALKER

Marton Medical Centre
1 Glastonbury Avenue, Blackpool FY1 6SF
Tel: 01253 761321 Fax: 01253 600370
(Blackpool Primary Care Trust)
Patient List Size: 12000

Practice Manager Marie Chambers

GP Michael John WILSON, Rajnish LUTHRA

The Medical Centre
25 South King Street, Blackpool FY1 4NF
Tel: 01253 626637 Fax: 01253 290315
(Blackpool Primary Care Trust)

GP Eric Michael BONSELL, Richard Jeffrey FEAKS, Peter John LAKE, Richard TEHI, Marie Elena WILLIAMS

North Shore Surgery
95-99 Holmfield Road, Blackpool FY2 9RS
Tel: 01253 593971 Fax: 01253 596039
(Blackpool Primary Care Trust)

Practice Manager Debbie Coleman

GP Stephen CUSHING, Ted FURNISS, Stephen John PARR-BURMAN

Oxford Medical Centre
406 Waterloo Road, Blackpool FY4 4BL
Tel: 01253 764444 Fax: 01253 838552
(Blackpool Primary Care Trust)
Patient List Size: 3300

GP Saroj ARYA, Subhash Chandra ARYA

St Mary's Surgery
467 Lytham Road, Blackpool FY4 1JH
Tel: 01253 345086 Fax: 01253 403363
(Blackpool Primary Care Trust)
Patient List Size: 3900

Practice Manager Audrey Ellis

GP Andrew R GARSTANG, Valsa GEORGE

St Paul's Medical Centre
Dickson Road, Blackpool FY1 2HH
Tel: 01253 623896 Fax: 01253 752818
Website: www.stpaulsmedicalcentre.nhs.uk
(Blackpool Primary Care Trust)
Patient List Size: 12000

Practice Manager A P Bagot-Moore

GP Christopher Graham EVANS, Philippe Francois Thomas BOISSIERE, Stephen Keith ELLIS, Terence Robert NIXON, M P POWER, Leanne Rose RUDNICK, Colin Wilson SCOTT

Vicarage Lane Surgery
189 Vicarage Lane, Blackpool FY4 4NG
Tel: 01253 838997 Fax: 01253 699375
(Blackpool Primary Care Trust)
Patient List Size: 2500

Practice Manager A Tun

GP Si Thu TUN

Waterloo Road Surgery
178 Waterloo Road, Blackpool FY4 3AD
Tel: 01253 348619 Fax: 01253 404330
(Blackpool Primary Care Trust)
Patient List Size: 10300

GP Mark Stephen PRESKEY, Michael Liam BUTLER, John Stuart CALVERT, Allison Noreen REES, Stephen William THOMPSON

Blakeney

The Surgery
Millend, Blakeney GL15 4ED
Tel: 01594 510225 Fax: 01594 516074
(West Gloucestershire Primary Care Trust)
Patient List Size: 3200

Practice Manager Ruth Wadley

GP Martin GIBBS, Jennifer ELLIS, John W LINSELL

Blandford Forum

Eagle House Surgery
Eagle House, White Cliff Mill Street, Blandford Forum DT11 7DQ
Tel: 01258 453171 Fax: 01258 459603
(North Dorset Primary Care Trust)

Practice Manager J Tory

GP David Aylmer BURLTON, Timothy Cameron Scott BLEVINS, James CLEMENTS, Jane Victoria DAVIES, Phillipa Diana SCOREY

The Milton Abbas Surgery
Catherines Well, Milton Abbas, Blandford Forum DT11 0AT
Tel: 01258 880210 Fax: 01258 881252
Email: postmaster@gp-J81035.nhs.uk
Website: miltonabbassurgery.com
(North Dorset Primary Care Trust)
Patient List Size: 3600

Practice Manager Val Lamb

GP Malcolm James Holman HILLIER, Ethel Weir HILLIER, Elizabeth JONES, Martin Charles LONGLEY

The Surgery
White Cliff Mill Street, Blandford Forum DT11 7DQ
Tel: 01258 452501 Fax: 01258 455675
(North Dorset Primary Care Trust)

GP N Y BERRY, Philip BOSWORTH, Jonathan Morgan EVANS, Dr FORD, Dr HENSHELWOOD, Dr KREEGER, Dr NIXON, Geoffrey Nigel PERCIVAL, Dr PRIOR, Anne Margaret THOMAS

Blaydon-on-Tyne

Chainbridge Medical Partnership
Chainbridge House, The Precinct, Blaydon-on-Tyne NE21 5BT
Tel: 0191 414 2856 Fax: 0191 499 0449
Email: chainbridge.gps@btinternet.com
(Gateshead Primary Care Trust)

Practice Manager J.Brian Donnelly

GP Desmond John MATHESON, Howard John INGRAM, Richard Michael JOHNSON, Jessica KATTAN, Peter John LOUGHRIDGE, Laura Margaret ROBERTSON, Sarah ROBSON

Hollyhurst Surgery
8 Front Street, Winlaton, Blaydon-on-Tyne NE21 4RD
Tel: 0191 499 0966 Fax: 0191 414 2891
(Gateshead Primary Care Trust)
Patient List Size: 2953

Practice Manager Helen Urwin

GP Rajendra Prasad DUGGAL, Thomas YELLOWLEY

Winlaton and Ryton Family Partnership
10 Front Street, Winlaton, Blaydon-on-Tyne NE21 4RD
Tel: 0191 414 2339 Fax: 0191 414 4779
(Gateshead Primary Care Trust)
Patient List Size: 8500

Practice Manager P Arthur, K Lumley

GP Patricia BRAGG, Martin Alan JOHNSON, Jacinta MANSHIP, Jane McWILLIAMS, Jane PURVIS, William Don WESTWOOD

Blyth

Bondicar Medical
Thoroton Street, Blyth NE24 1DX
Tel: 01670 396500 Fax: 01670 396516
(Northumberland Care Trust)
Patient List Size: 4500

Practice Manager Margaret Nesbit

GP Jayanti Kumar GHOSH, Richard William McCOLLUM

Marine Medical
Blyth Health Centre, Thoroton Street, Blyth NE24 1DX
Tel: 01670 396520 Fax: 01670 396537
(Northumberland Care Trust)

Practice Manager A Siddle

GP John Sydney ALLEN, Zahid HUSSAIN, David Christopher MORGAN, Julian Paul TURNER

Rawes
The Harbour Suite, Blyth Hospital, Blyth NE24 1DX
Tel: 01670 396550 Fax: 01670 396556
(Northumberland Care Trust)
Patient List Size: 2250

Practice Manager L M Murdy

GP Geoffrey Douglas RAWES

Station Medical Group
Gatacre Street, Blyth NE24 1HD
Tel: 01670 396540 Fax: 01670 396517
(Northumberland Care Trust)

GP David WESTGARTH, David Michael EYNON, Dr HENDERSON, Peter Anthony McEVEDY

Waterloo Surgery
Thoroton Street, Blyth NE24 1DX
Tel: 01670 396560 Fax: 01670 396579
Email: colin.maxwell@gp-A84009.nhs.uk
(Northumberland Care Trust)
Patient List Size: 13000

Practice Manager Colin Maxwell

GP Robert Alan MURPHY, Lynn COCHRAN, Samantha GITTINS, Marie IMLACH, Ranjit JOHRI, John KIMMITT, Peter David YEOMAN

Bodmin

Carnewater Practice
Dennison Road, Bodmin PL31 2LB
Tel: 01208 256200 Fax: 01208 256229
(North and East Cornwall Primary Care Trust)
Patient List Size: 10000

Practice Manager Henry Gallichan

GP Richard John EVANS-JONES, David Ian FARRAR, Stephen Patrick HIGNELL, Matthew Sumner STEAD, Martin STEAN, Harriet Teresa Wynn TULLBERG, Stephen John Owen WATKINS

Stillmoor House Surgery
Dennison Road, Bodmin PL31 2JJ
Tel: 01208 72489
(North and East Cornwall Primary Care Trust)

Practice Manager S Carthew

GP Joseph MAGUIRE, Julia Heather EDDY, James NOTMAN, Rebecca RUSHTON, Martyn WOODFIELD

Bognor Regis

Bersted Green Surgery
32 Durlston Drive, Bognor Regis PO22 9TD
Tel: 01243 821392 Fax: 01243 842590
(Western Sussex Primary Care Trust)
Patient List Size: 10300

Practice Manager Christine Smith

GP Michael Maurice SHAW, Matthew Roy BRADSTOCK-SMITH, Michaela Jane Spencer DORMER, Krzysztof Antoni FURLEPA, Nicola L GEOGHEGAN, Mark Loring WEEKS

Bognor Medical Practice
West Street, Bognor Regis PO21 1UT
Tel: 01243 823864 Fax: 01243 623800
(Western Sussex Primary Care Trust)

GP Ervine Allingham ELLIS, Paul Lawrence CALLAWAY, Hugh Charles CONDON, Maxwell Hilton FOX, Ciaran HYDES, Nick PLUMB, John Neville TREPESS

Felpham and Middleton Health Centre
109 Flansham Park, Felpham, Bognor Regis PO22 6DH
Tel: 01243 582384 Fax: 01243 584933
Email: fm.hc@gp-H82038.nhs.uk
(Western Sussex Primary Care Trust)
Patient List Size: 11600

Practice Manager Sue Edgar

GP Julian Neil McLOUGHLIN, Fiona BELL, Maria KIPLING, Alison LAVENDER, William John ROGERS, Mark TWIST, Helen WARTNABY

Grove House Surgery
80 Pryors Lane, Rose Green, Bognor Regis PO21 4JB
Tel: 01243 265222 Fax: 01243 268693
(Western Sussex Primary Care Trust)
Patient List Size: 12000

Practice Manager Jenny Richardson

GP Malcolm Gavin RIDLEY, James Sabastian BRAMALL, Peter Mark HANAN, Andrew Mark Antony NAYLOR, Fraser Neil PATERSON

Maywood Surgery
180 Hawthorn Road, Bognor Regis PO21 2UY
Tel: 01243 830872 Fax: 01243 842115
Website: www.maywoodsurgery.com
(Western Sussex Primary Care Trust)
Patient List Size: 9250

Practice Manager Tracey Osborne

GP Peter David SPURRIER

Norfolk Square Surgery
14 Aldwick Road, Bognor Regis PO21 2LJ
Tel: 01243 821404 Fax: 01243 841404
(Western Sussex Primary Care Trust)
Patient List Size: 2300

Practice Manager Jeanette Powell

GP Faiz Ur REHMAN

Boldon Colliery

Aitken, Thorniley-Walker, Lombard and Booth
Medical Centre, Gibson Court, Boldon Colliery NE35 9AN
Tel: 0191 519 3000 Fax: 0191 519 2020
(South Tyneside Primary Care Trust)
Patient List Size: 6500

Practice Manager Aidan W Berry

GP Gordon James AITKEN, Amanda Frances BOOTH, David Charles LOMBARD, Edward George Anthony THORNILEY-WALKER

Gibson Court Medical Centre
Gibson Court, Boldon Colliery NE35 9AN
Tel: 0191 519 0077 Fax: 0191 537 3559
(South Tyneside Primary Care Trust)
Patient List Size: 6700

Practice Manager Jackie Lambert

GP William HALL, Sarah J ASTBURY, Helen Rachel MACKLIN, Paul John NELLIST, Judy Hope SIMPSON

Bolton

Agarwal
Farnworth Health Centre, Frederick Street, Farnworth, Bolton BL4 9AL
Tel: 01204 795170 Fax: 01204 572787
(Bolton Primary Care Trust)
Patient List Size: 7000

GP S R AGARWAL, K C AGARWAL, C CHARIDEMOU, V I OGBO

Alastair Ross Health Centre
Breightmet Fold Lane, Bolton BL2 6NT
Tel: 01204 385206 Fax: 01204 364626
(Bolton Primary Care Trust)

GP Dr ARIFF

Alastair Ross Health Centre
Breightmet Fold Lane, Bolton BL2 6NT
Tel: 01204 364626 Fax: 01204 399920
(Bolton Primary Care Trust)
Patient List Size: 5800

Practice Manager D Crank, L Patel

GP Andrew CRANK, P A CROSS, K J PATEL

Avondale Health Centre
Avondale Street, Bolton BL1 4JP
Tel: 01204 843803 Fax: 01204 493751
(Bolton Primary Care Trust)

GP Dr GREENHALGH

Avondale Health Centre
Avondale Street, Bolton BL1 4JP
Tel: 01204 643070 Fax: 01204 493751
(Bolton Primary Care Trust)

GP Dr SIRR

Barua
Farnworth Health Centre, Frederick Street, Farnworth, Bolton BL4 9AH
Tel: 01204 795445 Fax: 01204 796889
(Bolton Primary Care Trust)

GP C BARUA

Bradshaw Brow
30 Bradshaw Brow, Bradshaw, Bolton BL2 3DH
Tel: 01204 302212 Fax: 01204 595559
(Bolton Primary Care Trust)
Patient List Size: 4500

Practice Manager Kath Seel

GP John Angus Lamont KIRBY, J E McMILLEN, K PAGE

Burnside Surgery
365 Blackburn Road, Bolton BL1 8DZ
Tel: 01204 528205 Fax: 01204 361165
(Bolton Primary Care Trust)

Practice Manager Anne Simister

GP Geraldine May HEARN, Sarah R GREEN, Philip John ORMISTON

Caswell
108 Crescent Road, Great Lever, Bolton BL3 2JR
Tel: 01204 550100 Fax: 01204 550101
(Bolton Primary Care Trust)
Patient List Size: 2300

GP S J CASWELL

Cornerstone Surgery
469 Chorley Old Road, Bolton BL1 6AH
Tel: 01204 495426 Fax: 01204 497423
(Bolton Primary Care Trust)
Patient List Size: 4150

Practice Manager Margaret Walsh

GP Robert James WALKER, C BEVERIDGE, Elizabeth PERRY

Dakshina-Murthi
Pikes Lane Centre, Deane Road, Bolton BL3 5HP
Tel: 01204 655319 Fax: 01204 655319
(Bolton Primary Care Trust)

GP M DAKSHINA-MURTHI

Dennard and Partners
Pikes Lane Centre, Deane Road, Bolton BL3 5HP
Tel: 01204 874310 Fax: 01204 874305
(Bolton Primary Care Trust)

GP Robert LITTLEWOOD, G COUNSELL, S GREENHALGH, S A HALL, M A MIRZA

Dr A Zarrouk
65 Bradford Street, The Haulgh, Bolton BL2 1HT
Tel: 01204 521061 Fax: 01204 392009
(Bolton Primary Care Trust)
Patient List Size: 2900

Practice Manager Cathryn Dwyer

GP A ZARROUK

Dr H A Duncalf
263 Wigan Road, Deane, Bolton BL3 5QX
Tel: 01204 657878 Fax: 01204 658734
(Bolton Primary Care Trust)

GP H A DUNCALF

Dr Hardman and partners
Tonge Moor Health Centre, Thicketford Road, Bolton BL2 2LW
Tel: 01204 521094 Fax: 01204 523849
(Bolton Primary Care Trust)
Patient List Size: 5300

Practice Manager M C Gawthorpe

GP J L HARDMAN, A C AL-ABADI, M S BENJAMIN, K J COLEMAN, A D HILL, G S LANCASHIRE, S A G SHAW

Dr Liversedge, Dr Carey and Dr McCurdie
Egerton & Dunscar Health Centr, Darwen Road, Bromley Cross, Bolton BL7 9RG
Tel: 01204 309525 Fax: 01204 596562
Website: www.bolton.nhs.uk/gp/liversedge
(Bolton Primary Care Trust)
Patient List Size: 4050

Practice Manager Gill Warburton

GP Stephen Nicholas LIVERSEDGE, Elizabeth Ann CAREY, Michael McCURDIE

Dunstan Medical Centre
284 Bury Road, Bolton BL2 6AY
Tel: 01204 531557 Fax: 01204 364407
(Bolton Primary Care Trust)
Patient List Size: 6224

Practice Manager Vera Bourn

GP Thomas LYNCH, Timothy ISAAC, Gillian RINIC

Edgworth Medical Centre
354 Bolton Road, Turton, Bolton BL7 0DU
Tel: 01204 852226
(Bolton Primary Care Trust)
Patient List Size: 2800

Practice Manager Anita Grundy

GP V C UMEBUANI, Dr FADRA

Falouji
Pikes Lane Centre, Deane Road, Bolton BL3 5HP
Tel: 01204 533846 Fax: 01204 388236
(Bolton Primary Care Trust)

GP R A M FALOUJI

Ghosh and Partner
Little Lever Health Centre, Mytham Road, Little Lever, Bolton BL3 1JF
Tel: 01204 578577 Fax: 01204 705711
(Bolton Primary Care Trust)

GP A K GHOSH, P K JAIN

The Halliwell Surgery
Lindfield Drive, Bolton BL1 3RG
Tel: 01204 523813 Fax: 01204 384204
(Bolton Primary Care Trust)

Practice Manager Sylvia Sangster

GP Robert Alan HUNT, Anne Marie ILIFF

Harwood Medical Centre
Hough Fold Way, Harwood, Bolton BL2 3HQ
Tel: 01204 591526 Fax: 01204 303368
(Bolton Primary Care Trust)
Patient List Size: 13300

Practice Manager Kalina Carey

GP John Leslie HARDMAN, Amira AL-ABADI, Marie Suzy BENJAMIN, Jane BRADFORD, Kenneth John COLEMAN, Diane DUGGAN, Andrew Derek HILL, Graham Stewart LANCASHIRE, Stuart Antony Graham SHAW

Heaton Medical Centre
2 Lucy Street, Bolton BL1 5PU
Tel: 01204 843677
(Bolton Primary Care Trust)

Practice Manager J L Lamb

GP Adrian Keith LAMB, Dr HAMILTON

Inglewood Surgery
676 Blackburn Road, Astley Bridge, Bolton BL1 7AD
Tel: 01204 301161 Fax: 01204 598156
(Bolton Primary Care Trust)
Patient List Size: 5300

Practice Manager Michelle C Gawthorpe

GP David Thomas BUNN, Julian Stuart TOMKINSON, Terry A WALMSLEY

Jones and Partner
374-376 St Helens Road, Bolton BL3 3RR
Tel: 01204 62418/654021 Fax: 01204 665588
(Bolton Primary Care Trust)

GP I JONES, M PATEL, J VARKER

Kent
12 Bolton Road, Farnworth, Bolton BL4 7JW
Tel: 01204 571178 Fax: 01204 708909
(Bolton Primary Care Trust)

GP L N KENT

Kildonan House
Ramsbottom Road, Horwich, Bolton BL6 5NW
Tel: 01204 468161 Fax: 01204 698186
(Bolton Primary Care Trust)
Patient List Size: 11700

Practice Manager Christine M Ellis

GP Pamela Ann DRYBURGH, Mark James HALL, Ian Edward HAMER, Isabel Joy POPE, John Edward TABOR, Zaheda WALSH

Ladybridge Surgery
10 Broadgate, Ladybridge, Bolton BL3 4PZ
Tel: 01204 653267 Fax: 01204 665350
(Bolton Primary Care Trust)

GP Andrew John WRIGHT, P J PARR, J W SMYTH

Little Lever Health Centre
Mytham Road, Little Lever, Bolton BL3 1JF
Tel: 01204 572611 Fax: 01204 862051
(Bolton Primary Care Trust)
Patient List Size: 2000

Practice Manager Samantha Taylor

GP Davendra KUMAR

Loomba
Lever Chambers Centre for Health, Ashburner Street, Bolton BL1 1SQ
Tel: 01204 360051/360050 Fax: 01204 385207
(Bolton Primary Care Trust)

GP Y LOOMBA

Mandalay Medical Centre
933 Blackburn Road, Bolton BL1 7LR
Tel: 01204 302228/301041 Fax: 01204 597949
(Bolton Primary Care Trust)
Patient List Size: 9200

Practice Manager Irene Russell

GP Martyn Steven FLETCHER, K L BIRKENSHAW, G R GHOSH, Jonathan Richard JONES, David Edward McAULEY, Colin Peter MERCER, S L QUELAULT

Market Surgery
103 Chorley New Road, Horwich, Bolton BL6 5QF
Tel: 01204 697696 Fax: 01204 699676
(Bolton Primary Care Trust)

Practice Manager C A Forrest

GP Stephen John DOYLE, Robert Anthony HAILWOOD, Eva MITCHELL

Mitchell
Great Lever Health Centre, Rupert Street, Bolton BL3 6RN
Tel: 01204 363785/525429 Fax: 01204 380221
(Bolton Primary Care Trust)
Patient List Size: 2400

GP R G MITCHELL, S H KHAN

Naqvi
46 Greenland Road, Great Lever, Bolton BL3 2EG
Tel: 01204 383052/388882 Fax: 01204 395810
(Bolton Primary Care Trust)

GP S M H NAQVI

Naqvi
279/283 St Helens Road, Daubhill, Bolton BL3 3QB
Tel: 01204 62919/62516 Fax: 01204 62919
(Bolton Primary Care Trust)

GP U NAQVI

Newgrosh
Great Lever Health Centre, Rupert Street, Bolton BL3 6RN
Tel: 01204 526955
(Bolton Primary Care Trust)

GP B S NEWGROSH

Parikh and Partner
Little Lever Health Centre, Mytham Road, Bolton BL3 1JF
Tel: 01204 791448/575333 Fax: 01204 579896
(Bolton Primary Care Trust)

GP S PARIKH, M PARIKH

Pike View Medical Centre
2-10 Albert Street, Horwich, Bolton BL6 7AS
Tel: 01204 699311 Fax: 01204 668387
(Bolton Primary Care Trust)

Practice Manager Yvonne Burgess

GP Krishnarao KORLIPARA, S M MALHOTRA, Arun Kumar MISHRA

Prasad and Partner
Lever Chambers Centre for Health, Ashburner Street, Bolton BL1 1SQ
Tel: 01204 360040 Fax: 01204 360043
(Bolton Primary Care Trust)

GP A PRASAD

Rout and Partners
Kearsley Medical Centre, Jackson Street, Kearsley, Bolton BL4 8EP
Tel: 01204 578825/573164 Fax: 01204 792161
(Bolton Primary Care Trust)

GP D A WALL, S A B MUNSHI, L A NATHA, G H OGDEN

Sabrine
Great Lever Health Centre, Rupert Street, Bolton BL3 6RN
Tel: 01204 399933 Fax: 01204 360061
(Bolton Primary Care Trust)

GP S F SABRINE

Shri-Kant and Partner
Spring View Medical Centre, Mytham Road, Little Lever, Bolton BL3 1HQ
Tel: 01204 578128/572939 Fax: 01204 795565
(Bolton Primary Care Trust)

Practice Manager Yvonne Burgess

GP A SHRI-KANT, A GUPTA

Silvert and Partners
Stonehill Medical Centre, Piggott Street, Farnworth, Bolton BL4 9QZ
Tel: 01204 574073/573445 Fax: 01204 791633
(Bolton Primary Care Trust)
Patient List Size: 11900

GP B D SILVERT, N BROWNE, A D HAWKRIDGE, H HEALEY, A KAY, M KINSEY, N ROBBIE, P A WHITE

Spring House
555 Chorley Old Road, Bolton BL1 6AF
Tel: 01204 848411 Fax: 01204 849968
(Bolton Primary Care Trust)

GP Peter Anthony SAUL, Ian Gordon Vizetelly JAMES, P J PRIEST, I A G SIDAT, Z I WALSH

Swan Lane Medical Centre
Swan Lane, Bolton BL3 6TL
Tel: 01204 655009/62129 Fax: 01204 660516
(Bolton Primary Care Trust)
Patient List Size: 6200

Practice Manager Margaret Carney

GP I D CALDWELL, Dr MARYA

Tonge Moor Road Surgery
398 Tonge Moor Road, Bolton BL2 2LA
Tel: 01204-385231 Fax: 01204-385231
(Bolton Primary Care Trust)
Patient List Size: 4200

Practice Manager Anita Jones

GP Ahmed ARIFF, M CHOWDHURY

The Unsworth Group Practice
Peter House, Captain Lees Road, Westhoughton, Bolton BL5 3UB
Tel: 01942 812525 Fax: 01942 813431
(Bolton Primary Care Trust)
Patient List Size: 18900

GP Allan NEEDHAM, W BHATIANI, Wirinder BHATIANI, M C BROWN, M R P DAVIES, J M HALL, J P NAGLE, F M ROWLANDS, R A SIMPSON, N WATTS

Victoria Road Surgery
27 Victoria Road, Horwich, Bolton BL6 5NA
Tel: 01204 668166 Fax: 0870 845 9049
(Bolton Primary Care Trust)

GP Shuba Rani PANJA

Wakefield and Partners
Lever Chambers Centre for Health, 1st Floor, Ashburner Street, Bolton BL1 1SQ
Tel: 01204 360030/31 Fax: 01204 360033
(Bolton Primary Care Trust)
Patient List Size: 6800

Practice Manager Anne Grundy

GP Christopher John WAKEFIELD, Christopher John EARNSHAW, Dawn Elizabeth HARRIS, Alison Lesley LYON

Bootle

Aintree Road Practice
2 Aintree Road, Bootle L20 9DN
Tel: 0151 922 1768
(South Sefton Primary Care Trust)

GP K K JHA, N K SINHA, S K SINHA

Glovers Lane Practice
Glovers Lane, Netherton, Bootle L30 5TA
Tel: 0151 524 2444 Fax: 0151 524 2880
(South Sefton Primary Care Trust)
Patient List Size: 7300

Practice Manager Gill Halpin

GP Andrew DILWORTH, Martina CORNWELL, Peter GOLDSTEIN, Dr SLADE

King's Park Surgery
83 Stanley RP, Bootle L20 7DA
Tel: 0151 4767962 Fax: 0151 4767985
(South Sefton Primary Care Trust)

GP David Owen GOLDBERG

Moore Street Health Centre
77 Moore Street, Bootle L20 4SE
Tel: 0151 944 1066 Fax: 0151 933 4715
(South Sefton Primary Care Trust)

GP Anthony Waldron ROBERTS, Carol Gillian Sheena McCORMICK, Kieran Edward MURPHY, Nicholas John ORME

North Park Health Centre
290 Knowsley Road, Bootle L20 5DQ
Tel: 0151 922 3841 Fax: 0151 933 7335
(South Sefton Primary Care Trust)
Patient List Size: 8400

Practice Manager Carole Westhead

GP P K ANTEN, Prabodh Kumar SRIVASTAVA, Adel BAKER, Shim Yan WONG CHING HWAI

Park Street Surgery
Park Street, Bootle L20 3DF
Tel: 0151 922 3577 Fax: 0151 933 6098
(South Sefton Primary Care Trust)

Practice Manager Mary Midonough

GP Barry John STANLEY, Kong Meng CHUNG, Annalie Elise MAIER

Stanley Road Surgery
204 Stanley Road, Bootle L20 3EW
Tel: 0151 922 5719 Fax: 0151 933 8600
Email: carol.taylor@gp-n84015.nhs.uk
(South Sefton Primary Care Trust)
Patient List Size: 6400

Practice Manager Dorothy Whelan

GP Terence Anthony NEWMAN, R E SIVORI, Sarah Jane STEPHENSON, A VINCHENZO

Strand Medical Centre
272 Marsh Lane, Bootle L20 5BW
Tel: 0151 922 1600 Fax: 0151 933 5300
(South Sefton Primary Care Trust)

GP Amjed ALI, Stephen Andrew MORRIS, Sharon Marie OLIVER

Bordon

Badgerswood Surgery
Mill Lane, Headley, Bordon GU35 8LH
Tel: 01428 713511 Fax: 01428 713812
(North Hampshire Primary Care Trust)

Practice Manager Dilys Williamson

GP Paul Andrew BEECH, Geoffrey BOYES, John Stuart ROSE, Frank Hugh WILLIAMS-THOMAS

Pinehill Surgery
Pinehill Road, Bordon GU35 0BS
Tel: 01420 472113 Fax: 01420 489471
(North Hampshire Primary Care Trust)
Patient List Size: 4100

Practice Manager Deirdre Warren

GP Piers Niel Paton McGREGOR-WOOD, K BEAUMONT, Paul CONLEY

Woolmer Surgery
Forest Road, Bordon GU35 0BJ
Tel: 01420 474135 Fax: 01420 476714
(North Hampshire Primary Care Trust)
Patient List Size: 4300

Practice Manager Brenda Taitt

GP Dale Carlton EGERTON, Charles Richard DAWSON

Borehamwood

Fairbrook Medical Centre
4 Fairway Avenue, Borehamwood WD6 1PR
Tel: 020 8953 7666
(Hertsmere Primary Care Trust)

Practice Manager Kathleen Ramsden

GP Leonard HIRSCH, Anthony John DRAKE, Michael Rex EDWARDS, Carolyn Jane HOWE, Miriam JAFFE, Catherine PAGE

Grove Road Surgery
25 Grove Road, Borehamwood WD6 5DX
Tel: 020 8953 2444 Fax: 020 8207 4060
(Hertsmere Primary Care Trust)
Patient List Size: 6100

Practice Manager Karen Story

GP Catherine Agnes NICHOLSON, Jane Deborah ROSE, Andrew SCHEPIRA

Manor Way Surgery
27 Manor Way, Borehamwood WD6 1QR
Tel: 020 8953 3095
(Hertsmere Primary Care Trust)

Practice Manager M Midson

GP Jennifer Thea SPRING

Schopwick Surgery
Everett Court, Romeland, Elstree, Borehamwood WD6 3BJ
Tel: 020 8953 1008 Fax: 020 8905 2196
(Hertsmere Primary Care Trust)

Practice Manager Sue Williams

GP Susan Carol ELLIOTT, Ann Varee McDOUGALL, Nicolas Mark Warren SMALL, Allison Lucy Blair SMITH, Joanna SZAFARYN, Andrew Thomas WILSON, Christine Elizabeth WILSON

Theobald Centre
119-121 Theobald Street, Borehamwood WD6 4PT
Tel: 020 8953 3355
(Hertsmere Primary Care Trust)

Practice Manager Janet Agnew

GP Dipak Rasiklal Chandulal KAPACEE, Salinder RAYAT

Boscastle

Bottreaux Surgery
Boscastle PL35 0BG
Tel: 01840 250209 Fax: 01840 250666
(North and East Cornwall Primary Care Trust)
Patient List Size: 4796

Practice Manager C J Pethick

GP Christopher Anthony Neville JARVIS, Paul Ralph ABBOTT, Graham David GARROD

Boston

Church Close Surgery
3 Church Close, Boston PE21 6NB
Tel: 01205 311133 Fax: 01205 358986
(East Lincolnshire Primary Care Trust)
Patient List Size: 9400

Practice Manager Alan Taylor

GP Jonathan Nigel SAVORY, Andrew Ian DODDRELL, Ian Edward LOWE, Lynne WOODS, Paul Julian WOODS

James Street Surgery
2 James Street, Boston PE21 8RD
Tel: 01205 362556 Fax: 01205 359050
(East Lincolnshire Primary Care Trust)
Patient List Size: 7500

Practice Manager Jill Kime

GP Michael Roy POLLING, G HARKER, Kiki Carolyn Mary STEEL

Liquorpond Street Surgery
10 Liquorpond Street, Boston PE21 8UE
Tel: 01205 362763 Fax: 01205 358918
(East Lincolnshire Primary Care Trust)

Practice Manager Elaine Lovell

GP Brian Eric Penny WOOKEY, John Richard BROCKLEHURST, Michael David GERMER, Henry Herbert MATITI, David Baskerville RANCE

The Medical Centre
Church End, Old Leake, Boston PE22 9LE
Tel: 01205 870666 Fax: 01205 870971
(East Lincolnshire Primary Care Trust)
Patient List Size: 6520

Practice Manager Karen Bruce, David Deegan

GP Ian Roger Braithwaite BLOOM, Charles Stuart BULL, Richard William LATCHEM, James Robert MACKIN

Parkside Surgery
Tawney Street, Boston PE21 6PF
Tel: 01205 365881 Fax: 01205 357583
(East Lincolnshire Primary Care Trust)

Practice Manager Les Viner

GP Christopher Roy Lewis ALLWOOD, Philip John HARRIS, Muna Salih Abdul RAZZAK, Martyn Ronald WALLING, David WILKINSON

Stickney Surgery
Main Road, Stickney, Boston PE22 8AA
Tel: 01205 480237 Fax: 01205 480987
(East Lincolnshire Primary Care Trust)
Patient List Size: 4250

Practice Manager Christine Morgan

GP Simon Tudur RHYS-DAVIES, Terence John BROWES, Thomas Andreas Heinrich BUSCH

Stuart House Surgery
Sleaford Road Medical Centre, Sleaford Road, Boston PE21 8EG
Tel: 01205 362173 Fax: 01205 365710
(East Lincolnshire Primary Care Trust)
Patient List Size: 6106

Practice Manager Wendy Brady

GP Clive Edwin John WARREN, Nicolas BULMER, Kathryn Mary GLENN, Peter Raymond HOLMES

The Surgery
Off Station Road, Kirton, Boston PE20 1LD
Tel: 01205 722437 Fax: 01205 724358
(East Lincolnshire Primary Care Trust)

Practice Manager Sandra Hall

GP N BUNTING

Sutterton Surgery
Spalding Road, Sutterton, Boston PE20 2ET
Tel: 01205 460254 Fax: 01205 460779
(East Lincolnshire Primary Care Trust)

Practice Manager S Allen

GP Philip John GRAY, Andrew Stephen HUGHES

Swineshead Medical Group
The Surgery, Church Lane, Swineshead, Boston PE20 3JA
Tel: 01205 820204 Fax: 01205 821034
Website: www.swinesheadmedicalgroup.co.uk
(East Lincolnshire Primary Care Trust)
Patient List Size: 9184

Practice Manager Suzanne Baxter

GP Peter John DAWSON, S DOUGLAS, Catherine Jane GRIFFITHS, Craig KELLY, S J SAVORY, K A ULRICH

Bourne

Bourne Galletly Practice Team
40 North Road, Bourne PE10 9BT
Tel: 01778 562200 Fax: 01778 562207
(Lincolnshire South West Teaching Primary Care Trust)
Patient List Size: 9070

Practice Manager Delia Ledner

GP Rajnikant Bhanabhai PATEL, Bettina Anne BRIGGS, Colin Richard BURR, Julie Claire HARRIS, Ian Gerard PACE, Antony Marcus WRIGHT

Hereward Medical Centre
Exeter Street, Bourne PE10 9XR
Tel: 01778 393366 Fax: 01778 391715
Email: hereward.practice@gp-C83035.nhs.uk
Website: www.herewardgp.co.uk
(Lincolnshire South West Teaching Primary Care Trust)
Patient List Size: 10300

Practice Manager Robert Brown

GP Nigel Bruce TURNBULL, Viven Lesley BEVERIDGE, Clive COLE, Rachel Alison ELDER, Carl Richard PEARS, Ian Michael WHEATLEY

Bourne End

Hawthornden Surgery
Wharf Lane, Bourne End SL8 5RX
Tel: 01628 522864 Fax: 01628 533226
(Wycombe Primary Care Trust)
Patient List Size: 6500

Practice Manager C Bradley

GP Sarah Helena BUXTON, Tanveer HUSSAIN, Peter William NEWMAN, Michael Benjamin WOLFIN

Bournemouth

Adeline Road Surgery
4 Adeline Road, Boscombe, Bournemouth BH5 1EF
Tel: 01202 309421 Fax: 01202 304893
(Bournemouth Teaching Primary Care Trust)

Practice Manager G Douch

GP David John POULTON, Ian Cambell BESWICK, Andrew BLASZCZYK, John Edward Clifford BRAY, Isobel Diana GANNON, Nermina SELIMOVIC, Susan Elizabeth WALKER-DATE

Alma Partnership
Winton Health Centre, Alma Road, Winton, Bournemouth BH9 1BP
Tel: 01202 519311 Fax: 01202 548532
(Bournemouth Teaching Primary Care Trust)
Patient List Size: 7200

Practice Manager Alan Gordon

GP Carol Anne LINNARD, Andrew Christopher BARRACLOUGH, Helen Margaret DUNKELMAN, Peter Richard HEARN

Banks Medical Centre
272 Wimborne Road, Bournemouth BH3 7AT
Tel: 01202 593444 Fax: 01202 548534
(Bournemouth Teaching Primary Care Trust)

Practice Manager Sue Price

GP Michael Gordon PATTEN, Clare DAVIES, Mark Simon HOCKEY, C MARSHALL, Martin Bellamy SHAW

Boscombe Manor Medical Centre
40 Florence Road, Boscombe, Bournemouth BH5 1HQ
Tel: 01202 303012/303013 Fax: 01202 303014
(Bournemouth Teaching Primary Care Trust)
Patient List Size: 2200

Practice Manager Linda Cluer

GP Linda Adrienne EVE, Richard Wordsworth HATTERSLEY

Crescent Surgery
3 The Crescent, Boscombe, Bournemouth BH1 4EX
Tel: 01202 393755 Fax: 01202 303511
Email: crescent@gp-j81624.nhs.uk
(Bournemouth Teaching Primary Care Trust)

Practice Manager Rachel Carter

GP Brian Omar MORELAND

Denmark Road Medical Centre
37 Denmark Road, Winton, Bournemouth BH9 1PB
Tel: 01202 521111 Fax: 01202 516761
Email: postmaster@gp-j81625.nhs.uk
(Bournemouth Teaching Primary Care Trust)
Patient List Size: 6080

Practice Manager Joy Collins

GP Nigel Mark COWLEY, Christina FILA, Nicholas KENNEDY

Durdells Avenue Surgery
1 Durdells Avenue, Kinson, Bournemouth BH11 9EH
Tel: 01202 573947 Fax: 01202 590021
(Bournemouth Teaching Primary Care Trust)
Patient List Size: 3500

Practice Manager Denise Homer

GP John Lawrence HUTCHINGS, Adrian HUTCHINGS

Gervis Road Surgery
14 Gervis Road, Bournemouth BH1 3EG
Tel: 01202 293418/317320/780324 Fax: 01202 317866
(Bournemouth Teaching Primary Care Trust)
Patient List Size: 9750

Practice Manager Nick J Thompson

GP Nicholas Timothy MacIver PANTON, David John Lewis BINTCLIFFE, Shelley CARTER, Irena DANIELS, Roberta Ann KING, Margaret Anne McKENNA, Adam Nicholas SAWYER, Fadia SOBHY, Mark SPRING

Harewood Crescent Surgery
Harewood Crescent, Littledown, Bournemouth BH7 7BU
Tel: 01202 309500 Fax: 01202 309565
(Bournemouth Teaching Primary Care Trust)
Patient List Size: 3975

Practice Manager S Smith

GP Paul Edward MECKLENBURGH, Karen LINDALL, Bernadette ROGERS

Holdenhurst Road Surgery
199 Holdenhurst Road, Bournemouth BH8 8DE
Tel: 01202 558337
(Bournemouth Teaching Primary Care Trust)

GP Giles TETLEY, Peter William Hammond BLICK, Anne Marie LEVITT, William Martyn SHAKESPEARE

J M Waters and Partners
21 Beaufort Road, Southbourne, Bournemouth BH6 5AJ
Tel: 01202 433081 Fax: 01202 430527
(Bournemouth Teaching Primary Care Trust)
Patient List Size: 11500

Practice Manager Jenny Osborne

GP John Mortimer WATERS, Tamar EL KHOLY, Douglas Gordon GREGORY, Oliver GUNSON, David LEONARD, Barbara LESLEY, Anne Marguerite THURSTON

James Fisher Medical Centre
4 Tolpuddle Gardens, Bournemouth BH9 3LQ
Tel: 01202 522622 Fax: 01202 548480
(Bournemouth Teaching Primary Care Trust)
Patient List Size: 12863

Practice Manager Maggie Dobson

GP Stephen THOMAS, David BELLAMY, Richard Anthony BENSON, Nadia Mary BRIDGMAN, David Angus CRICHTON, Mark Adrian GRAINGER, Joanne Elizabeth HARVEY, Janet Mary SLY

Kinson Road Surgery
440 Kinson Road, Bournemouth BH10 5EY
Tel: 01202 574604 Fax: 01202 590029
(Bournemouth Teaching Primary Care Trust)
Patient List Size: 9300

Practice Manager Denny Gill

GP Ian Dean GORDON, Andrew BREWER, Janet Elizabeth COOKE, Ian Hugh HEATLEY

Leybourne Surgery
1 Leybourne Avenue, Ensbury Park, Bournemouth BH10 6ES
Tel: 01202 527003 Fax: 01202 549339
(Bournemouth Teaching Primary Care Trust)
Patient List Size: 3710

Practice Manager Ian Wright

GP Gordon TURNER, Andrew Saville FOOT

Marine Surgery
29 Belle Vue Road, Southbourne, Bournemouth BH6 3DB
Tel: 01202 423377 Fax: 01202 424277
(Bournemouth Teaching Primary Care Trust)

Practice Manager V Whitham

GP Paul Frederic FRENCH, John HARRIS, Richard POWER, Sian SHAW, Fiona WHITWORTH, Deborah Elizabeth WILLIAMS, Kathryn Ann WILLIS

Moordown Medical Centre
2A Redhill Crescent, Moordown, Bournemouth BH9 2XF
Tel: 01202 516139 Fax: 01202 548525
(Bournemouth Teaching Primary Care Trust)
Patient List Size: 7450

Practice Manager C L Beezum

GP Subrata SEN, Linda Susan PRYCE, Stephen Andrew ROGERS

Northbourne Surgery
1368 Wimborne Road, Bournemouth BH10 7AR
Tel: 01202 574100 Fax: 01202 590030
(Bournemouth Teaching Primary Care Trust)

Practice Manager Melva Clifford

GP Ann Jennifer EDWARDS, Clifden John CROCKETT, Nigel Christopher IRWIN

Poole Road Medical Centre
7 Poole Road, Bournemouth BH2 5QR
Tel: 01202 761120 Fax: 01202 767271
(Poole Primary Care Trust)
Patient List Size: 5800

Practice Manager Nora Waygood

GP Nigel Carsley PRICE, Timothy ALDER, Tina Louise A'NESS, Karen TENNYSON

Providence Surgery
12 Walpole Road, Boscombe, Bournemouth BH1 4HA
Tel: 01202 395195 Fax: 01202 304293
(Bournemouth Teaching Primary Care Trust)
Patient List Size: 3500

Practice Manager Kim Herbert

GP Peter TURNBULL, Mufeed NI'MAN

Southbourne Surgery
17 Beaufort Road, Southbourne, Bournemouth BH6 5BF
Tel: 01202 427878 Fax: 01202 430730
(Bournemouth Teaching Primary Care Trust)
Patient List Size: 7850

Practice Manager Ruth Cragill

GP Peter Doré PERKINS, Jackie Mary HEAD, Daniel Nimalan JEYATHEVA, Sally LEWIS, Simon Craigen PENNELL

St Albans Medical Centre
26-28 St. Albans Crescent, Charminster, Bournemouth BH8 9EW
Tel: 01202 517333 Fax: 01202 517336
(Bournemouth Teaching Primary Care Trust)
Patient List Size: 10000

Practice Manager Sue Elston

GP Kevin Richard EAST, Katrina Anne HEATLEY, Stephen Paul KIDMAN, Ian NELEMANS, Corinne PAVY

Strouden Park Medical Centre
2A Bradpole Road, Bournemouth BH8 9NX
Tel: 01202 532253 Fax: 01202 548524
(Bournemouth Teaching Primary Care Trust)

Practice Manager Usha R Sekhar

GP Cheemala John Raja SEKHAR

Talbot Medical Centre
63 Kinson Road, Bournemouth BH10 4BX
Tel: 01202 523059 Fax: 01202 533239
Email: postmaster@gp-J81033.nhs.uk
Website: www.talbotmedicalcentre.co.uk
(Bournemouth Teaching Primary Care Trust)

Practice Manager Judith Young

GP Harold Alexander CHADWICK, Susan Nicola Allison COX, Elizabeth Sara CRAIG, Margaret Anne FARDON, Simon Thomas FLACK, Jonathan Hugh Giles FOULKES, Richard HOLMES, Martin Christopher HUGHES, Jon TURNER, Richard David WEAVER

Westbourne Medical Centre
Milburn Road, Bournemouth BH4 9HJ
Tel: 01202 752550 Fax: 01202 769700
Website: www.westbournemedical.com
(Poole Primary Care Trust)
Patient List Size: 13000

Practice Manager David Clippingdale

GP James Alan FISHER, Tessa Mair BEVAN JONES, Lawrence Duncan Ashley BRAD, Stephen MORGAN, Alistair Hugh SCALES, Robert Maurice Charles SCHUSTER BRUCE, Susan Elizabeth SYLVESTER

Woodlea House Surgery
1 Crantock Grove, Castle Lane West, Bournemouth BH8 0HS
Tel: 01202 300903 Fax: 01202 304826
(Bournemouth Teaching Primary Care Trust)

Practice Manager L Thomas

GP Fabio Roberto TORQUATI, Andrew George ROWLAND

Brackley

Halse Road Health Centre
Halse Road, Brackley NN13 6EJ
Tel: 01280 703460 Fax: 01280 703460
(Cherwell Vale Primary Care Trust)
Patient List Size: 5000

Practice Manager Pat A Rush

GP M A S S WIJAYAWARDENA, Lynne CARGILL, Charles Stephen PERROTT

Springfield Surgery
Springfield Way, Brackley NN13 6JJ
Tel: 01280 703431 Fax: 01280 703241
(Cherwell Vale Primary Care Trust)
Patient List Size: 8000

Practice Manager Deena Tomkinson

GP David Andrew CHIDWICK, C L BENNETT, H R CAMPBELL, D B NICHOLLS, Andrew Charles RATHBORNE

Washington House Surgery
77 Halse Road, Brackley NN13 6EQ
Tel: 01280 702436 Fax: 01280 701805
Email: surgery@washingtonhousesurgery.fsnet.co.uk
(Cherwell Vale Primary Care Trust)
Patient List Size: 8400

Practice Manager Soo Styles

GP Jane CASSIDY, John HARRISON, Paul PARSON, Philip John STEVENS

Bracknell

The Balfron Practice
Skimped Hill Health Centre, Skimped Hill Lane, Bracknell RG12 1LH
Tel: 01344 306613 Fax: 01344 306614
(Bracknell Forest Primary Care Trust)
Patient List Size: 3340

Practice Manager Helen Osborn

GP Marie WOODS, Lillian JOHNSTON

The Binfield Practice
Binfield Health Centre, Terrace Road North, Binfield, Bracknell RG42 5JG
Tel: 01344 425434 Fax: 01344 301843
Website: www.mygeneralpractice.co.uk/bingield
(Bracknell Forest Primary Care Trust)

Practice Manager Roland Cundy

GP Katherine Elizabeth CRISP, Robert James A M KOEFMAN, Neesha MOHAN, Jeremy Michael PLATT, William TONG

Boundary House Surgery
Boundary House, Mount Lane, Bracknell RG12 9PG
Tel: 01344 483900 Fax: 01344 862203
(Bracknell Forest Primary Care Trust)
Patient List Size: 7796

Practice Manager Wendy Miller

GP Margaret Christine SLEMP, Catherine Jane CAIRD, Martin Geoffrey Standford KNIGHT, Gordon WEIR

The Crown Wood Medical Centre
4A Crown Row, Bracknell RG12 0TH
Tel: 01344 310202 Fax: 01344 310303
(Bracknell Forest Primary Care Trust)

Practice Manager Janice Mitchell

GP Mallipeddi VENKATA-RAO

The Crown Wood Medical Centre
4A Crown Row, Bracknell RG12 0TH
Tel: 01344 310310 Fax: 01344 310300
(Bracknell Forest Primary Care Trust)

Practice Manager Annette O'Connor

GP Neelam VERMA

Easthampstead Practice
Easthampstead Surgery, 23 Rectory Lane, Bracknell RG12 7BB
Tel: 01344 457535 Fax: 01344 301862
(Bracknell Forest Primary Care Trust)

Practice Manager Tina Brown

GP Trevor John KEELING, David METSON

The Evergreen Practice
Skimped Hill Health Centre, Skimped Hill Lane, Bracknell RG12 1LH
Tel: 01344 306936 Fax: 01344 306966
(Bracknell Forest Primary Care Trust)
Patient List Size: 3400

Practice Manager Yun Tay

GP Kem Sing TAY

Forest End Medical Centre
Rinemead, Birch Hill, Bracknell RG12 7PG
Tel: 01344 421364 Fax: 01344 301812
(Bracknell Forest Primary Care Trust)
Patient List Size: 7300

Practice Manager Kevin Linsell

GP Sandra Karen BALL, David EVANS, Adam Peter GREIG

The Great Holland Practice
The Great Hollands Health Centre, Great Hollands Square, Bracknell RG12 8WY
Tel: 01344 426043 Fax: 01344 786910
(Bracknell Forest Primary Care Trust)
Patient List Size: 3140

Practice Manager Helen Osborne

GP Keemti Lal ARORA, Kanchan Lata ARORA

Ringmead Medical Practice
Great Hollands Health Centre, Great Hollands Square, Bracknell RG12 8WY
Tel: 01344 454338 Fax: 01344 861050
(Bracknell Forest Primary Care Trust)
Patient List Size: 14300

Practice Manager David Bathe

GP George KASSIANOS, David HOLMES, Dr LAYING, David Paul NORMAN, Anant Kumar SACHDEV, Dr SANKHARI, Dr TOBIN

The Waterfield Practice
Warfield Green Medical Centre, 1 County Lane, Whitegrove, Bracknell RG42 3JP
Tel: 01344 869771 Fax: 01344 869773
(Bracknell Forest Primary Care Trust)

Practice Manager Val Taylor, Janet Thrower

GP Alastair J MACHRAY, Paul Richard McBURNIE, James W I MURRAY, Kay Jocelyn Welsby NEWTON, Karin Schoubo NIELSEN, Sagarika SANKHARI, Rowan Elizabeth STEPHENS

The Waterfield Practice
Ralphs Ride, Harmanswater, Bracknell RG12 9LH
Tel: 01344 454626 Fax: 01344 404601
(Bracknell Forest Primary Care Trust)
Patient List Size: 11700

Practice Manager Wendy Miller

GP Paul Richard McBURNIE, Nuala B MORTON, James William Ian MURRAY, Kay Jocelyn Welsby NEWTON, Karin Schoubo NIELSEN, Shantamu S RAHMAN

Bradford

Ashwell Medical Centre
Ashwell Road, Manningham, Bradford BD8 9DP
Tel: 01274 490409 Fax: 01274 499112
Email: jdanby@bradford.nhs.uk
Website: www.ashwellmedicalcentre.co.uk
(Bradford City Teaching Primary Care Trust)
Patient List Size: 6700

Practice Manager Anne-Marie Pemberton

GP Judith DANBY, Ilyas HUSSAIN, Mugrat KHAN, Anne-Marie KILLEEN, David PEARSON, Ameen RASUL

Avicenna Medical Practice
14 Institute Road, Eccleshill, Bradford BD2 2HX
Tel: 01274 637417 Fax: 01274 640316
(Bradford City Teaching Primary Care Trust)
Patient List Size: 7255

Practice Manager Viven Bell

GP Akram KHAN, Binoy Kumar SINGH, Sarah BAILEY, Allison HUYTON, Janed REHMAN

Barkerend Health Centre
Barkerend Road, Bradford BD3 8QH
Tel: 01274 778400 Fax: 01274 770146
(Bradford City Teaching Primary Care Trust)
Patient List Size: 3000

Practice Manager Nadia Elbaz

GP Ahmed El Syed Ahmed EL AZAB

Barkerend Health Centre
Daffodil Building, Barkerend Road, Bradford BD3 8QH
Tel: 01274 663321 Fax: 01274 228019
(Bradford City Teaching Primary Care Trust)
Patient List Size: 3500

Practice Manager Christine Shackleton

GP Richard Duncan FALLS, T H HUSSAIN

Barkerend Health Centre
Bradford BD3 8QH
Tel: 01274 661341 Fax: 01274 775880
(Bradford City Teaching Primary Care Trust)

GP R S RAMAN, Jyoti Prakash SINGH

Barkerend Health Centre
Bradford BD3 8QH
Tel: 01274 663553
(Bradford City Teaching Primary Care Trust)

GP Nasar KHAN, Bhupat Ray KHARA

Beacon Road Surgery
71 Beacon Road, Wibsey, Bradford BD6 3ET
Tel: 01274 690008 Fax: 01274 690950
Email: ksinha2@bradford.nhs.uk
(Bradford South and West Primary Care Trust)
Patient List Size: 1500

Practice Manager K Sinha

GP Hemendra Kumar SINHA

Beckside Road Surgery
47 Beckside Road, Bradford BD7 2JN
Tel: 01274 576035
(Bradford City Teaching Primary Care Trust)
Patient List Size: 1350

Practice Manager Elaine Smith

GP Shoshanna GOWA

Bertram Road Surgery
21 Bertram Road, Bradford BD8 7LN
Tel: 01274 547763
(Bradford City Teaching Primary Care Trust)

GP Ahmed MASOOD

Bilton Medical Centre
120 City Road, Bradford BD8 8JT
Tel: 01274 782080
(Bradford City Teaching Primary Care Trust)

GP Mendhy Hussain KHAN

Bilton Medical Centre
Bradford BD8 8JT
Tel: 01274 782080
(Bradford City Teaching Primary Care Trust)

GP M ROSS

Birch Lane Medical Centre
Birch Lane, Bradford BD5 8PA
Tel: 01274 393392
(Bradford City Teaching Primary Care Trust)

Practice Manager Valerie Coley

GP Mohammad Idris ANSARI

Bradford Student Health Service
Laneisteridge Lane, Bradford BD5 0NH
Tel: 01274 234979 Fax: 01274 235940
(Bradford City Teaching Primary Care Trust)
Patient List Size: 8500

Practice Manager Val King

GP Raj CHANDER, Jane Cecilia GILL, Belinda Ann HORSMAN, Graham Donald SANDERSON

Carlton Medical Practice
252 Girlington Road, Bradford BD8 9PB
Tel: 01274 544742 Fax: 01274 483362
Email: enquiries@carltonmedical.co.uk
Website: wwwcarltonmedical.co.uk
(Bradford South and West Primary Care Trust)
Patient List Size: 5705

GP Gillian A RILEY, Andrew Charles BOOTH, James Richard Francis WELFORD

Chatham Street Surgery
2 Chatham Street, Bradford BD3 0JG
Tel: 01274 636434 Fax: 01274 776522
(Bradford City Teaching Primary Care Trust)

GP Karuna Kanta DAS

Cleckheaton Road Surgery
26 Cleckheaton Road, Odsal, Bradford BD6 1BE
Tel: 01274 672331
(Bradford South and West Primary Care Trust)

GP Louis Ronald D'ARCY

Dr Coley
Pollard Park Health Centre, 190 Otley Road, Bradford BD3 0DQ
Tel: 01274 306346
(Bradford City Teaching Primary Care Trust)

Practice Manager Elizebeth Webster

GP Kuldip COLEY

Dr Overend and Partners
Ashurst Surgery, 22 Sherwood Place, Undercliffe, Bradford BD2 3AG
Tel: 01274 637076 Fax: 01274 626979
(North Bradford Primary Care Trust)
Patient List Size: 8365

GP Sarah Elizabeth BROMLEY, Ashraf Mohammad KHAN, Vijay KUMAR, Ramesh MEHAY, Gillian Sydney OVEREND, Andreas WOLFF

Farrow Medical Centre
177 Otley Road, Bradford BD3 0HX
Tel: 01274 637031
(Bradford City Teaching Primary Care Trust)
Patient List Size: 5000

Practice Manager Heather Waite

GP John Howard BARGH, Wendy Glenys LEEDHAM, James Christopher Paul NEWMARK, Patricia Ann NEWMARK, Sarah REYNOLDS

Grange Lea
23 Hollingwood Lane, Bradford BD7 2RE
Tel: 01274 571437 Fax: 01274 571437
(Bradford South and West Primary Care Trust)
Patient List Size: 4500

GP John Christopher HARDAKER, Nigel George WALKER

Grange Practice
Allerton Health Centre, Bell Denie Road, Allerton, Bradford BD15 7WA
Tel: 01274 541696 Fax: 01274 491776
(Bradford South and West Primary Care Trust)
Patient List Size: 7500

Practice Manager Hauna Baran

GP Andrew Walter James WITHERS, Fernado FERNANDEZ-LLAMAZARES, Adele MADDY, David Michael THORNTON

Green Lane Surgery
6 & 8 Green Lane, Lumb Lane, Bradford BD8 7SP
Tel: 01274 724418
(Bradford City Teaching Primary Care Trust)
Patient List Size: 1860

GP Urmila GUPTA, E STEPHENS

Haigh Hall Medical Centre
Haigh Hall Road, Greengates, Bradford BD10 9AZ
Tel: 01274 613326 Fax: 01274 614769
(North Bradford Primary Care Trust)

Practice Manager Kate Bradley

GP Wendy Sharon Grey PASSANT, Emma DINTINGER, Fiona FLEMING

Harrogate Road Surgery
23 Harrogate Road, Bradford BD2 3DY
Tel: 01274 639857 Fax: 01274 627006
(North Bradford Primary Care Trust)
Patient List Size: 2800

GP Martin Richard SPIERS

Heaton Medical Centre
Haworth Road, Bradford BD9 6LL
Tel: 01274 541701 Fax: 01274 546533
(Bradford South and West Primary Care Trust)

GP Sally D BLACKBURN, Nilofer Fatima ABBAS, Neil Arthur Cameron BOWRING, James Arthur JENNINGS

Highfield Health Centre
2 Proctor Street, off Tong Street, Bradford BD4 9QA
Tel: 01274 227700 Fax: 01274 227900
(Bradford South and West Primary Care Trust)
Patient List Size: 12000

Practice Manager Bill McKenitt

GP Rushdi Shafiq SIDRA, Angela Jane MOULSON

Highfield Health Centre
2 Proctor Street, off Tong Street, Bradford BD4 9QA
Tel: 01274 227800 Fax: 01274 227900
(Bradford South and West Primary Care Trust)
Patient List Size: 7700

Practice Manager Bill McKevitt

GP Carmel MICALLEF, Tim CARVIN, Keith Philip FRASER, Angela MOURSON

Holmewood Clinic
Bradford BD4 9EJ
Tel: 01274 653365
(Bradford City Teaching Primary Care Trust)

GP Gunasiri AMBEPITIYA

Horton Bank Practice
1220 Great Horton Road, Bradford BD7 4PL
Tel: 01274 410666 Fax: 01274 521605
(Bradford South and West Primary Care Trust)

Practice Manager Kath Crabbe

GP Charles Andrew Harrower MICHIE, David Eric PICKERSGILL, Barbara Elizabeth SLOAN, Stephen Arthur YORK

Horton Grange Road Surgery
1 Horton Grange Road, Bradford BD7 3AH
Tel: 01274 502102
(Bradford City Teaching Primary Care Trust)

Practice Manager Lynne Garforth

GP Syed Mohammad IMTIAZ, Irshad Ali KHAN

Horton Park Surgery
99 Horton Park Avenue, Bradford BD7 3EG
Tel: 01274 394277
(Bradford City Teaching Primary Care Trust)

GP David Shemtob GAGUINE, Clare Mary CONNOLLY, Alun Owen GRIFFITHS, Michael LAWSON, Emma Frances Rowan SARGANT

Idle Medical Centre
440 Highfield ROAd, Idle, Bradford BD10 8RU
Tel: 01274 771999 Fax: 01274 772001
(North Bradford Primary Care Trust)
Patient List Size: 11500

Practice Manager Pat Suddards

GP Alison Margaret ROBERTS, Lynne HUGHES-GUY, M JAMIESON, R KASPER, S MATTHEWS, C McCORMACK, C MILLS, Matthew PARKER

Jandu and Partners
274 Keighley Road, Frizinghall, Bradford BD9 4LH
Tel: 01274 495577 Fax: 01274 480703
(Bradford City Teaching Primary Care Trust)
Patient List Size: 3500

Practice Manager Patricia Beddard

GP Jaspal JANDU, E HUBBARD, S WHITEHEAD

Kensington Street Health Centre
Whitefield Place, Girlington, Bradford BD8 9LB
Tel: 01274 499209
(Bradford City Teaching Primary Care Trust)

GP Valerie Elizabeth WILSON, Alastair John BAVINGTON, Irengbam Mohendra SINGH, David Brian STOUT, Martin George TAYLOR

Kensington Street Health Centre
Bradford BD8 9LB
Tel: 01274 496433
(Bradford City Teaching Primary Care Trust)

GP M ROSS

Killinghall Road Surgery
308 Killinghall Road, Bradford BD2 4SE
Tel: 01274 637115 Fax: 01274 637115
(Bradford City Teaching Primary Care Trust)

GP Mohammed Mehdi HOSSAIN

Laisterdyke Clinic
Moorside Lane, Bradford BD3 8DH
Tel: 01274 662441 Fax: 01274 661947
Email: laisterdykeclinic@braford.nhs.uk
Website: www.laisterdyke-clinic.co.uk
(Bradford City Teaching Primary Care Trust)
Patient List Size: 6700

Practice Manager Liz Webster

GP Paul Francis COTTERILL, Muhammad ASIF, Sandra Patricia BATEMAN, Stephen Giles MANCHESTER

Leylands Medical Centre
81 Leylands Lane, Bradford BD9 5PZ
Tel: 01274 770771 Fax: 01274 771088
(North Bradford Primary Care Trust)
Patient List Size: 8200

Practice Manager Christine Allen

GP Brian John KARET, Mark Darren BROOKE, Carole Jane LARSEN, Majella OKEAHIALAM

Little Horton Lane Surgery
407 Little Horton Lane, Bradford BD5 0LG
Tel: 01274 740400 Fax: 01274 726680
(Bradford City Teaching Primary Care Trust)
Patient List Size: 2000

Practice Manager Fiona Reid

Low Moor House
167 Netherlands Avenue, Low Moor, Bradford BD12 0TB
Tel: 01274 606818 Fax: 01274 693837
(Bradford South and West Primary Care Trust)
Patient List Size: 7300

Practice Manager Barbara Baker

GP J B COLLINS, Jonathan Brierley COLLINS, Frances Mary GAVIN, Charles Douglas Scott STRACHAN

Manchester Road Medical Centre
774 Manchester Road, Bradford BD5 7QP
Tel: 01274 392108
(Bradford City Teaching Primary Care Trust)

GP Ghulam Mohammad GILKAR

Mayfield Medical Centre
4 Glenholme Park, Clayton, Bradford BD14 6NF
Tel: 01274 880650 Fax: 01274 883256
(Bradford South and West Primary Care Trust)
Patient List Size: 6500

GP David John SHOESMITH, Alison Nicola MATTOCKS, Parmjit RAWAL, Craig SKEET, Sally WOOD

The Medical Centre
4 Craven Avenue, Thornton, Bradford BD13 3LG
Tel: 01274 832110/834387 Fax: 01274 831694
(Bradford South and West Primary Care Trust)
Patient List Size: 8000

Practice Manager Ann Riley

GP Roger CLARK, Andrew Timothy HANSEN, Bryan Francis PARKINSON, Christine TEMPERLEY

Moorside Surgery
1 Thornbridge Mews, Bradford BD2 3BL
Tel: 01274 626691 Fax: 01274 626195
Email: enquiries@moorsidesurgery.co.uk
Website: www.moorsidesurgery.co.uk
(North Bradford Primary Care Trust)
Patient List Size: 5932

Practice Manager Jenny Morris

GP R T VAN DER WERT, J A DIXON, Elizabeth Rebecca PENNINGTON, John Marcus SULLIVAN

Mughal Medical Centre
55 Ivanhoe Road, Bradford BD7 3HY
Tel: 01274 504425 Fax: 01274 414282
(Bradford City Teaching Primary Care Trust)

GP Zahir Ahmed MUGHAL

New Cross Street Health Centre
New Cross Street, Bradford BD5 7AW
Tel: 01274 728909 Fax: 01274 321823
(Bradford City Teaching Primary Care Trust)
Patient List Size: 3900

GP Maria Gerarda Wilhelmina DE HAAR, Michael LONGFIELD

New Cross Street Health Centre
New Cross Street, Bradford BD5 7AW
Tel: 01274 733232
(Bradford City Teaching Primary Care Trust)

GP Simon Haywood DEDRICK, Ian Ernest FENWICK, Michael Graham SCARLAND

Otley Road Medical Centre
Bradford BD3 0HX
Tel: 01274 632723
(Bradford City Teaching Primary Care Trust)

GP A BARUAH

Park Road Medical Centre
Bradford BD5 0SG
Tel: 01274 721924 Fax: 01274 776466
(Bradford City Teaching Primary Care Trust)

GP Keshaw Prasad MALL

The Parklands Medical Practice
Park Road, Bradford BD5 0SG
Tel: 01274 227575 Fax: 01274 693558
(Bradford South and West Primary Care Trust)

Practice Manager Kathleen Flynn

GP Hatim Shaikhadam MOOCHHALA, Roger Timothy CALLAGHAN, Saskia Susan DE MOWBRAY, Christopher Anthony JOHNSTON, Anne Brunton MONCRIEFF, Ian Rodney STINSON

Parklands Medical Practice
The Medical Centre, 30 Buttershaw Lane, Bradford BD6 2DD
Tel: 01274 678464 Fax: 01274 693558
(Bradford South and West Primary Care Trust)

Peel Park Surgery
3 Airedale Road, Bradford BD3 0LR
Tel: 01274 634989 Fax: 01274 627043
(Bradford City Teaching Primary Care Trust)
Patient List Size: 2800

Practice Manager A Malloy

GP Nihares CHAKRABARTI

Pemberton Drive Surgery
9 Pemberton Drive, Bradford BD7 1RA
Tel: 01274 721621
(Bradford City Teaching Primary Care Trust)

GP Mohammad AZAM

Phoenix Medical Practice
Allerton Clinic, Belldean Road, Allerton, Bradford BD15 7NJ
Tel: 01274 544749 Fax: 01274 546013
Website: www.phoenixmp.co.uk
(Bradford South and West Primary Care Trust)
Patient List Size: 3000

Practice Manager C Davidson

GP A A HENDERSON, S M ALI

Picton Medical Centre
161 Lumb Lane, Bradford BD8 7SW
Tel: 01274 734994 Fax: 01274 723174
(Bradford City Teaching Primary Care Trust)

GP Munir Ahmed KHAN

The Ridge Medical Practice
3 Paternoster Lane, Great Horton, Bradford BD7 3EE
Tel: 01274 322822 Fax: 01274 322833
Email: the.ridge@bradford.nhs.uk
Website: www.theridge@bradford.nhs.uk
(Bradford South and West Primary Care Trust)
Patient List Size: 17200

GP Robert ASHWORTH, Fliss BARNES, Vincenzo CAVALIERE, Anne Lesley CONNOLLY, John Michael CONNOLLY, Andrew HANSON, Christopher Paul HARRIS, Narejh KANURILLI, Susan RANAL, Susan TOWERS, Susan Marie TOWERS

Rooley Lane Medical Centre
Rooley Lane, Bradford BD4 7SS
Tel: 01274 223118 Fax: 01274 772661
(Bradford South and West Primary Care Trust)
Patient List Size: 6500

Practice Manager C Kestin

GP Robert David ANTROBUS, Dr ABAD, Dr BYRNE, H COLE, C PARNELL, Dr YOUNG

Rooley Lane Medical Centre
Rooley Lane, Bradford BD4 7SS
Tel: 01274 223118 Fax: 01274 772661
(Bradford South and West Primary Care Trust)

Practice Manager C Kestin

GP Cathrine PARNELL

Rooley Lane Medical Centre
Rooley Lane, Bradford BD4 7SS
Tel: 01274 224888 Fax: 01274 772661
(Bradford South and West Primary Care Trust)

Practice Manager C Kestin

GP Imtiaz Ali KHAN, H J DEWHIRST, P KAMILL

Royds Healthy Living Centre
20 Ridings Way, Bradford BD6 3UD
Tel: 01274 321888 Fax: 01274 322029
(Bradford South and West Primary Care Trust)

GP Cordelia Lynn PATERSON

Sai Medical Centre
59 St. Pauls Road, Manningham, Bradford BD8 7LS
Tel: 01274 543464 Fax: 01274 490003
(Bradford City Teaching Primary Care Trust)
Patient List Size: 2000

GP Sabanathan CHITSABESAN

Smith Lane Surgery
1 Smith Lane, Bradford BD9 5HE
Tel: 01274 544926
(Bradford City Teaching Primary Care Trust)
Patient List Size: 1600

Practice Manager Sultana Sayed

GP Gyasuddin Mohamed SAYED

St Paul's Road Surgery
50 St Paul's Road, Bradford BD8 7LP
Tel: 01274 543684 Fax: 01274 487674
(Bradford City Teaching Primary Care Trust)
Patient List Size: 2300

Practice Manager Sumitra Patel

GP C P SAHAY, Mohammed Tahir QURESHI

Sunnybank House Medical Centre
Towngate, Wyke, Bradford BD12 9NG
Tel: 01274 424111 Fax: 01274 424001
(Bradford South and West Primary Care Trust)

Practice Manager Susan Dawrant

GP Philip James ATHERTON, Catherine M BRADLEY, Karen DOHERTY, Graham Malcolm HILLARY, Louise KING, Andrew J McELLIGOTT, Ella K RUSSELL, Helen Garden SWAPP, Matthew WALSH

The Surgery
5 Alice Street, Off Lumb Lane, Bradford BD8 7RT
Tel: 01274 736996 Fax: 01274 726956
(Bradford City Teaching Primary Care Trust)
Patient List Size: 3700

Practice Manager G Phillips

GP A BINDU

The Surgery
4 Bertram Road, Bradford BD8 7LN
Tel: 01274 493345
(Bradford City Teaching Primary Care Trust)

GP Mohammad AZAM

The Surgery
1-3 White's Terrace, Bradford BD8 8NR
Tel: 01274 481600
(Bradford City Teaching Primary Care Trust)

GP M GUPTA

The Surgery
52 St Paul's Road, Bradford BD8 7LP
Tel: 01274 548117
(Bradford City Teaching Primary Care Trust)

GP M S ISLAM

White's Terrace Surgery
27 White's Terrace, Bradford BD8 8NR
Tel: 01274 544915 Fax: 01274 821999
(Bradford City Teaching Primary Care Trust)

Practice Manager Zida Khan

GP Mohammad MAHMOOD

Wibsey and Queensbury Medical Practice
Fair Road, Wibsey, Bradford BD6 1TD
Tel: 01274 677198 Fax: 01274 693389
(Bradford South and West Primary Care Trust)
Patient List Size: 10600

Practice Manager Nicola Costello

GP James Humphrey SAYWELL, Edward Owen BARTLE, Jennifer Susan CORBRIDGE, Barbara Ann HAKIN, Daniel George Royston HARDING, John Paul MAGUIRE, R NIGAM

Willows Medical Centre
Osbourne Drive, Queensbury, Bradford BD13 2GD
Tel: 01274 882008 Fax: 01274 818447
(Bradford South and West Primary Care Trust)
Patient List Size: 6000

GP Patrick Kevin DALTON, Yasmin KHAN, David John ROUT, Linda Anne YOUNG

Wilsden Health Centre
Ling Bob Court, Wilsden, Bradford BD15 0LP
Tel: 01535 273227 Fax: 01535 274860
Email: wilsdenmp@bradford.nhs.uk
(Bradford South and West Primary Care Trust)

GP G M BROWN, E BRAMWELL, J JAGGER, J LEE, M McKITTRIDE, M PURVIS, Andrew Richard WILSON

Wilsden Medical Practice
2 Ling Bob Court, Wilsden, Bradford BD15 0LP
Tel: 01535 273227 Fax: 01535 274860
(Bradford South and West Primary Care Trust)

Practice Manager Veronica Carrington

GP George Morris BROWN, Eleanor Ruth BRAMWELL, Janet Elizabeth LEE, Julie Anne PATTERSON, Mark Julian PURVIS, Andrew Richard WILSON

Woodhead Road Surgery
157 Woodhead Road, Bradford BD7 2BL
Tel: 01274 502050 Fax: 01274 414308
(Bradford City Teaching Primary Care Trust)

GP Dasharathlal Sankalchand MODI

Wrose Health Centre
Kings Road, Bradford BD2 1QG
Tel: 01274 638353 Fax: 01274 772899
(North Bradford Primary Care Trust)

Practice Manager Rachel Thompson

GP Cyril Derek PARKINSON, Neil Barrie WINN, Abdul Aziz QAZI, Sheila Elizabeth ROBERTS

Bradford-on-Avon

St Margarets Surgery
29 Bridge Street, Bradford-on-Avon BA15 1BY
Tel: 01225 863278 Fax: 01225 868648
Email: ethel-johnson@gp-J83620.nhs.uk
(West Wiltshire Primary Care Trust)
Patient List Size: 3332

Practice Manager Alda Sinclair

GP Ethel Barbara JOHNSON

Station Approach Health Centre
Station Approach, Bradford-on-Avon BA15 1DQ
Tel: 01225 866611 Fax: 01225 868493
(West Wiltshire Primary Care Trust)
Patient List Size: 13400

Practice Manager Angie Brown

GP Andrew Richard SNOW, Andrew CHISNALL, Nigel Anthony GOUGH, James Sidney HEFFER, Louise PATERSON, Janice PATRICK, Fiona TEES, Nell Victoria WYATT

Braintree

Blandford House Surgery
7 London Road, Braintree CM7 2LD
Tel: 01376 347100 Fax: 01376 349934
(Witham, Braintree and Halstead Care Trust)
Patient List Size: 14800

Practice Manager Alison Howett

GP Ian George Longrigg GIBSON, Carol Vivien GIBSON, E O JESSA, Robert Edmund Peter MAYO, Abdul RASHID, David Anthony WILLIAMS

Blyth's MeadowSurgery
9 Coggeshall Road, Braintree CM7 9DD
Tel: 01376 552508 Fax: 01376 552690
Email: blythsmeadowsurgery@fomail.net
(Witham, Braintree and Halstead Care Trust)
Patient List Size: 8200

Practice Manager June Mya Than Win

GP Kyaw HTUN, L DE VIVO, June Mya Than WIN

Freshwell Health Centre
Wethersfield Road, Finchingfield, Braintree CM7 4BQ
Tel: 01371 810328 Fax: 01371 811282
(Witham, Braintree and Halstead Care Trust)
Patient List Size: 5500

Practice Manager Anita Clapson

GP Andrew Charles Collingwood HILDREY, Adam Mark CUTTS, Richard Peter MEAKIN, Imogen Clare SHAW

Mount Chambers Surgery
92 Coggeshall Road, Braintree CM7 9BY
Tel: 01376 553415 Fax: 01376 552451
(Witham, Braintree and Halstead Care Trust)
Patient List Size: 13000

Practice Manager P Matthams

GP Martin David JACKSON, J MERRITT, Jeremy Robert PATERSON, Noel Bertram Michael PEREIRA, Paul John READ, Ann-Marie Rose SOARES, Susan Katharine SUMMERS, K WILBRAHAM

St Lawrence Medical Centre
4 Bocking End, Braintree CM7 9AA
Tel: 01376 552474 Fax: 01376 552417
(Witham, Braintree and Halstead Care Trust)
Patient List Size: 15853

Practice Manager Jenny Raymond

GP Roger Hugh MARTIN, Carol BLADEN, Robin CHESTERS, Rosemary Lynne KING, Henricus Joseph Raphael MEESTERS, Anne Veronica PURDIE, John Edward SLATER, Ravi VANUKURU

Brampton

Brampton Medical Practice
4 Market Place, Brampton CA8 1NL
Tel: 016977 2551 Fax: 016977 41944
Email: brampton.surgery.freeserve.co.uk
(Eden Valley Primary Care Trust)
Patient List Size: 14200

Practice Manager C Keen

GP Peter Geoffrey WEAVING, John Robert BESTWICK, Carol Agnes BRODIE, Mark BYERS, Patrick John GRAY, Andrew St John HOLLINGS, Christine Patricia KEHOE, Gordon Davidson LOW, Janice ROYLE

Brandon

Daley and Partners
Lakenheath Surgery, 135 High Street, Lakenheath, Brandon IP27 9EP
Tel: 01842 860400 Fax: 01842 862078
(Suffolk West Primary Care Trust)

Practice Manager Pat Turner

GP Timothy Patrick DALEY, E L BOWER, S M RATON-LUNN

The Forest Group Practice
The Surgery, Bury Road, Brandon IP27 0BU
Tel: 01842 813353 Fax: 01842 815221
(Suffolk West Primary Care Trust)

Practice Manager Kate Birrell

GP Guillermo Henrique CAMPMAN, Nicholas COOPER, Thomas Michael HICKS, Charles James PUGH, Angela Elizabeth WARREN

Braunton

Caen Health Centre
Braunton EX33 1LR
Tel: 01271 812005 Fax: 01271 814768
(North Devon Primary Care Trust)
Patient List Size: 11000

Practice Manager Suzanne Bennett

GP Susanna Ruth HILL, Brian BENNETT, Hugh Russell BRADFORD, Angela FLETCHER, John Richard Clement FRANCIS, David Gerald MOORE, Henry Arthur Chernocke PEARSE

Brentford

Brentford Group Practice
Boston Manor Road, Brentford TW8 8DS
Tel: 020 8321 3844 Fax: 020 8321 3862
(Hounslow Primary Care Trust)
Patient List Size: 7200

Practice Manager Linda Clubb

GP Stuart McDonald LANE, P GUPTA, Catherine (Katy) HUGH-JONES, Sudhan ROY

Brentford Health Centre
Boston Manor Road, Brentford TW8 8DS
Tel: 020 8321 3822 Fax: 020 8321 3808
(Hounslow Primary Care Trust)

Practice Manager Susie Smith

GP Khaled Mustafa YASIN

Brentford Health Centre
Boston Manor Road, Brentford TW8 8DS
Tel: 020 8321 3838 Fax: 020 8321 3814
(Hounslow Primary Care Trust)

Practice Manager Maureen Redington

GP Richard BAXTER, Annabel CROWE, Catherine LAWRENCE, Sukhdeu MATHARU

Brentwood

Avenue Road Surgery
2 Avenue Road, Warley, Brentwood CM14 5EL
Tel: 01277 212820 Fax: 01277 234169
(Billericay, Brentwood and Wickford Primary Care Trust)
Patient List Size: 11600

Practice Manager Kate Woolterton

GP Peter Ronald OUTEN, John GARRETT, Megan MULLINS, Dayanand Ramrao PANDIT, W SAINI, Jonathan James TUPPEN, Mark Clive WOOLTERTON

The New Surgery
8 Shenfield Road, Brentwood CM15 8AB
Tel: 01277 218393 Fax: 01277 201017
Website: www.thenewsurgery-brentwood.co.uk
(Billericay, Brentwood and Wickford Primary Care Trust)
Patient List Size: 11900

Practice Manager Sue Johnson

GP Rakesh GUPTA, Victor Douglas BRADBURY, Margaret Alicia HAMILTON, Ajaz Ahmed NAEEM, Mamsoon NASIF, Stephen John WATTS

The Surgery
Mount Avenue, Shenfield, Brentwood CM13 2NL
Tel: 01277 224612 Fax: 01277 201218
(Billericay, Brentwood and Wickford Primary Care Trust)

Practice Manager M Eringa, Deborah Fielding

GP Joanna DENNIS, M R LISSMAN, James John MURRAY, Jonathan Charles Willerton RICHARDSON

The Surgery
Outings Lane, Doddinghurst, Brentwood CM15 0LS
Tel: 01277 821699 Fax: 01277 821226
(Billericay, Brentwood and Wickford Primary Care Trust)
Patient List Size: 8500

Practice Manager C Bailey

GP Stuart John JENNINGS, Nigel Stephen BUTLER, Lesley Anne CLOUGH, Helen DEVONALD

The Surgery
Rockleigh Court, 136 Hutton Road, Shenfield, Brentwood CM15 8NN
Tel: 01277 223844 Fax: 01277 230136
(Billericay, Brentwood and Wickford Primary Care Trust)
Patient List Size: 6200

Practice Manager Steve Waters

GP David Philip AINSWORTH, Kevin Ian MEAD, Yasodhara SATHANANTHAN

Tile House Surgery
33 Shenfield Road, Brentwood CM15 8AQ
Tel: 01277 227711 Fax: 01277 200649
(Billericay, Brentwood and Wickford Primary Care Trust)
Patient List Size: 15000

Practice Manager Karen Smith

GP Graham William HILLMAN, Damian AUNG, Magda Maria DRYDEN, Jonathan David EVANS, Sarah Christine HILDEBRAND, Christopher VILLIERS, Sami YAQUB

Bridgnorth

Alveley Health Centre
Alveley, Bridgnorth WV15 6NG
Tel: 01746 780553 Fax: 01746 780976
(Shropshire County Primary Care Trust)
Patient List Size: 2150

Practice Manager Jane Hunt

GP Nirver Singh SANDHU, Elizabeth GUEST

Bridgnorth Medical Practices
Northgate House, 7 High Street, Bridgnorth WV16 4BU
Tel: 01746 767121
(Shropshire County Primary Care Trust)

GP William HAMMERTON, Michael Stewart GOODALL, Michael John MAGILL, Simon Lewis MARTIN, David Blair McDOWELL, Anthony John SEELEY, Stuart Lloyd WRIGHT, Pamela Mary YUILLE

Brown Clee Medical Practice
Station Road, Ditton Priors, Bridgnorth WV16 6SS
Tel: 01746 712672 Fax: 01746 712580
(Shropshire County Primary Care Trust)
Patient List Size: 2700

Practice Manager C Lewis

GP Richard Charles Cumming GROVES, William Lloyd BASSETT

New Medical Centre
Main Road, Highley, Bridgnorth WV16 6HG
Tel: 01746 861572 Fax: 01746 862295
(Shropshire County Primary Care Trust)
Patient List Size: 3400

Practice Manager R Patel

GP Yashvant Ashabhai PATEL

Bridgwater

Brent House Surgery
Brent House, 14 King Street, Bridgwater TA6 3ND
Tel: 01278 458551 Fax: 01278 431116
Email: dawn.underhill@brenthouse.nhs.uk
(Somerset Coast Primary Care Trust)
Patient List Size: 7535

Practice Manager Dawn Underhill

GP Roger John LAMBERT, Hilary Mavis ALLEN, Andrew William Rowe DOUGLASS, Shona GILMOUR-WHITE, M SMART

Cannington Health Centre
Mill Lane, Cannington, Bridgwater TA5 2HB
Tel: 01278 652335 Fax: 01278 652453
Email: moria.allen@canningtonhc.nhs.uk
(Somerset Coast Primary Care Trust)
Patient List Size: 4800

Practice Manager Moira Allen

GP Michael Fraser JOHNSON, Eleanor Lucy BRAY, Charles Francis MACADAM, John Lambert OGLE, W SEARLE

Church Street Surgery
17 Church Street, Bridgwater TA6 5AT
Tel: 01278 424901 Fax: 01278 437103
Email: sandy.jones@churchstsurgery.nhs.uk
(Somerset Coast Primary Care Trust)

Practice Manager Sandy Jones

GP Richard James LEE

East Quay Medical Centre
East Quay, Bridgwater TA6 5YB
Tel: 01278 444666 Fax: 01278 445448
Email: sandra.criddle@eastquaymc.nhs.uk
Website: www.eastquaymedicalcentre.com
(Somerset Coast Primary Care Trust)
Patient List Size: 12500

Practice Manager Rachel Stark

GP Paul Kenneth HANSFORD, Peter Malcolm AIRD, Jeremy David BUDD, Stephen GARDINER, Alison Mary GOLDIE, Richard Andrew Dermod O'BRIEN, Susan Elizabeth Kim ROBERTS, Hilary Jane SWINDALL

Quantock Medical Centre
Banneson Road, Nether Stowey, Bridgwater TA5 1NW
Tel: 01278 732696 Fax: 01278 733381
Email: qmcdrs@globalnet.co.uk
(Somerset Coast Primary Care Trust)
Patient List Size: 3050

Practice Manager Marion Maddison

GP David Thomas MATTHEWS, Christopher M STONE

Quarry Ground Surgery
Broadway, Edington, Bridgwater TA7 9JB
Tel: 01278 722077 Fax: 01278 722352
Website: http://extranet.somerset-health.org.uk/area16/Redg
(Somerset Coast Primary Care Trust)

Practice Manager Marina Turnbull

GP Peter Simon HAYNE, A J ROWLING, Anthony WRIGHT

Redgate Medical Centre
Westonzoyland Road, Bridgwater TA6 5BF
Tel: 01278 444411 Fax: 01278 446816
(Somerset Coast Primary Care Trust)

Practice Manager Neil Davies

GP S J AKHTER, Donal Morley HYNES, Roger David JOHNSON, J E SHACKLETON

The Surgery
Mill Street, North Petherton, Bridgwater TA6 6LX
Tel: 01278 662223 Fax: 01278 663727
Email: lesleymildren@northpetherton.nhs.uk
(Somerset Coast Primary Care Trust)
Patient List Size: 4250

Practice Manager Lesley Mildren

GP Nicholas John BRAY, N HAWKES, M HOWELL, Caroline Elizabeth LAWLER, Timothy Mark TILSLEY

Taunton Road Medical Centre
12-16 Taunton Road, Bridgwater TA6 3LS
Tel: 01278 720000 Fax: 01278 423691
Email: trmc@globalnet.co.uk
Website: www.trmc.co.uk
(Somerset Coast Primary Care Trust)

Practice Manager Ann Gass

GP John Dawson WROUT, S BRIDGMAN, G FERGUSSON, Jon PARRATT, Anne Elisabeth Ryder REED, Peter Dennis REED, David Kenneth ROOKE, Gregory Peter Gerrard TANNER, Helena TANNER, Timothy Michael Winn TAYLOR

Bridlington

Field House Surgery
18 Victoria Road, Bridlington YO15 2AT
Tel: 01262 673362 Fax: 01262 400218
(Yorkshire Wolds and Coast Primary Care Trust)
Patient List Size: 9900

Practice Manager Noel Parr

GP Dr BOWDEN, Dr BARANAUSKAS, Dr GARWOOD, James Ross GILLESPIE, Dr PICKERING, Dr THOMPSON

Manor House Surgery
Providence Place, Bridlington YO15 2QW
Tel: 01262 602661 Fax: 01262 400891
(Yorkshire Wolds and Coast Primary Care Trust)

Practice Manager Chris Colley

GP John Burgess BAYNE, Keith Thomas James FARLEY, Alan Christopher FRANCIS, Carolien LINO, Sergio Antonello RAISE, Alistair Stuart ROBERTSON

The Medical Centre
Station Avenue, Bridlington YO16 4LZ
Tel: 01262 670690
(Yorkshire Wolds and Coast Primary Care Trust)

GP Hamish Kellar MACNAB, David Edmund Graham HICKSON, Michael McKENNA

The Medical Centre
Station Avenue, Bridlington YO16 4LZ
Tel: 01262 670686 Fax: 01262 401685
(Yorkshire Wolds and Coast Primary Care Trust)
Patient List Size: 9677

Practice Manager Denise Shippey

GP Peter MUNDY, Ian Bell, Anthony John CLARKE, Paul Anthony HARRIS, Margaret Robertson

The Medical Centre - Practice One
Station Avenue, Bridlington YO16 4LZ
Tel: 01262 670683 Fax: 01262 401685
(Yorkshire Wolds and Coast Primary Care Trust)

GP Hamish Robin Peter MELDRUM, Elizabeth Ann BARTON

Bridport

Hollands and Partners
Bridport Medical Centre, North Allington, Bridport DT6 5DU
Tel: 01308 421896 Fax: 01308 420869
(South West Dorset Primary Care Trust)

Practice Manager P Hayter

GP Jeremy Jonathan de Carteret HOLLANDS, Joanna COTTON, Robert Lawrence NEAME, Colin Bryce WILSON

Littlehurst Surgery
The Street, Charmouth, Bridport DT6 6PE
Tel: 01297 560872 Fax: 01297 560584
Email: postmaster@gp-j81628.nhs.uk
(South West Dorset Primary Care Trust)
Patient List Size: 1860

GP Martin Joseph John BECKERS, Susan Rachel BECKERS

Skellern and Partners
Bridport Medical Centre, North Allington, Bridport DT6 5DU
Tel: 01308 421109 Fax: 01308 420869
(South West Dorset Primary Care Trust)

Practice Manager Pauline Hayter

GP George SKELLERN, Bridget May BURT, Alan Blair MILLAR, Ian Thomas PLATT, Philip Guy WEBB

Brierley Hill

Albion House Surgery
Albion Street, Brierley Hill DY5 3EE
Tel: 01384 70220 Fax: 01384 78284
(Dudley South Primary Care Trust)

Practice Manager M A Gregory

GP Margaret Anne BUNDRED, Ian Frank CRAGGS, Catherine Ruth EDWARDS, Dominic Hilary Richard FAUX, Ian Alan REED, Amanda Jane YOUNG

Brierley Hill Health Centre
Albion Street, Brierley Hill DY5 3EE
Tel: 01384 573771
Email: jamal.mary@dudley.nhs.uk
(Dudley South Primary Care Trust)
Patient List Size: 3000

GP Jamal Salman Georges MARY

Brierley Hill Health Centre
Albion Street, Brierley Hill DY5 3EE
Tel: 01384 77382 Fax: 01384 483931
Email: claire.ripper@dudley.nhs.uk
(Dudley South Primary Care Trust)
Patient List Size: 7500

GP Mahendra Kumar Mulchand SUMARIA, L BHARDWAJ, U.P. INGLE, K C JAIN, Ashok Kumar KHASGIWALE

Brierley Hill Health Centre
Albion Street, Brierley Hill DY5 3EE
(Dudley South Primary Care Trust)

GP Dr SAHNI, Dr SAHNI

Quarry Bank Medical Centre
165 High Street, Quarry Bank, Brierley Hill DY5 2AE
Tel: 01384 566651 Fax: 01384 829170
(Dudley South Primary Care Trust)
Patient List Size: 4146

Practice Manager Denise Hickman

GP Mohamed Rezaul KARIM, Hajera KARIM

The Surgery
30 Sandringham Way, Quincy Rise, Brierley Hill DY5 3JR
Tel: 01384 422698 Fax: 01384 860800
(Dudley South Primary Care Trust)

GP Sunil Kumar MEROTRA

Thorns Road Surgery
43 Thorns Road, Quarry Bank, Brierley Hill DY5 2JS
Tel: 01384 77524 Fax: 01384 486540
Email: c.williams@M87033.dudley-pcg.wmids.nhs.uk
(Dudley South Primary Care Trust)
Patient List Size: 2890

Practice Manager LindaChristine Williams

GP Jayantibhai Ashabhai PATEL

Withymoor Village Surgery
3 Turners Lane, Withymoor Village, Brierley Hill DY5 2PG
Tel: 01384 366740 Fax: 01384 350444
(Dudley South Primary Care Trust)
Patient List Size: 4500

Practice Manager Jackie Atkins

GP C FERNANDES, T E G JONES

Brigg

Church Street Surgery
Church Street, Hibaldstow, Brigg DN20 9ED
Tel: 01652 650580
(West Lincolnshire Primary Care Trust)
Patient List Size: 2900

GP Michael EDMONDSON-JONES, Annabel Louise YULE-SMITH

Riverside Surgery
Barnard Avenue, Brigg DN20 8AS
Tel: 01652 650131 Fax: 01652 651551
(North Lincolnshire Primary Care Trust)
Patient List Size: 12000

Practice Manager John Clarke

GP David William CHESTER, John Francis BURSCOUGH, Peter Edward NORRIS, Neerja RAI, Paul Adrian SUTTON, Allan William TENNANT

Whitaker and Partners
53 Bridge Street, Brigg DN20 8NS
Tel: 01652 657779 Fax: 01652 659440
Email: bridge.street@virgin.net
Website: www.53bridgestreet.net
(North Lincolnshire Primary Care Trust)
Patient List Size: 6300

Practice Manager Carole Corringham

GP Andrew Spencer WHITAKER, Benedicte Marie IUEL, Valerie Suzanne WHITAKER, E A WILLIS

Brighouse

Church Lane Surgery
24 Church Lane, Brighouse HD6 1AS
Tel: 01484 714349 Fax: 01484 720479
Email: churchln@globalnet.co.uk
(Calderdale Primary Care Trust)
Patient List Size: 11950

Practice Manager Eileen Todd

GP Patrick Joseph Anthony O'CARROLL, Steven John CHAMBERS, Julie Ann CROSSLAND, Josephine WAITE, Robert Malcolm WYLIE

Longroyde Surgery
38 Castle Avenue, Rastrick, Brighouse HD6 3HT
Tel: 01484 721102
(Calderdale Primary Care Trust)

GP Alan Charles BROOK, J P GRANT

Rastrick Health Centre
Chapel Croft, Rastrick, Brighouse HD6 3NA
Tel: 01484 710853/4 Fax: 01484 722983
(Calderdale Primary Care Trust)

Practice Manager Karen Saville

GP Peter Jeffrey GORMAN, S M FEATHERSTONE, Joanna WILKINSON

Rydings Hall Surgery
Church Lane, Brighouse HD6 1AT
Tel: 01484 715324 Fax: 01484 400847
(Calderdale Primary Care Trust)
Patient List Size: 9200

Practice Manager Margaret Bridges

GP John Richard GATECLIFF, Gregory Michael MATISCHEN, L REED, A WILKINSON

Brighton

Ardingly Court Surgery
Ardingly Court, 1 Ardingly Street, Brighton BN2 1SS
Tel: 01273 688333 Fax: 01273 671128
(Brighton and Hove City Teaching Primary Care Trust)

Practice Manager Dee French

GP Sharon DREWETT, Veronica Anne SUTCLIFFE, Mary FLYNN, Jo WARD

The Avenue Surgery
1 The Avenue, South Moulsecoomb, Brighton BN2 4GF
Tel: 01273 604220/606214 Fax: 01273 685507
(Brighton and Hove City Teaching Primary Care Trust)
Patient List Size: 6459

Practice Manager Jacqui Mason

GP Robert Stanley HACKING, Roger Andrew WINTER

Broadway Surgery
9 The Broadway, Whitehawk Road, Brighton BN2 5NF
Tel: 01273 600888 Fax: 01273 605664
(Brighton and Hove City Teaching Primary Care Trust)
Patient List Size: 2043

Practice Manager A Villani

GP Sudhakara Gupta SRIPURAM

Church Surgery
Saunders Park Rise, Lewes Road, Brighton BN2 4ES
Tel: 01273 684500 Fax: 01273 625581
(Brighton and Hove City Teaching Primary Care Trust)

Practice Manager H Elliott

GP R MITCHELL, S PARISH, D TIERNEY

Elm Grove Medical Centre
151 Elm Grove, Brighton BN2 3ES
Tel: 01273 604774 Fax: 01273 623281
(Brighton and Hove City Teaching Primary Care Trust)

Practice Manager Afsangh Chiang

GP Vince CHIANG

The Health Centre
University of Sussex, Falmer, Brighton BN1 9RW
Tel: 01273 249049 Fax: 01273 249040
(Brighton and Hove City Teaching Primary Care Trust)

Practice Manager Andrea Garidis

GP Rosemary McCONNELL, Jan AUSTERA, Philip Anthony DENIS LE SEVE, Christopher Anthony WATSON

Highcroft Villas Medical Practice
35a Chatsworth Road, Brighton BN1 5DA
Tel: 01273 552063 Fax: 01273 555836
(Brighton and Hove City Teaching Primary Care Trust)
Patient List Size: 3600

Practice Manager Karen Lintern

GP Nick HASLAM, David HEAL

Links Road Surgery
27-29 Links Road, Portslade, Brighton BN41 1XH
Tel: 01273 412585 Fax: 01273 885800
(Brighton and Hove City Teaching Primary Care Trust)
Patient List Size: 5800

Practice Manager Joan Shaw

GP Alexander Sharen Suresh KHOT, Peter ALDERMAN, Nicky COLEMAN

The Manor Practice
20 Southwick Street, Southwick, Brighton BN42 4TB
Tel: 01273 592723/596077 Fax: 01273 597938
(Adur, Arun and Worthing Primary Care Trust)

Practice Manager Hazel Donaldson

GP Graham Paul TUCKER, Timothy BUCK, Anna CRESSEY, A HOYLE, Ronald John NINES, S SRINIVASAN

The Manor Practice
20 Southwick Street, Southwick, Brighton BN42 4TE
Tel: 01273 596077 Fax: 01273 597938
(Adur, Arun and Worthing Primary Care Trust)

Practice Manager Johanna Gall

GP Timothy BUCK, A HOYLE, Ronald John NINES, S SRINIVASAN, Graham Paul TUCKER

Mile Oak Clinic
Chalky Road, Portslade, Brighton BN41 2WF
Tel: 01273 417390/419365 Fax: 01273 889192
(Brighton and Hove City Teaching Primary Care Trust)
Patient List Size: 6500

Practice Manager Ann Watson

GP Robert Allen WILLIAMS, Sarah Anne BARNARD, Christine Marie HABGOOD, Simon HARRIS, Avni PATEL, Barnaby TREDGOLD

The Montpelier Surgery
2 Victoria Road, Brighton BN1 3FS
Tel: 01273 328950 Fax: 01273 729767
(Brighton and Hove City Teaching Primary Care Trust)
Patient List Size: 5730

Practice Manager Amanda Page

GP Simon Lawrence SACKS, Paul GAYTON, Jane Elizabeth RODERIC-EVANS

Morley Street Surgery
Morley Street, Brighton BN2 2RA
Tel: 01273 385500 Fax: 01273 240956
(Brighton and Hove City Teaching Primary Care Trust)

Practice Manager Karen French

GP Christopher Frederick SARGEANT, Anne DEW

North Laine Medical Centre
12-14 Gloucester Street, Brighton BN1 4EW
Tel: 01273 601112 Fax: 01273 682408
(Brighton and Hove City Teaching Primary Care Trust)

Practice Manager Mike Stemp

GP Michael John Aubrey SHARP, Elain CLARKE

Park Crescent New Surgery
1A Lewes Road, Brighton BN2 3JJ
Tel: 01273 680135 Fax: 01273 698863
(Brighton and Hove City Teaching Primary Care Trust)

Practice Manager Carol Witney

GP Richard GRAY, Gregory John CLIFFORD, Richard Paul CROSSMAN, Sheila Margaret FIRTH, Ruediger GRIMM, Susan Lynn LIPSCOMBE

Portslade County Clinic
Old Shoreham Road, Portslade, Brighton BN41 1XR
Tel: 01273 411229 Fax: 01273 412078
(Brighton and Hove City Teaching Primary Care Trust)
Patient List Size: 3060

GP Brian KIRKLAND, Catherine BRYANT

Portslade Health Centre
Church Road, Portslade, Brighton BN41 1LX
Tel: 01273 422525/425342 Fax: 01273 413510
(Brighton and Hove City Teaching Primary Care Trust)
Patient List Size: 12800

Practice Manager Judi Davies

GP Richard DE SOUZA, Fiona Caroline LEVACK, Anne MINERS, Susan Rosemary ROCKWELL, Michael THOMPSON, Charles Mark Vernon WRIGHT

Preston Park Surgery
2A Florence Road, Brighton BN1 6DJ
Tel: 01273 559601/566033 Fax: 01273 507746
(Brighton and Hove City Teaching Primary Care Trust)
Patient List Size: 10500

Practice Manager Tricia Gibbons

GP David Lincoln SUPPLE, Catherine Frances BROWN, Jane Mary DEADY, Julian Alexander Handley GREAVES, Maria SLATTERY

Rock Sadens Surgery
42 Upper Rock Gardens, Brighton BN2 1QF
Tel: 01273 600103 Fax: 01273 620100
(Brighton and Hove City Teaching Primary Care Trust)
Patient List Size: 4369

Practice Manager Joyce Howfield

GP Linda Margaret ALLENBY, Sandra BURROW

School House Surgery
Hertford Road, Brighton BN1 7GF
Tel: 01273 551031 Fax: 01273 382036
(Brighton and Hove City Teaching Primary Care Trust)
Patient List Size: 2031

Practice Manager Helen Elliott

GP Stephen Peter Edward PARISH, Richard MITCHELL, Dawn TIERNEY

The Seven Dials Medical Centre
24 Montpelier Crescent, Brighton BN1 3JJ
Tel: 01273 773089 Fax: 01273 207098
(Brighton and Hove City Teaching Primary Care Trust)
Patient List Size: 9700

Practice Manager Valerie Leach

GP John Stephen Michael William Peter VAN RYSSEN, Andrew DUCKWORTH, Peter Frank MEADE

Ship Street Surgery
65-67 Ship Street, Brighton BN1 1AE
Tel: 01273 778622 Fax: 01273 776933
(Brighton and Hove City Teaching Primary Care Trust)

Practice Manager Mike Stemp

GP Alison Patricia HERMITAGE

St Lukes Surgery
Saltdean Oval Care Park, Saltdean Park Road, Saltdean, Brighton BN2 8SD
Tel: 01273 302638 Fax: 01273 307615
(Brighton and Hove City Teaching Primary Care Trust)
Patient List Size: 2100

Practice Manager Sue Ward

GP Rifaat AMIN

St Peter's Medical Centre
30-36 Oxford Street, Brighton BN1 4LA
Tel: 01273 606006 Fax: 01273 623896
(Brighton and Hove City Teaching Primary Care Trust)

Practice Manager Corinne Barnard

GP Howard Raymond CARTER, Katharine Rebecca JARVIS, Joanne Sara LAWRENCE, Maria NAGY, Xavier Philippe NALLETAMBY, Caroline Evelyn Ann ROBERTS, Jonathan WASTIE

The Surgery
4 Old Steine, Brighton BN1 1EJ
Tel: 01273 685588 Fax: 01273 624328
(Brighton and Hove City Teaching Primary Care Trust)
Patient List Size: 10000

Practice Manager Lin Martin

GP Rodney Temple TATE, Nigel John ADAMS, Judith Elizabeth ASTON, Catherine Susan BURGESS, Gary GILHOOLY, David WINDSOR-MARTIN

The Surgery
21 Queens Road, Brighton BN1 3XA
Tel: 01273 328080 Fax: 01273 725209
Email: qrsurgery@mistral.co.uk
Website: www3.mistral.co.uk/qrsurgery/index.html
(Brighton and Hove City Teaching Primary Care Trust)
Patient List Size: 4700

Practice Manager J Cox

The Surgery
10 Matlock Road, Brighton BN1 5BF
Tel: 01273 562356/562223 Fax: 01273 562137
(Brighton and Hove City Teaching Primary Care Trust)
Patient List Size: 3000

Practice Manager David Craeton

GP Yok Fun CHANG, Paul ALLAN

The Surgery
118/120 Stanford Avenue, Brighton BN1 6FE
Tel: 01273 506361 Fax: 01273 552483
Website: www.thegrouppractice.com
(Brighton and Hove City Teaching Primary Care Trust)
Patient List Size: 16000

Practice Manager David Drew

GP Elizabeth Jane EADIE, Calum Iain BARTLETT, Andrea Jane BHERMI, Clare GAREWAL, James Reid GRAHAM, Ali Nazim PUNJA, Jenanne SHAHEEN

The Surgery
100 Beaconsfield Villas, Brighton BN1 6HE
Tel: 01273 555999/557908 Fax: 01273 540990
(Brighton and Hove City Teaching Primary Care Trust)
Patient List Size: 3200

Practice Manager Jackie Stenning

GP Dermot Ian Francis KELLEHER

The Surgery
138 Beaconsfield Villas, Brighton BN1 6HQ
Tel: 01273 552212/555401 Fax: 01273 271148
(Brighton and Hove City Teaching Primary Care Trust)
Patient List Size: 7100

Practice Manager Ruth Field

GP David Richard HARPER, Nigel BIRD, Vanessa LYNCH, Fiona Mary PERRY

The Surgery
17B Warmdene Road, Brighton BN1 8NL
Tel: 01273 508811 Fax: 01273 559860
(Brighton and Hove City Teaching Primary Care Trust)
Patient List Size: 10000

Practice Manager Marian Legg

GP John Brian ELVIDGE, Michael COCKCROFT, Catriona GREENWOOD, Naseer Ahmad KHAN, Jyotsna LEWIS

The Surgery
114-116 Carden Avenue, Brighton BN1 8PD
Tel: 01273 500155 Fax: 01273 501193
(Brighton and Hove City Teaching Primary Care Trust)
Patient List Size: 5863

Practice Manager Barbara Neal

GP Ian Tyrie CRAIGIE, Jonathan HALFORD, Rekha SHAH

The Surgery
24 Eaton Place, Brighton BN2 1EH
Tel: 01273 686863 Fax: 01273 623402
(Brighton and Hove City Teaching Primary Care Trust)
Patient List Size: 7100

Practice Manager Jane Demario, Sue Yates

GP Malcolm John STALKER, Robert John MOCKETT

The Surgery
9 Albion Street, Brighton BN2 2PS
Tel: 01273 601122 Fax: 01273 623450
(Brighton and Hove City Teaching Primary Care Trust)

Practice Manager Betty Kirkbright

GP Michael John Patrick BIDDULPH, Nicholas H KESCHTKAR, Nicholas David PATTON

The Surgery
1 The Ridgway, Woodingdean, Brighton BN2 6PE
Tel: 01273 307555 Fax: 01273 304861
(Brighton and Hove City Teaching Primary Care Trust)

Practice Manager Christine Jarvis

GP Ashley Robert Crawford CRICHTON, Peter HOLLIS, Peter Jeremy SAGAR

The Surgery
75 Longridge Avenue, Saltdean, Brighton BN2 8LA
Tel: 01273 305723 Fax: 01273 300962
(Brighton and Hove City Teaching Primary Care Trust)
Patient List Size: 9700

Practice Manager Mary Wills

GP David Lynn PHILLIPS, Paul Ruxton BERESFORD-JONES, Gavin Michael SHANNON, Andrew David WOOLLONS

The Surgery
188/189 Lewes Road, Brighton BN2 3LA
Tel: 01273 603616 Fax: 01273 694101
(Brighton and Hove City Teaching Primary Care Trust)
Patient List Size: 2000

GP Amrut Chunilal SHAH

The Surgery
31 St James Avenue, Brighton BN2 1QD
Tel: 01273 675252 Fax: 01273 682405
(Brighton and Hove City Teaching Primary Care Trust)

Practice Manager Peta Martin

GP Martin Henry KNOTT

The Surgery
130 The Ridgeway, Woodingdean, Brighton BN2 6PB
Tel: 01273 304325 Fax: 01273 304496
(Brighton and Hove City Teaching Primary Care Trust)
Patient List Size: 2500

Practice Manager Nicola Banks

GP Jeremy BAKER, Dodie FAHMY

The Surgery
9 Beaconsfield Road, Brighton BN1 4QH
Tel: 01273 698666 Fax: 01273 672742
(Brighton and Hove City Teaching Primary Care Trust)

GP Jitinkumar Kanchanlal PARIKH

Whitehawk Surgery
Whitehawk Way, Brighton BN2 5NP
Tel: 01273 605438 Fax: 01273 605047
(Brighton and Hove City Teaching Primary Care Trust)

Practice Manager Margaret Cutts

GP Jean HAINING, Emma STANLEY

The Willow Surgery
50 Heath Hill Avenue, Lower Bevandean, Brighton BN2 4FH
Tel: 01273 606391 Fax: 01273 684880
(Brighton and Hove City Teaching Primary Care Trust)

Practice Manager Carol Hamilton

GP Hefin Wyn PRITCHARD

Bristol

Air Balloon Surgery
Kenn Road, St George, Bristol BS5 7PD
Tel: 0117 909 9914 Fax: 0117 908 6660
(Bristol North Primary Care Trust)
Patient List Size: 12500

Practice Manager Kate Francis

GP David Stephen MEMEL, Nicholas Peter GOYDER, Jonathan GUEST, Andrew KAYE, Berenice LOPEZ, Patricia Ann McQUONEY, Sandra MYERS

Almondsbury Surgery
Sundays Hill, Almondsbury, Bristol BS32 4DS
Tel: 01454 613161 Fax: 01454 615745
(South Gloucestershire Primary Care Trust)

Practice Manager Margaret Warren

GP Martin Stephen LOCKYER, Karen Elizabeth HILL

Avonmouth Medical Centre
Collins Street, Avonmouth, Bristol BS11 9JJ
Tel: 0117 982 4322 Fax: 0117 938 2677
(Bristol North Primary Care Trust)
Patient List Size: 2500

Practice Manager Carol Rhodes

GP Sarah Jane GOLDING, Jonathan Charles ROGERS

Blackhorse Medical Centre
St Lukes Close, District Centre, Emerson Green South, Bristol BS16 7AL
Tel: 0117 957 6000 Fax: 0117 957 6001
(South Gloucestershire Primary Care Trust)
Patient List Size: 6850

Practice Manager Karen Hill

GP Shaukat ALI, Sally ERNSLEY, Martin JENKINS

Blackwell Medical Centre
15 West Town Road, Backwell, Bristol BS48 3HA
Tel: 01275 850600
(North Somerset Primary Care Trust)

GP Robin George LAMBERT, Diana Elizabeth BLOSS, David Edward COX, Janet ELPHICK, Caroline Edwina Louise HADDY, Matthew Anthony Richard HOGHTON, Christopher John WATKINS

Bradgate Surgery
Ardenton Walk, Brentry, Bristol BS10 6SP
Tel: 0117 959 1920 Fax: 0117 983 9332
(Bristol North Primary Care Trust)

GP Nigel William Gervase TAYLOR, S A CHADWICK, Thomas Patrick Bernard FAHEY, Barbara Ilse Marie LAUE, Michael Dermot McCALDIN, Margaret Susan THOMAS

Bradley Road Surgery
38-46 Bradley Road, Patchway, Bristol BS34 5LD
Tel: 0117 969 2040 Fax: 0117 947 0440
(South Gloucestershire Primary Care Trust)

Practice Manager Sara Thorne

GP Mohammad Azizar RAHMAN

Bradley Stoke Surgery
Brook Way, Bradley Stoke North, Bristol BS32 9DS
Tel: 01454 616262 Fax: 01454 619155
Email: bss@pcgee.demon.co.uk
(South Gloucestershire Primary Care Trust)
Patient List Size: 12500

Practice Manager Julian Barge

GP Elizabeth Jane TODD, Norman Thomas Edward DOUGLAS, Dianne EDDISON, Timothy John GARROD, Sandra Anne KELLAND, Dylan SUMMERS, Carol TELFER

Brook Advisory Centre
1 Unity Street, Bristol BS1 5HH
Tel: 0117 929 0090 Fax: 0117 922 1293
Email: manager@brookavon.demon.co.uk
Website: www.brook.org.uk
Patient List Size: 5000

GP T MARTESS, A EGGINTON

Brooklea Clinic
Wick Road, Bristol BS4 4HU
Tel: 0117 971 1211
(Bristol South and West Primary Care Trust)

Practice Manager Kath Williamson

GP Peter Nicholas HARBORD

Brooklea Clinic
Wick Road, Bristol BS4 4HU
Tel: 0117 330 4223/4225
(Bristol South and West Primary Care Trust)
Patient List Size: 5200

Practice Manager Sue Tiley

GP Sylvia Anne CARLISLE, Hilary Krystyna FAREY, Peter SAUNDERS

Brooklea Health Centre
Wick Road, Brislington, Bristol BS4 4HU
(Bristol South and West Primary Care Trust)

Practice Manager Diane Pullin

GP P A PRIMROSE

Brooklea Health Centre
Wick Road, Brislington, Bristol BS4 4HU
(Bristol South and West Primary Care Trust)

GP C R STEPHENSON

Cadbury Heath Health Centre
Parkwall Road, Cadbury Heath, Bristol BS30 8HS
Tel: 0117 980 5700 Fax: 0117 980 5701
(South Gloucestershire Primary Care Trust)
Patient List Size: 5000

Practice Manager Helen Tillman

GP Mark Yves O'MAHONY, Elizabeth Ann SEPHTON, Dr GAUNT, Rachaael Mary KENYON

Cadbury Heath Health Centre
Parkwall Road, Bristol BS30 8HS
Tel: 0117 960 0129 Fax: 0117 947 7539
(South Gloucestershire Primary Care Trust)

GP Cheryl Clare ATTER, P R VALENTINE, Claire Louise WOODWARD

Cadbury Heath Health Centre
Parkwall Road, Cadbury Heath, Bristol BS30 8HS
Tel: 0117 980 5706 Fax: 0117 980 5707
Email: drcoote.partners@gp-l81130.nhs.uk
(South Gloucestershire Primary Care Trust)
Patient List Size: 5500

Practice Manager Mark Allon

GP Elizabeth Anne COOTE, Cheryl Clare ATTER, Austin CONNER, Anne Deborah SANDERS

Charlotte Keel Health Centre
Seymour Road, Easton, Bristol BS5 0UA
Tel: 0117 951 2244 Fax: 0117 951 2373
Website: www.surgeriesonline.com/drnormanandpartners
(Bristol North Primary Care Trust)
Patient List Size: 9480

Practice Manager Pat Denner

GP James Marcus NORMAN, Josephine Olwen FLEMING, Kate NICHOLLS, David Elliott SOODEEN

Charlotte Keel Health Centre
Seymour Road, Easton, Bristol BS5 0UA
Tel: 0117 951 2244 Fax: 0117 935 4447
(Bristol North Primary Care Trust)
Patient List Size: 6100

Practice Manager Suzanne Walpole

GP D M PRICE, Peter Leonard ALLEN, Ruth Margaret MUIR, J D M TAYLOR

Charlotte Keel Health Centre
Seymour Road, Easton, Bristol BS5 0UA
Tel: 0117 951 2244 Fax: 0117 952 3022
(Bristol North Primary Care Trust)

Practice Manager Caroline Robinson

GP Dr GODFREY, Dr MURPHY, Dr WINT

Clevedon Health Centre
Old Street, Clevedon, Bristol BS21 6DG
Tel: 01275 335534
(North Somerset Primary Care Trust)

GP D GREEN, P A HORRY, G C HOW, I S MILLER, C J PARFITT

Clifton Village Practice
52 Clifton Down Road, Clifton, Bristol BS8 4AH
Tel: 0117 973 2178 Fax: 0117 925 6178
(Bristol South and West Primary Care Trust)
Patient List Size: 3700

Practice Manager Juliet Bodman

GP T H FREWIN, V HIBBERT, W WALTER

Close Farm Surgery
47 Victoria Road, Warmley, Bristol BS30 5JZ
Tel: 0117 932 2108 Fax: 0117 987 3977
Email: close.farm@seglospcg.btinternet.com
(South Gloucestershire Primary Care Trust)

Practice Manager Clarie Harrill

GP Michael Kevin DARCY, Luke Robert Cowdy PARKER, R A TAYLOR

Coniston Medical Practice
The Parade, Coniston Road, Patchway, Bristol BS34 5TF
Tel: 0117 969 2508 Fax: 0117 969 0456
(South Gloucestershire Primary Care Trust)
Patient List Size: 8000

Practice Manager Peggy Phillips

GP Elizabeth Stewart SAUNDERS, R BERESFORD, Susan Margaret BLACK, I PAUL

Corbett House Surgery
Avonvale Road, Bristol BS5 9QS
Tel: 0117 955 7474 Fax: 0117 955 5402
(Bristol North Primary Care Trust)
Patient List Size: 6200

Practice Manager Rosemarie Ross

GP Christine Alice Elizabeth HOYTE, Peter Malcolm BRINDLE, Paul HUNT, Sarah Caroline JAHFAR

Courtside Surgery
Kennedy Way, Yate, Bristol BS37 4DQ
Tel: 01454 313874 Fax: 01454 327110
Email: postmaster@gp-l81024.nhs.uk
Website: www.courtside.nhs.uk
(South Gloucestershire Primary Care Trust)
Patient List Size: 12400

Practice Manager Barry King

GP Christopher Patrick Charles PAXTON, Andrew Stewart APPLETON, Robert James BALDWIN, Rachel Anne BAYLY, Judith Lavinia BYRNE, John Hamilton ENTRICAN, Brian Keith TOMLINSON, Jane TURNER

The Crest Family Practice
William Budd Health Centre, Knowle West Heath Park, Downton, Bristol BS4 1WH
Tel: 01179 449700 Fax: 0117 944 9799
(Bristol South and West Primary Care Trust)
Patient List Size: 5100

Practice Manager Mary Stork

GP D J MOON, C HILL, C WILLIAMS

Davies and Lawson
Station Road, Congresbury, Bristol BS49 5DX
Tel: 01934 832158 Fax: 01934 834165
(North Somerset Primary Care Trust)
Patient List Size: 3800

Practice Manager Chris Maurin

GP Vivian Mansel DAVIES, E M GRAHAM, Richard Hugh LAWSON

Dean Lane Family Practice
1 Dean Lane, Bedminster, Bristol BS3 1DE
Tel: 0117 966 3149 Fax: 0117 953 0699
(Bristol South and West Primary Care Trust)
Patient List Size: 9500

Practice Manager Helen Deverson

GP Susan Jacqueline HEROD, Jane COLLYER, Ian Trevor GARBUTT, Nicola HARKER, David PEEL, Gillian Adele RICE

Eastville Health Centre
East Park, Bristol BS5 6YA
Tel: 0117 951 0038 Fax: 0117 935 5056
(Bristol North Primary Care Trust)

Practice Manager Angela Toumi

GP Jeffrey Peter Stanley PARROTT, John Steven WRIGHT

Elm Hayes Surgery
High Street, Paulton, Bristol BS39 7QJ
Tel: 01761 413155 Fax: 01761 410573
Email: elm.hayes@gp-L81059.nhs.uk
(Bath and North East Somerset Primary Care Trust)
Patient List Size: 7500

Practice Manager Richard Bluden

GP Barbara Fulton ROY, Emily Ruth GILBERT, Andrew David STEPHENS, Jeremy Marcus Adrian TONGE, Philip John WHITAKER

Elm Lodge Surgery
43 Gloucester Road North, Filton, Bristol BS7 0SN
Tel: 0117 969 0909 Fax: 0117 983 9969
Website: www.elmlodgesurgery.nhs.uk
(Bristol North Primary Care Trust)
Patient List Size: 1800

GP John V REDMOND, Sian WALTERS

Fallodon Way Medical Centre
13 Fallodon Way, Henleaze, Bristol BS9 4HT
Tel: 0117 962 0652 Fax: 0117 962 0839
(Bristol North Primary Care Trust)
Patient List Size: 8000

Practice Manager Cath Sage

GP Elizabeth Ann FARNALL, Gillian CALLOW, Jeremy POLAND, Tom SMITH, Karl John STAINER

The Family Practice
Western College, Cotham Road, Bristol BS6 6DF
(Bristol South and West Primary Care Trust)
Patient List Size: 10600

Practice Manager David Redshaw

GP R W HEATH

Fishponds Health Centre
Beechwood Road, Fishponds, Bristol BS16 3TD
Tel: 0117 908 2365 Fax: 0117 908 2377
(Bristol North Primary Care Trust)

Practice Manager Rosemary Wyatt

GP Elizabeth Jane ANSTEY, Simon ATKINS, David William FELCE, Claire HATTON, David PORTEOUS, Moira Caroline SUTCLIFFE, Frances Katherine WATT

Fishponds Health Centre
Beechwood Road, Fishponds, Bristol BS16 3TD
Tel: 0117 965 2360 Fax: 0117 908 2354
(Bristol North Primary Care Trust)
Patient List Size: 11400

Practice Manager Rosemary Wyatt

GP Colin Andrew WALLACE, Nicholas Joseph GWILLIAM, Catherine Melly HALL, Philip Peter HARRIS, Sheila Mary MONTGOMERY, K PETTIT

Frome Valley Medical Centre
2 Court Road, Frampton Cotterell, Bristol BS36 2DE
Tel: 01454 772153 Fax: 01454 250078
Website: www.fromevalley.nhs.uk
(South Gloucestershire Primary Care Trust)
Patient List Size: 14000

Practice Manager Pamela Harwood

GP Charles Steven SELLICK, Elaine Gladys ANDERSON, Jennifer Lennox BOLT, Paul Andrew BUCKLEY, Jane GORAM, Lucy JOSLIN, Paula KENWRIGHT, Robert Quentin LAURENCE, Charles A RECORD

Gaywood House Surgery
North Street, Bedminster, Bristol BS3 3AZ
(Bristol South and West Primary Care Trust)

Practice Manager Jane Morris

GP C M ROBERTS

Gloucester Road Medical Centre
Tramway House, 1A Church Road, Horfield, Bristol BS7 8SA
Tel: 0117 949 7774 Fax: 0117 949 7730
(Bristol North Primary Care Trust)

Practice Manager Judy Holbrook

GP Paul Anthony Gulluck PAYNE, Michael John CLEMENT, Nicolette Mary DIXON, Jonathan Edward HOLDSWORTH, Jasmin KRISCHER, Edward Patrick LAVIN, Anne MITCHELL, Sarah SMITH

Grange Road Surgery
Grange Road, Bishopsworth, Bristol BS13 8LD
Tel: 0117 964 4343
Email: name@gp-L81054.nhs.uk
(Bristol South and West Primary Care Trust)
Patient List Size: 8600

Practice Manager Ros Banfield, Dennis Gaye

GP S N BRADLEY

Hanham Surgery
33 Whittucks Road, Hanham, Bristol BS15 3HY
Tel: 0117 967 5201 Fax: 0117 947 7749
(South Gloucestershire Primary Care Trust)
Patient List Size: 14200

Practice Manager Cath Nagle

GP Bernard Godfrey WHITESIDE, Ayo ADEROGBA, David John Godfrey BAILEY, Mark Thomas Gunn BIGWOOD, Stephen Charles ILLINGWORTH, Susan LOWREY, Sarah PEPPER, Joanna RICHARDS, Paul Anthony TAYLOR

Harbourside Family Practice
Harbourside Surgery, Harbour Road, Portishead, Bristol BS20 7DD
Tel: 01275 847474
(North Somerset Primary Care Trust)
Patient List Size: 3730

GP F ALLINSON, K CHAN, C CRILLY

Harptree Surgery
Bristol Road, West Harptree, Bristol BS40 6HF
Tel: 01761 221406 Fax: 01761 221882
(Bath and North East Somerset Primary Care Trust)
Patient List Size: 6250

Practice Manager Judy Robinson

GP T GOLLIN, W COPPOCK, P GUY

Hartcliffe Health Centre
Hareclive Road, Bristol BS13 0JP
Tel: 0117 964 2839 Fax: 0117 964 9628
Email: stubbs@phc.u-net.com
(Bristol South and West Primary Care Trust)
Patient List Size: 7653

Practice Manager L Brown

GP Peter Damian STUBBS, Dougal Robert DARVILL, Joy Annette MAIN, Paul Graeme Neilson MAIN, Tony STEELE, Diana WARNER, Susan Jane WILLIAMS

Helios Medical Centre
17 Stoke Hill, Stoke Bishop, Bristol BS9 1JN
Tel: 0117 962 6060 Fax: 0117 962 6663
(Bristol North Primary Care Trust)

Practice Manager Catherine Ward

GP A C J MAENDL, Dr GRUENEWALD, M HAMILTON, Dr WILSON

Heywood Family Practice
Heywood Surgery, Lodway Gardens, Pill, Bristol BS20 0DL
Tel: 01275 372105 Fax: 01275 373879
(North Somerset Primary Care Trust)
Patient List Size: 6850

Practice Manager Marlene Watkins

GP Jonathan Sydney FLIGELSTONE, Roger DENTON, Yvonne JACKSON, Nicholas Julian KENT, Emma MASON, Carol Ann NAUGHTON

Hillview Family Practice
Hareclive Road, Hartcliffe, Bristol BS13 0JP
Tel: 0117 964 5588 Fax: 0117 964 9055
(Bristol South and West Primary Care Trust)
Patient List Size: 6000

Practice Manager Ann Gleave

GP Gerard Harry Raleigh GIBBS, Wendy Barbara MITCHELL, Ray Ferguson MONTAGUE, Helen Elizabeth WEHNER

Horfield Health Centre
Lockleaze Road, Horfield, Bristol BS7 9RR
Tel: 0117 969 5391 Fax: 0117 931 5879
(Bristol North Primary Care Trust)

GP Arnold John MAYES, Alison Jane BOLAM, S K M CHAN, Andrew John CORDELL, Victoria Helen HARTNELL, Morris David JEWELL, Terence John KEMPLE, Elizabeth Charlotte LEE, Jane Louise OWEN-JONES

Kennedy Way Surgery
Kennedy Way, Yate, Bristol BS37 4AA
Tel: 01454 313849 Fax: 01454 329039
(South Gloucestershire Primary Care Trust)

Practice Manager Sue McSherry

GP David CAPEHORN, Duncan Stuart GOODLAND, Louise Ann POWELL, Jane Rosemary SAVAGE, Richard James SHERRIFF, Graham Russell WARD

Kingswood Health Centre
Alma Road, Kingswood, Bristol BS15 4EJ
Tel: 0117 961 1774 Fax: 0117 947 7419
(South Gloucestershire Primary Care Trust)
Patient List Size: 11000

Practice Manager Pat Lewis

GP Robert FIELDS, Janet Rosemary GORDON, Neil Edward KERFOOT, Stephen Richard KITSON, Peter John MOORE, H STODDART, Anna Marie WHEATLEY

Lawrence Hill Health Centre
Hassell Drive, Easton, Bristol BS2 0AN
Tel: 0117 955 5241 Fax: 0117 941 1162
(Bristol North Primary Care Trust)
Patient List Size: 8100

Practice Manager E Cameron

GP D S WALSH, Philip A G BAKKER, M J BARBER, C J COLES, P GARDINER, Dr WILLMOTT

Leap Valley Surgery
18 Fouracre Road, Bristol BS16 6PG
Tel: 0117 970 2033 Fax: 0117 956 4885
(South Gloucestershire Primary Care Trust)
Patient List Size: 11300

Practice Manager Helen Holbrook

GP Andrew Paul NASH, Jonathan EVANS, Richard Anthony HAYES, Caroline Mary JONES, Kathleen Clare NICHOLS, Philip Malcolm SMITH

The Lennard Surgery
1 Lewis Road, Bedminster Down, Bristol BS13 7JD
Email: lennard.surgery@ukonline.co.uk
(Bristol South and West Primary Care Trust)
Patient List Size: 7580

Practice Manager P Slade

GP S J PAGE

Lodgeside Surgery
22 Lodgeside Avenue, Kingswood, Bristol BS15 1NH
Tel: 0117 961 5666 Fax: 0117 947 6854
Website: www.lodgeside.nhs.uk
(Bristol North Primary Care Trust)

Practice Manager Martyn Nicholls

GP Michael John DOYLE, Julia Alice BARRY-BRAUNTHAL, Donna Louise DENNIS, Victoria Louise HIBBERT, Judith Flora LINDECK, Charilaos Petrou MINAS, Graham Vaughan RAWLINSON, Philippa Rosemary Joan STABLES

Long Ashton Surgery
55 Rayens Cross Road, Long Ashton, Bristol BS41 9DY
Tel: 01275 392134 Fax: 01275 394576
Email: info@physician.org.uk
(North Somerset Primary Care Trust)
Patient List Size: 5300

Practice Manager Eileen Butterworth

GP Peter Stephen FOREMAN, Jennifer GRENFELL-SHAW, Gaye Victoria HARDIMAN, Mark Dennis O'CONNOR

The Malago Surgery
40 St. Johns Road, Bedminster, Bristol BS3 4JE
Tel: 0117 966 5238
(Bristol South and West Primary Care Trust)
Patient List Size: 10500

Practice Manager John Gibson

GP George Thomas SMYTH, Susan CHAMBERS, Andrew John GREEN, Rosa HELLINGS, Alison JAMES, Judith Elizabeth JONES, Harriet Anne LUPTON, Brian McMANUS

Mangotsfield Surgery
26 Stockwell Drive, Mangotsfield, Bristol BS16 9DN
Tel: 0117 956 7831
(South Gloucestershire Primary Care Trust)

Practice Manager M Stambuli

GP P STAMBULI

The Merrywood Practice
William Budd Health Centre, Downton Road, Knowle, Bristol
(Bristol South and West Primary Care Trust)

GP T S DEAN

Monks Park Surgery
24 Monks Park Avenue, Horfield, Bristol BS7 0UE
Tel: 0117 969 3106 Fax: 0117 931 1546
Website: www.monksparksurgery.com
(Bristol North Primary Care Trust)
Patient List Size: 1900

Practice Manager Hilary Doxford

GP Francis Andrew LANGTON, Amanda WOOD

Monks Park Surgery
24 Monks Park Avenue, Horfield, Bristol BS7 0UE
Tel: 0117 696 3106 Fax: 0117 979 8011
Website: www.monksparksurgery.com
(Bristol North Primary Care Trust)
Patient List Size: 1900

Practice Manager Hilary Doxford

GP Mike DENNISON, Amanda WOOD

Montpelier Health Centre
Bath Buildings, Bristol BS6 5PT
Tel: 0117 942 6811 Fax: 0117 944 4182
(Bristol North Primary Care Trust)
Patient List Size: 13250

Practice Manager Marilyn Ellis

GP S P CEMBROWICZ, T A BAILWARD, A BLAKE, Dr BROWN, Dr HEARN, S MASHEDER, Dr MITCHELL, Dr OAKLEY, C ZOLLMAN

Nailsea Family Practice
Tower House Medical Centre, Stockway South, Nailsea, Bristol BS48 2XX
Tel: 01275 866700
(North Somerset Primary Care Trust)

GP Frank Bernard PAGE, Mary Frances BACKHOUSE, David Philip CHISNALL, P S GILBERT, Rosalind Penelope KENNEDY, L M PATERSON, Timothy Michael SOUTHWOOD

Northville Family Practice
521 Filton Avenue, Horfield, Bristol BS7 0LS
Tel: 0117 969 2164 Fax: 0117 931 5743
(South Gloucestershire Primary Care Trust)

Practice Manager Ros Banfield

GP Raymond William SAWFORD, Pun Hon CHANG, Lesley Margaret JORDAN, Carolyn Sarah SMITH

Oldland Surgery
192 High Street, Oldham Common, Bristol BS30 9QQ
Tel: 0117 932 4444 Fax: 0117 932 4101
(South Gloucestershire Primary Care Trust)
Patient List Size: 5800

Practice Manager Suzanne O'Loughlin

GP David Cyril HOGG, Jayne Louise CUNLIFFE, Jonathan Richard HAYES

Orchard Medical Centre
Macdonald Walk, Kingswood, Bristol BS15 8NJ
Tel: 0117 980 5100 Fax: 0117 980 5104
(South Gloucestershire Primary Care Trust)
Patient List Size: 11700

Practice Manager Caroline Pearmain

GP Philip Andrew YATES, Richard James BERKLEY, Patricia Mary FLANAGAN, J GORMAN, N JACKSON, Jonathan JEWKES, R JONES, Mark Adrian NORMAN

Overnhill Family Practice
14 Overnhill Road, Staple Hill, Bristol BS16 5DN
Tel: 0117 970 1656 Fax: 0117 987 2479
(South Gloucestershire Primary Care Trust)
Patient List Size: 7500

Practice Manager Sue Bailey

GP Timothy John COULSON, Diana Mary FOSTER, Roger Ernest GREEN

Portishead Health Centre
Victoria Square, Portishead, Bristol BS20 6AQ
Tel: 01275 847474 Fax: 01275 817516
(North Somerset Primary Care Trust)
Patient List Size: 15300

Practice Manager Lynn Parker

GP Jeremy Ian Halcro MITCHESON, Sarah BIRD, Paul John CONWAY, Carolyn Clare DONALD, Gerwyn OWEN, Phillip Edward PEMBERTON, Katharine Margaret RILEY, Anthony George RYAN, Richard THOMSON, Katherine WHYBREW, Jonathan David WILLIAMS

Ridingleaze Medical Centre
Ridingleaze, Bristol BS11 0QE
Tel: 0117 982 2693 Fax: 0117 938 1707
(Bristol North Primary Care Trust)
Patient List Size: 7400

Practice Manager Keith Minty

GP David Edward Balliol TARLETON, Keith Francis ERSKINE, Mary Geraldine O'CARROLL, Veronica PICKERING

Sea Mills Surgery
2 Riverleaze, Sea Mills, Bristol BS9 2HL
Tel: 0117 968 1182 Fax: 0117 908 3377
Email: seamills@gp-L81077.nhs.uk
(Bristol North Primary Care Trust)
Patient List Size: 6350

Practice Manager Jean Allchorne

GP Hugh Stuart SILVEY, Clare Siobhan ANDERSSON, Mervyn Thomas McGOWAN, Saffron REAVLEY, KATHRYN WATERS

Shirehampton Group Practice
Shirehampton Health Centre, Pembroke Road, Shirehampton, Bristol BS11 9SB
Tel: 0117 916 2226 Fax: 0117 916 2206
(Bristol North Primary Care Trust)
Patient List Size: 10100

Practice Manager Carole Brooke

GP Richard Geoffrey TAYLOR, Dr ADDISON, Paul St John ARCHER, Dr FOWLER, Susan Mary GREEN, Dr HELLIER, Iain David HINE, Deborah Janette SHARP, Lisabeth Lee WARD

Sneyd Park Surgery
Holly House, 8 Rockleaze Avenue, Bristol BS9 1NG
Tel: 0117 968 3284 Fax: 0117 968 7617
(Bristol North Primary Care Trust)

GP Christopher John SHARPLES

Southmead Health Centre
Ullswater Road, Bristol BS10 6DF
Tel: 0117 950 7750 Fax: 0117 959 1110
(Bristol North Primary Care Trust)

Practice Manager Irene Worrall

GP Eveline Dilys HARLOW, Rajesh JOBANPUTRA, David Michael Lawrence KERSHAW, Melanie Anne MACKINTOSH, Margaret Caroline NAYSMITH, Dr STEINER, William Arthur WARIN

Southmead Health Centre
Ullswater Road, Bristol BS10 6DF
Tel: 0117 950 7100 Fax: 0117 908 4673
(Bristol North Primary Care Trust)

GP Richard John HOFFMAN, Daniel Dallas BRETT, Barbara Anne Katherine KENNEY, Virginia ROYSTON

Southville Surgery
67 Coronation Road, Southville, Bristol BS3 1AS
Tel: 0117 966 9724 Fax: 0117 953 2604
(Bristol South and West Primary Care Trust)
Patient List Size: 6000

Practice Manager Andrew Bale

GP Annie SEMUGOMA, Robert Kingsley ADAMS, David Terence McCARTHY

Spence Group Practice
Westcliffe House, 48-50 Logan Road, Bishopston, Bristol BS7 8DR
Tel: 0117 944 0701 Fax: 0117 944 0707
(Bristol North Primary Care Trust)

Practice Manager Richard West

GP Richard William SPENCE, Janet Frances GRAY, William Roger PHILLIPS

St Augustines Medical Practice
4 Station Road, Keynsham, Bristol BS31 2BN
Tel: 0117 986 2343 Fax: 0117 986 1176
(Bath and North East Somerset Primary Care Trust)
Patient List Size: 9900

Practice Manager John Moon

GP Jane WYATT

St George Health Centre
Bellevue Road, St. George, Bristol BS5 7PH
Tel: 0117 961 2161 Fax: 0117 961 8761
(Bristol North Primary Care Trust)
Patient List Size: 8900

Practice Manager J May

GP Doron Lavee BOONE, R Mark EDDISON, Wanda Irena OWEN, Alison Jean WICKERT

St Johns Lane Health Centre
St Johns Lane, Bedminster, Bristol BS3 5AS
(Bristol South and West Primary Care Trust)

GP S C BASSI

St Martins Surgery
378 Wells Road, Knowle, Bristol BS4 2QR
Tel: 0117 977 5641 Fax: 0117 977 5490
(Bristol South and West Primary Care Trust)
Patient List Size: 5100

Practice Manager Ruth Cooper

GP William Brian Andrew BARWELL, Annabelle Jane CERVANTES, Karen Jayne HOUGHTON, Barry Alexander SCOTT

St Peters Hospice
St Agnes Avenue, Knowle, Bristol BS4 2DU

GP C M DACOMBE

Stockwood Medical Centre
Hollway Road, Stockwood, Bristol BS14 8PT
(Bristol South and West Primary Care Trust)

Practice Manager Paul Mugford

GP N MINORS

Stoke Gifford Medical Centre
Ratcliffe Drive, Stoke Gifford, Bristol BS34 8UE
Tel: 0117 979 9430 Fax: 0117 940 6966
(South Gloucestershire Primary Care Trust)
Patient List Size: 11300

Practice Manager Mary Nicholls

GP K E AITKEN, James Michael BRAGG, Graham John DEAKIN, Carolyn ELLIS, Jonathan Philip JELFS, Monica Mary WARNOCK

Stokes Medical Centre
Braydon Avenue, Little Stoke, Bristol BS34 6BQ
Tel: 01454 616767 Fax: 01454 616189
(South Gloucestershire Primary Care Trust)

Practice Manager Mandy Stewart

GP Anthony Richard COLMAN, Kathleen Elizabeth BOYD, Anne Marie CARSWELL, J W INGLESFIELD, T S J LE COYTE, J L RECORD, David Winthrop SWITHINBANK

Students Health Service
25 Belgrave Road, Clifton, Bristol BS8 2AA
(Bristol South and West Primary Care Trust)

Practice Manager Louise Jones

GP A V J BUTLER

The Surgery
St Mary Street, Thornbury, Bristol BS35 2AT
Tel: 01454 413691 Fax: 01454 411141
(South Gloucestershire Primary Care Trust)
Patient List Size: 6600

Practice Manager Callum Murray

GP Jacqueline Patricia GUMB, Nicholas Alan McCULLOCH, Mark David Ian HARRISON

The Surgery
Northwick Road, Pilning, Bristol BS35 4JF
Tel: 01454 632393 Fax: 01454 632802
(South Gloucestershire Primary Care Trust)
Patient List Size: 4300

Practice Manager Sue Prior

GP Terence Andrew PATERSON, Fiona ORMEROD

The Surgery
227 Lodge Causeway, Fishponds, Bristol BS16 3QW
Tel: 0117 965 3102 Fax: 0117 958 4272
(Bristol North Primary Care Trust)

Practice Manager Jeremy Lyons

GP Paul Robert HEPBURN, Dr ADAMSON, Dr BUCKLEY, William Damian CUSSEN

The Surgery
Madam's Paddock, Chew Magna, Bristol BS40 8PP
Tel: 01275 332420 Fax: 01275 331355
Email: chewmagnasurgery@gp-L81072.nhs.uk
(Bath and North East Somerset Primary Care Trust)
Patient List Size: 9000

Practice Manager Richard Blunden

GP R C RAFFETY, S E FENN, E W MORRIS, R J PRICE, Timothy James SEPHTON

The Surgery
233 Wells Road, Knowle, Bristol BS4 2DF
Tel: 0117 977 0018 Fax: 0117 972 8608
(Bristol South and West Primary Care Trust)

GP Ian James ROBERTSON, Michel Semir BONNET

The Surgery
58 Pembroke Road, Clifton, Bristol BS8 3DT
Tel: 0117 974 1452 Fax: 0117 923 8040
(Bristol South and West Primary Care Trust)
Patient List Size: 2100

Practice Manager G Penry

GP Victoria BOWLER, Nicholas Paul RING

The Surgery
111 Pembroke Road, Clifton, Bristol BS8 3EU
Tel: 0117 973 3790
(Bristol South and West Primary Care Trust)
Patient List Size: 9400

Practice Manager Mary Webb

GP Griselda Frances Clare GOODDEN, Anthony Steven FIELDING, Sarah GANLY, Sarah Winnifred LESLEY, Rhona Isabel MACPHERSON, Rohan PERERA, Michael George Philip ROSSDALE, Joanne WILKINS

The Surgery
Wellington Road, Yate, Bristol BS37 5UY
Tel: 01454 323366 Fax: 01454 315077
(South Gloucestershire Primary Care Trust)
Patient List Size: 1300

GP Sandhya SAHAY

The Surgery
13 Clarence Road East, Weston Super Mare, Bristol BS23 4BP
Tel: 01931 415080 Fax: 01934 612813
Patient List Size: 4917

Practice Manager Sue Christian

GP P MAKSIMCZYK, I R LONGHORN, M T WYATT

The Surgery
227 Lodge Causeway, Bristol BS16 3QW
Tel: 0117 958 3102 Fax: 0117 958 4272
(Bristol North Primary Care Trust)
Patient List Size: 6750

GP Paul HEPBURN, Brian David ADAMSON, Carole BUCKLEY, Damian CUSSEN

The Surgery
269 Stapleton Road, Fishponds, Bristol BS5 0PQ
Tel: 0117 951 0042
(Bristol North Primary Care Trust)

Practice Manager Sue Hyde

GP Dr MATIN

Sussex Place Surgery
63 Sussex Place, Bristol BS2 9QR
Tel: 0117 955 6275 Fax: 0117 941 4843
Email: doctor@gp-l81658.nhs.uk
(Bristol North Primary Care Trust)
Patient List Size: 2500

Practice Manager Tim Johaston

GP Sylvia Ann THOMPSON

Temple House Surgery
Temple House, Temple Street, Keynsham, Bristol BS31 1EJ
Tel: 0117 986 2406 Fax: 0117 986 5695
Email: templ.house@gp-l81064.nhs.uk
(Bath and North East Somerset Primary Care Trust)
Patient List Size: 6419

Practice Manager Sue Feltham

GP Nicholas Mark REYNOLDS, Kerensa Jane BRANFOOT, Helen Michelle ECCLES, Jennifer Susan LOCKYER

Thornbury Health Centre
Eastland Road, Thornbury, Bristol BS35 1DP
Tel: 01454 412599 Fax: 01454 416090
(South Gloucestershire Primary Care Trust)
Patient List Size: 10400

Practice Manager Valerie Verey

GP P J BURNEY, H BRADLEY, W H BURNHAM, G J CLARKE, W J FOUBISTER, A HARRIS, B LODGE

Thornbury Health Centre
Eastland Road, Thornbury, Bristol BS35 1DP
Tel: 01454 412167 Fax: 01454 419522
(South Gloucestershire Primary Care Trust)

Practice Manager Joy Martin

GP Paul Philippe MALE, Helen Jennifer LEWIS, Mark John THOMPSON

Wells Road Surgery
326 Wells Road, Knowle, Bristol BS4 2QJ
Tel: 0117 949 3958 Fax: 0117 987 2905
(Bristol South and West Primary Care Trust)
Patient List Size: 8600

Practice Manager Kay Madge

GP J E FORNEAR

West View Surgery
9 Park Road, Keynsham, Bristol BS31 1BX
Tel: 0117 986 3063 Fax: 0117 986 5061
(Bath and North East Somerset Primary Care Trust)
Patient List Size: 6400

Practice Manager Garry Smith

GP Wendy Jacqueline COE, Andrew Ralph HAVERS, Ernst SCHOLTE, Alison WHEELER

West View Surgery
9 Park Road, Keynsham, Bristol BS31 1BX
Tel: 0117 986 3063 Fax: 0117 986 5061
(Bath and North East Somerset Primary Care Trust)
Patient List Size: 6505

Practice Manager Garry Smith

GP W COE, O BOURKE, A HAVERS, E SCHOLTE, A WHEELER

West Walk Surgery
21 West Walk, Yate, Bristol BS37 4AX
Tel: 01454 272200 Fax: 01454 272220
(South Gloucestershire Primary Care Trust)

Practice Manager Mandy Gurr

GP Gillian Carolyn DEGENS, Edward EMMANUEL, Amanda Suzanne HIGGINS, N LLOYD POWIS, Nicholas Charles MANSFIELD, David Ernest MARSHALL, Andrew Charles MONCRIEF, Timothy John SPARE

The Westbury-on-Trym Practice
60 Falcondale Road, Westbury-on-Trym, Bristol BS9 3JY
Tel: 0117 962 3406 Fax: 0117 962 1404
(Bristol North Primary Care Trust)
Patient List Size: 6800

Practice Manager Gillian Johnson

GP Denise Margaret JOHNSON, Michael Adam Hart COHEN, Lulce KOUPPARIS, Philip Gerard McCARTHY

Whitchurch Health Centre
Armada Road, Whitchurch, Bristol BS14 0SU
Tel: 01275 832285
(Bristol South and West Primary Care Trust)
Patient List Size: 8000

GP A G NEGUS, G BADGER, Z BAKER, N CRICHTON, C JUDGE, J PIKE

Whitchurch Health Centre
Armada Road, Bristol BS14 0SU
Tel: 01275 835625 Fax: 01275 540035

(Bristol South and West Primary Care Trust)
Patient List Size: 4050

Practice Manager Denise Rodway

GP Marguerite Elisabeth CLARK, Jonathan Andrew BRIGGS, Katherine Emma LEWIS

Whiteladies Health Centre
Whatley Road, Clifton, Bristol BS8 2PU
Tel: 0117 9731201 Fax: 0117 9466850
(Bristol South and West Primary Care Trust)
Patient List Size: 21500

Practice Manager Lin Zerovali

GP David S CHESNEY, John A BAILEY, Rajan BOWRI, Andrew COULSON, Barbara DUNNING, Stephen K GRANIER, Gillian M JENKINS, Nina Elizabeth MOORMAN, Jane Ceridwen PARKER, Graham C PEGG, Elizabeth S POTTER, Knut SCHROEDER, Joanna WALSH

The Willow Surgery
Coronation Road, Downend, Bristol BS16 5DH
Tel: 0117 970 9500 Fax: 0117 970 9501
(South Gloucestershire Primary Care Trust)

Practice Manager Lyn Garraway

GP Jerzy Marek CONRAD, I BENAZON, Amanda Susan BOLTON, Georgina Ann EVANS, John Mervin KINGSTON, K PEARCE, P S SIMONS, Caroline Yelverton WARREN-BROWNE, Roger YEOMAN

Wrington Vale Medical Practice
Station Road, Wrington, Bristol BS40 5NG
Tel: 01934 862532 Fax: 01934 863568
(North Somerset Primary Care Trust)
Patient List Size: 9013

Practice Manager Jane Tarnowsky

GP Nicholas Robert Joseph HOOPER, Alan McCLATCHEY, Shruti Devyani PATEL, Charles David PORTAS, Janet SNOW, Charles David TRICKS

Yatton Family Practice
155 Mendip Road, Yatton, Bristol BS49 4ER
Tel: 01934 832277 Fax: 01934 876085
Website: www.yfpd.co.uk
(North Somerset Primary Care Trust)

Practice Manager Hilary Atkinson

GP Michael Fenner Hermann NELKI, Farooq FAHEEM, Ann Cordelia FEUCHTWANG, M J TAYLOR, Andrew David WARINTON, Anne Moya WILSON

Brixham

Compass House Medical Centres
25 Bolton Street, Brixham TQ5 9BZ
Tel: 01803 855897 Fax: 01803 855613
(Torbay Primary Care Trust)

Practice Manager David McIlrath

GP Douglas Gordon Howland ANSLEY, Peter Jonathan AVERY, Robert Michael BROMIGE, Margaret Bridget McCONNELL, Andrew Nicholas PATON

Greenswood Surgery
1 Greenwood Road, Brixham TQ5 9HN
Tel: 01808 853153 Fax: 01803 850001
Email: namedperson@nhs.net
(Torbay Primary Care Trust)
Patient List Size: 4200

Practice Manager Louise Lillicrap

GP Paul SHEENA, Michael GIBLIN

St Lukes Medical Centre
17 New Road, Brixham TQ5 8NA
Tel: 01803 852731 Fax: 01803 852637
Email: stlukesmedicalcentre@gp-l83078.nhs.uk
Website: www.stlukesmedicalcentre.co.uk
(Torbay Primary Care Trust)
Patient List Size: 6200

Practice Manager Fred Whalley

GP Paul Bernard JOHNSON, Lorraine HILL, Jane KNIGHT, Richard William MONTGOMERY, Iain WALKER

Broadstairs

Albion Road Surgery
30 Albion Road, St Peter's, Broadstairs CT10 2UP
Tel: 01843 862179 Fax: 01843 861317
(East Kent Coastal Teaching Primary Care Trust)

Practice Manager Margaret Atkins

GP Peter Edward WILSON

Broadstairs Health Centre
The Broadway, Broadstairs CT10 2AJ
Tel: 01843 861014 Fax: 01843 869177
(East Kent Coastal Teaching Primary Care Trust)

Practice Manager T De Silva

GP T DE SILVA

Broadstairs Health Centre
The Broadway, Broadstairs CT10 2AJ
Tel: 01843 862304 Fax: 01843 869177
(East Kent Coastal Teaching Primary Care Trust)
Patient List Size: 2200

Practice Manager L Miller

GP Ian R HODGINS

Broadstairs Health Centre
The Broadway, Broadstairs CT10 2AJ
Tel: 01843 861565 Fax: 01843 869177
(East Kent Coastal Teaching Primary Care Trust)
Patient List Size: 2210

GP S. SAHADEVAN

Mocketts Wood Surgery
Mocketts Wood House, Hopeville Avenue, St Peter's, Broadstairs CT10 2TR
Tel: 01843 862996 Fax: 01843 860126
(East Kent Coastal Teaching Primary Care Trust)

Practice Manager Joan Marshall

GP David Ian MARSHALL

Osborne Road Surgery
25 Osborne Road, Broadstairs CT10 2AF
Tel: 01843 863353 Fax: 01843 861412
(East Kent Coastal Teaching Primary Care Trust)
Patient List Size: 2350

Practice Manager Mrs Divers

GP Chander Dayaram KHEMANI, Shakuntala KHEMANI

Queens Road Surgery
17 Queens Road, Broadstairs CT10 1NX
Tel: 01843 862648 Fax: 01843 860739
(East Kent Coastal Teaching Primary Care Trust)

Practice Manager Hussania Shariff

GP Syed Yakub SHARIFF

St Peter's Surgery
6 Oaklands Avenue, Broadstairs CT10 2SQ
Tel: 01843 860777 Fax: 01843 866647
(East Kent Coastal Teaching Primary Care Trust)
Patient List Size: 4300

Practice Manager Tina Smith

GP Alan John Keith CUNARD, Morris DAVIES, Susan Marie GOLDBERG

Broadstone

Hadleigh House

20 Kirkway, Broadstone BH18 8EE
Tel: 01202 692268 Fax: 01202 658954
(Poole Primary Care Trust)
Patient List Size: 17500

Practice Manager M Besant

GP M BRIDGMAN, K FAWKNER, Joanne Lesley HADLEY, Christopher John McCALL, H MOLYNEUX, James Mark PHARAOH, A PURBRICK, Michael Ian RICHARDSON, E SANDERS, R TIMMIS, Alistair James WATKINS

Harvey Practice

18 Kirkway, Broadstone BH18 8EE
Tel: 01202 697307 Fax: 01202 658973
Email: drs@theharveypractice.co.uk
Website: theharveypractice.co.uk
(Poole Primary Care Trust)

Practice Manager Denise Hunter

GP Dr CARTWRIGHT, Dr DAVIES, Dr DUDDING, Dr JENKINS, Dr LAWRENCE, Dr STEPHENS, Dr TAYLOR

Broadway

Barn Close Surgery

38-40 High Street, Broadway WR12 7DT
Tel: 01386 853651 Fax: 01386 853982
Website: www.barnclose.co.uk
(South Worcestershire Primary Care Trust)
Patient List Size: 7400

Practice Manager Christine Payne

GP Thomas Peter Stephan BLOCH, John Lloyd HUGHES, Neil William Norman TOWNSHEND, Emma Jane VINCENT

Brockenhurst

Smith, Baynes, Orton and Fitzsimmons

The Surgery, Highwood Road, Brockenhurst SO42 7RY
Tel: 01590 622272 Fax: 01590 624009
(New Forest Primary Care Trust)
Patient List Size: 6990

Practice Manager Elizabeth Wingham

GP Sally Agnes Culver SMITH, Stephen Charles BAYNES, Ian FITZSIMMONS, Mark Alan ORTON

Bromley

Carisbrooke House Surgery

1A Pope Road, Bromley BR2 9SS
Tel: 020 8460 4611 Fax: 020 8460 9450
Email: poperoad.surgery@gp-g84024.nhs.uk
Website: carisbrookehousesurgery.co.uk
(Bromley Primary Care Trust)
Patient List Size: 8400

Practice Manager Kate Watney

GP Barbara Susan LEWIS, Stephanie Myra Louise BIRMINGHAM-McDONOGH, Anthony Richard CRAIGHILL, Christopher Simon STOTT

Court Farm Road Surgery

218 Court Farm Road, Mottingham, Bromley
(Bromley Primary Care Trust)

Dysart House Surgery

13 Ravensbourne Road, Bromley BR1 1HN
Tel: 020 8464 4138 Fax: 020 8466 9248
(Bromley Primary Care Trust)
Patient List Size: 9000

Practice Manager Wendy Ciel

GP Kim Peter FLANNERY, Elizabeth Mary DE COTHI, Stefan Pawel RAKOWICZ, Penolope RYBA, Gurmit SINGH

Forge Close Surgery

Forge Close, Hayes, Bromley BR2 7LP
Tel: 020 8462 1601 Fax: 020 8462 7410
(Bromley Primary Care Trust)
Patient List Size: 5425

Practice Manager Susan Perry

GP Wilhelmina Juliette Batson CASTLES, Peter George WRAGG, Sarah Louise YOUNG

Links Medical Practice

198 Court Farm Road, Mottingham, Bromley BR1
Tel: 020 8461 3333 Fax: 020 8695 5567
(Bromley Primary Care Trust)
Patient List Size: 5000

Practice Manager Rosie Church

GP James Nicholas MUIR, Catherine Michaela JENSON, Miranda Ruth SELBY, Margaret Rosemary SWIFT

London Lane Clinic

Kinnaird House, 37 London Lane, Bromley BR1 4HB
Tel: 020 8460 2661 Fax: 020 8464 5041
(Bromley Primary Care Trust)
Patient List Size: 16040

Practice Manager Allison Cannon

GP Ross McAndrew ELLICE, P A DJANGMAH, Mark HOMOLKA, E MacCANN, Phillipa Anne TAYLOR

Pickhurst Surgery

56 Pickhurst Lane, Bromley BR2 7JF
Tel: 020 8462 2880 Fax: 020 8462 9581
Website: www.pickhurstsurgery.co.uk
(Bromley Primary Care Trust)
Patient List Size: 6400

Practice Manager Barbara Hill

GP A MAHENDRARAJAH, R KIRBY, Mahendra KUMAR, E A PALLANT, Chandrakant Ranchhodbhai PATEL

Sundridge Medical Practice

84 London Lane, Bromley BR1 4HE
(Bromley Primary Care Trust)

The Surgery

Southview Lodge, South View, Bromley BR1 3DR
Tel: 020 8460 1945 Fax: 020 8323 1423
(Bromley Primary Care Trust)
Patient List Size: 5500

Practice Manager Sandie Thompson

GP Richard Norman WILLATT, James Anthony HEATHCOTE

The Surgery

356 Southborough Lane, Bromley BR2 8AA
Tel: 020 8468 7081 Fax: 020 8295 3575
(Bromley Primary Care Trust)
Patient List Size: 10000

Practice Manager Suzanne Beacom

GP Michael Edward COLLINS, Richard Anthony DE SOUZA, John Barrington KENYON, Sashi Kiran SEHMI, Natalie VOWLES

The Surgery

Southview Lodge, South View, Bromley BR1 3DR
Tel: 020 8460 1932 Fax: 020 8323 1423
(Bromley Primary Care Trust)
Patient List Size: 5500

Practice Manager Sandie Thompson

GP Mary Anne MATTHEWS, Nicola Margaret PAYNE

The Surgery
10 Highland Road, Bromley BR1 4AD
Tel: 020 8460 2368 Fax: 020 8313 9908
(Bromley Primary Care Trust)
Patient List Size: 3600

GP Sivagnanapragasam GNANACHELVAN, Koneswary GNANACHELVAN

The Surgery
46 Southlands Road, Bromley BR2 9QP
Tel: 020 8289 3981
(Bromley Primary Care Trust)

GP K JEGAMOHAN

Bromsgrove

Catshill Village Surgery
36 Woodrow Lane, Catshill, Bromsgrove B61 0PU
Tel: 01527 872426 Fax: 01527 870507
(Redditch and Bromsgrove Primary Care Trust)
Patient List Size: 4807

Practice Manager Wendy Goodchild

GP Oliver Paul JACK, Fiona BOWEN, David JACK, Christopher Howard KIMBERLEY

Churchfields Surgery
Recreation Road, Bromsgrove B61 8DT
Tel: 01527 872163 Fax: 01527 576401
Email: m81070.clinical@nhs.net
(Redditch and Bromsgrove Primary Care Trust)
Patient List Size: 12800

Practice Manager Anne Banner

GP Richard David WILKINSON, Barry BYWATER, Alison Clare GRIFFITHS, Claire Jeanette Salma LAXTON, Michael Keith LECI, Ian MORREY, David Simon Ewart PRYKE, Laura WOFFENDEN

Davenal House Surgery
28 Birmingham Road, Bromsgrove B61 0DD
Tel: 01527 872008
(Redditch and Bromsgrove Primary Care Trust)

GP Robert Michael JENKINS, Jacqueline Susan LEWIN, Charles E PARROTT, Marion Elaine RADCLIFFE, Ulrich Otto Erich SCHIRRMACHER, Pamela J SMITH

New Road Surgery
46 New Road, Bromsgrove B60 2JS
Tel: 01527 872027 Fax: 01527 574516
(Redditch and Bromsgrove Primary Care Trust)
Patient List Size: 11000

Practice Manager K Leech

GP William Giles Henry DOWLEY, John Patrick Drummond BLACKER, Sophia Penelope Marianne DOWLEY, Andrew Michael FAIRHURST, Kevin HOLLIER, Deborah Sian HOTHAM

St Johns Surgery
5 Kidderminster Road, Bromsgrove B61 7JJ
Tel: 01527 871706 Fax: 01527 576022
Email: practice.M81082@gp-M81082.nhs.uk
(Redditch and Bromsgrove Primary Care Trust)
Patient List Size: 8500

Practice Manager Chris Farrell

GP Mary Ann FELLOWES, Jonathan ASHLEY, Frederick John HALL, Rebecca Jayne HALL, Christopher David HEATH, Melanie HILL, Thomas TORRENCE

Bromyard

Nunwell Surgery
10 Pump Street, Bromyard HR7 4BZ
Tel: 01885 483412 Fax: 01885 488739
(Herefordshire Primary Care Trust)

Practice Manager Mark Simmons

GP John Kevin ILSLEY, Linda BULL, Mary Rosina CLEAR, Steven Fraser Owen SCOTT, Nicholas Adrian Albert SPICER, Ian James TAIT

Broseley

Broseley Medical Practice
Health Centre, Bridgnorth Road, Broseley TF12 5EL
Tel: 01952 882854
(Shropshire County Primary Care Trust)
Patient List Size: 4694

Practice Manager Marilyn Knight

GP Jan Dorian BHAGEERUTTY, Deborah WEST, Martin YEANDLE

Brough

Brough and South Cave Medical Practice
4 Centurion Way, Brough HU15 1AY
Tel: 01482 667450 Fax: 01482 665090
(East Yorkshire Primary Care Trust)
Patient List Size: 15900

Practice Manager Victoria Karnon

GP John Christopher KEEL, Stephen Paul ALLEN, Paul Barry CHARLSON, William Alexander HART, Naila LOQUEMAN, C L LYONS, Suzanne PARTRIDGE, Dr ROBERTS, Joanne WALTERS

The Health Centre
Thornton Dam Lane, Gilberdyke, Brough HU15 2UL
Tel: 01430 440225 Fax: 01430 440646
(East Yorkshire Primary Care Trust)
Patient List Size: 6000

Practice Manager John Scally

GP Robert Alexander FERGUSON, Joanne Hilary BRAY, Simon Richard MARSHALL

Upper Eden Medical Practice
The Medical Centre, Brough CA17 4AY
Tel: 017683 41294 Fax: 01768 341068
(Eden Valley Primary Care Trust)

GP Ian Alexander Arthur TOD, A MACDONALD

Broughton-in-Furness

Park Stile Cottage Surgery
Park Stile Cottage, Church Street, Broughton-in-Furness LA20 6HJ
Tel: 01229 716337 Fax: 01229 716928
(Morecambe Bay Primary Care Trust)

GP Trevor Hambleton BATES

Broxbourne

High Road Surgery
27 High Road, Wormley, Broxbourne EN10 6HT
Tel: 01992 440877
(South East Hertfordshire Primary Care Trust)

GP A T NAQVI

Park Lane Surgery
8 Park Lane, Broxbourne EN10 7NQ
Tel: 01992 465555 Fax: 01992 471160
(South East Hertfordshire Primary Care Trust)
Patient List Size: 11100

Practice Manager J Draper

GP Karen Heather ALLEN, Robert Nicholas Harford CONDON, Emma Marie DEMPSEY, Bridget Mary Veronica HISCOCK, Jacqueline Susan SHERIDAN, Alasdair Guy WOOD

The Surgery
Groom Road, Turnford, Broxbourne EN10 6BW
Tel: 01992 444203 Fax: 01990 478740

(South East Hertfordshire Primary Care Trust)
Practice Manager Cathleen Sewell
GP Aradhana MUKHERJEE

Bruton

Burton Surgery
Patwell Lane, Bruton BA10 0EG
Tel: 01749 812310 Fax: 01749 812938
(Mendip Primary Care Trust)
Patient List Size: 5950
Practice Manager Marcus Pawson
GP Mark Hort PLAYER, Lesley Helen CHAMBERS, Nick GOMPERTZ, Ulrike NAUMANN

Buckfastleigh

Buckfastleigh Medical Centre
7 Bossell Road, Buckfastleigh TQ11 0DE
Tel: 01364 42534 Fax: 01364 644057
(Teignbridge Primary Care Trust)
GP Peter Davey EDWARDS, Tessa Jane BARTON, James Roderick HEDGER, Jonathan Robert TOWERS

Buckhurst Hill

Kings Medical Centre
23 Kings Avenue, Buckhurst Hill IG9 5LP
Tel: 020 8504 0122 Fax: 020 8559 2984
Website: www.kingsmedicalcentre.co.uk
(Epping Forest Primary Care Trust)
Patient List Size: 6900
Practice Manager Suzann Channing
GP Christopher TRANMER, Iftikhar HUSSAIN, Fiona Margaret Anne OSBOROUGH

Palmerston Road Surgery
18 Palmerston Road, Buckhurst Hill IG9 5LT
Tel: 020 8504 1552
(Epping Forest Primary Care Trust)
Patient List Size: 4600
Practice Manager Brenda Woothipoom
GP John Stephen Garratt TAYLOR, Andrew Charles BRIGGS

River Surgery
16 Rous Road, Buckhurst Hill IG9 6BN
Tel: 020 8504 7364 Fax: 020 8559 0269
(Epping Forest Primary Care Trust)
Patient List Size: 3500
Practice Manager Tracy Beckley
GP Christine Elizabeth MOSS, Alexandra BARRETT

Buckingham

Horn Street Surgery
24 Horn Street, Winslow, Buckingham MK18 3AL
Tel: 01296 714504 Fax: 01296 715195
(Vale of Aylesbury Primary Care Trust)
Patient List Size: 2360
GP Anthony C NICOLAOU

Masonic House Surgery
26 High Street, Buckingham MK18 1NU
Tel: 01280 816450 Fax: 01280 823885
(Vale of Aylesbury Primary Care Trust)
Patient List Size: 7838
Practice Manager Mike Streten
GP Iain QUINEY, Elaine ROBB, Martin William AUSTIN, Tracey LARGENT, Tracey Anita LAVELL

Norden House Surgery
Avenue Road, Winslow, Buckingham MK18 3DW
Tel: 01296 713434
(Vale of Aylesbury Primary Care Trust)
Patient List Size: 7600
Practice Manager Mary Jacklin
GP Jonathan FAIRFIELD, Rodger Norman DICKSON, Margaret Ruth MASON, Diana Mary STRAKER

North End Surgery
High Street, Buckingham MK18 1NU
Tel: 01280 818600 Fax: 01280 818618
Email: northend-surgery@gp-K82007.nhs.uk
Website: www.northendsurgery.nhs.uk
(Vale of Aylesbury Primary Care Trust)
Patient List Size: 7800
Practice Manager D J Scott
GP Robert William WOODROFFE, Roger William Edward HARRINGTON, Jonathan Grant PRYSE, Rebecca PRYSE, Gregory SIMONS

North End Surgery
2 Vicarage Lane, Steeple Claydon, Buckingham MK18 2PR
Tel: 01296 733300 Fax: 01296 7333309
Website: www.northendsurgery.co.uk
(Vale of Aylesbury Primary Care Trust)
Patient List Size: 9000
Practice Manager Debbie Scott
GP Robert WOODROFFE, Roger HARRINGTON, Jonathan PRYSE, Rebecca PRYSE, Greg SIMONS

Verney Close Family Practice
Verney Close, Buckingham MK18 1JP
Tel: 01280 822777 Fax: 01280 823541
(Vale of Aylesbury Primary Care Trust)
Patient List Size: 8726
Practice Manager Lyn Bensley
GP Alison BANKS, Martina HENS, Stuart Robin MATHEWS, Tariq SADDIQUE

Bude

Stratton Medical Centre
Hospital Road, Stratton, Bude EX23 9BP
Tel: 01288 352133
(North and East Cornwall Primary Care Trust)
Patient List Size: 14500
Practice Manager Jenny Keane
GP David John SWEET, Philip Wright HADDON, Charles Ian MORWOOD, Andrew York Dobson MOSS, Michael TROWBRIDGE, Robert Arthur WATERHOUSE, David WEARDEN

Budleigh Salterton

Budleigh Salterton Medical Centre
1 The Lawn, Budleigh Salterton EX9 6LS
Tel: 01395 441200 Fax: 01395 441244
(East Devon Primary Care Trust)
Patient List Size: 7400
Practice Manager Wendy Matthews
GP Graham Errington TAYLOR, Tanas DAVIS, Simon FRANKLIN, Richard Hugh MEJZNER, H PARKES

Bungay

The Beeches
67 Lower Olland Street, Bungay NR35 1BZ
Tel: 01986 892055 Fax: 01986 895519
(Waveney Primary Care Trust)
Practice Manager Sarah Harris

GP Christopher Hillary HAND, Iain Gerald CROFTON BRIGGS, Andrew Robert EMERSON, Brian Michael GOSS, Marian Zelma LATCHMAN, Ann Elizabeth SELF, Gillian WILLIAMS

Buntingford

The Health Centre
White Hart Close, Buntingford SG9 9DQ
Tel: 01763 271362 Fax: 01763 272878
(Royston, Buntingford and Bishop's Stortford Primary Care Trust)
Patient List Size: 5400

Practice Manager S Taylor

GP Digby Paul WITHERS

Orchard Surgery
Baldock Road, Buntingford SG9 9DL
Tel: 01763 272410 Fax: 01763 273023
Email: sue.mills2@nhs.net
(Royston, Buntingford and Bishop's Stortford Primary Care Trust)
Patient List Size: 2800

Practice Manager Sue Mills

GP Josephine Gail BRYANT, Stuart HANDYSIDES

Burford

Burford Surgery
59 Sheep Street, Burford OX18 4LS
Tel: 01993 822176 Fax: 01993 822885
Email: debra.barnes@burfordsurgery.co.uk
Website: www.burfordsurgery.co.uk
(South West Oxfordshire Primary Care Trust)

Practice Manager Debra Barnes

GP Oliver John SHARPLEY, Simon Nigel ALBERT, Julian HANCOCK, Lesley WILLBY

Burgess Hill

Lyle and Partners
The Surgery, 4 Silverdale Road, Burgess Hill RH15 0EF
Tel: 01444 233450 Fax: 01444 230412
Website: www.silverdale-doctors.com
(Mid Sussex Primary Care Trust)
Patient List Size: 10700

Practice Manager Carol Collett

GP Peter Thomas Wreford LYLE, Robert William DENNEY, Ian Arthur HOLWELL, Simon Haddon PLANT, Elizabeth Patricia TAYLOR

The Meadows Surgery
Temple Grove, Gatehouse Lane, Sussex Way, Burgess Hill RH15 9XN
Tel: 01444 242860 Fax: 01444 870496
(Mid Sussex Primary Care Trust)
Patient List Size: 10000

Practice Manager Jenny Hizzey

GP Donal Francis Ellis ROCHE, Robert Michael CLARK, Alex DOMBROWE, Sue EDWARDS, Simon Alexander GANKERSEER

The Medical Centre
The Brow, Burgess Hill RH15 9BS
Tel: 01444 246162 Fax: 01444 232199
(Mid Sussex Primary Care Trust)

Practice Manager J Reiss

GP Mandy CLAIDEN, Karen EASTMAN, Portia Anne HUSSEY, Hans USHER

Park View Surgery
113A Church Road, Burgess Hill RH15 9AA
Tel: 01444 244294
(Mid Sussex Primary Care Trust)

GP T GRACE, R MIARKOWSKI

Burnham-on-Crouch

The Burnham Surgery
Foundry Lane, Burnham-on-Crouch CM0 8SJ
Tel: 01621 782054 Fax: 01621 785592
(Maldon and South Chelmsford Primary Care Trust)
Patient List Size: 9700

Practice Manager Elizabeth Mackenzie

GP Mohammed Hamid LATIF, Christine Janice COLLINS, Lisimoni KAMI, Fawzi Joseph KAMLOW

Burnham-on-Sea

Burnham Medical Centre
Love Lane, Burnham-on-Sea TA8 1EU
Tel: 01278 795445 Fax: 01278 793024
Website: www.burnhammedicalcentre.co.uk
(Somerset Coast Primary Care Trust)

Practice Manager Deborah Hale

GP Michael Roy THOMSON, Richard BOWLEY, David Andrew GAULD, Sally Gordon HOLL, Nicola MATTHEWS, Stephen MIELL, Harvey Charles Reginald SAMPSON, Adrian TYLER

Burnley

Briercliffe Road Surgery
357 Briercliffe Road, Burnley BB10 1TX
Tel: 01282 424720 Fax: 01282 429055
(Burnley, Pendle and Rossendale Primary Care Trust)
Patient List Size: 9000

Practice Manager M V Simpson

GP Subhash Ranjan Naha BISWAS, Syed Toufeeq ALI, Clive John BELL, Jawaid KHAN

Burnley Wood Medical Centre
50 Parliament Street, Burnley BB11 3JX
Tel: 01282 425521 Fax: 01282 832556
Email: bwmc@gp-P8113.nhs.uk
(Burnley, Pendle and Rossendale Primary Care Trust)

GP George Kunert CRUMBLEHOLME, Pauline PATRICK, Paul Charles RHODES

Colne Road Surgery
34-36 Colne Road, Burnley BB10 1LQ
Tel: 01282 456564 Fax: 01282 451639
(Burnley, Pendle and Rossendale Primary Care Trust)
Patient List Size: 4777

Practice Manager Gail Hayle

GP D T M BRENNAN, Andre GREENWOOD, Arnold James JENKINS

Danehouse Medical Centre
Old Hall Street, Burnley BB10 1BH
Tel: 01282 423288 Fax: 01282 422797
(Burnley, Pendle and Rossendale Primary Care Trust)
Patient List Size: 3020

Practice Manager Karen Clayton

GP Anil KUMAR

The Health Centre
Kiddrow Lane, Burnley BB12 6LH
Tel: 01282 426840 Fax: 01282 433252
(Burnley, Pendle and Rossendale Primary Care Trust)
Patient List Size: 4100

Practice Manager H Harrison

GP Dr SMITH, Dr BARSBY

Ightenhill Medical Centre
Tabor Street, Burnley BB12 0HL
Tel: 01282 424464 Fax: 01282 416327

(Burnley, Pendle and Rossendale Primary Care Trust)

GP Chaudry Kamruz Zaman HYDER

Manchester Road Surgery
187 Manchester Road, Burnley BB11 4HP
Tel: 01282 420680 Fax: 01282 456924
Email: manchesterroadsurgery@hotmail.com
Website: www.manchesterroadsurgery.co.uk
(Burnley, Pendle and Rossendale Primary Care Trust)
Patient List Size: 4300

Practice Manager Pauline Woodworth

GP Iftikhar Ali SYED, Nigel TATTERSALL

Oxford Road Medical Centre
25 Oxford Road, Burnley BB11 3BB
Tel: 01282 423603 Fax: 01282 832827
(Burnley, Pendle and Rossendale Primary Care Trust)
Patient List Size: 4300

Practice Manager Denise Hopkin

GP Longsobemo Mozhui LOTHA, Gwen Elizabeth Hodgson PHILLIPS, Chi Kuen WONG

Padiham Group Practice
Padiham Medical Centre, Burnley Road, Padiham, Burnley BB12 8BP
Tel: 01282 771298 Fax: 01282 777720
(Burnley, Pendle and Rossendale Primary Care Trust)
Patient List Size: 12800

Practice Manager Diane Holt

GP Ian Lewis MILNE, Charles Joseph Munro DONALD, Antony Peter MITCHELL, Barbara Frances SAVAGE, Barbara SEENEY

Rosegrove Surgery
225-227 Gannow Lane, Burnley BB12 6HY
Tel: 01282 423295 Fax: 01282 832609
Email: carol.nutter@gp-P81197.nhs.uk
(Burnley, Pendle and Rossendale Primary Care Trust)
Patient List Size: 3950

GP Janet Elizabeth SEAVERS, Peter SEAVERS

Rosehill Surgery
189 Manchester Road, Burnley BB11 4HP
Tel: 01282 428200 Fax: 01282 838492
(Burnley, Pendle and Rossendale Primary Care Trust)

Practice Manager C Tillotson

GP Gordon Barry DICKENS, Dr HAWKES, Alison SWANN, David John WHITE

Ruskin Health Care
38-40 Colne Road, Burnley BB10 1LG
Tel: 01282 448244 Fax: 01282 448282
(Burnley, Pendle and Rossendale Primary Care Trust)

GP Dr SINGH, Dr NAHEED, Dr SALIM

St Nicholas Health Centre
Saunder Bank, Burnley BB11 2EN
Tel: 01282 831249 Fax: 01282 425269
(Burnley, Pendle and Rossendale Primary Care Trust)
Patient List Size: 9900

Practice Manager J Bullas

GP Alison Elizabeth CRAIG, Michael DOHERTY, Ian Stewart MAUDSLEY, Michael William McDEVITT, Lucy Alice MERVIN, James Gordon Fergus ROBERTSON

St Nicholas Health Centre
Saunder Bank, Burnley BB11 2EN
Tel: 01282 422528 Fax: 01282 832834
(Burnley, Pendle and Rossendale Primary Care Trust)
Patient List Size: 4000

GP Michael Anthony DURKIN, Maurice Iskander HANNA

St Nicholas Health Centre
Saunder Bank, Burnley BB11 2EN
Tel: 01282 423677 Fax: 01282 832945
(Burnley, Pendle and Rossendale Primary Care Trust)

GP Desmond Hugh FLEMING, Maung MAUNG, Syed Safdar RAZA

Thursby Surgery
2 Browhead Road, Burnley BB10 3BF
Tel: 01282 422447 Fax: 01282 832575
(Burnley, Pendle and Rossendale Primary Care Trust)
Patient List Size: 7400

Practice Manager Phillipa Hill

GP Venkataswamy NARAYANA, David William BAILEY, Prabhavati SUNDARARAJAN, James Patrick TAYLOR

Yorkshire Street
80 Yorkshire Street, Burnley BB11 3BT
Tel: 01282 420141 Fax: 01282 832477
(Burnley, Pendle and Rossendale Primary Care Trust)
Patient List Size: 6000

GP Paul Christopher HARTLEY, Andrew David SIBSON, Mark Ronald WALTON

Burton-on-Trent

All Saints Surgery
28 All Saints Road, Burton-on-Trent DE14 3LS
Tel: 01283 510768 Fax: 01283 563058
(East Staffordshire Primary Care Trust)
Patient List Size: 6000

Practice Manager Lily Singh

GP R K SINGH, J NWEKE

Alrewas Surgery
Exchange Road, Alrewas, Burton-on-Trent DE13 7AS
Tel: 01283 790316 Fax: 01283 791863
(East Staffordshire Primary Care Trust)

GP R M HORTON, Janet MAGER-JONES, J F SEIGEL

Barton Health Centre
Short Lane, Barton-under-Needwood, Burton-on-Trent DE13 8LB
Tel: 01283 712207 Fax: 01283 712116
Website: www.surgeriesonline/bartonmp
(East Staffordshire Primary Care Trust)
Patient List Size: 6700

Practice Manager David Rose

GP Jonathan Celt WHITE, Declan MULVANAY, Mussarat SHER

Bridge Surgery
St Peters Street, Stapenhill, Burton-on-Trent DE15 9AW
Tel: 01283 563631 Fax: 01283 500896
Website: www.bridgesurgery.net
(East Staffordshire Primary Care Trust)
Patient List Size: 10150

Practice Manager Julie Woolliscroft

GP Marek Jerzy TRELINSKI, Dr GEORGLOU, Charles Godfrey Laurence PIDSLEY, Kathryn Fiona SELLENS, Elizabeth Mary WADDY, Dr WONG

Butchart
The Surgery, King Street, Burton-on-Trent DE14 3AG
Tel: 01283 741177 Fax: 01283 565657
(East Staffordshire Primary Care Trust)
Patient List Size: 2700

Practice Manager C M Winfindale

GP Graham David BUTCHART

Carlton Street Surgery
Carlton Street, Horninglow, Burton-on-Trent DE13 0TE
Tel: 01283 511387 Fax: 01283 517174
(East Staffordshire Primary Care Trust)

GP John Joseph Laurence CLEARY, George Andrew Nicholas LUFT, Andrew John PORTER, Stuart Ronald WINCHURCH

Gordon Street Surgery
72 Gordon Street, Burton-on-Trent DE14 2JA
Tel: 01283 563175 Fax: 01283 500638
(East Staffordshire Primary Care Trust)
Patient List Size: 10000

GP Hamid Ali KHAN, Stephen Leonard COLLIER, Christopher Charles GUNSTONE, Eileen Marie GUNSTONE, Brendan Thomas O'REILLY, Philip Norman ROBINSON

Peel Croft Surgery
Lichfield Street, Burton-on-Trent DE14 3RH
Tel: 01283 568405 Fax: 01283 515761
Website: www.peelcroftsurgery.co.uk
(East Staffordshire Primary Care Trust)
Patient List Size: 2690

Practice Manager Tim Hinchley

GP Cecil David FARRAR, Catherine Louise FAARUP

Stapenhill Surgery
Fyfield Road, Stapenhill, Burton-on-Trent DE15 9QD
Tel: 01283 565200 Fax: 01283 500617
(East Staffordshire Primary Care Trust)
Patient List Size: 10000

Practice Manager Tim Briers

GP Jeremy Augustus Frederick LOCKWOOD, Gregory BUTLER, Philip NEEDHAM, A ROBERTS, Naomi Marydell SPENCER, Mark Andrew YOUNG

Trent Meadows Medical Centre
87 Wood Street, Burton-on-Trent DE14 3AA
Tel: 01283 845555 Fax: 01283 845222
(East Staffordshire Primary Care Trust)
Patient List Size: 10300

Practice Manager M B Fildes

GP J M CROSSE, P L JONES, Tilo Albert Fritz Paul SCHEEL, P G L SMITH, John Michael TANSEY

Tutbury Health Centre
Monk Street, Tutbury, Burton-on-Trent DE13 9NA
Tel: 01283 812210 Fax: 01283 815810
(East Staffordshire Primary Care Trust)
Patient List Size: 3757

GP H SKINNER, E J GUNN, M SALWEY, Julia Mary SPENCER-JONES

Yoxall Health Centre
Savey Lane, Yoxall, Burton-on-Trent DE13 8PD
Tel: 01543 472202 Fax: 01543 472362
Website: www.yoxallhealthcentre.org
(East Staffordshire Primary Care Trust)
Patient List Size: 5100

Practice Manager Lorraine Stevens

GP Muhammad Arif KHAN, Martin Guy Wickham ATKINSON, Andrew TOMAN

Bury

Blackford House Medical Centre
137 Croft Lane, Hollins, Bury BL9 0QA
Tel: 0161 766 6622 Fax: 0161 786 2748
(Bury Primary Care Trust)
Patient List Size: 8000

Practice Manager Carol Armstrong

GP James Robert HURST, Stephen Laurence BOWERS, Jonathan Laurence GOLDING, Alison Kim McGOWAN

Garden City Surgery
1A Garden City, Holcombe Brook, Bury BL0 9TN
Tel: 01204 884710 Fax: 01204 888334
(Bury Primary Care Trust)
Patient List Size: 2900

Practice Manager Deborah Nolan

GP Chan Yoong CHUI YEW CHEONG

Greenmount Medical Centre
9 Brandlesholme Road, Greenmount, Bury BL8 4DR
Tel: 01204 885111 Fax: 01204 887431
Website: www.greenmountmc.nhs.uk
(Bury Primary Care Trust)
Patient List Size: 7760

Practice Manager Irene Lord

GP Janice Mary PRESSLER, John Roderick HAMPSON, Kiran P PATEL, Marie-Josee ROLLI

Huntley Mount Medical Centre
Huntley Mount Road, Bury BL9 6JA
Tel: 0161 761 6677 Fax: 0161 761 3283
Email: AndrewDemetriou@gp-P83621.nhs.uk
(Bury Primary Care Trust)
Patient List Size: 3700

Practice Manager Maria Stacy

GP Andrew DEMETRIOU

Knowsley Street Medical Centre
9-11 Knowsley Street, Bury BL9 0ST
Tel: 0161 764 1217
(Bury Primary Care Trust)

Practice Manager Joy Weaver

GP R K THAKER, P K JAIN, B K THAKER, Kantilal Kalidas THAKER

Mile Lane Health Centre
80 Mile Lane, Bury BL8 2JR
Tel: 0161 764 7804 Fax: 0161 763 1931
(Bury Primary Care Trust)
Patient List Size: 2100

Practice Manager Sandra Leaver

GP Kailash BHALLA

Minden Medical Centre
2 Barlow Street, Bury BL9 0QP
Tel: 0161 764 2651 Fax: 0161 761 5967
(Bury Primary Care Trust)

Practice Manager Barbara Gaskell

GP Derek Peter FLETCHER, D M COULTER, Patricia Florence FLETCHER

Minden Medical Centre
2 Barlow Street, Bury BL9 0QP
Tel: 0161 764 2652 Fax: 0161 761 5967
(Bury Primary Care Trust)

Practice Manager Barbara Gaskell

GP Peter Alan STANDING, Helen DEAKIN, Paul Richard NORMAN

Minden Medical Centre
2 Barlow Street, Bury BL9 0QP
Tel: 0161 764 2651 Fax: 0161 761 5967
(Bury Primary Care Trust)

Practice Manager Barbara Gaskell

GP Chandra SHEKAR, Simon Richard de VIAL, Audrey GIBSON, Neil JOSEPH

Peel Health Centre
Angouleme Way, Bury BL9 0BT
Tel: 0161 764 0311 Fax: 0161 761 7548
(Bury Primary Care Trust)

Practice Manager Pamela Casey

GP Irena Stanislawa KARWOWSKI, Pauline Mary CLEARY

Peel Health Centre
Angouleme Way, Bury BL9 0BT
Tel: 0161 763 7790 Fax: 0161 761 2392
(Bury Primary Care Trust)

Practice Manager Angela Coric

GP Paul Anthony JACKSON, J C JACSON

Peel Health Centre
Angouleme Way, Bury BL9 0BT
Tel: 0161 763 7613 Fax: 0161 763 9625
(Bury Primary Care Trust)

Practice Manager June Jennings

GP Sarah Anne SIEGLER, John Anthony HARBOTTLE

Peel Health Centre
Angouleme Way, Bury BL9 0BT
Tel: 0161 764 8700 Fax: 0161 764 8700
(Bury Primary Care Trust)

GP S SUD

Ramsbottom Health Centre
Carr Street, Ramsbottom, Bury BL0 9DD
Tel: 01706 824583 Fax: 01706 821196
(Bury Primary Care Trust)
Patient List Size: 2300

Practice Manager Shirley Candler

GP Masood Ali BAIG, Shakila BAIG

Ramsbottom Health Centre
Carr Street, Ramsbottom, Bury BL0 9DD
Tel: 01706 824413 Fax: 01706 821196
(Bury Primary Care Trust)
Patient List Size: 5760

Practice Manager Mary Sharkey

GP Gordon MACKINNON, Chet CHANRE, Veronica CHURREY, Ailie Serena Rosemary MACKINNON

Ramsbottom Health Centre
Carr Street, Ramsbottom, Bury BL0 9DD
Tel: 01706 824445 Fax: 01706 821196
(Bury Primary Care Trust)
Patient List Size: 1250

Practice Manager Maureen Anderton

GP Shyamal Kanti SARKAR

Ribblesdale House Medical Centre
Market Street, Bury BL9 0BU
Tel: 0161 764 7241 Fax: 0161 763 3557
(Bury Primary Care Trust)

Practice Manager Samamtha Hesketh

GP Edward Damian John STONE, Mark A McCOUDNEY, Shanmugam SUBBIAH

Ribblesdale House Medical Centre
Market Street, Bury BL9 0BU
Tel: 0161 764 7241 Fax: 0161 763 3557
(Bury Primary Care Trust)

Practice Manager Samamtha Hesketh

GP Peter James WOODCOCK, Cheryl Ann BRITTON, Douglas Neil KYFFIN

Ribblesdale House Medical Centre
Market Street, Bury BL9 0BU
Tel: 0161 764 7241 Fax: 0161 763 3557
(Bury Primary Care Trust)

Practice Manager Joan Richardson

GP Alfa ISMAN, Zia JALAL

Tottington Health Centre
16 Market Street, Tottington, Bury BL8 4AD
Tel: 01204 885106 Fax: 01204 887717
(Bury Primary Care Trust)
Patient List Size: 10500

Practice Manager Jean Fitzpatrick

GP Noel Jeremy Chisnall MARTIN, Carol Anne CORNMELL, Stephen Kenneth KIRKHAM, Charlotte McKINNON, Sandra QUENAULT, Robert Andrew STOKES, Jillian Patricia WATTS

Unsworth Medical Centre
Parr Lane, Unsworth, Bury BL9 8JR
Tel: 0161 766 4092 Fax: 0161 767 9811
(Bury Primary Care Trust)
Patient List Size: 7400

Practice Manager J Smith

GP Michael Lewis MATTISON, Jacqueline HAYDEN, Kathleen Mary O'CALLAGHAN, Rekha RALHAN, Brian Joseph SOPHER

Walmersley Road Surgery
110 Walmersley Road, Bury BL9 6DX
Tel: 0161 764 6100 Fax: 0161 764 0100
(Bury Primary Care Trust)
Patient List Size: 2885

Practice Manager Shahida Anjum

GP Iftikhar Ahmad ANJUM

Woodbank Surgery
2 Hunstanton Drive, Bury BL8 1EG
Tel: 0161 705 1630 Fax: 0161 763 3221
Website: www.woodbanksurgery.nhs.uk
(Bury Primary Care Trust)

Practice Manager M Bolton

GP Patrick David Roger NEININGER, Simon Richard CHILD, K CLARKE, J C SCOTT

Bury St Edmunds

Angel Hill Surgery
1 Angel Hill, Bury St Edmunds IP33 1LU
Tel: 01284 753008 Fax: 01284 724744
(Suffolk West Primary Care Trust)
Patient List Size: 14300

Practice Manager Judy Smith

GP Robert Keith BRADLEY, Paul David HARRISON, Brian Read JONES, Peter Brian KILNER, Jonathan Edward MASTERS, Janet RUTHERFORD, William John TASKER

Barrow Hill Surgery
Barrow Hill, Barrow, Bury St Edmunds IP29 5DX
Tel: 01284 810330 Fax: 01284 811388
(Suffolk West Primary Care Trust)
Patient List Size: 1560

Practice Manager David Busby

GP R C COOLEDGE

Ixworth Surgery
Peddars Close, Ixworth, Bury St Edmunds IP31 2HD
Tel: 01359 230252 Fax: 01359 232586
(Suffolk West Primary Care Trust)
Patient List Size: 9300

Practice Manager Keith Hoddy

GP John Clayton CANNON, Mary Theresa BROOKES, Nicholas Charles Wilfrid HARPUR, Calum HART, Matthew James LOCKYER, Anne TEBBIT

Market Cross Surgery
7 Market Place, Mildenhall, Bury St Edmunds IP28 7EG
Tel: 01638 713109 Fax: 01638 718615
(Suffolk West Primary Care Trust)

Practice Manager Maggie Lake

GP Godfrey REYNOLDS, Monica BELL, John Anthony BRUTON, Jacqueline Sarah COOLEDGE, M MISTRY, J SATISH

Mount Farm Surgery
Lawson Place, Bury St Edmunds IP32 7EW
Tel: 01284 769643 Fax: 01284 700833
Email: mountfm@epulse.net

(Suffolk West Primary Care Trust)
Patient List Size: 10800

Practice Manager Peter Knights

GP Graeme KELVIN, Susan Mary BROWN, Claire Elizabeth GILES, Christopher Charles HODGSON, Eugene LEWIS, John Bruce THOMPSON

Oliver and Partners

The Guildhall Surgery, Lower Baxter Street, Bury St Edmunds IP33 1ET
Tel: 01284 701601 Fax: 01284 702943
(Suffolk West Primary Care Trust)
Patient List Size: 9940

Practice Manager Christine Wragge

GP Stephen Francis OLIVER, Philip Rhys EVANS, Heather Margaret GRAHAM, Michael Robert Creswell JONES, Richard Conrad ROBINSON, B SENGUPTA

Swan Surgery

Northgate Street, Bury St Edmunds IP33 1AE
Tel: 01284 750011 Fax: 01284 723565
Email: swansurgery@cs.com
(Suffolk West Primary Care Trust)
Patient List Size: 6000

Practice Manager Rachel Helliar

GP Crispin Thomas Pereira DUNNE, Dr DERBYSHIRE, Kirsty Jane REID

Victoria Surgery

Victoria Street, Bury St Edmunds IP33 3BD
Tel: 01284 725550 Fax: 01284 725551
(Suffolk West Primary Care Trust)
Patient List Size: 11300

Practice Manager Kathryn Colsell

GP David Howard WATSON, Paul Richard DEAN, Kevin Roger GRACE, Paul Alexander HADLEY, Richard Henry SOPER

White House Surgery

10/10A Market Place, Mildenhall, Bury St Edmunds IP28 7EF
Tel: 01638 718177 Fax: 01638 718901
Email: admin@gp-D83078.nhs.uk
(Suffolk West Primary Care Trust)

Practice Manager Stuart Collis

GP George Patrick HOPKINSON, Richard Adrian HUTTON

Woolpit Health Centre

Heath Road, Woolpit, Bury St Edmunds IP30 9QU
Tel: 01359 240298 Fax: 01359 241975
(Suffolk West Primary Care Trust)
Patient List Size: 12200

Practice Manager Sallie Crouch

GP Anthony Robert BRAIN, Tin Tun AUNG, Alastair McCOLL, David Anthony PEARSON, William Patrick RIDSDILL SMITH, Richard John WEST

Buxton

Buxton Medical Practice

2 Temple Road, Buxton SK17 9BZ
Tel: 01298 24105 Fax: 01298 73227
(High Peak and Dales Primary Care Trust)

Practice Manager David Doig

GP Anthony Pattison BRIGGS, Charlotte Mary DOIG, Jeffrey HADDON, Anthony William HARTLEY, Ian Arthur SAUNDERS

Elmwood Medical Centre

7 Burlington Road, Buxton SK17 9AY
Tel: 01298 23019 Fax: 01298 24930
Website: www.elmwoodsurgery.co.uk
(High Peak and Dales Primary Care Trust)
Patient List Size: 8600

Practice Manager Lawrie Harding

GP Sean Frederick KING, Rosemary BERESFORD, Rachel Mary DULLEHAN, Sally GILMOUR, Timothy Charles HODGKINSON, David John SWINHOE, Karoline Mary WEIR

Hartington Surgery

Dig Street, Hartington, Buxton SK17 0AQ
Tel: 01298 84315 Fax: 01298 84899
(High Peak and Dales Primary Care Trust)
Patient List Size: 3300

Practice Manager Martin Bennett

GP Edward Malcolm BRADBURY, Graham Leslie HURST, Susan Elizabeth WOODS

Park Road Surgery

Park Road, Tideswell, Buxton SK17 8NS
Tel: 01298 871292 Fax: 01298 872580
(High Peak and Dales Primary Care Trust)
Patient List Size: 3200

Practice Manager Jayne Wharton

GP Philip John COX, Catherine Teresa MARK

The Stewart Medical Centre

15 Hartington Road, Buxton SK17 6JP
Tel: 01298 22338 Fax: 01298 72678
(High Peak and Dales Primary Care Trust)
Patient List Size: 8700

Practice Manager Louise Chipp

GP Brian Rees WILLIAMS, Andrew James COLLIER, Sheila Mary DALE, Lezli Ann PEARSON, Peter Richard David SHORT

Callington

Callington and Gunnislake Group Practice

The Health Centre, Haye Road, Callington PL17 7AW
Tel: 01579 382666 Fax: 01579 383345
(North and East Cornwall Primary Care Trust)
Patient List Size: 15700

Practice Manager Sue Duke, Elizabeth Scott

GP Adrian Philip KRATKY, Michael Charles BLEKSLEY, N D BUXTON, Simon CHAPLIN, J EARLY, A P FARR, A MASSEY, S M McCORMICK, F M PRENTICE, A P STEWART, J G TILBURY, E J WARREN

Calne

Church Street Surgery

15 Church Street, Calne SN11 0HY
Tel: 01249 821831 Fax: 01249 816020
(Kennet and North Wiltshire Primary Care Trust)
Patient List Size: 3500

Practice Manager K Martin

GP David Selwyn BISHOP, Averil Mary SANDFORD-HILL

Northlands Surgery

North Street, Calne SN11 0HH
Tel: 01249 812091 Fax: 01249 815343
(Kennet and North Wiltshire Primary Care Trust)
Patient List Size: 10500

Practice Manager Robert Baggs

GP Norman Ronald BEALE, Richard Maurice Cameron LEACH, Martin Anthony SEARLE, Andrew Shepherd THORNTON, Elizabeth Margaret Knox TULLY

Camberley

Ash Vale Health Centre

Wharf Road, Ash Vale, Camberley GU16 4QQ
(Surrey Heath and Woking Primary Care Trust)

GP Brett WHITBY-SMITH, David ANDERSON, Lawrence BURKE, Audrey INNES, Fiona KINGSTON, Claire WALTON, Philip WHATMOUGH

Camberley Health Centre
159 Frimley Road, Camberley GU15 2QA
Tel: 01276 20101 Fax: 01276 21661
(Surrey Heath and Woking Primary Care Trust)
Patient List Size: 10000

Practice Manager Carole Wingrove

GP Paul Laurence BUCHANAN, Brian Patrick BOOTH, Rebecca Elizabeth FISHER, John Roger HARRIS, David Lloyd HEARN

Frimley Green Medical Centre
1 Beech Road, Frimley Green, Camberley GU16 6QQ
Tel: 01252 835016 Fax: 01252 837908
Website: www.fgmc.org.uk
(Surrey Heath and Woking Primary Care Trust)
Patient List Size: 11700

Practice Manager Ian Friend

GP Michael John YATES, Catrin BEAVAN, Peter Charles CURETON, Richard James MacKenzie DE FERRARS, Catherine HILEY, Colin TANNER

Hartley Corner Surgery
51 Frogmore Road, Blackwater, Camberley GU17 0DB
Tel: 01252 872791 Fax: 01252 878910
(Blackwater Valley and Hart Primary Care Trust)

GP Stephen Roy JONES, Karl BENNETT, Rachel Helen BLACKMAN, Kathryn Barbara GRADY, Richard Mark HINTON, J MARTIN

Heatherside Surgery
73 Cumberland Road, Camberley GU15 1SE
Tel: 01276 64758
(Surrey Heath and Woking Primary Care Trust)
Patient List Size: 3587

Practice Manager M Williams

GP S A WILLIAMS, Fiona BUXTON, Nicola TOWNSEND

Old Dean Surgery
Berkshire Road Clinic, Berkshire Road, Camberley GU15 4DP
Tel: 01276 29119 Fax: 01276 676333
Website: www.surgeriesonline.com/olddeansurgery
(Surrey Heath and Woking Primary Care Trust)
Patient List Size: 2500

Practice Manager Wendy Hopkins

GP Shekhar LOHIA

The Surgery
143 Park Road, Camberley GU15 2NN
Tel: 01276 26171
(Surrey Heath and Woking Primary Care Trust)
Patient List Size: 12200

Practice Manager Gill Suter

GP Graham Beresford HEY, Andrew BROOKS, Rachel DARROCH, Susan DENTON, Dayantha Sunimal FERNANDO, Nigel John HAGUE, Mark PUGSLEY

The Surgery
4 Station Road, Frimley, Camberley GU16 7HG
Tel: 01276 62622 Fax: 01276 683908
(Surrey Heath and Woking Primary Care Trust)
Patient List Size: 7180

Practice Manager Denise Gubbins

GP Samuel Arthur COULTER, Rachell BENNETT, B FERGUSON, Jane SNEL

Upper Gordon Road Surgery
37 Upper Gordon Road, Camberley GU15 2HJ
Tel: 01276 459040
(Surrey Heath and Woking Primary Care Trust)
Patient List Size: 11000

Practice Manager Carrie Vincent

GP Geoffrey David ROBERTS, Ruth CURETON, John Murray FRASER, Karen Jane LOTHE, Jane Elizabeth Keppel ORR, Fenella PAMBAKIAN

Camborne

Pheonix Surgery
Health Office, Rectory Road, Camborne TR14 7DL
Tel: 01209 714876 Fax: 01209 886539
(West of Cornwall Primary Care Trust)
Patient List Size: 4859

Practice Manager Alison Butterill

GP Timothy Peter KEECH, Judith ADINKRA, Kenneth George WHITTLE

Praze Surgery
School Road, Praze-An-Beeble, Camborne TR14 0LB
Tel: 01209 831386 Fax: 01209 831885
Email: michele.brown@praze.cornwall.nhs.uk
(West of Cornwall Primary Care Trust)
Patient List Size: 4590

Practice Manager Michele Brown

GP Dr BENSA, Hugh Hunter FAIRLIE, Dr SMITH

Trevithick Surgery
Basset Road, Camborne TR14 8TT
Tel: 01209 886588 Fax: 01209 612488
Email: veronica.pascoe@trevithick.cornwall.nhs.uk
(West of Cornwall Primary Care Trust)
Patient List Size: 4756

Practice Manager Veronica Pascoe

GP Simon Langton WHITING, Anne BEABLE, Robert Anthony HARVEY

Veor Surgery
South Terrace, Camborne TR14 8SN
Tel: 01209 886555 Fax: 01209 886569
Email: ray.rounsevell@veor.cornwall.nhs.uk
(West of Cornwall Primary Care Trust)

Practice Manager Ray S Rounsevell

GP Peter John PERKINS, Jonathan Falcon NORRIS, Maria Juliette PATTEN

Cambourne

Monkfield Medical Practice
Monkfield Medical Practice, Sackville House, Sackville Way, Cambourne CB3 6HD
Tel: 01954 282153 Fax: 01954 282151
Website: www.mankfieldpractice.co.uk
(South Cambridgeshire Primary Care Trust)
Patient List Size: 2000

Practice Manager Joyleene Abrey

GP Peter BAILEY, A ANDERSON, C COOPER

Cambridge

Arbury Road Surgery
114 Arbury Road, Cambridge CB4 2JG
Tel: 01223 364433 Fax: 01223 315728
(Cambridge City Primary Care Trust)

Practice Manager H E Leah

GP Richard Michael GANT, Anna Friederike FISHER, Dr KETTLE, Ann Miriam MAHAFFEY, Andrew Brailsford WATSON, Eleanor Jane WITHERS

Bannold Road Surgery
Rosalind Franklin House, Bannold Road, Waterbeach, Cambridge CB5 9LQ
Tel: 01223 860387 Fax: 01223 576259

(South Cambridgeshire Primary Care Trust)

Practice Manager Barbara Brown

GP Janice Margaret MACHEN, Clare Gillian BURRELL, Nicola HOWARD

Bottisham Medical Practice

Tunbridge Lane, Bottisham, Cambridge CB5 9DU
Tel: 01223 810030 Fax: 01223 810031
(East Cambridgeshire and Fenland Primary Care Trust)

Practice Manager M Barrett-Small

GP Mark Hamilton TOWRISS, Peta Elisabeth CROUCHER, Margaret Louise ELLIOTT, Jonathan HIGHAM

Boxworth End Surgery

58 Boxworth End, Swavesey, Cambridge CB4 5RA
Tel: 01954 230202 Fax: 01954 206035
(South Cambridgeshire Primary Care Trust)
Patient List Size: 2800

Practice Manager Mark Thomas

GP Lakhbir Kaur TAYLOR

Bridge Street Surgery

67 Bridge Street, Cambridge CB2 1UU
Tel: 01223 355060 Fax: 01223 460812
(Cambridge City Primary Care Trust)
Patient List Size: 8500

Practice Manager A Turner

GP Sue HOLMES, Caroline Jane STEPHENS, Corinne BAKKER, Carol Nessa Margaret CONNOLLY, Anna DEVINE, Geraldine LINEHAN

Brookfields Health Centre

Seymour Street, Cambridge CB1 3DQ
Tel: 01223 723160 Fax: 01223 723089
Email: steve.leadbitter@gp-d81025.nhs.uk
Website: www.brookfields-health.co.uk
(Cambridge City Primary Care Trust)
Patient List Size: 11200

GP Christopher Bower HICKLING, Max BERENDS, Miranda BUCKLEY, Christine EMERSON, S MUKERJEE, Nessa WARD, Eileen WHITTLE

Brooklands Avenue Medical Centre

Brooklands Avenue Medical Centre, 7 Brooklands Avenue, Cambridge CB2 2BB
Tel: 01223 356715 Fax: 01223 357789
Website: www.brooklands-avenue-surgery.co.uk
(Cambridge City Primary Care Trust)
Patient List Size: 2300

Practice Manager Rachel Galloway

GP Richard PARKER, Elizabeth O'DONNELL

The Burwell Surgery

Newmarket Road, Burwell, Cambridge CB5 0AE
Tel: 01638 741234 Fax: 01638 743948
(East Cambridgeshire and Fenland Primary Care Trust)
Patient List Size: 7243

Practice Manager Aileen Allen

GP Anne SHNEERSON, Alex MANNING, James PARRY, Andrew J WILLS

Cornford House Surgery

364 Cherry Hinton Road, Cambridge CB1 8BA
Tel: 01223 247505 Fax: 01223 568187
(Cambridge City Primary Care Trust)
Patient List Size: 7957

Practice Manager Roger Carvell

GP Aleksander KUCZYNSKI, Catherine Margaret BENNETT, Richard Goronwy DAVIES, Christine Mary GASTON, Nigel Gregory HARRISON, Raji MADABHUSHI

Cottenham Surgery

Lewis House, 188 High Street, Cottenham, Cambridge CB4 8SE
Tel: 01954 250079 Fax: 01954 206078
(South Cambridgeshire Primary Care Trust)
Patient List Size: 3750

Practice Manager David Brammer

GP Juliet Mary GOULD, Anthony COLE

Drings Close Surgery

1 Drings Close, Over, Cambridge CB4 5NZ
Tel: 01954 231550 Fax: 01954 231573
(South Cambridgeshire Primary Care Trust)
Patient List Size: 4200

Practice Manager John Ritchie

GP Fiona Helen WATERS, Bamidele Olusola AMURE, Katrina Brown COOPE, Judith DAVIS

East Barnwell Health Centre

Ditton Lane, Cambridge CB5 8SP
Tel: 01223 728900 Fax: 01223 728901
(Cambridge City Primary Care Trust)
Patient List Size: 6500

Practice Manager Virginia Kalcev

GP Ronald Hugh KING, Stephen Ian Gurney BARCLAY, Stephen Ernest JONES, Fiona LECKIE, Virginia Jane LEGGATT

Firs House Surgery

Station Road, Histon, Cambridge CB4 9NP
Tel: 01223 234286 Fax: 01223 235931
(South Cambridgeshire Primary Care Trust)

Practice Manager Miriam McNally

GP Michael John GRANDE, Jo PRITCHARD, Emma BALDWIN, Rosemary Anne Veronica FREEMAN, Simon Benedict POOLE

Great Shelford Health Centre

Ashen Green, Great Shelford, Cambridge CB2 5EY
Tel: 01223 843661 Fax: 01223 844569
(South Cambridgeshire Primary Care Trust)

Practice Manager Dorothy Quayle

GP John Lindsay TWEEDALE, Colin HITCHCOCK, C Rebecca JONES, Sarah Frances RANN, Christoper SCHRAMM

Green End Surgery

58 Green End, Comberton, Cambridge CB3 7DY
Tel: 01223 262500 Fax: 01223 264401
(South Cambridgeshire Primary Care Trust)
Patient List Size: 8500

Practice Manager Jill Baden

GP P G R ALEXANDER, Christopher Jan KENT, Alan James David MILLS, Ian Richard PARKER, Barbara Catherine SHEPHERD

Haigh and Partners

11 Church Street, Harston, Cambridge CB2 5NP
Tel: 01223 870250 Fax: 01223 872741
(South Cambridgeshire Primary Care Trust)

Practice Manager Geraldine O'Leary

GP Elaine HAIGH, Fraser Stewart ALLEN, C GEE, Julia Margaret PURR

Hanover Close Health Centre

Hanover Close, Bar Hill, Cambridge CB3 8SE
Tel: 01954 780442 Fax: 01954 789590
(South Cambridgeshire Primary Care Trust)

Practice Manager Maureen Cundy

GP Jacob HASSAN, Dr RANASINGHE

Hills Road Surgery

Beechwood Practice, 41 Hills Road, Cambridge CB2 1NT
Tel: 01223 315541 Fax: 01223 301422
(Cambridge City Primary Care Trust)

Practice Manager Nicola Newton

GP Christine Gail KENNEY, Anita AMIN, Jenny NEWELL

Huntingdon Road Surgery
1 Huntingdon Road, Cambridge CB3 0DB
Tel: 01223 364127 Fax: 01223 322541
(Cambridge City Primary Care Trust)
Patient List Size: 12000

Practice Manager Sarah West

GP Peter David TOASE, Peter Daniel CONNAN, Philippa Margaret EVANS, Anthony John FLINN, Karen NEWMAN

The Laurels Surgery
20 Newmarket Road, Cambridge CB5 8DT
Tel: 01223 350513 Fax: 01223 300445
(Cambridge City Primary Care Trust)

Practice Manager K Caldwell

GP Geoffrey LEVINE, Mary Christine HUGH-JONES

Lensfield Medical Practice
48 Lensfield Road, Cambridge CB2 1EH
Tel: 01223 352779 Fax: 01223 566930
(Cambridge City Primary Care Trust)

Practice Manager Paul Carroll

GP Paul James PAXTON, Sui-Yen W AH-SEE, Ian Hugh Pudsey DAWSON, Susan Mary HOLMES, Veronica Josephine SPOONER, Antony Richard WARREN

Linton Health Centre
Coles Lane, Linton, Cambridge CB1 6JS
Tel: 01223 892555 Fax: 01223 890033
(South Cambridgeshire Primary Care Trust)
Patient List Size: 11000

Practice Manager S Griffiths

GP James Laurence HEWLETT, Miguel ARBIDE, Roger Charles Ricardo BERTRAM, Jennifer Anne BISSET, Joanna Elaine FARNELL, John Roger PETTER, Jonathan David SILVERMAN, Valerie Ann WHEELER

Milton Surgery
Coles Road, Milton, Cambridge CB4 6BL
Tel: 01223 420511 Fax: 01223 425078
(South Cambridgeshire Primary Care Trust)

Practice Manager Pam Vincett

GP Rebecca Jane STEWARD, Cain Rohan HUNT

Newmarket Road Surgery
125 Newmarket Road, Cambridge CB5 8HA
Tel: 01223 364116 Fax: 01223 366088
(Cambridge City Primary Care Trust)

Practice Manager J L Davies

GP Mary Ethna POLKINHORN, A E BROWN, J D A COOPER, D S CREED, Anthony George MALES, A G TAPNEY

Newnham Walk Surgery
Wordsworth Grove, Cambridge CB3 9HS
Tel: 01223 366811 Fax: 01223 302706
(Cambridge City Primary Care Trust)

Practice Manager Barbara Willis

GP Pauline Ruth BRIMBLECOMBE, Sally Ann BARNARD, Fiona Elizabeth CORNISH, Paul LINEHAN, Adrian James O'REILLY

Nuffield Road Medical Centre
Nuffield Road, Chesterton, Cambridge CB4 1GL
Tel: 01223 423424 Fax: 01223 566450
Website: www.nrmc.nhs.uk
(Cambridge City Primary Care Trust)
Patient List Size: 9800

Practice Manager Andrew Fowles

GP Thomas St John ALDERSON, Susan Chapman CHESTER, Robert DOBLER, Arnold FERTIG, Ruth GREEN, Katherine Margaret GRIMSHAW, Selma MALIK, John Rodham PERRY, Amanda Jane WHARTON

Petersfield Medical Practice
Dr Farrant & Partners, 25 Mill Road, Cambridge CB1 2AB
Tel: 01223 350647 Fax: 01223 576096
(Cambridge City Primary Care Trust)
Patient List Size: 6100

Practice Manager Mary E Miller

GP Colin Geoffrey Cameron FARRANT, Sebastian John Campbell ALEXANDER, Moya KELLY, Alison WEISSBERG, Jane WILSON

The Queen Edith Medical Practice
59 Queen Ediths Way, Cambridge CB1 8PJ
Tel: 01223 247288 Fax: 01223 213459
(Cambridge City Primary Care Trust)
Patient List Size: 5650

Practice Manager Barbara Green

GP Andrew Stephen HUSSEY, Jenny CLAPHAY, Alice HUDKINSON, Gruffydd John THOMAS

Red House Surgery
96 Chesterton Road, Cambridge CB4 1ER
Tel: 01223 365555 Fax: 01223 356848
(Cambridge City Primary Care Trust)
Patient List Size: 13000

Practice Manager Caroline Mason, Sylvia Prestwich

GP Martin HUGHES, John FOO, Samim KAPADIA, Richard MARRIOTT, Ralph Paul SALMON

Sawston Health Centre
Link Road, Sawston, Cambridge CB2 4LB
Tel: 01223 727555 Fax: 01223 836096
Website: www.sawstonmedicalcentre.co.uk
(South Cambridgeshire Primary Care Trust)
Patient List Size: 12800

Practice Manager Pauline Betts

GP Peter Joseph McKENNA, S J BALL, Susan Bernice BEHR, Carol EVANS, Alan David Norman GELSON, David KILLCOMMONS, Stephen Myles TAVARE

Smith, Niemczuk, Puuirajasingham
279-281 Mill Road, Cambridge CB1 3DG
Tel: 01223 247812 Fax: 01223 214191
(Cambridge City Primary Care Trust)

Practice Manager Zoe May

GP Tracy Amanda SMITH, Aileen LARBIE, Peter NIEMCZUK, Shiuanf PUNUIRAJASINGHAM

The Surgery
25 Alms Hill, Bourn, Cambridge CB3 7SH
Tel: 01954 719313 Fax: 01954 718012
(South Cambridgeshire Primary Care Trust)
Patient List Size: 5400

Practice Manager Tracey Wilson

GP Geoffrey Brian TOBIN, Leigh GORDON, Cynthia Ann LALLI, Michael David REDWOOD

The Surgery
Chequers Lane, Papworth Everard, Cambridge CB3 8QQ
Tel: 01480 830888 Fax: 01480 830001
(Huntingdonshire Primary Care Trust)
Patient List Size: 4354

Practice Manager Rob Johnson

GP David Wenyon BARTLETT, David Roger Harrison CRONK, Paula Jane NEWTON

Trumpington Street Medical Practice
56 Trumpington Street, Cambridge CB2 1RG
Tel: 01223 303048 Fax: 01223 356837
(Cambridge City Primary Care Trust)
Patient List Size: 9500

Practice Manager Wendy Manley

GP Anthony Redgewell DANSIE, Mark DOURISH, Inaam HAMDI, Caroline LEA-COX, Simon OWENS, Angus John STEWART, Mary Eileen Campbell WATSON

Willingham Medical Practice
52 Long Lane, Willingham, Cambridge CB4 5LB
Tel: 01954 260230 Fax: 01954 206204
(South Cambridgeshire Primary Care Trust)
Patient List Size: 5350

Practice Manager Cynthia Bidwell

GP Thomas Gordon HEWLETT, Matthew N S HUNT, Branko JANKOVIC, Catherine Mary SUTER

Camelford

Church Field Medical Centre
Church Field, Camelford PL32 9YT
Tel: 01840 213894 Fax: 01840 212986
(North and East Cornwall Primary Care Trust)

GP John Patrick Stuart RICHARDSON, Andrew Charles GARROD

The Medical Centre
Churchfield, Camelford PL32 9YT
Tel: 01840 213894 Fax: 01840 212276
(North and East Cornwall Primary Care Trust)

Practice Manager A Goodman

GP A NASH, Dr ROWLANDS

Cannock

Aungmingalar Surgery
46 Anglesey Street, Hednesford, Cannock WS12 1AA
Tel: 01543 422787 Fax: 01543 879128
Email: aung.yi@nhs.net
(Cannock Chase Primary Care Trust)
Patient List Size: 2813

Practice Manager Yinyin Myaing

GP Aung YI

Cannock Road Surgery
441 Cannock Road, Hednesford, Cannock WS12 4AE
Tel: 01543 422531 Fax: 01543 428531
(Cannock Chase Primary Care Trust)
Patient List Size: 2744

Practice Manager Linda Foster

GP T R K MURTY

Chadmoor Medical Practice
45 Princess St, Cannock WS11 2JT
Tel: 01543 571650 Fax: 01543 462304
(Cannock Chase Primary Care Trust)
Patient List Size: 4420

Practice Manager Louise Pike

GP Andiappan SELVAM, T M CAMPBELL, Catherine Alison SPEEDIE

Chapel Street Surgery
12 Chapel Street, Norton Canes, Cannock WS11 3NT
Tel: 01543 279232 Fax: 01543 450527
(Cannock Chase Primary Care Trust)
Patient List Size: 4500

Practice Manager Jenny Painter

GP B K SINGH, T M CAMPBELL, S PAREKH

Eskrett Street Surgery
Eskrett Street, Hednesford, Cannock WS12 5AR
Tel: 01543 422154 Fax: 01543 451120
(Cannock Chase Primary Care Trust)

GP V K SINGH

GP Suite
Cannock Chase Hospital, Brunswick Road, Cannock WS11 2XY
Tel: 01543 576660 Fax: 01543 576663
(Cannock Chase Primary Care Trust)
Patient List Size: 8105

Practice Manager Mary Aplin

GP Kyaw MYINT, K H MYINT, H NAING, K ZEYA

Hawks Green Medical Centre
Hawks Green, Heath Hayes, Cannock WS12 5XP
Tel: 01543 271313 Fax: 01543 271313
(Cannock Chase Primary Care Trust)
Patient List Size: 2200

Practice Manager Juliette Addis

GP S GONSALVES

Heath Hayes Health Centre
Gorsemoor Road, Heath Hayes, Cannock WS12 5TG
Tel: 01543 278461 Fax: 01543 271199
(Cannock Chase Primary Care Trust)
Patient List Size: 3000

Practice Manager K Gupta

GP Y K GUPTA

Hednesford Street Surgery
60 Hednesford Street, Cannock WS11 1DJ
Tel: 01543 503121 Fax: 01543 468024
Email: hednesford.street@sshawebmail.nhs.uk
(Cannock Chase Primary Care Trust)

Practice Manager Heather Brace

GP Lynne Veronica HULME, Jane Anne SAINSBURY, Paul Martin BALLINGER, Dr CONMEY, Judith HOLBROOK, Judith Margaret HOPPER, Jan HORSTINK

Moss Street Surgery
Chadsmoor, Cannock WS11 2DE
Tel: 01543 504477 Fax: 01543 504636
(Cannock Chase Primary Care Trust)

Practice Manager Clive Cropper

GP Stephen Roland GIBBINS, John Robert GALLIMORE, Sarah Jane HANDS, C WILEY

Newhall Street Surgery
14-16 Newhall Street, Cannock WS11 1AB
Tel: 01543 506511 Fax: 01543 462356
(Cannock Chase Primary Care Trust)
Patient List Size: 2087

Practice Manager S Kilgallon

GP Amarjit VERMA

Norton Canes Clinic
Brownhills Road, Norton Canes, Cannock WS11 3SE
Tel: 01543 450222 Fax: 01543 450014
(Cannock Chase Primary Care Trust)

Practice Manager Lindsey Guzowski

GP Dr MAW, Dr PO

Red Lion House
86 Hednesford Road, Cannock WS11 2LB
Tel: 01543 502391 Fax: 01543 573424
(Cannock Chase Primary Care Trust)
Patient List Size: 4036

Practice Manager Gill Clayton

GP Timothy John BERRIMAN, B CHILLALA, G FREE

St John's Surgery
437 Cannock Road, Cannock WS12 4AE
Tel: 01543 422307 Fax: 01543 425734
(Cannock Chase Primary Care Trust)
Patient List Size: 2300

Practice Manager Pat Carless

GP J S CHANDRA, D ISRAEL

Stafford Road Surgery
60 Stafford Road, Cannock WS11 2AQ
Tel: 01543 503332 Fax: 01543 503010
(Cannock Chase Primary Care Trust)
Patient List Size: 3000

Practice Manager Linda Protheroe

GP Andrew Jeffrey THOMPSON

The Surgery
24 Bideford Way, Cannock WS11 1QD
Tel: 01543 571055 Fax: 01543 574930
(Cannock Chase Primary Care Trust)
Patient List Size: 3599

Practice Manager Gill Harper-Potts

GP R D APTA, M EL-SEBAI

The Surgery
65 Church Street, Cannock WS11 1DS
Tel: 01543 577972 Fax: 01543 462520
(Cannock Chase Primary Care Trust)

Practice Manager Susan Farmer

GP P K THAKER, S M DAVENPORT

The Surgery
Rawnsley Road, Rawnsley, Cannock WS12 5JF
Tel: 01543 877842 Fax: 01543 423037
(Cannock Chase Primary Care Trust)
Patient List Size: 3426

Practice Manager Clive Cropper

GP M P WOO, S AL-HAKIM

Canterbury

Aylesham Health Centre
The Boulevard, Aylesham, Canterbury CT3 3DU
Tel: 01304 840233/840415 Fax: 01304 842797
(East Kent Coastal Teaching Primary Care Trust)

Practice Manager Alison Lynden

GP Jeyakumar ARIYARATNAM, Aravinthan SOMASUNDARAM

Canterbury Health Centre
26 Old Dover Road, Canterbury CT1 3JH
Tel: 01227 780437 Fax: 01227 784 979
(Canterbury and Coastal Primary Care Trust)
Patient List Size: 4000

Practice Manager Pat Roser

GP Robert SIMMONDS, Martin KUHNEN

Canterbury Health Centre
26 Old Dover Road, Canterbury CT1 3JH
Tel: 01227 452444 Fax: 01227 780646
(Canterbury and Coastal Primary Care Trust)

GP Kim STILLMAN, Susan Jane GREAVES, Joseph Paul MOLONY, Ian Ross SUTHERLAND

Chartham Surgery
Parish Road, Chartham, Canterbury CT4 7JU
Tel: 01227 738224 Fax: 01227 732115
(Canterbury and Coastal Primary Care Trust)
Patient List Size: 2100

Practice Manager C Barrett

GP Simon WHARFE, Lisa JOHNSON

College Medical Centre
Christ Church College, North Holmes Road, Canterbury CT1 1QU
Tel: 01227 767700
(Canterbury and Coastal Primary Care Trust)

GP Joseph Paul MOLONY, Susan Jane GREAVES, Denyer John KITTLE, Jane LILLEY, Kim STILLMAN

Cossington House Surgery
51 Cossington Road, Canterbury CT1 3HX
Tel: 01227 763377 Fax: 01227 786908
(Canterbury and Coastal Primary Care Trust)

Practice Manager D Hodgetts

GP Peter Gerard LIVESEY, Julie Anne FEGENT, William Lloyd HUGHES, Gregory MANSON, Madeleine Helen RICHARDSON

London Road Surgery
49 London Road, Canterbury CT2 8SG
Tel: 01227 463128 Fax: 01227 786308
(Canterbury and Coastal Primary Care Trust)
Patient List Size: 5000

Practice Manager Graham Martin

GP Anthony TASOU, Spyros Andrea ZINTILIS

New Dover Road Surgery
10 New Dover Road, Canterbury CT1 3AF
Tel: 01227 462197 Fax: 01227 786041
(Canterbury and Coastal Primary Care Trust)

Practice Manager Kevin Arthrell

GP Penelope BARLEY, David Laurence EAVES, Cecily FOLEY, Geoffrey Liddell JONES, Ronald Nigel McWILLIAMS, Gillian Mary ROBINSON

Northgate Medical Practice
1 Northgate, Canterbury CT1 1WL
Tel: 01227 463570 Fax: 01227 786147
(Canterbury and Coastal Primary Care Trust)
Patient List Size: 12397

Practice Manager Lisa Chapman, Alison Noble

GP Peter Edward BIGGS, Peter William BURROWES, Simon Brian Auckland ELLIS, Alice Louise FOORD, David John Preston GRICE, Jacqueline Eleanor Matilda McIVOR, Robert Paul Emmanuel WALKINGTON

The Old School Surgery
Bolts Hill, Chartham, Canterbury CT4 7JX
Tel: 01227 738282
(Canterbury and Coastal Primary Care Trust)

GP Dale Steven KINNERSLEY

Sturry Surgery
53 Island Road, Sturry, Canterbury CT2 0EF
Tel: 01227 710372 Fax: 01227 713060
(Canterbury and Coastal Primary Care Trust)

GP Paul MOLONY, Kim STILLMAN, Sue GREAVES, Jane LILLEY, Ian SUTHERLAND

The Surgery
The Corn Stores, 12 Nargate Street, Littlebourne, Canterbury CT3 1UH
Tel: 01227 721515
(Canterbury and Coastal Primary Care Trust)

GP David Mark JONES, Mary RAFLA, Peter Hugh SYKES

The Surgery
Chilton Place, Ash, Canterbury CT3 2HD
Tel: 01304 812227 Fax: 01304 813788
(East Kent Coastal Teaching Primary Care Trust)
Patient List Size: 5600

Practice Manager Pauline Marsh

GP Anthony Richard SMITH, Helene Elizabeth ARMSTRONG, Denyer KITTLE, Lilian LAMBIE

The Surgery
Old Road, Elham, Canterbury CT4 6UH
Tel: 01303 840213
(Shepway Primary Care Trust)

Practice Manager Jill Wood

GP Allan BEATON, Robert More STEWART

The Surgery
St Albans Road, Hersden, Canterbury CT3 4EX
Tel: 01227 710416 Fax: 01227 710288
(Canterbury and Coastal Primary Care Trust)

Practice Manager Kerry Quinney

GP A Murray McGREGOR, Ian William RITCHIE, Keren SHAW

The Surgery
Old Road, Elham, Canterbury CT4 6UH
Tel: 01303 840213
(Shepway Primary Care Trust)
Patient List Size: 6500

Practice Manager Jill Wood

GP Allan BEATON, Robert More STEWART

The University Medical Centre
Giles Lane, Canterbury CT2 7PB
Tel: 01227 823583 Fax: 01277 824466
Website: www.kent.ac.uk/medical
(Canterbury and Coastal Primary Care Trust)
Patient List Size: 11000

GP Alyson Ann BOWHAY, Jane Elizabeth DROUOT, Timothy Charles NOBLE, Michael Hugh NORMAN, Alan Peter TOLLINS

Wingham Surgery
2 Northcourt Road, Wingham, Canterbury CT3 1BN
Tel: 01227 720205 Fax: 01227 720699
(Canterbury and Coastal Primary Care Trust)
Patient List Size: 1980

Practice Manager Harry Turner

GP Shelagh Mary Grehan BLISS

Canvey Island

Canvey Village Surgery
391 Long Road, Canvey Island SS8 0JH
Tel: 01268 510520 Fax: 01268 684083
(Castle Point and Rochford Primary Care Trust)

GP Habib Ur RAHMAN, Dr BOWEN

Hawkesbury Road Surgery
1A Hawkesbury Road, Canvey Island SS8 0EX
Tel: 01268 682303
(Castle Point and Rochford Primary Care Trust)

GP Javed Bashir GHAURI

Long Road Surgery
409 Long Road, Canvey Island SS8 0JH
Tel: 01268 692959 Fax: 01268 690035
Email: umer.sulemanqureshi@gp-f81699.nhs.uk
(Castle Point and Rochford Primary Care Trust)
Patient List Size: 2927

Practice Manager Chris Hutchings

GP Dr SULEMAN-QURESHI

New Health Centre
Third Avenue, Canvey Island SS8 9UW
Tel: 01268 683758 Fax: 01268 684057
(Castle Point and Rochford Primary Care Trust)

Practice Manager Carole Seymour

GP Sithamparapillai KANAPATHIPPILLAI, Dr LEE, Steven John LIMAGE, Dr TAY ZA AUNG

Oak Road Surgery
1 Oak Road, Canvey Island SS8 7AX
Tel: 01268 692211 Fax: 01268 683138
(Castle Point and Rochford Primary Care Trust)
Patient List Size: 8600

Practice Manager Judith Buckingham

GP Mahesh KAMDAR, Mohammed MUJAHID, Dr SHASHIRAI

The Surgeries
Grafton Road, Canvey Island SS8 7BT
Tel: 01268 682277 Fax: 01268 685149
(Castle Point and Rochford Primary Care Trust)
Patient List Size: 7200

Practice Manager Ann-Marie Williams

GP Dr BROWN, Dr NOORAH, Dr WONG

Vanderwalt Avenue Surgery
1 Vanderwalt Avenue, Canvey Island SS8 7RW
Tel: 01268 690171 Fax: 01268 696781
(Castle Point and Rochford Primary Care Trust)
Patient List Size: 2700

Practice Manager C Vickery

GP Dr SODIPO

Carlisle

Ajai-Ajagbe
Outgang Barn, Outgang Road, Aspatria, Carlisle CA7 3HW
Tel: 016973 20367 Fax: 016973 23230
(Carlisle and District Primary Care Trust)
Patient List Size: 1565

Practice Manager Maggy Ajai-Ajagbe

GP Emmanuel Kunnuji Oluyinka AJAI-AJAGBE

Britton and Partners
10 Spencer Street, Carlisle CA1 1BP
Tel: 01228 29171
(Carlisle and District Primary Care Trust)

Practice Manager J Rogers

GP John Newton BRITTON, Michael Francis GOOLD, Angela Christine HERRICK, Katharine Mary HOLMES, Thomas Ian MACKAY, Clyde Paul MITCHELL

Brunswick House Medical Group
1 Brunswick Street, Carlisle CA1 1ED
Tel: 01228 515808 Fax: 01228 593048
(Carlisle and District Primary Care Trust)

Practice Manager S Cook

GP Diana Gwyneth HAYES, Christopher CORRIGAN, Andrew John EDGAR, Ian MARSHALL, Jane Ann NOLAN, Colin PATTERSON, Mark SIXSMITH, Robert WESTGATE

The Croft Surgery
The Croft, Kirkbridge, Carlisle CA7 5JH
(Carlisle and District Primary Care Trust)

GP John Joseph NOBLETT, Elspeth Anne SWAN

Dalston Medical Group
Townhead Road, Dalston, Carlisle CA5 7PZ
Tel: 01228 710451 Fax: 01228 711898
(Carlisle and District Primary Care Trust)
Patient List Size: 5190

Practice Manager Lorraine Errington, Ann Reay

GP Ruth Catherine REED, John FRENCH, Martin JOHN, Valerie Frances PALMER, Allister STROVER

Doctors Surgery
Townhead Road, Dalston, Carlisle CA5 7PZ
Tel: 01228 710451 Fax: 01228 711898
(Carlisle and District Primary Care Trust)

Practice Manager A Reay

GP George David DICKINSON, Martin Richard JOHN

Eden Medical Group
Port Road, Carlisle CA2 7AJ
Tel: 01228 24477

(Carlisle and District Primary Care Trust)
Patient List Size: 14000

Practice Manager Les Mardon

GP Richard Hugh MURRAY, Iain Michael GRAINGER, Paul Herbert Mark KING, John Forbes McDOWELL, Yvonne McKENZIE, Martin Frank Lytton SELLS

Grosvenor House Surgery
Grosvenor House, Warwick Square, Carlisle CA1 1LB
Tel: 01228 536561 Fax: 01228 515786
(Carlisle and District Primary Care Trust)
Patient List Size: 8000

Practice Manager Larry Brown

GP Jeremy Clive FROST, Graeme Peter ADAM, Duncan Brand WARD, Nicholas Paul WIGMORE

Grosvenor House Surgery
6 Warwick Square, Carlisle CA1 1LB
Tel: 01228 525041 Fax: 01228 515786
(Carlisle and District Primary Care Trust)

Practice Manager L Brown, B Stitt

GP Geoffrey Woodford STITT

London Road Surgery
46-48 London Road, Carlisle CA1 2EL
Tel: 01228 27559 Fax: 01228 594434
(Carlisle and District Primary Care Trust)
Patient List Size: 8200

Practice Manager Elizabeth Hays

GP Anthony Ronald HORNE, Charlotte Elaine ASQUITH, Claire Louise HIGGINS, G M Upani JAYAWONDER, Robert James LIGHTFOOT

Longtown Clinic
Burn Street, Longtown, Carlisle CA6 5TA
Tel: 01228 791328 Fax: 01228 791430
(Carlisle and District Primary Care Trust)

GP Christopher david BAKER

Prospect House Surgery
Prospect House, King Street, Aspatria, Carlisle CA7 3AH
Tel: 016973 20224 Fax: 016973 23624
(Carlisle and District Primary Care Trust)

Practice Manager K Fisher

GP Donald Stewart WHEATLEY

Silloth Group Medical Practice
Lanewn Terrace, Silloth, Carlisle CA7 4AH
Tel: 016973 31309 Fax: 016973 32834
(Carlisle and District Primary Care Trust)

Practice Manager A Hodgson

GP Martin Graham ROSS, Rodney Marshall JONES, Stephen Niall THORNHILL

St Pauls Medical Centre
St Pauls Square, Carlisle CA1 1DG
Tel: 01228 524354 Fax: 01228 616660
Email: admin@spmc.co.uk
(Carlisle and District Primary Care Trust)
Patient List Size: 13200

Practice Manager Tracey Scott

GP Ian Montgomery Scott KERSS, John Grant ANDERSON, Richard John BARNSLEY, John Arthur BONE, Louise DODGEON, Alan David EDWARDS, Lawrence Neil MARGERISON, Sally ROBERTS, Brian McGregor Reith SCROGGIE, Rosemary Anne Hamilton SWAIN

Stanwix Medical Practice
77-81 Scotland Road, Carlisle CA3 9HL
Tel: 01228 25768 Fax: 01228 592965
Website: www.northumbria.nhs.uk/stanwix
(Carlisle and District Primary Care Trust)
Patient List Size: 5850

Practice Manager H Hill

GP Michael Arthur KEWLEY, Celia Kay LEWIS, W J MEELAY

Swan Street Surgery
35-41 Swan Street, Longtown, Carlisle CA6 5UZ
Tel: 01228 791202 Fax: 016973 22333
(Carlisle and District Primary Care Trust)

GP Mohammad ZOBAIR

Warwick Road Surgery
65 Warwick Road, Carlisle CA1 1EB
Tel: 01228 536303 Fax: 01228 593606
(Carlisle and District Primary Care Trust)
Patient List Size: 6000

Practice Manager George S Thomson

GP Gangaprasad NAIR, Adrian G RIPPON, Hans L SCHMID

The White House Surgery
Court Thorn Surgery, Low Hesket, Carlisle CA4 0HP
Tel: 016974 73548 Fax: 016974 73781
Website: www.courrtthornsurgery.co.uk
(Eden Valley Primary Care Trust)

GP Ken SUTTON, Tim YOUNG

Carnforth

Arnside Medical Practice
The Surgery, Orchard Road, Arnside, Carnforth LA5 0DP
Tel: 01524 761311 Fax: 01524 762470
Email: arnside@gp-A82074.nhs.uk
(Morecambe Bay Primary Care Trust)
Patient List Size: 2500

Practice Manager Doreen Blacklee

GP Andrew Alexander MATCHETT, Monica Mary FLETCHER

Ash Trees Surgery
Market Street, Carnforth LA5 9JU
Tel: 01524 720000 Fax: 01524 720110
(Morecambe Bay Primary Care Trust)
Patient List Size: 13500

GP John SHAKESPEARE, Nicola ABRAHAN, Paul BATES, Gillian E HALHEAD, George Antony Talbot HOBBS, David Howard Francis KOPCKE, Judith Penelope LONGLEY, Richard Norman SEWELL

Green Close Surgery
Green Close, Kirkby Lonsdale, Carnforth LA6 2BS
Tel: 01524 271210 Fax: 01524 272713
(Morecambe Bay Primary Care Trust)

Practice Manager S M Howard

GP Philippa Jane Inglis HALL, Marion Marjorie BEAGAN, Sharon Marie KAYE, David Gareth THOMAS, Peter Julien WEEKS

Carshalton

Beeches Surgery
9 Hill Road, Carshalton SM5 3RB
Tel: 020 8647 6608/6609
(Sutton and Merton Primary Care Trust)

Practice Manager M Bland

GP Alan Francis FROLEY, Vidya Bhushan GHOORBIN, Maria-Danuta SIALA

Doctors Surgery
181 Carshalton Road, Carshalton SM1 4NJ
Tel: 020 8661 1505
(Sutton and Merton Primary Care Trust)

GP Mohamed Fasihuddin Siddique ALI KHAN, Nuzhat Fatima ALI KHAN

Goel
11 Crichton Road, Carshalton SM5 3LS
Tel: 020 8643 3030/9551 Fax: 020 8643 1013
(Sutton and Merton Primary Care Trust)
Patient List Size: 3558

Practice Manager Daphne Taylor

GP Raj Kumar GOEL

Green Wrythe Surgery
411A Green Wrythe Lane, Carshalton SM5 1JF
Tel: 020 8648 2022 Fax: 020 8646 6555
(Sutton and Merton Primary Care Trust)
Patient List Size: 7500

Practice Manager Marion Gower

GP K H YU, M SHETH, S THAYALAN

The Surgery
62 Waltham Road, Carshalton SM5 1PW
Tel: 020 8644 8989 Fax: 020 8661 9348
(Sutton and Merton Primary Care Trust)

GP Ramesh MODY

The Surgery
121 Wrythe Lane, Carshalton SM5 2RT
Tel: 020 8644 2727 Fax: 020 8644 6267
(Sutton and Merton Primary Care Trust)
Patient List Size: 7000

Practice Manager J Cooper

GP Anthony DITRI, J M R COCKBAIN, Irene HEALY

The Surgery
138 London Road, Hackbridge, Carshalton SM5 7HF
Tel: 020 8647 3711 Fax: 020 8773 8577
(Sutton and Merton Primary Care Trust)
Patient List Size: 3400

Practice Manager Caroline Hall

GP Turabul MADINA, Chendinka CARROLL

Wrythe Green Surgery
Wrythe Lane, Carshalton SM5 2RE
Tel: 020 8669 3232 Fax: 020 8773 2524
(Sutton and Merton Primary Care Trust)
Patient List Size: 11600

Practice Manager David Smithson

GP Alison GALLOWAY, Sophia Ann DEXTER, Soran SAEED, Makrkus SCHICHTEL, Alan Robert Clifton SMITH, Mark Philip Paul WELLS

Carterton

Wilkinson and Partners
Carterton Surgery, 17 Alvescot Road, Carterton OX18 3JL
Tel: 01993 844567 Fax: 01993 841551
(South West Oxfordshire Primary Care Trust)

Practice Manager Anthea Sadler

GP Andrew Richard WILKINSON, Christine Hannah Dorothy A'COURT, Fiona Constance CLOUGH, Nicholas Michael JONES

Castle Cary

Millbrook Gardens Surgery
Millbrook Gardens, Castle Cary BA7 7EE
Tel: 01963 350210 Fax: 01963 350366
(South Somerset Primary Care Trust)
Patient List Size: 4000

Practice Manager S Scott

GP Michael Kingsley ROYLANCE, Judith J SCULL

Castleford

Elizabeth Court Surgery
Elizabeth Drive, Airedale, Castleford WF10 3TG
(Eastern Wakefield Primary Care Trust)

Practice Manager Jane Holmes

GP Raymond Henry DUNPHY, Hans Raj BANCE, Stephen John BECKER, Russell John CROSS, Rosalind Anne DUNPHY, Debika MINOCHA

The Health Centre
Welbeck Street, Castleford WF10 1DP
Tel: 01977 465777 Fax: 01977 519342
(Eastern Wakefield Primary Care Trust)

Practice Manager Dorothy Penistone

GP Arjun PRASAD, Sabeeha JABEEN, Suresh Chandroth NAMBIAR

Henry Moore Clinic
26 Smawthorne Lane, Castleford WF10 4EN
Tel: 01977 552007 Fax: 01977 604176
(Eastern Wakefield Primary Care Trust)

Practice Manager Joan Calvert

GP John Henry Neil McCLINTOCK, Paul Alexander FOX, Janet Elizabeth McCLINTOCK, Antony Russell THOMAS

Nova Scotia Medical Centre
Leeds Road, Allerton Bywater, Castleford WF10 2DP
Tel: 01977 552193 Fax: 01977 518891
(East Leeds Primary Care Trust)

GP Bogdan Antony PIERECHOD, Kesavan Kodappilly GOPINATHAN, O D KHAN

Riverside Medical Centre
Savile Road, Castleford WF10 1PH
Tel: 01977 554831 Fax: 01977 603057
(Eastern Wakefield Primary Care Trust)
Patient List Size: 10500

Practice Manager C M Wilson

GP Graham Richard ALDRIDGE, J ISSAC, M MATHEWS, Nadim Ahmed NAYYAR

Tieve Tara
Rear of Park Dale, Airedale, Castleford WF10 2QT
Tel: 01977 552360 Fax: 01977 603470
(Eastern Wakefield Primary Care Trust)
Patient List Size: 5000

Practice Manager Celia Burnhope

GP Richard Ernest George SLOAN, Sarah BAKER, Anne Carol GODRIDGE

Caterham

Caterham Valley Medical Practice
Eothen House, Eothen Close, Caterham CR3 6JU
Tel: 01883 347811 Fax: 01883 342929
(East Surrey Primary Care Trust)
Patient List Size: 8300

Practice Manager Richard Dires

GP Pamela Fay ROBERTS, Paul Gareth HAMILTON, Jonathan Michael LEWIS, Richard Edward WRIGHT

Chaldon Road Surgery
Chaldon Road, Caterham CR3 5PG
Tel: 01883 345466 Fax: 01883 330942
Email: susan.goundry@gp-h81662.nhs.uk
(East Surrey Primary Care Trust)
Patient List Size: 4600

Practice Manager Susan Gomersall

GP Susan Ann CRISPIN, Patrick Donald RUST

Town End Medical Practice
41 Town End, Caterham CR3 5UJ
Tel: 01883 343333 Fax: 01883 330142
(East Surrey Primary Care Trust)
Patient List Size: 12500

Practice Manager Gill Vaughan

GP Andrew HUTCHINSON, Anthony Hugh Sydenham CLARKE, Kevin Paul DEFRIEND, Jane Louise HAMPSON, John Vincent HOWARD, Frances Clare O'BRIEN

Catterick Garrison

Harewood Medical Practice
Richmond Road, Catterick Garrison DL9 3JD
Tel: 01748 833904 Fax: 01748 834290
(Hambleton and Richmondshire Primary Care Trust)
Patient List Size: 4500

Practice Manager Graham Dickinson

GP V PLEYDELL, William LUMB, Ian Scot WATT, Sioban Elizabeth WATT

Chard

Essex House Medical Centre
59 Fore Street, Chard TA20 1QB
Tel: 01460 63071 Fax: 01460 66560
(South Somerset Primary Care Trust)

Practice Manager April Jeffopson

GP William FREESTON, John BEAVEN, Paul James DENNER, Ian M WILCOX, William WILSON

Glanvill and Partners
Springmead Surgery, Summerfields Road, Chard TA20 2EW
Tel: 01460 63380 Fax: 01460 66483
(South Somerset Primary Care Trust)
Patient List Size: 6000

Practice Manager Beverly Adams

GP Andrew Peter GLANVILL, Stephen William HARRIS, Martin HUGHES, Andrew Philip Tavender TRESIDDER

Tawstock Medical Centre
7 High Street, Chard TA20 1QF
Tel: 01460 67763 Fax: 01460 66044
Email: tawstock.medical@goL85619.nhs.uk
(Taunton Deane Primary Care Trust)
Patient List Size: 3600

Practice Manager Jan Lowe

GP Andrew Gerald DOWN, Inge Adriana ALBERT, Susan Jane DAVIES, Catharine Diana STAVELEY

Chatham

Churchill Clinic
94 Churchill Avenue, Chatham ME5 0DL
Tel: 01634 842397
(Medway Teaching Primary Care Trust)
Patient List Size: 2500

Practice Manager Nalini Vibhuti

GP Ravi VIBHUTI

The Halfway Surgery
68 New Road, Chatham ME4 4QR
Tel: 01634 828665
(Medway Teaching Primary Care Trust)

GP Imad Mohammed ALI

King George Road Surgery
52A King George Road, Walderslade, Chatham ME5 0TU
Tel: 01634 863305 Fax: 01634 671194
(Medway Teaching Primary Care Trust)

Practice Manager Margaret Gamble

GP Mohammad Mahbubul KARIM, Velupillai KUNASINGAM, S MAHESWARAN

Kings Family Practice
30-34 Magpie Hall Road, Chatham ME4 5JY
Tel: 01634 404632 Fax: 01634 843270
(Medway Teaching Primary Care Trust)
Patient List Size: 9500

Practice Manager D Clarke

GP C A KHAN, C D HUXHAM, H LADD, C NORWOOD, E SCHIRRMACHER

Kiran Virdee Medical Centre
Sultan Road, Lordswood, Chatham ME5 8TJ
Tel: 01634 669221 Fax: 01634 682220
(Medway Teaching Primary Care Trust)

GP B S VIRDEE, J V S RAO

Lordswood Health Centre
Sultan Road, Lordswood, Chatham ME5 8TJ
Tel: 01634 666996
(Medway Teaching Primary Care Trust)
Patient List Size: 2800

GP K S SETHI

Lordswood Health Centre
Sultan Road, Lordswood, Chatham ME5 8TJ
Tel: 01634 863168 Fax: 01634 671915
(Medway Teaching Primary Care Trust)
Patient List Size: 4000

Practice Manager Ann Griffin

GP O S SINGH, S P SINGH

Maidstone Road Surgery
262 Maidstone Road, Chatham ME4 6JL
Tel: 01634 842093 Fax: 01634 842151
Email: practice.manager@gp-g82139.nhs.uk
(Medway Teaching Primary Care Trust)
Patient List Size: 3300

Practice Manager K Shipp

GP Jill COHEN, Khalda Nasreen QURESHI

The Medical Centre
29 Bryant Street, Chatham ME4 5QS
Tel: 01634 848913
(Medway Teaching Primary Care Trust)
Patient List Size: 1779

Practice Manager Prafulla Modha

GP Priyavadan Girdharlal MODHA

The Medical Centre
29 Bryant Street, Chatham ME4 5QS
Tel: 01634 848912 Fax: 01634 407731
Email: keshav@kanekal.freeserve.co.uk
(Medway Teaching Primary Care Trust)
Patient List Size: 2100

Practice Manager A K Kanekal

GP Keshavrao Venkatrao KANEKAL

The Medical Centre
29 Bryant Street, Chatham ME4 5QS
Tel: 01634 848911
(Medway Teaching Primary Care Trust)

GP Muhammad Afzal CHAUDHRY

New Road Surgery
24 New Road, Chatham ME4 4QR
Tel: 01634 811463 Fax: 01634 840337
(Medway Teaching Primary Care Trust)
Patient List Size: 3800

Practice Manager Teresa Clare

GP Mohamed Adiluzzaman KHAN, A A PHIROZ

New Surgery
West Drive, Davis Estate, Chatham ME5 9XG
Tel: 01634 867587
(Medway Teaching Primary Care Trust)
Patient List Size: 1500

Practice Manager Marion Higgins

GP Nasrullah BALUCH, Shakira BALUCH, Jaishree RAO

Princes Park Medical Centre
Dove Close, Walderslade, Chatham ME5 7TD
Tel: 01634 201272 Fax: 01634 868159
(Medway Teaching Primary Care Trust)

Practice Manager Robert Penoer

GP Toqeer ASLAM

Stonecross Surgery
25 Street End Road, Chatham ME5 0AA
Tel: 01634 842334 Fax: 01634 817476
(Medway Teaching Primary Care Trust)
Patient List Size: 5500

Practice Manager Linda Dalliga

GP Kali Sankar MAHAPATRA, Edmund RUPASINGHE

Tunbury Avenue Surgery
16 Tunbury Avenue, Walderslade, Chatham ME5 9EH
Tel: 01634 668814/684981
(Medway Teaching Primary Care Trust)

GP A B JHA

Walderslade Medical Centre
Princes Avenue, Chatham ME5 7PQ
Tel: 01634 682611
Email: mehdi.d@virgin.net
(Medway Teaching Primary Care Trust)

Practice Manager Nancy Clark, Fereshteh Dabestani

GP Mehdi DABESTANI

Walderslade Medical Centre
Princes Avenue, Chatham ME5 7PQ
Tel: 01634 668160
(Medway Teaching Primary Care Trust)

Practice Manager K Loader

GP Kumari PADMA

Walderslade Village Surgery
62A Robin Hood Lane, Walderslade, Chatham ME5 9LD
Tel: 01634 687250
(Medway Teaching Primary Care Trust)
Patient List Size: 8250

Practice Manager Carole Neate

GP Jayantkumar Kantilal RAVAL, Fiona Charlotte DAVIS, Nathan NATHAN, Chau Ming SHUM

Wayfield Road Surgery
183B Wayfield Road, Chatham ME5 0HD
Tel: 01634 845613 Fax: 01634 813993
(Medway Teaching Primary Care Trust)
Patient List Size: 2500

Practice Manager P Fraser

GP A R MIR

Chatteris

George Clare Surgery
Swan Drive, New Road, Chatteris PE16 6EX
Tel: 01354 695888 Fax: 01354 695415
Email: georgeclare@dialpipex.com
(East Cambridgeshire and Fenland Primary Care Trust)
Patient List Size: 9840

Practice Manager Diane Clifford

GP Frances Helen SZEKELY, Paul Nicholas DARER, Dr HUGENHOLTZ, Alex NOOTEBOOM, Stephen James WATTS

Cheadle

Adshall Road Medical Practice
97 Adshall Road, (off Councillor Lane), Cheadle SK8 2JN
Tel: 0161 491 2291 Fax: 0161 491 3993
(Stockport Primary Care Trust)
Patient List Size: 5400

Practice Manager Jane Whitworth

GP Lindsay Joy WEBB, Dr GILBERT, Dr WILKINSON

Adshall Road Surgery
Adshall Road, Cheadle SK8 2JN
Tel: 0161 491 2292
(Stockport Primary Care Trust)

GP David John GILBERT

Cheadle Hulme Medical Centre
Smithy Green, Hulme Hall Road, Cheadle Hulme, Cheadle SK8 6LU
Tel: 0161 485 7272
(Stockport Primary Care Trust)

GP Teresa Isabel Maria MIRSKI, Alison Mary SHIPSTON

Cheadle Medical Practice
1-5 Ashfield Crescent, Cheadle SK8 1BH
Tel: 0161 428 7575 Fax: 0161 283 8884
(Stockport Primary Care Trust)

Practice Manager J Ralphs

GP John Robert ADAMS, Aubrey CAHILL, Stephen Charles GADUZO, Susan Rosamund GLICHER, Jane Patricia MAMELOK

Gatley Group Practice
Old Hall Road, Gatley, Cheadle SK8 4DG
Tel: 0161 428 8484 Fax: 0161 428 6333
(Stockport Primary Care Trust)
Patient List Size: 7813

Practice Manager A Wallis

GP Andrew HARDMAN, Peter Rudiger CARNE, Andrew John DAVISON, Sravoni Bonny NEEDHAM

Smithy Green Surgery
Hulme Hall Road, Cheadle Hulme, Cheadle SK8 6LU
Tel: 0161 4857272 Fax: 0161 4856567
(Stockport Primary Care Trust)

GP Dr MATHER

Wright and Partners
Heald Green Medical Centre, Finney Lane, Heald Green, Cheadle SK8 3JD
Tel: 0161 436 8448 Fax: 0161 493 9268
(Stockport Primary Care Trust)

Practice Manager C Nylan

GP Andrew Timothy WRIGHT, Kevin Malcolm DEAN, Emma Andree LEON, Tessa Caroline MILLER, Penelope Ann OWEN, Michael Anthony VON FRAUNHOFER

Cheddar

Cheddar Medical Centre
Roynon Way, Cheddar BS27 3NZ
Tel: 01934 742061 Fax: 01934 744374
(Somerset Coast Primary Care Trust)
Patient List Size: 7035

Practice Manager Diana Hill

GP Jonathan Richard HINCKS, Thomas Elwyn DAVIES, Jillian Claire HOWARD, Claire Loiuse LABAND, Simone Yvette Anne THOMAS

Chelmsford

Beauchamp House Surgery
37 Baddow Road, Chelmsford CM2 0DB
Tel: 01245 262255 Fax: 01245 262256
(Chelmsford Primary Care Trust)
Patient List Size: 12046

Practice Manager Linda Keeble

GP Jonathan Charles GARVEY, James Douglas Lyn BULKELEY, Sally Penelope DILLEY, Simon Philip SCHULTZ, Peter James Douglas WOOD

Brook Hill Surgery
30 Brook Hill, Little Waltham, Chelmsford CM3 3LL
Tel: 01245 360253 Fax: 01245 361343
(Witham, Braintree and Halstead Care Trust)
Patient List Size: 14500

Practice Manager Margaret Boddy

GP Sarah Michelle BAKEWELL, A AGARWAL, Peter DE MEZA, Dr FOX, Anthea Valerie LINTS, Dr WIJEKOOH

Broomfield Road Surgery
252 Broomfield Road, Chelmsford CM1 4DY
Tel: 01245 355460 Fax: 01245 344659
(Chelmsford Primary Care Trust)
Patient List Size: 1450

Practice Manager M I Middleton

GP Margaret Isobel MIDDLETON

Dickens Place Surgery
Dickens Place, Chelmsford CM1 4UU
Tel: 01245 442628 Fax: 01245 443647
(Chelmsford Primary Care Trust)
Patient List Size: 5900

Practice Manager Lesley Beale

GP Thomas Anthony CUMMINS, Timothy Martyn BAYLIS

Gloucester Avenue Surgery
158 Gloucester Avenue, Chelmsford CM2 9LG
Tel: 01245 353182 Fax: 01245 344479
(Chelmsford Primary Care Trust)

Practice Manager Sally Bevan

GP John Cumming LITTLE, David Ian FORBES, Jane Eleanor HARPUR, Elizabeth Anne MURPHY

Greenwood Surgery
Tylers Ride, South Woodham Ferrers, Chelmsford CM3 5XD
Tel: 01245 322443 Fax: 01245 321844
Email: postmaster@gp-F81185.nhs.uk
(Maldon and South Chelmsford Primary Care Trust)
Patient List Size: 5800

Practice Manager Debbie Morley

GP Carey CHAPMAN, John Francis CORMACK, Donald McGEACHY

Hawsted Medical Centre
1 The Drive, Maryland, Chelmsford CM3 6AB
Tel: 01621 740726 Fax: 01621 743428
(Maldon and South Chelmsford Primary Care Trust)
Patient List Size: 2248

Practice Manager Ann Montague-Brown

GP Herbert James MONTAGUE BROWN

High Street
16 High Street, Great Baddow, Chelmsford CM2 7HQ
Tel: 01245 473251 Fax: 01245 478394
(Chelmsford Primary Care Trust)
Patient List Size: 10050

Practice Manager Sue Finch

GP Stephen McCausland RUSSELL, Waseem AHMED, Elizabeth Tovani BARRON, M LANGDALE-BROWN, Peter Max STERN, Anja VERMEULEN

The Hoppit Surgery
Butts Lane, Danbury, Chelmsford CM3 4NP
Tel: 01245 222518 Fax: 01245 222116
(Maldon and South Chelmsford Primary Care Trust)
Patient List Size: 1825

Practice Manager Sally Barber

GP Ashley Nigel PAIN

Humber Road Surgery
27 Humber Road, Springfield, Chelmsford CM1 7PE
Tel: 01245 268635 Fax: 01245 344552
(Chelmsford Primary Care Trust)
Patient List Size: 10800

Practice Manager S Ardley, Margaret Brand

GP A J DAWTON, S L JENKINS, M R HOROBIN, M F McGREGOR

Lee House Surgery
Eves Corner, Danbury, Chelmsford CM3 4QA
Tel: 01245 225522 Fax: 01245 222196
(Maldon and South Chelmsford Primary Care Trust)
Patient List Size: 10500

Practice Manager Lindsey Scott

GP Nicholas Ian COOPER, Caroline DOLLERY, Somaly LACH, Patricia Dawn McALLISTER, Sai Sankar NAGAMANICKAM, Mervyn PATTERSON, Robert PLATE

Maldon Road Surgery
39 Maldon Road, Danbury, Chelmsford CM3 4QL
Tel: 01245 225868 Fax: 01245 224253
(Maldon and South Chelmsford Primary Care Trust)
Patient List Size: 2000

Practice Manager Mrs Wagle

GP Sudhir Ghanashyam WAGLE

Maylandsea Medical Centre
Imperial Avenue, Maylandsea, Chelmsford CM3 6AH
Tel: 01621 742233 Fax: 01621 742917
(Maldon and South Chelmsford Primary Care Trust)

Practice Manager Marilyn Bicheno

GP Michael Alan NORTH

Melbourne House Surgery
12 Napier Court, Queensland Crescent, Chelmsford CM1 2ED
Tel: 01245 354370 Fax: 01245 344476
(Chelmsford Primary Care Trust)
Patient List Size: 7000

Practice Manager Janet Burney

GP John Trygve BOOTH, Stephen CASS, Bronwen Mary PITT, Michael SARJUDEEN

Mountbatten House Surgery
1 Montgomery Close, North Springfield, Chelmsford CM1 6FF
Tel: 01245 467750 Fax: 01245 466192
(Chelmsford Primary Care Trust)
Patient List Size: 7367

Practice Manager Bernadette Curns

GP Premdat HARIRAM, Geeta DHAIRYAWAN, Ian FREED

Rivermead Gate Medical Centre
123 Rectory Lane, Chelmsford CM1 1TR
Tel: 01245 348688 Fax: 01245 458800
(Chelmsford Primary Care Trust)
Patient List Size: 10300

Practice Manager Pam Bishop

GP Christopher Frank DANN, Nigel Guy HUNT, Nigel Allen SAVAGE, Ruth Anne SQUIRE, Ann Philippa TETSTALL

The Surgery
Brickfields Road, South Woodham Ferrers, Chelmsford CM3 5XB
Tel: 01245 328855 Fax: 01245 329849
(Maldon and South Chelmsford Primary Care Trust)
Patient List Size: 5770

Practice Manager Janice Cheese

GP Ramesh PATEL, Anne Elizabeth DYSON, Suzanne Caroline EVERETT

The Surgery
42 Kings Way, South Woodham Ferrers, Chelmsford CM3 5QH
Tel: 01245 321391 Fax: 01245 325627
(Maldon and South Chelmsford Primary Care Trust)

Practice Manager George Piper

GP Dr PANDYA, Dr PATEL

The Surgery
Clement House, Knight Street, South Woodham Ferrers, Chelmsford CM3 5ZL
Tel: 01245 329996 Fax: 01245 327311
(Maldon and South Chelmsford Primary Care Trust)
Patient List Size: 3000

Practice Manager D P Patel

GP C. PRAFUL

Sutherland Lodge Surgery
115 Baddow Road, Chelmsford CM2 7QD
Tel: 01245 351351 Fax: 01245 494192
(Chelmsford Primary Care Trust)
Patient List Size: 12000

Practice Manager Carol Sands

GP Miriam EDELSTEN, Joanna BIRN-JEFFERY, Dr CLIMIE, Gerald Anthony CUNNIFFE, Azmi NADRA, Hilary Vanessa RAMSAY

Tennyson House Surgery
20 Merlin Place, Chelmsford CM1 4HW
Tel: 01245 260459 Fax: 01245 344287
Email: postmaster@gp.F81122.nhs.uk
(Chelmsford Primary Care Trust)
Patient List Size: 7833

Practice Manager Jenny Crook

GP Ellen MacINNES, Andrea Dionne PITT, Joanna Kathleen ROBERTS, Charlotte Helen STEAD

Towson and Partners
Juniper Road, Boreham, Chelmsford CM3 3DX
Tel: 01245 467364 Fax: 01245 465584
(Chelmsford Primary Care Trust)
Patient List Size: 10022

GP Nigel Bernard Dene TOWSON, Leslie Robert BRANN, John GUY, Lesley Mary GUY, Michael Jeremy SPURR

Whitley House Surgery
Moulsham Street, Chelmsford CM2 0JJ
Tel: 01245 347539 Fax: 01245 454600
(Chelmsford Primary Care Trust)
Patient List Size: 11500

Practice Manager Julie Price

GP Elizabeth TOWERS, Martin Peter BELL, Catherine Sheila BOON, Deanne HOOPER, Neil John MONSELL, Stuart NEWMAN

The Writtle Surgery
16A Lordship Road, Writtle, Chelmsford CM1 3EH
Tel: 01245 421205 Fax: 01245 422094
(Chelmsford Primary Care Trust)
Patient List Size: 8000

Practice Manager Anne Young

GP Michael Charles BAILEY, Nicholas Robert John VINCENT, Angela Dorothy WILSON, Edwin Charles WOOD

Cheltenham

Berkeley Place Surgery
11 High Street, Cheltenham GL52 6DA
Tel: 01242 513975 Fax: 01242 263787
(Cheltenham and Tewkesbury Primary Care Trust)
Patient List Size: 6600

GP Simon Philip RYLEY, Wendy Elizabeth ALLUM, Vanessa DANE, Michael ELLIS

Corinthian Surgery
St Paul's Medical Centre, 121 Swindon Road, Cheltenham GL50 4DP
Tel: 01242 707777 Fax: 01242 707776
Website: www.corinthian.surgery.co.uk
(Cheltenham and Tewkesbury Primary Care Trust)
Patient List Size: 8500

Practice Manager Morris Watt

GP Stephen Edmund WEST, Stephen Patrick COLLYER, Mary Geraldine HYATT WILLIAMS, Christopher St. John LAMDEN, Peter Thomas SMITH

James and Partners
Fortey Road, Northleach, Cheltenham GL54 3EQ
Tel: 01451 860247 Fax: 01451 860718
(Cotswold and Vale Primary Care Trust)
Patient List Size: 8900

Practice Manager David Winter

GP Bernard Guy JAMES, Ann COOPER, John Norton DISNEY, Paul Kenneth JOHNSON

Leckhampton Surgery
Lloyd Davies House, 17 Moorend Park Road, Cheltenham GL53 0LA
Tel: 01242 515363 Fax: 01242 253512
(Cheltenham and Tewkesbury Primary Care Trust)
Patient List Size: 12500

Practice Manager Sue Careswell

GP Robin Raymond HARROD, Ann-Marie COX, James Percy MOSS, Olivia MUNN, Nigel MUTLOW, Martin Edward NICHOLAS, Bridget Ruth NICOLSON, David PASCOE-WATSON

Moore Health Centre
Moore Health Centre, Moore Road, Bourton on the Water, Cheltenham GL54 2AZ
Tel: 01451 829242 Fax: 01451 820532
(Cotswold and Vale Primary Care Trust)
Patient List Size: 8900

Practice Manager David Winter

GP Bernard Guy JAMES, Timothy John CARTER, Ann COOPER, John DISNEY, Paul JOHNSON, Jonathan WREFORD

Overton Park Surgery
Overton Park Road, Cheltenham GL50 3BP
Tel: 01242 580511 Fax: 01242 253542
(Cheltenham and Tewkesbury Primary Care Trust)
Patient List Size: 8900

Practice Manager Sue Bradley

GP Stuart Angus Barrons NELSON, Ian Stephen ALCOCK, Annette Elizabeth BUGAIGHIS, Caroline Anne COPPS, Sarah MOLIVER, Julian Michael WILSON

The Portland Practice
St Paul's Medical Centre, 121 Swindon Road, Cheltenham GL50 4DP
Tel: 01242 707792
(Cheltenham and Tewkesbury Primary Care Trust)

Practice Manager Terry Saunders, Roger Tyrell

GP David John WATKINS, Colin Charles BURGESS, Sally Louise DAVIES, Shirley Ann ELLIOTT, William Robert MILES, Stephen Francis PRATT, Ian Duncan RAMSAY

Royal Crescent Surgery
11 Royal Crescent, Cheltenham GL50 3DA
Tel: 01242 580248 Fax: 01242 253618
(Cheltenham and Tewkesbury Primary Care Trust)
Patient List Size: 7500

Practice Manager Janet Stephens

GP Anthony Francis Dennis WITHERS, Valerie Ellen COGGER, James Gordon PEARSON, Roger John WILLIAMS

Royal Well Surgery
St Pauls Medical Centre, 121 Swindon Road, Cheltenham GL50 4DP
Tel: 01242 707701 Fax: 01242 707705
Website: www.royalwell.co.uk
(Cheltenham and Tewkesbury Primary Care Trust)
Patient List Size: 7020

Practice Manager Lynette Goode

GP Robert HYATT WILLIAMS, Phillip Donald FIELDING, David Gareth PRICE, Sarah-Louise YOUNGS

Sevenposts Surgery
326A Prestbury Road, Prestbury, Cheltenham GL52 3DD
Tel: 01242 244103
(Cheltenham and Tewkesbury Primary Care Trust)

Practice Manager Harry Curzon

GP David William LYLE, John Crighton BRAMWELL, Diane MARSON, Jillian Wendy VERNON-SMITH, Sarah WILKINSON, Nicholas James YOUNG

Sixways Clinic
London Road, Charlton Kings, Cheltenham GL52 6HS
Tel: 01242 583520
(Cheltenham and Tewkesbury Primary Care Trust)

Practice Manager N Hall

GP Kevin Richard CLARKSON, Susan Margaret DRING, Siobhan DURKIN, Douglas Joseph GIRALDI, Graham Shields MENNIE, Neil James MORISON

St Catherine's Surgery
St Pauls Medical Centre, 121 Swindon Road, Cheltenham GL50 4DP
Tel: 01242 580668 Fax: 01242 707699
(Cheltenham and Tewkesbury Primary Care Trust)
Patient List Size: 9200

Practice Manager Sue Johnson

GP David Michael GOODALL, John Henry BATTEN, Sarah Louise HUGHES, Isabel Joanna LIEBERT, Graham Miller WILSON

St George's Surgery
St Pauls Medical Centre, 121 Swindon Road, Cheltenham GL50 4DP
Tel: 01242 707755 Fax: 01242 707749
(Cheltenham and Tewkesbury Primary Care Trust)
Patient List Size: 10800

Practice Manager Sue Yost

GP Kenneth John MORPHEW, Alexander James CAMPBELL, Robert David CHAPPLE, Rosemary Jean DALTON, James Francis FLYNN, Christine Mary HASELER

The Surgery
2 Crescent Bakery, St. Georges Place, Cheltenham GL50 3PN
Tel: 01242 226336 Fax: 01242 253587
(Cheltenham and Tewkesbury Primary Care Trust)

Practice Manager Lyn Joy

GP Richard George MATHERS, Mark David TRUEMAN, Susan Elizabeth COURT, Linda Frances MEDLAND

The Surgery
4 Stoke Road, Bishops Cleeve, Cheltenham GL52 8RP
Tel: 01242 672007
(Cheltenham and Tewkesbury Primary Care Trust)

Practice Manager Beverley Beaman

GP Peter George SLIMMINGS, T J HARDWICK, James Brown MOORE, Yvette Marie PYGOTT, Finlay McLean ROBINSON

Underwood Surgery
139 St. Georges Road, Cheltenham GL50 3EQ
Tel: 01242 580644 Fax: 01242 253519
(Cheltenham and Tewkesbury Primary Care Trust)
Patient List Size: 9500

Practice Manager Pauline Upton

GP Clive Edward TIMLIN, Robin David HOLLANDS, T Mark JACKSON, Elizabeth Ann MURPHY

Well Lane Surgery
Well Lane, Stow on the Wold, Cheltenham GL54 1EQ
Tel: 01451 830625 Fax: 01451 830693
(Cotswold and Vale Primary Care Trust)
Patient List Size: 5580

Practice Manager Paula Evison

GP Timothy James George HEALY, Steven RAWSTORNE, Paul SHERRINGHAM, Judith Ann THORNETT

Winchcombe Medical Practice
Stone House, Abbey Terrace, Winchcombe, Cheltenham GL54 5LL
Tel: 01242 602307 Fax: 01242 603689
(Cheltenham and Tewkesbury Primary Care Trust)

Practice Manager David Cockram

GP Crispin George CUMMIN, Keith William CURTIS, Anthony Richard TRIBLEY

Yorkleigh Surgery
93 St. Georges Road, Cheltenham GL50 3ED
Tel: 01242 519049 Fax: 01242 253556
(Cheltenham and Tewkesbury Primary Care Trust)
Patient List Size: 10000

GP Simon Gregor Erskine McMINN, Andrew Robert GREEN, Christopher Geoffery John KINCHIN, Mark MALDEN, Isobel Fiona McKENZIE, Ian McPHERSON

Chertsey

The Abbey Practice
The Family Health Centre, Stepgates, Chertsey KT16 8HZ
Tel: 01932 565655 Fax: 01932 571842
(North Surrey Primary Care Trust)
Patient List Size: 10000

Practice Manager Cathy Hough

GP Peter Francis BRODRIBB, Nicola MANTEL-COOPER, Helen Sylvia MAXFIELD, Hugh Gerald TOWIE, Miriam Louise WYATT, Khalid Osman Abeer WYNE

The Bridge Practice
The Health Centre, Stepgates, Chertsey KT16 8HZ
Tel: 01932 561199 Fax: 01932 571732
(North Surrey Primary Care Trust)

Practice Manager Kathy Edwards

GP David Paul NORTH-COOMBES, Neville John BLEWITT, Marie Christine CANTY, E M LAWN, Amanda Meredith Barclay VINCENT-BROWN

New Ottershaw Surgery
3 Bousley Rise, Ottershaw, Chertsey KT16 0JX
Tel: 01932 875001/872261 Fax: 01932 873855
(North Surrey Primary Care Trust)
Patient List Size: 4600

Practice Manager Alan Titchener

GP Andrew John HARRIS, Judith Ann DONALDSON, Barbara JONES

Chesham

Aureole House Surgery
Market Square, 9 Church Street, Chesham HP5 1HS
Tel: 01494 792558
(Chiltern and South Bucks Primary Care Trust)
Patient List Size: 1992

Practice Manager Sylvia Morris

GP Alan Edward MORRIS

The New Surgery
Lindo Close, Chesham HP5 2JN
Tel: 01494 782262 Fax: 01494 785917
(Chiltern and South Bucks Primary Care Trust)
Patient List Size: 10500

Practice Manager Monica Lawernson

GP Peter John FLINT, Christopher DAVIES, Rachel Mary FIRTH, Ibramin HAMAMI, Geoffrey Paul Ingleby PAYNE, Diana Claire STEVENS

The Surgery
Gladstone Road, Chesham HP5 3AD
Tel: 01494 782884 Fax: 01494 792686
(Chiltern and South Bucks Primary Care Trust)
Patient List Size: 4400

Practice Manager Margaret Lee

GP Angela Phyllis BISHOP, Peter William BOAST, Sara WESTCOTT

Water Meadow Surgery
Red Lion Street, Chesham HP5 1ET
Tel: 01494 782241 Fax: 01494 782005
(Chiltern and South Bucks Primary Care Trust)

Practice Manager John Juniper

GP Robert Andrew JORDAN, Neil Christopher COOPER, Sandra Margaret KING, Alexandra MURRAY, Fiona Rosalind NEALE, Marlo OFFSIDE, Rosie SHOTTS

Chessington

Gosbury Hill Health Centre
Orchard Gardens, Chessington KT9 1AG
Tel: 020 8397 2142 Fax: 020 8974 2717
(Kingston Primary Care Trust)
Patient List Size: 10500

Practice Manager Denise Smith

GP Sivapragasam VISVA NATHAN, Siva BALASINGAM, John Edward GRAY, Michael Stannard UDAL

The Surgery
207 Hook Road, Chessington KT9 1EA
Tel: 020 8397 6361 Fax: 020 8973 1573
(Kingston Primary Care Trust)

Practice Manager Susan Burge

GP Alan John LYONS, Anne Lydia Helen BARUCH

The Surgery
270 Hook Road, Chessington KT9 1PF
Tel: 020 8397 3574
(Kingston Primary Care Trust)
Patient List Size: 6000

Practice Manager Dianne Gray

GP Prasun KUMAR, Ashism PAUL, Shanim RAHMAN, Rupinder SUMRA

Chester

Boughton Medical Group
Boughton Health Centre, Hoole Lane, Chester CH2 3DP
Tel: 01244 325421
(Cheshire West Primary Care Trust)
Patient List Size: 11000

Practice Manager Samantha Fletcher

GP Paul James DENNITTS, Amanda BERTRAM, Paula B M DAVIS, Mark David GRIFFITHS, Annabel Julia JONES, Stephen Nicholas KAYE, Sally Elizabeth NAYLOR

City Walls Medical Centre
St Martin's Way, Chester CH1 2NR
Tel: 01244 357800
(Cheshire West Primary Care Trust)
Patient List Size: 1800

Practice Manager Linda Leigh

GP Ian Samuel DANIELS, Rachel Teresa ARNOLD, Andrew DUNBAVAND, David Lawson FARRALL, Jayne HOLLAND, Isabelle Lois HUGHES, Daniel JONES, Kulai Narayana KINI, Christopher Ralph NEUKOM, Anthony SHANAHAN, Janice Mary STEPHENS

Elms Medical Centre
31 Hoole Road, Chester CH2 3NH
Tel: 01244 351000
(Cheshire West Primary Care Trust)
Patient List Size: 9000

Practice Manager Peta Murphy

GP Ian Alexander RUSSELL, Michael John Shaun LOWRIE, Ann Rosemary Josephine McNUTT, Bernard MILLS, James Edward RAMSDALE

Farndon Health Centre
Church Lane, Farndon, Chester CH3 6QD
Tel: 01829 270206 Fax: 01829 270803
(Cheshire West Primary Care Trust)
Patient List Size: 3700

Practice Manager Janet Crispin

GP David Neil DUFFIN, Linda Bettina DUFFIN

Garden Lane Medical Centre
19 Garden Lane, Chester CH1 4EN
Tel: 01244 346677 Fax: 01244 310094
(Cheshire West Primary Care Trust)

Practice Manager Roberta Mallett, Hayley Pashley

GP Lindsay Michael RILEY, Kathryn Elizabeth BUSHELL, John HODGSON, Susan Mary MEACHIM, David George NICHOLSON, Lee WALKER-BAKER

Handbridge Medical Centre
Greenway Street, Handbridge, Chester CH4 7JS
Tel: 01244 680169 Fax: 01244 680162
(Cheshire West Primary Care Trust)

Practice Manager J Jackson

GP Carole-Ann HOLME, Catrin CLWYD JONES, Susan O'DELL, Mark Wakefield THOMPSON

Heath Lane Medical Centre
Heath Lane, Chester CH3 5UJ
Tel: 01244 348844 Fax: 01244 351057
(Cheshire West Primary Care Trust)
Patient List Size: 7000

Practice Manager David Ellis

GP Frances Gillian EVANS-JONES, Christopher Paul FRYAR, Wanda Jane HARGREAVES, Timothy Philip SAUNDERS

Hoole Road Surgery
71 Hoole Road, Chester CH2 3NJ
Tel: 01244 325721 Fax: 01244 313836
Email: anthony.bland@gp-81102.nhs.uk
(Cheshire West Primary Care Trust)
Patient List Size: 2400

Practice Manager Tony Lambe

GP Anthony Kenmore BLAND

Lache Health Centre
Hawthorn Road, Lache, Chester CH4 8HX
Tel: 01244 671991 Fax: 01244 680729
(Cheshire West Primary Care Trust)
Patient List Size: 5800

Practice Manager Nick Blackledge

GP Patricia Mary OWENS, Nicola FOX, Kevin Thomas GUINAN, Susan Elizabeth MACDONALD

Northgate Medical Centre
10 Upper Northgate Street, Chester CH1 4EE
Tel: 01244 379906 Fax: 01244 379703
(Cheshire West Primary Care Trust)
Patient List Size: 6835

Practice Manager Margaret Freeburn

GP Nicholas Henry BRONNERT, Martin Miles ALLAN, Juliet Evelyn CAIN, Kath HENRY, Stewart LEITCH

Northgate Village Surgery
Northgate Avenue, Chester CH2 2DX
Tel: 01244 390396 Fax: 01244 370762
(Cheshire West Primary Care Trust)
Patient List Size: 5539

Practice Manager Brenda Waugh

GP Elizabeth Alison McCLURE, Robin Maelor DAVIES, Ian Roland MINSHALL

Park Medical Centre
Shavington Avenue, Newton Lane, Chester CH2 3RD
Tel: 01244 324136 Fax: 01244 317257
(Cheshire West Primary Care Trust)
Patient List Size: 8270

Practice Manager Patricia Harrison

GP Arthur Colin HUGHES, Neil Stewart BLACKLOCK, Gillian Elizabeth HOLLEY, Christopher Rimington LEWIS, Robert Curle STEWART

Rookery Surgery
Chester Road, Tattenhall, Chester CH3 9AH
Tel: 01829 770234 Fax: 01829 771136
(Cheshire West Primary Care Trust)
Patient List Size: 2175

Practice Manager Dawn Beeston

GP Philip Michael MILNER

Tattenhall Medical Practice
Mercury House, High St, Tattenhall, Chester CH3 9PX
Tel: 01829 770606 Fax: 01829 770144
(Cheshire West Primary Care Trust)
Patient List Size: 1300

Practice Manager Carole Goodinson

GP Pauline ROYLANCE

Upton Village Surgery
Wealstone Lane, Upton, Chester CH2 1HD
Tel: 01244 382238 Fax: 01244 381576
(Cheshire West Primary Care Trust)
Patient List Size: 5700

GP Rowan BROOKES, Andrew William Charles CLOUTING, David Charles INCHLEY

Western Avenue Medical Centre
Gordon Road, Blacon, Chester CH1 5PA
Tel: 01244 390755 Fax: 01244 383955
(Cheshire West Primary Care Trust)
Patient List Size: 3900

Practice Manager K Norman

GP Anthony Lawrence KAUFMAN, Raymond Mark ADAMS, Roman JIMENEZ-GIL

Chester-le-Street

Birtley Lane Surgery
4 Birtley Lane, Birtley, Chester-le-Street DH3 1AX
(Gateshead Primary Care Trust)

Birtley Medical Group Practice
Birtley Medical Group, Durham Road, Birtley, Chester-le-Street DH3 2QT
Tel: 0191 410 3421 Fax: 0191 410 9672
(Gateshead Primary Care Trust)
Patient List Size: 14500

Practice Manager Alan Griffin

GP James Paddon DERRICK, Jocelyn Alan BRAY, Joanna Margaret HUGHES, Philip Leon LE DUNE, James Wallace STEELE, Paul William VINCENT

Cestria Health Centre
Whitehill Way, Chester-le-Street DH2 3DJ
Tel: 0191 388 7771 Fax: 0191 387 1803
(Durham and Chester-le-Street Primary Care Trust)

Practice Manager Denise Hunter

GP Anne SULLIVAN, Christopher Jocelyn BENNETT, Sheila Jane BOWMAN, Adam Raoul Harvey DOUGLAS, James Lees McMICHAEL, Neil O'BRIEN

Group Practice Surgery
Middle Chare, Chester-le-Street DH3 3QD
Tel: 0191 3884857 Fax: 0191 388 7448
Website: www.middlecharesurgery.co.uk
(Durham and Chester-le-Street Primary Care Trust)
Patient List Size: 10500

Practice Manager Paul Weddle

GP Anthony John GOLLINGS, Geoffrey CRACKETT, Richard Stephen HALL, Karen Elizabeth HUBBARD, John Grainger PRESTON

Pelton Fell Surgery
21 Gardner Crescent, Pelton Fell, Chester-le-Street DH2 2NJ
Tel: 0191 368 0614 Fax: 0191 387 4644
(Durham and Chester-le-Street Primary Care Trust)
Patient List Size: 2150

GP Raveendran Raghavan NAIR

The Surgery
Front Street, Pelton, Chester-le-Street DH2 1DE
Tel: 0191 3826700 Fax: 0191 382 6715
(Durham and Chester-le-Street Primary Care Trust)
Patient List Size: 9724

Practice Manager Katie Davison

GP Anthony John TYSON, Jose MIRALLES, Anita Jacqueline TURNER, Robin WHEATLEY

The Surgery
Front Street, Great Lumley, Chester-le-Street DH3 4LE
Tel: 0191 388 5600 Fax: 0191 388 3912
Website: www.greatlumleysurgery.co.uk
(Durham and Chester-le-Street Primary Care Trust)
Patient List Size: 4656

Practice Manager Patricia Holland

GP Paul Thomas FLETCHER, Alex DOCTON, Michelle GOODING

The Surgery
Bridge End, Chester-le-Street DH3 3SL
Tel: 0191 3883236 Fax: 0191 389 0989
(Durham and Chester-le-Street Primary Care Trust)
Patient List Size: 9000

Practice Manager Peter Brown

GP Richard John LILLY, M A EARNSHAW, J S D FARROW, T P S JOHNSTON

Chesterfield

Ash Lodge Medical Centre
73 Old Road, Chesterfield S40 2RA
Tel: 01246 232962 Fax: 01246 231824
(Chesterfield Primary Care Trust)
Patient List Size: 9000

Practice Manager Wendy Torrinson

GP Iain Robert SERRELL, E O'DONNELL, John Brendan RYAN, Hugh William Fraser SCOTLAND, Catherine Ann SPOONER

Ashover Medical Practice
Milken Lane, Ashover, Chesterfield S45 0BA
Tel: 01246 590711 Fax: 01246 590528
(North Eastern Derbyshire Primary Care Trust)
Patient List Size: 1960

Practice Manager Rosemary Early

GP Nigel Edward EARLY, Gordon JONES

Avenue House Surgery
109 Saltergate, Chesterfield S40 1LE
Tel: 01246 272139 Fax: 01246 556336
(Chesterfield Primary Care Trust)

Practice Manager Carol Brannan

GP David Ian ANDERSON, Peter FLYNN, Catherine Anne MADDEN, Andrew Peter Marston MATTHEWS, Steven MURRAY

Avondale Surgery
5 Avondale Road, Chesterfield S40 4TF
Tel: 01246 232946 Fax: 01246 556246
(Chesterfield Primary Care Trust)

GP Stephen LANGAN, Anthony Joseph AINSWORTH, Martin Fergusson ANDREW, Mark David BLAGDEN, Cathryn A WORTHINGTON, Barry Stuart YOUNG

Barlborough Medical Practice
The Old Malthouse, 7 Worksop Road, Barlborough, Chesterfield S43 4TY
Tel: 01246 819994 Fax: 01246 812293
(North Eastern Derbyshire Primary Care Trust)
Patient List Size: 4100

Practice Manager Nigel Atkin

GP Andrew PALMER, Judith Anne GARDNER

Blue Dykes Surgery
Eldon Street, Clay Cross, Chesterfield S45 9NR
Tel: 01246 862468 Fax: 01246 861058
(North Eastern Derbyshire Primary Care Trust)
Patient List Size: 9000

Practice Manager Marianne Cox

GP Stephen Ernest DILLEY, Christine Sharon FOWLER, Charles William Peter JACKSON, John Richard MANN, Matthew J C WAYMAN

Brimington Surgery
Church Street, Brimington, Chesterfield S43 1JG
Tel: 01246 273224 Fax: 01246 556616
(Chesterfield Primary Care Trust)
Patient List Size: 7500

Practice Manager David Kee

GP Richard Robert LIVINGS, Michael Derek BANNING, Emma Jane FORDHAM, Mark John TORKINGTON

Calow and Brimington Practice
Brimington Medical Centre, Foljambe Road, Brimington, Chesterfield S43 1DD
Tel: 01246 220166 Fax: 01246 208221
(Chesterfield Primary Care Trust)
Patient List Size: 6000

Practice Manager Sheila Barrett

GP Richard Edward BULL, Christopher HEE, Kathryn MARKUS, Shantha Stephnie Arumaiammal TYLER

Castle Street Medical Centre
Castle Street, Bolsover, Chesterfield S44 6PP
Tel: 01246 822983 Fax: 01246 822265
(North Eastern Derbyshire Primary Care Trust)
Patient List Size: 3000

Practice Manager Pat Round

GP Swapan Kumar SENGUPTA, Renuka GADHVI

Chatsworth Road Medical Centre
Chatsworth Road, Brampton, Chesterfield S40 3PY
Tel: 01246 568065 Fax: 01246 567116
(Chesterfield Primary Care Trust)
Patient List Size: 8500

Practice Manager Amanda Raybould

GP Richard James NEEP, Christopher John PILCHER, David Alun PRICE, Elizabeth RICHES

Chawla
1A Welbeck Drive, Wingerworth, Chesterfield S42 6SN
Tel: 01246 276590 Fax: 01246 203453
(North Eastern Derbyshire Primary Care Trust)

Practice Manager Paula Richardson

GP Vimla CHAWLA

Chesterfield Road Medical Centre
Chesterfield Road, North Wingfield, Chesterfield S42 5ND
Tel: 01246 851035 Fax: 01246 856139
(North Eastern Derbyshire Primary Care Trust)
Patient List Size: 6300

Practice Manager Heather Leigh

GP Margaret Barron KELMAN, Timothy Keith KNOWLES, C S SINGH

Clowne Health Centre
Creswell Road, Clowne, Chesterfield S43 4LU
Tel: 01246 819444/819047 Fax: 01246 819010
(North Eastern Derbyshire Primary Care Trust)
Patient List Size: 7654

Practice Manager Janina Gawel

GP David COLLINS, Matthew DEXTER, Carolyn EMSLIE, Louise MERRIMAN

Eastwood House Surgery
10 Mill Street, Clowne, Chesterfield S43 4JN
Tel: 01246 810303 Fax: 01246 811483
(East Yorkshire Primary Care Trust)

Practice Manager Angela Gustason, Pat Quinn

GP A KAY, B McKENZIE

Friendly Family Surgery
Welbeck Road, Bolsover, Chesterfield S44 6DE
Tel: 01246 826815 Fax: 01246 822723
(North Eastern Derbyshire Primary Care Trust)
Patient List Size: 4650

Practice Manager Peter Strelley

GP Maureen Elizabeth HEHIR STRELLEY

Hasland Surgery
66 Storforth Lane, Hasland, Chesterfield S41 0PW
Tel: 01246 277973 Fax: 01246 203645
(Chesterfield Primary Care Trust)

GP Anjuman Diwan CHAND

High Street Medical Centre
19 High Street, Staveley, Chesterfield S43 3UU
Tel: 01246 472296 Fax: 01246 471665
Website: www.draldredandpartners.co.uk
(Chesterfield Primary Care Trust)

Practice Manager Jim Hindle

GP Philip Robert ALDRED, Nicholas James COOK, Nicholas Wayne DUNPHY, P GILL, Margie PETERSON, Emile WRIGHT

High Street Surgery
117 High Street, Clay Cross, Chesterfield S45 9DZ
Tel: 01246 862237 Fax: 01246 861384
(North Eastern Derbyshire Primary Care Trust)

Practice Manager P Allen

GP Stavros Kleopas Talliadoros NEOFYTOU, Michael GREEN, Philip Cook JACKSON

Holywell House Surgery
Holywell Street, Chesterfield S41 7SD
Tel: 01246 273075 Fax: 01246 555711
(Chesterfield Primary Care Trust)
Patient List Size: 9300

Practice Manager Valerie J Gascoyne

GP Michael George DORNAN, Nadine Jane KALE, Richard John MEREDITH, J M PAGE, John Whieldon THURSTAN

Leyfield Surgery
2 Eckington Road, Staveley, Chesterfield S43 3XZ
Tel: 01246 473321 Fax: 01246 477303
(Chesterfield Primary Care Trust)
Patient List Size: 3850

Practice Manager Christine Unwin

GP Thomas James Davison McCONNELL, Barbara Mary LOWER

The Maples Medical Centre
Barnfield Close, Staveley, Chesterfield S43 3UL
Tel: 01246 472309 Fax: 01246 470546
(Chesterfield Primary Care Trust)
Patient List Size: 5997

Practice Manager Josie Elliott

GP Basant Kumar SHRESTHA, P K RAI

Newbold Surgery
3 Windermere Road, Chesterfield S41 8DU
Tel: 01246 277381 Fax: 01246 239828
(Chesterfield Primary Care Trust)
Patient List Size: 12000

Practice Manager Wendy Tomlinson

GP David Martin ELMORE, Deirdre BIRKS, Martin Andrew BRADLEY, Ann Sarah GEDGE, John Hurst LOVEDAY, Peter John STEVENS

Newbold Surgery
3 Windermere Road, Newbold, Chesterfield S41 8DU
Tel: 01246 277381 Fax: 01246 239828
(Chesterfield Primary Care Trust)
Patient List Size: 12000

Practice Manager Wendy Tomlinson

GP D M ELMORE, Dr ABRAHAM, D M BIRKS, Dr BRADLEY, A S GEDGE, J H LOVEDAY, P J STEVENS

North Wingfield Road Surgery
186 North Wingfield Road, Grassmoor, Chesterfield S42 5ED
Tel: 01246 852995 Fax: 01246 855146
(North Eastern Derbyshire Primary Care Trust)

Practice Manager Elizabeth Roe

GP Khaja Azizuddin AHMED

St Lawrence Road Surgery
17-19 St. Lawrence Road, North Wingfield, Chesterfield S42 5LH
Tel: 01246 851029 Fax: 01246 853724
(North Eastern Derbyshire Primary Care Trust)
Patient List Size: 4220

Practice Manager Martin Barrett

GP Antony Leo NATT, Pauline MILLER

St Philips Drive Surgery
82 St. Philips Drive, Hasland, Chesterfield S41 0RG
Tel: 01246 278008 Fax: 01246 278008
(Chesterfield Primary Care Trust)

GP Catherine Kemp

Tennyson Avenue Medical Centre
1 Tennyson Avenue, Chesterfield S40 4SN
Tel: 01246 232339 Fax: 01246 209097
(Chesterfield Primary Care Trust)

GP Paul Stephen CROWTHER, K ALEXANDER, Elizabeth Frances CROWTHER

Welbeck Road Surgery
1A Welbeck Road, Bolsover, Chesterfield S44 6DF
Tel: 01246 823742 Fax: 01246 240781
Website: www.welbeckroadsurgery.co.uk
(North Eastern Derbyshire Primary Care Trust)
Patient List Size: 9400

Practice Manager Rosemary Adams

GP Michael Richard SPENCER, Angela BURSTOW, Joseph Paul COOK, Frances CRYAN, Frances Elizabeth FERMER, Thomas Alan HUMPHRIES, Catherine LONGSHAW, Simon Henry NISSENBAUM

The Whittington Medical Centre
High Street, Old Whittington, Chesterfield S41 9JZ
Tel: 01246 455440 Fax: 01246 261851
(Chesterfield Primary Care Trust)
Patient List Size: 3300

GP William Arthur Kenneth JONES

Whittington Moor Surgery
Scarsdale Road, Chesterfield S41 8NA
Tel: 01246 542549 Fax: 01246 454669
(Chesterfield Primary Care Trust)
Patient List Size: 7350

Practice Manager Margaret Dawson, Gillian Sykes

GP Richard Andrew MEE, Debra Jane ABELL, Elizabeth CHURCH, Peter WOODCOCK

Chichester

Cathedral Medical Group
15 Cawley Road, Chichester PO19 1XT
Tel: 01243 786666/781833 Fax: 01243 530042
(Western Sussex Primary Care Trust)
Patient List Size: 11850

GP David Martin HOARE, Tanya DEAVALL, Liz EVANS, Yvonne Edna HUNNIFORD, Fiona Jane LEWIS

Croft Surgery
Barnham Road, Eastergate, Chichester PO20 6RP
Tel: 01243 543240
(Western Sussex Primary Care Trust)
Patient List Size: 8200

Practice Manager Judith Walker

GP Philip Meyrick QUINNELL, Ian Yule BUCHANAN, Richard Graham PATERSON, Susan Louise ROSE

Johnson and Partners
Langley House, 27 West Street, Chichester PO19 1RW
Tel: 01243 782266/782955 Fax: 01243 779188
(Western Sussex Primary Care Trust)
Patient List Size: 9200

Practice Manager Victoria Hamer

GP Patrick Allingham JOHNSON, Madeleine BONSEY, Bruce Norman Burney DUNLOP, Michael Edward GILBERT, Sarah KING, Folliott Charles Edward WALKER

Parklands Surgery
4 Parklands Road, Chichester PO19 3DT
Tel: 01243 782819/786827 Fax: 01243 537923
(Western Sussex Primary Care Trust)
Patient List Size: 9500

Practice Manager Valerie Cooper

GP Alan COPSEY, Timothy John HAMMOND, Charlie LAVENDER, Margaret Jane ORR, David Neil PATIENT, James Michael PRICE

Seal Medical Group
Selsey Medical Centre, High Street, Selsey, Chichester PO20 0QG
Tel: 01243 604321 Fax: 01243 607996
Website: www.selseymedicalcentre.org
(Western Sussex Primary Care Trust)
Patient List Size: 5200

Practice Manager Lynn Cank

GP Mark HOWARTH, Katherine MILLER, Hilary PLATTS

Selsey Medical Centre
High Street, Selsey, Chichester PO20 0QC
Tel: 01243 608201 Fax: 01243 607996
(Western Sussex Primary Care Trust)

GP Richard HARRIS, Michael James LACEY, Alison PARRISH

The Surgery
8 Lavant Road, Chichester PO19 5RH
Tel: 01243 527264 Fax: 01243 530607

(Western Sussex Primary Care Trust)
Patient List Size: 9500

Practice Manager Lyn Heyward

GP Bryony Eleanor WHITTAKER, Amelia BARNETT, Justyn JACKSON, Grant Stuart-Black KELLY, Sara Katharine KELLY, Peter John Donald WHITTAKER, Linda Kennedy WILLIAMS

The Surgery
8 Lavant Road, Chichester, Chichester PO19 5RH
Tel: 01243 527264 Fax: 01243 530607
(Western Sussex Primary Care Trust)
Patient List Size: 9500

Practice Manager Lyn Heyward

GP Amelia BARNETT, Justin JACKSON, Linda WILLIAMS

Westgate Surgery
15 Westgate, Chichester PO19 3ET
Tel: 01243 782866 Fax: 01243 532436
Website: www.thewestgatesurgery.com
(Western Sussex Primary Care Trust)

GP William David Cave MALLAM, Slice CHISHICK, Robert James WILSON

The Witterings Health Centre
Cakeham Road, East Wittering, Chichester PO20 8BH
Tel: 01243 673434 Fax: 01243 672563
Email: witchdoc@ewitte.freeserve.co.uk
(Western Sussex Primary Care Trust)
Patient List Size: 7400

Practice Manager J E Nicholls

GP David Ronald NICHOLLS, Adrian Bede GREGORY, Michele Lesley LACEY, Gregory John TAMLYN, Graham Vincent WATTS

Witterings Health Centre
Cakeham Road, East Wittering, Chichester PO20 8BH
Tel: 01243 670707 Fax: 01243 672808
(Western Sussex Primary Care Trust)
Patient List Size: 2500

Practice Manager Tina Stephenson

GP Tina G EDWARDS

Chinnor

Church Road Surgery
Church Road, Chinnor OX39 4PG
Tel: 01844 351584 Fax: 01844 354350
(Vale of Aylesbury Primary Care Trust)

GP Christopher Allen HOOD

Station Road New Surgery
5 Station Road, Chinnor OX39 4PX
Tel: 01844 351230 Fax: 01844 354328
(Vale of Aylesbury Primary Care Trust)

Practice Manager J M Webb

GP Martin John KNIGHTLEY, Lowri KEW, Michael MULHOLLAND, Stephen Andrew STAMP

Chippenham

Hathaway Surgery
32 New Road, Chippenham SN15 1HP
Tel: 01249 447766 Fax: 01249 443948
Email: administrator@gp-J83007.nhs.uk
(Kennet and North Wiltshire Primary Care Trust)
Patient List Size: 10200

Practice Manager Andy Briggs

GP William Stuart HENRY, James Anthony BROSCH, Debbie GATUN, Susi GREGSON, Lorraine JEFFERY, Vicky JENNINGS, Tamara Anne TUREK, Anthony Thomas Stanley WRIGHT

Jubilee Field Surgery
Yation Keynell, Chippenham SN14 7EJ
Tel: 01249 782204 Fax: 01249 783110
Email: robin.while@J83603.nhs.uk
(Kennet and North Wiltshire Primary Care Trust)
Patient List Size: 4400

Practice Manager Tracy Harris

GP Robin Symington Armstrong WHILE, Fiona GILROY, Sanjeev POPLI

Lodge Surgery
Lodge Road, Chippenham SN15 3SY
Tel: 01249 660667 Fax: 01249 447350
(Kennet and North Wiltshire Primary Care Trust)
Patient List Size: 7694

Practice Manager Chantal Collins

GP Robert Francis MUIR, Melanie Jane BLACKMAN, Nicola Wyn McCORMACK, Darragh O'DRISCOLL

Marshfield Road Surgery
47 Marshfield Road, Chippenham SN15 1JT
Tel: 01249 654466
(Kennet and North Wiltshire Primary Care Trust)

Marshfield Surgery
2 Back Lane, Marshfield, Chippenham SN14 8NQ
Tel: 01225 891265 Fax: 01225 891909
(South Gloucestershire Primary Care Trust)
Patient List Size: 9000

Practice Manager Linda Beazer, Aurea Hart

GP P H BRUNYATE, R A C GREENWAY, C HORLEY, J E MORGAN, J D M SEDDON, Joanna SEDDON

Regional Medical Centre
RAF Lyneham, Chippenham SN15 4PZ
Tel: 01249 890381 Fax: 01249 890381
(Kennet and North Wiltshire Primary Care Trust)

GP F DIGNAN, J RUSSELL

Rowden Surgery
Rowden Hill, Chippenham SN15 2SB
Tel: 01249 444343 Fax: 01249 446797
(Kennet and North Wiltshire Primary Care Trust)
Patient List Size: 16200

Practice Manager Sheila Poulton

GP Ian Menmuir GRANDISON, John Arthur William BARTER, Nicholas Hugh BROWN, Alison Sarah CHALLENS, Gavin Michael DURRANT, Richard Martin Charles GAUNT, Anne Marie LASHFORD, Alistair Richard McKIBBIN

The Surgery
Chestnut Road, Sutton Benger, Chippenham SN15 4RP
Tel: 01249 720244 Fax: 01249 721165
(Kennet and North Wiltshire Primary Care Trust)
Patient List Size: 2070

Practice Manager John Palmer

GP Charles Edward WILKINSON

Chipping Campden

Campden Surgery
Back Ends, Chipping Campden GL55 6AU
Tel: 01386 840296 Fax: 01386 841919
(Cotswold and Vale Primary Care Trust)
Patient List Size: 3600

Practice Manager J Burn

GP Giles Basil Hardisty BOINTON, Fiona CAMPBELL, Jacquie WILLIAMS

Chipping Norton

Charlbury Medical Centre
Spendlove Centre, Enstone Road, Charlbury, Chipping Norton OX7 3PQ
Tel: 01608 810210 Fax: 01608 811636
(South West Oxfordshire Primary Care Trust)
Patient List Size: 4800

Practice Manager W Rouse

GP John Raymond GOVES, Helen Jane BAYLISS, Pippa BROOKES-WHITE

Walton and Partners
West Street Surgery, 12 West Street, Chipping Norton OX7 5AA
Tel: 01608 642529 Fax: 01608 645066
Email: weststreet@aol.com
(Cherwell Vale Primary Care Trust)
Patient List Size: 6800

Practice Manager Di Waller

GP John Alexander WALTON, Catherine Anne ELLIOTT, Wendy Lucy HALL, Jonathan Graeme MOORE, Jane Margaret PARGETER

White House Surgery
Horsefair, Chipping Norton OX7 5AL
Tel: 01608 642742 Fax: 01608 642794
(Cherwell Vale Primary Care Trust)
Patient List Size: 8000

Practice Manager A J Love

GP David Ronald EDWARDS, A AHMED, Stephen Charles BLAKE, Jill Elizabeth EDWARDS, Caroline KEENAN, Mary KEENAN, Stephen QUELCH

Wychwood Surgery
62 High Street, Milton-under-Wychwood, Chipping Norton OX7 6LE
Tel: 01993 830260 Fax: 01993 831867
Email: wychdocs@oxbox.com
(Cherwell Vale Primary Care Trust)
Patient List Size: 4967

Practice Manager Vanessa Newman

GP Gordon SCOTT, Christopher John DAWKINS, David Peter NIXON

Chislehurst

Chislehurst Medical Practice
42 High Street, Chislehurst BR7 5AQ
Tel: 020 8467 5551 Fax: 020 8468 7658
Website: www.chislehurstmedicalpractice.co.uk
(Bromley Primary Care Trust)
Patient List Size: 14500

Practice Manager Pam Scott

GP Roland Werner FRY, Caroline FRASER, Norman Charles HAMBLYN, Meena Anne KHARADE, Andrew Francis PARSON, Hasib-ur RUB, David STRANGE, Viral TANND

Red Hill Family Practice
11 Redhill, Chislehurst BR7 6DB
Tel: 020 8467 7419 Fax: 020 8295 1270
Email: Fam.doc@lineone.net
(Bromley Primary Care Trust)

Practice Manager Mandy Becker

GP Walter Graham Ellis BECKER, Elizabeth BRANDER, Michael Loke Onn CHOONG, Nicola PASCALL

Choppington

Guidepost Health Centre
North Parade, Guidepost, Choppington NE62 5RA
Tel: 01670 822071 Fax: 01670 531068
(Northumberland Care Trust)
Patient List Size: 9560

Practice Manager Susan Rowland

GP Peter William SANDERSON, Martin ECCLES, Jane FARNDALE, Eileen HIGGNS, William Paul MACDONALD, Barbara Louise PARKER, Geert VAN ZON, Ruth WHITE

Chorley

Acreswood Surgery
5 Acreswood Close, Coppull, Chorley PR7 5EN
Tel: 01257 793578 Fax: 01257 794005
(Chorley and South Ribble Primary Care Trust)
Patient List Size: 8200

Practice Manager Lynda Keeley

GP Andrew Keith BROWN, Leslie HARRIS, David Saleem Ahmed KHAN, Aneil RAWSON

Adlington Medical Centre
22-24 Babylon Lane, Anderton, Chorley PR6 9NW
Tel: 01257 482076 Fax: 01257 474770
Email: feda.khawaja@gp-P81740.nhs.uk
(Chorley and South Ribble Primary Care Trust)

GP Othman Abd El Rahman Shehde EL HALHULI

Chorley Health Centre
Collison Avenue, Chorley PR7 2TH
Tel: 01772 644184 Fax: 01257 232285
(Chorley and South Ribble Primary Care Trust)

Practice Manager Susan Hartley

GP Robert David HARTLEY, Raffi Boghos BAGHDJIAN, Peter Alexander Collins BAMFORD, Richard Mostyn LYONS

Chorley Health Centre
Collison Avenue, Chorley PR7 2TH
Tel: 01257 268955 Fax: 01257 241870
(Chorley and South Ribble Primary Care Trust)

Practice Manager Jayne Preston

GP Ian Howard JONES

Clayton Brook Surgery
Tunley House, Clayton Brook, Chorley PR5 8ES
Tel: 01772 313950 Fax: 01772 620467
(Chorley and South Ribble Primary Care Trust)

Practice Manager Carole Page

GP Vinod Kumar KHANNA, A KHANNA

Collison Avenue Health Centre
Collison Avenue, Chorley PR7 2TH
Tel: 01772 644194 Fax: 01257 232285
Email: practice@gp-p81127.nhs.uk
(Chorley and South Ribble Primary Care Trust)
Patient List Size: 3650

Practice Manager P Stringer

GP Matthew St. John GALE, Carlos IRIZAR

Cunliffe Medical Centre
41 Cunliffe Street, Chorley PR7 2BA
Tel: 01257 267127 Fax: 01257 234664
(Chorley and South Ribble Primary Care Trust)

Practice Manager Sheila Eckersley

GP Stephen Neil HILTON, Sara Elizabeth SHACKLETON

Eaves lane Surgery
311 Eaves Lane, Chorley PR6 0DR
Tel: 01257 272904 Fax: 01257 266821
(Chorley and South Ribble Primary Care Trust)
Patient List Size: 2100

Practice Manager Gillian Cutheroe

GP Dr PITALIA, Dr THORNLEY

Eccleston Health Centre
20 Doctors Lane, Eccleston, Chorley PR7 5RA
Tel: 01257 451221 Fax: 01257 450911
(Chorley and South Ribble Primary Care Trust)

Practice Manager June M Knock

GP Robert John Charles BENNETT, Helen Jane WHITAKER

Eccleston Health Centre
20 Doctors Lane, Eccleston, Chorley PR7 5RA
Tel: 01772 644765
(Chorley and South Ribble Primary Care Trust)
Patient List Size: 2383

Practice Manager Diana Heaton

GP Qamar AHMAD

Euxton Medical Centre
St Marys Gate, Euxton, Chorley PR7 6AH
Tel: 01257 267402 Fax: 01257 271501
(Chorley and South Ribble Primary Care Trust)

Practice Manager Christine Meredith

GP Stephen Rostron LORD, Robert David LETCH

Granville House Medical Centre
Granville Street, Adlington, Chorley PR6 9PY
Tel: 01257 481966 Fax: 01257 474655
(Chorley and South Ribble Primary Care Trust)
Patient List Size: 7800

Practice Manager Linda Kershaw

GP Patricia Anne MUMFORD, Rebecca BOYES, Michael COOPER, Daniel Martin McALLISTER

Library House Surgery
Avondale Road, Chorley PR7 2AD
Tel: 01257 262081 Fax: 01257 232114
(Chorley and South Ribble Primary Care Trust)

Practice Manager J A Parry

GP William Richard ALMOND, G NIRODI, Clive BARKER, Iain Munro HALL, Suzanne Jayne HEALD, Jane Anne LOFTHOUSE, Donovan ROSS, R YATES

Regent House Surgery
21 Regent Road, Chorley PR7 2DH
Tel: 01257 264842 Fax: 01257 231387
(Chorley and South Ribble Primary Care Trust)

Practice Manager S M Dempsey

GP Roy Anthony EVISON, Stephen James EDWARDS, Mark Edmund SAVAGE, Mark Anthony SLOAN

Whittle Surgery
199 Preston Road, Whittle-le-Woods, Chorley PR6 7PS
Tel: 01257 262383 Fax: 01257 261019
(Chorley and South Ribble Primary Care Trust)

Practice Manager Sally Cooke

GP Margaret Ann SERVICE, Hemlata DESI, Robin Richard SHAW, Mark A B TURNER

Withnell Health Centre
Railway Road, Withnell, Chorley PR6 8UA
Tel: 01254 830311 Fax: 01254 832337
(Chorley and South Ribble Primary Care Trust)
Patient List Size: 5100

Practice Manager Marilyn Clowes

GP Vincent Gerard MAINEY, Margaret Mary FRANCE, Hugh JONES

Christchurch

Barn Surgery
Christchurch Medical Centre, 1 Purewell Cross Road, Christchurch BH23 3AF
Tel: 01202 486456/486455 Fax: 01202 486678
(South and East Dorset Primary Care Trust)

Practice Manager Marion Ainge

GP Gerald Anthony RHODES, John Douglas COLLIER, Morag LIVINGSTONE, Neil Peter TALLANT, Roderick Lister THOMAS

Burton Medical Centre
Salisbury Road, Burton, Christchurch BH23 7JN
Tel: 01202 474311 Fax: 01202 484412
(South and East Dorset Primary Care Trust)
Patient List Size: 9000

Practice Manager Lorraine Trim

GP Nicholas Hunter GAMPER, Melanie Susan Lovell BREVITT, Angus Edgar HICKISH, Richard JENKINSON, Lynn Karen JOSEPHS, Michael Andrew LONGLEY

Farmhouse Surgery
Christchurch Medical Centre, 1 Purewell Cross Road, Purewell, Christchurch BH23 3AF
Tel: 01202 488487 Fax: 01202 486724
Website: www.farmhousesurgery.co.uk
(South and East Dorset Primary Care Trust)
Patient List Size: 7100

Practice Manager Marilyn Weaver

GP Barry John KELLY, Andrew Bruce BLAIKLEY, James Robert Stuart DAGUE, Melanie GRAEME-BARBER

The Grove Surgery
83 The Grove, Christchurch BH23 2EZ
Tel: 01202 481192 Fax: 01202 479732
(South and East Dorset Primary Care Trust)
Patient List Size: 3000

GP Juliet Pamela GREGSON, Stephen TOMKINS

Highcliffe Medical Centre
Hella House, 248 Lymington Road, Highcliffe, Christchurch BH23 5ET
Tel: 01425 272203 Fax: 01425 271086
(South and East Dorset Primary Care Trust)
Patient List Size: 9828

Practice Manager Pam Jones

GP John Edward Terence PILLINGER, Stephen Christopher Philip COLLINS, Lucy GODWIN, Joanne Melissa LEE, Anne LLOYD-THOMAS, Reginald Massey ODBERT, Naveed SAMI

Orchard Surgery
Christchurch Medical Centre, 1 Purewell Cross Road, Christchurch BH23 3AF
Tel: 01202 481902/481901 Fax: 01202 486887
(South and East Dorset Primary Care Trust)

GP David John ROGERS, Richard Joseph OLIVER, Wendy Margaret SCOTT-JUPP, Yeut Yee Mary TANG, Joanne Sally WHITE

Stour Surgery
49 Barrack Road, Christchurch BH23 1PA
Tel: 01202 464500 Fax: 01202 464529
Website: www.stoursurgery.co.uk
(South and East Dorset Primary Care Trust)

Practice Manager Cyril Bishop

GP Graham Eric ARCHARD, Nicola Frances CAREY, Simon Charles COUPE, Graeme KLEIN

Twin Oaks Medical Centre
Ringwood Road, Bransgore, Christchurch BH23 8AD
Tel: 01425 672741 Fax: 01425 674333
(New Forest Primary Care Trust)
Patient List Size: 4020

Practice Manager Merle Hatterslem

GP Jane BOWRY, Andrew Peter MacBryde BOYD, Nigel John SAVAGE, Catherine Margaret TERRY

Chulmleigh

Chulmleigh Health Centre
Three Crossways, Chulmleigh EX18 7AA
Tel: 01769 580269 Fax: 01769 581045
(North Devon Primary Care Trust)
Patient List Size: 6000

Practice Manager Hedley Lower

GP Christopher Richard BOWMAN, Barbara Anne BROWN, J E T BURKE, Will SHERLOCK, Roelien Cornelia Aliet Diana WIELINK

Church Stretton

Easthope Road Health Centre
Easthope Road, Church Stretton SY6 6BL
Tel: 01694 722127 Fax: 01694 724604
Email: csmedpra@yahoo.com
Website: www.churchstrettondoctors.co.uk
(Shropshire County Primary Care Trust)
Patient List Size: 7352

Practice Manager Julia Thompson

GP Jonathan William BEACH, Digby BENNETT, Jennifer A HOWARD, Timothy G PARKER, Sarah Margaret RIDING, Karen A ROBINSON

Cinderford

Cinderford Health Centre
Dockham Road, Cinderford GL14 2AN
Tel: 01594 598020
(West Gloucestershire Primary Care Trust)
Patient List Size: 6300

Practice Manager Lorraine Higgleton

GP Caroline Dorothy Margaret BURROWS, Ian Christopher GADSBY, Simon Nathan SILVER, Pervez ZAHEER

Forest Health Care
The Health Centre, Dockham Road, Cinderford GL14 2AN
Tel: 01594 598030 Fax: 01594 598040
Email: forest.helath@gp-l84028.nhs.uk
(West Gloucestershire Primary Care Trust)
Patient List Size: 7300

Practice Manager Sally Charlton

GP Andrew COOMBES, Deborah Marianne LANE, Donald Grant SHAW, Ian SMITH, Margaret WALLINGTON

Cirencester

The Avenue Surgery
1 The Avenue, Cirencester GL7 1EH
Tel: 01285 653122 Fax: 01285 650098
(Cotswold and Vale Primary Care Trust)

Practice Manager Lynn Marriott

GP Richard Ivor EVANS, Diana Jane EVANS, Christopher Richard HUTCHISON, Charles Michael MARRIOTT

Mitchell and Partners
The Park Surgery, Old Tetbury Road, Cirencester GL7 1UX
Tel: 01285 654733 Fax: 01285 641408
(Cotswold and Vale Primary Care Trust)
Patient List Size: 7500

Practice Manager Adrian Hunnisett

GP David Colin MITCHELL, Anton BORG, Roger Michael PAWSON, Elizabeth Ann SPARLING, Julian Griffith John TALLON

Phoenix Surgery
9 Chesterton Lane, Cirencester GL7 1XG
Tel: 01285 652056 Fax: 01285 641562
Email: phoenixsurgery@hotmail.com
Website: www.thephoenixsurgery.co.uk
(Cotswold and Vale Primary Care Trust)
Patient List Size: 10826

Practice Manager Moira McCall

GP Ian John SIMPSON, Christopher John GOLDIE, Gillian Margaret McINERNEY, Alison NICHOL, Philip REYNOLDS, Rohit SETHI, Nicola THURSTON

Rendcomb Surgery
Rendcomb, Cirencester GL7 7EY
Tel: 01285 831257 Fax: 01285 831679
(Cotswold and Vale Primary Care Trust)
Patient List Size: 3054

Practice Manager Maureen Brewer

GP Stuart William DRYSDALE, Ian DAVIS, Susan Eleanor WHITTLES

St Peter's Road Surgery
1 St. Peters Road, Cirencester GL7 1RF
Tel: 01285 653184 Fax: 01285 655795
(Cotswold and Vale Primary Care Trust)
Patient List Size: 7000

Practice Manager Laurella Parffrey

GP Martyn Frank HEWETT, Helen BROMWICH, Helen Elizabeth HEWETT, Michael Peter JACOB, James Edward MILLER

Clacton-on-Sea

East Lynne Medical Centre
3-5 Wellesley Road, Clacton-on-Sea CO15 3PP
Tel: 01255 220010 Fax: 01255 476350
(Tendring Primary Care Trust)
Patient List Size: 10867

Practice Manager P Mackenzie

GP Harvey Ingvald FAERESTRAND, Martin Patrick BARRY, Francine Marjorie BOWSHER, Diane Elizabeth HALSTEAD, Stuart James MACMILLAN

Epping Close Surgery
5-7 Epping Close, Clacton-on-Sea CO15 4UZ
Tel: 01255 222668 Fax: 01255 220946
(Tendring Primary Care Trust)

Practice Manager Alison Fityan

GP Zuhair Hamza Abdul Razak FITYAN

Frinton Road Surgery
68 Frinton Road, Holland-on-Sea, Clacton-on-Sea CO15 5UW
Tel: 01255 421778 Fax: 01255 812384
(Tendring Primary Care Trust)
Patient List Size: 5100

Practice Manager Andrea Apps

GP Amanda Grace Elizabeth Mary STEWART, Wolfgang SECKLER, Jane A SLAWSON

Grove Lodge Surgery
72 Queensway, Holland-on-Sea, Clacton-on-Sea CO15 5JU
Tel: 01255 815550
(Tendring Primary Care Trust)
Patient List Size: 2100

Practice Manager Jenny Bird

GP Andrew John LITTLEMORE

North Road Surgery
17 North Road, Great Clacton, Clacton-on-Sea CO15 4DA
Tel: 01255 423075 Fax: 01255 426215
(Tendring Primary Care Trust)
Patient List Size: 9800

Practice Manager B Mathias

GP Simon COX, Abdul K. GBLA, Vimala KARUNAKARAN, Padmini MISHRA, N PUVI

Old Road Surgery
147-149 Old Road, Clacton-on-Sea CO15 3AU
Tel: 01255 424334 Fax: 01255 475687

(Tendring Primary Care Trust)
Patient List Size: 6250

GP K U MIRZA, S M AL-NAJJAR

Ranworth Surgery
103 Pier Avenue, Clacton-on-Sea CO15 1NJ
Tel: 01255 421344 Fax: 01255 473581
Email: doctors@ransurg.demon.co.uk
(Tendring Primary Care Trust)
Patient List Size: 5644

Practice Manager Hazel Martin

GP Thomas James CULLEN, Gary Alan SWEENEY

St James Surgery
89 Wash Lane, Clacton-on-Sea CO15 1DA
Tel: 01255 222121 Fax: 01255 436479
(Tendring Primary Care Trust)
Patient List Size: 12500

Practice Manager H J Knappett

GP Michael MANN, Wendy Margaret FAERESTRAND, Anthony Robert GRANGE, John Philip Pius LINEEN, Alan John MORRISON, V M RAJA, G TABBONE

The Surgery
High Street, Thorpe-le-Soken, Clacton-on-Sea CO16 0EA
Tel: 01255 861850 Fax: 01255 860330
(Tendring Primary Care Trust)
Patient List Size: 2700

Practice Manager Stephanie Durrant

GP Linda Alison BUCHANAN, Alasdair David Colin MACKENZIE

The Surgery
Units 7-8, Crusader Bus Park, Stephenson Road West, Clacton-on-Sea CO15 4TN
Tel: 01255 688805 Fax: 01255 223169
(Tendring Primary Care Trust)
Patient List Size: 3000

Practice Manager Sharon Holding

GP John Leonard GUILLE

Cleckheaton

Drs Greenwood, Scrivings, Cameron and Davies
The Health Centre, Greenside, Cleckheaton BD19 5AP
Tel: 01274 872650 Fax: 01274 851871
(North Kirklees Primary Care Trust)
Patient List Size: 4900

Practice Manager Pam Fortune

GP Alan GREENWOOD, Andrew James CAMERON, Dr DAVIES, Belinda Ann SCRIVINGS

The Health Centre
Greenside, Cleckheaton BD19 5AN
Tel: 01274 872200
(North Kirklees Primary Care Trust)
Patient List Size: 6000

Practice Manager Carol Eastwood

GP Geoffrey Stewart FOX, Jane STRINGER

St Johns House Surgery
St Johns House, Cross Church Street, Cleckheaton BD19 3RQ
Tel: 01274 851188 Fax: 01274 851042
(North Kirklees Primary Care Trust)

Practice Manager Kathy Jowett

GP Muhammad Sayeed Akhtar KHAN, Sarah Louise NICHOLLS, Andrew John WOODHALL

Cleethorpes

Blundell Park Surgery
142-144 Grimsby Road, Cleethorpes DN35 7DL
Tel: 01472 699522 Fax: 01472 694652
(North East Lincolnshire Primary Care Trust)
Patient List Size: 1850

Practice Manager Karen Thickett

GP Dinabandhu SARKAR

Grimsby Road Medical Practice
18-20 Grimsby Road, Cleethorpes DN35 7AB
Tel: 01472 342859
(North East Lincolnshire Primary Care Trust)

GP Dr KUMAR, Dr KUMAR

Pembroke House
32 Albert Road, Cleethorpes DN35 8LU
Tel: 01472 691033 Fax: 01472 291516
(North East Lincolnshire Primary Care Trust)
Patient List Size: 1200

Practice Manager Gill Woodward

GP Iain Alexander SUTHERLAND, Sudip Kumar BHADURI, B BISWAS, Timothy John BRUNING, Dr FIRKIN, J HANSON, Philip HURST, Dr LAVIN, Dr OSBORNE

Purser and Partners
Clee Medical Centre, 323 Grimsby Road, Cleethorpes DN35 7XE
Tel: 01472 697257 Fax: 01472 690852
Website: www.cleemedicalcentre.co.uk
(North East Lincolnshire Primary Care Trust)
Patient List Size: 16100

Practice Manager David Hawley

GP Paul Cyril PURSER, Robert Nicolson CROMBIE, Dr DIJOUX, Craig DOBSON, Dr GUILAS, Jasmine MUNJAL, A D STEAD

Singh and Reddy
44 Grimsby Road, Cleethorpes DN35 7AB
Tel: 01472 342763 Fax: 01472 344490
(North East Lincolnshire Primary Care Trust)
Patient List Size: 4000

Practice Manager Mary Johnson

GP Narendra Pal SINGH, V R L REDDY

The Surgery
6-7 Aspen Court, Belvoir Park Road, Cleethorpes DN35 0SJ
Tel: 01472 291977
(North East Lincolnshire Primary Care Trust)

GP Mushtaq Ahmad ZARO

The Surgery
202 Grimsby Road, Cleethorpes DN35 7EZ
Tel: 01472 691040 Fax: 01472 290624
(North East Lincolnshire Primary Care Trust)
Patient List Size: 1685

Practice Manager Dawn Best

GP I K C HUNTER

The Surgery
64 St Peter's Avenue, Cleethorpes DN35 8HP
Tel: 01472 691606 Fax: 01472 290057
(North East Lincolnshire Primary Care Trust)

Practice Manager Christine Whitby

GP R JAISWAL

The Surgery
1 Isaacs Hill, Cleethorpes DN35 8JX
Tel: 01472 691162 Fax: 01472 290493
(North East Lincolnshire Primary Care Trust)
Patient List Size: 1900

GP R D P VEDUTLA

Clevedon

Clevedon Health Centre
Old Street, Clevedon BS21 6DG
Tel: 01275 335512
(North Somerset Primary Care Trust)

GP Robert Dean BULLOCK, A BYRNE, Martin Charles HIME, D K S IRVING, Stephen Howard Christopher PILL, Sophia Ann SANDFORD

Sunnyside Surgery
4 Sunnyside Road, Clevedon BS21 7TA
Tel: 01275 873588 Fax: 01275 875218
Email: sue.wilson@gp-L81102.nhs.uk
(North Somerset Primary Care Trust)
Patient List Size: 6520

Practice Manager Sue Wilson

GP John Jeffrey FORD, Emma C COORE, Glenda R HORNER, Samuel J PARTRIDGE, Elizabeth A S PATRICK

Clitheroe

Pendleside Medical Practice
Clitheroe Health Centre, Railway View Road, Clitheroe BB7 2JG
Tel: 01200 422674 Fax: 01200 443652
(Hyndburn and Ribble Valley Primary Care Trust)

Practice Manager David Priest

GP William John David McKINLAY, John Alasdair Fraser CARTER, Melanie Anne CRONIN, Alan CROWTHER, Henryk John ZAKRZEWSKI

Pendleside Medical Practice
Clitheroe Health Centre, Railway View Road, Clitheroe BB7 2JG
Tel: 01200 422674 Fax: 01200 443652
(Hyndburn and Ribble Valley Primary Care Trust)

GP Sheila BAILEY, Martin FLATLEY, Richard Antony FREEMAN, Ronald James HIGSON, Anne Sybil HUSON, John SAUNDERS

Pendleside Medical Practice
Clitheroe Health Centre, Railway View Road, Clitheroe BB7 2JG
Tel: 01200 425201
(Hyndburn and Ribble Valley Primary Care Trust)

Practice Manager Marjorie Saberton

GP Benjamin Torquil Neilson HUTCHISON, Ian James IBBOTSON, William George MACKEAN

Slaidburn Health Centre
Shay Lane, Slaidburn, Clitheroe BB7 3EP
Tel: 01200 446229 Fax: 01200 446258
(Hyndburn and Ribble Valley Primary Care Trust)
Patient List Size: 1050

GP Neil WILSON, Sheelagh DONNELLY

Coalville

Belvoir Road Surgery
99 Belvoir Road, Coalville LE67 3PH
Tel: 01530 831331 Fax: 01530 833985
Email: surgeryone@lineone.net
(Charnwood and North West Leicestershire Primary Care Trust)
Patient List Size: 8250

Practice Manager J Keane

GP David Patrick Vaughan HEWITT, Timothy Marcus HAMMOND, Christopher David HEWITT, Lynne Mary MORGAN, Nicholas Robert PULMAN

Broom Leys Surgery
Broom Leys Road, Coalville LE67 4DE
Tel: 01530 832095 Fax: 01530 815138
Email: broomleys@hotmail.com
(Charnwood and North West Leicestershire Primary Care Trust)
Patient List Size: 7500

Practice Manager Tony Dales

GP Ian Clive ROBINSON, Graham John HAZLEHURST, Colin HORSBURGH, Marcelle Wendy MORRIS, Katherine OLIVER

Coalville Health Centre
1 Market Street, Coalville LE67 3DX
Tel: 01530 835544
(Charnwood and North West Leicestershire Primary Care Trust)

GP M M DEVAIAH

Forest Road Health Centre
8 Forest Road, Hugglescote, Coalville LE67 3SH
Tel: 01530 832109
(Charnwood and North West Leicestershire Primary Care Trust)

Practice Manager J Cufflin

GP David John NEWMAN, P J CHAPMAN, David Mack WOODS

Whitwick Health Centre
North Street, Whitwick, Coalville LE67 5HX
Tel: 01530 838866 Fax: 01530 810581
(Charnwood and North West Leicestershire Primary Care Trust)
Patient List Size: 3800

Practice Manager C J Leeland

GP Alan GARLICK, E A HEPPLEWHITE

Whitwick Health Centre
North Street, Whitwick, Coalville LE67 5HX
Tel: 01530 839629 Fax: 01530 839065
(Charnwood and North West Leicestershire Primary Care Trust)

Practice Manager Pat Lee

GP Alan Mervyn LEWIS, R M PATEL

Whitwick Road Surgery
Whitwick Road, Coalville LE67 3FA
Tel: 01530 836507
(Charnwood and North West Leicestershire Primary Care Trust)

Practice Manager Suzanne Birkin

GP Pramod Mangesh KHIRWADKAR, Janet BAKER, Nilesh Jayantilal CHAWDA, Richard William LAWRENCE

Cobham

The Cobham Health Centre
168 Portsmouth Road, Cobham KT11 1HT
Tel: 01932 867231 Fax: 01932 866874
(East Elmbridge and Mid Surrey Primary Care Trust)

GP David Neill GLOVER, Maryse Ingrid Nilmini DESOR, Mark David Bedo HOBBS, Sarah Evelyn MACKAY, Michael Paul TRENT, Anthony WATSON, C A WRIGLEY

Cockermouth

Derwent House Surgery
Derwent House, Wakefield Road, Cockermouth CA13 0HZ
Tel: 01900 324100 Fax: 01900 324106
(West Cumbria Primary Care Trust)
Patient List Size: 6540

Practice Manager Pauline Bewley

GP Andrew RICHARD, David Gregory CLARKSON, Anne Elizabeth ELDRED, Jonathan MARSH, Alison Jane PEARSON

Fitz Road Surgery
24 Fitz Road, Cockermouth CA13 0AD
Tel: 01900 324124 Fax: 01900 324126
Website: www.northcumbriahealth.nhs.uk/fitzroad.nhs.uk
(West Cumbria Primary Care Trust)
Patient List Size: 2200

Practice Manager Greg Greenhalgh

GP John Paul HOWARTH, Annemieke Caroline NELIS

South Street Surgery
South Street, Cockermouth CA13 9QP
Tel: 01900 324123 Fax: 01900 827511
(West Cumbria Primary Care Trust)
Patient List Size: 7500

Practice Manager F Tibbitts

GP David Michael LEES, Gillian Lesley CAMPBELL, Nicholas Robert Laurence COWAN, Simon Andrew DESERT, Sian GILCHRIST

Colchester

Ambrose Avenue Surgery
76 Ambrose Avenue, Colchester CO3 4LN
Tel: 01206 549444 Fax: 01206 369910
(Colchester Primary Care Trust)
Patient List Size: 15248

Practice Manager Jean Smith

GP Joseph Pius HUBER, Lester CARLYON, Max Peter HICKMAN, Helen Margaret JAMES, Naila KARIM, Colin Roy MACALLAN, Madeleine Ann WILSON

The Avenue Surgery
71 The Avenue, Wivenhoe, Colchester CO7 9PP
Tel: 01206 824447 Fax: 01206 827973
(Colchester Primary Care Trust)
Patient List Size: 7600

Practice Manager Jane Ringland

GP John Clinton Parker HALE, Andrew Ian COPE, Anne Philippa HAWLEY

Bluebell Surgery
Jack Andrews Drive, Highwoods, Colchester CO4 9YU
Tel: 01256 855222 Fax: 01256 845681
(Colchester Primary Care Trust)
Patient List Size: 1677

Practice Manager Sue Poole

GP R T KURIAKOSE, M PARSONS

Castle Gardens Medical Centre
78 East Hill, Colchester CO1 2QS
Tel: 01206 866626 Fax: 01206 869575
(Colchester Primary Care Trust)
Patient List Size: 6905

Practice Manager Jane Frost

GP Stuart David RUDGE, Karen CHUMBLEY, Philippa GEAR, Barbara MURRAY

Coggeshall Surgery
Stoneham Street, Coggeshall, Colchester CO6 1UH
Tel: 01376 561242 Fax: 01376 563486
(Witham, Braintree and Halstead Care Trust)

Practice Manager Jane Chapman

GP Justin David Titus BARKHAM, E A BEVAN

Colne Medical Centre
40 Station Road, Brightlingsea, Colchester CO7 0DT
Tel: 01206 302522 Fax: 01206 305131
(Tendring Primary Care Trust)

Practice Manager Caroline Bowden

GP Graham David PARKER, Michael Forsyth HARE, Andrew Alexander JUSTICE, Philip Henry Jodrell LETTON

Creffield Road Surgery
19 Creffield Road, Colchester CO3 3HZ
Tel: 01206 570371 Fax: 01206 369908
(Colchester Primary Care Trust)

Practice Manager Pauline Emerson

GP Paul MARFLEET, Nicholas Thomas DIXON, Carol Elizabeth Branson JONES, Andrew Michael LENNARD-JONES, Anne Vivien ST JOSEPH

East Hill Surgery
78 East Hill, Colchester CO1 2RW
Tel: 01206 866133 Fax: 01206 869054
(Colchester Primary Care Trust)

Practice Manager Christine Owen

GP Alan James OGILVIE, Robert Charles CUTLER, David John HENDERSON, Pamela Louise WRIGHT

The Hawthorn Surgery
The St Edmunds Centre, Tamarisk Way, Greenstead, Colchester CO4 3YA
Tel: 01206 871157 Fax: 01206 869567
(Colchester Primary Care Trust)
Patient List Size: 3425

Practice Manager Isabelle Kendall

GP Beate W GRIMM, Anthony David CHYC

High Street Surgery
46 High Street, Kelvedon, Colchester CO5 9AG
Tel: 01376 572906 Fax: 01376 572484
(Witham, Braintree and Halstead Care Trust)
Patient List Size: 3600

Practice Manager Linda Wells

GP Cedric Francis Derek THOMPSON, E B IRWIN

Highwoods Square Surgery
Highwoods Square, Colchester CO4 4SR
Tel: 01206 752010 Fax: 01206 843280
(Colchester Primary Care Trust)

Practice Manager Diana Bates

GP Tirunelveli Lakshmanaswamy ASHOK KUMAR

The Hollies Surgery
The Green, Great Bentley, Colchester CO7 8PJ
Tel: 01206 250691 Fax: 01206 252496
Email: postmaster@gp-F81021.nhs.uk
(Tendring Primary Care Trust)
Patient List Size: 8250

Practice Manager Hugh Cronin

GP Freda BHATTI, Nicholas Francis CAVENAGH, Mathew John Nicholas HUNT, Debra Jane LETTON, Nicholas Brian Michael STEINER

Kelvedon Surgery
59 High Street, Kelvedon, Colchester CO5 9AE
Tel: 0870 417 3980 Fax: 01376 573602
Email: barbara.lord@gp-f81738.nhs.uk
(Witham, Braintree and Halstead Care Trust)
Patient List Size: 4100

Practice Manager Barbara Lord

GP R A ALSAYED, M CHESTERS, C J MACNAMARA

Layer Road Surgery
Layer Road, Colchester CO2 9LA
Tel: 01206 546494 Fax: 01206 369912
(Colchester Primary Care Trust)

Practice Manager Melanie Lodge

GP Antoine BANNA, Laurence Alfred William RUSHBROOK, Susan Lynda STEDMAN

Maltings Green Road Surgery
64 Maltings Green Road, Layer de la Haye, Colchester CO2 0JJ
Tel: 01206 734293 Fax: 01206 734070
(Colchester Primary Care Trust)
Patient List Size: 2500

Practice Manager Margaret Sadler

GP Christine Thelma TARALA

Mersea Road Surgery
272a Mersea Road, Colchester CO2 8QY
Tel: 01206 764374 Fax: 01206 765667
(Colchester Primary Care Trust)

Practice Manager Judy Watts

GP David WITHNALL, Richard William Stephen COULSON, Jonathan Christopher GATLAND, Huw MORGAN-DAVIES, Clive SOUTHGATE

Mill Road Surgery
61 Mill Road, Mile End, Colchester CO4 5LE
Tel: 01206 845900 Fax: 01206 844090
(Colchester Primary Care Trust)
Patient List Size: 6985

Practice Manager Mary Reynolds

GP Christopher Roy GILBERT, Clair CARPENTER, Tracey COPEMAN, Philippa Margaret TUCKER

North Hill Surgery
18 North Hill, Colchester CO1 1DZ
Tel: 01206 578070 Fax: 01206 769880
(Colchester Primary Care Trust)
Patient List Size: 12600

Practice Manager Carole Baldwin

GP David James Alexander BATEMAN, Stuart Peter BALDWIN, Susan DIXON, Vivian Edward Noel FOX, Kilian HOCHESTEIN-MINTZEI, David Robert Marmion MILNE, Louisa POLAK

North Station Road Surgery
78 North Station Road, Colchester CO1 1SE
Tel: 01206 574483 Fax: 01206 767558
(Colchester Primary Care Trust)
Patient List Size: 3000

Practice Manager Jayne Roe

GP Laurel Loveday Rosemary SPOONER

Parsons Heath Medical Practice
35A Parsons Heath, Colchester CO4 3HS
Tel: 01206 864395 Fax: 01206 869047
(Colchester Primary Care Trust)
Patient List Size: 11800

Practice Manager Janice Wood

GP Michael Henry MOORE, Jane Elizabeth BEAUCHAMP, Martin James HARGREAVES, Una Catherine O'CALLAGHAN, Peter Michael SAMPSON, Robert Eric THIBAUT

Portland Road Surgery
2 Portland Road, Colchester CO2 7EH
Tel: 01206 369936 Fax: 01206 766033
(Colchester Primary Care Trust)
Patient List Size: 2160

Practice Manager Marion Llewellyn

GP Erwin Alexander RODRIGUES

Rectory Road Surgery
7 Rectory Road, Rowhedge, Colchester CO5 7HP
Tel: 01206 728585 Fax: 01206 729262
(Colchester Primary Care Trust)
Patient List Size: 10156

Practice Manager Kevan Baker

GP Paul Andrew RASOR, Siobhan Maire O'REGAN, Roderick Peter ROSS-MARRS, M WALL

Richardson Road Surgery
56 Richardson Road, East Bergholt, Colchester CO7 6RR
Tel: 01206 298272 Fax: 01206 299010
(Central Suffolk Primary Care Trust)
Patient List Size: 12000

Practice Manager Lesley Hutchings

GP Sidney Albert Bruce FINCH, Fayez Khaled AYACHE, Paul Jeremy Alistair HALFHIDE, Richard Roy Graydon POOLE, Michael Dahlbom PULLEN

Shrub End Road Surgery
122 Shrub End Road, Colchester CO3 4RY
Tel: 01206 573605 Fax: 01206 200219
(Colchester Primary Care Trust)
Patient List Size: 8180

Practice Manager Paul Faber

GP Andrew William Russell LOTHIAN, Judith Anne BROWN, Linda Margareta Elisabeth MAHON-DALY, Richard Pearce WRIGHT

The Surgery
32 Kingsland Road, West Mersea, Colchester CO5 8RA
Tel: 01206 382015 Fax: 01206 385593
(Colchester Primary Care Trust)

Practice Manager Marion Harding

GP Austin Stephen MARSHALL, Penelope Ann MATTHES, Janis Ann MEANLEY, Philip Alan Michael WOODCOCK

The Surgery
Queens Road, Earls Colne, Colchester CO6 2RR
Tel: 01787 222022
(Witham, Braintree and Halstead Care Trust)
Patient List Size: 7500

Practice Manager Sylvia Hopkins, Jo Watson

GP Denis Paul BROGAN, Paul Martin SPOWAGE, Edward John STANNARD, Anthea Hilary YORK

The Surgery
Dedham Road, Ardleigh, Colchester CO7 7LD
Tel: 01206 230224 Fax: 01206 231602
Email: postmaster@gp-F81044.nhs.uk
Website: www.ardleighsurgery.nhs.uk
(Colchester Primary Care Trust)
Patient List Size: 4900

Practice Manager Fred Merrin

GP Paul J MANDERS, Vernon Selby BETTLE, Jane Mary OWENS

Tiptree Medical Centre
Church Road, Tiptree, Colchester CO5 0HB
Tel: 01621 816475 Fax: 01621 819902
Email: info@medcentre.co.uk
Website: tiptree-medcentre.co.uk
(Colchester Primary Care Trust)
Patient List Size: 1100

Practice Manager John Grover

GP Nicholas Arden TURNER, Philip David BROWN, Shane Anron GORDON

Wimpole Road Surgery
52 Wimpole Road, Colchester CO1 2DL
Tel: 01206 794794 Fax: 01206 790403
(Colchester Primary Care Trust)
Patient List Size: 9430

Practice Manager Sallyann Pamment

GP Patricia Margaret CLARIDGE, Andrew Graham Hunter DAVIDSON, John Dennis JEFFRIES, Imran RAMJAN

Winstree Road Surgery
84 Winstree Road, Colchester CO3 5PZ
Tel: 01206 572372 Fax: 01206 764412
(Colchester Primary Care Trust)

Practice Manager Alan Davis

GP Eamonn Gabriel O'CALLAGHAN, Lloyd GUNETILLEKE, Clive George MORRIS

Coleford

Brunston Surgery
Cinderhill, Coleford GL16 8HJ
Tel: 01594 833255 Fax: 01594 810971
(West Gloucestershire Primary Care Trust)
Patient List Size: 5500

Practice Manager Carol Hallam

GP Andrew John Merrill COATES, Eric PORTMAN, Gwyn ROBERTS

Coleford Health Centre
Railway Drive, Coleford GL16 8RH
Tel: 01594 832117
(West Gloucestershire Primary Care Trust)
Patient List Size: 7600

Practice Manager Bridget Docking

GP Nicholas Mark WILKINSON, Janet ADAMS, Barbara Danielle CUMMINS, Rupert Hillary LONGLEY

Colford Health Centre
Railway Drive, Coleford GL16 8RH
Tel: 01594 598068 Fax: 01594 810683
(West Gloucestershire Primary Care Trust)
Patient List Size: 1975

Practice Manager Susie D Nagle

GP Paul Joseph NAGLE, Janet M ADAMS, Barbara D CUMMINS, Rupert Hillary LONGLEY, Nicholas Mark WILKINSON

Colne

Colne Health Centre
Market Street, Colne BB8 0LJ
Tel: 01282 862451 Fax: 01282 871698
(Burnley, Pendle and Rossendale Primary Care Trust)

Practice Manager C Jackson

GP Thomas Varley COWPE, Fiona Jayne KERRIDGE, Cecil Samuel NORTHRIDGE, Bogdan Maciej PALMOWSKI, Caroline Mary SPENCER-PALMER

Harambee Surgery
27 Skipton Road, Trawden, Colne BB8 8QU
Tel: 01282 868482 Fax: 01282 862685
Email: david.molyneux@nhs.net
(Burnley, Pendle and Rossendale Primary Care Trust)
Patient List Size: 3500

Practice Manager Angela Emmott

GP David Harvey MOLYNEUX, Carien VILJOEN

Park Road New Surgery
Park Road, Barnoldswick, Colne BB18 5BG
Tel: 01282 812244 Fax: 01282 850220
(Burnley, Pendle and Rossendale Primary Care Trust)

Practice Manager A R Watson

GP Ian BOWER, Ian David BROWN, S BRYAN, Stuart Richard BRYAN, Geoffrey Harold COOPER, Angela Caroline HARE, Sheila Mary JACKSON, Robert KENNY

Congleton

Lawton House Surgery
Bromley Road, Congleton CW12 1QG
Tel: 01260 275454 Fax: 01260 298412
(Eastern Cheshire Primary Care Trust)
Patient List Size: 9200

Practice Manager Melanie Lyman

GP Adam Charles DUTTON, Miranda FARMER, David FRAY, Mary HESKETH, Richard Gibson POTTER, Caroline Margaret TAYLOR

Meadowside Medical Centre
Meadowside, Mountbatten Way, Congleton CW12 1DY
Tel: 01260 272331 Fax: 01260 294759
(Eastern Cheshire Primary Care Trust)

Practice Manager Beverley Griffiths, Mary Mobley

GP Clare Mary THOMSON, John Bradley Standish BROOKS, Ian HULME, Pamela JAMES, Mary LOUGHRAN, Christopher John STUDDS

Readesmoor Medical Group Practice
29-29A West Street, Congleton CW12 1JP
Tel: 01260 276161 Fax: 01260 297340
(Eastern Cheshire Primary Care Trust)
Patient List Size: 13250

Practice Manager Anita Harris

GP Timothy Holland BAKER, Warwick John BRINDLEY, Paul Thomas BROMLEY, Elizabeth Ann CARTER, Gillian Elizabeth KAY, Peter John RIGBY, Stuart Alan THOMAS

Coniston

Wraysdale House Surgery
Wraysdale House, Coniston LA21 8ES
Tel: 01539 441205 Fax: 01539 441205
Email: wraysdale@hotmail.com
(Morecambe Bay Primary Care Trust)
Patient List Size: 1100

GP Raymond Anthony Berry WOOD

Consett

Consett Medical Centre
Station Yard, Consett DH8 5YA
Tel: 01207 216116 Fax: 01207 216119
(Derwentside Primary Care Trust)
Patient List Size: 20000

Practice Manager Kathleen Robson

GP William John STEVENSON, Liam Frederick AINSWORTH, John Charlton ELLIOTT, Ernest James FLYNN, Pablo GARCIA, Claire HAMILTON, Judith Ann MOUNTFORD, Diane Margaret PETTERSON, L PLUNKETT, John TURNER, John Dewar YOUNG

Leadgate Surgery
George Ewen House, Watling Street, Consett DH8 6DP
Tel: 01207 583555 Fax: 01207 215150
(Derwentside Primary Care Trust)
Patient List Size: 4483

Practice Manager John Hall

GP David Adrian ASTLEY, John A J ELLIS, Susan LEVICK

Queens Road Surgery
10B Queens Road, Blackhill, Consett DH8 0BN
Tel: 01207 216432 Fax: 01207 216426
(Derwentside Primary Care Trust)

Practice Manager Alyson Marshall

GP John Roger HAMILTON, A J CLARKE, S P ENGLISH, Jonathan Frank LEVICK, J STUART, J N WORTHY

Corbridge

Corbridge Health Centre
Manor Court, Corbridge NE45 5JW
Tel: 01434 632011 Fax: 01434 633878
(Northumberland Care Trust)
Patient List Size: 6400

Practice Manager Norna White

GP William Francis CUNNINGHAM, Roger James DYKINS, David George HARLE, Robert William James KINGETT, Robin MULROY

Corby

Great Oakley Medical Centre
Barth Close, Great Oakley, Corby NN18 8LU
Tel: 01536 460046 Fax: 01536 461404
(Northamptonshire Heartlands Primary Care Trust)

Practice Manager Kay Taylor

GP Tristan John Nicholson HARRIS

Lakeside Surgery
Cottingham Road, Corby NN17 2UR
Tel: 01536 204154 Fax: 01536 748286
(Northamptonshire Heartlands Primary Care Trust)
Patient List Size: 16800

Practice Manager Linda Ward

GP Peter Joseph George WILCZYNSKI, Richard David BAXTER, D J BROWN, John Gregory MELLOR, Susan Margaret WADSWORTH, Russell Neil WHITTAKER

The Medical Centre
Forest Gate Road, Corby NN17 1TR
Tel: 01536 202507 Fax: 01536 206099
(Northamptonshire Heartlands Primary Care Trust)
Patient List Size: 15000

Practice Manager Murial Witt

GP Paul Vinton BUCKINGHAM, Ian Macleod BOWIE, Colin GRAHAM, David Allan PALMER, Christopher Terence PARTINGTON, Simon WADE

Norse Walk Surgery
66 Norse Walk, Corby NN18 9DG
Tel: 01536 743228 Fax: 01536 460092
(Northamptonshire Heartlands Primary Care Trust)

Practice Manager Sue Singh

GP Bimal Ranjan BHATTACHARYA

Studfall Medical Centre
Studfall Avenue, Corby NN17 1LG
Tel: 01536 401372 Fax: 01536 401300
(Northamptonshire Heartlands Primary Care Trust)

Practice Manager Gill M Weal

GP Buddhadeb SANYALL, P CAIN, David Ian MARSH

Studfall Medical Centre
Studfall Avenue, Corby NN17 1LG
Tel: 01536 401371 Fax: 01536 401300
(Northamptonshire Heartlands Primary Care Trust)

Practice Manager Judith Mathew

GP Roman Peter SUMIRA

Willowbrook Health Centre
Cottingham Road, Corby NN17 2UR
Tel: 01536 265311 Fax: 01536 403263
(Northamptonshire Heartlands Primary Care Trust)

Practice Manager Mrs Khan

GP Salahuddin KHAN

Willowbrook Health Centre
Cottingham Road, Corby NN17 2UR
Tel: 01536 406711/265311/400600 Fax: 01536 402153/403263
(Northamptonshire Heartlands Primary Care Trust)

Practice Manager Anne Amos

GP James Dermot O'NEILL, A R BROWN, S KHAN, K R WILLIAMS

Willowbrook Health Centre
Cottingham Road, Corby NN17 2UR
Tel: 01536 260303 Fax: 01536 406761
(Northamptonshire Heartlands Primary Care Trust)

Practice Manager Hazel Beaver

GP Ian Raymond TREHARNE, F M ROGERS

Woodsend Medical Centre
Woodsend Medical Centre, School Place, Corby NN18 0QP
Tel: 01536 407006 Fax: 01536 401711
(Northamptonshire Heartlands Primary Care Trust)
Patient List Size: 8000

Practice Manager Linda E Whitehead

GP M Akram KHALID, Cathryn Rebecca APPLETON, Angeli MAYE, David NEWMAN

Corsham

Box Surgery
London Road, Box, Corsham SN13 8NA
Tel: 01225 742361 Fax: 01225 742646
(Kennet and North Wiltshire Primary Care Trust)
Patient List Size: 6300

Practice Manager Jeni Leggat

GP John Anthony BULLEN, Kevin GRUFFYDD-JONES, Hannah Elizabeth LEYDEN, Susan Jane WALKER

Porch Surgery
Beechfield Road, Corsham SN13 9DL
Tel: 01249 712232 Fax: 01249 701389
(Kennet and North Wiltshire Primary Care Trust)
Patient List Size: 10500

Practice Manager Helen Paish

GP David John MacARTHUR, Heather Elizabeth BAKER, Simon James BURRELL, Andrew Simon COWIE, Margaret Jean HATHERELL, Tim MONELLE, Claire RIGBY, Eoin SPILLANER, Lesley Margaret STARR, Anne-Marie WILCOX

Cottingham

Cottingham Medical Centre
17-19 South Street, Cottingham HU16 4AJ
Tel: 01482 845078 Fax: 01482 845078
Website: www.cottinghammedicalcentre.co.uk
(East Yorkshire Primary Care Trust)
Patient List Size: 8750

Practice Manager Brian Harrison

GP John Christopher WILLSON, Diane BILLINGS, Lesley ELLIOTT, Diarmuid Niall Brian KIERAN, Michael MORGAN

Hallgate Surgery
123 Hallgate, Cottingham HU16 4DA
Tel: 01482 845832
(East Yorkshire Primary Care Trust)

Practice Manager Kate Webster

GP M E HANCOCKS

Thwaite Street Surgery
The Chestnuts, 45 Thwaite Street, Cottingham HU16 4QX
Tel: 01482 847250 Fax: 01482 848173
(East Yorkshire Primary Care Trust)
Patient List Size: 3270

Practice Manager Tracey Mulholland

GP J ROBSON

Coulsdon

Bramley Avenue Surgery
1B Bramley Avenue, Coulsdon CR5 2DR
Tel: 020 8660 0193 Fax: 020 8763 8952
(Croydon Primary Care Trust)
Patient List Size: 2160

Practice Manager Rizwana Baig

GP H KULARATNE

Chipstead Valley Road Surgery
48B Chipstead Valley Road, Coulsdon CR5 2RA
Tel: 020 8660 9400 Fax: 020 8645 9415
(Croydon Primary Care Trust)
Patient List Size: 4300

Practice Manager Jo McKay

GP P G SAMARAWICKRAMA

Coulsdon Medical Practice
66 Brighton Road, Coulsdon CR5 2BB
Tel: 020 8660 2700 Fax: 020 8763 2706
(Croydon Primary Care Trust)
Patient List Size: 3370

Practice Manager Penny Johnson

GP Jamil Ahmad KHAN

Coulsdon Road Practice
157A Coulsdon Road, Old Coulsdon, Coulsdon CR5 1EG
Tel: 01737 553660 Fax: 01737 550477
Email: mohammed.irfan@gp-H83614.nhs.uk
(Croydon Primary Care Trust)
Patient List Size: 1300

Practice Manager Sue Colomb

GP Mohammed IRFAN

Old Coulsdon Medical Practice
2A Court Avenue, Old Coulsdon, Coulsdon CR5 1HF
Tel: 01737 553393 Fax: 01737 550267
(Croydon Primary Care Trust)
Patient List Size: 10687

Practice Manager Richard Frier

GP Peter Benedict John BOFFA, Iain David CRUICKSHANK, M GALLAGHER, J HARCOURT, R MacCALLUM

Tollers Lane Surgery
59 Tollers Lane, Old Coulsdon, Coulsdon CR5 1BF
Tel: 01737 556880
(Croydon Primary Care Trust)
Patient List Size: 1650

Practice Manager Jan James

GP Subhash Chander CHITKARA

Woodcote Group Practice
140 Chipstead Valley Road, Coulsdon CR5 3BB
Tel: 020 8660 1305
Website: www.woodcotegrouppractice.co.uk
(Croydon Primary Care Trust)
Patient List Size: 15500

Practice Manager Nan Nobes

GP Kaleem KHAN, John Graham LINNEY, Peter William NEWLANDS, Fola SHOBOWALE, C WEBSTER-SMITH

Coventry

Allesley Park Medical Centre
Whitaker Road No.2, Coventry CV5 9JE
Tel: 024 7667 4123 Fax: 024 7667 2196
(Coventry Teaching Primary Care Trust)

Practice Manager A Boutall, Jeanette Udeshi

GP Richard James BALLANTINE, Matthew John BUTLER, Elizabeth Williamson Hunter COWAN, Robert David JONES, Sheila Deirdre SHIELDS, Daniele Alexandra THORNTON

Balliol Road Surgery
1 Balliol Road, Coventry CV2 3DR
Tel: 024 7644 911 Fax: 024 7663 6526
(Coventry Teaching Primary Care Trust)

Practice Manager Shirley Streeting

GP Patricia Margaret WEAVER, Ranjita ALLAN, Zaw MIN, Khin Myint MO

Bennetts Road North Surgery
2 Bennetts Road North, Keresley End, Coventry CV7 8LA
Tel: 024 7633 2636 Fax: 024 7633 7353
(Coventry Teaching Primary Care Trust)

Practice Manager Maxine Simmonds

GP Rodney Alan SWALLOW, Ruth Barbara GIRVAN, Peter Jeremy HORN, Ethel M Y MWALE, Andrew John SMITHERS

Brandon Road Surgery
108 Brandon Road, Binley, Coventry CV3 2JF
Tel: 024 7645 3634 Fax: 024 7663 6886
(Coventry Teaching Primary Care Trust)

Practice Manager Maureen Price

GP Peter Sylvanus KENYON, Dr GRIFFITHS, Mark Edward LAWTON, I McMORRAN, Mohammad SHAHABUDDIN

Bredon Avenue Surgery
232 Bredon Avenue, Binley, Coventry CV3 2FD
Tel: 024 7645 8777 Fax: 024 7643 1839
(Coventry Teaching Primary Care Trust)

Practice Manager V Smith

GP Danuta Bozena PERLIK-KOLACKI

Broad Lane Surgery
684 Broad Lane, Coventry CV5 7BB
Tel: 024 7646 6583 Fax: 024 7669 5972
(Coventry Teaching Primary Care Trust)
Patient List Size: 3100

Practice Manager D O'Brien

GP John Anthony O'BRIEN

Broad Street Surgery
129 Broad Street, Coventry CV6 5BD
Tel: 024 7666 3111
(Coventry Teaching Primary Care Trust)

GP Mansoor SOOMRO

Broomfield Park Medical Centre, Spon End
5 Albany Road, Earlsdon, Coventry CV1 3HQ
Tel: 024 7622 8606 Fax: 024 7622 9985
(Coventry Teaching Primary Care Trust)

Practice Manager Ann Boutall, Tim Morris, Anne Parsons

GP Colin Ernest PARKER, Christine Susanne DURR, Roger Nevill LEE, Fiona Anne RITCHIE, Peter Michael WHIDBORNE

Central Medical Centre
42 St. Pauls Road, Coventry CV6 5DF
Tel: 024 7668 1231 Fax: 024 7666 4935
(Coventry Teaching Primary Care Trust)
Patient List Size: 4900

Practice Manager I G Sheikh

GP Sheikh SAEED-AHMAD, Raj Kumar DUTTA

Copsewood Medical Centre
95 Momus Boulevard, Coventry CV2 5NB
Tel: 024 7645 7497 Fax: 024 7663 6395
(Coventry Teaching Primary Care Trust)

Practice Manager Brenda Stuart

GP Gurdip Singh JUDGE, Naheed T KAZMI

Crossley Practice
16 Henley Road, Coventry CV2 1LP
Tel: 024 7666 8401 Fax: 024 7666 7127
Website: www.thecrossleypractice.fsnet.co.uk
(Coventry Teaching Primary Care Trust)
Patient List Size: 6100

Practice Manager Pauline Smart

GP Stephen James WEBSTER, Joseph Martin BOOKER, Grant Jonathan INGRAMS

Daventry Road Surgery
281 Daventry Road, Coventry CV3 5HJ
Tel: 024 7650 3485 Fax: 024 7650 5730
(Coventry Teaching Primary Care Trust)
Patient List Size: 3280

Practice Manager T Briggs

GP Rashpal Singh DOSANJ

Doctors Surgery
2 Maidavale Crescent, Coventry CV3 6FZ
Tel: 024 7641 2372 Fax: 024 7641 1318
(Coventry Teaching Primary Care Trust)

GP Hugh Christopher EVANS, Maribasappa JAGADESHWARI

Engleton House Surgery
2 Villa Road, Coventry CV6 3HZ
Tel: 024 7659 2012 Fax: 024 7660 1913
(Coventry Teaching Primary Care Trust)

Patient List Size: 13500

Practice Manager Janet Hastings

GP Keith Thomas THOMSON, Jeremy DALE, David Laurence DAWES, Terence Joseph EATON, Moira Nancy HILL, Paul Graeme JOHNSON, Claire Catherine KEANE, Sandra THORNTON

Ezzat and Partners

Phoenix Family Care, 35 Park Road, Coventry CV1 2LE
Tel: 024 7622 7234 Fax: 024 7663 4816
(Coventry Teaching Primary Care Trust)
Patient List Size: 7200

Practice Manager Elizabeth C Cartwright, Andrea Reid

GP Ali Ahmed EZZAT, Susan Mary EXON, Ian James WARD

Foleshill Road Surgery

949 Foleshill Road, Coventry CV6 5HN
Tel: 024 7668 8482/8230 Fax: 024 76688230
(Coventry Teaching Primary Care Trust)
Patient List Size: 9500

Practice Manager Chris Bacon

GP Sewa Singh LYALL, Senarath BOGAHALANDE, Andrew Marshall HERD, Jennifer SNOWDON, Asadu SSEMWOGERERE

Forum Health Centre

1A Farren Road, Wyken, Coventry CV2 5EP
Tel: 024 7626 6370 Fax: 024 7663 6518
(Coventry Teaching Primary Care Trust)

Practice Manager Francis Dixon

GP Brian COLE, Dr CHOHAN, Trevor Jude DE SOUZA, W LOVATT, Sabaratnam THEVENDRA, Madeline WELLS

George Eliot Medical Centre

216 Foleshill Road, Coventry CV1 4JH
Tel: 024 7652 0183 Fax: 024 7623 0205
(Coventry Teaching Primary Care Trust)

Practice Manager Krisna Parnandi

GP Tribhovan Premjibhai JOTANGIA

Govind Health Centre

77c Moor Street, Coventry CV5 6EU
Tel: 024 7667 5016 Fax: 024 7671 7405
(Coventry Teaching Primary Care Trust)

GP Madhu GARALA

Harnall Lane Medical Centre

Harnall Lane East, Coventry CV1 5AE
Tel: 024 7622 4640 Fax: 024 7622 3859
(Coventry Teaching Primary Care Trust)

Practice Manager Pauline Smart

GP J V C MOHAN, Alison JACKSON, Usha JETTY, Jan Auke Aries KAPMA, Sarah MATTHEWS, Elaine Margaret SELWYN

Henley Green Medical Centre

Henley Road, Coventry CV2 1AB
Tel: 024 7661 4255 Fax: 024 7660 2699
(Coventry Teaching Primary Care Trust)

Practice Manager Ann John

GP Emmanuel Philip Domnal BELLAMY, David Charles FISH, Margaret Catherine Helen HARKNESS

Hillfields Health Centre

1 Howard Street, Coventry CV1 4GH
Tel: 024 7622 2527
(Coventry Teaching Primary Care Trust)

GP Malik Javed HUSSAIN

Hillfields Health Centre

1 Howard Street, Coventry CV1 4GH
Tel: 024 7622 0661 Fax: 024 7622 8300
(Coventry Teaching Primary Care Trust)

Practice Manager J M Court

GP P ROY, Michael Edward Nalder DOWNING, Dr SINGH

Hillfields Health Centre

1 Howard Street, Coventry CV1 4GH
(Coventry Teaching Primary Care Trust)

GP Dr AGARWAL

Hillsfield Health Centre

1 Howard Street, Coventry CV1 4GH
Tel: 024 7622 3446 Fax: 024 7622 5846
(Coventry Teaching Primary Care Trust)

GP George John KALLOOR, Paul Andrew BEAUMONT, Gareth John BLAND

Holbrook Lane Surgery

268 Holbrook Lane, Coventry CV6 4DD
Tel: 024 7668 8340 Fax: 024 7663 7526
(Coventry Teaching Primary Care Trust)
Patient List Size: 9000

Practice Manager J Mottram

GP Serena Janet CALDER, Bhavesh BODALIA, Rajesh BODALIA, E McDARMAID, Aderonke Adewunmi OKOJIE

Holbrooks Health Team

75-77 Wheelwright Lane, Holbrooks, Coventry CV6 4HN
Tel: 024 7636 6775 Fax: 024 7636 5793
Email: kerry.crutchion@nhs.uk
(Coventry Teaching Primary Care Trust)

Practice Manager Maria Spiward

GP Kenneth Martin HOLTON, Andrew James Gurney BARCLAY, David Russell EVANS, Bettina Uta KLEINE

Holyhead Surgery

1 Chester Street, Coventry CV1 4DH
Tel: 024 7622 4687 Fax: 024 7622 6652
(Coventry Teaching Primary Care Trust)
Patient List Size: 4802

Practice Manager Carol Drew

GP David Martin McALPINE, A G SHARMA

Jasmine Grove Surgery

64 Jasmine Grove, Coventry CV3 1EA
Tel: 024 7665 1188 Fax: 024 7651 1811
(Coventry Teaching Primary Care Trust)
Patient List Size: 1300

Practice Manager Carol Smolka

GP Kopparamachandra Rao MADHU

Jubilee Healthcare

41 Westminster Road, Coventry CV1 3GB
Tel: 024 7622 3565 Fax: 024 7623 0053
(Coventry Teaching Primary Care Trust)
Patient List Size: 7500

Practice Manager Karin Heidi Bruce

GP Antony Richard FELTBOWER, Elizabeth A LEIGH, Valerie A ROBSON, Robert Chad SMITH, Susan R VENN, Miriam R WIGGINS

Jubilee Healthcare

60 Station Avenue, Coventry CV4 9HS
Tel: 024 7646 6585 Fax: 024 7669 5944
(Coventry Teaching Primary Care Trust)

Practice Manager Christine Banfield

GP A FELTBOWER, E LEIGH, V ROBSON, R SMITH, S VENN, M WIGGINS

Kensington Road Surgery

148 Kensington Road, Coventry CV5 6HY
Tel: 024 7667 2466 Fax: 024 7671 7311
(Coventry Teaching Primary Care Trust)

GP Marcus John COCKERILL, I S NAGRA

Keresley Road

2 Keresley Road, Coventry CV6 2JD
Tel: 024 7633 2628 Fax: 024 7633 1326

(Coventry Teaching Primary Care Trust)
Patient List Size: 7800

Practice Manager K Furnival

GP Julius EBO, James Hector MACPHERSON, M PERERA, Jonathon PYWELL, N RAJAKUMARAN

Longford Medical Centre
18a Sydnall Road, Coventry CV6 6BW
Tel: 024 7664 4123 Fax: 024 7636 3157
(Coventry Teaching Primary Care Trust)
Patient List Size: 2350

GP Mohammed Aslam PATHAN

Mansfield Medical Centre
56 Binley Road, Coventry CV3 1JB
Tel: 024 7645 7551 Fax: 024 7644 2250
(Coventry Teaching Primary Care Trust)

Practice Manager Maureen Day

GP Ian Walter BAYMAN, Bhajan Singh KHARA, Jane Louise SMITH

Morris Avenue Surgery
36 Morris Avenue, Coventry CV2 5GX
Tel: 024 7644 7744 Fax: 024 7645 5363
(Coventry Teaching Primary Care Trust)
Patient List Size: 3600

Practice Manager J Holmes

GP M KASHOTY

Moseley Avenue Surgery
109 Moseley Avenue, Coventry CV6 1HS
Tel: 024 7659 2201 Fax: 024 7660 1226
(Coventry Teaching Primary Care Trust)
Patient List Size: 11250

Practice Manager S Brindley

GP John BATTEN, Maurice Roderick GOLD, Patrick John GRIFFIN, Richard John KEATING, Susanne MEYER

Mount Street Surgery
69 Mount Street, Coventry CV5 8DE
Tel: 024 7667 2277 Fax: 024 7671 7352
(Coventry Teaching Primary Care Trust)
Patient List Size: 10500

Practice Manager Mrs Pattison

GP Margaret Joan MASON, Judith Barbara LUCAS, P J O'BRIEN, Peter George PAIGE, Caroline Ann RHODES, Miriam Anne WOOD

Pai and Dillon
Tile Hill Primary Health Care, Jardine Crescent, Coventry CV4 9PN
Tel: 024 7646 0800 Fax: 024 7646 7512
(Coventry Teaching Primary Care Trust)
Patient List Size: 3700

Practice Manager Janice Brook

GP Manoj Sanathan PAI, Surjit Kaur DHILLON

Paradise Medical Centre
Broad Street, Coventry CV6 5BG
Tel: 024 7668 9343 Fax: 024 7663 8733
(Coventry Teaching Primary Care Trust)
Patient List Size: 6000

Practice Manager Balbir Bal

GP Dalpatram Karsan MISTRY, Mukesh MISTRY, Dharmesh PATEL

Park House Surgery
2 St. Georges Road, Stoke, Coventry CV1 2DL
Tel: 024 7622 4438 Fax: 024 7622 9782
(Coventry Teaching Primary Care Trust)
Patient List Size: 5000

Practice Manager Angela Gunton

GP Jagdishchandra Maganbhai PATEL, Dwijananda MAHANTA

Queen Mary's Road Surgery
2 Queen Mary's Road, Coventry CV6 5LL
Tel: 024 7668 5918
(Coventry Teaching Primary Care Trust)

GP Kumkum MISHRA, Vijay Kant MISRA

Quinton Road Surgery
74 Quinton Road, Coventry CV3 5FD
Tel: 024 7650 2255 Fax: 024 7650 5812
(Coventry Teaching Primary Care Trust)
Patient List Size: 5600

Practice Manager Keena Smith

GP N P MOTTRAM, M S JASPAL, Claire Elizabeth STEVENSON

Spring Hill Medical Centre
Spring Hill, Arley, Coventry CV7 8FD
Tel: 01676 40395
(North Warwickshire Primary Care Trust)

Practice Manager Heather Norgrove

GP John William BLAND

Spring Hill Medical Centre
Spring Hill, Arley, Coventry CV7 8FD
Tel: 01676 540395 Fax: 01676 540760
(North Warwickshire Primary Care Trust)
Patient List Size: 8250

Practice Manager Anne McCalon

GP Timothy David DICKSON, Linda Ann CRAGGS, R S ZUROB

St Georges Road Surgery
102 St Georges Road, Coventry CV1 2DL
Tel: 024 7655 5231 Fax: 024 7663 4813
(Coventry Teaching Primary Care Trust)
Patient List Size: 2040

Practice Manager Carol Warner

GP Mathurdas Ramji DADHANIA

Station Street West Surgery
100 Station Street West, Coventry CV6 5ND
Tel: 024 7666 2822 Fax: 024 7668 3076
(Coventry Teaching Primary Care Trust)

Practice Manager M Sheikh

GP S ALIJAH

Stoke Aldermoor Medical Centre
The Barley Lea, Coventry CV3 1EG
Tel: 024 7663 6972 Fax: 024 7665 0620
(Coventry Teaching Primary Care Trust)

Practice Manager Lesley Norman

GP P AGGARWAL

Stoney Stanton Medical Centre
475 Stoney Stanton Road, Coventry CV6 5EA
Tel: 024 7688 8484 Fax: 024 7658 1247
(Coventry Teaching Primary Care Trust)
Patient List Size: 4500

Practice Manager Kath Jenkins

GP Kantilal Liladhar KAKAD

Stretton Avenue Surgery
Stretton Avenue, Coventry CV3 3QA
Tel: 024 7630 4299 Fax: 024 7630 5504
(Coventry Teaching Primary Care Trust)
Patient List Size: 2459

Practice Manager Amanda Lanigan

GP S BANERJEE

The Surgery
Stretton Avenue, Willenhall, Coventry CV3 3QA
Tel: 024 7630 4330 Fax: 024 7669 7087
(Coventry Teaching Primary Care Trust)

Practice Manager Catherine Coleman

GP Kingsley Eric BOATENG

Swanswell Medical Centre
Swanswell Street, Coventry CV1 5FT
Tel: 024 7622 3250 Fax: 024 7655 3405
(Coventry Teaching Primary Care Trust)

Practice Manager S Baladurai

GP Mariampillai JAYARATNAM, Kamalambigai JAYARATNAM

Tanyfron
The Barley Lea, Coventry CV3 1DZ
Tel: 024 7645 8151 Fax: 024 7645 8881
(Coventry Teaching Primary Care Trust)

Practice Manager Julie Constable

GP Kollannur Sebastian FRANCIS

Telfer Road
190 Telfer Road, Coventry CV6 3DR
Tel: 024 7659 6060 Fax: 024 7660 1607
(Coventry Teaching Primary Care Trust)

GP Jagroop Singh SIHOTA, Hergeven Singh DOSANJH, Sukhdev Singh NAHL

Tile Hill Health Centre
Jardine Crescent, Coventry CV4 9PN
Tel: 024 7647 4744 Fax: 024 7646 9891
(Coventry Teaching Primary Care Trust)
Patient List Size: 2600

GP Pravin Jagjivandas SADRANI

Walsgrave Health Centre
50 Hall Lane, Coventry CV2 2SW
Tel: 024 7661 2004 Fax: 024 7660 3779
(Coventry Teaching Primary Care Trust)

Practice Manager Lyn Rowstron

GP K RAI, S J ALLEN

Walsgrave Road Surgery
59 Walsgrave Road, Coventry CV2 4HF
Tel: 024 7622 2094 Fax: 024 7663 3860
(Coventry Teaching Primary Care Trust)
Patient List Size: 2100

Practice Manager Val Rollason

GP Muhammad Zaimul Akhtar ANSARI

Westwood Medical Centre
298 Tile Hill Lane, Coventry CV4 9DR
Tel: 024 7646 6106 Fax: 024 7642 2475
(Coventry Teaching Primary Care Trust)

Practice Manager L McCullum

GP Amarjit Singh KUKREJA, Ravinder Kaur KUKREJA, Walter James McDONALD

Wheatley and Macdonald
163 Birmingham Road, Allesley Village, Coventry CV5 9BD
Tel: 024 7640 3250 Fax: 024 7640 5009
Email: macdonald.ian@talk21.com
(Coventry Teaching Primary Care Trust)
Patient List Size: 4000

Practice Manager Janet Saunders

GP Kathleen Anne WHEATLEY, Ian MACDONALD

Wheelwright Lane Surgery
25 Wheelwright Lane, Coventry CV6 4HF
Tel: 024 7668 8289
(Coventry Teaching Primary Care Trust)

Practice Manager G Halder

GP Sudhir Ranjan HALDER

Willenhall Oak Medical Centre
70 Remembrance Road, Coventry CV3 3DP
Tel: 024 7663 9909 Fax: 024 7630 5312
(Coventry Teaching Primary Care Trust)
Patient List Size: 3642

Practice Manager Carrie Dickinson

GP Maureen Elizabeth Hamilton WALLACE, Iqbal SAEED

Willenhall Primary Care Centre
Remembrance Road, Willenhall, Coventry CV3 3DG
Tel: 024 7630 2082 Fax: 024 7630 2402
(Coventry Teaching Primary Care Trust)
Patient List Size: 3980

Practice Manager J J Garforth

GP Robert Anthony HOGG, P J SHARMA

Windmill Road Health and Family
85 Windmill Road, Coventry CV6 7AT
Tel: 024 7663 7636 Fax: 024 7658 1412
(Coventry Teaching Primary Care Trust)

GP Shyam Sunder KATTI

Wood End Health Centre
67B Deedmore Road, Coventry CV2 1AX
Tel: 024 7661 2929 Fax: 024 7661 8665
(Coventry Teaching Primary Care Trust)

Practice Manager Sharon Dempsey

GP Mark William DUNN, Maria CEURSTEMONT, Rabindra Robin LAL-SARIN

Woodlands Surgery
24 Woodlands, Meeting House Lane, Balsall Common, Coventry CV7 7FX
Tel: 01676 532587 Fax: 01676 535154
Email: peter.lea@bcsc7.ms.solihull-ha.wmids.nhs.uk
(Solihull Primary Care Trust)
Patient List Size: 1200

Practice Manager Joanne Hope

GP Peter Martin LEA, Susan BARRATT, Mandeep BHANDAL, Martin John CAMM, Christopher John KIRKHAM, Michael John MATTHEWS, Elspeth Anne VALLET

Woodside Medical Centre
Jardine Crescent, Coventry CV4 9PL
Tel: 024 7669 4001 Fax: 024 7669 5639
(Coventry Teaching Primary Care Trust)
Patient List Size: 6843

Practice Manager Margaret Johnson

GP Robert Sidney TRENT, Gillian Mary COOPER, Christopher Michael TAGGART

Wyken Medical Centre
Brixham Drive, Coventry CV2 3LB
Tel: 024 7668 9149 Fax: 024 7666 5151
(Coventry Teaching Primary Care Trust)

GP Hemendra Kashinath PANDYA, Moinuddin SUBHANI

Cowes

Cowes Health Centre
8 Consort Road, Cowes PO31 7SH
Tel: 01983 295251 Fax: 01983 280461
(Isle of Wight Primary Care Trust)
Patient List Size: 13800

Practice Manager Karen Woodford

GP Gordon STAINER, Jagannadha Rao BOORLE, Rakesh CHOPRA, Eileen Anne Mary FINCH, Simon FORDHAM, Christine Ursula FREYTAG, Beate PARSONS, Mary Ruth STAINER

Cramlington

Ahmed
The Health Centre, Civic Precinct, Forum Way, Cramlington NE23 6QN
Tel: 01670 714581 Fax: 01670 730386
(Northumberland Care Trust)
Patient List Size: 2500

Practice Manager Denise Curtis

GP M Mohamed AHMED, Barry WARNER

Brockwell Medical Group
Brockwell Centre, Northumbrian Road, Cramlington NE23 1XZ
Tel: 01670 392700 Fax: 01670 392701
Website: www.brockwell.co.uk
(Northumberland Care Trust)
Patient List Size: 11500

Practice Manager Jill Dickson

GP Alan Peter DOVE, Dawn ADKIN, Gaye DICKINSON, Patricia Anne Tanya GREEN, Sarah JONES, Aamir MUNIR, Christopher John PRANK, Christopher Charles WARD, Rebecca WRIGHT

Cramlington Medical Group
The Health Centre, Civic Precinct, Forum Way, Cramlington NE23 6QN
Tel: 01670 713911 Fax: 01670 735958
(Northumberland Care Trust)
Patient List Size: 3938

GP Dr LEITH, Dr BELL, Dr BOURNE

Dr Foster, Ferguson and Orr
Civic Precinct, Forum Way, Cramlington NE23 6QN
Tel: 01670 713021 Fax: 01670 735880
(Northumberland Care Trust)
Patient List Size: 5200

Practice Manager Sally I Pern

GP Laura Anne FOSTER, Elizabeth Mary FERGUSON, Malcolm John ORR

Netherfield House
Station Road, Seghill, Cramlington NE23 7EF
Tel: 0191 237 0643 Fax: 0191 237 1091
Website: www.netherfieldhousesurgery.co.uk
(Northumberland Care Trust)
Patient List Size: 5800

Practice Manager Sue Cummings

GP David Michael Gellatly BROWN, Barbara Elizabeth HOLDING, Susan Elizabeth QUAYLE

Village Surgery
Dudley Lane, Cramlington NE23 6US
Tel: 01670 712821 Fax: 01670 730837
Email: village.surgery@gp-a84030.nhs.uk
(Northumberland Care Trust)
Patient List Size: 9250

Practice Manager David Shannon

GP Graeme DUNBAR, Dawn BENNETT, Jane Frances ERRIDGE, Alison GEORGE, John David Roderick MACMILLAN, Michelle PATTON, Linda THOMPSON

Cranbrook

The Crane Surgery
Rectory Fields, Cranbrook TN17 3JB
Tel: 01580 712260
(Maidstone Weald Primary Care Trust)

GP David John HINDMARSH, J HOWELL

Forge House Surgery
Frittenden, Cranbrook TN17 2EE
Tel: 01580 891220
(Maidstone Weald Primary Care Trust)

GP M C DAVIES

North Ridge Medical Practice
North Ridge, Rye Road, Hawkhurst, Cranbrook TN18 4EX
Tel: 01580 753935 Fax: 01580 754452
Email: practice.manager@gp-g82055.nhs.uk
(Maidstone Weald Primary Care Trust)
Patient List Size: 5800

Practice Manager Geoff Barry

GP Robert James BLUNDELL, Charles John Roderick LEWIS, Peter Val PLAYER, Ann Mabel WOOD

Old Parsonage Surgery
Balcombes Hill, Goudhurst, Cranbrook TN17 1AN
Tel: 01580 211241 Fax: 01580 211659
(Maidstone Weald Primary Care Trust)

GP Hilary LLEWELLYN, Jeremy Neil WATSON

Orchard End Surgery
Dorothy Avenue, Cranbrook TN17 3AY
Tel: 01580 713622 Fax: 01580 7515537
(Maidstone Weald Primary Care Trust)
Patient List Size: 1800

Practice Manager Rosemary Hoare

GP Hazel Jane BUTLER

Wish Valley Surgery
Talbot Road, Hawkhurst, Cranbrook TN18 4NB
Tel: 01580 753211 Fax: 01580 754612
(Maidstone Weald Primary Care Trust)
Patient List Size: 4700

Practice Manager Christine Paddock

GP Clive Richard DEWING, E LANOR, Kathryn Elliott VALE, Frank Peter VAN DER PLAS

Cranleigh

Cranleigh Health Centre
18 High Street, Cranleigh GU6 8AE
Tel: 01483 273951 Fax: 01483 275755
(Guildford and Waverley Primary Care Trust)
Patient List Size: 15000

Practice Manager Tina Hudson

GP Catherine Ann BRATTY, Michael John BUNDY, Diane CHRISTIE, Matthew Lucas CLARK, Dr DONAVAN, Robin FAWKNER-CORBETT, Ruth TURNER, Jonathon Hendley VERDON

Craven Arms

Jay Lane Health Centre
Jay Lane, Leintwardine, Craven Arms SY7 0LG
Tel: 01547 540355 Fax: 01547 540355
(Herefordshire Primary Care Trust)

Practice Manager R J Garlick

GP Martin John GARLICK

Shrewsbury Road Surgery
20 Shrewsbury Road, Craven Arms SY7 9PY
Tel: 01588 672309 Fax: 01588 673943
(Shropshire County Primary Care Trust)

GP Philippa Rachel Xanthe WINTER, David Jackson APPLEBY

Crawley

Bewbush Medical Centre
Bewbush Place, Bewbush, Crawley RH11 8XT
Tel: 01293 519420
(Crawley Primary Care Trust)
Patient List Size: 5500

Practice Manager M Roy

GP Arun ROY, Tajammul HUSAIN, Nigel Raymond STORER

Bridge Medical Centre
Wassand Close, Three Bridges Road, Crawley RH10 1LL
Tel: 01293 526025 Fax: 01293 538952
(Crawley Primary Care Trust)

Practice Manager Sharon Harrison

GP Jonathan Aidan ROYDS-JONES, Keith William Campbell TRUTER, Jill Patricia AVERY, Bronwin BARTMAN, Katherine BUCHAN, Alun Lewis COOPER, John Ireland O'Brien CRAIK, Elizabeth Anne HORNUNG, N A MOHABIR, William Cletus SMITH, Salvino XERRI

Caldbeck and Partners
Hurst Close, Gossops Green, Crawley RH11 8TY
Tel: 01293 527138 Fax: 01293 522571
(Crawley Primary Care Trust)
Patient List Size: 7250

Practice Manager Barbara Neal

GP Carole Rosemary CALDBECK, Rakesh Kumar NANDHA, Raj SINHA, Michael John WALDRON

The Health Centre
Bowers Place, Crawley Down, Crawley RH10 4HY
Tel: 01342 713031 Fax: 01342 718715
(Mid Sussex Primary Care Trust)
Patient List Size: 7300

Practice Manager Marguerite J Riley

GP Nicholas John CLEMENS, Alan David CLIFFORD, Lesley Caroline CROUCHER, Daniel William JEFFERIES

The Health Centre
Coachmans Drive, Broadfield, Crawley RH11 9YZ
Tel: 01293 531951
(Crawley Primary Care Trust)

Practice Manager Sarah Ruse

GP Ian Douglas McINTOSH, Richard Noel HAWORTH, Jeremy Russell LUKE, Amanda Jayne MOLLOY, Ellen Oi-Lun TOMLINSON

Leacroft Medical Practice
Ifield Road, Ifield, Crawley RH11 7BS
Tel: 01293 526441 Fax: 01293 619970
Website: www.leacroft.co.uk
(Crawley Primary Care Trust)
Patient List Size: 10070

Practice Manager Kate Harvey

GP Paul STILLMAN, Iman HANNA, Robert Charles HIAM, Laura HILL, Charlotte RUGLYS, Nyan Kyaw TIN

Pound Hill Medical Group
1 Crawley Lane, Pound Hill, Crawley RH10 7DX
Tel: 01293 549916 Fax: 01293 844222
(Crawley Primary Care Trust)
Patient List Size: 15000

Practice Manager John Wilkin

GP Susan Mary BOWER, Neil Warren JACKSON, Jurrien KUIPERS, Jennifer Ann LITCHFIELD, Malcolm Scott PROCTER, Aiyadurai SATTIANAYAGAM, Paul SPENSLEY, David James WILLIAMSON

Saxonbrook Medical
Maidenbower Square, Crawley RH10 7QH
Tel: 01293 450400 Fax: 01293 450401
(Crawley Primary Care Trust)
Patient List Size: 11000

Practice Manager Janet Norman

GP Richard PHILLIPS, Ian Paul ANDERSON, Geraint THOMAS

Southgate Surgery
2 Forester Road, Southgate, Crawley RH10 6EQ
Tel: 01293 522231 Fax: 01293 515655
(Crawley Primary Care Trust)
Patient List Size: 3500

Practice Manager Beryl Yeo

GP Amitabh BHARGAVA, John Christopher BLECHYNDEN, Anita Margaret WILKINSON

The Surgery
9 Woolborough Road, Northgate, Crawley RH10 8EZ
Tel: 01293 547315 Fax: 01293 613439
(Crawley Primary Care Trust)

GP Richard Charles PHILLIPS, Ian Paul ANDERSON, Geraint Huw THOMAS

The Surgery
50 The Glade, Furnace Green, Crawley RH10 6JN
Tel: 01293 612741 Fax: 01293 603802
Website: www.crawleygp.org.ik
(Crawley Primary Care Trust)
Patient List Size: 7258

Practice Manager Maureen Taylor

GP Kevin John HURRELL, Susan Jane CHORLEY, Paul Selby VINSON, Robert John WARD

The Surgery
218 Ifield Drive, Ifield, Crawley RH11 0EP
Tel: 01293 547846
(Crawley Primary Care Trust)

Practice Manager Mike Korab

GP Pothen ALEXANDER, Janet Elizabeth ARMSTRONG, Cherry Glesni BRIGHTWELL, Susan Janette DONNELLY, Jeffrey Enrique OLIVER

Woodlands/Clerklands Surgery
Tilgate Way, Tilgate, Crawley RH10 5BW
Tel: 01293 520001 Fax: 01293 514778
(Crawley Primary Care Trust)
Patient List Size: 16200

Practice Manager Anne Davies

GP Paul Michael WESTON-BURT, Leonardo ACUYO PASTOR, Jonathan Keith BIRCH, Amanda GREENGRASS, Ohar Abdulle PENNY, Richard Sheridan STANLEY, Sinnadurai SUNTHARANTHAN

Crediton

Bow Surgery
Fair Park, Bow, Crediton EX17 6EY
Tel: 01363 82333 Fax: 01363 82841
(Mid Devon Primary Care Trust)
Patient List Size: 2444

Practice Manager Peter John Selley

GP Peter John SELLEY, Roger Edwin STEPHENSON

Chiddenbrook Surgery
Threshers, Crediton EX17 3JJ
Tel: 01363 772227 Fax: 01363 775528
(Mid Devon Primary Care Trust)
Patient List Size: 6894

Practice Manager Paul Janion

GP Charles P KENT, Michael R BRADDICK, Martin Hugh MURPHY, Janet Susan SHORNEY, Peter James Golden TWOMEY

Newcombes Surgery
Newcombes, Crediton EX17 2AR
Tel: 01363 772263 Fax: 01363 775906
(Mid Devon Primary Care Trust)
Patient List Size: 6369

Practice Manager John Young

GP Paul Arthur WESTWOOD, Amanda Mary HALL, Ann C. HOMER, Elizabeth M J SAUNDERS

Crewe

Audlem Medical Practice
16 Cheshire Street, Audlem, Crewe CW3 0AH
Tel: 01270 811440 Fax: 01270 812382
(Cheshire West Primary Care Trust)
Patient List Size: 4000

Practice Manager Helen Matthews

GP Barrie Richard HUFTON, Russell MUIRHEAD

Brookland House
501 Crewe Road, Wistaston, Crewe CW2 6QP
Tel: 01270 567250 Fax: 01270 665829
(Central Cheshire Primary Care Trust)
Patient List Size: 14515

Practice Manager I C Jones

GP Harold Sydney DOBSON, John Maurice DIXON, Katharine Clare Verney HADRILL, P A HUNTER, Sanjiu SHRIDHAR, David Gordon SMITH, Carole WATSON

Cedars Medical Centre
Alsager, Crewe
(Central Cheshire Primary Care Trust)

Cobbs Lane Surgery
19 Cobbs Lane, Hough, Crewe CW2 5JN

GP William John PETTIT

Delamere Street Health Centre
45 Delamere Street, Crewe CW1 2ER
Tel: 01270 214046 Fax: 01270 251239
(Central Cheshire Primary Care Trust)
Patient List Size: 10027

Practice Manager C W Buckley

GP G C ARMSTRONG, Momtaz Parveen MATIN, Mark MITCHYN, Gerard Patrick O'SULLIVAN

Earnswood Medical Centre
92 Victoria Street, Crewe CW1 2JR
Tel: 01270 257255 Fax: 01270 501943
(Central Cheshire Primary Care Trust)
Patient List Size: 14589

Practice Manager A J Potter

GP John Cedric VICKERS, Peter Alan BOOTH, C BUNTE, Richard John CALDERHEAD, Austin Gerard DOHERTY, Andrew Lindsay RAEBURN, E SPENCER, June Elizabeth Alice WILLIAMS

Grosvenor Medical Centre
Grosvenor Street, Crewe CW1 3HB
Tel: 01270 256348 Fax: 01270 250786
(Central Cheshire Primary Care Trust)
Patient List Size: 14248

Practice Manager Lesley Meade

GP David Philip Harvey WILLIAMSON, James Graham COOPER, C FISHER, Andrea PIGGOTT, Nicola SIMPKIN, Andrew Lawrence SPOONER, Jonathan Mark WATSON

Haslington Surgery
Crewe Road, Haslington, Crewe CW1 5QY
Tel: 01270 581259 Fax: 01270 257958
(Central Cheshire Primary Care Trust)
Patient List Size: 7930

GP David Henry HANDS, Nicholas Anthony KING, Thomas Winfield SMIRK

Holmes Chapel Health Centre
London Road, Holmes Chapel, Crewe CW4 7BB
Tel: 01477 533100 Fax: 01477 532563
(Eastern Cheshire Primary Care Trust)
Patient List Size: 11585

Practice Manager L Sanchez

GP Stephen Richard TATE, Paul BAILEY, Michael John CLARKE, Nicola HULME, Clare TAYLOR, Robert Anthony Frederick THORBURN

Hungerford Medical Centre
School Crescent, Crewe CW1 5HA
Tel: 01270 582589 Fax: 01270 216330
Website: www.hungerfordmedicalcentre.co.uk
(Central Cheshire Primary Care Trust)
Patient List Size: 9813

Practice Manager Alan Rickards

GP Norman Graham Michael WILSON, Gemma BEEGAN, Gregory Paul Stanford HARDY, John Christopher HOWARD, Andrew WILSON

Merepark Medical Centre
Alsager, Crewe
Tel: 01270 882004 Fax: 01270 872404
Website: www.mereparkmedical.cjb.net
(Central Cheshire Primary Care Trust)
Patient List Size: 5811

Practice Manager R Chaudhury

GP N P RICKARDS, H M CORCORAN, C A DANIELS, A D WILLIAMSON

Mill Street Health Centre
Mill Street, Crewe CW2 7AQ
Tel: 01270 212725 Fax: 01270 216323
(Central Cheshire Primary Care Trust)
Patient List Size: 11656

Practice Manager Gill Flisher

GP Michael Russell FREEMAN, Angela PUGH, Jennifer FLOWER, Rayan HAMDY, Mark LAWRENCE, D SHACKLETON

Moss Lane Surgery
Moss Lane, Madeley, Crewe CW3 9NQ
Tel: 01782 750274 Fax: 01782 751835
(Newcastle-under-Lyme Primary Care Trust)
Patient List Size: 6200

Practice Manager Julie Cole

GP A W IRVINE, B A EDWARDS, J L GEAR, Christopher George OLESHKO

The Surgery
Main Road, Betley, Weinehill, Crewe CW3 9BL
Tel: 01270 620527 Fax: 01270 820527
(Newcastle-under-Lyme Primary Care Trust)

GP N PATEL

Crewkerne

Rosser and Partners
Crewkerne Health Centre, Middle Path, Crewkerne TA18 8BX
Tel: 01460 72435 Fax: 01460 77957
(South Somerset Primary Care Trust)
Patient List Size: 11500

Practice Manager Carol Kemp

GP Jeffrey Graham ROSSER, Berge Hagop BALIAN, Mark William FIELD, Roger Alfred James GILSON, John Justin HORNE, Maeve Anne McINERNEY, Carol Louise ZWARTOUW

Cromer

Canada Road Surgery
7 Canada Road, Cromer NR27 9AH
Tel: 01263 512157 Fax: 01263 515577
(North Norfolk Primary Care Trust)

Practice Manager Patricia Barrett

GP C D DING

Cromer Group Practice
48 Overstrand Road, Cromer NR27 0AJ
Tel: 01263 513148

(North Norfolk Primary Care Trust)

GP William Anthony NORMAN, Ferdinand BECKER, Alasdair Murray LENNOX, Simon Richard MAY, Pamela Dorothy RIPLEY, Michael Herbert Archibald SYMES

Crook

North House Surgery

North House, Hope Street, Crook DL15 9HU
Tel: 01388 762945 Fax: 01388 765333
(Durham Dales Primary Care Trust)
Patient List Size: 12700

Practice Manager Denise Simpson

GP John Alexander CLARKE, David Ian CATTERICK, Mark Alan GAYER, Gordan Thomas GOWANS, Donald Peter GUNNING, George David HOLBROOK, Catherine WILLIAMS, Derek William YOUNG

Willington Medical Group

Chapel Street, Willington, Crook DL15 0EQ
Tel: 01388 746342 Fax: 01388 747665
(Durham Dales Primary Care Trust)

Practice Manager Julia Steele

GP Enda Thomas CHADWICK, Mary Regine CARNEY, Ian Black GRANT, John Anthony JEWITT, Paul Patrick McGORAN

Crowborough

Beacon Surgery

Beacon Road, Crowborough TN6 1AF
Tel: 01892 652233 Fax: 01892 668840
(Sussex Downs and Weald Primary Care Trust)
Patient List Size: 9800

Practice Manager Carol Gent

GP Christopher Stuart SAMPSON, Vivienne Owen ANKRETT, Justin Vivian MORRIS, Maurice Charles O'CONNELL

Rotherfield Surgery

Rotherfield, Crowborough TN6 3QW
Tel: 01892 852415/853288 Fax: 01892 853499
(Sussex Downs and Weald Primary Care Trust)
Patient List Size: 6445

Practice Manager Adrienne Cooper

GP John Owen Greenland DAVIES, Sarah DAVIS, Michael John GOLTON, Vitoria J C PACE, Susan Jane TAYLOR

Saxonbury House

Croft Road, Crowborough TN6 1DL
Tel: 01892 652266 Fax: 01892 668607
(Sussex Downs and Weald Primary Care Trust)
Patient List Size: 10500

GP Philip John MARRIOTT, Peter Charles BIRTLES, Michael Anthony SPENCER, Cathryn Elizabeth STOKES

Crowthorne

Heath Hill Practice

Heath Hill Road South, Crowthorne RG45 7BN
Tel: 01344 777915
(Bracknell Forest Primary Care Trust)

Practice Manager Brenda Leighton

GP Richard Stephen Lloyd THOMAS, Anne CRAMPTON, Gordon Robert MACKAY, Carol Jane OAKLEY

New Wokingham Road Surgery

18 New Wokingham Road, Crowthorne RG45 6JL
Tel: 01344 773418 Fax: 01344 762753
(Wokingham Primary Care Trust)
Patient List Size: 6600

Practice Manager Jenny Hanna

GP Edmond Ping Wa CHAU, Susanne BETTNER, Elizabeth HARRIS

Croydon

Addiscombe Road Surgery

395A Addiscombe Road, Croydon CR0 7LJ
Tel: 020 8654 2200 Fax: 020 8655 1358
(Croydon Primary Care Trust)
Patient List Size: 3380

Practice Manager Alison Barnet

GP Bellanage Sunanda Sirimevan JAYARATNE

Ashburton Park Medical Centre

416 Lower Addiscombe Road, Croydon CR0 7AG
Tel: 020 8654 1068 Fax: 020 8654 0487
(Croydon Primary Care Trust)
Patient List Size: 1730

Practice Manager Shaku Desai

GP Indravadan Thakorbhai DESAI

Beddington Medical Centre

172 Croydon Road, Beddington, Croydon CR0 4PG
Tel: 020 8688 8486
(Sutton and Merton Primary Care Trust)
Patient List Size: 4000

GP D P PATTANI

Castle Hill Surgery

1A Castle Hill Avenue, New Addington, Croydon CR0 0TH
Tel: 01689 843636 Fax: 01689 844827
Email: hilary.ellis@gp-h83012.nhs.uk
(Croydon Primary Care Trust)
Patient List Size: 6100

Practice Manager Hilary Ellis

GP G RAVI-SHANKAR, Y CONTRACTOR

East Croydon Medical Centre

59 Addiscombe Road, Croydon CR0 6SD
Tel: 020 8688 1213 Fax: 020 8686 5818
(Croydon Primary Care Trust)
Patient List Size: 10500

Practice Manager Daphine Gibbs

GP D W K McCREA, Clive Vincent BAILEY, J N EDE, Paul RYBINSKI, S A SHAIKH

Fieldway Medical Centre

15A Danebury, New Addington, Croydon CR0 9EU
Tel: 01689 84166 Fax: 01689 800643
(Croydon Primary Care Trust)
Patient List Size: 4400

Practice Manager Jacqui Smith

GP Chandra Mohan PAWA, Richard Toluwalope BAMGBOYE

Friends Road Medical Practice

49 Friends Road, Croydon CR0 1ED
Tel: 020 8688 0532 Fax: 020 8688 2165
(Croydon Primary Care Trust)
Patient List Size: 8400

Practice Manager Karen Northwood

GP Griselda Nicolette ADCOCK, Kaushal KANSAGRA, Niaz Bin KARIM, Christian Jeremy WILCOCK

Greenside Surgery

88 Greenside Road, Croydon CR0 3PN
Tel: 020 8240 0072 Fax: 020 8240 0074
(Croydon Primary Care Trust)
Patient List Size: 3400

Practice Manager Susan Farrant

GP Nicholas Anthony CAMBRIDGE, Marc RAVETTO

Hartland Way Surgery

1 Hartland Road, Shirley, Croydon CR0 8RG
Tel: 020 8777 7215 Fax: 020 8777 7648
(Croydon Primary Care Trust)

Patient List Size: 3900

Practice Manager Sue Barner

GP Margaret Mary REILLY, David Alan GARDINER

Headley Drive Surgery

117A Headley Drive, New Addington, Croydon CR0 0QL
Tel: 01689 843036 Fax: 01689 843036
(Croydon Primary Care Trust)
Patient List Size: 2700

Practice Manager Linda Burchell

GP Jeyakumar SINGANAYAGAM

Heathfield Surgery

39 Heathfield Road, Croydon CR0 1EZ
Tel: 020 686 6655 Fax: 020 8686 8436
(Croydon Primary Care Trust)
Patient List Size: 3550

Practice Manager Peggy O'Brien

GP V E D BEAL, S HAMEED, A KARIM

Lennard Road Medical Practice

26 Lennard Road, Croydon CR0 2UL
Tel: 020 8680 2270 Fax: 020 8649 8763
(Croydon Primary Care Trust)
Patient List Size: 2550

Practice Manager A Murray

GP Charles Thomas Anthony MURRAY

Lower Addiscombe Road Surgery

188 Lower Addiscombe Road, Croydon CR0 6AH
Tel: 020 8654 1427 Fax: 020 8662 1272
(Croydon Primary Care Trust)
Patient List Size: 6700

Practice Manager Joanna Stone

GP Derrick Andrew CUTTING, Kamran Ahmed KHAN, Anne Geraldine STACEY

Mersham Medical Centre

30 Norbury Road, Thornton Heath, Croydon CR7 8JN
Tel: 020 8653 1869 Fax: 020 8771 4167
(Croydon Primary Care Trust)
Patient List Size: 3580

Practice Manager Jamil Cockar

GP N W KHINE, T KHINE-SMITH, M M LWIN

Morland Road Surgery

1 Morland Road, Croydon CR0 6HA
Tel: 020 8688 0434 Fax: 020 8649 8477
(Croydon Primary Care Trust)
Patient List Size: 7100

Practice Manager Debra Surallie

GP V SHAH, J C GOONERATNE, U PARAMESWARAN

Norman House

Brookside Way, Croydon CR0 7RR
Tel: 020 8656 3371 Fax: 020 8656 4916
(Croydon Primary Care Trust)
Patient List Size: 5000

Practice Manager Alan Walker

GP Indira BHAMBRI

Parchmore Medical Centre

97 Parchmore Road, Thornton Heath, Croydon CR7 8LY
Tel: 020 8251 4208 Fax: 020 8251 0550
(Croydon Primary Care Trust)
Patient List Size: 12700

Practice Manager Teresa Chapman

GP R K NAMASIVAYAM, D CHOWDHURY, A T FERNANDES, E Y HO, E PAULPILLAI, S S SHAIKH, S YUSUF

Parkway Health Centre 1

Parkway, New Addington, Croydon CR0 0JA
Tel: 01689 848939 Fax: 01689 841032
(Croydon Primary Care Trust)
Patient List Size: 7160

Practice Manager Linda Burchell

GP Balasubramaniam BASKARAN, Olajumoke ABILI, Thuraiappah SELVARAJAH, Sivapragasam THIRUCHANDRAN

Parkway Health Centre 2

Parkway, New Addington, Croydon CR0 0JA
Tel: 01689 846642 Fax: 01689 849729
(Croydon Primary Care Trust)
Patient List Size: 5000

Practice Manager Pauline Wellington

GP Ruwanpura Nandasena de Silva AMARASEKARA, L DE SILVA

Parkway Health Centre 3

Parkway, New Addington, Croydon CR0 0JA
Tel: 01689 841264
(Croydon Primary Care Trust)
Patient List Size: 2950

Practice Manager Sharon Nobes

GP Javier Oscar SALERNO

Sanderson and Partners

125 Holmbury Grove, Featherbed Lane, Croydon CR0 9AQ
Tel: 020 8657 8231
(Croydon Primary Care Trust)
Patient List Size: 11920

Practice Manager Gill Bashford

GP Robert Desmond Stuart SANDERSON, Mary Elizabeth CASHMAN, Jacqueline Lesley Beverley COCKELL, William Mark JASPER, David Alexander LYELL

Shirley Medical Centre

370 Wickham Road, Croydon CR0 8BH
Tel: 020 8777 2066 Fax: 020 8776 0441
(Croydon Primary Care Trust)
Patient List Size: 5000

Practice Manager Alan Walker

GP H P ABBOT, A ABBOT

South Way Surgery

2 South Way, Shirley, Croydon CR0 8RP
Tel: 020 8777 1876 Fax: 020 8776 2677
(Croydon Primary Care Trust)
Patient List Size: 3470

Practice Manager Barry Austin

GP Nicholas Talbot FORD

Spring Park Medical Practice

23 Broom Road, Croydon CR0 8NG
Tel: 020 8777 5511 Fax: 020 8777 9532
(Croydon Primary Care Trust)
Patient List Size: 4100

GP R SINGH, T WIN

St James's Medical Centre

189A St James' Road, Croydon CR0 2BZ
Tel: 020 8684 5353 Fax: 020 8665 1229
Email: hilary.ellis@gp-h83012.nhs.uk
(Croydon Primary Care Trust)
Patient List Size: 6100

Practice Manager Hilary Ellis

GP G RAVI-SHANKAR

Thornton Heath Health Centre

61A Gillett Road, Thornton Heath, Croydon CR7 8RL
Tel: 020 8689 5797 Fax: 020 8665 1195
(Croydon Primary Care Trust)
Patient List Size: 7380

Practice Manager John Pheasant

GP S E RAMSBOTHAM, C J BARRETTO, I L JAYAMANNE, M OGAKWU, V SAPATNEKAR

Thornton Road Surgery
299 Thornton Road, Croydon CR0 3EW
Tel: 020 8683 1255 Fax: 020 8251 0166
(Croydon Primary Care Trust)
Patient List Size: 3850

Practice Manager Catherine Boyce

GP John OGEAH, P PUVANENDRAN

Valley Park Surgery
Healthly Living Centre, Franklin Way, Croydon CR0 4YD
Tel: 020 8251 9470 Fax: 020 8251 9504
(Croydon Primary Care Trust)
Patient List Size: 750

Practice Manager Gazelle Howard

GP C R PATEL, A CHADHA

Violet Lane Medical Practice
231 Violet Lane, Croydon CR0 4HN
Tel: 020 8688 0333 Fax: 020 8688 9707
(Croydon Primary Care Trust)
Patient List Size: 8750

Practice Manager Lorraine Braithwaite

GP William Hugh BARCLAY, K ARORA, S T HAMA-RAHIM, N J WALLS

The Whitehorse Practice
87 Whitehorse Road, Croydon CR0 2JJ
Tel: 020 8684 1162 Fax: 020 8665 1454
(Croydon Primary Care Trust)
Patient List Size: 6700

Practice Manager Penny Spencer

GP Paul Philip CHARLTON, Nina Vijaya Lakshmi ARJUN, S KHAN, J NWUFOH

Cullompton

Bramblehaies Surgery
College Road, Cullompton EX15 1TZ
Tel: 01884 33536 Fax: 01884 35401
Email: brambly2@aol.com
Website: http://members.aol.com/brambly2
(Mid Devon Primary Care Trust)
Patient List Size: 6360

Practice Manager Tracey Pratt

GP Stephen James STRAUGHAN, Malcolm Alan BODGER, Richard HARPER, Ceinwen Jayne ROBERTS

College Surgery
College Road, Cullompton EX15 1TG
Tel: 01884 831300 Fax: 01884 831313
(Mid Devon Primary Care Trust)
Patient List Size: 13705

Practice Manager Wendy Evans

GP Neil Patrick RUSHTON, David Michael DIXON, H M HARRIS, J I JACOB, David Robert JENNER, Angela Mary MARTIN, C E MATTHEWS, J L ROWBURY, A G SMITH

The Surgery
Station Road, Heymock, Cullompton EX15 3SF
Tel: 01823 680206 Fax: 01823 680680
(Mid Devon Primary Care Trust)
Patient List Size: 7096

Practice Manager Wendy Eggleton

GP Donald McKenzie McLINTOCK, Susan Jennifer BROCKLESBY, Mark William COULDRICK, John Norman DAVIES, Amanda L M LEACH, Stuart MURRAY

Dagenham

Becontree Medical Centre
641-645 Becontree Avenue, Dagenham RM8 3HP
Tel: 020 8592 1778 Fax: 020 8595 2736
(Barking and Dagenham Primary Care Trust)
Patient List Size: 300

Practice Manager G Dack

GP Asma MOGHAL, S GYIMAH

Bennetts Castle Surgery
178 Bennetts Castle Lane, Dagenham RM8 3XP
Tel: 020 8592 0499 Fax: 020 8593 7566
(Barking and Dagenham Primary Care Trust)

GP Naseem Sehar KUNWAR

Five Elms Medical Practice
Five Elms Health Centre, Five Elms Road, Dagenham RM9 5TT
Tel: 020 8517 1175 Fax: 020 8592 0114
(Barking and Dagenham Primary Care Trust)
Patient List Size: 6595

Practice Manager Susan Hayes

GP Paul Anton HEININK, Ndalai Majiyebo ABANIWO, Rajbir Singh RANDHAWA

Goresbrook Medical Centre
50 Goresbrook Road, Dagenham RM9 6UR
Tel: 020 8593 7141 Fax: 020 8593 9853
(Barking and Dagenham Primary Care Trust)
Patient List Size: 2100

Practice Manager Hazel D Hook

GP Mir Mesbahuddin AHMED

Grosvenor Road Surgery
1 Grosvenor Road, Dagenham RM8 1NR
Tel: 020 8592 1082 Fax: 020 8593 2313
(Barking and Dagenham Primary Care Trust)
Patient List Size: 7300

GP Durga Prasad JAISWAL, Dr AHMAD, Dr HAIDER, Dr MONTEIRO

Halbutt Surgery
2 Halbutt Street, Dagenham RM9 5AS
Tel: 020 8592 1544 Fax: 020 8596 9833
(Barking and Dagenham Primary Care Trust)
Patient List Size: 4800

Practice Manager Sandra Beazley

GP Benjamin Bassaw QUANSAH, Adedayo ADEDEJI

Hatfield Road Surgery
104/106 Hatfield Road, Dagenham RM9 6JS
Tel: 020 8592 4011 Fax: 020 8220 0011
(Barking and Dagenham Primary Care Trust)

GP Asit Kumar MITRA, Thota Chandra MOHAN, Meghnath ROY

Heathway Surgery
585 Heathway, Dagenham RM9 5AZ
Tel: 020 8592 1771 Fax: 020 8592 1751
(Barking and Dagenham Primary Care Trust)
Patient List Size: 2100

Practice Manager Darayus Malefout

GP Syed Mohammed Mattinudin ASHRAFF

Hedgemans Surgery
The Medical Centre, 92 Hedgemans Road, Dagenham RM9 6HT
Tel: 020 8592 4242 Fax: 020 8593 2094
(Barking and Dagenham Primary Care Trust)
Patient List Size: 5100

Practice Manager Darayus Malekout

GP S N AHMAD, Dr HAIDER, Durga Prasad JAISWAL, Dr MONTEIRO

Julia Engwell Health Centre
Woodward Road, Dagenham RM9 4SU
Tel: 020 8592 5500 Fax: 020 8592 1127
(Barking and Dagenham Primary Care Trust)
Patient List Size: 4000

GP Sheela BAJPAI, Bijay Kumar JAISWAL

Laburnum Health Centre
George Crouch Centre, Althorne Way, Dagenham RM10 7DF
Tel: 020 8515 0222 Fax: 020 8596 9778
(Barking and Dagenham Primary Care Trust)
Patient List Size: 2700

Practice Manager Linda Franklin

GP Arun Kumar SHARMA

Lodge Avenue Nurse Led PMS Pilot
434 Lodge Avenue, Dagenham RM9 4QS
Tel: 020 8592 5251 Fax: 020 8592 1183
(Barking and Dagenham Primary Care Trust)
Patient List Size: 2400

Practice Manager Wendy Muhley

GP B DIXIT

Longbridge Road Surgery
620 Longbridge Road, Dagenham RM8 2AJ
Tel: 020 8517 3771/2 Fax: 020 8517 1448
(Barking and Dagenham Primary Care Trust)

GP Uddin Ahmed AFSER

Manor Road Surgery
65 Manor Road, Dagenham RM10 8BD
Tel: 020 8592 0868
(Barking and Dagenham Primary Care Trust)
Patient List Size: 3000

GP Asokananda KUMAR, Mina GOYAL

Markyate Road Surgery
50 Markyate Road, Dagenham RM8 2LD
Tel: 020 8592 2983 Fax: 020 8984 8500
(Barking and Dagenham Primary Care Trust)

Practice Manager Linda Harding

GP Alok Kumar MITTAL

Medical Centre
7 Felhurst Crescent, Dagenham RM10 7XT
Tel: 020 8592 2323 Fax: 020 8984 3732
(Barking and Dagenham Primary Care Trust)

Practice Manager Jackie Myers

GP Rabindia Bahadur BASNYAT

Naseby Road Surgery
61 Naseby Road, Dagenham RM10 7JS
Tel: 020 8592 1841 Fax: 020 8598 5514
(Barking and Dagenham Primary Care Trust)
Patient List Size: 3950

Practice Manager Jane Hannan

GP Rajendra Singh KALRA, Vasu Deo AGRAWAL, Abdul-Karim Saheb JAWAD

Rainham Surgery
598 Rainham Road South, Dagenham RM10 8YP
Tel: 020 8592 0049
Website: www.dagenhameastsurgery.co.uk
(Barking and Dagenham Primary Care Trust)
Patient List Size: 2450

GP Norman ELLAL

Stone Close Surgery
39 Stone Close, Dagenham RM8 3BT
Tel: 020 8592 1955 Fax: 01708 722645
(Barking and Dagenham Primary Care Trust)

GP Suresh Kumar PATHAK, Dr BEHESHTI, Dr SANOMI

The Surgery
872 Green Lane, Dagenham RM8 1BX
Tel: 020 8599 7151 Fax: 020 8983 8784
(Barking and Dagenham Primary Care Trust)
Patient List Size: 2400

Practice Manager June O'Toole

GP N P S TEOTIA

The Surgery
The Gables, 284 Porters Avenue, Dagenham RM8 2EQ
Tel: 020 8592 7679 Fax: 020 8593 8110
Email: gablessurgery@surgeriesonline.com
(Barking and Dagenham Primary Care Trust)
Patient List Size: 4554

Practice Manager F B Ghosh

GP Tushar Kanti GHOSH, Dr NAVARATNAM

The Surgery
563 Valence Avenue, Dagenham RM8 3RH
Tel: 020 8592 9111 Fax: 020 8593 6524
(Barking and Dagenham Primary Care Trust)
Patient List Size: 3300

GP Kubra Nahead JUNAID, Dr FINNEGAN, Z HAIDER

The Surgery
67-69 Langley Crescent, Dagenham RM9 6TB
Tel: 020 8592 5523 Fax: 020 8593 7235
(Barking and Dagenham Primary Care Trust)
Patient List Size: 3000

GP Subhash Chandra HORA, Seema HORA

The Surgery
36 Dewey Road, Dagenham RM10 8AR
Tel: 020 8517 8551 Fax: 020 8595 0100
(Barking and Dagenham Primary Care Trust)

GP Coopa MITRA

The Surgery
35 Maplestead Road, Dagenham RM9 4XH
Tel: 020 8595 0017 Fax: 020 8595 7741
Website: www.drmohanandpartners.co.uk
(Barking and Dagenham Primary Care Trust)
Patient List Size: 5447

Practice Manager Jennifer Phillips

GP Thota Chandra MOHAN, D ABAZIE, H R N SHAH

The Surgery
2 First Avenue, Dagenham RM10 9AT
Tel: 020 8592 4082 Fax: 020 8592 8182
(Barking and Dagenham Primary Care Trust)
Patient List Size: 1820

Practice Manager Cliff West

GP Mohammad FATEH

Tulasi Medical Centre
10 Bennetts Castle Lane, Dagenham RM8 3XU
Tel: 020 8590 1773 Fax: 020 8599 6604
(Barking and Dagenham Primary Care Trust)
Patient List Size: 4200

GP Venkatarao GORIPARTHI

Valence Wood Surgery
259 Valence Wood Road, Dagenham RM8 3AD
Tel: 020 8517 9416 Fax: 020 8517 9416
Email: sivapragarm.sivalingham@gp-f82667.nhs.uk
(Barking and Dagenham Primary Care Trust)
Patient List Size: 1500

Practice Manager Soma Sivalingam

GP Sivapragarm SIVALINGHAM

Dalton-in-Furness

Market Street Surgery
92 Market Street, Dalton-in-Furness LA15 8AB
Tel: 01229 462591 Fax: 01229 468217
(Morecambe Bay Primary Care Trust)

Practice Manager Louise Vine

GP Richard Noel JOHNSON, Phillip M BLAND, Jennifer A NEWMAN, James John O'DONOVAN, Joanna Ruth STANLEY

Nelson Street Surgery
18 Nelson Street, Dalton-in-Furness LA15 8AF
Tel: 01229 463999
(Morecambe Bay Primary Care Trust)

GP Carol Elizabeth AMOS

Darlington

Carmel Surgery
Nunnery Lane, Darlington DL3 8SQ
Tel: 01325 463149 Fax: 01325 381834
(Darlington Primary Care Trust)

Practice Manager G Carroll

GP Ahmet FUAT, Heather METCALFE, Basil Francis PENNEY

Felix House Surgery
Middleton Lane, Middleton St. George, Darlington DL2 1AE
Tel: 01325 332235 Fax: 01325 333626
(Darlington Primary Care Trust)
Patient List Size: 5400

Practice Manager Jane Saddington

GP Adrian John MARSHALL, Patrick John L HOLMES, Emma Jane PEART, Samantha S WOLFE

Felix House Surgery
Middleton Lane, Middleton St. George, Darlington DL2 1AE
Tel: 01325 332219
(Darlington Primary Care Trust)

GP Robert CARTER

Gainford Surgery
Main Road, Gainford, Darlington DL2 3BE
Tel: 01325 730204 Fax: 01325 730204
(Durham Dales Primary Care Trust)
Patient List Size: 3000

Practice Manager Annie Johnson

GP Michael James NEVILLE, Ian Ernest Gwynne WALDIN

Moorlands Surgery
139 Willow Road, Darlington DL3 9JP
Tel: 01325 469168 Fax: 01325 353695
(Darlington Primary Care Trust)
Patient List Size: 15776

GP Frank Clifford CARTER, Moira Joan HARGREAVES, Kenneth Dudley McKEOWN, Martin RHODES, Anthony SHAW, Robin WADE

Neasham Road Surgury
186 Neasham Road, Darlington DL1 4YL
Tel: 01325 461128 Fax: 01325 469123
(Darlington Primary Care Trust)
Patient List Size: 9500

Practice Manager K Crook

GP William Henry Thomas BYRNE, Sarah Marie FINNIE, Simon GULLIVER, Peter John LANGHAM, Susan Elizabeth McILHINNEY, Andreas RUSS

Netherlaw Surgery
28 Stanhope Road, Darlington DL3 7SQ
Tel: 01325 380640 Fax: 01325 350938
(Darlington Primary Care Trust)
Patient List Size: 8600

Practice Manager C Q Lees

GP David Anthony JEAVONS, Andrew John BAINES, Andrea Bronwen JONES, Andrew Forbes MICHIE, Susan Mary WATERWORTH

Orchard Court Surgery
Orchard Court, Orchard Road, Darlington DL3 6HS
Tel: 01325 465285 Fax: 01325 284034
(Darlington Primary Care Trust)
Patient List Size: 7400

GP Robert Stephen CHARLTON, Kate GORDON, David RUSSELL, Richard Charles Harrisson STEVENS, Sally Ann STONE

Parkgate Health Centre
Park Place, Darlington DL1 5LW
Tel: 01325 462762
(Darlington Primary Care Trust)

GP Charles Paul DAVISON, John Michael DAVISON, Andrew Frank KENT, Jennifer Margaret TOWNSHEND, Catherine Scott TREWBY

Parkgate Health Centre
Park Place, Darlington DL1 5LW
Tel: 01325 465646
(Darlington Primary Care Trust)

GP Aidan William LAVENDER, John SHEERAN

Parkgate Surgery
Park Place Health Centre, Darlington DL1 5LW
Tel: 01325 359585/389800 Fax: 01325 389801
(Darlington Primary Care Trust)
Patient List Size: 3500

Practice Manager Justine Watson

GP Ana Vilanova RAMOS, Caroline LENNOX

Parkgate Surgery
Park Place, Darlington DL1 5LW
Tel: 01325 389800 Fax: 01325 389801
(Darlington Primary Care Trust)

GP Caroline LENNOX, Ana Vilaneva RAMOS

The Surgery
Rockliffe Court, Hurworth Place, Darlington DL2 2DS
Tel: 01325 720605
(Darlington Primary Care Trust)
Patient List Size: 4930

GP Ian Michael Murray BAGSHAW, Gillian Barbara Glyn WILLIAMS

The Surgery
Denmark Street, Darlington DL3 0PD
Tel: 01325 460731 Fax: 01325 362183
(Darlington Primary Care Trust)

Practice Manager G Carroll

GP Roger David JAMES, Harold Hilton DIXON, John JEWITT, Shelagh Margaret NAISMITH, Geoffrey James Arthur POTTER, Martin UITENBOSCH, Anne Margaret WHITTAKER, Anna Catriona Micaela YOUNG

Whinfield Surgery
Whinbush Way, Darlington DL1 3RT
Tel: 01325 481321 Fax: 01325 380116
Email: admin@whinfield.co.uk
Website: www.whinfield.co.uk
(Darlington Primary Care Trust)
Patient List Size: 11875

Practice Manager Karol Curry

GP Robert Thomas Percy UPSHALL, Julia Lesley BROOKES, Elisabeth Maria Alberta BRUGGINK, Alessandro CALABRO, James William ELLIOT, Richard Anthony Gerard HARKER, Helen McLEISH

Dartford

Bean Village Surgery
High Street, Bean, Dartford DA2 8BS
Tel: 01474 707236
(Dartford, Gravesham and Swanley Primary Care Trust)
Patient List Size: 2150

GP S T S SOMASEGARAM

Crayford Medical Centre
4-6 Green Walk, Crayford, Dartford DA1 4JL
Tel: 01322 520100 Fax: 01322 520101
(Bexley Care Trust)

GP Jagadis Chandra SARKAR

Dartford East Health Centre
Pilgrims Way, Dartford DA1 1QY
Tel: 01322 274211 Fax: 01322 284329
(Dartford, Gravesham and Swanley Primary Care Trust)

GP Clive Henry WEST, Patricia Mary Claire BEAZLEY, Ishrat Khanum DHILLION, Charles John SHIMMINS, Shobha Jean WESTBROOK

Dartford West Health Centre
Tower Road, Dartford DA1 2HA
Tel: 01322 223600 Fax: 01322 292282
(Dartford, Gravesham and Swanley Primary Care Trust)
Patient List Size: 9000

Practice Manager Rita Whiting

GP David Richard JONES, Vibha MOHAN, Jane Frances SCOTT, David Hugh SHORT, Charis Ann SPENSLEY

Dartford West Health Centre
Tower Road, Dartford DA1 2HA
Tel: 01322 278818/220594
(Dartford, Gravesham and Swanley Primary Care Trust)
Patient List Size: 2500

Practice Manager Julia Carter

GP B S SHORA

Dartford West Health Centre
Tower Road, Dartford DA1 2HA
Tel: 01322 291636/292001
(Dartford, Gravesham and Swanley Primary Care Trust)
Patient List Size: 2100

Practice Manager Jean de Dulin

GP Nilmoni SIKDAR

Devon Road Surgery
32 Devon Road, South Darenth, Dartford DA4 9AB
Tel: 01322 862121 Fax: 01322 868794
(Dartford, Gravesham and Swanley Primary Care Trust)
Patient List Size: 6000

Practice Manager Barbara Westcott

GP John Andrew NICOLSON, Simon Peter ABURN, Anita Bernadette HUNT

Dr C H West and Partners
Dartford East Health Centre, Pilgrims Way, Dartford DA1 1QY
Tel: 01322 274211 Fax: 01322 284329
Email: practice.manager@gp-g82006.nhs.uk
(Dartford, Gravesham and Swanley Primary Care Trust)
Patient List Size: 11500

Practice Manager A D Cole

GP C H WEST, P M C BEAZLEY, I K DHILLON, C J SHIMMINS, S J WESTBROOK

Farningham Surgery
Braeside, Gorse Hill, Farningham, Dartford DA4 0JU
Tel: 01322 866038 Fax: 01322 862991
Email: practice.manager@gp-g82218.nhs.uk
Website: www.braesidesurgery.co.uk
(Dartford, Gravesham and Swanley Primary Care Trust)
Patient List Size: 5475

Practice Manager Maggie Burcham

GP Caroline DAVIES-WRAGG, John Andrew FRASER, Nigel PERRY

Horsman's Place Surgery
Instone Road, Dartford DA1 2JP
Tel: 01322 228363/277444
(Dartford, Gravesham and Swanley Primary Care Trust)
Patient List Size: 12000

Practice Manager A Mulville

GP John Bernard Lloyd SYMES, Anwara ALI, Nicholas Bosco FERNANDES, Andrew Antonio MEILAK, Gareth Michael PARRY

Lowfield Medical Centre
65-67 Lowfield Street, Dartford DA1 1HP
Tel: 01322 224550
(Dartford, Gravesham and Swanley Primary Care Trust)
Patient List Size: 5800

Practice Manager Bonny Bryan

GP David John LAWRENCE, Leonie Morgan BURROWS, Frances Mary HUNTER, Jennifer Mary RUSH

The Orchard Practice
Tower Road, Dartford DA1 2HA
Tel: 01322 228032/223960 Fax: 01322 290613
(Dartford, Gravesham and Swanley Primary Care Trust)
Patient List Size: 8285

Practice Manager June Foreman

GP David John Richard CORBETT, A P DOYLE, Vanessa Constance JEANS, Clare KING

The Surgery
Bennett Way, Darenth, Dartford DA2 7JU
Tel: 01474 707662 Fax: 01474 708940
(Dartford, Gravesham and Swanley Primary Care Trust)
Patient List Size: 2070

Practice Manager Cilla Armstrong

GP Amitabh MOHAN

Temple Hill Square Surgery
2 Temple Hill Square, Dartford DA1 5HY
Tel: 01322 226090 Fax: 01322 287655
(Dartford, Gravesham and Swanley Primary Care Trust)

GP A V KOTHARI, N A NUAMAN

Whitehill House Surgery
1 Crayford Road, Crayford, Dartford DA1 4AN
Tel: 01322 225603 Fax: 01322 293244
(Bexley Care Trust)
Patient List Size: 2700

GP Tarangini Purushottam PATEL

Dartmouth

Darmouth Medical Practice
Victoria Place, 35 Victoria Road, Dartmouth TQ6 9RT
Tel: 01803 832212 Fax: 01803 837917
Website: www.dartmedical.co.uk
(South Hams and West Devon Primary Care Trust)
Patient List Size: 8500

Practice Manager Angela Harris

GP John Sinton FENTON, Anthony Colin ANDERSON, Andrew John EYNON-LEWIS, Graham Dempster LOCKERBIE, Fiona MacKEACHAN

Darwen

Blackburn Road Surgery
153 Blackburn Road, Darwen BB3 1ET
Tel: 01254 701961 Fax: 01254 761233
(Blackburn with Darwen Primary Care Trust)

Practice Manager Carol Barr

GP Pulloori JAGADESHAM

Darwen Health Care 2000
Union Street, Darwen BB3 0DA
Tel: 01254 778366 Fax: 01254 778367
(Blackburn with Darwen Primary Care Trust)

Practice Manager Sheila Kendall

GP David Mark ANDREWS, Christopher Russell DALTON, Penelope Jane MORRIS, Mamen NWAN, Allan Alexander SINCLAIR, Raymond SUDELL

Darwen Health Centre
Union Street, Darwen BB3 0DA
Tel: 01254 706345 Fax: 01254 778388
(Blackburn with Darwen Primary Care Trust)
Patient List Size: 5669

Practice Manager Kathleen Gould

GP Ehsan AHMED, Ajeet GUPTA

Darwen Health Centre
Union Street, Darwen BB3 0DA
Tel: 01254 778377 Fax: 01254 778372
(Blackburn with Darwen Primary Care Trust)

Practice Manager Julie Price

GP Ahmed ZAMAN, Shaheed AHMED

Darwen Health Centre
Union Street, Darwen BB3 0DA
Tel: 01254 778379 Fax: 01254 778372
(Blackburn with Darwen Primary Care Trust)

Practice Manager Julie Price

GP Anthony Michael HIRST

Health Centre
Union Street, Darwen BB3 0DA
Tel: 01254 778350 Fax: 01254 778347
(Blackburn with Darwen Primary Care Trust)
Patient List Size: 3100

Practice Manager Lynda Crook

GP I M DERAR

Springfield Surgery
102 Bolton Road, Darwen BB3 1BZ
Tel: 01254 701000 Fax: 01254 761160
(Blackburn with Darwen Primary Care Trust)

GP Syed Khursheed ALAM

The Surgery
42 Railway Road, Darwen BB3 2RJ
Tel: 01254 675367 Fax: 01254 675367
(Blackburn with Darwen Primary Care Trust)

Practice Manager Ann Davis

GP A ALAM

Daventry

Byfield Medical Centre
Church Street, Byfield, Daventry NN11 6XN
Tel: 01327 260230 Fax: 01327 262243
Email: byfieldmc@dial.pipex.com
(Cherwell Vale Primary Care Trust)
Patient List Size: 7500

Practice Manager Sandra Stevens

GP Peter Howard MIDDLETON, A D BONE, Dennis Frederick BURTON

Danetre Medical Practice
The Health Centre, London Road, Daventry NN11 4EJ
Tel: 01327 703333 Fax: 01327 311221
(Daventry and South Northamptonshire Primary Care Trust)
Patient List Size: 11500

Practice Manager Ruth Farthing

GP Lesley Margaret JEFFERS, G J JAMES, Stuart KETCHIN, YU Jin SEOW, Judith VIIRA, F VOETEN

Monksfield Surgery
1 Wimbourne Place, Daventry NN11 5XY
Tel: 01327 706606 Fax: 01327 706656
(Daventry and South Northamptonshire Primary Care Trust)

Practice Manager Nigel Brown

GP Kevin Charles HERBERT, Alastair John CRAIG, Matthew Graham DAVIES, Susan Patricia DAVIES, Patricia Susan GARDINER, Thomas Michael LEYDEN, Christopher John LOVATT, Anne Margaret REDPATH, Charles David Lauchlan ROSE, Joanne Margaret SEWELL, Alexander WENNEKES

Dawlish

Barton Surgery
Barton Terrace, Dawlish EX7 9QH
Tel: 01626 888877 Fax: 01626 888360
(Teignbridge Primary Care Trust)

Practice Manager Janine Payne

GP Gerald Keith BROOK, Elizabeth Anne ALBOROUGH, Matthew FOX, Debra JEFFERY, Slav PAJOVIC, John Richard Edmund WHITEHEAD

Deal

Allen House Surgery
80 Middle Street, Deal CT14 6HL
Tel: 01304 369777 Fax: 01304 369888
(East Kent Coastal Teaching Primary Care Trust)
Patient List Size: 2250

Practice Manager J Hutchison

GP Victor John ALLEN

Balmoral Surgery
1 Victoria Road, Deal CT14 7AU
Tel: 01304 373444
(East Kent Coastal Teaching Primary Care Trust)
Patient List Size: 12000

Practice Manager L K Betts

GP Keith Leonard RAWLINGS, Tracey EASTBROOK, Frank HOFFMAN, Nicholas John SHARVILL, Arvind Kumar SINGH, Ian Robert Christopher SPARROW, Mark Trevor VINEY

The Ceders Surgery
24 Marine Road, Walmer, Deal CT14 7DN
Tel: 01304 373341 Fax: 01304 372864
(East Kent Coastal Teaching Primary Care Trust)

GP John Saunders SWALES, Marc Terence FEENEY, Elizabeth MILLS, Philip James RAWSON, Sally RUSSELL

Manor Road Surgery
38 Manor Road, Deal CT14 9BX
Tel: 01304 367495 Fax: 01304 239202
(East Kent Coastal Teaching Primary Care Trust)

GP Michael Edward HEELEY

Queen Street Surgery
13A Queen Street, Deal CT14 6ET
Tel: 01304 363181 Fax: 01304 381996
(East Kent Coastal Teaching Primary Care Trust)
Patient List Size: 9200

GP S J T WILLIAMS, H L BARROW, John Karl DYER, M J PARKS, Susan Jane RUTHERFORD, A M SCHULZ, S SCHULZ, N SWAPRASAD

Derby

Allen, Moore, Jackson and Ferrer
Wellside Medical Centre, 3 Burton Road, Derby DE1 1TH
Tel: 01332 737777 Fax: 01332 737778
(Central Derby Primary Care Trust)

Practice Manager Christine Inness

GP Geoffrey Robert ALLEN, Ian Royston FERRER, David John JACKSON, Jayne Karen MOORE

Alvaston Medical Centre
14 Boulton Lane, Alvaston, Derby DE24 0GE
Tel: 01332 571322
(Greater Derby Primary Care Trust)
Patient List Size: 11900

Practice Manager Nicola Boddy

GP Anthony Paul HARRIS, Sarah Jane ARCHER, Jane ASHBY, John Joseph SANFEY, Adrian SUMMERSCALES, Andrew URE

Appletree Medical Practice
47a Town Street, Duffield, Derby DE56 4GG
Tel: 01332 841219 Fax: 01332 841219
(Amber Valley Primary Care Trust)

Practice Manager Jayne Cooper

GP Barbara LEYLAND, Christopher John BRENTNALL, Paul Henry O'FLANAGAN, Claire Elizabeth STEVENS, Richard John WARD

Ascot Medical Centre
690 Osmaston Road, Derby DE24 8GT
Tel: 01332 348845 Fax: 01332 345726
(Central Derby Primary Care Trust)
Patient List Size: 5747

Practice Manager J Patel

GP Mohammed RAMZAN, Rameshchandra Chhotabhai PATEL

Brook Medical Centre
183 Kedleston Road, Derby DE22 1FT
Tel: 01332 291991/340576 Fax: 01332 207181
(Greater Derby Primary Care Trust)
Patient List Size: 3150

Practice Manager J Peach

GP Dr O'REILLY, Dr AITCHISON

Castle Donington Surgery
53 Borough Street, Castle Donington, Derby DE74 2LB
Tel: 01332 811480 Fax: 01332 811748
(Charnwood and North West Leicestershire Primary Care Trust)
Patient List Size: 8500

Practice Manager Kathy Wright

GP James WARD-CAMPBELL

Chapel Street Health Centre
10 Chapel Street, Spondon, Derby DE21 7RJ
Tel: 01332 674173 Fax: 01332 280387
(Greater Derby Primary Care Trust)

GP David GATES, Priscilla Shanti DAVID, T FRYATT, Ian William MATTHEWS, D J YOUNG

Charnwood Surgery
5 Burton Road, Derby DE1 1TH
Tel: 01332 737737 Fax: 01332 737738
(Central Derby Primary Care Trust)
Patient List Size: 12000

Practice Manager Judith Kirkland

GP David FARMER, Timothy Edward HEALEY, Ashish Ashok JOSHI, Sandeep KHOSLA, Philip George LACEY, Vivienne NOTLEY, Judith Mollie PARSONS

Chellaston Medical Centre
17 Derby Road, Chellaston, Derby DE73 1SA
Tel: 01332 700309 Fax: 01322 691499
(Central Derby Primary Care Trust)
Patient List Size: 1847

Practice Manager Sheila Bennett

GP Shah Mazharul Islam CHOWDHURY

Clarence Road Health Centre
63-65 Clarence Road, Normanton, Derby DE23 6LR
Tel: 01332 768912 Fax: 01332 271597
(Central Derby Primary Care Trust)
Patient List Size: 3100

Practice Manager M K Nagra

GP Mussaddaq IQBAL

The Dale Medical Centre
30 Lower Dale Road, Derby DE23 6WY
Tel: 01332 346226
(Central Derby Primary Care Trust)

GP R SEN, S K SEN

Derby Lane Medical Centre
30 Derby Lane, Derby DE23 8UA
Tel: 01332 773243
(Central Derby Primary Care Trust)
Patient List Size: 4000

Practice Manager A R Hamid

GP Arshid PIRACHA, Nasser Ali ZAMAN

Derwent Medical Centre
26 North Street, Derby DE1 3AZ
Tel: 01332 292939
Email: gm.e.gdp-pct.c81652-reception@nhs.net
(Greater Derby Primary Care Trust)
Patient List Size: 3800

Practice Manager Sarah Morcom

GP Inderjit Kaur EDYVEAN, Richard J F EDYVEAN

Derwent Valley Medical Practice
20 St Marks Road, Derby DE21 6AT
Tel: 01332 224588 Fax: 01332 224589
(Greater Derby Primary Care Trust)

Practice Manager Clive Reynolds

GP Philip Anthony DODGSON, Anna FRAIN, John Patrick James FRAIN, Andrew RATCLIFFE, Peter John WRIGGLESWORTH

Dr Doris and Partners
The medical Centre, Vicarage Road, Mickleover, Derby DE3 0HA
Tel: 01332 513283 Fax: 01332 518569
(Greater Derby Primary Care Trust)
Patient List Size: 11300

Practice Manager S Brundish

GP Edward Joseph DORIS, David Francis BOOTH, John Alexander CHARLTON, Carolyn Jean KEELING, Leszek REDLAFF

Dr N R Williams and Partners
Wellbrook Medical Centre, Welland Road, Hilton, Derby DE65 5GZ
Tel: 01283 731202 Fax: 01283 731200
Email: reception@gp-c81110.nhs.uk
(Derbyshire Dales and South Derbyshire Primary Care Trust)
Patient List Size: 7600

Practice Manager Catherine Jones

GP Neill Roger WILLIAMS, Helen L LEVER, Roger John NEWTON, Sarah Jane SMITH, Michael Harrison VICKERS

Friargate Surgery
Agard Street, Derby DE1 1DZ
Tel: 01332 294040 Fax: 01332 732026
(Greater Derby Primary Care Trust)

Practice Manager Anne Hutchinson

GP Denise Joy BINNIE, Murali GEMBALI, S S GIRN, S TRAFFORD

Hadfield Medical Centre
82 Brosscroft, Hadfield, Glossop, Derby SK13 1DS
Tel: 01457 868686 Fax: 01457 857739

(Tameside and Glossop Primary Care Trust)
Patient List Size: 3000

Practice Manager Mary Griffiths

GP Richard Peter FITTON

The Hema Medical Centre

Kledholme Lane, Alvaston, Derby DE24 0RY
Tel: 01332 571677 Fax: 01332 751302
Email: jbiswas@nhs.net
Website: www.hemamc.co.uk
(Central Derby Primary Care Trust)
Patient List Size: 2380

GP Anjan Kumar BISWAS

Hodson and Partners

Park Farm Medical Centre, Allestree, Derby DE22 2QN
Tel: 01332 559402 Fax: 01332 541001
Email: reception@gp-c81064.nhs.uk
Website: www.parkfarm-medical.net
(Greater Derby Primary Care Trust)
Patient List Size: 8760

Practice Manager L Bernthal

GP Paul Brian HODSON, Madhuri CHEEDELLA, Brian CROWLEY, Ruth LENEHAN, Christopher Brian TURNER, Paul Albert Avery WOOD

Hollybrook Medical Centre

Hollybrook Way, Heatherton Village, Derby DE23 7TU
Tel: 01332 523300
(Central Derby Primary Care Trust)

Practice Manager Daljit Shokur

GP Madeline Clare Hermina BLACKWALL, Melvyn HEAPPEY, Paul Andrew NATHAN

Jaybee Medical Centre

25 Charnwood Street, Derby DE1 2GU
Tel: 01332 342711 Fax: 01322 349004
(Central Derby Primary Care Trust)
Patient List Size: 1500

Practice Manager Wendy Bateman

GP Jogindra BAKSHI

Lister House Surgery

Lister House, 53 Harrington Street, Pear Tree, Derby DE23 8PF
Tel: 01332 271212 Fax: 01332 271939
(Central Derby Primary Care Trust)
Patient List Size: 15500

Practice Manager G Heard

GP John SPINCER, Andrew James BROOKS, William Mark HALE, Janet Alexis MILLAR CRAIG, Peter John MOSS, Simeon Sharratt RAYNER, Margaret Helen WICKS

Littleover Medical Centre

640 Burton Road, Littleover, Derby DE23 6EL
Tel: 01332 207100 Fax: 01332 342680
Email: k.patel@gp-C81112.nhs.uk
(Greater Derby Primary Care Trust)
Patient List Size: 2500

GP Kantilal Chhaganbhai PATEL, Pravina Kantilal PATEL

London Road Surgery

1149 London Road, Alvaston, Derby DE24 8QF
Tel: 01332 571344 Fax: 01332 757243
(Greater Derby Primary Care Trust)

Practice Manager Glenda Rudd

GP Prasanta Kumar CHAKRABORTI, Alaka CHAKRABORTI

Macklin Street Surgery

90 Macklin Street, Derby DE1 1JX
Tel: 01332 340381 Fax: 01332 345387
(Central Derby Primary Care Trust)
Patient List Size: 10500

Practice Manager Sue Threadgould

GP Thomas Alexander William Patrick BOLD, John Norman Heathcote EISENBERG, Sally Anne HANSON, Stuart Anthony HOLLOWAY, Martin Neil ROWAN-ROBINSON, Heather Joy SMITH

Melbourne Health Care Centre

Penn Lane, Melbourne, Derby DE73 1EF
Tel: 01332 862124 Fax: 01332 865154
Email: reception@gp-c81108.nhs.uk
(Greater Derby Primary Care Trust)
Patient List Size: 12400

Practice Manager Annette Jennison

GP Iain Laidlaw BLACK, P D DAS, James LONG, D O THOMAS, C VELTMAN, H E WRIGHT

Mickleover Surgery

10 Cavendish Way, Mickleover, Derby DE3 5BJ
Tel: 01332 519160 Fax: 01332 523054
(Greater Derby Primary Care Trust)
Patient List Size: 4958

Practice Manager Stephanie Shepherd

GP Nehad Philippe HANNA, Shoukry Latif GAYED

Normanton Medical Centre

151 St Thomas' Road, Normanton, Derby DE23 8RH
Tel: 01332 765100
Website: www.normantonmedicalcentre.co.uk
(Central Derby Primary Care Trust)
Patient List Size: 3500

Practice Manager Madhu Paul

GP J M PAUL

North Street Surgery

2 North Street, Littleover, Derby DE23 6BJ
Tel: 01332 346622 Fax: 01332 204266
(Greater Derby Primary Care Trust)

Practice Manager T Ibrahim

GP Farouk Riskalla IBRAHIM

Oakwood Surgery

380 Bishops Drive, Oakwood, Derby DE21 2DF
Tel: 01332 281220 Fax: 01332 677150
(Greater Derby Primary Care Trust)
Patient List Size: 4790

Practice Manager Kate McCall

GP Santha Kumari SREEVALSAN, M TAMPI

Orchard Surgery

The Dragwell, Kegworth, Derby DE74 2EL
Tel: 01509 672419 Fax: 01509 674196
(Rushcliffe Primary Care Trust)
Patient List Size: 7500

Practice Manager Denise Greenwood

GP Caroline Mary ANDERSON, Nigel Paul CARTWRIGHT, Helen Mara EGLITIS, Nicholas John FOSTER

Osmaston Road Medical Centre

212 Osmaston Road, Derby DE23 8JX
Tel: 01332 346433 Fax: 01332 345854
(Central Derby Primary Care Trust)
Patient List Size: 12500

Practice Manager Chris Hare

GP Ian Richard SHAND, Mark Nicholas Killin BROWNE, Ruth Isobel HEWITT, Stephen Peter STANLEY-SMITH, Christopher TOWER, Christopher Eric James WARNER, Theresa WHITTON

Overdale Medical Practice

207 Victoria Avenue, Borrowash, Derby DE72 3BH
Tel: 01332 680314 Fax: 01332 669256
Website: www.overdale.net
(Greater Derby Primary Care Trust)
Patient List Size: 10400

Practice Manager Mike Parnell

GP Alan RAYMENT, Brian Joseph BATES, R S GREGSON, Jackie HULL, Sheena LANYON, Janice LINDSAY, Xavier QULI

Park Lane Surgery
2 Park Lane, Allestree, Derby DE22 2DS
Tel: 01332 552461 Fax: 01332 541500
(Greater Derby Primary Care Trust)
Patient List Size: 5650

Practice Manager Irene Doody

GP John Edward BLISSETT, Geoffrey James NICHOLS, Isobel Rose PARKES

The Park Medical Practice
Maine Drive Clinic, Maine Drive, Chaddesden, Derby DE21 6LA
Tel: 01332 665522 Fax: 01332 678210
Website: www.parkmedical.org.uk
(Greater Derby Primary Care Trust)
Patient List Size: 20200

Practice Manager H Simpson

GP Jonathan COX, David James DISNEY, Margaret Lesley FIELDHOUSE, Roderick Alec JAMES, Martin KEELING, Jane Ann RIVERS, Douglas John THOMSON

Parkfields Surgery
1217 London Road, Alvaston, Derby DE24 8QJ
Tel: 01332 571602 Fax: 01332 758020
(Greater Derby Primary Care Trust)
Patient List Size: 5600

Practice Manager Val Hackett

GP Anthony D W GOULD, M J BAWDEN, A G BROWN

Peartree Medical Centre
159 Pear Tree Road, Derby DE23 8NQ
Tel: 01332 360692 Fax: 01332 368181
(Central Derby Primary Care Trust)
Patient List Size: 3500

Practice Manager S Rashid

GP Dhruva Narayan Prasad SINGH

The Vernon Street Medical Centre
13 Vernon Street, Derby DE1 1FW
Tel: 01332 332812 Fax: 01332 202698
(Greater Derby Primary Care Trust)
Patient List Size: 7000

Practice Manager Mike Kelly

GP Mohini Mohan BHOWMIK, Peter William IDDON, Paul McQUADE, Caroline Anne WILLIAMS

The Vernon Street Medical Centre
13 Vernon Street, Derby DE1 1FW
Tel: 01332 332812 Fax: 01332 202608
Email: mike.kew@gp-C81007.nhs.uk
(Greater Derby Primary Care Trust)

Practice Manager Mike Kelly

GP Mohini Mohan BHOWMIK, Peter IDDON, Paul McQUADE, Caroline WILLIAMS

Vidya Medical Centre
12 Charnwood Street, Derby DE1 2GT
Tel: 01332 345406 Fax: 01332 345863
Email: iffat.Khan@gp.C816501.nhs.uk
(Central Derby Primary Care Trust)
Patient List Size: 2500

Practice Manager Iffat Khan

GP Santosh SINHA

Village Surgery
233 Village Street, Derby DE23 8DD
Tel: 01332 766762 Fax: 01332 272084
(Central Derby Primary Care Trust)
Patient List Size: 10805

Practice Manager May Giordano

GP Peter Julian HORDEN, Kerryn Marie COTTON, Sara Elizabeth DEW, Peter James HOWELL, Joao Leonardo MONTEIRO, Adrian Leslie WHITEHALL

Willington Surgery
4 Repton Road, Willington, Derby DE65 6BX
Tel: 01283 703318 Fax: 01283 701457
Website: www.willingtonsurgery.co.uk
(Derbyshire Dales and South Derbyshire Primary Care Trust)
Patient List Size: 8300

Practice Manager Lisa Smith

GP Kyran Anthony FARRELL, Roslyn Joanne FARROW, Brian Gerard HANDS, Liam Michael O'HARA, Ramanathan RAJENDRAN

Wilson Street Surgery
11 Wilson Street, Derby DE1 1PG
Tel: 01332 344366 Fax: 01332 348813
Email: enquiries@wilsonstreetsurgery.co.uk
Website: www.wilsonstreetsurgery.co.uk
(Central Derby Primary Care Trust)

Practice Manager Valerie Winn

GP Nicholas COXON, James DANIELLS, Jill FLETCHER, Andrew FYALL, Helen JERVIS, Jabeen KHAN, Steven LITTLE, Mohammed MUNIT, Jayne NUTTALL, Andrew SOUMERS

Dereham

Elmham Surgery
Holt Road, Elmham, Dereham NR20 5JS
Tel: 01362 668215 Fax: 01362 668625
Email: elmsurgery@lineone.net
(Southern Norfolk Primary Care Trust)
Patient List Size: 7600

GP Paul John STRICKLAND, Simon Michael CARROLL, Simon Charles HIBBERD, Ian JENNINGS, C M MUELLER, T W WELLTON

The Orchard Surgery
Commercial Road, Dereham NR19 1AE
Tel: 01362 693029 Fax: 01362 698347
(Southern Norfolk Primary Care Trust)
Patient List Size: 8500

Practice Manager Rachel Crampton

GP Stephen Christopher MOORE, Katharine Gunilla LAVELLE, Andrew George MARCZEWSKI, Colin TRACEY

The Surgery
15 Dereham Road, Mattishall, Dereham NR20 3QA
Tel: 01362 850227 Fax: 01362 858466
(Southern Norfolk Primary Care Trust)

Practice Manager Stephen Smith

GP Richard John Rippon HUGHES, Adrian Laurence HODGE, Elizabeth Ann JONES, Hywel Wyn JONES, Kenneth Rhys WEBB

Theatre Royal Surgery
27 Theatre Street, Dereham NR19 2EN
Tel: 01362 852800 Fax: 01362 852819
Email: enquiries@theatresurgery.com
Website: www.theatresurgery.com
(Southern Norfolk Primary Care Trust)
Patient List Size: 9900

Practice Manager Val Harvey

GP Simon Freeth COOPER, Christopher Adrian ABELL, William Simon CARTLEDGE, M ROSBERGEN, Sandra Jane TAYLOR, Scott David TURNER

The Walker-Gregory Practice
2 Chapel Lane, Toftwood, Dereham NR19 1LD
Tel: 01362 691196 Fax: 01362 698091
Email: toftwoodmedicalcentre@gp-d82629.nhs.uk
(Southern Norfolk Primary Care Trust)
Patient List Size: 3500

Practice Manager Eve Barrett

GP A WALKER, A GREGORY

Devizes

Lansdowne Surgery
Waiblingen Way, Devizes SN10 2BU
Tel: 01380 722278 Fax: 01380 723790
Email: hansdowne@gp-J83034.nhs.uk
(Kennet and North Wiltshire Primary Care Trust)
Patient List Size: 8000

Practice Manager Jill Cross

GP David Anthony Neil TWINER, Charles Johnstone COWEN, Brian James JONES, Elizabeth Anne MADIGAN

Littleton Panell Surgery
78 High Street, Littleton Panell, Devizes SN10 4EX
Tel: 01380 813300
(Kennet and North Wiltshire Primary Care Trust)

Market Lavington Surgery
The High Street, Market Lavington, Devizes SN10 4AG
Tel: 01380 812500 Fax: 01380 818267
Email: dawn.edwards@gp-j83056.nhs.uk
(Kennet and North Wiltshire Primary Care Trust)
Patient List Size: 5400

Practice Manager Dawn Edwards

GP Jonathan David Temple MILLER, Anna COLLINGS, Mary Anne Barbara GOMPELS, Richard Charles Simon SANDFORD-HILL

Southbroom Surgery
15 Estcourt Street, Devizes SN10 1LQ
Tel: 01380 720909
(Kennet and North Wiltshire Primary Care Trust)

Practice Manager Viv Laing

GP Stephen Henton SIGGERS, Richard David John ARCHER, John Squire HEATON-RENSHAW, Rosemary Gaenor LINDON, Joanna Eve PULLEN, Ian WILLIAMS

St James Surgery
Gains Lane, Devizes SN10 1QU
Tel: 01380 722206 Fax: 01380 734541
Website: www.st-james-gp-surgery-devizes.com
(Kennet and North Wiltshire Primary Care Trust)
Patient List Size: 5500

Practice Manager Joss Green-Armytage

GP John Wickham NEW, A DAVIES, Anthony DOWNEY, Paul Duncan JACKSON, Minar PARSLEY

Dewsbury

Charles Street Surgery
25 Charles Street, Ravensthorpe, Dewsbury WF13 3LA
Tel: 01924 464909
(North Kirklees Primary Care Trust)

GP T UNNIKRISHNAN

Clarkson Street Surgery
42 Clarkson Street, Ravensthorpe, Dewsbury WF13 3DR
Tel: 01924 491096
(North Kirklees Primary Care Trust)
Patient List Size: 2000

Practice Manager Sandra Lachucik

GP Mushtaq AHMAD

Earlsheaton Medical Centre
252 Wakefield Road, Earlsheaton, Dewsbury WF12 8AH
Tel: 01924 465511
(North Kirklees Primary Care Trust)
Patient List Size: 12600

Practice Manager Lynn Batley

GP Abdulrehman Ibrahim RAJPURA, S N HASSAN, Yaqub HUSSAIN, M J KHAN, S KHAN, Mazhar KHURSHID, A SHAICH

Eightlands Surgery
Eightlands Road, Dewsbury WF13 2PA
Tel: 01924 465929 Fax: 01924 488740
(North Kirklees Primary Care Trust)
Patient List Size: 6600

Practice Manager Ann Bibey

GP John HICKS, Susan DHIR, Kollura Mudianselage Jayawickrama SENARATNE

Halifax Road Surgery
9 Halifax Road, Dewsbury WF13 2JH
Tel: 01924 463934 Fax: 01924 485800
Email: practice.manager@B85004.nhs.uk
(North Kirklees Primary Care Trust)
Patient List Size: 4500

Practice Manager Clare Towend, Susan Walker

GP Steven Neil MEDLEY, Christine Ann CONWAY, Heather Dawn SPENCER

Mountain Road Medical Centre
Thornhill, Dewsbury WF12 0BS
Tel: 01924 522100 Fax: 01924 522102
(North Kirklees Primary Care Trust)
Patient List Size: 2900

Practice Manager Louise Manders

GP Hanume THIMMEGOWDA, A T MERSON

The New Brewery Lane Surgery
Brewery Lane, Thornhill Lees, Dewsbury WF12 9DU
Tel: 01924 458787 Fax: 01924 458040
(North Kirklees Primary Care Trust)
Patient List Size: 2000

Practice Manager Janet Smith

GP Yunus Y ASMAL

North Road Surgery
27 North Road, Ravensthorpe, Dewsbury WF13 3AA
Tel: 01924 464492 Fax: 01924 452998
(North Kirklees Primary Care Trust)

GP Sabaratnam BALASUNDERAM, N CHANDRA, C G G KUMAR, M MUTHY

The Paddock Surgery
Chapel Lane, Thornhill, Dewsbury WF12 0DH
Tel: 01924 465343 Fax: 01924 455781
(North Kirklees Primary Care Trust)
Patient List Size: 5225

Practice Manager Irene Micklethwaite

GP Shelagh Patricia BULLIMORE, Christopher David ROBINSON, A SINGH

Slaithwaite Road Surgery
140 Slaithwaite Road, Thornhill Lees, Dewsbury WF12 9DW
Tel: 01924 461369
(North Kirklees Primary Care Trust)
Patient List Size: 6000

GP Yakub Valibhai Suleman PATEL, E F O'DALY

The Surgery
47 Albion Street, Dewsbury WF13 2AJ
Tel: 01924 450303 Fax: 01924 438200
(North Kirklees Primary Care Trust)
Patient List Size: 3200

Practice Manager Kathleen North

GP N A SALAM, A A SALAM

The Town Surgery
38 The Town, Dewsbury WF12 0QY
Tel: 01924 430386
(North Kirklees Primary Care Trust)

Practice Manager A Cross

GP K SHARMA

Warren Street Surgery
37 Warren Street, Savile Town, Dewsbury WF12 9LX
Tel: 01924 468686 Fax: 01924 520020
(North Kirklees Primary Care Trust)
Patient List Size: 2670

Practice Manager Rashida Pandor

GP Tariq Mahmood FAROOQUI

West Park Surgery
20 West Park Street, Dewsbury WF13 4LA
Tel: 01924 461735 Fax: 01924 507999
(North Kirklees Primary Care Trust)

Practice Manager June Hardy

GP Ebrahim Ismail DADIBHAI, M J KHAN

Windsor Medical Centre
2 William Street, Leeds Road, Dewsbury WF12 7BD
Tel: 01924 465699 Fax: 01924 456232
(North Kirklees Primary Care Trust)
Patient List Size: 2900

Practice Manager S Brown

GP Ajit Pratap MEHROTRA

Didcot

Didcot Health Centre
Britwell Road, Didcot OX11 7JH
Tel: 01235 512288 Fax: 01235 811473
Email: practice@didcothc.oxongps.co.uk
(South West Oxfordshire Primary Care Trust)
Patient List Size: 16250

Practice Manager Jackie Mercer

GP Keith Bryan James BESWICK, William Gerald Richard COULDRICK, David Henry George EBBS, William James FITCHFORD, Victoria Hazel HAMILTON, Sheelagh Elisabeth HAWTHORNE, David Henry STAINTHORP, Caroline Mary YORSTON

Oak Tree Health Centre
Tyne Avenue, Didcot OX11 7GD
Tel: 01235 810099 Fax: 01235 815181
Website: www.oaktreehc.nhs.uk
(South West Oxfordshire Primary Care Trust)
Patient List Size: 6800

Practice Manager Barry Coward

GP Ian Donald MACKENZIE, David CORPS, Justine GEDDES, Alyson LEE, Justine TURNBULL

Woodlands Medical Centre
Woodland Road, Didcot OX11 0BB
Tel: 01235 511355 Fax: 01235 512808
(South West Oxfordshire Primary Care Trust)
Patient List Size: 10660

Practice Manager L McGuigan

GP Nicholas George SALZMAN, Barbara Jean BATTY, John Brinley DELFOSSE, Jill Anne KERSHAW, Dona PATHINAYAKE, Peter RUBIN

Diss

Avicenna
High Street, Hopton, Diss IP22 2QX
Tel: 01953 681303 Fax: 01953 681305
(Suffolk West Primary Care Trust)
Patient List Size: 4079

Practice Manager Mavis Hunt

GP Andrew Gemmel HASSAN, Elisabeth Caroline WALLACE, Suzanne Margaret WHEBLE

Church Hill Surgery
Station Road, Pulham Market, Diss IP21 4TX
Tel: 01379 676227 Fax: 01379 608014
(Southern Norfolk Primary Care Trust)
Patient List Size: 4150

Practice Manager Brenda Beech

GP Philip Andrew LEFTLEY, Dr HARTLY BOOTH, Dr WISDOM

The Health Centre
Back Hills, Botesdale, Diss IP22 1DW
Tel: 01379 898295 Fax: 01379 890477
Email: docs.botesdale@btinternet.com
(Suffolk West Primary Care Trust)
Patient List Size: 7563

Practice Manager Mike South

GP Robert Humphrey Felix BAWDEN, Lauren BATE, Timothy David COOKE, Susan Elizabeth DRAKE, Monica KEEL, Timothey WATSON, Thomas Andrew YAGER

Mount Street Health Centre
The Lawns Medical Practice, Mount Street, Diss IP22 4QG
Tel: 01379 642021 Fax: 01379 641673
(Southern Norfolk Primary Care Trust)
Patient List Size: 6200

Practice Manager Ann Steele

GP Allan Desmond JONES, Andreas PANTAZIS, Martin SCHEDE, Nigel Stuart THOMSON

Mount Street Health Centre
The Parishfields Practice, Mount Street, Diss IP22 4QG
Tel: 01379 642023 Fax: 01379 643320
(Southern Norfolk Primary Care Trust)

Practice Manager Mike Daylion

GP Roger Michael GROGONO, Susan Mary CLARKE, Ian Martyn HUME, Michelle McCARTHY

Doncaster

Ali-Khan and Partners
128 High Street, Bentley, Doncaster DN5 0AT
Tel: 01302 874551 Fax: 01302 820920
(Doncaster West Primary Care Trust)
Patient List Size: 5850

Practice Manager Debbie Forbes

GP Mirza Kamran BAIG, Mir Vizarath ALI KHAN, Vanessa Louise BARRETT, Selina FOX

Askern Health Centre
Spa Pool Road, Askern, Doncaster DN6 0HZ
(Doncaster West Primary Care Trust)
Patient List Size: 1800

Practice Manager Beverley Sayer

GP A A KOUCHOUK

The Burns Medical Practice
4 Albion Place, Bennetthorpe, Doncaster DN1 2EQ
Tel: 01302 810888 Fax: 01302 812150
(Doncaster Central Primary Care Trust)

Practice Manager Sue Greenham

GP Kenneth Anthony KILVINGTON, David Henry CUBBON, Simon Nicholas FEARNS, Patrick O'HORAN

Carcroft Health Centre
Chestnut Avenue, Carcroft, Doncaster DN6 8AG
Tel: 01302 723510 Fax: 01302 337027
Email: carcrofthealthcentre@gp-c86001.nhs.uk
(Doncaster West Primary Care Trust)
Patient List Size: 10900

Practice Manager Kath Jones

GP Nicola Jane CZEPULKOWSKI, Alfredo ESPINA, Judith Mary FEARNS, Ian Peter KERR, Robin Francis PARDOE

Chestnut House Surgery
20 Field Road, Thorne, Doncaster DN8 4AF
Tel: 01405 741100 Fax: 01405 812937
(Doncaster East Primary Care Trust)
Patient List Size: 2170

Practice Manager Nic Burne

GP Julia Mary BURNE

The Clinic
Church Road, Denaby Main, Doncaster DN12 4AB
Tel: 01709 863302
(Doncaster West Primary Care Trust)
Patient List Size: 2000

Practice Manager Claire Davies

The Dove Primary Care Centre
Phoenix Medical Practice, 1A Cavendish Court, South Parade, Doncaster DN1 2DJ
Tel: 01302 762110
Email: reception@gp-C86030.nhs.uk
(Doncaster Central Primary Care Trust)

Practice Manager Jacqui Harper

GP Mohammed Aurangzeb KHAN, K BRENNAN, H D GODLEY, A GRAVES, M E HUGHES, A J INMAN, D MALSON, D SAVAGE

Dunsville Medical Centre
128 High Street, Dunsville, Doncaster DN7 4BY
Tel: 01302 890108 Fax: 01302 881425
(Doncaster East Primary Care Trust)

Practice Manager Joan Wright

GP Julia Helen JACKSON, Alison FISHER

Gardens Lane Health Centre
Gardens Lane, Conisborough, Doncaster DN12 3JW
Tel: 01709 862150 Fax: 01709 868322
Email: john@gilbert63.freeserve.co.uk
(Doncaster West Primary Care Trust)
Patient List Size: 2100

Practice Manager Susan Tarry

GP John GILBERT

Harworth Medical Centre
73A Bawtry Road, Harworth, Doncaster DN11 8NT
Tel: 01302 752798 Fax: 01302 742202
(Bassetlaw Primary Care Trust)

Practice Manager Andrea Hibberd

GP A RAHEEM

Hatfield Health Centre
Crookesbroom Lane, Hatfield, Doncaster DN7 6JN
Tel: 01302 841373 Fax: 01302 351862
(Doncaster East Primary Care Trust)
Patient List Size: 10336

Practice Manager Brian Ward

GP Lindsay Frances SIMMONITE, Jeremy Mark BRADLEY, Sara Edwina FARMER, R Z L SHAH, Ian Robert WEEKS

The Health Centre
Bridge Street, Thorne, Doncaster DN8 5QH
Tel: 01405 812121 Fax: 01405 741059
(Doncaster East Primary Care Trust)
Patient List Size: 12500

Practice Manager Pauline Dobson

GP Garry Nelson TOMLINSON, A GHOSH, Philip GLAVES, W GORMAN, R P LUND, A K RANA

The Health Centre
Broomhouse Lane, Edlington, Doncaster DN12 1LW
Tel: 01709 863256
(Doncaster West Primary Care Trust)

Practice Manager Jean Reynolds

GP M A ZAIDI, Gordon Raymond CORRIE, Prakash Rao JADHAV

Health Centre
Station Road, Bawtry, Doncaster DN10 6RQ
Tel: 01302 710210 Fax: 01302 710261
(Bassetlaw Primary Care Trust)

Practice Manager Richard Gilbert

GP A M JOHNSON, Dr STEWART

Health Clinic
Gardens Lane, Conisborough, Doncaster DN12 3JW
Tel: 01709 862150
(Doncaster West Primary Care Trust)

GP Tarikere Shanthappa JAGADISH

Health Clinic
Gardens Lane, Conisborough, Doncaster DN12 3JW
Tel: 01709 862150
(Doncaster West Primary Care Trust)

GP Muhammad Shamsul HAQ, Mohamed Badrul ISLAM

Health Clinic
Gardens Lane, Conisborough, Doncaster DN12 3JW
Tel: 01709 862150
(Doncaster West Primary Care Trust)
Patient List Size: 2400

Practice Manager Jean Ellor

GP Riyaz Ahmad GONI

Kingthorne Group Practice
83A Thorne Road, Doncaster DN1 2EU
Tel: 01302 342832 Fax: 01302 366995
(Doncaster Central Primary Care Trust)
Patient List Size: 9000

Practice Manager Jane A Windust

GP Martyn Crawford COLEMAN, R P CHAUDHARY, Anne Lesley FORBES, Neil Robert SELLARS, Carol Anne SHARPE, N A TUPPER

Lakeside Practice
The Health Centre, Off Station Road, Askern, Doncaster DN6 0JB
Tel: 01302 700212 Fax: 01302 707370
(Doncaster West Primary Care Trust)
Patient List Size: 6900

Practice Manager Eileen Gilmour

GP Melvyn Roy TAYLOR, Christopher Stephen BROPHY, Dominic Sean OTTEY

Mayflower Medical Practice
Bawtry Health Centre, Station Road, Bawtry, Doncaster DN10 6RQ
Tel: 01302 710326 Fax: 01302 719884
(Doncaster East Primary Care Trust)
Patient List Size: 7835

GP Laurence Malcombe ADAMS, Richard CROOKS, David MALIN, Helen OAKLEY, Jill SADDLER

The Medical Centre
2 Francis Street, Doncaster DN1 1JS
Tel: 01302 349431
Website: www.medicalcentredoncaster.co.uk
(Doncaster Central Primary Care Trust)
Patient List Size: 8900

Practice Manager Chris Simmonds

GP Leslie BRAIDWOOD, Patricia BARBOUR, Nicholas McKinley MIDDLETON, Charles William WRIGHT

The Nelson Practice
Amersall Road, Scawthorpe, Doncaster DN5 9PQ
(Doncaster West Primary Care Trust)

GP James Prestwich NELSON

The Oakwood Surgery
Masham Road, Cantley, Doncaster DN4 6BU
Tel: 01302 537611 Fax: 01302 371804
(Doncaster Central Primary Care Trust)
Patient List Size: 5800

Practice Manager Paul Byron

GP John Joseph HARRIS, Rosemary Ann HAMLIN, Michael Frederick HASENFUSS, Sharon Louise PHILLIPS

The Petersgate Medical Centre
99 Amersall Road, Scawthorpe, Doncaster DN5 9PQ
Tel: 01302 390490 Fax: 01302 390412
Website: www.petersgatemedicalcentre.nhs.uk
(Doncaster West Primary Care Trust)

GP Barry Joseph McKENNA, Carolyn Margaret BLOORE, Sheila Ann INGLIS, Marco PIERI, Stephan WELLER

Phoenix Surgery
10-12 Bradford Row, Doncaster DN1 3NF
Tel: 01302 323492 Fax: 01302 341008
(Doncaster Central Primary Care Trust)
Patient List Size: 2000

Practice Manager Cindy Shaw

GP Dr KHAN

Princess Medical Centre
Princess Street, Woodlands, Doncaster DN6 7LX
Tel: 01302 723406 Fax: 01302 723433
(Doncaster West Primary Care Trust)

GP Stephen Roderick INMAN, Michael Graeme POSKITT

Ransome Practice
Bentley Health Centre, Askern Road, Bentley, Doncaster DN5 0JX
Tel: 01302 874416 Fax: 01302 875820
(Doncaster West Primary Care Trust)
Patient List Size: 4400

Practice Manager Mary Hudson

GP Alfred ANIM-ADDO, Markkandu KULANTHAIVELU, Puvanasundaram UMAPATHEE

Regent Square Group Practice
8-9 Regent Square, Doncaster DN1 2DS
Tel: 01302 819999 Fax: 01302 369204
(Doncaster Central Primary Care Trust)
Patient List Size: 11800

Practice Manager Janet Hancock

GP Andrew John MARSHALL, Katherine Mary ADDEY, Don HEZSELTINE, Patrick John HURLEY, Lesley KIRKPATRICK

Rossington Practice
Grange Lane, New Rossington, Doncaster DN11 0LP
Tel: 01302 868421 Fax: 01302 863622
(Doncaster East Primary Care Trust)
Patient List Size: 11500

Practice Manager Jean Reynolds

GP Inderjeet Singh DUA, W D DAHANAYAKE, Promila DUA, S Z JAMALI, S T A SHAH

Saint Vincent Medical Centre
77 Thorne Road, Doncaster DN1 2ET
Tel: 01302 361318
Website: www.stvincentpractice.com
(Doncaster Central Primary Care Trust)
Patient List Size: 7500

Practice Manager Lynne Neale, Chris Rice

GP Alison Joy INMAN, Douglas SAVAGE, Kevin BRENNAN, Victoria Elise BURNETT, Peter Ronald DONK, Heather Daphne GODLEY, Alastair Clydesdale GRAVES, Deborah Jane MALSON

Sandringham Practice
Sandringham Road Health Centre, Sandringham Road, Intake, Doncaster DN2 5JH
Tel: 01302 321521 Fax: 01302 761792
(Doncaster Central Primary Care Trust)
Patient List Size: 8061

Practice Manager Margaret Forsyth

GP Peter William LOVE, Rebecca CLARK, Ibrahim HASSAN, Kerry STRACHAN, Kenneth Bryan SYKES

Scawsby Health Centre
Barnsley Road, Scawsby, Doncaster DN5 8QE
Tel: 01302 782208 Fax: 01302 390897
(Doncaster West Primary Care Trust)
Patient List Size: 6100

Practice Manager A Renney

GP A SYED, M ABBAS, V REHMAN

The Scott Practice
1 Greenfield Lane, Balby, Doncaster DN4 0TG
Tel: 01302 850546 Fax: 01302 851940
(Doncaster Central Primary Care Trust)
Patient List Size: 13500

Practice Manager Rose Fells

GP Anthony Martin LE VANN, Peter John BENSON, Lindsey Denise BRITTEN, John Robert CORLETT, C D HEAD, Kevin Michael Stewart LEE, Valerie Christine MARSH, P NDIR

Shelley House
King Edward Street, Belton, Doncaster DN9 1QN
Tel: 01427 872757
(North Lincolnshire Primary Care Trust)

GP J MATHEW

Spa Surgery
Portacabin off Spa Pool Road, Askern, Doncaster DN6 0HZ
Tel: 01302 700378 Fax: 01302 708006
(Doncaster West Primary Care Trust)

Practice Manager Jo Phipps

GP L A KIRKPATRICK

St John's Group Practice
1 Greenfield Lane, Balby, Doncaster DN4 0TH
Tel: 01302 854521 Fax: 01302 310823
(Doncaster Central Primary Care Trust)
Patient List Size: 9500

GP Howard William ORRIDGE, Margaret Anne COPE, Simon John de GROOT, Suzanne KIRBY, Duncan Sherwood MACKENZIE, Karen WAGSTAFF

The Surgery
25 St Mary's Road, Tickhill, Doncaster DN11 9NA
Tel: 01302 742503 Fax: 01302 752293
(Doncaster East Primary Care Trust)
Patient List Size: 9559

Practice Manager Angela Dean

GP Richard James BUCKLE, Peter Howard Ellis Gledhill COOK, David Charles FEARNS, Ian Michael SAUNDERS

The Surgery
54 Thorne Road, Doncaster DN1 2JP
Tel: 01302 361222 Fax: 01302 367833
(Doncaster Central Primary Care Trust)
Patient List Size: 12400

Practice Manager Joanne Gibbins

GP Aubrey Winston BERRY, John Charles FELTON, Sento KAR, Stephen MOORE, Bhupen Motibhai PATEL, Heinz ZAHUR

The Surgery
Marsh Lane, Misterton, Doncaster DN10 4DL
Tel: 01427 890206 Fax: 01427 891794
Website: www.mistertongrouppractice@'nhs.uk
(Bassetlaw Primary Care Trust)
Patient List Size: 5650

Practice Manager Graham Mickley

GP Robert John WYATT, Anthony Jonathan BROWNSON, Christopher McMAHON

The Surgery
4 Bungalow Road, Edlington, Doncaster DN12 1DL
Tel: 01709 868080
(Doncaster West Primary Care Trust)

Practice Manager Lin Webb

GP H B NAYAR, R K NAYAR

The Surgery
1 Wheatley Street, Denaby Main, Doncaster DN12 4AT
Tel: 01709 866175
(Doncaster West Primary Care Trust)

GP David Charles FITTON

The Surgery
Fox Lane, Barnburgh, Doncaster DN5 7ET
Tel: 01709 892059 Fax: 01709 888744
(Doncaster West Primary Care Trust)
Patient List Size: 1600

Practice Manager Deborah Leigh

GP Lisbeth Jane RODGERS

The Surgery
Field Road, Stainforth, Doncaster DN7 5AF
Tel: 01302 841202 Fax: 01302 351725
(Doncaster East Primary Care Trust)
Patient List Size: 9292

Practice Manager Paul Kemm

GP David John BROWN, Jonathan Charles BUNDY, Andrew Charles OAKFORD, Rachel Sarah SYKES, Paul Douglas WILSON

The Surgery
Lyndhurst, Church Road, Stainforth, Doncaster DN7 5PW
Tel: 01302 841507 Fax: 01302 350545
(Doncaster East Primary Care Trust)
Patient List Size: 2500

Practice Manager Rashida Islam

GP Gousul ISLAM

The Surgery
41 Ellers Lane, Auckley, Doncaster DN9 3HY
Tel: 01302 770327 Fax: 01302 771302
(Doncaster East Primary Care Trust)
Patient List Size: 2223

Practice Manager Elizabeth Walsh

GP Nabel Doss SALAMA

The Surgery
High Street, Epworth, Doncaster DN9 1EP
Tel: 01427 872232 Fax: 01427 874944
(North Lincolnshire Primary Care Trust)

Practice Manager Marilyn Bates

GP Niall Mackay SINCLAIR, Andrea DEXTER, Dr EALK, John Martin GALLAGHER, Karena Anne PLATTS, Rosemarie Felicity WEBB, Keith YOUNG

The Surgery
142 Marshland Road, Moorends, Doncaster DN8 4SU
Tel: 01405 740094 Fax: 01405 741063
(Doncaster East Primary Care Trust)
Patient List Size: 4000

Practice Manager Hilary Cook

GP Pradipkumar PRAMANIK, Asok Kumar SETH

The Village Practice
Mere Lane, Armthorpe, Doncaster DN3 2DB
Tel: 01302 300322 Fax: 01302 300737
Email: thevillagepractice@gpc-86039.nhs.uk
(Doncaster East Primary Care Trust)
Patient List Size: 6173

Practice Manager Deborah Velasco

GP Paul Fearnley EDDISON, Alan John BAKE, Jose VELASCO ALBENDEA

West End Clinic
West End Lane, Rossington, Doncaster DN11 0PQ
Tel: 01302 865865 Fax: 01302 868346
(Doncaster East Primary Care Trust)
Patient List Size: 3540

Practice Manager Yvonne Cave

GP Ashok TANEJA, Wendy BARKER, Kathryn KEMP

White House Farm Medical Centre
Church Street, Armthorpe, Doncaster DN3 3AH
Tel: 01302 831437 Fax: 01302 300623
(Doncaster East Primary Care Trust)
Patient List Size: 6356

Practice Manager Carole Brown

GP Shabbir AHMAD, Jahanna BENNEKERS, Sem DAHANAYAKE

Woodside Surgery
Woodside Road, Woodlands, Doncaster DN6 7JR
Tel: 01302 330212 Fax: 01302 330591
(Doncaster West Primary Care Trust)

Practice Manager Mrs Hinds

GP David Arnold GIBSON

Dorchester

Cornwall Road Surgery
15 Cornwall Road, Dorchester DT1 1RU
Tel: 01305 251128 Fax: 01305 250837
(South West Dorset Primary Care Trust)
Patient List Size: 5800

Practice Manager M E Johnson

GP Paul Francis WRIGHT, Stella Loraine BAWDEN, Charles Rollason CAMPION-SMITH, Andrew James RIDDOCH

Crosstree Close Surgery
Osmington Drove, Broadmayne, Dorchester DT2 8EN
Tel: 01305 852231 Fax: 01305 852999
Email: abowering@gp-j81623.nhs.uk
(South West Dorset Primary Care Trust)
Patient List Size: 1150

Practice Manager Linda Bollom

GP Anthony Richard BOWERING

Fordington Surgery
91-93 High Street, Fordington, Dorchester DT1 1LD
Tel: 01305 250505 Fax: 01305 262821
(South West Dorset Primary Care Trust)

Practice Manager R Southway

GP Adrian Michael George CLARKE, Andrew BAILEY, Sue FLOWERDEW

Grosvenor Road Surgery
4 Grosvenor Road, Dorchester DT1 2BB
Tel: 01305 251004 Fax: 01305 250684
(South West Dorset Primary Care Trust)

Practice Manager B Chesney

GP David CHESNEY

Long Street Practice
51 Long Street, Cerne Abbas, Dorchester DT2 7JG
Tel: 01300 341666 Fax: 01300 341090
(North Dorset Primary Care Trust)
Patient List Size: 4125

Practice Manager Lynne Dolder

GP Craig Timothy WAKEHAM, Jeremy Francis Roland DOBBS, Helen Murray TAYLOR, Jill Rachel VINES

Mill Street Surgery
Mill Street, Puddletown, Dorchester DT2 8SH
Tel: 01305 848333 Fax: 01305 848061
(South West Dorset Primary Care Trust)
Patient List Size: 3500

Practice Manager Carol Taylor

GP John S TAYLOR, Anne Mary Elizabeth BOYLE

Prince of Wales Road Surgery
6 Prince of Wales Road, Dorchester DT1 1PW
Tel: 01305 251762 Fax: 01305 251366
(South West Dorset Primary Care Trust)
Patient List Size: 3700

Practice Manager P Wallace

GP Christopher Brian Edwin MILLNER, F J QUICK, K E SCOTT, S M SCOTT

Queens Avenue Surgery
14 Queens Avenue, Dorchester DT1 2EW
Tel: 01305 262886 Fax: 01305 250607
(South West Dorset Primary Care Trust)
Patient List Size: 6750

Practice Manager T Bowden

GP Graham John FRANCIS, Jacqueline Clare FLEET, Rod LEWIS, Desmond LING

Trinity Street Surgery
20 Trinity Street, Dorchester DT1 1TU
Tel: 01305 251545 Fax: 01305 269707
Email: postmaster@gp-J81086.nhs.uk
(South West Dorset Primary Care Trust)
Patient List Size: 6200

Practice Manager Bev Knowlden

GP Elizabeth Anne WILLIAMS, Jonathan S EASTERBROOKE, Sian Sarah GRIFFITHS

Wiley, Sinclair and Kettell
The Surgery, Pound Piece, Maiden Newton, Dorchester DT2 0DB
Tel: 01300 320206 Fax: 01300 320399
Email: postmaster@gp-J81076.nhs.uk
(South West Dorset Primary Care Trust)
Patient List Size: 5600

Practice Manager Sheila McConnell

GP Paul Francis WILEY

Dorking

Health Building Surgery
1 Bentsbrook Close, North Holmwood, Dorking RH5 4HY
Tel: 01306 885802
(East Elmbridge and Mid Surrey Primary Care Trust)

Practice Manager John Short

GP Richard Hollis CHAPPELL, Justin Rhys THOMPSON

Leith Hill Practice
The Old Forge Surgery, 168 The Street, Capel, Dorking RH5 5EQ
Tel: 01306 711105 Fax: 01306 712751
(East Elmbridge and Mid Surrey Primary Care Trust)
Patient List Size: 8200

Practice Manager Jill Shankley

GP Richard Thomas Lees CURTIES, Anna BARHAM, Graham John BLOCKEY, Juliet BOWER, Stephen David Byron JEFFERIES, Louise KEENE

Medwyn Surgery
Moores Road, Dorking RH4 2BG
Tel: 01306 882422 Fax: 01306 742280
Website: www.medwynsurgery-homestead.com
(East Elmbridge and Mid Surrey Primary Care Trust)
Patient List Size: 6915

Practice Manager Marion Webb

GP Salvatore Christopher MONELLA, Louise Dawn TOMEI, Stewart TOMLINSON

New House Surgery
142A South Street, Dorking RH4 2QR
Tel: 01306 881313 Fax: 01306 877305
(East Elmbridge and Mid Surrey Primary Care Trust)
Patient List Size: 10172

Practice Manager Louise Watkins

GP Robert Marryat YOUNG, Giles Moir GUTHRIE, K HOFMANN, Susan Jane KOBER, R LEIGH, Stephen Robert LOVELESS, Muna QURESHI

Riverbank Surgery
Westcott Street, Westcott, Dorking RH4 3PA
Tel: 01306 875577 Fax: 01306 883230
(East Elmbridge and Mid Surrey Primary Care Trust)
Patient List Size: 2050

Practice Manager Elaine Guilder

GP Thomas Fergusson GUILDER

Dover

Abbey Practice
107 London Road, Temple Ewell, Dover CT16 3BY
Tel: 01304 821182 Fax: 01304 827673
Email: Stellon@btinternet.com
Website: www.abbeypractice.co.uk
(East Kent Coastal Teaching Primary Care Trust)
Patient List Size: 1900

Practice Manager J Stellon

GP Anthony John STELLON

Buckland Medical Centre
Brookfield Place, Buckland Avenue, Dover CT16 2AE
Tel: 01304 206353 Fax: 01304 209522
(East Kent Coastal Teaching Primary Care Trust)
Patient List Size: 3900

Practice Manager Jane Stoakes

GP Tej BAHADUR, Ingrid DODD, J WOOD

Dover Health Centre
Maison Dieu Road, Dover CT16 1RH
Tel: 01304 865544
(East Kent Coastal Teaching Primary Care Trust)

GP Thomas Charles TORRANCE, D THANGAVEL

The Health Centre
Maison Dieu Road, Dover CT16 1RH
Tel: 01304 865577 Fax: 01304 865501
(East Kent Coastal Teaching Primary Care Trust)
Patient List Size: 2600

Practice Manager Madhu Jain

GP Subhash Chander JAIN

Park Avenue Surgery
100 High Street, Dover CT16 1EQ
Tel: 01304 206463 Fax: 01304 216066
(East Kent Coastal Teaching Primary Care Trust)
Patient List Size: 7441

Practice Manager Lorraine Buckett

GP Sourja CHAUDHURI, Blathnaid Ann KELLY, T A KHAN, Z MYINT, M STEVENS

Pencester Surgery
10/12 Pencester Road, Dover CT16 1BW
Tel: 01304 240553 Fax: 01304 201773
(East Kent Coastal Teaching Primary Care Trust)
Patient List Size: 9300

Practice Manager Kim Horsford

GP Anthony Charles MOTTERSHEAD, Beata DUNNE, Kirsten FLOWER, J I J M MORRIS, David John TURNER

Peter Street Surgery
Peter Street, Dover CT16 1EF
Tel: 01304 216890 Fax: 01304 216891
Website: www.peterstreetsurgerydover.co.uk
(East Kent Coastal Teaching Primary Care Trust)
Patient List Size: 7500

Practice Manager Angie Scrivener

GP Michael COLLINS, Cris DUMITRESCU, Tracey HOPWOOD, Baldev KANG

River Surgery
110 London Road, River, Dover CT16 3AB
Tel: 01304 823039 Fax: 01304 827223
Email: riversurgery@g-gp82227.nhs.uk
(East Kent Coastal Teaching Primary Care Trust)
Patient List Size: 2460

Practice Manager Yvonne Green

GP Julian D S MEAD, Lynne M WRIGHT

St James Surgery
Harold Street, Dover CT16 1SF
Tel: 01304 225559 Fax: 01304 213070
Website: www.stjamessurgery.com
(East Kent Coastal Teaching Primary Care Trust)
Patient List Size: 8200

Practice Manager C J Mackenny

GP Stuart Scott WATERS, Stephen Francis HODNETT, Jonathan James NEYLON, Michael REINECKE

White Cliffs Medical Centre
143 Folkestone Road, Dover CT17 9SG
Tel: 01304 201705 Fax: 01304 216224
(East Kent Coastal Teaching Primary Care Trust)

GP Pankaj PREMNATH, Ramal PREMNATH

Downham Market

The Bridge Street Surgery
30-32 Bridge Street, Downham Market PE38 9DH
Tel: 01366 388888 Fax: 01366 383716
(West Norfolk Primary Care Trust)

Practice Manager Diane Burton

GP Alastair Hugh Tyrell MACKICHAN, Timothy Matthew GENT, Raymond Deryck SCOTT, Clive Thomas SHEPPARD

The Howdale Surgery
48 Howdale Road, Downham Market PE38 9AF
Tel: 01366 383405 Fax: 01366 383433
Website: http://howdalesurgery.gponline.com
(West Norfolk Primary Care Trust)
Patient List Size: 7300

Practice Manager Sally Chase

GP Jonathan Charles Alexander SCONCE, Paul GARNER, Nicholas HART, Graham Anthony HATCHER

Driffield

Bridge Street Practice
21 Bridge Street, Driffield YO25 6DB
Tel: 01377 253441 Fax: 01377 241962
Website: www.the-surgery.co.uk/bridge-street
(Yorkshire Wolds and Coast Primary Care Trust)
Patient List Size: 13575

Practice Manager Paula Snaith

GP David Fearnley WIGGLESWORTH, Guy Christopher CLARKSON, Susan Patricia DALE, Robin Craig FREEMAN, Michael Robert Charles HARDMAN, Catherine Helen HEATON, Simon John TOWERS, Cornelio VINCINI

The Medical Centre
Cranwell Road, Driffield YO25 6UH
Tel: 01377 208208 Fax: 01377 208200
(Yorkshire Wolds and Coast Primary Care Trust)
Patient List Size: 9850

Practice Manager Gillian Dowson

GP Alan David CLARKE, Sally Jane ANDERSON, Adrian Neil CRAWFORD, Andulne Claudine FATHGAZAM, Nigel PICKERING, Mark Brice WAKERLEY

Droitwich

Corbett Medical Practice
36 Corbett Avenue, Droitwich WR9 7BE
Tel: 01905 795566 Fax: 01905 796984
(South Worcestershire Primary Care Trust)
Patient List Size: 9600

Practice Manager Fran Westrop

GP Carl Robert ELLSON, Nicola Mary ELLIOTT, M J W PICKWORTH, Veronica Mary WILKIE, William Richard WOOF

Ombersley Medical Centre
Hastings House, Kidderminster Road, Ombersley, Droitwich WR9 0EL
Tel: 01905 620202 Fax: 01905 621188
(South Worcestershire Primary Care Trust)
Patient List Size: 4000

Practice Manager M Thompson

GP David Stanley BROWNRIDGE, Andrew Charles HORN, J POLE, C THORLEY

Salters Medical Practice
Droitwich Health Centre, Ombersley Street, Droitwich WR9 8RD
Tel: 01905 773535 Fax: 01905 794098
(South Worcestershire Primary Care Trust)
Patient List Size: 10700

Practice Manager C Parker

GP Ian Lindsay KERTON, Alison Fiona KAMEEN, Andrew Charles William KENYON, Ian LAWS, Richard George NEWSHOLME, Steven SIDAWAY

Spa Medical Practice
Ombersley Street, Droitwich WR9 8RB
Tel: 01905 772389 Fax: 01905 797386
(South Worcestershire Primary Care Trust)
Patient List Size: 6900

Practice Manager Margaret Forknell

GP Jenny BILLINGHAM, Alison BLAKE, Anthony John KELLY, Richard Inigo KINSMAN, Katherine TARR

Drybrook

Drybrook Surgery
Drybrook Road, Drybrook GL17 9JE
Tel: 01594 542239 Fax: 01594 544501
(West Gloucestershire Primary Care Trust)

Practice Manager Jane Smith

GP Christopher Douglas GOOD, P A KING, Angela Joy TOWNSEND

Dudley

Bath Street Surgery
73 Bath Street, Sedgley, Dudley DY3 1LS
Tel: 01902 882880 Fax: 01902 882880
(Dudley Beacon and Castle Primary Care Trust)

Practice Manager J Taylor

GP P K SARKAR

Bilston Street Surgery
25 Bilston Street, Sidgley, Dudley DY3 1JA
Tel: 01902 665700 Fax: 01902 688533

(Dudley Beacon and Castle Primary Care Trust)

GP Nabil Aziz SHATHER

Brook Street Surgery
7 Brook Street, Woodsetton, Dudley DY3 1AD
Tel: 01902 883346 Fax: 01902 673757
(Dudley Beacon and Castle Primary Care Trust)
Patient List Size: 5500

Practice Manager J Tong

GP Martyn Victor John BROAD, Sabah Francis AL-RABBAN, Julian RANDALL

Castle Meadows Surgery
100 Milking Bank, Dudley DY1 2TY
Tel: 01384 234737 Fax: 01384 350652
(Dudley Beacon and Castle Primary Care Trust)

GP Jaswant Singh RATHORE

Cross Street Health Centre
Cross Street, Dudley DY1 1RN
Tel: 01384 459044 Fax: 01384 232467
(Dudley Beacon and Castle Primary Care Trust)
Patient List Size: 5300

Practice Manager Lyn Conway

GP David Gratton PARRY, Gillian Lynda COX

Cross Street Health Centre
Cross Street, Dudley DY1 1RN
Tel: 01384 459090/459006 Fax: 01384 459090
(Dudley Beacon and Castle Primary Care Trust)

GP John Samuel BOOTH, B B SINGH, M H SMITH, S W WONG

Dr Z A Shaikh and Partners
Kent Street, Upper Gornal, Dudley DY3 1UX
Tel: 01902 882243 Fax: 01902 680777
(Rowley Regis and Tipton Primary Care Trust)
Patient List Size: 8900

Practice Manager Rachel C Parker

GP Zaheer Ahmed SHAIKH, Joanna COATES, H H O OGUNNAIKE, David Andrew ORAM, Ian James WALTON

Eve Hill Medical Practice
29-53 Himley Road, Dudley DY1 2QD
Tel: 01384 254423 Fax: 01384 254424
(Dudley Beacon and Castle Primary Care Trust)

GP Anthony Joseph BLACKMAN, Jayesh DESAI, L OMHEA, Victoria Mary SMART

Grange Road Surgery
74 Grange Road, Dudley DY1 2AW
Tel: 01384 252729 Fax: 01384 242109
(Dudley Beacon and Castle Primary Care Trust)

GP B D HILL, Bipan Kumar JALOTA

Grange Road Surgery
Dudley DY1 2AW
Tel: 01384 255387/252095 Fax: 01384 242109
(Dudley Beacon and Castle Primary Care Trust)

GP Ada Margaret PORTER, William Aubrey Blackwood PORTER

Irani, Dawes, Foster and Singh
The Ridgeway Surgery, 175 The Ridgeway, Sedgley, Dudley DY3 3UH
Tel: 01902 884343 Fax: 01902 882101
Email: s.irani@m87007.dudley-pcg.wmids.nhs.uk
(Dudley Beacon and Castle Primary Care Trust)
Patient List Size: 8600

Practice Manager Jean Clarke

GP Shahbehram IRANI, Kevin Richard DAWES, Helen Margaret FOSTER, Subhas C SINGH

Keelinge House Surgery
176 Stourbridge Road, Dudley DY1 2ER
Tel: 01384 77194 Fax: 01384 820210
(Dudley Beacon and Castle Primary Care Trust)

GP Stephen Terence CARTWRIGHT, James BULLOCK, Mona MAHFOUZ

Lower Gornal Health Centre
Bull Street, Gornal Wood, Dudley DY3 2NQ
Tel: 01384 459621 Fax: 01384 359495
(Dudley Beacon and Castle Primary Care Trust)
Patient List Size: 8600

Practice Manager Pauline Whitehouse

GP Richard William GEE, Naeem Mansoor MALIK, Mohsen NASSRALIA, Steven Peter WILD

Masefield Road Surgery
Masefield Road, Lower Gornal, Dudley DY3 3BU
Tel: 01922 882002 Fax: 01922 882002
(Dudley Beacon and Castle Primary Care Trust)
Patient List Size: 2600

Practice Manager A Jain

GP S K JAIN

Netherton Health Centre
Halesowen Road, Dudley DY2 9PU
Tel: 01384 254935 Fax: 01384 242468
(Dudley Beacon and Castle Primary Care Trust)

GP Delia Mary CONLON, Rohanta Kumar PERERA, Nigel John WARRINGTON

Netherton Health Centre
Halesowen Road, Dudley DY2 9PU
Tel: 01384 253673 Fax: 01384 457979
(Dudley Beacon and Castle Primary Care Trust)

Practice Manager Aileen Jensen

GP Margaret Anne Marie MacAVINEY

Netherton Surgery
84 Halesowen Road, Netherton, Dudley DY2 9PS
Tel: 01384 239657 Fax: 01384 458136
Email: ppurshotam.gupta@dudley.nhs.uk
Website: www.nethertonsurgery.co.uk
(Dudley Beacon and Castle Primary Care Trust)

Practice Manager David Lawrence

GP Purshotam Dass GUPTA

Northway Surgery
8 Alderwood Precinct, Dudley DY3 3QY
Tel: 01902 885180
(Dudley Beacon and Castle Primary Care Trust)
Patient List Size: 5200

Practice Manager S M Bytheway

GP William Trevor HAMPSON, S J PRITCHARD

Quarry Road Surgery
10 Quarry Road, Dudley DY2 0EF
Tel: 01384 569050 Fax: 01384 350321
(Dudley Beacon and Castle Primary Care Trust)

GP Prabhakar Rangnath INGLE, Urmila Prabhakar INGLE

St Thomas's Medical Practice
Beechwood Road, Dudley DY2 7QA
Tel: 01384 242973
(Dudley Beacon and Castle Primary Care Trust)

Practice Manager Una Hadlington

GP S BASU

Stepping Stones Medical Practice
Stafford Street, Dudley DY1 1RT
Tel: 01384 459966 Fax: 01384 459885
(Dudley Beacon and Castle Primary Care Trust)

Patient List Size: 7200

Practice Manager Joanne Green

GP Nigel Charles Cunningham WELCH, A R KHAN, Richard John SPIERS

The Surgery
Tinchbourne Street, Dudley DY1 1RH
Tel: 01384 235540 Fax: 01384 458135
(Dudley Beacon and Castle Primary Care Trust)

GP Joginder PALL

The Surgery
8 Alderwood Precinct, Northway, Sedgley, Dudley DY3 3QY
Tel: 01902 85180/880825
(Dudley Beacon and Castle Primary Care Trust)

Practice Manager Susan Bytheway

GP William Trevor HAMPSON, Alan Walton PARKES, S J PRITCHARD

The Surgery
Central Clinic, Hall Street, Dudley DY2 7BX
Tel: 01384 253616 Fax: 01384 253332
(Dudley Beacon and Castle Primary Care Trust)
Patient List Size: 2900

Practice Manager Michael Brettell

GP Paul Brian Varney BRETTELL

The Surgery
5 Bean Road, Dudley DY2 8TH
Tel: 01384 252229 Fax: 01384 458137
(Dudley Beacon and Castle Primary Care Trust)

GP S DAS GUPTA

Dukinfield

Davaar Medical Centre
20 Concord Way, Dukinfield SK16 4DB
Tel: 0161 343 6382 Fax: 0161 330 7326
(Tameside and Glossop Primary Care Trust)

GP Charles Anthony DOUGLAS

Hollies Surgery
83 Birch Lane, Dukinfield SK16 4AJ
Tel: 0161 330 2039 Fax: 0161 330 5149
(Tameside and Glossop Primary Care Trust)

Practice Manager Megan Thompson

GP Julian Christopher PROCTER, David Henderson MARR

King Street Medical Centre
96-98 King Street, Dukinfield SK16 4JZ
Tel: 0161 330 1142/2157 Fax: 0161 330 6569
Email: kingstreetmc@hotmail.com
(Tameside and Glossop Primary Care Trust)
Patient List Size: 3800

Practice Manager Jean Cadwallader

GP Siong S LEE

Town Hall Surgery
112 King Street, Dukinfield SK16 4LD
Tel: 0161 330 2125 Fax: 0161 330 6899
(Tameside and Glossop Primary Care Trust)
Patient List Size: 3750

Practice Manager J Wain

GP Aruna ASTHANA, Deepak MALIK

Dulverton

Dulverton Medical Practice
Trumpington House, 56 High Street, Dulverton TA22 9DW
Tel: 01398 323333 Fax: 01398 324030
(Somerset Coast Primary Care Trust)

Practice Manager Stephanie Martinez

GP D BERGER, C BIRD, Lee BURTON, C M MACKIE, A S TRILL

Dunmow

Angel Lane Surgery
Angel Lane, Great Dunmow, Dunmow CM6 1AQ
Tel: 01371 872105 Fax: 01371 873679
Website: www.angellanesurgery.co.uk
(Uttlesford Primary Care Trust)
Patient List Size: 8500

Practice Manager Glynis Bradley

GP Andrew HYND, Marit DUNN, Mark Andrew GRECH, Birgit KELLER, Peter LINN, Tara SINGH

John Tasker House Surgery
56 New Street, Great Dunmow, Dunmow CM6 1BH
Tel: 01371 872121 Fax: 01371 873793
(Uttlesford Primary Care Trust)
Patient List Size: 10800

Practice Manager Ann Taylor

GP Jonathan Simon Brindley JACKSON, Gillian Susan GRAVES, Sarah Anne RAYBOULD, Malcolm SLACK, Michael Kevin TEE, David TIDESWELL, John Gervase VERNON

Thaxted Surgery
Margaret Street, Thaxted, Dunmow CM6 2QN
Tel: 01371 830213 Fax: 01371 831278
(Uttlesford Primary Care Trust)
Patient List Size: 6700

Practice Manager Caroal Lewis

GP Michael John TAYLER, Jonna HALL, Robert William HOWLETT, Emma Caroline PUGH, Michelle RALPH

Dunstable

Dunstable Health Centre
Priory Gardens, Dunstable LU6 3SU
Tel: 01582 699622 Fax: 01582 663431
(Bedfordshire Heartlands Primary Care Trust)

Practice Manager Venetia Bunker

GP Michael John Ingram DAY, Harish Devjibhai BODHANI, Paul Christopher HASSAN

Eastgate Surgery
Eastgate House, 28-34 Church Street, Dunstable LU5 4RR
Tel: 01582 670050 Fax: 01582 607490
(Bedfordshire Heartlands Primary Care Trust)
Patient List Size: 2492

Practice Manager Shahida Haq

GP Mohamed Fazlul HAQ

Edlesborough Surgery
11 Cow Lane, Edlesborough, Dunstable LU6 2HT
Tel: 01525 221630 Fax: 01525 222961
(Vale of Aylesbury Primary Care Trust)
Patient List Size: 5665

Practice Manager Vicky Bath

GP Gordon DUNFORD, Martyn JONES

High Street South Surgery
47 High Street South, Dunstable LU6 3RZ
Tel: 01582 663406
(Bedfordshire Heartlands Primary Care Trust)

Practice Manager Sylvia Donald

GP Angus DONALD

High Street Surgery
108 High Street North, Dunstable LU6 1LN
Tel: 01582 608420 Fax: 01582 472857
(Bedfordshire Heartlands Primary Care Trust)

Practice Manager Denise Tearle

GP Jagdish Prasad DASHORE

Houghton Regis Medical Centre
Peel Street, Houghton Regis, Dunstable LU5 5EZ
Tel: 01582 866161 Fax: 01582 865483
(Bedfordshire Heartlands Primary Care Trust)
Patient List Size: 8500

Practice Manager Bina Beant

GP Pravin Kumar GOUTAM, Vinay Kumar BHALLA, Joy E JINNI, Arabinda Kumar MALLIK, Chandrakant Natverlal SHAH

Kingsbury Court Surgery
Church Street, Dunstable LU5 4RS
Tel: 01582 663218 Fax: 01582 476488
(Bedfordshire Heartlands Primary Care Trust)
Patient List Size: 7500

Practice Manager Margaret Godfrey

GP Katherine Mary HAWKING, Nicholas Alexander BENEDIKT, John FSADNI

Kirby Road Surgery
58 Kirby Road, Dunstable LU6 3JH
Tel: 01582 609121 Fax: 01582 472002
(Bedfordshire Heartlands Primary Care Trust)
Patient List Size: 8300

Practice Manager Steve Wilson

GP Oliver Bartholomew O'TOOLE, Nicholas Edwin CURT, Marcel SCHUTTE, Catherine SYKES

The Surgery
10 Matthew Street, Dunstable LU6 1SD
Tel: 01582 666660 Fax: 01582 667800
(Bedfordshire Heartlands Primary Care Trust)

Practice Manager Jane Brown

GP O H ORFALI

Toddington Medical Centre
Luton Road, Toddington, Dunstable LU5 6DE
Tel: 01525 872222 Fax: 01525 876711
(Bedfordshire Heartlands Primary Care Trust)

Practice Manager Mavis Doohan

GP Andrew Colin LONG, Roger Charles NEAL, Jane Deborah Alison PERKINS, Lindsay Jill REYNER

West Street Surgery
89 West Street, Dunstable LU6 1SF
Tel: 01582 664401 Fax: 01582 475766
(Bedfordshire Heartlands Primary Care Trust)
Patient List Size: 12000

Practice Manager Sue Dobson

GP Roger John CRO, Kathryn J ASTIN, Janet Elizabeth BERRY, Kathryn Ann FREEMAN, Joanne PETERS, Stephen V PRICE, Christopher Francis QUARTLY

Durham

Browney House Surgery
Front Street, Langley Park, Durham DH7 9YT
Tel: 0191 373 2860 Fax: 0191 373 0685
(Derwentside Primary Care Trust)
Patient List Size: 2900

Practice Manager Louise Young

GP Sukhwinder Singh NAGI, Catherine E BROMHAM

Burnhope Surgery
The Haven, Burnhope, Durham DH7 0BD
Tel: 01207 214707 Fax: 01207 214700
(Derwentside Primary Care Trust)
Patient List Size: 1640

Practice Manager Barbara Anderson

GP James Edward ANDERSON

Chastleton Surgery
Newton Drive, Framwellgate Moor, Durham DH1 5BH
Tel: 0191 384 6171 Fax: 0191 386 3743
Website: www.chastletonmedicalgroup.co.uk
(Durham and Chester-le-Street Primary Care Trust)
Patient List Size: 14000

Practice Manager Sue Roff

GP I A K SUTHERLAND, A CAMPBELL, David Graham CLIFFORD, Peter Jonathan Brian MATTINSON, D T THOMAS

Cheveley Park Medical Centre
Cheveley Park Shopping Centre, The Links, Belmont, Durham DH1 2UW
Tel: 0191 386 4285 Fax: 0191 386 5934
(Durham and Chester-le-Street Primary Care Trust)

Practice Manager Enid Miller

GP George MUNRO, James Herbert HARRISON

Claypath Medical Practice
26 Gilesgate, Durham DH1 1QW
Tel: 0191 333 2830 Fax: 0191 333 2836
(Durham and Chester-le-Street Primary Care Trust)
Patient List Size: 11267

Practice Manager Kenneth Crossman

GP Ian Richard UNDERWOOD, Rosemary COOPER, Patricia FLANAGAN, Edward John HOLMES, Fiona JONES, Andrew KENT, Vikram MAINI, Helen MARSDEN, Jan PANKE, Stephen James WHITFIELD

Coxhoe Medical Practice
1 Lansdowne Road, Cornforth Lane, Coxhoe, Durham DH6 4DH
Tel: 0191 377 0340 Fax: 0191 377 0604
(Durham and Chester-le-Street Primary Care Trust)

Practice Manager Sylvia Jessop

GP R WOODS, K C BARKER, H D TURNER

Dunelm Medical Practice
1-2 Victor Terrace, Bearpark, Durham DH7 7DF
Tel: 0191 373 2077 Fax: 0191 373 6216
(Durham and Chester-le-Street Primary Care Trust)
Patient List Size: 10600

Practice Manager D W Harris

GP David Wilson SMART, Cho Cho AYE, D J EGLINTON, James Martin IBBOTT, Alexander MacINTYRE, E E OSBOURNE, G WELSH

Khan
Brandon Lane Surgery, Stackgarth, Brandon, Durham DH7 8SJ
Tel: 0191 3782099 Fax: 0191 378 0898
(Durham and Chester-le-Street Primary Care Trust)
Patient List Size: 2276

Practice Manager Gillian Clare

GP Cliff Fazal KHAN

The Medical Group
McKenzie House, Newhouse Road, Esh Winning, Durham DH7 9LA
Tel: 0191 3734232 Fax: 0191 373 9619
(Derwentside Primary Care Trust)

GP Margaret Susan DEYTRIKH, Dr BEGGS, Dr BENN, Dr CHESTER, Dr CLARK, Dr FINNIGHAN, Dr HAND, Dr HAZELL, Dr KEMBALL, Dr MURRAY, Dr WHALLEY, Dr YULE

The Medical Health Centre
Gray Avenue, Sherburn, Durham DH6 1JE
Tel: 0191 3720441 Fax: 0191 372 1238
(Durham and Chester-le-Street Primary Care Trust)
Patient List Size: 8500

Practice Manager Teresa McNeill

GP John Ernest HARRISON, Kenneth James ARMSTRONG, Martin Roy GREEN, Patrick James WRIGHT

Park House Surgery
Station Road, Lanchester, Durham DH7 0PE
Tel: 01207 520877 Fax: 01207 521997
(Derwentside Primary Care Trust)

Practice Manager Doug Rossi

GP Catherine M BIDWELL, Ian G DAVIDSON

Patel and Partners
Thornley Road Surgery, Thornley Road, Wheatley Hill, Durham DH6 3NR
Tel: 01429 820233 Fax: 01429 823667
(Easington Primary Care Trust)
Patient List Size: 8011

Practice Manager Joyce Doyle

GP Kanubhai Mangalbhai PATEL, Nand Kishore MAHTO, Harbhahn MANGAT, Win MAUNG, Koko NAING

Romaine Square Surgery
4 Romaine Square, Bowburn, Durham DH6 5AE
Tel: 0191 377 2495 Fax: 0191 377 3379
(Durham and Chester-le-Street Primary Care Trust)

Practice Manager Wendy Graham

GP William Anton POLLARD

Rutherford House
Langley Park, Durham DH7 9XD
Tel: 0191 373 1386 Fax: 0191 373 4288
(Durham and Chester-le-Street Primary Care Trust)

Practice Manager Mike O'Hare

GP John Charles YULE, Graeme Cochrane BEGGS, Helen Mary BENN, Paul Giles CHESTER, John Adrian CLARK, Ellen-Ann FINNIGHAN, Robert Wilton HAND, Mark Jeremy HAZELL, Heather Jane KEMBALL, Robert William MURRAY, Ian Charles NEEDHAM, Francis Edward WHALLEY

South Hetton Surgery
Front Street, South Hetton, Durham DH6 2TH
Tel: 0191 5171055 Fax: 0191 5260001
(Easington Primary Care Trust)
Patient List Size: 3175

Practice Manager P Smith

GP Mohammad QUASIM, Mubarak SANGHERA

Southdene Medical Centre
Front Street, Shotton Colliery, Durham DH6 2LT
Tel: 0191 5265818 Fax: 0191 526 7740
(Easington Primary Care Trust)
Patient List Size: 2850

GP Samir Hassan Saleh MANSOUR

The Surgery
Station Road, Shotton Colliery, Durham DH6 2JL
Tel: 0191 5265913 Fax: 0191 526 2651
(Easington Primary Care Trust)

Practice Manager Anne Summerill

GP Richard George ABBOTT, Ambalal Shankerlal PATEL

The Surgery
Cross Road, Sacriston, Durham DH7 6LJ
Tel: 0191 3710232 Fax: 0191 371 8306
(Durham and Chester-le-Street Primary Care Trust)
Patient List Size: 9200

GP Paul Robert WALTON, Kirsti HARNOR, Martin Lawrence JUDSON, Fiona Kathryn McCONNELL, Alison PRITCHARD, Paul Robert SHEPHERD, Susan Elizabeth WALTON

The Surgery
Bevan Close, Shotton Colliery, Durham DH6 2LQ
Tel: 0191 5261643 Fax: 0191 517 2746
(Easington Primary Care Trust)

Practice Manager Mrs Gupta

GP Gupta Mudalagiri Dasappagupta RAMAKRISHNA

University of Durham
Student Health Centre, 42 Old Elvet, Durham DH1 3JF
Tel: 0191 386 5081 Fax: 0191 333 5001
(Durham and Chester-le-Street Primary Care Trust)

Practice Manager Kenneth Crossman

GP John William CHARTERS, Alice WALLING

Dursley

May Lane Surgery
May Lane, Dursley GL11 4JN
Tel: 01453 540540 Fax: 01453 540570
(Cotswold and Vale Primary Care Trust)

Practice Manager Susan Robinson, Marian Shaw

GP Timothy George FRANKAU, Jane MILSON, Tom Charles WARDELL-YERBURGH

The Orchard Medical Centre
Fairmead, Cam, Dursley GL11 5NE
Tel: 01453 548666 Fax: 01453 548124
(Cotswold and Vale Primary Care Trust)
Patient List Size: 6729

Practice Manager Rowena Gardner

GP Martin John FREEMAN, Graham John COLE, Peter James HARNEY, Marion Jane McDOWELL

The Street Surgery
42 The Street, Uley, Dursley GL11 5SY
Tel: 01453 860459 Fax: 01453 860972
(Cotswold and Vale Primary Care Trust)
Patient List Size: 3400

Practice Manager Ray Manghan

GP Stephen John ALVIS, Jonathan Andrew Paul STEEL

The Westgate Surgery
40 Parsonage Street, Dursley GL11 4AA
Tel: 01453 545981
(Cotswold and Vale Primary Care Trust)
Patient List Size: 4000

Practice Manager Susan Robinson, Marian Shaw

GP Damian KENNY, Katherine Sarah CURTIS HAYWARD, Simon Joseph OPHER

East Cowes

East Cowes Health Centre
Down House, York Avenue, East Cowes PO32 6RR
Tel: 01983 295611 Fax: 01983 280815
(Isle of Wight Primary Care Trust)

GP Martin Leonard Rees DAVIES, Christopher John Antony ANDREWS, Shaun Anthony GILLAN, Catherine Frances M O'CALLAGHAN

East Grinstead

Judges Close Surgery
Judges Close, East Grinstead RH19 3AA
Tel: 01342 324628 Fax: 01342 318055
(Mid Sussex Primary Care Trust)
Patient List Size: 9500

Practice Manager Jane Hemblade

GP Richard James Rowley DUNSTAN, Kathryn Jane BROOKS, Anthony Richard Derek ENSKAT, Mark LYTHGOE

Moatfield Surgery
St Michael's Road, East Grinstead RH19 3GW
Tel: 01342 327555 Fax: 01342 316240
Email: moatfield@mistral.co.uk
(Mid Sussex Primary Care Trust)
Patient List Size: 12500

Practice Manager Christa Wilson

GP Jeremy Jock VEVERS, David Robert BAINBRIDGE, Bryan Wilfrid Cosby Carmichael CHRISTOPHER, Julian Harry CLARKE, Veronique Anne Louise FOULGER, M PATEL, David Grant Machattie POWELL

Ship Street Surgery
Ship Street, East Grinstead RH19 4EE
Tel: 01342 325959 Fax: 01342 314681
(Mid Sussex Primary Care Trust)
Patient List Size: 11200

Practice Manager David Jamieson

GP Alistair Anthony James MACKENZIE, Stephen John BELLAMY, Ann Patricia BERKOVITCH, Maria BYRNE, Jean-Pierre DIAS, Jeremy Donald HILL

East Molesey

Glenlyn Medical Centre
115 Molesey Park Road, East Molesey KT8 0JX
Tel: 020 8979 3253 Fax: 020 8941 7914
(East Elmbridge and Mid Surrey Primary Care Trust)

GP Stephen Edward BRANT, Gordon Robin Walker BROWNE, Ian David COXON, Victoria ELVIN, Jane GRAY, Ashish KAPOOR, Brinda Navaluxmi PARAMOTHAYAN

Eastbourne

Green Street Clinic
118-122 Green Street, Eastbourne BN21 1RT
Tel: 01323 722908 Fax: 01323 723136
(Eastbourne Downs Primary Care Trust)
Patient List Size: 10500

Practice Manager Heather King

GP Ian Charles McNAUGHTON, Bernard Patrick Michael BRENNAN, Helen R DAGGETT, Peter DICKENS, Mark St John GAFFNEY, Daniela J PENGE

Park Practice
12 Brodrick Close, Hampden Park, Eastbourne BN22 9NQ
Tel: 01323 502200 Fax: 01323 500527
(Eastbourne Downs Primary Care Trust)
Patient List Size: 8000

Practice Manager Alan Packard

GP Paul Richard SHEPHERD, Idango Ibifuro ADOKI, Jo MARTYR, David THOMAS, Katta VERNON-HUNT, Martin Darren Levett WRITER

Princes Park Health Centre
Wartling Road, Eastbourne BN22 7PF
Tel: 01323 744644 Fax: 01323 736094
(Eastbourne Downs Primary Care Trust)

GP Jonathan ANDREWS, Karen Claire NORWOOD, Julian Paul RABUSZKO, Peter Hugh SCARISBRICK, Dr SOROOSHIAN, Martyn Graham STOCKTON

Seaside Medical Centre
18 Sheen Road, Eastbourne BN22 8DR
Tel: 01323 725667 Fax: 01323 417169
(Eastbourne Downs Primary Care Trust)

GP John Desborough BARNES, Timothy William GIETZEN, Stephen Timothy LYTTON, Stephen Robert MATHIAS, Carolyn Deborah SHEPHERD, Robert MacKenzie WICKS

The Surgery
1 Arlington Road, Eastbourne BN21 1DH
Tel: 01323 727531 Fax: 01323 417085
(Eastbourne Downs Primary Care Trust)
Patient List Size: 13500

GP Peter George WILLIAMS, Debra Ann DAVISON, Robert William DEERY, Paul Alexander FRISBY, David HIGGS, Pravin JAIN, Jane Anne LOFTS, Tvan RAJAP

The Surgery
5 Enys Road, Eastbourne BN21 2DQ
Tel: 01323 410088 Fax: 01323 644638
(Eastbourne Downs Primary Care Trust)
Patient List Size: 9500

Practice Manager Sharon McDavitt

GP John Arthur CLARKE, Gillian Mary COUTTS, Karen Elizabeth LEESON, William George MILLER, Alfred Patrick PARKER

The Surgery
10 Bolton Road, Eastbourne BN21 3JY
Tel: 01323 730537 Fax: 01323 412759
(Eastbourne Downs Primary Care Trust)
Patient List Size: 5971

GP Norman Andrew KINNIBURGH, Graeme Christopher BROWN, Thomas Noel Anthony RICHARDSON

The Surgery
6 College Road, Eastbourne BN21 4HY
Tel: 01323 735044 Fax: 01323 417705
(Eastbourne Downs Primary Care Trust)

Practice Manager Jon Early

GP John Keith PROSSER, Mark Rowland EVASON, Simon Jonathan EYRE, Gregory Anthony Joseph FOLWELL, Maia NICHOLLES, Andrew Norman STEWART, Hugh Falcon THOMAS, Benjamin TYRELL

Eastleigh

Boyatt Wood Surgery
Boyatt Wood Shopping Centre, Shakespeare Road, Boyatt Wood, Eastleigh SO50 4QP
Tel: 023 8061 2051 Fax: 023 8062 0679
(Eastleigh and Test Valley South Primary Care Trust)

Practice Manager Lynne Tibo

GP Anuka DAS, Peter Murray MUIR

The Brownhill Surgery
2 Brownhill Road, Chandlers Ford, Eastleigh SO53 2ZB
Tel: 023 8025 2414 Fax: 023 8036 6604
(Eastleigh and Test Valley South Primary Care Trust)
Patient List Size: 6100

Practice Manager Nicola Webb

GP James Frith WILLIAMSON, Ian Francis FARMER, K L GREGORY, Elizabeth Marguerite KAY

Eastleigh Health Centre
Newtown Road, Eastleigh SO50 9AG
Tel: 023 8061 2197 Fax: 023 8065 0786
Website: www.drdarcyandptnrs.co.uk
(Eastleigh and Test Valley South Primary Care Trust)
Patient List Size: 4800

Practice Manager Yvonne Young

GP Anthony Hugh Edward D'ARCY, James Howard GREENHALGH, Derrin Felicity WILKINS

Eastleigh Health Centre
Newtown Road, Eastleigh SO50 9AG
Tel: 023 8061 2123 Fax: 023 8039 9032
(Eastleigh and Test Valley South Primary Care Trust)

Practice Manager Denise Nason

GP Reefat Khurshid DRABU

Fryern and Millers Dale Partnership
Millers Dale Surgery, 9 Ormesby Drive, Chandlers Ford, Eastleigh SO53 1SH
Tel: 023 8026 2488 Fax: 023 8025 5524
(Eastleigh and Test Valley South Primary Care Trust)
Patient List Size: 9200

Practice Manager Christine Ireland Ireland

GP Stuart A P WARD, Mark Christopher ALEY, Dr BROUGH, Dr FOOTE, Philippa Kaye GODFREY

Fryern and Millers Dale Partnership
Fryern Surgery, Oakmount Road, Chandlers Ford, Eastleigh SO53 2LH
Tel: 023 8027 3252/3458 Fax: 023 8027 3459
(Eastleigh and Test Valley South Primary Care Trust)

GP S A P WARD, M C ALEY, Guinevere Ann FOOTE, P K GODFREY

The Fryern Surgery
Oakmount Road, Chandlers Ford, Eastleigh SO53 2LH
Tel: 023 8025 2122/2082
(Eastleigh and Test Valley South Primary Care Trust)

GP Barry Joseph BROUGH

The Old Anchor Inn
Riverside, Bishopstoke, Eastleigh SO50 6LQ
Tel: 023 8064 2538 Fax: 023 8065 2308
(Eastleigh and Test Valley South Primary Care Trust)

GP N C PATEL

Park Surgery
Hursley Road, Chandlers Ford, Eastleigh SO53 2ZH
Tel: 023 8026 7355 Fax: 023 8026 5394
(Eastleigh and Test Valley South Primary Care Trust)
Patient List Size: 14400

Practice Manager Robert Stangroom

GP Manfred Rudiger COLMSEE, Christopher Donald ARDEN, Simon Paul CHAPLIN ROGERS, Kathryn Margaret Anne FOWLER, Michella HOLSON, Jayne O'CONNOR, Mark Alan RICKENBACH, Julia M TERRY

Parkside Family Practice
Eastleigh Health Centre, Newtown Road, Eastleigh SO50 9AG
Tel: 023 8061 2032 Fax: 023 8062 9623
(Eastleigh and Test Valley South Primary Care Trust)

Practice Manager Judi Green

GP Margaret Catherine TANSLEY, George Harold BLACK, Thomas George FRANK, Geoffrey KELL, T McCARTHY

St Andrews Surgery
166 Market Street, Eastleigh SO50 5PT
Tel: 023 8061 2472 Fax: 023 8061 1717
(Eastleigh and Test Valley South Primary Care Trust)
Patient List Size: 7100

Practice Manager Jane Lee

GP Eileen Ross GORROD, Madelyn Ann DAKEYNE, John GAVIN, James McAULAY

Stokewood Surgery
Fair Oak Road, Fair Oak, Eastleigh SO50 8AU
Tel: 023 8069 2000 Fax: 023 8069 3891
(Eastleigh and Test Valley South Primary Care Trust)

Practice Manager Roger Greenwood

GP Patricia Margaret ACTON, Richard Charles CARTER, Andrew Clark HILLAM, William Alistair Fenton HOOD, Douglas Alexander MACLEAN, Marie Elizabeth McCARTHY

Edenbridge

Edenbridge Medical Practice
West View, Station Road, Edenbridge TN8 5ND
Tel: 01732 864442/865055 Fax: 01732 862376
(South West Kent Primary Care Trust)
Patient List Size: 11500

Practice Manager Caroline Dyer

GP Timothy Ralph Lowndes BAYLEY, Tara Yvette GARRETT, Mark Dorian ILSLEY, Kristina Brigid KELLY, Simon John MORRISON, Brian Scott SPEAR

Edgware

Bacon Lane Surgery
11 Bacon Lane, Edgware HA8 5AT
Tel: 020 8952 5073/7876
(Harrow Primary Care Trust)
Patient List Size: 9500

Practice Manager Julia Hynes

GP Maralyn Marcia PAMPEL, Laurence HOMMEL, Jacob KURIEN, J C NATHAN, Gillian Mary PARSONS, Rekha RAJA

Chandos Crescent
82 Chandos Crescent, Edgware HA8 6HL
Tel: 020 8952 7662
(Harrow Primary Care Trust)

GP Ella ROZEWICZ

Cressingham Road Surgery
36 Cressingham Road, Edgware HA8 0RW
Tel: 020 8959 1496 Fax: 020 8906 8713
(Barnet Primary Care Trust)

GP Thambimuttu GANESH, Muthulingam SATHANANTHAN

Dr C Chakraborty
Chakraborty, The Quadrant, Manor Park Crescent, Edgware HA8 7LU
Tel: 020 8952 0004
(Barnet Primary Care Trust)
Patient List Size: 1000

GP Chanchal CHAKRABORTY

Dr Sirisena
156 Deans Lane, Edgware HA8 9NT
Tel: 020 8906 3337
(Barnet Primary Care Trust)

GP Udawattage Nihal H SIRISENA

Lane End Medical Group
25 Edgwarebury Lane, Edgware HA8 8LJ
Tel: 020 8958 4233 Fax: 020 8905 4657
(Barnet Primary Care Trust)
Patient List Size: 7000

Practice Manager Barbara Fortune

GP Brian Henry John BRIGGS, Michelle FERRIS, Michelle Julia NEWMAN, Iftikhar Mahmood SARAF, Sarah Miriam SCAMBLER

Lane End Medical Group
25 Edgwarebury lane, Edgware HA8 8LJ
Tel: 020 8958 4233 Fax: 020 8905 4657
(Barnet Primary Care Trust)
Patient List Size: 4500

Practice Manager Barbara Fortune

GP Michael Trevor WYNDHAM, Lyndon WAGMAN

Oak Lodge Medical Centre
234 Burnt Oak Broadway, Edgware HA8 0AP
Tel: 020 8952 1202 Fax: 020 8381 1156
(Barnet Primary Care Trust)

Practice Manager B Duncan, L J Walters

GP Jean Catherine BENEY, Maureen Elizabeth BARNARD, Eleanor Jane SCOTT, Lauren Kristina STEPHENSON, Sapna SUBHANI

Penshurst Gardens Surgery
39 Penshurst Gardens, Edgware HA8 9TN
Tel: 020 8958 3141 Fax: 020 8905 4638
Website: www.penhurstsurgery.co.uk
(Barnet Primary Care Trust)
Patient List Size: 6500

Practice Manager Catherine Lau

GP Valerie BARD, David Henry KRASNER, Zoe Anne PINTO, Jasminder SETHI

The Surgery
46 SOUTH PARADE, Mollison Way, Edgware HA8 5QL
Tel: 020 8952 5788 Fax: 020 89525788
(Harrow Primary Care Trust)
Patient List Size: 4000

Practice Manager Nirmala Patel

GP J J GOLDSTEINE

The Surgery
82 Stag Lane, Edgware HA8 5LP
Tel: 020 8952 8484 Fax: 020 8952-8583
(Brent Teaching Primary Care Trust)

GP A K M SHAH, Husna BANO, K C BHATT

The Surgery
114 Edgwarebury Lane, Edgware HA8 8NB
Tel: 020 8958 3255 Fax: 020 8905 3538
(Barnet Primary Care Trust)
Patient List Size: 3600

GP D M DINSHAW, H MILLER

Watling Medical Centre
108 Watling Avenue, Burnt Oak, Edgware HA8 0NR
Tel: 020 8906 1711 Fax: 020 8201 1283
(Barnet Primary Care Trust)

Practice Manager Ian Petrie

GP Gerald Maurice MICHAEL, Seema NAGPAUL, Anup Madhusen PATEL, Maria Benicia Yvette SALDANHA, Susan Mary SUMNERS, Penelope Anne TRAFFORD, Camilla WRIGHT

Woodcroft Medical Centre
Gervase Road, Burnt Oak, Edgware HA8 0NR
Tel: 020 8906 0500 Fax: 020 8906 0700
(Barnet Primary Care Trust)

GP Peter Simon GUGENHEIM, Hasmukh MAKANJI

Woodcroft Medical Centre
Gervase Road, Burnt Oak, Edgware HA8 0NR
Tel: 020 8201 1812
(Barnet Primary Care Trust)

GP Peter Simon GUGENHEIM

Woodcroft Medical Centre
Gervase Road, Burnt Oak, Edgware HA8 0NR
Tel: 020 8906 8700 Fax: 020 8959 0718
(Barnet Primary Care Trust)

GP Devi MOODALEY

Zain Medical Centre
122 Turner Road, Edgware HA8 6BH
Tel: 020 8952 3721 Fax: 020 8952 8472
(Harrow Primary Care Trust)
Patient List Size: 2000

Practice Manager Nila Dashi

GP Syeda Sabera KIRMANI

Egham

The Grove Medical Centre
Church Road, Egham TW20 9QJ
Tel: 01784 433159 Fax: 01784 477208
Website: www.thegrovemedicalcentre.co.uk
(North Surrey Primary Care Trust)
Patient List Size: 12500

Practice Manager Carole Stock

GP John Vincent ELLIOTT, N A-ALI, Ruth Olivia MORRIS, Veronica Ruth PRIESTLEY, Rosemarie Philomena SALMON, Peter Maciej WARWICKER

Egremont

Beech House Group Practice
Beech House Medical Centre, St Bridgets Lane, Egremont CA22 2BD
Tel: 01946 820203 Fax: 01946 820372
(West Cumbria Primary Care Trust)
Patient List Size: 11200

Practice Manager Marie Shawcross

GP Jan HEIJNE den BAK, Michael BEWICK, Julie CARTER, Fiona Dorothy GALLOWAY, Richard Alexander JAKOBSON, Mary PHILIPS, John William VEITCH

Egremont Medical Centre
9 King Street, Egremont CH44 8AT
Tel: 0151 639 0777 Fax: 0151 637 0532
(Birkenhead and Wallasey Primary Care Trust)

Practice Manager Dot Molyneux

GP Anthony G CUMMINS, John Joseph Mary HICKEY

Westcroft Surgery
66 Main Street, Egremont CA22 2DB
Tel: 01946 820348 Fax: 01946 821611
(West Cumbria Primary Care Trust)

Practice Manager Janet Toole

GP Anthony Lowry Nicholson CREED, C D HALL, Andrew SANT

Elland

Bankfield Surgery
15 Huddersfield Road, Elland HX5 9BA
Tel: 01422 375537 Fax: 01422 370776
(Calderdale Primary Care Trust)
Patient List Size: 7555

Practice Manager J D Leslie

GP Pravinbhai Prahladbhai PARMAR, Susan Anne BRENNAN, Edward Peter BYLINA, Jane Elizabeth CLARKSON

Burley Street Surgery
Burley Street, Elland HX5 0AQ
Tel: 01422 372057 Fax: 01422 311563
(Calderdale Primary Care Trust)
Patient List Size: 3200

Practice Manager Sonia Heard

GP Falak NAZ, Evelyn Mary NAZ

Ellesmere

The Surgery
Ellesmere Medical Practice, Trimperley, Ellesmere SY12 0DB
Tel: 01691 622798 Fax: 01691 623294
(Shropshire County Primary Care Trust)
Patient List Size: 7200

Practice Manager Ed Manning

GP Evan Andrew Meredith GREVILLE, Victoria Jane MANNING, Sheelin Jane NEWTON, Yvonne Marie VIBISHANAN, Geoffrey Mark WILLIS

Ellesmere Port

Great Sutton Medical Centre
Old Chester Road, Great Sutton, Ellesmere Port CH66 3PB
Tel: 0151 339 3079 Fax: 0151 339 9225
(Ellesmere Port and Neston Primary Care Trust)
Patient List Size: 6000

Practice Manager Carol Gunn

GP Malcolm FRAZER COX, Geraint Wynn GRIFFITHS, Andrew John McALAVEY

Great Sutton Medical Centre
Old Chester Road, Great Sutton, Ellesmere Port CH66 3PB
Tel: 0151 339 3126 Fax: 0151 339 9225
(Ellesmere Port and Neston Primary Care Trust)
Patient List Size: 7745

Practice Manager Carol Gunn

GP Michael Richard KENNEDY, Aled Wyn GRIFFITH, Ann Patricia JUDGE, John Penrose WEARNE

Great Sutton Medical Centre
Old Chester Road, Great Sutton, Ellesmere Port CH66 3PB
Tel: 0151 339 2424 Fax: 0151 339 9225
(Ellesmere Port and Neston Primary Care Trust)
Patient List Size: 6189

Practice Manager Carol Gunn

GP Gerald FAULKS, Harriet Brigid FLATTERY, Nigel WOOD

Whitby Group Practice
114 Chester Road, Whitby, Ellesmere Port CH65 6TG
Tel: 0151 355 6151 Fax: 0151 355 6843
(Ellesmere Port and Neston Primary Care Trust)
Patient List Size: 5266

Practice Manager Jennifer Jackson

GP Geoffrey BURGESS, Richard Adam POWELL, Christina Mary WALL

Whitby Group Practice Surgery
Chester Road, Whitby, Ellesmere Port CH65 6TG
Tel: 0151 355 6144 Fax: 0151 355 6843
(Ellesmere Port and Neston Primary Care Trust)
Patient List Size: 6979

GP Geoffrey Bowerbank HAYLE, Steven Nigel BOWMAN, J STRINGER, Diane Michele TAYLOR

Whitby Group Practice Surgery
Chester Road, Whitby, Ellesmere Port CH65 6TG
Tel: 0151 355 6153 Fax: 0151 355 6843
(Ellesmere Port and Neston Primary Care Trust)
Patient List Size: 4610

GP Fiona Margaret WARREN, T BALW, Robert Nigel SHILLITO, Wendy Elizabeth SHILLITO

Ely

The Health Centre
Granby Street, Littleport, Ely CB6 1NE
Tel: 01353 860223 Fax: 01353 862198
(East Cambridgeshire and Fenland Primary Care Trust)
Patient List Size: 8000

Practice Manager H Setchfield

GP Stephen John MAHER, Alain GREEN, Richard William HEIGHTON, Shirin HOWELL, Susan KING

Priors Field Surgery
24 High Street, Sutton, Ely CB6 2RB
Tel: 01353 778208 Fax: 01353 777765
(East Cambridgeshire and Fenland Primary Care Trust)
Patient List Size: 9324

Practice Manager Christine Sparrow

GP Christopher Richard HORNE, Peter William BENNETT, Hannah DEAN, Sally Elizabeth HARDING, John McHUGH, Joanna PARRY, Derek Neil YULL

St Marys Surgery
37 St. Mary's Street, Ely CB7 4HF
Tel: 01353 665511 Fax: 01353 669532
(East Cambridgeshire and Fenland Primary Care Trust)
Patient List Size: 16000

Practice Manager Kathryn Green

GP David Granville WOODS, John CRAWFORD, Andrew Scott DOUGLAS, Deirdre Helen Pauline Tempany McCORMACK, Susan Elizabeth MEE, Kate NORRIS, Balraj SANGHERA, John Robert SHACKLETON, Katrina Mary YOUNG

Staploe Medical Centre
Brewhouse Lane, Soham, Ely CB7 5JD
Tel: 01353 624123 Fax: 01353 624203
(East Cambridgeshire and Fenland Primary Care Trust)
Patient List Size: 15000

Practice Manager Michael Wilde

GP Jagadish PARTHA, Sarah BURLING, Richard BURNFORD, Alun Michael GEORGE, Anthony GUNSTONE, James HOWARD, Sarah HUTCHINSON, J A JONES, Anne Heather MOLYNEUX

The Surgery
The Green, Haddenham, Ely CB6 3TA
Tel: 01353 740205 Fax: 01353 741364
(East Cambridgeshire and Fenland Primary Care Trust)
Patient List Size: 6662

Practice Manager Ann Enticknap

GP Pamela KENNY, Jan Stefan ANISKOWICZ, Stuart Charles FINDLAY, John LEVENTHORPE

Emsworth

North Street House Surgery
6 North Street, Emsworth PO10 7DD
Tel: 01243 372132 Fax: 01243 379080
(East Hampshire Primary Care Trust)

Practice Manager Peter Loveridge

GP David Longden INGRAM, James Stanhope COLLINGS-WELLS, S L GILES, Diana Judith Lucy HAWKER, Philippa Mary NEWMAN, J I O'BRIEN, Janet Elisabeth SUSSEX, Philip Graydon TIBBS

Southbourne Surgery
337 Main Road, Emsworth PO10 8JH
Tel: 01243 372623 Fax: 01243 379936
(Western Sussex Primary Care Trust)
Patient List Size: 8650

GP Ian A RICHARDSON, Kingsley C CHADWICK, Jo NASH, Justin B SMITH, Rophina O YELD

Enfield

Abernethy House
70 Silver Street, Enfield EN1 3EB
Tel: 020 8366 1314 Fax: 020 8364 4176
(Enfield Primary Care Trust)
Patient List Size: 12500

Practice Manager Tracey Jenkins

GP Michael Charles GOCMAN, Anjum IQBAL, Janet Elizabeth McQUEEN, Patrick Henry Michael O'MAHONY, Wendy Elizabeth WHITTAKER, Elaine Ruth YEO

Brick Lane Surgery
28 Brick Lane, Enfield EN3 5BA
Tel: 020 8443 0413 Fax: 020 8805 9097
(Enfield Primary Care Trust)
Patient List Size: 3800

Practice Manager Julia Reid

GP Josephine Theresa CONNAUGHTON, Lois BENJAMIN

Bush Hill Park Medical Centre
25 Melbourne Way, Bush Hill Park, Enfield EN1 1XG
Tel: 020 8366 5858 Fax: 020 8366 8514
(Enfield Primary Care Trust)
Patient List Size: 2000

Practice Manager Phillip Tegg

GP Carl Tsang Nin CHANG

Bush Hill Park Surgery
24 Amberley Road, Enfield EN1 2QY
(Enfield Primary Care Trust)

GP A NICHOLAS-PILLAI, C UWAGBOE

Carlton House Surgery
28 Tenniswood Road, Enfield EN1 3LL
Tel: 020 8363 7575 Fax: 020 8366 8228
(Enfield Primary Care Trust)

Practice Manager Christine Holder

GP Jarir Odeh AMARIN, Clare Mary JEPSON, Andrew Wing-Fung MOK, Peter Michael NEWTON, Alan Timothy RIDGE, John Richard SALMON

Carterhatch Lane Surgery
99 Carterhatch Lane, Enfield EN1 4LA
Tel: 020 8804 5312 Fax: 020 8804 5095
(Enfield Primary Care Trust)

GP Retnasabapathy Anantha ROOBAN

Curzon Avenue Surgery
74 Curzon Avenue, Ponders End, Enfield EN3 4UE
Tel: 020 8364 7846 Fax: 020 8443 0503
(Enfield Primary Care Trust)
Patient List Size: 4900

Practice Manager Alyson Hicks

GP Nivedita BOSE, Helen Margaret ELDON, Susan Valerie LOVE, Gloria OKAFOR-EZEJIOFOR

Dean House Surgery
193 High Street, Ponders End, Enfield EN3 4DZ
Tel: 020 8804 1060 Fax: 020 8804 9589
(Enfield Primary Care Trust)

GP SM CHOUDHRY

Eagle House Surgery
291 High Street, Ponders End, Enfield EN3 4DN
Tel: 020 8351 1000 Fax: 020 8351 1007
(Enfield Primary Care Trust)
Patient List Size: 12857

Practice Manager Bel Burns

GP Peter BARNES, Catherine AIMIUWU, M A BARNES, Anthony Simon MARKS, Ian David RUBENSTEIN, Isabella SNOWDEN

Enfield Island
c/o Cedar House, St. Michael's Stie, 19 Chase Side Crescent, Enfield EN2 0JA
Tel: 020 8967 5973 Fax: 020 8364 6442
(Enfield Primary Care Trust)
Patient List Size: 2750

Practice Manager Helen Robinson

GP D DUROJAIYE

Freezywater Primary Care Centre
2B Aylands Road, Enfield EN3 6PN
Tel: 01992 763794 Fax: 01992 764570
(Enfield Primary Care Trust)
Patient List Size: 10250

Practice Manager Kalpana Patel

GP Laurence John KNOTT, Nawroze Iqbal CHOWDHURY, Raj MAZUMDER, P P PATEL

Green Street Surgery
48 Green Street, Enfield EN3 7HW
Tel: 020 8804 3200 Fax: 020 8443 2615
(Enfield Primary Care Trust)

Practice Manager Susan Juriansz

GP Ponniah SUBANANDAN

Lincoln Road Medical Practice
Lincoln Road, Enfield EN1 1LJ
(Enfield Primary Care Trust)

Moorfield Road Health Centre
2 Moorfield Road, Enfield EN3 5PS
Tel: 020 8804 1522 Fax: 020 8443 1465
(Enfield Primary Care Trust)
Patient List Size: 4600

Practice Manager Carol Crick

GP Selambaram PALANIAPPAN, Abrahampillai Remy STANISLAUS

Ordnance Road Surgery
171 Ordnance Road, Enfield Lock, Enfield EN3 6AD
Tel: 01992 761185 Fax: 01992 760938
(Enfield Primary Care Trust)
Patient List Size: 4100

Practice Manager R A Wakelin

GP Pasapula Chinna SUBRAHMANYAM, Sajida CHOUDHRY

Riley House Surgery
413 Hertford Road, Enfield EN3 5PR
Tel: 020 8364 7400 Fax: 020 8805 8128
(Enfield Primary Care Trust)
Patient List Size: 9000

GP K CHATTERJEE, M N HOSSAIN, Kazi Kilsum HUQ, M S KABIR, K RAJENDRAN

Southbury Surgery
73 Southbury Road, Enfield EN1 1PJ
Tel: 020 8363 0305 Fax: 020 8364 4288
(Enfield Primary Care Trust)
Patient List Size: 3700

Practice Manager Marion Bacon

GP P G D KEATING, Helen APPLETON

The Surgery
11 Bincote Road, Enfield EN2 7RD
Tel: 020 8367 7315 Fax: 020 8366 0623
Email: bincote@ndirect.co.uk
(Enfield Primary Care Trust)
Patient List Size: 5200

Practice Manager Ann Williams

GP Hettiarachchige Ranjith Marcus DISSANAYAKE, M COFFEY, N N PATEL

The Surgery
24 Trinity Avenue, Enfield EN1 1HS
Tel: 020 8363 4493 Fax: 020 8363 4493
(Enfield Primary Care Trust)

Practice Manager P R Nathan

GP P RAMA-NATHAN

The Surgery
340 High Street, Ponders End, Enfield EN3 4DE
Tel: 020 8805 5972 Fax: 020 8292 3772
(Enfield Primary Care Trust)

Practice Manager Tahera Hussain

GP Razia Sultana MOOSVI

Town Surgery
37 Cecil Road, Enfield EN2 6TJ
Tel: 020 8342 0330 Fax: 020 8342 0330
(Enfield Primary Care Trust)
Patient List Size: 2100

GP Muttiah THEIVENDRA

White Lodge Medical Practice
68 Silver Street, Enfield EN1 3EW
Tel: 020 8363 4156 Fax: 020 8364 6295
(Enfield Primary Care Trust)
Patient List Size: 11000

Practice Manager C Morgan

GP Michael Albert Murad Baruch CARMI, Nipulkumar AMIN, A FENTON, Benjamin GARLAND, H GREWAL, A PATEL, S PATEL

Willow House Surgery
285 Willow Road, Enfield EN1 3AZ
Tel: 020 8363 0472 Fax: 020 8363 8936
(Enfield Primary Care Trust)

Practice Manager Theresa Smart

GP Sunil DHAR, V HITCHINGS, G KUMAR

Epping

High Street Surgery
301 High Street, Epping CM16 4DA
Tel: 01992 572012/571717 Fax: 01992 572956
(Epping Forest Primary Care Trust)
Patient List Size: 6000

Practice Manager Sue Surridge

GP Diana Margaret LOWRY, Rizwan Mohamedtaki PRADHAN

Limes Medical Centre
The Plain, Epping CM16 6TL
Tel: 01992 572727 Fax: 01992 574889
(Epping Forest Primary Care Trust)

Practice Manager Patricia Kirrane, Maureen Stuttard

GP Andrew Livingstone ASHFORD, Ahmed Tareq ABOUHARB, Emma Marie DEMPSEY, Dr DUGGINS, Susan Jane HANGER, N R JACKSON, R McCREA, Deirdre Mary Elizabeth O'CONNOR, Jane RICHES

Epsom

Ashley Centre Surgery
Ashley Square, Epsom KT18 5DD
Tel: 01372 723668 Fax: 01372 726796
(East Elmbridge and Mid Surrey Primary Care Trust)

Practice Manager R D Harmsworth

GP Jean Alexander CUNNINGHAM, James Arthur HOUGHTON, Sylvia Ann ROBERTS, Andrew Paul SHARPE

Bourne Hall Health Centre
Chessington Road, Ewell, Epsom KT17 1TG
(East Elmbridge and Mid Surrey Primary Care Trust)

GP John PIPER

Bourne Hall Health Centre
Spring Street, Ewell, Epsom KT17 1TG
(East Elmbridge and Mid Surrey Primary Care Trust)

Practice Manager Hanna Williams

GP Jane Susanne Almond SENHENN

Derby Medical Centre
8 Derby Square, Epsom KT19 8AG
Tel: 01372 726361
(East Elmbridge and Mid Surrey Primary Care Trust)
Patient List Size: 12500

Practice Manager H Harwood

GP Joan BROWN, John Francis FLOWER, Hilary Jean FLOYD, Dean Mark HARRIS, Nigel Duncan McKEE, Robert Lee WORMLEY

Dr Orton and Partners
Chessington Road, Ewell, Epsom KT17 1TG
Tel: 020 8394 1362
(East Elmbridge and Mid Surrey Primary Care Trust)

Practice Manager Mark O'Neill

GP Jonathan HOLBROOK, Julian Jasper ORTON

Glenwood Road Surgery
20 Glenwood Road, Stoneleigh, Epsom KT17 2LZ
Tel: 020 8393 6051 Fax: 020 8873 1059
(East Elmbridge and Mid Surrey Primary Care Trust)
Patient List Size: 2100

Practice Manager Evelyn Cupit

GP V K PATEL

Integrated Care Partnership
Fitznells Manor Surgery, 2 Chessington Road, Ewell, Epsom KT17 1TF
Tel: 020 8394 2365 Fax: 020 8393 9753
(East Elmbridge and Mid Surrey Primary Care Trust)
Patient List Size: 6250

Practice Manager V Parnell

GP Ralph Haight BURTON, Claire CRABTREE, Katherine DALE, Susan MITCHELL, Paul STEVENSON

Integrated Care Partnership
Fitznell Manor Surgery, Chessington Road, Ewell, Epsom KT17 1TF
Tel: 020 8394 1471 Fax: 020 8393 9753
(East Elmbridge and Mid Surrey Primary Care Trust)
Patient List Size: 6250

Practice Manager C Crossen

GP Susan Carolyn MITCHELL, Paul Nigel STEVENTON

Longmead Surgery
Norman Colyer Court, Hollymoor Lane, Epsom KT19 9JZ
Tel: 01372 743432 Fax: 01372 817595
(East Elmbridge and Mid Surrey Primary Care Trust)
Patient List Size: 2650

Practice Manager Cristina Silva

GP Francisco Briones SILVA

Old Cottage Hospital Surgery
Alexandra Road, Epsom KT17 4BL
Tel: 01372 724434 Fax: 01372 748171
Website: www.old-cottage-hospital.co.uk
(East Elmbridge and Mid Surrey Primary Care Trust)
Patient List Size: 13100

Practice Manager Susan Ebanks

GP Richard Anthony Philip STOTT, Catherine BRYCE, Michael Neal BUNN, Heather CARR-WHITE, Richard John COWLARD, S EMANUEL, Amanda Jane FREE, Joanna RENDELL, Timothy RICHARDSON, Michael Ron SEVENOAKS

Stoneleigh Medical Centre
24 The Broadway, Stoneleigh, Epsom KT17 2HU
(East Elmbridge and Mid Surrey Primary Care Trust)

GP N N SIDHOM

The Surgery
Cox Lane Centre, Cox Lane, West Ewell, Epsom KT19 9PS

GP Ashok Kumar KATIYAR

Tattenham Health Centre
Tattenham Crescent, Epsom KT18 5NU
Tel: 01737 371011 Fax: 01737 359641
(East Elmbridge and Mid Surrey Primary Care Trust)

GP Marjorie Joy BALDWIN, Elizabeth Louise BARR, Suzanne MOORE

Erith

Bulbanks Medical Centre
62 Battle Road, Erith DA8 1BJ
Tel: 01322 432997 Fax: 01322 442324
(Bexley Care Trust)
Patient List Size: 3700

Practice Manager Hazel Sharma

GP Ashok Kumar SHARMA, Kanwalpal Singh NANDRA

Dr K Manis
Erith Health Centre, 50 Pier Road, Erith DA8 1RQ
Tel: 01322 334237 Fax: 020 8298 7165
(Bexley Care Trust)
Patient List Size: 7300

GP Kostas MANIS

Le Geyt
Erith Health Centre, Queen Street, Erith DA8 1TT
Tel: 01322 332838 Fax: 01322 351559
(Bexley Care Trust)

GP John David LE GEYT

Northumberland Heath Medical Centre
Hind Crescent, Northumberland Heath, Erith DA8 3DB
Tel: 01322 336556 Fax: 01322 351475
(Bexley Care Trust)
Patient List Size: 9330

Practice Manager Pamela Waller

GP Malcolm Rowan McINTYRE, Wilson Wai Fung FOK, Mohan Hjertholm GHOSH, Surjit Singh KAILEY

Patel
Erith Health Centre, Queen Street, Erith DA8 1TT
Tel: 01322 330283 Fax: 01322 351504
Email: valsuni@hotmail.com
(Bexley Care Trust)
Patient List Size: 4500

Practice Manager Anna Wood

GP Valabh Shambhubhai PATEL

Slade Green Medical Centre
156 Bridge Road, Slade Green, Erith DA8 2HS
Tel: 01322 334884 Fax: 01322 351510
(Bexley Care Trust)
Patient List Size: 5940

GP Ramesh Chandra DHATARIYA

The Surgery
25 Mill Road, Erith DA8 1HW
Tel: 01322 332455 Fax: 01322 335754
Website: www.millroadsurgery.co.uk
(Bexley Care Trust)
Patient List Size: 2341

Practice Manager Rinoshini Jayakumar

GP Senathirajah SELLAPPAH

Esher

Capelfield Surgery
Elm Road, Claygate, Esher KT10 0EH
Tel: 01372 462501 Fax: 01372 470258
(East Elmbridge and Mid Surrey Primary Care Trust)
Patient List Size: 7300

Practice Manager Linda Kendall

GP Neil Macarthur MUNRO, S ASIRDAS, Alison JOHNSTON, Avtar Singh KAMBOJ, Heather Frances PATEL

Esher Green Surgery
Esher Green Drive, Esher KT10 8BX
Tel: 01372 462726 Fax: 01372 471050
(East Elmbridge and Mid Surrey Primary Care Trust)

Practice Manager Jackie Caldwell

GP Jill Catherine EVANS, Sharonn BULLEN, Joan Teresa MUNNELLY, Alison SHINE

Littleton Surgery
Buckland House, Esher Park Avenue, Esher KT10 9NY
Tel: 01372 462235 Fax: 01372 470622
(East Elmbridge and Mid Surrey Primary Care Trust)
Patient List Size: 4000

Practice Manager Lorraine Knapp

GP Anne Michele GOLDSACK, Philip William GAVINS

Etchingham

Woodgate, Packham and Thomas
Fairfield Surgery, High Street, Burwash, Etchingham TN19 7EU
Tel: 01435 882306 Fax: 01435 882064
(Bexhill and Rother Primary Care Trust)
Patient List Size: 4035

Practice Manager Stephen Fowler

GP Jane Elizabeth WOODGATE, Bruce Anthony PACKHAM, Matthew THOMAS

Evesham

Abbey Medical Practice
The Health Centre, Merstow Green, Evesham WR11 4BS
Tel: 01386 761111 Fax: 01386 769515
(South Worcestershire Primary Care Trust)
Patient List Size: 6350

Practice Manager Richard Allen

GP S C GRANT, Irene J HENRY, J H LLOYD, Christopher M OUNSTED

De Montfort Medical Centre
Burford Road, Bengeworth, Evesham WR11 3HD
Tel: 01386 443333 Fax: 01386 422884
(South Worcestershire Primary Care Trust)
Patient List Size: 5488

Practice Manager Nigel Higenbottam

GP David Andrew JONES, Paul Giles HELLER, Kathryn Margaret SHORE

Merstow Green Medical Practice
Merstow Green, Evesham WR11 4BS
Tel: 01386 765600 Fax: 01386 446807
(South Worcestershire Primary Care Trust)
Patient List Size: 10700

Practice Manager Nicola Bamber

GP John Christopher Geoffrey MILNER, Catriona Mary Ross D'ARCY, John EGAN, David FARMER, Yang Wern OOI, Ian Lennox Taylor SMITH

The Riverside Surgery
Waterside, Evesham WR11 6JP
Tel: 01386 40121 Fax: 01386 442615
(South Worcestershire Primary Care Trust)

Practice Manager Joe Icke

GP Geoffrey BURTON, Julie Ann EDWARDES, Lennox Fyfe GREGOROWSKI, David Charles HEROLD, Neville Reed JACKSON, David Ian JEFFREY, Anne Gwyneth SERENYI, Amanda Louise SWINDLEHURST

Exeter

Barnfield Hill Surgery
12 Barnfield Hill, Exeter EX1 1SR
Tel: 01392 432761 Fax: 01392 422406
Email: sally.ewings@fsmail.net
Website: www.barnfieldhillsurgery.co.uk
(Exeter Primary Care Trust)
Patient List Size: 6400

Practice Manager Elizabeth Deasy

GP Juliet Mary CAMPLING, Sally Ann EWINGS, Paul McDERMOTT, Michael David RAMELL, Neil Nicholas SMALLWOOD

Beacon Lane Surgery
109 Beacon Lane, Exeter EX4 8LT
Tel: 01392 73484 Fax: 01392 490135
(Exeter Primary Care Trust)

Practice Manager Mrs Anderson

GP Robert James ANDERSON

Chapel Platt Surgery
1901 Fore Street, Topsham, Exeter EX3 0HE
Tel: 01392 875777 Fax: 01392 875770
Email: chapelplatt@gp-l83661.nhs.uk
(Exeter Primary Care Trust)
Patient List Size: 2500

Practice Manager Sue Barnes

GP T J GOULDING, Adrian Charles Dominic RENOUF

Charters Surgery
38 Polsloe Road, Exeter EX1 2DW
Tel: 01392 273805
Email: info@charters.co.uk
Website: www.charters.co.uk
(Exeter Primary Care Trust)
Patient List Size: 3100

Practice Manager David Cobley

GP Charles Stuart REAVES, Elizabeth Chance REAVES

Cheriton Bishop Surgery
Cheriton Bishop, Exeter EX6 6JA
Tel: 01647 24272 Fax: 01647 24038
(Mid Devon Primary Care Trust)
Patient List Size: 4211

Practice Manager Margaret Brash

GP Simon Bryan DUDBRIDGE, Jason Matthew John CLUNIE, Josephine HERDMAN

Church Street Surgery
Church Street, Starcross, Exeter EX6 8PZ
Tel: 01626 890368 Fax: 01626 891330
(Exeter Primary Care Trust)
Patient List Size: 6800

Practice Manager Stephanie George

GP Rachel MANN, Paul Benjamin OSBORNE, John Hilmar PERKINS, Elke QUINN, Simon George Harding RAINS

Delph House Surgery
8 Pinhoe Road, Exeter EX4 7HL
Tel: 01392 72304 Fax: 01392 423819
(Exeter Primary Care Trust)
Patient List Size: 2500

Practice Manager Sue Power

GP John Derek Peter EGGLETON

Exwick Health Centre
New Valley Road, Exeter EX4 2AD
Tel: 01392 676600 Fax: 01392 676601
(Exeter Primary Care Trust)

GP J FOX, H PLUMMER, A SMITH

Fulford Way Surgery
Fulford Way, Woodbury, Exeter EX5 1NZ
Tel: 01395 232509 Fax: 01395 232065
(East Devon Primary Care Trust)
Patient List Size: 3200

Practice Manager Sandie Hampshire

GP Angela Margaret DOUGLAS, Elfred Noel LAWN

Heavitree Health Centre
South Lawn Terrace, Exeter EX1 2RX
Tel: 01392 431355 Fax: 01392 498305
(Exeter Primary Care Trust)
Patient List Size: 7545

Practice Manager M Chapple

GP Vaughan Charles Edgar ROSSER, Andrew Jeremy HARRISON, Alison Jane Renowden HUDSON, Dr RICHARD, Josephine Mary WITHEY

The Heavitree Practice
South Lawn Terrace, Heavitree, Exeter EX1 2RX
Tel: 01392 211511 Fax: 01392 499451
(Exeter Primary Care Trust)
Patient List Size: 6900

Practice Manager Len Young

GP Robert Henry MOODY, Niall MACLEOD, Anna MORRIS

Hill Barton Surgery
1 Lower Hill Barton Road, Exeter EX1 3EN
Tel: 01392 444242 Fax: 01392 446240
(Exeter Primary Care Trust)
Patient List Size: 3635

Practice Manager Wendy Jackson

GP Elizabeth Ann MAPSON, Steven A BARADA, Clare LASCELLES

Homefield Surgery
6 Homefield Road, Exeter EX1 2QS
Tel: 01392 214151 Fax: 01392 214217
Email: admin@homefieldsurgery.freeserve.co.uk
Website: www.homefieldsurgery.nhs.uk
(Exeter Primary Care Trust)
Patient List Size: 1990

Practice Manager David Cobley

GP Adrian Keith MIDGLEY, Alison SHELLOCK

Ide Lane Surgery
Ide Lane, Alphington, Exeter EX2 8UP
Tel: 01392 439868 Fax: 01392 428913
(Exeter Primary Care Trust)
Patient List Size: 6100

Practice Manager Imelda Liversage

GP Nicholas Cadbury Albert BRADLEY, William Leo CLARKE, David Colin Wood HILTON, Gillian Margaret STOWELL, Stephen VERCOE

Mount Pleasant Health Centre
Mount Pleasant Road, Exeter EX4 7BW
Tel: 01392 55262 Fax: 01392 270497
(Exeter Primary Care Trust)

Practice Manager Ken Stokes

GP Roger Martin ONYETT, Clare Margaret CLAREY, Nicholas Hares HELLIAR, David HOPKINS, Christopher Paul THORNE

Mount Pleasant Health Centre
Mount Pleasant Road, Exeter EX4 7BW
Tel: 01392 255722 Fax: 01392 270497
(Exeter Primary Care Trust)

Practice Manager Ken Stokes

GP Dr McFADYEN, Dr ROBERTS, Dr RUSSELL

Pinhoe Surgery
Pinn Lane, Exeter EX1 3SY
Tel: 01392 469666 Fax: 01392 464178
(Exeter Primary Care Trust)
Patient List Size: 8450

Practice Manager Alan Bennett

GP Malcolm Edward BIRD, Catherine Louise CLEMENTS, Martin John MEREDITH, Carol Marion SCOTT, Jonathon STRIDE, Anne Catherine WALKER

Southernhay House Surgery
30 Barnfield Road, Exeter EX1 1RX
Tel: 01392 211266/01392 425126 Fax: 01392 204407
(Exeter Primary Care Trust)
Patient List Size: 6000

Practice Manager Sue Montford

GP Dr LEGER, Dr AMHERST, Dr BATES, Dr KNOWLES

St. Leonards Medical Practice
34 Denmark Road, St Leonards, Exeter EX1 1SF
Tel: 01392 201790 Fax: 01392 201796
(Exeter Primary Care Trust)

Practice Manager Peter Sanderson

GP Philip EVANS, Harriet DICKSON, Adrian FREEMAN, Alex HARDING, Pip HAYES

St Thomas Health Centre
Cowick Street, St. Thomas, Exeter EX4 1HJ
Tel: 01392 676678 Fax: 01392 676677
Email: stthomas@nhs.net
(Exeter Primary Care Trust)
Patient List Size: 29500

Practice Manager Gill Heppell

GP Harpreet ARSHI, Guy Charles BRADLEY-SMITH, Lorna Jane COLEMAN, J FOX, David Penrose KERNICK, P MILLER, Ruth Patricia NORTHOVER, H PLUMMER, J RUTTER, A SMITH, K THOMAS, Mark Benjamin WATSON, Alexander WILLIAMS

The Surgery
The Bury, Thorverton, Exeter EX5 5NT
Tel: 01392 860273 Fax: 01392 860654
(Mid Devon Primary Care Trust)
Patient List Size: 1316

Practice Manager Richard Larouche

GP Amanda Jane WOODS, Jon Peter WRIDE

The Topsham Surgery
The White House, Holman Way, Topsham, Exeter EX3 0EN
Tel: 01392 874646 Fax: 01392 875261
(Exeter Primary Care Trust)
Patient List Size: 6200

Practice Manager Linda Kay

GP Gareth BROAD, Catherine Laura DICK, Elizabeth Ann FOSTER, Andrew KAY, David Stanley LEEDER, Robert John TURNER

The Whipton Surgery
378 Pinhoe Road, Whipton, Exeter EX4 8EG
Tel: 01392 462770 Fax: 01392 466220
(Exeter Primary Care Trust)
Patient List Size: 3200

Practice Manager Christine Howe

GP Sally Clare BUNKALL, Michael CULLEN, John Guy Marcus HARRILL

Wonford Green Surgery
Burnthouse Lane, Exeter EX2 6NF
Tel: 01392 250135 Fax: 01392 498572
(Exeter Primary Care Trust)
Patient List Size: 4800

Practice Manager Lynette Drew

GP Ian Trevor HOWARD, Barrie Margaret FERGUSON, Ben HOBAN, Lesley Elizabeth KEALEY, Monika KINTEH

Wyndham House Surgery
Fore Street, Silverton, Exeter EX5 4HZ
Tel: 01392 860034 Fax: 01392 861165
(Mid Devon Primary Care Trust)
Patient List Size: 3845

Practice Manager Clare Crocker

GP Richard John LEETE, Anthony T J O'BRIEN, Jonathan William STEAD

Exmouth

Claremont Medical Practice
Exmouth Health Centre, Claremont Grove, Exmouth EX8 2JF
Tel: 01395 273666 Fax: 01395 223301
(East Devon Primary Care Trust)

Practice Manager Hazel Hunt

GP P ACHESON, Elizabeth Jane Rosann DEBENHAM, Thomas Robert DEBENHAM, Kevin Michael DOUGLAS, R J GANNER, N F A JOHNSTON, Teresa Felicity NICHOLSON, Geoffrey Oliffe RICHMOND

Haldon House Surgery
37-39 Imperial Road, Exmouth EX8 1DQ
Tel: 01395 222777/222888 Fax: 01395 269769
Email: surgery@haldon-house.co.uk
Website: www.haldon-house.co.uk
(East Devon Primary Care Trust)
Patient List Size: 5500

Practice Manager Elizabeth Hopkins

GP Judyth Elizabeth AARONS, Robin John HOPKINS, Simon Robert KAY, Colin John MAY

Imperial Surgery
49 Imperial Road, Exmouth EX8 1DQ
Tel: 01395 224555 Fax: 01395 279282
Email: reception@gp-l83628.nhs.uk
(East Devon Primary Care Trust)

Practice Manager Bob Bryant

GP Susan Lynne POCKLINGTON, Antony Peter LEWIS, Mark Edward James NICHOLSON

Raleigh Surgery
33 Pines Road, Brixington, Exmouth EX8 5NH
Tel: 01395 222499 Fax: 01395 225493
(East Devon Primary Care Trust)
Patient List Size: 4200

Practice Manager Cindy Flatt

GP David SPIERS, V Jane CARTLEDGE, Alison PRUST

Rolle Medical Partnership
Exmouth Health Centre, Claremont Grove, Exmouth EX8 2JF
Tel: 01395 273001 Fax: 01395 273771
(East Devon Primary Care Trust)

Practice Manager June Berry

GP Helen Madeleine ENRIGHT, F J FERNANDEZ-GUILLEN, Stephen Rhys PRICE, Stephen David John ROSS, Lynne SANDERSON, Christopher Linton SCOTT, Clive Alan STUBBINGS, Susan Margaret STUBBINGS, Stephen WARD

Eye

Fressingfield Medical Centre
New Street, Fressingfield, Eye IP21 5PJ
Tel: 01379 586227 Fax: 01379 588265
(Central Suffolk Primary Care Trust)
Patient List Size: 4203

Practice Manager Maureen Edgeway

GP Sandra Joan HOLMES, James A C MORRIS, Gregory Martin READ

The Health Centre
Castleton Way, Eye IP23 7DD
Tel: 01379 870689
(Central Suffolk Primary Care Trust)

GP Michael ELLIS-JONES, Henry R A LEWIS, C PARTRIDGE

Fairford

Hilary Cottage Surgery
Keble Lawns, Fairford GL7 4BQ
Tel: 01285 712377 Fax: 01285 713084
(Cotswold and Vale Primary Care Trust)

Practice Manager David Forbes

GP Alexander Stewart BENZIE, Anne Elizabeth GARDINER, Martin John Guy KNIGHTS, Dorothy Christine LUNNEY, Andrew Cole SABOURIN

Fakenham

Fakenham Medical Practice
The Fakenham Medical Centre, Greenway Lane, Fakenham NR21 8ET
Tel: 01328 851321 Fax: 01328 851412
Email: doctors@fakenham-practice.freeserve.co.uk
(North Norfolk Primary Care Trust)
Patient List Size: 14700

Practice Manager John Smith

GP George Stafford ACHESON, David John Newland BENNETT, Janet Elizabeth CAMPBELL, Paolo de MARCO, Richard George GORROD, Carly Anna HUGHES, Manhar JOSHI, Patricia Alice KENDALL, Piers Hayward REINHOLD

Falmouth

Constantine Surgery
Bowling Green, Constantine, Falmouth TR11 5AP
Tel: 01326 340667 Fax: 01326 340968
(West of Cornwall Primary Care Trust)
Patient List Size: 2168

Practice Manager Neil Stevens

GP Adrian Brian ROBERTS, Paula ROBERTS

Falmouth Health Centre
Trevaylor Road, Falmouth TR11 2LH
Tel: 01326 434800 Fax: 01326 434829
Website: www.faldoc.co.uk
(Central Cornwall Primary Care Trust)
Patient List Size: 9400

Practice Manager Geoff Dennis

GP Philip Denis SLATER, Sophie CHIDDICK, Richard David Goronwy JAMES, Andrew Charles SEAMAN

Trescobeas Surgery
Trescobeas Road, Falmouth TR11 2UN
Tel: 01326 315615 Fax: 01326 434899
(Central Cornwall Primary Care Trust)
Patient List Size: 9100

Practice Manager R S Fox

GP George William DAVIS, Philip BURNETT, Dr DAVIS, Philip Granville DOMMETT, David George MILLER, Mark Andrew REEVES

Westover Surgery
Western Terrace, Falmouth TR11 4QJ
Tel: 01326 212120
(Central Cornwall Primary Care Trust)

Practice Manager M Hardman

GP Carolyn CHEETHAM, Mark CROUSE, Harold Adam STACPOOLE

Woodlane Surgery
Trelawney Road, Falmouth TR11 3GP
Tel: 01326 312091 Fax: 01326 311260
(Central Cornwall Primary Care Trust)
Patient List Size: 4000

Practice Manager D Cummins

GP Anthony DOWNEY, Katherine Sarah DOWNEY

Fareham

Fareham Health Centre
Osborn Road, Fareham PO16 7ER
Tel: 01329 822111 Fax: 01329 286636
(Fareham and Gosport Primary Care Trust)

GP Robert Arthur BELLENGER, Donal Ciaran COLLINS, Samantha DIGGINS, Katie Elizabeth DIXON, Grant John Clement DU FEU, Susan Jane GRIFFITHS, Barbara Louise JORDAN, Nicholas Maciej LEWKOWICZ

Gudgeheath Lane Surgery
187 Gudgeheath Lane, Fareham PO15 6QA
Tel: 01329 280887 Fax: 01329 513668
(Fareham and Gosport Primary Care Trust)
Patient List Size: 8000

Practice Manager Malcolm Board

GP Alexander Paul WOLPE, Nicholas John ALLEN, Ailsa MAGUIRE, Adrian MILLMAN, Elizabeth Judith MUSHENS

The Health Centre
Osborn Road, Fareham PO16 7ER
Tel: 01329 823456 Fax: 01329 285772
(Fareham and Gosport Primary Care Trust)

Practice Manager B Maw

GP Keith David BARNARD, F E HARRIS, Christine HENRY, B M PALMER, Lyndon John PALMER, Peter James SMITH, Eric Marshall WEBSTER

Jubilee Surgery
Barrys Meadow, High St Titchfield, Fareham PO14 4EH
Tel: 01329 844220 Fax: 01329 841484
Email: www.Jubileesurgery@hotmail.com
(Fareham and Gosport Primary Care Trust)
Patient List Size: 8900

Practice Manager M A Lessels

GP Peter William George EVANS, Janet Sarah NAYLOR, David James SINCLAIR, Nigel Ross WADE

Portchester Health Centre
West Street, Portchester, Fareham PO16 9TU
Tel: 023 9237 6913 Fax: 023 9222 1964
(Fareham and Gosport Primary Care Trust)
Patient List Size: 8400

Practice Manager Mark Birch

GP Timothy Guy Charles DOUGLAS, Simon David LARMER, Justine Shirley SIMS, Catherine J WAKEFIELD

The Surgery
Park Lane, Stubbington, Fareham PO14 2JP
Tel: 01329 664231 Fax: 01329 664958
(Fareham and Gosport Primary Care Trust)

Practice Manager Andrew Kern

GP H CANNON, Patrick Noel HOPKINS, Andrew James PATERSON, Judith Elizabeth REES, S J ROBINS, Michael Teodors TENTERS, James Robert WARNER

Westlands Medical Centre
20b Westlands Grove, Portchester, Fareham PO16 9AE
Tel: 023 9237 7514 Fax: 023 9221 4236
Website: www.westlandsmedicalcentre.co.uk
(Fareham and Gosport Primary Care Trust)
Patient List Size: 10000

Practice Manager Cathy Thomas

GP G SOMMERVILLE, Jennifer BATEMAN, Barry CULLEN, A J MUNDEN, J J O'BYRNE, A J TUCKER

Wickham Surgery
Station Road, Wickham, Fareham PO17 5JL
Tel: 01329 833121 Fax: 01329 832443
(Mid-Hampshire Primary Care Trust)
Patient List Size: 10743

Practice Manager Sylvia Hoskins

GP Peter RICHARDS, Anne BOWDEN, Alison CAREY, Deirdre DUNBAR, Jill FOOT, Jonathan MORRIS, Steve SMALLWOOD

Faringdon

Fern Hill Practice
Faringdon Medical Centre, Volunteer Way, Faringdon SN7 7YD
Tel: 01367 245425
(South West Oxfordshire Primary Care Trust)

Patient List Size: 4160

Practice Manager Lynda Smith

GP Faith Elizabeth HOLDSWORTH, Iain Bruce CRAIGHEAD

The White Horse Medical Practice
Volunteer Way, Faringdon SN7 7YU
Tel: 01367 242388 Fax: 01367 245401
(South West Oxfordshire Primary Care Trust)
Patient List Size: 9100

Practice Manager Virginia Bushell

GP Gavin John BARTHOLOMEW, Katrina BOUTIN, Simon Richard CARTWRIGHT, Anna Margaret Rosemary DOUGLAS, Lindsay O'KELLY, Malcolm David WARNER

Farnborough

Alexander House
2 Salisbury Road, Farnborough GU14 7AW
Tel: 01252 541155 Fax: 01252 370569
Website: www.salisburyroadsurgery.co.uk
(Blackwater Valley and Hart Primary Care Trust)
Patient List Size: 9324

Practice Manager S Watson

GP George Robert CAIRD, Albert Mark CAVE, Olive Jane FAIRBAIRN, Niall Robert FERGUSON

Doctors Surgery
Southwood Medical Centre, Links Way, Farnborough GU14 0NA
Tel: 01252 371715 Fax: 01252 524344
(Blackwater Valley and Hart Primary Care Trust)
Patient List Size: 5500

Practice Manager Rose Hopkins

GP William David KAY

Giffard Doctors Surgery
68 Giffard Drive, Cove, Farnborough GU14 8QB
Tel: 01252 541282 Fax: 01252 372159
(Blackwater Valley and Hart Primary Care Trust)

Practice Manager J Reed

GP Ian Michael STUART, Paul Dudley DRAPER, A TEO, E WARR

Heywood and Partners
Mayfield Medical Centre, Croyde Close, Farnborough GU14 8UE
Tel: 01252 541884 Fax: 01252 511410
(Blackwater Valley and Hart Primary Care Trust)
Patient List Size: 6200

Practice Manager S Scott

GP Stephanie Ann HEYWOOD, Christine Blyth MARSHALL, Tina Louise SUMNER

Jenner House Surgery
159 Cove Road, Farnborough GU14 0HH
Tel: 01252 548141 Fax: 01252 371516
(Blackwater Valley and Hart Primary Care Trust)
Patient List Size: 10500

Practice Manager Rose Allan

GP Charles Arthur HEADLEY, K V DUONG, Iain Terence EGGELING, Christopher John ISAACS, Kumuthini RAMACHANDRAN

Jenner House Surgery
159 Cove Road, Farnborough GU14 0HH
Tel: 01252 373738 Fax: 01252 373799
(Blackwater Valley and Hart Primary Care Trust)

Practice Manager Gilly Tullett

GP Mary Monica STACK

Milestone Surgery
208 Farnborough Road, Farnborough GU14 7JN
Tel: 01252 545078 Fax: 01252 370751
(Blackwater Valley and Hart Primary Care Trust)

Practice Manager Hazel Morgan

GP Stephen Paul LINTON, John Arthur DE VERTEUIL, Andrew Neil GIBBONS, Nicholas John HUGHES, Lorraine Susan Kendrick LINTON, Glen MICKLETHWAITE

North Camp Surgery
2 Queen's Road, Farnborough GU14 6DH
Tel: 01252 517734 Fax: 01252 551079
(Blackwater Valley and Hart Primary Care Trust)
Patient List Size: 3500

GP Vinod KUMAR

Farnham

Bentley Village Surgery
Hole Lane, Bentley, Farnham GU10 5LP
Tel: 01420 22106 Fax: 01420 520024
(North Hampshire Primary Care Trust)

Practice Manager Claire Moore

GP Jonathan W A MOORE, Melanie WAY

The Bourne Surgery
41 Frensham Road, Lower Bourne, Farnham GU10 3PZ
Tel: 01252 793141
(Guildford and Waverley Primary Care Trust)

GP William Jolly MAY, D BROWN, Rebecca REYNOLDS

Crondall New Surgery
Redlands Lane, Crondall, Farnham GU10 5RF
Tel: 01252 850292 Fax: 01252 850352
(Blackwater Valley and Hart Primary Care Trust)
Patient List Size: 2890

Practice Manager Edna Ranger

GP A H WILLIAMS, S A STEDMAN

Downing Street Surgery
4 Downing Street, Farnham GU9 7PA
Tel: 01252 716226
(Guildford and Waverley Primary Care Trust)
Patient List Size: 12800

GP Christopher William TIBBOTT, M BAUNRO, H C EVENNETT, V C RISHWORTH, Dr RUSSELL, J L STEED

Farnham Health Centre
Brightwells, East Street, Farnham GU9 7SA
Tel: 01252 723122 Fax: 01252 728302
(Guildford and Waverley Primary Care Trust)
Patient List Size: 11200

Practice Manager John de la Perrelle

GP Peter Charles ROBINSON, Sarmad AL-ASSADI, Margaret Catherine ARDACH, Fiona Jane BLUNDELL, Chen Siang Vincent KOH, Thomas David LUSCOMBE, Malini SPINK

Farnham Health Centre
Brightwells, Farnham GU9 7SA
Tel: 01252 723122
(Guildford and Waverley Primary Care Trust)

GP Agnes Jean IBRAHIM, Jane Beaumont DEMPSTER, Brenda Joyce HOLMES, Maxine Lida Leonie STURDY

Farnham Health Centre
Brightwells, Farnham GU9 7SA
Tel: 01252 723122
(Guildford and Waverley Primary Care Trust)

GP Hugh O'DONNELL, Susan Jennifer CLARKE, Christopher Ronald EVANS, Helen Judith Margaret ROBERTS

Hollytree Surgery
42 Boundstone Road, Wrecclesham, Farnham GU10 4TG
Tel: 01252 793183 Fax: 01252 795437
(Guildford and Waverley Primary Care Trust)

Practice Manager Sarah Shepherd

GP Paul John ADAMS, Amanda Jane ELLIOTT, Robert PRICE

Faversham

Boughton Surgery
60 The Street, Boughton-under-Blean, Faversham ME13 9AS
Tel: 01227 751217
(Canterbury and Coastal Primary Care Trust)

GP Mohendra Singh CHOPRA, Gargi CHOPRA

The Faversham Health Centre
Bank Street, Faversham ME13 8PR
Tel: 01795 536621
(Canterbury and Coastal Primary Care Trust)

GP Dr KNOWLES, Dr CORBLE, Dr CURRY

Faversham Health Centre
Bank Street, Faversham ME13 8QR
Tel: 01795-562011 Fax: 01795 562184
(Canterbury and Coastal Primary Care Trust)

Practice Manager Kevin Austin

GP Paul Richard DAWSON-BOWLING, Roderick Alexander KESSON, Laurence Charles LOGAN, Daniel Jeffery MOORE, Dr POTTER

The Faversham Health Centre
Bank Street, Faversham ME13 8QR
Tel: 01795-562004 Fax: 01795 590794
(Canterbury and Coastal Primary Care Trust)
Patient List Size: 6223

GP Philip Arthur KNOWLES, Gillian CORBLE, Richard David CURRY

Faversham Health Centre
Bank Street, Faversham ME13 8PR
Tel: 01795 562000 Fax: 01795 562014
(Canterbury and Coastal Primary Care Trust)

GP Dr DAWSON-BOWLING, Gillian CABLE, Richard David CURRY, Philip Arthur KNOWLES

Newton Place Surgery
Newton Road, Faversham ME13 8FH
Tel: 01795 530777
(Canterbury and Coastal Primary Care Trust)

GP Dr TAYLOR

Felixstowe

Hamilton Road Surgery
201 Hamilton Road, Felixstowe IP11 7DT
Tel: 01394 283197 Fax: 01394 270304
(Suffolk Coastal Primary Care Trust)
Patient List Size: 16300

Practice Manager J Molloy

GP Robert Anthony DAVENPORT, Stephen Robert James FELTWELL, T V LEICHENKO, David Nigel Lee MOON, Keith William PEARCE, William Alexander SUDELL, Lynda Carole TEMPEST

Haven Health Surgery
Grange Farm Avenue, Felixstowe IP11 2FB
Tel: 01394 670107 Fax: 01394 282872
(Suffolk Coastal Primary Care Trust)

GP Richard Lisle BENNETT, Timothy John REED, Karol SILOVSKY

Howard House Surgery
31 Orwell Road, Felixstowe IP11 7DD
Tel: 01394 282706 Fax: 01394 278955
(Suffolk Coastal Primary Care Trust)
Patient List Size: 6200

Practice Manager M Hingley

GP Fiona Jane ROWE, Maarten DE CLEEN, Fiona HOBDAY, Robert Stanley JAMES, Janet MASSEY, Michael Robert MINDHAM

Walton Surgery
301 High Street, Walton, Felixstowe IP11 9QL
Tel: 01394 278844 Fax: 01394 284438
(Suffolk Coastal Primary Care Trust)
Patient List Size: 4040

Practice Manager M Martin

GP William Bernard McKEE

Feltham

Dagg-Heston
Cleeve, Raleigh Way, Hanworth, Feltham TW13 7NX
Tel: 020 8384 2062 Fax: 020 8384 2063
(Hounslow Primary Care Trust)
Patient List Size: 2200

GP Roger DAGG-HESTON

Elm Road Surgery
2 Elm Road, Bedfont, Feltham TW14 8EW
Tel: 020 8890 7397 Fax: 020 8890 7397
Email: zahir.mecci@gp-e85698.nhs.uk
(Hounslow Primary Care Trust)
Patient List Size: 1600

Practice Manager Caz Marsh

GP Zahir Hasan MECCI

Grove Village Medical Centre
4 Cleeve Court, Grove Village, Bedfont, Feltham TW14 8SN
Tel: 020 8751 6281 Fax: 020 8751 0054
(Hounslow Primary Care Trust)

Practice Manager June Watmore

GP Baljit Kaur BHULLAR

Hatton Medical Practice
186 Hatton Road, Bedfont, Feltham TW14 9PY
Tel: 020 8893 2993 Fax: 020 8893 2889
Email: muzafer@cwcom.net
(Hounslow Primary Care Trust)
Patient List Size: 3500

GP Mohammad Hussain MUZAFER, Parveen MUZAFER

High Street Surgery
109 High Street, Feltham TW13 4HG
Tel: 020 8751 3394 Fax: 020 8890 0547
(Hounslow Primary Care Trust)
Patient List Size: 1391

GP Asim Kumar GHOSH

High Street Surgery
190 High Street, Feltham TW13 4HY
Tel: 020 8751 3404 Fax: 020 8890 4858
(Hounslow Primary Care Trust)

GP Lila NAVANI

Hounslow Road Surgery
112 Hounslow Road, Feltham TW14 0AX
Tel: 020 8890 3930 Fax: 020 8844 0760
(Hounslow Primary Care Trust)

GP Mohammed Gholi ETMINAN, Simria TANVIR

Hounslow Road Surgery
158 Hounslow Road, Feltham TW14 0BA
Tel: 020 8890 9376 Fax: 020 8890 9376
(Hounslow Primary Care Trust)

GP Padmanabh Dasu KOTIAN

Little Park Surgery
281 Hounslow Road, Hanworth, Feltham TW13 5JG
Tel: 020 8894 6588 Fax: 020 8894 6668
(Hounslow Primary Care Trust)

GP Carolyn Mary LYNCH, Lubomyr Mychajlo PASKA

Manor House Health Centre
Manor Lane, Feltham TW13 4JQ
Tel: 020 8321 3747 Fax: 020 8321 3749

(Hounslow Primary Care Trust)

GP A S JAY, M SATHANANTHAN

Manor House Health Centre
Manor Lane, Feltham TW13 4JQ
Tel: 020 8321 3737 Fax: 020 8321 3739
(Hounslow Primary Care Trust)

GP Vinodkumar Natubhai PATEL, Subathira RAJITHAKUMAR

Manor House Health Centre
Manor Lane, Feltham TW13 4JQ
Tel: 020 8321 3748 Fax: 020 8321 3749
(Hounslow Primary Care Trust)

GP Dr O'CONNOR

The Medical Centre
192 Twickenham Road, Hanworth, Feltham TW13 6HD
Tel: 020 8979 3058 Fax: 020 8979 8994
(Hounslow Primary Care Trust)
Patient List Size: 4450

Practice Manager Sheena Winayall

GP Varendar Kumar WINAYAK

Mount Medical Centre
7 Market Parade, Hampton Road West, Hanworth, Feltham TW13 6AJ
Tel: 020 8893 8699 Fax: 020 8893 8680
(Hounslow Primary Care Trust)

Practice Manager Frances Lee

GP Michael Augustine MEAGHER, J M BAKSHI

Pentelow Gardens Surgery
26 Pentelow Gardens, Bedfont, Feltham TW14 9EF
Tel: 020 8890 2029 Fax: 020 8893 2623
(Hounslow Primary Care Trust)

GP R MORAN

Queens Park Gardens
1 Queens Park Gardens, Feltham TW13 4JS
Tel: 020 8751 6057 Fax: 020 8751 4083
(Hounslow Primary Care Trust)
Patient List Size: 3200

GP Vallipuran Eliyathamby KUMARAN, Jeyagowry KUMARAN

The Surgery
12 Hanworth Road, Feltham TW13 5AD
Tel: 020 8890 2208 Fax: 020 8893 1399
(Hounslow Primary Care Trust)

GP Dr SEN, G T ASWANI

The Surgery
32 Harlington Road East, Feltham TW14 0AB
Tel: 020 8893 1160 Fax: 020 8893 1116
(Hounslow Primary Care Trust)

GP Dr GILL

Ferndown

Orchid House Surgery
Ferndown Medical Centre, St Marys Road, Ferndown BH22 9HF
Tel: 01202 897000 Fax: 01202 897888
(South and East Dorset Primary Care Trust)
Patient List Size: 8100

Practice Manager Karen Holcombe

GP Sarah Virginia CLARKE, Lesley Anne ADAMS, Elaine Justine DAVENPORT, Mark EVERY, Fran GRANA, Neale Mark Watcyn JENKINS

Penny's Hill Practice
Ferndown Medical Centre, St Marys Road, Ferndown BH22 9HB
Tel: 01202 897200 Fax: 01202 877753
Website: www.pennyshill.doctors.org.uk
(South and East Dorset Primary Care Trust)

Practice Manager Christine Vinnicombe

GP Charles Robert REES, Richard Kenneth GREEN, Geoffrey Bickersteth OTTLEY, Patricia Jane PILLING, Julian Paul STRAUSS

The Surgery
Corbin Avenue, Tricketts Cross, Ferndown BH22 8AZ
Tel: 01202 897989 Fax: 01202 877743
(South and East Dorset Primary Care Trust)
Patient List Size: 4500

Practice Manager Ken Broad

GP Albert Anthony BARCELLOS, William Jeremy FERGUSON

The Village Medical Practice
164 Station Road, West Moors, Ferndown BH22 0JB
Tel: 01202 877185/871999 Fax: 01202 892080
(South and East Dorset Primary Care Trust)
Patient List Size: 2297

Practice Manager Anna McKinstry

GP Thomas Herbert McKINSTRY

West Moors Group Practice
Heathlands House, 175 Station Road, West Moors, Ferndown BH22 0HX
Tel: 01202 872585 Fax: 01202 892155
(South and East Dorset Primary Care Trust)

Practice Manager Shirley Tedder

GP John Michael Seaverns BLACKMORE, Jonathan Ellis LADD, Mark Alistair SMITH

Ferryhill

Ferryhill Medical Practice
Durham Road, Ferryhill DL17 8JJ
Tel: 01740 651238 Fax: 01740 656291
(Sedgefield Primary Care Trust)
Patient List Size: 16000

Practice Manager Jennifer Wood

GP Andrew Gordon Perrin OAKENFULL, Anneke ALGERA, Derek Robert McGLADE, Peter James MERSON, Helen Elisabeth MOORE, Martin ORLANDI, Brigitte SCHNEELOCH, Gary STEVENSON, Andreas Charles TYSSELING, David Michael WILLIS

High Street Surgery
38 High Street, West Cornforth, Ferryhill DL17 9HR
Tel: 01740 656578 Fax: 01740 653928
(Sedgefield Primary Care Trust)

Practice Manager Linda McCann

GP Stephen Colin DREW

Filey

Filey Surgery
Station Avenue, Filey YO14 9AE
Tel: 01723 515881 Fax: 01723 515197
Website: fileysurgery.com
(Scarborough, Whitby and Ryedale Primary Care Trust)
Patient List Size: 8700

Practice Manager Carolyn Liddle

GP James Francis Philip GARNETT, Ricardo GARCIA-SANCHEZ, Bryan Roger NUNN, Christopher Michael SHEPHERD, Raoul WILHELMUS, Anna WYNANDS

Hunmanby Clinic
Hungate Lane, Hunmanby, Filey YO14 0NN
Tel: 01723 892336 Fax: 01723 892568
(Scarborough, Whitby and Ryedale Primary Care Trust)

Practice Manager Sue Thompson

Hunmanby Clinic
Hungate Lane, Hunmanby, Filey YO14 0NN
Tel: 01723 892336 Fax: 01723 892568
(Scarborough, Whitby and Ryedale Primary Care Trust)

Practice Manager Caroline Clarke

Fleet

Fleet Medical Centre
Church Road, Fleet GU51 4PE
Tel: 01252 613327 Fax: 01252 815156
Email: john.healey@gp-J8240.nhs.uk
(Blackwater Valley and Hart Primary Care Trust)
Patient List Size: 14000

GP John Charles HEALEY, David John Carver GARSED-BENNET, Christopher John Charles HIGGINS, Clifford John KIMBER, Helen Jessica McGINTY, Linda Ann SHIELLS, Barbara Joan TOLLETT

Richmond Surgery
Richmond Close, Fleet GU52 7US
Tel: 01252 811466 Fax: 01252 815031
(Blackwater Valley and Hart Primary Care Trust)

Practice Manager Maggie Richmond

GP Andrew Lance Howard SHARP, Anna CHAMBERLAIN, Timothy Brooks de GLANVILLE, Steven KING, Michelle SINCLAIR, Rachel TENNER

The Surgery
Branksomewood Road, Fleet GU51 4JX
Tel: 01252 613624 Fax: 01252 816489
(Blackwater Valley and Hart Primary Care Trust)

Practice Manager Jean Fox

GP Michael Andrew SWIFT, Nigel Andrew Denis CLARK, Steven Alexander CLARKE, Peita Joan CRISTOFANI, T W L MORGAN

Fleetwood

Belle Vue Surgery
419 Poulton Road, Fleetwood FY7 7JY
Tel: 01253 779113 Fax: 01253 770707
(Wyre Primary Care Trust)

GP Cobarsanellore D RAMESH

Broadway Medical Centre
65-67 Broadway, Fleetwood FY7 7DG
Tel: 01253 874222 Fax: 01253 874448
(Wyre Primary Care Trust)

Practice Manager B Summers

GP M AZIZ, Paul Graham CARPENTER, Susan FAIRHEAD, Sarah Jane KIRK, Robert Andrew Colhoun SMYTH

The Health Centre
London Street, Fleetwood FY7 6HD
Tel: 01253 875305 Fax: 01253 878417
(Wyre Primary Care Trust)
Patient List Size: 2293

Practice Manager Sheila Morris

GP Syed Maqbool ALI

Kwun
6 Waverley Avenue, Fleetwood FY7 8BN
Tel: 01253 778448
(Wyre Primary Care Trust)

Practice Manager Pat Lawrence

GP Pin Cheong TSE SAK KWUN

The Mount View Practice
London Street Medical Centre, London Street, Fleetwood FY7 6HD
Tel: 01253 873312 Fax: 01253 873130
Website: http://fyldemedical.com/mountview
(Wyre Primary Care Trust)
Patient List Size: 10250

Practice Manager Helen Dingle

GP Michael James Scott PAGE, Howard BROWN, Roger John CLARK, Helen Patricia GRENIER, G MEEHAN, M SAUNDERS, Mark SPENCER

Folkestone

Central Surgery
86 Cheriton Road, Folkestone CT20 2QH
Tel: 01303 220707 Fax: 01303 254292
(Shepway Primary Care Trust)
Patient List Size: 3000

Practice Manager V J Hooton

GP Yogesh Yeshvantlal AMIN

Denmark Street Surgery
1 Denmark Street, Folkestone CT19 6EJ
Tel: 01303 850216
(Shepway Primary Care Trust)
Patient List Size: 2400

Practice Manager J Reed

GP L PO-BA

Downs Road Surgery
2 Downs Road, Folkestone CT19 5PJ
Tel: 01303 253032 Fax: 01303 253032
Email: downsrd@gp-g82187.nhs.uk
(Shepway Primary Care Trust)
Patient List Size: 2400

Practice Manager Jan Bennett

GP Dr THAN HTUT

Folkestone Surgeries Group
65-69 Guildhall Street, Folkestone CT20 1EJ
Tel: 01303 851411 Fax: 01303 220443
(Shepway Primary Care Trust)
Patient List Size: 9500

Practice Manager Patrica Coxon

GP Mohammad Altaf HOSSAIN, V J ALLEN, A Y F KARIM, S MONTGOMERY, M R PATEL

The Manor Clinic
31 Manor Road, Folkestone CT20 2SE
Tel: 01303 851122 Fax: 01303 220914
(Shepway Primary Care Trust)
Patient List Size: 7200

Practice Manager Rosalind Keeler

GP Giles Richard BEACH, Manuel Agnelo Andrew Mario FERNANDES, Gregory Anthony ROBERTS, B ROBINSON

New Lyminge Surgery
Greenbanks, Lyminge, Folkestone CT18 8NS
Tel: 01303 863160 Fax: 01303 863492
(Shepway Primary Care Trust)

Practice Manager Pamela Clarke

GP Michael Philip BLINSTON JONES, Christopher Ewen CATTO

The New Surgery
128 Canterbury Road, Folkestone CT19 5SR
Tel: 01303 243516 Fax: 01303 244633
(Shepway Primary Care Trust)

Practice Manager Sue Chandler

GP Daniel Paul EVANS, Hugh ROBERTSON-RITCHIE, Kathryn Elizabeth ALLEN, James Peter de CAESTECKER

Park Farm Surgery
1 Alder Road, Folkestone CT19 5BZ
Tel: 01303 851021 Fax: 01303 226743
(Shepway Primary Care Trust)
Patient List Size: 3025

Practice Manager Diane Standen

GP D. K. MAITRA

Sandgate Road Surgery
180 Sandgate Road, Folkestone CT20 2HN
Tel: 01303 221133 Fax: 01303 251068
(Shepway Primary Care Trust)

Practice Manager Brian Cunningham

GP George Henry FINDLAY, Gary Dennis CALVER, David James FARROW, Karen HADDAFORD, Corrig HEAW, William Stephen WHITBY

The Surgery
Church Road, Lyminge, Folkestone CT18 8HY
Tel: 01303 862109 Fax: 01303 863643
(Shepway Primary Care Trust)

Practice Manager Helen Wilson

GP Thomas Maurice MICHAELS, R KORIA

White House Surgery
1 Cheriton High Street, Folkestone CT19 4PU
Tel: 01303 275434 Fax: 01303 271921
(Shepway Primary Care Trust)
Patient List Size: 9700

Practice Manager Janet Jones

GP John Anthony JEDRZEJEWSKI, Norman Wilson ANDERSON, Pia HOLWERDA, Nicholas Fredrick MORLEY-SMITH

Fordingbridge

Fordingbridge Surgery
Bartons Road, Fordingbridge SP6 1RS
Tel: 01425 652123 Fax: 01425 654393
Email: fbridge.surgery@gp-J82131.nhs.uk
(New Forest Primary Care Trust)
Patient List Size: 12400

Practice Manager Jacqueline Lydford

GP Hywel John Lloyd MORRIS, Philip DOWNES, Martin John GANNON, Caroline Elizabeth KNIGHT, Janet McGEE, Simon SMITH, Eamon Bernard STAUNTON

Forest Row

Ashdown Forest Health Centre
Lewes Road, Forest Row RH18 5AQ
Tel: 01342 822131 Fax: 01342 826015
Website: www.ashdownforesthealthcen.co.uk
(Sussex Downs and Weald Primary Care Trust)
Patient List Size: 9900

Practice Manager D R H Tucker

GP Steven Andrew MILLER, Justin A BASELEY, Richard John BAXTER, Alison L A FYTE, Louise C WISEMAN

Fowey

Fowey River Practice
Rawlings Lane, Fowey PL23 1DT
Tel: 01726 832451 Fax: 01726 833764
(Central Cornwall Primary Care Trust)
Patient List Size: 7200

GP Alan MIDDLETON, Margaret Hazel HAMILTON, Andrew PARTINGTON, Michael Jeremy WALDRON

Freshwater

Brookside Health Centre
Brookside Road, Freshwater PO40 9DT
Tel: 01983 753433 Fax: 01983 753662
(Isle of Wight Primary Care Trust)
Patient List Size: 10700

Practice Manager Christine Johnson

GP George Edward THOMSON, Richard John FOSTER, Marion HILL, Kenneth John MAGEE, Joy MARSHALL, Annette SCIVIER, Gordon McPherson WALKER, Dawn Helen WHITE

Frinton-on-Sea

Station Approach Surgery
Caradoc, Station Approach, Frinton-on-Sea CO13 9JT
Tel: 01255 850101 Fax: 01255 851004
(Tendring Primary Care Trust)
Patient List Size: 7551

Practice Manager Sue Mitson

GP Ian David HARRISON, Graham Stephen MOORE, Martyn Turner WALL

Frome

Beckington Family Practice
St Luke's Surgery, Beckington, Frome BA11 6SE
Tel: 01373 830316 Fax: 01373 831261
(Mendip Primary Care Trust)
Patient List Size: 7600

Practice Manager K Ferguson-Lees

GP J D BROOKS, P ARCHER, J T BEAVEN, K GIBBS, B G MANSFIELD

Frome Medical Practice
Health Centre, Park Road, Frome BA11 1EZ
Tel: 01373 301300 Fax: 01373 301313
Email: general@fromemedicalpractice.nhs.uk
Website: www.frommedicalpractice.co.uk
(Mendip Primary Care Trust)
Patient List Size: 27900

Practice Manager Malcolm Maggs, Susan Palmer

GP Nicholas Francis WHITEHEAD, D M BUNGAY, Thomas Edward CAHILL, Robert Lyn GRIFFITHS, Mark Atkinson HUNT, Helen Mary KINGSTON, W LIDDELL, Tina Louise MERRY, Mark Anthony VOSE

Locks Hill Surgery
95 Locks Hill, Frome BA11 1NG
Tel: 01373 454446 Fax: 01373 454447
(Mendip Primary Care Trust)

Practice Manager Carol Mead

GP Nick WHITEHEAD, Simon CAPP, R KAYE

Gainsborough

Caskgate Street Surgery
3 Caskgate Street, Gainsborough DN21 2DJ
Tel: 01427 612501 Fax: 01427 615459
(West Lincolnshire Primary Care Trust)
Patient List Size: 10100

Practice Manager L Juhos

GP Stephen Lee CLARKE, Dr DIETZEL, Dr EVERSHED, N GREEN, Gordon David WARNES

Cleveland House
16 Spital Terrace, Gainsborough DN21 2HE
Tel: 01427 613158 Fax: 01427 616644
(West Lincolnshire Primary Care Trust)

Practice Manager D M Prince

GP Christopher Simon HUNT, Simon Brian ANDERSON, Ian Duncan PERCIVAL, Richard Anthony WILKINS

Hawthorn Surgery
Scotton Road, Scotter, Gainsborough DN21 3SB
Tel: 01724 762204 Fax: 01724 764265
(West Lincolnshire Primary Care Trust)
Patient List Size: 3129

Practice Manager E Anderson

GP Peter Rodney HYDE, David Allan JOLLY

High Street Surgery
High Street, Willingham by Stow, Gainsborough DN21 5JZ
Tel: 01427 788277 Fax: 01427 787630
Website: www.willinghamsurgery.co.uk
(West Lincolnshire Primary Care Trust)
Patient List Size: 3000

Practice Manager Christine Taylor

GP Kathryn Ann FICKLING, Andrew WASS

Ropery Road Surgery
2A Ropery Road, Gainsborough DN21 2NL
Tel: 01427 612895 Fax: 01427 811763
(West Lincolnshire Primary Care Trust)

Practice Manager R Tomkins

GP Andrew Markham PROCTER, Gillian Sarah PROCTER

The Surgery
Traingate, Kirton Lindsey, Gainsborough DN21 4PQ
Tel: 01652 648214 Fax: 01652 648398
(North Lincolnshire Primary Care Trust)

GP Robert George PADLEY, Keith Leslie PILSWORTH, Dr TURNER

Gateshead

Beacon View Medical Centre
Beacon Lough, Gateshead NE9 6YS
(Gateshead Primary Care Trust)

Bensham Family Practice
Sydney Grove, Bensham, Gateshead NE8 2XB
Tel: 0191 477 6955 Fax: 0191 477 1554
(Gateshead Primary Care Trust)
Patient List Size: 5700

Practice Manager Pauline Tennant

Bewick Road Surgery
10 Bewick Road, Gateshead NE8 4DP
(Gateshead Primary Care Trust)

The Croft
Springwell Road, Gateshead NE9 6DT
(Gateshead Primary Care Trust)

Dewhurst Terrace Surgery
8 Dewhurst Terrace, Sunniside, Gateshead NE16 5LP
Tel: 0191 496 6477 Fax: 0191 488 2800
(Gateshead Primary Care Trust)

GP Alan James HUNT

Dr Ranu and Partners
23A Ravensworth Road, Dunston, Gateshead NE11 9AD
Tel: 0191 460 4354
(Gateshead Primary Care Trust)
Patient List Size: 5899

GP Harpal K RANU, Upkar S PANNU, David A ROBERTS

Fell Cottage
123 Kells Lane, Low Fell, Gateshead NE9 5XY
Tel: 0191 487 2656 Fax: 0191 491 0475
(Gateshead Primary Care Trust)
Patient List Size: 8700

Practice Manager S Harrigan

GP Dr BRYSON, Dr BOSE, Dr KINGSTON, Dr ROBINSON, Dr WARWICK

Fell Tower Medical Centre
575 Durham Road, Low Fell, Gateshead NE9 5EY
(Gateshead Primary Care Trust)

Gateshead Health Centre
Prince Consort Road, Gateshead NE8 1NB
(Gateshead Primary Care Trust)

Glenpark Medical Centre
61 Ravensorth Road, Dunston, Gateshead NE11 9AD
(Gateshead Primary Care Trust)

Practice Manager Jill Mark

GP P J ESPIE, A HOLMES, Dr PLUNKETT, K PRUDHOE, Caroline RICHARDSON, B E TASKER

High Street Medical Centre
91/91a High Street, Wrekenton, Gateshead NE9 7JR
(Gateshead Primary Care Trust)

Longrigg Medical Centre
Felling, Gateshead NE10 8QJ
Tel: 0191 469 2173 Fax: 0191 495 0893
(Gateshead Primary Care Trust)
Patient List Size: 11230

Practice Manager Gail White

GP Dr BRUMBY, Dr HARRISON, Dr METCALFE, Dr REEKIE, Dr ROWNTREE, Dr STREIT, Dr WISE

The Medical Centre
1 Rawling Road, Gateshead NE8 4QS
Tel: 0191 477 2180 Fax: 0191 477 6979
(Gateshead Primary Care Trust)
Patient List Size: 4078

Practice Manager Henny Carmichael

GP Runja MOHAMMED, Lee CANAVAN, Gordon ORRITT

Oxford Terrace Medical Group
Oxford Terrace, Gateshead NE8 1RQ
Tel: 0191 4772169 Fax: 0191 4775633
Website: www.oxfordterrace.com
(Gateshead Primary Care Trust)
Patient List Size: 10000

Practice Manager Ed Hinde

GP Jane CHALMERS, Zeba CHISTI, Paul GRAINGER, Kevin JONES, Neil MORRIS, Caroline SNELL, Peter YOUNG

Pelaw Medical Practice
7-8 Croxdale Terrace, Pelaw, Gateshead NE10 0RR
Tel: 0191 4692337 Fax: 0191 4386132
(Gateshead Primary Care Trust)
Patient List Size: 4850

Practice Manager Joan Carrick

GP MS SUCHDEV, H FOWNES, FL NAYLOR

Ravensworth Road Surgery
23a Ravensworth Road, Dunston, Gateshead NE11 9AB
(Gateshead Primary Care Trust)

Rawling Road Surgery
108 Rawling Road, Gateshead NE8 4QR
Tel: 0191 4203255 Fax: 0191 420 3253
(Gateshead Primary Care Trust)
Patient List Size: 2200

Practice Manager Hazel Blake

GP N M KRISHNAN

St Alban's Medical Group
Felling, Gateshead NE10 9QG
(Gateshead Primary Care Trust)

The Surgery
Second Street, Gateshead NE8 2UR
Tel: 0191 477 2430 Fax: 0191 978 6823
(Gateshead Primary Care Trust)
Patient List Size: 2294

GP A KUMAR

The Surgery
Johnson Street, Gateshead NE8 2PJ
(Gateshead Primary Care Trust)

Walker Terrace Surgery
5 Walker Terrace, Gateshead NE8 1HX
Tel: 0191 477 2033 Fax: 0191 478 2083
(Gateshead Primary Care Trust)
Patient List Size: 5500

Practice Manager Carole Crawford

GP S M IMAM

Gerrards Cross

Calcot Medical Centre
Hampden Road, Chalfont St. Peter, Gerrards Cross SL9 9SA
Tel: 01753 887311 Fax: 01753 891933
(Chiltern and South Bucks Primary Care Trust)

Practice Manager Lise Randell

GP Gina ALLAN, Simon James BAILEY, Sheila Joan BRAY, Andrew Edward DEAN, Gurjit Singh DHESI

The Hall Practice
Calcot Medical Centre, Hampden Road, Chalfont St. Peter, Gerrards Cross SL9 9SA
Tel: 01753 887311 Fax: 01753 890639
(Chiltern and South Bucks Primary Care Trust)
Patient List Size: 8600

Practice Manager Lorene Butcher

GP Simon James BUTCHER, Jonathon DAVEY, Richard Alan FOSKETT, Peter James Stephen PETRIE, Nicola Simone TURNER

The Misbourne Surgery
Church Lane, Chalfont St. Peter, Gerrards Cross SL9 9RR
Tel: 01753 891010 Fax: 01753 883312
(Chiltern and South Bucks Primary Care Trust)

Practice Manager Jackie Hampton

GP David Paul BRODIE, Adam Jan BARTKIEWICZ, John NASH, Sheila PAUL, Isabel TAYLOR, Andrew Mark WEBBER

Gillingham, Dorset

The Barn Surgery
Newbury, Gillingham SP8 4XS
Tel: 01747 824201 Fax: 01747 825098
(North Dorset Primary Care Trust)
Patient List Size: 9500

GP Matthew SHORT, Vicky COLES, Geoffrey David LEWIS, Hilary SAGE, Timothy Charles Anthony WOOD

Gillingham Road Surgery
Gillingham Road, Silton, Gillingham SP8 5DF
Tel: 01747 840226 Fax: 01747 840950
(South Wiltshire Primary Care Trust)

Practice Manager Jane Smith

GP Malcolm FREELAND, Elizabeth HILLS

Gillingham, Kent

Balmoral Road Surgery
12 Balmoral Road, Gillingham ME7 4PG
Tel: 01634 854933
(Medway Teaching Primary Care Trust)
Patient List Size: 2300

Practice Manager S Rahman

GP Mohammad RAHMAN, S M SONI

Birling Avenue Surgery
3 Birling Avenue, Rainham, Gillingham ME8 7HB
Tel: 01634 360390/361843 Fax: 01634 264061
(Medway Teaching Primary Care Trust)
Patient List Size: 5000

Practice Manager Sue Clarke

GP Lynn Vera FERRIN, Karen Lesley HAWORTH, Mary Concepta QUIGLEY

Byron House Surgery
30 Byron Road, Gillingham ME7 5QH
Tel: 01634 576347 Fax: 01634 570159
(Medway Teaching Primary Care Trust)
Patient List Size: 5900

Practice Manager Maureen Housden

GP P PATEL, J THACKRAY, Janet WATKIN

Canterbury Street Surgery
511 Canterbury Street, Gillingham ME7 5LG
Tel: 01634 573020 Fax: 01634 281287
(Medway Teaching Primary Care Trust)
Patient List Size: 1999

Practice Manager Iris Wells

GP Ranweer Baldevdutt SILHI

Canterbury Street Surgery
218 Canterbury Street, Gillingham ME7 5XL
Tel: 01634 852824
(Medway Teaching Primary Care Trust)

GP H R GHOSH

Eastcourt Lane Surgery
52 Eastcourt Lane, Gillingham ME8 6EY
Tel: 01634 232144 Fax: 01634 261811
(Medway Teaching Primary Care Trust)
Patient List Size: 2240

Practice Manager Lynn Gibson

GP Rajendra Pushpakrai DHOLAKIA

Garden Street Surgery
28A Garden Street, Brompton, Gillingham ME7 5AS
Tel: 01634 845898 Fax: 01634 871823
(Medway Teaching Primary Care Trust)
Patient List Size: 2474

Practice Manager S Singh

GP Bijendra Narayan SINGH

Gillingham Medical Centre
Woodlands Road, Gillingham ME7 2BU
Tel: 01634 854431
(Medway Teaching Primary Care Trust)
Patient List Size: 11994

Practice Manager H Ashok, Jo Nightingale

GP Nand Prakash RISHI, Chottakoriande Kalamaiah ASHOK, Prem BAKSHI, Noreen RASHI, F YAZAMAIDR

The Health Centre
Holding Street, Rainham, Gillingham ME8 7JP
Tel: 01634 262333
(Medway Teaching Primary Care Trust)
Patient List Size: 6500

Practice Manager Joan Keohane

GP John Leslie GRANT, Theo DE BIE, Timothy John WOODMAN

Kings Family Practice
Cleave Road Surgery, 91 Cleave Road, Gillingham ME7 4AX
Tel: 01634 850473
(Medway Teaching Primary Care Trust)
Patient List Size: 10000

Practice Manager D Wetherill

GP Edwin Roy JONES, Stephen LAWRENCE, Meindert Roger VERHEUL

Long Catlis Road Surgery
119 Long Catlis Road, Parkwood, Rainham, Gillingham ME8 9RR
Tel: 01634 360989
(Medway Teaching Primary Care Trust)

GP Subramaniyan Tamil SELVAN, S SIVAN

Maidstone Road Surgery
53B Maidstone Road, Rainham, Gillingham ME8 0DP
Tel: 01634 231423 Fax: 01634 261665
(Medway Teaching Primary Care Trust)

Practice Manager Veronica Brill

GP Lok Nath SHAUNAK, Vidosava SHAUNAK

Matrix Medical Practice
146A Hempstead Road, Hempstead, Gillingham ME7 3QE
Tel: 01634 363561 Fax: 01634 263768
(Medway Teaching Primary Care Trust)
Patient List Size: 2600

GP Anthony Nicholas STACEY

The Medical Centre
4a Waltham Road, Gillingham ME8 6XQ
Tel: 01634 231074
(Medway Teaching Primary Care Trust)

GP Jagga Chinna LAKSHMAN, Venkatesh LAKSHMAN

Napier Road Surgery
151 Napier Road, Gillingham ME7 4HH
Tel: 01634 580480 Fax: 01634 281851
(Medway Teaching Primary Care Trust)
Patient List Size: 2132

Practice Manager Gillian Attwell

GP Prathap Padmanabhan JANA

Nelson Road Surgery
105 Nelson Road, Gillingham ME7 4LT
Tel: 01634 582992
(Medway Teaching Primary Care Trust)

GP C K R CHITEOPKER, K. GHOSH

Nelson Road Surgery
156 Nelson Road, Gillingham ME7 4LU
Tel: 01634 850943
(Medway Teaching Primary Care Trust)

GP Naveen KARWAL

The Parkwood Health Centre
Long Catlis Road, Parkwood, Rainham, Gillingham ME8 9PR
Tel: 01634 233491
(Medway Teaching Primary Care Trust)

GP Michael Jeffrey FRANK

Parkwood Health Centre
Long Catlis Road, Rainham, Gillingham ME8 9PR
Tel: 01634 371535 Fax: 01634 263895
(Medway Teaching Primary Care Trust)
Patient List Size: 4000

Practice Manager Eila Ragab

GP Subramaniam SIVAN

Patel's Surgery
90-92 Malvern Road, Gillingham ME7 4BB
Tel: 01634 578333 Fax: 01634 852581
(Medway Teaching Primary Care Trust)
Patient List Size: 1830

GP Chandrakant Prabhudas PATEL, N PATEL, S K PATEL

Pump Lane Surgery
13 Pump Lane, Rainham Mark, Gillingham ME8 7AA
Tel: 01634 231856
(Medway Teaching Primary Care Trust)
Patient List Size: 24800

Practice Manager Barbara Allen

GP Sarita BHATIA

Railway Street Surgery
19 Railway Street, Gillingham ME7 1XF
Tel: 01634 853667 Fax: 01634 575006
(Medway Teaching Primary Care Trust)

GP Samuel Bhaskar BHASME

Railway Street Surgery
7 Railway Street, Gillingham ME7 1XG
Tel: 01634 851193 Fax: 01634 570948
(Medway Teaching Primary Care Trust)
Patient List Size: 5000

Practice Manager R Evans

GP M RAMESH, J V SUBBA-RAO

St Werburgh Medical Practice
1st Floor Kingsley House, Balmoral Road, Gillingham ME7 4PS
Tel: 01634 571740 Fax: 01634 380141
(Medway Teaching Primary Care Trust)
Patient List Size: 3500

Practice Manager S Bodle

GP G C J DAVIES, Geraldine McKEEVER, D O'DONNELL, D O'KANE

The Surgery
St Barnabas House, Duncan Road, Gillingham ME7 4LD
Tel: 01634 850067
(Medway Teaching Primary Care Trust)

GP Yasine KARIM, J AHMAD, S O SYED AHMAD

The Surgery
114 Woodside, Wigmore, Gillingham ME8 0PW
Tel: 01634 234131
(Medway Teaching Primary Care Trust)

The Surgery
44 Broadway, Twydall, Gillingham ME8 6BD
Tel: 01634 231364
(Medway Teaching Primary Care Trust)

GP Madhu Ganeshbhai PATEL

The Surgery
2 Thames Avenue, Rainham, Gillingham ME8 9BN
Tel: 01634 360486 Fax: 01634 375159
Website: www.thames-avenue-surgery.co.uk
(Medway Teaching Primary Care Trust)
Patient List Size: 4700

Practice Manager Sarah Hill

GP Warnakulasuriya Sudharman Bernard P. FERNANDO, Donna Renuka Camellia DIAS

The Surgery
114 Woodside, Wigmore, Gillingham ME8 0PW
Tel: 01634 231752
(Medway Teaching Primary Care Trust)

GP N R PATEL, S K C PATEL

Wigmore Road Surgery
23 Mierscourt Road, Rainham, Gillingham ME8 8JE
Tel: 01634 379555 Fax: 01634 325205
(Medway Teaching Primary Care Trust)
Patient List Size: 1800

GP M KANNAN

Wyvill Close Surgery
Rainham, Gillingham ME8 9NE
Tel: 01634 230461
(Medway Teaching Primary Care Trust)

GP Medhat Abdel Aziz EL-FARAMAWI

Glastonbury

Glastonbury Health Centre
1 Wells Road, Glastonbury BA6 9DD
Tel: 01458 834100 Fax: 01458 834371
(Mendip Primary Care Trust)
Patient List Size: 4800

Practice Manager Janet Hole

GP Roy Audus WELFORD, Mary Rachel HELSBY, Nicholas William MATTHEWS

Glastonbury Surgery
Feversham Lane, Glastonbury BA6 9LP
Tel: 01458 833666 Fax: 01458 834536
Website: www.glastonburysurgery.co.uk
(Mendip Primary Care Trust)
Patient List Size: 13000

Practice Manager Andrea Ball

GP Ian David STRAWFORD, Alastair Robert Henry CORFIELD, J HAZLEWOOD, R HUGHES, Philip Anthony JACKSON, David Keith Llewellyn JONES, Pauline Anne JONES, Catherine McELROY, Sarah Ann MONTAGNON, Hugh Culliford SHARP

Glossop

Cottage Lane Surgery
47 Cottage Lane, Gamesley, Glossop SK13 6EQ
Tel: 01457 861343 Fax: 01457 864301
(Tameside and Glossop Primary Care Trust)
Patient List Size: 2062

Practice Manager Kath Bailey

GP Alan James DOW

Group Practice Centre
Howard Street, Glossop SK13 7DE
Tel: 01457 854321 Fax: 01457 854439
(Tameside and Glossop Primary Care Trust)

GP V P RAO, S VUYYURU

Lambgates Doctors Surgery
1-5 Lambgates, Hadfield, Glossop SK13 1AW
Tel: 01457 869090 Fax: 01457 857367
(Tameside and Glossop Primary Care Trust)
Patient List Size: 6100

Practice Manager Veronica Frodsham

GP Kumbakonam Srinivasachar BHANUMATHI, Lindsay Anne PALMER, Andrew Peter THORNLEY

Manor House Surgery
Manor House Surgery, Manor Street, Glossop SK13 8PS
Tel: 01457 860860 Fax: 01457 860017
Email: admin@gp-C31081.nhs.uk
Website: www.manorhousesurgery.co.uk
(Tameside and Glossop Primary Care Trust)
Patient List Size: 10300

Practice Manager Gwynneth French

GP John OLDHAM, Jonathan EVANS, Margaret Anne TALBOT, Nicola THORLEY, Guy WILKINSON

Pennine Road Surgery
15A Pennine Road, Glossop SK13 6NN
Tel: 01457 862305 Fax: 01457 857010
(Tameside and Glossop Primary Care Trust)
Patient List Size: 3200

Practice Manager Joan Highley, Christine Wendon

GP Subhash Chandra BHATT

Rao and Vuyyuru
Howard Medical Practice, Howard Street, Glossop SK13 7DE
Tel: 01457 854321 Fax: 01457 854439
(Tameside and Glossop Primary Care Trust)
Patient List Size: 3600

Practice Manager Denise Fay

GP V Purnachandra RAO, Sivakumari VUYYURU

Gloucester

Barnwood Medical Practice
51 Barnwood Road, Gloucester GL2 0SE
Tel: 01452 523362 Fax: 01452 387931
(West Gloucestershire Primary Care Trust)
Patient List Size: 6600

Practice Manager Dottie Moore

GP David Ronald MARTIN, Judith Ann BROOKE, Robert James Fitzgerald BYRNE, Joseph Xaviar MORENS

Bartongate Surgery
115 Barton Street, Gloucester GL1 4HR
Tel: 01452 422944 Fax: 01452 387871
(West Gloucestershire Primary Care Trust)
Patient List Size: 7500

Practice Manager Veronica Walkins

GP Patrick St. Lawrence LUSH, Colin James GOLD, Gillian Jean JOHNSON, Shanta NAIR

Cheltenham Road Surgery
16 Cheltenham Road, Gloucester GL2 0LS
Tel: 01452 522709 Fax: 01452 304321
Email: crs@doctors.org.uk
Website: www.cheltenhamroadsurgery.co.uk
(West Gloucestershire Primary Care Trust)
Patient List Size: 8200

Practice Manager Simon J T Colbeck

GP Christopher John CHAMPION, Michael Harry Vivian DELHANTY, Michael Stead ELLIS, Lindsay Ann ROBERTS, Janet Lois WEBB

Dr M E Rouse and Partners
24 St John's Avenue, Churchdown, Gloucester GL3 2DB
Tel: 01452 713036 Fax: 01452 714726
(West Gloucestershire Primary Care Trust)
Patient List Size: 12940

Practice Manager Trudy James

GP Michael Edward ROUSE, M T BILLINGTON, Jeremy HALLIDAY, Robert Hope MACKAY, John Conal McCRUM, L PICKETT, A SNOW, N TOWLE, Peter Norman WHITEHEAD

Hadwen Medical Practice
Glevum Way Surgery, Abbeydale, Gloucester GL4 4BL
Tel: 01452 529933
(West Gloucestershire Primary Care Trust)

Practice Manager Eve Beard

GP William David Stafford HAYNES, James Royse MURPHY, Susan Frances PACK, Christopher John Charles REMFRY, S M YOUNG

The Health Centre
Rikenel, The Park, Gloucester GL1 1XR
Tel: 01452 891110 Fax: 01452 891111
(West Gloucestershire Primary Care Trust)
Patient List Size: 7200

Practice Manager Steve Long

GP John Fennell BUCKLEY, Nicholas Alexander McDOWALL, Walter John NOONAN, Carol Ruth PARSONS

Heathville Road Surgery
5 Heathville Road, Gloucester GL1 3DP
Tel: 01452 528299 Fax: 01452 522959
(West Gloucestershire Primary Care Trust)
Patient List Size: 10519

GP Rhys Mervyn WATKINS, Nicholas James GILBERT, Rachel LIMBRICK, Sarah Elizabeth RICHARDS, Andrew SEYMOUR

Kingsholm Surgery
Alvin Street, Gloucester GL1 3EN
Tel: 01452 522902 Fax: 01452 387819
(West Gloucestershire Primary Care Trust)
Patient List Size: 4500

Practice Manager Lorraine Pugh

GP Peter Michael BARROW, Jennie Mair BARROW, Luke Daniel CORRIGAN

London Road Medical Practice
97 London Road, Gloucester GL1 3HH
Tel: 01452 522079 Fax: 01452 387884
(West Gloucestershire Primary Care Trust)
Patient List Size: 6700

Practice Manager Philip Mellis

GP Garvin Kenneth James FALKUS, Karen Lesley CARR, Iain Stuart JARVIS, Nicholas Howard TAYLOR

Longlevens Surgery
19b Church Road, Longlevens, Gloucester GL2 0AJ
Tel: 01452 522695 Fax: 01452 525547
(West Gloucestershire Primary Care Trust)

Practice Manager Leslie Allen

GP Philip James DODWELL, Justine Elizabeth FOSTER, Richard Hugh WEBSTER

Miller and Mann
The College Yard Surgery, Mount Street, Westgate, Gloucester GL1 2RE
Tel: 01452 412888 Fax: 01452 387874
(West Gloucestershire Primary Care Trust)
Patient List Size: 3500

Practice Manager Carol A Hewlett

GP Helen Joy MILLER, Jane Elizabeth MANN

Pavilion Family Doctors
153A Stroud Road, Gloucester GL1 5JJ
Tel: 01452 385555 Fax: 01452 387905
(West Gloucestershire Primary Care Trust)

Practice Manager Val Dirken

GP Susan Carolyn BAILEY, Mark Kilsyth BANCROFT-LIVINGSTON, Andrew Edward BROOKE, Allan Richard HARRIS, Gary MARLOWE, Barbara Anne WILLIAMS

Quedgeley Clinic
Quedgeley Health Campus, St. James, Quedgeley, Gloucester GL2 4WD
Tel: 01452 728882 Fax: 01452 728885
Website: www.siva.org.uk
(West Gloucestershire Primary Care Trust)

Practice Manager Manju Siva

GP Nadarajah SIVANANTHAN

Rosebank Surgery
153B Stroud Road, Gloucester GL1 5JQ
Tel: 01452 543000 Fax: 01452 414862
Email: rosebankhealth.co.uk
(West Gloucestershire Primary Care Trust)
Patient List Size: 16700

Practice Manager Wyndham Parry

GP Robert James PATERSON, Vivienne Eileen BARRICK, Oliver James HIDSON, David Paul KNIGHT, Jonathan Mark LAYZELL, Rita REMFRY, David Michael ROBERTS, Jonathan UNWIN

Saintbridge Surgery
Askwith Road, Saintbridge, Gloucester GL4 4SH
Tel: 01452 500252 Fax: 01452 387844
(West Gloucestershire Primary Care Trust)
Patient List Size: 7900

Practice Manager Angela Maile

GP Andrew George SAMUEL-GIBBON, William Hugh FOSTER, Samantha KUOK, Jitumpa SARKAR

Staunton and Corse Surgery
Corse, Staunton, Gloucester GL19 3RB
Tel: 01452 840228
(West Gloucestershire Primary Care Trust)
Patient List Size: 6300

Practice Manager Iain Collinson

GP Alan David DOCHERTY, Ian Norman Clowes MACLEOD, Jayne Elizabeth MASON, Roger WHITTLE

Steinhardt and Partners
The Surgery, 5A Brookfield Road, Hucclecote, Gloucester GL3 3HB
Tel: 01452 617295 Fax: 01452 375536
(West Gloucestershire Primary Care Trust)
Patient List Size: 8818

Practice Manager Judy Page

GP Stephen Ian STEINHARDT, Rachael BAILEY, Paul HODGES, David Fleming MAXTED, Katherine Jane McINTOSH

The Surgery
Whitminster Lane, Frampton on Severn, Gloucester GL2 7HU
Tel: 01452 740213/741664 Fax: 01452 740989
Email: surgery@gp-l84078.nhs.uk
(Cotswold and Vale Primary Care Trust)
Patient List Size: 4945

Practice Manager Jane White

GP Charles Ian Wharton BUCKLEY, Anne Elizabeth SPARGO, Peter John Ralph SPARGO

The Surgery
Abbotswood Road, Brockworth, Gloucester GL3 4PE
Tel: 01452 863200 Fax: 01452 864993
(West Gloucestershire Primary Care Trust)

Practice Manager Mrs Jacques

GP Timothy George HARBOTTLE, Robert William BELL, Derek John CONATY, Godfrey Roy Henderson FAIRBAIRN

The Surgery
61 Wheatway, Abbeydale, Gloucester GL4 5ET
Tel: 01452 383323 Fax: 01452 525823
Website: www.drnicol.co.uk
(West Gloucestershire Primary Care Trust)

GP Andrew NICOL

Godalming

Binscombe Medical Centre
106 Binscombe Lane, Godalming GU7 3PR
Tel: 01483 415115 Fax: 01483 414925
Website: www.binscombe.com
(Guildford and Waverley Primary Care Trust)
Patient List Size: 10700

GP Christopher Roy JAGGER, Martin D BRUNET, Andrew Stephen COOK, Jessica Kirwan JAMESON, Karen A JONES, Peter Sean Richard O'DONNELL, Richard Iain SPRUELL

Chiddingfold Surgery
Woodside Road, Chiddingfold, Godalming GU8 4QD
Tel: 01428 683174 Fax: 01428 685780
(Guildford and Waverley Primary Care Trust)
Patient List Size: 4500

Practice Manager Jeremy Bradshaw

GP G M CAMERON-BLACKIE, Darren WATTS, Claire Jeanette WILLETT

Hurst Farm Surgery
Chapel Lane, Milford, Godalming GU8 5HU
Tel: 01483 415885
(Guildford and Waverley Primary Care Trust)

GP Susan RILEY, Joseph SAVUNDRA

Springfield Surgery
Elstead, Godalming GU8 6EG
Tel: 01252 703122 Fax: 01252 703215
(Guildford and Waverley Primary Care Trust)
Patient List Size: 3850

Practice Manager Elaine Barnes

GP Rachel BRAY, Dr JENKINSON, Dr RAYNER

Square Medical Centre
High Street, Godalming GU7 1AZ
Tel: 01483 415141 Fax: 01483 414881
(Guildford and Waverley Primary Care Trust)
Patient List Size: 15000

Practice Manager Barbara Pope

GP John Frederick Arthur BLOWERS, Ailsa BORTHWICK, Anthony CERULLO, Mary Elizabeth Loveband DAVIS, Colin Thomas FLEETCROFT, Klaus GREEN, Felicity Jane OVERINGTON, Steven Edward Danbolt SIMONS

Witley Surgery
Wheeler Lane, Witley, Godalming GU8 5QR
Tel: 01428 682218 Fax: 01428 682218
(Guildford and Waverley Primary Care Trust)

GP Peter Robert WILKS, Andrew Fullerton SEARS, Tanja Maria SHAH, James Alexander John WHITAKER

Godstone

Pond Tail Surgery
The Green, Godstone RH9 8DY
Tel: 01883 742279 Fax: 01883 742913
(East Surrey Primary Care Trust)
Patient List Size: 7200

Practice Manager Commy Roffey

GP Colin William HOWARD, Sheila Margaret FROST, Michael GLOVER, Mark HINDLE

Goole

Bartholomew Medical Group
The Health Centre, Bartholomew Avenue, Goole DN14 6AW
Tel: 01405 767711 Fax: 01405 768212
(East Yorkshire Primary Care Trust)
Patient List Size: 15500

Practice Manager Joy Dawson

GP P J CALDWELL, Balmiki KUMAR, Richard Edward KURTIS, R P SINGH, Francis Martin THORNTON, Lynne WRIGHTSON

Howden Medical Centre
Pinfold Street, Howden, Goole DN14 7DD
Tel: 01430 430318 Fax: 01430 432050
(East Yorkshire Primary Care Trust)
Patient List Size: 6600

Practice Manager Carol Hunt

GP R W HARRISON, D J HANLY

The Marshes
Butt Lane, Snaith, Goole DN14 9DY
Tel: 0870 890 2525 Fax: 0870 890 2626
Email: enquires@gp-b81029.nhs.uk
Website: www.themarshessurgery.co.uk
(East Yorkshire Primary Care Trust)
Patient List Size: 9282

Practice Manager Margaret Clark

GP John Edward CLARK, Frances Helen BOOTH, Andrew John BREWS, Susan Elizabeth FOSTER, Andrew Paul SUMMERS, Noel Richard TINKER

Montague Medical Centre
Fifth Avenue, Goole DN14 6JD
Tel: 01405 767600 Fax: 01405 726111
(East Yorkshire Primary Care Trust)
Patient List Size: 7977

Practice Manager Sandra Raspin

GP Gordon Findlay REID, Claire HENSBY, Caroline LAPWORTH, Anthony G MORAN, M S PATEL

Gosport

Brockhurst Medical Centre
139-141 Brockhurst Road, Gosport PO12 3AX
Tel: 023 9258 3564 Fax: 023 9251 0782
(Fareham and Gosport Primary Care Trust)
Patient List Size: 4800

Practice Manager Eve Kean

GP Peter Alexander LACEY, Martin Paul COOPER, Janet Elizabeth FORSTER

Gosport Health Centre
Bury Road, Gosport PO12 3PN
Tel: 023 9258 3302 Fax: 023 9250 1421
(Fareham and Gosport Primary Care Trust)

Practice Manager Jean Smith

GP Paul A BURGESS, Georg BURLEIN, David Anthony EVANS, Rosalind REID

Pennells and Partners
Gosport Health Centre, Bury Road, Gosport PO12 3PN
Tel: 023 9258 3344 Fax: 023 9260 2704
(Fareham and Gosport Primary Care Trust)
Patient List Size: 9800

Practice Manager J A Colebourne

GP Robert Arthur PENNELLS, David Michael CHILVERS, Matthew Charles DAVIS, David Bernard TRAYNOR, Hazel Eunice Dorothy YEO

Rowner Health Centre
143 Rowner Lane, Gosport PO13 9SP
(Fareham and Gosport Primary Care Trust)

The Surgery
66-68 Stoke Road, Gosport PO12 1PA
Tel: 023 9258 1529 Fax: 023 9250 1417
(Fareham and Gosport Primary Care Trust)
Patient List Size: 8600

Practice Manager Fiona Todd

GP Brendan COONAN, Peter Philip GARRATT, Declan Nigel LYNCH, Derek NORTH

The Surgery
148 Forton Road, Gosport PO12 3HH
Tel: 023 9258 6242 Fax: 023 9260 1107
(Fareham and Gosport Primary Care Trust)
Patient List Size: 11800

Practice Manager Lesley Green

GP Jane Ann BARTON, Peter Alexander BEASLEY, Michael James BRIGG, Sarah Jane BROOK, Anthony Charles KNAPMAN, Edward John PETERS

The Surgery
Bridgemary Medical Centre, 2 Gregson Avenue, Gosport PO13 0HR
Tel: 01329 232446 Fax: 01329 282624
Website: www.bridgemarymedicalcentre.co.uk
(Fareham and Gosport Primary Care Trust)
Patient List Size: 9000

Practice Manager Jill Wright

GP John Thomas Hughes ANDERSON, Janet Linda ANDERSON, Martin Scott ASBRIDGE, David Orr ERSKINE, David Alan YOUNG

The Surgery
1 Rowner Road, Gosport PO13 9UA
Tel: 023 9258 0093 Fax: 023 9250 4060
(Fareham and Gosport Primary Care Trust)
Patient List Size: 6600

Practice Manager Pamela Wayman

GP John Howard GROCOCK, Sheila Mary Elizabeth LYNCH, Stuart Robert Ewing MORGAN

The Surgery
69 Bury Road, Gosport PO12 3PR
Tel: 023 9258 0363 Fax: 023 9260 1346
(Fareham and Gosport Primary Care Trust)
Patient List Size: 5683

Practice Manager Ann Reeves

GP S W DAGOGO, Nicholas C HAJIANTONIS, Nicholas PETERS

Grange-over-Sands

Fairfield Surgery
Station Road, Flookburgh, Grange-over-Sands LA11 7JY
Tel: 01539 558307 Fax: 01539 558442
(Morecambe Bay Primary Care Trust)
Patient List Size: 4000

Practice Manager P Hickson

GP Sheila PHIZACKLEA, Diane RUELL, Timothy Clarke WHITE

Nutwood Surgery
Windermere Road, Grange-over-Sands LA11 6EG
Tel: 01539 532108 Fax: 01539 535986
(Morecambe Bay Primary Care Trust)

GP John Richard NORMAN, Jane Elizabeth IRWIN

Windy Nook Surgery
Cartmel, Grange-over-Sands LA11 6PJ
Tel: 01539 536366 Fax: 01539 536766
Email: pre.req@gp-q82647.nhs.uk
Website: www.mbpct.nhs.uk/cartmelsurgery
(Morecambe Bay Primary Care Trust)
Patient List Size: 1758

Practice Manager Janice Longmine

GP Heather May LOVATT, Simon David MILLIGAN

Grantham

Back Lane Surgery
Back Lane, Colsterworth, Grantham NG33 5NJ
Tel: 01476 860243 Fax: 01476 860200
(Lincolnshire South West Teaching Primary Care Trust)

GP Michael Gervase BAMBER, Ann McKECHNIE

Caythorpe Surgery
52-56 High Street, Caythorpe, Grantham NG32 3DN
Tel: 01400 272215 Fax: 01400 273608
Website: www.villagedoctor.co.uk
(Lincolnshire South West Teaching Primary Care Trust)
Patient List Size: 7500

Practice Manager Nigel Kenward

GP Roger Alan GEE, Samuel James Boyd GILMORE, Simon Lee ROBINSON, Anthony James WATTS, Wiktor Stanislaw ZBRZEZNIAK

Glenside Practice
Castle Bytham Surgery, 12b High Street, Castle Bytham, Grantham NG33 4RZ
Tel: 01780 410205 Fax: 01780 410817
(Lincolnshire South West Teaching Primary Care Trust)
Patient List Size: 5600

Practice Manager Vanessa Coates

GP George C CAMPBELL, Margaret Anne CAMPBELL, Keith F CROFT, Martin Howard WEBSTER

Harrowby Lane Surgery
Harrowby Lane, Grantham NG31 9NS
Tel: 01476 579494 Fax: 01476 579694
(Lincolnshire South West Teaching Primary Care Trust)

Practice Manager Tracey Berry

GP Ian ALLSEBROOK, Nicola ANDREWS, Donal Gerard Mary MORAN

Market Cross Surgery
The Market Place, Corby Glen, Grantham NG33 4HN
Tel: 01476 550056 Fax: 01476 550057
(Lincolnshire South West Teaching Primary Care Trust)
Patient List Size: 2660

Practice Manager Diane Faux

GP John Balfour ELDER

St Johns Medical Centre
62 London Road, Grantham NG31 6HR
Tel: 01476 590055 Fax: 01476 400042
(Lincolnshire South West Teaching Primary Care Trust)
Patient List Size: 10800

Practice Manager Julie Hadlow

GP Richard CALEY, Mark Thomas BOAST, Katrina Mary NICHOLSON, David John ROPER, Michael John TEDBURY, Jaqueline Ann WILSON

St Peters Hill Surgery
15 St. Peters Hill, Grantham NG31 6QA
Tel: 01476 590009 Fax: 01476 570898
(Lincolnshire South West Teaching Primary Care Trust)

GP Susan COOMBES, John Alexander CRUICKSHANK, Jonathan William DUNKIN, John Stevenson KERR, Stephen John MANISTRE, Michael Gerard PARKIN, James John SNEDDON, Joseph Gerard Anthony SOUTHALL

Trent Road Surgery
Trent Road, Grantham NG31 7XQ
Tel: 01476 571166 Fax: 01476 570397
(Lincolnshire South West Teaching Primary Care Trust)

Practice Manager Julie Beatty

GP Abraham Peter CUTAJAR, Deidre Mary GOULD

Vine House Surgery
Vine Street, Grantham NG31 6RQ
Tel: 01476 576851 Fax: 01476 591732
(Lincolnshire South West Teaching Primary Care Trust)

GP Martin Timothy Christopher HIGGINS, David John BAKER, Pamela HARGREAVES, Mukesh Narendra PATEL

Woolsthorpe Surgery
Main Street, Woolsthorpe, By Belvoir, Grantham NG32 1LX
Tel: 01476 870166 Fax: 01476 870560
Website: www.users.globalnet.co.uk/~chale/home1.htm
(Lincolnshire South West Teaching Primary Care Trust)
Patient List Size: 1200

Practice Manager Joan Linforth

GP Christopher HALE, Amber PORTER

Gravesend

Darnley Road Surgery
90 Darnley Road, Gravesend DA11 0SW
Tel: 01474 355331 Fax: 01474 324407
(Dartford, Gravesham and Swanley Primary Care Trust)
Patient List Size: 15000

Practice Manager A J Glaysher

GP Gutta Hanumanta RAO, Irshad AHMAD, Woj BIERNACKI, V JAYAPRAKASH, Stephen Geoffrey KING, Simon Gavin MORAN, Manpinder SAHOTA, Carol Ann Linda TELFER

Dene Holm and The Hill Surgeries
Hunt Road, Northfleet, Gravesend DA11 8JT
Tel: 01474 535445 Fax: 01474 564475
(Dartford, Gravesham and Swanley Primary Care Trust)

GP I CARNE ROSS, A H MORGAN, C OZUA, H W TAYLOR

Granby Place Surgery
Granby Place, 1 High Street, Northfleet, Gravesend DA11 9EY
Tel: 01474 352447/362252
(Dartford, Gravesham and Swanley Primary Care Trust)

GP Ian Pattison CARNE-ROSS, Patrick BOYLE, Andrew Howard MORGAN, Hugh William TAYLOR

Gravesend Medical Centre
No 1 New Swan Yard, Gravesend DA12 2EN
Tel: 01474 534123 Fax: 01474 333629
Website: www.gravesendmedicalcentre.org
(Dartford, Gravesham and Swanley Primary Care Trust)
Patient List Size: 8252

Practice Manager Margaret Lane

GP Janet HALL, Charles Bruce ARMSTRONG, Anna BRYANT, David SOILE

King's Drive Surgery
2 King's Drive, Gravesend DA12 5BG
Tel: 01474 560717
Email: kings.drive.surgery@cablenet.co.uk
(Dartford, Gravesham and Swanley Primary Care Trust)
Patient List Size: 2600

Practice Manager Mrs Shuttlewood

GP Bhargawa VASUDAVEN

Lamorna Surgery
Thomas Drive, Gravesend DA12 5PZ
Tel: 01474 363217 Fax: 01474 353746
(Dartford, Gravesham and Swanley Primary Care Trust)
Patient List Size: 4000

Practice Manager Lynne Otton

GP Mahendra Maganbhai PATEL, Jaishree RAO

Lower Higham Road Surgery
48 Lower Higham Road, Gravesend DA12 2NG
Tel: 01474 564575
(Dartford, Gravesham and Swanley Primary Care Trust)
Patient List Size: 2600

GP M ARANHA

Marling Way Surgery
117 Marling Way, Gravesend DA12 4RQ
Tel: 01474 533201
(Dartford, Gravesham and Swanley Primary Care Trust)

GP Navin Naran ZALA

Meopham Medical Centre
Wrotham Road, Meopham, Gravesend DA13 0AH
Tel: 01474 814811/814068 Fax: 01474 814699
(Dartford, Gravesham and Swanley Primary Care Trust)

GP Philip Harrison VICARAGE, Jane Anne BAILEY, Jane Helen HOWIE, Jonathan Paul MOUNTY, David Magnus John WOODHEAD

Old Road West Surgery
30 Old Road West, Gravesend DA11 0LL
Tel: 01474 352075/567799 Fax: 01474 333952
(Dartford, Gravesham and Swanley Primary Care Trust)
Patient List Size: 11400

Practice Manager Karen Hoadley

GP Lynfa PRICE, Julian Henry GILES, Jill Elizabeth KENT, Ian Stuart MILLAR, Dermot Charles O'CONNOR, David James SUMNER

Parrock Street Medical Centre
186 Parrock Street, Gravesend DA12 1EN
Tel: 01474 567888 Fax: 01474 536999
Email: surgery@kashmir.co.uk
(Dartford, Gravesham and Swanley Primary Care Trust)
Patient List Size: 3700

GP S U D SHAH, M TAHMASSEBI

Rochester Road Surgery
115 Rochester Road, Gravesend DA12 2HU
Tel: 01474 560346 Fax: 01474 356044
(Dartford, Gravesham and Swanley Primary Care Trust)
Patient List Size: 3220

GP J SINGH

The Shrubbery
65A Perry Street, Northfleet, Gravesend DA11 8RD
Tel: 01474 356661 Fax: 01474 534542
(Dartford, Gravesham and Swanley Primary Care Trust)
Patient List Size: 14700

Practice Manager Linda Barton, Beverley Shanks

GP Robert SHANKS, B BELLS, Olajumoke Masire KOSO-THOMAS, Nigel Bernard SEWELL, M TAHIR, Richard George TODD, John Crispin TOWNSEND, Mark Andrew WESTBROOK

The Surgery
The Forge, Old Perry Street, Northfleet, Gravesend DA11 8BT
Tel: 01474 564758 Fax: 01474 569575
(Dartford, Gravesham and Swanley Primary Care Trust)

GP V KARUNAHARAN

White and Partners
Downs Way Medical Practice, 34 Fairview Road, Istead Rise, Gravesham, Gravesend DA13 9DR
Tel: 01474 832999 Fax: 01474 832011
(Dartford, Gravesham and Swanley Primary Care Trust)

GP P R WHITE, C F HANDY, J R A PATEL, D J PAYNE

Grays

Balfour Medical Centre
2 Balfour Road, Grays RM17 5NS
Tel: 01375 373366 Fax: 01375 394562
Email: info@balfourmc.com
Website: www.balfourmc.com
(Thurrock Primary Care Trust)
Patient List Size: 4880

Practice Manager June Tobin

GP Anil BANSAL, Pradeep ARORA, Ruby PUNWANI

Chadwell Medical Centre
1 Brentwood Road, Chadwell St Mary, Grays RM16 4JD
Tel: 01375 842289/853404 Fax: 01375 840357
(Thurrock Primary Care Trust)
Patient List Size: 4454

Practice Manager Linda Moore

GP Rajan Vishwanath MOHILE, Sonny LIE

Chafford Hundred Medical Centre
Drake Road, Chafford Hundred, Grays RM16 6RS
Tel: 01375 480000 Fax: 01375 483084
(Thurrock Primary Care Trust)
Patient List Size: 12500

Practice Manager Colin Townsend

GP Tonio ABELA, Nada AIUB, Jeanette EVANS, Kouta GUNASEKERA, Sam OLATIGBE

The Dilip Sabnis Medical Centre
Linford Road, Chadwell St Mary, Grays RM16 4JD
Tel: 01375 851578 Fax: 01375 857539
(Thurrock Primary Care Trust)

Practice Manager Susan Rutland

East Thurrock Road Medical Centre
34 East Thurrock Road, Grays RM17 6SP
Tel: 01375 390575 Fax: 01375 384136
(Thurrock Primary Care Trust)
Patient List Size: 5400

Practice Manager Marilyn Spires

GP Nita YADAVA, Anjan BOSE

East Tilbury Medical Centre
85 Coronation Avenue, East Tilbury, Grays RM18 8SW
Tel: 01375 846232 Fax: 01375 840440
Email: practice.manager@gp-F81691.nhs.uk
(Thurrock Primary Care Trust)
Patient List Size: 3200

Practice Manager Shahid Mohd Khan

GP Roohi Shahid KHAN

East Tilbury Surgery
Princess Margaret Road, East Tilbury, Grays RM18 8RL
Tel: 01375 843217 Fax: 01375 840423
(Thurrock Primary Care Trust)
Patient List Size: 5000

Practice Manager Linda Clark

GP Colin George LAKE, Gabriel Paul BYRNE, Stephen Ronald JONES

Grays Health Centre
Brooke Road, Grays RM17 5BY
Tel: 01375 898345 Fax: 01375 394685
(Thurrock Primary Care Trust)

Practice Manager Thushara Collins

GP (Kankanige Pemasiri) Ranjith DAMBAWINNA

Grays Health Centre
Brooke Road, Grays RM17 5BY
Tel: 01375 898345 Fax: 01375 391254
(Thurrock Primary Care Trust)

Practice Manager Thushara Collins

GP R DAMBAWINNA

The Health Centre
Crammavill Street, Stifford Clays, Grays RM16 2AP
Tel: 01375 377127 Fax: 01375 394520
(Thurrock Primary Care Trust)

Practice Manager Steve Dance

GP Olivia Therese HEADON, Diane DANIEL, Michael David HURTER, Peter Alan Boddington MARTIN, Kevin Paul WATKINS

Milton Road Surgery
12 Milton Road, Grays RM17 5EZ
Tel: 01375 381612 Fax: 01375 392366
(Thurrock Primary Care Trust)
Patient List Size: 3640

Practice Manager Davinder Masson

GP Kamlesh Kumar MASSON, Harish MASSON

New Road Medical Surgery
22 New Road, Grays RM17 6NG
Tel: 01375 390717 Fax: 01375 383489
(Thurrock Primary Care Trust)

Practice Manager Jackie Smith

GP L JOSEPH, P A JOSEPH

Orsett Road Surgery
111 Orsett Road, Grays RM17 5HA
Tel: 01375 372135 Fax: 01375 394642
(Thurrock Primary Care Trust)
Patient List Size: 5340

GP Asoka Kumarraj ABEYEWARDENE, M A AMARASINGHA

The Surgery
63 Rowley Road, Orsett, Grays RM16 3ET
Tel: 01375 892082 Fax: 01375 892487
(Thurrock Primary Care Trust)
Patient List Size: 6700

Practice Manager Jan Mason

GP Murray COLBURN, Nigel BINGHAM, Jeanne Marie Therese D'MELLO, Audrey Helen MITCHELL

The Surgery
Primecare Family Medical Centre, 167 Bridge Road, Grays RM17 6DB
Tel: 01375 373322 Fax: 01375 375329
(Thurrock Primary Care Trust)
Patient List Size: 3445

Practice Manager Jean Burrows

GP Sangat Singh SIDANA

Great Missenden

The Chequers Surgery
1-3 Chequers Drive, Prestwood, Great Missenden HP16 9DU
Tel: 01494 863899 Fax: 01494 865202
(Chiltern and South Bucks Primary Care Trust)

Practice Manager Barbara A Renouf

GP Mary J MITCHELL, Lynette HYKIN, Amyn A KANJI, PENELOPE SUTCLIFFE, Simon J P WILSON

John Hampden Surgery
97 High Street, Prestwood, Great Missenden HP16 9EU
Tel: 01494 890900 Fax: 01494 866990
(Chiltern and South Bucks Primary Care Trust)
Patient List Size: 3000

Practice Manager Sue Suddards

GP Jonathan Douglas LYONS, Rebecca MALLARD-SMITH

Prospect House Surgery
High Street, Great Missenden HP16 0BG
Tel: 01494 862325 Fax: 01494 890510
Email: practice.M81608@gp-M81608.nhs.uk
(Chiltern and South Bucks Primary Care Trust)
Patient List Size: 3000

Practice Manager Angela Hough

GP Caroline Elizabeth JENKINS, Kate BARNES, Lyn Marshall JENKINS

Great Yarmouth

Central Surgery
Sussex Road, Gorleston-on-Sea, Great Yarmouth NR31 6QB
Tel: 01493 414141 Fax: 01493 656253
(Great Yarmouth Primary Care Trust)

Practice Manager S A Spooner

GP Norman Keith Ian McIVER, Christopher Henry BROOKINGS, Robert COLEMAN, Andrew Paul COLVIN, Neil Michael LIVINGSTONE, William John LOCKETT, Marius MAGSON, Thomas PACE, David Graham WATSON, Simon David WORSLEY

Coastal Villages Practice
Pippin Close, Ormesby St. Margaret, Great Yarmouth NR29 3RW
Tel: 01493 730205 Fax: 01493 733120
Email: thecoastalvillagespractice@freeserve.co.uk
(Great Yarmouth Primary Care Trust)
Patient List Size: 15100

Practice Manager C Thompson

GP Alan Zdenek Scott NOVAK, Michael Robert CRICK, William Thomas Garfield DALTON, Richard Andrew HEMS, Mark Roberts NEWSTEAD, Harry Macdonald TAYLOR

Falklands Surgery
Falkland Way, Bradwell, Great Yarmouth NR31 8RW
Tel: 01493 442233
(Great Yarmouth Primary Care Trust)

GP Richard Edward DEVONSHIRE, Hilary Ann BAKER, Adrian PENN, Geoffrey Lawrence PERRY

Family Health Care Centre
1 East Anglian Way, Gorleston-on-Sea, Great Yarmouth NR31 6TY
Tel: 01493 662130 Fax: 01493 441780
Email: winthan@fhcc.freeserve.co.uk

(Great Yarmouth Primary Care Trust)
Patient List Size: 5777

Practice Manager Lyn Nicholls

GP Swe Swe WIN, Kyan THAN, Ian YATES

Gorleston Medical Centre

Stuart Close, Gorleston-on-Sea, Great Yarmouth NR31 7BU
Tel: 01493 650490
(Great Yarmouth Primary Care Trust)

Practice Manager Deborah Lines

GP Ajay KUMAR, Ardyn ROSS, Ranjeet VERMA

King Street Surgery

55 King Street, Great Yarmouth NR30 2PW
Tel: 01493 855589 Fax: 01493 332824
Email: kingstreet.surgery@nhs.net
(Great Yarmouth Primary Care Trust)
Patient List Size: 4450

Practice Manager Christine Cornish

GP Nigel Stuart GOULD, Rekha LAL

Leonard Ley Surgery

Nathaniel Fish Row, 43 King Street, Great Yarmouth NR30 2PN
Tel: 01493 330338
(Great Yarmouth Primary Care Trust)

GP Mark RUMBLE

Leonard Ley Surgery

43 King Street, Great Yarmouth NR30 2PN
Tel: 01493 330338 Fax: 01493 844744
Email: mark.rumble@gp-D82630.nhs.uk
(Great Yarmouth Primary Care Trust)

Practice Manager J Rossage

GP Michael David John ROSSAGE, Mark RUMBLE

Mill Lane Surgery

Mill Lane, Fleggburgh, Great Yarmouth NR29 3AW
Tel: 01493 369232
(Great Yarmouth Primary Care Trust)

GP Gary ROGERS

Millwood Surgery

Mill Lane, Bradwell, Great Yarmouth NR31 8HS
Tel: 01493 661549 Fax: 01493 440187
Email: dooldeniya.and.partners@care4tree.net
(Great Yarmouth Primary Care Trust)
Patient List Size: 8600

Practice Manager Monica Barton

GP Vincent DOOLDENIYA, Paul Richard CONNELL, Jen Willem HELLENDOORN, Andrew McCALL, Peter John SHELTON

Newtown Surgery

147 Lawn Avenue, Great Yarmouth NR30 1QP
Tel: 01493 853191 Fax: 01493 331861
(Great Yarmouth Primary Care Trust)

Practice Manager G Smith

GP John Trevor DAWSON, David Edward ADAMS, Anthony Campbell ALLAN, Alan Frederick BETTS, Jeanette GOULD, Louise Bernadette SANTORI, Liam Francis STEVENS

The Park Surgery

4 Alexandra Road, Great Yarmouth NR30 2HW
Tel: 01493 855672
(Great Yarmouth Primary Care Trust)

Practice Manager Carol Charles

GP Neil Richard STATTER, Myles DUFFIELD, David John EKBERY, Paul Christopher NOAKES, Wendy Ruth OUTWIN

South Quay Surgery

35-36 South Quay, Great Yarmouth NR30 2RG
Tel: 01493 843196 Fax: 01493 331835
(Great Yarmouth Primary Care Trust)
Patient List Size: 5500

Practice Manager S J Smith

GP Sunita NAGPAL, Suman NAGPAL

Staithe Road Surgery

Staithe Road, Ludham, Great Yarmouth NR29 5AB
Tel: 01692 678611 Fax: 01692 678295
(North Norfolk Primary Care Trust)
Patient List Size: 5400

Practice Manager Frances McKenzie

GP James Smallwood SAVAGE, Simon MORRIS, Andrew Colin Buchanan SALE, Sheila SUDLOW

Greenford

Allendale Road Surgery

35 Allendale Road, Greenford UB6 0RA
Tel: 020 8902 8146 Fax: 020 8795 2385
(Ealing Primary Care Trust)

Practice Manager Theresa Allum

GP Surjit Singh GORAYA, J SEIMON

Conway Crescent Surgery

2 Conway Crescent, Perivale, Greenford UB6 8HU
Tel: 020 8997 2457 Fax: 020 8810 9489
(Ealing Primary Care Trust)

Practice Manager Linda Haywood

GP Sipra GUHA

Eastmead Surgery

20 Eastmead Avenue, Greenford UB6 9RB
Tel: 020 8578 1244 Fax: 020 8575 5927
(Ealing Primary Care Trust)
Patient List Size: 5600

Practice Manager Anne-Marie Black

GP Surinder Kaur GILL, Hemant PATEL, Bonna P K WASSAN

Elm Trees Surgery

2A Horsenden Lane North, Greenford UB6 0PA
Tel: 020 8869 7910 Fax: 020 8869 7911
(Ealing Primary Care Trust)
Patient List Size: 4300

Practice Manager Rashmi Bathia

GP Inderjit Kaur SANDHU, Dilip PATEL

Greenford Road Medical Centre

591 Greenford Road, Greenford UB6 8QH
Tel: 020 8575 8347 Fax: 020 8523 2773
(Ealing Primary Care Trust)
Patient List Size: 7524

Practice Manager Tina Carroll

GP Robert Clive MOORE, Rosalyn Anne LEWIS, Nayana PATEL, Jacqueline SWORDS

Greenford Road Surgery

1268 Greenford Road, Greenford UB6 0HJ
Tel: 020 8422 7970
(Ealing Primary Care Trust)

GP Jennifer Ann Scott Lendrum BROWN

Mansell Road Practice

73 Mansell Road, Greenford UB6 9EN
Tel: 020 8575 6866 Fax: 020 8813 1280
(Ealing Primary Care Trust)

Practice Manager Tina Streeter

GP David Adam JENKINS, Dennis John HEAVEY, S RAMPHUL

Oldfield Family Practice

285 Greenford Road, Greenford UB6 8RA
Tel: 020 8578 1914 Fax: 020 8575 6327
Email: ofp@gp-E85069.nhs.uk

(Ealing Primary Care Trust)

Practice Manager April Boyle

GP Norman Harold SEGALL, Susan Melanie SEGALL

Ribchester Medical Centre
31 Ribchester Avenue, Perivale, Greenford UB6 8TG
Tel: 020 8998 3598 Fax: 020 8998 4838
(Ealing Primary Care Trust)

Practice Manager Mrs Patel

GP N N PATEL

The Surgery
18 Kings Avenue, Greenford UB6 9BZ
Tel: 020 8578 6016 Fax: 020 8575 1141
(Ealing Primary Care Trust)
Patient List Size: 2600

Practice Manager S Urrinder Hunjan

GP Mohinder Singh HUNJAN, H SINGH

Greenhithe

Elmdene Surgery
273 London Road, Horns Cross, Greenhithe DA9 9DB
Tel: 01322 382010 Fax: 01322 381696
Email: practice.manager@gp-g8221.nhs.uk
(Dartford, Gravesham and Swanley Primary Care Trust)
Patient List Size: 4200

Practice Manager Jane Langley

GP Stephen Henry LANGLEY, Dr AHMED

Ivy Bower Surgery
Ivy Bower Close, London Road, Greenhithe DA9 9NF
Tel: 01322 382024
(Dartford, Gravesham and Swanley Primary Care Trust)

GP C R L WATTEGEDERA

Grimsby

Albion House Surgery
3 Hainton Avenue, Grimsby DN32 9EX
Tel: 01472 345411 Fax: 01472 269471
(North East Lincolnshire Primary Care Trust)
Patient List Size: 6200

Practice Manager Sheila Towler

GP Hasmukh JETHWA

Birkwood Surgery
Birkwood, 31-33 Laceby Road, Grimsby DN34 5BH
Tel: 01472 879529 Fax: 01472 278817
Email: birkwood@gp-B81087.nhs.uk
(North East Lincolnshire Primary Care Trust)
Patient List Size: 7500

Practice Manager Stephanie Pidgen

GP Robert Oswald BARTON, Dr CANTIN, Iain James INGRAM, Dr OJADI, O F WILSON

The Chantry Lane Health Group
Church View Health Centre, Catergate, Grimsby DN31 1QZ
Tel: 01472 264999 Fax: 01472 264999
Website: www.chantrylanehealth.nhs.uk
(North East Lincolnshire Primary Care Trust)
Patient List Size: 5000

Practice Manager John Noton

GP Thomas Dunstan CULSHAW, Ademola M BAMGBALA, Bhasker GHOSH, Dr HUSSAIN

Field House Medical Centre
13 Dudley Street, Grimsby DN31 2AE
Tel: 01472 350327
(North East Lincolnshire Primary Care Trust)
Patient List Size: 14500

Practice Manager Jenny Stevenson

GP Derek Edward HOPPER, Malcolm Richard EAST, Kim PEACOCK, Jonothan Stuart PLOTNEK, Dr PRIEUR, David Charles PYE

Healing Health Centre
97 Station Road, Healing, Grimsby DN37 7RB
Tel: 01472 280221
(North East Lincolnshire Primary Care Trust)

GP Kalwant Singh KOONAR, Dr CROMPTON

Highfield Road Surgery
Highfield Road, North Thoresby, Grimsby DN36 5RT
Tel: 01472 840202 Fax: 01472 840970
(East Lincolnshire Primary Care Trust)

Practice Manager L Wright

GP B D MASSEY, A ANDERSON, J F BALLANTYNE, F BLANCO, P HARRIS, H IRVING

New Waltham Surgery
Greenlands Park, Station Road, New Waltham, Grimsby DN36 4PN
Tel: 01472 220333
(North East Lincolnshire Primary Care Trust)
Patient List Size: 2800

Practice Manager K Ben

GP Narinder Pal Singh BEDI

Pelham Medical Group
Church View Health Centre, Cartergate, Grimsby DN31 1QZ
Tel: 01472 353303/4 Fax: 01472 267443
(North East Lincolnshire Primary Care Trust)
Patient List Size: 7672

GP Peter LAWLESS, David Campbell ELDER, Alastair FINCH, Caroline Janine Cameron HOBBES

Pilgrim Primary Care Centre
Pelham Road, Immingham, Grimsby DN40 1JW
Tel: 01469 574197 Fax: 01469 574198
(North East Lincolnshire Primary Care Trust)
Patient List Size: 2750

Practice Manager Anne Redding

GP S BANERJEE

The Roxton Practice
Pilgrim Primary Care Centre, Pelham Road, Immingham, Grimsby DN40 1JW
Tel: 01469 572058 Fax: 01469 573043
(North East Lincolnshire Primary Care Trust)
Patient List Size: 11700

GP Richard Montgomery BARR, Peter David BELCHER, Dr DAS, Dr LANSLEY, Peter John MELTON, Dr NAYYAR, Peter Michael OPIE, Dr SINGH, Anne Elizabeth SPALDING, Sean Arthur THRIPPLETON

Scartho Medical Centre
26 Waltham Road, Grimsby DN33 2QA
Tel: 01472 871747 Fax: 01472 276050
Email: steven.lewis@gp-b81030.nhs.uk
Website: scathomedicalcentre.nhs.uk
(North East Lincolnshire Primary Care Trust)
Patient List Size: 10100

Practice Manager Steven Lewis

GP Anthimos Char STERGIDES, Dr DIJOUX, Paul HEATH, Alan Francis PEEL, Dr SALISBURY, Catherine Ann TWOMEY, Paul Anthony TWOMEY

The Surgery
2 Littlefield Lane, Grimsby DN31 2LG
Tel: 01472 342250 Fax: 01472 251742
Website: www.littlefieldlanesurgery.com
(North East Lincolnshire Primary Care Trust)
Patient List Size: 5600

Practice Manager Carole Flecther

GP Keith Anthony COLLETT, Sanjay CHAUHAN, E ZOON

The Surgery
20 Heneage Road, Grimsby DN32 9DY
Tel: 01472 343067
(North East Lincolnshire Primary Care Trust)

GP Iain David Stewart CHALMERS, Dr MEIER

The Surgery
261 Hainton Avenue, Grimsby DN32 9JX
Tel: 01472 343071 Fax: 01472 362648
Email: benjamin.deodhar@gp-B81603.nhs.uk
(North East Lincolnshire Primary Care Trust)
Patient List Size: 2829

Practice Manager Raili Tuxworth

GP Dr DEODHAR, Dr PRIEUR

The Surgery
264 Laceby Road, Grimsby DN34 5SU
Tel: 01472 877978 Fax: 01472 753204
(North East Lincolnshire Primary Care Trust)
Patient List Size: 1985

Practice Manager L Yarborough

GP Kamala Pati SINGH

The Surgery
20 North Sea Lane, Humberston, Grimsby DN36 4UZ
Tel: 01472 211116 Fax: 01472 811832
(North East Lincolnshire Primary Care Trust)
Patient List Size: 3400

Practice Manager Deborah Landymore

GP Rajendra Prasad SHARMA, N SHARMA, Sushima SHARMA

The Surgery
Town Street, South Killingholme, Grimsby DN40 3HR
Tel: 01469 540786
(North East Lincolnshire Primary Care Trust)

GP Dr BHORCHI

The Surgery
19 Dudley Street, Grimsby DN31 2AW
Tel: 01472 344989 Fax: 01472 341449
(North East Lincolnshire Primary Care Trust)

GP Dr DE, R S N SAHA

The Surgery
30 Dudley Street, Grimsby DN31 2AB
Tel: 01472 356832
(North East Lincolnshire Primary Care Trust)

GP Egbert Nathalan HOPKINS

The Surgery
20 Heneage Road, Grimsby DN32 9DY
Tel: 01472 343067 Fax: 01472 340746
Website: www.heneageroad.co.uk
(North East Lincolnshire Primary Care Trust)

GP Iain David Stewart CHALMERS, Valentijn O MEIER

The Surgery
14 Eleanor Street, Grimsby DN32 9DT
Tel: 01472 355640 Fax: 01472 349394
(North East Lincolnshire Primary Care Trust)
Patient List Size: 1400

Practice Manager G Farren

GP Arun Kumar MAJUMDER

The Surgery
128 Chelmsford Avenue, Grimsby DN34 5BA
Tel: 01472 877227
(North East Lincolnshire Primary Care Trust)

GP S N KESHRI

The Surgery
307 Laceby Road, Grimsby DN34 5LP
Tel: 01472 872024 Fax: 01472 278758
(North East Lincolnshire Primary Care Trust)
Patient List Size: 2930

Practice Manager Joyce Kaveney

GP R P PATHAK

The Surgery
259 Hainton Avenue, Grimsby DN32 9JX
Tel: 01472 342570
(North East Lincolnshire Primary Care Trust)

Practice Manager Anna Sauke

GP Dr RAJESEKHARA, Dr SURESH-BABU

The Surgery
373 Hainton Avenue, Grimsby DN32 9QP
Tel: 01472 357050 Fax: 01472 267291
(North East Lincolnshire Primary Care Trust)

GP S K SARKAR

Woodford Surgery
29-31 Chantry Lane, Grimsby DN31 2LL
Tel: 01472 342325 Fax: 01472 251739
Website: www.woodfordmedicalcentre.nhs.uk
(North East Lincolnshire Primary Care Trust)
Patient List Size: 10150

Practice Manager David Holmes, Jo Molton

GP John Richard Crisop POTTER, Julian David CLARK, Paul Barry CLARSON, G T K JAFRI, Dr JOHN

Wyberswood Surgery
367 St Nicholas Drive, Wybers Wood, Grimsby DN37 9SF
Tel: 01472 328071 Fax: 01472 328072
(North East Lincolnshire Primary Care Trust)
Patient List Size: 2000

Practice Manager Rachel Everitt

GP R KUMAR

Guildford

Austen Road Surgery
1 Austen Road, Guildford GU1 3NW
Tel: 01483 564578 Fax: 01483 505368
(Guildford and Waverley Primary Care Trust)
Patient List Size: 7000

Practice Manager Martin Brown

GP Simon PIPER, Julia BLATCHLY, Ian Charles EWART, Helen FAWCETT, Cathy McMULLAN, Kay STEPHENSON

Dapdune House Surgery
Wharf Road, Guildford GU1 4RP
Tel: 01483 573336 Fax: 01483 306602
(Guildford and Waverley Primary Care Trust)
Patient List Size: 11200

Practice Manager Janet Luft

GP David George EYRE-BROOK, Diane ACKERLEY, Ian Foster CUNLIFFE, Fiona GROOM, Allison Elizabeth JUMP, Caroline Rosemary KARANJIA, Anthony Francis George RIMMER

Fairlands Medical Centre
Fairlands Avenue, Worplesdon, Guildford GU3 3NA
Tel: 01483 594250 Fax: 01483 598767
Email: fairlands@medprac.freeserve.co.uk
Website: www.fairlands.co.uk
(Guildford and Waverley Primary Care Trust)
Patient List Size: 11000

Practice Manager C M McDermott

GP Martin Stephen McKENDRY, Jonathan Scott NORRIS, Timothy David ARNOLD, Sarah Margaretha DOBBS, David Tarrant LAURENCE, Christopher Mark LUKASZEWICZ, Hilary Anne TRIGG

Merrow Park Surgery
Kingfisher Drive, Guildford GU4 7EP
Tel: 01483 503331 Fax: 01483 303457
Email: calvert@merrow.free-online.co.uk
(Guildford and Waverley Primary Care Trust)
Patient List Size: 10000

Practice Manager Anne Long

GP Alan Frederick TUTIN, S BOUCHER, H GRISEWOOD, Calvert F HAN, Jerome SENDER, Angela Myfanwy TUTIN

New Inn Surgery
202 London Road, Burpham, Guildford GU4 7JS
Tel: 01483 301091 Fax: 01483 453232
Email: leon.barbour@gp-h81647.nhs.uk
Website: www.newinnsurgery.co.uk
(Guildford and Waverley Primary Care Trust)

Practice Manager Jennifer Lusty

GP Leon Aldous Andrew BARBOUR, Robert BLUNDELL, Jill OLIVER

The Oaks Surgery
Guildowns Group Practice, Applegarth Avenue, Park Barn, Guildford GU2 8LZ
Tel: 01483 563424 Fax: 01483 563789
Email: s.carr-ballis@surrey.ac.uk
Website: www.guildowns.nhs.uk
(Guildford and Waverley Primary Care Trust)

GP Anne Gordon BRYETT, Stephen CARR-BAINS, David Michael COUPER, Oliver Hugh Basil FRANKS, Ann HENNELL, Colin Joo Eong OH, Helen M RESTORICK, Victoria WOOLLAM

Peaslake Surgery and Dispensary
Peaslake Lane, Peaslake, Guildford GU5 9RL
Tel: 01306 730875 Fax: 01306 731509
Email: ckeown@nhs.net
(Guildford and Waverley Primary Care Trust)
Patient List Size: 900

GP Christine Elizabeth KEOWN

Shere Surgery and Dispensary
Gomshall Lane, Shere, Guildford GU5 9DR
Tel: 01483 202066 Fax: 01483 202761
(Guildford and Waverley Primary Care Trust)

Practice Manager Jennifer Healey

GP Graham Robert TYRRELL, Malcolm Philip HARVEY, Catharine Mary HUMPHRYS, Charlotte Ann KNIGHT

St Lukes Surgery
Warren Road, Guildford GU1 3JH
Tel: 0870 471 3979 Fax: 0870 417 3978
(Guildford and Waverley Primary Care Trust)
Patient List Size: 9300

Practice Manager Sharon Rees

GP David Richard ELLIOTT, Jonathan Nicholas BARNARDO, Andrew Paul CROSS, Mary Catherine MORRISON, John Gordon WILLIAMS, S XAVIER

St Nicolas Surgery
Buryfields, Guildford GU2 4AZ
Tel: 01483 303200 Fax: 01483 452309
(Guildford and Waverley Primary Care Trust)
Patient List Size: 2550

Practice Manager Cordilia Ryan

GP Jonathan David BEAUMONT, Robert BLUNDELL, Patricia Mary PARKER

Wonersh Surgery
The Sheilings, Wonersh, Guildford GU5 0PE
Tel: 01483 898123 Fax: 01483 893104
Website: www.onershsurgery.org.uk
(Guildford and Waverley Primary Care Trust)
Patient List Size: 10500

Practice Manager P West

GP Graham Albert Wilfrid HORNETT, Susan BODGENER, Dominique Paul Henri DAULTON, Sian JONES, Shaun Phillip O'HANLON, Anne WILKINSON, Sidney WORTHINGTON

Woodbridge Hill Surgery
1 Deerbarn Road, Guildford GU2 8YB
Tel: 01483 562230 Fax: 01483 301132
(Guildford and Waverley Primary Care Trust)

Practice Manager Gaynor Hardy

GP Simon DE LUSIGNAN, William Page BEVINGTON, Angela Mary Elizabeth Tamsin CARLYON, Giles Edmund FIELD, Julia Lynne OXENBURY, John Donald George REES, Elizabeth Anne WHITELAW

Guisborough

The Garth Surgery
Rectory Lane, Guisborough TS14 7DJ
Tel: 01287 632206 Fax: 01287 635112
(Langbaurgh Primary Care Trust)
Patient List Size: 10500

Practice Manager John King

GP Joanna Mary Frances GILLIAT, Patrick GORDON, Donald Cochran MARR, Amanda Jean SMITH, Robert WHELAN, Stephen Morriss WILLIAMS

Springwood Surgery
Rectory Lane, Guisborough TS14 7DJ
Tel: 01287 619611 Fax: 01287 619613
Website: www.springwoodsurgery.co.uk
(Langbaurgh Primary Care Trust)
Patient List Size: 8330

Practice Manager Fiona Graham

GP David William HOBKIRK, Katherine ANTHONY, William FRANCIS, Angela Joy HALLOWAY, Sarah LEE, Nicola Jane THOMAS, Rachel Margaret Sarah THOMSON

Gunnislake

Gunnislake Health Centre
The Orchard, Gunnislake PL18 9JZ
Tel: 01822 836241 Fax: 01822 833757
(North and East Cornwall Primary Care Trust)

Practice Manager Sue Duke

GP Andrew Peter STEWART, Nicholas David BUXTON, Shelagh McCORMICK, Jon TILBURY, Jane WARREN

Hailsham

Bethany House Surgery
85 Battle Road, Hailsham BN27 1UA
Tel: 01323 848485 Fax: 01323 847988
(Eastbourne Downs Primary Care Trust)
Patient List Size: 3500

Practice Manager D Mitchell

GP Michael Charles HOPE-GILL

Bridgeside Surgery
1 Western Road, Hailsham BN27 3DG
Tel: 01323 441234 Fax: 01323 440970
(Eastbourne Downs Primary Care Trust)
Patient List Size: 4100

Practice Manager Lesley Stadasnes

GP Savvakis SAVVAS, A McGREGOR

Nicki West Memorial Surgery
The Health Centre, Vicarage Field, Hailsham BN27 1BE
Tel: 01323 440202 Fax: 01323 847410
(Eastbourne Downs Primary Care Trust)
Patient List Size: 2100

Practice Manager Liz Phillips

GP Peter Lyn HAYS, Patrick William DUNPHY

Quintins Medical Centre
Hawkswood Road, Hailsham BN27 1UG
Tel: 01323 845669 Fax: 01323 846653
(Eastbourne Downs Primary Care Trust)
Patient List Size: 5000

GP John Stuart Francis HOLDEN, Kerstin EDWARDS, Graz GARONER, Rosanne LOWE

Seaforth Farm Surgery
Vicarage Lane, Hailsham BN27 1BH
Tel: 01323 848494 Fax: 01323 849316
(Eastbourne Downs Primary Care Trust)
Patient List Size: 6014

GP Alan John PEARCE, Alison Jane GRIMSTON, Paul Christopher Brian HOLMES

The Surgery
West End, Herstmonceux, Hailsham BN27 4NN
Tel: 01323 833535 Fax: 01323 833998
(Eastbourne Downs Primary Care Trust)

Practice Manager A Walker

GP Guy Richard Hamilton BAKER

Vicarage Field Surgery
Vicarage Field, Hailsham BN27 1BE
Tel: 01323 441155 Fax: 01323 847209
(Eastbourne Downs Primary Care Trust)
Patient List Size: 5400

Practice Manager Jackie Letchford

GP N CERECEDA, Dr CROUCHER, Martin Derek CROUCHER, C McGREGOR, K THURSTON

Halesowen

Alexandra Medical Centre
1 Short Street, Halesowen B63 3UH
Tel: 0121 585 5188/8600 Fax: 0121 602 6737
(Dudley South Primary Care Trust)
Patient List Size: 3080

GP Nazir Ahmad SHAMEEM, Maheen SHAMEEM

Coombswood and Hawned Surgery
146-148 Coombs Road, Halesowen B62 8AF
Tel: 0121 5614275 Fax: 0121 5614275
(Dudley South Primary Care Trust)
Patient List Size: 2500

Practice Manager Carol Jones

GP Humphrey Narh AKUFO-TETTEH

Crestfield Surgery
39 Highfield Road, Halesowen B63 2DH
Tel: 01384 566789 Fax: 01384 567534
(Dudley South Primary Care Trust)

GP V K MITTAL

Feldon Lane Surgery
Feldon Lane, Halesowen B62 9DR
Tel: 0121 422 4703 Fax: 0121 422 3773
(Dudley South Primary Care Trust)
Patient List Size: 1500

Practice Manager Dawn Salt

GP C S BAMFORD, Timothy Bremner HORSBURGH, Rosemary THORNS

Halesowen Health Centre
14 Birmingham Street, Halesowen B63 3HL
Tel: 0121 550 1010 Fax: 0121 585 0993
(Dudley South Primary Care Trust)

Practice Manager Peter Timms

GP Richard Anthony JOHNSON, Bridget Penelope JOHNSON

Halesowen Medical Practice
St Margaret's Well Surgery, 2 Quarry Lane, Halesowen B63 4DW
Tel: 0121 550 4917 Fax: 0121 504 0140
(Dudley South Primary Care Trust)
Patient List Size: 6800

Practice Manager Malcolm Wallace

GP Jonathan Henry DARBY, Sarah ALLEN, Claire Fiona HALFORD, Gillian Mary LOVE

Lapal Medical Centre
95 Goodrest Avenue, Halesowen B62 0HP
(Dudley South Primary Care Trust)

GP R J SOUTHAM, Jane Elizabeth KEVERN, R A LEWIS

Lapal Medical Practice
95 Goodrest Avenue, Halesowen B62 0HP
Tel: 0121 422 2345 Fax: 0121 423 3099
Website: www.lapalmedicalpractice.co.uk
(Dudley South Primary Care Trust)
Patient List Size: 6000

Practice Manager D J Smith

GP Richard Alan LEWIS, J HALL, Clare HAWKINS, Alison MABLEY, Richard John SOUTHAM

Meadowbrook Road Surgery
4 Meadowbrook Road, Halesowen B63 1AB
Tel: 0121 550 1034 Fax: 0121 550 4758
(Dudley South Primary Care Trust)
Patient List Size: 8100

Practice Manager M Vansouwe

GP Michael J COOKE, Alan Clive CARR, Iqbal MORE

The Surgery
19 Long Lane, Halesowen B62 9LL
(Dudley South Primary Care Trust)

GP Lall Singh BASSAN

The Surgery
3 Tenlands Road, Halesowen B63 4JJ
(Dudley South Primary Care Trust)

GP Vinodini MODI

The Surgery
30 Hagley Road, Hayley Green, Halesowen B63 1DH
Tel: 0121 550 2872
(Dudley South Primary Care Trust)
Patient List Size: 1400

GP M J KHETANI, Dr TALATI

Halesworth

Cutlers Hill Surgery
Bungay Roaad, Halesworth IP19 8SG
Tel: 01986 874618 Fax: 01986 874908
(Waveney Primary Care Trust)

Practice Manager Jenny Doane

GP Catherine Sophia NORTHOVER, Annette Beatrix ABBOTT, Clare CRAIK, Richard KELL, Kevin MACLUSKY, Judith Mary SHAPLAND, Paul Stephen SQUIRES

Halifax

Beechwood Medical Centre
60a Keighley Road, Ovenden, Halifax HX2 8AL
Tel: 01422 345798 Fax: 01422 343049
(Calderdale Primary Care Trust)
Patient List Size: 6500

Practice Manager Caroline McLaughlin

GP Frederick Anthony MAYLAND, Mark Peter RASTALL, Caroline Louise TAYLOR

Boothtown Road Surgery
4 Boothtown Road, Boothtown, Halifax HX3 6HG
Tel: 01422 352096
(Calderdale Primary Care Trust)

GP A SINGH

Clare Road Surgery
51 Clare Road, Halifax HX1 2JP
Tel: 01422 365460 Fax: 01422 348706
(Calderdale Primary Care Trust)
Patient List Size: 2000

Practice Manager Sue Law

GP Moheb Choucri Aziz CHOUCRI

The Frank Swire Health Centre
Nursery Lane, Ovenden, Halifax HX3 5TE
Tel: 01422 355535
(Calderdale Primary Care Trust)

GP Suryagopal Obulisamy SUKUMARAN

Heath House Surgery
Free School Lane, Halifax HX1 2PS
Tel: 01422 365533 Fax: 01422 345851
(Calderdale Primary Care Trust)
Patient List Size: 8500

Practice Manager Vanessa Costello

GP Stephen THORNBER, Melinda BLACKMAN, Hazel Anne CARSLEY, Victor D'AMBROGIO

Keighley Road Surgery
Keighley Road, Illingworth, Halifax HX2 9LL
Tel: 01422 244397/248308 Fax: 01422 241101
(Calderdale Primary Care Trust)
Patient List Size: 11000

GP Catherine Margaret Scott ANDERSON, Kumbera Somaiah AIYAPPA, John Hari CHATTERJEE, Min Sein CHIANG, Michael Wynn HOUGHTON

King Cross Surgery
199 King Cross Road, Halifax HX1 3LW
Tel: 01422 330612 Fax: 01422 323740
(Calderdale Primary Care Trust)
Patient List Size: 7395

Practice Manager Sheila Barker

GP Rebecca Louise HARDY, John Victor TAYLOR, Helen M BOLLAND, Robert VAUGHAN

Kos Clinic
4 Roydlands Street, Hipperholme, Halifax HX3 8AF
Tel: 01422 205154 Fax: 01422 201443
(Calderdale Primary Care Trust)
Patient List Size: 11600

GP Kai Yoon NG, Roger Thomas BROWN, Ruth CAMERON, Dominic CHIN, Alex ROSS

Lord Street Surgery
10 Lord Street, Halifax HX1 5AE
Tel: 01422 353956
(Calderdale Primary Care Trust)

GP Krishan Chander SADOTRA, A K SARKER

Mixenden Stones Surgery
Mixenden Road, Halifax HX2 8RQ
Tel: 01422 249788 Fax: 01422 246189
(Calderdale Primary Care Trust)
Patient List Size: 3071

Practice Manager Catherine Gill

GP C BEITH, Peter DAVIES, R SUTCLIFFE

Plane Trees Group Practice
51 Sandbeds Road, Pellon, Halifax HX2 0QL
Tel: 01422 330860 Fax: 01422 364830
(Calderdale Primary Care Trust)
Patient List Size: 9000

Practice Manager Reg Tomkin

GP Habib ULLAH, David Stuart ELLWOOD, Susan Carole GARDINER, Ian Reginald ORMEROD

Queens Road Surgery
252 Queens Road, Halifax HX1 4NJ
Tel: 01422 330636 Fax: 01422 342105
(Calderdale Primary Care Trust)
Patient List Size: 5455

GP Surinder Kumar GOYAL, Dr AGBIR, Richard LON

Rosegarth Surgery
Rothwell Mount, Halifax HX1 2XB
Tel: 01422 353450/350420
(Calderdale Primary Care Trust)

GP Lesley LORD, Martin James FINDLAY, Paul Gabriel SAWCZYN, David Ian Hamilton SMITH, David Anthony TAYLOR

Shelf Health Centre
Shelf Moor Road, Shelf, Halifax HX3 7PQ
Tel: 01274 691159
(Calderdale Primary Care Trust)
Patient List Size: 3600

Practice Manager Julia Clayton-Stead

GP Andrew John CLAYTON-STEAD

Southowram Surgery
Law Lane, Southowram, Halifax HX3 9QB
Tel: 01422 344107
(Calderdale Primary Care Trust)
Patient List Size: 2050

Practice Manager Marilyn Greenwood

GP A D SIMMONS

Spring Hall Group Practice
Spring Hall Medical Centre, Spring Hall Lane, Halifax HX1 4JG
Tel: 01422 349501 Fax: 01422 322645
(Calderdale Primary Care Trust)

Practice Manager H E Langhorn

GP Christine Susan PARRY, S J CLEASBY, L HENSON, R T MANYEULA, S NAGPAUL, Felicity Margaret PRICE, S M TAHIR

Stannary House
Stainland Road, Stainland, Halifax HX4 9HA
Tel: 01422 374109 Fax: 01422 375174
(Calderdale Primary Care Trust)
Patient List Size: 7650

Practice Manager David Hibbert

GP Roderic Bruce BAIN, Keith D BEST, Tanya Louise DUNNING, Eilidh J GWNOON, Erika Lorraine HAMMOND, Stanley MARTIN, Catherine Margaret McMICHAEL

Stansfield House Surgery
305 Skircoat Green Road, Halifax HX3 0NA
Tel: 01422 353517 Fax: 01422 380799
Email: shama_hs@yahoo.com.uk
(Calderdale Primary Care Trust)
Patient List Size: 2476

Practice Manager S Hussain

GP I HUSSAIN

Victoria Street Surgery
3 Victoria Street, Greetland, Halifax HX4 8DF
Tel: 01422 372355
(Calderdale Primary Care Trust)

GP P S SEN

Halstead

The Castle Surgery
9-10 Falcon Square, Castle Hedingham, Halstead CO9 3BY
Tel: 01787 461465 Fax: 01787 462829
(Witham, Braintree and Halstead Care Trust)

Practice Manager Frances Carre

GP Nancy Jane SALMON, William LITTLER

ThE Elizabeth Courtauld Surgery
Factory Lane West, Halstead CO9 1EX
Tel: 01787 475944 Fax: 01787 474506
(Witham, Braintree and Halstead Care Trust)
Patient List Size: 16050

Practice Manager Joyce Smith

GP Michael Paul BRISTOL, Peter James DUFFUS, Timothy Ormond HEATH, Daniela KREIS, John Edward MARKHAM, Shan M NEWHOUSE, Jayne M SMITH, Bryan John SPENCER, Alan John Forsyth SYMINGTON

Hilton House Surgery
77 Swan Street, Sible Hedingham, Halstead CO9 3HT
Tel: 01787 460612 Fax: 01787 462754
(Witham, Braintree and Halstead Care Trust)
Patient List Size: 3422

Practice Manager Frances Carre

GP Paul Frank MARSHALL, Kathryn Lillian MORGAN

Haltwhistle

Haltwhistle Medical Group
Haltwhistle Health Centre, Greencroft Avenue, Haltwhistle NE49 9AP
Tel: 01434 320077 Fax: 01434 320674
Email: admin@gp-A84034.nhs.uk
(Northumberland Care Trust)
Patient List Size: 5800

Practice Manager Julie Johnston

GP Paul Henry BURNHAM, R J ADAMSON, M BAKER, Derek Adam THOMSON

Hampton

Hampton Hill Medical Centre
23 Wellington Road, Hampton TW12 1JP
Tel: 020 8977 0043 Fax: 020 8977 8691
Website: www.hhsurgery.co.uk
(Richmond and Twickenham Primary Care Trust)
Patient List Size: 6000

Practice Manager Christopher Toop

GP Andrew John WRIGHT, Karina KNIGHTS, Charlotte Frances PENNYCOOK

Hampton Medical Centre
Lansdowne, 49a Priory Road, Hampton TW12 2PB
Tel: 020 8979 5150 Fax: 020 8941 9068
Email: lewis.graham@gp.h84040.nhs.uk
(Richmond and Twickenham Primary Care Trust)
Patient List Size: 15000

Practice Manager Kader Zinat

GP Graham John LEWIS, Damon James ALEXANDER, Audrey BARRETO, Richard Montgomery HINTON, Michelle Doreen Anne NUNES, Una Catherina O'REILLY, Joy PILLAI

The Surgery
71 Broad Lane, Hampton TW12 3AX
Tel: 020 8979 5406 Fax: 020 8941 8838
(Richmond and Twickenham Primary Care Trust)
Patient List Size: 5118

Practice Manager Rita Stringer

GP Parvin DHALLA

Harleston

Harleston Doctors Surgery
Bullock Fair Close, Harleston IP20 9AT
Tel: 01379 853217 Fax: 01379 854082
(Southern Norfolk Primary Care Trust)

Practice Manager Jenny Anderson

GP Peter Wyndham KEMP, Patrick William FREW, Anne Helen KEMP, Alexander Maxim VALORI

Harlow

Addison House Surgery
Hamstel Road, Harlow CM20 1DS
Tel: 01279 692777 Fax: 01279 692760
(Harlow Primary Care Trust)

Practice Manager Geraldine Acriman

GP Mohammed Abul BASHER, Farida HAQUE

Addison House Surgery
Hamstel Road, Harlow CM20 1DS
Tel: 01279 692780 Fax: 01279 692781
(Harlow Primary Care Trust)

Practice Manager Wendy Tyler

GP Anne Marie VANNER, Z I KAWA, Hassanali Mohamedali Rajabali KHIMJI

Barbara Castle Health Centre
Broadley Road, Harlow CM19 5SJ
Tel: 01279 308888 Fax: 01279 308080
(Harlow Primary Care Trust)

Practice Manager Pat Somerfield

GP Nadira CHOWDHURY, C GOPINATH, Christopher Giles William LOXLEY

The Hamilton Practice
Keats House, Bush Fair, Harlow CM18 6LY
Tel: 01279 692720 Fax: 01279 692719
Website: www.hamiltonpractice.nhs.uk
(Harlow Primary Care Trust)
Patient List Size: 10000

Practice Manager George Shields

GP C Ann BEDFORD, Clifford William BISHOP, Austin Chibneze CHUKWU, Kathryn Anne JONES, Michael David LURKINS, Helen Elizabeth MEDHURST, Thambiah RADHAKRISHNAN

Lister Medical Centre
Lister House, Staple Tye, Harlow CM18 7LU
Tel: 01279 414882 Fax: 01279 439600
(Harlow Primary Care Trust)
Patient List Size: 17000

Practice Manager Tracy May

GP Clive Haskell RICHARDS, Trevor Hugh Gronow GEORGE, Martin Clive JACOBS, Beata KREISS, Pushpaben MISTRY, Richard NORRIS, Titilola Christine OGBONNAYA, Mukeshkumar Haridas RAJANI, Miranda Jane ROBERTS, Padma VEMPALI

Nuffield House Surgery
The Stow, Harlow CM20 3AX
Tel: 01279 425661 Fax: 01279 427116
(Harlow Primary Care Trust)
Patient List Size: 11600

Practice Manager Elaine Murr

GP Joanna Shaw SWAINSBURY, Sajive BANSAL, A ESTEKI, Elizabeth Joan INGHAM, C PARIKH, David Simon SMALLEY, K TULLY

Old Harlow Health Centre
Jenner House, Garden Terrace Road, Old Harlow, Harlow CM17 0AX
Tel: 01279 418136 Fax: 01279 429650
Email: postmaster@gp-f81056.nhs.uk
Website: www.oldharlowhealth.co.uk
(Harlow Primary Care Trust)
Patient List Size: 9100

Practice Manager Jan Dixon

GP William Norman Cecil NASH, Richard Ywan ANTHONY, Diane Maureen MEEHAN, Krish RADHAKRISHNAN, carolyn SMELLEY

Osler House Surgery
Potter Street, Harlow CM17 9BG
Tel: 01279 422664/629707 Fax: 01279 422576
(Harlow Primary Care Trust)
Patient List Size: 11200

Practice Manager Pat Kissane

GP M HUSSAIN, P LANCASTER

The Ross Practice
Keats House, Bush Fair, Harlow CM18 6LY
Tel: 01279 692747 Fax: 01279 692737
(Harlow Primary Care Trust)
Patient List Size: 8550

Practice Manager Jackie Kingdom

GP Janet Margaret BELLINGHAM, Karin Nina ASHAR, Robin David GERLIS, John Patrick PORTELLY, Kathryn Nicola TULLY

Sydenham House Surgery
Monkswick Road, Harlow CM20 3NT
Tel: 01279 422525 Fax: 01279 436210
(Harlow Primary Care Trust)

Practice Manager Tracey Mays

GP K SINGH, H MAND

Harpenden

Davenport House Surgery
Bowers Way, Harpenden AL5 4HX
Tel: 01582 767821 Fax: 01582 769285
Website: www.davenportsurgery.demon.co.uk
(St Albans and Harpenden Primary Care Trust)
Patient List Size: 12200

Practice Manager Anthea Doran

GP Alan Patrick O'Connell STRANDERS, Charles Arthur BARBER-LOMAX, Alka CASHYAP, Andrew Thomas Herbert CHAFER, Jayne HARRIS, Kirsten Mary LAMB, Mark SANDLER

Dr Stephens and Partners
The Village Surgery, Amenbury Lane, Harpenden AL5 2BT
Tel: 01582 712021 Fax: 01582 462414
(St Albans and Harpenden Primary Care Trust)

Practice Manager Margaret Gray

GP John STEPHENS, Roger John GIBBS, Deborah GILHAM, Tania GOODWIN, Stephen David INGRAM, Patrick Austen O'HARE, Katheryne SOLOMONS, Robert WALKER

Elms Medical Practice
5 Stewart Road, Harpenden AL5 4QA
Tel: 01582 769393 Fax: 01582 461735
(St Albans and Harpenden Primary Care Trust)
Patient List Size: 14000

Practice Manager Geoff Morgan

GP Dylan Gwynne Leyshon PHILLIPS, Catherine Mary ARGYLE, David Nicholas HEMSI, Jacqueline Anne IMPEY, Elizabeth Kirstie LONG, Keith Antony MANN, Bethan REES, Julian SMITH

Harrogate

Alexandra Road Practice
11 Alexandra Road, Harrogate HG1 5JS
Tel: 01423 503218 Fax: 01423 505512
(Craven, Harrogate and Rural District Primary Care Trust)
Patient List Size: 5500

Practice Manager Susan Marks

GP Euan Gavin Cooper McLUSKY, Stephen FOLEY, Mary Siobhan Gerandine O'NEILL, Carol Jane WRIGHT

Baker, Greenwood and Gammack
110 King's Road, Harrogate HG1 5HW
Tel: 01423 503035 Fax: 01423 562665
(Craven, Harrogate and Rural District Primary Care Trust)
Patient List Size: 4716

Practice Manager Jean Eames

GP Raymond Francis BAKER, Andrew GAMMACK, Sian GREENWOOD

Burton Leonard Surgery
Burton Leonard Village Hall, Burton Leonard, Harrogate HG3 3RW
(Craven, Harrogate and Rural District Primary Care Trust)

GP Alastair Scott GREEN, John William CROMPTON, Clare Sarah EISNER, Martin Arthur JONES

Burton Lodge Medical Centre
86 Station Parade, Harrogate HG1 1HH
Tel: 01423 503129 Fax: 01423 561820
(Craven, Harrogate and Rural District Primary Care Trust)
Patient List Size: 5500

GP Bernard Palandapatirage DIAS, Karen J EMMS, Mark D HAMMATT, E Lucy MAW, Mary-Jane PROWSE

Dr Moss and Partners
28-38 Kings Road, Harrogate HG1 5JP
Tel: 01423 560261 Fax: 01423 501099
(Craven, Harrogate and Rural District Primary Care Trust)

Practice Manager Rachel Simpson

GP George Alan CROUCH, Michelle Kimberley BRAY, Carol Margaret GOODMAN, Michael Andrew LEACH, Vivienne POSKITT, Richard Charles SWEENEY, Nicholas Patrick TAYLOR, James WOODS, James Crerar WOODS, James David YOUNG

East Parade Surgery
East Parade, Harrogate HG1 5LW
Tel: 01423 566574 Fax: 01423 568015
(Craven, Harrogate and Rural District Primary Care Trust)

Practice Manager Sue Elliott

GP Sarah CRAVEN, John Edward HENDERSON, Fiona Margaret ATKINSON, Robert Anthony PENMAN

Grange Medical Centre
Dacre Banks, Harrogate HG3 4DX
Tel: 01423 780436 Fax: 01423 781416
(Craven, Harrogate and Rural District Primary Care Trust)
Patient List Size: 9500

Practice Manager P A Berriman

GP Michael John BEER, John Michael Henry HAIN, David G B LAWSON, Iain Menzies McINTOSH, Carolyn Mary RYAN, John Robert SPAIN, Alison Margaret WATERWORTH

The Health Centre
80 Knaresborough Road, Harrogate HG2 7LU
Tel: 01423 557232 Fax: 01423 557234
(Craven, Harrogate and Rural District Primary Care Trust)
Patient List Size: 13000

Practice Manager P Reed

GP Timothy John THORNTON, J C ANDERSON, John Crispin Dunlop BANKS, Douglas Finlay BANNATYNE, Ian Andrew BARGH, James Henry BRADSHAW, Jonathan Newton IDDON, Derek George Hugh

JAMES, Sarah Jane MINTY, Margaret Anne PLOWMAN, Christine June SULLIVAN, Christopher John Lytham WALSH

Jennyfield Health Centre
Grantley Drive, Harrogate HG3 2XT
Tel: 01423 524605 Fax: 01423 524605
(Craven, Harrogate and Rural District Primary Care Trust)

Practice Manager Brenda Exall

GP Issa ASAAD, Lillian ASAAD

Jennyfield Health Centre
Jennyfield Drive, Harrogate HG3 2XQ
(Craven, Harrogate and Rural District Primary Care Trust)

GP Hugh Jackson HOUSTON, Evan Gavin Cooper McLUSKY, Mary Siobhan Gerandine O'NEILL

Jennyfield Health Centre
Jennyfield Drive, Harrogate HG3 2XT
(Craven, Harrogate and Rural District Primary Care Trust)

GP Stephen FOLEY

Kings Road Surgery
67 Kings Road, Harrogate HG1 5HJ
Tel: 01423 875875 Fax: 01423 875885
(Craven, Harrogate and Rural District Primary Care Trust)
Patient List Size: 6365

Practice Manager Annita Langley

GP Charles Leggett SCOTT-KNOX-GORE, David Anthony GILMORE, Ruth Elsbeth GLOVER, Andrew Ward STANWORTH

The Leeds Road Practice
49/51 Leeds Road, Harrogate HG2 8AY
Tel: 01423 566636 Fax: 01423 569208
(Craven, Harrogate and Rural District Primary Care Trust)
Patient List Size: 11700

Practice Manager A Given

GP Phyllis Ann JONES, Michael Alva SCATCHARD, Peter Charles BANKS, Richard Vernon CHAVE-COX, Richard Scott HALL, Anna Louise POWELL, Amanda WOODS

Leeds Road Practice
49-51 Leeds Road, Harrogate HG2 8AY
Tel: 01423 566636 Fax: 01423 569208
(Craven, Harrogate and Rural District Primary Care Trust)
Patient List Size: 11800

Practice Manager Alan Haines

GP Peter Charles BANKS, Richard Vernon CHAVE-COX, Richard Scott HALL, Phyllis Ann JONES, Anna Louise POWELL, Michael Alva SCATCHARD, Amanda Jayne WOODS

Nidderdale Group Practice
Feastfield Medical Centre, King Street, Pateley Bridge, Harrogate HG3 5AT
Tel: 01423 711369 Fax: 01423 712482
(Craven, Harrogate and Rural District Primary Care Trust)

Practice Manager P A Berriman

GP Michael John BEER, John Michael Henry HAIN, David LAWSON, Iain Menzies McINTOSH, Carolyn Mary RYAN, John Robert SPAIN, Alison Margaret WATERWORTH

Pannal Surgery
2A Hillside Road, Pannal, Harrogate HG3 1JP

GP Michael Ian GOULD

Park Parade Surgery
27-28 Park Parade, Harrogate HG1 5AG
Tel: 01423 502776 Fax: 01423 568036
(Craven, Harrogate and Rural District Primary Care Trust)
Patient List Size: 6163

Practice Manager Christabel Spink

GP Roger Martin CALVERT, Anne BIRD, A A CUNNINGHAM, Rachel Louise FALSHAW

Sanatorium
Harrogate Ladies College, Harrogate HG1 2QG
(Craven, Harrogate and Rural District Primary Care Trust)

GP Mary Siobhan Gerandine O'NEILL

Spring Gables Surgery
Clint Bank, Birstwith, Harrogate HG3 3AJ
Tel: 01423 770202 Fax: 01423 711403
(Craven, Harrogate and Rural District Primary Care Trust)

Practice Manager P A Berriman

GP Michael John BEER, John Michael Henry HAIN, David G B LAWSON, Patricia Rosalind MARSHALL, Iain Menzies McINTOSH, Carolyn Mary RYAN, Alison Margaret WATERWORTH

The Surgery
54 Church Avenue, Harrogate HG1 4HG
Tel: 01432 564168 Fax: 01432 501102
(Craven, Harrogate and Rural District Primary Care Trust)
Patient List Size: 13300

Practice Manager Jennifer Joyce

GP Dr THORNTON, J C ANDERSON, Dr BANNATYNE, Dr SULLIVAN

Thornton and Partners
The Surgery, 54 Church Avenue, Harrogate HG1 4HG
Tel: 01423 564168 Fax: 01423 501102
(Craven, Harrogate and Rural District Primary Care Trust)
Patient List Size: 13000

Practice Manager Jennifer Joyc

GP Timothy John THORNTON, J C ANDERSON, Douglas Finlay BANNATYNE, Ian Andrew BARGH, Derek George Hugh JAMES, R B KASPER, Christine June SULLIVAN

Harrow

Aspri Medical Centre
1-3 Long Elmes, Harrow Weald, Harrow HA3 5LE
Tel: 020 8427 9623 Fax: 020 8424 9136
Email: kaushik.karia@gp-E84658.nhs.uk
(Harrow Primary Care Trust)

GP Kaushikkumar KARIA, H JABBAL, Dr PARAMALINGHAM, R SHAH

Belmont Health Centre
516 Kenton Lane, Kenton, Harrow HA3 7LT
Tel: 020 8427 1213 Fax: 020 8424-0542
(Harrow Primary Care Trust)

GP L M ADLER, Rosalind LANDAU, Graham David SADO, Darwin TAM, Jyotsna VYAS

Charlton Medical Centre
223 Charlton Road, Kenton, Harrow HA3 9HT
Tel: 020 8294 2686
(Harrow Primary Care Trust)

GP Ramesh Yeshwant KELSHIKER, Kunda KELSHIKER

Civic Medical Centre
18 Bethecar Road, Harrow HA1 1SE
Tel: 020 8427 9445 Fax: 020 8424 0652
(Harrow Primary Care Trust)

GP Dilip Kumar Chhotabhai PATEL, M A C PERERA

Dukes Medical Centre
1 Lankers Drive, North Harrow, Harrow HA2 7PA
Tel: 020 8868 5268
(Harrow Primary Care Trust)

GP Rajendra Balkrishna SHUKLA

The Elmcroft Surgery
5 Elmcroft Crescent, North Harrow, Harrow HA2 6HL
Tel: 020 8863 1337 Fax: 020 8863 6826
(Harrow Primary Care Trust)

GP Kevin Edward PEARCE, Jonathan Samuel CHARLTON

GP Direct
5/7 Welback Road, West Harrow, Harrow HA2 0RQ
Tel: 020 8515 9300 Fax: 020 8515 9300
Email: info@gpdirecto.co.uk
Website: www.gpdirect.co.uk
(Harrow Primary Care Trust)
Patient List Size: 8105

Practice Manager Yvonne Lineen

GP Nizar Roshanali MERALI, S AHMAD, A NURMOHAMED, Tayyaba SHERIF, Rabia YAQOOB

Harold MacMillan Medical Centre
43 Butler Avenue, Harrow HA1 4EJ
Tel: 020 8423 6644 Fax: 020 8428 9782
(Harrow Primary Care Trust)
Patient List Size: 4000

Practice Manager Nicole Kniep

GP Mansur AHMAD

Headstone Lane Medical Centre
238 Headstone Lane, Harrow HA2 6LY
Tel: 020 8428 1211 Fax: 020 8428 9434
(Harrow Primary Care Trust)
Patient List Size: 3200

Practice Manager B Sutherland

GP V RAVIKUMAR, V PARAMALINQAM, G ROGERS

Kenton Bridge Medical Centre
155-175 Kenton Road, Kenton, Harrow HA3 0YX
Tel: 020 8907 6989 Fax: 020 89076003
Website: www.kbms.org.uk
(Harrow Primary Care Trust)
Patient List Size: 3600

GP Mark Lionel LEVY, Rekha RAJA

Kenton Bridge Medical Centre
155-175 Kenton Road, Harrow HA3 0XF
Tel: 020 8907 6013
(Brent Teaching Primary Care Trust)

Practice Manager Jenny Walker

GP Geraldine Anne GOLDEN

Kenton Clinic
533a Kenton Road, Harrow HA3 0UQ
Tel: 020 8204 2255 Fax: 020 8204 7589
(Brent Teaching Primary Care Trust)
Patient List Size: 3000

Practice Manager Naina Sodha

GP Peter Johnson DAVID

Kenton Medical Centre
7 Northwick Avenue, Harrow HA3 0AA
Tel: 020 8907 6105 Fax: 020 8907 8259
(Brent Teaching Primary Care Trust)

GP Purnendu Kumar DAS, Bindu DAS

Lanfranc Medical Practice
2 Lanfranc Court, Greenford Road, Harrow HA1 3QE
Tel: 020 8422 1813 Fax: 020 8423 7697
(Brent Teaching Primary Care Trust)
Patient List Size: 6800

Practice Manager Jean Higgs

GP Pravin Chandulal MEHTA, D C DATTANI, Sandhya P MEHTA

The Medical Centre
45 Enderley Road, Harrow Weald, Harrow HA3 5HF
Tel: 020 8863 3333
(Harrow Primary Care Trust)

Practice Manager L Cowens

GP Martin Trevor RHODES, Jyoti BHANDARI, Beverly Maralyn PETER, Leonard Harold PETER, Christopher Gurth Goland ROBINSON, Sonal Kantilal SHAH

P J Kaye and Partners
Northwick Surgery, 36 Northwick Park Road, Harrow HA1 2NU
Tel: 020 8427 1661 Fax: 020 8864 2737
(Harrow Primary Care Trust)
Patient List Size: 9000

Practice Manager Bali Kharay

GP Patrick John KAYE, Fergus James McCLOGHRY, Ruth TOPPER, George VARGHESE, Anjum ZAIDI

The Pinner Road Surgery
196 Pinner Road, Harrow HA1 4JS
Tel: 020 8427 0130 Fax: 020 8424 2509
(Harrow Primary Care Trust)
Patient List Size: 4900

Practice Manager M A McCarthy

GP Ghiasuddin KHAJA, G PALREDDY

The Primary Care Medical Centre
475 Kenton Road, Kenton, Harrow HA3 0UN
Tel: 020 8204 2650 Fax: 020 8204 3533
(Brent Teaching Primary Care Trust)
Patient List Size: 3000

Practice Manager Mary Manning

GP Ajit H SHAH

The Ridgeway Surgery
71 Imperial Drive, North Harrow, Harrow HA2 7DU
Tel: 020 8427 2470
(Harrow Primary Care Trust)

GP Ryszard Andrzej HERMASZEWSKI, David John LLOYD, Sandra OELBAUM, Kenneth Robert WALTON

Roxbourne Medical Centre
37 Rayners Lane, South Harrow, Harrow HA2 0UE
Tel: 020 8422 5602 Fax: 020 8422 3911
(Harrow Primary Care Trust)
Patient List Size: 6800

Practice Manager Sue Sullivan

GP Shah Masood Ahmed FAROOQI, Malita MIRZA, Wahid Asif SHAIDA, Sarmad ZAIDI

Shaftesbury Medical Centre
39 Shaftesbury Parade, South Harrow, Harrow HA2 0AH
Tel: 020 8423 5500
(Harrow Primary Care Trust)

GP Shamim AKHTAR, Shaukat HAYAT

Simpson House Medical Centre
255 Eastcote Lane, South Harrow, Harrow HA2 8RS
Tel: 020 8864 3466 Fax: 020 8864 1002
(Harrow Primary Care Trust)
Patient List Size: 13000

Practice Manager Lynda Miller

GP Guy Wayland Seymour GRAHAM, Helen BATES, John Macarthur JUSTICE, Michael John MALONE, Kusem PAUL, Deborah Phyllis ROZEWICZ, Sirjit Singh Atma Singh SEYAN

St Peters Medical Centre
Colbeck Road, West Harrow, Harrow HA1 4BS
Tel: 020 8864 4868
(Harrow Primary Care Trust)
Patient List Size: 4753

GP Elizabeth PRICE, Michael Edward DAVEY, Tamie DOWNES

The Surgery
48 Harrow View, Harrow HA1 1RQ
Tel: 020 8427 7172 Fax: 020 8424 9375
Email: docpan@aol.com
(Harrow Primary Care Trust)
Patient List Size: 3001

Practice Manager Surjit Bahra

GP Mukesh Dalpatbhai PANDYA

The Surgery
70 Minehead Road, Harrow HA2 9DS
(Harrow Primary Care Trust)

GP Shamsuddin SHAIKH

The Surgery
204 Kings Road, South Harrow, Harrow HA2 9JJ
Tel: 020 8422 2081
(Harrow Primary Care Trust)
Patient List Size: 7300

Practice Manager R Rawlinson

GP Michael Paul EDDINGTON, L WIJAYARATNA

The Surgery
1 Streatfield Road, Harrow HA3 9BP
Tel: 020 8907 0381 Fax: 020 8909 2134
(Harrow Primary Care Trust)

GP Alexander Charles SMART, Harishchandra Gandhabhai MISTRY, Katherine Elizabeth PARNELL

The Surgery
116 Sudbury Court Drive, Harrow HA1 3TG
Tel: 020 8904 6767 Fax: 020 8922 6579
(Brent Teaching Primary Care Trust)
Patient List Size: 3900

Practice Manager Maureen Jani

GP John AKUMABOR, M HATHTHOTUWA, U W OMODU

The Surgery
121 Preston Hill, Harrow HA3 9SN
Tel: 020 8905 0894 Fax: 020 8204 7440
(Brent Teaching Primary Care Trust)
Patient List Size: 1875

Practice Manager Carole Thurgood

GP Ryhana BATHOOL, Dr KHAMMAS, Dr KHAN

The Surgery
177 Streatfield Road, Kenton, Harrow HA3 9BL
Tel: 020 8204 5561
(Harrow Primary Care Trust)

GP K K VARA

Wasu Medical Centre
275A Kings Road, South Harrow, Harrow HA2 9LG
Tel: 020 8866 0920 Fax: 020 8426 1104
(Harrow Primary Care Trust)
Patient List Size: 3110

Practice Manager Harmander Wasu

GP Paramjit Singh WASU

Wijeratne and Partners
Belmont Health Centre, 516 Kenton Lane, Kenton, Harrow HA3 7LT
Tel: 020 8863 6863 Fax: 020 8863 9815
(Harrow Primary Care Trust)

Practice Manager Nick Highton

GP J J WIJERATNE, Hardeep Kaur MANGAT, O D RATNAYAKE, Somil Devendra WIJENDRA

Hartfield

The Surgery
Church Street, Hartfield TN7 4AQ
Tel: 01892 770402 Fax: 01892 770189
(Sussex Downs and Weald Primary Care Trust)

Practice Manager A J T Furneaux

GP Peter John Sidney FURNEAUX

Hartlepool

Bank House Surgery
The Health Centre, Victoria Road, Hartlepool TS26 8DB
Tel: 01429 274800 Fax: 01429 860811
(Hartlepool Primary Care Trust)
Patient List Size: 8000

Practice Manager R Tattersall

GP Roger B STONEY, Andrew Peter DOWNS, Christopher George HEGGS, Michael Inglis SMITH

Blackhall and Peterlee Group Practice
Blackhall Community Health Centre, Hesleden Road, Blackhall, Hartlepool TS27 4LQ
Tel: 0191 586 4331 Fax: 0191 586 4844
Email: gp-a83007.nhs.uk
(Easington Primary Care Trust)
Patient List Size: 9500

Practice Manager Marie Venners

GP Paul G BURRELL, R ARMSTRONG, P GALLAGHER, R LEIGH

Chadwick House Surgery
127 York Road, Hartlepool TS26 9DN
Tel: 01429 234646 Fax: 01429 861559
(Hartlepool Primary Care Trust)

Practice Manager J Sharpe

GP Zarina ANAM, Charles John Hamilton Greig BRASH, John HOWE, Chander PARKASH

The General Medical Centre
Surgery Lane, Hartlepool TS24 9DN
Tel: 01429 282600 Fax: 01429 282166
(Hartlepool Primary Care Trust)
Patient List Size: 4400

Practice Manager M Dawson

GP A R DAWSON, Miguel Alfonso LASA GALLEGO, W SALTISSI

Gladstone House Surgery
46 Victoria Road, Hartlepool TS26 8DD
Tel: 01429 297290 Fax: 01429 297291
(Hartlepool Primary Care Trust)

GP Sanjay Kumar RAY, Mala KALIA, Kai SANDER

Grange House Surgery
22 Grange Road, Hartlepool TS26 8JB
Tel: 01429 272679 Fax: 01429 861265
(Hartlepool Primary Care Trust)
Patient List Size: 5333

Practice Manager Michelle Martin

GP Alison Helen EATON, Patrick Francis McGOWAN, Rachel ROBERTS

Hart Lodge Surgery
Jones Road, Hartlepool TS24 9BD
Tel: 01429 267573 Fax: 01429 869027
(Hartlepool Primary Care Trust)

GP David KIPLING, Jane Hargreaves DUNSTONE, Frederick Robert Peter JOHNSTON

The Headland Surgery
113 Durham Street, Hartlepool TS24 0HU
Tel: 01429 288100 Fax: 01429 282500
(Hartlepool Primary Care Trust)

GP Fazal OMER, John SINCLAIR, R THAKUR

The Health Centre
Victoria Road, Hartlepool TS26 8DB
Tel: 01429 272000/274899 Fax: 01429 863877
(Hartlepool Primary Care Trust)
Patient List Size: 7320

Practice Manager C Neil

GP Malcolm Anthony AYRE, Simon John ACEY, Richard George MOODY, Boleslaw Marek POSMYK

The Health Centre
Victoria Road, Hartlepool TS26 8DB
Tel: 01429 273191 Fax: 01429 864006
(Hartlepool Primary Care Trust)
Patient List Size: 5000

Practice Manager Denise Corbett, Jane Harrington

GP Jeffrey Chin Hoe KOH, Graham TRORY

The Health Centre
Victoria Road, Hartlepool TS26 8DB
Tel: 01429 272945 Fax: 01429 867797
(Hartlepool Primary Care Trust)

GP S GUPTA, James GALLAGHER

The Health Centre
Victoria Road, Hartlepool TS26 8DB
Tel: 01429 262095 Fax: 01429 272374
(Hartlepool Primary Care Trust)
Patient List Size: 3800

Practice Manager M Errington

GP Stuart Kenneth HAZLE

McKenzie House Surgery
Kendal Road, Hartlepool TS25 1QU
Tel: 01429 233611 Fax: 01429 297713
(Hartlepool Primary Care Trust)
Patient List Size: 17000

Practice Manager Claudia Miller

GP Philip John Wesley BOLT, Steven Harry ANDELIC, S CUTLER, Paul Anthony PAGNI, Carl David PARKER, Catherine Sian PARKER, Nicholas Anthony Patrick TIMLIN, Edvige VCCELLI

The Surgery
Station Lane, Seaton Carew, Hartlepool TS25 1AX
Tel: 01429 278827 Fax: 01429 278827
(Hartlepool Primary Care Trust)
Patient List Size: 2300

Practice Manager Pauline Killick

GP J K B PATEL, M PENG

Wynyard Road Surgery
35-37 Wynyard Road, Hartlepool TS25 3LB
Tel: 01429 223195 Fax: 01429 296007
(Hartlepool Primary Care Trust)
Patient List Size: 1008

Practice Manager P Singh

GP Arun Kumar SINGH

Harwich

Fronks Road Surgery
77 Fronks Road, Dovercourt, Harwich CO12 3RS
Tel: 01255 556868 Fax: 01255 556969
(Tendring Primary Care Trust)

Practice Manager Jacky Whittle

GP Stuart William CHILD, David HARKNESS, John RANKIN

Harewood Surgery
Harwich Road, Great Oakley, Harwich CO12 5AD
Tel: 01255 880341 Fax: 01255 880815
(Tendring Primary Care Trust)

Practice Manager Ann Read

GP Graham Victor BALIN

Health Clinic
407 Main Road, Dovercourt, Harwich CO12 4EU
Tel: 01255 201299 Fax: 01255 201270
(Tendring Primary Care Trust)

Practice Manager Elizabeth Stovell

GP Arthur Richard ALLDRICK, Dr ANDREWS, Peter John NIGHTINGALE, James Christopher Marnan STRACHAN, Jillian Valerie SULLIVAN, Richard John WILSON, A T WYNNE

Haslemere

Haslemere Health Centre
Church Lane, Haslemere GU27 2BQ
Tel: 01483 783000 Fax: 01428 645065
Email: hasledocs@aol.com
(Guildford and Waverley Primary Care Trust)
Patient List Size: 17765

Practice Manager Melanie Baker

GP Christopher Paul TAYLOR, Rosalind BAILANCE, N BULL, Melanie Elizabeth CANT, Jeremy William Michael CORNISH, Nolan GEEVES, E HAMPSON, J HOBBS, Mark HURST, M McNEIL, Marcus Laurence Thomas PANCHAUD, Philip RIDSDILL SMITH, Sarah Patricia WHITAKER

Hassocks

Health Centre
Windmill Avenue, Hassocks BN6 8LY
Tel: 01273 843563 Fax: 01273 846500
(Mid Sussex Primary Care Trust)
Patient List Size: 3630

Practice Manager Helen Hatcher

GP Christopher Anthony SHEARN, Kay HANCOCK, Karen McGORRY

Mid Sussex Health Care
The Health Centre, Trinity Road, Hurstpierpoint, Hassocks BN6 9UQ
Tel: 01273 834388 Fax: 01273 834529
(Western Sussex Primary Care Trust)
Patient List Size: 14700

Practice Manager M Spires

GP Robert Norman JEFFERY, Peter Joseph Marten HEELEY, Dr MOORE, Joanna THOMSON

Hastings

Beaconsfield Road Surgery
21 Beaconsfield Road, Hastings TN34 3TW
Tel: 01424 422389 Fax: 01424 431500
(Hastings and St Leonards Primary Care Trust)

Practice Manager Christina Bowditch

GP Krishnakant RADIA, Jonathan MORRELL, Linda PARKER

Cornwallis Gardens Surgery
10 Cornwallis Gardens, Hastings TN34 1LP
Tel: 01424 722666 Fax: 01424 460951
(Hastings and St Leonards Primary Care Trust)

Practice Manager Jan Pearce

GP Glenis Grant BENNETT

Harold Road Surgery
164 Harold Road, Hastings TN35 5NH
Tel: 01424 720878 Fax: 01424 719525
(Hastings and St Leonards Primary Care Trust)
Patient List Size: 10200

Practice Manager Sharon Fairbrother, Carole Williams

GP Roger Edmund CHISHOLM-BATTEN, Richard TILL, Parvin DHALLA, Isobel HORSLEY, Gregory Eugene WILCOX

Priory Road Surgery
83 Priory Road, Hastings TN34 3JJ
Tel: 01424 430800 Fax: 01424 465555
(Hastings and St Leonards Primary Care Trust)

Practice Manager Linda Godden

GP Priyatosh DAS

Roebuck House
High Street, Hastings TN34 3EY
Tel: 01424 452800
(Hastings and St Leonards Primary Care Trust)

Practice Manager Caroline Thomas

GP Andrew Charles DUNFIELD-PRAYERO

Roebuck House
High Street, Hastings TN34 3EY
Tel: 01424 452802
(Hastings and St Leonards Primary Care Trust)

Practice Manager Gail Brooks

GP Ankur CHOPRA

Roebuck House
High Street, Hastings TN34 3EY
Tel: 01424 452803 Fax: 01424 719234
(Hastings and St Leonards Primary Care Trust)

Practice Manager Leanne Cordell

GP David Andrew John DUTCHMAN

Roebuck House
High Street, Hastings TN34 3EY
Tel: 01424 420378 Fax: 01424 719234
(Hastings and St Leonards Primary Care Trust)

Practice Manager Tracy White

GP John ROWAN

Roebuck House
High Street, Hastings TN34 3EY
Tel: 01424 452804
(Hastings and St Leonards Primary Care Trust)

Practice Manager Jan Phillips

GP Sally Elizabeth PAGET, Rosina KYU

Shankill Surgery
21 Fairlight Road, Hastings TN35 5ED
Tel: 01424 421046 Fax: 01424 425177
(Hastings and St Leonards Primary Care Trust)
Patient List Size: 5750

Practice Manager Sarah Farrant

GP Francis James Thomas HOWIE, Karl FRANCIS

Stone Street Surgery
4 Stone Street, Hastings TN34 1QD
Tel: 01424 427015 Fax: 01424 427633
(Hastings and St Leonards Primary Care Trust)

Practice Manager Marion Nicholson

GP Hugh Philip NICHOLSON

Wellington Square Medical Centre
45 Wellington Square, Hastings TN34 1PN
Tel: 01424 722066 Fax: 01424 718385
(Hastings and St Leonards Primary Care Trust)

Practice Manager Carole Kent

GP Mike COOPER, Paul SEAL

Wellington Square Medical Centre
45 Wellington Square, Hastings TN34 1PN
Tel: 01424 722262 Fax: 01424 718385
(Hastings and St Leonards Primary Care Trust)

Practice Manager Sally Moore

GP Hannah Eirlys HUGHES, Dr COOPER, Dr HIGGINSON, Dr SEAL

Wellington Square Medical Centre
45 Wellington Square, Hastings TN34 1PN
Tel: 01424 722866
(Hastings and St Leonards Primary Care Trust)
Patient List Size: 2530

Practice Manager Caz Taylor

GP Brian HIGGINSON

Hatfield

Burvill House Surgery
52 Dellfield Road, Hatfield AL10 8HP
Tel: 01707 269091 Fax: 01707 269300
(Welwyn Hatfield Primary Care Trust)
Patient List Size: 8300

Practice Manager Duncan Ferguson

GP Carol Ann RESTELL, Anne-Marie ANGUS, Geoffrey Stanley DAVIES, Neil Kevin DYTHAM, Vivian TANGANG, Thomas Hugh WILLSON

Lister House Surgery
The Common, Hatfield AL10 0NL
Tel: 01707 268822 Fax: 01707 263990
(Welwyn Hatfield Primary Care Trust)

Practice Manager Andrew McMenemy

GP Peter Edward OATES, Robert Vincent BROOKS, Lynn JAMES, Rachel KINSLER, Richard Charles William LAVELLE, Gareth Huw LEWIS, Gwen Katherine McDOWALL, Muralidharan RAJARATNAM

Potterells Medical Centre
Station Road, North Mymms, Hatfield AL9 7SN
Tel: 01707 273338 Fax: 01707 263564
(Welwyn Hatfield Primary Care Trust)
Patient List Size: 13500

Practice Manager Lillian Cross

GP Robert Anthony WIKNER, Claire HEATH, Sarah HOOLE, James RIDOUT, Mark Rider STEWARD

Wrafton House Surgery
Wrafton House, 9-11 Wellfield Road, Hatfield AL10 0BS
Tel: 01707 265454 Fax: 01707 272033
(Welwyn Hatfield Primary Care Trust)

Practice Manager Jenny Potton

GP Sek Chiew LIM, Dinesh Christopher Rex JAYESINGHE, Ann Marie KELLEY, Thamotheram NIMALARAJ

Havant

Greywells Surgery
15 Park Parade, Leigh Park, Havant PO9 5AA
Tel: 023 9247 4448 Fax: 023 9247 4458
(East Hampshire Primary Care Trust)

GP Carl Wyndham Robin ANANDAN

Havant Health Centre Suite A
PO Box 41, Civic Centre Road, Havant PO9 2AJ
Tel: 023 9245 1300 Fax: 023 9249 2524
Email: bosmeremedical@cs.com
Website: www.havanthealth.com
(East Hampshire Primary Care Trust)
Patient List Size: 15000

Practice Manager Sylvia Sowerby

GP Ronald Norman PEARSON, Terence Corduff ALLAN, Peter ALLEN, Felicity Jane BEDFORD, Caroline Jane KENNEDY-COOKE, Dirk KONIG, Michael John MACLEAN, David Harcourt MELVILLE, Brian Stuart ROBINSON

Havant Health Centre Suite C
PO Box 44, Havant PO9 2AT
Tel: 023 9247 4351 Fax: 023 9249 2104
(East Hampshire Primary Care Trust)
Patient List Size: 8000

Practice Manager Paula Russell

GP Cym Anthony RYLE, Claire BROADLEY, J A STOTT, Roger Malcolm SUTTON

Havant Health Centre Suite D
Suite D, Havant Health Centre, Havant PO9 2AP
Tel: 023 9247 5010 Fax: 023 9247 5570

(East Hampshire Primary Care Trust)
Patient List Size: 3170

Practice Manager Estelle Brans

GP Alan Ian Neil McNEILL, Karen SIZER

Havant Health Centre Suite E

PO Box 40, Havant PO9 2AG
Tel: 023 9247 5778 Fax: 023 9249 2392
(East Hampshire Primary Care Trust)

GP Mukul CHAUDHURI, Clare Elizabeth MORRISON, Damian Patrick TIMMS

The Homewell Practice

Havant Health Centre Suite B, PO Box 43, Havant PO9 2AQ
Tel: 023 9248 2124 Fax: 023 9247 5515
(East Hampshire Primary Care Trust)
Patient List Size: 12500

Practice Manager Avril Reynolds

GP John Richard HUGHES, Neil Antony BALL, Emma Caroline BOWLEY, Michael John CORBIN, Janier GARCIA, Brian MAGEE, Peter Richard WILLICOMBE

Middle Park Medical Centre

15 Middle Park Way, Leigh Park, Havant PO9 4AB
Tel: 023 9261 1055 Fax: 023 9278 2389
(East Hampshire Primary Care Trust)
Patient List Size: 3800

Practice Manager Susan Burbridge

GP Mohamed John HAZELDENE

Park Lane Medical Centre

82 Park Lane, Bedhampton, Havant PO9 3HN
Tel: 023 9247 4777 Fax: 023 9245 1394
(East Hampshire Primary Care Trust)

Practice Manager Tracy Elgar

GP Nigel Basil TORODE

Haverhill

Christmas Maltings Surgery

Camps Road, Haverhill CB9 8HF
Tel: 01440 702203 Fax: 01440 712198
(Suffolk West Primary Care Trust)
Patient List Size: 9600

Practice Manager Marion McLaine

GP Charles Andrew CORNISH, David Hugh DONOVAN, Nicola Mary MANN, Simon Timothy SMITH, Paul Seamus STEPHENSON

Christmas Maltings Surgery

Camps Road, Haverhill CB9 8HF
Tel: 01440 702010 Fax: 01440 714761
(Suffolk West Primary Care Trust)

Practice Manager Daphne Summers

GP Harry Bonthala MOHAN, Matthew Francis Martin LAWFIELD, Jonathan Neville SELBY, John Byron SERVANT

Clements Surgery

Greenfields Way, Haverhill CB9 8LU
Tel: 01440 702462 Fax: 01440 712112
(Suffolk West Primary Care Trust)

Practice Manager Yvonne Mayes

GP Bernard PIAT, Carolyn Louise PLATT, Robert WHELAN

Steeple Bumpstead Surgery

Bowers Hall Estate, Steeple Bumpstead, Haverhill CB9 7ED
Tel: 01440 730235 Fax: 01440 730379
(Uttlesford Primary Care Trust)
Patient List Size: 2500

Practice Manager Margaret Barrett

GP J E RIDLEY, W R SLADE

Stourview Medical Centre

Crown Passage, High Street, Haverhill CB9 8BB
Tel: 01440 761177 Fax: 01440 714688
(Suffolk West Primary Care Trust)
Patient List Size: 3200

Practice Manager Pauline Efford

GP Ross WORTHINGTON

Hawes

Central Dales Practice

The Health Centre, Hawes DL8 3QR
Tel: 01969 667200/667149 Fax: 01969 667149
Website: www.centraldalespractice.co.uk
(Hambleton and Richmondshire Primary Care Trust)
Patient List Size: 4600

Practice Manager Clive West

GP Pamela Karen Anne WEST, Jonathan Keith FRANCE, Adrian Clive Nicholas JONES, Jonathan Hugh PAIN

Hayes

Botwell Lane Surgery

238 Botwell Lane, Hayes UB3 2AP
Tel: 020 8573 0808 Fax: 020 8571 9199
(Ealing Primary Care Trust)

GP Raj Singh CHANDOK, Kawal MOHAN, Gulbash SINGH

Brookside Medical Centre

Brookside Road, Hayes UB4 0PL
Tel: 020 8848 4262 Fax: 020 8848 9263
(Hillingdon Primary Care Trust)

GP Michael Adesegun AKIN-TAYLOR

The Cedas Brook Practice

11 Kingshill Close, Hayes UB4 8DD
Tel: 020 8845 7100 Fax: 020 8842 4401
(Hillingdon Primary Care Trust)
Patient List Size: 7000

GP Brett Morgan THOMAS, Jane Margaret CARTER, Patricia Bernadette HURTON, James Gerard KENNEDY, Susan Kristina THURLOW

Elers Road Health Clinic

Elers Road, Hayes UB3 1NY
Tel: 020 8561 4473 Fax: 020 8569 0738
(Hillingdon Primary Care Trust)

GP Harhajan Kaur SIRA

Glendale Medical Centre

155 High Street, Harlington, Hayes UB3 5DA
Tel: 020 8897 8288/0724 Fax: 020 8754 1539
(Hillingdon Primary Care Trust)
Patient List Size: 5000

Practice Manager Margaret Mulhern

GP Heather Gail CAMPBELL, Kamlesh MEHTA, Mayur Kumar NANAVATI, David TRYTHALL

Heathrow Medical Centre

1 St Peters Way, Harlington, Hayes UB3 5AB
Tel: 020 8745 1555 Fax: 020 8754 1626
(Hillingdon Primary Care Trust)
Patient List Size: 4000

Practice Manager Devi Rajan

GP M N RAJAN

Kincora Practice

Kincora, 134 Coldharbour Lane, Hayes UB3 3HG
Tel: 020 8573 2092 Fax: 020 8573 4627
(Hillingdon Primary Care Trust)
Patient List Size: 3000

Practice Manager A K Marld

GP AtmakUr Narsimhulu GOUD

Kinsgway Surgery
17 Kingsway, Hayes UB3 2TT
Tel: 020 8573 3934 Fax: 020 8813 7034
(Hillingdon Primary Care Trust)
Patient List Size: 3500

Practice Manager Soraiya Rahmaan

GP Bashir M A DODHY

Lansbury Drive Practice
166 Lansbury Drive, Hayes UB4 8SG
Tel: 020 8848 3858 Fax: 020 8573 2082
(Hillingdon Primary Care Trust)

GP Syed Arif QUADRI, Reva GUDI, Amed KAMALUDDIN

North Hyde Road Surgery
167 North Hyde Road, Hayes UB3 4NF
Tel: 020 8573 8560 Fax: 020 8569 0551
(Hillingdon Primary Care Trust)

GP Simria TANVIR

Old Station Road Surgery
157 Old Station Road, Hayes UB3 4NA
Tel: 020 8573 2037/1200 Fax: 020 8813 7552
(Hillingdon Primary Care Trust)

GP Chandubhai Bhailalbhai PATEL, Mita MUKERJEE, Surendra K VERMA, Kshama Hemant VYAS

Shakespeare Avenue Surgery
75 Shakespeare Avenue, Hayes UB4 0BE
Tel: 020 8573 6042 Fax: 020 8569 3293
(Hillingdon Primary Care Trust)

Practice Manager Jenny Cook

GP Thekkinkattil MADHAVAN

Station Road Surgery
259 Station Road, Hayes UB3 4JE
Tel: 020 8573 9787 Fax: 020 8561 5152
(Hillingdon Primary Care Trust)

GP Padma Rekha KANTHAN

Townsfield Doctors Surgery
Hayes Community Campus, Uxbridge College, 34 College Way, Hayes UB3 3DZ
Tel: 020 8573 2365/0483 Fax: 020 8576 4461
(Hillingdon Primary Care Trust)
Patient List Size: 7200

Practice Manager Josh Ruparelia

GP Vrajlal Kalyanji RUPARELIA, Mohamed ADEM, Mehboobali I SALEH, Gurdas Rai SETHI, Krishna K SETHI

The Warren Practice
The Warren, Uxbridge Road, Hayes UB4 0SF
Tel: 020 8573 2476/1781 Fax: 020 8561 3461
(Hillingdon Primary Care Trust)

GP Hemlata Ashokkumar PATEL, Delair Hassan KHIDER, Rajany SIVANATHAN, Peter John STEPHENS

The Willow Tree Surgery
2 Jollys lane, Hayes UB4 9NS
Tel: 020 8842 1024 Fax: 020 8841 8030
(Hillingdon Primary Care Trust)
Patient List Size: 4200

GP Anita SINHA

Yadanabon Surgery
234 Coldharbour Lane, Hayes UB3 3HH
Tel: 020 8573 9101 Fax: 020 8573 5155
(Hillingdon Primary Care Trust)
Patient List Size: 2000

GP A Y E AYE NAING

Yeading Court Practice
1-2 Yeading Court, Masefield Lane, Hayes UB4 5AJ
Tel: 020 8845 1515 Fax: 020 8841 1171
(Hillingdon Primary Care Trust)

Practice Manager Lynne Casey

GP Thakur Das RAJU, Kolanu Anantha REDDY

Yeading Lane Practice
346 Yeading Lane, Hayes UB4 9AY
Tel: 020 8845 8866 Fax: 020 8845 4581
(Hillingdon Primary Care Trust)

Practice Manager Bhavna Joshi

GP Jayendra P JOSHI

Hayle

Bodriggy Health Centre
60 Queens Way, Bodriggy, Hayle TR27 4PB
Tel: 01736 753136 Fax: 01736 753467
Email: irene.luzmore@bodriggy-hayle.cornwall.nhs.uk
(West of Cornwall Primary Care Trust)
Patient List Size: 9520

Practice Manager Irene Luzmore

GP Michael James Edward HIGGS, J EVANS, Nicholas Henry GIBSON, C JONES, Anne Margaret MASKELL, Jane SLATER, Nigel John WHITEHOUSE

Hayling Island

The Health Centre
Elm Grove, Mengham, Hayling Island PO11 9AP
Tel: 023 9246 8413 Fax: 023 9263 7013
(East Hampshire Primary Care Trust)

Practice Manager Janice Matthews

GP Robert Henry Morrah WILLIAMS, James Duncan MITCHELL

The Health Centre
Elm Grove, Mengham, Hayling Island PO11 9AP
Tel: 023 9246 6216 Fax: 023 9263 7013
(East Hampshire Primary Care Trust)

Practice Manager Jane Austin

GP Andrew John STRATFORD, Colin TURNER

The Health Centre
Elm Grove, Mengham, Hayling Island PO11 9AP
Tel: 023 9246 6224 Fax: 023 9246 6079
(East Hampshire Primary Care Trust)
Patient List Size: 8500

Practice Manager Hazel Timms

GP Andrew Donald MOSSMAN, Gayle Avis CATTERALL, Sam Thomas DAVID, Richard John THOMAS

Haywards Heath

Cuckfield Medical Centre
Glebe Road, Cuckfield, Haywards Heath RH17 5BQ
Tel: 01444 458738 Fax: 01444 416714
(Mid Sussex Primary Care Trust)
Patient List Size: 6700

Practice Manager Cindy Franzel

GP Michael Robert HARVEY, Nicholas James BARRIE, Angie GURNER, Robert Alexander Hamilton HARVEY, Anita RAKHIT

Dumbledore Surgery
High Street, Handcross, Haywards Heath RH17 6BN
Tel: 01444 400243 Fax: 01444 401461
(Mid Sussex Primary Care Trust)
Patient List Size: 5200

Practice Manager Vivienne de Pemberton

GP Robert Philip MORRIS, Stephen Ronald COX, Janet Elizabeth HARDINGHAM, Louise McMINN, Caroline Margaret SMITH

The Medical Centre
High Street, Lindfield, Haywards Heath RH16 2HX
Tel: 01444 457666 Fax: 01444 483887
(Mid Sussex Primary Care Trust)

Practice Manager C Howard, Y McCulloch

GP Andrew Stephen HARDING, Stephen Robert ALDEN, J DONALD, Anthony James LAWRENCE, Andrew Graham Maxwell READER

Newtons
The Health Centre, Heath Road, Haywards Heath RH16 3BB
Tel: 01444 412280 Fax: 01444 416943
Email: val@newtons.mistral.co.uk
Website: www.newtonspractice.co.uk
(Mid Sussex Primary Care Trust)
Patient List Size: 11600

Practice Manager Mandy Day

GP Robert Bruce Hamilton LAMBERT, William George FULFORD, Philip Charles HART, Clare JONES, Francis John MITCHINSON, Kyle Hadley Victor NAGENDRA, Janet Anne WHILE

Northlands Wood Practice
7 Walnut Park, Haywards Heath RH16 3TG
Tel: 01444 458022 Fax: 01444 415960
(Mid Sussex Primary Care Trust)
Patient List Size: 5000

Practice Manager Stephanie Fisk

GP Elizabeth Mary JENKINS, Ian Michael ATKINSON, John SIMMONS

Heanor

Brooklyn Medical Practice
65 Mansfield Road, Heanor DE75 7AL
Tel: 01773 712552 Fax: 01773 531545
(Amber Valley Primary Care Trust)

GP G FINCH, Alastair Baker GRAHAM, Robert MANLEY, Marcus James WILKINSON

Kelvingrove Medical Centre
28 Hands Road, Heanor DE75 7HA
Tel: 01773 713201 Fax: 01773 534380
(Amber Valley Primary Care Trust)

GP James NOBLE, Lesley Anne FOSKETT, Stuart MELLOR, Alan WALKER

Park Surgery
60 Ilkeston Road, Heanor DE75 7DX
Tel: 01773 531011 Fax: 01773 534440
(Amber Valley Primary Care Trust)
Patient List Size: 7800

Practice Manager Jane Wharton

GP Ilyas AHMED, Jayne GOODLASS, Richard LODGE, John M TOMPKINSON

Heathfield

The Firs
Cross in Hand, Heathfield TN21 0LT
Tel: 01435 862021 Fax: 01435 867522
(Sussex Downs and Weald Primary Care Trust)

GP Charles Henry REID, Marilyn Elena CASARES

Manor Oak Surgery
Horebeech Lane, Horam, Heathfield TN21 0DS
Tel: 01435 812116 Fax: 01435 813737
(Sussex Downs and Weald Primary Care Trust)
Patient List Size: 4000

Practice Manager Jackie Smith

GP Sharon PALMER, Marilyn CASARES

The Surgery
96-98 High Street, Heathfield TN21 8JD
Tel: 01435 864999/862192 Fax: 01435 867449
(Sussex Downs and Weald Primary Care Trust)
Patient List Size: 12092

Practice Manager Brenda Pittman

GP Simon Mark WADMAN, Graham Neil McCONKEY, Richard PERTWEE, Martin Christopher ROGERS, Yvonne Margaret UNDERHILL, Marcus VAN ZUTPHEN, Caroline Mary WOODS

Hebburn

Campbell Park Surgery
Campbell Park Road, Hebburn NE31 2SP
Tel: 0191 451 6241 Fax: 0191 451 6252
(South Tyneside Primary Care Trust)

Practice Manager J Hitchson

GP S BOLL, L JOWETT

Hebburn Health Centre
Campbell Park Road, Hebburn NE31 2SP
Tel: 0191 4516233 Fax: 0191 4838652
(South Tyneside Primary Care Trust)
Patient List Size: 7500

GP Brian Richard WITHINGTON, Martin BRADY, Kit-Mei NICHOLLS, Christopher John OLIPHANT, J SYEPHERS

Mountbatten Medical Centre
12 Victoria Road West, Hebburn NE31 1LD
Tel: 0191 451 6266 Fax: 0191 451 6256
(South Tyneside Primary Care Trust)
Patient List Size: 6500

Practice Manager R Whitehead

GP Martin BURNS, Alison Hilary MINCHIN, Maxwell STEEL

Victoria Medical Centre
12-28 Glen Street, Hebburn NE31 1NU
Tel: 0191 483 2106 Fax: 0191 428 5270
(South Tyneside Primary Care Trust)
Patient List Size: 4100

Practice Manager June Thoresen

GP Inder Paul VINAYAK, Veena VINAYAK

Hebden Bridge

Valley Medical Centre
Valley Road, Hebden Bridge HX7 7BZ
(Calderdale Primary Care Trust)

Practice Manager Angela Worobell

GP Dr BURLEY, Dr DAVIES, Dr GOOCH, Dr GRAINGER, Dr HEBDEN, Dr MOORE, Dr SMITH-MOORHOUSE, Dr TAYLOR, Dr WILD

Heckmondwike

Albion Street Surgery
10 Albion Street, Heckmondwike WF16 9LQ
Tel: 01924 402073
(North Kirklees Primary Care Trust)
Patient List Size: 2800

Practice Manager Yvonne Warren

GP B AHMAD

Brookroyd House Surgery
Cook Lane, Heckmondwike WF16 9JG
Tel: 01924 403061 Fax: 01924 411687
Email: john.pickford@gpB85014.nhs.uk
(North Kirklees Primary Care Trust)

Patient List Size: 10006

GP David James YOUD, David John FINDLAY, David KELLY, Nigel Andrew MYERS

Helston

Helston Medical Centre

Helston Medical Centre, Trelawney Road, Helston TR13 8AU
Tel: 01326 572637 Fax: 01326 565525
Email: marisa.etwell@HMC.cornwall.nhs.uk
(West of Cornwall Primary Care Trust)
Patient List Size: 11547

Practice Manager Marisa Etwell

GP John Digby LANSDOWNE, Linda Ann DAVIES, Richard Charles DRUMMOND, Judith DUCKWORTH, Andrew HILLARY, Judith HINDLEY, Frances OLD, Rodney Stewart SMITH

Mengage Street Surgery

100 Mengage Street, Helston TR13 8RF
Tel: 01326 435888 Fax: 01326 563310
(West of Cornwall Primary Care Trust)
Patient List Size: 6105

Practice Manager Linda Granger

GP Brian LAWTON, Rosemary Anne SHELLEY, A THOMEY, Marion Siobhan WILLIAMS

Mullion Health Centre

Willis Vean, Mullion, Helston TR12 7DQ
Tel: 01326 240212 Fax: 01326 242102
Email: chris.gilbert@mullion.cornwall.nhs.uk
(West of Cornwall Primary Care Trust)
Patient List Size: 5229

Practice Manager Christopher Gilbert

GP Christopher Michael CUFF, Robert Ian EDGERLEY, James Philip OLIVER

Porthleven Surgery

Sunset Gardens, Porthleven, Helston TR13 9BT
Tel: 01326 562204 Fax: 01326 569222
Email: marisa.etwell@HMC.cornwall.nhs.uk
(West of Cornwall Primary Care Trust)
Patient List Size: 3216

Practice Manager Marisa Etwell

GP Richard C DRUMMOND, Judy DUCKWORTH

St Keverne Health Centre

St Keverne, Helston TR12 6PB
Tel: 01326 280205 Fax: 01326 280710
(West of Cornwall Primary Care Trust)
Patient List Size: 2835

Practice Manager Frances Hough

GP Penelope Ann BARTON, Kate GEARING

Hemel Hempstead

Archway Surgery

52 High Street, Bovingdon, Hemel Hempstead HP3 0HJ
Tel: 01442 833380 Fax: 01442 832093
Email: archway@careprovider.com
Website: www.archway.nhs.uk
(Dacorum Primary Care Trust)
Patient List Size: 2653

Practice Manager Mary McMinn

GP Gerard Vincent Mathias BULGER, Janet CRABTREE, Philip EDWARDS

Bennetts End Surgery

Gatecroft, Hemel Hempstead HP3 9LY
Tel: 01442 63511 Fax: 01442 235419
Website: www.besteam.co.uk
(Dacorum Primary Care Trust)
Patient List Size: 18000

GP Michael John DRAKE, Elisabeth Ann BRAZIER, Victoria Rosalina CRANE, Paul Trevor HEATLEY, Zuzanna Helena HURST, David Brian KERRY, Lian Sin LIM, Kathryn June Chantrell McFARLANE, James Henry NODDER

Coleridge Crescent Surgery

2 Coleridge Crescent, Woodhall Farm Estate, Hemel Hempstead HP2 7PQ
Tel: 01442 234220
(Dacorum Primary Care Trust)
Patient List Size: 2100

Practice Manager E Luke

GP Shailendra Kumar BHATT

Everest House Surgery

Everest Way, Hemel Hempstead HP2 4HY
Tel: 01442 240422 Fax: 01442 235045
(Dacorum Primary Care Trust)
Patient List Size: 12700

Practice Manager Margaret Ambrose

GP Ian McLean ROYSTON, Matthew John Gunton BUNN, Alison CARR, Paula COYLE, Harold Cheung Yin HA, Yera SHAH, Berndine Gesiene TIPPLE, David TURNER

Fernville Surgery

Midland Road, Hemel Hempstead HP2 5BL
Tel: 01442 213919 Fax: 01442 216433
(Dacorum Primary Care Trust)
Patient List Size: 12000

Practice Manager Mark Jones

GP Rajinder Singh BHAMRA, Joanne EGGLEDEN, Keith HODGE, Rajeshkumar MAPARA, Adrian Scott RICHARDSON, Ann Patricia SHIPLEY-ROWE, Janet Ruth WRIGHT

Grovehill Medical Centre

Kilbride Court, Hemel Hempstead HP2 6AD
Tel: 01442 212038
(Dacorum Primary Care Trust)
Patient List Size: 4455

Practice Manager Elizabeth Keenan

GP Fatehali Merali HIRJI, Hussein Issak KHATRI, Vimal TIMARI

Highfield Surgery

The Heights, Jupiter Drive, Hemel Hempstead HP2 5NU
Tel: 01442 265322 Fax: 01442 256641
(Dacorum Primary Care Trust)
Patient List Size: 4602

Practice Manager Kalyami Mishra

GP Krishna Mohan MISHRA, Elizabeth CRASKE, Meenakshi Premchand SAVLA

Lincoln House Surgery

Wolsey Road, Hemel Hempstead HP2 4TU
Tel: 01442 254366 Fax: 01442 244554
(Dacorum Primary Care Trust)

Practice Manager Linda Haskard

GP Lynne DYSON, Jill Carolyn ALLISTONE, G BENSON, Topan DUTTA, B LAWSON, T STRONGER

The Surgery

Parkwood Drive, Warners End, Hemel Hempstead HP1 2LD
Tel: 01442 250117 Fax: 01442 256185
(Dacorum Primary Care Trust)
Patient List Size: 16600

Practice Manager Colin Heal

GP Henrietta ANTSCHERL, Jonathan Charles BRAZIER, Trevor Don FERNANDES, Richard Jonathan GALLOW, Richard Jonathan GALLOW, Penelope Rachel OLIVER, Helena PATTISON, Mark Andrew PECK, Gary SOLOMONS, Susan STIER, Catherine Louise WARD, Genie Yasmin WHITE

Woodhall Health Centre
Valley Green, Off Shenley Road, Hemel Hempstead HP2 7RJ
Tel: 01442 61805 Fax: 01442 261750
(Dacorum Primary Care Trust)
Patient List Size: 3500

Practice Manager Anne Khan

GP Mir Alam Khan KHATTAK

Henfield

Henfield Medical Centre
Deer Park, Henfield BN5 9JQ
Tel: 01273 492255 Fax: 01273 495050
Website: www.henfieldmedicalcentre.co.uk
(Horsham and Chanctonbury Primary Care Trust)
Patient List Size: 8900

Practice Manager Katie Hill

GP Evelyn Patrick Edgeworth READE, Karen Elizabeth CRAWFORD-CLARKE, Jonathan Duncan DERRETT, Anna Catherine HAYLETT, Malcolm Stuart McLEAN, John Robin NORMAN

Henley-on-Thames

The Bell Surgery
York Road, Henley-on-Thames RG9 2DR
Tel: 01491 843250 Fax: 01491 411295
(South East Oxfordshire Primary Care Trust)
Patient List Size: 9000

Practice Manager Cathy Ronald

GP Terence Patrick DUDENEY, Peter Anthony ASHBY, Elizabeth COLLETT, Marie Clare CRAIK, Christopher Norman M LANGLEY, Virginia Joan STEPHENS

Dr Terris and Partners
The Hart Surgery, York Road, Henley-on-Thames RG9 2DR
Tel: 01491 843200 Fax: 01491 411296
(South East Oxfordshire Primary Care Trust)

Practice Manager Cathy Ronald

GP Alexander James McDonnell TERRIS, Clare ALSOP, Jenifer Ann Marie Ryan COPELAND, Juan A MARTINEZ, Julia Mary MILLIGAN, Roger Philip UNWIN

McWhirter, Barton and Silver
The Surgery, Wanbourne Lane, Nettlebed, Henley-on-Thames RG9 5AJ
Tel: 01491 641204 Fax: 01491 641162
Email: nettlebed.practice.manager@gp-k8405.nhs.uk
(South East Oxfordshire Primary Care Trust)
Patient List Size: 3600

Practice Manager Pat Ashmore

GP James Holman McWHIRTER, Julie Hilda BARTON, Lisa Rebecca SILVER

Henlow

The Surgery
109 Station Road, Lower Stondon, Henlow SG16 6JJ
Tel: 01462 850305 Fax: 01462 851858
(Bedfordshire Heartlands Primary Care Trust)
Patient List Size: 4748

GP R PURITZ, H COLLINS

Hereford

Belmont Medical Centre
Eastholme Avenue, Belmont, Hereford HR2 7XT
Tel: 01432 354366 Fax: 01432 340434
(Herefordshire Primary Care Trust)

Practice Manager S Matthews

GP Paul HARRIS, Elizabeth COOMBS, Andrew Grahame JONES, Richard Luke Westall KIPPAX

Cantilupe Surgery
49-51 St. Owen Street, Hereford HR1 2JB
Tel: 01432 268031 Fax: 01432 352584
(Herefordshire Primary Care Trust)
Patient List Size: 10850

Practice Manager Julie Burgens

GP Richard John HENDERSON, David GOODFELLOW, Jill Caroline GOODFELLOW, Mark Medlicott HELME, Susan Mary MARSDEN, Clare SCOTCHER, Mark Richard WATERS, Janie WILSON

Forest Road Medical Centre
Forest Road, Hay-on-Wye, Hereford HR3 5DS
Tel: 01497 822100 Fax: 01497 822110
(Herefordshire Primary Care Trust)
Patient List Size: 7800

Practice Manager Ros Gittoes

GP Sean O'REILLY, Antonia BRADLEY, Nansi-Wynne Davies EVANS, Julie GRIGG, Peter Alfred HORVATH-HOWARD, Mary Rothwell HUGHES, James WRENCH

Fownhope Medical Centre
Commonhill Lane, Fownhope, Hereford HR1 4PZ
Tel: 01432 860235 Fax: 01432 860900
(Herefordshire Primary Care Trust)
Patient List Size: 4390

Practice Manager Penny Crossley

GP Christopher John ALLEN, Alison WOOD

Greyfriars Surgery
25 St. Nicholas Street, Hereford HR4 0BH
Tel: 01432 265717 Fax: 01432 340150
(Herefordshire Primary Care Trust)
Patient List Size: 5422

Practice Manager Valerie Hinder

GP Christopher William FRITH, Stephen John ADAMS, Saadi HASAN, Pamela Ruth YOUNG

King Street Surgery
22A King Street, Hereford HR4 9DA
Tel: 01432 272181 Fax: 01432 344725
(Herefordshire Primary Care Trust)
Patient List Size: 8994

Practice Manager Janet Jennings

GP Adrian John EYRE, S CLEGG, Catherine Jane Frances LAIRD, Ian William Millward ROPER, Mark TURNBULL, A WILLIAMS

Moorfield House Surgery
35 Edgar Street, Hereford HR4 9JP
Tel: 01432 272175 Fax: 01432 341942
(Herefordshire Primary Care Trust)

Practice Manager Ann Hodges

GP Patrick John MATTHEWS, Timothy Charles BARLING, Jonathan Mark DUFFETT, Richard Baillie LAIRD, Diana MAJEED, Anthony McNeill ORR

Quay House Medical Centre
100 Westfaling Street, Hereford HR4 0JF
Tel: 01432 352600 Fax: 01432 340320
(Herefordshire Primary Care Trust)

Practice Manager Deborah Newman

GP David Paul LANGFORD, Martin John Murless KNIGHT, James George MACKIE

Sarum House Surgery
3 St. Ethelbert Street, Hereford HR1 2NS
Tel: 01432 265422 Fax: 01432 358440
(Herefordshire Primary Care Trust)
Patient List Size: 11000

Practice Manager Jean Harrison

GP Julian Guy WHEELER, Fiona CHATAWAY, Andrew John HEAL, Jennifer Ann LITCHFIELD, David Middlemore MALINS, Andrew Charles WATTS

The Surgery
Kingstone, Hereford HR2 9HN
Tel: 01981 250215 Fax: 01981 251189
(Herefordshire Primary Care Trust)

Practice Manager Ann Ellis

GP Jonathan Duncan SLEATH, Richard Graham WARNER

The Surgery
Ewyas Harold, Hereford HR2 0EU
Tel: 01981 240320 Fax: 01981 241023
(Herefordshire Primary Care Trust)
Patient List Size: 5680

Practice Manager Ruth Truelove

GP Benjamin Peter RICHARDSON, Carol BATHURST, Richard Lanfear GRIFFITHS, Nicholas John LATTEY

The Surgery
Much Birch, Hereford HR2 8HT
Tel: 01981 540310 Fax: 01981 540748
(Herefordshire Primary Care Trust)
Patient List Size: 4700

Practice Manager M C G M Willis

GP Peter Richard GARLICK, David Michael DAVIES, Vanessa ENGLAND, Andrea JOHNSON

The Surgery
Staunton-on-Wye, Hereford HR4 7LT
Tel: 01981 500227 Fax: 01981 500603
(Herefordshire Primary Care Trust)
Patient List Size: 5300

Practice Manager Sheila Devlin

GP Oliver James St. John PENNEY, Michael Charles BRACEBRIDGE, R CUTLER, R M PENNEY, R A SYKES

Watt and Partners
Wargrave House, 23 St. Owen Street, Hereford HR1 2JB
Tel: 01432 272285 Fax: 01432 344059
Website: www.wargravehousesurgery.co.uk
(Herefordshire Primary Care Trust)
Patient List Size: 9650

Practice Manager Carol Steele

GP Iain Douglas WATT, Nigel Bruce FRASER, Abigail Clare GOODWIN, Michael Leofric JOHNSON, Sarah Jane JOHNSON, C JONES, Michael John MASLEN, K SMITH

Herne Bay

The Coach House Surgery
27 Canterbury Road, Herne Bay CT6 5DQ
Tel: 01227 374040 Fax: 01227 741544
(Canterbury and Coastal Primary Care Trust)

Practice Manager P Perry

GP Simon Michael Webster WHARFE, Patrick John GARROD, Sabine Odette STUBGEN

The Park Surgery
116 Kings Road, Herne Bay CT6 5RE
Tel: 01227 742200 Fax: 01227 742277
Email: philip.murray@gp-g82119.nhs.uk
(Canterbury and Coastal Primary Care Trust)
Patient List Size: 13100

Practice Manager Philip Murray

GP Arthur Wilfred PRINCE, John Neville BROWN, Roxana DIDEHVAR, Georgette GERDES, Robin Michael Hamilton JENKINS, Hugh MATTHEWS, Marion J NICHOLS, Amanda SCARLETT, R G SIGURDSSON

St Annes Group Practice
161 Station Road, Herne Bay CT6 5NF
Tel: 01227 742226 Fax: 01227 741439
(Canterbury and Coastal Primary Care Trust)
Patient List Size: 14559

Practice Manager Dawn Simmons

GP Roger WHEELDON, Christopher John BRIAN, Huw Rhys CLEVERLEY, Simon John DUNN, S McLUCKIE, Justin Bruce Kingsley PARSLOE, Philip RANGER, John Paul RINE, Sallyanne ROBLIN

William Street Surgery
67 William Street, Herne Bay CT6 5NR
Tel: 01227 740000 Fax: 01227 742729
(Canterbury and Coastal Primary Care Trust)
Patient List Size: 5500

Practice Manager Kerry Gunney

GP Ian William RITCHIE, A Murray McGREGOR

Hertford

Castlegate Surgery
42 Castle Street, Hertford SG14 1HH
Tel: 01992 589928 Fax: 01992 501430
(South East Hertfordshire Primary Care Trust)

Practice Manager Liz Watson

GP Lawrence Joseph WATSON, Susan Joan GREATREX, Giles PRATT

Hanscombe House Surgery
52A St Andrew Street, Hertford SG14 1JA
Tel: 01992 582025 Fax: 01992 305511
(South East Hertfordshire Primary Care Trust)
Patient List Size: 9400

Practice Manager Janine Ellis

GP Katharine Joyce CORLETT, C BROWN, Ian Richardson McCLURE, Anita Paulette OATES, Philip John TAYLOR

Wallace House Surgery
5-11 St Andrew Street, Hertford SG14 1HZ
Tel: 01992 550541 Fax: 01992 557600
(South East Hertfordshire Primary Care Trust)
Patient List Size: 13000

Practice Manager Denise Dilley

GP Jan Antoni CEMBALA, Kathryn ATWILL, David Ian CROSSTHWAITE, John Ransford EAMES, G McCABE, David James Stuart McLEES, Richard John MOBLEY

Ware Road Surgery
77 Ware Road, Hertford SG13 7EE
Tel: 01992 414500 Fax: 01992 504623
(South East Hertfordshire Primary Care Trust)

Practice Manager Heather Wren

GP Catherine Mary STOTT, Dr HORSMAN, Jane Louisa Mary TITCOMBE, Andrew William WHITE

Watton Place Clinic
60 High Street, Watton-at-Stone, Hertford SG14 3TA
Tel: 01920 830232 Fax: 01920 830005
(South East Hertfordshire Primary Care Trust)
Patient List Size: 4800

Practice Manager Sue Meaker

GP David William HASLAM, Dilesh SHAH

Hessle

The Health Centre
11 Hull Road, Hessle HU13 9LU
Tel: 01482 645295 Fax: 01482 649513
(East Yorkshire Primary Care Trust)
Patient List Size: 13000

Practice Manager Denise Dukes

GP Alistair Charles ROBERTSON, Laurent M J BARÉ, Neuri MAGUET, Donal Ulick O'SULLIVAN, Janet Mary SHERMAN, Krishnaraj SIVARAJAN

Park View Surgery
87 Beverley Road, Hessle HU13 9AJ
Tel: 01482 648552 Fax: 01482 642600
(East Yorkshire Primary Care Trust)
Patient List Size: 3750

Practice Manager Pauline Marshall

GP J S HOWARD, D F TURPIN

The Surgery
80 Hull Road, Hessle HU13 9LU
Tel: 01482 646581 Fax: 01482 645509
(East Yorkshire Primary Care Trust)

Practice Manager Helena Hutchinson

GP Yassin ADHAMI

Hexham

Allendale Health Centre
Shilburn Road, Allendale, Hexham NE47 9LG
Tel: 01434 683280 Fax: 01434 683884
(Northumberland Care Trust)

GP M J I'ANSON, Gerald MORROW

Burn Brae Surgery
Hencotes, Hexham NE46 2ED
Tel: 01434 603627 Fax: 01434 606373
(Northumberland Care Trust)
Patient List Size: 8200

Practice Manager Simon Guy

GP Peter WILLIS, Timothy Alan CARNEY, Eleanor Jean GALLAGHER, David Thomas GRAHAM, Celia Dorothy HELLIWELL, Florence Mary Noreen POWELL

Haydon Bridge Health Centre
North Bank, Haydon Bridge, Hexham NE47 6HG
Tel: 01434 684216 Fax: 01434 684144
Email: sford-hb@dircon.co.uk
Website: www.sford-hb.dircon.co.uk/hc
(Northumberland Care Trust)
Patient List Size: 3295

Practice Manager Marion Wilson

GP Steven Duncan FORD, Michelle GEORGE, Mary Theresa HENDERSON, Gail YOUNG

Hlimshaugh and Wark Medical Group
The Surgery, Wark, Hexham NE48 3LS
Tel: 01434 230654 Fax: 01434 230059
(Northumberland Care Trust)
Patient List Size: 4100

Practice Manager Norah Phipps

GP Neville Kenneth KEEP, Trevor ALKON, John Parlane Kinloch McCOLLUM, Hayley WRIGHT

Middleton and Partners
Sele Gate Surgery, Hencotes, Hexham NE46 2EG
Tel: 01434 602237 Fax: 01434 609496
Email: admin@gp-A84033.nhs.uk
(Northumberland Care Trust)
Patient List Size: 6120

Practice Manager Norman Davidson

GP Christopher Stephen Hugh MIDDLETON, Janet Suzanne GOLD, Barrie Dudley HARTE, Matthew Craig WALKER

The Surgery
Bellingham, Hexham NE48 2HE
Tel: 01434 220203 Fax: 01434 220798
(Northumberland Care Trust)
Patient List Size: 2900

GP Derek Stewart BLADES, Lesley A DUKE, Amanda L GRAY, Iain James MUNGALL, Joanna J THOMPSON

Heywood

Argyle Street Surgery
141 Argyle Street, Heywood OL10 3SD
Tel: 01706 366135 Fax: 01706 627706
(Heywood and Middleton Primary Care Trust)

GP Susan Louise BUNTING, Christopher John DUFFY, Oscar NAVARRO SERRANO, Temujin ONON

Hopwood Medical Centre
1-3 Walton Street, Hopwood, Heywood OL10 2BS
Tel: 01706 369886 Fax: 01706 627619
(Heywood and Middleton Primary Care Trust)
Patient List Size: 3700

Practice Manager Adele Hardacre

GP Patricia Anne ADSHEAD, Elizabeth Sara OSBORNE

Longford Street Group Practice
Longford Street, Heywood OL10 4NH
Tel: 01706 621417 Fax: 01706 622915
(Heywood and Middleton Primary Care Trust)

Practice Manager Ray Guy

GP John Anthony GIBSON, Eamon Martin MOONEY, Myroslav Roman PARASHCHAK, Stefanie Katrina POKINSKYJ, Anthony WILLIAMS, Elizabeth WILLIAMS

York Street Surgery
19 York Street, Heywood OL10 4NN
(Heywood and Middleton Primary Care Trust)

GP M B TAYLOR

High Kelling

Holt Medical Practice
Kelling Hospital, Old Cromer Road, High Kelling NR25 6BH
Tel: 01263 712461 Fax: 01263 713211
Website: www.holt-practice.co.uk
(North Norfolk Primary Care Trust)
Patient List Size: 14000

Practice Manager Rosemary Scott

GP Andrew Charles CHAPMAN, Alison Clare BROOKS, Peter BRUEGGEMANN, Jayne Deborah COOPER, Henry Burton CRAWLEY, Peter Keith FRANKLIN, Steven John GROVE, P HARVEY, Andrew LATTEN

High Peak

Goyt Valley Medical Practice
Chapel Street, Whaley Bridge, High Peak SK23 7SR
Tel: 01663 732911 Fax: 01663 735702
(High Peak and Dales Primary Care Trust)
Patient List Size: 7700

Practice Manager Margaret Farrer

GP David John RIDDELL, Andrew David BARTHOLOMEW, Stuart John BOOTLE, Jane Alison HOLDERNESS

The Surgery
15 New Mills Road, Hayfield, High Peak SK22 2JG
Tel: 01663745030 Fax: 01663741248
(High Peak and Dales Primary Care Trust)
Patient List Size: 3500

Practice Manager Anna Houareau

GP Dr KARMUIRMISTRY, David POWELL

High Wycombe

Benjamin Road Surgery
22 Benjamin Road, High Wycombe HP13 6SR
Tel: 01494 534524
(Wycombe Primary Care Trust)
Patient List Size: 2200

Practice Manager J Allim

GP Raouf Masud ALLIM

Carrington House Surgery
19 Priory Road, High Wycombe HP13 6SL
Tel: 01494 526029 Fax: 01494 538299
(Wycombe Primary Care Trust)

Practice Manager Helen Morris-Khan

GP Mary BEGLEY, Dennis Gutteridge SMITH, Andrew James BURTON, Nicola Jill INMAN

Cherrymead Surgery
17 Straight Bit, Flackwell Heath, High Wycombe HP10 9LS
Tel: 01628 522838 Fax: 01628 529255
(Wycombe Primary Care Trust)
Patient List Size: 9400

GP Kirteen FRASER, Kristina KING, Graham LANG, June Christine MORETTO

Chiltern House Medical Centre
45-47 Temple End, High Wycombe HP13 5DN
Tel: 01494 450691 Fax: 01494 530483
(Wycombe Primary Care Trust)
Patient List Size: 10500

Practice Manager Steve Howard

GP Edward Charles BRAY, Wim AMIR, Pilar GARCIA, Mohamed MUBARAK, Jennifer Helen TAOR, Mark Hans TWEEDY

Desborough Avenue Surgery
65 Desborough Avenue, High Wycombe HP11 2SD
Tel: 01494 526006 Fax: 01494 473569
(Wycombe Primary Care Trust)

Practice Manager Angela Wilkie

GP Richard Nicholas REIDY, Zoe Anne BLAIR, Nadarajah NAVANEETHAM, Harjeev RAI, Pedro Jose VALVERDE LUQUE

The Health Centre
Stokenchurch, High Wycombe HP14 3TG
Tel: 01494 483633 Fax: 01494 483690
(Wycombe Primary Care Trust)

Practice Manager C Glenn

GP James Andrew WALTER, Geoffrey Nicholas David COWLAND, Josephine DUDLEY, Katie HANNAFORD

Highfield Surgery
Highfield Way, Hazlemere, High Wycombe HP15 7UW
Tel: 01949 813396 Fax: 01949 814107
(Wycombe Primary Care Trust)

GP Nigel James MASTERS, Jacqueline Susan MAXMIN, Jacqueline OPENSHAW

Hughenden Valley Surgery
Valley Road, Hughenden, High Wycombe HP14 4
Tel: 01494 563275 Fax: 01494 565165
(Chiltern and South Bucks Primary Care Trust)

Practice Manager Barbara A Renouf

GP Mary MITCHELL, Sara COTTAM, Joanne HERBERT, Lynnette HYKIN, Savelia SEVONA, Penny SUTCLIFFE

Kingswood Surgery
Hollis Road, Totteridge, High Wycombe HP13 7UN
Tel: 01494 474783 Fax: 01494 438424
(Wycombe Primary Care Trust)
Patient List Size: 7500

Practice Manager Lee Richardson

GP Elaine Niven BAXTER, Jane Frances BERRY, Annet Petrina GAMELL, Katherine Ann KUHN, David WALTON

Lynton House Surgery
43 London Road, High Wycombe HP11 1BP
Tel: 01494 527036/538811/510117 Fax: 01494 447070
(Wycombe Primary Care Trust)
Patient List Size: 6000

Practice Manager Alan R Titchener

GP Mohammed ANZAK, Shahid AMIN

Pound House Surgery
8 The Green, Wooburn Green, High Wycombe HP10 0EE
Tel: 01628 529633 Fax: 01628 810963
(Wycombe Primary Care Trust)
Patient List Size: 6930

Practice Manager Juliette Knott

GP Peter Brian HAVELOCK, Elizabeth BAILEY, Anne BISSELL, Raj THAKKAR, Sally WILLIAMS

Priory Avenue Surgery
24-26 Priory Avenue, High Wycombe HP13 6SH
Tel: 01494 448132 Fax: 01494 686407
Email: priory.surgery@virgin.net
(Wycombe Primary Care Trust)
Patient List Size: 12500

Practice Manager Susan Doricott

GP Allen William John MEDHURST, Francis Henderson ARMITAGE, Nigel Francis BACON, Jennifer Ruth CANDY, Duncan George GRAHAM, Keith George LETHBRIDGE, Alison Mary NICE

Riverside Surgery
George Street, High Wycombe HP11 2RZ
Tel: 01494 526500 Fax: 01494 450237
(Wycombe Primary Care Trust)
Patient List Size: 10300

Practice Manager Carol Wotherspoon

GP Daphne Margaret SCOTT, Angela May HART, John Roydon HORNER, Ajit Gordon Vimalendran KADIRGAMAR, Rosalind McALLISTER, Rashmi SAWHNEY, Thillaimpalam SIVARAMALINGAM

The Surgery
Finings Road, Lane End, High Wycombe HP14 3ES
Tel: 01494 881209
(Wycombe Primary Care Trust)
Patient List Size: 4500

GP Nicola Anne ELEY, Heather Mary Royston DAVIS, John EVANS

Tower House Surgery
169 West Wycombe Road, High Wycombe HP12 3AF
Tel: 01494 526840
(Wycombe Primary Care Trust)
Patient List Size: 8000

Practice Manager Hilary Smith

GP Peter John LOWE, Christopher Mark BINNS, Christopher David FOORD, Stephanie WHITEHEAD

Wye Valley Surgery
2 Desborough Avenue, High Wycombe HP11 2RN
Tel: 01494 521044 Fax: 01494 472770
Website: www.wyevalleysurgery.co.uk
(Wycombe Primary Care Trust)
Patient List Size: 10400

Practice Manager D Stallwood

GP Michael Henry BOWKER, Hasan ALY, Frances Clare CARTER, Azhar HAMEED, Bernadette HAYNES, Waquar HUSSAIN, Russell MANAPUZHA

Highbridge

Brent Area Medical Centre

Anvil House, Brent Road, East Brent, Highbridge TA9 4JD
Tel: 01278 760313 Fax: 01278 760753
Email: bamc@globalnet.co.uk
(Somerset Coast Primary Care Trust)
Patient List Size: 2700

Practice Manager Judy Dury

GP Siw Lwin AUNG, Carol Ann REYNOLDS

Highbridge Medical Centre

Pepperall Road, Highbridge TA9 3YA
Tel: 01278 783220 Fax: 01278 795486
Email: john.down@highbridgemc.nhs.uk
Website: www.hbmc.co.uk
(Somerset Coast Primary Care Trust)
Patient List Size: 12800

Practice Manager John Down

GP Mieczyslaw Jerzy BIZON, Stuart John ANDERSON, Ciaran Mary CLAPHAM, Martin Christopher EDWARDS, Richard Anthony GRIFFITH, Geoffrey Mark TROWELL

Hinckley

Burbage Surgery

Tilton Road, Burbage, Hinckley LE10 2SE
Tel: 01455 634879 Fax: 01455 619860
(Hinckley and Bosworth Primary Care Trust)
Patient List Size: 8500

Practice Manager Wendy J Shaw

GP Pulin Behari MAITY, D A JONES, Samir Kumar SIL, Wayne Mark TURNER

Castle Mead Medical Centre

Hill Street, Hinckley LE10 1DS
Tel: 01455 637659 Fax: 01455 238754
(Hinckley and Bosworth Primary Care Trust)
Patient List Size: 9107

GP Ralph Andrew YARDLEY, R GLASTONBURY, Fay Julie SUTTON, D TULL, Nicholas John WILLMOTT

Centre Surgery

Hinckley Health Centre, 27 Hill Street, Hinckley LE10 1DS
Tel: 01455 632277 Fax: 01455 890635
(Hinckley and Bosworth Primary Care Trust)
Patient List Size: 6000

Practice Manager E R Dale

GP Christopher GILBERTHORPE, Andrew DALE, Pragna SOLANKI

Dr A M Parkinson and Partners

Station View Health Centre, Southfield Road, Hinckley LE10 1UA
Tel: 01455 635362 Fax: 01455 619797
(Hinckley and Bosworth Primary Care Trust)
Patient List Size: 12700

Practice Manager Rod Prior

GP Adrian Michael PARKINSON, C ALEXANDER, Colleen Alston ALEXANDER, Helen HOWES, Sally JOHNSON, Rachel REID, Victor Laurie ROWE, Rodney Harry Lewen WARNER

Hollycroft Medical Centre

Clifton Way, Hollycroft, Hinckley LE10 0XN
Tel: 01455 234414
(Hinckley and Bosworth Primary Care Trust)
Patient List Size: 3100

Practice Manager Jean Caiger

GP Bhupinder Singh SACHA

Maples Family Medical Practice

35 Hill Street, Hinckley LE10 1DS
Tel: 01455 234576 Fax: 01455 250506
(Hinckley and Bosworth Primary Care Trust)
Patient List Size: 10944

Practice Manager Mary Newman

GP Ian Douglas CRACKNELL, Jane Elizabeth ALUN-JONES, John HARRISON, Ashitkumar Kantilal KOTHARI, Ganesh SHANBHAG, Anil Kumar SOOD

Hindhead

The Grayshott Surgery

Boundary Road, Grayshott, Hindhead GU26 6TY
Tel: 01428 604343
(Guildford and Waverley Primary Care Trust)

GP Keith Graham HANCOCK, Nigel John Douglas BALDOCK, Lance Christian CAVANNAGH, Simon John DUNBAR, Claire Brigitte PATTEN, David Edward TOBIN, Joanna Susan TOMES

Hitchin

High Street Surgery

60 High Street, Whitwell, Hitchin SG4 8AG
Tel: 01438 871398 Fax: 01438 871505
(North Hertfordshire and Stevenage Primary Care Trust)
Patient List Size: 2200

GP David Peter ARCHER

Larksfield Surgery

Arlesey Road, Stotfield, Hitchin SG5 4HB
Tel: 01462 732200 Fax: 01462 832715
(Bedfordshire Heartlands Primary Care Trust)

GP Dr SEAMAN, Dr HODGSON, Dr LEWIS, Dr LINCOLN, Dr RADFORD

Orford Lodge Surgery

100 Bancroft, Hitchin SG5 1ND
Tel: 01462 432042 Fax: 01462 436505
(North Hertfordshire and Stevenage Primary Care Trust)
Patient List Size: 8700

Practice Manager Eve Gibbins

GP Michael Anthony SLATTERY, Jeremy Patrick Halton COX, Margaret Claire GILVARRY, Subir ROHATGI

The Portmill Surgery

114 Queen Street, Hitchin SG4 9TH
Tel: 01462 434246 Fax: 01462 441246
(North Hertfordshire and Stevenage Primary Care Trust)
Patient List Size: 14000

Practice Manager E J Morrison

GP Gerald TIDY, Jehad Taha ALDEGHATHER, Robin Andrew Stark CHRISTIE, Felicity COOPER, Roger Martin INGRAM, Neil Philip KENDELL, Carol KENNY

Regal Chambers Surgery

50 Bancroft, Hitchin SG5 1LL
Tel: 01462 453232 Fax: 01462 631536
(North Hertfordshire and Stevenage Primary Care Trust)
Patient List Size: 12300

Practice Manager Jill T Berkley

GP John MACHEN, David J BARRATT, Alastair J CRUICKSHANK, K DAVY, Victoria G FRASER, A T HERBERT, Christine Noel RYECART, Joseph Edward TURNER, Mark A VORSTER

The Surgery

Marshall House, Bancroft Court, Hitchin SG5 1LH
Tel: 01462 420740
(North Hertfordshire and Stevenage Primary Care Trust)
Patient List Size: 6637

Practice Manager Denise Robson

GP Keith Brian GREENISH, Michael Shaun CARRAGHER, David Paul WILLIAMS

Hockley

Greensward Surgery
Greensward Lane, Hockley SS5 5HQ
Tel: 01702 202353 Fax: 01702 204535
(Castle Point and Rochford Primary Care Trust)
Patient List Size: 6600

Practice Manager Y A Dray

GP Trevor Percival REES, Martin George RICH, Lidya SARSAM, Nosheen WAHEED

Riverside Medical Centre
175 Ferry Road, Hullbridge, Hockley SS5 6JH
Tel: 01702 230555 Fax: 01702 231207
(Castle Point and Rochford Primary Care Trust)
Patient List Size: 7003

Practice Manager David Bell

GP Peter Stanley CORNES, Sylvia CONNER, Dr DONNELLY

Hoddesdon

Amwell Street Surgery
19 Amwell Street, Hoddesdon EN11 8TS
Tel: 01992 464147 Fax: 01992 708698
(South East Hertfordshire Primary Care Trust)
Patient List Size: 12000

GP Ian Michael Kelvin HISCOCK, Andrew Wallace DAVIES, J LAUBLE, Christopher Sean MAYS, Joanne Linda ROBERTS, Mary Ruth WENLEY

The Limes Surgery
8-14 Limes Court, Conduit Lane, Hoddesdon EN11 8EP
Tel: 01992 464533 Fax: 01992 470729
(South East Hertfordshire Primary Care Trust)
Patient List Size: 11227

Practice Manager Christine Price

GP Fiona Judith HENDERSON, Mark ANDREWS, Colin Philip BLANKFIELD, Rodney Frederick BRITTAN, Tessa Meriel DORMON, G PARKES

Ware Road Surgery
59 Ware Road, Hoddesdon EN11 9AB
Tel: 01992 463363 Fax: 01992 471108
(South East Hertfordshire Primary Care Trust)

Practice Manager Alison Stevens

GP Brenda BAXTER, Bhupendra Shambhuprasad VYAS, Christopher WADDINGTON, David Andrew WILLIS

Holsworthy

Bradworthy Surgery
The Square, Bradworthy, Holsworthy EX22 7SY
Tel: 01409 241215 Fax: 01409 241086
(North Devon Primary Care Trust)
Patient List Size: 3000

Practice Manager Belinda Waggett

GP John Bowring BETTS, Ranjan KANDASAMY

Holsworthy Medical Centre
Dobles Lane, Holsworthy EX22 6GH
Tel: 01409 253692 Fax: 01409 254184
(North Devon Primary Care Trust)

Practice Manager Peter McLean

GP Alan John EDWARDS, Jonathan COPE, Gretel Kathryn GREEN-ARMYTAGE, David Kenneth HILLEBRANDT, Richard James PAGE, Robert Frederick SHAW, Rosalind Mary WARDLE

Honiton

Honiton Surgery
Marlpits Lane, Honiton EX14 2NY
Tel: 01404 41141 Fax: 01404 46621
(East Devon Primary Care Trust)

Practice Manager Christine Baugh

GP David PENWARDEN, Paul C BARBER, Phil T COURTNEY, Sarah A EVANS, David S J RAMPERSAD, Anne P SAUNDERS, Clare P SEAMARK, David A SEAMARK, Fiona M SHORT, David G WARD, Janet A WARD

Hook

Hook and Hartley Wintney Medical Partnership
1 Chapter Terrace, Hartley Wintney, Hook RG27 8QJ
Tel: 01252 842087 Fax: 01252 843145
Website: www.hartleywintneysurgery@nhs.uk
(Blackwater Valley and Hart Primary Care Trust)
Patient List Size: 15300

Practice Manager Louise Greenwood

GP Howard Christopher Charles BARNS, Andrea Elizabeth CLAY, Andrew Mark FERNANDO, Edward Bernard GONCALVES-ARCHER, Christopher James HUNTER, Charlotte Anne HUTCHINGS, Sarah Frances LONGSTAFF, David Muir LOVE, Jane Louise THOMPSON

Odiham Health Centre
Deer Park View, Odiham, Hook RG29 1JY
Tel: 01256 702371 Fax: 01256 701180
(Blackwater Valley and Hart Primary Care Trust)
Patient List Size: 8500

Practice Manager Moira Clark

GP Anthony David WEAVER, Raffi ASSADOURIAN, N EBRAHIM, Isobel Joyce GOOLD, Claudia Ruth SHAND

Hope Valley

Evelyn Medical Centre
Marsh Avenue, Hope, Hope Valley S33 6RJ
Tel: 01433 621557 Fax: 01433 621745
(High Peak and Dales Primary Care Trust)
Patient List Size: 6062

GP D J MOSELEY, T J ADLER, B E HOWSON, D I HUTCHINSON

The Surgery
Church Street, Eyam, Hope Valley S32 5QH
Tel: 01433 630836 Fax: 01433 631832
(High Peak and Dales Primary Care Trust)

Practice Manager S L Murden

GP Dr JACKSON, Dr GOODWIN, Dr IZARD

Horley

The Health Centre
Kings Road, Horley RH6 7DG
Tel: 01293 772686 Fax: 01293 823950
(East Surrey Primary Care Trust)
Patient List Size: 15500

Practice Manager Christine Earwaker

GP Richard John OLLIVER, Sheila Georgina HOLE, James Humphry HOUSE

Smallfield Surgery
Wheelers Lane, Smallfield, Horley RH6 9PT
Tel: 01342 843382/22 Fax: 01342 844080
(East Surrey Primary Care Trust)
Patient List Size: 4800

Practice Manager Judith Brown

GP Terence Anthony CONATY, M BOSCH, Lucinda Anne COOK, H J DIACK, Elaine Margaret JENKINS, M MUELLER

Wayside Surgery
12 Russells Crescent, Horley RH6 7DN
Tel: 01293 782057 Fax: 01293 821809
(East Surrey Primary Care Trust)
Patient List Size: 4050

Practice Manager Helen Saunders

GP Jonathan Keith DORMER, Richard Douglas Charles WILLIAMSON

Horncastle

The Old Vicarage
Spilsby Road, Horncastle LN9 6AL
Tel: 01507 522477 Fax: 01507 522997
(East Lincolnshire Primary Care Trust)

GP Timothy WATKINS, Lee BURMAN, James Ranald Carr CAMPBELL, Keith GRUNDY, Simon Mihill READ

The Wolds Practice
Tetford, Horncastle LN9 6QP
Tel: 01507 533133 Fax: 01507 533489
(East Lincolnshire Primary Care Trust)
Patient List Size: 2300

Practice Manager Cereda Kemp

GP Yvonne Eleanor Mary OWEN, David SMITH

Hornchurch

Cosyhaven
Cecil Avenue, Hornchurch RM11 2LY
Tel: 01708 476011 Fax: 01708 471735
(Havering Primary Care Trust)

Practice Manager J Flasz

GP Malcolm Hyam FLASZ

Dr M M Rahman
The Surgery, 482 Southend Road, Hornchurch RM12 5PA
Tel: 01708 476036 Fax: 01708 471330
(Havering Primary Care Trust)
Patient List Size: 2810

Practice Manager Laila Rahman

GP Muhammad Mahbubur RAHMAN

Maylands Healthcare
300 Upper Rainham Road, Hornchurch RM12 4EQ
Tel: 01708 476411 Fax: 01708 620039
(Havering Primary Care Trust)
Patient List Size: 14500

Practice Manager Linda Ennis

GP Stuart BRANDMAN, Helen Jane CARRUTHERS, Keith Stanley KENDALL, Nikhil Ramananda RAO, Atul AGGARWAL, Pamela ARASU

Rosewood Medical Centre
30 Astra Close, Elm Park, Hornchurch RM12 5NJ
Tel: 01708 554557
(Havering Primary Care Trust)

Practice Manager L Shea, Norman Smith, J Thorogood

GP Parayath SETHU, Jennifer Anjali BARBOSA, Jonathan Joseph MANASCO, S OGANWU, Helen Margaret VIVERS

The Surgery
221 High Street, Hornchurch RM11 3XT
Tel: 01708 447747 Fax: 01708 451408
(Barking and Dagenham Primary Care Trust)
Patient List Size: 5300

Practice Manager Anila Dattani

GP Hamida ASADULLAH

The Surgery
58B Billet Lane, Hornchurch RM11 1XB
Tel: 01708 442377 Fax: 01708 447362
(Havering Primary Care Trust)
Patient List Size: 4415

Practice Manager Carole Osborne, Rita Walsh

GP Timothy Charles BLAND, Gopa MITRA, Ann QUAGHEBEUR

The Surgery
38 Easedale Drive, Elm Park, Hornchurch RM12 5HJ
Tel: 01708 451585 Fax: 01708 459287
Email: alaklata.jaiswal@nhs.net
(Havering Primary Care Trust)
Patient List Size: 2300

Practice Manager M Gleeson

GP Alak Lata JAISWAL

The Surgery
39 Wood Lane, Elm Park, Hornchurch RM12 5HX
Tel: 01708 450902 Fax: 01708 470875
(Havering Primary Care Trust)
Patient List Size: 4662

GP Janet Christine Edith CAIRA, Ashok Rangrao DESHPANDE

The Surgery
140 Station Lane, Hornchurch RM12 6LU
Tel: 01708 440780 Fax: 01708 455489
(Havering Primary Care Trust)

Practice Manager N S Gillet-Waller

GP Qurban Husain Abbasbha GILLET-WALLER

The Surgery
24 Suttons Avenue, Hornchurch RM12 4LF
Tel: 01708 442711 Fax: 01708 471756
(Havering Primary Care Trust)

Practice Manager Elaine Dawkins

GP Pravinkumar Maganbhai PATEL, Amy QUEGHEBEUR

The Surgery
9 Glanville Drive, Hornchurch RM11 3SZ
Tel: 01708 442117 Fax: 01708 620095
(Havering Primary Care Trust)
Patient List Size: 3800

Practice Manager Pat Williams

GP Vijaykumar Maganbhai PATEL

The Surgery
30 Dorian Road, Hornchurch RM12 4AN
Tel: 01708 470791 Fax: 01708 472737
(Havering Primary Care Trust)

Practice Manager Val Wickes

GP S UBEROY, V K UBEROY

The Surgery
106 Ardleigh Green Road, Hornchurch RM11 2LG
Tel: 01708 476455 Fax: 01708 479485
(Havering Primary Care Trust)

GP H McDONALD, D ACHESON, J LEE, A R McDONALD, K MINOCHA, S ZACHARIAH

Upminster Bridge Surgery
126 Upminster Road, Hornchurch RM12 6PL
Tel: 01708 440642 Fax: 01708 477329
Email: johnomoore@doctors.org.uk
(Havering Primary Care Trust)
Patient List Size: 2950

GP John O'MOORE

Hornsea

Eastgate Medical Group
37 Eastgate, Hornsea HU18 1LP
Tel: 01964 532212 Fax: 01964 535007
Email: jn86@dial.pipex.com
(Yorkshire Wolds and Coast Primary Care Trust)
Patient List Size: 11700

Practice Manager Carol Brocklebank

GP Paul Irving COLLINGWOOD, Emma Elizabeth DAWBER, David John GARWOOD, Colin Martin HANNA, Paul David PHILLIPS, Ian Clifford SIBLEY-CALDER

Horsham

Courtyard Surgery
The Courtyard, London Road, Horsham RH12 1AT
Tel: 01403 253100 Fax: 01403 267480
(Horsham and Chanctonbury Primary Care Trust)
Patient List Size: 6000

Practice Manager Diana Hartley

GP Ronald Innes WATSON, Mark René CHOPIN, Iain Donald McNEIL

Holbrook Surgery
Bartholomew Way, Horsham RH12 5JL
Tel: 01403 755900 Fax: 01403 755909
Email: holbrookgp@bigfoot.com
Website: www.horsham.co.uk/holbrook.htm
(Horsham and Chanctonbury Primary Care Trust)
Patient List Size: 13650

Practice Manager Heather Heatley

GP Jonathan Patrick HEATLEY, Christopher HEATH, H LIU, Aijaz Ahmed SHEIKH, Ann Elisabeth WILLIAMS, Paul Michael WOODS, N ZIYADA

Orchard Surgery
Lower Tanbridge Way, Horsham RH12 1PJ
Tel: 01403 253966 Fax: 01483 266237
(Horsham and Chanctonbury Primary Care Trust)

Practice Manager Clive Farringham

GP John Christopher DAWE, Sadhana BRYDIE, Joanna Merrill CLEMENT, Nigel David HILLS, Richard Jack William LEWIS

Orchards Surgery
Black Horse Way, Horsham RH12 1SG
(Horsham and Chanctonbury Primary Care Trust)

GP J C DAWE

Park Surgery
Albion Way, Horsham RH12 1BG
Tel: 01403 217100 Fax: 01409 214 639
Website: www.parksurgery.com
(Horsham and Chanctonbury Primary Care Trust)

Practice Manager Paula Salerno

GP David Gordon SKIPP, John Edward CLARKE, Simon John DEAN, Elizabeth FISHER, Stephen Robert FISHER, David William HOLWELL, Tariq JAHANGIR, Christina KING

Riverside Surgery
48 Worthing Road, Horsham RH12 1UD
Tel: 01403 264848 Fax: 01403 276386
(Horsham and Chanctonbury Primary Care Trust)
Patient List Size: 7750

Practice Manager Trica Brennan

GP Tanya Katherine Susan LAWSON, Josephine DEBONO, Michael Robert HOWARD, Sarah Jane WILLIAMS

Rudgwick Medical Centre
Station Road, Rudgwick, Horsham RH12 3HB
Tel: 01403 822103 Fax: 01403 823017
(Western Sussex Primary Care Trust)
Patient List Size: 3500

Practice Manager Mary Hamilton, S Knight

GP William James JARRATT, Susan Jane WIGHTMAN

The Surgery
St Peters Close, Cowfold, Horsham RH13 8DN
Tel: 01403 864204 Fax: 01403 864408
(Mid Sussex Primary Care Trust)
Patient List Size: 4609

Practice Manager Margaret Dolman

GP John Francis DARCY, Meera Elizabeth SMETHURST

Village Surgery
Station Road, Southwater, Horsham RH13 9HQ
Tel: 01403 730016 Fax: 01403 730660
(Horsham and Chanctonbury Primary Care Trust)
Patient List Size: 5950

Practice Manager Mary Compson

GP Gabrielle Joan WILLIAMS, Eileen GRAY, Nigel Jeremy Adrian KING-TOURS, Ian Colin POTHECARY

Houghton-le-Spring

Grangewood Surgery
Chester Road, Shiney Row, Houghton-le-Spring DH4 4RB
Tel: 0191 385 2898 Fax: 0191 385 82565
(Sunderland Teaching Primary Care Trust)
Patient List Size: 6010

Practice Manager Joan Moseby

GP Alan Stewart WALLACE, K L BAYLIS, Carol GRAY, John Charles Shafto MACKAY, Julia ROBSON

Herrington Medical Centre
Philadelphia Lane, Houghton-le-Spring DH4 4LE
Tel: 0191 584 2632 Fax: 0191 584 3786
(Sunderland Teaching Primary Care Trust)
Patient List Size: 6802

Practice Manager Julie Oxenham

GP Richard James LILLEY, Keith Graham BIRRELL, P HOWDEN, Jane Sarah PETERSEN, Mary Gerardine QUINN

Hetton Group Practice
Hetton Medical Centre, Francis Way, Hetton-le-Hole, Houghton-le-Spring DH5 9EZ
Tel: 0191 526 1177 Fax: 0191 517 3859
(Sunderland Teaching Primary Care Trust)
Patient List Size: 12601

Practice Manager Joan Smithson

GP Helen Mary PEPPER, Martin Anthony BALDASERA, J L BEM, T SLADEK, James Bennett STANCLIFFE, M E STANLEY, Caspar Maurits Dieuwert VAN BUUREN

Houghton Medical Group
Church Street, Houghton-le-Spring DH4 4DN
Tel: 0191 584 2154 Fax: 0191 584 1074
(Sunderland Teaching Primary Care Trust)
Patient List Size: 7629

Practice Manager Kim Christie

GP John Gerald WATTERS, Dr AITKEN, Dr CRAWFORD, Dr MORGAN

Kepier Medical Practice
Houghton le Spring, Leyburn Grove, Houghton-le-Spring DH4 4DN
Tel: 0191 584 2106 Fax: 0191 584 9493
(Sunderland Teaching Primary Care Trust)
Patient List Size: 9453

GP Sameh Kameel MISHREKI, H M ANCLIFF, J E ANCLIFF, Richard Angus GOUDIE, Paul Joseph LINNETT, S PARKS, Rosemary Houghton PRUDHOE

Westbourne Medical Group
Gill Crescent North, Fencehouses, Houghton-le-Spring DH4 6AW
Tel: 0191 385 2508 Fax: 0191 385 8243
(Sunderland Teaching Primary Care Trust)
Patient List Size: 6791

Practice Manager Giona Middleton

GP Dr MUTHU, M P HUBBARD, M THAIAYASINGHAM

Westbourne Surgery
Kelso Grove, Shiney Row, Houghton-le-Spring DH4 4RW
Tel: 0191 385 2512 Fax: 0191 385 8810
(Sunderland Teaching Primary Care Trust)
Patient List Size: 6791

Practice Manager Gloria Middleton

GP Bala Subramaniam MUTHU, Michael Patrick HUBBARD, Marie Edna Laleeni THALAYASINGAM

Woodland View Surgery
Woodland View, West Rainton, Houghton-le-Spring DH4 6RQ
Tel: 0191 584 3809 Fax: 0191 584 9177
(Durham and Chester-le-Street Primary Care Trust)
Patient List Size: 6500

Practice Manager Brenda Hall

GP Anthony SARTORIS, Sally Ann Pheasey CARMICHAEL, John Charles NICHOLSON, Graeme WYLIE

Hounslow

Basildene Road Surgery
26 Basildene Road, Hounslow TW4 7LE
Tel: 020 8570 9609 Fax: 020 8572 0935
(Hounslow Primary Care Trust)

GP Ujvala CAPOOR, Bhasker Chunibhai PATEL

Bath Road Surgery
303 Bath Road, Hounslow TW3 3DB
Tel: 020 8570 3620 Fax: 020 8569 4933
(Hounslow Primary Care Trust)
Patient List Size: 2704

GP Krishana Mohan SINGH

Bath Road Surgery
134 Bath Road, Hounslow TW3 3ET
Tel: 020 8577 9035 Fax: 020 8577 9200
(Hounslow Primary Care Trust)
Patient List Size: 5000

GP S K MAYOR

The Beaver's Centre for Health
117-119 Beavers Lane, Hounslow TW4 6HF
(Hounslow Primary Care Trust)
Patient List Size: 1382

Practice Manager Carey Musgrove

GP A KAVE, Dr NASIR

Clifford Road Surgery
65 Clifford Road, Hounslow TW4 7LR
Tel: 020 8577 5304 Fax: 020 8577 0626
(Hounslow Primary Care Trust)
Patient List Size: 3560

GP R K SINGH

Crane Park Medical Centre
748 Hanworth, Hounslow TW4 5NT
Tel: 020 8893 4567 Fax: 020 8893 8026
(Richmond and Twickenham Primary Care Trust)
Patient List Size: 2297

Practice Manager Savita Sinha

GP Vishwambhar Nath Prasad SINHA

Cranford Medical Centre
24 High Street, Cranford, Hounslow West, Hounslow TW5 9RG
Tel: 020 8564 8696 Fax: 020 8564 7891
(Hounslow Primary Care Trust)

GP Robert Mark CHAMBERS, S A MARWAHA, Alexander James MUNRO

Drs Coll, Patel and Kanani
Family Doctor Unit, 92 Bath Road, Hounslow TW3 3LN
Tel: 020 8577 9555 Fax: 020 8570 2266
(Hounslow Primary Care Trust)
Patient List Size: 8000

Practice Manager Emma Nicholls

GP Alison Jane COLL, Sanjay KANANI, Bijesh PATEL

Family Doctor Unit
92 Bath Road, Hounslow TW3 3LN
Tel: 020 8577 9666 Fax: 020 8577 0692
(Hounslow Primary Care Trust)

GP V PATEL, Dr JAIN, Dr THOMAS

Family Doctor Unit Surgery
92 Bath Road, Hounslow TW3 3LN
Tel: 020 8570 6271 Fax: 020 8570 3243
(Hounslow Primary Care Trust)

GP William Charles KING, Frances Mary MORAN, Avtar Singh NIJJAR

Family Doctor Unit Surgery
92 Bath Road, Hounslow TW3 3LN
Tel: 020 8577 9666 Fax: 020 8577 0692
(Hounslow Primary Care Trust)
Patient List Size: 4200

Practice Manager Satvir Kahlon

GP Payal JAIN, Vipin PATEL, Sarah THOMAS

Family Doctor Unit Surgery
92 Bath Road, Hounslow TW3 3LN
Tel: 020 8570 6270
(Hounslow Primary Care Trust)

GP Sukhpal Singh DHESI

Great West Road Surgery
222 Great West Road, Heston, Hounslow TW5 9AW
Tel: 020 8572 6859
(Hounslow Primary Care Trust)

GP J C A ARCHARD

Heston Health Centre
25 Cranford Lane, Heston, Hounslow West, Hounslow TW5 9ER
Tel: 020 8321 3414 Fax: 020 8321 3409
(Hounslow Primary Care Trust)

GP Tahir Javaid Nayeem BHATTI

Heston Health Centre
Cranford Lane, Heston, Hounslow West, Hounslow TW5 9ER
Tel: 020 8321 3411 Fax: 020 8321 3409
(Hounslow Primary Care Trust)
Patient List Size: 2000

Practice Manager Meera Sood

GP Sunil SOOD

Hibernia House Surgery
108 Hibernia Road, Hounslow East, Hounslow TW3 3RN
Tel: 020 8577 9697 Fax: 020 8577 2618
(Hounslow Primary Care Trust)
Patient List Size: 2890

GP U UPADHYAYA

The Jersey Practice
Heston Health Centre, Cranford Lane, Hounslow TW5 9ER
Tel: 020 8321 3434 Fax: 020 8321 3440
(Hounslow Primary Care Trust)

Patient List Size: 5700

GP D P TRIPATHI

Maswell Park Health Centre
Hounslow Avenue, Hounslow TW3 2DY
Tel: 020 8321 3482 Fax: 020 8893 4368
(Hounslow Primary Care Trust)
Patient List Size: 4800

Practice Manager Bridget Docking

GP Valerie Jane PHILIP, J P HOWES

Maswell Park Health Centre
Hounslow Avenue, Hounslow TW3 2DY
Tel: 020 8321 3488 Fax: 020 8893 4368
(Hounslow Primary Care Trust)
Patient List Size: 5200

Practice Manager Josie Martin

GP Paul Adrian SHENTON, Lesley SEDDON

Maswell Park Health Centre
Hounslow Avenue, Hounslow TW3 2DY
Tel: 020 8321 3476 Fax: 020 8893 4368
(Hounslow Primary Care Trust)
Patient List Size: 3400

Practice Manager Bridget Docking

GP Madeline Rose BAUM, Judith VICKERS

Maswell Park Health Centre
Maswell Park Health Centre, Hounslow Avenue, Hounslow TW3 2DY
Tel: 020 8321 3476 Fax: 020 8893 4368
(Hounslow Primary Care Trust)
Patient List Size: 3400

Practice Manager Anagi Rathasinghe

GP Mandy BAUM, J VICKERS

The Medical Centre
5 Cecil Road, Hounslow TW3 1NU
Tel: 020 8572 2536 Fax: 020 8570 3197
Email: dorismcmanu@gp-E85096.nhs.uk
(Ealing Primary Care Trust)
Patient List Size: 5900

Practice Manager K B McManus

GP Bhupinder Singh MANGAT, Surjit Kaur MANGAT

Parklands Parade Surgery
4 Parklands Parade, Bath Road, Hounslow TW5 9AX
Tel: 020 8570 4408 Fax: 020 8570 0669
(Hounslow Primary Care Trust)

GP K M THEIN

Skyways Medical Centre
2 Shelley Crescent, Hounslow TW5 9BJ
Tel: 020 8569 5688 Fax: 020 8577 9952
(Hounslow Primary Care Trust)
Patient List Size: 5000

Practice Manager Janet Griffith

GP Martin Robert TURNER, J H NEWMAN

The Surgery
77 Lampton Road, Hounslow TW3 4JX
Tel: 020 8572 1497 Fax: 020 8577 7322
(Hounslow Primary Care Trust)

GP Dr GARCHA

The Surgery
60 Broad Walk, Hounslow TW5 9AB
Tel: 020 8572 2324 Fax: 020 8571 9199
(Hounslow Primary Care Trust)
Patient List Size: 3722

Practice Manager I Nelson-Wright

GP Dr MELICHAR

The Surgery
Farnell House Practice, 25 Spring Grove Road, Hounslow TW3 4BE
Tel: 020 8577 7801/020 8577 2484 Fax: 020 8572 5272
Email: mohammed.anis@gp-E85062.nhs.uk
(Hounslow Primary Care Trust)
Patient List Size: 4000

GP H COPENHAGEN, B SHAH

Hove

Brunswick Surgery
18/19 Western Road, Hove BN3 1AE
Tel: 01273 772020 Fax: 01273 739851
(Brighton and Hove City Teaching Primary Care Trust)

Practice Manager Nula Kanal

GP Ruth BARKER, Christa BEESLEY

The Central Hove Surgery
3 Ventnor Villas, Hove BN3 3DD
Tel: 01273 744911 Fax: 01273 744929
(Brighton and Hove City Teaching Primary Care Trust)
Patient List Size: 4500

Practice Manager Gill Muncey

GP Paul Gabriel DALY, Geraldine ELCOMBE, Charlotte HALL

The Charter Medical Centre
88 Davigdor Road, Hove BN3 1RF
Tel: 01273 204059 Fax: 01273 220883
(Brighton and Hove City Teaching Primary Care Trust)

Practice Manager Margot Redwood

GP John Adrian CONDON, Paul Brian FORSDICK, Daniel JENKINSON, Jane JENKINSON, Jens PETZOLD, John ROGERS, Karina Louise TURNER, Katrina WATSON

Eaton Gardens Surgery
3 Eaton Gardens, Hove BN3 3TL
Tel: 01273 733620 Fax: 01273 774850
(Brighton and Hove City Teaching Primary Care Trust)

Practice Manager Annette Thornton

GP Lucy C FREE, T E GRACE, Nigel HIGSON, Milind R JANI, A A WELLS, J D WILLIAMSON

Goodwood Court Surgery
52 Cromwell Road, Hove BN3 3ER
Tel: 01273 328232/206911 Fax: 01273 207235
(Brighton and Hove City Teaching Primary Care Trust)

Practice Manager Annette Thornton

GP Nigel HIGSON, Tania GRACE, Milind JANI, Alec WELLS, John WILLIAMSON

Hove Medical Centre
West Way, Hove BN3 8LD
Tel: 01273 430088 Fax: 01273 430172
(Brighton and Hove City Teaching Primary Care Trust)
Patient List Size: 10000

Practice Manager Mary MacCabe

GP Michael John SHARMAN, Nicholas Liam BODKIN, Susan Jane MILLS

The Surgery
20 Sackville Road, Hove BN3 3FF
Tel: 01273 778585/736030 Fax: 01273 724648
(Brighton and Hove City Teaching Primary Care Trust)

Practice Manager Pamela Hadland

GP Edward James KING, Clive David BACH, Sunil Solomon EMMANUEL, Timothy Gavin McMINN

The Surgery
28 Wilbury Road, Hove BN3 3JP
Tel: 01273 733830 Fax: 01273 207424
(Brighton and Hove City Teaching Primary Care Trust)

Patient List Size: 850

Practice Manager Barbara Haywood

GP Duncan Bernard STEWART

The Surgery
124 New Church Road, Hove BN3 4JB
Tel: 01273 729194 Fax: 01273 881992
(Brighton and Hove City Teaching Primary Care Trust)
Patient List Size: 4300

Practice Manager Brian Smith

GP Nigel Adrian CHANNING, Paul Christopher EVANS, Sheryl Anne KNIGHT

The Surgery
145 Portland Road, Hove BN3 5QJ
Tel: 01273 734888 Fax: 01273 203232
(Brighton and Hove City Teaching Primary Care Trust)
Patient List Size: 1854

Practice Manager Lisa Waller

GP Krishna Sastrigal RUKMANI

The Surgery
18 Hove Park Villas, Hove BN3 6HG
Tel: 01273 776245 Fax: 01273 324202
(Brighton and Hove City Teaching Primary Care Trust)
Patient List Size: 3840

Practice Manager Jill Sinclair

GP Mary Helen STUART, William Alexander MANCEY-BARRATT

The Surgery
14 Burwash Road, Hove BN3 8GQ
Tel: 01273 739271 Fax: 01273 727786
(Brighton and Hove City Teaching Primary Care Trust)

Practice Manager Maureen Beech

GP Eric Joseph David HENDERSON

The Surgery
1 Onslow Road, Hove BN3 6TA
Tel: 01273 502379 Fax: 01273 502379
(Mid Sussex Primary Care Trust)

Practice Manager Jean Evans

GP David John Evan EVANS

The Surgery
39 Brunswick Street West, Hove BN3 1EL

GP John Brendan DONAGHY

Huddersfield

Almondbury Surgery
Westgate, Almondbury, Huddersfield HD5 8XJ
Tel: 01484 421391 Fax: 01484 532405
(Huddersfield Central Primary Care Trust)
Patient List Size: 5000

Practice Manager Carole Askham

GP Marcus Roman JABCZYNSKI, Jonathan Mark GURR, Susan Mary SPENCER

Bradford Road Surgery
93 Bradford Road, Huddersfield HD1 6DZ
Tel: 01484 300455 Fax: 01484 300455
(Huddersfield Central Primary Care Trust)
Patient List Size: 4600

Practice Manager Graham Jepson

GP M A BUTT, M S N AHMED

Church Lane Surgery
1 Church Lane, Newsome, Huddersfield HD4 6JE
Tel: 01484 514118
(Huddersfield Central Primary Care Trust)
Patient List Size: 6600

Practice Manager Sue Wilkinson

GP K CHATTOPADHYAY, Graeme EALES, Abdul Rahim Ahmed Said HAMID

Clifton House Surgery
1 Church Street, Golcar, Huddersfield HD7 4AQ
Tel: 01484 654100
(Huddersfield Central Primary Care Trust)
Patient List Size: 3000

GP Thayumanavar HARIHARAN, V HARIHARAN

Croft House Surgery
5 Croft House, 114 Manchester Road, Slaithwaite, Huddersfield HD7 5JY
Tel: 01484 842652 Fax: 01484 348223
(South Huddersfield Primary Care Trust)
Patient List Size: 6300

Practice Manager Josephine Anderson

GP Michael John WRIGHT, David John HINDLE, Susan Mary WALKER, Robert Barry WOODHEAD

Dalton Surgery
364A Wakefield Road, Dalton, Huddersfield HD5 8DY
Tel: 01484 530068
(Huddersfield Central Primary Care Trust)

GP Richard Douglas JENKINSON, Victoria Jane IVES, Christopher Paul MARTLAND

Dearne Valley Health Centre
Wakefield Road, Scissett, Huddersfield HD8 9JL
Tel: 01484 862793
(South Huddersfield Primary Care Trust)
Patient List Size: 3474

Practice Manager F G Draper

GP David SEELEY, Helen Clare ASH

Dr N Balendran
42 Westbourne Road, Marsh, Huddersfield HD1 4LE
Tel: 01484 426044 Fax: 01484 454541
(Huddersfield Central Primary Care Trust)
Patient List Size: 2119

Practice Manager Linda Hobson

GP Nadarajah BALENDRAN

Drs. O'Leary, Shortt, Littlewood and Mounsey
The Health Centre, Level 5, C S Building, University of Huddersfield, Queensgate, Huddersfield HD1 3DH
Tel: 01484 430386 Fax: 01484 473085
Email: health-centre@gp-B85062.nhs.uk
(South Huddersfield Primary Care Trust)
Patient List Size: 7100

Practice Manager Linda Uttley

GP M. A. O'LEARY, Jeff LITTLEWOOD, Sandy MOFFITT, Nicola L MOUNSEY, C V O'SHAUGHNESSY, Alan Martin SHORTT

Elmwood Health Centre
Huddersfield Road, Holmfirth, Huddersfield HD9 3TR
Tel: 01484 689111 Fax: 01484 689333
Website: www.elmwooddoctors.co.uk
(South Huddersfield Primary Care Trust)
Patient List Size: 7000

Practice Manager Ann Booker

GP John Richard CLAYDEN, James BUCKLE, Muhammad Yusuf Saleem SHAMSEE

Elmwood Health Centre
Huddersfield Road, Holmfirth, Huddersfield HD9 3TR
Tel: 01484 681777 Fax: 01484 689603
(South Huddersfield Primary Care Trust)

Practice Manager Roger Parkin

GP Philip Russell JENNISON, Robert Maurice AKAM, Gillian BRADLEY, Dawn Elizabeth HAZLEHURST, David Morgan HUGHES,

Cameron Douglas IRVING, Julie Elizabeth MANNING, Nicholas MARTIN

Fartown Green Road Surgery
34 Fartown Green Road, Fartown, Huddersfield HD2 1AE
Tel: 01484 534386
Email: smh@fartownsurgery.com
Website: www.fartownsurgery.com
(Huddersfield Central Primary Care Trust)

Practice Manager Asha Handa

GP Satish Mohan HANDA

Fieldhead Surgery
Fieldhead, Leymoor Road, Golcar, Huddersfield HD7 4QQ
Tel: 01484 654504 Fax: 01484 460296
Email: fieldhead@doctors.org.uk
(Huddersfield Central Primary Care Trust)
Patient List Size: 7350

Practice Manager Susan Robinson

GP Peter Patrick John FAULKNER, Sheila BENETT, Steven JOYNER

Greenhead Road Surgery
19 Greenhead Road, Huddersfield HD1 4EN
Tel: 01484 539088
(Huddersfield Central Primary Care Trust)
GP K REDDY

The Health Centre
Spaines Road, Fartown, Huddersfield HD2 2QA
Tel: 01484 544318
(Huddersfield Central Primary Care Trust)
Patient List Size: 10000

GP David George ANDERSON, Ailsa Elizabeth CARE, L M CONNOR, Jane Louise FORD, D H LATHAM, Shaun TUNSTALL

The Health Centre
Victoria Street, Marsden, Huddersfield HD7 6DF
Tel: 01484 844332 Fax: 01484 845779
(South Huddersfield Primary Care Trust)
Patient List Size: 4350

Practice Manager A Harmon

GP Andrew Robert DEACON, Helen Anne BENSON, Rachel Jane TOMLINSON

The Health Centre
Fieldhead, Shepley, Huddersfield HD8 8DR
Tel: 01484 602001 Fax: 01484 608125
(South Huddersfield Primary Care Trust)
Patient List Size: 6200

Practice Manager J R Kimberley

GP Richard Lees BUXTON, Leslie John ORME, Duncan Charles SHAW

The Health Centre
Spaines Road, Fartown, Huddersfield HD2 2QA
Tel: 01484 533314
(Huddersfield Central Primary Care Trust)

GP D DUTT

The Health Centre
Spaines Road, Fartown, Huddersfield HD2 2QA
Tel: 01484 530358
(Huddersfield Central Primary Care Trust)

GP Bhuyan BHUYAN

The Health Centre
Commercial Road, Skelmanthorpe, Huddersfield HD8 9DA
Tel: 01484 862239
(South Huddersfield Primary Care Trust)

GP Dr ANDERSON, Dr CASSIDY, Dr KAYE, Dr WADE, Michael Thomas Christopher WELCH

The Health Centre
Commercial Road, Skelmanthorpe, Huddersfield HD8 9DA
Tel: 01484 862239 Fax: 01484 863120
(South Huddersfield Primary Care Trust)

Practice Manager Jilian Thistlewood

GP N M KAYE, R SAMANATA, T C WELCH

Health Services Centre
Shelley Lane, Kirkburton, Huddersfield HD8 0SJ
Tel: 01484 602040 Fax: 01484 602012
(South Huddersfield Primary Care Trust)
Patient List Size: 6900

Practice Manager Janet Atkinson

GP John Frederick Walter PRIESTMAN, Karen Margaret Lesley DEAN, Mary KEMSHELL, Victoria LYNCH, Michael Anthony WALLWORK

Honley Surgery
Marsh Gardens, Honley, Huddersfield HD9 6AG
Tel: 01484 303366 Fax: 01484 303365
(South Huddersfield Primary Care Trust)
Patient List Size: 8174

Practice Manager E M Broadbent

GP Hilary PARKER, Deirdre Anne CASHIN, C F ISAAC, John Robert LORD, Jenny Georgina NANCARROW, Debra Samantha RAWCLIFFE, Mark Andrew TAYLOR, C J TILLOTSON

Keldregate Surgery
268 Keldregate, Deighton, Huddersfield HD2 1LE
Tel: 01484 532399
(Huddersfield Central Primary Care Trust)

GP Mohammed Nazrul ISLAM

Lepton Surgery
Highgate Lane, Lepton, Huddersfield HD8 0HH
Tel: 01484 606161
(Huddersfield Central Primary Care Trust)
Patient List Size: 7500

Practice Manager Yvonne Armstrong

GP Diarmuid BARNWELL, Adrian CLARKSON, Peter Holland FITTON, Neal Colin JOLLY, Helen Elizabeth PACE

The Lindley Group Practice
62 Acre Street, Lindley, Huddersfield HD3 3DY
Tel: 01484 342191
(Huddersfield Central Primary Care Trust)
Patient List Size: 8000

Practice Manager Janet Buck

GP Lynn Elizabeth MASON, Alan David MASON, Christopher Richard PARKER, Judith Alison PARKER

Lindley Village Surgery
Thomas Street, Lindley, Huddersfield HD3 3JD
Tel: 01484 651403 Fax: 01484 644198
(Huddersfield Central Primary Care Trust)
Patient List Size: 4150

Practice Manager Jo Markiewicz

GP Helen Margaret Radula Scott SPENCER, Joseph Anthony SCHEMBRI

Lockwood Surgery
3 Meltham Road, Lockwood, Huddersfield HD1 3XH
Tel: 01484 421580 Fax: 01484 480100
(Huddersfield Central Primary Care Trust)
Patient List Size: 4750

Practice Manager Peter Embling

GP Robin Andrew SHARMAN, Shona M ATKINSON, Owen DEMPSEY

Meltham Group Practice
1 The Cobbles, Meltham, Huddersfield HD9 4AH
Tel: 01484 347620 Fax: 01484 347621
Email: doctors@gp-B85032.nhs.uk
(South Huddersfield Primary Care Trust)
Patient List Size: 6000

Practice Manager Liz Turner

GP Robert Daniel MITCHELL, Sally Joanne HAIGH, Joanne Rachel HARDING, Anne Elizabeth TATTERSALL

Meltham Road Surgery
9 Meltham Road, Lockwood, Huddersfield HD1 3UP
Tel: 01484 432940 Fax: 01484 451423
(South Huddersfield Primary Care Trust)
Patient List Size: 7500

Practice Manager Shahda Chaudry

GP Anil AGGARWAL, Elizabeth BROOK, Naim Ul Haq HASANIE, Anne Marjory STEYN

Meltham Village Surgery
Parkin Lane, Meltham, Huddersfield HD9 4EN
Tel: 01484 850638 Fax: 01484 854891
(South Huddersfield Primary Care Trust)
Patient List Size: 2353

Practice Manager Patricia Yvonne Walker

GP Michael Kazimierz PACYNKO, Caroline BIGGS, James BUCKLE

Moor Hill Road Surgery
144 Moor Hill Road, Salendine Nook, Huddersfield HD3 3XA
Tel: 01484 644956 Fax: 01484 460825
(Huddersfield Central Primary Care Trust)

Practice Manager Susan Heuer

GP N BALAKUMAR

New Street Surgery
21 New Street, Milnsbridge, Huddersfield HD3 4LB
Tel: 01484 651622
(Huddersfield Central Primary Care Trust)
Patient List Size: 1400

GP Bharat Bhooshan BHASIN

Norwood Road Surgery
37 Norwood Road, Birkby, Huddersfield HD2 2YD
Tel: 01484 519911 Fax: 01484 546007
(Huddersfield Central Primary Care Trust)
Patient List Size: 2550

Practice Manager M K Singh

GP M SINGH

Park Road West Surgery
11 Park Road West, Crosland Moor, Huddersfield HD4 5RX
Tel: 01484 642020/642044 Fax: 01484 460774
(Huddersfield Central Primary Care Trust)
Patient List Size: 6700

Practice Manager P Lockwood

GP Michael TAYLOR, Vivien Hannah MARTIN

Scar Lane Surgery
31 Scar Lane, Milnsbridge, Huddersfield HD3 4QH
Tel: 01484 654108
(Huddersfield Central Primary Care Trust)
Patient List Size: 2000

Practice Manager V Gledhill

GP M N ALI

Skelmanthorpe Family Doctors
The Health Centre, Commercial Road, Skelmanthorpe, Huddersfield HD8 9DA
Tel: 01484 863542
(South Huddersfield Primary Care Trust)
Patient List Size: 8895

Practice Manager Maria Grayson

GP M T L WELCH, Elizabeth Jane ANDERSON, Paul Philip CASSIDY, N KAKE

Slaithwaite Health Centre
New Street, Slaithwaite, Huddersfield HD7 5AB
Tel: 01484 846674
(South Huddersfield Primary Care Trust)
Patient List Size: 3800

Practice Manager Elizabeth Williams

GP Amanda CURGENVEN, Fiona Jane Frances McCARTHY

Speedwell Surgery
1 Speedwell Street, Paddock, Huddersfield HD1 4TS
Tel: 01484 531786 Fax: 01484 424249
(Huddersfield Central Primary Care Trust)
Patient List Size: 6800

Practice Manager Susan France, Mary George

GP Timothy David SWIFT, Bharat Kumar JINDAL, Mark Andrew STILES

The Surgery
17 The Triangle, Paddock, Huddersfield HD1 4RN
Tel: 01484 422509 Fax: 01484 451212
(Huddersfield Central Primary Care Trust)
Patient List Size: 4000

Practice Manager Gill Jones

GP Matthew Peter BOULTON, Paul CULLINEY

Thornton Lodge Road Surgery
60 Thornton Lodge Road, Thornton Lodge, Huddersfield HD1 3SB
Tel: 01484 309991 Fax: 01484 309996
(Huddersfield Central Primary Care Trust)
Patient List Size: 2000

Practice Manager Anne Smith

GP M HANNAN

Trinity Street Surgery
124 Trinity Street, Huddersfield HD1 4DT
Tel: 01484 535152 Fax: 01484 532311
(Huddersfield Central Primary Care Trust)
Patient List Size: 1700

Practice Manager I Halstead

GP S H N GOWA

Waterloo Surgery
617 Wakefield Road, Waterloo, Huddersfield HD5 9XP
Tel: 01484 531461 Fax: 01484 467825
(Huddersfield Central Primary Care Trust)
Patient List Size: 8000

Practice Manager B Collinge

GP Michael John ADAM, Sheelagh KAY, Hubert Anthony Agnelo NAZARETH

Wentworth Street Surgery
15 Wentworth Street, Huddersfield HD1 5LJ
Tel: 01484 530834
(Huddersfield Central Primary Care Trust)
Patient List Size: 3200

Practice Manager D L Brook

GP Robin Wilfrid James WYBREW, Maria Elizabeth WYBREW

Westbourne Surgery
11A St. James Road, Marsh, Huddersfield HD1 4QR
Tel: 01484 531672 Fax: 01484 456463
(Huddersfield Central Primary Care Trust)
Patient List Size: 3700

Practice Manager Susan Ramsden

GP John Anthony BAIRSTOW, Sabita AGGARWAL

Woodhouse Hill Surgery
71A Woodhouse Hill, Fartown, Huddersfield HD2 1DH
Tel: 01484 533833 Fax: 01484 516966

(Huddersfield Central Primary Care Trust)
Patient List Size: 2800
Practice Manager Diane McFarlane
GP P K DAS, Pushpa DAS, M D HOOPER

Hull

Anlaby Road Surgery
263 Anlaby Road, Hull HU3 2SE
Tel: 01482 324650 Fax: 01482 326337
(West Hull Primary Care Trust)
Patient List Size: 3100
Practice Manager Norman Halliday
GP Aga Wajahat HUSSAIN, T ABRAHAM, Sherbanu Gulam HUSSAIN

Anlaby Road Surgery
497 Anlaby Road, Hull HU3 6DT
Tel: 01482 353997 Fax: 01482 575010
(West Hull Primary Care Trust)
Practice Manager Jane A. Macphie
GP Samuel MACPHIE, Kishni Kumari KOUL

Anlaby Road Surgery
561 Anlaby Road, Hull HU3 6SH
Tel: 01482 352981 Fax: 01482 561071
(West Hull Primary Care Trust)
Practice Manager Francis Rawcliffe
GP Stefan Horatio REISS

Anlaby Road Surgery
531 Anlaby Road, Hull HU3 6EP
Tel: 01482 351161 Fax: 01482 563384
(West Hull Primary Care Trust)
Practice Manager Francis Rawcliffe
GP A H TAK, S REISS

The Anlaby Surgery
7 Weeton Way, Anlaby, Hull HU10 6QH
Tel: 01482 658918 Fax: 01482 655205
(East Yorkshire Primary Care Trust)
GP Johnny George BEST

Beverley Road Surgery
840 Beverley Road, Hull HU6 7HP
Tel: 01482 853270 Fax: 01482 85323270
(West Hull Primary Care Trust)
Patient List Size: 4100
Practice Manager Pat Ruston
GP Malcolm David LENG

Bransholme South Health Centre
Goodhart Road, Bransholme, Hull HU7 4DW
Tel: 01482 831257 Fax: 01482 836167
(Eastern Hull Primary Care Trust)
Patient List Size: 3200
Practice Manager S Venugopal
GP Janardanan VENUGOPAL

Bransholme South Health Centre
Goodhart Road, Bransholme, Hull HU7 4DW
Tel: 01482 825496 Fax: 01482 836383
(Eastern Hull Primary Care Trust)
Patient List Size: 3700
Practice Manager Janet Whitby
GP Pradeep Chandra GHOSH, Krishna GHOSH

Bransholme South Health Centre
Goodhart Road, Bransholme, Hull HU7 4DW
Tel: 01482 823377 Fax: 01482 820707
(Eastern Hull Primary Care Trust)
Patient List Size: 7075
Practice Manager Julie Charles
GP P K GEORGE, V B ANIKHINDI, George PALOORAN

Bransholme South Health Centre
Goodhart Road, Bransholme, Hull HU7 4DW
Tel: 01482 825438 Fax: 01482 825438
Email: gabriel.hendow@gp-B81616.nhs.uk
(Eastern Hull Primary Care Trust)
Practice Manager Juliet Taylor
GP Gabriel Thomas HENDOW

Bransholme South Health Centre
Goodhart Road, Bransholme, Hull HU7 4DW
Tel: 01482 823232 Fax: 01482 836353
(Eastern Hull Primary Care Trust)
Patient List Size: 2937
Practice Manager Jennifer Lawrence
GP K V GOPAL

Bransholme South Health Centre
Goodhart Road, Bransholme, Hull HU7 4DW
Tel: 01482 835566 Fax: 01482 836214
(Eastern Hull Primary Care Trust)
Practice Manager Niki Dunlop
GP N A POULOSE

Chanterlands Avenue Surgery
149-153 Chanterlands Avenue, Hull HU5 3TJ
Tel: 01482 343614 Fax: 01482 492480
(West Hull Primary Care Trust)
Practice Manager Diane Jones
GP Winston George Theodore SANDE, Brian Francis COOK, S NANDI, Patricia WARRAN

Church View Surgery
5 Market Hill, Hedon, Hull HU12 8JE
Tel: 01482 899348
(Yorkshire Wolds and Coast Primary Care Trust)
Practice Manager Linda Riley
GP Malcolm WILKINSON, Peter St. John DAVIS, Ruth Katherine DRIVER, Andrew Duncan INNES, Caroline Jane LAMBERT, John Peter David LEWIS

Clifton House Medical Centre
263-265 Beverley Road, Hull HU5 2ST
Tel: 01482 341423 Fax: 01482 449373
(West Hull Primary Care Trust)
Patient List Size: 12600
Practice Manager Julia Smith
GP Medavaram Jagdish PRATAP VARMA, Ghanshyam Singh CHAUHAN, Koshy JOHNSON, Kah Wai LEE, Charlotte Mary Parker LEWIS, Peter THACKRAY

Cottingham Road Surgery
138 Cottingham Road, Hull HU6 7RY
Tel: 01482 335555 Fax: 01482 335558
(West Hull Primary Care Trust)
Practice Manager Jonathan Kutte
GP Paul Nicholas JONES, Donald COSTELLO

Dunvegan Road Surgery
174 Dunvegan Road, Chestnut Farm, Hull HU8 9LF
Tel: 01482 701090 Fax: 01482 708669
(Eastern Hull Primary Care Trust)
Practice Manager P Mahendra
GP K K MAHENDRA

Faith House Surgery
723 Beverley Road, Hull HU6 7ER
Tel: 01482 853296 Fax: 01482 855235
(West Hull Primary Care Trust)

Patient List Size: 6970

Practice Manager Maureen Robinson

GP David Louis Anthony CRICK, Helen BOWDEN, Amanda Jane MELVILLE, Justine SMITH, Adam Man Kit WONG

Ganstead Lane Surgery
5 Ganstead Lane, Hull HU11 4AS
Tel: 01482 811249 Fax: 01482 817602
(Eastern Hull Primary Care Trust)
Patient List Size: 3000

Practice Manager Bill Pyle

GP J AUSTIN

The Health Centre
Marmaduke Street, Hessle Road, Hull HU3 3BH
Tel: 01482 323449 Fax: 01482 610920
(West Hull Primary Care Trust)

Practice Manager Wendy Clapson

GP R Y AL-JUMAILY, John David BLOW, Marion Jane BROWN, P V JOSEPH, Ahmad Sayeed SIDDIQUI

Hedon Group Practice
4 Market Hill, Hedon, Hull HU12 8JD
Tel: 01482 899111 Fax: 01482 890967
(Yorkshire Wolds and Coast Primary Care Trust)

Practice Manager Roy Peckitt

GP Anne Vivienne Norah PEPPER, John BALSHAW, Peter ENGLISH, Andrew Martin GREEN, Ngozi PATRICK

Hessle Road Surgery
339 Hessle Road, Hull HU3 4EJ
Tel: 01482 214022 Fax: 01482 214760
(West Hull Primary Care Trust)
Patient List Size: 1350

Practice Manager Jenny Clayton

GP Bhushan Lal KOUL

Highlands Health Centre
Lothian Way, Bransholme, Hull HU7 5DD
Tel: 01482 835880 Fax: 01482 820926
(Eastern Hull Primary Care Trust)
Patient List Size: 3500

Practice Manager Anita Choudhary

GP C A KUMAR

Holderness Road Surgery
445 Holderness Road, Hull HU8 8JS
Tel: 01482 374255 Fax: 01482 715251
(Eastern Hull Primary Care Trust)
Patient List Size: 5700

Practice Manager Jim Doran

GP John Warlow RICHARDSON, Ian Andrew ASHWORTH, Colin Thomas FAIRHURST

Holderness Road Surgery
675 Holderness Road, Hull HU8 9AN
Tel: 01482 374644 Fax: 01482 784469
(Eastern Hull Primary Care Trust)
Patient List Size: 2530

Practice Manager Norman Halliday

GP Golam M CHOWDHURY

Holderness Road Surgery
733 Holderness Road, Hull HU8 9AR
Tel: 01482 711112 Fax: 01482 791766
(Eastern Hull Primary Care Trust)
Patient List Size: 2789

Practice Manager Gail Baynes

GP M E AHMED, R A ALI

Holderness Road Surgery
434 Holderness Road, Hull HU9 3DW
Tel: 01482 376425 Fax: 01482 715556
(Eastern Hull Primary Care Trust)

GP J DATTA

Holderness Road Surgery
1199 Holderness Road, Hull HU8 9EA
Tel: 01482 799139 Fax: 01482 787983
(Eastern Hull Primary Care Trust)

Practice Manager Susan Wilson

GP Mohammad Athar MANSOOR, Dr MALCZEWSKI

Holderness Road Surgery
1181 Holderness Road, Hull HU8 9EA
Tel: 01482 784966 Fax: 01482 374305
(Eastern Hull Primary Care Trust)

Practice Manager Mrs Shakh

GP Mutiullah SHAIKH

James Reckitt Avenue Surgery
356 James Reckitt Avenue, Hull HU8 0JA
Tel: 01482 796121 Fax: 01482 796996
(Eastern Hull Primary Care Trust)
Patient List Size: 1800

Practice Manager Sue Moody

GP R. D. YAGNIK

Kingston Medical Group
151 Beverley Road, Hull HU3 1TY
Tel: 01482 328861 Fax: 01482 321223
(West Hull Primary Care Trust)

Practice Manager Sara Emmett

GP P G R McALPIN, Henk DEVRIES, P E G NAGHTON-DOE, S NANDI, Jereon PINTO, M S SETIYA, Bart VANHOVE

Laurbel Surgery
14 Main Road, Bilton, Hull HU11 4AR
Tel: 01482 814121 Fax: 01482 817003
(Eastern Hull Primary Care Trust)
Patient List Size: 3264

GP G DAVE

Lomond Road Surgery
2 Lomond Road, Hull HU5 5BN
Tel: 01482 351956 Fax: 01482 351199
(West Hull Primary Care Trust)
Patient List Size: 3500

Practice Manager Lesley Bird

GP Eugene Glenn STRYJAKIEWICZ

Main Street Surgery
45 Main Street, Willerby, Hull HU10 6BY
Tel: 01482 652652 Fax: 01482 658376
(East Yorkshire Primary Care Trust)
Patient List Size: 7500

Practice Manager Sue Morris

GP Michael Ernest Arthur MOODY, Manel DVENAS, Anne PESTELL, R M TAYLOR

Marfleet Group Practice
350 Preston Road, Hull HU9 5HH
Tel: 01482 701834 Fax: 01482 784751
(Eastern Hull Primary Care Trust)

Practice Manager John Maffin

GP Patrick Fitzgerald NEWMAN, J M CHAPELA, Frederick Hal JORNA, P K SINHA, John Anthony David WEIR, Ling YU

Marfleet Lane Surgery
358 Marfleet Lane, Hull HU9 5AD
Tel: 01482 781032 Fax: 01482 781048
Email: drsetiya@gpexchange1.eridingha.northy.nhs.uk

(Eastern Hull Primary Care Trust)
Patient List Size: 3200

Practice Manager Judith Dyson

GP Leendert WITVLIET

Mizzen Road Surgery
5 Mizzen Road, Hull HU6 7AG
Tel: 01482 854574 Fax: 01482 854576
Email: goolamali.rangwala@gp-b81662.nhs.uk
(West Hull Primary Care Trust)
Patient List Size: 2359

Practice Manager Mrs Rangwala

GP Goolamali Dawoodbhai RANGWALA

Morrill Street Health Centre
Holderness Road, Hull HU9 2LJ
Tel: 01482 320046 Fax: 01482 589611
(Eastern Hull Primary Care Trust)

Practice Manager Vanessa Manning

GP Trevor BOLTON, A BUNTING, Russell William ELLWOOD, B B HAMAL, Dr HUSSAIN, M ISLAM, Stephen Alexander LEES, John Stephen PARKER, Kathryn Sarah TOMMINS

Morrill Street Health Centre
Morrill Street, Holderness Road, Hull HU9 2LJ
Tel: 01482 323398 Fax: 01482 217957
(Eastern Hull Primary Care Trust)
Patient List Size: 3980

Practice Manager M Pinder

GP Nassif T ABD-MARIAM, Kim Man TANG

Newhall Surgery
Oakfield Court, Cottingham Road, Hull HU6 8QF
Tel: 01482 343390 Fax: 01482 445858
(West Hull Primary Care Trust)
Patient List Size: 8000

Practice Manager Helen McAteer

GP Christopher Alan JARY, Vincent Anthony RAWCLIFFE, Diana Katharine GREENE, Lindsay GUEST, Sanjeev KAPUR

Newland Avenue Surgery
129 Newland Avenue, Hull HU5 2ES
Tel: 01482 343671 Fax: 01482 448839
(West Hull Primary Care Trust)
Patient List Size: 6850

Practice Manager Iain Swallow

GP Richard PERCIVAL, Peng Sang CHIA, Richard John WESTROP

Newland Group Practice
239-243 Newland Avenue, Hull HU5 2EJ
Tel: 01482 448456 Fax: 01482 449536
(West Hull Primary Care Trust)

Practice Manager Carole Robinson

GP Syed Mazhar HUSSAIN, Dr CLARK, James Robert LORENZ, Tolulola Olusesan Olusola OGUNLESI, Anne Elizabeth PARKIN

Newland Health Centre
187 Cottingham Road, Hull HU5 2EG
Tel: 01482 492219 Fax: 01482 441418
(West Hull Primary Care Trust)
Patient List Size: 6700

Practice Manager Andrew Newman

GP Janaky Kutty NAYAR, Petrus Leonardus VAN MAARSEVEEN

Oaks Medical Centre
Council Avenue, Hull HU4 6RT
Tel: 01482 354251 Fax: 01482 573987
(West Hull Primary Care Trust)
Patient List Size: 8000

Practice Manager Ellen Ransom

GP Abdul Aziz MATHER, Ivan Alexander GALEA, T KUNDU, John MILLER

Orchard 2000 Medical Centre
480 Hall Road, Hull HU6 9BS
Tel: 01482 854552 Fax: 01482 859900
(West Hull Primary Care Trust)

Practice Manager Patricia Nalton

GP Stephen Andrew SCARFE, Ramzan Khan AWAN

Orchard Park Health Centre
250 Ellerburn Avenue, Hull HU6 9RR
Tel: 01482 804555 Fax: 01482 610920
(West Hull Primary Care Trust)

Practice Manager Wendy Clapson

GP Dr BLOW, Dr AL-JUMAILY, Dr BROWN, P V JOSEPH, Dr SIDDIQUI

Princes Avenue Surgery
Princes Court, Princes Avenue, Hull HU5 3QA
Tel: 01482 342473 Fax: 01482 493382
(West Hull Primary Care Trust)
Patient List Size: 5138

Practice Manager Linda Tong

GP Jan MUSIL, Paul John QUEENAN

The Quays Medical Centre
35-39 Myton Street, Hull HU1 2PS
Tel: 01482 335335 Fax: 01482 335339
(West Hull Primary Care Trust)

Practice Manager Denise Wilkinson

GP Peter CAMPION, Ros DAVIES, Anita JAMAL, Noel TINKER, Mark WILLIAMSON

Shannon Road Surgery
329 Shannon Road, Hull HU8 9QA
Tel: 01482 815860 Fax: 01482 811616
(Eastern Hull Primary Care Trust)

GP J C JOSEPH

Southcoates Medical Centre
225 Newbridge Road, Hull HU9 2LR
Tel: 01482 708333 Fax: 01482 708336
(Eastern Hull Primary Care Trust)

Practice Manager Tracy Woodrow

GP Dr BANERJEE, Dr REJ

Spring Bank Group Practice
168 Spring Bank, Hull HU3 1QW
Tel: 01482 328581 Fax: 01482 221970
(West Hull Primary Care Trust)
Patient List Size: 7500

Practice Manager Pauline Dobson, Sandra Rock

GP Jainandan Jai Nandan SINGH, Jennifer Judith JONES, Carlos LORENCES RUIZ, J MILAZZO, Kanan PANDE

Spring Bank West Surgery
919 Spring Bank West, Hull HU5 5BE
Tel: 01482 351219 Fax: 01482 351930
(West Hull Primary Care Trust)

Practice Manager Barbara Smithson

GP Manas Kumar MALLIK

Springhead Medical Centre
376 Willerby Road, Hull HU5 5JT
Tel: 01482 352263 Fax: 01482 352480
(West Hull Primary Care Trust)
Patient List Size: 10800

Practice Manager Jean Holborn

GP John David PRICE, Gary James CURRAN, Elizabeth DOBSON, Rukhsana JAMALI, Daniel James ROPER, Glynnis TURNER

St Andrews Group Practice
Marmaduke Street, Hessle Road, Hull HU3 3BH
Tel: 01482 336812 Fax: 01482 336826
(West Hull Primary Care Trust)

Practice Manager Terri Wardell

GP A RAGHUNATH, Mark FINDLEY, Shama Uday JOSHI, Karel REINDERS

The Surgery
Greenwich Avenue, Hull HU9 4UX
Tel: 01482 335640 Fax: 01482 335665
(Eastern Hull Primary Care Trust)

Practice Manager P Haire

GP Neil Hamish McDONALD, David James BARNES, Christopher Alan HAMMERSLEY, Dr MAUNG, Peter John WRIGHT

The Surgery
Littondale, Sutton Park, Hull HU7 4BJ
Tel: 01482 825681 Fax: 01482 837591
(Eastern Hull Primary Care Trust)

GP Sushil Kumar RAY

Sutton Manor Surgery
Nanne Road, Hull HU7 4TT
Tel: 01482 826457 Fax: 01482 824182
(Eastern Hull Primary Care Trust)
Patient List Size: 6800

Practice Manager Barbara Young

GP Paul Charles MITCHELL, Jennifer Caroline HOLMQUIST, James Halyburton LOOSE, Lisa MARSHALL

Sydenham House Surgery
Boulevard, Hull HU3 2TD
Tel: 01482 326818 Fax: 01482 218267
(West Hull Primary Care Trust)

Practice Manager Caroline Wilson

GP Michael Hugh Anthony MARTIN-SMITH, Malcolm FOULDS, Margaret LOVETT, Michael Anthony RUSLING

Wheelerstreet Healthcare
Wheeler Street, Anlaby Road, Hull HU3 5QE
Tel: 01482 354933 Fax: 01482 355090
(West Hull Primary Care Trust)
Patient List Size: 5800

Practice Manager Judith Turner

GP Mohammad AYYUB, A M AHMED, Danny J Y YU

Hungerford

Bockhampton Road Surgery
Bockhampton Road, Lambourn, Hungerford RG17 8PS
Tel: 01488 71715 Fax: 01488 73569
(Newbury and Community Primary Care Trust)

Practice Manager Iris Seagar

GP Hugh Benedict POWELL, Norman CURRIE, John Richard JONES

Hungerford Surgery
The Croft, Hungerford RG17 0HY
Tel: 01488 682507 Fax: 01488 681018
Website: www.hungerford-surgery.org.uk
(Newbury and Community Primary Care Trust)
Patient List Size: 8000

Practice Manager Ian Barnes

GP Hugh Lynton PIHLENS, Jeremy Keith BRAY, Helen Mary DACE, Robin Jeremy DUNN, Peter le Geyt HETHERINGTON

The Kintbury Medical Practice
Kintbury Surgery, Newbury Street, Kintbury, Hungerford RG17 9UX
Tel: 01488 658294 Fax: 01488 657440
(Newbury and Community Primary Care Trust)

Practice Manager Louise Wilkin

GP Nicholas YATES, C MONTAGUE, U TREADGOLD, C WEST

Hunstanton

Valentine Road Surgery
Valentine Road, Hunstanton PE36 5DN
Tel: 01485 532859 Fax: 01485 534608
(West Norfolk Primary Care Trust)
Patient List Size: 5000

Practice Manager Melvyn Peveritt

GP Clive MACHIN, Robert MUNRO, Nigel Christopher THORPE

Huntingdon

Acorn Community Health Centre
California Road, Huntingdon PE29 1BJ
(Huntingdonshire Primary Care Trust)

Almond Road Surgery
Almond Road, St. Neots, Huntingdon PE19 1DZ
Tel: 01480 473413 Fax: 01480 406906
(Huntingdonshire Primary Care Trust)

GP Nicholas John TAYLOR, Niall Antony BACON, Barbara USZYOKA

Cedar House Surgery
14 Huntingdon Street, St. Neots, Huntingdon PE19 1BQ
Tel: 01480 406677 Fax: 01480 475167
(Huntingdonshire Primary Care Trust)
Patient List Size: 12000

Practice Manager Julie Boyles

GP John Victor TURNER, Ian Brian DUMBELTON, Anthony William SWINSCOE, Thekanady Mathew THOMAS, Malcolm Harold George WRIGHT

Charles Hicks Centre
75 Ermine Street, Huntingdon PE29 3EZ
Tel: 01480 453038 Fax: 01480 434104
(Huntingdonshire Primary Care Trust)
Patient List Size: 12875

Practice Manager A Robinson

GP Adelaide TURNILL, Harriet Maude Jennie PLATTEN, Robin John Roe STANGER, Ian Arthur SWEETENHAM, Richard Stanley WEYELL, Michael William WHITTON

Cromwell Place Surgery
Cromwell Place, St. Ives, Huntingdon PE27 5JD
Tel: 01480 462206 Fax: 01480 465313
Website: www.cromwellplacesurgery.nhs.uk
(Huntingdonshire Primary Care Trust)
Patient List Size: 9000

Practice Manager Marilyn Clark

GP Francis Geoffrey FERREIRA, Philip Simon BOWER, Kevin Francis DONNELLY, Christopher Hamilton JESSOP, Sine Morag KING

Eaton Socon Health Centre
274 North Road, Eaton Socon, St. Neots, Huntingdon PE19 8BB
Tel: 01480 477111 Fax: 01480 403524
Email: eshc@gp-D81032.nhs.uk
(Huntingdonshire Primary Care Trust)
Patient List Size: 12200

Practice Manager Gail Gunter

GP Martin Rodney NEWBY, Susan Patricia BABBINGTON, Timothy Paul MEARS, Michael John MOOR, Paul Jonathan SEARLE, Peter Howard WILLIAMS

Great Staughton Surgery
57 The Highway, Great Staughton, St. Neots, Huntingdon PE19 5DA
Tel: 01480 860770 Fax: 01480 862890
(Huntingdonshire Primary Care Trust)

Patient List Size: 3200

Practice Manager Barbara Wallis

GP David Hywel Griffith ROBERTS, Stephanie Ann JOHNSON, Christina MARSH

Harding
The Orchard Surgery, Constable Road, St. Ives, Huntingdon PE27 3ER
Tel: 01480 466611 Fax: 01480 492360
(Huntingdonshire Primary Care Trust)

Practice Manager J O'Brien

GP Phillip John HARDING, Helen JOHNSON, Carole Ann MILLS

Hunters Way Medical Centre
Hunters Way, Kimbolton, Huntingdon PE28 0JF
Tel: 01480 860205 Fax: 01480 861590
(Huntingdonshire Primary Care Trust)

GP John RAWLINSON, John Nicholas FELLS, Jane Margaret HORSNELL, Fiona Wallace McCULLOUGH

Jubilee Close Surgery
Jubilee Close, Little Paxton, Huntingdon PE19
Tel: 01480 219060 Fax: 01480 211776
(Huntingdonshire Primary Care Trust)
Patient List Size: 2250

Mayfield Surgery
Mayfield, Buckden St. Neots, Huntingdon PE19 5SZ
Tel: 01480 810216 Fax: 01480 810745
(Huntingdonshire Primary Care Trust)
Patient List Size: 5100

Practice Manager Bob Young

GP David Stephen Slade IRWIN, Paulo FRAGNOLI, Paul Richard GOODWIN

Northcote House Surgery
Northcote House, 8 Broad Leas, Huntingdon PE27 5PT
Tel: 01480 461873 Fax: 01480 460612
(Huntingdonshire Primary Care Trust)
Patient List Size: 4500

Practice Manager Phil Witherington

GP John Broadhurst HYDE, Roy Frederick CARLYLE, Andrew Francis GREATREX

Old Grammar School Surgery
Ramsey Road, St Ives, Huntingdon PE27 5BZ
(Huntingdonshire Primary Care Trust)

Old Telephone Exchange
East Street, St Ives, Huntingdon PE27 5PB
Tel: 01480 497477 Fax: 01480 497550
(Huntingdonshire Primary Care Trust)
Patient List Size: 2678

Practice Manager Carole Pollack

GP John Douglas CASWELL, Judith SOMERS HESLAM

Parkhall Surgery
Parkhall Road, Somersham, Huntingdon PE28 3EU
Tel: 01487 740888 Fax: 01487 843635
(Huntingdonshire Primary Care Trust)
Patient List Size: 4000

Practice Manager Anne Bailey

GP Derek James MARTIN, Robert ALLAN, Ravindra BARAPATRE, Susan CHENG, Kathryn Anne LUND

Priory Fields Surgery
Nursery Road, Huntingdon PE29 3RL
Tel: 01480 52361 Fax: 01480 434640
(Huntingdonshire Primary Care Trust)

Practice Manager Alan Chambers

GP Malav Yogesh BHIMPURIA, Duncan Edward BLAKE, Esther Mary GREEN, Nicola Thirza Anne POPPLEWELL, Edward REJ, Emma Jane TIFFIN, Andrew WRIGHT

Rainbow Surgery
Stocking Fen Road, Ramsey, Huntingdon PE26 1SA
Tel: 01487 710980 Fax: 01487 710982
(Huntingdonshire Primary Care Trust)
Patient List Size: 3200

GP Arun Kumar AGGARWAL, Rita AGGARWAL, Sandy NASHEF, John RICHMOND

Ramsey Health Centre
Mews Close, Ramsey, Huntingdon PE26 1BP
Tel: 01487 812611 Fax: 01487 711801
Email: ramseyhc@gp-D81059.nhs.uk
Website: www.freespace.virgin.net/ramsey.hc
(Huntingdonshire Primary Care Trust)

Practice Manager Carole Collier

GP David Antony HASLAM, Simon Jeremy BROWN, Martin William GLOVER, Adrian HAMILTON, John Luke TWELVES, Kate WISHART

The Spinney Surgery
The Spinney, Ramsey Road, St. Ives, Huntingdon PE27 3TP
Tel: 01480 492501 Fax: 01480 356159
Email: debbie.spinney@virgin.net
(Huntingdonshire Primary Care Trust)
Patient List Size: 8700

Practice Manager Debra Wheatley

GP George Robert SMERDON, Dennis Charles Anthony COX, Sean CULLOTY, Rosemary Helen LANE

St Mary's Surgery
6A Church Street, Somersham, Huntingdon PE28 3EG
Tel: 01487 841300 Fax: 01487 740765
(Huntingdonshire Primary Care Trust)

Practice Manager Ms Bevens

GP Chi Kee LIU, Naier Fahmy HABIB

The Surgery
School Lane, Alconbury, Huntingdon PE28 4EQ
Tel: 01480 890281 Fax: 01480 891787
(Huntingdonshire Primary Care Trust)
Patient List Size: 8000

Practice Manager David Cripps

GP Paul Albert SACKIN, Barbara Kathleen CHURMS, Francesca Camilla Anna LASMAN, Alexandra Jean NASHEF, Duncan Patrick REA

Warbrick-Smith and Partners
The Moat House Surgery, Beech Close, Warboys, Huntingdon PE28 2RQ
Tel: 01487 822230 Fax: 01487 823721
(Huntingdonshire Primary Care Trust)
Patient List Size: 6000

Practice Manager Kathryn How, Kathryn How

GP David WARBRICK-SMITH, Brendan Eugene BOYLE, Jennifer Ann BOYLE, Helen Margaret MACKAY, Jonathan Michael WILCOCK

Wellside Surgery
45 High Street, Sawtry, Huntingdon PE28 5SU
Tel: 01487 830340 Fax: 01487 832753
Website: www.wellside.org.uk
(Huntingdonshire Primary Care Trust)
Patient List Size: 6800

Practice Manager Claire Wright

GP Ian Grindon WILLIAMS, Charlotte Christian ARCHER, Abby RICHARDSON, Richard James SMITH

Hyde

Awburn House
Mottram Moor, Mottram, Hyde SK14 6LA
Tel: 01457 763263
(Tameside and Glossop Primary Care Trust)

Practice Manager G Clark

GP Michael Richard Simon CLARK, Darah Kevin BURKE, Helen MURPHY

The Brooke Surgery
20 Market Street, Hyde SK14 1AT
Tel: 0161 368 3312 Fax: 0161 368 5670
(Tameside and Glossop Primary Care Trust)
Patient List Size: 9800

GP Rajesh PATEL, Susan BOOTH, Jeremy DIRCZE, Alastair MacGILLIVRAY, Louise PRESTON

The Brooke Surgery
20 Market Street, Hyde SK14 1AT
Tel: 0161 368 3312 Fax: 0161 268 5670
(Tameside and Glossop Primary Care Trust)
Patient List Size: 10000

Practice Manager Geoff Ames

GP Alistair McGILLIVRAY, Jeremy M DIRCZKE, R GULATI, Rajesh PATEL, L PRESTON

Clarendon Medical Practice
Clarendon Street, Hyde SK14 2AQ
Tel: 0161 368 5224 Fax: 0161 366 6303
(Tameside and Glossop Primary Care Trust)

Practice Manager S C Gilks

GP Vikram Narandas Morarji TANNA, Jonathan Marcus HEPTONSTALL, Stephen Clifford PROCTOR, Eddie Wing Cheong THORNTON-CHAN

Donnybrook House Group Practice
Clarendon Street, Hyde SK14 2AH
Tel: 0161 368 3838 Fax: 0161 368 2210
(Tameside and Glossop Primary Care Trust)

GP Jeffery Osmer MOYSEY, Ian Gordon NAPIER, Vincent Patrick Joseph BRADY, Derek Henry CARROLL, Lisa Christine GUTTERIDGE, Keith Graeme John MacLAVERTY, David Andrew ROBERTS

Hattersley Group Practice
Hattersley Road East, Hyde SK14 3EH
Tel: 0161 368 4161 Fax: 0161 351 1989
(Tameside and Glossop Primary Care Trust)
Patient List Size: 5950

Practice Manager Margaret Taylor

GP Andrew HERSHON, F KHAN, Mukta SHAH

Nimaroy Surgery
20 -24 Great Norbury Street, Hyde SK14 1BR
Tel: 0161 366 6204
(Tameside and Glossop Primary Care Trust)

GP A M CUMMING, L GUTTERIDGE, M A HOSSAIN, G P SINGH

The Smithy Surgery
4 Market Street, Hollingworth, Hyde SK14 8LN
Tel: 01457 763558 Fax: 01457 766429
(Tameside and Glossop Primary Care Trust)

Practice Manager Wendy Swann

GP Simon James RUSHTON, Heather METCALFE

Hythe

The David Briggs Practice
Hythe Medical Centre, Beaulieu Road, Hythe SO45 4ZD
Tel: 023 8084 5955 Fax: 023 8084 1869
(New Forest Primary Care Trust)

Practice Manager Susan Saunders

GP Robert David BRIGGS

The Green Practice
Waterside Health Centre, Beaulieu Road, Hythe SO45 5WX
Tel: 023 8084 5955 Fax: 023 8084 1292
(New Forest Primary Care Trust)
Patient List Size: 13500

Practice Manager Peter Barnard

GP Francis Henry GREAVES, Charlie BESLEY, Chris COLE, Kenneth William DAVIDSON, Jeanette FARMER, Philipp Henry GREGORY, Susan Carolyn RIAL

High Street Surgery
116-118 High Street, Hythe CT21 5LE
Tel: 01303 266652 Fax: 01303 261711
(Shepway Primary Care Trust)
Patient List Size: 8000

Practice Manager Sarah Roseaman

GP John ALLINGHAM, Robert Edward IMMELMAN, Eunice KELLY, Alison Judith WILTSHIRE

The Red Practice
Waterside Health Centre, Beaulieu Road, Hythe SO45 5WX
Tel: 023 8084 5955 Fax: 023 8020 1292
(New Forest Primary Care Trust)
Patient List Size: 13500

Practice Manager Peter Barnard

GP Andrew Charles Edward HAMILTON, Anthony Phillip ALLEN, Bernard BEDFORD, Douglas Robert CAMPBELL, John Richard PITTS, Angela Dawn VARNEY, Margaret Evelyn WHITBY

Sun Lane Surgery
Sun Lane, Hythe CT21 5JY
Tel: 01303 267102 Fax: 01303 265861
(Shepway Primary Care Trust)
Patient List Size: 7810

Practice Manager Jill Blackman

GP M CHANDRAKUMAR, A N BANIK, S BORGHARDT

Waterfront Garden Surgery
Jones Lane, Hythe SO45 6AW
Tel: 023 8084 1841/8061 2451 Fax: 023 8084 8084
(New Forest Primary Care Trust)

Practice Manager Judith Willshire

GP David Puckle MARKBY, Paul Terence MENIN

Ibstock

Krishnan, Stack, Peden, Foster and Abo-Seido
Ibstock House, 132 High Street, Ibstock LE67 6JP
Tel: 01530 260216/260284/264900 Fax: 01530 261397
(Charnwood and North West Leicestershire Primary Care Trust)
Patient List Size: 9650

Practice Manager Charles Jones

GP Ramachandra KRISHNAN, Hussam ABO-SEIDO, Adam M FOSTER, Alan T PEDEN, Michael Maurice STACK

Ilford

Balfour Road Surgery
92 Balfour Road, Ilford IG1 4JE
Tel: 020 8478 0209 Fax: 020 8220 8777
(Redbridge Primary Care Trust)
Patient List Size: 3910

Practice Manager Mrs Davda

GP Shyana SINILA

Belmont Road Surgery
69 Belmont Road, Ilford IG1 1YW
Tel: 020 8478 0555 Fax: 020 8220 3377

(Redbridge Primary Care Trust)

GP Aturu Bhaskara REDDY

Castleton Road Surgery
19-21 Castleton Road, Goodmayes, Ilford IG3 9QW
Tel: 020 8599 9951 Fax: 020 8597 9974
(Redbridge Primary Care Trust)
Patient List Size: 4000

GP Mohammad Aslam QURAISHI, Zebunnisa QURAISHI

Cedar Medical Centre
4 Granville Road, Ilford IG1 4JY
Tel: 020 8270 0440 Fax: 020 8270 0402
(Newham Primary Care Trust)
Patient List Size: 8500

GP Malvinder Singh SOHI, Chandar Prabha RAINA, Harjit SINGH

Chigwell Medical Centre
300 Fencepiece Road, Hainault, Ilford IG6 2TA
Tel: 020 8500 0066 Fax: 020 8559 8670
(Redbridge Primary Care Trust)
Patient List Size: 8200

GP Kamal Ragheb Tewfilx BISHAI, Nadia CROKER, Jiri PECHAN, Raza RASHID

Clayhall Clinic
14 Clayhall Avenue, Ilford IG5 0LG
Tel: 020 8550 5050 Fax: 020 8551 6393
(Redbridge Primary Care Trust)

GP Michael John HODGES, Munis Abdul Hameed KASHIN

Courtand Avenue Surgery
62 Courtland Avenue, Ilford IG1 3DP
Tel: 020 8554 2700 Fax: 020 8518-5757
(Redbridge Primary Care Trust)

GP Surinder Kumar BABBAR

Cranbrook Road Surgery
700 Cranbrook Road, Barkingside, Ilford IG6 1HP
Tel: 020 8551 2341 Fax: 020 8551 1479
(Redbridge Primary Care Trust)
Patient List Size: 4500

GP Undinti David SHUBHAKER, Urmila SHUBHAKER

The Doctor's House
40 Cameron Road, Seven Kings, Ilford IG3 8LF
Tel: 020 8590 1134 Fax: 020 8599 0282
(Redbridge Primary Care Trust)

Practice Manager J Zeff

GP Maximillian Peter SEGAL, Hector Paul SPITERI

The Drive Surgery
22 The Drive, Ilford IG1 3HT
Tel: 020 8554 1961
(Redbridge Primary Care Trust)

GP Mohinder SINGH, Dr SAKTHIBALAN

Eastern Avenue Surgery
167 Eastern Avenue, Redbridge, Ilford IG4 5AW
Tel: 020 8550 4532 Fax: 020 8551 2199
(Redbridge Primary Care Trust)
Patient List Size: 5000

Practice Manager H Bakahi

GP Rameshchandra Premjibhai BAKHAI, Maheswaralingam SAKTHIBALAN

Fencepiece Road Surgery
83 Fencepiece Road, Hainault, Ilford IG6 2NB
Tel: 020 8500 3526 Fax: 020 8924 1188
(Redbridge Primary Care Trust)

GP Naheed BUKHARI

Forest Edge Practice
Manford Way Health Centre, 53 Foremark Close, Hainault, Ilford IG6 3HS
Tel: 020 8500 9938 Fax: 020 8559 9319
Email: rob.orange@gp-f86007.nhs.uk
(Redbridge Primary Care Trust)
Patient List Size: 8900

Practice Manager Robert Orange

GP Rowena Jane CAMERON-MOWAT, H SALIH, Muhammad TAHIR, Sharon THOMPSON

The Fullwell Avenue Surgery
272 Fullwell Avenue, Clayhall, Ilford IG5 0SB
Tel: 020 8550 9988 Fax: 020 8551 1241
(Redbridge Primary Care Trust)

GP Rajesh Bhailalbhai PATEL

Fullwell Cross Health Centre
1 Tomswood Hill, Barkingside, Ilford IG6 2HG
Tel: 020 8500 0231 Fax: 020 8559 9657
(Redbridge Primary Care Trust)

GP Ali Tekin ATALAR, Elizabeth Julia COLGATE, Sugirthavalli DAVIE, Gerardo Gustavs STEINBERGS

Gants Hill Medical Centre
63-65 Ethelbert Gardens, Ilford IG2 6UW
Tel: 020 8550 3740 Fax: 020 8550 4300
(Redbridge Primary Care Trust)
Patient List Size: 4780

Practice Manager Shirley Suker

GP Upendra Nath SAHU, Ramzan Mohamed MUGHAL

Goodmayes Medical Centre
4 Eastwood Road, Goodmayes, Ilford IG3 8XB
Tel: 020 8590 1169 Fax: 020 8590 1170
(Redbridge Primary Care Trust)
Patient List Size: 6000

GP Ambrish Kumar SHAH, Sushma SHAH

Granbrook Surgery
465 Granbrook Road, Gants Hill, Ilford IG2 6EW
Tel: 020 8554 7111 Fax: 020 8491 6374
(Redbridge Primary Care Trust)
Patient List Size: 2600

Practice Manager K Wilson

GP Palapillai MAHENDRA-YOGAM

Green Lane Surgery
595 Green Lane, Goodmayes, Ilford IG3 9RN
Tel: 020 8590 6600 Fax: 020 8983 8992
(Redbridge Primary Care Trust)

Practice Manager Kim Nicholls

GP Anthony Ewen PRUSS, Mark Richard BEAVER

Hampton Road Surgery
120-122 Hampton Road, Ilford IG1 1PR
Tel: 020 8553 1774 Fax: 020 8514 4622
(Redbridge Primary Care Trust)
Patient List Size: 4242

GP Mrudula Vinodchandra SHAH

Ilford Lane Surgery
165 Ilford Lane, Ilford IG1 2RS
Tel: 020 8478 1366 Fax: 020 8491 9066
(Redbridge Primary Care Trust)
Patient List Size: 3000

Practice Manager S Nandu

GP Nirendra Nath DUTTA, M P SAHU

Ilford Lane Surgery
281 Ilford Lane, Ilford IG1 2SF
Tel: 020 8553 9577 Fax: 020 8478 5652

(Redbridge Primary Care Trust)

GP Suresh Jivrajbhai MATHUKIA

Ilford Medical Centre
61-63 Cleveland Road, Ilford IG1 1EE
Tel: 020 8514 7761/8478 0367 Fax: 020 8478 4448
(Redbridge Primary Care Trust)
Patient List Size: 11500

Practice Manager Janice Fields, Marilyn Thomas

GP Brian James GREENAWAY, Barzan Akram IZZAT, Najib SEEDAT, Shahrokh Moaddab SHABESTARY, Narinder Kumar SHARMA

Ilford Medical Practice
112 Henley Road, Ilford IG1 2TS
Tel: 020 8478 0764 Fax: 020 8478 6566
(Redbridge Primary Care Trust)
Patient List Size: 2500

GP Nirmal Kumar BOSE

Ilford Medical Practice
3rd Floor, Ilford Chambers, 11 Chapel Road, Ilford IG1 2DR
Tel: 020 8491 1821 Fax: 020 8491 1981
(Redbridge Primary Care Trust)
Patient List Size: 2692

GP Sanjeev SINGH, Elizabeth WEBSTER

Longwood Gardens Surgery
150 Longwood Gardens, Clayhall, Ilford IG5 0BE
Tel: 020 8550 6362
(Redbridge Primary Care Trust)
Patient List Size: 2600

Practice Manager L Howlett

GP Philip Orlando Bosco SOARES

New North Road Surgery
563 New North Road, Hainault, Ilford IG6 3TF
Tel: 020 8500 3054 Fax: 020 8501 3025
(Redbridge Primary Care Trust)
Patient List Size: 1900

Practice Manager Kuljit Kaur

GP Avinash Chander SURI

Newbury Park Health Centre
40 Perrymans Farm Road, Ilford IG2 7LE
Tel: 020 8518 2414 Fax: 020 8518 3194
(Redbridge Primary Care Trust)
Patient List Size: 3950

Practice Manager Hilary Powell

Newbury Park Health Centre
Newbury Park Health Centre, 40 Perrymans Farm Road, Barkingside, Ilford IG2 7LE
Tel: 020 8554 3944/1094 Fax: 020 8518 5911
(Redbridge Primary Care Trust)
Patient List Size: 8300

Practice Manager K Wilson

GP Hansraj Ravji PARMAR, Ahlam AL MOUSANI, Fitzroy CLARKE, Syed SHAH

Oak Tree Medical Centre
273-275 Green Lane, Seven Kings, Ilford IG3 9TJ
Tel: 020 8599 3474 Fax: 020 8590 8277
(Redbridge Primary Care Trust)
Patient List Size: 7500

Practice Manager Colleen Atkinson

GP Ann Elizabeth O'BRIEN, Henry AKPABHO, H AKPABIO, Aynkaran KANAGASUNDREM

Palms Medical Centre
97-101 Netley Road, Newbury Park, Ilford IG2 7NW
Tel: 020 8554 9551 Fax: 020 8518 2045
(Redbridge Primary Care Trust)
Patient List Size: 4900

Practice Manager E Allen

GP Ian Frank CRABBE, Shabir HUSSEIN, Graham Douglas MACKENZIE

Salisbury Road Surgery
1 Salisbury Road, Seven Kings, Ilford IG3 8BG
Tel: 020 8597 0924 Fax: 020 8598 8254
(Redbridge Primary Care Trust)
Patient List Size: 2000

Practice Manager Linda Curry

GP Dean Robert Gregory PRICE, Geeta Devi PATEL

Spearpoint Gardens Surgery
1 Spearpoint Gardens, Aldborough Road North, Newbury Park, Ilford IG2 7SX
Tel: 020 8590 3048 Fax: 020 8983 8241
(Redbridge Primary Care Trust)
Patient List Size: 2720

Practice Manager Lorraine Brett

GP Ghulam MUSTFA, Matthew ONYEKWELI, Radha PRABHAKAR

St Clement's Surgery
38 Bathurst Road, Ilford IG1 4LA
Tel: 020 8554 1371 Fax: 020 8491 3345
(Redbridge Primary Care Trust)
Patient List Size: 2800

Practice Manager Valerie O'Sullivan

GP Winston Christadoss Asir SOLOMON

The Surgery
68 The Drive, Ilford IG1 3PW
Tel: 020 8554 3014 Fax: 020 8518 0863
(Redbridge Primary Care Trust)
Patient List Size: 3500

Practice Manager Harsha Popat

GP Satyapaul SHARMA, Sanjay KUMAR

Windermere Gardens Surgery
49 Windermere Gardens, Redbridge, Ilford IG4 5BZ
Tel: 020 8550 9195 Fax: 020 8550 3746
(Redbridge Primary Care Trust)
Patient List Size: 1800

Practice Manager D Vasishtha

GP Kamini SUBBERWAL

York Road Surgery
55 York Road, Ilford IG1 3AF
Tel: 020 8514 0906
(Redbridge Primary Care Trust)

GP Guhaeni THURAIRAJAH

Ilfracombe

St Brannocks Road Medical Centre
St Brannocks Road, Ilfracombe EX34 8EG
Tel: 01271 863119 Fax: 01271 867839
(North Devon Primary Care Trust)
Patient List Size: 9100

Practice Manager Helen Tanner

GP David Ian Ross WALLACE, Sally Ann BEVAN, Richard Michael CULLEN, Anne FRANCIS, Gillian Frances KILNER, Sean David ROSS, John Samuel Bassett WOMERSLEY

Waterside Primary Care
Combe Martin Health Centre, Castle Street, Combe Martin, Ilfracombe EX34 0JA
Tel: 01271 882406 Fax: 01271 883821
(North Devon Primary Care Trust)
Patient List Size: 3000

Practice Manager J Rose

GP Michael Thomas FENNER, Adrian Clifford FREEMAN, Brian John GRIFFITHS, Stephen James HUNT, Martin James Cossor MATHER, Sarah Louise STAMPFLI

Ilkeston

The Arthur Medical Centre

Four Lane Ends, Horsley Woodhouse, Ilkeston DE7 6AX
Tel: 01332 880249
(Amber Valley Primary Care Trust)

Practice Manager V Foulke

GP Francis James Fraser BINNIE, L E CROWDER, Gregory Simon CROWLEY, Andrew John McKENZIE, Julie Elaine OSBORNE

Dr M F McGhee and Partners

Borough Street Surgery, 53 Borough Street, Castle Donington, Ilkeston DE74 2LB
Tel: 01332 810241 Fax: 01332 811748
(Charnwood and North West Leicestershire Primary Care Trust)
Patient List Size: 8800

Practice Manager Simon Atkinson

GP Michael McGHEE, Helen GODRIDGE, Marilyn Elizabeth Anne HORNER, Carol Mary Philomena McGRATH, Keith Robert SUMNER, Gordan James WARD-CAMPBELL

Eden Surgery

Cavendish Road, Ilkeston DE7 5AN
Tel: 0115 944 4081
(Erewash Primary Care Trust)
Patient List Size: 3000

Practice Manager Jayne Suthers

GP Richard Derek ADAMS, Neerunjun JOOTUN

Gladstone House Surgery

Gladstone Street West, Ilkeston DE7 5QS
Tel: 0115 932 0248 Fax: 0115 944 7347
(Erewash Primary Care Trust)
Patient List Size: 6400

Practice Manager Glen Pickering

GP Judith Anne DONOVAN, Amanda HANCOCK, Arvind Khandubhai MISTRY, Anita NATHAN, Ammini TAMPI

Ilkeston Health Centre

South Street, Ilkeston DE7 5PZ
Tel: 0115 932 2933 Fax: 0115 944 5496
(Erewash Primary Care Trust)

Practice Manager Gill Cresswell

GP Jesbir Kaur JOHAL, Amanda Elizabeth PORTNOY, David PORTNOY, Carol Louise WEBB

Ilkeston Health Centre

South Street, Ilkeston DE7 5PZ
Tel: 0115 932 2968
(Erewash Primary Care Trust)

GP Erica BAILEY, Stephen John MILLER, Simon Leslie PURNELL

Littlewick Medical Centre

42 Nottingham Road, Ilkeston DE7 5PR
Tel: 0115 932 5229 Fax: 0115 932 5413
Email: littlewick@btinternet.com
(Erewash Primary Care Trust)
Patient List Size: 16000

Practice Manager Dawn Campbell

GP Catharine Jane PARFITT, Katherine Jane BAGSHAW, Nigel Malcolm DOWNES, Patrick John HALLS, Markus HENN, Victoria Susan MOK, Emma Louise PIZZEY, Paul David TRAVELL, Gail Margaret WALTON, Paul Andrew WESTON SMITH

Old Station Surgery

Heanor Road, Ilkeston DE7 8ES
Tel: 0115 930 1055 Fax: 0115 944 5496
(Erewash Primary Care Trust)
Patient List Size: 13700

Practice Manager Dawn Douglas

GP Douglas Marshall HAMILTON, John S ASHCROFT, Andrew DAVIES, Vanessa Mary FOOT, Simon T KELLY, Miles D LANGDON, Janice THOMSON, Karen J WILSON

West Hallam Medical Centre

The Village, West Hallam, Ilkeston DE7 6GR
Tel: 0115 932 5462
(Erewash Primary Care Trust)

GP Lily Maclennan GAME, Stephen Christopher HOULTON, A W SWORD

Ilkley

Dr Rawling and Partners

Springs Lane, Ilkley LS29 8TH
Tel: 01943 604455 Fax: 01943 604466
Email: rawlingpartners@hotmail.com
Website: www.ilkleydoctors.org.uk
(Airedale Primary Care Trust)

GP Roger Graham RAWLING, David COCKSHOOT, Angela Heather RAWLING

Grange Park Surgery

Grange Road, Burley in Wharfedale, Ilkley LS29 7HG
Tel: 01943 862108 Fax: 01943 864997
(Airedale Primary Care Trust)
Patient List Size: 6495

Practice Manager Bridget McIntyre

GP Roger Banwell GOODWIN-JONES, S DAY, H GREEN, L JOWETT, E NEWTON, C RAYMENT

Ilkley Moor Doctors Group

Springs Lane, Ilkley LS29 8TH
Tel: 01943 604999 Fax: 01943 430005
(Airedale Primary Care Trust)

Practice Manager Wendy Ribbands

GP S DICKSON, Mark Jeremy Richard FRENCH, Robin Arcot POULIER, Helena Clare ROLFE, H D WATSON

Ilkley Moor Medical Practice

The Health Centre, Springs Lane, Ilkley LS29 8TH
Tel: 01943 604999 Fax: 01943 886307
(Airedale Primary Care Trust)

Practice Manager Wendy Ribbands

GP Mark FRENCH, Rosemary Elizabeth HARGREAVES, Robin Arcot POULIER, Helena Clare ROLFE, Graeme C SUMMERS, Helen Deborah WATSON

The Surgery

103 Main Street, Addingham, Ilkley LS29 0PD
Tel: 01943 830367 Fax: 01934 831287
(Airedale Primary Care Trust)
Patient List Size: 2980

Practice Manager Pat Smith

GP Eugene RAUBITSCHEK

Ilminster

North Street Surgery

22 North Street, Ilminster TA19 0DG
Tel: 01460 52284/52469 Fax: 01460 57233
(Taunton Deane Primary Care Trust)
Patient List Size: 2993

Practice Manager Katie Packham

GP Antony David Leigh AUSTIN, Julie Frances PATUCK

Summervale Medical Centre
Wharf Lane, Ilminster TA19 0DT
Tel: 01460 52354 Fax: 01460 52652
Email: first.lastname@summervaleilm.nhs.uk
(South Somerset Primary Care Trust)
Patient List Size: 6600

GP Robin Norman BARBER, Sally Jane GAYER, David Fram PATUCK, Alan Graham McTurk WILSON, Jillian Elizabeth WILSON

Ingatestone

The Coach House Surgery
High Street, Stock, Ingatestone CM4 9BD
Tel: 01277 840267 Fax: 01277 841568
(Chelmsford Primary Care Trust)

Practice Manager Shelley Scott-Horne

GP John Pennell COFFIN, David Jan ACORN

Ipswich

Barrack Lane Medical Practice
1 Barrack Lane, Ipswich IP1 3NQ
Tel: 01473 252827 Fax: 01473 250463
(Ipswich Primary Care Trust)
Patient List Size: 11000

Practice Manager Penny Ashbee

GP Michael David FREESTONE, Anthony Juno JESUTHASAN, C MAMUJEE, Anthony James REIDY, Dipika THAKERAR, Christopher UZOKWE

Birches Medical Centre
Twelve Acre Approach, Kesgrave, Ipswich IP5 1JF
Tel: 01473 624800
(Suffolk Coastal Primary Care Trust)

Practice Manager C Malpass

GP Nicholas John EDWARDS, Darren CAVE, N DE SILVA, Kusum Himatlal MEHTA

Burlington Road Surgery
14 Burlington Road, Ipswich IP1 2EU
Tel: 01473 211661 Fax: 01473 289187
(Ipswich Primary Care Trust)
Patient List Size: 15306

Practice Manager C Heath

GP Donald James McELHINNEY, Denis John ALLEN, Anthony COLLINS, Alastair Eric FLETT, Steven Washington HALL, Peter HOLLOWAY, Hubert Anthony Benedict Maria LELIJVELD, Peter David POORE, Rajiv SAMARASINGHE

County Practice
Barking Road, Needham Market, Ipswich IP6 8EZ
Tel: 01449 720666 Fax: 01449 720030
(Central Suffolk Primary Care Trust)

Practice Manager P Goodrum

GP Thomas Durward MARSH, Sarah Elizabeth CARROLL, Catherine May HELPS, Christopher W LEWIS, Christine Jill ROBERTS, Michael WATSON, Paul WYTHE

Deben Road Surgery
2 Deben Road, Ipswich IP1 5EN
Tel: 01473 741152 Fax: 01473 743237
(Ipswich Primary Care Trust)

Practice Manager Marlene Robinson

GP Stephen John ROBERTS, Martin BARRY, Ulrike DATAN, Simon Clifford Llewelyn HARLEY, Sukhi JOHAL

Derby Road Practice
52 Derby Road, Ipswich IP3 8DN
Tel: 01473 728121 Fax: 01473 718810
(Ipswich Primary Care Trust)
Patient List Size: 12000

Practice Manager Lesley Summers

GP Verity Jane BROWN, Jasper Richard GOODWYN, John Stuart HAGUE, Stephen JONES, Julie Elizabeth KITE, T D MARSH, Gerard TRAVERS, Sarah TRIGG, Robin Joseph WATSON

Felixstowe Road Surgery
235 Felixstowe Road, Ipswich IP3 9BN
Tel: 01473 719112 Fax: 01473 270148
(Ipswich Primary Care Trust)

Practice Manager Yvonne Reeve

GP Robert John COLLINS, Stephen BADCOCK, Cornelius Gerrard Mary McCARTHY, Andrew John PENKETHMAN, Neil David RENSHAW

Gipping Valley Practice
Norwich Roade, Barham, Ipswich IP6 0DJ
Tel: 01473 832832 Fax: 01473 830200
Email: email@gippingvalleypractice.co.uk
Website: www,grippingvalleypractice.co.uk
(Central Suffolk Primary Care Trust)

GP Paul David THOMAS

Hatfield Road Surgery
70 Hatfield Road, Ipswich IP3 9AG
Tel: 01473 272828 Fax: 01473 273515
(Ipswich Primary Care Trust)

Practice Manager Christine Watts

GP Brian Emlyn Burney WILLIAMS, Rebecca BALL, Emily BALME, Jane CAMPBELL, Madhu DOSHI, Mark LLOYD, David Alexander TURNER

Hawthorn Drive Surgery
206 Hawthorn Drive, Ipswich IP2 0QQ
Tel: 01473 685070 Fax: 01473 688707
(Ipswich Primary Care Trust)
Patient List Size: 7800

Practice Manager Kevin Bernard

GP James Newell DUNCAN, David BAGLEY BAGLEY, Pamela BARCELLA, Moira PINKNEY, Olive Joyce POWELL, Iraide SAGARNA, Danny SHOWELL

Health Centre
High Street, Bildeston, Ipswich IP7 7EX
Tel: 01449 740254 Fax: 01449 740903
(Central Suffolk Primary Care Trust)

GP Michael James BROWNE, David G C CLARK, Jane FAIRWEATHER, Mark Aelred HAINSWORTH

Ivry Street Medical Practice
5 Ivry Street, Ipswich IP1 3QW
Tel: 01473 254718 Fax: 01473 287790
(Ipswich Primary Care Trust)
Patient List Size: 10400

Practice Manager Paul D Kinlan

GP Christopher Mark Danton BROWN, Andrew BARNES, A DOIG, Lynne JAMES, Trevor John LOCKWOOD, Richard Jack PEARCE, Mary Vinnien Thomson WYBORN

Lattice Barn Surgery
14 Woodbridge Road East, Ipswich IP4 5PA
Tel: 01473 726836 Fax: 01473 273567
(Ipswich Primary Care Trust)
Patient List Size: 12000

Practice Manager Sarah Page

GP Charles Bernard WELLINGHAM, Paul Anthony BETHELL, Christopher Ian Murray COOK, Lucy Anne Helen HENSHALL, Jonathan Clive KNIGHT, Rajesh Manubhai PATEL

Norwich Road Surgery
199 Norwich Road, Ipswich IP1 4BX
Tel: 01473 289777 Fax: 01473 289545
(Ipswich Primary Care Trust)
Patient List Size: 9361

Practice Manager Linda Broughton

GP Susan Jane SMITH, Patricia CAHILL, Thomas KADICHEENI, Peter MACKENZIE, Peter William McKAY, Adam John MOWLES, Deborah SWINGLEHURST

Orchard Medical Practice
Orchard Street, Ipswich IP4 2PU
Tel: 01473 213261 Fax: 01473 287741
(Ipswich Primary Care Trust)

Practice Manager Andrea Clarke

GP Jane Anne PAVITT, Uma Devi ADAPA, David George Hubert CHITTICK, Michael Gerard McCULLAGH, denise PATTISON, Sally Anne WILLIAMS

Orchard Street Health Centre
Orchard Street, Ipswich IP4 2PU
Tel: 01473 213261 Fax: 01473 287741
(Ipswich Primary Care Trust)

Practice Manager Kim Coe

GP Benjamin Thomas SOLWAY, S A WHALE

Orchard Street Health Centre
Orchard Street, Ipswich IP4 2PU
Tel: 01473 213261 Fax: 01473 287741
(Ipswich Primary Care Trust)

Practice Manager Sue Stagg

GP A CRAGGS

The Ravenswood Surgery
Freston Road, Ipswich IP3 9UJ
Tel: 01473 274495 Fax: 01473 727642
(Ipswich Primary Care Trust)
Patient List Size: 3700

Practice Manager Sheila Shingler

GP Ishwar Lal BHATIA, Jane CAMPBELL, Baribefe Jephthah VITE

Squire and Partners
Market Place, Hadleigh, Ipswich IP7 5DN
Tel: 01473 822961 Fax: 01473 824895
Website: www.btinternet.com/~hadleigh
(Central Suffolk Primary Care Trust)
Patient List Size: 13000

Practice Manager Peter Larner

GP John Nicholas FLATHER, Elizabeth Mary COPE, Gillian CROOT, Christopher Patrick CULLEN, Carrie EVERITT, Matthew Sean Lawrence GLASON, Peter Thomas John IRWIN, Ruth NABARRO, Nikki SEXTON

The Surgery
29 Chesterfield Drive, Ipswich IP1 6DW
Tel: 01473 741349 Fax: 01473 744492
(Ipswich Primary Care Trust)

Practice Manager Hilary Bowen

GP James Cotton HENDERSON, Peter Andrew BUSH, Penelope EXLEY, Sarah Jane TAYLOR, David Michael WARD

The Surgery
23 The Square, Martlesham Heath, Ipswich IP5 3SL
Tel: 01473 610028 Fax: 01473 610791
(Suffolk Coastal Primary Care Trust)
Patient List Size: 5300

Practice Manager Lynne Marsh

GP Andrew Jaroslav Vlcek SCHURR, Anne Elizabeth Christina TESH

The Surgery
The Street, Holbrook, Ipswich IP9 2QS
Tel: 01473 328263 Fax: 01473 327185
(Central Suffolk Primary Care Trust)
Patient List Size: 8000

Practice Manager Barbara Galloway

GP Simon Jonathan DINEEN, John Michael CAREY, David Robert KING, Jane Elizabeth MIDFORTH, John Richard WILLIAMS

Wadera and Chhabra
478 Landseer Road, Ipswich IP3 9LU
Tel: 01473 274494 Fax: 01473 727742
Email: satish.wadera@gp-d83614.nhs.uk
(Ipswich Primary Care Trust)
Patient List Size: 3000

Practice Manager Sandra Last

GP Satish Prakash WADERA, Rajiv CHHABRA

Woodbridge Road Surgery
165-167 Woodbridge Road, Ipswich IP4 2PE
Tel: 01473 256251 Fax: 01473 286667
(Ipswich Primary Care Trust)
Patient List Size: 10900

Practice Manager Simon Eagle

GP Owen Anthony THURTLE, Peter William BURN, Nigel Christopher GIBBONS, Anne Elisabeth Pauline LAUKENS, Stephen W McCARTHY, James Patrick MOORE-SMITH, Jennifer Mary SHEEHAN, Roy Raymond STEINER

Isleworth

The Grove Medical Centre
103 The Grove, Isleworth TW7 4JE
Tel: 020 8560 2069 Fax: 020 8560 1284
(Hounslow Primary Care Trust)

GP Dr HO

The Isleworth Centre
146 Twickenham Road, Isleworth TW7 7DJ
Tel: 020 8321 3604 Fax: 020 8321 3607
(Hounslow Primary Care Trust)

GP John EDWARDS, Ros OLIVER

Spring Grove Road Surgery
215 Spring Grove Road, Isleworth TW7 4AG
Tel: 020 8560 7750 Fax: 020 8560 1284
(Hounslow Primary Care Trust)

Practice Manager Margaret Croucher

GP M DONAGH, Susanne HEFFERNAN, Dr LOOMBA

The Surgery
19 Harvard Road, Isleworth TW7 4PA
Tel: 020 8560 4841 Fax: 020 8568 5548
(Hounslow Primary Care Trust)

GP Dr KAIKINI

Iver

Iver Medical Centre
High Street, Iver SL0 9NU
Tel: 01753 653008 Fax: 01753 650890
(Chiltern and South Bucks Primary Care Trust)

Practice Manager Robert Skinner

GP Moji GILANI, Helen CORLETT, Christopher NOWERS, Tina PATEL

Ivybridge

Highlands Health Centre
Fore Street, Ivybridge PL21 9AE
Tel: 01752 897111 Fax: 01752 691477
(South Hams and West Devon Primary Care Trust)
Patient List Size: 3650

Practice Manager J Oaken

GP Trevor Neil GRIFFITHS, Gillian BEDFORD, Marian Joan LANGSFORD

Morris, Harker, Bleiker and Partners
Ivybridge Health Centre, Station Road, Ivybridge PL21 0AJ
Tel: 01752 690777 Fax: 01752 690252
Email: postmaster@gp-l83100.nhs.uk
(South Hams and West Devon Primary Care Trust)
Patient List Size: 11480

Practice Manager Janet Mallett

GP John Rhidian MORRIS, Philip Francois BLEIKER, Leslie CAMPBELL, Gary DAVIES, Ruth Jasmine HARKER, Sally Christine SHEPPARD

Poundwell Meadow Health Centre
Poundwell Meadow, Modbury, Ivybridge PL21 0QL
Tel: 01548 830666 Fax: 01548 831085
(South Hams and West Devon Primary Care Trust)
Patient List Size: 4000

Practice Manager Angela Clarke

GP Robert Miles WYATT, Helen Clare DAY, Peter James HOLLEY

Jarrow

Albert Road Surgery
118 Albert Road, Jarrow NE32 5AG
Tel: 0191 489 7002 Fax: 0191 428 5640
(South Tyneside Primary Care Trust)
Patient List Size: 3800

Practice Manager Carol Craggs

GP Winifred Helen McMANUS, Ezzat Rageh Mahmoud HASSAN

GP Surgery
East Wing, Palmer Community Hospital, Jarrow NE32 3UX
Tel: 0191 451 6075 Fax: 0191 451 6019
(South Tyneside Primary Care Trust)

Practice Manager Rachel Sisterson

GP F A NIXON, S S M ZAIDI

Mayfield Medical Centre
Park Road, Jarrow NE32 5SE
Tel: 0191 489 7183 Fax: 0191 483 2001
(South Tyneside Primary Care Trust)
Patient List Size: 8700

GP Bernard Francis DIAS, Elizabeth ASH, Ajay Kumar BEDI, Duane Edward Stuart CORDNER

Palmer Community Hospital GP Suite
Wear Street, Jarrow NE32 3UX
Tel: 0191 451 6078 Fax: 0191 451 6088
(South Tyneside Primary Care Trust)

Practice Manager L Miller

GP Angus Oldfield DOWSETT, Kevin GRIFFITHS, Karen OVERS

Wear Street Medical Centre
Wear Street, Jarrow NE32 3JN
Tel: 0191 489 7320 Fax: 0191 483 8876
(South Tyneside Primary Care Trust)

Practice Manager Carol Kirton

GP S SINGH

Keighley

Alim and Partners
151 North Street, Keighley BD21 3AU
Tel: 01535 607444 Fax: 01535 691247
(Airedale Primary Care Trust)
Patient List Size: 7200

Practice Manager Yasmeen Alim

GP Shaik Abdul ALIM, Jane Margaret HORNSEY, E G NAGARAJA

Farfield Group Practice
St Andrew's Surgeries, West Lane, Keighley BD21 2LD
Tel: 01535 607333 Fax: 01535 611818
(Airedale Primary Care Trust)
Patient List Size: 13150

Practice Manager Arlene Woollard

GP Stuart Michael GABBITAS, Sally Ann HUNTER, Jo HUXLEY, John Richard KENNEDY, Gordon Stephen Moore McLELLAN, Philip PUE, William Stuart THORBURN, Penelope Kate WEBSTER, Sarah WHITFIELD

Health Centre
Holme Lane, Cross Hills, Keighley BD20 7LG
Tel: 01535 632147 Fax: 01535 637576
(Craven, Harrogate and Rural District Primary Care Trust)
Patient List Size: 11800

Practice Manager Hazel Painter

GP Adrian Michael DUNBAR, Sean EMMOTT, Rosemary E HILL, Rosemary Elizabeth HILL, Elizabeth Ellen McCULLOCH, John Stephen PICKLES, Catherine SMITH, Anna WOODHAMS

Holycroft Surgery
The Health Centre, Oakworth Road, Keighley BD21 1SA
Tel: 01535 602010 Fax: 01535 691313
(Airedale Primary Care Trust)

Practice Manager Marion Ackroyd

GP John Hilary PARRY, Gerald William PARTRIDGE, Alison BROWN, Damian James RILEY, Louise RILEY, C WARD, Gaynor Caroline WILLIAMS

Kilmeny Surgery
50 Ashbourne Road, Ingrow, Keighley BD21 1LA
Tel: 01535 606415 Fax: 01535 669895
(Airedale Primary Care Trust)
Patient List Size: 12600

Practice Manager Mavis Clarkson, Sharon Ward

GP John Keith ENGLAND, Judith Elizabeth ALDRED, Margaret Alison ENGLAND, David Terence GOPAL, James Denis HODGSON, Brendan KENNEDY, Ronald McGILL, Andrew PARSONS, John Mulligan PRESHAW

Ling House Surgeries
49 Scott Street, Keighley BD21 2JH
Tel: 01535 605747 Fax: 01535 672576
(Airedale Primary Care Trust)
Patient List Size: 9572

Practice Manager Carole Short

GP Gordon CUNLIFFE, Margaret Frances HELLIWELL, Jacquilyn AITKEN, Margaret BUSHBY, Beth DEVLIN, Jean Carolyn Spear GILL, Pauline Helen SKARROTT, Neil Robert SMITH, Richard Edgar Bethel SOLOMONS

Oakworth Health Centre
3 Lidget Mill, Oakworth, Keighley BD22 7HN
Tel: 01535 643306 Fax: 01535 645832
(Airedale Primary Care Trust)
Patient List Size: 3200

Practice Manager Linda Grimshaw

GP Martin Kitson HOYLE, Carol Anne WALSHAW

Silsden Health Centre
Elliott Street, Silsden, Keighley BD20 0DG
Tel: 01535 652447 Fax: 01535 657296
(Airedale Primary Care Trust)
Patient List Size: 10350

Practice Manager Christine Glen

GP Brian John TONES, Elizabeth Jocelyn CLEMENTS, David HEPPELL, Matthew Robert MILBOURN, Neil Andrew Leighton SMITH, Helen Jane WALKER

Station Road Surgeries
Station Road, Haworth, Keighley BD22 8NL
Tel: 01535 642255 Fax: 01535 645380
Email: collinsn@bradford-ha.northy.nhs.uk
(Airedale Primary Care Trust)

Patient List Size: 9057

Practice Manager Jim Spencer

GP Andrew COLLINSON, Ross BROWN, John Howard William BURTON, Hella COX, Graham CRUICKSHANK, Ian Gordon FERGUSON, Anne Pamela SIDES

Kendal

The James Cochrane Practice
Maude Street, Kendal LA9 4QE
Tel: 01539 722124 Fax: 01539 734995
(Morecambe Bay Primary Care Trust)
Patient List Size: 14800

Practice Manager Susan Blonsky

GP Philip Wilkinson BUCKLER, Jennifer BUCKLER, Michael Lewis HOWSE, Alistair Grant MACKENZIE, Maria MARTIN, Robert Sven William MILNES, Susan OSTICK, Romola STRINGER

Station House Surgery
Station Road, Kendal LA9 6SA
Tel: 01539 722660 Fax: 01539 734845
(Morecambe Bay Primary Care Trust)

GP Martin Robert Palmer MEYRICK, Geraldine Anne Marr DAVIES, Mark ELLIOTT, Richard William MITCHELL, Jacqueline PAYNE, R SCOTT, Paul David SIMPSON

The Surgery
Captain French Lane, Kendal LA9 4HR
Tel: 01539 720241 Fax: 01539 725048
(Morecambe Bay Primary Care Trust)
Patient List Size: 8200

Practice Manager Andy Robinson

GP Michael John BRENNAN, Catherine BRENNAN, Simon EDGECOMBE, Simon James Nicholas GARDNER, Amy LEE, Julia Elizabeth PIGOTT, Elizabeth C WILLIAMS

Kenilworth

Abbey Medical Centre
42 Station Road, Kenilworth CV8 1JD
Tel: 01926 853142 Fax: 01926 851746
(South Warwickshire Primary Care Trust)
Patient List Size: 12500

GP Paul Christopher MILLER, Elaine Helen ARCHIBALD, Roger Neil DAVIES, Andrew James DELANEY, Peter JOHN, Susan Elizabeth PROSSER

The Castle Medical Centre
22 Bertie Road, Kenilworth CV8 1JP
Tel: 01926 857331 Fax: 01926 851070
(South Warwickshire Primary Care Trust)

Practice Manager Kimberley Dodd, Gabrielle Harris

GP Stephen George HARVEY, Karen APPLEYARD, Louise NEWSON, David Michael RAPLEY, David Thomas SPRAGGETT, Clare STODDART

Kenley

Moorings Medical Practice
Valley Road, Kenley CR8 5DG
(Croydon Primary Care Trust)
Patient List Size: 5470

GP F M COLLINS, A R KEATING, F SAMI

Keswick

Bank Street Surgery
9 Bank Street, Keswick CA12 5JY
Tel: 01768 772438 Fax: 01768 772454
(Eden Valley Primary Care Trust)
Patient List Size: 2100

Practice Manager Christine Harper

GP Judith Ann ATACK, Michael John EVANS

Castlehead Medical Centre
Ambleside Road, Keswick CA12 4DB
Tel: 01768 772025 Fax: 01768 773862
(Eden Valley Primary Care Trust)
Patient List Size: 6200

Practice Manager Yvonne Craig

GP Peter Malcolm WHITE, P E HEMINGWAY, Timothy Michael HOOPER, G P WHITE

Kettering

Burton Latimer Health Centre
High Street, Burton Latimer, Kettering NN15 5RH
Tel: 01536 723566 Fax: 01536 420226
(Northamptonshire Heartlands Primary Care Trust)

Practice Manager Sandra Morrison

GP Michael Charles SPENCER, Anne Frances CRAVEN, Richard Kenneth DEMPSTER, David Nicholas HERBERT, Martin Godfrey JAMES

Dryland Surgery
1 Field Street, Kettering NN16 8JZ
Tel: 01536 518951 Fax: 01536 486200
(Northamptonshire Heartlands Primary Care Trust)
Patient List Size: 13500

Practice Manager Elaine Nicholson, Dawn Savage

GP John Herbert Knowles FITTON, Luz Stella BRAYBROOKS, Hadrian MOSS, Adrian PERKINS, Leszek PIECHOWSKI, Alastair David WILDGOOSE

Eskdaill Medical Centre
Eskdaill Street, Kettering NN16 8RA
Tel: 01536 522633 Fax: 01536 417572
Website: www.eskdaill.co.uk
(Northamptonshire Heartlands Primary Care Trust)
Patient List Size: 10700

Practice Manager Carol M Bryceland

GP Leslie Gary NEILL, Katherine Mary BLAND, Kathryn Muriel BRYANT, R K KAPUR, Matthew James MAYE, Clive David SHACKLETON, E SMITH

Headlands Surgery
20 Headlands, Kettering NN15 7HP
Tel: 01536 518886 Fax: 01536 527757
(Northamptonshire Heartlands Primary Care Trust)
Patient List Size: 10200

Practice Manager Claire Mee

GP Michael John BRITTON, John HART, Sam MYERS, Anthony James Barter RUSSELL, Michael SLIP

Linden Medical Group
Linden Medical Centre, Linden Avenue, Kettering NN15 7NX
Tel: 01536 512104 Fax: 01536 415930
(Northamptonshire Heartlands Primary Care Trust)
Patient List Size: 13300

Practice Manager Peter Billingham

GP Robin James WHITBY, Paul BARCLAY, S HAUGHNEY, Nigel LOVEDAY, Jennifer Susan MOORE, Tony Martin PENNEY, Christopher Francis ROSE, Simon SPOONER

Midland Road Surgery
Midland Road, Thrapston, Kettering NN14 4JR
Tel: 01832 734444 Fax: 01832 734426
(Northamptonshire Heartlands Primary Care Trust)
Patient List Size: 5000

Practice Manager Jane Sheppard

GP Hossam Mohamed Hassaballah ABDALLAH, John SHEPPARD

Nene Valley Surgery
Green Lane, Thrapston, Kettering NN14 4QL
Tel: 01832 732456 Fax: 01832 736939
Email: nene.valley@gp-k83065.nhs.uk
Website: www.nenevalleysurgery.co.uk
(Northamptonshire Heartlands Primary Care Trust)
Patient List Size: 5150

Practice Manager Gordon Shone

GP Stephen John COTTERELL, Geoffrey Philip NICHOLSON, Lynn Margaret WARREN

Rothwell Health Centre
Bridge Street, Rothwell, Kettering NN14 6JW
Tel: 01536 418518 Fax: 01536 418373
(Northamptonshire Heartlands Primary Care Trust)
Patient List Size: 17300

Practice Manager Norman Gray

GP John Michael HOLDEN, William Paul ASPINALL, Paul Richard Stanley AYTON, Karim Michael KHAN, Timothy Ian MYHILL, Miciel VAAL

Weavers Medical Centre
50 School Lane, Kettering NN16 0DH
Tel: 01536 513494 Fax: 01536 526330
(Northamptonshire Heartlands Primary Care Trust)
Patient List Size: 14600

Practice Manager Maureen Heath

GP John Joseph Aloysius AHERNE, Clark Balfour BALLOCH, Lynne Sylvia GRAHAM, John Brendan McMANUS, Narendra Hirabhai MISTRY, Raffaella V POGGI, Jonathan David Woodruff SANSOME

Kidderminster

Aylmer Lodge Surgery
Broomfield Road, Kidderminster DY11 5PA
Tel: 01562 822015 Fax: 01562 827137
Website: www.aylmerlodge.nhs.uk
(Wyre Forest Primary Care Trust)
Patient List Size: 10833

Practice Manager Diane Millett

GP Christopher Michael Dodds SMITH, Timothy Michael Williams ALLEN, Janine Mair BURRIDGE, Anthony Graham CARTER, Francis Brendan MORGAN, Christine Rosemary SMITH, Loanne Kay STANLEY

The Church Street Practice
David Corbet House, 2 Callows Lane, Kidderminster DY10 2JG
Tel: 01562 822051 Fax: 01562 827251
(Wyre Forest Primary Care Trust)

Practice Manager Heather Park

GP John Marston WILNER, Timothy Charles CAMPION, Caroline Anne IRLAM, David Herbert MALCOMSON, Elizabeth Jane MALCOMSON, Parveen MANN, Baron MENDES DA COSTA, John Gowen TUDOR, Timothy Mayow WADSWORTH, Paul William WILLIAMS

Cookley Surgery
1 Lea Lane, Cookley, Kidderminster DY10 3TA
Tel: 01562 850770
(Wyre Forest Primary Care Trust)
Patient List Size: 2300

Practice Manager Valerie Hinton

GP Therese Manel SAVERYMUTTU, Stoyko KOLEV

Forest Glades Medical Centre
Bromsgrove Street, Kidderminster DY10 1PG
Tel: 01562 822509 Fax: 01562 827046
(Wyre Forest Primary Care Trust)

Practice Manager Alison Field

GP Paul Alexander STEWART, Gillian Frances BLANCHARD, Alistair JACKSON

Health Centre Practice
Bromsgrove Street, Kidderminster DY10 1PG
Tel: 01562 822077 Fax: 01562 823733
(Wyre Forest Primary Care Trust)
Patient List Size: 6588

Practice Manager Pamela Whitehead

GP Richard Alexander DAVIES, Lynne Hazel BUTCHER, David William STARKIE, Clive Graham THORLEY

The Medical Centre
Pinkham, Cleobury Mortimer, Kidderminster DY14 8QE
(Shropshire County Primary Care Trust)

GP Dr HOLZMAN

Northumberland House Surgery
437 Stourport Road, Kidderminster DY11 7BL
Tel: 01562 745715 Fax: 01562 863010
Website: www.northumberlandhousesurgery.co.uk
(Wyre Forest Primary Care Trust)
Patient List Size: 11500

Practice Manager D Beckett

GP Victor Philip SCHRIEBER, Bhaskar APPANNA, Anthony John DE COTHI, Judith M HARDWICK, Sally RUMLEY, Fiona SIMPSON, Paul THOMPSON, Clare TURNER, Christopher D WILKINSON

Stanmore House Surgery
Linden Avenue, Kidderminster DY10 3AA
Tel: 01562 822647 Fax: 01562 827255
(Wyre Forest Primary Care Trust)

Practice Manager Eunice Hoare

GP Neil Curtis JARVIE, Hilary BOYLE, Nigel Brian COCKRELL, Graeme Jackson WILCOX

The Surgery
Hemming Way, Chaddesley Corbett, Kidderminster DY10 4SF
Tel: 01562 777239 Fax: 01562 777196
(Wyre Forest Primary Care Trust)

Practice Manager C Ward, J Westwood

GP John Philip SPALDING, Stuart WILKIE

Wolverley Surgery
Wolverley, Kidderminster DY11 5TH
Tel: 01562 850800 Fax: 01562 852575
Email: practice.M81608@gp-M81608.nhs.uk
Website: www.wolverleysurgerykidderminster.co.uk
(Wyre Forest Primary Care Trust)
Patient List Size: 2950

Practice Manager Paul R Copsey

GP Kevin Hugh O'CONNOR, Claire BOLTON

Kidlington

Exeter Surgery
Exeter Close, Oxford Road, Kidlington OX5 1AP
Tel: 01865 375215 Fax: 01865 848148
(North East Oxfordshire Primary Care Trust)
Patient List Size: 10500

Practice Manager Caroline Jones

GP Simon Haswell STREET, Kate JOHNSON, Claire NESLING

Gosford Hill Medical Centre
167 Oxford Road, Kidlington OX5 2NS
Tel: 01865 374242 Fax: 01865 377826
(North East Oxfordshire Primary Care Trust)
Patient List Size: 7300

Practice Manager Sally Mackie

GP Martin Andrew STUBBINGS, Joanna Mary HEAF, Heidi LUCKHURST, Suzanne STEWART, Mark Jonathan WALLACE

Islip Medical Practice
Bletchingdon Road, Islip, Kidlington OX5 2TQ
Tel: 01865 371666 Fax: 01865 842475
Email: enquiries@islipsurgery.org.uk
(North East Oxfordshire Primary Care Trust)

Practice Manager Beverley Turner

GP Neil Henry Learmont BRYSON, Lisa IBBS, Heeny PAUL, alexandra THRELFAIL, Julie TRANTER

Kings Langley

Haverfield Surgery
34 High Street, Kings Langley WD4 9HT
Tel: 01923 262514
(Dacorum Primary Care Trust)

GP Saifu-Allah KANANI, Mary Patricia FAY

The New Surgery
The Nap, Kings Langley WD4 8ET
Tel: 01923 261035 Fax: 01923 269629
(Dacorum Primary Care Trust)
Patient List Size: 11200

Practice Manager Sheila Burgess

GP Stephen Jeremy COHEN, Mark Owen Newton BROWNFIELD, Claire EL-BORAI, Deborah KERR, Jean Marion McLELLAN, Jitendra PATEL, Elspeth Gordon WALLIS

King's Lynn

Broughton Surgery
Chapel Road, Boughton, King's Lynn PE33 9AG
Tel: 01366 500331 Fax: 01366 501375
(West Norfolk Primary Care Trust)
Patient List Size: 3470

Practice Manager Pauline Whitehead

GP Hugh Cameron SIMPSON, S R G KNOTT

Burnham Market Surgery
Church Walk, Burnham Market, King's Lynn PE31 8DH
Tel: 01328 737000 Fax: 01328 730104
(West Norfolk Primary Care Trust)
Patient List Size: 4485

Practice Manager Pat Layton

GP Richard Carlyle REDMAN, Marcus BRUDENELL, Helen CASWELL, Sarah-Jane Rosalind GORROD

Carole Brown Healthcentre
Saxon Way, Dersingham, King's Lynn PE31 6LY
Tel: 01553 692333 Fax: 01485 543259
Website: www.thehealthcentre.org.uk
(West Norfolk Primary Care Trust)
Patient List Size: 6000

Practice Manager C Gyton

GP M A BALUCH, Ian Keith CAMPBELL, Simon HAMBLING, M T KENNY, Jeremy Johnston RUSSELL

Centre Point Surgery
Centre Point, Fairstead, King's Lynn PE30 4SR
Tel: 01553 772063 Fax: 01553 771463
Email: doc@surgery95.freeserve.co.uk
(West Norfolk Primary Care Trust)
Patient List Size: 3900

Practice Manager Margaret Titmarsh

GP Kirtikumar Kalyanji SUCHAK, S AHMED

Dr Campbell and Partners
Heacham Group Practice, 45 Station Road, Heacham, King's Lynn PE31 7EX
Tel: 01485 572769 Fax: 01485 579255
(West Norfolk Primary Care Trust)
Patient List Size: 8000

GP Ian Keith CAMPBELL, Adrian George CLIFTON, Andrew Kevin LAKE, Jeremy Johnston RUSSELL

Gayton Road Health and Surgical Centre
Gayton Road, King's Lynn PE30 4DY
Tel: 01553 962333 Fax: 01553 696819
Website: www.thehealthcentre.org.uk
(West Norfolk Primary Care Trust)
Patient List Size: 16500

Practice Manager G R Dickerson, Hilary Judd

GP Gareth Bennett ALLEN, David Lewis BARTLETT, R BIRAN, Gerald Arthur CUPPER, Leena DEOL, Rajendra Govind DHUMALE, Colin Charles ELSTON, Bryan Ronald JELFS, Martin Thomas KENNY, Stephen Robert SUMMERS, Elizabeth VAUGHAN-WILLIAMS

Grimston Medical Centre
Congham Road, Grimston, King's Lynn PE32 1DW
Tel: 01485 600341 Fax: 01485 601411
(West Norfolk Primary Care Trust)

Practice Manager Sandra Brock

GP Michael Inigo ARCHER, Angela CLIFTON, Judy Monica SCOTT

Koopowitz and Partners
Watlington Medical Centre, Rowan Close, Watlington, King's Lynn PE33 0TU
Tel: 01553 810253 Fax: 01553 811629
(West Norfolk Primary Care Trust)
Patient List Size: 5300

Practice Manager Scilla Ash

GP Philip KOOPOWITZ, Charlotte-Sue BUCKLAND, Clare HAMBLING, Ian James MACK

Litcham Health Centre
Manor Drive, Litcham, King's Lynn PE32 2NW
Tel: 01328 701568 Fax: 01328 700632
Website: www.litchamhealthcentre.co.uk
(West Norfolk Primary Care Trust)
Patient List Size: 3500

Practice Manager Sarah Meek

GP Alan COLLETT, Julian BROWN

Southgates Medical Centre
41 Goodwins Road, King's Lynn PE30 5QX
Tel: 01553 819460 Fax: 01553 819466
(West Norfolk Primary Care Trust)
Patient List Size: 9200

Practice Manager Noel McGivern

GP Alan Laurie HEATH, S ATCHESON, Laurence Kingsley ATKINSON, Catherine Anne CONNOLLY, F HILL, Ian Keith HOTCHIN, Hilary Ira LAZARUS, Christopher McKENZIE

St Clement's Surgery
24 Marshland Street, Terrington St. Clement, King's Lynn PE34 4NE
Tel: 01553 828475/827051 Fax: 01553 827594
(West Norfolk Primary Care Trust)
Patient List Size: 4950

GP Beryl DUNCAN, V BHUPATHI, D G TIERNAN

St James House Surgery
County Court Road, King's Lynn PE30 5SY
Tel: 01553 774221 Fax: 01553 692181
Website: www.stjamessurgery.co.uk
(West Norfolk Primary Care Trust)
Patient List Size: 17000

Practice Manager Elizabeth Batstone

GP John David MARTIN, Michael Denis CUNNINGHAM, John Murray GALLOWAY, Andreas HOLNSBEIN, Elizabeth NICHOLLS, Aruna PATEL, Keith Andrew REDHEAD, Andrew Nicholas SHERWOOD, Peter Roy William TASKER, Eibert Frank TIGCHELAAR

The Surgery
Station Road, Great Massingham, King's Lynn PE32 2JQ
Tel: 01485 518336 Fax: 01485 518725

(West Norfolk Primary Care Trust)
Patient List Size: 5600

GP Charles Gethyn BARBER, Anthony Stuart BURGESS, Suzanne PHILLIPS, Robert Brian PRYN

The Woottons Surgery
Priory Lane, North Wooton, King's Lynn PE30 3PT
Tel: 01553 631469 Fax: 01553 631011
(West Norfolk Primary Care Trust)
Patient List Size: 5000

Practice Manager Nicki Simpson

GP Robert OUTRED, Mohammed EDRIS, Deborah HOPKIN

Kingsbridge

McIntosh, Harvey and STUBBS
Health Centre, Orchard Way, Chillington, Kingsbridge TQ7 2LB
Tel: 01548 580214 Fax: 01548 581080
(South Hams and West Devon Primary Care Trust)
Patient List Size: 3600

Practice Manager Kathy Burn

GP Christopher Gordon McINTOSH, Alison Jane HARVEY, Benjamin STUBBS

Norton Brook Medical Centre
Cookworthy Road, Kingsbridge TQ7 1AE
Tel: 01548 853551 Fax: 01548 857741
(South Hams and West Devon Primary Care Trust)
Patient List Size: 10000

Practice Manager Louise Killick

GP Brian John REEVE, Dr BALDWIN, Dr BEST, Dr HAMPSON, Simon James HARGREAVES, Elizabeth Carolyn HASLAM, Margaret Anne SMITH, Dr WILLIAMS

Kingston upon Thames

Canbury Medical Centre
1 Elm Road, Kingston upon Thames KT2 6HR
Tel: 020 8549 8818 Fax: 020 8547 0058
Website: www.canburymedicalcentre.co.uk
(Kingston Primary Care Trust)
Patient List Size: 10300

Practice Manager Louise Naidu

GP Josephine Celia BOXER, Michael Francis D'SOUZA, Sean Robert HILTON, Judith Anne KANE, Sagayamary LOURUDUSAMY, Isabel REBOLLO, Dhiren Shantila SHAH

Churchill Medical Centre
Clifton Road, Kingston upon Thames KT2 6PG
Tel: 020 8546 1809 Fax: 020 8549 4297
(Kingston Primary Care Trust)

Practice Manager Susan Puffett

GP Duncan Millroy CLEMENTS, Ann Eleri GIBBONS, Haythem NASEEF, Carmel William SAMMUT ALESSI, Peter Samuel SMITH, Margaret Julia WALKER

Fairhill Medical Practice
81 Kingston Hill, Kingston upon Thames KT2 7PX
Tel: 020 8546 1407 Fax: 020 8547 0075
(Kingston Primary Care Trust)
Patient List Size: 15900

Practice Manager Carole Robinson

GP Paul Anthony BOWSKILL, Carol Amanda MYERS, Michael Anthony Bryan CROW, Sarah FODDY, Elizabeth Ildiko KATAY, Alec KENNAUGH

Hampton Wick Surgery
1 Upper Teddington Road, Kingston upon Thames KT1 4DL
Tel: 020 8977 2638 Fax: 020 8977 2434
(Richmond and Twickenham Primary Care Trust)

Practice Manager Lynn Roylance

GP June BETTS, Katherine MOORE, Kieran O'FLYNN

Richmond Road Medical Centre
95 Richmond Road, Kingston upon Thames KT2 5BT
Tel: 020 8546 1961 Fax: 020 8974 9008
(Kingston Primary Care Trust)

GP Michael BARRIE, Julie Catherine BEATTIE, Alexandra Jane CHESWORTH, David Nicholas JEBB

The Surgery
15 Brackendale, 25 Gloucester Road, Kingston upon Thames KT1 3RL
Tel: 020 8546 8864 Fax: 020 8541 0217
(Kingston Primary Care Trust)

GP Charles Gabriel STEER

The Surgery
212 Richmond Road, Kingston upon Thames KT2 5HF
Tel: 020 8546 0400 Fax: 020 8974 5771
(Kingston Primary Care Trust)
Patient List Size: 7300

Practice Manager Pat Owen

GP Patricia Mary NORRIS, Vistasp Jal PAREKH, John Richard PARRISH

The Surgery
192 Tudor Drive, Kingston upon Thames KT2 5QH
Tel: 020 8549-0061 Fax: 020 8549 9488
(Kingston Primary Care Trust)
Patient List Size: 4250

Practice Manager Maureen Bertorelli

GP Jayendra Gordhandas THAKERAR, Hans Raj YADAV

Kingswinford

Kingswinford Health Centre
Standhills Road, Kingswinford DY6 8DN
Tel: 01384 271241 Fax: 01384 297530
(Dudley South Primary Care Trust)
Patient List Size: 8800

Practice Manager Sanora Jones

GP Anthony Bernard SKILBECK, Louise BUTLER, Judith Frances CARR, Neil Andrew KITELEY, Albert John THORNTON

Moss Grove Surgery
15 Moss Grove, Kingswinford DY6 9HS
Tel: 01384 277377 Fax: 01384 402329
(Dudley South Primary Care Trust)

Practice Manager Sonia G Clark

GP David Frank CRIPPS, Sandra Mary BRINDLEY, Mark Jeffrey HOPKIN, Mark KULIGOWSKI, Stephen John PARNELL, Susan Jane POTTER

Rangeways Road Surgery
33 Rangeways Road, High Acres, Kingswinford DY6 8PN
Tel: 01384 280111 Fax: 01384 401157
(Dudley South Primary Care Trust)
Patient List Size: 4320

Practice Manager Sandra Wilkinson

GP Terence HOLLINGWORTH, Judith Alison BLOOR, Samia SAROUFEEM

The Surgery
84 Market Street, Kingswinford DY6 9LN
Tel: 01384 402327
(Dudley Beacon and Castle Primary Care Trust)
Patient List Size: 2576

Practice Manager M Chisholm

GP Ian Thomas CHISHOLM

The Surgery
Summerhill, Kingswinford DY6 9JG
Tel: 01384 273275 Fax: 01384 833366
(Dudley South Primary Care Trust)
Patient List Size: 6500

GP Nicholas Anthony PLANT, Edward Thomas Michael COOKE, Peter Graham DALTON, J WISEMAM

Kington

The Meads Surgery
The Meads, Kington HR5 3DQ
(Herefordshire Primary Care Trust)

Practice Manager Rose Hopwood

GP M LIAS, S BROOKES, R KING, B MURPHY, G RANNIE, A WILLIAMS

The Surgery
The Meads, Kington HR5 3DQ
Tel: 01544 230302 Fax: 01544 230824
(Herefordshire Primary Care Trust)

Practice Manager Debbie Pritchard

GP Philip Ralph CLELAND, Malcolm LIAS, David John Owen GRIFFITH, Billie Joanne Mary MURPHY, Gordon Hugh RANNIE

Kirkby-in-Furness

The Surgery
Askew Gate House, Askew Gate, Kirkby-in-Furness LA17 7TE
Tel: 01229 889247 Fax: 01229 889097
(Morecambe Bay Primary Care Trust)

Practice Manager C Marcus-Cromwell

GP Helen CLAYSON, Philomena Mary SWARBRICK

Kirkby Stephen

Upper Eden Medical Practice
The Health Centre, Silver Street, Kirkby Stephen CA17 4RB
Tel: 01228 71369 Fax: 01768 372385
(Eden Valley Primary Care Trust)

GP Carl Samuel Milton HALLAM, Stephen HUCK, Jacqueline Claire MERCKEL

Knaresborough

Beech House Surgery
1 Ash Tree Road, Knaresborough HG5 0UB
Tel: 01423 542580 Fax: 01423 864450
(Craven, Harrogate and Rural District Primary Care Trust)
Patient List Size: 8600

Practice Manager John Gutherie

GP Jane Suzannah CARRADINE, Claire Lindsay KEENLESIDE, Anthony Joseph KEOGH, Amal Raj RAMDEEHOL, William Forbes WATSON

Eastgate Surgery
31B York Place, Knaresborough HG5 0AD
Tel: 01423 867451
(Craven, Harrogate and Rural District Primary Care Trust)
Patient List Size: 11078

Practice Manager Sue Ward

GP Jonathan Newton IDDON, John Crispin Dunlop BANKS, James Henry BRADSHAW, Sarah Jane MINTY, Margaret Anne PLOWMAN, Christopher John Lytham WALSH

Stockwell Road Surgery
21 Stockwell Road, Knaresborough HG5 0JY
Tel: 01423 867433 Fax: 01423 869633
(Craven, Harrogate and Rural District Primary Care Trust)

Practice Manager S K Massey

GP C A J DIXON, David Ian JOBLING, Rachael Marie ROBINSON, Stephen Frederick WALTON

The Village Hall Surgery
Staveley, Knaresborough HG5 9LD
Tel: 01423 322309 Fax: 01423 360296

Practice Manager Mary Guest

GP Alastair Scott GREEN, Stella Jane CALDWELL-RIDER, John William CROMPTON, Michelle Suzanne DAY, Clare Sarah EISNER, Martin Arthur JONES, Ronald John NIXON, Helen Mary REES

Knebworth

The Surgery
Station Road, Knebworth SG3 6AP
Tel: 01438 812494 Fax: 01438 816497
(North Hertfordshire and Stevenage Primary Care Trust)
Patient List Size: 12350

Practice Manager Marion Watson

GP David Cecil WOOD, Rosemary Anne DANIEL, Ian Gordon EDMUNDS, Eckart LOEFRLER, Katherine McMANNS

Knottingley

Ash Grove Surgery
Cow Lane, Knottingley WF11 9BZ
Tel: 01977 673141 Fax: 01977 677054
(Eastern Wakefield Primary Care Trust)

Practice Manager Joyce Harland

GP Prabir Kumar BRAHMA, Probhat Chandra BARUAH, S R JOYNER, Lesley Ann NEWLAND, G SAHAY, Nripendra Kumar SAIKIA, Paul Martin WAKEFIELD

Ferrybridge Medical Centre
8-10 High Street, Ferrybridge, Knottingley WF11 8NQ
Tel: 01977 672109 Fax: 01977 635032
Website: www.ferrybridgemedicalcentre.com
(Eastern Wakefield Primary Care Trust)
Patient List Size: 9200

Practice Manager Alan Grimes

GP Carole Ann PINDER, Phillip EARNSHAW, John Anthony HIGGINS, Arthur Denis MONE, Kate SCOFFINGS, Patrick WYNN

Knutsford

Annandale Medical Centre
Mobberley Road, Knutsford WA16 8HR
Tel: 01565 755222 Fax: 01565 652049
(Eastern Cheshire Primary Care Trust)
Patient List Size: 5230

Practice Manager Janet Loynton

GP James William BILLINGHAM, Gerant ALLEN, Joy Lesley DAVIES, Timothy John MALLON

Manchester Road Medical Centre
27-31 Manchester Road, Knutsford WA16 0LY
Tel: 01565 633101 Fax: 01565 750135
Website: www.mrmc-online.co.uk
(Eastern Cheshire Primary Care Trust)
Patient List Size: 6620

Practice Manager Joan Carpenter

GP Gail LEICESTER, Sally HARRIS, Alastair Keith Ian HOLT, Patrick James KEARNS, Susan Mary REEVES, Robin Nicholas STONES

Toft Road Surgery
Toft Road, Knutsford WA16 9DX
Tel: 01565 632681 Fax: 01565 632630
Website: www.toftroadsurgery.co.uk
(Eastern Cheshire Primary Care Trust)
Patient List Size: 9225

GP Martyn Hugh BERRISFORD, David Kilpatrick ARTHUR, Lesley Anne BAYLISS, Jennifer Anne LAWN, Robert John STEPHENSON

Lancaster

Bentham Medical Practice
Grasmere Drive, High Bentham, Lancaster LA2 7JP
Tel: 01524 261202 Fax: 01524 262905
(Craven, Harrogate and Rural District Primary Care Trust)
Patient List Size: 7500

Practice Manager S Macdonald

GP Clive Alwyn STORY, Jane BURNETT, Nick HOWLETT, Mairi McKIRDY, Peter Bryan NIGHTINGALE, Ralph SULLIVAN, Bernard Hugh WALKER

Dalton Square Surgery
8 Dalton Square, Lancaster LA1 1PN
Tel: 01524 842200 Fax: 01524 585411
(Morecambe Bay Primary Care Trust)
Patient List Size: 13600

Practice Manager Sandy Clark

GP David John LONGDEN, Kathryn E BRECKON, Nigel Kenneth COOK, Neil Geoffrey ECKERSLEY, Howard John FAIRHURST, Andrew Lindsay PATON, T J REYNARD, Neal VAUGHAN-JONES

King Street Surgery
38 King Street, Lancaster LA1 1RE
Tel: 01524 32294 Fax: 01524 848412
(Morecambe Bay Primary Care Trust)

Practice Manager Jean Kendall

GP Robin Henry BURR, Clifford Mark ELLEY, Duncan HALLAM, Helen Christine HALSTEAD, Paul Francis TYNAN, Kirsten Elizabeth WONG, Micheal-Kwai Yew WONG

Meadowside Medical Practice
1-3 Meadowside, Lancaster LA1 3AQ
Tel: 01524 32622 Fax: 01524 846353
Email: msidesurg@aol.com
Website: www.go.to/meadowside
(Morecambe Bay Primary Care Trust)
Patient List Size: 6500

Practice Manager Vicky Jameson

GP Morna Janet MURGATROYD, Andrew John CRAVEN, Mark David DENVER, David Stephen McDONNELL

Mechie and Partners
67 Owen Road, Lancaster LA1 2LG
Tel: 01524 846999 Fax: 01524 385424
(Morecambe Bay Primary Care Trust)

Practice Manager Susan Jackson

GP Graeme Lawrence MECHIE, Michael Robert KINGSTON, Andrew PARTINGTON, Alison Jane TOY, Andrew Dean Charles WHITTON

Queen Square Surgery
2 Queen Square, Lancaster LA1 1RP
Tel: 01524 843333 Fax: 01524 580980
(Morecambe Bay Primary Care Trust)
Patient List Size: 12800

GP D M ELLIOTT, Alison Margaret BATEMAN, S J CONNELL, Nicholas Alan JOHNSTONE, Jeremy David MARRIOTT, Kamlesh SIDHU, Simon Charles WETHERELL, David John YARNALL

Rosebank Surgery
Ashton Road, Road, Lancaster LA1 4JS
Tel: 01524 842284 Fax: 01524 844839
(Morecambe Bay Primary Care Trust)

GP Robin Geoffrey JACKSON, Philip David BATTY, Patricia T CARVILL, Andrew Robert GALLAGHER, Averil McCLELLAND, P NIGHTINGALE, John Kingsley NORTH

Lancing

Ball Tree Surgery
Western Road North, Sompting, Lancing BN15 9UX
Tel: 01903 752200 Fax: 01903 768317
(Adur, Arun and Worthing Primary Care Trust)
Patient List Size: 8300

Practice Manager R Hayes

GP John Howard YOUNG, Chris HAYSOM, David Godwin HOBSON, Paula IRVING, Jennifer Margaret YOUNG

Kingfisher Surgery
19 Culver Road, Lancing BN15 9AX
Tel: 0870 890 2535 Fax: 0870 890 2536
(Adur, Arun and Worthing Primary Care Trust)
Patient List Size: 3300

Practice Manager Sue Cristofoli

GP Anja GOOSSENS, Ton VON BIEL

Lancing Health Centre
Penstone Park, Lancing BN15 9AG
Tel: 01903 843298 Fax: 01903 843301
(Adur, Arun and Worthing Primary Care Trust)
Patient List Size: 2178

Practice Manager Stella Manning

GP Peter Ian BRUMMITT

New Pond Row Surgery
35 South Street, Lancing BN15 8AN
Tel: 0870 890 2515 Fax: 0870 890 2516
(Adur, Arun and Worthing Primary Care Trust)
Patient List Size: 5800

Practice Manager B Storm

GP David Paul STARBUCK, James BARTLETT, Gillian K WEBB, Bethan W WILLIAMS

The Orchard Surgery
Penstone Park, Lancing BN15 9AG
Tel: 01903 843333 Fax: 01903 843332
(Adur, Arun and Worthing Primary Care Trust)
Patient List Size: 6600

Practice Manager Mary Feeney

GP Patrick Joseph FEENEY, Christopher Paul VARTY, Caroline WILTON

Peskett
38 Old Shoreham Road, Lancing BN15 0QT
Tel: 01903 754358 Fax: 01903 754358
Email: heather.carrigan@nhs.net
(Adur, Arun and Worthing Primary Care Trust)
Patient List Size: 1925

Practice Manager Heather Carrigan

GP David John PESKETT

Langport

Richards and Partners
The Surgery, North Street, Langport TA10 9RH
Tel: 01458 250464 Fax: 01458 253246
(Taunton Deane Primary Care Trust)
Patient List Size: 11400

Practice Manager Brigitie Teuber

GP Michael Lindsay RICHARDS, Richard BALAI, David William Ramsay GIBSON, Myriam GROESSENS, Elizabeth Anne Esslemont NIGHTINGALE, Peter John NIGHTINGALE, Adrian STEWART

Launceston

Launceston Medical Centre
Landlake Road, Launceston PL15 9HH
Tel: 01566 772131 Fax: 01566 772223
(North and East Cornwall Primary Care Trust)
Patient List Size: 14500

Practice Manager Judy Cole

GP Robert Geoffrey de GLANVILLE, Patrick Terence COLLIER, James Loman FITZGERALD, Robert Owen MORICE, Michelle Lesley WELLS, John Derek WHEAL

Leamington Spa

Clarendon Lodge Medical Practice
16 Clarendon Street, Leamington Spa CV32 5SS
Tel: 01926 422094 Fax: 01926 331400
Website: www.leamington-gp.org.uk
(South Warwickshire Primary Care Trust)
Patient List Size: 12000

Practice Manager P E Fitzgerald

GP John Fabian WILMOT, Evelyn April CHAN, K CHAPMAN, John Edward FULLBROOK, Maeve Jocelyn GREEN, J O MULLEY, A PARSONS

Croft Medical Centre
Calder Walk, Leamington Spa CV31 1SA
Tel: 01926 421153 Fax: 01926 832343
(South Warwickshire Primary Care Trust)
Patient List Size: 9600

Practice Manager Jennifer Creighton

GP Malcolm Lawrence EYKYN, Veronica Mary Egerton HYLAND, Susan Michele INMAN, Peter Francis SHIPTON, Nicholas TAIT, Andrew WARNER

Cubbington Road Surgery
115 Cubbington Road, Leamington Spa CV32 7AT
Tel: 01926 425131 Fax: 01926 427254
(South Warwickshire Primary Care Trust)

GP Christopher Tobias CLOWES, Peter Alexander BONSALL, Rupert Jamie Christopher COLLINS, Lindsay Margaret FOSTER

Harbury Surgery
Mill Street, Harbury, Leamington Spa CV33 9HR
Tel: 01926 612232 Fax: 01926 612991
Website: www.harburysurgery.co.uk
(South Warwickshire Primary Care Trust)
Patient List Size: 6400

Practice Manager B M Andrews

GP John Lovatt HANCOCK, Colin Maxwell SNOWDON, Jonathan James Arthur WILKINSON

Lisle Court Medical Centre
Brunswick Street, Leamington Spa CV31 2ES
Tel: 01926 425436 Fax: 01926 427257
(South Warwickshire Primary Care Trust)
Patient List Size: 3612

Practice Manager J M Easter

GP Nigel MADAGAN, Angela BRADY

Park Street Surgery
33 Park Street, Leamington Spa CV32 4QN
Tel: 01926 422580 Fax: 01926 410338
(South Warwickshire Primary Care Trust)

GP Andrew Martin TEMPLETON, John Christopher CARTER, Timothy James CROSS, Susan LAIRD

Sherbourne Medical Centre
40 Oxford Street, Leamington Spa CV32 4RA
Tel: 01926 424736 Fax: 01926 470884
(South Warwickshire Primary Care Trust)
Patient List Size: 10300

Practice Manager Veronica Ward

GP Christopher David MOFFATT, Paul AINSWORTH, Richard Treloar COURTENAY, Geoffrey HAWKES, Lorna OLIVER

Spa Medical Centre
81 Radford Road, Leamington Spa CV31 1NE
Tel: 01926 421214 Fax: 01926 421217
(South Warwickshire Primary Care Trust)

GP Dr KNIGHT, Kirit Kashinath PANDYA

Waterside Medical Centre
Court Street, Leamington Spa CV31 2BB
Tel: 01926 428321 Fax: 01926 458350
(South Warwickshire Primary Care Trust)
Patient List Size: 9000

Practice Manager Karen Baxter

GP Yvonne WILKINSON, Clare Manda BOOTHROYD, Anthony THOMAS, Alastair McEwan WATT

Whitnash Medical Centre
110 Coppice Road, Whitnash, Leamington Spa CV31 2LT
Tel: 01926 316711 Fax: 01926 427260
(South Warwickshire Primary Care Trust)
Patient List Size: 5400

GP Peter John Montague DAVIS, Richard Michael Waldo DUNN, John Christopher EMERY

Leatherhead

Ashlea Medical Practice
30 Upper Fairfield Road, Leatherhead KT22 7HH
Tel: 01372 375666 Fax: 01372 360117
Website: www.ashlea.nhs.uk
(East Elmbridge and Mid Surrey Primary Care Trust)
Patient List Size: 17113

Practice Manager Janet Palfreeman

GP Geoffrey Braham CLARIDGE, Alison ANDERSON, Gillian CARVER, James Brooks CLOSE, Lynne Coralie DAVIES, Gill EVANS, John Jordan LOWES, Peta-Ann TEAGUE, Sharon WILLIAMS, John Soo Kiam WONG

Fairfield Medical Centre
Lower Road, Bookham, Leatherhead KT23 4DH
Tel: 01372 455450 Fax: 01372 455456
Website: www.fairfield.com
(East Elmbridge and Mid Surrey Primary Care Trust)
Patient List Size: 12000

Practice Manager Chris Boughey

GP Graham Lester CHINN, Carol Margaret BLOW, Aoife Mary EVANS, Sabina GEORGE, Sarah HAYDON, Jeremy David STEPHENSON

Martin and Barr
Eastwick Park Medical Practice, Eastwick Park Avenue, Great Bookham, Leatherhead KT23 3ND
Tel: 01372 452081 Fax: 01372 451680
Website: www.eastwickpark.co.uk
(East Elmbridge and Mid Surrey Primary Care Trust)
Patient List Size: 6000

Practice Manager A Compton

GP William Stephen Ramsey BARR, Christine MARTIN, P DEGAITAS, Cathy GUEST, E HORROCKS

The Medical Centre
Kingston Avenue, East Horsley, Leatherhead KT24 6QT
Tel: 01483 284151 Fax: 01483 285814
(Guildford and Waverley Primary Care Trust)
Patient List Size: 9690

Practice Manager Michael Gilbert

GP Vincent Preston FINNAMORE, Caroline Jane DEANE, Clifford William GOSDEN, Philip John Michael MARAZZI, Jane SPURGEON

Molebridge Practice
The North Leatherhead Medical Practice, 148-154 Kingston Rd, Leatherhead KT22 7PZ
Tel: 01372 362099 Fax: 01372 361179
(East Elmbridge and Mid Surrey Primary Care Trust)
Patient List Size: 6500

Practice Manager Lesley Meredith

GP Jane Rosamund MOORE, F FLORIDO-SANTANA, Justine ROSE, Simon WILLIAMS

Oxshott Medical Centre
Holtwood Road, Oxshott, Leatherhead KT22 0QJ
Tel: 01372 844000
(East Elmbridge and Mid Surrey Primary Care Trust)
Patient List Size: 5850

GP Nicholas Adrian Collett DOWN, Richard John DRAPER, Jacqueline Heidi PICKIN

Lechlade

Thomson and Partners
The Medical Centre, Oak Street, Lechlade GL7 3RY
Tel: 01367 252264 Fax: 01367 253180
Website: www.leachlademedical.nhs.uk
(Cotswold and Vale Primary Care Trust)
Patient List Size: 4475

Practice Manager Justin Clark

GP Ian Andrew THOMSON, Veronica Helena SAWICKI, Henry Michael Alcwyn STEPHENS

Ledbury

Ledbury Market Surgery
Market Street, Ledbury HR8 2AQ
Tel: 01531 632423 Fax: 01531 631560
(Herefordshire Primary Care Trust)
Patient List Size: 4079

Practice Manager Carolyn Barlow

GP Christopher David HILEY, Robert Hugh DAVIES

St Katherines Surgery
High Street, Ledbury HR8 1DZ
Tel: 01531 633271 Fax: 01531 632410
(Herefordshire Primary Care Trust)
Patient List Size: 8700

Practice Manager David Lloyd

GP Robert Dean SCHOLEFIELD, Kathryn Rachel CONWAY, Martin Clifford CROOK, Wendy Jane HUNTER, Nicholas MEYER

Lee-on-the-Solent

Lee on Solent Health Centre
Manor Way, Lee-on-the-Solent PO13 9JG
Tel: 023 9255 0220
(Fareham and Gosport Primary Care Trust)
Patient List Size: 5700

Practice Manager J Carty

GP John Howard BASSETT, Gillian Helen ASHBY, Ian Stuart BELL, Deidre A E DURRANT

Lee on Solent Health Centre
Manor Way, Lee-on-the-Solent PO13 9JG
Tel: 023 9255 3161 Fax: 023 9255 4135
(Fareham and Gosport Primary Care Trust)
Patient List Size: 2704

GP Evelyn Alice BEALE, Felicity SHAW

Leeds

Abbey Medical Centre
Norman Street, Leeds LS5 3JN
Tel: 0113 295 1844 Fax: 0113 295 1845
(Leeds North West Primary Care Trust)
Patient List Size: 5555

Practice Manager Margaret Pollard

GP Judith CARTER, John KIRKHAM, Shi Ming LIU, J WATSON

Allerton Medical Centre
6 Montreal Avenue, Leeds LS7 4LF
Tel: 0113 295 3460
(Leeds North East Primary Care Trust)
Patient List Size: 6000

Practice Manager S Simm

GP Geoffrey LIPMAN, F LAWRENSON, Janet Margaret SIMM

Armley Medical Centre
16 Church Road, Armley, Leeds LS12 1TZ
Tel: 0113 295 3800/3802 Fax: 0113 295 3810
(Leeds West Primary Care Trust)
Patient List Size: 9700

Practice Manager Susan Robinson

GP Ping Siang LEE, Craig Anthony ADCOCK, Gary Andrew LEES, Maureen Amanda LINDSAY, Robin Richard MUIR-COCHRANE, N SIMPSON

Arthington Medical Centre
5 Moor Road, Hunslet, Leeds LS10 2JJ
Tel: 0113 270 5645 Fax: 0113 270 0927
(South Leeds Primary Care Trust)
Patient List Size: 4150

Practice Manager D Handley-Fawcett

GP Rajgopalan MENON, Alison Kathleen HOUSE, S K MENON

Ashfield Medical Centre
15 Austhorpe Road, Cross Gates, Leeds LS15 8BA
Tel: 0113 295 1820 Fax: 0113 295 1822
(East Leeds Primary Care Trust)
Patient List Size: 6139

Practice Manager Marcus Collumb

GP Raphael Francis CATHERWOOD, Peter George EASTWOOD, Christopher Paul HOLMES

Ashton View Medical Centre
7 Ashton View, Leeds LS8 5BS
Tel: 0113 295 3880 Fax: 0113 295 3881
(East Leeds Primary Care Trust)
Patient List Size: 1800

Practice Manager Janet Burton

GP David Cecil George FIRTH, Y F S WONG

Austhorpe View Surgery
5 Austhorpe View, Leeds LS15 8NN
Tel: 0113 260 2262 Fax: 0113 232 8090
(East Leeds Primary Care Trust)

Practice Manager Sue Grant

GP Daniel Murray ROSE, Christine Ann CLYDE

Avenue Crescent Surgery
47 Avenue Crescent, Leeds LS8 4HD
Tel: 0113 262 4630 Fax: 0113 262 4630
(Leeds North East Primary Care Trust)
Patient List Size: 1040

GP Emmanuel Samuel ASIEDU-OFEI

Avenue Surgery
24 The Avenue, Alwoodley, Leeds LS17 7BE
Tel: 0113 295 3788 Fax: 0113 295 3781
(Leeds North East Primary Care Trust)
Patient List Size: 5000

Practice Manager Carole Holmes

GP Simon Morris FELLERMAN, Carolyn HUSTON, Linsey PEARSON

Beech Tree Medical Centre
178 Henconner Lane, Leeds LS13 4JH
Tel: 0113 295 4250 Fax: 0113 295 4251
(Leeds West Primary Care Trust)
Patient List Size: 2200

Practice Manager Stephen Simm

GP Santokh Singh MATHARU

Beeston Hill Health Centre
Beeston Hill, Beeston, Leeds LS11 8BS
Tel: 0113 270 5131 Fax: 0113 272 0722
(South Leeds Primary Care Trust)
Patient List Size: 7800

Practice Manager Heather Ball

GP Alexander IWANTSCHAK, Simon Kevin HOGAN, David Patrick MITCHELL, Hilary PUNTIS

Beeston Village Surgery
Beeston District Centre, Town Street, Leeds LS11 8PN
Tel: 0113 272 0720 Fax: 0113 277 7778
(South Leeds Primary Care Trust)
Patient List Size: 3500

Practice Manager H R Thompson

GP John Michael BERRIDGE, Helen M LOVELL

Bellbrooke Surgery
395-397 Harehills Lane, Leeds LS9 6AP
Tel: 0113 249 4848 Fax: 0113 248 4993
(East Leeds Primary Care Trust)
Patient List Size: 6500

Practice Manager Tony Heywood

GP Adrian Simon BOONIN, Celia ALLAN, Helen Rachel ALPIN, Alison ROBERTS

Belle Isle Medical Centre
Middleton Road, Leeds LS10 3DZ
Tel: 0113 270 9139 Fax: 0113 270 9139
(South Leeds Primary Care Trust)

GP Birendra PRASAD

Blomfield Practice
Nursery Lane Surgery, 150 Nursery Lane, Leeds LS17 7AQ
Tel: 0113 293444 Fax: 0113 295 3440
(Leeds North East Primary Care Trust)

Practice Manager V C Cameron

GP Ian Anthony BLOMFIELD, R A MURRAY, Angela Frances RICKARDS, John Baden SUTTON

Burley Park Doctors
Burley Park Medical Centre, 273 Burley Road, Leeds LS4 2EL
Tel: 0113 295 3250 Fax: 0113 295 3864
(Leeds North West Primary Care Trust)
Patient List Size: 11501

Practice Manager Heather Reid

GP Angela Elizabeth BIRKIN, Kirsty Ann BALDWIN, Michael John BERRIDGE, Amanda Susan DWYER, Catherine Joan KIRKWOOM, Jonathan Nigel David MAYERS, Julie Catherine STANTON

Burmantofts Health Centre
Cromwell Mount, Leeds LS9 7TA
Tel: 0113 295 3700 Fax: 0113 295 3701
(East Leeds Primary Care Trust)

Practice Manager Mrs Nash

GP Andrew Edward COHEN, M GOPAL

Burton Croft Surgery
5 Burton Crescent, Leeds LS6 4DN
Tel: 0113 274 4777 Fax: 0113 230 4219
(Leeds North West Primary Care Trust)

GP Ian Graham ALLMAN, Carole GREGORY, James William David MOXON, Fiona Clare PECKHAM, Gordon SINCLAIR

Butt Lane Surgery
58 Butt Lane, Leeds LS12 5AZ
Tel: 0113 295 4350/4334 Fax: 0113 295 4355
(Leeds West Primary Care Trust)

Practice Manager Ann Jafrate

GP Elizabeth Honor JARVIS, Pablo MILLARES-MARTIN, Amanda Susan Ann ROBINSON

Carlton Gardens Surgery
27 Carlton Gardens, Leeds LS7 1JL
Tel: 0113 295 2678 Fax: 0113 295 2679
(Leeds North East Primary Care Trust)
Patient List Size: 7671

GP Janice PRITLOVE, Carol Angela BROWNING, Christine CARR, Nigel MOODY, Simon Charles OTTMAN

Chapeloak Practice
347 Oakwood Lane, Leeds LS8 3HA
Tel: 0113 240 9999 Fax: 0113 235 9233
(Leeds North East Primary Care Trust)

Practice Manager Paul Storey

GP Stephen John BLACK, Charles Bryan FREEMAN, Julia Mary ALEXANDER, Anne Frances COHEN, T A FITZGERALD, Anne Louise WESTON

Chapeltown Health Centre
Spencer Place, Leeds LS7 4BB
Tel: 0113 240 7000 Fax: 0113 240 8623
(Leeds North East Primary Care Trust)
Patient List Size: 5940

Practice Manager N C Brown

GP Jennifer Bernadette MANUEL, Mary Teresa FEENEY, Gulrez Shah KHAN

Chapeltown Road Surgery
178 Chapeltown Road, Leeds LS7 4HP
Tel: 0113 262 1239 Fax: 0113 262 1239
(Leeds North East Primary Care Trust)
Patient List Size: 2300

Practice Manager Julie Smith

GP Constance Mary HUNTER

Charles Street Surgery
Otley, Leeds LS21 1BJ
Tel: 01943 466124
Website: www.charlesstreet.org.uk
(Leeds North West Primary Care Trust)
Patient List Size: 6650

Practice Manager S Morris

GP N J ALLEN

Church Street Surgery
57 Church Street, Hunslet, Leeds LS10 2PE
Tel: 0113 271 1884 Fax: 0113 272 0008
(South Leeds Primary Care Trust)

GP Sadiq Ahmed ALI

Commercial Road Surgery
75 Commercial Road, Leeds LS5 3AT
Tel: 0113 2951380 Fax: 0113 295 1381
(Leeds North West Primary Care Trust)
Patient List Size: 4800

Practice Manager Jackie Credland

GP Lynne Mary OGDEN, Ian McDERMOTT, Kate Antonia WELCH

Conway Medical Centre
51-53 Conway Place, Leeds LS8 5DE
Tel: 0113 249 0535 Fax: 0113 235 0144

(East Leeds Primary Care Trust)

GP S M ALI, S MANSOOR

Craven Road Medical Centre
60 Craven Road, Leeds LS6 2RX
Tel: 0113 295 3530 Fax: 0113 295 3542
(Leeds North West Primary Care Trust)

Practice Manager S Lunn

GP Takis CHRISTOU, Leonard Arie BIRAN, Helen Elizabeth BOLLAND, Philip Mark DYER, Trilok Bercharbhai PATEL, Gaye Lynn SHEERMAN-CHASE

The Croft and Tinshill Medical Practice
8 Tinshill Lane, Leeds LS16 7AP
Tel: 0113 267 3462 Fax: 0113 230 0402
(Leeds North West Primary Care Trust)
Patient List Size: 22500

Practice Manager Christine Gaughran

GP Paul Francis TAYLOR, Andrew John BOLTON, Simon BOYLE, Mark Andrew BROWN, Sarah HUTCHINSON, Martin Roy ISLIP, Kevin Alan JACKSON, Kirsten Jane MANOCK, Paul Frank ROBINSON, Christian Werner WACHSMUTH

Danks, Smith, Sykes and Farrell
134 Beeston Road, Beeston Hill, Leeds LS11 8BS
Tel: 0113 276 0717 Fax: 0113 270 3727
(South Leeds Primary Care Trust)

Practice Manager Clare Dean, Kelly Watson

GP Jonathan Francis DANKS, Peter FARRELL, Katie Jane GAUNT, Nicholas Anthony Gould SMITH, Rod SUTCLIFFE, Steven John SYKES

The Dekeyser Group Practice
The Fountain Medical Centre, Little Fountain, Leeds LS27 9EN
Tel: 0113 295 1600 Fax: 0113 238 1901
(South Leeds Primary Care Trust)

GP Stephen James LEDGER, Alison BEST, Stephen Mark FELDMAN, Sabodh Chander GOGNA, Daniel Clive HURWITZ, K L LOGAN, Francis PEREZ-CARRAL

Dib Lane Practice
112A Dib Lane, Leeds LS8 3AY
Tel: 0113 295 4650 Fax: 0113 295 4663
(East Leeds Primary Care Trust)

Practice Manager Richard Harrison

GP Arnold Geoffrey ZERMANSKY, Denise HUGHES, Zelia Karen MUNCER, Christakis Kyriacos VARNAVIDES

Dixon Lane Medical Centre
102 Dixon Lane, Lower Wortley, Leeds LS12 4AD
Tel: 0113 279 7234 Fax: 0113 295 3873
(Leeds West Primary Care Trust)

Practice Manager Alison Gaskell

GP Christopher ELLISON

Dr Janik and Partners
The Surgery, High Street, South Milford, Leeds LS25 5AA
Tel: 01977 682202 Fax: 01977 681628
(Selby and York Primary Care Trust)
Patient List Size: 9200

Practice Manager Lisa Furness

GP Antoni Jerzy JANIK, William St John HIRST, Stefano Girgorio LOUISETTO, Anne Catherine Mary MACKENZIE, Susan Frances MURPHY, Susan STUTTARD

East Park Parade Surgery
1 East Park Parade, Leeds LS9 9NQ
Tel: 0113 248 2454 Fax: 0113 248 2454
(East Leeds Primary Care Trust)

Practice Manager Jane Guckian

GP Damian Michael Francis GUCKIAN

Fieldhead Surgery
65 New Road Side, Horsforth, Leeds LS18 4JY
Tel: 0113 295 3410 Fax: 0113 295 3417
(Leeds North West Primary Care Trust)
Patient List Size: 4960

Practice Manager Linda Fergusson

GP Graham LONGBOTTOM, J SCHALLAMACH, Jennifer Anne SNELL

Garden Surgery
78A Osmondthorpe Lane, Leeds LS9 9BL
Tel: 0113 248 2291 Fax: 0113 240 5362
(East Leeds Primary Care Trust)

Practice Manager Doreen Sheppard

GP David Guy DOWSON, Paula HOWDEN, K KAIN

Garforth Medical Centre
Church Lane, Garforth, Leeds LS25 1ER
Tel: 0113 286 5311 Fax: 0113 287 5864
(East Leeds Primary Care Trust)
Patient List Size: 11914

Practice Manager Dawn Harrison

GP Nigel Rowden MATTHEWS, Samantha Jane BROWNING, Diana Elizabeth DRIFE, Kevin Greaves PORTER, Jonathan Paul RICHOLD, Andrew ROBINSON

Gildersome Health Centre
Finkle Lane, Gildersome, Morley, Leeds LS27 7HL
Tel: 0113 253 5134 Fax: 0113 253 4899
(South Leeds Primary Care Trust)

Practice Manager Margaret Elsworth

GP Prakash Narain MEHROTRA, John Lawrence SINGH

Gilsyke House
212A Selby Road, Halton, Leeds LS15 0LF
Tel: 0113 295 2710 Fax: 0113 295 2713
(East Leeds Primary Care Trust)
Patient List Size: 7400

GP Malcolm Bernard ADDLESTONE, Mohammad ILYAS, Sheila Jane Kerr RENWICK, A C SMITH

Grange Medical Centre
Seacroft Crescent, Leeds LS14 6NX
Tel: 0113 295 1801 Fax: 0113 295 1799
Email: reception1@gp-B86075.nhs.uk
(East Leeds Primary Care Trust)
Patient List Size: 8700

Practice Manager Pamela Spetch

GP Anne Marie HOUGHTON, Thomas Peter FOX, David Grahame HIGGINS, Janet Elizabeth KENNEDY

Harrogate Road Surgery
355 Harrogate Road, Leeds LS17 6PZ
Tel: 0113 268 0066 Fax: 0113 288 8643
(Leeds North East Primary Care Trust)

Practice Manager Coleen Maltby

GP Elizabeth Margaret PEARSON, Marcus JULLER, Elizabeth Maria MARTIN, Nargas NAZIR, Manjit S PUREWAL

Hawthorn Surgery
Wilfrid Terrace, Branch Road, Lower Wortley, Leeds LS12 5NR
Tel: 0113 295 4770/4772 Fax: 0113 295 4771
(Leeds West Primary Care Trust)
Patient List Size: 3200

Practice Manager Amanda Nelson

GP Peter Vincent SHEVLIN, Kenyatta GIBBS

The Health Centre
Gibson Lane, Kippax, Leeds LS25 7JN
Tel: 0113 287 0870 Fax: 0113 232 0746
(East Leeds Primary Care Trust)

Practice Manager Celia Watkinson

GP Helen Jane McGRATH, Judith Elise Lawson BEATY, Diana JAMES, Atulkumar PATEL, Philip Simon TOWNSEND, Andrew Derek WATERS

Highfield Medical Centre
16 Highfield Road, Bramley, Leeds LS13 2BL
Tel: 0113 2563250 Fax: 0113 236 0606
(Leeds West Primary Care Trust)

Practice Manager K Kripal

GP H SINGH, K KRIPAL

Highfield Surgery
Holtdale Approach, Leeds LS16 7ST
Tel: 0113 295 3600 Fax: 0113 295 3602
(Leeds North West Primary Care Trust)

Practice Manager Lorraine Brown

GP Janusz Andrzej ZOLTOWSKI, Rosa BOBET, Carol Ann KITCHEN, John David SHAW, Ian WHITELEY

Hunslet Health Centre
24 Church Street, Leeds LS10 2PE
Tel: 0113 270 5620 Fax: 0113 276 5595
(South Leeds Primary Care Trust)

GP Kaushal Kumar GUPTA, Muhammad NASEEM

Hyde Park Surgery
3 Woodsley Road, Leeds LS6 1SG
Tel: 0113 295 1235 Fax: 0113 295 1220
(Leeds North West Primary Care Trust)
Patient List Size: 8100

Practice Manager L Quashie

GP Thomas Stephen O'SHEA, Anne Patricia BELL, Julie Helen MARSDEN, John David RUSSELL, Farakh Jamil SADIQ, David Lyndon WATSON

Kinghorn and Partners
Woodhouse Health Centre, Woodhouse Street, Leeds LS6 2NS
Tel: 0113 295 3500 Fax: 0113 295 3503
(Leeds North East Primary Care Trust)
Patient List Size: 6300

Practice Manager Janet Brocklebank

GP Susan Hall KINGHORN, Catriona Jane BRENT, Michelle Jean HUME, Carole Elizabeth LEE

Kippax Hall Surgery
54 High Street, Kippax, Leeds LS25 7AB
Tel: 0113 286 2044 Fax: 0113 287 3970
(East Leeds Primary Care Trust)

GP Andrew David PEARLMAN, Paul HUNT, Sue WILLIAMS

Kirkstall Lane Medical Centre
216B Kirkstall Lane, Leeds LS6 3DS
Tel: 0113 295 3666 Fax: 0113 295 3650
(Leeds North West Primary Care Trust)
Patient List Size: 6500

Practice Manager Eve Clitheroe

GP Paul MOXON, Paul KAYE, Sarah Louise LAWTON

Laurel Bank Surgery
216B Kirkstall Lane, Leeds LS6 3DS
Tel: 0113 295 3900 Fax: 0113 295 3901
Email: lbs.secretary@nhs.net
(Leeds North West Primary Care Trust)
Patient List Size: 6100

Practice Manager Chad Chaplin

GP Mary Frances WALKER, Naweed Ali Shah BUKHARI, Claire Amanda SAMUEL

Leeds Student Medical Practice
4 Blenheim Court Walk, Leeds LS2 9AE
Tel: 0113 295 4488 Fax: 0113 295 4499
Email: lsmp@leeds.ac.uk
Website: www.leeds.ac.uk/lsmp
(Leeds North West Primary Care Trust)

Practice Manager Carrie Ellison

GP Julie GREENWAY, Jeremy Nicholas John ANDERSON, Daryl Margaret HAYWARD, Paul HUDSON, Michael Andrew JANULEWICZ, David MURRAY, Simon Gregory PEACOCK, Maureen REYNOLDS, Deborah Anne SMITH

Lingwell Croft Surgery
Ring Road, Middleton, Leeds LS10 3LT
Tel: 0113 270 4848 Fax: 0113 272 0030
(South Leeds Primary Care Trust)

Practice Manager Ruth M Long

GP Angelo M CALLIATO, Jacqueline Anne CAMPBELL, Terry Lee CRYSTAL, Paul Michael GLYNN, Richard Anthony LESTNER, Lucinda Elizabeth RUSSELL, Anne Lesley WEISS

The Lodge Medical Centre
Grange Park Avenue, Leeds LS8 3BA
Tel: 0113 265 6454 Fax: 0113 295 3710
(East Leeds Primary Care Trust)

GP A L GREEN

Manor Park Surgery
Bell Mount Close, Bramley, Leeds LS13 2UP
Tel: 0113 295 4302/4319 Fax: 0113 295 4321
(Leeds West Primary Care Trust)

Practice Manager Ruth Wood

GP Jennifer Mary TOLLEY, Katherine Michelle BIRNAGE, Nigel Philip CALAGHAN, John Allen CUNNINGHAM, Susan Mary ELTON, Russell David GILMORE, Rosemary YARWOOD

Manston Surgery
72-76 Austhorpe Road, Leeds LS15 8DZ
Tel: 0113 264 5455 Fax: 0113 232 6181
(East Leeds Primary Care Trust)
Patient List Size: 7000

Practice Manager Elizabeth Holmes

GP Martin John SWABY, Jane Elizabeth GILBEY, Peter David LEWIS, O O'DUCHON

Market Cross Surgery
103 Commercial Street, Rothwell, Leeds LS26 0QD
Tel: 0113 282 2119 Fax: 0113 282 5170
(South Leeds Primary Care Trust)
Patient List Size: 2607

Practice Manager Pat Lavin

GP Nighat SULTAN

Meanwood Group Practice
548 Meanwood Road, Leeds LS6 4JN
Tel: 0113 295 1737/295 1730 Fax: 0113 295 1736
(Leeds North East Primary Care Trust)
Patient List Size: 12443

Practice Manager A D Newbound

GP Andrew David NEWBOUND, A M C BEARPARK, Andrew D BEARPARK, Ruth J CUNLIFFE, Stephen Daniel HUMPHRIS, Sheena Stuart McMAIN, Richard Mark VAUTREY

Medical Centre
Beech Grove, Sherburn in Elmet, Leeds LS25 6ED
Tel: 01977 682208 Fax: 01977 681665
(Selby and York Primary Care Trust)

Practice Manager Margaret Britton

GP David Frederick HARRISON, Jonathan Kellman BYNOE, Roger Downend PARKIN

The Medical Centre
143 Rookwood Avenue, Leeds LS9 0NL
Tel: 0113 249 3011 Fax: 0113 240 1958
(East Leeds Primary Care Trust)

Practice Manager Paul Barry

GP Faye WALDEN, Mary Margaret BOLAND, Harry BROWN, Susan Mary LAYBOURN, David Gerrard MOORE, Kenneth David SHENDEREY

The Medical Centre
Station Road, Drighlington, Leeds BD11 1JU
Tel: 0113 285 2115
(South Leeds Primary Care Trust)

Moorcroft Surgery
646 King Lane, Leeds LS17 7AN
Tel: 0113 295 2750 Fax: 0113 295 2761
(Leeds North East Primary Care Trust)

Practice Manager Melanie Keane

GP Geoffrey Ian HALL, Debra NEWELL, Richard Andrew STACEY

Moorfield House Surgery
11 Wakefield Road, Garforth, Leeds LS25 1AN
Tel: 0113 286 2214 Fax: 0113 287 4371
(East Leeds Primary Care Trust)
Patient List Size: 4200

Practice Manager J Darwell

GP Stuart Mark DAVIS, John Mark TAYLOR

Moresdale Lane Surgery
95 Moresdale Lane, Leeds LS14 6GG
Tel: 0113 295 1200 Fax: 0113 295 1210
(East Leeds Primary Care Trust)
Patient List Size: 5600

Practice Manager Maureen Atkinson

GP Sarah Fiona FROST, Simon Kieran HALL, Robert Edmund PEARSON

Morley Health Centre
Corporation Street, Morley, Leeds LS27 9NB
Tel: 0113 295 4060 Fax: 0113 295 4062
(South Leeds Primary Care Trust)
Patient List Size: 2980

Practice Manager Liz Lloyd

GP Mohammad Ejazul HAQUE

Newton Surgery
305 Chapeltown Road, Leeds LS7 3JT
Tel: 0113 295 3737 Fax: 0113 295 3738
Email: newton.surgery@nhs.net
(Leeds North East Primary Care Trust)
Patient List Size: 2100

GP Manjit Singh HUNJIN

Oakley Terrace Surgery
12 Oakley Terrace, Leeds LS11 5HT
Tel: 0113 272 0900 Fax: 0113 270 7300
(South Leeds Primary Care Trust)

GP Howard Arthur LAST, Stewart Irwin MANNING

Oakwood Surgery
Glenhow Rise, Leeds LS8 4AA
Tel: 0113 295 1515 Fax: 0113 295 1500
(Leeds North East Primary Care Trust)

Practice Manager Marilyn Ingram

GP Gurminder Pal SINGH

Oulton Medical Centre
Quarry Hill, Oulton, Leeds LS26 8SZ
Tel: 0113 282 1571 Fax: 0113 282 4720
(South Leeds Primary Care Trust)
Patient List Size: 11600

Practice Manager J Beatson

GP John LYNAGH, Lesley FREEMAN, Canice James GARRETT, Jocelyn HUDSON, Robert Ian MARSHMAN, Yvonne Margaret RAYNOR, Roderick I SUTCLIFFE

Park Road Medical Centre
44 Park Road, Guiseley, Leeds LS20 8AR
Tel: 01943 873332 Fax: 01943 878294
(Leeds North West Primary Care Trust)
Patient List Size: 9600

Practice Manager Nicholas Bush

GP Colin Menzies ALEXANDER, Graham John SHERWOOD, Hilary Elizabeth TAYLOR, Andrew John THOMPSON

Primary Healthcare Team for Homeless
68 York Street, Leeds LS9 8AA
Tel: 0113 295 4840 Fax: 0113 247 0290
Website: www.nfahealthteam.org
(East Leeds Primary Care Trust)
Patient List Size: 6000

GP Sally READ

Priory View Medical Centre
2a Green Lane, Leeds LS12 1HU
Tel: 0113 295 4260/4267 Fax: 0113 295 4278
(Leeds West Primary Care Trust)
Patient List Size: 10800

Practice Manager Sandra Kaye

GP Andrew David BURKILL, Carl Andrew FOSTER, Susan NELSON, Bernard SHORT

Radsham Medical Centre
33-35 Butt Hill, Kippax, Leeds LS25 7JU
Tel: 0113 286 1891 Fax: 0113 286 2550
(East Leeds Primary Care Trust)

GP Aruna MALHOTRA, Prem Krishan MALHOTRA

Rawdon Surgery
11 New Road Side, Rawdon, Leeds LS19 6DD
Tel: 0113 295 4234 Fax: 0113 295 4228
Email: melissa.dexter@nhs.net
(Leeds North West Primary Care Trust)
Patient List Size: 7200

Practice Manager M J Dexter

GP Chand Karan MADAN, Katherine Isabel BERRIDGE, Sarah E GARDINER, Timothy Simon SHEARD, Janet SOUYAVE

Richmond Medical Centre
15 Upper Accommodation Road, Leeds LS9 8RZ
Tel: 0113 248 0948 Fax: 0113 240 9898
(East Leeds Primary Care Trust)

GP Sunil Kumar SRIVASTAVA

Rothwell Health Centre
Stonebrig Lane, Rothwell, Leeds LS26 0UE
Tel: 0113 282 1938 Fax: 0113 282 9195
(South Leeds Primary Care Trust)

GP Iqbal AHMED

Roundhay Road Surgery
209 Roundhay Road, Leeds LS8 4HQ
Tel: 0113 249 0504 Fax: 0113 248 0330
(Leeds North East Primary Care Trust)

Practice Manager Camilla Hawkes

GP G P SINGH, Helen HAYWOOD, Catherine LOUGH, Emma STORR

Shadwell Medical Centre
137 Shadwell Lane, Leeds LS17 8AE
Tel: 0113 293 9999 Fax: 0113 203 4276
(Leeds North East Primary Care Trust)

Practice Manager Colin Bateman

GP Roger Karl POTTS, Warren Reuben GOLDING, Jeremy Marshall SAGER

Shaftesbury Medical Centre
480 Harehills Lane, Leeds LS9 6DE
Tel: 0113 248 5631 Fax: 0113 235 0658

(East Leeds Primary Care Trust)
Patient List Size: 16000

Practice Manager Jenny Taylor

GP Arthur Walter ALLEN, Nicholas BISHOP, Brendan Thomas CAHILL, Peter Gordon DARBYSHIRE, Donald Wylie FORRESTER, Andrew Michael HARRIS, Nicholas KOSLOWSKY, Naomi Kathryn PENN, Joyce Elaine PIERONI

Shaftesbury Medical Centre
480 Harehills Lane, Leeds LS9 6DE
Tel: 0113 248 0392 Fax: 0113 235 1585
(East Leeds Primary Care Trust)

GP John Lawrence SINGH

Shafton Lane Surgery
20A Shafton Lane, Holbeck, Leeds LS11 9RE
Tel: 0113 295 4393 Fax: 0113 295 4390
(South Leeds Primary Care Trust)
Patient List Size: 3500

Practice Manager Penny Young

GP Lata Vasanth BHANDARY, Panambur Vasanth BHANDARY

Shaw House
11 Shaw Lane, Headingley, Leeds LS6 4DH
Tel: 0113 278 4914 Fax: 0113 274 5822
(Leeds North West Primary Care Trust)
Patient List Size: 3500

Practice Manager Rita Wright

GP Rachel Mary Elizabeth LANGFORD, Philip John ILES

Sherburn Group Practice
The Old Hungate Hospital, Finkle Hill, Sherburn in Elmet, Leeds LS25 6EB
Tel: 01977 682208
(Selby and York Primary Care Trust)

GP David HARRISON

Silver Lane Surgery
1 Suffolk Court, Yeadon, Leeds LS19 7JN
Tel: 0113 250 4953 Fax: 0113 250 9804
(Leeds North West Primary Care Trust)

Practice Manager Resemary Jay

GP Cheuk Hung Peter Ching CHU, Duncan James ROBSON, Hilary Caroline LUSCOMBE, Bernadette Ann O'LOUGHLIN, Martin Anthony SHELLY

Spencer Place Medical Practice
Chapeltown Health Centre, Spencer Place, Leeds LS7 4BB
Tel: 0113 240 9090 Fax: 0113 249 8480
(Leeds North East Primary Care Trust)
Patient List Size: 3250

Practice Manager Ann Cant

GP Pranjit Kumar BHATTACHARYYA, Myra Caroline SLOAN, Sally WALLACE

St Martins Practice
319 Chapeltown Road, Leeds LS7 3JT
Tel: 0113 262 1013 Fax: 0113 23 74747
(Leeds North East Primary Care Trust)

Practice Manager A Walker

GP Susanna Lucy LAWRENCE, Jonathan Mark ADAMS, Allison Margaret FIELD, Urfi SULAIMAN, Jeremy Charles THOMPSON, Caroline Mallorie Irwin TURNER

Stratford Street Surgery
9 Stratford Street, Leeds LS11 6JP
Tel: 0113 277 7914 Fax: 0113 237 4758
(Leeds North East Primary Care Trust)

GP Sheo Narayan PRASAD

The Street Lane Practice
12 Devonshire Avenue, Leeds LS8 1AY
Tel: 0113 295 3838 Fax: 0113 295 3842
(Leeds North East Primary Care Trust)
Patient List Size: 11650

Practice Manager Sue Clayton

GP John Michael APPS, Guy BAKER, Nigel Martin BEW, Margaret Lowri COOKE, Shaun Michael O'CONNELL, Lesley Anne SUNDERLAND

The Surgery
67 St James Street, Wetherby, Leeds LS22 6RS
Tel: 01937 585669 Fax: 01937 522703
(Leeds North East Primary Care Trust)
Patient List Size: 3400

Practice Manager Liz Webster

GP Stephen EDWARDS, Jacqueline KNIGHT

The Surgery
South Queen Street, Morley, Leeds LS27 9EW
Tel: 0113 253 4863 Fax: 0113 238 3564
Email: linda.brown2@nhs.net
(South Leeds Primary Care Trust)
Patient List Size: 4400

Practice Manager Linda Brown

GP Carole Anne HICKS, Joseph James McPEAKE

The Surgery
179 York Road, Leeds LS9 7RD
Tel: 0113 248 0268 Fax: 0113 248 8490
(East Leeds Primary Care Trust)
Patient List Size: 1250

GP Abdool Rajack SOOLTAN

The Surgery
67 Hilton Road, Chapeltown, Leeds LS8 4HA
(Leeds North East Primary Care Trust)

GP A BASU-RAY

Tempest Road Surgery
230 Tempest Road, Leeds LS11 7DH
Tel: 0113 2706555/2350379 Fax: 0113 2489597
(Leeds North East Primary Care Trust)
Patient List Size: 2500

GP Sita Ram SINGH, Arun RAI

Thakur and Partners
Silver Lane Surgery, 1 Suffolk Court, Yeadon, Leeds LS19 7JN
Tel: 0113 250 5988 Fax: 0113 250 3298
(Leeds North West Primary Care Trust)
Patient List Size: 3100

Practice Manager Jenny Thakur

GP Makhan Chandra THAKUR, Peter LINDSAY, Karen NAYLOR

Thornton Medical Centre
Green Lane, New Wortley, Leeds LS12 1JE
Tel: 0113 231 0626/201 5070 Fax: 0113 231 5079
(Leeds West Primary Care Trust)
Patient List Size: 8532

Practice Manager Pamela Wilson

GP Robert Irving ADDLESTONE, Shalini Rebecca DEVARAJ, Nicolaos MOURMOURIS, Gail Elizabeth ORME, Andrew M SIXSMITH

Thorpe Road Surgery
8 Thorpe Road, Middleton, Leeds LS10 4BA
Tel: 0113 270 5221 Fax: 0113 249 0261
(South Leeds Primary Care Trust)
Patient List Size: 2158

Practice Manager Sabiha Khan

GP Abida Shah Noor KHAN, Shah Noor KHAN

Vesper Road Surgery
43 Vesper Road, Leeds LS5 3QT
Tel: 0113 275 1248 Fax: 0113 274 9090
(Leeds North West Primary Care Trust)
Patient List Size: 6400

Practice Manager Liz Jackson

GP Patrick Gerard Mary GERAGHTY, Tracey FITZGERALD, Sue LYONS, B PAUSE

Victoria House Surgery
228 Dewsbury Road, Leeds LS11 6HQ
Tel: 0113 270 4754 Fax: 0113 272 0561
Website: www.victoriahousesurgery.gponline.com
(South Leeds Primary Care Trust)

Practice Manager Mary Whitehead

GP Carolyn Grace ABBOTT, Litsa EVANGELOU, Jason JONES

Westfield Medical Centre
2 St Martin's Terrace, Chapeltown Road, Leeds LS7 4JB
Tel: 0113 295 4750 Fax: 0113 295 4755
(Leeds North East Primary Care Trust)
Patient List Size: 2908

Practice Manager Margaret Lee

GP Pandichary Chandra PRAKASH-BABU, Sarojini SHARMA

Whinmoor Surgery
White Laithe Approach, Whinmoor, Leeds LS14 2EH
Tel: 0113 295 3295 Fax: 0113 295 3291
(East Leeds Primary Care Trust)

Practice Manager Elaine Mossad

GP Makram Gabra MOSSAD

The Whitfield Practice
Hunslet Health Centre, 24 Church Street, Leeds LS10 2PE
Tel: 0113 270 5194 Fax: 0113 270 2795
(South Leeds Primary Care Trust)
Patient List Size: 6800

Practice Manager J Roper

GP Daniel John ALBERT, Sally Jane BROWN, Michael MORRIS, Christine ROONEY, Simal Chandra SAHA

Windmill Health Centre
Mill Green, Leeds LS14 5JS
Tel: 0113 273 3733 Fax: 0113 232 3202
(East Leeds Primary Care Trust)
Patient List Size: 9000

Practice Manager Malcolm Scanun

GP Clive Mitchell SAFFER, Andrew FRIEND, Antonia FRIEND, James William GERRARD, Pathima KHAN, Jon Hilton ROBERTS

Windsor House Surgery
Corporation Street, Morley, Leeds LS27 9NB
Tel: 0113 252 5223 Fax: 0113 238 1262
(South Leeds Primary Care Trust)

Practice Manager W E Lawson

GP Richard James ADAMS, Robert ARNOLD, John Anthony BROWNE, Fiona Anne McNeil PINDER, Keith Douglas POLLOCK, Jeanette Marie TURLEY

Yeadon Health Centre
17 South View Road, Yeadon, Leeds LS19 7PS
Tel: 0113 295 4040 Fax: 0113 295 4044
(Leeds North West Primary Care Trust)
Patient List Size: 10600

Practice Manager M Cole, A Williams

GP Paul Robert JACQUES, Lisa BECKWITH, Robert Stuart EDWARDSON, Andrew Martin MARSHALL, D STACEY, Jennifer Anne STANTON, Andrew Leslie WRIGHT

Leek

The John Kelso Practice
Park Medical Centre, Ball Haye Road, Leek ST13 6QR
Tel: 01538 399007 Fax: 01538 370014
(Staffordshire Moorlands Primary Care Trust)
Patient List Size: 7300

Practice Manager Joyce Hird

GP Mark Ernest Paul PORCHERET, David James EVANS, Julie Dawn OXTOBY, Simon James SOMERVILLE, Susan Eve TURNER

Leek Health Centre
Fountain Street, Leek ST13 6JB
Tel: 01538 381022 Fax: 01538 398638
Website: www.leekhealthcentre.co.uk
(Staffordshire Moorlands Primary Care Trust)
Patient List Size: 7800

Practice Manager Maria Slack

GP Barrie Edward SCRIVEN, Jonathan HILL, Suzzane Elizabeth HOPKINS, James Talbot LEE, David Edward SHIERS

Moorland Medical Centre
Dyson House, Regent Street, Leek ST13 6LU
Tel: 01538 399008 Fax: 01538 398228
(Staffordshire Moorlands Primary Care Trust)
Patient List Size: 8100

Practice Manager Fiona Edridge

GP Gordon Roy CARPENTER, L COAR, Jane GREIG, David Hywel HUGHES

Stockwell Surgery
Park Medical Centre, Ball Haye Road, Leek ST13 6QP
Tel: 01538 399398/384213 Fax: 01538 399523
(Staffordshire Moorlands Primary Care Trust)
Patient List Size: 5000

Practice Manager Glenys Gallon

GP Simon James ELSDON, Alyson Frances REES, Matthew George STEPHENSON

Leicester

Anstey Surgery
21A The Nook, Anstey, Leicester LE7 7AZ
Tel: 0116 236 2531 Fax: 0116 235 7867
(Charnwood and North West Leicestershire Primary Care Trust)
Patient List Size: 6300

Practice Manager Kathy Platts

GP Nigel William OSBORNE, David Christopher ANDREW, H J HUGHES, S SCOTT

Arrazi Medical Centre
1 Evington Lane, Leicester LE5 5PQ
Tel: 0116 249 0000 Fax: 0116 249 0088
Email: vania_ak@gp-c82105.nhs.uk
(Eastern Leicester Primary Care Trust)
Patient List Size: 4000

GP Abdul-Kader VANIA

The Assist Project
Clyde Street Medical Practice, 1A Clyde Street, Leicester LE1 2BG
Tel: 0116 295 1400
(Eastern Leicester Primary Care Trust)

Practice Manager June Kennel

GP John Graham ASTLES, Stephen Robert BORLEY, Anna Louise HILEY, Nitin Harilal JOSHI, Dermot Martin McAULEY

Austin and Partners
4 Market Place, Billesdon, Leicester LE7 9AJ
Tel: 0116 259 6206 Fax: 0116 259 6388
(Melton, Rutland and Harborough Primary Care Trust)
Patient List Size: 6136

Practice Manager Wendy Reece

GP Margaret Wendy Elizabeth AUSTIN, Richard WHITELEY, Stephen David Sigrist COOKE, Gerald John NEVITT, Simeon RAYNER

Aylestone Road Medical Centre
705 Aylestone Road, Leicester LE2 8TG
Tel: 0116 283 2325
(Leicester City West Primary Care Trust)

GP Dhiren Shantilal SHAH, Dr NOLAN

Aylestone Road Medical Centre
705 Aylestone Road, Leicester LE2 8TG
Tel: 0116 283 5582 Fax: 0116 283 3963
(Leicester City West Primary Care Trust)
Patient List Size: 2700

GP Eileen Mary NOLAN, Michelle HARRISON

Barclay Street Health Centre
36 Barclay Street, Leicester LE3 0JA
Tel: 0116 254 7684
(Leicester City West Primary Care Trust)
Patient List Size: 1500

Practice Manager L Dyer

GP Sushilkumar Kundanlal DAVE

Barwell Medical Centre
39 Jersey Way, Barwell, Leicester LE9 8HR
Tel: 01445 842981
(Hinckley and Bosworth Primary Care Trust)
Patient List Size: 5500

Practice Manager J London, A M Tuttiett

GP S S A SHAH, Shauna McGIBBON, Nigel Paul SCARBOROUGH

Baxters Close Surgery
2 Baxters Close, Beaumont Leys, Leicester LE4 0QR
Tel: 0116 235 3579
(Leicester City West Primary Care Trust)
Patient List Size: 6456

GP Graham Clive ACKERLEY, V F ASHMAN, Dara Singh VIRDEE

Beaumont Leys Health Centre
1 Little Wood Close, Beaumont Leys, Leicester LE4 0UZ
Tel: 0116 235 0435
(Leicester City West Primary Care Trust)
Patient List Size: 2600

Practice Manager Jillian Brown

GP Virendra Kumar AGARWAL

Birstall Medical Centre
4 Whiles Lane, Birstall, Leicester LE4 4EE
Tel: 0116 267 5255 Fax: 0116 267 1108
(Charnwood and North West Leicestershire Primary Care Trust)

Practice Manager Surinder Sher

GP Karnail Singh SHER, Carol FURLONG

Briton Street Medical Centre
5 Briton Street, Leicester LE3 0AA
Tel: 0116 233 7744
(Leicester City West Primary Care Trust)

Practice Manager Neeta B Manek

GP K N GADHIA

Broadhurst Street Medical Centre
10 Broadhurst Street, Leicester LE4 6NF
Tel: 0116 226 2662 Fax: 0116 266 9109
(Eastern Leicester Primary Care Trust)

GP K S MORJANA

Canon Street Medical Centre
122 Canon Street, Leicester LE4 6NL
Tel: 0116 266 1247
(Leicester City West Primary Care Trust)

GP Bhupendra Vanravan MODI

Central Surgery
Brooksby Drive, Oadby, Leicester LE2 5AA
Tel: 0116 271 2175 Fax: 0116 271 4015
(South Leicestershire Primary Care Trust)
Patient List Size: 8250

Practice Manager Jackie Cotton

GP Christopher Donald YOUNG, Andrew Grant COOK, Michael John DAVIES, Susan Elisabeth HADLEY, Victoria JAMESON, Izabelina Rosaline KUNCEWICZ

Charnwood Health Centre
1 Spinney Hill Road, Leicester LE5 3GH
Tel: 0116 262 5102
(Eastern Leicester Primary Care Trust)
Patient List Size: 3100

GP T K CHOWDHURY

Charnwood Health Centre
1 Spinney Hill Road, Leicester LE5 3GH
(Eastern Leicester Primary Care Trust)

GP P C PATEL

Churchward and Partners
Croft Medical Centre, 2 Glen Road, Oadby, Leicester LE2 4PE
Tel: 0116 271 2564 Fax: 0116 272 9000
Website: www.croftmedical.com
(South Leicestershire Primary Care Trust)
Patient List Size: 8500

GP Hedley Cole Vickers CHURCHWARD, Nigel Geoffrey DADGE, Dr DALBY, Alison Elizabeth Jennifer MOORE, Daniel Finnbarr O'KEEFFE

Clarendon Park Road Health Centre
296 Clarendon Park Road, Leicester LE2 3AG
Tel: 0116 270 5049 Fax: 0116 270 0188
(Eastern Leicester Primary Care Trust)
Patient List Size: 5300

GP Balwant CHAUHAN, Avinashi PRASAD

Countesthorpe Health Centre
Central Street, Countesthorpe, Leicester LE8 5QJ
Tel: 0116 277 6336 Fax: 0116 278 0851
Website: www.countesthorpe.clara.net
(South Leicestershire Primary Care Trust)
Patient List Size: 9100

Practice Manager Isobel Wells

GP Michael John WRIGHT, Gary Eric ARAM, Robert BROWNE, Catherine GITTINS, Aly RASHID, Susan Jane RING

Derwent Street Surgery
68 Derwent Street, Leicester LE2 0GD
Tel: 0116 251 5095 Fax: 0116 253 2535
(Eastern Leicester Primary Care Trust)
Patient List Size: 3000

Practice Manager Hawabibi Pandor

GP Andrea WILKINSON

Desford Surgery
13 Cottage Lane, Desford, Leicester LE9 9GF
Tel: 01455 828947 Fax: 01455 828994
(Hinckley and Bosworth Primary Care Trust)
Patient List Size: 1550

GP John S GAUNTLETT, Madhukar AMBEKAR, Vidula AMBEKAR

The East Leicester Medical Practice
131 Uppingham Road, Leicester LE5 4BP
Tel: 0116 276 7145 Fax: 0116 246 1637
Email: elmp@dial.pipex.com
(Eastern Leicester Primary Care Trust)
Patient List Size: 13293

Practice Manager Amit Rawal

GP Stephen LONGWORTH, J BARETTO, A FAROOQI, Louis Steven LEVENE, Robert Kee McKINLEY, Richard John MORIARTY, S K SAHOTA, T STOKES, S WARD-BOOTH

East Park Road Health Centre
352 East Park Road, Leicester LE5 5AY
Tel: 0116 273 7569 Fax: 0116 273 7443
(Eastern Leicester Primary Care Trust)
Patient List Size: 3450

Practice Manager Asma Sader

GP S N CHOUDARY

East Park Road Medical Centre
264 East Park Road, Leicester LE5 5FD
Tel: 0116 273 7700
(Eastern Leicester Primary Care Trust)

Practice Manager Shantaben Mistry, Meina Patel

GP C KUMAR, Rajesh Parmanand PANDYA, J S PARMA, I N PATEL

Enderby Surgery
80 King Street, Enderby, Leicester LE9 5NT
Tel: 0116 286 6088
(South Leicestershire Primary Care Trust)

Practice Manager Usha Bhutani

GP Harish Chander BHUTANI, N MUGHAL, W O PRICHARD

Evington Road Medical Centre
71 Evington Road, Leicester LE2 1QH
Tel: 0116 212 0212
(Eastern Leicester Primary Care Trust)

GP Kevin Peter NEWLEY

Forest House Medical Centre
2A Park Drive, Leicester Forest East, Leicester LE3 3FN
Tel: 0116 289 8111
(South Leicestershire Primary Care Trust)

GP Robin Kenneth ADKINSON, Richard Martin CARR, Donald William Francis MAY, Michael Gordon MEAD, Marcus Christian David WOOLFORD

Fosse Medical Centre
344 Fosse Road North, Leicester LE3 5RR
Tel: 0116 253 8988 Fax: 0116 242 5178
(Leicester City West Primary Care Trust)
Patient List Size: 6950

Practice Manager Ellen Weir

GP Gopal Krishan SHARMA, Simon HUGH-JONES, Hafiz MUKADAM, Neel-Kumari SHARMA

Freemen's Common Health Centre
161 Welford Road, Leicester LE2 6BF
Tel: 0116 255 4776 Fax: 0116 254 9518
(Eastern Leicester Primary Care Trust)
Patient List Size: 13968

Practice Manager Samantha Spencer

GP Pratima KHUNTI, Linda Esther BROWNE, Paul DAVIES, Ashok Arjan JETHWA

Glenfield Surgery
111 Station Road, Glenfield, Leicester LE3 8GS
Tel: 0116 2333600 Fax: 0116 2332674/2333602
(South Leicestershire Primary Care Trust)
Patient List Size: 12000

Practice Manager Rob C S Davies

GP Nainesh CHOTAI, John Graham COOPER, Michael John SALT, Justin William TRAYNER

Greengate Medical Centre
1 Greengate Lane, Birstall, Leicester LE4 3JF
Tel: 0116 267 7901 Fax: 0116 267 7504
(Charnwood and North West Leicestershire Primary Care Trust)
Patient List Size: 13316

Practice Manager Duncan Mann

GP Stephen James HARDCASTLE, Richard George ACKERLEY, Susan Elizabeth FORD, B J GODDARD, Andrew John GREER, M PATEL

Groby Road Medical Centre
9 Groby Road, Leicester LE3 9ED
Tel: 0116 253 8185 Fax: 0116 2624180
(Leicester City West Primary Care Trust)
Patient List Size: 8000

Practice Manager J Peake

GP Ian Douglas PATCHETT, Paul John DANAHER, Michael Charles C HUNTER, Linda LUCRAFT, Caroline Jayne RABBITT

Health Centre
Melton Road, Syston, Leicester LE7 2EQ
Tel: 0116 260 9161 Fax: 0116 269 8388
(Melton, Rutland and Harborough Primary Care Trust)

Practice Manager Dawn Adcock

GP Richard Sells HURWOOD, Gareth Graham CHIDLOW, Linda Mary DICKINSON, Timothy Robin JENNINGS, Lesley Judith TWIGG

Heath Lane Surgery
Earl Shilton, Leicester LE9 7PB
Tel: 01455 844431 Fax: 01455 442297
Website: www.heathlanesurgery.co.uk
(Hinckley and Bosworth Primary Care Trust)
Patient List Size: 12800

Practice Manager Julie Price

GP Philip Andrew THOMAS, Maxine CLEAVER, Anne GREAVES, Gethin JENKINS, Colin James MONCRIEFF, Steven John MORGAN, Jenny Elizabeth TURA

Heatherbrook Surgery
Beaumont Leys, Leicester LE4 1EF
Tel: 0116 235 6324 Fax: 0116 234 0333
(Leicester City West Primary Care Trust)
Patient List Size: 2900

Practice Manager Shenna Charlton

GP Robert Paul ARCHER, Caroline Kvetoslava ARCHER

Hedges Medical Centre
Pasley Road, Eyres Monsell, Leicester LE2 9BU
Tel: 0116 225 1227 Fax: 0116 225 1477
(Leicester City West Primary Care Trust)
Patient List Size: 3923

Practice Manager Carol Timson

GP Sally Anne BAILEY, Fiona PARTRIDGE, Emma RITCHIE

Highfield Surgery
25 Severn Street, Leicester LE2 0NN
Tel: 0116 254 3253
(Eastern Leicester Primary Care Trust)
Patient List Size: 4670

Practice Manager R Bapodra

GP Vijoy Kumar SINGH, Sarman Vajshi BAPODRA

Humberstone Park Surgery
190 Uppingham Road, Leicester LE5 0QG
Tel: 0116 276 6605 Fax: 0116 2760754
(Eastern Leicester Primary Care Trust)
Patient List Size: 7050

Practice Manager L Merricks

GP Ian Philip JONES, Agnes Mary MONTAGUE, Lisa NEVILLE, David Stephen SALKIN, Tanya Lesley Helen SPERRY, Aileen TINCELLO

Kingsway Medical Centre
23 Kingsway, Narborough Road South, Leicester LE3 2JN
Tel: 0116 289 5081 Fax: 0116 263 0145
(South Leicestershire Primary Care Trust)

GP Paul Anthony LAZARUS, Julia BOWDEN, Joseph Chi Kong CHAN, Angela Marjorie HOLLINGTON, Sean LAMBERT, Leigh MARTIN

Limeleigh Medical Centre
169 Narborough Road, Leicester LE3 0PE
Tel: 0116 255 2688
(Leicester City West Primary Care Trust)

GP John Christopher GOODIER

Limeleigh Medical Group
434 Narborough Road, Leicester LE3 2FS
Tel: 0116 282 7070 Fax: 0116 289 3805
Email: doctors@dircon.co.uk
(Leicester City West Primary Care Trust)
Patient List Size: 10000

GP Geoffrey David COOK, Rachel CLARKE, Janeen MLNER, Robert Patrick TEW

The Limes Medical Centre
65 Leicester Road, Narborough, Leicester LE9 5DU
Tel: 0116 284 1347 Fax: 0116 275 2447
(South Leicestershire Primary Care Trust)
Patient List Size: 13428

Practice Manager Ann Pickering

GP Graham David Windsor PROWSE, Richard John BENNETTS, Andrew Peter MOLTU, Michael John ROWE, Hungerford Aboyne Thomas ROWLEY, Caroline Jane RUDDOCK

Lutterworth Road Medical Centre
58 Lutterworth Road, Blaby, Leicester LE8 4DN
Tel: 0116 247 7828
(South Leicestershire Primary Care Trust)

Practice Manager S J Uprichard

GP William Owen UPRICHARD, Syed AHMAD, Helen Jennifer WATSON

Mahavir Medical Centre
10 Chestnut Way, East Goscote, Leicester LE7 3QQ
Tel: 0116 260 1007 Fax: 0116 260 1008
(Charnwood and North West Leicestershire Primary Care Trust)
Patient List Size: 1500

Practice Manager Natasha Draycott

GP Bipinchandra Jaysukhlal SHAH

Malabar Road Medical Centre
60 Malabar Road, Leicester LE1 2PD
Tel: 0116 251 8047
(Eastern Leicester Primary Care Trust)

GP Harkishan Kanji VAGHELA

Melbourne Road Medical Centre
47 Melbourne Road, Leicester LE2 0GT
Tel: 0116 255 9869
(Eastern Leicester Primary Care Trust)

GP Indira Ghanshyam PATEL

Melbourne Road Surgery
71 Melbourne Road, Leicester LE2 0GU
Tel: 0116 253 9479 Fax: 0116 242 5602
(Eastern Leicester Primary Care Trust)

Practice Manager Hazra Sidat

GP Jatin Kumar Vishnooprasad PATEL, Rajendra PATEL, Vishnubhai Rambhai PATEL

Melbourne Street Medical Centre
56 Melbourne Street, Leicester LE2 0AS
Tel: 0116 262 2721
(Eastern Leicester Primary Care Trust)

Practice Manager Cliff Davey

GP Stuart Muir Findlay FRASER, Julian DACIE, Richard Charles NICHOLAS, Patrick Anthony O'CALLAGHAN

Narborough Health Centre
Narborough, Leicester LE9 5GX
Tel: 0116 286 6859
(South Leicestershire Primary Care Trust)

GP Sudhirbhai Prabhudas DESAI

Narborough Health Centre
Narborough, Leicester LE9 5GX
Tel: 0116 286 2386
(South Leicestershire Primary Care Trust)
Patient List Size: 1800

GP S T RAJA

Newbold Verdon Medical Practice
St George's Close, Newbold Verdon, Leicester LE9 9PZ
Tel: 01445 822171 Fax: 01445 824968
(Hinckley and Bosworth Primary Care Trust)
Patient List Size: 10200

Practice Manager Eileen Coupe

GP David Michael JONES, Paul Geoffrey DAVENPORT, Caroline Fiona KING, Uche NGWU, Ian REES, Julie Ann TAYLOR

Northfield Road Medical Centre
Northfield Road, Blaby, Leicester LE8 4NS
Tel: 0116 277 1705 Fax: 0116 277 9961
(South Leicestershire Primary Care Trust)

Practice Manager Arthur Binns

GP T BLOUNT, Nicholas Alexander Joseph GLOVER, Robert HOLLINGWORTH, D G JONES, Nicholas Wilson LAWRENCE, Andrew Frank Robert ST JOHN

Oakmeadow Surgery
87 Tatlow Road, Glenfield, Leicester LE3 8NF
Tel: 0116 287 7911 Fax: 0116 287 7911
Website: wwwoakmeadowsurgery.co.uk
(Leicester City West Primary Care Trust)
Patient List Size: 8846

Practice Manager Frank Hunter

GP Ian Robert PANTON, Perry JONES, Robert Andrew LEACH, Peter NEWSTEAD

Old Elms Surgery
72A Lutterworth Road, Aylestone, Leicester LE2 8PG
Tel: 0116 244 0010 Fax: 0116 282 4734
(Leicester City West Primary Care Trust)
Patient List Size: 1600

Practice Manager M A C Buck

GP Robert Graham BUCK

The Old School Surgery
2A Station Street, Kibworth, Leicester LE8 0LN
Tel: 0116 279 2422 Fax: 0116 279 6251
(Melton, Rutland and Harborough Primary Care Trust)
Patient List Size: 10900

Practice Manager David Winter

GP J M WILSON, John Ranald Burt KILPATRICK, M G MASON, S MONTGOMERIE, Dr WHITE

The Old School Surgery
Hinckley Road, Stoney Stanton, Leicester LE9 4LJ
Tel: 01455 271445 Fax: 01445 274526
(Hinckley and Bosworth Primary Care Trust)
Patient List Size: 6400

GP Kay ROTHWELL, Nigel BENTON, Garry DARLINGTON

Orchard Medical Practice
Orchard Road, Broughton Astley, Leicester LE9 6RG
Tel: 01445 282599 Fax: 01445 286772
(Hinckley and Bosworth Primary Care Trust)
Patient List Size: 10440

Practice Manager Justine Watkinson

GP Barbara Eugenia LEES, Karen BRUNT, Dr CHAN, Adele Louise JEFFERIES-BECKLEY, Arshad Mahmood KHALID, Dr MAJOR

Parker Drive Medical Centre
122 Parker Drive, Leicester LE4 0JF
Tel: 0116 235 3148 Fax: 0116 235 4816
(Leicester City West Primary Care Trust)
Patient List Size: 13300

Practice Manager Rebecca Degia

GP Hemant Vishvanath TRIVEDI, Suhas Madhusudan AROLKER, Durairaj JAWAHAR, K NATARAJAN, V D PATEL

The Parks Medical Centre
340 Aikman Avenue, Leicester LE3 9PW
Tel: 0116 287 1230 Fax: 0116 287 3724
(Leicester City West Primary Care Trust)

Practice Manager S Allden

GP Basil Hadi Amin HAINSWORTH

Pasley Road Health Centre
Pasley Road, Eyres Monsell, Leicester LE2 9BU
Tel: 0116 278 6112
(Leicester City West Primary Care Trust)

GP Teck Keong KHONG

Pasley Road Health Centre
Pasley Road, Eyres Monsell, Leicester LE2 9BU
Tel: 0116 278 5182
(Leicester City West Primary Care Trust)

GP Frank Emilio Godfrey GATTONI, James Joseph HAMILL, Paul Anthony WILLIAMS

Petworth Drive Medical Centre
5 Petworth Drive, Leicester LE3 9RF
Tel: 0116 255 0030
(Leicester City West Primary Care Trust)

GP Gunvantrai Dalabhai PATEL

The Queens Road Medical Centre
220 Queens Road, Leicester LE2 3FT
(Eastern Leicester Primary Care Trust)

GP Jonathan LENTEN

Queens Road Surgery
108 Queens Road, Leicester LE2 3FL
Tel: 0116 270 7067 Fax: 0116 270 1892
(Leicester City West Primary Care Trust)

GP S K DEY, S MANSINGH

Ratby Surgery
122-124 Station Road, Ratby, Leicester LE6 0JP
(Hinckley and Bosworth Primary Care Trust)

Practice Manager Saeeda Parwatz

GP Paul PARWAIZ

Rookery Lane Health Centre
26 Rookery Lane, Groby, Leicester LE6 0GL
Tel: 0116 231 3331
(Hinckley and Bosworth Primary Care Trust)

GP Surjeet Singh GAJEBASIA

Roper and Partners
Syston Health Centre, Melton Road, Syston, Leicester LE7 2EQ
Tel: 0116 260 9111 Fax: 0116 260 9025
(Melton, Rutland and Harborough Primary Care Trust)

Practice Manager Sue Johnstone

GP Paul Winnard ROPER, Phillip Neil GREEN, Philip Graham HUSSEY, John Kingsley INMAN, Cheryl METCALFE, Elizabeth Mary SELLEN

Rosemead Drive Health Centre
103 Rosemead Drive, Oadby, Leicester LE2 5PP
Tel: 0116 271 3020
(South Leicestershire Primary Care Trust)

Practice Manager A Parker

GP S Z HUSAIN, Shamsher Singh CHOHAN, Janette Margaret WAKE

Roy
Fosse Road South, Leicester LE3 0QD
Tel: 0116 285 7329 Fax: 0116 285 7329
(Leicester City West Primary Care Trust)

Practice Manager D Roy

GP U K ROY

Rushey Mead Health Centre
8 Lockerbie Walk, Leicester LE4 7ZX
Tel: 0116 266 9616
(Eastern Leicester Primary Care Trust)

GP Elizabeth Frances HAMPSON, John Mervyn FRY, Jan Willem HELLENDOORN, Parimal PATEL

Saffron Group Practice
509 Saffron Lane, Leicester LE2 6UL
Tel: 0116 244 0888 Fax: 0116 283 1405
(Leicester City West Primary Care Trust)
Patient List Size: 9900

Practice Manager Patricia Brookhouse

GP Catherine Helen DUNCAN, Haider BHOGADIA, Adrian Michael HASTINGS, David Gary KERBEL, Sophie RICHARDS, David James SHEPHERD, Andrew Douglas WILSON

Severn Surgery
159 Uplands Road, Oadby, Leicester LE2 4NW
Tel: 0116 271 9042
(South Leicestershire Primary Care Trust)

GP Michael Peter SHANKS, Alison Katharine BAKER, Sue Patricia LONDON

Sheikh
91 St. Peters Road, Leicester LE2 1DJ
Tel: 0116 254 3003 Fax: 0116 270 0743
(Eastern Leicester Primary Care Trust)

Practice Manager Davinder Ruprai

GP Saeed Ahmed SHEIKH, Shahida Bokhari SHEIKH

Silverdale Drive Health Centre
6 Silverdale Drive, Thurmaston, Leicester LE4 8NN
Tel: 0116 260 0640 Fax: 0116 260 1640
(Charnwood and North West Leicestershire Primary Care Trust)
Patient List Size: 3381

Practice Manager Caroline Roberts

GP Yogeshkumar Bhagwatilal SHAH, Annette May RIISNAES

Smeeton Road Health Centre
Smeeton Road, Kibworth, Leicester LE8 0LG
Tel: 0116 279 3308 Fax: 0116 279 3320
(Melton, Rutland and Harborough Primary Care Trust)
Patient List Size: 7000

Practice Manager Maureen Barr

GP Miriam Ann WILLIAMS, N CHOUDHURY, Saskia FREESTONE, Nigel Alexander STOLLERY

Spinney Hill Medical Centre
143 St. Saviours Road, Leicester LE5 3HX
Tel: 0116 251 7870 Fax: 0116 262 9816
(Eastern Leicester Primary Care Trust)
Patient List Size: 16800

Practice Manager K Lorgat

GP Ashok Jashbhai AMIN, L MEHTA, Arvindkumar Dahyabhai MISTRY, Harish Ranchhod MISTRY, Prakash PANCHOLI, S D PATEL, Shyamsundar Jagannath PUROHIT, Surinder Singh SIAN

St Matthew's Medical Centre
Prince Philip House, Malabar Road, Leicester LE1 2NZ
Tel: 0116 224 4700 Fax: 0116 295 4627
(Eastern Leicester Primary Care Trust)

Patient List Size: 4500

Practice Manager Julie Harris

GP Angela Isabela Agnes LENNOX, T CHEESEMAN, George St. John LEATHER, J WRIGHT

St Peter's Health Centre
Sparkenhoe Street, Leicester LE2 0TA
Tel: 0116 251 8276 Fax: 0116 251 8276
(Eastern Leicester Primary Care Trust)

Practice Manager S Reid

GP Robert Chee Loong AU-YONG

St Peters Health Centre
Sparkenhoe Street, Leicester LE2 0TA
(Eastern Leicester Primary Care Trust)

Station Road Medical Centre
152 Station Road, Wigston, Leicester LE18 2DL
Tel: 0116 281 3722 Fax: 0116 281 3774
Email: shaffu_bg@gp-c82641.nhs.uk
(South Leicestershire Primary Care Trust)
Patient List Size: 2030

Practice Manager Julie Loach

GP Badi SHAFFU

Student Health Centre
De Montfort University, The Gateway, Leicester LE1 9BH
Tel: 0116 257 7594 Fax: 0116 257 7614
(Leicester City West Primary Care Trust)
Patient List Size: 12750

Practice Manager Bev Hallett

GP Alison Jane RHODES, Sarah Jane CHAPPLE, Ian Beresford CROSS, Ruth Mary DURKAN, Michael John GOULD

The Surgery
2-6 Halsbury Street, Leicester LE2 1QA
Tel: 0116 2730044
(Eastern Leicester Primary Care Trust)

Practice Manager Dolini Patel

GP Ranjit Sinh THAKOR, Indira Ravji MANDALIA, Babubhai MISTRY, H NANDHA

The Surgery
612 Saffron Lane, Leicester LE2 6TD
Tel: 0116 291 1212 Fax: 0116 291 0300
(Leicester City West Primary Care Trust)
Patient List Size: 6000

Practice Manager Julia Hikhman

GP Nancy Elizabeth THOMAS, Denise CHATTERIS, Shailesh Somabhai PATEL, Bharat Keshavji SHIKOTRA

The Surgery
4 Cross Street, Leicester LE4 5BA
Tel: 01162681242 Fax: 0116 268 1070
(Eastern Leicester Primary Care Trust)
Patient List Size: 3500

Practice Manager Eileen Moorhouse

GP Kishan Kumar PANJA

The Surgery
155 Downing Drive, Evington, Leicester LE5 6LP
Tel: 0116 241 3801
(Eastern Leicester Primary Care Trust)
Patient List Size: 7200

Practice Manager Lois P Parker

GP Anthony John James BENTLEY, Philip Andrew DOWNS, Simon Paul GIBBON

The Surgery
10 Broadhurst Street, Leicester LE4 6NF
(Eastern Leicester Primary Care Trust)

GP J N JANSARI

The Surgery
25 Buller Road, Leicester LE4 5GB
(Eastern Leicester Primary Care Trust)

Practice Manager Tara Gandecha

GP Dr GANDECHA

Uppingham Road Medical Centre
46-48 Uppingham Road, Leicester LE5 0QD
Tel: 0116 276 7133 Fax: 0116 276 4464
(Eastern Leicester Primary Care Trust)

Practice Manager Hazel Goodchild

GP Jeremy GOODCHILD

Walnut Street Medical Centre
110 Walnut Street, Leicester LE2 7LE
Tel: 0116 285 5300 Fax: 0116 285 5577
(Eastern Leicester Primary Care Trust)
Patient List Size: 3078

Practice Manager Jyoti Lodhia

GP Bhanuchandra Rugnath LODHIA

Welford Road Health Centre
693 Welford Road, Leicester LE2 6FQ
Tel: 0116 288 4450 Fax: 0116 288 4436
(Eastern Leicester Primary Care Trust)
Patient List Size: 2500

Practice Manager B S Byer

GP Lionel David BYER

Westcotes Family Practice
2 Westcotes Drive, Leicester LE3 0QR
Tel: 0116 255 8588
(Leicester City West Primary Care Trust)

GP Dharmamitra JUGESSUR

Westcotes Family Practice
2 Westcotes Drive, Leicester LE3 0QR
Tel: 0116 254 7887
(Leicester City West Primary Care Trust)
Patient List Size: 1800

Practice Manager Maureen Cooper

GP Nabil George SHAFFU

Westcotes Health Centre
Fosse Road South, Leicester LE3 0LP
Tel: 0116 254 0547 Fax: 0116 2540547
(Leicester City West Primary Care Trust)
Patient List Size: 4500

Practice Manager Geraldine Stokes

GP Richard Lawrence HAZELDINE, Kenneth Mark TAYLOR

Westcotes Health Centre
Fosse Road South, Leicester LE3 0LP
Tel: 0116 254 8568
(Leicester City West Primary Care Trust)

GP Neil Jeffrey GRUNDY, Sheelagh Brigid BOLT, Vindo GOHIL, Mark Jonathn REUBEN

Wigston Central Surgery
48 Leicester Road, Wigston Magna, Leicester LE18 1DR
Tel: 0116 288 2566 Fax: 0116 257 3314
(South Leicestershire Primary Care Trust)

Practice Manager Christine Elthernngton

GP Keith BAKER, Rakesh DESOR, Brenda Joan GRIFFIN, Sangita RAVAT

Willowbrook Medical Centre
195 Thurcourt Road, Thurnby Lodge, Leicester LE5 2NL
(Eastern Leicester Primary Care Trust)

Winstanley Drive Surgery
138 Winstanley Drive, Leicester LE3 1PB
Tel: 0116 285 8435 Fax: 0116 275 5416
(Leicester City West Primary Care Trust)
Patient List Size: 9600

Practice Manager Mary Carr

GP Ivor Ashby AMBUS, Kamlesh KHUNTI, Brendan William KINSELLA, Susan J McLOUGHLIN, Maria Anna Theresia NICHOLLS-VAN VLIET

Leigh

Brook Mill Medical Centre
College Street, Leigh WN7 2RB
Tel: 01942 681880 Fax: 01942 262578
(Ashton, Leigh and Wigan Primary Care Trust)

Practice Manager Sheila Gardener

GP Mark Richard Bruce COTTRILL, Balwinder DUPER, Gillian FELLOWS, Rachel HILTON, John Michael PICKIN

College Street Health Centre
College Street, Leigh WN7 2RF
Tel: 01942 684343 Fax: 01942 680477
Email: suren.tomar@gp-p92035.nhs.uk
(Ashton, Leigh and Wigan Primary Care Trust)
Patient List Size: 2800

GP Surendra Singh TOMAR, Anand DESHPANDE

Direct Access Surgery
79 Church Street, Leigh WN7 1AZ
Tel: 01942 680909/82991 Fax: 01942 673188
(Ashton, Leigh and Wigan Primary Care Trust)

Practice Manager Mina Das

GP Dhirendra Nath DAS

Drs Trivedi and Trivedi
4-12 Westleigh Lane, Leigh WN7 5JE
Tel: 01942 607627 Fax: 01942 261747
(Ashton, Leigh and Wigan Primary Care Trust)

Practice Manager Jeff Villiers

GP Dr TRIVEDI, Dr TRIVEDI

Foxleigh Family Surgery
Henry Street, Leigh WN7 2PE
Tel: 01942 602020 Fax: 01942 609039
(Ashton, Leigh and Wigan Primary Care Trust)
Patient List Size: 1990

Practice Manager Elaine Cowley

GP Stephen FOX

Grasmere Street Health Centre
Grasmere Street, Leigh WN7 1XB
Tel: 01942 672811 Fax: 01942 680883
(Ashton, Leigh and Wigan Primary Care Trust)
Patient List Size: 3051

Practice Manager R Cadman

GP John Lester LEWIS

Grasmere Street Health Centre
Grasmere Street, Leigh WN7 1XB
Tel: 01942 672811 Fax: 01942 680883
(Ashton, Leigh and Wigan Primary Care Trust)
Patient List Size: 2700

Practice Manager R Cadman

GP Susan Mary MARTIN

Grasmere Street Health Centre
Grasmere Street, Leigh WN7 1XB
Tel: 01942 672881 Fax: 01942 680883
(Ashton, Leigh and Wigan Primary Care Trust)
Patient List Size: 2521

Practice Manager R Cadman

GP Ahsan Masud SIDDIQUI

The Health Centre
Grasmere Street, Leigh WN7 1XB
Tel: 01942 673831 Fax: 01942 680883
(Ashton, Leigh and Wigan Primary Care Trust)
Patient List Size: 2475

Practice Manager R Cadman

GP Anil Sadashivrao DONGRE

The Health Centre
Grasmere Street, Leigh WN7 1XB
Tel: 01942 672811 Fax: 01942 680883
(Ashton, Leigh and Wigan Primary Care Trust)
Patient List Size: 2767

Practice Manager R Cadman

GP Morris Patrick Hugh DOUBLET-STEWART

The Health Centre
College Street, Leigh WN7 2RF
Tel: 01942 678600 Fax: 01942 261179
(Ashton, Leigh and Wigan Primary Care Trust)
Patient List Size: 2950

Practice Manager Clare M Hitchen

GP David CLIFT, Thomas Stanley FLETCHER, Alastair WILSON

The Surgery
Bengal Street, Leigh WN7 1YA
Tel: 01942 605506 Fax: 01942 680109
(Ashton, Leigh and Wigan Primary Care Trust)
Patient List Size: 9000

Practice Manager M Canty

GP M SPEILMANN, Paul Stuart RICHARDSON

The Surgery
95-97 Railway Road, Leigh WN7 4AD
Tel: 01942 673900 Fax: 01942 605812
(Ashton, Leigh and Wigan Primary Care Trust)
Patient List Size: 4000

Practice Manager Lynne Hodges

GP Dr HIND, Barooah JAINS, Dr RAABE

Leigh-on-Sea

Blenheim Chase Surgery
9 Blenheim Chase, Leigh-on-Sea SS9 3BZ
Tel: 01702 470336 Fax: 01702 476210
(Southend-on-Sea Primary Care Trust)

Practice Manager Jenny Anderson

GP Sankarakumaran SATHANANDAN

Cranleigh Drive Surgery
33 Cranleigh Drive, Leigh-on-Sea SS9 1SX
Tel: 01702 75485 Fax: 01702 471365
(Southend-on-Sea Primary Care Trust)

GP Nirmalendu KONGAR

Eastwood Surgery
348 Rayleigh Road, Eastwood, Leigh-on-Sea SS9 5PU
Tel: 01702 525289 Fax: 01702 520134
(Southend-on-Sea Primary Care Trust)

GP Sarwat ZAIDI

Elm Road Surgery
84 Elm Road, Leigh-on-Sea SS9 1SJ
Tel: 01702 711559 Fax: 01702 471447
(Southend-on-Sea Primary Care Trust)

Practice Manager Jackie Hunter

GP Michael Hassan ALAWI

Elmsleigh Drive Surgery
203 Elmsleigh Drive, Leigh-on-Sea SS9 4JH
Tel: 01702 712666 Fax: 01702 471163
(Southend-on-Sea Primary Care Trust)
Patient List Size: 1650

Practice Manager Alexandra Bowman

GP Amjad Abdul Latif PURI

Elmsleigh Drive Surgery
194 Elmsleigh Drive, Leigh-on-Sea SS9 4JQ
Tel: 01702 470705 Fax: 01702 471153
(Southend-on-Sea Primary Care Trust)
Patient List Size: 2148

Practice Manager Jean Joughin

GP George Kingsley JAYATILAKA

Fairway Medical Centre
7 The Fairway, Leigh-on-Sea SS9 4QN
Tel: 0870 417 6543 Fax: 01702 528300
(Southend-on-Sea Primary Care Trust)
Patient List Size: 3155

Practice Manager Joan Doshi

GP Harish Vrajlal DOSHI

Highlands Surgery
1643 London Road, Leigh-on-Sea SS9 2SQ
Tel: 01702 710131 Fax: 01702 471154
(Southend-on-Sea Primary Care Trust)
Patient List Size: 9800

Practice Manager Denis Tilbrook

GP Brian Richard Mason HOUSTON, Fred FISHER, Basil GARO-FAILIDES, Jamie GRANT, Paul HUSSELBEE, Heather Ruth KENNEDY, Michael SMITH

Kent Elms Health Centre
Rayleigh Road, Eastwood, Leigh-on-Sea SS9 5UU
Tel: 01702 522012 Fax: 01702 512375
(Southend-on-Sea Primary Care Trust)
Patient List Size: 6000

Practice Manager Margaret Darragh

GP A C KRISHNAN, N KRISHNAN

Kent Elms Health Centre
Rayleigh Road, Leigh-on-Sea SS9 5UU
Tel: 01702 421888 Fax: 01702 421818
(Southend-on-Sea Primary Care Trust)

Practice Manager Jenny Bailey

GP Habib ZAIDI, Syeda Talat Abbas ZAIDI

Kent Elms Medical Centre
1 Rayleigh Road, Leigh-on-Sea SS9 5UU
Tel: 01702 529333 Fax: 01702 522696
Email: practicemanager@gp-f81223.nhs.uk
(Southend-on-Sea Primary Care Trust)

Practice Manager Shaheen Malik

GP S A MALIK

Lydia House Surgery
8 Sutherland Boulevard, Leigh-on-Sea SS9 3PS
Tel: 01702 552900 Fax: 01702 553474
(Southend-on-Sea Primary Care Trust)

Practice Manager Anne Walker

GP Lawrence SINGER

Pall Mall Surgery
178 Pall Mall, Leigh-on-Sea SS9 1RB
Tel: 01702 478338 Fax: 01702 471294
(Southend-on-Sea Primary Care Trust)
Patient List Size: 10200

Practice Manager Marguerite Whybrow

GP Leonard Anthony DICKENS, Alison BEHN, Martin James BEVERTON, Heather KENNEDY, Lionel Richard NAGLE

The Surgery
348 Rayleigh Road, Eastwood, Leigh-on-Sea SS9 5PU
Tel: 01702 525289 Fax: 01702 520134
(Southend-on-Sea Primary Care Trust)

Practice Manager Jenny Bailey

GP Syed Habib Haider ZAIDI

Leighton Buzzard

Ashcroft Surgery
Stewkley Road, Wing, Leighton Buzzard LU7 0NE
Tel: 01296 688201 Fax: 01296 681421
(Vale of Aylesbury Primary Care Trust)
Patient List Size: 4232

Practice Manager Joanna Griffiths

GP Gordon DUNFORD, Martin GIBBY

Bassett Road Surgery
29 Bassett Road, Leighton Buzzard LU7 1AR
Tel: 01525 373111 Fax: 01525 853767
(Bedfordshire Heartlands Primary Care Trust)
Patient List Size: 12500

GP Roger Geoffrey CHAPMAN, John Lawrence HENDERSON, Mary Carole HORKAN, John Anthony SCUDAMORE, Henry TOOMEY, Ingrid Maria WALLACE, Tushara WICKRAMANAYAKA

Europa House
West Street, Bassett Road, Leighton Buzzard LU7 1DD
Tel: 01525 851888 Fax: 01525 853319
(Bedfordshire Heartlands Primary Care Trust)

Practice Manager Dorothy Squires

GP Alan Morgan MEADE, Joseph Enebieni ANA, Shankini SILAKUMAR

Lake Street Surgery
20-22 Lake Street, Leighton Buzzard LU7 1RT
Tel: 01525 851995 Fax: 01525 374783
(Bedfordshire Heartlands Primary Care Trust)
Patient List Size: 1500

Practice Manager Jennifer Gent

GP Miheengar Mohamad SHAFI

Leighton Road Surgery
1 Leighton Road, Linslade, Leighton Buzzard LU7 1LB
Tel: 01525 372571 Fax: 01525 850414
Email: docs@buzzmedic.freeserve.co.uk
Website: www.leightonroadsurgery.fsnet.co.uk
(Bedfordshire Heartlands Primary Care Trust)
Patient List Size: 9300

Practice Manager Liz Selby

GP Michael BUTTERISS, Nicola HUTCHESON, Bryce TAYLOR, Ann R TURNER

Mentmore Road Surgery
30 Mentmore Road, Linslade, Leighton Buzzard LU7 2NZ
Tel: 01525 383202 Fax: 01525 851740
(Bedfordshire Heartlands Primary Care Trust)
Patient List Size: 2762

Practice Manager Margaret Timothy

GP Edward Zygmunt George EVERSHED

Pitstone Surgery
Yardley Avenue, Pitstone, Leighton Buzzard LU7 9BE
Tel: 01296 668800
(Vale of Aylesbury Primary Care Trust)

Salisbury House Surgery
Lake Street, Leighton Buzzard LU7 1RS
Tel: 01525 373139/ 373288 Fax: 01525 853006

(Bedfordshire Heartlands Primary Care Trust)
Patient List Size: 9600

Practice Manager C Deane

GP Fiona Jane DRY, Mazedul HOQUE, Marios JOSEPHIDOU, Christopher Duncan Ward MARSHALL, K SMITH, R SRINIVASAN

The Surgery
46 Stewkley Road, Wing, Leighton Buzzard LU7 0NE
Tel: 01296 688949
(Vale of Aylesbury Primary Care Trust)
Patient List Size: 4450

Practice Manager Sue Ford

GP Myra JONES, John LILLEY, Elizabeth PEEL

Leiston

The Surgery
Main Street, Leiston IP16 4ES
Tel: 01728 830526 Fax: 01728 832029
(Suffolk Coastal Primary Care Trust)
Patient List Size: 7000

Practice Manager Ben O'Dwyer

GP Kay OSLER, Kevork HOPAYIAN, Geraint Vernon JONES, Sally-Jane SIMMONDS

Leominster

The Croase Orchard Surgery
Kingsland, Leominster HR6 9QL
Tel: 01568 708214 Fax: 01568 708188
(Herefordshire Primary Care Trust)
Patient List Size: 7200

Practice Manager Mary Shepphard

GP Thomas Grayson MATHIAS, Andrew BLACK, Richard DALES, Marian DAVIS, Jeremy GRAY

Marches Surgery
Westfield Walk, Leominster HR6 8HD
Tel: 01568 614141 Fax: 01568 610293
(Herefordshire Primary Care Trust)
Patient List Size: 8100

Practice Manager Eleanor Brookes-Owen

GP Roger Martin THOMPSON, Jennie EDWARDS, Crispin FISHER, Andrew Leslie KNIGHT, Carolyn KNIGHT, I WALL

Westfield Surgery
Westfield Walk, Leominster HR6 8HD
Tel: 01568 612084 Fax: 01568 610340
(Herefordshire Primary Care Trust)
Patient List Size: 8900

Practice Manager Chris Williams

GP Gareth James BOWEN, Clare CATHCART, Lizabeth GWILLIAM, William Andrew JAMES, Andrew SENIOR

Letchworth

Birchwood Surgery
232-240 Nevells Road, Letchworth SG6 4UB
Tel: 01462 683456 Fax: 01462 483567
(North Hertfordshire and Stevenage Primary Care Trust)
Patient List Size: 14250

GP Graham HEELIS, Christopher George ASHWOOD, Anthea Mary BOND, Carole Anne BROOKS, Robert James Ogle GRAHAM, R NEWBY, F RAYMOND

Garden City Surgery
59 Station Road, Letchworth SG6 3BJ
Tel: 01462 624000 Fax: 01462 624004
(North Hertfordshire and Stevenage Primary Care Trust)

GP Raj Pardeep CHAND, Paul VOOGHT

The Sollershott Surgery
44 Sollershott East, Letchworth SG6 3JW
Tel: 01462 683637 Fax: 01462 481348
(North Hertfordshire and Stevenage Primary Care Trust)
Patient List Size: 5000

Practice Manager J Mills

GP Nes Stewart IRVINE, S EMSLEY, Richard Spencer Charles NEVARD

The Surgery
Nevells Road, Letchworth SG6 4TS
Tel: 01462 683051 Fax: 01462 485650
(North Hertfordshire and Stevenage Primary Care Trust)

GP Michael Geoffrey KIRBY, Simon CHATFIELD, Rodney James LANGSTAFF, Timothy RAMSBOTTOM, Andrew YOUNG

Lewes

Newick Health Centre
The Green, Newick, Lewes BN8 4LR
Tel: 01825 722272 Fax: 01825 724391
(Sussex Downs and Weald Primary Care Trust)
Patient List Size: 8300

Practice Manager J Morton

GP Peter Geoffrey ESTCOURT, Peter Hereward ASHBY, John Vincent ELLIOT, Jane Christina HILL

River Lodge Surgery
Malling Street, Lewes BN7 2RD
Tel: 01273 472233 Fax: 01273 486879
(Sussex Downs and Weald Primary Care Trust)

Practice Manager Valerie Jenkins, Valerie Jenkins

GP Ian Noel HEMPSHALL, L BUTTI, Frauke DINGELSTAD, Robert Alan FERNS, S RICHARDS, Gabor SZEKELY

St Andrews Surgery
The Old Central School, Southover Road, Lewes BN7 1US
Tel: 01273 476216 Fax: 01273 487587
(Sussex Downs and Weald Primary Care Trust)
Patient List Size: 8200

Practice Manager Susan Henderson

GP Ernest Eugene CREAN, Gail BALL, Andrew James HEATH, Helen PRICE, Richard Anthony ROSS

The Surgery
School Hill House, 33 High Street, Lewes BN7 2LU
Tel: 01273 480 888 Fax: 01273 486 368
Email: schoolhill@fastnet,co.uk
(Sussex Downs and Weald Primary Care Trust)

Practice Manager Pamela Burgh

GP Martin John HEATH, Elizabeth Francis LAMB, Katie McINTOSH, Olvia SNAPE, David J SWAINE, Bernard Philip James WAY

Leyburn

Aysgarth Medical Practice
Dyke Hollins Lane, Aysgarth, Leyburn DL8 3AA
Tel: 01969 663222 Fax: 01969 663051
Website: www.centraldalespractice.co.uk
(Hambleton and Richmondshire Primary Care Trust)
Patient List Size: 4600

Practice Manager John West

GP J K FRANCE

Leyburn Medical Practice
The Nurseries, Leyburn DL8 5AU
Tel: 01969 622391 Fax: 01969 624446
(Hambleton and Richmondshire Primary Care Trust)

Practice Manager Margaret White

GP George Richard WALKER, Debbie ASHCROFT, Julia Mary BROWN, Adrian Michael DAWSON, Stephen WILD

Lichfield

Langton Medical Group

St Chads Health Centre, Dimbles Lane, Lichfield WS13 7HT
Tel: 01543 258983 Fax: 01543 414776
Email: lmgdoc@lmgobc.co.uk
(Burntwood, Lichfield and Tamworth Primary Care Trust)
Patient List Size: 8600

Practice Manager Jane Ball

GP Jeremy Rea Duncan BROWN, Geoffrey Ian HACKETT, Andrew Clinton HALL, Linda Janet HALLIFAX, Christopher Mark LOCKWOOD, Jacqueline Gail WAKEMAN

The Minster Practice

Greenhill Health Centre, Church Street, Lichfield WS13 6JL
Tel: 01543 255511 Fax: 01543 418668
Email: mailroom@minster.org.uk
(Burntwood, Lichfield and Tamworth Primary Care Trust)
Patient List Size: 10500

Practice Manager Sylvia D Bailey

GP Michael CAUSER

The Spires Practice

St Chads Health Centre, Dimbles Lane, Lichfield WS13 7HT
Tel: 01543 258987 Fax: 01543 410162
(Burntwood, Lichfield and Tamworth Primary Care Trust)
Patient List Size: 8170

Practice Manager Sue Rogers

GP Richard William HENSHAW, Leslie Thomas HARRINGTON, Gerrit Boudewijn HUISMAN, Helen LAW, Koy MOHANNA

Westgate Practice

Greenhill Health Centre, Church Street, Lichfield WS13 6JL
Tel: 01543 414311 Fax: 01543 256364
Website: www.westgate.practice@sshawwebmail.nhs.uk
(Burntwood, Lichfield and Tamworth Primary Care Trust)
Patient List Size: 16000

Practice Manager K Tompkinson

GP Trefor John HERBERT, Peter Henry COOPER, Nicola Jane FLANAGAN, John Douglas JAMES, Elizabeth Jean MULLER, D NEWSON, Clare Joanne PILKINGTON, James W ROCKETT, Graham John SOUTHALL, Richard Nicholas WALSH

Lifton

Lifton Surgery

North Road, Lifton PL16 0EH
Tel: 01566 784788
(South Hams and West Devon Primary Care Trust)
Patient List Size: 3000

GP Michael Anthony SPARROW

Lightwater

Lightwater Surgery

All Saints House, 39 All Saints Road, Lightwater GU18 5SQ
Tel: 01276 472248 Fax: 01276 473873
(Surrey Heath and Woking Primary Care Trust)
Patient List Size: 10200

Practice Manager Allison Guary, Julia Southern

GP Barry NEWPORT, Stephen John LANDER, Susan Mary McFARLANE, Nicola Ann TOWNSEND, Andrew John WHITFIELD

Lincoln

Abbey Medical Practice

95 Monks Road, Lincoln LN2 5HR
Tel: 01522 530334 Fax: 01522 569442
(West Lincolnshire Primary Care Trust)
Patient List Size: 5200

Practice Manager Pauline L. Mardle

GP Peter Richard STURTON, Phillipa BIRCH, Elmer Ramos MOLAVE

Arboretum Surgery

76 Monks Road, Lincoln LN2 5HU
Tel: 01522 524274 Fax: 01522 525355
(West Lincolnshire Primary Care Trust)

GP Francis David BEER, Lucy Sarah HINDOCHA, Patrick Joseph TWOMEY

Barton Road Surgery

181 Burton Road, Lincoln LN1 3LT
Tel: 01522 544222/544333 Fax: 01522 560665
(West Lincolnshire Primary Care Trust)
Patient List Size: 2633

Practice Manager Carys Riley

GP J F BREW, B ECHEVERRIA

Bassingham Surgery

16 Torgate Lane, Bassingham, Lincoln LN5 9HF
Tel: 01522 788250 Fax: 01522 788180
(West Lincolnshire Primary Care Trust)
Patient List Size: 3708

Practice Manager Diane Lord

GP Susan Lilian MARRIS, Peter BRIDGWOOD, Marie Clare FARRELL

Billinghay Medical Practice

39 High Street, Billinghay, Lincoln LN4 4AU
Tel: 01526 860490 Fax: 01526 869800
(Lincolnshire South West Teaching Primary Care Trust)
Patient List Size: 4150

Practice Manager Steve Illingworth

GP Kenneth Charles LEEPER, Robert John HINCHCLIFFE

Birchwood Medical Practice

Jasmin Road, Lincoln LN6 0QQ
Tel: 01522 501111 Fax: 01522 682793
(West Lincolnshire Primary Care Trust)
Patient List Size: 7650

Practice Manager John Walkley

GP Martin John LATHAM, C PORTER, Richard Nicholas Evans SMITH, R P WILLIAMS

Boultham Park Medical Practice

Boultham Park Road, Lincoln LN6 7SS
Tel: 01522 874444 Fax: 01522 874466
(West Lincolnshire Primary Care Trust)

Practice Manager Stuart Edwards

GP William Michael WHITLOW, John Francis COFFEY, Damian John JACKSON, Michelle B McGOWAN, Julian J SAGGIURATO

Branston Surgery

Station Road, Branston, Lincoln LN4 1LH
Tel: 01522 793081 Fax: 01522 793562
(West Lincolnshire Primary Care Trust)
Patient List Size: 5157

Practice Manager Lynne Ivatt

GP Paul Robert Stuart BURNS, John Lewis PARKIN

The Brant Road Surgery

291 Brant Road, Lincoln LN5 9AB
Tel: 01522 722853 Fax: 01522 722195
(West Lincolnshire Primary Care Trust)
Patient List Size: 6500

Practice Manager Diane Dickens

GP Wilfred Alvyn BELL, Sadie AUBREY, Peter Henry CALVELEY, Abigail HURST, Catherine Ann Grace PERRY

Brayford Medical Practice
34 Newland, Lincoln LN1 1XP
Tel: 01522 543943 Fax: 01522 538088
(West Lincolnshire Primary Care Trust)
Patient List Size: 4000

Practice Manager David Beresford

GP George Li Tin Niam LI WAN PO

Burton Road Surgery
82 Burton Road, Lincoln LN1 3LJ
Tel: 01522 513895 Fax: 01522 525660
(West Lincolnshire Primary Care Trust)

GP Shahid Mahmood ANSARI

Church Walk Surgery
Drury Street, Metheringham, Lincoln LN4 3EZ
Tel: 01526 320522 Fax: 01526 322210
(West Lincolnshire Primary Care Trust)
Patient List Size: 3753

Practice Manager Sue Richardson

GP Christine Ann FERNLEY, Nicholas DAVID

Cliff Road Health Centre
4 Cliff Road, Welton, Lincoln LN2 3JH
Tel: 01673 860203 Fax: 01673 862888
(West Lincolnshire Primary Care Trust)
Patient List Size: 8650

Practice Manager Sallie Stead

GP Graham Malcolm INDER, Andrew BARBER, Stephen John BARTON, Mark HOWARD, Margaret Mary LENNON

Cliff Villages Medical Practice
Mere Road, Waddington, Lincoln LN5 9NX
Tel: 01522 720277 Fax: 01522 729174
(West Lincolnshire Primary Care Trust)
Patient List Size: 7500

Practice Manager A Freeman

GP Liam John BROUGHTON, Catherine Elizabeth FUSSEY, John Gerard McLOUGHLIN

Crossroads Medical Practice
Lincoln Road, North Hykeham, Lincoln LN6 8NH
Tel: 01522 682848 Fax: 01522 697930
Website: www.crossroadsmedicalpractice.co.uk
(West Lincolnshire Primary Care Trust)
Patient List Size: 3000

Practice Manager Alison Lowerson

GP Adam Guy PAXTON, Matthew C POSTER

Drs Abbas, Ash, Attrup, Azar and Gopee
85 Sykes Lane, Saxilby, Lincoln LN1 2NU
Tel: 01522 702236 Fax: 01522 703132
(West Lincolnshire Primary Care Trust)
Patient List Size: 8300

GP Edgar Munir ABBAS, Catherine Elizabeth ASH, Martin ATTRUP, Ned AZAR, Aaaron GOPEE

Ingham Practice
Lincoln Road, Ingham, Lincoln LN1 2XF
Tel: 01522 730269 Fax: 01522 730192
Email: inghamsurgery@hotmail.com
(West Lincolnshire Primary Care Trust)
Patient List Size: 2900

Practice Manager Ruth Piper

GP Radi SULTAN

Lindeem Medical Practice
1 Cabourne Court, Cabourne Avenue, Lincoln LN2 2JP
Tel: 01522 569033 Fax: 01522 576713
(West Lincolnshire Primary Care Trust)

GP John Daniel William KAAR, Kathryn Barbara Louise HANSON, Mark RICHARDSON, Kanwaljit Kaur ROSSA

Minster Medical Practice
Cabourne Court, Cabourne Avenue, Lincoln LN2 2JP
Tel: 01522 568838 Fax: 01522 546740
(West Lincolnshire Primary Care Trust)
Patient List Size: 7700

Practice Manager Liz Stephenson

GP Alyson Jane PONTIN, Christopher John BATTY, Jonathan Crispin GIBBS, Aurelia MORENO-BETETA

Montaigne Crescent Surgery
17 Montaigne Crescent, Glebe Park, Wragby Road, Lincoln LN2 4QN
(West Lincolnshire Primary Care Trust)

GP Malcolm LOCKER

Nettleham Medical Practice
14 Lodge Lane, Nettleham, Lincoln LN2 2RS
Tel: 01522 751717 Fax: 01522 754474
(West Lincolnshire Primary Care Trust)
Patient List Size: 10974

Practice Manager Mally Daubney

GP John Rennie CRAVEN, Peter Francis ATKINS, Simon BAKER, Ian Robert LACY, Mark Christopher PROTHEROE, Sally Louise WALLER

New Coningsby Surgery
20 Silver Street, Coningsby, Lincoln LN4 4SG
Tel: 01526 344544 Fax: 01526 345540
(East Lincolnshire Primary Care Trust)

Practice Manager C Loughe

GP Simon LOUGHE, Amos Jehoshua RAMON

Newark Road Surgery
501 Newark Road, South Hykeham, Lincoln LN6 8RT
Tel: 01522 537944 Fax: 01522 510932
(West Lincolnshire Primary Care Trust)

Practice Manager Karen Watson

GP Paul STRATTON, Maureen BAKER, K HANSON, Clive Charles WARE

Portland Medical Centre
60 Portland Street, Lincoln LN5 7LB
Tel: 01522 876800 Fax: 01522 876803
(West Lincolnshire Primary Care Trust)

Practice Manager Mrs Bali

GP H S BALI, S HINDOCHA, Tej Bahadur Singh MEHTA, A THURKETTLE

RAF Medical Centre
RAF Coningsby, Conningsby, Lincoln LN4 4SY
Tel: 01526 347216 Fax: 01526 343713
(East Lincolnshire Primary Care Trust)
Patient List Size: 2500

GP J ONUORAH

Richmond Medical Centre
Moor Lane, North Hykeham, Lincoln LN6 9AY
Tel: 01522 500240 Fax: 01522 500232
(West Lincolnshire Primary Care Trust)
Patient List Size: 6031

Practice Manager Dianne Taylor

GP Margaret Anne MAGEE, Matthew FREEMAN, Thomas Angus MacDonald LOUGH

School Lane Surgery
School Lane, Washingborough, Lincoln LN4 1BN
Tel: 01522 792360 Fax: 01522 794144
(West Lincolnshire Primary Care Trust)
Patient List Size: 6985

Practice Manager A Dale

GP Hugh GOLDSTEIN, David GRANT, Dorothy Anne WOOD, Monica Jane WOOD

Silver Street Surgery
19 Silver Street, Coningsby, Lincoln LN4 4SG
Tel: 01526 342348 Fax: 01526 345255
(East Lincolnshire Primary Care Trust)

GP Ian David RAWLINGS

Springcliffe Surgery
42 St. Catherines, Lincoln LN5 8LZ
Tel: 01522 520443 Fax: 01522 543430
(West Lincolnshire Primary Care Trust)
Patient List Size: 2700

Practice Manager Jan May

GP Ved Brat SOOD

St Catherine Surgery
19 St. Catherines, Lincoln LN5 8LT
Tel: 01522 871771 Fax: 01522 871773
(West Lincolnshire Primary Care Trust)

Practice Manager Rosemary Hogg

GP Ashfaq Husain QURESHI, H Z QURESHI

Sturton Road Surgery
12 Sturton Road, Saxilby, Lincoln LN1 2PG
Tel: 01522 702791 Fax: 01522 704434
(West Lincolnshire Primary Care Trust)
Patient List Size: 2900

Practice Manager Yvonne Whitelock

GP Anthony Martin ROBBINS-CHERRY

Swallowbeck Grange
320 Hykeham Road, Lincoln LN6 8BW
Tel: 01522 681400 Fax: 01522 697663
(West Lincolnshire Primary Care Trust)

Practice Manager Pat Smith

GP Mark Edward FALLON, F POUNDER

The Woodland Medical Practice
Jasmin Road, Birchwood, Lincoln LN6 0QQ
Tel: 01522 683590 Fax: 01522 695666
(West Lincolnshire Primary Care Trust)
Patient List Size: 7243

Practice Manager Janice White

GP Alan Stanley Guy USHER, Keith BAILEY, Paul Xavier DONNELLY, Rachel SOWERBY

Lingfield

NCYPE Lingfield Surgery
St Piers Lane, Lingfield RH7 6PW

Practice Manager Hugh Roberts

GP Peter A CLIFFE

The Surgery
East Grinstead Road, Lingfield RH7 6ER
Tel: 01342 833456 Fax: 01342 836347
(East Surrey Primary Care Trust)
Patient List Size: 10000

Practice Manager Hugh Roberts

GP Andrew James ROBERTSON, Fiona Jane ALLEN, Peter Andrew Harvey CLIFFE, James Edward GARDNER

Liphook

Ship House Surgery
The Square, Liphook GU30 7AQ
Tel: 01428 723296 Fax: 01420 724022
(North Hampshire Primary Care Trust)
Patient List Size: 5200

Practice Manager Betty McClure

GP T CHUNG, A HALLATT, S JUDGE

Liskeard

The Health Centre
Station Road, East Looe, Liskeard PL13 1HA
Tel: 01503 756970 Fax: 01503 265680
(North and East Cornwall Primary Care Trust)

Practice Manager J K Price

GP Peter John Jeaffreson BREWER, G N DAVIES, Christopher Guy Coombs FAGG, Douglas Royston GOSS, D M JEFFERY, Michael John PALMER, Ian Gordon ROY

Parade Surgery
The Parade, Liskeard PL14 6AF
Tel: 01579 342667 Fax: 01579 340650
(North and East Cornwall Primary Care Trust)
Patient List Size: 10500

Practice Manager Romayne Sichel

GP John CRITCHLEY, Geoffrey Douglas AUCKLAND, Stephen Bowcott JEFFERIES, Catriona Margaret Burn THORNTON, Graham Ralph TOMS, Jonathan Howard USSHER

Pensilva Health Centre
School Road, Pensilva, Liskeard PL14 5RP
Tel: 01579 362249 Fax: 01579 363323
Email: practicemanager@pensilva.cornwall.nhs.uk
(North and East Cornwall Primary Care Trust)
Patient List Size: 4800

Practice Manager Catherine Pickstone

GP Jan Lennox MACFARLANE, Mark Robert McCARTNEY, Martin Gerard RONCHETTI

Rose Dean Surgery
8 Dean Street, Liskeard PL14 4AQ
Tel: 01579 343133 Fax: 01579 344933
(North and East Cornwall Primary Care Trust)
Patient List Size: 9000

Practice Manager Richard Matthews

GP Anthony Richard PIPER, Iain Michael CHARLTON, David John HARGADON, Leela Anne KALRA, Carol Ann KNEEBONE, Andrew Dennis SMALLEY

Liss

Hillbrow Surgery
Hill Brow Road, Liss GU33 7LE
Tel: 01730 892262 Fax: 01730 895779
(East Hampshire Primary Care Trust)

Practice Manager Sue Kent

GP John Rich SEDGWICK, J BOTHAM, Patrick Michael CRAIG-McFEELY, Suzy HOLDEN, Barbara Elizabeth Anne RUSHTON

Kelsey's Surgery
Mill Road, Liss GU33 7AZ
Tel: 01730 892184 Fax: 01730 893634
(East Hampshire Primary Care Trust)
Patient List Size: 2200

Practice Manager Lucy Panton

GP David John PANTON

Littleborough

Church Street Surgery
11 Church Street, Littleborough OL15 8AA
(Rochdale Primary Care Trust)

GP David Terence BRAZIER

Littleborough Health Centre
Featherstall Road, Littleborough OL15 8HF
(Rochdale Primary Care Trust)

GP Biswanath BHATTACHARJEE, Ruth CHEW, Simon Duncan HOWSON, Antony Paul ROBERTS

Littleborough Health Centre
Featherstall Road, Littleborough OL15 8HF
Tel: 01706 374990 Fax: 01706 371648
(Rochdale Primary Care Trust)
Patient List Size: 2800

Practice Manager J Dimery

GP Ian Philip DIMERY

The Village Medical Centre
Market Square, Peel Street, Littleborough OL15 8AQ
(Rochdale Primary Care Trust)

GP C DATTA

Littlehampton

East Street Medical Centre
18-20 East Street, Littlehampton BN17 6AW
Tel: 01903 731111 Fax: 01903 732295
Website: www.familydoctors.co.uk
(Adur, Arun and Worthing Primary Care Trust)

Practice Manager Wendy Pratt

GP Jill ADAM, Timothy Arlingham DAVIES, Ann DEY, Brian FITZGERALD

Littlehampton Health Centre
Fitzalan Road, Littlehampton BN17 5JR
Tel: 01903 732453/690111 Fax: 01903 843601
(Adur, Arun and Worthing Primary Care Trust)

Practice Manager Anne Scott

GP Douglas William McLEOD, Yvonne Anna Maria GRANT, Michael Richard David MILLER, Dr SHLOSBERG, Martin WISEMAN

The Park Surgery
St Flora's Road, Littlehampton BN17 6BF
Tel: 01903 717154 Fax: 01903 732908
(Adur, Arun and Worthing Primary Care Trust)
Patient List Size: 6543

Practice Manager Robyn Clark

GP Gordon Keir BYARS, Timothy David ATKINSON, Timothy John KIMBER, Mary Philomena LISTON

The Surgery
The Coppice, Herne Lane, Rustington, Littlehampton BN16 3BE
Tel: 01903 783178 Fax: 01903 859027
(Adur, Arun and Worthing Primary Care Trust)
Patient List Size: 6250

Practice Manager Janet Rogers

GP Derek Joseph HANDLEY, Timothy Owen CRITCHFIELD, Belinda CROEBIE, Martina HOUSKA, Sandra JONES, Peter LOVELL, Geoffrey Arthur Gillard STAPLETON

Westcourt
12 The Street, Rustington, Littlehampton BN16 3NX
Tel: 01903 784311 Fax: 01903 850907
(Adur, Arun and Worthing Primary Care Trust)
Patient List Size: 12000

Practice Manager Sylvia Sene

GP Craig Kerr BROWN, Gregory Duncan MIDDLETON, Matthew Giles William TAYLOR-ROBERTS, Emma Jane TILLEY, Daniel Glyn WILLIAMS, Susan Jane WORMSLEY

Willow Green Surgery
Station Road, East Preston, Littlehampton BN16 3AH
Tel: 01903 758152 Fax: 01903 859986
Website: www.willowgreensurgery.co.uk
(Adur, Arun and Worthing Primary Care Trust)
Patient List Size: 8600

Practice Manager Sandy Maslen, Janet Williamson

GP David FARRER-BROWN, Sally CAMPBELL, Sarah PLEDGER, Roma Elizabeth ROBERTS, Rajesh SANGHANI, Sindy WILLIAMS, Stewart John WRIGHT

Liverpool

30 Hillside Road Surgery
30 Hillside Road, Huyton, Liverpool L36 8BJ
Tel: 0151 480 4205 Fax: 0151 489 2204
(Knowsley Primary Care Trust)
Patient List Size: 2138

Practice Manager Lisa O'Brien

GP Arun Kumar SINGHAL

Abbeystead Road Surgery
4 Abbeystead Road, Liverpool L15 7JF
Tel: 0151 722 1080
(Central Liverpool Primary Care Trust)

GP Hitesh Pranlal KOTHARI, Galina ARTIOUKH

Abercromby Health Centre
Grove Street, Edge Hill, Liverpool L7 7HG
Tel: 0151 709 2806
(Central Liverpool Primary Care Trust)

GP Ritar Kulasegaram SAVERIMUTTU

Abercromby Health Centre
Grove Street, Edge Hill, Liverpool L7 7HG
Tel: 0151 708 9370
(Central Liverpool Primary Care Trust)

GP Gorakanage Basil GOMES DERANIYAGALA, D N LAKHANI

Abingdon Family Health Centre
361-365 Queens Drive, Walton, Liverpool L4 8SJ
Tel: 0151 226 1501 Fax: 0151 256 0593
(North Liverpool Primary Care Trust)
Patient List Size: 2651

Practice Manager Irene M Bush

GP F E H EL-SAYED

Aintree Park Group Practice
46 Moss Lane, Orrell Park, Liverpool L9 8AL
Tel: 0151 525 2736 Fax: 0151 524 1037
(North Liverpool Primary Care Trust)

GP Kay EARLY, Anil Kumar BOSE, Christopher Frank DOWRICK, Catherine Marian HUBBERT, Nigel Edward Brian JONES, Fiona Marie LEMMENS, David William READE

Albion Street Surgery
1 Albion Street, Liverpool L5 3QN
Tel: 0151 263 1176 Fax: 0151 261 1295
(North Liverpool Primary Care Trust)
Patient List Size: 1800

GP A T KEYSAER, Lisa RAYNER

Anfield Medical Centre
117 Priory Road, Liverpool L4 2SG
Tel: 0151 263 1081 Fax: 0151 260 7470
(North Liverpool Primary Care Trust)
Patient List Size: 1950

Practice Manager Bridget Richards

GP Mirza Ahref Ali BAIG

Ash Surgery
1 Ashfield Road, Liverpool L17 0BY
Tel: 0151 727 1155 Fax: 0151 726 0018
(South Liverpool Primary Care Trust)

GP Elisabeth Marjorie COTTON, Paul Philip JOHNSON, Karen Louise LYNN, Peter SPOFFORTH, C V WALKER

Baycliffe Family Health Care Centre
Baycliffe Road, Liverpool L12 6QX
Tel: 0151 228 4272
(Central Liverpool Primary Care Trust)
Patient List Size: 2300

Practice Manager J Price

GP Sayed Abdel Kader Mohamed HAMAD

Belle Vale Health Centre
Hedgefield Road, Liverpool L25 2XE
Tel: 0151 487 0514 Fax: 0151 488 6601
(South Liverpool Primary Care Trust)
Patient List Size: 9000

Practice Manager Paul Smith

GP I G BUTLER, Penelope Jane ALLEN, C GRAAS, F OGDEN-FURDE, S ROSE, John Winston TAYLOR-ROBINSON

Benim Medical Centre
2 Penvalley Crescent, Liverpool L6 3BY
Tel: 0151 263 6588 Fax: 0151 263 4723
(Central Liverpool Primary Care Trust)
Patient List Size: 3600

Practice Manager Sandra Fildes

GP B DAS, B THIMMIAH

Blue Bell Lane Surgery
2 Blue Bell Lane, Huyton, Liverpool L36 7TN
Tel: 0151 489 1422 Fax: 0151 489 8599
(Knowsley Primary Care Trust)
Patient List Size: 4012

Practice Manager J E Brown

GP Gillian Patricia BEVAN, Helen WEST

Bluebell Lane Surgery
79 Bluebell Lane, Huyton, Liverpool L36 7XX
Tel: 0151 489 2499 Fax: 0151 489 8708
(Knowsley Primary Care Trust)
Patient List Size: 1906

Practice Manager F Hossain

GP M M HOSSAIN

Bousfield Health Centre
Westminster Road, Liverpool L4 4PP
Tel: 0151 207 0813
(North Liverpool Primary Care Trust)

GP Peter BUSE, John Wynne ROBERTS

Bousfield Health Centre
Westminster Road, Liverpool L4 4PP
Tel: 0151 207 1468 Fax: 0151 284 6864
(North Liverpool Primary Care Trust)
Patient List Size: 4000

Practice Manager D Murray

GP Dilip Kumar SHAH, A KUMAR

Breckfield Road North Surgery
141 Breckfield Road North, Liverpool L5 4QT
Tel: 0151 263 6534 Fax: 0151 260 7446
Email: riaz@liverpooldoctors.co.uk
Website: www.liverpooldoctors.co.uk
(North Liverpool Primary Care Trust)
Patient List Size: 4496

GP A RIAZ, Joseph John GODFREY

Bridge Road Surgery
66-88 Bridge Road, Litherland, Liverpool L21 6PH
Tel: 0151 949 0249 Fax: 0151 928 2008
(South Sefton Primary Care Trust)
Patient List Size: 8100

Practice Manager Gwyneth Roden

GP Alan Keith CANTER, Dr CARROLL, Martin John VICKERS

Camberley Medical Centre
11b Camberley Drive, Halewood, Liverpool L25 9PS
Tel: 0151 486 1178 Fax: 0151 486 1108
(Knowsley Primary Care Trust)

Practice Manager S Kelly

GP J HEATH

Chapel Lane Surgery
13 Chapel Lane, Formby, Liverpool L37 4DL
Tel: 01704 876363 Fax: 01704 833808
Email: chapel.lane@gp-n84006.nhs.uk
Website: www.chapellanesurgery.co.uk
(Southport and Formby Primary Care Trust)
Patient List Size: 8000

Practice Manager Roy Boardman

GP L M JONES, D M CALLOW, C J JACKSON, J L PROCTER

Childwall Valley Road Surgery
70 Childwall Valley Road, Liverpool L16 4PE
Tel: 0151 722 7321
(Central Liverpool Primary Care Trust)

Practice Manager Irene Glendinning

GP David Anthony ORLANS, Marian ORLANS

Claremont Medical Centre
171-173 Liverpool Road, Maghull, Liverpool L31 8AA
Tel: 0151 520 3060 Fax: 0151 520 3080
(South Sefton Primary Care Trust)

GP Fabrizio EQUIZI

Cornerways Medical Centre
27 Woolfall Heath Avenue, Huyton, Liverpool L36 3TH
Tel: 0151 489 4444 Fax: 0151 489 0528
(Knowsley Primary Care Trust)
Patient List Size: 3414

Practice Manager Pauline Titherington

GP Robert John CASHIN, S K VERMA

Derby Lane Surgery
88 Derby Lane, Liverpool L13 3DN
Tel: 0151 228 5868 Fax: 0151 259 6996
(Central Liverpool Primary Care Trust)
Patient List Size: 4500

Practice Manager Karen Wynne

GP Parveen Lata GUPTA, Shakti Kumar GUPTA

Dinas Lane Medical Centre
149 Dinas Lane, Huyton, Liverpool L36 2NW
Tel: 0151 489 2298 Fax: 0151 489 4332
(Knowsley Primary Care Trust)

Practice Manager Pat Puddifer

GP Narayani Prasad SINGH, Paul Gerard CONWAY, Gul Sarah DARABSHAW, G MOORE, Andrew Charles William PRYCE

Dovecot Health Centre
Longreach Road, Liverpool L14 0NL
Tel: 0151 228 3336
(Central Liverpool Primary Care Trust)

GP Graham Alexander CORRIGHAN, N C CURPEN

Dr D M Flanagan and Partners
Liverpool Road Surgery, 133 Liverpool Road, Crosby, Liverpool L23 5TE
Tel: 0151 931 3197 Fax: 0151 931 4006
(South Sefton Primary Care Trust)
Patient List Size: 7000

Practice Manager Maureen Guy

GP David Michael FLANAGAN, Graham John BIRD, Gokul Kumar MISRA

Dr D P O'Hara and Partners
46-48 Grey Road, Liverpool L9 1AY
Tel: 0151 525 3533 Fax: 0151 523 4958
(North Liverpool Primary Care Trust)
Patient List Size: 5200

Practice Manager Jean Howgate

GP Dermot Patrick O'HARA, J L BLISS, K L FINN

Dr S K Pande
14 North View, Edge Hill, Liverpool L7 8TS
Tel: 0151 709 3779 Fax: 0151 709 6349
(Central Liverpool Primary Care Trust)
Patient List Size: 1600

Practice Manager Jenny Hale

GP Shiv Kumar PANDE

Earle Road Medical Centre
131 Earle Road, Liverpool L7 6HD
Tel: 0151 733 7172
(Central Liverpool Primary Care Trust)

GP Gurcharan Singh ARORA, John Leslie BLAKEBOROUGH, M N CHANDRASHEKHAR

Earle Road Medical Centre
131 Earle Road, Liverpool L7 6HD
Tel: 0151 734 3535 Fax: 0151 734 1769
(Central Liverpool Primary Care Trust)
Patient List Size: 4500

Practice Manager Bernadette McLennan, Lisa Taylor

GP F A A MAJEED

Earle Road Medical Centre
131 Earle Road, Liverpool L7 6HD
Tel: 0151 733 5538 Fax: 0151 733 6914
(Central Liverpool Primary Care Trust)
Patient List Size: 2100

Practice Manager Pushpa Yadav

GP J K YADAV

Eastview Surgery
81-83 Crosby Road North, Liverpool L22 4QD
Tel: 0151 928 8849 Fax: 0151 928 2090
(South Sefton Primary Care Trust)
Patient List Size: 7500

Practice Manager L Brown

GP Ivor William HUGHES, Rebecca Katherine DYE, Mark Ivor HUGHES, Andrew Patrick MIMNAGH

Eaton Road Surgery
276 Eaton Road, West Derby, Liverpool L12 2AW
Tel: 0151 228 3768 Fax: 0151 259 7008
(Central Liverpool Primary Care Trust)
Patient List Size: 11700

Practice Manager J Keeley

GP Barry Jack MINTZ, Helen Jane AVANN, Philip Robert BURNS, David Richard ECCLES, Margaret EDWARDS, Colin David WELSH

Edge Hill Health Centre
Crosfield Road, Liverpool L7 5QL
Tel: 0151 260 2777
(Central Liverpool Primary Care Trust)

Practice Manager S Horton

GP Oskar DOVER, Nadim Akhtar FAZLANI, Anne Cecilia GALTREY, Gopal GOENKA, Birendra Kumar SINHA, Ponnudurai SIVABALAN

Edge Lane Medical Centre
1-5 Marmaduke Street, Liverpool L7 1PA
Tel: 0151 260 5335
(Central Liverpool Primary Care Trust)

Practice Manager L Tomlinson

GP S R DARLA

Ellergreen Medical Centre
24 Carr Lane, Norris Green, Liverpool L11 2YA
Tel: 0151 256 9800 Fax: 0151 256 5765
(North Liverpool Primary Care Trust)
Patient List Size: 11800

Practice Manager Terence Johnson

GP Melvyn SNYDER, Mary Paula FINNERTY, David KEWN, Peter Vincent Stephen REDMOND, Stephen James REDMOND, Ian Felix SHIFFMAN

Everton Road General Practice
70 Everton Road, Liverpool L6 2EW
Tel: 0151 260 5050 Fax: 0151 260 4498
(North Liverpool Primary Care Trust)
Patient List Size: 2300

GP Bernard THOMAS, Jill THOMAS

Fairfield Medical Centre
10 Hampstead Road, Liverpool L6 8NG
Tel: 0151 263 1323 Fax: 0151 263 8263
(Central Liverpool Primary Care Trust)
Patient List Size: 2510

Practice Manager V P Singh

GP S B P SINGH

Freshfield Surgery
61 Gores Lane, Formby, Liverpool L37 3NU
Tel: 01704 879430 Fax: 01704 833883
(Southport and Formby Primary Care Trust)

Practice Manager Bernice Fisher

GP Alison Catherine NEWMAN, Geoffrey Philip WELCH

Fulwood Green Medical Centre
Fulwood Green Medical Centre, Jericho Lane, Liverpool L17 5AR
Tel: 0151 727 2440 Fax: 0151 726 1936
(South Liverpool Primary Care Trust)
Patient List Size: 5900

Practice Manager P Currie

GP J V GONSALVES, S BOWERS, David Edward O'Connell BOX

Gateacre Brow Surgery
1 Gateacre Brow, Liverpool L25 3PA
Tel: 0151 428 1851
(South Liverpool Primary Care Trust)

GP John CALDWELL, Margaret Mary REID, Peter Charles REILLY, Richard Neil Ashley WOOD

Gateacre Medical Centre
49 Belle Vale Road, Liverpool L25 2PA
Tel: 0151 487 8660
(South Liverpool Primary Care Trust)

GP A K JAIN

Gillmoss Medical Centre
48 Petherick Road, Liverpool L11 0AG
Tel: 0151 546 3867
(North Liverpool Primary Care Trust)

GP Tej Krishan RASTOGI, K LWIN

Gorsey Lane Surgery
93 Gorsey Lane, Ford, Liverpool L21 0DF
Tel: 0151 928 7757 Fax: 0151 928 9125
(South Sefton Primary Care Trust)

Practice Manager J Merrilees

GP Thomas MAWDSLEY, Brian Joseph FRASER, Noreen Helen WILLIAMS

Grassendale Medical Practice
23 Darby Road, Liverpool L19 9BP
Tel: 0151 427 1214 Fax: 0151 427 0611
(South Liverpool Primary Care Trust)

Practice Manager Lyn Bateson

GP Paul Michael BATESON, Robert Patrick BOYCE, George Robert COOK, David Peter Michael RYAN

Great Homer Street Health Centre
Great Homer Street, Liverpool L5 3SF
Tel: 0151 207 6077 Fax: 0151 207 3016
Email: docabrams@aol.com
(North Liverpool Primary Care Trust)
Patient List Size: 2500

Practice Manager Catherine Campbell

GP Simon Eliot ABRAMS

Green Lane Medical Centre
15 Green Lane, Stoneycroft, Liverpool L13 7DY
Tel: 0151 228 9101 Fax: 0151 228 2472
(Central Liverpool Primary Care Trust)

Practice Manager Norma Harris

GP Moira Ann BAIRD, Nicola Jane CARTER, Timothy James FITZSIMONS, James Christopher GRAHAM

Greenbank Drive Surgery
8 Greenbank Drive, Sefton Park, Liverpool L17 1AW
Tel: 0151 733 5703
(Central Liverpool Primary Care Trust)

GP Colin Douglas McKEAN, Vivienne Helen CRAWFORD, Brian Dominic O'CONNOR

Greenbank Road Surgery
29 Greenbank Road, Liverpool L18 1HG
Tel: 0151 733 3224 Fax: 0151 5221121
(Central Liverpool Primary Care Trust)

GP Robert Nigel BARNETT, Helen Elizabeth CLARKE, Karen O'HANLON, Claire POLLARD, Janet Louise SIDDELL, Jonathan Mark THOMAS

Gresford Medical Centre
Pilch Lane, Huyton, Liverpool L14 0JE
Tel: 0151 489 2020 Fax: 0151 449 3892
(Knowsley Primary Care Trust)
Patient List Size: 5020

Practice Manager Marion Cooper

GP Martin Stewart FELD, Carmen GARCIA, M J HAMPSON, Fui Boon LO

Halewood Health Centre
Roseheath Drive, Halewood, Liverpool L26 9UH
Tel: 0151 486 5848
(Knowsley Primary Care Trust)
Patient List Size: 2025

Practice Manager Gaynor Stubbs

GP D S IQBAL, J IQBAL

Halifax Crescent Surgery
4 Halifax Crescent, Thornton, Liverpool L23 1TH
Tel: 0151 924 3532 Fax: 0151 924 3171
(South Sefton Primary Care Trust)
Patient List Size: 2157

GP H K SINGH, M J KENT

The Health Centre Surgery
60 Roseheath Drive, Halewood, Liverpool L26 9UH
Tel: 0151 486 3780 Fax: 0151 448 0650
(Knowsley Primary Care Trust)
Patient List Size: 5143

Practice Manager Lynda Bolton

GP Thomas Scott KINLOCH, Brendan Patrick MORAN

High Pastures
138 Liverpool Road North, Maghull, Liverpool L31 2HW
Tel: 0151 526 2161 Fax: 0151527 2377
(South Sefton Primary Care Trust)
Patient List Size: 12000

Practice Manager Lisa Morrissey

GP Adrian Rowland BALL, Dr ANDREWS, Dr CLARKSON, Gary Taylor SIMPSON, P S THOMAS, Carolyn Margaret THOMSON, Philip John WESTON, Dr WOODWARD

Hightown Village Surgery
1 St Georges Road, Hightown, Liverpool L38 3RY
Tel: 0151 929 3603 Fax: 0151 929 3226
(South Sefton Primary Care Trust)
Patient List Size: 2000

Practice Manager Ann Marie Jameson

GP Judith Anne WELCH

Hillside House
Hillside Road, Huyton, Liverpool L36 8BJ
Tel: 0151 489 4539 Fax: 0151 489 4409
(Knowsley Primary Care Trust)
Patient List Size: 3805

Practice Manager Pam McCaffery

GP Rachel MARTIN, Pervez Muhammad SADIQ

Hollies Surgery
Elbow Lane, Formby, Liverpool L37 4AF
Tel: 01704 877600 Fax: 01704 833811
(Southport and Formby Primary Care Trust)

Practice Manager Collette Riley

GP Andrea Mary TREE, Janice Ann ELDRIDGE, Deborah Jane SUMNER

Hornspit Medical Centre
Hornspit Lane, Liverpool L12 5LT
Tel: 0151 256 5755
(Central Liverpool Primary Care Trust)

GP K PRAMANIK

Hunts Cross Group Practice
Hunts Cross Health Centre, 70 Hillfoot Road, Hillfoot, Liverpool L25 0ND
Tel: 0151 486 1428 Fax: 0151 448 0233
(South Liverpool Primary Care Trust)

Practice Manager Cathy Hogan

GP Alan Milne Webster FORBES, Barbara Elisabeth SCHMIDT

Huyton Primary Care Resource Centre
Nutgrove Villa, Westmorland Road, Huyton, Liverpool L36 6GA
Tel: 0151 489 2276 Fax: 0151 489 7577
(Knowsley Primary Care Trust)
Patient List Size: 4005

Practice Manager Madeline Bolton

GP Neelakantapuram JAYARAM, A L SHANTHA

Islington Square Surgery
3 Islington Square, Liverpool L3 8DD
Tel: 0151 207 0848
(North Liverpool Primary Care Trust)
Patient List Size: 2800

GP Mary Collette Blaise Leah RENTON, C KENNEDY

Jubilee Medical Centre
52 Croxteth Hall Lane, Croxteth, Liverpool L11 4UG
Tel: 0151 546 3956 Fax: 0151 546 3221
Email: info@jubileemc.co.uk
Website: www.jubileemc.co.uk
(North Liverpool Primary Care Trust)
Patient List Size: 6787

Practice Manager M Hitchott

GP Jonathan David Thomas LOCK, Jane Elizabeth FOSTER, Ian Robert GILCHRIST, Susan HARDING, J P REYNOLDS

Kensington Medical Centre
17 Fielding Street, Liverpool L6 9AP
Tel: 0151 263 3085 Fax: 0151 261 1435
(Central Liverpool Primary Care Trust)
Patient List Size: 2300

Practice Manager Jean Sutton

GP S RASTOGI

Kingsway Surgery
20 Kingsway, Waterloo, Liverpool L22 4RQ
Tel: 0151 920 9000 Fax: 0151 928 2411
(South Sefton Primary Care Trust)
Patient List Size: 3500

Practice Manager Elaine McDonald

GP Margaret Elizabeth TATAM, Clare Louise DORAN, Maura MURPHY

Kirkdale Medical Centre
63 Walton Road, Liverpool L4 4AF
Tel: 0151 207 0950
(North Liverpool Primary Care Trust)

GP Raj Kumar BAJAJ, Veena BAJAJ

Knotty Ash Medical Centre
411-413 East Prescot Road, Liverpool L14 2DE
Tel: 0151 228 4369 Fax: 0151 252 0030
(Central Liverpool Primary Care Trust)

GP Sabyasachi SARKER

Lance Lane Medical Centre
19 Lance Lane, Liverpool L15 6TS
Tel: 0151 737 2882 Fax: 0151 737 2883
(Central Liverpool Primary Care Trust)

Practice Manager Angela Holligan

GP Susan Valerie CRAIG, A P FISKE, Paul Brian HAYWARD

Langbank Medical Centre
Broad lane, Norris Green, Liverpool L11 1AD
Tel: 0151 226 1976 Fax: 0151 270 2873
(North Liverpool Primary Care Trust)
Patient List Size: 8700

Practice Manager Mary Crear

GP M N MEHTA, Sundar MUTHU, N M PATEL

Leathers Lane Surgery
155 Leathers Lane, Liverpool L26 1XG
Tel: 0151 281 4041 Fax: 0151 281 8797
(Knowsley Primary Care Trust)
Patient List Size: 1828

Practice Manager S Kelly

GP J HEATH

Leathers Lane Surgery
90 Leathers Lane, Halewood, Liverpool L26 0TU
Tel: 0151 448 1040 Fax: 0151 448 1215
Email: peter.swinhoe@sthkhealth.nhs.uk
(Knowsley Primary Care Trust)
Patient List Size: 1879

Practice Manager Julia Parkinson

GP P J SWINHOE, Rose JOHNSTON

Long Lane Medical Centre
Long Lane, Liverpool L9 6DQ
Tel: 0151 530 1009
(North Liverpool Primary Care Trust)

Practice Manager Julie Woods

GP John Trevor BENTLEY, Judith Mary CALLAGHAN, Ian Malcolm McClure WOODS

Long Lane Surgery
15 Long Lane, Liverpool L19 6PE
Tel: 0151 494 1445 Fax: 0151 494 182
(South Liverpool Primary Care Trust)

GP H.R. KAUR, Mark Richard BROOKES

Longview Health Care Centre
132 Longview Drive, Huyton, Liverpool L36 6EQ
Tel: 0151 489 2833 Fax: 0151 480 1133
(Knowsley Primary Care Trust)
Patient List Size: 3840

Practice Manager Celia Dickson

GP Manu ALEXANDER, Ann ALEXANDER

MacMillan Surgery
10 Dulas Road, Kirkby, Liverpool L32 8TL
Tel: 0151 546 2908 Fax: 0151 548 0704
(Knowsley Primary Care Trust)
Patient List Size: 2323

Practice Manager M Thong

GP Kok Foon THONG

Manor Farm Medical Centre
Manor Farm Road, Huyton, Liverpool L36 0UB
Tel: 0151 480 1244 Fax: 0151 480 6047
(Knowsley Primary Care Trust)
Patient List Size: 7000

Practice Manager Sue Kelly

GP A ALI, A ARAIN, G ARORA, D HEATH, J HEATH, B M JOHNSTON, N LELTY, S McNALLY, G THOMAS, C TOME, P WEBSTER, N WRIGHT

Margaret Thompson Medical Centre
105 East Millwood Road, Speke, Liverpool L24 6TH
Tel: 0151 425 3331 Fax: 0151 425 2272
(South Liverpool Primary Care Trust)
Patient List Size: 4371

Practice Manager Olive Fagan

GP Marian BOGGILD, Albert DORR, Punam RAWAL, Kathrin Jane THOMAS

Mather Avenue Practice
584 Mather Avenue, Liverpool L19 4UG
Tel: 0151 427 6239 Fax: 0151 427 8876
(South Liverpool Primary Care Trust)
Patient List Size: 9000

Practice Manager Ida Ellwood

GP Frank Thomas HARGREAVES, John Charles BIRCH, Pamela McCROSSAN, Maurice Raymond SMITH

Max Road Surgery
4-6 Max Road, Liverpool L14 4BH
Tel: 0151 259 2549
(Central Liverpool Primary Care Trust)
Patient List Size: 4000

Practice Manager Betty Brannan

GP H AKHTER, S H ASKARI

McElroy, Thompson and Thomas
15 Sefton Road, Litherland, Liverpool L21 9HA
Tel: 0151 928 4820
(South Sefton Primary Care Trust)

Practice Manager Alison Harkin

GP Colette Alicia McELROY, Paul S THOMAS, Terence Joseph THOMPSON

Meldrum, Vitty and Pfeiffer
40-42 Kingsway, Waterloo, Liverpool L22 4RQ
Tel: 0151 928 2415 Fax: 0151 928 3775
Email: mvp@gp-N84001.nhs.uk
(South Sefton Primary Care Trust)

Practice Manager Mary McDonough

GP David MELDRUM, U PFEIFFER, Frederick Peeter VITTY

Mersey Medical Centre
First Floor, Port of Liverpool Building, Liverpool L3 1BY
Tel: 0151 236 6031

(Central Liverpool Primary Care Trust)

GP Iftikhar AHMED

Moss Way Surgery
53 Moss Way, Liverpool L11 0BL
Tel: 0151 549 2127
(North Liverpool Primary Care Trust)

Practice Manager Olive Kinsella

GP Dr KUKASAWADIA

Netherley Health Centre
Middlemass Hey, Liverpool L27 7AF
Tel: 0151 234 1240 Fax: 0151 487 5767
(South Liverpool Primary Care Trust)

Practice Manager G Bullen

GP Vallikalayil Verghese ABRAHAM, Stephanie GALLARD, Hilary KEVAN

Oak Vale Medical Centre
158-160 Edge Lane Drive, Liverpool L13 4AQ
Tel: 0151 259 1551 Fax: 0151 252 1121
(Central Liverpool Primary Care Trust)
Patient List Size: 6500

Practice Manager Sarah Wilkins

GP Moya Frances DUFFY, Michael Stephen CRANNEY, Monica Devi KHURAIJAM

Old Swan Health Centre
St Oswalds Street, Liverpool L13 2BY
Tel: 0151 228 2216 Fax: 0151 228 2216
(Central Liverpool Primary Care Trust)
Patient List Size: 7000

Practice Manager Margaret Webster

GP Rajendra Prasad AGARWAL, Vinci Wan Che HO, G R JESUDASON

Old Swan Health Centre
St Oswalds Street, Liverpool L13 2BY
Tel: 0151 228 2216 Fax: 0151 228 2216
(Central Liverpool Primary Care Trust)

GP G R R JESUDASON

Old Swan Health Centre
Crystal Close, Old Swan, Liverpool L13 2GA
Tel: 0151 285 3716 Fax: 0151 285 3754
(Central Liverpool Primary Care Trust)

Practice Manager Patricia Tinsley

GP George Robert PARRY

Orrell Lane Surgery
47 Orrell Lane, Liverpool L9 8BX
Tel: 0151 525 3051 Fax: 0151 525 1568
(South Sefton Primary Care Trust)
Patient List Size: 2050

Practice Manager Dorothy Aindow

Page Moss Health Centre
603 Princess Drive, Huyton, Liverpool L14 9ND
Tel: 0151 489 2888 Fax: 0151 489 8382
(Knowsley Primary Care Trust)
Patient List Size: 2390

Practice Manager S Kelly

GP J HEATH

Park Road Group Practice
The Elms Medical Centre, 3 The Elms, Dingle, Liverpool L8 3SS
Tel: 0151 727 5555 Fax: 0151 288 5016
Email: theelms@prgp.demon.co.uk
(Central Liverpool Primary Care Trust)
Patient List Size: 9265

Practice Manager Linda Footer

GP John Anthony HUSSEY, Kate EVANS, Anne KAZICH, Kathryn Sylvia MOORE, Denis Joseph O'BRIEN, Christopher PETERSON, Patricia Ann SMITH

Peatwood Medical Centre
2 Peatwood Avenue, Southdene, Kirkby, Liverpool L32 7PR
Tel: 0151 546 2881 Fax: 0151 548 3286
(Knowsley Primary Care Trust)
Patient List Size: 2051

GP S P SINHA

Penny Lane Surgery
7 Smithdown Place, Liverpool L15 9EH
Tel: 0151 733 2800
(Central Liverpool Primary Care Trust)

GP Ashok Kumar AGGARWAL, Nancy Elizabeth GIBSON, Paul Francis MULLEN, Maria Therese WINSTANLEY

Photiou and Partners
1 Warren Road, Blundellsands, Liverpool L23 6TZ
Tel: 0151 924 6464 Fax: 0151 932 0663
(South Sefton Primary Care Trust)

GP Sophocles PHOTIOU, Simon Robert JOHNSON, Nigel Anthony TONG, Jean Louise WYATT

Picton Road Surgery
194 Picton Road, Liverpool L15 4LL
Tel: 0151 733 1347 Fax: 0151 735 1411
(Central Liverpool Primary Care Trust)
Patient List Size: 3000

GP Joseph Edward Gerard O'RIORDAN

Pilch Lane Surgery
Pilch Lane, Huyton, Liverpool L14 0JE
Tel: 0151 489 1806 Fax: 0151 489 0920
(Knowsley Primary Care Trust)
Patient List Size: 4820

Practice Manager Lyn Grue

GP M SUARES, Albert MENDEZ-CLUNY BELMONT

Poulter Road Medical Centre
34 Poulter Road, Liverpool L9 0HJ
Tel: 0151 525 5792
(North Liverpool Primary Care Trust)
Patient List Size: 1700

GP Somendra Lal GHOSE

Princes Park Health Centre
Bentley Road, Liverpool L8 0SY
Tel: 0151 728 8313 Fax: 0151 728 8417
(Central Liverpool Primary Care Trust)
Patient List Size: 7700

Practice Manager Val Ravenscroft

GP Mark Simon BURNS, Elisabeth Grace DAVIDSON, Michael EJUONEATSE, George FAIRBAIRN, Katy GARDNER, Martin Clive SMITH

Princes Road Surgery
116 Princes Road, Liverpool L8 2UL
Tel: 0151 727 3434
(Central Liverpool Primary Care Trust)

GP M S RAO

Princess Drive Surgery
485 Princess Drive, Huyton, Liverpool L14 8XE
Tel: 0151 228 2036 Fax: 0151 228 0031
(Knowsley Primary Care Trust)
Patient List Size: 2875

Practice Manager H Messing

GP Zvi Ram MESSING, R K TAGORE

Queens Drive Surgery
73 Queens Drive, Mossley Hill, Liverpool L18 2DU
Tel: 0151 733 2812 Fax: 0151 733 4922
Email: snsingh@gp-m82107.nhs.uk
(Central Liverpool Primary Care Trust)
Patient List Size: 2330

GP Shambhu Nath SINGH

Queens Drive Surgery
339 Queens Drive, Liverpool L4 8SJ
Tel: 0151 226 6024
(North Liverpool Primary Care Trust)

GP Rajesh Kumar GERG

Radnor Place Surgery
2 Radnor Place, Liverpool L6 4BD
Tel: 0151 263 3100 Fax: 0151 263 2850
(North Liverpool Primary Care Trust)
Patient List Size: 2000

Practice Manager Sara Shaw

GP Bilquis AHMAD, J DILLON

Riverside Centre for Health
Park Street, Liverpool L8 6QP
Tel: 0151 706 8313
(Central Liverpool Primary Care Trust)

Practice Manager Pat Nelson

GP Alan Alastair FINCH

Riverside Centre for Health
Park Street, Liverpool L8 6QP
Tel: 0151 706 8317
(Central Liverpool Primary Care Trust)

GP Ragchandra Naganna HEDGE, Y K GOEL

Riverside Centre for Health
Park Street, Liverpool L8 6QP
Tel: 0151 706 8310
(Central Liverpool Primary Care Trust)

GP Roy Charles LUNT

Riverside Centre for Health
Park Street, Liverpool L8 6QP
Tel: 0151 706 8306
(Central Liverpool Primary Care Trust)

GP H M SULAIMAN

Robson Street Medical Centre
54 Robson Street, Liverpool L5 1TG
Tel: 0151 263 2295
(North Liverpool Primary Care Trust)

GP D R MALIK

Roby Medical Centre
70-72 Pilch Lane East, Roby, Liverpool L36 4NP
Tel: 0151 449 1972 Fax: 0151 489 4020
(Knowsley Primary Care Trust)
Patient List Size: 2392

Practice Manager Debbie Guy

GP Geeta Prashant NAYAK

Rock Court Surgery
Rock Court, Old Swan, Liverpool L13 2BY
Tel: 0151 228 0672 Fax: 0151 228 0298
(Central Liverpool Primary Care Trust)

GP Pramod ARORA, Margaret ALTY, R M ARORA

Rutherford Medical Centre
1 Rutherford Road, Mossley Hill, Liverpool L18 0HL
Tel: 0151 722 1803 Fax: 0151 738 0083
(Central Liverpool Primary Care Trust)

Practice Manager Jacqueline Westcott

GP Peter Martin GRIFFITHS, James Anthony CUTHBERT, B I GAZE, Mary Catherine LEYLAND

Sandringham Medical Centre
1A Aigburth Road, Liverpool L17 4JP
Tel: 0151 727 1352
(Central Liverpool Primary Care Trust)
Patient List Size: 3200

Practice Manager Indira Mohanan

GP Koratty Swaroopam MOHANAN, Manu ALEXANDER, Jessica DOCKRELL, Jamie HAMPSON, Kanila Seetharam MELANTA

Sefton Park Medical Centre
Smithdown Road, Liverpool L15 2LQ
Tel: 0151 734 5666 Fax: 0151 734 1321
(Central Liverpool Primary Care Trust)

GP Ian David RODGERS, Lyn BERRY, Michael FLYNN

Sefton Road Surgery
129 Sefton Road, Litherland, Liverpool L21 9HG

GP Selwyn Brendon GOLDTHORPE

Shaw and Partners
30 Kingsway, Waterloo, Liverpool L22 4RQ
Tel: 0151 928 8668 Fax: 0151 949 1117
(South Sefton Primary Care Trust)
Patient List Size: 5500

Practice Manager E Lonorgan

GP Martin B MORAN, Clive Richard SHAW, Fiona J WRIGHT

Sidney Powell Avenue Family Health Centre
Sidney Powell Avenue, Westvale, Kirkby, Liverpool L32 0TL
Tel: 0151 546 5103 Fax: 0151 547 2729
(Knowsley Primary Care Trust)
Patient List Size: 4048

Practice Manager Tricia Woosey

GP Christine Rebecca WYCHERLEY, Nigel John WYCHERLEY

Snaefell Avenue Surgery
14 Snaefell Avenue, Liverpool L13 7HA
Tel: 0151 228 2377
(Central Liverpool Primary Care Trust)

GP Ruth SINGER

Southdene Primary Care Resource Centre
Bewley Drive, Kirkby, Liverpool L32 9PF
Tel: 0151 546 2480 Fax: 0151 548 3474
(Knowsley Primary Care Trust)
Patient List Size: 9445

Practice Manager Edna Jones

GP Ruth WINTERBURN, P DAFFARA, Paul Martyn ELLIS, Michael Gerard MERRIMAN, M SEGAR

Speke Health Centre
North Parade, Speke, Liverpool L24 2XP
Tel: 0151 486 1695
(South Liverpool Primary Care Trust)

GP Elvira Cecilia ARYA, S C THAKUR

Speke Health Centre
North Parade, Liverpool L24 2XP
Tel: 0151 448 1293
(South Liverpool Primary Care Trust)

GP P CHOUDHARY

Speke Health Centre
North Parade, Liverpool L24 2XP
Tel: 0151 486 2694
(South Liverpool Primary Care Trust)

Practice Manager Ritha Mangarai

GP Kishan Rao MANGARAI

St James Health Centre
29 Great George Square, Liverpool L1 5DZ
Tel: 0151 709 1120
(Central Liverpool Primary Care Trust)

GP T PRASAD, N SATCHITHANANTHAN

St John's Surgery
2 Greenfield Walk, Huyton, Liverpool L36 0XP
Tel: 0151 489 9067 Fax: 0151 489 2838
(Knowsley Primary Care Trust)
Patient List Size: 2248

Practice Manager P Khandavalli

GP K SUDHAKAR

St Joseph's Medical Centre
350 Upper Parliament Street, Liverpool L8 7QL
Tel: 0151 709 3985 Fax: 0151 708 5367
(Central Liverpool Primary Care Trust)
Patient List Size: 2800

Practice Manager Bernadette McLennan

GP F A A MAJEED

St Laurence's Medical Centre
32 Leeside Avenue, Kirkby, Liverpool L32 9QU
Tel: 0151 549 0000 Fax: 0151 547 4747
(Knowsley Primary Care Trust)
Patient List Size: 5934

Practice Manager Kay Convey

GP F DE GIOVANNI, A FELL, Robert Ian KING, David STOKOE

Stafford Street Surgery
21 Stafford Street, Liverpool L3 8LX
Tel: 0151 207 0921 Fax: 0151 207 0921
(North Liverpool Primary Care Trust)

GP Andrew Ademoye BADERIN

Stanley Medical Centre
60 Stanley Road, Kirkdale, Liverpool L5 2QA
Tel: 0151 207 1076
(North Liverpool Primary Care Trust)
Patient List Size: 2500

Practice Manager Manju Sharma

GP Suraj Prakash SHARMA

Stanley Medical Centre
60 Stanley Road, Kirkdale, Liverpool L5 2QA
Tel: 0151 207 3113 Fax: 0151 207 3800
(North Liverpool Primary Care Trust)
Patient List Size: 2548

Practice Manager Rajni Gupta

GP S K GUPTA

Stanley Medical Centre
60 Stanley Road, Kirkdale, Liverpool L5 2QA
Tel: 0151 207 0126
(North Liverpool Primary Care Trust)

Practice Manager Irene Harvey

GP Vincent Anderson HARVEY

Stockbridge Village Health Centre
Leachcroft, Waterpark Drive, Stockbridge Village, Liverpool L28 1ST
Tel: 0151 489 9924 Fax: 0151 489 8298
(Knowsley Primary Care Trust)
Patient List Size: 8491

Practice Manager Dot Blacklee

GP Philip Leslie JONES, Dr BARRY, Terence MULLIN, Paul RIGBY

Stoneycroft Medical Centre
Stoneville Road, Liverpool L13 6QD
Tel: 0151 228 1138 Fax: 0151 228 1653
(Central Liverpool Primary Care Trust)

GP Elizabeth Anne BAINBRIDGE, Ernst BUHRS, Rita Veronica CASSIDY

Student Services Centre
150 Mount Pleasant, Liverpool L69 3BX
Tel: 0151 794 4720
(North Liverpool Primary Care Trust)

GP Diane EXLEY, Deborah FAINT, Edward Sebastian GAYNOR, Deborah Jane NOLAND

Tarbock Health Centre
104 Tarbock Road, Huyton, Liverpool L36 5TH
Tel: 0151 489 1444 Fax: 0151 481 0042
(Knowsley Primary Care Trust)
Patient List Size: 3424

Practice Manager S Graham

GP S K DESAI, S SINGH

Tarbock Road Surgery
133 Tarbock Road, Huyton, Liverpool L36 5TE
Tel: 0151 449 3020 Fax: 0151 489 9375
(Knowsley Primary Care Trust)
Patient List Size: 3305

Practice Manager S Kelly

GP J HEATH

Taylor, Parsons, Donnelly, Kuruvilla and Mulrine
Woolton House Medical Centre, 4/6 Woolton Street, Woolton, Liverpool L25 5JA
Tel: 0151 428 4184 Fax: 0151 428 4598
(South Liverpool Primary Care Trust)
Patient List Size: 9200

Practice Manager Gail Tyrer

GP Andrew Spencer TAYLOR, George KURUVILLA, Catriona Helen MULRINE, Julie OWEN, David WEBSTER

Tower Hill Health Centre
Highfield, Towerhill, Kirkby, Liverpool L33 1DX
Tel: 0151 546 9955 Fax: 0151 549 1037
(Knowsley Primary Care Trust)
Patient List Size: 3755

Practice Manager Colin Maassarani

GP Faisal MAASSARANI, Hassan Ali MAASSARANI

Towerhill Health Centre
82-84 Waddicar Lane, Melling, Liverpool L31 1DY
Tel: 0151 549 1583 Fax: 0151 548 5711
(Knowsley Primary Care Trust)
Patient List Size: 2936

Practice Manager P Kakati

GP Benudhar KAKATI

Townsend Lane Surgery
263 Townsend Lane, Clubmoor, Liverpool L13 9DG
Tel: 0151 226 1358
(North Liverpool Primary Care Trust)

GP S KUMAR, S SINGH

Trentham Road Surgery
37 Trentham Road, Kirkby, Liverpool L32 4UB
Tel: 0151 546 3711 Fax: 0151 548 4625
(Knowsley Primary Care Trust)
Patient List Size: 4502

Practice Manager V Tewari

GP V K TEWARI, A AWI, S PRABHU

Upper Parliament Street Surgery
334 Upper Parliament Street, Liverpool L8 7QL
Tel: 0151 709 1263
(Central Liverpool Primary Care Trust)

GP V KISHAN RAO, V USHA-RANI

The Valley Medical Centre
14 Waller Close, Liverpool L4 4QJ
Tel: 0151 207 3447 Fax: 0151 2867909
(North Liverpool Primary Care Trust)

GP Jill Frances O'DONNELL

Valley Medical Centre
14 Waller Close, Liverpool L4 4QJ
Tel: 0151 207 3447
(Central Liverpool Primary Care Trust)

GP Mary Penelope NEWSON, Denis Dominic BUCKLEY, Rosaleen Mary BUCKLEY, Andrew David NOBLE

Vauxhall Health Centre
Limekiln Lane, Liverpool L5 8XR
Tel: 0151 207 2274
(North Liverpool Primary Care Trust)

GP Vinod KUMAR

Vauxhall Health Centre
Limekiln Lane, Liverpool L5 8XR
Tel: 0151 298 2246
(North Liverpool Primary Care Trust)

GP Kit Oi CHUNG, Catherine HOPKINS, Helen Margaret McKENDRICK

Village Medical Centre
20 Quarry Street, Liverpool L25 6HE
Tel: 0151 428 4282 Fax: 0151 421 0884
(South Liverpool Primary Care Trust)
Patient List Size: 3575

Practice Manager Lynn Robinson

GP Edward James Henry BYRNE, Hugh John NIELSEN

The Village Surgery
Elbow Lane, Formby, Liverpool L37 4AW
Tel: 01704 878661 Fax: 01704 832488
(Southport and Formby Primary Care Trust)

Practice Manager Sheila Ainsworth

GP Charles Forbes INNES, G J ALLWRIGHT, Stephen John CROSBY, Dr HOUGH, Jacqueline Anne REDDINGTON

Walton Breck Road Practice
291 Walton Breck Road, Liverpool L4 0SX
Tel: 0151 260 2760
(North Liverpool Primary Care Trust)

GP M A DAR

Walton Hall Avenue Medical Centre
12 Walton Hall Avenue, Liverpool L4 6UF
Tel: 0151 524 0267 Fax: 0151 525 9989
(North Liverpool Primary Care Trust)
Patient List Size: 3300

Practice Manager Janet Peppard

GP Bhaskar CHAKRABARTI

Walton Medical Centre
2-4 Bedford Road, Liverpool L4 5PX
Tel: 0151 525 6438 Fax: 0151 530 1748
(North Liverpool Primary Care Trust)
Patient List Size: 8100

Practice Manager Linda Stewart

GP Susan Elizabeth LUCK, John ARMSTRONG, Dirk BODE, Stephen Geoffrey WRIGHT

Walton Village Medical Centre
172 Walton Village, Liverpool L4 6TW
Tel: 0151 525 8254 Fax: 0151 525 6448
(North Liverpool Primary Care Trust)

GP Syed Ahmed Hussain RAZVI

Walton Village Medical Centre
172 Walton Village, Liverpool L4 6TW
Tel: 0151 525 1700 Fax: 0151 525 6448
(North Liverpool Primary Care Trust)
Patient List Size: 2330

Practice Manager Tracy Fagan

GP Mohamad Ali DIAB

Westminster Medical Centre
Aldams Grove, Liverpool L4 3TT
Tel: 0151 922 3510 Fax: 0151 902 6071
(North Liverpool Primary Care Trust)

Practice Manager Dorothy Gibson

GP A K SHARMA, Yashwant SINGH

The Westmoreland GP Centre
Fazakerley Hospital, Aintree, Liverpool L9 7AL
Tel: 0151 525 6286
(North Liverpool Primary Care Trust)

GP James Michael FORREST, Margaret Linda GODDARD, Sian ALEXANDER-WHITE, Anthony Peter BARKER, Margaret Patricia BROWN, Andrew CAVADINO, Julie Margaret COLEMAN

Westway Medical Centre
Westway, Maghull, Liverpool L31 0DJ
Tel: 0151 526 1121 Fax: 0151 531 2631
(South Sefton Primary Care Trust)
Patient List Size: 8300

Practice Manager S M Brigden

GP John Robert Edward WRAY, E A AINSWORTH, S P GOUGH, Kathryn Bernadette HULME

Wingate Medical Centre
79 Bigdale Drive, Northwood, Liverpool L33 6YJ
Tel: 0151 546 2958 Fax: 0151 546 2914
(Knowsley Primary Care Trust)
Patient List Size: 15435

Practice Manager Susan Winter

GP Colin David FORD, Hilary Janice BRINKSMAN, Jeffrey GOLDSTONE, John Edward HUGHES, Christopher James MIMNAGH, Paul Robert MORRIS, John Desmond O'DONNELL, S PERRITT, John Anthony Cooper WINTER

Liversedge

Liversedge Health Centre
Valley Road, Liversedge WF15 6DF
Tel: 01924 407771 Fax: 01924 411727
(North Kirklees Primary Care Trust)
Patient List Size: 2405

Practice Manager Wendy Stead

GP Hamidullah KHAN

Liversedge Health Centre
Valley Road, Liversedge WF15 6DF
Tel: 01924 404900
(North Kirklees Primary Care Trust)

GP Partha SARATHY

London, E1

Albion Health Centre
333 Whitechapel Road, London E1 1BU
Tel: 020 7247 1730 Fax: 020 7247 2589
(Tower Hamlets Primary Care Trust)
Patient List Size: 7280

Practice Manager J F Dale

GP D C HICK, I KAYES, Dr RASHID, Tessa Mary STURT, D A R TOLLISS

Brayford Square Surgery
5 Brayford Square, Stepney, London E1 0SG
Tel: 020 7790 2136 Fax: 020 7790 0802
(Tower Hamlets Primary Care Trust)

GP Chandrashekhar Mohenlal VARMA

East One Health
14 Deancross Street, London E1 2QA
Tel: 020 7790 2978
(Tower Hamlets Primary Care Trust)

GP Richard Thomas Carlyle MITCHELL

Jubilee Street Practice
Commercial Road, London E1 0LR
Tel: 020 7335 4900 Fax: 020 7335 4701
Website: www.jubileestreet.org
(Tower Hamlets Primary Care Trust)
Patient List Size: 9416

Practice Manager Jean Trollope

GP Salma AHMED, Naomi Rosemary BEER, Nicola Anne Lee COWAP, Mary Ewins EDMONDSON, Nicola HAGDRUP, Sarah Ann HULL, Andrew WARSOP

London Hospital Medical College Staff Clinics
Turner Street, London E1 2AD

GP Alan McEWAN

Shahjalal Medical Centre
44-56 Hessel Street, London E1 2LP
Tel: 020 7702 2063 Fax: 020 7748 2323
(Tower Hamlets Primary Care Trust)
Patient List Size: 10520

Practice Manager C H Stears

GP K N ISLAM, M G HOSSAIN, M A SAMAD

Spitalfields Practice
20 Old Montague Street, London E1 5PB
Tel: 020 7247 7070 Fax: 020 7650 1920
(Tower Hamlets Primary Care Trust)
Patient List Size: 11800

Practice Manager Hasmukh Sanghvi

GP Jeffrey Gerald SAFIR, Stuart James BINGHAM, Peter BUCKMAN, Saida DESAI, Christopher Janson HANBURY, Hosne Ara HAQ, Olusegun Abayomi ODETOYINBO

Stepney Green Medical Practice
45-47 Ben Jonson Road, London E1 4SA
Tel: 020 7790 1059 Fax: 020 7702 7454
(Tower Hamlets Primary Care Trust)
Patient List Size: 7500

Practice Manager Evelyn Galbraith

GP Gita DEB, Richard Bryan HABERSHON, Tai OKUN, Michael Arthur Farnham ST JOHN

The Surgery
12-14 Nightingale House, St Katherines Dock, Thomas More Street, London E1W 1UA

GP M R YOUNG

The Surgery
1 Barnardo Gardens, Barnardo Street, London E1 0LN

GP Sekhar Nath BASU

Tower Medical Centre
129 Cannon Street Road, London E1 2LX
Tel: 020 7488 4240 Fax: 020 7702 2443
(Tower Hamlets Primary Care Trust)

GP John Anthony PRINCE, Sanjay BATRA, S A J STANLEY

The Wapping Group Practice
Wapping Health Centre, 22 Wapping Lane, London E1W 2RL
Tel: 020 7481 9376 Fax: 020 7488 4246
(Tower Hamlets Primary Care Trust)

Practice Manager Gwen Sawyer

GP Martha Frances Margaret LEIGH, Daniel James MOONEY, Adam Bernard STERN, Para THAYALASEKARAN

London, E2

Bethnal Green Health Centre
60 Florida Street, London E2 6LL
Tel: 020 7739 4837 Fax: 020 7729 2190
(Tower Hamlets Primary Care Trust)

Practice Manager K Ahamed

GP Ganesh Chandra DUTT, Roseanna Mary POLLEN, J N HARDY, A KHANAM, Rajesh Manubhai PATEL, Vivien Mary TAYLOR

The Blithehale Medical Centre
3 Jersey Street, Bethnal Green, London E2 0AW
Tel: 020 7739 5497
(Tower Hamlets Primary Care Trust)
Patient List Size: 6500

Practice Manager Ruth Castle

GP Siobhan Dolores COOKE

Globe Town Surgery
82-86 Roman Road, London E2 0PG
Tel: 020 8980 3023 Fax: 020 8983 4627
Email: firstname.lastname@nhs.net
(Tower Hamlets Primary Care Trust)

Practice Manager Isabel Cossar

GP Alison Susan ARNOTT, Lisa GODDARD, Robert A KIELTY

Medical Centre
3 Strouts Place, London E2 7QU
Tel: 020 7739 8859 Fax: 020 7739 6906
(Tower Hamlets Primary Care Trust)
Patient List Size: 5043

Practice Manager Beverley Fraser-Davis

GP Shamsuddin AHMED, Rezaur RAHMAN

The Mission Practice
208 Cambridge Heath Road, London E2 9LS
Tel: 020 8983 7300 Fax: 020 8983 6800
(Tower Hamlets Primary Care Trust)
Patient List Size: 8400

Practice Manager David Billingham

GP Gillian Kelso WEBSTER, Paul JAKEMAN, Judith LITTLEJOHNS, Andrew Guy MEAD, Mary Eleanor Beatrice NUNNS, Timothy ROWELL, Margaret STALEY, David Antony WHITTINGTON

Silk Court Surgery
47 Pollard Row, London E2 6NA

GP S N M KHAN

The Surgery
167 Kingsland Road, London E2 8AL
Tel: 020 7739 3600 Fax: 020 7613 5345
(City and Hackney Teaching Primary Care Trust)

GP Fouad A M RIZK, Adeyemi Abiodun ADEKANMI

London, E3

Bhaiwala
St Paul's Way Medical Centre, 99 St Paul's Way, London E3 4AJ
(Tower Hamlets Primary Care Trust)

Practice Manager Alia Rahman

GP Batul Zoeb BHAIWALA, ZZoeb Shaikhadambhai BHAIWALA

Bromley-by-Bow Health Centre
St Leonards Street, London E3 3BT
(Tower Hamlets Primary Care Trust)

GP Angela Claire BURNETT, Julia Elizabeth DAVIS, Anthony Herbert (Sam) EVERINGTON

Harley Grove Medical Centre
15 Harley Grove, Bow, London E3 2AT
Tel: 020 8980 3130 Fax: 020 89831255
(Tower Hamlets Primary Care Trust)
Patient List Size: 4211

Practice Manager A Afzal

GP Selladurai SHANMUGADASAN, Thanaluxmy SHANMUGDASAN

Jain
St Paul's Way Medical Centre, St Paul's Way, London E3 4AJ
(Tower Hamlets Primary Care Trust)

GP Alok Suta JAIN, Anil Kumar JAIN

Ruston Street Clinic
Ruston Street, London E3 2LR
Tel: 020 8980 1652
Email: naimish.amin@nhs.nst
(Tower Hamlets Primary Care Trust)
Patient List Size: 2412

Practice Manager Barbara Carter

GP N B AMIN, A O'CONNELL

St Stephens Health Centre
Bow Community Hall, William Place, London E3 5ED
Tel: 020 8980 1760 Fax: 020 8980 6619
(Tower Hamlets Primary Care Trust)
Patient List Size: 8700

Practice Manager Patricia Sharp

GP Soraya BOOMLA, Suzanne BURNS, Ricardo CABOT, Michael Stuart David CALLAGHAN, Philippa Jane COCKMAN, Sian Rowena HOWELL

Strooudley Walk Health Centre
38 Stroudley Walk, London E3 3EW
Tel: 020 8981 4742 Fax: 020 8981 9165
(Tower Hamlets Primary Care Trust)
Patient List Size: 3900

Practice Manager Debbie Russell

GP O AMULUDUN, L EMOHARE, R GOEL

The Surgery
5 Merchant Street, London E3 4LJ
Tel: 020 8980 3676 Fax: 020 89833009
(Tower Hamlets Primary Care Trust)

GP A K RANA

The Surgery
1-3 Birchdown House, Devons Road, Bow, London E3 3NS
Tel: 020 8980 1888 Fax: 020 8980 2753
(Tower Hamlets Primary Care Trust)

GP Vijaya Kumar NISCHAL

The Surgery
3 Ivanhoe House, 130 Gore Road, London E3 5TW
Tel: 020 8980 1767 Fax: 020 8980 1793
(Tower Hamlets Primary Care Trust)
Patient List Size: 3387

GP K SHAH

The Surgery
35 St Stephen's Road, London E3 5JD
(Tower Hamlets Primary Care Trust)

GP I HODKINSON

The Tredegar Practice
35 St Stephen's Road, London E3 5JD
Tel: 020 8980 1822 Fax: 020 8983 7131
(Tower Hamlets Primary Care Trust)

GP George Allen FARRELLY, Isabel HOOKINSON

London, E4

Chingford Health Centre
109 York Road, Chingford, London E4 8LF
Tel: 020 8529 1541 Fax: 020 8559 4091
(Waltham Forest Primary Care Trust)
Patient List Size: 2158

Practice Manager Bobbie Shepherd

GP Mohammad Saeed KHALAF

Chingford Health Centre
109 York Road, Chingford, London E4 8LF
Tel: 020 8524 8422 Fax: 020 8559 3538
(Waltham Forest Primary Care Trust)

Practice Manager Susan Harden

GP Claudia Anne LLOYD ROE

Chingford Mount Road Surgery
107-109 Chingford Mount Road, Chingford, London E4 8LT
Tel: 020 8524 1230 Fax: 020 8559 3004
Email: medandson@aol.com
(Waltham Forest Primary Care Trust)

Practice Manager Mahmooda Dadabhoy

GP Mohamed Ebrahim DADABHOY, Shahid Mohamed DADABHOY

Chingford Surgery
197 Chingford Mount Road, Chingford, London E4 8LR
Tel: 020 8529 1290 Fax: 020 8504 5544
(Waltham Forest Primary Care Trust)

Practice Manager Mr Kumar

GP Shashi Surjit KUMAR, S J KUMAR, B PATEL, H SOHAIL

Churchill Medical Centre
1 Churchill Terrace, Chingford, London E4 8DA
Tel: 020 8524 1777 Fax: 020 8559 4142
(Waltham Forest Primary Care Trust)

Practice Manager Seizin Osman

GP Phillip James KOCZAN, Carol Morag BATCHELOR, A KHAN, E SINGER

Dr B C Nandi Surgery
93 The Ridgeway, Chingford, London E4 6QW
Tel: 020 8529 6479 Fax: 020 8523 7341
(Waltham Forest Primary Care Trust)
Patient List Size: 3500

Practice Manager Janet Wright

GP Bipul Chandra NANDI

Hampton Practice
57 Hampton Road, London E4 8NH
Tel: 020 8529 8588 Fax: 020 8523 7054
(Waltham Forest Primary Care Trust)

Practice Manager Tara Khare

GP Kailash Chandra KHARE, R BHATNAGAR

Health Centre
Handsworth Avenue, Highams Park, London E4 9PD
Tel: 020 8527 0913 Fax: 020 8527 6583
(Waltham Forest Primary Care Trust)
Patient List Size: 13500

Practice Manager Josie Camplin

GP Ann Marysia TELESZ, A A BASHIR, Christopher Paul BRITT, Gordon BROWN, Tonia Rosalind MYERS, Simon James ORMEROD, Mark Kevin SCOWEN

Kings Head Hill Surgery
178 Kings Head Hill, Chingford, London E4 7NX
Tel: 020 8529 3501 Fax: 020 8559 4456
(Waltham Forest Primary Care Trust)
Patient List Size: 3500

Practice Manager R Shepherd

GP David DRAKE, P LAWRENCE

Larkshall Medical Centre
1 Larkshall Road, Chingford, London E4 7HS
Tel: 020 8524 6355 Fax: 020 8524 0605
(Waltham Forest Primary Care Trust)
Patient List Size: 4000

Practice Manager Surjit Kumar

GP Shashi Surjit KUMAR, S J KUMAR, B PATEL, H SOHAIL

New Road Clinic
114 New Road, Chingford, London E4 9SY
Tel: 020 8524 8124 Fax: 020 8529 4801
(Waltham Forest Primary Care Trust)
Patient List Size: 8300

Practice Manager Ray Wydell

GP David John McDonald AITCHISON, Ruth Mary HARVEY, Christopher Mark PUTT, Kauser Jabeen WARRIS

The Old Church Surgery
99 Chingford Avenue, Chingford, London E4 6RG
Tel: 020 8529 5543 Fax: 020 8553 4149
(Waltham Forest Primary Care Trust)
Patient List Size: 2866

Practice Manager Annette Fisher

GP Paul Anthony DAVIS, Michal GRENVILLE

The Old Hall Surgery
237 Hall Lane, Chingford, London E4 8HX
Tel: 020 8524 3410 Fax: 020 8524 6424
(Waltham Forest Primary Care Trust)

Practice Manager Yvonne Garwood

GP Alfred GARWOOD

Park House Surgery
1 Cavendish Road, Highams Park, London E4 9NQ
Tel: 020 8523 1401
(Waltham Forest Primary Care Trust)

GP S BASHIR, Christopher Paul BRITT, Gordan BROWN, Tonia Rosalind MYERS, Simon James ORMEROD, Mark Kevin SCOWEN, Ann Marysia TELESZ

The Ridgeway Surgery
1 Mount Echo Avenue, Chingford, London E4 7JX
Tel: 020 8529 2233 Fax: 020 8529 4484
(Waltham Forest Primary Care Trust)
Patient List Size: 4700

Practice Manager Yvonne Davey

GP Susan Elizabeth WEST, G CAVE, M MOFFAT

London, E5

Athena Medical Centre
21 Atherden Road, London E5 0QP
Tel: 020 8985 6675 Fax: 020 8533 7775
(City and Hackney Teaching Primary Care Trust)
Patient List Size: 5000

GP Affia Chidi OKOREAFFIA

Clapton Surgery
154 Upper Clapton Road, London E5 9JZ
(City and Hackney Teaching Primary Care Trust)

GP Tauqir AHMAD

Healy Medical Centre
200 Upper Clapton Road, London E5 9DH
Tel: 020 8806 1611
(City and Hackney Teaching Primary Care Trust)

GP Manjeet Singh DUGGAL, Balvinder DUGGAL, C S DUGGAL, S DUGGAL

Lower Clapton Group Practice
36 Lower Clapton Road, London E5 0PD
Tel: 020 8986 7111 Fax: 020 8986 8140
(City and Hackney Teaching Primary Care Trust)

Practice Manager Deb L'Aimable

GP Robert Charles Heard LYLE, Miriam Sybil BEEKS, Nick BREWER, Gene Solomon FEDER, Christopher John GRIFFITHS, Clare HIGHTON, P KATONA, Tessa KATZ

Median Road Surgery
28 Median Road, Clapton, London E5 0PL
Tel: 020 8985 2664
(City and Hackney Teaching Primary Care Trust)

GP Melvyn Alan OSEN

Nightingale Practice
10 Kenninghall Road, Clapton, London E5 8BY
Tel: 020 8985 8388 Fax: 020 8986 6004
(City and Hackney Teaching Primary Care Trust)
Patient List Size: 7000

Practice Manager Deborah Rose

GP Victoria Janet HOLT, Jasper Nicholas MAHON, Thomas Christopher PAYNE, Mark RICKETS, Joanna Mary SUDELL, Sarah Anne-Marie WILLIAMS

Sorsby Health Centre
3 Mandeville Street, Clapton, London E5 0DH
Tel: 020 8986 5613 Fax: 020 8986 8072
(City and Hackney Teaching Primary Care Trust)
Patient List Size: 7984

GP Devanaboina RAMA MOHANA RAO

The Surgery
83 Clifden Road, Clapton, London E5 0LJ
Tel: 020 8985 4554 Fax: 020 8986 0667
(City and Hackney Teaching Primary Care Trust)
Patient List Size: 3200

Practice Manager Margaret Philpot

GP Karam Vir KAPUR, Andrew MITCHEL

The Surgery
144-150 Upper Clapton Road, London E5 9JZ
(City and Hackney Teaching Primary Care Trust)

GP Paul RUBNER, Joseph Reuben HOROWITZ, Atef Tawfik IBRAHIM

The Surgery
83 Clifden Road, Clapton, London E5 0LJ
(City and Hackney Teaching Primary Care Trust)

London, E6

Barking Road Surgery
533 Barking Road, East Ham, London E6 2LN
Tel: 020 8472 3080 Fax: 020 8552 3706
(Newham Primary Care Trust)

GP Pratap Rai DUBAL, Niran Janbhal Ratilal PATEL, Anthony Trevor SEATON

East Ham Surgery
154 High Street South, East Ham, London E6 3RW
Tel: 020 8472 9260 Fax: 020 8552 3307
(Newham Primary Care Trust)

GP Inayat INAYATULLAH

Market Street Health Group
52 Market Street, East Ham, London E6 2RA
Tel: 020 8548 2200 Fax: 020 8548 2288
(Newham Primary Care Trust)

GP Hilary Gaye MEADOWS, O DARAMOLA, Clare Meriel DAVISON, G HALL, Adekola ORIMOLOYE, Robert Edward Michael WAUGH

Royal Docks Medical Centre
21 East Ham, Manor Way, Beckton, London E6 5NA
Tel: 020 7511 4466 Fax: 020 7511 1492
(Newham Primary Care Trust)
Patient List Size: 6000

Practice Manager Lynne Evans

GP James Alexander LAWRIE, Stuart GRECON, Handeol HAMERD-NASRAT, Sashi NANDRAKUMAR, Chris RIFFORD

St Bartholomews Surgery
292A Barking Road, London E6 3BA
Tel: 020 8472 0669/1077 Fax: 020 8471 9122
(Newham Primary Care Trust)
Patient List Size: 8300

Practice Manager Carol Robinson

GP Hasmukh Shivabhai PATEL, Adefolane AJANLEKOKO, Nnaemeka Jonathan OJUKWU, Trevor Adrian POWELL

St John's Road Medical Centre
1-3 St. Johns Road, East Ham, London E6 1NW
Tel: 020 8503 5783 Fax: 020 8503 5784
(Newham Primary Care Trust)

GP Nejat CHALABI, Abdul-Razaq MONSIN ABDULLA

The Surgery
27 Burges Road, East Ham, London E6 2BJ
Tel: 020 8472 0421 Fax: 020 8552 9912
(Newham Primary Care Trust)

Practice Manager Raj Bhaker

GP Anthony Trevor SEATON, Pratap Rai DUBAL, Niranjanbhai Ratilal PATEL

The Surgery
34 Barking Road, East Ham, London E6 3BP
Tel: 020 8472 1347 Fax: 020 8470 5244
(Newham Primary Care Trust)
Patient List Size: 4000

Practice Manager Parveen Akhtar

GP I INAYATULLAH

The Surgery
159 Wakefield Street, East Ham, London E6 1LG
Tel: 020 8472 0208 Fax: 020 8471 0794
(Newham Primary Care Trust)
Patient List Size: 1800

GP Archibald Jasper BARNABAS

The Surgery
1 Clements Road, East Ham, London E6 2DS
Tel: 020 8472 0603 Fax: 020 8553 0211
(Newham Primary Care Trust)

GP Samuel MANDAVILLI, P SHUKLA

The Surgery
19-21 High Street South, Eastham, London E6 6EN
Tel: 020 8472 2474 Fax: 020 8586 0902
(Newham Primary Care Trust)

GP K AZAD, A AZAD

Tollgate Health Centre
220 Tollgate Road, London E6 5JS
Tel: 020 7445 7700 Fax: 020 7445 7715
(Newham Primary Care Trust)

Practice Manager Malcolm Vincent

GP P EIJSENBURG, David Erickson WATT, K J COCHRANE, Gillian Lesley GOOSE, Chander Kiran SIKKA, Robert STANOWSKI

London, E7

Birchdale Road Medical Centre
2 Birchdale Road, London E7 8AR
Tel: 020 8472 1600 Fax: 020 8471 7712
(Newham Primary Care Trust)

GP Bhupendra Kumar SINHA

Claremont Clinic
459-463 Romford Road, Forest Gate, London E7 8AB
Tel: 020 8522 0222 Fax: 020 8522 0444
(Newham Primary Care Trust)
Patient List Size: 6472

Practice Manager S Rattu

GP Sarah Augusta WOOD, Ciaran JOYCE, Atmaji MANAM, K SINHA, Sarah TREEASKES

Katherine Road Medical Centre
511 Katherine Road, London E7 8DR
Tel: 020 8472 7029
(Newham Primary Care Trust)

GP Govind BAPNA

Lord Lister Health Centre
121 Woodgrange Road, Forest Gate, London E7 0EP
Tel: 020 8250 7510 Fax: 020 8250 7515
(Newham Primary Care Trust)
Patient List Size: 7000

Practice Manager Pritdal Kallah, Natasha Rae

GP Nowshir Ratanshaw DRIVER, Catherine Mary FRIEL, Leung Ting LAM KIN TENG

Lord Lister Health Centre
121 Woodgrange Road, Forest Gate, London E7 0EP
Tel: 020 8250 7550 Fax: 020 8250 7553
(Newham Primary Care Trust)
Patient List Size: 2896

Practice Manager Lola Mazarelo

GP P ABIOLA

Lord Lister Health Centre
121 Woodgrange Road, Forest Gate, London E7 0EP
Tel: 020 8250 7530 Fax: 020 8250 7535
(Newham Primary Care Trust)
Patient List Size: 3000

Practice Manager Hesham Farghaly

GP Sawsan Kamel Selim SWEDAN

Shrewsbury Road Health Centre
Shrewsbury Road, London E7 8QP
Tel: 020 8586 5111 Fax: 020 8586 5046
(Newham Primary Care Trust)
Patient List Size: 10500

Practice Manager Carol Lowrie

GP Sandra IVINSON, Anita Parish BHASI, Sinnadurai MAHENDRAN, G PURUSHOTAMAN, M SRI-GANESHAN

The Surgery
45 Westbury Road, Forest Gate, London E7 8BU
Tel: 020 8472 4123 Fax: 020 8552 5329
(Newham Primary Care Trust)

GP Alauddin AHMED, Mohammed Matiar RAHMAN

The Surgery
279 Katherine Road, Forest Gate, London E7 8PP
Tel: 020 8586 6555 Fax: 020 8470 1318
(Newham Primary Care Trust)

Practice Manager K L Satchi

GP Thyaqarajagopalan Krishna MURTHY

The Surgery
2 Jephson Road, London E7 8LZ
Tel: 020 8470 6429 Fax: 020 8470 5383
(Newham Primary Care Trust)

GP C M PATEL

The Surgery
162 Boleyn Road, London E7 9QJ
Tel: 020 8503 5656 Fax: 020 8586 9028
(Newham Primary Care Trust)

GP Saeeda Sultana RAFIQ

Upton Lane Medical Centre
75-77 Upton Lane, London E7 9PB
Tel: 020 8471 6912 Fax: 020 8471 3845
(Newham Primary Care Trust)
Patient List Size: 8000

GP P G SHANKER, Baljeet Kaur SALUJA

Woodgrange Medical Practice
40 Woodgrange Road, Forest Gate, London E7 0QH
Tel: 020 8250 7585 Fax: 020 8250 7587
(Newham Primary Care Trust)
Patient List Size: 3750

Practice Manager A Mahatma

GP V I PATEL, S J PARMAR

London, E8

Dalston Practice
1 Madinah Road, London E8 1PG
(City and Hackney Teaching Primary Care Trust)

GP S K KAWALE, J D PATEL

Kingsland Medical Centre
414 Kingsland Road, London E8 4AA
Tel: 020 7249 8732 Fax: 020 7254 6878
(City and Hackney Teaching Primary Care Trust)
Patient List Size: 3000

GP Ramniklal Tribhovandas DATTANI

The London Fields Medical Centres
38-44 Broadway Market, London E8 4QJ
Tel: 020 7254 2883 Fax: 020 7254 2066
(City and Hackney Teaching Primary Care Trust)

Practice Manager Mike Kiely

GP May Frances Anne CAHILL, Sarah Jane COWLEY, Mary Clodagh MURPHY

Queensbridge Group Practice
24 Holly Street, London E8 3XP
Tel: 020 7254 1101 Fax: 020 7923 1541
Email: gp@f84117.nhs.ujude.kidd@nhs.net
(City and Hackney Teaching Primary Care Trust)
Patient List Size: 6300

Practice Manager Jude Kidd

GP Lewis CAPLIN, Sally COOPER, Gemma KELVIN, Janet Louise KIRTON, Anna D PILKINGTON

Richmond Road Medical Centre
136 Richmond Road, London E8 3HN
Tel: 020 7254 2298
(City and Hackney Teaching Primary Care Trust)

GP Suresh Prasad TIBREWAL

Richmond Road Medical Centre
136 Richmond Road, London E8 3HN
(City and Hackney Teaching Primary Care Trust)

GP Krishan Chandra GUPTA

Richmond Road Surgery
119 Richmond Road, Dalston, London E8 3AA
Tel: 020 8254 2298 Fax: 020 7923-9247
(Newham Primary Care Trust)

GP Sanjay GUPTA, Dr TIBREWAL

Sandringham Practice
The Medical Centre, 1 Madinah Road, London E8 1PG
Tel: 020 7275 0022 Fax: 020 7923 2622
(City and Hackney Teaching Primary Care Trust)
Patient List Size: 5500

Practice Manager Emel Yaltirik

GP Godfrey Vukile MDINGI, Ndubuisi Linus EMEAGI

London, E9

Elsdale Street Surgery
28 Elsdale Street, London E9 6QY
Tel: 020 8985 2719
(City and Hackney Teaching Primary Care Trust)
Patient List Size: 4000

Practice Manager Keren Fisher

GP Heather Jane CHARLES, Alison GIBB, Jems RUHBACH, Kathleen WENADEN

Homerton Surgery
139 Homerton High Street, Homerton, London E9 6AS
Tel: 020 8985 3444 Fax: 020 8985 8108
(City and Hackney Teaching Primary Care Trust)

GP Devanaboina RAMA MOHANA RAO, A K KHATRI

Kingsmead Healthcare
4 Kingsmead Way, London E9 5QG
Tel: 020 8985 1930 Fax: 020 8533 3951
(City and Hackney Teaching Primary Care Trust)
Patient List Size: 7000

Practice Manager Deepak Sinha

GP V S P ADIREDDI, G R ANANTHAPADMANABAN

Patel
Latimer Health Centre, 4 Homerton Terrace, off Morning Lane, Hackney, London E9 6RT
Tel: 020 8985 2249 Fax: 020 8985 7333
(City and Hackney Teaching Primary Care Trust)
Patient List Size: 5000

Practice Manager Amanda Waite

GP Geeta Harendra PATEL, Harendra Gordhanbhai PATEL

The Surgery
74 Brooksby's Walk, London E9 6DA
Tel: 020 8985 2797 Fax: 020 8985 0999
(City and Hackney Teaching Primary Care Trust)

Practice Manager A Prasad

GP Raghureshwar PRASAD

Well Street Surgery
52B Well Street, London E9 7PX
Tel: 020 8985 2050 Fax: 020 8985 5780
(City and Hackney Teaching Primary Care Trust)

GP Paul Anthony Collyer JULIAN, Fiona Deborah BERNARD, J HAYMAN, Catherine Ruth HIGHTON, Gabriela Jill TOBIAS, Sotirios ZALIDIS

The Wick Health Centre
200 Wick Road, Homerton, London E9 5AN
Tel: 020 8986 6341
(City and Hackney Teaching Primary Care Trust)

GP Melvyn Alan OSEN

London, E10

Crawley Road Medical Centre
479 High Road, Leyton, London E10 5EL
Tel: 020 8539 1880 Fax: 020 8556 1318
(Waltham Forest Primary Care Trust)

GP Sisir Kanti SEN, Tej Kamal Kaur KALRA

Francis Road Surgery
94 Francis Road, Leyton, London E10 6PP
Tel: 020 8539 3131 Fax: 020 8539 7875
(Waltham Forest Primary Care Trust)
Patient List Size: 3600

Practice Manager Rayan Vimal

GP Vimalathevi HARIHARAN

Grange Park Medical Centre
24 Grange Park Road, Leyton, London E10 5EP
Tel: 020 8539 2962 Fax: 020 8539 7940
(Waltham Forest Primary Care Trust)
Patient List Size: 6500

Practice Manager Caroline Paul

GP Dinesh KAPOOR, D FERNANDIS, Ranjana KAPOOR, F LASHID, E LEVENE

High Road Surgery
706-708 High Road, Leyton, London E10 6JP
Tel: 020 8539 4707 Fax: 020 8539 1690
(Waltham Forest Primary Care Trust)

GP Krishna Bhusan MALLICK, Golap MALLICK

Kapoor Surgery
234 Francis Road, Leyton, London E10 6NQ
Tel: 020 8539 2542
(Waltham Forest Primary Care Trust)

GP D A FERNANDES, Dinesh KAPOOR, Ranjana KAPOOR

Lea Bridge Road Surgery
266 Lea Bridge Road, Leyton, London E10 7LD
Tel: 020 8539 1221 Fax: 020 8539 2303
(Waltham Forest Primary Care Trust)

GP Maheskumar Ramanlal PATEL, Spencer PHILLIPS

Leyton Green Neighbourhood Health Service
180 Essex Road, Leyton, London E10 6BT
Tel: 020 7539 0756 Fax: 020 7556 6902
(Waltham Forest Primary Care Trust)

GP Maria Christina ZAMORA EGUILUZ, Mary Bernadette CROWE

Lyndhurst Drive Surgery
53 Lyndhurst Drive, Leyton, London E10 6JB
Tel: 020 8539 1663 Fax: 020 8556 1977
(Waltham Forest Primary Care Trust)

GP Kishori ZADOO, Bansi Lal GURTU

The Manor Practice
Lea Bridge Road Surgery, 454 Lea Bridge Road, Leyton, London E10 7DY
Tel: 020 8539 5000 Fax: 020 8556 9082
(Waltham Forest Primary Care Trust)
Patient List Size: 5200

GP Martin James HUDDART, Prasanta Kumar DAS, Ratna DAS

SMA Medical Centre
693-695 High Road, Leyton, London E10 6AA
Tel: 020 8539 2078 Fax: 020 8558 3833
(Waltham Forest Primary Care Trust)

Practice Manager Elean Ali

GP Syed Masroor ALI, N GIRIJA, T B SHEIKH

SMA Medical Centre
693-695 High Road, Leyton, London E10 6RA
Tel: 020 8539 2078 Fax: 020 8558 3833
(Waltham Forest Primary Care Trust)

GP Syed Masroor ALI, T B N SHEIKH

London, E11

Allum Medical Centre
Fairlop Road, Leytonstone, London E11 1BN
Tel: 020 8539 2513 Fax: 020 8558 0525
(Waltham Forest Primary Care Trust)

GP Kanyalal ASWANI, Mary Elizabeth HOTTON, Dapinder Singh RATTAN, Surinder Singh SEEHRA

Cann Hall Road Surgery
135 Cann Hall Road, Leytonstone, London E11 3NJ
Tel: 020 8534 1882 Fax: 020 8555 7109
(Waltham Forest Primary Care Trust)

Practice Manager Vandana Roy

GP Baidya Nath MUKHERJEE, Sanjay KUMAR

Chadwick Road Surgery
33 Chadwick Road, Leytonstone, London E11 1NE
Tel: 020 8989 2936 Fax: 020 8530 8540
(Waltham Forest Primary Care Trust)

Practice Manager Bernadette Siggins

GP Paul Charles SIGGINS

Goodall Medical Centre
2-4 Goodall Road, Leytonstone, London E11 4EP
Tel: 020 8539 5050 Fax: 020 8539 9527
(Waltham Forest Primary Care Trust)

GP Gurmeet Kaur BAURA, Dr UMOH

Green Man Medical Centre
1 Hanbury Drive, Leytonstone, London E11 1HR
Tel: 020 8989 2606 Fax: 020 8989 2610
(Waltham Forest Primary Care Trust)
Patient List Size: 3000

GP Mohamed Abdul Mohssin MOHAMED

Hainault Road Surgery
226 Hainault Road, Leytonstone, London E11 1EP
Tel: 020 8539 0261 Fax: 020 8556 1417
(Waltham Forest Primary Care Trust)
Patient List Size: 4600

Practice Manager Sally Stevens

GP Arani Sreeramulu CHALAPATHY, Anna SIPAN

Harrow Road Surgery
110 Harrow Road, Leytonstone, London E11 3QE
Tel: 020 8519 5627 Fax: 020 8519 9879
(Waltham Forest Primary Care Trust)

Practice Manager J Samuel

GP John SAMUEL, Mary Margaret SAMUEL

High Road Surgery
287 High Road, Leytonstone, London E11 4HH
Tel: 020 8532 8460 Fax: 020 8532 8458
(Waltham Forest Primary Care Trust)
Patient List Size: 2400

GP Sanjay KUMAR

High Street Surgery
26 High Street, Wanstead, London E11 2AQ
Tel: 020 8989 0407 Fax: 020 8518 8435
(Redbridge Primary Care Trust)

Practice Manager Shelly Gillan

GP Anthony HUTCHINGS, Sarah AMINI, Elizabeth Joan ASHLEY

Kumar
135 Cann Hall Road, Leytonstone, London E11 3NJ
(Waltham Forest Primary Care Trust)

GP S KUMAR

Kumar
135 Cann Hall Road, Leytonstone, London E11 3NJ
(Waltham Forest Primary Care Trust)
GP S KUMAR

Langthorne Health Centre
13 Langthorne Road, Leytonstone, London E11 4HX
Tel: 020 8558 5858 Fax: 020 8539 3865
(Waltham Forest Primary Care Trust)
GP Shobha AGARWAL

Langthorne Health Centre
13 Langthorne Road, Leytonstone, London E11 4HX
Tel: 020 8556 9550 Fax: 020 8532 8274
(Waltham Forest Primary Care Trust)
GP RAM PRAKASH

Langthorne Health Centre
13 Langthorne Road, Leytonstone, London E11 4HX
Tel: 020 8558 5858 Fax: 020 8539 2768
(Waltham Forest Primary Care Trust)
Practice Manager Anne Bloor
GP Tahir Maqsood KIYANI

Langthorne Health Centre
13 Langthorne Road, Leytonstone, London E11 4HX
Tel: 020 8539 1513 Fax: 020 8539 7769
(Waltham Forest Primary Care Trust)
GP Poonam Chand SHARMA

Lime Tree Surgery
38 Cann Hall Road, Leytonstone, London E11 3HZ
Tel: 020 8519 9914
(Waltham Forest Primary Care Trust)
Practice Manager Joy Glasgow
GP Alison Barbara Jane STABLES, L ALI

Pretoria Road Surgery
4 Goodall Road, Leytonstone, London E11 4EP
Tel: 020 8539 3232
(Waltham Forest Primary Care Trust)
GP Gurmeet Kaur BAURA, R BHATNAGER

Pretoria Road Surgery
1 Pretoria Road, Leytonstone, London E11 4BB
Tel: 020 8539 3232 Fax: 020 8558 9096
(Waltham Forest Primary Care Trust)
Patient List Size: 2400
Practice Manager R T Amin
GP Ameena SUDDERUDDIN

The Shieling
24 Spratt Hall Road, Wanstead, London E11 2RQ
Tel: 020 8989 0585 Fax: 020 8518 8977
Email: drmuirtaylor@aol.com
Website: www.theshielingsurgery.spyw.com
(Redbridge Primary Care Trust)
Patient List Size: 2000
Practice Manager P Hutchinson
GP Jane Helen MUIR-TAYLOR

The Surgery
36 Harvey Road, Leytonstone, London E11 3DB
Tel: 020 8539 7414 Fax: 020 8518 7977
(Waltham Forest Primary Care Trust)
GP Syed Anwar HUSSAIN

Wanstead Place Surgery
45 Wanstead Place, Wanstead High Street, Wanstead, London E11 2SW
Tel: 020 8989 2019 Fax: 020 8532 1124
(Redbridge Primary Care Trust)
Patient List Size: 7200
Practice Manager Sheree Horsey
GP Susan Elizabeth ROBINSON, Pradeep SHARMA, Louise Solange TRANMER

London, E12

Aldersbrook Road Medical Centre
65 Aldersbrook Road, Manor Park, London E12 5DL
Tel: 020 8518 8080 Fax: 020 8518 8227
(Redbridge Primary Care Trust)
Patient List Size: 3500
GP Indu SINHA

Byron Avenue Surgery
151 Byron Avenue, Manor Park, London E12 6NQ
Tel: 020 8471 5037
(Newham Primary Care Trust)
GP Perrumal ALAGRAJAH

Church Road Health Centre
30 Church Road, Manor Park, London E12 6AQ
Tel: 020 8478 8797 Fax: 020 8478 7660
(Newham Primary Care Trust)
GP Girija KUGAPALA

Dr Singh Surgery
1 Sibley Grove, Manor Park, London E12 6SD
Tel: 020 8472 3828 Fax: 020 8472 4025
(Newham Primary Care Trust)
GP Mohinder SINGH

E12 Health Centre
97 Browning Road, Manor Park, London E12 6RB
Tel: 020 8472 0744 Fax: 020 8470 4086
(Newham Primary Care Trust)
GP Lise HERTEL, Bhupinder KOHLI

The Medical Centre
Church Road, Manor Park, London E12 5PJ
Tel: 020 8478-0686 Fax: 020 8478-1666
(Newham Primary Care Trust)

Romford Road Surgery
780 Romford Road, Manor Park, London E12 5JG
Tel: 020 8478 4080
(Newham Primary Care Trust)
GP N B BHADRA

Shelley Avenue Surgery
59 Shelley Avenue, Manor Park, London E12 6PX
Tel: 020 8472 9332
(Newham Primary Care Trust)
Patient List Size: 2400
GP Aturu B REDDY

The Surgery
997 Romford Road, Manor Park, London E12 5JR
Tel: 020 8478 2711 Fax: 020 8553 4696
Website: www.drmkshetty.co.uk
(Newham Primary Care Trust)
Patient List Size: 2500
Practice Manager Nailh Shah
GP Manjaya Kaliyur SHETTY

The Surgery
57 Gladstone Avenue, Manor Park, London E12 6NR
Tel: 020 8471 4764 Fax: 020 8472 3378
(Newham Primary Care Trust)
Practice Manager Susan Byrne
GP Malvinder Singh SOHI, Chandar Prabha RAINA, H SINGH

The Surgery
778 Romford Road, Manor Park, London E12 5JG
Tel: 020 8478 0533 Fax: 020 8514 5403
(Newham Primary Care Trust)
Patient List Size: 3700

Practice Manager Rina Bhadra

GP Nirode Baran BHADRA

The Surgery
315 High Street North, London E12 6SL
Tel: 020 8470 5520 Fax: 020 8470 1506
(Newham Primary Care Trust)

GP M PILLAI

The Surgery
30 Church Road, Manor Park, London E12 6AQ
Tel: 020 8478 0686 Fax: 020 8478 1666
(Newham Primary Care Trust)

GP Jadeng Mani ZAMANTHANGI

The Surgery
688 Romford Road, Manor Park, London E12 5AJ
Tel: 020 8478 0757 Fax: 020 8478 2416
(Newham Primary Care Trust)

GP Surendra Kumar DHARIWAL

Wordsworth Health Centre
19 Wordsworth Avenue, Manor Park, London E12 6SU
Tel: 020 8548 5960 Fax: 020 8548 5983
(Newham Primary Care Trust)
Patient List Size: 7000

Practice Manager Jenny Mazarelo

GP Peter GRAHAM, Petre Timothy Cedric JONES, Abdul Husain Kadhim NASRALLA, Andrew Robert POPLE

London, E13

Esk Road Medical Centre
12 Esk Road, London E13 8LJ
Tel: 020 7474 9002 Fax: 020 7473 1917
(Newham Primary Care Trust)
Patient List Size: 3800

Practice Manager P Venugopal

GP Ramaswamysetty S VENUGOPAL

Essex Lodge
94 Greengate Street, Plaistow, London E13 0AS
Tel: 020 8472 4888 Fax: 020 8472 5777
(Newham Primary Care Trust)

Practice Manager Sue Perry

GP Raymond George HIGGINS, Abu KHAN, Hardip Singh NANDRA, Anne PAULEAU

Glen Road Medical Centre
1-9 Glen Road, London E13 8RU
Tel: 020 7476 3434 Fax: 020 7473 6092
(Newham Primary Care Trust)

Practice Manager Judith Harkin

GP Madipalli Venkateswara RAO, Sudha MADIPALLI

Newham Medical Centre
576 Green Street, London E13 9DA
Tel: 020 8470 7859 Fax: 020 8552 2161
(Newham Primary Care Trust)
Patient List Size: 3900

GP Altaf Uddin AHMED

The Surgery
85 Stopford Road, Plaistow, London E13 0NA
Tel: 020 8472 3901 Fax: 020 8503 4818
(Newham Primary Care Trust)

GP Benu Bhushon CHAUDHURI, Reddy ATURU

The Surgery
97 Stopford Road, Plaistow, London E13 0NA
Tel: 020 8472 3846 Fax: 020 8552 1442
(Newham Primary Care Trust)

Practice Manager V Gilbert

GP Malkit Singh BHAGRATH, R SAMUEL, R B P SAXENA

The Surgery
61 Plashet Road, London E13 0QA
Tel: 020 8470 8186 Fax: 020 8503 4989
(Newham Primary Care Trust)
Patient List Size: 4800

Practice Manager Jennifer Alvares

GP Ila BASU, Suniti Kumar BASU

The Surgery
113 Balaam Street, London E13 8AF
Tel: 020 8472 1238 Fax: 020 8470 1739
(Newham Primary Care Trust)
Patient List Size: 5580

Practice Manager Hilda Coe

GP Ghassan Basim AL-MUDALLAL, Barry SULLMAN

The Surgery
309 Barking Road, London E13 8EE
Tel: 020 7511 6009 Fax: 020 7474 9151
(Newham Primary Care Trust)

GP P P SOOD

The Surgery
152 Plashet Road, Upton Park, London E13 0QT
Tel: 020 8472 0473 Fax: 020 8471 2243
(Newham Primary Care Trust)
Patient List Size: 4891

GP Wali Mohummed UMRANI, M A QURESHI

The Surgery
17 Stopford Road, London E13 0LY
Tel: 020 8552 6858 Fax: 020 8472 8532
(Newham Primary Care Trust)
Patient List Size: 2400

Practice Manager Z Fitzgerald

GP S QURESHI

The Surgery
104 Plashet Road, London E13 0RQ
Tel: 020 8471 7239 Fax: 020 8471 8699
(Newham Primary Care Trust)

GP M H RAHMAN

The Surgery
509 Barking Road, London E13 8QB
Tel: 020 8470 7448 Fax: 020 8470 7448
(Newham Primary Care Trust)

GP Indu Busan SARKAR

The Surgery
487 Barking Road, Plaistow, London E13 8PS
Tel: 020 8471 7160 Fax: 020 8652 0794
(Newham Primary Care Trust)
Patient List Size: 5000

Practice Manager Ruby Sarwar

GP S KALHORO, A GOPINATHAN

The Surgery
179 Cumberland Road, London E13 8LS
Tel: 020 7476 1029 Fax: 020 7476 6616
(Newham Primary Care Trust)

GP Ramnikgiri Bachugiri GONSAI

Upper Road Medical Centre
50 Upper Road, London E13 0DH
Tel: 020 8552 2129 Fax: 020 8471 4180
(Newham Primary Care Trust)
Patient List Size: 3700

Practice Manager Rosemary Rezia-Khanom

GP Abul Kashem Mohd ZAKARIA

London, E14

Aberfeldy Practice
50 Aberfeldy Street, London E14 0NU
Tel: 020 7515 5622 Fax: 020 7538 3462
(Tower Hamlets Primary Care Trust)
Patient List Size: 3074

Practice Manager Moriom Ullah

GP Phillip John BENNETT-RICHARDS, Robin CARTWRIGHT, Sarah PITKANEN

Chrisp Street Health Centre
100 Chrisp Street, London E14 6PG
Tel: 020 7515 4860 Fax: 020 7515 3055
Website: www.crispstreetpractice.org
(Tower Hamlets Primary Care Trust)
Patient List Size: 10500

Practice Manager Simon Robinson

GP Kambiz Roointan Faridoon BOOMLA, Benjamin Tudor HART, Jacqueline Brenda KETLEY, Ferhat KHWAJA, Luise PARSONS, John Peter ROBSON, Alison Martha SMAILES, William Andrew TWIST

Docklands Medical Centre
100 Spindrift Avenue, Isle of Dogs, London E14 9WU
Tel: 020 7537 1444
(Tower Hamlets Primary Care Trust)

GP Vitthal Das MAHAJAN, R S AMIRTHANATHAR

Gill Street Health Centre
11 Gill Street, London E14 8HQ
Tel: 020 7515 2211
(Tower Hamlets Primary Care Trust)
Patient List Size: 8200

Practice Manager Melanie Grant

GP Laura Jean EPSTEIN, David Anthony KIRBY, Anna Eleri LIVINGSTONE, Vanda Jane PLAYFORD, Alison Ruth VICKERS

Island Health
145 East Ferry Road, London E14 3BQ
Tel: 020 7363 1111 Fax: 020 7363 1112
Website: www.islandh.demon.co.uk
(Tower Hamlets Primary Care Trust)

Practice Manager Stacey Franks

GP Josephine Elizabeth ALLRED, Shera L CHOK, Neil Alexander DOUGLAS, Mike FITCHETT, Antonia LILE, Sudip NANDY, Joanna Rachel RICHARDSON

The Island Medical Centre
Roserton Street, London E14 3PG
(Tower Hamlets Primary Care Trust)

Practice Manager Sheila Dod

GP S YOGADEVA, Dr MAHMOOD

Newby Place Centre
21 Newby Place, London E14 0EY
(Tower Hamlets Primary Care Trust)

Practice Manager Patricia Duggan

GP Deepak Dinkar KHOPKAR

Newby Place Centre
21 Newby Place, London E14 0EY
Tel: 020 7515 5525 Fax: 020 7538 1719
Email: mostafa.farook@nhs.net
(Tower Hamlets Primary Care Trust)
Patient List Size: 2250

Practice Manager Mostafa Farook

GP Sourendra Nath DUTTA

Sai Medical Centre
12 Robin Hood Lane, Poplar, London E14 0HN
Tel: 020 7987 3536 Fax: 020 7536-9549
(Tower Hamlets Primary Care Trust)

Practice Manager Margaret King

GP Chandrakant Vrajlal KOTHARI

The Surgery
74-78 Gough Walk, Canton Street, London E14 6HR
Tel: 020 7515 4701 Fax: 020 7515 2414
(Tower Hamlets Primary Care Trust)
Patient List Size: 3000

Practice Manager Breda Bower

GP N SELVAN

London, E15

Abbey Road Health Centre
28A Abbey Road, Stratford, London E15 3LT
Tel: 020 8534 2515 Fax: 020 8555 0197
(Newham Primary Care Trust)

GP H YATES, Miriam Sarah Anne BARKER, R TAYLOR, Kenny UKOKA

High Road Surgery
136 High Road, Leytonstone, London E15 1UA
Tel: 020 8534 1671 Fax: 020 8519 7577
(Waltham Forest Primary Care Trust)

Practice Manager Anita Verma

GP Upender Kumar VERMA

Knight
125 The Grove, Stratford, London E15 1EN
Tel: 020 8519 6009 Fax: 020 8519 9669
(Newham Primary Care Trust)
Patient List Size: 2450

Practice Manager Razia Antria

GP P C L KNIGHT

Stephens Road Surgery
60/62 Stephens Road, West Ham, London E15 3JL
Tel: 020 8534 2040
(Newham Primary Care Trust)

GP Malkit Singh BHARGARTH, Roseline SAMUEL, RBR SAXENA

Stratford Health Centre
121-123 The Grove, Stratford, London E15 1EN
Tel: 020 8534 5300 Fax: 020 8534 3273
(Newham Primary Care Trust)

GP Mathew Khai Laing CHANG

Stratford Village Practice
50C Romford Road, London E15 4BZ
Tel: 020 8534 4133 Fax: 020 8534 3860
(Newham Primary Care Trust)
Patient List Size: 5444

Practice Manager A Bearwisn

GP Ashwin Mukund SHAH, S A SHAH

The Surgery
401 Corporation Street, London E15 3DJ
Tel: 020 8555 0428 Fax: 020 8555 0641
(Newham Primary Care Trust)

GP Prasanta Ranjan BHOWMIK

The Surgery
60 Leytonstone Road, London E15 1SQ
Tel: 020 8534 1533 Fax: 020 8534 4283
(Newham Primary Care Trust)
Patient List Size: 2500

Practice Manager Nasrin Brohi

GP Abdul Qayoom BROHI

The Surgery
157 Leytonstone Road, Stratford, London E15 1LH
Tel: 020 8534 1026 Fax: 020 8534 4415
(Newham Primary Care Trust)

GP Abdul Qayoom QADRI

The Surgery
69 Water Lane, London E15 4NL
Tel: 020 8519 6780 Fax: 020 8592 0591
(Newham Primary Care Trust)
Patient List Size: 2356

GP Arindam Rafiqur RAHMAN

London, E16

Comyns Close Clinic
1 Comyns Close, Hermit Road, Canning Town, London E16 4JJ
Tel: 020 7476 4862 Fax: 020 7473 6400
(Newham Primary Care Trust)
Patient List Size: 9373

Practice Manager Irene Glover

GP Malcolm John COMYNS, H A EDUNG, Carolyn Rosalie FANG, Sarojini Sharad PALAV, B P PATEL

Custom House Surgery
16 Freemasons Road, London E16 3NA
Tel: 020 7476 2255 Fax: 020 7511 8980
(Newham Primary Care Trust)

Practice Manager Sylvia Nicholas

GP Zuhair Khalil ZARIFA, F F H AL SHAVIK, Rotimi Olusegun BAKARE, Dirk Frederic Franciscus DE COCQ, Lise HERTEL, Eleanor SHORE

Kennard Street Health Centre
1 Kennard Street, North Woolwich, London E16 2HR
Tel: 020 7473 1971 Fax: 020 7473 2042
(Newham Primary Care Trust)
Patient List Size: 2700

Practice Manager Christine Quincey

GP Minakshi SAHA

Kennard Street Health Centre
1 Kennard Street, North Woolwich, London E16 2HR
Tel: 020 7473 1948 Fax: 020 7511 2040
(Newham Primary Care Trust)

GP Ravi Tej SEHRA

St Luke's Health Centre
2 St Luke's Square, Tabling Road, London E16 1HT
Tel: 020 7366 6440 Fax: 020 7366 6441
(Newham Primary Care Trust)
Patient List Size: 2500

Practice Manager Kamaideep Sahota

GP B BANERJEE

St Luke's Health Centre
2 St Luke's Square, Tarling Road, London E16 1HT
Tel: 020 7366 6430 Fax: 020 7366 6431
(Newham Primary Care Trust)

GP M F HAQUE

The Surgery
343 Prince Regent Lane, London E16 3JL
Tel: 020 7511 2980 Fax: 020 7474 7816
Email: t2lwin@england.com
(Newham Primary Care Trust)

Practice Manager D Narlar

GP Tun LWIN

London, E17

Addison Road Medical Practice
12-14 Addison Road, Walthamstow, London E17 9LT
Tel: 020 8520 4708 Fax: 020 8520 6266
(Waltham Forest Primary Care Trust)
Patient List Size: 5800

Practice Manager M Cooney

GP Seamus COONEY, S MUHUNDHA-KUMAR, R RAYANI

Boundary Road Surgery
273 Boundary Road, Walthamstow, London E17 8NE
Tel: 020 8521 7086 Fax: 020 8521 7086
(Waltham Forest Primary Care Trust)
Patient List Size: 2400

Practice Manager Saima Arzf

GP Nuzhat MUNAWER

Carisbrooke Road Surgery
41 Carisbrooke Road, Walthamstow, London E17 7EE
Tel: 020 8520 8284 Fax: 020 8520 7077
(Waltham Forest Primary Care Trust)
Patient List Size: 2700

Practice Manager U N Qazi

GP Arifa Moin SIDDIQUI

Central Surgery
8 Corbett Road, Walthamstow, London E17 3JZ
Tel: 020 8503 6700
(Waltham Forest Primary Care Trust)

Practice Manager H Monteiro

GP Robert Flage MONTEIRO

Claremont Medical Centre
29-31 Claremont Road, Walthamstow, London E17 5RJ
Tel: 020 8527 1888 Fax: 020 8527 8111
(Waltham Forest Primary Care Trust)
Patient List Size: 3356

GP Hisham Ibrahim SWEDAN

Dr Anachebi Surgery
Forest Road Medical Centre, 354-368 Forest Road, Walthamstow, London E17 5JL
(Waltham Forest Primary Care Trust)

GP C ANACHEBI

Dr F N O Oraelosi and Partners
Warwick Terrace, Lea Bridge Road, London E17 9DP
Tel: 020 8539 2077 Fax: 020 8556 1723
(Waltham Forest Primary Care Trust)
Patient List Size: 7100

Practice Manager Pauline Smith

GP A J WITTINE, Florence Nwakaego Obiamaka ORAELOSI, George Morounfolu SOWEMIMO

Dr Ivbijaro Surgery
Forest Road Medical Centre, 354-368 Forest Road, Walthamstow, London E17 5JL
Tel: 020 8520 6060 Fax: 020 8520 6505
Email: chinaeme.anachebe@gp-f86602.nhs.uk
(Waltham Forest Primary Care Trust)
Patient List Size: 3025

GP C I A ANACHEBE, Dr IVBIJARO

Dr Shantir Surgery
Forest Road Medical Centre, 354-368 Forest Road, Walthamstow, London E17 5JL
Tel: 020 8520 7115 Fax: 020 8923 1199
(Waltham Forest Primary Care Trust)
Patient List Size: 3012

Practice Manager A Shantir

GP Daoud Yosuf Abdul-Rahman SHANTIR

The Firs
Stephenson Road, London E17 7JT
Tel: 020 8520 9286 Fax: 020 8521 1751
(Waltham Forest Primary Care Trust)
Patient List Size: 8700

Practice Manager Rehana Vadivelu

GP Festus AKINGBALA, Terry Martin JOHN, Anwar YAQUB

The Firs
Stephenson Road, Walthamstow, London E17 7JT
Tel: 020 8520 9286 Fax: 020 8521 1751
(Waltham Forest Primary Care Trust)

Practice Manager Rehana Vadivelu

GP Festus AKINGBALA, Nilofer ARASTU, Terry JOHN, Anwar YAQUB

Forest Road Medical Centre
354-358 Forest Road, Walthamstow, London E17 5JL
Tel: 020 8520 6060 Fax: 020 8521 6505
(Waltham Forest Primary Care Trust)
Patient List Size: 4000

Practice Manager Ann Woodrow

GP G IVBIJARO

Forest Surgery
2 MacDonald Road, Walthamstow, London E17 4BA
Tel: 020 8527 2569/5434 Fax: 020 8523 4077
(Waltham Forest Primary Care Trust)

Practice Manager Annetta Dawson

GP Nasma Abdul Jabber ABDUL-RAZAK, Sohaib Mahmud Ali AHMAD, Tharmalingen SIVARAJAH

Fulbourne Road Surgery
117 Fulbourne Road, Walthamstow, London E17 4HA
Tel: 020 8527 6373 Fax: 020 8503 3877
(Waltham Forest Primary Care Trust)

GP Jagadis Chandra RAY

Grove Surgery
103-105 Grove Road, Walthamstow, London E17 9BU
Tel: 020 8521 2221 Fax: 020 8503 7773
(Waltham Forest Primary Care Trust)
Patient List Size: 7300

Practice Manager Irene Placks

GP Mayank Ramanlal SHAH, Ratap DAS, Rita PUSHPARAJAH, S SHARMA

Higham Hill Medical Centre
258-260 Higham Hill Road, Walthamstow, London E17 5RQ
Tel: 020 8527 2677 Fax: 020 8527 3636
(Waltham Forest Primary Care Trust)
Patient List Size: 3500

GP Ravindra Kumar GUPTA, Hanife DERVISH, Usha GUPTA

Hurst Road Health Centre
Hurst Road, Walthamstow, London E17 3BL
Tel: 020 8503 6710 Fax: 020 8521 8293
(Waltham Forest Primary Care Trust)

GP Pallipuram Bharathan SUBRAMANIAN

Hurst Road Health Centre
Hurst Road, Walthamstow, London E17 3BL
Tel: 020 8520 5571 Fax: 020 8509 1659
(Waltham Forest Primary Care Trust)

GP Raghav Prasad DHITAL

Palmerston Road Surgery
148 Palmerston Road, Walthamstow, London E17 6PY
Tel: 020 8520 3059
(Waltham Forest Primary Care Trust)

GP Anil Kumar MALHOTRA

Penrhyn Surgery
2A Penrhyn Avenue, Walthamstow, London E17 5DB
Tel: 020 8527 2563 Fax: 020 8527 6583
(Waltham Forest Primary Care Trust)
Patient List Size: 6500

Practice Manager J Streight

GP Steven LINDALL, Patrick Anthony BELTON, Amird NASSEM

Peterhouse Surgery
122 Forest Rise, Walthamstow, London E17 3PW
Tel: 020 8521 4743 Fax: 020 8521-1876
(Waltham Forest Primary Care Trust)

GP Dr DAS, Dr PUSHPARAJ, Mayank Ramanlal SHAH, Dr SHARMA

Queens Road Surgery
48 Queens Road, Walthamstow, London E17 8PX
Tel: 020 8520 2625 Fax: 020 8925 4195
(Waltham Forest Primary Care Trust)

GP Abdul Qayyum SHEIKH, Abu Taleb Sabbir AHMED, Naheed KHAN-LODHI

Shernhall Street Surgery
103 Shernhall Street, Walthamstow, London E17 9HS
Tel: 020 8520 5138
(Waltham Forest Primary Care Trust)

GP Jennifer BAILEY

St James Health Centre
47 St. James Street, Walthamstow, London E17 7NH
Tel: 020 8521 6138 Fax: 020 8521 4931
(Waltham Forest Primary Care Trust)

Practice Manager Sue Crabbe

GP Prakash Mal KAWAR, Evan JAMES

St James Health Centre
47 St. James Street, Walthamstow, London E17 7NH
Tel: 020 85209 9308
(Waltham Forest Primary Care Trust)

GP Ameya DEVA, Samarendra Satyendra Chandra DEVA

Stainforth Road Surgery
33 Stainforth Road, Walthamstow, London E17 9RB
Tel: 020 8521 8050 Fax: 020 8520 2464
(Waltham Forest Primary Care Trust)
Patient List Size: 1500

Practice Manager M Kanth

GP Zafar Iqbal MALIK

The Surgery
117 Fulbourne Road, Walthamstow, London E17 4HA
(Waltham Forest Primary Care Trust)

GP Jagandis Chandra RAY, G SALUJA

The Surgery
12B Sinnott Road, Walthamstow, London E17 5QB
Tel: 020 8531 8272 Fax: 020 8531 3999
(Waltham Forest Primary Care Trust)
Patient List Size: 2250

Practice Manager Christine Smith

GP Dr SHUI, Renu RAYANI

Wood Street Medical Centre
39 Wood Street, Walthamstow, London E17 3JX
Tel: 020 8503 6111 Fax: 020 8520 7385

(Waltham Forest Primary Care Trust)
Patient List Size: 2300

Practice Manager Leona Adams

GP Laxmi GUPTA

London, E18

Eastwood Medical Centre

Eastwood Road, South Woodford, London E18 1BN
Tel: 020 8530 4108 Fax: 020 8518 8728
(Redbridge Primary Care Trust)

Practice Manager Elaine Edwards

GP Kenneth Charles HINES

Glebelands Avenue Surgery

2 Glebelands Avenue, South Woodford, London E18 2AB
Tel: 020 8989 6272 Fax: 020 8518 8783
(Redbridge Primary Care Trust)

Practice Manager Norma Cracknell

GP Sean Frederick Joseph HOWLETT, Sri Rajini ARAVINDHAN, J COHEN

The Health Centre

114 High Road, South Woodford, London E18 2QS
Tel: 020 8491 3310 Fax: 020 8491 3307
(Redbridge Primary Care Trust)

Practice Manager Ruth Coombes

GP Margaret Lawson STAPLEY, T BOWLEY, Maureen CROWN, Beverley PENFIELD

South Woodford Health Centre

114 High Road, South Woodford, London E18 2QS
Tel: 020 8491 3303 Fax: 020 8559 2451
(Redbridge Primary Care Trust)

Practice Manager Susan Fitzpatrick

GP Elizabeth HACKETT, Yaseen SIDDIQUE

Southdene Surgery

The Shrubberies, George Lane, London E18 1BD
Tel: 020 8530 3731 Fax: 020 8518 8157
(Redbridge Primary Care Trust)

GP John Geoffrey EDWARDS, P ELLIOTT, Mary Lucia HANLEY

London, EC1

City House Medical Centre

Unit 1-3 Ground Floor, City House, 190-196 City Road, London EC1V 2QH
Tel: 020 7530 2750
(Islington Primary Care Trust)

Practice Manager Stephen Coleman

GP Katherine COLEMAN, Patrick GLACKIN, Josephine SAUVAGE

City University Health Centre

20 Sebastian Street, London EC1V 0JA
Tel: 020 7253 4454
(Islington Primary Care Trust)

GP Dr RAJAH

Clerkenwell Medical Practice

Finsbury Health Centre, Pine Street, London EC1R 0JH
(Islington Primary Care Trust)

GP Peter Scott BAINES, Sarah Gillian GREENHOUGH

Finsbury Health Centre

Pine Street, London EC1R 0JH
Tel: 020 7713 5256
(Islington Primary Care Trust)

GP Paul Maciej Peter JUREK

The Surgery

66 Long Lane, London EC1A 9RQ
(City and Hackney Teaching Primary Care Trust)

GP Gillian Mary NEAMAN, Rachel LEVENE, Caron Phaik Lin LOH, David VASSERMAN

London, EC3

The Surgery

H. M. Tower of London, 2 Tower Green, London EC3N 4AB

GP Michael Geoffrey O'DONOGHUE

London, N1

Bamsbury Medical Practice

153 Copenhagen Street, London N1 0SR
Tel: 020 7833 4981 Fax: 020 7713 8649
(Islington Primary Care Trust)
Patient List Size: 3500

GP Tahir HAFFIZ

Elizabeth Ave Group Practice

2 Elizabeth Avenue, London N1 3BS
Tel: 020 7226 6363
(Islington Primary Care Trust)
Patient List Size: 7500

Practice Manager Pamela Welson

GP Anthony Gaskell FURNESS, Justin Patrick LIVINGSTON, Anna SKALICKA, Heather Cullenbel SUCKLING, Anne Lesley WEISS

Englefield Road Surgery

6-8 Englefield Road, London N1 4LN
Tel: 020 7254 1324 Fax: 020 7923 9248
(City and Hackney Teaching Primary Care Trust)

Englefield Road Surgery

6-8 Englefield Road, London N1 4LN
Tel: 020 7241 3380 Fax: 020 7923 9242
(City and Hackney Teaching Primary Care Trust)
Patient List Size: 4000

GP Singh MARLOWE

Hoxton Medical Practice

12 Rushton Street, London N1 5DR
Tel: 020 7739 8990 Fax: 020 7729 3197
Email: hhc@dircon.uk
(City and Hackney Teaching Primary Care Trust)
Patient List Size: 2700

Practice Manager Mike Search

GP Sadie TAYLOR

Killick Street Health Centre

75 Killick Street, London N1 9RH
Tel: 020 7833 9939 Fax: 020 7427 2740
Website: www.killickstreethelathcentre.co.uk
(Islington Primary Care Trust)
Patient List Size: 6000

Practice Manager Bernadette Edwards

GP Karen Jane SENNETT, James HICKLING, Polly HOOTTON, Rachel Julia HOPKINS

The Lawson Practice

85 Nuttall Street, London N1 5HZ
Tel: 020 7739 9701
(City and Hackney Teaching Primary Care Trust)

GP Deborah Rosalind COLVIN, Jonathan Henry Shaw FULLER, Jonathan Charles Patrick GORE, Gary Teejpaul Singh MARLOWE

Prebend Street Surgery

15 Prebend Street, London N1 8PG
Tel: 020 7226 9090 Fax: 020 7354 3330
(Islington Primary Care Trust)

Patient List Size: 3000

Practice Manager M Brakes

GP Marion Evelyn FLEETWOOD, Dr SKELLY

Ritchie Street Group Practice
34 Ritchie Street, London N1 0DG
Tel: 020 7837 1663
Email: ritchiestreet@gp-f83021.nhs.uk
(Islington Primary Care Trust)
Patient List Size: 9500

Practice Manager Jacky Willett

GP L SPEIGHT, R G GOLDBERG, S R HAZELWOOD, S V LIMAYE, S M MILLS

River Place Group Practice
River Place, Essex Road, London N1 2DE
Tel: 020 7530 2100 Fax: 020 7530 2102
(Islington Primary Care Trust)
Patient List Size: 8300

Practice Manager Katy Watts

GP Robert James BUNT, David EGERTON, Lis HANSON, Jane TENNICK, Sophie Leonora WOLLASTON

Shoreditch Park Surgery
10 Rushton Street, London N1 5DR
Tel: 020 7739 8525 Fax: 020 7739 5352
(City and Hackney Teaching Primary Care Trust)
Patient List Size: 3873

Practice Manager Lorraine Warner

GP J BODDINGTON, C IDRIS-EVANS, Paul KELLAND, Lucy O'ROURKE

Shoreditch Park Surgery
10 Rushton Street, London N1 5DR
(City and Hackney Teaching Primary Care Trust)

GP Dr O'ROURKE

St Pauls Road Medical Centre
248 St Pauls Road, London N1 2LJ
(Islington Primary Care Trust)

GP Judith Ann DIXON, D R HAI, Jeremy Simon MARSHALL, S M WISEMAN, K YOUNG

St Peters Street Medical Practice
16 St Peters Street, London N1 8JG
Tel: 020 7226 7131 Fax: 020 7354 9120
(Islington Primary Care Trust)

Practice Manager J Jones

GP Michael John Kenneth TIBBLE, Caroline Ann CATTELL, Olga GORODETSKAIA, Sarah Josephine HAUGHEY, Peter Russell McCARTNEY, Karen Elizabeth SUMMERFIELD

The Surgery
2 Mitchison Road, London N1 3NG
Tel: 020 7226 6016
(Islington Primary Care Trust)
Patient List Size: 4950

GP Berenice Ruth BEAUMONT, Imogen Ann Meriel BLOOR, Brian Simon HURWITZ, Terence John WELSH

The Surgery
8 Rushton Street, London N1 5DR
(City and Hackney Teaching Primary Care Trust)

GP C M VARMA

The Surgery
172 Pitfield Street, London N1 6JP
(City and Hackney Teaching Primary Care Trust)

Practice Manager Sonali Roy

GP Radha Binode ROY, Sucheta ROY

The Surgery
6-8 New North Road, London N1 6JE

GP Ravi VARMA

The Surgery
8 Rushton Street, London N1 5DR
Tel: 020 7739 5164 Fax: 020 7739 5166
(City and Hackney Teaching Primary Care Trust)
Patient List Size: 2000

GP Zouhair KHAZNE CHARIMO

The Surgery
30 Huntington Street, London N1 1BS
Tel: 020 7607 3681 Fax: 020 7609 7968
(Islington Primary Care Trust)
Patient List Size: 2800

Practice Manager Alison Parr

GP H FLINDERS

The Surgery
337 Caledonian Road, London N1 1DW
(Islington Primary Care Trust)

GP A BHARGAVA

Surgery 1
Rushton Medical Centre, 6 Rushton Street, London N1 5DR
(City and Hackney Teaching Primary Care Trust)

Whiston Practice
St Leonards, Nuttall Street, London N1 5LZ
(City and Hackney Teaching Primary Care Trust)

GP R KUMAR, K P S SABHARWAL, C J SHIVNANI, R P TAHALANI

London, N2

Baronsmere Road Surgery
39 Baronsmere Road, East Finchley, London N2 9QD
Tel: 020 8883 1458 Fax: 020 8883 8854
(Barnet Primary Care Trust)

Practice Manager Pam Batchelor

GP Trixie KELLY, Diane Michelle TWENA

Cherry Tree Surgery
26 Southern Road, London N2 9JG
Tel: 020 8444 7478 Fax: 020 8444 7628
(Barnet Primary Care Trust)
Patient List Size: 2200

Practice Manager Aui Joshi

GP Sergio DE CESARE, Joanna RUSTIN

Heathfield Medical Centre
Lyttelton Road, Hampstead Garden Suburb, London N2 0EE
Tel: 020 8458 9262 Fax: 020 8458 0300
Email: heathfieldemedicalcentre@yahoo.com
(Barnet Primary Care Trust)
Patient List Size: 8000

Practice Manager B Samanta

GP Simon GIBEON, Lisa Deborah ANDERSON, Joshua Alec GOLDIN, Michael LAURINO, Rachel Anne MELLINS, Judith Ann TOBIN

London, N3

Ballards Lane Surgery
209 Ballards Lane, London N3 1LY
Tel: 020 8346 0726
(Barnet Primary Care Trust)
Patient List Size: 3400

GP Dharmendra Kantilal VYAS, Su Su THWE

Church Crescent Surgery
50 Church Crescent, Finchley, London N3 1BJ
Tel: 020 8346 1323 Fax: 020 8343 4026

(Barnet Primary Care Trust)

Practice Manager H Wilson

GP Ann Eleri ROWLANDS, Kenneth Stephen DODANWATAWANA

Cornwall House Surgery
Cornwall Avenue, London N3 1LD
Tel: 020 8346 1976 Fax: 020 8343 3809
(Barnet Primary Care Trust)
Patient List Size: 6200

GP Celia Elizabeth BANGHAM, Amelia Helen CHAN, Avril Louise SEFTEL

Dr Prasad and Partners
2 Rosemary Avenue, Finchley, London N3 2QN
Tel: 020 8346 1997
(Barnet Primary Care Trust)
Patient List Size: 3000

Practice Manager M Prasad

GP Sudama PRASAD, Nitu JONES

Lichfield Grove Surgery
64 Lichfield Grove, Finchley, London N3 2JP
Tel: 020 8346 3123 Fax: 020 8343 4919
(Barnet Primary Care Trust)
Patient List Size: 3000

Practice Manager Maja Djordjic

GP Nicholas Peter DURDEN, Anne ARNOLD, Peter DIN

The Mountfield Surgery
55 Mountfield Road, Finchley, London N3 3NR
Tel: 020 8346 4271 Fax: 020 8371 0187
Email: patrick.keane@gp-e83638.nhs.uk
(Barnet Primary Care Trust)
Patient List Size: 4000

Practice Manager Lisa Clark

GP Patrick Martin KEANE, Carmel MOND, Ann Chany ROBINSON, Natalie WOODWARD

Squires Lane Medical Practice
2 Squires Lane, Finchley, London N3 2AU
Tel: 020 8346 1516 Fax: 020 8343 2537
(Barnet Primary Care Trust)
Patient List Size: 6050

Practice Manager Liz Matthews

GP Eileen Mary GIBBONS, David Edward HAGUE, Debratna SIRKER

Supreme House
300 Regents Park Road, Finchley, London N3 2JX
Tel: 020 8346 3291/0446
(Haringey Teaching Primary Care Trust)

GP Judith Ann CAVENDISH, Roma FERNANDEZ

Wentworth Medical Practice
38 Wentworth Avenue, Finchley, London N3 1YL
Tel: 020 8346 1242 Fax: 020 8343 3614
(Barnet Primary Care Trust)
Patient List Size: 6700

Practice Manager Marian Nash

GP A S PATEL, K COOPER, A DALEY, L A ISENBERG, H R NATARAJU, C WESTERMANN

London, N4

The 157 Medical Practice
157 Stroud Green, London N4 3PF

GP H RAMNANI

Bridge House Healthcare Centre
96 Umfreville Road, London N4 1TL
Tel: 020 8482 9670 Fax: 020 8372 2096
(Haringey Teaching Primary Care Trust)
Patient List Size: 5000

Practice Manager Christine Pittman

GP J SINGER, Joanna Marion HAAS

The Cedar Practice
John Scott Health Centre, Green Lanes, London N4 2NU
Tel: 020 8800 0111 Fax: 020 8809 6900
(City and Hackney Teaching Primary Care Trust)

GP R T CARVER, Dr JEGANATHAN, Dr SHIER, Dr STANLEY

Ferme Park Road Surgery
18 Ferme Park Road, Hornsey Vale, London N4 4ED
Tel: 020 7340 6050
(Haringey Teaching Primary Care Trust)

GP Abul Kalam RUHUL AMIN

Heron Practice
John Scott Health Centre, Green Lanes, London N4 2NU
Tel: 020 7690 1172 Fax: 020 8809 0999
Website: www.theheronpractice.co.uk
(City and Hackney Teaching Primary Care Trust)
Patient List Size: 8001

Practice Manager Diane Goodwins

GP Meena KRISHNAMURTHY, Samantha BIGGS, Sian Jessica Anne HARRIS, Laura Katherine LYTTELTON, Fiona Elizabeth SANDERS, Carmel SHER

The Heron Practice
Green Lanes, Clapton, London N4 2NU
Tel: 020 7690 1172 Fax: 020 8809 0999
(City and Hackney Teaching Primary Care Trust)

Practice Manager Diane Goodwins

GP Meena KRISNAMURTHY, Samantha BIGGS, Sian HARRIS, Laura Katherine LYTTELTON, Fiona SAUNDERS

John Scott Health Centre
Woodbury Down, Green Lanes, London N4 2NU
Tel: 020 8800 0111
(City and Hackney Teaching Primary Care Trust)

GP V N PATEL

New Stroud Surgery
16 Upper, London N4 3EL

GP William Ajibola Olusegun NUBI

The Surgery
48 Wilberforce Road, London N4 2SR
Tel: 020 7226 4865 Fax: 020 7226 7161
(City and Hackney Teaching Primary Care Trust)
Patient List Size: 2038

Practice Manager Beverley Allen

GP H BEGUM

Tollington Court Surgery
1 Tollington Court, Tollington Park, London N4 3QT
Tel: 020 7272 2121
(Islington Primary Care Trust)

GP P C PATEL

London, N5

Highbury Grange Health Centre
Highbury Grange, London N5 2QB
Tel: 020 7226 2462
(Islington Primary Care Trust)

GP Alan TROSSER

Highbury New Park Surgery
49 Highbury New Park, London N5 2ET
Tel: 020 7354 1972 Fax: 020 7704 1932
(Islington Primary Care Trust)
Patient List Size: 10650

Practice Manager David Gorman

GP Valerie June DOCK, Sharon Denise BENNETT, Nicholas BRAND, Jeanine Elizabeth SMIRL, Kathleen TUCK

Highbury Park
94 Highbury Park, London N5 2XE
Tel: 020 7226 5360 Fax: 020 7354 3090
Email: jitendra.patel2@nhs.net
(Islington Primary Care Trust)
Patient List Size: 2600

Practice Manager Fateha Khaturi

GP Jitendrakumar Dahyabhai PATEL

The Surgery
30B Drayton Park, London N5 1PB
Tel: 020 7609 2692
(Islington Primary Care Trust)

GP Franklyn JACOBS

London, N6

Highgate Group Practice
44 North Hill, London N6 4QA
Tel: 020 8340 6628 Fax: 020 8342 8428
(Haringey Teaching Primary Care Trust)
Patient List Size: 16500

Practice Manager Frances Kaufhan

GP Matthew Henry CHESSHYRE, S DICKIE, Nikita GROVER, Richard JAYLOR, Robert David MAYER, W McINTYRE, Jonathan Douglas RIDDELL, S M ROBERTSON

The Surgery
18 Ferne Park, London N6 4ED
(Haringey Teaching Primary Care Trust)

GP M A K M RUHUL AMIN

London, N7

Andover Medical Centre
270-282 Hornsey Road, London N7 7QZ
Tel: 020 7281 6956 Fax: 020 7561 1515
(Islington Primary Care Trust)
Patient List Size: 4400

Practice Manager Kelly Poole

GP Dilipkumar Jashbhai AMIN, U S MISHRA, Amish PATEL

Family Practice
117 Holloway Road, London N7 8LT
Tel: 020 7607 4322 Fax: 020 7619 0112
(Islington Primary Care Trust)
Patient List Size: 4007

Practice Manager Shamsa Karmali

GP H N BOWRY, U BOWRY, C M SCERIF

Goodinge Health Centre
Goodinge Close, North Road, London N7 9EW
Tel: 020 7530 4940
(Islington Primary Care Trust)
Patient List Size: 10100

Practice Manager Sarah Hayward

GP Gregory Noel BATTLE, Michael Trease CRIPWELL, Mary DAVIES, Dr HAINES, Susan Teresa HUNT, Michael David SILLS, Margaret Elizabeth TATHAM

Holloway Road Surgery
94 Holloway Road, London N7 8JG
Tel: 020 7607 2323 Fax: 020 7607 3391
(Islington Primary Care Trust)

GP Dr MORRIS-DAVIES, Dr WOOLF

Hornsey Road Surgery
80 Hornsey Road, London N7 7NN
Tel: 020 7609 3488
(Islington Primary Care Trust)

GP Bipin Ratilal DESAI

Isledon Road Medical Centre
115 Isledon Road, London N7 7JJ
Tel: 020 7700 4383
(Islington Primary Care Trust)

GP Dr SYED

Isledon Road Surgery
115 Isledon Road, London N7 7JJ
Tel: 020 7700 6464 Fax: 020 7700 6464
(Islington Primary Care Trust)

Practice Manager Sue Doris

GP R M M MA, P McDAID, Dr SYED

Medical Centre
140 Holloway Road, London N7 8DD
Tel: 020 7607 8259 Fax: 020 7609 8803
(Islington Primary Care Trust)
Patient List Size: 3850

Practice Manager L Edoman

GP Simon EDOMAN, R PATEL

Medical Practice
58 Roman Way, London N7 8XF
Tel: 020 7607 7502
(Islington Primary Care Trust)

GP Maria de Lourdes Pamela COUTINHO, Stanley Wangtat HO, Bina SHAH

Medicine House
143 Seven Sisters Road, London N7 7QE
Tel: 020 7272 2585 Fax: 020 7561 0506
(Islington Primary Care Trust)
Patient List Size: 6000

GP Dr NANDI, Dr SAHA

Northern Medical Centre
594 Holloway Road, London N7 6LB
Tel: 020 7445 8100
(Islington Primary Care Trust)

GP Lawrence Michael Joseph KINSELLA, Geraldine McCULLAGH, N H SHAH, R VUREVIC

Sobell Medical Centre
272 Holloway Road, London N7 6NE
Tel: 020 7609 3050
(Islington Primary Care Trust)
Patient List Size: 2000

Practice Manager Maria Valente

GP Virender Kumar GUPTA

The Surgery
Fairweather House, London N7 0NS
Tel: 020 7607 1339
(Islington Primary Care Trust)

GP Diane ROSENTHAL

London, N8

Allenson House Practice
Allenson House, Weston Park, London N8 9TB

GP E L YOUNG

Christchurch Hall Surgery
20 Edison Road, London N8 8AE
Tel: 020 8340 2877 Fax: 020 8340 0896
Website: www.christchurchhallsurgery.co.uk

(Haringey Teaching Primary Care Trust)
Patient List Size: 4400

GP Telesilla GUERET-WARDLE

The Clock Tower Practice
50-66 Park Road, Crouch End, London N8 8SU
Tel: 020 8348 7711
(Haringey Teaching Primary Care Trust)

GP Doris Mina BLASS, Dina DHORAJIWALA, Margaret Jean ELLERBY, David MASTERS, Mervyn John Paul RODRIGUES

Crouch End Health Centre
45 Middle Lane, Crouch End, London N8 8PH
Tel: 020 8340 3295 Fax: 020 8347 6997
Patient List Size: 6000

GP H F N HENDERSON, Amina KARIM, Richard David STOCK, Kazimierz Julian STRYCHARCZYK

Crouch Hall Surgery
48 Crouch Hall Road, Hornsey, London N8 8HJ
Tel: 020 8340 7736 Fax: 020 8455 3384
(Haringey Teaching Primary Care Trust)
Patient List Size: 6800

Practice Manager Margaret Maciejczek

GP Karen Judith BENSON, M S GOR

Hornsey Park Surgery
114 Turnpike Lane, London N8 0PH
Tel: 020 8888 2227 Fax: 020 8889 4715
Email: patricia.binns@gp-f85046.nhs.uk
(Haringey Teaching Primary Care Trust)
Patient List Size: 2600

Practice Manager Patricia Binns

GP Manikam DORMISINGHAM

The Park Lane Medical and Surgical Services
625 Green Lane, Hornsey, London N8 0RE
Tel: 020 8340 6898 Fax: 020 8340 8191
(Haringey Teaching Primary Care Trust)
Patient List Size: 2500

GP Aman Ullah Khan RAJA, Andreas SAMPSON

The Surgery
98 Turnpike Lane, Hornsey, London N8 0PH
Tel: 020 8889 6770 Fax: 020 8889 3131
(Haringey Teaching Primary Care Trust)
Patient List Size: 5000

Practice Manager B Clark

GP S EL KINANI

The Surgery
153 Park Road, London N8 8JJ
Tel: 020 8340 7940 Fax: 020 8348 1530
(Haringey Teaching Primary Care Trust)
Patient List Size: 4080

Practice Manager Elaine Knight

GP Enid GREENBURY, Diane ROSENTHAL, Jonathan Joseph ROSENTHAL

The Surgery
49 Tottenham Lane, Hornsey, London N8 9BD

GP I A K SARDAR, Mahe TALAT

The Surgery
42 Haringey Park, Hornsey, London N8 9JD

GP R S PATEL, S R PATEL

The Surgery
572 Green Lanes, Hornsey, London N8 0RP
Tel: 020 8802 6250
(Haringey Teaching Primary Care Trust)
Patient List Size: 2300

GP Anna HASSIOTOU

The Surgery
618 Green Lanes, Hornsey, London N8 0SD
Tel: 020 8888 6459
(Haringey Teaching Primary Care Trust)
Patient List Size: 2800

Practice Manager Emilia Zoplakkis

GP A P ANSARI

The Surgery
2 Willoughby Road, Haringey, London N8 0HR
Tel: 020 8348 5466 Fax: 020 8341 6500
Email: Berk.cahit@gp.F85655.nhs.uk
(Haringey Teaching Primary Care Trust)
Patient List Size: 2560

Practice Manager Sabiha Basaran

GP Cahit BERK

London, N9

Boundary House Surgery
459 Hertford Road, Edmonton, London N9 7DU
Tel: 020 8804 2190 Fax: 020 8805 8755
Email: kanapathi.pillai@gp-F85676.nhs.uk
(Enfield Primary Care Trust)

Practice Manager M Jones

GP Kanapathipillai Oppilamani PILLAI

Chalfont Surgery
2 Chalfont Road, Edmonton, London N9 9LW
(Enfield Primary Care Trust)

GP Shee Hung YU

The Health Centre
2A Forest Road, Edmonton, London N9 8RZ
Tel: 020 8804 0121
(Enfield Primary Care Trust)

GP Dilis CLARE, Syed HIKMATULLAH, S A JOWETT, John Martin Nicholas LAUNER, Mary Bridget LOGAN, Ronald Victor Julius SINGER

Keats Surgery
290A Church Street, Edmonton, London N9 9HJ
Tel: 020 8807 2051 Fax: 020 8887 0003
(Enfield Primary Care Trust)
Patient List Size: 4700

GP George Victor KATTAN, Jayanthy GNANANANDAN

Nightingale Road Surgery
1-3 Nightingale Road, London N9 8AJ
Tel: 020 8804 3333 Fax: 020 8805 7776
(Enfield Primary Care Trust)

Practice Manager Marilyn Davis

GP Jonathan Sidney WARREN, D ABIDOYE, J M THOMAS

The Surgery
27-29 Bounces Road, Edmonton, London N9 8JB
Tel: 020 8807 0532 Fax: 020 8884 3399
(Enfield Primary Care Trust)
Patient List Size: 5800

Practice Manager V Slade

GP O M Prakash SHARMA, Suresh PANJWANI

The Surgery
277 Fore Street, Edmonton, London N9 0PD
(Enfield Primary Care Trust)

GP Daulat Khanum Nooredin RESHAMWALLA

The Surgery
62 Church Street, Edmonton, London N9 9PA
Tel: 020 8807 5027 Fax: 020 8807 2815
(Enfield Primary Care Trust)
Patient List Size: 3000

Practice Manager M Colaro

GP Tuljaram PATALAY

The Surgery
252 Church Street, Edmonton, London N9 9HQ
Tel: 020 8884 0541 Fax: 020 8841974
(Enfield Primary Care Trust)
Patient List Size: 2150

GP P G PATEL

The Surgery
2A Latymer Road, Edmonton, London N9 9PU
(Enfield Primary Care Trust)

GP R T B MAKULOLUWE, Alyson Susan JONES, S VIJERATNAM

The Surgery
60 Market Square, Edmonton Green, London N9 0TZ
Tel: 020 8807 7393 Fax: 020 8807 9247
(Enfield Primary Care Trust)
Patient List Size: 4500

Practice Manager Diane Williams

GP Rajnikant Khushaldas BAVISHI, Sandip Ramkrishna HEREKAR

London, N10

Colney Hatch Lane Surgery
192 Colney Hatch Lane, Muswell Hill, London N10 1ET
Tel: 020 8883 5555
(Barnet Primary Care Trust)
Patient List Size: 8000

Practice Manager Kathleen Barry

GP Victoria Elmire KNOCK

Dukes Avenue Surgery
1 Dukes Avenue, London N10 2PS
Tel: 020 8883 9149 Fax: 020 8883 0194
Website: www.lukesavenuesurgery.co.uk
(Haringey Teaching Primary Care Trust)
Patient List Size: 10500

Practice Manager Lesley Mayo

GP Peter Kevin CHRISTIAN, C M GALLAGHER, Timothy John GERRARD, Rosemarie HEALY, Amanda SUTTON

Grosvenor Road Surgery
23 Grosvenor Road, Muswell Hill, London N10 2DR
Tel: 020 8883 5600 Fax: 020 8815 0980
Email: grosvenor.surgery@gp-F85658.nhs.uk
(Haringey Teaching Primary Care Trust)
Patient List Size: 3685

Practice Manager S Moodey

GP Dayantha Christopher Premalal KARUNARATNE, Adel George ISAAK, Samera Haseeb PUTRIS

Queens Avenue Surgery
46 Queens Avenue, Muswell Hill, London N10 3BJ
Tel: 020 8883 1846 Fax: 020 8365 2265
(Haringey Teaching Primary Care Trust)

GP John DEMADES, Batia FRIEDMANN, Thaiman SIVAKUMAR

Rutland House Surgery
40 Colney Hatch, Muswell Hill, London N10 1DU
Tel: 020 8883 5412 Fax: 020 8883 3382
(Barnet Primary Care Trust)

Practice Manager Janine Ross

GP Rebecca HATJIOSIF, Andreas MARIANNOU

The Surgery
57 Curzon Road, Muswell Hill, London N10 2RB

GP Mohanlal Nathoobhai GUDKA

London, N11

Bounds Geen Group Practice
Bounds Green Group Practice, Gordon Road, New Southgate, London N11 2PF
Tel: 020 8889 1961 Fax: 020 8889 7844
Email: info@bggp.co.uk
(Haringey Teaching Primary Care Trust)
Patient List Size: 11000

Practice Manager Breda Nugent, Nicola Wright

GP Lionel Maurice SHERMAN, Jacqueline Diane MANSFIELD, Susan RAMSELL, Paul SALOMON, Alan Jeffrey SCHAMROTH

Brownlow Medical Centre
140 Brownlow Road, Southgate, London N11 2BD
Tel: 020 8888 7775
(Enfield Primary Care Trust)

Practice Manager Margaret Colaco

GP Agha HAIDAR

Friern Barnet Road Surgery
79 Friern Barnet Riad, London N11 3EH
Tel: 020 8368 9874
(Barnet Primary Care Trust)

GP Joakin Apeadu Bosompra OFORI

Health Centre
Brunswick Park Road, London N11 1EY
Tel: 020 8368 1568
(Barnet Primary Care Trust)
Patient List Size: 4500

Practice Manager E Abel

GP Stella Ifeoma OKONKWO

Health Centre
Brunswick Park Road, London N11 1EY
Tel: 020 8368 0813 Fax: 020 8361 0288
(Barnet Primary Care Trust)
Patient List Size: 2250

Practice Manager Sue O'Keefe

GP G DURU

Health Centre
Gordon Road, London N11 2PA

GP Colin Henry DICKIE

St Johns Villas Surgery
16 St Johns Villas, Friern Barnet Road, London N11 3BU
Tel: 020 8368 1707
(Barnet Primary Care Trust)
Patient List Size: 5000

Practice Manager Karen Lowry

GP Snehlata Mukundchandra PATEL, H R SHAH

London, N12

Guindi
16 Nether Street, London N12 7NL
Tel: 020 8445 6582
(Barnet Primary Care Trust)
Patient List Size: 2500

Practice Manager Eileen Magna Vacca

GP George GUINDI

Torrington Park Group Practice
16 Torrington Park, North Finchley, London N12 9SS
Tel: 020 8445 7622/4127 Fax: 020 8445 3043
(Barnet Primary Care Trust)
Patient List Size: 12500

Practice Manager Amanda Reilly

GP Charles John Scott BRETT, Peter Basil BEZUIDENHOUT, Allan Richard DAITZ, Monica Hedy LEIGHTON, Carole Melanie PEISACH, Noëmi Joan WEINGARTEN

Torrington Park Health Centre
Torrington Park, North Finchley, London N12 9SS
Tel: 020 8445 7261 Fax: 020 8343 9122
Email: mailuser@gp-E83010.nhs.uk
(Barnet Primary Care Trust)

Practice Manager Rogar Tumor

GP Angela Mary PARKER, Ralph ABRAHAMS, John Stephen CORCORAN, Philomena DARDIS, Clare STEPHENS

London, N13

Connaught Surgery
144 Hedge Lane, Palmers Green, London N13 5ST
Tel: 020 8886 2284 Fax: 020 8372 7246
(Enfield Primary Care Trust)
Patient List Size: 3600

Practice Manager Anne Winkworth

GP Thakorlal Bhailalbhai PATEL, Ina Sok Mon FOO, A PATEL

Gillan House Surgery
457 Green Lanes, Palmers Green, London N13 4BS
Tel: 020 8882 9393 Fax: 020 88862569
(Enfield Primary Care Trust)

GP Alan Robertson DICK, S KARTHIKESALINGAM

Grenoble Gardens Surgery
1 Grenoble Gardens, Palmers Green, London N13 6JE
Tel: 020 8889 5423 Fax: 020 8881 4656
Email: chandra.patalay@gp-F85077.nhs.uk
(Enfield Primary Care Trust)
Patient List Size: 2600

Practice Manager Elaine Walsh

GP Chandra PATALAY

Grovelands Medical Centre
1 Grovelands Road, Palmers Green, London N13 4RJ
(Enfield Primary Care Trust)
Patient List Size: 5200

Practice Manager Angela Wass

GP R SINGH, V SINGH

Kolman and Partners
Rochdale Surgery, Broomfield Avenue, Palmers Green, London N13 4JJ
Tel: 020 8886 3631 Fax: 020 8882 8345
(Enfield Primary Care Trust)
Patient List Size: 5200

Practice Manager Gabriella C Esposito

GP Pia Cornelia KOLMAN, Howard DAITZ

Palm Medical Centre
Ulster Gardens, London N13 5DP
Tel: 020 8807 2045 Fax: 020 8807 1417
Email: jan@palmmedical-c.co.uk
(Enfield Primary Care Trust)
Patient List Size: 2521

Practice Manager N J Khan

GP Jameel Ullah KHAN

Park Lodge Medical Centre
3 Old Park Road, Palmers Green, London N13 4RG
Tel: 020 8886 6866 Fax: 020 8882 8884
Website: www.parklodgemedicalcentre.co.uk
(Enfield Primary Care Trust)
Patient List Size: 7300

Practice Manager Sue Spencer

GP Janet Elizabeth HIGH, Deborah GILL, Anne GRIFFIN, George KOULOUMAS, Stephen PARKINSON, Angela PATEL

London, N14

Hampden Medical Centre
22 Hampden Square, Southgate, London N14 5JR
Tel: 020 8361 4403
(Barnet Primary Care Trust)

Practice Manager Ann Collins

GP Mariya Sithi Mirza HAMID

Jaina House Surgery
66 Arnos Grove, Southgate, London N14 7AR
Tel: 020 8886 4035 Fax: 020 8882 7024
Email: dshah30@hotmail.co.uk
(Enfield Primary Care Trust)
Patient List Size: 2600

GP Dilip Kumar Liladhar Raishi SHAH

Oakwood Medical Centre
Malcolms Way, Reservoir Road, Southgate, London N14 4AQ
Tel: 020 8886 1115 Fax: 020 8866 6166
(Enfield Primary Care Trust)
Patient List Size: 6300

Practice Manager Samita Mookerjee

GP A K MUKHOPADHYAY, Lynn Rebecca D'SOUZA, A C MITCHELL

Osidge Medical Centre
182 Osidge Lane, Southgate, London N14 5DR
Tel: 020 8368 2800
(Barnet Primary Care Trust)

GP Nitin Nanji LAKHANI

Southgate Surgery
270 Chase Side, Southgate, London N14 4PR
Tel: 020 8440 9301 Fax: 020 8449 9349
(Enfield Primary Care Trust)
Patient List Size: 7200

Practice Manager Denise Leech

GP Basil Brian GEFFIN, Rajendran John ANNARADNAM, Selvia NITHIYANANATHAN

London, N15

Aarogya Medical Centre
270-274 West Green Road, Tottenham, London N15 3QR
Tel: 020 8365 7282 Fax: 020 8374 7770
Email: ruth.truelove@gp-m81009.nhs.uk
(Haringey Teaching Primary Care Trust)
Patient List Size: 3000

Practice Manager Raka Mukhopadhyay

GP Dipendra Nath MUKHOPADHYAY

Fernlea Surgery
114 High Road, London N15 6JR
Tel: 020 8809 6445 Fax: 020 8800 4224
(Haringey Teaching Primary Care Trust)
Patient List Size: 5600

Practice Manager V. Henry

GP Russell Simon CAPLAN, Julian Martin CHADWICK, Sandra Carole RACHMAN

Havergal Surgery
9-10 Havergal Villas, Green Lanes, London N15 3DY
Tel: 020 8888 6662 Fax: 020 8881 3650
(Haringey Teaching Primary Care Trust)
Patient List Size: 4700

Practice Manager Tracey Christodoulou

GP Amrish GOR

Lawrence House
107 Philip Lane, Tottenham, London N15 4JR
Tel: 020 8801 6640
(Haringey Teaching Primary Care Trust)

Practice Manager Sila Makoon

GP Hasan Tahsin BILGINER, Rini PAUL, John Stephen ROHAN

St Anns Medical Centre
198 St Anns Road, Tottenham, London N15 5RP
Tel: 020 8800 7060 Fax: 020 8442 8066
(Haringey Teaching Primary Care Trust)
Patient List Size: 5500

GP D K SHAH

The Surgery
37 High Road, London N15 6DS
Tel: 020 8809 3091 Fax: 020 8809 2640
Email: tanvir.afghan@gp-f85674.nhs.uk
(Haringey Teaching Primary Care Trust)
Patient List Size: 2095

Practice Manager Tanvir Afghan

GP K AFGHAN

The Surgery
326 Philip Lane, Tottenham, London N15 4AB
Tel: 020 8808 0322 Fax: 020 8801 5093
(Haringey Teaching Primary Care Trust)

Practice Manager Gulen Hussein

GP Kathiravellupillai SIVASINMYANANTHAN, P THIRUVUDAIYAN

The Surgery
9 Fladbury Road, Tottenham, London N15 6SB
Tel: 020 8802 1091
(Haringey Teaching Primary Care Trust)
Patient List Size: 3500

Practice Manager Katriye Ahmet

GP K C C REDDY

The Surgery
18 St Johns Road, Tottenham, London N15 6QP
Tel: 020 8442 8220 Fax: 020 8802 8539
(Haringey Teaching Primary Care Trust)
Patient List Size: 3200

GP Dilip Kumar KUNDU

The Surgery
1 Grove Road, Tottenham, London N15 5HJ
Tel: 020 8800 9781 Fax: 020 8800 3196
(Haringey Teaching Primary Care Trust)
Patient List Size: 3000

Practice Manager Zalike Osman

GP Jerome Kaine IKWUEKE

The Surgery
1 Spur Road, Tottenham, London N15 4AA

GP P DAS GUPTA

The Surgery
339-341 West Green Road, Tottenham, London N15 3PB
Tel: 020 8881 9606 Fax: 020 8881 4204
(Haringey Teaching Primary Care Trust)
Patient List Size: 4600

Practice Manager Matthew Zornenky

GP Muhammad Shahjahan Ali AKUNJEE

London, N16

Abney House Medical Centre
2 Defoe Road, Stoke Newington, London N16 0EP
Tel: 020 7254 6820
(City and Hackney Teaching Primary Care Trust)

GP Michael John Thomson DALTON

Allerton Road Surgery
34A Allerton Road, London N16 5UF
Tel: 020 8802 2882
(City and Hackney Teaching Primary Care Trust)

GP Heschil LEWIN

Barretts Grove Surgery
6 Barretts Grove, Stoke Newington, London N16 8AR
Tel: 020 8254 1661 Fax: 020 7275 8777
(City and Hackney Teaching Primary Care Trust)
Patient List Size: 3139

GP Rajendra Lal GANGOLA, Milan GANGOLA

Barton House Health Centre
233 Albion Road, London N16 9JT
Tel: 020 7249 5511 Fax: 020 7254 8985
(City and Hackney Teaching Primary Care Trust)
Patient List Size: 11545

Practice Manager Kay Sutton

GP Matthew Tytherleigh BENCH, Patricia Mary BOHN, Gabriela CLOUTER, Christopher John DERRETT, Michael John FITZPATRICK, Janet WILLIAMS

The Fontayne Road Health Centre
1a Fontayne Road, Stoke Newington, London N16 7EA
Tel: 020 8806 8514
(City and Hackney Teaching Primary Care Trust)

GP Mulubhai Raja GADHVI

Fountayne Road Health Centre
1A Fountayne Road, London N16 7EA
Tel: 020 8806 3311 Fax: 020 8806 9197
(City and Hackney Teaching Primary Care Trust)

GP Susan Jaqueline Rachel KIERNAN, A J V JENKINS, Abdul Hafiz PATHAN, S SHARIFF, David WOLFSON

Mildmay Medical Practice
2a Green Lanes, London N16 9NF
Tel: 020 7923 1999 Fax: 020 7923 1616
(Islington Primary Care Trust)
Patient List Size: 6200

Practice Manager Judy Banks

GP A HOSSAIN, D V WHEELER, B WOODHATCH

Oldhill Medical Centre
19-21 Oldhill Street, London N16 6LD
Tel: 020 8806 6993 Fax: 020 8806 6008
(City and Hackney Teaching Primary Care Trust)
Patient List Size: 8700

Practice Manager Sanjiv Gupta

GP Satya Prakash GUPTA, Kumud TRIVEDI

Somerford Grove Practice
Somerford Grove Health Centre, Somerford Grove, London N16 7UA
Tel: 020 7241 9700 Fax: 020 7275 7198
(City and Hackney Teaching Primary Care Trust)
Patient List Size: 10000

Practice Manager Jan Harley-Doyle

GP Anthony David KEENE, Mark Christopher HINDLEY, Shirley HOPPER, Peter Teiksoon KAY, Christopher MALONEY

Stamford Hill Group Practice
2 Egerton Road, Stamford Hill, London N16 6UA
Tel: 020 8800 1000 Fax: 020 8880 2402
(City and Hackney Teaching Primary Care Trust)

Practice Manager Jane Telfer

GP (H) James CARNE, Charlotte Sarah FOSTER, Clifton Michael MARKS, Louise Jane WALDMAN, Dan Shannon WILLIAMS

Stamford Hill Group Practice
2 Egerton Road, Stamford Hill, London N16 6UA
Tel: 020 8800 1000 Fax: 020 8880 2402
(City and Hackney Teaching Primary Care Trust)

GP L BLUMBERG, Adrian Jules DELL

Statham Grove Surgery
Statham Grove, London N16 9DP
Tel: 020 7254 4327 Fax: 020 7241 4098
(City and Hackney Teaching Primary Care Trust)
Patient List Size: 7500

Practice Manager Claire Lister

GP Rhiannon ENGLAND, Leon CLARK, Declan Richard PHELAN, Melissa SAYER, Ruth SILVERMAN, Nicki SINGER

The Surgery
62 Cranwich Road, London N16 5JF
Tel: 020 8802 2002 Fax: 020 8880 2112
(City and Hackney Teaching Primary Care Trust)

Practice Manager S Neville

GP Joseph SPITZER, Anthony Lionel LEVY

The Surgery
40-42 Brooke Road, London N16 7LR
Tel: 020 7254 5652
(City and Hackney Teaching Primary Care Trust)

GP Sachida Nand PRASAD

The Surgery
100 Church Street, Stoke Newington, London N16 0AP
Tel: 020 7254 3807 Fax: 020 7923 9260
(City and Hackney Teaching Primary Care Trust)
Patient List Size: 2700

GP Nwabueze John OGBUEHI

The Surgery
71 Amhurst Park, London N16 5DL
(City and Hackney Teaching Primary Care Trust)

GP Mehrbanoo FARUHAR

The Surgery
271 Amhurst Road, London N16 7UP
(City and Hackney Teaching Primary Care Trust)

GP P DASGUPTA

The Surgery
2-3 Batley Place, London N16 7NS
(City and Hackney Teaching Primary Care Trust)

London, N17

Broadwater Surgery
Willan Road, Tottenham, London N17 6BF

GP D L JONES

Bruce Grove Primary Health Care Centre
461-463 High Road, Tottenham, London N17 6QB
Tel: 020 8808 4710 Fax: 020 8885 3745
(Haringey Teaching Primary Care Trust)
Patient List Size: 10060

Practice Manager V S Mani

GP M PAL, A AUGUST, M S HOQUE, N KADIR, Q M RAHMAN, S SENGUPTA

Castleview Surgery
119 Lordship Lane, London N17 6XE
Tel: 020 8801 1565 Fax: 020 8493 8750
(Haringey Teaching Primary Care Trust)

Charlton House Medical Centre
581 High Road, Tottenham, London N17 6SB
Tel: 020 8808 2837 Fax: 020 8801 4179
(Haringey Teaching Primary Care Trust)
Patient List Size: 7200

Practice Manager Susan Darbo

GP Charles Melvin MORRISON, K AGYEMAN, Anoma Hemantha RANMUTHU

Morris House Surgery
Waltheof Gardens, Tottenham, London N17 7EB
Tel: 020 8801 1277 Fax: 020 8801 8228
(Haringey Teaching Primary Care Trust)
Patient List Size: 10000

Practice Manager N C Fellowes

GP Gino Antonio AMATO, Sally Anne DOWLER, J HILL, Sue MOORTHY, Usna THILLAIAMBALAM

Somerset Gardens Family Health
4 Creighton Road, Tottenham, London N17 8NW
Tel: 020 8493 9090 Fax: 020 8493 6000
(Haringey Teaching Primary Care Trust)
Patient List Size: 12000

GP Paul BARNETT, Loretta Shryanthi Keshini BASTIANPILLAI, W R GOONERATNE, Martin Stephen LINDSAY, B MUKHOPADHYAY, Kate REES

The Surgery
57 Dowsett Road, Tottenham, London N17 9DL

GP Morvarid WOOLLACOTT

The Surgery
104-108 Park Lane, Tottenham, London N17 0JP

GP K NAGARAJAH

The Surgery
1A Landsdowne Road, Tottenham, London N17 0LL
Tel: 020 8808 9891 Fax: 020 4938 047
Patient List Size: 3672

GP K R JEYARAJAH, K JEYARAJAH

The Surgery
1A St Paul's Road, Tottenham, London N17 0NJ
(Haringey Teaching Primary Care Trust)

GP D K SURI

London, N18

Dover House
28 Bolton Road, Edmonton, London N18 1HR
(Enfield Primary Care Trust)

GP M DHARMARAJAH, S N VERMA

Fore Street Surgery
234 Fore Street, Edmonton, London N18 2LY
Tel: 020 8803 6705
(Enfield Primary Care Trust)
Patient List Size: 4000

GP Michael Ellman SILVER, Dr CLAFF, Dr MASTERS, N OWINJ

Silver Street Medical Centre
159 Silver Street, London N18 1PY
Tel: 020 8807 1057 Fax: 020 8345 5259
(Enfield Primary Care Trust)
Patient List Size: 6700

Practice Manager V Thapar

GP Rama THAPAR, Hope BELL-GAM, Stephen Chee Cheung HIEW, S THEYMOZHI

The Surgery
20 Kendal Parade, Silver Street, Edmonton, London N18 1ND
Tel: 020 8803 0020
(Enfield Primary Care Trust)

GP Manickam VISWANATHAN, A H Y RAJENDRAM

The Surgery
29 Folkestone Road, Edmonton, London N18 2ER
Tel: 020 8807 2176
(Enfield Primary Care Trust)
Patient List Size: 4200

Practice Manager Berrin Buyukarslan

GP Brendan Patrick O'BRIEN, K RATNARAJAN

The Surgery
1 Boundary Court, Fore Street, Snells Park, Edmonton, London N18 2TB
Tel: 020 8807 3126 Fax: 020 8556 1821
(Enfield Primary Care Trust)

GP Ayesha Ashma SULTANA

The Surgery
112 Ingleton Road, Edmonton, London N18 2RT
(Enfield Primary Care Trust)

GP S NATKUNARAJAH

London, N19

Archway Medical Centre
652 Holloway Road, London N19 3NU
Tel: 020 7272 2877 Fax: 020 7561 0744
(Islington Primary Care Trust)
Patient List Size: 5500

Practice Manager Kalpna Parekh

GP Milan KOYA, Susannah BARNES, Robert BRADY, Brigid Sarah SHEPPARD

Hornsey Rise Health Centre
Hornsey Rise, London N19 3YU
Tel: 020 7530 2484 Fax: 020 7530 2491
(Islington Primary Care Trust)
Patient List Size: 7200

Practice Manager James Stuart Knox

GP Liane Celia Regina Bertha TAYLOR, Jyotsna HIRA, Stephen ROGERS, Susan SALKIND

Hornsey Rise Health Centre
Hornsey Rise, London N19 3YU
Tel: 020 7530 2455
(Islington Primary Care Trust)

GP Dr MONEEB

Hornsey Road Surgery
510 Hornsey Road, London N19 3QW
Tel: 020 7272 0765
(Islington Primary Care Trust)

GP Soraya Parvin RAHAMAN

Ko
244 Tufnell Park Road, London N19 5EW
Tel: 020 7272 8747 Fax: 020 7272 2030
(Islington Primary Care Trust)

Practice Manager R Ko

GP Aaron Hoi Nam KO

St Johns Way Medical Centre
96 St. Johns Way, London N19 3RN
Tel: 020 7272 1585 Fax: 020 7561 1237
(Islington Primary Care Trust)
Patient List Size: 11500

Practice Manager Penny Borrow

GP Anthony Charles Michael INWALD, Stephen David AARONS, Susan Mary BLAKE, Dr COOPER, Kate DURRANT, Mark JOHNSON, Kate JOLOWICZ

Tufnell Park Road Surgery
244 Tufnell Park Roa, London N19 5EW
Tel: 020 7272 9105 Fax: 020 7272 8996
(Islington Primary Care Trust)
Patient List Size: 4200

Practice Manager Cristina Kateb

GP Heskel Joseph KATEB, Juliet BROWN

Wedmore Gardens Surgery
5 Wedmore Gardens, Upper Holloway, London N19 4DL
Tel: 020 7263 2794
(Islington Primary Care Trust)

GP Dr HUSSAIN

London, N20

Derwent Crescent Surgery
20 Derwent Crescent, Whetstone, London N20 0QQ
Tel: 020 8446 0171 Fax: 020 8446 0073
(Barnet Primary Care Trust)
Patient List Size: 4898

Practice Manager Sue Lendon

GP Jonathan Richard LUBIN, Daniel BEATUS, Katherine BOODLE, Attiya KHAN, Irene LIU

Dr Lumley and Partners
Oakleigh Road Clinic, 280 Oakleigh Road North, Whetstone, London N20 0DH
Tel: 020 8361 1996 Fax: 020 8361 3638
(Barnet Primary Care Trust)

GP Daniel George Charles FREE, Claire Naheed HASSAN, Jane HOWELLS, Kim LUMLEY, John Roslyn MAXWELL

The Health Centre
Oakleigh Road North, Whetstone, London N20 0DH
Tel: 020 8368 6550 Fax: 020 8361 4116
(Barnet Primary Care Trust)
Patient List Size: 8000

Practice Manager Virginia Wood

GP Kim LUMLEY, Daniel George Charles FREE, Claire HASSAN, Jane (Helina) HOWELLS, John MAXWELL

St Andrews Medical Practice
50 Oakleigh Road North, Whetstone, London N20 9EX
Tel: 020 8445 0475 Fax: 020 8446 0179
Email: firstname.surname@gp-e83024.nhs.uk
(Barnet Primary Care Trust)
Patient List Size: 10000

GP Paul Michael BRAY, WanNei NG, Anita Givindji PATEL, Hillas Rodney SMITH, Sandeep TANNA, Alexandra WHITER

St Andrews Medical Practice
50 Oakleigh Road North, Whetstone, London N20 9EX
Tel: 020 8445 0475 Fax: 020 8446 0179
(Barnet Primary Care Trust)
Patient List Size: 9800

Practice Manager Michele Eshmene

GP Dr BRAY, Dr PATEL, Dr SMITH, Dr WHITER

London, N21

The Surgery
939 Green Lanes, Winchmore Hill, London N21 2PB
Tel: 020 8360 2228 Fax: 020 8360 5702
(Enfield Primary Care Trust)
Patient List Size: 7800

Practice Manager Sandra Marshall

GP Glenn Marvin STERN, R NOOR, Sanjay PATEL

The Surgery
939 Green Lanes, Winchmore Hill, London N21 2PB
Tel: 020 8360 2228 Fax: 020 9360 5702
(Enfield Primary Care Trust)
Patient List Size: 6000

Practice Manager Sandra Marshall

GP Frances Carmel NOLAN, Ian Harris FLETCHER, Rakesh PARBHOO

The Surgery
939 Green Lanes, Winchmore Hill, London N21 2PB
Tel: 020 8360 2228 Fax: 020 9360 5702
(Enfield Primary Care Trust)
Patient List Size: 1800

Practice Manager Malcolm Bull

GP Janusz Stanley MACIOLEK

The Woodberry Practice
1 Woodberry Avenue, Winchmere Hill, London N21 3LE
(Enfield Primary Care Trust)

Practice Manager Sebastian D'Souza

GP Raymond Clive HUME, Raju RAITHATHA, Jane Elizabeth SELWOOD

Woodberry Surgery
1 Woodberry Avenue, London N21 3LE
Tel: 020 8886 2751 Fax: 020 8882 2891
(Enfield Primary Care Trust)
Patient List Size: 8030

Practice Manager Sebastian D'Souza

GP Raymond Clive HUME, Raju RAITHATHA, Jane Elizabeth SELWOOD

London, N22

Alexandra Surgery
125 Alexandra Park Road, London N22 7UN
Tel: 020 8888 2518
(Haringey Teaching Primary Care Trust)

Practice Manager J H Ross

GP Nalliah SIVANANTHAN

Arcadian Gardens Surgery
1 Arcadian Gardens, Bowes Park, London N22 5AB
Tel: 020 8888 4142 Fax: 020 8829 9337
(Haringey Teaching Primary Care Trust)
Patient List Size: 4496

Practice Manager Lisa Woods

GP Sadguna Manharlal PAUN, A T PATEL, D T RAJPOPAT

The High Road Surgery
391 High Road, Wood Green, London N22 8JB
Tel: 020 8889 1115 Fax: 020 8881 4372
(Haringey Teaching Primary Care Trust)
Patient List Size: 5000

Practice Manager V J Holt

GP Lionel SAMARASINGHE, M F JURANGPATHY

Staunton Group Practice
3-5 Bounds Green Road, Wood Green, London N22 8HE
Tel: 020 8889 4311 Fax: 020 8826 9100
(Haringey Teaching Primary Care Trust)
Patient List Size: 15500

Practice Manager Cindy O'Garro

GP Vivienne Helen MANHEIM, R J ACHARYA, Kansar M ALI, Hoda BOTROS, Nicholas William GRAHAM, Carol Jane HIGGINS, Thomas STROMMER, Mary Frances WINDLE

Stuart Crescent Health Centre
8 Stuart Crescent, Wood Green, London N22 5NJ
Tel: 020 8889 1001
(Haringey Teaching Primary Care Trust)
Patient List Size: 3800

Practice Manager Bharti M Dave

GP Mahendra Shantilal DAVE, R G MANGALESWARADEVI

The Surgery
26 Westbury Avenue, Wood Green, London N22 6RS
Tel: 020 8888 3227 Fax: 020 8829 9642
(Haringey Teaching Primary Care Trust)

GP Abu Taher Mohammed Mozammel HOQUE, Jayaratnam VARATHARAJ

The Surgery
27 Cheshire Road, Wood Green, London N22 8JJ

GP A PELENDRIDES

The Surgery
53 Myddleton Road, Wood Green, London N22 8LZ

GP D PRASAD

The Surgery
730 Lordship Lane, Wood Green, London N22 5JN

GP Harvey Stewart COHEN

Westbury Medical Centre
205 Westbury Avenue, Wood Green, London N22 6RX
Tel: 020 8888 3021 Fax: 020 8888 6898
Website: www.westbury.nhs.uk
(Haringey Teaching Primary Care Trust)
Patient List Size: 7500

Practice Manager Linda Potter

GP Mukund Kanubhai PATEL, Harshadaben Maheshkumar PATEL, Mark STEINBERG

London, NW1

Ampthill Square Medical Centre
219 Evershott Street, London NW1 1DE
Tel: 020 7387 6161 Fax: 020 7387 0420
(Camden Primary Care Trust)

Practice Manager Margaret Heals

GP Dilys Ann COWAN, Richard Nigel ALLINSON, Dr BRENNAN, Penelope Eugenie ELPHINSTONE

Camden Road Surgery
142 Camden Road, London NW1 9HR
Tel: 020 7284 0384 Fax: 020 7428 0493
(Camden Primary Care Trust)

Practice Manager Liam Doherty

GP Wendy ABRAMS, Robert Braith HARBORD, Dr WOODCROFT

Cliff Road Surgery
10A Cliff Road, London NW1 9AN
Tel: 020 7485 2276 Fax: 020 7428 9602
(Camden Primary Care Trust)
Patient List Size: 3500

Practice Manager Carol Barrett, Lynn O'Connor

GP Devi FATNANI

Crowndale Road Surgery
53 Crowndale Road, London NW1 1TN
Tel: 020 7387 7762
(Camden Primary Care Trust)
Patient List Size: 3200

GP Petros Panoyiotis PETROU

Kings Cross Road Surgery
79 Camden Road, London NW1 9ES
Tel: 020 7278 5657 Fax: 020 7278 3337
(Camden Primary Care Trust)

Practice Manager Amanda Lord

Marylebone Health Centre
17 Marylebone Road, London NW1 5LT
Tel: 020 7935 6328
(Westminster Primary Care Trust)
Patient List Size: 8500

Practice Manager Amanda Lawrence

GP Harriet FRASER, Andrew GOODSTONE, Richard MORRISON, Susan Christine MORRISON, Tom MTANDABARI, B PATEL

Regents Park Medical Centre
Cumberland Market, London NW1 3RH
Tel: 020 7387 3653
(Camden Primary Care Trust)

Practice Manager Suzanne Collins

GP Dr GHOSH

Regents Park Medical Centre
Cumberland Market, London NW1 3RH
Tel: 020 7387 4576 Fax: 020 7387 2331
(Camden Primary Care Trust)

GP Marian Zelma LATCHMAN, Harbikramjit S. CHANDOK, Christine Alice Margaret PICKARD

Regents Park Road Surgery
99 Regents Park Road, London NW1 8UR
Tel: 020 7722 0038 Fax: 020 7722 9724
(Camden Primary Care Trust)

Practice Manager Tracy Chapman

GP John Sutherland BARLOW, Paula Mildred DRUMMOND, Katharine Victoria HECKER

Somers Town Medical Centre
77-83 Charlton Street, London NW1 1HY
Tel: 020 7387 6855 Fax: 020 7388 3325
(Camden Primary Care Trust)
Patient List Size: 3600

Practice Manager Carol Murphy

GP C L PARRY, E PARSONS

London, NW2

Crest Medical Centre
157 Crest Road, London NW2 7NA
Tel: 020 8452 5155
(Brent Teaching Primary Care Trust)
Patient List Size: 3800

GP Anil Velji DALSANIA, Rajan Anil DALSANIA

Cricklewood Broadway Surgery
60 Cricklewood Broadway, London NW2 3ET
Tel: 020 8452 9904 Fax: 020 8208 0509
(Brent Teaching Primary Care Trust)

Practice Manager Bhavani Maheswaran

GP W T MAHESWARAN

Gladstone Medical Centre
5 Dollis Hill, London NW2 6JH
Tel: 020 8452 1616 Fax: 020 8452 0446
(Brent Teaching Primary Care Trust)
Patient List Size: 5800

Practice Manager Katrina Johnson

GP Nigel Stuart de KARE-SILVER, Iklinno ONWHANBE

Greenfield Medical Centre
143-145 Cricklewood Lane, London NW2 1HS
Tel: 020 8450 5454
(Barnet Primary Care Trust)

Practice Manager Martin Sinon

GP Kokila Atul MEHTA, Antonia Clare BRIFFA, Barry SUBEL

Neasden Medical Centre
21 Tanfield Avenue, London NW2 7SA
Tel: 020 8450 2834 Fax: 020 8452 4324
(Brent Teaching Primary Care Trust)

GP Raphael RASOOLY, Manubhai Kevaldas PATEL

Pennine Drive Surgery
6-8 Pennine Drive, London NW2 1PA
Tel: 020 8455 9977
(Barnet Primary Care Trust)

Practice Manager Sunita Miles

GP Margaret Phyllis McCOLLUM, Barbara Jayne FROSH, Clare June HALSTED, Michael Adam JOLLES, Peter John RUDGE

Staverton Surgery
51 Staverton Road, London NW2 5HA
Tel: 020 8459 6865 Fax: 020 8451 6897
(Brent Teaching Primary Care Trust)

Practice Manager Jenny Poole

GP Anthony Martin BURCH, Amanda Polly CRAIG, Encarnacion FERNANDEZ

The Surgery
19 Chichele Road, London NW2 3AH
Tel: 020 8452 3232 Fax: 020 8452 9812
(Brent Teaching Primary Care Trust)

Practice Manager Y DeSouza

GP Uttamchand Raishi SHAH, Usha Uttamchand SHAH

The Surgery
25 Chichele Road, London NW2 3AN
Tel: 020 8452 4666 Fax: 020 8450 3680
(Brent Teaching Primary Care Trust)

GP Joothica Ulhas RANADE, Prakesh R JAGADAMBE

The Surgery
131 Dartmouth Road, London NW2 4ES
Tel: 020 8450 0403 Fax: 020 8450 3355
(Brent Teaching Primary Care Trust)
Patient List Size: 2200

GP Jyotika Gyandev SHETH

The Surgery
114 Walm Lane, London NW2 4RT
Tel: 020 8452 0366 Fax: 020 8450 3816
(Brent Teaching Primary Care Trust)
Patient List Size: 8500

Practice Manager Maria O'Brien

GP Sheila Margaret COATES, Jennifer IMESON, Miriam ONYEADOR, Montserrat REDRADO

The Surgery
81 Oxgate Gardens, London NW2 6EA
Tel: 020 8208 0291 Fax: 020 8208 1753
(Brent Teaching Primary Care Trust)

Practice Manager Jacqui Tonge

GP Ruth Elizabeth JONES, Katharine Gurney HAYNES, Judith M KELLERMAN, Jacqueline Ruth MARSHALL

The Surgery
59 Anson Road, London NW2 3UY
Tel: 020 8208 4141 Fax: 020 8208 3536
(Brent Teaching Primary Care Trust)
Patient List Size: 4100

Practice Manager K L Bhattee

GP Zahair Nahi NAJIM

The Surgery
9 Dollis Hill Lane, London NW2 6JH
Tel: 020 8450 4040 Fax: 020 8450 7334
(Brent Teaching Primary Care Trust)

GP Isis Fouad Zaki NEOMAN

Windmill Medical Practice
65 Shoot Up Hill, London NW2 3PS
Tel: 020 8452 7646 Fax: 020 8450 2319
(Brent Teaching Primary Care Trust)
Patient List Size: 8200

Practice Manager Elaine Clements, Jane Watson

GP Max Trahearn OLIVER, Susan Elizabeth MITCHLEY, Ann Louise ROBINSON, Miriam Hilary SKELKER

London, NW3

Adelaide Medical Centre

111 Adelaide Road, London NW3 3RY
Tel: 020 7722 4135 Fax: 020 7586 7558
(Camden Primary Care Trust)
Patient List Size: 10000

Practice Manager Monika Cleaver

GP Frances Anne LOUGHRIDGE, Marcus CRAVEN, Cathryn KATZ, Karen MILLER, Helen MOOR, Caroline SAYER, Ian Kazimierz SIENKOWSKI

Belsize Lane Surgery

37 Belsize Lane, Hampstead, London NW3 5AS
Tel: 020 7794 5787
(Camden Primary Care Trust)

GP Thomas Stephen Vladimir BOSTOCK

Daleham Practice

5 Daleham Gardens, London NW3 5BY
Tel: 020 7530 2510 Fax: 020 7530 2511
(Camden Primary Care Trust)
Patient List Size: 2400

Practice Manager Margaret Guilfayne

GP G WONG, C McGRATH

Hampstead Group Practice

75 Fleet Road, London NW3 2QU
Tel: 020 7435 4000 Fax: 020 7435 9000
(Camden Primary Care Trust)
Patient List Size: 10500

Practice Manager M Coppens

GP Sylvia Ruth LAQUEUR, Kathy HOFFMANN, Sarah Louise MORGAN, Jeremy Mark SANDFORD, Paul George WALLACE

The Keats Group Practice

1B Downshire Hill, London NW3 1NR
Tel: 020 7435 1131 Fax: 020 7431 8501
(Camden Primary Care Trust)
Patient List Size: 8000

Practice Manager Michael Calahan

GP Lucia GRUN, Eunice Modupe Oluwemimo Abimbola LALEYE, Irwin NAZARETH, Jonathan Howard SHELDON

The Park End Surgery

3 Park End, South Hill Park, London NW3 2SE
Tel: 020 7435 7282
(Camden Primary Care Trust)

Practice Manager Christine Hayward

GP Annette Michal BENDOR, John Paul HORTON, Dr SHAW, Andrew Brian Douglas STUART

Rosslyn Hill Surgery

20 Rosslyn Hill, London NW3 1PD
Tel: 020 7435 1132
(Camden Primary Care Trust)

Practice Manager M Roche

GP Dr DODDS, Gillian GERTNER

The Surgery

543 Finchley Road, London NW3 7BJ
Tel: 020 7431 5991 Fax: 020 7431 4663
(Camden Primary Care Trust)

Practice Manager Marilyn Phillips

GP Bryan David SHEINMAN

London, NW4

Beaufort Gardens Surgery

2 Beaufort Gardens, Hendon, London NW4 3QP
Tel: 020 8202 1990/2141 Fax: 020 8203 3638
(Barnet Primary Care Trust)

GP Sisir RAY

Boyne Avenue Surgery

57 Boyne Avenue, Hendon, London NW4 2JL
Tel: 020 8203 2230 Fax: 020 8202 7900
(Barnet Primary Care Trust)
Patient List Size: 2200

Practice Manager Gabrielle O'Doherty

GP Saramma SAMUEL

Grovemead Health Partnership

67 Elliot Road, Hendon, London NW4 3EB
Tel: 0870 417 6560 Fax: 020 8203 1682
(Barnet Primary Care Trust)
Patient List Size: 7300

GP Karen FRASER, Sanavia ABDULLA, Nayeem AZIM, Douglas BALDY-GRAY

Hillview Practice

114 Finchley Lane, Hendon, London NW4 1DG
Tel: 020 8203 0546 Fax: 020 8203 2963
Website: www.surgeriesonline.co.uk/hillu.eu114
(Barnet Primary Care Trust)
Patient List Size: 2700

GP S SAMUEL

St Georges Medical Centre

7 Sunningfields Road, Hendon, London NW4 4QR
Tel: 020 8202 6232 Fax: 020 8202 3906
(Barnet Primary Care Trust)
Patient List Size: 8000

Practice Manager J D Hall

GP Patricia Ann THROWER, Caroline HOFFBRAND, Rohan MAILOO, Michael Stuart MUSGRAVE, Jonathan Stephen SCHWARTZ

Station Road Surgery

42 Station Road, London NW4 3SU
Tel: 020 8202 3733 Fax: 020 8203 8096
(Barnet Primary Care Trust)
Patient List Size: 8000

Practice Manager Beverley Clark

GP Vina Meden CHATRATH, Abdul Kalma Rashid HASAN, J T POPAT

The Surgery

4 Raleigh Close, Hendon, London NW4 2TA
Tel: 020 8202 8302 Fax: 020 8203 7295
(Barnet Primary Care Trust)

Practice Manager M Dryer

GP Victoria Murad AZIZ

The Surgery

86 Audley Road, Hendon, London NW4 3HB
Tel: 020 8203 5150 Fax: 020 8202 5682
(Barnet Primary Care Trust)
Patient List Size: 2000

GP Surendra Ambalal PATEL

Watford Way Surgery

278 Watford Way, London NW4 4UR
Tel: 020 8203 1166/7 Fax: 020 8203 0430
(Barnet Primary Care Trust)

GP Safder Ali Lalji DATOO

London, NW5

Brookfield Park Surgery
2 Brookfield Road, London NW5 1ER
Tel: 020 7485 7363 Fax: 020 7485 6506
(Camden Primary Care Trust)
Patient List Size: 4762

Practice Manager Shoba Sinha

GP Sudhir Kumar SINHA, Shobha SINHA

Caversham Practice
4 Peckwater Street, London NW5 2UP
Tel: 020 7530 6500 Fax: 020 7530 6530
Email: caversham.practice@gp-f83022.nhs.uk
(Camden Primary Care Trust)

Practice Manager George Moorcroft

GP Stephen Michael AMIEL, Judy BENNETT, Caroline Margaret DICKINSON, Iona Caroline HEATH, Mohammad Azhar MALIK, Jane MYAT, Daniel TOEG

Dr Dow and Partners
87-89 Prince of Wales Road, London NW5 3NT
Tel: 020 7267 0067 Fax: 020 7485 8211
(Camden Primary Care Trust)

GP Nigel Paul ASHWORTH, Alison Margaret DOW, Sarah Catherine PALMER, Richard Ian WALTHEW

Dr Turvill Surgery
76 Queens Crescent, London NW5 4EB
Tel: 020 7485 6104 Fax: 020 7485 5277
(Camden Primary Care Trust)

Practice Manager Debbie Richards

GP P TURVILL

Four Trees Surgery
118 Malden Road, London NW5 4BY
Tel: 020 7813 1600 Fax: 020 7813 1395
(Camden Primary Care Trust)

Practice Manager Isata Fullah

GP Ardeshir MEHTA, Gillian ALLISON

James Wigg Group Practice
Kentish Town Health Centre, 2 Bartholomew Road, London NW5 2AJ
Tel: 020 7530 4747 Fax: 020 7530 4750
(Camden Primary Care Trust)
Patient List Size: 14800

Practice Manager Renata Johnstone

GP Marek Tadeusz KOPERSKI, Eric Lance BRITTON, Donald Roy MACGREGOR, Philip Joseph POSNER, Jane SACKVILLE-WEST

Parliament Hill Surgery
113-117 Highgate Road, London NW5 1TR
Tel: 020 7482 9280 Fax: 020 7284 4677
(Camden Primary Care Trust)

GP S H GRAHAM, T M SMITH

Prince of Wales Road Surgery
87-89 Prince of Wales Road, London NW5 3NT
Tel: 020 7284 3888 Fax: 020 7267 6067
(Camden Primary Care Trust)

GP Philip John MATTHEWMAN

London, NW6

Belsize Priory Health Centre
208 Belsize Road, London NW6 4DX
Tel: 020 7625 6181 Fax: 020 7530 2661
(Camden Primary Care Trust)
Patient List Size: 1100

Practice Manager Susan Aaron, Monica Jankel

GP Susannah Rose LUKSENBERG

Belsize Priory Medical Practice
208 Belsize Road, London NW6 4DX
Tel: 020 7530 2666 Fax: 020 7372 2404
Email: reception.bpmp@nhs.uk
(Camden Primary Care Trust)
Patient List Size: 5300

Practice Manager Maryla Wood

GP M V SHAH, D S GREENHOW, K W MAN

Belsize Priory Medical Practice
208 Belsize Road, London NW6 4DX
Tel: 020 7530 2666 Fax: 020 7530 2645
Email: reception.bpmp@nhs.net
(Camden Primary Care Trust)
Patient List Size: 5057

Practice Manager M Wood

GP Mansukhlal Vershi SHAH, Aythen ELKINDI, K W MAN

Brondesbury Medical Centre
279 Kilburn High Road, Kilburn, London NW6 7JQ
Tel: 020 7624 9853 Fax: 020 7372 3660
(Camden Primary Care Trust)
Patient List Size: 13000

Practice Manager E Orr

GP Helen Sharon HALPERN, Richard Charles MENDALL, Alan Frederick ROSENFELDER, Tag El Baha'a Ahmed Fathi SHERIF, Adrian Nicholas WAYNE

Cambridge Gardens Surgery
18 Cambridge Gardens, London NW6 5AY
Tel: 020 7624 1034 Fax: 020 7328 8193
(Brent Teaching Primary Care Trust)

GP John Michael LUCAS, S L MEHRA

Cholmley Gardens Surgery
1 Cholmley Gardens, Mill Lane, London NW6 1AE
Tel: 020 7794 6256 Fax: 020 7794 0540
(Camden Primary Care Trust)
Patient List Size: 3500

Practice Manager Gail Green

GP Eric ANSELL, Miranda ABRAHAM

Compayne Gardens Surgery
Flat 1, 10 Compayne Gardens, London NW6 3DH
Tel: 0870 890 2440 Fax: 0870 890 2441
(Camden Primary Care Trust)
Patient List Size: 6500

Practice Manager John Orr

GP C R EDMONDSON, D M KANSAGRA, S C SMITH

Fortune Green Road Surgery
80 Fortune Green Road, London NW6 1DS
Tel: 020 7794 9566 Fax: 020 7431 0789
(Camden Primary Care Trust)

Practice Manager Jacky Carby

GP Dr MAHMUD, Sumara NADEEM

Kilburn Park Medical Centre
12 Cambridge Gardens, London NW6 5AY
Tel: 020 7624 2414 Fax: 020 7624 2489
(Brent Teaching Primary Care Trust)

Practice Manager Julie Finnigan

GP Gillian Anne BRAUNOLD, Alison HILL, Fabia Melanie SHAW, Andrew Lawson TATE

Lonsdale Medical Centre
24 Lonsdale Road, London NW6 6RR
Tel: 020 7328 8331 Fax: 020 7328 8630
Website: www.lonsdalemedicalcentre.com

(Brent Teaching Primary Care Trust)
Patient List Size: 13300

Practice Manager Roger Bailey

GP Stephen Roger ILIFFE, Frances Louise CUNNINGHAM, Levin Anthony Timon DAVID, Heather DAVIS, Daniel DIETCH, Christine Helen FORD, Lisa Jane MILLER, Elizabeth MURRAY, Tajoin Alibhai PRADHAN

Malvern Surgery
105 Malvern Road, London NW6 5PU
Tel: 020 7328 3625 Fax: 020 7328 3326
(Brent Teaching Primary Care Trust)
Patient List Size: 1500

Practice Manager Debbie Nimblette

GP Margaret OBIEKWE

The Medical Centre
17-19 Clarence Road, London NW6 7TG
Tel: 020 7624 1345 Fax: 020 7624 7292
(Brent Teaching Primary Care Trust)

GP M F HUSSAIN, Saravanamuthu MUTHULINGAM, Max SKOBLO

Mill Lane Medical Centre
112 Mill Lane, London NW6 1XQ
Tel: 020 7431 1588 Fax: 020 7431 8919
(Camden Primary Care Trust)
Patient List Size: 8000

Practice Manager Amanda Ure

GP Ivan OSRIN, Jonathan BARNETT, Marion NEWMAN

Park House Medical Centre
18 Harvist Road, London NW6 6SE
Tel: 020 8969 7711 Fax: 020 8969 8880
(Brent Teaching Primary Care Trust)
Patient List Size: 5600

Practice Manager Loris Guerguis

GP Barbara TOOTH, Sally C LANDAU

Peel Precinct Surgery
3 Peel Precinct, London NW6 5RE
Tel: 020 7372 2172
(Brent Teaching Primary Care Trust)
Patient List Size: 1920

GP A I SHAIKH

Solent Road Health Centre
9 Solent Road, London NW6 1TP
Tel: 020 7530 2588 Fax: 020 7530 2591
(Camden Primary Care Trust)

The Surgery
Chippenham Gardens, 2-8 Malvern Road, London NW6 5PP
Tel: 020 7328 3836 Fax: 020 7328 3839
(Westminster Primary Care Trust)
Patient List Size: 2500

GP Myrto ANGELOGLOU

The Surgery
341 Kilburn High Road, London NW6 7QB
Tel: 020 7624 4414 Fax: 020 7328 5158
(Brent Teaching Primary Care Trust)

GP K MAHMOOD

West End Lane Surgery
125 West End Lane, London NW6 2PB
Tel: 020 7624 1769
(Camden Primary Care Trust)

GP Michael Ellerston Muir GRASSE

London, NW7

Millway Medical Practice
Hartley Avenue, Mill Hill, London NW7 2HX
Tel: 020 8959 0888 Fax: 020 8959 7050
Website: www.millwaymedical.com
(Barnet Primary Care Trust)
Patient List Size: 15000

Practice Manager David Watson

GP Susan Valerie THWAITES, Daniela AMASANTI, Kay CHAN, Philip John Charles CUTTELL, Simon Adrian FIGA, Deborah Karen FROST, Stephanie Claire HITCHCOCK, Justin Luke Timothy PETER, Mahesh SAINI

Salcombe Gardens
8 Salcombe Gardens, Mill Hill, London NW7 2NT
Tel: 020 8959 6592 Fax: 020 8959 0112
(Barnet Primary Care Trust)
Patient List Size: 4000

Practice Manager Laura Rogers

GP Gabriella CLAASEN, Yew Cheen TANG

Sefton Avenue Surgery
3 Sefton Avenue, London NW7 3QB
Tel: 020 8959 1868 Fax: 020 8906 0595
(Barnet Primary Care Trust)
Patient List Size: 3900

Practice Manager Elene Wildman

GP Maria De Fatima Almeida GOMES, Anthony JOBIAS

London, NW8

Abbey Medical Centre
87-89 Abbey Road, London NW8 0AG
Tel: 020 7624 9383 Fax: 020 7328 2147
Email: abbeymedical@hotmail.com
(Camden Primary Care Trust)
Patient List Size: 8800

Practice Manager Susan Ings

GP Antonios Kyriacou ANTONIOU, B FASHOLA, Doris Anne LISTER, Asma SIDDIQI, P SUPER

Bakker, Brown, Jacobs and Wormell
Lisson Grove Health Centre, Gateforth Street, London NW8 8EG
Tel: 020 7723 2213 Fax: 020 7723 4961
(Westminster Primary Care Trust)

GP Adam Antoni BAKKER, Ruth Alicia BROWN, Leonard JACOBS, H MINTZ, Robert Hugh Dillon WORMELL

Lisson Grove Health Centre
Gateforth St, London NW8 8EG
Tel: 020 7262 1366 Fax: 020 7258 1943
(Westminster Primary Care Trust)

GP Brian JARMAN, Andrew Hill ELDER, Gillian Frances EVANS, Naomi Susan GILLINGHAM, Henry Gilbert MINTZ, Neville Richard PURSSELL, Sally Margaret TAYLOR, Joseph Frederick WILTON

St Johns Wood Medical Practice
22 St. Anne's Terrace, London NW8 6PJ
Tel: 020 7722 7389 Fax: 020 7722 9722
(Westminster Primary Care Trust)

Practice Manager Sue Nicholson

GP Steven Mark CHARKIN, Dennis Isaac ABADI, Naomi CRAFT, Rhian JONES, Judith MILLER

Wellington Health Centre
16 Wellington Road, St John's Wood, London NW8 9SP
Tel: 020 7722 3382 Fax: 020 7722 2390
(Westminster Primary Care Trust)
Patient List Size: 6000

Practice Manager Carole Bartholomew

GP Maria CONSTANTINIDOU, Edward LEIGH, Alex TOILEGKENDIS

London, NW9

Colindeep Lane Surgery
61 Colindeep Lane, Colindale, London NW9 6DJ
Tel: 020 8205 6798 Fax: 020 8200 5242
(Barnet Primary Care Trust)
Patient List Size: 2200

GP Manubhai Karsanbhai LAMBA

Dr Rashid
25 Sheaveshill Avenue, Colindale, London NW9 6SE
Tel: 020 8205 2336
(Barnet Primary Care Trust)

GP Badr Ur RASHID

Fryent Medical Centre
331 Church Lane, London NW9 8JD
Tel: 020 8205 6262/1687 Fax: 020 8200 3088
(Barnet Primary Care Trust)

GP K H LEVERE, R K BABU-NARAYAN

Grahame Park Health Centre
The Concourse, Grahame Park Estate, London NW9 5XT
Tel: 020 8205 2301 Fax: 020 8200 9173
(Barnet Primary Care Trust)
Patient List Size: 8900

Practice Manager P Halfteck

GP Alan Stuart FOX, Robert Neil LIPMAN, Halima MIRZA, Ila Dushyant THAKKAR

Kings Edge Medical Centre
132 Stag Lane, Kingsbury, London NW9 0QP
Tel: 020 8204 0151
(Brent Teaching Primary Care Trust)
Patient List Size: 4500

Practice Manager Pragna Damani

GP Pratapnarain Vishnudatt KUMAR, M AK, T GHOSH, N QUREST

Stag Lane Medical Centre
245 Stag Lane, London NW9 0EF
Tel: 020 8204 0777
(Harrow Primary Care Trust)
Patient List Size: 2900

Practice Manager R K Gorsia

GP Amritlal Jinabhai MODI

The Surgery
46 Girton Avenue, London NW9 9SU
Tel: 020 8206 1490 Fax: 020 8206 1490
Email: neena.banerjeec@gp-e84662.nhs.uk
(Harrow Primary Care Trust)
Patient List Size: 2200

Practice Manager Izabella Bakhshi

GP Neena BANERJEE

The Surgery
22 Fryent Way, Kingsbury, London NW9 9SB
Tel: 020 8204 8228
(Brent Teaching Primary Care Trust)

GP A G E FUNG, Peter David KRAUS, Kumud A PATEL, Ajit Hirji SHAH

The Surgery
5 Brampton Road, Kingsbury, London NW9 9BX
Tel: 020 8204 6919 Fax: 020 8206 0883
Website: upender.sobti@gp-E84049.nhs.uk
(Brent Teaching Primary Care Trust)
Patient List Size: 2190

GP Upender Kaur SOBTI

Willow Tree Family Doctors
301 Kingsbury Road, London NW9 9PE
Tel: 020 8204 6464 Fax: 020 8905 0946
(Brent Teaching Primary Care Trust)
Patient List Size: 10500

Practice Manager Jo Dunkley-Hughes

GP Alan SELWYN, Rhiannon Vaughan LLOYD, Claire Patricia MITCHELL, Upma SHAH, Rebecca ZAMIR

London, NW10

Banerjee
Craven Park Health Centre, Shakespeare Crescent, London NW10 8XW
Tel: 020 8965 0151 Fax: 020 8838 3579
(Brent Teaching Primary Care Trust)

Practice Manager Carole Thurgood

GP Kajali BANERJEE, S K BANERJEE, A MONDAL

Bowman and Khan
Craven Park Health Centre, Shakespeare Crescent, London NW10 8XW
Tel: 020 8965 0151 Fax: 020 8965 4921
(Brent Teaching Primary Care Trust)
Patient List Size: 3975

Practice Manager Joyce Popely

GP Pearl BOWMAN, Mulbagal Afzal Ali KHAN

Brentfield Medical Centre
10 Kingfisher Way, Brentfield Road, London NW10 8TF
Tel: 020 8459 8833 Fax: 020 8459 9599
(Brent Teaching Primary Care Trust)
Patient List Size: 10000

Practice Manager Caroline Kerby

GP Selina Louise GELLERT, Carole Ann Ebiwari AMOBI, Andrew Ronald GELLERT, Rowland HUGHES, Dharmesh SHAH

Chamberlayne Road Surgery
124 Chamberlayne Road, London NW10 3JP
(Brent Teaching Primary Care Trust)

GP Dr PATEL

Church End Medical Centre
66 Mayo Road, Church End Estate, Willesden, London NW10 9HP
Tel: 020 8930 6262 Fax: 020 8930 6260
Email: cemc@gp-E84013.nhs.uk
(Brent Teaching Primary Care Trust)
Patient List Size: 7500

Practice Manager Cathy Allcard

GP Lucille KAY, Jonathan AGRANOFI, Cyril EVBUOMWAN, Etheldreda Kee Ching KONG, Ijeoma UKACHUKWU

Craven Park Health Centre
Shakespeare Crescent, London NW10 8XW
Tel: 020 8965 0151 Fax: 020 8965 4921
(Brent Teaching Primary Care Trust)
Patient List Size: 4200

Practice Manager Carole Thurgood

GP S K BANERJEE

Craven Park Medical Centre
6 Craven Park, London NW10 8SY
Tel: 020 8965 3396 Fax: 020 8965 7457
(Brent Teaching Primary Care Trust)

GP Ramesh Ramanlal DHARIA

Dr Deshmukh and Partners
The Medical Centre, 144-150 High Road, Willesden, London NW10 2PJ
Tel: 020 8459 5550 Fax: 020 8451 7268
Website: www.willesdenmedicalcentre.co.uk

(Brent Teaching Primary Care Trust)
Patient List Size: 14222

Practice Manager Patsy Campbell

GP Sheela B DESHMUKH, Mukesh DATTANI, Ameeta GAJJAR, Pushpa KUMARAN, Antonypillai Manuelpillai PETER, Sangeeta RAMDAHEN-GOPAL, Smita SAMANI

Freuchen Medical Centre
190 High Street, Harlesden, London NW10 4ST
Tel: 020 8965 5174 Fax: 020 8838 0255
(Brent Teaching Primary Care Trust)
Patient List Size: 6300

Practice Manager Pearl Curran

GP Soma PANCH, Kalyani KIRUBAHARAN, Kuga PADIKALINGHAM

Greenhill Park Medical Centre
Greenhill Park, Harlesden, London NW10 9AR
Tel: 020 8965 7128 Fax: 020 8838 1303
Email: gurdas.israni@gp-e84650.nhs.uk
(Brent Teaching Primary Care Trust)
Patient List Size: 2783

GP Gurdas Kewalram ISRANI

Law Medical Group Practice
9 Wrottesley Road, London NW10 5UY
Tel: 020 8965 8011 Fax: 020 8961 6239
(Brent Teaching Primary Care Trust)
Patient List Size: 11850

Practice Manager Carole Khiari

GP Jennifer SHIELDS, Lucille Naomi ABRAHAMS, Derek Anthony COFFMAN, Anita KAPOOR, Andrew MILNE, Adrian RICHARDSON

Mathew, George and Murugesu
2-4 Buckingham Road, Harlesden, London NW10 4RR
Tel: 020 8965 6078 Fax: 020 8961 9315
(Brent Teaching Primary Care Trust)
Patient List Size: 7000

Practice Manager M Harriott

GP K S MATHEW, R K GEORGE, Indrani MURUGESU

Roundwood Park Medical Centre
Pound Lane Clinic, 63 Pound Lane, London NW10 2HH
Tel: 020 8459 0336 Fax: 020 8451 8810
(Brent Teaching Primary Care Trust)

Practice Manager J Wicks

GP Godafreed Sorab IRANI, Prakash Thakurdas CHATLANI

Singh
Craven Park Health Centre, Shakespeare Crescent, London NW10 8XW
Tel: 020 8965 0151 Fax: 020 8965 4921
(Brent Teaching Primary Care Trust)
Patient List Size: 3000

Practice Manager Peter Anand

GP Shatrughna Prasad SINGH, S V BUSHAN

The Surgery
77 Burnley Road, London NW10 1EE
Tel: 020 8452 7689
(Brent Teaching Primary Care Trust)

GP Samuel Chinatu WOKO

The Surgery
99 High Road, Willesden Green, London NW10 2SL
Tel: 020 8459 0579 Fax: 020 8830 1992
(Brent Teaching Primary Care Trust)

Practice Manager Judy Fazal

GP Osita Godfrey AGBIM

The Surgery
26A Park Road, Harlesden, London NW10 8TA
Tel: 020 8965 5255 Fax: 020 8965 9080
(Brent Teaching Primary Care Trust)

Practice Manager Denise Woolich

GP John Gevenson WOOLICH, Bachubhai Bhogilal PATEL

The Surgery
85-87 Acton Lane, Harlesden, London NW10 8UT
Tel: 020 89611183 Fax: 020 89614785
(Brent Teaching Primary Care Trust)

GP I P PATEL

The Village Medical Centre
20 Braemar Avenue, Neasden, London NW10 0DJ
Tel: 020 8450 5405 Fax: 020 8450 5405
(Brent Teaching Primary Care Trust)
Patient List Size: 2660

Practice Manager Padma Bhargava

GP Sandhya BHARGAVA

Willesden Green Surgery
125 High Road, Willesden, London NW10 2SR
Tel: 020 8459 7755 Fax: 020 8459 7809
(Brent Teaching Primary Care Trust)

GP Stephen Daniel FLETCHER, Satnam Kaur BAURA

London, NW11

Beechcroft Avenue Surgery
20 Beechcroft Avenue, Golders Green, London NW11 8BL
Tel: 020 8455 9994
(Barnet Primary Care Trust)

GP Joseph Samuel ADLER

Dr Cavendish
73 Hodford Road, London NW11 8NH
Tel: 020 8905 5234
(Barnet Primary Care Trust)

Practice Manager Carole Carlton

GP Michael Neil CAVENDISH

The Drive Surgery
90 The Drive, London NW11 9UL
Tel: 020 8455 5901 Fax: 020 8731 9517
(Barnet Primary Care Trust)

GP Jayantilal Chhaganlal SHAH

Finchley Road Surgery
999 Finchley Road, London NW11 7HB
Tel: 020 8458 5708
(Barnet Primary Care Trust)

GP Emma MUKHERJEE

Finchley Road Surgery
682 Finchley Road, Golders Green, London NW11 7NP
Tel: 020 8455 9994 Fax: 020 8458 9183
Email: manager@gp-e83600.nhs.uk
(Barnet Primary Care Trust)
Patient List Size: 4500

Practice Manager Avava Adler

GP Joseph Samuel ADLER, Richard Henry Marshall TELLER

Golders Green Road Surgery
188 Golders Green Road, London NW11 9AY
Tel: 020 8455 1907
(Barnet Primary Care Trust)
Patient List Size: 7561

Practice Manager John Bentley

GP Tina GRIMBLE, John BENTLEY

Northway Surgery
41 Northway, London NW11 6PB
Tel: 020 8458 2751

(Barnet Primary Care Trust)

GP Natasha ROSE

Ravenscroft Medical Centre
166-168 Golders Green Road, London NW11 8BB
Tel: 020 8455 2477 Fax: 020 8201 8298
Email: jane.davis@gp-e83039.nhs.uk
(Barnet Primary Care Trust)
Patient List Size: 7000

Practice Manager J Davis

GP Brian Jonathan GOLDEN, Paul Stephen BLOM, Stuart Samuel WOLFMAN

Temple Fortune Health Centre
23 Temple Fortune Lane, London NW11 7TE
Tel: 020 8458 4431 Fax: 020 8731 8257
(Barnet Primary Care Trust)

GP Karen Ruth GROSSMARK, Christopher Murray PAGE, Peter Jeremy HERBERT

Temple Fortune Health Centre
23 Temple Fortune Lane, London NW11 7TE
Tel: 020 8458 4431 Fax: 020 8731 8257
(Barnet Primary Care Trust)

GP Martin HARRIS

Temple Fortune Health Centre
23 Temple Fortune Lane, London NW11 7TE
Tel: 020 8458 4431 Fax: 020 8731 8257
(Barnet Primary Care Trust)
Patient List Size: 2150

Practice Manager June Kavanagh

GP L HARVERD, Dr GROSSMARK, Dr HERBERT, Dr PAGE

Temple Fortune Health Centre
23 Temple Fortune Lane, London NW11 7TE
Tel: 020 8458 4431 Fax: 020 8731 8257
(Barnet Primary Care Trust)

Practice Manager L Fogg

GP Laurence BUCKMAN

Temple Fortune Health Centre
23 Temple Fortune Lane, London NW11 7TE
Tel: 020 8458 4431
(Barnet Primary Care Trust)

GP Karen Ruth GROSSMARK, Peter Jeremy HERBERT, Christopher Murray PAGE

London, SE1

Abu-Nijaila
182-184 Old Kent Road, London SE1 5TY
Tel: 020 7252 6272 Fax: 020 7252 6474
(Southwark Primary Care Trust)
Patient List Size: 4100

Practice Manager Jill Capeless

GP A A ABU-NIJAILA, M DABIKIKHAH, M C VILLARD

Bermondsey and Lansdowne Medical Centre
The Surgery, Decima Street, London SE1 4QX
Tel: 020 7407 0752 Fax: 020 7378 8209
(Southwark Primary Care Trust)

Practice Manager Lin Clark

GP Christopher Oliver PAYNE, Carol LEE, Kathryn Dorothy McADAM-FREUD, Rebecca TORRY

Blackfriars Medical Practice
45 Columbo Street, London SE1 8EE
Tel: 020 7928 6216 Fax: 020 7928 7958
(Southwark Primary Care Trust)
Patient List Size: 4550

Practice Manager Mr Mehta

GP S S CHUDHA, I BENARD, P WALL

Borough Medical Centre
1-5 Newington Causeway, London SE1 6ED
Tel: 020 7357 0288 Fax: 020 7378 0865
(Southwark Primary Care Trust)

GP Kaushal Kishore MISRA

Falmouth Road Surgery
78 Falmouth Road, London SE1 4JW
Tel: 020 7407 4101/0945 Fax: 020 7357 6170
(Southwark Primary Care Trust)
Patient List Size: 9000

Practice Manager Anne Morabito

GP Thomas Bradley CLARK, Margaret GUINEY, Hilary Anne LAVENDER, G RAANA, Ian Mitchell STONE, Alison Po Ling WONG

The Grange Road Practice
108 Grange Road, London SE1 3BW
Tel: 020 7237 1078 Fax: 020 7771 3550
(Southwark Primary Care Trust)
Patient List Size: 7200

Practice Manager June Robinson

GP M BROOKS

Guys and St Thomas' Group Practice
Guys Hospital, St Thomas Street, London SE1 7EH
Tel: 020 7955 2851 Fax: 020 7407 6112
(Southwark Primary Care Trust)

GP Dr SHAPIRO

Lee
249 Old Kent Road, London SE1 5LU
Tel: 020 7237 2492 Fax: 020 7237 1076
(Southwark Primary Care Trust)

GP Sarah Lian Choo LEE

Mill Street Clinic
1 Wolseley Street, London SE1 2BP
Tel: 020 7252 1817 Fax: 020 7394 6312
(Southwark Primary Care Trust)

GP Alan CAMPION

Parkers Row Family Practice
2 Wade House, Parkers Row, London SE1 2DN
Tel: 020 7237 1517 Fax: 020 7231 4275
(Southwark Primary Care Trust)
Patient List Size: 6800

Practice Manager Sue Connelly

GP Shabir Ahmad BHATTI, Ranjan DAS, Nancy KUTCHEMAN, Patna SOMALINGHAM

Princess Street Group Practice
2 Princess Street, London SE1 6JP
Tel: 020 7928 0253 Fax: 020 7261 9804
(Southwark Primary Care Trust)
Patient List Size: 12100

Practice Manager T L Bennett

GP Steven CURSON, Sarah Jane DOHERTY, Claire Pepita LLOYD, Raymond Allan Yves PIETRONI, S S S SOO

Waterloo Health Centre
5 Lower Marsh, London SE1 7RJ
Tel: 020 7928 4049 Fax: 020 7928 2644
(Lambeth Primary Care Trust)

Practice Manager Maureen Watson

GP Jane BECKLEY, Eithne Rose BRENNER, Richard WRIGLEY, Patrick William HARBOROW

London, SE2

Basildon Road Surgery
111 Basildon Road, Abbey Wood, London SE2 0ER
Tel: 020 8311 3917 Fax: 020 8310 3969
(Greenwich Teaching Primary Care Trust)

Practice Manager Joan Christer

GP M CHAND, R RAHMAN

Lakeside Health Centre
Tavy Bridge, Thamesmead, London SE2 9LH
Tel: 020 8310 3281 Fax: 020 8312 3867
(Bexley Care Trust)
Patient List Size: 13000

GP A G McCULLAGH, P K ANAND, F P GREGORY, T F W KOELMEL, P A MILSTEIN, L M ROBERTS, E SLATER, V A TODD

The Surgery
9 Godstow Road, Abbey Wood, London SE2 9AT
Tel: 020 8310 7066 Fax: 020 8311 8867
(Greenwich Teaching Primary Care Trust)
Patient List Size: 8000

Practice Manager Tara Armsby

GP David Robert PULSFORD, Abdul Karim AL-ZAIDY, S G KERUR, H E ONEYEKWELU

London, SE3

Apurba House Surgery
154a Shooters Hill Road, Blackheath, London SE3 8RP
Tel: 020 8856 4990 Fax: 020 8856 1056
(Greenwich Teaching Primary Care Trust)

Practice Manager Geeta Borooah

GP Pabitra Ram BOROOAH, Katharine MURI

The Blackheath Standard Surgery
11-13 Charlton Road, Blackheath, London SE3 7HB
Tel: 0870 417 6555 Fax: 020 8293 9286
(Greenwich Teaching Primary Care Trust)
Patient List Size: 8400

Practice Manager Rose Cork

GP Grace Patricia WHITFIELD, Liman Mahamoud MUHAMMAD, Nayan PATEL, Suresh Kanubhai PATEL

Henley Cross Medical Practice
115 Tudway Road, Ferrier Estate, Kidbrooke, London SE3 9YX
Tel: 020 8856 4167 Fax: 020 8856 1269
(Greenwich Teaching Primary Care Trust)

Practice Manager Carol Streek

GP Satish Kumar BASSI

Manor Brook Medical Centre
117 Brook Lane, London SE3 0EN
Tel: 020 8856 5678 Fax: 020 8856 8632
(Greenwich Teaching Primary Care Trust)
Patient List Size: 11000

Practice Manager Sharon Kelly

GP J LONG, Ruth Carol MARCHANT, Cornelia Ann McCARTHY, Juliet MILLWATERS, Martin Barry POWELL, Richard John WOOLLETT

The Surgery
20 Lee Road, Blackheath, London SE3 9RT
Tel: 020 8852 1235/8018 Fax: 020 8297 2193
(Lewisham Primary Care Trust)
Patient List Size: 10000

Practice Manager Janet Fitzgerald

GP Robert Alan LUMB, Penelope Jane MILNER, Alan Brian Robert THOMPSON, Desmond George THOMPSON, Jacqueline Eleanor URWIN

The Surgery
10-12 Carnbrook Road, London SE3 8AE
Tel: 020 8319 3303 Fax: 020 8319 3265
Email: tsnathanhs@hotmail.com
(Greenwich Teaching Primary Care Trust)
Patient List Size: 1530

Practice Manager Growey Nathan

GP T SITHAMPARANATHAN

The Surgery
30-31 Telemann Square, Ferrier Estate, London SE3 9YR
Tel: 020 8856 1800 Fax: 020 8319 0500
(Greenwich Teaching Primary Care Trust)

Practice Manager Devinda Guram

GP Nardip Singh GURAM

The Surgery
115 Tudway Road, Ferrier Estate, Kidbrooke, London SE3 9YX
Tel: 020 8856 4167 Fax: 020 8856 1269
(Greenwich Teaching Primary Care Trust)

Practice Manager Carol Streek

GP D MAHESH

The Surgery
67 Charlton Road, Blackheath, London SE3 8TJ
Tel: 020 8858 8513 Fax: 020 8293 9615
(Greenwich Teaching Primary Care Trust)

Practice Manager Lin Findley

GP S J RATNARAJAN

London, SE4

Dr Kahlon Surgery
228 Lewisham Way, London SE4 1XL
Tel: 020 8692 2707
(Lewisham Primary Care Trust)

GP Karnail Singh KAHLON

Hilly Fields Medical Centre
172 Adelaide Avenue, London SE4 1JN
Tel: 020 8314 5552 Fax: 020 8314 5557
(Lewisham Primary Care Trust)
Patient List Size: 11102

Practice Manager Smita Malde, Michael Sharpe

GP Girish Mulchandbhai MALDE, Michael A ADESI, Faruk MAJID, Paula S O'DONNELL, Olek Andrew SOBOLEWSKI

Honor Oak Health Centre
20 Turnham Road, London SE4 2LA
Tel: 020 7639 9797
(Lewisham Primary Care Trust)
Patient List Size: 6880

Practice Manager Linda Swinden

GP Frank Richard NEAL, C DE SILVA, Eric William FELLOWS, Andrew Mark WATTS

O Khan and Shanmugasundaram
467 Brockley Road, London SE4 2PJ
Tel: 020 8291 4249 Fax: 020 8699 6291
(Lewisham Primary Care Trust)
Patient List Size: 5000

GP R SHANMUGASUNDARAM, O KHAN

St Johns Medical Centre
287A Lewisham Way, London SE4 1XF
(Lewisham Primary Care Trust)

GP Jean Helen PARKER, Elzbieta PAWLOWSKA

The Surgery
58 Vesta Road, Lewisham, London SE4 2NH
Tel: 020 7639 0654 Fax: 020 7358 9930

(Lewisham Primary Care Trust)
Patient List Size: 4620

Practice Manager Sue Flemming, Alex Gietzen, Rita Knight

GP Ralph BERMAN, Khaled ABOKARSH

London, SE5

Corner Surgery
99 Coldharbour Lane, London SE5 9NS
Tel: 020 7274 4507 Fax: 020 7733 6545
(Lambeth Primary Care Trust)
Patient List Size: 4000

Practice Manager J Tsoneva

GP Helen Jane Whiston BAKER, Stephanie KLEIN, David Harold WICKSTEAD

Dickinson
3 Sir John Kirk Close, London SE5 0BB
Tel: 020 7703 2046 Fax: 020 7277 2240
Email: reception@gp-G85050.hns.uk
Website: www.sirjohnkirkclosesurgery@nhs.uk
(Southwark Primary Care Trust)
Patient List Size: 3200

Practice Manager Mandy Lochrane

GP Lewis DICKINSON

The Hambleden Clinic
Blanchedown, Dulwich, London SE5 8HL
Tel: 020 7274 3939 Fax: 020 7274 6007
Email: peter.mccreedy-may@gp-g85112.nhs.uk
Website: www.hambledenclinic.nhs.uk
(Southwark Primary Care Trust)
Patient List Size: 3000

GP Patricia CRITCHLEY, H MBIANDJI

Parkside Medical Centre
52 Camberwell Green, London SE5 7AQ
Tel: 020 7703 0596 Fax: 020 7701 0044
(Southwark Primary Care Trust)
Patient List Size: 5000

Practice Manager Diane Gayle

GP Sarah LEDINGHAM, George VARUGHESE, Azra Parveen PARVEZ

St Giles Surgery
40 St. Giles Road, London SE5 7RF
Tel: 020 7252 5936
(Southwark Primary Care Trust)

GP Azad Jashbhai PATEL, Elizabeth Anne BEGLEY, Joan Jemima ROSEMEN, Kishorchandra VASANT, A N VIRJI

St Giles Surgery
40 St Giles Road, London SE5 7RF
Tel: 020 7252 5936 Fax: 020 7701 6199
(Southwark Primary Care Trust)

GP Dr VIRJI

The Surgery
13 Camberwell Green, London SE5 7AF
Tel: 020 7703 3788 Fax: 020 7701 2361
(Southwark Primary Care Trust)

Practice Manager Sue Kingham

GP Roger Stephen DURSTON, Christopher Edward BROWNSDON, Helen Margaret COTTON, Jonathan Mark Patrick MORTIMER, Andrew Martin ROWELL, Yvonne YUHAZ

The Surgery
144 Grove Lane, London SE5 8BP
Tel: 020 7274 3762 Fax: 020 7274 3762
(Southwark Primary Care Trust)
Patient List Size: 1600

GP Umapati BISWAS

London, SE6

Bellingham Green Surgery
24 Bellingham Green, London SE6 3JB
Tel: 020 8697 7285 Fax: 020 8695 6094
(Lewisham Primary Care Trust)
Patient List Size: 6200

Practice Manager Rosie Colwell

GP David Paul MISSELBROOK, Wendy Gillian GASKELL, Janet Elizabeth McCREDIE, David Stephen SHARPE, Nicholas John SURRIDGE

Boundfield Medical Centre
103 Boundfield Road, London SE6 1PG
Tel: 020 8697 2920 Fax: 020 8697 2920
(Lewisham Primary Care Trust)

Practice Manager Maureen Spencer

GP Jayashri Sreenivasarao PAVAR

Mani-Babu
50 Muirkirk Road, London SE6 1BQ
Tel: 020 8697 2810
(Lewisham Primary Care Trust)

GP A MANI-BABU

Perry Hill Surgery
145 Perry Hill, London SE6 4LR
Tel: 020 8699 1062
(Lewisham Primary Care Trust)
Patient List Size: 6500

Practice Manager Marie Ah Moye

GP Hilary Jane ENTWISTLE, Nan DOBLE, Karen Margaret MacAUSLAN

South Lewisham Group Practice
50 Conisborough Crescent, London SE6 2SP
Tel: 020 8698 8921 Fax: 020 7771 4025
Email: slhc@gp-G85005.nhs.uk
Website: www.southlewishamgp.co.uk
(Lewisham Primary Care Trust)
Patient List Size: 12823

Practice Manager Sandra Evans

GP K ISMAIL, Arun GUPTA, R JETHA, R KANPATHAPPILLAI, James Francis LEE, Russell James O'BRIEN

The Surgery
186 Brownhill Road, London SE6 1AT
Tel: 020 8698 6566
(Lewisham Primary Care Trust)

GP L N DAS, L SAVARY

Torridon Road Medical Practice
80 Torridon Road, London SE6 1RA
Tel: 020 8698 5281 Fax: 020 8695 1841
(Lewisham Primary Care Trust)
Patient List Size: 10500

Practice Manager Mike Munns

GP Markandu RAGUPATHY, Tan Dung NGUYEN, Esther Suganthaleela SELVANATHAN

London, SE7

The Fairfield Centre
Fairfield Grove, Charlton, London SE7 8TX
Tel: 020 8858 5738 Fax: 020 8305 3005
(Greenwich Teaching Primary Care Trust)

Practice Manager Karen James

GP Stephen John PALMER, Derek Colvin ABEL, Diane Gustavia BROWNE, Sarah Helen CORSTON, Elizabeth Jane DICKSON, Karen FRANKIS

London, SE8

Grove Medical Centre
Windlass Place, London SE8 3QH
Tel: 020 8692 1882 Fax: 020 8691 1703
(Lewisham Primary Care Trust)
Patient List Size: 7300

Practice Manager A Davis

GP Akber MOHAMEDALI, Ann RILEY

The Kingfisher Medical Centre
3 Kingfisher Square, Staunton Street, London SE8 5DA
Tel: 020 8692 7373 Fax: 020 8691 6572
Email: kingfisher@gp-G85020.nhs.uk
(Lewisham Primary Care Trust)

Practice Manager Liam Doherty

GP Ashok Kumar Motilal JAIN, Asha JAIN, Lionel SAVARY, Robert WOLFF

The Surgery
309 Evelyn Street, Deptford, London SE8 5RA
Tel: 020 8469 3090 Fax: 020 8691 2525
(Greenwich Teaching Primary Care Trust)

Practice Manager F Hormasji

GP Khalida Zia HASHMI

Waldron Health Centre
Stanley Street, London SE8 4BG
Tel: 020 8692 2314
(Lewisham Primary Care Trust)

GP I HASSAN, M IRVING, S SINGH

Waldron Health Centre
Stanley Street, London SE8 4BG
Tel: 020 8692 3952 Fax: 020 8692 0606
(Lewisham Primary Care Trust)

Waldron Health Centre
Stanley Street, London SE8 4BG
Tel: 020 8691 0144 Fax: 020 8692 5094
(Lewisham Primary Care Trust)
Patient List Size: 4000 approx

Practice Manager Urmila Batra

GP Bhupinder Kumar BATRA

Waldron Health Centre
Stanley Street, Deptford, London SE8 4BG
Tel: 020 8692 3152 Fax: 020 8692 0606
Email: drjamil@gp-G85043.nhs.uk
(Lewisham Primary Care Trust)
Patient List Size: 3500

Practice Manager Debby Boulton

GP M A Q JAMIL

London, SE9

The Coldharbour Surgery
79 William Barefoot Drive, Eltham, London SE9 3JD
Tel: 020 8857 3472 Fax: 020 8851 6471
Email: m.baksh@gp-G83003.nhs.uk
(Greenwich Teaching Primary Care Trust)
Patient List Size: 4150

Practice Manager Len Franklin

GP Madhu BAKSH, Ramesh A PATEL

The Coldharbour Surgery
79 William Barefoot Drive, Eltham, London SE9 3JD
Tel: 020 8857 1900 Fax: 020 8857 7778
(Greenwich Teaching Primary Care Trust)
Patient List Size: 4200

GP Suppiah RATNESWAREN

Court Yard Surgery
John Evans House, 28 Court Yard, London SE9 5QA
Tel: 020 8850 5141 Fax: 020 8294 2380
(Greenwich Teaching Primary Care Trust)
Patient List Size: 10523

Practice Manager J Haill

GP Phyllis Irene CAMPBELL, Arbjit CHAUHAN, Dermot Alexander KENNY

Eltham Park Surgery
46 Westmount Road, London SE9 1JE
Tel: 020 8850 1030 Fax: 020 8859 2036
(Greenwich Teaching Primary Care Trust)
Patient List Size: 5000

Practice Manager Jennifer Coates

GP Aklakun Nesa KHANAM, John Stuart LIVINGSTONE

The Mound Medical Centre
4-6 The Mound, William Barefoot Drive, Eltham, London SE9 3AZ
Tel: 020 8857 1957 Fax: 020 8857 0386
Website: www.themoundmedicalcentre.co.uk
(Greenwich Teaching Primary Care Trust)
Patient List Size: 1800

Practice Manager Suzanne Francis

GP Veena AGARWAL

Sherard Road Medical Centre
71 Sherard Road, Eltham, London SE9 6ER
Tel: 020 8850 2120 Fax: 020 8850 1220
(Greenwich Teaching Primary Care Trust)
Patient List Size: 6000

Practice Manager Helen Oakley

GP Martin Frank HYATT, Vibha Rohit RAO

The Surgery
480 Footscray Road, New Eltham, London SE9 3UA
Tel: 020 8850 2458 Fax: 020 8859 5763
(Greenwich Teaching Primary Care Trust)
Patient List Size: 3500

Practice Manager Linda Batten

GP Jawahar LAL, K L SHAHAB

The Surgery
21 Shawbrooke Road, Eltham, London SE9 6AE
Tel: 020 8850 1613 Fax: 020 8859 5199
(Greenwich Teaching Primary Care Trust)

GP Victor Lartey ACQUAAH, Benedict KAWOOYA

The Surgery
1 Alderwood Road, Eltham, London SE9 2JY
Tel: 020 8850 4008 Fax: 020 8859 3361
(Greenwich Teaching Primary Care Trust)
Patient List Size: 3000

Practice Manager N Peiris

GP Pushpa PEIRIS, Nandin Ariyamithra DE SILVA

The Surgery
Briset Corner, 591 Westhorne Avenue, Eltham, London SE9 6JX
Tel: 020 8850 5022 Fax: 020 8859 6096
(Greenwich Teaching Primary Care Trust)
Patient List Size: 3000

Practice Manager J Lankester

GP Surinder Kumar SENNIK

The Surgery
118 Restons Crescent, Eltham, London SE9 2JJ
Tel: 020 8859 7941 Fax: 020 8859 2382
(Greenwich Teaching Primary Care Trust)
Patient List Size: 2100

Practice Manager Irene Preston

GP Clarence Dayasiri THENUWARA

Well Hall Surgery
174-180 Well Hall Road, Eltham, London SE9 6SR
Tel: 020 8850 1615 Fax: 020 8294 1486
(Greenwich Teaching Primary Care Trust)

Practice Manager Janet Smith

GP Kevin McCARTHY

Westmount Surgery
191 Westmount Road, London SE9 1XY
Tel: 020 8850 1540 Fax: 020 8859 4737
(Greenwich Teaching Primary Care Trust)
Patient List Size: 3300

Practice Manager Lynda Forbes

GP Vasanti SANDRASAGRA

London, SE10

Burney Street Practice
48 Burney Street, London SE10 8EX
Tel: 020 8858 0631 Fax: 020 8293 9616
(Greenwich Teaching Primary Care Trust)

GP Gordon Oliver COCHRAN, Rashida AMIN, Andrew Paul BROWN, Helen Margaret PHILLIPS

South Street Medical Centre
71a Greenwich South Street, Greenwich, London SE10 8NT
Tel: 020 8293 3330 Fax: 020 8293 3303
(Greenwich Teaching Primary Care Trust)
Patient List Size: 9600

Practice Manager Tanya Greenland

GP Marko ANTTILA, Nageswary RATNESWAREN, L RUSSO, Suppiah THIRUKKANESAN

Vanbrugh Group Practice 2000
Vanbrugh Hill Health Centre, Vanbrugh Hill, Greenwich, London SE10 9HQ
Tel: 020 8312 6095 Fax: 020 8293 1226
(Greenwich Teaching Primary Care Trust)
Patient List Size: 9300

Practice Manager Christine Benford

GP Christine Barbara CHALLACOMBE, Zsuzsanna CASSIDY, Micaela GOSSLAU, Ellen Sylvia WRIGHT

Woodlands Surgery
Woodlands Walk, Off Trafalgar Road, London SE10 9UB
Tel: 020 8858 0689 Fax: 020 8293 9615
(Greenwich Teaching Primary Care Trust)

GP Nadarajan RATNARAJAN, Subathira Thevy RATNARAJAN

London, SE11

The Hurley Clinic
Ebenezer House, Kennington Lane, London SE11 4HJ
Tel: 020 7735 7918 Fax: 020 7587 5296
(Lambeth Primary Care Trust)
Patient List Size: 14000

GP David POOLE, Mark ASHWORTH, Frances Linda DUDLEY, Clare GERADA, Arvind Kumar MADAN, Cynthia Oi San YIU

Irani
204 Kennington Lane, London SE11 5DN
Tel: 020 7735 1770 Fax: 020 7582 4697
(Lambeth Primary Care Trust)

Practice Manager Kathy Lambert

GP Bejan Aspandiar IRANI

Lambeth Walk Group Practice
5 Lambeth Walk, London SE11 6SP
Tel: 020 7735 4412 Fax: 020 7840 9489
Email: firstname.surname@gp-g85054.nhs.uk
Website: www.lambethwalkgppractice.co.uk
(Lambeth Primary Care Trust)
Patient List Size: 8200

Practice Manager Sue Brown

GP Raj MITRA, Nird AMIN, D BIVONA, Alasdair HONEYMAN, James MAY

Shah
8 Jonathan Street, London SE11 5NH
Tel: 020 7735 1971 Fax: 020 7735 6619
(Lambeth Primary Care Trust)
Patient List Size: 2750

GP Kirit SHAH

London, SE12

Baring Road Medical Centre
282 Baring Road, Grove Park, London SE12 0DS
Tel: 020 8857 5682 Fax: 020 8851 6978
(Lewisham Primary Care Trust)
Patient List Size: 4000

Practice Manager Sharon Anderson, Steve Williams

GP Shashi B ARORA

Dr Sarker's Surgery
147 Baring Road, South Lee, London SE12 0LA
Tel: 020 8857 6333 Fax: 020 8516 0168
Email: sarker.osman@gp-g85718.nhs.uk
(Lewisham Primary Care Trust)
Patient List Size: 2400

GP O A SARKER

Lee Health Centre
2 Handen Road, London SE12 8NP
Tel: 020 8852 2611 Fax: 020 8297 8221
(Lewisham Primary Care Trust)
Patient List Size: 8300

Practice Manager F Syres

GP Ian Robert Joseph MacDONAGH, Leonardo Stelian ANTONY, John Christopher Patrick BENTHAM, P D MORGAN

Marvels Lane Health Centre
37 Marvels Lane, London SE12 8PN
Tel: 020 8857 4145
(Lewisham Primary Care Trust)

GP S LINGARAJAH

Nightingdale Surgery
2 Handen Road, Lewisham, London SE12 8NP
Tel: 020 8852 8074 Fax: 020 7771 4840
(Lewisham Primary Care Trust)
Patient List Size: 3000

Practice Manager Amanda Collins

GP Gnanapragasam Anton Joseph SELVANATHAN

The Surgery
32 Chinbrook Road, London SE12 9TH
Tel: 020 8857 4660 Fax: 020 8857 6374
(Lewisham Primary Care Trust)
Patient List Size: 2400

Practice Manager Isabel Jorquera

GP Yog Darshan MALIK, N BEGUM

Whitworth
234 Baring Road, London SE12 0UL
Tel: 020 8851 5212
(Lewisham Primary Care Trust)

GP Magda WHITWORTH

London, SE13

Abraham and Partners
21 Morden Hill, Lewisham, London SE13 7NN
Tel: 020 8469 2880 Fax: 020 8692 9399
(Lewisham Primary Care Trust)
Patient List Size: 8200

Practice Manager Sandy Seward

GP David Melville ABRAHAM, Michael BANNON, Siobhan Ellen Marie GIBBS, Anthony Charles GOSTLING, Catherine Margaret ROE

Campshill Surgery
Campshill Road, London SE13 6QU
Tel: 020 8852 1384
(Lewisham Primary Care Trust)

GP William Charles LETTINGTON

Hill and Partners
36 Belmont Hill, London SE13 5AY
Tel: 020 8852 8357 Fax: 020 8297 2011
(Lewisham Primary Care Trust)
Patient List Size: 6500

Practice Manager Sandy Cunningham

GP Michael David HILL, Marilyn Eileen ALISTER, Gail HOLLOWAY, Steven PIERPOINT

Lewisham Medical Centre
164 Lee High Road, London SE13 5PL
Tel: 020 8852 0079 Fax: 020 8297 0763
(Lewisham Primary Care Trust)
Patient List Size: 3500

Practice Manager Valerie Ayres

GP Benedict KAWOOYA

New Surgery
2 Morley Road, London SE13 6DQ
Tel: 020 8297 7999 Fax: 020 8297 7880
Email: uduku.newsurg@shaw.lslha.sthames.nhs.uk
(Lewisham Primary Care Trust)
Patient List Size: 3400

Practice Manager Beverley Moore

GP Catriona BRODIE, Ngozi Ola-Adetokunbo UDUKU

The Rushey Green Group Practice
Central Lewisham Clinic, 410 Lewisham High Street, London SE13 6LJ
Tel: 020 8314 5440
Email: rggp@gp-G85633.nhs.uk
(Lewisham Primary Care Trust)
Patient List Size: 6700

Practice Manager Charlotte Blyth

GP Richard Norman BYNG, J K C CHEN, Abbey GERSTEN, M MULLER

The Surgery
231 Algernon Road, London SE13 7AG
Tel: 020 8690 0333
(Lewisham Primary Care Trust)

GP A ST GEORGE

The Surgery
25 Lewisham Road, London SE13 7QS
Tel: 020 8692 7591 Fax: 020 8694 9947
(Greenwich Teaching Primary Care Trust)
Patient List Size: 2710

Practice Manager Tajinder Bajwa

GP M HASHIM

The Surgery
7 Lewisham Road, Lewisham, London SE13 7QS
Tel: 020 8691 0079 Fax: 020 8692 8677
(Greenwich Teaching Primary Care Trust)

Practice Manager A Mann

GP G KASINATHAN

Triangle Group Practice
2 Morley Road, London SE13 6DQ
Tel: 020 8318 7272 Fax: 020 8297 9519
(Lewisham Primary Care Trust)
Patient List Size: 7500

Practice Manager Joe Warner-Johnson

GP Barbara Ruth JACOBS, H HAMA, A McNAIR, H PANESHAR

London, SE14

Clifton Rise Medical Centre
27 Clifton Rise, London SE14 6ER
Tel: 020 8692 1387
(Lewisham Primary Care Trust)
Patient List Size: 5508

Practice Manager Antonia Makinde

GP Ratnam KANDAVEL, Sangarapillai JEYANATHAN

Dr H Bulter
42 Gellatly Road, London SE14 5TT
Tel: 020 7639 1027 Fax: 020 7639 2178
Email: gellatly.surgery@nhs.net
(Lewisham Primary Care Trust)

GP H BUTLER, S LAMB

Jayram Surgery
502-504 New Cross Road, London SE14 6TJ
(Lewisham Primary Care Trust)

GP Ram Nain TIWARY

The Medical Centre
24 Laurie Grove, London SE14 6NH
Tel: 020 8692 6427 Fax: 020 8691 9698
Email: recep.1@gp-g85076.nhs.uk
(Lewisham Primary Care Trust)
Patient List Size: 5200

Practice Manager L Gladding

GP Anne Elizabeth MACFARLANE, Maria Ghoula CHARMANTAS

Mornington Surgery
433 New Cross Road, London SE14 6TD
Tel: 020 8692 8299 Fax: 020 8691 2081
(Lewisham Primary Care Trust)
Patient List Size: 6000

Practice Manager Fiona Osborne

GP Saravanapalasuriyar SHRI KRISHNAPALASURIYAR, Md Osman Ghani SARDER

Queens Road Partnership
387 Queens Road, London SE14 5JN
Tel: 020 7635 2170 Fax: 020 7635 2175
Email: frances.andrews@gp-g85015.nhs.uk
Website: www.queensroadpartnership.co.uk
(Lewisham Primary Care Trust)
Patient List Size: 9567

Practice Manager F Andrews

GP P J RODRIGUES, M AQUILINA, C CHUNG, S KHAWADA, Pamela MARTIN, Kamran SAYYAH-SINA

London, SE15

Acorn Surgery
136 Meeting House Lane, London SE15 2TT
Tel: 020 7639 5055 Fax: 020 7732 4225
Website: www.acornsurgery.co.uk
(Southwark Primary Care Trust)
Patient List Size: 7445

Practice Manager David Jones

GP Anna Stefania RAKOWICZ, K AMUSAN, D V DAVE, A KHANDERIA

Hossain
Lister Health Centre, 25 Commercial Way, London SE15 6DP
Tel: 020 7277 1067 Fax: 020 7771 3810
(Southwark Primary Care Trust)

GP Dr HOSSAIN

Isidore Crown Medical Centre
60 Chadwick Road, London SE15 4PU
Tel: 020 7639 9622 Fax: 020 7732 0849
(Southwark Primary Care Trust)
Patient List Size: 7500

GP Michael Alan Kenneth DUGGAN

Kumar and Mehta
12 Queens Road, London SE15 2PT
Tel: 020 7639 1133
(Southwark Primary Care Trust)

GP Sanjay KUMAR, Prem Prakash MEHTA

Lister Health Centre
1 Camden Square, London SE15 3LW
Tel: 020 7708 5413 Fax: 020 7771 3810
(Southwark Primary Care Trust)
Patient List Size: 3800

Practice Manager S Stephenson

GP A MADAN, A ULLAH

The Nunhead Surgery
58 Nunhead Grove, London SE15 3LY
Tel: 020 7639 2715 Fax: 020 7635 6942
(Southwark Primary Care Trust)
Patient List Size: 6780

Practice Manager C Landrei

GP Yvonneke Olivia Walton ROE, Dominic ANDERSON, Martin LU

Peckham Hill Street Surgery
143 Peckham Hill Street, London SE15 5JZ
Tel: 020 7639 1133 Fax: 020 7277 7858
(Southwark Primary Care Trust)

GP Dr KUMAR

Sekweyama and Pratt
10 Trafalgar Avenue, London SE15 6NR
Tel: 020 7703 9271 Fax: 020 7252 7209
(Southwark Primary Care Trust)
Patient List Size: 4100

Practice Manager Laura Nagi

GP Silvanus Godfrey Galiwango SEKWEYAMA, Tunde PRATT

Sternhall Lane Surgery
12 Sternhall Lane, London SE15 4NT
Tel: 020 7639 3553 Fax: 020 7639 0835
(Southwark Primary Care Trust)

GP Dr VUKOTIC

The Surgery
Lister Health Centre, 25 Commercial Way, London SE15 6DP
Tel: 020 7277 1067 Fax: 020 7771 3810
(Southwark Primary Care Trust)

Practice Manager Rita Fletcher

GP Mahmood HOSSAIN, David Michael LOMAS

Ullah
Lister Health Centre, 25 Commercial Way, London SE15 6DP
Tel: 020 7708 4211 Fax: 020 7771 3810
(Southwark Primary Care Trust)

GP Dr ULLAH

London, SE16

The Alfred Salter Medical Centre
6 Drummond Road, London SE16 4BU
Tel: 020 7237 1857
(Southwark Primary Care Trust)

GP Ronald Arthur EASTER

The Avicenna Health Centre
2 Verney Way, London SE16 3HA
Tel: 020 7237 1685 Fax: 020 7394 7200
(Southwark Primary Care Trust)

GP Rashid Yahya KADHIM

Donmall and Partners
87 Albion Street, London SE16 7JX
Tel: 020 7237 2092 Fax: 020 7231 1435
(Southwark Primary Care Trust)
Patient List Size: 10100

Practice Manager Denise Griffin

GP Richard Clinton DONMALL, Judith Katharine FERGUSON, T HUMPHREY, B MARSH, Valerie O'NEILL, Catherine Joy OTTY

North Aisle Medical Centre
St Jaemes' Church, Thurland Road, London SE16 4AA
Tel: 020 7237 4066 Fax: 020 7740 1031
(Southwark Primary Care Trust)
Patient List Size: 2000

GP David ZIGMOND

Park Medical Centre
57 Hawkstone Road, London SE16 2PE
Tel: 020 7237 3414 Fax: 020 7231 9425
(Southwark Primary Care Trust)
Patient List Size: 5500

Practice Manager Sandra Constantino

GP J K GANDHI, Jayesh Narendra BHATT

The Surgery
34 Rotherhithe New Road, London SE16 2PS
Tel: 020 7237 4091 Fax: 020 7231 8944
(Southwark Primary Care Trust)

GP Prasanta Kumar DAS, David Vijaya Kumar MOSES

Surrey Docks Health Centre
Downtown Road, London SE16 6NP
Tel: 020 7231 0207
(Southwark Primary Care Trust)
Patient List Size: 7400

Practice Manager Carol McPaul

GP Noel BAXTER, Patrick James HOLDEN, Pamela Jane Mary Martin MARRINAN, Kerstin Birgit O'CONNOR

London, SE17

Aylesbury Partnership
Aylesbury Medical Centre, Taplow House, Thurlow Street, London SE17 2XE
Tel: 020 7703 2205
(Southwark Primary Care Trust)
Patient List Size: 23000

Practice Manager Allan Stibbs

GP Stewart KAY, Christopher Ivor DAVENPORT-JONES, Emma Jane KIERNAN, Cornelius MURPHY, Leslie ROUND, Olugbenga Oluseun SANGOWAWA, William Kenneth THOMAS, Amr ZEINELDENE

The Health Centre
301 East Street, London SE17 2SX
Tel: 020 7703 4550 Fax: 020 7703 1888
(Southwark Primary Care Trust)

GP A T BRADFORD, Timothy St John TROUGHTON

The Surgery
1 Richmond House, East Street, London SE17 2DU
Tel: 020 7703 7393 Fax: 020 7708 3077
(Southwark Primary Care Trust)
Patient List Size: 4964

Practice Manager Diana Braithwaite

GP Frances Sara DIFFLEY, A BABALOLA, Emmeline Harriet BREW-GRAVES, Julia Marion HODGES

The Surgery
1 Manor Place, London SE17 3BD
Tel: 020 7703 3988 Fax: 020 7252 4002
(Southwark Primary Care Trust)
Patient List Size: 10600

Practice Manager Paul Hillman

GP Roger Hubert HIGGS, Carola Seward HAIGH, Venetia J HERZMARK, Alison Jane MAYCOCK, Susan Joanna NIXON, Olufemi OSONUCIA

The Surgery
33 Penrose Street, London SE17 3DW
Tel: 020 7703 3677
(Southwark Primary Care Trust)
Patient List Size: 4000

GP Meheboob Fhakaruddin SAMUDRI, Abdulkhadir NOOHU KANNU

The Surgery
7 Maddock Way, London SE17 3NH
Tel: 020 7735 3644 Fax: 020 7582 2565
Email: rhksinha@hotmail.com
(Southwark Primary Care Trust)
Patient List Size: 2700

Practice Manager R Sinha

GP R H K SINHA

London, SE18

Anglesea Medical Centre
4a Anglesea Avenue, Woolwich, London SE18 6EH
Tel: 020 8317 2120 Fax: 020 8317 3488
(Greenwich Teaching Primary Care Trust)

Practice Manager Indi Briah

GP B LAKSHMINARAYANA

Char and Aggarwal
Plumstead Health Centre, Tewson Road, Plumstead, London SE18 1BH
Tel: 020 8854 8027 Fax: 020 8317 3030
(Greenwich Teaching Primary Care Trust)
Patient List Size: 5300

Practice Manager Anita Raipal

GP Dwarka Nath CHAR, Ram Paul AGGARWAL

The Clarendon Surgery
213 Burrage Road, London SE18 7JZ
Tel: 020 8854 0356 Fax: 020 8855 5484
(Greenwich Teaching Primary Care Trust)

Practice Manager Brenda Webber

GP Clare Eileen RODEN, Azuka AYORINDE, Susan COLVIN, M J COUTINHO, Yann LEFEYVRE, L VUKOTIC

Corelli Surgery
374 Shooters Hill Road, Woolwich, London SE18 4LS
Tel: 020 8319 0074 Fax: 020 8319 8952
(Greenwich Teaching Primary Care Trust)

Practice Manager Angela Chenery

GP Wurvokonda Sarojini RAO

Ferryview Health Centre
25 John Wilson Street, Woolwich, London SE18 6PZ
Tel: 020 8319 5400 Fax: 020 8319 5404
Email: doctors@valentine-health.org.uk
(Greenwich Teaching Primary Care Trust)
Patient List Size: 13000

GP Robert Kieron Frederick HUGHES, Jane DEACON, Georgina DEIGHTON, Sarah Elizabeth DIVALL, William MORGAN, Sami Toufic RACHED, Rebecca ROSEN, Kara Rosemary McKenna TANEGA

Plumstead Health Centre
Tewson Road, Plumstead, London SE18 1BB
Tel: 020 8854 1898 Fax: 020 8855 9958
(Greenwich Teaching Primary Care Trust)

Practice Manager Karen Powell

GP Sisir Kumar GHOSH

St Marks Medical Centre
24 Wrottesley Road, Plumstead, London SE18 3EP
Tel: 020 8854 6262 Fax: 020 8317 3098
(Greenwich Teaching Primary Care Trust)
Patient List Size: 5380

Practice Manager Susan Raphael, Tracey Wahba

GP Nabil Fekry RAPHAEL, Hany Fahmy WAHBA

The Surgery
76 Herbert Road, London SE18 3PR
Tel: 020 8854 3964 Fax: 020 8317 8512
(Greenwich Teaching Primary Care Trust)
Patient List Size: 5500

Practice Manager L Ayliffe

GP Rama SRI KRISHNA, Chandra Mohan Raju CHINDULURI

The Surgery
110 Sandy Hill Road, Plumstead, London SE18 7BA
Tel: 020 8854 3736 Fax: 020 8854 4381
Email: karen.powell@gp-g83636.nhs.uk
(Greenwich Teaching Primary Care Trust)
Patient List Size: 3800

Practice Manager Karen Powell

GP Sisir Kumar GHOSH, Shah RAHMAN

The Surgery
4 Kirkham Street, Plumstead, London SE18 2JU
Tel: 020 8854 3206 Fax: 020 8316 1187
Website: www.hussain. phc.co.uk
(Greenwich Teaching Primary Care Trust)
Patient List Size: 1700

Practice Manager Jenny Cheetham

GP A YONES, P M YOUNG, Dr HUSSAIN, Dr RAUINDRAM, Dr SABAT

The Surgery
37 Waverley Crescent, Plumstead, London SE18 7QU
Tel: 020 8317 7258 Fax: 020 8316 6353
(Greenwich Teaching Primary Care Trust)
Patient List Size: 5500

Practice Manager Mohini Sohal

GP Sajiv Kumar GUPTA, Rashmi GOEL

The Surgery
12 The Slade, Plumstead, London SE18 2NB
Tel: 020 8317 9327 Fax: 020 8855 8075
(Greenwich Teaching Primary Care Trust)

GP Parviz Fredoon IRANI

The Surgery
12 The Slade, Plumstead, London SE18 2NB
Tel: 020 8317 3031 Fax: 020 8317 2536
(Greenwich Teaching Primary Care Trust)

Practice Manager Kate Minter

GP Asha SEN

The Surgery
141 Plumstead High Street, Plumstead, London SE18 1SE
Tel: 020 8855 0052 Fax: 020 8855 7672
(Greenwich Teaching Primary Care Trust)

Practice Manager A. Saleem

GP Sabiha SALEEM, S M SHARIFF

The Surgery
20-22 Bannockburn Road, Plumstead, London SE18 1ES
Tel: 020 8855 5540 Fax: 020 8855 4970
(Greenwich Teaching Primary Care Trust)
Patient List Size: 3000

Practice Manager Heather Mustafa

GP Bharati Amritlal SHAH

The Surgery
44 Conway Road, Plumstead, London SE18 1AH
Tel: 020 8854 2042 Fax: 020 8855 1938
(Greenwich Teaching Primary Care Trust)

Practice Manager Jennie Humphreys, Naina Patel

GP C L GUPTA

London, SE19

Auckland Surgery
84A Auckland Road, Upper Norwood, London SE19 2DF
Tel: 020 8653 5146 Fax: 020 8653 1195
(Croydon Primary Care Trust)
Patient List Size: 5250

Practice Manager Nicky Garnham

GP Lesley Ann HICKIN, Catherine Janet GRAY, Anne HOLDEN, Paul NUNN

Crown Dale Medical Centre
61 Crown Dale, London SE19 3NY
Tel: 020 8670 2414 Fax: 020 8670 0277
Website: www.crowndalemedicalcentre.co.uk
(Lambeth Primary Care Trust)
Patient List Size: 10700

Practice Manager Yvonne Everett

GP Maria Krisztina ELLIOTT, Mark CHAMLEY, Colin Christopher GATWARD, Caroline Louise TAYLOR, Patrick Thomas WHITE

Upper Norwood Group Practice
60 Central Hill, London SE19 1DT
Tel: 020 8670 7117 Fax: 020 8670 1671
(Croydon Primary Care Trust)
Patient List Size: 7400

Practice Manager Maggie Fidler

GP Andrew Oliver DIVER, Cheryl HARTLEY-BROWN, Sivalingam SIVATHASAN, Deshminder Singh VIRDI

London, SE20

The Park Group Practice
113 Anerley Road, Anerley, Penge, London SE20 8AJ
Tel: 020 8778 8027 Fax: 020 8289 1418
(Bromley Primary Care Trust)

GP Alan FISHTAL, Margaret FAGBOHUN, Sarah Jane STONER

Robin Hood Surgery
94 Croydon Road, Penge, London SE20 7AB
Tel: 020 8778 8651 Fax: 020 8778 5529
(Bromley Primary Care Trust)

GP Charles Richard MOZLEY, Olusegun Emmanuel OBAFEMI

The Surgery
182 Anerley Road, Anerley, London SE20 8BL
(Bromley Primary Care Trust)

GP Dr DAVDA

The Surgery
21 High Street, Penge, London SE20 7HJ
(Bromley Primary Care Trust)
Patient List Size: 2700

GP S.K. HAZRA

The Surgery
224 Anerley Road, Anerley, Penge, London SE20 8TJ
Tel: 020 8659 9343
(Bromley Primary Care Trust)

GP Dissanayake Mudiyanselage Cyril Wijeratne Ban PATTAPOLA

The Surgery
33 Croydon Road, Penge, London SE20 7TJ
Tel: 020 8778 5135/4897 Fax: 020 8402 1919
Email: croydonroad.surgery@gp-684022.nhs.uk
(Bromley Primary Care Trust)
Patient List Size: 6400

GP M K SAHI, P N PRASAD, S SAHI

The Surgery
161 Croydon Road, Penge, London SE20 7TY
(Bromley Primary Care Trust)

GP Ponnudurai THILLAIVASAN

London, SE21

Paxton Green Health Centre
1 Alleyn Park, London SE21 8AU
Tel: 020 8670 6878 Fax: 020 8766 7057
(Lambeth Primary Care Trust)
Patient List Size: 18500

Practice Manager Kevin Trott

GP Tyrrell George John Robert EVANS, Malcolm ARTLEN, Gillian ELLSBURN, Wendy FLIZMAN, John Charles FRENCH, Isobel Louise MICHELL, Stephen Charles MILLER, Caroline QUVM

The Rosendale Surgery
103a Rosendale Road, West Dulwich, London SE21 8EZ
Tel: 020 8670 3292 Fax: 020 8761 7310
Email: Thames.chabuk@gp-G85706.nhs.uk
(Lambeth Primary Care Trust)
Patient List Size: 6600

Practice Manager Carolyn Lornie

GP Thamer Mahmoud CHABUK, Kerry HOWARD, Matthew Robert KILN, Rosemary LEONARD

London, SE22

3-Zero-6 Medical Centre
306 Lordship Lane, London SE22 8LY
Tel: 020 8693 4704 Fax: 020 8693 3034
Website: www.306medicalcentre.nhs
(Southwark Primary Care Trust)
Patient List Size: 3000

Practice Manager Mr Dawood

GP Hassanali DEWJI

Doha
417 Lordship Lane, London SE22 8JN
Tel: 020 8693 2912 Fax: 020 8693 8041
(Southwark Primary Care Trust)
Patient List Size: 3800

GP S A K M S DOHA

Dulwich Medical Centre
163-169 Crystal Palace Road, London SE22 9EP
Tel: 020 8693 2727 Fax: 020 8693 2121
(Southwark Primary Care Trust)

GP Ram Prashad GUPTA, Tanja GORDINSKY, R GUPTA, Sarah HAWXWELL

Forest Hill Group Practice
1 Forest Hill Road, London SE22 0SQ
Tel: 020 8693 2264 Fax: 020 8299 0200
(Southwark Primary Care Trust)

Practice Manager Pat Claxton

GP Alan David ROGERS, George ADAM, S CROSLAND, Helen Judith GRAHAM, C L MCCOLL, Rebecca Mowbray SCORER, Henry TEGNER, S WOODS

Melbourne Grove Medical Practice
Melbourne Grove, London SE22 8QN
Tel: 020 8299 0499 Fax: 020 8299 1954
(Southwark Primary Care Trust)
Patient List Size: 9100

Practice Manager Lynn Newman

GP Sheila Anne GRANT, Peter Julien ILVES, David Arthur Reginald LIDGEY, A MADAN

Sarma
East Dulwich Primary Care Centre, East Dulwich Grove, London SE22 8PT
Tel: 020 8693 6205 Fax: 020 8693 6205
(Southwark Primary Care Trust)
Patient List Size: 3000

GP R SARMA

The Surgery
The Gardens, London SE22 9QU
Tel: 020 8693 4715 Fax: 020 8299 4418
(Southwark Primary Care Trust)
Patient List Size: 6300

Practice Manager Jenny Shearer

GP Jane Margaret CLIFFE, Mary Cecilia COSTELLO, Helen Marie FOWLER

London, SE23

Jenner Health Centre
201 Stanstead Road, London SE23 1HU
Tel: 020 7771 4209 Fax: 020 7771 4210
Website: www.jennerpractice.co.uk
(Southwark Primary Care Trust)
Patient List Size: 14500

Practice Manager Jeanette Garforth

GP Raymond Marc ROWLAND, A S AUGUSTINE, Antionette AUGUSTINE, Martin Varnam EDWARDS, Maurice Anthony Jerome HICKEY, Christopher LAMPTEY, Anne SYKES, S E VAN-COOTEN, Sarah VAN COUTEN, P WHITE

Vale Medical Centre
195-197 Perry Vale, Forest Hill, London SE23 2JF
Tel: 020 8291 7007 Fax: 020 8291 5111
Email: vale@gp-g85696.nhs.uk
Website: www.valemedical.nhs.uk
(Lewisham Primary Care Trust)
Patient List Size: 8000

Practice Manager Jean Yull

GP Jaipal ISRAEL, Jacky McLEOD, Awai RAMANANANDAN, Nilu VAJPEYI, Uma VAJPEYI, Rashmi VARMA

London, SE24

Deerbrook Surgery
114-116 Norwood Road, London SE24 9BB
Tel: 020 8674 4623 Fax: 020 8678 6236
(Lambeth Primary Care Trust)
Patient List Size: 3800

Practice Manager Julia O'Hara

GP Christopher John George WRIGHT

Elm Lodge Surgery
2 Burbage Road, London SE24 9HJ
Tel: 020 7274 2820 Fax: 020 7924 0710
(Southwark Primary Care Trust)
Patient List Size: 7000

Practice Manager Peter Hall

GP David Howard LEDGER, John NOUR, Luke O'FLAFHERTY

Herne Hill Group Practice
74 Herne Hill, London SE24 9QP
Tel: 020 7274 3314 Fax: 020 7738 6025
(Lambeth Primary Care Trust)
Patient List Size: 9850

Practice Manager Ms Eustace, Mary McColl

GP Gerard DICKINSON, David Ian TOVEY, Melanie Anne HOUGHTON, Sadrudin KHERAJ, Denise Elexia ROBERTSON, Siyana SHAFFI

Herne Hill Road Medical Practice
1-3 Herne Hill Road, London SE24 0AU
Tel: 020 7737 3928 Fax: 020 7501 9191
Email: hernehillrd.practice@06.lslha.sthames.nhs.uk
(Lambeth Primary Care Trust)
Patient List Size: 5700

Practice Manager B Johnson

GP Surinder Kumar ARORA, Dr DEVILLIENS, Dr MOREL

The Surgery
117 Norwood Road, Herne Hill, London SE24 9AE
Tel: 020 8674 5400 Fax: 020 8678 5405
(Lambeth Primary Care Trust)
Patient List Size: 4200

Practice Manager Patricia Dolar

GP Brian Paul FINE, Sarah BRUML, Miriam Rachel ISH-HOROWICZ

London, SE25

Portland Medical Centre
184 Portland Road, London SE25 4QB
Tel: 020 8662 1233 Fax: 020 8662 1223
(Croydon Primary Care Trust)
Patient List Size: 8250

Practice Manager Vicky Bernard

GP S O'HARA, R DABO, P M JACKSON, Ravindra SONDHI

Selhurst Medical Centre
27 Selhurst Road, South Norwood, London SE25 5QA
Tel: 020 8684 2010 Fax: 020 8665 1228
(Croydon Primary Care Trust)
Patient List Size: 1960

Practice Manager S Parulekar

GP N S PARULEKAR

South Norwood Hill Medical Centre
103A South Norwood Hill, London SE25 6BY
Tel: 020 8771 0742 Fax: 020 8771 6097
(Croydon Primary Care Trust)
Patient List Size: 5800

Practice Manager Richard McDonough

GP Nicola Ann Louise CUTLER, Adrian Carmel ATTARD, J O OJO, K A OKUBOYEJO

South Norwood Hill Surgery
21B South Norwood Hill, London SE25 6AA
Tel: 020 8653 0635 Fax: 020 8771 8013
(Croydon Primary Care Trust)
Patient List Size: 2340

Practice Manager Elaine handover

GP P K SRIVASTAVA, Geeta SRIVASTAVA

South Norwood Medical Centre
93 Whitehorse Lane, London SE25 6RA
Tel: 020 8771 9779 Fax: 020 8771 3779
(Croydon Primary Care Trust)
Patient List Size: 3870

Practice Manager Ellen Patel

GP Jasjeet Singh DHOAT, Narinder DHOAT

Whitworth Road Surgery
9 Whitworth Road, South Norwood, London SE25 6XN
Tel: 020 8653 1414 Fax: 020 8771 8666
(Croydon Primary Care Trust)
Patient List Size: 7950

Practice Manager David Brown

GP T T LWIN, T T MYINT

Woodside Health Centre 1
3 Enmore Road, London SE25 5NS
Tel: 020 8656 5790 Fax: 020 8656 7984
Email: administrator@gp-H83025.sthames.nhs.uk
(Croydon Primary Care Trust)
Patient List Size: 5930

Practice Manager Anne Churchill

GP J ALLERTON, K CHATTERJEE, Duncan Roderick Edward JONES, F MCRZA, John Edmund Andrew SPICER

Woodside Health Centre 2
3 Enmore Road, London SE25 5NS
Tel: 020 8655 1410
(Croydon Primary Care Trust)
Patient List Size: 2400

Practice Manager Diane Johnson, Sara Lowe

GP Kevin William BARBER

Woodside Health Centre 3
3 Enmore Road, London SE25 5NS
Tel: 020 8655 1223 Fax: 020 8656 1229
Email: terry.callaghan@gp-h83026.nhs.uk
(Croydon Primary Care Trust)
Patient List Size: 4830

Practice Manager Terri Callaghan

GP Ruth CLERY, S AJAYI, H PLETSCH

Woodside Health Centre 4
3 Enmore Road, London SE25 5NS
Tel: 020 8656 5790 Fax: 020 8656 7984
(Croydon Primary Care Trust)
Patient List Size: 2770

Practice Manager Sheha Morjaria

GP H D S NORONHA

London, SE26

Sydenham Green Group Practice
26 Holmshaw Close, London SE26 4TH
Tel: 020 8676 8836 Fax: 020 7771 4710
(Lewisham Primary Care Trust)
Patient List Size: 12500

Practice Manager P Jenkins

GP Benjamin John ESSEX, Julia Margaret CAMPBELL, Andrew Maurice PLATMAN, James Jan SIKORSKI, Sian Elizabeth THOMAS

Sydenham Surgery
2 Sydenham Road, London SE26 5QW
Tel: 020 8778 8552 Fax: 020 8776 9027
(Southwark Primary Care Trust)
Patient List Size: 5500

Practice Manager Barry Gent

GP Patrick George Vivian MORANT, Kanapathipillai KANGESAN, Neimat MOHAMED

Wells Park Practice
1 Wells Park Road, Sydenham, London SE26 6JQ
Tel: 020 8699 2840 Fax: 020 8699 2552
Email: name.surname@gp-G85114.nhs.uk
(Lewisham Primary Care Trust)
Patient List Size: 7200

Practice Manager Jayne Hampson

GP Anthony Oladeji ADEGOKE, (Angela) Carol CHEAL, Brian Henry FISHER, Shona LIDGEY, Adrian MUNN, Ruth WILLIAMS

London, SE27

Norwood Surgery
483 Norwood Road, London SE27 9NJ
Tel: 020 8670 1000 Fax: 020 8766 7557
(Lambeth Primary Care Trust)

Practice Manager Alba Dourado

GP N C FERNANDES

The Surgery
130 Knights Hill, London SE27 0ST
Tel: 020 8670 2940
(Lambeth Primary Care Trust)

GP Jonathan CHOYCE

The Surgery
130 Knights Hill, London SE27 0ST
Tel: 020 8670 2940
(Lambeth Primary Care Trust)

Practice Manager Marian Leahy

GP Y HU

London, SE28

Gallions Reach Health Centre
Bentham Road, Thamesmead, London SE28 8BE
Tel: 020 8333 5001 Fax: 020 8333 5020
(Greenwich Teaching Primary Care Trust)

GP John Myles KENNEDY, Lia Elizabeth CRISTOFOLI, Peter Guy LEWINS, Charles Frederick Martyn LOBLEY, Anjaua TEMPLE, David Michael WHEELER

London, SW1

Belgrave Medical Centre
13 Pimlico Road, London SW1W 8NA
Tel: 020 7730 5171 Fax: 020 7730 6092
Email: firstname.lastname@gp-E87753.nhs.uk
(Kensington and Chelsea Primary Care Trust)

Practice Manager Caroline Hazlerigg

GP Victoria Robin-Jane MUIR, Maher AL SHAKARCHI

The Belgravia Surgery
24-26 Eccleston Street, London SW1W 9PY
Tel: 020 7590 8000 Fax: 020 7590 8010
Email: belgravia-surgery@gp-E87005.nhs.uk
(Kensington and Chelsea Primary Care Trust)
Patient List Size: 5500

Practice Manager Margaret Burton

GP Peter John TLUSTY, David Loyd PARRY

The Cambridge Street Surgery
93 Cambridge Street, London SW1V 4PY
Tel: 020 7834 5502 Fax: 020 7834 2350
(Kensington and Chelsea Primary Care Trust)

Practice Manager Caroline Nelson

GP Andrew Pearce DICKER, Niro Kaniz Fatema AMIN, Djanan Meryem MANIERA

Cowen and Ashe
51 Sloane Street, London SW1X 9SW
Tel: 020 7838 9422 Fax: 020 7259 5409
(Kensington and Chelsea Primary Care Trust)

Practice Manager Susannah Nicholas

GP John COWEN

Knightsbridge Medical Centre
71-75 Pavilion Road, London SW1X 0ET
Tel: 020 8237 2600
(Kensington and Chelsea Primary Care Trust)
Patient List Size: 6250

Practice Manager Rajni Sanga

GP Mark Gerard SWEENEY, Katherine BRUNTON

Marven Medical Practice
45-50 Lupus Street, London SW1V 3EB
Tel: 020 7834 1160 Fax: 020 7834 0147
(Kensington and Chelsea Primary Care Trust)

Practice Manager Coral Parker

GP Jack Christopher JERJIAN

The Surgery
141-143 Lupus Street, London SW1V 3HQ
Tel: 020 7828 9252
(Kensington and Chelsea Primary Care Trust)
Patient List Size: 1800

Practice Manager Esther Forder

GP Hege MOSTAD

Victoria Medical Centre
Victoria Medical Centre, 7 Longmoore Street, London SW1V 1JH
Tel: 020 7821 1531 Fax: 020 7233 5995
Website: www.vicmedcentre.com
(Westminster Primary Care Trust)
Patient List Size: 9500

Practice Manager Susan Lauder

GP Fiona ALEXANDER, Samir ALVI, Frank FOGELMAN, Howard MANUEL, Susan Elizabeth RANKINE

Westminster and Pimlico General Practice
15 Denbigh Street, London SW1V 2HF
Tel: 020 7834 6969 Fax: 020 7931 7747
(Kensington and Chelsea Primary Care Trust)
Patient List Size: 10000

Practice Manager Dixie Coombs

GP Alastair John MITCHELL, Jonathan Eric Lewis MUNDAY, Jeremy Simon TEW

London, SW2

Brixton Hill Group Practice
22 Raleigh Gardens, London SW2 1AE
Tel: 020 8674 6376
(Lambeth Primary Care Trust)

Practice Manager Jackie Morley

GP Dudley Stratford BENNETT, Louise HOPKINS, Annu LAL, Marian Sophia MANCEY-JONES, Clare STANNARD, Clare Elizabeth WILKIE, Richard Tudor Humphrey WILLIAMS

Edith Cavell Practice
41a-c Streatham Hill, London SW2 4TP
Tel: 020 8243 2224 Fax: 020 8243 2237
(Lambeth Primary Care Trust)
Patient List Size: 4200

Practice Manager G Collins

GP S BELL, W DEEN

Palace Road Surgery
3 Palace Road, London SW2 3DY
Tel: 020 8674 2083 Fax: 020 8674 6040
(Lambeth Primary Care Trust)

Practice Manager Helen Cop

GP Christopher David ROBERTS, Emmanuel HOPE, Arumugan PAVIMATHAN, Lee Nigel WINTER

Singh and Singh
28 Streatham Place, London SW2 4QY
Tel: 020 8671 6191/8674 8500 Fax: 020 8678 1055
Email: streathamplace.surgery@ob.islha.sthomas.nhs.uk
(Lambeth Primary Care Trust)
Patient List Size: 7500

Practice Manager Anjali Singh

GP A K SINGH, J SINGH

The Surgery
4 Hardell Rise, Tulse Hill, London SW2 3DX
Tel: 020 8674 6586 Fax: 020 8674 6043
(Lambeth Primary Care Trust)
Patient List Size: 9500

GP Guy René AH-MOYE, Lisa CROWE, Rachael KILNER, Patricia KIRKMAN, Adrienne Ashley Tina NEWTON, Yvonne TURNER

The Surgery
93 Streatham Hill, London SW2 4UD
Tel: 020 8671 9424
(Lambeth Primary Care Trust)

Practice Manager Carl Prendergast

GP Mildred Rosemary ANDLAW

Ung
56 Blairderry Road, Streatham, London SW2 4SB
Tel: 020 8671 3340
(Lambeth Primary Care Trust)

GP I C UNG

Water Lane Surgery
48 Brixton Water Lane, London SW2 1QE
Tel: 020 7274 1521 Fax: 020 7738 3258
(Lambeth Primary Care Trust)
Patient List Size: 7500

Practice Manager Sarah Vallotton

GP Vipinchandra Chhotabhai PATEL, Maha Rosa SAIF, Sarah Michelle UTTING

London, SW3

The Chelsea Practice
Violet Melchett Clinic, 30 Flood Walk, London SW3 5RR
Tel: 020 8237 2544 Fax: 020 7352 7105
(Kensington and Chelsea Primary Care Trust)

Practice Manager John Miller

GP Claire Caroline SCUDDER

The Surgery
5 Sloane Avenue, London SW3 3JD
Tel: 020 7581 3187 Fax: 020 7225 0034
Email: chelsea.medical@gp-E87705.nhs.uk
(Kensington and Chelsea Primary Care Trust)
Patient List Size: 3100

Practice Manager P E Rose

GP Andrew John ROSE

The Surgery
57 Sydney Street, London SW3 6PX
Tel: 020 7362 8031 Fax: 020 7351 3726
(Kensington and Chelsea Primary Care Trust)

GP Ashok MAINI

London, SW4

Clapham Family Practice
51 Clapham High Street, London SW4 7TL
Tel: 020 7622 4455 Fax: 020 7622 4466
(Lambeth Primary Care Trust)

GP Paul Nicholas HEENAN, Desmond Patrick COFFEY, Victoria LAMB, Greg J McEWAN, Angela MUNDEN, Redmond WALSH

Clapham Park Surgery
72 Clarence Avenue, London SW4 8JP
Tel: 020 8674 4436
(Lambeth Primary Care Trust)
Patient List Size: 6000

Practice Manager Barbara Christopher

GP Thomas Anthony GLANVILLE, Penelope Anne GILHAM, Gita SUNTHANKAR

The Clapham Park Surgery
72 Clarence Avenue, London SW4 8JP
Tel: 020 8674 0101 Fax: 020 8674 2941
(Lambeth Primary Care Trust)
Patient List Size: 7100

Practice Manager Stewart Casimir

GP Carole GLASSON, Simon Tobias SHEPHERD, Elizabeth Jane WILLIAMS

Courtyard Surgery
1 Poynders Road, London SW4 8NU
Tel: 020 8673 1386 Fax: 020 8673 3312
(Lambeth Primary Care Trust)
Patient List Size: 4000

Practice Manager Karen Woodvine

GP Pamela Susan ASHTON

Curran and Partners
Manor Health Centre, 86 Clapham Manor Street, London SW4 6EB
Tel: 020 7411 6866 Fax: 020 7411 6857
Email: curran.manorhc@ob.lslha.sthames.nhs.uk
Website: www.claphamhealth.org.uk
(Lambeth Primary Care Trust)
Patient List Size: 9000

Practice Manager Murray King

GP David Patrick Mary CURRAN, Farrukh A MAJEED, Rebecca Jane McKENZIE, Edward SMYTHE

Gupta and Ball
10 Sandmere Road, London SW4 7QJ
Tel: 020 7274 6366 Fax: 020 7738 5172
(Lambeth Primary Care Trust)

Practice Manager Puneet Gupta

GP Gauri Shankar GUPTA, Reena BALL, Harpal Singh HARRAR

The Hetherington Group Practice
18 Hetherington Road, London SW4 7NU
Tel: 020 7274 4220 Fax: 020 7737 0205
Email: office@gp-G85045.nhs.uk
Website: www.hetheringtongp.co.uk
(Lambeth Primary Care Trust)
Patient List Size: 9900

Practice Manager Judy Cook

GP Catherine Anne Lucy BURTON, Dianne Marie AITKEN, Miranda COOK, Adrian James McLACHLAN, Catherine MISKIN, Stephen MOWLE, Harpreet SHARIF, Suzy SHAW

The Nightingale Surgery
11A Nightingale Lane, London SW4 9AH
Tel: 020 8673 4289 Fax: 020 8673 4912
(Wandsworth Primary Care Trust)
Patient List Size: 2250

Practice Manager Linda Banks

GP Dr QAIYUM

Santamaria
Manor Health Centre, 86 Clapham Manor Street, London SW4 6EB
Tel: 020 7411 6877 Fax: 020 7411 6867
Email: santamaria.manor@gp-g85010.nhs.uk
(Lambeth Primary Care Trust)
Patient List Size: 3168

Practice Manager Carol Mitchum

GP Sheila SANTAMARIA

The Surgery
1 Binfield Road, London SW4 6TB
Tel: 020 7622 1424 Fax: 020 7978 1436
(Lambeth Primary Care Trust)
Patient List Size: 7400

Practice Manager Belinda Anderson, Neil Suttie

GP Sally Elizabeth WHITTET, Tom ASLAN, John Robert BALAZS, Neil VASS

London, SW5

Brompton Medical Centre
237 Old Brompton Road, London SW5 0EA
Tel: 020 7373 4102 Fax: 020 7835 0041
(Kensington and Chelsea Primary Care Trust)
Patient List Size: 6000

Practice Manager Sana Rabbani

GP Mohamed ALI

Courtfield Medical Centre
73 Courtfield Gardens, London SW5 0NL
Tel: 020 7370 2453 Fax: 020 7244 0018
(Kensington and Chelsea Primary Care Trust)
Patient List Size: 4600

GP Jill Diane HARLING, Timothy Eric LADBROOKE, Kathrine Mary O'BRIEN

El Borai
32 Eardley Crescent, London SW5 9JZ
Tel: 020 7373 0140 Fax: 020 7244 6617
(Kensington and Chelsea Primary Care Trust)
Patient List Size: 3800

Practice Manager Fatima Kassab

GP Mohamed Rimah EL BORAI, Burthan ADIB

Om Sai Clinic
248 Earls Court Road, London SW5 9AD
Tel: 020 7935 1455 Fax: 020 7370 7497
(Kensington and Chelsea Primary Care Trust)
Patient List Size: 8000

Practice Manager M Lhahir

GP Sinnadurai NATHAN, Subraya NAYAK, Thiyagarajah PERIYASAMY

The Surgery
269 Old Brompton Road, London SW5 9JA
Tel: 020 7370 2643 Fax: 020 7370 5970
(Kensington and Chelsea Primary Care Trust)

GP S PARAMESHWARAN

London, SW6

Ashville Surgery
Swan House, Parsons Green Lane, London SW6 4US
Tel: 020 7371 7171 Fax: 020 7331 0101
(Hammersmith and Fulham Primary Care Trust)
Patient List Size: 5300

Practice Manager Martin Bennett

GP Stephen Francis ARAS, Tamsin GRAHAM, Carolyn HALL

Cassidy Medical Centre
651A Fulham Road, London SW6 5PX
Tel: 020 7731 2511 Fax: 020 7371-7857
(Hammersmith and Fulham Primary Care Trust)

GP C I DELLAPORTAS, Dr MUKHERJEE, Dr SHAREEF

Fulham Clinic
82 Lillie Road, London SW6 1TN
Tel: 020 7386 9299 Fax: 020 7610 0635
Email: c.bailey@virgin.net
(Hammersmith and Fulham Primary Care Trust)
Patient List Size: 10000

Practice Manager Pauline Patterson

GP David Milne COWPER, Grant BLAIR, Wendy June CHRISTIAN, George Kenneth FREEMAN, Jane Louise HARROP-GRIFFITHS, Andrew WESTERN

Fulham Medical Centre
446 Fulham Road, London SW6 1BG
Tel: 020 7385 6001 Fax: 020 7385 3755
(Hammersmith and Fulham Primary Care Trust)
Patient List Size: 8000

Practice Manager Tessa Newby

GP Adriana MANTAFOUNIS, Gustav Nils AHRENS, Timothy McNICHOLAS

Fulham Road Surgery
630 Fulham Road, London SW6 5RS
Tel: 020 7736 4344 Fax: 020 7736 4985
(Hammersmith and Fulham Primary Care Trust)

Practice Manager Linda Gilson

GP Michael Adrian Lloyd EVANS, Kay Frances DEEMING, Robert Tudor JENKINS, Richard Ingham LAWSON

Fulham Road Surgery
714 Fulham Road, London SW6 5SB
Tel: 020 7736 6305 Fax: 020 7384 3153
(Hammersmith and Fulham Primary Care Trust)

GP Krishan Lal MANGWANA, Dr VILATHGAMUWA

Hurlingham Road Surgery
34A Hurlingham Road, Fulham, London SW6 3RF
Tel: 020 7371 8472
(Hammersmith and Fulham Primary Care Trust)

GP Judith Anne ATKINSON

Lillie Road Surgery
328-330 Lillie Road, London SW6 7PP
Tel: 020 7385 1964 Fax: 020 73816 1071
(Hammersmith and Fulham Primary Care Trust)

GP Zaheer HUSSAIN

Lillie Road Surgery
139 Lillie Road, Fulham, London SW6 7SX
Tel: 020 7385 7101
(Hammersmith and Fulham Primary Care Trust)

GP Luis Albert Candon Placida DE SOUSA

Munster Road Surgery
292 Munster Road, Fulham, London SW6 6BQ
Tel: 020 7385 1965 Fax: 020 7610 3765
(Hammersmith and Fulham Primary Care Trust)

GP S M JEFFRIES, Mark Howard DOWNS, E MAHMOOD, M ROUSSEAU

The Salisbury Surgery
178 Dawes Road, Fulham, London SW6 7AS
Tel: 020 7381 9195
(Hammersmith and Fulham Primary Care Trust)

GP Ravindrasena Navaratnam MUTHIAH, Suzanne Elizabeth HALLIDAY

The Sands End Health Clinic
170 Wandsworth Bridge Road, London SW6 2UQ
Tel: 020 7371 8472 Fax: 020 7371 8473
Email: Lawley@setic.prestel.co.uk
(Hammersmith and Fulham Primary Care Trust)

Practice Manager Alexandra Von Hengel

GP Guy Charles LAWLEY, Gemma CRITTENDEN, S EDWARDS

Wandsworth Bridge Road Surgery
29 Wandsworth Bridge Road, London SW6 2TA
Tel: 020 7736 9341 Fax: 020 7384 1493
(Hammersmith and Fulham Primary Care Trust)
Patient List Size: 2800

GP Bright Selvadurai SELVARAJAN

Wansdworth Bridge Road Surgery
172 Wandsworth Bridge Road, London SW6 2UQ
Tel: 020 7731 3498
(Hammersmith and Fulham Primary Care Trust)

GP B DAS, B BASU

London, SW7

Emperor's Gate Centre for Health
First Floor, 49 Emperors Gate, London SW7 4HJ
Tel: 020 8237 5333 Fax: 020 8237 5344
(Kensington and Chelsea Primary Care Trust)
Patient List Size: 5200

Practice Manager Sarah Welch

GP Hilary Lucina KING, Caroline STOTT

Imperial College Health Centre
Southside, Watt's Way, London SW7 1LU
Tel: 020 7584 6301 Fax: 020 7594 9390
(Kensington and Chelsea Primary Care Trust)

GP Peter Stewart DORWARD, Sarah Anne FREEDMAN, Dr GILLON, Irene Rachel WEINREB

The Surgery
18 Thurloe Street, London SW7 2SU
Tel: 020 7225 2424 Fax: 020 7225 1874
(Kensington and Chelsea Primary Care Trust)
Patient List Size: 2230

Practice Manager Deborah Boreham

GP Jonathan James Campbell BOREHAM, Peter David ROWLEY

The Surgery
45 Rosary Gardens, London SW7 4NQ
Tel: 020 7373 6557 Fax: 020 7373 6426
(Kensington and Chelsea Primary Care Trust)

GP Hooshand GHADIMI

The Surgery
29 Thurloe Street, London SW7 2LQ
Tel: 020 7584 6771 Fax: 020 7589 1591
(Kensington and Chelsea Primary Care Trust)

GP Terence Horton Walker DEANE

The Surgery
7 Kynance Place, Gloucester Road, London SW7 4QS
Tel: 020 7581 3040 Fax: 020 7584 0506
(Kensington and Chelsea Primary Care Trust)

GP Michael David McKEOWN

West, Gillies and Steeden
7 Stanhope Mews West, London SW7 5RB
Tel: 020 7835 2600 Fax: 020 7835 0979
(Kensington and Chelsea Primary Care Trust)

Practice Manager Anita Ladd

GP Katherine Mary GILLIES, Andrew Louis STEEDEN, John Ronald Crook WEST

London, SW8

Dr Ala's Surgery
514 Wandsworth Road, London SW8 3LT
Tel: 020 7622 5642 Fax: 020 7978 1927
Email: reception@gp-g85674.nhs.uk
(Lambeth Primary Care Trust)

Practice Manager Rosemarie Callaghan

GP Abul Jamil Khursheed ALA, Michael Joseph HOLLOWAY, Peter Anthony JACKSON, Claire McMAHON

Dr Moussa and Partner
178a Wandsworth Road, London SW8 2JR
Tel: 020 7622 5947 Fax: 020 7622 7095
(Lambeth Primary Care Trust)

GP R MOUSSA, P N SOYSA

Mawbey Brough Health Centre
39 Wilcox Close, London SW8 2UD
Tel: 020 7622 3827 Fax: 020 7498 1069
(Lambeth Primary Care Trust)

Practice Manager Chrissie Carson

GP Patricia Jane Alison LOGAN, Jennifer Esmee LAW, Mohammed Iqbal SEDAR, Sandra Jean TAYLOR

Mawbey Brough Health Centre
39 Wilcox Close, London SW8 2UD
Tel: 020 7627 5541 Fax: 020 7411 5726
(Lambeth Primary Care Trust)

Practice Manager Dolina Redjimi

GP Joginder Singh CHEEMA

Muhammad
455 Wandsworth Road, London SW8 4NX
Tel: 020 7622 2808 Fax: 020 7498 1073
Email: gpsurgery@aol.com
(Lambeth Primary Care Trust)
Patient List Size: 3000

Practice Manager Yvonne Muhammad

GP Haroon Ali MUHAMMAD

South Lambeth Road Practice
1 Selway House, 272 South Lambeth Road, London SW8 1UL
Tel: 020 7622 1923 Fax: 020 7498 5530
(Lambeth Primary Care Trust)

Practice Manager Victoria Churchill

GP Dominic COSTA, Claudia HANSO, Angela Margaret SKUCE, Dominic STEVENS

The Surgery
14 Queenstown Road, Battersea, London SW8 3RX
Tel: 020 7622 9295 Fax: 020 7498 5206
(Wandsworth Primary Care Trust)
Patient List Size: 8000

Practice Manager Sharon Higgins

GP Sian Angharad JOB, Helen EAKIN, Ilias GAVRIELIDES, Ian William SMITH, Jonathan WHARRAM

London, SW9

Berlyn and Whitmey
Myatts Fields Health Centre, Patmos Road, London SW9 7RX
Tel: 020 7411 3593 Fax: 020 7411 3583
(Lambeth Primary Care Trust)
Patient List Size: 5500

Practice Manager Debbie Berlyn

GP Roger Andrew David BERLYN, Robert James WHITMEY

Ferreira
134-136 Landor Road, London SW9 9JB
Tel: 020 7737 7550 Fax: 020 7733 4531
Email: ivor.ferreira@gp-g85700.nhs.uk
(Lambeth Primary Care Trust)
Patient List Size: 4120

Practice Manager Vanda Joaquim

GP Ivor FERREIRA

Grantham Health Centre
Grantham Road, London SW9 9DL
Tel: 020 7733 6191 Fax: 020 7737 2870
(Lambeth Primary Care Trust)

Practice Manager Pat Evans

GP Marie Joyce CROCOMBE, Elizabeth Priscilla McGINN, Joannes Catharine VAN DEN BERK, Sunanda Srilal WICKREMESINGHE

Hawthorne
Myatts Field Health Centre, Foxley Square Surgery, London SW9 7RX
Tel: 020 7411 3553 Fax: 020 7411 3557
(Lambeth Primary Care Trust)
Patient List Size: 3784

Practice Manager Jean Treadwell

GP Abdul MUKADAM

Iveagh House Surgery
Iveagh House, Loughborough Road, London SW9 7SE
Tel: 020 7274 8850 Fax: 020 7733 2102
Email: paul.wallington@gp-g85135.nhs.uk
(Lambeth Primary Care Trust)
Patient List Size: 8000

Practice Manager Paul Wallington

GP Nigel Ian KONZON, Nicola Anne BECK, Herman LAI, Louise MEDFORTH, Nupur VERMA

McCarthy
328 Clapham Road, London SW9 9AE
Tel: 020 7622 2006
(Lambeth Primary Care Trust)

GP Daniel Peter Justin McCARTHY

Patel and Cresswell
Myatts Field Health Centre, Patmos Road, London SW9 6SE
Tel: 020 7411 3573 Fax: 020 7411 3583
(Lambeth Primary Care Trust)
Patient List Size: 7200

Practice Manager Debbie Berlyn

GP H PATEL, B E CRESSWELL

Pavilion Practice
9 Brighton Terrace, London SW9 8DJ
Tel: 020 7274 9252 Fax: 020 7274 0740
(Lambeth Primary Care Trust)

GP D C PATEL, Samir Niranjan PATEL

Stockwell Group Practice
107 Stockwell Road, London SW9 9TJ
Tel: 020 7274 3225/3223 Fax: 020 7738 5005
(Lambeth Primary Care Trust)
Patient List Size: 16000

Practice Manager Jenny Hoggins

GP Richard Anthony SAVAGE, Rosalind Susan CHURCH, Helen EDWARDS, John HITCHENS, Katherine Anne HOPKINSON, Christopher John Russell JENKINS, Hung Kee Pantalen LEE, Stephanie Diana MAY

London, SW10

The Redcliffe Surgery
10 Redcliffe Street, London SW10 9DT
Tel: 020 7460 2222 Fax: 020 7460 0116
(Kensington and Chelsea Primary Care Trust)

Practice Manager Maggie Holleran

GP Suzanne Elizabeth FARRAR

The Redcliffe Surgery
10 Redcliffe Street, London SW10 9DT
Tel: 020 7460 2222 Fax: 020 7460 0116
(Kensington and Chelsea Primary Care Trust)
Patient List Size: 11000

Practice Manager Maggie Holleran

GP Karen Claire NAPIER

The Surgery
409 Kings Road, Chelsea, London SW10 0LR
Tel: 020 7351 1766 Fax: 020 7352 2240
(Kensington and Chelsea Primary Care Trust)

GP Elizabeth Anne SINCLAIR

The Surgery
4 Drayton Gardens, London SW10 9SA
Tel: 020 7373 3356 Fax: 020 7370 3738
(Kensington and Chelsea Primary Care Trust)

GP Joseph CAVANAGH, Patricia Agnes CAVANAGH

The Surgery
10 Redcliffe Street, London SW10 9DT
Tel: 020 7460 2222
(Kensington and Chelsea Primary Care Trust)

GP Fiona BUTLER

Worlds End Health Centre
529 Kings Road, London SW10 0UD
Tel: 020 7351 0357 Fax: 020 8846 6399
(Kensington and Chelsea Primary Care Trust)

GP Dr EMILIANI

London, SW11

Bridge Lane Health Centre
20 Bridge Lane, Battersea, London SW11 3AD
Tel: 020 7585 1499 Fax: 020 7978 4707
(Wandsworth Primary Care Trust)
Patient List Size: 11000

Practice Manager Theresa Campbell

GP Caroline ELLIN, Sheila Frances FITZGERALD, Simon MILLS, Helen Mary PUGH, Elizabeth Elaine SNAPE, Elizabeth Patricia Fay WOLFF

Dr N A Shakir
Bridge Lane Health Centre, 20 Bridge Lane, Battersea, London SW11 3AD
Tel: 020 7978 6737 Fax: 020 7228 7373
(Wandsworth Primary Care Trust)
Patient List Size: 2500

Practice Manager Rachel Shakir

GP Naseer Ahmad SHAKIR

Falcon Road Surgery
47 Falcon Road, Battersea, London SW11 2PH
Tel: 020 7228 1619/3399 Fax: 020 7924 3375
(Wandsworth Primary Care Trust)
Patient List Size: 10900

Practice Manager Karl Arato

GP Augustine O OKONMAH, Rehana BUTT, Shaheen HAQ, Amer SALIM, Rosemary Anne SAVAGE

Huitt Square Surgery
Carmichael Close, Winstanley Estate, Battersea, London SW11 2DH
Tel: 020 7228 8988 Fax: 020 7978 4550
(Wandsworth Primary Care Trust)

Practice Manager Mary Howard

GP Joanna Alice GAZZARD, Andrew Gordon DICKS, Michelle Glynis DURHAM, A E ENO, Claire WINSTANLEY

Lavender Hill Group Practice
19 Pountney Road, Battersea, London SW11 5TU
Tel: 020 7228 4042 Fax: 020 7738 9346
(Wandsworth Primary Care Trust)

Practice Manager Phil Evans

GP Simon Philip FREEMAN, Catherine Mary KROLL, Jeremy Pieter GRAY, Helen LUCAS, Susan Caroline ROBINSON

The Surgery
17 Battersea Rise, London SW11 1HG
Tel: 020 7228 0195 Fax: 020 7978 5119
(Wandsworth Primary Care Trust)

Practice Manager Lilian Fitzerald

GP Andrzej Jerzy SURAWY, David WHOOLEY

The Surgery
263 Lavender Hill, London SW11 1JD
Tel: 020 7223 5520 Fax: 020 7228 1067
(Wandsworth Primary Care Trust)

Practice Manager Mohammad Sibai

GP Abul Basher Mohamed Mosharraf HOSSAIN

The Surgery
3 Austin Road, Battersea, London SW11 5JP
Tel: 020 7498 0232 Fax: 020 7498 0271
(Wandsworth Primary Care Trust)
Patient List Size: 8900

Practice Manager P Dennemont

GP Julian Duncan CHURCHER, Jonathan CHAPPELL, David Graham FINCH, Jonathan GRANNELL, Rosalind GREEN, Emma GRIFFIN, Janet LAI-FOOK, Serena NORTH

The Surgery
87 Northcote Road, London SW11 6PL
Tel: 020 7223 2417 Fax: 020 7924 6722
(Wandsworth Primary Care Trust)

Practice Manager Mr Baig

GP Daud Basharat Akbar KHAN

The Surgery
100 Lavender Hill, Battersea, London SW11 5RE
Tel: 020 7738 0070 Fax: 020 7207 3302
(Wandsworth Primary Care Trust)

GP Sita B FERNANDO

The Surgery
162A St Johns Hill, London SW11 1SW
Tel: 020 8874 1691 Fax: 020 8871 9132
(Wandsworth Primary Care Trust)
Patient List Size: 2000

Practice Manager Muna Al-Hashimi

GP Saad Mohamed Jawad HAIDER

The Surgery
7 Farrant House, Winstanley Road, Battersea, London SW11 2EJ
Tel: 020 7228 4172 Fax: 020 7924 5737
(Wandsworth Primary Care Trust)

GP Mustafa Hussain ANSARI

The Surgery
123 St Johns Hill, Battersea, London SW11 1SZ
Tel: 020 7223 5308 Fax: 020 7207 1757
Email: margaret.beavis@gp.H85659.nhs.uk
(Wandsworth Primary Care Trust)

Patient List Size: 2600

GP Khalida BEGG

The Surgery
119 Northcote Road, Battersea, London SW11 6PW
Tel: 020 7228 6762 Fax: 020 7801 0748
Email: practice.admin@gp-H85077.nhs.uk
(Wandsworth Primary Care Trust)
Patient List Size: 6000

GP R GULATI, H PUVINATHAN, Rasiah RAMANATHAN

The Surgery
20 Lavender Road, Battersea, London SW11 2UG
Tel: 020 7223 1056 Fax: 020 7978 4112
(Wandsworth Primary Care Trust)
Patient List Size: 3500

Practice Manager Susan Haynes

GP Jayanidhi PATTABHI

London, SW12

Balham Health Centre
120 Bedford Hill, London SW12 9HS
Tel: 020 8673 1720 Fax: 020 8673 1549
(Wandsworth Primary Care Trust)
Patient List Size: 10900

GP Robert Anthony OULTON, A KANGATHARAN, Ai LECHI, Cedric Albert RIBELRO, Feirooz Sinbad Bedros TOROSSIAN

Balham Health Centre
120 Bedford Hill, London SW12 9HS
Tel: 020 8673 8268
(Wandsworth Primary Care Trust)
Patient List Size: 2700

GP Naseem AKBAR

Dr Kumar and Partners
143-145 Balham Hill, London SW12 9DL
Tel: 020 8673 1776 Fax: 020 8673 1198
(Wandsworth Primary Care Trust)
Patient List Size: 3500

GP Anjana KUMAR, Pradeep KUMAR, Cecil Emile LOBO

Sai Medical Centre
17B Balham Park Road, Balham, London SW12 8DT
Tel: 020 8673 9693 Fax: 020 8675 3636
Email: smsree@nhs.net
(Wandsworth Primary Care Trust)
Patient List Size: 2300

GP Mathiaparanam SREETHARAN

The Surgery
47 Boundaries Road, Balham, London SW12 8EU
Tel: 020 8673 1476 Fax: 020 8675 9757
(Wandsworth Primary Care Trust)
Patient List Size: 6359

Practice Manager Nirmal Mittal

GP Virendra Kumar MITTAL

The Surgery
77 Thurleigh Road, Balham, London SW12 8TZ
Tel: 020 8675 3521 Fax: 020 8675 3800
(Wandsworth Primary Care Trust)

Practice Manager Sandra Reeves

GP Christopher John David PEACH, Nicola Jill SALT, Roger Paul SCHOFIELD

The Surgery
298 Cavendish Road, Balham, London SW12 0PL
Tel: 020 8675 2029 Fax: 020 8673 5113
(Wandsworth Primary Care Trust)
Patient List Size: 12941

GP M FRANKLIN, M S MUGHAL, N J MUGHAL, Paul Lindsay NICHOLAS, P SHAH, M SZOLACH, Susan WALLAT-VAGO

London, SW13

Flood and Partners
Essex House Surgery, Station Road, Barnes, London SW13 0LW
Tel: 020 8876 1033 Fax: 020 8878 5894
(Richmond and Twickenham Primary Care Trust)
Patient List Size: 8413

Practice Manager Alison MacLeod

GP Rosemarie Jane FLOOD, Patrick Wilfred GIBSON, Elizabeth Anne HOCKNEY

The Surgery
1 Glebe Road, Barnes, London SW13 0DR
Tel: 020 8748 1065 Fax: 020 8741 8665
(Richmond and Twickenham Primary Care Trust)
Patient List Size: 18148

Practice Manager Sue Bell, Soraya Dizia, Christine Tompson

GP Jennifer LEBUS, Jonathan Paul BOTTING, Elizabeth BURCHER, Owen EVANS, Rosemary NAUNTON-MORGAN, Caroline OLIVER, Shelagh Mary OLNEY, Marilyn Jane PLANT, Claire QUIGGIN, Matilda Claire RICE-JONES, Benjamin YORKE-BARBER

The Surgery
74 Castelnau, London SW13 9EX

GP David Rowland JONES

The Surgery
22 Castelnau, Barnes, London SW13 9RU
Tel: 020 8748 7574 Fax: 020 8563 8821
(Richmond and Twickenham Primary Care Trust)
Patient List Size: 4000

Practice Manager Diana Elsdon, Lily Fitzgerald

GP Alain Edward PALACCI, Rachel WOOLRYCH

London, SW14

Deanhill Surgery
2 Deanhill Road, London SW14 7DF
Tel: 020 8876 2424 Fax: 020 8876 3249
(Richmond and Twickenham Primary Care Trust)
Patient List Size: 2825

Practice Manager Eileen Murr

GP Roger Lewis WEEKS, Carina SALAZAR

Jezierski and Partners
The Health Centre, Sheen Lane, London SW14 8LP
Tel: 020 8876 3901 Fax: 020 8878 9620
(Richmond and Twickenham Primary Care Trust)
Patient List Size: 7839

Practice Manager Laura jones

GP Marek Riszard JEZIERSKI, Christina Elizabeth Alice GRAYSON, Sophie JUKES, Dorren TYMENS

Sheen Lane Health Centre
70 Sheen Lane, London SW14 8LP
Tel: 020 8876 4086 Fax: 020 8878 9620
(Richmond and Twickenham Primary Care Trust)
Patient List Size: 8920

Practice Manager Linda Halstead

GP Ian Andrew JOHNSON, Catriona Ashley Scott BEARD, Denise DAVIES, Sarah Ruth Muluskha SAMPSON

London, SW15

The Alton Practice
208 Roehampton Lane, London SW15 4LE
Tel: 020 8788 4844 Fax: 020 8788 4844
(Wandsworth Primary Care Trust)

Patient List Size: 3900

Practice Manager Amar Alissa

GP A M J ALISSA, V MOUDGIL

Ashburton Medical Practice
105 Carslake Road, London SW15 3DD
Tel: 020 8785 6440 Fax: 020 8788 2063
(Wandsworth Primary Care Trust)

GP P L BOWEN, R NIRMALAN

Balmuir Surgery
Balmuir Gardens, London SW15 6NG
Tel: 020 8788 0818/8735 9313 Fax: 020 8780 1737
(Wandsworth Primary Care Trust)
Patient List Size: 4400

Practice Manager Julie Pomeroy

GP Rosemary Francesca Alice DE BOER, Alison Jane BRADSHAW, Alison Ann Louise KIRKLAND

Heathbridge Practice
327D Upper Richmond Road, London SW15 6SU
Tel: 020 8788 6002 Fax: 020 8789 8568
(Wandsworth Primary Care Trust)
Patient List Size: 12300

Practice Manager Shushima Jani

GP Virginia Margaret BEARN, Richard John ESTALL, Fiona Margaret PAYNE, Kyi TUN

Mayfield Surgery
246 Roehampton Lane, London SW15 4AA
Tel: 020 8780 5770/5650 Fax: 020 8780 5649
(Wandsworth Primary Care Trust)
Patient List Size: 6000

Practice Manager Jenny Ridge

GP Lindsay BURT, Lauren G BLOCH, Stephen Cameron DEAS, A EDWARDS

Putney Surgery
4 Disraeli Road, London SW15 2DS
Tel: 020 8788 4836 Fax: 020 8780 2961
Email: docbma@aol.com
(Wandsworth Primary Care Trust)
Patient List Size: 4650

Practice Manager Karen Segal

GP Brian Michael AARONS

Putneymead Medical Centre
350 Upper Richmond Road, London SW15 6TL
Tel: 020 8788 0686 Fax: 020 8780 0831
(Wandsworth Primary Care Trust)
Patient List Size: 11500

Practice Manager Karen Harris

GP Sarah Melody NORTH, Nichola Claire Joanne LLOYD, Donald James McKENZIE, Susan Mary PLUMLEY, Anna REIDY, Jacqueline Mary ROBERTS

Richardson and Ilves
351 Danebury Avenue, London SW15 4DU
Tel: 020 8876 6666 Fax: 020 8878 2629
(Wandsworth Primary Care Trust)

Practice Manager Marja Moffat

GP Hazel Joan RICHARDSON, Peter Julian ILVES

The Roehampton Surgery
191 Roehampton Lane, London SW15 4HN
Tel: 020 8788 1188 Fax: 020 8789 9914
(Wandsworth Primary Care Trust)
Patient List Size: 5400

GP Philippa Louise BOWEN, Rajanayagam NIRMALAN

The Surgery
30 Chartfield Avenue, London SW15 6HG
Tel: 020 8788 6442
(Richmond and Twickenham Primary Care Trust)

Practice Manager Valerie Clements

GP Owen Gwynfor EVANS, Jennifer Catherine Morris LEBUS, Rosemary Ann MORGAN

The Surgery
351 Danebury Avenue, Upper Richmond Road, London SW15 4DU
Tel: 020 8788 0952
(Wandsworth Primary Care Trust)

Practice Manager Sheila Mayes

GP Raymond Leonard COTTEE, S R SAMSON

London, SW16

The Exchange Surgery
136 Streatham High Road, London SW16 1BW
Tel: 020 8769 2844 Fax: 020 8769 0638
(Lambeth Primary Care Trust)

Practice Manager Suzanne Long

GP Nuala GALAZKA, Leandro CASTRO

Greyswood Practice
66 Eastwood Street, London SW16 6PX
Tel: 020 8769 0845 Fax: 020 8677 2960
(Wandsworth Primary Care Trust)
Patient List Size: 7500

Practice Manager Bev Atkins, Sam Frewin

GP Peter Gifford THOMSON, Sarah Jane MACKENZIE, Penelope Pauline OSBORNE

Jayaratnam and Ramanan
106 Greyhound Lane, London SW16 5RW
Tel: 020 8677 4488
(Lambeth Primary Care Trust)
Patient List Size: 3700

GP T RAMANAN, W JAYARATNAM

Masterton Thomson and Bolade
2 Prentis Road, Streatham, London SW16 1XU
Tel: 020 8769 5002 Fax: 020 8677 1800
Website: www.2prentisroadsurgery
(Lambeth Primary Care Trust)

Practice Manager Ruth James-More

GP I O BOLADE, J MASTERTON, K R THOMSON

Norbury Health Centre (1)
2B Pollards Hill North, Norbury, London SW16 4NL
Tel: 020 8679 6591 Fax: 020 8679 9435
(Croydon Primary Care Trust)

Practice Manager Rasik Shah

GP S K HANDA, N CHAUDERY, K SHAH

Norbury Health Centre (2)
2B Pollards Hill North, Norbury, London SW16 4NL
Tel: 020 8679 1700 Fax: 020 8764 6873
Email: sushil.newatia@gp-h3003.nhs.uk
(Croydon Primary Care Trust)
Patient List Size: 2600

Practice Manager Sue Marley

GP Sushil M NEWATIA

The Rowans Surgery
1 Windermere Road, Streatham, London SW16 5HF
Tel: 020 8764 0407 Fax: 020 8679 4149
(Sutton and Merton Primary Care Trust)

Practice Manager Dorrie Carmichael

GP Harriet Catherine BLACKLAY, Mubeen AFZAL, Alan Charles COHEN, Sanjay KUMAR, Karen Anne WORTHINGTON

Streatham Park Surgery
91 Mitcham lane, Streatham, London SW16 6LY
Tel: 020 8769 0705 Fax: 020 8677 3505
(Wandsworth Primary Care Trust)

Practice Manager Helen Wolak Lloyd

GP Dr GHUFOOR, Dr HUSSAIN

The Surgery
1-4 The High Parade, Streatham High Road, London SW16 1EX
Tel: 020 8769 8753 Fax: 020 8769 8704
Email: peter.ashley@gp-G85002.nhs.uk
(Lambeth Primary Care Trust)
Patient List Size: 3100

Practice Manager A J Rawson

GP Peter Maxted ASHBY, Friedrich HANSEN

The Surgery
31 Prentis Road, London SW16 1QB
Tel: 020 8769 3308 Fax: 020 8769 4855
(Lambeth Primary Care Trust)
Patient List Size: 3180

Practice Manager Rajini Gunasuntharam

GP Thambirajah GUNASUNTHARAM

The Surgery
9 Drakewood Road, London SW16 5DT
Tel: 020 8679 6126
(Lambeth Primary Care Trust)

GP Mustafa SADEK

The Surgery
St Andrews Hall, Guildersfield Road, London SW16 5LS
Tel: 020 8765 4901
(Lambeth Primary Care Trust)

Practice Manager Astrid Hill

GP Suzanne Jane SAVAGE, Ambar GOEL, U G PARATIAN, Carys SONNENBERG, Dora WAITT

The Surgery
142 Mitcham Lane, Streatham, London SW16 6NS
Tel: 020 8769 0635 Fax: 020 8664 6434
(Wandsworth Primary Care Trust)

Practice Manager Darsha De Almeida

GP P D DE ALMEIDA, Suresha Therese Lakmalie DE ALMEIDA

Valley Road Surgery
139 Valley Road, London SW16 2XT
Tel: 020 8769 2566 Fax: 020 8769 5301
(Lambeth Primary Care Trust)

GP Audrey Barbara PECK, Justin HAYES

London, SW17

Ashvale Medical Centre
4 Ashvale Road, London SW17 8PW
Tel: 020 8672 2085 Fax: 020 8682 2993
(Wandsworth Primary Care Trust)
Patient List Size: 3858

GP Qurrat-ul-Aen KHAN

Garratt Lane Surgery
657 Garratt Lane, London SW17 0PB
Tel: 020 8944 6827 Fax: 020 8894 7357
(Wandsworth Primary Care Trust)
Patient List Size: 3671

Practice Manager Dakeha Makhecha

GP Hertha VONSCHACK, Veronica SALH

The Surgery
886 Garratt Lane, London SW17 0NB
Tel: 020 8672 1948
(Sutton and Merton Primary Care Trust)

GP Ghazi Shafiqul Alam CHOUDHURY, Sarla Tharumal FATNANI, N S KHAN

The Surgery
Waterfall House, 223 Tooting High Street, London SW17 0TD
Tel: 020 8672 1327 Fax: 020 8767 5615
(Wandsworth Primary Care Trust)
Patient List Size: 5296

Practice Manager Wendy Williams

GP Thambirajah ANANDARAJAH, Judit Sarlay HANSPAL

The Surgery
127 Trinity Road, Tooting, London SW17 7HJ
Tel: 020 8672 3331
(Wandsworth Primary Care Trust)
Patient List Size: 12941

Practice Manager Agnes Downing

GP Mary FRANKLIN, Mohammed Shariff MUGHAL, Nafees Jahan MUGHAL, Paul NICHOLAS, P K SHAH, Maria Regina SZOLACH, Susan WALLAT-VAGO

The Surgery
62 Upper Tooting Road, London SW17 7PB
Tel: 020 8672 3133 Fax: 020 8767 8904
(Wandsworth Primary Care Trust)
Patient List Size: 3652

Practice Manager Nirmal Mittal

GP Virendra Kumar MITTAL

The Surgery
80 Bickersteth Road, London SW17 9SJ
Tel: 020 8682 0521 Fax: 020 8672 6532
(Wandsworth Primary Care Trust)
Patient List Size: 2365

Practice Manager M Shirazoddullah

GP Mahfel SHIRAZ, F HENNESSEY

The Surgery
226 Mitcham Road, Tooting, London SW17 9NN
Tel: 020 8672 7868 Fax: 020 8672 8630
(Wandsworth Primary Care Trust)
Patient List Size: 3000

Practice Manager Uzma Mirza

GP Mohamed Sabji SULTAN

The Surgery
218 Franciscan Road, Tooting, London SW17 8HG
Tel: 020 8672 5191
Email: shobha.singh@gp-h85688.nhs.uk
(Wandsworth Primary Care Trust)
Patient List Size: 4902

GP Ran Vijai Prasad SINGH

Tooting Bec Surgery
313 Balham High Road, London SW17 7BA
Tel: 020 8682 0352
(Wandsworth Primary Care Trust)

GP Bipin Chimanbhai AMIN, Melville Alade SEMAO

London, SW18

Brocklebank Health Centre
249 Garratt Lane, London SW18 4UE
Tel: 020 8870 1341/871 4448
(Wandsworth Primary Care Trust)

Practice Manager Theresa Nahanandi

GP Barbara Ann DAVIES, Elizabeth Philippa CHAPMAN, Thomas Anthony COFFEY, Nicola JONES, Neil Charles ROUSSEAU, Grant Bruce Milo WINSTOCK

Dr Sharma and Partners
The Medical Centre, 90-92 Garratt Lane, Wandsworth, London SW18 4DD
Tel: 020 8874 4984 Fax: 020 8877 0732
(Wandsworth Primary Care Trust)
Patient List Size: 5500

Practice Manager Nick Shimmin

GP Omkar Parmanand SHARMA, Roderick Alistair EWEN

Elborough Street Surgery
81-83 Elborough Street, Southfields, London SW18 5DS
Tel: 020 8874 7113 Fax: 020 8874 3682
(Wandsworth Primary Care Trust)
Patient List Size: 4100

GP Carolynne Leslie CHRISTIE, Susan Carol WHITEHEAD

Patel
Brocklebank Health Centre, 249 Garrett Lane, London SW18 4UE
Tel: 020 8870 1341
(Wandsworth Primary Care Trust)

Practice Manager Amrita Patel

GP Lalitkumar Chaturbhai PATEL, D PATEL

Southfields Group Practice
14 Elsenham Street, London SW18 5NJ
Tel: 020 8947 0061 Fax: 020 8944 8694
(Wandsworth Primary Care Trust)
Patient List Size: 12000

Practice Manager Blanche Simmons

GP Ann Allister PHILLIPS, Frank Thomas AUTY, Andrew James DEUCHAR, H S KOONER, Kate Sarah McINTYRE, M H NEIL, C P WONG

The Surgery
2-4 Steerforth Street, Earlsfield, London SW18 4HH
Tel: 020 8946 5681
(Wandsworth Primary Care Trust)
Patient List Size: 8000

Practice Manager Lyn Hawes

GP D H GORDON, N BAMPURD, I LLEWELLYN

The Surgery
78 Granville Road, London SW18 5SG
Tel: 020 8874 2471
(Wandsworth Primary Care Trust)

GP Mujib-ul Haq KHAN

Triangle Surgery
Triangle House, 2 Broomfield Road, London SW18 4HX
Tel: 020 8874 1700 Fax: 020 8870 7695
(Wandsworth Primary Care Trust)
Patient List Size: 4900

GP D PATEL

Wandle Valley Group Practice
249 Garratt Lane, London SW18 4UE
(Wandsworth Primary Care Trust)

GP M RASHID

London, SW19

Alexandra Surgery
39 Alexandra Road, Wimbledon, London SW19 7JZ
Tel: 020 8946 7578 Fax: 0845 330 8569
Email: alexandra-surgery@hotmail.com
(Sutton and Merton Primary Care Trust)
Patient List Size: 5000

Practice Manager Shiela Leach

GP Narendra SORNALINGAM, Mayura MAHADEVAN, Abdul Hussain Asgar Ali Abdul NABIJEE

Church Lane Practice
2 Church Lane, Merton Park, London SW19 3NY
Tel: 020 8542 1174 Fax: 020 8544 1583
(Sutton and Merton Primary Care Trust)

Practice Manager Paula McCarthy

GP Patricia Mary GREENFIELD, Sarah Frances CUNNINGHAM, Angela Mary FIELD, Francis Charles Andrew MILLS, Trevor Gordon STAMMERS, Angela Margaret WAKE, Martyn Charles WAKE

Colliers Wood Surgery
58 High Street Colliers Wood, London SW19 2BY
Tel: 020 8540 6303 Fax: 020 8544 9337
(Sutton and Merton Primary Care Trust)
Patient List Size: 8000

Practice Manager Jeanette Chomiczewski

GP Zuhair Matti YACOB, Dr ARMAD, M S AYUB, S SHAN

Fairview Medical Centre
69 Fairview Road, Norbury, London SW19 5PX
Tel: 020 8764 6666 Fax: 020 8764 4659
(Croydon Primary Care Trust)
Patient List Size: 3970

Practice Manager Kathy Coughlan

GP M GRAHAM

The Merton Medical Practice
12-17 Abbey Parade, Merton High Street, London SW19 1AZ
Tel: 020 8540 1109 Fax: 020 8543 3353
(Sutton and Merton Primary Care Trust)

Practice Manager Frank Fitzmaurice

GP Ernest NORTLEY, Nicola WALDMAN

Morden Hall Medical Centre
256 Morden Road, London SW19 3DA
Tel: 020 8540 0585 Fax: 020 8542 4480
(Sutton and Merton Primary Care Trust)
Patient List Size: 13200

Practice Manager Lynda Robinson

GP Thomas Peter Ferrari RHIND, Rukhshunda Naheed AHMAD, Syed Amir Arshad AKHTAR, Paul Frederick ALFORD, Robert Frank BETTRIDGE, Cathrine Fiona GIBBS, Ravindrabhai PATEL

Princes Road Surgery
51 Princes Road, London SW19 8RA
Tel: 020 8542 2827/2407 Fax: 020 8296 9505
(Sutton and Merton Primary Care Trust)
Patient List Size: 9350

Practice Manager Sandra Chapman

GP Elizabeth Maureen EMERSON, A ADEYEMI, Soumyen MAITRA, J RANAWEERA, L SHARIFFI, V SHARMA

Queens Road Surgery
27 Queens Road, Wimbledon, London SW19 8NW
Tel: 020 8944 5916 Fax: 020 8947 8677
(Sutton and Merton Primary Care Trust)

Practice Manager Jane Fisk, Diana Ljubic

GP C J BAILLIE, Sarah BLAKE, Wendy Kathryn BULMAN, Ian Dominic Richard HARPER, J D NELSON

Riverhouse Surgery
East Road, Wimbledon, London SW19 1YG
(Sutton and Merton Primary Care Trust)

St Paul's Cottage Surgery
88a Augustus Road, London SW19 6EW
Tel: 020 8788 8880 Fax: 020 8287 8905
(Wandsworth Primary Care Trust)

GP Morag Eleanor McKINNON, Ashleigh HELM

The Surgery
24 High Street, Colliers Wood, London SW19 2AE
Tel: 020 8542 1483 Fax: 020 8543 9104

(Sutton and Merton Primary Care Trust)
Patient List Size: 1900

Practice Manager K K Garg

GP Vasundhara PAGADALA

The Surgery, The Inner Park Road Health Centre
86-88 Inner Park Road, Wimbledon, London SW19 6DA
Tel: 020 8788 2578 Fax: 020 8788 2404
(Wandsworth Primary Care Trust)
Patient List Size: 3700

Practice Manager Alison Marks

GP Madliavan Ganesan IYER

Thurairatnam
Tudor Lodge Health Centre, 8c Victoria Drive, London SW19 6AE
Tel: 020 8780 0125 Fax: 020 8788 9445
(Wandsworth Primary Care Trust)
Patient List Size: 4650

Practice Manager Pat Hennessy

GP Arulnathan THURAIRATNAM, P SELVAPAT

Vineyard Hill Road Surgery
67 Vineyard Hill Road, London SW19 7JL
Tel: 020 8947 2579
(Sutton and Merton Primary Care Trust)
Patient List Size: 5700

Practice Manager Beverley Snell

GP John Robert JONES, K LITTLE, Gillian Claire PROVOST, G SCHIFFER

Wimbledon Village Practice
35A High Street, Wimbledon, London SW19 5BY
Tel: 020 8946 4820 Fax: 020 8944 9794
(Sutton and Merton Primary Care Trust)

Practice Manager Laura Bond

GP Andrew Peter Tudor TUDOR MILES, Jane Margaret Shaw ALLEN, Paul Robert CUNDY, Robin Philip Colm MULCAHY, Timothy David TAYLOR-ROBERTS

London, SW20

The Cannon Hill Lane Medical Practice
153 Cannon Hill Lane, Raynes Park, London SW20 9DA
Tel: 020 8542 5201 Fax: 020 8540 9049
(Sutton and Merton Primary Care Trust)
Patient List Size: 6800

Practice Manager Alison Kirk

GP Sarah Jane WOROPAY, Katharine CHILDS, Sonya IBRAHIM, Marek Kazimierz JARZEMBOWSKI, Graham John MASON

Dr H M Freeman and Partners
12 Durham Road, Raynes Park, London SW20 0TW
Tel: 020 8946 0069 Fax: 020 8944 2927
(Sutton and Merton Primary Care Trust)
Patient List Size: 21000

Practice Manager Diana Iribar

GP Howard Michael FREEMAN, Helen ALLISON, Revathy ARUNASALAM, Susan Doris BORTHWICK, Elizabeth CLEWING, Stephen James DE WILDE, Nicola DOWLING, Michael LANE, A RANG, Judith Alison ROBERTS, Simon Peter ROHDE, Penelope Elaine SMITH, Bernadette VEIRAS, Cheong WONG

Grand Drive Surgery
132 Grand Drive, London SW20 9EA
Tel: 020 8542 5555 Fax: 020 8542 6969
(Sutton and Merton Primary Care Trust)
Patient List Size: 7200

Practice Manager Debra Kirton

GP Joanna Clare KINGSMILL, Lawrence Martin WEBBER, Alka CHANDI, Janusz KOLENDO

Pepys Road Surgery
20 Pepys Road, Raynes Park, London SW20 8PF
Tel: 020 8946 3074/8249 Fax: 020 8296 0145
(Sutton and Merton Primary Care Trust)
Patient List Size: 7600

Practice Manager Linda Bradley

GP Ian Charles Rowley HARTLEY, Caroline Samantha CHILL, Nazirahmed Hassanali Kassam DHALLA, Conor John MOLONY

The Surgery
153 Cannon Hill Lane, London SW20 9DA
Tel: 020 8543 5581 Fax: 020 8540 9049
(Sutton and Merton Primary Care Trust)
Patient List Size: 1700

Practice Manager Brenda Hill

GP Richard John Donald CHEGWIDDEN

London, W1

Cavendish Health Centre
53 New Cavendish Street, London W1G 9TQ
Tel: 020 7487 5244 Fax: 020 7487 1500
Email: derek.chase@gp-E87745.nhs.uk
Website: www.cavendishhealth.nhs.uk
(Westminster Primary Care Trust)

Practice Manager Liz Chapple

GP Harold Derek CHASE, Sarah ANDERSON, Clare HEATH, Asma KHAN, Claire McMULLEN

The Crawford Street Surgery
95-97 Crawford Street, London W1H 2HJ
Tel: 020 7723 6324 Fax: 020 7616 0350
(Westminster Primary Care Trust)

Practice Manager Kevin McDonald

GP Janet AMAKYE, Soo Kim WONG

Mayfair Medical Centre
3-5 Weighhouse, London W1K 5LS
Tel: 020 7493 1647 Fax: 020 7493 3169
(Westminster Primary Care Trust)
Patient List Size: 2300

Practice Manager Valerie Tilleke

GP Shaukat NAZEER

Murphy
Soho Centre for Health and Care, First Floor, 1 Frith Street, London W1D 3QS
Tel: 020 7534 6570 Fax: 020 7534 6566
(Westminster Primary Care Trust)
Patient List Size: 2400

Practice Manager Marjorie Kelly

GP Helen Mary MURPHY

Soho Square General Practice
Soho Centre for Health and Care, First Floor, 1 Frith Street, London W1D 3QS
Tel: 020 7534 6575 Fax: 020 7534 6607
(Westminster Primary Care Trust)
Patient List Size: 2500

Practice Manager Brenda Neville

GP Dr CHEUNG

The Surgery
55 Wimpole Street, London W1G 8YL
Tel: 020 7935 9795 Fax: 020 7486 3934
(Westminster Primary Care Trust)
Patient List Size: 1600

Practice Manager Jeanette Challier

GP Anna Eva SZABOLCSI

The Surgery
2 Hanway Place, London W1T 1HB
Tel: 020 7323 0760 Fax: 020 7580 5063
(Westminster Primary Care Trust)

Practice Manager M Kelly

GP Nancy Elizabeth LEE

The Surgery
3 Fitzroy Square, London W1T 5HG
Tel: 020 7387 5798 Fax: 020 7387 2497
(Westminster Primary Care Trust)
Patient List Size: 4200

Practice Manager Lucienne Bruderlin

GP John Simon Henry COHEN, Caroline Jane EVANS

London, W2

The Bayswater Surgery
46 Craven Road, London W2 3QA
Tel: 020 7402 2073 Fax: 020 7723 8579
(Westminster Primary Care Trust)

Practice Manager Mouna Allam

GP Daya SILVA

Crompton Medical Centre
1 Crompton Street, London W2 1ND
Tel: 020 7723 7789
(Kensington and Chelsea Primary Care Trust)
Patient List Size: 3400

Practice Manager Beverley Moore

GP Gulzar AHMED

Harrow Road Health Centre
263-265 Harrow Road, London W2 5EZ
Tel: 020 7286 1231 Fax: 020 7266 1253
Email: dan.redsull@gp-E87637.nhs.uk
(Westminster Primary Care Trust)
Patient List Size: 5800

Practice Manager Dan Redsull

GP Jonathan Derek FLUXMAN, Philip Bandele OLUFUNWA

Lancaster Gate Medical Centre
20-21 Leinster Terrace, London W2 3ET
Tel: 020 7479 9750 Fax: 020 7479 9751
(Westminster Primary Care Trust)
Patient List Size: 3800

Practice Manager Joyce Brown

GP Sunil MAINI, Soraya MEER

Little Venice Medical Centre
2 Crompton Street, London W2 1ND
Tel: 020 7723 1314 Fax: 020 7723 8580
(Westminster Primary Care Trust)
Patient List Size: 4500

Practice Manager Frances Dunkley

GP Robert Emmett David HENEBURY, Thomas Charles BARNWELL, Elizabeth Iona COBB

The Newton Medical Centre
14-18 Newton Road, London W2 5LT
Tel: 020 7229 4578 Fax: 020 7229 7315
(Westminster Primary Care Trust)

GP Thomas KADAS, Therese Nicolette SHORTNALL, Georges SIMONS

Paddington Green Health Centre
4 Princess Louise Close, London W2 1LQ
Tel: 020 7887 1600 Fax: 020 7887 1635
(Westminster Primary Care Trust)
Patient List Size: 8300

Practice Manager Alison Dalal

GP Andrew ELDER, Melinda CREME, Thomas ESTCOURT, Neville Richard PURSSELL, Sally TAYLOR

Paddington Surgery
11 Praed Street, London W2 1NJ
Tel: 020 7262 4123 Fax: 020 7262 4107
(Westminster Primary Care Trust)

GP Htay KYWE

The Surgery
41 Connaught Square, London W2 2HL
Tel: 020 7723 3338 Fax: 020 7402 3342
(Westminster Primary Care Trust)

Practice Manager Raheelah Ahmad

GP Ruth O'HARE

The Surgery
2 Garway Road, London W2 4NH
Tel: 020 7221 8803/020 8962 4400 Fax: 020 7792 9923
(Westminster Primary Care Trust)

GP Sheena Jill BUCHANAN-BARROW, Michael CORNELL, Louise Simone HEGGESSEY, Yung Lung HUANG, Gary WILLIAMS

The Surgery
Basement Flat, 160 Gloucester Terrace, London W2 6HR
Tel: 020 7706 2504 Fax: 020 7706 3870
(Westminster Primary Care Trust)
Patient List Size: 1250

Practice Manager M Saxena

GP Surya Prakash SAXSENA

West Two Health Centre
33-35 Praed Street, London W2 1NR
Tel: 020 7262 1307 Fax: 020 7402 3013
(Westminster Primary Care Trust)

GP Nicola LANGDON

London, W3

Acton Health Centre
35-61 Church Road, London W3 8QE
Tel: 020 8992 6768 Fax: 020 8896 2908
(Ealing Primary Care Trust)

Practice Manager Mandy Huxley

GP Patricia Margaret BABER, Napolion Evan ISSAC

Acton Town Medical Centre
122 Gunnersbury Lane, London W3 9BA
Tel: 020 8993 1314 Fax: 020 8896 2786
(Ealing Primary Care Trust)
Patient List Size: 2400

Practice Manager Maureen Cousins

GP Wafik Mohamed MOUSTAFA

Crown Street Surgery
2 Lombard Court, Crown Street, Acton, London W3 8SA
Tel: 020 8992 1963 Fax: 020 8896 2791
(Ealing Primary Care Trust)
Patient List Size: 7600

Practice Manager Jacqui Hawkins

GP Nazaret Haig PAMBAKIAN, Sarah BULL, Rekha GARG, Michael KENNY

Datta
64 Churchfield Road, Acton, London W3 6DL
Tel: 020 8992 3854 Fax: 020 8896 2380
(Ealing Primary Care Trust)

Practice Manager Mrs Datta

GP Satyendra Nath DATTA

Eastfields Road Surgery
1 Eastfields Road, Acton, London W3 0AA
Tel: 020 8922 4331 Fax: 020 8990 7585
(Ealing Primary Care Trust)
Patient List Size: 4000

Practice Manager Malgorzata Kramarzyk

GP Ewa Maria ROBINSKA, Claire SILLITOE

Hillcrest Surgery
337 Uxbridge Road, Acton, London W3 9RA
Tel: 020 8993 0982 Fax: 020 8993 0164
Email: hillcrest.surgery@gp-E85028.nhs.uk
(Ealing Primary Care Trust)
Patient List Size: 7100

Practice Manager Gill Cunningham

GP Sarah Jane McKEIGUE, Madhuri DHATT, Stephen Mark SPENCER, Vijay TAILOR

Horn Lane Surgery
156 Horn Lane, Acton, London W3 6PH
Tel: 020 8992 4722 Fax: 020 8992 2650
(Ealing Primary Care Trust)

Practice Manager Aruna Saujani

GP Arvind Vallabhdas SAUJANI

Mill Hill Surgery
111 Avenue Road, Acton, London W3 8QH
Tel: 020 8992 9955 Fax: 020 8896 0941
(Ealing Primary Care Trust)

Practice Manager Barbara Brunswick

GP Kate Lucy CABOT, J DURANDT, Imogen Frances MEASDAY, Anne SCULLY

The Surgery
2 Burlington Gardens, Acton, London W3 6BA
Tel: 020 8992 0346 Fax: 020 8993 1636
(Ealing Primary Care Trust)

GP H M MAMDANI

The Surgery
118 Old Oak Road, London W3 7HG
Tel: 020 8740 7328 Fax: 020 8743 2235
(Hammersmith and Fulham Primary Care Trust)
Patient List Size: 5600

GP C ANYIAH-OSIGWE, D C NIRIELLA, P TARABA

The Vale Surgery
97 The Vale, Acton, London W3 7RG
Tel: 020 8743 4086 Fax: 020 8746 0346
(Ealing Primary Care Trust)

Practice Manager Pramila C Reddy

GP Challa S Prabhakar REDDY, P V REDDY

Western Avenue Surgery
56 Western Avenue, Acton, London W3 7TY
Tel: 020 8743 4133 Fax: 020 8743 3574
(Ealing Primary Care Trust)
Patient List Size: 3000

Practice Manager Surjeet Panesar

GP Bharat Prasad SINHA

London, W4

Bedford Park Surgery
55 South Parade, Chiswick, London W4 5LH
Tel: 020 8742 1331 Fax: 020 8742 1246
Email: admin@beford-park.co.uk
(Ealing Primary Care Trust)
Patient List Size: 3600

Practice Manager Les Cook

GP John KEEN, Eileen Gertrude DALY

Chiswick Family Practice
89 Southfield Road, Bedford Park, Chiswick, London W4 1BB
Tel: 020 8995 8948/1 Fax: 020 8747 8968
Email: aw@keystone.demon.co.uk
(Ealing Primary Care Trust)
Patient List Size: 3000

Practice Manager Helen Burkitt

GP Andrzej Marek WEBER

Chiswick Family Practice
89 Southfield Road, Bedford Park, Chiswick, London W4 1BB
Tel: 020 8995 8948 Fax: 020 8747 8968
(Ealing Primary Care Trust)

Practice Manager Eunice Hayes, Andy Kolendo

GP Andrzej Marek WEBER

Chiswick Family Practice
89 Southfield Road, Bedford Park, Chiswick, London W4 1BB
Tel: 020 8995 6707 Fax: 020 8995 0750
Email: reception@gp-E85130.nhs.uk
(Ealing Primary Care Trust)
Patient List Size: 3500

Practice Manager Barbara Bilski

GP Vikram Batukrai BHATT, Janina SZYSZKO

Chiswick Health Centre
Fishers Lane, London W4 1RX
Tel: 020 8321 3551 Fax: 020 8321 3556
(Hounslow Primary Care Trust)
Patient List Size: 3923

Practice Manager V Venkatesham

GP Guduguntla VENKATESHAM, Jayantilal Popatlal SONI

Chiswick Health Centre
Fishers Lane, London W4 1RX
Tel: 020 8321 3518/9 Fax: 020 8321 3568
(Hounslow Primary Care Trust)
Patient List Size: 11500

Practice Manager Vernon Sexton

GP Stephen Leon HIRST, Jennifer Margaret CHISHOLM, Yolanda Mary HOLDERNESS, Graham Victor HUGHES, Mark Jon KAPLAN, Vanessa O'MARA

Chiswick Health Centre
Fishers Lane, London W4 1RX
Tel: 020 8994 4482 Fax: 020 8742 7816
(Hounslow Primary Care Trust)

Practice Manager Brenda Moussa

GP R MOUSSA, B A ADIB, Priyantha Naomal SOYSA

Chiswick Health Centre
Fishers Lane, London W4 1RX
Tel: 020 8994 2465 Fax: 020 8994 9497
(Hounslow Primary Care Trust)

Practice Manager Jackie Corless

GP Ruth Janet HEINSHEIMER, Debdas CHOUDHURI, E A DENNIS

Crossley House Surgery
Crossley House, Sutton Lane North, Chiswick, London W4 4HF
Tel: 020 8994 0342 Fax: 020 8994 6927
(Hounslow Primary Care Trust)
Patient List Size: 2500

Practice Manager Angela Belcher

GP Zygmunt KUKULSKI

Glebe Street Surgery
1 Glebe Street, Chiswick, London W4 2BD
Tel: 020 8747 4800 Fax: 020 8995 4388
(Hounslow Primary Care Trust)
Patient List Size: 4200

Practice Manager Caroline Wilson

GP Christine Ann GARDINER, Mumkush PATEL

Grove Park Surgery
95 Burlington Lane, Chiswick, London W4 3ET
Tel: 020 8747 1549 Fax: 020 8995 9529
Email: groveparksurgery@gp-E85693.nhs.uk
(Hounslow Primary Care Trust)
Patient List Size: 6000

Practice Manager Shaheen Hamid

GP Sheila Moira HUNT, Andrew DEVINE, Shantha SETHURAJAN

Grove Park Terrace Surgery
25 Grove Park Terrace, Chiswick, London W4 3JL
Tel: 020 8995 1743 Fax: 020 8742 1590
Email: recep.one@gp-e85639.nhs.uk
(Hounslow Primary Care Trust)
Patient List Size: 2500

Practice Manager Antre Buchanan

GP G M WILLIAMS, L S DAVID

Holly Road Medical Centre
2A Holly Road, Chiswick, London W4 1NU
Tel: 020 8994 0976 Fax: 020 8994 3685
(Hounslow Primary Care Trust)
Patient List Size: 2600

GP Navinchandra Amarshi THAKRAR

Southfield Medical Centre
89 Southfield Road, Bedford Park, Chiswick, London W4 1BB
Tel: 020 8994 4644 Fax: 020 8747 8968
(Ealing Primary Care Trust)

GP Sally Elizabeth EDMUNDS, Janina Maria SZYSZKO

The Surgery
253 Acton Lane, Chiswick, London W4 5DG
Tel: 020 8995 5706 Fax: 020 8995 5706
(Ealing Primary Care Trust)

Practice Manager Peter Lwin

GP S M YIN

Wellesley Road Surgery
7 Wellesley Road, Chiswick, London W4 4BJ
Tel: 020 8995 4396 Fax: 020 8994 4314
(Hounslow Primary Care Trust)

Practice Manager S Sanders

GP Nicola Vivien BURBIDGE, Elizabeth MORRIS, Katherine O'BRIEY

London, W5

Boileau Road Surgery
104 Boileau Road, London W5 3AJ
Tel: 020 8997 6604 Fax: 020 8998 0452
(Ealing Primary Care Trust)

Practice Manager Vicky Stiff

GP Margaret Rosaleen JONES

Ealing Park Health Centre
195A South Ealing Road, Ealing, London W5 4RH
Tel: 020 8758 0570 Fax: 020 8560 5182
Email: ephc@gp-e85657.nhs.uk
(Ealing Primary Care Trust)
Patient List Size: 6634

Practice Manager Carol Saunders

GP Lucy Katherine FARLEY, F ISLAM, R J NORBURY, Jacqueline Dawn PIGGOTT

The Florence Road Surgery
26 Florence Road, Ealing, London W5 3TX
Tel: 020 8567 2111 Fax: 020 8840 5768
(Ealing Primary Care Trust)

Practice Manager Sarah Townsend

GP David Charles Michael EVANS, G AZIZ-SCOTT, G JONES, Sarbjit Singh KALER, S WHITEHURST

Junction Road Surgery
20 Junction Road, London W5 4XL
Tel: 020 8560 8529
(Ealing Primary Care Trust)

GP N MITRA, S K MITRA

Pitshanger Lane Surgery
209 Pitshanger Lane, Ealing, London W5 1RQ
Tel: 020 8997 4747 Fax: 020 8566 7422
Website: www.pitshangerfamilypractice.fsnet.co.uk
(Ealing Primary Care Trust)
Patient List Size: 3200

Practice Manager Valerie Kennedy

GP Simon Hugh Charles VALENTINE, Luna DAS

Queens Walk Surgery
6 Queens Walk, Ealing, London W5 1TP
Tel: 020 8997 3041 Fax: 020 8566 9100
Email: debra.fleetwood@gp-n85029.nhs.uk
(Ealing Primary Care Trust)
Patient List Size: 9600

Practice Manager Margaret Mathias

GP Susan Elizabeth ALLAN, Cornelius Joseph CROWLEY, Jeremy Charles GITTINS

St David's Clinic
2 Bramley Road, Ealing, London W5 4SS
Tel: 020 8579 0165 Fax: 020 8579 0424
Email: m.karu@medix-uk.com
(Hounslow Primary Care Trust)
Patient List Size: 3500

Practice Manager I Hathaway

GP Mudhitha KARUNARATNE

The Surgery
75 Brunswick Road, Ealing, London W5 1AQ
Tel: 020 8810 5545 Fax: 020 8997 4880
(Ealing Primary Care Trust)
Patient List Size: 2700

Practice Manager Jurate Baziene

GP N F LEWIS

The Surgery
10 Crofton Road, Ealing, London W5 2HS
Tel: 020 8997 4215 Fax: 020 8991 9574
(Ealing Primary Care Trust)

Practice Manager Mike Fitzgerald

GP Allan David LAUDER, Mary Margaret LAUDER

The Surgery
9 Lynwood Road, Ealing, London W5 1JQ
Tel: 020 8997 7522 Fax: 020 8997 9429
(Ealing Primary Care Trust)
Patient List Size: 1500

Practice Manager Elizabeth Abrahamian

GP Haider Hasan Mohamad Ali AL-HASANI

London, W6

The Brook Green Medical Centre
Bute Gardens, London W6 7EG
Tel: 020 8237 2800 Fax: 020 8237 2811
(Hammersmith and Fulham Primary Care Trust)
Patient List Size: 8000

Practice Manager Paul Aston

GP Doreen Diana Rachel SHAOUL, Edward SHAOUL, David John Charles WINGFIELD

Hammersmith Surgery
1 Hammersmith Road, London W6 9DU
(Hammersmith and Fulham Primary Care Trust)

GP Paula Francesca Rosemarie FERNANDES, H COLEMAN, H THOMAS

Ravenscourt Road Surgery
34 Ravenscourt Road, London W6 0UG
Tel: 020 8748 4842 Fax: 020 8563 2779
(Hammersmith and Fulham Primary Care Trust)

GP Terence Joseph MULLIGAN

Richford Gate Medical Practice
49 Richford Gate, Richford Street, London W6 7HY
Tel: 020 8846 7555 Fax: 020 8846 7538
Website: www.grovemedicalpractice.co.uk
(Hammersmith and Fulham Primary Care Trust)
Patient List Size: 11000

Practice Manager Renos Pittarides

GP Jozef Ivan KOPPEL, Alan Neil Lee FRAZER, Sarah Caroline JARVIS, B A McDONALD, Claire SLEIGHT, R D THOMSON, Tony WILLS

Shepherds Bush Road Surgery
3 Shepherds Bush Road, Hammersmith, London W6 7NA
Tel: 020 7610 4292 Fax: 020 7602 9596
(Hammersmith and Fulham Primary Care Trust)

GP B K DHAR, F B MALIK

The Surgery
15 Brook Green, London W6 7BL
Tel: 020 8603 7563 Fax: 020 8602 6840
(Hammersmith and Fulham Primary Care Trust)

GP Sarah CLARK-MAXWELL, V M LYNCH, L SLATER

The Surgery
89 Fulham Palace Road, London W6 8JA
Tel: 020 8748 3197 Fax: 020 8563 1661
(Hammersmith and Fulham Primary Care Trust)

GP R N SRIVASTAVA

London, W7

Cuckoo Lane Surgery
14 Cuckoo Lane, Hanwell, London W7 3EY
Tel: 020 8567 4315 Fax: 020 8567 7950
(Ealing Primary Care Trust)

Practice Manager Nicolette Boyce

GP Felicity Wendy LIGHT, Z ROGERS

Elthorne Park Surgery
106 Elthorne Park Road, Hanwell, London W7 2JJ
Tel: 020 8567 0447 Fax: 020 8567 0984
(Ealing Primary Care Trust)
Patient List Size: 6952

Practice Manager Gill Butler

GP Colin John LEONARD, Sally Ann PINNEY, P J REYNOLDS, R SHAH, M WATERS

Family Health Practice
20 Church Road, Hanwell, London W7 1DR
Tel: 020 8579 7338 Fax: 020 8840 9928
(Ealing Primary Care Trust)
Patient List Size: 2900

Practice Manager Linda Williams

GP Onkar Singh SAHOTA

Greenford Avenue Medical Centre
322 Greenford Avenue, Hanwell, London W7 3AH
Tel: 020 8578 1880 Fax: 020 8357 6585
(Ealing Primary Care Trust)

Practice Manager Lola A Freeman

GP Anthony Leon FREEMAN, Rodney Maxwell WALDES

Hanwell Health Centre
20 Church Road, Hanwell, London W7 1DR
Tel: 020 8579 7337 Fax: 020 8579 7337
(Ealing Primary Care Trust)
Patient List Size: 3300

Practice Manager Gurmeet Virdee

GP Rosamund Chad STEWART, Alexandra Louise HALLUMS

Hanwell Health Centre
20 Church Road, Hanwell, London W7 1DR
Tel: 020 8567 5738 Fax: 020 8567 7472
(Ealing Primary Care Trust)
Patient List Size: 5800

Practice Manager Maureen Ham

GP Richard NAISH, Andrew Robert LEES, Sandy True Vijeyasingam PERINPANAYAGAM

The Surgery
438 Greenford Avenue, Hanwell, London W7 3DD
Tel: 020 8578 1430 Fax: 020 8575 6625
(Ealing Primary Care Trust)
Patient List Size: 2800

Practice Manager Linda Thomson

GP B R PATEL

The Surgery
161 Grenford Avenue, London W7 1HA
Tel: 020 8567 1497
(Ealing Primary Care Trust)

GP V MATHUR

London, W8

Abingdon Medical Centre
88-92 Earls Court Road, London W8 6EG
Tel: 020 8746 5959 Fax: 020 7746 5960
(Kensington and Chelsea Primary Care Trust)

GP Dr CHUA, Patricia Clare CORBETT, Dr KILDUFF, Teresa Rosalia Barbara PAWLIKOWSKA

Scarsdale Place Medical Centre
2 Scarsdale Place, London W8 5SX
Tel: 020 7938 1887 Fax: 020 8376 2784
(Kensington and Chelsea Primary Care Trust)
Patient List Size: 4200

Practice Manager L French

GP Patrick Joseph KIERNAN, Dr RABY

The Surgery
2 Scarsdale Villas, London W8 6PR
Tel: 020 7937 3343 Fax: 020 7937 3949
(Kensington and Chelsea Primary Care Trust)
Patient List Size: 3600

GP Mazen Haider MALHAS, Susan Margaret MALHAS

The Surgery
90 1/2 Lexham Gardens, (Rear 17 Marloes Road), London W8 6JQ
Tel: 020 7370 0180 Fax: 020 8672 9799
(Kensington and Chelsea Primary Care Trust)

GP Muhammad Akhtar Ali SHAH

The Surgery
5 Kensington Place, London W8 7PT
Tel: 020 7229 7111 Fax: 020 7221 3069
(Kensington and Chelsea Primary Care Trust)
Patient List Size: 6800

Practice Manager Clare Parker

GP Carole Eve BRONSDON, James Reid THOMPSON

London, W9

Elgin Partnership
38 Elgin Avenue, London W9 3QT
Tel: 020 7286 0747 Fax: 020 7286 9773
(Westminster Primary Care Trust)

GP Caroline Jane BEARSTED, Neil Richard PERRETT

Lanark Medical Centre
Ground Floor, 165 Lanark Road, London W9 1NZ
Tel: 020 7328 1128 Fax: 020 7328 0605
(Westminster Primary Care Trust)
Patient List Size: 3000

GP Yousry Abdel Shaffy EL-GAZZAR

Maida Vale Medical Centre
40 Biddulph Mansions, Elgin Avenue, London W9 1HT
Tel: 020 7286 6464 Fax: 020 7266 1017
(Westminster Primary Care Trust)

Practice Manager S Joffe

GP David Michael SPIRO, Hugh Edward WRIGHT

The Medical Centre
7E Woodfield Road, London W9 3XZ
Tel: 020 7266 1449 Fax: 020 7266 1449
(Westminster Primary Care Trust)
Patient List Size: 5200

Practice Manager Leiola Jefferson

GP Susan Elizabeth HONEY, Mark GILES

The Medical Centre
165 Lanark Road, Third Floor, London W9 1NZ
Tel: 020 7624 8616 Fax: 020 7372 0244
(Westminster Primary Care Trust)

GP L M ABOUZEKRY

New Elgin Practice
44 Chippenham Road, London W9 2AF
Tel: 020 7266 2431 Fax: 020 7289 6275
Email: quilliam@dircon.co.uk
(Westminster Primary Care Trust)
Patient List Size: 5000

Practice Manager Joan Newman

GP Robert Paul QUILLIAM, Judith TATE

Randolph Surgery
235A Elgin Avenue, London W9 1NH
Tel: 020 7286 6880 Fax: 020 7286 9787
(Westminster Primary Care Trust)
Patient List Size: 5500

Practice Manager Linda Duncan

GP Abigail Jane BERGER, Robert Anthony HICKS

The Surgery
56 Maida Vale, London W9 1PP
Tel: 020 7624 4433 Fax: 020 7624 0803
(Westminster Primary Care Trust)

GP Selwyn Leon DEXTER

The Surgery
321 Shirland Road, London W9 3JJ
Tel: 020 8969 2626 Fax: 020 8964 0353
(Westminster Primary Care Trust)
Patient List Size: 5200

Practice Manager Bernard Hatswell, A Joseph

GP Anna Maria GARFIELD, Marek Anthony SARNICKI

London, W10

Ahmed
Queens Park Health Centre, Dart Street, London W10 4LD
Tel: 020 8964 9990 Fax: 020 8964 0436
(Westminster Primary Care Trust)

GP Nazeer AHMED

The Exmoor Surgery
Exmoor Street, London W10 6DZ
Tel: 020 8962 4245 Fax: 020 8962 4252
(Westminster Primary Care Trust)

GP Mohammad Lutfor RAHMAN, Hanan YOUSIF

The Golborne Medical Centre
12-16 Golborne Road, London W10 5PE
Tel: 020 8964 4801 Fax: 020 8964 5702
(Westminster Primary Care Trust)

Practice Manager D Tasneem

GP Hamid Hussain Mohamadali DATHI

Latimer Surgery
1 Waynflete Square, London W10 6UX
Tel: 020 8969 1242 Fax: 020 8968 3045
(Westminster Primary Care Trust)

GP A NIJHAR, M MARKS, L SASH

The Meanwhile Garden Medical Centre
Unit 5, 1-31 Elkstone Road, London W10 5NT
Tel: 020 8960 5620 Fax: 020 8964 1964
(Westminster Primary Care Trust)
Patient List Size: 5000

Practice Manager Esre Knowles

GP Nalini JASANI, Hugh Michael GILLESPIE, Dr KRAEMER

Queens Park Health Centre
Dart Street, London W10 4LD
Tel: 020 8960 5252 Fax: 020 8964 3266
(Westminster Primary Care Trust)

GP Risiyur Krishnaswamy NAGARAJAN

Queens Park Health Centre
Dart Street, London W10 4LD
Tel: 020 8969 1490 Fax: 020 8964 0436
(Westminster Primary Care Trust)

GP Dr LAI CHUNG FONG

St Quintins Health Centre
St Quintin Avenue, London W10 6NX
Tel: 020 8960 5677 Fax: 020 8968 5933
(Kensington and Chelsea Primary Care Trust)

Practice Manager Carole Proctor

GP Elizabeth Patricia DENSHAM, Ian KELSO, Shelley Naomi SWADE

The Surgery
12-14 Golborne Road, London W10 5PG
Tel: 020 8969 2058 Fax: 020 8964 4156
(Westminster Primary Care Trust)
Patient List Size: 5000

Practice Manager P Grey

GP Wedad Soliman ABBAS, Nirmalan RAMASAMY

The Surgery
80 Cambridge Gardens, London W10 6HS
Tel: 020 8969 5517 Fax: 020 8964 4766
(Westminster Primary Care Trust)
Patient List Size: 1900

Practice Manager Cath Esbester

GP Martin Gerard Daniel O'RAWE, Stella BAKER

The Surgery
85 St Quintin Avenue, London W10 6PB
Tel: 020 8969 2563/020 8354 3836 Fax: 020 8969 2563
(Westminster Primary Care Trust)

Practice Manager S Higgs

GP George Dawson SADLER

The Surgery
574 Harrow Road, London W10 4NJ
Tel: 020 8960 5499 Fax: 020 8968 1947
(Westminster Primary Care Trust)

GP Kumara SRIKRISHNAMURTHY

London, W11

Chung
Colville Health Centre, 51 Kensington Park Road, London W11 1PA
Tel: 020 7727 8212 Fax: 020 7460 1631
(Kensington and Chelsea Primary Care Trust)

GP Margaret Mary CHUNG

The Foreland Medical Centre
188 Walmer Road, London W11 4ES
Tel: 020 7727 2604 Fax: 020 7792 1261
(Kensington and Chelsea Primary Care Trust)
Patient List Size: 4500

GP Lisa CRAM, Bradley Andrew PEARL

Jackson
17 Pembridge Road, London W11 3HG
Tel: 020 7221 0174 Fax: 020 7229 0774
(Westminster Primary Care Trust)

Practice Manager Barrie Waugh

GP Gaye Diana Mary JACKSON

The Pembridge Villas Surgery
45A Pembridge Villas, London W11 3EP
Tel: 020 7727 2222 Fax: 020 7792 2867
(Westminster Primary Care Trust)
Patient List Size: 3500

Practice Manager Gordana Stojanovska

GP Simon Steve RAMSDEN, Philip John REID

Pettifer and Mok
Colville Health Centre, 51 Kensington Park Road, London W11 1PA
Tel: 020 7727 4592 Fax: 020 7221 4613
(Kensington and Chelsea Primary Care Trust)
Patient List Size: 4500

Practice Manager Karin Frowd

GP Brenda Jane PETTIFER, Catherine Ann Kit Yee MOK

The Portland Road Practice
16 Portland Road, London W11 4LA
Tel: 020 7727 7711 Fax: 020 7226 6755
(Westminster Primary Care Trust)
Patient List Size: 5000

Practice Manager Yvonne Fraser

GP Krystyna Maria Teresa SOBONIEWSKA, Diane WATSON

Portobello Medical Centre
14 Codrington Mews, London W11 2EH
Tel: 020 7727 5800/2326 Fax: 020 7792 9044
(Westminster Primary Care Trust)

Practice Manager Ray Read

GP John Stanley Charles STRIDE, Stephen Jeremy HOLDEN, Susan Anne SALKELD, Annette Christa STEELE

The Surgery
241 Westbourne Grove, London W11 2SE
Tel: 020 7229 5800 Fax: 020 7243 2058
(Kensington and Chelsea Primary Care Trust)
Patient List Size: 8500

Practice Manager Terry Brown

GP William Chung Wing CHENG, Pearl CHIN, Catherine Mary Ita O'CONNOR

The Surgery
73 Holland Park, London W11 3SL
Tel: 020 7221 4334 Fax: 020 7792 8517
(Kensington and Chelsea Primary Care Trust)
Patient List Size: 8414

Practice Manager Anne Barnes

GP Christopher Roy CALMAN, Caroline Anna BLOOM, Richard Chenoweth HOOKER, Evelyn Mary LEWIS

The Surgery
112 Princedale Road, London W11 4NH
Tel: 020 7727 2022 Fax: 020 7727 2022
(Westminster Primary Care Trust)

GP Valerie Odette DIAS, Lucy OWENS

The Surgery
96 Sirdar Road, London W11 4EG
Tel: 020 7727 9238 Fax: 020 7460 7305
(Westminster Primary Care Trust)

GP Druseela WIJAYSINGHE

London, W12

Ashchurch Surgery
134 Askew Road, Shepherd Bush, London W12 9BP
Tel: 020 8743 2920 Fax: 020 8743 1545
(Hammersmith and Fulham Primary Care Trust)
Patient List Size: 6300

Practice Manager Jana Rajah

GP Kamal WINAYAK, Mary BEST, Indira COLEMAN

The Bush Doctors
16-17 The Links, Shepherds Bush Centre, London W12 8PP
Tel: 020 8749 1882 Fax: 020 8749 4278
(Hammersmith and Fulham Primary Care Trust)

GP F SAMJI, S CHATTOO, C S CUMMINGS, J M M HUDDY, S McGOLDRICK

The Medical Centre
13 Ollgar Close, Uxbridge Road, Shepherds Bush, London W12 0NS
Tel: 020 8740 7407 Fax: 020 8743 0220
(Hammersmith and Fulham Primary Care Trust)

GP R KUKAR

Ollgar Close Surgery
13 Ollgar Close, Askew Estate, Uxbridge Road, London W12 0NF
Tel: 020 8743 4541
(Hammersmith and Fulham Primary Care Trust)

GP R K KUKAR

Rylett Road Surgery
45A Rylett Road, Shepherds Bush, London W12 9ST
Tel: 020 8749 7863 Fax: 020 8743 5161
(Hammersmith and Fulham Primary Care Trust)
Patient List Size: 6900

Practice Manager Evelyn Baud

GP Angela Elizabeth PITT, Vincenzo Matteo GRIPPAUDO

Rylett Road Surgery
45A Rylett Road, Shepherds Bush, London W12 9ST
Tel: 020 8749 7863 Fax: 020 8743 5161
(Hammersmith and Fulham Primary Care Trust)
Patient List Size: 6900

Practice Manager Evelyn Baud

GP Deirdre Mary Bernadette O'GALLAGHER

Rylett Road Surgery
42A Rylett Road, Shepherds Bush, London W12 9ST
Tel: 020 8749 7863 Fax: 020 8743 5161
(Hammersmith and Fulham Primary Care Trust)
Patient List Size: 6900

Practice Manager Evelyn Baud

GP Peter Guy FERMIE

Shepherds Bush Medical Centre
336 Uxbridge Road, London W12 7LS
Tel: 020 8743 5153 Fax: 020 8742 9070
Email: ahmedbadat@aol.com
(Hammersmith and Fulham Primary Care Trust)
Patient List Size: 4400

GP Ahamed Adamjee BADAT, K SHAH

The Surgery
143A Uxbridge Road, London W12 9RD
Tel: 020 8743 1511 Fax: 020 8740 0310
(Hammersmith and Fulham Primary Care Trust)

GP George MOSES, Ronda Verina JOLLY, Stuart MILLER

The Surgery
13 Westway, London W12 0PT
Tel: 020 8743 3704 Fax: 020 8742 9500
(Hammersmith and Fulham Primary Care Trust)
Patient List Size: 3700

Practice Manager Neena Dasgupia

GP S DASGUPTA, J A KEYANI

White City Health Centre
Australia Road, Shepherds Bush, London W12 7PH
Tel: 020 8749 4145
(Hammersmith and Fulham Primary Care Trust)

GP Gurjeet Singh UPPAL, Sheila UPPAL

White City Health Centre
Australia Road, Shepherds Bush, London W12 7PH
Tel: 020 8743 3090
(Hammersmith and Fulham Primary Care Trust)
Patient List Size: 5000

Practice Manager D Dandapat

GP Raja DANDAPAT, Dona Sabina Dushanthi CANISIUS

White City Health Centre
Australia Road, Shepherds Bush, London W12 7PH
Tel: 020 8749 4141
(Hammersmith and Fulham Primary Care Trust)
Patient List Size: 3000

GP N S MIRZA

London, W13

The Argyle Surgery
128 Argyle Road, Ealing, London W13 8ER
Tel: 020 8601 2500 Fax: 020 8601 2503
Email: argyle.surgery@gp-E85120.nhs.uk
Website: www.argylesurgery.nhs.uk
(Ealing Primary Care Trust)
Patient List Size: 5263

Practice Manager Kristina Borowicz

GP Gouri DHILLON, S D SHARMA

Coldershaw Road Surgery
168 Coldershaw Road, West Ealing, London W13 9DT
Tel: 020 8567 0970
(Ealing Primary Care Trust)

GP R DASOJU, B SNEHALATHA, G YIANGOU

Gordon House Surgery
78 Mattock Lane, Ealing, London W13 9NZ
Tel: 020 8799 5683 Fax: 020 8840 0533
(Ealing Primary Care Trust)

Practice Manager Fionnuala O'Donnell

GP Ian BERNSTEIN, Joanne HARRIS, Naeem QURESHI, Vicki RAMAGE, Ravi RAMANATHAN, A SANTODIROCCO, Marcus John Francesco SOLDINI

Grosvenor House
147 Broadway, West Ealing, London W13 9BJ
Tel: 020 8567 0165 Fax: 020 8810 0902
(Ealing Primary Care Trust)

Practice Manager Heather McNally

GP Ramulu DASOJU, B SNEHALATHA, G YIANGOU

Grosvenor House
147 Broadway, West Ealing, London W13 9BE
Tel: 020 8567 0165/5172 Fax: 020 8810 0902
(Ealing Primary Care Trust)
Patient List Size: 6400

Practice Manager Heather McNally, Anita Suratwala

GP R DASOJU, K MANKOO, B SNEHALATHA, Georgia YIANGOU

The Surgery
102 The Avenue, Ealing, London W13 8LA
Tel: 020 8997 2525 Fax: 020 8991 8074
(Ealing Primary Care Trust)
Patient List Size: 9800

Practice Manager Ann Soiza

GP Jane LIVINGSTON, Jacqueline Mary BAYER

The Surgery
61 Northfield Avenue, West Ealing, London W13 9QP
Tel: 020 8567 1612 Fax: 020 8579 2593
(Ealing Primary Care Trust)
Patient List Size: 9000

Practice Manager Denise Hunt

GP David Stephen COWEN, Susan Margaret JAMES, Sally Joanne MASON, Christina WARREN

The Surgery
55 Coldershaw Road, Ealing, London W13 9EA
Tel: 020 8840 1757 Fax: 020 8840 2088
(Ealing Primary Care Trust)
Patient List Size: 1900

Practice Manager Marie Imosen

GP Patrick Hon-Hing LAU

The Surgery
147 The Broadway, London W13 9BE
(Ealing Primary Care Trust)

GP Dr SNEHALATHA

London, W14

Kensington Park Medical Centre
75 Russell Road, London W14 8HW
Tel: 020 7603 5206 Fax: 020 7602 0417
(Kensington and Chelsea Primary Care Trust)

Practice Manager Alexandra Womphrey

GP Jasjeet Singh DUA, P NOCHOLAS

Milson Road Health Centre
1-13 Milson Road, London W14 0LJ
Tel: 020 8846 6262 Fax: 020 8846 6263
(Hammersmith and Fulham Primary Care Trust)

GP Mustafa Akanni OSHODI

Milson Road Health Centre
1-13 Milson Road, London W14 0LJ
Tel: 020 8846 6262/6251 Fax: 020 8846 6239
(Hammersmith and Fulham Primary Care Trust)

Practice Manager M Living

GP M A OSHODI

Milson Road Surgery
1-13 Milson Road, London W14 0LJ
Tel: 020 8846 6262 Fax: 020 8846 6263
(Hammersmith and Fulham Primary Care Trust)

Patient List Size: 2500

GP Musstaffa A OSHODI

North End Medical Centre
211 North End Road, West Kensington, London W14 9NP
Tel: 020 7385 7777 Fax: 020 7386 9612
Website: www.the-medical-centre.com
(Hammersmith and Fulham Primary Care Trust)
Patient List Size: 12748

Practice Manager Paul Ferguson

GP Sally Hutcheon IND, Richard Anthony CLUBB, Michele Mary DAVISON, C LYONS, Hemma SIMS, Peter Nicholas WILSON

Sterndale Surgery
74a Sterndale Road, London W14 0HX
Tel: 020 8746 5972 Fax: 020 8371 3347
(Hammersmith and Fulham Primary Care Trust)

GP M CLARK, C ELLIOTT

London, WC1

Amwell Practice
4 Naoroji Street, London WC1X OGB
Tel: 020 7837 2020 Fax: 020 7278 7135
Website: amwellpractice.co.uk
(Islington Primary Care Trust)

Practice Manager Peter Floyd

GP David William DAVIES, Kevin DEWHIRST, Sonia MANNELLY, Paul ROGERS, Liam SMEETH, Victoria TZORTZIOU, Karina Mary UPTON

Bloomsbury Street Surgery
60 Bloomsbury Street, London WC1B 3QU
Tel: 020 7437 4467 Fax: 020 7580 2062
(Camden Primary Care Trust)
Patient List Size: 5000

Practice Manager E Wieczorek

GP Dr GRECO

The Bloomsbury Surgery
1 Handel Street, London WC1N 1PD
Tel: 020 7837 8559 Fax: 020 7837 3562
(Camden Primary Care Trust)

Practice Manager Nasim Rehman

GP A M REHMAN

Brunswick Medical Centre
53 Brunswick Centre, London WC1N 1BP
Tel: 020 7837 3811 Fax: 020 7833 8408
(Camden Primary Care Trust)

Practice Manager Jenny Fisher

GP Peter Justin SKOLAR, Michelle Linda LANGDON

Gower Place Practice
3 Gower Place, London WC1E 6BN
Tel: 020 7387 6306 Fax: 020 7387 3645
Email: gpp@gp-f83043.nhs.uk
(Camden Primary Care Trust)
Patient List Size: 11000

Practice Manager Carol Shiels

GP Peter Anthony ANDERSEN, Ali Amijee ALIBHAI, Mark BARRETT, Claire Alexandra ELLIOTT

Gray's Inn Medical
79 Grays Inn Road, London WC1X 8TT
Tel: 020 7405 9360 Fax: 020 7831 1964
(Camden Primary Care Trust)

Practice Manager Brian Eastwood

GP S M E SOLOMON, A FLEISHMAN

Great Russell Street Surgery
58 Great Russell Street, London WC1B 3BE
Tel: 020 7405 2739 Fax: 020 7404 1642
(Camden Primary Care Trust)
Patient List Size: 2660

Practice Manager Roseana McCabe

GP Denise Jacqueline BAVIN

Holborn Medical Centre
64 Lambs Conduit Street, London WC1N 3NA
Tel: 020 7405 3541 Fax: 020 7404 8198
(Camden Primary Care Trust)
Patient List Size: 5545

Practice Manager Christina Tucker

GP Richard Toralf Longdon HALVORSEN, Alexander James MOGHISSI

The Surgery
20 Gower Street, London WC1E 6DP
Tel: 020 7636 7628 Fax: 020 7580 2497
(Camden Primary Care Trust)

Practice Manager Peter Edmonds

GP C CUSACK, A GILLIBRAND, R MURTHI

London, WC2

Convent Garden Medical Centre
47 Shorts Gardens, London WC2H 9AA
Tel: 020 7379 7209
(Westminster Primary Care Trust)

Practice Manager Lila Bently

GP Kandiah PATHAMANATHAN, Neveen Aly RADY, Sockalingham SENTHIL KUMAR

St Phillips Health Centre
Houghton Street, London WC2A 2AE
Tel: 020 7955 7016 Fax: 020 7955 6818
(Camden Primary Care Trust)
Patient List Size: 8000

Practice Manager Kay Duggan

GP Elisabeth FENDER, John David KELT, Rathini RATNAVEL

Longfield

Kent House Surgery
36 Station Road, Longfield DA3 7QD
Tel: 01474 702127 Fax: 01474 704735
(Dartford, Gravesham and Swanley Primary Care Trust)

GP David John REBEL, Paul Robert DAVIES, Yvonne Mary DAVIES, Andrew Graham DOTT, Naimish GANDHI, Jeanne HERRING, John Noel LUFFINGHAM, Susan Mary PIMENTA, Peter Karl Edward SMITH

Lostwithiel

Lostwithiel Medical Practice
North Street, Lostwithiel PL22 0EF
Tel: 01208 872589 Fax: 01208 873710
Email: losteng@lostwithiel.cornwall.nhs.uk
(North and East Cornwall Primary Care Trust)
Patient List Size: 4700

Practice Manager Amanda Bone, Alison Howe

GP Robert William HOWE, Hannah Patricia BOWEN, Iestyn Rhys BOWEN

Loughborough

Alpine House Surgery
86 Rothley Road, Mountsorrel, Loughborough LE12 7JU
Tel: 0116 230 3062 Fax: 0116 237 4218

(Charnwood and North West Leicestershire Primary Care Trust)

Practice Manager Kate Walker

GP Ian Richard SCHOFIELD, J A ELLISON, Peter John FURBER, Karen Tracy Ann MATTHEWS

The Banks Surgery

9 The Banks, Sileby, Loughborough LE12 7RD
Tel: 01509 812343 Fax: 01509 815992
(Charnwood and North West Leicestershire Primary Care Trust)
Patient List Size: 5200

GP Richard PALIN, Sujata GOPAL, Stephen JONES

Barrow Health Centre

27 High Street, Barrow on Soar, Loughborough LE12 8PY
Tel: 01509 413525 Fax: 01509 620664
(Charnwood and North West Leicestershire Primary Care Trust)

Practice Manager Christine Spencer

GP Nicholas Harold Randell SIMPSON, Dipak Raman DAYAH, Susan Angela DUFFY, Sarah Caroline PARKER

Bridge Street Medical Practice

20 Bridge Street, Loughborough LE11 1NQ
Tel: 01509 263018 Fax: 01509 211427
Website: www.bsmp.co.uk
(Charnwood and North West Leicestershire Primary Care Trust)
Patient List Size: 8700

Practice Manager Pauline Sealy

GP Philip Ronald Hopkin GIBSON, Peter Mark CANNON, Sarah EVESON, Satbir Singh JASSAL, EMILY TERRELL

Charnwood Surgery

39 Linkfield Road, Mountsorrel, Loughborough LE12 7DJ
Tel: 0116 237 5089 Fax: 0116 237 5089
(Charnwood and North West Leicestershire Primary Care Trust)
Patient List Size: 2700

Practice Manager Liz Robinson

GP R K HIRANI

Cross Street Surgery

5 Cross Street, Hathern, Loughborough LE12 5LB
Tel: 01509 646326 Fax: 01509 646098
(Charnwood and North West Leicestershire Primary Care Trust)

Practice Manager Karen Pearce

GP Balvinder KAUR, Narinder Singh SAUND, Balbir SINGH

East Leake Health Centre

Gotham Lane, East Leake, Loughborough LE12 6JG
Tel: 01509 852181 Fax: 01509 852099
(Rushcliffe Primary Care Trust)
Patient List Size: 8400

Practice Manager Nicola Tyler

GP Alan Robert BARLOW, Peter David GORDON, Anthony Thomas KELLY, Stephen SHORTT

Forest House Surgery

25 Leicester Road, Shepshed, Loughborough LE12 9DF
Tel: 01509 508412
(Charnwood and North West Leicestershire Primary Care Trust)
Patient List Size: 11900

Practice Manager I M Stackhouse

GP Keith James EVANS, Kamlesh Nanji BADIANI, Elizabeth Angela HALL, Trevor Duke HALL, Gurmeet SINGH, Aidan Robert SKEOCH, Katherine Fiona SOUTHWELL

Highgate Medical Centre

5 Storer Close, Sileby, Loughborough LE12 7UD
Tel: 01509 816364 Fax: 01509 815528
(Charnwood and North West Leicestershire Primary Care Trust)
Patient List Size: 2500

Practice Manager May Lakhani

GP Mayur K LAKHANI

Loughborough University Medical Centre

Loughborough University of Technology, Loughborough LE11 3TU
Tel: 01509 222061 Fax: 01509 223996
(Charnwood and North West Leicestershire Primary Care Trust)
Patient List Size: 12500

Practice Manager N King

GP Mohammed Asghar BHOJANI, Kate E COLEMAN, Harinder Kaur GILL, Naresh Narshi VAGHELA

Manor House Medical Centre

Manor House, Mill Lane, Belton, Loughborough LE12 9UJ
Tel: 01530 222368 Fax: 01530 2242273
(Charnwood and North West Leicestershire Primary Care Trust)

GP John Charles William JOLLEYS, Melanie Jayne ARAM, Bevis Michael HEAP

Park View Surgery

24-28 Leicester Road, Loughborough LE11 2AG
Tel: 01509 230717 Fax: 01509 236891
(Charnwood and North West Leicestershire Primary Care Trust)
Patient List Size: 7000

Practice Manager Sue Melling

GP William John AUST, Edward George CLODE-BAICER, Kim Daniel NEUBERG, Diane Elizabeth WALLIS

Pinfold Medical Practice

Loughborough Health Centre, Pinfold Gate, Loughborough LE11 1DQ
Tel: 01509 568880 Fax: 01509 568879
(Charnwood and North West Leicestershire Primary Care Trust)
Patient List Size: 9800

Practice Manager Samantha Spencer

GP Leslie BORRILL, Janice BRUNSKILL, David Gerard JEWSON, Roger John Anthony PRICE, Sharon SCOTT

Quorn Medical Centre

1 Station Road, Quorn, Loughborough LE12 8BP
Tel: 01509 412232 Fax: 01509 620652
(Charnwood and North West Leicestershire Primary Care Trust)
Patient List Size: 9030

Practice Manager L Baker

GP Susan Ann CULLIS, Christopher Robert BARLOW, Stephen John Charles CLAY, Michael Fisher FROST

Shepshed Health Centre

Field Street, Shepshed, Loughborough LE12 9AL
Tel: 01509 601201 Fax: 01509 651311
(Charnwood and North West Leicestershire Primary Care Trust)
Patient List Size: 1745

GP P S GHATORA

Soar Valley Surgeries

45 Orchard Close, Loughborough LE12 5NF
Tel: 01509 672229 Fax: 01509 670426
(Rushcliffe Primary Care Trust)
Patient List Size: 2600

Practice Manager Diane Webster

GP Gopal PATEL

Storer Road Medical Centre

2A Storer Road, Loughborough LE11 5EQ
Tel: 01509 212120
(Charnwood and North West Leicestershire Primary Care Trust)

GP John Francis MIDDLETON, Helen COX, Paul Stuart GOFFIN, Margaret Clare HALE, Geoffrey Peter HANLON, Joan Margaret STEED, Simon Marcus WILDE

Town Surgery

Baxter Lane, Loughborough LE11 1TT
Tel: 01509 568840 Fax: 01509 568841
(Charnwood and North West Leicestershire Primary Care Trust)
Patient List Size: 1800

Practice Manager B R Patel

GP Rajnikant Shambhubhai PATEL, Stuart KIRKPATRICK

Woodbrook Medical Centre
28 Bridge Street, Loughborough LE11 1NH
Tel: 01509 239166 Fax: 01509 238747
(Charnwood and North West Leicestershire Primary Care Trust)
Patient List Size: 8600

Practice Manager Simon Bardsley

GP Marie Ginette KOK-SHUN, Dermot Patrick RYAN, Melvinderpal Singh GHALY, Angela Francesca NEWTON, Andrew P TAYLOR, Helen UNITT

Loughton

High Road Surgery
113 High Road, Loughton IG10 4JA
Tel: 020 8508 9949 Fax: 020 8508 9961
(Epping Forest Primary Care Trust)
Patient List Size: 2100

Practice Manager C Hasan

GP Abul HASAN

Loughton Health Centre
The Drive, Loughton IG10 1HW
Tel: 020 8508 8117 Fax: 020 8508 7895
(Epping Forest Primary Care Trust)
Patient List Size: 11500

Practice Manager Hazel Harbour

GP Tasneem KANAMIA, Anwar Ali KHAN, Hameed Ullah KHAN, David LUKEY, Meenu Vasdev MIRCHANDANI, David WONG

Pradhan and Partners
Traps Hill Surgery, 25 Traps Hill, Loughton IG10 1SZ
Tel: 0870 417 3100 Fax: 020 8508 7269
(Epping Forest Primary Care Trust)
Patient List Size: 6200

Practice Manager Julie Walsh

GP Abhay Madhav PRADHAN, C BROCKBANK, K KANAGASABAI

Pyrles Lane Surgery
26 Pyrles Lane, Loughton IG10 2NW
Tel: 020 8508 4580 Fax: 020 8508 7269
(Epping Forest Primary Care Trust)

Practice Manager Julie Walsh

GP Dr PRAJAPATI

Rectory Lane Health Centre
Rectory Lane, Loughton IG10 3RU
Tel: 020 8272 4650 Fax: 020 8272 4651
(Epping Forest Primary Care Trust)

Practice Manager Ann Nugent

GP B LAWRENCE

Station Road Surgery
26 Pyrles Lane, Loughton IG10 4NH
Tel: 020 8508 4580 Fax: 020 8508 4383
(Epping Forest Primary Care Trust)
Patient List Size: 10100

Practice Manager Laura Ford

GP Joanna Elizabeth IDE, Siobhan BARNES, K S DOGRA, B KEVAI, Rachel Penelope Ludmilla ROBERTS

Louth

James Street Family Practice
49 James Street, Louth LN11 0JN
Tel: 01507 611122 Fax: 01507 610435
Email: malcolm.taylor@jamesstreet.co.uk
Website: www.jamesstreet.co.uk
(East Lincolnshire Primary Care Trust)
Patient List Size: 8100

Practice Manager Malcolm Taylor

GP Jutta MEIWALD, Andrew John MOWAT, Lawrence Charles PIKE, Simon Paul TOPHAM

Kidgate Surgery
32 Queen Street, Louth LN11 9AU
Tel: 01507 602421 Fax: 01507 601700
(East Lincolnshire Primary Care Trust)
Patient List Size: 3775

Practice Manager J Cox

GP Donal STAUNTON, Patricia Helen STOVIN

Marsh Medical Practice
Keeling Street, North Somercotes, Louth LN11 7QU
Tel: 01507 358623 Fax: 01507 358746
(East Lincolnshire Primary Care Trust)
Patient List Size: 6200

Practice Manager Lorraine Valance

GP Nigel Henry Thomas KING, Graham Stuart PARKER, Paul Bernard STANHOPE, James Richard YOUNG

Newmarket Medical Practice
153 Newmarket, Louth LW11 9EH
Tel: 01507 603121 Fax: 01507 605916
(East Lincolnshire Primary Care Trust)
Patient List Size: 10050

Practice Manager Michael Peacock

GP John Julian BIRCH, Michael John Adrian DWYER, Neal Richard Quine PARKES, Dorothy Jean REYNOLDS, Kerry TYERMAN

Lowestoft

Alexandra Road Surgery
Alexandra Road, Lowestoft NR32 1PL
Tel: 01502 574524 Fax: 01502 531526
(Waveney Primary Care Trust)
Patient List Size: 13000

Practice Manager Barbara Craddock

GP Douglas Robert HENDERSON, James Leon ATKINS, F BOHNCKE, Ravinder Singh LALL, Vidyasagar VALMIKI

Andaman Surgery
303 Long Road, Lowestoft NR33 9DF
Tel: 01502 517346 Fax: 01502 531450
(Waveney Primary Care Trust)
Patient List Size: 4250

Practice Manager Bridget Aitken

GP Mark Stephen BUTT, Sarah BUTT, Mariella ELISSAN, Susan LOCK

Beach Road Surgery
15 Beach Road, Lowestoft NR32 1EA
Tel: 01502 572000 Fax: 01502 508892
(Waveney Primary Care Trust)

Practice Manager Helen Clarke

GP Frederick Michael Retna KERRY, Savirimuthu Rayappu PERISELNERIS

Bridge Road Surgery
1A Bridge Road, Oufton Broad, Lowestoft NR32 3LJ
Tel: 01502 565936 Fax: 01502 567359
Website: www.bridgeroadsurgery.nhs.uk
(Waveney Primary Care Trust)
Patient List Size: 11200

Practice Manager Ann Handley

GP Richard Ian BOND, Martin John AYLWARD, Kay BOUCH, Michael Thomas LLOYD, Mark Andrew NETTLETON

Field Lane Surgery
42 Field Lane, Kessingland, Lowestoft NR33 7QA
Tel: 01502 740203 Fax: 01502 742368
(Waveney Primary Care Trust)
Patient List Size: 6400

Practice Manager Kash Gopee

GP Nigel Rodney DRANE, Aysha Mary COCKSHOTT, Robert Andrew COLEMAN, David JOHNSTON, Julian Lorimer SANGER

High Street Surgery
High Street, Lowestoft NR32 1JE
Tel: 01502 589151 Fax: 01502 566719
(Waveney Primary Care Trust)
Patient List Size: 11000

Practice Manager Drena Black

GP Robert DAKIN, Andrew H DRUMMOND, Renee Lata KATHURIA, Gavin James Simon LOCKYER, Simon Richard PRINCE, Manjeet Singh SEEHRA

London Road South Surgery
366 London Road South, Lowestoft NR33 0BQ
Tel: 01502 573333 Fax: 01502 581590
(Waveney Primary Care Trust)
Patient List Size: 6000

Practice Manager Sue Gooding

GP Howard John Ferdinand VAN PELT, Bart E DE LIGT, Kathleen GUNN, John Francis KELLY

Oulton Village Medical Centre
Meadow Road, Oulton, Lowestoft NR32 3AZ
Tel: 01502 501535 Fax: 01502 512388
Website: www.marine-oultonsurgeries.co.uk
(Waveney Primary Care Trust)
Patient List Size: 5500

Practice Manager Brenda Fitzgerald

GP Susan Mary COX, Mustafa RAFIQUE

Rosedale Surgery
Ashburnam Way, Carlton Colville, Lowestoft NR33 8LG
Tel: 01502 505100
(Waveney Primary Care Trust)

Victoria Road Surgery
82 Victoria Road, Oulton Broad, Lowestoft NR33 9LU
Tel: 01502 572369 Fax: 01502 537035
(Waveney Primary Care Trust)
Patient List Size: 9500

Practice Manager Doug Riley

GP Alexander Ritchie ANDERSON, Andrew Russell BIGG, Sandeep CHANDRA, Gomathy Anandan MOORTHIE, Jennifer Mary MORRISON

Westwood Surgery
45-47 Westwood Avenue, Lowestoft NR33 9RW
Tel: 01502 588854
(Waveney Primary Care Trust)
Patient List Size: 2270

GP Fergal Alexander O'DRISCOLL

Ludlow

Orleton Surgery
Millbrook Way, Orleton, Ludlow SY8 4HW
Tel: 01584 831300 Fax: 01584 831186
(Shropshire County Primary Care Trust)

GP Dr DAVIS, Dr GRAY, Dr MATHIAS

Portcullis Surgery
Portcullis Lane, Ludlow SY8 1GT
Tel: 01584 872939 Fax: 01584 879031
Email: anne.bairdz@nhs.nst
(Shropshire County Primary Care Trust)
Patient List Size: 7200

Practice Manager Anne Baird

GP Thomas James BOOG-SCOTT, Nicholas FARNELL, Dorian David YARHAM

Station Drive Surgery
Station Drive, Ludlow SY8 2AB
Tel: 01584 872461 Fax: 01584 877971
(Shropshire County Primary Care Trust)
Patient List Size: 8500

Practice Manager Brian Canfer

GP James Desmond CULLEN, Graham Patrick COOK, Roger Donald DAVIES, Caron MORTON

Luton

Ashcroft Road Medical Centre
170 Ashcroft Road, Stopsley, Luton LU2 9AY
Tel: 01582 727192
(Luton Teaching Primary Care Trust)

Practice Manager I K Shah

GP Kantilal Devshi SHAH

Barton Hills Medical Group
Whitehorse Vale, Barton Hills, Luton LU3 4AD
Tel: 01582 490087 Fax: 01582 499640
Website: www.bartonhillsdoctor.co.uk
(Luton Teaching Primary Care Trust)
Patient List Size: 6000

Practice Manager Susan Godsmark

GP Peter Clive WAKEFIELD, Aasim SIDDIQUE, M B V STRATFORD, Gillian Margaret TOWLER

Bell House Medical Centre
163 Dunstable Road, Luton LU1 1BW
Tel: 01582 723553/ 429 009 Fax: 01582 487686
(Luton Teaching Primary Care Trust)
Patient List Size: 9607

Practice Manager Yvonne Quantrill

GP Saumitra Kumar Paul CHOUDHURY, Talib ABUBACKER, Joanne CAMPBELL, Una DUFFY, Kuldip SULE

Biscot Road Medical Centre
177 Biscot Road, Luton LU3 1AP
Tel: 01582 737917 Fax: 01582 593631/457876
Email: ghanshyam.sukhani@nhs.uk
(Luton Teaching Primary Care Trust)
Patient List Size: 2500

Practice Manager Jenny Beck

GP Ghanshyam SUKHANI

Biscot Road Surgery
21 Biscot Road, Luton LU3 1AH
Tel: 01582 732697 Fax: 01582 402554
(Luton Teaching Primary Care Trust)
Patient List Size: 4300

Practice Manager Susan Izod

GP Raj KHANCHANDANI, Iqbal HUSSAIN

Caddington Surgery
33 Manor Road, Caddington, Luton LU1 4EE
Tel: 01582 25673 Fax: 01582 726672
Website: www.caddingtonsurgery.co.uk
(Bedfordshire Heartlands Primary Care Trust)
Patient List Size: 5100

Practice Manager Marie Dunn

GP Susannah Virginia HOWARD, Kay Elizabeth ELLIOTT, T H VERITY

Cardiff Road Surgery
12 Cardiff Road, Luton LU1 1QG
Tel: 01582 722148 Fax: 01582 485721
Email: rieger60@hotmail.com
Website: www.gpinternet.co.uk
(Luton Teaching Primary Care Trust)
Patient List Size: 6631

Practice Manager Kath Gerrard

GP Christopher Andrew RIEGER, Martin KUNZEMANN, Heather LINEHAN, Abdul NASIR-KHAN

Castle Street Surgery
39 Castle Street, Luton LU1 3AG
Tel: 01582 729242 Fax: 01582 725192
(Luton Teaching Primary Care Trust)
Patient List Size: 14000

Practice Manager Deborah McBeard

GP Peter Graham WILLIAMS, Kathryn Joyce COCKERILL, Stuart Harris DAVEY, Helen Lesley McGILL, D OWUSU, E SALIK

Conway Medical Centre
49 Westbourne Road, Luton LU4 8JD
Tel: 01582 429953 Fax: 01582 487500
(Luton Teaching Primary Care Trust)
Patient List Size: 7700

Practice Manager A Sinha

GP K PRASAD, S PRASAD, K SANJAY, Angeeta THIRUCHELVAM

The Crossway Health Centre
31 The Crossway, Farley Hill, Luton LU1 5LY
Tel: 01582 728826 Fax: 01582 732999
(Luton Teaching Primary Care Trust)
Patient List Size: 1450

GP Navnitlal Dahyabhai DHABUWALA

Foley
Bute House Medical Centre, Ground Floor, Grove Road, Luton LU1 1QJ
Tel: 01582 725740 Fax: 01582 485517
(Luton Teaching Primary Care Trust)
Patient List Size: 2300

Practice Manager Maureen Turner

GP Mark Anthony FOLEY

Leagrave Road Surgery
16 Leagrave Road, Luton LU4 8HZ
Tel: 01582 413331 Fax: 01582 482204
Email: naomi.chauhan@nhs.net
Website: www.16leagraveroaddoctor.co.uk
(Luton Teaching Primary Care Trust)
Patient List Size: 2250

Practice Manager Sylvia Rankin

GP M A JABBAR

Leagrave Surgery
37A Linden Road, Luton LU4 9QZ
Tel: 01582 572817 Fax: 01582 494675
Email: leagrave.surgery@nhs.net
Website: www.leagravedoctor.co.uk
(Luton Teaching Primary Care Trust)
Patient List Size: 7950

Practice Manager Lisa Harris

GP Wassim Helmy Mikhael MATTA, Paul DEELEY, Ian RALPH

Lister House
473 Dunstable Road, Luton LU4 8DG
Tel: 01582 571565 Fax: 01582 582074
(Luton Teaching Primary Care Trust)
Patient List Size: 6800

Practice Manager C Lavin

GP Laila Boshra YANNY, A IHONOR, C ODONG, J SIVASORUBAN

Liverpool Road Health Centre
9 Mersey Place, Liverpool Road, Luton LU1 1HH
Tel: 01582 722525 Fax: 01582 421602
(Luton Teaching Primary Care Trust)
Patient List Size: 14500

Practice Manager Bernie Naughton

GP Peter John WARD, Howard Martin Graham CALOW, Audrey Helen DORMAN, Steve GILLAM, Nina PEARSON, Paul Ashley SINGER

Liverpool Road Health Centre
Mersey Place, Luton LU1 1HH
Tel: 01582 731321 Fax: 01582 481224
(Luton Teaching Primary Care Trust)
Patient List Size: 7700

Practice Manager Janice Naish

GP Petros Pavlou EROTOCRITOU, R JAIN, A VERGHESE

MacBrayne and Partners
The Oakley Surgery, Addington Way, Luton LU4 9FJ
Tel: 0870 417 3989 Fax: 01582 561808
Website: www.oakleydoctor.co.uk
(Luton Teaching Primary Care Trust)
Patient List Size: 5000

GP John Thom MacBRAYNE, Vinod SHAMPRASADH

Malzeard Road Health Centre
2A Malzeard Road, Luton LU3 1BD
Website: www.malzeardroaddoctor.co.uk
(Luton Teaching Primary Care Trust)
Patient List Size: 3005

Practice Manager Binita Ray Chandhuri

GP A ZAMAN, L BHATT

Marsh Farm Health Centre
Purley Centre, The Moakes, Luton LU3 3SR
Tel: 01582 502336 Fax: 01582 494541
(Luton Teaching Primary Care Trust)
Patient List Size: 2800

Practice Manager Marion Layton

GP Muhammad Younus KHAN

The Medici Practice
37 Castle Street, Luton LU1 3AG
Tel: 01582 726123 Fax: 01582 731150
(Luton Teaching Primary Care Trust)
Patient List Size: 8200

Practice Manager Carole Welham

GP Ashok Kumar SAHDEV, Omar RAHIM, Jackie RATNE

Medina Medical Centre
3 Medina Road, Luton LU4 8BD
Tel: 01582 722475 Fax: 01582 722474
Email: u_kumar@talk21
(Luton Teaching Primary Care Trust)
Patient List Size: 3500

Practice Manager Paluinder Dhillon

GP U KUMAR, R SINGH

Neville Road Surgery
5 Neville Road, Luton LU3 2JG
Tel: 01582 563373 Fax: 01582 705085
(Luton Teaching Primary Care Trust)
Patient List Size: 1900

Practice Manager Ekram Ar-Rikaby

GP Hussain Amber AR-RIKABY

Rainbow Medical Centre
265 Dunstable Road, Luton LU4 8BS
Tel: 01582 411628 Fax: 01582 725083
(Luton Teaching Primary Care Trust)

Patient List Size: 4168

GP Paratha Sarathi HALDAR

Shah and Thomson
Bute House Medical Centre, Ground Floor, Grove Road, Luton LU1 1QJ
Tel: 01582 723357 Fax: 01582 417762
(Luton Teaching Primary Care Trust)
Patient List Size: 4922

Practice Manager T Simpson

GP Margaret THOMSON, Hasmukh Mohanlal SHAH

Stopsley Group Practice
Wigmore Lane Health Centre, Luton LU2 8BG
Tel: 01582 481294 Fax: 01582 456259
Email: lynne.russell@gp-e81075.nhs.uk
Website: www.elliswlhcdoctor.co.uk
(Luton Teaching Primary Care Trust)
Patient List Size: 6200

Practice Manager Lorraine Dakin

GP Christopher David Winter ELLIS, Ian HILL-SMITH, Georgina Mary JOHNSON

Stopsley Village Practice
26 Ashcroft Road, Stopsley Green, Luton LU2 9AU
Tel: 01582 722555 Fax: 01582 418145
(Luton Teaching Primary Care Trust)
Patient List Size: 9151

Practice Manager Geoff Phillips

GP Sara Elizabeth WARRINER, Edmund RUPASINGHE, Diane Wendy SEMARK, Piers TOMLINSON

Sundon Medical Centre
142-144 Sundon Park Road, Sundon Park, Luton LU3 3AH
Tel: 01582 571130 Fax: 01582 564452
(Luton Teaching Primary Care Trust)
Patient List Size: 7555

Practice Manager Deborah Porter

GP Kathleen Mary SWAN, KHALID MAHMOOD, Haydn WILLIAMS, Richard Ying Wai YIP

Sundon Park Clinic
Tenth Avenue, Sundon Park, Luton LU3 3EP
(Luton Teaching Primary Care Trust)
Patient List Size: 6700

Practice Manager S Ali-Khan

GP Adil ALI KHAN, I U ALI KHAN, Mir Askar ALI KHAN

The Surgery
49 Ashcroft Road, Stopsley, Luton LU2 9AU
Tel: 01582 391831 Fax: 01582 488052
(Luton Teaching Primary Care Trust)

Practice Manager Sheelagh Toomey

GP Pritpal Singh BATH

The Surgery
30 The Green, Hockwell Ring, Luton LU4 9PG
Tel: 01582 505355 Fax: 01582 443126
(Luton Teaching Primary Care Trust)

Practice Manager G Mirza

GP Irshad Ali MIRZA

The Surgery
53 Leagrave Road, Luton LU4 8HT
Tel: 01582 404967 Fax: 01582 421291
Email: shahina.54@hotmail.com
(Luton Teaching Primary Care Trust)
Patient List Size: 1853

Practice Manager Shahina Kada

GP Muhammad Qamarul HODA

The Surgery
Pastures Way, Lewsey Farm, Luton LU4 0PF
Tel: 01582 667017 Fax: 01582 660525
(Luton Teaching Primary Care Trust)

Practice Manager Evette Singh

GP D V SHAH, B S VIRK

Ward, Seery, Ahmad, Shakoor
Gardenia Surgery, 2A Gardenia Avenue, Luton LU3 2NS
Tel: 01582 572612 Fax: 01582 494553
(Luton Teaching Primary Care Trust)
Patient List Size: 8717

GP Eileen Mary Claire WARD, Zulfquar AHMAD, James Alexis SEERY, Abdul SHAKOOR

Wenlock Street Surgery
40 Wenlock Street, Luton LU2 0NN
Tel: 01582 727094
Email: isam.saleh@nhs.net
(Luton Teaching Primary Care Trust)
Patient List Size: 2980

Practice Manager Regina Saleh

GP I SALEH

Wheatfield Surgery
60 Wheatfield Road, Lewsey Farm, Luton LU4 0SY
Tel: 01582 601116 Fax: 01582 666421
(Bedfordshire Heartlands Primary Care Trust)
Patient List Size: 13300

Practice Manager W G Parsley

GP Keith John BRIGHT, Khairul Abul Kassem Mohammed ANAM, Fiona Ann Ruth HARRIS, R C ROBINSON, Sanjay SHARMA, Torrick SOLOMON, Edward Thomas WATTS

Wigmore Lane Health Centre
Wigmore Lane, Luton LU2 8BG
Tel: 01582 481301, 434026 Fax: 01582 481298
(Luton Teaching Primary Care Trust)
Patient List Size: 3850

Practice Manager S Shankar

GP Navin SHANKAR

Woodland Avenue Practice
30 Woodland Avenue, Luton LU3 1RW
(Luton Teaching Primary Care Trust)
Patient List Size: 11600

Practice Manager Susan Doherty

GP Margaret Delyth ROBERTS, Manraj BARHEY, Manoj CHANDRON, Christiane Gay Maxine HARRIS, Julian Kay MARSDEN, Shahid RAHMAN, Vasanthy RAWICHANDRAN, Abbas ZAIDI

Lutterworth

Lutterworth Health Centre
Gilmorton Road, Lutterworth LE17 4EB
Tel: 01455 553531 Fax: 01455 559653
Website: www.lutterworthhealthcentre.org
(South Leicestershire Primary Care Trust)

GP William John WIGGINS, Penelope Ann FLAXMAN, Judith Margaret GREAVES, Robert HAMPTON, Zoe HUGHES, Graham JOHNSON, Louise KIRK, V MASHARANI, John Clifford REYNOLDS, Jane TAYLOR

Lutterworth Health Centre
Gilmorton Road, Lutterworth LE17 4EB
Tel: 01455 552346
(South Leicestershire Primary Care Trust)

GP Vipul MASHARANI

The Surgery
Kilworth Road, Husbands Bosworth, Lutterworth LE17 6JZ
Tel: 01858 880522 Fax: 01858 880111

(Melton, Rutland and Harborough Primary Care Trust)

GP Christopher George DOWELL, Dr MAXWELL

Lydbrook

Lydbrook Health Centre

Lydbrook GL17 9LG
Tel: 01594 860219/860650 Fax: 01594 860987
(West Gloucestershire Primary Care Trust)
Patient List Size: 5500

Practice Manager Carol Hallam

GP Andrew John Merrill COATES, Eric PORTMAN, Gwyn ROBERTS

Lydney

Miller and Partners

The Health Centre, Albert Street, Lydney GL15 5NQ
Tel: 01594 842167 Fax: 01594 845550
Website: www.lydneygp.co.uk
(West Gloucestershire Primary Care Trust)
Patient List Size: 7200

Practice Manager Linda Vaughan

GP M D MILLER, P BENNETT, R BOUNDS, S SHARMA

Severnbank Surgery

Tutnalls Street, Lydney GL15 5PQ
Tel: 01594 845222 Fax: 01594 845637
Website: www.severnbanksurgery.co.uk
(West Gloucestershire Primary Care Trust)
Patient List Size: 3898

Practice Manager Carolyn Thomas

GP Peter Richard FELLOWS, Jonathan CHAMBERS, Rowena CHRISTMAS, K HAMILTON, D JONES

Yorkley Health Centre

Bailey Hill, Yorkley, Lydney GL15 4RS
Tel: 01594 562437 Fax: 01594 564319
(West Gloucestershire Primary Care Trust)
Patient List Size: 6850

Practice Manager Yvonne A Smith

GP Robin Blair JONES, Michael ANDREW, Andrew EDWARDS, Michelle HAYES

Lyme Regis

The Lyme Bay Surgery

View Road, Lyme Regis DT7 3AA
Tel: 01297 443399 Fax: 01297 442340
(South West Dorset Primary Care Trust)
Patient List Size: 2000

Practice Manager E Rowe

GP Forbes Gordon WATSON

Lyme Practice

Lyme Regis Medical Centre, Uplyme Road, Lyme Regis DT7 3LS
Tel: 01297 445777 Fax: 01297 444917
Email: dministrator@lymepractice.nhs.uk; administratoe@gp-j81088.nhs.uk
Website: www.lymepractice.nhs.uk
(South West Dorset Primary Care Trust)

Practice Manager Anita Wright

GP Barry John ROBINSON, Ian Michael CONWAY

Lymington

Chawton House Surgery

St Thomas Street, Lymington SO41 9ND
Tel: 01590 672953 Fax: 01590 674137
(New Forest Primary Care Trust)

Practice Manager P Dudley

GP Thomas Hamilton McEWEN, Annabel Jane ARNOLD, Sally JOHNSTON, E R J REEVES

The Wistaria Surgery

Wistaria Court, 18 Avenue Road, Lymington SO41 9PJ
Tel: 01590 672212 Fax: 01590 679930
(New Forest Primary Care Trust)
Patient List Size: 8800

Practice Manager Anne Metcalf

GP David Stephen BADHAM, Anthea Margaret MacALISTER, Gareth John MORRIS, David Edward READ, Angela J SIZER, Neale WHITLEY

Lymm

Brookfield Surgery

Whitbarrow Road, Lymm WA13 9AD
Tel: 01925 756969 Fax: 01925 756173
(Warrington Primary Care Trust)
Patient List Size: 8000

Practice Manager Brenda Daniels

GP Paul Nicholas John COTTRILL, Anthony Harvey JOHNSTONE, Aparna Ananthakrishna RAO, Claire Pamela REVELL, Alan Irvin SKRZYPIEC-ALLEN

Lyndhurst

Lyndhurst Surgery

2 Church Lane, Lyndhurst SO43 7EW
Tel: 023 8028 2689 Fax: 023 8028 2918
(New Forest Primary Care Trust)

Practice Manager Louise Overton

GP David Melville BALFOUR, Sarah Ellen CHINN, Jonathon James LYON-MARIS

Lynton

Burvill Street Health Centre

Burvill Street, Lynton EX35 6HA
Tel: 01598 753226
(North Devon Primary Care Trust)
Patient List Size: 2562

Practice Manager Val Pugsley

GP Glen ALLAWAY, John Barry FRANKISH

Lytham St Annes

Church Road Surgery

261 Church Road, St Annes on Sea, Lytham St Annes FY8 3NP
Tel: 01253 728911 Fax: 01253 732114
(Fylde Primary Care Trust)
Patient List Size: 6800

Practice Manager C Bonney

GP Richard John HELLIER, Trevor CLARKE, Pamela Ann FRENCH, James REID, Andrew Macgregor WILMINGTON

Clifton Drive South

300 Clifton Drive South, Lytham St Annes FY8 1LJ
Tel: 01253 723194
(Fylde Primary Care Trust)

Practice Manager Carol Foulkes

GP Peter BENETT, Catherine JEPSON, Philip John MOORHOUSE

Derbe Road Surgery

43 Derbe Road, Lytham St Annes FY8 1NJ
Tel: 01253 725811 Fax: 01253 720001
(Fylde Primary Care Trust)
Patient List Size: 1670

Practice Manager Joyce Whatmough

GP Robert Neil CURZON

Dr Dempsey and Partners
24 St Annes Road East, Lytham St Annes FY8 1UR
Tel: 01253 722121 Fax: 01253 789211
(Fylde Primary Care Trust)

Practice Manager Amanda Emery

GP Howard Francis Matthew DEMPSEY, Colin BAMFORD, Kathryn Mary GREENWOOD, Richard William WILLIAMS

Fernbank Surgery
18 Church Road, Lytham, Lytham St Annes FY8 5LL
Tel: 01253 736453 Fax: 01253 732987
(Fylde Primary Care Trust)
Patient List Size: 9025

Practice Manager Diane Eaton

GP John David FIELDING, Catherine Veronica CONNOLLY, Simon Timothy ELLWOOD, Ruth MASON, Keith Michael McLENNAN

Holland House
31 Church Road, Lytham, Lytham St Annes FY8 5LL
Tel: 01253 794999 Fax: 01253 795744
(Fylde Primary Care Trust)
Patient List Size: 9800

Practice Manager Duncan McGrath

GP Christopher Michael Barrett REID, Nicholas Charles LOWE, Richard William REED, Steven Patrick John REID, Morag Elizabeth SLOAN

The Old Links Surgery
104 Highbury Road East, Lytham St Annes FY8 2LY
Tel: 01253 713621
(Fylde Primary Care Trust)

Practice Manager Amanda Emery

GP Russell John THORPE

Park Road Medical Centre
17 Park Road, St. Annes on Sea, Lytham St Annes FY8 1PW
Tel: 01253 727938 Fax: 01253 780992
(Fylde Primary Care Trust)

Practice Manager Alan Cooper

GP Michael ZARYCKYJ, Martin Tristram Colin ATHERTON, Eileen BAMBER

Mablethorpe

Marisco Medical Practice
Seacroft Road, Mablethorpe LN12 2DT
Tel: 01507 473483 Fax: 01507 478865
(East Lincolnshire Primary Care Trust)
Patient List Size: 13000

Practice Manager Janet Goult, Ann-Marie Steadman, Julie Worshop

GP Steven CARTER, Irene CARTER, Steven LIMAGE, Roger NORTH

Park Road East Surgery
1 Park Road East, Sutton-on-Sea, Mablethorpe LN12 2NL
Tel: 01507 441245 Fax: 01507 443700
(East Lincolnshire Primary Care Trust)

GP Irene Martha CARTER, Eddys Elizabeth AMAKU

Macclesfield

Bollington Medical Centre
Wellington Road, Bollington, Macclesfield SK10 5JH
Tel: 01625 572481 Fax: 01625 575650
(Eastern Cheshire Primary Care Trust)
Patient List Size: 10700

Practice Manager Janie Staley

GP Gerald Arrowsmith COOPE, Tom LOSEL, Deborah Ann MAXWELL, Valerie Marie RAMSDEN, Sian STOKES, Sharon WASSON, Peter WILSON

Broken Cross Surgery
Fallibroome Road, Macclesfield SK10 3LA
Tel: 01625 617300 Fax: 01625 617300
(Eastern Cheshire Primary Care Trust)

Practice Manager Annie Lowe

GP William Paul Douglas FORD-YOUNG

Cumberland House
Jordangate, Macclesfield SK10 1EG
Tel: 01625 428081 Fax: 01625 503128
(Eastern Cheshire Primary Care Trust)
Patient List Size: 14700

Practice Manager A Pollitt

GP Stewart Allen HIGGINS, Elizabeth Louise FINCH, Jeffrey Mark HODGSON, Shelly MAUND, Jeffrey Brereton RICHARDS, Anne Whitehead STIRLING, James Richard USHER

High Street Surgery
2 High Street, Macclesfield SK11 8BX
Tel: 01625 423692
(Eastern Cheshire Primary Care Trust)

GP Martin Mills BLUCK, Patricia Margaret COCKER, John Roger HANSON, Andrew Makepeace NUTTALL

Park Green Surgery
Sunderland Street, Macclesfield SK11 6HW
Tel: 01625 429555 Fax: 01625 502950
(Eastern Cheshire Primary Care Trust)

GP Stephen Edward BECKETT, Ruth Hannah KENNY, Kim Nina MONAGHAN, David Robert MORRIS, Christopher Alan RATCLIFFE, Rosemary VAN ROSS, David Robert Bernard Mackinlay YOUNG

Park Lane House Medical Centre
187 Park Lane, Macclesfield SK11 6UD
Tel: 01625 422893 Fax: 01625 424870
(Eastern Cheshire Primary Care Trust)
Patient List Size: 8939

Practice Manager Chris Campbell-Kelly

GP Robert Charles Frederick HEYWORTH, John CARTER, Louise HASTINGS, Helen MACLEOD, Valerie Ann PICKLES

Roycroft, Madden and Thomas
Chelford Surgery, Elmstead Road, Chelford, Macclesfield SK11 9BS
Tel: 01625 861316 Fax: 01625 860075
(Eastern Cheshire Primary Care Trust)
Patient List Size: 3650

Practice Manager Anne Evans, Katie Harding, Kate O'Callaghan, Julia Slater

GP Peter Lawrence MADDEN, Helen Joan THOMAS

Smith and Partners
South Park Surgery, 250 Park Lane, Macclesfield SK11 8AD
Tel: 01625 422249 Fax: 01625 502169
Email: name@gp-N81029.nhs.uk
Website: www.southparksurgery.com
(Eastern Cheshire Primary Care Trust)
Patient List Size: 13255

Practice Manager M C Halligan

GP Lorna Katherine Ritchie SMITH, D ALEXANDER, G BERGER, C BROOKS, R CALVER, David Kevin CRAGG, A K MOAR, Gillian Dorne PLANT

Maidenhead

Cedars Surgery
8 Cookham Road, Maidenhead SL6 8AJ
Tel: 01628 620458 Fax: 01628 633270
Email: cedars.surgery@gp-K81036.nhs.uk
Website: www.cedarsdoctors.co.uk
(Windsor, Ascot and Maidenhead Primary Care Trust)
Patient List Size: 10500

Practice Manager Lesley Cresta

GP Marek Jerzy STAWARZ, Stuart Charles BLACKMORE, Mandy LAMBTON, Paul LAYNE, Steve PRATT, Joanne Marie RUSHTON

Claremont Surgery
Wilderness Medical Centre, 2 Cookham Road, Maidenhead SL6 8AN
Tel: 01628 673033 Fax: 01628 673432
Website: www.claremontdoctor.co.uk
(Windsor, Ascot and Maidenhead Primary Care Trust)
Patient List Size: 12500

Practice Manager David Taylor

GP Richard FLEW, Perihan Eva COLYER, Henry Nicholas Christopher MAWSON, Myra NEWMAN, Ian David NOCK, Alison Mary POUNTNEY, Huw THOMAS

Dr J E Barker and Partners
85 Ross Road, Maidenhead SL6 2SR
Tel: 01628 623767 Fax: 01628 789623
(Windsor, Ascot and Maidenhead Primary Care Trust)
Patient List Size: 21300

Practice Manager Pat Poulson

GP Jean Elizabeth BARKER, Sanjiv Kumar MATA, Bernard Chukwura OBI, Charlotte SMYTH

The Holyport Surgery
Stroud Farm Road, Holyport, Maidenhead SL6 2LP
Tel: 01628 624469 Fax: 01628 778869
Website: www.holyportdoctor.co.uk
(Windsor, Ascot and Maidenhead Primary Care Trust)
Patient List Size: 5019

Practice Manager Carol Buckland

GP Jennifer Ann LANGDON, Christopher Guy LANGDON

Linden Medical Centre
9A Linden Avenue, Maidenhead SL6 6HD
Tel: 01628 20846 Fax: 01628 789318
(Windsor, Ascot and Maidenhead Primary Care Trust)

GP Robert Julian HABERSHON, Geoffrey Charles FRANCIS, William Harold Cooke GUTTERIDGE, Judith Ann KINDER, Robert Duncan SMITH, Jane Louise VALENTINE

Lower Road Medical Health Centre
Lower Road, Cookham Rise, Maidenhead SL6 9HX
Tel: 01628 524646 Fax: 01628 810201
(Windsor, Ascot and Maidenhead Primary Care Trust)
Patient List Size: 8300

Practice Manager D Yerburgh

GP Azmy Vispi BIRDI, Julia Compton MERCER, Peter ROBERTS, Joseph SANTOS, Cathie SCOTHORNE, Matthew John SOUTHGATE

Maudgil
Doctors Surgery, 1 Cordwallis Road, Maidenhead SL6 7DQ
Tel: 01628 27284 Fax: 01628 32432
(Windsor, Ascot and Maidenhead Primary Care Trust)

GP Bhagwan Dass MAUDGIL

Redwood House Practice
Redwood House, Cannon Lane, Maidenhead SL6 3PH
Tel: 01628 826227 Fax: 01628 829426
(Windsor, Ascot and Maidenhead Primary Care Trust)

Practice Manager E Haynes

GP John Charles SIDERY, Sarah Joanne SPIER

Rosemead Surgery
8A Ray Park Avenue, Maidenhead SL6 8DS
Tel: 01628 622023 Fax: 01628 639495
Website: www.rosemeaddoctor.co.uk
(Windsor, Ascot and Maidenhead Primary Care Trust)
Patient List Size: 4600

GP Muriel Veronica Trilby JOHNSON, Catherine Mary HUTCHINGS, Julius PARKER

The Symons Medical Centre
25 All Saints Avenue, Maidenhead SL6 6EL
Tel: 01628 626131 Fax: 01628 410051
(Windsor, Ascot and Maidenhead Primary Care Trust)

GP David James LLOYD-WILLIAMS, Michael Ruffley MULLINEUX, Peter John SHAW, Rory Charles Francis SYMONS, Jeremy Stuart WHEELER

Woodlands Park Surgery
15 Woodlands Park Road, Maidenhead SL6 3NW
Tel: 01628 825674 Fax: 01628 829036
(Windsor, Ascot and Maidenhead Primary Care Trust)

Practice Manager Susan Cordey

GP David John HASLAM, Patricia Mary HEMMINGS

Maidstone

Allington Park Surgery
1C Newbury Avenue, Allington, Maidstone ME16 0RB
Tel: 01622 683257 Fax: 01622 677365
(Maidstone Weald Primary Care Trust)

Practice Manager Lesley Larman

GP Robert Harold MENNIE

Blackthorn Medical Centre
St Andrews Road, Barming, Maidstone ME16 9AN
Tel: 01622 726277 Fax: 01622 725774
(Maidstone Weald Primary Care Trust)
Patient List Size: 7300

Practice Manager Maureen Bortolozzo

GP Jennifer Rosemary Macfarlane BINGHAM, Martin GERHARDS, David McGAVIN, Jacqueline Middleton WITT

Brewer Street
4 Brewer Street, Maidstone ME14 1RU
Tel: 01622 755401/755402
(Maidstone Weald Primary Care Trust)

Practice Manager Jane Glancey

GP Robin Francis Anson GARDNER, Edward GARRETT, Steven Richard JOHNSON

Cobtree Medical Practice
Southways, Sutton Valence, Maidstone ME17 3HT
Tel: 01622 843800 Fax: 01622 844184
(Maidstone Weald Primary Care Trust)
Patient List Size: 2050

Practice Manager Suzanne Orchin

GP M HEBER

College Road Surgery
50/52 College Road, Maidstone ME15 6SB
Tel: 01622 752345 Fax: 01622 758133
(Maidstone Weald Primary Care Trust)
Patient List Size: 12500

Practice Manager Marie Gilbert

GP Ian Fortescue McLEAN, Steven CHRISTMAS, Renuka Lilanthi FERNANDO, John GREEN, Protichi MALLICK, Michael Charles STRACHAN, Deborah Hannah TAYLOR

Forsythe and Gaule
14 Pelican Court, Wateringbury, Maidstone ME18 5SS
Tel: 01622 814466

(Maidstone Weald Primary Care Trust)

Practice Manager Michael Byrne

GP David Tristram FORSYTHE, Edward William GAULE

Grove Park Surgery

116 Sutton Road, Maidstone ME15 9AP
Tel: 01622 753211 Fax: 01622 756722
(Maidstone Weald Primary Care Trust)

GP Gopal Chandra SINHA

Holland Road Surgery

97 Holland Road, Maidstone ME14 1UW
Tel: 01622 754874 Fax: 01622 688676
(Maidstone Weald Primary Care Trust)
Patient List Size: 6500

Practice Manager Margaret Hobbs

GP S A PATEL, J GASTON, P SZWEDZIUK

King Street Surgery

84 King Street, Maidstone ME14 1DZ
Tel: 01622 756721/756722/3
(Maidstone Weald Primary Care Trust)
Patient List Size: 10000

Practice Manager Marion Wilson

GP Elizabeth Carolyn HARLAND, Timothy Gowan HARLAND, Alan Bremner MASON, Linda Vivien MORGAN, David Anthony NEWMAN

Len Valley Practice

Tithe Yard, Church Square, Lenham, Maidstone ME17 2PJ
Tel: 01622 858341 Fax: 01622 859659
(Maidstone Weald Primary Care Trust)
Patient List Size: 7000

Practice Manager Janet Gleadall

GP Martin Herdman PORTER, Graham Clive HAGAN, Ian Douglas Halliburton McMULLEN, Anupama RAO

Marsham Street Surgery

1 Marsham Street, Maidstone ME14 1EW
Tel: 01622 752615/756129
(Maidstone Weald Primary Care Trust)
Patient List Size: 6400

Practice Manager Wendy Wilkins

GP John Gethin THOMAS, Maria Luisa ARAGONES ARROYO, Bruce Ian POLLINGTON

The Medical Centre

10A Northumberland Court, Shepway, Maidstone ME15 7LN
Tel: 01622 753920 Fax: 01622 692747
(Maidstone Weald Primary Care Trust)

Practice Manager Bhupi Singh

GP Kulvinder SINGH, Gordon McEWAN

The Mote Medical Practice

St Saviours Road, Maidstone ME15 9FL
Tel: 01622 756888 Fax: 01622 672573
(Maidstone Weald Primary Care Trust)

Practice Manager Emma Couch

GP Peter John WILFORD, Heather Emily ANDERSON, Stephen Hilary MEECH, Hannah REECE-JONES, David Mark WHISTLER

New Grove Medical Centre

Unit 1, Minor Centre, Grove Green, Maidstone ME14 5TQ
Tel: 01622 743775 Fax: 01622 730493
(Maidstone Weald Primary Care Trust)
Patient List Size: 4081

Practice Manager Susan Smith

GP Zubeda BANO, S T RAHMAN

The Orchard Medical Centre

146 Heath Road, Coxheath, Maidstone ME17 4PL
Tel: 01622 744994 Fax: 01622 741162
Website: www.orchardmedicalcentre.org.uk
(Maidstone Weald Primary Care Trust)
Patient List Size: 3300

Practice Manager Viv Cassell

GP Nicola Lesley PULHAM, Jackie C GASTON

The Orchard Surgery

Horseshoes Lane, Langley, Maidstone ME17 3JY
Tel: 01622 863030 Fax: 01622 862912
Email: practice.manager@gp-g82691.nhs.uk
(Maidstone Weald Primary Care Trust)
Patient List Size: 2323

Practice Manager Mette Unsworth

GP Andrew Antoni Patrick CZAYKOWSKI

Senacre Wood Surgery

Reculver Walk, Senacre, Maidstone ME15 8SW
Tel: 01622 761963
(Maidstone Weald Primary Care Trust)

GP Helen Patricia RING

Stockett Lane Surgery

3 Stockett Lane, Coxheath, Maidstone ME17 4PS
Tel: 01622 745585 Fax: 01622 743346
(Maidstone Weald Primary Care Trust)
Patient List Size: 6700

Practice Manager S Bradburn

GP Paul Lothian LEWIS, Astrid Coreen Elizabeth CUNNINGHAM, Edward Mark Royle REYNOLDS, Helen Mary TERRELL, Anne Elizabeth WALKER

The Surgery

Bearsted Medical Centre, Yeoman Lane, Bearsted, Maidstone ME14 4DS
Tel: 01622 737326/738344/738345 Fax: 01622 730745
(Maidstone Weald Primary Care Trust)
Patient List Size: 10700

Practice Manager June Jarrett

GP Peter Richard BONDS, P R BONDS, Lisa Jane DOLMAN, Christopher GODSMARK, Richard Jacques LAURENT, Alison Jane MILROY, Martin Leslie MOSS

The Surgery

Burgess Bank, Benover Road, Yalding, Maidstone ME18 6ES
Tel: 01622 814380 Fax: 01622 814549
(Maidstone Weald Primary Care Trust)
Patient List Size: 5500

Practice Manager Irene Welch

GP Anthony Clive FINCHAM, Kevin George MILLER, Joy Collins VIRDEN

Sutton Valence Surgery

South Lane, Sutton Valence, Maidstone ME17 3BD
Tel: 01622 842212 Fax: 01622 844396
Email: practice.manager@g82229.nhs.uk
(Maidstone Weald Primary Care Trust)
Patient List Size: 3550

Practice Manager Joanina Lambe

GP Paul Jeremy HOBDAY, Caroline Rosemary JESSEL, Paul LEWIS, Marion ZEHNTER

Tichborne Close Surgery

26 Tichborne Close, Allington, Maidstone ME16 0RY
Tel: 01622 679020 Fax: 01622 679020
(Maidstone Weald Primary Care Trust)

Practice Manager Marina Simmons

GP Munjandira Ayyapa MUTHANA

Tichborne Close Surgery

26 Tichborne Close, Allington, Maidstone ME16 0RY
Tel: 01622 679020 Fax: 01622 720928
(Maidstone Weald Primary Care Trust)

Practice Manager Angela Muthana

GP M A MUTHANA

The Vine Medical Centre
166 Tonbridge Road, Maidstone ME16 8SS
Tel: 01622 754898 Fax: 01622 751611
(Maidstone Weald Primary Care Trust)
Patient List Size: 8000

Practice Manager Lynn Coles

GP Helen Mary DOWNING, Anthony Mason JONES, Fiona Mary MEIHUIZEN, Jonathan Leslie WENTZEL

Wallis Avenue Surgery
Wallis Avenue, Parkwood, Maidstone ME15 9JJ
Tel: 01622 686963 Fax: 01622 695622
(Maidstone Weald Primary Care Trust)
Patient List Size: 3100

GP Petrus Hendrikus Jozef HANRATH, Jacqueline DENNISON

White House Surgery
Mackenders Lane, Eccles, Maidstone ME20 7HX
Tel: 01622 718558 Fax: 01622 791076
(Medway Teaching Primary Care Trust)
Patient List Size: 1200

Practice Manager Joy Vidler

GP Nasrullah BALUCH, Shakira BALUCH

Maldon

Blackwater Medical Centre
Princes Road, Maldon CM9 7DS
Tel: 01621 854204 Fax: 01621 850246
Email: blackwatermedical@compuserve.com
(Maldon and South Chelmsford Primary Care Trust)
Patient List Size: 14500

Practice Manager Karen Wheelhouse

GP Robin James Martin MACDONALD, Catherine Lucy CARGILL, Aubrey Bruce Carey CHAPMAN, Martin Peter HAEGER, Linda LIM, Robin Mark ROPER, Elisabeth Mary SMALE, Dr TEATINO

High Street Surgery
25 High Street, Tollesbury, Maldon CM9 8RG
Tel: 01621 869204 Fax: 01621 869023
(Maldon and South Chelmsford Primary Care Trust)

GP Edward Harvey BOZMAN, Richard John FURZE

Longfield Medical Centre
Princes Road, Maldon CM9 5DF
Tel: 01621 856811 Fax: 01621 852627
(Maldon and South Chelmsford Primary Care Trust)
Patient List Size: 13650

Practice Manager Janice Betts

GP Richard Frank DE SOUZA, Linda Margaret BROWN, Michael Joseph Temple CARR, Marianne CRONIN, Jane Marie DEASY, Simon Gideon MANN, Simon John STACEY

Malmesbury

Gable House
46 High Street, Malmesbury SN16 9AT
Tel: 01666 825825
(Kennet and North Wiltshire Primary Care Trust)
Patient List Size: 13800

Practice Manager David Grogan

GP Kathleen (Kate) BADCOCK, David Lindsay CHARLES, Victoria GRAHAM, John HARRISON, Anna LE, Jacqueline Suzanne NEALE, John Gregory PETTIT, Nigel John PICKERING, Chris TOWNSEND

The Tolsey Surgery
High Street, Sherston, Malmesbury SN16 0LQ
Tel: 01666 840270 Fax: 01666 841074
(Kennet and North Wiltshire Primary Care Trust)
Patient List Size: 3300

GP John Philip HEATHCOCK, Lorna HARRIS, Philippa Clare PETTIT

Malpas

Hulbert, Price, Hulbert and Davies
Laurel Bank Surgery, Old Hall Street, Malpas SY14 8PS
Tel: 01948 860205 Fax: 01948 860142
(Cheshire West Primary Care Trust)
Patient List Size: 6200

Practice Manager Lynn Suckley

GP Christopher Courtenay HULBERT, Louise Mary Claire DAVIES, Grace Miriam HULBERT, Michael Leslie PRICE, Emma TAYLOR

Malton

Derwent Practice
Norton Road, Norton, Malton YO17 9RF
Tel: 01653 600069 Fax: 01653 698014
(Scarborough, Whitby and Ryedale Primary Care Trust)
Patient List Size: 18900

Practice Manager Lorraine Akers

GP Warren Carnegie GRANT, Hilary CLARKE, Clive John DIGGORY, Andrew HARPER, Christopher JONES, David LONGWORTH, Michael LYNCH, Stephen POPE, Martin Lamont SLEEMAN, Douglas Frederick TAYLOR-HELPS, Helen Patricia TAYLOR, Julian WADSWORTH

The Sherburn and Rillington Surgery
50 St Hilda's Street, Sherburn, Malton YO17 8PH
Tel: 01944 710226 Fax: 01944 710817
(Scarborough, Whitby and Ryedale Primary Care Trust)
Patient List Size: 4576

Practice Manager Anne Raper

GP Donald Raymond CARRIE, J L CAINE, A T KEMPSTON, S M THORNTON

Malvern

The Court Road Surgery
Court Road, Malvern WR14 3BW
Tel: 01684 573161 Fax: 01684 561593
(South Worcestershire Primary Care Trust)
Patient List Size: 9150

Practice Manager Linda Norman

GP Michael Charles COLQUHOUN, David Kingsley PAYLER, James McLeod MATHER, S D ROBERTS, G M WILLIAMS

Inchgarth
369 Worcester Road, Malvern Link, Malvern WR14 1AR

GP John Langwill HUNTER

Link End Surgery
39 Pickersleigh Road, Malvern WR14 2RP
Tel: 01684 568466 Fax: 01684 891064
(South Worcestershire Primary Care Trust)

Practice Manager Sara Edwards

GP Jill SEFTON-FIDDIAN, Christopher Gordon ADENEY, David John FULLER

Malvern Health Centre
Victoria Park Road, Malvern Link, Malvern WR14 2JY
Tel: 01684 612703 Fax: 01684 612779
(South Worcestershire Primary Care Trust)
Patient List Size: 9750

Practice Manager David Jago

GP Kenneth William JARRETT, J BENNETT, Guy Louis BUSHER, Julia EDWARDS, A S MEREDITH, David James RADLEY

St Saviours Surgery
Merick Road, Malvern Link, Malvern WR14 1DD
Tel: 01684 572323 Fax: 01684 891067
(South Worcestershire Primary Care Trust)

Practice Manager S Grigg

GP Marc HINCHLIFFE, Iain Robb MACLEOD, Barbara-Anne WARD

The Surgery
28A Avenue Road, Malvern WR14 3BG
Tel: 01684 561333/574773 Fax: 01684 893664
(South Worcestershire Primary Care Trust)
Patient List Size: 7500

Practice Manager Pauline Smith

GP Adrian Lees McCRACKEN, Alison FINDLAY, James Bernard LAVIN, Stephanie LAVIN, Nicholas Richard Humber MILLARD, Barry Austin TUCK

Manchester

Ailsa Craig Medical Centre
270 Dickenson Road, Longsight, Manchester M13 0YL
Tel: 0161 224 5555 Fax: 0161 248 9112
(Central Manchester Primary Care Trust)

Practice Manager Eileen Corry

GP Bharatkumar Anant NANAVATI, Anne Elizabeth MAW

Alexandra Park Health Centre
2 Whitswood Close, Manchester M16 7AP
Tel: 0161 226 2710 Fax: 0161 226 0340
(Central Manchester Primary Care Trust)

Practice Manager Anita Baral

GP Farakh Rehana CHAUDURY, L DASS, S SINHA

Alexandra Park Health Centre
2 Whitswood Close, Manchester M16 7AP
Tel: 0161 226 4616
(Central Manchester Primary Care Trust)

Practice Manager L Dass

GP Lakshman DASS

Alexandra Park Health Centre
2 Whitswood Close, Manchester M16 7AP
Tel: 0161 226 3620 Fax: 0161 226 4918
(Central Manchester Primary Care Trust)

Practice Manager Anita Baral

GP Sanjay SINHA

Alexandra Practice
365 Wilbraham Road, Manchester M16 8NG
Tel: 0161 860 4400 Fax: 0161 860 7324
Email: Ivan.Benett@Mchester-ha.nwest.nhs.uk
(Central Manchester Primary Care Trust)
Patient List Size: 4500

Practice Manager Karen Wood

GP Ivan John BENETT, Avril Franciszka DANCZAK, Timothy James GREENAWAY

Alfeshan Medical Centre
3 Shirley Road, Cheetham, Manchester M8 0WB
Tel: 0161 795 0200 Fax: 0161 795 4908
(North Manchester Primary Care Trust)

Practice Manager Hashim Khan

GP Gul Muhammad KHAN

Alliston Medical Centre
28 Crofts Bank Road, Urmston, Manchester M41 0UH
Tel: 0161 747 2411 Fax: 0161 747 8841
(Trafford North Primary Care Trust)
Patient List Size: 3400

Practice Manager D Summers

GP Michael John CALLANDER, P LAVILLE

Artane Medical Centre
1 Middleton Road, Higher Crumpsall, Manchester M8 5SA
Tel: 0161 740 2785 Fax: 0161 740 0399
(North Manchester Primary Care Trust)

GP Mohammed Shamsul ISLAM

Ashcroft Surgery
803 Stockport Road, Levenshulme, Manchester M19 3BS
Tel: 0161 224 1329 Fax: 0161 224 0095
(Central Manchester Primary Care Trust)

Practice Manager Jodi Kelly

GP Subhash Chandra ARORA, Donald MacLennan COUPER, A Craig FRAME, C E WHITE

Ashton New Road Surgery
863 Ashton New Road, Clayton, Manchester M11 4PB
Tel: 0161 370 7115/6 Fax: 0161 371 1548
(North Manchester Primary Care Trust)

GP Nur SAEED, Riaz SAEED, D SHANKER, Kishen SHANKER

Ashton Road Surgery
58 Ashton Road, Droylsden, Manchester M43 7BW
Tel: 0161 370 1610 Fax: 0161 371 1258
(Tameside and Glossop Primary Care Trust)

GP Anthony Simon BUTLER, Andrew Edward COX, Stephen Anthony CROOK, Rodney WILLIAMSON

Ashville Surgery
171 Upper Chorlton Road, Manchester M16 9RT
Tel: 0161 881 4293 Fax: 0161 860 5265
(Central Manchester Primary Care Trust)
Patient List Size: 5150

Practice Manager Stephan Voysey

GP Philip Geoffrey FYANS, Carole Anne BOWLEY, Susan Rowena HILTON

Avenue Medical Centre
51-53 Victoria Avenue, Blackley, Manchester M9 6BA
Tel: 0161 720 8282 Fax: 0161 740 7991
(North Manchester Primary Care Trust)

Practice Manager Pauline Davies

GP Abdul MOMEN, Denise Mary HENNESSY, Wendy Jane KITCHING, Liam Patrick McGROGAN

Bag Lane Surgery
32 Bag Lane, Atherton, Manchester M46 0EE
Tel: 01942 896489 Fax: 01942 888793
(Ashton, Leigh and Wigan Primary Care Trust)

GP Esther Chandrika VASANTH, Vasanth SESHAPPA

Balayogi, Hussain and Sreenivasan
Doctors Surgery, 76 Market Street, Droylsden, Manchester M43 6DE
Tel: 0161 370 2626 Fax: 0161 371 0888
(Tameside and Glossop Primary Care Trust)
Patient List Size: 7912

Practice Manager M Barlow

GP Komakula Krishna BALAYOGI, Iftikhar HUSSAIN, Pudiya V SREENIVASAN

Barlow Medical Centre
8 Barlow Moor Road, Didsbury, Manchester M20 6TR
Tel: 0161 445 2101 Fax: 0161 445 9560
Website: www.barlowmed.com
(South Manchester Primary Care Trust)
Patient List Size: 12300

Practice Manager Jayne Cooney

GP Ian Donald BURTON, Tariq M CHAUHAN, Claudia Ceridwen DORNAN, Z L HODSON, Douglas E JEFFERY, See KWOK, S MUDDLESTON

Bellott Street Practice
63 Bellott Street, Cheetham, Manchester M8 0PQ
Tel: 0161 205 3847 Fax: 0161 205 2515
Email: richh@manchester.nwest.nhs.uk
(North Manchester Primary Care Trust)
Patient List Size: 4000

Practice Manager Rubina Ullah

GP N ALI-NAWAZ, Q ZAMAN

Benchill Medical Practice
127 Woodhouse Lane, Benchill, Wythenshawe, Manchester M22 9WP
Tel: 0161 998 4304 Fax: 0161 945 4028
(South Manchester Primary Care Trust)

Practice Manager Siobhan O'Malley-Butler

GP Nedi Nicou SMYRNIOU

Bennett Street Surgery
Bennett Street, Stretford, Manchester M32 8SG
Tel: 0161 865 1100 Fax: 0161 865 7710
(Trafford North Primary Care Trust)
Patient List Size: 3500

Practice Manager M Grange

GP M H WROBLEWSKA

Birches Medical Centre
Polefield Road, Prestwich, Manchester M25 2GN
Tel: 0161 773 3037 Fax: 0161 773 3640
(Bury Primary Care Trust)
Patient List Size: 3600

Practice Manager Linda Brosnan

GP R D BROSNAN, S PADMA

Blackburn Street Health Centre
Blackburn Street, Radcliffe, Manchester M26 1WS
Tel: 0161 723 2062 Fax: 0161 724 5628
(Bury Primary Care Trust)
Patient List Size: 6793

Practice Manager Irene Abbott

GP Mohammad Iqbal QURESHI, A J BEHRANA, Rosemary May PRICE

Bodey Medical Centre
363 Wilmslow Road, Fallowfield, Manchester M14 6XU
Tel: 0161 248 6644 Fax: 0161 224 4228
(South Manchester Primary Care Trust)

Practice Manager Elaine Parkinson

GP Christopher STEELE, Jean Elizabeth Anderson FULLER, Peter GILL, Sheila HOLLINGSHEAD, Harry LOWE, Tarik RASHID

Bollington Road Surgery
126 Bollington Road, Ancoats, Manchester M40 7HD
Tel: 0161 205 2979 Fax: 0161 205 6368
(North Manchester Primary Care Trust)
Patient List Size: 4000

Practice Manager Anne Harrison

GP Syed Ziauddin AHMAD, Bashir Ahmad PATTOO

Borcharot Medical Centre
62 Whitchurch Road, Withington, Manchester M20 1EB
Tel: 0161 445 7475 Fax: 0161 448 0466
(South Manchester Primary Care Trust)

Practice Manager Jom Bond

GP William Patrick TAMKIN, M BROOK, Janet CHARNLEY, Christopher Edward George MARTIN, Lynn Patricia NORBURY, Nicholas Stephen SMITH

Boundary Medical Practice
63 Booth Street West, Hulme, Manchester M15 6PR
Tel: 0161 227 9785 Fax: 0161 226 0471
(Central Manchester Primary Care Trust)
Patient List Size: 2200

Practice Manager Sue Copper

GP Gregory Robert Edward KEYNES, K M FLETCHER

Bowland Road
52 Bowland Road, Baguley, Manchester M23 1JX
Tel: 0161 998 2014 Fax: 0161 945 6354
(South Manchester Primary Care Trust)

Practice Manager Pat Gregory

GP Kenneth SHEARER, Timothy L FRANK, Claire GOODING, Jennifer Isabel HAWORTH, Susan Margaret HYDE

Bowness Road Surgery
133 Bowness Road, Middleton, Manchester M24 4EN
(Heywood and Middleton Primary Care Trust)

GP James Timothy ANGLIN

Brookdale Surgery
202 Droyldsden Road, Newton Heath, Manchester M40 1NZ
Tel: 0161 681 4265 Fax: 0161 947 0112
(North Manchester Primary Care Trust)
Patient List Size: 3000

Practice Manager S Karim

GP M KARIM

Brooklands Medical Practice
594 Altrincham Road, Brooklands, Manchester M23 9JH
Tel: 0161 998 3818 Fax: 0161 946 0716
Email: sdudley103@aol.com
Website: www.brooklandsmedicalpractice.freeserve.co.uk
(South Manchester Primary Care Trust)
Patient List Size: 4400

Practice Manager Elaine Reynolds

GP Hilary Jean HARRIS, Hilary THOMPSON

Brooks Bar Medical Centre
162-164 Chorlton Road, Old Trafford, Manchester M16 7WW
Tel: 0161 226 7777 Fax: 0161 232 9963
(Trafford North Primary Care Trust)
Patient List Size: 8000

Practice Manager Jackie Garvey

GP Vijay Kumar TREHAN, Robert Ian EDEN, Madhuri KHURANA, Derek Michael SEEX

Brunswick Health Centre
Hartfield Close, Manchester M13 9YA
Tel: 0161 273 4901 Fax: 0161 273 5952
(Central Manchester Primary Care Trust)
Patient List Size: 17000

Practice Manager Judith A Harris

GP C T CHUI, Maria Bernadette CUNNINGHAM, C NGAN, Kamprath SREEDHARAN, H BARRETT, Sandip SHROFF, J C WILLIAMSON

Burnage Primary Care Resource Centre
347 Burnage Lane, Manchester M19 1EW
Tel: 0161 432 1404 Fax: 0161 442 7900
(South Manchester Primary Care Trust)

Practice Manager David Whitehouse

GP Peter Charles CHADWICK, M C DAINTON

Canterbury Road Surgery
186 Canterbury Road, Davyhulme, Manchester M41 0GR
Tel: 0161 748 5559 Fax: 0161 747 1997
(Trafford North Primary Care Trust)

Practice Manager K Fraser

GP Rachel Elsa HOWARD, Niall JORDAN, Anthony Howard KAYE, Elizabeth LANG-SADLER, David Geoffrey Michael LEE, Rowena Ann RUTTER, Kamani WISEYLSEKENA

Capitol Road Surgery
2-6 Capitol Road, Higher Openshaw, Manchester M11 1LA
Tel: 0161 370 2133 Fax: 0161 371 0737

(North Manchester Primary Care Trust)

GP Stephen William FARRAR, Barry Joseph O'DRISCOLL, Susan Catherine O'DRISCOLL

Chapel Medical Centre
220 Liverpool Road, Irlam, Manchester M44 6FE
Tel: 0161 775 7373 Fax: 0161 775 5603
(Salford Primary Care Trust)

Practice Manager Kate Upton

GP Vijaya JOSHI

Charlestown Health Centre
Charlestown Road, Blackley, Manchester M9 7ED
Tel: 0161 740 7414 Fax: 0161 795 3162
(North Manchester Primary Care Trust)
Patient List Size: 2400

Practice Manager Ann Darby

GP Shahid Munir AHMAD

Cherry Medical Centre
478-482 Manchester Road East, Little Hulton, Manchester M38 9NS

GP Than KYAW, Tun TAUK

Chester Road Surgery
864-866 Chester Road, Stretford, Manchester M32 0PA
Tel: 0161 865 5556 Fax: 0161 866 8688
(Trafford North Primary Care Trust)
Patient List Size: 3960

Practice Manager S Mann

GP Ravindra MENE

Chorlton Health Centre
1 Nicolas Road, Chorlton, Manchester M21 9NJ
Tel: 0161 881 7941 Fax: 0161 861 7567
(Central Manchester Primary Care Trust)

Practice Manager Christine Henderson

GP N N SARMAH, D S RATCLIFFE

Chorlton Health Centre
1 Nicolas Road, Chorlton, Manchester M21 9NJ
Tel: 0161 881 6131 Fax: 0161 860 7290
(Central Manchester Primary Care Trust)

Practice Manager Paula Langley

GP Volker Walter Martin SIEBERT, Gill EDMONDSON

Chorlton Health Centre
1 Nicolas Road, Chorlton, Manchester M21 9NJ
Tel: 0161 881 4545 Fax: 0161 860 4565
(Central Manchester Primary Care Trust)
Patient List Size: 3185

Practice Manager C Meredith

GP N N SARMAH, D S RATCLIFFE

Church Lane Surgery
77 Church Lane, Harpurhey, Manchester M9 5BH
Tel: 0161 205 2714 Fax: 0161 205 2716
(North Manchester Primary Care Trust)

GP Vijay Bhaskarrao SOMAN, Tindivanam BHISHMA, Varshit SHAH

Church Street Surgery
169 Church Street, Eccles, Manchester M30 0LU
Tel: 0161 787 8880 Fax: 0161 787 8864
(Salford Primary Care Trust)
Patient List Size: 3800

GP Pralhad Laxmanrao GANVIR

Churchgate Surgery
119 Manchester Road, Denton, Manchester M34 3RA
Tel: 0161 336 2114 Fax: 0161 320 7045
(Tameside and Glossop Primary Care Trust)
Patient List Size: 7800

Practice Manager Bob Gregg

GP Pamela Ruth JOYCE, David Brian RONEY, Efren German SANCHEZ, Kaye WARD

City Road Surgery
204 City Road, Hulme, Manchester M15 4EA
Tel: 0161 872 8129 Fax: 0161 877 0321
(Central Manchester Primary Care Trust)

Practice Manager Margaret Matthews

GP Mary Georgina GIBBS, S HODSON

Clayton Health Centre
89 North Road, Clayton, Manchester M11 4EJ
Tel: 0161 223 9229 Fax: 0161 223 1116
(North Manchester Primary Care Trust)
Patient List Size: 6000

Practice Manager Monica Monaco

GP Andrew Lewis GLASS, Brian GOODALL

Clayton Health Centre
89 North Road, Clayton, Manchester M11 4EJ
Tel: 0161 223 1658 Fax: 0161 231 6977
(North Manchester Primary Care Trust)

Practice Manager Dorothy Rothwell

GP Hasan Khurshid MAZHARI

Clayton Health Centre
89 North Road, Clayton, Manchester M11 4EJ
Tel: 0161 223 8388 Fax: 0161 223 9390
(North Manchester Primary Care Trust)
Patient List Size: 6000

Practice Manager D Gallagher

GP Ashok Venkatesh MOKASHI, G KIELY, D KUMAR

Cleggs Lane Surgery
81-85 Cleggs Lane, Little Hulton, Manchester M38 9WU
Tel: 0161 799 4988 Fax: 0161 799 5271
(Salford Primary Care Trust)
Patient List Size: 3000

Practice Manager Karen Fleming

GP N PAWAR

Collegiate Medical Centre
Brideoak Street, Manchester M8 0AT
Tel: 0161 205 4364 Fax: 0161 203 5511
(North Manchester Primary Care Trust)
Patient List Size: 9300

GP Avril Felice MATTISON, Jane Mary FORD, Richard GUY, Sohail Bashir MUNSHI, Linda Henrietta SANDLE, Martin WHITING

Corkland Road Surgery
10 Corkland Road, Chorlton, Manchester M21 2UR
Tel: 0161 881 6223
(Central Manchester Primary Care Trust)

Practice Manager Shameem Chaudhury

GP Mahendra Prasad JAISWAL, Judith CURRAN

Cornishway Medical Centre
37 Cornishway, Woodhouse Park, Manchester M22 6LE
Tel: 0161 437 1467 Fax: 0161 493 9043
(South Manchester Primary Care Trust)

Practice Manager Janice Langley

GP David Graham WATERHOUSE, Judith Ann REAM, C SEENAN, Pathma Jani SUKUMAR

Crescent Road Surgery
72 Crescent Road, Crumpsall, Manchester M8 9NT
Tel: 0161 740 9864 Fax: 0161 740 0524
(North Manchester Primary Care Trust)

Practice Manager Elizabeth Haigh

GP Surinder Singh JOLLY

Dam Head Medical Centre
1020 Rochdale Road, Blackley, Manchester M9 7HD
Tel: 0161 720 9744 Fax: 0161 720 9755
(North Manchester Primary Care Trust)

GP H GATOFF

David Medical Centre
274 Barlow Moor Road, Chorlton, Manchester M21 8HA
Tel: 0161 881 1681 Fax: 0161 860 7071
(South Manchester Primary Care Trust)

Practice Manager Shamim Khan

GP Surendra Kumar SHARMA, Punam PARIHAR, Sukhbir Singh PARIHAR

Dearden Avenue Surgery
1A Dearden Avenue, Little Hulton, Manchester M38 9GH
Tel: 0161 799 2784 Fax: 0161 799 1889
(Salford Primary Care Trust)

GP Amarjeet AHUJA

Denton Medical Practice
100 Ashton Road, Denton, Manchester M34 3JE
Tel: 0161 336 2324 Fax: 0161 336 1161
(Tameside and Glossop Primary Care Trust)
Patient List Size: 5200

GP Sumita GUPTA, Raj KHIROYA

Didsbury Medical Centre
645 Wilmslow Road, Didsbury, Manchester M20 6BA
Tel: 0161 445 1957 Fax: 0161 434 9931
(South Manchester Primary Care Trust)
Patient List Size: 10300

Practice Manager Lynn Cordock

GP Henry Mark ASHWORTH, Mark John WHITAKER, Dr BAXTER, Alison VICKERS

The Docs
55-59 Bloom Street, Manchester M1 3LY
Tel: 0161 237 9490 Fax: 0161 228 3164
(Central Manchester Primary Care Trust)

Practice Manager Sue Sheridan

GP Timothy William John WORDEN, Barbara Kathryn ALLAN

Dr Juma
145 Elliott Street, Tyldesley, Manchester M29 8FL
Tel: 01942 892727 Fax: 01942 888847
(Ashton, Leigh and Wigan Primary Care Trust)

Practice Manager Christina Cooney

GP Najaff JUMA, Urmila SHAH

Dr Metzger Surgery
20-24 Park Hill Avenue, Crumpsall, Manchester M8 4RA
Tel: 0161 702 1311 Fax: 0161 795 1811
(North Manchester Primary Care Trust)

GP Dr METZGER

Droylsden Road Surgery
125 Droylsden Road, Newton Heath, Manchester M40 1NT
Tel: 0161 681 1956 Fax: 0161 681 2039
(North Manchester Primary Care Trust)

GP Partha Sarathi BASU, Dr AKHTAR, M GAMAGE

Durnford Medical Centre
113 Long Street, Middleton, Manchester M24 6DL
Tel: 0161 643 2011 Fax: 0161 653 6570
Email: doctor.g@gconnect.com
(Heywood and Middleton Primary Care Trust)
Patient List Size: 9000

Practice Manager Susan Mayo

GP Paul Justin GRIFFITHS, Nigel Peter BARBER, Andrew Paul BRACEGIRDLE, Matthew John JUDAH, Fiona Jane McINTYRE

Elliott Street Surgery
145 Elliott Street, Tyldesley, Manchester M29 8FL
Tel: 01942 892727 Fax: 01942 888847
(Ashton, Leigh and Wigan Primary Care Trust)

Practice Manager Christina Cooney

GP Najaf JUMA

Elms Medical Centre
Green Lane, Whitefield, Manchester M45 7FD
Tel: 0161 766 2311 Fax: 0161 767 9544
(Bury Primary Care Trust)
Patient List Size: 6300

Practice Manager Amanda Williams

GP John Francis NOONE, Laura FREED, Latha JAYAKUMAR, Adrian Gerard Mary O'HARE

Failsworth Group Practice
Ashton Road West, Failsworth, Manchester M35 0HN
Tel: 0161 682 6297 Fax: 0161 683 5861
(Oldham Primary Care Trust)

Practice Manager L Clemens

GP Linda CRYER, B ABDUL-KARIM, S AL-KAMIL, M FAULKNER, K JEFFERY, N MORRIS, Y WILLIAMS

Fairview Medical Centre
131-133 Flixton Road, Urmston, Manchester M41 5ZZ
Tel: 0161 748 2021 Fax: 0161 748 7974
(Trafford North Primary Care Trust)

Practice Manager Mrs Wellbelove

GP Amarjit Kaur GILL, Har Mohander Singh GILL, L GILL

Fallowfield Medical Centre
75 Ladyburn Lane, Fallowfield, Manchester M14 6YL
Tel: 0161 224 4503 Fax: 0161 256 4292
(South Manchester Primary Care Trust)

GP A KAKKAR

Fallsworth Health Centre
Ashton Road West, Fallsworth, Manchester M35 0HN
Tel: 0161 681 1401 Fax: 0161 681 8651
(Oldham Primary Care Trust)

GP Dr HOSSAIN

Fernclogh Surgery
1 Tavistock Square, Manchester M9 5RD
Tel: 0161 205 1638 Fax: 0161 205 1638
Email: sion.saleh@gpp84605.nhs.uk
(North Manchester Primary Care Trust)
Patient List Size: 2000

Practice Manager Frances Saleh

GP Sion SALEH

Fernclogh Surgery
1 Tavistock Square, Harpurhey, Manchester M9 5RD
Tel: 0161 205 1638 Fax: 0161 205 1638
Email: sion@saleh48.freeserve.co.uk
(North Manchester Primary Care Trust)
Patient List Size: 1700

Practice Manager F Saleh

GP Sion SALEH

Five Oaks Family Practice
47 Graham Street, Beswick, Manchester M11 3BB
Tel: 0161 223 4293 Fax: 0161 230 6728
Email: fiveoaks@themutual.net
(North Manchester Primary Care Trust)
Patient List Size: 7396

Practice Manager Helen Denn

GP Rameshchandra Hiralaji RATHI, J BARROW, S DEAN, Vijay NATHOO

Gill Medical Centre
5 Harriet Street, Walkden, Worsley, Manchester M28 3DR
Tel: 0161 790 3033 Fax: 0161 702 9544
(Salford Primary Care Trust)
Patient List Size: 5000

Practice Manager Maureen Seddon

GP Pamela Jean CLEATOR, Ian Thomas TASKER

Gloucester House Medical Centre
17 Station Road, Urmston, Manchester M41 9JS
Tel: 0161 748 7115 Fax: 0161 749 8032
(Trafford North Primary Care Trust)
Patient List Size: 2700

Practice Manager Salam Prodhan

GP Masud Salam PRODHAN, Farah AZAM

Gorse Hill Medical Centre
879 Chester Road, Stretford, Manchester M32 0RN
Tel: 0161 864 3037 Fax: 0161 864 3066
(Trafford North Primary Care Trust)
Patient List Size: 5400

Practice Manager H Bedi, A Taylor

GP Satnam KAUR, A KHAN, M MAYANS

Gorton Medical Centre
46 Wellington Street, Gorton, Manchester M18 8LJ
Tel: 0161 223 1113 Fax: 0161 223 8639
(Central Manchester Primary Care Trust)

Practice Manager Sylvia Clarke

GP Martin Robert GRIFFITHS, S KANE, J T KIDD, A F SIDDIQUI, G J WATT

Greenbrow Road Surgery
379 Greenbrow Road, Newall Green, Manchester M23 2XP
Tel: 0161 437 3164/0975 Fax: 0161 498 8010
(South Manchester Primary Care Trust)
Patient List Size: 3000

Practice Manager Melaine Lomas

GP Sheikh Yawar HUSAIN

Greyland Medical Centre
468 Bury Old Road, Prestwich, Manchester M25 1NL
Tel: 0161 798 7850 Fax: 0161 773 9219
(Bury Primary Care Trust)
Patient List Size: 3000

Practice Manager J Firestone

GP Laurence Howard SHERMAN, Bethel ROSENBERG

Haber and Partners
250 Langworthy Road, Salford, Manchester M6 5WW
Tel: 0161 736 7422 Fax: 0161 736 4816
(Salford Primary Care Trust)
Patient List Size: 12500

Practice Manager Jackie Rowan

GP Shinga HABER, Lawrence Spencer ADDLESTONE, Karen Louise GOODMAN, Phyllis Anne LEVENTHALL, Magaret McPHILLIPS, Susan Elaine ROSENBERG

Haque and Partner
Blackburn Street Health Centre, Blackburn Street, Radcliffe, Manchester M26 1WS
Tel: 0161 724 9030 Fax: 0161 723 3313
(Bury Primary Care Trust)
Patient List Size: 3988

GP Iftikhar-ul HAQUE, Irshad-ul HAQUE

Harpurhey Health Centre
1 Church Lane, Harpurhey, Manchester M9 4BE
Tel: 0161 205 1541 Fax: 0161 202 3700
Website: www.ranote.co.uk
(North Manchester Primary Care Trust)
Patient List Size: 3800

Practice Manager J Sabuldihin

GP Amar Singh RANOTE, Sushima Rani RANOTE

Haughton Vale Surgery
Tatton Road, Denton, Manchester M34 7PL
Tel: 0161 336 3005 Fax: 0161 320 3884
Email: surgery@haughtonvale.tsnet.co.uk
(Tameside and Glossop Primary Care Trust)
Patient List Size: 9000

Practice Manager Brian Jones

GP Amy Montgomery CUMMING, Lisa Christine GUTTERIDGE, Mohammed HOSSAIN, Gyan Prakash SINGH

The Hazeldene Medical Centre
97 Moston Lane East, New Moston, Manchester M40 3HD
Tel: 0161 681 7287 Fax: 0161 681 7438
(North Manchester Primary Care Trust)

GP E E WESTON, Susan Elizabeth MARTIN, Bernard Leslie POSTON, P TAYLOR

High Street Surgery
High Street, Astley Tyldesley, Manchester M29 8AL
Tel: 01942 882950 Fax: 01942 886611
(Ashton, Leigh and Wigan Primary Care Trust)

GP Ajit BURMAN, C P KHATRI, R S SHAH

Higher Blackley Medical Centre
156 Victoria Avenue, Manchester M9 0FN
Tel: 0161 740 2106 Fax: 0161 720 6384
(North Manchester Primary Care Trust)
Patient List Size: 6000

GP Marvin Raymond LEWIS, S MEONCICAR, N SINHA

Hodge Road Surgery
2 Hodge Road, Worsley, Manchester M28 3AT
Tel: 0161 790 3615 Fax: 0161 703 7638
(Salford Primary Care Trust)
Patient List Size: 9500

Practice Manager Denise Carroll

GP Clive Trevor BOYCE, Nigel Aubrey HYAMS, Bruce SUTHERLAND, Simon Andrew WRIGHT

Hulme Medical Centre
175 Royce Road, Hulme, Manchester M15 5TJ
Tel: 0161 226 0606 Fax: 0161 226 5644
Website: www.hulmemedicalptc.4dw.com
(Central Manchester Primary Care Trust)
Patient List Size: 10200

Practice Manager Danuta Hopwood

GP Shiv Kumar Jagannath CHOUKSEY, Kuen Po CHAN, Ruth HAWTING, Tracey LEIGH, Sian Lois SEGAR, Christopher John WOODHOUSE

Hulme Medical Centre
175 Royce Road, Hulme, Manchester M15 5TJ
Tel: 0161 226 1804 Fax: 0161 226 3421
(Central Manchester Primary Care Trust)

GP A KAPOOR

Hulton District Health Centre
Haysbrook Avenue, Worsley, Manchester M28 0AY
Tel: 0161 790 3276 Fax: 0161 703 7948
(Salford Primary Care Trust)

GP Syed Ahmed Ali GILANI

Hyde Road Surgery
119 Hyde Road, Denton, Manchester M34 3BB
Tel: 0161 336 2835
(Tameside and Glossop Primary Care Trust)

GP Ashoke Kumar RAY

Junction Surgery
346 Grimshaw Lane, Middleton Junction, Middleton, Manchester M24 2AU
Tel: 0161 643 2063
(Heywood and Middleton Primary Care Trust)

GP Joan Esmé MARTIN, Frederic William THOMASON

Kenyon Lane Surgery
152 Kenyon Lane, Moston, Manchester M40 9DF
Tel: 0161 681 3383 Fax: 0161 681 3383
(North Manchester Primary Care Trust)

GP Mythili IYENGAR

Khan
Blackburn Street Health Centre, Blackburn Street, Radcliffe, Manchester M26 1WS
Tel: 0161 724 9737 Fax: 0161 723 0008
(Bury Primary Care Trust)

GP Zarrar Aqueel KHAN

King's Medical Centre
7 Kings Road, Old Trafford, Manchester M16 7RT
Tel: 0161 226 1288 Fax: 0161 232 7973
(Central Manchester Primary Care Trust)
Patient List Size: 1815

Practice Manager Amanda Stewart

GP Shabbir Ahmed RAHUJA

Kingsway Medical Centre
655 Kingsway, Burnage, Manchester M19 1RD
Tel: 0161 432 2725 Fax: 0161 947 9192
(South Manchester Primary Care Trust)
Patient List Size: 6500

Practice Manager Evelyn Grayshon

GP Gillian Susan ALEXANDER, Margaret Mary CANT, Jonathan Edward KAYE, B McCARTHY

Ladybarn Group Practice
177 Mauldeth Road, Fallowfield, Manchester M14 6SG
Tel: 0161 224 2873 Fax: 0161 225 3276
(South Manchester Primary Care Trust)
Patient List Size: 9700

Practice Manager Bronwen Cox

GP Helen BURGESS, Ahmed ABBAS, D FOX, R LINDLEY, Joan Mary O'CONNOR, Clare Mary RONALDS, Jullien Hardie Caton WALKLEY

The Lance Medical Centre
121 Witington Road, Whalley Range, Manchester M16 8EE
Tel: 0161 226 1567/9717/8030 Fax: 0161 226 6469/232 5418
(Central Manchester Primary Care Trust)
Patient List Size: 6500

Practice Manager Keith Myhill

GP A S FISHER, L CAMPBELL, M COOPER, Slobodan MIHAJLOVIC

Langley Surgery
109-111 Windermere Road, Langley, Middleton, Manchester M24 5WF
Tel: 0161 6553834 Fax: 0161 6553815
(Heywood and Middleton Primary Care Trust)
Patient List Size: 2500

Practice Manager Mandy Pearson

GP Farhat Jabeen AHMAD

Levenshulme Health Centre
Dunstable Street, Levenshulme, Manchester M19 3BX
Tel: 0161 225 4033 Fax: 0161 248 8020
(Central Manchester Primary Care Trust)
Patient List Size: 6500

Practice Manager Margaret Baldwin

GP Milton David BALLON, S SHEEHAN, Alison I DICKSON, Debra WARD

The Limes Medical Centre
8-12 Hodge Road, Worsley, Manchester M28 3AT
Tel: 0161 790 8621 Fax: 0161 703 8670
(Salford Primary Care Trust)
Patient List Size: 6500

Practice Manager J Marsh, J Solomon

GP Paul ELEMENT, Gabby GREGORY, Denis Kevin McCARTHY, M TRAN

Liverpool Road Surgery
523 Liverpool Road, Irlam, Manchester M44 6ZS

Practice Manager Joan Haines

GP Ravindra Vishwanath APTE

Liverpool Road Surgery
523 Liverpool Road, Irlam, Manchester M44 6ZS

GP Colin Ian MALCOMSON, Nigel Philip MALLOY, Jonathan Neil ROLFE

Longsight Health Centre
528 Stockport Road, Longsight, Manchester M13 0RR
Tel: 0161 256 4488 Fax: 0161 225 0505
(Central Manchester Primary Care Trust)
Patient List Size: 3500

Practice Manager Linda Connors

GP P MOYO, C MOYO

Ma-Fat
Woodlands Surgery, 9 Maple Road, Brooklands, Manchester M23 9RL
Tel: 0161 962 1332 Fax: 0161 905 1099
(South Manchester Primary Care Trust)
Patient List Size: 2020

Practice Manager Gloria Davenport

GP Roger MA-FAT

MacDonald Road Medical Centre
MacDonald Road, Irlam, Manchester M44 5LH
Tel: 0161 775 5421 Fax: 0161 775 2568
(Salford Primary Care Trust)
Patient List Size: 7250

Practice Manager S Anderson

GP Brian HOPE, Neil Graham BATES

Manchester Road Practice
391A Manchester Road, Astley, Tyldesley, Manchester M29 7BY
Tel: 01942 876339 Fax: 01942 889914
(Ashton, Leigh and Wigan Primary Care Trust)

Practice Manager P Rawlinson

GP M T ALVA, N ALVA

Manchester Road Surgery
63 Manchester Road, Swinton, Manchester M27 5FX
Tel: 0161 794 4343 Fax: 0161 736 0669
(Salford Primary Care Trust)

GP K ARMSHAW, Dr COPPOCK, Martin John HAYES, Hamish Gordon Blair STEDMAN

Manchester Road Surgery
39 Manchester Road, Walkden Worsley, Manchester M28 3NS
Tel: 0161 702 8595 Fax: 0161 702 8592
(Salford Primary Care Trust)

Practice Manager Lorna Brownsey

GP Enid Antoinette NORONHA, James William McCORKINDALE, Sheila McCORKINDALE, Howard MILLIGAN

Manchester Road Surgery
11 Manchester Road, Audenshaw, Manchester M34 5PZ
Tel: 0161 370 9539
(Tameside and Glossop Primary Care Trust)

GP D K SHAH, V AGGARWAL, N U MISTRY

The Maples Medical Centre
2 Scout Drive, Newall Green, Manchester M23 2SY
Tel: 0161 498 8484 Fax: 0161 428 9411
(South Manchester Primary Care Trust)

GP Geraint ALLEN, Petula Christine CHATTERJEE, Peter Robert FINK, P HUNTER

Mauldeth Medical Centre
112 Mauldeth Road, Fallowfield, Manchester M14 6SQ
Tel: 0161 434 6678 Fax: 0161 438 0602
(South Manchester Primary Care Trust)
Patient List Size: 5000

Practice Manager Catherine Forrester

GP Meir GARSON, J LOCHAM

Medical Centre
Bee Fold Lane, Atherton, Manchester M46 0BD
Tel: 01942 876011 Fax: 01942 873905
(Ashton, Leigh and Wigan Primary Care Trust)

GP N HATI-KAKOTY

Mersey Bank Avenue Surgery
38A Mersey Bank Avenue, Chorlton, Manchester M21 7NN
Tel: 0161 445 5559 Fax: 0161 445 9725
(South Manchester Primary Care Trust)
Patient List Size: 3100

Practice Manager Gaynor Whitelock

GP Iain Livingstone Mackay HOTCHKIES

Mill Street Surgery
439 Mill Street, Bradford, Manchester M11 2BL
Tel: 0161 223 0637 Fax: 0161 220 6728
(North Manchester Primary Care Trust)
Patient List Size: 6300

Practice Manager Bernadette Buckley

GP Navinchandra Uttambhai MISTRY, Vimal AGGARWAL, William NLUBE

Mitford Street Surgery
Mitford Street, Stretford, Manchester M32 8AG
Tel: 0161 866 8556 Fax: 0161 865 4937
(Trafford North Primary Care Trust)
Patient List Size: 3960

Practice Manager Sue Mann

GP R P MENE

Mohammad
6 Copson Street, Withington, Manchester M20 3HE
Tel: 0161 445 2181
(South Manchester Primary Care Trust)

GP Dost MOHAMMAD, S SIDDIQI

Monton Medical Centre
Canal Side, Monton Green, Eccles, Manchester M30 8AR
(Salford Primary Care Trust)

GP David Henry ALLAUN, Joseph M BORG COSTANZI, Manju KHANNA, Geoffrey LEECH

Moss Side Health Centre
Monton Street, Moss Side, Manchester M14 4GP
Tel: 0161 226 1849 Fax: 0161 226 1849
(Central Manchester Primary Care Trust)

GP Zahid HUSSAIN

Moss Side Medical Centre
Monton Street, Moss Side, Manchester M14 4GP
Tel: 0161 226 5053
(Central Manchester Primary Care Trust)

GP Z HUSSAIN, M PASHA

Mount Road Surgery
110 Mount Road, Gorton, Manchester M18 7BQ
Tel: 0161 231 4997 Fax: 0161 230 6227
(Central Manchester Primary Care Trust)

Practice Manager Jackie Lewis-Hughes

GP Francis Aden BERESFORD, Colin Edward HODDES, Alison Jane Fletcher HUTTON

Mount Road Surgery
62 Mount Road, Alkrington, Middleton, Manchester M24 1DZ
(Heywood and Middleton Primary Care Trust)

GP Venkataswamy NAMMALWAR

Naylor Street Surgery
4 Naylor Street, Miles Platting, Manchester M40 7JH
Tel: 0161 205 3177 Fax: 0161 205 7270
(North Manchester Primary Care Trust)

Practice Manager Sheila Wiseman

GP Nicholas Paul VITES

Newton Heath Health Centre
2 Old Church Street, Manchester M40 2JF
Tel: 0161 681 1353 Fax: 0161 682 1728
(North Manchester Primary Care Trust)
Patient List Size: 5900

Practice Manager Joanne McCullam

GP M ELLIS, S AHMED, Muhammad FAROOQ

Northenden Health Centre
489 Palatine Road, Northenden, Manchester M22 4DH
Tel: 0161 998 3206
(South Manchester Primary Care Trust)

GP Peter Hugh WILLIAMS, Marion Ann GOODMAN, Catherine Sylvia WHITE

Northern Moor Medical Practice
216A Wythenshawe Road, Northern Moor, Manchester M23 0PH
Tel: 0161 998 2503 Fax: 0161 945 0695
(South Manchester Primary Care Trust)
Patient List Size: 2326

Practice Manager Sue Gregson

GP Dr BURNS, Michael Edward Yaron CAPEK

Oakleigh Medical Centre
58 Ash Tree Road, Crumpsall, Manchester M8 5SA
Tel: 0161 740 1226 Fax: 0161 795 8611
(North Manchester Primary Care Trust)

Practice Manager Catherine Gallagher

GP Charles Julius SIMENOFF

Oswald Medical Centre
4 Oswald Road, Chorlton, Manchester M21 9LH
Tel: 0161 881 4744 Fax: 0161 861 7027
(Central Manchester Primary Care Trust)

Practice Manager Tracy Kirby

GP Jennifer Elaine Barrington BLACK, Ann SMALLDRIDGE

Park Medical Centre
434 Altrincham Road, Manchester M23 9AB
Tel: 0161 998 5538 Fax: 0161 945 8026
(South Manchester Primary Care Trust)
Patient List Size: 5064

Practice Manager B A Gatley

GP Shahla HANNAN, S J PATEL

Park View Medical Centre
5 Delauneys Road, Crumpsall, Manchester M8 4QS
Tel: 0161 795 5667 Fax: 0161 702 3225
(North Manchester Primary Care Trust)

GP Mandy CAPLAN, Dr FARNHAM

Parkside Surgery
187 Northmoor Road, Longsight, Manchester M12 5RU
Tel: 0161 257 3338 Fax: 0161 257 3338
(Central Manchester Primary Care Trust)

Practice Manager Auzma Rehman

GP Fatima Ahmed NAQUI

Partington Health Centre
Central Road, Partington, Manchester M31 4FL
Tel: 0161 775 7033 Fax: 0161 775 8411
(Trafford North Primary Care Trust)

Practice Manager A Clemens

GP Anthony DEWEEVER, Rebecca CONNELL, Anne Michele KINNEY

Partington Health Centre
Central Road, Partington, Manchester M31 4FL
Tel: 0161 775 7032 Fax: 0161 777 8003
(Trafford North Primary Care Trust)
Patient List Size: 4000

GP S FARHAN, M LINKER-TROOST

Peel Hall Medical Centre
2 Bleak Hey Road, Peel Hall, Manchester M22 5ES
Tel: 0161 437 2661 Fax: 0161 437 8332
(South Manchester Primary Care Trust)

Practice Manager J M Crean

GP William John PETTIT, A BAKAT

Pendlebury Health Centre
The Lowry Medical Centre, 659 Bolton Road, Pendlebury, Manchester M27 8HP
Tel: 0161 793 8686 Fax: 0161 727 8011
(Salford Primary Care Trust)

Practice Manager Andrea Simpson

GP Harbhajan Shah G SINGH, Ian Andrew BALLIN, David John WILCOCK, Jane WILCOCK

Pendlebury Health Centre
Nelson Fold Medical Centre, 659 Bolton Road, Pendlebury, Manchester M27 8HP
Tel: 0161 950 4545 Fax: 0161 950 4546
(Salford Primary Care Trust)
Patient List Size: 4200

Practice Manager Jackie Smith

GP Madan Mohan SHARMA, I C McCALL, Spencer NICHOLSON

Pensby Walk Practice
8 Pensby Walk, Miles Platting, Manchester M40 8GN
Tel: 0161 205 2867 Fax: 0161 205 2972
(North Manchester Primary Care Trust)
Patient List Size: 3300

Practice Manager Diane Stansfield

GP G O'SHEA, Shaun JACKSON, Kay PHILLIPS

Peterloo Medical Centre
133 Manchester Old Road, Middleton, Manchester M24 4DZ
Tel: 0161 643 5005
(Heywood and Middleton Primary Care Trust)
Patient List Size: 9600

GP Dr CLARK, David BROOKS, Dr CALDWELL, M JIVA, Gillian TONGE, Dr WALKER

Platt Lane Surgery
204 Platt Lane, Manchester M14 7BS
Tel: 0161 224 2468 Fax: 0161 256 4094
(Central Manchester Primary Care Trust)

Practice Manager Pauline Bancroft

GP Steven Douglas ELLIOT

Poplars Medical Centre
202 Partington Lane, Swinton, Manchester M27 0NA
Tel: 0161 794 6287 Fax: 0161 728 3415
(Salford Primary Care Trust)
Patient List Size: 9500

Practice Manager Margaret Mullin

GP Winston Michael FORMAN, Colin BRUNT, Jacqueline HARRIS, Sarah Louise HAUGHNEY, Anne Rosemarie STEWART, William WHEELDIN

Prestwich Health Centre
Fairfax Road, Prestwich, Manchester M25 1BT
(Bury Primary Care Trust)

Practice Manager S Evason

GP Dr RALPH

Prestwich Health Centre
Fairfax Road, Prestwich, Manchester M25 1BT
Tel: 0161 773 2483 Fax: 0161 773 9218
(Bury Primary Care Trust)
Patient List Size: 5500

Practice Manager Vickie Waters

GP Deepak Trilok Chand PRABHAKAR, Margaret COLTER, Nigel William DIXON

Prestwich Health Centre
Fairfax Road, Prestwich, Manchester M25 1BT
Tel: 0161 773 0525 Fax: 0161 773 9218
(Bury Primary Care Trust)

Practice Manager Jan Rogers

GP Dudley Arthur MOSS

Primrose Avenue Surgery
1 Primrose Avenue, Urmston, Manchester M41 0TY
Tel: 0161 747 2424 Fax: 0161 749 9719
(Trafford North Primary Care Trust)
Patient List Size: 6500

Practice Manager M Halliday

GP Peter David BAZLEY, Maria A DIMITRAKOS, Cecilia Mary McGAWLEY

Princess Road Surgery
471-475 Princess Road, Withington, Manchester M20 1BH
Tel: 0161 445 7805 Fax: 0161 448 2419
(Central Manchester Primary Care Trust)
Patient List Size: 4000

Practice Manager Joyce Duncan

GP Michael Richard UNWIN, Margaret Louise WILLIAMS

Quayside Medical Practice
Ashton Road West, Fallsworth, Manchester M35 0HN
Tel: 0161 681 1818 Fax: 0161 681 8596
(Oldham Primary Care Trust)
Patient List Size: 4000

Practice Manager Vivien Dawber

GP Deborah C BAYMAN, Balsam ABDUL-KARIM, Sarmid A K A AL-KAMIL, Linda Margaret CRYER, Michele Anne FAULKNER, Keith Frederick Key JEFFERY, D McMASTER, Neil A MORRIS, Yvonne WILLIAMS

Rectory Lane Surgery
44 Rectory Lane, Prestwich, Manchester M25 1BL
Tel: 0161 773 1803 Fax: 0161 773 3292
(Bury Primary Care Trust)
Patient List Size: 4200

GP Michael David CRANE, Seema MUNJAL

Red Bank Group Practice
Red Bank Health Centre, Unsworth Street, Radcliffe, Manchester M26 3GH
Tel: 0161 724 0777 Fax: 0161 724 8288
(Bury Primary Care Trust)
Patient List Size: 10100

Practice Manager Bernard Carroll

GP Stephen Michael FLASCHER, D S KOUVARELLIS, Anna MIRANDA, Janet Suzanne NEWTON, Peter Walter Vaughan THOMAS

Reddish Lane Surgery
63 Reddish Lane, Gorton, Manchester M18 7JH
Tel: 0161 223 0031 Fax: 0161 223 7282
(Central Manchester Primary Care Trust)

Practice Manager Mrs Barker

GP Kala TIWARI

RK Medical
283 Hollyhedge Road, Wythenshawe, Manchester M22 4QR
Tel: 0161 428 9411 Fax: 0161 428 9116
(South Manchester Primary Care Trust)

GP David John KAMINSKI, J RANDHAWA

The Robert Darbishire Practice
Rusholme Health Centre, Walmer Street, Rusholme, Manchester M14 5NP
Tel: 0161 225 6699 Fax: 0161 248 4580
(Central Manchester Primary Care Trust)

Practice Manager Pat Lockton

GP Carolyn Anne CHEW-GRAHAM, Martin Oliver ROLAND, N R CURTIS, Aneez Bahadurali ESMAIL, A JACKSON, K LIM, M S MIAN, Amanda MYERSCOUGH, Mark Stephen PERRY, Sarah Elizabeth SMITHSON, Rosemary Margaret TELFORD, Robert Michael VARNAM

Rochdale Road Surgery
48A Rochdale Road, Middleton, Manchester M24 2PU
Tel: 0161 643 9131
(Heywood and Middleton Primary Care Trust)

GP Sajid Saeed KHAN, S F AHMED, Ian Trevor HEATHCOTE

Seven Brooks Medical Centre
21 Church Street, Atherton, Manchester M46 9DE
Tel: 01942 882799 Fax: 01942 873859
(Ashton, Leigh and Wigan Primary Care Trust)
Patient List Size: 7000

Practice Manager T Cooper

GP John Clifford THOMPSON, A RAWSON

Sevenways Surgery
The Delamere Centre, Delamere Avenue, Stretford, Manchester M32 0DF
Tel: 0161 864 0200 Fax: 0161 864 0200
(Trafford North Primary Care Trust)
Patient List Size: 7000

Practice Manager Maureen Lowther

GP Marilyn Elizabeth KERR, M D BANGURA, George David Niman KISSEN

Seymour Grove Health Centre
70 Seymour Grove, Old Trafford, Manchester M16 0LW
Tel: 01612 877 9230 Fax: 0161 877 7103
(Trafford North Primary Care Trust)
Patient List Size: 2000

Practice Manager D Rigby

GP K KUNA

Seymour Grove Health Centre
70 Seymour Grove, Old Trafford, Manchester M16 0LW
Tel: 0161 848 7563 Fax: 0161 876 7805
(Trafford North Primary Care Trust)

Practice Manager A Baral

GP Syamal BARAL

Seymour Grove Health Centre
70 Seymour Grove, Old Trafford, Manchester M16 0LW
Tel: 0161 872 1870 Fax: 0161 877 1041
(Trafford North Primary Care Trust)

Practice Manager Ben Ward

GP Koteswarawma KUNA

Shiv Lodge Medical Centre
357-359 Dickenson Road, Longsight, Manchester M13 0WQ
Tel: 0161 224 6522/224 9465/225 5372 Fax: 0161 225 5366
Email: ramesh.gulati@gp-p84026.nhs.uk/padmini.gulati@gp-p84026.nhs.uk/
(Central Manchester Primary Care Trust)
Patient List Size: 7649

Practice Manager Deborah Coombes

GP Ramesh Chandra GULATI, P GULATI

The Sides Medical Centre
Moorside Road, Swinton, Manchester M27 0EW
Tel: 0161 794 1604 Fax: 0161 727 3615
Email: Michael.Nmoore@gp-P87016.nhs.uk
(Salford Primary Care Trust)
Patient List Size: 12500

Practice Manager A R Howell

GP Michael Allan MOORE, David Ian BUTTERWORTH, Gursharan Kaur JOLLY, John Edwin MARGINSON, Girish PATEL, Patricia Mary RUSSELL, Karan Vir SINGH

Spring Lane Surgery
15-17 Spring Lane, Radcliffe, Manchester M26 2TQ
Tel: 0161 724 6938 Fax: 0161 724 0172
(Bury Primary Care Trust)

Practice Manager Barbara Birnie

GP Kumar Shamrao KOTEGAONKAR, Manju Kumar KOTEGAONKAR, Ajay KOTEGAONKAR

Springfield House
New Lane, Patricroft, Eccles, Manchester M30 7JE
Tel: 0161 789 5858 Fax: 0161 707 7747
Email: springfield@mckernanm.fsnet.co.uk
(Salford Primary Care Trust)

Practice Manager Sarah Talbot

GP Michael Francis McKERNAN, John Hedley PURSER, Jarjisur RAHMAN, Linda Fay STALLEY, Elaine Jean TAMKIN

St Andrews Medical Centre
30 Russell Street, Eccles, Manchester M30 0NU
Tel: 0161 707 5500 Fax: 0161 787 9159
(Salford Primary Care Trust)

GP Barry ALLWEIS, Jacqueline Solveig BROXTON, Eva Mary JACOBS, Stephen Douglas LINDSAY, Nicolette Marie TYRRELL, John Yehia BEHARDIEN, Peter Duncan BUDDEN, Helen SUTHERLAND, Mhairi Stewart YATES

St Bees Surgery
34-36 St Bees Close, Moss Side, Manchester M14 4GG
Tel: 0161 226 7615 Fax: 0161 226 0413
(Central Manchester Primary Care Trust)

Practice Manager Vera Herring

GP Mufta Mohammed DRAH

St Gabriels Medical Centre
4 Bishops Road, Prestwich, Manchester M25 0HT
(Bury Primary Care Trust)

Practice Manager Ann Stewart

GP Olive Margaret DUDDY

St Gabriels Medical Centre
4 Bishops Road, Prestwich, Manchester M25 0HT
(Bury Primary Care Trust)

GP David Louis HIBBERT, J H LIEBERMAN

St Georges Medical Centre
St Georges Drive, Moston, Manchester M40 5HP
Tel: 0161 681 2127 Fax: 0161 684 8709
(North Manchester Primary Care Trust)

Practice Manager Carole Moran

GP Raquel DELGADO, Dawn NARHLYA, Mark NORTHFIELD

The Surgery
239 Mosley Common Road, Boothstown, Worsley, Manchester M28 1BZ
Tel: 0161 790 2192 Fax: 0161 799 5046
(Ashton, Leigh and Wigan Primary Care Trust)
Patient List Size: 4836

Practice Manager D Try

GP Michael David YATES

The Surgery
Tyldesley Health Centre, Poplar Street, Tyldesley, Manchester M29 8AX
Tel: 01942 881960 Fax: 01942 881961
(Ashton, Leigh and Wigan Primary Care Trust)

Practice Manager Lynn Avison

GP Dr COWLAND, Dr GILL

The Surgery
3 Formby Avenue, Atherton, Manchester M46 0EX
Tel: 01942 883044 Fax: 01942 888777
(Ashton, Leigh and Wigan Primary Care Trust)
Patient List Size: 2580

Practice Manager Karen Holgate

The Surgery
8 Elmfield Avenue, Atherton, Manchester M46 0HW
Tel: 01942 882001 Fax: 01942 886707
(Ashton, Leigh and Wigan Primary Care Trust)

GP Ajoy Kumar GHOSH, Dr SHARMA

The Surgery
Meadowview Medical Centre, 3 Formby Avenue, Atherton, Manchester M46 0EX
Tel: 01942 883330 Fax: 01942 877748
(Ashton, Leigh and Wigan Primary Care Trust)
Patient List Size: 2800

Practice Manager Sharon Fairbrother

GP Ashok Kumar ATREY, Neela ATREY

The Surgery
10 Higher Green Lane, Astley, Tyldesley, Manchester M29 7HG
Tel: 01942 883794 Fax: 01942 889830
(Ashton, Leigh and Wigan Primary Care Trust)
Patient List Size: 3000

Practice Manager Ann Atherton

GP H A CLUTTON, K KHATRI

The Surgery
885 Chester Road, Stretford, Manchester M32 0RN
Tel: 0161 865 3807 Fax: 0161 865 4964
(Trafford North Primary Care Trust)
Patient List Size: 2300

GP Quamer Ahmed KHAN

The Surgery
1 Coldalhurst Lane, Astley, Tyldesley, Manchester M29 7BS
Tel: 01942 878711 Fax: 01942 878714
(Ashton, Leigh and Wigan Primary Care Trust)

Practice Manager Janet Welch

GP Rakshaben PATEL, Ramesh PATEL

The Surgery
1 Smedley Street, Cheetham Hill, Manchester M8 8UN
Tel: 0161 205 4777 Fax: 0161 203 5861
(North Manchester Primary Care Trust)

GP Dr BOKHARI

The Surgery
60 Ayres Road, Old Trafford, Manchester M16 9WH
Tel: 0161 226 3449 Fax: 0161 226 7440
(Trafford North Primary Care Trust)

GP A HASAN

Surrey Lodge Practice
11 Anson Road, Victoria Park, Manchester M14 5BY
Tel: 0161 224 2471 Fax: 0161 257 2264
(Central Manchester Primary Care Trust)

Practice Manager Michael Maxwell

GP Lynne Ceris ENOCH, Henry Peterson PETRIE, Steven Frederick RILEY, Tracey Jayne VELL

Talbot Court Medical Practice
The Delamere Centre, Stretford, Manchester M32 0AF
Tel: 0161 865 1197 Fax: 0161 864 1966
Email: nicholas.singleton@nhs.net
(Trafford North Primary Care Trust)
Patient List Size: 3600

Practice Manager Judith Collinson

GP Amal DEAN, Nicholas Andrew SINGLETON

Tregenna Group Practice
399 Portway, Woodhouse Park, Manchester M22 0EP
Tel: 0161 499 3777 Fax: 0161 493 9119
(South Manchester Primary Care Trust)
Patient List Size: 6900

Practice Manager Linda Wright

GP Ian Mark BUCHALTER, Claire Margaret HUGHES, David Jonathan NEEDHAM, Hoi Shing WONG

Urmston Group Practice
154 Church Road, Urmston, Manchester M41 9DL
Tel: 0161 755 9870 Fax: 0161 755 9896
(Trafford North Primary Care Trust)
Patient List Size: 11250

Practice Manager Deborah Darlington

GP Wallace Robert FRASER, Ann Margaret HARRISON, Iain Michael MACLEAN, Dermot Martin REGAN, Frances Maxine WEBB, Raymond Gerrard WILSON

Urmston Lane Surgery
Delamer Centre, Delamere Avenue, Stretford, Manchester M32 0DF
Tel: 0161 865 3400 Fax: 0161 865 4429
(Trafford North Primary Care Trust)
Patient List Size: 2960

Practice Manager Kathleen Mulrooney

GP Anthony John CLARK

Vaishali Medical Centre
13 Corkland Road, Chorlton, Manchester M21 8UP
Tel: 0161 881 5074 Fax: 0161 881 8242
(Central Manchester Primary Care Trust)

Practice Manager P Prasad

GP S N PRASAD

Valentine House
2 Smethurst Street, Blackley, Manchester M9 8PP
Tel: 0161 202 4100 Fax: 0161 202 4202
(North Manchester Primary Care Trust)

Practice Manager Julie Brobbin

GP Donald Stuart CLEGG, John Stephen FALLON, Fiona Margaret HARGREAVES, Julie Louise RICHARDS, Alan Brett STOREY

Victoria Medical Centre
16-18 Victoria Parade, Urmston, Manchester M41 9BP
Tel: 0161 746 7088 Fax: 0161 746 7162
Email: m.seely@btinternet.com
(Trafford North Primary Care Trust)
Patient List Size: 2500

Practice Manager Eileen Corbishley

GP Martin Francis SEELY

Victoria Road Surgery
122 Victoria Road, Stretford, Manchester M32 0AD
Tel: 0161 865 1651

(Trafford North Primary Care Trust)

GP Azad FIROZE, Katherine Vivian FIROZE

The Village Surgery
25 Old Market Street, Blackley, Manchester M9 3DT
Tel: 0161 721 4865 Fax: 0161 740 6532
(North Manchester Primary Care Trust)
Patient List Size: 4000

GP Thomas Eugene NEVILLE, John HUGHES

Wellfield Surgery
53-55 Crescent Road, Crumpsall, Manchester M8 9JT
Tel: 0161 740 2213 Fax: 0161 720 9311
(North Manchester Primary Care Trust)

GP Peter Anthony DIXON, Arthur Samuel FINKE

West Gorton Medical Centre
6A Wenlock Way, West Gorton, Manchester M12 5LH
Tel: 0161 223 5226 Fax: 0161 230 6305
Website: www.westgortonmedical
(Central Manchester Primary Care Trust)
Patient List Size: 6200

Practice Manager Julie Jefferson

GP Pauline Louise HARRIS, Michael Charles William EECKELAERS, I S FRASER, D J HYLAND

West Point Medical Centre
167-169 Slade Lane, Levenshulme, Manchester M19 2AF
Tel: 0161 248 5100 Fax: 0161 225 6258
(Central Manchester Primary Care Trust)
Patient List Size: 6768

GP David Michael FOX, Graeme ASKEW, Jill DEAS, K P MORGAN

Whitefield Health Centre
Bury New Road, Whitefield, Manchester M45 8GH
Tel: 0161 766 8221
(Bury Primary Care Trust)

GP Nicholas Jesse WOODHEAD, Vivien Patricia ADDIS, Deborah Ann FERGUSON, Nicolas WALTON

Whitley Road Medical Centre
1 Whitley Road, Collyhurst, Manchester M40 7QH
Tel: 0161 205 4407 Fax: 0161 203 5269
(North Manchester Primary Care Trust)

Practice Manager Barbara McLaughlin

GP Harold Steven WEINSTOCK, Denis COLLIGAN, Rachel Irma GORDON, Kenneth VICKERS

Whittaker Lane Medical Centre
Daisy Bank, Whittaker Lane, Prestwich, Manchester M25 5EX
Tel: 0161 773 1580
(Bury Primary Care Trust)

GP Jeffrey SCHRYER, A B BROMLEY, S J TAYLOR

Wilbraham Road Surgery
515 Wilbraham Road, Chorlton, Manchester M21 1UF
Tel: 0161 881 6120 Fax: 0161 861 7796
(Central Manchester Primary Care Trust)
Patient List Size: 4004

Practice Manager Marion Murray

GP Michael John COOKE, G B WILSON

Willow Bank Surgery
1 Willow Bank, Church Lane, Harpurhey, Manchester M9 4WH
Tel: 0161 205 9240 Fax: 0161 202 4690
(North Manchester Primary Care Trust)

GP M L SAHA

Wilmslow Road Medical Centre
156 Wilmslow Road, Rusholme, Manchester M14 5LQ
Tel: 0161 224 2452 Fax: 0161 248 9261
(Central Manchester Primary Care Trust)
Patient List Size: 2900

Practice Manager Christine Henderson

GP Prem Lata PATHAK, A KAKKAR

Wilmslow Road Surgery
599 Wilmslow Road, Didsbury, Manchester M20 3QD
Tel: 0161 445 1952 Fax: 0161 448 1764
(South Manchester Primary Care Trust)

GP P FINK, P KALLIS, E LEON

Windmill Medical Practice
Ann Street, Denton, Manchester M34 2AJ
Tel: 0161 320 3131 Fax: 0161 337 8250
(Tameside and Glossop Primary Care Trust)
Patient List Size: 12500

Practice Manager Sue Kelly

GP Richard William GARDNER, Jennifer Margaret CASSIDY, M JOHNSON, Philip KERSHAW, Dr MADDOCK, William A ROGERS

Woodsend Road Surgery
14 Woodsend Road, Flixton, Manchester M41 8QT
Tel: 0161 747 4975 Fax: 0161 747 4446
(Trafford North Primary Care Trust)
Patient List Size: 3500

Practice Manager A Catterall

GP Peter Arnot BUTLER

Woodside Medical Centre
247 Wood Street, Middleton, Manchester M24 5QL
Tel: 0161 643 5385 Fax: 0161 653 6430
(Heywood and Middleton Primary Care Trust)

GP Stephen Michael MAYNARD, Stephen David BRADY, Jonathan Geoffrey HYMAN, David John MANCHESTER, Manthravadi VIDYAVATHI

Worsley Road North Surgery
90 Worsley Road North, Walkden Worsley, Manchester M28 3QW

GP Raghavendra Prasad SINHA

Manningtree

Edgefield Avenue Surgery
2 Edgefield Avenue, Lawford, Manningtree CO11 2HD
Tel: 01206 392617 Fax: 01206 391148
(Tendring Primary Care Trust)

Practice Manager Maureen Lines

GP John Christopher KELLY, Humayun AHMAD, Khadim Hussain BALOCH

Riverside Health Centre
Station Road, Manningtree CO11 1AA
Tel: 01206 397070 Fax: 01206 391570
(Tendring Primary Care Trust)
Patient List Size: 3700

Practice Manager Melanie Lodge

GP John HOSKYNS, Marc LE ROUX

Mansfield

Bull Farm Surgery
112A Chesterfield Road North, Mansfield NG19 7HZ
Tel: 01623 621059 Fax: 01623 648621
(Mansfield District Primary Care Trust)
Patient List Size: 2700

Practice Manager Natasha Lomas

GP N KARUNARAKAE

Churchside Medical Practice
Wood Street, Mansfield NG18 1QB
Tel: 01623 664877 Fax: 01623 664878
(Mansfield District Primary Care Trust)

Practice Manager Sandra Chatwin

GP Simon Jeremy WARD, Patrick LAW, Gaynor MONKCOOK, Vanessa Lynne PEARCE

Court View Surgery
Rosemary Street, Mansfield NG19 6AB
Tel: 01623 623600 Fax: 01623 635460
Website: www.courtview.co.uk
(Mansfield District Primary Care Trust)

Practice Manager Reg Murray

GP William Malcolm POWELL, Martin Rainer ANKENBAUER, Janet Taylor DORNAN, F M KHALIL

Health Centre
Church Street, Warsop, Mansfield NG20 0BP
Tel: 01623 843521 Fax: 01623 844040
(Mansfield District Primary Care Trust)

Practice Manager Karen Howe

GP J BARUAH

Health Centre
Church Street, Warsop, Mansfield NG20 0BP
Tel: 01623 844421 Fax: 01623 847642
(Mansfield District Primary Care Trust)
Patient List Size: 4190

Practice Manager Philippa Hutchinson

GP Balwant Singh BANGA, G ASHMORE, K CHAUDHURI, G DROWN

Hillview
Sherwood Parade, Kirklington Road, Rainworth, Mansfield NG21 0JP
Tel: 01623 795562 Fax: 01623 798879
(Newark and Sherwood Primary Care Trust)
Patient List Size: 3300

Practice Manager E Winter

GP G HUNT

Major Oak Medical Practice
22 High Street, Edwinstowe, Mansfield NG21 9QS
Tel: 01623 822303 Fax: 01623 825216
Email: firstname.surname@gp-c84113.nhs.uk
(Newark and Sherwood Primary Care Trust)
Patient List Size: 9780

Practice Manager C Roberts

GP R M JOSHI, Michael Gerard GLAZIER

Meden Vale Medical Centre
Egmanton Road, Meden Vale, Warsop, Mansfield NG20 9QN
Tel: 01623 845694 Fax: 01623 844550
(Mansfield District Primary Care Trust)
Patient List Size: 6200

Practice Manager J Jones

GP Christopher Joseph SUDELL, S ALLEN, J D J TOIT

Millview Surgery
1A Goldsmith Street, Mansfield NG18 5PF
Tel: 01623 649528 Fax: 01623 624595
Website: www.millviewsurgery.co.uk
(Mansfield District Primary Care Trust)
Patient List Size: 7900

Practice Manager Pauline Harrison

GP A CLARKIN, John Hinton DALE, H E FIELD, Simon John Rokeby MADDOCK, C MANN

Oak Tree Lane Surgery
Jubilee Way South, Mansfield NG18 3SF
Tel: 01623 649991
(Mansfield District Primary Care Trust)

GP P R GHOSH

Oakwood Surgery
Church Street, Mansfield Woodhouse, Mansfield NG19 8BL
Tel: 01623 633111 Fax: 01623 423480
(Mansfield District Primary Care Trust)
Patient List Size: 15100

Practice Manager Rosalyn Reavill

GP Subarna Man SHRESTHA, Khalid Shafiq BUTT, Peter John Bradshaw FRITH, Antoinette Elizabeth Aldegonde LUCASSEN, Thant SYN

Orchard Medical Practice
Innisdoon, Crow Hill Drive, Mansfield NG19 7AE
Tel: 01623 400100/ 424824 Fax: 01623 400101
(Mansfield District Primary Care Trust)
Patient List Size: 9000

Practice Manager Carole Wheaterof

GP Raian Rahmat SHEIKH, Walter FREEMAN, C J MACGREGOR, J E MILLS, K PHIPPS, Dean Russell TEMPLE

Pleasley Surgery
Chesterfield Road, Pleasley, Mansfield NG19 7PE
Tel: 01623 810249 Fax: 01623 811414
(Mansfield District Primary Care Trust)

Practice Manager Marilyn Wallis

GP K R PATEL

Pollard, Bilas, Jack and Smith
Clipstone Health Centre, First Avenue, Clipstone Village, Mansfield NG21 9DA
Tel: 01623 626132 Fax: 01623 420578
(Newark and Sherwood Primary Care Trust)
Patient List Size: 8000

Practice Manager Ros Irwin

GP Valerie Audrey POLLARD, Zenko BILAS, Kate JACK, Justin SMITH

Rainworth Health Centre
Warsop Lane, Rainworth, Mansfield NG21 0AD
Tel: 01623 794293 Fax: 01623 799218
(Newark and Sherwood Primary Care Trust)
Patient List Size: 6164

Practice Manager Julie Hoyes

GP Kirsten J BOLSHER, Christopher Norman CORBYN, Susan Emily HUGGARD, Kerrie WILKINS

Roundwood Surgery
Wood Street, Mansfield NG18 1QQ
Tel: 01623 648880 Fax: 01623 631761
Email: roundwood.surgery@gp-c84069.nhs.uk
(Mansfield District Primary Care Trust)
Patient List Size: 10510

Practice Manager Pam Clarke

GP Eduard Samuel STEINER, Elizabeth BAYLIS, Simon CAPPIN, Laura CARTER, John Patrick MURPHY, Vanessa PEACOCK, Milind TADPATRIHAN, Meryl WATKINS

Sandy Hills Practice
Sandy Lane, Mansfield NG18 2LT
Tel: 01623 659229 Fax: 01623 621557
(Mansfield District Primary Care Trust)
Patient List Size: 1800

Practice Manager Sharon McGachan

GP N VAN DER MEER

Sandy Lane Surgery
77 Sandy Lane, Mansfield NG18 2LT
Tel: 01623 656055 Fax: 01623 424898
(Mansfield District Primary Care Trust)
Patient List Size: 5000

Practice Manager Jackie Shirley

GP Hamid MASUD, Matoug Moh AGHEL

Shires Health Care
18 Main Street, Shirebrook, Mansfield NG20 8DG
Tel: 01623 742464 Fax: 01623 743921
(North Eastern Derbyshire Primary Care Trust)
Patient List Size: 14000

Practice Manager Zoe Tennant

GP John J HENNESSY, Elizabeth D BARRETT, Francis BARRETT, Shyamal CHATTERJEE, Susan Patricia DAY, Robert SUCHETT-KAYE

The Surgery
59 Mansfield Road, Blidworth, Mansfield NG21 0RB
Tel: 01623 795461 Fax: 01623 490514
(Newark and Sherwood Primary Care Trust)
Patient List Size: 11934

Practice Manager C J Brill

GP Timothy John BUTLER, Caroline Louise AHRENS, Eich CHUI, Martin James DALTON, Virupaki GOLSHETTI, Janet Elsie LOKER, James Alexander MATTICK

The Surgery
Health Centre, St. John Street, Mansfield NG18 1RH
Tel: 01623 622541 Fax: 01623 661313
(Mansfield District Primary Care Trust)
Patient List Size: 3107

Practice Manager Sally Haywood

GP Mohammed Anwarul HAQUE, B KHAN

The Surgery
Health Centre, St. John Street, Mansfield NG18 1RH
Tel: 01623 622541 Fax: 01623 622541
(Mansfield District Primary Care Trust)

Practice Manager Linda Moore

GP R S SHARMA

Marazion

Marazion Surgery
Gwallon Lane, Marazion TR17 0HW
Tel: 01736 710505 Fax: 01736 711205
Email: jackie.brown@marazion.cornwall.nhs.uk
(West of Cornwall Primary Care Trust)
Patient List Size: 7074

Practice Manager Jackie Brown

GP Alistair Byrne HAMILTON, Deirdre KILLEEN, David SUGRUE, Simon John THACKER, Neil Patrick Michael WALDEN

March

Addison Road Surgery
Wimblington Village Hall, Addison Road, Wimblington, March PE15 0QT
(East Cambridgeshire and Fenland Primary Care Trust)

Practice Manager Elizabeth Welcher

GP Tapas Kumar GOSWAMI

The Cornerstone Practice
26 Clwyn Road, March PE15 9BT
Tel: 01354 606300 Fax: 01354 606302
(East Cambridgeshire and Fenland Primary Care Trust)
Patient List Size: 8500

Practice Manager Bill Ridley

GP Martin John TAYLOR, Brian Roy COLLINGS, Wendy Nicola HARRISON, Elizabeth Ann MATHER, Robert Stuart David SHIELDS

East Street Surgery
East Street, Manea, March PE15 0JJ
Tel: 01354 680774 Fax: 01354 688222
Email: richard.hirson@nhs.net
Website: www.mantasurgery.org.uk
(East Cambridgeshire and Fenland Primary Care Trust)
Patient List Size: 2200

GP Richard Bernard HIRSON

Mercheford House Surgery
Mercheford House, Elwyn Road, March PE15 9BT
Tel: 01354 656841 Fax: 01354 660788
(East Cambridgeshire and Fenland Primary Care Trust)
Patient List Size: 6300

Practice Manager Pauline M Whitehead

GP Thomas Stuart WARRENDER, John Derek LISHMAN, Eamonn John WALSH

The Riverside Practice
40 Burrowmoor Road, March PE15 9RP
Tel: 01354 661922 Fax: 01354 650926
Email: www.ley@freeserve.co.uk
(East Cambridgeshire and Fenland Primary Care Trust)
Patient List Size: 5680

Practice Manager June Garford

GP Martyn Geoffry THOMAS, Christopher Charles LEY

Margate

Cecil Square Surgery
1 Cecil Square, Margate CT9 1BD
Tel: 01843 232222 Fax: 01843 232205
(East Kent Coastal Teaching Primary Care Trust)

Practice Manager D A Jarvis

GP Tariq Akhtar RAHMAN

Cliftonville Surgery
5 Cliftonville Avenue, Margate CT9 2AL
Tel: 01843 292873
(East Kent Coastal Teaching Primary Care Trust)

Practice Manager M Kazmie

GP M. KAZMIE

Cornwall Gardens Surgery
77 Cornwall Gardens, Cliftonville, Margate CT9 2JF
Tel: 01843 209300 Fax: 01843 209301
(East Kent Coastal Teaching Primary Care Trust)
Patient List Size: 12700

Practice Manager Lynn Shaw

GP David Edward Ferguson TUMATH, Graham John Aston JOY, Stephen Hunter LILLICRAP, Tony Stuart MARTIN, Gregory James ROGERS, Heather Wynne SCOTT, Richard Alexander SCOTT

Garlinge Surgery
Westbrook Centre, 150 Canterbury Road, Margate CT9 5DD
Tel: 01843 255693 Fax: 01843 255695
(East Kent Coastal Teaching Primary Care Trust)

Practice Manager Wendy Blake

GP Z MYINT

Northdown Surgery
St Anthony's Way, Cliftonville, Margate CT9 2TR
Tel: 01843 296413 Fax: 01843 231231
(East Kent Coastal Teaching Primary Care Trust)
Patient List Size: 10500

Practice Manager Jennifer Cartier

GP Jeffrey Eric RYDER, Dr BRAGA, Dr GEEVARGHESE, John Derek HEATHER, Jonathan Norton Deane LANGWORTHY, Clive Munro MARTIN

The Surgery
The Limes Medical Centre, Trinity Square, Margate CT9 1QY
Tel: 01843 227567 Fax: 01843 222720
(East Kent Coastal Teaching Primary Care Trust)
Patient List Size: 8100

Practice Manager Julie Sandum

GP Brian John SUMMERFIELD, Oak Soe KHA, Hugh McCAFFREY

Union Row Surgery
Union Row, Margate CT9 1PP
Tel: 01843 296980 Fax: 01843 280188
(East Kent Coastal Teaching Primary Care Trust)

GP S HENRY

Market Drayton

Ashley Surgery
School Lane, Ashley, Market Drayton TF9 4LF
Tel: 01630 672225 Fax: 01630 673863
(Newcastle-under-Lyme Primary Care Trust)

Practice Manager Nicky Adams

GP Richard James ADAMS

Drayton Medical Practice
Cheshire Street, Market Drayton TF9 3BS
Tel: 01630 652158
(Shropshire County Primary Care Trust)

GP Robert Alan HARES, Anthony James Thomas WILSON

Drayton Medical Practices
The Health Centre, Cheshire Street, Market Drayton TF9 3BS
Fax: 01630 652322
(Shropshire County Primary Care Trust)
Patient List Size: 16000

Practice Manager Dawn Jones

GP Robert Alan HARES, Colin Gerald BATES, Grahame Philip COLEMAN, Charlotte Jessop GREEN, Michael Robert MATTHEE, Robert William RICHARDS, Sally Louise RODGE, Anthony James WILSON, Robin Gaythorn Bramma WOOD

Hodnet Medical Centre
18 Drayton Road, Hodnet, Market Drayton TF9 3NF
Tel: 01630 685230 Fax: 01630 685770
(Shropshire County Primary Care Trust)

GP N RAICHURA, S MEHTA

Vicarage Surgery
Old Vicarage, Cheswardine, Market Drayton TF9 2RN
Tel: 01630 661650
(Shropshire County Primary Care Trust)

GP Naresh RAICHURA

Market Harborough

Market Harborough Medical Centre
67 Coventry Road, Market Harborough LE16 9BX
Tel: 01858 464242 Fax: 01858 462929
(Melton, Rutland and Harborough Primary Care Trust)
Patient List Size: 23789

Practice Manager A P Bagot-Moore

GP Anthony Paul BENNETT, Fiona Mary BISHOP, Thomas Michael BLAKE, Jonathan Mark Golland CROWLEY, Hugh James DELARGY, Phil HEALEY, Nicholas Terence LEACH, Hamant Kumar MISTRY, B A WILLIAMS, Mark YATES

Market Rasen

Binbrook Surgery
Back Lane, Binbrook, Market Rasen LN8 6ED
Tel: 01472 398202 Fax: 01472 398795
(East Lincolnshire Primary Care Trust)
Patient List Size: 2525

Practice Manager Trish Bee

GP David Michael BEE

Dale View Health Centre
Dale View, Caistor, Market Rasen LN7 6NX
Tel: 01472 851203 Fax: 01472 852495
(West Lincolnshire Primary Care Trust)
Patient List Size: 4800

Practice Manager Judith Neal

GP Geoffrey Campbell WOOD, Catherine BACKHOUSE, David Michael McKINLAY

Mill Road Surgery
Mill Road, Market Rasen LN8 3BP
Tel: 01673 843556 Fax: 01673 844388
(West Lincolnshire Primary Care Trust)
Patient List Size: 8650

Practice Manager Rachael Simpson

GP Michael Ronald EAMES, Margaret HORNS, Therese MAXWELL, James Robert TELFER, Robert Victor WEEKS

Wragby Surgery
Old Grammar School Way, Wragby, Market Rasen LN8 5DA
Tel: 01673 858206 Fax: 01673 857622
(East Lincolnshire Primary Care Trust)
Patient List Size: 3053

Practice Manager Jan Swinton

GP Rhoderick Peter WHITBREAD, M RHODES, David Ian Andrew SMITH

Markfield

Markfield Surgery
The Green, Markfield LE67 9WU
Tel: 01530 242313 Fax: 01530 245668
(Charnwood and North West Leicestershire Primary Care Trust)

Practice Manager Diane Thompson

GP Elizabeth Suzanne EATON, Helen Dawn FERNANDEZ, Thomas Robert HAILSTONE, Christopher John TRZCINSKI

Marlborough

Marlborough Medical Practice
The Surgery, George Lane, Marlborough SN8 4BY
Tel: 01672 512187 Fax: 01672 516809
(Kennet and North Wiltshire Primary Care Trust)
Patient List Size: 11900

Practice Manager Michael Reynolds

GP Jonathan GLOVER, Sally Marguerite HANSON, Richard William HOOK, David Pierce MAURICE, Ralph ROSALIE, Pamela Mary Buchanan TULLOCH, John Henry WILLIAMS, Deborah Margaret YEARSLEY

The Old School Surgery
Church Street, Great Bedwyn, Marlborough SN8 3PF
Tel: 01672 870388 Fax: 01672 870664
(Kennet and North Wiltshire Primary Care Trust)
Patient List Size: 2700

Practice Manager Keith Marshall

GP Timothy Harold BALLARD

Ramsbury Surgery
High Street, Ramsbury, Marlborough SN8 2QT
Tel: 01672 520366 Fax: 01672 520180
(Kennet and North Wiltshire Primary Care Trust)
Patient List Size: 8000

Practice Manager A C Flesher

GP Rodney James Ferguson OWEN-JONES, Graham Stephen MULLER, Jonathan Machan Hockin RAYNER, Rosemary SYMON, Rachel Zoe WARDLEY

Sprays Surgery
9 The Sprays, Burbage, Marlborough SN8 3TA
Tel: 01672 810566 Fax: 01672 811329
(Kennet and North Wiltshire Primary Care Trust)
Patient List Size: 2400

GP Trevor John KING

Marlow

The Doctors House
Victoria Road, Marlow SL7 1DN
Tel: 01628 484666 Fax: 01628 891206
(Chiltern and South Bucks Primary Care Trust)

Practice Manager Sue Wale

GP James Meynell Ingram HAYTER, Roger Hyde MOSTON, Vivien Margaret BURGESS, Anne Margaret GALVIN, Andrew Michael Birkby HOBBS, Thomas James MORROW, Christopher Ivan NORTH, John Patrick Gerard SWIETOCHOWSKI, Elizabeth Clare VINCENT, Hilary Margaret WALSH, Helen Francis WILLSDON

Martock

Church Street Surgery
Church Street, Martock TA12 6JL
Tel: 01935 822541 Fax: 01935 826116
(South Somerset Primary Care Trust)
Patient List Size: 11000

Practice Manager John Hayes

GP James Richard BUCKLE, Alistair David McLennan BARCLAY, John Keith BEATTIE, Adrian Read BRIDGE, Julie Mildred CAMSEY, Andrew John McMullan QUAYLE

Maryport

Maryport Group Practice
Alneburgh House, Ewanrigg Road, Maryport CA15 8EL
Tel: 01900 815544 Fax: 01900 816626
Email: maryportgrouppractice@gp-A82032.nhs.uk
(West Cumbria Primary Care Trust)
Patient List Size: 13800

Practice Manager Sarah Cousins

GP Terence McQueen COLLINS, Fayyaz Latif CHAUDHRI, Jonathan David Clayden GROVE, Josephine HEWSON, Brian Ironside MONEY, Andrea MULGREW, Alison Jane OVEREND, Keith Michael Aldren SLINGER, George Mark STEEL

Matlock

Crich Medical Practice
Bulling Lane, Crich, Matlock DE4 5DX
Tel: 01773 852966 Fax: 01773 853919
(Amber Valley Primary Care Trust)
Patient List Size: 7200

Practice Manager Sheila Jones

GP Malcolm Gordon WARD, Alexandra Marian KNIGHT, B MORLAND, C E M SHEARER, Robert Ian SMALLMAN

The Darley Dale Medical Centre
Two Dales, Darley Dale, Matlock DE4 3FD
Tel: 01629 734277
(High Peak and Dales Primary Care Trust)
Patient List Size: 7400

Practice Manager Horton S

GP D C PICKWORTH, David M CLARK, Ben C MILTON, David C PICKWORTH, Jonathan P SMITH

Hannage Brook Medical Centre
Hannage Way, Wirksworth, Matlock DE4 4DZ
Tel: 01629 822434 Fax: 01629 821788
(Derbyshire Dales and South Derbyshire Primary Care Trust)
Patient List Size: 8048

Practice Manager Stephen Hewitt

GP Jill RAPOPORT

Imperial Road Surgery
8 Imperial Road, Matlock DE4 3NL
Tel: 01629 583249
(High Peak and Dales Primary Care Trust)

GP James Falkland MACFARLANE, Carole Ann CHAMBERLAIN, Ralph Colin EMMERSON, Peter John Pashley HOLDEN, Anthony David SINNOTT

Lime Grove Medical Centre
Lime Grove Walk, Matlock DE4 3FD
Tel: 01629 583223
(High Peak and Dales Primary Care Trust)

GP Paul Sheldon LINGARD, James Thomas BATHGATE

Lime Grove Medical Centre
Lime Grove Walk, Matlock DE4 3FD
Tel: 01629 582241
(High Peak and Dales Primary Care Trust)

GP Rodney Allan Parry CURTIS

Wirksworth Centre
St John's Street, Wirksworth, Matlock DE4 4DT
(Derbyshire Dales and South Derbyshire Primary Care Trust)

Mayfield

Woodhill Surgery
Station Road, Mayfield TN20 6BW
Tel: 01435 873000 Fax: 01435 873807
(Sussex Downs and Weald Primary Care Trust)
Patient List Size: 3200

Practice Manager J Smith

GP A COATES

Melksham

Giffords Primary Care Centre
Spa Road, Melksham SN12 7EA
Tel: 01225 703370 Fax: 01225 898200
(West Wiltshire Primary Care Trust)
Patient List Size: 15800

Practice Manager Sharan White

GP Richard Martin KAHANE, Maeve Ann DUIGNAN, Rowena Mary EAST, Mark HARRISON-SMITH, James HILL, Peter James PHILLIPS, Sally Anne ROSSER

Spa Surgery
6 Spa Road, Melksham SN12 7NS
Tel: 01225 703236
(West Wiltshire Primary Care Trust)

GP Jeremy Paul SIMMONS, Rupert James GABRIEL, Robert John MATTHEWS, D M THOMAS

St Damiens Surgery
1 Place Road, Melksham SN12 6JN
Tel: 01225 791212
(West Wiltshire Primary Care Trust)

Practice Manager Clare Hardie

GP Robert Alastair HARDIE, Susan Margaret FRANKLAND

Melton Mowbray

Latham House Medical Practice
Latham House, Sage Cross Street, Melton Mowbray LE13 1NX
Tel: 01664 854949 Fax: 01664 501825
(Melton, Rutland and Harborough Primary Care Trust)
Patient List Size: 34500

Practice Manager Alison Hipkin

GP Ronald James THEW, David Arthur BARROW, Dean Perry BENNISON, David Maurice BRIGGS, Darach Joseph CORVIN, Jessie Louise HARRIS, John Michael HARVEY, Geetisha HIRANI, Sacheen HIRANI, Brian KIRKUP, Elizabeth Ann LOUGHRIDGE, Diane Margaret LOVETT, Peter RILEY, Paul Gerard SLEVIN, Timothy Donald Weston

SMITH, Igone Pena UGARTE, Mary Fiona Ming Chi WONG, Thomas Andrew WYATT

Long Clawson Medical Practice
The Surgery, The Sands, Long Clawson, Melton Mowbray LE14 4PA
Tel: 01664 822214/5 Fax: 01664 823486
(Melton, Rutland and Harborough Primary Care Trust)
Patient List Size: 5200

Practice Manager Cherry Lawrence

GP Amanda Joy GALLOP, Philip Sean RATHBONE, Simon Charles WOODING

Somerby Surgery
53 High Street, Somerby, Melton Mowbray LE14 2PZ
Tel: 01664 454204 Fax: 01664 454879
(Melton, Rutland and Harborough Primary Care Trust)
Patient List Size: 1100

Practice Manager G Pearson

GP J FENBY-TAYLOR, H REES

Mexborough

Crown Street Surgery
17 Crown Street, Swinton, Mexborough S64 8NB
Tel: 0845 122 1665
(Rotherham Primary Care Trust)

Practice Manager J France

GP Garry CHAMBERS, Ian M TURNER, Malcolm VENABLES, Clive Bernard WALLIS

Health Centre
Adwick Road, Mexborough S64 0BY
Tel: 01709 590590 Fax: 01709 578166
(Doncaster West Primary Care Trust)
Patient List Size: 7220

Practice Manager Liz Dawson

GP D L AGRAWAL, P KIRUPANANTH, A T R KRISHNA RAO, V NAGARAJ

Health Centre
Adwick Road, Mexborough S64 0BY
Tel: 01709 590231 Fax: 01709 577376
(Doncaster West Primary Care Trust)

The New Surgery
Health Centre, Adwick Road, Mexborough S64 0BY
Tel: 01709 590707 Fax: 01709 511800
(Doncaster West Primary Care Trust)

Practice Manager D Gillott

GP Molly Christine LEACH, V V SASTRY

Middlesbrough

Albert House Clinic
101 Normanby Road, South Bank, Middlesbrough TS6 6SE
Tel: 01642 453049 Fax: 01642 464343
(Middlesbrough Primary Care Trust)

Practice Manager Marilyn Barrett

GP Krishna Prasad BHANDARY, R N BATTACHARYYA, Shaukat Akberally MAMUJEE

Borough Road and Nunthorpe Medical Group
167a Borough Road, Middlesbrough TS1 3RY
Tel: 01642 243668 Fax: 01642 222252
Email: helen.bell@nhs.net
(Middlesbrough Primary Care Trust)
Patient List Size: 11800

Practice Manager Helen Bell

GP John Michael LAKEMAN, Mandy Jane BROWNLEE, Helena Mary Frances CONNOLLY, John Richard GELDART, Fiona Joy HOULDSWORTH, Nicholas John JACOTT, Edward Michael SELBY

The Cambridge Medical Group
10A Cambridge Road, Linthorpe, Middlesbrough TS5 5NN
Tel: 01642 851177 Fax: 01642 851176
(Middlesbrough Primary Care Trust)
Patient List Size: 7600

Practice Manager Alan Jackson

GP Dennis William HERBERT, Christopher DITCHBURN, Andrew PHELLAS, James Douglas Alexander ROBERTSON

Coulby Medical Practice
Cropton Way, Coulby Newham, Middlesbrough TS8 0TL
Tel: 01642 590500 Fax: 01642 579049
(Middlesbrough Primary Care Trust)

Practice Manager Jenny Eggett

GP Philip John INCH, Stewart CHILTON, Stephen Norman GOWLAND, Heather Caroline WETHERELL, Catherine Jane WILLIAMSON

Crossfell Health Centre
Berwick Hills, Middlesbrough TS3 7RL
Tel: 01642 296777 Fax: 01642 296851
(Middlesbrough Primary Care Trust)

Practice Manager Gillian Nodding

GP Margaret Vicki NATH, Nicky MAYES, P T McCARTHY, Yamuna MUDDAPPA, Enrique PERON

Great Ayton Health Centre
Rosehill, Great Ayton, Middlesbrough TS9 6BL
Tel: 01642 723421 Fax: 01642 724575
Email: health@great-ayton.org
Website: www.great-ayton.org
(Hambleton and Richmondshire Primary Care Trust)
Patient List Size: 5500

Practice Manager Ann Howard

GP John Leslie DAVIES, Brian BLACKLIDGE, Peter Andrew GREEN

The Health Centre
20 Cleveland Square, Middlesbrough TS1 2NX
Tel: 01642 246138 Fax: 01642 222291
(Middlesbrough Primary Care Trust)
Patient List Size: 7200

Practice Manager Barbara Gannon

GP Jeremiah George MURPHY, Helen Boswell BURKE, Elizabeth Mary CHAPPELOW, John Charles DOLAN, Anne Margaret HARRISON

The Health Centre
20 Cleveland Square, Middlesbrough TS1 2NX
Tel: 01642 242746 Fax: 01642 220766
(Middlesbrough Primary Care Trust)
Patient List Size: 8800

Practice Manager S A Binks

GP Satish KHAIR, F D AL-KHABASS, K SANDRASEGARAN

The Health Centre
20 Cleveland Square, Middlesbrough TS1 2NX
Tel: 01642 245069 Fax: 01642 230388
(Middlesbrough Primary Care Trust)

GP P GEISER, Stephen William McILHINNEY, Anne Mary TOWNEND, Jane Fulton McIlwaine WASSON

The Health Centre
North Road, Stokesley, Middlesbrough TS9 5DY
Tel: 01642 710748 Fax: 01642 713037
Email: doctors@stokeleyhc.freeserve.co.uk
(Hambleton and Richmondshire Primary Care Trust)
Patient List Size: 9450

Practice Manager Paul Siddons

GP Michael Huntley FAULKNER, Michaela Elisabeth AMANN, Mark Robert DUGGLEBY, George Edwin PARK, Stephen Barclay TAWSE

The Health Centre
PO Box 101(a), The Health Centre, 20 Cleveland Square, Middlesbrough TS1 2NX
Tel: 01642 242192 Fax: 01642 231809
(Middlesbrough Primary Care Trust)
Patient List Size: 7000

Practice Manager Jackie Landells

GP Teresa Agnes FOSTER, John Timothy CANNING, Janice Irene KIBIRIGE, Melanie Anne MALDEN, Nigel Timothy ROWELL

Hirsel Medical Centre
58a Kings Road, North Ormesby, Middlesbrough TS3 6EG
Tel: 01642 242880 Fax: 01642 251494
(Middlesbrough Primary Care Trust)

Practice Manager Sue Carter

GP J MUKHERJEE, M MUKHERJEE, R K MUKHOPADYAY

Kings Road Medical Centre
73 Kings Road, North Ormesby, Middlesbrough TS3 6HA
Tel: 01642 244766/ 631033 Fax: 01642 246243
(Middlesbrough Primary Care Trust)
Patient List Size: 5500

Practice Manager Marlene Allick

GP Ramesh Chander PRASAD, Sangeeta SHAH

Linthorpe Road Surgery
378 Linthorpe Road, Middlesbrough TS5 6HA
Tel: 01642 817166 Fax: 01642 824094
Website: www.linthorpesurgery.com
Patient List Size: 13500

Practice Manager T Garbutt

GP John BLAKEY, Tony CHAHAL, Paul Edward ELLENGER, Penny NEWMAN, Raj PANDEY, Mark PETTIT, Anne Jacqueline PHELLAS, John Richard WOOD

Manor House Surgery
Braidwood Road, Normanby, Middlesbrough TS6 0HA
Tel: 01642 453338 Fax: 01642 468915
Email: christopher.mckeown@gp-A81043.nhs.uk
(Middlesbrough Primary Care Trust)
Patient List Size: 8000

Practice Manager Helen Price

GP Christopher Owen McKEOWN, Richard John BARKER, J MULGREW, David Mark St John ROYAL, Janet Elizabeth WALKER

Martonside Medical Centre
1a Martonside Way, Middlesbrough TS4 3BU
Tel: 01642 812266 Fax: 01642 828722
(Middlesbrough Primary Care Trust)
Patient List Size: 8000

GP H R BARTON, John Edwin BOOTH, D T DONOVAN, S T MORENO, Roger John WHEELER

Newlands Medical Centre
Borough Road, Middlesbrough TS4 2EJ
Tel: 01642 247029 Fax: 01642 223803
Website: www.shpal.mcmail.com
(Middlesbrough Primary Care Trust)

Practice Manager Collette Shipley

GP Stephen Hunter PALCZYNSKI, Anthony Ronald John BOGGIS, Charles Stanley CORNFORD, Lawrence Edward DUNN, Jennifer Mary DYCKHOFF, Jacqueline GRAINGER, George HARGATE, Susan WHITE

Normanby Road Surgery
502-508 Normanby Road, Normanby, Middlesbrough TS6 9BZ
Tel: 01642 452727/440501 Fax: 01642 466723
(Middlesbrough Primary Care Trust)

Practice Manager F Craven, T Laughton

GP Iftikhar Ahmed LONE, R N BLYTH, Alan DUNNING, Susan Barbara JONES, Ajai MAJUPURIA

Oakfield Road Surgery
1 Oakfield Road, North Ormesby, Middlesbrough TS3 6EZ
Tel: 01642 244990 Fax: 01642 248714
(Middlesbrough Primary Care Trust)

GP Bhupinder Singh CHAUDHRY, Nicola Jacqueline MAYES, B K MITRA

Park Surgery
2 Park Road North, Middlesbrough TS1 3LF
Tel: 01642 247008 Fax: 01642 245748
Email: parksurgery@lineone.net
(Middlesbrough Primary Care Trust)
Patient List Size: 9500

Practice Manager Stephen Doyle

GP I S BASSON, Ignacio GARCIA, Gillian HODGSON, M W LAU, Mohammed SHAFIQ, Richard SMITH

Parkway Medical Centre
Cropton Way, Coulby Newham, Middlesbrough TS8 0TL
Tel: 01642 270033 Fax: 01642 270055
(Middlesbrough Primary Care Trust)
Patient List Size: 3900

Practice Manager Christine Savill

GP William James BEEBY, Dr GARCIA, Dr TOLLES

Queens Court Surgery
7 Harris Street, Middlesbrough TS1 5EF
Tel: 01642 253234 Fax: 01634 246737
(Middlesbrough Primary Care Trust)

GP S S KHAIR

South Grange Medical Centre
Trunk Road, Eston, Middlesbrough TS6 9QG
Tel: 01642 467001 Fax: 01642 463334
(Middlesbrough Primary Care Trust)

Practice Manager Gwenda Kyte-Powell

GP Narayan Ram JOSHI, Dilip Basant ACQUILLA, R KHATUN, Hanif MOHAMMED, Shafquth RASOOL

The Surgery
10-12 Jubilee Road, Eston, Middlesbrough TS6 9ER
Tel: 01642 455524 Fax: 01642 454883
(Middlesbrough Primary Care Trust)

GP Chris MOLL, Nigel James ROBSON

Thorntree Surgery
11 Beresford Buildings, Thorntree, Middlesbrough TS3 9NB
Tel: 01642 248127 Fax: 01642 248261
(Middlesbrough Primary Care Trust)
Patient List Size: 2285

GP I S BASSON, M W LAU, R SMITH

Village Medical Centre
400-404 Linthorpe Road, Middlesbrough TS5 6HF
Tel: 01642 851234 Fax: 01642 820821
(Middlesbrough Primary Care Trust)
Patient List Size: 11000

Practice Manager T A Doyle, T Laughton

GP Henry John WATERS, Brian Patrick CORBETT, Marion Jill HOWITT, Helen LAND, Kiran SINGH

Woodlands Road Surgery
6 Woodlands Road, Middlesbrough TS1 3BG
Tel: 01642 247982 Fax: 01642 241636
(Middlesbrough Primary Care Trust)

GP Howard LEIGH, Christopher Thomas ANKCORN, Robert HANDYSIDE, Richard Stewart MURPHY, William Gary SCOTT

Middlewich

The Acorns Surgery
85 Wheelock Street, Middlewich CW10 9AE
Tel: 01606 837400 Fax: 01606 837500
(Central Cheshire Primary Care Trust)
Patient List Size: 4467

Practice Manager Paula Costello

GP Peter George CURBISHLEY, Jerome CONRAD, Kathryn E TEBAY

Oaklands
Middlewich Medical Centre, St. Anns Walk, Middlewich CW10 9BE
Tel: 01606 836481 Fax: 01606 834828
(Central Cheshire Primary Care Trust)
Patient List Size: 10061

Practice Manager Lorraine Carter

GP Martin Richard CLIFTON, John Alexander CROFTS, Deborah Louise FORD, Janice Elizabeth GILMOUR, S HYDER, T JOHNSON

Midhurst

Riverbank Medical Centre
Dodsley Lane, Midhurst GU29 9AW
Tel: 01730 812121 Fax: 01730 811400
(Western Sussex Primary Care Trust)
Patient List Size: 12000

GP Alexander Gordon MacCALLUM, Richard EDWARDS, Paul FLUDDER, Rowena HILL, Timothy John HILL, Sue MacCALLUM, Lorena RODRIGUEZ

Millom

Waterloo House Surgery
Waterloo House, 42-44 Wellington Street, Millom LA18 4DE
Tel: 01229 772123 Fax: 01229 771300
(Charnwood and North West Leicestershire Primary Care Trust)

Practice Manager Denise Cloudsdale

GP Elizabeth Ann JOHNSON, Graham Philip POGREL, Paul Anthony PATCHETT, Richard Charles Michael WALKER, Philip John WALTERS

Milnthorpe

Park View Surgery
Haverflatts Lane, Milnthorpe LA7 7PS
Tel: 01539 563327 Fax: 01539 564059
(Morecambe Bay Primary Care Trust)
Patient List Size: 5400

GP Judith Ann IRVING, Jim HACKING, Jon RYLANCE, Julia SMITH

Stoneleigh Surgery
Police Square, Milnthorpe LA7 7PW
Tel: 01539 563307 Fax: 01539 562005
(Morecambe Bay Primary Care Trust)

Practice Manager A Cookson

GP Michael Robert WARREN, Carl Terence DARBY, John Hippolyte GORRIGAN, Elaine Janet PEARSON, Sarah J THORNTON

Milton Keynes

Asplands Medical Centre
Apslands Close, Woburn Sands, Milton Keynes MK17 8QP
Tel: 01908 582069 Fax: 01908 281597
(Bedfordshire Heartlands Primary Care Trust)
Patient List Size: 10600

Practice Manager Robert Squair

GP John LOGAN, Fiona ANDERSON, John MUIR, James NOTT, Madeline ROGERS

Central Milton Keynes Medical
1 North Sixth Street, Saxon Gate West, Milton Keynes MK9 2NR
Tel: 01908 605775 Fax: 01908 295657
(Milton Keynes Primary Care Trust)
Patient List Size: 10200

Practice Manager Alyson Taylor

GP Adrian John PRISK, Shahid AMIN, Emma Frances HUISH, Stephen NORMAN, Susan Margaret WEATHERHEAD, Jolly ZACHARIAH

Drayton Road Surgery
20 Drayton Road, Bletchley, Milton Keynes MK2 3EJ
Tel: 01908 371481 Fax: 01908 378700
(Milton Keynes Primary Care Trust)

Practice Manager Jo Smekens

GP Prababhar KUSRE, Qamar Ali KHAN

Eaglestone Health Centre
Standing Way, Eaglestone, Milton Keynes MK6 5AZ
Tel: 01908 679111 Fax: 01908 230601
(Milton Keynes Primary Care Trust)
Patient List Size: 11673

Practice Manager Ann Hurry

GP Anwar YAHYA, Michael Patrick CASSIDY, Hamdy Hussein HILMY, Manatosh ROY, Abdulrahim SULEMAN, Arshad WAHEED

Fishermead Medical Centre
Fishermead Boulevard, Fishermead, Milton Keynes MK6 2LR
Tel: 01908 609240 Fax: 01908 695674
(Milton Keynes Primary Care Trust)

Practice Manager Christine Smith

GP Arnold Bernard BERGER, Mokshad Harilaz KANSGRA, Aye Aye (Lily) WIN

Ganguli
Wolverton Health Centre, Gloucester Road, Wolverton, Milton Keynes MK12 5DF
Tel: 01908 317825
(Milton Keynes Primary Care Trust)

Practice Manager Margaret J Short

GP Satyabrata GANGULI

Grafton Medical Centre
208A-208B North Row, Buckingham Square, Central Milton Keynes, Milton Keynes MK9 3LQ
Tel: 01908 695070 Fax: 01908 694911
(Milton Keynes Primary Care Trust)
Patient List Size: 2900

Practice Manager Mary Welsh

GP Leonard Ian Michael Cameron McILWAIN, Dr NICOLAOU

The Grove Surgery
Farthing Grove, Netherfield, Milton Keynes MK6 4NG
Tel: 01908 668453 Fax: 01908 695064
(Milton Keynes Primary Care Trust)

Practice Manager Sue Dixon

GP Stephen Simon ANAMAN, Asha SHARMA

Hanslope Surgery
1 Western Drive, Hanslope, Milton Keynes MK19 7LA
Tel: 01908 510230
(Daventry and South Northamptonshire Primary Care Trust)

GP Dr SUTTON

Hilltops Medical Centre
Kensington Drive, Great Holm, Milton Keynes MK8 9HN
Tel: 01908 568446
(Milton Keynes Primary Care Trust)

GP Anthony WATSON, Adeline AFONG, Mohamed Raza Merali DEWJI, Sophie ELLIS, Bryony Anne HILDICK-SMITH, Andrea Helen KINGSTON, Bipin PATEL, Maria TANG

Milton Keynes Village Practice

Griffith Gate, Middleton, Milton Keynes MK10 9BQ
Tel: 01908 393979 Fax: 01908 393774
Email: enquiries@mkvillagepractice.co.uk
Website: www.mkvillagepractice.co.uk
(Milton Keynes Primary Care Trust)

Practice Manager Deb Williams

GP Eric ROSE, Darren MOORE

Neath Hill Health Cente

1 Tower Crescent, Neath Hill, Milton Keynes MK14 6JY
Tel: 01908 663300
(Milton Keynes Primary Care Trust)

Practice Manager Denise Moreton

GP Mulukutla PRASAD

Parkside Medical Centre

Whalley Drive, Bletchley, Milton Keynes MK3 6EN
Tel: 01908 375341 Fax: 01908 374975
(Milton Keynes Primary Care Trust)
Patient List Size: 9750

Practice Manager Bryan Steiner

GP Allan ALLSOPP, Martin CAVE, Paul Conrad MINNEY, Melanie Fiona MUNRO, Nicola Lisbeth SMITH

Patel and Partners

4 Bedford Street, Bletchley, Milton Keynes MK2 2TX
Tel: 01908 377101 Fax: 01908 645903
(Milton Keynes Primary Care Trust)
Patient List Size: 11300

Practice Manager Christine Zscherpel

GP Bhaskerrai PATEL, Motaz GASHI, Rameshchandra Harmanbhai PATEL, Sarah STRANKS, Hadayat ULLAH

Purbeck Health Centre

Purbeck, Stantonbury, Milton Keynes MK14 6BL
Tel: 01908 318989 Fax: 01908 319493
(Milton Keynes Primary Care Trust)
Patient List Size: 7500

Practice Manager Harry Willcox

GP Joy Matthew THALAKOTTUR, Paul IYAMABO, Victor OKUZU

The Red House Surgery

241 Queensway, Bletchley, Milton Keynes MK2 2EH
Tel: 01908 375111 Fax: 01908 370977
Email: jane.hanlon@mkpct.nhs.uk
(Milton Keynes Primary Care Trust)

Practice Manager Jane Hanlon

GP Nigel George BUNTING, Janet Chessher EWART, Nigel Anthony FAGAN, Janet Christine GOODMAN, Paul STATEN

Sovereign Medical Centre

Sovereign Drive, Pennyland, Milton Keynes MK15 8AJ
Tel: 01908 661166 Fax: 01908 233921
(Milton Keynes Primary Care Trust)

Practice Manager Rosemary Smith

GP Samuel MUTHUVELOE, Ahmed Zafar NASIRI, Margaret OWOLABI, Gregory WILLIAMS

Stantonbury Health Centre

Purbeck, Stantonbury, Milton Keynes MK14 6BL
Tel: 01908 316262 Fax: 01908 221432
(Milton Keynes Primary Care Trust)
Patient List Size: 8600

Practice Manager Steve Pratt

GP Prabha KHURANA, Mohammed AHAD, Muttucumarasamy MAHENDRAN, Vatrapu Laxmi Narayana REDDY, Arun Dev SHARDA

Stonedean Practice

Health Centre, Market Square, Stony Stratford, Milton Keynes MK11 1YA
Tel: 01908 261155
(Milton Keynes Primary Care Trust)

Practice Manager J H Bradley

GP Julian Henry BRADLEY, Neil DOUSE

Stony Stratford Health Centre

Market Square, Stony Stratford, Milton Keynes MK11 1YA
Tel: 01908 565555 Fax: 01908 575815
(Milton Keynes Primary Care Trust)

Practice Manager P A Thurling

GP Kenneth Henry CHAMBERS, Michael John BRAMLEY, Lara Ann GRIMES, Sarah Ann GRINYER, Christina Mary KENNY, Julian Charles Gordon LAMBLEY, Peter David MILES

Walnut Tree Health Centre

Blackberry Court, Walnut Tree, Milton Keynes MK7 7NR
Tel: 01908 691123 Fax: 01908 691120
(Milton Keynes Primary Care Trust)
Patient List Size: 10000

Practice Manager Penny Giraudeau

GP Elizabeth Ann HOWARD, Sue BAXTER, Cathy BRUCE, Nessan CARSON, Dorothy Josephine MORRISON, Keith THOMAS

Water Eaton Health Centre

Fern Grove, Bletchley, Milton Keynes MK2 3HN
Tel: 01908 371318 Fax: 01908 643843
(Milton Keynes Primary Care Trust)
Patient List Size: 5700

Practice Manager Sharon Rust

GP Arvindchandra Velji KARIA, Islar p KAWJEE, Mira SINGH

Watling Vale Medical Centre

Burchard Crescent, Shenley Church End, Milton Keynes MK5 6EY
Tel: 01908 501177 Fax: 01908 504916
(Milton Keynes Primary Care Trust)

GP Peter Laurence BERKIN, Susan CORBISHLGY, Maxine EDWARDSON, John Slippe QUARTEY, Margaret Elizabeth WYKE

Westcroft Health Centre

1 Savil Lane, Westcroft, Milton Keynes MK4 4EN
Tel: 01908 520545 Fax: 01908 520975
Email: westcrofthc@aol.com
Website: www.westcrofthealthcentre.com
(Milton Keynes Primary Care Trust)
Patient List Size: 6000

GP Rowena Antoinette LIESCHING, Jawad AHMAD, J MALIK

Westfield Road Surgery

11 Westfield Road, Bletchley, Milton Keynes MK2 2DJ
Tel: 01908 377103 Fax: 01908 374427
(Milton Keynes Primary Care Trust)
Patient List Size: 5370

Practice Manager Sandra White

GP Richard Gordon HO-YEN, Sarah Anne GRINYER, Stephan Gerrard JOHANNES

Whaddon House Surgery

221 Whaddon Way, Bletchley, Milton Keynes MK3 7EA
Tel: 01908 373058 Fax: 01908 630076
(Milton Keynes Primary Care Trust)
Patient List Size: 10500

Practice Manager John Parnell

GP John Christopher PHILBIN, Hopeson ALIFOE, Christine Jane BRADLEY, Pauline Margaret Mary CLERKIN, Naguib Mounir Halim HILMY, Tahmina SIDDIQUI

Willen Village Surgery

Beaufort Drive, Willen, Milton Keynes MK15 9ET
Tel: 01908 230888 Fax: 01908 230885
(Milton Keynes Primary Care Trust)

Practice Manager Lisa Judd

GP Ronald Charles CARTER, Agnela LOBB

Wolverton Health Centre
Gloucester Road, Wolverton, Milton Keynes MK12 5DF
Tel: 01908 316633 Fax: 01908 225397
(Milton Keynes Primary Care Trust)
Patient List Size: 13500

Practice Manager Elizabeth J McMillan

GP Satya MURTHY, S BANNERJEE, S GUPTA, Ganeschandra HALDAR, Barbara Anne KING, S MUSHTAQ, Nathalal ODEDRA, P SEN

Minehead

Harley House Surgery
2 Irnham Road, Minehead TA24 5DL
Tel: 01643 703441 Fax: 01643 704867
Email: hhsurg@globalnet.co.uk
Website: www.harleyhouse.nhs.uk
(Somerset Coast Primary Care Trust)
Patient List Size: 7074

Practice Manager Lesley Struck

GP Alan Rache NELSON, John Morris Munro HIGGIE, Philippa Susan NEVILLE, John Gerald O'DOWD, Simon Sebastian VALE

Irnham Lodge Surgery
Townsend Road, Minehead TA24 5RG
Tel: 01643 703289 Fax: 01643 707921
Email: kate.atkins@irnhamlodge.nhs.uk
Website: www.irnhamlodgesurgery.nhs.uk
(Somerset Coast Primary Care Trust)
Patient List Size: 6700

Practice Manager Kate Atkins

GP Paul Jonathan Baker SLADE, Jonathan Mark DRISCOLL, T E GRONOW, C L NETTLETON, Huw Gerwyn THOMAS

Porlock Medical Centre
The Old Tannery, High Street, Porlock, Minehead TA24 8PJ
Tel: 01643 862575 Fax: 01643 862571
Email: portlock@globalnet.co.uk
(Somerset Coast Primary Care Trust)
Patient List Size: 1680

Practice Manager G Langley

GP Ian KELHAM

The Surgery
3 Park Street, Dunster, Minehead TA24 6SR
Tel: 01643 821244 Fax: 01643 821770
(Somerset Coast Primary Care Trust)
Patient List Size: 2200

Practice Manager Katheen Marshall

GP Michael Alastair CURRIE, Anne Louise CURRIE

Mirfield

The Health Centre
Doctor Lane, Mirfield WF14 8DU
Tel: 01924 495721 Fax: 01924 480605
Website: www.mirfieldhealthcentre.co.uk
(North Kirklees Primary Care Trust)
Patient List Size: 17500

Practice Manager P Auty

GP Roger PARKER, Michael Ronald BEDFORD, Elizabeth Sara EABRY, Howard Graeme GRASON, Farhad KOHI, Milos LUKIC, Stephen Terence WARNER

Mitcham

Church Road Surgery
1 Church Road, Mitcham CR4 3YU
Tel: 020 8648 0822 Fax: 020 8640 4013
(Sutton and Merton Primary Care Trust)

Practice Manager Gillian Frost

GP Philip Jennings WHITEHEAD, Navnit Singh CHANA, Margaret Elizabeth Mary COCHRANE, Janet Susan GOUGH, Andrew OTLEY

Figges Marsh Surgery
41 Streatham Road, Mitcham CR4 2AD
Tel: 020 8648 2611 Fax: 020 8640 4617
(Sutton and Merton Primary Care Trust)
Patient List Size: 3642

Practice Manager Judith Dedman

GP Roderick COLBORN, Tana BAJWA

Mitcham Medical Centre
81 Haslemere Avenue, Mitcham CR4 3PR
Tel: 020 8648 3234 Fax: 020 8646 7632
Website: www.mitchammedicalcentre.co.uk
(Sutton and Merton Primary Care Trust)
Patient List Size: 10500

Practice Manager Lynn McGovern

GP Ghazi Shafiqul Alam CHOUDHURY, Naem KHAN, Bishwajit NAHA

The Surgery
42 Graham Road, Mitcham CR4 2HA
Tel: 020 8648 2432/8249 Fax: 020 8646 8249
(Sutton and Merton Primary Care Trust)
Patient List Size: 3600

Practice Manager Mrs Savita

GP Raghunath LALL, Abdul KARIM

Tamworth House Medical Centre
341 Tamworth Lane, Mitcham CR4 1DL
Tel: 020 8764 2666 Fax: 020 8679 3621
(Sutton and Merton Primary Care Trust)
Patient List Size: 9500

Practice Manager Jill McAndrew

GP Geoffrey Paul HOLLIER, Sonya IBRAHIM, Santina LA PORTA, Patrick MANSFIELD, Jane WILLIAMS, Aric WONG

Wandle Valley Health Centre
1 Miller Close, Mitcham CR4 4AX
Email: practice.manager@gp-h85086.nhs.uk
(Sutton and Merton Primary Care Trust)
Patient List Size: 2229

Wideway Medical Centre
Wide Way, Mitcham CR4 1BP
Tel: 020 8764 7612 Fax: 020 8765 1043
(Sutton and Merton Primary Care Trust)
Patient List Size: 6700

Practice Manager Louise M Aitken

GP Mina PATEL, Sellappah GANESARATNAM, Colin Michael JONES

Mitcheldean

Mitcheldean Surgery
Brook Street, Mitcheldean GL17 0AU
Tel: 01594 542270 Fax: 01594 544897
(West Gloucestershire Primary Care Trust)
Patient List Size: 5650

Practice Manager Ann Richards

GP Roger Ellis MARTIN, Andrew Francis RODGETT, Paul David WEISS

Morden

Faccini House Surgery
64 Middleton Road, Morden SM4 6RS
Tel: 020 8646 4282 Fax: 020 8646 2848
(Sutton and Merton Primary Care Trust)
Patient List Size: 5500

Practice Manager Beverley Moore

GP Javed Hassan SHEIKH, M E ERSKINE, Iram ZAIDI

The Surgery
191 Bishopsford Road, Morden SM4 6BH
Tel: 020 8648 3187 Fax: 020 8648 3157
Email: chandra.perera@gp-H85023.nhs.uk
Website: www.drperera-drpiyasena.co.uk
(Sutton and Merton Primary Care Trust)
Patient List Size: 4000

Practice Manager Lynne Murray

GP C PERERA, C PIYASENA

The Surgery
107 Seymour Avenue, Morden SM4 4RA
Tel: 020 8337 3112
(Sutton and Merton Primary Care Trust)

Practice Manager Valerie Stone

GP Jerome Joseph JEPHCOTT, S D K IYER

The Surgery
42 Central Road, Morden SM4 5RT
Tel: 020 8648 9126 Fax: 020 8646 4682
(Sutton and Merton Primary Care Trust)

Practice Manager Evelyn Cupit

GP Chatchithananantham VIVEKANANDA, Kanagalingam SUGUMAR

The Wandle Road Surgery
161 Wandle Road, Morden SM4 6AA
Tel: 020 8648 1877 Fax: 020 8648 4737
Email: chris.arulrajah@nhs.net
(Sutton and Merton Primary Care Trust)
Patient List Size: 5200

Practice Manager Ruth Steines

GP Selvaratnam ARULRAJAH, H CHONG, E R LAWRENCE

Morecambe

Heysham Health Centre
Middleton Way, Heysham, Morecambe LA3 2LL
Tel: 01524 853851 Fax: 01524 855388
(Morecambe Bay Primary Care Trust)

GP Thomas Douglas Samuel BELL, Hira Lal KAPUR

Lansdowne Road Surgery
6 Lansdowne Road, Morecambe LA4 6AL
Tel: 01524 418871 Fax: 01524 400185
(Morecambe Bay Primary Care Trust)

GP Malcolm Heywood SEVILLE

Morecambe Health Centre
Hanover Street, Morecambe LA4 5LY
Tel: 01524 418418 Fax: 01524 832584
(Morecambe Bay Primary Care Trust)
Patient List Size: 10000

Practice Manager Lorraine McLoskrie

GP Roger DILLON, Roger Kenneth Edward DOCTON, Robert Ward GILL, David Orme KNAPPER, Stephanie WILLIAMS

Morecambe Health Centre
Hanover Street, Morecambe LA4 5LY
Tel: 01524 418418 Fax: 01524 832584
(Morecambe Bay Primary Care Trust)
Patient List Size: 5300

Practice Manager Sue Brimelow

GP Christopher David EVANS, Alison Jane MACLEOD, Robin Alastair SYKES

Strawberry Gardens Medical Practice
377 Heysham Road, Morecambe LA3 2BP
Tel: 01524 850999 Fax: 01524 855688
(Morecambe Bay Primary Care Trust)

GP Alexander Smith FORSYTH, Anne Marie GREENWOOD, Dominic James INGRAM

West End Medical Practice
1 Heysham Road, Heysham, Morecambe LA3 1DA
Tel: 01524 831931 Fax: 01524 832516
(Morecambe Bay Primary Care Trust)
Patient List Size: 9600

Practice Manager Kim Jones

GP Paul Andrew TOWNLEY, W J CHASE, Alexander Richard GAW, Gwen M HERD, A J MADDOX

Westgate Medical Practice
Braddon Close, Morecambe LA4 4UZ
Tel: 01524 832888 Fax: 01524 832722
(Morecambe Bay Primary Care Trust)
Patient List Size: 7900

Practice Manager Helen Freschini

GP Philip John Wright WINFIELD, Timothy GARTSIDE, Mark Gerard GREALY, Sarah Patricia MAHER

York Bridge Surgery
5 James Street, Morecambe LA4 5TE
Tel: 01524 831111 Fax: 01524 832493
(Morecambe Bay Primary Care Trust)

Practice Manager Rosaleen Wallbank

GP Richard ROUTLEDGE, Sarah Elizabeth BREAR, Ian GUINAN, Jonathan Mark WIMBORNE

Moreton-in-Marsh

Mann Cottage Surgery
Oxford Street, Moreton-in-Marsh GL56 0LA
Tel: 01608 650764 Fax: 01608 650996
(Cotswold and Vale Primary Care Trust)
Patient List Size: 3638

Practice Manager Linda Mantella

GP Rosemary Gillian (Jill) BARLING, Hywel FURN-DAVIES

White House Surgery
High Street, Moreton-in-Marsh GL56 0AT
Tel: 01608 650317 Fax: 01608 650071
(Cotswold and Vale Primary Care Trust)

Practice Manager Heather Knight

GP Paul Stephen LUTTER, Christopher Charles MORTON

Morpeth

Albion Terrace Surgery
13 Albion Terrace, Lynemouth, Morpeth NE61 5SY
Tel: 01670 860212 Fax: 01670 860669
(Northumberland Care Trust)
Patient List Size: 3350

Practice Manager Valerie Brotherton

GP Isobel CRAFT

Coquet Medical Group
Amble Health Centre, Percy Drive, Amble, Morpeth NE65 0HD
Tel: 01665 710481 Fax: 01665 513009
(Northumberland Care Trust)
Patient List Size: 11000

Practice Manager M McAndrew

GP Paul Anthony CREIGHTON, Alan Robert FRASER, Ian Patrick Martin McELHINNEY, Matthew William PETTIFER, Gareth David WATKINS, Scott WILKES

Dr J A Farndale
Hernspeth House, Harbottle, Morpeth NE65 7DQ
Tel: 01669 650280 Fax: 01669 650439
(Northumberland Care Trust)

Patient List Size: 1000

GP John Anthony FARNDALE, Jane Elizabeth FARNDALE

Grange Road Welfare Centre
Grange Road, Widdrington, Morpeth NE61 5LX
Tel: 01670 790229 Fax: 01670 791312
Email: admin@gp-a84029.nhs.uk
(Northumberland Care Trust)

Practice Manager Pamela Mountain

GP Finnbarr Hugh O'DRISCOLL, C J WAITE

Greystoke Surgery
Kings Avenue, Morpeth NE61 1JA
Tel: 01670 511393 Fax: 01670 503282
(Northumberland Care Trust)

GP Thomas Bell SCOTT, Sally Jane ELPHICK, Stephen Paul GRAY, Stuart JOBLING, David Curtis RIDLEY

Middle Farm Surgery
51 Main Street, Felton, Morpeth NE65 9PR
Tel: 01670 787353 Fax: 01670 787353
Email: admin@gp-a84609.nhs.uk
(Northumberland Care Trust)
Patient List Size: 1597

Practice Manager Margaret Askew

GP Mark Stephen HORNER

Morpeth Health Centre
Gas House Lane, Morpeth NE61 1SR
Tel: 01670 513657 Fax: 01670 511966
(Northumberland Care Trust)

Practice Manager S Gutherson

GP John Martin MYERS, Patricia Anne COLVER, John Paul O'NEILL, G L PEARSON

The Rothbury Practice
3 Market Place, Rothbury, Morpeth NE65 7UW
Tel: 01669 620339 Fax: 01669 620583
(Northumberland Care Trust)

Practice Manager Trine Bonsnes

GP Alistair Gordon CAMERON, Frances Helen DOWER, Rebecca ELLIOT, Peter Geoffrey HUNT, Elizabeth WALSH

Scots Gap Surgery
Scots Gap, Morpeth NE61 4EG
Tel: 01670 774216 Fax: 01670 774388
(Northumberland Care Trust)

GP Catherine Mary MENAGE, Nicholas Robert WINSLOW

Wellway Medical Group
The Surgery, Wellway, Morpeth NE61 6TB
Tel: 01670 517300 Fax: 01670 511931
Email: firstname.lastname@gp-A84036.nhs.uk
(Northumberland Care Trust)
Patient List Size: 8500

Practice Manager Gillian Slaughter

GP Peter ANDERSON, Stephen Andrew HINCHLIFFE, Justin John LAWSON, Christopher MARR

Much Hadham

The Health Centre
Ash Meadow, High Street, Much Hadham SG10 6DE
Tel: 01279 842242 Fax: 01279 843973
(South East Hertfordshire Primary Care Trust)
Patient List Size: 6600

Practice Manager Rosemary Golds

GP Colin Francis Gordon BROOKBANKS, Paul Francis HAIMES, Robert Lewis MAYSON

Nantwich

Kiltearn Medical Centre
33-35 Hospital Street, Nantwich CW5 5RN
Tel: 01270 610200 Fax: 01270 610637
(Central Cheshire Primary Care Trust)
Patient List Size: 11064

Practice Manager Emma Ashley

GP John Humphrey KNAPMAN, Susanne Ruth CAESAR, Peter James FLATTERY, Jane Louise HOWELL, Katherine Frances C HUTCHINSON, Annabel Aulene Mary LONDON, Marie McKAVANAGH, Carolyn Ann PAUL

Nantwich Health Centre
Beam Street, Nantwich CW5 5NX
Tel: 01270 610181 Fax: 01270 610511
(Central Cheshire Primary Care Trust)
Patient List Size: 5600

Practice Manager Liz Tipping

GP Alan Alexander BARRON, Josephine BUTCHER, L GURNANI, A PARK

The Surgery
The Green, Nantwich Road, Wrenbury, Nantwich CW5 8EW
Tel: 01270 780210 Fax: 01270 780658
(Cheshire West Primary Care Trust)
Patient List Size: 2290

Practice Manager Marion Mortimer

GP Graham John DAVENPORT, Sarah ROWE

The Tudir Surgery
The Health Centre, Beam Street, Nantwich CW5 5NX
Tel: 01270 610686 Fax: 01270 625770
(Central Cheshire Primary Care Trust)
Patient List Size: 4000

Practice Manager Debbie Howarth

GP C NEWBROOK, A INNES, I C MALONE

Nelson

Barrowford Surgery
Ridgeway, Barrowford, Nelson BB9 8QP
Tel: 01282 612621 Fax: 01282 611958
(Burnley, Pendle and Rossendale Primary Care Trust)
Patient List Size: 3410

Practice Manager Lisa Topham

GP Iain Richard ASHWORTH, Samantha GOLDING, Angus SCOTT

Brierfield Health Centre
Arthur Street, Brierfield, Nelson BB9 5SQ
Tel: 01282 615175 Fax: 01282 698157
(Burnley, Pendle and Rossendale Primary Care Trust)
Patient List Size: 2225

Practice Manager B L McWhinney

GP Rafiz Ahmad QAZI

Nelson Health Centre
Leeds Road, Nelson BB9 9TG
Tel: 01282 698036
(Burnley, Pendle and Rossendale Primary Care Trust)

Practice Manager Pat Bennett

GP Prosanto Kumar GUHA, David Robert Murray FLEMING, Julia Melissa PEARSON, Jayashree Rajnikant SHAH, Graeme Thomas Russell SPENCER, Peter Darcy WALSH

Nelson Health Centre
Leeds Road, Nelson BB9 9TG
Tel: 01282 615216 Fax: 01282 619514
(Burnley, Pendle and Rossendale Primary Care Trust)

Practice Manager Deborah Almond

GP Mirza Muhammad Idrees BAIG, Suleman VOHRA

Nelson Health Centre
Leeds Road, Nelson BB9 9TG
Tel: 01282 613592 Fax: 01282 619771
Email: arshad.haque@gp-P81174.nhs.uk
(Burnley, Pendle and Rossendale Primary Care Trust)
Patient List Size: 2730

Practice Manager Lucinda M Hopkins

GP Mohammad Arshadul HAQUE

Nelson Health Centre
Leeds Road, Nelson BB9 9TG
Tel: 01282 615577 Fax: 01282 619402
(Burnley, Pendle and Rossendale Primary Care Trust)
Patient List Size: 2700

GP Qazi Mohammad JEHANGIR

Nelson Health Centre
Leeds Road, Nelson BB9 9TG
Tel: 01282 699995
(Burnley, Pendle and Rossendale Primary Care Trust)

GP Asiz-Ur-Rahman KHAN

Nelson Health Centre
Leeds Road, Nelson BB9 9TG
Tel: 01282 614157
(Burnley, Pendle and Rossendale Primary Care Trust)

Practice Manager Joyce Knight

GP Mohammad Ikram MALIK, Raisa Ikram MALIK

Nelson Health Centre
Leeds Road, Nelson BB9 9TG
Tel: 01282 614878
(Burnley, Pendle and Rossendale Primary Care Trust)

GP Muhammad SAEED

Nelson Health Centre
Leeds Road, Nelson BB9 9TG
Tel: 01282 613192
(Burnley, Pendle and Rossendale Primary Care Trust)

GP Om Prakash TANDON, Usha TANDON

Pendle View Surgery
Arthur Street, Brierfield, Nelson BB9 5RZ
Tel: 01282 614599
(Burnley, Pendle and Rossendale Primary Care Trust)
Patient List Size: 6500

GP William Michael IONS, Ursula Margaret HUTCHINSON, David John WEBBORN

Neston

Willaston Surgery
Neston Road, Willaston, Neston CH64 2TN
Tel: 0151 327 4593 Fax: 0151 327 8618
Email: geff.meyer@gp-n81104.nhs.uk
(Ellesmere Port and Neston Primary Care Trust)
Patient List Size: 4300

Practice Manager Susan King

GP Geffrey MEYER

New Malden

The Groves Medical Centre
72 Coombe Road, New Malden KT3 4QS
Tel: 020 8336 2222 Fax: 020 8336 0297
Website: www.thegrovesmedicalcentre.co.uk
(Kingston Primary Care Trust)
Patient List Size: 9100

GP Jeremy Nicholas HARRIS, Susan Elizabeth BROWN, Vince GRIPPAUDO, Joan Hannah MAY, Leonard Adrian SHERSKI

Holmwood Corner Surgery
134 Malden Road, New Malden KT3 6DR
Tel: 020 8942 0066 Fax: 020 8336 1377
(Kingston Primary Care Trust)

GP Nicholas Hanson SHELDON, Christine Michele CHAPMAN, Philippa CRAWFORD, Jonathan Peter LUCKETT

New Malden Health Centre
4 Blagdon Road, New Malden KT3 4AD
Tel: 020 8942 2660 Fax: 020 8336 0378
(Kingston Primary Care Trust)
Patient List Size: 4000

Practice Manager Sheila Petrohilos

GP Nazim Amirali JIVANI, Amirali Kassam JIVANI

Roselawn Surgery
Roselawn, 149 Malden Road, New Malden KT3 6AA
Tel: 020 8949 0555 Fax: 020 8395 5666
(Kingston Primary Care Trust)
Patient List Size: 4000

Practice Manager S Fraser, G Halsley, J Mohan

GP G S GOEL, M GOEL

The Surgery
157 High Street, New Malden KT3 4BH
Tel: 020 8942 0094 Fax: 020 8269 0065
(Kingston Primary Care Trust)

Practice Manager Karin Al-Yaqubi

GP Nabil Najib AL-YAQUBI

The Surgery
98a Westbury Road, New Malden KT3 5AN
Tel: 020 8949 6778 Fax: 020 8336 0103
(Kingston Primary Care Trust)

GP Bernadette Mary Susan GRIMMETT

West Barnes Surgery
229 West Barnes Lane, New Malden KT3 6JD
Tel: 020 8336 1773 Fax: 020 8395 4797
(Kingston Primary Care Trust)

Practice Manager Pat Dodson

GP S L CHANG, A R HUGHES, N IQBAL, M S S KUMAR, S MAKAR

New Milton

Arnewood Practice
Milton Medical Centre, Avenue Road, New Milton BH25 5JP
Tel: 01425 620393 Fax: 01425 624219
Email: doctors@gp-j82007.nhs.uk
Website: www.arnewoodpractice.nhs.uk
(New Forest Primary Care Trust)
Patient List Size: 12400

Practice Manager Jayne C Tabor

GP Michael Puttrell THACKER, Philip BREWER, Mark Wayne KYDD-COUTTS, Brian MARSH, Jane Burnaby McLEOD, Amanda WALDEN, Nigel Frank WATSON

Barton Surgery
1 Edmunds Close, Barton Court Avenue, Barton-on-Sea, New Milton BH25 7EN
Tel: 01425 620830 Fax: 01425 629812
(New Forest Primary Care Trust)
Patient List Size: 10200

Practice Manager Hugh Rowlands

GP David James PARKER, Donald Miles BARGH, Geraint Alyn DAVIES, Jacqueline Fiona DAVIES, Delyth JENKINS, Lawrence Carteret MAULE

New Milton Health Centre
Spencer Road, New Milton BH25 6EN
Tel: 01425 621188 Fax: 01425 620646

(New Forest Primary Care Trust)

Practice Manager Margot Whitehorn

GP Timothy John THURSTON, Karen Dorothea BENTLEY, Paul Jonathan CAMPBELL, Bridget D CRACKNELL, Jeremy William Haydn DAVIES, Annie N RUTHERFORD

New Romney

Oak Hall Surgery

41-43 High Street, New Romney TN28 8BW
Tel: 01797 362106 Fax: 01797 366495
(Shepway Primary Care Trust)
Patient List Size: 5500

Practice Manager Angela Cochrane

GP Paul Telford COCHRANE, Steven John SWOFFER

Newark

Birkwood

35 Mickledale Lane, Bilsthorpe, Newark NG22 8QB
Tel: 01623 870230 Fax: 01623 411407
(Newark and Sherwood Primary Care Trust)

Practice Manager A Cullum

GP Paul HORMIS, Michael JOHNSON

Collingham Health Centre

High Street, Collingham, Newark NG23 7LB
Tel: 01636 892156 Fax: 01636 893391
Website: www.collinghammedicalcentre.co.uk
(Newark and Sherwood Primary Care Trust)
Patient List Size: 6200

Practice Manager Julie Reid

GP Derek Alan HUTTON, Anne de GAY, Peter Julian DENNIS, Michael Alexander Leary PRINGLE, Lisa M TERRILL

de Gay and Partners

The Surgery, 50 Barnaby Gate, Newark NG24 1QD
Tel: 01636 704225 Fax: 01636 613044
(Newark and Sherwood Primary Care Trust)
Patient List Size: 12200

Practice Manager L Macmillan

GP Nigel Robert de GAY, Julie Anne BARKER, Lesley Anne CAMPBELL, Mark HUNTER, David Jonathan MILE, B L SINGLETON

Eborall and Partners

Fountain Medical Centre, Sherwood Avenue, Newark NG24 1QH
Tel: 01636 704378/9 Fax: 01636 610875
(Newark and Sherwood Primary Care Trust)
Patient List Size: 13000

Practice Manager Alistair Wood

GP John Frederick Saywell EBORALL, John Philip CHARLESWORTH, Alan Davidson GARROW, James Glynn McGILL, Jane Elizabeth SELWYN, Susan Mary WARD

Middleton Lodge Surgery

Church Circle, New Ollerton, Newark NG22 9SZ
Tel: 01623 860668 Fax: 01623 836073
(Newark and Sherwood Primary Care Trust)
Patient List Size: 11200

Practice Manager Lynne Baxter

GP Richard Martin CHALMERS, Stephen HEAD, Peter BARBER, Walden Howard EFFINGHAM, Helen Emily WARD

The Surgeries

Lombard Street, Newark NG24 1XG
Tel: 01636 702363 Fax: 01636 613037
(Newark and Sherwood Primary Care Trust)

Practice Manager Diana Kirk

GP David Edward Roger BRITTON, Simon BRENCHLEY, Alex CHAMBERS, Elizabeth HULL, Andrew John PARKIN, Joanne SEEDHOUSE, Ram Chand VOHRAH, David John WATHEN, Timothy Peter WEST

The Surgery

Faraday Avenue, Tuxford, Newark NG22 0HT
Tel: 01777 870203 Fax: 01777 872221
(Bassetlaw Primary Care Trust)

Practice Manager June Simpson

GP Michael Blair ASHTON, Ian William DAVIES, Malcolm Edwin FINCH

The Surgery

Station Lane, Farnsfield, Newark NG22 8LA
Tel: 01623 882289 Fax: 01623 882286
(Newark and Sherwood Primary Care Trust)

Practice Manager A Colquhoun

GP James Maurice HEALY, John David PORTER

The Surgery

Hounsfield Way, Sutton-on-Trent, Newark NG23 6PX
Tel: 01636 821023 Fax: 01636 822308
(Newark and Sherwood Primary Care Trust)
Patient List Size: 3100

Practice Manager C Davison

GP Charles Philip Lawrence CLAYTON, Fiona Gray NELSON

The Surgery

9A Bullpit Road, Balderton, Newark NG24 3PT
Tel: 01636 705826 Fax: 01636 605222
(Newark and Sherwood Primary Care Trust)
Patient List Size: 2700

Practice Manager F Canning

GP P D JONES, S K KHARKONGOR

The Surgery

15 Winters Lane, Long Bennington, Newark NG23 5DW
Tel: 01400 281220
(Lincolnshire South West Teaching Primary Care Trust)
Patient List Size: 4918

Practice Manager Evelyn Ryan

GP C J LAWRENSON, S R W LONGFIELD, S PULLINGER

Newbury

Chapel Row Surgery

The Avenue, Bucklebury, Newbury RG7 6NS
Tel: 0118 971 3252 Fax: 0118 971 4161
Website: www.crsurgery.co.uk
(Newbury and Community Primary Care Trust)
Patient List Size: 6750

Practice Manager Paul Gomm

GP C MARKHAM, M EDWARDS-MOSS, J LENNOX, P WESTLAR

Downland Practice

East Lane, Chieveley, Newbury RG20 8UY
Tel: 01635 248251 Fax: 01635 247261
Website: www.downlanpractice.org
(Newbury and Community Primary Care Trust)
Patient List Size: 9400

Practice Manager Liz Saxton

GP Leslie Mark LOWENTHAL, James Alan Harvard CAVE, Christine Elizabeth DAVIES, Mary DYSON, Alison Elizabeth HUNTER, Andrew Roger WARDLE

Eastfield House Surgery

6 St. Johns Road, Newbury RG14 7LW
Tel: 01635 41495 Fax: 01635 522751
(Newbury and Community Primary Care Trust)

Practice Manager Laura Hutchinson

GP Richard John Greenhill WELLER, Diana Joy DAVIES, Bruce Baird LETHAM, Jennifer PATON, Geoffrey Norman SHILLAM, Helen Kristi WALLIS

The Falkland Surgery
Monks Lane, Newbury RG14 7DF
Tel: 01635 279972 Fax: 01635 279973
Website: www.falklandsurgery.co.uk
(Newbury and Community Primary Care Trust)

Practice Manager Sally Sutton

GP Stephen CHAPMAN, Patrick Nicholas Russell BROOKE, Charlotte CHANDLER, Keith ENDERSBY, Ruth LAMBERT, Susan Elizabeth Halstead RENDEL, Louise TITCOMB, Timothy Neil WALTER

Kingsclere Medical Practice
Kingsclere, Newbury RG20 5QX
Tel: 01635 296000 Fax: 01635 299282
(North Hampshire Primary Care Trust)

Practice Manager Winnie Harfield

GP David J POLLARD, Sarah Elizabeth Louise BOND, Mark G WOTHERSPOON

Northcroft Surgery
Northcroft Lane, Newbury RG14 1BU
Tel: 01635 31575 Fax: 01635 551857
(Newbury and Community Primary Care Trust)

Practice Manager Sarah Arnold

GP Michael Eric YOUDAN, Ann-Marie FAULKNER, Ruth HILLMAN, Madeline Georgina NORMAN, Angela Jane SULLIVAN

St Marys Road Surgery
St Marys Road, Newbury RG14 1EQ
Tel: 01635 31444 Fax: 01635 551316
(Newbury and Community Primary Care Trust)
Patient List Size: 10981

Practice Manager Denise Griffiths

GP Robert Doré WATSON, Maria Frances HYDE, Judith JONES, Paul Malcolm Ronald MILLARD, Graham Howard STIFF, Meg THOMAS

Newcastle, Staffordshire

Castletown Surgery
123 Liverpool Road, Cross Heath, Newcastle ST5 9ER
Tel: 01782 637082 Fax: 01782 710421
(Newcastle-under-Lyme Primary Care Trust)
Patient List Size: 2013

Practice Manager Christine Mason

GP Latif Mohammed HUSSAIN

Higherland Surgery
3 Orme Road, Poolfields, Newcastle ST5 2UE
Tel: 01782 717044 Fax: 01782 715447
(Newcastle-under-Lyme Primary Care Trust)
Patient List Size: 4000

Practice Manager Pamela Cox

GP Kevan John THORLEY, Richard Andrew HAYWARD, Shamid JAVAID

Kingsbridge Medical Practice
Kingsbridge Avenue, Clayton, Newcastle ST5 3HP
Tel: 01782 427361 Fax: 01782 427369
(Newcastle-under-Lyme Primary Care Trust)
Patient List Size: 6600

Practice Manager Sue Beckett

GP Marcus Llewellyn GRIFFITHS, W J COOPER, M ENDALL, S W LEE

Loomer Road Surgery
Loomer Road, Chesterton, Newcastle ST5 7JS
Tel: 01782 565000 Fax: 01782 565666
(Newcastle-under-Lyme Primary Care Trust)
Patient List Size: 2000

Practice Manager Jackie Cooke

GP Napoleon Enninful ACQUAH

Lyme Valley Medical Centre
Lyme Valley Road, Newcastle ST5 3TF
Tel: 01782 615367 Fax: 01782 713355
(Newcastle-under-Lyme Primary Care Trust)
Patient List Size: 5700

Practice Manager S M Smith

GP Michael Stuart SMITH

Miller Street Surgery
Miller Street, Off Kings Street, Newcastle ST5 1JD
Tel: 01782 711618 Fax: 01782 713940
(Newcastle-under-Lyme Primary Care Trust)
Patient List Size: 13800

Practice Manager Linda Fox

GP Geoffrey Ian GARDNER, Paul William COX, Stephen DUKES, Michael Ernest LLOYD, Martin Frederick TOMMEY

Silverdale Medical Centre
Vale Pleasant, Silverdale, Newcastle ST5 6PS
Tel: 01782 612375 Fax: 01782 714036
(Newcastle-under-Lyme Primary Care Trust)

Practice Manager Muriel Goode

GP Michael Peter HOLLINS, Gerald Palmer MORGANS, A SACKEY, Paul Robert David SCOTT, Jonathan Mark WRIGHT

The Surgery
2 Heathcote Street, Newcastle ST5 7EB
Tel: 01782 561057 Fax: 01782 563907
(Newcastle-under-Lyme Primary Care Trust)
Patient List Size: 9100

Practice Manager Sharon Shottom

GP Keith Sloan DICK, H SINGH, James Murray SMITH, Simon Roy WALSH, Sharif ZULFIKER

The Surgery
132 Liverpool Road, Cross Heath, Newcastle ST5 9EQ
Tel: 01782 616573
(Newcastle-under-Lyme Primary Care Trust)

Practice Manager Fiona MacNamara

GP Peter John FRANKLIN

The Village Surgery
49 High Street, Wolstanton, Newcastle ST5 0ET
Tel: 01782 626172
(Newcastle-under-Lyme Primary Care Trust)
Patient List Size: 6400

Practice Manager J Wright

GP Varsha Vasant MANUDHANE, Krishna Kumar AGARWAL, Subra MANIAN

Wolstanton Medical Centre
Palmerston Street, Newcastle ST5 8BN
Tel: 01782 627488 Fax: 01782 662313
(Newcastle-under-Lyme Primary Care Trust)
Patient List Size: 10000

Practice Manager Lynne Cooper

GP Michael John Yair FISHER, John J EDWARDS, Alwyn Thomas Raynor RALPHS, Mark SHAPLEY

Newcastle-under-Lyme

Keele Practice
University Medical Centre, University of Keele, Keele, Newcastle-under-Lyme ST5 5BG
Tel: 01782 753550 Fax: 01782 753555
(Newcastle-under-Lyme Primary Care Trust)
Patient List Size: 5710

Practice Manager Jan Documes

GP Philippa DOVE, Thomas David MAIRS, Even O'BYRNE, J SHAHAB

Liverpool Road Surgery
128 Liverpool Road, Cross Heath, Newcastle-under-Lyme ST5 9EQ
(Newcastle-under-Lyme Primary Care Trust)

GP Richard Bryce FRANKLIN

Newcastle upon Tyne

Adelaide Medical Centre
Adelaide Terrace, Benwell, Newcastle upon Tyne NE4 8BE
Tel: 0191 219 5599 Fax: 0191 219 5596
(Newcastle Primary Care Trust)
Patient List Size: 3750

Practice Manager Veronica Christie

GP Helen Ruth WHITEMAN, Claire POPELY, Adam SANDELL, Winnie STACK

Armstrong Road Health Centre
460 Armstrong Road, Scotswood, Newcastle upon Tyne NE15 6BY
Tel: 0191 228 0960
(Newcastle Primary Care Trust)

GP F MAHMOOD

Avenue Medical Practice
5 Osborne Avenue, Jesmond, Newcastle upon Tyne NE2 1JQ
Tel: 0191 281 0041 Fax: 0191 281 1474
(Newcastle Primary Care Trust)
Patient List Size: 3100

Practice Manager Pamela A Patterson

GP Konrad Wladislaw CONRAD, Dr CARR, Gillian Patricia RYE

The Avenues Medical Group
27-29 Roseworth Avenue, Gosforth, Newcastle upon Tyne NE3 1NS
Tel: 0191 285 8035
(Newcastle Primary Care Trust)

GP Andrew Christopher John BURDON, Dr TOMASZCZYK, Stephen Anthony TURLEY

Bentinck Road Medical Centre
2 Bentinck Road, Arthur's Hill, Newcastle upon Tyne NE4 6UT
Tel: 0191 273 3919 Fax: 0191 2736323
(Newcastle Primary Care Trust)
Patient List Size: 2500

Practice Manager Patricia Prendergast

GP Tapan Chandra SARMA

Betts Avenue Medical Centre
2 Betts Avenue, Benwell, Newcastle upon Tyne NE15 6TQ
Tel: 0191 274 2767/2842 Fax: 0191 274 0244
(Newcastle Primary Care Trust)
Patient List Size: 10000

Practice Manager Marion Hurst, Riba Noble

GP David Allan BLACK, Margaret BONE, G I M BUERSTEDDE, Dr KERRY, Dr PODOGROCKI

Biddlestone Health Group
1 Biddlestone Road, Heaton, Newcastle upon Tyne NE6 5SL
Tel: 0191 265 5755 Fax: 0191 275 5500
(Newcastle Primary Care Trust)

Practice Manager Liz Jepson

GP David John ROBSON, Peter Matthew CARRINGTON, Mary Kathleen PEARSTON, Elizabeth WATERSTON

Brenkley Avenue Health Centre
Brenkley Avenue, Shiremoor, Newcastle upon Tyne NE27 0PR
Tel: 0191 219 5700 Fax: 0191 219 5706
(North Tyneside Primary Care Trust)
Patient List Size: 5061

Practice Manager J Bradley

GP Christopher David BOWMAN, C S NAIR, Simon John YOUNG

Brenkley Avenue Health Centre
Brenkley Avenue, Shiremoor, Newcastle upon Tyne NE27 0PR
Tel: 0191 251 6151
(North Tyneside Primary Care Trust)

GP Susan Frances BAKER, Kathleen Mary BURNS, Desmond Murray SMITH

Brenkley Avenue Health Centre
Brenkley Avenue, Shiremoor, Newcastle upon Tyne NE27 0PR
Tel: 0191 219 5708
(North Tyneside Primary Care Trust)
Patient List Size: 3000

GP Parayil Mohan THARAKAN

Broadway Medical Centre
164 Great North Road, Gosforth, Newcastle upon Tyne NE3 5JP
Tel: 0191 219 6900 Fax: 0191 219 6910
(Newcastle Primary Care Trust)

Practice Manager Ruth Eskdale

GP H G COOKEY, D K DALAL, A P THICK

Cruddas Park Surgery
178 Westmorland Road, Cruddas Park, Newcastle upon Tyne NE4 7JT
(Newcastle Primary Care Trust)

GP Sheelagh Maria TURNER, Philip Charles ANTOUN, Carol Anne BROUGHAM, Dr CROFT, Dr PILKINGTON, Ilva STAFFORD

Denton Park Medical Group
Denton Park Centre, West Denton Way, Newcastle upon Tyne NE5 2QZ
Tel: 0191 267 2751 Fax: 0191 264 1588
(Newcastle Primary Care Trust)

Practice Manager P Johnson

GP Mary Geraldine PATTMAN, Susan Nicola ANDERSON, Michael MEINEN, Jonathan Henry PAYNE, Katherine Margaret SOWARD

Denton Turret Medical Centre
10 Kenley Road, Slatyford, Newcastle upon Tyne NE5 2UY
Tel: 0191 274 1840
(Newcastle Primary Care Trust)

GP David John HOWARTH, Rosemary Erica NYHOLM, Caroline SHARP, Philip James Steevens TAYLOR

Elmfield Health Group
18 Elmfield Road, Gosforth, Newcastle upon Tyne NE3 4BP
Tel: 0191 285 1663 Fax: 0191 284 7015
(Newcastle Primary Care Trust)
Patient List Size: 4600

Practice Manager Yvonne Froldi, Sue Kirkby

GP Dr ANAND, Atoosa RABET-NEJAD, Rajkumar Hukumchand SAIGAL

Ethel Street Surgery
88-90 Ethel Street, Benwell, Newcastle upon Tyne NE4 8QA
Tel: 0191 219 5456 Fax: 0191 226 0300
(Newcastle Primary Care Trust)
Patient List Size: 3200

GP Gerard REISSMANN, Colette Catherine Pauline ANDERSON, Gina Pinucia CONGERA, Helen MURRELL, Timothy Clive OWEN

Falcon House Surgery
17-19 Heaton Road, Heaton, Newcastle upon Tyne NE6 1SA
Tel: 0191 265 3361 Fax: 0191 224 3209
(Newcastle Primary Care Trust)
Patient List Size: 6000

Practice Manager Lorna Todd

GP T A WHITE, Shelagh Jean SCOTT, Stephen STEEL

Fenham Hall Surgery
Fenham Hall Drive, Fenham, Newcastle upon Tyne NE4 9XD
Tel: 0191 274 3724 Fax: 0191 274 5674
(Newcastle Primary Care Trust)

Practice Manager John Allan

GP Brian Dermot Michael COGAN, Kate ASHLEY, Carolyn Helen BURTON, Martin WAUGH

Forest Hall Health Centre
Station Road, Forest Hall, Newcastle upon Tyne NE12 9BQ
(North Tyneside Primary Care Trust)

Practice Manager A Leighton

GP Dr COYNE

Gosforth Memorial Medical Centre
Church Road, Gosforth, Newcastle upon Tyne NE3 1TX
Tel: 0191 285 1119 Fax: 0191 213 2611
(Newcastle Primary Care Trust)
Patient List Size: 6000

Practice Manager Margaret Robertson

GP Ian Stewart WINTERTON, Helen M McCLELLANS, Philip TAYLOR, Sarah C TAYLOR, Sandra WINTERTON

Grove Medical Group
1 The Grove, Gosforth, Newcastle upon Tyne NE3 1NU
Tel: 0191 210 6680 Fax: 0191 210 6682
(Newcastle Primary Care Trust)
Patient List Size: 11200

Practice Manager Cynthia Jackson

GP Stephen Michael BLADES, Justin Thomas BURDON, Robin DOUGLAS, Cheong Keong FOO, Karen Chinedu NIELSEN, Fiona Anne Eileen SCHWABE

Heaton Road Surgery
41 Heaton Road, Heaton, Newcastle upon Tyne NE6 1TP
Tel: 0191 265 5509 Fax: 0191 224 1824
(Newcastle Primary Care Trust)
Patient List Size: 7356

Practice Manager Helen R Hislop

GP Robert Hugh MORRISON, Christopher Irvin EMMERSON, Eileen Margaret HIGGINS, Joanne Nicola LEE

High Laws Surgery
5 High Laws, South Gosforth, Newcastle upon Tyne NE3 1RQ

GP Bryonie Susan GALLAGHER

Holmside Medical Group
142 Armstrong Road, Benwell, Newcastle upon Tyne NE4 8QB
Tel: 0191 273 4009 Fax: 0191 273 2745
(Newcastle Primary Care Trust)
Patient List Size: 11660

Practice Manager Carol Broughton

GP Brian Trevor SPENCER, Simone HAASE, Sarjit Singh MARWAHA, Geoffrey Kenneth NEEDHAM, Timothy John PEARSON, Andrew Frederick PRICE, Sarah Margaret PRICE

Jesmond Clinic
48 Osborne Road, Jesmond, Newcastle upon Tyne NE2 2AL
Tel: 0191 281 4060 Fax: 0191 281 0231
(Newcastle Primary Care Trust)
Patient List Size: 3400

Practice Manager Maureen Lillie

GP V A WADGE, T R H PRICE, M F L SELLS

Knight, Todd, Jackson and Mather
Hawthorn House Medical Centre, 28-30 Heaton Road, Newcastle upon Tyne NE6 1SD
Tel: 0191 265 5543/6246 Fax: 0191 276 2985
(Newcastle Primary Care Trust)
Patient List Size: 6600

Practice Manager Doreen Brown

GP Nicholas Francis KNIGHT, Ian David JACKSON, Martin F MATHER, Kim Paula TODD

Lane End Surgery
2 Manor Walk, Benton, Newcastle upon Tyne NE7 7XX
Tel: 0191 266 5246 Fax: 0191 266 6241
Email: laneendsurgery@aol.com
Website: www.laneendsurgery.co.uk
(North Tyneside Primary Care Trust)
Patient List Size: 8100

Practice Manager Lin Murray

GP C M SPRAKE, Ashley LISTON, Rachel LUNNEY, Linda MASSON, Mark SMITH

The Medical Centre
37A Heaton Road, Heaton, Newcastle upon Tyne NE6 1TH
Tel: 0191 265 8121 Fax: 0191 276 6085
(Newcastle Primary Care Trust)
Patient List Size: 7300

Practice Manager Angela James

GP Dr LOVEDALE, Dr LEEDER, Dr NETTS, Dr WOOLLEY

Newburn Road Surgery
4 Newburn Road, Newcastle upon Tyne NE15 8LX
Tel: 0191 229 0090 Fax: 0191 267 4830
(Newcastle Primary Care Trust)

GP Michael Edwin SCOTT, Elspeth Mary Strathie ADAMS, Kim Janet FIRSTBROOK, Julian Nicholas Scott HARGREAVES, Kathleen HARGREAVES

Oakfield House Surgery
Low Westwood, Hamsterley Colliery, Newcastle upon Tyne NE17 7PT
Tel: 01207 560206 Fax: 01207 560172
Email: terence.drought@gp-A83618.nhs.uk
(Derwentside Primary Care Trust)
Patient List Size: 2300

Practice Manager Jenny Drought

GP Terence Kenneth DROUGHT

Osborne Road Surgery
17 Osborne Road, Newcastle upon Tyne NE2 2AH
Tel: 0191 281 4588 Fax: 0191 212 0379
(Newcastle Primary Care Trust)

Practice Manager T Stuchlik

GP Richard Blair EDMUNDS, Relton Alexander CUMMINGS, Susan Claire HUGHES, Antony Richard MOORE, Susan PINNINGTON

The Park Medical Group
Fawdon Park Road, Newcastle upon Tyne NE3 2PE
Tel: 0191 285 1763 Fax: 0191 284 2374
(Newcastle Primary Care Trust)
Patient List Size: 11000

Practice Manager John Johnson

GP Alison Mary CHARLEWOOD, Christina COCK, Andrew Lilwall RAMSHAW, Gordon McIntyre SHIELLS, Jill Elaine SMITH, Stephen Paul SUMMERS, Victoria Louise WILLIAMS

Parkway Medical Centre
2 Frenton Close, Chapel House Estate, Newcastle upon Tyne NE5 1EH
Tel: 0191 267 1313 Fax: 0191 229 0630
(Newcastle Primary Care Trust)
Patient List Size: 6900

Practice Manager Donna Aydon

GP John Michael Hugh JACKSON, Catherine Jane DIAS, Nicholas Charles POSNER, Alison RICHARDSON, Daphne THORNTON, Nicola Frances WEAVER

Ponteland Medical Group
Thornhill Road, Ponteland, Newcastle upon Tyne NE20 9PZ
Tel: 01661 825513 Fax: 01661 860755
(Northumberland Care Trust)

Practice Manager Eileen Smith

GP Denise Margaret ADAMS, Sue CLUGSTON, Graham Hamilton HUBBARD, Anthony John Noblet KAY, A McCAWOIN, Nigel TWELVES

Preston and Austin
Killingworth Health Centre, Citadel East, Killingworth, Newcastle upon Tyne NE12 6UR
Tel: 0191 216 0061 Fax: 0191 268 5360
(North Tyneside Primary Care Trust)

Practice Manager Dr Preston

GP Mark Richard PRESTON, Angela Helen AUSTIN

Primary Health Care Centre
South Road, Chopwell, Newcastle upon Tyne NE17 7BU
Tel: 01207 561736 Fax: 01207 563610
(Gateshead Primary Care Trust)
Patient List Size: 3384

Practice Manager R Hassan

GP Mohammad Sabit HASSAN, Iqbal Ahmed ANSARI

Proctor and Partners
Doctors Surgery, 42 Heaton Road, Heaton, Newcastle upon Tyne NE6 1SE
Tel: 0191 265 5911 Fax: 0191 265 6974
(Newcastle Primary Care Trust)
Patient List Size: 5600

Practice Manager Julie Bullen

GP Isobel Stewart PROCTOR, Philip Hedley BROOKES, Graham Alan RUTT, Denise Elizabeth Maria WILKINS

Prospect House Medical Group
Prospect House, Prospect Place, Newcastle upon Tyne NE4 6QD
Tel: 0191 219 6444 Fax: 0191 273 0129
(Newcastle Primary Care Trust)
Patient List Size: 13000

Practice Manager E M Liddle

GP Keith ARCHER, Jane Frances CARMAN, Leonie Elizabeth COATES, Bryonie Susan GALLAGHER, Valerie Ann HALL, Jeremiah Joseph KELLIHER, Dr RAY-CHADHURI, Graeme WILKES

Saville Medical Group
7 Saville Place, Newcastle upon Tyne NE1 8DQ
Tel: 0191 232 4274 Fax: 0191 233 1050
Website: www.savillemed.co.uk
(Newcastle Primary Care Trust)

Practice Manager Debbie Grey

GP Richard John GRAY, Jatinder S BRATCH, Julian Christopher BROMLY, Natalie A CROWE, Duncan CUMBERLIDGE, Rupert Adam FLINT, Brian KENT, Jane KIDD, Philip LAMBALLE, Philip LAMBALLE, Mari McGEEVER, Katherine MOORE, Roanna MORRISON, Louise Ann ROBINSON, Judith Victoria SALKELD, Dr WAITE

Shieldfield Health Centre
Stoddart Street, Shieldfield, Newcastle upon Tyne NE2 1AL
Tel: 0191 232 4872
(Newcastle Primary Care Trust)
Patient List Size: 4600

Practice Manager Sue Shone

GP Anne Vera SMITH, Alan Jonathan SILVER

Shiremoor Health Centre
Brenkley Avenue, Shiremoor, Newcastle upon Tyne NE27 0PR
Tel: 0191 219 5708 Fax: 0191 219 5711

Practice Manager K Kewen

GP Dr THARAKAN

Shiremoor Health Centre
Brenkley Avenue, Shiremoor, Newcastle upon Tyne NE27 0PR
(North Tyneside Primary Care Trust)

GP C S NAIR

Shiremoor Health Centre
Brenkley Avenue, Shiremoor, Newcastle upon Tyne NE27 0PR
(North Tyneside Primary Care Trust)

GP D M SMITH

St Anthony's Medical Group
Thomas Gaughan House, Pottery Bank, Newcastle upon Tyne NE6 3SW
Tel: 0191 219 6100
(Newcastle Primary Care Trust)

GP Wendy Elizabeth ROSS, Jonathan Reed CAUDLE, Christine Agnes JONES-UNWIN, Penelope Jane SCHOFIELD

St Anthony's Medical Group
St Anthony's Road, Walker, Newcastle upon Tyne NE6 2NN

GP Dr SCHOFIELD

Stoneleigh Avenue Surgery
98A Stoneleigh Avenue, Longbenton, Newcastle upon Tyne NE12 8NT
Tel: 0191 266 2271
(North Tyneside Primary Care Trust)
Patient List Size: 1190

Practice Manager Margaret Glover

GP Kottoruge Gilbert SILVA

The Surgery
200 Osborne Road, Jesmond, Newcastle upon Tyne NE2 3LD
Tel: 0191 281 4777 Fax: 0191 281 4309
Website: www.thesurgey.org
(Newcastle Primary Care Trust)

Practice Manager Linda Moore

GP Dr BORTHWICK, Dr BROWELL, Dr DARLING, Dr LOVEDALE

Swarland Avenue Surgery
2 Swarland Avenue, Benton, Newcastle upon Tyne NE7 7TD
Tel: 0191 215 0141 Fax: 0191 266 1358
(North Tyneside Primary Care Trust)

Practice Manager Anita Mayhew

GP C MEARS, M N IQBAL, John Charles O'KEEFFE

Throckley Surgery
Tilmouth, Throckley, Newcastle upon Tyne NE15 9PA
Tel: 0191 210 6700 Fax: 0191 210 6702
(Newcastle Primary Care Trust)
Patient List Size: 6050

Practice Manager Marie Bottomley

GP Douglas John BOOKLESS, David Nicholas GRAINGER, David William JONES, Brigid Margot JOUGHIN

University Medical Centre
Claremont Road, Newcastle upon Tyne NE2 4AN
Tel: 0191 232 2973 Fax: 0191 230 3631
Email: university.medical@gp-a86027.nhs.uk
Website: www.umc-newscastle.co.uk
(Newcastle Primary Care Trust)

Practice Manager Suzanne Bosworth

GP Neil Daniel LLOYD-JONES, Carolyn Jane FRASER

Walker Medical Group
Church Walk, Walker, Newcastle upon Tyne NE6 3BS
Website: www.walkermedicalgroup.co.uk
(Newcastle Primary Care Trust)
Patient List Size: 11250

Practice Manager Dianne Moran

GP Dr PEARSTON, T K BINMORE, Dr COYNE, Dr NABI, Dr TASKER

Welbeck Road Medical Centre
495 Welbeck Road, Walker, Newcastle upon Tyne NE6 2PB
Tel: 0191 224 3795
(Newcastle Primary Care Trust)

GP Dr KHADRI

Wellspring Medical Practice
381 West Farm Avenue, Longbenton, Newcastle upon Tyne NE12 8UT
Tel: 0191 266 1728 Fax: 0191 270 1488
(North Tyneside Primary Care Trust)
Patient List Size: 4800

Practice Manager Liz Brittlebank

GP Dr BOGUES, Dr FINDLAY, Dr GEDNEY, Dr RITCHIE

West Road Surgery
170 West Road, Fenham, Newcastle upon Tyne NE4 9QB
Tel: 0191 273 6364
(Newcastle Primary Care Trust)
Patient List Size: 9100

Practice Manager Sue Shone

GP Barbara Ann PALMER, Vivien FERRIER, Anthony John FRANCIS, Carl HANRATTY, Martin James HEARDMAN

Westerhope Medical Group
377 Stamfordham Road, Westerhope, Newcastle upon Tyne NE5 2LH
Tel: 0191 243 7000 Fax: 0191 243 7006
(Newcastle Primary Care Trust)
Patient List Size: 12000

Practice Manager Jane Moore

GP Alison Jane SMITH, Sue CLASPER, Pamela Marie COIPEL, David Toby LIPMAN, John O'KEEFE, Ruth Margaret REES, Andrew Philip THOMPSON, Nicholas James WILD

Whickham Health Centre
Rectory Lane, Whickham, Newcastle upon Tyne NE16 4PD
Tel: 0191 488 5555 Fax: 0191 496 0424
(Gateshead Primary Care Trust)

GP Graeme OLIVER, Lynne Eileen BLOXHAM, Sarah Joanna HUNT, Stephen Francis KIRK, Ian Christopher LEE, Malcolm MACE, John Francis McNULTY, Malcolm John SMITH

White Medical Group
Thornhill Road, Ponteland, Newcastle upon Tyne NE20 9PZ
Tel: 01661 822222 Fax: 01661 821994
(Northumberland Care Trust)

Practice Manager Janet Boakes

GP John Paul McHUGH, Gillian Margaret NOBLE, Thomas SCRATCHERD

Wideopen Medical Centre
Great North Road, Wideopen, Newcastle upon Tyne NE13 6LN
Tel: 0191 236 2115 Fax: 0191 236 2116
(North Tyneside Primary Care Trust)

GP Dr D'SILVA, Dr LIDDLE, Dr MAY

Woodlands Park Health Centre
Canterbury Way, Wideopen, Newcastle upon Tyne NE13 6JL
Tel: 0191 236 2366 Fax: 0191 236 7619
(North Tyneside Primary Care Trust)
Patient List Size: 5800

Practice Manager Margaret Maxwell

GP James Francis TURLEY, Paul Thomas MORRIS, Hazel Joan NEEDHAM

Newent

Holts Health Centre
Watery Lane, Newent GL18 1BA
Tel: 01531 820689
(West Gloucestershire Primary Care Trust)
Patient List Size: 10100

Practice Manager P Moreton

GP Ian Adrian COCKS, Kathlyn Anne DREWETT, Andrew HENSON, David Norman SILLINCE, David Gareth WILLIAMS

Newhaven

Chapel Street Surgery
Chapel Street, Newhaven BN9 9PW
Tel: 01273 517000 Fax: 01273 515845
(Sussex Downs and Weald Primary Care Trust)

GP Anthony BRADBURY, Rosalind DAINTREE, George KNOX

Quayside Medical Practice
Chapel Street, Newhaven BN9 9PW
Tel: 01273 615000 Fax: 01273 611527
(Sussex Downs and Weald Primary Care Trust)

Practice Manager Ryan Christina

GP Roger FIGGINS, Alan Marcus BARKER, Mary Jeanne Patricia KAVANAGH, Paul Nicholas MOORE, Deborah June SHARP

Newmarket

Dr Polkinhorn and Partners
The Surgery, Boyden Close, Nunnery Green, Wickhambrook, Newmarket CB8 8XU
Tel: 01440 820140/820140 Fax: 01440 823809
(Suffolk West Primary Care Trust)
Patient List Size: 4300

Practice Manager Libby Hoffman

GP John Skewes POLKINHORN, Angela Florence CLIFTON-BROWN, Paul Hayes COOPER, Philip Martin LLOYD-JONES

Oakfield Surgery
Vicarage Road, Newmarket CB8 8JF
Tel: 01638 662018 Fax: 01638 660294
(Suffolk West Primary Care Trust)

Practice Manager Zena Cornell

GP Simon ARTHUR, Andrea BARKLEY, Deepa GUPTA, Paul SILVERSTON

Orchard House Surgery
Fred Archer Way, Newmarket CB8 8NU
Tel: 01638 663322 Fax: 01638 561921
(Suffolk West Primary Care Trust)
Patient List Size: 8800

Practice Manager Gill Burry

GP John William CALVERT, Theodore Robert Simon BAILEY, Judith Amanda LOMAS, Judith McLAREN, Dr PULLAN, Rupert Orlando WACE, Warwick Jeremy Stephen WEBB

Rookery Medical Centre
Rookery House, Newmarket CB8 8NW
Tel: 01638 665711 Fax: 01638 561280
(Suffolk West Primary Care Trust)
Patient List Size: 14000

Practice Manager Jane Taylor

GP Anthony John Simon WHITE, Melanie JACKSON, Richard James LONGMAN, Emma RAMSAY, Paul SABAW, Mary SELBY, Michael Robert Ian SLOWE, Kumar SRISKANDAN, Malini WACE

Newnham

The Surgery
High Street, Newnham GL14 1BE
Tel: 01594 516241 Fax: 01594 516801
(West Gloucestershire Primary Care Trust)
Patient List Size: 3300

Practice Manager Sharon Head

GP Raj Vasan BHAGEERUTTY, Anthea Louise BEE, Chris NANCOLLAS

Newport, Isle of Wight

Carisbrooke Health Centre
22 Carisbrooke Road, Newport PO30 1NR
Tel: 01983 522150 Fax: 01983 825902
Email: carisbrooke@gp-J84011.nhs.uk
(Isle of Wight Primary Care Trust)
Patient List Size: 8600

Practice Manager Ivor Warlow

GP Hugh Cameron Muir MACLEAN, David Henry ISAAC, Ide McCARTHY, Judith Sarah MOORE, Patrick WILLS

The Dower House Surgery
27 Pyle Street, Newport PO30 1JW
Tel: 01983 523525 Fax: 01983 535710
(Isle of Wight Primary Care Trust)

GP H L CLARKE, R J KNIGHT, C N A MOBBS, F S B NEGRO, M H SIMMONS, Timothy R WHELAN

South Wight Medical Practice
The Surgery, New Road, Brighstone, Newport PO30 4BB
Tel: 01983 740219 Fax: 01983 741399
Email: brightstone@gp-J84016.nhs.uk
(Isle of Wight Primary Care Trust)
Patient List Size: 5500

Practice Manager Jean Kennett

GP Alan Kenneth HAYES, Gabi T FRITZSCHE, Ashley Robert GORDON, Peter J HILL

West Street Surgery
16 West Street, Newport PO30 1PR
Tel: 01983 522198 Fax: 01983 524258
(Isle of Wight Primary Care Trust)
Patient List Size: 6500

GP Maurice Ronald BROOKS, Alasdair Roy GOVE, Gert Martin KAISER, Ilona TOBEY

Newport, Shropshire

Linden Hall Surgery
Station Road, Newport TF10 7EN
Tel: 01952 820400 Fax: 01952 825149
(Telford and Wrekin Primary Care Trust)

Practice Manager Janet Brotherton

GP Christopher Henry LISK, Roger J HENDERSON, S WALDENHORF

Wellington Road Surgery
Wellington Road, Newport TF10 7HG
Tel: 01952 811677 Fax: 01952 825981
(Telford and Wrekin Primary Care Trust)
Patient List Size: 12500

Practice Manager Lynn Kupiec

GP Nicholas John TINDALL, Joanna BALDCOCK, Aidan A EGLESTON, Jonathan S FITZGERALD-FRAZER, Jane Anne METCALF, Stephen William POWELL, Michael STAITE

Newport Pagnell

Kingfisher Surgery
26 Elthorne Way, Newport Pagnell MK16 0JR
Tel: 01908 618265 Fax: 01908 217804
(Milton Keynes Primary Care Trust)
Patient List Size: 8200

Practice Manager Elizabeth A Webber

GP Alexander Campbell PATON, Pedro MORAN-RASCHIO, Catherine Anne PATON

Newport Pagnell Medical Centre
Queens Avenue, Newport Pagnell MK16 8QT
Tel: 01908 611767 Fax: 01908 615099
Website: www.npmc.nhs.uk
(Milton Keynes Primary Care Trust)
Patient List Size: 16000

Practice Manager Helen Core

GP Ian Spencer CARTER, James Norman Gray GILCHRIST, Christopher Robert HERMAN, Caroline Katherine Rose HICKSON, Dr HOLOWKA, L JAMES, Peter John SKINNER

Newquay

Dalton House Surgery
66 Edgcumbe Avenue, Newquay TR7 2NN
Tel: 01637 873209
(Central Cornwall Primary Care Trust)
Patient List Size: 2116

Practice Manager J Boulton

GP John Victor William BOULTON

Narrowcliff Surgery
Narrowcliff, Newquay TR7 2QF
Tel: 01637 873363 Fax: 01637 850735
(Central Cornwall Primary Care Trust)
Patient List Size: 10500

Practice Manager Georgina Curtin

GP John Howard INGLE, Lloyd Gary KERSH, Douglas MACREADY, Justin RANDELL, Charles STEPHENS, Vivien WIGHT

St Thomas Road Health Centre
St Thomas Road, Newquay TR7 1RU
Tel: 01637 878599/872956 Fax: 01637 878937
(Central Cornwall Primary Care Trust)
Patient List Size: 6200

GP Thomas Michael ETTLING, David A HOOD, Christine Bryden Johnson HUNTER, Nicholas D WALKER

Newton-le-Willows

Bridge Street Surgery
48 Bridge Street, Newton-le-Willows WA12 9QS
Tel: 01925 225755
(St Helens Primary Care Trust)

GP H R MAHAJAN, Narendra Vithal SHETTY

Market Street Surgery
102 Market Street, Newton-le-Willows WA12 9BP
Tel: 01925 221457
(St Helens Primary Care Trust)

Practice Manager Irene Cullen

GP Antony JAMES, Jane CROMPTON, Zaheer HUSSAIN, Patricia Anne MALHAM

Patterdale Lodge Medical Centre
Legh Street, Newton-le-Willows WA12 9NA
Tel: 01925 227111 Fax: 01925 294701
(St Helens Primary Care Trust)

Practice Manager Pat Shepherd

GP Shah Mohammed Siddique RAHMAN, Stephen Harcourt LOWE, Andrew William OSBORNE, Julie Anne Teresa WHITTAKER, Ian Charles WYNNE

Primary Health Care Medical Centre
31 Wargrave Road, Newton-le-Willows WA12 9QN
Tel: 01925 220469 Fax: 01925 229114
(St Helens Primary Care Trust)

Practice Manager Linda Raza

GP Mohsin RAZA

Newton Abbot

Albany Surgery
Albany Street, Newton Abbot TQ12 2TX
Tel: 01626 334411 Fax: 01626 335663
Website: www.albanysurgery.co.uk
(Teignbridge Primary Care Trust)
Patient List Size: 10307

Practice Manager Robert Elliott

GP Richard Geoffrey Huddart WADE, Norman Harold DOIDGE, Barry Perkins HENWOOD, Michael John RICHARDS, Andrew John ROBINSON

Ashburton Surgery
1 Eastern Road, Ashburton, Newton Abbot TQ13 7AP
Tel: 01364 652440 Fax: 01364 654273
Website: www.ashburtonsurgery.co.uk
(Teignbridge Primary Care Trust)
Patient List Size: 5600

Practice Manager Richard Mitchell

GP Peter BELLAMY, Stephanie DYER, Kate FIELD, Richard John HOPKINS, Paul Michael THOMAS

Buckland Surgery
1 Raleigh Road, Buckland, Newton Abbot TQ12 4HG
Tel: 01626 332813 Fax: 01626 332814
(Teignbridge Primary Care Trust)

Practice Manager Louise Cooke

GP Jill Patricia MILLAR, Richard PERRETT

Chagford Health Centre
Chagford, Newton Abbot TQ13 8BW
Tel: 01647 433320 Fax: 01647 432425
(Mid Devon Primary Care Trust)
Patient List Size: 3075

Practice Manager Judi Fowler

GP Peter Trevor WOOD, Maria-Teresa CLARIDGE, Sarah WOLLASTON

Cricketfield Surgery
Cricketfield Road, Newton Abbot TQ12 2AS
Tel: 01626 208020 Fax: 01626 333356
(Teignbridge Primary Care Trust)
Patient List Size: 11000

Practice Manager Loraine Chudley

GP Robin Neil ASHWORTH, Sue C BINNING, Harriet Mary EVERY, Thomas Arthur Watkin MORRIS, John Richard STACKHOUSE, Richard William George WARD, Kavin John WRIGHT

Devon Square Surgery
Devon Square Surgery, Newton Abbot TQ12 2HH
Tel: 01626 332182 Fax: 01626 334986
Email: devon.square@which.net
(Teignbridge Primary Care Trust)
Patient List Size: 7500

Practice Manager Mike Stewart

GP Aidan Ronald DUNN, Richard Neil BRYANT, Susan Janette CRONSHAW, Michael James Curtis LEE

Kingsteignton Surgery
Whiteway Road, Kingsteignton, Newton Abbot TQ12 3HN
Tel: 01626 883312 Fax: 01626 336406
(Teignbridge Primary Care Trust)

Practice Manager Clare Randall

GP Adrian John ALMOND, Philip James Douglas ARTHUR, Charles Malcolm AVERY, Karen BATES, Mark Christian CLARVIS, Derek George GREATOREX, Diane MILBURN, Nicola Sarah SOFFE

Moretonhampstead Health Centre
Embleford Crescent, Moretonhampstead, Newton Abbot TQ13 8LW
Tel: 01647 440591 Fax: 01647 440089
Email: moretonhampstead.surgery@gp-L83049.nhs.uk
(Mid Devon Primary Care Trust)
Patient List Size: 3030

Practice Manager Ros Carr

GP Timothy Alastair DUDGEON, Vivienne Kay BEDDOE, David D E ROGERS

Riverside Surgery
Le Molay Littry Way, Bovey Tacey, Newton Abbot TQ13 9QP
Tel: 01626 832666
(Teignbridge Primary Care Trust)
Patient List Size: 12700

Practice Manager Justine Scott

GP Peter Hugh STANLEY, Neville Peter Richard BROWN, Alan HALE, John Douglas HEATHER, Douglas Ernest Leonard HOWES, Keith MAYBIN, Felicity Anne PARKER

School Road Health Centre
School Road, Kingskerwell, Newton Abbot TQ12 3HN
Tel: 01803 873551 Fax: 01803 875774
(Teignbridge Primary Care Trust)
Patient List Size: 8500

Practice Manager Robert Anthony Hooper

GP Nicholas John D'ARCY, Peter Richard GALLI, Rowena NICHOLSON, Emma ORAM, Nicholas Ian ROBERTS, Sally Ann ROBERTS

Newton Aycliffe

Bewick Crescent Surgery
27 Bewick Crescent, Newton Aycliffe DL5 5LH
Tel: 01325 313289 Fax: 01325 301428
(Sedgefield Primary Care Trust)
Patient List Size: 14810

Practice Manager Mike McDermott

GP Mark Richard BAMFORD, Gordon FERGUSON, Martin Glynne JONES, Robert Martin McKINTY, Peter Denis RAMSAY, Frank Coutts SAUNDERS, Christopher John STEPHENSON, Mark WELSH

The Jubilee Medical Group
Cobblers Hall Surgery, Cobblers Hall, Burn Lane, Newton Aycliffe DL5 4SE
Tel: 01325 311300 Fax: 01325 301389
(Sedgefield Primary Care Trust)

Practice Manager M Kersley

GP Howard MARTIN, Julian Vincent FOX, Hilary Jane LUDER

The Pease Way Medical Centre
2 Pease Way, Newton Aycliffe DL5 5NH
Tel: 01325 301888 Fax: 01325 304396
(Sedgefield Primary Care Trust)
Patient List Size: 10300

Practice Manager David Lowe

GP David Maxwell SHELDON, Andrew Stuart CLARKE, Craig HEATH, Ronald POUNDER

Normanton

High Street Surgery
High Street, Normanton WF6 1AA
Tel: 01924 893277 Fax: 01924 223535
(Eastern Wakefield Primary Care Trust)

Practice Manager Sue Garratt

GP Paul DEWHIRST

Newland Surgery
Newland Lane, Normanton WF6 1QD
Tel: 01924 220256 Fax: 01924 220558
(Eastern Wakefield Primary Care Trust)
Patient List Size: 4450

Practice Manager Lynn Mears

GP P K VENU, Ram Prasad GUPTA

Patience Lane Surgery
Patience Lane, Altofts, Normanton WF6 2JZ
Tel: 01924 890729 Fax: 01924 896546
(Eastern Wakefield Primary Care Trust)
Patient List Size: 2588

Practice Manager Pam Moss

GP Gokaraju ARUNA PRASAD

Princess Street Surgery
63 Princess Street, Normanton WF6 1AB
Tel: 01924 892132 Fax: 01924 898168
(Eastern Wakefield Primary Care Trust)
Patient List Size: 9550

Practice Manager Christine Sanderson

GP E BARBER, Marc Louis Francois BAZIN, David William BROWN, P MOONEY, J M WALSH

The Surgery
148 Castleford Road, Normanton WF6 2EP
Tel: 01924 223636 Fax: 01924 220252
(Eastern Wakefield Primary Care Trust)

Practice Manager Anne Golby

GP R WUNNA

North Ferriby

The Surgery
15 School Lane, North Ferriby HU14 3DB
Tel: 01482 634004
(East Yorkshire Primary Care Trust)

Practice Manager Karen Mitchell

GP Robert Grieg MITCHELL

West End Surgery
10 West End, Swanland, North Ferriby HU14 3PE
Tel: 01482 633570 Fax: 01482 632507
(East Yorkshire Primary Care Trust)

Practice Manager C Clarke

GP Ronald Gibb CLARKE

North Shields

Appleby Surgery
Hawkeys Lane, North Shields NE29 0SF
Tel: 0191 296 1770 Fax: 0191 296 1770
(North Tyneside Primary Care Trust)

Practice Manager Maureen Lilley

GP Andrew Michael BATES, Kathryn Margaret CURRY, Rachel Jane FIRTH, S PROCTOR

Collingwood Surgery
Hawkeys Lane, North Shields NE29 0SF
Tel: 0191 257 1779 Fax: 0191 226 9909
(North Tyneside Primary Care Trust)
Patient List Size: 12000

Practice Manager Alice Southern

GP William George TAPSFIELD, L A ASHTON, Amit Kumar CHATTERJEE, Liz HARRISON, Diana Mary JELLEY, Dawn Vanessa LINFORD, jane PERRY, David Peter Carey TOMSON, Timothy David VAN ZWANENBERG

Nelson Health Centre
Cecil Street, North Shields NE29 0DZ
Tel: 0191 257 1204/4001 Fax: 0191 258 7191
(North Tyneside Primary Care Trust)

Practice Manager Vivien Cairns

GP Pratima MEHRA, David Richard PARKINSON, Gillian PARKINSON, Thomas John WESTGARTH

Nelson Health Centre
Cecil Street, North Shields NE29 0DZ
Tel: 0191 257 1191 Fax: 0191 258 4961
(North Tyneside Primary Care Trust)

GP Ram Krishna TIWARI, Manju MALIK

New York Surgery
Brookland Terrace, New York, North Shields NE29 8EA
Tel: 0191 258 5316 Fax: 0191 257 8231
(North Tyneside Primary Care Trust)

Practice Manager George Sallie

The Priory Medical Group
19 Albion Road, North Shields NE29 0HT
(North Tyneside Primary Care Trust)

Practice Manager E Smith

GP J B ROBERTS

Rose, Walker, Chaudhei and Scarlett
Spring Terrace Health Centre, Spring Terrace, North Shields NE29 0HQ
Tel: 0191 296 1588 Fax: 0191 296 2901
(North Tyneside Primary Care Trust)
Patient List Size: 6500

Practice Manager Janet Robson

GP Kathleen Fionuala ROSE, S M B CHAUDHRI, C E SCARLETT, Sally Elizabeth WALKER

Spring Terrace Health Centre
Spring Terrace Health Centre, Spring Terrace, North Shields NE30 1PW
Tel: 0191 296 1366 Fax: 0191 257 4050
(North Tyneside Primary Care Trust)

Practice Manager C Lilley

Tynemouth Medical Centre
Percy Street, North Shields NE30 4HD
(North Tyneside Primary Care Trust)

Wallsend Road Medical Centre
34 Wallsend Road, North Shields NE29 7BJ
Tel: 0191 296 1456 Fax: 0191 2573127
(North Tyneside Primary Care Trust)
Patient List Size: 3700

Practice Manager Louise New

GP Christine Barbara TOSE, Alexis Sharon GANDY, Timothy PEARSON

North Walsham

Birchwood Surgery
Park Lane, North Walsham NR28 0BQ
Tel: 01692 402035 Fax: 01692 409609
Email: birchwoodsurgery@fsmail.net
Website: www.birchwoodsurgery.co.uk
(North Norfolk Primary Care Trust)
Patient List Size: 10500

Practice Manager Linda Leavold

GP Paul Ralph EVERDEN, Patricia BUNNING, Stuart Leighton DAVIDSON, James Donald GAIR, John LUCK, Sian Angharad TYRYNIS-THOMAS

Paston Surgery
9-11 Park Lane, North Walsham NR28 0BQ
Tel: 01692 403015 Fax: 01692 500619
(North Norfolk Primary Care Trust)

GP Graham Anthony Roscoe PRICE, Simon Mark Andrew VAVASOUR, Frances WHITFIELD, Richard John YOUNG

Northallerton

Mayford House Surgery
Boroughbridge Road, Northallerton DL7 8AW
Tel: 01609 772105 Fax: 01609 778553
(Hambleton and Richmondshire Primary Care Trust)

Practice Manager Graham Espiner

GP Andrew Watson CURRY, Hilary Jane ENEVOLDSON, Georgina Dawn JACKSON, Christopher Glyn OATES, Peter Andrew RAMSDEN, Antony WALTERS

Mowbray House
Malpas Road, Northallerton DL7 8FW
Tel: 01609 775281 Fax: 01609 778029
(Hambleton and Richmondshire Primary Care Trust)
Patient List Size: 15800

Practice Manager Richard Rodley

GP Andrew George BRERETON, Lorraine Jane BURTON, Amanda Mary EAMES, Peter James EDON, Simon William Percy MIERS, Nick PALMERLEY, Duncan Paul Evans ROGERS, Catherine Louise TODD, John Henry WALDRON

RAF Medical Centre
RAF Leeming, Northallerton DL7 9NJ
Tel: 01677 457141 Fax: 01677 457001
(Hambleton and Richmondshire Primary Care Trust)

Regional Medical Centre
Royal Air Force, Leeming, Northallerton DL7 9NJ
Tel: 01677 457567 Fax: 01677 457001
(Hambleton and Richmondshire Primary Care Trust)
Patient List Size: 2743

Practice Manager D E McLeish

GP M REYNOLDS, J BROWN, D NICOLL

Whorlton Village Hall Surgery
Swainby, Northallerton DL6 3HT

GP B H DAVIES

Northampton

Abington Health Complex
Doctors Surgery, 51A Beech Avenue, Northampton NN3 2JG
Tel: 01604 791999 Fax: 01604 450155
(Northampton Primary Care Trust)
Patient List Size: 12250

Practice Manager Lorna McMillan

GP Michael KIRWAN, William Gerard ASKEW, David George Warwick BUCKLER, Peter Bertwistle MEDCALF, Simon THOMPSON

Abington Park Surgery
Christchurch Medical Centre, Ardington Road, Northampton NN1 5LT
Tel: 01604 630291 Fax: 01604 603524
Email: aps.patients@gp-K83029.nhs.uk
Website: www.abingtonparksurgery.co.uk
(Northampton Primary Care Trust)
Patient List Size: 10630

Practice Manager Ian Watson

GP David Maxwell GILLAM, Hilary Edith HALSTEAD, Catherine MASSEY, Stephanie Jane Evans SMITH, Kamal Kumar SOOD, Liezl SULLIVAN

Brook Medical Centre
Ecton Brook Road, Northampton NN3 5EN
Tel: 01604 401185 Fax: 01604 403268
(Northampton Primary Care Trust)
Patient List Size: 6200

Practice Manager Gordon Baxter

GP Mukul SWAROOP, Patrick Kevin BYRNE, Deepa SWAROOP

Clarence Avenue Surgery
14 Clarence Avenue, Northampton NN2 6NZ
Tel: 01604 718464 Fax: 01604 721589
(Northampton Primary Care Trust)

Practice Manager Rita Allen

GP Thomas John WHITE, Richard VALENTINE

County Surgery
202-204 Abington Avenue, Northampton NN1 4QA
Tel: 01604 632918 Fax: 01604 601578
(Northampton Primary Care Trust)
Patient List Size: 4400

Practice Manager Sian McLennan

GP David Charles WADE, Santiago DARGALLO NIETO

Crescent Medical Centre
2 The Crescent, Northampton NN1 4SB
Tel: 01604 713434 Fax: 01604 717689
(Northampton Primary Care Trust)
Patient List Size: 7600

Practice Manager Julie Pavitt

GP Rick F FREEMAN, Christopher WALDRUM

Danes Camp Surgery
Rowtree Road, East Hunsbury, Northampton NN4 0NY
Tel: 01604 709426 Fax: 01604 709427
(Northampton Primary Care Trust)
Patient List Size: 6500

Practice Manager Marilyn Hodges

GP Martin Charles COOMBS, Jennifer Marianne JOHNSON, Peter John WALTERS

Delapre Medical Centre
Gloucester Avenue, Northampton NN4 8QF
Tel: 01604 761713 Fax: 01604 708589
(Northampton Primary Care Trust)
Patient List Size: 10850

Practice Manager Mark Leonald

GP Richard Ian Reid WILLOWS, Mark Derek BARROWCLOUGH, Jagtar CHHINA, Charlotte Fiona DUNCAN, Nicholas David HEWITT, Jacqueline Elizabeth KING, Carolyn Jane PERRYER

Dr A Willis and Partners
King Edward Road Surgery, Christchurch Medical Centre, King Edward Road, Northampton NN1 5LY
Tel: 01604 633466/634593 Fax: 01604 603227
Email: firstname.lastname@gp-K83012.nhs.uk
(Northampton Primary Care Trust)
Patient List Size: 8700

Practice Manager Margaret Hoppitt

GP Andrew William WILLIS, Simon David GREGORY, Claire JENKS, Allan Edwin LEROY, Judith Alison REEDER, John RICKERBY, Ann-Marie WOOD

Dr Blackman and Partners
28 West Street, Earls Barton, Northampton NN6 0EW
Tel: 01604 810219 Fax: 01604 810401
(Northamptonshire Heartlands Primary Care Trust)

Practice Manager Lyn Brook

GP Catherine P BLACKMAN

Flore Surgery
Bricketts Lane, Flore, Northampton NN7 4LU
(Daventry and South Northamptonshire Primary Care Trust)

GP R GARDNER

Greenview Surgery
129 Hazeldene Road, Northampton NN2 7PB
Tel: 01604 791002 Fax: 01604 721822
(Northampton Primary Care Trust)

Practice Manager Pat Jakeman

GP Peter James HALSTEAD, Tiffany Elizabeth CRAWFORD, Nuala Marie KELLY, Helen Janet SPENCER

Guilsborough Surgery

High Street, Guilsborough, Northampton NN6 8PU
Tel: 01604 740210/740142 Fax: 01604 740869
(Daventry and South Northamptonshire Primary Care Trust)
Patient List Size: 6700

Practice Manager Kathryn Baines

GP Catherine Mary MOSS, Julia Elizabeth BOON, Neil MENON, Simon Frank TWIGG

Harborough Road Surgery

Harborough Road North, Northampton NN2 8LL
Tel: 01604 845144 Fax: 01604 820241
(Northampton Primary Care Trust)

Practice Manager Jo Stroud

GP Peter Bruce LITTLEWOOD, Vivienne Jane ABBOTT, R BOWATER, L R LAD

Harlestone Road Surgery

117 Harlestone Road, Northampton NN5 7AQ
Tel: 01604 751832 Fax: 01604 586065
Website: www.drgillandpartners.co.uk
(Northampton Primary Care Trust)
Patient List Size: 15000

Practice Manager Debbie Green

GP Thomas John GILL, Martin ADAMS, Philip ASTBURY, Sinead Mary ROGERS, Caroline Elizabeth SAYNOR, John Frederic TANQUERAY

Kingsthorpe Medical Centre

Eastern Avenue South, Northampton NN2 7JN
Tel: 01604 713823 Fax: 01604 721996
(Northampton Primary Care Trust)
Patient List Size: 6000

Practice Manager Wendy Davies

GP Firozali Abdulhusein MAKHANI, Diana Catherine BUCK, Dr PARDHAN

Langham Place Surgery

11 Langham Place, Northampton NN2 6AA
Tel: 01604 38162
(Northampton Primary Care Trust)
Patient List Size: 8500

Practice Manager Jenny Mills

GP Dominic SEFTON, Armed AJAZ, Naomi Eliza COLDWELL, Judith Patricia DAWSON, Sarah Lindsay GREENING, Brian Andrew WILSON

Leicester Terrace Health Care Centre

8 Leicester Terrace, Northampton NN2 6AL
Tel: 01604 633682 Fax: 01604 233408
Email: miriam.muller@-K83014.nhs.uk
(Northampton Primary Care Trust)
Patient List Size: 10800

Practice Manager Susan Hart

GP John Leaver WALTON, Sue COTES, Andrew GILMORE, Fiona Catherine MOORE, Ahmed SHURRAB, David John SMART

Levitts Surgery

Levitts Road, Bugbrooke, Northampton NN7 3QN
Tel: 01604 830348 Fax: 01604 832785
(Daventry and South Northamptonshire Primary Care Trust)

Practice Manager Barbara Auburn

GP Dipak Kumar DUTTA, David William Joseph MILLER, Jonathan Howard SHRIBMAN, Helen Marie WARWICK

Long Buckby Practice

24 Station Road, Long Buckby, Northampton NN6 7QB
Tel: 01327 842360 Fax: 01327 842302
Email: longbuckby.practice@gp-K83019.nhs.uk
(Daventry and South Northamptonshire Primary Care Trust)
Patient List Size: 5900

Practice Manager David Billingham

GP Graham William CRADDUCK, Sean Graham GOWER, Julia Anne KENDALL, Sara Anne THOMPSON

Mounts Medical Centre

Campbell Street, Northampton NN1 3DS
Tel: 01604 631952 Fax: 01604 634139
(Northampton Primary Care Trust)
Patient List Size: 11000

Practice Manager Vivien Vials

GP J A G RAPHAEL, S S DALE, Donovan Glyndyr Frederick JEFFREYS, S SADEK, Anthony James WILLIAMS

New Croft Surgery

57 New Croft, Weedon, Northampton NN7 4RX
Tel: 01327 340212 Fax: 01327 349728
(Daventry and South Northamptonshire Primary Care Trust)

Practice Manager Elizabeth Perry

GP Jonathan Henry Woodiwiss HILL, Richard Ronan GARDNER, Katherin Elizabeth HILL, E N WILLIAMS

Northampton Lane North Surgery

120 Northampton Lane North, Moulton, Northampton NN3 7QP
Tel: 01604 790108 Fax: 01604 670827
(Northampton Primary Care Trust)
Patient List Size: 9100

Practice Manager Sue Saunders

GP Jonathan Peter IRELAND, Roger David BAILEY, J POPE, Darin Guy SEIGER, A STEPHEN, T VASKOVIC

Orchard Lane Surgery

Orchard Lane, Denton, Northampton NN7 1HT
Tel: 01604 890313 Fax: 01604 890143
(Northampton Primary Care Trust)
Patient List Size: 4600

Practice Manager Barbara White

GP Anthony Jean-Marie Coutin PICKERING, Richard James ABBATT, Helen Mary COGHILL

Park Avenue Medical Centre

166-168 Park Avenue North, Northampton NN3 2HZ
Tel: 01604 716500 Fax: 01604 721685
(Northampton Primary Care Trust)
Patient List Size: 9800

Practice Manager Cheryl Harrald

GP Nigel John BIRD, Patricia Elaine AITCHESON, David John CLEAL, Julia Kate FLETCHER, Helen Margaret MEAD, Desmin Pierce O'CALLAGHAN

Park Slope Surgery

32 Stoke Road, Blisworth, Northampton NN7 3BT
Tel: 01604 858237 Fax: 01604 859437
(Daventry and South Northamptonshire Primary Care Trust)

Practice Manager Marilyn Hodges

GP Anthony Robert HILLIER, Jonathan Breck TAYLOR

Penvale Park Medical Centre

Hardwick Road, East Hunsbury, Northampton NN4 0GP
Tel: 01604 700660 Fax: 01604 700772
(Northampton Primary Care Trust)

Practice Manager Jane Smith

GP Shashikant Ratilal PATEL

Pytchley Court Health Centre

5 Northampton Road, Brixworth, Northampton NN6 9DX
Tel: 01604 880228 Fax: 01604 880467
(Daventry and South Northamptonshire Primary Care Trust)
Patient List Size: 6400

Practice Manager Sue Salmon

GP Michael Robert SOUTHCOTT, David Joseph ALSTON, Estelle BRIGGS

Queensview Medical Centre
Thornton Road, Northampton NN2 6LS
Tel: 01604 713315 Fax: 01604 714378
Email: **@gpk8003.nhs.uk
(Northampton Primary Care Trust)
Patient List Size: 9700

Practice Manager Margaret Keegan

GP David John THORNTON, Daniel Fritz Robert DE BRAUW, Brian Richard RIGDEN, Alex J SWAN

Rillwood Medical Centre
Tonmead Road, Lumbertubs, Northampton NN3 8HZ
Tel: 01604 405006 Fax: 01604 410826
(Northampton Primary Care Trust)
Patient List Size: 4300

Practice Manager Patrick Morgan

GP Chekka KRISHNA RAO, P ARUMUGAM

Roade Medical Centre
16 London Road, Roade, Northampton NN7 2NN
Tel: 01604 862218 Fax: 01604 862129
Website: www.mydoc-online.com
(Daventry and South Northamptonshire Primary Care Trust)

Practice Manager Muriel Tucker

GP Alison Dawn OTTO, M R SHAH, Naeem YOUNUS

The Surgery
16 Watford Road, Crick, Northampton NN6 7TT
Tel: 01788 822203 Fax: 01788 824177
(Daventry and South Northamptonshire Primary Care Trust)
Patient List Size: 4150

Practice Manager Shirley Silvester

GP Alan Robert Godfrey WARD, Annette Isobel TWIGG

Weston Favell Health Centre
Weston Favell Centre, Northampton NN3 8DW
Tel: 01604 409631 Fax: 01604 786738
(Northampton Primary Care Trust)
Patient List Size: 3400

Practice Manager Gill Taylor

GP Abu Layes MOLLA, Venkata Rao KESANI

Weston Favell Health Centre
Weston Favell Centre, Billing Brook Road, Northampton NN3 8DW
Tel: 01604 785027 Fax: 01604 414880
(Northampton Primary Care Trust)
Patient List Size: 3840

Practice Manager Fay Hinton

GP Azim Abdulkarim LAKHA

Weston Favell Health Centre
Weston Favell Centre, Northampton NN3 8DW
Tel: 01604 409002 Fax: 01604 407034
(Northampton Primary Care Trust)

Practice Manager Jenny Ryan

GP Barbara Lois MORRANT

Weston Favell Health Centre
Weston Favell Centre, Northampton NN3 8DW
Tel: 01604 415157 Fax: 01604 407472
(Northampton Primary Care Trust)

Practice Manager Mrs Andreoli

GP S M HASSAN, K S LAMBA

Whitefields Surgery
Hunsbury Hill Road, Camp Hill, Northampton NN4 9UW
Tel: 01604 760171 Fax: 01604 708528
Website: www.whitefields-surgery.co.uk
(Northampton Primary Care Trust)

Practice Manager Dana Ball

GP Andrew Thomas STOCKLEY, Judith HUNT, Pieter WALSMA

Woodview Medical Centre
26 Holmecross Road, Thorplands, Northampton NN3 8AW
Tel: 01604 670780 Fax: 01604 646208
(Northampton Primary Care Trust)

Practice Manager Chrisi Burns

GP Kenneth Stephen ELLAM, John Alexander BOLLAND, Ruth Eileen DAVIES, Virendra Kumar DOGRA, Royston Frank WILLIAMS, (Mary) Philippa WOOD

Wootton Medical Centre
36-38 High Street, Wootton, Northampton NN4 6LW
Tel: 01604 709933 Fax: 01604 709944
(Northampton Primary Care Trust)
Patient List Size: 5458

Practice Manager Shirley Connolly

GP Christopher John Frost MOORE, Elizabeth Shan DAVIES, Hilary Anne PENFOLD

Northolt

The Barnabas Medical Centre
Girton Road, Northolt UB5 4SR
Tel: 020 8864 4437 Fax: 020 8423 6929
(Ealing Primary Care Trust)
Patient List Size: 8200

Practice Manager Paul Ranken

GP M G PARMAR, Harj K BHATOA, K W HUI, David Graham KNIGHT, Harpreet Singh KOONER

The Grove Medical Practice
81 Danemead Grove, Petts Hill, Northolt UB5 4NY
Tel: 020 8423 8423 Fax: 020 8423 5578
(Ealing Primary Care Trust)
Patient List Size: 3200

Practice Manager Surinder Allum

GP Rameshchandra Kantilal BHATT

The Medical Centre
45 Doncaster Drive, Northolt UB5 4AT
Tel: 020 8864 8133 Fax: 020 8423 2963
(Ealing Primary Care Trust)
Patient List Size: 5000

GP Govindasamy BALACHANDRAN

The Surgery
3 Mandeville Road, Northolt UB5 5HB
Tel: 020 8845 3275 Fax: 020 8845 1804
(Ealing Primary Care Trust)
Patient List Size: 3600

Practice Manager Jean Scott

GP S C SEIMON, P SENEVIRATNE

The Surgery
45 Islip Manor Road, Northolt UB5 5DZ
Tel: 020 8845 4911 Fax: 020 8845 9543
(Ealing Primary Care Trust)
Patient List Size: 3000

Practice Manager Tahera Khan

GP K M LATIF, Mohammed Abdul LATIF

The Surgery
38 Petts Hill, Northolt UB5 4NL
Tel: 020 8422 6113 Fax: 020 8908 0118
(Ealing Primary Care Trust)

Practice Manager Suresh Shah

GP K S SHAH

The Surgery
337 Ruislip Road, Northolt UB5 6AS
Tel: 020 8578 1537 Fax: 020 8813 2169
(Ealing Primary Care Trust)
Patient List Size: 2500

Practice Manager Jane Maclauglin

GP Bakul V JOSHI, V P JOSHI

The Surgery
141 Mandeville Road, Northolt UB5 4LZ
Tel: 020 8422 3181 Fax: 020 8621 3437
(Ealing Primary Care Trust)
Patient List Size: 3400

Practice Manager Anju Patel

GP G SIVARAJAH, T SIVARAJAH

The Surgery
296 Church Road, Northolt UB5 5AP
Tel: 020 8248 2609 Fax: 020 8723 3302
(Ealing Primary Care Trust)
Patient List Size: 3260

Practice Manager Graham Hodges

GP Fazlur Rehman QUADRI

Yeading Medical Centre
18 Hughenden Gardens, Northolt UB5 6LD
Tel: 020 8841 8222 Fax: 020 8841 6402
(Ealing Primary Care Trust)
Patient List Size: 6500

Practice Manager Flavio Gracias

GP R HASAN, S G KASSAM, P M PATEL, N R SARNA

Northwich

Castle Surgery
5 Darwin Street, Castle, Northwich CW8 1BU
Tel: 01606 74863 Fax: 01606 784847
(Central Cheshire Primary Care Trust)
Patient List Size: 7875

Practice Manager Lynda Thornley

GP John Malcolm TORRANCE, Susan Jean BROWN, Joanne HARDIE, Alan Sellers NORMAN

Danebridge Medical Centre
29 London Road, Northwich CW9 5HR
Tel: 01606 338100 Fax: 01606 331977
Email: danebridge@gp-N81087.nwest.nhs.uk
(Central Cheshire Primary Care Trust)
Patient List Size: 20915

Practice Manager Kathryn Cook

GP Christopher John BARRATT, Alan Sidney ADAMS, Mark Alexander James DICKINSON, William James FORSYTH, Lynda Kay HAENEY, Nigel Graham MATTHEWS, Fiona Ann McGREGOR-SMITH, Michael Scott MULLIN, David Andrew PERRY, Adrian Michael ROSSALL, Nichola Antonia RUSSELL

Middlewich Street Surgery
163-165 Middlewich Street, Northwich CW9 7DB
Tel: 01606 43850 Fax: 01606 41337
(Central Cheshire Primary Care Trust)
Patient List Size: 6671

Practice Manager Linda Mercer

GP Vijay Mani ANTHWAL, M ALASADI, Fiona Kathryn KILBY

Oakwood Medical Centre
Oakwood Lane, Barnton, Northwich CW8 4HE
Tel: 01606 74718 Fax: 01606 784529
(Central Cheshire Primary Care Trust)
Patient List Size: 7273

Practice Manager Ann Stringer

GP John Charles KERSLAKE, Robert Oliver CHAPMAN, Rachel HARDING, Jane PARKER, T STREFFORD

Watling Medical Centre and Riverside Medical Practice
Watling Street, Northwich CW9 5EX
Tel: 01606 42445
(Central Cheshire Primary Care Trust)

Practice Manager Mandy Wright

GP Andrew BRETTELL, Robert John HUGHES, Garry Victor BARTLETT, Elizabeth Jane BILL

Weaverham Surgery
Northwich Road, Weaverham, Northwich CW8 3EU
Tel: 01606 853106 Fax: 01606 854980
Website: www.weaverhamsurgery.co.uk
(Central Cheshire Primary Care Trust)
Patient List Size: 8009

Practice Manager Frieda O'Connor

GP Paul Douglas OLDFIELD, Aileen Catherine Mary JENNINGS, Martin Brett LLEWELLYN, Robert Arthur ROYLE

Witton Street Surgery
162 Witton Street, Northwich CW9 5QU
Tel: 01606 42007 Fax: 01606 350659
Website: www.wittonstreetsurgery.co.uk
(Central Cheshire Primary Care Trust)
Patient List Size: 7500

Practice Manager Ann Jacks

GP Richard John MURPHY, Rebekah McINTOSH, Jenneth Mary PATRICK, Graham James SAUNDERS

Northwood

Northwood Health Centre
Neal Close, Acre Way, Northwood HA6 1TQ
Tel: 01923 829608 Fax: 01923 840593
(Hillingdon Primary Care Trust)
Patient List Size: 2414

Practice Manager L Levy

GP Sara Jane HARING

Northwood Health Centre
Neal Close, Acre Way, Northwood HA6 1TQ
Tel: 01923 821821 Fax: 01923 840891
(Hillingdon Primary Care Trust)

GP Syed Imad HAIDER, Malvika DALAL

Northwood Health Centre
Neal Close, Acre Way, Northwood HA6 1TQ
Tel: 01923 820866 Fax: 01923 840891
(Hillingdon Primary Care Trust)
Patient List Size: 2200

Practice Manager H Ellis

GP Christopher Anthony G STERN, Malvika DAZAL

Northwood Health Centre
Neal Close, Acre Way, Northwood HA6 1TQ
Tel: 01923 820844/833736 Fax: 01923 820648
(Hillingdon Primary Care Trust)

GP Farah HUSSAIN, Shilpa Jayantilal PATEL, Daviash Narendra THAKRAR

Norwich Road Practice
35 Norwich Road, Northwood Hills, Northwood HA6 1ND
Tel: 01923 820770 Fax: 01923 820770
(Hillingdon Primary Care Trust)
Patient List Size: 1200

Practice Manager Farida Malik

GP Anil Goverhandas GANDHI

Steven Shackman Practice
Northwood Health Centre, Neal Close, Acre Way, Northwood HA6 1TQ
Tel: 01923 828488 Fax: 01923 835548
Website: www.stevenshackmanpractice
(Hillingdon Primary Care Trust)
Patient List Size: 9300

Practice Manager Max Black

GP Ian Lawrence GOODMAN, Farida AHMAD, Elizabeth Jane HERMASZEWSKA, Subodh Rambhai KANT, Susan J PUGH, Suzanne SAIDMAN

The Surgery
3 Eastbury Road, Northwood HA6 3AB
Tel: 01923 824588 Fax: 01923 840534
(Hillingdon Primary Care Trust)

GP Paul Raymond GOODWIN, Timothy Michael BURFORD, Ewa CUMMING, Mario DI MONACO, Kuldhir K JOHAL

Norwich

Acle Medical Centre
Bridewell Lane, Acle, Norwich NR13 3RA
Tel: 01493 750888 Fax: 01493 751652
(Broadland Primary Care Trust)
Patient List Size: 8500

Practice Manager Grace Yorke

GP Nicholas John IRELAND, John Martin APPLEGATE, Michael John NOBLE, Nigel Paul ROLLS, Roger Francis TIMMS

Adelaide Street Health Centre
19 Adelaide Street, Norwich NR2 4JL
Tel: 01603 625015 Fax: 01603 766820
Email: wvmpas@aol.com
(Norwich Primary Care Trust)
Patient List Size: 12650

Practice Manager Julie Spurgeon, Mary Taylor

GP John Michael FINNEY, Andrew CHEESBROUGH, Mohamed CHILENGE, Suzannah Jane FISKE

Bacon Road Medical Centre
16 Bacon Road, Norwich NR2 3QX
Tel: 01603 503917 Fax: 01603 458793
Email: baconrd@aol.com
(Norwich Primary Care Trust)
Patient List Size: 5000

Practice Manager Angela Dew

GP Michael Desmond LAURENCE, Toni ALDERTON, Sheilini BOWRY, Christopher Richard Thomas FRANCIS

Baxter and Conway
The Surgery, Hardingham Street, Hingham, Norwich NR9 4JB
Tel: 01953 850237 Fax: 01953 850581
(Southern Norfolk Primary Care Trust)
Patient List Size: 3800

Practice Manager Joyce Halstead

GP Lawson Derek BAXTER, Shaun CONWAY

Blofield Surgery
Plantation Road, Blofield, Norwich NR13 4PL
Tel: 01603 712337 Fax: 01603 712899
(Broadland Primary Care Trust)

Practice Manager Monica Long

GP Philip Rodney HARRIS, Mark Andrew GASKIN, Mary Patricia MILLER, David John Fuller PILCH

Brundall Medical Centre
The Dales, Brundall, Norwich NR13 5RP
Tel: 01603 712255 Fax: 01603 712156
(Broadland Primary Care Trust)
Patient List Size: 8200

Practice Manager Andy Gray

GP David Adrian VARVEL, Anthony George ASHMAN, Ian Stewart GIBSON, Philip John Richard HARSTON, Anthony John RIGBY

Church Plain Surgery
Church Plain, Loddon, Norwich NR14 6EX
Tel: 01508 520222 Fax: 01508 528579
Email: loddon.doctors@nhs.net
(Southern Norfolk Primary Care Trust)

Practice Manager Christine Harris

GP Peter Mudie BARRIE, Graham Stuart CLARK, Alasdair DUTHIE, Andrew William Helm GODFREY, Anna Dilys GUY, Sharon PHILLIPS, Linda VALENTINE

Coltishall Medical Centre
St John's Close, Rectory Road, Coltishall, Norwich NR12 7HL
Tel: 01603 737593 Fax: 01603 737067
(Broadland Primary Care Trust)
Patient List Size: 7100

Practice Manager Jackie Cunington

GP Robert Montague LEANEY, Christopher Andrew MALPAS, Sanjay KUMAR, Timothy Guy Robert MANSFIELD, Neil Michael TAYLOR

Cringleford Surgery
Cantley Lane, Norwich NR4 6TA
Tel: 01603 54678 Fax: 01603 58287
(Southern Norfolk Primary Care Trust)

GP Christine BUCKTON, David John MUNSON, Siobhan ROWE

Doctors Surgery
Great Melton Road, Hethersett, Norwich NR9 3AB
Tel: 01603 810250 Fax: 01603 812402
(Broadland Primary Care Trust)

Practice Manager S Collinge

GP Dr BAYLISS-BROWN, Dr BEEBY, Dr BRANTIGAN, Dr BUCKTON, Dr HARWOOD, Dr LEAMAN, Dr MORRIS, Nicola Mary MORRIS, Dr MUNSON, Dr OVERY, Dr PRESS, Anthony Martin PRESS, Dr ROWE

Dr Harris's Surgery
Adelaide Street Health Centre, 19 Adelaide Street, Norwich NR2 4JL
Tel: 01603 622044 Fax: 01603 767289
(Norwich Primary Care Trust)
Patient List Size: 1700

Practice Manager Sarah Innes

GP Paul Rupert HARRIS

Drayton and St Faiths Medical Practice
8 Manor Farm Close, Drayton, Norwich NR8 6EE
Tel: 01603 867532 Fax: 01603 261497
(Broadland Primary Care Trust)
Patient List Size: 12800

Practice Manager Mike Scott

GP David John LEEMING, Roderick Paul BARCLAY, Ferdinand BECKON, James Samuel Oxenham DALRYMPLE, Stephen Michael DAYKIN, Alan LEE, Sarah MARTIN, James Frederick RIVETT

East Harling Surgery
Market Street, East Harling, Norwich NR16 2AD
Tel: 01953 717204 Fax: 01953 718116
(Southern Norfolk Primary Care Trust)
Patient List Size: 6700

Practice Manager Wayne Rawlings

GP Peter Timothy LOCK, Andrew Paul HAYWARD, Dr HAZELL, Dr MAIR

Gurney Surgery
101-103 Magdalen Street, Norwich NR3 1LN
Tel: 01603 448800
(Norwich Primary Care Trust)

Practice Manager Mike Trett

GP Michael CLARIDGE, Sally Louise BARNARD, Richard Frederick Tracey GILBERT, Caimin Martin HARDIMAN, Christopher Tom

HUTCHINSON, Irene Margaret McCARTNEY, Carol Ann MORETON, Hitesh PATEL, Martin SCHEDE, David Atkinson VAUGHAN

Heathgate Surgery
The Street, Poringland, Norwich NR14 7JT
Tel: 01508 494343 Fax: 01508 495423
(Southern Norfolk Primary Care Trust)
Patient List Size: 8000

Practice Manager Garry Whiting

GP John Stephen SAMPSON, Joanne Mary GILSON, Andrea MEYERHOFF, Anthony PALFRAMAN, Claire Elizabeth THIRKELL

Hellesdon Medical Practice
343 Reepham Road, Hellesdon, Norwich NR6 5QJ
Tel: 01603 486602 Fax: 01603 401389
(Broadland Primary Care Trust)

Practice Manager Simon Farrow

GP Robert STONE, Anne Carol CHEETHAM, George Nicholas DUNCAN, James Kenneth MATHEWS, Dr THORNTON, Ian Philip TOLLEY

High Green Surgery
High Green, Brooke, Norwich NR15 1JD
Tel: 01508 50204
(Southern Norfolk Primary Care Trust)

Practice Manager Hamida Sattar

GP Mohammad Abdus SATTAR

Horning Road Surgery
Horning Road West, Hoveton, Norwich NR12 8QH
Tel: 01603 782155 Fax: 01603 782189
Email: wrox.sur@paston.co.uk
(North Norfolk Primary Care Trust)
Patient List Size: 8000

Practice Manager S Taylor

GP John THURLOW, Simon Muir DOWNS, Vivienne Hazel FOWLER, Linda Christine HUNTER, James Shanklin POWELL, Clare SINGH

Horsford Medical Centre
205 Holt Road, Horsford, Norwich NR10 3DX
Tel: 01603 898300 Fax: 01603 891818
Email: horsmed@netcom.co.uk
(Broadland Primary Care Trust)
Patient List Size: 2350

Practice Manager Rachel Dave

GP Hugh Blaise O'NEILL

King's Ride Surgery
Quidenham Road, Kenninghall, Norwich NR16 2EF
Tel: 01953 887208 Fax: 01953 887515
(Southern Norfolk Primary Care Trust)

Lakenham Surgery
1 Ninham Street, Norwich NR1 3JJ
Tel: 01603 765550 Fax: 01603 766790
(Norwich Primary Care Trust)
Patient List Size: 9800

Practice Manager Philip Gainsborough

GP David Kirk BRYCE, Mark Richard Morgan FERRIS, Abraham GEORGE, Derek James GUY, Ian PHIPP, David Roger THORN

Long Stratton Health Centre
Swan Lane Surgery, Swan Lane, Thurston, Norwich NR15 2UY
Tel: 01508 530781 Fax: 01508 530700
(Southern Norfolk Primary Care Trust)

Practice Manager Mike Trett

GP Philip Gordon Patrick MANSON-BAHR, Stephen Christopher BAMBER, Kathryn Johnson KESTIN, Malcolm David Fergus WILLIS

Longwater Lane Medical Centre
Longwater Lane, Old Costessey, Norwich NR8 5AH
Tel: 01603 742021 Fax: 01603 740271
(Broadland Primary Care Trust)
Patient List Size: 7000

Practice Manager Jan Hardinge

GP James Derek TORRENS, Michael George CHERRY, Judith Mary THOMAS

Magdalen Medical Practice
Lawson Road, Norwich NR3 4LF
Tel: 01603 475555 Fax: 01603 787210
(Norwich Primary Care Trust)

Practice Manager Bert Bustin

GP John Cranston BENNETT, Charles Stewart FRASER, Donald Ormsby McGOVERN, Sunil PINTO, Anne Elizabeth RICHARDS, David Alastair ROBERTSON, Katrina Elizabeth YOUNG

Market Surgery
26 Norwich Road, Aylsham, Norwich NR11 6BW
Tel: 01263 733331 Fax: 01263 735879
(Broadland Primary Care Trust)

Practice Manager Ian Barker

GP Keith Raymond HARRISON, Nazia AHMED, Kevin Paul ELSBY, Peter Robert LAWSON, James Walter MUMFORD

Mulbarton Surgery
The Common, Mulbarton, Norwich NR14 8JG
Tel: 01508 570212 Fax: 01508 570042
(Southern Norfolk Primary Care Trust)

Practice Manager Cyril Lindsey

GP Pamela Dawn BRANTIGAN, Dr BUCKTON, Andrew Michael Stanley LEAMAN, Richard Douglas OVERY

Mundesley Medical Centre
Munhaven Close, Mundesley, Norwich NR11 8AR
Tel: 01263 724500 Fax: 01263 720165
(North Norfolk Primary Care Trust)
Patient List Size: 5300

Practice Manager Linda Horne

GP John James HARRIS-HALL, Rebecca ABBOTT, Pete HENLEY

Newmarket Road Surgery
7 Newmarket Road, Norwich NR2 2HL
Tel: 01603 621006
(Norwich Primary Care Trust)

Practice Manager Rosemary Moore

GP Julia Mary LEACH, Paul Bannister BARNARD, Steven Grant COPSON, Miles Richard FERRARI

Oak Street Medical Practice
1 Oak Street, Norwich NR3 3DL
Tel: 01603 613431 Fax: 01603 767209
(Norwich Primary Care Trust)

Practice Manager Frank Mitchell

GP Peter Marten LENEY, Brian Stephen COLE, Brian Leslie ELVY, Martin Jonathon GILLINGS, Catherine Rose ROBINSON

Old Catton Surgery
55 Lodge Lane, Old Catton, Norwich NR6 7HQ
Tel: 01603 423341 Fax: 01603 486445
(Broadland Primary Care Trust)

Practice Manager Jan Wright

GP David Newton CARLYLE, Diane Lesley BOOL, Robert KEANE, Robert MINNS

Old Mill Surgery
Stoke Road, Poringland, Norwich NR14 7JL
Tel: 01508 492929 Fax: 01508 495371
(Southern Norfolk Primary Care Trust)
Patient List Size: 6800

Practice Manager Mary Parker

GP Jeffrey John FOX, Elizabeth Rose MASCARENHAS, Roy John NEWMAN, Clive WATERHOUSE

Old Palace Medical Practice
148 Old Palace Road, Norwich NR2 4JA
Tel: 01603 663363 Fax: 01603 664173
(Norwich Primary Care Trust)
Patient List Size: 2526

Practice Manager Donna Laws-Chapman

GP Dr LISTER

Prospect Medical Practice
95 Aylsham Road, Norwich NR3 2HW
Tel: 01603 488477 Fax: 01603 485989
(Norwich Primary Care Trust)

Practice Manager Michael Hall

GP Sophie BENNET, Kathryn GREEN, William Jeffrey MIRZA

Reepham Surgery
Smugglers Lane, Reepham, Norwich NR10 4QT
Tel: 01603 870271 Fax: 01603 872995
(Broadland Primary Care Trust)
Patient List Size: 8400

Practice Manager Chris Tippett

GP Barbara Kathleen KELLY, Dr COTTON, Christopher Patrick PEARCE, Frances Mary PRICE, Michael Ernest PRICE, Carl Albert STUTTARD

The Sprowston-Thorpe Medical Partnership
Thorpe Health Centre, St. Williams Way, Norwich NR7 0AJ
Tel: 01603 701010 Fax: 01603 701942
(Broadland Primary Care Trust)

Practice Manager Arda Lambert

GP Yvonne WATTS, Gordon James Graham BASTABLE, John EFSTRATIOU, Andrew FEW, Gil Jonathan RATTNER, Sabine SCHERZINGER

Staithe Surgery
Lower Staithe Road, Stalham, Norwich NR12 9BU
Tel: 01692 582000 Fax: 01692 580428
(North Norfolk Primary Care Trust)

Practice Manager Martin Langdon

GP David Glen WILLITS, Hilary Lynn COYSH, Anoop Singh DHESI, Diana Hilary Jacqueline HOOD

The Surgery
Norwich Road, Saxlingham Nethergate, Norwich NR15 1TP
Tel: 01508 499208 Fax: 01508 498207
(Southern Norfolk Primary Care Trust)

Practice Manager Ann Lee

GP Andrew Gilmore GIBSON, Gillian R TEWSON

Taverham Surgery
Sandy Lane, Taverham, Norwich NR8 6JR
Tel: 01603 867481 Fax: 01603 261781
(Broadland Primary Care Trust)
Patient List Size: 12900

Practice Manager Scott McKenzie

GP Simon Richard LOCKETT, Henry Albert KASZUBOWSKI, Jonathan MOULD, Angela Mary PENNELL, Philip PINNEY, Gregory QUINN, Sharon Janet SMITH

Thorpe Health Centre
St William's Way, Thorpe St. Andrew, Norwich NR7 0AJ
Tel: 01603 701010 Fax: 01603 701942
(Broadland Primary Care Trust)

Practice Manager Arde Lambert

GP Cameron Robb Dixon CAMPBELL, Gordon James Graham BASTABLE, John EFSTRATIOU, Gil Jonathan RATTNER, Sabine H SCHERZINGER, Yvonne WATTS

Thorpewood Medical Group
140 Woodside Road, Thorpe St Andrew, Norwich NR7 9QL
Tel: 01603 701477 Fax: 01603 701512
Email: stephen.edwards@gp-d82048.nhs.uk
Website: www.thorpewood.co.uk
(Broadland Primary Care Trust)
Patient List Size: 12600

GP Kevin Orion THOMPSON, Helene BARCLAY, Peter John BURROWS, C GREEN, Richard HAMPSHEIR, Christine Ann LESLEY, Spiridion MACRIS, John MALCOLM, S RAOSINGHE

Tilford, Rash and Burrell
Health Centre, Lawson Road, Norwich NR3 4LE
Tel: 01603 427096 Fax: 01603 403704
(Norwich Primary Care Trust)
Patient List Size: 6200

Practice Manager Diane Rose

GP Maureen Patricia TILFORD, Mark Andrew BURRELL, Guy RASH

Trinity Street Surgery
1 Trinity Street, Norwich NR2 2BG
Tel: 01603 624844 Fax: 01603 766829
(Norwich Primary Care Trust)
Patient List Size: 9000

Practice Manager Don Chapman

GP Susan Jacqueline VAUGHAN, Maire Siobhan BEALES, Jane CRAIG, Johannes DE VRIJER, Klaus KOCH, Ian Nicholas MORTON, Helene SIMPER

University of East Anglia Health Centre
University of East Anglia, Earlham Road, Norwich NR4 7TJ
Tel: 01603 592172 Fax: 01603 506579
Email: uhs@uea.ac.uk
(Norwich Primary Care Trust)
Patient List Size: 11036

Practice Manager Christina Fielding

GP Paul Alexander COATHUP, Bernadette CANT, Suzanne Mary EDMONDS, Kathleen Frances HAYDN, Rob JAMES, Keith LIGHTFOOT, Nick RAITHATHA, Helen TABBERER, Charlotte TURNER

Unthank Road Surgery
38 Unthank Road, Norwich NR2 2RD
Tel: 01603 624715
(Norwich Primary Care Trust)

Practice Manager Bryan Oldman

GP Alan Ronald GALL, Sally Joanne BUTT, Andrew James PYPER

Victoria Street Surgery
1 Victoria Street, Norwich NR1 3QX
Tel: 01603 620872 Fax: 01603 766812
(Norwich Primary Care Trust)
Patient List Size: 3020

Practice Manager Sylvia MacDonald

GP Andrew Ayton FAIRCLOUGH, Richard LARSSON

West Pottergate Health Centre
137 West Pottergate, Norwich NR2 4BX
Tel: 01603 628705 Fax: 01603 766789
(Norwich Primary Care Trust)
Patient List Size: 4100

Practice Manager Brenda Varnava

GP David Stephen GOLDSER, Karen HEATON, Frances SCOULLER

Willow Wood Surgery
Aslake Close, Sprowston, Norwich NR7 8TT
Tel: 01603 427153 Fax: 01603 787341
(Broadland Primary Care Trust)
Patient List Size: 4800

Practice Manager Heather Watts

GP Haydar S ABDELMUTTI, Lisa JACKSON, Maike JUERGENS, T MOORE

Wood and Dawson
The Surgery, Chapel Road, Aldborough, Norwich NR11 7NN
Tel: 01263 768602 Fax: 01263 761340
Email: philip.wood@nhs.net
(North Norfolk Primary Care Trust)
Patient List Size: 2336

Practice Manager Ruth Lambert

GP Philip Milton WOOD, Sarah DAWSON

Woodcock Road Surgery
29 Woodcock Road, Norwich NR3 3UA
Tel: 01603 425989 Fax: 01603 425989
(Norwich Primary Care Trust)

Practice Manager Cherry Tythcott

GP Alan Andrew ROBINSON, Jonathan Charles Blackwell SHUTES, David Andrew LING

Yare Valley Medical Practice
202 Thorpe Road, Norwich NR1 1TJ
Tel: 01603 437559 Fax: 01603 701773
(Norwich Primary Care Trust)

Practice Manager Mary Osborne

GP Joseph Onyekachi OKORO, Francoise GRUNSTEIN, Richard PANNETT, Sidha SAMBANDAN

Nottingham

Abbey Medical Centre
63 Central Avenue, Beeston, Nottingham NG9 2QP
Tel: 0115 925 0862 Fax: 0115 922 0522
(Broxtowe and Hucknall Primary Care Trust)
Patient List Size: 5500

Practice Manager Shirley Lynch

GP Nicholas Charles BROWNE, Irena JARAM, R T N ROGERS

Adam House Medical Centre
Sandiacre, Nottingham NG10 5HZ
Tel: 01159 491194 Fax: 0115 949 1522
(Erewash Primary Care Trust)
Patient List Size: 8600

Practice Manager Wendy Abbott

GP Dr ALI, Dr COLEMAN, Dr HOLMAN, Dr ROYAL, Dr SAAD, Dr ULLAH

Aitune Medical Practice
The Health Centre, Midland Street, Long Eaton, Nottingham NG10 1NY
Tel: 0115 973 2157 Fax: 0115 946 5420
Email: reception@c81023.nhs.uk
(Erewash Primary Care Trust)
Patient List Size: 9500

Practice Manager L J Hogg

GP J NICHOLSON, A ALLAN, A ASKEW, P DENNY, B PLAYFOR, K ROTCHFORD

Appletree Medical Practice
4 Wheatsheaf Court, Burton Joyce, Nottingham NG14 5EA
Tel: 0115 931 2929 Fax: 0115 931 2267
(Gedling Primary Care Trust)

Practice Manager Janet Cottee

GP Claire JAMES, Arun SHETTY

Ashfield House
Forest Road, Annesley Woodhouse, Kirkby in Ashfield, Nottingham NG17 9JB
Tel: 01623 752295 Fax: 01623 759350
Email: reception.kirkby@gp-c84067.nhs.uk
(Ashfield Primary Care Trust)

Practice Manager Pat Hardstaff

GP Peter William MACDOUGALL, Gregory Francis PLACE, Mark Adrian REDFERN

Aspley Medical Centre
511 Aspley Lane, Aspley, Nottingham NG8 5RW
Tel: 0115 929 2700 Fax: 0115 929 8276
(Nottingham City Primary Care Trust)

GP Simon Ronald WRIGHT, Jonathan Henry HARTE, Carol Ann MICHEL, Penny Alice SHIELDS

Baldwin and Partners
Hucknall Road Medical Centre, off Kibworth Close, Nottingham NG5 1FX
Tel: 0115 960 6652 Fax: 0115 969 1746
(Nottingham City Primary Care Trust)
Patient List Size: 10000

Practice Manager Anne Horsley

GP Peter Martin BALDWIN, Michael Andrew BUTLER, Fiona-May EMERSON, Anne FELSTEAD, Alastair Neil McLACHLAN

Beaumont Practice
Sneinton Health Centre, Beaumont Street, Sneinton, Nottingham NG2 4PJ
Tel: 0115 950 1941
(Nottingham City Primary Care Trust)
Patient List Size: 1670

GP Robyn Adele SCOTT

Beechdale Surgery
439 Beechdale Road, Nottingham NG8 3LF
Tel: 0115 929 0754 Fax: 0115 929 6843
(Nottingham City Primary Care Trust)

Practice Manager Marion Widdison

GP Marius Ainsley BICKNELL, Marinus Dirk HAGE

Belvoir Vale
17A Walford Close, Bottesford, Nottingham NG13 0AN
(Lincolnshire South West Teaching Primary Care Trust)

GP G ENNIS

Belvoir Vale
17A Walford Close, Bottesford, Nottingham NG13 0AN
Tel: 01949 842341 Fax: 01949 844209
(Lincolnshire South West Teaching Primary Care Trust)

GP S J GLENCROSS

Bestwood Park Health Centre
Pedmore Valley, Bestwood Park, Nottingham NG5 5PB
Tel: 0115 920 8597 Fax: 0115 967 1910
(Nottingham City Primary Care Trust)
Patient List Size: 3250

Practice Manager H Goodwin

GP Kalyana Rao BHAJANTRI

Bilborough Medical Centre
Bracebridge Drive, Bilborough, Nottingham NG8 4PN
Tel: 0115 929 2354 Fax: 0115 929 1656
(Nottingham City Primary Care Trust)

Practice Manager A Khalique

GP Abraze KHALIQUE, Roderick James WILLIAMS

Bilborough Surgery
112 Graylands Road, Bilborough, Nottingham NG8 4FD
Tel: 0115 929 2358 Fax: 0115 929 5878
(Nottingham City Primary Care Trust)

GP N V PHILLIPS

Black and Partners
Sherwood Health Centre, Elmswood Gardens, Sherwood, Nottingham NG5 4AD
Tel: 0115 985 8822/9607127 Fax: 0115 933 9050
(Nottingham City Primary Care Trust)
Patient List Size: 8800

Practice Manager Mary Simpson

GP Douglas George BLACK, Penelope Jane DEXTER, Rosalind Leonie KING, Irfin Ahmed MALIK, Jane MILBURN, Ian Michael Geoffrey TRIMBLE

Bramcote Surgery
2A Hanley Avenue, Bramcote, Beeston, Nottingham NG9 3HF
Tel: 0115 922 4960 Fax: 0115 922 9050
(Broxtowe and Hucknall Primary Care Trust)

Practice Manager Michael Salt

GP Martin SOOLE, Eliz JORDAN

Bulwell Health Centre
Main Street, Bulwell, Nottingham NG6 8QJ
Tel: 0115 927 9119 Fax: 0115 977 1236
(Nottingham City Primary Care Trust)

GP Andrew David ADAMS, Helen Clarissa Sian MASON, Rosemary Lovann ROSSER

Bulwell Health Centre
Main Street, Bulwell, Nottingham NG6 8QJ
Tel: 0115 977 1181 Fax: 0115 977 1377
(Nottingham City Primary Care Trust)

GP Una CAROLAN, Herbel Singh PABLA, George Salvarani RIPLEY, Maurice Ian RIPLEY

The Calverton Practice
2A St. Wilfrids Square, Calverton, Nottingham NG14 6FP
Tel: 0115 965 2294 Fax: 0115 965 5898
(Gedling Primary Care Trust)

GP Louise Jane MAILE, Kesten Barbara CHALLEN, J R HOPKINSON, Philip Michael Charles RAYNER, James Donald SIMPSON

Charlton House Medical Centre
Long Eaton, Nottingham NG10 2BU
(Erewash Primary Care Trust)

GP Dr HENDERSON SMITH

Church House Surgery
Church House, Shaw Street, Ruddington, Nottingham NG11 6HF
Tel: 0115 984 7101 Fax: 0115 984 7404
(Rushcliffe Primary Care Trust)
Patient List Size: 3000

Practice Manager Lynne E Burnett

GP Michael David EATON, Ruth Jane GREAVES

Church Street Medical Centre
11B Church Street, Eastwood, Nottingham NG16 3BP
Tel: 01773 712065 Fax: 01773 534295
(Broxtowe and Hucknall Primary Care Trust)
Patient List Size: 8600

Practice Manager Janis Lynch

GP Adam Kazimierz SMEREKA, Peter Michael EXLEY, Rowan Kaye LATIMER, Jeremy David Saunders WALKER

Churchfields Medical Practice, Old Basford Health Centre
1 Bailey Street, Old Basford, Nottingham NG6 0HD
Tel: 0115 978 1231 Fax: 0115 979 0419
Email: julie.frankish@gp-c84034.nhs.uk
(Nottingham City Primary Care Trust)
Patient List Size: 11000

Practice Manager Juli Frankish

GP Patrick Joseph KEAVNEY, Lewis HALL, Dorothy Jane HARRISON, Trevor Anthony MILLS, Kate ROY

Clifton Medical Centre
571 Farnborough Road, Clifton, Nottingham NG11 9DN
Tel: 0115 921 1288
(Nottingham City Primary Care Trust)
Patient List Size: 8000

Practice Manager Marilyn Brooks

GP Ernest David GREGSON, James Bruce HAMILTON, Paul Nicholas Stuart PARKEN, Helen Denise TAYLOR

Compton Acres Medical Centre
Compton Acres, Nottingham NG2 7PA
Tel: 0115 984 6767 Fax: 0115 945 5888
Email: amu.sharma@gp-C84666.nhs.uk
(Rushcliffe Primary Care Trust)
Patient List Size: 3058

GP N K SHARMA, A LATA

The Cripps Health Centre
University Park, Nottingham NG7 2QW
Tel: 0115 950 1654
(Nottingham City Primary Care Trust)
Patient List Size: 22500

Practice Manager P O'Connor

GP Angela WHITE, Tim BAKER, Elaine Ruth GIBBS, Claire MANKTELOW, Dylan Llywelyn NASH, John Francis Hugh PORTER

Dale Surgery
67 Sneinton Dale, Nottingham NG2 4LG
Tel: 0115 911 0256 Fax: 0115 911 0256
(Nottingham City Primary Care Trust)
Patient List Size: 2800

Practice Manager Margaret Smith

GP Pritpal Singh CHAHAL

Daybrook Health Centre
Salop Street, Daybrook, Nottingham NG5 6HP
(Gedling Primary Care Trust)

Practice Manager B G Lee

GP Gerard Michael GALLAGHER, Lisa Ann BORUCH, Param Jit SINGH

Department of General Practice
Queens Medical Centre, Derby Road, Nottingham NG7 2UH
Tel: 0115 970 9901
(Nottingham City Primary Care Trust)

GP Richard David CHURCHILL, Kathryn Ann DUNN

Dewar and Randerson
The Health Centre, 1 Bridgeway Centre, Meadows, Nottingham NG2 2JG
(Nottingham City Primary Care Trust)

Practice Manager M Craske

GP Jane Rosemary DEWAR, Jonathan Michael RANDERSON

Dr Yus Rao
Greenfields Medical Centre, 12 Terrace Street, Hyson Green, Nottingham NG7 6ER
Tel: 0115 942358 Fax: 0115 900 2330
(Nottingham City Primary Care Trust)

Practice Manager Sheila Davis

GP Yella Veera Venkata Satya RAO

Earwicker and Partners
The Health Centre, 97 Derby Road, Stapleford, Nottingham NG9 7AT
Tel: 0115 939 2444 Fax: 0115 939 5625
(Broxtowe and Hucknall Primary Care Trust)
Patient List Size: 5400

Practice Manager Tony Oram

GP Stephen Charles EARWICKER, Julie BIGNELL, Ruth BOOTH, Helen Alison O'NEIL, Michael John O'NEIL, Helen PERCIVAL

East Bridgford Medical Centre
2 Butt Lane, East Bridgford, Nottingham NG13 8NY
Tel: 01949 20216 Fax: 01949 21283
(Rushcliffe Primary Care Trust)
Patient List Size: 6000

Practice Manager Glenda Pearson

GP Andrew Thomas HARRISON, Roberto Agostino SCAFFARDI, Ann-Marie STEWART

Family Medical Centre
171 Carlton Road, Nottingham NG3 2FW
Tel: 0115 504068 Fax: 0115 950 9844
Email: anyone@pmcnottm.freeserve.co.uk
(Nottingham City Primary Care Trust)
Patient List Size: 7500

Practice Manager E M Pain

GP Naresh Chander SOOD, Jonathan Richard ARDEN-JONES, Kenneth Paul Hudson BROWN, Julie Simone DAY, Dili SATHA

Family Medical Centre
56A Low Moor Road, Kirkby in Ashfield, Nottingham NG17 7BG
Tel: 01623 757219 Fax: 01623 751578
(Ashfield Primary Care Trust)

GP A G SIDDIQUI, M G SIDDIQUI

Farndon Green Medical Centre
1 Farndon Green, Wollaton Park, Nottingham NG8 1DU
Tel: 0115 928 8666 Fax: 0115 928 8343
(Nottingham City Primary Care Trust)
Patient List Size: 5000

Practice Manager Jackie Cowley

GP Nicholas Andrew SILCOCK, Judith Sarah AMBROSE, Alice Margaret DUFFY, Elizabeth Helen McVICAR, Melanie Jane ROTHERHAM

Gamston Medical Centre
Gamston District Centre, Gamston, Nottingham NG2 6PS
Tel: 0115 945 5946 Fax: 0115 969 6217
(Rushcliffe Primary Care Trust)
Patient List Size: 3300

Practice Manager Sue Hughes

GP Linda Hermesh Kaur KANDOLA

Gideon Medical Centre
10 Chapel Lane, Arnold, Nottingham NG5 7DR
Tel: 0115 920 7988 Fax: 0115 926 3883
(Gedling Primary Care Trust)
Patient List Size: 1750

Practice Manager Ruth Cutler

Greenwood and Sneinton Family Medical Centre
249 Sneinton Dale, Sneinton, Nottingham NG3 7DQ
Tel: 0115 950 1854 Fax: 0115 958 0044
Email: bruce.smith@gp-c84063.nhs.uk
(Nottingham City Primary Care Trust)
Patient List Size: 6100

Practice Manager Bruce Smith

GP Graham David Ross MARTIN, Simon Oakley FRADD, Sarah LAYZELL, Mark Edward SMITH

Hama Medical Centre
11A Nottingham Road, Kimberley, Nottingham NG16 2NB
Tel: 0115 939 2101 Fax: 0115 945 9208
(Broxtowe and Hucknall Primary Care Trust)
Patient List Size: 4700

Practice Manager Martin Rowlatt

GP Tariq Mahmood HAMA, Zahida Ansari HAMA

Hartley Road Medical Centre
91 Hartley Road, Radford, Nottingham NG7 3AQ
Tel: 0115 942 2622 Fax: 0115 924 9150
Email: mahipal.verma@gp-C84632.nhs.uk
(Nottingham City Primary Care Trust)
Patient List Size: 3100

Practice Manager Jai Verma

GP Mahipal Singh VERMA, Vilas DIGHE, Jennifer GRAY, Ramesh ROY

Health Care Complex
52 Low Moor Road, Kirkby in Ashfield, Nottingham NG17 7BG
Tel: 01623 752312 Fax: 01623 723700
(Ashfield Primary Care Trust)

GP N J OZA, P OZA

The Health Centre
Main Road, Radcliffe-on-Trent, Nottingham NG12 2GD
Tel: 0115 933 3737
(Rushcliffe Primary Care Trust)

GP Felicity Elizabeth ARMITAGE, Jaswant Singh BILKHU, Rameshbhai Ramubhai PATEL, Gillian Mary THOMPSON

The Health Centre
Bunny Lane, Keyworth, Nottingham NG12 5JU
Tel: 0115 937 3527 Fax: 0115 937 6781
Website: www.keyworthhealthcentre.co.uk
(Rushcliffe Primary Care Trust)
Patient List Size: 11800

Practice Manager Michele Broutta

GP Clive Howard LEDGER, Douglas JENKINSON, Jill LANGRIDGE, Corinna SMALL, Andrew Michael WOOD

The Health Centre
High Street, Arnold, Nottingham NG5 7BQ
Tel: 0115 926 7257 Fax: 0115 956 3232
(Gedling Primary Care Trust)

GP Genowefa BAJEK, Michael Edmund ELLIOTT, Philip David GARD, John Richard HOWARD, Fiona Margaret McCRACKEN, Suresh R PATEL, Peter Colin PAVIER

The Health Centre
1 Ilkeston Road, Nottingham NG7 3GW
Tel: 0115 919 6662 Fax: 0115 919 6663
(Nottingham City Primary Care Trust)

GP A S GHATTAORA

The Health Centre
Low Moor Road, Kirkby in Ashfield, Nottingham NG17 7LG
Tel: 01623 752454 Fax: 01623 755750
(Ashfield Primary Care Trust)

GP K AYE

Highfield Medical Centre
86 College Street, Long Eaton, Nottingham NG10 4NP
(Erewash Primary Care Trust)

GP Dr MORLEY

Howson and Partner
Mary Potter Health Centre, Gregory Boulevard, Hyson Green, Nottingham NG7 5HY
Tel: 0115 942 0330
(Nottingham City Primary Care Trust)

Practice Manager S Khan

GP Anthony Neville HOWSON, Helen Frances PARKEN

Ibrahim
St Anns Health Centre, St Anns, Well Road, Nottingham NG3 3PX
Tel: 0115 950 1883 Fax: 0115 950 1865
(Nottingham City Primary Care Trust)
Patient List Size: 2200

GP Pamela IBRAHIM

John Ryle Health Centre
Southchurch Drive, Clifton, Nottingham NG11 8EW
Tel: 0115 921 2970
(Nottingham City Primary Care Trust)
Patient List Size: 6800

Practice Manager Marion Tongue

GP Roger Michael O'SHEA, Peter LAVELLE, Stephen Peter RILEY

Khan
Mary Potter Health Centre, Gregory Boulevard, Hyson Green, Nottingham NG7 5HY
Tel: 0115 942 3216 Fax: 0115 970 4640
(Nottingham City Primary Care Trust)
Patient List Size: 2700

Practice Manager Di Brammer

GP Zahoor KHAN

Lady Bay Surgery
195A Trent Boulevard, West Bridgford, Nottingham NG2 5BX
Tel: 0115 981 6100 Fax: 0115 981 7709
(Rushcliffe Primary Care Trust)

Practice Manager Bev Browitt

GP Christopher Thomas CLARK

Lambley Lane Surgery
6 Lambley Lane, Burton Joyce, Nottingham NG14 5BG
Tel: 0115 931 2500 Fax: 0115 931 3899
(Gedling Primary Care Trust)
Patient List Size: 4600

Practice Manager Elaine Bell

GP Nigel Paul McHALE

Lenton Medical Centre
266 Derby Road, Nottingham NG7 1PR
Tel: 0115 941 1208
(Nottingham City Primary Care Trust)

GP D MAINI

Limetree Surgery
1 Limetree Avenue, Cinderhill, Nottingham NG8 6AB
Tel: 0115 979 1281 Fax: 0115 979 2864
Email: linda.barron@gp-c84694.nhs.uk
(Nottingham City Primary Care Trust)

Practice Manager Linda Barron

GP Raja Safiy KARIM, Rubina KARIM

The Linden Medical Group
205 Russell Drive, Wollaton, Nottingham NG8 2BD
Tel: 0115 928 3201 Fax: 0115 985 4981
(Nottingham City Primary Care Trust)
Patient List Size: 15000

Practice Manager Don Gardner

GP P A JONES, Grant DEX, Philippa GALLIVAN, Simon GREGORY, Christopher PERKO, Michael STANLEY, Larysa Oksana WERCHOLA

The Linden Medical Group
The Health Centre, 97 Derby Road, Stapleford, Nottingham NG9 7AT
Tel: 0115 939 2444 Fax: 0115 949 1751
(Broxtowe and Hucknall Primary Care Trust)
Patient List Size: 15000

Practice Manager Don Gardner

GP Peter Alan JONES, Grant DEX, Philippa Rachael GALLIVAN, Simon Andrew GREGORY, Christopher Darko PERKO, Michael Joseph SHANLEY, Larysa Oksana WERCHOLA

Long Eaton Health Centre
Long Eaton, Nottingham
(Erewash Primary Care Trust)

GP Dr GOULD

Lowdham Medical Centre
Francklin Road, Lowdham, Nottingham NG14 7BG
(Newark and Sherwood Primary Care Trust)

Ludlow Hill Surgery
152 Melton Road, West Bridgford, Nottingham NG2 6ER
Tel: 0115 9143366/68 Fax: 0115 914 3375
(Rushcliffe Primary Care Trust)
Patient List Size: 4870

GP Nicholas Philip Freeman PAGE, Jeremy Paul GRIFFITHS, Joanne HOBSON

Malvern House
41 Mapperley Road, Nottingham NG3 5AQ
Tel: 0115 841 2022 Fax: 0115 841 2022
(Gedling Primary Care Trust)
Patient List Size: 2200

GP Mark Andrew John STEVENS

The Manor Surgery
Middle Street, Beeston, Nottingham NG9 1GA
Tel: 0115 925 6127 Fax: 0115 967 8612
(Broxtowe and Hucknall Primary Care Trust)

Practice Manager Josephine Woods

GP Elizabeth Mary PHILLIPSON, Peter John BARRETT, David CHARLES, Lorraine EASSON, Jean Roberta MADELEY

Marsh, Kennedy, Chapman, Wilde and Pathy
Netherfield Medical Practice, 2A Forester Street, Netherfield, Nottingham NG4 2NJ
Tel: 0115 940 3775 Fax: 0115 961 4069
(Gedling Primary Care Trust)
Patient List Size: 8200

Practice Manager Jacqueline Newman

GP Anthony James MARSH, Joanne Elizabeth CHAPMAN, Caitriona Mary KENNEDY, Harish PATHY, Stephen Marek Julius Jozefowicz WILDE

The Medical Centre
Valley House, St. Anns, Well Road, Nottingham NG3 3HR
Tel: 0115 950 2703
(Nottingham City Primary Care Trust)

Practice Manager Karl Routledge-Wilson

GP Prem Prakash TIWARI, Shobhi Rani TIWARI

Medical Centre
Main Road, Jacksdale, Nottingham NG16 5JW
Tel: 01773 608760 Fax: 01773 541121
(Ashfield Primary Care Trust)
Patient List Size: 2455

Practice Manager Mel Lindley

GP K S S RAJAH, E McLOGHLIN

Medical Centre
2a Zulu Road, Basford, Nottingham NG7 7DS
(Nottingham City Primary Care Trust)

GP S BALENDRAN

Melbourne Park Medical Centre
Melbourne Road, Aspley, Nottingham NG8 5HL
Tel: 0115 978 6114 Fax: 0115 924 9334
(Nottingham City Primary Care Trust)
Patient List Size: 9000

Practice Manager Lynda Cotton

GP Christopher John RYAN, Alison Clare BEST, Stephen Andrew COX, Diane RIDLEY, Audrey Serena RUSSELL

Moir Medical Centre
Long Eaton, Nottingham NG10 1QQ
Tel: 0115 973 5820 Fax: 0115 946 0197
Email: reception@gp-C81010.nhs.uk
(Erewash Primary Care Trust)

Practice Manager Steve McHale

GP Dr JOWETT, Dr BHATIA, Dr DUNN, Dr JORDAN, Dr LAKHANI, Dr WARD

Musters Medical Practice
214 Musters Road, West Bridgford, Nottingham NG2 7DR
Tel: 0115 981 4124 Fax: 0115 981 3117
(Rushcliffe Primary Care Trust)
Patient List Size: 9000

Practice Manager Judy Bigham, Catherine Wilkinson

GP Ian William Lindsay McCULLOCH, Richard BARNSLEY, Gavin DERBYSHIRE, Elizabeth Margaret SMITH

NDU Surgery
St Anns Health Centre, St Anns, Well Road, Nottingham NG3 3PX
Tel: 0115 950 5455 Fax: 0155 958 8493
(Nottingham City Primary Care Trust)
Patient List Size: 1725

Practice Manager Lorna Taylor

GP Rosemary ROSSER, Christopher Chukwuekelua UDENZE

Newthorpe Medical Centre
Chewton Street, Eastwood, Nottingham NG16 3HB
Tel: 01773 760202 Fax: 01773 710951
(Broxtowe and Hucknall Primary Care Trust)
Patient List Size: 4682

Practice Manager Sue Sharp

GP Nigel James SPARROW, Sarah Louise BAMFORD, Denise KENDRICK, Ian Keith TEDSTONE

The Nirmala Surgery
112 Pedmore Valley, Bestwood Park, Nottingham NG5 5NN
Tel: 0115 920 8501 Fax: 0115 967 1910
(Nottingham City Primary Care Trust)
Patient List Size: 2500
GP Pulak Kanti G RAY

Oakenhall Medical Practice
Bolsover Street, Hucknall, Nottingham NG15 7UA
Tel: 0115 963 3511 Fax: 0115 968 0947
(Broxtowe and Hucknall Primary Care Trust)
Patient List Size: 6700

Practice Manager Mary Maggs

GP David MYERS, Nicholas Mark Stanhope GILMORE, Helen Clare ROUGHTON, S STURROCK

The Oaks Medical Centre
18-20 Villa Street, Beeston, Nottingham NG9 2NY
Tel: 0115 925 4566 Fax: 0115 967 7470
(Broxtowe and Hucknall Primary Care Trust)

Practice Manager Kathryn Mercer

GP Mary Elizabeth CARR, Paul John JACKLIN, Guy MANSFORD

Parkview Surgery
89 Plumptre Way, Eastwood, Nottingham NG16 3LQ
Tel: 01773 714414 Fax: 01773 533306
Email: sagar@nottinghamgp.nhs.uk
(Broxtowe and Hucknall Primary Care Trust)
Patient List Size: 2600

Practice Manager Sarah Petter

GP Mark DICKSON, Thankam DICKSON

Patrick and Partners
Rise Park Surgery, Revelstoke Way, Nottingham NG5 5EB
Tel: 0115 927 2525 Fax: 0115 979 7056
(Nottingham City Primary Care Trust)
Patient List Size: 5700

Practice Manager Marian Harris

GP Paul Richard PATRICK, Lynn Margaret BROWN, Margaret Ceredwen JONES, Nadeem QURESHI

The Peacock Practice
577 Carlton Road, Carlton, Nottingham NG3 7AF
Tel: 0115 958 0415 Fax: 0115 950 9245
(Nottingham City Primary Care Trust)
Patient List Size: 4000

Practice Manager D Jones

GP Paul Anthony David OLIVER, Heena PATEL, Peter Courtenay SAUNDERS

Portland Medical Practice
The Health Centre, Curtis Street, Hucknall, Nottingham NG15 7JE
Tel: 0115 963 2535 Fax: 0115 963 2885
(Broxtowe and Hucknall Primary Care Trust)
Patient List Size: 6100

Practice Manager Elizabeth Swainson

GP Myra Teresa D'MELLO, Kevin Anthony D'MELLO, Thomas Michael McHUGH

Radford Health Centre
Ilkeston Road, Nottingham NG7 3GW
Tel: 0115 979 1313 Fax: 0115 979 1470
(Nottingham City Primary Care Trust)
Patient List Size: 4400

Practice Manager Margaret Goodband

GP Ramesh ROY, Naomi Noble Vinayakumar PHILLIPS

Radford Medical Practice
1 Ilkeston Road, Nottingham NG7 3GW
Tel: 0115 979 2691 Fax: 0115 942 2619
(Nottingham City Primary Care Trust)
Patient List Size: 12000

Practice Manager Karen Murch, Hazel Taylor

GP K KAUR, Helen Margaret EARWICKER, Susan KINGDON, F O LIAU, R E LONSDALE, Karen Vivien WORTH

RHR Medical Centre
Calverton Drive, Strelley, Nottingham NG8 6QN
Tel: 0115 975 3666 Fax: 0115 975 3888
(Nottingham City Primary Care Trust)
Patient List Size: 3060

Practice Manager Karen Bolton

GP Kalpana SHARMA

Rivergreen Medical Centre
106 Southchurch Drive, Clifton, Nottingham NG11 8AD
Tel: 0115 9211566 Fax: 0115 9405579
Website: www.rivergreenmc.co.uk
(Nottingham City Primary Care Trust)

Practice Manager Mark Milnes, J Tomlinson

GP Howard Anthony LEWIS, Elizabeth HAMPSON, Catherine LEWIS, S McGIBBON

Riverlyn Medical Centre
Station Road, Bulwell, Nottingham NG6 9AA
Tel: 0115 927 3222 Fax: 0115 927 3444
(Nottingham City Primary Care Trust)
Patient List Size: 5056

Practice Manager B Prince

GP Michael Charles GRANT DE LONGUEUIL, Christopher BLANSHARD, Venessa DOEL

Ruddington Medical Centre
Church Street, Ruddington, Nottingham NG11 6HD
Tel: 0115 921 1144 Fax: 0115 940 5139
(Rushcliffe Primary Care Trust)
Patient List Size: 6500

Practice Manager David Cole

GP Clifford Michael SPENCER, Linda CHAPMAN, Jagjit RAI

Rudrashetty and Partners
Mary Potter Health Centre, Gregory Boulevard, Hyson Green, Nottingham NG7 5HY
(Nottingham City Primary Care Trust)

GP Sarojani RUDRASHETTY, Frances Mary RHODEN, Susan Mary TAYLOR

Ryecroft Street Health Centre
Ryecroft Street, Stapleford, Nottingham NG9 8PN
Tel: 0115 939 5555 Fax: 0115 939 8652
(Broxtowe and Hucknall Primary Care Trust)
Patient List Size: 3300

Practice Manager A Humphreys

GP John Anthony DODDY, Cecilia CHAN

Selston Surgery
139 Nottingham Road, Selston, Nottingham NG16 6BT
Tel: 01773 810226 Fax: 01773 863957
(Ashfield Primary Care Trust)
Patient List Size: 4500

Practice Manager Pat Bell

GP S R BASSI, S M R KARIM

Shankar and Rao
The Health Centre, 1 Bridgeway Centre, Meadows, Nottingham NG2 2JG
Tel: 0115 9861128 Fax: 0115 9851836
(Nottingham City Primary Care Trust)
Patient List Size: 3500

GP R S C SHANKAR, D RAO

Sharma
Mary Potter Health Centre, Gregory Boulevard, Hyson Green, Nottingham NG7
(Nottingham City Primary Care Trust)

GP Om Prakash SHARMA

Sherrington Park Medical Practice
402 Mansfield Road, Nottingham NG5 2EJ
Tel: 0115 985 8552 Fax: 0115 985 8553
Email: sherringtonpark@doctor.com
(Nottingham City Primary Care Trust)

Practice Manager Mrs Rubbins

GP William Francis HOLMES, Andrew Peter FLEWITT, Mona VINDLA

Sherwood Rise Surgery
31 Nottingham Road, Sherwood, Nottingham NG7 7AD
Tel: 0115 962 3080 Fax: 0115 962 2989
(Nottingham City Primary Care Trust)
Patient List Size: 4300

GP Sardar Mohammad QURESHI, Gerrard F FINNAGAN

Snapewood Medical Centre
Snapewood Road, Bulwell, Nottingham NG6 7GH
Tel: 0115 975 2810 Fax: 0115 977 0731
(Nottingham City Primary Care Trust)

GP S H SHARMA

Southview Surgery
178 Musters Road, West Bridgford, Nottingham NG2 7AA
Tel: 0115 981 4472 Fax: 0115 981 2812
(Rushcliffe Primary Care Trust)
Patient List Size: 6200

Practice Manager Sheila Braithwaite

GP Kevin Graham BRATT, Sarah Catherine Anne JORDAN, Oonagh Michaela LIVESEY, Lynn Anne OVENDEN

Sparrow and Partners
Torkard Hill Medical Centre, Farleys Lane, Huckhall, Nottingham NG15 6DY
Tel: 0115 963 3676 Fax: 0115 968 1957
(Broxtowe and Hucknall Primary Care Trust)
Patient List Size: 12000

GP Ian Michael SPARROW, Mary Elizabeth BROWN, Maria DALTON, J FRENCH, David William HANNAH, Victoria Mary KARNEY, Maryan Ryszard WIECEK

St Mary's Medical Centre
Old Farm Road, Top Valley, Nottingham NG5 9AJ
Tel: 0115 927 6038 Fax: 0115 927 8941
(Nottingham City Primary Care Trust)
Patient List Size: 1626

GP S ARYA

Stenhouse Medical Centre
Furlong Street, Arnold, Nottingham NG5 7BP
Tel: 0115 967 3877 Fax: 0115 967 3838
(Gedling Primary Care Trust)

GP Stephen John BOLSHER, Ann Patricia COCKBURN, Brian William HAMMERSLEY, Christine Anne LEIPER, Elaine Faith MADDOCK, John David THORNHILL

Strelley Health Centre
116 Strelley Road, Strelley, Nottingham NG8 6LN
Tel: 0115 929 9219 Fax: 0115 929 6522
(Nottingham City Primary Care Trust)

GP John COCKRILL, Helen Ruth HOLLIS

Sugden and Ndirika
The Health Centre, Curtis Street, Hucknall, Nottingham NG15 7JE
Tel: 0115 963 3580 Fax: 0115 963 3733
(Broxtowe and Hucknall Primary Care Trust)

Practice Manager Pat Gisborne, Jacqueline Plenty

GP Brian David SUGDEN, Amelia Chinwe NDIRIKA

Sunrise Medical Practice
Ilkeston Road, Radford, Nottingham NG7 3GW
Tel: 0115 919 6662 Fax: 0115 919 6663
(Nottingham City Primary Care Trust)

Practice Manager Sukhi Ghattaora

GP A S GHATTAORA, R S GHATTAORA

The Surgery
Church Walk, Eastwood, Nottingham NG16 3BH
Tel: 01773 712951 Fax: 01773 534160
(Broxtowe and Hucknall Primary Care Trust)

Practice Manager Alison Rance

GP Hirendra Chandra BARKATAKI, Caroline ASHWORTH, Thomas David LESTER, Kelvin Kwok Jin LIM

The Surgery
57 Plains Road, Mapperley, Nottingham NG3 5LB
Tel: 0115 962 1717 Fax: 0115 962 5824
(Gedling Primary Care Trust)
Patient List Size: 5300

Practice Manager Ann Pillai

GP Chittaranjan Narayana PILLAI, Angela Maria Clare JONES, Maeve Moira MEREDITH

The Surgery
318 Westdale Lane, Mapperley, Nottingham NG3 6EU
Tel: 0115 987 7604 Fax: 0115 956 8592
(Gedling Primary Care Trust)
Patient List Size: 4000

Practice Manager Margaret Shaw

GP Alan Ross FORD, Shelagh Ann FORD

The Surgery
319 Westdale Lane, Carlton, Nottingham NG3 6EW
Tel: 0115 952 5320 Fax: 0115 952 5321
(Gedling Primary Care Trust)

Practice Manager Suzanne Howard

GP Benedicte Lawrence PARSONS, Graham John COX

The Surgery
20-22 Westdale Lane, Carlton, Nottingham NG4 3JA
Tel: 0115 961 9401
(Gedling Primary Care Trust)
Patient List Size: 10300

GP John Howard Michael MOREWOOD, Brian W CROSS, U F KHALIQ

The Surgery
292 Derby Road, Lenton, Nottingham NG7 1QG
Tel: 0115 947 4002 Fax: 0115 924 0783
(Nottingham City Primary Care Trust)

Practice Manager S Budd

GP John Darcus TEMPLE, Alan David BIRCHALL, Karen Lesley HAMBLETON, Peter HORSEFIELD, Jill Elizabeth JONES, Judith Joan MASKERY, K K MORAR

The Surgery
201 Queensbower Road, Bestwood Park, Nottingham NG5 5RB
Tel: 0115 920 8615 Fax: 0115 966 6073
(Nottingham City Primary Care Trust)
Patient List Size: 4000

Practice Manager A V Dove

GP Barbara COLLINSON, Andrew H BOWMAN

The Surgery
30 Beeston Fields Drive, Beeston, Nottingham NG9 3DB
(Nottingham City Primary Care Trust)
Patient List Size: 5500

GP Balvinder Singh MEHAT, Suzanna VAN SCHAICK

The Surgery
1 Hankin Avenue, Underwood, Nottingham NG16 5FU
Tel: 01773 764444 Fax: 01773 535532
(Ashfield Primary Care Trust)
Patient List Size: 1600

GP J A SIRUR

The Surgery
Low Moor Road, Kirkby in Ashfield, Nottingham NG17 7BG
Tel: 01623 759447 Fax: 01623 750906
(Ashfield Primary Care Trust)

GP Noreen M SOAR, S RAHMAN, Kalasyam Kochayyappan WHITE

The Surgery
492 Nottingham Road, Giltbrook, Nottingham NG16 2GE
Tel: 0115 938 3191 Fax: 0115 945 9556
(Broxtowe and Hucknall Primary Care Trust)
Patient List Size: 3600

Practice Manager N Khalique

GP P KHALIQUE

The Surgery
12-14 Regent Street, Kimberley, Nottingham NG16 2LW
Tel: 0115 938 4453 Fax: 0115 945 9923
(Broxtowe and Hucknall Primary Care Trust)
Patient List Size: 2236

Practice Manager Julie Thurlby

GP R S SANDHU

The Surgery
38 Cockington Road, Bilborough, Nottingham NG8 4BZ
Tel: 0115 928 2231 Fax: 0115 928 4917
(Nottingham City Primary Care Trust)

GP Ian David SKLAR

Trent Bridge Family Medical Practice
28A Henry Road, West Bridgford, Nottingham NG2 7NA
Tel: 0115 914 6600 Fax: 0115 914 6604
(Rushcliffe Primary Care Trust)
Patient List Size: 3300

Practice Manager L Davis

GP Richard John MASCARI, Angela Mary Josephine FOULDS

Tudor House Medical Practice
138 Edwards Lane, Sherwood, Nottingham NG5 3HU
Tel: 0115 966 1233 Fax: 0115 967 0017
(Nottingham City Primary Care Trust)

Practice Manager Karen Maher

GP Donald James HENRY, Richard Ian Faulkner HENRY, Julian Kenneth HENRY

Tudor Square Medical Practice
1st Floor, Barclays Bank Chambers, Tudor Square, West Bridgford, Nottingham NG2 6BT
Tel: 0115 914 3200 Fax: 0115 914 3201
(Rushcliffe Primary Care Trust)
Patient List Size: 6750

Practice Manager Wenda Broadbery

GP Roger Michael LIVESEY, D S HAPGOOD, Matthew Francis Dawson JELPKE

The Valley Surgery
81 Bramcote Lane, Chilwell, Nottingham NG9 4ET
Tel: 0115 943 0530 Fax: 0115 943 1958
(Broxtowe and Hucknall Primary Care Trust)

Practice Manager Joyce Batchelor

GP Arunavema Sathyadatta NAIDOO, Anthony John AVERY, Susanne Jane BOND, Ann Lewis BRIDGEWATER, Richard David CHURCHILL

Victoria Health Centre
Glasshouse Street, Nottingham NG1 3LW
Tel: 0115 948 3030 Fax: 0115 911 1074
(Nottingham City Primary Care Trust)
Patient List Size: 7200

Practice Manager Alison Parker

GP Mary HEPDEN, Timothy Philip CONNERY, George Michael LEUTY, Jean Margaret SHAW

The Village Surgery
108 Victoria Road, Pinxton, Nottingham NG16 6NH
Tel: 01773 810207 Fax: 01773 863700
(North Eastern Derbyshire Primary Care Trust)
Patient List Size: 7300

Practice Manager Joan Melbourne

Welbeck Surgery
481-491 Mansfield Road, Nottingham NG5 2JJ
Tel: 0115 962 0932 Fax: 0115 962 0065
(Nottingham City Primary Care Trust)

Practice Manager D W Sayers

GP John Denton SAYERS, Martin James DENNIS, Susan Mary FOX

Wellspring Surgery
St Anns Health Centre, St Anns, Well Road, Nottingham NG3 3PX
Tel: 0115 950 5907/8 Fax: 0115 988 1582
(Nottingham City Primary Care Trust)

Practice Manager J Sherwood

GP Richard John WILSON, Ruth BOOTH, Peter John CANSFIELD, Sally Ann CAPLIN, Amanda Joyce NEVILLE, Alison Rhona TEED

West Bridgford Health Centre
97 Musters Road, West Bridgford, Nottingham NG2 7PX
Tel: 0115 981 1858/5666 Fax: 0115 982 6448
(Rushcliffe Primary Care Trust)

Practice Manager Hazel Wynaghan

GP Michael John WOODS

West End Surgery
19 Chilwell Road, Beeston, Nottingham NG9 1EH
Tel: 0115 925 4443 Fax: 0115 922 1255
Email: doctors@19chilwell.freeserve.co.uk
(Broxtowe and Hucknall Primary Care Trust)
Patient List Size: 7100

Practice Manager Debs Marsh

GP Stephen John BUNNAGE, Shelagh Frances BROWN, Gillian Ruth CALDER, Robin HUNTER

Western Boulevard Surgery
635 Western Boulevard, Nottingham NG8 5GS
Tel: 0115 9786557
(Nottingham City Primary Care Trust)

GP M K KACHROO

Wharfedale Surgery
41 Wharfendale, Road, Nottingham NG10 3HG
Tel: 0115 946 2690 Fax: 0115 946 2690
Email: trudi.cockayne@gp-c81642.nhs.uk
(Erewash Primary Care Trust)
Patient List Size: 3050

GP S GOKHALE, N GOKHALE

Willows Medical Centre
Church Street, Carlton, Nottingham NG4 1BJ
Tel: 0115 940 4252 Fax: 0115 956 9976
Email: npbhanji@bigfoot.com
(Gedling Primary Care Trust)
Patient List Size: 2500

GP Nasheer Pyarally BHANJI, Ian Wallace CAMPBELL, M B CHAUDRI

Windmill Practice
Sneinton Health Centre, Beaumont Street, Sneinton, Nottingham NG2 4PJ
Tel: 0115 950 5426 Fax: 0115 950 5404
Email: michael@windmillpractice.com
(Nottingham City Primary Care Trust)
Patient List Size: 5300

Practice Manager Robert White

GP Michael Adrian VARNAM, Margaret Daphne ABBOTT, Steve Gerard KNIGHTS, Helen SPERRY, Stephen WILLOTT

The Woll Surgery
The Welby Practice, Walford Close, Bottesford, Nottingham NG13 0AN
Tel: 01949 842325 Fax: 01949 844211
(Lincolnshire South West Teaching Primary Care Trust)
Patient List Size: 4700

Practice Manager Gill Bullimore

GP Karel MEUWISSEN, Julia REBSTEIN, Julia REBSTEIN, Laura SKINNER

Wollaton Vale Health Centre
Wollaton Vale, Nottingham NG8 2GR
Tel: 0115 928 1151 Fax: 0115 928 8703
(Nottingham City Primary Care Trust)
Patient List Size: 2800

GP Binay Kumar PATHAK

Wollaton Vale Health Centre
Wollaton Vale, Wollaton, Nottingham NG8 2GR
Tel: 0115 928 2216 Fax: 0115 928 0590
(Nottingham City Primary Care Trust)

GP Kamini Kumar ARANDHARA, John Richard MERRY, Pamela SAUNDERS

Wollaton Vale Health Centre
Wollaton Vale, Nottingham NG8 2GR
Tel: 0115 928 1842 Fax: 0115 916 6064
(Nottingham City Primary Care Trust)
Patient List Size: 2400

GP Khahayar GHAHARIAN

Nuneaton

Arbury Medical Centre
Cambridge Drive, Stockingford, Nuneaton CV10 8LW
Tel: 024 7638 8555 Fax: 024 7635 2396
(North Warwickshire Primary Care Trust)

Practice Manager John Holmes

GP James JACOB, Lisa Jayne BARFIELD, Michael GUEST, Rachael Mary GUMMERY, Martin Neil JORDAN

Camphill Road Surgery
10 Camp Hill Road, Nuneaton CV10 0JH
Tel: 024 7639 3111 Fax: 024 7639 7911
(North Warwickshire Primary Care Trust)
Patient List Size: 2425

Practice Manager G Ganapathi

GP Erode Nallathambi GANAPATHI

Camphill Road Surgery
10 Camp Hill Road, Nuneaton CV10 0JH
Tel: 024 7639 3388 Fax: 024 7639 7907
(North Warwickshire Primary Care Trust)

Practice Manager M Price

GP Anup Kumar CHAUDHURI

The Chaucer Surgery
Off School Walk, Attleborough, Nuneaton CV11 4UZ
Tel: 024 7638 3784 Fax: 024 7635 4958
Email: lynn.slater@gp-M84057.nhs.uk
(North Warwickshire Primary Care Trust)
Patient List Size: 2000

GP Mahesh Kumar ARORA

The Grange Medical Centre
39 Leicester Road, Nuneaton CV11 6AB
Tel: 024 7632 2810 Fax: 024 7632 2820
(North Warwickshire Primary Care Trust)

GP Arun KUMAR, Christopher Nicholas GRAHAM, James Ian HOPE, Karen Lynn JONES, John Gareth WILLIAMS

The Health Centre
High Street, Bedworth, Nuneaton CV12 8NQ
Tel: 024 7631 5827 Fax: 024 7631 0580
(North Warwickshire Primary Care Trust)

Practice Manager Catherine Henchcliffe

GP Clive Michael REILY, Vicente CASTELLS, Iain James CLAMP

Health Centre
High Street, Bedworth, Nuneaton CV12 8NQ
Tel: 024 7631 5432 Fax: 024 7631 0038
(North Warwickshire Primary Care Trust)
Patient List Size: 13700

Practice Manager Hilary Jackson

GP Susan Vicky PHELPS, Kirit GARALA, Andrew John GODFREY, Peter John HICKSON, Sukhdev Sanghera SINGH, Amer Ahmad ZURUB

Leicester Road Surgery
57 Leicester Road, Bedworth, Nuneaton CV12 8AB
Tel: 024 7631 2288 Fax: 024 7631 3502
(North Warwickshire Primary Care Trust)
Patient List Size: 3100

GP Dr WARKS

Manor Court Surgery
5 Manor Court Avenue, Nuneaton CV11 5HX
Tel: 024 7638 1999 Fax: 024 7632 0515
(North Warwickshire Primary Care Trust)

GP Harjit SINGH, Karim KHAN, Guner NECATI

The Old Cole House
41 Park Road, Bedworth, Nuneaton CV12 8LH
Tel: 024 7631 1200 Fax: 024 7631 2311
(North Warwickshire Primary Care Trust)

GP Richard Neil HYSLOP

Old Mill Surgery
Marlborough Road, Nuneaton CV11 5PQ
Tel: 024 7638 2554 Fax: 024 7635 0047
(North Warwickshire Primary Care Trust)
Patient List Size: 10000

Practice Manager Sharon Roberts

GP Robin Philip Donovan TOONE, Karen MARLOW, Steve MARSON, Mark WILLETT

Queens Road Surgery
88A Queens Road, Nuneaton CV11 5LE
Tel: 024 7664 2368 Fax: 024 7632 7204
(North Warwickshire Primary Care Trust)

GP Betty Lorraine Clare HENDERSON

Red Roofs
31 Coton Road, Nuneaton CV11 5TW
Tel: 024 7635 7100 Fax: 024 7664 2036
(North Warwickshire Primary Care Trust)
Patient List Size: 14600

Practice Manager Terry Salter

GP Roger GADSBY, Peter Eric BRUCK, Michael George BURNETT, Heather Rosemary GORRINGE, Elizabeth HODGES, Nigel JOHNSON, Stephen Howlett JONES, June Lorraine TODD, Michael Ting Chung WOO

Rugby Road Surgery
18 Rugby Road, Bulkington, Nuneaton CV12 9JE
Tel: 024 7664 3243 Fax: 024 7664 3918
(North Warwickshire Primary Care Trust)
Patient List Size: 3410

Practice Manager Lesley Davies

GP Christian Yogendradeva Theivendrasena MUTHIAH, Mankaiatkarasi MUTHIAH

Stockingford Medical Centre
13 Northumberland Avenue, Stockingford, Nuneaton CV10 8EJ
Tel: 024 7638 6344 Fax: 024 7638 4512
(North Warwickshire Primary Care Trust)
Patient List Size: 5625

Practice Manager Megna Boffin

GP Vijay Kumar AGRAWAL, Bishnodeo Narayan SINGH

The Surgery
Chancery Lane, Chapel End, Nuneaton CV10 0PB
Tel: 024 7639 4766 Fax: 024 7639 6870
(North Warwickshire Primary Care Trust)
Patient List Size: 5700

Practice Manager Lynn Gibson

GP Balwinder Singh SIDHU, Ram Paul BATRA, Jeremy MENAGE

The Surgery
Riversley Road, Nuneaton CV11 5QT
Tel: 024 7638 2239/7664 2409 Fax: 024 7632 5623
(South Warwickshire Primary Care Trust)

Practice Manager Rebecca Egan

GP Bhavinchandra Govindlal KACHHIA, Kishorchandra Lalji THANKEY

The Surgery
18 Bracebridge Street, Nuneaton CV11 5PA
Tel: 024 7664 1979 Fax: 024 7664 1911
(North Warwickshire Primary Care Trust)
Patient List Size: 2060

GP P KUMAR

Woodlands Surgery
301 New Town Road, Bedworth, Nuneaton CV12 0AJ
Tel: 024 7649 0909 Fax: 024 7631 0565
(North Warwickshire Primary Care Trust)
Patient List Size: 2400

Practice Manager Nalini Patel

GP Chandresh Ratilal PATEL

Oakham

Empingham Medical Centre
37 Main Street, Empingham, Oakham LE15 8PR
Tel: 01780 460202 Fax: 01780 460283
(Melton, Rutland and Harborough Primary Care Trust)

Practice Manager Alison Bairsto

GP Noel Richard SEYMOUR, Michael EAVES, Alison Elizabeth GUTHRIE, Susan Elizabeth SELMES

London Road Medical Centre
2 London Road, Uppingham, Oakham LE15 9JT
Fax: 01572 821145
(Melton, Rutland and Harborough Primary Care Trust)

Practice Manager Bonnie Shortt

GP Hugh Edward Gordon REES, Jeremy David CROSTHWAITE, Jennifer Palmer JONES, David Robert MAY

Oakham Medical Practice
Cold Overton Road, Oakham LE15 6NT
Tel: 01572 722621 Fax: 01572 722257
(Melton, Rutland and Harborough Primary Care Trust)
Patient List Size: 16000

Practice Manager Elga Zivtins

GP Timothy John GRAY, Sian G CHEVERTON, A DAVISON, David Andrew James KER, Susan Grace MARTIN, Graham Eugene McCORMACK, Helen SADLER, S J YOUNG

The Surgery
Thistleton Road, Market Overton, Oakham LE15 7PP
Tel: 01572 767229 Fax: 01572 767153
(Melton, Rutland and Harborough Primary Care Trust)

Practice Manager Gillian Pearson

GP Jeremy William FENBY TAYLOR

Okehampton

Devonshire House Surgery
Essington, North Tawton, Okehampton EX20 2EX
Tel: 01837 82204 Fax: 01837 82459
(Mid Devon Primary Care Trust)
Patient List Size: 2151

Practice Manager Linda Warre

GP John Henry WARRE, Karen RASAIAH

Hatherleigh Medical Centre
Pipers Meadow, Okehampton EX20 3JT
Tel: 01837 810283 Fax: 01837 810876
(Mid Devon Primary Care Trust)
Patient List Size: 2000

Practice Manager Michelle Downie

GP Malcolm Campbell DOWNIE

Okement Primary Care Centre
Okehampton Hospital, Cavell way, Okehampton EX20 1PN
Tel: 01837 658051 Fax: 01837 658072
(Mid Devon Primary Care Trust)
Patient List Size: 709

Practice Manager Felicity Barry

GP Keith GILLESPIE, Susan M TAHERI

Okethampton Medical Centre
East Street, Okehampton EX20 1AY
Tel: 01837 52233 Fax: 01837 54950
(Mid Devon Primary Care Trust)
Patient List Size: 11775

Practice Manager David Seward Seward

GP David Roland Tyeth GUNDRY, Thomas Richard Douglas BELL, Amanda Louise COX, Ian GOULT, Nigel PADFIELD, Ruth L TAYLOR, Kathryn Sarah Marjorie VILE, Timothy Martin WATSON, Nick WOODALL

Oldbury

Hill Top Medical Centre
15 Hill Top Road, Oldbury B68 9DU
Tel: 0121 422 2146 Fax: 0121 422 9235

(Oldbury and Smethwick Primary Care Trust)
Patient List Size: 7600

Practice Manager Carol Dugmore

GP Hany Sadek Fahmi HANNA, S J HOUSE, M M KHAN

Oakham Surgery
213 Regent Road, Tividale, Oldbury B69 1RZ
Tel: 01384 252274 Fax: 01384 240088
(Rowley Regis and Tipton Primary Care Trust)
Patient List Size: 9100

Practice Manager A J Cooper

GP J FINCH, A S NAGRA, A J NANKERVIS, B PATEL, I R SYKES, A J WRIGHT

Oldbury Health Centre
Old Bus Station Site, Halesowen Street, Oldbury B69 2AJ
Tel: 0121 552 6747 Fax: 0121 552 2999
(Oldbury and Smethwick Primary Care Trust)
Patient List Size: 10400

Practice Manager Jean Price

GP Basil Andreas ANDREOU, Alison Claire BEVERIDGE, Keith HOLTOM, Bryan Peter ROTHWELL, Karamvir Singh THANDI

Oldbury Health Centre
Albert Street, Oldbury B69 4DE
Tel: 0121 552 6665 Fax: 0121 544 8580
(Oldbury and Smethwick Primary Care Trust)

Practice Manager Lin Hill

GP Nicholas John GRIGGS

The Surgery
Pound Close, Oldbury B68 8LZ
Tel: 0121 552 1632 Fax: 0121 552 0848
(Oldbury and Smethwick Primary Care Trust)

Practice Manager Lyn Wharton

GP Shyam Hariram BATHIJA, Christine BINKS, Susan Jennifer COLLIER, Dalip Singh GAHLE, Nikhil MEWAR, Helen Mary NUTBEAM, John Edward TYLER

The Surgery
464 Hagley Road West, Oldbury B68 0DJ
Tel: 0121 422 2267 Fax: 0121 422 4808
(South Birmingham Primary Care Trust)

GP Karim LADHA

The Surgery
158 Causeway Green Road, Oldbury B68 8LJ
Tel: 0121 552 1968 Fax: 0121 544 2042
(Oldbury and Smethwick Primary Care Trust)
Patient List Size: 2300

Practice Manager Sue Pace

GP Mashi Sunder MASHICHARAN

The Surgery
Vicarage Road, Oldbury B68 8HL
Tel: 01922 626692 Fax: 0121 544 6075
(Oldbury and Smethwick Primary Care Trust)

Practice Manager Donna Cattell

GP Ismail Abdul-Latif MEHREZ

The Surgery
64 Dog Kennel Lane, Oldbury B68 9LZ
Tel: 0121 552 1713 Fax: 0121 552 9980
(Oldbury and Smethwick Primary Care Trust)

Practice Manager Margaret Ely

GP Abdul NAEEM

The Surgery
273 Tat Bank Road, Oldbury B68 6NP
Tel: 0121 544 8666 Fax: 0121 544 7666
(Oldbury and Smethwick Primary Care Trust)
Patient List Size: 1850

Practice Manager Mrs Menon

GP A G M MENON

Tividale Medical Centre
51A New Birmingham Road, Tividale, Oldbury B69 2JQ
Tel: 0121 552 1854 Fax: 0121 544 1927
(Oldbury and Smethwick Primary Care Trust)

Practice Manager Louise Merrick

GP Carl Francis PRIME

Walford Street Surgery
19 Walford Street, Tividale, Oldbury B69 2LD
Tel: 0121 557 1328 Fax: 0121 557 2274
(Rowley Regis and Tipton Primary Care Trust)
Patient List Size: 2400

Practice Manager Carol Adney

GP A C INDWAR, Elizabeth TAYLOR

Warley Road Surgery
118 Warley Road, Oldbury B68 9SZ
Tel: 0121 544 5681 Fax: 0121 544 0155
(Oldbury and Smethwick Primary Care Trust)

GP S KAUR, Dr HALLAN

Oldham

Alexandra Group Medical Practice
Glodwick Health Centre, 137 Glodwick Road, Oldham OL4 1YN
Tel: 0161 909 8370 Fax: 0161 909 8414
(Oldham Primary Care Trust)

Practice Manager Jpaul Cunningham

GP Peter Norman WRIGHT, Dianne Elizabeth SMITH

Alexandra Group Medical Practice
Glodwick Health Centre, 137 Glodwick Road, Oldham OL4 1YN
Tel: 0161 909 8377 Fax: 0161 909 8414
(Oldham Primary Care Trust)

Practice Manager Lesley Rajkovic

GP Fiona COOPER, William NCUBE

Alexandra Group Medical Practice
Glodwick Health Centre, 137 Glodwick Road, Oldham OL4 1YN
Tel: 0161 909 8391 Fax: 0161 909 8414
(Oldham Primary Care Trust)

Practice Manager V Nield

GP Anne Moira ROTHERY, Jennifer Anne ADDY

Alexandra Group Medical Practice
Glodwick Health Centre, Glodwick Road, Oldham OL4 1YN
Tel: 0161 909 8350 Fax: 0161 909 8354
(Oldham Primary Care Trust)
Patient List Size: 8975

Practice Manager June Hunt

GP Denise Irene MUNRO, Zuber AHMED, Phillip BLAND, Raj CHAUHAN, Ralph Michael HAMPSON

Block Lane Surgery
158 Block Lane, Chadderton, Oldham OL9 7SG
Tel: 0161 620 2321 Fax: 0161 628 5604
(Oldham Primary Care Trust)

GP J S BAILEY, C A McINTOSH, David A MENZIES, Janet Kay WREGLESWORTH

Cannon Street Health Centre
Cannon Street, Oldham OL9 6EP
Tel: 0161 909 8228 Fax: 0161 909 8226
(Oldham Primary Care Trust)

Practice Manager Elizabeth Chamley

GP Geoffrey ALLEN, Douglas Ian FLEMING, Roger McINNES

Chadderton and Hollinwood Medical Group
370 Manchester Road, Hollinwood, Oldham OL9 7PG
Tel: 0161 624 1287 Fax: 0161 620 9466
Website: www.ch-medical.co.uk
(Oldham Primary Care Trust)
Patient List Size: 6500

Practice Manager Sue Grant

GP Richard James ORR, Naseem Tariq GILL, Jane Elizabeth ROTHWELL, Dianne SMITH

Chadderton Health Centre
Middleton Road, Chadderton, Oldham OL9 0LH
Tel: 0161 652 5432
(Oldham Primary Care Trust)

GP Shahid AHMED, Saddat ALAM

Chadderton South Health Centre
Eaves lane, Chadderton, Oldham OL9 8RT
Tel: 0161 652 1876 Fax: 0161 909 8121
(Oldham Primary Care Trust)
Patient List Size: 2905

Practice Manager Julie Rose

GP Anita SHARMA

Chadderton (Town) Health Centre
Middleton Road, Chadderton, Oldham OL9 0LH
Tel: 0161 909 8131 Fax: 0161 909 8133
(Oldham Primary Care Trust)
Patient List Size: 9700

Practice Manager Pauline McGonigle, Beverly Thompson

GP Ian WILKINSON, J EVANS, Susan Jane KENYON, Attupaskam KUMAR, Adam SIMON

The Chowdhury Practice
Majory Lees Health Centre, Egerton Street, Oldham OL1 3SF
Tel: 0161 909 8444 Fax: 0161 909 8464
(Oldham Primary Care Trust)

Practice Manager Rez Chowdhury

GP Delowar Hussain CHOWDHURY

Compton Health Centre
High Street, Shaw, Oldham OL2 8ST
Tel: 01706 842511 Fax: 01706 847106
(Oldham Primary Care Trust)

GP Pahlaj Rai JETHANI, John Alan DUMSDAY, Sally Elizabeth HALL, Vijayan Ratnaraj ISAACS, Mark Noel WOODHOUSE

Crofton Street Surgery
1 Crofton Street, Oldham OL8 3BZ
Tel: 0161 624 4716 Fax: 0161 628 9513
(Oldham Primary Care Trust)
Patient List Size: 4800

Practice Manager Patricia Davis

GP John Francis GRAY

Crompton Health Centre
High Street, Shaw, Oldham OL2 8ST
Tel: 01706 842511 Fax: 01706 290751
(Oldham Primary Care Trust)

GP Syed AHMAD, Michael John BEARD, Pamela HEYES, John KELLY, Helena Mary Jane THORNTON, Carolyn Anne WALKER

Donald Wilde Medical Centre
283 Rochdale Road, Oldham OL1 2HG
Tel: 0161 652 3184 Fax: 0161 620 2101
(Oldham Primary Care Trust)
Patient List Size: 6000

Practice Manager M D Rimmer

GP Asimes CHAKRABARTI, Bipin Chimanbhai AMIN, Krishna PANIGRAHI, Dipak ROY

Doyle Moorside Medical Practice
3 Doyle Close, Sholver, Oldham OL1 4RG
Tel: 0161 652 0302 Fax: 0161 633 6547
(Oldham Primary Care Trust)
Patient List Size: 2000

Practice Manager Margaret Burgess

Dr Rajesh Saraf's Surgery
Glodwick Health Centre, 137 Glodwick Road, Oldham OL4 1YN
Tel: 0161 909 8388 Fax: 0161 909 8581
Email: thema.clarke@nhs.uk
(Oldham Primary Care Trust)
Patient List Size: 1850

Practice Manager Thelma Clark

GP Rajesh SARAF

Edward Street Surgery
2 Edward Street, Oldham OL9 7QW
Tel: 0161 624 1285 Fax: 0161 620 5914
(Oldham Primary Care Trust)

Practice Manager Linda Greenbank

GP John DANSON

Edward Street Surgery
2 Edward Street, Oldham OL9 7QW
Tel: 0161 627 0339 Fax: 0161 627 2437
(Oldham Primary Care Trust)

Practice Manager Anne Callow

GP Paul John CALLOW

Hollins Road Surgery
796 Hollins Road, Oldham OL8 4SA
Tel: 0161 682 2512
(Oldham Primary Care Trust)

Practice Manager Niharbala Mohanty

GP Artatran MOHANTY

Hopwood House
The Vineyard, Lees Road, Oldham OL4 1JN
Tel: 0161 628 3628 Fax: 0161 628 4970
(Oldham Primary Care Trust)
Patient List Size: 5700

Practice Manager Val Wild

GP Kathleen Grace BUCKLEY, Alan David NYE, Hugh STURGESS

Hopwood House
The Vineyard, Lees Road, Oldham OL4 1JN
Tel: 0161 633 2988 Fax: 0161 678 6266
(Oldham Primary Care Trust)
Patient List Size: 2700

Practice Manager Lilian Dalloway

Jarvis House Surgery
Jarvis Street, Oldham OL4 1DT
Tel: 0161 2728 Fax: 0161 628 8876
(Oldham Primary Care Trust)
Patient List Size: 2500

Practice Manager Yasmin Akttar

GP Nasreen SIKANDER

Leesbrook Surgery
Mellor Street, Lees, Oldham OL4 3DG
Tel: 0161 621 4800 Fax: 0161 628 6717
(Oldham Primary Care Trust)

GP John Whittaker KELSO, Fiona Margaret COGAN, Andrew William TAYLOR, Ian Graeme WHITLEY

The Medical Practice
53 Manchester Road, Oldham OL8 4LR
Tel: 0161 682 2120 Fax: 0161 620 2924
(Oldham Primary Care Trust)
Patient List Size: 4600

Practice Manager Jonquilyn Horton

GP Mohammed ALI, Ramaswamy RAJAN

The Orchards
2 Westfield Drive, Grasscroft, Oldham OL4 4HT

GP Catherine Hamilton CAMPBELL

The Perkins Practice
Marjory Lees Health Centre, Egerton Street, Oldham OL1 3SF
Tel: 0161 909 8425 Fax: 0161 909 8426
(Oldham Primary Care Trust)
Patient List Size: 2264

Practice Manager Helen Peel

GP Brian PERKINS

Royton Medical Centre
Market Street, Royton, Oldham OL2 5QA
Tel: 0161 652 6336 Fax: 0161 620 3986
Website: meta.dave@gp-p80159.nhs.uk
(Oldham Primary Care Trust)
Patient List Size: 4000

Practice Manager Meeta Dave

GP Vidya DHANAWADE

Royton Medical Centre
Rochdale Road, Royton, Oldham OL2 5QB
Tel: 0161 624 4857 Fax: 0161 628 5010
(Oldham Primary Care Trust)
Patient List Size: 7300

Practice Manager C Cenci

GP Saphal Kanti PAL, Anthony DEVINE, Rakesh KOHLI

Saddleworth Medical Practice
The Clinic, Smithy Lane, Uppermill, Oldham OL3 6AH
Tel: 01457 872228 Fax: 01457 876520
Website: www.saddleworthmedicalpractice.com
(Oldham Primary Care Trust)
Patient List Size: 12700

Practice Manager Tracy Jenkinson

GP Judith Margaret WRIGHT, Alison FLETCHER, Sarah Helen GARSIDE, Adam Matthew GIBBONS, Rus HARTLEY, Ian MILNES, Ian WATSON

Springfield House Medical Centre
275 Huddersfield Road, Oldham OL4 2RJ
Tel: 0161 633 2333 Fax: 0161 628 6682
(Oldham Primary Care Trust)
Patient List Size: 8500

Practice Manager Debbie Garside

GP Michael Colin BRADY, Matthew Henry MILTON, Michael Bernard KOSTECKY, Saroj SARAF

St Thomas Street South Surgery
2 St. Thomas Street South, Oldham OL8 1SG
Tel: 0161 665 3488 Fax: 0161 620 5510
(Oldham Primary Care Trust)
Patient List Size: 6500

GP Jagdish Chander KHURANA, Anand KHURANA

The Surgery
4 Collinge Street, Shaw, Oldham OL2 8AA
Tel: 01706 881028
(Oldham Primary Care Trust)

GP E A MKANDAWIRE

The Surgery
284 Lees Road, Oldham OL4 1PA
Tel: 0161 652 1285
(Oldham Primary Care Trust)
Patient List Size: 3895

Practice Manager Alison Wallace

GP P REID, N MISTRY

The Surgery
St. Chads Centre, Lime Green Parade, Limehurst, Oldham OL8 3HH
Tel: 0161 620 1611 Fax: 0161 627 2377
(Oldham Primary Care Trust)
Patient List Size: 2800

Practice Manager Karen Arundell

GP Dr MONKS

Sydney and Partners
St Mary's Medical Centre, Rock St, Oldham OL1 3UL
Tel: 0161 6206667 Fax: 0161 6262499
(Oldham Primary Care Trust)
Patient List Size: 4900

Practice Manager Ann Galbraith

GP John Paul Martin SYDNEY, Susan Elaine DIXON, Brian LEWIS

The Trewinnard Practice
Majory Lees Health Centre, Egerton Street, Oldham OL1 3SF
Tel: 0161 909 8454 Fax: 0161 909 8464
(Oldham Primary Care Trust)
Patient List Size: 2300

Practice Manager April Hall

GP Dr TREWINNARD

Werneth Hall Road Surgery
94 Werneth Hall Road, Oldham OL8 4BD
Tel: 0161 624 9856 Fax: 0161 633 4663
(Oldham Primary Care Trust)
Patient List Size: 3600

Practice Manager Kath Oldham

GP Jagjit Kumar KAPUR, Janet Ruth DAY

Westwood Medical Centre
Winterbottom Street, Westwood, Oldham OL9 6TS
Tel: 0161 633 3395 Fax: 0161 627 5809
(Oldham Primary Care Trust)

Practice Manager Margaret Wilkinson

GP Pradip PAUL

Windsor Road Surgery
76A Windsor Road, Oldham OL8 4AL
Tel: 0161 620 5677 Fax: 0161 620 2236
(Oldham Primary Care Trust)
Patient List Size: 3300

Practice Manager I Shah

GP M SHAH

Olney

Cobbs Garden Surgery
West Street, Olney MK46 5QG
Tel: 01234 711344 Fax: 01234 711883
(Milton Keynes Primary Care Trust)
Patient List Size: 8500

Practice Manager Emma L Barter

GP David Robin BARTLETT, Brian Edward PARTRIDGE, Jayne ADAMS, Suzanne Elizabeth BEAL, Stuart SHORT

Ongar

Great Bansons Surgery
Bansons Lane, Ongar CM5 9AR
Tel: 01277 363028 Fax: 01277 365264
(Epping Forest Primary Care Trust)

Practice Manager Brian Anderson

GP Hugh Fraser TAYLOR, Alwyn Ruth Noelle LLOYD, David Andrew ROGERS, Simon WHITEHEAD, Zia YAQUB

The Ongar Surgery
High Street, Ongar CM5 9AA
Tel: 01277 363976 Fax: 01277 365115
(Epping Forest Primary Care Trust)

Practice Manager Jean Harris

GP Nimal Kenneth MENON

Ormskirk

Aughton Surgery
19 Town Green Lane, Aughton, Ormskirk L39 6SE
Tel: 01695 422384
(West Lancashire Primary Care Trust)

Practice Manager Barbara Stubley

GP Michael Walter STUBLEY

Burscough Health Centre
Stanley Court, Lord Street, Burscough, Ormskirk L40 4LA
Tel: 01704 892254 Fax: 01704 897182
(West Lancashire Primary Care Trust)
Patient List Size: 4915

Practice Manager Audrey Meek

GP Barbara Lynne HAWKES, Christine SIMPSON, Rachel WOODALL

Burscough Health Centre
Stanley Court, Lord Street, Burscough, Ormskirk L40 4LA
Tel: 01704 894997
(West Lancashire Primary Care Trust)

Practice Manager Linda Roberts

GP Sushil SURI, Shobha SURI

County Road Surgery
109 County Road, Ormskirk L39 1NL
Tel: 01695 572714
(West Lancashire Primary Care Trust)

GP Ranjit RAY

Elms Surgery
5 Derby Street, Ormskirk L39 2BJ
Tel: 01695 571560 Fax: 01695 578300
(West Lancashire Primary Care Trust)
Patient List Size: 6400

Practice Manager Pam Greaves

GP Charles David TRAVIS, Richard T CORKE, Christine RANDALL, Ruth E THOMASSON

Latham House Surgery
Latham House Surgery, 31 Lord Street, Burscough, Ormskirk L40 4BZ
Tel: 01704 895566 Fax: 01704 897510
(West Lancashire Primary Care Trust)
Patient List Size: 4000

Practice Manager Margaret Draper

GP Andrew Gordon KIPPAX, Alison Mary STATHAM

Leyland House Surgery
18 Derby Street, Ormskirk L39 2BY
Tel: 01695 579501 Fax: 01695 571724
(West Lancashire Primary Care Trust)

GP Hugh Robert Lee BISHOP-CORNET, Simon Peter FRAMPTON, Susan Rose MARSHALL

Park Gate Surgery
28 St. Helens Road, Ormskirk L39 4QR
Tel: 01695 72561 Fax: 01695 571709
(West Lancashire Primary Care Trust)
Patient List Size: 7000

Practice Manager Vi Holland

GP Alfred Joseph CUNNINGTON, Alistair John GARDINER, Betty UNDERWOOD

Railway Road Surgery
11 Railway Road, Ormskirk L39 2DN
Tel: 01695 572096 Fax: 01695 570049
(West Lancashire Primary Care Trust)
Patient List Size: 2170

Practice Manager M Hardman-Welsh, Lisa Jackson

GP Sujoy BISWAS, R BONSOR, S PANIKKER

Rose Allod Surgery
21 Knowsley Road, Ormskirk L39 4RB
Tel: 01695 577215 Fax: 01695 572886
Email: simondarley@yahoo.co.uk
(West Lancashire Primary Care Trust)
Patient List Size: 1450

Practice Manager Judy Darley

GP Simon Nicolas DARLEY

Stanley Street Surgery
6 Stanley Street, Ormskirk L39 2DH
Tel: 01695 572085
(West Lancashire Primary Care Trust)

GP Akhilesh Kumar VARMA

Orpington

Bank House Surgery
84 High Street, Farnborough, Orpington BR6 7BA
Tel: 01689 857691 Fax: 01689 850042
(Bromley Primary Care Trust)

Practice Manager Dorothy Bain

GP Jan BLACK

Broomwood Road Surgery
41 Broomwood Road, St Paul's Cray, Orpington BR5 2JP
Tel: 01689 832454 Fax: 01689 826165
(Bromley Primary Care Trust)
Patient List Size: 10500

Practice Manager Marion Mundy

GP Jonathan Ashley PALIN

The Crescent Surgery
38 Marion Crescent, St Mary Cray, Orpington BR5 2DD
Tel: 01689 818696 Fax: 01689 609634
(Bromley Primary Care Trust)
Patient List Size: 2500

Practice Manager Carole Howell

GP Kathleen Patricia RING

Crofton Surgery
109A Crofton Road, Orpington BR6 8HU
Tel: 01689 822266 Fax: 01689 891790
(Bromley Primary Care Trust)

Practice Manager Gill Howes

GP John William BRENNAN, J LAMB, F LYONS

Cross Hall Surgery
31 High Street, St Mary Cray, Orpington BR5 3NL
Tel: 01689 831949 Fax: 01689 833595
(Bromley Primary Care Trust)

GP S BALACHANDRAN

The Doctors Centre
41 Broomwood Road, Orpington BR5 2JP
Tel: 01689 832454 Fax: 01689 826165
(Bromley Primary Care Trust)

Practice Manager Marion Mundy

GP Oonagh Rosemary WOOTTON, Diane Clare BAMBERGER, S T H CHEUNG, Kurunandan Rathawrsingh COONJOBEEHARRY, Jonathan Ashley PALIN, Marian Elizabeth ROBERTS

The Family Surgery
7 High Street, Green Street Green, Orpington BR6 6BG
Tel: 01689 850231 Fax: 01689 862746
(Bromley Primary Care Trust)

Practice Manager Sandra Simmons

GP Christopher Iain MACKENZIE, Veinan PARKER

Green Street Green Medical Centre
21A High Street, Green Street Green, Orpington BR6 6BG
Tel: 01689 850012 Fax: 01689 862247
Website: www.gsgmc.co.uk
(Bromley Primary Care Trust)

Practice Manager Louise Hussey

GP Geoffrey Robin BARKER, Peter Ralph BARKER, C LEWIS

Knoll Rise Surgery
1 Knoll Rise, Orpington BR6 0EJ
Tel: 01689 824563 Fax: 01689 820712
(Bromley Primary Care Trust)
Patient List Size: 5000+

Practice Manager Dorothy Banning

GP Rengaswami SELVARANGAN, Christeta Ratnakumari PUSHPARAJAH

Poverest Medical Centre
42 Poverest Road, St Mary Cray, Orpington BR5 2DQ
Tel: 01689 833645 Fax: 01689 891976
(Bromley Primary Care Trust)

Practice Manager Sandra Peek

GP A BANJOKO, Kevin Sidney DENNIS, E EDWARDS, A MUSTAPHA, W OVIONJI, Anna Louise WILKINSON

Summerlands Surgery
Starts Hill Road, Farnborough, Orpington BR6 7AR
Tel: 01689 861098 Fax: 01689 852165
Email: enquiries@summerlandssurgery.com
(Bromley Primary Care Trust)
Patient List Size: 6800

Practice Manager Frank McNichol

GP Simon Jack TURLEY, Joseph Henry Lewis BAILEY, Mark DAVIS, Colin Mark FINCHAM

The Surgery
322 High Street, St. Mary Cray, Orpington BR5 4AR
Tel: 01689 820523 Fax: 01689 821145
(Bromley Primary Care Trust)
Patient List Size: 3500

Practice Manager Susan Robinson

GP Mosammat Jarina BEGUM

The Surgery
29 Derry Downs, Orpington BR5 4DU
Tel: 01689 820036 Fax: 01689 819768
(Bromley Primary Care Trust)
Patient List Size: 5350

Practice Manager Bhama Mahesuaran

GP Catharine Helen WAGNER, Amrit Pal Singh BINDRAN, Seluadurai MAHESWARAN

The Surgery
108 Chislehurst Road, Orpington BR6 0DP
Tel: 01689 826664 Fax: 01689 890795
(Bromley Primary Care Trust)

Practice Manager Joan Wallis-Norton

GP Abdolah TAVABIE, Jacqueline Ann TAVABIE

The Surgery
62 Windsor Drive, Orpington BR6 6HD
Tel: 01689 852204 Fax: 01689 857122
(Bromley Primary Care Trust)

Practice Manager David Powis

GP Janet Catherine Murray LEGGETT, Vernon Lester PARKER, Jalal SHARIF, Gail Allison WALKER

The Surgery
59 Sevenoaks Road, Orpington BR6 9JN
Tel: 01689 820159 Fax: 01689 835367
(Bromley Primary Care Trust)
Patient List Size: 8900

Practice Manager Mike Smith

GP Penelope Kim LESTER, Dr MERCER, Martyn John NICHOLLS, Lesley TAOR, Robert Tester THOMPSON, David Lloyd WILLIAMS

The Surgery
8 Oakleigh Gdns, Orpington BR6 9PL

GP Anne Elizabeth GANCKE

The Surgery
44 Sevenoaks Road, Orpington BR6 9JR
Tel: 01689 821179 Fax: 01689 832579
(Bromley Primary Care Trust)
Patient List Size: 2600

Practice Manager V Purwar

GP Ram Manohar GUPTA

The Surgery
1 Gillmans Road, Orpington BR5 4LA
Tel: 01689 822022 Fax: 01689 897929
(Bromley Primary Care Trust)

Practice Manager Bhama Maheswaran

GP S MAHESWARAN

The Surgery
74 Perry Hall Road, Orpington BR6 0HS
Tel: 01689 837366 Fax: 01689 872990
(Bromley Primary Care Trust)

Practice Manager Stella Orphanides

GP D ORPHANIDES

The Surgery
2B Tile Farm Road, Orpington BR6 9RZ
Tel: 01689 855022 Fax: 01689 860355
(Bromley Primary Care Trust)

Practice Manager S Moosvi

GP Syed Kazim MOOSVI

Tudor Way Surgery
42 Tudor Way, Orpington BR5 1LH
Tel: 01689 820268 Fax: 01689 839414
(Bromley Primary Care Trust)
Patient List Size: 5600

Practice Manager Linda Lugg

GP S RAJASUNDARAM, Selene JAISRI, Nadarajah NAVARATNARAJAH

The Whitehouse Surgery
123 Towncourt Lane, Petts Wood, Orpington BR5 1EL
Tel: 01689 821551 Fax: 01689 818692
Email: whitehouse.surgery@gp-g84621.nhs.uk
(Bromley Primary Care Trust)
Patient List Size: 3300

Practice Manager Carol Rogers

GP A D PERERA, A F FENUYI

Ossett

The Group Surgery
Church Street, Ossett WF5 9DE
Tel: 01924 217999 Fax: 01924 217676
(Wakefield West Primary Care Trust)
Patient List Size: 11100

Practice Manager Janice Burnley

GP Simon J DYSON, Paul Nicholas FARRIMOND, Frank FURNESS, Christopher Scott JONES, Michael John LANGTON, A RASHID

Prospect Road Surgery
22 Prospect Road, Ossett WF5 8AN
Tel: 01924 274123 Fax: 01924 263350
(Wakefield West Primary Care Trust)
Patient List Size: 7300

Practice Manager Marion Dickinson

GP Jane Elizabeth SENIOR, Graham COLE, Adrian NORTH

Oswestry

Cae Glas Doctors Surgery
34 Church Street, Oswestry SY11 2SP
Tel: 01691 652929 Fax: 01691 670175
(Shropshire County Primary Care Trust)
Patient List Size: 5300

Practice Manager Sheila Jones

GP Ian Frank RUMMENS, Sarah ESLAVA, Simon Haydn ROBINSON

The Caxton Surgery
Oswald Road, Oswestry SY11 1RD
Tel: 01691 654646 Fax: 01691 670994
(Shropshire County Primary Care Trust)

Practice Manager Helen Owens

GP David Lister CAMPBELL, Michael ARTHUR, Joanna BEACH-THOMAS, Jacqueline LEATHER, Alastair Ian MACKERETH, Paul Ian MIDDLETON, Joanne REES

Knockin Surgery
Knockin, Oswestry SY10 8HL
Tel: 01691 682203 Fax: 01691 682700
(Shropshire County Primary Care Trust)

GP Mark Douglas JOHNSON, William GRECH

Plas Ffynnon Medical Centre
Middleton Road, Oswestry SY11 2RB
Tel: 01691 655844
(Shropshire County Primary Care Trust)
Patient List Size: 8400

Practice Manager R J Roden

GP Richard Anthony Robert TREASURE, Wendy DYKE, David LOVEDAY, Raymond Grant McMURRAY, Helen WILLOWS

Willow Street Medical Centre
81-83 Willow Street, Oswestry SY11 1AJ
Tel: 01691 653143 Fax: 01691 679130
(Shropshire County Primary Care Trust)

Practice Manager R A Clarke

GP Peter Seymour Lorraine BARLING, Harry Timothy Richard BREESE, Rosemary POWELL, Anthony St. John TAYLOR

Otley

Chevin Medical Practice
3 Bridge Street, Otley LS21 1BQ
Tel: 01943 858300 Fax: 01943 858333
Email: dave.kendall@gp-B86032.nhs.uk
(Leeds North West Primary Care Trust)

Practice Manager M C Moryson

GP Charan Jeev GOGNA, Dave KENDALL, Jennifer Anne LUND, Emily MUIRHEAD, Nicholas John NATHAN, Simon David North O'HARA, Claire RENWICK, Marcus SMITH

Westgate Surgery
Westgate, Otley LS21 3HD
Tel: 01943 465406 Fax: 01943 468363
(Leeds North West Primary Care Trust)
Patient List Size: 4910

Practice Manager Deborah Hollings

GP Pauline SPENCER, Victoria McKEEVER, Simon David ROBINSON, Oliver SYKES

Ottery St Mary

Coleridge Medical Centre
Canaan Way, Ottery St Mary EX11 1EQ
Tel: 01404 814447 Fax: 01404 816716
Email: reception@gp-l83095.nhs.uk
(East Devon Primary Care Trust)
Patient List Size: 15000

Practice Manager Anne Maher

GP John Turner ACKROYD, Jean Margaret BROWN, Timothy John COX, Nigel Antoninus DE SOUSA, Christopher John DILLEY, Katharine Jane GURNEY, S J KERR, Matthew Raymond KING, Emma Louise STUART

Oxford

Banbury Road Surgery
172 Banbury Road, Oxford OX2 7BT
Tel: 01865 515731 Fax: 01865 510711
(Oxford City Primary Care Trust)
Patient List Size: 8000

Practice Manager Richard Hamilton

GP Jane Elizabeth MORRIS, Helen GASKELL, Christopher HORNBY, Antony MADDISON, Catherine Teresa McDONNELL

Beaumont Street Surgery
19 Beaumont Street, Oxford OX1 2NA
Tel: 01865 240501 Fax: 01865 240503
(Oxford City Primary Care Trust)

Practice Manager Angie Eachus

GP Donald Neil MacLENNAN, Christopher Mark KENYON, Ann McPHERSON, Simon John PLINT, Meriel RAINE, N M RAINE, Richard Donald SILVESTER, Deborah Jane WALLER

Beaumont Street Surgery
28 Beaumont Street, Oxford OX1 2NP
Tel: 01865 311811 Fax: 01865 310327
(Oxford City Primary Care Trust)
Patient List Size: 5000

Practice Manager Susie Hyde-Smith

GP John Henry Sylvester SICHEL, Diana Elizabeth Jane FERGUSON, Cecilia GOULD

Beaumont Street Surgery
27 Beaumont Street, Oxford City, Oxford OX1 2NR
Tel: 01865 311500 Fax: 01865 311720
Email: practice@gp-k84049.nhs.uk
(Oxford City Primary Care Trust)
Patient List Size: 8500

Practice Manager Meriel Redknap

GP Hugo Neville HAMMERSLEY, Catharine Alice BENSON, Sarah LEDINGHAM, Jane Alison MORTENSEN

Blackbird Leys Health Centre
63 Blackbird Leys Road, Oxford OX4 6HL
Tel: 01865 778244
(Oxford City Primary Care Trust)

Practice Manager Geoff Price

GP Fergus George Rose BURTENSHAW, Stuart William CRAIG, Fiona Ruth Caroline Gordon DUXBURY, E Jane MOORE, Matthew WILKINSON

Botley Medical Centre
Elms Road, Botley, Oxford OX2 9JS
Tel: 01865 248719 Fax: 01865 728116
(Oxford City Primary Care Trust)

Practice Manager Penny Harris

GP John Norman SLATER, Leszek Wladyslaw BLAZEWICZ, John David Henry CHADWICK, Robert Barnby MARSDEN

Bury Knowle Health Centre
207 London Road, Headington, Oxford OX3 9JA
Tel: 01865 761651 Fax: 01865 768559
Website: www.buryknowle.org
(Oxford City Primary Care Trust)
Patient List Size: 11000

Practice Manager Stuart MacFarlane

GP Cecilia Mary Meredyth PYPER, Justin Mark AMERY, Debra BLYTHE, Robert Thompson WALTON

Donnington Health Centre
1 Henley Avenue, Oxford OX4 4DH
Tel: 01865 771207
(Oxford City Primary Care Trust)

Practice Manager Jo Gleed

GP Paresh Suryaprasad MEHTA

Donnington Health Centre
1 Henley Avenue, Oxford OX4 4DH
Tel: 01865 771207 Fax: 01865 770781
(Oxford City Primary Care Trust)
Patient List Size: 2625

Practice Manager Linda Gardiner

GP P S MEHTA, Marion K ANSCOMBE, Richard Arthur GREEN, Jane HEMPSON-BROWN, Susan Patricia HOPE, Peter Martin SAUNDERS, Stephen Arthur WILLIS, Stephen J WOOD

Donnington Health Centre
1 Henley Avenue, Oxford OX4 4DH
Tel: 01865 771313
(Oxford City Primary Care Trust)

Practice Manager John Folley

GP Stephen WOOD, Marion Katharine ANSCOMBE, Richard Arthur GREEN, Jane HEMPSON BROWN, Peter Martin SAUNDERS

Dr Rajakulendran
Woodfarm Health Centre, Leiden Road, Oxford OX3 8RZ
Tel: 01865 762500 Fax: 01865 762511
Email: thambimuthu.raj@gp-k84620.nhs.uk
(Oxford City Primary Care Trust)
Patient List Size: 2225

Practice Manager S Rajakulendran

GP Thambimuthu RAJAKULENDRAN

Dr Robson and Partners
Manzil Way, Cowley Road, Cowley, Oxford OX4 1XD
Tel: 01865 242109
Website: www.home.clara.net/eichstorff
(Oxford City Primary Care Trust)

Practice Manager Maggie Perrin

GP Georgina Mary Willett ROBSON, Thomas John Francis NICHOLSON-LAILEY, Tarrant Robert STEIN, Peter Daniel George VON EICHSTORFF, Kathryn WARD

East Oxford Health Centre
Manzil Way, Cowley Road, Cowley, Oxford OX4 1XD
Tel: 01865 791850 Fax: 01865 727358
(Oxford City Primary Care Trust)
Patient List Size: 4500

Practice Manager David Carthy

GP Richard Murray STEVENS, Alana Jane FAWCETT, Helen GROOM

High Street Surgery
48 High Street, Chalgrove, Oxford OX44 7SS
Tel: 01865 890760
(South East Oxfordshire Primary Care Trust)
Patient List Size: 7400

Practice Manager Gerry Davidson

GP Ian Andrew NEALE, Eileen Maura McMANUS

Hollow Way Medical Centre
58 Hollow Way, Cowley, Oxford OX4 2NJ
Tel: 01865 777495 Fax: 01865 771472
(Oxford City Primary Care Trust)
Patient List Size: 7000

GP Martin FLEMINGER, Robert BENNETT, David Eric CHAPMAN, Deborah Lynne GOLDMAN, Louise Joy HICKS

Jericho Health Centre
Walton Street, Oxford OX2 6NW
Tel: 01865 311234 Fax: 01865 311087
(Oxford City Primary Care Trust)

Practice Manager Senga Allen

GP James Michael KENWORTHY-BROWNE, Judith Evelyn BOGDANOR, Laurence Bradley LEAVER, Mark Patrick O'SHEA, Colin Richard TIDY

Jericho Health Centre
Walton Street, Oxford OX2 6NW
Tel: 01865 558861 Fax: 01865 311884
(Oxford City Primary Care Trust)
Patient List Size: 2210

Practice Manager Nicky White

GP Charles Andrew CHIVERS, Claire PARKER

Kendall Crescent Health Centre
Templer Road Estate, Oxford OX2 8NE
Tel: 01865 512288 Fax: 01865 310046
Email: diana.young@gp-K84623.nhs.uk
(Oxford City Primary Care Trust)
Patient List Size: 2198

GP Mark Reinhardt HUCKSTEP

Kennington Health Centre
200 Kennington Road, Kennington, Oxford OX1 5PY
Tel: 01865 730911 Fax: 01865 327759
(Oxford City Primary Care Trust)
Patient List Size: 6500

Practice Manager Yvonne Milward

GP Stuart Charles FRANKUM, Mary O AKINOLA, Janet Mary DARLING, Richard John ERIN, Rosamond Maria HALL, Linda Ann JONES

King Edward Street Surgery
9 King Edward Street, Oxford City, Oxford OX1 4JA
Tel: 01865 242657
(Oxford City Primary Care Trust)

GP Gordon GANCZ

Luther Street Primary Care Ltd
Luther Street, PO Box 7, Oxford OX1 1TD
Tel: 01865 726008 Fax: 01865 204133
Email: sallyreynolds@lutherstreet.freeserve.co.uk
(Oxford City Primary Care Trust)
Patient List Size: 1250

Practice Manager Fiona Grove

GP Sally REYNOLDS, Angela JONES, James PORTER, Sue PRITCHARD, Charles RISTIC

Manor Surgery
Osler Road, Headington, Oxford OX3 9BP
Tel: 01865 762535
(Oxford City Primary Care Trust)

Practice Manager Sue Smith

GP Gerald Edmund SACKS, Richard Jeremy BARNETT, David Balfour BULLOCK, Honor Mary MERRIMAN, (Karen) Jane ROBLIN, David Michael STERN

Marston Medical Centre
24 Cherwell Drive, Headington, Oxford OX3 0LY
Tel: 01865 761234 Fax: 01865 744066
(Oxford City Primary Care Trust)

Practice Manager Wendy Greenberg

GP Robert ARMSTRONG, Margaret Susan DENMAN, Paul GALLOWAY, David Robert SCARFE

Morland House Surgery
2 London Road, Wheatley, Oxford OX33 1YJ
Tel: 01865 872448 Fax: 01865 874158
(South East Oxfordshire Primary Care Trust)

Practice Manager Carol Cripps

GP Lynda Maria WARE, David COPPING, Catherine GOTHARD, Anthony Richard HARNDEN, Stephen HARPER, Amanda HART, Elinor Myles PRICE

North Oxford Medical Centre
96 Woodstock Road, Oxford OX2 7NE
Tel: 01865 311005 Fax: 01865 311257
(Oxford City Primary Care Trust)
Patient List Size: 5800

Practice Manager Karen Rhodes

GP Robert John MATHER, Karen Lesley HOWIE, Helen Clare STEEL, Peter Randall WILLIAMS

South Oxford Health Centre
Lake Street, Oxford OX1 4RP
Tel: 01865 244428 Fax: 01865 200985
(Oxford City Primary Care Trust)
Patient List Size: 3300

Practice Manager Tricia Smith

GP Anthony Alexander Stephen RANDALL, Maggie BUDDEN, Gillian Shirley DEAN

St Bartholomew's Medical Centre
Manzil Way, Cowley Road, Cowley, Oxford OX4 1XB
Tel: 01865 242334 Fax: 01865 204018
Website: www.sbmc.org
(Oxford City Primary Care Trust)
Patient List Size: 15750

Practice Manager Jane Marshall

GP Ann BEVAN, Peter David BURKE, Roger BURNE, Rachel BUTLER, Alison FAIRLEY, Jeanne FAY, Mohamad Hanif RAHIM

St Clements Surgery
39 Temple Street, Oxford OX4 1JS
Tel: 01865 248550
(Oxford City Primary Care Trust)

Practice Manager Elizabeth Wheeler

GP Donald Edward MILLAR, William Stanley CRONAN, Helen Alexandra McBEATH

Summertown Group Practice
160 Banbury Road, Oxford OX2 7BS
Tel: 01865 515552 Fax: 01865 311237
Website: www.summertownhc.co.uk
(Oxford City Primary Care Trust)
Patient List Size: 13500

Practice Manager Jessica Newman

GP Judith Mary SHAKESPEARE, Siobhan BECKER, Richard Alban BRIGGS, Simon Philip CURTIS, Carolyn Jane GODLEE, Roisin McCLOSKEY, Penelope Jane MOORE

Temple Cowley Health Centre
Templar House, Temple Road, Oxford OX4 2HL
Tel: 01865 777024 Fax: 01865 777548
(Oxford City Primary Care Trust)

Practice Manager Carole Barnes

GP Anthony Hugh ABRAHAMS, David Michael DORLING, Ian Quarmby EASTWOOD, Barbara Helen PORTER, Laura Marion TURBERFIELD, Andrew Stuart Parker WILSON, Ruth Pauline Elspeth WILSON

Williamson and Partners
Jericho Health Centre, Walton Street, Oxford OX2 6NW
Tel: 01865 429993 Fax: 01865 458410
(Oxford City Primary Care Trust)
Patient List Size: 6100

Practice Manager K Whitehead

GP Kenneth Noel Bamford WILLIAMSON, Karen Elizabeth KEARLEY, Helen SALISBURY, Dave TRIFFITT

Wolvercote Surgery
73 Godstow Road, Wolvercote, Oxford OX2 8PE
Tel: 01865 556044
(Oxford City Primary Care Trust)

GP Nina Valerie CARTWRIGHT

Oxted

The Health Centre
10 Gresham Road, Oxted RH8 0BQ
Tel: 01883 832850 Fax: 01883 832851
(East Surrey Primary Care Trust)
Patient List Size: 15900

Practice Manager H Marriott

GP Michael John MYERS, Cynthia ÉCLAIR-HEATH, David Jonathan HILL, T N JONES, Carolyn Kendrick MARSH, Peter Keith MORLEY, N D SATHANANTHAN, Richard Wallace SPILLER, John Sheldon WILLIAMS

Padstow

Padstow Medical Centre
Boyd Avenue, Padstow PL28 8ER
Tel: 01841 532346 Fax: 01841 532602
(Central Cornwall Primary Care Trust)
Patient List Size: 14400

Practice Manager Sheila Morgan

GP Gareth John Hughes EMRYS-JONES, Christina HUNT, Fiona MACKINNON, Ian Alexander McKELVEY, Sean O'SHEA, Martin Stuart PRIEST, Mark STEPHEN

Paignton

Bishops Place Surgery
1 Bishops Place, Paignton TQ3 3DZ
Tel: 01803 559421 Fax: 01803 663381
(Torbay Primary Care Trust)
Patient List Size: 3800

Practice Manager Ingrid Marsh

GP Veronica Eileen DEAKIN, Ian Paul DEAKIN, Richars DEAKIN

Cherry Brook Medical Centre
Hookhills Road, Paignton TQ4 7SH
Tel: 01803 844566 Fax: 01803 845244
Email: enquiries.cherrybrookenhs.net
Website: www.cherrybrookmedicalcentre.co.uk
(Torbay Primary Care Trust)
Patient List Size: 3400

Practice Manager T Blackburn

GP David Cameron MILLS, B JAMES, David Laurence WILLIAMS

Corner Place Surgery
46A Dartmouth Road, Paignton TQ4 5AH
Tel: 01803 557458 Fax: 01803 524844
(Torbay Primary Care Trust)
Patient List Size: 11550

Practice Manager Brenda van den Berg

GP Peter John MacLOUGHLIN, Gillian Anne RICHARDS, Ian Michael RICHARDS

Grosvenor Road Surgery
17 Grosvenor Road, Paignton TQ4 5LB
Tel: 01803 559308 Fax: 01803 526702
(Torbay Primary Care Trust)
Patient List Size: 5550

Practice Manager Hazel Cook

GP William Morison WATT, Simon Robert Poole LANSDOWN, Jonathan Patrick Tristram SHAW, Yvette Elizabeth STEELE

Mayfield Medical Centre
37 Totnes Road, Paignton TQ4 5LA
Tel: 01803 558257 Fax: 01803 663353
(Torbay Primary Care Trust)

Practice Manager Laurette M E Ackland

GP Deborah Anne AVERY, Lorraine Patricia FOREMAN, Andrew Giles HAMMERSLEY, Robin Fellows HYDE, Jonathan David Vaughan ROBERTS, Edward SOUTHALL

Old Farm Surgery
67 Foxhole Road, Paignton TQ3 3TB
Tel: 01803 556403 Fax: 01803 665588
Email: oldfarm@gp-6836007.nhs.uk
Website: www.oldfarmsurgery.co.uk
(Torbay Primary Care Trust)
Patient List Size: 3750

Practice Manager Madeline Way

GP James Gerard BULLEN, Sarah HANROOT, Anne Judith LOWES

Pembroke House Surgery
1 Fortescue Road, Paignton TQ3 2DA
Tel: 01803 553558 Fax: 01803 663180
(Torbay Primary Care Trust)

Practice Manager Louise Glover, Louise Killick

GP Philip Anthony GREEN, William Peter Fowler HOWITT, Peter Geoffrey HUNT, Carol Rosemary KUUR

Upper Manor Road Surgery
95 Upper Manor Road, Paignton TQ3 2TQ
Tel: 01803 558034 Fax: 01803 523339
(Torbay Primary Care Trust)
Patient List Size: 1500

Practice Manager Diane Radford

GP John Robert BRIDGE

Withycombe Lodge Surgery
123 Torquay Road, Paignton TQ3 2SG
Tel: 01803 525525 Fax: 01803 550314
Email: withycombe.lodge:gp-L83637.nhs.uk
Website: www.withycombelodgesurgery.co.uk
(Torbay Primary Care Trust)
Patient List Size: 2050

Practice Manager Lesley Jones

GP Henryk SLOMKA, Nicola SPICER

Par

Middleway Surgery
Middleway, St. Blazey, Par PL24 2JL
Tel: 01726 812019 Fax: 01726 816464
(Central Cornwall Primary Care Trust)
Patient List Size: 6250

Practice Manager Yvonne Endean

GP Bernard Francis HANNETT, J A HAYWOOD, C L McGUINNESS, Penelope Elizabeth MONK

Peacehaven

Central Surgery
1 Central Court, Central Avenue, Telscombe Cliffs, Peacehaven BN10 7LU
Tel: 01273 588777 Fax: 01273 588522
Email: lal.mandel@nhs.net
(Sussex Downs and Weald Primary Care Trust)
Patient List Size: 2177

GP Lal B MANDAL

Foxhill Medical Centre
10-11 Foxhill, Peacehaven BN10 7SE
Tel: 01273 583637 Fax: 01273 580586
Email: reception.foxhill@nhs.net
(Sussex Downs and Weald Primary Care Trust)
Patient List Size: 2800

Practice Manager L Alliston

GP Virendra Kumar GUPTA

Meridian Surgery
Meridian Way, Peacehaven BN10 8NF
Tel: 01273 581999 Fax: 01273 589025
(Sussex Downs and Weald Primary Care Trust)
Patient List Size: 7000

Practice Manager Sarah Uron

GP John Edward ETHERTON, Andrew James STARLING, Christopher John GURTLER, Ron WHITE

Rowe Avenue Surgery
17 Rowe Avenue, Peacehaven BN10 7PE
Tel: 01273 579500/579505 Fax: 01273 579501
(Sussex Downs and Weald Primary Care Trust)
Patient List Size: 6000

Practice Manager Geraldine Anscombe

GP Graham John MILNE, Liam Geoffrey BYRNE, Helen Anne JEFFORD

Penrith

Birbeck Medical Group
Penrith Health Centre, Bridge Lane, Penrith CA11 8HW
Tel: 01768 245200 Fax: 01768 245295
(Eden Valley Primary Care Trust)

Practice Manager A P Bowmer

GP Anthony REED, Robert BARR, Josephine DUNLOP, Michael Stewart DUNLOP, John Alexander ELLERTON, James Peter Gordon HODKIN, Helen Ann LONG, Ian Paul PRITCHARD, V L PURDY, Theodore Paul WESTON

Bishopyards Medical Group
Penrith Health Centre, Bridge Lane, Penrith CA11 8HW
Tel: 01768 245219 Fax: 01768 891052
(Eden Valley Primary Care Trust)
Patient List Size: 5500

GP Graham BUCKLE, R M PRESTON, C BROOK, Caroline Jane HALLE, Ian William MITCHELL

Corney Place Medical Group
The Health Centre, Bridge Lane, Penrith CA11 8HW
Tel: 01768 245226 Fax: 01768 245229
(Eden Valley Primary Care Trust)
Patient List Size: 4200

Practice Manager J McLeod

GP Paul Gerard Ruthven GOULDING, A C ECKERSALL, Richard William HALL

Doctors Surgery
Shap Medical Practice, West Lane, Shap, Penrith CA10 3LT
Tel: 01931 716230 Fax: 01931 716231
(Eden Valley Primary Care Trust)
Patient List Size: 2900

GP H DUNNING, M McCABE, Dr STENHOUSE

Glenridding Health Centre
Glenridding, Penrith CA11 0PD
Tel: 01768 482383 Fax: 01768 482145

(Eden Valley Primary Care Trust)
Patient List Size: 600

Practice Manager Lynn Iredale

GP J K SMITH

The Surgery
Ravenghyll, Kirkoswald, Penrith CA10 1DQ
Tel: 01768 898560 Fax: 01768 898905
(Eden Valley Primary Care Trust)
Patient List Size: 2200

Practice Manager G M Unwin

GP David Edmund John UNWIN

The Surgery
Cottage Hospital, Alston, Penrith CA9 3QY
Tel: 01434 381214 Fax: 01434 382210
(Eden Valley Primary Care Trust)

Practice Manager Kathleen Walton

GP Sarah Louise MILLS, Michael Timothy HANLEY

Temple Sowerby Medical Practice
Temple Sowerby, Penrith CA10 1RZ
Tel: 01768 361232 Fax: 01768 361980
Email: essurgery@gp-982038.nhs.uk
(Eden Valley Primary Care Trust)
Patient List Size: 3500

Practice Manager Alan Dunn

GP Gavin Leslie YOUNG, Julia Elizabeth BARR, Josephine Amanda THOMPSON, Timothy Stuart Staveley YOUNG

Penryn

The Penryn Surgery
Saracen Way, Penryn TR10 8HX
Tel: 01326 372502 Fax: 01326 378126
Email: docs@penryn.co.uk
(Central Cornwall Primary Care Trust)
Patient List Size: 13000

Practice Manager Ann Kerr

GP Anthony John SEDDON, Robert James BECKETT, Ian Stuart BISHOP, Ian Michael Campbell BROWN, Helen BURNS, Michael Frederick ELLIS, Jonathan KATZ, Michael John PAXTON

Penzance

Alverton Practice
The Alverton Practice, 7 Alverton Terrace, Penzance TR18 4JH
Tel: 01736 351014/363741 Fax: 01736 330776
Email: chris.thomas@alverton.cornwall.nhs.uk
(West of Cornwall Primary Care Trust)
Patient List Size: 6805

Practice Manager Chris Thomas

GP John RYAN, richard CHEYNE, Mark RUSSELL, Sue TURNER

Alverton Surgery
7 Alverton Terrace, Penzance TR18 4JH
Tel: 01736 363741 Fax: 01736 330776
Email: john.ryan@alverton.cornwall.nhs.uk
(West of Cornwall Primary Care Trust)
Patient List Size: 6805

Practice Manager Christine Thomas

GP John Francis RYAN, Richard CHEYNE, Fijke MIDDENDROP, Mark RUSSELL, Sarah SHAW, Sue TURNER

Cape Cornwall Surgery
Market Street, St. Just-in-Penwith, Penzance TR19 7HX
Tel: 01736 788306 Fax: 01736 786288
Email: elisabeth.thomas@cape-cornwall.cornwall.nhs.uk
(West of Cornwall Primary Care Trust)
Patient List Size: 4784

Practice Manager Elisabeth Thomas

GP Elizabeth CLEGG, David Michael CARRUTHERS, Adam ELLERY

Marrab Surgery
Morrab Surgery, 2 Morrab Road, Penzance TR18 4EL
Tel: 01736 363866 Fax: 01736 367809
Email: jayne.hocking@morrab.cornwall.nhs.uk
(West of Cornwall Primary Care Trust)
Patient List Size: 11097

Practice Manager Jayne Hocking

GP William Neil ARMSTRONG, Andrew Huw MARSHALL, Janet Susan POWER, Carla Jane ROWE, Stewart Ferguson RUTHERFURD, Susan Jane WILLIAMS

Penalverne Surgery
Penalverne Drive, Penzance TR18 2RE
Tel: 01736 363361 Fax: 01736 332118
Email: lesley.searie@penalverne.cornwall.nhs.uk
(West of Cornwall Primary Care Trust)
Patient List Size: 5500

Practice Manager Lesley J Searle

GP Marcus Henry LONG, Peter John CORMIE, Norman John FLETCHER

Sunnyside Surgery
Sunnyside Surgery, Hawkins Road, Penzance TR18 4LT
Tel: 01736 363340 Fax: 01736 332116
Email: jim.payne@sunnyside.cornwall.nhs.uk
(West of Cornwall Primary Care Trust)
Patient List Size: 6800

Practice Manager Jim Page

GP Angela Jane BONNAR, Ian David Campbell CURRIE, Malcolm Rosser JONES, Patrick Pownall WILSON

Perranporth

The Perranporth Surgery
Perranporth TR6 0PS
Tel: 01872 572255 Fax: 01872 573022
Email: enquiries@perraporth.cornwall.nhs.uk
(Central Cornwall Primary Care Trust)
Patient List Size: 6600

Practice Manager Lisa Fogg

GP Mary Elizabeth TURFITT, Peter Kieran MERRIN, Charles F SIDEBOTHAM, Shane TELLAM

Pershore

Abbotswood Medical Centre
Defford Road, Pershore WR10 1HZ
Tel: 01386 552424 Fax: 01386 561400
(South Worcestershire Primary Care Trust)
Patient List Size: 9600

Practice Manager Julia Moore

GP Felix Jacques BORCHARDT, Alison Clare ATKINSON, Peter Mark EVANS, Niall Anthony O'LOGHLEN, Glenn John Gareth RALPHS, Kathryn Patricia THOMAS, Claire Margaret WUNSCH

The Health Centre
Priest Lane, Pershore WR10 1RD
Tel: 01386 502030 Fax: 01386 502058
(South Worcestershire Primary Care Trust)
Patient List Size: 10400

Practice Manager P Ford

GP Tom PITTS-TUCKER, Katherine EDWARDS, Gill JOHNSTONE, Chris PERKS, John PRITCHARD, James RANKIN, Catherine YOUNG

Pershore Health Centre
Priest Lane, Pershore WR10 1RD
Tel: 01386 502030 Fax: 01386 502058
(South Worcestershire Primary Care Trust)

Practice Manager Sophie Guarneri

GP Christopher Nigel PAINE, Timothy John ALDER, Katharine Meriel Rosina EDWARDS, Gillian Eileen JOHNSTONE, Christian Edward PERKS, Thomas John PITTS-TUCKER, James Sinnett RANKIN, Catherine Margaret YOUNG

Peterborough

The Abbey View Surgery
Thorney Road, Crowland, Peterborough PE6 0AL
(Lincolnshire South West Teaching Primary Care Trust)

GP V A B ROBERTS

Abbeyview Surgery
Thorney Road, Crowland, Peterborough PE6 0AL
Tel: 01733 210254 Fax: 01733 210256
(Lincolnshire South West Teaching Primary Care Trust)
Patient List Size: 5600

GP Vab ROBERTS

Ailsworth Surgery
32 Main Street, Ailsworth, Peterborough PE5 7AF
Tel: 01733 380686 Fax: 01733 380400
(South Peterborough Primary Care Trust)
Patient List Size: 1360

Practice Manager C Brown

GP Mohsin Ahmed Hussain LALIWALA

Bretton Medical Practice
Rightwell, Bretton, Peterborough PE3 8DT
Tel: 01733 264506 Fax: 01733 266728
(North Peterborough Primary Care Trust)

Practice Manager Dragomir Crnomarkovic

GP Sterlin NAVAMANI, Alla Pitchai Sahib Sheik Mian Sahib ABDUL KARIM, Michael Charles North HENCHY, Elaine Rosemary HUNT, Venkatesha MURTHY, John Edward Bentley YOUENS

The Deepings Practice
2 Godsey Lane, Market Deeping, Peterborough PE6 8OD
Tel: 01778 319000 Fax: 01778 319009
Website: www.deepingspractice.co.uk
(Lincolnshire South West Teaching Primary Care Trust)
Patient List Size: 22150

GP N W MARSHALL

Dogsthorpe Medical Centre
Poplar Avenue, Peterborough PE1 4QF
Tel: 01733 560061
(North Peterborough Primary Care Trust)
Patient List Size: 4200

Practice Manager Vivian Tyler

GP J B KHAN, G PETANGODA, J R SELWYN

Eye Road Surgery
144 Eye Road, Off Welland Estate, Peterborough PE1 4SG
Tel: 01733 563515
(North Peterborough Primary Care Trust)

Practice Manager Richard Jordan

GP Ranjit Kumar MAZUMDAR, S SRINIVASAN

Gordon and Partners
1 North Street, Peterborough PE1 2RA
Tel: 01733 312731 Fax: 01733 311447
(North Peterborough Primary Care Trust)
Patient List Size: 6500

Practice Manager J Stancombe

GP Ross Barclay GORDON, Zbigniew Jerzy MYSZKA, Anne Isabel FOWLIE, Peter HADFIELD, Laurence JACOBS, Helen JOHNSTON, David Wright MITCHELL, Rodney Thomas PURCELL, Keith SAMPSON, Paul Jacques VAN DEN BENT

Hampton Health
Unit 6B, Serpentine Green Shopping Centre, Hampton, Peterborough PE7 8DR
Tel: 01733 556900
(South Peterborough Primary Care Trust)

GP C DOBBING

Hodgson Centre Surgery
Hodgson Centre, Hodgson Avenue, Werrington, Peterborough PE4 5EG
Tel: 01733 573232 Fax: 01733 328355
(North Peterborough Primary Care Trust)

Practice Manager Pauline Scott

GP Vijay Kumar Subrahmanium IYER, P IYER

Huntly Grove Practice
Thomas Walker Medical Centre, Peterborough PE1 2QP
Tel: 01753 551789/551771 Fax: 01733 556260
(North Peterborough Primary Care Trust)
Patient List Size: 2200

GP B K SHOBAN

Jenner Health Centre
Turners Lane, Whittlesey, Peterborough PE7 1EJ
Tel: 01733 203601 Fax: 01733 206210
(South Peterborough Primary Care Trust)

Practice Manager Paul Limming

GP Robert Alexander RENNIE, Andrew Alexander ANDERSON, Gillian Elizabeth EVANS, Clifford Graham SCOTT, Mark Andrew TYLER

Lincoln Road Practice
63 Lincoln Road, Peterborough PE1 2SF
Tel: 01733 565511 Fax: 01733 569230
(North Peterborough Primary Care Trust)

Practice Manager Jacqui A Cotton

GP Hanna Fouad SAYEGH, Frederick Richard FLORES, Susan Joy GRANT, Sohrab PANDAY, Richard Fleming TROUNCE, Stephen John WATSON

London Road Surgery
79 London Road, Peterborough PE2 9BS
Tel: 01733 343139 Fax: 01733 341945
(North Peterborough Primary Care Trust)
Patient List Size: 1850

Practice Manager S Mbanu

GP Alfred MBANU

Millfield Medical Centre
St Martins Street, Peterborough PE1 3BF
Tel: 01733 310095 Fax: 01733 892356
(North Peterborough Primary Care Trust)
Patient List Size: 5052

Practice Manager Sarah Harrison

GP M J KENNEDY

The Millfield Surgery
10 Serjeant Street, Peterborough PE1 2LR
Tel: 01733 563051 Fax: 01733 563051
(North Peterborough Primary Care Trust)

Practice Manager Usha Joshi

GP Kaushik Madhavji JOSHI

Minster Medical Practice
Thomas Walker Medical Centre, Peterborough PE1 2QP
(North Peterborough Primary Care Trust)

Nene Valley Medical Centre
Clayton, Orton Goldhay, Peterborough PE2 5GP
Tel: 01733 366600 Fax: 01733 366677
Email: admin@nenevalleysurgery.org.uk
Website: www.nenevalleysurgery.org.uk

(South Peterborough Primary Care Trust)
Patient List Size: 8800

Practice Manager D Mucklin

GP Nicolas John FLETCHER, David John MARR, Kevin David STANTON-KING, Stephen Eric WALKER, Sanath Naresh YOGASUNDRAM

Old Fletton Surgery
Rectory Gardens, Old Fletton, Peterborough PE2 8AY
Tel: 01733 343137/315141 Fax: 01733 894739
(South Peterborough Primary Care Trust)
Patient List Size: 11554

Practice Manager Maria Hoskin

GP D L CHINN, Martina BARRETT, Howard Lister BLATCHFORD, T C COXON, John Hamilton GEMMELL, C C NNOCHIRI

Orton Medical Practice
Orton Centre, Orton Goldhay, Peterborough PE2 5RQ
Tel: 01733 391022 Fax: 01733 391034
Website: www.ortonmedical.org
(South Peterborough Primary Care Trust)
Patient List Size: 4045

Practice Manager Katrina Murray

GP Kampta Persaud OUTAR, O Jonathan OKOWKWO

Park Medical Centre
164 Park Road, Peterborough PE1 2UF
Tel: 01733 552801 Fax: 01733 425015
(North Peterborough Primary Care Trust)
Patient List Size: 8000

Practice Manager David Sheppard

GP Michael John CASKEY, Ruth BEAMAN, Nikki JAMES, Simon MULLA, Jacqueline Susan THOMPSON

Parnwell Health Centre
Unit 3, Saltersgate, Peterborough PE1 4YL
Tel: 01733 896112 Fax: 01733 892286
(North Peterborough Primary Care Trust)

Practice Manager Barry Salter

GP Myint THEIN

Paston Health Centre
Chadburn, Peterborough PE4 7DH
Tel: 01733 572584 Fax: 01733 328131
(North Peterborough Primary Care Trust)
Patient List Size: 12250

Practice Manager Kim Robinson

GP Mukund Jayavadan MEHTA, Ramesh Chandra PATEL, Mansukhlal Lakhamshi SHAH, Amber SIGGS, Sunil Kumar SOOD

Prasad and Partners
Westwood Clinic, Wicken Way, Peterborough PE3 7JW
Tel: 01733 265535 Fax: 01733 264263
(North Peterborough Primary Care Trust)
Patient List Size: 4500

Practice Manager Karen McNally

GP Koneru Satya PRASAD, Usha KONERU

Queen Street Surgery
9-11 Queen Street, Whittlesey, Peterborough PE7 1AY
Tel: 01733 204611 Fax: 01733 208926
(South Peterborough Primary Care Trust)
Patient List Size: 13758

Practice Manager Helena R Ayre

GP Malcolm Glyn SADLER, Anthony John BOND, Katharine Mary EADIE, Manohar Rao MADDULA, Paula Anne O'DONNELL, Christopher David SCARISBRICK, Richard McKerchar SCOTT

Thistlemoor Road Medical Centre
6-8 Thistlemoor Road, Peterborough PE1 3HP
Tel: 01733 551988 Fax: 01733 707702
Email: jdmodha@virginnet.co.uk
(North Peterborough Primary Care Trust)
Patient List Size: 6000

GP Jitendra Dayaram MODHA, Nalini Jitendra MODHA

Thomas Walker Surgery
Thomas Walker Medical Centre, Peterborough PE1 2QP
(North Peterborough Primary Care Trust)

Thorney Medical Practice
Wisbech Road, Thorney, Peterborough PE6 0SD
Tel: 01733 270219 Fax: 01733 270860
(South Peterborough Primary Care Trust)

Practice Manager Lisa Butcher

GP Nicholas Raymond JACKSON, Joanne Mary HOBBIS, Andrew John KNIGHTS, Simon David RICHARDS

Thorpe Road Surgery
64 Thorpe Road, Peterborough PE3 6AP
Tel: 01733 310070 Fax: 01733 554834
Email: janet.martyr@nhs.net
(South Peterborough Primary Care Trust)
Patient List Size: 3550

Practice Manager Janet Martyr

GP Malcolm Clive BISHOP, A A BASHIR, S P H PINDAR

Wansford Surgery and Kings Cliffe Practice
Yarwell Road, Wansford, Peterborough PE8 6PL
Tel: 01780 782342 Fax: 01780 783434
Website: www.wansford.com
(South Peterborough Primary Care Trust)
Patient List Size: 5881

Practice Manager Jennie Gatheral

GP Gillian TUCK, David COWIE, Rhiannon NALLY, Amrit TAKHAR

Westgate Surgery
60 Westgate, Peterborough PE1 1RG
Tel: 01733 562420 Fax: 01733 311780
(North Peterborough Primary Care Trust)
Patient List Size: 6000

Practice Manager Geoff Tinson

GP Nader Khalil MORGAN, Jose LOPPER, Neil Peter SANDERS

Wittering (Royal Air Force)
The Medical Centre, RAF Wittering, Peterborough PE8 6HB
Tel: 01780 783838
(South Peterborough Primary Care Trust)

GP Jackie BARNEY

Yaxley Group Practice
Yaxley Health Centre, Landsdowne Road, Yaxley, Peterborough PE7 3JL
Tel: 01733 240478 Fax: 01733 244645
(South Peterborough Primary Care Trust)
Patient List Size: 13227

Practice Manager Shirley Drawwater

GP Thomas Meredith DAVIES, JASDEEP BHARI, Beryl DENNIS, Alison Jayne GRAHAM, Christopher Mark GRANT, Audrey Daphne HAMMERSLEY, Philip HARTROPP, Richard Alan WITHERS

Peterlee

Blackhills Surgery
16 Blackhills Road, Horden, Peterlee SR8 4DW
Tel: 0191 5183646 Fax: 0191 5862773
(Easington Primary Care Trust)
Patient List Size: 1970

Practice Manager Chanda Choudary

GP Sita Ram CHOUDHARY

Horden Group Practice
The Surgery, Sunderland Road, Horden, Peterlee SR8 4QP
Tel: 0191 5864210 Fax: 0191 586 9725

(Easington Primary Care Trust)
Patient List Size: 7660

Practice Manager Angela Fisher

GP Pundarik Kumar BANNERJEE, Alistair Rory Sutherland BURLEIGH, Gordon PEARSON, Ajoy Kumar SIL

Shinwell Medical Centre
Fourth Street, Horden, Peterlee SR8 4LE
Tel: 0191 5863859 Fax: 0191 5860748
(Easington Primary Care Trust)
Patient List Size: 3650

Practice Manager Joseph Chandy

GP Joseph CHANDY, G R SETTY

Sukumaran
Jupiter House Surgery, Sunderland Road, Horden, Peterlee SR8 4PF
Tel: 0191 5872488 Fax: 0191 5861995
(Easington Primary Care Trust)
Patient List Size: 3400

Practice Manager Gill Johnson

GP Othayoth SUKUMARAN

William Brown Centre
Manor Way, Peterlee SR8 5TW
Tel: 0191 5544544 Fax: 0191 554 4552
(Easington Primary Care Trust)

Practice Manager Glenn Carroll

GP William James Derek BROWN, David Guy ANDERSON, Dr ATKINSON, Peter BARLOW, Gerard FROST, Dr HAWES, Kathryn Jane HAYS, Alun Hugh THOMAS

Petersfield

Douglas and Partners
The Grange Surgery, The Causeway, Petersfield GU31 4JR
Tel: 01730 267722 Fax: 01730 233526
Website: www.thegrangesurgery.org.uk
(East Hampshire Primary Care Trust)
Patient List Size: 5200

Practice Manager Beryl Ely

GP Andrew Rutter DOUGLAS, Hugh John Adolphus CONI, Madeleine Ann LITCHFIELD, Penny MILEHAM

The Surgery
Doctors Lane, West Meon, Petersfield GU32 1LR
Tel: 01730 829333 Fax: 01730 829229
(Mid-Hampshire Primary Care Trust)

GP Anne Elizabeth YOUNG

Swan Surgery
Swan Street, Petersfield GU32 3AB
Tel: 01730 264011 Fax: 01730 231093
(East Hampshire Primary Care Trust)

Practice Manager C Giles

GP Brian Gareth ELLIS, Stephen John BUCKLEY, Andrew William CAIRNS, Catherine CHRISTIE, Claire Margaret COX, Guy CUNLIFFE, Andrew Francis Harold HOLDEN, Fiona JACKLIN

West Meon Surgery
Doctors Lane, West Meon, Petersfield GU32 1LR
Tel: 01730 829666 Fax: 01730 829229
(Mid-Hampshire Primary Care Trust)
Patient List Size: 2600

Practice Manager Mike Lish

GP Stuart CHRISTIE, Anne YOUNG

Petworth

The Surgery
Grove Street, Petworth GU28 0LP
Tel: 01798 342248 Fax: 01798 343987
(Western Sussex Primary Care Trust)
Patient List Size: 6500

Practice Manager John Venner

GP Graham Mark LYONS, Simon PETT, Martin ROLPH, Seonaid SIMPSON

Pevensey

The Medical Centre
10 Richmond Road, Pevensey Bay, Pevensey BN24 6AQ
Tel: 01323 465100 Fax: 01323 461180
(Eastbourne Downs Primary Care Trust)

GP Mirza Ilyas BAIG, Ajaib BANSEL, Jeffrey Paul DARWENT, Ramin TASHARROFI

Pewsey

Avon Valley Practice
Fairfield, Upavon, Pewsey SN9 6DZ
Tel: 01980 630221 Fax: 01980 630393
(South Wiltshire Primary Care Trust)

Practice Manager Hilary Jenkins

GP Peter David JENKINS, I GREEN, Fiona Mary ROSS RUSSELL

Pewsey Surgery
High Street, Pewsey SN9 5AQ
Tel: 01672 563511 Fax: 01672 563004
(Kennet and North Wiltshire Primary Care Trust)
Patient List Size: 6700

Practice Manager Shirley Hatt

GP Phillip James VICKERS, Stephen Walter PHILLIPS, E POTTER, Jonathan Paul George RING, Teresa Ann SHIREHAMPTON

Pickering

The Old School Surgery
Brook Lane, Thornton Dale, Pickering YO18 7RZ
Tel: 01751 472441 Fax: 01751 475400
(Scarborough, Whitby and Ryedale Primary Care Trust)
Patient List Size: 10080

Practice Manager John Fletcher

GP D E CAPES, M CASTLE, J S COPPACK, D COTTINGHAM

Pickering Medical Pratice
Southgate, Pickering YO18 8BL
Tel: 01751 472441 Fax: 01751 475400
Email: pickering.admin@gp-b82033.nhs.uk
Website: www.surgeriesonline.co.uk/pickering
(Scarborough, Whitby and Ryedale Primary Care Trust)
Patient List Size: 10300

Practice Manager John Fletcher

GP David Edward CAPES, James Samuel COPPACK, Daniel COTTINGHAM, Martha DUDDINGTON, Fran JACOBS, Kate LEE, Timothy James THORNTON

The Surgery
Rosedale Abbey, c/o Pickering Medical Practice, Southgate, Pickering YO18 8BU
Tel: 01751 472441 Fax: 01751 475400

Practice Manager John Fletcher

GP T THORNTON

Pinner

Elliott Hall Medical Centre
165-167 Uxbridge Road, Hatch End, Pinner HA5 4EA
Tel: 020 8428 4019
(Harrow Primary Care Trust)
Patient List Size: 7000

Practice Manager Denise Lavey

GP Alan Howard BYERS, Christopher Stanley JENNER, Ashok KELSHIKER, Reena MAJUS

Hatch End Medical Centre
577 Uxbridge Road, Hatch End, Pinner HA5 4RD
Tel: 020 8428 0272 Fax: 020 8421 4109
(Harrow Primary Care Trust)

GP Brigitte Caroline RUDD, Riadh Botrous DAWOOD

Milne Feild Surgery
168 Uxbridge Road, Hatch End, Pinner HA5 4DR
Tel: 020 8421 3277 Fax: 020 8421 3277
(Harrow Primary Care Trust)

GP Rosemary Elaine ALEXANDER

Pinn Medical Centre
8 Eastcote Road, Pinner HA5 1HF
Tel: 020 8866 5766 Fax: 020 8429 0251
(Harrow Primary Care Trust)
Patient List Size: 11500

Practice Manager Marjorie Condie

GP Anthony Jeffery Stephen NICHOLLS, Isobel Susan BLEEHEN, Andrea EDWARDS, Amol Sharad KELSHIKER, Jonathan Kevin RUDOLPH, Shashikant Zaverchand SHAH

The Village Surgery
5 Barrow Point Avenue, Pinner HA5 3HQ
Tel: 020 8429 3777 Fax: 020 8429 4413
(Harrow Primary Care Trust)

Practice Manager Sonal Somaiya

GP Niall Allan Rider DOVE, Ann HARDMAN, Suni PERERA, Paul David SHERIDAN

Plymouth

Adelaide Street Surgery
20 Adelaide Street, Stonehouse, Plymouth PL1 3JF
Tel: 01752 667623 Fax: 01752 315553
Email: practicemanager@gp-L83651.nhs.uk
(Plymouth Teaching Primary Care Trust)
Patient List Size: 2646

Practice Manager Andrea Smyth

GP Trevor Thomas AUGHEY, Ellen Marjolein LOOPSTRA

Armada Surgery
28 Oxford Place, Western Approach, Plymouth PL1 5AJ
Tel: 01752 665805 Fax: 01752 220056
Email: practicemanager@gp-L83064.nhs.uk
(Plymouth Teaching Primary Care Trust)
Patient List Size: 2500

Practice Manager Jo Skinner

GP Graham John WALSH, Nicholas BURDETT

Barton Surgery
Horn Lane, Plymstock, Plymouth PL9 9BR
Tel: 01752 407129 Fax: 01752 482620
Email: practicemanager@gp-L83125.nhs.uk
(Plymouth Teaching Primary Care Trust)
Patient List Size: 3934

Practice Manager Jan Chapman

GP John MAHONY, Steven NIMMO, Diana Elizabeth SIMS

Beaumont Villa Surgery
23 Beaumont Road, Plymouth PL4 9BL
Tel: 01752 663776 Fax: 01752 261520
Email: jamie.stabb@nhs.net
Website: www.beaumont-villa.co.uk
(Plymouth Teaching Primary Care Trust)
Patient List Size: 8200

Practice Manager Felicity Barry

GP John Gimson PICKARD, Sarah Jane COLE, Paul Hartshorne HARDY, David Newton JONES

Budshead Health Centre
433 Budshead Road, Whitleigh, Plymouth PL5 4DU
Tel: 01752 206002 Fax: 01752 206005
(Plymouth Teaching Primary Care Trust)
Patient List Size: 5507

Practice Manager Elaine Boardman

GP David James McEWING, Nicholas Paul CHIAPPE, Preston Maurice Simplicio de MENDONCA

Chard Road Surgery
Chard Road, St Budeaux, Plymouth PL5 2UE
Tel: 01752 363111 Fax: 01752 363611
Email: kayslater@nhs.uk
(Plymouth Teaching Primary Care Trust)
Patient List Size: 8426

Practice Manager Kay Slater

GP Rory O'NEILL, Mike BURDON, Philip David OLIVER, Georgina SOWMAN, Rachel TYLER

Church View Surgery
30 Holland Road, Plymstock, Plymouth PL9 9BW
Tel: 01752 403206 Fax: 01752 482293
Email: practicemanager@gp-L83064.nhs.uk
(Plymouth Teaching Primary Care Trust)

Practice Manager Amanda Sharp

GP Justin Alexander Baird ROBBINS, Charles Mark HAYWARD, Rosamund Mary HEATH, Jacqueline MOORCROFT, Anthony SHARPLES, Robert Rex WOODS

Collings Park Medical Centre
57 Eggbuckland Road, Hartley, Plymouth PL3 5JR
Tel: 01752 771500 Fax: 01752 769946
Email: practicemanager@gp-L83132.nhs.uk
(Plymouth Teaching Primary Care Trust)
Patient List Size: 5500

Practice Manager L Rickard

GP John HAMBLY, Ian HODGINS, Jane KINGSNORTH, Susan Gillian OVERAL

Crownhill Surgery
103 Crownhill Road, Plymouth PL5 3BN
Tel: 01752 771713
Email: practicemanager@gp-L83107.nhs.uk
(Plymouth Teaching Primary Care Trust)
Patient List Size: 3872

Practice Manager Jennifer Langman

GP Ahmed GASIM, Kouros TORABI

The Cumberland Surgery
Cumberland Centre, Damerel Close, Devonport, Plymouth PL1 4JZ
Tel: 01752 562802/561054 Fax: 01752 551219
(Plymouth Teaching Primary Care Trust)
Patient List Size: 5100

Practice Manager Lynn Moy

GP R C PRIOR, R A FORD, William Arthur KNIGHT

Dean Cross Surgery
21 Radford Park Road, Plymstock, Plymouth PL9 9DL
Tel: 01752 404743 Fax: 01752 480212
Email: practicemanager@gp-L83021.nhs.uk
(Plymouth Teaching Primary Care Trust)
Patient List Size: 9450

Practice Manager Patricia Bowsher

GP Marcos Freddy VITAL, Julia Elizabeth HAMPSHIRE, Maldwyn Henry OWEN, Timothy James PADLEY, Grant J WILLS

Elm Surgery
Leypark Walk, Estover, Plymouth PL6 8UE
Tel: 01752 776772 Fax: 01752 785108
Email: practicemanager@gp-L83019.nhs.uk
(Plymouth Teaching Primary Care Trust)
Patient List Size: 4750

Practice Manager Anna Rodgers

GP Richard St. John HAROLD, Timothy ALEXANDER, Anne Katherine Jean ROGERS

Estover Health Centre
Leypark Walk, Estover, Plymouth PL6 8UE
Tel: 01752 788778 Fax: 01752 779905
Email: practicemanager@gp-L83144.nhs.uk
(Plymouth Teaching Primary Care Trust)

Practice Manager Sandra Howard

GP Christopher Harwood HUGHES, Karen Nicola CHIAPPE

Estover Health Centre
Leypark Walk, Estover, Plymouth PL6 8UE
Tel: 01752 789030 Fax: 01752 772665
Email: practicemanager@gp-L83642.nhs.uk
(Plymouth Teaching Primary Care Trust)
Patient List Size: 2700

GP Ernest ARCHER-KORANTENG

Freedom Health Centre
78 Lipson Road, Plymouth PL4 8RH
Tel: 01752 674494 Fax: 01752 263365
Email: practicemanager@gp-L83006.nhs.uk
(Plymouth Teaching Primary Care Trust)
Patient List Size: 1800

Practice Manager Gail Fletcher

GP Hugh Malcolm CAMPBELL

Friary House Surgery
Friary House, 2a Beaumont Road, St Judes, Plymouth PL4 9BH
Tel: 01752 663138 Fax: 01752 675805
Email: practicemanager@gp-L83019.nhs.uk
(Plymouth Teaching Primary Care Trust)
Patient List Size: 12400

Practice Manager Sue Wilson

GP Muhammad Sakhawat Husain CHOWDHURY, Howard Graham ACKFORD, T M BERTIE, David William FISHER, Pamela Nemone LENDEN, Carmel Ann SHALES

Glendower Road Surgery
54 Glendower Road, Peverell, Plymouth PL3 4LD
Tel: 01752 673336 Fax: 01752 267130
Email: practicemanager@gp-L83093.nhs.uk
(Plymouth Teaching Primary Care Trust)
Patient List Size: 4993

Practice Manager Lynn Moy

GP Roderick Clive PRIOR, Ralph Alan FORD, William Arthur KNIGHT

Glenside Medical Centre
Glenside Rise, Plympton, Plymouth PL7 4DR
Tel: 01752 341340 Fax: 01752 348913
Email: practicemanager@gp-L83138.nhs.uk
(Plymouth Teaching Primary Care Trust)

Practice Manager Kath Dix

GP Brian Harvey GURRY, Jane Elisabeth MELHUISH, William James Crawford MURPHY

Honicknowle Green Medical Centre
Guy Miles Way, Honicknowle Green, Plymouth PL5 3PY
Tel: 01752 777207 Fax: 01752 775556
Email: practicemanager@gp-L83672.nhs.uk
(Plymouth Teaching Primary Care Trust)
Patient List Size: 1520

Practice Manager Veena Rai

GP Kundadka RAI

Hyde Park Surgery
2 Hyde Park Road, Mutley, Plymouth PL3 4RJ
Tel: 01752 224437 Fax: 01752 315495
Email: yolanda.wood@nhs.net
(Plymouth Teaching Primary Care Trust)
Patient List Size: 1790

Practice Manager Yolanda Wood

GP Stephen John WARREN, Ju;iette WHITFIELD

Knowle House Surgery
4 Meavy Way, Crownhill, Plymouth PL5 3JB
Tel: 01752 771895 Fax: 01752 766510
Email: practicemanager@gp-L83089.nhs.uk
(Plymouth Teaching Primary Care Trust)
Patient List Size: 10600

Practice Manager Craig Smith-Avery

GP Matthew James WESTHEAD, Peter Ronald BROOKS, Keith GILLESPIE, Timothy HALL, L HILLMAN, S MACARTNEY

Laira Surgery
95 Pike Road, Laira, Plymouth PL3 6HG
Tel: 01752 663473
(Plymouth Teaching Primary Care Trust)

Practice Manager B Lewin

GP A CALKOEN, James Colin CAMPBELL, Maria Jane EARLEY, G T HART, Hugh Graham WILLS, Christopher Edward WILSON

Lisson Grove Medical Centre
3-5 Lisson Grove, Mutley, Plymouth PL4 7DL
Tel: 01752 205555 Fax: 01752 205558
Email: practicemanager@gp-L83138.nhs.uk
(Plymouth Teaching Primary Care Trust)

Practice Manager Suzanne Brown

GP Paul Michael SHEWRING, Christopher Paul FLETCHER, John FOTHERINGHAM, Charlotte Elizabeth Orgill MASSEY, Helen Catherine THOMAS, Brian John THURSTON

The Mannamead Surgery
22 Eggbuckland Road, Mannamead, Plymouth PL3 5HE
Tel: 01752 223652 Fax: 01752 253875
Email: practicemanager@gp-L83061.nhs.uk
(Plymouth Teaching Primary Care Trust)

Practice Manager Susan Smith

GP Meriel Perpetua KITSON, Colin Francis BANNON, Colin Alan DONALDSON, Claire HARNETT, Peter LEMAN, Christopher LLOYD

Marlborough Street Surgery
1 Marlborough Street, Devonport, Plymouth PL1 4AE
Tel: 01752 568864 Fax: 01752 606974
Email: practicemanager@gp-L83642.nhs.uk
(Plymouth Teaching Primary Care Trust)
Patient List Size: 2870

Practice Manager Jennifer Coombes

GP S JASH

Milehouse Surgery
21 Milehouse Road, Milehouse, Plymouth PL3 4AD
Tel: 01752 207930 Fax: 01752 207931
Email: practicemanager@gp-L83048.nhs.uk
(Plymouth Teaching Primary Care Trust)

Practice Manager Carol Peters

GP Philip Kim LAWRENCE

North Road West Medical Centre
167 North Road West, Plymouth PL1 5BZ
Tel: 01752 662780 Fax: 01752 254541
Email: nrw@gp-L83030.nhs.uk
(Plymouth Teaching Primary Care Trust)

Practice Manager Jenny Haynes

GP Janet Mary PERKS, Carmel Rose BOYHAN, Andrew POTTER, Elizabeth WESTON-BAKER

The Nova Surgery
Leypark Walk, Estover, Plymouth PL6 8UE
Tel: 01752 315476
Email: practicemanager@gp-L83671.nhs.uk
(Plymouth Teaching Primary Care Trust)

Practice Manager Tracey May

GP Nigel William SCOTT

Park View Surgery
34 Ford Park Road, Mutley, Plymouth PL4 6NU
Tel: 01752 663795 Fax: 01752 253465
(Plymouth Teaching Primary Care Trust)

GP Vijay KANDAMPULLY

Pathfields Practice
Plympton Health Centre, Mudgeway, Plymouth PL7 1AD
Tel: 01752 341474 Fax: 01752 345757
Email: practicemanager@gp-L83008.nhs.uk
(Plymouth Teaching Primary Care Trust)
Patient List Size: 7600

Practice Manager Bernice Lewin

GP James Colin CAMPBELL, A CALKOEN, Michelle EARLEY, Gerard HART, Christopher Edward WILSON

Peverell Park Surgery
162 Outland Road, Peverell, Plymouth PL2 3PR
Tel: 01752 791438 Fax: 01752 783623
Email: practicemanager@gp-L83028.nhs.uk
(Plymouth Teaching Primary Care Trust)

Practice Manager Damaris Stiles

GP Richard George BENJAFIELD, Christine LAURENS, Sarah Judith MURRAY, Philip ROWLAND, Kim Johanna STORROW, Peter WILLIAMS

Plym River Practice
Plympton Health Centre, Mudge Way, Plymouth PL7 1AD
Tel: 01752 348884 Fax: 01752 345443
Email: practicemanager@gp-L83133.nhs.uk
(Plymouth Teaching Primary Care Trust)
Patient List Size: 6400

Practice Manager Lynn Langridge

GP John Sager MAKIN, Sadie JONES, Steven William MILLARD, David SIMPSON

Ridgeway Practice
Plympton Health Centre, Mudgeway, Plymouth PL7 1AD
Tel: 01752 346634 Fax: 01752 341444
Email: polly.ellison@nhs.net
Website: www.ridgeway.org.uk
(Plymouth Teaching Primary Care Trust)
Patient List Size: 16000

Practice Manager Polly Ellison

GP Christopher Norman WESTWOOD, Paul Richard GILES, Anthony GOLDING-COOK, Sarah Jane HARRIS, Jane PITMAN, Roger William PRICE, Jennifer Barbara RICHARDSON, Frances ROBERSON, Stephen John ROBINSON

Roborough Surgery
1 Eastcote Close, Southway, Plymouth PL6 6PH
Tel: 01752 701659 Fax: 01752 201410
(Plymouth Teaching Primary Care Trust)
Patient List Size: 9900

Practice Manager Claire Hansell

GP Keith McBRIDE, John Howard ARKLE, C D BREITHEYER, Rupert Charles Marshall JONES, Charles LLOYD, Roger John STEVENS, Helen WRIGHT

Salisbury Road Surgery
43 Salisbury Road, St Judes, Plymouth PL4 8QU
Tel: 01752 665879 Fax: 01752 226343
Email: practicemanager@gp-L83037.nhs.uk
(Plymouth Teaching Primary Care Trust)
Patient List Size: 1700

Practice Manager Justine Payton

GP Janice Lesley LONGWORTH

Saltash Road Surgery
218 Saltash Road, Keyham, Plymouth PL2 2BB
Tel: 01752 562843 Fax: 01752 607024
Email: practicemanager@gp-L83671.nhs.uk
(Plymouth Teaching Primary Care Trust)

Practice Manager B W R Moore

GP Robert John GARDNER

Southway Surgery
2 Bampfylde Way, Southway, Plymouth PL6 6TA
Tel: 01752 776650 Fax: 01752 770249
Email: vivallen@nhs.net
(Plymouth Teaching Primary Care Trust)
Patient List Size: 5000

Practice Manager Viv Allen

GP David Anthony EVANS, Marc Timothy EPPS, Deborah Jayne TAYLER

St Barnabas Surgery
St Barnabas Terrace, Stoke, Plymouth PL1 5NN
Tel: 01752 607006 Fax: 01752 560166
Email: practicemanager@gp-L83074.nhs.uk
(Plymouth Teaching Primary Care Trust)
Patient List Size: 2050

Practice Manager Brenda Netherton

GP Jonathan Ennion Sadler GALE

St Budeaux Health Centre
Stirling Road, St Budeaux, Plymouth PL5 1PL
Tel: 01752 361010/362070 Fax: 01752 350675
Email: practicemanager@gp-L83074.nhs.uk
(Plymouth Teaching Primary Care Trust)
Patient List Size: 10700

Practice Manager Rosemary Davies

GP Donald John PALIN, Joanna Lydia BUTCHER, Henrietta Dawn EPPS, Stephen John Frederick HOBBS, Rory Michael McGILL, James William Buchan ROSS

St Neots Surgery
47 Wolseley Road, Plymouth PL2 3BJ
Tel: 01752 561305 Fax: 01752 605565
Email: practicemanager@gp-L83028.nhs.uk
(Plymouth Teaching Primary Care Trust)
Patient List Size: 10300

Practice Manager Paul Davies

GP William Tennison HILL, Edward Leslie BROWN, Ben DAWSON, Angela LAWRENCE, Jacqueline Margaret RANCE, Michael TUTTY

Stoke Surgery
Belmont Villas, Stoke, Plymouth PL3 4DP
Tel: 01752 562569 Fax: 01752 607299
Email: practicemanager@gp-L83071.nhs.uk
(Plymouth Teaching Primary Care Trust)
Patient List Size: 5000

Practice Manager Lesley McCreery

GP John Rafe FRANKLIN, Simon Richard ANDERSON, Margaret Jane LONGHURST

The Surgery
54/56 Ernesettle Green, Plymouth PL5 2SX
Tel: 01752 314958 Fax: 01752 314959
Email: practicemanager@gp-L83006.nhs.uk
(Plymouth Teaching Primary Care Trust)
Patient List Size: 3600

GP Gary LENDEN, Peter RUDGE

Sutherland Road Surgery
44 Sutherland Road, Mutley, Plymouth PL4 6BN
Tel: 01752 662992 Fax: 01752 265538
Email: practicemanager@gp-L83089.nhs.uk
(Plymouth Teaching Primary Care Trust)
Patient List Size: 2700

Practice Manager Shirley Carey

GP Jim Hamish Nicholas COLLIER

Tothill Surgery
10 Tothill Avenue, St Judes, Plymouth PL4 8PH
Tel: 01752 315594 Fax: 01752 315407
Email: practicemanager@gp-L83123.nhs.uk
(Plymouth Teaching Primary Care Trust)

Practice Manager Sharon Kershaw

GP Jonathan Neil Rutherford CARLSON, Amanda BOASLEY

Trelawny Surgery
45 Ham Drive, Plymouth PL2 2NJ
Tel: 01752 350700 Fax: 01752 315505
Email: practicemanager@gp-L83660.nhs.uk
(Plymouth Teaching Primary Care Trust)
Patient List Size: 1500

GP Apparao NAGABHYRU

Waterloo Surgery
191 Devonport Road, Stoke, Plymouth PL1 5RN
Tel: 01752 563147 Fax: 01752 563304
(Plymouth Teaching Primary Care Trust)
Patient List Size: 6000

Practice Manager Elizabeth Brimacombe

GP Martin Alan WATTS, Mark ADAMS, Mary EMBLETON, Hilary Ann NEVE

Wembury Surgery
51 Hawthorn Drive, Wembury, Plymouth PL9 0BE
Tel: 01752 862118 Fax: 01752 862075
(South Hams and West Devon Primary Care Trust)

Practice Manager A Treagust

GP Seán Garfield BENNETT

West Hoe Surgery
2 Cliff Road, Plymouth PL1 3BP
Tel: 01752 660105 Fax: 01752 260135
(Plymouth Teaching Primary Care Trust)

Practice Manager Audrey Gibbs

GP Anthony Edward MURRAY, Andrew CRAIG, Amanda Jane HARRY

Wycliffe Surgery
Elliott Road, Prince Rock, Plymouth PL4 9NH
Tel: 01752 660648 Fax: 01752 261468
(Plymouth Teaching Primary Care Trust)
Patient List Size: 5100

Practice Manager Kathy Perrett

GP John Edward BIGGS, Julia Karen BERESFORD, Gillian Briony EADIE, Raj PATEL, Brian John POLLARD

Yealm Medical Centre
Market Street, Yealmpton, Plymouth PL8 2EA
(South Hams and West Devon Primary Care Trust)

Practice Manager Alex Cherry

GP Dr PAGE, Robert S HIRST, William F THOMADD, Nicola J TOYNTON

Polegate

Downlands Medical Centre
77 High Street, Polegate BN26 6AE
Tel: 01323 482323 Fax: 01323 488497
(Eastbourne Downs Primary Care Trust)
Patient List Size: 10150

Practice Manager A Piper

GP Christopher Mark BEDFORD-TURNER, Stephen Richard DICKSON, Alistair Ian HAMMETT, Sally Belinda HOLME, Michael Philip SHARP

Manor Park Medical Centre
High Street, Polegate BN26 5DJ
Tel: 01323 482301 Fax: 01323 484848
(Eastbourne Downs Primary Care Trust)
Patient List Size: 5000

Practice Manager Norma Hitt

GP Dr BRIERLEY, Russell D BROWN, Harry DESMOND

The Surgery
The Furlongs, Alfriston, Polegate BN26 5XT
Tel: 01323 870244 Fax: 01323 870244
(Eastbourne Downs Primary Care Trust)

GP Richard James ADCOCK

Pontefract

College Lane Surgery
Barnsley Road, Ackworth, Pontefract WF7 7HZ
Tel: 01977 611023 Fax: 01977 612146
(Eastern Wakefield Primary Care Trust)

Practice Manager B J Ward

GP Ivan Paschal Gerard HANNEY, Jonathan Mark EASTWOOD, Elizabeth Alison MOULTON, Karen Lesley NEEDHAM, Lisa Jane YELLOP

Friarwood Surgery
Carleton Glen, Pontefract WF8 1SU
Tel: 01977 703235 Fax: 01977 600527
(Eastern Wakefield Primary Care Trust)
Patient List Size: 13200

Practice Manager J M Beech

GP Martin Thomas JOHNSON, Elizabeth de DOMBAL, Arit HASHMI, Martin Gabriel LANNON, Anne Mary Eileen MARTIN, Kirsty Jane SANDERSON, Graeme Barrie SLACK, David Bruce WATSON

The Grange
Highfield Road, Hemsworth, Pontefract WF9 4DP
Tel: 01977 610009 Fax: 01977 617182
(Eastern Wakefield Primary Care Trust)

Practice Manager Angela Marwood

GP Lutfe Rabbi Mustafa KAMAL, Linda Carol CRAWLEY, Anne Elizabeth HAWKINS, Ramniklal KANANI, Anthony Niall SWEENEY

Greenview Medical Centre
Waggon Lane, Upton, Pontefract WF9 1JS
(Eastern Wakefield Primary Care Trust)

GP R PRASAD

Health Centre
Little Lane, South Elmsall, Pontefract WF9 2NJ
Tel: 01977 465331 Fax: 01977 645832
Email: douglas.diggle@wakeha.nhs
(Eastern Wakefield Primary Care Trust)
Patient List Size: 4350

Practice Manager Jean Thornton

GP Douglas Phillip DIGGLE, Emmanuel Ashaley OKINE

Northgate Surgery
Northgate, Pontefract WF8 1NG
Tel: 01977 703635 Fax: 01977 702562
(Eastern Wakefield Primary Care Trust)
Patient List Size: 8950

Practice Manager Maureen Sharp

GP John Richard WARING, G J DAVENPORT, David ECCLES, Alul PATEL, Grahame David SMITH, Lambert VAN DEN ENDE, Gillian WILSON

Southmoor Surgery
Southmoor Road, Hemsworth, Pontefract WF9 4DP
Tel: 01977 615153
(Eastern Wakefield Primary Care Trust)

St Thomas Road Surgery
St Thomas Road, Featherstone, Pontefract WF7 5HF
Tel: 01977 792212 Fax: 01977 600278
(Eastern Wakefield Primary Care Trust)
Patient List Size: 7800

Practice Manager John Taylor

GP Philip George GORDON, David Geoffrey ROBERTS, Robert Christopher HILLS

Station Lane Medical Centre
Station Lane, Featherstone, Pontefract WF7 6JL
Tel: 01977 600381 Fax: 01977 600776
(Eastern Wakefield Primary Care Trust)
Patient List Size: 5772

Practice Manager Sue Jodrell

GP Martin Paul SHUTKEVER, Karen Anne Louise EDRIDGE, Hans Nico MEULENDIJK, Beverley Anne SOAN

Stuart Road Surgery
Stuart Road, Pontefract WF8 4PQ
Tel: 01977 703437 Fax: 01977 602334
(Eastern Wakefield Primary Care Trust)
Patient List Size: 8650

Practice Manager I Connolly

GP Andrew PERKINS, Jennifer Susan MONTGOMERY, Velayudham SYAM, John Mark TAYLOR

The Surgery
69 Stockingate, South Kirkby, Pontefract WF9 3PE
Tel: 01977 642251 Fax: 01977 645515
(Eastern Wakefield Primary Care Trust)
Patient List Size: 9600

Practice Manager Ken Cross

GP Joseph CHANDY, Lisa BERRIDGE, Andrew Martin HUGGETT, Dhirubhai MISTRY, Surendra Pratap SINGH

The White Rose Surgery
Exchange Street, South Elmsall, Pontefract WF9 2RD
Tel: 01977 642412 Fax: 01977 641290
(Eastern Wakefield Primary Care Trust)
Patient List Size: 7850

Practice Manager Karen Whitfield

GP Raj Kumar AGGARWAL, R BUCKLEY, Roger Graham Stuart QUARTLEY, Ruth Elizabeth ROCHE, Caoimhin Padraig TOBIN, Deborah Ann WAKEFIELD

Poole

Adam Practice
306 Blandford Road, Poole BH15 4JQ
Tel: 01202 679234 Fax: 01202 667127
(Poole Primary Care Trust)
Patient List Size: 28500

Practice Manager C J Steele

GP Dr MORGAN, David Anthony GRAHAM, Dr MOWBRAY-WEBB, Graham Alan MOYSE, Dr NEAVE

Adam Practice
Upton Health Centre, Blandford Road North, Poole BH16 5PW
Tel: 01202 622339
(Poole Primary Care Trust)
Patient List Size: 8000

Practice Manager Carol Steele

GP George Stratton LIDDIARD, Nicholas BRITTON, Christopher James PLAYFAIR, Charles Edward POWELL, Jacqueline Anne RAY

Birchwood Practice
Birchwood Medical Centre, Northmead Drive, Poole BH17 7XZ
Tel: 01202 697639 Fax: 01202 659323
Website: www.birchwoodpractice.co.uk
(Poole Primary Care Trust)
Patient List Size: 7200

Practice Manager Vanessa Kerrigan

GP Martin William BRIGGS, Christopher C COLE, David Jeremy GOODWORTH, Susan Jacqueline WARREN

Canford Heath Group Practice
9 Mitchell Road, Canford Heath, Poole BH17 8UE
Tel: 01202 672474 Fax: 01202 777778
Email: anthony.howe@gp-j81013.nhs.uk
(Poole Primary Care Trust)
Patient List Size: 11523

Practice Manager Hazel Clarke

GP Anthony Harry HOWE, Patrica AIZPITARTE, Phillip Howard ATKINSON, David Alan BAKER, Christine Mary GADD, Duncan Peter Rennie MUIR, Sarah Margaret PRIMAVESI, David Peter RICHARDSON

Carlisle House
53 Lanegland Street, Poole BH15 1QD
Tel: 01202 678484 Fax: 01202 660507
(Poole Primary Care Trust)
Patient List Size: 5560

Practice Manager J Andrews

GP John Simon Coleridge SCOTT, Mark Thomas NELMS, Sharon REDPATH, Alison Mary ROGERS

Evergreen Oak Surgery
43 Commercial Road, Parkstone, Poole BH14 0HU
Tel: 01202 747496 Fax: 01202 743624
(Poole Primary Care Trust)
Patient List Size: 4500

Practice Manager Rosemarie Brown

GP Rosalind Ruth MAYCOCK, Geraldine Marjorie BRAY

Heath Cottage Surgery
High Street, Lytchett Matravers, Poole BH16 6DB
Tel: 01202 632764
(Poole Primary Care Trust)

GP Anne Catherine LINLEY-ADAMS, Dr BALLINGER, Dr BRITTON, Dr GRAHAM, Dr LEVITT, Dr LIDDIARD, K F LITTLE, Dr MORGAN, Dr MOWBRAY, Dr MOYSE, Dr NEAVE, Dr PLAYFAIR, Dr POWELL, Dr RAY, Dr SEAL, Dr WEBBS

Heatherview Medical Centre
Alder Road, Parkstone, Poole BH12 4AY
Tel: 01202 743678 Fax: 01202 739960
(Poole Primary Care Trust)
Patient List Size: 9580

Practice Manager Pam Braid

GP Derek Joseph HOBBS, Steven MORRIS, Alastair William Gordon PONTON, John E PROSSER, Rita PROSSER

Herbert Avenue Surgery
268 Herbert Avenue, Poole BH12 4HY
Tel: 01202 743333 Fax: 01202 738998
(Poole Primary Care Trust)
Patient List Size: 3063

Practice Manager Nigel Hansford

GP Iain Samuel FULLERTON, Nicky DAWSON, Judy GORDON

Lilliput Surgery
Elms Avenue, Lindisfarne, Poole BH14 8EE
Tel: 01202 741310 Fax: 01202 739122
(Poole Primary Care Trust)
Patient List Size: 8500

Practice Manager Julie Williams

GP Geoffrey Peter WALDER, Karen BAYLEY, Andrew Frank Knowles RUTLAND, Tanya SMITH, Susan Marguerite THOMAS

Longfleet House Surgery
56 Longfleet Road, Poole BH15 2JD
Tel: 01202 666677 Fax: 01202 660319
(Poole Primary Care Trust)
Patient List Size: 4800

Practice Manager Pat Meen

GP David John WILLIAMS, Christopher Mark JONES, Gillian Deborah SMITH

Longfleet Road Surgery
117 Longfleet Road, Poole BH15 2HX
Tel: 01202 676111
Email: adampractice@gp-J81006.nhs.uk
(Poole Primary Care Trust)

Practice Manager Carol Steele

GP David Frederick MORGAN, Fiona Carol BALLINGER, Richard Julian LEVITT, Patrick James SEAL

Madeira Road Surgery
1A Madeira Road, Parkstone, Poole BH14 9ET
Tel: 01202 741345 Fax: 01202 739794
Email: maderiamedicalcentre@gp-J81065.nhs.uk
(Poole Primary Care Trust)
Patient List Size: 8300

GP Desmond Francis McCANN, Mark BETTLEY-SMITH, Christopher Adrian MURCOTT, Gerard William ROBERTS

Parkstone Health Centre
Mansfield Road, Poole BH14 0DJ
Tel: 01202 741370 Fax: 01202 730952
(Poole Primary Care Trust)
Patient List Size: 9000

Practice Manager Alison Blenign

GP John David COLLINSON, Sarah Rosemary ATKINSON, Fiona MITFORD-SLADE, John Francis PRIMAVESI, Edward Ashley SHERIDAN, Richard Naylor SMITH

Poole Town Surgery
36 Parkstone Road, Poole BH15 2PG
Tel: 01202 670111 Fax: 01202 660718
(Poole Primary Care Trust)
Patient List Size: 4000

Practice Manager Gail Morton

GP Ian John HAYWARD, Hilary Lottie Maria CLARK, Matthew James GREEN

Rosemary Medical Centre
2 Rosemary Gardens, Parkstone, Poole BH12 3HF
Tel: 01202 741300 Fax: 01202 721868
Email: rosemarymedicalcentre@gp-j81036.nhs.uk
Website: www.freespace.virgin.net/rmmc.poole
(Poole Primary Care Trust)

Practice Manager Shirley Blackmore

GP James John LOVEJOY, Susan GARLAND, Colin Gareth PUGH, Steven WARLOW, Jo WISELY

The Surgery
36 Parkstone Road, Poole BH15 2PG
Website: doctornewman.co.uk
(Poole Primary Care Trust)

Practice Manager Emma Rogers

GP Dr NEWMAN

Village Surgery
Gillett Road, Talbot Village, Poole BH12 5BF
Tel: 01202 525252 Fax: 01202 533956
(Bournemouth Teaching Primary Care Trust)
Patient List Size: 8500

Practice Manager M Brown

GP Howard Irving REIN, Douglas CLARKE, Anthony John SHEARMAN, James WHITTICASE

Wessex Road Surgery
Wessex Road, Parkstone, Poole BH14 8BQ
Tel: 01202 734924 Fax: 01202 738957
(Poole Primary Care Trust)

GP Patrick Joseph FORBES, Sian Elspeth LEWIS, Steven Howard WHALEN

West Canferd Medical Centre
8-12 Ryath Road, Canford Heath, Poole BH17 9FA
Tel: 01202 658767 Fax: 01202 659189
(Poole Primary Care Trust)
Patient List Size: 1766

Practice Manager Ann Wilkinson

GP Ralph Attila VADAS

Port Isaac

Port Isaac Practice
Hillson Close, Port Isaac PL29 3TR
Tel: 01208 880222 Fax: 01208 880633
(North and East Cornwall Primary Care Trust)
Patient List Size: 7300

Practice Manager Anne Boney

GP David Kelsey Stuart DAVISON, Paul COOK, James Joseph LUNNY, Malcolm McKENDRICK, Eileen Patricia PARTINGTON, Alan David SAINSBURY

Portland

Royal Manor Health Centre
Gatehouse Medical Centre, Portland Hospital, Castle Road, Portland DT5 1AU
Tel: 01305 820422 Fax: 01305 823849
(South West Dorset Primary Care Trust)
Patient List Size: 11927

Practice Manager Wendy Milverton

GP David Bowen HARGRAVE, Matthew Ian BROOK, Sarah GOODMAN, Robert JANSSEN, Paul John MASON, Sarah NEWMAN, Mark NINHAM, Richard SAMOUELLE, Mark TOWNSEND

Portsmouth

Buckland Medical Centre
24 Gamble Road, Portsmouth PO2 7BN
Tel: 023 9266 0910/92661257 Fax: 023 9267 8175
(Portsmouth City Teaching Primary Care Trust)
Patient List Size: 6050

Practice Manager Sue Crowley

GP R C PATEL, U W MO, S A MUNRO, V R RANDALL

Chichester Road Surgery
34 Chichester Road, Portsmouth PO2 0AD
(Portsmouth City Teaching Primary Care Trust)

GP Colin Arthur OLFORD

Copnor Road Surgery
111 Copnor Road, Portsmouth PO3 5AF
Tel: 023 9266 3368 Fax: 023 9278 3203
(Portsmouth City Teaching Primary Care Trust)
Patient List Size: 7800

Practice Manager T L Till

GP Mark Charles GLASGOW, S P EVANS, Catherine Ann FOLEY, Susan Peta JAMES, John Noel Dickson THORNTON

Cosham Health Centre
Vectis Way, Portsmouth PO6 3AW
Tel: 023 9238 1117 Fax: 023 9237 4183

(Portsmouth City Teaching Primary Care Trust)
Patient List Size: 9500

Practice Manager Pauline Cook

GP Roger Melvyn GRINDROD, Bettyanne CHARLTON, Alexander McLaren GALLOWAY, Richard SAWYER, Simon Paul WERNICK

Hanway Road Surgery
2 Hanway Road, Buckland, Portsmouth PO1 4ND
Tel: 023 9281 5317 Fax: 023 9289 9926
(Portsmouth City Teaching Primary Care Trust)
Patient List Size: 10500

Practice Manager L L McNulty

GP Richard Michael HUGHES, Fiona Jane GAUGHT, Ian Hugh MORRIS, Amir NESSIM, David James Garfield SMART, Ranjani THAMBU

The Health House
1 Wootton Street, Cosham, Portsmouth PO6 3AP
Tel: 023 9238 1118 Fax: 023 9232 6379
(Portsmouth City Teaching Primary Care Trust)
Patient List Size: 4500

Practice Manager S A Haithwaite

GP Alan Charles ALLCOCK, Mary Shelagh WILSON

John Pounds Surgery
John Pounds Medical Centre, 3 Aylward Street, Portsea, Portsmouth PO1 3AP
Tel: 023 9281 2033 Fax: 023 9287 1077
(Portsmouth City Teaching Primary Care Trust)
Patient List Size: 3100

Practice Manager Julie Youseman

GP Luis CASTILLA, Anthea NORMAN

Lake Road Health Centre
Nutfield Place, Portsmouth PO1 4JT
Tel: 023 9282 1201 Fax: 023 9287 5658
(Portsmouth City Teaching Primary Care Trust)
Patient List Size: 10500

Practice Manager Helen Tiller, Joan Wright

GP Geoffrey John ROBINSON, James Patrick Rinaldo HOGAN, David Ronald PLENTY, Marcus Lee SAUNDERS, Andrew William SCOTT-BROWN, Andrew Ivor WILLIAMS

McLaughlin and Partners
27-29 Derby Road, North End, Portsmouth PO2 8HW
Tel: 023 9266 3024 Fax: 023 9265 4991
(Portsmouth City Teaching Primary Care Trust)
Patient List Size: 10600

Practice Manager Karen Merritt

GP Neil Philip McLAUGHLIN, Catherine Anne CAUSER, Andrew Mark Edward RICHARDSON, Micheala WHYTE-VENABLES, Timothy John WILKINSON

Northern Road Surgery
56 Northern Road, Cosham, Portsmouth PO6 3DS
Tel: 023 9237 3321 Fax: 023 9232 7595
Email: surgery.staff@gp-j82086.nhs.uk
(Portsmouth City Teaching Primary Care Trust)
Patient List Size: 5000

Practice Manager Sandra Jordan

GP Bernard KLEMENZ, Nicholas DOLL, Nathan MOSS

Queens Road Surgery
8 Queens Road, Portsmouth PO2 7NX
Tel: 023 9266 5134 Fax: 023 9265 5305
(Portsmouth City Teaching Primary Care Trust)

Practice Manager Clare Petfield

GP Talat KHAN, David Gerald ATCHISON, F NEGRO, Adrian Patrick RILEY

Sunnyside Doctors Surgery
150 Fratton Road, Portsmouth PO1 5DH
Tel: 023 9282 4725 Fax: 023 9281 2905
(Portsmouth City Teaching Primary Care Trust)
Patient List Size: 11034

Practice Manager D Lock

GP David Stuart RAW, Charles Howat LEWIS, Jane Elizabeth LOXTON, Fiona MOSS, David Charles ORAM, Judith Ann THOMPSON, Anthony Richard TOLLAST

The Surgery
134 Baffins Road, Portsmouth PO3 6BH
Tel: 023 9282 7132 Fax: 023 9282 7025
(Portsmouth City Teaching Primary Care Trust)
Patient List Size: 8200

Practice Manager Mike Turner

GP Simon Ward MITCHELL, Stephen Hugh FRANKS, David Charles ROGERS, Jill Mary STONER, Catherine Mary SWEATMAN

The Surgery
280 Havant Road, Drayton, Portsmouth PO6 1PA
Tel: 023 9237 0422 Fax: 023 9261 8383
(Portsmouth City Teaching Primary Care Trust)

Practice Manager Mary Gale

GP Hillary Ashton BAGSHAW, Susan Margaret DAKIN, S J EGELSTAFF, Richard John GILL, Nicholas Peter O'ROURKE, Barry Neil RUSSELL, Richard Anthony SANDERSON

The Surgery
281 London Road, North End, Portsmouth PO2 9HE
Tel: 023 9237 7006 Fax: 023 9237 4263
(Portsmouth City Teaching Primary Care Trust)

Practice Manager Maggie Waldren

GP John HILL, Ko Ko LAING

The Surgery
131 Goldsmith Avenue, Milton, Portsmouth PO4 8QZ
(Portsmouth City Teaching Primary Care Trust)

GP Martin Philip RANDLE, Elizabeth Jane FELLOWS

The Surgery
194 Allaway Avenue, Paulsgrove, Portsmouth PO6 4HJ
Tel: 023 9237 7006 Fax: 023 9237 4263
Email: stephen.mckenning@gp-j82635.nhs.uk
(Portsmouth City Teaching Primary Care Trust)
Patient List Size: 1900

Practice Manager Georgina Lale

GP Stephen Thomas McKENNING

University Surgery
The Nuffield Centre, St Michael's Centre, Portsmouth PO1 2BH
Tel: 023 9273 6006 Fax: 023 9277 8939
(Portsmouth City Teaching Primary Care Trust)
Patient List Size: 9600

Practice Manager Stephanie Murray

GP Kathleen Mary PRIMROSE, Anne LAWSON, Janet Elisabeth SUSSEX

Potters Bar

Annandale Surgery
239 Mutton Lane, Potters Bar EN6 2AS
Tel: 01707 644451 Fax: 01707 655583
(Hertsmere Primary Care Trust)
Patient List Size: 6800

Practice Manager Annette Barnes

GP Brian Terence WOODS, Sally DERRICK, Nicola Jane RAMSELL, Shubha SETTY

Cuffley Village Surgery
Maynard Place, Cuffley, Potters Bar EN6 4JA
Tel: 01707 875201 Fax: 01707 876756
(South East Hertfordshire Primary Care Trust)
Patient List Size: 6723

Practice Manager Teresa Bird

GP Robert Paul Lloyd DAVIES, G FULLES, Michael Christopher STONE, Cynthia Pauline Janet TAYLOR

Highview Surgery
20 Southgate Road, Potters Bar EN6 5DZ
Tel: 01707 871980 Fax: 01707 871995
Website: www.highviewmedicalcentre.co.uk
(Hertsmere Primary Care Trust)
Patient List Size: 8107

Practice Manager Andy Cole

GP Richard Frank CIEZAK, Robert Gravely Benson CLARKE, Rosemary Jane ELDER, Catherine Mary MUNRO, Alison Frances RITCHIE, Bernadette Frances STURRIDGE

Parkfield Medical Centre
The Walk, Potters Bar EN6 1QH
Tel: 01707 651234 Fax: 01707 660452
(Hertsmere Primary Care Trust)
Patient List Size: 12500

Practice Manager Brian Eastwood

GP Alan Richard FERRIS, Caroline Jennifer DAIN, Pang NG, Sai RAMANATHAN, Barry John SMALL, Sally TREVOR, Adwoa YEBOAH

Poulton-le-Fylde

Carleton Surgery
Castle Gardens Crescent, Carleton, Poulton-le-Fylde FY6 7NJ
Tel: 01253 895545 Fax: 01253 899350
(Wyre Primary Care Trust)
Patient List Size: 4000

Practice Manager Paul Dempsey

GP Martin Charles COOK, Vivien Jane DEMPSEY, Catherine Lisa DIDSBURY

The Medical Centre
Queensway, Poulton-le-Fylde FY6 7ST
Tel: 01253 890219 Fax: 01253 894222
(Wyre Primary Care Trust)
Patient List Size: 9224

Practice Manager Jacqueline Tipton

GP Richard Ronald RHODES, Gillian Taylor AU, John Anthony EAST, T LOWSON, R MITCHELL, John Newton WATT

Over Wyre Medical Centre
Wilkinson Way, Off Pilling Lane, Preesall, Poulton-le-Fylde FY6 0EX
Tel: 01253 810722 Fax: 01253 812039
(Wyre Primary Care Trust)
Patient List Size: 10500

Practice Manager Lynda Steven

GP John Philip LEWIN, Francis Thomas COSTELLO, Stephen LYNCH, Angela Katherine NOBLETT, John Edward QUALTROUGH

The Surgery
Westbourne Court, Lockwood Avenue, Poulton-le-Fylde FY6 7AB
Tel: 01253 886878 Fax: 01253 896670
(Wyre Primary Care Trust)

Practice Manager Nathalie Draper

GP Ian Charles KIRKHAM, Stephen J R HORTON, Dawn ISHERWOOD

Prescot

Cedar Cross Medical Centre
42 Cedar Road, Prescot L35 2XA
Tel: 0151 426 5569 Fax: 0151 426 5969
(Knowsley Primary Care Trust)
Patient List Size: 2825

Practice Manager Heather Baker

GP T M AUNG

Cross Lane Surgery
148 Cross Lane, Prescot L35 5DU
Tel: 0151 426 5345 Fax: 0151 426 6017
(Knowsley Primary Care Trust)
Patient List Size: 2125

Practice Manager Cynthia Finney

GP Mohammad Khaledur RAHMAN, N N RAHMAN

The Crossroads Surgery
449 Warrington Road, Rainhill, Prescot L35 4LL
Tel: 0151 430 9989
(St Helens Primary Care Trust)

Practice Manager Mr Som Chana

GP Lorna Valerie CHANA

Longton Medical Centre
451 Warrington Road, Rainhill, Prescot L35 4LL
Tel: 0151 430 0333 Fax: 0151 431 0017
(St Helens Primary Care Trust)
Patient List Size: 5000

Practice Manager Elizabeth Ward

GP Deborah Anne TREE, Michael CLAYTON, Raquel HERRAIZ MORILLAS

McNeilly, McKenna and Fearon
529 Warrington Road, Rainhill, Prescot L35 4LP
Tel: 0151 426 2141 Fax: 0151 430 6210
(St Helens Primary Care Trust)

GP George William McKENNA, Julia Helen FEARON, Paul McNEILLY

Prescot Primary Care Resource Centre
SewellStreet, Prescot L34 1ND
Tel: 0151 426 5253 Fax: 0151 431 0652
(Knowsley Primary Care Trust)
Patient List Size: 6250

Practice Manager Pam Lee

GP M AHAMED, N ALSAYED, Leslie John BRINDLEY, R H DEACON

Preston

Ash Tree House
Church Street, Kirkham, Preston PR4 2SE
Tel: 01772 686688 Fax: 01772 672054
(Fylde Primary Care Trust)
Patient List Size: 10859

Practice Manager Claire Chapman

GP Paul REES, Gillian A BREESE, Jonathan Charles Myers BROWN, Thomas JOHNSON, Jacky PANESAR, Mark SLASKI

Ashton Health Centre
67-69 Pedders Lane, Ashton-on-Ribble, Preston PR2 1HR
Tel: 01772 726839
(Preston Primary Care Trust)

GP Henry Paul CONWAY

Ashton Health Centre
67-69 Pedders Lane, Ashton-on-Ribble, Preston PR2 1HR
Tel: 01772 726535
(Preston Primary Care Trust)

GP Ken TAYLOR

Ashton Health Centre
67-69 Pedders Lane, Ashton-on-Ribble, Preston PR2 1HR
Tel: 01772 726169
(Preston Primary Care Trust)

GP Kailash NATH

Ashton Health Centre
67-69 Pedders Lane, Ashton-on-Ribble, Preston PR2 1HR
Tel: 01772 726500
(Preston Primary Care Trust)

GP Ennis Ignatius O'DONNELL

Ashton Street Surgery
34 Ashton Street, Ashton-on-Ribble, Preston PR2 2PP
Tel: 01772 726588 Fax: 01772 760788
(Preston Primary Care Trust)
Patient List Size: 1900

Practice Manager Karen Baron

GP Bipad Taran DAS, A LATIFF

Beechdrive Surgery
17-19 Beechdrive, Fulwood, Preston PR2 3NB
Tel: 01772 863033
(Preston Primary Care Trust)

Practice Manager Carol Molyneux

GP Ramachandra Krishna NAIK

Beeches Medical Centre
Liverpool Road, Longton, Preston PR4 5AB
Tel: 01772 613123 Fax: 01772 616311
(Chorley and South Ribble Primary Care Trust)
Patient List Size: 1600

GP Ashok Kumar TANDON

Briarwood Medical Centre
514 Blackpool Road, Ashton-on-Ribble, Preston PR2 1HY
Tel: 01772 726186 Fax: 01772 768823
(Preston Primary Care Trust)

Practice Manager Mrs Janson

GP Manjit Singh JANDU, P Neil HARTLEY-SMITH, Nimalendran Jayantha MUTTUCUMARU

Broadway Surgery
2 Broadway, Fulwood, Preston PR2 9TH
Tel: 01772 717261 Fax: 01772 787652
(Preston Primary Care Trust)
Patient List Size: 6850

Practice Manager Anne Fairclough

GP Dineshchandra PATEL, Kaiser CHAUDHRI, Melanie Frances WALSH, Stephen Robert WHITE

Central Park Surgery
Balfour Street, Leyland, Preston PR25 2TD
Tel: 01772 623110 Fax: 01772 623885
Email: centralpark.surgery@gp-P81117.nhs.uk
(Chorley and South Ribble Primary Care Trust)
Patient List Size: 4250

Practice Manager Anne Marie Miller

GP K PATEL, A R PATEL

Chakrabarti
110 Deepdale Road, Preston PR1 5AR
Tel: 01772 884308 Fax: 01772 887735
(Preston Primary Care Trust)
Patient List Size: 2900

Practice Manager Pamela Allen

GP Hara Prosad CHAKRABARTI

Croston Medical Centre
30 Brookfield, Croston, Preston PR26 9HY
Tel: 01772 600081 Fax: 01772 601612
Email: kamlesh.garg@GP-P8.nhs.uk
(Chorley and South Ribble Primary Care Trust)
Patient List Size: 3800

Practice Manager Glennys Parr

GP Kamlesh Kumar GARG, Archana GARG

Deepdale Road Healthcare Centre
Deepdale Road, Preston PR1 5AF
Tel: 01772 655533 Fax: 01772 653414
(Preston Primary Care Trust)

Practice Manager Pam Grogan

GP Antony Charles MAWSON, David Arthur Lincoln BROOKS, Dr FAHIM, Ashok Nanubhai PATEL, Cameron MacKinnon WILSON

Deepdale Road Surgery
98 Deepdale Road, Preston PR1 5AR
Tel: 01772 821069
(Preston Primary Care Trust)
Patient List Size: 2020

Practice Manager K M Thompson

GP Boota SINGH

Deepdale Road Surgery
228-232 Deepdale Road, Preston PR1 6QB
Tel: 01772 555733 Fax: 01772 885406
(Preston Primary Care Trust)
Patient List Size: 3200

Practice Manager Pat Bracken

GP Saiyed Zakaullah SHAHID

Doclands Medical Centre
Blanche Street, Ashton-on-Ribble, Preston PR2 2RL
Tel: 01772 723222 Fax: 01772 726619
(Preston Primary Care Trust)
Patient List Size: 6300

Practice Manager S Chikhaliker

GP Malcolm CRAIG, Michael John EVES

Fishergate Hill Surgery
50 Fishergate Hill, Preston PR1 8DN
Tel: 01772 254484 Fax: 01772 881835
(Preston Primary Care Trust)
Patient List Size: 5700

Practice Manager Wendy Sutton

GP Hardev SINGH, Julia Alexandra JOHNSON, Alyson JONES, Ronnie LOWE

Forrester, Bowman and Rowlandson
Berry Lane Medical Centre, Berry Lane, Longridge, Preston PR3 3JJ
Tel: 01772 783021 Fax: 01772 785809
(Hyndburn and Ribble Valley Primary Care Trust)
Patient List Size: 8700

Practice Manager Sue Carr

GP Ian Robert FORRESTER, Ann BOWMAN, Stephen John GRIFFIN, George ROWLANDSON, Margaret Lilian SMALL

Frenchwood Avenue Surgery
49 Frenchwood Avenue, Preston PR1 4ND
Tel: 01772 254173
(Preston Primary Care Trust)
Patient List Size: 2400

Practice Manager Barbara Parker

GP Mark WEBSTER

Garstang Road Surgery
63-65 Garstang Road, Preston PR1 1LB
Tel: 01772 253554 Fax: 01772 909131
Email: surgery@gp-p81152.nhs.uk
(Preston Primary Care Trust)
Patient List Size: 5800

Practice Manager Joanne Nicholas

GP Graeme Anthony ROBB, Angela ROBB

Geoffrey Street Health Centre
Geoffrey Street, Preston PR1 5NE
Tel: 01772 401760 Fax: 01772 401766
(Preston Primary Care Trust)
Patient List Size: 6000

Practice Manager Sally Thornton

GP Martin Julian COAKER, Simon John SHAW, Usha SOBTE

The Health Centre
Raikes Road, Great Eccleston, Preston PR3 0ZA
Tel: 01995 670066 Fax: 01995 671054
Website: www.gehc.co.uk
(Wyre Primary Care Trust)
Patient List Size: 7287

Practice Manager Sylvia Welberry

GP Sean Patrick COUGHLIN, M AHMED, Hilary Theresa CASSELS, Stephen Nicholas COTTAM, Christina J HYNES, Rachel H MOLLOY, L TAYLOR

Ingol Health Centre
87 Village Green Lane, Ingol, Preston PR2 7DS
Tel: 01772 729730 Fax: 01772 769733
(Preston Primary Care Trust)

GP D PATEL, K CHAUDHRI, M WALSH, S WHITE

Kingsfold Medical Centre
Woodcroft Close, Penwortham, Preston PR1 9BX
Tel: 01772 746492 Fax: 01772 909141
Website: www.kingsfoldmedicalcentre.co.uk
(Chorley and South Ribble Primary Care Trust)
Patient List Size: 4173

Practice Manager W Bate

GP Ramaprasad DAS GUPTA, Tina AMBURY, Gautam Tukaram CHIKHALIKAR

Kirkham Health Centre
Moor Street, Kirkham, Preston PR4 2DL
Tel: 01772 683420 Fax: 01776 672251
(Fylde Primary Care Trust)
Patient List Size: 8400

Practice Manager Nadine Woodmason

GP Douglas Milne WRIGHT, Nigel Vincent CARTMELL, Stephen Anthony HARDWICK, Tara Amelia LOWSON

The Landscape Surgery
High Street, Garstang, Preston PR3 1FA
Tel: 01995 603355 Fax: 01995 601810
(Wyre Primary Care Trust)
Patient List Size: 5500

Practice Manager Patricia A Pearson

GP Margaret Mary ASHCROFT, F CARTER, Melvyn Edward JOHN

Longton Health Centre
Liverpool Road, Longton, Preston PR4 5HA
Tel: 01772 615429 Fax: 01772 611094
(Chorley and South Ribble Primary Care Trust)
Patient List Size: 10500

Practice Manager Kath Swain

GP Samuel David MOSS, Teresa CEPEDA-LUCAS, Anthony James COCKERAM, Dawn Marie EDGE, John Reginald LOUDONSACK, Peter William ROBINSON

Lostock Hall Medical Centre
410 Leyland Road, Lostock Hall, Preston PR5 5SA
Tel: 01772 518080 Fax: 01772 518086
(Chorley and South Ribble Primary Care Trust)

Practice Manager Patricia Cook

GP Roopendra Kumar PRASAD, K M SINGH

Lytham Road Surgery
2 Lytham Road, Fulwood, Preston PR2 8JB
Tel: 01772 716033 Fax: 01772 715445
(Preston Primary Care Trust)
Patient List Size: 10900

Practice Manager Pamela Tabeth

GP Raymond John Hambleton CHESWORTH, John Henry Procter CARTER, Alison Mary Yule PARSON, John Byron William WIGNALL

Meadow Street Surgery
57-59 Meadow Street, Preston PR1 1TS
Tel: 01772 252414 Fax: 01772 254101
(Preston Primary Care Trust)

Practice Manager Glenda Sanaham

GP Qudratulla Omar KHAN, Krishna Lal GUPTA

Medicare Unit
1 Croston Road, Lostock Hall, Preston PR5 5RS
Tel: 01772 330724 Fax: 01772 620160
(Chorley and South Ribble Primary Care Trust)
Patient List Size: 2654

Practice Manager Janet Gallagher

GP Gigurawa Gamage Khemananda WIJETHILLEKE

Moor Park Surgery
49 Garstang Road, Preston PR1 1LB
Tel: 01772 252077 Fax: 01772 885451
(Preston Primary Care Trust)
Patient List Size: 4650

Practice Manager Gwen Davy

GP Edward Maxim SMITH, Ina Shelagh Joan PAVEY, Nichola WILLIAMS

Moss Side Medical Centre
16 Moss Side Way, Leyland, Preston PR26 7XL
Tel: 01772 623954 Fax: 01772 622897
(Chorley and South Ribble Primary Care Trust)
Patient List Size: 4000

Practice Manager Janet McGrath

GP Hem Dattatray SULE, Sulabha Hem SULE

New Hall Lane Practice
The Health Centre, Geoffrey Street, Preston PR1 5NE
Tel: 01772 401730 Fax: 01772 401731
(Preston Primary Care Trust)
Patient List Size: 9300

Practice Manager Gill Fraser

GP Andrew Harold James PRITCHETT, Stephen Nicholas HIRST, Seema MARROTT, Andrew Colin MAYOR, Nigel David PIDGEON

New Hall Lane Surgery
330 New Hall Lane, Preston PR1 4SU
Tel: 01772 794172 Fax: 01772 703365
(Preston Primary Care Trust)
Patient List Size: 1100

Practice Manager Pushpa Patel

GP Mohammad Zahurul Hoque BHUIYA

Plungington Road Surgery
100 Plungington Road, Preston PR1 7UE
Tel: 01772 250574
(Preston Primary Care Trust)

GP Baleshwar THAKUR

The Porta-Kabin
The Village Surgery, William Street, Preston PR5 5RZ
Tel: 01772 697666
(Preston Primary Care Trust)

GP Karim MASHAYEKHI

Preston Road Surgery
5 Preston Road, Leyland, Preston PR25 4NT
Tel: 01772 622505
(Preston Primary Care Trust)

GP Sylvia Grace BOWKER

Ribble Village Surgery
200 Miller Road, Ribbleton, Preston PR2 6NH
Tel: 01772 792864
(Preston Primary Care Trust)

GP Ghassan BAROUDI

Ribblesdale Place Surgery
23 Ribblesdale Place, Preston PR1 3NA
Tel: 01772 258474
(Preston Primary Care Trust)

GP Philip Arthur BIRD, David Ward HOLDEN, John Alexander Rogers LUSK

Riverside Medical Centre
194 Victoria Road, Walton-le-Dale, Preston PR5 4AY
Tel: 01772 556703 Fax: 01772 880861
(Chorley and South Ribble Primary Care Trust)
Patient List Size: 9405

Practice Manager Jane Holmes

GP Alexander Blackwood PHILLIPS, A BUCKLEY, Alexander Scott FORBES, Shireen KENNEDY

Roslea Surgery
51 Station Road, Bamber Bridge, Preston PR5 6PE
Tel: 01772 335128 Fax: 01772 492248
Website: www.roseleasurgery.co.uk
(Chorley and South Ribble Primary Care Trust)
Patient List Size: 10000

Practice Manager M Callaghan, V Callaghan

GP D R BALL, K L ASHTON, John Mansfield BREARLEY, Helen R KING, David Robert MOORE, J M SMITH

Sandy Lane Surgery
Sandy Lane, Leyland, Preston PR25 2EB
Tel: 01772 909915 Fax: 01772 909911
(Chorley and South Ribble Primary Care Trust)

Practice Manager Anne Strangeways

GP Janet EVERISS, Peter Ronald CURTIS, Pauline May GRACE, Jane Margaret HUDSON, David Stuart JONES, Linda Jane MASSEY, Brian Vishnu RAMBIHAR, Stephen Thomas WARD

St Fillan's Medical Centre
2 Liverpool Road, Penwortham, Preston PR1 0AD
Tel: 01772 745427 Fax: 01772 752562
(Chorley and South Ribble Primary Care Trust)
Patient List Size: 8542

Practice Manager L A Dickinson

GP Terence Patrick O'CONNOR, Alison Pamela GREENING, Isobel Tracy Ann HILES, Alan Ronald WILKINSON

St Marys Health Centre
Cop Lane, Penwortham, Preston PR1 0SR
Tel: 01772 744404 Fax: 01772 752967
(Chorley and South Ribble Primary Care Trust)
Patient List Size: 15000

Practice Manager Gwen Adams

GP Nicholas Stuart McCRAITH, Penelope Jane BERENDS-SHERIFF, Edward Ian James BUCKLEY, Ian Philip JONES, C Adrian ROBINSON

St Pauls Surgery
36-38 East Street, Preston PR1 1UU
Tel: 01772 252409 Fax: 01772 885509
(Preston Primary Care Trust)
Patient List Size: 2800

Practice Manager Valerie Wiles

GP Binoy KUMAR

Station Surgery
8 Golden Hill Lane, Leyland, Preston PR25 3NP
Tel: 01772 622505 Fax: 01772 457718
(Chorley and South Ribble Primary Care Trust)

GP George Wadie AHAD

Station Surgery
8 Golden Hill Lane, Leyland, Preston PR25 3NP
Tel: 01772 622808 Fax: 01772 457718
(Chorley and South Ribble Primary Care Trust)
Patient List Size: 3000

Practice Manager Glennys Parr

GP George W AHAD, Tripuraneni LEELAKUMARI

Stonebridge Surgery
Preston Road, Longridge, Preston PR3 3AP
Tel: 01772 783271 Fax: 01772 782836
(Hyndburn and Ribble Valley Primary Care Trust)
Patient List Size: 7450

Practice Manager Lynda Williams

GP Kevin Michael Francis Gordon PAVEY, Natalya EVANS, Elaine Claire HAWARD, Andrew Peter HICKS

The Surgery
310 St Georges Road, Deepdale, Preston PR1 6NR
Tel: 01772 254546 Fax: 01772 254546
(Preston Primary Care Trust)
Patient List Size: 2100

Practice Manager Marie Dean

GP Jib Narayan JHA

The Surgery
652 Preston Road, Clayton-le-Woods, Preston PR6 7EH
Tel: 01772 323021 Fax: 01772 620078
(Chorley and South Ribble Primary Care Trust)

Practice Manager Lorraine Parkinson

GP El-Said Moustafa Hamid DAWOUD, Ghadeer Mohamed El-Solaih Ali HAMAD

Village Surgery
William Street, Lostock Hall, Preston PR5 5RZ
Tel: 01772 697666 Fax: 01772 697888
(Chorley and South Ribble Primary Care Trust)

Practice Manager Beverley Masheyakhy

GP K MASHEYAKHY

Village Surgery
2 Churchside, New Longton, Preston PR4 4LU
Tel: 01772 613804 Fax: 01772 617812
(Chorley and South Ribble Primary Care Trust)

Practice Manager Geraldine Helm

GP Susan Elizabeth LEWIS, Peter BLAKE

The Windsor Road Surgery
Windsor Road, Garstang, Preston PR3 1ED
Tel: 01995 603350 Fax: 01995 601301
(Wyre Primary Care Trust)
Patient List Size: 11200

Practice Manager Catherine Thornton

GP L BRADDOCK, Colin James DANIELS, David Philip Ward DEAKIN, Michael Brian GILES, F LAING, S J McKIMMIE, Elizabeth TEW, Jonathan WILLIAMSON

Woodplumpton Road Surgery
104 Woodplumpton Road, Fulwood, Preston PR2 3TF
Tel: 01772 729756 Fax: 01772 760862
(Preston Primary Care Trust)
Patient List Size: 3000

Practice Manager Margaret Ghori

GP Shabbir Salim GHORI

Worden Medical Centre
West Paddock, Leyland, Preston PR25 1HW
Tel: 01772 423555 Fax: 01772 623878
(Chorley and South Ribble Primary Care Trust)

GP Colin John CAMPBELL, S BEDFORD, Alan Richard KELSALL, Alastair John KILGOUR, John PARKER, Anthony Donald REID, Karen Lesley WARNER

Worden Medical Centre
West Paddock, Leyland, Preston PR25 1HR
Tel: 01772 423555 Fax: 01772 623878
(Chorley and South Ribble Primary Care Trust)

Patient List Size: 12500

Practice Manager Tracy Williams

GP Sarah BEDFORD, John PARKER, Colin John CAMPBELL, A R KELSALL, Alastair John KILGOUR, Anthony Donald REID, Karen Lesley WARNER

Young and Partners

The Ryan Medical Centre, St Marys Road, Bamber Bridge, Preston PR5 6JD
Tel: 01772 335136 Fax: 01772 626701
(Chorley and South Ribble Primary Care Trust)
Patient List Size: 11800

Practice Manager Julie Howarth

GP David William YOUNG, Anne Hamilton ALLISTER, Ian Alan CLELLAND, Stephen Alexander HOWELL, Joegy Kunjbihari SHAH

Princes Risborough

Cross Keys Practice

High Street, Princes Risborough HP27 0AX
Tel: 01844 344488 Fax: 01844 274714
(Vale of Aylesbury Primary Care Trust)
Patient List Size: 15500

Practice Manager Ann Poote

GP Janet DURBAN, Peter Norman John APPLETON, John Francis Bosco CAHILL, Lucy GUEST, Annabel HOWELL, Malcolm Howard JONES, Anthony Robin MAISEY, T W NEALE

Wellington House Practice

Aylesbury Road, Princes Risborough HP27 9HG
Tel: 01844 344281 Fax: 01844 274719
(Vale of Aylesbury Primary Care Trust)
Patient List Size: 9000

Practice Manager Karen Washbourn

GP Richard Alexander McKENZIE, Lowri KEW, Martin John KNIGHTLEY, Michael MULHOLLAND, Carolyn Rosemary-Anne PARTRIDGE, Stephen Andrew STAMP

Prudhoe

Adderlane Surgery

Adderlane Road, West Wylan, Prudhoe NE42 5HR
Tel: 01661 836386 Fax: 01661 831353
Email: admin@gp-a84614.nhs.uk
(Northumberland Care Trust)
Patient List Size: 2000

Practice Manager Julie Haywood

GP Stephen Clifford HAYWOOD, Laura ANDERSON

Castle Surgery

Kepwell Bank Top, Prudhoe NE42 5PW
Tel: 01661 832209 Fax: 01661 836338
(Northumberland Care Trust)

Practice Manager Elizabeth Robinson

GP A EGAN, J IRVINE, Steven Juan QUILLIAM, H THORNTON

Pudsey

The Gables

231 Swinnow Road, Pudsey LS28 9AP
Tel: 0113 257 4730 Fax: 0113 255 8644
(Leeds West Primary Care Trust)
Patient List Size: 4100

Practice Manager Joanne Robinson

GP Dr DARIGALA

Hillfoot Surgery

126 Owlcotes Road, Pudsey LS28 7QR
Tel: 0113 257 4169 Fax: 0113 236 3380
(Leeds West Primary Care Trust)
Patient List Size: 6342

Practice Manager Patricia Lawrence

GP Paul James MADDY, E W HUTCH, H M LONGDON, Kathleen Anne STEWARD

K J Watson and Partners

West Lodge Surgery, New Street, Farsley, Pudsey LS28 5DL
Tel: 0113 239 4573 Fax: 0113 236 2509
(Leeds West Primary Care Trust)
Patient List Size: 16018

Practice Manager Linda Harrison

GP Michael Barry COHEN, Nicholas Stewart BALL, Cathryne Anne Sisson HEARNSHAW, Timothy Ian HUDSON, Adrian Vincent LEE, Susan Margaret SMITH, Kevin John WATSON

Pudsey Health Centre

18 Mulberry Street, Pudsey LS28 7XP
Tel: 0113 257 0711/236 3926 Fax: 0113 295 4168
(Leeds West Primary Care Trust)

Practice Manager Jenny Bell

GP Robert Jeremy ROSS, Jeremy Francis HALL, Christopher Michael MASON, Bernadette Marie TAWSE

Robin Lane Medical Centre

Robin Lane, Pudsey LS28 7RR
Tel: 0113 295 1444/1449 Fax: 0113 295 1440
(Leeds West Primary Care Trust)
Patient List Size: 9300

Practice Manager Samual Forbes

GP Peter John LINDSAY, Linda BELDERSON, Rosemary DALY, Kristan Celia TOFT, Francesco Luigi ZICCHIERI

Sunfield Medical Centre

Sunfield Place, Stanningley, Pudsey LS28 6DR
Tel: 0113 257 0361/255 5263 Fax: 0113 236 3822
(Leeds West Primary Care Trust)
Patient List Size: 5900

Practice Manager Derrick Allen

GP Carolyn BROOM, Kenneth Wilson McGECHAEN, Phillip RICHARDS

Pulborough

The Glebe Surgery

Monastery Lane, Storrington, Pulborough RH20 4LR
Tel: 01903 742942 Fax: 01903 740700
(Horsham and Chanctonbury Primary Care Trust)

Practice Manager S Smith

GP Martin Edward KALAHER, Gillian LEWIS, Bonnie Si-Wang TSE, David Mark WHITEHEAD

Mill Stream Medical Centre

North Street, Storrington, Pulborough RH20 4DH
Tel: 01903 743083 Fax: 01903 740959
Website: www.millstreammedical.co.uk
(Horsham and Chanctonbury Primary Care Trust)
Patient List Size: 4800

Practice Manager Jane Royal

GP Ian H CREEK, Carolyn Ann EVANS, Jo BAILEY

Pulborough Medical Group

Barnhouse Surgery, Barnhouse Close, Pulborough RH20 2HQ
Tel: 01798 872815 Fax: 01798 872123
(Western Sussex Primary Care Trust)
Patient List Size: 12000

Practice Manager Elizabeth Coulthard

GP Michael John SHILLINGFORD, Timothy FOOKS, Edward A A GIBBON, Peter HARD, Christopher John KING, David S PULLAN

Purley

The Keston House Medical Practice
70 Brighton Road, Purley CR8 2LJ
Tel: 020 8660 8292 Fax: 020 8763 2142
(Croydon Primary Care Trust)
Patient List Size: 8600

Practice Manager Graham Merry

GP Patricia Coulson PHILLIPS, S BHARTIYA, Katherine Mary HOPKINS JONES, C MACKENZIE, Robert David Charles OVERTON, K PAVKOVICH, K REDMAN

Purley Medical Practice
73 Lansdowne Road, Purley CR8 2PE
Tel: 020 8660 4130 Fax: 020 8645 9071
(Croydon Primary Care Trust)
Patient List Size: 4300

Practice Manager Jo McKay

GP Padma Grace SAMARAWICKRAMA

Woodcote Group Practice
32 Foxley Lane, Purley CR8 3EE
Tel: 020 8660 1304 Fax: 020 8660 0721
Email: woodcote.practice@gp-H83024.nhs.uk
(Croydon Primary Care Trust)
Patient List Size: 15000

Practice Manager Nan Nobes

GP Peter William NEWLANDS, Kaleem KHAN, John Graham LINNEY, Fola SHOBOWALE, C WEBSTER-SMITH

Radlett

Gateways Surgery
Andrew Close, Porters Park Drive, Shenley, Radlett WD7 9LP
Tel: 01923 857146 Fax: 01923 857145
(Hertsmere Primary Care Trust)
Patient List Size: 1962

Practice Manager Anne O'Grady

GP Michael Downton CROFT

Red House Surgery
124 Watling Street, Radlett WD7 7JQ
Tel: 01923 855606 Fax: 01923 853577
(Hertsmere Primary Care Trust)
Patient List Size: 14720

Practice Manager Kenneth Spooner

GP Craig William MAXWELL, Stephen Benedict FITZGERALD, Ian David GOLD, Michael Jeremy INGRAM, Peter Martin SWEENEY

Radstock

St Chads Surgery
Gullock Tyning, Midsomer Norton, Radstock BA3 2UH
Tel: 01761 413585 Fax: 01761 411176
Email: stchads@gp-L81025.nhs.uk
(Bath and North East Somerset Primary Care Trust)

Practice Manager David Carter

GP G E JACKSON, E HERSH, N C R JONES, C H KENDRICK, Lucy MACKENZIE, A A G MORRICE, J P VALENTINE, E J WIDDOWSON

Rainham

Dr A Abdullah
Rainham Health Centre, Upminster Road, Rainham RM13 9AB
Tel: 01708 796579 Fax: 01708 796577
(Havering Primary Care Trust)

Practice Manager Jackie Whitney

GP A R M ABDULLAH

Integrated Medical Care Rainham
17 Berwick Road, Rainham RM13 9QU
Tel: 01708 520830 Fax: 01708 522137
Email: dr.adur@lineone.net
(Havering Primary Care Trust)

Practice Manager Val Nicholls

GP Ranjan Mohan ADUR, S ALAM, B DIXIT, D C KAKATI

South Hornchurch Clinic
Southend Road, Rainham RM13 7XR
Tel: 01708 557601 Fax: 01708 555945
(Havering Primary Care Trust)
Patient List Size: 2130

GP Mustaq Ahmad WANI

The Surgery
382 Upminster Road North, Rainham RM13 9RZ
Tel: 01708 553120 Fax: 01708 550666
Email: ajawad@nhs.net
(Havering Primary Care Trust)
Patient List Size: 2300

Practice Manager Debra Copsey

GP Abdul-Karim JAWAD

The Surgery
39 Mungo Park Road, Rainham RM13 7PB
Tel: 01708 554797 Fax: 01708 525571
(Havering Primary Care Trust)

GP Sickan SUBRAMANIAM

The Surgery
106 Cowper Road, Rainham RM13 9TS
Tel: 01708 550276 Fax: 01708 552620
(Havering Primary Care Trust)

GP Eric Edward TONI

The Surgery
1 Harlow Road, Rainham RM13 7UP
Tel: 01708 552072 Fax: 01708 524408
(Havering Primary Care Trust)

GP K A SUBRAMANIAN

The Surgery
39 Frederick Road, Rainham RM13 8NJ
Tel: 01708 552738 Fax: 01708 551463
(Havering Primary Care Trust)
Patient List Size: 1910

Practice Manager C West

GP M FATEH, G BARCLAY

Ramsey

Ramsey Road Health Centre
Mews Close, Whytefield Road, Ramsey PE27 5BZ
Tel: 01480 466466
(Huntingdonshire Primary Care Trust)

GP David Jon RODGERS

Ramsgate

Addington Street Surgery
69 Addington Street, Ramsgate CT11 9JH
Tel: 01843 593544 Fax: 01843 594310
(East Kent Coastal Teaching Primary Care Trust)
Patient List Size: 5400

Practice Manager Marion O'Grady

GP Alyson Maxine MACPHERSON, Christine Sabina ARNOLD

Dashwood House Surgery
24 South Eastern Road, Ramsgate CT11 9DU
Tel: 01843 593252

(East Kent Coastal Teaching Primary Care Trust)

Practice Manager Lisa Webb

GP Michael David CARDWELL, Anthony Carlyle KNEATH, F RAHIMI

The Grange Medical Centre
West Cliff Road, Ramsgate CT11 9LJ
Tel: 01843 595051 Fax: 01843 591999
Website: www.thegrangemedicalcentre.co.uk
(East Kent Coastal Teaching Primary Care Trust)
Patient List Size: 10060

Practice Manager R W Thompson

GP Alan David KITCHENER, John Daniel BEALE, Sabine BOHNER, Jean Rosemary JOHNSTONE, Richard Clive MORCOM, Nicholas Charles WARD

High Street Surgery
75 High Street, Minster, Ramsgate CT12 4AB
Tel: 01843 821333 Fax: 01843 823146
(East Kent Coastal Teaching Primary Care Trust)
Patient List Size: 6700

GP Caroline Eleanor CROSFIELD, M D ELLIOTT, Carol Ann Mary RICKENBACH, B STROMDVIK, M J VAN VUUREN

Mildmay Court Surgery
Mildmay Court, Bellevue Road, Ramsgate CT11 8JX
Tel: 01843 592576 Fax: 01843 852980
Email: mail@mildmaysurgery.co.uk
Website: www.mildmaysurgery.co.uk
(East Kent Coastal Teaching Primary Care Trust)
Patient List Size: 8500

Practice Manager Ian Macdougald

GP John Michael HARDAKER, Catherine Anne NEDEN, John Wilfred David NEDEN, Michael John PICK, Robert Owen SADLER

Newington Road Surgery
100 Newington Road, Ramsgate CT12 6EW
Tel: 01843 595951 Fax: 01843 853387
Email: administrator@gp-G82150.nhs.uk
(East Kent Coastal Teaching Primary Care Trust)
Patient List Size: 8600

Practice Manager P McGurk

GP Malcolm Thomas REEVES, Susanna Felicity TIMMINS

Summerhill Surgery
243 Margate Road, Ramsgate CT12 6SU
Tel: 01843 591758 Fax: 01843 580370
(East Kent Coastal Teaching Primary Care Trust)
Patient List Size: 7300

Practice Manager Christina Cleworth

GP O B PETERS, K W AFRIDI, Simon Paul GROVER, M S ROSS-PARKER

Wickham Surgery
1 Wickham Avenue, Ramsgate CT11 8AY
Tel: 01843 593420 Fax: 01843 591799
(East Kent Coastal Teaching Primary Care Trust)

Practice Manager Tina Milham

GP Paul Robert Arthur ATTWOOD

Rayleigh

Audley Mills Surgery
57 Eastwood Road, Rayleigh SS6 7JF
Tel: 01268 774981
(Castle Point and Rochford Primary Care Trust)

GP Robert Miles SWINBURNE, Dr BELTRAN, Carol Cameron DAYSON, Alan Peter KERRY, Dr LEWIS, Dr TAYLOR, Dr THOMAS, Jennifer Susan THORP

Church View Surgery
Burley House, 15 High Street, Rayleigh SS6 7DY
Tel: 01268 774477 Fax: 01268 771293
(Castle Point and Rochford Primary Care Trust)
Patient List Size: 16000

Practice Manager A M Marriott

GP Geoffrey Peter KITTLE, Richard ARCHER, Dr CRYRUS, Peter GLOVER, James Eric NICHOLLS, Susan E TUCKER

Rawreth Lane Surgery
49 Rawreth Lane, Rayleigh SS6 9QD
Tel: 01268 780408 Fax: 01268 784088
(Castle Point and Rochford Primary Care Trust)
Patient List Size: 2626

Practice Manager Susan Grant

GP Indra JAYAWEERA

William Harvey Surgery
83 London Road, Rayleigh SS6 9HR
Tel: 01268 784003 Fax: 01268 782131
(Castle Point and Rochford Primary Care Trust)
Patient List Size: 4800

Practice Manager Rita Redfern

GP Dr RAMANATHAN, Dr THARMARATNAM

Reading

Alexandra Road Surgery
31 Alexandra Road, Reading RG1 5PG
Tel: 0118 935 2121 Fax: 0118 935 9420
(Reading Primary Care Trust)
Patient List Size: 5200

Practice Manager Rosemary Tilbury

GP Gerard Lionel D'CRUZ, Jude Egbert Maurice D'CRUZ

Balmore Park Surgery
59A Hemdean Road, Caversham, Reading RG4 7SS
Tel: 0118 946 4025 Fax: 0118 946 1766
(Reading Primary Care Trust)
Patient List Size: 14300

Practice Manager R A Redpath

GP Patrick McCormick Donald ANDERSON, Fiona Jean AITKEN, Andrew BREWSTER, Gwendolen Maria DELANY, Graham John PAIGE, Helen PAIGE, Samantha POTTER, Roderick Andrew SMITH

Brookside Group Practice
Brookside Close, Gipsy Lane, Earley, Reading RG6 7HG
Tel: 0118 966 9222 Fax: 0118 935 3174
(Wokingham Primary Care Trust)
Patient List Size: 26500

Practice Manager Lizzie Page

GP Derek Charles MUNDAY, Stephen Gerald Edward BROWN, Cleve CHEVASSUT, Bernard CHOI, Philip David HAYNES, Rosalind Margaret HISLOP, Stephen Alan MADGWICK, Peter Jonathan MARSHALL, James Tait PIMM, Rodney Charles SHARPE, Matthew Byrom SHAW, Rachel Mary WEEKS, Katherine Sarah WHATMORE

Chancellor House Surgery
6 Shinfield Road, Reading RG2 7BW
Tel: 0118 931 0006 Fax: 0118 975 7194
(Reading Primary Care Trust)
Patient List Size: 8600

Practice Manager Jan Charlton

GP Trevor Alan UNDERWOOD, Tarek MOHEIM, Volodimir Alexander PIZURA

Chatham Street Surgery
121 Chatham Street, Reading RG1 7JE
Tel: 0118 950 5121 Fax: 0118 959 0545
(Reading Primary Care Trust)

Practice Manager J Caston

GP Raj Pal SHARMA, Ali ASGHAR, Catherine LAWRANCE, Shobhana PATEL

Christchurch Road Practice
81 Christchurch Road, Reading RG2 7BD
Tel: 0118 975 5788 Fax: 0118 926 3230
(Reading Primary Care Trust)
Patient List Size: 4260

Practice Manager S Nirgude

GP Harjeet Singh BINDRA, Satpal KAUR

Circuit Lane Surgery
53 Circuit Lane, Reading RG30 3AN
Tel: 0118 958 2537 Fax: 0118 957 6115
(Reading Primary Care Trust)
Patient List Size: 10900

Practice Manager Jenny Marnock

GP Philip Arthur SIMMONS, J A ADAMS, Malcolm John DODSON, Peter James GARSIDE, David Kenneth HORNE, Susan Joy JARMAN, Derek John PEMBERTON

Eldon Square Surgery
9 Eldon Square, Reading RG1 4DP
Tel: 0118 957 4891
(Reading Primary Care Trust)

Practice Manager Rosemarie Tilbury

GP Ramnath NARAYAN

Emmer Green Surgery
4 St Barnabas Road, Caversham, Reading RG4 8RA
Tel: 0118 948 6900 Fax: 0118 946 3341
Email: surgery.mail@gp-K81041.nhs.uk
Website: www.emmergreensurgery.co.uk
(Reading Primary Care Trust)
Patient List Size: 9500

Practice Manager Pauline Cook

GP Andy CIECIERSKI, Isabel Jane COOK, Julie Alice GORING, Kathryn Margaret HOOKWAY, Ian Charles KEMP, Charles Robert MARTIN-BATES

Goring and Woodcote Medical Practice
Red Cross Road, Goring on Thames, Reading RG8 9HG
Tel: 01491 872372 Fax: 01491 875908
(South East Oxfordshire Primary Care Trust)
Patient List Size: 9600

Practice Manager Clare Wagner

GP Rhys William HAMILTON, Andrew GOODE, Angela LAMB, Stephen RICHARDS, Gordon ROBERTSON, Angela ROWE

Grovelands Medical Centre
701 Oxford Road, Reading RG30 1HG
Tel: 0118 958 2525 Fax: 0118 950 9284
Website: www.grovelandsmc.co.uk
(Reading Primary Care Trust)
Patient List Size: 13100

GP Antony Sylvester COOMBER, Majidah ALI, Ighacio ESCAMILLA, Ian Robert Morris JACOBS, Ishak NADEEM, Stephen PICK, Deborah Anne RILEY

Loddon Vale Practice
Hurricane Way, Woodley, Reading RG5 4UX
Tel: 0118 969 0160 Fax: 0118 969 9103
Email: info@gp-K81069.nhs.uk
Website: www.loddonvale.com
(Wokingham Primary Care Trust)
Patient List Size: 18000

Practice Manager W John

GP Charles Robert Sabine TAIT, Christine Valerie BYRNE, David John CLAYTON, Omid Entekhasi FARD, Michael Richard KITCHING, Jeremy Charles LADE, David MARSHALL, Jennifer Mary MILLER, Deborah Dawn MILLIGAN, David Manfred WESTON

London Road Practice
172 London Road, Reading RG1 3PA
Tel: 0118 926 4992 Fax: 0118 926 3231
(Reading Primary Care Trust)
Patient List Size: 2200

Practice Manager Beverly Manton

GP Satish Manibhai PATEL

London Street Practice
72 London Street, Reading RG1 4SJ
Tel: 0118 957 4640 Fax: 0118 959 7613
(Reading Primary Care Trust)

Practice Manager Jim Kidd

GP Michael Andrew JACOBS, Najat Isaac Shamas ESSA, Marianne HARROLD, Elizabeth Isabella TINTO

Longbarn Lane Surgery
22 Longbarn Lane, Reading RG2 7SZ
Tel: 0118 987 1377 Fax: 0118 975 0375
(Reading Primary Care Trust)

GP Susan Elizabeth WILLIAMS, Charles Bell SLATER

Melrose Surgery
73 London Road, Reading RG1 5BS
Tel: 0118 950 7950 Fax: 0118 959 4044
(Reading Primary Care Trust)

GP Frank Aldwyn Benedict WILLIAMS

Melrose Surgery
73 London Road, Reading RG1 5BS
Tel: 0118 959 5200 Fax: 0118 950 7726
(Reading Primary Care Trust)

GP Lionel Jeremy DEAN

Milman Road Health Centre
Milman Road, Reading RG2 0AR
Tel: 0118 987 1297
(Reading Primary Care Trust)

GP Prakash KUMAR

Milman Road Health Centre
Milman Road, Reading RG2 0AR
Tel: 0118 968 2285/6 Fax: 0118 975 5033
Email: drparker.mrhc@gp-k81040.nhs.uk
(Reading Primary Care Trust)
Patient List Size: 9850

Practice Manager John McKenzie

GP Brendon Anthony LISTER, Andrew John CHAPMAN, Rabinder Kumar MITTAL, Janice Gwendoline RICHARDS, Simone Andrea SLATER

Mortimer Surgery
Victoria Road, Mortimer Common, Reading RG7 3SQ
Tel: 0118 933 2436 Fax: 0118 933 3801
(Reading Primary Care Trust)

GP Derrick Alan LANDER, Joan Frances CRAWFORD, Alasdair Robert DUTHIE, Gillian Samantha FRENCH, Sarah Margaret MILLER, Iain William ROCK, Christopher James Ballantyne STRANG

Oxford Road Surgery
101 Oxford Road, Reading RG1 7UD
Tel: 0118 957 4687
(Reading Primary Care Trust)

GP Pran Nath JOLLY

Oxford Road Surgery
292 Oxford Road, Reading RG30 1AD
Tel: 0118 957 4614 Fax: 0118 959 5486
(Reading Primary Care Trust)
Patient List Size: 3000

Practice Manager Jennie Hawkins

GP Natwarlal Gangjibhai PATEL, Shobhana PATEL

Pangbourne Medical Practice
The Boat House Surgery, Whitchurch Road, Pangbourne, Reading RG8 7DP

Tel: 0118 984 2234 Fax: 0118 984 3022
(Reading Primary Care Trust)
Patient List Size: 10360

Practice Manager Ann Wells

GP Willem Barend WESTERMANN, Ian Douglas COX, Christopher Martin KEAST, Matilda Magdalen Grenville OPPENHEIMER, Hazel Morag POWELL, Michael Pearce POWELL

Parkside Family Practice

Green Road Surgery, 224 Wokingham Road, Reading RG6 1JT
Tel: 0118 935 1653 Fax: 0118 926 3269
(Wokingham Primary Care Trust)
Patient List Size: 12600

Practice Manager Michael Kennedy

GP Nicola Jane BROCK, Aaron GOLD, Judith JAMES, Medhat MIKHAIL, Richard PERRY, Julia Belinda THILO, Alison Margaret WATSON

Peppard Road Surgery

45 Peppard Road, Caversham, Reading RG4 8NR
Tel: 0118 946 2224
(Reading Primary Care Trust)

GP Harold Nordin CHADWICK

Priory Avenue Surgery

2 Priory Avenue, Caversham, Reading RG4 7SE
Tel: 0118 947 2431 Fax: 0118 946 3340
Email: practice.reception@gp-k81054.nhs.uk
(Reading Primary Care Trust)
Patient List Size: 7500

Practice Manager Trish Selby

GP Jonathan Philip ROUT, Mahnaz ALI, Helen Mary Shingler GEORGE, Peter A McFARLANE

Russell Street Surgery

79 Russell Street, Reading RG1 7XG
Tel: 0118 959 2131 Fax: 0118 959 3112
(Reading Primary Care Trust)

Practice Manager Sandra Ashton

GP Manohar Lal SWAMI, Sadhana SWAMI

Russell Street Surgery

41 Russell Street, Reading RG1 7XD
Tel: 0118 957 3752 Fax: 0118 956 0381
(Reading Primary Care Trust)

Practice Manager Smita Nirgude

GP Subhashchandra Vasant NIRGUDE

Sonning Common Health Centre

Wood Lane, Sonning Common, Reading RG4 9SW
Tel: 0118 972 2188 Fax: 0118 972 4633
(South East Oxfordshire Primary Care Trust)

Practice Manager Glen Higgins

GP Andrew BURNETT, Ralph DRURY, Kim EMERSON, Evelyn O'CONNOR, Susan RONAY

Swallowfield Medical Practice

The Surgery, Swallowfield, Reading RG7 1QT
Tel: 0118 988 3134 Fax: 0118 988 5759
(Wokingham Primary Care Trust)

GP Graham David BUSFIELD, Helen Margaret Mary HEGARTY, Niall Jervis RIDDELL, Martin Daniel SMITH, David Richard Tudor THOMAS

Theale Medical Centre

Englefield Road, Theale, Reading RG7 5AS
Tel: 0118 930 2513 Fax: 0118 930 4419
(Reading Primary Care Trust)

Practice Manager David Davies

GP Robin Mathieson BORTHWICK, Sarah Judith Russell BROOKE, James Rawdon BYWATER, Clare Louise ROCK, Elizabeth Jeanne STONE, John Paul WINCHESTER

Tilehurst Surgery

Tylers Place, Pottery Road, Tilehurst, Reading RG30 6BW
Tel: 0118 942 7528 Fax: 0118 945 2405
Website: www.tilehurstsurgery.freeserve.co.uk
(Reading Primary Care Trust)
Patient List Size: 12500

Practice Manager Alan Wiseman

GP Abul Hazeque Mohammad Husnul KARIM, Ian BARROW, George Bushra BOULOS, Richard CROFT, Christopher Ross HOWLETT, Anna MAGNUSSON, Nikolas MARKERT, Joanne McCONNELL, Judith WESTON

Tilehurst Village Surgery

92 Westwood Road, Tilehurst, Reading RG31 5PP
Tel: 0118 945 2612
(Reading Primary Care Trust)

GP T UNDERWOOD

Twyford Surgery

Loddon Hall Road, Twyford, Reading RG10 9JA
Tel: 0118 934 6680 Fax: 0118 934 6690
(Wokingham Primary Care Trust)
Patient List Size: 10500

Practice Manager Theresa Date

GP Robert William Cecil COLLETT, John William CHISHOLM, Helen Susan CRAWLEY, Michael Glyn DAVIES, Vincent Alpe Mark GRANTHAM, Carol JAMES, Vivienne Margaret ROBERTS, S RUFFLE

University Health Centre

9 Northcourt Avenue, Reading RG2 7HE
Tel: 0118 987 4551
(Reading Primary Care Trust)

GP Peter P JOHNSON, Jillian BIRD, Judith Rosemary FELTON, Emma JARVIS, Elizabeth JOHNSTON, Bethan JONES, Irme RASHID, Robert Aidan Rodney SMITH

Wargrave Surgery

Victoria Road, Wargrave, Reading RG10 8BP
Tel: 0118 940 3939 Fax: 0118 940 1357
(Wokingham Primary Care Trust)
Patient List Size: 6500

Practice Manager Maria Goddard

GP Michael Daniel BOYLE, Mark Richard PUDDY, Sandra Elizabeth SWAN, Julia Sarah THURSTON

Western Elms Surgery

317 Oxford Road, Reading RG30 1AT
Tel: 0118 959 0257 Fax: 0118 959 7950
(Reading Primary Care Trust)
Patient List Size: 13900

Practice Manager Scott Trathen

GP Neil LATCHFORD, Lynette BERMINGHAM, John Haslett CONNOR, Penny CUNINGHAM, Jeff LUNT, Jonathan MILLAR, John NASH, Julie NEWSHAM, Geoff WILLIAMS

Westwood Road Practice

66 Westwood Road, Tilehurst, Reading RG31 5PR
Tel: 0118 942 7421 Fax: 0118 945 3537
(Reading Primary Care Trust)

GP Archana GARGAV

Whitley Villa Surgery

1 Christchurch Road, Reading RG2 7AB
Tel: 0118 986 0794 Fax: 0118 931 4046
(Reading Primary Care Trust)

Practice Manager M Kay

GP Sunil Kumar MODI, Kiran MODI, Kishore B NARAN

Whitley Wood Lane Surgery

96 Whitley Wood Lane, Reading RG2 8PP
Tel: 0118 987 6522 Fax: 0118 975 7067

(Reading Primary Care Trust)

GP Ashok Kumar GARGAV

Whitley Wood Road Practice
257 Whitley Wood Road, Whitley Wood, Reading RG2 8LE
Tel: 0118 975 3621 Fax: 0118 975 7065
(Reading Primary Care Trust)

GP Neena GROVER

Wilderness Road Surgery
1 Wilderness Road, Earley, Reading RG6 7RU
Tel: 0118 926 1613 Fax: 0118 926 3300
(Wokingham Primary Care Trust)

GP Rajinder Kumar CHADHA

Woodley Centre Surgery
106 Crockhamwell Road, Woodley, Reading RG5 3JY
Tel: 0118 969 5011 Fax: 0118 944 0382
(Wokingham Primary Care Trust)
Patient List Size: 8850

GP David John BUCKLE, Mary Gwyneth CRACKNELL, Rupa JOSHI, Gurpreet Singh KALRA, C J REEDER

Redcar

The Coatham Surgery
18 Coatham Road, Redcar TS10 1RJ
Tel: 01642 483495 Fax: 01642 759959
(Langbaurgh Primary Care Trust)
Patient List Size: 7713

GP Anthony John Hubert STOCKING, John Hill LYLE, Donna Rachel MOORE, Edward James SUMMERS

Dr Davidson and Partners
Redcar Health Centre, Coatham Road, Redcar TS10 1SX
Tel: 01642 475157 Fax: 01642 470885
Email: julia.speight@nhs.net
Website: www.healthcentre.uk.com
(Langbaurgh Primary Care Trust)
Patient List Size: 7600

Practice Manager Julia Speight

GP Robert Cameron DAVIDSON, Keith Michael BARKER, Julie COWSER

The Health Centre
Coatham Road, Redcar TS10 1SX
Tel: 01642 482647 Fax: 01642 489166
(Langbaurgh Primary Care Trust)
Patient List Size: 5762

Practice Manager Jean Somerset

GP James BENTLEY, B K LAL, Ali TAHMASSEBI

The Health Centre
Coatham Road, Redcar TS10 1SX
Tel: 01642 475222 Fax: 01642 477751
(Langbaurgh Primary Care Trust)
Patient List Size: 2208

GP Mohammed Anwarul ISLAM, Nigel ROBINSON

The Lagan Surgery
20 Kirkleatham Street, Redcar TS10 1TZ
Tel: 01642 488128 Fax: 01642 485063
(Langbaurgh Primary Care Trust)

GP Colin WILSON, Kim Caroline SUTCLIFFE

The Medical Centre
Hall Close, Marske-by-the-Sea, Redcar TS11 6BW
Tel: 01642 482725 Fax: 01642 483334
(Langbaurgh Primary Care Trust)

Practice Manager C Hurst

GP William Peter Francis MOORE, Gillian COLECLOUGH, J STURMAN, S C YATES

Park Avenue Surgery
13 Park Avenue, Redcar TS10 3LA
Tel: 01642 470692 Fax: 01642 480163
(Langbaurgh Primary Care Trust)

GP John Christopher DOHERTY

The Saltscar Surgery
22 Kirkleatham Street, Redcar TS10 1UA
Tel: 01642 484495/471388 Fax: 01642 488701
(Langbaurgh Primary Care Trust)
Patient List Size: 8300

Practice Manager Susan Bastiman

GP Ian Frederick JOHN, Derek Charlton INGLEDEW, William Joseph Dominic O'FLANAGAN, Roger SMITH

The Wynd Surgery
9 The Wynd, Marske-by-the-Sea, Redcar TS11 7LD
Tel: 01642 477133 Fax: 01642 475150
(Langbaurgh Primary Care Trust)
Patient List Size: 5200

Practice Manager Les Boyd

GP Kakkar MACHENDER, James GOSSON, Raj SAHA

Redditch

Bridge Surgery
8 Evesham Road, Redditch B97 4LA
Tel: 01527 550131 Fax: 01527 547074
(Redditch and Bromsgrove Primary Care Trust)
Patient List Size: 5450

Practice Manager S M Knowles

GP Norman Charles DAWES, Giovanni Antonio CARANCI, Tessa Susan Mary FRANKLIN

Church Hill Medical Centre
Tanhouse Lane, Church Hill, Redditch B98 9AA
Tel: 01527 591927 Fax: 01527 597679
(Redditch and Bromsgrove Primary Care Trust)
Patient List Size: 3550

Practice Manager Jackie Crossland

GP Javid Akther HAKEEM, Farooq AHMAD

Crabbs Cross Surgery
38 Kenilworth Close, Crabbs Cross, Redditch B97 5JX
Tel: 01527 544610 Fax: 01527 540286
Email: rachel.herring@gp-m81617.nhs.uk
(Redditch and Bromsgrove Primary Care Trust)
Patient List Size: 3250

Practice Manager Rachel Hemin

GP Zan THA, Patricia Agnes WONG

Dow Surgery
William Street, Redditch B97 4AJ
Tel: 01527 62285 Fax: 01527 596260
Email: dowsurgery@doctors.org.uk
(Redditch and Bromsgrove Primary Care Trust)
Patient List Size: 10200

Practice Manager Pauline Waddy

GP Susan Jane JENKINS, Helen Mary BOON, John James CASSIDY, Richard William DAVENPORT, John Duncan Campbell DOW, Darren HUDSON

Elgar House Surgery
Church Road, Redditch B97 4AB
Tel: 01527 69261 Fax: 01527 596856
(Redditch and Bromsgrove Primary Care Trust)

Practice Manager Dawn lane

GP Ronald Norman FORD, Gillian Ruth COOPER, Alastair Roger DIOR, Charles Mark JOHNSTONE, Shaun Hugo PIKE, Adrian John WILLIAMS

Hillview Medical Centre
60 Bromsgrove Road, Redditch B97 4RN
Tel: 01527 66511
(Redditch and Bromsgrove Primary Care Trust)
Patient List Size: 8500

Practice Manager Linda Pratt

GP Jonathan Joseph WELLS, E L GILES, Belinda Patricia KEOGH, Penelope Ruth LOCKE, William Joseph Samuel Thomas SHAW

The Medical Centre
39 Kenilworth Close, Crabbs Cross, Redditch B97 5JX
Tel: 01527 402149 Fax: 01527 540183
(Redditch and Bromsgrove Primary Care Trust)

Practice Manager Hilary Jordan

GP Mohamad Riaz HAQQANI

The Medical Centre
Tanhouse Lane, Church Hill, Redditch B98 9AA
Tel: 01527 67715
(Redditch and Bromsgrove Primary Care Trust)

Practice Manager S M Roberts

GP John David COCHRANE, Sylvia Irene Joyce CHANDLER, Catherine Helen McGREGOR

Ridgeway Surgery
6-8 Feckenham Road, Astwood Bank, Redditch B96 6DS
Tel: 01527 892418
(Redditch and Bromsgrove Primary Care Trust)

Practice Manager R Tobbell, R Tobbell

GP John Edward COWBURN, D H BLACKWELL, Inske B F SEYLER

Smallwood Health Centre
Church Green West, Redditch B97 4DJ
(Redditch and Bromsgrove Primary Care Trust)

GP Edwin Thomas MELLEY, T RUSSELL

St Stephens Surgery
Adelaide Street, Redditch B97 4AL
Tel: 01527 65444 Fax: 01527 69218
(Redditch and Bromsgrove Primary Care Trust)
Patient List Size: 10900

Practice Manager L Luke

GP Helena AMEY, Julia Felicity BROWN, Richard BURLING, Rosemarie BYRNES, Anil JOSHI, Simon John PARKINSON, Mark TALBOT

Winyates Health Centre
Winyates, Redditch B98 0NR
Tel: 01527 525274 Fax: 01527 517969
(Redditch and Bromsgrove Primary Care Trust)

Practice Manager Julie Ingram

GP Niall Patrick DOHERTY, Euripides William BORASTERO, Gillian CLARKE, Julian Warwick DAVEY, Jean Mary OUNSTED, Vattakkat PREMCHAND, Gillian Rachel PRYKE

Woodrow Medical Centre
Woodrow, Redditch B98 7RY
Tel: 01527 526824 Fax: 01527 501787
(Redditch and Bromsgrove Primary Care Trust)
Patient List Size: 3700

Practice Manager Julie Haresign

GP Sabarathnam ANANTHRAM, Urmila Ravjibhai AMIN

Redhill

Greyston House Surgery
99 Station Road, Redhill RH1 1EB
Tel: 01737 761201 Fax: 01737 780510
(East Surrey Primary Care Trust)
Patient List Size: 11500

Practice Manager Penny Binns

GP Mary Elana WATKINS, Penelope ARNOLD, David John ASLETT, Joseph McGILLIGAN, Phillipa PIPER, John Russell WILSON

The Hawthorns
1 Oxford Road, Redhill RH1 1DT
Tel: 01737 762902 Fax: 01737 762902
Email: valerie.gould@gp-h81055.nhs.uk
(East Surrey Primary Care Trust)
Patient List Size: 8700

GP Diana Louise Empain BULLOCK, Richard William ANSELL, John Cornelius DOYLE, Cathryn Sian McINTOSH, Jessica Claire RYDER

Homhurst Medical Centre
17 Hatchlands Road, Redhill RH1 6AA
Tel: 01737 766602/761614 Fax: 01737 780608
(East Surrey Primary Care Trust)
Patient List Size: 7350

Practice Manager Jeanette Beales

GP Marilyn Susan HIEATT, Jane Katherine HAMMOND, Caroline HART, Sharmila KAR, Rachel McGILLIGAN

The Moat House Surgery
Worsted Green, Merstham, Redhill RH1 3PN
Tel: 01737 642207 Fax: 01737 642209
(East Surrey Primary Care Trust)

GP Kalpita GORDGE, Victoria Anne HILDRETH, Christopher Alon HUGHES, Matthew Owen KING, Christopher H WARWICK, Alastair James WELLS

Woodlands Surgery
5 Woodlands Road, Redhill RH1 6EY
Tel: 01737 761343 Fax: 01737 770804
(East Surrey Primary Care Trust)

GP David Michael Bankes TOMPKIN, Dr ADAMS, Angela Elizabeth FERGUSON, Arthur James FERGUSON

Redruth

Clinton Road Surgery
19 Clinton Road, Redruth TR15 2LN
Tel: 01209 216507 Fax: 01209 218262
Email: joy.adamson@clintonroad.cornwall.nhs.uk
(West of Cornwall Primary Care Trust)
Patient List Size: 4390

Practice Manager Joy Adamson

GP Paula Marie HAYES, Deborah BUGG, Geraint Brierley HUGHES

Harris Memorial Surgery
Harris Memorial Surgery, Robartes Terrace, Illogan, Redruth TR16 4RX
Tel: 01209 842449 Fax: 01209 842380
Email: robert.boyce@harrismemorial.cornwall.nhs.uk
(West of Cornwall Primary Care Trust)
Patient List Size: 5171

Practice Manager Bob Boyce

GP Warren Adrian DAVIES, Ian Paris GETHIN, Simon R F KNOWLES

Homecroft Surgery
Voguebeloth, Illogan, Redruth TR16 4ET
Tel: 01209 843843 Fax: 01209 842027
Email: di.daniels@homecroft.cornwall.nhs.uk
(West of Cornwall Primary Care Trust)
Patient List Size: 6053

Practice Manager Di Daniels

GP Christopher William WILSON, Dr KINDER, David Neil PHILPOTT, Martin Charles SPITTLE, Evelyn Mary WELLER

Manor Surgery
Forth Noweth, Chapel Street, Redruth TR15 2BY
Tel: 01209 313313 Fax: 01209 313813
Email: mercedes.kelly-madden@manor.cornwall.nhs.uk
(West of Cornwall Primary Care Trust)

Patient List Size: 12455

Practice Manager Mercedes Kelly-Madden

GP John Edwin DAVIES, Clive Edward BLAKE, Andron Lesile CRAZE, Tamsin Mary CRAZE, Thomas Charles EDMUNDS, John Stuart FOSTER, Timothy Alexander ROGERS

Pool Health Centre

Station Road, Pool, Redruth TR15 3DU
Tel: 01209 717471 Fax: 01209 612160
Email: stephen.holby@pool.cornwall.nhs.uk
(West of Cornwall Primary Care Trust)
Patient List Size: 9996

Practice Manager Stephen Holby

GP Rowland JOSEPH, Timothy John Stuart BAKER, Mark DANIELSEN, Helen Miriam JONES, Peter Benjamin Turnley JONES, Philip Roy TREVAIL

Reigate

South Park Surgery

42A Prices Lane, Reigate RH2 8AX
Tel: 01737 240022 Fax: 01737 244660
(East Surrey Primary Care Trust)

Practice Manager Susan Meyer

The Wall House Surgery

Yorke Road, Reigate RH2 9HG
Tel: 01737 224432 Fax: 01737 244616
(East Surrey Primary Care Trust)

Practice Manager John Chambers

GP Paul LAMBOURNE, Keith BARROW, Deanna Christine JENNINGS, Patrick David KERR

Retford

Bridgegate Surgery

43 Bridgegate, Retford DN22 7UX
Tel: 01777 702381 Fax: 01777 711880
(Bassetlaw Primary Care Trust)
Patient List Size: 7200

Practice Manager Jane Beattie

GP Albertus Antony WEENINK, Joel Edward CHAPMAN, Louise Sandra DALE, Claire Magdalene HURREN, Helen Mary SCOTT

Crown House Surgery

Chapelgate, Retford DN22 6NX
Tel: 01777 703672 Fax: 01777 710534
(Bassetlaw Primary Care Trust)

Practice Manager A Milne

GP Phillip FOSTER, Adrian Robert ANDERSON, Gary CHERRILL, M GIMENEZ-BURGOS, Clive Henry PEARSON, Julian ROBERTS, John Reginald SKEAVINGTON

Riverside Health Centre

Riverside Walk, Retford DN22 6AA
Tel: 01777 706661 Fax: 01777 711966
(Bassetlaw Primary Care Trust)
Patient List Size: 6250

Practice Manager Anne Clark, Gillian Wainwright

GP John TONGE, Paul Richard John HARDMAN, M T H HO, Elizabeth ROBERTS

The Surgery

Sturton Road, North Leverton, Retford DN22 0AB
Tel: 01427 880223 Fax: 01427 880927
Email: northlowertonsurgery@gp-C84692.nhs.uk
(Bassetlaw Primary Care Trust)
Patient List Size: 2500

Practice Manager Peter Nixon

GP G M BROWNSON

Tall Trees Surgery

Rectory Road, Retford DN22 7AY
Tel: 01777 701637 Fax: 01777 710619
(Bassetlaw Primary Care Trust)
Patient List Size: 5770

Practice Manager P Bacon

GP Richard Lingard BROWN, Ivan John GILBERT, David Henry JARVIS

Richmond, North Yorkshire

Bridge House Surgery

Aldbrough St. John, Richmond DL11 7SU
Tel: 01325 374332 Fax: 01325 374063
(Hambleton and Richmondshire Primary Care Trust)

Practice Manager Anne Roberts

GP Mark David HODGSON, Michael KEAVNEY

Catterick Garrison Medical Centre

Horne Road, Catterick Garrison, Richmond DL9 4DF
Tel: 01748 832521 Fax: 01748 873132
(Hambleton and Richmondshire Primary Care Trust)

Practice Manager Eileen Harkness

GP P N GILLESPIE

Friary Surgery

Queens Road, Richmond DL10 4UJ
Tel: 01748 822306 Fax: 01748 850356
(Hambleton and Richmondshire Primary Care Trust)

Practice Manager D C Robinson

GP R C GIBSON, Alistair Graham PATERSON, Timothy PEARSON

The Health Centre

High Street, Catterick Village, Richmond DL10 7LD
Tel: 01748 811475 Fax: 01748 818284
(Hambleton and Richmondshire Primary Care Trust)
Patient List Size: 5711

Practice Manager Glenn Carroll

GP Thomas William Eric TROUGHTON, Andrew Luke CHALLIS, Christopher David WEBB

The Quakers Lane Surgery

Quakers Lane, Richmond DL10 4BB
Tel: 01748 850440 Fax: 01748 850802
(Hambleton and Richmondshire Primary Care Trust)

Practice Manager J Woodkock

GP Anthony David GINNS, Paul Thomas KIPLING, Timothy MAWER, J A MOON

Reeth Surgery

Reeth, Richmond DL11 6SU
Tel: 01748 884396 Fax: 01748 884250
Email: paul.bond@gp-b82622.nhs.uk
(Hambleton and Richmondshire Primary Care Trust)
Patient List Size: 1536

Practice Manager Kathleen Harker

GP Paul Robert BOND

Scorton Surgery

High Row, Scorton, Richmond DL10 6QD
Tel: 01748 811320 Fax: 01748 812004
(Hambleton and Richmondshire Primary Care Trust)

Practice Manager Kathy Bellas

GP Nigel Stuart Parker ENEVOLDSON, John Howard MOUNTJOY

Richmond, Surrey

Cooper

Queens Medical Centre, 109 Queens Road, Richmond TW10 6HF
Tel: 020 8255 1144 Fax: 020 8255 0300

(Richmond and Twickenham Primary Care Trust)
Patient List Size: 3000

Practice Manager Lee Dolan

GP Joseph Emery COOPER

Kew Gardens Surgery
1 Kew Gardens Road, Kew, Richmond TW9 3HN
Tel: 020 8940 1048/1812 Fax: 020 8332 7644
(Richmond and Twickenham Primary Care Trust)
Patient List Size: 3679

Practice Manager Samantha Lawrence

GP John David LAWRENCE

Kew Medical Practice
14 High Park Road, Kew, Richmond TW9 4BH
Tel: 020 8487 8292 Fax: 020 8878 9621
(Richmond and Twickenham Primary Care Trust)
Patient List Size: 1291

Practice Manager Frank Fitzmaurice

GP Moj FITZMAURICE, Diane MILLAR, Siegfried TREVZER

North Road Surgery
77 North Road, Richmond TW9 4HQ
Tel: 020 8876 4442 Fax: 020 8392 2311
(Richmond and Twickenham Primary Care Trust)
Patient List Size: 4850

Practice Manager H Harrison

GP Joanna Mary CROWLEY, Warwick BEALES, Alexandra STRACHAN

Paradise Road Practice
37 Paradise Road, Richmond TW9 1SA
Tel: 020 8940 2423 Fax: 020 8332 6363
(Richmond and Twickenham Primary Care Trust)
Patient List Size: 4000

Practice Manager Susan Gates

GP William Edward GRIFFITHS

Queens Medical Centre
109 Queens Road, Richmond TW10 6HF
Tel: 020 8255 1144 Fax: 020 8255 0300
(Richmond and Twickenham Primary Care Trust)

Practice Manager Lee Dolan

GP J E COOPER, Samara LEWIS, P J HUGHES

Richmond Green Medical Centre
19 The Green, Richmond TW9 1PX
Tel: 020 8332 7515 Fax: 020 8332 0026
(Richmond and Twickenham Primary Care Trust)
Patient List Size: 2000

Practice Manager Miguele Bocti

GP Antoine SAYER

Seymour House Surgery
154 Sheen Road, Richmond TW9 1UU
Tel: 020 8940 2802 Fax: 020 8332 7877
(Richmond and Twickenham Primary Care Trust)
Patient List Size: 13500

Practice Manager Gill Russell

GP Justin Wynne BLAKE JAMES, Maria Helena GAWLINSKA, Patrick Timothy Pilkington HUDSON, A M KAYZAKIAN, K J MACKIE, A NAVAMANI

The Surgery
36 Pagoda Avenue, Richmond TW9 2HG
Tel: 020 8948 4217 Fax: 020 8332 7639
(Richmond and Twickenham Primary Care Trust)

Practice Manager Cherry Coote

GP Frances Mary BATES, Nicholas Clive Greenwood JACKMAN, Alan STARCK

The Vineyard Surgery
35 The Vineyard, Richmond TW10 6PP
Tel: 020 8948 0404 Fax: 020 8332 7598
(Richmond and Twickenham Primary Care Trust)
Patient List Size: 4178

Practice Manager Lynne Price

GP Garth Arnold Rajachandra EZEKIEL, Lourenco Jose Rosario DA COSTA

Rickmansworth

Baldwins Lane Surgery
266 Baldwins Lane, Croxley Green, Rickmansworth WD3 3LG
Tel: 01923 774732 Fax: 01923 711933
(Watford and Three Rivers Primary Care Trust)
Patient List Size: 4400

Practice Manager T Fletcher

GP Ian David FLUDE, Monique AURORA, Claire DYER, Pauline HERNANDEZ

Chorleywood Health Centre
15 Lower Road, Chorleywood, Rickmansworth WD3 5EA
Tel: 01923 287100 Fax: 01923 287120
(Watford and Three Rivers Primary Care Trust)
Patient List Size: 5448

GP Russell Wynn JONES, Sadwana KULKARNI, Edin LAKASING

Colne House Surgery
99A Uxbridge Road, Rickmansworth WD3 7DJ
Tel: 01923 776295 Fax: 01923 777744
(Watford and Three Rivers Primary Care Trust)

Practice Manager J A Fraser

GP Jeffrey Neil ZANE, Nicholas Edward FOREMAN, Malcolm Robert GOLIN, Sukhjit SANGHA, Alena Charlotta Konstancie SAVANI, Narendra SAVANI

Gade House Surgery
99B Uxbridge Road, Rickmansworth WD3 7DJ
Tel: 01923 775291 Fax: 01923 711790
(Watford and Three Rivers Primary Care Trust)
Patient List Size: 11950

Practice Manager Mandy Carr

GP Frederick BENNETT, Timothy Peter AIREY, William James HINTON, Deborah KEMP, Annette Patricia SLADE, Rosemary TOY

The Surgery
166 New Road, Croxley Green, Rickmansworth WD3 3HD
Tel: 01923 778277
(Watford and Three Rivers Primary Care Trust)

Practice Manager Peter Lilywhite

GP Nigel CORP, Kevin BARRETT, Claire Jan CHESWORTH, Andrew John LARKWORTHY

Ringwood

Cornerways Medical Centre
Parkers Close, Gorley Road, Poulner, Ringwood BH24 1SD
Tel: 01425 472515 Fax: 01425 470030
Email: cornerways.surgery@gp-J82150.nhs.uk
(New Forest Primary Care Trust)
Patient List Size: 10500

Practice Manager John Wyatt

GP Gregory Douglas ANSELL, S BALDRY, Yvonne Louise DENMAN, Robert John GEMMELL, J H A JONES, T J KNIGHT, C H SHAW

Ringwood Health Centre
The Close, Ringwood BH24 1JY
Tel: 01425 478901 Fax: 01425 478239
(New Forest Primary Care Trust)

Practice Manager Steve Antill

GP David Chester Cranmer HUGHES, Timothy William Owen BRIGSTOCKE, Maria Teresa Ann CARY, Fiona Helen McKAY, Nigel Boyd SHIELD, Simon Patrick THOMPSON

Ripley

Ivy Grove Surgery
1 Ivy Grove, Ripley DE5 3HN
Tel: 0845 456 7789 Fax: 01773 749812
(Amber Valley Primary Care Trust)

Practice Manager Charmagne Stephenson

GP Dr HORTON, Martin David JONES, Sheila Mary NEWPORT, Michael Stuart SMALL, Michael WONG, Anthony Richard WORDLEY

Ripley Medical Centre
Derby Road, Ripley DE5 3HR
Tel: 01773 742170/747486 Fax: 01773 513470
(Amber Valley Primary Care Trust)

Practice Manager Jackie Dowler

GP A HORSFIELD, Sarah Louise MILNER, David William TAYLOR, I R TOOLEY

Ripon

Ashfield House Surgery
Main Street, Kirkby Malzeard, Ripon HG4 3SE
Tel: 01765 658298 Fax: 01765 658846
(Craven, Harrogate and Rural District Primary Care Trust)
Patient List Size: 5200

Practice Manager G R Hyde

GP Michael HARFORD-CROSS, Helen Alexandra AKESTER, Elizabeth Shelagh HARFORD-CROSS, Roger Heyworth HIGSON

The Mechanics Institute Surgery
Main Street, Kirkby Malzeard, Ripon HG4 3QL
(Craven, Harrogate and Rural District Primary Care Trust)

Practice Manager Kathleen Swan

GP Angus Muir LIVINGSTONE, Hilary Vivien BURTON

North House Surgery
28 North Street, Ripon HG4 1HL
Tel: 01765 690666 Fax: 01765 690249
(Craven, Harrogate and Rural District Primary Care Trust)
Patient List Size: 8785

Practice Manager Jane Baldwin

GP Christopher Julian BENNETT, Graham Richard ABBOTT, Stephen Paul GRANDISON, Derek JEARY, Morag Shelagh McDOWALL, Sarah Louise MOSS

Park Street Practice
Park Street, Ripon HG4 2BE
Tel: 01765 692366 Fax: 01765 606440
(Craven, Harrogate and Rural District Primary Care Trust)
Patient List Size: 7001

Practice Manager Carolyn Paterson

GP Angus Muir LIVINGSTONE, Hilary Vivien BURTON, Patricia Rosemary LIVINGSTONE, Clyde Bernard WEBB

The Surgery
7-8 Park Street, Ripon HG4 2AX
Tel: 01765 692337 Fax: 01765 601757
(Craven, Harrogate and Rural District Primary Care Trust)

Practice Manager Robert Gammon

GP Penelope Jane Lesley DICKSON, Charles Henry FLETCHER, Joy Valerie FLETCHER, Alistair James INGRAM

Robertsbridge

Oldwood Surgery
Station Road, Robertsbridge TN32 5DG
Tel: 01580 880790 Fax: 01580 882192
(Bexhill and Rother Primary Care Trust)

Practice Manager Pamela Golding

GP Elizabeth Mary ELLIOT-PYLE, L PARKER

Rochdale

Ashworth Street Surgery
85 Spotland Road, Rochdale OL12 6RT
Tel: 01706 346767 Fax: 01706 346800
(Rochdale Primary Care Trust)
Patient List Size: 9700

Practice Manager Pauline Mayor

GP John Stephen DOYLE, Shalini Vinod GADIYAR, David Jeffrey HUDSON, Jenny Jane NELSON, David Carl OSBORNE, Hazel Florence Mary PLATTS

Baillie Street Health Centre
Baillie Street, Rochdale OL16 1XS
Tel: 01706 525384 Fax: 01706 861625
(Rochdale Primary Care Trust)
Patient List Size: 4500

Practice Manager Rachael Chambers

GP M B GHAFOOR, Abdul SAEED

Baillie Street Health Centre
Baillie Street, Rochdale OL16 1XS
Tel: 01706 525322 Fax: 01706 713246
(Rochdale Primary Care Trust)
Patient List Size: 5500

Practice Manager Janet Perkins

GP I K BABAR, F KHAN, K MAHMOOD, S K MORIJAWALA

Bulwer Street Surgery
1-3 Bulwer Street, Rochdale OL16 2EU
(Rochdale Primary Care Trust)

GP Purnendu Kumar SEN

Castleton Health Centre
2 Elizabeth Street, Castleton, Rochdale OL11 3HY
Tel: 01706 658905 Fax: 01706 343990
(Rochdale Primary Care Trust)

Practice Manager Janet Grant

GP Alvin BODNER, Barry LEWIS, Parmjit Singh MAMMAN, Timothy Simon PLATTS, Elizabeth Vanda Mary TUTTON

Dawes Family Practice
83 Spotland Road, Rochdale OL12 6RX
Tel: 01706 644040 Fax: 01706 750808
(Rochdale Primary Care Trust)
Patient List Size: 6000

Practice Manager Margaret Swann

GP S BABBS, N J DAWES, S A DAWES, E GREENWOOD, C LAL

Drake Street Surgery
134 Drake Street, Rochdale OL16 1PS
(Rochdale Primary Care Trust)

GP Deborah Mary DENCH

East Street Surgery
1 East Street, Rochdale OL16 2EG
Tel: 01706 639002 Fax: 01706 713256
(Rochdale Primary Care Trust)

Practice Manager Kalsum Ahmed

GP Sukanti TARAPHDAR, Niranjan GHOSH

Edenfield Road Surgery
Cutgate Shopping Precinct, Edenfield Road, Rochdale OL11 5AQ
Tel: 01706 344044 Fax: 01706 526882
Email: janie.priestley@edenfieldsurgery.nhs.uk
(Rochdale Primary Care Trust)

GP Richard Henry VERITY, Martin DRANSFIELD, Sarah JONES, Darren John MANSFIELD, Alexander Roberts Telfer McFARLANE, Simon Mitchell RHODES, Ann Elizabeth THRELFALL

Healey Surgery
Whitworth Road, Rochdale OL12 0SN
(Rochdale Primary Care Trust)
Patient List Size: 7000

Practice Manager Carole Hand

GP Abdul RAUF, M. HUSSAIN, B KAFLE, A VAN DEN BOS

Milnrow Health Centre
21 Stonefield Street, Milnrow, Rochdale OL16 4HZ
Tel: 01706 527752 Fax: 01706 713221
(Rochdale Primary Care Trust)
Patient List Size: 1850

GP B K CHAKRABARTI

Milnrow Village Practice
44-48 Newhey Road, Milnrow, Rochdale OL16 4EG
(Rochdale Primary Care Trust)

GP Andrew Christopher GUNN, Jane KEIGHLEY, Surendra Balwantray THAKOR

Oldham Road Surgery
244-246 Oldham Road, Rochdale OL11 2ER
Tel: 01706 356464 Fax: 01706 713253
(Rochdale Primary Care Trust)
Patient List Size: 2300

Practice Manager S Asif

GP H B SYED

Stonefield Street Surgery
21 Stonefield Street, Milnrow, Rochdale OL16 4JQ
Tel: 01706 46234 Fax: 01706 527946
(Rochdale Primary Care Trust)
Patient List Size: 8300

Practice Manager Irene Longhurst

GP Stephen Philip ROTHERY, Lynn Alison HAMPSON, Andrew John PENROSE, Jennifer Anne RANSOME

The Strand Medical Centre
The Strand, Kirkholt, Rochdale OL11 2JG
(Heywood and Middleton Primary Care Trust)

GP Gowri Narayana SWAMY

The Surgery
2 Mark Street, Rochdale OL12 9BE
Tel: 01706 43183 Fax: 01706 526640
(Rochdale Primary Care Trust)
Patient List Size: 9800

Practice Manager Lesley Tickle

GP Peter Crawford Banks FORMAN, Jennifer Anne BIRKETT, Andrew Brian PARTON, Jacqueline Ann ROSE

Triple H PMS Pilot
175-177 Yorkshire Street, Rochdale OL12 0DR
Tel: 01706 708120 Fax: 01706 708 123
(Rochdale Primary Care Trust)
Patient List Size: 320

GP W ASHWORTH

Tweedale Street Surgery
65 Tweedale Street, Rochdale OL11 1HH
(Rochdale Primary Care Trust)

GP J V RANE

Vicars Drive Surgery
1 Vicars Drive, Rochdale OL16 1UR
Tel: 01706 643189 Fax: 01706 711617
(Rochdale Primary Care Trust)
Patient List Size: 2010

Practice Manager Maureen Smith

GP George Wilfred Dedan BHIMA

Wellfield Surgery
291 Oldham Road, Rochdale OL16 5HX
Tel: 01706 355111
(Rochdale Primary Care Trust)

Practice Manager Alison Flannery

GP Anthony James CROOK, Barry Martin CALDWELL, Stephen Anthony CROOK, James Ernest HORROCKS, Maria Antoinette O'REILLY, Anthony Royston STONE, Susan Elisabeth TRAVIS

Yorkshire Street Surgery
190 Yorkshire Street, Rochdale OL16 2DN
Tel: 01706 644973/5
(Rochdale Primary Care Trust)
Patient List Size: 6300

Practice Manager Diane Nelson

GP Alan Stuart EASTWOOD, Peter Eugene JONES, Vincent Martin Christopher MEAGHER

Rochester

City Way Surgery
67 City Way, Rochester ME1 2AY
Tel: 01634 843351 Fax: 01634 830421
Email: practice.manager@gp-g82051.nhs.uk
(Medway Teaching Primary Care Trust)
Patient List Size: 9700

Practice Manager D M R Ashby

GP Shahab SYED, Timothy Simon COLBERT, Mohan KAKADE, Glen MARTIN, Abd El Azim Abd El Monem OSMAN

Court View Surgery
2A Darnley Road, Strood, Rochester ME2 2HA
Tel: 01634 290333 Fax: 01634 295131
(Medway Teaching Primary Care Trust)
Patient List Size: 8100

GP Arthur Paul BOARD, Graham Robert Sinclair DOLMAN, Jane Kathryn LONSDALE, Julian Thomas William SPINKS

The Elms Medical Centre
Tilley Close, Main Road, Hoo, Rochester ME3 9AE
Tel: 01634 250142 Fax: 01634 255029
(Medway Teaching Primary Care Trust)

GP Kim Wah LEE, Jasminder Singh BIRDI, Helen Kit-Man MARA, John David WOODFIELD

Halling Medical Centre
Ferry Road, Halling, Rochester ME2 1NP
Tel: 01634 240238
(Medway Teaching Primary Care Trust)

Practice Manager N.M.K. Malradi

GP Vyakaranam Padmavathi RAO, Malladi Ravindranatha SASTRY

The Health Centre
Delce Road, Rochester ME1 2EL
Tel: 01634 401111
(Medway Teaching Primary Care Trust)
Patient List Size: 2100

GP N ELAPATHA

Hoo St Werburgh Practice
98 Bells Lane, Hoo Street, Werburgh, Rochester ME3 9HU
Tel: 01634 250523 Fax: 01634 255272
(Medway Teaching Primary Care Trust)

Patient List Size: 10000

GP G C J DAVIES, Geraldine McKEEVER, D O'DONNELL, D O'KANE

Marlowe Park Medical Centre
Wells Road, Strood, Rochester ME2 2PW
Tel: 01634 719692
(Medway Teaching Primary Care Trust)

GP Joseph Vincent BROPHY

The Medical Centre
Gun Lane, Strood, Rochester ME2 4UW
Tel: 01634 726555 Fax: 01634 296404
(Medway Teaching Primary Care Trust)
Patient List Size: 2100

Practice Manager P Linehan

GP Vasantika AGARWAL

The Medical Centre
Gun Lane, Strood, Rochester ME2 4UW
Tel: 01634 290644
(Medway Teaching Primary Care Trust)

Practice Manager Linda Markwell

GP Mohd Anwar SIDDIQI

The Medical Centre
Gun Lane, Strood, Rochester ME2 4UW
Tel: 01634 720220
(Medway Teaching Primary Care Trust)

GP Don Walwin Somasiri MUNASINGHE, Robolge Vijayalakshmi PREMARATNE

The Medical Centre
Gun Lane, Strood, Rochester ME2 4UW
Tel: 01634 727888
(Medway Teaching Primary Care Trust)
Patient List Size: 1560

GP Jyoti Narayan RAY

The Medical Centre
Gun Lane, Strood, Rochester ME2 4UW
Tel: 01634 290655 Fax: 01634 296404
(Medway Teaching Primary Care Trust)
Patient List Size: 1968

GP Peter Sean STORY

The Medical Centre
Gun Lane, Strood, Rochester ME2 4UW
Tel: 01634 720722
(Medway Teaching Primary Care Trust)

GP N MYO

Phoenix Surgery
33 Bell Lane, Burham, Rochester ME1 3SX
Tel: 01634 367982 Fax: 01634 864513
(Maidstone Weald Primary Care Trust)
Patient List Size: 2800

Practice Manager R J Langridge

GP Nicholas Richard PILE, Trudy Ann FITZWATER

Rochester Health Centre
Delce Road, Rochester ME1 2EL
Tel: 01634 401111
(Medway Teaching Primary Care Trust)

GP Amarjit Singh DHINDSA

Rochester Health Centre
Delce Road, Rochester ME1 2EL
Tel: 01634 401111
(Medway Teaching Primary Care Trust)

GP Sneh Lata TANDON

St Mary's Medical Centre
Vicarage Road, Strood, Rochester ME2 4DG
Tel: 01634 291299/291266 Fax: 01634 295752
(Medway Teaching Primary Care Trust)
Patient List Size: 8400

Practice Manager Julie Allen

GP Brian Rawdon BANNAR-MARTIN, John David CLARKE, Festus OJAGBEMI

The Surgery
1 The Esplanade, Rochester ME1 1QE
Tel: 01634 843142
(Medway Teaching Primary Care Trust)
Patient List Size: 200

GP James Houston REDMAN

The Surgery
25 Wouldham Road, Borstal, Rochester ME1 3JY
Tel: 01634 408765
(Medway Teaching Primary Care Trust)

GP Chidambaram Sundram BALACHANDER, Yin YAU

The Surgery
The Parks Medical Practice, Miller Way, Wainscott, Rochester ME2 4LP
Tel: 01634 717450 Fax: 01634 716300
(Medway Teaching Primary Care Trust)

GP Peter Huw GREEN, Clare HAWARDEN, Rosemary Christine LOFTUS, Reza MEHR-GHERBANI, Anne Karen WHEELER

The Thorndike Centre
Longley Road, Rochester ME1 2TH
Tel: 01634 817217
(Medway Teaching Primary Care Trust)

GP Jashpal Singh TANDAY, Thu Anh BUI, Gillian FARGHER, Peter Huw GILBERT, Francis Alexander YEATES

Rochford

Ashingdon Medical Centre
57 Lascelles Gardens, Ashingdon, Rochford SS4 3BW
Tel: 01702 544959 Fax: 01702 530160
(Castle Point and Rochford Primary Care Trust)
Patient List Size: 3400

Practice Manager Valerie Wallis

GP Bupinder SINGH

Rochford Surgery
1 Leecon Way, Ashingdon Gardens, Rochford SS4 1TU
Tel: 01702 547828 Fax: 01702 530139
(Castle Point and Rochford Primary Care Trust)
Patient List Size: 3400

Practice Manager D Morgan

GP A K SEN, D AGGARWAL

Southwell House Surgery
Southwell House, Back Lane, Rochford SS4 1AY
Tel: 01702 545241 Fax: 01702 546390
(Castle Point and Rochford Primary Care Trust)
Patient List Size: 13200

Practice Manager Tim Curtis

GP Angela Jane PUZEY, Jose BAJEN, Imigo BLASCO, Chanda KOTHARI, Deepak NANDA

Romford

Annie Prendergash Health Centre
Ashton Gardens, Romford RM6 6RT
Tel: 020 8590 1461 Fax: 020 8597 7819
(Havering Primary Care Trust)

Practice Manager P Snelling

GP James Andrew HAMILTON-SMITH, Vijaychandra Jashbhai PATEL

Annie Prendergast Health Centre
Ashton Gardens, Chadwell Heath, Romford RM6 6RT
Tel: 020 8590 1401 Fax: 020 8590 1350
(Havering Primary Care Trust)

Practice Manager C Hart, M Wells

GP Aarron Neil PATEL, Ruth Shahami PATEL

Annie Prendergast Health Centre
Ashton Gardens, Chadwell Heath, Romford RM6 6RT
Tel: 020 8599 8499 Fax: 020 8599 9314
(Havering Primary Care Trust)

Practice Manager J Innes

GP S J HASKELL

Chadwell Heath Surgery
72 Chadwell Heath Lane, Chadwell Heath, Romford RM6 4AF
Tel: 020 8590 2800 Fax: 020 8599 1454
(Havering Primary Care Trust)
Patient List Size: 7000

GP Dhirendra KANA

Chase Cross Medical Centre
13-15 Chase Cross Road, Collier Row, Romford RM5 3PJ
Tel: 01708 749918 Fax: 01708 742692
(Havering Primary Care Trust)
Patient List Size: 2500

Practice Manager Joyce Watson

GP S KULENDRUN

Collier Row Lane Surgery
250 Collier Row Lane, Romford RM5 3NJ
Tel: 01708 764991 Fax: 01708 722377
(Havering Primary Care Trust)

Practice Manager Mary Ladner

GP P A JOSEPH

Collier Row Lane Surgery
36 Collier Row Lane, Collier Row, Romford RM5 3BJ
Tel: 01708 741510 Fax: 01708 742328
(Havering Primary Care Trust)
Patient List Size: 4000

Practice Manager Alison Lipman

GP M MAHMOOD, V KUHAN

Gubbins Lane Surgery
89 Gubbins Lane, Harold Wood, Romford RM3 0DR
Tel: 01708 346666 Fax: 01708 381300
(Havering Primary Care Trust)

GP Donald Christopher ACHESON, John LEE, A R McDONALD, Henry Francis McDONALD, Kuldeep MINOCHA, Samuel Raymond ZACHARIAH

Harold Hill Centre
Gooshays Drive, Romford RM3 9SU
Tel: 01708 341188 Fax: 01708 346784
(Havering Primary Care Trust)
Patient List Size: 2129

Practice Manager R Jabbar

GP A JABBAR

Harold Hill Health Centre
Gooshays Drive, Romford RM3 9SU
Tel: 01708 343991 Fax: 01708 346795
(Havering Primary Care Trust)
Patient List Size: 7000

Practice Manager Angela Keeley

GP Nazir Ahmad KUCHHAI, Behnam Saeed SAHEECHA

Harold Hill Health Centre
Gooshays Drive, Romford RM3 9SU
Tel: 01708 341188 Fax: 01708 346784
(Havering Primary Care Trust)

GP Abdul JABBAR

Ingrebourne Medical Centre
135 Straight Road, Harold Hill, Romford RM3 7JJ
Tel: 01708 372021 Fax: 01708 378161
(Havering Primary Care Trust)
Patient List Size: 2900

Practice Manager Pauline Trinder

GP Manzur AHMAD, Fahima Bano Shamima AHMAD

Lynwood Medical Centre
Lynwood Drive, 4 Collier Row, Romford RM5 3QL
Tel: 01708 743244 Fax: 01708 736783
(Havering Primary Care Trust)
Patient List Size: 10200

Practice Manager Mrs Grimmet

GP Harshadrao Dahyabhai PATEL, Sanjit PALIT, Lata Manojkumar PATEL, Gurdev Singh SAINI, Manisha SIRCAR

Marks Gate Health Centre
Lawn Farm Grove, Chadwell Heath, Romford RM6 5LL
Tel: 020 8590 7066 Fax: 020 8597 0313
(Havering Primary Care Trust)
Patient List Size: 2700

Practice Manager S Kashyap

GP Kuldip Prasad KASHYAP

Mawney Medical Centre
34 Mawney Road, Romford RM7 7HD
Tel: 01708 743627 Fax: 01708 738244
Email: mawneymed@aol.com
(Havering Primary Care Trust)
Patient List Size: 10000

Practice Manager Valerie Kaleda

GP Smita Hasmukh PATEL, Asha DARMASSEELANE, David Martin HAMILTON, Mohammed Nazmul HOSSAIN, Dr SHAH

Mawney Road Surgery
206 Mawney Road, Romford RM7 8BU
Tel: 01708 739379 Fax: 01708 780457
(Havering Primary Care Trust)
Patient List Size: 3000

Practice Manager Pramila Gupta

GP Nagendra Kumar GUPTA

Mill Lane Surgery
135 Mill Lane, Chadwell Heath, Romford RM6 6RS
Tel: 020 8599 6835
(Barking and Dagenham Primary Care Trust)
Patient List Size: 3800

Practice Manager S Teotia

GP Narendra Pal Singh TEOTIA

Modern Medical Centre
195 Rush Green Road, Romford RM7 0PX
Tel: 01708 741872 Fax: 01708 722103
(Havering Primary Care Trust)
Patient List Size: 3360

Practice Manager F Davey

GP P KUKATHASAN

New Medical Centre
264 Brentwood Road, Romford RM2 5SU
Tel: 01708 478800 Fax: 01708 471422
(Havering Primary Care Trust)
Patient List Size: 10000

Practice Manager Teresa Mayer

GP Mini Mary EDISON, Lanre Caroline AKWENUICE, Lanre Caroline AKWENUKE, Ayodele Olusegun OLA

North Street Medical Centre
274 North Street, Romford RM1 4QJ
Tel: 01708 764477 Fax: 01708 757656/757712
(Havering Primary Care Trust)
Patient List Size: 12600

Practice Manager L Turner

GP Eric Martin SAUNDERSON, Robert John BEDDOE, Richard Jonathan BURACK, Kazimierz FUKS, Stephen John NEWELL, Helen Rose Mary PURDIE

Oak Lodge Medical Centre
Oak Lodge, 6 Oak Road, Harold Wood, Romford RM3 0PT
Tel: 01708 342139
(Havering Primary Care Trust)

GP Rana Surajit CHOWDHURY

Padnall Road Surgery
48 Padnall Road, Marks Gate, Chadwell Heath, Romford RM6 5BJ
Tel: 020 8599 0735
(Barking and Dagenham Primary Care Trust)

GP Kishor Jechand MEHTA

Petersfield Surgery
70 Petersfield Avenue, Harold Hill, Romford RM3 9PD
Tel: 01708 343113 Fax: 01708 384672
Website: www.petersfield@msn.com
(Havering Primary Care Trust)
Patient List Size: 8000

GP Mark Roslyn FELDMAN, Philippa Margaret FELDMAN, Ketheeswary RABINDRA-ANANDH, Paul SHARMA, Olujimi SOLANKE

Roles Grove Surgery
Panacea House, 18 Roles Grove, Marks Gate, Romford RM6 5LT
Tel: 020 8590 4030 Fax: 020 8597 1727
Email: mohamed.ali@gp-F82629.nhs.uk
(Havering Primary Care Trust)
Patient List Size: 2000

Practice Manager Teresa Harris

GP Muhammad Matleb ALI

Rush Green Medical Centre
Dr Poolo's Surgery, 261 Dagenham Road, Romford RM7 0XR
Tel: 01708 740730 Fax: 01708 725388
(Havering Primary Care Trust)
Patient List Size: 2600

Practice Manager J Ward

GP Saravanamuthu POOLOGANATHAN, Parameswari POOLOGANATHAN

Rush Green Medical Centre
261 Dagenham Road, Romford RM7 0XR
Tel: 01708 728261 Fax: 01708 722645
(Havering Primary Care Trust)

Practice Manager Mary Manson

GP Madhu Lata PATHAK, Badiullah BEHESHTI, M SANOMI

The Surgery
107 Brentwood Road, Romford RM1 2SH
Tel: 01708 740244 Fax: 01708 740272
(Havering Primary Care Trust)

Practice Manager Jane ward

GP Colin Timothy Cyril MARKS

The Surgery
137 Straight Road, Harold Hill, Romford RM3 7JJ
Tel: 01708 343281 Fax: 01708 345386
(Havering Primary Care Trust)

Practice Manager Sandra Jepson

GP Jwala PRASAD

The Surgery
Gidea Park, Romford RM2 6PS
Tel: 01708 740660 Fax: 01708 722632
(Havering Primary Care Trust)

Practice Manager M Aye

GP Prem Nath SATSANGI, A O OLA

The Surgery
37 Ongar Road, Abridge, Romford RM4 1UD
Tel: 01992 761387 Fax: 01992 716163
(Epping Forest Primary Care Trust)
Patient List Size: 3942

Practice Manager Jane Witham

GP Robert CHEW, Douglas Abraham COLVIN

Western Road Medical Centre
99 Western Road, Romford RM1 3LS
Tel: 01708 746495 Fax: 01708 737936
Website: www.westernroad.co.uk
(Havering Primary Care Trust)
Patient List Size: 13600

Practice Manager S J Buffoni

GP David James BASS, Sylvia Louise BOND, Katherine Jane HASKELL, Neil LEIGH-COLLYER, Paul Charles MYERS, Ian Graeme QUIGLEY

Romney Marsh

Orchard House Surgery
Bleak Road, Lydd, Romney Marsh TN29 9AE
Tel: 01797 320307
(Shepway Primary Care Trust)

Practice Manager Janice Stanley

GP Paul Leonard DOWNIE

Orgarswick Avenue Surgery
9 Orgarswick Avenue, Dymchurch, Romney Marsh TN29 0NX
Tel: 01303 872245 Fax: 01303 872610
(Shepway Primary Care Trust)
Patient List Size: 10000

Practice Manager Keith Nicholas

GP V G KANEGAONKAR, Robert Francis CULLEN, James Frederick SHARP, Ruth SMITH, Mark Richard TOWNDROW

Thomas House Surgery
12A Eastbridge Road, Dymchurch, Romney Marsh TN29 0PF
Tel: 01303 873156 Fax: 01303 874885
(Shepway Primary Care Trust)

Practice Manager Alison Webster-Kell

Romsey

Abbey Mead Surgery
Abbey Mead, Romsey SO51 8EN
Tel: 01794 512218 Fax: 01794 514224
(Eastleigh and Test Valley South Primary Care Trust)

Practice Manager Linda Bent

GP Peter James BURROWS, Roger Martin ABBOTT, Sharon Mary ALLEN, Alexandra Jane MANSELL, Martin Leigh MITCHELL, Angela MOONEY

Alma Road Surgery
Alma Road, Romsey SO51 8ED
Tel: 01794 513422 Fax: 01794 518668
Website: www.almaroad.nhs.uk
(Eastleigh and Test Valley South Primary Care Trust)
Patient List Size: 12000

Practice Manager Cheryl Tucker

GP James Anthony BARRATT, Neil GAVINS, Sarah JOHNSON, Margaret Ann KEIGHTLEY, Ian Alistair KEITH, Inma ROS, Caroline SNELL, Christopher Peter THOMAS

Nightingale Surgery
Greatwell Drive, Cupernham Lane, Romsey SO51 7QN
Tel: 01794 517878 Fax: 01794 514236
Website: www.nightingalesurery.com
(Eastleigh and Test Valley South Primary Care Trust)
Patient List Size: 9200

GP Peter James WHITE, Paul LITTLE, Richard Henry PEACE, Susan Anne TIPPETT, Gregory WARNER, Katharine Jane WARNER

Ross-on-Wye

Alton Street Surgery
Alton Street, Ross-on-Wye HR9 5AB
Tel: 01989 563646 Fax: 01989 769438
Email: admin@gp-M81044.nhs.uk
Website: www.altonstreet.nhs.uk
(Herefordshire Primary Care Trust)
Patient List Size: 8750

Practice Manager Shirley Hallett

GP Clive Richard HARTSHORN, Philip Frank CLAYTON, Richard John COOK, Nichola Benedicte JANIS, Sasha Clare ROBINSON

Pendeen Surgery
Kent Avenue, Ross-on-Wye HR9 5AL
Tel: 01989 763535 Fax: 01989 768288
(Herefordshire Primary Care Trust)
Patient List Size: 8800

Practice Manager Valerie Finney

GP Andrew John ROGERS, Susan Jane CROSLAND, Paul Francis DOWNEY, Ruth KING, Andrew John LEEMAN, Russell John MELLOR

Rossendale

Haslingden Health Centre
7-9 Manchester Road, Haslingden, Rossendale BB4 5SL
Tel: 01706 212518 Fax: 01706 218112
(Burnley, Pendle and Rossendale Primary Care Trust)

Practice Manager M Berry

GP Patricia RISHTON, Thomas Hunter Maclauchlan MACKENZIE, Sally Jane QUINN, Graham Stuart SELLENS, Stephen TOWERS

Haslingden Health Centre
Health Centre Manchester Road, Haslingden, Rossendale BB4 5SL
Tel: 01706 214281 Fax: 01706 214831
(Burnley, Pendle and Rossendale Primary Care Trust)
Patient List Size: 1931

Practice Manager Karen Wilde

GP Abd El-Fatah Mahmoud MOUSTAFA

Haslingden Health Centre
Manchester Road, Haslingden, Rossendale BB4 5SL
Tel: 01706 226705 Fax: 01706 225705
(Burnley, Pendle and Rossendale Primary Care Trust)

GP Kumarakulatungam RAJASEKERAN

Manchester Road Health Centre
7-9 Manchester Road, Haslingden, Rossendale BB4 5SL
Tel: 01706 215208 Fax: 01706 221130
(Burnley, Pendle and Rossendale Primary Care Trust)

Practice Manager Elaine Badr

GP Mahmoud Momtaz Ahmed BADR, Dr MOUJAES

Medical Centre
Market Street, Whitworth, Rossendale OL12 8QS
Tel: 01706 852238 Fax: 01706 853877
(Burnley, Pendle and Rossendale Primary Care Trust)

GP E TIERNEY, S FARROW, J C V GILLINGHAN, J ORMROD

Rawtenstall Health Centre
Bacup Road, Rawtenstall, Rossendale BB4 7PL
Tel: 01706 213060 Fax: 01706 213060
(Burnley, Pendle and Rossendale Primary Care Trust)
Patient List Size: 16000

Practice Manager Caron Harrison

GP John BUNTING, Christopher James AINSWORTH, Malcolm Liddle BURNIE, Tanzila Waheed CHOUDHRY, William Stuart HINCHLIFFE, Brian MOTTERSHEAD, Rhys Morgan SAYES

Rawtenstall Health Centre
Bacup Road, Rawtenstall, Rossendale BB4 7PL
Tel: 01706 211217
(Burnley, Pendle and Rossendale Primary Care Trust)

GP Jalal-ud-Din BACHH, Mumtaz Nawaz KHAN, Khalid MAHMOOD

Waterfoot Health Centre
Cowpe Road, Waterfoot, Rossendale BB4 7DN
Tel: 01706 215178
(Burnley, Pendle and Rossendale Primary Care Trust)

GP Diana Mary DOHERTY, Sumit Kumar KAR, Michael Patrick POWER, Md. Abdur RAZZAQUE

Rotherham

Badsley Moor Lane Surgery
292 Badsley Moor Lane, Rotherham S65 2QW
Tel: 0845 122 2276
(Rotherham Primary Care Trust)

Practice Manager J Gibson

GP Hilal Abdulla JARJIS

Blyth Road Medical Centre
8 Blyth Road, Maltby, Rotherham S66 8JD
Tel: 01709 812827 Fax: 01709 798623
(Rotherham Primary Care Trust)

Practice Manager C Jones

GP R W SHELTON, Geoffrey Charles AVERY, Peter Alan CONTARDI

Brinsworth Medical Centre
171 Bawtry Road, Brinsworth, Rotherham S60 5ND
Tel: 01709 828806
(Rotherham Primary Care Trust)

Practice Manager J Venkotroman

GP Thondiculum Bhaskaran VENKATRAMAN, M SINGH, J P S VOHRA, S M WRIGLEY

Broom Lane Medical Centre
70 Broom Lane, Rotherham S60 3EW
Tel: 01709 364470 Fax: 01709 820009
(Rotherham Primary Care Trust)
Patient List Size: 11800

Practice Manager B Highfield

GP Naresh Ambalal PATEL, Richard CULLEN, N W GEORGE, Angela GILES, Ramul KACKER, Philip Louis MARTIN, Judith SANDERS, David Rowland STOTT, Dorothy THOMAS

Canklow Road Surgery
245/247 Canklow Road, Canklow, Rotherham S60 2JH
Tel: 01709 363398
(Rotherham Primary Care Trust)

Practice Manager Lynn Hazeltine

GP Ashim GANGULI

Central Surgery
Welfare Road, Thurnscoe, Rotherham S63 0JZ
Tel: 01709 890501 Fax: 01709 889689
Email: practice.manager@gp-85023.nhs.uk
(Barnsley Primary Care Trust)
Patient List Size: 3592

Practice Manager R Foster

GP Graham John LEESE, Matthew William AMOS

Central Surgery
Welfare Road, Thurnscoe, Rotherham S63 0JZ
Tel: 01709 892249 Fax: 01709 892202
(Barnsley Primary Care Trust)
Patient List Size: 7000

Practice Manager David Burns

GP Chandra Nath NEOGY, Mukund Gopal DEHADRAY, A N DUTTA

Clifton Medical Centre
Rotherham Health Village, Doncaster Gate Hospital, Doncaster Gate, Rotherham S65 1DA
Tel: 01709 382315 Fax: 01709 512646
(Rotherham Primary Care Trust)

Practice Manager Linda Green

GP Gavin Beattie PECKITT, Alison Elizabeth ASHTON, John William BYRNE, Matthew Stephen CAPEHORN, Karen Denise CLEMINSON, Catherine Anne COOPER, Karol KAPELLER, Adrian David OGDEN, Amy Jane WRIGHT

Dr S H M Kadarsha
Doncaster Road, Goldthorpe, Rotherham S63 9JB
Tel: 01709 893678 Fax: 01709 893652
(Barnsley Primary Care Trust)
Patient List Size: 2800

GP S H M I KADARSHA

Greasbrough Medical Centre
Munsbrough Rise, Greasbrough, Rotherham S61 4RB
Tel: 01709 559955 Fax: 01709 512152
(Rotherham Primary Care Trust)

Practice Manager B J Vickerage

GP Mohammed Hamid HUSAIN, M SUHAIL

Greenside Surgery
Greasbrough, Rotherham S61 4PT
Tel: 0845 124 0887
(Rotherham Primary Care Trust)

Practice Manager Carole Dalling

GP Robert Charles Adair COLLINSON, N C KELLY, Christopher Peter MYERS

The Health Centre
Magna Lane, Dalton, Rotherham S65 4HH
Tel: 0845 124 4746 Fax: 01709 578691
(Rotherham Primary Care Trust)

Practice Manager Steve Hindle

GP T AHMED, K M BOLSTER, N NAZIR, S VON SCHREIBER, H L WEBSTER

The Health Centre
Magna Lane, Dalton, Rotherham S65 4HH
Tel: 01709 851414 Fax: 01709 852882
(Rotherham Primary Care Trust)
Patient List Size: 3901

Practice Manager Paul Hardstaff, Steve Hindle

GP Tariq ALI, Noor HUSSAIN, Tariq Mahmoud AHMED, Sarah JONES, Simon von SCHREIBER

The Health Centre
Braithwell Road, Maltby, Rotherham S66 8JE
Tel: 01709 812615
(Rotherham Primary Care Trust)

GP Birbal KAPUR

The Health Centre
Braithwell Road, Maltby, Rotherham S66 8JE
Tel: 0845 121 9932
(Rotherham Primary Care Trust)

Practice Manager T Gibbons

GP Mohammad Bankole ZUBAIRU

Houghton Road Medical Centre
Welfare Road, Thurnscoe, Rotherham S63 0JZ
Tel: 01709 894653
(Barnsley Primary Care Trust)

GP D SHANKAR

The Manor Field Surgery
The Health Centre, Braithwell Road, Maltby, Rotherham S66 8JE
Tel: 0845 122 3231
(Rotherham Primary Care Trust)

Practice Manager J Small

GP R VAN DER LIJN, D C BELLAMY, A MELLOR, P J STASZEK

Market Surgery
Warehouse Lane, Wath-On-Dearne, Rotherham S63 7RA
Tel: 0870 428 0772
(Rotherham Primary Care Trust)

Practice Manager B Lee

GP David Gareth POLKINGHORN, Sarah Jane JORDAN, Philip Peter OLIVER, David Julian PLEWS, Malcolm Bryan SWALLOW

Morthen Road Surgery
2 Morthen Road, Wickersley, Rotherham S66 1EU
Tel: 0845 122 7423
(Rotherham Primary Care Trust)

Practice Manager C Lowery

GP Terence MOORE, Katherine Jane BALCH, M M BROWN, Richard David FULBROOK, H MILLS, Vetrivel VELAMAIL

Parkgate Medical Centre
Netherfield Lane, Parkgate, Rotherham S62 6AW
Tel: 0845 125 2336
(Rotherham Primary Care Trust)

Practice Manager Patricia Dearden

GP M C ALEXANDER, M J IQBAL, Puthenparampil George THOMAS

Queens Medical Centre
Muglet Lane, Maltby, Rotherham S66 7NA
Tel: 01709 817755
(Rotherham Primary Care Trust)

Practice Manager Zahida Khan

GP Zulfikar Ali KHAN

Rawmarsh Health Centre
Barbers Avenue, Rawmarsh, Rotherham S62 6AD
Tel: 01709 514448 Fax: 01709 526277
(Rotherham Primary Care Trust)

Practice Manager Sasi Viswesvaraiah

GP Bhalchandra Chhaganlal THAKKAR, Manickam VISWESVARAIAH

Rosehill Medical Centre
52 Rosehill Road, Rawmarsh, Rotherham S62 7BT
Tel: 01709 522595
(Rotherham Primary Care Trust)

Practice Manager K Bhimpuria

GP Yogesh Rajendraprasad BHIMPURIA

Shakespeare Road Surgery
50 Shakespeare Road, Eastwood, Rotherham S65 1QY
Tel: 0845 121 3122 Fax: 01709 837000
(Rotherham Primary Care Trust)
Patient List Size: 3550

Practice Manager Derrick Small

GP Ahsan-Ul-Haq GONI, M S CHAUHDRY

St Ann's Medical Centre
Rotherham Health Village, Doncaster Gate Hospital, Doncaster Gate, Rotherham S65 1DW
Tel: 01709 379283

(Rotherham Primary Care Trust)

Practice Manager Dorothy Hardcastle

GP John Eric FEARNSIDE, C G ALTON, A FORRESTER, A J HUDSON, A S JUBB, R P KENNY, Julie Anne KITLOWSKI, Simon Timothy MACKEOWN, Gareth OWEN, John Edward POWELL, Judith Ann SANDERS, Susan Ann START

Stag Medical Centre
162 Wickersley Road, Rotherham S60 4JW
Tel: 0845 122 3121
(Rotherham Primary Care Trust)

Practice Manager Karl Rex

GP Martin Clifford CLARK, Susan Jennifer ABBEY, Stephen Brian BURNS, Robert N McWHINNIE, Gorul R R MUTHOO, John Charles Christopher PROCTOR

The Surgery
High Street, Rawmarsh, Rotherham S62 6LW
Tel: 01709 522888
(Rotherham Primary Care Trust)

Practice Manager T Gibbons

GP R I HIRST, S DEL POZO, M J HILLIER, H O UCHEGBU

The Surgery
York Road, Rotherham S65 1PW
Tel: 0845 125 5084
(Rotherham Primary Care Trust)

Practice Manager Pam Abbott

GP Srini VASAN, U ANAND, M KRISHNATHASAN

The Surgery
Photopia, Limesway, Maltby, Rotherham S66 8JF
Tel: 01709 812714 Fax: 01709 817320
(Rotherham Primary Care Trust)
Patient List Size: 3500

Practice Manager B Wiles

GP Om Prakash SHRIVASTAVA, Rani SHRIVASTAVA

The Surgery
142 Furlong Road, Bolton on Dearne, Rotherham S63 8HA
Tel: 01709 890771 Fax: 01709 889704
(Barnsley Primary Care Trust)

GP Mulayil Krishnan GOPINATH

The Surgery
96 Barnsley Road, Goldthorpe, Rotherham S63 6DQ
Tel: 01709 890686 Fax: 01709 888347
(Barnsley Primary Care Trust)

Practice Manager S Hollingworth

GP S R SEN, R K DATTA

The Surgery
Sough Hall Avenue, Thorpe Hesley, Rotherham S61 2QP

GP T K MUKHOPADHYAY

Surgery of Light
Hungerhill Lane, Whiston, Rotherham S60 4BD
Tel: 0845 124 0441
(Rotherham Primary Care Trust)

GP Muzahim Salih BADER

Thrybergh Medical Centre
21 Park Lane, Thrybergh, Rotherham S65 4BT
Tel: 0845 122 0669
(Rotherham Primary Care Trust)

Practice Manager A E Redmond

GP Leonard JACOB

Treeton Medical Centre
10 Arundel Street, Treeton, Rotherham S60 5PW
Tel: 0114 269 2600 Fax: 0114 269 3296
(Rotherham Primary Care Trust)
Patient List Size: 6000

Practice Manager Trevor C Ledger

GP Kameshwar PRASAD, Bipin CHANDRAN, Carl Andrew HUTSON

The Village Surgery
24-28 Laughton Road, Thurcroft, Rotherham S66 9LP
Tel: 0845 122 0821
(Rotherham Primary Care Trust)

Practice Manager Mo Jameson

GP Eric Walter SIMPSON, Johnathan James COBB, Gail CROWLEY, Duncan Henry WILSON

Wath Health Centre
35 Church Street, Wath-On-Dearne, Rotherham S63 7RF
Tel: 01709 877886 Fax: 01709 877886
(Rotherham Primary Care Trust)

Practice Manager M Stone

GP Christopher St. John KEAR

Wath Health Centre
35 Church Street, Wath-On-Dearne, Rotherham S63 7RF
Tel: 01709 873233
(Rotherham Primary Care Trust)

Practice Manager C Ramsey

GP Hari Das RAHA

West House Surgery
West Street, Wath-On-Dearne, Rotherham S63 7QX
Tel: 0845 124 4749 Fax: 01709 873858
(Rotherham Primary Care Trust)

Practice Manager Susan Khidir

GP Zein E S KHIDIR

Wickersley Health Centre
Poplar Glade, Wickersley, Rotherham S66 2JQ
Tel: 0845 121 1740
(Rotherham Primary Care Trust)

Practice Manager Paula Davies

GP Sathineni Venkateshwar REDDY, Peter John CLARKE, S B JESPERSEN, H E SIMPSON

Woodgrove Surgery
2 Doncaster Road, Wath on Dearne, Rotherham S63 7AL
Tel: 01709 763400 Fax: 01709 872899
(Barnsley Primary Care Trust)

Practice Manager Martyn Smith

GP Martin Richard SICS, A MELLOR, K PHIPPS

Woodstock Bower Group Practice
1 Kimberworth Road, Rotherham S61 1AH
Tel: 01709 561442/562319 Fax: 01709 740690
(Rotherham Primary Care Trust)

Practice Manager Mike Austin

GP Adrian John COLE, Russell Mark BRYNES, S CHATTERJEE, S J DOWSETT, Bernard James EVERETT, S J IQBAL, Bethan Alison JONES, Alan James KEITH

Rowlands Castle

The Surgery
12 The Green, Rowlands Castle PO9 6BN
Tel: 023 9241 2846 Fax: 023 9241 3070
(East Hampshire Primary Care Trust)
Patient List Size: 3500

Practice Manager I Kent

GP John Robert HARRISON, Ian Robert CALDWELL

Rowlands Gill

Medical Centre
The Grove, Rowlands Gill NE39 1PW
Tel: 01207 542136 Fax: 01207 543340
(Gateshead Primary Care Trust)
Patient List Size: 7784

Practice Manager Evelyn Mee

GP Robert Thomas DAWSON, Mary IMLAH, Alexander Brian Gant LIDDLE

Rowley Regis

Rowley Medical Practice
165 Hawes Lane, Rowley Regis B65 9AF
Tel: 0121 559 2449 Fax: 0121 559 6579
(Rowley Regis and Tipton Primary Care Trust)
Patient List Size: 4000

GP J P M RILEY, I J SUMNER

Royston

The Health Centre
Melbourn Street, Royston SG8 7BS
Tel: 01763 242981 Fax: 01763 249197
Email: enquiries.roystoncenhs.net
Website: roystonhealthcentre.com
(Royston, Buntingford and Bishop's Stortford Primary Care Trust)
Patient List Size: 10200

Practice Manager Yvonne West

GP John Roderick HEDGES, Melita Rose BROWNRIGG, Theresa LEIGHTON, Kenneth Malcolm René VAN TERHEYDEN, John Francis WRIGHT

Orchard Surgery
New Road, Melbourn, Royston SG8 6BX
Tel: 01763 260 220 Fax: 01763 262 968
(South Cambridgeshire Primary Care Trust)

Practice Manager Vikki George-Hutt

GP R E G MAXIM, Dr COLGATE, Dr EASTON, Dr RICHTER

Roysia Surgery
Burns Road, Royston SG8 5PT
Tel: 01763 243166 Fax: 01763 245315
Website: www.rbbs-pct.nhs.uk/roysiasurgery
(Royston, Buntingford and Bishop's Stortford Primary Care Trust)
Patient List Size: 6500

Practice Manager Yvonne Buckley

GP Richard Norman HAY, Christopher Mark POLGE, Anne Theresa RIGNEY, Jean SEYMOUR

The Surgery
High Street, Barley, Royston SG8 8HY
Tel: 01763 848244 Fax: 01763 848677
(Royston, Buntingford and Bishop's Stortford Primary Care Trust)
Patient List Size: 6700

Practice Manager Nikki Foster

GP Peter GOUGH, Timothy Colin CLUBB, Adrian WOOD

Rugby

Ahluwhalia and Partner
31 Overslade Lane, Rugby CV22 6DY
Tel: 01788-811259
(Rugby Primary Care Trust)

Practice Manager D Bedi

GP Dr AHLUWALIA, Dr BALASUBRAMANIAM

Albert Street Surgery
63 Albert Street, Rugby CV21 2SN
Tel: 01788 573366 Fax: 01788 573473
(Rugby Primary Care Trust)

Practice Manager Lynne Booth

GP Martha Sebastian D'MELLO, Seshu Babu KAVURI

Brookside Surgery
Stretton-on-Dunsmore, Rugby CV23 9NH
Tel: 024 7654 2525 Fax: 024 7654 5617
(Rugby Primary Care Trust)

GP Michael Ponting HOUGHTON, Kay BRIDGEMAN

Central Surgery
Corporation Street, Rugby CV21 3SP
Tel: 01788 574335 Fax: 01788 547693
(Rugby Primary Care Trust)

Practice Manager Linda Ashmore

GP Jacqueline Susan BARNEY, David BLACK, Nicholas James COOK, Jeffery William COTTERILL, Emma Katherine EEDLE, John HAM

Clifton Road Surgery
22 Clifton Road, Rugby CV21 3QF
Tel: 01788 544744/544718 Fax: 01788 553902
(Rugby Primary Care Trust)
Patient List Size: 8000

Practice Manager Avril Hurt

GP Betty GALLAGHER, John Charles Anthony DERRICK, Mark LINDSEY, Denise MARTYR

Clifton Road Surgery
26 Clifton Road, Rugby CV21 3QF
Tel: 01788 543088 Fax: 01788 551496
(Rugby Primary Care Trust)
Patient List Size: 12000

Practice Manager C H Pollock

GP Norman BYRD, Adrian CANALE-PAROLA, Lesli DAVIES, Helen Elizabeth DOUSE, William James FIELDING, Hilary Jane Bethea GAMMELL, Glynis ISORESRU

Clifton Road Surgery
95 Clifton Road, Rugby CV21 3QQ
Tel: 01788 578800/568810 Fax: 01788 541063
(Rugby Primary Care Trust)
Patient List Size: 5000

Practice Manager S Merrell

GP Colin Andrew WEST, Enid Jane CUMMING, Katharine Jane LEACH

Dunchurch Surgery
Dunsmore Heath, Dunchurch, Rugby CV22 6AP
Tel: 01788 522448 Fax: 01788 814609
Email: office@gp.m84046.nhs.uk
(Rugby Primary Care Trust)
Patient List Size: 7500

Practice Manager Susan Evans

GP Ian Wojciech David CZERNIEWSKI, David Ronald CARNE, Kate Margaret REYNOLDS, Elizabeth June ROBERTS

Medical Practice
1 Whitehall Road, Rugby CV21 3AE
Tel: 01788 562749 Fax: 01788 543665
(Rugby Primary Care Trust)

GP Jagmohan Singh AHLUWALIA, Tamboo Shanmugampillai BALASUBRAMANIAM

The Surgery
Barr Lane, Brinklow, Rugby CV23 0LU
Tel: 01788 832994 Fax: 01788 833021
(Rugby Primary Care Trust)

Practice Manager Anne Davey

GP Steven Leonard BROWN, Keith Joseph EDGAR, David James SHORE

The Surgery
School Street, Wolston, Rugby CV8 3HG
Tel: 024 7654 2192 Fax: 024 7654 4075
(Rugby Primary Care Trust)

GP Wayne Albert DUCHARME, Anna Louise DUCHARME

Warwick Street Surgery
18 Warwick Street, Rugby CV21 3DH
Tel: 01788 540860 Fax: 01788 560988
(Rugby Primary Care Trust)
Patient List Size: 6740

Practice Manager G White

GP Barrie Vernon BEMAND, Nick J DOHERTY, Robyn Dorothy CRIGHTON

Whitehall Medical Practice
Morton Gardens, Rugby CV21 3AQ
Tel: 01788 544264 Fax: 01788 575783
(Rugby Primary Care Trust)
Patient List Size: 14500

GP Ruth Mary BRYANT, Isabel Barbara DRAPER, Richard Killingbeck HOLDSWORTH, Michael Norman Jack JACOBY, Peter John KILVERT, Ashok Parshottam KORIA, Peter MORRIS

Whitehall Road Surgery
1 Whitehall Road, Rugby CV21 3AE
Tel: 01788 561319 Fax: 01788 553762
(Rugby Primary Care Trust)

Practice Manager Norma Elliott

GP Kantilal Bhagoobhai PARMAR, J S AHLUWALIA, T BALASUBRAMANIAM

Rugeley

Brereton Surgery
88 Main Street, Brereton, Rugeley WS15 1DU
Tel: 01889 575560 Fax: 01889 575560
(Cannock Chase Primary Care Trust)
Patient List Size: 3756

Practice Manager S. Sivanesan

GP Vaithilingam Nagalingam SIVANESAN, N DAVIES

Hillsprings Portacabin Surgery
Glen Haven, Off Green Lane, Rugeley WS15 2GS
Tel: 01889 585502 Fax: 01889 582958
(Cannock Chase Primary Care Trust)
Patient List Size: 2598

Practice Manager Faiza Kayani

GP Shahpur KAYANI

Horsefair Practice
Horse Fair, Rugeley WS15 2EL
Tel: 01889 582244 Fax: 01899 582244
(Cannock Chase Primary Care Trust)
Patient List Size: 19318

Practice Manager Patsi Hemmingsley

GP A S I BAGHDADY, Sekhar DEB, Subhas Chandra DEY, Ibrahim Habib IBRAHIM, Navin Chandra RASTOGI, M P SINGH, P E STAITE, Michael John STOKES

The Surgery
School House Lane, Abbots Bromley, Rugeley WS15 3BT
Tel: 01283 840228 Fax: 01283 840919
(East Staffordshire Primary Care Trust)

GP Richard Vincent Hope ALDRIDGE, Judith Susan BELL

Ruislip

Cedars Medical Centre
118 Elliott Avenue, Ruislip HA4 9LZ
Tel: 020 8429 9595 Fax: 020 8429 9596
(Hillingdon Primary Care Trust)

GP Elzbieta KOSCIESZCA, Ritu PRASAD

Devonshire Lodge Practice
Eastcote Health Centre, Abbotsbury Gardens, Eastcote, Pinner, Ruislip HA5 1TG
Tel: 020 8866 0200/8981 Fax: 020 8429 3087
(Hillingdon Primary Care Trust)
Patient List Size: 7450

Practice Manager Linda Jones

GP Jennifer Alexis ALLEN, Jonathan Michael BREWERTON, Martin Dennis HALL

Eastcote Health Centre
Abbotsbury Gardens, Eastcote, Pinner, Ruislip HA5 1TG
Tel: 020 8866 8382/0121 Fax: 020 8866 1028
(Hillingdon Primary Care Trust)
Patient List Size: 6700

Practice Manager Susan Dransfield

GP Christopher Grant TIMMIS, Peter Felix JOSEPH, Sheila Dorothy SAVILLE

Field End Road Practice
700 Field End Road, South Ruislip, Ruislip HA4 0QR
Tel: 020 8422 5900 Fax: 020 8423 8405
(Hillingdon Primary Care Trust)
Patient List Size: 2555

Practice Manager Susan Fossett

GP Khandubhai G MISTRY

Field End Road Surgery
81 Field End Road, Eastcote, Pinner, Ruislip HA5 1TD
Tel: 020 8866 1238 Fax: 020 8423 7901
(Harrow Primary Care Trust)
Patient List Size: 7552

Practice Manager R Rawlinson

GP Michael Paul EDDINGTON, L WIJAYARATNA

King Edward's Medical Centre
19 King Edwards Road, Ruislip HA4 7AE
Tel: 01895 632021/632114 Fax: 01895 623828
(Hillingdon Primary Care Trust)

GP Mahendra Kumar MASHRU

Ladygate Lane Surgery
22 Ladygate Lane, Ruislip HA4 7QU
Tel: 01895 632741 Fax: 01895 637343
(Hillingdon Primary Care Trust)

GP Amina KARIM, Marie Teresa TSO

The Medical Centre
69 Queens Walk, Ruislip HA4 0NT
Tel: 020 8842 2991 Fax: 020 8842 2245
(Hillingdon Primary Care Trust)

GP Cedric Matthew SOLOMON, Jacob Israel SOLOMON, Judith Alexis LIVINGSTONE

The Medical Centre
2A Wood Lane, Ruislip HA4 6ER
Tel: 01895 632677 Fax: 01895 634020
(Hillingdon Primary Care Trust)

Practice Manager L Willoughby

GP Alison Margaret MARRIOTT, Myrna LIBERMAN, Philip Alfred ROSE, Steven Maurice SHAPIRO

Oxford Drive Medical Centre
1 Oxford Drive, Eastcote, Ruislip HA4 9EY
Tel: 020 8866 3430 Fax: 020 8868 3317
(Hillingdon Primary Care Trust)

GP Ravinder Paul AURORA, Fiona Elizabeth McCRIMMON, Sarah Ruth NEWBERY

RAF Medical Centre
RAF Northolt, West End Road, Ruislip HA4 6NG
Tel: 020 8845 2300
(Hillingdon Primary Care Trust)

GP R JAYAKUMAR, S BILLINGTON

Southcote Clinic
Southcote Rise, Ruislip HA4 7LJ
Tel: 01895 679800 Fax: 01895 625044
(Hillingdon Primary Care Trust)

GP John David HENDLEY, Eve SPEIGHT

St Martins Medical Centre
21 Eastcote Road, Ruislip HA4 8BE
Tel: 01895 632410 Fax: 01895 675058
(Hillingdon Primary Care Trust)

GP Nag RAJ, Jacob JOSEPH, Latha RAJ

Walnut Way Surgery
21 Walnut Way, Ruislip HA4 6TB
Tel: 020 8845 4400 Fax: 020 8845 4403
(Hillingdon Primary Care Trust)
Patient List Size: 2700

Practice Manager Asfia Siddiqui

GP Mohammed Lutfur Rehman SIDDIQUI, Yousuf Ullah SIDDIQUI

Runcorn

Brookvale Practice
Hallwood Health Centre, Hospital Way, Runcorn WA7 2UT
Tel: 01928 718182 Fax: 01928 750209
(Halton Primary Care Trust)
Patient List Size: 8000

Practice Manager Bernie Haskayne

GP Karin Maria CORRADO, Patricia Mary ABBOTT, David John O'BRIEN, Clifford RICHARDS

Castlefields Health Centre
Chester Close, Castlefields, Runcorn WA7 2HY
Tel: 01928 566671 Fax: 01928 581631
(Halton Primary Care Trust)
Patient List Size: 12000

Practice Manager Kelly Atkins

GP David Geoffrey COLIN-THOME, Anthony George Bradshaw FRITH, Matthew KEARNEY, David LYON, Rachel MILLERCHIP, Shashangka OTIV, Zoe ROG, Anne-Marie WILD

Grove House Practice
St Pauls Health Centre, High St, Runcorn WA7 1AB
Tel: 01928 566561 Fax: 01928 590212
(Halton Primary Care Trust)
Patient List Size: 11500

Practice Manager Christine Leadbetter

GP David Harold WILSON, N R FILDES, Catherine HYATT, Carol MANLEY, S THOMAS, Carole Anne WATSON

Heath Road Medical Centre
Heath Road, Runcorn WA7 5TJ
Tel: 01928 565881 Fax: 01928 566748
(Halton Primary Care Trust)

Practice Manager Doris Chimes

GP Mukesh Kumar SAKSENA

Murdishaw Health Centre
Gorsewood Road, Murdishaw, Runcorn WA7 6ES
Tel: 01928 712061 Fax: 01928 791988
(Halton Primary Care Trust)
Patient List Size: 8100

Practice Manager Suzy Angeluk

GP Gareth MORGAN, Maria EASAW, John FOX, John HAWKSWELL, Elizabeth Barbara MIRSKI

Tower House Practice
St Pauls Health Centre, High Street, Runcorn WA7 1AB
Tel: 01928 567404
(Halton Primary Care Trust)
Patient List Size: 13200

Practice Manager Sarah Larkin, Davina Morrell

GP Madeleine Mary ORPIN, Andrew Basil BARENDT, Blyth Taylor BELL, Madeleiene GIBSON, John GRIFFIN, Damian McDERMOTT, Harjinder Singh SANDHU

Weaver Vale Practice
Hallwood Health Centre, Hospital Way, Runcorn WA7 2UT
Tel: 01928 711911 Fax: 01928 717368
(Halton Primary Care Trust)
Patient List Size: 9400

Practice Manager Maureen Marriott

GP James Arthur NEWEY, Johnathon BEYNON, Fenella Mary COTTIER, Heather Penelope FEARON, Richard Andrew William FROOD, Peter JOHNSON

Rushden

Dr Wingfield and Partners
Adnitt Road, Rushden NN10 9TR
Tel: 01933 412444 Fax: 01933 317666
(Northamptonshire Heartlands Primary Care Trust)
Patient List Size: 10900

Practice Manager Martin Clifford

GP S A WINGFIELD, James Joseph KELLY, Jonathan LANCASTLE-SMITH, Anna Margaret PASSMORE, D R THOMAS

Higham Ferrers Surgery
5 College Street, Higham Ferrers, Rushden NN10 8DX
Tel: 01933 412777 Fax: 01933 419013
(Northamptonshire Heartlands Primary Care Trust)
Patient List Size: 4500

GP Peter David CLIFFORD, Mary DELL, Jonathan David WALI

Rushden Medical Centre
Parklands, Wymington Road, Rushden NN10 9EB
Tel: 01933 396000
(Northamptonshire Heartlands Primary Care Trust)

Practice Manager Tony Byles

GP Adrian John BURCH, Roger William COLES, Anne Maria DUNCAN, Steven John HOGG, Joannes Wilibrordus Gerardus LANGENDIJK, Alison Frances LEE, Muruga Kumar SUBRAMANIAM

Rushden Medical Practice
Adnitt Road, Rushden NN10 9TR
Tel: 01933 412666 Fax: 01933 317666
(Northamptonshire Heartlands Primary Care Trust)

Practice Manager Lesley Legg

GP Amrik Singh HANSPAUL, James Black FINDLAY, Rose Maria Brenda MURRAY, David Glyn WILLIAMS

Ryde

Argyll House
78 West Street, Ryde PO33 2QJ
Tel: 01983 562955 Fax: 01983 618130
(Isle of Wight Primary Care Trust)

GP Avril MARTIN, Allan John GREEN, Christine SIEGER

Dr Manning and Partners
The Surgery, Tower House, Rink Road, Ryde PO33 1LP
Tel: 01983 811431 Fax: 01983 817215
(Isle of Wight Primary Care Trust)
Patient List Size: 9400

Practice Manager K Draper

GP Christopher James Ford MANNING, Mark DENMAN-JOHNSON, Susan Caroline GRIFFITHS, Richard HUDSON, Catherine O'CALLAGHAN, Bryn Spencer James REES, Richard Charles WILLIAMS

Esplanade Surgery
19 Esplanade, Ryde PO33 2EH
Tel: 01983 611444 Fax: 01983 811548
(Isle of Wight Primary Care Trust)

GP Pamela Georgina SIM, Eugene Joseph HUGHES, Jean Eileadh MELTZER, Julian Mark Courtenay ROGERS

Garfield Road Surgery
18 Garfield Road, Ryde PO33 2PT
Tel: 01983 565103 Fax: 01983 617288
(Isle of Wight Primary Care Trust)
Patient List Size: 2564

GP Kallol MAJUMDAR, Bhaswati MAJUMDAR

High Street Surgery
94 High Street, Wootton Bridge, Ryde PO33 4PR
Tel: 01983 883520 Fax: 01983 883538
(Isle of Wight Primary Care Trust)

Practice Manager Mary Long

GP Anne Elizabeth BEABLE

Upper Green Road Medical Centre
Upper Green Road, St Helens, Ryde PO33 1UG
Tel: 01983 872772 Fax: 01983 874800
(Isle of Wight Primary Care Trust)

Practice Manager Catherine Barton

GP John PARTRIDGE, Kieron Daniel COONEY, Matthew John Keith de BELDER, Hein FERREIRA, Yvonne Elizabeth HAZELL

Rye

Postern Gate Surgery
Cinque Ports Street, Rye TN31 7AP
Tel: 01797 224924 Fax: 01797 226858
(Bexhill and Rother Primary Care Trust)
Patient List Size: 7418

Practice Manager Lizzie Stern

GP Norman James FERGUSON, Harry Benjamin James CHISHICK, Andrea Louise GRIFFIN, George TAGGART

The Surgery
Main Street, Northiam, Rye TN31 6ND
Tel: 01797 252140 Fax: 01797 252077
(Bexhill and Rother Primary Care Trust)
Patient List Size: 5200

Practice Manager Linda Cox

GP John CARROLL, Philip Margrave JAMES, Janet Fiona DINWIDDIE

The Surgery
Cinque Ports House, Cinque Ports Street, Rye TN31 7AN
Tel: 01797 223230 Fax: 01797 227234
(Bexhill and Rother Primary Care Trust)

Practice Manager Georgina Cooke

GP Mohammad Sultan Wali JEELANI, Ruqia Akhtar JEELANI

Ryton

Crawcrook Medical Centre
Back Chamberlain Street, Crawcrook, Ryton NE40 4TZ
Tel: 0191 413 2243 Fax: 0191 413 8098
(Gateshead Primary Care Trust)

GP Malcolm Kenneth PHILLIPS, Stanley Waters CHAPMAN, Anil DOSHI

Doctors Surgery
Grange Road, Ryton NE40 3L
(Gateshead Primary Care Trust)

Elvaston Road Surgery
7 Elvaston Road, Ryton NE40 3NT
Tel: 0191 413 3459 Fax: 0191 413 3459
(Gateshead Primary Care Trust)

GP Dr HILTON

The Surgery
7 Elvaston Road, Ryton NE40 3NT
Tel: 0191 4133459 Fax: 0191 41 33580
(Gateshead Primary Care Trust)
Patient List Size: 2500

GP Stephen Mark HILTON

Saffron Walden

Borough Lane Surgery
2 Borough Lane, Saffron Walden CB11 4AF
Tel: 01799 524224 Fax: 01799 524830
(Uttlesford Primary Care Trust)
Patient List Size: 4700

Practice Manager Linda Ainscough

GP Christopher John EATON, Ryszard BIETZK, Catherine BROWN

Gold Street Surgery
Gold Street, Saffron Walden CB10 1EJ
Tel: 01799 525325 Fax: 01799 524042
(Uttlesford Primary Care Trust)
Patient List Size: 9800

Practice Manager Jacky Porter

GP Christopher David CLAYTON-PAYNE, Bjorn ALSOS, C IQBAL, David John LORT

Newport Surgery
Frambury Lane, Newport, Saffron Walden CB11 3PY
Tel: 01799 540570 Fax: 01799 542126
(Uttlesford Primary Care Trust)
Patient List Size: 8000

Practice Manager Gillian Clapperton

GP Mark Norton STEVENS, S S BASRA, Elizabeth Ann LORT, J WEST, E WOKO

Rectory Surgery
18 Castle Street, Saffron Walden CB10 1BP
Tel: 01799 522327 Fax: 01799 525436
(Uttlesford Primary Care Trust)

Practice Manager Jan Millard

GP Philip Radcliffe SILLS, Clive Conrad PAUL, Andrew Edward Rodney SMITH, Jane Jackson WEIR

Salcombe

Redfern Health Centre
Shadycombe Road, Salcombe TQ8 8DJ
(South Hams and West Devon Primary Care Trust)

Practice Manager S Sharp

GP Eric Winston McLARTY, Dr BAXTER, Helen Jane BLOOMER, Dr DEVLIN

Salcombe Health Centre
Shadycombe Road, Salcombe TQ8 8DJ
(South Hams and West Devon Primary Care Trust)

Sale

Bodmin Road Health Centre
Bodmin Road, Ashton on Mersey, Sale M33 5JH
Tel: 0161 962 4625 Fax: 0161 905 3317
(Trafford South Primary Care Trust)
Patient List Size: 6599

Practice Manager J Marks

GP Peter John WELSH, Deborah POLE, Peter Michael Andrew SIMPSON, Stephanie YARNELL

Boundary House
462 Northenden Road, Sale M33 2RH
Tel: 0161 972 9999
(Trafford South Primary Care Trust)
Patient List Size: 9000

Practice Manager Alison Overton

GP Jonathan Peter BERRY, Paul Anthony GRAY, Dion HUTCHINSON, Frances Mary MOLEY, Alison PALMER, Janet Elizabeth WEBB

Conway Road Health Centre
Conway Road, Sale M33 2TB
Tel: 0161 962 7321 Fax: 0161 973 1151
(Trafford South Primary Care Trust)
Patient List Size: 6800

GP Clive Jeffrey Bruce MARCHI, Sally Rachel FRIER, Anthony Brian GALLAGHER, Oonagh Josephine McKAIGUE

Conway Road Health Centre
80a Conway Road, Sale M33 2TB
Tel: 0161 905 1933 Fax: 0161 905 2847
(Trafford South Primary Care Trust)
Patient List Size: 3600

GP M B A McGARRY

Derbyshire Road South Surgery
12 Derbyshire Road South, Sale M33 3JP
(Trafford South Primary Care Trust)
Patient List Size: 3400

GP Richard George CLARE

Meadway Health Centre
Meadway, Sale M33 4PS
Tel: 0161 905 2850
(Trafford South Primary Care Trust)

GP David Lynne EDWARDS, Linda ASHCROFT, Karnen DRABBLE, Robert JENYO

Meadway Health Centre
Meadway, Sale M33 4PS
Tel: 0161 905 2850
(Trafford South Primary Care Trust)

GP Peter Anthony JACKSON, Michael Joseph HOLLOWAY, Clare McMAHON

Meadway Health Centre
Meadway, Sale M33 4PS
Tel: 0161 905 2850 Fax: 0161 969 0225
(Trafford South Primary Care Trust)

GP Philip Jonathan LUKEMAN, Katherine Jane SUTTON, D J TRAGEN

Norris Road Surgery
356 Norris Road, Sale M33 2RL
Tel: 0161 962 5464
(Trafford South Primary Care Trust)

GP Dr PLATT

Norris Road Surgery
356 Norris Road, Sale M33 2RL
Tel: 0161 962 5464
(Trafford South Primary Care Trust)

GP Graham PLATT

St John's Medical Centre
St John's Road, Sale WA14 2NW
Tel: 0161 928 8727 Fax: 0161 929 8550
(Trafford South Primary Care Trust)

GP N P LORD

St John's Medical Centre
St John's Road, Sale WA14 2NW
Tel: 0161 928 8727 Fax: 0161 929 8550
(Trafford South Primary Care Trust)

GP M S SANGHA

Washway Road Medical Centre
67 Washway Road, Sale M33 7SS
Tel: 0161 962 4354 Fax: 0161 905 4706
(Trafford South Primary Care Trust)

Practice Manager J Davis

GP James Barry Tunstall TEBB, Joanna BURGESS, Elizabeth CLARKE, Mark Alfred JARVIS, Geraldine O'MALLEY, Robert John PARKS, Hilary Frances SIMONTON, Helen WILKINSON

Salford

Claremont Medical Centre
91 Claremont Road, Salford M6 7GP
Tel: 0161 743 0453 Fax: 0161 743 9141
(Salford Primary Care Trust)

Practice Manager Susan Wilkinson

GP Pamela Ann COLLIER, Mark Andrew AUSTIN, Muhammad Ehsanul HAGUE

The Daruzzaman Care Centre
3 Derby Road, Salford M5 5NZ
Tel: 0161 736 4037 Fax: 0161 743 9384
(Salford Primary Care Trust)
Patient List Size: 2160

Practice Manager Shelly Dunn

GP S BEDI, C MALCOMSON

Higher Broughton Health Centre
Bevendon Square, Salford M7 4TP
Tel: 0161 792 5111 Fax: 0161 708 8944
(Salford Primary Care Trust)
Patient List Size: 3500

GP Badal Krishna DASS, Christopher Brian WARBURTON

Higher Broughton Health Centre
Bevendon Square, Salford M7 4TP
Tel: 0161 792 2142/2582 Fax: 0161 792 9203
(Salford Primary Care Trust)

GP Deborah LARAH, Laurence BACALL, Simon JOSEPH

Higher Broughton Health Centre
Bevendon Square, Salford M7 4TP
Tel: 0161 792 6888 Fax: 0161 708 8510
(Salford Primary Care Trust)

Practice Manager Sangamitra Ghosh

GP Purab Ratan GHOSH

Lanceburn Health Centre
Clarendon Surgery, Churchill Way, Salford M6 5QX
Tel: 0161 736 4529 Fax: 0161 736 2724
(Salford Primary Care Trust)

Practice Manager Linda Brown

GP Jeremy William TANKEL, Wendy Anne OWEN

Lanceburn Health Centre
Churchill Way, Salford M6 5QX
Tel: 0161 745 9241 Fax: 0161 745 9241

(Salford Primary Care Trust)

Practice Manager Barbara Aherne

GP Ahmed Ataul HUQ

Lanceburn Health Centre
Churchill Way, Salford M6 5QX
Tel: 0161 745 9239 Fax: 0161 736 2387
(Salford Primary Care Trust)

Practice Manager Amina Bakhshi

GP Nisar Ahmad BAKHSHI

Lanceburn Health Centre
Churchill Way, Salford M6 5QX
Tel: 0161 745 9237
(Salford Primary Care Trust)

Practice Manager Anita Baral

GP Dhirendra Nath DAS

Langworthy Road Surgery
250 Langworthy Road, Salford M6 5WW
Tel: 0161 736 7422 Fax: 0161 736 4816
(Salford Primary Care Trust)

Practice Manager Jackie Sedgwick

GP Shraga HABER, Karen Louise GOODMAN, Phyllis Anne LEVENTHALL, Susan Elaine ROSENBERG

Langworthy Road Surgery
195 Langworthy Road, Salford M6 5PW
Tel: 0161 736 2338 Fax: 0161 737 2415
(Salford Primary Care Trust)
Patient List Size: 2000

Practice Manager Susan Watson

GP Rai Mohan BAISHNAB

Leicester Road Surgery
53 Leicester Road, Salford M7 4AS
Tel: 0161 708 9992 Fax: 0161 792 9800
(Salford Primary Care Trust)
Patient List Size: 2300

Practice Manager Veronica Clayhills

GP Wayne Sefton DAVIS

Limefield Medical Centre
8 Limefield Road, Salford M7 4LZ
Tel: 0161 721 4845 Fax: 0161 720 6494
(Salford Primary Care Trust)
Patient List Size: 3000

Practice Manager Glenda Marks

GP Samuel LEVENSON

Littleton Road Surgery
29 Littleton Road, Salford M6 6ED
Tel: 0161 736 7333 Fax: 0161 737 5199
(Salford Primary Care Trust)
Patient List Size: 3500

Practice Manager Ann Watt

GP Ambalang Odage K L DE SILVA

Lower Broughton Health Centre
Great Clowes Street, Salford M7 1RD
Tel: 0161 839 2730 Fax: 0161 832 1210
(Salford Primary Care Trust)
Patient List Size: 2800

Practice Manager Lyndsay Rodway

GP Mohammad SULTAN

Lower Broughton Health Centre
Great Clowes Street, Salford M7 1RD
Tel: 0161 839 2725 Fax: 0161 832 1210
(Salford Primary Care Trust)
Patient List Size: 2300

Practice Manager Joanne Faulkner

GP Hari Ranjan CHOWDHURY

Lower Broughton Health Centre
Great Clowes Street, Salford M7 1RD
Tel: 0161 839 2723 Fax: 0161 832 1210
(Salford Primary Care Trust)

Practice Manager Deborah Regan

GP Inder JEET, Dr KALRA

Lower Broughton Health Centre
Great Clowes Street, Salford M7 1RD
Tel: 0161 832 4915 Fax: 0161 832 1210
(Salford Primary Care Trust)

Mocha Parade Surgery
4-5 Mocha Parade, Salford M7 1QE
Tel: 0161 839 2721 Fax: 0161 819 1191
(Salford Primary Care Trust)
Patient List Size: 3850

Practice Manager Tania Kernaghan

GP Nooralla Noormohamed KASSAM, Almas PIRA

Ordsall Health Centre
Regent Park Surgery, Belfort Drive, Salford M5 3PP
Tel: 0161 872 2021 Fax: 0161 877 3592
Email: mandy.b.chall@gp-p87035.nhs.uk
(Salford Primary Care Trust)

Practice Manager Amanda Birchall

GP Jana ROBINSON, Susan COULSON, Katharine Maria SAXBY

Ordsall Health Centre
Belfort Drive, Salford M5 3PP
(Salford Primary Care Trust)

Practice Manager John Gregson

GP Neville Hyman FLETCHER

Ordsall Health Centre
Belfort Drive, Salford M5 3PP
(Salford Primary Care Trust)

GP Mahmood AZAM, Akhtar HASAN

Ordsall Health Centre
Belfort Drive, Salford M5 3PP
Tel: 0161 877 0564
(Salford Primary Care Trust)

Practice Manager Ruth Wilkins

GP Geoffrey Selwyn WILKINS

Salford Medical Centre
194 Langworthy Road, Salford M6 5PP
Tel: 0161 736 2651 Fax: 0161 745 8955
(Salford Primary Care Trust)
Patient List Size: 4000

Practice Manager Nicola Meachin

GP Abdul SALIM, Shamim-ur REHMAN, Zeb REHMAN

Sorrel Group Practice
Bolton Road Surgery, 23 Bolton Road, Salford M6 7HL
Tel: 0161 736 1616 Fax: 0161 737 1878
(Salford Primary Care Trust)

Practice Manager Rachel Bell

GP Niall Anthony FINEGAN, P F KALLIS, Luciano PICARDO, J SARA-RIVERO

The Willows Surgery
Lords Avenue, Salford M5 2JR
Tel: 0161 736 2356 Fax: 0161 737 2265
(Salford Primary Care Trust)
Patient List Size: 2500

Salisbury

A R Newton Dunn and Partners
61 New Street, Salisbury SP1 2PH
Tel: 01722 334402 Fax: 01722 410473
(South Wiltshire Primary Care Trust)
Patient List Size: 5500

Practice Manager Ann Rooney

GP Alan Richard NEWTON DUNN, Richard Gregory MANN, Paul McKINLEY

Barcroft Medical Practice
Barcroft Medical Centre, Amesbury, Salisbury SP4 7DL
Tel: 01980 623983 Fax: 01980 625530
(South Wiltshire Primary Care Trust)
Patient List Size: 9000

Practice Manager Jeremy Morris

GP Fionee Gail COLLINS, Helen Clare ADAMS, Andrew George MANTON, Katherine Mary MASH, Neil Harry MEARDON, Adrian John YULE

Bechers Brook Surgery
High Street, Fovant, Salisbury SP3 5JL
Tel: 01722 714789 Fax: 01722 714702
Email: gordonmorse@yahoo.com
(South Wiltshire Primary Care Trust)
Patient List Size: 1670

Practice Manager Stella Thake

GP Gordon Ridding MORSE

Bemerton Heath Surgery
Pembroke Road, Salisbury SP2 9DJ
Tel: 01722 411691 Fax: 01722 415047
Email: joy.underwood@gp-j83627.nhs.uk
Website: www.southwilts.co.uk/site/bemerton-heath-surgery
(South Wiltshire Primary Care Trust)
Patient List Size: 3298

Practice Manager J Underwood

GP Christine de Chair BAKER, Olivia CHAPPLE, John JAMESON

Castle Street Surgery
67 Castle Street, Salisbury SP1 3SP
Tel: 01722 322726 Fax: 01722 410315
(South Wiltshire Primary Care Trust)

Practice Manager Doris Grant

GP Kenneth Andrew CLARK, Graham Mark Higgins JAGGER, Margaret Elizabeth ROBERTSON, Jennifer Ann Stracey STONE, Gea VANDER ZEE

Cross Plain Surgery
84 Bulford Road, Durrington, Salisbury SP4 8DH
Tel: 0844 415 7959 Fax: 01980 655178
Email: ruth.freeman@gp-j83632.nhs.uk
(South Wiltshire Primary Care Trust)
Patient List Size: 3300

Practice Manager Ruth Freeman

GP William Morrow GRUMMITT, Paul Stuart MASLIN, Fiona Jane PEACH, Julia Vanessa WRIGHT

Dean Lane Surgery
Dean Lane, Sixpenny Handley, Salisbury SP5 5PA
Tel: 01725 552500 Fax: 01725 552029
(North Dorset Primary Care Trust)

GP Mark Christopher MORGAN, Elizabeth Mary Louise NODDER, Hugh John Wordsworth PELLY

Endless Street Doctors Surgery
72 Endless Street, Salisbury SP1 3UH
Tel: 01722 336441 Fax: 01722 410319
(South Wiltshire Primary Care Trust)
Patient List Size: 9000

Practice Manager Gillian Ibberson

GP Jane Elizabeth BOWDEN, Sherwood Major ELCOCK, Nazmul KAMAL, Kerry Michael O'CONNOR, Marek Thomas PODKOLINSKI, Frances Judith WALTERS

Grove House Surgery
18 Wilton Road, Salisbury SP2 7EE
Tel: 01722 333034 Fax: 01722 410308
Email: grove.house@gp-J83021.nhs.uk
(South Wiltshire Primary Care Trust)
Patient List Size: 6800

Practice Manager Barbara Tomlinson

GP Judith Vida BURNS, Robert Philip HEWETSON, Charles Alistair Newton SEARS, Peter SHARPE

Harcourt Medical Centre
Crane Bridge Road, Salisbury SP2 7TD
Tel: 01722 333214 Fax: 01722 421643
(South Wiltshire Primary Care Trust)
Patient List Size: 12500

Practice Manager S Kuczera

GP Christopher John NETTLE, Jeffrey Anthony EASTON, Timothy Edward MARKEY, Margaret Ruth MORRIS, John Peter Richard RAULT, Bernadette Mary THORNE

Howgrave-Graham and Partners
The Surgery, Moot Lane, Downton, Salisbury SP5 3QD
Tel: 01725 510296 Fax: 01725 513119
(South Wiltshire Primary Care Trust)

Practice Manager Monica Hales

GP Antony John HOWGRAVE-GRAHAM, Paul Brierley BORRELLI, Peter Charles DAVIES, Jayne Victoria KING

The Old Orchard Surgery
South Street, Wilton, Salisbury SP2 0JU
Tel: 01722 744775 Fax: 01722 746616
(South Wiltshire Primary Care Trust)
Patient List Size: 6300

Practice Manager Michael Cooney

GP Andy HALL, John FISHWICK, Sally HOUGHTON, Lynne MACREADY, Harriet MEADER

St Ann Street Surgery
82 St. Ann Street, Salisbury SP1 2PT
Tel: 01722 322624 Fax: 01722 410624
(South Wiltshire Primary Care Trust)

Practice Manager Michael Wilson

GP Robert Graham COLLIER, Christopher Michael Robert GLAYSHER, Catherine Susan HIGGINS, A P M REEVE, Nicholas Robert Yorke STANGER, Julian E TOTMAN

St Melor Surgery
St Melor House, Edwards Road, Amesbury, Salisbury SP4 7LT
Tel: 01980 622474 Fax: 01980 622475
(South Wiltshire Primary Care Trust)
Patient List Size: 5500

Practice Manager J Jones

GP Peter John THOMPSON, Jennifer Anne CALDER-SMITH, Stuart Vincett EASTMAN

The Surgery
High Street, Hindon, Salisbury SP3 6DJ
Tel: 01747 820222 Fax: 01747 820736
(South Wiltshire Primary Care Trust)
Patient List Size: 1900

Practice Manager Judith Tame

GP Patrick Michael CRAIG-McFEELY, Sally Ann HAYES

The Three Swans Surgery
Rollestone Street, Salisbury SP1 1DX
Tel: 01722 333548 Fax: 01722 503626
Website: www.3swanssurgery.nhs.uk
(South Wiltshire Primary Care Trust)

Patient List Size: 7400

Practice Manager Tessa Wakeman

GP Elizabeth STANGER, Hugh Robertson Lester BOND, Helena Maria McKEOWN, Michael Vivian MOORE, Matther TURNER

Till Valley Surgery

High Street, Shrewton, Salisbury SP3 4BZ
Tel: 01980 620259 Fax: 01980 620060
(South Wiltshire Primary Care Trust)

Practice Manager Liz Thomas

GP M THOMAS

Tisbury Surgery

Park Road, Tisbury, Salisbury SP3 6LF
Tel: 01747 870204 Fax: 01747 871023
(South Wiltshire Primary Care Trust)

Practice Manager Rosemary Eacott

GP John DALTON, Laurence CARTER

Whiteparish Surgery

Common Road, Whiteparish, Salisbury SP5 2SU
Tel: 01794 884269 Fax: 01794 885271
(South Wiltshire Primary Care Trust)
Patient List Size: 6200

Practice Manager E A Carter

GP Christopher Ronald GOTHAM, Rachel CLAPTON, Isabelle Anne Margaret DEAN, Martin ESSIGMAN, Rosemary Margaret PARRY

Wilton Health Centre

Wilton, Salisbury SP2 0HT
Tel: 01722 742404 Fax: 01722 744116
(South Wiltshire Primary Care Trust)
Patient List Size: 3500

Practice Manager David Browne

GP Richard BROWN, Jill BURNETT, Karen IRWIN

Saltash

Jackson and Partners

Port View Surgery, Higher Port View, Saltash PL12 4BU
Tel: 01752 847131 Fax: 01752 847124
(North and East Cornwall Primary Care Trust)
Patient List Size: 6100

Practice Manager Jean Ackrell

GP Sarah JACKSON, Christopher BOOTH, Susanne Christa CHARLTON, Philip John WEBSTER-HARRISON

The Lynher Surgery

St Germans, Saltash PL12 5LT
Tel: 01503 230358 Fax: 01503 230133
(North and East Cornwall Primary Care Trust)

Practice Manager Erith Amanda

GP Michael John ERITH

Quay Lane Surgery

Old Quay Lane, St Germans, Saltash PL12 5LH
Tel: 01503 230088 Fax: 01503 230713
(North and East Cornwall Primary Care Trust)
Patient List Size: 4200

Practice Manager Judy Carpenter

GP James Richard Armstrong MOORE, Simon FULLALOVE, Pennt THOMSON

Saltash Health Centre

Callington Road, Saltash PL12 6DL
Tel: 01752 842281 Fax: 01752 844651
(North and East Cornwall Primary Care Trust)
Patient List Size: 12500

Practice Manager Lynn Chenery

GP Robert Charles COOK, Alistair David BROADHEAD, Christine BROWN, Neville John DEVONPORT, Caroline Louise FOX, Robert Christopher Beresford KNEEN

Saltburn-by-the-Sea

Dundas Street West Surgery

6 Dundas Street West, Saltburn-by-the-Sea TS12 1BL
Tel: 01287 622207 Fax: 01287 623803
(Langbaurgh Primary Care Trust)
Patient List Size: 5900

Practice Manager John King

GP Michael Lloyd MILNER, Kevin Peter Francis FISH

East Cleveland Hospital

Alford Road, Brotton, Saltburn-by-the-Sea TS12 2FF
Tel: 01287 676215 Fax: 01287 678121
(Langbaurgh Primary Care Trust)
Patient List Size: 5360

Practice Manager Linda Campbell

GP Brian William CLEMENTS, Lisa Helen ROBERTS, John Christopher Robert SAXTON

The Health Centre

Byland Road, Skelton-in-Cleveland, Saltburn-by-the-Sea TS12 2NN
Tel: 01287 650430 Fax: 01287 651268
(Langbaurgh Primary Care Trust)
Patient List Size: 10800

Practice Manager S Bladen

GP Richard Anthony PARKIN, Allison ARMITAGE, Michael James BETTERTON, Jesus GONZALEZ-CASTRO, Alison Kate HARVIE, Fran HOOD, Peter Henry LAVELLE, Roger Fairfax NEVILLE-SMITH

Staithes Surgery

Seaton Crescent, Staithes, Saltburn-by-the-Sea TS13 5AY
Tel: 01947 840480 Fax: 01947 841034
(Scarborough, Whitby and Ryedale Primary Care Trust)

Practice Manager Jean Clennan

GP Graham CROFT, Stephen Alan JOHNSON

Woodside Surgery

High Street, Loftus, Saltburn-by-the-Sea TS13 4HW
Tel: 01287 640385 Fax: 01287 644071
(Langbaurgh Primary Care Trust)
Patient List Size: 7500

Practice Manager Joanne Westcott

GP Martin Stephen GLASBY, Roberto Giuseppe DALL'ARA, Christopher Michael DUNN, Carolyn Jane RIGBY, Richard Christopher RIGBY

Sandbach

Ashfields Primary Care Centre

Middlewich Road, Sandbach CW10 1EQ
Tel: 01270 275050 Fax: 01270 275055
(Central Cheshire Primary Care Trust)
Patient List Size: 20443

Practice Manager Christine Lanton

GP John Derrick ARMITAGE, David Lindsay BAKER, Peter John BROADBENT, S BROOME, Elizabeth Jane CUTTELL, Michael John OLVER, N PAUL, C ROBERTS, Amanda Kate ROSSON, Michael John TATE

The Commons Surgery

Sandbach CW11 1HR
Tel: 01270 764151 Fax: 01270 759944
(Central Cheshire Primary Care Trust)
Patient List Size: 7200

GP Robert Thomas BAXTER, Rachel S BROOME, Neil R PAUL, Charles Andrew ROBERTS

Sandhurst

Sandhurst Group Practice
72 Yorktown Road, Sandhurst GU47 9BT
Tel: 01252 872455 Fax: 01252 872456
(Bracknell Forest Primary Care Trust)
Patient List Size: 19500

Practice Manager Pam Watts

GP John Rhodes THING, Simon Nicholas BROWN, Izabela Zofia DAVIES, John FEATHERSTONE, Roger Paul HALLIWELL, Emma JOYNES, Nilesh KANJARIA, Rohail MALIK, Colleen Alison PIDGEON, James Robert Middleton SEDDON, Anita VAKIL

Sandown

Beech Grove Surgery
Mall Road, Brading, Sandown PO36 0DE
Tel: 01983 407775 Fax: 01983 406277
(Isle of Wight Primary Care Trust)

GP Peter BRAND, Jane Vivienne BRAND, Richard Simon LOACH, Christine Paula SEIGER

Sandown Medical Centre
Melville Street, Sandown PO36 8LD
Tel: 01983 402464 Fax: 01983 405781
(Isle of Wight Primary Care Trust)
Patient List Size: 11013

Practice Manager Karen Hermans

GP Peter James SUMMERHAYES, Hayley Louise ELSMORE, David John McMULLEN, Peter Graham RANDALL, Linda Mary REID, Hugh Miles TROWELL

Sandwich

The Butchery Surgery
7 The Butchery, Sandwich CT13 9DL
Tel: 01304 612138 Fax: 01304 620614
Email: the.surgery@gp-g82148.nhs.uk
(East Kent Coastal Teaching Primary Care Trust)
Patient List Size: 4000

Practice Manager Susan Harding

GP David Michael Julian GEEWATER, Patricia Mary MILLIGAN

The Market Place Surgery
Cattle Market, Sandwich CT13 9ET
Tel: 01304 613436/612589 Fax: 01304 613877
(East Kent Coastal Teaching Primary Care Trust)

Practice Manager Linda Wood

GP Alastair Moir CARNEGIE, Clare Elizabeth BIRCHALL, Anne Elise DAVIS, David John GREAVES, Christopher John HEALY

Sandy

Dr Reddy
12 St Neot's Road, Sandy SG19 1LB
Tel: 01767 683322 Fax: 01767 681161
(Bedfordshire Heartlands Primary Care Trust)
Patient List Size: 2860

Practice Manager Gerald Wells

GP Dr REDDY

Greensands Medical Practice
Brook End Surgery, Potton, Sandy SG19 2QS
Tel: 01767 260260 Fax: 01767 261777
(Bedfordshire Heartlands Primary Care Trust)
Patient List Size: 11200

Practice Manager Carole Peters

GP Michael BAKER, Laurence Karsten DRAKE, David Anthony HESLOP, Daniel JACKSON, Catherine JARVIS, Diana Landon TAINE, Hubertus VON BLUMENTHAL

Kings Road Surgery
27b Kings Road, Sandy SG19 1EJ
Tel: 01767 682277 Fax: 01767 691436
(Bedfordshire Heartlands Primary Care Trust)

Practice Manager Joyce Thirkell

GP Peter Donald GLEDHILL, Bridget Elizabeth BOURKE

Sandy Health Centre Medical Practice
Northcroft, Sandy SG19 1JQ
Tel: 01767 682525 Fax: 01767 681600
(Bedfordshire Heartlands Primary Care Trust)
Patient List Size: 7600

Practice Manager R Morris

GP Ajit Kumar KAPUR, Dr BAXTER, Steven HIGGINS, Dr PATEL, Gillian Denise SUMMERS

Sawbridgeworth

Central Surgery
Bell Street, Sawbridgeworth CM21 9AQ
Tel: 01279 724757 Fax: 01279 600717
(Royston, Buntingford and Bishop's Stortford Primary Care Trust)
Patient List Size: 11185

Practice Manager Sheila Keller

GP Peter Hans KELLER, Raquel Begona GONZALEZ CONTRERAS, Lloyd GUNETILLEKE, Deborah Margaret KEARNS

Saxmundham

The Surgery
Lambsale Meadow, North Entrance, Saxmundham IP17 1AS
Tel: 01728 602022
(Suffolk Coastal Primary Care Trust)

Practice Manager Jan Cameron

GP David William FOREMAN, Julie Anne EVANS, John Spencer HAVARD, Paul Michael Woodliffe MURPHY

Scarborough

Albemarle Surgery
27 Albemarle Crescent, Scarborough YO11 1XX
Tel: 01723 360098 Fax: 01723 501546
(Scarborough, Whitby and Ryedale Primary Care Trust)
Patient List Size: 4000

Practice Manager Carol Beswick

GP Ian Fraser FETTES, Ann Lucy Philippa BRENTNALL, Ian Robert HAMP, Patricia HUGHES

Belgrave Surgery
Lawrence House Medical Centre, 1 Belgrave Crescent, Scarborough YO11 1UB
Tel: 01723 361279 Fax: 01723 501589
Website: www.belgravesurgery.co.uk
(Scarborough, Whitby and Ryedale Primary Care Trust)
Patient List Size: 3665

Practice Manager Julianne Randji

GP Ruth Mary LALJEE, Andrew DAVIDSON, Nigel Charles FRASER

Claremont Surgery
56-60 Castle Road, Scarborough YO11 1XE
Tel: 01723 375050 Fax: 01723 378241
(Scarborough, Whitby and Ryedale Primary Care Trust)
Patient List Size: 6500

Practice Manager C Titley

GP David John KNOWELDEN, Fiona Jane BEARDSLEY, Gordon HAYES, Jane Ann TAYLOR, Alison Clare WILLIAMS

Danes Dyke Surgery
463A Scalby Road, Newby, Scarborough YO12 6UA
Tel: 01723 375343 Fax: 01723 501582
Email: sylvia.roche@gp-b82054.nhs.uk
Website: www.danesdykesurgery.com
(Scarborough, Whitby and Ryedale Primary Care Trust)
Patient List Size: 7400

Practice Manager Sylvia Roche

GP Nicholas Hugh WHELAN, Malcolm James ABRINES, Mark George LAWS, A POLKEY

Eastfield Group Practice
1 Eastway, Eastfield, Scarborough YO11 3LS
Tel: 01723 582297 Fax: 01723 582528
(Scarborough, Whitby and Ryedale Primary Care Trust)

Practice Manager Fay Ellis

GP Alan WALKER, Philip John HUGHES, Elizabeth Patricia NOBLE, Charles Michael SAFFMAN, Dipankar SENGUPTA

Falsgrave Surgery
Lawrence House Medical Centre, Belgrave Crescent, Scarborough YO11 1UB
Tel: 01723 360835 Fax: 01723 503220
(Scarborough, Whitby and Ryedale Primary Care Trust)
Patient List Size: 10000

Practice Manager Steve Greatorex

GP David Anthony OLDROYD, James ADAMSON, Susan Jane ADAMSON, Mark Andrew SCARBOROUGH, Sarah SCARBOROUGH, Sarah UTTING

Hackness Road Surgery
19 Hackness Road, Newby, Scarborough YO12 5DS
Tel: 01723 859302/506706 Fax: 01723 380920
(Scarborough, Whitby and Ryedale Primary Care Trust)

Practice Manager Lindsey Barker

GP Alison Judith HARK, Paul ROBINSON

Norwood House Surgery
Belle Vue Street, Scarborough YO12 7EJ
Tel: 01723 374485 Fax: 01723 501517
(Scarborough, Whitby and Ryedale Primary Care Trust)
Patient List Size: 7600

GP Jeremy John COPPACK, Lesley BARRON, Sunniva Anna Maria Theresia DE PONT, P M HIRSCHOWITZ, Anna L KING, Sarah LIVESEY

Peasholme Surgery
98 Tennyson Avenue, Scarborough YO12 7RE
Tel: 01723 378461 Fax: 01723 501335
(Scarborough, Whitby and Ryedale Primary Care Trust)
Patient List Size: 4200

Practice Manager Dagmar Moederle-Lumb

GP Douglas Andrew MOEDERLE-LUMB

Prospect Road Surgery
174 Prospect Road, Scarborough YO12 7LB
Tel: 01723 360178 Fax: 01723 501807
(Scarborough, Whitby and Ryedale Primary Care Trust)
Patient List Size: 8118

Practice Manager Pat Dunn

GP Judith Ann DAWES, Colette BROADHURST, Ronald Francis DIFFEY, Gaynor THOMPSON

Queens Corner Surgery
1 New Queen's Street, Scarborough YO12 7HL
Tel: 01723 378078 Fax: 01723 378010
(Scarborough, Whitby and Ryedale Primary Care Trust)
Patient List Size: 1996

Practice Manager Margaret Germaine

GP Isabella Deri PITTS

South Cliff Surgery
56 Esplanade Road, Scarborough YO11 2AU
Tel: 01723 360451 Fax: 01723 353518
(Scarborough, Whitby and Ryedale Primary Care Trust)
Patient List Size: 5200

Practice Manager Su Hutchcroft, Doreen Walsh

GP Shashi CHAWLA, Andrew John DAVIDSON, Kathleen Mary HALLORAN

The Surgery
53 Pickering Road, West Ayton, Scarborough YO13 9JF
Tel: 01723 863100 Fax: 01723 862902
(Scarborough, Whitby and Ryedale Primary Care Trust)
Patient List Size: 7649

Practice Manager Pam Saltmer

GP Paul John ROBINSON, David Samuel AMES, Louise Jane Clare BARTLETT, T A CAPPLEMAN, L HOBKINSON, John Mark Ridley REAY, James ROBERTSON

The Surgery
8A Denison Avenue, Seamer, Scarborough YO12 4QU
(Scarborough, Whitby and Ryedale Primary Care Trust)

GP Ronald Wilfred WARD, David Samuel AMES, John Mark Ridley REAY

Scunthorpe

Ashby Clinic
Collum Lane, Scunthorpe DN16 2SZ
Tel: 01724 281552 Fax: 01724 822580
Email: drghayes@epulse.net
(North Lincolnshire Primary Care Trust)
Patient List Size: 2200

Practice Manager Joy Mosey

GP Graham James HAYES

Ashby Clinic
Collum Lane, Scunthorpe DN16 2SZ
Tel: 01724 271877
(North Lincolnshire Primary Care Trust)

GP S BALASANTHIRAN

Ashby Turn Primary Care Centre
The Link, Scunthorpe DN16 2UT
Tel: 01724 842051 Fax: 01724 280346
Email: ashbyturnsurgery@compuserve.com
(North Lincolnshire Primary Care Trust)

Practice Manager C J Hazle

GP Michael Francis STANFORD, Trevor James GRATTAGE, Alan Marshall LEES, Francisco TERREROS-BERRUTE, Christopher John TRUEMAN, Jane WIDDERS

Church Lane Medical Centre
Orchid Rise, Off Church Lane, Scunthorpe DN15 7AN
Tel: 01724 864341 Fax: 01724 876441
(North Lincolnshire Primary Care Trust)

Practice Manager Cynthia Brown

GP John Robert MELROSE, Joanna MORRIS, Nicholas STEWART, Rekha WORAH

The Medical Centre
78 Oswald Road, Scunthorpe DN15 7PG
Tel: 01724 843168
(North Lincolnshire Primary Care Trust)
Patient List Size: 4000

Practice Manager Mary Raha

GP Arun Kumar RAHA, Shivnathram RAJKUMAR

Medical Centre
Cambridge Avenue, Bottesford, Scunthorpe DN16 3LG
Tel: 01724 842415 Fax: 01724 271437

(North Lincolnshire Primary Care Trust)
Patient List Size: 15000

Practice Manager Judith Muir

GP Alistair Scott KERSS, Frank George BAKER, Mono BHADRA, Thennavan ELANGO, Gordon McGLASHAM, Clive George NEWMAN, Diana Elizabeth WHITE

Shambhulingappa and Ugargol
58E Cottage Beck Road, Scunthorpe DN16 1LE
Tel: 01724 843744 Fax: 01724 843748
(North Lincolnshire Primary Care Trust)
Patient List Size: 4375

GP Dr SHAMBHULINGAPPA, Dr UGARGOL

The Surgery
20 - 22 Doncaster Road, Scunthorpe DN15 7RQ
Tel: 01724 842852 Fax: 01724 866187
(North Lincolnshire Primary Care Trust)
Patient List Size: 2230

Practice Manager Elaine Southern Gore

GP Rakhi BASU

The Surgery
Manlake Avenue, Winterton, Scunthorpe DN15 9TA
Tel: 01724 732202 Fax: 01724 734992
(North Lincolnshire Primary Care Trust)

Practice Manager Jenny Burgon

GP John Rodney MITCHELL, John Alexander ISAACS, M A SARVESVARAN, Nicholas SUMMERTON, Russell John WALSHAW, Patricia Anne WEBSTER

The Surgery
275 Ashby Road, Scunthorpe DN16 2AB
Tel: 01724 843375 Fax: 01724 270101
Email: surgery.ashbyrd@virgin.net
(North Lincolnshire Primary Care Trust)
Patient List Size: 4900

Practice Manager Patricia Hill

GP Martin J DWYER, PAUAN TANDON

The Surgery
291 Ashby Road, Scunthorpe DN16 2AB
Tel: 01724 864426/7/8 Fax: 01724 282570
Email: drkapil@globalnet.co.uk
(North Lincolnshire Primary Care Trust)
Patient List Size: 14800

Practice Manager Christine Tandy

GP Gyan Prakash KAPIL, Girgis HENALLA, John KENNEDY, Patricia McCORMACK, Lalitha RAMAN, Eugene Paul Mary RYAN

The Surgery
27 Comforts Avenue, Scunthorpe DN15 6PN
Tel: 01724 842377 Fax: 01724 842350
(North Lincolnshire Primary Care Trust)
Patient List Size: 2870

GP Dipak Kumar BASU

Trent View Medical Practice
45 Trent View, Keadby, Scunthorpe DN17 3DR
Tel: 01724 782209 Fax: 01724 784472
(North Lincolnshire Primary Care Trust)

Practice Manager Wendy Buttrick

GP Omma AYE, Brian Francis BARBIER, Dr BHADRA, Andrea Jean FRASER, Ernest Prabhu Kumar PHILLIPS, Margaret Lily SANDERSON, John ZACHARIAS

West Common Lane Medical Centre
West Common Lane, Dorchester Road, Scunthorpe DN17 1YH
Tel: 01724 870414 Fax: 01724 877730
(North Lincolnshire Primary Care Trust)
Patient List Size: 4500

Practice Manager Wendy High

GP Andrew William LEE, C J HALL, P STRINA, O TERREROS

Seaford

Old School Surgery
Church Street, Seaford BN25 1HH
Tel: 01323 890072 Fax: 01323 492340
(Eastbourne Downs Primary Care Trust)
Patient List Size: 6600

Practice Manager Gail Whiting

GP Shan Kumar PALIT, Ian BAYLES, Joanna Mary BAYLES, Francis NICHOLLS

Seaford Health Centre
Dane Road, Seaford BN25 1DH
Tel: 01323 490022 Fax: 01323 492156
(Eastbourne Downs Primary Care Trust)
Patient List Size: 17500

Practice Manager S Smith

GP John Michael COCKBURN, Mark Hodson BARNES, George Murray BAYNE, Daniel Henry ELLIOTT, Roger William HARVEY, John Gerard JONES, Caroline Jane LEWIS, Kenneth James McGHEE, Craig Stanley MELLOR, Brian James PICKERING, Mary-Rose Byars SHEARS

Seaham

Adelaide Row Medical Centre
1-2 Adelaide Row, Seaham SR7 7EF
Tel: 0191 5817661 Fax: 0191 513 0548
(Easington Primary Care Trust)
Patient List Size: 4300

Practice Manager Gillian Moyle

GP Raj Kumar DUSAD, Usha DUSAD

Deneside Medical Centre
The Avenue, Deneside, Seaham SR7 8LF
Tel: 0191 5130884 Fax: 0191 581 1855
(Easington Primary Care Trust)

Practice Manager Tracey Milburn

GP Asha Lata KAPOOR, Kulbhushan Rai KAPOOR

Deneside Medical Centre
The Avenue, Deneside, Seaham SR7 8LF
Tel: 0191 513 0202 Fax: 0191 581 6764
Website: www.reddy-surgery.co.uk
(Easington Primary Care Trust)
Patient List Size: 4500

Practice Manager Patricia Jobson

GP C Narayana REDDY, Kaukutla Venkat REDDY

Murton Medical Centre
20 Woods Terrace East, Murton, Seaham SR7 9AB
Tel: 0191 5170170 Fax: 0191 5264289
(Easington Primary Care Trust)
Patient List Size: 7200

Practice Manager L A Williams

GP John INGHAM, Clare LAZENBY, Stephen Mark MUSCAT, Daljit Singh RANGAR

The Surgery
Marlborough, Seaham SR7 7TS
Tel: 0191 5812866 Fax: 0191 5130393
(Easington Primary Care Trust)

Practice Manager Maureen Hudson

GP Mohan Edward GEORGE, Nripen BARKATAKI, Jane Veronica GUSTAFSSON, B K MITRA, David Charles NAPIER

Seascale

Dr B Walker and Partners
Health Centre, Gosforth Road, Seascale CA20 1PN
Tel: 01946 728101 Fax: 01946 727895
(West Cumbria Primary Care Trust)

Practice Manager Jane Blinco

GP Barrie WALKER, Paul Adrian CARHART, Kathryn Margaret ILLSLEY, Sheena Anne JAY, Michael Denis STEVENSON

Seaton

The Seaton and Colyton Medical Practice
Seaton Health Centre, Harepath Road, Seaton EX12 2DU
Tel: 01297 20877 Fax: 01297 23031
(East Devon Primary Care Trust)
Patient List Size: 6550

Practice Manager David Flatman

GP Michael Frederick ASKEW, Christopher John BASTIN, Roger BRAMLEY, John Alexander COOP, Peta Sedgley WEBB

Townsend House Medical Centre
49 Harepath Road, Seaton EX12 2RY
Tel: 01297 20616 Fax: 01297 20810
(East Devon Primary Care Trust)
Patient List Size: 6800

Practice Manager Annette Mungean

GP Patrick Jonathon Scott FARRELL, Robert J DANIELS, Julian Richard HURST, Giles Hugh PITT

Sedbergh

Brantgarth
Guldrey Lane, Sedbergh LA10 5DS
Tel: 015396 20239
(Morecambe Bay Primary Care Trust)

GP John Ralph SYRED

The Health Centre
Loftus Hill, Sedbergh LA10 5RX
Tel: 01539 620218 Fax: 01539 620265
(Morecambe Bay Primary Care Trust)

Practice Manager Anne Benville

GP Pauline Ann ORR, William Graham ORR

Selby

Beech Tree Surgery
68 Doncaster Road, Selby YO8 9AJ
Tel: 01757 703933 Fax: 01757 213473
(Selby and York Primary Care Trust)
Patient List Size: 14500

Practice Manager Richard Gregory

GP Patrick John McGRANN, David HEPWORTH, Nicholas JACKSON, Stephanie Patricia MERRIFIELD, Else Jane SCOTT, Mark Edward WILLIAMS

Dr A J Janik and Partners
12 Fox Lane, Thorpe Willoughby, Selby YO8 9NA
Tel: 01977 682202 Fax: 01977 681628
(Selby and York Primary Care Trust)
Patient List Size: 9000

Practice Manager Lisa Furness

GP Antoni Jerzy JANIK, William St John HIRST, Stefano Girgorio LOVISETTO, Anne Catherine Mary MACKENZIE, Susan Frances MURPHY, Susan STUTTARD

Portland Lodge Surgery
Main Street, Hemingbrough, Selby YO8 7QT

Practice Manager Mary McLellan Jackson

GP Alan John BROWN, Simon Richard HAWORTH

Posterngate Surgery
Portholme Road, Selby YO8 4QH
Tel: 01757 702561 Fax: 01757 213295
Email: enquiries@posterngate.co.uk
Website: www.posterngate.co.uk
(Selby and York Primary Care Trust)
Patient List Size: 14000

Practice Manager Mary Jackson

GP David William EDWARDS, Julia A BATTY, Paul Richard DAVIS, Simon Richard HAWORTH, Lisa Margaret HILDORE, John David REID, Andrew James STANFORD

Scott Road Medical Centre
Scott Road, Selby YO8 4BL
Tel: 01757 700231 Fax: 01757 213647
(Selby and York Primary Care Trust)
Patient List Size: 10000

Practice Manager David Addinall

GP Ian Adrian LEWIS, Graham BOND, Mary Audrey CHATWORTHY, Caroline DOCHERTY, Paul Francis DOCHERTY, Ernest Renny LORD

Settle

Townhead Surgeries
Townhead, Settle BD24 9JA
Tel: 01729 822611 Fax: 01729 892916
(Craven, Harrogate and Rural District Primary Care Trust)
Patient List Size: 9250

Practice Manager Elizabeth Wrigley

GP Eric WARD, Ashley DAVIES, William Walton HALL, Dr KING, John Malcolm LEWIS, Clare Imogen LITTLEJOHN, Hilary MOAKES, Colin Jeffrey RENWICK

Sevenoaks

Amherst Medical Practice
21 St Botolphs Road, Sevenoaks TN13 3AQ
Tel: 01732 459255 Fax: 01732 450751
(South West Kent Primary Care Trust)
Patient List Size: 13700

Practice Manager Wendy Bardell

GP Neil David ARNOTT, Ferella HARRLET, Richard G HUSBAND, Cathryn Jane LAY, Francese LYCAS, Alison LYNAM, Andrew Cathcart ROXBURGH

Borough Green Medical Practice
Quarry Hill Road, Borough Green, Sevenoaks TN15 8RQ
Tel: 01732 883161 Fax: 01732 886319
(South West Kent Primary Care Trust)
Patient List Size: 12500

Practice Manager Jude Unwin

GP David Gordon THOMAS, Antony Michael DIBBLE, Caroline GRANT, Celina KEENOR, Mark PASOLA

Otford Medical Practice
Leonard Avenue, Otford, Sevenoaks TN14 5RB
Tel: 01959 524633 Fax: 01959 525086
(South West Kent Primary Care Trust)
Patient List Size: 10200

Practice Manager W Anae

GP David Kelk EVANS, Nicholas John FARRAWAY, Gillian Margaret HAWORTH, Simon Charles HAWORTH, Meriel Jennifer Claire WYNTER

South Park Medical Practice
South Park, Sevenoaks TN13 1ED
Tel: 01732 744200 Fax: 01732 744206
Email: pblandy@aol.com
Website: www.southparkmedical.com
(South West Kent Primary Care Trust)
Patient List Size: 1300

Practice Manager Christine Dean

GP Paul Barrie LANDY, Nitika APPLEBY, Kevin BLEWETT

St John's Medical Practice
39 St. John's Hill, Sevenoaks TN13 3NT
Tel: 01732 747202 Fax: 01732 747218
Website: www.stjohnsmedicalpractice.co.uk
(South West Kent Primary Care Trust)
Patient List Size: 8284

Practice Manager Julia Gilliat-Smith

GP Keren Elizabeth HULL, A ROBSON, S SHAW, Susan Valerie TOOTHILL

Town Medical Centre
25 London Road, Sevenoaks TN13 1AR
Tel: 01732 454545 Fax: 01732 462181
Website: www.townmedicalcentre.freeserve.co.uk
(South West Kent Primary Care Trust)
Patient List Size: 5800

Practice Manager M Robinson

GP Philip John RAZZELL, Jennifer Anne COX, Olaf Uwe HOFMANN, Andrea Jane TAYLOR

West Kingsdown Medical Centre
London Road, West Kingsdown, Sevenoaks TN15 6EJ
Tel: 01474 855000 Fax: 01474 855001
(Dartford, Gravesham and Swanley Primary Care Trust)
Patient List Size: 2000

Practice Manager J Walker

GP Richard Paul DUNN

West Kingsdown Medical Centre
London Road, West Kingsdown, Sevenoaks TN15 6EJ
Tel: 01474 855000 Fax: 01474 855015
(Dartford, Gravesham and Swanley Primary Care Trust)

GP A MacDONNELL

Shaftesbury

The Shaftesbury Practice
Abbey View Medical Centre, Salisbury Road, Shaftesbury SP7 8DH
Tel: 01747 856700 Fax: 01747 856701
(North Dorset Primary Care Trust)
Patient List Size: 13250

Practice Manager Penny Foster

GP Christopher Tooth HEWETSON, Suzanne DADDY, Richard Joseph EMMS, Simon Scadding HORNER, Simone Melinda WALTERS, Andrew Wickham WEIR, David Michael WYNN-MACKENZIE

Shanklin

Shanklin Medical Centre
1 Carter Road, Shanklin PO37 7HR
Tel: 01983 862245 Fax: 01983 862310
(Isle of Wight Primary Care Trust)

GP Brian Edwin STONE, Alan Gibson FRAME, Graham Michael GENT, Rajiv Shantaram GHURYE, John William RIVERS, Janet Margaret WILLETTS

Sheerness

Alexandra Villa
19 Marine Parade, Sheerness ME12 2AP
Tel: 01795 585058 Fax: 01795 585158
(Swale Primary Care Trust)
Patient List Size: 5193

Practice Manager Marcia Packer

GP Fiona Jane ARMSTRONG, Michael Peter ROWE

Crescent Surgery
8 The Crescent, Halfway, Sheerness ME12 3BQ
Tel: 01795 662941
(Swale Primary Care Trust)
Patient List Size: 2838

GP Valiyakalayil Kesavan RAMU

Dr Chandran
231-235 High Street, Sheerness ME12 1UR
Tel: 01795 585001 Fax: 01795 663949
(Swale Primary Care Trust)
Patient List Size: 4186

Practice Manager Sheila Reynolds

GP Subash CHANDRAN, V RANGASWAMY, R RAY

Dr Murthy
Healthy Living Centre, Royal Road, Sheerness
Tel: 01795 585105
(Swale Primary Care Trust)
Patient List Size: 2522

Practice Manager Lesley Cockell

GP S R S MURTHY

High Street Surgery
231-235 High Street, Sheerness ME12 1UR
Tel: 01795 580909 Fax: 01795 665656
(Swale Primary Care Trust)
Patient List Size: 4459

Practice Manager Shaheen Ahmed

GP M AHMED, Mohsen Mohamed El-Sayed FAHMY

Minster Medical Centre
Abbey Ward, Sheppey Community Hospital, Wards Hill Road, Minster-on-Sea, Sheerness ME12 2LN
Tel: 01795 877714
(Swale Primary Care Trust)
Patient List Size: 2081

Practice Manager Juliet Henderson

GP O FERDINAID

The 'Om' Medical Centre
Wood Street, Sheerness ME12 1UA
Tel: 01795 580402 Fax: 01795 461318
Website: ommedicalcentre.co.uk
(Swale Primary Care Trust)
Patient List Size: 5631

Practice Manager Caroline Howard

GP K N PRASAD, G B SAHU

St Georges Medical Centre
55 St Georges Avenue, Sheerness ME12 1QU
Tel: 01795 663481
(Swale Primary Care Trust)
Patient List Size: 12142

Practice Manager Dawn Benjamin

GP Patrick Pearse D'ARCY, U OTA, A S PANNU, M PATEL, B N PRASAD, D S UPPAL, J K UPPAL

Sheffield

Abbey Lane Surgery
23 Abbey Lane, Sheffield S8 0BJ
Tel: 0114 274 5360 Fax: 0114 274 9580
(Sheffield South West Primary Care Trust)
Patient List Size: 2700

Practice Manager Sandra Street

GP John DAVIES, Helen TALLANTYRE

Avenue Medical Practice
7 Reney Avenue, Sheffield S8 7FH
Tel: 0114 237 7649
(Sheffield South West Primary Care Trust)
Patient List Size: 8700

Practice Manager Anne Sharpe

GP R G JOHNS, Richard John BARNES, Joseph Gerald BENJAMIN, Sally Elizabeth COLVER, David St John LIVESEY, Brigitta Elizabeth NORRIS

Barnsley Road Surgery
899 Barnsley Road, Sheffield S5 0QJ
Tel: 0845 242 2496 Fax: 0114 226 2997
(North Sheffield Primary Care Trust)
Patient List Size: 3000

Practice Manager Janette Burger

GP Anil GROVER, Wigdan ISSA

Baslow Road Surgery
148-150 Baslow Road, Totley, Sheffield S17 4DR
Tel: 0114 236 9957 Fax: 0114 262 0756
(Sheffield South West Primary Care Trust)
Patient List Size: 8800

GP Michael Anthony COLLINS, Scot Peter DARLING, Gerard LEIGH, John Fraser McKENNA, Stephen MOORHEAD, Tracy SHAW, Patrica STRODE

Beighton Health Centre
Queens Road, Beighton, Sheffield S20 1BJ
Tel: 0114 269 5061
Email: beighton@aol.com
(South East Sheffield Primary Care Trust)

Practice Manager Jackie Ashton

GP Trefor John ROSCOE, Julia Caroline BOWERS, S J ELLIS, Sandra Jane NEHRING, Alison RAINFORD, Rosemary Ann WELCH

Belgrave Medical Centre
22 Asline Road, Sheffield S2 4UJ
Tel: 0114 255 1184
(South East Sheffield Primary Care Trust)

Practice Manager G Ehiteley

GP R J M PASCOE, Robert Desmond WEIR, V A BOWRY, Christine KELL, Lucy Victoria MANNING, R J PARTINGTON, R J TAYLOR, M J F TOMSON

Bents Green Surgery
98 Bents Road, Sheffield S11 9RL
Tel: 0114 236 0641 Fax: 0114 262 1069
Website: www.bentsgreensurgery.org.uk
(Sheffield South West Primary Care Trust)
Patient List Size: 2492

Practice Manager Kathryn Parkin

GP Christine ANSONS, Sarah Ann WHITE

Birley Health Centre
120 Birley Lane, Sheffield S12 3BP
Tel: 0114 239 2541 Fax: 0114 264 5814
Email: birley.hc@gp-c88025.nhs.uk
(South East Sheffield Primary Care Trust)
Patient List Size: 8300

Practice Manager John Dixon

GP Dilys Ann NOBLE, Sarah Theresa ALLEN, Michael Simon BOYLE, Gawain Pennant DAVIES, Charles Thomas HEATLEY

Bluebell Medical Centre
356 Bluebell Road, Sheffield S5 6BS
Tel: 0845 120 9944 Fax: 0114 261 8074
Email: bluebellsurgery@gp-c88033.nhs.uk
(North Sheffield Primary Care Trust)
Patient List Size: 3920

Practice Manager Christine Hitchmough

GP Jessica Cornelia St. Helier TWENEY, N J MATHERS, Rachel PETTINGER, Robert Alan SHIRLEY

Buchanan Road Surgery
72 Buchanan Road, Sheffield S5 8AL
Tel: 0845 1222 582 Fax: 0114 257 7369
(North Sheffield Primary Care Trust)
Patient List Size: 4800

Practice Manager Michelle Richards

GP Sandra BURGOYNE, Gaynor Louise FLETCHER, Helen Elizabeth STOCKDALE, W H VENNELLS

Burncross Surgery
1 Bevan Way, Chapeltown, Sheffield S35 1RN
Tel: 0114 246 6052 Fax: 0114 245 0276
(North Sheffield Primary Care Trust)
Patient List Size: 16900

Practice Manager Mary Burbidge

GP Gary CHAMBERS, Richard Timothy KEMP, Caroline Ann MILLS, Amar Nath RUGHANI, Eugene Augustyn RYBINSKI, W A SHAW, William Edward WARREN

Burngreave Road Surgery
5 Burngreave Road, Sheffield S3 9DA
Tel: 0114 272 2858 Fax: 0114 279 8004
(North Sheffield Primary Care Trust)
Patient List Size: 6078

Practice Manager Carol Ward

GP Bryan HOPWOOD, Margaret Ann HOBDEN, Peter Nicholas MOONEY

Carrfield Medical Centre
Carrfield Street, Sheffield S8 9SG
Tel: 0114 258 4724
(South East Sheffield Primary Care Trust)

GP Sweeta SIVARAJAN

Carteknowle and Dore Medical Practice
1 Carterknowle Road, Sheffield S7 2DW
Tel: 0114 255 1218 Fax: 0114 258 4418
(Sheffield South West Primary Care Trust)

GP Michael John Yarnton RUCK, Brendan Marcus CHARLES, Nicholas Eric GREEN, Barbara Caroline Anne KING, Frances Patricia O'CONNOR, Dominic Sean OTTEY, Anthony John SHAW

The Crookes Practice
203 School Road, Sheffield S10 1GN
Tel: 0114 268 6928 Fax: 0114 266 4526
(Sheffield West Primary Care Trust)
Patient List Size: 7400

Practice Manager Martyn Heeley

GP Annabelle MASCOTT, Ellie CARR, Claire REYNOLDS, Alison RIDSDALE, Mark ROGERS

Crookes Valley Medical Centre
1 Barber Road, Sheffield S10 1EA
Tel: 0114 266 0703 Fax: 0114 267 8354
(Sheffield West Primary Care Trust)
Patient List Size: 3550

Practice Manager Margaret Bailey

GP Smad S GABRAWI

Crystals Peaks Medical Centre
Crystal Peaks, 15 Peaks Mount, Sheffield S20 7HZ
Tel: 0114 251 0040 Fax: 0114 251 0954
(South East Sheffield Primary Care Trust)
Patient List Size: 7200

Practice Manager Alan Hancock

GP Mark ANDVZEJOWSKI, Susan BOWMAN, George Scott DAVISON, Catherine May JEFFCOATE, Wasif Daood KITTO

Darnall Community Health
246 Darnall Road, Darnall, Sheffield S9 5AN
Tel: 0114 226 2600 Fax: 0114 221 2618
Email: darnallcommh.admin@gp-C88069.nhs.uk
(South East Sheffield Primary Care Trust)
Patient List Size: 5250

GP Jack Maciej CZAUDERNA, Rhada GRIMSHAW, Jane HEATHCOTE, Mike NUTT, Merriel Victoria REID

Darnall Health Centre
2 York Road, Sheffield S9 5DH
Tel: 0114 244 1681 Fax: 0114 242 1160
(South East Sheffield Primary Care Trust)
Patient List Size: 3500

Practice Manager Pat Spyve

GP Jane Ellen CHAPMAN, Stephen John SWINDEN

Deepcar Medical Centre
241-245 Manchester Road, Deepcar, Sheffield S36 2QZ
Tel: 0114 288 2146 Fax: 0114 283 1131
(Sheffield West Primary Care Trust)
Patient List Size: 4500

Practice Manager Sue Lambert

GP Kadicheeni Jacob DAVIS, Gillian DASENT-ALI, Thottungal Antony FRANCIS

Derbyshire Lane Practice
213 Derbyshire Lane, Sheffield S8 8SA
Tel: 0114 255 0972 Fax: 0114 255 0298
(Sheffield South West Primary Care Trust)
Patient List Size: 5500

Practice Manager Barbara Crowther

GP Philip John DEAKIN, Jeremy Ian CRITCHLOW, Margaret E DUNCAN, Wendy Yvonne HUGHES

Devonshire Green Medical Centre
126 Devonshire Street, Sheffield S3 7SF
Tel: 0114 272 1626 Fax: 0114 272 8637
(Sheffield West Primary Care Trust)
Patient List Size: 6200

GP Paul Ransome HARVEY, Elizabeth Sarah ALLSOPP, Helen Rhoda BRIDDON, Penelope Jane HARVEY, Graham Lonsdale Gerald McALL, Graham PETTINGER

The Dovercourt Surgery
309 City Road, Sheffield S2 5HJ
Tel: 0114 270 0997 Fax: 0114 276 6786
(South East Sheffield Primary Care Trust)
Patient List Size: 2350

Practice Manager Paul Wike

GP Maria Grazyna READ, Jane Elizabeth GORDON, Michael Neil NUTT

Dronfield Health Centre
High Street, Dronfield, Sheffield S18 1PY
Tel: 01246 419040 Fax: 01246 290882
(North Eastern Derbyshire Primary Care Trust)

Practice Manager Christine Stanley

GP Beverley TURNER, Richard BULL

Duke Medical Centre
28 Talbot Road, Sheffield S2 2TD
Tel: 0114 272 0689 Fax: 0114 275 1916
(South East Sheffield Primary Care Trust)

GP Patrick Niall BRYSON, Amir AFZAL, Diana Margaret LIGHTFOOT, Michael Damien MURTON

Dunninc Road Surgery
28 Dunninc Road, Shiregreen, Sheffield S5 0AE
Tel: 0845 124 2289 Fax: 0114 257 0069
Email: dunninc.pmanager@gp-C88643.nhs.uk
(North Sheffield Primary Care Trust)
Patient List Size: 3100

Practice Manager S M Barrett

GP D K CHATTERJEE

Dykes Hall Medical Centre
156 Dykes Hall Road, Sheffield S6 4GQ
Tel: 0114 232 3236 Fax: 0114 281 2108
(Sheffield West Primary Care Trust)

Practice Manager Barbara Bannister

GP Bronwen Myfanwy WHITE, John Scott BENNS, Gary BUTLER, Robert Hedley PURDY, Rosemary RAFFERTY, Jane SCHOLEFIELD, Steven THOMAS

Ecclesfield Group Practice
96A Mill Road, Ecclesfield, Sheffield S35 9XQ
Tel: 0845 120 4443 Fax: 0114 257 1935
(North Sheffield Primary Care Trust)
Patient List Size: 7600

Practice Manager S Kirby

GP Paul JEAVONS, Geoffrey Michael BUTCHER, Margaret Ann HACKNEY, Stephanie Nanette LEDINGHAM, Richard OLIVER

Elm Lane Surgery
104 Elm Lane, Sheffield S5 7TW
Tel: 0845 124 2624 Fax: 0114 257 1260
(North Sheffield Primary Care Trust)
Patient List Size: 5155

Practice Manager Margaret Turner

GP Desmond Andrew KEATING, Claire Elaine PINCHES, Valerie Susan SWALES

Emmett Carr Surgery
Abbey Place, Renishaw, Sheffield S21 3TY
Tel: 01246 430200 Fax: 01246 430203
(North Eastern Derbyshire Primary Care Trust)
Patient List Size: 4000

Practice Manager Margaret Fry

GP Hazel McMURRAY, Andrew HILTON, Steven LLOYD

Falkland House Surgery
2a Falkland Road, Sheffield S11 7PL
Tel: 0114 266 0285
(Sheffield South West Primary Care Trust)

GP Susan Catherine EILBECK, Thomas Robert COSSHAM

Far Lane Medical Centre
1 Far Lane, Sheffield S6 4FA
Tel: 0114 234 3229
(Sheffield West Primary Care Trust)

GP Peter John KING, Clive Pearson HERDMAN, Ravin Dinesh NAIK, Richard Alexander SWANN

Firth Park Road Surgery
400 Firth Park Road, Sheffield S5 6HH
Tel: 0114 242 6406 Fax: 0114 242 1966
Email: firthpark.surgery@gp-C88035.nhs.uk
(North Sheffield Primary Care Trust)
Patient List Size: 7200

Practice Manager Julian Stevens

GP Colin Stuart SHAWCROSS, Kathryn Elizabeth BROWN, Andrew FERGUSON, Andrew John GODDEN, Joanne HOPKINS, Leigh SORSBIE

Foxhill Medical Centre
363 Halifax Road, Sheffield S6 1AF
Tel: 0114 232 2055 Fax: 0114 285 5963
(North Sheffield Primary Care Trust)

Practice Manager Mandy Neville

GP Ian Wallace DAVIDSON, Thomas David HELLER, Ian David Janardan NERURKAR, Karine NOHR, Amanda Jane ROSARIO, Rachel WALSH

Gleadless Medical Centre
636 Gleadless Road, Sheffield S14 1PQ
Tel: 0114 239 6475 Fax: 0114 264 2277
(South East Sheffield Primary Care Trust)
Patient List Size: 8800

Practice Manager Denise Wilson

GP Christopher Joseph DAVIS, Sally BROWN, Robert Michael GORDON, Geoffrey Martin Kenneth SCHRECKER, Mary Catherine WREN

Gomersall Lane Surgery
2 Gomersall Lane, Dronfield, Sheffield S18 1RU
Tel: 01246 296600 Fax: 01246 296613
(North Eastern Derbyshire Primary Care Trust)

Practice Manager Michelle Batty

GP Peter ALLAMBY, Miles DAVIDSON

Granville Road Surgery
296 Granville Road, Sheffield S2 2RT
Tel: 0114 272 3638
(South East Sheffield Primary Care Trust)
Patient List Size: 2000

Practice Manager Johanne Shirt

GP Samuel John BLOWER, Mary Helen RAMSAY

Green Lane Surgery
18 Green Lane, Dronfield, Sheffield S18 2LZ
Tel: 01246 412332 Fax: 01246 411956
(North Eastern Derbyshire Primary Care Trust)

Practice Manager Kathleen Maufe

GP Susan ALLSOP

Greenhill Health Centre
482 Lupton Road, Sheffield S8 7NQ
Tel: 0114 237 2961 Fax: 0114 283 9962
(Sheffield South West Primary Care Trust)

Practice Manager Carole Burley

GP John REVILL, Deborah Celia TURNER

Greystones Medical Centre
33 Greystones Road, Sheffield S11 7BJ
Tel: 0114 266 6528 Fax: 0114 266 0801
Email: greystones.surgery@gp-C88652.nhs.uk
(Sheffield South West Primary Care Trust)

Practice Manager Elizabeth Ann Fisher

GP Christopher John ATKINS, Edward John SNELSON

Hackenthorpe Medical Centre
Main Street, Hackenthorpe, Sheffield S12 4LA
Fax: 0114 251 0539
(South East Sheffield Primary Care Trust)
Patient List Size: 6900

Practice Manager Richard Wingfield

GP C K DA SILVA, Joanne Pamela BECKETT, Andrew Michael PARKES, Julie Elizabeth PYCOCK

Handsworth Grange Medical Centre
432 Handsworth Road, Sheffield S13 9BZ
Tel: 0114 269 7505 Fax: 0114 269 8535
(South East Sheffield Primary Care Trust)
Patient List Size: 5500

GP Abdul Mannan SHAIKH, J R HASAN, A R SUAIKU

Handsworth Medical Centre
1 Fitzalan Road, Sheffield S13 9AW
Tel: 0114 269 3044
(South East Sheffield Primary Care Trust)

Practice Manager D Hicks

GP Chhama SETH, Pramod Chandra SETH

Harold Street Surgery
2 Harold Street, Sheffield S6 3QW
Tel: 0114 233 5930
(Sheffield West Primary Care Trust)

GP Thakur Sukdeo SINGH, Trichur Sundaram GANAPATHY

The Health Care Surgery
63 Palgrave Road, Sheffield S5 8GS
Tel: 0114 234 1200 Fax: 0114 231 4591
(North Sheffield Primary Care Trust)
Patient List Size: 4475

Practice Manager S A Birkby

GP Edward Anthony BIRKBY, Heather Margaret CHARLTON, Sandra EMERSON

The Health Centre
High Street, Dronfield, Sheffield S18 1PY
Tel: 01246 419040 Fax: 01246 291780
Website: www.turner-bull.co.uk
(North Eastern Derbyshire Primary Care Trust)
Patient List Size: 3000

Practice Manager Chris Stanley

GP Stuart SAUNDERS, Jill BETHELL, R E BULL, Gillian HARVEY, B A TURNER

Heeley Green Surgery
302 Gleadless Road, Sheffield S2 3AJ
Tel: 0114 250 0309 Fax: 0114 250 7185
(South East Sheffield Primary Care Trust)
Patient List Size: 5550

Practice Manager P D Barker

GP Jillian Margaret CREASY, Paul Harry DRISCOLL, Karen Ruth O'CONNOR

Highgate Surgery
Highgate, Tinsley, Sheffield S9 1WN
Tel: 0114 244 2256
(South East Sheffield Primary Care Trust)

GP Prem Prakash KACKER, Satya KACKER

The Hollies Medical Centre
20 St. Andrews Road, Sheffield S11 9AL
Tel: 0114 255 0094 Fax: 0114 258 2863
(Sheffield South West Primary Care Trust)

Practice Manager D Roe

GP Cyril William Kendall Handley GREAVES, Vanessa Mary FISHER, Simon Philip John O'CONNOR, June SMAILES

Jaunty Springs Health Centre
53 Jaunty Way, Sheffield S12 3DZ
Tel: 0114 239 9453
(South East Sheffield Primary Care Trust)
Patient List Size: 4000

Practice Manager Maggie Bowden, Julia Openshaw

GP Nigel Ian WOOD, Alison FOX, Deirdre HENDRA

Kingswell Surgery
40 Shrewsbury Road, Penistone, Sheffield S36 6DY
Tel: 01226 765300 Fax: 01226 763753
(Barnsley Primary Care Trust)

Practice Manager Mark Schofield

GP J G DAVIES

Lawson Road Surgery
5 Lawson Road, Broomhill, Sheffield S10 5BU
Tel: 0114 266 5180
(Sheffield West Primary Care Trust)
Patient List Size: 8000

Practice Manager V Taylor

GP David Ian TAYLER, Martin John FRANCE, Kay Lesley FRANCIS, David Anthony SAVAGE

Lowedges Surgery
127a Lowedges Road, Sheffield S8 7LE
Tel: 0114 283 9839 Fax: 0114 283 9983
(Sheffield South West Primary Care Trust)
Patient List Size: 2850

Practice Manager P Ledbury

GP H M METCALF, S L BRADFORD, D P McALLISTER

Manchester Road Surgery
484 Manchester Road, Sheffield S10 5PN
Tel: 0114 266 8411 Fax: 0114 268 7158
(Sheffield South West Primary Care Trust)
Patient List Size: 3770

Practice Manager Pauline Horton

GP Michael John THEWLES, Caroline CROWTHER, Nicholas KEARSLEY, Andrew Stephen MARSHALL

Manor Park Medical Centre
204 Harborough Avenue, Sheffield S2 1QU
Tel: 0114 239 8602 Fax: 0114 265 8010
(South East Sheffield Primary Care Trust)
Patient List Size: 4600

Practice Manager Wendy Muttram

GP R ADDISON, Julie Sian HACKNEY, Helen JARVIS, T MOTHERSDALE

Manor Top Medical Centre
Rosehearty, Ridgeway Road, Sheffield S12 2SS
Tel: 0114 239 8324
(South East Sheffield Primary Care Trust)

Practice Manager Chris Nicol

GP U K SAVANI, S S SHARMA

The Medical Centre
New Street, Dinnington, Sheffield S25 2EZ
Tel: 01909 562207
(Rotherham Primary Care Trust)

Practice Manager J Donohoe

GP J A BARLEY, M G ALMEDA, R J ANGIER, Alan Philip BIRKS, D M CURRAN, T J DOUGLAS, J A EVERSDEN, S M MITCHELL, B J ROBERTSON, L K SLATER

Meersbrook Medical Centre
243-245 Chesterfield Road, Sheffield S8 0RT
Tel: 0114 258 3997
(Sheffield South West Primary Care Trust)

GP Ghanashyambhai Umedbhai PATEL

Mill Road Surgery
98A Mill Road, Ecclesfield, Sheffield S35 9XQ
Tel: 0845 124 1123 Fax: 0114 2577386
(North Sheffield Primary Care Trust)
Patient List Size: 4900

GP Martin John CALEY, Jane Mary FITZGERALD, M J GAMSU

Montgomery House Medical Centre
83 Infirmary Road, Sheffield S6 3BZ
Tel: 0114 272 5244 Fax: 0114 276 6288
(Sheffield West Primary Care Trust)
Patient List Size: 2200

Practice Manager Avis Barker

GP A MOHIT

Mosborough Health Centre
34 Queen Street, Mosborough, Sheffield S20 5BQ
Tel: 0114 248 7488
(South East Sheffield Primary Care Trust)
Patient List Size: 6000

Practice Manager A J Ward

GP David GELIPTER, Andrew Beverley Cawood COULDWELL, Sara Louise KELLOCK, Elizabeth Anne WOODS

Moss Valley Medical Practice
Gosber Road, Eckington, Sheffield S21 4BZ
Tel: 01246 432131 Fax: 01246 439104
(North Eastern Derbyshire Primary Care Trust)
Patient List Size: 8482

Practice Manager Michelle Slimm

GP Sheila KINGHORN, Martin McSHANE, Louise MOSS, Rachel TINKER, Michael UNDERWOOD

Nethergreen Road Surgery
34-36 Nethergreen Road, Sheffield S11 7EJ
Tel: 0114 230 2952
(Sheffield South West Primary Care Trust)

GP Gay FORSTER, Christopher Stewart BARCLAY, Virginia Ruth BENNETT, Patricia Anne BROADBENT, Adrian Henry Lampard SMITH, Rachel Olwyn YATES

Norfolk Park Health Centre
Tower Drive, Sheffield S2 3RE
Tel: 0114 276 9661 Fax: 0114 276 9471
(South East Sheffield Primary Care Trust)

Practice Manager M Gregory

GP Martin John FRANCE, Alexandra Mary Elizabeth BRINKLEY, Margaret Mary McKENNA, Frank William WRIGHT

Northern Avenue Surgery
141 Northern Avenue, Sheffield S2 2EJ
Tel: 0114 239 8686 Fax: 0114 253 1929
(South East Sheffield Primary Care Trust)
Patient List Size: 3500

Practice Manager Sharon Turner

GP Susan Elizabeth Haslam LUMB, Timothy Kevin HODSON, Anthony Michel KEMPLEN

Norwood Medical Centre
360 Herries Road, Sheffield S5 7HD
Tel: 0845 124 2498 Fax: 0114 261 9243
(North Sheffield Primary Care Trust)
Patient List Size: 7649

Practice Manager Samantha Grundy

GP Peter Gateshill HARDY, Sue LUPTON, Deborah Ann PARKER, Simon SHERRY

Oakhill Medical Practice
Oakhill Road, Dronfield, Sheffield S18 3EJ
Tel: 01246 296900 Fax: 01246 296903
(North Eastern Derbyshire Primary Care Trust)

Practice Manager Janet Turner

GP Alistair PARK, Arthur McFARLANE, Claire PARSONS

Okorie
The Medical Centre, 1a Ingfield Avenue, Sheffield S9 1WZ
Tel: 0114 261 0623 Fax: 0114 261 0949
(South East Sheffield Primary Care Trust)

GP N M OKORIE

Old School Medical Centre
School Lane, Greenhill, Sheffield S8 7RL
Tel: 0114 237 8866/ 237 8855 Fax: 0114 237 3400
Website: oldschoolmedical.co.uk
(Sheffield South West Primary Care Trust)
Patient List Size: 5100

Practice Manager Lynda Liddament

GP Janet HALL, Andrew BROWN, John PLATT

Oughtibridge Surgery
Church Street, Oughtibridge, Sheffield S35 0FW
Tel: 0114 286 2145 Fax: 0114 286 4031
(Sheffield West Primary Care Trust)

GP David Eden Rayner OATES, Philippa CREHAN, Timothy MOORHEAD

Owlthorpe Medical Centre
Moorthorpe bank, Sheffield S20 6PD
Tel: 0114 247 7852 Fax: 0114 248 3691
(South East Sheffield Primary Care Trust)
Patient List Size: 3606

Practice Manager Marilyn Bakewell

GP Stephen James ROWLAND, Jacqueline Anne TOOTH

Page Hall Medical Centre
101 Owler Lane, Sheffield S4 8GB
Tel: 0844 415 7999 Fax: 0114 261 1643
Email: allison.leonce@gp-c88051.nhs.uk
(North Sheffield Primary Care Trust)
Patient List Size: 6608

Practice Manager Allison Leonce

GP David Christopher BRINKLEY, Margaret Clare AINGER, Kate BELLINGHAM, Chris BRONSDON, Julian CREASY, Cathy EVANS, Heulwen EVANS

Park Health Centre
190 Duke Street, Sheffield S2 5QQ
Tel: 0114 272 7768
(South East Sheffield Primary Care Trust)
Patient List Size: 5800

Practice Manager Lynda Hall

GP David Reginald William BOTTOMLEY, Catherine Dierdre ELPHINSTONE, Linda GREENWOOD, Jane SEARLE, Elizabeth Helen STORY, Paul Julian THORPE, Christopher WALKER

Pitsmoor Surgery
151 Burngreave Road, Sheffield S3 9DL
Tel: 0845 122 2231 Fax: 0114 276 0169
(North Sheffield Primary Care Trust)
Patient List Size: 7000

Practice Manager David Emmas

GP Patricia EDNEY, William Wilson CARLILE, A R HOBBS, Alison HOBBS, Hugh Clement McCULLOUGH, Clare Denise RICHARDSON

Porter Brook Medical Centre
9 Sunderland Street, Sheffield S11 8HN
(Sheffield West Primary Care Trust)

GP A N JONES

Primary Care Centre
Chapel Way, Kiveton Park, Sheffield S26 6QU
Tel: 01909 770213
(Rotherham Primary Care Trust)

Practice Manager J Kaus

GP D T SAY, A GRAFTON, M A GRAFTON, J J REID, H M SPEIGHT, N A THORMAN, D R TOOTH, J WALLIS

Prince of Wales Road Medical Centre
Kuaerner Site, Sheffield S9 4EX
Tel: 0114 244 1384
(South East Sheffield Primary Care Trust)
Patient List Size: 1700

Practice Manager P Usherwood

GP Mary RAMSEY

Richmond Medical Centre
462 Richmond Road, Sheffield S13 8NA
Tel: 0114 239 9291 Fax: 0114 253 0737
(South East Sheffield Primary Care Trust)

Practice Manager Graham Daniel

GP Nicholas John KEARSLEY, Anita Merle CAMPBELL, Caroline Elizabeth WALTON

Richmond Road Surgery
400 Richmond Road, Sheffield S13 8LZ
Tel: 0114 239 9803
(South East Sheffield Primary Care Trust)
Patient List Size: 3890

Practice Manager Anne Riley

GP V B MEHROTRA, Vishwa Nath MEHROTRA

Rustlings Road Medical Centre
105 Rustlings Road, Sheffield S11 7AB
Tel: 0114 266 0726 Fax: 0114 267 8394
(Sheffield South West Primary Care Trust)

Practice Manager S Berwick, Louise Bland

GP Mandy Sharon SHARPE, David John WIGHT

Selborne Road Medical Centre
1 Selborne Road, Sheffield S10 5ND
Tel: 0114 268 4422 Fax: 0114 266 9892
(Sheffield South West Primary Care Trust)

GP Richard John HOARE, Gaynor Susan CARTER, Sarah Anne ZADIK

Sharrow Lane Surgery
129 Sharrow Lane, Sheffield S11 8AN
Tel: 0114 255 6600 Fax: 0114 250 8995
Email: sharrow.surgery@gp-g-88060.nhs.uk
Website: www.sharrowlanemc.co.uk
(Sheffield South West Primary Care Trust)
Patient List Size: 3966

GP Satish Chandra SAXENA, Savita SAXENA, Badrul ISLAM

Sheffield Medical Centre
21 Spital Street, Sheffield S3 9LB
Tel: 0845 121 5399 Fax: 0114 275 4254
(North Sheffield Primary Care Trust)
Patient List Size: 2500

Practice Manager Julie King

GP C S NWAFOR, N W EZI

Sheffield Road Surgery
209 Sheffield Road, Killamarsh, Sheffield S21 1DX
Tel: 0114 251 0000 Fax: 0114 248 9380
(North Eastern Derbyshire Primary Care Trust)

GP James SUTHERLAND, Hena BRAR, Paul CRACKNELL, Stephen SHAW

Shiregreen Medical Centre
492 Bellhouse Road, Sheffield S5 0RG
Tel: 0845 121 1232 Fax: 0114 257 0964
(North Sheffield Primary Care Trust)
Patient List Size: 7000

Practice Manager T Strong

GP Muhammed SALEEM, Gillian Norma NORTH, Martin John STARBUCK, Edward Charles TURNER

Sloan Practice
251 Chesterfield Road, Sheffield S8 0RT
Tel: 0114 255 1164 Fax: 0114 258 9006
(Sheffield South West Primary Care Trust)
Patient List Size: 9500

Practice Manager Lesley Carnall, Helen Proud

GP Marion Edith SLOAN, Clare FREEMAN, David GREENSTREET, Dominic John Walter SHIRT, Linda Margaret SLOAN, Sara Barbara SLOAN

Southey Green Medical Centre
281 Southey Green Road, Sheffield S5 7QB
Tel: 0114 232 6401 Fax: 0114 285 4402

(North Sheffield Primary Care Trust)
Patient List Size: 4000

Practice Manager Janet Scott

GP Navnitbhai Hargovindbhai PATEL

The Stannington Health Centre
Uppergate Road, Stannington, Sheffield S6 6BX
Tel: 0114 234 8779 Fax: 0114 285 4778
(Sheffield West Primary Care Trust)
Patient List Size: 2800

Practice Manager Mary Wood

GP Angela Mary BAIRD, David Milne SHURMER

Stonecroft Medical Centre
871 Gleadless Road, Sheffield S12 2LJ
Tel: 0114 39 8575 Fax: 0114 265 0001
(Sheffield South West Primary Care Trust)
Patient List Size: 8000

Practice Manager Carol Sayers

GP Penelope Anne BRADBURY, Victoria Anne HOLDEN, Robert John MUGGLETON, Stephen Robert WALTON

The Surgery
19 High Street, Penistone, Sheffield S36 6BR
Tel: 01226 762257 Fax: 01226 762984
(Barnsley Primary Care Trust)

Practice Manager Mary McEnhill

GP P M BROWN, S E BALL, C CALLADINE, D GALLAGHER, G R GIBBONS, J J GRIFFIN, D J LINDOP, S McCARTHY, H D MORRIS

Swallownest Health Centre
Hepworth Drive, Aston, Sheffield S26 2BG
Tel: 0114 287 2486
(Rotherham Primary Care Trust)

Practice Manager S Carr

GP R U WATSON, R DALY, R C EARL, R EVANS, B HILLMAN, P HOLMES, J KAVANAGH, P SCORAH, P TATTON

Totley Rise Medical Centre
96 Baslow Road, Sheffield S17 4DQ
Tel: 0114 236 5450 Fax: 0114 262 0942
(Sheffield South West Primary Care Trust)
Patient List Size: 3100

Practice Manager N Crowther

GP Kieran Joseph PRESSLEY, Carol Joan SHAWCROSS

Tramways Medical Centre
54 Holme Lane, Sheffield S6 4JQ
Tel: 0114 234 3418 Fax: 0114 285 5958
(Sheffield West Primary Care Trust)
Patient List Size: 8500

Practice Manager Jenny M Faulding

GP Alan Frederick MORLEY, Alastair Russell BRADLEY, K E BRADLEY, John Paul O'CONNELL, P J WILKIE

Tramways Medical Centre
54a Holme Lane, Sheffield S6 4JQ
Tel: 0114 233 9462 Fax: 0114 232 5620
Email: tramways54a@gp-c88043.nhs.uk
(Sheffield West Primary Care Trust)
Patient List Size: 6500

GP John POYSER, Eurgain BAKER, Fiona LLOYD, Neil Andrew MILNER

University Health Service
2 Claremont Place, Sheffield S10 2TB
Tel: 0114 222 2100 Fax: 0114 276 7223
(Sheffield West Primary Care Trust)

GP Melvyn Ambrose OSBORNE, Bernadette Marie Therese D'MELLO, Michael JAKOBOVIC, Alison Frances JAMES, Jennifer Ann KING, Vivien Frances LEIGH, Derek Frank PICKERING, Karen TAYLOR

Upperthorpe Medical Centre
Addy Street, Sheffield S6 3FT
Tel: 0114 234 3904
(Sheffield West Primary Care Trust)
Patient List Size: 9600

Practice Manager Gill Hides

GP John RUSSELL, Nicholas William HUDSON, Jacqueline Anne POXON, G F RUSSELL, Brendan Joseph SWALES

Upwell Street Surgery
93 Upwell Street, Sheffield S4 8AN
Tel: 0845 120 2826 Fax: 0114 226 2636
Email: johanne.shirt@gpc88027.nhs.uk
(North Sheffield Primary Care Trust)

Practice Manager Johanne Shirt

GP Joanna Sarah CANNON, Jackie BURTON, Janet CHELLIAH, Howard KEY, Lyn Julia PROSSER

Valley Medical Centre
Johnson Street, Stocksbridge, Sheffield S36 1BX
Tel: 0114 288 3841 Fax: 0114 288 7896
(Sheffield West Primary Care Trust)
Patient List Size: 10300

Practice Manager Paul Hancock

GP Paul Gorvin NORTON, Christine Elizabeth ATKIN, Mark ATKIN, David Edward BARON, Sandra LEICESTER, Julian Miles PEACE

Wadsley Bridge Medical Centre
103 Halifax Road, Sheffield S6 1LA
Tel: 0845 124 4662
(North Sheffield Primary Care Trust)
Patient List Size: 7200

Practice Manager Anita Jayne Warner

GP Richard Michael PANNIKER, Jean Alison BOLDY, Mark Edmund DURLING, Jo L HAZELL, James E NOODY

Walkley House Medical Centre
23 Greenhow Street, Walkley, Sheffield S6 3TN
Tel: 0114 234 3716 Fax: 0114 231 3326
(Sheffield West Primary Care Trust)
Patient List Size: 10040

Practice Manager Julia Openshaw

GP Richard George LEDINGHAM, David Michael FITZGERALD, Sarah Jane Stringer HUNTER, Andrew Jerzy KITLOWSKI, Jennifer Ann STEPHENSON

Westfield Health Centre
Westfield Northway, Westfield, Sheffield S20 8NZ
Tel: 0114 248 2498 Fax: 0114 251 3383
Email: westfield.hc@gp-c88013.nhs.uk
(South East Sheffield Primary Care Trust)
Patient List Size: 2740

GP Gurchuran Singh CHADHA, Pushpinder CHADHA

Whitehouse Surgery
189 Prince of Wales Road, Sheffield S2 1FA
Tel: 0114 239 7229 Fax: 0114 253 1650
(South East Sheffield Primary Care Trust)
Patient List Size: 5300

Practice Manager Ken Staniland

GP Richard John WATTON, Brian James HOPKINS, Ruth KENNEDY, Helen Margaret McDONOUGH

Wincobank Medical Centre
16 Chapman Street, Sheffield S9 1NG
Tel: 0114 242 6411 Fax: 0114 244 8571
(South East Sheffield Primary Care Trust)

Practice Manager Roy Wary

GP Dr COSKERY, Deborah Elizabeth CRAWLEY, Nicholas John FIELD, Dr MAHER

Woodhouse Medical Centre
5 Skelton Lane, Woodhouse, Sheffield S13 7LY
Tel: 0114 269 2049 Fax: 0114 269 6539
(South East Sheffield Primary Care Trust)

GP Margaret Jane SPINKS, Jonathan David KEEL, Callum James McLEAN, Zachary William McMURRAY

Woodhouse Medical Centre
7 Skelton Lane, Woodhouse, Sheffield S13 7LY
Tel: 0114 269 0025
(South East Sheffield Primary Care Trust)
Patient List Size: 6245

Practice Manager Allison Ward

GP Caroline Anne MITCHELL, Ngozi ANUMBA, Paula JONES, Christopher ROBERTS, Nicholas SMITH

Woodseats Medical Centre
4 Cobnar Road, Woodseats, Sheffield S8 8QB
Tel: 0114 274 0202 Fax: 0114 274 6835
(Sheffield South West Primary Care Trust)
Patient List Size: 8500

Practice Manager Sheila Gilbert

GP Stephen John WRIGHT, Helen Elizabeth JOESBURY, Jonathan Neil RODDICK, Roger THOMPSON

Shefford

The Health Centre
Iveldale Drive, Shefford SG17 5AD
Tel: 01462 814899 Fax: 01462 815322
(Bedfordshire Heartlands Primary Care Trust)

Practice Manager V Kinch-Jameson

GP Charles Anthony Richard BALDOCK, Dr BAXTER, Ryszard Geraint BIETZK, Dr BLACKSHAW, Stephen Robert CAKEBREAD, Sarah Katherine Waldron GRIFFITH, Dr O'BRIEN

Shepperton

Shepperton Health Centre
Shepperton Court Drive, Laleham Road, Shepperton TW17 8EJ
Tel: 01932 220524 Fax: 01932 244948
(North Surrey Primary Care Trust)
Patient List Size: 10000

Practice Manager Nikki Leonard

GP Claire Mary ATKIN, Simon John BELLAMY, David Julian Michael CHOAT, Hardeep KULLAR, Frances Anne Louise ROGERS, D SIDHU, T TURVEY

Upper Halliford Medical Centre
270 Upper Halliford Road, Shepperton TW17 8SY
Tel: 01932 785496 Fax: 01932 779277
(North Surrey Primary Care Trust)

GP Nihal Joseph Camillus CANDAPPA

Shepton Mallet

Evercreech Medical Centre
Prestleigh Road, Evercreech, Shepton Mallet BA4 6JY
Tel: 01749 830325 Fax: 01749 830604
(Mendip Primary Care Trust)
Patient List Size: 2000

Practice Manager Marion Rossiter

GP James David Ian LINDSAY

Grove House Surgery
West Shepton, Shepton Mallet BA4 5UH
Tel: 01749 342314 Fax: 01749 344016
Email: reception@grovehousesurgery.nhs.uk
(Mendip Primary Care Trust)
Patient List Size: 6000

Practice Manager Tracy Hole

GP Christopher Malcolm HOWES, Josephine Kate CUDMORE, Robert Christopher KENYON, Janet Mary MILLAR

The Park Medical Practice
Cannands Grave Road, Shepton Mallet BA4 5RT
Tel: 01749 334383 Fax: 01749 334393
(Mendip Primary Care Trust)

Practice Manager Thelma Thompson

GP Christopher Stewart NORRIS, Stephen HOLMES, Fiona KNIGHT, Geoffrey SHARP, Timothy Richard Wolfe WALKER

Sherborne

Apples Medical Centre
East Mill Lane, Sherborne DT9 3DG
Tel: 01935 812633 Fax: 01935 817484
(North Dorset Primary Care Trust)
Patient List Size: 5200

Practice Manager Jayne Ashworth

GP Gregory MILES, Carolyn Susan GRIFFITHS, Robert Arthur LEWIS, Stephen Reynolds Seymour MORRIS

Bute House
Grove Medical Centre, Wootton Grove, Sherborne DT9 4DL
Tel: 01935 810900 Fax: 01935 810901
(North Dorset Primary Care Trust)
Patient List Size: 5000

Practice Manager Olive Lynch

GP David William TOWNSEND, Isabel Anne Cooper BARTLETT, Robert Austin CHILDS, Charles Edward MIDDLE

Gaymer, Gledhill and Burke
The Cross, Milborne Port, Sherborne DT9 5DF
Tel: 01963 250334 Fax: 01963 251180
Email: carol.hunt@milborneportsurgery.co.uk
(South Somerset Primary Care Trust)
Patient List Size: 4950

GP Adrian R GAYMER, Dr BRIFFA, Dr BURKE, Dr GLEDHILL, Dr WYER

New Land Surgery
Grove Medical Centre, Wooton Grove, Sherborne DT9 4DL
Tel: 01935 813438 Fax: 01935 817470
(North Dorset Primary Care Trust)

Practice Manager Jane Crocker

GP Simon Gay Furneaux CAVE, Christine Anne FOSTER, Neil Stuart FRASER, Simon Nicholas MOTTRAM

Yetminster Health Centre
Church Street, Yetminster, Sherborne DT9 6LG
Tel: 01935 872530 Fax: 01935 873484
(North Dorset Primary Care Trust)
Patient List Size: 3350

Practice Manager Sue Thring

GP Ian Anthony LATHAM, Christopher Patrick CLEAVER, Kathryn DIXON

Sheringham

Sheringham Medical Practice
Health Centre, Cromer Road, Sheringham NR26 8RT
Tel: 01263 822066 Fax: 01263 823890
(North Norfolk Primary Care Trust)
Patient List Size: 9985

Practice Manager Charlotte Pike

GP Peter William SAMPSON, Catherine ASHWORTH, Daryl FREEMAN, Paul David ROEBUCK, Ian Charles SMITH

Shifnal

Shifnal Medical Practice
Shrewsbury Road, Shifnal TF11 8AJ
Tel: 01952 460414 Fax: 01952 463192
(Shropshire County Primary Care Trust)
Patient List Size: 8290

Practice Manager Dave Price

GP Stephen William WHITING, Mark Alan BRINKLEY

Shildon

Hallgarth Surgery
Cheapside, Shildon DL4 2HP
Tel: 01388 772362 Fax: 01388 774150
(Sedgefield Primary Care Trust)
Patient List Size: 7000

Practice Manager G Carroll

GP Ian Thomas WALTON, Anne Jeanette CLARIDGE, Lee Karen GRIMES

Shildon Health Clinic
Church Street, Shildon DL4 1DU
Tel: 01388 772829 Fax: 01388 770426
(Sedgefield Primary Care Trust)

Practice Manager Janet Stephenson

GP Surendra Kallianpur BALIGA

Shipley

Dr K Hickey's Surgery
Alexandra Road, Shipley BD18 3EG
Tel: 01274 589160 Fax: 01274 321865
(North Bradford Primary Care Trust)

Practice Manager Beryl Handley

GP Kevin HICKEY

Eisner, Goldman and Ship
Shipley Health Centre, Alexandra Road, Shipley BD18 3EG
Tel: 01274 531153 Fax: 01274 770882
(North Bradford Primary Care Trust)
Patient List Size: 4100

Practice Manager Paula Guiry

GP Margaret Claire EISNER, Leslie Harry GOLDMAN, Rebecca Harriet SHIP

Newton Way Surgery
Newton Way, Baildon, Shipley BD17 5NH
Tel: 01274 581979 Fax: 01274 532426
(North Bradford Primary Care Trust)
Patient List Size: 9207

Practice Manager Janet McNiffe

GP Sally Anne ALLARD, Nigel CARAGHAN, Nicholas John DRIVER, Patricia Mary GOMERSALL, Stephen PATTERSON, Lucy SYKES

Saltaire Medical Centre
Richmond Road, Shipley BD18 4RX
Tel: 01274 593101 Fax: 01274 772588
(North Bradford Primary Care Trust)
Patient List Size: 9700

Practice Manager Kath Murray

GP Wendy Stella TONKS, Alison BARKER, Asma FARUQUE, Ian LIVINGSTONE, S A MILLNS SIZER

Westcliffe Medical Centre
Westcliffe Road, Shipley BD18 3EE
Tel: 01274 580787 Fax: 01274 532210
(North Bradford Primary Care Trust)

Practice Manager Susan Tear

GP John Gray CRAIG, Mary Margaret CUTHBERT, Matthew FAY, Sara Helen HUMPHREY, Ian Paul RUTTER

Windhill Green Medical Centre
2 Thackley Old Road, Shipley BD18 1QB
Tel: 01274 584223 Fax: 01274 530182
(North Bradford Primary Care Trust)

Practice Manager Janet Saunders

GP Clare Margaret BROOKE, John Allan BIBBY, Colin Charles PASSANT, Jane PETTY, Stephen URWIN

Shipston-on-Stour

The Medical Centre
Badgers Crescent, Shipston-on-Stour CV36 4BQ
Tel: 01608 661845 Fax: 01608 663614
(South Warwickshire Primary Care Trust)
Patient List Size: 10450

Practice Manager Pamela Hole

GP Theo Perry Calwell SCHOFIELD, Jane Elizabeth GILDER, Caroline Meryl NIXON, Sue PRITCHARD, Christopher THOROGOOD, Andrew Micheal WHITELEY, David Brian Kenneth WILLIAMS

Shoreham-by-Sea

The Health Centre
Pond Road, Shoreham-by-Sea BN43 5US
Tel: 01273 466052/3 Fax: 01273 462109
(Adur, Arun and Worthing Primary Care Trust)

Practice Manager Alison Ellis

GP Jon MORGAN, Marisa DEGGNAAR, Natasha GILANI, Simon HOWARD, Aranzazu VAZQUEZ-SALAZAR

Lyons and Partners
Shoreham Health Centre, Pond Road, Shoreham-by-Sea BN43 5US
Tel: 01273 440550 Fax: 01273 462109
(Adur, Arun and Worthing Primary Care Trust)
Patient List Size: 6200

Practice Manager Rosemary Carter

GP Nigel Stephen LYONS, Howard BENTLEY, Christopher HUCKSTEP, Roslyn Mary MACLINTOCK

Northbourne Medical Centre
Eastern Avenue, Shoreham-by-Sea BN43 6PE
Tel: 01273 464640 Fax: 01273 440913
(Adur, Arun and Worthing Primary Care Trust)
Patient List Size: 9300

Practice Manager J Grey

GP Alison Doreen SMITH, Hugo John BEARDMORE, Alice BUTLER, Michael Ian LEVY, Alistair Charles RAIMAN, Reggie SANGHA

Shrewsbury

Albert Road Medical Centre
60 Albert Road, Shrewsbury SY1 4HY
Tel: 01743 352343 Fax: 01743 369540
(Shropshire County Primary Care Trust)
Patient List Size: 7400

GP John Evan MATTHIAS, Gary V BRANFIELD, David MARTIN, Diana Frances WESTWELL

Beeches Medical Practice
1 Beeches Road, Bayston Hill, Shrewsbury SY3 0PF
Tel: 01743 874565 Fax: 01743 873696
(Shropshire County Primary Care Trust)
Patient List Size: 4950

Practice Manager R Jewsbury

GP Peter William BARRITT, Teresa Linda GRIFFIN, Robert Jonathan LAYCOCK

Belvidere Medical Practice
23 Belvidere Road, Shrewsbury SY2 5LS
Tel: 01743 363640 Fax: 01743 363692
(Shropshire County Primary Care Trust)
Patient List Size: 5200

Practice Manager Caroline Davis

GP Mary Ursula McCARTHY, Paul Anthony Evelyn MOTT, John Mark PEPPER

Claremont Bank Surgery
Claremont Bank, Shrewsbury SY1 1RL
(Shropshire County Primary Care Trust)

GP Dr KENDALL

Clive Surgery
20 High Street, Clive, Shrewsbury SY4 5PS
Tel: 01939 220295
(Shropshire County Primary Care Trust)

GP Julia Margaret BENNETT

Marden Medical Practice
25 Sutton Road, Shrewsbury SY2 6DL
Tel: 01743 241313 Fax: 01743 360725
(Shropshire County Primary Care Trust)
Patient List Size: 6500

Practice Manager Joy Baker

GP Peter BOTTOMLEY, J EDEN, M MOSELHI, Wendy Jane WALTON

Marysville Medical Practice
1 Burlington Place, Belle Vue, Shrewsbury SY3 7LF
Tel: 01743 244000 Fax: 01743 244788
Website: www.marysville.gpwebsite.com
(Shropshire County Primary Care Trust)
Patient List Size: 4365

Practice Manager Ann Barrett

GP Richard EVANS, Elizabeth FENNELLY, James MUIR

Mount Pleasant Medical Centre
Ditherington Road, Shrewsbury SY1 4DQ
Tel: 01743 235111
(Shropshire County Primary Care Trust)
Patient List Size: 6800

Practice Manager M Herbert

GP Peter CLOWES, Simon COCKILL, Gaynor O'GRADY, Helen WHITWORTH

Mytton Oak Medical Practice
Racecourse Lane, Shrewsbury SY3 5LZ
Tel: 01743 362223 Fax: 01743 2445811
(Shropshire County Primary Care Trust)
Patient List Size: 10400

GP Peter Shepherd BENNETT, Hilary CLARKE, Paul GARDNER, William John GOWANS, Tim HILL, Angela JONES, Alan OTTER

Pontesbury Surgery
Pontesbury, Shrewsbury SY5 0RF
Tel: 01743 790325 Fax: 01743 792851
(Shropshire County Primary Care Trust)
Patient List Size: 6300

Practice Manager Heather Brown

GP P BLAND, Steven John EDMUNDS, Helen HAWKRIDGE, J POVEY

Prescott Surgery
Prescott Road, Prescott, Baschurch, Shrewsbury SY4 2DR
Tel: 01939 260210 Fax: 01939 260752
(Shropshire County Primary Care Trust)
Patient List Size: 5630

Practice Manager Kay Gowrie

GP David Gilchrist Ross LOWDON, M GUILDFORD, Sarah Josephine TILEY

Radbrook Green Surgery
Bank Farm Road, Shrewsbury SY3 6DU
Tel: 01743 231816 Fax: 01743 344099
(Shropshire County Primary Care Trust)
Patient List Size: 9600

Practice Manager Michael B Carver

GP Simon Charles REID, H M CALLAHAN, Peter Gordon CROW, Rachel Mary PALMER, Nigel Charles RUSSELL, Rachel WILLS

Riverside Medical Practice
Roushill, Shrewsbury SY1 1PQ
Tel: 01743 352371 Fax: 01743 244055
Website: www.gpsurgery.co.uk
(Shropshire County Primary Care Trust)
Patient List Size: 12500

Practice Manager Martin Cousins

GP Desmond John CLESHAM, Michael Christopher LOVETT, Charles David Jacques MAURICE, Robert PARK, Julian STRINGER, Philippa May WALKER

The Surgery
South Hermitage, Belle Vue, Shrewsbury SY3 7JS
Tel: 01743 343148 Fax: 01743 357772
Website: www.southhermitagesurgery.co.uk
(Shropshire County Primary Care Trust)
Patient List Size: 7350

Practice Manager Richard Jewsbury

GP Sandra Eunice HALLATT, Laurie Russell DAVIS, Timothy John GOULD, V LEWIS, Susan Mary MURPHY, S OGILVIE

The Surgery
Poynton Road, Shawbury, Shrewsbury SY4 4JS
Tel: 01939 250237 Fax: 01939 250093
(Shropshire County Primary Care Trust)
Patient List Size: 3200

Practice Manager Rose Pain

GP David Michael B LATTO, Alistair C W CLARK

Wem and Prees Medical Practice
New Street, Wem, Shrewsbury SY4 5AF
Tel: 01939 233476
(Shropshire County Primary Care Trust)

Practice Manager P M Davies

GP Richard Graham Morant SMITH, James Ian Cowell BARTLETT, Patrick Mark BERESFORD, Ruth Elizabeth OLDROYD

Westbury Medical Centre
Westbury, Shrewsbury SY5 9QX
Tel: 01743 884727 Fax: 01743 884955
(Shropshire County Primary Care Trust)
Patient List Size: 3800

Practice Manager Frances E Williams

GP John Arthur WILLIAMS, Alison ADAMS, David Christopher LEWIS, Katy A LEWIS

Worthen Medical Practice
Worthen, Shrewsbury SY5 9HT
(Shropshire County Primary Care Trust)

GP Kieran L McCORMACK, S McCORMACK

Sidcup

Barnard Medical Centre
43 Granville Road, Sidcup DA14 4TA
Tel: 020 8302 7721 Fax: 020 8309 6579
(Bexley Care Trust)
Patient List Size: 11200

Practice Manager Gill Collins

GP B J OLIVER, Dr HUTSON, Dr MARTIN, Dr MEDHURST, Dr MILLARD, Dr MILNE, Dr SCOTT, Dr VIRDEE

Marlborough Park Avenue Surgery
82 Marlborough Park Avenue, Sidcup DA15 9DX
Tel: 020 8300 1197 Fax: 020 8309 7187
(Bexley Care Trust)
Patient List Size: 4588

Practice Manager Marilyn Beadle

GP Christopher John NEAL

Oaklands Avenue
30 Oaklands Avenue, Sidcup DA15 8NB
Tel: 020 8300 1798 Fax: 020 8309 1727
(Bexley Care Trust)

Practice Manager Doris Harley

GP Felicia Josephine MASCARENHAS

Sidcup Medical Centre
2 Church Avenue, Sidcup DA14 6BU
Tel: 020 8302 1114 Fax: 020 8309 6350
(Bexley Care Trust)
Patient List Size: 7000

GP Hiralal Laxminarayan BHATTAD, Ahjan BANDYOPADHYAY, Sidharh DESHMUKH, Shraddha KARKARE

Station Road Surgery
69 Station Road, Sidcup DA15 7DS
Tel: 020 8309 0201 Fax: 020 8309 9040
(Bexley Care Trust)
Patient List Size: 10500

Practice Manager Judy Kent

GP Roger William Townsend NICHOLS, Tamsin Ann ELSEY, Timothy Michael HARDING, Britta F S KNIGGE, Andrew Christopher LANG, Richard Peter MONEY

Woodlands Surgery
146 Halfway Street, Sidcup DA15 8DF
Tel: 020 8300 1680 Fax: 020 8309 7020
(Bexley Care Trust)

Practice Manager Mena Williams

GP K A RITCHIE

Sidmouth

Sid Valley Practice
Blackmore Health Centre, Blackmore Drive, Sidmouth EX10 8ET
Tel: 01395 512601 Fax: 01395 578408
Website: www.siddoc.co.uk
(East Devon Primary Care Trust)
Patient List Size: 14300

Practice Manager Rob Spargo

GP Andrew Hughes RIDLER, Ross DELL, P J FUNG, C S L HADFIELD, Duncan Philip HALL, Joanna J KINDER, Edmund Noel MORRIS, Nicholas John READ, Michael Joseph William SLOT

Sittingbourne

Canterbury Road Surgery
111 Canterbury Road, Sittingbourne ME10 4JA
Tel: 01795 423300
(Swale Primary Care Trust)
Patient List Size: 1785

Practice Manager Allyson Beerstecher

GP H J BEERSTECHER

Chestnuts Surgery
70 East Street, Sittingbourne ME10 4RU
Tel: 01795 423197 Fax: 01795 430179
(Swale Primary Care Trust)
Patient List Size: 10003

Practice Manager Tracy Bridge

GP Frank Michael CANTOR, Caroline Jane BROWN, Lawrence EYO, Adrian Patrick HALL, Paul STAKER

Grovehurst Surgery
Grovehurst Road, Kemsley, Sittingbourne ME10 2ST
Tel: 01795 430444 Fax: 01795 410539
Email: practice.manager@gp-G82026.nhs.uk
(Swale Primary Care Trust)
Patient List Size: 6149

Practice Manager Lisa Vandepeer

GP Christine Marion MARSH, Paul COUSINS, Megan Jane PHILPOTT, Simon James WITTS

High Street Surgery
95 High Street, Milton Regis, Sittingbourne ME10 2AR
Tel: 01795 426640
(Swale Primary Care Trust)
Patient List Size: 2664

Practice Manager Yvonne Deacon

GP C RAMU

Hollybank Surgery
31 London Road, Sittingbourne ME10 1NQ
Tel: 01795 472534/425439 Fax: 01795 473886
(Swale Primary Care Trust)
Patient List Size: 3755

GP Claude Hugh Francis MORRISH, Dhanvanti Narayan VENKATACHALAM

Lakeside Medical Centre
Todd Crescent, Church Milton, Sittingbourne ME10 2TZ
Tel: 01795 424315
(Swale Primary Care Trust)
Patient List Size: 2979

Practice Manager J D'Olivera

GP Bijan Kumar SAHA

London Road Surgery
9 London Road, Sittingbourne ME10 1NQ
Tel: 01795 472018
(Swale Primary Care Trust)
Patient List Size: 2215

The Medical Centre
32 London Road, Sittingbourne ME10 1ND
Tel: 01795 472109/472100 Fax: 01795 471400
Email: practice.manager@gp-g82231.nhs.uk
(Swale Primary Care Trust)
Patient List Size: 9317

Practice Manager Cheryl Wood

GP Kay Elizabeth WILCOX, Fateh Saeed AMER, Malcolm James FARQUHARSON

Memorial Medical Centre
Bell Road, Sittingbourne ME10 4XX
Tel: 01795 477764 Fax: 01795 475138
(Swale Primary Care Trust)
Patient List Size: 8010

Practice Manager Michelle Coomber

GP M D BREW, J M GILL, K C HIPKINS, J H HOWIE, A R McLEOD

Oak Lane Surgery
58 Oak Lane, Upchurch, Sittingbourne ME9 7AU
Tel: 01634 231423 Fax: 01634 261665
(Medway Teaching Primary Care Trust)

Practice Manager Veronica Brill

GP Lok Nath SHAUNAK, Vidosava SHAUNAK

Saffron Way Health Centre
Saffron Way, Sittingbourne ME10 2TX
Tel: 01795 475882
(Swale Primary Care Trust)
Patient List Size: 2721

Practice Manager Sharon Kennedy

GP David Gareth JONES, Mark PASOLA, B SZPUNT

The Surgery
London Road, Teynham, Sittingbourne ME9 9QL
Tel: 01795 521205 Fax: 01795 522795
(Swale Primary Care Trust)
Patient List Size: 2648

Practice Manager Sharon Moss

GP Ravi Bhushan KUMAR

The Surgery
31 London Road, Sittingbourne ME10 1NQ
Tel: 01795 422269
(Swale Primary Care Trust)
Patient List Size: 1870

GP S K MAHTHA

Teynham Medical Centre
The Surgery, 72 Station Road, Teynham, Sittingbourne ME9 9SN
Tel: 01795 521948 Fax: 01795 520785
(Swale Primary Care Trust)
Patient List Size: 1994

GP Atindra Nath SIKDAR

Skegness

Beacon Medical Practice
Chuchill Avenue, off Burgh Road, Skegness PE25 2AN
Tel: 01754 897000 Fax: 01754 761024
(East Lincolnshire Primary Care Trust)

Practice Manager Richard Johns

GP Stephen Roger BAXTER, Jagdish Singh CHAGGAR, Patrick Anthony COTTON, Derek Davidson DEWAR, James Nicholas LAYFIELD, Oluropo Ebenezer OJO, Regina RASHID, Robert Leonard SEAL, John Kieran SHARROCK, Claudius Bola TAIWO, Louise TAYLOR-KAVANAGH

Dr Baxter and Partners
The Surgery, Ancaster Avenue, Chapel St Leonards, Skegness PE24 5SL
Tel: 01754 872541/897000 Fax: 01754 871598/750071
(East Lincolnshire Primary Care Trust)
Patient List Size: 4300

Practice Manager Linda Sanchez

GP Stephen Roger BAXTER, Jagdish Singh CHAGGER, Patrick Anthony COTTON, Derek Davidson DEWAR, James Nicholas LAYFIELD, Jose Luis QUEVEDOSORIANO, Robert Leonard SEAL, John Kieran Clive SHARROCK, Claudius Bola TAIWO, Louise TAYLOR-KAVANAGH

Hawthorn Medical Practice
Hawthorn Road, Skegness PE25 3TD
Tel: 01754 896350 Fax: 01754 896366
(East Lincolnshire Primary Care Trust)
Patient List Size: 13600

Practice Manager Steve O'Dare

GP William Ross GOOD, Stephen BAIRD, Matthew Burra JORDAN, Susan Anne LAWSON, Raj NAIR, Vincent Joseph ROGERS, Torsten STUMPF

The Surgery
Wainfleet Road, Burgh Le Marsh, Skegness PE24 5ED
Tel: 01754 810205
(East Lincolnshire Primary Care Trust)

GP Seth Alexander Greer SYKES

William Way Doctors Surgery
William Way, Wainfleet All Saints, Skegness PE24 4DE
Tel: 01754 880212 Fax: 01754 880788
(East Lincolnshire Primary Care Trust)
Patient List Size: 3400

Practice Manager Kirsty Garrill

GP Usman GHANI, Chithriki RUDRAPPA

Skelmersdale

Ashurst Health Centre
Lulworth, Ashurst, Skelmersdale WN8 6QS
Tel: 01695 732468 Fax: 01695 555365
(West Lancashire Primary Care Trust)
Patient List Size: 5000

Practice Manager Janice Higgins

GP Mohamed QAMRUDDIN, Iyassu TEKLE

Beacon Primary Care
Sandy Lane, Skelmersdale WN8 8LA
Tel: 01695 555566
(West Lancashire Primary Care Trust)
Patient List Size: 9600

Practice Manager M Hardman-Welsh

GP Sujoy BISWAS, Meena BISWAS, Ros BONSOR, R R GANGAKHEDKAR, G HENRY, S PANIKKER

Birleywood Health Centre
Birleywood, Skelmersdale WN8 9BW
Tel: 01695 723333 Fax: 01695 556193
(West Lancashire Primary Care Trust)

GP Sujit Kumar SUR, Alaric John HICKS, George Alfred ORR

Birleywood Health Centre
Birleywood, Skelmersdale WN8 9BW
Tel: 01695 725555
(West Lancashire Primary Care Trust)

GP Jawahar Lal JAIN

Birleywood Health Centre
Birleywood, Skelmersdale WN8 9BW
Tel: 01695 728073 Fax: 01695 556172
(West Lancashire Primary Care Trust)

GP Upendra SINGH

Hall Green Surgery
164 Ormskirk Road, Upholland, Skelmersdale WN8 0AB
Tel: 01695 624331
(West Lancashire Primary Care Trust)

GP Patrick Gerard RYDER

Hall Green Surgery
164 Ormskirk Road, Upholland, Skelmersdale WN8 0AB
Tel: 01695 622268
(West Lancashire Primary Care Trust)

GP Gerard FLOOD, Daniel See Kuan CHANG, Steven Gary HEATON

Hillside Health Centre
Tanhouse Road, Tanhouse, Skelmersdale WN8 6DS
Tel: 01695 722424
(West Lancashire Primary Care Trust)

Practice Manager Sue Hagan

GP Usha SHARMA, Hanuman Prasad SHARMA

Hillside Health Centre
Tanhouse Road, Tanhouse, Skelmersdale WN8 6DS
Tel: 01695 726888 Fax: 01695 556330
(West Lancashire Primary Care Trust)
Patient List Size: 2500

Practice Manager C Matthew

GP Bir Bahadur SINGH

Hillside Health Centre
Tanhouse Road, Tanhouse, Skelmersdale WN8 6DS
Tel: 01695 725553
(West Lancashire Primary Care Trust)

GP Ratnakar Ramchandrarao GANGAKHEDKAR

Sandy Lane Health Centre
Sandy Lane, Skelmersdale WN8 8LA
Tel: 01695_ 727772 Fax: 01695 727771
(West Lancashire Primary Care Trust)

Practice Manager Christine Halliwell

GP Asha BISARYA, Anand Kumar BISARYA

Sandy Lane Health Centre
Sandy Lane, Skelmersdale WN8 8LA
Tel: 01695 723279 Fax: 01695 556143
(West Lancashire Primary Care Trust)
Patient List Size: 2500

Practice Manager J M Littler

GP Andrew David LITTLER

Sandy Lane Health Centre
Sandy Lane, Skelmersdale WN8 8LA
Tel: 01695 559558 Fax: 01695 726691
(West Lancashire Primary Care Trust)
Patient List Size: 2700

GP Jaisukh Shamjibhai MODHA

Skipton

Dyneley House Surgery
Newmarket Street, Skipton BD23 2HZ
Tel: 01756 799311 Fax: 01756 707203
(Craven, Harrogate and Rural District Primary Care Trust)

Practice Manager Lynn Knowles

GP Christopher Joseph CRAIG, Bruce Andrew WOODHOUSE, Julian Peter ALLEN, Andrew David BUNDOCK, Lucy CHECKER, Sally Jane CHURCHER, Gail M JONES, Andrew Gordon SUMNALL

Fisher Medical Centre
Millfields, Coach Street, Skipton BD23 1EU
(Craven, Harrogate and Rural District Primary Care Trust)

Practice Manager Jenny Hutchinson

GP Bernard Martin HOLMES, Judith CLARKE, Jeremy Rees GOODALL, G Alan HASSEY, David John PEARSON, Thomas Milnes WHITE, Helen Sarah WILKINSON

Grassington Medical Centre
9 Station Road, Grassington, Skipton BD23 5LS
Tel: 01756 752313 Fax: 01756 753320
Website: www.grassingtonmedicalcentre.co.uk
(Craven, Harrogate and Rural District Primary Care Trust)
Patient List Size: 4053

Practice Manager Elizabeth Henfrey

GP Ian Keith KINNISH, Andrew Jonathan JACKSON, Ellyn S McCULLOCH

Hellifield Surgery
15 Brook Street, Hellifield, Skipton BD23 4EX
(Craven, Harrogate and Rural District Primary Care Trust)

Practice Manager Elizabeth Wrigley

GP Eric WARD, William Walton HALL, John Malcolm LEWIS, Clare Imogen LITTLEJOHN

Sleaford

Manor Street Surgery
Manor Street, Ruskington, Sleaford NG34 9EN
Tel: 01526 832204
(Lincolnshire South West Teaching Primary Care Trust)

GP Gregory DENTON, Malcolm Edward JONES, Paul Terence PRICE

Parry
The Surgery, Spring Wells, Billingborough, Sleaford NG34 0QQ
Tel: 01529 240234 Fax: 01529 240520
(East Lincolnshire Primary Care Trust)
Patient List Size: 3777

Practice Manager Caroline Parry

GP Jonathan Edward PARRY

Sleaford Medical Group
Riverside Surgery, 47 Boston Road, Sleaford NG34 7HD
Tel: 01529 303301 Fax: 01529 415401
(Lincolnshire South West Teaching Primary Care Trust)
Patient List Size: 15800

Practice Manager E Owen

GP John Deane COLLINGE, Sukhvinder Kaur BHANDAL, Marc Andrew CARTWRIGHT, William Graham Hickey GAMBLE, Nicholas John Craig HUMPHRY, David Alan MURPHY, Julie Anne WEBSTER

Sleaford Road Surgery
1 Sleaford Road, Heckington, Sleaford NG34 9QP
Tel: 01529 460213 Fax: 01529 460087
(Lincolnshire South West Teaching Primary Care Trust)

GP Sri VARAH, Ratnam GOWRIBALAN, Kasiraman MALATHY, Kesava Pillai VIJAYAN

Slough

Avenue Medical Centre
Wentworth Avenue, Slough SL2 2DG
Tel: 01753 524549 Fax: 01753 552537
(Slough Primary Care Trust)

Practice Manager Steve Gowing

GP John Gerard Mary O'DOWD, Neil Samuel COLEMAN, Christine LEWIS, Julius Clifford PARKER, Diana Joan PURVIS

Bharani Medical Centre
450 Bath Road, Cippenham, Slough SL1 6BB
Tel: 01628 602564 Fax: 01628 660122
(Slough Primary Care Trust)
Patient List Size: 6000

Practice Manager Rokha Kumar

GP Malu L Hemantha KUMAR, Arumugam UMAPATHY

Burlington Avenue Surgery
32 Burlington Avenue, Slough SL1 2LD
Tel: 01753 530548 Fax: 01753 552376
(Slough Primary Care Trust)

GP Joginder S BUMBRA

Burnham Health Centre
Minniecroft Road, Burnham, Slough SL1 7DE
Tel: 01628 605333 Fax: 01628 663743
(Chiltern and South Bucks Primary Care Trust)

Practice Manager Roger Herbert

GP Robert GREEN, Antony BARRETT, Patrick CLARKE, Simon DAILY, Hilary FRYER, Patricia GREWAL, Muhammad JAMIL, Hilary THOMSON

Cippenham Surgery
261 Bath Road, Cippenham, Slough SL1 5PP
Tel: 01753 532006 Fax: 01753 554987
(Slough Primary Care Trust)

GP Qamar SHAFIQ

Crosby House Surgery
91 Stoke Poges Lane, Slough SL1 3NY
Tel: 01753 520680 Fax: 01753 552780
(Slough Primary Care Trust)

GP Gurdip Singh HEAR, Farouk JAMAL, Margaret Valerie ROBINSON

The Datchet Health Centre
4 Green Lane, Datchet, Slough SL3 9EX
Tel: 01753 541268 Fax: 01753 582324
Website: www.datchetdoctor.co.uk
(Windsor, Ascot and Maidenhead Primary Care Trust)
Patient List Size: 7250

Practice Manager Jane Cockley

GP Adrian Neil DALTON, Martin CHAN, Nicola Jane WALLBANK, Michael Barrett WATTS

Farnham Road Surgery
301 Farnham Road, Slough SL2 1HD
Tel: 01753 520917 Fax: 01753 550680
Email: drjimodonnell@farnhamroadsurgery.freeserve.co.uk
(Slough Primary Care Trust)
Patient List Size: 20800

GP Leonard Bernard Christopher GILFEATHER, Emma Jane Charlotte BAMBRIDGE, Jacqueline Mary BULGER, Amanda GILLILAND, Peter JAMES, Susan Lucetta LOUGHLIN, David Ian McILROY, Christopher David MORRIS, Katherine MOWAT, James Gerard O'DONNELL, David Marcus RODGERS, Usha SHARMA, David William WARD

Grasmere Avenue Surgery
59 Grasmere Avenue, Slough SL2 5JE
Tel: 01753 579803 Fax: 01753 553745
(Slough Primary Care Trust)

Practice Manager Poonam Kumar

GP Harsh KUMAR

Herschel Medical Centre
45 Osborne Street, Slough SL1 1TT
Tel: 01753 520643 Fax: 01753 554964
(Slough Primary Care Trust)
Patient List Size: 10500

GP Richard John Horace NEALE, Rafath BHARGAVA, Roderic Lawrance CLARK, Qamar Ara KHAN, Bharat PATEL, Rachel Trixie POPE

Langley Health Centre
Common Road, Slough SL3 8LE
Tel: 01753 544288 Fax: 01753 592415
(Slough Primary Care Trust)

GP Norman GORDON, Phoebe Joyce Arach ABE, Nazaff Shah E ADAM, Raymond Roy BAIN, Elizabeth Janet CAMPBELL, Mohinder Singh DHATT, William Malcolm Isaac EVANS, John McCARTHY, Stella Madeleine READINGS

Leeds Road Surgery
3 Leeds Road, Slough SL1 3PX
Tel: 01753 538741 Fax: 01753 553137
(Slough Primary Care Trust)

GP Joginder K MAINI

Manor Park Medical Centre
2 Lerwick Drive, Off Granville Avenue, Slough SL2 1JT
Tel: 01753 526625 Fax: 01753 552962
(Slough Primary Care Trust)
Patient List Size: 10000

Practice Manager Sheila Sunner

GP Sudesh KUMAR, Mahendra AMIN, Maria EASAW, Kilvinder JANGHERA, Kesar Singh SADHRA

Shreeji Medical Centre
22 Whitby Road, Slough SL1 3DQ
Tel: 01753 527988 Fax: 01753 530269
(Slough Primary Care Trust)
Patient List Size: 5200

Practice Manager M J Trivedi

GP Jitendrakumar TRIVEDI

Southmead Surgery
Southmead House, Blackpond Lane, Farnham Common, Slough SL2 3ER
Tel: 01753 643195 Fax: 01753 642157
(Chiltern and South Bucks Primary Care Trust)
Patient List Size: 7000

Practice Manager Susan Hazell, Susan Salmon

GP John Geoffrey David SALMON, Tilly SIVARAMALINGA, Kate STAVELEY

Threeways
84 Roger Lane, Stoke Poges, Slough SL2 4LF
Tel: 01753 643445 Fax: 01753 646906
(Chiltern and South Bucks Primary Care Trust)

Practice Manager Lyn Carle

GP S LYNCH, S ALLEN, A BRODIE, C HASSIN

Trelawney Avenue Surgery
425 Trelawney Avenue, Langley, Slough SL3 7TT
Tel: 01753 775545 Fax: 01753 775545
(Slough Primary Care Trust)
Patient List Size: 3800

Practice Manager Sonia Lunn

GP Graham John BURDEN, Jeremy Neil THOMPSON

Upton Medical Partnership
18 Sussex Place, Slough SL1 1NS
Tel: 01753 522713 Fax: 01753 552790
(Slough Primary Care Trust)

GP John Gilbert EYERS, Marion Ruth OVERTON, Barbara Wendy PECK, Julie STRAWFORD

Wexham Road Surgery
242 Wexham Road, Slough SL2 5JP
Tel: 01753 552255 Fax: 01753 219100
(Slough Primary Care Trust)
Patient List Size: 3500

GP Mohanlal AGGARWAL, Sivakumari SIZHIRAPATHY

Wexham Road Surgery
240 Wexham Road, Slough SL2 5JP
Tel: 01753 517360 Fax: 01753 552365
(Slough Primary Care Trust)

Practice Manager E Haverley

GP Veena SHARMA

Smethwick

Bearwood Medical Centre
176 Milcote Road, Smethwick B67 5BP
Tel: 0121 429 1572 Fax: 0121 434 4518
(Oldbury and Smethwick Primary Care Trust)
Patient List Size: 3900

Practice Manager Kathleen Harris

GP Harpal Singh CHAWLA, Suman CHAWLA

Cape Hill Medical Centre
Raglan Road, Smethwick B66 3NR
Tel: 0121 558 0871 Fax: 0121 558 6125
Website: www.capehillmc.co.uk
(Oldbury and Smethwick Primary Care Trust)
Patient List Size: 9200

Practice Manager Stuart Tilsley

GP David Laurie CHILD, G GARDNER, Richard Alan LOVELESS, Roderick MACRORIE, Lionel MILLS, D MORRIS, M PHILP

Marshall Street Surgery
45-46 Marshall Street, Smethwick B67 7NA
Tel: 0121 558 4446 Fax: 0121 555 5832
(Oldbury and Smethwick Primary Care Trust)

Practice Manager S Rahman

GP Abul Kalam Mohammed Raziur RAHMAN

Sarephed Medical Centre
Arden Road, Smethwick B67 6AJ
Tel: 0121 558 0263 Fax: 0121 558 9071
(Oldbury and Smethwick Primary Care Trust)
Patient List Size: 2500

Practice Manager Glen Taylor

GP Binod Prasad CHOUDHARY

Snodland

Central Surgery
Queens Avenue, Snodland ME6 5BP
Tel: 01634 240295 Fax: 01634 245820
(Maidstone Weald Primary Care Trust)

Practice Manager E Mannoolh

GP John Geoffrey Hazlitt BURLAND, David Duncan COLIN-JONES, Sheila KHEHAR, Hesanth PEIRIS, Sanjay SINGH

Solihull

Arden Medical Centre
Downing Close, Station Road, Knowle, Solihull B93 0OA
Tel: 01564 739194 Fax: 01564 771224
(Solihull Primary Care Trust)
Patient List Size: 4350

Practice Manager V Tabb

GP Michael John BLEBY, Jennifer Ann HAGON, Jane Alison HOLT, S HOUGHTON

Arran Medical Centre
Arran Way, Chelmsley Wood, Solihull B36 0PU
Tel: 0121 770 8484 Fax: 0121 770 9991
(Solihull Primary Care Trust)
Patient List Size: 4200

Practice Manager N Sandhu

GP V A BHASKAR

Avenue Road Surgery
3 Avenue Road, Dorridge, Solihull B93 8LH
Tel: 01564 776262 Fax: 01564 779599
Website: www.dorridgesurgery.co.uk
(Solihull Primary Care Trust)
Patient List Size: 10850

Practice Manager Michael Collins

GP William Stuart UPTON, John Allan DAVENPORT, Julia MARKHAM, Annette Mary PICKERING, Daniel Vernon REID, Simon George Thomas WATTS

Blossomfield Road Surgery
308 Blossomfield Road, Solihull B91 1TF
Tel: 0121 705 5339 Fax: 0121 709 0239
(Solihull Primary Care Trust)

Practice Manager J Parrington

GP Michael S ABDOU

Blythe Practice
1500 Warwick Road, Knowle, Solihull B93 9LE
Tel: 01564 779280 Fax: 01564 772010
(Solihull Primary Care Trust)
Patient List Size: 6000

Practice Manager A Hatfield

GP Irvine Renfrew STUART, Richard Hugh MORGAN, William Geoffrey NAYLOR

Fentham Hall Surgery
Marsh Lane, Hampton-in-Arden, Solihull B92 0AH
Tel: 01675 442510 Fax: 01675 443353
(Solihull Primary Care Trust)

Practice Manager C Macnair

GP Rodger Clement CHARLTON

Grafton Road Surgery
11 Grafton Road, Solihull Lodge, Solihull B90 1NG
Tel: 0121 474 4686 Fax: 0121 608 4900
(Solihull Primary Care Trust)
Patient List Size: 2800

Practice Manager Karen Page

GP Dibyendu SENGUPTA

Grove Road Surgery
3 Grove Road, Solihull B91 2AG
Tel: 0121 705 1105 Fax: 0121 711 4098
Email: name@gp-M89017.nhs.uk
(Solihull Primary Care Trust)
Patient List Size: 19000

Practice Manager Christiane E Bates

GP Peter James TRAVIS, Maria Del Mar FONT OLIVE, Sunil Babulal KOTECHA, Eli LEYTON, Ian David Paul MORGAN, Dilys Jane O'DRISCOLL, Thomas STENHOUSE, Mark Julian Gwyn STERRY, Robert Christopher STOCKDALE

Haslucks Green Road Surgery
287 Haslucks Green Road, Shirley, Solihull B90 2LW
Tel: 0121 744 6663 Fax: 0121 733 6895
Email: hasluck.surgery@aol.com
(Solihull Primary Care Trust)
Patient List Size: 7000

Practice Manager J L Clews, T J Hancox

GP S W DABYDEEN, K R DUNN, E A KONDRATOWICZ, Peter John McLean SLOAN

Hobs Moat Medical Centre
Ulleries Road, Solihull B92 8ED
Tel: 0121 742 5211 Fax: 0121 743 4217
Email: drs@mmcb.ms.solihull-ha.wmids.nhs.uk
(Solihull Primary Care Trust)
Patient List Size: 7700

Practice Manager T Cooper

GP Rachel Anne BAYLY, Stephen Michael COWLES, Brian Eric CRICHTON, Alison Jayne MATTHEWS, Y ZAKARIA

Lapworth Surgery
Old Warwick Road, Lapworth, Solihull B94 6LH
(South Warwickshire Primary Care Trust)

GP Barbara Jane NICOL, Rhoderic Eion NICOL

Meadowside Family Health Centre
30 Winchcombe Road, Solihull B92 8PJ
Tel: 0121 743 2560/742 5666 Fax: 0121 743 4216
(Solihull Primary Care Trust)
Patient List Size: 8700

Practice Manager M Handy

GP Martin David POWIS, Michael A H BAKER, Elizabeth EDWARDS, Carolyne Dawn SMITH, Sheila Hazel VANHOUSE, John Patrick Dinsmore WILKINSON

Monkspath Surgery
27 Farmhouse Way, Monkspath, Shirley, Solihull B90 4EH
Tel: 0121 711 1414 Fax: 0121 711 3753
Website: www.monkspathsurgery.co.uk
(Solihull Primary Care Trust)
Patient List Size: 11500

Practice Manager Rebecca Friend

GP Stanley Gleason DARLING, Beverley J DICKINSON, Simon Lomas GREEN, Arturo LUPOLI, Louise ROWE, Johama RUSSELL, Elizabeth Louise STOKES

Northbrook Group Practice
93 Northbrook Road, Shirley, Solihull B90 3LX
Tel: 0121 746 5000 Fax: 0121 746 5020
(Solihull Primary Care Trust)
Patient List Size: 10950

Practice Manager Christine Burr

GP Graham COGBILL, Rosalind ANFILOGOFF, Wendy Margaret MILLIGAN, Anessa OTTE, Shereen ZAKI

Northbrook Health Centre
93 Northbrook Road, Shirley, Solihull B90 3LX
Tel: 0121 744 5441 Fax: 0121 733 6891
(Solihull Primary Care Trust)

Practice Manager J Atkins

GP Gordon Arthur Wycliffe COLEMAN

Northbrook Health Centre
93 Northbrook Road, Shirley, Solihull B90 3LX
Tel: 0121 744 1872 Fax: 0121 733 6892
(Solihull Primary Care Trust)

Practice Manager J A Farmer

GP Gerald Stanley FARMER, Julia Louise LAWLEY

Northbrook Health Centre
93 Northbrook Road, Shirley, Solihull B90 3LX
Tel: 0121 745 9181 Fax: 0121 733 6893
(Solihull Primary Care Trust)

Practice Manager P A Grillage

GP Michael George GRILLAGE

Park Surgery
278 Stratford Road, Shirley, Solihull B90 3AF
Tel: 0121 241 1700 Fax: 0121 241 1710
(Solihull Primary Care Trust)
Patient List Size: 6760

Practice Manager Lindsey Kirby

GP Michael Robert TINCOMBE, Ela Dayalji PATEL, Marina THOMAS, Andrew Michael WADDELL

Richmond Medical Centre
179 Richmond Road, Olton, Solihull B92 7SA
Tel: 0121 743 7802 Fax: 0121 743 7802
(Solihull Primary Care Trust)
Patient List Size: 5430

Practice Manager Hazel Fields

GP Gordon Roy JARRETT, David Charles O'BRIEN, Z SOLEMAN

St Margarets Surgery
8 St. Margarets Road, Solihull B92 7JS
Tel: 0121 706 9796 Fax: 0121 765 0161
(Solihull Primary Care Trust)
Patient List Size: 6800

Practice Manager C Johnson

GP John George Barsley BAXTER, Catherine Anne LEWIS, Peter Stuart LOVE, Philip Andrew MELROSE

Tanworth Lane Surgery
2 Tanworth Lane, Shirley, Solihull B90 4DR
Tel: 0121 744 2025 Fax: 0121 733 6890
(Solihull Primary Care Trust)

Practice Manager J Gibson

GP Janet Patricia CLARKE, Brian Edward McCARTHY, Louise STACEY

Village Surgery
Cheswick Green, Solihull B90 4JA
Tel: 01564 703311 Fax: 01564 703794
(Solihull Primary Care Trust)
Patient List Size: 4044

Practice Manager J Evans

GP Janet LEESE, Janet Elizabeth BARRACLOUGH

Yew Tree Medical Centre
100 Yew Tree Lane, Solihull B91 2RA
Tel: 0121 705 8787 Fax: 0121 709 0240
(Solihull Primary Care Trust)
Patient List Size: 7500

Practice Manager Marion A Mann

GP Jeremy Andrew CROFT, Gurdeep LALL, Carolyn Ruth NAYLOR, Rosemary Rose SMITH

Somerton

Somerton Surgery
Cox's Yard, West Street, Somerton TA11 7PR
Tel: 01458 272473 Fax: 01458 274461
(South Somerset Primary Care Trust)
Patient List Size: 5700

Practice Manager Romy Wrangham

GP Andrew BAVERSTOCK, Sarah FREEMAN, Rosalind Elaine GRIFFITHS, Anthony LEAK, James NICHOLLS

South Brent

Plymouth Road Health Centre
Plymouth Road, South Brent TQ10 9HT
Tel: 01364 72394 Fax: 01364 72922
(South Hams and West Devon Primary Care Trust)
Patient List Size: 4500

Practice Manager Jenny Alexander

GP Tony BORN, James David HILL, Catherine Mary OLDERSHAW

South Croydon

The Birdhurst Medical Practice
1 Birdhurst Avenue, South Croydon CR2 7DX
Tel: 020 8686 2070 Fax: 020 8686 0824
(Croydon Primary Care Trust)
Patient List Size: 5670

Practice Manager Hazel Goodbody

GP James William GILLGRASS, Camilla CHAMBERS, Suveer GUPTA, K A OKUBOYE

Farley Road Medical Practice
53 Farley Road, Selsdon, South Croydon CR2 7NG
Tel: 020 8651 1222 Fax: 020 8657 9297
(Croydon Primary Care Trust)
Patient List Size: 11920

Practice Manager Gill Bashford

GP Robert Desmond Stuart SANDERSON, Penelope Charlotte BURGESS, Mary Elizabeth CASHMAN, J L B COCKELL, William Mark JASPER, David Alexander LYELL

Mitchley Avenue Surgery
116 Mitchley Avenue, Sanderstead, South Croydon CR2 9HH
Tel: 020 8657 6565 Fax: 020 8651 1701
(Croydon Primary Care Trust)
Patient List Size: 3250

GP Simon WOOLF, Franceso LENTCNI

Parkside Group Practice
27 Wyche Grove, South Croydon CR2 6EX
Tel: 020 8680 2588 Fax: 020 8680 1415
(Croydon Primary Care Trust)
Patient List Size: 11400

Practice Manager Jean McPhail

GP Martin Frederick JOHNSON, Michael Richard CLEMENTSON, L COLVIN, Sarah Margaret FOUND, K A KHAN, R MUHUNDAN

Queenhill Medical Practice
31 Queenhill Road, South Croydon CR2 8DU
Tel: 020 8651 1141 Fax: 020 8651 5011
Email: drbrzezicki@gp-l83014.nhs.uk
(Croydon Primary Care Trust)
Patient List Size: 7960

Practice Manager Mary Mitchell

GP Wendy June WALLACE, Anthony John BRZEZICKI, J HUGHES, M SIMMONDS

Selsdon Park Medical Practice
95 Addington Road, South Croydon CR2 8LG
Tel: 020 8657 0067 Fax: 020 8657 0037

(Croydon Primary Care Trust)
Patient List Size: 10000

Practice Manager Pat Davey

GP Alexander TROMPETAS, Ross Alan BAVERSTOCK, Peter CAMPBELL, Valerie Anne GALLAGHER, Henk PARMENTIER

South Croydon Medical Centre
226 Brighton Road, South Croydon CR2 6AH
Tel: 020 8688 8987 Fax: 020 8776 1911
(Croydon Primary Care Trust)
Patient List Size: 1890

Practice Manager Anil Nene

GP Ashwini Anil NENE, A KARIM

South Croydon Medical Practice
96 Brighton Road, South Croydon CR2 6AD
Tel: 020 8688 0875
(Croydon Primary Care Trust)
Patient List Size: 3850

Practice Manager Jane Bullman-Wood

GP Peadar M OHUIGINN, Stephen Robert GOLDING

South Molton

East Street Surgery
East Street, South Molton EX36 3BU
Tel: 01769 573811
(North Devon Primary Care Trust)

GP Michael John HAWKINS, Caroline Sara Louise HADFIELD, Deborah MORRIS, Richard Howson WESTCOTT

South Molton Health Centre
9-10 East Street, South Molton EX36 3BZ
Tel: 01769 573101 Fax: 01769 574371
Email: receptionL83137@gp-L83137.nhs.uk
Website: www.southmoltonhealth.com
(North Devon Primary Care Trust)
Patient List Size: 5011

Practice Manager Brenda McCamley

GP Rosemary Ann DODDINGTON, Christopher Alan GIBB, Jonathan David GILLARD, Helena Jane MURCH

South Ockendon

Aveley Medical Centre
22 High Street, Aveley, South Ockendon RM15 4AD
Tel: 01708 865640 Fax: 01708 865801
Email: occhealthnet@demon.co.uk
(Thurrock Primary Care Trust)
Patient List Size: 11000

Practice Manager John Patient

GP Luis Fernando Almeida LEIGHTON, Dirar Mustafa Muhammad Said KHRAISHI, Mohammed SADEHURA, Mark WILLIAMS

Fortin Path Surgery
2 Fortin Path, South Ockendon RM15 5NL
Tel: 01708 855009 Fax: 01708 851532
(Thurrock Primary Care Trust)

GP K R DEY

The Health Centre
Darenth Lane, South Ockendon RM15 5LP
Tel: 01708 853113 Fax: 01708 851265
(Thurrock Primary Care Trust)

Practice Manager Jan Beard

GP Muhammad Azizul HAQUE

The Health Centre
Darenth Lane, South Ockendon RM15 5LP
Tel: 01708 853113
(Thurrock Primary Care Trust)

GP M A HAQUE

Pear Tree Surgery
4 West Road, South Ockendon RM15 6PP
Tel: 01708 852318 Fax: 01708 853216
(Thurrock Primary Care Trust)

GP Stefan Dominic GARNER, Amanda Mary DAVIES, Chinnamma Sadasivan JAYAKUMAR

Sancta Maria Centre
Daiglen Drive, South Ockendon RM15 5SZ
Tel: 01708 851888 Fax: 01708 856570
(Thurrock Primary Care Trust)
Patient List Size: 5500

Practice Manager June Mason

GP Susan Valsa BELLWORTHY, Andrew HELLYAR

South Shields

Coronation Street Surgery
6A Coronation Street, South Shields NE33 1AZ
Tel: 0191 456 2856 Fax: 0191 427 0630
(South Tyneside Primary Care Trust)

Practice Manager Anne Grimmer

GP Asraf Uddin BORA

Farnham Medical Centre
435 Stanhope Road, South Shields NE33 4JE
Tel: 0191 455 4748 Fax: 0191 455 8573
(South Tyneside Primary Care Trust)

Practice Manager Ann Bull

GP Christopher Sutherland HARGREAVES, Dr CURTIS, Michelle EVANS, Dr GRAINGER, Christopher Shaun SANDBACH, Charles Nicholas WILSON

Flagg Court Health Centre
Flagg Court, South Shields NE33 2PG
Tel: 0191 456 2612 Fax: 0191 454 9131
(South Tyneside Primary Care Trust)

Practice Manager L Howe

GP Shaukat Hussain ANSARI

Flagg Court Health Centre
Wenlock Road Surgery, Flagg Court, South Shields NE33 2PG
Tel: 0191 456 0463 Fax: 0191 454 5525
(South Tyneside Primary Care Trust)

Practice Manager Sharon Richards

GP Mohammad Abrarul HAQUE, Mohammad Anwarul HAQUE

Imeary Street Surgery
78 Imeary Street, South Shields NE33 4EG
Tel: 0191 456 3824 Fax: 0191 427 5145
(South Tyneside Primary Care Trust)
Patient List Size: 3000

Practice Manager E Miller

GP Stephen Geoffrey MILLER

Marsden Road Surgery
The Health Centre, Marsden Road, South Shields NE34 6RE
Tel: 0191 454 0457 Fax: 0191 427 1793
(South Tyneside Primary Care Trust)
Patient List Size: 11100

Practice Manager Kathy Robinson

GP Arthur James MUCHALL, Colin BRADSHAW, Louise DUNCAN, Judith Margaret EGGLESTON, Alison HEATON, Niel SOULSBY, Matthew WALMSLEY

Perrins and Partners
Trinity Medical Centre, New George Street, South Shields NE33 5DU
Tel: 0191 454 7775 Fax: 0191 454 6787

(South Tyneside Primary Care Trust)
Patient List Size: 6200

Practice Manager M Weaver

GP John Kenneth PERRINS, Neil DOWDEN, Jane Ruth JENKINSON, Jyotsna Bhanuvilas PATTEKAR

Ravensworth Surgery
Horsley Hill Road, South Shields NE33 3ET
Tel: 0191 455 2093 Fax: 0191 427 6159
(South Tyneside Primary Care Trust)
Patient List Size: 4500

Practice Manager Irene McConnachie

GP Sreeni VIS-NATHAN, Ursuld HEIDENREICH

South Tyneside Health Care Trust
Flagg Court Health Centre, Flagg Court, South Shields NE33 2PG
Tel: 0191 456 0791 Fax: 0191 451 6447
(South Tyneside Primary Care Trust)
Patient List Size: 2200

GP Somesh CHANDER

Stanhope Parade Health Centre
Gordon Street, South Shields NE33 4HX
Tel: 0191 451 6143 Fax: 0191 451 6146
(South Tyneside Primary Care Trust)

Practice Manager Joy Curry

GP Suresh Govan DAYA

Stanhope Parade Health Centre
Gordon Street, South Shields NE33 4JP
Tel: 0191 456 4611 Fax: 0191 454 5103
(South Tyneside Primary Care Trust)

Practice Manager M Jennings

GP Jaya DEVIDAS

Stanhope Parade Health Centre
Gordon Street, South Shields NE33 4HX
Tel: 0191 455 4621 Fax: 0191 427 3180
(South Tyneside Primary Care Trust)

Practice Manager David Barnes

GP John Wallace MUNCASTER, Dianne Lesley BAINES, Dr BARNARD, Thomas Trenham BLAIR, Morris GALLAGHER, Dr MALONE, Dr TOSE

Talbot Medical Centre
Stanley Street, South Shields NE34 0AF
Tel: 0191 455 3867 Fax: 0191 454 3825
(South Tyneside Primary Care Trust)
Patient List Size: 9200

Practice Manager Dianne Burton

GP Michael Stewart CRAIG, Lorna J CARTER, Richard Ian HOLMES, Anthony William STONE

Trinity Medical Centre
New George Street, South Shields NE33 5DU
Tel: 0191 427 0338 Fax: 0191 456 5828
(South Tyneside Primary Care Trust)
Patient List Size: 8500

Practice Manager R Long

GP Nabil Awadalla NAROZ, Hung Song KOR, Nay WIN

Wawn Street Surgery
Wawn Street, South Shields NE33 4DX
Tel: 0191 451 6767 Fax: 0191 454 9428
(South Tyneside Primary Care Trust)
Patient List Size: 9300

Practice Manager Joan Carr-Lawton

GP Rajesh BHALLA, Rakesh BHALLA, Terry OWEN, Caroline GILL

Westoe Road Surgery
17 Westoe Road, South Shields NE33 4LS
Tel: 0191 456 2814 Fax: 0191 454 2424
(South Tyneside Primary Care Trust)
Patient List Size: 3200

Practice Manager L Sankar

GP Ramkrishna SANKAR

South Wirral

Hope Farm Medical Centre
Hope Farm Road, Great Sutton, South Wirral CH66 2WW
Tel: 0151 357 3777 Fax: 0151 357 1444
(Ellesmere Port and Neston Primary Care Trust)
Patient List Size: 11660

Practice Manager Margaret Freeburn

GP Jane Louise BROCKI, Geraldine M HOGAN, Karen L JONES, Susan Pamela KINGSTON, Simon G POWELL, Peter John TOWNSON

Neston Medical Centre
14-20 Liverpool Road, Neston, South Wirral CH64 3RA
Tel: 0151 336 4121 Fax: 0151 353 0151
(Ellesmere Port and Neston Primary Care Trust)
Patient List Size: 7800

Practice Manager Dot Stevenson

GP Roger Norman SNOOK, Sarah ASTON, Christopher Edwin STEERE, Teresa STREFFORD

Neston Surgery
Mellock Lane, Little Neston, South Wirral CH64 4BN
Tel: 0151 336 3951 Fax: 0151 353 0173
(Ellesmere Port and Neston Primary Care Trust)
Patient List Size: 8293

GP Mohammed Tahir Sultan AWAN, J M M PERKINS, A K TUCKER, Mark Ian WASHINGTON, Richard WILLCOX

Old Hall Surgery
26 Stanney Lane, Ellesmere Port, South Wirral CH65 9AD
Tel: 0151 355 1191 Fax: 0151 356 2683
Website: www.oldhallsurgery.co.uk
(Ellesmere Port and Neston Primary Care Trust)
Patient List Size: 5100

Practice Manager Jennifer Susan Roberts

GP Alan David BIRCH, Martyn Richard PHIPPS, Sally Anne SHAW

Westminster Surgery
Poole Community Centre, New Grosvenor Road, Ellesmere Port, South Wirral CH65 2HB
Tel: 0151 335 4864
(Ellesmere Port and Neston Primary Care Trust)

GP U A VELTKAMP

York Road Group Practice Surgery
York Road, Ellesmere Port, South Wirral CH65 0DB
Tel: 0151 355 2112 Fax: 0151 356 5512
(Ellesmere Port and Neston Primary Care Trust)

Practice Manager Catherine Mary Bedford

GP Nigel Christopher BARBER, Rodney Andrew DARLING, Richard Denis Joseph HODGES, B C LONGSTAFFE, Christopher James MACDONALD, A L SUDLOW, J F WILKINSON

Southall

Abbotts Road Surgery
42 Abbotts Road, Southall UB1 1HT
Tel: 020 8574 7746
(Ealing Primary Care Trust)

Practice Manager Amarjit Gill

GP K T MAW, H HTOO, M WYNN

Beaconsfield Road Surgery
23 Beaconsfield Road, Southall UB1 1BW
Tel: 020 8572 2536 Fax: 020 8570 3197
(Ealing Primary Care Trust)

Practice Manager Doris McManus

GP B S MANGAT, S K MANGAT

The Belmont Medical Clinic
18-20 Western Road, Southall UB2 5DU
Tel: 020 8574 0137 Fax: 020 8571 9683
(Ealing Primary Care Trust)
Patient List Size: 3200

Practice Manager Gursharan Sian

GP Ajaib Kaur SANDHU

The Guru Nanak Medical Centre
1 Woodlands Road, Southall UB1 1EE
Tel: 020 8574 1246 Fax: 020 8571 9199
(Ealing Primary Care Trust)

Practice Manager Mandip Duhra

GP G SINGH, R CHANOOK, K MOHAN

The Medical Centre
2-4 West End Road, Southall UB1 1JH
Tel: 020 8843 2000
(Ealing Primary Care Trust)

GP Dr PELT, Dr TAN, G S UPPAL, S UPPAL

Norwood Road Surgery
70 Norwood Road, Southall UB2 4EY
Tel: 020 8571 2182
(Ealing Primary Care Trust)

GP J S SANGHERA, V SANGHERA

Norwood Road Surgery
70A Norwood Road, Southall UB2 4EY
Tel: 020 8574 4454 Fax: 020 8571-2175
(Ealing Primary Care Trust)

GP J S SANGHERA, V K SANGHERA, Ann Elizabeth WALKER

Rutland Road Surgery
59 Rutland Road, Southall UB1 2UR
Tel: 020 8578 8255
(Ealing Primary Care Trust)
Patient List Size: 3000

Practice Manager Jayshree Patel

GP O S SAHOTA

The Saluja Clinic
36A Northcote Avenue, Southall UB1 2AY
Tel: 020 8574 5136 Fax: 020 8571 6816
(Ealing Primary Care Trust)
Patient List Size: 5500

Practice Manager Balbir Saluja

GP Rajinder Singh SALUJA

Southall Medical centre
128 Northcote Avenue, Southall UB1 2BA
Tel: 020 8574 4381 Fax: 020 8571 2531
(Ealing Primary Care Trust)
Patient List Size: 40500

Practice Manager Kuldip Sanghera

GP Jaswir Singh SANGHERA, V K SANGHERA

Sunrise Medical Centre
9 Abbotts Road, Southall UB1 1HS
Tel: 020 8843 9584 Fax: 020 8571 9934
(Ealing Primary Care Trust)

Practice Manager Jayshree Patel

GP F HAYAT

The Surgery
57 Lady Margaret Road, Southall UB1 2PH
Tel: 020 8547 5186 Fax: 020 8574 3202
(Ealing Primary Care Trust)
Patient List Size: 4780

Practice Manager Gurmeet K Lally

GP Sabiha RIZKI, Mohammed ALZARRAD

The Surgery
33 Dormers Wells Lane, Southall UB1 3HY
Tel: 020 8574 3986 Fax: 020 8893 6188
(Ealing Primary Care Trust)
Patient List Size: 5500

Practice Manager C Shah

GP Kamlesh KORPAL, Shri Kumar GAUTAM

The Surgery
95 Hammond Road, Southall UB2 4EH
Tel: 020 8574 5057 Fax: 020 8574 8459
(Ealing Primary Care Trust)

Practice Manager Jatinder Matharu

GP Avninder Singh SANDHU, Param Jeet Singh SANDHU

The Surgery
70 Norwood Road, Southall UB2 4EY
Tel: 020 8574 4454 Fax: 020 8813 9821
(Ealing Primary Care Trust)
Patient List Size: 3000

Practice Manager Joseph Andrew

GP Jamil RAHMAN, Huda WADIDDI

The Surgery
70a Norwood Road, Southall UB2 4EY
Tel: 020 8574 1822 Fax: 020 8571 2175
(Ealing Primary Care Trust)
Patient List Size: 4300

Practice Manager Bobby Chodha

GP Alan Jacob DAVIS, Valoria Mary Clare KENNEDY

The Surgery
64 Somerset Road, Southall UB1 2TS
Tel: 020 8578 1903 Fax: 020 8578 9213
Email: dr.qureshi@virgin.net
(Ealing Primary Care Trust)
Patient List Size: 2200

Practice Manager Hanifa Qureshi

GP S A QURESHI

The Surgery
21 St Georges Avenue, Southall UB1 1PZ
Tel: 020 8813 8122 Fax: 020 8574 1916
(Ealing Primary Care Trust)

Practice Manager Faye Bartel

GP Suganthamala RADHAKRISHNAN

The Surgery
423 Allenby Road, Southall UB1 2HG
Tel: 020 8578 1662
Email: malti.garg@gp.E85105.nhs.uk
(Ealing Primary Care Trust)

Practice Manager Pamela Bradbury

GP Malti GARG

The Surgery
2 Northcote Avenue, Southall UB1 2AX
Tel: 020 8571 3289 Fax: 020 8574 8222
(Ealing Primary Care Trust)
Patient List Size: 2000

Practice Manager Marlar Aye

GP S LWIN

The Surgery
276 Lady Margaret Road, Southall UB1 2RX
Tel: 020 8578 2421 Fax: 020 8747 7979
Email: ash_max@hotmail.com
(Ealing Primary Care Trust)

Practice Manager Varsha Chohan

GP A M BOTROS

The Surgery
150 Lady Margaret Road, Southall UB1 2RL
Tel: 020 8574 2812 Fax: 020 8571 5074
(Ealing Primary Care Trust)
Patient List Size: 2900

Practice Manager Manjit Kundi

GP M G MIKHAIL

The Surgery
1 Crosslands Avenue, Norwood Green, Southall UB2 5QY
Tel: 020 8574 1906 Fax: 020 8813 9718
(Hounslow Primary Care Trust)

GP Dr MENDEL, Dr SHARMA

The Surgery
128 Dormers Wells Lane, Southall UB1 3JB
Tel: 020 8571 0078 Fax: 020 8574 4952
(Ealing Primary Care Trust)
Patient List Size: 3600

Practice Manager Aysel Qadan

GP H QADAN

The Surgery
58 Carlyle Avenue, Southall UB1 2BH
Tel: 020 8843 9390 Fax: 020 8843 2219
(Ealing Primary Care Trust)
Patient List Size: 4700

Practice Manager Babita Ram

GP S CHATTERJEE, A KARUNALINGAM

The Surgery
243 Western Road, Southall UB2 5HS
Tel: 020 8571 5094 Fax: 020 8571 1415
(Ealing Primary Care Trust)

Practice Manager Babita Ram

GP K LAHON

The Surgery
95 Hammond Road, Southall UB2 4EY
(Ealing Primary Care Trust)

GP P J SANDHU

The Surgery
70 Norwood Road, Southall UB2 4EY
(Ealing Primary Care Trust)

GP Kim Yong NG

Southam

The Surgery
Stowe Drive, Southam CV47 1NY
Tel: 01926 812577 Fax: 01926 817447
Website: www.thesouthamsurgery.co.uk
(South Warwickshire Primary Care Trust)
Patient List Size: 8300

Practice Manager Ann Beadle

GP Alastair Malcolm ROBSON, Lesley Jane ADAMS, Larvinder MADAN, Michael John WRIGHT

The Surgery
High Street, Fenny Compton, Southam CV47 2YG
Tel: 01295 770855 Fax: 01295 770858
(South Warwickshire Primary Care Trust)

GP Peter Miles CHRISTOPHER, Richard Quentin MANN, Janet Rachel MARSHALL, Richard Andrew Stephen TAYLOR

Southampton

Aldermoor Health Centre
Aldermoor Close, Southampton SO16 5ST
Tel: 023 8079 7700 Fax: 023 8079 7767
(Southampton City Primary Care Trust)

Practice Manager Diana Mills

GP Marion Josephine DYER, Jennifer FIELD, Jennifer Helen GREENLAND, Patrick Michael St Quintin TERRY, Ian George WILLIAMSON

Alma Road Surgery
68 Alma Road, Portswood, Southampton SO14 6UX
Tel: 023 8067 2666 Fax: 023 8055 0972
Website: www.almamedcen.nhs.uk
(Southampton City Primary Care Trust)
Patient List Size: 11300

Practice Manager Paul T Clements

GP Robert David LEE, Louise Sarah BRADING, Ian Sinclair LAWRENCE, Chukwuma Ugwoeze Chugozare ONYEKWERE, Gail Celia ORD-HUME, Wilma WESTENSEE, Denis Noel YARDLEY

Atherley House Surgery
143-145 Shirley Road, Shirley, Southampton SO15 3FH
Tel: 023 8022 1964/0763 Fax: 023 8022 0763
(Southampton City Primary Care Trust)
Patient List Size: 3990

Practice Manager Jean Parker

GP Susan Isabel DAVIDSON, Angela Mary BLOUNT, Michael John BROOKE

Bath Lodge Practice
Bitterne Health Centre, Commercial Street, Bitterne, Southampton SO18 6BT
Tel: 023 8044 2111 Fax: 023 8042 1316
Email: bathlodge@aol.com
(Southampton City Primary Care Trust)
Patient List Size: 12800

Practice Manager Sue Wright

GP Philip John GRAY, Allison BUDGE, Christopher John BUDGE, Dawn Sheena GODWIN, Nicholas Richard HAYES, Fiona Jean MACKAY, Alexander McKAY, David John PAYNTON

Bishops Waltham Surgery
Lower Lane, Bishops Waltham, Southampton SO32 1GR
Tel: 01489 892288 Fax: 01489 894402
(Mid-Hampshire Primary Care Trust)
Patient List Size: 12300

Practice Manager Gina Daniels

GP Paul HEMMING, Jane COLLYER, Nicola EVANS, Ian FORSTER, Stephen HILLIER, S HUNTER, David IBBITSON, K O'REILLY, Susan WADE-WEST

Bitterne Park Surgery
28 Cobden Avenue, Bitterne Park, Southampton SO18 1BW
Tel: 023 8058 5655/6 Fax: 023 8055 5216
Website: www.bitterneparksurgery.nhs.uk
(Southampton City Primary Care Trust)
Patient List Size: 6400

Practice Manager Helen Whatmore

GP Stephen John TOWNSEND, Peter Alan LITTLEJOHNS, Richard McDERMOTT

Blackthorn Surgery
73 Station Road, Netley Abbey, Southampton SO31 5AE
Tel: 023 8045 3110 Fax: 023 8045 2747
Website: www.netleyhamblesurgeries.co.uk
(Eastleigh and Test Valley South Primary Care Trust)
Patient List Size: 10835

Practice Manager Anne Heathorn

GP David WILSON, Simon James Findlay GOODISON, Judy HARRIS, Hugh Christopher LAING, Ann Josephine LENNON, Emma MISCHEL, Christopher Mark Calder TOMSON

Botley Health Care Centre
Mortimer Road, Botley, Southampton SO32 2UG
Tel: 01489 783422 Fax: 01489 781919
(Eastleigh and Test Valley South Primary Care Trust)

Practice Manager Diane Taylor

GP Andrew William HILL, Grace Shannon MARSHALL, A MAYERS, Sheila Mary Mittell SORBY

Brook House Surgery
98 Oakley Road, Shirley, Southampton SO16 4NZ
Tel: 023 8077 4853 Fax: 023 8032 2357
(Southampton City Primary Care Trust)
Patient List Size: 4300

Practice Manager Adrienne Ely

GP Roland Lee SIMPSON, Katherine BARNES, Rosalind Margaret SIMPSON

Brook Lane Surgery
233a Brook Lane, Sarisbury Green, Southampton SO31 7DQ
Tel: 01489 575191 Fax: 01489 570033
(Fareham and Gosport Primary Care Trust)
Patient List Size: 9500

Practice Manager Carolyn Hill

GP G NEWMAN, C BERRY, A McFARLANE, T M TAYLER

Burgess Road Surgery
357a Burgess Road, Southampton SO16 3BD
Tel: 023 8067 6233 Fax: 023 8067 2909
(Southampton City Primary Care Trust)
Patient List Size: 7600

Practice Manager June Conklin

GP Chandrakant Shankerlal THAKER, Hemant Batukrai BHATT, Bhasker-Rai Pravinchandra DAVE, Angela Mary HALL

Bursledon Surgery
7 Manor Crescent, Bursledon, Southampton SO31 8DQ
Tel: 023 8040 4671 Fax: 023 8040 7417
(Eastleigh and Test Valley South Primary Care Trust)
Patient List Size: 3394

Practice Manager Anne Cutler

GP Anne BAUCHOP, Ann Elizabeth Alexandra ASHBURN

Canute Surgery
66A Portsmouth Road, Woolston, Southampton SO19 9AL
Tel: 023 8043 6277 Fax: 023 8039 9751
(Southampton City Primary Care Trust)

Practice Manager Carole Penney

GP Josephine Lynne WALSH, John GAY

Chessel Surgery - Bitterne Branch
4 Chessel Avenue, Bitterne, Southampton SO19 4AA
Tel: 023 8044 7777 Fax: 023 8042 5429
(Southampton City Primary Care Trust)

Practice Manager Patricia Crates

GP Michael Stuart FISHER, Ugochi C ADAMS, Kilian Jennifer BUTE, Maged Mourad Ramsis GIRGIS, Adrian Peter HIGGINS, David J MAGEE, Alfred Jeremy MEADOWS, Kenneth Ian SHAW

Cheviot Road Surgery
1 Cheviot Road, Millbrook, Southampton SO16 4AH
Tel: 01703 774040 Fax: 01703 702748
(Southampton City Primary Care Trust)

GP Anthony George KELPIE, Timothy James PATTEN, Caroline WHITEHOUSE

College Street Surgery
College Street, Southampton SO14 3EJ
Tel: 023 8033 3729 Fax: 023 8022 7233
(Southampton City Primary Care Trust)
Patient List Size: 1230

Practice Manager Jennifer Xavier

GP Alfredo Bruno XAVIER

Forest Gate Surgery
Hazel Farm Road, Totton, Southampton SO40 8WU
Tel: 023 8066 3839 Fax: 023 8066 7090
(New Forest Primary Care Trust)
Patient List Size: 12400

Practice Manager Lynne Penzer

GP Keith Teasdale PARRY, Nicolas Peter ARNEY, Cameron Michael AYRES, Clare Louise DETSIOS, Simon Paul FOWLER, Christopher John NEWMAN

Forestside Medical Practice
Beaulieu Road, Dibden Purlieu, Southampton SO45 4JA
Tel: 023 8087 7900 Fax: 023 8087 7909
(New Forest Primary Care Trust)
Patient List Size: 9,600

Practice Manager Angie May

GP S G HUDSON, Catherine June DAVIES, Stephen Paul Adrian HILL-COUSINS, R G MILLS, David John NEWTON

Grove Medical Practice
Shirley Health Centre, Grove Road, Shirley, Southampton SO15 3UA
Tel: 023 8078 3611 Fax: 023 8078 3156
(Southampton City Primary Care Trust)
Patient List Size: 10050

Practice Manager Kim Foster

GP Peter George Robin MAY, Carole Angela CLOUTER, Simon Douglas Stafford FRASER, John Halkon NIGHTINGALE, Peter McLay SHORT, Robert John WALTON

The Health Centre
Testwood Lane, Totton, Southampton SO40 3ZN
Tel: 023 8086 5051 Fax: 023 8086 5050
(New Forest Primary Care Trust)

Practice Manager Chris Brown

GP Terence Alwyn WOOD, Christopher George ALVEYN, Una Barrie BOYD, Malcolm Henry DARCH, Mary Anne FALLE, Simon Peter GAUNT, Sonia Jane GODFREY, Ian Peter STOBBS

Highfield Health
31 University Road, Highfield, Southampton SO17 1BJ
Tel: 023 8059 5545 Fax: 023 8059 5844
Email: health@soton.ac.uk
(Southampton City Primary Care Trust)
Patient List Size: 4920

GP Dr URSELL, Dr LOWE

Hill Lane Surgery
162 Hill Lane, Shirley, Southampton SO15 5DD
Tel: 023 8022 3086 Fax: 023 8023 5487
(Southampton City Primary Care Trust)
Patient List Size: 7900

Practice Manager Michelle Lombardi

GP Iain James LANG, Ian Spencer BENTLEY, Simon Charles HUNTER, Cecilia Mary THOMPSON

Homeless Healthcare Team PMS Pilot
30 Cranbury Avenue, Southampton SO14 0LT
Tel: 023 8033 6991 Fax: 023 8023 8596
(Southampton City Primary Care Trust)

Practice Manager Ann Duell

GP Louise Adele DUBRAS

Linfield Surgery
7 Belmont Road, Portswood, Southampton SO17 2GD
Tel: 023 8058 5858 Fax: 023 8039 9858
(Southampton City Primary Care Trust)
Patient List Size: 3900

GP John Michael GALLAGHER, Claire Louise HACKETT, Elizabeth PALMER

Lockswood Surgery
Centre Way, Locks Heath, Southampton SO31 6DX
Tel: 01489 885637 Fax: 01489 576185
(Fareham and Gosport Primary Care Trust)
Patient List Size: 13120

Practice Manager Heather Paul

GP Alan F A P COOPER, Adrian M COLE, Samuel HEAL, Colin MARTIN

Lordshill Health Centre
Lordshill District Centre, Lordshill, Southampton SO16 8HY
Tel: 023 8073 8144 Fax: 023 8073 0722
(Southampton City Primary Care Trust)
Patient List Size: 10100

Practice Manager Jennifer Gingell

GP Bruce John MANSBRIDGE, Beatrice Mary BAINBRIDGE, Michael BARNFIELD, Timothy Roy Markby BILLINGTON, Stephen Giles CRAWFORD, Beverley Anne GRAY

The Medical Centre
24-28 Lower Northam Road, Hedge End, Southampton SO30 4FQ
Tel: 01489 785722 Fax: 01489 799414
(Eastleigh and Test Valley South Primary Care Trust)
Patient List Size: 13200

Practice Manager Lynda Langford

GP John Templeton BUSH, Susan Frances COOKSON, Tina Louise CROOK, Elizabeth CROPLEY, Karl GRAHAM, Mark Daniel HOLLANDS, Ruth PADDAY, Richard Edward PERCIVAL, Corrin PHILLIPS

Midanbury Surgery
1 Woodmill Lane, Midanbury, Southampton SO18 2PA
Tel: 023 8055 5407 Fax: 023 8067 1491
(Southampton City Primary Care Trust)

Practice Manager Hazel Smith

GP Christopher John LUCKENS, Jeba J GNANAPRAGASAM

Mulberry House Surgery
38 Highfield Road, Highfield, Southampton SO17 1PJ
Tel: 023 8055 4549 Fax: 023 8055 3151
(Southampton City Primary Care Trust)
Patient List Size: 3300

Practice Manager Ann Beckett

GP Hugh Wollaston HADFIELD, Anne Amelia HADFIELD

North Baddesley Surgery
Norton Welch Close, Fleming Avenue, North Baddesley, Southampton SO52 9EP
Tel: 023 8074 3400/3401 Fax: 023 8074 3434
(Eastleigh and Test Valley South Primary Care Trust)
Patient List Size: 6650

Practice Manager Eileen Board

GP Stuart John SKEATES, Peter Stuart HAIG, Clare HARRIS, Sarah Patricia SCHOFIELD

Old Fire Station Surgery
68A Portsmouth Road, Woolston, Southampton SO19 9AN
Tel: 023 8044 8558/8901 Fax: 023 8043 5569
(Southampton City Primary Care Trust)
Patient List Size: 8100

Practice Manager Jill Dampier

GP William David GORROD, Fiona Ruth BABER, Hilary Marie CALLAHAN, Philip Gareth Wheyman MEAKINS, Anna Mark PURCELL

Portswood Road Surgery
186-188 Portswood Road, Portswood, Southampton SO17 2NJ
Tel: 023 8055 5181 Fax: 023 8036 6416
Email: portrdsurg@aol.com
(Southampton City Primary Care Trust)
Patient List Size: 2350

Practice Manager J Atkinson, Pauline Fillis

GP Peter Leslie THOMAS, Carol Adelaide THOMAS

Raymond Road Surgery
34 Raymond Road, Upper Shirley, Southampton SO15 5AL
Tel: 023 8022 7559 Fax: 023 8033 4028
(Southampton City Primary Care Trust)
Patient List Size: 3600

Practice Manager Nicola McKenzie

GP Yashvir SUNAK, Rosemary BAYLY, Alexandra FREEMAN

Regents Park Surgery
Park Street, Shirley, Southampton SO16 4RJ
Tel: 023 8078 3618 Fax: 023 8070 3103
(Southampton City Primary Care Trust)
Patient List Size: 5450

Practice Manager Kelvin Rush

GP Susan Jane ROBINSON, Timothy MORGAN, Patricia Jacqueline PORTER

Shirley Avenue Surgery
1 Shirley Avenue, Shirley, Southampton SO15 5RP
Tel: 023 8077 3258/1356 Fax: 023 8070 3078
(Southampton City Primary Care Trust)

Practice Manager David Lentle

GP Anthony Overbeck Cureton KNIGHT, Cormac Rowland Coman MURPHY, Jonathan James Austen PRINGLE, Michael John STRINGFELLOW

Six Dials Surgery
130-131 St. Marys Road, Southampton SO14 0BB
Tel: 023 8033 5151 Fax: 023 8033 9677
(Southampton City Primary Care Trust)

Practice Manager Janet Waghorn

GP Sankar Prosad PAL, Rama PAL

Spitfire Court Surgery
39 Spitfire Court, Mitchell Close, Woolston, Southampton SO19 7TN
Tel: 023 8042 0467 Fax: 023 8043 3050
(Southampton City Primary Care Trust)
Patient List Size: 2351

Practice Manager Frank Dix

GP David Francis William ADEY

St Denys Surgery
7 St Denys Road, Portswood, Southampton SO17 2GN
Tel: 023 8055 4161 Fax: 023 8055 4853
Email: nigel.dickson@gp-J82612.nhs.uk
Website: stdenyssurgery.nhs.uk
(Southampton City Primary Care Trust)
Patient List Size: 2850

Practice Manager Janet Waghorn

GP Nigel Keith DICKSON, Angus FERGUSON, Moria RUSSELL, David STREDDER

St Mary's Surgery
1 Johnson Street, Southampton SO14 1LT
Tel: 023 8033 3778 Fax: 023 8021 1894
(Southampton City Primary Care Trust)
Patient List Size: 14000

Practice Manager Barbara Clark

GP Kevin Vaughan REYNOLDS, Ingela CARRINGTON, George Bruce Seymour HOGHTON, Tim PEPPIATT, George Oliver PERCIVAL, Pauline Poh Lin YONG

St Peters Surgery
49-55 Portsmouth Road, Woolston, Southampton SO19 9RL
Tel: 023 8043 4355 Fax: 023 8043 4195
(Southampton City Primary Care Trust)
Patient List Size: 5247

Practice Manager Janet Knights

GP Graham Bentley SALMON, Hilary Jane BODDINGTON, Amyn Zahur KADRI

Stoneham Lane Surgery
6 Stoneham Lane, Swaythling, Southampton SO16 2AB
Tel: 023 8055 5776 Fax: 023 8039 9723
(Southampton City Primary Care Trust)
Patient List Size: 7200

Practice Manager Sue Roman

GP Gerald Eugene WADDINGTON, Lesley Marie CUNNINGHAM, William John FITZPATRICK, Amanda Nell HARMAN, Ceri Nigel LLOYD

The Surgery
2 Oxford Street, Southampton SO14 3DJ
Tel: 023 8033 5158/1366 Fax: 023 8033 5158
(Southampton City Primary Care Trust)

Practice Manager Carol O'Sullivan, Vivian Vine

GP Patrick Neville MORRIS, Bernadette Mary O'SULLIVAN

The Surgery
51 Locks Road, Locks Heath, Southampton SO31 7ZL
Tel: 01489 583777 Fax: 01489 571374
Email: dianne.heffer@gp-j82023.nhs.uk
Website: www.locksroadsurgery.co.uk
(Fareham and Gosport Primary Care Trust)
Patient List Size: 11800

Practice Manager Dianne Heffer

GP Stephen Gerard WHITAKER, Mark Lewis DENNISON, Camilla B HEYES, Paul Elliott HOWDEN, Andrew Anthony Rowland MOSTYN, Judy B PELL, Richard Marcus ROOPE

Testvale Surgery
12 Salisbury Road, Totton, Southampton SO40 3PY
Tel: 023 8086 6999/6990 Fax: 023 8066 3992
(New Forest Primary Care Trust)
Patient List Size: 12218

Practice Manager Linda Millard

GP John Frederick DRACASS, Suzanne BEAUMONT, Ian David ENTWISLE, Simon Lindsay HUNTER, Alison Louise THRELFALL, Michalakis Chris ZARDIS

Thornhill Park Road Surgery
90 Thornhill Park Road, Thornhill, Southampton SO18 5TR
Tel: 023 8047 4207 Fax: 023 8047 0004
(Southampton City Primary Care Trust)

Practice Manager Cheryl Domone

GP Wendy Margaret GARMAN, Samantha Denise Tonya DAVIES, Martin Norman LEWIS, Carol SMART

Townhill Surgery
Townhill District Centre, Southampton SO18 3RA
Tel: 023 8047 2232 Fax: 023 8046 5107
(Southampton City Primary Care Trust)
Patient List Size: 5244

Practice Manager Judith Pegram

GP Melissa J M JUDD, Douglas CAMPBELL, Alexander MUIR

University Health Service
University of Southampton, Building 48, Highfield, Southampton SO17 1BJ
Tel: 023 8055 7531 Fax: 023 8059 3259
Email: unidocs@cix.co.uk
Website: www.unidocs.co.uk
(Southampton City Primary Care Trust)
Patient List Size: 12500

Practice Manager Wendy Mills

GP Heather Norah WILSON, Sarah Jane Radley ARMSTRONG, Theresa Mary CREAGH, H EDWARDS, Christopher John JAMES

Victor Street Surgery
Victor Street, Shirley, Southampton SO15 5SY
Tel: 023 8077 4781 Fax: 023 8039 0680
(Southampton City Primary Care Trust)
Patient List Size: 14000

Practice Manager Andy Lopez

GP Alister Kenneth Mackinlay HUTCHIN, Sue BIRCH, David John Ker GIBSON, John Alan GLASSPOOL, Jill GRAHAM, Taina JEWSON, Ian PITT, Matthew RALL

West End Road Surgery
62 West End Road, Bitterne, Southampton SO18 6TG
Tel: 023 8044 9162 Fax: 023 8039 9742
(Southampton City Primary Care Trust)
Patient List Size: 9800

Practice Manager Jackie Spridgeon

GP Amrik Singh BENNING, Janet Elizabeth McFarlane MILLN, Alison ROBINS, Alexander Demetrius WALTERS

West End Surgery
Moorgreen Road, West End, Southampton SO30 3PY
Tel: 023 8047 2126/8039 9200 Fax: 023 8039 9201
(Eastleigh and Test Valley South Primary Care Trust)
Patient List Size: 7311

Practice Manager Barbara-Ann Harvell

GP Susan Victoria REES-JONES, Peter DAS, Simon Edward Morey LE BESQUE, Olivia RODRIGUES

White House Surgery
Weston Lane, Weston, Southampton SO19 9HJ
Tel: 023 8044 9913 Fax: 023 8044 6617
(Southampton City Primary Care Trust)

Practice Manager Harry Williamson

GP Barry Francis TREWINNARD, Anna Catherine ATKINSON, Philip James CLARKE, Stephen Francis HAYES, Martin David HUGHES, Melanie WHITEHORN

Wilton Lodge Surgery
56 Bedford Place, Southampton SO15 2DT
Tel: 023 8033 3326 Fax: 023 8033 3008
(Southampton City Primary Care Trust)

Practice Manager Janine Freemantle

GP Peter Charles Anthony GOODALL

Woolston Lodge Surgery
66 Portsmouth Road, Woolston, Southampton SO19 9AL
Tel: 023 8044 6733/6735 Fax: 023 8036 3568
Email: jayne.cruise@gp-j82076.nhs.uk
Website: www.woolstonlodge.co.uk
(Southampton City Primary Care Trust)
Patient List Size: 7243

Practice Manager Jayne Cruise

GP Edwin John ELLIOTT, Samantha HUMPHRIES, Peter Gaunt UPTON

Southend-on-Sea

Carnarvon Road Surgery
7 Carnarvon Road, Southend-on-Sea SS2 6LR
Tel: 01702 466340 Fax: 01702 603179
(Southend-on-Sea Primary Care Trust)
Patient List Size: 5500

Practice Manager Rita Barber

GP Fahim KHAN, Gigi Sara VERGHESE

Central Surgery
23 Boston Avenue, Southend-on-Sea SS2 6JH
Tel: 01702 342589 Fax: 01702 437015
(Southend-on-Sea Primary Care Trust)

Practice Manager Tina Wiseman

GP Azhar BAQAI, Varghese Kanisseril GEORGE

Dr N Elapatha and Partner
65 Warrior Square, Southend-on-Sea SS1 2JJ
Tel: 01702 467679 Fax: 01702 603207
Email: admin.mailbox@gp-F81159.nhs.uk
(Southend-on-Sea Primary Care Trust)
Patient List Size: 3802

Practice Manager Priyanti Manukularatne

GP I DHANAPALA, N ELAPATHA

Eagle Way Surgery
129 Eagle Way, Shoeburyness, Southend-on-Sea SS3 9YA
Tel: 01702 298109
(Southend-on-Sea Primary Care Trust)

GP K J K DHILLON

The Health Centre
55 High Street, Great Wakering, Southend-on-Sea SS3 0EF
Tel: 01702 577850 Fax: 01702 577853
(Castle Point and Rochford Primary Care Trust)
Patient List Size: 10170

Practice Manager Sandra Sheppard

GP Clifford Ernest OSBORNE, John Francis FREEL, Michael SAAD, Kenneth Ross SEATH, Rashti SRIYASTAVA

Health Centre
Campfield Road, Shoeburyness, Southend-on-Sea SS3 9BX
Tel: 01702 577702
(Southend-on-Sea Primary Care Trust)
Patient List Size: 6300

GP Navin KUMAR, Asha SINHA

Health Centre
Campfield Road, Shoeburyness, Southend-on-Sea SS3 9BX
Tel: 01702 577702 Fax: 01702 577726
Email: practice.manager@f81613.nhs.uk
(Southend-on-Sea Primary Care Trust)
Patient List Size: 6500

Practice Manager Christine Christmas, Benny Martine

GP N KUMAR, A SINHA

North Avenue Surgery
332 North Avenue, Southend-on-Sea SS2 4EQ
Tel: 01702 467215 Fax: 01702 603160
(Southend-on-Sea Primary Care Trust)

Practice Manager Peggy Byfield

GP Natverlal Kantilal SHAH

North Shoebury Surgery
Frobisher Way, Shoeburyness, Southend-on-Sea SS3 8UT
Tel: 01702 297976 Fax: 01702 290131
(Southend-on-Sea Primary Care Trust)
Patient List Size: 2500

Practice Manager Beverley Barns

GP Paul Nicholas Bolton MOSS

Prince Avenue Surgery
3 Prince Avenue, Southend-on-Sea SS2 6RL
Tel: 01702 349293 Fax: 01702 553244
(Southend-on-Sea Primary Care Trust)

Practice Manager Monica Mandalia, Stella Threadgold

GP K SANTHAKUMAR, Velaiuthar SOORIAKUMARAN

Queensway Surgery
75 Queensway, Southend-on-Sea SS1 2AB
Tel: 01702 463333 Fax: 01702 603026
Website: www.queenswaysurgery.co.uk
(Southend-on-Sea Primary Care Trust)

Practice Manager Carole Pelta

GP David Elliott PELTA, Anthony Robert Warrell BOWRING, Beverley HART, Michael Ernest William JACK, Kathryn JUPP, Phillip LAFFERTY, Diana RIGBY, David William SILLS, Eric WATKINS

Rochford Road Surgery
6A Rochford Road, Southend-on-Sea SS2 6SP
Tel: 01702 346615 Fax: 01702 437152
(Southend-on-Sea Primary Care Trust)

GP H H SHAH

Scott Park Surgery
205 Western Approaches, Southend-on-Sea SS2 6XY
Tel: 01702 420642 Fax: 01702 527852
(Southend-on-Sea Primary Care Trust)

Practice Manager Nancy Ng

GP H W NG

Shaftesbury Avenue
119 Shaftesbury Avenue, Southend-on-Sea SS1 3AN
Tel: 01702 582687 Fax: 01702 589143
(Southend-on-Sea Primary Care Trust)

Practice Manager Rosemary Weeks

GP William Thomas WEEKS

Southchurch Boulevard Surgery
27 Southchurch Boulevard, Southend-on-Sea SS2 4UB
Tel: 01702 468443 Fax: 01702 603281
(Southend-on-Sea Primary Care Trust)

Practice Manager R Crozier

GP Christopher Alan Vivian GOODCHILD, Uwe Christian HUTTER, Aidan Charles IRLAM

The Surgery
101 West Road, Shoeburyness, Southend-on-Sea SS3 9DT
Tel: 01702 293535 Fax: 01702 291282
(Southend-on-Sea Primary Care Trust)

Practice Manager Sandra Rider

GP A A KHAN

Tyrone Road Surgery
99 Tyrone Road, Thorpe Bay, Southend-on-Sea SS1 3HD
Tel: 01702 582670 Fax: 01702 589146
Email: doctor@thorpe-bay.surgery.co.uk
Website: www.thorpe-bay-surgery.co.uk
(Southend-on-Sea Primary Care Trust)
Patient List Size: 5200

Practice Manager R Y Siddique

GP Dr AGHA, Dr SIDDIQUE, Amah YEE

Warrior Square Surgery
61 Warrior Square, Southend-on-Sea SS1 2JJ
Tel: 01702 618411 Fax: 01702 464163
(Southend-on-Sea Primary Care Trust)
Patient List Size: 2740

Practice Manager Margaret Routledge

GP Sohan Lal VASHISHT

Southminster

Tillingham Medical Centre
61 South Street, Tillingham, Southminster CM0 7TH
Tel: 01621 778383 Fax: 01621 778034
(Maldon and South Chelmsford Primary Care Trust)
Patient List Size: 2800

Practice Manager Chris Shaw

GP Andrew George BARCLAY, Julie Elizabeth McGEACHY

The William Fisher Medical Centre
High Street, Southminster CM0 7AY
Tel: 01621 772360 Fax: 01621 773880
(Maldon and South Chelmsford Primary Care Trust)

Practice Manager Jo Farrell

GP Patricia Ann BOWTON, Trevor James SOUTHEY

Southport

Ainsdale Medical Centre
66-68 Station Road, Ainsdale, Southport PR8 3HW
Tel: 01704 574137 Fax: 01704 573875
Website: www.ainsdale-mc.co.uk
(Southport and Formby Primary Care Trust)
Patient List Size: 12800

Practice Manager Pamela Tabchi

GP Stuart Keith BENNETT, Stephan Joseph BONNET, Sara Hoghton BURNS, Simon Charles FOSTER, Colette Marie NUGENT, Elizabeth Ann QUINLAN, Robert McCulloch RUSSELL

Ainsdale Village Surgery
2 Leamington Road, Southport PR8 3LB
Tel: 01704 577866 Fax: 01704 576644
(Southport and Formby Primary Care Trust)
Patient List Size: 3400

Practice Manager Chris Taylor

GP Paul SMITH

Church Street Practice
8 Church Street, Southport PR9 0QT
Tel: 01704 533666 Fax: 01704 539239
(Southport and Formby Primary Care Trust)
Patient List Size: 10000

Practice Manager Paul Cheston, M Hamilton

GP Geoffrey Stuart HEDLEY, Graeme Muir ALLAN, Keith BOARDMAN, Ian Michael JOLLY, Elizabeth Anne ROSTRON, Gillian STUBBENS

Churchtown Medical Centre
137 Cambridge Road, Southport PR9 7LT
Tel: 01704 224416 Fax: 01704 507168
(Southport and Formby Primary Care Trust)

Practice Manager Ruth Shrubsole

GP Gregory Michael FIRTH, Paolo Biagio Luigi GIANNELLI, D R GRENYER, Dr KIDD, Mary Patricia McCORMACK, Dr SCOTT

The Corner Surgery
180 Cambridge Road, Southport PR9 7LW
Tel: 01704 506055 Fax: 01704 505818
(Southport and Formby Primary Care Trust)
Patient List Size: 3000

Practice Manager Pat Parry

GP Peter Brian ENTWISTLE, Georgina Helen Maimie SHARPE

The Corner Surgery
180 Cambridge Road, Southport PR9 7LW
Tel: 01704 505555 Fax: 01704 505818
(Southport and Formby Primary Care Trust)

Practice Manager Sally Fenton

GP Patricia Margaret TURNER, Elizabeth Ann WAINWRIGHT

Cumberland House Surgery
58 Scarisbrick New Road, Southport PR8 6PQ
Tel: 01704 501500 Fax: 01704 549382
Website: www.cumberlandhousesurgery.co.uk
(Southport and Formby Primary Care Trust)

Practice Manager Sue Critchlow

GP Hugh Peter MILLIGAN, Dr BURROWS, Olga EYRE, Ian Mark HUGHES, Dr RANDALL, Peter Lawrence WILLIAMS

Devi Surgery
13 Scarisbrick New Road, Southport PR8 6PX
Tel: 01704 531114 Fax: 01704 533794
(Southport and Formby Primary Care Trust)

Practice Manager Kath Harrington

GP Devyani Vipin TRIVEDI, Vipin Ambalal TRIVEDI

Family Surgery
107 Liverpool Road, Southport PR8 4DB
Tel: 01704 566646 Fax: 01704 550858
(Southport and Formby Primary Care Trust)

Practice Manager J Cox-Pridmore

GP Kebalanandha Ramamurthie NAIDOO

The Grange Surgery
41 York Road, Southport PR8 2AD
Tel: 01704 560506 Fax: 01704 563108
(Southport and Formby Primary Care Trust)
Patient List Size: 9700

Practice Manager Veronica Meethan

GP F CURRIE, M DRIJFHOUT, Martin David EVANS, Ian Michael KILSHAW, Alan James RYAN

Kew Medical Centre
70A Folkstone Road, Kew, Southport PR8 5PH
Tel: 01704 546800 Fax: 01704 540486
(Southport and Formby Primary Care Trust)

Practice Manager Linda Roberts

GP Halina OBUCHOWICZ

Norwood Surgery
11 Norwood Avenue, Southport PR9 7EG
Tel: 01704 226973 Fax: 01704 505758
(Southport and Formby Primary Care Trust)

Practice Manager Judy Cranshaw

GP Mark Charles CUSHING, John David SEARSON, Simon David Manning TOBIN, David John UNWIN

Richmond Surgery
147 Liverpool Road, Birkdale, Southport PR8 4NT
Tel: 01704 566277 Fax: 01704 563007
(Southport and Formby Primary Care Trust)
Patient List Size: 3000

Practice Manager Stephanie Perrett

GP P J RAO

Roe Lane Surgery
172 Roe Lane, Southport PR9 7PN
Tel: 01704 228439 Fax: 01704 506878
(Southport and Formby Primary Care Trust)
Patient List Size: 2300

Practice Manager Sue Lockyer

GP Jennifer Ann FOX, Wendy HEWITT, Niall Joseph LEONARD, Alison TREVOR

Sussex Road Surgery
125 Sussex Road, Southport PR8 6AF
Tel: 01704 536778 Fax: 01704 532838
(Southport and Formby Primary Care Trust)

Practice Manager Aileen Dinsdale

GP Leszek Andrzej SZCZESNIAK

Terrace End Surgery
57 Manchester Road, Southport PR9 9BN
Tel: 01704 532314 Fax: 01704 539740
(Southport and Formby Primary Care Trust)

Practice Manager Margaret Innes

GP Christine Elizabeth CORDER, Rajesh Rasikbhai PATEL, Julia Anne RONSON

Southsea

Campbell Surgery
2A Campbell Road, Southsea PO5 1RN
Tel: 023 9281 1275
(Portsmouth City Teaching Primary Care Trust)
Patient List Size: 2700

GP Barbara Joan DALE, Karen Ann SIZER

Doctors Surgery
Salisbury Road, Southsea PO4 9QX
Tel: 023 9273 1458
(Portsmouth City Teaching Primary Care Trust)

Practice Manager M. Beattie

GP David Gerald Roger PEARSON, F CRAWFORD, Joanne Elizabeth GIDDENS, Helen Rosemary HARPER, Andrew Paul PRESTON

Eastney Health Centre
Highland Road, Southsea PO4 9HU
Tel: 023 9287 1999 Fax: 023 9283 2832
(Portsmouth City Teaching Primary Care Trust)

Practice Manager Marie Skinner

GP Richard Francis TYRRELL, Rebecca LAKE, Laura PROCTER, Jane Louise RICHBELL

Milton Park Surgery
131 Goldsmith Avenue, Southsea PO4 8QZ
Tel: 023 9273 2578 Fax: 023 9281 1057
(Portsmouth City Teaching Primary Care Trust)

Practice Manager Lesley Randle

GP Elizabeth Jane FELLOWS, Stephanie Ann SCHOFIELD

Osborne Practice Surgery
25 Osborne Road, Southsea PO5 3ND
Tel: 023 9282 1371 Fax: 023 9229 1076
(Portsmouth City Teaching Primary Care Trust)

Practice Manager P Harrison

GP Brian David MITCHELL, S MACANOVIE, Jonathan Paul David PRICE, Margaret ROBINSON

Somers Town Health Centre
Blackfriars Close, Southsea PO5 4NJ
Tel: 023 9285 1202 Fax: 023 9229 6380
(Portsmouth City Teaching Primary Care Trust)
Patient List Size: 4000

Practice Manager Fran White

GP Christopher Vawer WILLIAMS, Elizabeth Mary SPOLTON

Somers Town Health Centre
Blackfriars Close, Southsea PO5 4NJ
Tel: 023 9285 1199 Fax: 023 9281 4626
Website: www.drsbarrontutteminay.co.uk
(Portsmouth City Teaching Primary Care Trust)
Patient List Size: 5400

Practice Manager Carol White

GP Geoffrey Robert BARRON, Ian Frederick MINAY, Kevin Philip TUTTE

The Surgery
3 Heyward Road, Southsea PO4 0DY
Tel: 023 9273 7373 Fax: 023 9229 6380
(Portsmouth City Teaching Primary Care Trust)

Practice Manager Viv Baker

GP Anne Jean WHITE, Catherine WELLS, Jane WINFIELD

The Surgery
262 Devonshire Avenue, Southsea PO4 9EH
Tel: 023 9273 1358 Fax: 023 9275 0091
(Portsmouth City Teaching Primary Care Trust)

Practice Manager Sue Crock

GP Douglas Paul PRYCE, Bella Noel CAIGER, Nicolas David O'DONOVAN

The Surgery
12 Victoria Road South, Southsea PO5 2BZ
Tel: 023 9282 3857 Fax: 023 9235 8944
(Portsmouth City Teaching Primary Care Trust)
Patient List Size: 6300

Practice Manager Elizabeth Berridge

GP Gordon Tallyn PARKIN, Michael CAIGER, Lisa HALL

The Surgery
36 Waverley Road, Southsea PO5 2PW
Tel: 023 9282 8281 Fax: 023 9282 2275
(Portsmouth City Teaching Primary Care Trust)

Practice Manager Marion Bedford

GP Angela Mary SISSONS, Alice Catherine EMERSON, Richard David FOORD

Southwell

Fenton and Partners
Medical Centre, Burgage Green, Southwell NG25 0EW
Tel: 01636 813561 Fax: 01636 816453
(Newark and Sherwood Primary Care Trust)

Practice Manager David Philip Mellor

GP Patrick Richard DANBY, Henry Colin COTTELL, D FENTON, Sarah Kathryn GROOME, Victoria Jane HILL, Simon David REEVES

Southwold

Southwold Surgery
York Road, Southwold IP18 6AN
Tel: 01502 722326 Fax: 01502 724708
(Waveney Primary Care Trust)
Patient List Size: 5200

Practice Manager A A Wilson

GP Andrew Nathaniel EASTAUGH, C R CASTLE, Mary HARLAND, J B STAMMERS

Sowerby Bridge

Brig Royd Surgery
Brig Royd, Ripponden, Sowerby Bridge HX6 4AN
Tel: 01422 822209
(Calderdale Primary Care Trust)
Patient List Size: 8500

Practice Manager Isobel Fletcher

GP Roger Watson POOL, Mary Louise KNOWLES, Carl Raymond LITTLEWOOD, Lisa Jane PICKLES, Ben Timothy WYATT

Station Road Surgery
Station Road, Sowerby Bridge HX6 3AB
Tel: 01422 831453/831457 Fax: 01422 835958
Email: office@stationsurgery.co.uk
(Calderdale Primary Care Trust)

Practice Manager Maureen Pitchforth

GP Paul James HINTON, Stephen Irving CATLOW, Arif Marzook Maqbul Ahmed KAZI, M C SOWDEN

Spalding

Church Street Surgery
Church Street, Spalding PE11 2PB
Tel: 01775 722189 Fax: 01775 712164
(East Lincolnshire Primary Care Trust)

Practice Manager P Slater

GP Philip Frederic Ewing RODGERS, David John CORLETT, Caroline Elisabeth MANNERS, David John RILEY, Andrew David Royston STONE

Lowgate Surgery
19 Lowgate, Gosberton, Spalding PE11 4NL
Tel: 01775 840204 Fax: 01775 841108
(East Lincolnshire Primary Care Trust)

GP Robert Henry BROOKES, Nicholas James LOW

Medical Centre
Gosberton, Spalding PE11 4NL
(East Lincolnshire Primary Care Trust)

Munro Medical Centre
West Elloe Avenue, Spalding PE11 2BY
Tel: 01775 725530 Fax: 01775 766168
(East Lincolnshire Primary Care Trust)
Patient List Size: 16700

Practice Manager E Holmes

GP James Malcolm COWELL, Alexander WALTON, Richard Mark BEATTY, Catherine Anne HAMBLIN, Charles Patrick Brian LENNON, Peter McCOMBIE, Graham WHEATLEY, Kieron Aubrey Raymond WISCOMBE

Pennygate Surgery
210 Pennygate, Spalding PE11 1LT
Tel: 01775 710133
(East Lincolnshire Primary Care Trust)

GP Azmeena NATHU

Price and Partners
The Surgery, Park Road, Holbeach, Spalding PE12 7EE
Tel: 01406 423288 Fax: 01406 426284
(East Lincolnshire Primary Care Trust)

GP Michael PRICE, Alastair Ian BELL, Shaun RAYNER

Sutton Medical Group
Allenby's Chase, Sutton Bridge, Spalding PE12 9SY
Tel: 01406 362081 Fax: 01406 351005
(East Lincolnshire Primary Care Trust)
Patient List Size: 14800

Practice Manager Andy Mills

GP John Brian JACKLIN, Christopher Charles BOOTH, Caroll Chee-Chiu FUNG, Alan Robert GLEAVE, Richard Huw JONES, Alistair James RUDD

Sykes and Menzies
Littlebury Medical Centre, Fishpond Lane, Holbeach, Spalding PE12 7DE
Tel: 01406 22231 Fax: 01406 425008
(East Lincolnshire Primary Care Trust)
Patient List Size: 6000

Practice Manager Paula Clark

GP Andrew SYKES

Thorpe, Burgess and Menzies
Moulton Medical Centre, High St, Moulton, Spalding PE12 6QB
Tel: 01406 370265 Fax: 01406 373219
(East Lincolnshire Primary Care Trust)

GP Douglas Anderson BURGESS, Scott Hamilton MENZIES, Richard William THORPE

Spennymoor

Sanderson and Partners
Adan House Surgery, St. Andrews Lane, Spennymoor DL16 6QA
Tel: 01388 817777 Fax: 01388 811700
(Sedgefield Primary Care Trust)
Patient List Size: 10000

Practice Manager Tracey Martin

GP Andrew Alexander Fleck SANDERSON, Naomi Elizabeth IBBOTT, Anthony James LONG, Sanjay Kumar PATEL, Alan Eric SENSIER

Spennymoor Health Centre
Bishops Close, Spennymoor DL16 6ED
Tel: 01388 811455 Fax: 01388 812034
(Sedgefield Primary Care Trust)
Patient List Size: 8900

Practice Manager Marie Carfoot

GP Michael Richard Duncan WOOD, Andrew John HENDERSON, Andrew Nicholas HERD, James Edward STAINES, Karen Ann VAN DEN BRUL

The Surgery
Oxford Road, Spennymoor DL16 6BQ
Tel: 01388 815081 Fax: 01388 815100
Email: dvroy@gp-A38603.nhs.uk
(Sedgefield Primary Care Trust)
Patient List Size: 2392

Practice Manager Michelle Bailey, Glenn Carroll

GP Dinah Venetia ROY

Spilsby

The Surgery
Bull Yard, Simpson Street, Spilsby PE23 5LG
Tel: 01790 752555 Fax: 01790 754457
Website: www.thespilsbysurgery.co.uk
(East Lincolnshire Primary Care Trust)
Patient List Size: 7500

Practice Manager Jeannie Bee

GP David Ernest CARTWRIGHT, Michael GERMER, Noel Ignatius O'KELLY, Mark Owen WAIN

St Agnes

Pengarth Road Surgery
Pengarth Road, St Agnes TR5 0TN
Tel: 01872 553881 Fax: 01872 553885
Email: enquiries@st-agnes.cornwall.nhs.uk
(Central Cornwall Primary Care Trust)
Patient List Size: 7200

Practice Manager Elizabeth Wills

GP John Trevor JULIAN, Ian James FUSSELL, Dr HENDERSON, Jane M NAYLOR, Christopher Martin WHITWORTH

St Albans

Colney Medical Centre
45-47 Kings Road, London Colney, St Albans AL2 1ES
Tel: 01727 822138 Fax: 01727 822130
Website: www.colneymedicalcentre.co.uk
(St Albans and Harpenden Primary Care Trust)

GP Pushpa KEDIA, Kapil KEDIA, Nitil KEDIA

Grange Street Surgery
2 Grange Street, St Albans AL3 5NF
Tel: 01727 833550 Fax: 01727 847961
Email: grangesurgery@gp.nhs.uk
(St Albans and Harpenden Primary Care Trust)
Patient List Size: 10000

Practice Manager Linda Ward

GP Anthony Richard HASELER, Anne Catherine ALLISTONE, Gemma CAVAITTHER, Iain Alasdair McNeill DOW, Hugh Alistair Daniel MARTIN

Harvey Group Practice
13-15 Russell Avenue, St Albans AL3 5HB
Tel: 01727 831888 Fax: 01727 845520
(St Albans and Harpenden Primary Care Trust)
Patient List Size: 11800

Practice Manager Philip Eaton

GP Jonathan Peter CLEGG, Angela Lesley ANDERSON, Sonia Mary ELSTOW, Ian Alexander HAMILTON, Satpal SINGH, Ruth Helen SUTTON, Mike WALTON

Hatfield Road Surgery
61 Hatfield Road, St Albans AL1 4JE
Tel: 01727 853079
(St Albans and Harpenden Primary Care Trust)
Patient List Size: 3700

Practice Manager Helen Tovey

GP Rukn Uddin HAIDER, Gauri SINHA

The Health Centre
High Street, Redbourn, St Albans AL3 7LZ
Tel: 01582 792356 Fax: 01582 793899
(St Albans and Harpenden Primary Care Trust)
Patient List Size: 5500

Practice Manager Maggie Raeburn

GP Kathryn Elizabeth DEXTER, Nirmal Kishore BAGUANT, Rosemary RAMSAY

Lattimore Surgery
1 Upton Avenue, St Albans AL3 5ER
Tel: 01727 855160 Fax: 01727 839617
(St Albans and Harpenden Primary Care Trust)

GP Josephine Mary BALDERAMOS-PRICE, Itrat Hazur KHAN

Lodge Surgery
Normandy Road, St Albans AL3 5NP
Tel: 01727 853107 Fax: 01727 862657
(St Albans and Harpenden Primary Care Trust)
Patient List Size: 10080

Practice Manager S Waldron

GP Anthony Hugh DAVIES, Mark Andrew BEVIS, Philip Leslie GRIFFIN, Amanda MARGERESON, Harriet STRAIN, Laura WASSON, Ruth Laura WILLIAMS

The Maltings Surgery
10 Victoria Street, St Albans AL1 3JB
Tel: 01727 855500 Fax: 01727 898164
(St Albans and Harpenden Primary Care Trust)
Patient List Size: 16600

Practice Manager Linda Cosgrove

GP Hilary SMITH, Mark William ALLEN, Alison DAVIES, Sarah Elizabeth DOWLING, Grant ELIAS, Julian Raymond Lister GODLEE, Paula Michelle LIVESEY, Philip Raymond MOORE, Philip Edmund SKELTON, Alan Robert THOMSON

Midway Surgery
93 Watford Road, St Albans AL2 3JX
Tel: 01727 832125 Fax: 01727 836384
(St Albans and Harpenden Primary Care Trust)
Patient List Size: 10000

Practice Manager Lynn Lamond

GP James Wellwood FERGUSON, Jill Annette BARTLETT, Michael Charles Stewart CANNELL, Elin JONES, Susan LOFTHOUSE

Parkbury House Surgery
St Peters Street, St Albans AL1 3HD
Tel: 01727 851589
(St Albans and Harpenden Primary Care Trust)
Patient List Size: 17000

GP Roger Edmund Maitland SAGE, Margaret Ethel BLANSHARD, Bruce Robert COVELL, Lisa DAY, Jonathan Elliot FREEDMAN, Steven LAITNER, Philippa Jane MAINWARING, Richard PILE, Amanda Jill PLATTS, Philip SAWYER

The Surgery
1 Hicks Road, Markyate, St Albans AL3 8LJ
Tel: 01582 840288
(Dacorum Primary Care Trust)

GP Julie Janina KUZEL

The Surgery
1 Hicks Road, Markyate, St Albans AL3 8LJ
Tel: 01582 841559 Fax: 01582 840083
(Dacorum Primary Care Trust)
Patient List Size: 2400

Practice Manager Gill Foskett

GP Tehmton Meherwan SEPAI

The Village Surgery
283 High Street, London Colney, St Albans AL2 1EU
Tel: 01727 823245
(St Albans and Harpenden Primary Care Trust)
Patient List Size: 4000

Practice Manager Sue Cannell

GP I KHAN, Sian EDWARDS, Easan KRISHNANANDAN, Antia PATEL

St Austell

Belmont Surgery
12 Belmont Road, St Austell PL25 4UJ
Tel: 01726 69444
(Central Cornwall Primary Care Trust)
Patient List Size: 5230

GP Rupert Brian ADKINS, Anthony Charles HEREWARD, Colan Denis ROBINSON

Brannel Surgery
58 Rectory Road, St. Stephen, St Austell PL26 7RL
Tel: 01726 822254 Fax: 01726 824450
Email: brannel.cornwall.nhs.uk
(Central Cornwall Primary Care Trust)
Patient List Size: 4600

Practice Manager Liz Cox

GP Francis Edmund BURKE, John Richard CECIL

Fore Street Surgery
Fore Street, St Dennis, St Austell PL26 8AG
Tel: 01726 822254
(Central Cornwall Primary Care Trust)

GP Heiko COOPER, Paul Bentham FOSTER, Susannah Maria JENKIN, Karl Wayne ROBINSON, Paul Michiel SCHENK

The New Surgery
River Street, Mevagissey, St Austell PL26 6UE
Tel: 01726 843701 Fax: 01726 842565
Website: www.mevagisseysurgery.co.uk
(Central Cornwall Primary Care Trust)
Patient List Size: 5390

GP Thomas Howard Edward HOTTON, Michael Francis DOWLING, K J JAMES, Christopher George TILEY

Park Medical Centre
19 Bridge Road, St Austell PL25 5HE
Tel: 01726 73042 Fax: 01726 74349
(Central Cornwall Primary Care Trust)
Patient List Size: 6575

Practice Manager D Marshall

GP Stephen John FORSDICK, Alan DAVIS, Rosalind HENNIG

Polkyth Surgery
14 Carlyon Road, St Austell PL25 4EG
Tel: 01726 75555 Fax: 01726 71217
(Central Cornwall Primary Care Trust)
Patient List Size: 10000

GP Anthony Richard WHITEHOUSE, Martin BROOKE, David Charles DEELEY, Angus SENIOR, Pernell TEMPEST, Paul TRAVIS

Woodland Road Surgery
20 Woodland Road, St Austell PL25 4QY
Tel: 01726 63311 Fax: 01726 74140
Email: woodland.enquiries@woodlandroad.cornwall.nhs.uk
Website: www.woodlandroad.f9.co.uk
(Central Cornwall Primary Care Trust)
Patient List Size: 7500

Practice Manager Sally Leigh

GP Jonathan Rupert Oliver LEIGH, Alistair Mark JAMES, David Robert MACKRELL, Martyn Gerald ROBINSON

St Helens

Acorn Surgery
39 Junction Lane, St Helens WA9 3JN
Tel: 01744 813065 Fax: 01744 819441
(St Helens Primary Care Trust)

Practice Manager Julie Fyles

GP Paul Gerard MARKEY

Bethany Medical Centre
151 Grafton Street, St Helens WA10 4GW
Tel: 01744 734128 Fax: 01744 759978
Email: bethany.reception@sthkhealth.nhs.uk
Website: www.bethanymedical.co.uk
(St Helens Primary Care Trust)

Practice Manager S Hodgetts

GP Laurence MILES, Christine Margaret MILES

The Bowery Medical Centre
Elephant Lane, St Helens WA9 5PR
Tel: 01744 816837 Fax: 01744 850800
(St Helens Primary Care Trust)
Patient List Size: 3600

Practice Manager Paula Alderson

GP Ritu MAINI, Shikha PITALIA, V K SAKSENA

Central Surgery
22 Cowley Hill Lane, St Helens WA10 2AE
Tel: 01744 24849 Fax: 01744 456497
(St Helens Primary Care Trust)

Practice Manager K E Thomson

GP Peter Anthony DILWORTH, Kenneth Noel MARRIOTT, Barbara Ann McCOURT, Minaxi SHAH

Ferguson Family Medical Practice
Berrymead Medical Centre, 140 Berrys Lane, Parr, St Helens WA9 3RP
Tel: 01744 25533 Fax: 01744 734752
(St Helens Primary Care Trust)
Patient List Size: 8500

Practice Manager Pam Lee

GP Jonathan Robert D'ARCY, Nicola Joy FERGUSON, Christopher PATTULLO, Andrew SMITH

Fingerpost Surgery
117 Higher Parr Street, St Helens WA9 1AG
Tel: 01744 21867 Fax: 01744 23342
(St Helens Primary Care Trust)

GP Karen BEEBY, Dr WHITTAKER

Four Acre Health Centre
Burnage Avenue, Clock Face, St Helens WA9 4QB
Tel: 01744 819884 Fax: 01744 850382
(St Helens Primary Care Trust)

Practice Manager H M Hesketh

GP John Andrew KURZEJA, Olawale Hakeen JUNAID, Katrina Maria O'DONNELL, Jarrod SCHOFIELD

Hall Street Surgery
28-30 Hall Street, St Helens WA10 1DW
Tel: 01744 733133 Fax: 01744 615982
(St Helens Primary Care Trust)

Practice Manager Edith Prescott

GP Terence Edward KENNY, Bina BANSAL

Haydock Medical Centre
Station Road, Haydock, St Helens WA11 0JN
Tel: 01744 734419 Fax: 01744 454875
(St Helens Primary Care Trust)

Practice Manager Marie Faulkner

GP Paul Howard VAUGHAN, Martin BREACH, John Duncan HOLDEN, Peter WEBB, Pamela Edith WILSON

The Health Centre
Station Road, Haydock, St Helens WA11 0JN
Tel: 01744 734419
(St Helens Primary Care Trust)
Patient List Size: 8400

Practice Manager Sharon Greenwood

GP Paul Howard VAUGHAN, martin BREACH, John Duncan HOLDEN, Peter WEBB, Pamela Edith WILSON

Kenneth Macrae Medical Centre
32 Church Road, Rainford, St Helens WA11 8HJ
Tel: 01744 882606 Fax: 01744 883546
(St Helens Primary Care Trust)

GP Eithne Maire Rosaleen MACRAE, Rosemary Anne Duncan MACRAE

Kumar
Irwin Road Health Centre, Irwin Road, St Helens WA9 3UG
Tel: 01744 816889 Fax: 01744 850483
(St Helens Primary Care Trust)
Patient List Size: 1700

Practice Manager Jacky Draycott

GP Dr KUMAR

Lancaster House Medical Centre
24-28 North Road, St Helens WA10 2TL
Tel: 01744 617000 Fax: 01744 451072
(St Helens Primary Care Trust)
Patient List Size: 3650

Practice Manager Helen Edwards

GP David Owen EDWARDS, Raj JAIN, Laura POGUE

Lingholme Health Centre
Atherton Street, St Helens WA10 2HT
Tel: 01744 22612 Fax: 01744 454493
(St Helens Primary Care Trust)

GP Dr LAGHARI, Dr ROY, John WOTHERSPOON, Carl YOUNG

Mill Street Medical Centre
2 Mill Street, St Helens WA10 2BD
Tel: 01744 23641 Fax: 01744 28398
(St Helens Primary Care Trust)
Patient List Size: 9500

Practice Manager Valerie Armstrong

GP Michael GAFFNEY, Hilary FLETT, Simon HARGREAVES, Jacqueline HOUGHTON, Z SKELLAND, Vanessa WOODCOCK

Old Whint Road Surgery
21A Old Whint Road, Haydock, St Helens WA11 0DN
Tel: 01744 612555 Fax: 01744 454619
(St Helens Primary Care Trust)

Practice Manager Dianne Rahil

GP Hussein Mohammad RAHIL

Ormskirk Street Surgery
51A Ormskirk Stret, St Helens WA10 2TB
Tel: 01744 29209 Fax: 01744 454491
(St Helens Primary Care Trust)
Patient List Size: 9029

Practice Manager E. Halsall

GP Pierino FILLETTI, Vivienne Theresa GILLANDERS, David SWORD, Robert William WRIGHT

Park House Surgery
55 Higher Parr Street, St Helens WA9 1BP
Tel: 01744 23705 Fax: 01744 454601
(St Helens Primary Care Trust)
Patient List Size: 7650

Practice Manager Madeline Marlow

GP James Joseph O'DONNELL, Joseph John BANAT, Susan GREEN, Prem SAGAR

Park Road Surgery
25 Park Road, St Helens WA9 1DG
Tel: 01744 738735 Fax: 01744 454624
(St Helens Primary Care Trust)

GP Dr CONSIGLIO, Jean Margaret SUTTON

Rainbow Medical Centre
333 Robins Lane, St Helens WA9 3PN
Tel: 01744 811211
(St Helens Primary Care Trust)
Patient List Size: 11620

Practice Manager Julie Hall

GP Barbara Anne BAINBRIDGE, John Michael HANRAHAN, Feroz SAYED, Graham Lawrence SMITH, Robert Stephen THOMAS, Andrew WHITTAKER

Sandfield Medical Centre
81 Liverpool Road, St Helens WA10 1PN
Tel: 01744 22378
(St Helens Primary Care Trust)

GP P GUPTA, M R VARMA

The Spinney Medical Centre
23 Whittle Street, St Helens WA10 3EB
Tel: 01744 758999 Fax: 01744 758322
(St Helens Primary Care Trust)
Patient List Size: 6300

Practice Manager B Carney

GP Michael Gerard VAN DESSEL, Stephen James COX, Susan Wendy HYDE

Spray Street Surgery
1 Spray Street, St Helens WA10 2NN
Tel: 01744 22006/29501 Fax: 01744 615972
(St Helens Primary Care Trust)

Practice Manager Lynn Sandford

GP Momosir ALI, Michael Philip ROSEN

Station Road Health Centre
Station Road, Haydock, St Helens WA11 0JN
Tel: 01744 22272
(St Helens Primary Care Trust)

GP Ian ROBERTS, Susan JOHNSON, Louise Ann MERCER, Peter Neil RUSSELL

Webster and Twomey
Rainford Health Centre, Higher Lane, Rainford, St Helens WA11 8AZ
Tel: 01744 882855 Fax: 01744 886559
(St Helens Primary Care Trust)
Patient List Size: 4500

Practice Manager Helen Sansbury

GP John WEBSTER, R METCALFE, Michael James TWOMEY

St Ives

The Stennack Surgery
The Old Stennack School, St Ives TR26 1RU
Tel: 01736 796413 Fax: 01736 796245
Email: jane.richards@stennacks.cornwall.nhs.uk
(West of Cornwall Primary Care Trust)
Patient List Size: 4008

Practice Manager Jane Richards

GP John Norman SELL, Christine Margaret Isabel MAY, Timothy Savile PARDOE

The Stennack Surgery
The Old Stennack School, St Ives TR26 1RU
Tel: 01736 793333 Fax: 01736 793746
Email: sue.hall@stennackr.cornwall.nhs.uk
(West of Cornwall Primary Care Trust)

Practice Manager Sue Hall

GP Ashley M ROYSTON, Simon Peter FREEGARD, Daniel RAINBOW

The Stennack Surgery
The Stennack Surgery, The Old Stennack School, St Ives TR26 1RU
Tel: 01736 795237 Fax: 01736 795362
Email: celia.mcintosh@stennackp.cornwall.nhs.uk
(West of Cornwall Primary Care Trust)
Patient List Size: 4200

Practice Manager Celia McIntosh

GP Colin John PHILIP, Rupert MANLEY, Michele Claire SHARKEY

St Leonards-on-Sea

Carisbrooke Surgery
Marlborough House, 19-21 Warrior Square, St Leonards-on-Sea TN38 6BG
Tel: 01424 423190 Fax: 01424 460473
(Hastings and St Leonards Primary Care Trust)
Patient List Size: 7500

Practice Manager Rosemary Loughton

GP Nicholas Eugene MacCARTHY, Alex ABTAHI, Robert Andrew CAMERON-WOOD, Willemyn DE HAAN, Elizabeth Anne FURLEY SMITH

Churchwood Medical Practice
Tilebarn Road, St Leonards-on-Sea TN38 9QU
Tel: 01424 853888
(Hastings and St Leonards Primary Care Trust)

Practice Manager Christine Smith

GP Mark Peter FREEMAN, Michael John HEBER, David Emlyn JONES

Essenden Road Surgery
49 Essenden Road, St Leonards-on-Sea TN38 0NN
Tel: 01424 720866 Fax: 01424 445580
(Hastings and St Leonards Primary Care Trust)
Patient List Size: 3600

Practice Manager Annette Tayan

GP Gautam SENGUPTA, David Rodney KINLOCH

Hollington Surgery
355 Battle Road, St Leonards-on-Sea TN37 7BE
Tel: 01424 851706 Fax: 01424 853210
(Hastings and St Leonards Primary Care Trust)

Practice Manager Rose Mowat

GP Pratibha Ajay MEHTA

Little Ridge Avenue Surgery
38 Little Ridge Avenue, St Leonards-on-Sea TN37 7LS
Tel: 01424 755355 Fax: 01424 755560
(Hastings and St Leonards Primary Care Trust)
Patient List Size: 2672

Practice Manager Atiya Rajbee

GP Tariq Yusuf RAJBEE, Faisal RAJBEE

Lower Glen Family Practice
174 Lower Glen Road, St Leonards-on-Sea TN37 7AR
Tel: 01424 721616 Fax: 01424 854812
(Hastings and St Leonards Primary Care Trust)
Patient List Size: 3670

Practice Manager Patricia Jasinski, Julie Swaffer

GP Peter James BRYDEN, Monica WONG

Sedlescombe House
8 Sedlescombe Road South, St Leonards-on-Sea TN38 0TA
Tel: 01424 720574 Fax: 01424 440199
(Hastings and St Leonards Primary Care Trust)
Patient List Size: 3960

Practice Manager Elizabeth Joyce

GP Jerzy Pawel Julian KALINIECKI

Silver Springs Practice
Beaufort Road, St Leonards-on-Sea TN37 6PP
Tel: 01424 422300 Fax: 01424 436400
(Hastings and St Leonards Primary Care Trust)

Practice Manager Malcolm Wright

GP Duncan James CAMERON, Elizabeth PRONGER, Ruediger SCHNEIDER, Andrew John YOUNG

South Saxon House Surgery
150A Bexhill Road, St Leonards-on-Sea TN38 8BL
Tel: 01424 441361 Fax: 01424 461799
(Hastings and St Leonards Primary Care Trust)

Practice Manager Avril Chambers

GP Miriam Esho SAPPER, Muthanna Abdul Wahed AL-SALEEM

Warrior Square Surgery
Marlborough House, 19-21 Warrior Square, St Leonards-on-Sea TN37 6BG
Tel: 01424 430123/423190 Fax: 01424 433706/460473
(Hastings and St Leonards Primary Care Trust)
Patient List Size: 6400

Practice Manager Diana Reddie

GP James William SEARSON, Ali-Reza ABTAHI, Robert Andrew CAMERON-WOOD, Elizabeth Anne FURLEY-SMITH, Nicholas Eugene MACCARTHY

St Mary's

The Health Centre
The Health Centre, King Edward Lane, St Mary's TR21 0HE
Tel: 01720 422628 Fax: 01720 423160
(West of Cornwall Primary Care Trust)
Patient List Size: 2446

Practice Manager Marian Harvey

GP Toby DALTON, Dougal JEFFRIES

Stafford

The Crown Surgery
23 High Street, Eccleshall, Stafford ST21 6BW
Tel: 01785 850226
(South Western Staffordshire Primary Care Trust)

Practice Manager Lyn Martin

GP Joseph Mark BLAND, David Maxwell CARR, William Alexander Douglas DAVIES

Harper, Munslow and Holden
Castlefields Surgery, Castle Way, Stafford ST16 1BS
Tel: 01785 223012
(South Western Staffordshire Primary Care Trust)
Patient List Size: 6500

Practice Manager Cate Lockley

GP Norman Nigel HARPER, Samuel W HOLDEN, Debra Jane MUNSLOW, David A SHARP

Holmcroft Surgery
Holmcroft Road, Stafford ST16 1JG
Tel: 01785 242172
(South Western Staffordshire Primary Care Trust)

Practice Manager Mavis Bishop

GP David John WHEELER, Charles Nicholas BARNES, Caron BRAMLEY, John Patrick HANNIGAN, Keith PRINGLE

John Amery Drive Surgery
14 John Amery Drive, Rising Brook, Stafford ST17 9LZ
Tel: 01785 252244
(South Western Staffordshire Primary Care Trust)

GP Bipinchandra Trikamlal NANAVATI, Cuckoo Bipinchandra NANAVATI

Mill Bank Surgery
Water Street, Stafford ST16 2AG
Tel: 01785 258348 Fax: 01785 227144
(South Western Staffordshire Primary Care Trust)
Patient List Size: 9850

Practice Manager Kate Tomkins

GP Michael Stirling RAWLE, Jason Alan DAVIES, John Stephen HEARN, Brian Raymond HODGKINSON, James Martin SPIERS

Penkridge Medical Practice
St Michael's Road, Penkridge, Stafford ST19 5AJ
Tel: 01785 712300 Fax: 01785 713696
(South Western Staffordshire Primary Care Trust)
Patient List Size: 10345

Practice Manager A J Page

GP Michael ALLBESON, Dawn Beverley ALLEN, David Sydney BLANCHARD, Anthony GROCOTT, Margaret Carol JONES, Sharma ZAIDI

Rising Brook Surgery
Merrey Road, Stafford ST17 9LY
Tel: 01785 251134 Fax: 01785 222441
(South Western Staffordshire Primary Care Trust)
Patient List Size: 11000

Practice Manager Ruth Buckenham

GP P K BASU, R M BEAL, A EL-ALFY, David Richard HAIG-FERGUSON, Michael Edward STAITE, Helga WAGNER

The Surgery
Sandy Lane, Brewood, Stafford ST19 9ES
Tel: 01902 850206 Fax: 01902 851360
(South Western Staffordshire Primary Care Trust)
Patient List Size: 10000

Practice Manager Gill Hughes

GP Richard Charles Henry TAYLOR, Alexander Robert HOULDER, Andrew James HUSSELBEE, Brenda Mary LUCK, Ian Maxwell TURNER

The Surgery
Hazeldene House, Great Haywood, Stafford ST18 0SU
Tel: 01889 881206 Fax: 01889 883083
Website: www.hazeldenehousesurgery.org.uk
(South Western Staffordshire Primary Care Trust)
Patient List Size: 8000

Practice Manager Pam Bishop

GP David Edward MERRIOTT, Fiona Frances Rose BURRA, Martin DAVIS, Helen McWILLIAMS, Guy Henry Stewart SKILTON

The Surgery
Wharf Road, Gnosall, Stafford ST20 0DB
Tel: 01785 822220 Fax: 01785 822776
(South Western Staffordshire Primary Care Trust)
Patient List Size: 7168

Practice Manager Jane Johnson

GP I C GREAVES, Bhupinder Singh COONER, Michael John Christopher MULLIGAN, T M WESTWOOD

The Surgery
Wildwood, Stafford ST17 4RA
Tel: 01785 662808
(South Western Staffordshire Primary Care Trust)

GP M D PATIL

The Surgery
10 Browning Street, Stafford ST16 3AT
Tel: 01785 258249 Fax: 01785 253119
Website: www.browningstsurgery.co.uk
(South Western Staffordshire Primary Care Trust)
Patient List Size: 9400

Practice Manager David J Griffiths

GP Linda JONES, Peter GLENNON, Sue KNIGHT, Tony LAMB, Mark OLIVER, David PALMER

Weeping Cross Heath Centre
Weeping Cross, Bodmin Avenue, Stafford ST17 0EG
Tel: 01785 662505 Fax: 01785 661064
(South Western Staffordshire Primary Care Trust)
Patient List Size: 9000

Practice Manager Steve Powell

GP Reginald Stuart LLOYD, A GOBEL, M R LISS, Clare Elizabeth NEWELL, E H PATERSON, G SKILTON

Wolverhampton Road Surgery
13 Wolverhampton Road, Stafford ST17 4BP
Tel: 01785 258161 Fax: 01785 224140
Website: www.wolverhamptonroadsurgery.co.uk
(South Western Staffordshire Primary Care Trust)
Patient List Size: 10200

Practice Manager Valerie D'Arcy

GP Ian WILSON, Faith M AIREY, Elizabeth Jessie ALBRIGHT, M E FREEMAN, Sharon M HILEY, Helen Mary MARTIN, Masood RAZA, Peter David Frederick SMITH

Staines

Chertsey Lane Surgery
5 Chertsey Lane, Staines TW18 3JH
Tel: 01784 454164 Fax: 01784 464360
(North Surrey Primary Care Trust)
Patient List Size: 4620

Practice Manager M Humphrey

GP John Barry PITTARD, Seda BOGHOSSIAN-TIGHE, Susan Jane DAWSON, Fiona Munro WILSON

Knowle Green Surgery
Staines Health Centre, Knowle Green, Staines TW18 1XD
Tel: 01784 883654 Fax: 01784 441244
Email: knowle.green@gp-H81002.nhs.uk
Website: www.knowlegreen.free-online.co.uk
(North Surrey Primary Care Trust)
Patient List Size: 4700

Practice Manager Elaine Burgess

GP Christopher David MILLS, Vineet THAPAR

St Davids Health Centre
Hadrian Way, Stanwell, Staines TW19 7HT
Tel: 01784 883930
(North Surrey Primary Care Trust)

GP Bhavneet OBERAI, Gabriel Teik Kiew OH, Jagjit RAI, Paul SODHI

Staines Health Centre
Knowle Green, Staines TW18 1XD
Tel: 01784 465229 Fax: 01784 464360
(North Surrey Primary Care Trust)
Patient List Size: 11600

GP John Peter PALMER, Rohit SHAUNAK, Deborah Miriam SILVER, Michael Graham WALLIS, Jean Mary WELLS

Staines Health Centre
Staines TW18 1XD
Tel: 01784 454965 Fax: 01784 441244
(North Surrey Primary Care Trust)

GP Mobin SALAHUDDIN, Joseph Robert Chan BLACKBURN

Staines Health Centre
Knowle Green, Staines TW18 1XD
Tel: 01784 883670 Fax: 01784 441244
(North Surrey Primary Care Trust)

GP Nasser JADALIZADEH

Wraysbury Medical Centre
45 Station Road, Wraysbury, Staines TW19 5ND
Tel: 01784 483243
(Windsor, Ascot and Maidenhead Primary Care Trust)

GP Nabil Abd El Wahab Gabr HASSAN

Stalybridge

Acres Lane Surgery
50 Acres Lane, Stalybridge SK15 2JU
Tel: 0161 338 4567
(Tameside and Glossop Primary Care Trust)

Practice Manager Rita Bassi

GP V K BASSI

Grosvenor Medical Centre
62 Grosvenor Street, Stalybridge SK15 1RZ
Tel: 0161 303 7250 Fax: 0161 303 8377
(Tameside and Glossop Primary Care Trust)
Patient List Size: 6000

Practice Manager Denise Fay

GP Stephen CARR, Herman ISERLOH

Lockside Medical Centre
85 Huddersfield Road, Stalybridge SK15 2PT
Tel: 0161 303 7200 Fax: 0161 304 9216
Website: www.locksidemedical.co.uk
(Tameside and Glossop Primary Care Trust)
Patient List Size: 5125

Practice Manager Christine Keyworth

GP Richard BIRCHER, Rachel EDWARDS, Joanna BIRCHER, Thomas JONES

St Andrews House
Waterloo Road, Stalybridge SK15 2AU
Tel: 0161 338 3181 Fax: 0161 303 1208
(Tameside and Glossop Primary Care Trust)
Patient List Size: 5500

Practice Manager Sharon Neal

GP Aideen Frances McNEIL, Neil Charles Hood McNEIL

Staveleigh Medical Centre
King Street, Stalybridge SK15 2AE
Tel: 0161 304 8009 Fax: 0161 303 7207
(Tameside and Glossop Primary Care Trust)
Patient List Size: 9000

Practice Manager Barbara Walsh

GP Anthony Edward JOHNSON, Susan Anne NELSON, Raymond WALSH, Timothy WARD

Stamford

The Little Practice
21 St. Mary Street, Stamford PE9 2DH
Tel: 01780 763308 Fax: 01780 755878
Website: www.littlesurgery.co.uk
(Lincolnshire South West Teaching Primary Care Trust)
Patient List Size: 3350

Practice Manager G Windsor

GP John Richard FIELDS, Melanie DENTON, Ruth Keren LIVINGSTONE

New Sheepmarket Surgery
Ryhall Road, Stamford PE9 1YA
Tel: 01780 758123 Fax: 01780 758102
(Lincolnshire South West Teaching Primary Care Trust)
Patient List Size: 11900

Practice Manager N Kelley

GP John Vincent MITCHELL, H M LITTLE, S R LOWRY, A G MACDONALD, A L MANN, Katharine Louise NOBLE, Stephen Butts REISS, John Penfold WILLIAMS

St Marys Medical Centre
Wharf Road, Stamford PE9 2DH
Tel: 01780 64121/765300 Fax: 01780 756515/761301
(Lincolnshire South West Teaching Primary Care Trust)
Patient List Size: 13000

Practice Manager V Coates

GP Gavin Edward KELLY, David John BABBS, Catherine Sarah FITT, Barbara Gail GLYNN, Sara Jane HALL, Andrew Watkin JONES, Steven Craig MANN

Stanford-le-Hope

Ash Tree Surgery

33 Fobbing Road, Corringham, Stanford-le-Hope SS17 9BG
Tel: 01375 643000 Fax: 01375 677150
Email: reception.mailbox@gp-F81644.nhs.uk
(Thurrock Primary Care Trust)

Practice Manager Vivienne Page

GP Mansukh Gordhandas KOTECHA

Hassengate Medical Centre

Southend Road, Stanford-le-Hope SS17 0PH
Tel: 01375 673064 Fax: 01375 675196
(Thurrock Primary Care Trust)
Patient List Size: 7985

Practice Manager Russell J Vine

GP Nicholas John TRESIDDER, Katherine Jane HANSON, Andrew O'DOHERTY, Judith Mary PUSEY

Neera Medical Centre

2 Wharf Road, Stanford-le-Hope SS17 0BY
Tel: 01375 672109 Fax: 01375 671724
(Thurrock Primary Care Trust)
Patient List Size: 3000

Practice Manager Isabel Mathers

GP A M DESHPANDE

The Sorrels Surgery

7 The Sorrels, Stanford-le-Hope SS17 7DZ
Tel: 01375 644740 Fax: 01375 678285
(Thurrock Primary Care Trust)
Patient List Size: 4361

GP G DEVARATA, V C DEVARATA

Southend Road Surgery

271A Southend Road, Stanford-le-Hope SS17 8HD
Tel: 01375 679316 Fax: 01375 679335
Email: practice.manager@gp-f81088.nhs.uk
(Thurrock Primary Care Trust)
Patient List Size: 5000

Practice Manager Barry Trewern

GP B B ROY

The Surgery

High Road, Horndon-on-the-Hill, Stanford-le-Hope SS17 8LB
Tel: 01375 642362 Fax: 01375 641747
(Thurrock Primary Care Trust)
Patient List Size: 2100

Practice Manager B A Richardson

GP Alexander Joseph PATTARA

Tudor Lodge Surgery

229 Southend Road, Stanford-le-Hope SS17 7AB
Tel: 01375 641740 Fax: 01375 678285
(Thurrock Primary Care Trust)

Practice Manager M Khan

GP M H ALI KHAN, M W ALI KHAN

Stanley

Annfield Plain Surgery

Durham Road, Annfield Plain, Stanley DH9 7TD
Tel: 01207 215005 Fax: 01207 281281
(Derwentside Primary Care Trust)
Patient List Size: 3000

Practice Manager Christine Serifoglu

GP Rangasamy HARIKRISHNAN

Craghead Medical Centre

The Middles, Craghead, Stanley DH9 6AN
Tel: 01207 232698 Fax: 01207 235774
(Derwentside Primary Care Trust)

Practice Manager Anne Finlayson

GP Pathikonda Viswambara NATH

Craghead Medical Centre

The Middles, Graghead, Stanley DH9 6AN
Tel: 01207 290032 Fax: 01207 290504
(Derwentside Primary Care Trust)

Practice Manager Angela Perryman

GP Abdool Rashid DHUNY

Dipton Surgery

Browns Buildings, Front Street, Dipton, Stanley DH9 9AB
Tel: 01207 571222 Fax: 01207 570070
(Derwentside Primary Care Trust)

Practice Manager Jeanette McGeary

GP A GOMATHINAYAGAM

Front Street Surgery

16 Front Street, Annfield Plain, Stanley DH9 8HY
Tel: 01207 214849 Fax: 01207 214847
(Derwentside Primary Care Trust)

Practice Manager Katherine Storey

GP Doraisamy PARTHASARATHY, Mallika PARTHASARATHY

Stanley Health Centre

Clifford Road, Stanley DH9 0XE
Tel: 01207 232696 Fax: 01207 239066
(Derwentside Primary Care Trust)
Patient List Size: 600

Practice Manager Wendy Graham

GP Mohammad Abul QUASEM, Ahmed Rushdi Ahmed HIJAB, Mohammad Masudur RAHMAN

Tanfield View Surgery

Scott Street, Stanley DH9 8AD
Tel: 01207 232384 Fax: 01207 237763
(Derwentside Primary Care Trust)

Practice Manager kate Pickering

GP Michael John HARBINSON, Catherine Mary BIDWELL, Ian Gordon DAVIDSON, Dolores Margaret Katrina MANSOUR, Peter David RILEY, Peter James WATSON

West Road Surgery

9 West Road, Annfield Plain, Stanley DH9 7XT
Tel: 01207 214925 Fax: 01207 214926
(Derwentside Primary Care Trust)

Practice Manager Audrey Allan

GP Brian LAMBERT, Ian William BRUNT

Stanmore

Elm Park Clinic

69 Elm Park, Stanmore HA7 4AU
Tel: 020 8954 8181 Fax: 020 8420 7027
(Harrow Primary Care Trust)
Patient List Size: 1200

Practice Manager Sylvia Forster

Honeypot Medical Centre

404 Honeypot Lane, Stanmore HA7 1JP
Tel: 020 8204 1363 Fax: 020 8903 0286
(Harrow Primary Care Trust)
Patient List Size: 6500

GP Chaand NAGPAUL, Alka PATEL, Meenakshi THAKUR

The Stanmore Medical Centre
85 Crowshott Avenue, Stanmore HA7 1HS
Tel: 020 8951 3888 Fax: 020 8952 8035
(Harrow Primary Care Trust)
Patient List Size: 6200

Practice Manager Susan Young

GP Lawrence Nigel GOULD, Julia GERRARD, S HASSAN, Sanjay LAKHANI

The Stanmore Surgery
9 Church Road, Stanmore HA7 4AR
Tel: 020 8954 4151
(Harrow Primary Care Trust)

GP Gloria Rita SEGAL

Stansted

Stansted Surgery
86 St Johns Road, Stansted CM24 8JS
Tel: 01279 813200 Fax: 01279 812426
(Uttlesford Primary Care Trust)
Patient List Size: 8000

Practice Manager Anabel Howard

GP Philip Godfrey JONES, Catherine HIGHAM, Susan Marie HUMPHREY, Christopher LEEMAN, Maria MYINT

Stevenage

Bedwell Medical Centre
Sinfield Close, Bedwell Crescent, Stevenage SG1 1LYU
Tel: 01438 355551 Fax: 01438 749704
(North Hertfordshire and Stevenage Primary Care Trust)
Patient List Size: 12750

Practice Manager Jennifer Darlow

GP Ramesh BAXANI, Sarah Valentine BAIRD-SMITH, Anthony Robert KOSTICK, Dana OGILVIE, Mg Mg OO

Canterbury Way Surgery
91A Canterbury Way, Stevenage SG1 4LQ
Tel: 01438 316646
(North Hertfordshire and Stevenage Primary Care Trust)
Patient List Size: 2050

Practice Manager Susan Lincoln

GP Mary Ananthavathy SELVADURAI

Chells Way Surgery
265 Chells Way, Stevenage SG2 0HN
Tel: 01438 313001 Fax: 01438 362322
(North Hertfordshire and Stevenage Primary Care Trust)
Patient List Size: 14000

Practice Manager Michelle Myers

GP Charles Andrew GOGBASHIAN, Susan Jane COXALL, Jeremy Charles EVANS, Russell HALL, Swah HOSKINS, Sarah Anne-Marie IRVINE, Adesola Olugbemiga OSINDERO

The Health Centre
Canterbury Way, Stevenage SG1 4QH
Tel: 01438 357411 Fax: 01438 720523
(North Hertfordshire and Stevenage Primary Care Trust)

Practice Manager Susan Shambrook

GP Syed Hasnain SHAREEF, Christopher John SAUNDERS, Amanda Jane WILSON

King George Surgery
135 High Street, Stevenage SG1 3HT
Tel: 01438 361111
(North Hertfordshire and Stevenage Primary Care Trust)

Practice Manager Gill Nicholson

GP Stephen James LACEY, Martinus Jacobus Johannes BRUGMAN, Lorraine EKONG, Anthony Emanuel LIPNER, R MAHALINGAM, Gillian Rosemary OSBORN, Teresa Catherine ROBERTS, John Erskine David STEVENSON

Manor House Surgery
Emperors Gate, Chells Manor, Stevenage SG2 7QX
Tel: 01438 742639
(North Hertfordshire and Stevenage Primary Care Trust)

GP Michael John DUGGAN

Shephall Way Surgery
29 Shephall Way, Stevenage SG2 9QN
Tel: 01438 312097
(North Hertfordshire and Stevenage Primary Care Trust)

GP Brian Richard ROUSE, Andrew Sutherland CORMACK, Penelope PRESTON, Andrew William George SAVAGE

St Nicholas Health Centre
Canterbury Way, Stevenage SG1 4LH
Tel: 01438 357411 Fax: 01438 72053
Email: docjamesbrooke@hotmail.com
Website: www.stnicholashc.co.uk
(North Hertfordshire and Stevenage Primary Care Trust)
Patient List Size: 9700

GP Syed Ishrat Ali ZAIDI, Angus James BROOKE, Michael Gerard DELANY, Annoj PATEL, Christopher SAUNDERS, Amanda WILSON

Wallis and Partners
The Health Centre, 5 Stanmore Road, Stevenage SG1 3QA
Tel: 01438 313223 Fax: 01438 749734
Email: m.d.wallisptnrs@tesco.net
(North Hertfordshire and Stevenage Primary Care Trust)
Patient List Size: 16500

Practice Manager Mary Bishop

GP Michael Owen WALLIS, Rekha BHATIANI, Rebecca Marie-Christine BOLS, Sally Ann GALE, Clare Helen GRIMSELL, R K JAYASEKARA, T NIKOLOVA, Claire Elaine POWELL, John Duff WARNER-SMITH

Steyning

Steyning Health Centre
Tanyard Lane, Steyning BN44 3RJ
Tel: 01903 843400 Fax: 01903 843440
(Horsham and Chanctonbury Primary Care Trust)

Practice Manager Diane Taylor, Susan Vaughan

GP Ronald Ernest WETSON, Jennifer Isabel FERRIE, Asmara GOODWIN, Jacqueline HOLDAWAY, Claes Eric NOREN, Alexander RAINBOW, Justine WOODCOCK

Stockbridge

The Surgery
New Street, Stockbridge SO20 6HG
Tel: 01264 810524 Fax: 01264 810591
Email: stockbridge.surgery@gp-j82016.nhs.uk
(Mid-Hampshire Primary Care Trust)
Patient List Size: 8150

Practice Manager Pauline Webster

GP Gareth EVANS, Paul MANCHETT, David Creffield SIMPSON, Adrian Philip TOWNSEND, C WARD

Stockport

Adswood Road Surgery
270 Adswood Road, Adswood, Stockport SK3 8PN
Tel: 0161 483 5155 Fax: 0161 419 9984
(Stockport Primary Care Trust)
Patient List Size: 3700

Practice Manager Vivienne Hallworth

GP Jill Barbara JEFFS, Eileen Anne EECKELAERS, Arun MOHINDRA

Alvanley
160 Buxton Road, Heaviley, Stockport SK2 6HA
Tel: 0161 483 3068 Fax: 0161 419 9554
(Stockport Primary Care Trust)

GP David Laurence HERBERT, H LLOYD

Alvanley Surgery
1 Auburn Avenue, Bredbury, Stockport SK6 2AH
Tel: 0161 430 2727 Fax: 0161 406 7999
(Stockport Primary Care Trust)

GP John Edwin MILSON, Robert Sidney BEARDSELL, Biswa Nath GHOSH

The Archways Surgery
86 Stockport Road, Romiley, Stockport SK6 3AA
Tel: 0161 494 5337 Fax: 0161 406 7884
Email: enquiries@archways.info
Website: www.archways.info
(Stockport Primary Care Trust)
Patient List Size: 3000

Practice Manager Carol Hall

GP Graham PARKER, Alison BUCKLEY

Arden House Surgery
15-17 New Mills Road, Hayfield, Stockport SK12 2JG
Tel: 01663 745030 Fax: 01663 741248
(High Peak and Dales Primary Care Trust)

Practice Manager Anna Houareau

GP David J POWELL, Karmvir MISTRY

Beech House Group Practice
Beech House, Beech Avenue Hazel Grove, Stockport SK7 4QR
Tel: 0161 483 6222 Fax: 0161 419 9244
(Stockport Primary Care Trust)

GP Michael John STONE, Philip James ALLAN, Caroline Ann HULL, Stephen Franklin LEVY, Jane Elizabeth MILNES, Philip James RILEY

Bents Lane Medical Practice
100 Lower Bents Lane, Bredbury, Stockport SK6 2NL
Tel: 0161 430 8708 Fax: 0161 406 6528
(Stockport Primary Care Trust)
Patient List Size: 2500

Practice Manager Pam Young

GP Abdul GHAFOOR

Birchfield Road Surgery
2 Birchfield Road, Cheadle Heath, Stockport SK3 0SY
Tel: 0161 428 7768
(Stockport Primary Care Trust)
Patient List Size: 2100

GP Kenneth Coid MARSHALL

Bracondale House Medical Centre
141 Buxton Road, Heaviley, Stockport SK2 6EQ
Tel: 0161 483 2811 Fax: 0161 487 4221
(Stockport Primary Care Trust)

Practice Manager Rosemary Hyde

GP Steven Michael HOPE, Rebecca Louise BARON, Jasmine LAPSIA

Bramhall Health Centre
66 Bramhall Lane South, Bramhall, Stockport SK7 2DY
Tel: 0161 439 8213 Fax: 0161 439 6398
(Stockport Primary Care Trust)

GP Javaid ALI, John Adrian GEARY, William Bryce GRAHAM, Harry Fraser HILL, Helen Grant SINGER, Derek Vernon SNOWDON, Diana WILKS

Bramhall Park Medical Centre
235 Bramhall Lane South, Bramhall, Stockport SK7 3EP
Tel: 0161 440 7669 Fax: 0161 440 7671
(Stockport Primary Care Trust)

Practice Manager F Oates

GP Nicholas Joseph DEVINE, Kanwalprit Singh GILL, Susan Mary JENKINS, Ashwin Mukesh PATEL, Michael Joseph ROONEY, Jane WHITTAKER

The Bredbury Medical Centre
1 Auburn Avenue, Bredbury, Stockport SK6 2AH
Tel: 0161 494 8884 Fax: 0161 494 5855
(Stockport Primary Care Trust)

GP Michael Hugh ARMSTRONG, Robert Sidney BEARDSELL

Brinnington Health Centre
Brinnington Road, Stockport SK5 8BS
Tel: 0161 430 4002 Fax: 0161 430 2918
(Stockport Primary Care Trust)
Patient List Size: 4500

Practice Manager David Whitehead

GP David BOSTOCK, Saroja DE SILVA, Alan Richard GILMAN

Brinnington Health Centre
Brinnington Road, Stockport SK5 8BS
Tel: 0161 430 4002 Fax: 0161 430 7918
(Stockport Primary Care Trust)
Patient List Size: 4300

Practice Manager David Whitehead

GP Janice Wendy ALLISTER, Natasha FRASER, Thomas HOWLING

Buxton Road Surgery
77 Buxton Road, High Lane, Stockport SK6 8DX
Tel: 01663 762551 Fax: 01633 763970
(Stockport Primary Care Trust)

GP Robert Charles Lavens MATHEWSON

The Congregational Hall
Town Street, Marple Bridge, Stockport SK6 5AA
Tel: 0161 427 2049/1074 Fax: 0161 427 8389
(Stockport Primary Care Trust)
Patient List Size: 7050

Practice Manager M R Roules

GP Judith Anne FRENCH, Patricia Jane HEDLEY, Morag Jane NEEDHAM, Martin RODGERS

Dean Lane Medical Centre
95 Dean Lane, Hazel Grove, Stockport SK7 6EJ
Tel: 01625 874664 Fax: 01625 858136
(Stockport Primary Care Trust)
Patient List Size: 2650

GP Brian Kenneth Wright LIGHTOWLER

Dial House Medical Centre
131 Mile End Lane, Offerton, Stockport SK2 6BZ
Tel: 0161 456 9905 Fax: 0161 456 7127
(Stockport Primary Care Trust)
Patient List Size: 6200

Practice Manager Pauline Kelly

GP Jonathan Richard OLDHAM, Kanwalprit Singh GILL, Stewart Thomas LUND, Jane WHITTAKER

Dulmer Drive Surgery
Fulmer Drive, Offerton, Stockport SK2 5JL
Tel: 0161 483 3363
(Stockport Primary Care Trust)

GP Yogendra Dutt SHARMA

Eastholme Surgery
2 Heaton Moor Road, Stockport SK4 4NT
Tel: 0161 443 1177 Fax: 0161 442 2521
(Stockport Primary Care Trust)
Patient List Size: 4300

Practice Manager Ann McClelland

GP Peter Geoffrey HICK, Barbara Jill CHAMBERS, Joanne HERD

Edgeley Medical Practice
1 Avondale Road, Edgeley, Stockport SK3 9NX
Tel: 0161 477 8230 Fax: 0161 4761915
(Stockport Primary Care Trust)

Practice Manager Lynne Garnor

GP Ranjit Singh GILL, Lucy HOUSLEY, Naomi Catherine LALLOO

Ellesmere Medical Centre
262 Stockport Road, Cheadle Heath, Stockport SK3 0RQ
Tel: 0161 428 6729 Fax: 0161 428 0710
(Stockport Primary Care Trust)

Practice Manager Gillian Miller

GP Patricia Margaret BERRY, Carolyn Ann DAY, Abigail Louise WEBSTER

Gorton Road Family Surgery
306 Gorton Road, Reddish, Stockport SK5 6RN
Tel: 0161 432 1235 Fax: 0161 442 2495
(Stockport Primary Care Trust)
Patient List Size: 7000

Practice Manager Joanne Cliff, Paul Stevens

GP Gnanamurthy MURUGAN, Ian Wallace DICKIE, Lesley PONTEFRACT

The Guywood Practice
Romiley Health Centre, Chichester Road, Romiley, Stockport SK6 4QR
Tel: 0161 430 3579 Fax: 0161 406 9528
(Stockport Primary Care Trust)
Patient List Size: 2900

Practice Manager Jeff Krell

GP Raina PATEL, Teresa MIRSKI

Haider Medical Centre
Jackson's Lane, Hazel Grove, Stockport SK7 5JW
Tel: 0161 440 8181 Fax: 0161 440 8253
(Stockport Primary Care Trust)
Patient List Size: 2000

Practice Manager Sue McDiarmio

GP Shafia SIDDIQI

Heald Green Health Centre
Heald Green, Stockport

GP Penelope Ann OWEN

Heald Green Health Centre
Finney lane, Heald Green, Stockport SK8 3JD
Tel: 0161 4368384 Fax: 0161 4939268
(Stockport Primary Care Trust)

GP Dr WRIGHT

Heaton Moor Medical Centre
32 Heaton Moor Road, Stockport SK4 4NX
Tel: 0161 432 0671
(Stockport Primary Care Trust)

Practice Manager G Edwards

GP Andrew David SHEPHERD, Margaret Geraldine May ADAIR, Constance ANDERSON, Timothy Nicholas BILLINGTON

Heaton Moor Medical Centre
32 Heaton Moor Road, Stockport SK4 4NX
Tel: 0161 432 0671
(Stockport Primary Care Trust)

GP Mahomed Ismail MOOLA, Moira Catherine CARMODY, David Leslie DAWSON, Barbara Maria JORASZ

Heaton Norris Health Centre
Cheviot Close, Heaton Norris, Stockport SK4 1JX
Tel: 0161 480 3338 Fax: 0161 429 9369
(Stockport Primary Care Trust)
Patient List Size: 7100

Practice Manager Gill Bufton

GP Christopher MARSHALL, Nelum DHARMAPRIYA, Richard George HARDMAN, Amanda LARGE, Julia Elizabeth MORRISON

Heaton Norris Health Centre
Cheviot Close, Heaton Norris, Stockport SK4 1JX
Tel: 0161 480 3338 Fax: 0161 477 0581
(Stockport Primary Care Trust)
Patient List Size: 2500

Practice Manager Lynn Bennett

GP Arepalli Padmaja MURTHY

Houldsworth Medical Centre
1 Rowsley Grove, Stockport SK5 7AY
Tel: 0161 442 3322 Fax: 0161 442 2594
(Stockport Primary Care Trust)

Practice Manager Elaine Arbuckle

GP Alan Frederick WILD

Longshut Lane West Surgery
24 Longshut Lane West, Stockport SK2 6SF
Tel: 0161 480 2373 Fax: 0161 480 2660
(Stockport Primary Care Trust)
Patient List Size: 1960

Practice Manager Margaret Smith

GP Michael James TRAVENEN

Lowfield Road
5 Lowfield Road, Shaw Heath, Stockport SK2 6RW
Tel: 0161 480 8249 Fax: 0161 474 0290
(Stockport Primary Care Trust)
Patient List Size: 3700

Practice Manager Meryl Davies

GP Heather PROCTOR, Ray HARRISON

Marple Cottage Surgery
50 Church Street, Marple, Stockport SK6 6BW
Tel: 0161 426 0011 Fax: 0161 427 8160
(Stockport Primary Care Trust)
Patient List Size: 6000

Practice Manager Johan Taylor

GP Keith WELLS, Katherine Harriet CHECKLAND, Andrew JOHNSON

Marple Medical Practice
50 Stockport Road, Marple, Stockport SK6 6AB
Tel: 0161 426 0299 Fax: 0161 427 8112
Email: srmp@gp.P88021.nhs.uk
(Stockport Primary Care Trust)
Patient List Size: 8504

GP Melanie Louise WYNNE-JONES, Gregory CARTER, John David HALL, Helen Jane HEWETSON

Maxwell and Bainbridge
The School House Surgery, Buxton Old Road, Disley, Stockport SK12 2BB
Tel: 01663 764488 Fax: 01663 766028
Email: carole@schoolhouse-surgery.co.uk
(Eastern Cheshire Primary Care Trust)
Patient List Size: 4900

Practice Manager C A Evans

GP Mary BAINBRIDGE, Wayne Ollyn MAXWELL

McIlvride Medical Practice
5 Chester Road, Poynton, Stockport SK12 1EU
Tel: 01625 872134 Fax: 01625 859748
Email: McIlvride@hotmail.com
(Eastern Cheshire Primary Care Trust)
Patient List Size: 6500

Practice Manager Helen Hughes, Jill Warburton

GP John Charles COLEY, Andrew Nicholas COLEY, Dannielle Maree FARRELL, Phillip Clive WALLACE

Meyer Street Surgery
20 Meyer Street, Cale Green, Stockport SK3 8JE
Tel: 0161 480 2882 Fax: 0161 480 0583
(Stockport Primary Care Trust)

GP Jacqueline Margaret CHANG, Helen Margaret TINSLEY

Offerton Health Centre
10 Offerton Lane, Offerton, Stockport SK2 5AR
Tel: 0161 480 0324
(Stockport Primary Care Trust)

GP George COWIE, Kevin James HIGGINBOTHAM-JONES, Michael John PARKINSON, Ronald Owen VASEY

Offerton Health Centre
10 Offerton Lane, Offerton, Stockport SK2 5AR
Tel: 0161 480 0326
(Stockport Primary Care Trust)

GP Martin Thomas LUNDY, Ursula Mary McCAUGHAN, William Francis RUSSELL

Ovoca
460 Didsbury Road, Heaton Mersey, Stockport SK4 3BT
Tel: 0161 432 2032 Fax: 0161 947 9689
(Stockport Primary Care Trust)
Patient List Size: 8000

Practice Manager Valerie Clements

GP Geryl Anne REES, Shehzana KHALID, Iain Cameron SEMPLE, Ian Richard WARBURTON, Helen Margaret WILKINS, Jeremy Benet WYNN

Park View Group Practice
2 Longford Road West, Stockport SK5 6ET
Tel: 0161 431 9339
(Stockport Primary Care Trust)

GP Satish Chander MEHTA, Lucinda Mary COCKAYNE, Najabat HUSSAIN, Sean Henry MAGUIRE, Sikander Khan MALIK

Priorslegh Medical Centre
Civic Centre, Park Lane, Poynton, Stockport SK12 1GP
Tel: 01625 872299
(Eastern Cheshire Primary Care Trust)

Practice Manager Julia Oldham

GP William Eric HELLIWELL, John Patrick BURNETT, Sylvia Ethel GLASS, Mark Whitmore GRADWELL, Clare Hazel STANLEY, Nigel Anthony STONES

Romiley Health Centre
Chichester Road, Romiley, Stockport SK6 4QR
Tel: 0161 430 2573 Fax: 0161 406 7237
(Stockport Primary Care Trust)

Practice Manager Jennifer Gordon

GP Ian MACLURE

Romiley Health Centre
Chichester Road, Romiley, Stockport SK6 4QR
Tel: 0161-494-2002 Fax: 0161 406-8932
(Stockport Primary Care Trust)

Practice Manager Debbie Flitcroft

GP Roger Simon BRIGGS

Romily Health Centre
Chichester Road, Romily, Stockport SK6 4QR
Tel: 0161 494 1234 Fax: 0161 406 8932
(Stockport Primary Care Trust)

GP Dr MORGAN

Sett Valley Medical Centre
Hyde Bank Road, New Mills, Stockport SK22 4BP
Tel: 01663 743483 Fax: 01663 741524
(High Peak and Dales Primary Care Trust)
Patient List Size: 11000

Practice Manager Pauline Richmond

GP David Edward WILLIAMS, John Kevin DOUGLAS, James Francis McCARTHY, Deborah Tracy ROYLE, Neil John START

South Reddish Medical Centre
The Surgery, Reddish Road, Stockport SK5 7QU
Tel: 0161 476 6030/480 8393
(Stockport Primary Care Trust)

GP Stella Josephine Ayodele COLE, Amarendra Mohan MISHRA, Sigmund Jenkins BENJAMIN, Jane Elizabeth MILNES

Springfield Surgery
24-28 Commercial Road, Hazel Grove, Stockport SK7 4AA
Tel: 0161 487 1200 Fax: 0161 483 6183
(Stockport Primary Care Trust)
Patient List Size: 2960

Practice Manager Doreen Henbrey

GP Jeffrey Stuart MORTIMER, Rosalind B DEERING

Stockport Medical Group
Delamere Practice, 257 Dialstone Lane, Great Moor, Stockport SK2 7NA
Tel: 0161 483 3175 Fax: 0161 456 4992
(Stockport Primary Care Trust)
Patient List Size: 3650

Practice Manager Laura Higginbotham

GP Jeannette WILKES, Leonie PRICE

The Surgery
30 Brinnington Road, Stockport SK1 2EX
Tel: 0161 480 4164 Fax: 0161 476 1996
Email: hany.azmy@gp-p88600.nhs.uk/drazmy@msn.com
Website: www.patientweb.co.uk/thesurgery30brinngtom.html
(Stockport Primary Care Trust)

Practice Manager E Allenson

GP Hany Helmy AZMY

Thornbrook Surgery
Thornbrook Road, Chapel-en-le-Frith, Stockport SK23 0RH
Tel: 01298 812725 Fax: 01298 816221
(High Peak and Dales Primary Care Trust)
Patient List Size: 8250

Practice Manager J Ralphs

GP Deborah AUSTIN, Graham BRODIE, Simon Hugh COCKSEDGE, John Nicholas FRANCIS

Village Surgery
31 Bramhall Lane South, Bramhall, Stockport SK7 2DN
Tel: 0161 439 3322 Fax: 0161 439 0794
(Stockport Primary Care Trust)
Patient List Size: 3654

Practice Manager Christine Whitfield

GP David Noel RILEY, David Rufus GOLDSPINT, Ingrid Ann WHITEMAN

Woodley Health Centre
Hyde Road, Woodley, Stockport SK6 1ND
Tel: 0161 430 2466 Fax: 0161 406 8217
(Stockport Primary Care Trust)

Practice Manager Sarah Kennedy

GP R A LEIVIVOX, Brian Patrick COGHLAN, John Rodney MANTON

Woodley Health Centre
Hyde Road, Woodley, Stockport SK6 1ND
Tel: 0161 430 4166 Fax: 0161 406 8218
(Stockport Primary Care Trust)
Patient List Size: 1962

Practice Manager Alison Westley

GP Monica CHANDA

Stocksfield

Branch End Surgery
Stocksfield NE43 7LL
Tel: 01661 842626 Fax: 01661 844392
(Northumberland Care Trust)

Practice Manager Anne Kennedy

GP Lynn CORBETT, Denis Patrick FEENEY, Alan Antony MAGUIRE

Stockton-on-Tees

Alma Street Medical Centre
Alma Street, Stockton-on-Tees TS18 2AP
Tel: 01642 607248 Fax: 01642 612968
(North Tees Primary Care Trust)
Patient List Size: 6000

Practice Manager Angela Clarke

GP Paul Joseph McGOWAN, Alexander Paul BARLOW, Jane H ROBERTS, Antonia Margaret STEPHENSON

Beckfields Medical Centre
Beckfields Avenue, Ingleby Barwick, Stockton-on-Tees TS17 0QA
Tel: 01642 765789 Fax: 01642 750872
(North Tees Primary Care Trust)

Practice Manager Jackie Gibson

GP David LEVAN, S CHOUDHRY

Harbinson House Surgery
Front Street, Sedgefield, Stockton-on-Tees TS21 3BN
Tel: 01740 620300 Fax: 01740 622075
Email: firstname.surname@gp-a83054.nhs.uk
(Sedgefield Primary Care Trust)
Patient List Size: 14000

Practice Manager Colin Campbell Miller

GP Peter Robert Mason JONES, D J ANDERSON, C BROWN, Christine Jane HEARMON, James Hugh LARCOMBE, Dr MACDOUGALL, William Edward Guy ROBERTSHAW, D E ROBINSON, M SHAMI

The Health Centre
Sunningdale Drive, Eaglescliffe, Stockton-on-Tees TS16 9EA
Tel: 01642 780113 Fax: 01642 791020
Website: www.eaglescliffemedical.co.uk
(North Tees Primary Care Trust)
Patient List Size: 8043

Practice Manager Angela Mackereth

GP David Leslie LEECH, Krystyna ELLENGER, Amritpal Singh HUNGIN, Fiona SMITH, Simon Nicholas STOCKLEY, Angela WATERHOUSE

The Health Centre
Trenchard Avenue, Thornaby, Stockton-on-Tees TS17 0DD
Tel: 01642 762636 Fax: 01642 766464
(North Tees Primary Care Trust)
Patient List Size: 13325

Practice Manager Jenny Barrett

GP Bhadresh Ramanlal CONTRACTOR, Sally Elizabeth KENYON, Thomas KIVAN, Rachel Yvonne LITSTER, Rajendra Bhailalbhai PATEL, Mohammed Nayar Iqbal QUASIM

The Health Centre
Trenchard Avenue, Thornaby, Stockton-on-Tees TS17 0DD
Tel: 01642 762921 Fax: 01642 760608
(North Tees Primary Care Trust)

Practice Manager Liz Hegarty

GP Gregory Paul RUBIN, Robin Nicholas ADAMS, Susan Marie BUCKLE, Andrew Paul COOK, Graham Kenneth DAYNES, Triona Treasa de BURCA, Leng Chuan NEOH, Ruth Vivien TURNER

The Health Centre
Lawson Street, Stockton-on-Tees TS18 1HX
Tel: 01642 672351 Fax: 01642 618112
(North Tees Primary Care Trust)
Patient List Size: 6200

Practice Manager Paula Clarke

GP Stephen Richard WILLIAMS, Gillian OLIVER

The Health Centre
Lawson Street, Stockton-on-Tees TS18 1HX
Tel: 01642 676520 Fax: 01642 614720
(North Tees Primary Care Trust)
Patient List Size: 4600

Practice Manager Chris Malloy

GP Kevin Patrick O'BYRNE, Ritendra Nath SINHA

The Health Centre
Lawson Street, Stockton-on-Tees TS18 1HX
Tel: 01642 607435 Fax: 01642 634694
(North Tees Primary Care Trust)

GP S A Z M I HAQUE

Norton Medical Centre
Billingham Road, Norton, Stockton-on-Tees TS20 2UZ
Tel: 01642 360111 Fax: 01642 558672
(North Tees Primary Care Trust)
Patient List Size: 16400

Practice Manager Victoria Laing

GP John Rodger THORNHAM, J M WYLIE, Richard Alan HORNE, A D MORTON, Cyril Patrick O'NEILL, Nigel ROBINSON, David Harper WHITE, C M WORTH

Norton Road Surgery
137 Norton Road, Stockton-on-Tees TS18 2BG
Tel: 01642 602222 Fax: 01642 604444
(North Tees Primary Care Trust)

GP Y SYED

Park Lane Surgery
Stillington, Stockton-on-Tees TS21 1JS
Tel: 01740 630208 Fax: 01740 631201
(North Tees Primary Care Trust)

GP Robert Philip REYNOLDS, Katharine Anne DEWHIRST

Queens Park Medical Centre
Farrer Street, Stockton-on-Tees TS18 2AW
Tel: 01642 679681 Fax: 01642 677124
(North Tees Primary Care Trust)

Practice Manager G Wynn

GP Thomas Francis POYNER, Elizabeth Mary BUDGE, Sue BURROWS, Richard CRAVEN, Michael Lawrence ELDER, Kevin George HALL, David Christopher HAZELTON, Mark HULYER, Ian Richard KIRKBRIDE, Timothy James McCARTHY, John Richard NICHOLAS, Charlotte SAHA

Riverside Medical Practice
25 Bridge Road, Stockton-on-Tees TS18 3AA
Tel: 01642 604117 Fax: 01642 604602
(North Tees Primary Care Trust)
Patient List Size: 1900

Practice Manager Lisa Elliott

GP Alagappan RAMASWAMY, Karen SNOWDEN

The Surgery
Tennant Street, Stockton-on-Tees TS18 2AT
Tel: 01642 613331 Fax: 01642 675612
(North Tees Primary Care Trust)
Patient List Size: 13050

Practice Manager R. White

GP Raghbir Singh SAGOO, Jonathan BERRY, Iain Charles BONAVIA, Rhiannon LEYSHON, Anthony McKENNA, Mary NAISBY, Barbara SCOTT, Rupert SMITH

The Surgery
Elm Tree Medical Centre, Elm Tree Avenue, Stockton-on-Tees TS19 0UW
Tel: 01642 603330 Fax: 01642 675656
(North Tees Primary Care Trust)
Patient List Size: 2000

Practice Manager Norma Hardie

GP Fazal TUNIO

The Surgery
Community Centre, Long Newton, Stockton-on-Tees TS21 1BX
Tel: 01642 580031
(North Tees Primary Care Trust)

GP A J MARSHALL, Dr HOLMES, Dr PEART

The Surgery
74 Norton Road, Stockton-on-Tees TS18 2DE
Tel: 01642 676906 Fax: 01642 674781
(North Tees Primary Care Trust)
Patient List Size: 1651

Practice Manager J H McLone

GP A K BANERJEE

Woodlands Medical Centre
106 Yarm Lane, Stockton-on-Tees TS18 1YE
Tel: 01642 607398 Fax: 01642 604603
(North Tees Primary Care Trust)
Patient List Size: 13538

Practice Manager Sue Browne

GP Richard Anthony DOUGLASS, Mark N UPTON, John Joseph HARLEY, Jonathan ROBINSON, Jonathan Andrew Nicholas SLADE, Lorna Doris Elspeth SLOAN

Stoke-on-Trent

Abbey Surgery
77 Woodhead Road, Abbey Hulton, Stoke-on-Trent ST2 8DH
Tel: 01782 542671 Fax: 01782 544365
(North Stoke Primary Care Trust)

GP Rajendra Singh BOLIA

Apsley House
188 Waterloo Road, Burslem, Stoke-on-Trent ST6 3HF
Tel: 01782 837498 Fax: 01782 833440
(North Stoke Primary Care Trust)
Patient List Size: 2400

Practice Manager M A Marathe

GP Ramesh Mahader MARATHE

Audley Health Centre
Church Street, Audley, Stoke-on-Trent ST7 8EW
Tel: 01782 721000 Fax: 01782 723808
(Newcastle-under-Lyme Primary Care Trust)
Patient List Size: 8450

Practice Manager Julie Stokes

GP R J PAGE, K HALL, M RAMPLING, E SUTTON, A SWEET, S A TURNER

Baddeley Green Surgery
988 Leek New Road, Stoke-on-Trent ST9 9PB
Tel: 01782 533777 Fax: 01782 533333
(North Stoke Primary Care Trust)
Patient List Size: 4200

GP Keith Thomas TATTUM

Birches Head Medical Centre
Diana Road, Birches Head, Stoke-on-Trent ST1 6RS
Tel: 01782 286843 Fax: 01782 535291
(North Stoke Primary Care Trust)
Patient List Size: 6200

Practice Manager Hilary Samal

GP Kamdev SAMAL, Mohammad NAYEEMUDDIN

Brook Medical Centre
98 Chell Heath Road, Bradeley, Stoke-on-Trent ST6 7NN
Tel: 01782 838355 Fax: 01782 836245
(North Stoke Primary Care Trust)
Patient List Size: 5991

Practice Manager Alyson Turner

GP Kenneth PARKINSON, John Arthur GILBY, S VELLENOWETH

Cambridge House
124 Werrington Road, Bucknall, Stoke-on-Trent ST2 9AJ
Tel: 01782 219075 Fax: 01782 279047
(North Stoke Primary Care Trust)
Patient List Size: 2900

GP Anwar HAIDAR, Narayanan PRABHAKARAN

Cinderhill Lane Surgery
95 Cinderhill Lane, Scholar Green, Stoke-on-Trent ST7 3HR
(Central Cheshire Primary Care Trust)

Combined Health Centre
Dunning Street, Stoke-on-Trent ST6 5AP
Tel: 01782 577822
(North Stoke Primary Care Trust)

GP V P MANUDHANE, C N VENKATASUBRAHMANIAN

Eardley and Partners
Biddulph Medical Centre, Well Street, Biddulph, Stoke-on-Trent ST8 6HD
Tel: 01782 512822 Fax: 01782 510331
(Staffordshire Moorlands Primary Care Trust)

Practice Manager Jill Eardley

GP Richard Clive EARDLEY, Catherine Mary AITKEN, Adrian Bruce BUTCHER, Claire Elizabeth GLIDDEN, John Graham JOHNSTON, Philip James TURNER

Furlong Medical Centre
Furlong Road, Tunstall, Stoke-on-Trent ST6 5UD
Tel: 01782 577388 Fax: 01782 838610
(North Stoke Primary Care Trust)
Patient List Size: 11100

Practice Manager Peter Whittingham

GP Philip John MASTERS, Michael Ibe AOILIH, Sharon Margaret BELL, Alistair David PULLAN, Paul Edward SCHUR

Good Hope Medical Practice
Dunning Street, Tunstall, Stoke-on-Trent ST6 5AP
Tel: 01782 425837 Fax: 01782 425842
(North Stoke Primary Care Trust)
Patient List Size: 1600

GP Dr CARLIN, Dr SMITH

Hanley Health Centre
Upper Huntbach Street, Hanley, Stoke-on-Trent ST1 2BN
Tel: 01782 262299 Fax: 01782 776711
(North Stoke Primary Care Trust)

GP M K ROHATGI, S ROHATGI

Hanley Health Centre
Upper Huntbach Street, Hanley, Stoke-on-Trent ST1 2BN
Tel: 01782 202422 Fax: 01782 205441
(North Stoke Primary Care Trust)

GP Mohamed Ossama Amin Mohamed SOLIMAN

Harley Street Medical Centre
Harley Street, Hanley, Stoke-on-Trent ST1 3RX
Tel: 01782 212305 Fax: 01782 201326
(North Stoke Primary Care Trust)
Patient List Size: 12200

Practice Manager Yvonne Bell

GP David Gerard Martin LOUGHNEY, Joseph S A HAPUARACHI, Catherine Marie HOBSON, Francis Richard PRZYSLO, David Alan SHEPPARD

The Health Centre

Dunning Street, Tunstall, Stoke-on-Trent ST6 5AP
Tel: 01782 577822 Fax: 01782 811024
(North Stoke Primary Care Trust)

Practice Manager Julie Bailey

GP Vasant Shivanarayan MANUDHANE

The Health Centre

Dunning Street, Stoke-on-Trent ST6 5BE
Tel: 01782 425834 Fax: 01782 577599
(North Stoke Primary Care Trust)
Patient List Size: 9800

Practice Manager Sonia Beckett

GP Ian Dennis LEESE, Catherine Elizabeth FOSTER, Colin Andrew SCOTT, Munawar Saleem SHAIKH, Duncan Neil YOUNG

The Health Centre

Dunning Street, Stoke-on-Trent ST6 5AP
Tel: 01782 425839 Fax: 01782 425844
(North Stoke Primary Care Trust)

GP Dr SINGH

Jary, Yates and Brown

Well Street Medical Centre, Well Street, Cheadle, Stoke-on-Trent ST10 1EY
Tel: 01538 753114 Fax: 01538 751485
(Staffordshire Moorlands Primary Care Trust)
Patient List Size: 7044

Practice Manager Julie Downie

GP Stephen Robert JARY, Michael Alan Irvine BROWN, David Owen YATES

Kidsgrove Medical Centre

Mount Road, Kidsgrove, Stoke-on-Trent ST7 4AY
Tel: 01782 784221 Fax: 01782 781703
(Staffordshire Moorlands Primary Care Trust)

GP Syed SHARAF-UD-DIN, Peter Charles DALLOW, Janice HOLLAND, David Nicholas McVERRY, Sabah Merzi Mahmoud RABIE, Michael ROBINSON, Ian TATTERSALL, Gillian Margaret WAKLEY

Leek Road Surgery

1441 Leek Road, Abbey Hulton, Stoke-on-Trent ST2 8BY
Tel: 01782 542266 Fax: 01782 544191
(North Stoke Primary Care Trust)
Patient List Size: 7600

Practice Manager Elaine Wilkinson

GP Venkata Subba Rao CHADALAVADA, U CHADALAVADA

Lucie Wedgewood Health Centre

Chapel Lane, Burslem, Stoke-on-Trent ST6 2AD
Tel: 01782 834488 Fax: 01782 837738
(North Stoke Primary Care Trust)

GP Calathur Nataraja VENKATA SUBRAHMA

Lucy Wedgwood Health Centre

Chapel Lane, Burslem, Stoke-on-Trent ST6 2AD
Tel: 01782 834488 Fax: 01782 811024
(North Stoke Primary Care Trust)

GP Dr MANUDHANE

Malgwa and Malgwa

RJ Mitchell Medical Centre, 19 Wright Street, Butt Lane, Kidsgrove, Stoke-on-Trent ST7 1NY
Tel: 01782 782215 Fax: 01782 774184
(Newcastle-under-Lyme Primary Care Trust)
Patient List Size: 4616

Practice Manager Derrath Lachin

GP Arvind MALGWA, Pushpa Rani MALGWA

Milton Surgery

Millrise Road, Milton, Stoke-on-Trent ST2 7BN
Tel: 01782 545444 Fax: 01782 570135
(North Stoke Primary Care Trust)

Practice Manager Linda Allen

GP Paul Anthony MAYLAND, Andrew Shaun BARTLAM, Andrew David CRESSWELL, Elaine DOMVILLE, Timothy Michael HARRISON

Moorcroft Medical Centre

10 Botteslow Street, Hanley, Stoke-on-Trent ST1 3NJ
Tel: 01782 281806 Fax: 01782 205755
(North Stoke Primary Care Trust)
Patient List Size: 6700

Practice Manager Gail Stanyer

GP Julie Maria McGOWAN, Jane Mary BARBER, Stephen FAWCETT, Hilary Elizabeth MORRISON, I M TOMLINSON

New Ford Health Centre

2 Baden Road, Smallthorne, Stoke-on-Trent ST6 1SA
Tel: 01782 834288
(North Stoke Primary Care Trust)
Patient List Size: 5500

Practice Manager Agnes Gohil

GP Kishor Bhimji GOHIL, Michael Loraine MEATON

The New Surgery

Old Road, Tean, Stoke-on-Trent ST10 4EG
Tel: 01538 722323 Fax: 01538 722215
(Staffordshire Moorlands Primary Care Trust)
Patient List Size: 7000

Practice Manager Dawn Forrester

GP Bernard Anthony SHEVLIN, Caroline Ann DONOGHUE, James Malcolm PILPEL

Orchard Surgery

Knypersley Road, Norton-in-the-Moors, Stoke-on-Trent ST6 8HY
Tel: 01782 534241 Fax: 01782 541068
(North Stoke Primary Care Trust)
Patient List Size: 10500

Practice Manager Angela Manley

GP Paul GOLIK, Ian Stuart BAILEY, Susan Mary BRADBURY, Medhat GUINDY, Maureen Joy MAJEKODUNMI

Page and Partners

Health Centre, Church Street, Audley, Stoke-on-Trent ST7 8EW
Tel: 01782 721345 Fax: 01782 723808
(Newcastle-under-Lyme Primary Care Trust)
Patient List Size: 8300

Practice Manager Julie Stokes

GP Richard John PAGE, Kenneth Henry HALL, Emma Jane SUTTON, Sharon Ann TURNER

Potteries Medical Centre

Beverley Drive, Bentilee, Stoke-on-Trent ST2 0JG
Tel: 01782 208755
(North Stoke Primary Care Trust)
Patient List Size: 4660

GP Rajiv Balkrishna TALATHI, Harshad Shantilal PARIKH

Sita Medical Centre

High Street, Goldenhill, Stoke-on-Trent ST6 5QJ
Tel: 01782 772242 Fax: 01782 776711
(North Stoke Primary Care Trust)

GP Mahindra Kumar ROHATGI, Shakuntla ROHATGI

Somerset Surgery

Somerset Road, Stoke-on-Trent ST1 2BH
Tel: 01782 212192 Fax: 01782 205078
(North Stoke Primary Care Trust)

GP Dr AHMED

The Stone House
Alton, Stoke-on-Trent ST10 4AG
Tel: 01538 702210 Fax: 01538 703500
(Staffordshire Moorlands Primary Care Trust)
Patient List Size: 1900

Practice Manager Julie Downie

GP Vincent George WEBSTER

The Surgery
117 Knypersley Road, Norton-in-the-Moors, Stoke-on-Trent ST6 8JA
Tel: 01782 545728 Fax: 01782 570069
(North Stoke Primary Care Trust)

Practice Manager Glennis Bates

GP Vinodchandra Ambalal PATEL, Chandra Vinodchandra PATEL

The Surgery
205A High Lane, Burslem, Stoke-on-Trent ST6 7BS
Tel: 01782 819925 Fax: 01782 824733
(North Stoke Primary Care Trust)

GP Surraya KHANAM

The Surgery
Allen Street, Cheadle, Stoke-on-Trent ST10 1HJ
Tel: 01538 752674 Fax: 01538 753265
(Staffordshire Moorlands Primary Care Trust)
Patient List Size: 4538

Practice Manager Jenny Manley

GP Paul CRAVEN, Nick CUNNINGHAM

The Surgery
5 Rupert Street, Biddulph, Stoke-on-Trent ST8 6EB
Tel: 01782 514674 Fax: 01782 523044
(Staffordshire Moorlands Primary Care Trust)

GP Ashok Kumar RATHI

Talke Clinic
High Street, Talke Pits, Stoke-on-Trent ST7 1QQ
Tel: 01782 783565 Fax: 01782 771686
(Newcastle-under-Lyme Primary Care Trust)

Practice Manager Andrea Conway

GP P M UNYOLO, A H HARVEY

The Tardis Surgery
9 Queen Street, Cheadle, Stoke-on-Trent ST10 1BH
Tel: 01538 753771 Fax: 01538 752557
(Staffordshire Moorlands Primary Care Trust)
Patient List Size: 6138

Practice Manager Margaret Ellis

GP Kevin Stephen UPTON, B L RATCLIFFE, Christine Mary TATTUM

Victoria Surgery
Victoria Square, 134 Broad Street, Hanley, Stoke-on-Trent ST1 4EQ
Tel: 01782 271996
(North Stoke Primary Care Trust)

Practice Manager S N Wahie

GP Kenneth William BENSON, Saroj Sudhir SHAH

Victoria Surgery
Victoria Square, 134 Broad Street, Hanley, Stoke-on-Trent ST1 4EQ
Tel: 01782 271882 Fax: 01782 570795
(North Stoke Primary Care Trust)

GP Shyamendra Narayan WAHIE

Waterhouses Medical Practice
Waterfall Lane, Waterhouses, Stoke-on-Trent ST10 3HT
Tel: 01538 308207 Fax: 01538 308653
(Staffordshire Moorlands Primary Care Trust)
Patient List Size: 3025

Practice Manager Kate Robotham

GP Sunil ANGRIS, Vincent COOPER, Dawn LAIN

Waterloo Road Surgery
279 Waterloo Road, Cobridge, Stoke-on-Trent ST6 3HR
Tel: 01782 279915
(North Stoke Primary Care Trust)

GP Uday Atmaram PATHAK

Well Street Medical Centre
Well Street, Biddulph, Stoke-on-Trent ST8 6HD
Tel: 01782 513939 Fax: 01782 523085
(Staffordshire Moorlands Primary Care Trust)
Patient List Size: 9100

Practice Manager Val Wooton

GP Andrew Nicholas Faulkner GREEN, John Matthew KING, Philippa Jane LIGHTFOOT, Neil John RUSSELL

Werrington Surgery
Ash Bank Road, Werrington, Stoke-on-Trent ST9 0JS
Tel: 01782 304611 Fax: 01782 302987
(Staffordshire Moorlands Primary Care Trust)

GP Dr BENNETT

Stoke-sub-Hamdon

Bulley and Partners
Hamdon Medical Centre, Matts Lane, Stoke-sub-Hamdon TA14 6QE
Tel: 01935 822236 Fax: 01935 826565
(South Somerset Primary Care Trust)

Practice Manager Kerne Inglett, Margaret Murray

GP Roger John BULLEY, Harriet Frances COLLINS, Paul James SCOTT

Stone

High Street Surgery
Cumberland House, 8 High Street, Stone ST15 8AP
Tel: 01785 813538 Fax: 01785 812208
(South Western Staffordshire Primary Care Trust)

Practice Manager S E McDowall

GP Ashoke Kumar CHATTERJEE, Norma Elizabeth CARLIN, Hilary DAVIS, Peter Gordon HAMILTON, Malcolm David MACKINNON, Paul Edward SCHUR, Angela Marie WATERHOUSE

Mansion House Surgery
Abbey Street, Stone ST15 8YE
Tel: 01785 815555 Fax: 01785 815541
(South Western Staffordshire Primary Care Trust)
Patient List Size: 13000

Practice Manager Sylvia Evans

GP Ian Arthur TAYLOR, Nicholas Anthony ALDRIDGE, Jonathan Peter BALLINGER, Janet Kathleen EAMES, Victor Robert KIMBER, Anthony James STAFFORD

Stonehouse

Regent Street Surgery
73 Regent Street, Stonehouse GL10 2AA
Tel: 01453 822145 Fax: 01453 821663
Email: pauline.cobb@tesco.net
Website: www.regentstreetsurgery.co.uk
(Cotswold and Vale Primary Care Trust)
Patient List Size: 4200

Practice Manager Pauline Beard

GP Susan Rowena Felicity ANSLOW, Ian Denis LAKE, Lucy Aileen LAKE, Janet Elizabeth SIVYER

Stonehouse Health Clinic
High Street, Stonehouse GL10 2NG
Tel: 01453 823144 Fax: 01453 821393
Email: esmail.esmailji@gp-L84613.nhs.uk
(Cotswold and Vale Primary Care Trust)

Practice Manager Joan Selwyn

GP Esmail Anverali ESMAILJI

Stourbridge

Chapel Street Surgery
87 Chapel Street, lye, Stourbridge DY9 8BT
Tel: 01384 897668
(Dudley South Primary Care Trust)

GP Braham Kumar PRASHARA

The Glebeland Surgery
The Glebe, Belbroughton, Stourbridge DY9 9TH
Tel: 01562 730303 Fax: 01562 731220
(Redditch and Bromsgrove Primary Care Trust)
Patient List Size: 3600

Practice Manager Teressa Price

GP Anne Fiona PHILLIPS, Robert Charles Berrisford KRICK

Greenfield Avenue Surgery
11 Greenfield Avenue, Stourbridge DY8 1SU
Tel: 01384 442111
(Dudley South Primary Care Trust)

GP Isobel Margaret DINGWALL, Ashok MALHOTRA

Hagley Surgery
1 Victoria Passage, Hagley, Stourbridge DY9 0NH
Tel: 01562 881700 Fax: 01562 887185
(Wyre Forest Primary Care Trust)
Patient List Size: 6500

Practice Manager G Clarke

GP John Nicholas HYDE, Louise Charlotte EVANS, Timothy Richard HEYWOOD, David Stephen RICHARDS

The Limes Surgery
172 High Street, Lye, Stourbridge DY9 8LL
Tel: 01384 422234
(Dudley South Primary Care Trust)

GP Michael Norman ROSE, David John GALLIMORE, Trudy Kathlyn JOY, Sally Joy PARTRIDGE, Mitchel PRICE

Meriden Avenue Surgery
1 Meriden Avenue, Wollaston, Stourbridge DY8 4QL
Tel: 01384 392563
(Dudley South Primary Care Trust)

Practice Manager Sylvia Marsh

GP John FIRTH

Pedmore Road Surgery
22 Pedmore Road, Lye, Stourbridge DY9 8DJ
Tel: 01384 422591
(Dudley South Primary Care Trust)
Patient List Size: 4108

Practice Manager Ann Powell

GP William Peter KILLIN, Michael John STONE

The Surgery
4-6 High Street, kinver, Stourbridge DY7 6HG
Tel: 01384 873311 Fax: 01384 877328
(South Western Staffordshire Primary Care Trust)
Patient List Size: 3800

Practice Manager Lynda Dunkerley

GP Kevin Paul RILEY

Three Villages Medical Practice
Audnam Lodge, Wordsley, Stourbridge DY8 4AL
Tel: 01384 395054 Fax: 01384 390969
Email: d.powell@dudley.nhs.uk
(Dudley South Primary Care Trust)
Patient List Size: 9300

Practice Manager Ann Sprague

GP David Fred POWELL, Robin Paul HIGGINS, John Stewart ISSITT, Adrian Graham WILD

Whittington Road Surgery
9 Whittington Road, Norton, Stourbridge DY8 3DB
Tel: 01384 393120 Fax: 01384 353636
(Dudley South Primary Care Trust)
Patient List Size: 6200

Practice Manager Rosemary F Pardoe

GP David Jolyan Stroud POWELL, Ronald Joseph BRINDLEY, Beverley Joy WATKINS

Worcester Street Surgery
24 Worcester Street, Stourbridge DY8 1AW
Tel: 01384 371616 Fax: 01384 444310
(Dudley South Primary Care Trust)
Patient List Size: 20000

Practice Manager Cathryn Bateman

GP Alastair James McCurrach WATT, Steven BERWICK, Simon CARVELL, John David CHALONER, Paul Simon FARLEY, Carol Ann GRIFFITHS, Heidi KERR, Stephen James MANN, James Ormonde NANCARROW, Glenys Ruth WILSON

Wordsley Green Health Centre
Wordsley Green, Wordsley, Stourbridge DY8 5PD
Tel: 01384 277591 Fax: 01384 401156
(Dudley South Primary Care Trust)
Patient List Size: 9000

GP David Alun REES, Stephen LIM, Craig MUNRO, Rosemary OLIVER, John Kenneth SPEAKMAN

Wychbury Medical Centre
121 Oakfield Road, Wollescote, Stourbridge DY9 9DS
Tel: 01562 882277
(Dudley South Primary Care Trust)
Patient List Size: 11700

Practice Manager Christine Penn

GP Susan Rosemary ANDERSON, David Michael HEGARTY, Karen Anne HEGARTY, Susan Jean HYNE, Stella PINTO, Colin Hugh YARWOOD-SMITH

Stourport-on-Severn

Areley Kings Surgery
The Bridge, Dunley Road, Stourport-on-Severn DY13 0AX
Tel: 01299 822103 Fax: 01299 827350
(Wyre Forest Primary Care Trust)
Patient List Size: 1750

Practice Manager Catherine Pedersen

GP Mahmoud Abdul Rahman Mahmoud AL-KHAYAT

The Health Centre
Worcester Street, Stourport-on-Severn DY13 8EH
Tel: 01299 827141 Fax: 01299 879074
(Wyre Forest Primary Care Trust)
Patient List Size: 7800

Practice Manager Clare Nock

GP Richard Jeremy HORTON, Gary John PARSONS, James Stewart Henry PATON, Rachel Ann WARD

York Street Medical Centre
20-21 York Street, Stourport-on-Severn DY13 9EH
Tel: 01299 827171 Fax: 01299 827910
(Wyre Forest Primary Care Trust)

GP Peter Ferens BATTY, Timothy Martin CHEW, James Stuart GOODMAN, Joanna Frances Mary GOODMAN, Lesley Jane HICKMAN, Wendy Elaine KINGSTON, Simon L RUMLEY

Stowmarket

Combs Ford Surgery
Combs Lane, Stowmarket IP14 2SY
Tel: 01449 678333 Fax: 01449 614535
(Central Suffolk Primary Care Trust)
Patient List Size: 9300

GP Adam Franciszek WANKOWSKI, David Malcolm Taylor CAMPBELL, C DUNMORE, Alistair David GORDON-BROWN, Jacqueline Elizabeth MUIR, J RATH

The Health Centre
Chapel Road, Mendlesham, Stowmarket IP14 5SQ
Tel: 01449 767722
(Central Suffolk Primary Care Trust)
Patient List Size: 6730

Practice Manager Val Baker

GP Paul Harvey HEAD, Anne Helen FENNING, John Rupert GILL, Jonathan Mark HERMAN

Stowhealth
Violet Hill House, Violet Hill Road, Stowmarket IP14 1NL
Tel: 01449 776000 Fax: 01449 776005
(Central Suffolk Primary Care Trust)
Patient List Size: 14000

Practice Manager Penny Flack

GP Michael Charles John HELLIWELL, Lynn DAILEY, Ian Anthony Rowland JENKINS, Veronica Maria KUBIS, Neil MACEY, Simon Victor RUDLAND, Mark Irving SHENTON, J Louise SKIOLDEBRAND, Baber YUSAF

The Surgery
20 Low Road, Debenham, Stowmarket IP14 6QU
Tel: 01728 860248 Fax: 01728 861300
(Central Suffolk Primary Care Trust)
Patient List Size: 7764

Practice Manager Mary Davey

GP John Patrick Seymour FIELDER, David John EGAN, Teresa Bernadette JENNINGS, Helen Mary MACPHERSON, Luke Conrad MORGAN

Stratford-upon-Avon

Arden Medical Centre
Albany Road, Stratford-upon-Avon CV37 6PG
Tel: 01789 414942 Fax: 01789 296427
(South Warwickshire Primary Care Trust)

GP Nigel Charles WOOD, Jacqueline FOX

Bridge House Medical Centre
Scholars Lane, Stratford-upon-Avon CV37 6HE
Tel: 01789 292201 Fax: 01789 262087
(South Warwickshire Primary Care Trust)
Patient List Size: 8400

Practice Manager Marie Tew

GP Jean Patricia Anne HODSON, Ian ALLWOOD, Eithne Mary BATT, Elaine Margaret ROSS, James William RUDGE, James SCRIVENS

Rother House Medical Centre
Alcester Road, Stratford-upon-Avon CV37 6PP
Tel: 01789 269386 Fax: 01789 298742
(South Warwickshire Primary Care Trust)

Practice Manager Tom Ganner

GP Charles George Anderson PHALP, Timothy George CROOK, Terence Malcolm GASPER, Rosalind Mary HENDERSON, Katharine Jane KING, Rebecca Jane LEWIS, Andrew Cameron Knight LOCKIE, Rosemary Jane THORNE

The Surgery
Chestnut Walk, Stratford-upon-Avon CV37 6HQ
Tel: 01789 292895 Fax: 01789 414721
(South Warwickshire Primary Care Trust)
Patient List Size: 13500

Practice Manager Jean Walker

GP Martin POPPLEWELL, Joanne Elizabeth ALLISTON, David Michael BUCKLEY, William FITCHFORD, Martyn GILL, Jennifer GOWANS, Julia Anne JONES, Gillian LEYLAND

The Surgery
Lower Quinton, Stratford-upon-Avon CV37 8SJ
Tel: 01789 720820 Fax: 01789 720052
(South Warwickshire Primary Care Trust)
Patient List Size: 2680

GP Ivan Martin CARRINGTON

Street

Monro and Vriend
Hindhayes Lane, Street BA16 0ET
Tel: 01458 841122 Fax: 01458 840044
(Mendip Primary Care Trust)
Patient List Size: 3400

GP Alexander James MONRO, R VRIEND

Vine Surgery
Hindhayes Lane, Street BA16 0ET
Tel: 01458 841122 Fax: 01458 840044
(Mendip Primary Care Trust)
Patient List Size: 7200

Practice Manager Peter Moran

GP John MERRICK, Susan Lynn DAVIES, Carole Ann RUSHFORD, Richard Nicholas SEYMOUR, Carey Spencer WOLFE

Vine Surgery
Hindhayes Lane, Street BA16 0ET
(Mendip Primary Care Trust)

Practice Manager David Moran

GP John MERRICK, Susan Lynn DAVIES, Robert LEVANTINE, Beatriz MOLINA, James MONRO, Carole Ann RUSHFORD, Stephen TALBOT, Robert VRIEND, Carey Spencer WOLFE

Stroud

Frithwood Surgery
45 Tanglewood Way, Bussage, Stroud GL6 8DE
Tel: 01453 884646 Fax: 01453 731302
(Cotswold and Vale Primary Care Trust)

Practice Manager Ruth Henney

GP Timothy CROUCH, Graeme Douglas HALL, Bridget Sinikka Christine JORRO, Patricia PEARSON

The Health Centre
Beeches Green, Stroud GL5 4BH
Tel: 01453 764696
(Cotswold and Vale Primary Care Trust)
Patient List Size: 4200

Practice Manager Hilary French

GP Christopher STANIFORTH, Anne HAMPTON, Dr LINSELL

The Health Centre
Beeches Green, Stroud GL5 4BH
Tel: 01453 763980
(Cotswold and Vale Primary Care Trust)

Practice Manager Lynne Geoghegan

GP Peter Gordon KELLY, Robert Patrick Hunter HOLMES, Graham John ISAAC, John Charles SALTER, Pamela Joy SWINDELL

Hoyland House Surgery
Hoyland House, Gyde Road, Painswick, Stroud GL6 6RD
Tel: 01452 812545
(Cotswold and Vale Primary Care Trust)

Practice Manager Keith Jones

GP Candace April Marie JANSEN, Roderick David JAQUES, Kevin BARRACLOUGH, Jennifer Ann DU TOIT

Locking Hill Surgery
Locking Hill, Stroud GL5 1UY
Tel: 01453 764222 Fax: 01453 756278
(Cotswold and Vale Primary Care Trust)

Practice Manager Kathy M Tomkins

GP James Logan DOD, Robin Nigel BLENKARN, Ian Michael BYE, Gillian DOD, Ewart David LEWIS, Christopher James WOODS

Marlow and Partners
The Surgery, Bell Lane, Minchinhampton, Stroud GL6 9JF
Tel: 01453 883793 Fax: 01453 731670
(Cotswold and Vale Primary Care Trust)
Patient List Size: 7000

Practice Manager John Raggett

GP Anne-Marie MARLOW, Anne CAIN, David Anthony Columba Godwin POUNCEY, Andrew Paul Forsythe SIMPSON, David Michael THOMAS, Susanne WEIR

Prices Mill Surgery
New Market Road, Nailsworth, Stroud GL6 0DQ
Tel: 01453 832424 Fax: 01453 833833
(Cotswold and Vale Primary Care Trust)
Patient List Size: 9000

Practice Manager Colin Rudall

GP Andrew Hugh Cecil BODDAM-WHETHAM, Nigel Jeremy BOOKER, Michael Joseph LATTER, Ros MULHALL

Rowcroft Medical Centre
Rowcroft Retreat, Stroud GL5 3BE
Tel: 01453 764471 Fax: 01453 755247
(Cotswold and Vale Primary Care Trust)
Patient List Size: 10000

Practice Manager Kay Badham

GP Ralph Harry STEPHENSON, Deborah Kate HAFFENDEN, Thornton John MacCALLUM, James Thomas QUEKETT, Richard David WALDON

St Lukes Medical Centre
53 Cainscross Road, Stroud GL5 4EX
Tel: 01453 763755 Fax: 01453 756573
(Cotswold and Vale Primary Care Trust)
Patient List Size: 3350

Practice Manager Adam Beard

GP Marianne ALLAN, Ricahrd BARRY, Michael Russell EVANS

Studley

The Pool Medical Centre
Pool Road, Studley B80 7QU
Tel: 01527 852133/853671 Fax: 01527 853072
(South Warwickshire Primary Care Trust)

GP Peter John HARRIS, Mary Francella Rebecca TONGE, Stephen WALTER

Studley Health Centre
40 High Street, Studley B80 7HJ
Tel: 01527 853311 Fax: 01527 854520
(South Warwickshire Primary Care Trust)

Practice Manager S Bosworth, S Rollings, Deborah Sydenham

GP Margaret Patricia BUCKLEY, Derek BROWN

Sturminster Newton

Station Road Surgery
Station Road, Stalbridge, Sturminster Newton DT10 2RQ
Tel: 01963 362363 Fax: 01963 362866
Email: dispensary@gp-j81040.nhs.uk
Website: www.stalbridgesurgery.co.uk
(North Dorset Primary Care Trust)
Patient List Size: 4359

Practice Manager Keith Holden

GP Geoffrey Edward Alan SPARROW, Stephen John CLAYTON, Deborah Alexandra GONPERTZ

Sturminster Newton Medical Centre
Barnes Close, Sturminster Newton DT10 1BN
Tel: 01258 474500 Fax: 01258 471547
(North Dorset Primary Care Trust)
Patient List Size: 7230

GP Matthew Graham CRIPPS, Elizabeth Carol BURTON, James Hendrik Reginald EDWARDS, Jonathon MUDSON, Joanna Patricia Jane ROBINSON

Sudbury

Guildhall Surgery
High Street, Clare, Sudbury CO10 8NY
Tel: 01787 277523 Fax: 01787 278628
Website: www.guildhallsurgery.co.uk
(Suffolk West Primary Care Trust)
Patient List Size: 4900

Practice Manager Carole Ovenden

GP Richard Paterson CHASE, Timothy Richard GARRETT-MOORE, Jonathan David HUCK

Hardwicke House Surgery
Hardwicke House, Stour Street, Sudbury CO10 2AY
Tel: 01787 370011 Fax: 01787 376521
(Suffolk West Primary Care Trust)
Patient List Size: 26600

Practice Manager Denise Chittenden

GP Bryan HAYHOW, Michael John Mowbray BARKER, Edward BENKE, David Carus Peploe BEVAN, Andrew Douglas Kenneth CROUCH, Marcello DEL TORRE, Sultan JETHA, Simon LOVEGROVE, Jacqueline RAE, Rakesh RAJA, James SHERIFI, Susan Catherine Johan SILLS, Sally Suzanne WILLIAMSON

Little Roseworthy Surgery
Little Roseworthy, 22 Meadow Lane, Sudbury CO10 2TD
Tel: 01787 310000 Fax: 01787 75245
(Suffolk West Primary Care Trust)

GP Kailash SARDA

The Long Melford Practice
Cordell Road, Long Melford, Sudbury CO10 9EP
Tel: 01787 378226 Fax: 01787 311287
Email: lmlav@epulse.net
(Suffolk West Primary Care Trust)
Patient List Size: 9800

Practice Manager Elizabeth Oakley

GP Charles David GOODLIFFE, Christopher John BROWNRING, Mark Edwin Wigfield CHAMBERS, Ralph Anthony HUGHES, Tessa Carolyn Margaret NORRIS

Pot Kiln Road Surgery
67 Pot Kiln Road, Great Cornard, Sudbury CO10 0DH
Tel: 01787 880337
(Suffolk West Primary Care Trust)

GP D P HARSHADRAI, S K JETHA

Siam Surgery
Siam Place, Sudbury CO10 1JH
Tel: 01787 370444 Fax: 01787 880322
(Suffolk West Primary Care Trust)
Patient List Size: 8100

Practice Manager Jean Coote

GP Roderick DONNELLY, Adrian Roy KEMP, Anthony P O'NEILL, David Lynton TAYLOR

Stonehall Surgery
Nethergate Street, Clare, Sudbury CO10 8NP
Tel: 01787 278999 Fax: 01787 278522
(Suffolk West Primary Care Trust)
Patient List Size: 2200

Practice Manager Hepy Wiley

GP Dr BARKER, Dr BEVAN, Dr CROUCH, Dr HAYHOW, Dr SILLS, Dr WILLIAMSON

The Surgery
Lion Road, Glemsford, Sudbury CO10 7RF
(Suffolk West Primary Care Trust)
Patient List Size: 5080

Practice Manager Jo Brown, Dennis Gray

GP Dr HELLER, Dr GIBLIN, Dr LESSER

Sunbury-on-Thames

Homewaters Surgery
Green Street, Sunbury-on-Thames TW16 6QB
Tel: 01932 784004
(North Surrey Primary Care Trust)

GP Kulwant Kaur SEEHRA

Sunbury Health Centre Group Practice
Green Street, Sunbury-on-Thames TW16 6RH
Tel: 01932 713399 Fax: 01932 713354
(North Surrey Primary Care Trust)
Patient List Size: 17000

Practice Manager Varsha Mandalia

GP Richard BARNETT, Jennifer Jane PEARCE, Nicholas Ricardo PEARCE, Glyn Bradley CHAPMAN, John R A DUCKWORTH, Susan HODSON, Anne Patricia SAUNDERS

Sunderland

Ashburne Medical Centre
74-75 Toward Road, Sunderland SR2 8JG
Tel: 0191 567 4397 Fax: 0191 514 3740
(Sunderland Teaching Primary Care Trust)
Patient List Size: 5560

Practice Manager A Porteous

GP Bipin Chandra Ramniklal SHETH, H PARRY, R PILAPITIYA, C WOHLRAB

Castletown Medical Centre
6 The Broadway, Castletown, Sunderland SR5 3EX
Tel: 0191 549 5113 Fax: 0191 516 0041
Website: www.sunderland.nhs.uk/castletown
(Sunderland Teaching Primary Care Trust)
Patient List Size: 2826

Practice Manager Amanda Holey

GP Roshan Lal DHAR, Oma KAUL

Central Surgery
27 Norfolk Street, Sunderland SR1 1EE
Tel: 0191 565 3040 Fax: 0191 514 0833
(Sunderland Teaching Primary Care Trust)
Patient List Size: 2060

Practice Manager Alison Heslin

GP Jairam Rama NATHAN

Chhabra's Surgery
3 Eden Terrace, Durham Road, Sunderland SR2 7PF
Tel: 0191 567 5673 Fax: 0191 514 7462
(Sunderland Teaching Primary Care Trust)
Patient List Size: 2106

Practice Manager Janice Poulton

GP Dev Raj CHHABRA

Church View Medical Centre
Silksworth Terrace, Silksworth, Sunderland SR3 2AW
Tel: 0191 521 1753 Fax: 0191 521 3884
(Sunderland Teaching Primary Care Trust)
Patient List Size: 6050

Practice Manager June Foster

GP Pamela Mary WORTLEY, Melaine BROWN, Ashar HUSSAIN, Rachael MYERS

Deerness Park Medical Centre
Suffolk Street, Sunderland SR2 8AD
Tel: 0191 567 0961 Fax: 0191 565 0075
(Sunderland Teaching Primary Care Trust)
Patient List Size: 13289

Practice Manager Eric Harrison

GP Priti Sadhan DATTA, Iain Merry GILMOUR, Ali IDRISSISBAI, A I JONES, Robert Blair MURRAY, Neil Macarthur OWEN, H C SCHOFIELD, Topti SINHARAY, Paula STIDOLPH

Drs Glass, Mekkawy, Parson and Steel
Aid Jack Cohen Health Centre, Springwell Road, Sunderland SR3 4HG
Tel: 0191 522 9908/9927 Fax: 0191 528 8294/4295
(Sunderland Teaching Primary Care Trust)
Patient List Size: 5739

Practice Manager Elizabeth Hamilton

GP Leslie George GLASS, E I MEKKAWY, Fiona PARSON, A M STEEL

Fulwell Medical Centre
Ebdon Lane, Fulwell, Sunderland SR6 8DZ
Tel: 0191 548 3635 Fax: 0191 516 0109
(Sunderland Teaching Primary Care Trust)
Patient List Size: 8607

Practice Manager J Rutherford

GP Robert Gordon RUTHERFORD, Dr ATCHISON, Dr BLAKE, Dr BOONHAM, Claire Joyce BROWN, Christopher James WALTON

Happy House Surgery
Durham Road, Sunderland SR3 4BY
Tel: 0191 528 2222 Fax: 0191 528 2626
(Sunderland Teaching Primary Care Trust)
Patient List Size: 2867

Practice Manager Steven Harder

GP Kevin Nicholas John WEAVER

Hendon Health Centre
Meaburn Terrace, Sunderland SR1 2ND
Tel: 0191 567 3393 Fax: 0191 510 3417
(Sunderland Teaching Primary Care Trust)
Patient List Size: 3639

Practice Manager Lisa Richardson

GP Shashank Madhav BHATE, Dr EL-SHAKANKERY

Millfield Medical Centre
63-83 Hylton Road, Sunderland SR4 7AF
Tel: 0191 567 9179 Fax: 0191 514 7452
(Sunderland Teaching Primary Care Trust)
Patient List Size: 13428

Practice Manager S J Sly

GP William WRIGHT, Jacqueline GILLESPIE, Lynn J HARNESS, Julia LEE, Dr LYNDON, Dr RUSSELL, Lehmbar SINGH, S Richard SMITHSON, Ian Douglas WATSON

Monkwearmouth Health Centre
Dundas Street, Sunderland SR6 0AB
Tel: 0191 567 4293 Fax: 0191 514 7889
(Sunderland Teaching Primary Care Trust)
Patient List Size: 2458

Practice Manager Judith Taylor

GP Arthur James McCracken CRUMMIE

Monkwearmouth Health Centre
Dundas Street, Sunderland SR6 0AB
Tel: 0191 567 8023 Fax: 0191 565 3336
(Sunderland Teaching Primary Care Trust)
Patient List Size: 2009

Practice Manager Suzanne Gilmour

GP Hazel OAKLEY

The New City Medical Centre
Tatham Street, Hendon, Sunderland SR1 2QB
Tel: 0191 567 5571 Fax: 0191 510 2746
(Sunderland Teaching Primary Care Trust)
Patient List Size: 7658

Practice Manager Denise S Elliott

GP Sangramsinha Gudleppa HALLIKERI, John Stanley PARTINGTON, Surya Narayan PATNAIK

The Old Forge Surgery
Pallion Park, Pallion, Sunderland SR4 6QE
Tel: 0191 510 9393 Fax: 0191 510 9595
(Sunderland Teaching Primary Care Trust)
Patient List Size: 8366

Practice Manager Vera Marshall

GP Lalldhar PAWAROO, Philip Mark PEVERLEY, Erio Aldo SPAGNOLI, Ian John WILSON

Pallion Health Centre
Hylton Road, Sunderland SR4 7XF
Tel: 0191 567 4673 Fax: 0191 565 0489
(Sunderland Teaching Primary Care Trust)
Patient List Size: 9936

Practice Manager Janet Willoughby

GP Alistair Martin Davidson BROWN, Dr LEFLEY, Dr McCANN, Dr SOMOZA, Dr WILDERMANN

Pallion Health Centre
Hylton Road, Sunderland SR4 7XF
Tel: 0191 567 2995 Fax: 0191 514 3516
(Sunderland Teaching Primary Care Trust)
Patient List Size: 2101

GP Shiv Prasad BAGCHI

Pallion Health Centre
Hylton Road, Sunderland SR4 7XF
Tel: 0191 565 8598 Fax: 0191 514 7467
(Sunderland Teaching Primary Care Trust)
Patient List Size: 5456

Practice Manager Christine Boston

GP Mohamed Ahmed Aboul ELA, Basim Gamal Othman AL-KHALIDI

Pallion Health Centre
Hylton Road, Sunderland SR4 7XF
Tel: 0191 657 1319 Fax: 0191 510 3558
(Sunderland Teaching Primary Care Trust)
Patient List Size: 4938

Practice Manager Enid Fairs

GP Bola Krishna Kishore SHETTY, Thirumalappa Sampangi RAMAN, Dr URSU

Pegari Practice
Hendon Health Centre, Meaburn Terrace, Sunderland SR1 2ND
Tel: 0191 510 1865
(Sunderland Teaching Primary Care Trust)

Practice Manager Lynn Calder

GP Dr WOHLRAB

Red House Surgery
127 Renfrew Road, Hylton Red House, Sunderland SR5 5PS
Tel: 0191 548 1269 Fax: 0191 549 8998
(Sunderland Teaching Primary Care Trust)
Patient List Size: 5995

Practice Manager Joan Reilly

GP Gaddam Madhusudan REDDY, Lim Chung Hwee WIN

Ryhope Health Centre
Black Road, Sunderland SR2 0RY
Tel: 0191 521 0210 Fax: 0191 521 4235
(Sunderland Teaching Primary Care Trust)
Patient List Size: 4837

Practice Manager J V Haswell

GP Martin Joseph WALKER, K BENTON, I W LAWTHER, I PATTISON

Ryhope Health Centre
Ryhope, Sunderland SR2 0RY
Tel: 0191 521 0559 Fax: 0191 521 3854
(Sunderland Teaching Primary Care Trust)
Patient List Size: 3049

Practice Manager Peter Gunn

GP Clifford FERNANDES

Silksworth Health Centre
Silksworth, Sunderland SR3 2AN
Tel: 0191 521 2282 Fax: 0191 523 5827
(Sunderland Teaching Primary Care Trust)
Patient List Size: 3950

Practice Manager Anne Lilley

GP Navajeevan Achyutrao JOSHI, Dr BRUCKMANN, Z RIZWI

Silksworth Health Centre
Silksworth, Sunderland SR3 2AN
Tel: 0191 521 0252 Fax: 0191 521 1288
(Sunderland Teaching Primary Care Trust)
Patient List Size: 5881

Practice Manager Margaret Hodgkinson

GP Kevin STEPHENSON, Dr WILSON

South Hill Crescent Surgery
4 South Hill Crescent, Durham Road, Sunderland SR2 7PA
Tel: 0191 567 6828 Fax: 0191 510 2810
(Sunderland Teaching Primary Care Trust)
Patient List Size: 4676

Practice Manager Linda Berry

GP Selwyn Brian BOLEL, Jane Rosemary MACKRELL

South Hylton Surgery
3-5 Cambria Street, South Hylton, Sunderland SR4 0LT
Tel: 0191 534 7386 Fax: 0191 534 1970
(Sunderland Teaching Primary Care Trust)
Patient List Size: 3455

Practice Manager Jacqui Wylie

GP Andrew David LEEKS, Ian Harry WIDDRINGTON

Southwick Health Centre
The Green, Southwick, Sunderland SR5 2LT
Tel: 0191 548 6634 Fax: 0191 549 4384
(Sunderland Teaching Primary Care Trust)
Patient List Size: 9480

Practice Manager Georgie Gilfillan

GP Brian Joseph CLOAK, Henry Yuk Chuen CHOI, Dr CLARK, Dr FIRTH, Gavin John MILLIGAN, Dr SCHOFIELD, Dr SHEPHERD

Southwick Health Centre
The Green, Southwick, Sunderland SR5 2LT
Tel: 0191 548 6944 Fax: 0191 5488055
(Sunderland Teaching Primary Care Trust)
Patient List Size: 2437

Practice Manager Christina Rayner

GP Rex OBONNA

Southwick Health Centre
The Green, Southwick, Sunderland SR5 2LT
Tel: 0191 548 6550 Fax: 0191 548 0867
(Sunderland Teaching Primary Care Trust)

Patient List Size: 2945

Practice Manager Wendy Atkinson

GP Martin Paul WEATHERHEAD, Emma Calre HEPPLE, Victoria Courtney MIDDLETON

Springwell House Surgery
Durham Road, North Moor, Sunderland SR3 1RN
Tel: 0191 528 3251 Fax: 0191 528 3100
(Sunderland Teaching Primary Care Trust)
Patient List Size: 2578

Practice Manager Clare Jenkinson

GP Hem Chandra SINGH

Springwell Medical Group
iAlderman Jack Cohen Health Centre, Springwell Road, Sunderland SR3 4HG
Tel: 0191 528 2727 Fax: 0191 528 3262
(Sunderland Teaching Primary Care Trust)
Patient List Size: 6326

Practice Manager V Hepplewhite

GP Kavindra Nath SHARMA, James P BELL, Rachel BERNADI, David Graeme GOUGH, Greg RUBIN

St Bede's Medical Centre
Lower Dundas Street, Sunderland SR6 0QQ
Tel: 0191 567 5335 Fax: 0191 510 2495
(Sunderland Teaching Primary Care Trust)
Patient List Size: 7747

Practice Manager Brenda Dawson

GP Roger Norman FORD, Ann CLARK, Kieran DULSON, Sarah JACKSON, Gerard Patrick McBRIDE

The Surgery
51-52 Roker Avenue, Sunderland SR6 0HT
Tel: 0191 567 8023 Fax: 0191 514 7430
(Sunderland Teaching Primary Care Trust)
Patient List Size: 2174

Practice Manager Ethel Barker

GP Jonathan Alfred MAIR

Villette Surgery
Suffolk Street, Hendon, Sunderland SR2 8AX
Tel: 0191 567 9361 Fax: 0191 514 7476
(Sunderland Teaching Primary Care Trust)
Patient List Size: 6216

Practice Manager Doreen Nicholson

GP Mohamadbhai Noorbhai MAREDIA, John David BRIGHAM, Dr PINTO-WRIGHT, Dr TAYLOR

Whitburn Surgery
3 Bryers Street, Whitburn, Sunderland SR6 7EE
Tel: 0191 529 3039 Fax: 0191 529 5436
(South Tyneside Primary Care Trust)

Practice Manager C Wagner

GP Pauline Veronica GOLDSMITH, Robert Francis Edward CERVENAK, K R O'NEIL

Surbiton

Berrylands Surgery
Howard Road, Surbiton KT5 8SA
Tel: 020 8399 6362 Fax: 020 8339 5700
(Kingston Primary Care Trust)
Patient List Size: 3652

Practice Manager Vicki Merrall

GP Carol Ann BARLIN, Jane Celia Hopton D'SOUZA

Brunswick Surgery
Oak Hill Health Centre, Oak Hill Road, Surbiton KT6 6EN
Tel: 020 8390 5321 Fax: 020 8390 3223
Email: dave.potton@gp-h84015.nhs.uk
Website: www.brunswicksurgery.co.uk
(Kingston Primary Care Trust)
Patient List Size: 6380

Practice Manager David J Potton

GP Judy Caroline Ann MUNBY, Paul DHILLON, Melinda O'DRISCOLL, M TURNER

Claremont Medical Centre
2A Glenbuck Road, Surbiton KT6 6BS
Tel: 020 8399 3516 Fax: 020 8390 0371
(Kingston Primary Care Trust)
Patient List Size: 6100

GP Martin Stephen WOLFSON, Anne Maureen HINSLEY, Arun KOCHHAR

Evesham Medical Practice
1 Evesham Terrace, St Andrews Road, Surbiton KT6 4DS
Tel: 020 8399 1837 Fax: 020 8399 5791
(Kingston Primary Care Trust)
Patient List Size: 1900

GP D CLEMENTS, Adel KARTAS, Haytheni NASEEF

Kingsdowne Surgery
34 Kingsdowne Road, Surbiton KT6 6LA
Tel: 020 8399 9032 Fax: 020 8390 2122
(Kingston Primary Care Trust)
Patient List Size: 3900

GP Junaid Ali SYED

Langley Medical Practice
Oak Hill Health Centre, Oak Hill Road, Surbiton KT6 6EN
Tel: 020 8390 9996 Fax: 020 8390 4057
(Kingston Primary Care Trust)
Patient List Size: 7100

GP Caroline ALDOYS, Sarah Amanda Jane BENNEY, John DALZELL, Siyana SHAFFI

Maypole Surgery
8 Hook Road, Surbiton KT6 5BH
Tel: 020 8390 3396 Fax: 020 8390 3396
(Kingston Primary Care Trust)

Practice Manager Carol Pateman

GP Stuart MACKIE

Oak Hill Health Centre
Oak Hill Road, Surbiton KT6 6EN
Tel: 020 8399 6622 Fax: 020 8390 4470
(Kingston Primary Care Trust)

Practice Manager Peter Hoy

GP David Lloyd ROBERTS, Jonathan Michael EDWARDS, Mandeep KOONER, Nassif Samuel Nassif MANSOUR, Philip Daniel MOORE, Vineet THAPAR, Judith Mary TOPP

Sunray Surgery
97 Warren Drive South, Surbiton KT5 9QD
Tel: 020 8330 4056 Fax: 020 8335 4080
(Kingston Primary Care Trust)

GP Thilagavathy Chandra MOHAN

The Surgery
1A Red Lion Road, Tolworth, Surbiton KT6 7QG
Tel: 020 8399 1779
(Kingston Primary Care Trust)

Practice Manager Marion Farrow

GP Rajendra Kumar AGRAWAL, Kusum AGRAWAL

Sutton

Benhill and Belmont
54 Benhill Avenue, Sutton SM1 4EB
Tel: 020 8770 0587 Fax: 020 8770 0586
Website: www.BenhillBelmontGPC.co.uk
(Sutton and Merton Primary Care Trust)
Patient List Size: 10070

Practice Manager Barbara Shaddock

GP Christopher James ELLIOTT, Jeffrey J CROUCHER, Anna KAYE, Padmalata Priyadarshini LIYANAGE, Adnan MALIK

Brennan and Neylan
The GP Centre, 322 Malden Road, North Cheam, Sutton SM3 8EP
Tel: 020 8644 0224 Fax: 020 8288 1012
Website: www.gpcentre.co.uk
(Sutton and Merton Primary Care Trust)

GP Cecilia Agnes Mary BRENNAN, Catherine Margaret Mary Angela NEYLAN

Cheam Family Practice
The Knoll, Parkside, Cheam, Sutton SM3 8BS
Tel: 020 8770 2014 Fax: 020 8770 1864
(Sutton and Merton Primary Care Trust)

Practice Manager Heather Arscott

GP Richard Andrew COOLING, Diana Muriel KAY, Gareth Antony RUSE, Joseph SCERRI, Alison SHEPHERD, Mark John TYLER

Elliott
The Health Centre, Robin Hood Lane, Sutton SM1 2RJ
Tel: 020 8642 2229/2220 Fax: 020 8642 2226
(Sutton and Merton Primary Care Trust)
Patient List Size: 3500

Practice Manager Jean Scaddan

GP Simon Denis Cotton ELLIOTT

The Grove Road Practice
83 Grove Road, Sutton SM1 2DB
Tel: 020 8642 1721/643 9366 Fax: 020 8288 1460
(Sutton and Merton Primary Care Trust)

GP David V P THOMAS, Brendan HUDSON, Jyotika RATHOD

Leghari, Lodge and Muktar
The GP Centre, 322 Malden Road, North Cheam, Sutton SM3 8EP
Tel: 020 8644 0224 Fax: 020 8288 1012
Website: www.gpcentre.co.uk
(Sutton and Merton Primary Care Trust)
Patient List Size: 5200

GP Jamil Ahmed Khan LEGHARI, June Winifred LODGE, Dan MUKTAR

Longley and Jolly
The GP Centre, 322 Malden Road, North Cheam, Sutton SM3 8EP
Tel: 020 8644 0224 Fax: 020 8288 1012
Website: www.gpcentre.co.uk
(Sutton and Merton Primary Care Trust)

GP Juliana Michal LONGLEY, Alexander William JOLLEY

The Old Court House
4 Throwley Way, Sutton SM1 4AF
Tel: 020 8643 8866
(Sutton and Merton Primary Care Trust)

GP Stephen John GRICE, G T COLDREY, Jane Evelyn VERNON, George Thomas WILLS

Seyan, Saffar and Rodin
The Health Centre, Robin Hood Lane, Sutton SM1 2RJ
Tel: 020 8642 2010/3848 Fax: 020 8286 1010
Email: robinhoodclinic@gp-h85095.nhs.uk
Website: www.robinhoodclinic.co.uk
(Sutton and Merton Primary Care Trust)
Patient List Size: 6500

Practice Manager Elaine Richmond

GP Marian RODIN, Ammer SAFFAR, Rabinder Singh Atma Singh SEYAN, B SUBASHINI

Stonecot Surgery
115 Epsom Road, Sutton SM3 9EY
Tel: 020 8644 5187 Fax: 020 8644 7003
(Sutton and Merton Primary Care Trust)
Patient List Size: 9020

Practice Manager Hilary Stoddart

GP Karen Louise JOHN, Claire Elisabeth DAVIES, Mark Christopher FREE, Vasa GNANAPRAGASAM

The Surgery
133 Reigate Avenue, Sutton SM1 3JR
Tel: 020 8644 7610 Fax: 020 8644 4403
(Sutton and Merton Primary Care Trust)
Patient List Size: 1900

Practice Manager Kumari Jayasena

GP A K M JAYASENA

The Surgery
48 Mulgrave Road, Belmont, Sutton SM2 6LX
Tel: 020 8642 2050
(Sutton and Merton Primary Care Trust)

Practice Manager Daphne Lewis

GP John Seymour PEMBREY, Anthony John FREE, Clare Jennifer O'SULLIVAN, Anne Mary THOMPSON

The Surgery
6 Well Court, 740 London Road, North Cheam, Sutton SM3 9BX
Tel: 020 8644 8400
(Sutton and Merton Primary Care Trust)
Patient List Size: 2200

GP Kangaratnam Kathirgama KANTHAN, Sukirthalojini KATHIRGAMAKANTHAN

The Surgery
92 Westmead Road, Sutton SM1 4HX
Tel: 020 8643 9830
(Sutton and Merton Primary Care Trust)

Practice Manager A Huggett

GP Syed Mustafa MOHIUD-DIN, Fouzia MOHIUD-DIN

The Surgery
23 Carshalton Road, Sutton SM1 4LF
Tel: 020 8642 0396
(Sutton and Merton Primary Care Trust)

GP D S PRASAD

Sutton-in-Ashfield

Healdswood Surgery
Mansfield Road, Skegby, Sutton-in-Ashfield NG17 3EE
Tel: 01623 513553 Fax: 01623 550753
(Ashfield Primary Care Trust)

Practice Manager Lesley Perry

GP Richard Alan HOOK, John Richard WILLIAMSON

Huthwaite Health Centre
New Street, Huthwaite, Sutton-in-Ashfield NG17 2LR
Tel: 01623 513147 Fax: 01623 515574
(Ashfield Primary Care Trust)
Patient List Size: 7900

Practice Manager Karen Mellors

GP George Stanley Alfred EWBANK, Kevin John HILL, Hilary Ann LOVELOCK, Philip George SMITH, Elaine Elizabeth Jane ULLIOTT

The Pantiles Medical Centre
Church Street, Sutton-in-Ashfield NG17 1EX
Tel: 01623 557646 Fax: 01623 440300
(Ashfield Primary Care Trust)

Practice Manager Carlin Jill

GP Qudsia CHANDRAN, Thambiturai Raj CHANDRAN

Robertson, McKenzie, Creedon and Pound
Woodlands Medical Practice, Bluebell Wood Way, Sutton-in-Ashfield NG17 1JW
Tel: 01623 528748 Fax: 01623 528747
(Ashfield Primary Care Trust)
Patient List Size: 8250

Practice Manager Patricia Brown

GP Neil Malcolm ROBERTSON, Jane CREEDON, Alison LAIRD, F J McKENZIE, N POUND

The Surgery
Harwood Close, Skegby Road, Sutton-in-Ashfield NG17 4PD
Tel: 01623 551015 Fax: 01623 443339
(Ashfield Primary Care Trust)
Patient List Size: 3408

GP D M SHARMA

Sutton Health Centre
New Street, Sutton-in-Ashfield NG17 1BW
Tel: 01623 559992 Fax: 01623 559943
(Ashfield Primary Care Trust)
Patient List Size: 2600

Practice Manager Jackie Brittlebank

GP Sibapriya MUKHOPADHYAY

Willowbrook Medical Practice
Brook Street, Sutton-in-Ashfield NG17 1ES
Tel: 01623 440018
(Ashfield Primary Care Trust)
Patient List Size: 13500

Practice Manager Linda Allum

GP George STEIN, Deborah Fortune BLISS, Jeremy Roland Furneaux JENKINS, Celestine JOHN, Arthur James LACEY, Thazathedathu Koshy MATHEW

Sutton Coldfield

Ashfield Surgery
8 Walmley Road, Sutton Coldfield B76 1QN
Tel: 0121 351 7955 Fax: 0121 313 2509
(North Birmingham Primary Care Trust)
Patient List Size: 13700

Practice Manager Marie Donoghue

GP Andrew Philip BLIGHT, Ian Peter COLLIER, Sally Jane COPE, A M KING, Christopher David LENTON, Huw David Edward LESTER, Lynn Joy SHELDRAKE, Sarabjit Singh SOORAE

Ashfurlong Health Centre
233 Tamworth Road, Sutton Coldfield B75 6DX
Tel: 0121 308 6311 Fax: 0121 323 3830
(North Birmingham Primary Care Trust)
Patient List Size: 7000

Practice Manager Ron Heaton

GP Peter John INGHAM, Joyce Barbara COLLIER, Herjinder DALL, Morag Jane DUGAS

Blackwood Health Centre
Blackwood Road, Streetly, Sutton Coldfield B74 3PL
Tel: 0121 353 7558 Fax: 0121 353 7056
(Walsall Teaching Primary Care Trust)

Practice Manager Sue Abdo

GP Osman Ahmed ABDO

The Falcon Medical Centre
93 Carhampton Road, Sutton Coldfield B75 7PG
Tel: 0121 686 9990
(North Birmingham Primary Care Trust)

Practice Manager Sally Hookes

GP Joginder BAINS

Four Oaks Medical Centre
Carlton House, Mere Green Road, Sutton Coldfield B75 5BS
Tel: 0121 308 2080 Fax: 0121 323 4694
(North Birmingham Primary Care Trust)
Patient List Size: 10500

Practice Manager Sylvia Bailey

GP Alexander Charles Iain SHEARER, Alan Stuart COJTTS, Alison Joy CUTHBERT, Roger John GENT, Carol Louise HOOPER

Hawthorns Surgery
331 Birmingham Road, Sutton Coldfield B72 1DL
Tel: 0121 373 2211 Fax: 0121 382 1274
(North Birmingham Primary Care Trust)
Patient List Size: 12400

Practice Manager Janet Marjoram

GP Charles Robert Matthew BROOMHEAD, Margaret Patricia CLARKE, John Melvyn DIVALL, Trevor William REES, O VAN LOON

Jockey Road Medical Centre
519 Jockey Road, Sutton Coldfield B73 5DF
Tel: 0121 354 1749 Fax: 0121 355 1840
(North Birmingham Primary Care Trust)
Patient List Size: 8000

Practice Manager Sonia Cox

GP Diana Patricia SPIERS, John Philip Oakley CHAPMAN, R GABRIEL, Marie Ellen ISZATT, A MANNAN, Joanne SMITH

Ley Hill Surgery
228 Lichfield Road, Sutton Coldfield B74 2UE
Tel: 0121 308 0359 Fax: 0121 323 2682
(North Birmingham Primary Care Trust)
Patient List Size: 12500

Practice Manager Alma Geary

GP David William WALL, Anne Louise BEAUMONT, Anne Christina DAVIES, Vineet KUNDRA, Alan John McDONALD, Pamela Joy MUNDY, Edward Kok Hun NG, Cathryn Patricia THOMAS

Manor Practice
James Preston Health Centre, 61 Holland Road, Sutton Coldfield B72 1RL
Tel: 0121 354 2032 Fax: 0121 321 1779
Website: www.manorpractice.co.uk
(North Birmingham Primary Care Trust)

Practice Manager Christine Bartlett

GP Stephen Charles MARTIN, Nirmali Sandra CAVE, Robert Michael FLACKS, Mark Lewis FORSHAW, Judith Mary RIMMER, Nigel James SPEAK

Mere Green Clinic
Mere Green Road, Sutton Coldfield B75 5BL
Tel: 0121 308 2137
(North Birmingham Primary Care Trust)

GP Henryk Bronislaw SLOMINSKI

Robinson, Ashton, Leung, Solari and Thompson
James Preston Health Centre, 61 Holland Road, Suttcn Coldfield B72 1RL
Tel: 0121 355 5150
(North Birmingham Primary Care Trust)

Practice Manager Lynn Willetts

GP William Henry ROBINSON, Christopher John ASHTON, Anthony Yin-Tuen LEUNG, Timothy John SOLARI, Anne Rosemary THOMPSON

Streetly Surgery
250A Chester Road, Streetly, Sutton Coldfield B74 3NB
Tel: 0121 353 3212
(North Birmingham Primary Care Trust)

Practice Manager Vasantha Kanagaratnam

GP S K RATNAM

The Surgery
149 Chester Road, Streetly, Sutton Coldfield B74 3NE
Tel: 0121 352 0570 Fax: 0121 353 7057
(Walsall Teaching Primary Care Trust)
Patient List Size: 1400

Practice Manager Nicky Ranu

GP Benoy Lal BANERJEA

Sutton Park Surgery
34 Chester Road North, Sutton Coldfield B73 6SP
Tel: 0121 353 2586 Fax: 0121 353 5289
(North Birmingham Primary Care Trust)
Patient List Size: 6200

Practice Manager Ellen Pearce

GP Earl Ivor John MORETON, Peter John HAYWARD, Livleen Kamal KAMAL, Gillian Dianne WALSH

Swadlincote

Goodacre and Partners
Swadlincote Surgery, Darklands Road, Swadlincote DE11 0PP
Tel: 01283 551717 Fax: 01283 211905
(Derbyshire Dales and South Derbyshire Primary Care Trust)
Patient List Size: 13400

Practice Manager Pauline Holmes

GP Andrew Stuart DAVIDSON, Andrew Stuart CALVEST, Roger Lindsey FOLLOWS, Selwyn Hugh GOODACRE, Jane Sheila KIRK, Kenneth John PATTON, Robin Fenwick TROTTER

Measham Medical Unit
High Street, Measham, Swadlincote DE12 7HR
Tel: 01530 270667 Fax: 01530 271433
(Charnwood and North West Leicestershire Primary Care Trust)
Patient List Size: 13000

Practice Manager G Benson

GP John Martin VAUGHAN, Carol A. ASHTON, Nicholas GRAVESTOCK, Teresa Mary KENNY, Kirk A. MOORE, Orest Peter MULKA, Clare I. SWAEBE, Donna M. TURFREY

Newhall Surgery
46-48 High Street, Newhall, Swadlincote DE11 0HS
Tel: 01283 217092 Fax: 01283 551997
(Derbyshire Dales and South Derbyshire Primary Care Trust)
Patient List Size: 11000

Practice Manager G Williams

GP Geoffrey Paul DAVIES, Andrew William HIGNETT, Robert William JAMISON, Wilma KNOWLES, Andrew MARSHALL

The Poplars
13 Linton Road, Castle Gresley, Swadlincote DE11 9HU
(Derbyshire Dales and South Derbyshire Primary Care Trust)

Prestwood House Surgery
74 Midway Road, Midway, Swadlincote DE11 7PG
Tel: 01283 212375 Fax: 01283 551923
(Derbyshire Dales and South Derbyshire Primary Care Trust)
Patient List Size: 7500

Practice Manager J Wainwright, W Wileman

GP Nigel STAREY, Bukhtawar DHADDA, Rebecca EVANS, Surendra PATEL

The Surgery
1 Hallcroft Avenue, Overseal, Swadlincote DE12 6JF
Tel: 01283 760595 Fax: 01283
(Derbyshire Dales and South Derbyshire Primary Care Trust)
Patient List Size: 1600

GP V P PARMAR

Taleb and Partners
The Surgery, Burton Road, Woodville, Swadlincote DE11 7JG
Tel: 01283 217036 Fax: 01283 552308
(Derbyshire Dales and South Derbyshire Primary Care Trust)
Patient List Size: 8000

GP Anthony CLEGG, Monica Catherine HANNON, Paul Leslie HARRISON, Sidi Mohammed TALEB

Swaffham

Barton and Partners
Campingland Surgery, Swaffham PE37 7RD
Tel: 01760 721211 Fax: 01760 720009
(West Norfolk Primary Care Trust)

Practice Manager Peter Wrighton

GP David Ian BARTON, Iain James CROMARTY, Mark Julian George HOLMES, Nicola Karen HOLMES, Richard Ian MUSSON

Plowright Surgery
Market Place, Swaffham PE37 7LQ
Tel: 01760 722797 Fax: 01760 720025
(West Norfolk Primary Care Trust)

Practice Manager David Cockayne

GP Robert Frank DORLING, Grace Elisabeth BARLOW, David John SORENSEN-POUND

Skinner and Partners
Manor Farm Medical Centre, Mangate Street, Swaffham PE37 7QN
Tel: 01760 721786 Fax: 01760 723703
Email: sallycross.skinner@virgin.net
(West Norfolk Primary Care Trust)
Patient List Size: 6000

Practice Manager Carol Bantick

GP John Malcolm SKINNER, Ian HACZEWSKI, John HATFIELD, Diana RAYNER, Robin Arthur RAYNER

Swanage

The Health Centre
Railway Station Approach, Station Road, Swanage BH19 1HB
Tel: 01929 422231
Website: www.swanagemedical.org.uk
(South and East Dorset Primary Care Trust)
Patient List Size: 12600

Practice Manager Phil Dowding

GP Peter Richard LEIGH, Robert William BAKER, Michael Paul CARUANA, Jason Charles Derwent CLARK, Christopher John ELFES, David Alexander HAINES, David KNOTT, Jeremy Nigel Roderick MUNDAY

Swanley

The Cedars Surgery
26 Swanley Centre, Swanley BR8 7AH
Tel: 01322 663111 Fax: 01322 614867
(Dartford, Gravesham and Swanley Primary Care Trust)
Patient List Size: 11000

Practice Manager Debbie Saunders

GP Mahendra GOPINATHAN, Don Julian HETTERIACHCHI, David Ian JONES, S MacDERMOTT, Amal RAMDEEHUL, Werner Robert RUMFELD

Main Road Surgery
31A Main Road, Hextable, Swanley BR8 7RB
Tel: 01322 666001/279288 Fax: 01322 669722
(Dartford, Gravesham and Swanley Primary Care Trust)
Patient List Size: 2400

GP A K MUTHAPPAN

Manzoori Clinic
322 Claremont Road, Hextable, Swanley BR8 7QZ
Tel: 01322 668900 Fax: 01322 660024
(Dartford, Gravesham and Swanley Primary Care Trust)

GP Dr SHAHNAWAZ

The Oaks
Nightingale Way, Swanley BR8 7UP
Tel: 01322 668775 Fax: 01322 668010
(Dartford, Gravesham and Swanley Primary Care Trust)
Patient List Size: 8500

Practice Manager Helen Parish

GP Ian Charles BROOMAN, Helen Mary CLAYTON, Barend Cilliers DELPORT, Stephen Neil GREGSON, W S POMEROY

Swanscombe

Swanscombe Health Centre
Southfleet Road, Swanscombe DA10 0GF
Tel: 01322 427447 Fax: 01322 422770
(Dartford, Gravesham and Swanley Primary Care Trust)
Patient List Size: 8400

Practice Manager H Borrow

GP Y S DESAI, J P PATEL, M K SAHOTA, A A SHAH, Alasdair James THOMSON

Swindon

Ashington House
Ashington Way, Westlea, Swindon SN5 7XY
Tel: 01793 614840 Fax: 01793 491191
Email: reception@gp-j83036.nhs.uk
Website: www.ashingtonhousesurgery.co.uk
(Swindon Primary Care Trust)
Patient List Size: 10000

Practice Manager Sandra Walklett

GP Robert Giles NIXON, Neil Godfrey James FARNHAM, Michelle MARTIN, Peter Michael STEPHENSON, Adele Marjorie STEPTOE, David Spencer TOMBOLINE

Cricklade Surgery
113 High Street, Cricklade, Swindon SN6 6AE
Tel: 01793 750645 Fax: 01793 752331
(Kennet and North Wiltshire Primary Care Trust)

Practice Manager Karen De Silva

GP Lanil Wimal DE SILVA

Crossroads Surgery
478 Cricklade Road, Swindon SN2 7BG
Tel: 01793 725113 Fax: 01793 701205
(Swindon Primary Care Trust)
Patient List Size: 3800

Practice Manager Christine Gill

GP Lynn Carol BRADING, Martin J STAGLES

Eldene Surgery
Eldene Health Centre, Eldene Centre, Swindon SN3 3RZ
Tel: 01793 522710 Fax: 01793 513217
Email: sec.eldene@gp-J83047.nhs.uk
Website: www.eldenesurgery.co.uk
(Swindon Primary Care Trust)
Patient List Size: 7200

GP Adam Michael KOWALCZYK, Parvin FARKHANI, Eric HOLLIDAY, Michael PETERS

Eldene Surgery
Eldene Health Centre, Eldene Centre, Swindon SN3 3RZ
Tel: 01793 522710 Fax: 01793 513217
Email: christine.mott@gp-j83047.nhs.uk
Website: www.eldenesurgery.co.uk
(Swindon Primary Care Trust)
Patient List Size: 7300

GP A KOWALCZYK, P FARKHANI, E HOLLIDAY

Elm Tree Surgery
High Street, Shrivenham, Swindon SN6 8AG
Tel: 01793 782207 Fax: 01793 784429
(Swindon Primary Care Trust)
Patient List Size: 7000

Practice Manager Clive Gill

GP John CLEMENTS, Margaret S ANDREWS, Anthony William Basil CROCKETT, Sian EDWARDS, Richard FISHER

Fan and Partners
Great Western Surgery, Farriers Close, Swindon SN1 2QU
Tel: 01793 421311 Fax: 01793 431412
(Swindon Primary Care Trust)
Patient List Size: 5700

Practice Manager Siobhan Timms

GP Siu Fai FAN

Freshbrook Surgery
Freshbrook Village, Freshbrook, Swindon SN5 8PY
Tel: 01793 870494
(Swindon Primary Care Trust)

GP G Y REDDY

Hawthorn Medical Centre
May Close, Swindon SN2 1UU
Tel: 01793 536541 Fax: 01793 421049
(Swindon Primary Care Trust)

Practice Manager V A Gibbons, L M Smith

GP Geoffrey Charles Hugh FREAKLEY, Anthony Michael DANCYGER, William Richard JANSON, Naga Panender Prasad KILARU, Elizabeth Anne MEARNS, Elizabeth OLIVER, Julian Francis WRIGHT

Kingswood Surgery
Kingswood Avenue, Swindon SN3 2RJ
Tel: 01793 534699
(Swindon Primary Care Trust)
Patient List Size: 9300

GP Jonathan Christopher ELLIMAN, Janet BENTLEY. Linda JACOBS, Philip John MAYES, Z MILEUSNIC

Marlborough Road Surgery
143 Marlborough Road, Swindon SN3 1NJ
Tel: 01793 431303 Fax: 01793 495779
(Swindon Primary Care Trust)

GP Daphne Elizabeth GREEN, Robert Frederick ROHLFING

Merchiston Surgery
Highworth Road, Swindon SN3 4BF
Tel: 01793 823307 Fax: 01793 820923
(Swindon Primary Care Trust)
Patient List Size: 13340

Practice Manager Angela Hirst

GP Stephen Christopher PIGOTT, Susan ADMAS, David Durairatnam JOHN, Susan LAVELLE, Elzbieta M MACIEJEWSKA, Kathryn MAITLAND-WARD, Anthony Simon NEWTON, Anna Mary Louise SMITH

Myatt and Rhodes
Hermitage Surgery, Dammas Lane, Old Town, Swindon SN1 3EF
Tel: 01793 522492 Fax: 01793 512520
(Swindon Primary Care Trust)
Patient List Size: 3800

Practice Manager Renne wheeler

GP Ivan William MYATT, Steven RHODES

New Court Surgery
Borough Fields, Wootton Bassett, Swindon SN4 7AX
Tel: 01793 852302 Fax: 01793 851119
(Kennet and North Wiltshire Primary Care Trust)

Practice Manager E Smitht

GP Simon NELSON, M K O'BRIEN, Mary Josephine VALENTINE, Nicholas Olyffe YERBURY

North Swindon Practice
Home Ground Surgery, Thames Avenue, Haydon Wick, Swindon SN25 1QQ
Tel: 01793 705777
(Swindon Primary Care Trust)
Patient List Size: 9000

Practice Manager Chris Gebel

GP Howard Glyn THOMAS, Barbara Elisabeth CLUETT, Deirdre Margaret GODFRAY, Alan Graham WHITWORTH

Old Town Surgery
10 Bath Road, Old Town, Swindon SN1 4BA
Tel: 01793 616165
(Swindon Primary Care Trust)
Patient List Size: 6600

GP Miles Fraser WIGFIELD, David Charles HEATON, J A WRIGHT

Park Lane Practice
7-8 Park Lane, Swindon SN1 5HG
Tel: 01793 523176 Fax: 01793 535080
(Swindon Primary Care Trust)
Patient List Size: 5800

Practice Manager Barry Mercer

GP Christopher Gerard HOLDEN, Andrew GOULD, N LLOYD

Phoenix Surgery
Dunwich Drive, Toothill, Swindon SN5 8SX
Tel: 01793 600440 Fax: 01793 600410
(Swindon Primary Care Trust)
Patient List Size: 6117

Practice Manager C A Swinyard

GP Peter William SWINYARD, Anke LEHMKUHL

Priory Road Surgery
Priory Road, Park South, Swindon SN3 2EZ
Tel: 01793 521154 Fax: 01793 512562
Email: prioryroadsurgery@freeserve.co.uk
(Swindon Primary Care Trust)
Patient List Size: 8400

Practice Manager Brian G Strachan

GP Jonathan Peter FLEW, David Anthony Haydon BIRLEY, Antonia Gay NEWELL, Mari RITSON, Alastair Martin STRONG

Purton Surgery
High Street, Purton, Swindon SN5 4BD
Tel: 01793 770207 Fax: 01793 772662
(Kennet and North Wiltshire Primary Care Trust)

GP Glynis Jacqueline EVANS, Andrew Reuben Mark BAKER, Gordon John BARRON, Carita Julia Boyd GOMARA, Michael John McKEMEY, Philip Alfred REYNOLDS

Queens Park and Moredon Surgeries
146 Drove Road, Swindon SN1 3AG
Tel: 01793 342000 Fax: 01793 342011
(Swindon Primary Care Trust)
Patient List Size: 14000

Practice Manager Christine Morgan

GP Peter Robert MACK, J R BESTWICK, R G LEE, Derek Keith ROBINSON, Eleanor Frances STANTON

Ridge Green Medical Centre
Ramleaze Drive, Shaw, Swindon SN5 5PY
Tel: 01793 874894 Fax: 01793 877711
(Swindon Primary Care Trust)
Patient List Size: 3150

Practice Manager J Margerum

GP D NOWOTZIN, M BHAMBRA, A DWIVEDI

Ridge Green Surgery
Ramlegze Drive, Shaw, Swindon SN5 5PX
Tel: 01793 874894
(Swindon Primary Care Trust)
Patient List Size: 5200

GP Dr NOWOTZIN, Dr DWIVEDI

Ridgeway View Family Practice
Barrett Way, Wroughton, Swindon SN4 9LW
Tel: 01793 812221 Fax: 01793 845526
(Swindon Primary Care Trust)
Patient List Size: 10000

Practice Manager Karen Cox

GP Nicola Ann CROSSLEY, A DAWSON, S FOZDAR, R E HALL, S MATA, Stephen Peter SEWELL, K J THOMSON, G WALLIS

Sparcells Surgery
Midwinter Close, Peatmoor, Swindon SN5 5AN
Tel: 01793 881928 Fax: 01793 879264
(Swindon Primary Care Trust)
Patient List Size: 3100

Practice Manager Jane Cremin

GP Ayakannu KANDIAH

Swindon Health Centre
Carfax Street, Swindon SN1 1ED
Tel: 01793 619955
(Swindon Primary Care Trust)

Practice Manager Cathy Rooke

GP Irshad Ahmad SHAD

Swindon Health Centre
Carfax Street, Swindon SN1 1ED
Tel: 01793 692062
(Swindon Primary Care Trust)

GP Gwylfa Idloes JOHN, Cherry Ann Beatrice HALL, Julian Paul Justin HAWKINS, Stephen Christopher HICKS, Stuart Alexander MACOUSTRA, Josephine Margaret Sarah OWEN-JONES

Taw Hill Practice
Queen Elizabeth Drive, Swindon SN25 1WL
Tel: 01793 709500 Fax: 01793 723875
Email: enquiries@tawhillsurgery.nhs.uk
Website: www.tawhillsurgery.nhs.uk
(Swindon Primary Care Trust)
Patient List Size: 2563

GP June MORRIS, Peter CROUCH

Tinkers Lane Surgery
High Street, Wootton Bassett, Swindon SN4 7AT
Tel: 01793 852131 Fax: 01793 848891
(Kennet and North Wiltshire Primary Care Trust)
Patient List Size: 9340

Practice Manager Sue Thornton

GP Peter Douglas Alexander FUDGE, Ceri Mark DAVIES, Jeremy Michael Holt MARSHALL

Victoria House Surgery
33 Victoria Road, Swindon SN1 3AW
Tel: 01793 536515
(Swindon Primary Care Trust)
Patient List Size: 3800

Practice Manager Lucy Stewart

GP Frances Mary KILLICK, Jonathan Henry MERCER, Judy Caroline ROBBINS

Victoria Road Surgery
168-169 Victoria Road, Swindon SN1 3BU
Tel: 01793 535584 Fax: 01793 497526
Email: alan.mason@gp-J83633.nhs.uk
(Swindon Primary Care Trust)
Patient List Size: 6450

GP Stephen Richard Mark BROOKE, Christine Elizabeth DUNCUMB, John Hedworth SLEGGS

Victoria Road Surgery
Nythe, Swindon SN3 3NN
Tel: 01793 522479
(Swindon Primary Care Trust)
Patient List Size: 6150

GP Stephen Richard Mark BROOKE, Christine Elizabeth DUNCUMB, Dr SLEGGS

Westrop Surgery
Newburgh Place, Highworth, Swindon SN6 7DN
Tel: 01793 762218 Fax: 01793 766073
Website: www.westropsurgery.co.uk
(Swindon Primary Care Trust)
Patient List Size: 10000

Practice Manager M Stephens

GP Jennifer Ann METCALFE, Peter Andrew BARNES, J BESTWICK, Simon CLARE, Julie FROST, Christopher Robert LLOYD, A WOODWORTH

Whalebridge Practice
Health Centre, Carfax Street, Swindon SN1 1ED
Tel: 01793 692933 Fax: 01793 524621
(Swindon Primary Care Trust)
Patient List Size: 9199

GP Alison Ruth MacINTYRE, Richard CARTER, Gauin JAMIE, Fintan James LONERGAN

Yew Tree Lane Surgery
5 Yew Tree Lane, Broad Hinton, Swindon SN4 9RH

GP Graham George ADKINS

Tadcaster

The Chapel Schoolroom Surgery
Main Street, Church Fenton, Tadcaster LS24 9PR

Practice Manager Margaret Britton

GP David Frederick HARRISON, Jonathan Kellman BYNOE, Roger Downend PARKIN, Andrew James PEEL

The Methodist Chapel Surgery
Ulleskelf, Tadcaster LS24 9DJ

Practice Manager Margaret Britton

GP David Frederick HARRISON, Andrew James PEEL

Tadcaster Medical Centre
Crab Garth, Tadcaster LS24 9HD
Tel: 01937 530082 Fax: 01937 530192
(Selby and York Primary Care Trust)
Patient List Size: 8000

Practice Manager Linda Coombs

GP Mark HAYES, Andrew Erskine INGLIS, Wendy Jane REEVES, Catherine Louise TURTON

Tadley

Clift Surgery
Minchens Lane, Bramley, Tadley RG26 5BH
Tel: 01256 881228
(North Hampshire Primary Care Trust)

Practice Manager Pam Hurley-Morris

GP Nigel J FISHER, Diana Helen KENSHOLE, Anne M Y PERKINS

Tadley Medical Partnership
Holmwood Health Centre, Franklin Avenue, Tadley RG26 4ER
Tel: 0118 981 4166 Fax: 0118 981 1432
(North Hampshire Primary Care Trust)
Patient List Size: 20000

Practice Manager Alison Jenner

GP Peter Robert BROUGH, Vivienne ADLER, Sunil Dutt BHANOT, Christine Anne CAREN, Stephen John COLLEY, Anne Marie HOGAN, D R NEWMAN, Jonathan PETERS, Rosemary WADDINGHAM, H K WALFORD

Tadworth

Heathcote Medical Centre
Heathcote, Tadworth KT20 5TH
Tel: 01737 360202
(East Elmbridge and Mid Surrey Primary Care Trust)

Practice Manager Leslie Trewinnard

GP Joanna WEBB, Mark JENKINS, Niki KIRBY, Nicola PARKER, Andreas Plisi PITSIAELI, Henry John VERITY

The Surgery
1 Troy Close, Tadworth Farm, Tadworth KT20 5JE
Tel: 01737 362327 Fax: 01737 373469
Website: www.tadworthmedicalcentre.co.uk
(East Elmbridge and Mid Surrey Primary Care Trust)
Patient List Size: 10000

Practice Manager Wilma O'Connor

GP Peter Charles STOTT, Azita JONES, Pedram SHABROKH, Clare STEPHENSON

Tamworth

The Aldergate Medical Practice
The Mount, Salters Lane, Tamworth B79 8BH
Tel: 01827 54775 Fax: 01827 62835
(Burntwood, Lichfield and Tamworth Primary Care Trust)
Patient List Size: 12500

Practice Manager Ann Musticone

GP Bruce Magnus MAIR, Vivienne Christine BOSS, Grahame James Crosbie BRUCE, Garth Peter DEACON, Arup Albert DESHPANDE, Martyn Ian KING, Elizabeth Anne ODBER

Amington Surgery
130 Tamworth Road, Amington, Tamworth B77 3BZ
Tel: 01827 54777 Fax: 01827 59539
(Burntwood, Lichfield and Tamworth Primary Care Trust)

GP Singu SREEHARI RAO, Y VEERAYYA

Anchor Practice
Glascote Heath Health Centre, Caledonian, Glascote Heath, Tamworth B77 2ED
Tel: 01827 251251 Fax: 01827 287486
(Burntwood, Lichfield and Tamworth Primary Care Trust)
Patient List Size: 2300

Practice Manager Patricia Darley

GP Ebrahim DABESTANI, S MAHANTA

Belgrave Surgery
108 Medway, Belgrave, Tamworth B77 2JW
Tel: 01827 285414 Fax: 01827 262316
(Burntwood, Lichfield and Tamworth Primary Care Trust)
Patient List Size: 2102

GP Ashok Kumar BAGRI

Crown Medical Practice
Tamworth Health Centre, Upper Gungate, Tamworth B79 7EA
Tel: 01827 315355 Fax: 01827 63873
(Burntwood, Lichfield and Tamworth Primary Care Trust)

Practice Manager Pat Murphy

GP K L PASCOE, Stephan T BENKERT, M M STANDEN

Dosthill and Wilnecote Street Surgery
45 Cadogan Road, Dosthill, Tamworth B77 1PQ
Tel: 01827 283487 Fax: 01827 261569
(Burntwood, Lichfield and Tamworth Primary Care Trust)
Patient List Size: 7600

Practice Manager Julie Devlin

GP Rais Ahmed RAJPUT, Rais KHAN, S Satish MAHANTA

Heath View Practice
Glascote Health Centre, Caledonian, Glascote Heath, Tamworth B77 2ED
Tel: 01827 281000 Fax: 01827 262048
(Burntwood, Lichfield and Tamworth Primary Care Trust)

Practice Manager M Russell

GP Rajnikant Manibhai PATEL

Hollies Medical Practice
Tamworth Health Centre, Upper Gungate, Tamworth B79 7EA
Tel: 01827 68511 Fax: 01827 51163
(Burntwood, Lichfield and Tamworth Primary Care Trust)
Patient List Size: 15500

Practice Manager Lynn Willetts

GP Jacqueline Marcelle STABLER, Graham Milton BARKER, Derek Peter BOSS, Yvonne Mary BOWEN, Steve DAVIES, David Charles HALPIN, Joanne Mary KING, Adrian PARKES, Mark David POPPLE

Laurel House Surgery
12 Albert Road, Tamworth B79 7JN
Tel: 01827 69283 Fax: 01827 318029
(Burntwood, Lichfield and Tamworth Primary Care Trust)

Practice Manager David Hicken

GP P S HARRISON, S R V BAGLEY, K CHAPMAN, David Lennard CUTTING, Helen Mary FITZGERALD, Roger Andrew HAWKES, Philip Damian KILLEEN, Philip Meldrum WOOD

Lichfield Street Surgery
267 Lichfield Street, Fazeley, Tamworth B78 3QF
Tel: 01827 289512 Fax: 01827 262244
(Burntwood, Lichfield and Tamworth Primary Care Trust)

GP Dr TAJUDDIN

Pear Tree Surgery
28 Meadow Close, Kingsbury, Tamworth B78 2NR
Tel: 01827 872755 Fax: 01827 874700
(North Warwickshire Primary Care Trust)
Patient List Size: 10200

Practice Manager Carol Cleeve

GP Michael Jan FOIST, Jana Marie Eva FOIST, John Bernard HAWKINS, Desmond Ronald LAWRENCE, Paul THORNTON

The Peel Medical Practice
Peel Croft, 2 Aldergate, Tamworth B79 7DJ
Tel: 01827 50575 Fax: 01827 318911
(Burntwood, Lichfield and Tamworth Primary Care Trust)

GP Philip BALLARD, Mark C CLAYSON, Malin S K DAVIS, Christopher J JONES, Sue RUDDLE, Julie D SHERLOCK

Pilesworth and Dordon Group Practice
162 Long Street, Dordon, Tamworth B78 1QA
Tel: 01827 892893
(North Warwickshire Primary Care Trust)

Practice Manager Deborah L J Pogorzelski

GP S C BIRD, G BROWN, A R GUMMERY, C A MARTIN, S R SPENCELEY

Riverside Surgery
41-42 Balfour, Riverside Surgery, New Street, Tamworth B79 7BH
Tel: 01827 66676 Fax: 01827 313095
(Burntwood, Lichfield and Tamworth Primary Care Trust)
Patient List Size: 2150

Practice Manager Jayne Belford

GP K W BEVAN

Stoneydelph Health Centre
Ellerbeck, Stoneydelph, Tamworth B77 4JA
Tel: 01827 897484 Fax: 01827 896945
(Burntwood, Lichfield and Tamworth Primary Care Trust)
Patient List Size: 1950

Practice Manager Jayne Darby

GP S R YANNAMANI

Stoneydelph Medical Centre
Ellerbeck, Stoneydelph, Tamworth B77 4JA
Tel: 01827 899919 Fax: 01827 897036
(Burntwood, Lichfield and Tamworth Primary Care Trust)

Practice Manager Sue Warmington

GP V K RAJPUT

Tarporley

Bunbury Medical Practice
The Surgery, Bunbury, Tarporley CW6 9PJ
Tel: 01829 260218 Fax: 01829 260411
(Cheshire West Primary Care Trust)
Patient List Size: 4800

Practice Manager Roz Gillot

GP Antony Nicholas HOY, John BERRY, Helen Elizabeth Warren BLACK

Kelsall Medical Centre
Church Street, Kelsall, Tarporley CW6 0QG
Tel: 01829 751252 Fax: 01829 752593
(Cheshire West Primary Care Trust)
Patient List Size: 3976

Practice Manager Diane Bird

GP Martin Andrew DURRANT, Patricia Mary MANN

Park Road Health Centre
Park Road, Tarporley CW6 0BE
Tel: 01829 732401 Fax: 01829 732404
(Cheshire West Primary Care Trust)

Practice Manager Liz Kilgannon

GP Kenneth ROWLAND, Robin Nigel Harrison GLEEK, Kay Vivienne TAYLOR

Sowerby and Partners
The Health Centre, Park Road, Tarporley CW6 0BE
Tel: 01829 733456 Fax: 01829 730124
(Cheshire West Primary Care Trust)
Patient List Size: 7600

Practice Manager Joyce Adams

GP Roy George SOWERBY, Peter Andrew CAMPBELL, Gillian Margaret CHAPPELL, Nigel Graham O'CALLAGHAN

Taunton

Blackbrook Surgery
Lisieux Way, Taunton TA1 2LB
Tel: 01823 259444 Fax: 01823 250200
Email: blackbrook.surgery@gp-L85014.nhs.uk
(Taunton Deane Primary Care Trust)

Practice Manager Gale Berryman

GP James Henry YOXALL, Michael GORMAN, Anne Adele Paterson HICKS, Lisa HORMAN, Alison Nicola Clare PRICE, John Gerard SCANLON, Mark Paul SMITH, Ruth WELLS

Creech Medical Centre
Creech St Michael, Taunton TA3 5QQ
Tel: 01823 442357 Fax: 01823 444287
(Taunton Deane Primary Care Trust)
Patient List Size: 2708

Practice Manager Elizabeth Tacchi

GP Barry Colin MOYSE, Willemijn BALDER

Drs Cotterell, Pfeiffer and Partners
College Way Surgery, Comeytrowe Centre, Taunton TA1 4TY
Tel: 01823 259333 Fax: 01823 259336

(Taunton Deane Primary Care Trust)
Patient List Size: 11400

Practice Manager J Kirkby

GP D P BADHAM, Paul William Arnold COTTRELL, Gabrielle Anne DE COTHI, David John DOWNS, A C HESFORD, Christine Zdenka PFEIFER, John Robert SKENE, Jonathan Michael SLADDEN

French Weir Health Centre
French Weir Avenue, Taunton TA1 1NW
Tel: 01823 331381 Fax: 01823 323689
Email: French.Weir@frenchweirhealth.nhs.uk
(Taunton Deane Primary Care Trust)
Patient List Size: 14600

Practice Manager Peter Taylor

GP James Edward DAVIDSON, David Francis BIRD, Stuart Ronald McDonald CAIRNS, William CHANDLER, Catherine FENLON, Hilda Kathryn Josephine GORMLEY, Timothy HOWES, Timothy Mark Gordon WARD

Harrison and Partners
The Surgery, Mount Street, Bishops Lydeard, Taunton TA4 3LH
Tel: 01823 432361 Fax: 01823 433864
(Taunton Deane Primary Care Trust)
Patient List Size: 4650

Practice Manager Chris Nelson

GP Simon Richard Barnard HARRISON, Roger Edmund CRABTREE, Rianne SEWELL

Hickman and Hickman
The Health Centre, Greenway, North Curry, Taunton TA3 6NQ
Tel: 01823 490505 Fax: 01823 491024
(Taunton Deane Primary Care Trust)
Patient List Size: 3810

Practice Manager Julia Mercer

GP James HICKMAN, Nicholas CHAPMAN

Lister House Surgery
Lister House Surgery, Bollams Mead, Wiveliscombe, Taunton TA4 2PH
Tel: 01984 623471 Fax: 01984 624357
Email: practice.manager@gp-L85038.nhs.uk
Website: www.wiveliscombsurgery.co.uk
(Taunton Deane Primary Care Trust)
Patient List Size: 6600

Practice Manager Peter Moran

GP Sarah BINFORD, Monica Denise DEVINE, Jacqueline Anne JAMES, Michael Gordon ROSTRON, J N TREPESS

Luson Surgery
Fore Street, Wellington, Taunton TA21 8AB
Tel: 01823 662836 Fax: 01823 660955
(Taunton Deane Primary Care Trust)

Practice Manager Martin Ellacott

GP Gordon James SCOTT, Barbara Jane CRABTREE, David John McCANN, R E M YATES

Lyngford Park Surgery
Fletcher Close, Taunton TA2 8SQ
Tel: 01823 333355 Fax: 01823 257022
(Taunton Deane Primary Care Trust)

Practice Manager Jane Evans

GP Vaughan Pearson SMITH, Helen Lyn BURTON, John Douglas TOLLIDAY, Julie Jane VODDEN, Michael Hilton YARDLEY

St James Medical Centre
St James Street, Taunton TA1 1JP
Tel: 01823 285400 Fax: 01823 285404
Website: www.stjamesmedicalcentre.co.uk
(Taunton Deane Primary Care Trust)
Patient List Size: 10600

Practice Manager Guy Patey

GP Madeleine BILBROUGH, Yvonne Louise DUTHIE, Adrian Francis Courtenay FULFORD, Rosmarie Anne GENNEYWORTH, Phillip James SKINNER, Philip Legh Brinsmead SQUIRE

Victoria Gate Surgery
East Reach, Taunton TA1 3EX
Tel: 01823 275656 Fax: 01823 321883
Email: patient.info@gp-l85616.nhs.uk
Website: www.victoriagate.co.uk
(Taunton Deane Primary Care Trust)
Patient List Size: 2650

Practice Manager Linda Willis

GP David Brayshay EDMONDSON, R HASAN

Warwick House Medical Centre
Holway, Taunton TA1 2QA
Tel: 01823 282147 Fax: 01823 338181
Email: reception@warwickhousemc.nhs.uk
Website: warwickhouse.org.uk
(Taunton Deane Primary Care Trust)
Patient List Size: 7150

Practice Manager Anne Ellis

GP Shura L ASHWORTH, Simon P HAMMERTON, Dr HANSON, Andrew C PAISLEY, Dr PERRY, Lorrie C SYMONS

Warwick House Medical Centre
Holway Green, Upper Holway Road, Taunton TA1 2QA
Tel: 01823 282147 Fax: 01823 338181
(Taunton Deane Primary Care Trust)
Patient List Size: 7200

Practice Manager Anne Ellis

GP Sian Deborah HANSON, Shura Louise ASHWORTH, Simon HAMMERTON, Andrew Charles PAISLEY, Andrew John PERRY, Lorrie SYMONS

Williton and Watchet Surgeries
Robert Street, Williton, Taunton TA4 4QE
Tel: 01984 632701 Fax: 01984 633933
Email: williton.surgery@willitonsurgery.nhs.uk
(Somerset Coast Primary Care Trust)
Patient List Size: 10000

Practice Manager Alison Foulkes

GP Nigel James HALLIDAY, Alistair BARCLAY, Robin DAVIES, Andrew DAYANI, David Edward GOVER, Shirley Margaret GOVER, Charles Richard PASCALL, Anne RIVETT, Robert RIVETT

Tavistock

Abbey Surgery
28 Plymouth Road, Tavistock PL19 8BU
Tel: 01822 612247 Fax: 01822 618771
(South Hams and West Devon Primary Care Trust)
Patient List Size: 10000

Practice Manager Heather Oliver

GP Rupert Adrian GUDE, Mark Simon CULLEN, Isobel Louise DAVIES, John Anthony Lodwick EVANS, Mary Annette ROBERTS, Peter John RODGERS, Robin John WILSON

Stannery Surgery
Abbey Rise, Whitchurch, Tavistock PL19 9BB
Tel: 01822 613517 Fax: 01822 618294
Email: health@stannerysurgery.org.uk
(South Hams and West Devon Primary Care Trust)
Patient List Size: 4800

Practice Manager Terry Rose

GP W J ALLENBY, V L EVANS, G A JOHNSON, Philip Norman PORTERFIELD

Wharfside Surgery
1 Canal Road, Tavistock PL19 8AR
Tel: 01822 616131 Fax: 01822 616404
(South Hams and West Devon Primary Care Trust)

Patient List Size: 3269

Practice Manager Lyn Baker

GP Philip VICARAGE, Mark EGGLETON, Jennifer GRAY

Teddington

The Surgery
37 Park Road, Teddington TW11 0AU
Tel: 020 8977 5481 Fax: 020 8977 7882
(Richmond and Twickenham Primary Care Trust)

Practice Manager Sue Desmond

GP Julian Andre BRADLEY, James BROCKBANK, Alexandra PATTON, Nicolette POTTS

The Surgery
Thameside Medical Practice, Thames House, 180 High Street, Teddington TW11 8HU
Tel: 020 8614 4930 Fax: 020 8977 1855
(Richmond and Twickenham Primary Care Trust)
Patient List Size: 3200

Practice Manager Sally Trainis

GP Amanda Jillian CHILDS, Victoria DE BRUYNE, Anne Marie KENDALL

Teignmouth

Channel View Surgery
Seacroft Court, 3 Courtenay Place, Teignmouth TQ14 8AY
Tel: 01626 774656 Fax: 01626 779266
(Teignbridge Primary Care Trust)

Practice Manager Susan Hedley

GP Paul Richard RABY, Caroline Anne KARAKUSEVIC, Clive Arnold LONG, Philip George MELLUISH

Richmond House Surgery
26 Brunswick Street, Teignmouth TQ14 8AF
Tel: 01626 773339 Fax: 01626 777811
(Teignbridge Primary Care Trust)
Patient List Size: 3500

Practice Manager Simon Bates

GP Karen BATES

Teign Estuary Medical Group
Glendevon Medical Centre, 3 Carlton Place, Teignmouth TQ14 8AB
Tel: 01626 770955 Fax: 01626 772107
(Teignbridge Primary Care Trust)
Patient List Size: 4000

Practice Manager John Pearce, Beverly Stretton

GP Julian Patrick SQUIRES, Melanie HOUGHTON, Clive Ronald PEIRCE, Tamsin Jayne VENTON

Teignmouth Medical Practice
2 Den Crescent, Teignbridge, Teignmouth TQ14 8BG
Tel: 01626 770297 Fax: 01626 777331
(Teignbridge Primary Care Trust)
Patient List Size: 7500

Practice Manager Michelle Jones

GP Denis Vincent KEANE, Kathryn ALLEN, Elizabeth BROWN, Rachel COOKSLEY, Martin KING, Emma PALMER

Telford

Aqueduct Surgery
Majestic Way, Aqueduct, Telford TF4 3RB
Tel: 01952 591555 Fax: 01952 660090
(Telford and Wrekin Primary Care Trust)

Practice Manager Rita Jinks

GP Mushtaq AHMAD

Bethesda Surgery
Church Road, Malinslee, Telford TF3 2JZ
Tel: 01952 502836 Fax: 01952 505182
(Telford and Wrekin Primary Care Trust)
Patient List Size: 2775

Practice Manager Irene Smith

GP Sam G S RAO

Charlton Medical Practice
Lion Street, Oakengates, Telford TF2 6AQ
Tel: 01952 620138 Fax: 01952 615282
Website: www.charltonmedical.co.uk
(Telford and Wrekin Primary Care Trust)
Patient List Size: 10000

Practice Manager Peter Leigh

GP Patrick John KIRBY, Jane BRIGHT, Martin Stuart COOPER-CRUMP, Denise Anne LEES, Albert James WHITING

Church Close Surgery
Church Close, Madeley, Telford TF7 5BP
Tel: 01952 586616 Fax: 01952 586324
(Telford and Wrekin Primary Care Trust)

Practice Manager Jackie Roberts

GP Rick W HAILEY, Jonathan HOAR, Teresa C McDONNELL

Dawley Medical Practice
Webb House, King Street, Dawley, Telford TF3 2AA
Tel: 01952 630500 Fax: 01952 630501
(Telford and Wrekin Primary Care Trust)

Practice Manager Sandra Taylor

GP Paul K SPENCER, Peter L ACKROYD, Hannah J BUFTON, Paul A CHANDLER, David J PARRISH

Donnington Medical Practice
Wrekin Drive, Donnington, Telford TF2 8EA
Tel: 01952 605252 Fax: 01952 677010
(Telford and Wrekin Primary Care Trust)

Practice Manager Maureen Prestwood

GP Timothy Bruce GOODE, James MILLIGAN, Rachel TAYLOR, Graham David THOMPSON, Lynette WILLIAMS, David John WRIGHT

The Hadley Medical Practice
Hadley Health Centre, High Street, Hadley, Telford TF1 5NG
Tel: 01952 249251 Fax: 01952 250013
(Telford and Wrekin Primary Care Trust)
Patient List Size: 3200

Practice Manager Murium Begum

GP Chelliah BALASUBRAMANIAM

Hollinswood Surgery
Downmead, Hollinswood, Telford TF3 2EW
Tel: 01952 201144 Fax: 01952 201125
(Telford and Wrekin Primary Care Trust)

Practice Manager Mala Mishra

GP Sudhar K MISHRA

Holliwell Practice
Deercote, Hollinswood, Telford TF3 2BH
Tel: 01952 293949 Fax: 01952 299319
Email: holliwell.practice@gp-m82612.wmids.nhs.uk
(Telford and Wrekin Primary Care Trust)
Patient List Size: 2400

Practice Manager Sarah Ghosh

GP Ratan K GHOSH

Ironbridge Medical Practice
Trinity Hall, Dale Road, Coalbrookdale, Telford TF8 7DT
Tel: 01952 432568 Fax: 01952 432012
(Telford and Wrekin Primary Care Trust)

Practice Manager Janine Laming

GP Glenn Paul RICHARDS, Louise A L WARBURTON

Kingsway Lodge
King Street, Much Wenlock, Telford TF13 6BL
(Bristol South and West Primary Care Trust)

GP C STANFORD

Lawley Medical Practice
Farriers Green, Lawley Bank, Telford TF4 2LL
Tel: 01952 560012/560039 Fax: 01952 501502
(Telford and Wrekin Primary Care Trust)

Practice Manager Romayne Wainwright

GP Adam J PRINGLE, Fiona WRIGHT

Leegomery Surgery
27 Lawton Farm Way, Leegomery, Telford TF1 6PP
Tel: 01952 255855 Fax: 01952 260381
(Telford and Wrekin Primary Care Trust)

Practice Manager Rashed Chowdhury

GP Barkat A CHOWDHURY, Saema CHOWDHURY

Madeley Medical Practice
Madeley Health Centre, Church Street, Madeley, Telford TF7 5BU
Tel: 01952 585566 Fax: 01952 684507
(Telford and Wrekin Primary Care Trust)

Practice Manager Ishrath Qureshi

GP Mujahid M QURESHI

Malinslee Surgery
Church Road, Malinslee, Telford TF3 2JZ
Tel: 01952 501234 Fax: 01952 630021
(Telford and Wrekin Primary Care Trust)
Patient List Size: 2000

Practice Manager Karen Denton

GP Syed Mohammad ZAKI AHMED

Oakengates Medical Practice
27 Limes Walk, Oakengates, Telford TF2 6JJ
Tel: 01952 620077/618817 Fax: 01952 620209
Website: www.limeswalle.info
(Telford and Wrekin Primary Care Trust)
Patient List Size: 17000

Practice Manager Keith L Rogers

GP Geoffrey Anson WAINWRIGHT, Tim J HUGHES, Ellen Mary NOLAN, David Graham Frank NORTHERN, Paul OGILVIE, Damien THOMPSON, Trevor Dawson WILLIAMS

Shawbirch Medical Centre
5 Acorn Way, Shawbridge, Telford TF5 0LW
Tel: 01952 641555 Fax: 01952 260913
(Telford and Wrekin Primary Care Trust)

Practice Manager Bet Wilkes

GP Christopher I BROWN, Peter J COVENTRY, Caroline Judith FREEMAN, Elizabeth Jean HERD, Nicholas John KING

Stirchley Medical Practice
Stirchley Health Centre, Sandino Road, Stirchley, Telford TF3 1FB
Tel: 01952 660444/599000 Fax: 01952 415139
(Telford and Wrekin Primary Care Trust)

Practice Manager Tracie Craddock

GP Patrick John CHUTER, Eve Olga CLEVENGER, Michael John DAWSON, Stephen Edward John HUGH, Mike A INNES, Christopher Alan Robert PEARSON, Peter Quentin SHAW, Lindsay Stuart WARD

Sutton Hill Medical Practice
The Medical Centre, Maythorne Close, Sutton Hill, Telford TF7 4DH
Tel: 01952 586471 Fax: 01952 588029
Website: www.suttonhillmedical.co.uk
(Telford and Wrekin Primary Care Trust)
Patient List Size: 8700

Practice Manager Sue D Bates

GP Jeremy Peter Allan RICHARDSON, Raja A BANDAK, Andrew Ronald INGLIS, James Mark William JAMES, Zoe Elizabeth ROSS

Wellington Medical Practice
The Health Centre, Wellington, Telford TF1 1PZ
Tel: 01952 226000/226012 Fax: 01952 226019
(Telford and Wrekin Primary Care Trust)

Practice Manager Allan Ress

GP Michael William LANE, Maggie H BARTLETT, David P HENDERSON, Roger Mark JOY, Timothy O'BRIEN, Mark O'TOOLE, Christopher Ian PELTON, James William SWALLOW, Christopher John Percy YATES

Woodside Medical Practice
Woodside Health Centre, Wensley Green, Woodside, Telford TF7 5NR
Tel: 01952 586691 Fax: 01952 587007
(Telford and Wrekin Primary Care Trust)
Patient List Size: 7022

Practice Manager Glenis Shimmon

GP Malcolm W AWTY, David I ADNITT, Ian M DONNELLAN, Charlotte N HART

Tenbury Wells

The Surgery
34 Teme Street, Tenbury Wells WR15 8AA
Tel: 01584 810343 Fax: 01584 819734
(South Worcestershire Primary Care Trust)
Patient List Size: 9000

Practice Manager Magdalen Graham

GP Nicholas John FOSTER, S FOSTER, C GUNTHER, Roger John Anthony LEAR, Richard Frederick William TINKLER, Andrew Martin WRIGHT

Tenterden

Ivy Court Surgery
Ivy Court, Tenterden TN30 6RB
Tel: 01580 763666/764022 Fax: 01580 766194
(Ashford Primary Care Trust)
Patient List Size: 14500

Practice Manager Jolyon Vickers

GP Alan Richard LLOYD-SMITH, Dineli Nirmaleen CHARLESWORTH, Stephen Philip COX, David Harold Hainsworth DODDS, Jonathan More DOWLING, Fiona INGLE-FINCH, Neil Lawrence MANUELPILLAR

Tetbury

Romney House Surgery
39-41 Long Street, Tetbury GL8 8AA
Tel: 01666 502303 Fax: 01666 504549
(Cotswold and Vale Primary Care Trust)
Patient List Size: 7500

Practice Manager Jean Henderson

GP Anthony WALSH, Malcolm Terence GERALD, Angela Kristel KIRBY, Christopher WOODS

Tewkesbury

Bredon Hill Surgery
Kemerton Road, Bredon, Tewkesbury GL20 7QN
Tel: 01527 526824 Fax: 01527 501787
(South Worcestershire Primary Care Trust)

GP Dr ASHBRIDGE, Dr PAWLEY, Kim Diane TRIBLEY

Church Street Surgery
77 Church Street, Tewkesbury GL20 5RY
Tel: 01684 292343 Fax: 01684 274305
(Cheltenham and Tewkesbury Primary Care Trust)

Practice Manager Barbara Lloyd

GP Andrew Nicholas CROWTHER, Robert William DAVIS, Elspeth Marilyn DUNLOP, Janice Lynn KNOTT-CRAIG, Michael John MULRENAN, Andrew Neil RIGBY, Sanjay SHYMAPANT

Jesmond House Practice
Chance Street, Tewkesbury GL20 5RF
Tel: 01684 292813 Fax: 01684 274910
(Cheltenham and Tewkesbury Primary Care Trust)
Patient List Size: 4040

Practice Manager Bridget Derrett

GP Stuart Rankine HUTCHISON, G D BOGLE, A E BRAND, Frances DORE-GREEN

Watledge Surgery
Barton Road, Tewkesbury GL20 5QQ
Tel: 01684 293278
(Cheltenham and Tewkesbury Primary Care Trust)
Patient List Size: 5900

Practice Manager Ann Blakey

GP Christopher Sydney James SHERVEY, Robert Guy BUCKLEY, Simon FEARN, Alison Wendy TUCK

Thame

Thame Health Centre
East Street, Thame OX9 3JZ
Tel: 01844 261066 Fax: 01844 260347
(Vale of Aylesbury Primary Care Trust)
Patient List Size: 11200

Practice Manager Alan Bone

GP Kenneth William BURCH, Charles CHUBB, Richard Vincent Manley HARRINGTON, Duncan James KEELEY, Dorothy Margaret LISTER, Katja SUCHY

Thames Ditton

Giggs Hill Surgery
14 Raphael Drive, Thames Ditton KT7 0EB
Tel: 020 8398 8619 Fax: 020 8398 8874
(East Elmbridge and Mid Surrey Primary Care Trust)
Patient List Size: 6788

GP David John MATTHEWS, Dr CROW, Gillian Aida JEBB, Dr KEATING, Katie KENYON

Thorkhill Road Surgery
115A Thorkhill Road, Thames Ditton KT7 0UW
Tel: 020 8398 3141 Fax: 020 8398 7836
(East Elmbridge and Mid Surrey Primary Care Trust)
Patient List Size: 5000

GP Catherine Mary GARDNER, Teresa Jane MITCHELL, Caroline Anne ROBERTS

Thatcham

Burdwood Surgery
Wheelers Green Walk, Thatcham RG19 4YF
Tel: 01635 868006 Fax: 01635 867484
(Newbury and Community Primary Care Trust)

Practice Manager Peter Dallison

Thatcham Medical Practice
Bath Road, Thatcham RG18 3HD
Tel: 01635 867171 Fax: 01635 876395
(Newbury and Community Primary Care Trust)

Practice Manager Linda Vousden

GP Robert Geoffrey TAYTON, Barbara BARRIE, Jonathan McLean HAYWARD, A L MACKINNON, Richard John RUDGLEY, Clifford Corbett SMITH, R SYLVESTER, Timothy Mark THOMPSON, Geoffrey William Gwynne VEVERS, Vivien Nicola WILLIAMS

Thetford

Grove Surgery
Grove Lane, Thetford IP24 2HY
Tel: 01842 752285 Fax: 01842 751316
(Southern Norfolk Primary Care Trust)
Patient List Size: 13098

Practice Manager Steve Poynter

GP Giles Rowan SMITH, Sarah EVANS, Paul Stephen Leslie GRAY, P A HALLIWELL, Michael LEPPER, Christopher William RIDDELL, Robert John WILLIAMS

Old Brandon Road Surgery
Old Brandon Road, Feltwell, Thetford IP26 4AW
Tel: 01842 828481 Fax: 01842 828172
(West Norfolk Primary Care Trust)

Practice Manager Deanne Nisbet

GP Ian Gardner NISBET, Michael HUGHES, Giselle Annette SAGAR

School Lane Surgery
School Lane, Thetford IP24 2AG
Tel: 01842 753115 Fax: 01842 751242
(Southern Norfolk Primary Care Trust)

Practice Manager Janet Hill

GP Martin HADLEY BROWN, Martin Peter BELSHAM, Jonathan Learmont BRYSON, Dr SCHUEM, Dr SCOTT

Shipdham Surgery
Chapel Street, Shipdham, Thetford IP25 7LB
Tel: 01362 820225 Fax: 01362 821189
Email: wissey@doctors.net.uk
(Southern Norfolk Primary Care Trust)
Patient List Size: 3000

Practice Manager Margot Harris

GP Stuart Anderson MARTIN, Ines Rachel HAHN

Walton Medical Practice
The Surgery, St Giles Road, Watton, Thetford IP25 6XG
Tel: 01953 889134/881247 Fax: 01953 885167
(Southern Norfolk Primary Care Trust)
Patient List Size: 11500

Practice Manager Stephanie Spooner

GP John TAYLOR, Victoria Mary AMIES, Timothy John GIBBS, William Benzie HENDERSON, Devendra Amol Shradhanand MAHATME, Dr ROBINSON

Thirsk

The Health Centre
Chapel Street, Thirsk YO7 1LG
Tel: 01845 523154 Fax: 01845 526213
(Hambleton and Richmondshire Primary Care Trust)
Patient List Size: 7500

Practice Manager S E Pick

GP Philip Anthony CASEY, Louise ALLEN, Jane RAJAN, Andrzej Wladyslaw TRZECIAK

Lambert Medical Centre
2 Chapel Street, Thirsk YO7 1LU
Tel: 01845 523157 Fax: 01845 524508
(Hambleton and Richmondshire Primary Care Trust)
Patient List Size: 7500

Practice Manager David Dodsworth

GP Jack DONALD, Fiona BELLAS, Elaine Julie COOK, Richard Joseph HILES, Simon Francis POOLEY

The Surgery
Long Street, Topcliffe, Thirsk YO7 3RP
Tel: 01845 577297 Fax: 01845 577128
(Hambleton and Richmondshire Primary Care Trust)

Practice Manager Brian Anderson

GP Christine Jane SHAW, Charles Marcus PARKER

Thornton

Beechwood Surgery

23 Beechwood Drive, Thornton FY5 5EJ
Tel: 01253 824288
(Wyre Primary Care Trust)
Patient List Size: 1980

Practice Manager V Bellamy

GP Charles Stewart FULTON

The Medical Centre

Church Road, Thornton FY5 2TZ
Tel: 01253 852287 Fax: 01253 863478
(Wyre Primary Care Trust)

GP L SNOWDEN

The Thornton Practice

Church Road, Thornton FY5 2TZ
Tel: 01253 827231 Fax: 01253 863478
Website: www.thedoctors.co.uk
(Wyre Primary Care Trust)
Patient List Size: 8000

Practice Manager Janet Bullock

GP Anthony NAUGHTON, Wendy Laura FORD, J FRANKLIN, Sheryl LORIMER, A MACBETH, William David MORRISON, P O'SULLIVAN

The Village Practice

Church Road, Thornton FY5 2TZ
Tel: 01253 854321 Fax: 01253 862854
(Wyre Primary Care Trust)
Patient List Size: 8500

Practice Manager Irene Broten

GP Philip HORSFIELD, Stephen Robert William DOEL, T FLEET, Alison J MACBETH, Louise Patricia NEWISS, Preeti PANDY, F YOUNG

Thornton-Cleveleys

Cleveleys Group Practice

Kelso Avenue, Thornton-Cleveleys FY5 3LF
Tel: 01253 853992 Fax: 01253 822649
(Wyre Primary Care Trust)

GP David John LLEWELLYN, Andreas ARVANITIS, J KERRANE, Catherine SCOTT, Andrew David WHITTLE

The Crescent Surgert

Kelso Avenue, Thornton-Cleveleys FY5 3LF
Tel: 01253 823215 Fax: 01253 860640
(Wyre Primary Care Trust)

Practice Manager Janis Holloway

GP Ian Michael ECCLESTON, S HAMMOND, J MATTHEWS, David John PILLING

Thornton Heath

Brigstock Family Practice

83 Brigstock Road, Thornton Heath CR7 7JH
Tel: 020 8689 7800 Fax: 020 8665 1315
Email: christian.lyons@gp-h3608.nhs.uk
(Croydon Primary Care Trust)
Patient List Size: 3100

Practice Manager Christian Lyons

GP Nilu VAJPEYI

Brigstock Medical Practice

141 Brigstock Road, Thornton Heath CR7 7JN
Tel: 020 8684 1128 Fax: 020 8689 3647
Website: www.brigstockmedical.co.uk
(Croydon Primary Care Trust)
Patient List Size: 10700

Practice Manager Maureen Banks

GP Mary Anne WHITEHEAD, Samuel Nathan HOLT, Dev Kumar MALHOTRA, Shoby SATHANANTHAN, Shamit ROY, Kevin Nigel TARRANT

Broughton Corner Medical Centre

87 Thornton Road, Thornton Heath CR7 6BH
Tel: 020 8683 1277 Fax: 020 8665 1365
(Croydon Primary Care Trust)
Patient List Size: 4720

Practice Manager A Sennik

GP Avinash Kumar SENNIK

Eversley Medical Centre

501 London Road, Thornton Heath CR7 6AR
Tel: 020 8684 1172 Fax: 020 8684 4515
(Croydon Primary Care Trust)
Patient List Size: 9700

Practice Manager Dawn van Couten

GP Rita Anne NEWLAND, Olayinka AJAYI-OBE, John CHAN, Veronica MONTGOMERY, Samantha NEWNHAM, Priya PARULEKAR, Norman Felix RODRIGUES

Galpins Road Practice

6 Galpins Road, Thornton Heath CR7 6EA
Tel: 020 8684 3450 Fax: 020 8683 0439
(Croydon Primary Care Trust)
Patient List Size: 5000

Practice Manager Lutfiye Gurses

GP H GOONERATNE, A R SIDDIQUI

Linden Lodge Medical Practice

519 London Road, Thornton Heath CR7 6AR
Tel: 020 8684 2161 Fax: 020 8665 0743
(Croydon Primary Care Trust)
Patient List Size: 7260

Practice Manager Usha Patel

GP Chandrakant Rambhai PATEL, A CHADA, H KHAN, N KHAN

London Road Medical Centre

Cavendish House, 515 London Road, Thornton Heath CR7 6AR
Tel: 020 8239 9002 Fax: 020 8239 9003
(Croydon Primary Care Trust)
Patient List Size: 7260

Practice Manager Usha Patel

GP Damal Pathangi SUGANTHI

North Croydon Medical Centre

518 London Road, Thornton Heath CR7 7HQ
Tel: 020 8684 2190 Fax: 020 8665 1156
(Croydon Primary Care Trust)
Patient List Size: 4450

Practice Manager Maureen Bouthemy

GP Rotimi O BAKARE

Tidworth

The Queen Elizabeth Memorial Health Centre

St Michael's Avenue, Tidworth SP9 7EA
Tel: 01980 602620 Fax: 01980 602780
(Kennet and North Wiltshire Primary Care Trust)
Patient List Size: 7775

GP Anil KUBER

Tilbury

Calcutta Road Surgery

57 Calcutta Road, Tilbury RM18 7QZ
Tel: 01375 859535 Fax: 01375 850095

(Thurrock Primary Care Trust)

Practice Manager Coral Wood

GP P K MUKHOPADHYAY

The Health Centre
London Road, Tilbury RM18 8EB
Tel: 01375 842028 Fax: 01375 840358
(Thurrock Primary Care Trust)

Practice Manager Mary Brady

GP R SUNTHARALINGAM

Medic House Surgery
Ottawa Road, Tilbury RM18 7RJ
Tel: 01375 855288 Fax: 01375 850366
(Thurrock Primary Care Trust)

Practice Manager R Ramachandran

GP Mannath Kulangara RAMACHANDRAN

Sai Medical Centre
105 Calcutta Road, Tilbury RM18 7QA
Tel: 01375 855643 Fax: 01375 857664
(Thurrock Primary Care Trust)

Practice Manager S Patel

GP Prasant Jeshangbhai PATEL

St Chad's Medical Centre
4 St Chad's Road, Tilbury RM18 8LA
Tel: 01375 842396 Fax: 01375 840448
Email: reception.mailbox@gp-f81206.nhs.uk
(Thurrock Primary Care Trust)
Patient List Size: 3000

Practice Manager J Mallagh

GP E SHEHADEH

Tilbury Surgery
4 Commonwealth House, Montreal Road, Tilbury RM18 7QX
Tel: 01375 855755 Fax: 01375 857673
(Thurrock Primary Care Trust)

Practice Manager Kay Saha

GP Pijush Kumar SAHA

Tipton

The Black Country Family Practice
Health Centre, Queens Road, Tipton DY4 8PH
Tel: 0121 557 6397
(Rowley Regis and Tipton Primary Care Trust)
Patient List Size: 11867

Practice Manager A P Bishop

GP Colin John BROWNE, Anthony John ROBINSON, Mohan Bhadoor SINGH, George SOLOMON, Catherine Mary SWAIN

Dr Z A Shaikh and Partners
14 Horseley Heath, Tipton DY4 7QU
Tel: 0121 522 2201 Fax: 0121 520 2038
(Rowley Regis and Tipton Primary Care Trust)
Patient List Size: 8900

Practice Manager Rachel Parker

GP Zaheer Ahmed SHAIKH, Joanne COATES, Harry Henry OGUNNAIKE, David Andrew ORAM, Ian James WALTON

Glebefields Health Centre
St Marks Road, Tipton DY4 0UB
Tel: 0121 557 2323 Fax: 0121 520 9562
(Rowley Regis and Tipton Primary Care Trust)

GP L N DAYANI

Great Bridge Partnerships for Health
Sai Surgery, 10 Slater Street, Tipton DY4 7EY
Tel: 0121 557 1467 Fax: 0121 557 7826
(Rowley Regis and Tipton Primary Care Trust)
Patient List Size: 3300

GP A HARLOW

Swanpool Medical Centre
St Marks Road, Tipton DY4 0UB
Tel: 0121 557 2581 Fax: 0121 520 9475
(Rowley Regis and Tipton Primary Care Trust)
Patient List Size: 3000

Practice Manager Wendy Turner

GP C M LEADBEATER, Yusuf Suleman BHIMJI

Swanpool Medical Centre
St Marks Road, Tipton DY4 0SZ
Tel: 0121 557 5310
(Rowley Regis and Tipton Primary Care Trust)

Practice Manager C Paxton

GP Surendra Kumar SHARMA

The Victoria Surgery
Victoria Road, Tipton DY4 8SS
Tel: 0121 557 3422
(Rowley Regis and Tipton Primary Care Trust)

GP Amarjeet Kaur DHODY

Tiverton

Bampton Medical Practice
The Surgery, Barnhay, Bampton, Tiverton EX16 9NB
Tel: 01398 331304 Fax: 01398 332067
(Mid Devon Primary Care Trust)
Patient List Size: 3715

GP Christopher John MEW, Paul Jonathan BACKHOUSE, H JOHNSON-FERGUSON

Castle Place Practice
Kennedy Way, Tiverton EX16 6NP
Tel: 01884 252333 Fax: 01884 252152
(Mid Devon Primary Care Trust)
Patient List Size: 13842

Practice Manager May Hindson, Helen Kingdon, Christine Tidborough

GP Alexander David REVOLTA, Jeremy DAVIES, Simon JOHNSON-FERGUSON, Alison Jane MILLER, Patrick McCutcheon MILLER, Rachel Mary MOUNSEY, Peter Bertram RUMBLE, Hugh SAVILL

Clare House Practice
Clare House Surgery, Newport Street, Tiverton EX16 6NJ
Tel: 01884 252337 Fax: 01884 254401
(Mid Devon Primary Care Trust)
Patient List Size: 9751

Practice Manager Linda Bent

GP John Nicholas Alexander BLOOM, E T R FITZHERBERT, Ingrid R HALFYARD, Francis Patrick O'KELLY, Graeme Kearley PETERS, Michael Thomas James SEYMOUR, Sarah-Jane SEYMOUR

Sampford Peverell Surgery
29 Lower Town, Sampford Peverell, Tiverton EX16 7BJ
Tel: 01884 820304 Fax: 01884 821188
(Mid Devon Primary Care Trust)
Patient List Size: 1343

Practice Manager Jean Saunders

GP John Hugh SHERIDAN, Robert H SEAL

School Surgery
Fore Street, Witheridge, Tiverton EX16 8AH
Tel: 01884 860205 Fax: 01884 860887
(Mid Devon Primary Care Trust)
Patient List Size: 4680

Practice Manager Sally Smyth

GP Peter Maxwell BULL, Lynne ANDERSON, Christopher Elles CLARK, Clare J COLEMAN

Todmorden

Hirst Street Surgery
9 Hirst Street, Cornholme, Todmorden OL14 8NX
Tel: 01706 817474
(Calderdale Primary Care Trust)

GP Amrit Pal Singh GREWAL

Todmorden Health Centre
Rose Street, Todmorden OL14 5AT
Tel: 01706 815126 Fax: 01706 812693
(Calderdale Primary Care Trust)
Patient List Size: 13800

Practice Manager Susan Haggerstone

GP Gerallt WILLIAMS, Ailsa Susan CORMACK, Nigel Peter DAVEY, Andrew Jeffrey HARRISON, Sarah Jane MINTER, David Andrew RYLAND

Tonbridge

Church House Surgery
Church Lane, Tonbridge TN9 1DA
Tel: 01732 353225/352450 Fax: 01732 367977
Email: practice.manager@gp-G82132.nhs.uk
Website: www.churchhousesurgery.com
(South West Kent Primary Care Trust)
Patient List Size: 4350

Practice Manager Helen Mary Smith

GP Mary Jane DAWSON, David STEPHENS

Dunorlan Medical Group
64 Pembury Road, Tonbridge TN9 2JG
Tel: 01732 352907 Fax: 01732 367408
(South West Kent Primary Care Trust)
Patient List Size: 10333

Practice Manager Karen Kelsall

GP Ian George Caton JUTTING, Pauline JOSHI, Anne Mary NIDA, Timothy Allan PALMER, Rebecca Mary SANDYS, Charles Derek STUART-BUTTLE, Karen Jane THOMAS

Guelder Rose Medical Centre
Headcorn Road, Staplehurst, Tonbridge TN12 0BU
Tel: 01580 893045 Fax: 01580 890252
(Maidstone Weald Primary Care Trust)
Patient List Size: 2300

Practice Manager D Gildeh

GP Penny KEFFORD, Botros GILDEH

Hadlow Medical Centre
Doctors Surgery, School Lane, Hadlow, Tonbridge TN11 0ET
Tel: 01732 850248 Fax: 01732 850089
(South West Kent Primary Care Trust)
Patient List Size: 3300

Practice Manager Darren Hasell

GP Stephen LLOYD-DAVIES, Anissa BALDWIN

The Hildenborough Medical Group
Westwood, Tonbridge Road, Hildenborough, Tonbridge TN11 9HL
Tel: 01732 838777 Fax: 01732 838297
(South West Kent Primary Care Trust)

Practice Manager Peter Nicholas

GP John Bradley KELYNACK, Peter Dominic BENCH, Kenneth Andrew CASTRO, Catherine Eleanor DEVENPORT, Kenneth Gordon Cathcart EVANS, Nicola Janet EVANS, Paul Royston GOOZEE, Rahul JOSHI, Nicole PERRY, Jocelyn Ann WILSON

Howell Surgery
High Street, Brenchley, Tonbridge TN12 7NQ
Tel: 01892 722007 Fax: 01892 722007
(Maidstone Weald Primary Care Trust)
Patient List Size: 4300

Practice Manager Jennifer Foulser

GP Mark Rex IRONMONGER, Sian THOMAS, Robert WEIGHELL

Marden Medical Centre
Church Green, Marden, Tonbridge TN12 9HP
Tel: 01622 831257 Fax: 01622 832840
(Maidstone Weald Primary Care Trust)
Patient List Size: 5500

Practice Manager David Shaw

GP Nigel Paul MINETT, Neil David M POTTER, Graham Stuart STREETER

Rose Cottage Surgery
High Street, Staplehurst, Tonbridge TN12 0AP
Tel: 01580 891220
(Maidstone Weald Primary Care Trust)
Patient List Size: 3700

Practice Manager S Lynch

GP V J DUNNE

The Surgery
The Pond, East Peckam, Tonbridge TN12 8LP
Tel: 01622 871540
(Maidstone Weald Primary Care Trust)

Practice Manager Susan Greenhalgh

GP John Stewart Nicholas ANDERSON, Nicholas Alexander CHEALES, K L POTTERTON, Cedric Martin WARNER, V WHILLER, David Edward WHILLIER

Warders Medical Centre
47 East Street, Tonbridge TN9 1LA
Tel: 01732 770088 Fax: 01732 770033
Email: neil@warders.co.uk
(South West Kent Primary Care Trust)
Patient List Size: 15830

Practice Manager C M Burgess

GP Jenny ALTON, David Martin Gostwyck GOODRIDGE, Alistair John HOWITT, Moya Elizabeth LOVE, John Philip MOORE, Michael John MORRIS

Woodlands Health Centre
Paddock Wood, Tonbridge TN12 6AX
Tel: 01892 833331 Fax: 01892 838269
(Maidstone Weald Primary Care Trust)
Patient List Size: 11088

Practice Manager Wendy Glover

GP John Stewart Nicholas ANDERSON, Nicholas Alexander CHEALES, K POTTERTON, Cedric Martin WARNER, David Edward WHILLIER

Torpoint

Antony Road Surgery
16 Antony Road, Torpoint PL11 2JW
Tel: 01752 813277 Fax: 01752 815733
(North and East Cornwall Primary Care Trust)
Patient List Size: 6500

Practice Manager Frances White

GP Anthony John DAVIS, Lawrence BARNES, Brenda Leoda MALLETT, Paul Charles McELENY

Greenland Surgery
Greenland, Millbrook, Torpoint PL10 1DE
Tel: 01752 822576 Fax: 01752 823155
(North and East Cornwall Primary Care Trust)
Patient List Size: 2500

Practice Manager Pat Beckett

GP Francesco Guiseppe SCAGLIONI, Dawn JEFFERY

St James Road Surgery
22 St. James Road, Torpoint PL11 2BH
Tel: 01752 812404 Fax: 01752 816436
Email: philly.jones@stjamesroad.cornwall.nhs.uk
(North and East Cornwall Primary Care Trust)
Patient List Size: 3100

Practice Manager Christine Cross

GP Kevin Mark MATTHOLIE, Mary Wendover STEWART

Torquay

Barton Surgery
Lymington House, Barton Hill Way, Torquay TQ2 8JG
Tel: 01803 323761 Fax: 01803 316920
Email: barton.surgery@gp-83032.nhs.uk
Website: www.bartonsurgery-torquay.co.uk
(Torbay Primary Care Trust)
Patient List Size: 8200

Practice Manager David Pratley

GP Nicholas FISHER, Paul Michael Benson BARTON, Philip Alan SHUTE, Vivenne THORN, Jennifer Mary WILLMER

Chilcote Surgery
104 Chatto Road, Torquay TQ1 4HY
Tel: 01803 314277 Fax: 01803 323967
Email: chatto@eclipse.co.uk
(Torbay Primary Care Trust)

Practice Manager Yvonne Bagg

GP Peter Lionel MOORE

Croft Hall Medical Practice
19 Croft Road, Torquay TQ2 5UA
Tel: 01803 298441 Fax: 01803 296104
(Torbay Primary Care Trust)
Patient List Size: 8500

Practice Manager P D Vooght

GP John Nicholas STAINFORTH, Stuart CROWE, David Julian LAW, Eleanor ROWE, Steven Jonathan SMITH

Dewerstone Surgery
Hampton Avenue, St Marychurch, Torquay TQ1 3LA
Tel: 01803 316333 Fax: 01803 316393
Email: firstname.lastname@gp-L83111.nhs.uk
(Torbay Primary Care Trust)
Patient List Size: 10979

GP Charles Henry Lee DANIELS, Alan Christopher FITTER, Andrew RYAN, Elizabeth Ann THOMAS, Jolyon David YOUNG

Kirkham Medical Practice
St Albans Road, Torquay TQ1 3SL
Tel: 01803 323541 Fax: 01803 313411
(Torbay Primary Care Trust)
Patient List Size: 10300

Practice Manager Alison Alderson

GP Peter Alan ROVIRA, Peter Vaughan BOSLEY, Michael Joseph HAUGH, Judith Anne KEANE, Andrew John TUCKER, Nicholas William WILDGOOSE

The Medical Centre
The Medical Centre, Fore Street, St Marychurch, Torquay TQ1 4QX
Tel: 01803 325123 Fax: 01803 322136
Email: medical.centre@nhs.net
(Torbay Primary Care Trust)
Patient List Size: 6000

Practice Manager Tracey Kerslake

GP Christopher Joseph MOLAN, Ian Michael BAXENDALE, John Graham SPEAKE

Old Mill Surgery
19 Old Mill Road, Chelston, Torquay TQ2 6AU
Tel: 01803 605939 Fax: 01803 606525
Website: www.oldmillsurgery.co.uk
(Torbay Primary Care Trust)
Patient List Size: 2300

Practice Manager Lis Bridgeman

GP Paul Franklin HUTCHINSON

Park Hill Medical Practice
3 Park Hill Road, Torquay TQ1 2AL
(Torbay Primary Care Trust)

Practice Manager Catherine Perring

GP Daniel Anthony McCARTHY, Roger Haworth FEARNLEY, Peter John FORWARD, Simon James MURRAY, Gary Paul TUDOR

Sherwell Valley Road Surgery
Chelston, Torquay TQ2 6EJ
Tel: 01803 605123
(Torbay Primary Care Trust)

Practice Manager Catherine Perring

GP Daniel Anthony McCARTHY, Roger Haworth FEARNLEY, Peter John FORWARD, Simon James MURRAY, Gary Paul TUDOR

Shiphay Manor
37 Shiphay Lane, Torquay TQ2 7DU
Tel: 01803 615059 Fax: 01803 614545
(Torbay Primary Care Trust)
Patient List Size: 5800

Practice Manager Julia Ellis

GP Alexander Walmsley ELLIS, Ian Richard MORRELL, David William SPEAR

Southover Medical Practice
Bronshill Road, Torquay TQ1 3HD
Tel: 01803 327100 Fax: 01803 316295
(Torbay Primary Care Trust)
Patient List Size: 5240

Practice Manager Sue Clay

GP David George GREENWELL, John Martin RIDGE, Ian Robert TRESIDDER

Walnut Lodge Surgery
Walnut Road, Chelston, Torquay TQ2 6HP
Tel: 01803 605359 Fax: 01803 605772
Email: admin@walnutlodge.co.uk
Website: www.walnutlodge.co.uk
(Torbay Primary Care Trust)
Patient List Size: 4750

Practice Manager Mark Thomas

GP Helen PALEY, Stefano CANNIZZARO, Louise Ann SOLARI

Torrington

Castle Gardens Surgery
Castle Hill Gardens, Torrington EX38 8EU
Tel: 01805 623222 Fax: 01805 625069
(North Devon Primary Care Trust)
Patient List Size: 5400

Practice Manager Susan Crane

GP Arthur Paul Dorrington BANGAY, Alastair Eric BREMNER, Nicholas Charles LAMB, Jennifer Gay MARTINEAU

Torrington Health Centre
New Road, Torrington EX38 8EL
Tel: 01805 622247 Fax: 01805 625083
(North Devon Primary Care Trust)
Patient List Size: 5200

Practice Manager Brian Butland

GP Helen FROW, Malcolm David PATTERSON, Rafik Ismail Mohammed SADEK, Rosemary Ann Natalie THOMAS

Totnes

Catherine House Surgery
New Walk, The Plains, Totnes TQ9 5HA
Tel: 01803 862073 Fax: 01803 862056
(South Hams and West Devon Primary Care Trust)
Patient List Size: 2500

Practice Manager Anthea Scholefield

GP Nicolas Anthony COOPER, Andrew John PETTINGER

Leatside Surgery
Babbage Road, Totnes TQ9 5JA
Tel: 01803 862671
(South Hams and West Devon Primary Care Trust)

Practice Manager Andrew Moore

GP Timothy Ivor MANSER, Andrew William FRANKLAND, Dr GELDER, Dr GRANT, Beverley Jean INGOLDSBY, Michael LOVEROCK, Dr MORRIS, Dr PERRETT

Leatside Surgery
Babbage Road, Totnes TQ9 5JA
(South Hams and West Devon Primary Care Trust)

Towcester

Towcester Medical Centre
Link Way, Towcester NN12 6HH
Tel: 01327 359953 Fax: 01327 358929
(Daventry and South Northamptonshire Primary Care Trust)
Patient List Size: 8079

Practice Manager Sharon Hennell

GP Andrew Neil HOOKER, Nicola ODDWELL, Andrew ODWELL, John Robert SUNDERLAND, Nicholas John WARD

Towcester Medical Centre
Link Way, Towcester NN12 6HH
Tel: 01327 359339 Fax: 01327 358944
(Daventry and South Northamptonshire Primary Care Trust)

Practice Manager Madeleine Clark

GP Leslie Vincent SANGER

Towcester Medical Centre
Link Way, Towcester NN12 6HH
(Daventry and South Northamptonshire Primary Care Trust)

Practice Manager June Shaw

GP Mohammed Arif SUPPLE

Trimdon Station

Dr Jones and Partners
Medical Centre, Grosvenor Terrace, Trimdon Colliery, Trimdon Station TS29 6DH
Tel: 01429 880284 Fax: 01429 881405
(Sedgefield Primary Care Trust)

Practice Manager C C Miller

GP P R M JONES, D J ANDERSON, C BROWN, C J HEARMON, J H LARCOMBE, B K MACDOUGALL, G ROBERTSHAW, D E ROBINSON, M SHAMI

Tring

The New Surgery
St Peters House, Chursch Yard, Tring HP23 5AE
Tel: 01442 890661 Fax: 01442 824874
(Dacorum Primary Care Trust)
Patient List Size: 3300

Practice Manager Jan Hearn

GP Anthony Hugh HALL-JONES

Rothschild House Surgery
Chapel Street, Tring HP23 6PU
Tel: 01442 822468 Fax: 01442 825889
(Dacorum Primary Care Trust)
Patient List Size: 14700

Practice Manager Pat James

GP David John OGDEN, Romit CHOUDHURY, Avinash GUPTA, Jonathan HYKIN, Susas OSBOND, Ralph Neville Frank ROBERTS, Panikos SISSOU, Alexandra Jeannette Rosalind WAINWRIGHT, Alison Jane WOODWARD

Trowbridge

Adcroft Surgery
Prospect Place, Trowbridge BA14 8QA
Tel: 01225 755878 Fax: 01225 775445
(West Wiltshire Primary Care Trust)
Patient List Size: 9587

Practice Manager Eugenie Burne

GP Huw Powell WILLIAMS, Karamjeet Singh BIMBH, John Gregory HOLE, Stephen Matthew LOCKE, Linda Susan PARR

Bradford Road Medical Centre
60 Bradford Road, Trowbridge BA14 9AR
Tel: 01225 754255 Fax: 01225 774391
(West Wiltshire Primary Care Trust)
Patient List Size: 9300

Practice Manager Christina Fowler

GP Raymond Neil JONES, Toby COOKSON, Brenda NYE, Stephen Charles ROWLANDS, Ian Robert SWAN

Lovemead Group Practice
Roundstone Surgery, Polebarn Circus, Trowbridge BA14 7EH
Tel: 01225 752752 Fax: 01225 776388
Email: lovemead@lovemead.co.uk
Website: www.lovemead.co.uk
(West Wiltshire Primary Care Trust)
Patient List Size: 15000

Practice Manager Lesley Morris

GP Elizabeth REECE, Keith Anthony SMALES, Gareth BRYANT, Katherine DOWNEY, Michael John Bowness DUCKWORTH, Marianne Wilson HALES, Joanne HARDEN, Janet Elizabeth SLACK, Lucy THOMPSON

Widbrook Surgery
72 Wingfield Road, Trowbridge BA14 9EN
Tel: 01225 752412
(West Wiltshire Primary Care Trust)
Patient List Size: 6287

Practice Manager Jenny Collis

GP S R NATH, Richard Andrew COLLINS, Carolyn FOGGETT

Truro

The Health Centre
Chacewater, Truro TR4 8QS
Tel: 01872 560346 Fax: 01872 562203
(Central Cornwall Primary Care Trust)
Patient List Size: 5600

Practice Manager L Janet Trestrail

GP John Shaw CRAN, James Anthony Russell BOLTON, Jean-Anne Galbraith EVERS, Mark Bradley GRIPPER

Lemon Street Surgery
18 Lemon Street, Truro TR1 2LZ
Tel: 01872 73133 Fax: 01872 260900
(Central Cornwall Primary Care Trust)

Practice Manager L Dennis

GP Stuart Cooper VOWLES, Hasnain Mohamed DALAL, Sarah Jane GRAY, Andrew James MAY, Martyn Charles Davidson PROCTOR, Peter SHORT, Mark SULLIVAN

Portscatho Surgery
Gerrans Hill, Portscatho, Truro TR2 5EE
Tel: 01872 580345 Fax: 01872 580788
(Central Cornwall Primary Care Trust)
Patient List Size: 3800

Practice Manager Jackie Dunstan

GP Adam Stainton PRICE, Michael BLACK, Gordon Forbes CAMPBELL, Dr JERVIS

The Surgery
Bissoe Road, Carnon Downs, Truro TR3 6JD
Tel: 01872 863221 Fax: 01872 864113
(Central Cornwall Primary Care Trust)
Patient List Size: 5000

Practice Manager Susan Horswill

GP David John MALING, Mark Lawrence CALDICOTT, Edward Paul Simon FFRENCH-CONSTANT, Joanna NICHOLLS, Linda SIMPSON

Tregony Road Surgery
Tregony Road, Probus, Truro TR2 4JZ
Tel: 01726 882745 Fax: 01726 883945
(Central Cornwall Primary Care Trust)

GP Howard John BALL, Victoria Jane BRIDGER, Alan Norton REDINGTON, Keith William ROUND, John Bartholomew TISDALE

The Upper Surgery
27 Lemon Street, Truro TR1 2LS
Tel: 01872 74931 Fax: 01872 260339
(Central Cornwall Primary Care Trust)

Practice Manager Liz Wilson

GP Barry PETTIT, Martin John FALKNER, Gyl Valerie GRUNDY, Anthony Trevan HAMBLY, Stephen Jeremy HAWKINS, Adam Wearne PAYNTER, Ian Stanley RADFORD

Tunbridge Wells

Clanricarde House Surgery
Clanricarde Road, Tunbridge Wells TN1 1PJ
Tel: 01892 546422 Fax: 01892 533987
(South West Kent Primary Care Trust)

GP Kenneth Edgar Gabriel REEVES, Eric Nicholas BENSON, Deborah Frances FLUTE, Andrew James MACDONALD-BROWN

Grosvenor Medical Centre
23 Upper Grosvenor Road, Tunbridge Wells TN1 2DX
Tel: 01892 544777 Fax: 01892 544733
(South West Kent Primary Care Trust)
Patient List Size: 8500

Practice Manager Susan Stewart

GP Graham John CHARLWOOD, Matthew James BULL, Gillean Penelope CHARLWOOD, Stephen Addison HALL, Helen Anne YATES

Hill House Surgery
Clanricarde Road, Tunbridge Wells TN1 1PJ
Tel: 01892 543516 Fax: 01892 536594
(South West Kent Primary Care Trust)
Patient List Size: 2700

Practice Manager Marguerite E. Jenner

GP Michael Robert JENNER, Kay SASADA

The Kingswood Surgery
Kingswood Road, Tunbridge Wells TN2 4UJ
Tel: 01892 511833 Fax: 01892 517597
Email: practice.manager@gp-g82016.nhs.uk
(South West Kent Primary Care Trust)
Patient List Size: 9000

GP Robert John BOWES, P ROOME, N STONE, J THALLON, S WILLIAMS

The Lonsdale Medical Centre
1 Clanricarde Road, Tunbridge Wells TN1 1PE
Tel: 01892 530329 Fax: 01892 536583
(South West Kent Primary Care Trust)
Patient List Size: 3500

Practice Manager Kate Harlow

GP Anthony Graham BUCKLAND, A STEWART

Medical Centre
12A Greggs Wood Road, Tunbridge Wells TN2 3JL
Tel: 01892 541444 Fax: 01892 511157
Email: practice.manager@gp-g82022.nhs.uk
(South West Kent Primary Care Trust)
Patient List Size: 8040

Practice Manager Gillian Orrin

GP Alexander James GRIEVE, Kathlyn Rae HEDLEY, Christopher SAWYER, Ian WILLIAMS

The Nook Surgery
Withyham Road, Groombridge, Tunbridge Wells TN3 9QP
Tel: 01892 863326 Fax: 01892 863985
(Sussex Downs and Weald Primary Care Trust)
Patient List Size: 4300

Practice Manager Mike Simms

GP Andrew Donald WOLFLE, Helen BARNABY, Julian BARNABY, Sara BEATTIE, Karen WHICHELLO

Queens Road Surgery
7 Queen's Road, Tunbridge Wells TN4 9LL
Tel: 01892 520027 Fax: 01892 540833
(South West Kent Primary Care Trust)
Patient List Size: 3500

Practice Manager Lorna Liggett

GP Lalta SACHDEVA, Swadesh Kumar SACHDEVA

Rowan Tree Surgery
Rowan Tree Road, Tunbridge Wells TN2 5PX
Tel: 01892 515658 Fax: 01892 526271
(South West Kent Primary Care Trust)
Patient List Size: 1700

Practice Manager E Ramm

GP Usha ARON, Dr JENNER

Rusthall Medical Centre
Nellington Road, Rusthall, Tunbridge Wells TN4 8UW
Tel: 01892 515142 Fax: 01892 532256
(South West Kent Primary Care Trust)
Patient List Size: 5500

Practice Manager J Martin

GP Michael Robert LAWES, Katharine Jane DISMORR, Karen Denise FINLAY

St Andrews Medical Centre
Pinewood Gardens, Southborough, Tunbridge Wells TN4 0LZ
Tel: 01892 515455 Fax: 01892 514019
(South West Kent Primary Care Trust)
Patient List Size: 7200

Practice Manager Gill Nunn

GP Paul Charles BOWDEN, Alison Stella BOWDEN, Peter Richard COTTRELL, Elizabeth ROBSON

St James Medical Centre
11 Carlton Road, Tunbridge Wells TN1 2HW
Tel: 01892 541634 Fax: 01892 545170
(South West Kent Primary Care Trust)

Practice Manager Ian Milton

GP Anthony Richard EDWARDS, Donald James GREEN, Andrew Lionel Johnson TAYLOR

The Surgery
The Down, Lamberhurst, Tunbridge Wells TN3 8EX
Tel: 01892 890800 Fax: 01892 891187
Email: practice.manager@gp-g82170.nhs.uk
(Maidstone Weald Primary Care Trust)
Patient List Size: 2710

Practice Manager Mica Macey

GP Neil ELLWOOD, Clare KENDAL, Nicole TRACEY

Upper Grosvenor Road Surgery
150 Upper Grosvenor Road, Tunbridge Wells TN1 2ED
Tel: 01892 515542 Fax: 01892 532247
(South West Kent Primary Care Trust)
Patient List Size: 3270

GP Richard Thomas CROFT, Helen CREED

Waterfield House Surgery
186 Henwood Green Road, Pembury, Tunbridge Wells TN2 4LR
Tel: 01892 825488
(Maidstone Weald Primary Care Trust)

GP Peter Richard Merriman PATTISSON, Andrew John CAMERON, Nina Mary WELCH

Yew Tree Road Surgery
8 Yew Tree Road, Tunbridge Wells TN4 0BA
Tel: 01892 529601 Fax: 01892 527610
(South West Kent Primary Care Trust)

GP Jonathan Mark Howard BOLTON

Twickenham

Acorn Practice Group
29-35 Holly Road, Twickenham TW1 4EA
Tel: 020 8891 0073 Fax: 020 8744 0060
(Richmond and Twickenham Primary Care Trust)
Patient List Size: 7332

Practice Manager Michele Hawksworth

GP Gillian Patricia ROWLANDS, Barbara Anne CHRISTIE, Neil Allen JACKSON, Branko MOMIC

Cole Park Surgery
224 London Road, Twickenham TW1 1EU
Tel: 020 8892 1858 Fax: 020 8607 9577
(Hounslow Primary Care Trust)

Practice Manager Alma Chisholm

GP Ravinder Kaur KOONER

Cross Deep Surgery
4 Cross Deep, Twickenham TW1 4QP
Tel: 020 8892 8124 Fax: 020 8744 9801
(Richmond and Twickenham Primary Care Trust)
Patient List Size: 9500

Practice Manager Jean Nash

GP Jean EDMONDS, Alison LLOYD, Andrew Graeme ROBERTSON, Ting Hoi TO

Crown Road Surgery
66 Crown Road, Twickenham TW1 3ER
Tel: 020 8892 2543 Fax: 020 8744 3055
(Richmond and Twickenham Primary Care Trust)
Patient List Size: 5200

Practice Manager Yvonne Joseph

GP Christopher John SMITH, Phillipa Jane HUGHES, Penelope Anne SOWDEN

The Green Surgery
1B The Green, Twickenham TW2 5TU
Tel: 020 8894 6870 Fax: 020 8893 8579
(Richmond and Twickenham Primary Care Trust)
Patient List Size: 7200

Practice Manager Gregor Swann

GP Venetia STENT, Sarah HUNTER, Archana SOOD, Rosemary SORLEY

Jubilee Avenue Surgery
24 Jubilee Avenue, Whitton, Twickenham TW2 6JB
Tel: 020 8893 8464 Fax: 020 8893 3954
(Richmond and Twickenham Primary Care Trust)
Patient List Size: 4070

Practice Manager Sally Young

GP Edward St. leger WARREN, Tara Louise BOOHAN

Oak Lane Medical Centre
Oak Lane, Twickenham TW1 3PA
Tel: 020 8744 0094 Fax: 020 8892 1332
(Richmond and Twickenham Primary Care Trust)
Patient List Size: 4800

Practice Manager Jo Walker

GP M M UNADKAT

St Margaret's Practices
237 St. Margarets Road, Twickenham TW1 1NE
Tel: 020 8892 1986 Fax: 020 8891 6466
(Hounslow Primary Care Trust)

Practice Manager Sarah Baird, Maggie Hayward

GP William John Lyth BADGETT, Jill Kathryn PUGH, S SAINI, Justine Katharine Lloyd SETCHELL, G TAYLOR

The Surgery
325 Staines Road, Twickenham TW2 5AX
Tel: 020 8894 2722 Fax: 020 8287 2829
(Richmond and Twickenham Primary Care Trust)

Practice Manager Indira Devaraj

GP S DEVARAJ

The Surgery
131 Warren Road, Whitton, Twickenham TW2 7DJ
Tel: 020 8894 0797 Fax: 020 8894 0797
(Richmond and Twickenham Primary Care Trust)

GP Bodh Sagar KANCHAN

Twickenham Park Surgery
17 Rosslyn Road, Twickenham TW1 2AR
Tel: 020 8892 1991 Fax: 020 8744 0533
(Richmond and Twickenham Primary Care Trust)
Patient List Size: 5700

Practice Manager Chris groves

GP Baljit Singh JOHAL, Jennie BEACH, Manisha KOTECHA

York Medical Practice
St John's Health Centre, Oak Lane, Twickenham TW1 3PH
Tel: 020 8744 0220 Fax: 020 8892 6855
(Richmond and Twickenham Primary Care Trust)
Patient List Size: 11500

Practice Manager Paul Lardner

GP Margaret Norah HARPER, Mary Lynn GARDNER, Quentin PARSONS, P E RICHARDS, Frank Melville THOMAS

Uckfield

Bird-In-Eye Surgery
Uckfield Community Hospital, Framfield Road, Uckfield TN22 5AW
Tel: 01825 763196 Fax: 01825 760039
(Sussex Downs and Weald Primary Care Trust)

Practice Manager Mercedes Moddern

GP Nicholas Anthony ARGYROU, Christopher John Philip MEIKLE, Robert James STEPHENS

The Meads Surgery
Grange Road, Uckfield TN22 1QU
Tel: 01825 765777 Fax: 01825 766220
(Sussex Downs and Weald Primary Care Trust)
Patient List Size: 10200

Practice Manager L A Van Blerk

GP Ian Leslie Colin SLY, Dr DUCKWORTH, Richard Andrew MERRITT, James OLIVER, Emma Elizabeth WALBROOK

The Surgery
April Cottage, High Street, Buxted, Uckfield TN22 4LA
Tel: 01825 732333 Fax: 01825 732072
(Sussex Downs and Weald Primary Care Trust)
Patient List Size: 6800

Practice Manager Jackie Smith

GP Clarissa Dorothy FABRE, Fiona Karen STEWART, David Sheldon WRIGHT

The Surgery
Lydford Mews, 23 High Street, East Hoathly, Uckfield TN22 4LA
Tel: 01825 840943 Fax: 01825 841309
(Sussex Downs and Weald Primary Care Trust)

GP C FABRE

Ulverston

The Croft Surgery
Penny Bridge, Ulverston LA12 7TD
Tel: 01229 861249
(Morecambe Bay Primary Care Trust)

GP Geoffrey John MOORE

Haverthwaite Surgery
Backbarrow, Ulverston LA12 8QF
Tel: 01539 531619 Fax: 01539 531495
(Morecambe Bay Primary Care Trust)
Patient List Size: 1300

Practice Manager D Rockliffe

GP Robert Francis CALLINGHAM

The Health Centre
Victoria Road, Ulverston LA12 0EW
Tel: 01229 582223
(Morecambe Bay Primary Care Trust)
Patient List Size: 3450

Practice Manager Paula Bell, Sarah J M Saunders

GP Jonathan Paul GRAHAM, Lewis Andrew WILSON

Ulverston Health Centre
Victoria Road, Ulverston LA12 0EW
Tel: 01229 582588
(Morecambe Bay Primary Care Trust)

Practice Manager Hazel Kennaugh

GP William Duncan Bright DARBISHIRE, Ewen Duncan FRASER, Gerald Richard MURRAY, Pamela Joan REDMAN

Ulverston Health Centre
Victoria Road, Ulverston LA12 0EW
Tel: 01229 583732 Fax: 01229 588769
(Morecambe Bay Primary Care Trust)

Practice Manager Sheila Gibbs, Janet Parratt

GP Jorg SCHMIDT, P M SWARBRICK, E J WATKIN

Ulverston Health Centre
Victoria Road, Ulverston LA12 0EW
Tel: 01229 583238 Fax: 01229 588769
(Morecambe Bay Primary Care Trust)

Practice Manager Jamir Parratt

Upminster

Beech Avenue Surgery
41 Beech Avenue, Upminster RM14 2HF
Tel: 01708 220478 Fax: 01708 641549
(Havering Primary Care Trust)

GP Douglas Kee Yat KWAN

Branfill Road Surgery
17 Branfill Road, Upminster RM14 2YX
Tel: 01708 220022 Fax: 01708 640526
(Havering Primary Care Trust)

GP Pratima CHAKRAVARTY

Cranham Health Centre
117 Marlborough Gardens, Upminster RM14 1SR
Tel: 01708 222722 Fax: 01708 640961
Website: www.thesurgerycranham.co.uk
(Havering Primary Care Trust)
Patient List Size: 2950

Practice Manager Lucy Rouse

GP Immaneni Kanaka SUDHA, Michelle GOULDIE

Cranham Surgery
143 Ingrebourne Gardens, Cranham, Upminster RM14 1BJ
Tel: 01708 228888 Fax: 01708 641479
(Havering Primary Care Trust)

Practice Manager Shona Henlen

GP Christina DAHS, John Roslyn ANTHONY, I HUMBERSTONE

Dr P Chopra
75 Sunnyside Gardens, Upminster RM14 3DP
Tel: 01708 223156 Fax: 01708 640967
Email: drpushpachopra@gp-F82643.nhs.uk
(Havering Primary Care Trust)
Patient List Size: 2200

Practice Manager Manju Arora

GP Pushpa Kumari CHOPRA

Haiderian Medical Centre
181 Corbets Tey Road, Upminster RM14 2YN
Tel: 01708 225161 Fax: 01708 641477
Website: www.haiderian.co.uk
(Havering Primary Care Trust)
Patient List Size: 4900

GP Syed Iftikhar HAIDER, K F ABBAS, N AL-HOLO, S BABAR, Shehnaz Sami HAIDER, N MALIK

St Marys Lane Health Centre
226 St Marys Lane, Upminster RM14 3DH
Tel: 01708 251407 Fax: 01708 221878
(Havering Primary Care Trust)

Uttoxeter

Balance Street Practice
36 Balance Street, Uttoxeter ST14 8JG
Tel: 01889 562145 Fax: 01889 568164
(East Staffordshire Primary Care Trust)

Practice Manager M Jefferies

GP Anthony Alfred BURLINSON, D J ATHERTON, Owen Philip BARRON, Roger Christopher BURTON, Peter John Heselton TREWIN

Newcroft Surgery
Mill Street, Rocester, Uttoxeter ST14 5JX
Tel: 01889 590208 Fax: 01889 590196
(East Staffordshire Primary Care Trust)
Patient List Size: 1725

GP Nigel Charles Harding WEBSTER

Northgate Surgery
Church Street, Uttoxeter ST14 8AG
Tel: 01889 562010 Fax: 01889 568948
(East Staffordshire Primary Care Trust)
Patient List Size: 4600

Practice Manager Pauline Boden

GP Marenka Anna SICHA, Ann Frances JOHNSON, Simon George William JONES

Uxbridge

Acorn Medical Centre
149 Long Lane, Hillingdon, Uxbridge UB10 9JN
Tel: 01895 237474 Fax: 01895 232039
(Hillingdon Primary Care Trust)

Practice Manager Patricia Campbell

GP Ajay BIRLY

The Belmont Medical Centre
53-57 Belmont Road, Uxbridge UB8 1SD
Tel: 01895 233211 Fax: 01895 812099
(Hillingdon Primary Care Trust)

Practice Manager Pauline Collins

GP Derek Robert COPLAND, Cathy Marie DONNER, Mitcholl Douglas GARSIN, Minoo MADHOK

Church Road Surgery
4a Church Road, Cowley, Uxbridge UB8 3NA
Tel: 01895 233736 Fax: 01895 256881
(Hillingdon Primary Care Trust)

GP Stephen John A MORT, M Siobhan STAPLETON

Denham Green Surgery
2 Ashcroft Surgery, Ashcroft Drive, Denham, Uxbridge UB9 5JF
Tel: 01895 831377 Fax: 01895 835031
(Chiltern and South Bucks Primary Care Trust)

Practice Manager Sue King

GP John LEES

Denham Medical Centre
Tilehouse Way, Denham, Uxbridge UB9 5JA
Tel: 01895 832012 Fax: 01895 834704
(Chiltern and South Bucks Primary Care Trust)

Practice Manager Janice Lee

GP Anna ASSAF

Harefield Health Centre
Rickmansworth Road, Harefield, Uxbridge UB9 6JY
Tel: 01923 822944 Fax: 01923 823755
(Hillingdon Primary Care Trust)

Practice Manager Janice Alder

GP Gillian Christine DALE, Richard George GILL, Michael HOGARTH, Anne Kathryne JAMES, Sarah KIRKHAM

Harlington Road Practice
198 Harlington Road, Hillingdon, Uxbridge UB8 3HA
Tel: 01895 233881 Fax: 01895 812773
(Hillingdon Primary Care Trust)

Practice Manager Jennifer Cook

GP Muhammad MUSAWWIR ALI

Hillingdon Health Centre
4 Freezeland Way, Hillingdon, Uxbridge UB10 9QR
Tel: 01895 234440 Fax: 01895 252471
(Hillingdon Primary Care Trust)

Practice Manager A Harper

GP Thomas James Wyndham DAVIES, Atul MEHTA

King Edwards and Swakeleys Medical Centre
93 Swakeleys Road, Ickenham, Uxbridge UB10 8DQ
Tel: 01895 632114 Fax: 01895 639987
(Hillingdon Primary Care Trust)
Patient List Size: 6000

GP Mahendra Kumar MASHRU

The Medical Centre
Brunel University, Kingston Lane, Uxbridge UB8 3PH
Tel: 01895 234426/235907 Fax: 01895 270964
(Hillingdon Primary Care Trust)
Patient List Size: 8900

Practice Manager Bill Darvill

GP Baldev Singh JASSAL, Sabah AHMAD, Marion Jacqueline MARSHALL

Oakland Medical Centre
344 Long Lane, Hillingdon, Uxbridge UB10 9PN
Tel: 01895 237411/234373 Fax: 01895 812875
(Hillingdon Primary Care Trust)

GP Sally Ann MADER, Vinod DABAS, Sukhvinder JOHAL

The Timbers Surgery
St Laurence Church Hall, Shepherds Close, Cowley, Uxbridge UB8 2EZ
Tel: 01895 234585/234092 Fax: 01895 233659
(Hillingdon Primary Care Trust)

Practice Manager T J Daily

GP Haydn Ronald DAILY-JONES

Uxbridge Medical Centre
George Street, Uxbridge UB8 1UB
Tel: 01895 231925 Fax: 01895 813190
(Hillingdon Primary Care Trust)

GP Murray McEWEN, Jeyan ABDUL-KARIM, Robert ASHER, Kiranjit PITROLA, Alison Joy RACKHAM, Rozina SARWAR, Stephen VAUGHAN-SMITH

Wallasey Crescent Practice
1 Wallasey Crescent, Ickenham, Uxbridge UB10 8SA
Tel: 01895 674156 Fax: 01895 623334
(Hillingdon Primary Care Trust)
Patient List Size: 1600

GP Kalpana Prakash PATEL

West Drayton Road Practice
60 West Drayton Road, Hillingdon, Uxbridge UB8 3LA
Tel: 020 8573 7674/3656 Fax: 020 8573 7498
(Hillingdon Primary Care Trust)

GP Graham Nigel STEARNES, Ajay MEHTA, Hanna STERA

Yiewsley Health Centre
High Street, Yiewsley, Uxbridge UB7 7DP
Tel: 01895 435377/435382 Fax: 01895 444672
(Hillingdon Primary Care Trust)
Patient List Size: 6002

Practice Manager Pamela Lemesre

GP Gurvinder Singh CHANA, Luisa J C CORBRIDGE, nderjeet RAJ

Ventnor

Grove House Surgery
102 Albert Street, Ventnor PO38 1EU
Tel: 01983 852427 Fax: 01983 852185
(Isle of Wight Primary Care Trust)

GP Steven Michael PORTER, Stephen Jeremy DOGGETT

Ventnor Medical Centre
3 Albert Street, Ventnor PO38 1EZ
Tel: 01983 852787 Fax: 01983 855447
(Isle of Wight Primary Care Trust)
Patient List Size: 5300

Practice Manager Daniel McMeechan

GP David Paul TURNER, Rebecca Julianna Angela ASHTON, Peter Alan COLEMAN, Martin William LOCK

Verwood

The Verwood Surgery
15 Station Road, Verwood BH31 7PY
Tel: 01202 825353 Fax: 01202 829697
(South and East Dorset Primary Care Trust)
Patient List Size: 7800

Practice Manager Dawn Jennings

GP Nigel Kirkham SANDY, Helen DEVEREUX, Raj KARKERA, Maeve O'DRISCOLL, A POLKINGHORN, Jonathan Michael Lance SEGAL

Virginia Water

Packers Surgery
Christchurch Road, Virginia Water GU25 4RL
Tel: 01344 842951 Fax: 01344 845121
(North Surrey Primary Care Trust)
Patient List Size: 4000

Practice Manager Linda Smit

GP Paul Maxwell LOXTON, Adam ROSEN

Wadebridge

Wadebridge and Camel Estuary Practice
Brooklyn, Wadebridge PL27 7BS
Tel: 01208 812222 Fax: 01208 815907
(North and East Cornwall Primary Care Trust)
Patient List Size: 7650

Practice Manager Sonia Geach

GP Charles Mark Bolton HEWITT, Alan Norman David AGNEW, James Benedict ASHBY, Christopher David SAITCH, Oliver John SCOTT, Clare Louise TYLER

Wadhurst

Belmont Surgery
St James Square, Wadhurst TN5 6BJ
Tel: 01892 782121 Fax: 01892 783989
(Sussex Downs and Weald Primary Care Trust)
Patient List Size: 8000

GP Antony James COLLIS, Andrew Michael Thomas BLACKBURN, Catherine Mary OFFORD, David ROCHE

Wakefield

The Almshouse Surgery
Trinity Medical Centre, Thornhill Street, Wakefield WF1 1PG
Tel: 01924 327150 Fax: 01924 327165
(Wakefield West Primary Care Trust)
Patient List Size: 12000

Practice Manager Liz Stead

GP Stephen Edward Poynton BIRKINSHAW, Philip Nigel BARKER, Susan Jean CRABBE, C R GLEAVE, Rolf RAUCH

Alverthorpe Surgery
Balne Lane, Wakefield WF2 0DP
Tel: 01924 372584 Fax: 01924 239383
(Wakefield West Primary Care Trust)
Patient List Size: 3500

Practice Manager Beverley Jeffery

GP Alasdair Barry MACLEAN, Kathryn L CHADWICK

Chapelthorpe Medical Centre
Standbridge Lane, Chapelthorpe, Wakefield WF2 7GP
Tel: 01924 255166 Fax: 01924 257653
(Wakefield West Primary Care Trust)
Patient List Size: 11000

Practice Manager Cheryl Wilden

GP Malcolm McDONALD, M F BENNETT, T CHERRY, Jane Lesley COOPER, C J HARRIES, Kevin Andrew JACKSON, M NADEEM, Jane Louise SCHINDLER

Crofton Health Centre
Slack Lane, Crofton, Wakefield WF4 1HJ
Tel: 01924 862612 Fax: 01924 865519
(Wakefield West Primary Care Trust)
Patient List Size: 9980

Practice Manager Carol Perkins

GP Alan Derrick LEADING, Edmond FERDINANDUS, Carolyn Joyce HALL, Gerald HANCOCK, Andrew SYKES, Joanne TAYLOR

Eastmoor Health Centre
Windhill Road, Wakefield WF1 4SD
Tel: 01924 327625 Fax: 01924 298488
Website: www.surgeriesonline.com/eastmoorhc
(Wakefield West Primary Care Trust)
Patient List Size: 2800

Practice Manager Anne Walker

GP Victor LABOR, Swaroop Kumar MAHANTY

The Grove Surgery
Trinity Medical Centre, Thornhill Street, Wakefield WF1 1PG
Tel: 01924 398009 Fax: 01924 398019
(Wakefield West Primary Care Trust)

Practice Manager Elizabeth Stead

GP James Anthony TABNER, Dorothea BROWN-DOBLHOFF-DIER, Mazin DADAH, Christos HADJICHARITOU, David Andrew SMITH, Mair TUNSTALL

Health Centre
Lake Lock Road, Stanley, Wakefield WF3 4HS
Tel: 01924 822328 Fax: 01924 870052
(Wakefield West Primary Care Trust)
Patient List Size: 7600

Practice Manager Pat Foster

GP Janice Marian WOODROW, David Christopher BRIGHTMAN, Joyce Kathleen BUTTERFIELD, Alison DANIEL, Robert John HUMPHRY, Daniel Maitland JEFFERY

Homestead Clinic
Homestead Drive, Wakefield WF2 9PE
Tel: 01924 384498 Fax: 01924 239775
(Wakefield West Primary Care Trust)
Patient List Size: 5000

Practice Manager Sarah Hubbard

GP Cecil Clifford Anthony DE SOUZA, Oye IRELEWUYI

Leigh View Medical Centre
Bradford Road, Tingley, Wakefield WF3 1RQ
Tel: 0113 253 7629 Fax: 0113 238 1286
(South Leeds Primary Care Trust)

Practice Manager Robert Campbell

GP Judith Anne LOWE, Geoffrey John BELL, Nicholas ELLIOTT, Catherine Ann LIMB, Peter NICHOLLS, Philippa Jane SCHOFIELD, Andrew Neil SMITH

Lofthouse Surgery
2 Church Farm Close, Lofthouse, Wakefield WF3 3SA
Tel: 01924 822273 Fax: 01924 825168
(South Leeds Primary Care Trust)
Patient List Size: 8959

Practice Manager Jenny Ramsden

GP Steven Alan Christopher CLEMENTS, Lynne Tracy BLAKEMORE, Benjamin Sacheverel BROWNING, Catherine LLOYD, Mark Antony PALMER, Ian Antony SANDERSON

Lupset Health Centre
off Horbury Road, Lupset, Wakefield WF2 8RE
Tel: 01924 373377 Fax: 01924 201649
Website: www.lupsetsurgery.co.uk
(Wakefield West Primary Care Trust)
Patient List Size: 12500

Practice Manager Josie Rhodes

GP Joseph TOSH, Sallie Elizabeth CARPENTER, H DEMPSEY, Shahid HANIF, Rosemarie JONES, Louise LOMAX, Mark NAPPER, Toby O'DONNELL, Adam Peter SHEPPARD, David Anselm TREE-BOOKER

Maybush Medical Centre
Belle Isle Health Park, Portobello Road, Wakefield WF1 5PN
Tel: 01924 328132 Fax: 01924 328130

(Wakefield West Primary Care Trust)
Patient List Size: 8750

Practice Manager Joan Huskisson

GP Margaret Elizabeth SCOTT, Neale Hudson CLARK, J L HAWKHEAD, Shane McALINDON

Middlestown Medical Centre
New Road, Middlestown, Wakefield WF4 4PA
Tel: 01924 237100 Fax: 01924 237107
(Wakefield West Primary Care Trust)
Patient List Size: 7300

Practice Manager Susan Gilbert

GP James Stevenson DONNAN, Terence GAIR, Antony John KIDD, A MACNAB, Philippa Fredericka WILLIAMS

New Southgate Surgery
Buxton Place, off Leeds Road, Wakefield WF1 3JQ
Tel: 01924 334400 Fax: 01924 334439
(Wakefield West Primary Care Trust)
Patient List Size: 11400

Practice Manager Susan Garton

GP Deborah Elizabeth HALLOTT, M AHMED, Gillian Anne BRAIN, David Richard FYFE, Keith Moray SOUTER, Stephen John WROE

Orchard Croft Medical Centre
Cluntergate, Horbury, Wakefield WF4 5BY
Tel: 01924 271016 Fax: 01924 279459
(Wakefield West Primary Care Trust)

Practice Manager Gill Cunningham

GP David Gordon MAYNARD, Gillian BENNETT, S DE SILVA, Brian Andrew HILL, David A HUNTER, Lawrence KING, Emma SAUNDERS

Outwood Park Medical Centre
Potovens Lane, Outwood, Wakefield WF1 2PE
Tel: 01924 786226 Fax: 01924 786248
(Wakefield West Primary Care Trust)
Patient List Size: 13000

Practice Manager Glennis Rhodes

GP George Peter Nicholas DUBLON, Ann-Marie CARROLL, Adrian Grant CLARKSON, John Philip Foster EDMONDS, Alison Mary JEPSON, John Peter Jeremy LAWN, Helen Rose PUTMAN

Rashid and Partners
Rycroft Primary Care Centre, Madeley Road, Havercroft, Wakefield WF4 2QG
Tel: 01226 725555 Fax: 01226 700051
(Eastern Wakefield Primary Care Trust)

Practice Manager A Fowler

GP Sheikh Abdur RASHID, Adam Leighton COOPER, Mohammad FAROOQ DAR, Rachel Elizabeth PHILLIPS

The Surgery
46 Montague Street, Wakefield WF1 5BB
Tel: 01924 251811 Fax: 01924 242140
(Wakefield West Primary Care Trust)
Patient List Size: 1042

Practice Manager Mavis Turner

GP Ahmed Ali QARSHI

Warrengate Medical Centre
Upper Warrengate, Wakefield WF1 4PR
Tel: 01924 371011 Fax: 01924 379567
(Wakefield West Primary Care Trust)
Patient List Size: 8500

Practice Manager Marie Smith

GP Patrick Francis O'CONNELL, C ABBOTT, J BATES, S JEYASUNDARAM, Simon J McGRAW, Myint Kyam OO

Wallasey

Central Park Medical Centre
132-134 Liscard Road, Wallasey CH44 0AB
Tel: 0151 638 8833 Fax: 0151 637 0208
Email: gp.cpmc@lineone.net
(Birkenhead and Wallasey Primary Care Trust)
Patient List Size: 7900

Practice Manager Joan Rogers

GP S K MUKHERJEE, Robert BROADBELT, M K LODH, A MUKHERJEE

Earlston Road Surgery
1 Earlston Road, Wallasey CH45 5DX
Tel: 0151 639 2635 Fax: 0151 638 7008
(Birkenhead and Wallasey Primary Care Trust)
Patient List Size: 3071

Practice Manager Monika Doyle

GP Neville Alan BRADLEY, Amrit MAHAI

Field Road Health Centre
Field Road, New Brighton, Wallasey CH45 5LN
Tel: 0151 639 7054 Fax: 0151 637 0581
(Birkenhead and Wallasey Primary Care Trust)
Patient List Size: 3475

Practice Manager Margaret Goodwin

GP David Charles DOWNWARD, Margaret Gwendoline HAYES

Grove Medical Centre
27 Grove Road, Wallasey CH45 3HE
Tel: 0151 691 1112 Fax: 0151 637 0266
(Birkenhead and Wallasey Primary Care Trust)

Practice Manager Rosanne Jones

GP David John PRICE, Alan ROBERTS

Liscard Group Practice
Croxteth Avenue, Liscard, Wallasey CH44 5UL
Tel: 0151 638 4764 Fax: 0151637 0579
(Birkenhead and Wallasey Primary Care Trust)

GP Allan Frederick CARGILL, Peter Hegarty JOHNSON, Elizabeth Irene REILLY

Manor Health Centre
Liscard Village, Wallasey CH45 4JG
Tel: 0151 638 8221 Fax: 0151 639 6512
(Birkenhead and Wallasey Primary Care Trust)

Practice Manager Melanie Peters

GP Sean Patrick Michael MAGENNIS, Ann COULSON, Cerys HUMPHREYS

Martins Lane Medical Centre
2 Martins Lane, Wallasey CH44 1BA
Tel: 0151 630 4747 Fax: 0151 639 7395
(Birkenhead and Wallasey Primary Care Trust)
Patient List Size: 2900

Practice Manager Wendy Fullard

GP William Thomas DUNNE

Seabank Road Surgery
213/215 Seabank Road, Wallasey CH45 1HE
Tel: 0151 630 6577 Fax: 0151 639 7477
(Birkenhead and Wallasey Primary Care Trust)

Practice Manager Marie Moorhouse, Gillian Piercy

GP H R PATEL

Somerville Medical Practice
64 Gorsey Lane, Wallasey CH44 4AA
Tel: 0151 638 9333 Fax: 0151 637 0291
(Birkenhead and Wallasey Primary Care Trust)

GP Victor-Elie Pepe Dimitri C. CHERIDJIAN, S M EVANS, A MAHAI, Richard Anthony SMYE, Paul Stewart Trevor WILSON

St George's Medical Centre
Field Road, New Brighton, Wallasey CH45 5LN
Tel: 0151 630 2080 Fax: 0151 637 0370
(Birkenhead and Wallasey Primary Care Trust)

Practice Manager Doreen Phoenix

GP Surendra Chimanlal SHAH, Lesley Margaret HODGSON, Ramesh Govindji PATEL, Jean QUINN, Steven Phillip RUDNICK, Dr TAYLOR

St Hilary Brow Group Practice
204 Wallasey Road, Wallasey CH44 2AG
Tel: 0151 638 2216 Fax: 0151 638 9097
(Birkenhead and Wallasey Primary Care Trust)
Patient List Size: 5500

Practice Manager Susan Davies

GP James Patrick KINGSLAND, Mark Stuart GREEN, Maureen Shannon RICHMOND, Christine Margaret THOMAS

Tandon
71 Grove Road, Wallasey CH45 3HF
Tel: 0151 639 4616 Fax: 0151 637 0182
(Birkenhead and Wallasey Primary Care Trust)
Patient List Size: 3000

Practice Manager Eve Evans

GP Pradip Kumar TANDON, R TANDON

Wallingford

Berinsfield Health Centre
Fane Drive, Berinsfield, Wallingford OX10 7NE
Tel: 01865 340558/340559 Fax: 01865 341973
Website: www.berinsfieldhealthcentre.nshs.uk
(South East Oxfordshire Primary Care Trust)
Patient List Size: 5200

Practice Manager Sandy Wetherall

GP Martyn John Benjamin AGASS, Julie Anne ANDERSON, Henry HOY, Claudia Ann JONES

Mill Stream Surgery
Mill Stream, Benson, Wallingford OX10 6RL
Tel: 01491 838286
(South East Oxfordshire Primary Care Trust)
Patient List Size: 4400

Practice Manager Margaret Wiggall

GP Peter William ROSE, Karen BATEMAN, Lucy JENKINS, Daniel Timothy Richardson WILSON

Wallingford Medical Practice
Reading Road, Wallingford OX10 9DU
Tel: 01491 835577 Fax: 01491 824034
Email: walingford.practice@gp-k84037.nhs.uk
Website: www.wallingfordmedicalpractice.co.uk
(South East Oxfordshire Primary Care Trust)
Patient List Size: 14540

Practice Manager Janet Newman

GP Anthony Richard VERNON, Tahra Melanie AKRAM-CHAUDRY, Elizabeth Ann ELEY, Andrew Lawrence HENRY, Charles Patteson HUGHES, Hans PAUL, Elizabeth Harriet WALKER

Wallington

Lings and Partners
Shotfield Health Centre, Shotfield, Wallington SM6 0HY
Tel: 020 8647 0031 Fax: 020 8773 1801
(Sutton and Merton Primary Care Trust)
Patient List Size: 9150

Practice Manager Susan Coulson

GP Heather Ruth LINGS, Bernard Patrick LEWIS, Joanna MUNDEN, Sayeda Salma Banu UDDIN

Maldon Road Surgery
35 Maldon Road, Wallington SM6 8BL
Tel: 020 8647 4622 Fax: 020 8288 8684
(Sutton and Merton Primary Care Trust)

GP Michael Edward ERSKINE, U KAR GUPTA

Manor Practice
57 Manor Road, Wallington SM6 0DE
Tel: 020 8647 1818 Fax: 020 8647 6699
(Sutton and Merton Primary Care Trust)
Patient List Size: 7200

Practice Manager S Kavanagh

GP K KO, Dr AKINMADE, M AMJAD

Park Road Surgery
Walpole Court, 1A Park Road, Wallington SM6 8AW
Tel: 020 8647 4485/2992 Fax: 020 8773 4838
(Sutton and Merton Primary Care Trust)
Patient List Size: 3000

Practice Manager Janet Boud

GP Tahir Hafeez TOOSY

Shotfield Health Centre
Shotfield, Wallington SM6 0HY
Tel: 020 8647 0031
(Sutton and Merton Primary Care Trust)
Patient List Size: 10700

GP Saradiadu BASU, Andrew Charles HILLYARD, M M AHMED, Ian Martin WILSON

The Surgery
19 Bandon Rise, Wallington SM6 8PT
Tel: 020 8647 3894/6959
(Sutton and Merton Primary Care Trust)

GP M R MOOLA

Wallington Medical Centre
52 Mollison Drive, Wallington SM6 9BY
Tel: 020 8647 0811 Fax: 020 8647 4574
(Sutton and Merton Primary Care Trust)

Practice Manager B R Bhattacharyya

GP Tapan Kumar HALDER

Wallsend

Bewicke Health Centre
51 Tynemouth Road, Wallsend NE28 0AD
Tel: 0191 262 3036 Fax: 0191 295 1663
(North Tyneside Primary Care Trust)

Practice Manager May Rodgers

GP Robert David THORNTON, Sarah L COOKE, Simon John Strudwick COOMBER, Deirdre Mary KELLY, Alison M PETRIE, Gerard Joseph VAUGHAN

Churchill Street Surgery
12 Churchill Street, Wallsend NE28 7SZ
Tel: 0191 262 3379 Fax: 0191 262 3209
(North Tyneside Primary Care Trust)

Practice Manager Bernie Caffrey

GP Alok Kumar GHOSH

Ferndale Avenue Surgery
24 Ferndale Avenue, Wallsend NE28 7NE
Tel: 0191 262 3505 Fax: 0191 262 4976
(North Tyneside Primary Care Trust)

GP Murari Lal AGGARWAL

Garden Park Surgery
225 Denbigh Street, Howdon, Wallsend NE28 0PP
Tel: 0191 289 2525 Fax: 0191 289 2526
(North Tyneside Primary Care Trust)
Patient List Size: 7500

Practice Manager Ann Crosby

GP Kelachandra Philip ABRAHAM, Vini DEWAN, Anis RAMLI, Priadarsh SANDHU

Park Road Surgery
93 Park Road, Wallsend NE28 7LP
Tel: 0191 262 5680 Fax: 0191 262 3646
(North Tyneside Primary Care Trust)

Practice Manager S Dowling

GP Beverley Jane KENNY, Katharine Anne CARDING, John David MATTHEWS

The Portugal Place Health Centre
Portugal Place, Wallsend NE28 6RZ
(North Tyneside Primary Care Trust)
Patient List Size: 13000

Practice Manager Karen Iliades

GP Dr SWEETMAN

The Village Green Surgery
The Green, Wallsend NE28 6BB
Tel: 0191 295 8500 Fax: 0191 295 8519
Email: david.gare@nhs.net
(North Tyneside Primary Care Trust)
Patient List Size: 9800

Practice Manager D Yare

GP Stephen Eric BLAIR, Ruth Linda EVANS, Aliya NAEEM SOOMRO, Peter William OLLEY, James Martin PAGE, Fiona Jane RIDDLE, Kirsty UTTRELL, Mark Anthony WESTWOOD

Walsall

Anand and Anand
The Health Centre, Bilston Street, Darlaston, Walsall WS10 8EY
Tel: 0121 526 2845 Fax: 0121 568 8034
(Walsall Teaching Primary Care Trust)
Patient List Size: 3137

Practice Manager Barbara Colley

GP Makhan Singh ANAND, Harkirat ANAND

Beechdale Centre
Edison Road, Walsall WS2 7HS
Tel: 01922 775200 Fax: 01922 775203
(Walsall Teaching Primary Care Trust)
Patient List Size: 4000

Practice Manager Jean Kadodwala

GP B MITRA, Gian SINGH

Birchills Health Centre
23-23 Old Birchills, Walsall WS2 8QH
Tel: 01922 614896/724279 Fax: 01922 635973
Email: pali.suri@walsall.nhs.uk
(Walsall Teaching Primary Care Trust)
Patient List Size: 3800

Practice Manager S P K Suri

GP Avtar Singh SURI, Basanti MITRA

Bloxwich Medical Practice
Field Road, Bloxwich, Walsall WS3 3JP
Fax: 01922 775161
(Walsall Teaching Primary Care Trust)
Patient List Size: 5200

GP T COLEMAN, D JOHNSON

Brace Street Clinic
Brace Street, Caldmore, Walsall WS1 3PS
Tel: 01922 858960 Fax: 01922 858937
(Walsall Teaching Primary Care Trust)

GP B C PAL

Brace Street Clinic
Brace Street, Caldmore, Walsall WS1 3PS
Tel: 01922 858979 Fax: 01922 858976
(Walsall Teaching Primary Care Trust)

Brace Street Health Centre
63 Brace Street, Caldmore, Walsall WS1 3PS
Tel: 01922 858963 Fax: 01922 858964
(Walsall Teaching Primary Care Trust)
Patient List Size: 4200

Practice Manager Jacqueline Harrison

GP Dipak Kumar BANERJEE, S DE

Brickiln Street Surgery
10 Brickiln Street, Brownhills, Walsall WS8 6AU
Tel: 01543 372390 Fax: 01543 454583
(Walsall Teaching Primary Care Trust)

Practice Manager Lilian Addis

GP Chandrakanta DEWADA

Broadstone Avenue Surgery
59-61 Broadstone Avenue, Leamore, Walsall WS3 1ER
Tel: 01922 476277 Fax: 01922 403208
Email: kaulp@gp.walsall-ha.wmids.nhs.uk
(Walsall Teaching Primary Care Trust)
Patient List Size: 3200

Practice Manager V Hayward

GP Pyre Lal KAUL, G K GILL

Broadway Medical Centre
213 Broadway, Walsall WS1 3HD
Tel: 01922 22064 Fax: 01922 613544
(Walsall Teaching Primary Care Trust)

GP Alakshendra Pal Singh KUSHWAHA

Burntwood Health Centre
Hudson Drive, Walsall WS7 0EW
Tel: 01543 682655
Email: burntwood.healthc@sshawebmail.nhs.uk
(Burntwood, Lichfield and Tamworth Primary Care Trust)

GP M SALEEM

Burntwood Health Centre
Hudson Drive, Walsall WS7 0EW
Tel: 01543 674477
Email: burntwood.medical@sshawebmail.nhs.uk
(Burntwood, Lichfield and Tamworth Primary Care Trust)

Practice Manager L Eales

GP C KING, J G WHARTON

Chapel Street Surgery
1 Chapel Street, Pelsall, Walsall WS3 4LN
Tel: 01922 685858 Fax: 01922 694763
(Walsall Teaching Primary Care Trust)
Patient List Size: 3065

Practice Manager Carol Winwood

GP Lakshmanan Sumathy NAMBISAN

Chasetown Medical Centre
29/31 High Street, Chasetown, Burntwood, Walsall WS7 8XE
Tel: 01543 671705 Fax: 01543 670475
Email: chasetown.medical@sshawebmail.nhs.uk
(Burntwood, Lichfield and Tamworth Primary Care Trust)

GP Indravadan B BHATT

Coalpool Clinic
Ross Road, Coalpool, Walsall WS3 1RE
Fax: 01922 723499
(Walsall Teaching Primary Care Trust)

GP A H M GATRAD

Doctors Surgery
Short Street, Brownhills, Walsall WS8 6AD
Tel: 01543 373222 Fax: 01543 454640
(Walsall Teaching Primary Care Trust)
Patient List Size: 3850

Practice Manager Jackie Hopkins

GP Natwar Gopal PANSARI, Har Bhajan Singh MANGAT

Great Wyrley Health Centre
Landy Wood Lane Great Wyrley, Walsall WS6 6JX
Tel: 01922 414315 Fax: 01922 416016
(Cannock Chase Primary Care Trust)

Practice Manager Margaret Broome

GP K A DESAI

Health Centre
Wardles Lane, Great Wyrley, Walsall WS6 6EW
Tel: 01922 415515
(Cannock Chase Primary Care Trust)
Patient List Size: 3753

Practice Manager Kim Cyster

GP Elaine WILSON, T K CHIAM

Health Centre
Wardles Lane, Great Wyrley, Walsall WS6 6EW
Tel: 01922 411948 Fax: 01922 412994
(Cannock Chase Primary Care Trust)
Patient List Size: 2207

Practice Manager Tina Taylor

GP Arunbhai Bhagwanbhai PATEL

High Street Surgery
High Street, Pelsall, Walsall WS3 4LX
Tel: 01922 682450 Fax: 01922 682644
(Walsall Teaching Primary Care Trust)

Practice Manager Angela Bevan

GP William John BEVAN

High Street Surgery
High Street, Pelsall, Walsall WS3 4LX
Tel: 01922 694186 Fax: 01922 682644
(Walsall Teaching Primary Care Trust)
Patient List Size: 2365

Practice Manager Jane Robinson

GP Shamim Ibrahim SAMEJA

Lichfield Road Surgery
77 Lichfield Road, Walsall Wood, Walsall WS9 9NP
Tel: 01543 361452 Fax: 01543 454587
(Walsall Teaching Primary Care Trust)

Practice Manager Munns Margaret

GP Ravi Baburao LATTHE

Lichfield Street Surgery
19 Lichfield Street, Walsall WS1 1UG
Tel: 01922 20532 Fax: 01922 616605
(Walsall Teaching Primary Care Trust)
Patient List Size: 7281

Practice Manager Estelle Powell

GP Angela Kathleen HAIRE, Salim ISMAIL, Cormac DENIHAN, Anthony Winston NEWTON, Joo Ee TEOH

Limes Medical Centre
5 Birmingham Road, Walsall WS1 2LX
Tel: 01922 620303 Fax: 01922 649526
(Walsall Teaching Primary Care Trust)
Patient List Size: 7837

GP A MANDOHA, K CONOO, R JARRAMS, R MANDER

Longfellow Road Surgery
11 Longfellow Road, Boney Hay, Walsall WS7 8EY
Tel: 01543 674503
(Burntwood, Lichfield and Tamworth Primary Care Trust)

GP M S AHMAD

Lower Farm Health Centre
109 Buxton Road, Bloxwich, Walsall WS3 3RT
Tel: 01922 476640 Fax: 01922 491836
(Walsall Teaching Primary Care Trust)
Patient List Size: 2500

Practice Manager Katrina Walker

GP Taj Mohammad KHATTAK

Luqman Medical Centre
75 Countess Street, Walsall WS1 4JZ
Tel: 01922 621659 Fax: 01922 621702
(Walsall Teaching Primary Care Trust)
Patient List Size: 7000

Practice Manager S Thoams

GP Mirza Azher SIDDIQ, Fasihuddin AHMED, Dr SIKKHA

The Medical Centre
2a Southfield Way, Great Wyrley, Walsall WS6 6JZ
Tel: 01922 415151 Fax: 01922 415152
Email: ganeskuki@hotmail.com
(Cannock Chase Primary Care Trust)
Patient List Size: 2994

Practice Manager Jayanthi Kukathasan

GP Ganesharatnam KUKATHASAN

The Medical Centre
2a Southfield Way, Great Wyrley, Walsall WS6 6JZ
(Cannock Chase Primary Care Trust)

GP G KUKUTHASAN

The Nile Practice
Park Street, Off Station Street, Cheslyn Hay, Walsall WS6 7EF
Tel: 01922 413209 Fax: 019220 413 209
(Cannock Chase Primary Care Trust)
Patient List Size: 4979

Practice Manager Lynda Bradbury

GP H ZEIN-ELABDIN, A ONABOLU

Northgate Medical Centre
Anchor Meadow Health Centre, Aldridge, Walsall WS9 8AJ
Tel: 01922 450900 Fax: 01922 450910
(Walsall Teaching Primary Care Trust)

Practice Manager Glover Paul

GP David Martin HOSKISSON, Lynne ELLIS, Christine Elizabeth LLOYD, Arun Kumar SINGAL, Wilfrid Denys Edward WELLS

Pelsall Road Surgery
26/26a Pelsall Road, Brownhills, Walsall WS8 7JE
Fax: 01543 372066

GP V T V JOSE

Pinfold Health Centre
Field Road, Bloxwich, Walsall WS3 3JP
Fax: 01922 775132
(Walsall Teaching Primary Care Trust)

GP Roger THRUSH

Pinfold Health Centre
Field Road, Bloxwich, Walsall WS3 3JP
Fax: 01922 775132
(Walsall Teaching Primary Care Trust)

GP Thomas Francis DENT

Pinfold Health Centre
Field, Bloxwich, Walsall WS3 3JP
Fax: 01922 775132
(Walsall Teaching Primary Care Trust)

GP Richard Guy JARRAMS

Pinfold Health Centre
Field Road, Bloxwich, Walsall WS3 3JP
Fax: 01922 775132
(Walsall Teaching Primary Care Trust)

GP Debra Christina JOHNSON

Pinfold Health Centre
Field Road, Bloxwich, Walsall WS3 3JP
Fax: 01922 775132
(Walsall Teaching Primary Care Trust)

GP Arthur Richard THOMAS

Pinfold Health Centre
Field Road, Bloxwich, Walsall WS3 3JP
Fax: 01922 775132
(Walsall Teaching Primary Care Trust)

GP Paul Frederick LAKER

Pinfold Health Centre
Field Road, Bloxwich, Walsall WS3 3JP
Fax: 01922 775132
(Walsall Teaching Primary Care Trust)

GP S KRISHNA MURTHY

Pinfold Health Centre
Field Road, Bloxwich, Walsall WS3 3JP
Fax: 01922 775132
(Walsall Teaching Primary Care Trust)

GP R M SUNKARANENI

Pinfold Health Centre
Field Road, Bloxwich, Walsall WS3 3JP
Fax: 01922 775132
(Walsall Teaching Primary Care Trust)

GP Trevor Douglas COLEMAN

Pleck Health Centre
16 Oxford Street, Pleck, Walsall WS2 9HY
Tel: 01922 647660 Fax: 01922 629251
(Walsall Teaching Primary Care Trust)
Patient List Size: 10000

Practice Manager P Paw

GP Jayantilal Devji PAW, Dr GHOSH, Surendra Prasad SAHU, Murli SINHA

Portland Medical Practice
Anchor Meadow Health Centre, Aldridge, Walsall WS9 8AJ
Tel: 01922 450950 Fax: 01922 450960
(Walsall Teaching Primary Care Trust)

GP Colin Kerbotson FLENLEY, Julie Michelle HARRISON, Dr RUFFLES

Rushall Medical Centre
107 Lichfield Road, Rushall, Walsall WS4 1HB
Tel: 01922 622212 Fax: 01922 637015
(Walsall Teaching Primary Care Trust)
Patient List Size: 11000

Practice Manager John Brett

GP A G IRVINE, Andrea Donna Mary BLIGH, A H M GATRAD, Robin Nigel KELLY, Satvinder SANDILANDS, Joanna Patricia TURNER

Saddlers Medical Centre
133 Hatherton Street, Walsall WS1 1YB
Fax: 01922 33239
(Walsall Teaching Primary Care Trust)

GP O S MANOCHA, J P MATHIAS-DUBASH

Sai Medical Centre
Forrester Street Precinct, Walsall WS2 8RE
Tel: 01922 633817 Fax: 01922 614088
(Walsall Teaching Primary Care Trust)
Patient List Size: 3010

GP Kartik Chandra RAY

Salters Meadow Health Centre
Rugeley Road, Chase Terrace, Walsall WS7 8AQ
Tel: 01543 682611 Fax: 01543 675391
(Burntwood, Lichfield and Tamworth Primary Care Trust)

Practice Manager Linda Miller

GP John Malcolm WINTER, P J GREGORY, Gordon Trevor HADFIELD, Trevor OWEN, Bruce Alfred Norman READ, P M YOUNG

Sandwell Street Surgery
130 Sandwell Street, Walsall WS1 3EG
Tel: 01922 634598 Fax: 01922 32145
(Walsall Teaching Primary Care Trust)
Patient List Size: 3000

GP S THAWAIT

Shelfield Surgery
144 Lichfield Road, Shelfield, Walsall WS4 1PW
Fax: 01922 694069

GP Martyn Howard NORTON

Springhill Medical Centre
154 Cannock Road, Burntwood, Walsall WS7 0BG
Tel: 01543 684696
(Burntwood, Lichfield and Tamworth Primary Care Trust)

GP Pulkit Indravadan BHATT

St John's Medical Centre
High Street, Walsall Wood, Walsall WS9 9LP
Tel: 01543 364500 Fax: 01543 364510
(Walsall Teaching Primary Care Trust)

Practice Manager Angela C Timms

GP Stephen Thomas GREEN, Andrew Timothy ASKEY, Rashmi CHAUHAN, Michael Anthony EDWARDS, Anne PETERS

St Peter's Surgery
58 Leckie Road, Walsall WS2 8DA
Tel: 01922 623755 Fax: 01922 746477
(Walsall Teaching Primary Care Trust)

Practice Manager J A Emery

GP Diarmuid Patrick Joseph HOULAHAN, Martin Francis CROWTHER, Zofia Wanda NEEVES, Naresh TANDON

The Surgery
Little London, Caldmore, Walsall WS1 3EP
Tel: 01922 628280/622898 Fax: 01922 623023
(Walsall Teaching Primary Care Trust)
Patient List Size: 7905

GP Subhas Chandra SEN, Albert Emanuel BENJAMIN, Kevin HARRISON, Mo Sam Yan MO-SZU-TI

The Surgery
Abbey Square, Walsall WS3 2RH
Tel: 01922 408416 Fax: 01922 400372
(Walsall Teaching Primary Care Trust)

Practice Manager Angela Lyons

GP Abdul GHAFFAR, Dr RIFAT-GHAFFAR

The Surgery
79-81 Lichfield Road, Walsall Wood, Walsall WS9 9NP
Tel: 01543 377285 Fax: 01543 454004
(Walsall Teaching Primary Care Trust)
Patient List Size: 6630

GP Sujan Kumar KUNDU, G KUNDU, S K PAL

The Surgery
High Street, Cheslyn Hay, Walsall WS6 7AB
Tel: 01922 701280 Fax: 01922 701280
(Cannock Chase Primary Care Trust)
Patient List Size: 5691

Practice Manager Lynda Kirkham

GP Wykeham Andrew LOCHEE BAYNE, Antony Roger WEBB, Ian Joseph WELDING

The Surgery
New Road, Brownhills, Walsall WS8 6AT
Tel: 01543 373214 Fax: 01543 454591
(Walsall Teaching Primary Care Trust)
Patient List Size: 1845

Practice Manager Shyamala Rajeshwar

GP Kasam RAJESHWAR

The Surgery
Berkley Close, Bentley, Walsall WS2 0LG
Fax: 01922 637378
(Walsall Teaching Primary Care Trust)

GP C BAGCHI, Amrik Singh GILL

The Surgery
22 Maple Drive, Yew Tree Estate, Walsall WS5 4JJ
Tel: 01922 620961 Fax: 01922 637387
(Wednesbury and West Bromwich Primary Care Trust)

GP R GHATGE

Sycamore House Medical Centre
111 Birmingham Road, Walsall WS1 2NL
Tel: 01922 624320 Fax: 01922 646744
(Walsall Teaching Primary Care Trust)
Patient List Size: 3600

Practice Manager Irene Brown

GP Bryan FEHILLY, M N DUGAS, K PORTLOCK

Walker Road Surgery
168 Walker Road, Harden, Walsall WS3 1BZ
Tel: 01922 711578 Fax: 01922 403486
(Walsall Teaching Primary Care Trust)
Patient List Size: 3000

GP A J DESAI

Waltham Abbey

Abbey Surgery
36 Howard Business Park, Howard Close, Waltham Abbey EN9 1XE
Tel: 01992 715755 Fax: 01992 716537
(South East Hertfordshire Primary Care Trust)
Patient List Size: 6200

Practice Manager Christine Adkins

GP Kalpana MISRA, Dr CHANDAK, Dev Raj SAHNI

Maynard Court Surgery
17-18 Maynard Court, Waltham Abbey EN9 3DU
Tel: 01992 761387 Fax: 01992 716163
(Epping Forest Primary Care Trust)

GP Bharat Bhushan BERRY, P KANDASAMY

Medical Centre
Greenyard, Waltham Abbey EN9 1RD
Tel: 01992 714088 Fax: 01992 763866
(Epping Forest Primary Care Trust)
Patient List Size: 2505

Practice Manager Jean Lawrence

GP Frederick Edward PYMONT

Old Society House Surgery
Church Street, Waltham Abbey EN9 1DX
Tel: 01992 719000 Fax: 01992 788457
(Epping Forest Primary Care Trust)

Practice Manager Mrs David-John

GP C DAVID-JOHN

Sun Street Surgery
34 Sun Street, Waltham Abbey EN9 1EJ
Tel: 01992 718711 Fax: 01992 788943
(Epping Forest Primary Care Trust)

Practice Manager P White

GP Amirali Gulamhusein Nassar LAKHA

The Surgery
61 Farmhill Road, Waltham Abbey EN9 1NG
Tel: 01992 713891 Fax: 01992 714278
(Epping Forest Primary Care Trust)
Patient List Size: 1700

Practice Manager Dawn Alison

GP A NZEWI

Waltham Cross

Abbey Road Surgery
63 Abbey Road, Waltham Cross EN8 7LJ
Tel: 01992 762082 Fax: 01992 717746
(South East Hertfordshire Primary Care Trust)
Patient List Size: 9300

Practice Manager Jayne Wells

GP Robin James HODGE, Lisa J ELLIS, William Thomas NEVILLE, Kelvyn PEYSNER, Ana Maria STUTTARD

Cromwell Medical Centre
11-11A Cromwell Avenue, Cheshunt, Waltham Cross EN7 5DL
Tel: 01992 624732 Fax: 01992 625401
(South East Hertfordshire Primary Care Trust)

Practice Manager Faisal Ijaz

GP Ahmad Tunveer NAQVI, N SENGUPTA, S V SINGH

Crossbrook Street Surgery
126 Crossbrook Street, Cheshunt, Waltham Cross EN8 8JH
Tel: 01992 622908 Fax: 01992 624756
(South East Hertfordshire Primary Care Trust)
Patient List Size: 9000

Practice Manager Catherine Church

GP Isabel Jean KING, Vivienne Elizabeth EMMETT, Entesar HADAD, Olusola Benjamin ISINKAYE, Dr JACKSON, D ROBERTS

High Street Surgery
13-15 High Street, Cheshunt, Waltham Cross EN8 0BX
Tel: 01992 642446 Fax: 01992 631777
(South East Hertfordshire Primary Care Trust)
Patient List Size: 6400

Practice Manager Christine Adkins

GP Kalpana MISRA, B CHANDAK, Dev Raj SAHNI

Stanhope Surgery
Stanhope Road, Waltham Cross EN8 7DJ
Tel: 01992 635300 Fax: 01992 624292
(South East Hertfordshire Primary Care Trust)
Patient List Size: 5100

Practice Manager Toulia Trupia

GP Kanval Kant NAGPAL, Mohammed HOSSAIN, Paul Richard WEADICK

Stockwell Lodge Medical Centre
Rosedale Way, Cheshunt, Waltham Cross EN7 6QQ
Tel: 01992 624408 Fax: 01992 626206
(South East Hertfordshire Primary Care Trust)
Patient List Size: 16300

Practice Manager G Clarke

GP John Clifford CONWAY, Chuba CHIGBO, Angela Margaret DAVIES, Marek DOBROWOLSKI, Lena QUIST-THERSON, Navina SULLIVAN

Warden Lodge Surgery
Albury Ride, Cheshunt, Waltham Cross EN8 8XE
Tel: 01992 622324 Fax: 01992 636900
(South East Hertfordshire Primary Care Trust)

Practice Manager Anne Barrett

GP Angela Mary GOODWIN, Alison BLAKELEY, Melvin JONES, Joanne SOUTHERTON, Lisa STEEN, Diana WOOD

Walton-on-Thames

Ashley Medical Practice
1A Crutchfield Lane, Walton-on-Thames KT12 1LF
Tel: 01932 252425 Fax: 01932 886912
Email: ashmed@bigfoot.com
Website: www.ashmed.co.uk
(North Surrey Primary Care Trust)
Patient List Size: 2360

Practice Manager Tracy Lewis

GP Layth DELAIMY

Fort House Surgery
32 Hersham Road, Walton-on-Thames KT12 1UX
Tel: 01932 253055 Fax: 01932 225910
(North Surrey Primary Care Trust)
Patient List Size: 6500

Practice Manager Liz Reynolds

GP David Malcolm RATCLIFFE, Hilary AUDSLEY, Kalpee MALDE, Richard REDFERN

The Health Centre
Rodney Road, Walton-on-Thames KT12 3LB
Tel: 01932 228999 Fax: 01932 225586
(North Surrey Primary Care Trust)
Patient List Size: 3800

GP Erle Rodney LITTLEWOOD, Gaynor Elizabeth LEWIS

The Health Centre
Rodney Road, Walton-on-Thames KT12 3LB
Tel: 01932 228999 Fax: 01932 225586
(North Surrey Primary Care Trust)

GP L GIBSON

The Surgery
Pleasant Place, Hersham, Walton-on-Thames KT12 4HT
Tel: 01932 229033 Fax: 01932 254706
(North Surrey Primary Care Trust)
Patient List Size: 8000

Practice Manager K Harvey

GP Christopher Charles NOON, Paul Jasper DANCE, Deepak DESOR, Susan FOTHERGILL

Walton Health Centre
Rodney Road, Walton-on-Thames KT12 3LB
Tel: 01932 228999 Fax: 01932 225586
(North Surrey Primary Care Trust)

GP Peter Frederick ARNOLD, Suzanne Jane BOWSKILL, Jennifer Mabel SILLICK, Adam SURMAN, Helen Victoria TILLY

Walton Health Centre
Rodney Road, Walton-on-Thames KT12 3LB
Tel: 01932 228999 Fax: 01932 225586
Email: waltonhealth@waltonhealth.idps.co.uk
(North Surrey Primary Care Trust)
Patient List Size: 4837

Practice Manager Lorraine Chandler

GP Peter Owen MEECHAN, Dzung Manh NGUYEN

Walton on the Naze

The Surgery
Vicarage Lane, Walton on the Naze CO14 8PA
Tel: 01255 674373 Fax: 01255 851005
(Tendring Primary Care Trust)
Patient List Size: 9060

Practice Manager Martin Durrand

GP Jonathan Andrew Frederick GELDARD, Charles Lee Michael BEARDMORE, Gregory Guy Randall GOUNDRY, Nigel David King ROPER, Joanne Helen THOMPSON

Wantage

Grove Medical Centre
3 Vale Avenue, Grove, Wantage OX12 7LU
Tel: 01235 770140 Fax: 01235 760027
(South West Oxfordshire Primary Care Trust)
Patient List Size: 4648

Practice Manager Ann Scott

GP David Graham Denham WISE, Andrew William Douglas ALLEN

Newbury Street Practice
The Health Centre, Mabey Way, Wantage OX12 9BN
Tel: 01235 763451 Fax: 01235 771829
Email: sandy.fisken@gp-kb4019.nhs.uk
Website: www.newburystreetpractice.co.uk
(South West Oxfordshire Primary Care Trust)
Patient List Size: 10300

Practice Manager Alexander Fiskin

GP Peter David KYLE, Jo BRODIE, George Andrew DINNIS, Patricia HEAKINS, John Charles ROBINSON, Sarah Caroline SHACKLETON, Frances WATT

Wantage Health Centre
Church Street, Wantage OX12 7AY
Tel: 01235 770245 Fax: 01235 770727
(South West Oxfordshire Primary Care Trust)

Practice Manager Helen Toms

GP Celia Margaret Lila TEARE, Phillip John AMBLER, Eleanor Joy ARTHUR, Paul Lancelot Dominic BRYAN, Victor Mark DRURY, Rickman James Philip GODLEE

Ware

Church Street Surgery
St Mary's Courtyard, Church Street, Ware SG12 9EF
Tel: 01920 468941 Fax: 01920 465531
(South East Hertfordshire Primary Care Trust)

Practice Manager Janice Seymour

GP Ian Howard BRIDGES, Stephen Harvey GIBSON, Debra GILBERT, Stephen Clive HARRIS, Nicolette WILLIAMS, Janet Margaret Seivwright YOUNG

Dolphin House Surgery
6-7 East Street, Ware SG12 9HJ
Tel: 01920 468777 Fax: 01920 484892
(South East Hertfordshire Primary Care Trust)
Patient List Size: 8900

Practice Manager John Thompson

GP Michael William John BAVERSTOCK, Martyn Watkin DAVIES, David John MADDAMS, Ruth Esther MORGAN, Jane Christine WATSON

Health Centre
Station Road, Puckeridge, Ware SG11 1TF
Tel: 01920 821404 Fax: 01920 821538
(South East Hertfordshire Primary Care Trust)
Patient List Size: 7300

Practice Manager Geoff Kemp

GP Timothy Henry REYNOLDS, J FOSTER, Michael James PARTINGTON

The Maltings Surgery
15 Amwell End, Ware SG12 9HP
Tel: 01920 469977 Fax: 01920 484619
(South East Hertfordshire Primary Care Trust)
Patient List Size: 2971

Practice Manager Penny Coggan

GP Wimala CHANDRASEGARAM

Wareham

Corfe Castle Surgery
East Street, Corfe Caste, Wareham BH20 5EE
Tel: 01929 480441 Fax: 01929 480804
(South and East Dorset Primary Care Trust)

Practice Manager J E Ingarfield

GP Dr HORSNELL

Sandford Surgery
Tyneham Close, Sandford, Wareham BH20 7BQ
Tel: 01929 554493 Fax: 01929 550661
(South and East Dorset Primary Care Trust)

Practice Manager Mary Barber

GP Timothy Stewart BROWN, Anne Margaret BROWN

The Surgery
Manor Farm Road, Bere Regis, Wareham BH20 7HB
Tel: 01929 471268 Fax: 01929 472098
(South and East Dorset Primary Care Trust)
Patient List Size: 3631

Practice Manager Wendy Nelson

GP Raymond Michael GREENFIELD, Timothy Gerald HARLEY, A L SALTER

Wareham Surgery
Streche Road, Wareham BH20 4PG
Tel: 01929 553444 Fax: 01929 550703
(South and East Dorset Primary Care Trust)

Practice Manager B C Vane

GP James Richard BENNETT, Carolyn Tracy CRICKMORE, Alastair McPHAIL, James RICHARD, Alastair WARD, Mark Gill WILLIAMS

Wool Surgery
Folly Lane, Wool, Wareham BH20 6DS
Tel: 01929 462376
(South and East Dorset Primary Care Trust)
Patient List Size: 5350

Practice Manager Jan Burt

GP Christopher Sidney IRWIN, Allison FRENCH, Nicholas Twyford LYONS, Richard MUGFORD, Christian VERRINDER

Warley

Church View Surgery
239 Halesowen Road, Cradley Heath, Warley B64 6JE
Tel: 01384 566929 Fax: 01384 561923
(Rowley Regis and Tipton Primary Care Trust)

GP M R EVELEIGH, S R GRAY, N M HARTE

Cradley Road Surgery
62 Cradley Road, Cradley Heath, Warley B64 6AG
Tel: 01382 569586
(Dudley South Primary Care Trust)

GP Stanley Trevor BLOXHAM, Frank William JONES, G A MUIR, D NEALE, Stella Matilda PINTO

Haden Road Surgery
8 Haden Road, Cradley Heath, Warley B64 6ER
Tel: 01384 466479 Fax: 01384 566836
(Rowley Regis and Tipton Primary Care Trust)

GP Alfred Beresford ABAYOMI-COLE

Haden Vale Surgery
Barrs Road, Cradley Heath, Warley B64 7HG
Tel: 01384 634511 Fax: 01384 410716
Website: www.hadenvale.org
(Rowley Regis and Tipton Primary Care Trust)

Practice Manager Nicola Bendall

GP D W MUTHUVELOE, L MUTHUVELOE

Hawthorns Medical Centre
94 Lewisham Road, Smethwick, Warley B66 2DD
Tel: 0121 555 5635 Fax: 0121 565 0293
(Oldbury and Smethwick Primary Care Trust)
Patient List Size: 4300

Practice Manager Yvonne Edwards

GP Kazi Ataur RAHMAN, M ALAM, C P DUNN

Holly Lane Clinic
Holly Lane, Smethwick, Warley B66 1QW
Tel: 0121 558 5117 Fax: 0121 555 6938
(South Warwickshire Primary Care Trust)
Patient List Size: 1500

Practice Manager Diane Crump

GP Eric HARRIS

Regis Medical Centre
Darby Street, Rowley Regis, Warley B65 0BA
Tel: 0121 559 3957 Fax: 0121 502 9117
(Rowley Regis and Tipton Primary Care Trust)

Practice Manager J M Pilipenko

GP Walter Rostron PRICE, Christopher John BALL, David John Fitzroy COLLIER, Virginia Margaret CORNISH, Rebecca A GIBBS, David Gilmour HAMILTON, J E LENNIE, Simon Keith MITCHELL

The Smethwick Medical Centre
Regent Street, Smethwick, Warley B66 3BQ
Tel: 0121 558 0105 Fax: 0121 555 7206
(Oldbury and Smethwick Primary Care Trust)
Patient List Size: 9500

Practice Manager Sandra Such

GP Krishna Kumar SRIVASTAVA, Peter Lindsay GIBSON, Mina GUPTA, Navnit Kaur PALL, Jacquelyn SHARP, Frauke WONG, Isabella Noble YOUNG

The Surgery
153 Bearwood Road, Smethwick, Warley B66 4LN
Tel: 0121 558 1840 Fax: 0121 565 0422
(Oldbury and Smethwick Primary Care Trust)

Practice Manager Freda Hudson

GP Jyoti AHUJA, Devendra K AHUJA

The Surgery
Lodge Road, Smethwick, Warley B67 7LU
Tel: 0121 558 0499 Fax: 0121 555 5348
(Oldbury and Smethwick Primary Care Trust)
Patient List Size: 5000

Practice Manager Margaret Thomas

GP Viney Kumar JHANJEE

The Surgery
348 Bearwood Road, Smethwick, Warley B66 4ES
Tel: 0121 429 1345 Fax: 0121 429 2535
(Oldbury and Smethwick Primary Care Trust)

Practice Manager Catherine McCleod

GP Yahiya IQBAL, Syed Muhammad ANWAR-FARID, Kanjana PARAMANATHAN

Victoria Health Centre
5 Suffrage Street, Smethwick, Warley B66 3PZ
Tel: 0121 558 0216 Fax: 0121 558 4732
(Oldbury and Smethwick Primary Care Trust)
Patient List Size: 8200

Practice Manager Lynne George

GP Faheem A KHAN, Mirza Mohammed Abid BAIG, David Anthony HARRINGTON, Kathleen Elizabeth ROBERTS, Paul Tong Yin WONG

Whiteheath Clinic
Hartlebury Road, Oldbury, Warley B69 1BG
Tel: 0121 552 2353 Fax: 0121 544 2232
(Rowley Regis and Tipton Primary Care Trust)
Patient List Size: 7100

Practice Manager Ray Wood

GP Prakashkumar Manubhai DESAI, Bhasker SHARMA

Warlingham

Church Road Surgery
Crossmount, 1 Church Road, Warlingham CR6 9NW
Tel: 01883 624686 Fax: 01883 625677
(East Surrey Primary Care Trust)
Patient List Size: 2500

Practice Manager Margaret Wilkinson

GP David BECKITT, Alex TROMPETAS

Hamsey Green Surgery
85A Limpsfield Road, Warlingham CR6 9RH
Tel: 01883 625022
(East Surrey Primary Care Trust)

GP Catherine Joyce TARRANT

Limpsfield Road Surgery
515 Limpsfield Road, Warlingham CR6 9LF
Tel: 01883 265262 Fax: 01883 627893
(East Surrey Primary Care Trust)

GP Philip Charles Vincent RAMAGE, Derrick Andrew HINKES

Warminster

The Avenue Surgery Partnership
14 The Avenue, Warminster BA12 9AA
Tel: 01985 224600 Fax: 01985 847059
Website: www.avanuesurgery.co.uk
(West Wiltshire Primary Care Trust)
Patient List Size: 20000

GP Alan GREENWOOD, Rebecca AUSTIN, Reva BULLEN, Oran Isabel Mary COREY, David James LITTLE, Kevin Niels McBRIDE, Vivian John Rodier STEVENS, Caroline Ann WINGFIELD

Cherry Orchard Surgery
Codford St Mary, Warminster BA12 0PN
Tel: 01985 850298
(South Wiltshire Primary Care Trust)

Practice Manager Michael Cooney

GP A J HALL, John FISHWICK, Sarah Rebecca Anne HOUGHTON

Mere Surgery
Dark Lane, Mere, Warminster BA12 6DT
Tel: 01747 860001 Fax: 01747 860119
(South Wiltshire Primary Care Trust)
Patient List Size: 4079

Practice Manager M E Honnywill

GP William James Pembroke PRICE, Isabel ANDREWS, Eve McBRIDE

Smallbrook Surgery
48 Boreham Road, Warminster BA12 9JR
Tel: 01985 846700 Fax: 01985 846700
(West Wiltshire Primary Care Trust)

GP Mark Adrian THORPE, Carol Ann SHEPPARD

Warrington

Appleton Primary Care
43-45 Dudlow Green Road, Appleton, Warrington WA4 5EQ
Tel: 01925 600068
(Warrington Primary Care Trust)

Practice Manager Helen Billson

GP Aida MIKHAIL, Richard Neil Ashley WOOD

Bewsey Street Medical Centre
40-42 Bewsey Street, Warrington WA2 7JE
Tel: 01925 635837 Fax: 01925 630353
(Warrington Primary Care Trust)
Patient List Size: 5790

Practice Manager Lorraine Stratulis

GP Peter John BANYARD, Susan Lesley BURKE, Anthony Joseph RIMMER

Birchwood Medical Centre
15 Benson Road, Birchwood, Warrington WA3 7PJ
Tel: 01925 823502 Fax: 01925 852422
(Warrington Primary Care Trust)
Patient List Size: 12000

Practice Manager Kath Longden

GP Anthony Michael DIXON, N MADAN, H O'SHEA, Anthony Keiron PATINIOTT, Francis PATINOTT, Simon William REDFEARN, David Andrew ROYLE

The Bold Street Medical Centre
25-29 Bold Street, Warrington WA1 1HH
Tel: 01925 244655 Fax: 01925 241855
(Warrington Primary Care Trust)
Patient List Size: 2132

Practice Manager Leela Kumaraswamy

GP Sri Pathmajothy KUMARASWAMY

Causeway Medical Centre
166-170 Wilderspool Causeway, Warrington WA4 6QA
Tel: 01925 635024/630282 Fax: 01925 655113
(Warrington Primary Care Trust)
Patient List Size: 5600

Practice Manager Jean Evans

GP V R HANUMANTHU, Roisin COLQUHOUN, Yvonne DOUGLAS

Chapelford Primary Health Care Centre
Burtonwood Road, Gt Sankey, Warrington WA5 3AN
Tel: 01925 574165 Fax: 01925 576048
(Warrington Primary Care Trust)

Practice Manager Sue Bloomfield

GP Dr DOWNES

Culcheth Practice
466 & 472 Warrington Road, Culcheth, Warrington WA3 5QX
Tel: 01925 765349 Fax: 01925 767118
(Warrington Primary Care Trust)
Patient List Size: 2000

Practice Manager Lynda Kennedy

GP G P SCOTT

Culcheth Surgery
Thompson Avenue, Culcheth, Warrington WA3 4EB
Tel: 01925 765101 Fax: 01925 765102
(Warrington Primary Care Trust)
Patient List Size: 6022

Practice Manager Helen Philbin

GP Lena BASMA, N D FISHER, G S GHAZAWY, Thomas TENNENT

Davis and Partners
274 Manchester Road, Warrington WA1 4PS
Tel: 01925 631132 Fax: 01925 630079
(Warrington Primary Care Trust)
Patient List Size: 9633

Practice Manager Pauline Millington

GP Paul Anthony DAVIS, Judith Ann BOOTH, Andrew Stuart DAVIES, Jane Margaret LEACH, Philippa ROY, David George TRENCHARD

Dennis and Partners
The Medical Centre, Folly Lane, Bewsey, Warrington WA5 0LU
Tel: 01925 417247 Fax: 01925 444319
(Warrington Primary Care Trust)
Patient List Size: 9789

Practice Manager John Rainford

GP Michael William DENNIS, Dale Antony COX, Rebecca LEECH, William Gordon MILLER, Elizabeth Anne PLUMB, Malcolm TYRER

Eric Moore Health Centre
Tanners lane, Warrington WA2 7LY
Tel: 01925 417252 Fax: 01925 417729
(Warrington Primary Care Trust)
Patient List Size: 3470

Practice Manager Eileen Walker

GP Tayyaba Tasnim AWAN, Malpica Gontad MALPICA

Eric Moore Partnership
Eric Moore Health Centre, 1 Tanners Lane, Warrington WA2 7LY
Tel: 01925 417248/411210/244225/650771 Fax: 01925 632868
Email: julie.mccann@gp-N81628.nhs.uk
(Warrington Primary Care Trust)
Patient List Size: 6600

Practice Manager Julie McCann

GP Chellatturai PARANJOTHY, A S RAJKUMAR, M NORONHA, C PARANJOTHY

Family Medical Practice
98 High Street, Golborne, Warrington WA3 3DA
Tel: 01942 272737 Fax: 01942 273321
Email: reception@gp-p92639.nhs.uk
(Ashton, Leigh and Wigan Primary Care Trust)

Practice Manager May Barker

GP Abid SHAHBAZI

Four Seasons Medical Centre
Orford Clinic, Capesthrone Road, Orford, Warrington WA2 9AR
Tel: 01925 419784 Fax: 01925 234221
(Warrington Primary Care Trust)
Patient List Size: 1687

Practice Manager Cheryl Owen

GP A D MALKHANDI

Guardian Street Medical Centre
Guardian Street, Warrington WA5 1UD
Tel: 01925 650226 Fax: 01925 240633
(Warrington Primary Care Trust)
Patient List Size: 8546

Practice Manager Brenda Smith

GP Graham Douglas SMITH, Catharine HYLAND, Margaret Anne KERR, Michael D THOMAS, Ian Stuart WILSON

Helsby Health Centre
Lower Robin Hood Lane, Helsby, Warrington WA6 0BW
Tel: 01928 723676 Fax: 01928 725677
(Cheshire West Primary Care Trust)

Practice Manager Chris Ashbrook

GP Teresa ADAIR, Richard BROOK, Elizabeth Marguerite AGNEW, Branwen Anne MARTIN, Samuel Peter SMITH

Helsby Street Medical Centre
2 Helsby Street, Warrington WA1 3AW
Tel: 01925 637304 Fax: 01925 570430
(Warrington Primary Care Trust)
Patient List Size: 8750

Practice Manager Jane Coulson

GP Richard Thomas JOHNSON, Sarah DIXON, Matthew PETCH, Alan Samuel Gregory PLATTS, David Allan STORRAR

Jackson Avenue Health Centre
Jackson Avenue, Culcheth, Warrington WA3 4DZ
Tel: 01925 763077
(Warrington Primary Care Trust)

Practice Manager Caroline O'Loan

GP John O'LOAN

Jarvis and Partners
Westbrook Medical Centre, 301-302 Westbrook Centre, Westbrook, Warrington WA5 8UF
Tel: 01925 654152 Fax: 01925 632612
(Warrington Primary Care Trust)
Patient List Size: 10400

Practice Manager Maureen Marsden

GP Simon James Fenwick JARVIS, Andrew Nigel BEARE-WINTER, Mary COUGHLIN, Alison Clare RITTER, Steven Michael WINTER

John Street Medical Centre
John Street, Golborne, Warrington WA3 3AS
Tel: 01942 729009 Fax: 01942 270903
(Ashton, Leigh and Wigan Primary Care Trust)

Practice Manager Valerie Dean

GP Abubaker ANIS, Yasmin Farzana ANIS

The Knoll Surgery
46 High Street, Frodsham, Warrington WA6 7HF
Tel: 01928 733249 Fax: 01928 739367
(Cheshire West Primary Care Trust)
Patient List Size: 11600

Practice Manager Barry W Jobber

GP John Edward LENEGHAN, Iola COLEMAN-SMITH, Heather Patricia HATT, Patrick John Murray MILROY, Steven Mark POMFRET, D STANAWAY

Lakeside Surgery
Lakeside Road, Lymm, Warrington WA13 0QE
Tel: 01925 755050
(Warrington Primary Care Trust)
Patient List Size: 8000

Practice Manager Jane Peers

GP Gordon Newman MILLS, David William PARKINSON, Susan Christine LYNCH

Latchford Medical Centre
5 Thelwall Lane, Latchford, Warrington WA4 1LJ
Tel: 01925 637508 Fax: 01925 654384
(Warrington Primary Care Trust)
Patient List Size: 4980

Practice Manager Jenny Hawthorne

GP C P M ALI, Max LEVY, Elspeth Alice MACKIN

Manchester Road Surgery
280 Manchester Road, Warrington WA1 3RB
Tel: 01925 230022 Fax: 01925 575069
(Warrington Primary Care Trust)

Practice Manager Pamela Peers

GP Janet Elizabeth NAPIER, John William BRASSILL, Jean Lindsay Lyle CROTON, L SAEID, Jade TRAVERS

O'Colmain and Partners
Fearnhead Cross Medical Centre, 25 Fearnhead Cross, Fearnhead, Warrington WA2 0HD
Tel: 01925 847000 Fax: 01925 818650
(Warrington Primary Care Trust)
Patient List Size: 13000

Practice Manager Maggie Bowen

GP Brendan Paul O'COLMAIN, David Joseph CARR, Valerie Margaret HORTON, Jasminder Singh SOKHI, Edmund TAYLOR, David John WALTON, Ian Norman WATSON

O'Leary Street Surgery
4 O'Leary Street, Warrington WA2 7RH
Tel: 01925 571640/634994 Fax: 01925 634297
(Warrington Primary Care Trust)

Patient List Size: 5600

GP C SHOME, M BHATNAGAR

Padgate Medical Centre
12 Station Road South, Padgate, Warrington WA2 0RX
Tel: 01925 815333 Fax: 01925 813650
(Warrington Primary Care Trust)
Patient List Size: 6200

Practice Manager Kate Broadbent

GP Philip Arthur REYNOLDS, Jonathan CLARKE, Elizabeth Anne ILES, Joanne Ruth Sarah McCORMACK, Louise Elizabeth NAPIER-HEMY

Penketh Health Centre
Honiton Way, Penketh, Warrington WA5 2EY
Tel: 01925 725644 Fax: 01925 791017
Email: general.enquiries@gp-N81020.nhs.uk
Website: www.penkethhealthcentre.co.uk
(Warrington Primary Care Trust)
Patient List Size: 15900

Practice Manager Pat Tavender

GP Harish Prasad TANDON, John Joseph Edward BANNON, Vijay Kumar BANSAL, Susan Jane CURETON, Robert KNILL, Jayne Angela PALIN, Colin Thomas PRIESTLEY, Mark RATHE

The Rock Surgery
50 High Street, Frodsham, Warrington WA6 7HG
Tel: 01928 732110 Fax: 01928 739273
(Cheshire West Primary Care Trust)
Patient List Size: 6156

Practice Manager Pauline A Sweeney

GP Richard John ADAIR, Helen ASTERIADES, Simon Jay HALL, Kathy RYAN

Slag Lane Medical Centre
John Street Medical Centre, Golborne, Warrington WA3 3AS
Tel: 01942 729009
(Ashton, Leigh and Wigan Primary Care Trust)

Practice Manager Parel Sarker

GP Dr BAJAJ

Stockton Heath Medical Centre
The Forge, London Road, Stockton Heath, Warrington WA4 6HJ
Tel: 01925 604427 Fax: 01925 210501
Email: general.enquiries@gp-N81075.nhs.uk
Website: www.stocktonhealthmedicalcentre.co.uk
(Warrington Primary Care Trust)
Patient List Size: 16300

Practice Manager Barbara West

GP Trevor GOODWIN, June Daphne HUNTER, Ashvinderjit AHULWAHA, Richard BROOKS, Clive Anthony Martin FREEMAN, Justin Peter MCCARTHY, Graham Robert PALMER, Menna REES, Janet Elizabeth STOTT

Stretton Medical Centre
5 Hatton Lane, Stretton, Warrington WA4 4NE
Tel: 01925 730412 Fax: 01925 730960
(Warrington Primary Care Trust)
Patient List Size: 3300

Practice Manager Ann Pass

GP Subbiah SATHIYASEELAN, V LETCHUMANAN

The Surgery
28 Holes Lane, Woolston, Warrington WA1 4NE
Tel: 01925 653218 Fax: 01925 244767
(Warrington Primary Care Trust)
Patient List Size: 11200

Practice Manager Janet Tomlin

GP Anthony John BATES, T A ASHTON, Ernest Patrick FRANCIS, Norma May ICETON, L UMNUS, Mark Ronald WADSWORTH

The Surgery
36 Braithwaite Road, Lowton, Warrington WA3 2HY
Tel: 01942 718221 Fax: 01942 728834
(Ashton, Leigh and Wigan Primary Care Trust)
Patient List Size: 5700

Practice Manager Jeff Villiers

GP V KADIYALA, Dr NARASIMHACHARLU

The Surgery
213 Slag Lane, Lowton, Warrington WA3 2EZ
(Ashton, Leigh and Wigan Primary Care Trust)

Practice Manager Margaret Riley

GP V BAJAJ

The Surgery
230C Newton Road, Lowton, Warrington WA3 2AD
Tel: 01942 605135 Fax: 01942 680593
(Ashton, Leigh and Wigan Primary Care Trust)
Patient List Size: 6500

Practice Manager I Notton

GP Dr XAVIER

The Surgery
107 High Street, Golborne, Warrington WA3 3BZ
Tel: 01942 270524 Fax: 01942 276100
(Ashton, Leigh and Wigan Primary Care Trust)
Patient List Size: 4000

GP D PAL, M PAL

Warwick

Budbrooke Medical Centre
Slade Hill, Hampton Magna, Warwick CV35 8SA
Tel: 01926 403881 Fax: 01926 403855
(South Warwickshire Primary Care Trust)
Patient List Size: 3790

GP Henry Gordon WHITE, June Shazeela Shanaaz ALLIM

Cape Road Surgery
3 Cape Road, Warwick CV34 4JP
Tel: 01926 499988 Fax: 01926 498956
(South Warwickshire Primary Care Trust)
Patient List Size: 4300

GP Richard William MEADEN, Sarah Jane INCHLEY

Hastings House
Kineton Road, Wellesbourne, Warwick CV35 9NF
Tel: 01789 840245 Fax: 01789 470993
(South Warwickshire Primary Care Trust)
Patient List Size: 10480

Practice Manager Maureen Buckle

GP Henry MEADOWS, Stephen Howard DESBOROUGH, Joanna Robson DOWELL, Helen Jane GUNTON, Ian Philip KILLEEN, David Somers RIVERS, Martin WHITTAKER

Kineton Surgery
The Old School, Market Square, Kineton, Warwick CV35 0LP
Tel: 01926 640471 Fax: 01926 640390
(South Warwickshire Primary Care Trust)
Patient List Size: 4000

Practice Manager Helen Mason

GP John WOODWARD, Frances DAVIES, Richard Philip MELTON

The Old Dispensary
8 Castle Street, Warwick CV34 4BP
Tel: 01926 494137 Fax: 01926 410348
(South Warwickshire Primary Care Trust)
Patient List Size: 4800

Practice Manager Christine Rogers

GP Stephen George CLARKSON, Barbara Anne HARLAND, Jacqueline Anne HATTON

Priory Medical Centre Partnership
Cape Road, Warwick CV34 4UN
Tel: 01926 494411 Fax: 01926 402394
(South Warwickshire Primary Care Trust)
Patient List Size: 12800

Practice Manager Yvonne Yates

GP Martin Charles Lainé LE TOCQ, Tajinder Singh BHANDAL, Mark Jolyon BOX, Catherine Mary DALLAWAY, Claire LEWIS, Susan Jennifer MARTIN, Hank MULDER, Dilys O'DRISCOLL

The Surgery
Station Road, Claverdon, Warwick CV35 8PH
Tel: 01926 842205 Fax: 01926 843467
(South Warwickshire Primary Care Trust)

GP Gillian Ruth LEYLAND, J E ALLISTON, D M BUCKLEY, W J FITCHFORD, M D GILL, J GOWANS, J A JONES, M POPPLEWELL

Warwick Gates Family Health Centre
Cressida Close, Heathcote, Warwick CV34 6DZ
Tel: 01926 461800 Fax: 01926 461803
Email: surgery@warwickgates.co.uk
(South Warwickshire Primary Care Trust)
Patient List Size: 5858

GP Francis CAMPBELL, Andrew Gerard KENNEDY, Moira ROSE, Josie SWINDEN

Washington

Barmston Medical Centre
Westerhope Road, Barmston, Washington NE38 8JF
Tel: 0191 419 0333 Fax: 0191 419 0444
(Sunderland Teaching Primary Care Trust)
Patient List Size: 5204

Practice Manager Sue Carmody

GP Nayan Arvindbhhai NANAVATI, Kamalakar Narayanrao YELNOORKAR

Galleries Health Centre
Washington Centre, Washington NE38 7NQ
Tel: 0191 416 1841 Fax: 0191 417 0531
(Sunderland Teaching Primary Care Trust)
Patient List Size: 5918

Practice Manager Gillian Webster

GP Bipin Ramaniklat VAKHARIA, Ayitha Kumar Kodyadke HEGDE

Galleries Health Centre
Encompass Health Care, Washington Centre, Washington NE38 7NQ
Tel: 0191 416 6130 Fax: 0191 416 6344
(Sunderland Teaching Primary Care Trust)
Patient List Size: 3535

Practice Manager Doreen Galloway, M Warden

GP Dr LISTEN

Galleries Health Centre
Washington Centre, Washington NE38 7NQ
Tel: 0191 416 7032
(Sunderland Teaching Primary Care Trust)
Patient List Size: 5000

Practice Manager Susan Carmody

GP Nayan A NANAVATI, Jane PETERSEN, Kamalakar YELNOORKAR

Harraton Surgery
3 Swiss Cottages, Vigo Lane, Harraton, Washington NE38 9AB
Tel: 0191 416 1641 Fax: 0191 415 7753
(Sunderland Teaching Primary Care Trust)
Patient List Size: 2606

Practice Manager Elaine Rose

GP Kannankara Mathew THOMAS

Rickleton Medical Centre
Vigo Lane, Rickleton, Washington NE38 9EH
Tel: 0191 415 0576 Fax: 0191 416 6286
(Sunderland Teaching Primary Care Trust)
Patient List Size: 2120

Practice Manager Auriel Blair

GP Nibedita NANDA

Victoria Road Health Centre
Victoria Road, Washington NE37 2PU
Tel: 0191 416 2578 Fax: 0191 416 6091
(Sunderland Teaching Primary Care Trust)
Patient List Size: 12348

Practice Manager Kim Hair

GP Geoffrey STEPHENSON, Emile Alexander BRANDES, J LEIGH, Dr SWINBURNE

Victoria Road Health Centre
Victoria Road, Washington NE37 2PU
Tel: 0191 415 4477 Fax: 0191 417 7500
(Sunderland Teaching Primary Care Trust)
Patient List Size: 2842

Practice Manager Anita Sykes

GP K SARAVANAMATTU

Victoria Road Health Centre
Victoria Road, Washington NE37 2PU
Tel: 0191 417 3557 Fax: 0191 415 7382
(Sunderland Teaching Primary Care Trust)
Patient List Size: 5673

Practice Manager Robert Douglas

GP Joseph Orlando MAZARELO, Dr DEWAN, Dr FAIRS, Dr SEN

Victoria Road Health Centre
Victoria Road, Washington NE37 2PU
Tel: 0191 416 8567 Fax: 0191 416 6274
(Sunderland Teaching Primary Care Trust)
Patient List Size: 2324

Practice Manager Trish O'Brien

GP C V BHATT, Dr BENN

Victoria Road Health Centre
Victoria Road, Washington NE37 2PU
Tel: 0191 415 5656 Fax: 0191 417 8100
(Sunderland Teaching Primary Care Trust)

Practice Manager Michelle Payne

GP Narendra Kumar RAY, Dr THOMAS

Watchet

Brendon Hills Surgery
Torre, Washford, Watchet TA23 0LA
Tel: 01984 640454 Fax: 01984 641164
Website: www.brendonhillssurgery.nhs.uk
(Somerset Coast Primary Care Trust)

GP Margaret Lynne WILSON, Philip Andrew WILSON

Waterlooville

Denmead Health Centre
Hambledon Road, Denmead, Waterlooville PO7 6NR
Tel: 023 9225 7111 Fax: 023 9225 7113
Website: www.denmeaddoctorssurgery.co.uk
(East Hampshire Primary Care Trust)
Patient List Size: 8600

Practice Manager Debora Wigley

GP David Gweirydd GRIFFITHS, Hilary Anne BROWNLIE, Timothy John GOULDER, Richard Vivian MILLARD, Janet Margaret WARWICK-BROWN

Doctors Surgery
2 Padnell Road, Cowplain, Waterlooville PO8 8DZ
Tel: 023 9226 3138 Fax: 023 9261 8100
(East Hampshire Primary Care Trust)
Patient List Size: 7200

Practice Manager Alex Thompson

GP Michael GREGORI, Michael JOHNS, Nicola Jane MILLEN, Tim WRIGHT

Forest End Surgery
Forest End, Waterlooville PO7 7AH
Tel: 023 9226 3089 Fax: 023 9223 1582
(East Hampshire Primary Care Trust)

Practice Manager Peter Radcliffe

GP David Andrew SPRUELL, Roderick Dougal BOWERMAN, Jane Elizabeth CLARKE-WILLIAMS, Hamish La Mont REID, Nicola Jane ROBERTS, Patrick Benedict RYAN

Horndean Surgery
Blendworth Lane, Horndean, Waterlooville PO8 0AA
Tel: 023 9259 2138 Fax: 023 9257 1628
(East Hampshire Primary Care Trust)
Patient List Size: 4300

Practice Manager Ian Crawford

GP Mark David COOMBE, Graham Howie CROKER

Portsdown Group Practice
Crookhorn Lane Surgery, Purbrook, Waterlooville PO7 5XP
Tel: 023 9226 3078 Fax: 023 9223 0316
(East Hampshire Primary Care Trust)
Patient List Size: 14450

Practice Manager Linda Bradley

GP Julian Rupert NEAL, Martin Christopher GADD, Jayeschandra GOHIL, Karen KYD, Richard Arthur Dacres MANNINGS, Robin Daniel Christopher MOATE, Andrew PLANE, Elizabeth SHEPHERD

Stakes Lodge Surgery
3A Lavender Road, Waterlooville PO7 8NS
Tel: 023 9225 4581 Fax: 023 9235 8867
(East Hampshire Primary Care Trust)
Patient List Size: 7946

Practice Manager Margaret Coker

GP Patrick Douglas BOYLE, Alastair Michael Scrymgoeur BATEMAN, Katherine Linden BURTON, Alan Philip Unna KING, Michael Joseph WHITE

The Surgery
223 London Road, Waterlooville PO8 8DA
Tel: 023 9226 3491 Fax: 023 9234 0504
(East Hampshire Primary Care Trust)
Patient List Size: 4000

Practice Manager Carole Ann McQuillan

GP Susan Patricia STANLEY, Sarah J HOBSON, John R WARWICK

The Surgery
133 London Road, Cowplain, Waterlooville PO8 8XL
Tel: 023 9226 2387
(East Hampshire Primary Care Trust)

GP Peter Anthony COX, Rupert CRISPIN, Mark David HARGREAVES, Andrew PURNELL

The Surgery
26 London Road, Cowplain, Waterlooville PO8 8DL
Tel: 023 9225 3844 Fax: 023 9223 2029
Email: drdaniel@d-daniel.screaming.net
(East Hampshire Primary Care Trust)
Patient List Size: 1800

Practice Manager Sandy Daniel

GP Richard John Earnshaw DANIEL

Waterlooville Health Centre
Dryden Close, Waterlooville PO7 6AL
Tel: 023 9225 7321 Fax: 023 9223 0739
(East Hampshire Primary Care Trust)
Patient List Size: 8400

Practice Manager K Hillman

GP H M PENFOLD, T KENNY, L M MARTIN, K McNICOL, Mark Anthony SAVILLE

Watford

Attenborough Surgery
Bushey Health Centre, London Road, Bushey, Watford WD23 2NN
Tel: 01923 231633
(Watford and Three Rivers Primary Care Trust)

Practice Manager R. Pybus

GP Christine Dora SINGLETON, Parvez Saeed KHAN, Soon Chye LIM, Loretto Mary McHUGH, Susan PURBRICK

Cassio Surgery
62-68 Merton Road, Watford WD18 0WL
Tel: 01923 226011 Fax: 01923 817342
Email: cassiodocs@watford.net
(Watford and Three Rivers Primary Care Trust)
Patient List Size: 10722

Practice Manager Valerie Streater

GP Manoranjan Kaur GUJRAL, Michael Jonathan KEEN, Richard David REUBIN, Timothy William ROBSON, Mark Edward James WATSON

Coach House Surgery
12 Park Avenue, Watford WD18 7LX
Tel: 01923 223178 Fax: 01923 816464
(Watford and Three Rivers Primary Care Trust)
Patient List Size: 8676

Practice Manager Lisa O'Sullivan

GP Sarah Jane WEIDMANN, Eivind James DULLFORCE, Simon HODES, Jeannette Anne KING, Deborah Anne SHEPHERD, Jeremy SHINDLER

The Consulting Rooms
Oxhey Drive, South Oxhey, Watford WD19 7RU
Tel: 020 8428 2292 Fax: 020 8421 1431
(Watford and Three Rivers Primary Care Trust)
Patient List Size: 10300

GP Dinesh Kumar Kantibhai PATEL, Ann BOLITHO-JONES, Philip Victor BOLITHO-JONES, Zia-Ul HUSSAIN, Bharat Gunvantray THACKER

The Elms Surgery
36 The Avenue, Watford WD17 4NT
Tel: 01923 224203 Fax: 01923 247341
(Watford and Three Rivers Primary Care Trust)

GP Bharat Prabhashanker JOSHI, Simonee Tara ALLEN

Garston Medical Centre
6a North Western Avenue, Watford WD25 9GP
Tel: 01923 672086 Fax: 01923 681980
(Watford and Three Rivers Primary Care Trust)
Patient List Size: 7969

Practice Manager Pam Dagnell

GP Michael Frank Alan APPLE, Rami Albert ELIAD, Anuja SHAH, Anthony STIMMLER

The Heath Surgery
104A High Road, Bushey Heath, Watford WD23 1GE
Tel: 020 8950 1285 Fax: 020 8950 4533
(Hertsmere Primary Care Trust)
Patient List Size: 2400

Practice Manager Michaela Campbell

GP Simon CATS

Holywell Surgery
83B Tolpits Lane, Holywell Estate, Watford WD18 6NT
Tel: 01923 243130 Fax: 01923 219396
Email: stephanie.hart@watford3r-pct.nhs.uk
(Watford and Three Rivers Primary Care Trust)
Patient List Size: 2100

GP Stephanie Margaret HART

Leavesden Road Surgery
141A Leavesden Road, Watford WD24 5DG
Tel: 01923 225128
(Watford and Three Rivers Primary Care Trust)

GP Thomas Vladimir NOVAK, Peter Michael ARON, Nigel Richard INESON, Wendy Barbara LEVISON, Clair Fiona MORING, Nicola RATTON

Little Bushey Surgery
California Lane, Bushey, Watford WD23 1EZ
Tel: 020 8386 8888 Fax: 020 8386 8898
Email: drlan@dial.pipex.com
(Hertsmere Primary Care Trust)

Practice Manager Frances Agnew

GP Ian David James FURBANK

Manor View Practice
Bushey Health Centre, London Road, Bushey, Watford WD23 2NN
Tel: 01923 225224 Fax: 01923 213270
(Watford and Three Rivers Primary Care Trust)
Patient List Size: 11000

Practice Manager Jackie Grieves

GP Thomas Jan BOYD, Brian John BINTCLIFFE, Michelle BUIST, Christopher Joseph CATES, Paul Jeremy DAVIS, Jenifer Imogen GLOVER, Sarbani RAY

Prestwick Road Surgery
259 Prestwick Road, Oxhey, Watford WD19 6XU
Tel: 020 8428 2432 Fax: 020 8386 2488
(Watford and Three Rivers Primary Care Trust)

Practice Manager Joan Minihan

GP Razia Sultana MIR, Saboor Ahmed MIR

Rickmansworth Road Surgery
35 Rickmansworth Road, Watford WD18 7HD
Tel: 01923 223232 Fax: 01923 235028
Email: gps.35rickmansworthroad.nhs.net
Website: www..nickyrd.demon.co.uk
(Watford and Three Rivers Primary Care Trust)
Patient List Size: 12900

Practice Manager Jacki Collett

GP Margaret Denise MURRAY, Hannah Emily COWLING, Airlie Linda Macdonald Brooksbank DYSON, Simon Joseph McCANN, Philip William David MEAGER, Peter Francis MOORE, Wendy Alison SAINSBURY, Clare Hilary SEARLE

Sheepcot Medical Centre
80 Sheepcot Lane, Garston, Watford WD25 0EA
Tel: 01923 672451 Fax: 01923 681404
(Watford and Three Rivers Primary Care Trust)
Patient List Size: 9800

Practice Manager Liz Lythaby

GP Alan Peter JACKSON, Nicholas John BROWN, Marie Anne ESSAM, Kim LANGER, Teck Leong LEE, Kathleen Anne MACKELL

South West Herts Health Centre
Oxhey Drive, South Oxhey, Watford WD19 7SF
Tel: 020 8421 5224
(Watford and Three Rivers Primary Care Trust)
Patient List Size: 1350

GP Monwar Shariar YAZDANI

Suthergrey House Surgery
37A St. Johns Road, Watford WD17 1LS
Tel: 01923 224424 Fax: 01923 243710
(Watford and Three Rivers Primary Care Trust)
Patient List Size: 12400

Practice Manager Barbara Mott

GP William Henry BULMAN, Gary GRIFFITH, Eva HELLER, Smita Chimanbhai PATEL, Peter Mark READER, Edward Christopher RIEU

Tudor Surgery
139 Bushey Mill Lane, Watford WD24 7PH
Tel: 01923 223724 Fax: 01923 237327
(Watford and Three Rivers Primary Care Trust)
Patient List Size: 6000

Practice Manager Cecile Pons

GP Vivienne Rosalind LAZZERINI, David LEWIS, David Paul MOSS

Upton Road Surgery
30 Upton Road, Watford WD18 0JS
Tel: 01923 226266 Fax: 01923 222324
(Watford and Three Rivers Primary Care Trust)
Patient List Size: 5834

Practice Manager Janet Dare

GP Thambipillai RATNAVEL, Thevaky JOGARAJAH, Hamid MAHMOOD, Regina ZAKANI

Watlington

Chiltern Surgery
Hill Road, Watlington OX49 5AF
Tel: 01491 612444 Fax: 01491 613988
(South East Oxfordshire Primary Care Trust)

Practice Manager Gerry Davidson

GP Robert Stephen NICHOLSON, Grace DING, Nigel Angus Patrick GREGORY

Wednesbury

Alexander Road Surgery
32 Alexander Road, Darlaston, Wednesbury WS10 9LJ
Fax: 0121 526 2546
(Walsall Teaching Primary Care Trust)

GP P KASLIWAL, Sundar Jaishi VAID

Church Street Surgery
67 Church Street, Darlaston, Wednesbury WS10 8DY
Tel: 0121 526 2924 Fax: 0121 568 8045
(Walsall Teaching Primary Care Trust)
Patient List Size: 2800

Practice Manager Barbara Severn

GP J SHAH, R J SHAH

Crankhall Lane Surgery
156 Crankhall Lane, Friar Park, Wednesbury WS10 0EB
Tel: 0121 556 3412 Fax: 0121 556 1529
(Wednesbury and West Bromwich Primary Care Trust)

GP N U HAQUE, A U RAHMAN

Darlaston Medical Centre
Birmingham Street, Darlaston, Wednesbury WS10 9JS
Tel: 0121 526 2466 Fax: 0121 568 6384
Email: syedfaud.ali@walsall.nhs.uk
(Walsall Teaching Primary Care Trust)
Patient List Size: 3500

Practice Manager F Ali

GP S F ALI

Jubilee Health Centre
1 Upper Russell Street, Wednesbury WS10 7AR
Tel: 0121 556 4615 Fax: 0121 506 2914
(Wednesbury and West Bromwich Primary Care Trust)

Patient List Size: 4250

Practice Manager Keith Eden

GP S GHOSH, T K SASARU

Moxley Medical Centre
10 Queen Street, Moxley, Wednesbury WV14 8TF
Tel: 01922 409515 Fax: 01922 404276
(Walsall Teaching Primary Care Trust)
Patient List Size: 3548

Practice Manager Karen Woodcroft

GP M P H VITARANA

Oakeswell Health Centre
Brunswick Park Road, Wednesbury WS10 9HP
Tel: 0121 556 2114 Fax: 0121 505 1843
(Wednesbury and West Bromwich Primary Care Trust)
Patient List Size: 9800

GP M B TAYLOR, David Millar HUEY, C D E MORRIS, Avtar Singh SAINI, Charanpal SIKKA

Rough Hay Surgery
44b Rough Hay Road, Darlaston, Wednesbury WS10 8NQ
Tel: 0121 526 2233 Fax: 0121 568 8206
(Walsall Teaching Primary Care Trust)
Patient List Size: 3482

Practice Manager Lesley Taff

GP Mohamad Zainul ABEDIN

Russell Medical Centre
Upper Russell Street, Wednesbury WS10 7AR
Tel: 0121 556 5470 Fax: 0121 505 1157
(Wednesbury and West Bromwich Primary Care Trust)
Patient List Size: 1600

Practice Manager Pamela Hickman

GP Gulam Ali TAYYEBI

The Surgery
96 Crankhall Lane, Friar Park, Wednesbury WS10 0EQ
Tel: 0121 556 2233 Fax: 0121 502 6358
(Wednesbury and West Bromwich Primary Care Trust)

Practice Manager Chris Gibbons

GP S A AHMED, S F AHMED

The Surgery
Jubilee Health Centre, 1 Upper Russell Street, Wednesbury WS10 7AR
Tel: 0121 502 5757 Fax: 0121 566 3361
(Wednesbury and West Bromwich Primary Care Trust)
Patient List Size: 2000

Practice Manager Christine Hand

GP B S BHADAURIA

Upper High Street Medical Centre
34 Upper High Street, Wednesbury WS10 7HJ
Tel: 0121 556 3500
(Wednesbury and West Bromwich Primary Care Trust)
Patient List Size: 4700

Practice Manager Tanya Cooper

GP Biplab DASGUPTA, J DAS

Welling

Doctors Surgery
2 Danson Crescent, Welling DA16 2AT
Tel: 020 8303 4204 Fax: 020 8298 1192
(Bexley Care Trust)
Patient List Size: 15115

GP Peter Christopher Jude OXFORD, P ELLIOTT, Lakhbir Kaur KAILEY, C MASI

The Surgery
84 Ingleton Avenue, Welling DA16 2JZ
Tel: 020 8303 1655 Fax: 020 8298 9228
(Bexley Care Trust)
Patient List Size: 4700

Practice Manager Ann Leach, Julie Steward

GP Gurdave Singh GILL, Michael Christian GERUM

The Surgery
2 Falconwood Parade, The Green, Welling DA16 2PL
Tel: 020 8304 7662 Fax: 020 8855 1938
(Greenwich Teaching Primary Care Trust)
Patient List Size: 2000

Practice Manager Jennifer Humphreys

GP Chaman Lall GUPTA, Narada WIJAYATILAKE

The Surgery
73 Upper Wickham Lane, Welling DA16 3AF
Tel: 020 8854 1910 Fax: 020 8317 3711
(Bexley Care Trust)

GP Apurba Chandra BARUAH, Jagjit Kaur CHAHAL, Achyut Prasad DHITAL

The Surgery
174 Bellegrove Road, Welling DA16 3RE
Tel: 020 8856 1770 Fax: 020 8319 8951
(Bexley Care Trust)
Patient List Size: 7100

Practice Manager A Rice

GP William Anthony COTTER, Jacqueline C J M BOHMER-LAUBIS, ANAYA FOCES

Westwood Surgery
24 Westwood Lane, Welling DA16 2HE
Tel: 020 8303 5353 Fax: 020 8298 0346
(Bexley Care Trust)
Patient List Size: 7500

Practice Manager P Siberry

GP Manfred Kwabena ANTO, Peter David FISH, Hemlata PATEL

Wellingborough

Albany House Medical Centre
3 Queen Street, Wellingborough NN8 4RW
Tel: 01933 222309 Fax: 01933 229236
(Northamptonshire Heartlands Primary Care Trust)
Patient List Size: 13500

Practice Manager Max hand

GP Stephen KOWNACKI, Warwick James COULSON, Judy Howard CRAIG, David Kenneth LAWRENCE, E A MONTAGUE, Aileen Patricia ROBERTSON, John TOWNSEND

Gold Street Medical Centre
106 Gold Street, Wellingborough NN8 4ES
Tel: 01933 224678 Fax: 01933 229240
(Northamptonshire Heartlands Primary Care Trust)

Practice Manager Karen Edwards

GP D DATTA, P PATEL, R S PRABHU

Gold Street Medical Centre
106 Gold Street, Wellingborough NN8 4ES
Tel: 01933 223429 Fax: 01933 229240
(Northamptonshire Heartlands Primary Care Trust)

Practice Manager Mel Smith

GP Peter INNS, Kate Louise HUGHES, Natalia IRISO, Geoffrey Richard KING, John Brian McMAHON, Vinodbhai Khushalbhai MISTRY, F POWELL

Marshall's Road Surgery
7 Marshall's Road, Raunds, Wellingborough NN9 6ET
Tel: 01933 622349 Fax: 01933 625421

(Northamptonshire Heartlands Primary Care Trust)

Practice Manager Andrea Haseldine

GP Komath NANDAKUMAR, Payoor NANDAKUMAR

Pepperman and Partners
The Cottons, Meadow Lane, Raunds, Wellingborough NN9 6YA
Tel: 01933 623327 Fax: 01933 623370
(Northamptonshire Heartlands Primary Care Trust)
Patient List Size: 8700

Practice Manager David Schumskit

GP Mark Andrew PEPPERMAN, Daniel Mark BLINDT, Kenneth Leo McGARITY, H NWOSU

The Redwell Medical Centre
1 Turner Road, Wellingborough NN8 4UT
Tel: 01933 400777 Fax: 01933 671959
(Northamptonshire Heartlands Primary Care Trust)
Patient List Size: 12500

Practice Manager Jenny Wyles

GP Peter John GORDON, Sabrah AL-HARDAN, Lynne Elizabeth BYLES, Ken CHUNG, Patrick Vincent LEYDEN, Joanna Clare LOUGHTON, Roger Malcolm PERRY, Main Ching YEE

Spinney Brook Medical Centre
59 High Street, Irthlingborough, Wellingborough NN9 5GA
Tel: 01933 650593 Fax: 01933 653641
(Northamptonshire Heartlands Primary Care Trust)
Patient List Size: 9500

Practice Manager Anna Barrett, Frances Hokins

GP Jonathan Morgan BEVAN, Jason ENGLISH, Iqbalhusein Abdulmalek Mohamed JASANI, Anne Margaret LAMBERT, M D MITCHELL, Nick G REED

Staff and Partners
Queensway Medical Centre, Olympic Way, Wellingborough NN8 3EP
Tel: 01933 678767 Fax: 01933 676657
(Northamptonshire Heartlands Primary Care Trust)

Practice Manager Julie Passmore

GP David Malcolm STAFF, Zoe ALEXANDER, Thomas Robert COWAN, Christopher Charles DENT, N LOVEDAY, Andrew Tristan WAINWRIGHT

Summerlee Medical Centre
Summerlee Road, Finedon, Wellingborough NN9 5LJ
Tel: 01933 682203 Fax: 01933 682205
(Northamptonshire Heartlands Primary Care Trust)
Patient List Size: 1410

Practice Manager J French

GP N G SEGAREN

The Surgery
163 London Road, Wollaston, Wellingborough NN29 7QS
Tel: 01933 664214 Fax: 01933 664132
(Northamptonshire Heartlands Primary Care Trust)

Practice Manager Pauline James

GP S S MARATHE, S V MARATHE

Wellington

Wellington Medical Centre
Bulford, Wellington TA21 8PW
Tel: 01823 663551 Fax: 01823 660650
Email: firstname.lastname@gp-L85059.nhs.uk
(Taunton Deane Primary Care Trust)
Patient List Size: 12646

Practice Manager Dorothy King

GP Paul William BEVAN, Caroline BETT, Mike MICHAELS, Kathryn PORTER, John Stuart WYNNE

Wells

Priory Medical Centre
Priory Park, Glastonbury Road, Wells BA5 1XJ
Tel: 01749 672137 Fax: 01749 836641
(Mendip Primary Care Trust)
Patient List Size: 11097

Practice Manager Julia Ewart

GP Roger ASHMAN, Jonathan Justin BENCH, Christopher Michael BRIDSON, Helen Elizabeth CRAWLEY, Rachel Bridget GATRILL, Andrew Spencer NORMAN

Wells City Practice
22 Chamberlain Street, Wells BA5 2PF
Tel: 01749 673356 Fax: 01749 670031
Email: hugh.goddard@gp-l85034.nhs.uk
(Mendip Primary Care Trust)
Patient List Size: 6500

Practice Manager Carol Judd

GP Robert Hugh GODDARD, Tristan John MARTIN, Jo NEWTON, Anthony Alastair PRYER

Wells-next-the-Sea

Wells Health Centre
Bolts Close, Wells-next-the-Sea NR23 1JP
Tel: 01328 710741 Fax: 01328 711825
(North Norfolk Primary Care Trust)
Patient List Size: 3200

GP Charles Sidney Thomas EBRILL, Gordon Campbell McANSH

Welwyn

Bridge Cottage Surgery
41 High Street, Welwyn AL6 9EF
Tel: 01438 715044 Fax: 01438 714013
(Welwyn Hatfield Primary Care Trust)
Patient List Size: 15600

Practice Manager Annette Macchia, Sally White

GP Royce Cubitt ABRAHAMS, Elaine ADAMS, Nicholas Brandon DANSIE, Ann DREW, Hilary Barbara NAPIER, Celia Anne PARDOE, Hari PATHMANATHAN, Anthony REED, E WALTER

Welwyn Garden City

Garden City Practice
11 Guessens Road, Welwyn Garden City AL8 6QW
Tel: 01707 330522 Fax: 01707 391629
Website: www.gardencitypractice.sageweb.co.uk
(Welwyn Hatfield Primary Care Trust)
Patient List Size: 7500

Practice Manager S J Humphreys

GP Barbara Ann HANAK, Sandra Jane CONROY, Martin Gerard RIMMER, Caroline Anne SHAW, Peter Frame SHILLIDAY

Hall Grove Surgery
4 Hall Grove, Welwyn Garden City AL7 4PL
Tel: 01707 328528 Fax: 01707 373139
(Welwyn Hatfield Primary Care Trust)
Patient List Size: 16500

Practice Manager Kate Thurman

GP Christopher David LUND, Anthea J CORSER, Frances Mary CRANFIELD, Jonathan Geoffrey EVISON, Philip Michael HOLT, John Humphrey Michael MERCER, Alister Richard John PARRY, Geoffrey PUGH

Peartree Lane Surgery
110 Peartree Lane, Welwyn Garden City AL7 3UJ
Tel: 01707 328919 Fax: 01707 391299
(Welwyn Hatfield Primary Care Trust)

Practice Manager Ann Dorman

GP Robert John DUNSTER, Robert Paul BREWIS, Rachel CLARKE, David Robert CREAK, Robin Paul DAVIES, Shona HYDE, Alastair George McGHEE, Michael Jeremy RULE, Simon John Shipley TURNER

Wembley

Alperton Medical Centre
32 Stanley Avenue, Wembley HA0 4JB
Tel: 020 8903 2379 Fax: 020 8903 3027
(Brent Teaching Primary Care Trust)
Patient List Size: 5500

Practice Manager Samir Parekh

GP Nikunj Shantilal MALDE, S CHANDRASEKARI, A DEB-BARMAN

Beechcroft Medical Centre
34 Beechcroft Gardens, Wembley HA9 8EP
(Brent Teaching Primary Care Trust)

GP Jonathan Frank BERNSTEIN, Helen McGOVERN

Chalkhill Health Centre
Chalkhill Road, Wembley HA9 9BQ
Tel: 020 8904 0911 Fax: 020 8908 0623
Email: rama.gopal@gp-e84032.nhs.uk
(Brent Teaching Primary Care Trust)
Patient List Size: 6600

GP John Victor SALINSKY

Dr D Rapp and Dr M Hussain
Chalkhill Health Centre, Rook Close, Off Chalkhill Road, Wembley HA9 9ER
Tel: 020 8901 1144 Fax: 020 8908 6945
Email: rapphussain@gp-e84033.nhs.uk
(Brent Teaching Primary Care Trust)
Patient List Size: 4300

Practice Manager Valerie Blustin

GP David Andrew RAPP, M HUSSAIN

Forty Willows Surgery
46 Forty Lane, Wembley HA9 9HA
Tel: 020 8385 0011 Fax: 020 8385 0411
(Brent Teaching Primary Care Trust)
Patient List Size: 6151

Practice Manager Esther Spicer

GP Max Mosche BAYER, Maura FLEMING, Jude MILLS

Hazeldene Medical Centre
Hazeldene, 1B Wyld Way, Wembley HA9 6PW
Tel: 020 8902 4792
(Brent Teaching Primary Care Trust)

GP Mahendra Babubhai AMIN, Nalini AMIN

Oakington Medical Centre
41 Oakington Avenue, Wembley HA9 8HX
Tel: 020 8904 3021
(Brent Teaching Primary Care Trust)
Patient List Size: 3296

Practice Manager Jasu Datiani

GP Sobhagchandra Mohanlal SHAH

Preston Medical Centre
23 Preston Road, Wembley HA9 8JZ
Tel: 020 8904 3263
(Brent Teaching Primary Care Trust)
Patient List Size: 4600

Practice Manager Saroj Patel

GP Ashwinkumar Rambhai PATEL

Preston Road Surgery
56 Preston Road, Wembley HA9 8LB
Tel: 020 8904 6442 Fax: 020 8908 1040
(Brent Teaching Primary Care Trust)
Patient List Size: 3600

Practice Manager Barbara Cohen

GP Kanagasingham NANDHABALAN, Nanthini BALACHANDRAN

Stanley Corner Medical Centre
1-3 Stanley Avenue, Wembley HA0 4JF
Tel: 020 8902 3887 Fax: 020 8903 0973
Email: manager@gp.E8405.nhs.uk
(Brent Teaching Primary Care Trust)
Patient List Size: 5300

Practice Manager Karen Harrison

GP Tejinder Gurmit SINGH, Laurence Ashley KROTOSKY, Monica Maria VLOEMANS

The Surgery
267 Ealing Road, Wembley HA0 1EU
Tel: 020 8997 3486 Fax: 020 8810 6171
(Brent Teaching Primary Care Trust)

GP Sharadchandra Mansukhlal MEHTA, H PATEL, N SRISKANTHARAJAH, G THANKI

The Surgery
1 Uxendon Crescent, Wembley HA9 9TW
Tel: 020 8904 3883 Fax: 020 8904 3899
(Brent Teaching Primary Care Trust)
Patient List Size: 6300

Practice Manager Wendy Mobbs

GP Carole Irene WILLS, Tariq KALEEM, Jyotsana Suresh PATEL

The Surgery
95 Grasmere Avenue, Wembley HA9 8TF
Tel: 020 8904 8045 Fax: 020 8908 5363
(Brent Teaching Primary Care Trust)
Patient List Size: 2250

Practice Manager Pramila Patel

GP Manilal Madhavji RAICHURA, Mukesh Jamnadas DATTANI

The Surgery
19 Lancelot Road, Wembley HA0 2AL
Tel: 020 8903 0609
(Brent Teaching Primary Care Trust)

GP Narindar Nath SABHARWAL, Chander Kanta SABHARWAL

The Surgery
26 Eagle Road, Wembley HA0 4SH
(Brent Teaching Primary Care Trust)

GP S C PATEL

The Surgery
262 Harrow Road, Wembley HA9 6QL
Tel: 020 8902 0055
(Brent Teaching Primary Care Trust)

GP M C PATEL

The Tudor House Medical Centre
1 Chalkhill Road, Wembley HA9 9DS
Tel: 020 8904 3673 Fax: 020 8904-9638
(Brent Teaching Primary Care Trust)

GP Roop Kawal GOSAIN, D COOPER

Wembley Centre for Health and Care
116 Chaplin Road, Crawford Avenue, Wembley HA0 4UZ
Tel: 020 8795 6200 Fax: 020 8795 6196
(Brent Teaching Primary Care Trust)
Patient List Size: 3233

Practice Manager Sudha Amin

GP N C AMIN

Wembley Centre for Health and Care
116 Chaplin Road, Wembley HA0 4UZ
Tel: 020 8451 8338 Fax: 020 8451 8365
(Brent Teaching Primary Care Trust)

Practice Manager Celia Dale

GP Malakumari Pursotam MAMTORA, Rita BHARDWAJ

Wembley Centre for Health and Care
Chaplin Road, Wembley HA0 4UZ
Tel: 020 8795 6180 Fax: 020 8795 6190
(Brent Teaching Primary Care Trust)

Practice Manager Veena Rawal

GP Premila B PATEL

Wembley Centre for Health and Care
Chaplin Road, Wembley HA0 4UZ
(Brent Teaching Primary Care Trust)

GP C D NOTANEY

Wembley Park Medical Centre
21 Wembley Park Drive, Wembley HA9 8HD
Tel: 020 8902 4411 Fax: 020 8795 2987
(Brent Teaching Primary Care Trust)
Patient List Size: 6500

Practice Manager Sue Richardson

GP Juliette ROSS, Vivian Colman HYMAN

West Bromwich

Bassan
Cronehills Health Centre, Cronehills Linkway, West Bromwich B70 8TJ
Tel: 0121 553 0277 Fax: 0121 580 1874
(Wednesbury and West Bromwich Primary Care Trust)
Patient List Size: 1800

Practice Manager K K Bassan

GP Tarlochan Singh BASSAN

Crampton and Partners
Carters Green Medical Centre, 396-400 High Street, West Bromwich B70 9LB
Tel: 0121 553 0385 Fax: 0121 525-9770
(Wednesbury and West Bromwich Primary Care Trust)
Patient List Size: 6700

Practice Manager Linda Hall

GP Gillian Mary CRAMPTON, Mohammed HANIF, Janet MERRON, Joanne WELLER

Cronehills Health Centre
Cronehills Linkway, West Bromwich B70 8TJ
Tel: 0121 525 0506
(Wednesbury and West Bromwich Primary Care Trust)

GP Dr DEWAN

Dartmouth Medical Centre
1 Richard Street, West Bromwich B70 9JL
Tel: 0121 553 1144 Fax: 0121 580 1914
(Wednesbury and West Bromwich Primary Care Trust)

Practice Manager Margaret Holder

GP Ramubhai Mitthalbhai PATEL, D R PATEL, J N PATEL

Gabbitas
Cronehills Health Centre, Cronehills Linkway, West Bromwich B70 8TJ
Tel: 0121 500 6455 Fax: 0121 580 1813
(Wednesbury and West Bromwich Primary Care Trust)

Practice Manager Carol Kiever

GP David Graham GABBITAS, R K ARORA

Gilbert and Partners
Cronehills Health Centre, Cronhills Walkway, West Bromwich B70 8TJ
Tel: 0121 553 0287 Fax: 0121 580 1821
Email: postmaster@gp-M88038.nhs.uk
Website: www.drgilbertandpartners.co.uk
(Wednesbury and West Bromwich Primary Care Trust)
Patient List Size: 8300

Practice Manager Linda Lloyd, Beverley Woodward

GP John Edward GILBERT, Brian Henry DEXTER, Anne LARGIE, Mark McGEOWN

Group Pratice Centre
291 Walsall Road, West Bromwich B71 3LN
Tel: 0121 588 2286 Fax: 0121 567 5435
(Wednesbury and West Bromwich Primary Care Trust)
Patient List Size: 6050

Practice Manager Puni Patel

GP P K PATEL, Bhavinkumar Sammukhlal MEHTA

Hill Top Surgery
68 Hill Top, West Bromwich B70 0PU
Tel: 0121 502 5818 Fax: 0121 502 5818
(Wednesbury and West Bromwich Primary Care Trust)

GP O J A R HASSOUNA

Oakwood Surgery
40 Izohs Road, West Bromwich B70 8PG
Tel: 0121 553 0757 Fax: 0121 553 0757
(Wednesbury and West Bromwich Primary Care Trust)

GP G K AGGRAWAL, K G AGGRAWAL

Stone Cross Medical Practice
293 Walsall Road, West Bromwich B71 3LN
Tel: 0121 588 3672 Fax: 0121 567 5838
(Wednesbury and West Bromwich Primary Care Trust)

Practice Manager Maureen Taphouse

GP U DASGUPTA

The Surgery
New Street, Hill Top, West Bromwich B70 0HN
Tel: 0121 556 0190 Fax: 0121 505 3705
(Wednesbury and West Bromwich Primary Care Trust)
Patient List Size: 2450

Practice Manager Christine Scully

GP Ram Vishnu KARANDIKAR

The Surgery
68 Hill Top, West Bromwich B70 0PU
Tel: 0121 556 0455 Fax: 0121 556 8664
(Wednesbury and West Bromwich Primary Care Trust)
Patient List Size: 4362

Practice Manager Debbie Morris

GP Pratibha Vitthal GUDI, W S GUDI

The Surgery
35 Herbert Street, West Bromwich B70 6HZ
Tel: 0121 525 1481
(Wednesbury and West Bromwich Primary Care Trust)

Practice Manager Kamla Devi

GP Subhash BAJAJ

The Surgery
216 Birmingham Road, West Bromwich B70 6QJ
Tel: 0121 580 0558
(Wednesbury and West Bromwich Primary Care Trust)

Practice Manager Gil Plimmer

GP Nisha Dattatray PATHAK

The Surgery
1A Cordley Street, West Bromwich B70 9NQ
Tel: 0121 553 3646 Fax: 0121 580 1908
(Wednesbury and West Bromwich Primary Care Trust)
Patient List Size: 2042

Practice Manager H. Bardha

GP Harbhajan Singh BARDHA, Anuradha Shyam BATHIJA

The Surgery
Clifton Lane, Stone Cross, West Bromwich B71 3AS
Tel: 0121 588 7989 Fax: 0121 567 5418
(Wednesbury and West Bromwich Primary Care Trust)

Practice Manager Karen Greavey

GP Neel Kamal AGARWAL, Shail AGARWAL

The Surgery
130 Lodge Road, West Bromwich B70 8PL
Tel: 0121 553 3780 Fax: 0121 553 7372
(Wednesbury and West Bromwich Primary Care Trust)

Practice Manager L Adma

GP Lakshmi Narayan ADMA, U R AMIN

The Surgery
1 Cambridge Street, West Bromwich B70 8HQ
Tel: 0121 525 9257 Fax: 0121 582 2015
(Wednesbury and West Bromwich Primary Care Trust)

Practice Manager J Kair

GP M SINGH

West Byfleet

Parishes Bridge Medical Practice
Madeira Road, West Byfleet KT14 6DH
Tel: 01932 336933 Fax: 01932 355681
(Surrey Heath and Woking Primary Care Trust)
Patient List Size: 11500

Practice Manager Elisabeth Hawkey

GP Antony Charles SHEPHEARD, Richard J BARKER, Christopher John Douglas DUNSTAN, Joanne Louise HORGAN, Helen Mary McEVOY, Auya NASIM

West Byfleet Health Centre
Madeira Road, West Byfleet KT14 6DH
Tel: 01932 340484 Fax: 01932 355681
(Surrey Heath and Woking Primary Care Trust)
Patient List Size: 7700

Practice Manager Janet Lake

GP Philip John Comyn CUMMIN, Jim BRAIDEN, Annette Lesley CUMMIN, Mark Thomas LYNCH

West Byfleet Health Centre
Madeira Road, West Byfleet KT14 6DH
Tel: 01932 336933 Fax: 01932 355681
(Surrey Heath and Woking Primary Care Trust)
Patient List Size: 9700

Practice Manager Liz Reynolds

GP Richard Stephen LAWRENCE, Martin CHURCHILL, Clive CODDINGTON, Sara Maxwell COE, Sarah Elizabeth Jean McKAY

West Drayton

Harmondsworth Road Surgery
114 Harmondsworth Road, Hayes, West Drayton UB7 9JW
Tel: 0870 417 3197 Fax: 01895 421766
(Hillingdon Primary Care Trust)

GP Tarjinder SINGH

The Medical Centre
6 The Green, West Drayton UB7 7PJ
Tel: 01895 442026/447627 Fax: 01895 430753
(Hillingdon Primary Care Trust)
Patient List Size: 8800

Practice Manager William Bramble

GP Anthony GREWAL, Christopher Stephen JOWETT, Joseph MONTGOMERY, Catherine Ellison PICTON, Pinkinder K SAHOTA

Otterfield Road Medical Centre
25 Otterfield Road, Yiewsley, West Drayton UB7 8PE
Tel: 01895 422611 Fax: 01895 431309
Email: surgery@otterfield.swinternet.co.uk
(Hillingdon Primary Care Trust)
Patient List Size: 5800

Practice Manager J Nijjar

GP Veluppillai PARAMANATHAN, Fazal Ur Rahman MIAN, Natasha PAUL-CASSEL, Harmeet SABHARWAL

Yiewsley Health Centre
High Street, Yiewsley, West Drayton UB7 7DP
Tel: 01895 422292 Fax: 01895 422134
(Hillingdon Primary Care Trust)
Patient List Size: 5000

Practice Manager Tom Johnson

GP Patrick ANDREWS, Latika CHANDRA

West Malling

Avicenna Medical Centre
Oxley Shaw Lane, Leybourne, West Malling ME19 5PU
Tel: 01732 841561/844676 Fax: 01732 872949
(Maidstone Weald Primary Care Trust)
Patient List Size: 2100

Practice Manager S Sargeant

GP Sheikh Dharvesh Mohammad CASSIM

West Malling Group Practice
116 High Street, Milverton, West Malling ME19 6LX
Tel: 01732 870212 Fax: 01732 742437
(Maidstone Weald Primary Care Trust)

Practice Manager Margaret Osborn

GP Richard James MUSGRAVE, John Bradley ASHTON, Richard Jonathan NEWELL, Thomas REICHHELM, Juliet Margaret ROBERTS, Michael John RUSHTON

West Wickham

Addington Road Surgery
33 Addington Road, West Wickham BR4 9BW
Tel: 020 8462 5771 Fax: 020 8462 8526
(Bromley Primary Care Trust)
Patient List Size: 8900

Practice Manager Marian Wade

GP Stuart Hamish ROBERTSON, Richard James DILLEY, Anna Beatrice LANGTRY, Oluseye Ayodeji LOKULO-SODIPE, Pamela PATRE, Manickauasagam SUNDARESAN

Station Road Surgery
74 Station Road, West Wickham BR4 0PU
Tel: 020 8777 8245
Website: www.wwdoc.co.uk
(Bromley Primary Care Trust)
Patient List Size: 12000

GP Ian David WHITTAKER, Sita Monica CARTER, Susan Antonietta HILL, Vijay PURWAR, Ranjit Kandadai SRINIVAS, Anabella STANFORTHY, Tania VENISON

The Surgery
315 Pickhurst Lane, West Wickham BR4 0HW
Tel: 020 8460 2264
(Bromley Primary Care Trust)

GP S JHALLY

Wickham Park Surgery
2 Manor Road, West Wickham BR4 9PS
Tel: 020 8777 1293 Fax: 020 8776 1977
Email: wickhampark@gp-g84607.nhs.uk
(Bromley Primary Care Trust)

Patient List Size: 4300

GP Donya Carolyn Denise YOUNG, Adelaja MUSTAPHA

Westbury

Eastleigh Surgery

Station Road, Westbury BA13 3JD
Tel: 01373 822807 Fax: 01373 828904
(West Wiltshire Primary Care Trust)
Patient List Size: 16800

Practice Manager Debbie Riddiford

GP Deborah Angharyd BEALE, S CONNELL, Richard Mark EDWARDS, E EVANS, Stephen FRANS, M GUMBLEY, Diana Joan SIGGERS, J C TAYLOR

Westcliff on Sea

Argyll Road Surgery

48 Argyll Road, Westcliff on Sea SS0 7HN
Tel: 01702 432040
(Southend-on-Sea Primary Care Trust)
Patient List Size: 2600

Practice Manager N Siani

GP Nanjit SIANI

Southbourne Grove Surgery

314 Southbourne Grove, Westcliff on Sea SS0 0AF
Tel: 01702 344074 Fax: 01702 435712
(Southend-on-Sea Primary Care Trust)

Practice Manager Rita Chaturvedi

GP Krishna Kant CHATURVEDI

Valkyrie Road Surgery

20 Valkyrie Road, Westcliff on Sea SS0 8BX
Tel: 01702 331255 Fax: 01702 437050
Email: practice.managerf81097@nhs.net
(Southend-on-Sea Primary Care Trust)
Patient List Size: 9500

Practice Manager Andrew Metcalf

GP Paul Thomas CHISNELL, Susan Mary CALLAGHAN, Sudeshna DUTTA, Rupert Michael HALLIDAY, Atika MUSTAFA, Tony Feuko NASAH, Peter Frank SUBRT

West Road Surgery

12 West Road, Westcliff on Sea SS0 9DA
Tel: 01702 344492 Fax: 01702 437051
(Southend-on-Sea Primary Care Trust)
Patient List Size: 8065

Practice Manager P J Adey

GP Colin ADEY, Wendy CORDESS, Beverley Sue DAVIES, Julian Seymour FRANKLIN, Martin Barry KENT

Westborough Road Surgery

6 Westborough Road, Westcliff on Sea SS0 9DR
Tel: 01702 349957 Fax: 01702 437048
(Southend-on-Sea Primary Care Trust)

Practice Manager Anita Hall

GP Javed GUL

Westborough Road Surgery

258 Westborough Road, Westcliff on Sea SS0 9PT
Tel: 01702 348800 Fax: 01702 338638
(Southend-on-Sea Primary Care Trust)
Patient List Size: 3950

GP V CROWHURST

Westborough Road Surgery

401 Westborough Road, Westcliff on Sea SS0 9TW
Tel: 01702 346442 Fax: 01702 437153
(Southend-on-Sea Primary Care Trust)

Practice Manager Janet Velmurugan

GP Marimuthu VELMURUGAN

Westerham

The Surgery

Stock Hill, Biggin Hill, Westerham TN16 3TJ
Tel: 01959 573352 Fax: 01959 570785
(Bromley Primary Care Trust)
Patient List Size: 11500

Practice Manager Barry Gent

GP John Francis Xavier RAWCLIFFE, Aslam AKHTAR, Bridget HOPKINS, Janet LEGGETT, Sylvia STEFANOVA, Selena WONG

The Surgery

14a Norheads Lane, Bigginhill, Westerham TN16 3XS
Tel: 01959 574488 Fax: 01959 570560
Email: drsingh.surgery@gp.G84039.nhs.uk
(Bromley Primary Care Trust)
Patient List Size: 2700

Practice Manager Carol Dorman

GP S SINGH, K SINGH

Winterton Surgery

Market Square, Westerham TN16 1RB
Tel: 01732 744200
(South West Kent Primary Care Trust)

GP Adam John SKINNER, Duncan BURNS, Angela KAPADIA, Vivien Elizabeth KNOX, Nicola Jane PARKER

Westgate-on-Sea

Westgate Bay Avenue Surgery

60 Westgate Bay Avenue, Westgate-on-Sea CT8 8SN
Tel: 01843 831335 Fax: 01843 835279
(East Kent Coastal Teaching Primary Care Trust)

Practice Manager Carole Perkins

GP James Audley TURTLE, Andrew John Philip DEAN, C G M LEIRE, David Richard MEAKIN, Andrew Neil WALTON

Weston Super Mare

The Cedars Surgery

87 New Bristol Road, Worle, Weston Super Mare BS22 6AJ
Tel: 01934 515878 Fax: 01934 520263
(North Somerset Primary Care Trust)
Patient List Size: 2500

Practice Manager Yvonne Allen

GP Michael Henry James PIMM, Caroline DAILLEY, Susan MACRAE

Graham Road Surgery

22 Graham Road, Weston Super Mare BS23 1YA
Tel: 01934 628111 Fax: 01934 645842
(North Somerset Primary Care Trust)

Practice Manager A Tancock

GP Clive Victor GILLIS, Miriam Kay AINSWORTH, Gerard Nicholas GARVEY, Duncan HUGH, Peter Derek MILNTHORPE

The Milton Surgery

232-234 Milton Road, Weston Super Mare BS22 8AG
Tel: 01934 625022 Fax: 01934 612470
(North Somerset Primary Care Trust)
Patient List Size: 8200

Practice Manager Charlie MacWilliams

GP Paul Bryan WILSON, Ozleny CILASUN, Paul D DAVIES, Nigel Peter LAKIN, Peter Robin SMITH

New Court Surgery

39 Boulevard, Weston Super Mare BS23 1PF
Tel: 01934 624242 Fax: 01934 642608

(North Somerset Primary Care Trust)

Practice Manager Carol Jones

GP Peter Martin WATKINSON, John Robert CHITTY, Christopher William CLARKE, Catherine Mary ENGLAND, David John EVANS, Catherine Wray PRESTON

Riverbank Medical Centre
Walford Avenue, Worle, Weston Super Mare BS22 7YZ
Tel: 01934 521133
(North Somerset Primary Care Trust)
Patient List Size: 8000

GP Roderick John Bertram BOWERING, Richard Mark DARLING, Jane Louise GODBEHERE, Mahavir Prasad VARSHNEY

Stafford Place Surgery
4 Stafford Place, Weston Super Mare BS23 2QZ
Tel: 01934 415212 Fax: 01934 612463
Email: stafford.place@virgin.net
Website: http://freespace.virgin.net/stafford.place
(North Somerset Primary Care Trust)
Patient List Size: 7250

Practice Manager Richard Harrison

GP Annette BRADLEY, Phillip CARMAN, Michael Joseph LEONARD, Emma STUART

The Surgery
9 Ebdon Road, Worle, Weston Super Mare BS22 6UB
Tel: 01934 514145 Fax: 01934 521345
(North Somerset Primary Care Trust)

GP Steven Christian PEARSE-DANKER, E G STALLWORTHY

The Surgery
6 Longton Grove Road, Weston Super Mare BS23 1LT
Tel: 01934 628118 Fax: 01934 645893
(North Somerset Primary Care Trust)

GP Roger Clifford PRESTON, K M HAGGERTY, Peter George LUMB

The Surgery
13 Clarence Road East, Weston Super Mare BS23 4BP
Tel: 01934 415080 Fax: 01934 612813
(North Somerset Primary Care Trust)
Patient List Size: 4700

Practice Manager J Porter

GP M T WYATT, I R LONGHORN, Peter MAKSIMCZYK

Tudor Lodge Health Centre
3 Nithsdale Road, Weston Super Mare BS23 4JP
Tel: 01934 622665 Fax: 01934 644332
(North Somerset Primary Care Trust)
Patient List Size: 10800

Practice Manager William Edwards

GP Philip Graham MURDIN, John Francis BIRKETT, Nizar Ibrahim HASHAM, Diane MATHISAN, Andrew Clive MATHISON, Jeremy MAYNARD, Ian WARING

The Village Surgery, Worle
Hill Road East, Worle, Weston Super Mare BS22 9HF
Tel: 01934 516671 Fax: 01934 520664
(North Somerset Primary Care Trust)
Patient List Size: 4200

Practice Manager M Rahman

GP Nila Dilip PATEL

Weston PMS Pilot
Bournville Locality Centre, Coniston Crescent, Weston Super Mare BS23 3RX
Tel: 01934 624942 Fax: 01934 637639
(North Somerset Primary Care Trust)

GP P W SEVIOUR, J R ROBERTSON, E STALLWORTHY

Wetherby

Bramham Medical Centre
Clifford Road, Bramham, Wetherby LS23 6RN
Tel: 01937 845854 Fax: 01937 844480
Email: john.nicholls2@nhs.net
(Leeds North East Primary Care Trust)
Patient List Size: 3700

GP John A J NICHOLLS, F LESSELS, M PEPPER

Church View Surgery
School La, Collingham, Wetherby LS22 5BQ
Tel: 01937 573848 Fax: 01937 574754
(Leeds North East Primary Care Trust)

Practice Manager Gillian Cottam

GP Andrew MAWSON, Rachel Mary Gomer CRABBE, Richard William DRAYSON, Stephen Roger LIGHTFOOT, Alison SMITH

Lynton Medical Centre
1 Lynton Avenue, Boston Spa, Wetherby LS23 6BL
Tel: 01937 842115 Fax: 01937 541657
(Leeds North East Primary Care Trust)

GP John Richard JEFFERY

New Medical Centre
Crossley Street, Wetherby LS22 6RT
Tel: 01937 543200 Fax: 01937 588689
(Leeds North East Primary Care Trust)
Patient List Size: 10949

Practice Manager Jane Foster

GP John Derek MATE, Maria D Sylvia FRITH, Robert WEBSTER

Spa Surgery
205 High Street, Boston Spa, Wetherby LS23 6PY
Tel: 01937 842842 Fax: 01937 841095
(Leeds North East Primary Care Trust)

Practice Manager Fay Jebson

GP John Maclachlan McARDLE, Michael David BRADY, Teresa ROSE

Weybridge

Church Street Practice
Weybridge Primary Care Centre, 22 Church Street, Weybridge KT13 8DW
Tel: 01932 853366 Fax: 01932 844902
(North Surrey Primary Care Trust)
Patient List Size: 12200

Practice Manager V Millis

GP Dr BROWN, Darren Philip COCKER, Lindy Anne FOZARD, Anne Marie GREEN, Dr LANGTON, Dr MENZIES-GOW, Clive Reece WALKER

Weybridge Health Centre
Church Street, Weybridge KT13 8DW
Tel: 01932 853366 Fax: 01932 859851
(North Surrey Primary Care Trust)

Practice Manager K A Rose

GP Emile Antonion Janim DE SOUZA, Ravdip Singh BUMRAH, Edward COMBER, Krzysztof Andrzej JAKUBOWSKI, Loraine Marie LAWRENCE, Wendy Sharon PAYNE

Weymouth

Abbotsbury Road Surgery
24 Abbotsbury Road, Weymouth DT4 0AE
Tel: 01305 786257 Fax: 01305 760532
(South West Dorset Primary Care Trust)
Patient List Size: 9000

GP Michael Morris KILLOCH, Christine BROWN, Peter John HEWETT, Peter Jonathan HULL, Hugh Stephen PRIESTLEY, Rachel TURBERVILLE-SMITH

Cross Road Surgery
Cross Road, Rodwell, Weymouth DT4 9QX
Tel: 01305 768844 Fax: 01305 760686
(South West Dorset Primary Care Trust)

Practice Manager Jayne Trevett

GP Alban John BLUNT, Ian CHAPMAN, Alexander MAN

Dorchester Road Surgery
179 Dorchester Road, Weymouth DT4 7LE
Tel: 01305 766472 Fax: 01305 766499
(South West Dorset Primary Care Trust)
Patient List Size: 3753

Practice Manager G Davidson

GP Steven Anthony BICK, Emma CASSON, Monica Ann HENDRICKS, Wayne Robert KNIGHT

Frederick Place Surgery
11 Frederick Place, Weymouth DT4 8HQ
Tel: 01305 774411 Fax: 01305 760417
Email: gary@fredplaceway.com
(South West Dorset Primary Care Trust)
Patient List Size: 13000

Practice Manager Paul Edgar

GP David Michael EVANS, David John BLEASE, Ivan Ross HALL, Karen Valerie KIRKHAM, Huw David LLEWELLYN, Prudence Jennifer MITCHELL, Martha Juliet O'NEILL, Rupert John TURBERVILLE SMITH

Lanehouse Surgery
Ludlow Road, Weymouth DT4 0HB
Tel: 01305 785681 Fax: 01305 760418
(South West Dorset Primary Care Trust)
Patient List Size: 2943

Practice Manager Tess Smith

GP Kenneth Caldwell HOUSTON, Sally Elizabeth HODDER

Preston Road Surgery
102 Preston Road, Weymouth DT3 6BB
Tel: 01305 832203 Fax: 01305 833805
(South West Dorset Primary Care Trust)
Patient List Size: 7000

Practice Manager K Meacham

GP Nicholas James STALLEY, William Barrett BOWDITCH, Brigid Mary GREENUP

Royal Crescent Surgery
25 Crescent Street, Weymouth DT4 7BY
Tel: 01305 774466 Fax: 01305 760538
(South West Dorset Primary Care Trust)
Patient List Size: 11000

Practice Manager Kate Meacham

GP David Richard SLATER, Sarita CHOPRA, Jonathon DE KRETSER, Alwyn Guy Wethered DICKINSON, Madeleine Jane KEYWORTH, Jonathan Martin ORRELL, Richard Andrew SALES

The Surgery
Malthouse Meadow, Portesham, Weymouth DT3 4NS
Tel: 01305 871468 Fax: 01305 871977
Email: postmaster@gp-j81609.nhs.uk
(South West Dorset Primary Care Trust)
Patient List Size: 2800

Practice Manager M Cantrille

GP Catherine Margaret Godwin POUNCEY, Paul Wayne BAIRD, Nevil Howard FOWLER

Wyke Regis Health Centre
Portland Road, Wyke Regis, Weymouth DT4 9BE
Tel: 01305 728886 Fax: 01305 760549
Email: fay.morris@gp-j81051.nhs.uk
(South West Dorset Primary Care Trust)
Patient List Size: 8000

Practice Manager Fay E Morris

GP John Hedley MANN, David Carson BOYD, Katharine GROGONO, Alison LAIRD, Graham David LAIRD, Anthony Philip ROBERTS

Whitby

Churchfield Surgery
14 Iburndale Lane, Sleights, Whitby YO22 5DP
Tel: 01947 810466 Fax: 01947 811375
(Scarborough, Whitby and Ryedale Primary Care Trust)
Patient List Size: 3629

Practice Manager Diane Shaw

GP Farhad EMAD, Margaret JACKSON, Richard Roderick NEWMAN

Dale End Surgery
Danby, Whitby YO21 2JE
Tel: 01287 660739 Fax: 01287 660069
(Scarborough, Whitby and Ryedale Primary Care Trust)
Patient List Size: 2200

GP Ruth Elizabeth PEARCE, Marcus VAN DAM

Sandsend Surgery
East Row, Sandsend, Whitby YO21 3SU
Tel: 01947 895356 Fax: 01947 895581
(Scarborough, Whitby and Ryedale Primary Care Trust)
Patient List Size: 1600

Practice Manager Jean Clennan

GP Ian Gerard SUCKLING

The Surgery
Egton, Whitby YO21 1TX
(Scarborough, Whitby and Ryedale Primary Care Trust)

Practice Manager Madge McQue

GP Paul William METCALFE, Julian Simon FESTER

Whitby Group Practice
Spring Vale Medical Centre, Whitby YO21 1SD
Tel: 01947 820888 Fax: 01947 824100
Website: www.whitbygp.com
(Scarborough, Whitby and Ryedale Primary Care Trust)
Patient List Size: 15400

Practice Manager Trish Rutland

GP George Bremner Buchanan CAMPBELL, William Jonathan CHADWICK, David CUNION, Caroyn J FISHER, Paul Charles JOHNSON, Martin John Henry LINTON, John Joseph McAULEY, Terence McCORMACK, Antoni NACZK, Nigel OSWALD, Amanda Lucy SMART, Alistair Paul SUTCLIFFE, David VASEY, Paul John WARD, Bryony Pauline WILLIAMS

Whitchurch, Hampshire

Whitchurch Surgery
Bell Street, Whitchurch RG28 7AE
Tel: 01256 892113 Fax: 01256 895610
Email: manager@witchdoctors.fsnet.co.uk
(Mid-Hampshire Primary Care Trust)
Patient List Size: 5250

Practice Manager Margaret Oakton

GP Richard STYLES, Audrey BOUCHER, Rachel HANNETT

Whitchurch, Shropshire

Dodington Surgery
29 Dodington, Whitchurch SY13 1EL
Tel: 01948 662033 Fax: 01948 663428
(Shropshire County Primary Care Trust)

GP Paul Frederick WILSON, John Sunderland CLAYTON

Richmond House Surgery
Richmond Terrace, Station Road, Whitchurch SY13 1RH
Tel: 01948 662870

(Shropshire County Primary Care Trust)

GP Stephen John TEATHER, Robin Eric TERRY

Sandy Lane Surgery
Hanmer, Whitchurch SY13 3DL
Tel: 01948 830223 Fax: 01948 830103
(Shropshire County Primary Care Trust)

GP James David McCARTER

The Surgery
Sandy Lane, Whitchurch SY13 3DL
Tel: 01948 830223 Fax: 01948 830103
(Shropshire County Primary Care Trust)
Patient List Size: 2200

GP James David McCARTER

Walford House Surgery
Shrewsbury Street, Prees, Whitchurch SY13 2DH
Tel: 01948 840206 Fax: 01948 840765
(Shropshire County Primary Care Trust)

Practice Manager H Chawla

GP Guy Stephen Edwards CARTER, Fintan LAST

Whitehaven

Catherine Street Surgery
3 Catherine Street, Whitehaven CA28 7PD
Tel: 01946 693094 Fax: 01946 592597
(West Cumbria Primary Care Trust)

Practice Manager Mary McClusky

GP Ronald Thomas PROUDFOOT, Julie Davina RUDMAN

Church Street Surgery
27-28 Church Street, Whitehaven CA28 7EB
Tel: 01946 693660 Fax: 01946 592215
(West Cumbria Primary Care Trust)

Practice Manager Linda Smith

GP Stanley Alfred BAGSHAW, Maxine Virginia ENGLISH, Joanne Margaret HULL-DAVIES, Richard TRANTER

Flatt Walks Health Centre
3 Castle Meadows, Catherine Street, Whitehaven CA28 7QE
Tel: 01946 692173 Fax: 01946 590606
(West Cumbria Primary Care Trust)
Patient List Size: 10800

Practice Manager Mark Megan

GP Michael Aidan SYDNEY, Catriona Elizabeth Largent BOYLE, Michael John GODDEN, Michael Andrew LEWIS, David John ROGERS, Valerie Joan SULLIVAN

Irish Street Surgery
22 Irish Street, Whitehaven CA28 7BU
Tel: 01946 694457 Fax: 01946 590613
(West Cumbria Primary Care Trust)

Practice Manager Angus Christie

GP Graham John IRONSIDE, Fiona Claire IRONSIDE

Lowther Medical Centre
1 Castle Meadows, Whitehaven CA28 7RG
Tel: 01946 692241 Fax: 01946 590617
(West Cumbria Primary Care Trust)
Patient List Size: 10100

GP Nicola Jane STEVENSON, Jose Luis FERNANDEZ-FIDALGO, G M MACKENZIE, J G TELFORD, Joyce WOFFINDIN

Trinity House Surgery
17 Irish Street, Whitehaven CA28 7BU
Tel: 01946 693412 Fax: 01946 592046
(West Cumbria Primary Care Trust)
Patient List Size: 2600

Practice Manager Margaret Thorpe

GP Aidan Patrick TIMNEY, John Neil WESTHEAD

Whitley Bay

Beaumont Park Surgery
Hepscott Drive, Beaumont Park, Whitley Bay NE25 9XJ
Tel: 0191 251 4548 Fax: 0191 251 5805
Email: info@gp-A87011.nhs.uk
(North Tyneside Primary Care Trust)
Patient List Size: 8000

Practice Manager David Beck

GP Dr CHALMERS, Dr INGRAM, Dr LEE, Dr RAE

Drs Inglis, Isher, Norman and Falconer
49 Marine Avenue, Whitley Bay NE26 1NA
Tel: 0191 252 4527
(North Tyneside Primary Care Trust)
Patient List Size: 6561

Practice Manager F Robinson

GP Dr FALCONER, Dr INGLIS, Dr ISHER, Dr NORMAN

Dunelm
1 Delaval Avenue, Whitley Bay NE25 0EF
Tel: 0191 237 1555 Fax: 0191 298 0290
(Northumberland Care Trust)
Patient List Size: 5040

Practice Manager M C Atkinson

GP Daniel MacDonald KERR, L UNDERWOOD

Dunelm
1 Delaval Avenue, Seaton Delaval, Whitley Bay NE25 0EF
Tel: 0191 2372299 Fax: 0191 298 0290
(Northumberland Care Trust)

GP Peter McDAID

Marine Avenue Medical Centre
64 Marine Avenue, Whitley Bay NE26 1NQ
(North Tyneside Primary Care Trust)

GP Dr CRITCHLOW

Monkseaton Medical Centre
Cauldwell Avenue, Whitley Bay NE25 9PH
Tel: 0191 252 1616 Fax: 0191 252 2151
Email: linda.willis@nhs.net
(North Tyneside Primary Care Trust)
Patient List Size: 8725

Practice Manager Linda Willis

GP Charles Nicholas LAWSON, Helen COUNDON, Kathryn Ann CROSS, John Hugh FERRIMAN, Andrew James LAWSON

Park Parade Surgery
69 Park Parade, Whitley Bay NE26 1DU
Tel: 0191 252 3135 Fax: 0191 253 3566
(North Tyneside Primary Care Trust)

Practice Manager Gill Swan

GP Katherine Annette REAY, Christopher Joseph LEE, Brian Thomas SMITH

Westbourne Terrace Health Centre
Westbourne Terrace, Seaton Delaval, Whitley Bay NE25 0BE
Tel: 0191 237 2244
(North Tyneside Primary Care Trust)

GP C D BOWMAN, C S NAIR, S YOUNG

Whitley Bay Health Centre
Whitley Road, Whitley Bay NE26 2ND
(North Tyneside Primary Care Trust)

Practice Manager Alan Leslie

GP Dr OLSBURGH

Whitstable

Saddleton Road Surgery

32 Saddleton Road, Whitstable CT5 4JQ
Tel: 01227 272809
(Canterbury and Coastal Primary Care Trust)

GP Mohamed Bahgat SHAR

The Whitstable Medical Practice

Whitstable Health Centre, Harbour Street, Whitstable CT5 1BZ
Tel: 01277 594400/794555 Fax: 01277 771474/266352/794677
Website: www.whitstablemedicalpractice.co.uk
(Canterbury and Coastal Primary Care Trust)
Patient List Size: 30729

Practice Manager Lesley King

GP John Edward TURNER, Vernon BROWN, Sandra Jane CHANDLER, Gerhard ESSER, Helen GLYNN, Jacinta HILLS, Mary Anne JARDINE, Gunalakshman Mohan Hensman KANAGASOORIAM, Edward M LEE, Sally OSBORNE, Ronald PIETERS, Hilary Joan PINNOCK, John Rees PUCKETT, John Martin RIBCHESTER, Terence Antony STEFANI, Michael Louis WAIN

Whyteleafe

Whyteleafe Surgery

19 Station Road, Whyteleafe CR3 0EP
Tel: 01883 624181 Fax: 01883 622498
(East Surrey Primary Care Trust)
Patient List Size: 5000

Practice Manager Theresa Archibald

GP Victor TUN, Ann ROBERTS, Alison SLATER

Wickford

The Dental Suite

Wickford Health Centre, 2 Market Road, Wickford SS12 0AG
Tel: 01268 562444 Fax: 01268 733854
(Billericay, Brentwood and Wickford Primary Care Trust)

GP R P S SAHOTA

London Road Surgery

64 London Road, Wickford SS12 0AH
Tel: 01268 765533 Fax: 01268 570762
(Billericay, Brentwood and Wickford Primary Care Trust)
Patient List Size: 10754

Practice Manager Barbara Firmin

GP Mark Andrew BEECHAM, Rebecca O'REILLY, Janki PERSAUD, Paul RICHARDS, Anthony WALTON

Robert Frew Medical Centre

Silva Island Way, Salcott Crescent, Wickford SS12 9NR
Tel: 01268 578800 Fax: 01268 578825
(Billericay, Brentwood and Wickford Primary Care Trust)
Patient List Size: 13200

Practice Manager Colleen Shelley

GP Oluremi Akin AGBAJE, J C BROWN, Shoab IBRAHIM, Shirin NIMMO, O A OGUNSANYA, A TAYO, Atef Halim WISSA

Shotgate Surgery

340 Southend Road, Shotgate, Wickford SS11 8QS
Tel: 01268 561888 Fax: 01268 570850
(Billericay, Brentwood and Wickford Primary Care Trust)
Patient List Size: 2200

Practice Manager C Fernando

GP J T FERNANDO

Swan Lane Surgery

66 Swan Lane, Wickford SS11 7DD
Tel: 01268 735951 Fax: 01268 570849
(Billericay, Brentwood and Wickford Primary Care Trust)
Patient List Size: 3500

Practice Manager Jennifer Nash

GP Perumal CHANDRA REDDY

Wickford Health Centre

2 Market Road, Wickford SS12 0AG
Tel: 01268 766222 Fax: 01268 572756
(Billericay, Brentwood and Wickford Primary Care Trust)
Patient List Size: 2200

Practice Manager Paul Hancock

GP Kim CHEUNG

Wickford Health Centre

2 Market Road, Wickford SS12 0AG
Tel: 01268 766222 Fax: 01268 853216
(Billericay, Brentwood and Wickford Primary Care Trust)

GP S PATEL

Widnes

Appleton Village Surgery

2-6 Appleton Village, Widnes WA8 6DZ
Tel: 0151 423 2990 Fax: 0151 424 1032
(Halton Primary Care Trust)
Patient List Size: 10600

Practice Manager Linda Norton

GP Indra Datt SHARMA, Miles Jonathan BRINDLE, Ursula Bernadette BURKE, Christopher Ian SCHOFIELD, Christopher John TIERNEY

Beaconsfield Road Surgery

1 Beaconsfield Road, Widnes WA8 9LB
Tel: 0151 424 3232/3986 Fax: 0151 424 1009
(Halton Primary Care Trust)

Practice Manager Yvonne Leather

GP Neil Leslie MARTIN, Adrian Gerard McLAUGHLIN, Shanila ROOHI, Man Hong TSEUNG

Beeches Medical Centre

20 Ditchfield Road, Widnes WA8 8QS
Tel: 0151 424 3101/423 6632 Fax: 0151 495 2925
(Halton Primary Care Trust)
Patient List Size: 7600

Practice Manager Wendy Lightfoot

GP Mary GIBBONS, Calvin BUTTON, Melanie FORREST, Rebecca MAGUIRE, Serge NUGENT

Blundell Road Surgery

56 Blundell Road, Widnes WA8 8SS
Tel: 0151 420 2404 Fax: 0151 420 7717
Email: s.cox@nhs.net
(Halton Primary Care Trust)
Patient List Size: 2712

Practice Manager Sue Cox

GP Mahima PANDEY, A AMBROSINO, William ROBERTS

Highfield Medical Centre

Highfield Road, Widnes WA8 7DJ
Tel: 0151 424 3646 Fax: 0151 422 6499
(Halton Primary Care Trust)
Patient List Size: 2200

Practice Manager Amanda Crank

GP Mohammad Hussain SALEEMI

Newtown Health Care Centre

18 Lugsdale Road, Widnes WA8 6DS
Tel: 0151 424 2178/5273 Fax: 0151 257 9681
Email: debbie.coombes@nhs.net
(Halton Primary Care Trust)
Patient List Size: 7600

Practice Manager Debbie Coombes

GP Alan Christopher STANLEY, C H K CHAN, Maha MUSTAFA

Peelhouse Lane Surgery
1 Peelhouse Lane, Widnes WA8 6TW
Tel: 0151 424 6221 Fax: 0151 420 5436
(Halton Primary Care Trust)
Patient List Size: 13500

Practice Manager Donna Hunt

GP Stuart John EDWARDS, Charles Philip HALLAM, Paul Laurence HURST, Michael McLAUGHLIN, Christopher Simon John WOODFORDE

Upton Medical Centre
Bechers, Hough Green, Widnes WA8 4TE
Tel: 0151 424 9518 Fax: 0151 420 4979
(Halton Primary Care Trust)
Patient List Size: 2600

Practice Manager Bernie Mitchell

GP Surendra KUMAR, Santosh KUMAR

Upton Rocks Primary Care Centre
Cronton Lane, Widnes WA8 9AR
Tel: 0151 422 9794 Fax: 0151 422 9795
Email: paula.mcgarry@gp-N81651.nhs.uk
(Halton Primary Care Trust)

GP Sharon Jane CHAPELHOW

West Bank Medical Centre
2 Lower Church Street, Widnes WA8 0NG
Tel: 0151 424 3113 Fax: 0151 420 2969
(Halton Primary Care Trust)
Patient List Size: 2765

Practice Manager Olive Fagan

GP M LAKSHMINARAYANA

Wigan

Aspull Surgery
Haigh Road, Aspull, Wigan WN2 1XH
Tel: 01942 831263 Fax: 01942 832065
(Ashton, Leigh and Wigan Primary Care Trust)

GP Christopher John LYONS, Maurice REID, Thomas Andrew SEDDON

Beech Hill Medical Practice
278 Gidlow Lane, Wigan WN6 7PD
Tel: 01942 821899 Fax: 01942 821752
(Ashton, Leigh and Wigan Primary Care Trust)
Patient List Size: 14500

Practice Manager Stephanie Byrom

GP Alexander David TURNBULL, Anthony Richard Pieter GRAHAM, Robin Charles Pieter GRAHAM, Christopher Peter LORD, Timothy Peter MARWICK, Helen Margaret UNWIN

Dicconson Terrace Surgery
Dicconson Terrace, Wigan WN1 2AF
Tel: 01942 239525 Fax: 01942 826552
(Ashton, Leigh and Wigan Primary Care Trust)

GP Salma MUGHAL, Nicola HACKING, Katherine HOSIE, Peter John SOUTHERN

Dr M Pal
Morden Avenue, Ashton-in-Makerfield, Wigan WN4 9PT
Tel: 01942 715667 Fax: 01942 711252
(Ashton, Leigh and Wigan Primary Care Trust)

GP D PAL

Dr Ollerton
Hawkley Brook Surgery, Highfield Grange Avenue, Marus Bridge, Wigan WN3 6SU
Tel: 01942 234298 Fax: 01942 826548
(Ashton, Leigh and Wigan Primary Care Trust)

Practice Manager Susan Hiley

GP Dr OLLERTON

Dr Zaman and Partner
Highfield grange Avenue, Marus Bridge, Wigan WN3 6SU
Tel: 01942 243776 Fax: 01942 496111
(Ashton, Leigh and Wigan Primary Care Trust)

Practice Manager Janet Margerison

GP Kazi Ansaru ZAMAN, Dr ZAMAN

Fallon and Partners
1 Houghton Lane, Shevington, Wigan WN6 8ET
Tel: 01257 253311 Fax: 01257 251081
Website: www.shoughton-surgery.co.uk
(Ashton, Leigh and Wigan Primary Care Trust)
Patient List Size: 12500

Practice Manager Alison Cheetham

GP Jonathan Paul Ian TRACE, Lisa Madaline Jharna BOSE, Allan John FAIRHURST-WINSTANLEY, Christopher J LANCASTER, Louise A MERCER, Catriona Jane MUNRO, Michael POLLARD

Gill and Partners
Alexander House Health Centre, 600-602 Liverpool Road, Platt Bridge, Wigan WN2 5BB
Tel: 01942 866137 Fax: 01942 866891
(Ashton, Leigh and Wigan Primary Care Trust)
Patient List Size: 8000

Practice Manager Catherine Burgess

GP Kelvin Charles GILL, G G GRIESS, A F GUNDA

Hawkley Brook Surgery
Highfield Grange Avenue, Marus Bridge, Wigan WN3 6SU
Tel: 01942 234740 Fax: 01942 820037
Email: dr.mohankumar@gp-P92024.nhs.uk
(Ashton, Leigh and Wigan Primary Care Trust)

Practice Manager Penny Sudworth

GP S MOHANKUMAR, Bill RUSSELL

Kirk, Jacks, Gerlach and Lippett
Marus Bridge Health Centre, Highfield Grange Avenue, Wigan WN3 6SU
Tel: 01942 246099 Fax: 01942 496705
(Ashton, Leigh and Wigan Primary Care Trust)
Patient List Size: 4900

Practice Manager Sharon Freeman

GP Robert Stewart KIRK, Andreas GERLACH, Ruth Dawson JACKS, Stephanie LIPPETT

Liverpool Road Health Centre
Liverpool Road, Hindley, Wigan WN2 3HQ
Tel: 01942 255189 Fax: 01942 526217
(Ashton, Leigh and Wigan Primary Care Trust)
Patient List Size: 9170

Practice Manager Barbara Tymen

GP Nazir Ahmad BURZA, Dr AGARWALA, M NAWAZ, D NINAN

Longshoot Health Centre
Scholes, Wigan WN1 3NH
Tel: 01942 242610 Fax: 01942 826612
(Ashton, Leigh and Wigan Primary Care Trust)

GP Manu Khandubhai PATEL, B V PRABHU, Caroline Ann RAYNER, Surathkal VASUDEVA KAMATH

Lord Street Surgery
2 Lord Street, Ince, Wigan WN2 2AJ
Tel: 01942 242403 Fax: 01942 242403
(Ashton, Leigh and Wigan Primary Care Trust)

GP Rao CHALASANI

Lower Ince Surgery
238 Ince Green Lane, Ince, Wigan WN3 4RP
Tel: 01942 246263 Fax: 01942 824084
(Ashton, Leigh and Wigan Primary Care Trust)

Market Street Medical Centre
112-114 Market Street, Hindley, Wigan WN2 3AZ
Tel: 01942 256221 Fax: 01942 522479
Website: www.marketstreetmedical.co.uk
(Ashton, Leigh and Wigan Primary Care Trust)
Patient List Size: 16000

Practice Manager Kath Fenney

GP Jacqueline GUKENBY, R F HART, David George BRODIE, Sally Anne HART, Catherine Anne HOLME, Victoria Jane HOLME, Justin Graham TANKARD

Mesnes View Surgery
Mesnes Street, Wigan WN1 1ST
Tel: 01942 242350 Fax: 01942 826431
Email: jean.lowe@gp-P92634.nhs.uk
(Ashton, Leigh and Wigan Primary Care Trust)
Patient List Size: 4800

Practice Manager Jean Lowe

GP Anthony John ELLIS, Peter Richard KREPPEL

Newtown Medical Centre
205/207 Ormskirk Road, Newtown, Wigan WN5 9DP
Tel: 01942 494711 Fax: 01942 826240
(Ashton, Leigh and Wigan Primary Care Trust)
Patient List Size: 7200

Practice Manager Angela Abbott

GP Charles L BEZZINA, Philippe Francois Dominique D'ARIFAT, Dr EL ISLAM, D LOEPTIEN

Orrell Road Practice
Bradshaw Street, Orrell, Wigan WN5 0AB
Tel: 01942 222321 Fax: 01942 620327
(Ashton, Leigh and Wigan Primary Care Trust)

GP Adam BAJKOWSKI, P A SMITH, Richard Frederick STRETCH, Sinnathurai SUNTHA, A H WENG

Pemberton Primary Care Resource Centre
Sherwood Drive, Pemberton, Wigan WN5 9QX
Tel: 01942 775880 Fax: 01942 775882
Email: esther.jackson@gp-p92019.nhs.uk
(Ashton, Leigh and Wigan Primary Care Trust)
Patient List Size: 8800

Practice Manager Ester Jackson

GP Penelope Grace ANGIOR, N CROSS, K DONALDSON, I G OWEN, D E ROSE, S J SHAW

Pemberton Primary Care Resource Centre
Sherwood Drive, Pemberton, Wigan WN5 9QX
Tel: 01942 775880
(Ashton, Leigh and Wigan Primary Care Trust)
Patient List Size: 8650

Practice Manager Esther Jackson, Nancy Whittaker

GP Penelope Grace ANGIOR, Ian Glyn OWEN, Sheila Joan SHAW

Platt House Surgery
60 Warrington Road, Platt Bridge, Wigan WN2 5JA
Tel: 01942 866565/6 Fax: 01942 867846
Email: m.ullah@gp-P92031.nhs.uk
(Ashton, Leigh and Wigan Primary Care Trust)
Patient List Size: 3500

Practice Manager M Faroogue, June Telford

GP M ULLAH

Shakespeare Grove Surgery
2-4 Shakespeare Grove, Worsley Mesnes, Wigan WN3 5YA
Tel: 01942 241209 Fax: 01942 241209
(Ashton, Leigh and Wigan Primary Care Trust)

GP T M DALTON

Standish Medical Practice
Rodenhurst, Church Street, Standish, Wigan WN6 0JP
Tel: 01257 421909 Fax: 01257 424259
(Ashton, Leigh and Wigan Primary Care Trust)
Patient List Size: 10990

Practice Manager A O'Brien

GP Norma Agnes ARTHUR, Paul Raymond BURKINSHAW, Marwan GHALAYINI, Joanne Sarah HALL, Andrew D LANE, Johannes Franciscus Petrus VAN SPELDE

Sullivan Way Surgery
Sullivan Way, Scholes, Wigan WN1 3TB
Tel: 01942 243649 Fax: 01942 826476
(Ashton, Leigh and Wigan Primary Care Trust)
Patient List Size: 7600

Practice Manager Elaine Sharples

GP Mark Christopher SMITH, Yvette Karen LEWIS, Fiona Theresa MACMILLAN, Andrew Nicholas SUTTON

Walthew Lane Surgery
180 Walthew Lane, Platt Bridge, Wigan WN2 5AW
Tel: 01942 866925
(Ashton, Leigh and Wigan Primary Care Trust)

GP S C GUPTA

Warrington Road Surgery
429A Warrington Road, Abram, Wigan WN2 5XB
Tel: 01942 866277 Fax: 01942 866198
(Ashton, Leigh and Wigan Primary Care Trust)
Patient List Size: 4050

Practice Manager J Villiers

GP Deepak TRIVEDI, A O'CONNOR, Alka Deepak TRIVEDI

Wigan Road Medicentre
185 Wigan Road, Ashton-in-Makerfield, Wigan WN4 9SL
Tel: 01942 726325 Fax: 01942 272137
(Ashton, Leigh and Wigan Primary Care Trust)
Patient List Size: 6300

GP L D ARYA, Anandamoy MUKHERJEE, M SHARMA

Wigan Road Surgery
246 Wigan Road, Bryn, Ashton-in-Makerfield, Wigan WN4 0AR
Tel: 01942 727270 Fax: 01942 272197
(Ashton, Leigh and Wigan Primary Care Trust)
Patient List Size: 5500

Practice Manager Mark Durden

GP Michael Robert ASHWORTH, Fiona Bernadette JONES, David Thomas VALENTINE

Wigan Road Surgery
120 Wigan Road, Ashton-in-Makerfield, Wigan WN4 9SU
Tel: 01942 727325 Fax: 01942 709081
(Ashton, Leigh and Wigan Primary Care Trust)
Patient List Size: 7200

GP M ASLAM, J M CADMAN, G DEAN, P L PITALIA, Sanjay Kumar PITALIA, V K SAKSENA

Wigan Road Surgery
233 Wigan Road, Bryn, Ashton, Wigan WN4 9SR
Tel: 01942 727107 Fax: 01942 727146
(Ashton, Leigh and Wigan Primary Care Trust)

Practice Manager Brendan Ratcliffe

GP John Harris Anthony LEVINE

Winstanley Medical Centre
Holmes House Avenue, Winstanley, Wigan WN3 6JN
Tel: 01942 221100 Fax: 01942 214372
(Ashton, Leigh and Wigan Primary Care Trust)
Patient List Size: 3100

Practice Manager Julie Hurst
GP Leena SAXENA

Wrightington Street Surgery
1 Wrightington Street, Wigan WN1 2AZ
Tel: 01942 231965 Fax: 01942 826427
(Ashton, Leigh and Wigan Primary Care Trust)
Patient List Size: 3700
Practice Manager Joyce Lewis
GP Satish Kumar AHUJA, Jonathan Derek SEABROOK

Wigston

Bushloe End Surgery
48 Bushloe End, Wigston LE18 2BA
Tel: 0116 288 3477
(South Leicestershire Primary Care Trust)
Patient List Size: 10300
Practice Manager Lynn Towers
GP Michael Neville CHAMBERLAIN, V BOLARUM, Peter Kenneth BUCK, Sarah Margaret DAUNCEY, Christopher Patrick PRIDEAUX, Tracy TOBIN

Long Street Medical Centre
24 Long Street, Wigston LE18 2AH
Tel: 0116 288 3314 Fax: 0116 288 6711
Email: longstreet@msn.com
(South Leicestershire Primary Care Trust)
Patient List Size: 3100
Practice Manager M Cashmore
GP Anantt Ramanlal DAYAH, V MANNAN

South Wigston Health Centre
80 Blaby Road, Wigston LE18 2SE
(South Leicestershire Primary Care Trust)
Practice Manager K A Jelley
GP Paul PLATTS, Michael Henry DRUCQUER, Andrew John Hughdeburg SHARP, Jacqueline Frances SHAW

Wigston Central Surgery
48 Leicester Road, Wigston LE18 1DR
Tel: 0116 288 2566
(South Leicestershire Primary Care Trust)
GP Keith BAKER, Rakesh DESOR, Brenda Joan GRIFFIN, Sangita RAVAT

Wigton

Doctors Surgery
Friar Row, Caldbeck, Wigton CA7 8DS
Tel: 01697 478254 Fax: 01697 478661
(Carlisle and District Primary Care Trust)
Patient List Size: 4720
Practice Manager Deborah Harman
GP Philip Mark SPENCER, Natalie HAWKRIGG, Kate KEOHANE, Rachel WICKS

Doctors Surgery
Half Moon Lane, Wigton CA7 9NQ
Tel: 016973 42254 Fax: 016973 45464
(Carlisle and District Primary Care Trust)
Practice Manager Lin Baillie
GP George Watson BROWN, John Pattison HONEYMAN, Christina Joan RUSSELL, Robin Fraser Cawley SWINDELLS, Anna Therese Mary TURNBULL

Willenhall

Bloxwick Road South Surgery
63 Bloxwich Road South, Willenhall WV13 1AZ
Tel: 01902 608838 Fax: 01902 604866
(Walsall Teaching Primary Care Trust)
Practice Manager Sangeeta Prasad
GP A K PRASAD

Kingfisher Medical Centre
65 Fisher Street, Willenhall WV13 2HT
Tel: 01902 606303 Fax: 01902 606333
(Walsall Teaching Primary Care Trust)
Patient List Size: 3500
Practice Manager Lisa Davison
GP Narinder Singh SAHOTA, A ASHRAF, R SANDHU

New Invention Health Centre
66 Cannock Road, Willenhall WV12 5RZ
Tel: 01922 475100 Fax: 01922 712934
(Walsall Teaching Primary Care Trust)
Practice Manager R Mehta
GP Arunkumar Revulal SHAH, A MANDAL

Portobello Medical Centre
33 Dilloways Lane, Portobello, Willenhall WV13 3EY
Tel: 01902 601150 Fax: 01902 366737
(Wolverhampton City Primary Care Trust)
Practice Manager B Badh
GP Fayez TADROS

Rose Hill Surgery
2 Bilston Street, Willenhall WV13 2AW
Tel: 01902 608163 Fax: 01902 606287
(Walsall Teaching Primary Care Trust)
Patient List Size: 2050
Practice Manager June Jones
GP Galaa E FAYED

Stroud Avenue Medical Centre
250 Stroud Avenue, Willenhall WV12 4EG
Tel: 01902 609500 Fax: 01902 603625
(Walsall Teaching Primary Care Trust)
Patient List Size: 4700
GP Rameshchandra Maganbhai PATEL, P R PATEL

Willenhall Health Centre
Croft Street, Willenhall WV13 2DR
Fax: 01902 634448
(Walsall Teaching Primary Care Trust)
GP Shadia Zaky ABDALLA, Kallolikkal Meeran AMIRUDDIN, Neerampuzha Devasia DEVASIA, P GANDI, I WARIYAR

Willenhall Medical Centre
Croft Street, Willenhall WV13 2DR
Tel: 01902 600933 Fax: 01902 600835
(Walsall Teaching Primary Care Trust)
Patient List Size: 4600
Practice Manager Amanda Murrell
GP Celia Lesley PLATT, Thoppil Antony VARKEY

Willenhall Medical Centre
Croft Street, Willenhall WV13 2DR
Fax: 01902 600904
(Walsall Teaching Primary Care Trust)
GP A THOMAS

Wolverhampton Surgery
Wolverhampton Street, Willenhall WV13 2NF
Tel: 01902 635177 Fax: 01902 635727
(Walsall Teaching Primary Care Trust)
Patient List Size: 3000

Practice Manager Elizabeth Sconce

GP C R PANDIT, R SANDHU

Wilmslow

Handforth Health Centre
The Green, 166 Wilmslow Road, Handforth, Wilmslow SK9 3HL
Tel: 01625 529421
(Eastern Cheshire Primary Care Trust)

Practice Manager J A Quigley

GP E R HUDSON, Stafford Martin JOHNSON, Judith Pamela McDONALD, Ruth Elizabeth NEWHOUSE, Eleanor Jill PATTERSON, James Edward SHIPSTON

Hawthorn Lane Surgery
23 Hawthorn Lane, Wilmslow SK9 5DD
Tel: 01625 523902 Fax: 01625 522112
(Eastern Cheshire Primary Care Trust)
Patient List Size: 1300

Practice Manager Derran Castellani

GP Wai Kui CHUNG

Kenmore Medical Centre
60-62 Alderley Road, Wilmslow SK9 1PA
Tel: 01625 532244 Fax: 01625 549024
(Eastern Cheshire Primary Care Trust)
Patient List Size: 13000

Practice Manager Mike Evans

GP William David STOCKLEY, Jamie BUTLER, Leslie Robb HENDRY, Julia Elizabeth HUDDART, Stephen Robert MAXWELL, Gillian SCOTT

Wilmslow Health Centre
Chapel Lane, Wilmslow SK9 5HX
Tel: 01625 548555 Fax: 01625 548287
(Eastern Cheshire Primary Care Trust)
Patient List Size: 7800

Practice Manager E Robinson

GP Kathleen Mary Thérèse CASE, Amar AHMED, Mark BRENNAN

Wimborne

The Old Dispensary
32 East Borough, Wimborne BH21 1PL
Tel: 01202 880786 Fax: 01202 880736
(South and East Dorset Primary Care Trust)
Patient List Size: 3083

Practice Manager Denise Morgan

GP Alice Mary PHARAOH, Mark DEVERELL

The Quarter Jack Surgery
Rodways Corner, Wimborne BH21 1AP
Tel: 01202 882112/843626 Fax: 01202 882368
Email: doctors@quarterjacksurgery.co.uk
Website: www.quarterjacksurgery.co.uk
(South and East Dorset Primary Care Trust)
Patient List Size: 13000

Practice Manager Christine Clark

GP Paul Joseph LOXTON, Philippa Jane Nicola DICKINS, Brian Lawrence LEAR, Christopher Joseph REID, Hayley SANKSON, Torleif Rene SKULE, John Bu Leong TAN

The Surgery
Pennys Lane, Cranborne, Wimborne BH21 5QE
Tel: 01725 517272 Fax: 01725 517746
(South and East Dorset Primary Care Trust)
Patient List Size: 8721

Practice Manager Jo Morris

GP Sandi MALPAS, Colin Mark DAVIDSON, Andrew Robert LEVINSON, Bruce Pargeter WOOLLARD

Walford Mill Medical Centre
Knobcrook Road, Wimborne BH21 1NL
Tel: 01202 886999 Fax: 01202 840049
(South and East Dorset Primary Care Trust)
Patient List Size: 6407

Practice Manager C Rainsford

GP David CRAIGMYLE, Anne Margaret ELDER, Kate Evans, Mark Jonathan LINLEY-ADAMS

Wincanton

Wincanton Health Centre
Carrington Way, Wincanton BA9 9JY
Tel: 01963 32000 Fax: 01963 32146
(South Somerset Primary Care Trust)
Patient List Size: 7800

Practice Manager Janet Loe

GP Colin Frank FARRANT, Marcus John FELLOWS, Robert Glyn JONES, Iain Geoffrey PHILLIPS, Helena SMITH

Winchester

Friarsgate Practice
Friarsgate Medical Centre, Friarsgate, Winchester SO23 8EF
Tel: 01962 854091 Fax: 01962 854956
(Mid-Hampshire Primary Care Trust)
Patient List Size: 20000

Practice Manager Linda Cooper

GP James Roderick Campbell MORTON, Lorraine Melony COLE, Amanda Veronica Heather DAVIS, Martyn David DIAPER, Michael Glenn Barnard LAMBERT, Kanwarinder Singh MANN, Timothy John STANNARD, Nigel Charles SYLVESTER, Nicola Jane WRIGHT

The Gratton Surgery
Sutton Scotney, Winchester SO21 3LE
Tel: 01962 760267 Fax: 01962 761138
Email: enquiries@gp-J82106.nhs.uk
(Mid-Hampshire Primary Care Trust)
Patient List Size: 6500

Practice Manager J Roberts

GP David Aylmer John FIREBRACE, Peter James LEE, James Adam Poole READ, Henrietta Anne ROSIE, Anna Stephenie WILSON

The Riverside Practice
Friarsgate Medical Centre, Winchester SO23 8EF
Tel: 01962 853599 Fax: 01962 849982
(Mid-Hampshire Primary Care Trust)

GP Frank David Charles BURROWS, Joselyn BURROWS, Timothy George COTTON, Michael George MOORE, Judith Helen MYERS, Juliet Anne THOMPSON

St Clements Partnership
Tanner Street, Winchester SO23 8AD
Tel: 01962 852211 Fax: 01962 856010
(Mid-Hampshire Primary Care Trust)
Patient List Size: 17000

Practice Manager Kathy Bracher

GP Robert Julius REICHENBACH, Anne Elizabeth BAVISTER, S CHAPMAN, T COURTENAY, Anthony David CRAWFORD, John Colin DAVIES, Alexander William James FITZGERALD-BARRON, Kim Elizabeth ROBERTS, James William Peter ROSE, Peter Charles TOONE

St Paul's Surgery
Oram's Mount, Winchester SO22 5DD
Tel: 01962 853599 Fax: 01962 849982
(Mid-Hampshire Primary Care Trust)
Patient List Size: 14000

Practice Manager Diane Lester

GP Frank BURROWS, Joselyn BURROWS, Jason COLLINS, Timothy George COTTON, Helen MYERS, Juliet Anne THOMPSON, Deborah WHITE

Twyford Surgery
Hazeley Road, Twyford, Winchester SO21 1QY
Tel: 01962 712202 Fax: 01962 715158
(Mid-Hampshire Primary Care Trust)
Patient List Size: 9040

Practice Manager Adrian Kirsop

GP John Laurence O'SULLIVAN, Michael Roland Witold EVANS, Sandra Mary Ruth JAY, Deborah Jane LOCK, Miles Howard ROBERTS

Windermere

The Health Centre
Goodly Date, Windermere LA23 2EG
Tel: 01539 445159 Fax: 01539 446029
(Morecambe Bay Primary Care Trust)

GP Edward William Ralph OAKDEN, Christopher Simon STOKES, Sarah Margaret WATSON

St Mary's Surgery
Applethwaite, Windermere LA23 1BA
Tel: 01539 488484 Fax: 01539 442838
(Morecambe Bay Primary Care Trust)
Patient List Size: 6000

Practice Manager C.A. Sutton

GP Pagan BURNS, J H ROBERTS, John Paul WINTER-BARKER

Windermere Health Centre
Goodly Dale, Windermere LA23 2EG
Tel: 01539 442496 Fax: 01539 448329
(Morecambe Bay Primary Care Trust)

GP John Philip HAWSON

Windsor

Clarence Medical Centre
Vansittart Road, Windsor SL4 5AS
Tel: 01753 865773 Fax: 01753 833694
(Windsor, Ascot and Maidenhead Primary Care Trust)
Patient List Size: 13500

Practice Manager Jane Thompson

GP Gero BAIARDA, Mark Richard Leslie DENNY, Louise Elizabeth HUNTLEY, Stephen Ian LEWIS, Alan Patrick Graham MILLS

Dedworth Road Surgery
300 Dedworth Road, Windsor SL4 4JR
Tel: 01753 864545 Fax: 01753 620272
(Windsor, Ascot and Maidenhead Primary Care Trust)

Practice Manager J. Kirk

GP David Edward EVANS, Alexander John FRASER

Lee House Surgery
84 Osborne Road, Windsor SL4 3EW
Tel: 01753 861612 Fax: 01753 833695
(Windsor, Ascot and Maidenhead Primary Care Trust)
Patient List Size: 7900

Practice Manager Sandra Smith

GP Isabel M MOWER, Basab Kumar BARUA, Deborah SMITH

Runnymede Medical Practice
Newton Court Medical Centre, Burfield Road, Old Windsor, Windsor SL4 2QF
Tel: 01753 863642 Fax: 01753 832180
(Windsor, Ascot and Maidenhead Primary Care Trust)
Patient List Size: 4500

Practice Manager Janet Webster

GP Robert George Hankin BETHEL, Adrian Patrick HAYTER, Julian Bruce HOWELLS, Gwen Marles LEWIS, Manjinder Singh UPPAL, Charles WALKER

Sheet Street Surgery
21 Sheet Street, Windsor SL4 1BZ
Tel: 01753 860334 Fax: 01753 833696
Email: firstname.lastname@gp-k81068.nhs.uk
(Windsor, Ascot and Maidenhead Primary Care Trust)
Patient List Size: 11000

Practice Manager Anne Cox

GP Michael Frank DENNY, Roger Kenneth GOULDS, Christian Young-Myoung SHIN, John Peter William STONE, Catherine Mary WELLINGTON

South Meadow Surgery
3 Church Close, Eton, Windsor SL4 6AP
Tel: 01753 833777 Fax: 01753 833689
(Windsor, Ascot and Maidenhead Primary Care Trust)
Patient List Size: 5800

Practice Manager Judy Foulks

GP Jonathan James Cornelius HOLLIDAY, Jonathan Keith BRUDNEY, Malcolm Thomas SMITH-WALKER

Wingate

Church Street Surgery
4 Church Street, Wingate TS28 5AQ
Tel: 01429 838217
(Easington Primary Care Trust)

Practice Manager Dawn Nelson

GP Christopher Paul FAIRLAMB, Amanda Maxine SIMPSON, Nicola Jane STIRK

Wingate Surgery
Medical Centre, Front West Street, Wingate TS28 5PZ
Tel: 01429 838203 Fax: 01429 836928
(Easington Primary Care Trust)
Patient List Size: 2460

GP Prithwiraj SINHA

Winscombe

Winscombe Surgery
Hillyfields Way, Winscombe BS25 1AF
Tel: 01934 842211
(North Somerset Primary Care Trust)
Patient List Size: 7800

GP D H JOHN, Wendy FLETCHER, John Charles JACKSON, M L H PAUL, Kathryn Brenda Louise RUDDELL

Winsford

High Street Medical Centre
High St, Winsford CW7 2AS
Tel: 01606 862767 Fax: 01606 550876
(Central Cheshire Primary Care Trust)
Patient List Size: 4399

Practice Manager Tina Birkby

GP Ranadhir TALUKDER, P LARMOUR

Launceston Close Surgery
9-10 Launceton Close, Winsford CW7 1LY
Tel: 01606 861200 Fax: 01606 592778
(Central Cheshire Primary Care Trust)
Patient List Size: 4600

Practice Manager B Lyons

GP Selva RASAIAH, Neil Rhys THOMAS

Swanlow Medical Centre
60 Swanlow Lane, Winsford CW7 1JF
Tel: 01606 862868 Fax: 01606 550245
(Central Cheshire Primary Care Trust)
Patient List Size: 10000

Practice Manager Margaret Smith

GP Ihsan-ul WADOOD, S BUSSOLO, A DAMANIA, S KEMSLEY, A KRISHNA, Vidyanand PRASAD, Mohammad SHUAIB

Weavervale Surgery
High Street, Winsford CW7 2AS
Tel: 01606 862767
(Central Cheshire Primary Care Trust)

Willow Wood Surgery
Crock Lane, Wharton, Winsford CW7 3GY
Tel: 01606 861120 Fax: 01606 863354
(Central Cheshire Primary Care Trust)
Patient List Size: 4909

Practice Manager Linda Williams

GP Judith-Ann PRICE, Peter SEFTON-FIDDIAN

Wirral

Allport Surgery
Treetops PHCC, 43 Bridle Road, Bromborough, Wirral CH62 6EE
Tel: 0151 334 3621 Fax: 0151 328 5635
Website: www.allportsurgery.nhs.uk
(Bebington and West Wirral Primary Care Trust)
Patient List Size: 3900

Practice Manager John Issott

GP Heather Ann Stewart WALTON, Santiago PUIG

Church Road Medical Centre
64 Church Road, Bebington, Wirral CH63 3EY
Tel: 0151 645 1020 Fax: 0151 643 8891
(Bebington and West Wirral Primary Care Trust)
Patient List Size: 2427

GP D Y PATWALA

Civic Medical Centre
Civic Way, Bebington, Wirral CH63 7RX
Tel: 0151 645 6936 Fax: 0151 643 1698
Email: allan.stewart@gp-N85006.nhs.uk
Website: www.civicmc.nhs.uk
(Bebington and West Wirral Primary Care Trust)
Patient List Size: 8900

Practice Manager Allan M Stewart

GP Stephen John PILLOW, Susan Mary BRENNAN, Helen Elizabeth DOWNS, Philip Solomon HARRIS, Emma Louise HAYWARD, Emma Jane LAWRENCE, James O'CONNOR

Greasby Group Practice
Greasby Primary CareCentre, Greasby, Wirral CH49 3AT
Tel: 0151 678 3000 Fax: 0151 604 1813
(Bebington and West Wirral Primary Care Trust)
Patient List Size: 8000

Practice Manager Linda Hulse

GP Paul James Randle CUTHBERTSON, Jill BLACKLIN, Phillipa Jane COPPOCK, Angelo John PILLITTERI

Heatherlands Medical Centre
Newhay Road, Woodchurch, Wirral CH49 9DA
Tel: 0151 677 2169/1034 Fax: 0151 677 4013
Website: www.heatherlands.net
(Birkenhead and Wallasey Primary Care Trust)
Patient List Size: 4900

Practice Manager Barbara Cavanagh

GP Ivan Ajay CAMPHOR

Heswall Health Centre
270 Telegraph Road, Heswall, Wirral CH60 7SG
Tel: 0151 342 2230 Fax: 0151 342 7706
(Bebington and West Wirral Primary Care Trust)

Practice Manager Bob Spencer

GP Susan Kay BOUSFIELD, Stephen Douglas FORSTER, David Hywel JONES, Keith Stuart NICHOLAS, Elizabeth Margaret RULE, Martin John WOOLLONS

Hoylake and Meols Medical Centre
53 Birkenhead Road, Meols, Wirral CH47 5AF
Tel: 0151 632 6660 Fax: 0151 632 5073
(Bebington and West Wirral Primary Care Trust)

Practice Manager C M Bell

GP Malcolm Battersby BURGESS, Jane Alison WIGHT

Hoylake Road Surgery
314 Hoylake Road, Wirral CH46 6DE
Tel: 0151 677 2425 Fax: 0151 604 0482
(Birkenhead and Wallasey Primary Care Trust)

Practice Manager Ken Lovell

GP Akhtar ALI, Vijay SHARMA

Kings Lane Medical Centre
100 Kings Lane, Wirral CH63 5LY
Tel: 0151 608 4347 Fax: 0151 608 9095
(Bebington and West Wirral Primary Care Trust)
Patient List Size: 3600

Practice Manager Susan Ryder

GP Denyse KERSHAW, Thomas NEIL

Leasowe Primary Care Centre
Hudson Road, Leasowe, Wirral CH46 2QQ
Tel: 0151 630 0354 Fax: 0151 638 0627
(Birkenhead and Wallasey Primary Care Trust)

Practice Manager Claire Brand

GP N D SWIFT, A P POWELL

Moreton Health Clinic
Ashton House, 8-14 Chadwick Street, Moreton, Wirral CH46 7XA
Tel: 0151 677 1207 Fax: 0151 677 1207
(Birkenhead and Wallasey Primary Care Trust)

Practice Manager John Haddow

GP S M J S JANIKIEWICZ, J O'MALLEY, J E M WRIGHT

Moreton Health Clinic
8-10 Chadwick Street, Wirral CH46 7XA
Tel: 0151 677 1207 Fax: 0151 604 0372
(Birkenhead and Wallasey Primary Care Trust)

Practice Manager John Haddow

GP Stefan Maria Joseph Stanislaus JANIKIEWICZ, John Anthony O'MALLEY, Jane Elizabeth Mary WRIGHT

Moreton Medical Centre
27 Upton Road, Wirral CH46 0PE
Tel: 0151 677 2327 Fax: 0151 677 8181
Email: mme@moretonmc.force9.co.uk
Website: www.moreton.force9.co.uk
(Birkenhead and Wallasey Primary Care Trust)
Patient List Size: 6016

Practice Manager L Coulthard

GP Jeremy HENRY, Fiona Annette COWIE, Arthur Stephen MELLORS, Albert Anthony Lazarus PEREIRA

The Orchard
Village Road, Bromborough, Wirral CH62 7EU
Tel: 0151 334 2084 Fax: 0151 343 9437
(Bebington and West Wirral Primary Care Trust)

Practice Manager Muriel Hawkins

GP Brian George LANNIGAN, B A CONLON, Anne Patricia TOMLINSON

Park Medical Centre
2 Park Road, West Kirby, Wirral CH48 4DW
Tel: 0151 625 6128
(Bebington and West Wirral Primary Care Trust)
Patient List Size: 4900

Practice Manager S Preston

GP Phillip David BARNARD, Simon E DELANEY

Parkfield Medical Centre
Sefton Road, New Ferry, Wirral CH62 5HS
Tel: 0151 644 6665 Fax: 0151 643 1679
(Birkenhead and Wallasey Primary Care Trust)
Patient List Size: 6500

Practice Manager Julie Mckeown

GP Ellen Mary HAWTHORNTHWAITE, Marian BOGGILD, William Chew Coon CHONG, Maluusha GOKHALE, John Gordon OATES

Parkfield Medical Centre
Sefton Road, New Ferry, Wirral CH62 5HS
Tel: 0151 644 0055 Fax: 0151 643 1679
(Birkenhead and Wallasey Primary Care Trust)
Patient List Size: 7400

Practice Manager P Rutherford

GP Susan Ann CHESTERS, Fiona Jane BOOTH, Caroline Margaret JONES, Christopher John RAYMOND, Paul WATSON

Pensby Road Surgery
349 Pensby Road, Pensby, Wirral CH61 9NL
Tel: 0151 648 1193 Fax: 0151 648 2934
(Bebington and West Wirral Primary Care Trust)
Patient List Size: 6100

GP Elizabeth Margaret RULE, Dr FORSTER, David Hywel JONES, Martin John WOOLLONS

Plymyard Avenue Surgery
170 Plymyard Avenue, Eastham, Wirral CH62 8EH
Tel: 0151 327 1391 Fax: 0151 327 8670
(Bebington and West Wirral Primary Care Trust)

Practice Manager K Gately

GP Stephen WILLIAMS, Michael BURKE, Karalie Jane BUSH, Karen COOKE, Paula DEEGAN, Susan Jane PIGOTT, Dr PORTEOUS

Silverdale Medical Centre
Mount Avenue, Heswall, Wirral CH60 4RH
Tel: 0151 342 6128 Fax: 0151 342 2435
Email: postmaster@gp-n85058.nhs.uk
(Bebington and West Wirral Primary Care Trust)
Patient List Size: 5000

Practice Manager Julia Winstanley

GP Thomas Daniel HENNESSY, D M LANG, Roger Llewellyn PICKLES

Spital Surgery
1 Lancelyn Precinct, Spital Road, Wirral CH63 9JP
Tel: 0151 334 4019 Fax: 0151 346 1063
(Bebington and West Wirral Primary Care Trust)
Patient List Size: 4000

GP Gillian Gwyneth FRANCIS, Jane HORTOP

Teehey Lane Surgery
66-68 Teehey Lane, Bebington, Wirral CH63 2JN
Tel: 0151 608 2519 Fax: 0151 608 9249
(Bebington and West Wirral Primary Care Trust)

Practice Manager Alison Godsil

GP A HUSSAIN, A SAGAR

Twickenham Drive Surgery
63 Twickenham Drive, Leasowe, Wirral CH46 2QA
Tel: 0151 677 8882 Fax: 0151 604 0122
(Birkenhead and Wallasey Primary Care Trust)

GP V M SHIRALKAR

Upton Group Practice
32 Ford Road, Wirral CH49 0TF
Tel: 0151 677 0486 Fax: 0151 604 0635
(Birkenhead and Wallasey Primary Care Trust)

Practice Manager Peta Muray

GP Richard Brian PICKIN, Peter Stephen LARKIN, Thomas Murray PARTRIDGE, Eunice Edith RICHMOND, Anthony Bernard SMITH

West Kirby Health Centre
The Concourse, Grange Road, West Kirby, Wirral CH48 4HZ
Tel: 0151 625 9171 Fax: 0151 625 9499
(Bebington and West Wirral Primary Care Trust)

Practice Manager Leslie Isaacs

GP John Howard CLARK, John Stephen Hulton BRIGGS, Deborah Louise FORSDYKE, Susan Margaret M WELLS, Patricia Clare WHITE

West Kirby Health Centre
The Concourse, West Kirby, Wirral CH48 4HZ
Tel: 0151 625 9171 Fax: 0151 625 9499
(Bebington and West Wirral Primary Care Trust)

Practice Manager Leslie Isaacs

GP J S BRIGGS, J H CLARK, D FORSDYKE, S M M WELLS, P C WHITE

West Kirby Health Centre
Grange Road, Wirral CH48 4HZ
(Bebington and West Wirral Primary Care Trust)

GP Alan Richard PRICE, Marion Elizabeth SMETHURST, Jonathan Andrew Richard THOMPSON

West Wirral Group Practice
33 Thingwall Road, Irby, Wirral CH61 3UE
Tel: 0151 648 1846 Fax: 0151 648 0362
(Bebington and West Wirral Primary Care Trust)
Patient List Size: 15081

Practice Manager Christine Brennan

GP David John VINE, Janet Marie HUGHES, Christine Dinah SANSOM

West Wirral Group Practice
530 Pensby Road, Thingwall, Wirral CH61 7UE
Tel: 0151 648 1174 Fax: 0151 648 0644
(Bebington and West Wirral Primary Care Trust)

Practice Manager John Davies

GP Alan Robert JOHNSTON, Dr MAY

West Wirral Group Practice
Winterdyne, Rocky Lane, Heswall, Wirral CH60 0BY
Tel: 0151 342 2557 Fax: 0151 342 9384
(Bebington and West Wirral Primary Care Trust)

Practice Manager John L Davies

GP John Alan WRIGHT, Dr CHARLES, Victoria Margaret de HOXAR, Dr LOUW, Vivienne Elisabeth MAY

Wisbech

Clarkson Surgery
De-Havilland Road, Wisbech PE13 3AN
Tel: 01945 583133 Fax: 01945 464465
(East Cambridgeshire and Fenland Primary Care Trust)
Patient List Size: 12300

Practice Manager Barbara R Mews

GP Nigel Christopher WILLIAMS, David Brian FORSTER, Iain Harold MASON, Glenn Macgregor MOFFAT, Michael Phillip Lorimer PRYER, Nicholas Charles Ian ROSIER

Main Road Surgery
Main Road, Parson Drove, Wisbech PE13 4LF
Tel: 01945 700223 Fax: 01945 700915
Website: www.parsondrovesurgery.com
(East Cambridgeshire and Fenland Primary Care Trust)

Patient List Size: 5650

GP Bharatkumar Narshidas Jagjivan KHETANI, Andrew CHANDLER, Paul WRIGHT

North Brink Practice
7 North Brink, Wisbech PE13 1JR
Tel: 01945 585121 Fax: 01945 476423
Email: marg@nbrink.freeserve.co.uk
Website: www.northbrink.com
(East Cambridgeshire and Fenland Primary Care Trust)
Patient List Size: 16750

Practice Manager Margaret Burton

GP John LINES, Angela Jane CULSHAW, Peter GODBEHERE, Nilesh Rajnikant PATEL, Michael John RICHARDSON, M S SIRA, Paul WHYMAN, Quintin Kwing Kee WONG

St John's Surgery
Main Road, Terrington St. John, Wisbech PE14 7RR
Tel: 01945 880471 Fax: 01945 880677
(West Norfolk Primary Care Trust)
Patient List Size: 6500

Practice Manager Jenny Taylor

GP Christopher John Michael WOOD, Tina ARIFFIN, Weeraman Maithra KARUNARATNE

Trinity Surgery
Norwich Road, Wisbech PE13 3UZ
Tel: 01945 476999 Fax: 01945 476900
Email: info@trinity-surgery.co.uk
Website: www.trinity-surgery.co.uk
(East Cambridgeshire and Fenland Primary Care Trust)
Patient List Size: 6300

Practice Manager Bridget Dalziel

GP Ray Talbot WEBB, Ziad BITAR, Ruth EARL, Andrew WORDSWORTH

Upwell Health Centre
Townley Close, Upwell, Wisbech PE14 9BT
Tel: 01945 773671 Fax: 01945 773152
(East Cambridgeshire and Fenland Primary Care Trust)
Patient List Size: 9000

Practice Manager Mike Greenbank

GP Stephen Paul MILLARD, David Rhys BEVAN, Clare BLUNDELL, Eamonn James CLARKE, Paul Raymond WILLIAMS

Witham

Collingwood Road Surgery
40 Collingwood Road, Witham CM8 2DZ
Tel: 01376 502264 Fax: 01376 502474
(Witham, Braintree and Halstead Care Trust)

Practice Manager Bernadette Piper

GP Nagalingam Kathirgamalingam CHANDRALINGHAM

Douglas Grove Surgery
Douglas Grove, Witham CM8 1TE
Tel: 01376 512827 Fax: 01376 502463
(Witham, Braintree and Halstead Care Trust)
Patient List Size: 4000

Practice Manager Lesley Lagden

GP Nicholas Owen PARRY-JONES, Roy MELAMED

Fern House Surgery
125-129 Newland Street, Witham CM8 1BH
Tel: 01376 502108 Fax: 01376 502281
(Witham, Braintree and Halstead Care Trust)
Patient List Size: 16400

Practice Manager Lesley Turner

GP Richard Charles GREW, David Eugene BEATTY, Brian Robert GOUGH, Joanne Paula HOPCROFT, Richard Thomas SUMMERS, Eric TEVERSON, Caroline WRIGHT

Health Centre
4 Mayland Road, Witham CM8 2UX
Tel: 01376 302746 Fax: 01376 502393
(Witham, Braintree and Halstead Care Trust)

Practice Manager Jean Mills

GP B AHMED

Witham Health Centre
4 Mayland Road, Witham CM8 2UX
Tel: 01376 302747 Fax: 01376 502411
(Witham, Braintree and Halstead Care Trust)

Practice Manager Joy Minton

GP Dr AHMED, Kalpana KRISHNAMURTHY, Magadi Ramaswarmy KRISHNAMURTHY, Krishna MURTHY

Withernsea

St Nicholas Surgery
Queen Street, Withernsea HU19 2PZ
Tel: 01964 613221 Fax: 01964 613960
(Yorkshire Wolds and Coast Primary Care Trust)
Patient List Size: 11800

Practice Manager Kathy Sherwood

GP Robert Daniel FOURACRE, Robert James BLACKBOURN, Robert Stephen FRENCH, Graham David HEATON, Fawaz KHOURY, Satpaul UBHI

Witney

Chalmers and Partners
Cogges Surgery, Cogges Hill Road, Witney OX28 3FS
Tel: 01993 700505 Fax: 01993 706610
(South West Oxfordshire Primary Care Trust)
Patient List Size: 5000

Practice Manager Beth Sinclair

GP Catherine Ann CHALMERS, Andrew DOUGLAS, Brian George GREEN

Deer Park Medical Centre
6 Edington Square, Witney OX28 5YT
Tel: 01993 700088 Fax: 01993 700140
Email: practice@deerpark.oxongps.nhs.uk
(South West Oxfordshire Primary Care Trust)
Patient List Size: 4500

Practice Manager Shirley Moon

GP Carol Ann LOLE-HARRIS, Karen GRIFFITHS

Eynsham Medical Group
Eynsham Medical Centre, Conduit Lane, Eynsham, Witney OX29 4QB
Tel: 01865 881206 Fax: 01865 881342
Email: firstname.lastname@gp-k4006.nhs.uk
Website: www.eynshammedicalgroup.org.uk
(South West Oxfordshire Primary Care Trust)
Patient List Size: 12850

Practice Manager Andy Benford

GP David John Maxwell PETERSON, Ian Hamlyn BINNIAN, Paul Patrick COFFEY, Helen Wynne EVANS, Philippa Claire JACKSON, Neil David RUST, Victoria Charlotte Standish STANSFIELD, Philip Bernard Ommanney STEPHENSON

Nuffield Health Centre
Welch Way, Witney OX28 6JQ
Tel: 01993 703641 Fax: 01993 773899
(South West Oxfordshire Primary Care Trust)

Practice Manager Moira Gardiner

GP Oliver Martin BOLAND, Stephen BRYLEWSKI, John Lawrence DERRY, Susanna GRAHAM-JONES, Connor Edward MORRIS, Nirmala Kausilya NAIDOO, Patricia Delphine PROSSER, Margaret STEWART

Windrush Health Centre
Welch Way, Witney OX28 6JS
Tel: 01993 702911 Fax: 01993 700931
Website: www.windrushhealthcentre.org
(South West Oxfordshire Primary Care Trust)
Patient List Size: 12000

Practice Manager Morag Keen

GP Jeremy Ronald JARVIS, Angela Nicole CADDICK, Peter Robert GRIMWADE, Stephen Michael Vincent SMITH, Rosemary Ann THORLEY, Paul Anthony WATSON

Woking

College Road Surgery
4-6 College Road, Woking GU22 8BT
Tel: 01483 771309
(Surrey Heath and Woking Primary Care Trust)

Practice Manager Edith Betts

GP Ghylam-Mustafa PANHWAR

Dr Close and Partners
St John's Health Centre, Hermitage Road, St John's, Woking GU21 1TD
Tel: 01483 723451 Fax: 01483 751879
(Surrey Heath and Woking Primary Care Trust)

Practice Manager Georgina Curtin

GP W H ANDERSEN, Sian LEWIS, Mohammed RAHMAN, Dafydd Huw Vaughan THOMAS, Anthony Robert James WALL

Greenfield Surgery
1 Claremont Avenue, Woking GU22 7SF
Tel: 01483 771171 Fax: 01483 725808
(Surrey Heath and Woking Primary Care Trust)
Patient List Size: 2820

Practice Manager Jane Pool

GP Richard John POOL

Hillview Medical Centre
3 Heathside Road, Woking GU22 7QP
Tel: 01483 766333 Fax: 01483 757067
(Surrey Heath and Woking Primary Care Trust)
Patient List Size: 10880

Practice Manager Carole Randall

GP Peter John Roland SMITH, Richard Peter EVANS, Henry Daniel KNIGHTS, Helena NEWMAN, Deborah Anne SHIEL

Maybury Surgery
Alpha Road, Maybury, Woking GU22 8HF
Tel: 01483 728757 Fax: 01483 729169
(Surrey Heath and Woking Primary Care Trust)
Patient List Size: 1500

Practice Manager Beverley Howard

GP Imtiaz Ahmed YUSUF, Shada Shane PARVEEN

Pirbright Surgery
The Old Vicarage, The Green, Pirbright, Woking GU24 0JE
Tel: 01483 474473 Fax: 01483 488727
(Surrey Heath and Woking Primary Care Trust)
Patient List Size: 2800

Practice Manager Bridget Martin

GP Yvonne Moira BISHOP, Paul VAN DEN BOSCH

Sheerwater Health Centre
Devonshire Avenue, Sheerwater, Woking GU21 5QJ
Tel: 01932 343524 Fax: 01932 355908
(Surrey Heath and Woking Primary Care Trust)

Practice Manager Sandra Dudman

GP Munira S MOHAMED

Southview Surgery
Guildford Road, Woking GU22 7RR
Tel: 01483 763186 Fax: 01483 821526
Email: doctors@gp-H81041.nhs.uk
Website: www.southviewsurgery.freeserve.co.uk
(Surrey Heath and Woking Primary Care Trust)
Patient List Size: 8400

Practice Manager Lorraine Knapp

GP Anthea Elizabeth HENDRY, Clare Louise BENHAM, David James HINDLEY, Paul John KUZMIN, Bernard John RUMBALL

Sunny Meed Surgery
15-17 Heathside Road, Woking GU22 7EY
Tel: 01483 772760 Fax: 01483 730354
Email: doctors@sunnymeed-surgery.freeserve.co.uk
(Surrey Heath and Woking Primary Care Trust)
Patient List Size: 9000

Practice Manager Fillipa Dilena

GP Michael Joseph BOURKE, Sara GIL RIVAS, Carmel Ann KELLY, Paul Vincent RANKIN

The Surgery
16 Windsor Road, Chobham, Woking GU24 8NA
Tel: 01276 857117 Fax: 01276 855668
(Surrey Heath and Woking Primary Care Trust)
Patient List Size: 10900

Practice Manager Lee Taylor

GP Paul Clifford BATES, Caroline BARKER, Paul CARTY, David JOHNSON, Susan Kay MICHELMORE, Sanjeeu SERON, Michael WALKER

The Villages Medical Centre
Send Barns Lane, Send, Woking GU23 7BP
Tel: 01483 226330 Fax: 01483 225253
(Guildford and Waverley Primary Care Trust)
Patient List Size: 6500

Practice Manager Veronica Payne

GP Anne BURNS, Yassir Mohamed Shaker AL-AARAJI, J KUNZ, K J NEVIN

York House Medical Centre
Heathside Road, Woking GU22 7XL
Tel: 01483 760014 Fax: 01483 766042
Email: practice@lytton.free-online.co.uk
(Surrey Heath and Woking Primary Care Trust)

Practice Manager Barbara Vaughan

GP Yvonne Dorothy COLLINS, C R CLAYTON, U S GAUR, Clare E GROVE, Nigel Henry Leighton SELLARS

York House Medical Centre
Heathside Road, Woking GU22 7XL
Tel: 01483 761100 Fax: 01483 751185
(Surrey Heath and Woking Primary Care Trust)
Patient List Size: 10900

Practice Manager Angela Grimshaw

GP James Philip MELLOR, Tracey M COLLINS, Neman KHAN, Nicholas Stephen LANCE, Sarah Maria LENO, Linda ROBERTS, Rakesh SHARMA

Wokingham

Burma Hills Surgery
Ashridge Road, Wokingham RG40 1PH
Tel: 0118 978 5854 Fax: 0118 989 3902
(Wokingham Primary Care Trust)

GP Dr WIN HLAING

Cedar House Surgery
269A Nine Mile Ride, Finchampstead, Wokingham RG40 3NS
Tel: 0118 932 8966 Fax: 0118 973 4710
(Wokingham Primary Care Trust)

Patient List Size: 3300

Practice Manager Sheila Stickland

GP Ian James HOSSACK, Rosemary Anne LATHAM

Finchampstead Road Surgery
474 Finchampstead Road, Finchampstead, Wokingham RG40 3RG
Tel: 0118 973 2678 Fax: 0118 973 3689
Email: bryan.woollatt@gp-k81025.nhs.uk
(Wokingham Primary Care Trust)
Patient List Size: 12328

Practice Manager Bryan Woollatt

GP Michael Hamilton CORFIELD, Jeremy BAILY-GIBSON, Susan Marie BIRD, Robin John MELLOWS, Karla Amanda WEIR, Heinrich Johan ZYLSTRA

Shute End Medical Centre
34 Reading Road, Wokingham RG41 1EH
Tel: 0118 978 2299 Fax: 0118 977 0284
(Wokingham Primary Care Trust)

GP Gopendra Gopal MITRA THAKUR

Tudor House and Rectory Road Medical Practice
14 Rectory Road, Wokingham RG40 1DH
Tel: 0118 978 3544 Fax: 0118 977 0420
(Wokingham Primary Care Trust)
Patient List Size: 23500

Practice Manager Adrian Wise

GP Martin Brooke HASLAM, Ranjit Singh BAHRA, Gillian Alexandra BEARD, Jane Rosemary DORAN, Robin Clive EDWARDS, Gerard Peter FOLEY, Charles John GALLAGHER, John David KERR, Moira Elizabeth MACDOUGALL, Deborah Anne STACKWOOD

Woosehill Surgery
Emmview Close, Woosehill, Wokingham RG41 3DA
Tel: 0118 978 8266/978 8689 Fax: 0118 979 3661
Website: www.woosehillsurgery.co.uk
(Wokingham Primary Care Trust)
Patient List Size: 9600

Practice Manager Jean Young

GP Mark Colin LEE, Richard Norman BLYTH, Susan Mary HELM, Philip Adrian Jocelyn SMYLY, Elizabeth Anne WATSON

Wolverhampton

Albrighton Medical Practice
Shaw Lane, Albrighton, Wolverhampton WV7 3DT
(Shropshire County Primary Care Trust)
Patient List Size: 8600

GP M PERRY

Alfred Squire Road Health Centre
Alfred Squire Road, Wednesfield, Wolverhampton WV11 1XU
Tel: 01902 731904
(Wolverhampton City Primary Care Trust)

Practice Manager Ian Currie

GP Sarah Josepha CURRIE

Alfred Squire Road Health Centre
Wednesfield, Wolverhampton WV11 1XU
(Wolverhampton City Primary Care Trust)

GP Dr OLDHAM

All Saints Surgery
17 Cartwright Street, Wolverhampton WV2 1EU
Tel: 01902 457617 Fax: 01902 351021
(Wolverhampton City Primary Care Trust)

GP J S KAINTH, Pravin KAINTH

Ashfield Road Surgery
39 Ashfield Road, Fordhouses, Wolverhampton WV10 6QX
Tel: 01902 783372 Fax: 01902 784671
(Wolverhampton City Primary Care Trust)
Patient List Size: 2950

Practice Manager Mrs Paul

GP Dr DHILLON, Dr PAUL

Ashmore Park Clinic
Griffiths Drive, Ashmore Park, Wolverhampton WV11 2LH
Tel: 01902 732442 Fax: 01902 729048
(Wolverhampton City Primary Care Trust)

Practice Manager Mandy Wilkinson

GP Mohamed Abdur RAHMAN, Mohammad Haseebur RAHMAN

Barry and Flynn
97 Blackhalve Lane, Wednesfield, Wolverhampton WV11 1BB
Tel: 01902 731902 Fax: 01902 307966
(Wolverhampton City Primary Care Trust)

Practice Manager Anne Barry

GP Kevin John BARRY, Aidan Gerard FLYNN

Bilbrook Medical Centre
Brookfield Road, Bilbrook, Wolverhampton WV8 1DX
Tel: 01902 847313 Fax: 01902 842322
(South Western Staffordshire Primary Care Trust)
Patient List Size: 7500

Practice Manager Diane Hall

GP Peter Richard MAIDMENT, Marisa COPPOLO, Jonathan GRIFFITHS, Susan KEMSLEY

Brooklands Parade Surgery
2 Brooklands Parade, Wolverhampton WV1 2ND
Tel: 01902 453345 Fax: 01902 452141
(Wolverhampton City Primary Care Trust)
Patient List Size: 1856

Practice Manager Chris Wainwright

GP Nathaniel DJAN

Cannock Road Surgery
60 Cannock Road, Wednesfield, Wolverhampton WV10 8PJ
Tel: 01902 739973 Fax: 01902 731958
(Wolverhampton City Primary Care Trust)
Patient List Size: 2802

Practice Manager Pat Arnold

GP M P LINNEMANN

Castlecroft Medical Practice
104 Castlecroft Road, Castlecroft, Wolverhampton WV3 8LU
Tel: 01902 761629 Fax: 01902 765660
(Wolverhampton City Primary Care Trust)
Patient List Size: 9500

Practice Manager A J Leighton, Cherry A Walton

GP Richard Stuart WALTON, Peter James DUNCAN, Vina PATEL, Richard ROBERTS, Joanna SHAW, Peter John WAGSTAFF

Coalway Road Surgery
119 Coalway Road, Penn, Wolverhampton WV3 7NA
Tel: 01902 341409 Fax: 01902 620527
(Wolverhampton City Primary Care Trust)
Patient List Size: 4990

Practice Manager Wendy Hollis

GP Stuart Victor COWEN, Elizabeth GUEST, Miles Ewan Pearce MANLEY

Cromwell Road Surgery
60 Cromwell Road, Bushbury, Wolverhampton WV10 8UT
Tel: 01902 784784
(Wolverhampton City Primary Care Trust)

Practice Manager Janet Beason

GP Kewal Singh KRISHAN

Dale Medical Practice
Planks Lane, Wombourne, Wolverhampton WV5 8DX
Tel: 01902 892209 Fax: 01902 892441

(South Western Staffordshire Primary Care Trust)

Practice Manager S A Brookes

GP Linda Helen BRYAN, Christopher Rhys HADLEY, A D JONES

Duncan Street Surgery

Duncan Street, Wolverhampton WV2 3AN
Tel: 01902 458193 Fax: 01902 458193
(Wolverhampton City Primary Care Trust)

Practice Manager Louise Phillips

GP Barbara Sylvia NOBLE, Dr KHAN, Wendy Sheila RYLANCE, Dr WELDING

Duncan Street Surgery

Blakenhall, Wolverhampton WV2 3AN
(Wolverhampton City Primary Care Trust)

GP J E DAVIES

Ednam Road Surgery

14 Ednam Road, Goldthorn Park, Wolverhampton WV4 5BL
Tel: 01902 340200 Fax: 01902 349715
(Wolverhampton City Primary Care Trust)
Patient List Size: 2690

GP P K CHAKRABARTI

Featherstone Family Health Centre

Old Lane, Hilton Lane, Featherstone, Wolverhampton WV10 7BS
Tel: 01902 305899 Fax: 01902 735577
(South Western Staffordshire Primary Care Trust)
Patient List Size: 3300

Practice Manager Maureen Lee

GP Edward Fong-Yin LEE

Goldthorn Medical Centre

130a Park Street South, Off Goldthorn Hill, Wolverhampton WV2 3JF
Tel: 01902 339283 Fax: 01902 339283
(Wolverhampton City Primary Care Trust)
Patient List Size: 5150

Practice Manager Munish Pahwa

GP Mahendra Kumar PAHWA, Ved Kumari PAHWA

Gravel Hill Surgery

Wombourne, Wolverhampton WV5 9HA
Tel: 01902 893375 Fax: 01902 896616
(South Western Staffordshire Primary Care Trust)

Practice Manager Christine Davis

GP Andrew Ernest John VYSE, Ian Timothy DUKES, Kenneth Brian FRANKLIN, Kirsten Jane HADLINGTON

Griffiths Drive Surgery

75 Griffiths Drive, Wednesfield, Wolverhampton WV11 2JN
Tel: 01902 731250 Fax: 01902 307193
(Wolverhampton City Primary Care Trust)

Practice Manager June Bond

GP Dr BILAS, Dr THOMAS

Grove Medical Centre

175 Steel House Lane, Wolverhampton WV2 2AU
Tel: 01902 455771 Fax: 01902 457594
Email: suneetjulka@freeserve.co.uk
(Wolverhampton City Primary Care Trust)
Patient List Size: 3650

Practice Manager Joanne Round

GP Surinder Kumar JULKA, Manjit KAINTH

The Health Centre

Alfred Squire Road, Wednesfield, Wolverhampton WV11 1XU
Tel: 01902 575033 Fax: 01902 575013
(Wolverhampton City Primary Care Trust)
Patient List Size: 9000

Practice Manager Julie Maiden

GP James William CLEWS, Davinder BAGARY, Rachael HOGG, Srayan LUCKRAFT, Julian David PARKES, Robert STOVES

Heath Town Medical Centre

Chervil Rise, Heath Town, Wolverhampton WV10 0HP
Tel: 01902 456211 Fax: 01902 688145
(Wolverhampton City Primary Care Trust)

Practice Manager Mrs Christopher

GP Dr CHRISTOPHER

Jeffcock Road Surgery

163 Jeffcock Road, Penn Fields, Wolverhampton WV3 7AQ
Tel: 01902 332994
(Wolverhampton City Primary Care Trust)

GP S VIJ

Lakeside Medical Centre

Church Road, Perton, Wolverhampton WV6 7QL
Tel: 01903 755329 Fax: 01902 755224
(South Western Staffordshire Primary Care Trust)

Practice Manager Jill McHale

GP Paul Douglas NIGHTINGALE, Kiaran ASTHANA, Anthony David BALDWIN

Lea Road Surgery

35 Lea Road, Pennfields, Wolverhampton WV3 0LS
Tel: 01902 23064 Fax: 01902 657800
(Wolverhampton City Primary Care Trust)
Patient List Size: 6150

Practice Manager David C Easy

GP Ho Hoi LEUNG, Nenry ORZ, Mona SIDHU

Leicester Street Medical Centre

Leicester Street, Wolverhampton WV6 0PS
Tel: 01902 424118 Fax: 01902 310087
(Wolverhampton City Primary Care Trust)
Patient List Size: 7000

GP Uma PASSI, Sudhir Inderraj HANDA, Man Mohan Lal PASSI

Low Hill Medical Centre

191 First Avenue, Low Hill, Wolverhampton WV10 9SX
Tel: 01902 731319 Fax: 01902 822883
(Wolverhampton City Primary Care Trust)

Practice Manager Takya Khan

GP Mohammad Irshad KHAN

Low Hill Medical Centre

191 First Avenue, Low Hill, Wolverhampton WV10 9SX
Tel: 01902 728861 Fax: 01902 822883
(Wolverhampton City Primary Care Trust)

Practice Manager Tracey Sutcliffe

GP Dr RYAN

Lower Street Health Centre

Lower Street, Tettenhall, Wolverhampton WV6 9LL
Tel: 01902 444551
(Wolverhampton City Primary Care Trust)

Practice Manager Susan Sephton

GP Mark WILSON, Martin ASHTON, Jeremy John BRIGHT, Timothy Nevil JACKSON, Robbert SMISSAERT

Marsh Lane Surgery

68 Marsh Lane, Fordhouses, Wolverhampton WV10 6RU
Tel: 01902 398111 Fax: 01902 680078
(Wolverhampton City Primary Care Trust)

GP Sankarprasad MAJI

Masefield Road Surgery

17 Keat's Grove, Wolverhampton WV10 8LY
Tel: 01902 731907 Fax: 01902 733309
(Wolverhampton City Primary Care Trust)
Patient List Size: 6000

Practice Manager Carol Kenney

GP Uwe KEHLER, Win AUNG

The Newbridge Surgery
255 Tettenhall Road, Wolverhampton WV6 0ED
Tel: 01902 751420 Fax: 01902 747936
(Wolverhampton City Primary Care Trust)
Patient List Size: 4500

Practice Manager S Hickman

GP Jane Sally WILKINSON, Gillian PICKAVANCE, Ian QUANCE

Northwood Park Road Surgery
85 Northwood Park Road, Bushbury, Wolverhampton WV10 8EX
Tel: 01902 831500 Fax: 01902 831996
(Wolverhampton City Primary Care Trust)
Patient List Size: 1900

Practice Manager Barbara Harper

GP Valli GRANDHI, Dr GRANDHI

Oxley Health Centre
Probert Road, Oxley, Wolverhampton WV10 6UF
Tel: 01902 444035 Fax: 01902 444944
(Wolverhampton City Primary Care Trust)

Practice Manager T Taylor

GP Dr HENDERSON, Dr JONES

Parkfield Medical Centre
255 Parkfield Road, Wolverhampton WV4 6EG
Tel: 01902 342152 Fax: 01902 620868
(Wolverhampton City Primary Care Trust)

Practice Manager S Thornhill

GP Henry Nicholas HALL, Helen Macpherson HIBBS, Alison JOHNSON, Akinwumi Adewale LATUNJI, Helen Elizabeth MEREDITH

Pendeford Health Centre
Whitburn Close, Wolverhampton WV9 5NJ
Tel: 01902 781728 Fax: 01902 781728
(Wolverhampton City Primary Care Trust)
Patient List Size: 1800

GP Ranjit PRASAD

Pendeford Health Centre
Whitburn Close, Pendeford, Wolverhampton WV9 5NJ
Tel: 01902 788177 Fax: 01902 575006
(Wolverhampton City Primary Care Trust)

Practice Manager Ann Hughes

GP Nejatollah TAHERI

Pendeford Health Centre
Whitburn Close, Pendeford, Wolverhampton WV9 5NJ
Tel: 01902-789080 Fax: 01902 781728
(Wolverhampton City Primary Care Trust)

GP Dr VIJ

Penn Manor Medical Centre
Manor Road, Penn, Wolverhampton WV4 5PY
Tel: 01902 331166 Fax: 01902 575078
(Wolverhampton City Primary Care Trust)
Patient List Size: 10800

Practice Manager Aileen Dain

GP Jonathan Francis Middleton WHITE, John Timothy BURRELL, Gordon Andrew FORREST, Huw Francis Bernard GLOVER, Manjeet Kaur SAMRA

Penn Surgery
2 Coalway Road, 2a Coalway Road, Penn, Wolverhampton WV3 7LR
Tel: 01902 332040 Fax: 01902 621540
(Wolverhampton City Primary Care Trust)

GP David MacKenzie BUSH, Peter GEE

Poplars Medical Centre
Third Avenue, Low Hill, Wolverhampton WV10 9PG
Tel: 01902 7331195 Fax: 01902 656466
(Wolverhampton City Primary Care Trust)
Patient List Size: 2500

Practice Manager Sandra Russon

GP Gurmit Ram MAHAY

Prestwood Road Surgery
279 Prestwood Road, Wednesfield, Wolverhampton WV11 1RF
Tel: 01902 305322 Fax: 01902 575016
(Wolverhampton City Primary Care Trust)

Practice Manager Sandra Griffins

GP Pranab Kumar GHOSH

Prestwood Road West Surgery
81 Prestwood Road West, Wednesfield, Wolverhampton WV11 1HT
Tel: 01902 721021 Fax: 01902 306225
(Wolverhampton City Primary Care Trust)
Patient List Size: 9700

Practice Manager Margaret Moses

GP Christopher WALKER, Elizabeth Susan BALL, Julian HICKMAN, Nasreen ILYAS, Clude LUIS, Julian Palmer MORGANS

Primrose Lane Health Centre
Primrose Lane, Wolverhampton WV10 8RN
Tel: 01902 731583 Fax: 01902 305789
(Wolverhampton City Primary Care Trust)

Practice Manager Pat Lewis

GP Michael John RUSSON, Andrew Michael SHARDLOW

Ravindran
East Park Medical Practice, Jonesfield Crescent, Wolverhampton WV1 2LW
Tel: 01902 455422/451983 Fax: 01902 454137
(Wolverhampton City Primary Care Trust)
Patient List Size: 3721

Practice Manager Lisa Homfray

GP Thambar Sabaratnam RAVINDRAN, Roger RAMSAY

Raynor Road Medical Centre
19 Raynor Road, Fallings Park, Wolverhampton WV10 9QY
Tel: 01902 307400 Fax: 01902 307406
(Wolverhampton City Primary Care Trust)
Patient List Size: 3000

Practice Manager J Roberts

GP Dr WARIYAR

Raynor Road Surgery
21 Raynor Road, Fallings Park, Wolverhampton WV10 9QU
Tel: 01902 307033 Fax: 01902 561722
(Wolverhampton City Primary Care Trust)
Patient List Size: 2440

Practice Manager Gerada Pemberton

GP Dr GANGULY

Ruskin Road Surgery
30-32 Ruskin Road, The Scotlands, Wolverhampton WV10 8DJ
Tel: 01902 731839 Fax: 01902 731839
Email: urszula.winiewicz@gp-m92637.nhs.uk
(Wolverhampton City Primary Care Trust)

Practice Manager Karen Withington

GP Urszula WINIEWICZ

Russell House Surgery
Bakers Way, Codsall, Wolverhampton WV8 1HD
Tel: 01902 842488
(South Western Staffordshire Primary Care Trust)

GP A J WAKEMAN, L JONES, J M LARKIN, D J WILLIAMS

Russell House Surgery
Russell House, Bakers Way, Codsall, Wolverhampton WV8 1HD
Tel: 01902 842488 Fax: 01902 846170
(South Western Staffordshire Primary Care Trust)

Practice Manager Renee White

GP Anne Juanita WAKEMAN, Leslie JONES, Joanna LARKIN, D J WILLIAMS

Stafford Road Surgery
470 Stafford Road, Oxley, Wolverhampton WV10 6AR
Tel: 01902 783103 Fax: 01902 575114
(Wolverhampton City Primary Care Trust)

GP Joseph Moelwyn FOWLER

The Surgery
Woden Road, Wolverhampton WV10 0BD
Tel: 01902 454242 Fax: 01902 352438
(Wolverhampton City Primary Care Trust)
Patient List Size: 5300

Practice Manager Julie Smith

GP Stephen Richard PEACOCK, Robert GRINSTED, Helen GRUBB, Fiona JONES

The Surgery
Spicers Close, Claverley, Wolverhampton WV5 7BY
Tel: 01746 710223 Fax: 01746 710744
(South Western Staffordshire Primary Care Trust)
Patient List Size: 4318

Practice Manager Linda Hanson

GP Michael George HALL, Richard COMMANDER, Peter Neville JONES

Tamar Medical Centre
Severn Drive, Perton, Wolverhampton WV6 7QL
Tel: 01902 755053 Fax: 01902 751744
Email: tamer.medical@nshawebmail.nhs.uk
(South Western Staffordshire Primary Care Trust)
Patient List Size: 2800

Practice Manager S M Cockerham

GP Harpal Singh DHINGRA

Tettenhall Road Surgery
80 Tettenhall Road, Wolverhampton WV1 4TF
Tel: 01902 22677
(Wolverhampton City Primary Care Trust)
Patient List Size: 3500

GP Dr MURRAY

Tettenhall Road Surgery
24 Tettenhall Road, Wolverhampton WV1 4SL
Tel: 01902 422055 Fax: 01902 711244
(Wolverhampton City Primary Care Trust)

Practice Manager Barbara Gallear

GP Dr VAGHJIANI, Dr VAGHJIANI

Tettenhall Road Surgery
199 Tettenhall Road, Wolverhampton WV1 0DD
Tel: 01902 21005
(Wolverhampton City Primary Care Trust)

GP Dr WHITEHOUSE

Thornley Street Surgery
40 Thornley Street, Wolverhampton WV1 1JP
Tel: 01902 26843 Fax: 01902 688500
(Wolverhampton City Primary Care Trust)

GP Timothy Martin CROSSLEY, Damayanthi Ruckmala CROSSLEY, Stephen William McCARTHY, Hanora Bernadette Mary RICHARDSON, Alison Mary WATSON

Tudor Road Surgery
Tudor Road, Heath Town, Wolverhampton WV10 0LS
Tel: 01902 731330 Fax: 01902 306406
(Wolverhampton City Primary Care Trust)

Practice Manager Christine Smith

GP Shiva Ram AGRAWAL

Warstones Health Centre
Pinfold Grove, Wolverhampton WV4 4PS
(Wolverhampton City Primary Care Trust)

GP S MITTAL

Warstones Health Centre
Pinfold Grove, Wolverhampton WV4 4PS
Tel: 01902 575012 Fax: 01902 575037
(Wolverhampton City Primary Care Trust)
Patient List Size: 4500

GP Dante DE ROSA, Anne E WILLIAMS

Warstones Health Clinic
Pinfold Grove, Warstones, Wolverhampton WV4 4PS
Tel: 01902 331300
(Wolverhampton City Primary Care Trust)

GP William Henry CUTHBERT

Waterloo Medical Centre
41 Dunkley Street, Wolverhampton WV1 4AN
Tel: 01902 23559
(Wolverhampton City Primary Care Trust)

GP Irshad Ali SHAH

Whitmore Reans Health Centre
Lowe Street, Whitmore Reans, Wolverhampton WV6 0QL
Tel: 01902 421679
(Wolverhampton City Primary Care Trust)
Patient List Size: 2550

GP Dr RAM

Whitmore Reans Health Centre
Lowe Street, Whitmore Reans, Wolverhampton WV6 0QL
Tel: 01902 422269 Fax: 01902 711394
(Wolverhampton City Primary Care Trust)
Patient List Size: 3498

Practice Manager Rita Lal

GP Dr RIKHI, Dr RIKHI

Woodbridge

Doctors Surgery
Pembroke Road, Framlingham, Woodbridge IP13 9HA
Tel: 01728 723627 Fax: 01728 621064
(Suffolk Coastal Primary Care Trust)
Patient List Size: 9000

Practice Manager Denise Guy

GP Linda CROSS, Philip Robert GETTING, Susan HOPTON, Robert John MOFFATT, Stephen Charles NORTON, Geoffrey Humphery Robin ROWELL, Charles Edward WRIGHT

Framfield House Surgery
42 St. Johns Street, Woodbridge IP12 1ED
Tel: 01394 382157
(Suffolk Coastal Primary Care Trust)

Practice Manager Lorriane Foster

GP Jonathan William HAIGH, Deborah FAIRWEATHER, John Peter William LYNCH, Tim REED, Chris RUFFORD, Richard Peter VERRILL, Phil WEEKS

The Health Centre
Mill Hoo, Alderton, Woodbridge IP12 3DA
Tel: 01394 411641 Fax: 01394 410183
(Suffolk Coastal Primary Care Trust)
Patient List Size: 4200

Practice Manager Denise Thorpe

GP K P YATES, S P BALL, Judith S SHELLEY

Little St John Street Surgery
7 Little St. John Street, Woodbridge IP12 1EE
Tel: 01384 382046 Fax: 01394 388457
(Suffolk Coastal Primary Care Trust)
Patient List Size: 5850

Practice Manager Kate Fox

GP Gareth Henry Fisher TAYLOR, Rajinder Singh SIDHU, Joanna WATTS

Wickham Market Medical Centre
Chapel Lane, Wickham Market, Woodbridge IP13 0SB
Tel: 01728 747101 Fax: 01728 747580
Email: jane.wallace@gp-d83061.nhs.uk
(Suffolk Coastal Primary Care Trust)
Patient List Size: 8900

Practice Manager Jane Wallace

GP John Graham JONES, Anna Elizabeth ALDEN, Charles William ELSON, Alison Margaret GLAISTER, Kathryn Mary JONES, Mark LAL

Woodford Green

Barnabas Road Surgery
4 St Barnabas Road, Woodford Green IG8 7DA
Tel: 020 8504 0032 Fax: 020 8599 2247
(Redbridge Primary Care Trust)
Patient List Size: 1300

Practice Manager C Burnell

GP Alan Kenneth BEAVIS

The Broadway Surgery
3 Broadway Gardens, Monkhams Avenue, Woodford Green IG8 0HL
Tel: 020 8491 3344 Fax: 020 8491 0116
(Redbridge Primary Care Trust)

Practice Manager Sandra Purchese

GP Robert Hugh JONES, Sanjeeda AHMED, Naz ALI

Dr F N O Oraelosi and Partners
178 Snakes Lane East, Woodford Green IG8 7JQ
Tel: 020 8505 7631/8504 2126
(Waltham Forest Primary Care Trust)
Patient List Size: 7100

Practice Manager Pauline Smith

GP Graham Albert William TAYLOR, Florence Nwakaego Obiamaka ORAELOSI, George Morounfolu SOWEMIMO

Ferndale Surgery
76 Snakes Lane East, Woodford Green IG8 7QQ
Tel: 020 8505 1603 Fax: 020 8505 1136
(Redbridge Primary Care Trust)
Patient List Size: 2045

Practice Manager Jayne Skeels

GP Elankootil Girija MENON

Roding Lane North Surgery
2 Roding Lane North, Woodford Bridge, Woodford Green IG8 8NR
Tel: 020 8559 0280 Fax: 020 8559 1349
(Redbridge Primary Care Trust)

Rydal
375 High Road, Woodford Green IG8 9QJ
Tel: 020 8504 0532 Fax: 020 8559 1503
(Redbridge Primary Care Trust)
Patient List Size: 11500

Practice Manager Liz Townrow

GP Alexander George LYONS, Susan E ILES, William George INNES, Victoria NEWMAN, Richard Vaughan PRICE, S S SANDHU

Woodhall Spa

Tasburgh Lodge
Victoria Avenue, Woodhall Spa LN10 6TX
Tel: 01526 352466 Fax: 01526 354462
(East Lincolnshire Primary Care Trust)
Patient List Size: 2650

Practice Manager Joy Dowsett

GP Keith Charles BUTTER

Woodhall Spa New Surgery
The Broadway, Woodhall Spa LN10 6SQ
Tel: 01526 353888 Fax: 01526 354445
(East Lincolnshire Primary Care Trust)

Practice Manager Tessa Clark

GP Colin Stewart CAMPBELL, James Edward DALTON, Mairi Catrina MURRAY

Woodstock

Park Lane Surgery
Park Lane, Woodstock OX20 1UD
Tel: 01993 811452 Fax: 01993 812554
(North East Oxfordshire Primary Care Trust)
Patient List Size: 9700

Practice Manager Margaret Adkins

GP Helen Georgina VAN OSS, Deborah BARRINGTON-WARD, Duncan BECKER, Sally Louise HOPE, Trevor TURNER

Wooler

Burnhouse Surgery
15 Burnhouse Road, Wooler NE71 6BJ
Tel: 01668 281575 Fax: 01668 282442
(Northumberland Care Trust)
Patient List Size: 3000

Practice Manager Caroline Douglas

GP Roderic CRAIG, Kathleen Mary SPOOR

Glendale Surgery
6 Glendale Road, Wooler NE71 6DN
Tel: 01668 281740 Fax: 01668 281514
(Northumberland Care Trust)
Patient List Size: 1500

Practice Manager Christine James

GP Charles Richard DEAN

Worcester

Albany House Surgery
Albany Terrace, Barbourne, Worcester WR1 3DU
Tel: 01905 26086 Fax: 01905 26888
(South Worcestershire Primary Care Trust)
Patient List Size: 6920

Practice Manager Sharon Tompkins

GP Margaret Cecilia DAVIES, Andrew Peter BROTHERWOOD, William David NORTON

Berwyn House Surgery
13 Shrubbery Avenue, Worcester WR1 1QW
Tel: 01905 22888 Fax: 01905 617352
(South Worcestershire Primary Care Trust)
Patient List Size: 10100

Practice Manager I Large

GP Michael Harry SORENSEN, Charles R HARRIS, John Christopher JONES, Margaret Mary KEEBLE

The Bull Ring Surgery
5 The Bull Ring, St. John's, Worcester WR2 5AA
Tel: 01905 422883 Fax: 01905 423639
Email: practice.M81006@gp-M81006.nhs.uk
(South Worcestershire Primary Care Trust)
Patient List Size: 19200

Practice Manager Martin Lewis

GP Julie Elizabeth SMITH, William BELLAMY, Alex BRENNAN, David LEWIS, I M MAWBY, B J McCAFFREY, C MILNER, J E MONTERO, Philip Francis Louis PENNOCK, L M W PICKERELL, L S SHORT

Haresfield House Surgery
6-10 Bath Road, Worcester WR5 3EJ
Tel: 01905 763161 Fax: 01905 767016
(South Worcestershire Primary Care Trust)
Patient List Size: 13500

Practice Manager Helen Hartley

GP David CAIRNS, Jim ALDIS, Louise BROWN, Peter CROOKALL, Alison Mary GEORGIOU, Carol GOLDSMITH, Roderick Ian MACKICHAN, Sarah NEWEY, David Mark SMITH

The Hawthorns
Stonepit Lane, Inkberrow, Worcester WR7 4ED
Tel: 01386 792784 Fax: 01386 792637
(South Worcestershire Primary Care Trust)
Patient List Size: 2700

Practice Manager Jill Paton

GP Richard Stewart PATON

Knightwick Surgery
Knightwick, Worcester WR6 5PH
Tel: 01886 21279 Fax: 01886 821516
(South Worcestershire Primary Care Trust)
Patient List Size: 3700

Practice Manager Angela Woodhall

GP Antony Thomas Gurney COLLIS, Andrew John BYWATER, Anne Margaret LEWIS

Lowesmoor Medical Centre
93 Lowesmoor, Worcester WR1 2SA
Tel: 01905 727874 Fax: 01905 724987
(South Worcestershire Primary Care Trust)
Patient List Size: 12000

Practice Manager T K Loveday

GP Eurfyl RICHARDS, David Julian ALLEN, Magda Gillian CULLEN, Glyn Morgan HAYES, Gerald MORROW, Andrew Frere TURNER

Lowesmoor Medical Centre
93 Lowesmoor, Worcester WR1 2SA
Tel: 01905 723441
(South Worcestershire Primary Care Trust)

Practice Manager T K Loveday

GP Dr ALLEN, Dr CULLEN, Dr MADDEN, Dr THOMPSON, Andrew Frere TURNER

Shrubbery Avenue Surgery
13 Shrubbery Avenue, Worcester WR1 1QW
Tel: 01905 22888
(South Worcestershire Primary Care Trust)

GP Elizabeth Joan PROSSER

St Johns House Surgery
28 Bromyard Road, St Johns, Worcester WR2 5BU
Tel: 01905 421688 Fax: 01905 740003
(South Worcestershire Primary Care Trust)

Practice Manager Roger Davidson

GP Stuart Geoffrey KING, Julie BUTLER, Geoffrey Douglas Thurston HOLEHOUSE, Robert Alan INGLES, Trevor John Duncan JONES, Ruth KING, Claire WEBSTER, Mark YOUNG

The Surgery
Worcester Road, Great Witley, Worcester WR6 6HR
Tel: 01299 896370 Fax: 01299 896873
(South Worcestershire Primary Care Trust)
Patient List Size: 5700

Practice Manager M L Bell

GP Simon Peter Atter WATSON, John Stuart JONES, Isabel TEAGUE

The Surgery
School Lane, Upton-upon-Severn, Worcester WR8 0LF
Tel: 01684 592696 Fax: 01684 593122
(South Worcestershire Primary Care Trust)
Patient List Size: 10000

Practice Manager A D Oliver

GP George Morrison WILSON, Julian Paul BARRELL, Susanna Margaret Alice EVERITT, Andrew Richard HAVERCROFT, C HOGGARTH, J MACLEOD, David Anthony WEBSTER

Thorneloe Lodge Surgery
29 Barbourne Road, Worcester WR1 1RU
Tel: 01905 22445 Fax: 01905 610963
(South Worcestershire Primary Care Trust)

Practice Manager Jim Shaw

GP Robert David MORRISON, Kathryn Mary COTTELL, Mark Jeremy DAVIS, Kelvin Alexander Mair LAIDLAW, Caroline Lois ROBERTSON

Worcester Health Centre
Spring Gardens, Worcester WR1 2BS
Tel: 01905 681681 Fax: 01905 681699
(South Worcestershire Primary Care Trust)

Practice Manager Joy Cox

GP John Andrew THOMPSON, Patricia Anne ALLEN, John William JEFFERSON-LOVEDAY, Maher Guirguis Guindy MORGAN, John Cochrane MORRISON, John Patrick O'DRISCOLL, Jonathan PRATLEY, Rowland Michael Hamilton SMITH

Worcester Health Centre
Spring Gardens, Worcester WR1 2BS
Tel: 01905 681781 Fax: 01905 681766
(South Worcestershire Primary Care Trust)
Patient List Size: 9876

Practice Manager Meg Richards

GP Anthony Noel Brace SIMPSON, Michael James DEIGHAN, Richard HOLDING, Kathryn Anne SOLESBURY, Ian Richard WHITMORE

Worcester Park

Manor Drive Surgery
3 The Manor Drive, Worcester Park KT4 7LG
Tel: 0870 417 3900 Fax: 020 8335 3281
(Kingston Primary Care Trust)
Patient List Size: 6800

Practice Manager Christine Blandford

GP Clive Timothy Malcolm BRADY, J DOUGHERTY, Susanne RADIG

The Medical Unit
3 Manor Drive, Worcester Park KT4 7LG
(Kingston Primary Care Trust)

GP W J GREENE

Workington

The Ann Burrow Thomas Health Centre
South William Street, Workington CA14 2EW
Tel: 01900 605258 Fax: 01900 871420
Email: mike.mort@gp-A82648.nhs.uk
(West Cumbria Primary Care Trust)
Patient List Size: 1800

Practice Manager Yvonne Tinnion

GP Michael John Lightbody MORT

Beechwood Group Practice
57 John Street, Workington CA14 3BT
Tel: 01900 64866 Fax: 01900 871561
(West Cumbria Primary Care Trust)

Practice Manager J O'Hagan

GP John David Charles WILMOT, Richard Michael GOODWIN, Andrew Peter JONES

James Street Group Practice
James Street, Workington CA14 2DL
Tel: 01900 62241 Fax: 01900 603385
(West Cumbria Primary Care Trust)
Patient List Size: 10000

Practice Manager Andrea Wilson

GP Christine Elizabeth JONES, Peter HOWARTH, Victoria Catherine Bronislawa JAY, Jennifer LAW, Niall Gerard McGREEVY, Michael RUSMAN

Oxford Street Surgery
20 Oxford Street, Workington CA14 2AJ
Tel: 01900 603302 Fax: 01900 871604
Email: linda.steel@gp-a82050.nhs.uk
(West Cumbria Primary Care Trust)
Patient List Size: 7258

Practice Manager Linda Steel

GP Michael Victor GOURLAY, Andrew Charles BUTLER, Mary MACBETH, Nicholas Alastair SHAW

Solway Health Services
11 Roper Street, Workington CA14 3BY
Tel: 01900 602997 Fax: 01900 870142
Website: www.northcumbriahealth.co.uk/solway
(West Cumbria Primary Care Trust)
Patient List Size: 3800

Practice Manager Mike Eddy

GP Pappu Bhogeswara RAO, Maxine ENGLISH

The Surgery
Hinnings Road, Distington, Workington CA14 5UR
Tel: 01946 830207 Fax: 01946 833793
(West Cumbria Primary Care Trust)
Patient List Size: 4000

Practice Manager Kirsty Savage

GP Robert Jeffrey RUDMAN, Eric John BATER, Heather Ann NAYLOR

Workington Health Centre
South William Street, Workington CA14 2ED
Tel: 01900 603985 Fax: 01900 871761
(West Cumbria Primary Care Trust)
Patient List Size: 4612

Practice Manager Julie Harris

GP Philip CROSBY, T JOHNSON, R SCHRADER, A SCOTT

Worksop

The Health Centre
The Square, Whitwell, Worksop S80 4QR
Tel: 01909 720236 Fax: 01909 720236
(North Eastern Derbyshire Primary Care Trust)
Patient List Size: 4872

Practice Manager Gaenor Tyler

GP William Stuart RIDDELL, Robert SUCHETT-KAYE

Lakeside Surgery
Church Street, Langold, Worksop S81 9NW
Tel: 01909 732933
(Bassetlaw Primary Care Trust)

Practice Manager Karen Harrison

GP Dr SHARMACHARJA

Larwood Health Centre
56 Larwood Avenue, Worksop S81 0HH
Tel: 01909 500233 Fax: 01909 479722
(Bassetlaw Primary Care Trust)
Patient List Size: 16200

Practice Manager Karen Harrison

GP Nihar Ranjan SHARMACHARJA, Gerard AUSTIN, Lisa Ann COLLINS, Richard DAVEY, Stephen Carlton DAVIES, Therese JORDAN, Dr McQUIRKE, Philip John MOXON, Christopher Paul STANLEY, Dr TEASDALE

Manor Lodge
Worksop Road, Whitwell, Worksop S80 4ST

GP Susan STILLWELL

The Newgate Medical Group
Newgate Street, Worksop S80 1HP
Tel: 01909 500266/500288 Fax: 01909 478014
(Bassetlaw Primary Care Trust)

Practice Manager Sheila Smith

GP Lenox Jardine MILLAR, Joas Carlos CALINAS-CORREIA, Martin Gerard CORBETT, William Maurice Mary DELANEY, Claire EASON, Juidth EDBROOKE, Martin Charles EMERY, Kathryn Louise FAIRHOLME, John Alexander FULTON, Ian Michael HALL, David P MAUNDERS, Kenneth Roger ROBINSON, Steve ROSSI, Charlotte Anna Melissa SLATER, Sven Nicholas Banks WARNER

Newgate Medical Group
Newgate Street, Worksop S80 1HP
Tel: 01909 500288 Fax: 01909 479564
(Bassetlaw Primary Care Trust)
Patient List Size: 7418

Practice Manager Shelia Smith

GP Martin Charles EMERY, Dr CALINAS-CORREIA, Martin Gerard CORBETT, Dr DAVIES, Dr DELANEY, Dr EASON, Dr EDBROOKE, Dr FAIRHOLME, Dr FULTON, Dr HALL, Dr HAMMOND-EVANS, Dr MILLAR, Dr ROBINSON, Dr ROSSI, Dr WARNER

The Surgery
2A Berne Square, Dinnington Road, Woodsetts, Worksop S81 8RJ

GP Gita HALDAR

The Surgery
1 The Archway, High Street, Blyth, Worksop S81 8EQ

GP Andrew Michael JOHNSON, Denis John Alexander STEWART

The Surgery
Welbeck Street, Creswell, Worksop S80 4HA
Tel: 01909 721206 Fax: 01909 722011
(North Eastern Derbyshire Primary Care Trust)
Patient List Size: 8800

Practice Manager Linda Mosley

GP Imtiaz Ahmad KHAN, Subhash Chandrakant PATEL, Tolu TAYLOR

Whitwell Health Centre
Health Centre, The Square, Whitwell, Worksop S80 4QR
Tel: 01909 720278 Fax: 01909 724113
(North Eastern Derbyshire Primary Care Trust)
Patient List Size: 5000

GP W S RIDDELL, Chayda WILKINS

Worthing

Barn Surgery
22 Ferring Street, Ferring, Worthing BN12 5HJ
Tel: 01903 242638 Fax: 01903 700574
(Adur, Arun and Worthing Primary Care Trust)
Patient List Size: 3700

Practice Manager Janine Martin

GP John Murray LONGMORE, Judith Annette Boyer COLLIER, Claire FARRER

Broadwater Surgery
24 Broadwater Road, Worthing BN14 8AB
Tel: 01903 231701 Fax: 01903 232023
(Adur, Arun and Worthing Primary Care Trust)

Practice Manager Ruth Windsor

GP Michael Anthony LYONS, Stephen Thomas KELLEY, Mark Mukund RAVAL

Cornerway Surgery
Cornerways, 145 George V Avenue, Worthing BN11 5RZ
Tel: 01903 247740/241997 Fax: 01903 242110
Email: rosalind.pickering@gp-h82076.nhs.uk
(Adur, Arun and Worthing Primary Care Trust)
Patient List Size: 4012

Practice Manager Rosalind Pickering

GP Robert David SAYERS, Bernard HARDWICK

Heene and Goring Practice
145 Heene Road, Worthing BN11 4NY
Tel: 01903 235344/288610
(Adur, Arun and Worthing Primary Care Trust)
Patient List Size: 12800

Practice Manager Gillian Eves

GP Nicholas David TROUNCE, Amarendra Nath DAS, Martha Irene VAN VOLLEVELDE

Highdown Surgery
1 Highdown Avenue, Worthing BN13 1PU
Tel: 01903 265656 Fax: 01903 830450
(Adur, Arun and Worthing Primary Care Trust)
Patient List Size: 3200

Practice Manager Felicity Belkin

GP Nicholas Rae McCARTHY, Dennis Gordon CRUTCHLEY

Lime Tree Surgery
Lime Tree Avenue, Findon Valley, Worthing BN14 0DL
Tel: 01903 264101 Fax: 01903 695494
(Adur, Arun and Worthing Primary Care Trust)

Practice Manager Pat Conway

GP Edwin Arthur Balfour CAMERON, James DUDDY, Mila GARCIA, David John MANNINGS, Katja PALAN, Karen Elizabeth PATEL, Iwona POGODA, Rebecca RICHARDS, Maurice Richard SHIPSEY, Marion SMITH

The Pheonix Surgery
64 Sea Lane, Goring-by-Sea, Worthing BN12 4PY
Tel: 01903 240568 Fax: 01503 247099
(Adur, Arun and Worthing Primary Care Trust)

Practice Manager Michael Lickiss

GP A FUNNELL, R WOODWARD-COURT

Queen Alexandra Hospital Home
Boundary Road, Worthing BN11 4LJ
Tel: 01903 213458 Fax: 01903 219151
Email: ceo@qahh.org.uk
Website: www.qahh.org.uk
(Adur, Arun and Worthing Primary Care Trust)

Practice Manager John Paxman

GP Richard ORPIN, Michael TWITCHEN

Selden Medical Centre
6 Selden Road, Worthing BN11 2LL
Tel: 01903 234962 Fax: 01903 214531
(Adur, Arun and Worthing Primary Care Trust)
Patient List Size: 7950

Practice Manager Lindsay Coleman

GP Alistair Malcolm Westwood HOLMES, Neelu GARG, Stephen Charles PIKE

Shelley Surgery
23 Shelley Road, Worthing BN11 4BS
Tel: 01903 234844 Fax: 01903 219744
(Adur, Arun and Worthing Primary Care Trust)
Patient List Size: 11512

Practice Manager Sue Parton

GP James Gebbie Ferguson ANDERSON, Bruce William ALLAN, Clare Michelle ANDERSON, E McCREANOR, E MEPHAM, Richard Peter Ian ORPIN, Lynne SULLIVAN, Michael TWITCHEN, Brian Keith YOUNG

Springfields Surgery
Durrington Health Centre, Durrington Lane, Worthing BN13 2RX
Tel: 01903 843810 Fax: 01903 843801
(Adur, Arun and Worthing Primary Care Trust)
Patient List Size: 4700

Practice Manager Christine Weller

GP Lionel X MENDES, Marianne HOWELL

The St Lawrence Surgery
79 St Lawrence Avenue, Worthing BN14 7JL
Tel: 01903 237346 Fax: 01903 219284
(Adur, Arun and Worthing Primary Care Trust)

Practice Manager Gillian Pearson

GP Andrew John CAIRNS, David Stewart CLARKE, Jennifer DUCKERING, Marian Margaret ENGLISH, Charles Andrew MacKenzie HILL, Martin James William ROLPH

The Strand Practice
2 The Strand, Goring-by-Sea, Worthing BN12 6DN
Tel: 01903 243351 Fax: 01903 705804
(Adur, Arun and Worthing Primary Care Trust)
Patient List Size: 15250

Practice Manager Mandy Colbourne

GP Michael EPSOM, James BURCH, Alistair Ian McCLUMPHA, Sarah Ann NELSON, Peter Gerald SEARLE-BARNES, Robert Nicholas Francics SPENCE, Andrew Maurice THOMPSON

Victoria Road Surgery
50 Victoria Road, Worthing BN11 1XB
Tel: 01903 230656 Fax: 01903 520094
(Adur, Arun and Worthing Primary Care Trust)

GP David Richard HOPKINS, Lionel Xavier MENDES, Johanna MONTGOMERY, John Alan NEWNHAM, Andrew Ronald WEBB, Birgit WOOLLEY

Wotton-under-Edge

Chipping Surgery
1 Symn Lane, Wotton-under-Edge GL12 7BD
Tel: 01453 842214 Fax: 01453 521558
Website: www.thechippingsurgery.co.uk
(Cotswold and Vale Primary Care Trust)
Patient List Size: 8200

Practice Manager D Phillips

GP William John BURROWS, Rachael Sarah HAMPSON, Jonathan Joseph KABLER, Michael Basil McCARTHY, Christine Louise THOMPSON

Culverhay Surgery
Culverhay, Wotton-under-Edge GL12 7LS
Tel: 01453 843893 Fax: 01453 512557
(Cotswold and Vale Primary Care Trust)

Practice Manager Maureen Brewer

GP James Kennedy ROBERTS, Susan Margaret GREEN, Philip Leslie James PRITCHARD, R PROBERT

Wylam

Riversdale Surgery
51 Woodcroft Road, Wylam NE41 8DH
Tel: 01661 852208 Fax: 01661 853779
(Northumberland Care Trust)
Patient List Size: 6338

Practice Manager Pauline Henderson

GP John KNAPTON, R W DONALDSON, A M MILLER, Catherine Jane ROBERTS

Wymondham

Windmill Surgery
30 Melton Road, Wymondham NR18 0DB
Tel: 01953 607607 Fax: 01953 606482
(Southern Norfolk Primary Care Trust)
Patient List Size: 2600

Practice Manager Elaine Howell

GP Jane Anne CALNE, Rachel McSHANE

Wymondham Medical Partnership
Postmill Close, Wymondham NR18 0RF
Tel: 01953 602118 Fax: 01953 605313
(Southern Norfolk Primary Care Trust)

Practice Manager Alan Scott-Davies

GP David George French SEATON, Steven Russell BROWN, Adrian Laurence GENT, Julie GLENN, Kathleen Mary GRANTHAM, James Daniel Frank GREEN, Celina PEREIRA, Robert SLOCOMBE, Christopher Andrew Laird THORMAN, Stephen Charles THURSTON

Yarm

Eastside Surgery
7-8 Eastside, Hutton Rudby, Yarm TS15 0DB
Tel: 01642 700993 Fax: 01642 701857
(Hambleton and Richmondshire Primary Care Trust)

Practice Manager Barbara Hodgson

GP Bruce Henry DAVIES, Diane CRAWFORD

Yarm Medical Centre
1 Worsall Road, Yarm TS15 9DD
Tel: 01642 786422 Fax: 01642 785617
(North Tees Primary Care Trust)
Patient List Size: 12650

GP Andrew John RAWLINSON, Sally BASTIMAN, Alison BONAVIA, Liza Jane LACK, William Stephen Michael ORR, Neil George REYNOLDS

Yateley

Monteagle Surgery
Tesimond Drive, Monteagle Park, Yateley GU46 6FE
Tel: 01252 878992 Fax: 01252 860677
(Blackwater Valley and Hart Primary Care Trust)
Patient List Size: 5500

Practice Manager Rita Crowch

GP David LISTER, Kathleen SANT, Patrick Gilbert Noel Godolphin WILLIAMS

The Oaklands Practice
Yateley Medical Centre, Oaklands, Yateley GU46 7LS
Tel: 01252 872333 Fax: 01252 890084
Website: www.ymcentre.freeserve.co.uk
(Blackwater Valley and Hart Primary Care Trust)
Patient List Size: 11000

Practice Manager Lorna Ormond

GP Margaret Anne PALMER, Ravinder AULAKH, Neil BHATIA, Sophie Louise HULME, Gareth Mark ROBINSON, Michael Anthony VINER

Yelverton

Bere Alston Medical Practice
Station Road, Bere Alston, Yelverton PL20 7EJ
Tel: 01822 840269 Fax: 01882 841104
Email: beremedics@aol.com
(South Hams and West Devon Primary Care Trust)
Patient List Size: 3150

Practice Manager John Bartlett

GP William Edmund Joseph LEVERTON, Elizabeth DICKSON, Harriet DOYLE, Neil John HARMSWORTH

Yelverton Surgery
Westella Road, Yelverton PL20 6AS
Tel: 01822 852202 Fax: 01822 852260
(South Hams and West Devon Primary Care Trust)
Patient List Size: 7000

Practice Manager June Chamberlaine, Pam Smith

GP David Neal LONGDON, Anthony Gerard Kenneth FINNIGAN, Elizabeth MALLABAND, Mary Elizabeth NICHOLS, Peter Gareth David SMITH

Yeovil

Hendford Lodge Medical Centre
74 Hendford, Yeovil BA20 1UJ
Tel: 01935 470200 Fax: 01935 470202
Website: www.hendford.co.uk
(South Somerset Primary Care Trust)
Patient List Size: 12700

Practice Manager Sian Brammer

GP M ARIARATNAM, Gerald Patrick CROWLEY, Maxwell James BALL, Robert Francis Miller FORWARD, John David Goronwy GOWER, Stephen HOLDEN, Susan LATIMER, Richard Edward Alexander MORE, Anne SALKIND, Andrew SUMMERS

Ilchester Surgery
17 Church Street, Ilchester, Yeovil BA22 8LN
Tel: 01935 840207 Fax: 01935 840002
(South Somerset Primary Care Trust)
Patient List Size: 3602

Practice Manager Jane Burrell

GP Michael John HOLMES, David ARATHOON, Sarah DENNIS

Oaklands Surgery
Birchfield Road, Yeovil BA21 5RL
Tel: 01935 473068 Fax: 01935 412307
(South Somerset Primary Care Trust)
Patient List Size: 4750

Practice Manager Sandra Jones

GP Richard Mark HOGBEN, Simon BONNINGTON, Helen Elizabeth DAY, Jonathan Martin ORRELL

Penn Hill Surgery
St Nicholas Close, Yeovil BA20 1SB
Tel: 01935 470800 Fax: 01935 470802
(South Somerset Primary Care Trust)

Practice Manager Neil Dyer

GP Martin Jeffrey O'Brien MINOGUE, Michael John Merrett COLLINS, Jeremy IMMS, William George NOTT-BOWER, Martyn James RICHARDS, Prosenjit SARKER

Preston Grove Medical Centre
Preston Grove, Yeovil BA20 2BQ
Tel: 01935 474353 Fax: 01935 425171
Email: preston.grove@gp-l85015.nhs.uk
(South Somerset Primary Care Trust)
Patient List Size: 13000

Practice Manager Karen Lashly

GP Anthony John SIMMONDS, Iris AGNEW, Rosemarie CORNISH, Allen Gwyn Russell EVANS, Simon FILOSE, Jemma HORSLEY, John

Charles Kenneth NADIN, Joanne Louise NICHOLL, Michael ROBINSON

Queen Camel Medical Centre
West Camel Road, Queen Camel, Yeovil BA22 7LT
Tel: 01935 850225 Fax: 01935 851247
(South Somerset Primary Care Trust)

Practice Manager Clare Hodgson

GP Julian Frank HART, Simon James HUINS, David Robert TAYLOR

Ryalls Park Medical Centre
Marsh Lane, Yeovil BA21 3BA
Tel: 01935 434000 Fax: 01935 473531
Website: www.surgeriesonline.com/ryallspark
(South Somerset Primary Care Trust)
Patient List Size: 5800

Practice Manager Rowena M Turner

GP Robin Grainger CARR, Andrew James ALLEN, Hilary Winnifred DEVONSHIRE, Alison Jane GREED

Westlake Surgery
High Street, West Coker, Yeovil BA22 9AH
Tel: 01935 862212 Fax: 01935 865105
(South Somerset Primary Care Trust)
Patient List Size: 3400

Practice Manager Jenny Shepperd

GP John Parry COX, Lindsay Frederick Paul SMITH

York

Acomb Health Centre
1 Beech Grove, Acomb, York YO26 5LD
Tel: 01904 791094
(Selby and York Primary Care Trust)
Patient List Size: 4200

Practice Manager Susan Petty

GP Stephen John SCHOFIELD, Meike DUX, Catherine WALLACE

Almsford House Surgery
1 Almsford House, Beckfield Lane, Acomb, York YO26 5PA
Tel: 01904 799000 Fax: 01904 789407
(Selby and York Primary Care Trust)
Patient List Size: 3300

Practice Manager J A Deamer

GP Graham David WATSON, Brian McGREGOR

Ampleforth Surgery
Back Lane, Ampleforth, York YO62 4EF
Tel: 01439 788215 Fax: 01439 788002
Email: e.mail@gp-B32609.nhs.uk
(Scarborough, Whitby and Ryedale Primary Care Trust)

Practice Manager Alison Redhead

GP Kaye MECHIE, G C BLACK, Peter TICEHURST

Church Lane Surgery
Church Lane, Boroughbridge, York YO51 9BD
Tel: 01423 322309 Fax: 01423 324458
Email: church.jane@gp-b82032.nhs.uk
Website: www.churchlane.surgery.co.uk
(Craven, Harrogate and Rural District Primary Care Trust)
Patient List Size: 9500

Practice Manager Wndy Dowson

GP Alastair Scott GREEN, John William CROMPTON, Michelle S DAY, Clare Sarah EISNER, Ronald John NIXON, Christopher Martin PREECE, Helen M REES

Drs Calder, Ashley and Geddes
The Clifton Health Centre, Water Lane, Clifton, York YO30 6PS
Tel: 01904 623259
(Selby and York Primary Care Trust)

Practice Manager D G Symes

GP Alexander Stuart Carmichael CALDER, Philippa Mary ASHLEY, David Robert GEDDES

Dunnington Surgery
Petercroft Lane, Dunnington, York YO19 5NQ
(Selby and York Primary Care Trust)

GP Peter Richard BURNETT, Pauline CARNEY, Graham Cornelius GIBSON, Christopher Ian HIRST

East Parade Medical Practice
89 East Parade, Heworth, York YO31 7YD
Tel: 01904 423666 Fax: 01904 431329
(Selby and York Primary Care Trust)

GP Andrew Christopher MURRAY, Catherine TURNBULL

The Escrick Surgery
Escrick, York YO19 6LE
Tel: 01904 728243/728826 Fax: 01904 728826
(Selby and York Primary Care Trust)
Patient List Size: 5680

Practice Manager CarolSue Harrison

GP William Henry SMITHSON, Sarah Jane BUTLIN, Francis EYRE, Jeanette LENTHALL

The Escrick Surgery
Escrick, York YO19 6LE
Tel: 01904 728243 Fax: 01904 728826
(Sedgefield Primary Care Trust)
Patient List Size: 5680

Practice Manager Sue Harrison

GP William Henry SMITHSON, Dr BUTLIN, Dr EYRE, Jeanette LENTHALL

Front Street Surgery
14 Front Street, Acomb, York YO24 3BZ
Tel: 01904 794141 Fax: 01904 788304
(Selby and York Primary Care Trust)
Patient List Size: 4800

Practice Manager Erica Rogers

GP Manuela FONTEBASSO, Gordon David ORR, John Paul REED

Fulford Surgery
2 Fulford Park, Fulford, York YO10 4QE
Tel: 01904 625566 Fax: 01904 671539
(Selby and York Primary Care Trust)
Patient List Size: 5400

Practice Manager Peter Speck

GP Andrew John DENT, Katherine Alison BILL, Stephen Herbert BILLSBOROUGH, Shona Bridget GILLEGHAN

Gale Farm Surgery
109-119 Front Street, Acomb, York YO24 3BU
Tel: 01904 798329 Fax: 01904 798329
(Selby and York Primary Care Trust)

Practice Manager Hilda Caldwell

GP Gerald Bruce JACKSON, Philip William MOGER, Claire Jennifer ANDERTON, Jonathan Wansborough BELL-SYER, John Kendall BUSH, Simon Paul WATSON

Gillygate Surgery
28 Gillygate, York YO31 7WQ
Tel: 01904 624404 Fax: 01904 651813
(Selby and York Primary Care Trust)
Patient List Size: 6000

Practice Manager K E Ten

GP Richard William Maylin WRIGHT, Robert John O'Sullivan MARKHAM, David MAZZA, Alison Anne Alexandra McLAREN, Alan Keith SCOTT, Catherine SNARE

Glentworth Surgery
Dalton Terrace, York YO24 4DB
Tel: 01904 658542 Fax: 01904 671979
(Selby and York Primary Care Trust)

Patient List Size: 8000

Practice Manager Mike Cutterson

GP Graham Peter FOSTER, Hazel Anne BROWN, David John COOP, Rury ELLIS-HOLLING, Christopher Mark Lloyd JONES

Haxby Group Practice
Haxby & Wigginton Health Centre, The Village, Wigginton, York YO32 2LL
Tel: 01904 724600 Fax: 01904 750168
(Selby and York Primary Care Trust)

Practice Manager Peter Thirsk, Peter Thirsk

GP Kenneth William MYERS, Richard Morley CARPENTER, Paul Frederick FALLER, Elizabeth Veronica FOWLER, Allan Leonard HARRIS, David HAYWARD, William Fenwick LAUGHEY, Alexander James MACFIE, Anne Elisabeth PRIEST, Charles Dominic RISTIC, Peter Stewart SMITH, Alfred Malcolm WISEMAN, Sheila YOUNG

Helmsley Medical Centre
Carlton Road, Helmsley, York YO62 5HD
Tel: 01439 770288 Fax: 01439 771169
(Scarborough, Whitby and Ryedale Primary Care Trust)
Patient List Size: 3100

Practice Manager Heather White

GP Nigel Stewart WALTERS, Nicholas J WILSON

Hull Road Surgery
289 Hull Road, York YO10 3LB
(Selby and York Primary Care Trust)

GP Keith Gerrard PRICE, Kathryn Elizabeth GRIFFITH, Alison Jane HUNTER, John Allan LETHEM, Keith John MacDERMOTT

Huntington Surgery
Garth Road, Huntington, York YO32 9QJ

GP Peter Richard BURNETT, Pauline CARNEY, Christopher Ian HIRST, Neil MORAN

The Jorvik Medical Practice
6 Peckitt Street, York YO1 9WF
Tel: 01904 639171 Fax: 01904 633881
(Selby and York Primary Care Trust)
Patient List Size: 9100

Practice Manager Alison Frankland, D Homer

GP J M ALEXANDER, Sarah Frances Evelyn BOTTOM, Margaret Wendy EVANS, David Stuart FAIR, N J GILL, David Charles HARTLEY, W J LOCKETT, Brian John ORMSTON

Kirkbymoorside Surgery
Tinley Garth, Kirkbymoorside, York YO62 6AR
Tel: 01751 431254 Fax: 01751 432980
(Scarborough, Whitby and Ryedale Primary Care Trust)
Patient List Size: 5900

Practice Manager Heather Bell

GP Andrew Michael MOULSON, Helen FORTUNE-JONES, Timothy Richard John HUGHES, Jackie A LODGE

Lonsborough Road Surgery
4 Lonsborough Road, Market Weighton, York YO4 3AY
(Yorkshire Wolds and Coast Primary Care Trust)

GP Dr WEBSTER

Main Street Surgery
Main Street, Helperby, York YO61 2NT
Tel: 01423 360296 Fax: 01423 324458
Patient List Size: 2000

Practice Manager Wendy Dowson

GP C M PREECE, H M REES

The Medical Centre
3A Whitby Drive, York YO31 1EX
Tel: 01904 416541 Fax: 01904 416541
(Selby and York Primary Care Trust)
Patient List Size: 1300

GP Peter John BURGESS

Millfield Surgery
Millfield Lane, Easingwold, York YO61 3JR
Tel: 01347 821557
(Selby and York Primary Care Trust)

GP Roger WESTERMAN, Lorraine Marie BOYD, S A PARKER

Minster Health
35 Monkgate, York YO31 7WE
Tel: 01904 626234 Fax: 01904 691699
(Selby and York Primary Care Trust)

Practice Manager Di Ruston

GP Michael Howard JONES, Martin Hugh ASHLEY, Pauline BOLTER, Fiona FORSYTHE, John Daniel MORONEY

The Old School Medical Practice
Horseman Lane, Copmanthorpe, York YO23 3UA
Tel: 01904 706455 Fax: 01904 705341
(Selby and York Primary Care Trust)

Practice Manager Adgan Ferdinand

GP John Ernest RILEY, Walter HRYCAICZUK, John Leslie IREDALE, Andrea NIGHTINGALE, Felicity WALDRON

Parkview Surgery
28 Millfield Avenue, Hull Road, York YO10 3AB
Tel: 01904 413644 Fax: 01904 431436
(Selby and York Primary Care Trust)

Practice Manager Lynn Owen

GP John Cosbie HAMILTON, Julianne Dorothy HEWITSON, James MACLEOD

Pocklington General Practice
Barmby Road, Pocklington, York YO42 2DL
(Yorkshire Wolds and Coast Primary Care Trust)

GP Dr DILLON

Poppleton Health Centre
The Green, Upper Poppleton, York YO26 6EQ
Tel: 01904 794322 Fax: 01904 788084
(Selby and York Primary Care Trust)

GP Philip William MOGER, Claire Jennifer ANDERTON, J W BELL-SYER, J K BUSH, J E SIMPSON

Priory Medical Group
Cornlands Road, Acomb, York YO24 3WX
Tel: 01904 781423 Fax: 01904 784886
Email: dag@priory-medical.org.uk
(Selby and York Primary Care Trust)
Patient List Size: 25500

Practice Manager David Gill

GP David Anthony WALSH, Peter Ian ANDERSON, Michael Raymond Francis BARRY, Carol Ann COLLINS, Derek Geoffrey COLLINSON, Robert Holdrich FISHER, Jacqueline Lesley Ruth GODFREY, William GRAY, Padraig KRAMER, Jonathan LLOYD, Sally Joan MEAKINS, Sadia MUHAMMED, Richard THOMPSON

Reading Room Surgery
Front Street, Naburn, York YO1 4RR
Tel: 01904 728243/728826
(Selby and York Primary Care Trust)

Practice Manager Sue Harrison

GP William Henry SMITHSON, Sarah Jane BUTLIN, Jeanette LENTHALL

Rusholme Surgery
Rusholme Road, Holme-on-Spalding Moor, York YO43 4BJ
(Yorkshire Wolds and Coast Primary Care Trust)

GP Dr MOORE

South Bank Medical Centre
175 Bishopthorpe Road, York YO23 1PD
Tel: 01904 635116 Fax: 01904 672938
(Selby and York Primary Care Trust)

Practice Manager D Homer

GP J M ALEXANDER, Sarah Frances Evelyn BOTTOM, M W EVANS, David Stuart FAIR, N J GILL, W J LOCKETT, Brian John ORMSTON

Springbank Surgery
York Road, Green Hammerton, York YO26 8BN
Tel: 01423 330030 Fax: 01423 331433
(Craven, Harrogate and Rural District Primary Care Trust)
Patient List Size: 5414

Practice Manager Anne Massheder

GP Sheila Kathleen TAIT, Ralph Nelson Robert SIMPSON, David WHITTLE

Stamford Bridge Medical Centre
Viking Road, Stamford Bridge, York YO41 1BR

GP Thomas John DONALDSON, Graham Cornelius GIBSON, Christopher Ian HIRST, Ian McClelland LYALL, Neil MORAN, Lesley Jayne WELCH

Strensall Medical Centre
Southfields Road, Strensall, York YO32 5UA
Tel: 01904 490532 Fax: 01904 491927
(Selby and York Primary Care Trust)
Patient List Size: 16622

GP Peter Richard BURNETT, Frances ATANG, Thomas John DONALDSON, Graham Cornelius GIBSON, Christopher Ian HIRST, Ian McClelland LYALL, Neil MORAN, Russell SAXBY, Mark J STENTON, Alison TRAVIS, Lesley Jayne WELCH

The Surgery
Church Lane, Elvington, York YO41 4AD
Tel: 01904 608 224 Fax: 01904 608 710
(Selby and York Primary Care Trust)
Patient List Size: 6350

Practice Manager Julie Lund

GP Urszula DUDEK, David LIGHTWING, T LONGMORE, Rome SIGSWORTH

The Surgery
32 Clifton, York YO30 6AE
Tel: 01904 653834 Fax: 01904 651442
(Selby and York Primary Care Trust)
Patient List Size: 7100

Practice Manager L P Harrison

GP David Stuart KEMP, Kirsten Isobel COE, Andrew FIELD, Rebeccca FIELD, Robert RUSTON

The Surgery
Back Lane, Stillington, York YO61 1LL
Tel: 01347 810332
(Selby and York Primary Care Trust)
Patient List Size: 3380

GP Peter Roscoe JONES, Susan MACKENZIE, Barbara McPHERSON

The Surgery
The Chantry, Coxwold, York YO61 4BB
Tel: 01347 868426 Fax: 01347 868782
(Selby and York Primary Care Trust)
Patient List Size: 800

Practice Manager Dawn Bainbridge

GP Saumen Kanti SEN

The Surgery
White Rose Avenue, Huntington, York YO32 4AD

Practice Manager Peter Thirsk

GP Kenneth William MYERS, Richard Morley CARPENTER, David HAYWARD, William Fenwick LAUGHEY, Anne Elisabeth PRIEST, Peter Stewart SMITH

The Surgery
32 The Village, Stockton on Forest, York YO32 9UQ

Practice Manager Peter Thirsk

GP Kenneth William MYERS, Richard Morley CARPENTER, Paul Frederick FALLER, David HAYWARD, William Fenwick LAUGHEY, Anne Elisabeth PRIEST, Charles Dominic RISTIC, Sheila YOUNG

The Surgery
Main Street, Ricall, York YO19 6QD

Practice Manager Richard Gregory

GP Andrew Richard TAYLOR, Nicholas JACKSON, S MERRIFIELD, Else Jane SCOTT, Mark Edward WILLIAMS

Tang Hall Surgery
190 Tang Hall Lane, York YO10 3RL
Tel: 01904 411139 Fax: 01904 431224
(Selby and York Primary Care Trust)

GP Jonathan TAMS, Carmel Frances Maria PARRY, Anthony Martin SWEENEY

Terrington Surgery
Church Lane, Terrington, York YO60 6PS
Tel: 01653 648260 Fax: 01653 648267
Email: terrington.surgery@gpB82619.nhs.uk
Website: www.terrington.com/gpsurgery
(Scarborough, Whitby and Ryedale Primary Care Trust)
Patient List Size: 1363

Practice Manager Elaine Dooley

GP Elizabeth Margaret BRADLEY

The Tollerton Surgery
5-7 Hambleton View, Tollerton, York YO61 1QW
Tel: 01347 838231 Fax: 01347 838699
(Selby and York Primary Care Trust)
Patient List Size: 3400

Practice Manager Shirley Shepherd

GP David Martin WHITCHER, Michael POTRYKUS

Wenlock Terrace Surgery
18 Wenlock Terrace, Fulford, York YO10 4DU
Tel: 01904 646861
(Selby and York Primary Care Trust)

GP Keith Gerrard PRICE, Kathryn Elizabeth GRIFFITH, Alison Jane HUNTER, John Allan LETHEM, Keith John MacDERMOTT, Timothy David WALLAM

York Medical Group
199 Acomb Road, Acomb, York YO24 4HD
Tel: 01904 342999 Fax: 01904 342990
Website: www.yourkmedicalgroup.nhs.uk
(Selby and York Primary Care Trust)

Practice Manager Shelagh Sheila Kirkby

GP R DOSWELL, Jonathan Charles Hedley EVANS, Paula Antoinette EVANS, A HENCKEL, Olga KALISZER, John MORRISON, William OVENDEM, Mark Victor ROMAN, Graham Peter SAUNDERS

Walk-in Centres (England)

Barking and Dagenham Walk-in Centre
The centre is open Monday-Sunday 0900-1900. There is a GP available weekdays 1000-1200 and 1600-1900; weekends 1000-1300.

132 Upney Lane, Barking IG11 9YD
Tel: 020 8924 6262

Nurse-in-Charge Linda Dinis
Centre Administrator Ann Rogers

Bath NHS Walk-in Centre
The centre is open Monday-Sunday 0900-2200.
4 Cambridge House, Henry Street, Bath BA1 1JT

Birmingham NHS Walk-in Centre
The centre is open Monday-Saturday 0800-2000; Sunday 1100-1700.

Boots The Chemists Ltd, Lower Ground Floor, 66 High Street, Birmingham B4 7TA
Tel: 0121 255 4500 Fax: 0121 200 1024

Nurse-in-Charge Gerry Peake

Bitterne NHS Walk-in Centre
The centre is open Monday-Friday 0730-2100; weekends 1000-2000.

Bitterne Health Centre, Commercial Street, Southampton SO18 6BT
Tel: 023 8042 6356

Blackpool NHS Walk-in Centre
The centre is open Monday-Friday 0700-2200; weekends 0900-2200.

26 Talbot Road, Blackpool FY1 1LF
Tel: 01253 655871

Lead Nurse Alison Unsworth

Bolton NHS Walk-in Centre
The centre is open Monday-Friday 0830-1900.

Lever Chambers, 27 Ashburner Street, Bolton BL1 1SQ

Nurse Clinician Lisa Phillips

Bristol (City Gate) NHS Walk-in Centre
The centre is open Monday-Saturday 0800-2000; Sunday 1000-1800.

33 Broad Street, Bristol BS1 2EZ
Tel: 0117 906 9600 Fax: 0117 906 9611

Nurse-in-Charge Ita Connolly

Bristol (South) NHS Walk-in Centre
The centre is open Monday-Sunday 0900-2100.

5 Knowle West Health Park, Downton Road, Knowle West, Bristol BS4 1WH

Burnage Drop-in Centre
The centre is open Monday-Friday 0830-1630.

Burnage Health Care Centre, 347 Burnage Lane, Manchester M19 1EW

Bury NHS Walk-in Centre
The centre is open Monday-Friday 0700-2200; weekends and bank holidays 0900-2200.

18 Parsons Lane, Bury BL9 0JZ

Centre Manager Amanda Pearce

Colchester NHS Walk-in Centre
The centre is open Monday-Sunday 0700-2200.

Suite B, Ground Floor, Middlesborough, The Octagon Building, Colchester CO1 1TR
Tel: 01206 744300 Fax: 01206 744324

Lead Nurse Nicola Cottington

Coventry NHS Walk-in Centre
The centre is open Monday-Sunday 0700-2400.

Stoney Stanton Road, Coventry CV1 4FH
Tel: 024 7624 6789

Nurse-in-Charge Sarah Crowther

Crawley NHS Walk-in Centre
The centre is open Monday-Sunday 0000-2400.

Crawley Hospital, West Green Drive, Crawley RH11 7DH
Tel: 01293 600300 Fax: 01239 600420

Nurse-in-Charge Dee Monk

Croydon NHS Walk-in Centre
The centre is open Monday-Friday 0700-2200; weekends and bank holidays 0900-2200.

45 High Street, Croydon CR0 1QD

Acting Lead Nurse Lorna Fowler

Edgware NHS Walk-in Centre
The centre is open Monday-Sunday 0700-2200.

Edgware Community Hospital, Burnt Oak Broadway, Edgware HA8 0AD

Emergency Primary Care Access Service (EPCAS)
The centre is open Monday-Friday 0800-2200; weekends and bank holidays 0900-1700.

Charing Cross Hospital, Fulham Palace Road, London W6 8RF
Tel: 020 8383 0904

Lead Nurse Sue Stubberfield

Exeter (City) NHS Walk-in Centre
The centre is open Monday-Friday 0730-1800; Saturday 0830-1800; Sunday 1030-1630.

31D Sidwell Street, Exeter EX4 6NN
Tel: 01392 276892

Lead Nurse Sue Vining

Exeter (Wonford) NHS Walk-in Centre
The centre is open Monday-Sunday 0700-2200.

Royal Devon and Exeter Hospital, Barrack Road, Exeter EX2 5DW

Lead Nurse Sue Vining

Finchley NHS Walk-in Centre
The centre is open daily from 0900-1900.

Finchley Memorial Hospital, Granville Road, London N12 0JE
Tel: 020 8349 6371

Hackney NHS Walk-in Centre
The centre is open from Monday-Friday 0800-2200; weekends and bank holidays 0900-2200.

Homerton University Hospital, Homerton Row, London E9 6SR
Tel: 020 8510 5342

Harlow (North) NHS Walk-in Centre
The centre is open Monday-Friday 0700-2200; weekends and bank holidays 0900-2200.

1A Wych Elm, Harlow CM20 1QP
Tel: 01279 694775

Lead Nurse Carole Woods

Leigh NHS Walk-in Centre
The centre is open Monday-Sunday 0700-2100.

Leigh Infirmary, The Avenue, Leigh WN7 1HS
Tel: 01942 264000 Fax: 01942 264007
Email: walkin.centre@wiganlhs-tr.nwest.nhs.uk

Lead Nurse Gail Gaskell

Leytonstone NHS Walk-in Centre
The centre is open Monday-Friday 0700-2300; weekends and bank holidays 0900-2300.

Whipps Cross Hospital, Whipps Cross Road, London E11 1NR
Tel: 020 8558 8965

Liverpool (City) NHS Walk-in Centre
The centre is open Monday-Sunday 0700-2200.

Unit 4, 53 Great Charlotte Street, Charlotte Row, Liverpool L1 1HU
Tel: 0151 285 3535

Clinical Lead Sharon Jackson

Liverpool (Old Swan) NHS Walk-in Centre
The centre is open Monday-Friday 0700-2200; weekends 0900-2200.

Old Swan Health Centre, St Oswalds Street, Liverpool L13 2BY

Tel: 0151 285 3565
Lead Nurse Dot Haworth

Loughborough NHS Walk-in Centre
The centre is open Monday-Sunday 0000-2400.
Loughborough Health Centre, Pinfold Gate, Loughborough LE11 1BE
Tel: 01509 553998
Centre Manager Frank Durning

Luton NHS Walk-in Centre
The centre is open Monday-Friday 0700-2200; weekends and bank holidays 0900-2200.
14-16 Chapel Street, Luton LU1 2SE
Tel: 01582 556400
Nurse-in-Charge Wendy Cunningham
Centre Manager Marie Simon

Maidstone NHS Walk-in Centre
The centre is open Monday-Friday from 0800-2000 or 1000-2200.
Maidstone Hospital, Hermitage Lane, Maidstone ME16 9QQ
Tel: 01622 729000

Manchester Airport NHS Walk-in Centre
The centre is open Monday-Friday 0800-1600.
Terminal 1, Manchester Airport plc, Manchester M90 1QX
Tel: 0161 489 2109

New Cross NHS Walk-in Centre
The centre is open Monday-Friday 0700-2200; weekends and bank holidays 0800-2000.
Henderson House, 40 Goodwood Road, New Cross, London SE14 6BL
Tel: 020 7206 3100
Lead Nurse Sue Smith

Newcastle (Westgate) NHS Walk-in Centre
The centre is open Monday-Sunday 0800-2200.
Newcastle General Hospital, Westgate Road, Newcastle upon Tyne NE4 6BE
Tel: 0191 256 3163
Lead Nurse Julie Gilson

Newham NHS Walk-in Centre
The centre is open Monday-Friday 0700-2200; weekends and bank holidays 0900-2200.
Glen Road, London E13 8SH
Tel: 020 7363 9200 Fax: 020 7363 9210

North Middlesex NHS Walk-in Centre
The centre is open Monday-Friday 0700-2200; weekends 0900-2200.
North Middlesex Hospital, Sterling Way, Edmonton, London N18 1QX
Tel: 020 8887 2680
Lead Nurse Marie Pearman
Manager Amal Wicks

Norwich NHS Walk-in Centre
The centre is open Monday-Saturday 0700-2200; Sunday 0900-2200.
Dussindale Centre, Pound Lane, Norwich NR7 0SR
Tel: 01603 300122
Lead Nurse Christine Hawkins

Nottingham NHS Walk-in Centre
The centre is open Monday-Sunday 0700-2100.
Seaton House, London Road, Nottingham NG2 4LA
Website: www.nottingham.nhs.uk/nhs-services/walk-in-centre
Nurse-in-Charge Ann Simpson

Oldham NHS Walk-in Centre
The centre is open Monday-Sunday 0730-2230.
Lindley House, 1 John Street, Oldham OL1 8DF

Parsons Green Walk-in Centre (WWC)
The centre is open Monday-Friday 0800-2000.
5-7 Parsons Green, London SW6 4UL
Tel: 020 8846 6758
Lead Nurse Emma Flewers, Claire Halkyard, Sue Stubberfield

Peterborough NHS Walk-in Centre
The centre is open Monday-Sunday 0700-2200.
Rivergate Primary Care Centre, Viersen Platz, Peterborough PE1 1SE
Tel: 01733 293800

Prestwich NHS Walk-in Centre
The centre is open Monday-Friday 0800-2100; weekends and bank holidays 0900-1700.
Fairfax Road, Prestwich, Manchester M25 1BT
Tel: 0161 773 7832
Nurse-in-Charge Amanda Pierce

Redbridge NHS Walk-in Centre
Expected to open 09/2005. It will be open Monday-Sunday 0000-2400.
King George Hospital, Barley Lane, Ilford IG3 8YB
Tel: 020 8983 8696

Rochdale NHS Walk-in Centre
The centre is open Monday-Friday 0700-2130; weekends and bank holidays 1000-1730.
90 Whitehall Street, Rochdale OL12 0ND
Tel: 01706 708051
Nurse-in-Charge Nicola Rigby

St Helens NHS Walk-in Centre
The centre is open Monday-Saturday 0700-2200; Sundays 0900-2200.
Millennium Building, Bickerstaffe Street, St Helens WA10 1DH
Tel: 01744 627405
Lead Nurse Christine Horrocks, Barbara Scanlon

Sheffield NHS Walk-in Centre
The centre is open Monday-Friday 0700-2200.
B Floor, Royal Hallamshire Hospital, Glossop Road, Sheffield S10 2JF
Tel: 0114 271 2340

Skelmersdale NHS Walk-in Centre
The centre is open Monday-Friday 0700-2200; weekends and bank holidays 0900-1700 for the treatment of minor injuries and ailments.
116-118 The Concourse, Skelmersdale WN8 6LJ
Tel: 01695 554260

Slough NHS Walk-in Centre
The centre is open Monday-Friday 0700-2200; weekends 0900-2200.
Upton Hospital, Albert Street, Slough SL1 2BJ
Tel: 01753 635505
Lead Nurse Sally Patrick

Soho NHS Walk-in Centre
The centre is open Monday-Friday 0800-2000; weekends and bank holidays 1000-2000.
1 Frith Street, London W1D 3HZ
Tel: 020 7534 6500 Fax: 020 7534 6550
Nurse-in-Charge Jill Cull

Southampton (Shirley) NHS Walk-in Centre
The centre is open Monday-Friday 0730-2100; weekends 1000-2000.

1A Howards Grove, Southampton SO15 5PR
Tel: 023 8079 0000

Centre Manager Sandra Attrill

Stoke (Haywood) NHS Walk-in Centre
The centre is open Monday-Friday 0700-2200; weekends and bank holidays 0900-2200.

High Lane, Stoke-on-Trent ST6 7AG
Tel: 01782 581112

Centre Manager Karen Dawson

Sunderland NHS Walk-in Centre
The centre is open from 0800-2200.

Sunderland Royal Hospital, Kayll Road, Sunderland SR4 7TP

Swindon NHS Walk-in Centre
The centre is open Monday-Sunday 0700-2200.

4 Cambridge House, Carfax Streeet, Swindon SN1 1ED
Tel: 01793 428524

Teddington NHS Walk-in Centre
The centre is open Monday-Friday 0700-2200; weekends and bank holidays 0800-2100.

Teddington Memorial Hospital, Hampton Road, Teddington TW11 0JL

Nurse Consultant Liza Coghill
Clinical Nurse Manager Joan Santos

Tooting NHS Walk-in Centre
The centre is open Monday-Sunday 0700-2200.

Clare House, St George's Hospital, Blackshaw Road, London SW17 0QT
Tel: 020 8700 0505 Fax: 020 8700 0525

Lead Nurse Kate Carter

Wakefield NHS Walk-in Centre
The centre is open Monday-Friday 0700-2000; weekends 0900-2000.

Trinity Medical Centre, Thornhill Street, Wakefield WF1 1PG

Walsall NHS Walk-in Centre
The centre is open Monday- Friday 0700-2000; weekends and bank holidays 0800-1700.

The Market Square, Unit 19-21, Digbeth, Walsall WS1 1QZ
Tel: 01922 858550 Fax: 01922 858849

Weybridge NHS Walk-in Centre
The centre is open Monday-Friday 0700-2200; weekends and bank holidays 0900-2200.

Weybridge Hospital and Primary Centre, 22 Church Street, Weybridge KT13 8DY
Tel: 01932 826013

Whitechapel Walk-in Centre
The centre is open Monday-Friday 0700-2200; weekends and bank holidays 0900-2200.

174 Whitechapel Road, London E1 1BZ
Tel: 020 7943 1333

Nurse Practitioner Sonia Hall

Whittington NHS Walk-in Centre
The centre is open daily 0800-2300.

Whittington Hospital, Highgate Hill, London N19 5NF
Tel: 020 7288 5216

Wirral Arrowe Park NHS Walk-in Centre
The centre is open Monday-Friday 0700-2200; weekends 0900-2200.

Arrowe Park Hospital, Arrowe Park Road, Wirral CH49 5PE
Tel: 0151 488 3706

Wirral NHS Walk-in Centre
The centre is open Monday-Friday 0700-2200; weekends 0900-2200.

Victoria Central Hospital, Mill Lane, Wallasey CH44 5UF
Tel: 0151 604 7296

Woking NHS Walk-in Centre
The centre is open Monday-Friday 0700-2200; weekends and bank holidays 0900-2200.

Woking Community Hospital, Heathside Road, Woking GU22 7HS
Tel: 01483 776080 Fax: 01483 722280

Clinical Manager Lou Major

Wythenshawe NHS Walk-in Centre
The centre is open Monday-Friday 0830-1630.

Wythenshawe Health Care Centre, Stancliffe Road, Manchester M22 4PJ
Tel: 0161 946 9400

York NHS Walk-in Centre
The centre is open Monday-Sunday 0700-2200.

31 Monkgate, York YO31 7WA
Tel: 01904 725401 Fax: 01904 674558

Nurse-in-Charge Veronica Gray

Scotland

Aberdeen

Albyn Medical Practice
30 Albyn Place, Aberdeen AB10 1NW
Tel: 01224 586829 Fax: 01224 213238
(NHS Grampian, Primary Care Division)

Practice Manager Claire Nicholl

GP Peter Ross Sinclair DUFFUS, Chris ALLAN, Graeme CORNWELL, Mary Catherine CRAIK, Kristin EFSKIND, Judith Margaret FARQUHARSON, William James HARRISON, William Simpson Younie STEPHEN

Brimmond Medical Group
106 Inverurie Road, Bucksburn, Aberdeen AB21 9AT
Tel: 01224 713869 Fax: 01224 716317
(NHS Grampian, Primary Care Division)

Practice Manager Val Malhan

GP Ivan Charles Fraser WISELY, Yvonne AIKEN, Neil S KENNEDY, Lesley MALCOLM, Roy Duncan McKERACHER, Malcolm Jack VALENTINE

Bucksburn Medical Practice
Kepplehills Road, Bucksburn, Aberdeen AB21 9DG
Tel: 01224 713927 Fax: 01224 715586
(NHS Grampian, Primary Care Division)
Patient List Size: 1475

Practice Manager Shonagh Swan

GP Pamela Margaret McMANN

Calsayseat Medical Group
44 Powis Place, Aberdeen AB25 3TS
Tel: 01224 634345 Fax: 01224 562220
(NHS Grampian, Primary Care Division)

Practice Manager Jackie Cairns

GP Colin David SINCLAIR, Shona Patricia DEANS, Lindsay Isobel GRANT, Kate Louise IRVINE, Moira Ellen JOHNSTON, Stephen John LYNCH, Carol STEWART

Camphill Medical Practice
St John's, Murtle House, Bieldside, Aberdeen AB15 9EP
Tel: 01224 868935 Fax: 01224 868971
(NHS Grampian, Primary Care Division)

Practice Manager Jane Masson

GP Stefan GEIDER, J R HOGENBOOM

Cults Medical Group
Cults Medical Centre, South Avenue, Cults, Aberdeen AB15 9LQ
Tel: 01224 867740 Fax: 01224 861392
(NHS Grampian, Primary Care Division)

GP Robert Marshall MILNE, Derek MATHIESON, John McKEOWN, Moira MORTON, Naomi SMITH

Danestone Medical Centre
Fairview Street, Danestone, Aberdeen AB22 8ZP
Tel: 01224 822866 Fax: 01224 707532
(NHS Grampian, Primary Care Division)

Practice Manager Anne Coombes

GP Peter Alexander KIEHLMANN, Stella ANDERSON, Caroline HAMPTON, Tricia Ann KIEHLMANN

Elmbank Group
Foresterhill Health Centre, Westburn Road, Aberdeen AB25 2AY
Tel: 01224 696949 Fax: 01224 691650
(NHS Grampian, Primary Care Division)
Patient List Size: 10000

Practice Manager Fiona Dalziel, Joanne Jack

GP Fraser RICHARDSON, Alexis CRAIG, Christopher David PROVAN, James Alexander REPPER, Morag STEWART, William Edwin TAYLOR, Ruby Margaret Julie WATT

Ferryhill Practice
193 Bon Accord Street, Aberdeen AB11 6UA
Tel: 01224 587484 Fax: 01224 574424
(NHS Grampian, Primary Care Division)

Practice Manager M Brown

GP Richard James LEGG

Gilbert Road Medical Group
39 Gilbert Road, Bucksburn, Aberdeen AB21 9AN
Tel: 01224 712138 Fax: 01224 712239
(NHS Grampian, Primary Care Division)

Practice Manager Jane Harvie

GP Murdoch John SHIRREFFS, John Douglas ORR, Linda Jane SANDILANDS, James SCOTT, David TAYLOR, Sheena TUTTLE, Jane Caroline WHITE, John Gordon WILSON

Great Western Road Medical Group
327 Great Western Road, Aberdeen AB10 6LT
Tel: 01224 571318 Fax: 01224 573865
Email: administrator@gtwesternrd.grampian.scot.nhs.uk
(NHS Grampian, Primary Care Division)
Patient List Size: 10800

Practice Manager Stephen Proctor

GP Alistair Thomas WILKINSON, Gillian Anne Macdonald BRUCE, Elaine HOWE, Kenneth LAWTON, Valerie MORRIS, Gary RITCHIE, Ewan Donaldson WALLACE

Hamilton Medical Group
4 Queens Road, Aberdeen AB15 4ZT
Tel: 01224 622345 Fax: 01224 627426
Email: administrator@hamilton.grampian.scot.nhs.uk
(NHS Grampian, Primary Care Division)
Patient List Size: 6958

Practice Manager Diane M Gordon

GP John Howard MAWDSLEY, Pamela ALDERSON, Frank CHARLESON, Wilma Marie COLLIE, John Gordon PATERSON, Lynne WALLWORK, David Paul Bartram WATSON

Holburn Medical Group
7 Albyn Place, Aberdeen AB10 1YE
Tel: 01224 400800 Fax: 01224 407777
(NHS Grampian, Primary Care Division)

Practice Manager Donna Dickson

GP Alison Doreen GLENESK, Andrew David HAY, Dorothy Jean Lambie LYNCH, Dr McGUIGAN, Cameron MUNRO, Stuart Thomas SCOTT

Homelessness Surgery
187 King Street, Aberdeen AB24 5AH
Tel: 01224 644465 Fax: 01224 644465
(NHS Grampian, Primary Care Division)

Practice Manager Eileen Bean

GP Richard LEGG, Tracy TAYLOR

Kincorth Medical Centre
26 Abbotswell Crescent, Aberdeen AB12 5JW
Tel: 01224 876000 Fax: 01224 899182
Email: administrater@kincorth.grampian.scot.nhs.uk
(NHS Grampian, Primary Care Division)

Practice Manager John Sefton

GP Anne Margaret Skinner DOUGLAS, Henry Finlayson FORBES, David FOWLER, Andrew HENDERSON, Craig HEWITT, Alasdair Duncan JAMIESON, Lynne MACKENZIE

Links Medical Practice
City Hospital, Park Road, Aberdeen AB24 5AU
Tel: 01224 644201 Fax: 01224 611090
(NHS Grampian, Primary Care Division)

North Wing
Denburn Health Centre, Rosemount Viaduct, Aberdeen AB25 1QB
Tel: 01224 643333/642757 Fax: 01224 555239
Email: administrator@denburnnorth.grampian.scot.nhs.uk
(NHS Grampian, Primary Care Division)
Patient List Size: 5300

GP Campbell MACGREGOR, Michael Alexander PRATT, Karyn WEBSTER

Northfield/Mastrick Clinic
Quarry Road, Northfield, Aberdeen AB16 5UU
Tel: 01224 662911 Fax: 01224 699825
Email: administrator@northfield.grampion.scot.nhs.uk
(NHS Grampian, Primary Care Division)
Patient List Size: 5200

Practice Manager Brenda McIntosh

GP Margaret E KNIGHT, Jenny FINLAYSON, Alistair McEWAN, Fraser Tullis SUTHERLAND

Old Machar Medical Practice
526 King Street, Aberdeen AB24 5RS
Tel: 01224 480324 Fax: 01224 276121
(NHS Grampian, Primary Care Division)

Practice Manager Margaret Mackie

GP Iain Robert AFFLECK, James Mackie COSGROVE, Torquil Neil Nicolson MACLEOD, Alexander Roland McKAY, Thomas William SIMPSON, Alison Susan Mary SNEDDON, Rorie John Gordon STEWART

Peterculter Medical Practice
Coronation Road, Aberdeen AB14 0RQ
Tel: 01224 733535 Fax: 01224 739979
(NHS Grampian, Primary Care Division)

Portlethen Group Practice
Portlethen Medical Centre, Bruntland Road, Portlethen, Aberdeen AB12 4QP
Tel: 01224 780223 Fax: 01224 781317

(NHS Grampian, Primary Care Division)
Patient List Size: 12300

Practice Manager Lyn King

GP George STEPHEN, Jonathan George BLAKE, Ewan Dryden CLARK, Christine GUTTERIDGE, Hilary Margaret Gail JOHNSTONE, Graeme Dunsmore MILLER, Moira Rosalind MILNE, Fiona Lindsay Mary OGG

Queens Road Medical Group
6 Queens Road, Aberdeen AB15 4NU
Tel: 01224 641560 Fax: 01224 659629
Email: administrator@qrmg.grampian.scot.nhs.uk
Website: www.queensmedical.co.uk
(NHS Grampian, Primary Care Division)
Patient List Size: 10600

GP Fiona Mary GARTON, Geoffrey Johnston CLARKE, Eunice Ann Farquhar CONNON, Paul Edward DAVIDSON, Theresa Jane MORWICK, Valerie STEREN, M Stuart WATSON

Rosemount Medical Practice
1 View Terrace, Aberdeen AB25 2RS
Tel: 01224 638050 Fax: 01224 627308
Email: administrator@rosemount.grampian.scot.nhs.uk
(NHS Grampian, Primary Care Division)
Patient List Size: 4100

Practice Manager Irene Barnett

GP Stephen John WILSON, C COOPER, James Macdonald MAITLAND

Rubislaw Place Medical Group
7 Rubislaw Place, Aberdeen AB10 1QB
Tel: 01224 641968 Fax: 01224 627159
Email: administrator@rpmg.grampian.scot.nhs.uk
(NHS Grampian, Primary Care Division)
Patient List Size: 10500

Practice Manager D Francis

GP Hugh Farquhar GIBSON, Tim R JONES, David Milne MARWICK, Linda Alison McKEE, Rebecca SEDDON, Lesley M VASS, Stephen WEDDERBURN

Rubislaw Terrace Surgery
23 Rubislaw Terrace, Aberdeen AB10 1XE
Tel: 01224 643665 Fax: 01224 625197
(NHS Grampian, Primary Care Division)
Patient List Size: 6048

Practice Manager Jean Grant

GP John Gregory Gordon DAVIDSON, Sandra Anne McINTOSH, Harold Bailey SMITH, Alasdair Neil WESTON

Scotstown Medical Centre
Cairnfold Road, Bridge of Don, Aberdeen AB22 8LD
Tel: 01224 702149 Fax: 01224 706688
(NHS Grampian, Primary Care Division)

Practice Manager Wendy Parslow

GP David John BELL, Alasdair Anderson FORBES, Robert Brown LAMBERTON, Dorothy Elizabeth McMURRAY, Paul Martin RHODES

Spa Well Medical Group
Denburn Health Centre, Rosemount Viaduct, Aberdeen AB25 1QB
Tel: 01224 640952 Fax: 01224 555285
Email: firstname.lastname@spawell.grampian.scot.nhs.uk
(NHS Grampian, Primary Care Division)
Patient List Size: 4500

Practice Manager J Grant

GP Alan Keill FRASER, Katrina DAVEY, Sandra Gail DAVIDSON, Julia Margaret HOUSE

Spital Medical Practice
119-121 Spital, Aberdeen AB24 3HX
Fax: 01224 639015
Email: administrator@spital.grampian.scot.nhs.uk
(NHS Grampian, Primary Care Division)

Practice Manager Carol Lesley

GP Alexandra Marion BARRETT-AYRES

University Medical Practice
University of Aberdeen, Block E, Taylor Buildings, Old Aberdeen, Aberdeen AB24 3UB
Tel: 01224 276655 Fax: 01224 272394
Email: administrator@university.grampian.scot.nhs.uk
(NHS Grampian, Primary Care Division)
Patient List Size: 9000

GP Dawn CHALMERS, Margaret Elizabeth HAMILTON, Walter MOUAT, David Ernest RAIT, Fiona Mary SPENCE

The Viaduct Medical Practice
Denburn Health Centre, Rosemount Viaduct, Aberdeen AB25 1QB
Tel: 01224 644744 Fax: 01224 555232
(NHS Grampian, Primary Care Division)

Practice Manager Lavinia Langan

GP Rita Pasqua Rosa DI MASCIO, Alison Morag RITCHIE, David I WINTOUR

Victoria Street Medical Group
7 Victoria Street, Aberdeen AB10 1QW
Tel: 01224 641930 Fax: 01224 656915
(NHS Grampian, Primary Care Division)
Patient List Size: 5300

Practice Manager S Lennox

GP Gavin Peter STARK, Sandra Helen GRANT, Gregor William Bell HOWE, Carmel Anne MURPHY

West Denburn Medical Practice
West Wing, Denburn Health Centre, Rosemount Viaduct, Aberdeen AB25 1QB
Tel: 01224 642955 Fax: 01224 637736
Email: marcia.robertson@nhs.net
(NHS Grampian, Primary Care Division)
Patient List Size: 4200

Practice Manager Marcia Robertson

GP Inthu SRIKATHARAJAN, Graham Douglas GAULD

Westburn Medical Group
Foresthill Health Centre, Westburn Road, Aberdeen AB25 2AY
Tel: 01224 559595 Fax: 01224 559597
Email: administrator@westburn.grampian.scot.nhs.uk
(NHS Grampian, Primary Care Division)
Patient List Size: 3550

Practice Manager John Forrest

GP William REITH, Sarah MACKENZIE, Katherine SNOWDEN, Pauline STRACTON

Westburn Medical Group A
Foresterhill Health Centre, Westburn Road, Aberdeen AB25 2AY
Tel: 01224 696848 Fax: 01224 696753
(NHS Grampian, Primary Care Division)

GP Ross Jenkins TAYLOR

Woodside Medical Group
80 Western Road, Aberdeen AB24 2SU
Tel: 01224 492631 Fax: 01224 276173
(NHS Grampian, Primary Care Division)
Patient List Size: 13000

GP Alexander BARBER, Linda DEMPSEY, Alison DOUGLAS, John DUNCAN, Brett FINLAYSON, Peter C FOGIEL, Kerry JACK, Matthew JACK, Walter T STEPHEN, Julia WALLACE

Aberfeldy

Inzievar Surgery
2 Kenmore Street, Aberfeldy PH15 2BL
Tel: 01887 820366 Fax: 01887 829566
(NHS Tayside, Primary Care Division)

GP Anthony Edmund PITCHFORTH, Hamish McNeil McBRIDE, David Smethhurst WRIGHT, Helen Mary WRIGHT

Aberlour

Aberlour Health Centre
Queens Road, Aberlour AB38 9PR
Tel: 01340 871210 Fax: 01340 871814
(NHS Grampian, Primary Care Division)

Practice Manager Karen Moir

GP Adrian Edward CAMMACK, Duncan John McDOWALL, Alan McGHEE, D MILLAR

Aboyne

Aboyne Health Centre
Bellwood Road, Aboyne AB34 5HQ
Tel: 01339 886345
(NHS Grampian, Primary Care Division)

Practice Manager Angela Beresford

GP Jack Lorimer TAYLOR, John GLASS, Judith K SCOTT, Mary Buchanan TAYLOR

The Surgery
Ailsa Muir, The Market Stance, Tarland, Aboyne AB34 4UB
Tel: 01339 881281 Fax: 01339 881077
Email: medical@tarland.com
Website: www.tarland.com/medical
(NHS Grampian, Primary Care Division)

Practice Manager L Fouguharson

GP David Raynor STARRITT

Acharacle

Pines Medical Centre
Acharacle PH36 4JU
Tel: 01967 431231 Fax: 01967 431396
Email: administrator@gp55662.highland-hb.scot.nhs.uk
(NHS Highland, Primary Care)
Patient List Size: 1231

Practice Manager Emma Moss

GP Maris Elizabeth BUCHANAN, Richard HOUSTON

Achnasheen

Torridon Medical Practice
Torridon, Achnasheen IV22 2EZ
Tel: 01445 791223 Fax: 01445 791401
Email: administrator@gp55446.highland-hb.scot.nhs.uk
(NHS Highland, Primary Care)
Patient List Size: 430

GP Caroline J BROWN, Helen STEWART

Airdrie

Adam Avenue Medical Centre
1 Adam Avenue, Airdrie ML6 6DN
Tel: 01236 763581 Fax: 01236 750507
Email: administrator@gp61061.low.lanark-hb.scot.nhs.uk
(NHS Lanarkshire, Primary Care Division)
Patient List Size: 8311

Practice Manager B Robertson

GP Aftabuddin AHMED, Patricia Elizabeth CARGO, Robert CLEMENTS, Catherine Findlay LEVEN, Mark Gordon SMYTH

Airdrie Health Centre
Monskcourt Avenue, Airdrie ML6 0JU
Tel: 01236 768900 Fax: 01236 750456
(NHS Lanarkshire, Primary Care Division)

Practice Manager Lorna Gilmour

GP John Lloyd LWANDA, Ailish Ann GLEN

Airdrie Health Centre
Monkscourt Avenue, Airdrie ML6 0JU
Tel: 01236 748488 Fax: 01236 770669
(NHS Lanarkshire, Primary Care Division)
Patient List Size: 3500

Practice Manager Linda Harley

GP Fiona Elizabeth JARVIE, James Richardson Murray LOUGH, Kathleen YIP

Airdrie Health Centre
Monkscourt Avenue, Airdrie ML6 0JU
Tel: 01236 766446 Fax: 01236 766513
(NHS Lanarkshire, Primary Care Division)

Practice Manager Elizabeth McCloskey

GP David WALKER

Airdrie Health Centre
Monkscourt Avenue, Airdrie ML6 0JU
Tel: 01236 769333
(NHS Lanarkshire, Primary Care Division)

GP John ATKINSON, Grace CAMPBELL, Rosemary Jane COOK, Joseph Neil DARROCH, James FEENEY, Sheena Law JARDINE, Colin Torrens Wilson LEES, John Edward Adetokubo ONI-ORISAN

Airdrie Health Centre
Monkscourt Avenue, Airdrie ML6 0JU
Tel: 01236 769388
(NHS Lanarkshire, Primary Care Division)

GP Joan Margaret Macpherson POLLOCK

Aitken Street Surgery
5 Aitken Street, Airdrie ML6 6LS
Tel: 01236 748900 Fax: 01236 748900
(NHS Lanarkshire, Primary Care Division)
Patient List Size: 840

Practice Manager Margaret Hailstones

GP Baharul Mulk Kazi Ahmed ASHRAFUZZAMAN

Bank House Medical Centre
East High Street, Airdrie ML6 6LF
Tel: 01236 766983 Fax: 01236 750471
(NHS Lanarkshire, Primary Care Division)

Practice Manager Donna Byrne

GP Anne Shona Sneddon HAMILTON, H S BIJRAL

Chapelhall Practice
30 Lauchope Street, Chapelhall, Airdrie ML6 8SR
Tel: 01236 762144 Fax: 01236 765411
(NHS Lanarkshire, Primary Care Division)

Practice Manager Ann Mackie

GP Margot McLAUGHLIN, Margaret Muir McLean ANGUS, Graeme David BROUGH, Maureen FERRIE

Clarkson Medical Centre
114 Forrest Street, Airdrie ML6 7AG
Tel: 01236 747611 Fax: 01236 754388
(NHS Lanarkshire, Primary Care Division)
Patient List Size: 1006

GP Tahira IDREES

Doctors Surgery
East High Street, Airdrie ML6 6LF
Tel: 01236 764722 Fax: 01236 750444
(NHS Lanarkshire, Primary Care Division)

GP Geoffrey Francis CARLIN

The Surgery
45 Main Street, Calderbank, Airdrie ML6 7JG
Tel: 01236 767704 Fax: 01236 759186

(NHS Lanarkshire, Primary Care Division)

GP Archibald Neil MacINNES

Alexandria

Alexandria Medical Centre

46-62 Bank Street, Alexandria G83 0LS
Tel: 01389 752419 Fax: 01389 710521
(NHS Argyll and Clyde, Lomond and Argyll Community Services Division)

GP Patrick TRUST, David CLARK, Philip GORDON, Nadja GUNNEBERG, Jean SHAND

Alexandria Medical Centre

46-62 Bank Street, Alexandria G83 0LS
Tel: 01389 752650 Fax: 01389 752361
(NHS Argyll and Clyde, Lomond and Argyll Community Services Division)

GP Gillian DREWERY, Euan GLEN, Christine HUNTER, Edwin ROBERTSON, James STEVENSON

Alexandria Medical Centre

46-62 Bank Street, Alexandria G83 0LS
Tel: 01389 752020 Fax: 01389 755549
(NHS Argyll and Clyde, Lomond and Argyll Community Services Division)

GP James FURNEAUX, Kathryn McLACHLAN, Alan STEPHEN

Alexandria Medical Centre

46-62 Bank Street, Alexandria G83 0LS
Tel: 01389 756029 Fax: 01389 710049
(NHS Argyll and Clyde, Lomond and Argyll Community Services Division)

Practice Manager J Biddulph

GP Malcolm Macdonald MACRAE, Rosemary COOK, Mark Edward Kaye GARTHWAITE, Gordon William HERD

The Surgery

75 Bank Street, Alexandria G83 0NB
Tel: 01389 752626 Fax: 01389 752169
Email: administrator@gp85230.ac.hscot.nhs.ukb.
Website: www.lochlomonddoctors.com
(NHS Argyll and Clyde, Lomond and Argyll Community Services Division)

Practice Manager Jane McNiven

GP Andrew Duncan BAXTER, Mary-Jo COFFIELD, Moira FABLING, Khalid HASSAN, Gary JOHNSON, Neil Sinclair Davis MACKAY, Michael SCULLION

Alford, Aberdeenshire

Alford Medical Practice

2 Gordon Road, Alford AB33 8AL
Tel 01975 562253 Fax: 01975 562613
(NHS Grampian, Primary Care Division)
Patient List Size: 5050

Practice Manager Audrey Thompson

GP George Stuart PAYNE, John Smith Hall REID, Nicholas Roland SHANKS

Alloa

Alloa Health Centre

Marshill, Alloa FK10 1AQ
Tel 01259 216701 Fax: 01259 724790
Email: administrator@gp26031.forth-hb.scot.nhs.uk
(NHS Forth Valley, Primary Care Operating Division)
Patient List Size: 6775

Practice Manager Pauline Dyer

GP David Stuart BORLAND, Fergus Robinson GREEN, Catriona Buchanan LAMB, Graham RIDDLE

Alloa Health Centre

Marshill, Alloa FK10 1AB
Tel: 01259 724181 Fax: 01259 724788
(NHS Forth Valley, Primary Care Operating Division)
Patient List Size: 9000

Practice Manager Katrina Dunbar

GP David Patterson KIRK, Jennifer Elizabeth Wood GREIG, James E SHARPE, Linda Anne SIME, Adrian Lawrence WARD, Nicholas M WARD

Alloa Health Centre

Marshill, Alloa FK10 1AQ
Tel: 01259 216476
(NHS Forth Valley, Primary Care Operating Division)

Practice Manager S Clinton

GP Brian Charles Andrew DULLEA, Graham James HOOD, Pauline MacINNES, Jean MacINTYRE, Shirley Joyce Rennet PROCTOR, Kenneth Whyte STIRLING

Alness

Alness/Invergordon Medical Group

Robertson Health Centre, High Street, Alness IV17 0UN
Tel: 01349 882229 Fax: 01349 884004
(NHS Highland, Primary Care)

Practice Manager P J Rolffe-Budd

GP Peter DOLAN, Peter Anthony BARKER, Peter Nicholas BAXTER, Shirley Jane CARRACHER, James Frederick HUTTON, Jeremy Dawson JACKSON, Stephen KELLY, Margaret McKENNA, John McRORIE, Kim MILLER

Alva

Alva Medical Practice

Alva Medical Practice, West Johnstone Street, Alva FK12 5BD
Tel: 01259 760331 Fax: 01259 769991
(NHS Forth Valley, Primary Care Operating Division)
Patient List Size: 11400

Practice Manager Carol Broadfoot

GP John Archibald YOUNG, Graeme Anderson ABEL, Joan Margaret CLARK, Fiona COLLIER, Graeme Ian HAY, Roderick Alfred HURRY, David Cowan MUSK, Claire Holly RUSSELL

Annan

Greencroft Medical Centre (North)

Greencroft Wynd, Annan DG12 6GN
Tel: 01461 202745 Fax: 01461 201492

Greencroft Medical Centre (North)

Greencroft Wynd, Annan DG12 6GN
Tel: 01461 202745 Fax: 01461 201492
(NHS Dumfries and Galloway; NHS Dumfries and Galloway)

Practice Manager Claire Carswell, Claire Carswell, Claire Carswell, Claire Carswell

GP Jeffrey Stewart KERR, Jeffrey Stewart KERR, Fergus DONACHIE, Fergus DONACHIE, Neil Grant KELLY, Neil Grant KELLY, Terence MAGGIORI, Terence MAGGIORI, Eileen MacFarlane McCALLUM, Eileen MacFarlane McCALLUM

Greencroft Medical Centre (South)

Greencroft Wynd, Annan DG12 6GS
Tel: 01461 202244 Fax: 01461 205401

Greencroft Medical Centre (South)

Greencroft Wynd, Annan DG12 6GS
Tel: 01461 202244 Fax: 01461 205401
(NHS Dumfries and Galloway; NHS Dumfries and Galloway)
Patient List Size: 6460
Patient List Size: 6460

Practice Manager Hazel Gracie, Hazel Gracie, Hazel Gracie, Hazel Gracie

GP Boguslaw Adam LAPKA, Boguslaw Adam LAPKA, David Laing BYERS, David Laing BYERS, Margo L DONACHIE, Margo L DONACHIE, William John Gerard KIERAN, William John Gerard KIERAN, Bronwyn McCALL, Bronwyn McCALL

Anstruther

Dr Hall and Partners

Anstruther Medical Practice, Skeith Health Centre, Crail Road, Anstruther KY10 3FF
Tel: 01333 310352 Fax: 01333 312525
(NHS Fife, Primary Care Division)
Patient List Size: 6400

Practice Manager Ann Jackson

GP Laura Anne BUMBRA, David James HALL, Alistair Forbes MITCHELL, Julia Anne SOMMERVILLE

Pittenweem Surgery

2 Routine Row, Pittenweem, Anstruther KY10 2LG
Tel: 01333 311307 Fax: 01333 312520
(NHS Fife, Primary Care Division)

Practice Manager Jean Bell

GP Andrew Watson KYLE, C FRANCIS, Ingeborg Clasina Martina Maria GUERTS VAN KESSEL, Derek John Wilson MARSTON

Appin

The Surgery

Port Appin, Appin PA38 4DE
Tel: 01631 730271 Fax: 01631 730533
Email: administrator@gp84006.ac.hb.scot.nhs.uk
(NHS Argyll and Clyde, Lomond and Argyll Community Services Division)
Patient List Size: 880

Practice Manager Linda A Magillivray

GP Iain David McNICOL, Kate E HOWLETT

Arbroath

Abbey Health Centre

East Abbey Street, Arbroath DD11 1EN
Tel: 01241 872692 Fax: 01241 872976
(NHS Tayside, Primary Care Division)
Patient List Size: 6000

Practice Manager Kath Ross

GP Allan Edward WARD, Alistair John ACHESON, Ching-Wa CHUNG, Anne C NOLTIE

Abbey Health Centre

East Abbey Street, Arbroath DD11 1EN
Tel: 01241 870307 Fax: 01241 431414
(NHS Tayside, Primary Care Division)

GP James Douglas Angus INGLIS, Michael Andrew LEDSON, Richard Bradley SPEIRS, Graeme Munro SUTHERLAND, Rebecca A WHEATER

Abbey Health Centre

East Abbey Street, Arbroath DD11 1EN
Tel: 01241 870311 Fax: 01241 875411
(NHS Tayside, Primary Care Division)

Practice Manager M Crabb

GP Arnold Hampshire HORNSBY, Stephen Peter Glover BIRD, Neil RAITT

Friockheim Health Centre

Westgate, Friockheim, Arbroath DD11 4TX
Tel: 01241 828444 Fax: 01241 828565
Email: administrator@friockheim.finix.org.uk
(NHS Tayside, Primary Care Division)
Patient List Size: 2700

Practice Manager Ann Carrie

GP Ronald James WALKER, Karen Christina SCALLAN

The Medical Centre

7 Hill Place, Arbroath DD11 1AE
Tel: 01241 431144 Fax: 01241 430764
(NHS Tayside, Primary Care Division)

GP John Stewart CHERRY, Charles FAGAN, Carolyn Mary McKAY, Graeme Lee MOFFAT, James Robertson OGILVIE, William Russell SMITH

Ardgay

Bonar Bridge Surgery

Library Buildings, Lairg Road, Bonar Bridge, Ardgay IV24 3DH
Tel: 01863 766383 Fax: 01863 766671
(NHS Highland, Primary Care)

GP Godfrey Reynold CRABB

Creich Surgery

Cherry Grove, Bonar Bridge, Ardgay IV24 3ER
Tel: 01863 766379 Fax: 01863 766768
(NHS Highland, Primary Care)

Practice Manager Margaret Ross

GP Christopher Jeffery MAIR, Sheila CARBARNS, Janet Mary MAIR

Ardrossan

Dr Haggerty, Adams and Sword

Central Avenue, Ardrossan KA22 7DX
Tel: 01294 463838 Fax: 01294 462798
(NHS Ayrshire and Arran, Community Health Division)

GP Gerard HAGGERTY, Steven ADAMS, L SWORD

South Beach Practice

17 South Crescent, Ardrossan KA22 8EA
Tel: 01294 463011 Fax: 01294 462790
(NHS Ayrshire and Arran, Community Health Division)

Practice Manager S J Clinton

GP Afzal MONIR, D AROKIANATHAN, Maureen McGUIRE, Allan John MERRY, John G NORTON, Gordon PORTEOUS

Arisaig

Arisaig Medical Practice

Rhu Road, Arisaig PH39 4NU
Tel: 01687 450258 Fax: 01687 450385
Email: ADMINISTRATOR@GP55588.HIGHLAND-HB.SCOT.NHS.UK
(NHS Highland, Primary Care)
Patient List Size: 570

Practice Manager Jane Foster

GP Shina Ann YOUNG, Iain GARTSHORE

Arrochar

Arrochar Surgery

Kirkfield Place, Arrochar G83 7AE
Tel: 01301 702531 Fax: 01301 702746
Email: administrator@gp85009.ac-hb.scot.nhs.uk
(NHS Argyll and Clyde, Lomond and Argyll Community Services Division)
Patient List Size: 1000

GP David Farquharson TROUP, Peter H FETTES

Auchterarder

St Margaret's Health Centre

St Margaret's Drive, Auchterarder PH3 1JH
Tel: 01764 662614 Fax: 01764 664178
Email: cduncan@auchterarder.tayside.scot.nhs.uk

(NHS Tayside, Primary Care Division)
Patient List Size: 8000

Practice Manager Carol Duncan

GP Jonathan D DICKSON, Alistair G FISKEN, James Alexander GRANT, James Colville LAIRD, Gordon F McLEAY, Roger Wellwood PATERSON, Fiona Jane PRICE, Susan WYLIE

Aviemore

Aviemore Medical Practice

Aviemore PH22 1SY
Tel: 01479 810258 Fax: 01479 810067
Email: gp@ski-injury.com
Website: www.ski-injury.com
(NHS Highland, Primary Care)
Patient List Size: 4202

Practice Manager C Malcolm

GP Angus MacNEILL, Gillian Elizabeth IRVINE, George Bogdan JACHACY, Gilly KIRKWOOD, Michael LANGRAN, E P MARTIN

Ayr

Barns Street Surgery

40 Dalblair Road, Ayr KA7 1UL
Tel: 01292 281439 Fax: 01292 288268
Email: kathleen.muirhead@aapct.scot.nhs.uk
Website: www.medicayr.co.uk
(NHS Ayrshire and Arran, Community Health Division)
Patient List Size: 8100

Practice Manager Jan McCulloch

GP James Logan NIBLOCK, P HULME, Thomas Walter HUNTER, Jennifer Garth LAWRIE, Thomas Campbell McGEE

The Cathcart Street Medical Practice

3 Cathcart Street, Ayr KA7 1BJ
Tel: 01292 264051 Fax: 01292 293803
(NHS Ayrshire and Arran, Community Health Division)
Patient List Size: 8700

GP James Brawn MILLER, Lindsay R MILLER, Claire A E OLDFIELD, Pauleen Elizabeth SHEARER, Archibald Craig SIMPSON, Paul George STEVENS

Dalblair Medical Practice

56 Dalblair Road, Ayr KA7 1UQ
Tel: 01292 267432 Fax: 01292 264871
(NHS Ayrshire and Arran, Community Health Division)

Practice Manager Amanda Crawley

GP John William WILSON, Suellen HILLS

Dalmellington Medical Practice

The Health Centre, 33 Main Street, Dalmellington, Ayr KA6 7QL
Tel: 01292 550238 Fax: 01292 551342
(NHS Ayrshire and Arran, Community Health Division)
Patient List Size: 3700

Practice Manager Kevin Lang

GP Anne Elizabeth FERGUSON, Michael ADAMSON, Hugh Coulter BROWN

Dr David Stevenson

Cornhill Surgery, Kincaidston, Ayr KA7 3YF
Tel: 01292 264080 Fax: 01292 269731
(NHS Ayrshire and Arran, Community Health Division)
Patient List Size: 1350

Practice Manager M Lancester

GP David STEVENSON

Dr Marie Forsyth

The Surgery, 3 Alloway Place, Ayr KA7 2AA
Tel: 01292 610682 Fax: 01292 263322
(NHS Ayrshire and Arran, Community Health Division)

Practice Manager Gail Dunlop

GP Marie Therese FORSYTH

Drongan Surgery

74 Mill O'Shields Road, Drongan, Ayr KA6 7AY
Tel: 01292 591345 Fax: 01292 590782
(NHS Ayrshire and Arran, Community Health Division)

GP Ian Fraser McNICOL, Niall Fraser Thomson MACKIE, Dr McKELVIE, Wilson Alexander McTAGGART

The Fullarton Medical Practice

40 Dalblair Road, Ayr KA7 1UL
Tel: 01292 264260 Fax: 01292 292160
(NHS Ayrshire and Arran, Community Health Division)

Practice Manager Jane McAusland

GP James Stuart Macpherson HOLMS, Joanne Lynne ASHCROFT, Adam Cook HANNAH, Ian David REWHORN, Alan Anthony James WHITE

Lennox and Partners

9 Alloway Place, Ayr KA7 2AA
Tel: 01292 611835 Fax: 01292 284982
(NHS Ayrshire and Arran, Community Health Division)
Patient List Size: 5500

Practice Manager Lorraine Bridson

GP Brian LENNOX, Karen Louise COULTER, Stuart William HENDRY, Helen HUNTER, David LINDEN

Racecourse Road Surgery

3 Racecourse Road, Ayr KA7 2DF
Tel: 01292 886622 Fax: 01292 269774
(NHS Ayrshire and Arran, Community Health Division)

Practice Manager Julie McGinley

GP Alexander Millar MARTIN, Calvin CHAPE, Brendan John DUNNE, Anne Julie Campbell KENNEDY, David Iain MATTHEWSON, Hans PIEPER

Riverside Medical Practice

27 Dalvennan Avenue, Patna, Ayr KA6 7NA
Tel: 01292 531367 Fax: 01292 531033
(NHS Ayrshire and Arran, Community Health Division)
Patient List Size: 7141

Practice Manager Marjorie McCubbin

GP Nicholas J F HUNTER, Carolyn Margaret LINTON, Samuel Wesley MARTIN, Brian Columbanus O'SULLIVAN, Gary John WHITE

Tams Brig Surgery

107 New Road, Ayr KA8 8DD
Tel: 01292 262697 Fax: 01292 265926
(NHS Ayrshire and Arran, Community Health Division)

GP Raymond James DOUGLAS, John BOWBEER, Malcolm Hugh FRASER, Calum George McCABE, Margaret Amelia SMOLLETT, D TAYLOR

Ballachulish

Bellachulish Medical Practice

Loan Fern, Ballachulish PH49 4JB
Tel: 01855 811226 Fax: 01855 811777
(NHS Highland, Primary Care)

GP Morag CALDUR

Ballater

Braemar Health Clinic

St Andrews Terrace, Braemar, Ballater AB35 5WR
Tel: 01339 741202 Fax: 01339 741450
(NHS Grampian, Primary Care Division)
Patient List Size: 600

Practice Manager M Jolly

GP Donald Murray CRUICKSHANK

Glass and McLeod
13 Provost Craig Road, Ballater AB35 5NN
Tel: 013397 55686 Fax: 013397 55839
(NHS Grampian, Primary Care Division)
Patient List Size: 2000

Practice Manager Elizabeth Simpson

GP Douglas James Allan GLASS, Ewen Donald John McLEOD

Ballindalloch

Glenlivet Community Surgery
Drumin, Glenlivet, Ballindalloch AB37 9AN
Tel: 01807 590273 Fax: 01807 590411
Patient List Size: 700

GP John Nubar DEROUNIAN

Banchory

Banchory Group Practice
The Surgery, Bellfield, Banchory AB31 5XS
Tel: 01330 822121 Fax: 01330 825265
(NHS Grampian, Primary Care Division)
Patient List Size: 11500

GP Frank Fentie MAIR, Derek George BARCLAY, Kate FINDLAY, Martin Gerrard McCRONE, Katrina Mary MORTON, Sandy ROUGH, Tracey SECRETT, Nicola SHOWELL, Mike STEVEN

Station Road Surgery
22 Station Road, Torphins, Banchory AB31 4JF
Tel: 01339 882221 Fax: 01339 882699
(NHS Grampian, Primary Care Division)

Practice Manager D Bruce

GP Iain Malcolm FERGUSON, K MALONE

Banff

Banff and Gamrie Medical Practice
Clunie Street, Banff AB45 1HY
Tel: 01261 812221 Fax: 01261 813929
(NHS Grampian, Primary Care Division)
Patient List Size: 3109

Practice Manager Ruth Hepburn

GP Roderick MACRAE, Babatope POPOOLA

Deveron Medical Group
Banff Health Centre, Clunie Street, Banff AB45 1HY
Tel: 01261 812027 Fax: 01261 813929
(NHS Grampian, Primary Care Division)
Patient List Size: 4000

Practice Manager Moyra Duncan

GP Janet Elizabeth ANDERSON, Rosalind CAMPBELL, George David Duncan INNES, Douglas B SCOTT, Blair Hamilton SMITH, Craig THOMPSON

Portsoy Surgery
16 Seafield Terrace, Portsoy, Banff AB45 2GB
Tel: 01261 842336 Fax: 01261 843959
Email: administrator@portsoy.grampian.scot.nhs.uk
(NHS Grampian, Primary Care Division)
Patient List Size: 2600

Practice Manager Aileen Wilson

GP Marguerita SMITH

Bathgate

Armadale Group Practice
18 North Street, Armadale, Bathgate EH48 3QB
Tel: 01501 730432 Fax: 01501 730262
(NHS Lothian, West Lothian Healthcare Division)
Patient List Size: 10900

GP Bryan Kenneth David JAMES, Philip Crane BELL, Innes Douglas DUNCAN, Douglas MacGILLIVRAY, J R McEWEN, Catriona Edith WILSON

Ashgrove Group Practice
Ashgrove, Blackburn, Bathgate EH47 7LL
Tel: 01506 652956 Fax: 01506 634790
(NHS Lothian, West Lothian Healthcare Division)

Practice Manager Jean Plowright

GP Donald MACAULAY, Sally BLACK, Brian Hubert McKINSTRY, Hugh Forbes MERRILEES

Blackridge Surgery
Fleming Place, Blackridge, Bathgate EH48 3SS
(NHS Lothian, West Lothian Healthcare Division)
Patient List Size: 1965

GP Alan J SRANT

Carlaw and Partners
Newland Medical Practice, Mid Street, Bathgate EH48 2QS
Tel: 01506 655155 Fax: 01506 636263
(NHS Lothian, West Lothian Healthcare Division)
Patient List Size: 5300

Practice Manager Theresa Cameron

GP William Greig CARLAW, Jacqueline Susan LEES, James Marshall MCCALLUM

Health Centre
Blackfaulds Place, Fauldhouse, Bathgate EH47 9AS
Tel: 01501 770282 Fax: 01501 772515
(NHS Lothian, West Lothian Healthcare Division)
Patient List Size: 3400

Practice Manager Ann Beuken

GP Vaughn RITCHIE, Ian Andrew JONES

Kingsgate Medical Practice
Bathgate Primary Care Centre, Whitburn Road, Bathgate EH48 2SS
Tel: 01506 653134 Fax: 01506 683134
(NHS Lothian, West Lothian Healthcare Division)
Patient List Size: 6700

GP Andrew FERGUSON, Kathryn Jane BROWN, Keith WARSHOW

Simpson Medical Group
Bathgate Primary Care Centre, Whitburn Road, Bathgate EH48 2SS
Tel: 01506 654444 Fax: 01506 635931
(NHS Lothian, West Lothian Healthcare Division)
Patient List Size: 6200

GP Deirdre Jane HAY, Clare HAYWARD, Robert W HOLDEN, Andrew Paul William McNUTT, Julie THOMSON

Stoneyburn Health Centre
73 Main Street, Stoneyburn, Bathgate EH47 8BY
Tel: 01501 762515 Fax: 01501 763174
(NHS Lothian, West Lothian Healthcare Division)
Patient List Size: 4500

Practice Manager Elizabeth Currie

GP Sheena Margaret MILNE, Fiona BRADSHAW, Quintin BRADSHAW, John Hatrick STEWART

Weavers Lane Surgery
1 Weavers Lane, Whitburn, Bathgate EH47 0SD
Tel: 01501 740297 Fax: 01501 745190
(NHS Lothian, West Lothian Healthcare Division)

Practice Manager John Martin

GP Liam BROWNE, Tracey GRAY, Alastair Magnus KERR, John Kristian MOONEY, Lynn Joyce PORTER, Neil POWER, Christoph Barthold TOELLNER

Beauly

Croyard Road Surgery
Croyard Road, Beauly IV4 7DT
Tel: 01463 782794 Fax: 01463 782111
(NHS Highland, Primary Care)
Patient List Size: 4890

Practice Manager Effie MacLeod

GP Muriel Joan HAWCO, R S FORSYTH, Kathryn Frances McKECHAN, Nigel PAUL

High Street Medical Practice
1 High Street, Beauly IV4 7BY
Tel: 01463 782214 Fax: 01463 782129
(NHS Highland, Primary Care)

GP James McLARDY, Lesley Ann FULLERTON, Alistair James McINTYRE

Beith

Beith Health Centre GP Practice
Reform Street, Beith KA15 2AE
Tel: 01505 502683 Fax: 01505 504151
(NHS Ayrshire and Arran, Community Health Division)

GP David Anderson PEGGIE, I K GRAHAM, Gordon Ian ISBISTER, Sheila Elizabeth McCARROLL

Bellshill

Bruce Medical Centre
388 Main Street, Bellshill ML4 1AX
Tel: 01698 747666 Fax: 01698 740363
(NHS Lanarkshire, Primary Care Division)
Patient List Size: 9483

Practice Manager Ellen Speedie

GP David John PARK, Stephen GADDIS, Catherine Anne KELLY, Edward Andrew McKENNA, Stewart RAEBURN

Main Street Surgery
494 Main Street, Bellshill ML4 1DQ
Tel: 01698 748421
(NHS Lanarkshire, Primary Care Division)

GP Allen Hodges BLINCOW, Anne-Marie BRANDON, Christine Ann JEFFRIES, Philip Gerard SHERIDAN

The Surgery
John Street, Bellshill ML4 1RJ
Tel: 01698 747195
(NHS Lanarkshire, Primary Care Division)
Patient List Size: 10100

Practice Manager Sandra Gibson

GP Colin Midgley McKIBBIN, Grant LECKIE, Alan Ross LIDDELL, Kirsteen MILLER, Elaine RUTHVEN, Lorraine WALKER

Berwick-upon-Tweed

Union Brae Surgery
Union Brae, Tweedmouth, Berwick-upon-Tweed TD15 2HB
Tel: 01289 330333 Fax: 01289 302556
(Northumberland Care Trust)
Patient List Size: 6400

GP Richard Andrew KNIGHT, Neil Duncan FORSTER, Vanessa Jane PEACOCK, Sarah H RUFFE, Philip Fraser Anderson WOOD

Well Close Square Surgery
Well Close Square, Berwick-upon-Tweed TD15 1LL
Tel: 01289 356920 Fax: 01289 356939
(Northumberland Care Trust)
Patient List Size: 10700

Practice Manager Hilary Lock

GP Brent Charles Howden SMITH, Adrienne Clare BROMLY, Bradley Norman CHEEK, Stephen Brendan DOCHERTY, Barry WARNER, John Maxwell WATSON, Regan Mary Susan WOODING

Biggar

Biggar Health Centre
South Croft Road, Biggar ML12 6BE
Tel: 01899 220383 Fax: 01899 221583
Email: frances.wallace@biggar.lanpct.scot.nhs.uk
(NHS Lanarkshire, Primary Care Division)
Patient List Size: 6500

Practice Manager Lilian K Browning

GP Robert Gourlay LEITCH, David CARVEL, Andrew Martin David GOLDIE, Pamela Gail McGREGOR, Peter STRIGNER

Bishopton

Bishopton Health Centre
Greenock Road, Bishopton PA7 5AW
Tel: 01505 863223 Fax: 01505 862798
(NHS Argyll and Clyde, Renfrewshire and Inverclyde Community Services Division)
Patient List Size: 6500

Practice Manager Janet Grngor

GP Jean Gilmour MASTERTON, Alan Michael BENNIE, Christine Anne BRADFORD, Fiona Barbara DOWNIE, Anne FRASER

Blairgowrie

Alyth Health Centre
New Alyth Road, Alyth, Blairgowrie PH11 8EQ
Tel: 01828 632317 Fax: 01828 633272
Email: administrator@alyth.finix.org.uk
(NHS Tayside, Primary Care Division)
Patient List Size: 4200

Practice Manager Anna Hughes

GP Alexander Muir Morton YOUNG, Keith FALOON, Fergus Buchanan GILMOUR

Ardblair Medical Practice
Ann Street, Blairgowrie PH10 6EF
Tel: 01250 872033 Fax: 01250 874517
Email: administrator@ardblair.finix.org.uk
(NHS Tayside, Primary Care Division)
Patient List Size: 7800

Practice Manager E M Simpson

GP Alexander Duncan SHAW, Andrew James BUIST, John Murray MACKAY, Morag McHoull MARTINDALE, Jessie Marion Anderson SHAW, Ivor John SIM

Strathmore Surgery
19 Jessie Street, Blairgowrie PH10 6BT
Tel: 01250 872552 Fax: 01250 874504
(NHS Tayside, Primary Care Division)
Patient List Size: 3300

GP Karalyn Elizabeth McLaren McNEILL, Richard David HUMBLE

Trades Lane Health Centre
Causewayend, Coupar Angus, Blairgowrie PH13 9DP
Tel: 01828 627318
(NHS Tayside, Primary Care Division)

GP Nico GRUNENBERG, James Ford Borrowman JACK

Trades Lane Health Centre
Causewayend, Coupar Angus, Blairgowrie PH13 9DP
Tel: 01828 627312 Fax: 01828 628105
(NHS Tayside, Primary Care Division)

GP John Walter WILLIAMS, George Charles GREIG, A MILNE

Bo'ness

Forth View Practice
Dean Road, Bo'ness EH51 0DQ
Tel: 01506 822466 Fax: 01506 826216
(NHS Forth Valley, Primary Care Operating Division)
Patient List Size: 4236

Practice Manager Anne Wylie

GP Mark Frank Winstan GILMOUR, Anne-Marie CRICHTON, Janet PATON, Robert PROUDLOVE

Kinglass Medical Practice
Kinglass Centre, Gauze Road, Bo'ness EH51 9UE
Tel: 01506 822556 Fax: 01506 828818
Email: administrator@gp25099.forth-hb.scot.nhs.uk
(NHS Forth Valley, Primary Care Operating Division)
Patient List Size: 2987

Practice Manager Linda Marshall

GP Elizabeth P IRELAND, Victoria H CARGILL, Morag H L REID

The Richmond Practice
Health Centre, Dean Road, Bo'ness EH51 0DH
Tel: 01506 822665 Fax: 01506 825939
(NHS Forth Valley, Primary Care Operating Division)

Practice Manager Janice Bennett

GP Thomas Stewart Pitt SARGENT, Alena KROSNAR, Graham LYONS, Kathleen Margaret ONORI, Deryn Joyce PARK, John PARK

Bonnybridge

Bonnybridge Health Centre
Larbert Road, Bonnybridge FK4 1ED
Tel: 01324 812315 Fax: 01324 814696
(NHS Forth Valley, Primary Care Operating Division)
Patient List Size: 4000

Practice Manager Morag Spinks

GP John Alexander WEIR, Sheena Cameron ANDERSON, Bridget McCALISTER, Peter William McCALISTER

Bonnybridge Health Centre
Larbert Road, Bonnybridge FK4 1ED
Tel: 01324 812315 Fax: 01324 814540
(NHS Forth Valley, Primary Care Operating Division)
Patient List Size: 8350

Practice Manager Julie Cunningham

GP Edward William Wright BRIGGS, Catherine Frieda DYER, Richard Stanbrook DYER, June Vivienne EDMUND, Samuel Stirling MORRISON

Bonnyrigg

Bonnyrigg Health Centre
35-37 High Street, Bonnyrigg EH19 2DA
Tel: 0131 536 8965 Fax: 0131 536 8909
(NHS Lothian, Primary and Community Division)

GP Iain Seymour Mackintosh SMART, S BARRETT, Gary George John THOMSON, Hilary Leith WATKINSON

Bonnyrigg Health Centre
35-37 High Street, Bonnyrigg EH19 2DA
Tel: 0131 536 8910 Fax: 0131 536 8909
(NHS Lothian, Primary and Community Division)

GP Ian Dempster BROWN, J D R HARDMAN, Marion Anne KEITH, Carole McALISTER

Strathesk Medical Group
The Health Centre, 35-37 High Street, Bonnyrigg EH19 2DA
Tel: 0131 536 8989 Fax: 0131 536 8909
(NHS Lothian, Primary and Community Division)

GP Andrew McNeill NORTON, John Roderick COMBE, Gillian Christine DICKSON, Terrina Clare DICKSON, Peter DOYLE, Felicity Margaret Hay DYSON, Linda Jane HEGGIE, Graham Norton HERBERT, Rosamund Bridget INNES, Penelope ROTHER

Brechin

Brechin Medical Practice
Infirmary Street, Brechin DD9 7AN
Tel: 01356 624411 Fax: 01356 666059
(NHS Tayside, Primary Care Division)
Patient List Size: 9600

GP Robert William Young MARTIN, Angus Ross DUFF, Simon Anthony Hyde FROST, Hamish David GREIG, Irene Marie MAHON, Archibald McCallum McINNES

Edzell Surgery
Lindsay Place, Edzell, Brechin DD9 7TR
Tel: 01356 648209 Fax: 01356 648824
(NHS Tayside, Primary Care Division)
Patient List Size: 1740

Practice Manager Gail Graham

GP Marc JACOBS

Bridge of Weir

The Surgery
Station Road, Bridge of Weir PA11 3LH
Tel: 01505 612555 Fax: 01505 615032
(NHS Argyll and Clyde, Renfrewshire and Inverclyde Community Services Division)

GP Aileen VAN DER LEE, William AITCHISON, George McLAREN, Janet SMITH, Mark STOREY

Brodick

Drs Kerr and Guthrie
Brodick Health Centre, Shore Road, Brodick KA27 8AJ
Tel: 01770 302175 Fax: 01770 302040
Email: brodickmedical@sol.co.uk
(NHS Ayrshire and Arran, Community Health Division)
Patient List Size: 1196

Practice Manager Carolyn Jameson

GP Malcolm Macfarlane KERR, Elizabeth Lindsay GUTHRIE

Drs Tinto and Campbell
Lamlash, Brodick KA27 8NS
Tel: 01770 600516 Fax: 01770 600132
(NHS Ayrshire and Arran, Community Health Division)
Patient List Size: 2500

Practice Manager Gill Gregory

GP Richard Graham TINTO, Donald Angus CAMPBELL

Shiskine Surgery
Inglewood, Shiskine, Brodick KA27 8EW
Tel: 01770 860247 Fax: 01770 860298
(NHS Ayrshire and Arran, Community Health Division)

GP Alistair Duncan GRASSIE

Brora

Brora Health Centre
Station Square, Brora KW9 6QJ
Tel: 01408 621320 Fax: 01408 621535
(NHS Highland, Primary Care)

GP Monica Maitland MAIN, Mary Hall FORTUNE, Willem Adriaan STRAUSS

Broxburn

Dr Wood and Partners
Strthbrook Partnership Centre, Broxburn EH52 5LH
Tel: 01506 771800 Fax: 01506 771820
(NHS Lothian, West Lothian Healthcare Division)

GP N R WOOD, Judith KEIGHLEY, Barbara KENT, Fergus McRAE, Fiona REID, John C RUSSELL, Patricia M SANTER

Ferguson Medical Practice
Strathbrock Partnership Centre, 189A West Main Street, Broxburn EH52 5LH
Tel: 01506 852678 Fax: 01506 858430
(NHS Lothian, West Lothian Healthcare Division)
Patient List Size: 5500

Practice Manager E Day

GP Thomas Hume FERGUSON, Clare Margaret CAMPBELL, David CUTHBERT, A E HAIGH

The Health Centre
Holmes Road, Broxburn EH52 5JZ
Tel: 01506 852008 Fax: 01506 856859
(NHS Lothian, West Lothian Healthcare Division)

GP John Fraser GUNN, Kathleen Margaret LESSELLS, Douglas Stewart McGOWN, David MORRISON

Winchburgh Health Centre
Niddry Road, Winchburgh, Broxburn EH52 6RX
Tel: 01506 890210
(NHS Lothian, West Lothian Healthcare Division)

GP A REID

Buckie

Ardach Health Centre
Highfield Road, Buckie AB56 1JE
Tel: 01542 831555 Fax: 01542 835799
(NHS Grampian, Primary Care Division)

Practice Manager Anne Sim

GP Gordon Mitchell PRINGLE, Alison DOUGLAS, William Angus GALLACHER, William George Anderson JAFFREY, Colin MENZIES, Lewis WALKER, B WELSH

Cullen Medical Centre
1 Reidhaven Street, Cullen, Buckie AB56 4SZ
Tel: 01542 840272 Fax: 01542 840799
(NHS Grampian, Primary Care Division)
Patient List Size: 2678

Practice Manager Pam Williams

GP R STOKER, Kathryn ARNOULD, S HAUNSCHMIDT

Seafield Medical Centre
Barhill Road, Buckie AB56 1FP
Tel: 01542 835577 Fax: 01542 835092
(NHS Grampian, Primary Care Division)
Patient List Size: 1926

Practice Manager Heather Pirie

GP James Gerard TUCKERMAN, Nicole BURGE

Burntisland

Kinghorn Medical Practice
Rossland Place, Kinghorn, Burntisland KY3 9RT
Tel: 01592 890217 Fax: 01592 890456
(NHS Fife, Primary Care Division)
Patient List Size: 3000

Practice Manager Fay Paterson

GP Philippe Tacklam CHUE HONG, Alison DUNN, Joan YULE

Masterton Health Centre
74 Somerville Street, Burntisland KY3 9DF
Tel: 01592 872761
(NHS Fife, Primary Care Division)

Practice Manager Roslyn Duncan

GP Michael David BELL, Lorna Elisabeth Mary FLEMING, Iain Macdonald HALLIDAY, Wendy Margaret HART

Masterton Health Centre
74 Somerville Street, Burntisland KY3 9DF
Tel: 01592 872761
(NHS Fife, Primary Care Division)

Practice Manager Elizabeth Whitby

GP James Hugh Budge MACDONALD

Cairndow

Dalnacraig Surgery
Dalnacraig, Strachur, Cairndow PA27 8BX
Tel: 01369 860224 Fax: 01369 860225
Email: TKBasu@btinternet.com
(NHS Argyll and Clyde, Lomond and Argyll Community Services Division)

GP Tapas BASU

The Surgery
Lochgoilhead, Cairndow PA24 8AQ
Tel: 01301 703258 Fax: 01301 703258
(NHS Argyll and Clyde, Lomond and Argyll Community Services Division)

GP Robert James KILPATRICK

The Surgery
Lochgoilhead, Cairndow PA24 8AA
Tel: 01301 703258 Fax: 01301 703400
(NHS Argyll and Clyde, Lomond and Argyll Community Services Division)

GP Robert KILPATRICK

Caithness

Dunbeath Health Centre
Achorn Road, Dunbeath, Caithness KW6 6EZ
Tel: 01593 731205 Fax: 01593 731378
Website: www.dunbeathsurgery.co.uk
(NHS Highland, Primary Care)
Patient List Size: 600

Practice Manager Andrew Usher

GP Natasha USHER

Callander

Main Street Surgery
171 Main Street, Callander FK17 8BJ
Tel: 01877 331000 Fax: 01877 330864
Email: administrator@gp25121.forth-ht.nhs.uk
(NHS Forth Valley, Primary Care Operating Division)
Patient List Size: 2388

Practice Manager Diana Bishop

GP Kerry George MATHEWSON, Isobel Margaret GIBSON

The Medical Centre
4 Bracklinn Road, Callander FK17 8EJ
Tel: 01877 331001 Fax: 01877 331720
Email: administrator@gp25116.forth-b.nhs.scot.uk
(NHS Forth Valley, Primary Care Operating Division)
Patient List Size: 1900

Practice Manager Margaret Davis

GP Graham Duncan Macgregor STRANG, Robert Mackie SCOTT

Campbeltown

Campbeltown Health Centre
Stewart Road, Campbeltown PA28 6AT
Tel: 01586 552105 Fax: 01586 554997
(NHS Argyll and Clyde, Lomond and Argyll Community Services Division)
Patient List Size: 6700

GP Michael Drummond HALL, Malcolm LAZARUS, James Thomas Smith LEASK, Dr NORRIE

Southend Medical Practice
Teapot Lane, Southend, Campbeltown PA28 6RW
Tel: 01586 830635 Fax: 01586 830322
Email: mail@southendmedicalpractice.co.uk
(NHS Argyll and Clyde, Lomond and Argyll Community Services Division)
Patient List Size: 490

Practice Manager Marion McDonald

GP James FINLAYSON

The Surgery
Carradale, Campbeltown PA28 6QG
Tel: 01583 431376 Fax: 01583 431237
Website: www.argyllnhs.org.uk/practices/carradale
(NHS Argyll and Clyde, Lomond and Argyll Community Services Division)
Patient List Size: 700

Practice Manager Gail McIntosh

GP Malcolm ELDER, Eric LIVINGSTON

Canonbie

Rose, Tinker and Healy
The Surgery, Bowholm, Canonbie DG14 0UX
Tel: 01387 371313 Fax: 01387 371244

Rose, Tinker and Healy
The Surgery, Bowholm, Canonbie DG14 0UX
Tel: 01387 371313 Fax: 01387 371244
(NHS Dumfries and Galloway; NHS Dumfries and Galloway)
Patient List Size: 2162
Patient List Size: 2162

Practice Manager Margaret Young, Margaret Young, Margaret Young, Margaret Young

GP Andrew John ROSE, Andrew John ROSE, Kieran D HEALY, Kieran D HEALY

Carluke

Health Centre
14 Market Place, Carluke ML8 4BP
Tel: 01555 771012
(NHS Lanarkshire, Primary Care Division)

GP Alexander James Gordon WORKMAN, Iain Rochford CHRISTIE, Elaine M CROSSAN, Dr MACLEOD

Health Centre
14 Market Place, Carluke ML8 4AZ
Tel: 01555 752150 Fax: 01555 751703
(NHS Lanarkshire, Primary Care Division)
Patient List Size: 10000

Practice Manager S Wilson

GP Alastair Cameron INNES, James Francis Norman STEWART, Susan ARNOTT, John Cameron BOYD, Susan GEMMILL, Lesley Ann MACDONALD

Carnoustie

Carnoustie Medical Group
Dundee Street, Carnoustie DD7 7RB
Tel: 01241 859888 Fax: 01241 852080
(NHS Tayside, Primary Care Division)

Practice Manager Isabel McKee

GP Anderson Dan McKENDRICK, Francis Robert Gordon CROSBY, Elaine McNAUGHTON

Carnoustie Medical Group
Dundee Street, Carnoustie DD7 7RB
Tel: 01241 859888 Fax: 01241 852080
(NHS Tayside, Primary Care Division)

Practice Manager Isabel McKee

GP Hamish LESLIE, Alasdair Iain McLellan EASTON, Lynda Jane MORTON, Peter William THORNTON

Castle Douglas

Castle Douglas Medical Group
Castle Douglas Health Centre, Academy Sreett, Castle Douglas DG7 1EE
Tel: 01556 503888 Fax: 01556 504550
Email: administrator@y18184.dghb.scot.nhs.uk
Website: www.castledouglasmedicalgroup.co.uk

Castle Douglas Medical Group
Castle Douglas Health Centre, Academy Sreett, Castle Douglas DG7 1EE
Tel: 01556 503888 Fax: 01556 504550
Email: administrator@y18184.dghb.scot.nhs.uk
Website: www.castledouglasmedicalgroup.co.uk
(NHS Dumfries and Galloway; NHS Dumfries and Galloway)
Patient List Size: 6500
Patient List Size: 6500

Practice Manager Mandy Neilson, Mandy Neilson, Mandy Neilson, Mandy Neilson

GP Iain Alexander CARMICHAEL, Iain Alexander CARMICHAEL, James Lechler DUCK, James Lechler DUCK, Gregor PURDIE, Gregor PURDIE, Kenneth Balfour SCOTT, Kenneth Balfour SCOTT, Peter John SCOTT, Peter John SCOTT, Lois Mary Elizabeth SPROAT, Lois Mary Elizabeth SPROAT, Mhari WILLIAMSON, Mhari WILLIAMSON

Castle Douglas Medical Group
Castle Douglas Health Centre, Academy Street, Castle Douglas DG7 1EE

Castle Douglas Medical Group
Castle Douglas Health Centre, Academy Street, Castle Douglas DG7 1EE
(NHS Dumfries and Galloway; NHS Dumfries and Galloway)

Practice Manager Aileen Garrett, Aileen Garrett, Aileen Garrett, Aileen Garrett

GP Andrew Peter Descarrieres WILKINSON, Andrew Peter Descarrieres WILKINSON, Elizabeth Anne CARSON, Elizabeth Anne CARSON, N OLIVER, N OLIVER

Glenkens Medical Practice
The Surgery, High Street, New Galloway, Castle Douglas DG7 3RN
Tel: 01644 420234 Fax: 01644 420493
Email: bjones@g18235.dghb.scot.nhs.uk

Glenkens Medical Practice
The Surgery, High Street, New Galloway, Castle Douglas DG7 3RN
Tel: 01644 420234 Fax: 01644 420493
Email: bjones@g18235.dghb.scot.nhs.uk
(NHS Dumfries and Galloway; NHS Dumfries and Galloway)
Patient List Size: 1700
Patient List Size: 1700

GP Bernard George JONES, Bernard George JONES, Shelagh Patricia NEIL, Shelagh Patricia NEIL

The Surgery
Garden Street, Gatehouse of Fleet, Castle Douglas DG7 2JU
Tel: 01557 814437

The Surgery
Garden Street, Gatehouse of Fleet, Castle Douglas DG7 2JU
Tel: 01557 814437
(NHS Dumfries and Galloway; NHS Dumfries and Galloway)

Practice Manager Fiona Donald, Fiona Donald, Fiona Donald, Fiona Donald

GP William Henry ARMSTRONG, William Henry ARMSTRONG, Isobel HAY, Isobel HAY

Castlebay

Clach Mhile Surgery
Castlebay HS9 5XD
Tel: 01871 810282 Fax: 01871 810333
(NHS Western Isles)

GP David John BICKLE, David MUNRO

Clackmannan

Clackmannan and Kincardine Medical Practice
Health Centre, Main Street, Clackmannan FK10 4QX
Tel: 01259 723725 Fax: 01259 724791
(NHS Forth Valley, Primary Care Operating Division)
Patient List Size: 6000

Practice Manager Mary Dunlop

GP Donald Ian MACPHAIL, Neil John DUTHIE, Valerie Anne SCOTT, Ian Bruce THOMSON

Clydebank

Clydebank Health Centre
Kilbowie Road, Clydebank G81 2TQ
Tel: 0141 531 6400 Fax: 0141 531 6336
Website: www.glasgow-hb.scot.nhs.uk
(NHS Greater Glasgow, Primary Care Division)
Patient List Size: 6600

Practice Manager Beverley H McCartney

GP Gordon MacDonald CRAWFORD, Eddie G CRAWFORD, David Ross HOUSTON, Katrina Jean MOFFAT, Amanda M WILSON

Clydebank Health Centre
Kilbowie Road, Clydebank G81 2TQ
Tel: 0141 531 6400 Fax: 0141 531 6413
(NHS Greater Glasgow, Primary Care Division)
Patient List Size: 1610

Practice Manager Anne Burrows

GP Donald Greer WALLACE, Anthony KEARNEY, Gillian MACIVER, Fiona McLEOD

Clydebank Health Centre
Kilbowie Road, Clydebank G81 2TQ
Tel: 0141 531 6400 Fax: 0141 531 6490
(NHS Greater Glasgow, Primary Care Division)

GP Malcolm Ross DOVERTY, William Neil CHALMERS, Michael HARKINS, Caroline Susan STEPHENS

Clydebank Health Centre
Kilbowie Road, Clydebank G81 2TQ
Tel: 0141 531 6465 Fax: 0141 531 6387
(NHS Greater Glasgow, Primary Care Division)

GP Debdas GOSWAMI, Pratibha GOSWAMI

Clydebank Health Centre
Kilbowie Road, Clydebank G81 2TQ
Tel: 0141 531 6400 Fax: 0141 531 6419
(NHS Greater Glasgow, Primary Care Division)

GP Abdul Quader Mohammed Hamidir RAHMAN

Clydebank Health Centre
Kilbowie Road, Clydebank G81 2TQ
Tel: 0141 531 6400 Fax: 0141 531 6336
(NHS Greater Glasgow, Primary Care Division)

GP Mohammed S. HAQUE

Clydebank Health Centre
Kilbowie Road, Clydebank G81 2TQ
Tel: 0141 531 6475 Fax: 0141 531 6478
Email: manager@gp0046-glasgow-hb.scot.nhs.uk
(NHS Greater Glasgow, Primary Care Division)
Patient List Size: 9750

Practice Manager Marion Mccleod

GP Dhia Wadie JABEROO, David Railton BELL, Patricia Isobel HARPER, Janice Margaret McCALL, Alexander Wilson POTTER, Alison Mary WILDING

Clydebank Health Centre
Kilbowie Road, Clydebank G81 2TQ
Tel: 0141 531 6400 Fax: 0141 531 6465
(NHS Greater Glasgow, Primary Care Division)

GP Brian Douglas CLEGG

The Health Centre
Kilbowie Road, Clydebank G81 2TQ
Tel: 0141 531 6400 Fax: 0141 531 6433
(NHS Greater Glasgow, Primary Care Division)

GP Grace Gilmour ROGERSON, Craig Alexander LENNOX, Alan Gregory McDEVITT, Joyce McDEVITT, Alan MCDOUGALL

The Health Centre
Kilbowie Road, Clydebank G81 2TQ
Tel: 0141 531 6400
(NHS Greater Glasgow, Primary Care Division)

Wallace and Partners
Blue Wing, Clydebank Health Centre, Kilbowie Road, Clydebank G81 2TQ
Tel: 0141 531 6410 Fax: 0141 531 6413
Email: administrator@gp40262.glasgow-hb.scot.nhs.uk
(NHS Greater Glasgow, Primary Care Division)
Patient List Size: 7800

Practice Manager Gordon Menzies

GP Agnes Dunlop WALLACE, Michael Antony FLETCHER, Elizabeth Anne HEADDEN, James Craig MILLER, Elaine Isabella MITCHELL

Coatbridge

Centenary Surgery
9 Centenary Gardens, Coatbridge ML5 4BY
Tel: 01236 423355 Fax: 01236 606345
Website: www.centenarysurgery.co.uk
(NHS Lanarkshire, Primary Care Division)
Patient List Size: 2000

Practice Manager Helen Ooi

GP Kao Hua OOI

Centre Street Surgery
8 Centre Street, Glenboig, Coatbridge ML5 2RY
Tel: 01236 872617 Fax: 01236 875585
(NHS Lanarkshire, Primary Care Division)

Practice Manager S Bawa

GP Sarabjit Singh BAWA

Church Street
7 Church Street, Coatbridge ML5 3EE
Tel: 01236 422678
(NHS Lanarkshire, Primary Care Division)
Patient List Size: 6700

Practice Manager Sheila Glen

GP Paul Damien FLANIGAN, Eamonn BRANKIN, David KILGOUR

Coatbridge Health Centre
1 Centre Park Court, Coatbridge ML5 3AP
Tel: 01236 422311 Fax: 01236 437787
(NHS Lanarkshire, Primary Care Division)

GP Simon Andrew CONNOLLY, Natalino Sergio MARCUCCILLI, Claire McCOLGAN, Eamon McLAUGHLIN, Brian Christopher O'NEILL, Lynn WRIGHT

Coatbridge Health Centre
1 Centre Park Court, Coatbridge ML5 3AP
Tel: 01236 422492
(NHS Lanarkshire, Primary Care Division)

Practice Manager Lesley Vickers

GP Liaquat A HAZARIKA, William SCULLION, James THOMPSON

Coatbridge Health Centre
1 Centre Park Court, Coatbridge ML5 3AP
Tel: 01236 433300
(NHS Lanarkshire, Primary Care Division)
Patient List Size: 6600

Practice Manager June Canning

GP Alexander STEWART, John Val DOCHERTY, John FIFE

Coatbridge Health Centre
1 Centre Park Court, Coatbridge ML5 3AP
Tel: 01236 421434 Fax: 01236 437831
(NHS Lanarkshire, Primary Care Division)
Patient List Size: 2438

Practice Manager Beatrice Goodfellow

GP Krishna Ballabh Prasad SINGH, Jeyalakshmi SETHURAMAN

Coatbridge Medical Practice
Coatbridge Health Centre, 1 Centre Park Court, Coatbridge ML5 3AP
Tel: 01698 422950 Fax: 01698 437787
(NHS Lanarkshire, Primary Care Division)

Practice Manager Jan Javidan

GP John David McGOWAN, Carlos BENARAN, Fiona Alexandra CHALMERS, James Michael CURLE, Helen Gabrielle JOHNSTON, Peter Martin JOHNSTON, Judith Susan McCALLION, Margaret MURPHY, John Brian REGAN

Coldstream

Coldstream Health Centre
Kelso Road, Coldstream TD12 4LQ
Tel: 01890 882711 Fax: 01890 883547
(NHS Borders, Primary Care Division)
Patient List Size: 3700

GP Martin HADSHAR, Paul MARYNICZ, Mary VEITCH

Cowdenbeath

Cowdenbeath Medical Practice
173 Stenhouse Street, Cowdenbeath KY4 9DH
Tel: 01383 518500 Fax: 01383 518509
Email: cmp@gp20305.fife-hb.scot.nhs.uk
(NHS Fife, Primary Care Division)

Practice Manager Marion Clacken

GP Ian William Young GALLOWAY, Marion Ann JOHNSTON, Ian Andrew McROBBIE, Dr ROY, Dr STEELE, Forbes MacKenzie STUART, Dr THOMPSON

Crossgates Medical Practice
94 Main Street, Crossgates, Cowdenbeath KY4 8DF
Tel: 01383 511398 Fax: 01383 611586
Email: administrator@gp20358.fife-hb.scot.nhs.uk
(NHS Fife, Primary Care Division)

Practice Manager Yousaf Rose

GP Mohammad Tahir YOUSAF, Frank David Holmes DOWNIE

Crieff

Comrie Medical Centre
Strowan Road, Comrie, Crieff PH6 2LW
Tel: 01764 670217 Fax: 01764 679125
Email: administrator:dundas.finix.org.uk
(NHS Tayside, Primary Care Division)
Patient List Size: 2400

Practice Manager Jane Johnson

GP Catherine Mary CARROLL, Ronald PAYNE, Philip TIPPING

Crieff Health Centre
King Street, Crieff PH7 3SA
Tel: 01764 652283 Fax: 01764 655756
(NHS Tayside, Primary Care Division)

Practice Manager Sheena Walker

GP Andrew Edward MARTIN, Elizabeth BRADLEY, C CORMACK, Hamish T DOUGALL, Stuart EVANS, Alan E MATTHEWS, David Gordon MITCHELL, Alastair MORRISON

Crieff Medical Centre
King Street, Crieff PH7 3SA
Tel: 01764 652456 Fax: 01764 657060
(NHS Tayside, Primary Care Division)
Patient List Size: 3527

Practice Manager Michael Archibald

GP George SAVAGE, Sarah CARTER, Peter A EWING, Helen Lightbody Steven KIRKWOOD

Cromarty

Allan Square Surgery
Allan Square, Cromarty IV11 8YF
Tel: 01381 600224 Fax: 01381 600223
(NHS Highland, Primary Care)
Patient List Size: 1200

GP Helen Grace CHARLEY, Susan HUSSEY

Cumnock

Auchinleck Health Centre
Main Street, Auchinleck, Cumnock KA18 2AY
Tel: 01290 421903
(NHS Ayrshire and Arran, Community Health Division)

Practice Manager Doris Bhatkar

GP Rajaninath Laxmanrao BHATKAR, Dr LATORIA, Dr MAHMOOD

Auchinleck Health Centre
Main Street, Auchinleck, Cumnock KA18 2AY
Tel: 01290 424713 Fax: 01290 426192
(NHS Ayrshire and Arran, Community Health Division)

Practice Manager Sally Brown

GP Jagdish Kumar LATORIA, T MAHMOOD

Dr Christie and partners
2 The Tanyard, Cumnock KA18 1BF
Tel: 01290 422723 Fax: 01290 425444
Website: www.cumnockhealthcentre.co.uk
(NHS Ayrshire and Arran, Community Health Division)
Patient List Size: 12800

Practice Manager Dennis J R Stroud

GP Iain Thomson CHRISTIE, Paul DUNLOP, Rosalind LOCKENS, J LYALL, Janet LYALL, Christine Fraser MACNAIR, James Malcolm MACNAIR, F McMURTRIE, Ian RAMSAY, Gordon STRACHAN

Muirkirk Clinic
Glasgow Road, Muirkirk, Cumnock KA18 3RQ
Tel: 01290 661286 Fax: 01290 661007
(NHS Ayrshire and Arran, Community Health Division)

GP Antoni Joseph KONDOL

New Cumnock Surgery
67 Afton Bridgend, New Cumnock, Cumnock KA18 4BA
Tel: 01290 338242 Fax: 01290 332010
Email: smith.barbara@gp-pct-scot.nhs.uk
(NHS Ayrshire and Arran, Community Health Division)
Patient List Size: 4260

Practice Manager Sandy Stevenson

GP Barbara Anne SMITH, Ross ADAMS, Monna AUMMRAN, J Stewart GILESPIE

Cupar

Auchtermuchty Health Centre
12 Carswell Wynd, Auchtermuchty, Cupar KY14 7AW
Tel: 01337 828262 Fax: 01337 828986
(NHS Fife, Primary Care Division)
Patient List Size: 6300

Practice Manager Dorothy Munro

GP Mary McEwan BROWN, Anne Helen INCE, John Alexander KERR, Graham David POLLINGTON

The Health Centre
11 Main Street, Newburgh, Cupar KY14 6DA
Tel: 01337 840462 Fax: 01337 840996
(NHS Fife, Primary Care Division)

Practice Manager Brenda Friel

GP Robert Donald Currie LENDRUM, David John Wilton BOOTH, H MURRAY

Health Centre
Bank Street, Cupar KY15 4JN
Tel: 01334 654945 Fax: 01334 657306
(NHS Fife, Primary Care Division)
Patient List Size: 8500

Practice Manager Lisa Prudom

GP Ann Campbell BLYTH, Gerald McKenzie BURNETT, Peter Nicholas HARGREAVES, Michael David HENDRY, Dorothy Beatrice SULLIVAN

Health Centre
Bank Street, Cupar KY15 4JN
Tel: 01334 653478 Fax: 01334 657305
(NHS Fife, Primary Care Division)

Practice Manager Mary Robertson

GP Annette CRUICKSHANK, Alasdair James GRAY, Niav Mary KENNY, William John KING, Elizabeth Anne Harvey SCOTT

Howe of Fife Medical Practice
27 Commercial Road, Ladybank, Cupar KY15 7JS
Tel: 01337 830765 Fax: 01337 831658
(NHS Fife, Primary Care Division)
Patient List Size: 4181

Practice Manager Lisa Arthur

GP Helen Mary McGREGOR, John BANKS, Alan Neil Morton PRYDE

Currie

Pentland Medical Centre
44 Pentland View, Currie EH14 5QB
Tel: 0131 449 2142 Fax: 0131 451 5855
(NHS Lothian, Primary and Community Division)

Practice Manager Diane Allan

GP Peter Paul McGAVIGAN, Diane ANDREWS, N A BAILLIE, John P GORDON, Jacqueline METCALF, Elaine Christine SCOTT, N SIMPSON, William Forbes WALLACE

Riccarton Practice
Heriot-Watt University Health Centre, The Avenue, Riccarton, Currie EH14 4AS
Tel: 0131 451 3010 Fax: 0131 451 3503
(NHS Lothian, Primary and Community Division)

Practice Manager Jacqueline Mann

GP Victor Robert Francis DE LIMA, Janette McKay CLINKENBEARD, Susan COBBETT, Shelia WARNOCK

Dalbeattie

The Clinic
Mill Isle, Craignair Street, Dalbeattie DG5 4HE
Tel: 01556 610331

The Clinic
Mill Isle, Craignair Street, Dalbeattie DG5 4HE
Tel: 01556 610331
(NHS Dumfries and Galloway; NHS Dumfries and Galloway)

Practice Manager C Watt, C Watt, C Watt, C Watt

GP Linda COWE, Linda COWE, Ronan BRANNIGAN, Ronan BRANNIGAN, Suzanne CHRISTIE, Suzanne CHRISTIE, Sebastian PFLANZ, Sebastian PFLANZ

Dalkeith

Dalkeith Medical Practice
24 St Andrew Street, Dalkeith EH22 1AP
Tel: 0131 561 5500 Fax: 0131 561 5555
(NHS Lothian, Primary and Community Division)
Patient List Size: 9750

GP Michael Stewart WILSON, Keith Alexander CHAPMAN, Vivien McKenzie Elliot IRELAND, William Dean MARSHALL, Mary Elizabeth Duncan MURRAY, Derek ROBERTSON, Dawn Lesley WESTWOOD

Newbattle Group Practice
Mayfield, Dalkeith EH22 4AD
Tel: 0131 663 1051 Fax: 0131 654 0665
(NHS Lothian, Primary and Community Division)

Practice Manager Sheena Hogg

GP Ralph Roderick Gardner WARWICK, Hilary ANSELL, Avril Harriet GLENCROSS, J GLIDDEN, Ann McCLELLAND, John Norman MILLER, R MORRISON, Michael J MURRAY, Lesley SMART

The Robertson Medical Centre
Danderhall Medical Practice, 85 Newton Chruch Road, Danderhall, Dalkeith EH22 1LX
Tel: 0131 654 1079 Fax: 0131 660 5038
(NHS Lothian, Primary and Community Division)
Patient List Size: 3000

Practice Manager Michelle Lawrie

GP Hedley Guy PHILPOTT, Hilary EGGO, Sue SPARROW

Dalmally

The Surgery
Dalmally PA33 1AX
Tel: 01838 200204 Fax: 01838 200376
(NHS Argyll and Clyde, Lomond and Argyll Community Services Division)

Dalry

Dalry Medical Practice
50 Vennel Street, Dalry KA24 4AF
Tel: 01294 832523 Fax: 01294 835771
Website: www.dalrymc.co.uk
(NHS Ayrshire and Arran, Community Health Division)
Patient List Size: 6250

Practice Manager Janice McPhail

GP James Aitken TAYLOR, Michael LAW, Jillie TAYLOR, Martin Thomson WILSON

Darvel

Dr A J Kondol and partners

East Donnington Street, Darvel KA17 0JR
Tel: 01560 320205 Fax: 01560 321643
(NHS Ayrshire and Arran, Community Health Division)
Patient List Size: 9000

Practice Manager I Morton

GP Antoni Joseph KONDOL, L NIXON, Elizabeth Anne RAIT, William RAMSAY, Margaret Alison ROBERTSON, Mark Frederick Robert SARGAISON

Denny

Carronbank Medical Practice

Denny Health Centre, Carronbank House, Denny FK6 6GD
Tel: 01324 822382 Fax: 01324 826675
Email: doctors@carronbank.co.uk
Website: www.carronbank.co.uk
(NHS Forth Valley, Primary Care Operating Division)
Patient List Size: 8100

Practice Manager Lesley Hamilton

GP Gillian Elizabeth RYRIE, Iain Kerr CAMPBELL, Stuart William DONALDSON, Andrew Stanley James McELHINNEY, Kenneth Fraser McLEAN

Dennycross Medical Centre

Duke Street, Denny FK6 6DB
Tel: 01324 822330 Fax: 01324 824415
(NHS Forth Valley, Primary Care Operating Division)
Patient List Size: 5100

Practice Manager Karin Deuchar

GP Robert Andrew DEUCHAR, Iain Fergusson CRAIG, Frances Mary SHIELS

Dingwall

Dingwall Medical Group

The Health Centre, Ferry Road, Dingwall IV15 9QS
Tel: 01349 863034 Fax: 01349 862022
Email: administrator@gp55376.highland-hb.sct.nhs.uk
(NHS Highland, Primary Care)
Patient List Size: 11206

Practice Manager Mark Gordan

GP Duncan Kerr Mather BLACK, Alan John Lawson DAVIDSON, Keith William EAGLESON, James Douglas HAYWARD, Miles Bradley MACK, Moira Fay McKENNA, John Simpson MILLAR, Paul RASDALE, Lindsey ROSS, S E THOMPSON

Dollar

Dollar Health Centre

Park Place, Dollar FK14 7AA
Tel: 01259 742120 Fax: 01259 743053
(NHS Forth Valley, Primary Care Operating Division)
Patient List Size: 4500

Practice Manager Roslynne O'Connor

GP Neil Mowat HOUSTON, Paul BAUGHAN, Gyda MEETEN, Helen Ferrars RANDFIELD

Dornoch

Dornoch Medical Practice

Shore Road, Dornoch IV25 3LS
Tel: 01862 810213 Fax: 01862 811066
(NHS Highland, Primary Care)
Patient List Size: 2300

Practice Manager Lillian Macrae

GP Kenneth James AITCHISON, Deirdre Elizabeth CAMPBELL, Deirdre Elizabeth CAMPBELL, Catherine HIGGOTT, Rod SAMPSON

Glan y Mor Surgery

Poles, Dornoch IV25 3HZ
(NHS Highland, Primary Care)

GP John Hugh SUTHERLAND

Doune

Doune Health Centre

Castlehill, Doune FK16 6DR
Tel: 01786 841213 Fax: 01786 842053
(NHS Forth Valley, Primary Care Operating Division)
Patient List Size: 3340

GP Philip Francis ROSE, Patricia Mary Napier HENDERSON, Charles Kenneth Herbert JARDINE

Dumbarton

Dumbarton Health Centre

Station Road, Dumbarton G82 1PW
Tel: 01389 602611 Fax: 01389 602621
Email: administrator@gp85032.ac-hb.scot.nhs.uk
(NHS Argyll and Clyde, Lomond and Argyll Community Services Division)
Patient List Size: 2700

Practice Manager Morag McGinley

GP Derek LOGAN, Anne MITCHELSON

The Health Centre

Station Road, Dumbarton G82 1PW
Tel: 01389 602644 Fax: 01389 602624
(NHS Argyll and Clyde, Lomond and Argyll Community Services Division)

Practice Manager William Dickson

GP Elizabeth CAIRNS, Stephen HAGGERTY, Katharin LENNOX, Raymund McNAMEE

The Health Centre

Station Road, Dumbarton G82 1PW
Tel: 01389 602662 Fax: 01389 602625
(NHS Argyll and Clyde, Lomond and Argyll Community Services Division)

GP Lawrence BIDWELL, Jennifer MACKENZIE, Robert McGONIGLE, Thomas McMASTER, Jane McMICHAEL

The Health Centre

Station Road, Dumbarton G82 1PW
(NHS Argyll and Clyde, Lomond and Argyll Community Services Division)
Patient List Size: 3862

Practice Manager Christine M Dawson

GP Stephen DUNN, Julia DUNN, Judith McGLINCHEY

The Health Centre

Station Road, Dumbarton G82 1PW
Tel: 01389 602655 Fax: 01389 602622
(NHS Argyll and Clyde, Lomond and Argyll Community Services Division)

GP Kenneth LYNN, Raymond WALES

Dumfries

Charlotte Street Surgery

1 Charlotte Street, Dumfries DG1 2AQ
Tel: 01387 267626 Fax: 01387 266824

Charlotte Street Surgery

1 Charlotte Street, Dumfries DG1 2AQ
Tel: 01387 267626 Fax: 01387 266824
(NHS Dumfries and Galloway; NHS Dumfries and Galloway)

Patient List Size: 11000
Patient List Size: 11000

GP John Brian Thompson CATHCART, John Brian Thompson CATHCART, John Wilson CLYDE, John Wilson CLYDE, Robert Alexander CURRIE, Robert Alexander CURRIE, Ronald Iain McGROUTHER, Ronald Iain McGROUTHER, Jean Elizabeth ROBSON, Jean Elizabeth ROBSON, Margaret Cunningham Gibb WILSON, Margaret Cunningham Gibb WILSON, William Adamson Melvin WILSON, William Adamson Melvin WILSON

Clayton and Partners
45 Castle Street, Dumfries DG1 1DU
Tel: 01387 252848 Fax: 01387 248096

Clayton and Partners
45 Castle Street, Dumfries DG1 1DU
Tel: 01387 252848 Fax: 01387 248096
(NHS Dumfries and Galloway; NHS Dumfries and Galloway)
Patient List Size: 6450
Patient List Size: 6450

Practice Manager Hayley Peden, Hayley Peden, Hayley Peden, Hayley Peden

GP Philip CLAYTON, Philip CLAYTON, Sheila Joy HANLIN, Sheila Joy HANLIN, Stephen MORRIS, Stephen MORRIS, Dr WILLIAMSON, Dr WILLIAMSON

George Street Surgery
99 George Street, Dumfries DG1 1DS
Tel: 01387 253333 Fax: 01387 253301

George Street Surgery
99 George Street, Dumfries DG1 1DS
Tel: 01387 253333 Fax: 01387 253301
(NHS Dumfries and Galloway; NHS Dumfries and Galloway)

Practice Manager Robert Scott-Brown, Robert Scott-Brown, Robert Scott-Brown, Robert Scott-Brown

GP Edmund Christopher FELLOWES, Edmund Christopher FELLOWES, Christopher Guy BEAUMONT, Christopher Guy BEAUMONT, Robert Wilson PARK, Robert Wilson PARK, Joseph McKinstry REID, Joseph McKinstry REID, David Donaldson TAYLOR, David Donaldson TAYLOR, Susan Barrie TAYLOR, Susan Barrie TAYLOR

Greyfriars Medical Centre
33-37 Castle Street, Dumfries DG1 1DL
Tel: 01387 257752 Fax: 01387 257020

Greyfriars Medical Centre
33-37 Castle Street, Dumfries DG1 1DL
Tel: 01387 257752 Fax: 01387 257020
(NHS Dumfries and Galloway; NHS Dumfries and Galloway)
Patient List Size: 13500
Patient List Size: 13500

Practice Manager Jacqui Little, Jacqui Little, Jacqui Little, Jacqui Little, P Sayers, P Sayers, P Sayers, P Sayers

GP David FLOCKHART, David FLOCKHART, Craig Arbuthnot BROWN, Craig Arbuthnot BROWN, Glidden CHALMERS, Glidden CHALMERS, Bruce William HALLIDAY, Bruce William HALLIDAY, Peter George HUTCHISON, Peter George HUTCHISON, Dawn PHILIP, Dawn PHILIP, Tomas TRUEBA-YANES, Tomas TRUEBA-YANES

Lochthorn Medical Centre
Heathhall, Dumfries DG1 1TR
Tel: 01387 259944 Fax: 01387 264932

Lochthorn Medical Centre
Heathhall, Dumfries DG1 1TR
Tel: 01387 259944 Fax: 01387 264932
(NHS Dumfries and Galloway; NHS Dumfries and Galloway)
Patient List Size: 3000
Patient List Size: 3000

GP Riyazali Yusufali SABUR, Riyazali Yusufali SABUR, F G M O'BRIEN, F G M O'BRIEN

Lowry, Bonn and Desai
Cairn Valley Medical Practice, Kirkgate, Dunscore, Dumfries DG2 0SZ
Tel: 01387 820266 Fax: 01387 820562

Lowry, Bonn and Desai
Cairn Valley Medical Practice, Kirkgate, Dunscore, Dumfries DG2 0SZ
Tel: 01387 820266 Fax: 01387 820562
(NHS Dumfries and Galloway; NHS Dumfries and Galloway)

Practice Manager Elaine Cool, Elaine Cool, Elaine Cool, Elaine Cool

GP William Shields LOWRY, William Shields LOWRY, Gillian BONN, Gillian BONN, Nitin Manubhai DESAI, Nitin Manubhai DESAI

Shebburn Surgery
Main Street, New Abbey, Dumfries DG2 8BY
Tel: 01387 850263 Fax: 01387 850468

Shebburn Surgery
Main Street, New Abbey, Dumfries DG2 8BY
Tel: 01387 850263 Fax: 01387 850468
(NHS Dumfries and Galloway; NHS Dumfries and Galloway)
Patient List Size: 2690
Patient List Size: 2690

Practice Manager Jane White, Jane White, Jane White, Jane White

GP Jane Angela Grace FALCONER, Jane Angela Grace FALCONER, David Andrew STRACHAN, David Andrew STRACHAN

Waite, McFadden and Brown
35 George Street, Dumfries DG1 1EA
Tel: 01387 53724 Fax: 01387 259780
Patient List Size: 4600

Practice Manager Jane McQuillen

GP Craig Arbuthnott BROWN, Patricia Mary McFADDEN, Frank Thomas John WAITE

Dunbar

Dunbar Medical Centre
Abbey Road, Dunbar EH42 1JP
Tel: 01368 862327 Fax: 01368 865646
(NHS Lothian, Primary and Community Division)
Patient List Size: 3600

GP Thomas Reginald BADGER, Charles Neil BLACK

Dunbar Medical Centre
Abbey Road, Dunbar EH42 1JP
Tel: 01368 863226 Fax: 01368 865646
(NHS Lothian, Primary and Community Division)

Practice Manager Paddy Wood

GP David Alasdair CASSELLS, Aileen Mary BREWSTER, Beverley MEE

Dunbar Medical Centre
Queens Road, Dunbar EH42 1JP
Tel: 01368 862227 Fax: 01368 865646
(NHS Lothian, Primary and Community Division)

GP Alan Ian GORDON, Christopher Ronald HORN, Pamela McCLAREN

Dunblane

Dunblane Medical Practice
Heatlh Centre, Well Place, Dunblane FK15 9BQ
Tel: 01786 822595 Fax: 01786 825298
(NHS Forth Valley, Primary Care Operating Division)
Patient List Size: 9600

Practice Manager W McLaren

GP William Gordon SWAN, Mary ABERCROMBIE, Graeme CLARK, Linda Janice McSHANE, Anne Maclean POLLOCK, Robert Graham WATSON, Fraser George WRIGHT

Dundee

Ancrum Medical Centre

12-14 Ancrum Road, Dundee DD2 2HZ
Tel: 01382 669316 Fax: 01382 660787
(NHS Tayside, Primary Care Division)
Patient List Size: 4200

Practice Manager Frances Young

GP Iain Douglas ARTHUR, Sarah Jane ARTHUR, Robin Wellesley SMITH

Ancrum Medical Centre

12-14 Ancrum Road, Dundee DD2 2HZ
Tel: 01382 669316 Fax: 01382 660787
Email: administrator@ancrum.finix.org.uk
(NHS Tayside, Primary Care Division)

Practice Manager Frances Young

GP Mary-Elizabeth ALLEN, Michael GRAY, Jean KER, Alison Jean Marin THOMSON

Ardler Surgery

Turnberry Avenue, Dundee DD2 3TP
Tel: 01382 833399 Fax: 01382 832484
Email: administrator@ardler.finix.org.uk
(NHS Tayside, Primary Care Division)
Patient List Size: 2000

Practice Manager Betty McGregor

GP Dennis Charles MILLER, Julie Ann ANDERSON

Blue Wing Medical Practice

Wallacetown Medical Centre, 3 Lyon Street, Dundee DD4 6RB
Tel: 01382 458333 Fax: 01382 461833
Email: administrator@blue.finix.org
(NHS Tayside, Primary Care Division)

Practice Manager Carol Watson

GP Katherine Mary EMSLIE-SMITH, Rodney Andrew FLEMING, Christine MAPLE, Andrew Gordon RUSSELL, David Michael SHAW, Peter Wright SLANE

Coldside Medical Practice

129 Strathmartine Road, Dundee DD3 8DB
Tel: 01382 826724 Fax: 01382 884129
(NHS Tayside, Primary Care Division)

Practice Manager A McGuckin

GP Michael Graham HAYES, Gordon Wales MACMILLAN, Elizabeth Seonag MACPHERSON, Robert ROSBOTTOM, Andrew TAYLOR

Downfield Medical Practice

325 Strathmartine Road, Dundee DD3 8NE
Tel: 01382 812111 Fax: 01382 858315
(NHS Tayside, Primary Care Division)
Patient List Size: 6400

Practice Manager Jeanette Anderson

GP Doris Susan VINCENT, Rebecca DUFFY, Kenneth Dickson JONES, Salahuddin MALIK, Joyce Nicoll MEIKLE

Dr MacLean and Partners

Monifieth Health Centre, Victoria Street, Monifieth, Dundee DD5 4LX
Tel: 01382 534301 Fax: 01382 535959
Email: administrator@monifieth.finix.org.uk
(NHS Tayside, Primary Care Division)
Patient List Size: 7737

Practice Manager Dorothy Brough

GP Malcolm Hugh MACLEAN, Rebecca Mary LOCKE, David Patterson STEWART, Susan Cobb WHYTE

Grove Health Centre

129 Dundee Road, Broughty Ferry, Dundee DD5 1DU
Tel: 01382 778881 Fax: 01382 731884
Email: administrator@broughty.finix.org.uk
(NHS Tayside, Primary Care Division)
Patient List Size: 5000

Practice Manager Gina Douglas

GP Estelle CHESTERS, Nicholas CONSTANCE, Louise DILLON, Alan George WOODLEY

Hawkhill Medical Centre

Hawkhill, Dundee DD1 5LA
Tel: 01382 669589 Fax: 01382 645526
(NHS Tayside, Primary Care Division)
Patient List Size: 11700

Practice Manager Elaine Hendry

GP Jane Tait BRUCE, Andrew James Henderson COWIE, Alan James DAWSON, Shaun James SCAHILL, John Parry VERNON, Margaret Mathews VERNON

The Health Centre

103 Brown Street, Broughty Ferry, Dundee DD5 1EP
Tel: 01382 731331 Fax: 01382 737966
(NHS Tayside, Primary Care Division)
Patient List Size: 8900

Practice Manager Kim O'Donnell

GP Niall ELLIOTT, Marta Joy Anna GEORGE, Christine Ann HANKINSON, Colin Andrew LEVIN, Lynda T SCULLION

Hillbank Health Centre

1A Constitution Street, Dundee DD3 6NF
Tel: 01382 221976 Fax: 01382 201980
Email: bharvie@hillbank.tayside.scot.nhs.uk
(NHS Tayside, Primary Care Division)
Patient List Size: 8450

Practice Manager Brian Harvie

GP Thomas DYMOCK, Charles John CARNEY, Stanley Robert HANNAH, Joan Skeoch LAMB, David James PROUDFOOT

Inverbervie Medical Centre

Church Street, Inverbervie, Dundee DD10 0RU
Tel: 01561 361260 Fax: 01561 361448
(NHS Grampian, Primary Care Division)

GP C J JOLLY, S McPHEE, P M WILSON, D YOUNG

Lochee Health Centre

1 Marshall Street, Lochee, Dundee DD2 3BR
Tel: 01382 611283 Fax: 01382 624480
Email: swhyte@lochee.finix.org.uk
(NHS Tayside, Primary Care Division)
Patient List Size: 4800

Practice Manager Sheila Whyte

GP Christopher James ROBSON, W A Iain PROCTOR, Morag Christine WARD

Maryfield Medical Centre

9 Morgan Street, Dundee DD4 6QE
Tel: 01382 462292 Fax: 01382 461052
Email: creid@maryfield.finix.org.uk
(NHS Tayside, Primary Care Division)
Patient List Size: 8133

Practice Manager Christine Reid

GP Kenneth Haughan FRESHWATER, Lesley Evans ELLISON, Charlotte PEART, Anne McIntyre WATSON, Graham Charles WATSON, Esther Teresa WILSON

The Mill Practice

Arthurstake Medical Centre, Dundee DD4 6QY
Tel: 01382 457629 Fax: 01382 450365
(NHS Tayside, Primary Care Division)
Patient List Size: 8574

GP Donald Fraser GEMMELL, Alistair Mark EMSLIE-SMITH, Moira Steele KENNEDY, Penny LOCKWOOD, Claire Louise MOIR, Nicola Clare SMEATON, Francis M SULLIVAN

Muirhead Medical Centre
Muirhead, Dundee DD2 5NH
Tel: 01382 580264 Fax: 01382 585200
(NHS Tayside, Primary Care Division)
Patient List Size: 6723

Practice Manager Jane Bruce

GP David John WALLACE, Jane Alison HARROLD, Brian KILGALLON, Ruth LEESE, Tanya VEITCH

Nethergate Medical Centre
2 Tay Square, Dundee DD1 1PB
Tel: 01382 221527 Fax: 01382 226772
Email: administrator@nethergate.tayside.scot.nhs.uk
(NHS Tayside, Primary Care Division)
Patient List Size: 9000

Practice Manager Douglas S Smith

GP Surendra Laxmanrao NARSAPUR, Sharon L COULL, Stuart DOIK, Gisela W SMITH, Edward S WOODWARD

Park Avenue Medical Centre
Park Avenue, Dundee DD4 6PP
Tel: 01382 462222 Fax: 01382 452866
Email: administrator@parkavenue.tayside.nhs.uk
(NHS Tayside, Primary Care Division)
Patient List Size: 5100

Practice Manager B H Glet

GP Colin Cameron AFFLECK, Michael Crawford DUFFY, Clare WOOD

Princes Street Surgery
155 Princes Street, Dundee DD4 6DG
Tel: 01382 461090 Fax: 01382 461091
(NHS Tayside, Primary Care Division)
Patient List Size: 7981

Practice Manager Sally Steelman

GP John FOSTER, Sheila BENNET, David Anderson BRUCE, Michelle Rosalynd DUNCAN, Jane Margaret MacINTYRE, Evan MALKIN

Ryehill Health Centre
St Peter Street, Dundee DD1 4JH
Tel: 01382 644466 Fax: 01832 646302
(NHS Tayside, Primary Care Division)

GP Hamish Arthur Scott MacCOWAN, Malcolm Norman MacDonald BUCKNEY, Katherine Elizabeth OGILVIE

Stobswell Medical Centre
153 Albert Street, Dundee DD4 6PX
Tel: 01382 461363 Fax: 01382 453423
(NHS Tayside, Primary Care Division)
Patient List Size: 2900

Practice Manager Heather Lindsay

GP Peter FOX, Mary O'BRIEN

Tay Court Surgery
50 South Tay Street, Dundee DD1 1PF
Tel: 01382 228228 Fax: 01382 202606
(NHS Tayside, Primary Care Division)

Practice Manager Frances Lavery

GP Margaretha BADENHORST, Catherine FLAVAHAN, Stephen GARDINER, Beren J HOLLINS, Alistair John MONTGOMERY

Taybank Medical Centre
10 Robertson Street, Dundee DD4 6EL
Tel: 01382 461588 Fax: 01382 452121
(NHS Tayside, Primary Care Division)

Practice Manager Agnes Ramsay

GP Anne Elizabeth RAMSAY, Keith Henry ALLEN, Rebecca Katherine MARTIN, Pascal Henry SCANLAN

Taybank Medical Centre
10 Robertson Street, Dundee DD4 6EL
Tel: 01382 461588 Fax: 01382 452121
(NHS Tayside, Primary Care Division)

GP Graham SUMMERS, Wendy Jane TAYLOR

Terra Nova House Medical Practice
43 Dura Street, Dundee DD4 6SW
Tel: 01382 451100 Fax: 01382 453679
(NHS Tayside, Primary Care Division)
Patient List Size: 5745

Practice Manager A. Kelly

GP David Archer RORIE, Joseph John MAGRO, Derek Keith RITCHIE

Terra Nova House Medical Practice
43 Dura Street, Dundee DD4 6SW
Tel: 01382 451100 Fax: 01382 453679
(NHS Tayside, Primary Care Division)
Patient List Size: 2300

Practice Manager A Kelly

GP John Kenneth Macdonald HULBERT, Subhalaxmi DAS

Wallacetown Health Centre
3 Lyon Street, Dundee DD4 6RF
Tel: 01382 459519 Fax: 01382 453110
(NHS Tayside, Primary Care Division)
Patient List Size: 10200

Practice Manager Linda Evans

GP Andrew Bruce BUCHAN, John Duncan FLETCHER, Lynda Margaret HENDERSON, James William LOCKE, Jane Hunt TAYLOR, Elaine Sheila THOMSON

West Gate Health Centre
Charleston Drive, Dundee DD2 4AD
Tel: 01382 667408 Fax: 01382 644807
(NHS Tayside, Primary Care Division)
Patient List Size: 9325

GP Alexander Davidson WATSON, Barclay Munro GOUDIE, Diana Winifred RUSSELL

West Gate Health Centre
Charleston Drive, Dundee DD2 4AD
Tel: 01382 668189 Fax: 01382 665943
Email: administrator@westgate.org.uk
Website: www.westgate.org.uk
(NHS Tayside, Primary Care Division)
Patient List Size: 7250

Practice Manager Sam Riddell

GP Robin Ford SCOTT, David Watt Torrance DORWARD, Ronald Gilmour NEVILLE, Lorna May NICOLL, James Peter ROBSON

Whitfield Surgery
123 Whitfield Drive, Dundee DD4 0DX
Tel: 01382 508410 Fax: 01382 508410
(NHS Tayside, Primary Care Division)

GP Mani RAJ

Dunfermline

Bellyeoman Surgery
Bellyeoman Road, Dunfermline KY12 0AE
Tel: 01383 721266 Fax: 01383 625068
(NHS Fife, Primary Care Division)
Patient List Size: 9600

Practice Manager James Anderson

GP Tierna Mary BROWNE, William Alexander CROSS, Estelle Marie HOLLIGAN, Gordon JOHNSTON, Robert Boyd LESTER, John Gardiner PIGGOT

Boggon and Laggan
The Health Centre, Wardlaw Way, Oakley, Dunfermline KY12 9QH
Tel: 01383 850293 Fax: 01383 851912

(NHS Fife, Primary Care Division)
Patient List Size: 3800

Practice Manager Christine Holliday

GP David Graham BOGGON, C HILL, Michael J LAGGAN

The Health Centre
Wardlaw Way, Oakley, Dunfermline KY12 9QH
Tel: 01383 850212 Fax: 01383 851841
Email: administrator@gp21651.fife-hb.scot.nhs.uk
(NHS Fife, Primary Care Division)
Patient List Size: 3600

Practice Manager C Harrison

GP Iain Hugh MATHIE, Yvonne MATHIE, Charles Scott McMINN

Hospital Hill Surgery
7 Izatt Avenue, Dunfermline KY11 3BA
Tel: 01383 731721 Fax: 01383 623352
Email: administrator@gp20471.fife-hb.scot.nhs.uk
Website: www.hospitalhillsurgery.co.uk
(NHS Fife, Primary Care Division)

Practice Manager S C Reid

GP Graham Forrest BURT, Gerard Desmond GILLESPIE, Kenneth Mackenzie MACKAY, Patricia Anne PEYTON, Michael Crawford PROUDFOOT

Limekilns Surgery
The Old Orchard, Limekilns, Dunfermline KY11 3HS
Tel: 01383 872201 Fax: 01383 873121
Email: dryukchan@yahoo.co.uk
(NHS Fife, Primary Care Division)
Patient List Size: 2200

GP Yuk Keun CHAN, Ian Logan MASON

Nethertown Surgery
Elliot Street, Dunfermline KY11 4TF
Tel: 01383 623516 Fax: 01383 624254
(NHS Fife, Primary Care Division)

Practice Manager G Givens

GP Alan Crawford Adam ALEXANDER, David ALEXANDER, Thomas James ANDERSON, Dr DUTHIE, Alison Brewster MacISAAC, Alan Watson McGOVERN, Mary Reid SCOTT, Dr SCULLY

New Park Medical Practice
163 Robertson Road, Dunfermline KY12 0BL
Tel: 01383 629200 Fax: 01383 629203
Email: administrator@gp20466.fife-hb.scot.nhs.uk
Website: www.newpark.org.uk
(NHS Fife, Primary Care Division)
Patient List Size: 10600

Practice Manager Gillian Stubbs

GP David Robert SHAW, Alison Elizabeth AUSTIN, Robin William DUNCAN, David Richard GILMORE, Richard Nan Pin KAO, Gail Elizabeth MURDOCH, Sara WILSON

Oliver and Partners
Millhill Surgery, 87 Woodmill Street, Dunfermline KY11 4JW
Tel: 01383 621222 Fax: 01383 622862
(NHS Fife, Primary Care Division)

Practice Manager S Hogarth

GP John Robert Fyffe BURT, Sandra Mary Thomson GRANT, James C MACKENZIE, Christopher John Russell OLIVER, Margaret Elizabeth PHILLIPS, Fiona Margaret SEAMAN

Park Road Surgery
Park Road, Rosyth, Dunfermline KY11 2SE
Tel: 01383 418931 Fax: 01383 419007
(NHS Fife, Primary Care Division)
Patient List Size: 5700

Practice Manager N McCorquodale

GP John Scott CHALMERS, Joanna Katherine HADOKE, Kenneth Edwin Charles MACAULAY, Suzanne Kathleen MACKAY

Primrose Lane Medical Centre
29 Primrose Lane, Rosyth, Dunfermline KY11 2UR
Tel: 01383 414874 Fax: 01383 418686
Website: www.primroselanemc.org.uk
(NHS Fife, Primary Care Division)
Patient List Size: 8296

Practice Manager S C Barratt

GP John Richard MOY, Susan Margaret FARRAR, Colin Edward FIRTH, Martin I HAMILTON, Joanne E MOXEY

Valleyfield Health Centre
Chapel Street, High Valleyfield, Dunfermline KY12 8SJ
Tel: 01383 880511 Fax: 01383 881848
Email: administrator@gp20729.fife-hb.scot.nhs.uk
(NHS Fife, Primary Care Division)
Patient List Size: 4500

Practice Manager Marjory Simpson

GP Robert BROWNLIE, Steven James GARVIE, Lesley-Ann PRENTICE

Dunkeld

Lagmhor Surgery
Little Dunkeld, Dunkeld PH8 0AD
Tel: 01350 727269 Fax: 01350 727772
(NHS Tayside, Primary Care Division)
Patient List Size: 3000

Practice Manager Fiona Gibson

GP David Stewart BINNIE, Janice Nancy SILBURN, Graham Alexander WRIGHT

Dunoon

Argyll Street Surgery
246 Argyll Street, Dunoon PA23 7HW
Tel: 01369 703252 Fax: 01369 706880
Email: administrator@gp8423Y.ac-hb.scot.nhs.uk
(NHS Argyll and Clyde, Lomond and Argyll Community Services Division)
Patient List Size: 3600

Practice Manager Isobel Nicol

GP David Thomas HERBERT, Sandra Mary JOHNSTON, John Gordon Hume STEWART

Church Street Surgery
30 Church Street, Dunoon PA23 8BG
Tel: 01369 703482 Fax: 01369 704502
(NHS Argyll and Clyde, Lomond and Argyll Community Services Division)
Patient List Size: 4832

Practice Manager Jane Williams

GP John PEARCE, Geoffrey HORTON, Melanie KING, Alan STEWART, Alison TURNER

Dr Campbell and Partners
246 Argyll Street, Dunoon PA23 7HW
Tel: 01369 703279 Fax: 01369 704430
(NHS Argyll and Clyde, Lomond and Argyll Community Services Division)

GP Peter CAMPBELL, David JOHNSTONE, Fiona MURDOCH, Alan THOMSON

Osbourne Lodge Surgery
121 Alexandra Parade, Dunoon PA23 8AW
Tel: 01369 705079
(NHS Argyll and Clyde, Lomond and Argyll Community Services Division)

Riverbank Surgery
Kilmun, Dunoon PA23 8SE
Tel: 01369 840279 Fax: 01369 840664

(NHS Argyll and Clyde, Lomond and Argyll Community Services Division)
Patient List Size: 1200

Practice Manager Gill McCormick

GP William Joseph WILKIE

Duns

Chirnside Medical Practice

South Crofts, Chirnside, Duns TD11 3XP
Tel: 01890 818253 Fax: 01890 818595
(NHS Borders, Primary Care Division)
Patient List Size: 2750

Practice Manager Sheila Trotter

GP Richard Gregory FOWLES, Donald James MACALLISTER

Duns Medical Practice

The Knoll, Station Road, Duns TD11 3EL
Tel: 01361 883322 Fax: 01361 882186
(NHS Borders, Primary Care Division)
Patient List Size: 5700

Practice Manager Margaret Squires

GP Bruce Milner AULD, Laura MACFARLANE, Simon Robert McCANN, P MORALEE, Gordon SIM

Greenlaw Surgery

Duns Road, Greenlaw, Duns TD10 6XJ
Tel: 01361 810216 Fax: 01361 810799
(NHS Borders, Primary Care Division)

Practice Manager Margaret Mitchell

GP David Livingstone MITCHELL, Dr TAYLOR

Earlston

Leader Health

Kidgate, Earlston TD4 6DW
Tel: 01896 848333 Fax: 01896 848349
(NHS Borders, Primary Care Division)
Patient List Size: 5000

Practice Manager Glynis Smyth

GP Ian Douglas BOND, Paul CORMIE, Jenny LOWLES, Sheena MACDONALD

East Linton

East Linton Surgery

Station Road, East Linton EH40 3DP
Tel: 01620 860204 Fax: 01620 860318
(NHS Lothian, Primary and Community Division)

Practice Manager Elayne Burley

GP Kenneth HARE

East Molesey

Vine Medical Centre

69 Pemberton Road, East Molesey KT8 9LJ
Tel: 020 8979 4200 Fax: 020 8941 9827
(East Elmbridge and Mid Surrey Primary Care Trust)
Patient List Size: 6200

Practice Manager Janette Hyde

GP Jonathan Samuel HAMILL, Kathy LARK, Tracey Louise ROWE, Peter John TAPPING

East Renfrewshire

Medical Centre

1 High Street, Neilston, East Renfrewshire G78 3HJ
Tel: 0141 880 6505 Fax: 0141 881 9266
(NHS Argyll and Clyde, Renfrewshire and Inverclyde Community Services Division)
Patient List Size: 2194

Practice Manager Theresa Millar

GP Agnes Dougan CAPALDI, John DUDGEON

Edinburgh

Bangholm Medical Centre

21-25 Bangholm Loan, Edinburgh EH5 3AH
Tel: 0131 552 7676 Fax: 0131 552 8145
(NHS Lothian, Primary and Community Division)
Patient List Size: 4000

Practice Manager Sandra Brady

GP Anne STEVENSON, Steven ALLAN, Kathryn Anne SUTHERLAND

Bangholm Medical Centre

21-25 Bangholm Loan, Edinburgh EH5 3AH
Tel: 0131 552 6363 Fax: 0131 552 8145
(NHS Lothian, Primary and Community Division)

GP Nigel Michael Jan OSTROWSKI, Laura J STOBIE

Baronscourt Surgery

89 Northfield Broadway, Edinburgh EH8 7RX
Tel: 0131 657 5444 Fax: 0131 669 8116
Email: reception.s70658@lothian.sccot.nhs.uk
(NHS Lothian, Primary and Community Division)
Patient List Size: 6300

Practice Manager Val Thomson

GP Frederick Owens GEORGE, Carola Mary BRONTE-STEWART, Michael Francis RYAN, Lucy Anne THOMSON

Bellevue Medical Centre

26 Huntingdon Place, Edinburgh EH7 4AT
Tel: 0131 556 8196 Fax: 0131 557 0535
(NHS Lothian, Primary and Community Division)
Patient List Size: 4500

Practice Manager Michelle Scott

GP Heather Clare GRAY, Joanne GARDINER, Jane MILLAR, Gregor VENTERS

Bellevue Medical Centre

26 Huntingdon Place, Edinburgh EH7 4AT
Tel: 0131 556 2642 Fax: 0131 557 4430
(NHS Lothian, Primary and Community Division)
Patient List Size: 5070

Practice Manager Gail Delworth

GP Martin Stephen TOLLEY, Nicola GRANT, Graham Thomas RUSSELL, Maria TORRES

Blackhall Medical Centre

51 Hillhouse Road, Edinburgh EH4 3TH
Tel: 0131 332 7696 Fax: 0131 315 2884
(NHS Lothian, Primary and Community Division)

Practice Manager Margaret Livingstone

GP John Peter STEYN, Maria GALEA, Helen Lindsay MACKINNON, C McFARLANE, Archibald Colin McNIVEN, Dorothy Elizabeth WALKER

Braids Medical Practice

6 Camus Avenue, Edinburgh EH10 6QT
Tel: 0131 445 5999 Fax: 0131 445 3553
(NHS Lothian, Primary and Community Division)
Patient List Size: 8600

Practice Manager Marie Watt

GP Clive Alan David BEACH, Helen Suzanne Coldwell HORSFALL, Kerr William NOBLE, Margaret Joy Crerar ROBERTSON, Samuel Alastair THOMSON

Brown and Partners
35 Saughton Crescent, Edinburgh EH12 5SS
Tel: 0131 337 2166 Fax: 0131 313 5059
Email: mmc@mmc.org.uk
(NHS Lothian, Primary and Community Division)
Patient List Size: 7000

Practice Manager Mairi Davidson

GP David Robertson BROWN, Christopher Ewan Hamish CRAWFORD, Linda Ritchie FINNIE, Theresa Mary TURNEY, Andrew Gordon WILSON

Brunton Place Surgery
9 Brunton Place, Edinburgh EH7 5EG
Tel: 0131 557 5545 Fax: 0131 557 4679
(NHS Lothian, Primary and Community Division)
Patient List Size: 7575

Practice Manager Alice Ewing

GP John Henderson DREVER, Alistair Edward DOBBIN, Richard HENDERSON, Alison M McLEAN, Suzanne Cathryn WATERER

Bruntsfield Medical Practice
11 Forbes Road, Edinburgh EH10 4EY
Tel: 0131 228 6081 Fax: 0131 229 4330
(NHS Lothian, Primary and Community Division)
Patient List Size: 11300

Practice Manager Cherylin Robertson

GP Kenneth James Anderson BROWN, Michael Peter CASH, Susan McLaren GALLOWAY, Stephen George Martin ILLINGWORTH, Ian J KEW, Elizabeth Dorothy Anne McCALL-SMITH, Judith M PENNY

Colinton Road Surgery
163 Colinton Road, Edinburgh EH14 1BE
(NHS Lothian, Primary and Community Division)

GP Kailash Behari VARMA, Meena VARMA

Colinton Surgery
296B Colinton Road, Edinburgh EH13 0LB
Tel: 0131 441 4555 Fax: 0131 441 3963
(NHS Lothian, Primary and Community Division)
Patient List Size: 10800

Practice Manager Rachel McArthur

GP Fiona Helen LOSSOCK, Margo McDERMOTT, Colin James McGREGOR, Thomas Mowbray McMILLAN, Janet OSWALD, Duncan Andrew REID

Craiglockhart Surgery
161 Colinton Road, Edinburgh EH14 1BE
Tel: 0131 455 8494 Fax: 0131 444 0161
(NHS Lothian, Primary and Community Division)

Practice Manager Dianne Reynolds

GP Iain Shing Hee CHEW, Henry Mercer BURNETT, Ann Lee CURRIE, Jacquelyn Ross ERRINGTON, Colin Drummond MACKENZIE, Alison Meta Elizabeth TORRANCE, Lynda Joyce TULLOCH

Craigmillar Medical Group
106 Niddrie Mains Road, Edinburgh EH16 4DT
Tel: 0131 536 9500 Fax: 0131 536 9545
Email: reception.rs70215@lothian.scot.nhs.uk
(NHS Lothian, Primary and Community Division)
Patient List Size: 8300

Practice Manager Anette I Thomson

GP Brian Robert WOOD, Mandy Elizabeth ALLISON, Carl Brian BICKLER, David William EWART, Walter Saggar JAMIESON, Catriona Margaret MORTON, Rachel Jane WOOD

Crewe Medical Centre
135 Boswall Parkway, Edinburgh EH5 2LY
Tel: 0131 552 5544 Fax: 0131 551 5364
(NHS Lothian, Primary and Community Division)
Patient List Size: 6900

Practice Manager J Campbell

GP Bernard Von KUENSSBERG, Lesley Jane ADAMS, Juli DALGLEISH, Graham John FENTIMAN, Lesley Anne MACDONALD

Dalkeith Road Medical Practice
145 Dalkeith Road, Edinburgh EH16 5HQ
Tel: 0131 667 1289 Fax: 0131 667 7051
(NHS Lothian, Primary and Community Division)

GP Irene PATERSON, Christopher Land HUBY, Teresa Josephine QUINN

Davidson's Mains Medical Centre
5 Quality Street, Edinburgh EH4 5BP
Tel: 0131 336 2291 Fax: 0131 336 1886
(NHS Lothian, Primary and Community Division)

Practice Manager E Kecheran

GP Patrick Stephen McGUIGAN, Y WALKER

Dr A Wilson and Partners
Sighthill Health Centre, 380 Calder Road, Edinburgh EH11 4AU
Tel: 0131 537 7060 Fax: 0131 537 7005
(NHS Lothian, Primary and Community Division)

Practice Manager Emma Nelson

GP Robert Alistair Mackay WATSON, Anthony Richard HARRISON, Pamela C LESLIE, Diana Mary WHITWORTH, Nigel WILLIAMS

Dr I H McKee and Partners
Wester Hailes Health Centre, 7 Murrayburn Gate, Edinburgh EH14 2SS
Tel: 0131 537 7300 Fax: 0131 537 7337
(NHS Lothian, Primary and Community Division)
Patient List Size: 6200

Practice Manager Kevin Lawrie

GP Ian Hume McKEE, Colin James COOPER, Marte Maria COWELL, Daniel James Nelson DREWITT, Penelope Ann WATSON

Dr Lang and Partners
Sighthill Health Centre, 380 Calder Road, Edinburgh EH11 4AU
Tel: 0131 537 7040 Fax: 0131 537 7005
(NHS Lothian, Primary and Community Division)
Patient List Size: 3096

GP John Anderson LANG, D PUTTA, F SHARPE

Durham Road Medical Group
25 Durham Road, Edinburgh EH15 1NY
Tel: 0131 669 1153 Fax: 0131 669 3633
(NHS Lothian, Primary and Community Division)
Patient List Size: 7047

Practice Manager Anne White

GP Kenneth Maurice O'NEILL, Mark Alister GRUBB, Jean Elizabeth Brawn LEITCH, Nesta MACKENZIE, Gordon James McCULLOCH, Rosalind WIGHT

Edinburgh Homeless Practice
The Access Point, 17 Leith Street, Edinburgh EH1 3AT
Tel: 0131 529 7747 Fax: 0131 557 9918
(NHS Lothian, Primary and Community Division)
Patient List Size: 1500

Practice Manager Kirsty Hogg

GP M P DONNELLY, Jennifer FORBES, Digby THOMAS, Mike WINTER

Eyre Crescent Surgery
31 Eyre Crescent, Edinburgh EH3 5EU
Tel: 0131 556 8842 Fax: 0131 557 2177
Email: reception.s70018@lothian.scot.nhs.uk
(NHS Lothian, Primary and Community Division)
Patient List Size: 2055

GP Peter Jonathon Pringle HOLLAND

Eyre Medical Practice
31 Eyre Crescent, Edinburgh EH3 5EU
Tel: 0131 556 8842 Fax: 0131 557 2177
Email: reception.s70018@lothian.scot.nhs.uk

(NHS Lothian, Primary and Community Division)
Patient List Size: 2150

GP Donald J M ALLAN

Eyre Medical Practice
31 Eyre Crescent, Edinburgh EH3 5EU
Tel: 0131 556 8842 Fax: 0131 557 2177
Email: reception.s70018@lothian.scot.nhs.uk
(NHS Lothian, Primary and Community Division)

GP Ian F DAVEY, Helen FAULDING-BIRD, Claire PEDDER

Eyre Medical Practice
31 Eyre Crescent, Edinburgh EH3 5BU
Tel: 0131 556 8842 Fax: 0131 557 2177
Email: reception.s700018@lothian.scot.nhs.uk
(NHS Lothian, Primary and Community Division)

GP Philip A GASKELL

Ferniehill Road Surgery
8 Ferniehill Road, Edinburgh EH17 7AB
Tel: 0131 664 2166 Fax: 0131 666 1075
(NHS Lothian, Primary and Community Division)

GP William Cameron MACKENZIE, Gavin BOYD, Judith Alison BUCHAN, Laura DICKSON, Alan Hugh WILLIAMS

Firrhill Medical Centre
167 Colinton Mains Drive, Edinburgh EH13 9AF
Tel: 0131 441 3119 Fax: 0131 441 4122
(NHS Lothian, Primary and Community Division)
Patient List Size: 4300

Practice Manager Eleanor MacDonald

GP James Temple COWAN, Julie FORSEY, Sarah Anne McMILLAN, Barbara STEWART

Grange Medical Group
1 Beaufort Road, Edinburgh EH9 1AG
Tel: 0131 447 1646 Fax: 0131 447 8192
(NHS Lothian, Primary and Community Division)
Patient List Size: 7300

Practice Manager Carrie Anderson

GP Alistair David MACLEOD, Gordon BLACK, Susan Margaret BUCK, Robert Martin MACFARLANE, Claire Fiona McDONALD

Hermitage Terrace Surgery
5 Hermitage Terrace, Edinburgh EH10 4RP
Tel: 0131 447 6277 Fax: 0131 447 9866
(NHS Lothian, Primary and Community Division)

Practice Manager Sheillah Smith

GP Keith DONALDSON, Susan COUPE, Elizabeth MORRIS

The Hermitages Medical Practice
5 Hermitage Terrace, Edinburgh EH10 4RP
Tel: 0131 447 6277 Fax: 0131 447 9866
Email: hermitage-medical-practices@hotmail.com
(NHS Lothian, Primary and Community Division)
Patient List Size: 1800

Practice Manager Sheillah Smith

GP Anthony Charles Murray AYLES, Rita Charlotte RIGG

The Hermitages Medical Practice
5 Hermitage Terrace, Edinburgh EH10 4RP
Tel: 0131 447 6277 Fax: 0131 447 9866
(NHS Lothian, Primary and Community Division)

GP James Frederick FAIR

Howdenhall Surgery
57 HowdenHall Road, Edinburgh EH16 6PL
Tel: 0131 664 2377 Fax: 0131 672 2114
(NHS Lothian, Primary and Community Division)
Patient List Size: 6000

Practice Manager Ian Cochrane

GP Linda Elizabeth DUNCAN, J Hugh AINSWORTH, Gail T CORBETT, Colin William JONES, Catherine Mary SIMMONS

Inchpark Surgery
10 Marmion Crescent, Edinburgh EH16 5QU
Tel: 0131 666 2121 Fax: 0131 666 0806
(NHS Lothian, Primary and Community Division)
Patient List Size: 5736

Practice Manager Cathy Wishart

GP Donald Rankin Kerr FRASER, Anne Veronica CAMERON, Katarina Cecilia FORSYTH, Stephen Dominic MURRAY

Inverleith Row Surgery
43 Inverleith Row, Edinburgh EH3 5PY
Tel: 0131 552 3369 Fax: 0131 552 5343
Email: isabel.smith@lothian.scot.nhs.uk
(NHS Lothian, Primary and Community Division)
Patient List Size: 3030

Practice Manager Isabel Smith

GP Peter Thomas STEWART, John Maxwell INWOOD

Ladywell Medical Centre
26 Featherhall Road, Edinburgh EH12 7UN
Tel: 0131 334 5000 Fax: 0131 334 8410
(NHS Lothian, Primary and Community Division)

Practice Manager Elaine Fairbairn

GP Hugh V EDWARDS, Robert ELSWOOD, Alexander E S MAIR, D MITCHELL, Jane MOORE, Henry J RODGERS, H Elizabeth ROSS, Alice TRAVERS

Ladywell Medical Centre (West)
Ladywell Road, Edinburgh EH12 7TB
Tel: 0131 334 3602 Fax: 0131 316 4816
(NHS Lothian, Primary and Community Division)
Patient List Size: 10500

Practice Manager Maris Munro

GP Iain Macalpine Macrae MACMILLAN, Donald BAIN, David William HOLTON, C Jane MILLER, Ianthe Elizabeth Lee MURRAY, Catherine J SYKES, Sally Anne TOTHILL, Martin J WILLIAMS

Lauriston Place Surgery
32 Lauriston Place, Edinburgh EH3 9EZ
Tel: 0131 229 7652 Fax: 0131 221 9563
Email: lauristonsurgery@aol.com
(NHS Lothian, Primary and Community Division)

Practice Manager Charlie Sclater

GP Linda MacCALLUM, Calum MACKENZIE

Leith Mount
46 Ferry Road, Edinburgh EH6 4AE
Tel: 0131 554 2958 Fax: 0131 555 6911
(NHS Lothian, Primary and Community Division)

GP George Brian MACKINLAY, Andrew Edward BRIMELOW, George CRAIG, Patricia Mary DONALD, Andrew DUNLOP, Julie M C GALLAGHER, Sara Cathryn HORNIBROOK, David W JOLLIFFE, Douglas I H LAMB, Gillian M PRICE, Fiona Margaret SKINNER, Laura STEVENSON

Leith Walk Surgery
60 Leith Walk, Edinburgh EH6 5HB
Tel: 0131 554 6471 Fax: 0131 555 4964
(NHS Lothian, Primary and Community Division)

GP Ian Angus MOFFAT, R McBAIN, D F McCORMICK, Roderick John SCOTT

Leven Medical Practice
Tollcross Health Centre, 10 Ponton Street, Edinburgh EH3 9QQ
(NHS Lothian, Primary and Community Division)
Patient List Size: 4500

GP Mary Pelc BLACK, Michael David BROUGH, Susan NICKERSON

Liberton Medical Group
65 Liberton Gardens, Edinburgh EH16 6JT
Tel: 0131 664 3050 Fax: 0131 672 1952
Website: www.libertonmedical.co.uk
(NHS Lothian, Primary and Community Division)

Practice Manager Dawn Saltman

GP Andrew MORRISON, Julie CATNACH, Orla MAYER, Angus Edward McVEAN, Lynne PHILIP

Links Medical Centre
4 Hermitage Place, Edinburgh EH6 8BW
Tel: 0131 554 1036 Fax: 0131 555 3995
(NHS Lothian, Primary and Community Division)

GP Simon Hony TROTTER, Andrew HESLOP, Fergus John MACPHERSON, John William PATERSON, Mary SCOTT

The Long House
73 East Trinity Road, Edinburgh EH5 3EL
Tel: 0131 552 4919 Fax: 0131 551 3965
(NHS Lothian, Primary and Community Division)

GP Alan Ninian Murray HEWITT, Catharine Mary GEORGE, Ian Michael McCULLOCH, Susan Barbara MOIR, Stephen Gordon TAYLOR

Marchmont Medical Practice
10 Warrender Park Terrace, Edinburgh EH9 1JA
Tel: 0131 229 6314 Fax: 0131 221 0551
Email: trea.webster@lothian.scot.nhs.uk
(NHS Lothian, Primary and Community Division)
Patient List Size: 1750

Practice Manager Trea Webster

GP Richard RACZKOWSKI

Mayfield Road Surgery
125 Mayfield Road, Edinburgh EH9 3AJ
Tel: 0131 668 1095 Fax: 0131 662 1734
(NHS Lothian, Primary and Community Division)
Patient List Size: 9300

Practice Manager Y. McBeth

GP Alexander Graham REID, Linda J BERTRAM, Genevieve Ann COMISKEY, Alexandra Louise CONNAN, Michael John FERGUSON, Ramon Alexander McDERMOTT, Lorna Margaret TAYLOR

McIntosh, Gourlay and Partners
Stockbridge Health Centre, 1 India Place, Edinburgh EH3 6EH
Tel: 0131 225 9191 Fax: 0131 226 6549
(NHS Lothian, Primary and Community Division)
Patient List Size: 8500

Practice Manager Susan Duncan

GP Alastair Hogg McINTOSH, Kathryn Anne GOURLAY, Roderick John SHAW, Peter Jonathan TWIDDY, Lynn Margaret WILSON

McKenzie Medical Centre
20 West Richmond Street, Edinburgh EH8 9DX
Tel: 0131 667 2955 Fax: 0131 650 2681
(NHS Lothian, Primary and Community Division)
Patient List Size: 5200

Practice Manager Fay Johnstone

GP David WELLER, Robert Edward BOLTON, Karen FAIRHURST, Scott Anderson MURRAY, Alison Alexandra SINCLAIR, Donald McDonald THOMSON

Meadows Medical Practice
9 Brougham Place, Edinburgh EH3 9HW
Tel: 0131 229 7709 Fax: 0131 229 0765
(NHS Lothian, Primary and Community Division)
Patient List Size: 4770

Practice Manager Elaine Murray

GP Robert Gavin DOWNIE, Susan M GRANT, Dr HOMER

Milton Surgery
132 Mountcastle Drive South, Edinburgh EH15 3LL
Tel: 0131 669 6101 Fax: 0131 669 0269
(NHS Lothian, Primary and Community Division)

GP Gavin Foster Crerar BRYDONE, Gordon CAMERON, Sarah Rosalind CHALMERS, Fiona Margaret MORRISON, Thomas Charles SCHOFIELD, Catherine Jane SCOTT

Morningside Medical Practice
2 Morningside Place, Edinburgh EH10 5ER
Tel: 0131 452 8406 Fax: 0131 447 3020
(NHS Lothian, Primary and Community Division)
Patient List Size: 8000

Practice Manager Anne Crandles

GP Roderick Kenneth John MACKINNON, Wilma Annabel CUPPLES, Jane Helen Rowand EDINGTON, William Richard UTTLEY, Isobel Margaret WILSON

Muirhouse Medical Group
1 Muirhouse Avenue, Edinburgh EH4 4PL
Tel: 0131 537 4343 Fax: 0131 537 4344
(NHS Lothian, Primary and Community Division)

GP James Roy ROBERTSON, D DAVIDSON, John Leo DUNN, Paul Alexander HEPPLE, Jane HILL, Peter SHISHODIA, Wilfrid TREASURE

Murrayfield Medical Practice
13B Riversdale Crescent, Edinburgh EH12 5QX
Tel: 0131 337 6151 Fax: 0131 313 5450
(NHS Lothian, Primary and Community Division)
Patient List Size: 6800

Practice Manager S Brown

GP William Alexander CAMPBELL, Robin Francis BALFOUR, Denise COLEIRO, Angela Mary HAMILL, Sarah L MORAN, Alan Inglis SMITH

Newington Surgery
14 East Preston Street, Edinburgh EH8 9QA
Tel: 0131 662 4400 Fax: 0131 662 4400
(NHS Lothian, Primary and Community Division)
Patient List Size: 3500

Practice Manager Michelle Scott

GP John Douglas McCALLUM, Liliana LAIRD

Parkgrove Terrace Surgery
22B Parkgrove Terrace, Edinburgh EH4 7NX
Tel: 0131 312 6600 Fax: 0131 312 7798
(NHS Lothian, Primary and Community Division)

Practice Manager C Crookes

GP Anne CURTIS, Lisa CARTER, David Paul CROOKES, Adrian Kenneth CULLEN, Rose Elizabeth Brown HAINING

Polwarth Surgery
72 Polwarth Gardens, Edinburgh EH11 1LL
Tel: 0131 229 5914 Fax: 0131 221 9897
(NHS Lothian, Primary and Community Division)
Patient List Size: 4740

Practice Manager Linda Blackmoore

GP Alexander McCallum MILLAR, Rosemary DIXON, Catherine GATES, Kenneth KNOX, Thomasin MACKIE

Restalrig Park Medical Centre
40 Alemoor Crescent, Edinburgh EH7 6UJ
Tel: 0131 554 2141 Fax: 0131 554 5363
(NHS Lothian, Primary and Community Division)
Patient List Size: 6600

GP Michael Patrick BYRNE, Geoffrey Arthur DOBSON, Jane MARSHALL, Helen I RICHES, Richard John WILLIAMS

Rose Garden Medical Centre
4 Mill Lane, Edinburgh EH6 6TL
Tel: 0131 554 1274 Fax: 0131 555 2159
Email: monoh.markens:lothian.scot.nhs.uk
(NHS Lothian, Primary and Community Division)

Patient List Size: 6500

Practice Manager Marion Martens

GP Ian Ronald Francis ROSS, Jennifer BENNISON, Ian Innes McKAY, Ewen Andrew STEWART, Celia Margaret TEMPLE

Sighthill Health Centre
380 Calder Road, Edinburgh EH11 4AU
Tel: 0131 537 7090 Fax: 0131 537 7005
(NHS Lothian, Primary and Community Division)
Patient List Size: 7500

Practice Manager Elayne Gilmartin

GP Gordon James Clelland SCOTT, Keith Johnson BLAIKIE, C B NICKERSON, N J RENNIE, Charlotte Dorothy WILDGOOSE

Sighthill Health Centre
380 Calder Road, Edinburgh EH11 4AU
Tel: 0131 537 7030 Fax: 0131 537 7005
(NHS Lothian, Primary and Community Division)
Patient List Size: 1700

Practice Manager Lorna Rosie

GP Guy Andrew JOHNSON, Helga REIN

Slateford Road Surgery
79 Slateford Road, Edinburgh EH11 1QW
Tel: 0131 313 2211 Fax: 0131 313 1667
(NHS Lothian, Primary and Community Division)
Patient List Size: 7500

Practice Manager Jacky Pitcairn

GP Alfred Edward Paul CHADWICK, Geraldine DENNIS, A J HOLLOWAY, Jill Sheelagh Maureen TIDMAN, F WELLS

Southern Medical Group
322 Gilmerton Road, Edinburgh EH17 7PR
Tel: 0131 664 2148 Fax: 0131 664 8303
(NHS Lothian, Primary and Community Division)

GP Howard Stanton MORLEY, Alexander Stuart BLAIR, Alexander Donald McKAIN, Dawn Margaret TAYLOR

Southfield Surgery
132 Mountcastle Drive South, Edinburgh EH15 3LL
Tel: 0131 669 0686
(NHS Lothian, Primary and Community Division)
Patient List Size: 3800

GP Malcolm Macleod MORRISON, Stuart J BLAKE, Sylvia Victoria MERINO LLORENS

Southside Surgery
17 Bernard Terrace, Edinburgh EH8 9NU
Tel: 0131 667 2240 Fax: 0131 662 1633
(NHS Lothian, Primary and Community Division)
Patient List Size: 5500

GP Alexander PATERSON, Penny REID, Alyson REIVE, Eileen Patricia SANDERSON

Springwell Medical Practice
24 Ardmillan Terrace, Edinburgh EH11 2JL
Tel: 0131 537 7500 Fax: 0131 537 7505
(NHS Lothian, Primary and Community Division)
Patient List Size: 8500

GP Archie BALLANTYNE, R Ian DICKSON, Ruth LIDDLE

St Leonard's Medical Centre
145 Pleasance, Edinburgh EH8 9RU
Tel: 0131 668 4547 Fax: 0131 667 5092
(NHS Lothian, Primary and Community Division)

Practice Manager Anne Ritchie

GP Ian BURNS-BROWN, Louise ILIFFE, David John McKIRDY

St Triduana's Medical Practice
54 Moira Park, Edinburgh EH7 6RU
Tel: 0131 657 3341 Fax: 0131 669 6055
(NHS Lothian, Primary and Community Division)
Patient List Size: 10200

Practice Manager Susan Sewell

GP Michael William WHITLEY, Hannah Mary Bernadette CRONIN, John Angus McVicar GARNER, Mairi Margaret MACARTNEY, Andrew R MACKAY, Gerald Maurice McPARTLIN, Aman Deep SINGH

Stockbridge Health Centre
1 India Place, Edinburgh EH3 6EH
Tel: 0131 225 9191 Fax: 0131 226 6549
(NHS Lothian, Primary and Community Division)

GP Peter Nigel Esmond BERREY, John Anderson McLAREN, Edith Fiona NICOL, James Barry PARKER, Alison Joan Cumming RODGERS, Janet Marion SAYERS

Summerside Medical Centre
29B Summerside Place, Edinburgh EH6 4NY
Tel: 0131 554 3533 Fax: 0131 554 9722
(NHS Lothian, Primary and Community Division)

Practice Manager Jill Calder

GP Gary McGREGOR, Wendy Teresa EDMUNDS, John Raymond KIRKUP, Hannah Mary ROYLE

The Surgery
651 Ferry Road, Edinburgh EH4 2TX
Tel: 0161 332 6130 Fax: 0161 332 6130
(NHS Lothian, Primary and Community Division)

GP Balkishan AGRAWAL

University Health Service
University of Edinburgh, Richard Verney Health Centre, 6 Bristo Square, Edinburgh EH8 9AL
Tel: 0131 650 2777 Fax: 0131 662 1813
Email: health.service@ed.ac.uk
(NHS Lothian, Primary and Community Division)
Patient List Size: 24000

Practice Manager Val Dunn

GP Nadine HARRISON, Timothy Simon BROWN, William Ross DONOVAN, Norma KING, William David McGRATH, Graeme Robert MILLIGAN, Judith Mary RICHARDSON, Sharon Moiran Midgley YOUNG

West End Medical Practice
21 Chester Street, Edinburgh EH3 7RF
Tel: 0131 225 5220 Fax: 0131 226 1910
(NHS Lothian, Primary and Community Division)

GP Peter Gardner WHITE, Thomas HEPBURN, Kirsten Lesley MACDONALD, Dean Granville POPE, John Frederick Gunn ROSS, Margaret Helen. STANSFIELD

Whinpark Medical Centre
6 Saughton Road, Edinburgh EH11 3RA
Tel: 0131 455 7999 Fax: 0131 455 8800
(NHS Lothian, Primary and Community Division)

Practice Manager Hilary Scott

GP Donald Henderson DOULL, John Richard CRISPIN, Alison Jean Catherine HUNTER, Alan Gordon Henry MACPHERSON, Robert Crawford MARCHANT WINK, Sharon Joy McHALE, Lyndsey Morag MYSKOW, Norman Walker WALLACE

Elgin

Elgin Community Surgery
Highfield House, Northfield Terrace, Elgin IV30 1NE
Tel: 01343 542234 Fax: 01343 562101
Email: administrator@elgincs.grampian.scot.nhs.uk
(NHS Grampian, Primary Care Division)
Patient List Size: 3125

Practice Manager Fiona Houliston

GP Mark David HOULISTON, Denise Elaine McFARLANE

Elgin Medical Centre
10 Victoria Crescent, Elgin IV30 1RQ
Tel: 01343 547512 Fax: 01343 546781
(NHS Grampian, Primary Care Division)
Patient List Size: 11500

Practice Manager Gillian Jacques, Iain Sinclair

GP William Macaskill MORRISON, Donald Farquhar BROWN, Rachel Jane LOWE, Alex McCLURE, David Robert MICKEL, Robin Lochrie PEARSON, John Trevor WILSON

Maryhill Practice
Elgin Health Centre, Maryhill, Elgin IV30 1AT
Tel: 01343 543788 Fax: 01343 551604
Email: administrator@elginhc.grampian.scot.nhs.uk
(NHS Grampian, Primary Care Division)
Patient List Size: 14590

Practice Manager Anna Cunningham, Eileen Rae

GP Jacquelyn Mary MOBBS, Elizabeth Malcolm ALBISTON, Charles Alistair HORNSBY, Andrew McPHERSON, John William NICOL, Ronald Dawson Miller STEWART, Graham Roy TAYLOR

Ellon

Ellon Group Practice
Health Centre, Schoolhill, Ellon AB41 9JH
Tel: 01358 720333 Fax: 01358 721578
(NHS Grampian, Primary Care Division)

Practice Manager Caroline Cumming

GP Rosamund Mary Routledge BELL, Peter James BROWN, Alan Eunson DONALDSON, H KAM, Donald Ian MACKAY, Duncan James McKERCHAR, Pilar Anne MURPHY, Martin John PUCCI, Ian Taylor SIMPSON

The Old School Surgery
The Old School, The Square, Tarves, Ellon AB41 7GX
Tel: 01651 851777 Fax: 01651 852090
(NHS Grampian, Primary Care Division)
Patient List Size: 4300

Practice Manager V Tanner

GP Helen Janet STEPHEN, Roy James BURNETT, Donna EVANS, Fiona MUNRO, Marion TAYLOR

Erskine

Bridgewater Medical Centre
Bridgewater Shopping Centre, Erskine PA8 7AA
Tel: 0141 812 2022 Fax: 0141 812 2023
(NHS Argyll and Clyde, Renfrewshire and Inverclyde Community Services Division)
Patient List Size: 2600

Practice Manager Mary Pitman

GP Jacob Kwadwo AFUAKWAH, Amarjit Singh NIJJAR

Erskine Health Centre
Barrgarran, Erskine PA8 6BS
Tel: 0141 812 4044/4422 Fax: 0141 812 3053
(NHS Argyll and Clyde, Renfrewshire and Inverclyde Community Services Division)
Patient List Size: 4300

Practice Manager Diane Stuart

GP D GRIFFITH, P.M. ASBURY, A J STOUT

Mains Medical Centre
300 Mains Drive, Park Mains, Erskine PA8 7JQ
Tel: 0141 812 3230 Fax: 0141 812 5226
(NHS Argyll and Clyde, Renfrewshire and Inverclyde Community Services Division)

GP Winifred TABONY, Tracey HANLEY, Murray MACPHERSON, William MURRAY, Janet WILLS

Eyemouth

Eyemouth Medical Practice
Houndlaw Park, Eyemouth TD14 5DD
Tel: 01890 750383 Fax: 01890 751749
(NHS Borders, Primary Care Division)
Patient List Size: 6100

Practice Manager Gitte Blackley

GP Ishbel Margaret DORWARD, John Alexander DORWARD, Michael Alexander FENTY, Charles HOLT, Alan Peter MASON

Falkirk

Ark Medical Practice
9 Booth Place, Falkirk FK1 1BA
Tel: 01324 621113 Fax: 01324 633456
(NHS Forth Valley, Primary Care Operating Division)
Patient List Size: 1820

Practice Manager K Ure

GP Satnam Singh ARK

Camelon Medical Practice
3 Baird Street, Camelon, Falkirk FK1 4PP
Tel: 01324 622854 Fax: 01324 633858
(NHS Forth Valley, Primary Care Operating Division)

GP Thomas William NIMMO, Kirsten Anne GLEN, Heather Alison HAYWOOD, Paul Chong-Kui LIM, J Kenneth NELSON, Ruth ROGERSON

Carron Medical Centre
Ronades Road, Bainsford, Falkirk FK2 7TA
Tel: 01324 619940 Fax: 01324 619941
Email: manager@carronmc.freeserve.co.uk
(NHS Forth Valley, Primary Care Operating Division)
Patient List Size: 2030

Practice Manager Caroline Buchanan

GP Gordon MUIRCROFT

Graeme Medical Centre
1 Western Avenue, Falkirk FK2 7HR
Tel: 01324 624437 Fax: 01324 633737
(NHS Forth Valley, Primary Care Operating Division)

GP Gavin James HICKFORD, Carolyn Margaret McNEILL, Brian Malcolm MERRICK, Susan May WALDRON

Meadowbank Health Centre
3 Salmon Inn Road, Polmont, Falkirk FK2 0XF
Tel: 01324 715540 Fax: 01324 716723
(NHS Forth Valley, Primary Care Operating Division)
Patient List Size: 6927

Practice Manager Lorna Brown

GP Howard Greig BROWN, Elizabeth BROWN, Angela ROBERTSON, William Graham WHITE

Meadowbank Health Centre
3 Salmon Inn Road, Falkirk FK2 0XF
Tel: 01324 715446 Fax: 01324 717986
(NHS Forth Valley, Primary Care Operating Division)

GP Ian HUNTER, Keith ORR, Ronnie SYDNEY, Robert Cunningham Glen THOMSON, Catherine Anne WHITELAW

Meadowbank Health Centre
3 Salmon Inn Road, Falkirk FK2 0XF
Tel: 01324 715753 Fax: 01324 717565
(NHS Forth Valley, Primary Care Operating Division)

GP Susan Anne MIDDLEMISS, Charles Keith OGILVIE, Stewart Thomas OLIVER, Keith Matthew ORR

Meadowbank Health Centre
3 Salmon Inn Road, Polmont, Falkirk FK2 0XF
Tel: 01324 722454 Fax: 01324 722458
(NHS Forth Valley, Primary Care Operating Division)

Patient List Size: 1850

GP Stephen BROWN, Suzanne WOOD

Meeks Road Surgery
10 Meeks Road, Falkirk FK2 7ES
Tel: 01324 619930 Fax: 01324 627266
(NHS Forth Valley, Primary Care Operating Division)
Patient List Size: 11700

Practice Manager P Wisdom

GP Gillian NICOL, James Douglas STEWART, James AULD, Colin BARTH, Patricia Lesley DUNCAN, Alastair Charles McCALL

Park Street Surgery
6 Park Street, Falkirk FK1 1RE
Tel: 01324 623577 Fax: 01324 633636
(NHS Forth Valley, Primary Care Operating Division)

GP George Philip EDWARDS, James BOYD, Teresa H CANNAVINA

The Surgery
Bank Street, Slamannan, Falkirk FK1 3EZ
Tel: 01324 851288 Fax: 01324 851622
(NHS Forth Valley, Primary Care Operating Division)
Patient List Size: 1800

Practice Manager Nicola Jayne McIntyre

GP John Hugh Stephen AINSWORTH, Suzanne WOOD

The Wallace Medical Centre
254 Thornhill Road, Falkirk FK2 7AZ
Tel: 01324 622826 Fax: 01324 633447
(NHS Forth Valley, Primary Care Operating Division)
Patient List Size: 7780

Practice Manager Linda Murhead

GP Warren Munro LUKE, Andrew Michael CROWE, John Dalton LEONARD, Mary Margaret PEDDIE

Fochabers

Medical Centre
12 High Street, Fochabers IV32 7EP
Tel: 01343 820247 Fax: 01343 820132
Email: administrator@fochabers.grampian.scot.nhs.uk
(NHS Grampian, Primary Care Division)
Patient List Size: 4295

GP Janis TAIT, Edwin BORROWMAN, Angus SIM

Forfar

Green Street Surgery
Green Street, Forfar DD8 3AR
Tel: 01307 462316 Fax: 01307 463623
Email: administrator@greenst.finix.org
(NHS Tayside, Primary Care Division)
Patient List Size: 10300

Practice Manager E Markowski

GP Alexander John Anthony MACDONALD, Douglas Peebles BURT, Finlay John Matheson Macdonald DAVIES, Kay Storm MacCALLUM, Robert William Elliot MELLISH, Ann Helen Margaret MORRIS, Caroline Frances Louise THOMAS

Lour Road Group Practice
3 Lour Road, Forfar DD8 2AS
Tel: 01307 463122 Fax: 01307 465278
Email: administrator@lour.finix.org.uk
(NHS Tayside, Primary Care Division)
Patient List Size: 5800

Practice Manager Lorna Batchelor, Catriona Milne

GP William Thomas Malcolm SMITH, Peter Reid DICK, Jon S DOWELL, Jonathan M D FAGERSON, Abigail A PATERSON

Ravenswood Surgery
New Road, Forfar DD8 2AE
Tel: 01307 463558 Fax: 01307 468900
(NHS Tayside, Primary Care Division)
Patient List Size: 3200

GP Guy Campbell WOODROFFE, Nico GRUNEBERG

Forres

Castlehill Health Centre
Castlehill, Forres IV36 1QF
Tel: 01309 672221 Fax: 01309 678870
(NHS Grampian, Primary Care Division)
Patient List Size: 7716

GP David Thomas SNEDDON, James Q G T HOGG, Peter Anthony KELLY, Richard Johnston KENNEDY, Margaret Ann NELSON, Alan Sinclair THOMSON

Castlehill Health Centre
Castlehill, Forres IV36 1QF
Tel: 01309 672233
(NHS Grampian, Primary Care Division)

Practice Manager Mary Dingwall

GP James Adam ANDERSON, Graeme GOVAN, Louise Kathryn Mackay ROY, David STEVENSON, Simon James WILLETTS

Fort Augustus

Cill Chuimein Medical Centre
Fort Augustus PH32 4BH
Tel: 01320 366216 Fax: 01320 366649
(NHS Highland, Primary Care)

GP Iain David FARMER, J SKEOCH

Fort William

Craig Nevis Surgery
Belford Road, Fort William PH33 6BU
Tel: 01397 702947 Fax: 01397 700655
Email: administrator@gp55605.highland-hb.scot.nhs.uk
(NHS Highland, Primary Care)
Patient List Size: 3560

Practice Manager Irene Burns

GP Michael Ewen MacDonald FOXLEY, Elizabeth Charlotte MACDONALD, John SHIRLEY, Alison Duff SMITH, Mike WOODBRIDGE

High Street Surgery
99 High Street, Fort William PH33 6DG
Tel: 01397 703773 Fax: 01397 701068
Email: highst@lochaber.almac.co.uk
(NHS Highland, Primary Care)
Patient List Size: 4700

Practice Manager Ena Hutchison

GP Christopher ROBINSON, Elisabeth Catriona MERRY, Hiresh Lal ROY, David Joseph TANGNEY

Tweeddale Medical Practice
High Street, Fort William PH33 6EU
Tel: 01397 703136 Fax: 01397 700139
Email: admin@tweeddale.com
Website: www.tweeddale.com
(NHS Highland, Primary Care)
Patient List Size: 5200

Practice Manager Joan MacLennan

GP James David MacDonald DOUGLAS, Neil ARNOTT, Alan MASSIE, Craig Andrew McARTHUR, Dorothy Jane MUNRO

Fortrose

Fortrose Medical Practice
Station Road, Fortrose IV10 8SY
Tel: 01381 620909 Fax: 01381 620505
Email: administrator@gp55381.highland-hb.scot.nhs.uk
(NHS Highland, Primary Care)
Patient List Size: 5000

Practice Manager Mary P Perrins

GP Alexander MacNaught MACGREGOR, Uilleam Somerled FRASER, David Edward GASKELL

Fraserburgh

Central Buchan Medical Group
The Surgery, School Street, New Pitsligo, Fraserburgh AB43 6NE
Tel: 01771 653205 Fax: 01771 653294
(NHS Grampian, Primary Care Division)

GP Andrew George Colin ROBERTSON, Sylvia Margaret GREIG, Gavin Bruce PACKHAM

Crimond Medical Centre
Crimond, Fraserburgh AB43 8QJ
Tel: 01346 532215 Fax: 01346 531808
Email: administrator@crimond.grampian.scot.nhs.uk
(NHS Grampian, Primary Care Division)
Patient List Size: 2900

Practice Manager Ada Brown

GP John Fraser KINNON, Helen GAULD, Robert Samuel Miller MURRAY

Finlayson Street Practice
33 Finlayson Street, Fraserburgh AB43 9JW
Tel: 01346 518088 Fax: 01346 510015
(NHS Grampian, Primary Care Division)

Practice Manager K Robertson

GP Alexander Barclay WISLEY, Alan Gordon BEATTIE, Dawn Mary TWEEDIE, Andrew Niall WATT

Saltoun Surgery
Lochpots Road, Fraserburgh AB43 9NH
Tel: 01346 514154 Fax: 01346 585228
Email: administrator@saltoun.grampian.scot.nhs.uk
(NHS Grampian, Primary Care Division)
Patient List Size: 8600

Practice Manager Ian M Alexander

GP William Murray STEELE, Michael James William DICK, Robert DUTHIE, Francesca Victoria Anne LEE-MASON, Helen TOBIN

Gairloch

Aultbea and Gairloch Medical Practice
The Health Centre, Auchtercairn, Gairloch IV21 2BP
Tel: 01445 712229 Fax: 01445 712092
Email: administrator@gp55357.highland-hb.scot.nhs.uk
(NHS Highland, Primary Care)
Patient List Size: 2200

Practice Manager Andrew Vickerstaff

GP Allan Logie MARSHALL, Gerard Philip BAPTIST, Grahame Alistair MITCHELL, Kirsty Moraich VICKERSTAFF

Galashiels

Currie Road Health Centre
Currie Road, Galashiels TD1 2UA
Tel: 01896 661350 Fax: 01896 661357
(NHS Borders, Primary Care Division)
Patient List Size: 4700

Practice Manager Norman Kellett

GP Malcolm Kerr LINDSAY, Gillian Mary ARBUCKLE, Fiona Roselynne Catriona MEGAHY, Robert SOUTTER

Currie Road Health Centre
Currie Road, Galashiels TD1 2UA
Tel: 01896 661355 Fax: 01896 661357
(NHS Borders, Primary Care Division)
Patient List Size: 3173

Practice Manager Mary Cockburn

GP David John OWEN, Anne V JOHNSTONE, Robert Reekie SMITH

Currie Road Health Centre
Currie Road, Galashiels TD1 2UA
Tel: 01896 752419 Fax: 01896 753876
(NHS Borders, Primary Care Division)

Practice Manager Aileen Anderson

GP Robert Lockhart JOHNSTON, Patricia Mary CRAMOND, Judith Rosemary JOHNSTON, Paul D JORDAN

Roxburgh Street Surgery
10 Roxburgh Street, Galashiels TD1 1PF
Tel: 01896 752557 Fax: 01896 755374
(NHS Borders, Primary Care Division)

Practice Manager George Ainslie

GP Dorothy AINSLIE, Richard John LEAVER, Alistair Kenneth John WRIGHT

Galston

Galston Medical Practice
5A Henrietta Street, Galston KA4 8HW
Tel: 01563 820424 Fax: 01563 822380
(NHS Ayrshire and Arran, Community Health Division)
Patient List Size: 6500

Practice Manager Graham Dobbie

GP James Stein McCALL, Gillian Catherine COLLISTER, James Wyllie McWHIRTER, William Sim NICOLL, Dawn Anne TAYLOR

Girvan

Back Road Surgery
7 Back Road, Dailly, Girvan KA26 9SH
Tel: 01465 811224 Fax: 01465 811518
(NHS Ayrshire and Arran, Community Health Division)

GP Edmund Paul McFADYEN, Thomas MALLOCH

Ballantrae Medical Practice
30 Main Street, Ballantrae, Girvan KA26 0NB
Tel: 01465 831302 Fax: 01465 831583
Email: hal.maxwell@aapct.scot.nhs.uk
(NHS Ayrshire and Arran, Community Health Division)
Patient List Size: 1485

Practice Manager Julie Callan

GP Haldane Lindsay MAXWELL, Kathleen SLOAN

Drs Barr, Anderson and McCulloch
Henrietta Street, Girvan KA26 9AN
Tel: 01465 712281 Fax: 01465 712187
(NHS Ayrshire and Arran, Community Health Division)
Patient List Size: 4300

Practice Manager Anne Bush

GP Gavin William BARR, David Gavin ANDERSON, T Scott McCULLOCH

Drs McMaster, Moore and Brooksbank
109A Henrietta Street, Girvan KA26 9AN
Tel: 01465 713343 Fax: 01465 714591
(NHS Ayrshire and Arran, Community Health Division)

Practice Manager Lynne Browne

GP Bruce W McMASTER, Kenneth L BROOKSBANK, Catherine Dawn MOORE

Glasgow

Aberfeldy Street Surgery
12 Aberfeldy Street, Glasgow G31 3NW
Tel: 0141 554 8054 Fax: 0141 554 2638
(NHS Greater Glasgow, Primary Care Division)
Patient List Size: 2200

Practice Manager K Cupplies

GP Leslie Forrester CUPPLES

Abronhill Health Centre
Pine Road, Cumbernauld, Glasgow G67 3BE
Tel: 01236 723223 Fax: 01236 781426
(NHS Lanarkshire, Primary Care Division)

GP Jugal Kishore ALLAHABADIA, John Steven TWADDLE

Abronhill Health Centre
Pine Road, Cumbernauld, Glasgow G67 3BE
Tel: 01236 727654
(NHS Lanarkshire, Primary Care Division)

GP Denis Joseph CLIFFORD

Alison Lea Medical Centre
Calderwood, East Kilbride, Glasgow G74 3BE
Tel: 01355 261666
(NHS Lanarkshire, Primary Care Division)

GP John Andrew Francis HAUGHNEY, Helen McNEIL

Alison Lea Medical Centre
Calderwood, East Kilbride, Glasgow G74 3BE
Tel: 01355 227220 Fax: 01355 276664
(NHS Lanarkshire, Primary Care Division)
Patient List Size: 3400

Practice Manager Lynne McKechnie, Anne Noble

GP Archana ALLAHABADIA, Linda Catherine McKERLIE, Anne Marie MEGGS, James William Simon WALKER

Alison Lea Medical Centre
Calderwood, East Kilbride, Glasgow G74 3BE
Tel: 01355 236444 Fax: 01355 239711
Website: www.alisonlea.co.uk
(NHS Lanarkshire, Primary Care Division)
Patient List Size: 5100

Practice Manager Karen Morrison

GP Astrid BENNETT, Ian McGregor CHISHOLM, Gabrielle Agnes GALLAGHER, Karen Moore GEDDES

Allander Street Surgery
124 Allander Street, Glasgow G22 5JH
Tel: 0141 336 8038 Fax: 0141 336 3440
(NHS Greater Glasgow, Primary Care Division)

GP Linda CHERRY, Margaret Barbour CRAIG, Alastair Macdonald DOUGLAS, Susan McKEAN

Allison and Partners
Maryhill Health Centre, 41 Shawpark Street, Glasgow G20 9DR
Tel: 0141 531 8840 Fax: 0141 531 8848
Email: administrator@g43011-glasgow-hb.scot.nhs.uk
(NHS Greater Glasgow, Primary Care Division)
Patient List Size: 6500

Practice Manager Lynn Baird

GP Andrew George ALLISON, Hugh Alexander CAMERON, Alison Catherine Ethel GARVIE, Wendy Jane LEEPER, John Anderson MACLEAN

Annfield Medical Centre
16 Annfield Place, Glasgow G31 2XE
Tel: 0141 554 2989 Fax: 0141 550 3965
(NHS Greater Glasgow, Primary Care Division)

GP Bruce Yew Wai TANG, Wendy Jane LEEPER

Anniesland Medical Practice
778 Crow Road, Glasgow G13 1LU
Tel: 0141 954 8860 Fax: 0141 954 0870
(NHS Greater Glasgow, Primary Care Division)

Practice Manager Lesley Cameron

GP David Logan BLAIR, Jane Love CAMPBELL, Helen Mary IRVINE, Janet Jennifer LEITCH

Apsley Street Surgery
14 Apsley Street, Glasgow G11 7SY
Tel: 0141 339 2960 Fax: 0141 334 6377
(NHS Greater Glasgow, Primary Care Division)

Practice Manager Janis McKenzie

GP David GAFFNEY, Alison Cameron McALPINE, John RAESIDE

Arden Medical Centre
74 Kyleakin Road, Arden, Glasgow G46 8DH
Tel: 0141 638 1464
Email: office@gp52147.glasgow-hb.scot.nhs.uk
(NHS Greater Glasgow, Primary Care Division)

Practice Manager Stephanie McKinnon

GP Raheela BHATTI

Ardoch Medical Centre
6 Ardoch Grove, Cambuslang, Glasgow G72 8HA
Tel: 0141 641 1255 Fax: 0141 646 1988
Email: administrator@g49657.glasgow-hb.scot.nhs.uk
(NHS Greater Glasgow, Primary Care Division)

Practice Manager Rosina Dunlop

GP Anoop Kumar GAJREE

Ardoch Medical Centre
6 Ardoch Grove, Cambuslang, Glasgow G72 8HA
Tel: 0141 641 3827
(NHS Greater Glasgow, Primary Care Division)
Patient List Size: 1600

GP Clare Marie McCANN

Ardoch Medical Centre
6 Ardoch Grove, Cambuslang, Glasgow G72 8HA
Tel: 0141 641 3729 Fax: 0141 641 4339
(NHS Greater Glasgow, Primary Care Division)

Practice Manager Margaret Anderson

GP Kamal Mohan OHRI, Chandrika K OHRI

Argyle Street Surgery
1119 Argyle Street, Glasgow G3 8ND
Tel: 0141 248 3698 Fax: 0141 221 5144
Email: administrator@gp40455.glasgow-hb.scot.nhs.uk
(NHS Greater Glasgow, Primary Care Division)

Practice Manager Janice Muirhead

GP Christine McCallum CRAWFORD, Alison Anne LAWSON, Dugald Roderick MacNEILL

Arran Surgery
40 Admiral Street, Glasgow G41 1HU
Tel: 0141 429 2626 Fax: 0141 429 2331
Email: administrator@gp52128.glasgow.hb.scot.nhs.uk
(NHS Greater Glasgow, Primary Care Division)
Patient List Size: 11000

Practice Manager Helen Ormiston

GP William Martin DOAK, Seonaid Anne CHIAH, Robert James FERGUSON, Douglas William McKNIGHT, Alan James MILLAR, Elaine Marjory ROXBY, Jennifer Mary SHARP, Frances Ann SWAN

Ashfield House Surgery
Ashfield House, 1 Ashfield Road, Milngavie, Glasgow G62 6BT
Tel: 0141 956 1339 Fax: 0141 956 7098
(NHS Greater Glasgow, Primary Care Division)
Patient List Size: 7752

Practice Manager Annerine Glen

GP Vincent CUDDIHY, Marjorie Ann FRASER, Lynette HARKINS, William R LIVINGSTONE, John Murchison LOVETT

Auchinairn Road Surgery
127/129 Auchinairn Road, Bishopbriggs, Glasgow G64 1NF
Tel: 0141 772 1808 Fax: 0141 762 1274
(NHS Greater Glasgow, Primary Care Division)
Patient List Size: 6600

Practice Manager Myra Liddle

GP Maher MANSOURI, Rhona RAEBURN, Raymund John WHITE, Christine Shearer WILSON

Baillieston Health Centre
20 Muirside Road, Baillieston, Glasgow G69 7AD
Tel: 0141 531 8040
(NHS Greater Glasgow, Primary Care Division)

GP Carolyn Brown CALDER, Alastair Cant HARPER, Alan D M MACKINNON, Alison Margaret TOUGH

Baillieston Health Centre
20 Muirside Road, Baillieston, Glasgow G69 7AD
Tel: 0141 531 8050 Fax: 0141 531 8067
(NHS Greater Glasgow, Primary Care Division)

Practice Manager Anne Gorman, Anne Taylor

GP Jennifer Sandra Margaret DOW, June GOLDIE, Charles E LANGAN, John J LANGAN, Moira Catherine Mary MACLEOD, Michelle Carmel McGLONE, Gerard Arthur McKAIG, Margaret Philomena McKENNA, Elaine Elizabeth POLLOCK

Baker Street Surgery
9 Baker Street, Glasgow G41 3YA
Tel: 0141 632 4962 Fax: 0141 636 6651
Email: administrator@gp49318.glasgow-hb.scot.nhs.uk
(NHS Greater Glasgow, Primary Care Division)

Practice Manager Jean Stuart

GP Roderick John MACLEOD

Balmore Road Surgery
138-142 Balmore Road, Glasgow G22 6LJ
Tel: 0141 531 9393 Fax: 0141 531 9389
Email: balmorsur@hotmail.com
(NHS Greater Glasgow, Primary Care Division)

Practice Manager Roseleen McKenzie

GP Allison Anna REID, Anne CONNELL, Lynsay CRAWFORD

Barnes and Graham
230 Dalmellington Road, Glasgow G53 7FY
Tel: 0141 883 8887 Fax: 0141 891 4400
(NHS Greater Glasgow, Primary Care Division)
Patient List Size: 4589

Practice Manager E Don

GP Dr BARNES, Dr GRAHAM, S FORD, J Shakur SALARIED

Barrhead Health Centre
201 Main Street, Barrhead, Glasgow G78 1SD
Tel: 0141 880 6161
(NHS Argyll and Clyde, Renfrewshire and Inverclyde Community Services Division)

GP M B MITCHELL, Charles O'DONOGHUE

Barrhead Health Centre
201 Main Street, Barrhead, Glasgow G78 1SA
Tel: 0141 880 6161 Fax: 0141 881 5636
(NHS Argyll and Clyde, Renfrewshire and Inverclyde Community Services Division)

GP Martin DOWNEY, Wilma GEMMELL, James MACRITCHIE, Matthew McALEER, Anne ROBERTSON, David WONG

Barrhead Health Centre
201 Main Street, Barrhead, Glasgow G78 1SA
Tel: 0141 880 6161 Fax: 0141 881 7636
(NHS Argyll and Clyde, Renfrewshire and Inverclyde Community Services Division)

GP Charles O'DONOGHUE, Mary MITCHELL

Bath Street Surgery
196 Bath Street, Glasgow G2 4HH
Tel: 0141 227 6767 Fax: 0141 227 6920
(NHS Greater Glasgow, Primary Care Division)

GP Patricia Agnes FITZSIMONS

Battlefield Road Surgery
148 Battlefield Road, Glasgow G42 9JT
Tel: 0141 632 6310 Fax: 0141 636 1180
(NHS Greater Glasgow, Primary Care Division)
Patient List Size: 4200

Practice Manager Gillian J Duffy

GP Lynn JACOBS, Carl McGIVERN, Philip Michael John WILSON

Battlefield Road Surgery
208 Battlefield Road, Glasgow G42 9HN
Tel: 0141 649 5878 Fax: 0141 636 6690
(NHS Greater Glasgow, Primary Care Division)

Practice Manager Pamela Jauhar

GP Virinder Kumar MADHOK

Blackwoods Medical Centre
8 Station Road, Muirhead, Glasgow G69 9EG
Tel: 0141 779 2228 Fax: 0141 779 3225
(NHS Greater Glasgow, Primary Care Division)
Patient List Size: 10800

Practice Manager Maureen Whelehan

GP James PENDER, Mary Teresa EASSON, David George JAMIESON, Kenneth Milroy LEE, Heidi PARKINSON, Indira Yashvant POLE, Angela Mary STURROCK

Blantyre Health Centre
64 Victoria Street, Blantyre, Glasgow G72 0BS
Tel: 01698 823260
(NHS Lanarkshire, Primary Care Division)

Practice Manager M McLean

GP Norman Edward SUCKLE, Satya R CHAKRABARTI, C GILCHRIST, Janis Marie JAMES

Blantyre Health Centre
Victoria Street, Blantyre, Glasgow G72 0BS
Tel: 01698 828868 Fax: 01698 823678
(NHS Lanarkshire, Primary Care Division)

GP Graeme Paul BINGHAM, Philip COTTON, Rosalie Therese DUNN, Mary Josephine SOMMERVILLE

Blantyre Health Centre
64 Victoria Street, Blantyre, Glasgow G72 0BS
Tel: 01698 826331
(NHS Lanarkshire, Primary Care Division)

GP Mary Veronica CHURCH, Iain Andrew Peter GROM, Lesley Gladys UNWIN

Bothwell Medical Centre
3 Uddingston Road, Bothwell, Glasgow G71 8ET
Tel: 01698 852299 Fax: 01698 854283
(NHS Lanarkshire, Primary Care Division)
Patient List Size: 10050

Practice Manager Marion Watt

GP Margaret Cynthia D'SILVA, Roy D'SILVA, Marie R McDOUGALL, John David McGARRITY, Gerard Anthony MURPHY

Braidcraft Medical Centre
200 Braidcraft Road, Glasgow G53 5QD
Tel: 0141 882 3396 Fax: 0141 883 3224
Email: administrator@gp52043.glasgow-hb.scot.nhs.uk
(NHS Greater Glasgow, Primary Care Division)
Patient List Size: 7600

Practice Manager Elaine Wilson

GP Robina HENDERSON, Jouda Singh JHEETA, Alan Anderson McARTHUR, Leslie Helen Ferguson RUSSELL, Graham Tweedie WHITHAM

Bridgeton Health Centre

201 Abercromby Street, Glasgow G40 2DA
Tel: 0141 550 3822
(NHS Greater Glasgow, Primary Care Division)
Patient List Size: 2300

Practice Manager Margaret Tarbert

GP Kevin Joseph CONNAUGHTON, Elaine Margaret McLELLAN

Bridgeton Health Centre

201 Abercromby Street, Glasgow G40 2DA
Tel: 0141 531 6500 Fax: 0141 531 6505
(NHS Greater Glasgow, Primary Care Division)

GP Mohammed Pervaiz HAMAYUN

Bridgeton Health Centre

201 Abercromby Street, Glasgow G40 2DA
Tel: 0141 531 6600 Fax: 0141 531 6616
(NHS Greater Glasgow, Primary Care Division)
Patient List Size: 2160

Practice Manager S Goold

GP Robert Ross JAMIESON

Bridgeton Health Centre

201 Abercromby Street, Glasgow G40 2DA
Tel: 0141 531 6670 Fax: 0141 531 6505
(NHS Greater Glasgow, Primary Care Division)

Practice Manager Rosemary McNulty

GP Pierre TSANG

Bridgeton Health Centre

210 Abercromby Street, Glasgow G40 2DA
Tel: 0141 531 6630 Fax: 0141 531 6626
(NHS Greater Glasgow, Primary Care Division)

Practice Manager Beth Mail

GP Leonard Alan ROSENGARD, Angela Mary Elizabeth DINGWALL, Anne Marie MAGUIRE

Bridgeton Health Centre

210 Abercromby Street, Glasgow G40 2DA
Tel: 0141 531 6650 Fax: 0141 531 6639
(NHS Greater Glasgow, Primary Care Division)
Patient List Size: 3200

Practice Manager Kath McNeil

GP John James DUNN, Gerard John LYNAS

Bridgeton Health Centre

201 Abercromby Street, Glasgow G40 2DA
Tel: 0141 531 6500 Fax: 0141 531 6505
(NHS Greater Glasgow, Primary Care Division)
Patient List Size: 3400

Practice Manager Kath McNeil

GP Ashis K BANERJEE, Pinaki GHOSH

Broomhill Practice

41 Broomhill Drive, Glasgow G11 7AD
Tel: 0141 339 3626 Fax: 0141 334 2399
Email: administrator@gp40121.glasgow-hb.scot.nhs.uk
(NHS Greater Glasgow, Primary Care Division)
Patient List Size: 4628

Practice Manager Elizabeth Robb

GP Bryan Lawrence WHITTY, Helen Toni JAMIESON, Andrew John MARSHALL

Buchanan Street

41-47 Buchanan Street, Balfron, Glasgow G63 0TS
Tel: 01360 440515 Fax: 01360 440831
(NHS Forth Valley, Primary Care Operating Division)

Practice Manager S McColl

GP Brian Douglas KEIGHLEY, B J ROEMMELE

Buckingham Terrace Medical Practice

31 Buckingham Terrace, Glasgow G12 8ED
Tel: 0141 211 6210 Fax: 0141 211 6232
Email: administrator@gp40012.glasgow-hb.scot.nhs.uk
(NHS Greater Glasgow, Primary Care Division)

Practice Manager Payman Javidan

GP Arthur David Warden ARNOT, Andrew J BLAIR, Thomas Patrick CUDDIHY, Iain George SCORGIE, Myra McInnes WADDELL

Budhill Medical Practice

2 Budhill Avenue, Glasgow G32 0PN
Tel: 0141 211 1585 Fax: 0141 211 1583
(NHS Greater Glasgow, Primary Care Division)
Patient List Size: 5000

GP Nelson CHEUNG, Alan WINTER

Busby Road Surgery

75 Busby Road, Clarkston, Glasgow G76 7BW
Tel: 0141 644 2666 Fax: 0141 644 5171
(NHS Greater Glasgow, Primary Care Division)

GP Colin Michael TAIT, Elaine Margaret FRASER, Michael Sutherland MORRICE

Busby Road Surgery

75 Busby Road, Clarkston, Glasgow G76 7BP
Tel: 0141 644 2669 Fax: 0141 644 5171
(NHS Greater Glasgow, Primary Care Division)

GP Edward Arthur CASTLE, Angela Dorothy FORD, William SIMMONS

Cairns Practice

Shettleston Health Centre, 420 Old Shettleston Road, Glasgow G32 7JZ
Tel: 0141 531 6220 Fax: 0141 531 6206
(NHS Greater Glasgow, Primary Care Division)

Practice Manager Susan McPhillie

GP Stirling James BRUCE, Katherine Anne GROSSET, Una MACLEOD, Paula ROGERS, Gerald George SPENCE, Donald George STODDART

Cairntoul Drive Surgery

9 Cairntoul Drive, Glasgow G14 0XT
Tel: 0141 959 5519 Fax: 0141 950 1028
(NHS Greater Glasgow, Primary Care Division)

GP Mairi Gray Browning SCOTT, Ahmed Charif ABBAS

Carolside Medical Centre

1 Carolside Gardens, Clarkston, Glasgow G76 7BX
Tel: 0141 644 3511 Fax: 0141 644 5525
(NHS Greater Glasgow, Primary Care Division)
Patient List Size: 7200

Practice Manager Stuart Fraser

GP Susan Elaine CAMPBELL, Janette Isobel MARSH, John Scott ROSS, Malcolm Alexander Dunn PICKARD

Castlemilk Health Centre

71 Dougrie Drive, Glasgow G45 9AW
Tel: 0141 531 8585 Fax: 0141 531 8596
(NHS Greater Glasgow, Primary Care Division)

Practice Manager Deborah Hamilton

GP Stanley Victor STEINBERG, Allan Russell YOUNG, Carol McKINNON, Richard James MULLEN, Peter Sidney WIGGINS

Castlemilk Health Centre

71 Dougrie Drive, Glasgow G45 9AW
Tel: 0141 531 8500 Fax: 0141 531 8505
(NHS Greater Glasgow, Primary Care Division)

GP Radha G SARKER

Central Health Centre
North Carbrain Road, Cumbernauld, Glasgow G67 1BJ
Tel: 01236 731738
(NHS Lanarkshire, Primary Care Division)

Practice Manager Marion McLaughlin

GP Ronald KIRKPATRICK, Margaret Gillian EARLEY, Arthur Stevenson GRAHAM, Palvinder Singh MAHAL, George Breton MORRISON, May Pettigrew WALKER-LOVE

Central Health Centre
North Carbrain Road, Cumbernauld, Glasgow G67 1BJ
Tel: 01236 737214 Fax: 01236 781699
(NHS Lanarkshire, Primary Care Division)
Patient List Size: 10850

Practice Manager Joyce Symon

GP Alan NORRIS, Ronald Leslie BERGIN, Geraldine CARROLL, Kareen GALLACHER, Julie Margaret MALLON, Edmund STEWART

Condorrat Health Centre
16 Airdrie Road, Cumbernauld, Glasgow G67 4DN
Tel: 01236 733221 Fax: 01236 457512
Email: kelly.caughey@core.lanpct.scot.nhs.uk
(NHS Lanarkshire, Primary Care Division)
Patient List Size: 4777

GP Urmil HANDA, Mohandas S NAIR, Jackton W O ODENY

Craigallian Avenue Surgery
11 Craigallian Avenue, Cambuslang, Glasgow G72 8RW
Tel: 0141 641 3129
(NHS Greater Glasgow, Primary Care Division)

Practice Manager J Brownlie

GP Iain William ROBERTSON, Helen Mary SKEOCH, Richard James WATSON

Crail Medical Practice
245 Tollcross Road, Glasgow G31 4UW
Tel: 0141 554 3199 Fax: 0141 551 9950
Email: administrator@gp46131.nhs.greaterglasgowHB.scot.nhs.uk
(NHS Greater Glasgow, Primary Care Division)
Patient List Size: 4500

GP Gail M ADDIS, Ian Clark AITKEN, Harjinder Singh BHACHU

The Crescent Medical Practice
12 Walmer Crescent, Glasgow G51 1AT
Tel: 0141 427 0191 Fax: 0141 427 1581
Email: administrator@gp52058.glasgow-hb.scot.nhs.uk
(NHS Greater Glasgow, Primary Care Division)

Practice Manager Mary Freel

GP Brendan SWEENEY, George BARLOW, Murray Farris Lyall BARNES, Donna Elizabeth NAPIER

Croftfoot Road Surgery
30 Croftfoot Road, Glasgow G44 5JT
Tel: 0141 531 8600 Fax: 0131 633 5284
(NHS Greater Glasgow, Primary Care Division)

GP Ronald Andrew GORDON, John ALBISTON, Elizabeth Jane GARWOOD, Sheila Campbell HENDERSON, Susan May MUTCH, John Francis TRAVERS

Croftfoot Road Surgery
44 Croftfoot Road, Glasgow G44 5JT
Tel: 0141 634 6333
(NHS Greater Glasgow, Primary Care Division)

GP Christine Jean Fairley BLEASBY, David George Addison WILLOX, Paul James McEVINNEY, Barbara Jane ROEMMELE

Crookfur Medical Practice
3 Corrour Road, Crookfur, Newton Mearns, Glasgow G77 6TR
Tel: 0141 639 8833 Fax: 0141 616 2486
(NHS Greater Glasgow, Primary Care Division)
Patient List Size: 2800

GP Subrata GHOSH

Crownpoint Medical Practice
201 Abercromby Street, Glasgow G40 2DA
Tel: 0141 531 6600 Fax: 0141 531 6655
(NHS Greater Glasgow, Primary Care Division)
Patient List Size: 4580

Practice Manager Morag Hoolachan

GP Carolynn Louise McDonald BRUCE, James KIDDIE, Jan VAN DEN HOVEN

Cumbernauld Road Surgery
804 Cumbernauld Road, Glasgow G33 2EH
Tel: 0141 770 5234 Fax: 0141 770 0850
(NHS Greater Glasgow, Primary Care Division)

GP Graham Barbour STRAIN

Cumbernauld Road Surgery
148 Cumbernauld Road, Glasgow G33 6HA
Tel: 0141 779 4445 Fax: 0141 779 4445
(NHS Greater Glasgow, Primary Care Division)

GP John KENNEDY

Cumbernauld Road Surgery
144-146 Cumbernauld Road, Stepps, Glasgow G33 6HA
Tel: 0141 779 2330 Fax: 0141 7799905
(NHS Greater Glasgow, Primary Care Division)
Patient List Size: 3000

Practice Manager Rae Dick

GP Robert James McNEILL, Agnes Anne Orr BARRIE

Denbridge Surgery
96 Drymen Road, Bearsden, Glasgow G61 2SY
Tel: 0141 942 9494 Fax: 0141 931 5496
Email: administrator@gp40402.glasgow-hb.scot.nhs
(NHS Greater Glasgow, Primary Care Division)
Patient List Size: 4076

Practice Manager Margaret Lindsay

GP Kenneth Alistair McGREGOR, Kathryn CAMPBELL-SHAW, Pauline Mary STEWART

Doctors Surgery
18 Union Street, Kirkintilloch, Glasgow G66 1DH
Tel: 0141 776 1238 Fax: 0141 775 2786
Email: practice@union-docs.co.uk
(NHS Greater Glasgow, Primary Care Division)
Patient List Size: 9100

Practice Manager Stuart Lennie

GP Gary Preston MACFARLANE, Norris Ferguson THOMPSON, Alastair Brian APPLEBY, David Mark McAULEY, Rhona Catherine McKEOWN, Elizabeth SWAIN

Dr H J and A P Jackson
91 Hyndland Road, Glasgow G12 9JE
Tel: 0141 339 7869 Fax: 0141 334 3207
(NHS Greater Glasgow, Primary Care Division)
Patient List Size: 4300

Practice Manager Marianne Wightman

GP Helen Jane JACKSON, Alexander Paul JACKSON, Mairi ROSS

Drumchapel Health Centre
80-90 Kinfauns Drive, Glasgow G15 7TS
Tel: 0141 211 6100 Fax: 0141 211 6104
(NHS Greater Glasgow, Primary Care Division)

GP Susan Catherine LYON, John Columba NUGENT, Alexander Provan SCOTT, Barbara Anne Kathleen WEST

Drumchapel Health Centre
80-90 Kinfauns Drive, Glasgow G15 7TS
Tel: 0141 211 6120 Fax: 0141 211 6128
Email: administrator@gp40205.glasgow-hb.soct.nhs.uk
(NHS Greater Glasgow, Primary Care Division)
Patient List Size: 5000

Practice Manager Susie Wyburn

GP Malachy DUFFY, Anne Helen MORGAN, Katherine Jane TURNER

Drumchapel Health Centre
80-90 Kinfauns Drive, Glasgow G15 7TS
Tel: 0141 211 6115
(NHS Greater Glasgow, Primary Care Division)

GP Jane Anne CONNELLY, Gordon McDONALD

Drumchapel Health Centre
80-90 Kinfauns Drive, Glasgow G15 7TS
Tel: 0141 211 6110 Fax: 0141 211 6140
(NHS Greater Glasgow, Primary Care Division)

Practice Manager Christine Bonar

GP David James ROBERTSON, Christine GRIEVE

Drumchapel Road Surgery
250 Drumchapel Road, Glasgow G15 6EG
Tel: 0141 944 3534 Fax: 0141 944 4534
(NHS Greater Glasgow, Primary Care Division)
Patient List Size: 3500

Practice Manager Roslyn Anderson

GP Jean McCrorie LINDSAY, Connie C SIMPSON

Drumchapel Road Surgery
242 Drumchapel Road, Glasgow G15 6EG
Tel: 0141 944 4453
(NHS Greater Glasgow, Primary Care Division)

Practice Manager Catriona Paton

GP Caroline CHRISTIE, Haradhan DATTA, Inderjit SINGH

Drymen Health Centre
2 Old Gartmore Road, Drymen, Glasgow G63 0DP
Tel: 01360 660203 Fax: 01360 660409
(NHS Forth Valley, Primary Care Operating Division)
Patient List Size: 1500

Practice Manager Loraine McLachlan

GP Jennifer Elizabeth FOSTER, Wm Kyle LIFSON

Drymen Road Surgery
96 Drymen Road, Bearsden, Glasgow G61 2SY
Tel: 0141 942 9494 Fax: 0141 931 5496
(NHS Greater Glasgow, Primary Care Division)

Practice Manager Margaret Lindsay

GP Alison Joyce BLAIR, Robert George DRYSDALE, Raymond Grant WALKER

Dumbarton Road Surgery
1264 Dumbarton Road, Glasgow G14 9PS
Tel: 0141 959 6311 Fax: 0141 954 9759
(NHS Greater Glasgow, Primary Care Division)

GP Alan Neilson LAURIE, Pamela Anne LEGGATE, Stuart Fotheringham WOOD

Dumbarton Road Surgery
1483 Dumbarton Road, Glasgow G14 9XL
Tel: 0141 211 9040 Fax: 0141 211 9043
(NHS Greater Glasgow, Primary Care Division)

Practice Manager Isobel Kearney

GP Moses Tako APILIGA

Dumbarton Road Surgery
1398 Dumbarton Road, Glasgow G14 9DR
Tel: 0141 959 1520 Fax: 0141 959 8463
(NHS Greater Glasgow, Primary Care Division)

GP Elaine FELL, Andrew William McCALL, John Philip WEIR

Dumbarton Road Surgery
1232 Dumbarton Road, Glasgow G14 9PY
Tel: 0141 211 9045 Fax: 0141 211 9047
(NHS Greater Glasgow, Primary Care Division)
Patient List Size: 2800

Practice Manager Moira Harvey

GP Maria Alexandra WIRTH, Jennifer McATEAR, Bridie O'DOWDS

Dyke Road Surgery
361 Dyke Road, Glasgow G13 4SQ
Tel: 0141 959 1074
(NHS Greater Glasgow, Primary Care Division)

GP Garry DICKSON, Pat ASBURY, May ROUSHDY-GEMIE

Eaglesham Surgery
30 Gilmour Street, Eaglesham, Glasgow G76 0AT
Tel: 01355 302221 Fax: 01355 302907
(NHS Greater Glasgow, Primary Care Division)

Practice Manager Lindsay Falconer

GP Sarah ANDERSON, Catriona Murray MACRAE, Valerie Margaret McDOUGALL, Douglas David McLACHLAN, James PHILLIPS

Easterhouse Health Centre
9 Auchinlea Road, Glasgow G34 9HQ
Tel: 0141 531 8150 Fax: 0141 531 8110
(NHS Greater Glasgow, Primary Care Division)

GP Mary Ellen BLATCHFORD, Marie Elizabeth WILSON

Easterhouse Health Centre
9 Auchinlea Road, Glasgow G34 9HQ
Tel: 0141 531 8170 Fax: 0141 531 8110
(NHS Greater Glasgow, Primary Care Division)

Practice Manager Elizabeth Graham

GP Eric BROWN, Catherine CAHILL, Andrew Timothy COLE, John Gerard Scott GOLDIE, Kristeen Ann LINDSAY, Andrew TOWNSLEY

Easterhouse Health Centre
9 Auchinlea Road, Glasgow G34 9HQ
Tel: 0141 531 8180 Fax: 0141 531 8186
(NHS Greater Glasgow, Primary Care Division)

GP Wilma Mary McArthur MUTCH, John Francis SCULLION, Derek Bertram SMITH

Edenkiln Surgery
Dumbrock Road, Strathblane, Glasgow G63 9EG
Tel: 01360 770340 Fax: 01360 771112
(NHS Forth Valley, Primary Care Operating Division)
Patient List Size: 2500

Practice Manager Karen Brown

GP Eric LIVINGSTON, David Nicholas PUGH

Eglinton Street Surgery
658-660 Eglinton Street, Glasgow G5 9RP
Tel: 0141 429 1421 Fax: 0141 429 8394
(NHS Greater Glasgow, Primary Care Division)
Patient List Size: 4000

Practice Manager Neera Bhasker

GP Vinod BHASKER, Mahammoud AKHTAR, Dr MONA-EL-AUMMRAN

Elmwood Avenue Surgery
3 Elmwood Avenue, Newton Mearns, Glasgow G77 6EH
Tel: 0141 639 2478 Fax: 0141 639 6708
(NHS Greater Glasgow, Primary Care Division)

Practice Manager J Williams

GP John Avrom TOBIAS, Gillian Dickson LOCKHART

Erskine View Clinic
Old Kilparick, Glasgow G60 5JG
Tel: 01389 872575 Fax: 01389 890919
(NHS Greater Glasgow, Primary Care Division)
Patient List Size: 3610

Practice Manager Anne Burrows

GP Donald Greer WALLACE, Anthony KEARNEY, Fiona McLEOD

Farne Drive Surgery
59 Farne Drive, Glasgow G44 5DQ
Tel: 0141 637 9828 Fax: 0141 633 5284
(NHS Greater Glasgow, Primary Care Division)

GP Ann Stirling ANDERSON, Sandra Karen MACCUISH

Fenwick Road Surgery
261 Fenwick Road, Giffnock, Glasgow G46 6JX
Tel: 0141 531 6993 Fax: 0141 531 6997
(NHS Greater Glasgow, Primary Care Division)
Patient List Size: 6200

Practice Manager Elizabeth Simpson

GP Ian Donald Mackintosh JAMIESON, Susan Margaret COOPER, Ann Kinsey FINCH, David Wilson FRAME

Fernbank Medical Centre
194 Fernbank St, Glasgow G22 6BD
Tel: 0141 589 8000 Fax: 0141 589 8004
Email: iaingbrown@aol.com
(NHS Greater Glasgow, Primary Care Division)
Patient List Size: 7500

Practice Manager Margaret Hanlon

GP Iain Grant BROWN, Silke BANNUSCHE, Annette BARNES, Graeme DRUMMOND, Vijay KUMAR, Gillian MILLER, Peter VON KAEHNE

Ferness Road Surgery
8 Ferness Road, Glasgow G21 3SH
Tel: 0141 558 6178 Fax: 0141 557 3405
(NHS Greater Glasgow, Primary Care Division)
Patient List Size: 1800

GP Mary Elizabeth SWEENEY, Margaret O'FARRELL

Fulton Street Surgery
94 Fulton Street, Glasgow G13 1JE
Tel: 0141 959 3391 Fax: 0141 950 2692
(NHS Greater Glasgow, Primary Care Division)
Patient List Size: 5100

Practice Manager Gillian Conn

GP Janet Hopes LAND, Gordon J CAMPBELL, Philip Albert EWART, Clare STILLMAN

Gardner Street Surgery
11 Gardner Street, Glasgow G11 5NR
Tel: 0141 334 2215 Fax: 0141 338 8197
(NHS Greater Glasgow, Primary Care Division)

GP Ursula KAUFMANN, Jenette ROBERTSON

Gilbertfield Street Surgery
67 Gilbertfield Street, Glasgow G33 3TU
Tel: 0141 774 5987 Fax: 0141 774 5210
(NHS Greater Glasgow, Primary Care Division)

GP William K CARLE, William C Y LAM, John Cameron SPENCE

Glenmanor Avenue Surgery
69 Glenmanor Avenue, Moodiesburn, Glasgow G69 0LB
Tel: 0141 787 2276
(NHS Greater Glasgow, Primary Care Division)

GP Antoninus Felician Sugitharaj JOHNPULLE

Glenmill Medical Centre
1191 Royston Road, Glasgow G33 1EY
Tel: 0141 770 4052 Fax: 0141 770 4255
(NHS Greater Glasgow, Primary Care Division)

GP Paul Francis RYAN, Iain Martin KENNEDY, Pauline Susan McALAVEY

Glenmore Avenue Surgery
33 Glenmore Avenue, Glasgow G42 0EH
Tel: 0141 647 3020
(NHS Greater Glasgow, Primary Care Division)

GP Rosaleen Margaret BEATTIE

Gorbals Health Centre
45 Pine Place, Glasgow G5 0BQ
Tel: 0141 531 8290 Fax: 0141 531 8208
(NHS Greater Glasgow, Primary Care Division)

GP Jonathan Samuel GORDON, Eric David LIVINGSTONE, Wilma Andrea BEST, Diane WATSON

Gorbals Health Centre
45 Pine Place, Glasgow G5 0BQ
Tel: 0141 531 8275 Fax: 0141 531 8208
(NHS Greater Glasgow, Primary Care Division)

GP Hugh J DONNACHIE

Govan Health Centre
5 Drumoyne Road, Govan, Glasgow G51 4BJ
Tel: 0141 531 8470 Fax: 0141 531 8471
(NHS Greater Glasgow, Primary Care Division)

GP Donald Lauder BLACKWOOD, William MacVicar DUNWOODIE, Elizabeth MASTERSON, John Gerard MONTGOMERY

Govan Health Centre
5 Drumoyne Road, Glasgow G51 4BJ
Tel: 0141 531 8400 Fax: 0141 531 8404
(NHS Greater Glasgow, Primary Care Division)

GP Niall MacLaine CAMERON, Brenda Alison McCaig DUTHIE, John James HERRON, Jane Margaret MARSHALL

Govan Health Centre
5 Drumoyne Road, Glasgow G51 4BJ
Tel: 0141 531 8490 Fax: 0141 531 8487
(NHS Greater Glasgow, Primary Care Division)
Patient List Size: 4076

Practice Manager Margaret Beggs

GP Robert Euan PATERSON, Carolyn GILLIES, John McGUINNESS, Marianne SCOTT

Govanhill Health Centre
233 Calder Street, Glasgow G42 7DR
Tel: 0141 531 8370 Fax: 0141 531 4431
(NHS Greater Glasgow, Primary Care Division)
Patient List Size: 10700

Practice Manager Patricia Donnelly

GP Maura Magdalene BERRY, Daniel Anthony CUMMING, John Gerald DYSART, Ruth MACDONALD, Anne Marie McNALLY, Fiona O'DONOGHUE, John SHARP

Govanhill Health Centre
233 Calder Street, Glasgow G42 7DR
Tel: 0141 531 8385 Fax: 0141 531 4432
(NHS Greater Glasgow, Primary Care Division)
Patient List Size: 5600

Practice Manager Diane MacDonald

GP Janet Findlay MacBRAYNE, Keong Seng CHIAH, Gillian E MacARTHUR, Graham Y SMITH

Govanhill Health Centre
233 Calder Street, Glasgow G42 7DR
Tel: 0141 531 8361 Fax: 0141 531 8375
(NHS Greater Glasgow, Primary Care Division)

Practice Manager Joan Hamilton

GP Kevin Peter FELLOWS, Anne Christine BUSH, Christopher Paul FRASER, Sheila Maria O'NEILL

Grantley Street Surgery
1 Grantley Street, Glasgow G41 3PT
Tel: 0141 632 4698 Fax: 0141 649 6671
Email: administrator@gp49553.glasgow.hb.scot.nhs.uk
(NHS Greater Glasgow, Primary Care Division)
Patient List Size: 3600

Practice Manager Ann Young

GP Eileen Margaret Cartner DUKE, Jacqueline BARR, Andrew Adam FITCHETT

Great Western Medical
1980 Great Western Road, Glasgow G13 2SW
Tel: 0141 959 1196 Fax: 0141 950 1811
(NHS Greater Glasgow, Primary Care Division)

Practice Manager Ann Fergus

GP Gillian Anne Crawford HOSIE, James HOSIE

Greenhills Health Centre
20 Greenhills Square, East Kilbride, Glasgow G75 8TT
Tel: 01355 236331 Fax: 01355 234977
Website: www.surgeriesonline.com/greenhillshc
(NHS Lanarkshire, Primary Care Division)
Patient List Size: 7650

Practice Manager M M Wilson

GP Glyn Michael PHILLIPS, Iain Andrew HATHORN, Jacqueline Ann LOGUE, Angela Macrae MOSLEY, Kuljinder SINGH

Guthrie and Guthrie
1448 Dumbarton Road, Glasgow G14 9DN
Tel: 0141 959 2023 Fax: 0141 950 1822
(NHS Greater Glasgow, Primary Care Division)
Patient List Size: 2000

Practice Manager Harriet Conner

GP Colin Ivar GUTHRIE, Eleanor GUTHRIE

Hunter Health Centre
Andrew Street, East Kilbride, Glasgow G74 1AD
Tel: 01355 906611 Fax: 01355 906615
(NHS Lanarkshire, Primary Care Division)
Patient List Size: 7200

Practice Manager Jacqueline Brownlie

GP Christopher John MACKINTOSH, Monica CANNING, Doreen WATSON, Jason WHITE, Susan Forsyth YOUNG

Hunter Health Centre
Andrew Street, East Kilbride, Glasgow G74 1AD
Tel: 01355 906622 Fax: 01355 906629
(NHS Lanarkshire, Primary Care Division)
Patient List Size: 7500

Practice Manager Valerie Matthews

GP Rosaleen Clare DOCHERTY, Brendan William CUNNING, Audrey FINNEGAN, Karen Anne MACRAE, Colin Alexander WILSON

Hunter Health Centre
Andrew Street, East Kilbride, Glasgow G74 1AD
Tel: 01355 906676 Fax: 01355 906676
(NHS Lanarkshire, Primary Care Division)
Patient List Size: 8300

GP Iain Cameron CAMPBELL, Olive LEITCH, Alan William George MOFFETT, Antony Edward Reid WILKINSON, Anne Margaret WYLIE

Hunter Health Centre
Andrew Street, East Kilbride, Glasgow G74 1AD
Tel: 01355 906632
(NHS Lanarkshire, Primary Care Division)

GP Lorne A M McADIE, John Bankier SLOAN, Vijay B SONTHALIA, Lesley Anne THOMSON

Hunter Health Centre
Andrew Street, East Kilbride, Glasgow G74 1AD
Tel: 01355 906643
(NHS Lanarkshire, Primary Care Division)

Practice Manager B Paterson

GP Barry COOPER, A Louise E SIMMONS

Hunter Health Centre
Andrew Street, East Kilbride, Glasgow G74 1AD
Tel: 01355 906655
(NHS Lanarkshire, Primary Care Division)

GP Marie Clare DAVIDSON, Michael DOUGAN, Helen McTAGGART, James Andrew SLAVIN

Hyndland Road Surgery
130 Hyndland Road, Glasgow G12 9PN
Tel: 0141 339 1298 Fax: 0141 334 0991
Email: isabelle.cullen@gp40188.glasgow-hb.scot.nhs.uk
(NHS Greater Glasgow, Primary Care Division)
Patient List Size: 2400

Practice Manager Margaret Weir

GP Isabelle Anne Skinnider CULLEN

Kausar
26 Bank Street, Glasgow G12 8ND
Tel: 0141 339 5513 Fax: 0141 357 5554
(NHS Greater Glasgow, Primary Care Division)
Patient List Size: 3100

Practice Manager M Aggarwal

GP Muhammad Shafi KAUSAR

Keddie
91 Kirkintilloch Road, Bishopbriggs, Glasgow G64 2AA
Tel: 0141 772 2241 Fax: 0141 762 3482
(NHS Greater Glasgow, Primary Care Division)
Patient List Size: 2100

Practice Manager Dierdre Bryson

GP James KEDDIE

Keir Street Surgery
42 Keir Street, Glasgow G41 2LA
Tel: 0141 423 3335 Fax: 0141 423 9883
(NHS Greater Glasgow, Primary Care Division)

GP Sohail Raza CHAUDHRY

Kelso Street Surgery
6 Kelso Street, Glasgow G14 0JZ
Tel: 0141 211 6999 Fax: 0141 211 6990
Email: administrator@gp40525.glasgow.hb.scot.nhs.uk
(NHS Greater Glasgow, Primary Care Division)

Practice Manager Micael Enkvist

GP Clare McCORKINDALE, John McDERMOTT

Kelvin Medical Centre
96 Napiershall Street, Maryhill, Glasgow G20 6GH
Tel: 0141 211 9597 Fax: 0141 331 0071
(NHS Greater Glasgow, Primary Care Division)
Patient List Size: 3800

Practice Manager Yvonne Sweeney

GP Fiona Anne DAVIDSON, M BROWN, Valerie Elaine KIDD, Susan E PERRYER

Kenilworth Medical Centre
1 Kenilworth Court, Greenfields, Cumbernauld, Glasgow G67 1BP
Tel: 01236 727816 Fax: 01236 726306
(NHS Lanarkshire, Primary Care Division)
Patient List Size: 15500

Practice Manager Eileen McBride

GP James REAVEY, Brian Grant ANDERSON, Maria HORGAN, Alexander JOHNSTONE, Catherine LEVEN, Emma McPHERSON, Catherine RAE, Roger Rajendra SOCKALINGAM

Kenmure Medical Practice
7 Springfield Road, Bishopbriggs, Glasgow G64 1PJ
Tel: 0141 772 6309 Fax: 0141 762 2018
Email: administrator@gp43171.glasgow-hb.scot.hns.uk
(NHS Greater Glasgow, Primary Care Division)
Patient List Size: 6375

Practice Manager Angela Thompson

GP Brian Joseph PAICE, Valerie Gibb BERG, Ann M DOUBAL, Ian Mitchell Hendry GORDON

Keppoch Medical Practice
85 Denmark Street, Glasgow G22 5EG
Tel: 0141 531 6170 Fax: 0141 531 6177
(NHS Greater Glasgow, Primary Care Division)

Patient List Size: 3625

Practice Manager Fiona McKinlay

GP Robert Parnell MANDEVILLE, Krystyna Ada Teresa GRUSZECKA, Ewen Cameron HARLEY, Petra SAMBALE

Kersland House Surgery
37 Station Road, Milngavie, Glasgow G62 8BT
Tel: 0141 956 1005 Fax: 0141 955 0342
Website: www.kerslandhouse.co.uk
(NHS Greater Glasgow, Primary Care Division)
Patient List Size: 7400

Practice Manager Sandra J Cunningham

GP Michael KENT, Steven GOLDTHORP, Graham MORRISON, MAIRI STANLEY, Fiona THOMSON

Kildrum Health Centre
Afton Road, Cumbernauld, Glasgow G67 2EU
Tel: 01236 721354
(NHS Lanarkshire, Primary Care Division)
Patient List Size: 5500

GP Prem Nath NAHAR, Victoria Agnes FAKHOURY, Eileen Mary FLYNN, Graeme Alistair MACLEOD

Killearn Health Centre
Balfron Road, Killearn, Glasgow G63 9NA
Tel: 01360 50339 Fax: 01360 550176
Email: administrator@gp95347.foeth-hb.scot.nhs.uk
(NHS Forth Valley, Primary Care Operating Division)
Patient List Size: 4500

Practice Manager Marta Emmerson

GP Stephen Thomas ELMS, Stuart Allan CUMMING, Caryn Margaret SIMMS

Kilmarnock Road Surgery
123 Kilmarnock Road, Glasgow G41 3YT
Tel: 0141 649 6231 Fax: 0141 632 2012
(NHS Greater Glasgow, Primary Care Division)
Patient List Size: 5200

Practice Manager A Murphy

GP Tanusree Mistu GRAY, Sharon BIRNEY, Ian C GEDDES, Morris James LEONARD

Kilsyth Medical Partnership
Kilsyth Health Centre, Burngreen Park, Kilsyth, Glasgow G65 0HU
Tel: 01236 822081 Fax: 01236 826231
(NHS Lanarkshire, Primary Care Division)
Patient List Size: 14220

Practice Manager Joyce Morrison

GP Sandra Milne Ross BROWN, Douglas Hamilton DICK, Patricia Mary DOVE, Allyson GAWN, Murray Robert William HARDIE, Fiona McGHIE, Ann Marie McGREGOR, Philip McMENEMY, Philip Michael RANKIN

Kings Park Surgery
274 Kings Park Avenue, Glasgow G44 4JE
Tel: 0141 632 1824 Fax: 0141 632 0461
(NHS Greater Glasgow, Primary Care Division)
Patient List Size: 1918

GP Philip Leo McNAUGHT

Kings Park Surgery
274 Kings Park Avenue, Glasgow G44 4JE
Tel: 0141 632 1824 Fax: 0141 632 0461
(NHS Greater Glasgow, Primary Care Division)
Patient List Size: 2015

GP Josephine Mary BELL

Kings Park Surgery
274 Kings Park Avenue, Glasgow G44 4JE
Tel: 0141 632 1824 Fax: 0141 632 0461
(NHS Greater Glasgow, Primary Care Division)

GP Mohammed Mahmood SHARIF

Kingsway Medical Practice
12Kingsway Court, Glasgow G14 9SS
Tel: 0141 959 6000 Fax: 0141 954 6971
(NHS Greater Glasgow, Primary Care Division)
Patient List Size: 3800

GP Roderick Watson SHAW, Elaine CAMERON, William Iain Fleming HENDERSON

Kinning Park Medical Centre
42 Admiral Street, Glasgow G41 1HU
Tel: 0141 429 0913 Fax: 0141 429 8491
Website: www.ar/sa-surgery.co.uk
(NHS Greater Glasgow, Primary Care Division)

Practice Manager Sandra Grant

GP George McKEEVE, Anne Caroline Hay PLENDERLEITH

Laurel St Patrick Surgery
4 Laurel St Patrick, Glasgow G3 6JB
Tel: 0141 332 5553 Fax: 0141 332 5557
(NHS Greater Glasgow, Primary Care Division)

GP Marion RICHMOND

Lennoxtown Clinic
103 Main Street, Lennoxtown, Glasgow G66 7DB
Tel: 01360 310357 Fax: 01360 311740
(NHS Greater Glasgow, Primary Care Division)

Practice Manager Isabelle Duidek

GP Allan James RAE, James Roger HENDERSON

Lightburn Medical Centre
930 Carntyne Road, Glasgow G32 6NB
Tel: 0141 778 0440 Fax: 0141 778 0143
(NHS Greater Glasgow, Primary Care Division)

GP James Edward Gerard O'NEIL, Elizabeth Ann CAVEN, Christine Isabella Margaret McNEISH

Lightburn Medical Centre
930 Corntyne Road, Glasgow G32 6NB
Tel: 0141 778 0111 Fax: 0141 778 0143
(NHS Greater Glasgow, Primary Care Division)

Practice Manager Deirdre Bryson

GP Alan George MACKENZIE, Mary McCULLUM

Lincluden Surgery
53 Bellshill Road, Uddingston, Glasgow G71 7PA
Tel: 01698 813873 Fax: 01698 816374
(NHS Lanarkshire, Primary Care Division)
Patient List Size: 6708

GP John S BOWMAN, A KING, Diane MELROSE, U SCHUTZ, Bruce Forsyth Morrison THOMSON

Lindsay and Partners
1413 Pollokshaws Road, Glasgow G41 3RG
Tel: 0141 632 9141 Fax: 0141 636 0414
(NHS Greater Glasgow, Primary Care Division)
Patient List Size: 5100

Practice Manager Barbara Watson

GP Margaret DODDS, David William LESLIE, Norman John Forrest LINDSAY, Margo Fraser McNICOL

Main Street Surgery
25 Main Street, Cambuslang, Glasgow G72 7EX
Tel: 0141 641 1663 Fax: 0141 641 9807
(NHS Greater Glasgow, Primary Care Division)

GP G HENRY

Maryhill Health Centre
41 Shawpark Street, Glasgow G20 9DR
Tel: 0141 531 8811 Fax: 0141 531 8808
(NHS Greater Glasgow, Primary Care Division)

Practice Manager Sandra Fisher

GP David BAILLIE, David Malcolm BYFORD, Noreen HAGGERTY, Jon MEREDITH, Desmond Frederick SPENCE

Maryhill Health Centre

41 Shawpark Street, Glasgow G20 9DR
Tel: 0141 531 8800 Fax: 0141 531 8851
Email: administrator@gp43241.glasgow-hb.scot.nhs.uk
(NHS Greater Glasgow, Primary Care Division)
Patient List Size: 4500

Practice Manager Elizabeth Thom

GP Margaret Cunningham HARRIS, Susan GIBSON-SMITH, James Anderson Boyd MACKENZIE

Maryhill Health Centre

41 Shawpark Street, Glasgow G20 9DR
Tel: 0141 531 8897 Fax: 0141 531 8863
Email: administrator@gp43311.glasgow-hb.scot.nhs.uk
Website: www.redarea.co.uk
(NHS Greater Glasgow, Primary Care Division)
Patient List Size: 6400

Practice Manager Irene Gunn

GP Gordon MacVicar MARTIN, Roland LESLIE, Avril Christina McMILLAN, Susanne Alcorn RUSSELL, Alisdair WEBB

Maryhill Health Centre

41 Shawpark Street, Glasgow G20 9DR
Tel: 0141 531 8700 Fax: 0141 531 8773
(NHS Greater Glasgow, Primary Care Division)

GP Charlotte Mary TOLMIE

Meadowpark Street Surgery

214 Meadowpark Street, Glasgow G31 2TE
Tel: 0141 554 0464
(NHS Greater Glasgow, Primary Care Division)

GP Ellen Jean BRUCE, Robert John Arthur FIFE, Morag Campbell GILMORE

Mearns Medical Centre

30 maple Avenue, Newton Mearns, Glasgow G77 5BQ
Tel: 0141 639 2753 Fax: 0141 616 2403
(NHS Greater Glasgow, Primary Care Division)
Patient List Size: 9000

Practice Manager M Hume

GP Leslie Murray QUIN, Roderick Walker IRELAND, Lesley MACAULAY, Fiona MARSHALL

Mearns Road Surgery

259 Mearns Road, Newton Mearns, Glasgow G77 5LU
Tel: 0141 639 3644
(NHS Greater Glasgow, Primary Care Division)

GP Michael Gerard Joseph HAUGHNEY

Merrylee Medical Centre

142-144 Clarkston Road, Glasgow G44 4EG
Tel: 0141 633 2345 Fax: 0141 633 5262
(NHS Greater Glasgow, Primary Care Division)

GP Douglas Anderson HUTCHISON, John Stephen HUTCHISON, John McKAY, Julie Alison PENNYCOOK

Midlock Medical Centre

7 Midlock Street, Glasgow G51 1SL
Tel: 0141 427 4271 Fax: 0141 427 1401
(NHS Greater Glasgow, Primary Care Division)

Practice Manager Aileen Campbell

GP Kenneth Edward COLLINS, Barry Jonathan ADAMS-STRUMP, Mark FAWCETT, Lesley Alison HAY, Kenneth Francis O'NEILL, Caitriana PARK, Alison Joyce THOMSON

Mill Street Surgery

81 Mill Street, Rutherglen, Glasgow G73 2LD
Tel: 0141 647 6294
(NHS Greater Glasgow, Primary Care Division)

GP Richard James AFUAKWAH

Mills and Marshall

Gorbals Health Centre, 45 Pine Place, Glasgow G5 0BQ
Tel: 0141 531 8250 Fax: 0141 531 8248
Email: administrator@gp69074.glasgow-hb.scot.nhs.uk
(NHS Greater Glasgow, Primary Care Division)

Practice Manager Rena Ruiz

GP Catherine MILLS, Graeme MARSHALL

Milngavie Road Surgery

85 Milngavie Road, Bearsden, Glasgow G61 2DN
Tel: 0141 211 5621 Fax: 0141 211 5625
(NHS Greater Glasgow, Primary Care Division)

Practice Manager Elspeth McKay

GP Judith M CHAPMAN, Jean Charlotte POWELL, Aileen Margaret Elizabeth PATERSON, Alastair TAYLOR

Milton Medical Centre

109 Egilsay Street, Glasgow G22 7JL
Tel: 0141 772 1183 Fax: 0141 772 2331
(NHS Greater Glasgow, Primary Care Division)
Patient List Size: 3500

Practice Manager Karen Stewart

GP Robert Michael TROLLEN, Pamela Mary GEDDES

Mount Florida Medical Centre

183 Prospecthill Road, Glasgow G42 9LQ
Tel: 0141 632 4004 Fax: 0141 636 6036
(NHS Greater Glasgow, Primary Care Division)

GP Jacqueline Angele CARRUTHERS, John Watson CRORIE, Sheila Anne McKECHNIE, Alan William ROBERTSON, Louise Jane SHEIL

Mull, Admiral Road Surgery

36 Admiral Road, Glasgow G41 1HU
Tel: 0141 429 0943
(NHS Greater Glasgow, Primary Care Division)
Patient List Size: 1800

GP Muhammad Fazlul ALAM

Murray Road Surgery

50 The Murray Road, East Kilbride, Glasgow G75 0RT
Tel: 01355 225374 Fax: 01355 239475
(NHS Lanarkshire, Primary Care Division)

Practice Manager Anee McKay

GP Alistair Stevenson MacCORMICK, Thomas Mark BONNES, Alan Laurie BOYD, Mary Ann BOYD, Simon Clifford MACQUIRE, Thomas Barrie MATTHEW

Nithsdale Road Surgery

162 Nithsdale Road, Glasgow G41 5RU
Tel: 0141 424 1831 Fax: 0141 423 7422
(NHS Greater Glasgow, Primary Care Division)
Patient List Size: 11000

Practice Manager Maggie MacFadden

GP Ian Martin MACDONALD, Vimal Sharad AMIN, Angela Justine DUNN, Jill Elizabeth FOWLIE, Eileen Margaret McAULAY, William Patrick McKEAN, Lindsay Stewart McMENEMIN

North Avenue Surgery

18 North Avenue, Cambuslang, Glasgow G72 8AT
Tel: 0141 641 3037 Fax: 0141 646 1905
(NHS Greater Glasgow, Primary Care Division)
Patient List Size: 9520

Practice Manager Marguerite McLean

GP Leslie Ronald Nimmo SMITH, Elaine Allison CARTLIDGE, Keith John McINTYRE, Ian Andrew NOTMAN

Northcote Surgery

2 Victoria Circus, Glasgow G12 9LD
Tel: 0141 339 3211 Fax: 0141 357 4480
(NHS Greater Glasgow, Primary Care Division)
Patient List Size: 12500

Practice Manager Patrick Clarke

GP Ian Leslie REID, Peter Frederick Hume DAWES, Iain KENNEDY, Catherine Patricia PICKERING, Siobhan Maire Michelle WALSH, Marni WILLENS

The Oaks Medical Centre
1 Paisley Road, Barrhead, Glasgow G78 1HG
Tel: 0141 580 1001 Fax: 0141 580 1002
(NHS Argyll and Clyde, Renfrewshire and Inverclyde Community Services Division)

GP David MEIGHAN, Thomas NAVEN

Old Mill Surgery
100 Old Mill Road, Uddingston, Glasgow G71 7JB
Tel: 01698 817219
(NHS Lanarkshire, Primary Care Division)
Patient List Size: 10500

Practice Manager Liz Reilly

GP Anne MacALISTER, William Proctor BOYD, Lindsay Ann CLARK, Malachy Peter LARKIN, William Gilmour MARTIN, Helen Murray PARK

Paisley Road West Surgery
1314 Paisley Road West, Glasgow G52 1DB
Tel: 0141 882 4567 Fax: 0141 882 4548
(NHS Greater Glasgow, Primary Care Division)
Patient List Size: 3100

Practice Manager P Warren

GP Robert Maclean MAIR, William Henry PITT

Paisley Road West Surgery
1841 Paisley Road West, Glasgow G52 3SU
Tel: 0141 211 6666 Fax: 0141 211 6668
(NHS Greater Glasgow, Primary Care Division)
Patient List Size: 1650

Practice Manager L Donald

GP Lorna VENTRY

Paisley Road West Surgery
532 Paisley Road West, Glasgow G51 1RN
Tel: 0141 427 2504
(NHS Greater Glasgow, Primary Care Division)
Patient List Size: 2900

Practice Manager Helen Eadie

GP Chiara Elizabeth BERARDELLI, Balbir Singh CHITA

Paisley Road West Surgery
1808 Paisley Road West, Glasgow G52 3TS
Tel: 0141 211 6660 Fax: 0141 211 6662
(NHS Greater Glasgow, Primary Care Division)

GP Gibson FLEMING, Sheila Margaret THOMSON

The Park Surgery
7 Baker Street, Glasgow G41 3YA
Tel: 0141 632 0203 Fax: 0141 636 5349
(NHS Greater Glasgow, Primary Care Division)
Patient List Size: 3182

Practice Manager Elizabeth McColl

GP Ilyas HUSSAIN, Marie Frances PIRRET

Parkhead Health Centre
101 Salamanca Street, Glasgow G31 5BA
Tel: 0141 531 9070 Fax: 0141 531 9020
(NHS Greater Glasgow, Primary Care Division)
Patient List Size: 3300

Practice Manager Maria Morris

GP Barry J McCUSKER, Barbara Anne MILLAR

Parkhead Health Centre
101 Salamanca Street, Glasgow G31 5BA
Tel: 0141 531 9050 Fax: 0141 531 9026
(NHS Greater Glasgow, Primary Care Division)

GP Thomas Gerard LAFFERTY, William Peter MacPHEE

Parkhead Health Centre
101 Salamanca Street, Glasgow G31 5BA
Tel: 0141 531 9060 Fax: 0141 531 9042
Email: adminstrator@gp46146.glasgow-hb.scot.nhs.uk
(NHS Greater Glasgow, Primary Care Division)
Patient List Size: 4800

Practice Manager Patricia Donnelly

GP Thomas C GIHOOLY, Jayne MORRISON, Norman Walter POOLE

Peel Street Surgery
11 Peel Street, Glasgow G11 5LL
Tel: 0141 334 9331 Fax: 0141 334 9332
(NHS Greater Glasgow, Primary Care Division)

GP Nayeem Ahmed GHOURI

Peelview Medical Centre
45-53 Union Street, Kirkintilloch, Glasgow G66 1DN
Tel: 0141 211 8270 Fax: 0141 211 8279
(NHS Greater Glasgow, Primary Care Division)

Practice Manager Helen Boyle

GP Elizabeth G ROURKE, Simon J BEARDSLEY, Ian Alistair Neville CANNON, Andrew Paul FITZPATRICK, Mary Isabel HARRIS, John Hamilton McLAUCHLAN

Pennan Place Surgery
20 Pennan Place, Glasgow G14 0EA
Tel: 0141 959 1704 Fax: 0141 958 1100
(NHS Greater Glasgow, Primary Care Division)

GP Douglas Kerr ROBERTSON

Pollok Health Centre
21 Cowglen Road, Glasgow G53 6EQ
Tel: 0141 531 6860 Fax: 0141 531 6808
(NHS Greater Glasgow, Primary Care Division)

GP Patricia BOYLE, Maria DUFFY, Nicholas John TREADGOLD

Pollok Health Centre
21 Cowglen Road, Glasgow G53 6EQ
Tel: 0141 531 6880 Fax: 0141 531 6808
(NHS Greater Glasgow, Primary Care Division)

GP K M Wasil SIDDIQUI

Pollokshaws Doctors Centre
26 Wellgreen, Glasgow G43 1RR
Tel: 0141 649 2836 Fax: 0141 649 5238
(NHS Greater Glasgow, Primary Care Division)
Patient List Size: 1020

GP Malcolm Roy BROWN, Sandra Jane SPILG

Pollokshaws Doctors Centre
26 Wellgreen, Glasgow G43 1RR
Tel: 0141 649 2836 Fax: 0141 649 5238
(NHS Greater Glasgow, Primary Care Division)
Patient List Size: 7350

GP Harvey William LIVINGSTONE, James GALBRAITH, Bridgid MOLLOY, Simon Christopher OSBORNE, Freya Marion SMITH

Possilpark Health Centre
85 Denmark Street, Glasgow G22 5EG
Tel: 0141 531 6150 Fax: 0141 531 6152
(NHS Greater Glasgow, Primary Care Division)
Patient List Size: 2643

Practice Manager Liz Graham

GP Erich Werner Brunton LAMB, Luis ALGUERO

Provanmill Road Surgery
228 Provanmill Road, Glasgow G33 1DQ
Tel: 0141 770 4763 Fax: 0141 770 6770
(NHS Greater Glasgow, Primary Care Division)

GP Thevasundrai LOGENDRA

Queens Crescent Surgery
10 Queens Cresent, Glasgow G4 9BL
Tel: 0141 332 3526 Fax: 0141 332 1150
(NHS Greater Glasgow, Primary Care Division)

GP Jonathan Harvey COSSAR, Kenneth Richmond McCLURE, Brian Galbraith SHAW

Queens Drive Surgery
181 Queens Drive, Glasgow G42 8QD
Tel: 0141 423 3474
Email: administrator@g49286glasgow-hb.scot.nhs.uk
(NHS Greater Glasgow, Primary Care Division)
Patient List Size: 2714

Practice Manager Helen Minto

GP Gillian Patricia MACLEAN, Catriona Anne O'NEILL

Radnor Street Surgery
3 Radnor Street, Glasgow G3 7UA
Tel: 0141 334 6111
(NHS Greater Glasgow, Primary Care Division)

GP Sheila Carrick HARRISON, Jeremy Christopher ROBERTS

Rutherglen Health Centre
130 Stonelaw Road, Rutherglen, Glasgow G73 2PQ
Tel: 0141 531 6020 Fax: 0141 531 6070
(NHS Greater Glasgow, Primary Care Division)

Practice Manager Linda Carson

GP Colin Francis BARRETT, Rosemary BARRETT, Michael Daniel KELLY

Rutherglen Health Centre
130 Stonelaw Road, Rutherglen, Glasgow G73 2PQ
Tel: 0141 531 6065
(NHS Greater Glasgow, Primary Care Division)

GP Douglas John BRUCE, Alasdair CAMPBELL, William Allan Cooper SPEIR

Rutherglen Health Centre
130 Stonelaw Road, Rutherglen, Glasgow G73 2PQ
Tel: 0141 531 6030 Fax: 0141 531 6031
(NHS Greater Glasgow, Primary Care Division)

GP Richard James Callon WALLACE, Declan Joseph CAMPBELL, Douglas Robert COLVILLE, Amr Hussein FAWZI, Anne Elizabeth Margaret FORREST, Andrew John MANCHIP

Rutherglen Health Centre
130 Stonelaw Road, Rutherglen, Glasgow G73 2PQ
Tel: 0141 531 6020 Fax: 0141 531 4130
Email: administrator@gp49021.glasgow-hb.scot.nhs.uk
Website: www.rutherglenhealthcentre.co.uk
(NHS Greater Glasgow, Primary Care Division)
Patient List Size: 5600

Practice Manager R D Cairns

GP Alison Cameron BIRKMYRE, Jackie ABERNETHY, Arnold Neill JOHNSTON

Rutherglen Primary Care Centre
130 Stonelaw Road, Rutherglen, Glasgow G73 2PQ
Tel: 0141 531 6010 Fax: 0141 613 3460
(NHS Greater Glasgow, Primary Care Division)
Patient List Size: 5000

Practice Manager Heather Patterson

GP David Mark REID, Linda HENDERSON, Janis LYNCH

Rutland Place Surgery
21 Rutland Place, Glasgow G51 1TA
Tel: 0141 427 3121 Fax: 0141 427 7600
(NHS Greater Glasgow, Primary Care Division)

GP Mairie Annabella ROSS, Mary Frances SHIELDS, Ronald WOLFE

Semple and Partner
436 Mosspark Boulevard, Glasgow G52 1HX
Tel: 0141 882 5494
(NHS Greater Glasgow, Primary Care Division)

GP Linsey Charlotte SEMPLE

Shaftesbury Medical Practice
1265 Dumbarton Road, Glasgow G14 9UU
Tel: 0141 959 5500 Fax: 0141 954 4864
Email: shaftesbury@gp40210-hb.scot.nhs.uk
(NHS Greater Glasgow, Primary Care Division)
Patient List Size: 1800

Practice Manager Linda Honeyman, Jacqueline Young

GP Maureen Elizabeth HEPBURN, Janice Elizabeth OLIVER

The Sheddens Medical Practice
5a Eaglesham Road, Clarkston, Glasgow G76 6BU
Tel: 0141 644 2356 Fax: 0141 644 1721
(NHS Greater Glasgow, Primary Care Division)

GP Irene COLQUHOUN, Fraser MACLEOD

Shettleston Health Centre
Shettleston Health Centre, 420 Old Shettleston Road, Glasgow G32 7JZ
Tel: 0141 531 6250 Fax: 0141 531 6216
(NHS Greater Glasgow, Primary Care Division)
Patient List Size: 4000

GP Animesh Chandra DAS, Nicola MARTIN, Muniyal Aravinda SHETTY, Marjory Frances TAYLOR

Southbank Road Surgery
17-19 Southbank Road, Kirkintilloch, Glasgow G66 1NH
Tel: 0141 776 2183 Fax: 0141 777 8321
(NHS Greater Glasgow, Primary Care Division)

Practice Manager Ann O'Brien

GP Lawrence Malcolm CAMPBELL, Diane Rutherford KELLY, Allison LAW, Isabel McCARLIE, John McKAY, Diane MEEK

Springburn Health Centre
200 Springburn Way, Glasgow G21 1TR
Tel: 0141 531 9631 Fax: 0141 531 9543
(NHS Greater Glasgow, Primary Care Division)

GP John William DONNELLY, Anila Narendra DAVDA, Colin Sinclair Stuart MacKELVIE, Richard Andrew MILBURN

Springburn Health Centre
200 Springburn Way, Glasgow G21 1TR
Tel: 0141 531 9671 Fax: 0141 531 6705
(NHS Greater Glasgow, Primary Care Division)

GP Linda Elsa Kathleen COPELAND, Jean Marie GRAHAM, Dr ROBERTSON

Springburn Health Centre
200 Springburn Way, Glasgow G21 1TR
Tel: 0141 531 9661 Fax: 0141 531 9666
(NHS Greater Glasgow, Primary Care Division)

GP Ronald PATTERSON, Deirdre Patricia O'DRISCOLL, David WATSON

Springburn Health Centre
200 Springburn Way, Glasgow G21 1TR
Tel: 0141 531 9611 Fax: 0141 531 6706
(NHS Greater Glasgow, Primary Care Division)

Practice Manager Ann Zuk

GP Henry Thomson BRUCE, Graeme William BROWN, Anna Frances PETTIGREW

Springburn Health Centre
200 Springburn Way, Glasgow G21 1TR
Tel: 0141 531 9691 Fax: 0141 531 6705
(NHS Greater Glasgow, Primary Care Division)

GP Jean McGiven TURNER, Fiona Ellen HARRIS

Springburn Health Centre
200 Springburn Way, Glasgow G21 1TR
Tel: 0141 531 9600 Fax: 0141 531 9605

(NHS Greater Glasgow, Primary Care Division)

GP Roger T A BOYLE

Springburn Health Centre
200 Springburn Way, Glasgow G21 1TR
Tel: 0141 531 9641 Fax: 0141 531 9642
(NHS Greater Glasgow, Primary Care Division)

GP Dr CANDY, Alison Mary CRON, Colin HOWAT, Mary Pauline McGOWAN, I McKINLAY, Michael Robert McLAUGHLIN

Springburn Health Centre
200 Springburn Way, Glasgow G21 1TR
Tel: 0141 531 9620 Fax: 0141 531 9623
(NHS Greater Glasgow, Primary Care Division)
Patient List Size: 1350

GP Chittaranjan BURMAN

Springfield Medical Practice
9 Springfield Road, Bishopbriggs, Glasgow G64 1PN
Tel: 0141 772 4744 Fax: 0141 772 3035
(NHS Greater Glasgow, Primary Care Division)
Patient List Size: 8140

Practice Manager Irene McChlery

GP Margaret Smith COWAN, Mary EASSON, William Austin JOHNSTONE, Robert MACMILLAN, Gerry MURDOCH

Springfield Road Surgery
86 Springfield Road, Glasgow G40 3ET
Tel: 0141 554 3546
(NHS Greater Glasgow, Primary Care Division)

GP Adnan M AL ZUBAIRI

St George's Medical Centre
137 St George's Road, Glasgow G3 6JB
Tel: 0141 332 5553 Fax: 0141 332 5557
Email: chowdry@gp40441.glasgow.hb.scot.nhs.uk
(NHS Greater Glasgow, Primary Care Division)

GP Akhund S CHOWDRY

Stewartville Street Surgery
5 Stewartville Street, Glasgow G11 5PE
Tel: 0141 339 0902 Fax: 0141 339 0132
Email: administrator@gp40070.glasgow-hb.scot.nhs.uk
(NHS Greater Glasgow, Primary Care Division)
Patient List Size: 1920

Practice Manager Angela Green

GP Joseph Matthew McCONNELL

Struthers and Partners
436 Mosspark Boulevard, Glasgow G52 1HX
Tel: 0141 882 5494 Fax: 0141 883 1015
(NHS Greater Glasgow, Primary Care Division)
Patient List Size: 1100

GP Ian Robertson STRUTHERS

The Surgery
10 Union Street Surgery, York Place, Kirkintilloch, Glasgow G66 1DG
Tel: 0141 776 1273 Fax: 0141 776 4060
(NHS Greater Glasgow, Primary Care Division)
Patient List Size: 2564

Practice Manager Catherine Campbell

GP Kenneth McGlashan MACK

The Surgery
Castlemilk Health Centre, 71 Dougrie Drive, Castlemilk, Glasgow G45 9AW
Tel: 0141 531 8538 Fax: 0141 630 1883
(NHS Greater Glasgow, Primary Care Division)
Patient List Size: 1515

Practice Manager Elizabeth Emslie

GP Purnendu CHAKRABARTI

The Surgery
Calder Street, Blantyre, Glasgow G72 0AU
Tel: 01689 854767
(NHS Lanarkshire, Primary Care Division)

GP C ROWLANDS

The Terrace Medical Practice
160 Drymen Road, Bearsden, Glasgow G61 3RD
Tel: 0141 942 6644 Fax: 0141 942 2210
Email: administrator@gb40027.glasgow-hb.scot.nhs.uk
Website: www.terracemedicalpractice.co.uk
(NHS Greater Glasgow, Primary Care Division)
Patient List Size: 6300

Practice Manager A Downie

GP Robert Daniel LEVY, Brian William RITCHIE, Dr SEFRE, Rona WOTHERSPOON

Thornliebank Health Centre
20 Kennishead Road, Thornliebank, Glasgow G46 8NY
Tel: 0141 531 6979 Fax: 0141 531 6910
(NHS Greater Glasgow, Primary Care Division)

GP Gerard John CANNING, Fiona Campbell DORWARD, Richard Francis QUIGLEY, Iain Wilson WALLACE

Thornliebank Health Centre
20 Kennishead Road, Thornliebank, Glasgow G46 8NY
Tel: 0141 531 6901 Fax: 0141 638 7113
Email: administrator@gp52255.glasgow-hb.scot.nhs.uk
(NHS Greater Glasgow, Primary Care Division)
Patient List Size: 5023

Practice Manager Lorraine Griffiths

GP Yvonne TAYLOR, Iain C McCOLL

Thurston Road Surgery
140 Thurston Road, Glasgow G52 2AZ
Tel: 0141 883 8838 Fax: 0141 810 1511
(NHS Greater Glasgow, Primary Care Division)

GP Jane Alison GORDON, Alasdair Nicolson RITCHIE, Anne Marie Helene WILLIAMS

Tollcross Medical Centre
1101-1105 Tollcross Road, Glasgow G32 8UH
Tel: 0141 778 2717 Fax: 0141 778 2747
(NHS Greater Glasgow, Primary Care Division)
Patient List Size: 5700

Practice Manager Anne Campbell

GP Morag CAMPBELL, Lesley Elizabeth CONNELL, Richard Elliot GRODEN, Rosalind HOPKINS, Keith MERCER

Tollcross Road Surgery
304 Tollcross Road, Tollcross, Glasgow G31 4UR
Tel: 0141 554 0441 Fax: 0141 554 1906
Email: administrator@gp46862.glasgow-hb.scot.nhs.uk
(NHS Greater Glasgow, Primary Care Division)
Patient List Size: 816

GP Khwaja J ABEDIN

Townhead Health Centre
16 Alexandra Parade, Glasgow G31 2ES
Tel: 0141 531 8940 Fax: 0141 531 8935
(NHS Greater Glasgow, Primary Care Division)

Practice Manager Julie Martin

GP Rashid AHMED, Mairi Cameron CASSELS, Caroline Jane DELY, Alan Geoffrey ROLLO

Townhead Health Centre
16 Alexandra Parade, Glasgow G31 2ES
Tel: 0141 531 8972 Fax: 0141 531 8980
(NHS Greater Glasgow, Primary Care Division)

Practice Manager Morag Trench

GP Daniel Patrick McGHEE, Amanda CAMPBELL, Alexander David DOWERS, Owen Christopher McHUGH

Tullis Street Surgery
12-14 Tullis Street, Glasgow G40 1HN
Tel: 0141 531 6595 Fax: 0141 557 3405
(NHS Greater Glasgow, Primary Care Division)

GP Mohammed Abdur RASHID

Turret Medical Centre
3 Catherine Street, Kirkintilloch, Glasgow G66 1JB
Tel: 0141 211 8260 Fax: 0141 211 8264
(NHS Greater Glasgow, Primary Care Division)

GP Narendra S DAVDA, Mary J DEIGHAN, Stuart Gerard McPHEE, Lisa WILLIAMS

Viewpark Health Centre
Burnhead Street, Uddingston, Glasgow G71 5SU
Tel: 01698 813753 Fax: 01698 812062
(NHS Lanarkshire, Primary Care Division)
Patient List Size: 2600

Practice Manager E Aitken

GP Kenneth Alfred RUSSELL, Christine Anne YOUNG

Waverley Park Practice
19 Dinmont Road, Shawlands, Glasgow G41 3UJ
Tel: 0141 632 8883 Fax: 0141 636 0654
(NHS Greater Glasgow, Primary Care Division)
Patient List Size: 4600

Practice Manager Lesley Ann Dowens

GP Grace BALLANTYNE, Ronald Alexander FAIRWEATHER, Paul NEWMAN

Westmuir Medical Centre
109 Crail Street, Glasgow G31 5RA
Tel: 0141 554 4253 Fax: 0141 550 0177
(NHS Greater Glasgow, Primary Care Division)

Practice Manager P Sennauth

GP Nadeem BHATTI, Yasin MOHAMMED

Whitevale Medical Group
30 Whitevale Street, Glasgow G31 1QS
Tel: 0141 554 4536 Fax: 0141 554 3979
(NHS Greater Glasgow, Primary Care Division)

Practice Manager Sheila Waddell

GP Roger Anthony Lester BLACK, Roger J HARDMAN, Lee Gek TEH

Williamwood Practice
Williamwood Medical Centre, 85 Seres Road, Clarkston, Glasgow G76 7NW
Tel: 0141 620 0333 Fax: 0141 638 8827
Email: williamwood_practice@hotmail.com
Website: www.williamwood.co.uk
(NHS Greater Glasgow, Primary Care Division)
Patient List Size: 4900

Practice Manager Christine Sneddon

GP Helen Nicola GILMOUR, Moya Helen KELLY, Lesley Norah Margaret MACKINTOSH, Nigel Frederick PEXTON

Woodeside Health Centre
Barr Street, Glasgow G20 7LR
Tel: 0141 531 9570 Fax: 0141 531 9572
(NHS Greater Glasgow, Primary Care Division)
Patient List Size: 5300

Practice Manager John McIldowie

GP Graham David WEBSTER, Carol Ann SMITH, Stewart James WHYTE

Woodside Health Centre
Barr Street, Glasgow G20 7LR
Tel: 0141 531 9585 Fax: 0141 531 9339
(NHS Greater Glasgow, Primary Care Division)
Patient List Size: 2050

Practice Manager Duncan Elder

GP Susan Jane LANGRIDGE

Woodside Health Centre
Barr Street, Glasgow G20 7LR
Tel: 0141 531 9510 Fax: 0141 531 9515
(NHS Greater Glasgow, Primary Care Division)

Practice Manager Joy Carswell

GP Alastair John MUIR

Woodside Health Centre
Barr Street, Glasgow G20 7LR
Tel: 0141 531 9556 Fax: 0141 531 9555
(NHS Greater Glasgow, Primary Care Division)

Practice Manager Alex Harris

GP Barnet Melvyn GLEKIN, Louis Allan GLEKIN, David Findlay SUTHERLAND

Woodside Health Centre
Barr Street, Glasgow G20 7LR
Tel: 0141 531 9560 Fax: 0141 531 9572
(NHS Greater Glasgow, Primary Care Division)
Patient List Size: 4500

GP Graham Hamilton LOVE, Sheila Mary LAWRIE, Gillian LESLIE

Woodside Health Centre
Barr Street, Glasgow G20 7LR
Tel: 0141 531 9530 Fax: 0141 331 9545
(NHS Greater Glasgow, Primary Care Division)

Practice Manager Marie Furey

GP Albert Edward BURTON, Wilma RENFREW

Woodside Health Centre
Barr Street, Glasgow G20 7LR
Tel: 0141 531 9507 Fax: 0141 531 9509
(NHS Greater Glasgow, Primary Care Division)

Practice Manager Kathleen Diamond

GP David James ESLER, Norman James GAW

Woodside Health Centre
Barr Street, Glasgow G20 7LR
Tel: 0141 531 9521 Fax: 0141 531 9545
(NHS Greater Glasgow, Primary Care Division)
Patient List Size: 5900

Practice Manager J Harris

GP John Francis MULHEARN, Patricia Agnes FITZSIMONS, Geraldine Mary KELLY, Gerard Patrick WEST

Woodside Health Centre
Barr Street, Glasgow G20 7LR
Tel: 0141 531 9200
(NHS Greater Glasgow, Primary Care Division)

GP Thomas Stuart MURRAY

York Place Surgery
12 Union Street, Kirkintilloch, Glasgow G66 1DG
Tel: 0141 776 2468 Fax: 0141 775 3341
Email: administrator@gp43345.glasgow-hb.scot.nhs.uk
(NHS Greater Glasgow, Primary Care Division)
Patient List Size: 3000

Practice Manager Grace Wilson

GP Marion Elizabeth Bolton BUCHANAN, Hilary Gregg MELROSE, Douglas J MURPHY

Glenrothes

Cos Lane Medical Practice
Woodside Road, Glenrothes KY7 4AQ
Tel: 01592 752100 Fax: 01592 612692
(NHS Fife, Primary Care Division)
Patient List Size: 10000

Practice Manager Jim McAllister

GP Iain Milne McBRIDE, Duncan BROWN, Chris CONLON, Norman Gilbert MacDIARMID, Douglas SCOTT, Jacqueline SMITH, Helen Suzanne SOPPITT, Anne Margaret THOMPSON

Glenwood Health Centre
Napier Road, Glenrothes KY6 1HL
Tel: 01592 611171 Fax: 01592 611931
(NHS Fife, Primary Care Division)
Patient List Size: 5400

Practice Manager Jacqueline Wilson

GP Catherine Grace COLLIE, Martyn Keith CLAYTON, Malcolm Kenneth HEELES, Jonathan MacGregor PAISLEY

The Lomond Practice
Napier Road, Glenrothes KY6 1HL
Tel: 01592 611000 Fax: 01592 611639
(NHS Fife, Primary Care Division)
Patient List Size: 8000

Practice Manager E Smollett

GP Susanne BOYCE, Robert Granger CAMPBELL, Cecilia Helen DOWNIE, George Mark GORDON, Samir Youssef ISKANDER

Markinch Medical Practice
Markinch Health Centre, 19 High Street, Markinch, Glenrothes KY7 6ER
Tel: 01592 610640 Fax: 01592 761080
(NHS Fife, Primary Care Division)
Patient List Size: 5350

Practice Manager Anthony Routledge

GP Harold STEWART, David ANDERSON, Helen HELLEWELL, Niall HYNDMAN

North Glen Medical Practice
1 Huntsmans Court, Glenrothes KY7 6SX
Tel: 01592 620062 Fax: 01592 620465
(NHS Fife, Primary Care Division)

Practice Manager P Moir

GP Bangarpet Ramarao KRISHNASWAMY, Mohammed Faisal Mohammed FAWZI, Doris Sarah Te-Yung MACLEOD, John Hartley McELHINNEY, Dr MICHAEL, Robert Chapman Gibson ROBERTSON

Rothes Medical Practice
Glamis Centre, Glenrothes KY7 4RH
Tel: 01592 771177 Fax: 01592 631208
(NHS Fife, Primary Care Division)
Patient List Size: 8400

Practice Manager Anne McCormick

GP John Malcolm BELL, B Elaine CARLYLE, David L CARLYLE, Ginette FERGUSON, John Perryman GALLOWAY, Niall GARVEY

The Surgery
Anderson Drive, Leslie, Glenrothes KY6 3LQ
Tel: 01592 620222 Fax: 01592 620553
(NHS Fife, Primary Care Division)

Practice Manager C Laing

GP John Alexander MILNE, William Duncan CARR, Fiona Marie DE SOYZA, Frank Andrew REGLINSKI

Golspie

Golspie Medical Practice
Golspie KW10 6TH
Tel: 01408 633221/633444 Fax: 01408 633303
Email: administrator@gp55220.highland-hb.scot.nhs.uk
(NHS Highland, Primary Care)
Patient List Size: 2040

Practice Manager Angela MacBeath

GP Alister Brims BEGG, Ernest R MILLARD

Gorebridge

Newbyres Medical Group
Gorebridge Health Centre, 15 Hunterfield Road, Gorebridge EH23 4TP
Tel: 01875 820405 Fax: 01875 820269
(NHS Lothian, Primary and Community Division)
Patient List Size: 8200

Practice Manager Su Boyd

GP Elizabeth Anne MATEAR, Marion Pettigrew STORRIE, Andrew CREMONA, M PEAT, Elizabeth Anna SCALES

Gourock

Gourock Health Centre
181 Shore Street, Gourock PA19 1AQ
Tel: 01475 634617 Fax: 01475 636009
(NHS Argyll and Clyde, Renfrewshire and Inverclyde Community Services Division)

GP Robert MURRAY-LYON, Jane ADAMS, David BLAIR, James CRAIG, David RUSSELL

Grangemouth

Bo'ness Road Medical Practice
31-33 Bo'ness Road, Grangemouth FK3 8AN
Tel: 01324 482653
(NHS Forth Valley, Primary Care Operating Division)

GP Brian George ANDERSON, Gregor CRAWFORD, Leslie James William CRUICKSHANK, Allyson de Voy GAWN, Ian Brown MURDOCH

Grange Medical Group
21A Kersiebank Avenue, Grangemouth FK3 9EL
Tel: 01324 665533 Fax: 01324 665693
(NHS Forth Valley, Primary Care Operating Division)

GP Ian Robert HAMILTON, Bakrabile Dinkar HEGDE, Jennifer Anne LIM, Duncan Roy MURRAY

Group Medical Practice
Kersiebank Avenue, Grangemouth FK3 9EL
Tel: 01324 471511
(NHS Forth Valley, Primary Care Operating Division)

GP David Ian SELFRIDGE, Donald Ingram BALLANTINE, John Grant DUGGIE

Grantown-on-Spey

Grantown-on-Spey Health Centre
Castle Road East, Grantown-on-Spey PH26 3HR
Tel: 01479 872484 Fax: 01479 873503
(NHS Highland, Primary Care)

Practice Manager Marilyn Neal

GP Frances Watt BURNS, Peter Francis GRANT, Stephen Bruce MATHERS, Samuel Boyd PETERS, Lesley Kathryn PIRIE

Greenock

Ardgowan Medical Practice
2 Finnart Street, Greenock PA16 8HW
Tel: 01475 888155 Fax: 01475 785060
(NHS Argyll and Clyde, Renfrewshire and Inverclyde Community Services Division)
Patient List Size: 9500

Practice Manager Angela Owens

GP Patrick BARR, Anne PETTIGREW, Alan DICKSON, Owen GALLAGHER, Robert GRAY, Eleanor HAMILTON

Balmer and Partners
Greenock Health Centre, 20 Duncan Street, Greenock PA15 4LY
Tel: 01475 724477 Fax: 01475 727140
(NHS Argyll and Clyde, Renfrewshire and Inverclyde Community Services Division)
Patient List Size: 4965

Practice Manager Rosemary Nolan

GP Francis Joseph BALMER, Geraldine Marie MACNAB, Robert Craig SPEIRS, James Peter WARD

Blyth and Partners
Greenock Health Centre, 20 Duncan Street, Greenock PA15 4LY
Tel: 01475 724477 Fax: 01475 727140
(NHS Argyll and Clyde, Renfrewshire and Inverclyde Community Services Division)
Patient List Size: 7620

Practice Manager Phyllis M Arthur

GP Angus Campbell BLYTH, William Barber HENDERSON, Brian Andrew KERR, Anne RUTHERFORD, Glen Campbell SYKES

Campbell and Partners
Greenock Health Centre, 20 Duncan Street, Greenock PA15 4LY
Tel: 01475 724477 Fax: 01475 727140
(NHS Argyll and Clyde, Renfrewshire and Inverclyde Community Services Division)

GP Andrew MALLOCH, Ian CAMPBELL, Sheila FISHER, William McNEIL, Aileen ROSS, Judith SEMPLE

Foster and Partners
Greenock Health Centre, 20 Duncan Street, Greenock PA15 4LY
Tel: 01475 724477 Fax: 01475 731244
(NHS Argyll and Clyde, Renfrewshire and Inverclyde Community Services Division)

Practice Manager Mary Lynn

GP Douglas FOSTER, Alan HULME

Kapasi
Greenock Health Centre, 20 Duncan Street, Greenock PA15 4LY
Tel: 01475 724477 Fax: 01475 723450
(NHS Argyll and Clyde, Renfrewshire and Inverclyde Community Services Division)
Patient List Size: 3440

Practice Manager Hilda McLeese

GP Mustafa KAPASI, Isabella HOGAN, Francis J PALMER

Thompson and Partners
Greenock Health Centre, 20 Duncan Street, Greenock PA15 4LY
Tel: 01475 724477 Fax: 01475 731697
(NHS Argyll and Clyde, Renfrewshire and Inverclyde Community Services Division)
Patient List Size: 6400

GP Alan J BARTHOLOMEW, John Brian THOMPSON, M KOHLHAGEN

Wing F Group Medical Practice
Greenock Health Centre, 20 Duncan Street, Greenock PA15 4LY
Tel: 01475 724477 Fax: 01475 727140
(NHS Argyll and Clyde, Renfrewshire and Inverclyde Community Services Division)
Patient List Size: 76100

Practice Manager Margaret C House

GP Kenneth Andrew HAGGERTY, Nripren GANAI, Andrew GIBSON, Kathleen McGARRITY, Susan McKINNON, Ruth WARD

Wing F Group Medical Practice
Greenock Health Centre, 20 Duncan Street, Greenock PA15 4LY
Tel: 01475 724477 Fax: 01475 656187
(NHS Argyll and Clyde, Renfrewshire and Inverclyde Community Services Division)
Patient List Size: 4700

Practice Manager Margaret House, Janice McCulloch

GP Kenneth Andrew HAGGERTY, N K GANAI, Andrew GIBSON, Kathleen McGARRITY, Susan McKINNON, R WARD

Gretna

The Surgery
Central Avenue, Gretna DG16 5NA
Tel: 01461 338317 Fax: 01461 339244
Email: administrator@718428dghb.scot.nhs.uk

The Surgery
Central Avenue, Gretna DG16 5NA
Tel: 01461 338317 Fax: 01461 339244
Email: administrator@718428dghb.scot.nhs.uk
(NHS Dumfries and Galloway; NHS Dumfries and Galloway)
Patient List Size: 4437
Patient List Size: 4437

GP Philip Richard HERRICK, Philip Richard HERRICK, Alastair William RIGG, Alastair William RIGG, Shirley McLean STENHOUSE, Shirley McLean STENHOUSE

Gullane

Broadgait Green
Broadgait Green, Gullane EH31 2DW
Tel: 01620 842171 Fax: 01620 843020
(NHS Lothian, Primary and Community Division)

Practice Manager Elma Wood

GP Charles James CUSWORTH, Agnes Wallace DURIE, Andrew SMITH

Haddington

Drs Langlands, Holton and Wright
Newton Port, Haddington EH41 3NF
Tel: 01620 825051 Fax: 01620 824622
(NHS Lothian, Primary and Community Division)

Practice Manager Marion Bisset

GP Ross William Duff LANGLANDS, Diana Elizabeth HOLTON, Henry William WRIGHT

Newton Port Surgery
Newton Port, Haddington EH41 3NF
Tel: 01620 823183 Fax: 01620 824622
(NHS Lothian, Primary and Community Division)
Patient List Size: 5500

Practice Manager Carol Orr

GP Graham ALEXANDER, Peter Douglas HASTINGS, C MILES, Fionn Mary Mercer NAIRN, L WILSON

The Surgery
Newton Port, Haddington EH41 3NF
Tel: 01620 825497 Fax: 01620 824622
(NHS Lothian, Primary and Community Division)

Practice Manager Janis Gill

GP Sheila Mary Rose GLENDINNING, James Finlay FULTON, Vera Jane HOGG, Robert James LAWSON

Hamilton

Burnbank Medical Centre
18 Burnbank Road, Hamilton ML3 0NQ
Tel: 01698 286555 Fax: 01698 286686
(NHS Lanarkshire, Primary Care Division)
Patient List Size: 7400

Practice Manager Claire Murdoch

GP David Stevenson MATHIE, Joseph Scott HACKETT, Lorna MARSHALL, Robert TOBIN

Cadzow Health Centre
187 Low Waters Road, Hamilton ML3 7QQ
Tel: 01698 327028 Fax: 01698 327344
(NHS Lanarkshire, Primary Care Division)
Patient List Size: 4100

Practice Manager Anne Bonnyman

GP Peter John Marian BARTON, Gillian DAMES, Sharon Lesley RUSSELL

Douglas Street Surgery
1 Douglas Street, Hamilton ML3 0DR
Tel: 01698 286262 Fax: 01698 283367
(NHS Lanarkshire, Primary Care Division)
Patient List Size: 6809

GP William Morrison YOUNG, Lorna Margaret HAMILTON, John Alexander Matheson HANNAH, Sheila Catherine SMYTH

Low Waters Medical Centre
11 Mill Road, Hamilton ML3 8AA
Tel: 01698 283626 Fax: 01698 282839
(NHS Lanarkshire, Primary Care Division)
Patient List Size: 7352

Practice Manager Veronica Travers

GP David Allan BROWN, C CAVOURA, Douglas Stuart NAISMITH, J M SIMPSON

Oak Lodge Surgery
32 Miller Street, Hamilton ML3 7EN
Tel: 01698 282350 Fax: 01698 282502
(NHS Lanarkshire, Primary Care Division)
Patient List Size: 6800

Practice Manager Lorna Dalziel, Phyllis Gilroy

GP David Rowatt BROWN, Kirsten HENDERSON, David McCRUM, Mark Eian PATERSON

Portland Park Medical Centre
51 Portland Park, Hamilton ML3 7JY
Tel: 01698 284353 Fax: 01698 891101
(NHS Lanarkshire, Primary Care Division)
Patient List Size: 6677

Practice Manager H Neilson

GP David Thompson DOBBIE, Pamela CRAWFORD, Alasdair GRAHAM, Murray MacRae HERBERT

The Surgery
53 Burnbank Road, Hamilton ML3 9AQ
Tel: 01698 281407 Fax: 01698 286004
(NHS Lanarkshire, Primary Care Division)
Patient List Size: 8500

Practice Manager Patricia Coggans

GP Desmond BANCEWICZ, Kevin Gerard IRVINE, Brian Robert LYNAS, C S NAIR

Wellhall Medical Centre
4 Hillhouse Road, Hamilton ML3 9TZ
Tel: 01698 285818
(NHS Lanarkshire, Primary Care Division)
Patient List Size: 9437

GP Anthony Weldon BABOOLAL, James McLellan FULTON, Roderick Kerr McLAY, James McKellar SANDILANDS, Gillian Anne TWEDDELL

Hawick

O'Connell Street Medical Practice
6 O'Connell Street, Hawick TD9 9HU
Tel: 01450 372276 Fax: 01450 371564
(NHS Borders, Primary Care Division)
Patient List Size: 6930

Practice Manager Christine Scott

GP Geoffrey M J ROSS, Graeme BIANCHI, Linda Margaret BRUCE, John Maxwell MACDONALD, Emma WOLFENDEN

Teviot Medical Practice
Hawick Health Centre, Teviot Road, Hawick TD9 9DT
Tel: 01450 370999 Fax: 01450 371025
Email: administrator@teviot.borders.nhs.uk
(NHS Borders, Primary Care Division)
Patient List Size: 11200

Practice Manager Margaret Landles

GP Charles H OLIVER, Rachel BOON, Catherine S C ELLIOTT, Jonathon KIRK, Paul LOCKIE, Patrick G C MANSON, Lesley MORRISON, Alistair A PALMER, Douglas M ROLLAND

Helensburgh

Calder
12 East King Street, Helensburgh G84 7QL
Tel: 01436 673366
Email: administrator@gp85141.ac-hb.scot.nhs.uk
(NHS Argyll and Clyde, Lomond and Argyll Community Services Division)
Patient List Size: 10373

Practice Manager Alice Ball

GP Brian Downie CALDER

Doyle and Falconer
The Surgery, Shore Road, Kilcreggan, Helensburgh G84 0JL
Tel: 01436 842156 Fax: 01436 842259
(NHS Argyll and Clyde, Lomond and Argyll Community Services Division)
Patient List Size: 2750

Practice Manager Susan Aitchison

GP Anthony John DOYLE

The Medical Centre
Feorlin Way, Garelochhead, Helensburgh G84 0DG
Tel: 01436 810370 Fax: 01436 810909
(NHS Argyll and Clyde, Lomond and Argyll Community Services Division)

Practice Manager Alison Holland

GP Charles BROWN, James McKELVIE

The Medical Centre
12 East King Street, Helensburgh G84 7QL
Tel: 01436 672277 Fax: 01436 674526
(NHS Argyll and Clyde, Lomond and Argyll Community Services Division)

Practice Manager Morag Philips

GP Wendy FLATMAN, Catherine MACLEOD, Brian McLACHLAN, Alison RAM, John ROBIN, Kim STARK

Medical Centre
12 East King Street, Helensburgh G84 7QL
Tel: 01436 673366 Fax: 01436 679715
(NHS Argyll and Clyde, Lomond and Argyll Community Services Division)
Patient List Size: 10055

Practice Manager Alice Bell

GP Brian Downie CALDER, William Roger Harron BROWN, Margaret Elizabeth Evans MORRISON, Teresa REITANO, Elizabeth UNDERWOOD, Alastair George WOODBURN

Helmsdale

Helmsdale Health Centre
Rockview Place, Helmsdale KW8 6LF
Tel: 01431 821225 Fax: 01431 821567
(NHS Highland, Primary Care)
Patient List Size: 700

Practice Manager M Mitchell

GP M MAIN, M FORTUNE, W STRAUSS

Huntly

Aberchirder Medical Practice
The Surgery, Parkview, Aberchirder, Huntly AB54 7SW
Tel: 01466 780213 Fax: 01466 780580
Email: administrator@aberchirder.grampian.scot.nhs.uk
(NHS Grampian, Primary Care Division)
Patient List Size: 2300

Practice Manager Aileen Wilson

GP Robin Alix Bronte GATENBY, Kathleen Anne LYONS

Bydand Medical Group
Jubilee Hospital, Bleachfield Street, Huntly AB54 8EX
Tel: 01466 792116 Fax: 01466 794699
Email: administrator@huntly.grampion.scot.nhs.uk
(NHS Grampian, Primary Care Division)
Patient List Size: 300

Practice Manager Jackie Elvidge

GP Eileen Elizabeth COSGROVE, Gordon CARTER, David Alan Halliday EASTON, Dominic HORNE, R KIT, Barry WATT

Rhynie Medical Practice
Manse Road, Rhynie, Huntly AB54 4WA
Tel: 01464 861271 Fax: 01464 861486
(NHS Grampian, Primary Care Division)
Patient List Size: 1100

Practice Manager Kate Hunter

GP Graham Stewart GORDON, K E SCHRADER

Innerleithen

St Ronan's Health Centre
Angle Park, Innerleithen EH44 6QE
Tel: 01896 830203 Fax: 01896 831202
(NHS Borders, Primary Care Division)
Patient List Size: 4000

Practice Manager Margaret Blyth

GP Robert Loudon CUMMING, Frances SOUTTER, Gregor WATT

Insch

Insch Health Centre
Rannes Street, Insch AB52 6JJ
Tel: 01464 821500 Fax: 01464 821527
(NHS Grampian, Primary Care Division)

Practice Manager Lorraine Simpson

GP George Mitchell MORRICE, Douglas Michael KAY, K SIMPSON, Stephen James TEAL

Inveraray

The Surgery
Furnace, Inveraray PA32 8XN
Tel: 01499 500207
(NHS Argyll and Clyde, Lomond and Argyll Community Services Division)
Patient List Size: 1270

Practice Manager Rajinder Kaur Bijral

GP Keval BIJRAL

Inverkeithing

Inverkeithing Medical Group
5 Friary Court, Inverkeithing KY11 1NU
Tel: 01383 413234 Fax: 01383 427527
(NHS Fife, Primary Care Division)
Patient List Size: 18385

Practice Manager Diana Hamilton

GP Kenneth Brian RITCHIE, John James ALLAN, Allan Johnstone COCHRANE, Dr DONALDSON, Lesley Elizabeth DUNCAN, Dr GARMANY, Maan JALIL, Mary Ringrose LAPRAIK, Dr LEE, John PHILLIPS, Dr SHEEHAN, Dr SOMERVILLE, David McIntyre TAYLOR

Inverness

Adlarich Medical Practices
Ardlarich, 15 Culduthel Road, Inverness IV2 4AG
Tel: 01463 712233 Fax: 01463 240541
(NHS Highland, Primary Care)

Practice Manager M H Farr

GP Ian Robertson SMITH, Ruth Janet GILMOUR, Jeremiah Gerard O'ROURKE, Alexander Buchan THAIN, Joanne Clare WILSON

Adlarich Medical Practices
Ardlarich, 15 Culduthel Road, Inverness IV2 4AG
Tel: 01463 712233 Fax: 01463 240541
(NHS Highland, Primary Care)

Practice Manager M H Farr

GP Ronald MacVICAR, A MACIVER, Keith WYCLIFFE-JONES

Adlarich Medical Practices
Ardlarich, 15 Culduthel Road, Inverness IV2 4AG
Tel: 01463 712233 Fax: 01463 240541
(NHS Highland, Primary Care)

Practice Manager M H Farr

GP Michael James Peter MACPHERSON, Shona Roseanne HAGGERTY

Ardersier Medical Practice
142 Manse Road, Ardersier, Inverness IV2 7SR
Tel: 01667 462240 Fax: 01667 462912
(NHS Highland, Primary Care)

GP Jonathan Lewis BALL, Linsey Margaret BALL, Helen S PIKE

Balmacaan Road Surgery
Balmacaan Road, Drumnadrochit, Inverness IV63 6UR
Tel: 01456 450577 Fax: 01456 450799
Email: hmacdonald@gp55728.highland-hb.scot.nhs.uk
Website: www.nhsscotland.com/dmp
(NHS Highland, Primary Care)
Patient List Size: 2122

GP Peter Richard WILKES, Pik CHUN, Anne ROSSER, Duncan Edward THOM, Amanda WALKER

Burnfield Medical Practice
Harris Road, Inverness IV2 3PF
Tel: 01463 220077 Fax: 01463 714588
(NHS Highland, Primary Care)
Patient List Size: 3786

Practice Manager Ishbel MacDonald

GP Freda Kelman CHARTERS, John McFADDEN, Tilman VON DIELFT

Crown Avenue Surgery
12 Crown Avenue, Inverness IV2 3NF
Tel: 01463 710777 Fax: 01463 714511
(NHS Highland, Primary Care)

Practice Manager Francis Russell

GP Henry Ian McNAMARA, Iain Cairns RUSSELL, Hilary Margaret Christine STRACHAN, John Fraser SWEENIE

Culloden Medical Practice
Keppoch Road, Culloden, Inverness IV2 7LL
Tel: 01463 793777 Fax: 01463 792143
(NHS Highland, Primary Care)
Patient List Size: 4019

Practice Manager A MacKenzie, R Philip

GP Donald MacVICAR, Claire Julie ENNIS, Roderick Samuel MACLEOD, A SNOW

Culloden Surgery
Keppoch Road, Culloden, Inverness IV2 7LL
Tel: 01463 793400 Fax: 01463 793060
(NHS Highland, Primary Care)

Practice Manager Charlotte Leggatt

GP Calum URQUHART, Jean Alison ALEXANDER, Christina Isabella CHANCELLOR, H MACDONALD

Fairfield Medical Practice
22A Abban Street, Inverness IV3 8HH
Tel: 01463 713939 Fax: 01463 667860
Email: fairfieldsurgery@tesco.net
(NHS Highland, Primary Care)
Patient List Size: 4300

Practice Manager Marie Scicluna

GP John Robert MARTIN, Diane MALONE, William Alexander ROSS

Foyers Medical Centre
Foyers, Inverness IV2 6YB
Tel: 01456 486224 Fax: 01456 486425
(NHS Highland, Primary Care)

GP Gregor James MACKINTOSH, Lesley Elizabeth MACKINTOSH

Kingsmills Medical Practice
18 Southside Road, Inverness IV2 3BG
Tel: 01463 235245 Fax: 01463 714400
(NHS Highland, Primary Care)

Practice Manager Caron Morrison

GP Carol Ann BROWN, Neil William GILLIES, Brian Neil MACLEAN, Susan Kathleen MACLEOD, Malcolm John MACRAE, M L TAYLOR

Kinmylies Medical Practice
Assynt Road, Kinmylies, Inverness IV3 8PB
Tel: 01463 239865 Fax: 01463 711218
Email: administrator@gp.55860.highland-hb.scot.nhs.uk
Website: www.surgeriesonline.com/kinmyliesmp
(NHS Highland, Primary Care)
Patient List Size: 2638

Practice Manager Moira MacRae

GP Anthony Derek SMITH, Christine McLeod MARTIN

The Medical Centre
Foyers, Inverness IV2 6YB
Tel: 01456 486224 Fax: 01456 486425
Email: administrator@gp.highland-hb.scot.nhs.uk
(NHS Highland, Primary Care)

GP G J MACKINTOSH, L E MACKINTOSH

Riverside Medical Practice
Ballifeary Lane, Ness Walk, Inverness IV3 5PW
Tel: 01463 715999 Fax: 01463 718763
(NHS Highland, Primary Care)

GP Ingrid Catherine FERGUSON, Andrea HENDERSON, Iain KENNEDY, John KENNEDY, Philip Andrew KILN, Sally MARTIN, Adam Iain Cameron SYME

Southside Road Surgery
43 Southside Road, Inverness IV2 4XA
Tel: 01463 710222 Fax: 01463 714072
(NHS Highland, Primary Care)

GP Christopher John JONES, Constance Anne GRIFFITHS, Ian Graham SCOTT, Agnes Dykes STRUTHERS

Inverurie

Inverurie Medical Group
Health Centre, 1 Constitution Street, Inverurie AB51 4SU
Tel: 01467 621345 Fax: 01467 625374
(NHS Grampian, Primary Care Division)

Practice Manager Doreen Restall

GP James Alexander Gordon BEATTIE, James Elder BLACK, Sally Marianne HARKNESS, David Blair HOOD, Victor William JOHNSTON, Fiona Margaret Anne McKAY, David George Alexander RUTLEDGE

Kemnay Medical Group
High Street, Kemnay, Inverurie AB51 5NB
Tel: 01467 642289 Fax: 01467 643100
Email: administrator@kemnay.grampian.scot.nhs.uk
(NHS Grampian, Primary Care Division)
Patient List Size: 6200

Practice Manager Marjorie Gordon

GP Graham YOUNG, Janet DEAN, Paul GREEN, David Stanton HAWSON, Karen LEFEVRE, Helen Noel MACK

Oldmeldrum Medical Centre
The Meadows, Oldmeldrum, Inverurie AB51 0BF
Tel: 01651 872239 Fax: 01651 872968
(NHS Grampian, Primary Care Division)
Patient List Size: 6500

Practice Manager S Yule

GP R M WALLACE, D G CONNELL, S B ROBERTSON, C WATSON, T D WILSON

Irvine

Bourtreehill Medical Practice
Cheviot Way, Bourtreehill South, Irvine KA11 1JU
Tel: 01294 211993 Fax: 01294 218461
Email: Bourtreehill.admin@aapct.scot.nhs.uk
Website: www.bourtreehillmedicalpractice.co.uk
(NHS Ayrshire and Arran, Community Health Division)
Patient List Size: 8000

Practice Manager R C Faulks

GP Robert Michael WAGNER, Barbara Kathleen ALEXANDER, William David CAMPBELL, Colin Patterson JOHNSTON, Jagbir NELSON

Eglinton Medical Practice
The Cabins, Ayrshire Central Hospital, Kilwinning Road, Irvine KA12 8ST
Tel: 01294 279178 Fax: 01294 313095
(NHS Ayrshire and Arran, Community Health Division)
Patient List Size: 4500

Practice Manager Anne McGunnigle

GP Satyesh C SHARMA, Iain JAMIESON, Lindsay Marian PARK

Frew Terrace Surgery
9 Frew Terrace, Irvine KA12 9DY
Tel: 01294 272326 Fax: 01294 312614
(NHS Ayrshire and Arran, Community Health Division)

Practice Manager Marioin McCallum

GP Gerard Joseph McSHERRY, David CUNNINGHAM, Paul KERR, P MACKAY, Catriona McHUGH, D McNAB, Garry WALKER

Townhead Surgery
Townhead Surgery, 6-8 High St., Irvine KA12 0AY
Tel: 01294 273131 Fax: 01294 312832
Email: enquiries@townleadsurgery.co.uk
Website: www.townleadsurgery.com
(NHS Ayrshire and Arran, Community Health Division)
Patient List Size: 16710

Practice Manager Alison Douglas

GP James Peter Stephen McELHONE, H SIMPSON, James Alexander CAMPBELL, Martin Frank DOIG, Charles Ewing MACDONALD, R MELVILLE, Alexander Allan NIXON, Susan Gillian RUSSELL, Amanda Jane STIRLING, Alison Jane TURNER, Andrea Flynn WARDELL

Isle of Benbecula

Benbecula Medical Practice

Griminish Surgery, Griminish, Isle of Benbecula HS7 5QA
Tel: 01870 602215 Fax: 01870 602630
(NHS Western Isles)
Patient List Size: 2500

Practice Manager Sheena Mackinnon

GP Susannah Katharine DAWSON, Mark JOHNSON, Andrew John SENIOR, Francis TIERNEY

Isle of Coll

Coll Medical Practice

Aringour, Isle of Coll PA78 6SY
Tel: 01879 230326 Fax: 01879 230418
Email: mbshb@aol.com
(NHS Argyll and Clyde, Lomond and Argyll Community Services Division)
Patient List Size: 160

Practice Manager Alison McVey

GP Michael BOYLE

Isle of Colonsay

The Surgery

Benoran, Isle of Colonsay PA61 7YW
Tel: 01951 200328 Fax: 01951 200328
Email: drjohncurrie@yahoo.com
(NHS Argyll and Clyde, Lomond and Argyll Community Services Division)

Practice Manager Marion Main

GP John CURRIE

Isle of Eigg

Small Isles Medical Practice

Grianan, Isle of Eigg PH42 4RL
Tel: 01687 482427 Fax: 01687 482415
Email: rachelweldon@cs.com
(NHS Highland, Primary Care)
Patient List Size: 160

Practice Manager Eileen Ferguson

GP Rachel H WELDON

Isle of Islay

Geirhilda Surgery

Geirhilda, Back Street, Port Ellen, Isle of Islay PA42 7DR
Tel: 01496 302103 Fax: 01496 302112
(NHS Argyll and Clyde, Lomond and Argyll Community Services Division)
Patient List Size: 1320

Practice Manager Kay Whitelaw

GP Jean Mary KNOWLES

The Rhinns Medical Centre

Port Charlotte, Isle of Islay PA48 7UD
Tel: 01496 850210 Fax: 01496 850511
(NHS Argyll and Clyde, Lomond and Argyll Community Services Division)

Practice Manager Gill Chasemore

GP Grace GIBSON, Kitty WATT

The Rhinns Medical Centre

Port Charlotte, Isle of Islay PA48 7UD
Tel: 01496 850210 Fax: 01496 850511
Patient List Size: 900

Practice Manager Gill Chasemore

GP Grace GIBSON, Kitty WATT

The Surgery, Windsor

Main Street, Bowmore, Isle of Islay PA43 7JH
Tel: 01496 810273 Fax: 01496 810607
(NHS Argyll and Clyde, Lomond and Argyll Community Services Division)
Patient List Size: 1265

GP David LATTA

Isle of Jura

Glencairn Surgery

Glencairn, Craighouse, Isle of Jura PA60 7XG
Tel: 01496 820218 Fax: 01496 820111
(NHS Argyll and Clyde, Lomond and Argyll Community Services Division)
Patient List Size: 180

Practice Manager Fiona McChee

GP L B HAWKER, E HOLLOWAY

Isle of Lewis

North Lochs Medical Practice

Surgery, Levcbost, Lochs, Isle of Lewis HS2 9JP
Tel: 01851 860222 Fax: 01851 860611
(NHS Western Isles)
Patient List Size: 1890

Practice Manager Chris Macaulay

GP Laura Scott MARSHALL, David Jeffrey RIGBY

Pairc Medical Centre

The Surgery, Gravir, Isle of Lewis HS2 9QX
Tel: 01851 880272 Fax: 01851 880201
(NHS Western Isles)
Patient List Size: 390

Practice Manager Susan Barker

GP Jack Anthony BARKER

The Surgery

Upper Carloway, Isle of Lewis HS2 9AG
Tel: 01851 643333 Fax: 01851 643293
Email: administrator@gp90026.wihb.scot.nhs.uk
(NHS Western Isles)
Patient List Size: 1175

GP John SMITH, B ECHAUARRAN

The Surgery

Miaraig, Uig, Isle of Lewis HS2 9HE
Tel: 01851 672283 Fax: 01851 672233
(NHS Western Isles)

GP Colin Alexander MACDONALD

Isle of Mull

Rockfield Road Surgery

Rockfield Road, Tobermory, Isle of Mull PA75 6PN
Tel: 01688 302013 Fax: 01688 302092
(NHS Argyll and Clyde, Lomond and Argyll Community Services Division)
Patient List Size: 1403

Practice Manager Joanne MacPhail

GP Jennifer JACK, Victor LINNEMANN

Salen Surgery

Pier Road, Salen, Aros, Isle of Mull PA72 6JL
Tel: 01680 300327 Fax: 01680 300312
(NHS Argyll and Clyde, Lomond and Argyll Community Services Division)

GP Anthony CHARLIER

The Surgery
Bunessan, Isle of Mull PA67 6DG
Tel: 01681 700261 Fax: 01681 700261
(NHS Argyll and Clyde, Lomond and Argyll Community Services Division)

GP Maureen DOUGLAS, Louise McADAM

Isle of Skye

Broadford Medical Practice
High Road, Broadford, Isle of Skye IV49 9AA
Tel: 01471 822460 Fax: 01471 822860
(NHS Highland, Primary Care)
Patient List Size: 1860

GP Alasdair CLARK, Helen JOHNSON, Helen STEWART, Cameron TALLACH, Sheila Anne TURVILLE

Carbost Medical Practice
Trien, Carbost, Isle of Skye IV47 8SR
Tel: 01478 640202 Fax: 01478 640464
(NHS Highland, Primary Care)
Patient List Size: 580

GP Frank TEUNISSE

Dunvegan Medical Practice
Dunvegan, Isle of Skye IV55 8GU
Tel: 01470 521203 Fax: 01470 521328
Email: administrator@gp55535.highlands-hb.scot.nhs.uk
Website: www.dunveganpractice.org
(NHS Highland, Primary Care)

GP Pat ARNOLD, Sally GODWARD, Rachel McKENZIE, Stephen MORAN, Kirsty SHAW

Portree Medical Centre
Portree, Isle of Skye IV51 9BZ
Tel: 01478 612013 Fax: 01478 612340
(NHS Highland, Primary Care)

Practice Manager Colin Kneen

GP Charles Lachlan CRICHTON, Thomas Wilson Forrest BANKS, Angus Norman MACDONALD, Stephen David McCABE, Carroll Anthony O'DOLAN, Julian Stanley Martyn TOMS

Sleat Medical Practice
Ferrindonald, Sleat, Isle of Skye IV44 8RF
Tel: 01471 844283 Fax: 01471 844234
(NHS Highland, Primary Care)

GP Angus Dougall VENTERS

Isle of Tiree

Baugh House Surgery
Baugh House, Scarinish, Isle of Tiree PA77 6UN
Tel: 01879 220323 Fax: 01879 220893
(NHS Argyll and Clyde, Lomond and Argyll Community Services Division)

GP John HOLLIDAY

Jedburgh

The Health Centre
Queen Street, Jedburgh TD8 6EN
Tel: 01835 863361 Fax: 01835 864273
(NHS Borders, Primary Care Division)
Patient List Size: 6200

Practice Manager Ian Duncan

GP Edward Summerfield MUIR, Graham Alexander COOK, Catriona Ruth DORWARD, Ross James MITCHELL

Johnstone

Johnstone Health Centre
60 Quarry Street, Johnstone PA5 8DZ
Tel: 01505 324348 Fax: 01505 323875
(NHS Argyll and Clyde, Renfrewshire and Inverclyde Community Services Division)

GP Avril CAMPBELL, Alison COATS, Gordon FORREST, Tej-Narayan SINGH

Quarry Street Surgery
16-24 Quarry Street, Johnstone PA5 8EB
Tel: 01505 321733/324249 Fax: 01505 322181
Email: administrator@gp87305.ac-hb.scot.nhs.uk
(NHS Argyll and Clyde, Renfrewshire and Inverclyde Community Services Division)

GP Margaret BORTHWICK, Graham HARRIS, Eilidh RENWICK, Clemency SHADBOLT

Quarry Street Surgery
22 Quarry Street, Johnstone PA5 8DZ
Tel: 01505 331673
(NHS Argyll and Clyde, Renfrewshire and Inverclyde Community Services Division)
Patient List Size: 2600

GP Daya KHANNA

Ravenswood Doctors Surgery
Thomson Avenue, Johnstone PA5 8SU
Tel: 01505 331979 Fax: 01505 323444
(NHS Argyll and Clyde, Renfrewshire and Inverclyde Community Services Division)
Patient List Size: 6150

Practice Manager Lesley Stewart

GP Andrew WRIGHT, Barbara BIGGART, Martin INNES, Christine JONES

Riverview Medical Centre
6/8 George Street, Johnstone PA5 8SL
Tel: 01505 320208 Fax: 01505 322543
(NHS Argyll and Clyde, Renfrewshire and Inverclyde Community Services Division)

GP Clare CUNNING, Lorna DUNLOP, Gerald O'KANE

Riverview Medical Centre
6/8 George Street, Johnstone PA5 8SL
Tel: 01505 320151 Fax: 01505 322543
(NHS Argyll and Clyde, Renfrewshire and Inverclyde Community Services Division)

GP Margaret MITCHELL, Joseph CASSIDY, Daniel McBRYAN

Westfield Surgery
Westfield, Graham Street, Johnstone PA5 8QY
Tel: 01505 337888 Fax: 01505 337700
Email: administrator@gp87288.ac-hb.scot.nhs.uk
(NHS Argyll and Clyde, Renfrewshire and Inverclyde Community Services Division)
Patient List Size: 3700

GP Luway DHIYA, Dr COATS

Keith

Dufftown Medical Group
Health Centre, Stephen Avenue, Dufftown, Keith AB55 4FJ
Tel: 01340 820888 Fax: 01340 821614
Email: administrator@dufftown.grampian.scot.nhs.uk
(NHS Grampian, Primary Care Division)
Patient List Size: 2352

Practice Manager Karen Moir

GP Thomas Terence HENEGHAN, Samuel MacKay SHAW

Keith Medical Group
Keith Health Centre, Turner Street, Keith AB55 5DJ
Tel: 01542 882244 Fax: 01542 881002
Email: administrator@keith.grampian.scot.nhs.uk
(NHS Grampian, Primary Care Division)
Patient List Size: 7201

Practice Manager K Moir

GP William Melvin MORRISON, David Charles GOULD, C GREEN, John Hendry HARRINGTON, Robert Brown HUTCHISON, Janie THOMASON

Kelso

Kelso Medical Group Practice
Health Centre, Inch Road, Kelso TD5 7LF
Tel: 01573 224424 Fax: 01573 226388
(NHS Borders, Primary Care Division)
Patient List Size: 11000

Practice Manager Penny Fleming

GP Robert Ian CUTTING, Ian Gordon FINGLAND, Carol Anne JOHNSTON, John Roberton MAGUIRE, James Anderson MILLAR, Alexander Russell MORRIS, Ruth NISBET, Sarah Frances POTTER, Andrew Sharp SUTHERLAND

Kelty

Kelty Medical Practice
80 Main Street, Kelty KY4 0AE
Tel: 01383 831281 Fax: 01383 831825
(NHS Fife, Primary Care Division)
Patient List Size: 6600

Practice Manager Vicki Cunningham

GP Alan William Thomas MELVILLE, Romilly Grace CARTER, Conrad Paul EWING, Louise Anne PRYDE, Patrick Alan SHEIL

Kilbirnie

Kilbirnie Medical Practice
2 Kirkland Road, Kilbirnie KA25 6HS
Tel: 01505 683591 Fax: 01505 681512
(NHS Ayrshire and Arran, Community Health Division)

Practice Manager Jackie Graham

GP Anne Brodie COLQUHOUN, David Drummond COLBURN, David Alexander FERRY, Robert George HILLMAN, Gerard McAFEE

Killin

Killin Medical Practice
Laggan Leigheas, Ballechroisk, Killin FK21 8TQ
Tel: 01567 820213 Fax: 01567 820805
Email: administrator:gp25351.forthhb.scot.nhs.uk
(NHS Forth Valley, Primary Care Operating Division)
Patient List Size: 1600

Practice Manager Fiona Buchanan

GP David McBride SYME, Antonia M DE LAAT, Christopher J HOLDEN

Kilmacolm

Dorema Surgery
Dorema, Bridge of Weir Road, Kilmacolm PA13 4AP
Tel: 01505 872155 Fax: 01505 874191
(NHS Argyll and Clyde, Renfrewshire and Inverclyde Community Services Division)

Practice Manager Jean Irvine

GP Iain McLELLAN, Laura S SIMPSON

New Surgery
Bridge of Weir Road, Kilmacolm PA13 4AP
Tel: 01505 872844 Fax: 01505 872299
Email: administrator@gp86209.ac-hb.scot.nhs.uk
(NHS Argyll and Clyde, Renfrewshire and Inverclyde Community Services Division)
Patient List Size: 3575

Practice Manager Petrena McCann

GP Russell Philip WOOTTON, Euthymia MANASSES

Kilmarnock

Academy Street Surgery
2 Academy Street, Hurlford, Kilmarnock KA1 5BU
Tel: 01563 525314 Fax: 01563 573561
(NHS Ayrshire and Arran, Community Health Division)

Practice Manager E Gold

GP Iain Lockhart GOLD, D McKAY

Dr Drummond and partners, Crosshouse surgery
The Surgery, Gatehead Road, Crosshouse, Kilmarnock KA2 0HU
Tel: 01563 521506 Fax: 01563 573695
(NHS Ayrshire and Arran, Community Health Division)
Patient List Size: 7600

Practice Manager David Johnston

GP John Wilson DRUMMOND, Joseph Robert MAGEE, William Arthur McALPINE, Jane McBRIDE, Ruksiana STEVEN

Dundonald Medical Practice
9 Main Street, Dundonald, Kilmarnock KA2 9HF
Tel: 01563 850496 Fax: 01563 850426
(NHS Ayrshire and Arran, Community Health Division)
Patient List Size: 5000

Practice Manager Diane Fletcher

GP John David WATTS, David Marshall ILLINGWORTH, Sheena Ruth McADAM, Lynne McDOUGALL, Michael Johnson WOOD

London Road Medical Practice
12 London Road, Kilmarnock KA3 7AE
Tel: 01563 523593 Fax: 01563 573552
Email: londonroad.admin@aapct.scot.nhs.uk
Website: www.londonroadmedicalpractice.co.uk
(NHS Ayrshire and Arran, Community Health Division)
Patient List Size: 13000

Practice Manager Leslie M Wilson

GP Ian Ross BUCHANAN, Robert David BEVERIDGE, Paul CLARK, Melanie HORNE, Anne McTAGGART, J S MORTON, Elaine PRENTICE, Michael Joseph TIMMONS

Portland Medical Practice
34 Portland Road, Kilmarnock KA1 2DL
Tel: 01563 522411 Fax: 01563 545499
(NHS Ayrshire and Arran, Community Health Division)
Patient List Size: 8000

Practice Manager Fiona Shearer

GP Calum DOBBIE, Paul Gerard GAFFNEY, Frank McGUIRE, Lesley Anne McINTYRE

Portland Road Surgery
31 Portland Road, Kilmarnock KA1 2DJ
Tel: 01563 522118 Fax: 01563 573562
(NHS Ayrshire and Arran, Community Health Division)

Practice Manager Boyd Elizabeth

GP Roderick Morris PUGH, J COURTNEY, W A FREN, Iain McKay RICHARDS, Sohail Aabud SARDAR, John MacLeod SOMMERVILLE

Stewarton Medical Practice
45 High Street, Stewarton, Kilmarnock KA3 5BP
Tel: 01560 482011 Fax: 01560 485483
(NHS Ayrshire and Arran, Community Health Division)

Patient List Size: 9200

Practice Manager Allison Bird

GP W J COSTLEY, John Dempster DUKE, S GALBRAITH, Colin Andrew HUNTER, F WATT, G WILKIE

The Surgery
4-6 Old Irvine Road, Kilmarnock KA1 2BD
Tel: 01563 522413 Fax: 01563 573559
(NHS Ayrshire and Arran, Community Health Division)

Practice Manager John Lamont

GP John David CURRAN, Dr DUNN, Kenneth Henry IRVINE, Dr McGREGOR, Allan Stewart LOCHRIE

Wards Medical Practice
25 Dundonald Road, Kilmarnock KA1 1RU
Tel: 01563 526514 Fax: 01563 573558
(NHS Ayrshire and Arran, Community Health Division)
Patient List Size: 13000

Practice Manager Ann McAughtrie

GP James Paterson BLACK, Sarah COY, Lynda Helen DEAN, Raymond Thomas DEAN, Ann HAMILTON, Kessar KHALIQ, George Clifford PAXTON, Michael James SMYTH, Alastair STEWART

Kilwinning

Kilwinning Medical Practice
15 Almswall Road, Kilwinning KA13 6BL
Tel: 01294 554591 Fax: 01294 557300
Website: www.kilwinningmedicalpractice.co.uk
(NHS Ayrshire and Arran, Community Health Division)
Patient List Size: 13500

Practice Manager Eileen Singleton

GP Peter CLARKE, Peter FERRIS, Thomas GROVES, D LAMBE, Janet Anderson McCARLIE, William James McCARLIE, Tim McCLURE, Bruce McINROY, David James MILLER

Oxenward Surgery
3 Oxenward Road, Kilwinning KA13 6EH
Tel: 01294 551555 Fax: 01294 559505
(NHS Ayrshire and Arran, Community Health Division)

GP Patricia MUIRHEAD, R WHYTE, C WOODBURN

Kingussie

Kingussie Medical Practice
Ardvonie Park, Kingussie PH21 1ET
Tel: 01540 661233 Fax: 01540 661277
(NHS Highland, Primary Care)
Patient List Size: 2885

Practice Manager Denise Frost

GP Alastair Ross MICHIE, Mary Elizabeth Margaret ANDERSON, Alistair CONVERY, H IRELAND

Kinlochleven

The Surgery
Kearan Road, Kinlochleven PH50 4QQ
Tel: 01855 831225 Fax: 01855 831494
(NHS Highland, Primary Care)
Patient List Size: 850

GP Geoffrey Dewar HEADDEN

Kinross

Loch Leven Health Centre
Kinross KY13 8SY
Tel: 01577 862112 Fax: 01577 862515
(NHS Tayside, Primary Care Division)
Patient List Size: 10500

Practice Manager John Litster

GP Alistair John McCRACKEN, Evelyn M MENZIES

Loch Leven Health Centre
Lathro, Kinross KY13 8SY
Tel: 01577 862112 Fax: 01577 862515
(NHS Tayside, Primary Care Division)

GP Patrick James CARRAGHER, Claire A DAWSON, Victor J JACK, David William RICHMOND

Kirkcaldy

Bennochy Medical Centre
65 Bennochy Road, Kirkcaldy KY2 5RB
Tel: 01592 263332 Fax: 01592 644288
Email: administrator@gp20979.fife-hb.scot.nhs.uk
(NHS Fife, Primary Care Division)
Patient List Size: 7,300

Practice Manager Heather Fleming

GP James Douglas ROBERTSON, Graham Moreland BROWN, Pamela Freda CAIRNS, Alison Elizabeth McCALLUM, Rajasingham PRIYADHARSHAN

Health Centre
Whyteman's Brae, Kirkcaldy KY1 2NA
Tel: 01592 642902 Fax: 01592 644814
(NHS Fife, Primary Care Division)
Patient List Size: 6500

Practice Manager Audrey Meek

GP William Keith OATES, Lynda Jane ANDERSON, Gary George BARKER, Karl McKENNA, Ruth Louise MORRIS

The Health Centre
Whyteman's Brae, Kirkcaldy KY1 2NA
Tel: 01592 642178 Fax: 01592 644782
(NHS Fife, Primary Care Division)

Practice Manager June Reid

GP Richard ROBERTSON, Jean EGERTON, Ann Marie FLYNN, Gordon Eric GREIG, Victor John LINNEMANN

The Health Centre
Whyteman's Brae, Kirkcaldy KY1 2NA
Tel: 01592 641203 Fax: 01592 642796
(NHS Fife, Primary Care Division)

Practice Manager C Low

GP David John KENDALL, Michael Collins MITCHELL, Dr MORRIS

The Health Centre
Whyteman's Brae, Kirkcaldy KY1 2NA
Tel: 01592 640600 Fax: 01592 641462
(NHS Fife, Primary Care Division)

Practice Manager Sheena Turpie

GP C M J M MacGLONE

Nicol Street Surgery
48 Nicol Street, Kirkcaldy KY1 1PH
Tel: 01592 642969 Fax: 01592 643526
Email: administrator@gp20950.fife-hb.scot.nhs.uk
(NHS Fife, Primary Care Division)

Practice Manager Grace Kennedy, Elizabeth Stuart

GP Keith Duncan FERGUSON, Lesley Ann FERGUSON, Brian Ernest Richard WILSON

Path House Medical Practice
Path House, 7 Nether Street, Kirkcaldy KY1 2PG
Tel: 01592 644533 Fax: 01592 644550
(NHS Fife, Primary Care Division)
Patient List Size: 10300

Practice Manager Elizabeth McLaren

GP Alan Gilchrist BLACK, J BERY, Grant CAMPBELL, Elspeth Ann MACDONALD, R SACHDEU, Andrew Gourdie SMITH

St Brycedale Surgery
St Brycedale Road, Kirkcaldy KY1 1ER
Tel: 01592 640800 Fax: 01592 644944
(NHS Fife, Primary Care Division)

Practice Manager Carol Lawson

GP Allan Peter LEES, David Edward BEE, Andrew Douglas Graham DUNCAN, Fiona Jane McGOWAN

Kirkcudbright

Health Centre
St Marys Place, Townend, Kirkcudbright DG6 4BJ
Tel: 01557 330755 Fax: 01557 330917

Health Centre
St Marys Place, Townend, Kirkcudbright DG6 4BJ
Tel: 01557 330755 Fax: 01557 330917
(NHS Dumfries and Galloway; NHS Dumfries and Galloway)
Patient List Size: 4800
Patient List Size: 4800

Practice Manager Sandra Christie, Sandra Christie, Sandra Christie, Sandra Christie

GP Robert Henry MACK, Robert Henry MACK, Catriona Corrine BUCHAN, Catriona Corrine BUCHAN, Robert Gordon GRIEVE, Robert Gordon GRIEVE, William John LOCKE, William John LOCKE, Jeannette Margaret MORTON, Jeannette Margaret MORTON

Kirkliston

Health Centre
The Glebe, Kirkliston EH29 9AS
Tel: 0131 333 3215 Fax: 0131 333 4993
(NHS Lothian, West Lothian Healthcare Division)
Patient List Size: 4000

Practice Manager Margaret Mactavish

GP Robert MacGregor MILNE, William Scott SIMPSON

Kirkwall

Scapa Practice
Health Centre, New Scapa Road, Kirkwall KW15 1BQ
Tel: 01856 885445 Fax: 01856 873556

GP Martyn HARVEY, Susan MacALISTER, Duncan Jack MacINNES, Marjolein VAN SCHAYK, Timothy Freeman WRIGHT

Skerryvore Practice
Health Centre, New Scapa Road, Kirkwall KW15 1BX
Tel: 01856 888 240 Fax: 01856 888 068
Website: www.skerryvorepractice.co.uk

Practice Manager Paula Craigie

GP Steven Robert BEAVEN, William James Douglas DEANS, Peter John FAY, Mhari LINKLATER, Anne Law NICOLSON

Kirriemuir

Kirriemuir Health Centre
Tannage Brae, Kirriemuir DD8 4DL
Tel: 01575 573333 Fax: 01575 577000
(NHS Tayside, Primary Care Division)

GP Andrew Bertram Guthrie LENDRUM, Jane A DELANEY, Alan Maxwell FARQUHAR, Michelle C WATTS, Alan Duncan WEIR, Andrew P WILMHURST

Kyle

Church Road Surgery
Church Road, Kyle IV40 8DD
Tel: 01599 534257 Fax: 01599 534107
(NHS Highland, Primary Care)
Patient List Size: 2700

GP Peter John Patrick MORGAN, Julian C LAW, Rebecca Eleanor MACKINNON, Morag MACLEAN, Lesley UNWIN

Glenelg Health Centre
Allt Ruadh, Glenelg, Kyle IV40 8JD
Tel: 01599 522272 Fax: 01599 522377
(NHS Highland, Primary Care)
Patient List Size: 300

Practice Manager J A Zelaya

GP Simon Bartholomew HURDING, Kathryn MACRAE

Lairg

Assynt Medical Practice
The Health Centre, Lochinver, Lairg IV27 4JZ
Tel: 01571 844226 Fax: 01571 844476
(NHS Highland, Primary Care)
Patient List Size: 1000

Practice Manager Margaret Macleod

GP Richard John VINE, David Anthony SLATOR

Durness Surgery
Durness, Lairg IV27 4PH
Tel: 01971 511273 Fax: 01971 511325
(NHS Highland, Primary Care)

GP Alan Hunter BELBIN

Lairg Health Centre
Main Street, Lairg IV27 4DD
Tel: 01549 402007 Fax: 01549 402511
Email: alexander.dickson@gp55249.highland-hb.scot.nhs.uk
(NHS Highland, Primary Care)
Patient List Size: 1100

GP Alexander DICKSON, Aline MARSHALL

St Andrew's Glebe Health Centre
St Andrew's Glebe, Tongue, Lairg IV27 4XB
Tel: 01847 611213 Fax: 01847 611382
(NHS Highland, Primary Care)
Patient List Size: 550

GP Marion MACDOUGALL

The Surgery
Scourie, Lairg IV27 4SX
Tel: 01971 502002 Fax: 01971 502399
(NHS Highland, Primary Care)

Practice Manager Judith Cadamy

GP Anthony Roger CADAMY

Lanark

Ayr Road Surgery
69 Ayr Road, Douglas, Lanark ML11 0PX
Tel: 01555 851226
(NHS Lanarkshire, Primary Care Division)
Patient List Size: 5440

GP William Sinclair SCOTT, Robert James FLOWERDEW, Doris IKES, Iain McEwan KANE, Ann Elizabeth LANG, Margaret McARTHUR

Carlisle Road Surgery
125 Carlisle Road, Kirkmuirhill, Lanark ML11 9RT
Tel: 01555 893961
(NHS Lanarkshire, Primary Care Division)

GP Peter V BOWMAN

Carnwarth Health Centre
7 Biggar Road, Carnwath, Lanark ML11 8HJ
Tel: 01555 840214
(NHS Lanarkshire, Primary Care Division)
Patient List Size: 3492

GP Louise CHRISTIE, Fiona MACGREGOR, Michael John TILEY

Carstairs Health Centre
The School House, School Road, Carstairs, Lanark ML11 8QF
Tel: 01555 870512
(NHS Lanarkshire, Primary Care Division)

GP Charles Morrison ANDERSON, Frances Elizabeth McKNIGHT

Glebe Medical Centre
Abbeygreen, Lesmahagow, Lanark ML11 0EF
Tel: 01555 892328 Fax: 01555 894094
(NHS Lanarkshire, Primary Care Division)
Patient List Size: 5500

GP Alexander James CHRISTIE, Zia Ul ISLAM, Alistair Thomas KERR

Lanark Doctors
Health Centre, South Vennel, Lanark ML11 7JT
Tel: 01555 665522 Fax: 01555 666857
(NHS Lanarkshire, Primary Care Division)

Practice Manager Frank Caddell

GP William Robert CRIGGIE, John COPLAND, Craig Morrison DUNCAN, James Geoffrey HILL, Allyson June MATTHEWS, Jill MURIE, Jean Isobel YOUNG

The Surgery
40 Manse Road, Forth, Lanark ML11 8AJ
Tel: 01555 811200 Fax: 01555 811200
(NHS Lanarkshire, Primary Care Division)
Patient List Size: 2890

Practice Manager Sybil McGinty

GP Donald Malcolm MACRITCHIE, Pamela Agnes MACRITCHIE

Langholm

The Health Centre
Charles Street, Langholm DG13 0JY
Tel: 01387 380355 Fax: 01387 381211
Email: administrator@y18447.dghb.scot.nhs.uk

The Health Centre
Charles Street, Langholm DG13 0JY
Tel: 01387 380355 Fax: 01387 381211
Email: administrator@y18447.dghb.scot.nhs.uk
(NHS Dumfries and Galloway; NHS Dumfries and Galloway)

Practice Manager J E Henderson, J E Henderson, J E Henderson, J E Henderson

GP H C PHILLIPS, H C PHILLIPS, Mark Leslie Clifford PHILLIPS, Mark Leslie Clifford PHILLIPS, E Jeanne TAUDEVIN, E Jeanne TAUDEVIN

Larbert

Health Centre
Park Drive, Stenhousemuir, Larbert FK5 3BB
Tel: 01324 552200 Fax: 01324 553623
(NHS Forth Valley, Primary Care Operating Division)
Patient List Size: 5400

GP John Allan LEEMING, Dr MARTIN, Mary Jane Walker McNAB

Health Centre
Park Drive, Stenhousemuir, Larbert FK5 3BB
Tel: 01324 554136 Fax: 01324 553622
(NHS Forth Valley, Primary Care Operating Division)

GP Stephen Thomas Coleman BROWN, Lila Russell HILLAN

Health Centre
Park Drive, Stenhousemuir, Larbert FK5 3BB
Tel: 01324 554411 Fax: 01324 553629
Email: KAY.TOTTEN@GP25402.FORTH-HBSCOT.NHS.UK
(NHS Forth Valley, Primary Care Operating Division)
Patient List Size: 3114

Practice Manager Kay Totten

GP David Peter ELLISON, Onsi Samuel GHOBRIAL

Health Centre
Park Drive, Stenhousemuir, Larbert FK5 3BB
Tel: 01324 570570 Fax: 01324 553632
(NHS Forth Valley, Primary Care Operating Division)

GP Alexander CROOKSTON, Catherine Robertson THOMSON

Tryst Medical Centre
431 King Street, Stenhousemuir, Larbert FK5 4HT
Tel: 01324 551555 Fax: 01324 551925
Email: administrator@gp25648.forth-hb.scot.nhs.uk
(NHS Forth Valley, Primary Care Operating Division)
Patient List Size: 6130

Practice Manager Jennifer Douglas

GP David Hill PATON, Ian George MACGREGOR, Gayle Henderson PATERSON, Jill ROBINSON

Largs

Aitken Street Surgery
20 Aitken Street, Largs KA30 8AU
Tel: 01475 674545 Fax: 01475 689645
(NHS Ayrshire and Arran, Community Health Division)
Patient List Size: 9300

GP Thomas CLARK, Andrew AULD, Maureen Ruth GREENFIELD, Stuart Gilbert LEWIS, James Anthony TIMMONS

Fraser Street Surgery
10/14 Fraser Street, Largs KA30 9HP
Tel: 01475 673380 Fax: 01475 674149
Email: valeriemcnicol@aapct.scot.nhs.uk
(NHS Ayrshire and Arran, Community Health Division)
Patient List Size: 4800

GP Douglas Alistair SOUTTER, Rosalind Elizabeth BARNES, Maeve Margaret DOCHERTY, Andrew JONES

Larkhall

Avon Medical Centre
Academy Street, Larkhall ML9 2BJ
Tel: 01698 882547 Fax: 01698 888138
(NHS Lanarkshire, Primary Care Division)
Patient List Size: 11500

Practice Manager Kay Danks

GP John Robertson WILSON, N C CAMPBELL, Elena FAWCETT, Alasdair Robert MARTIN, P F J SKEHAN, Anne Tait THOMPSON

Gallowhill Surgery
4-6 Gallowhill, Larkhall ML9 1EX
Tel: 01698 884082 Fax: 01698 889211
(NHS Lanarkshire, Primary Care Division)
Patient List Size: 2400

Practice Manager Jean Gorniak

GP Naresh BALKRISHNA

Union Street Surgery
75 Union Street, Larkhall ML9 1DZ
Tel: 01698 882105 Fax: 01698 886332
(NHS Lanarkshire, Primary Care Division)
Patient List Size: 10600

Practice Manager Elizabeth Moyes

GP James Finlayson SMART, Diane Elizabeth KINNIBURGH, Esther Adesomo OFILI, Colin Robert RUSSELL, Gregor Ian SMITH

Lauder

Leader Medical Group
1 Factors Park, Lauder TD2 6QW
Tel: 01578 718670 Fax: 01578 718744
(NHS Borders, Primary Care Division)

Patient List Size: 5300

GP Cath CORMIE, Paul Julian CORMIE, Jennifer Margaret LOWLES

Memorial Medical Centre
2 Edinburgh Road, Lauder TD2 6TW
Tel: 01578 722267 Fax: 01578 718667
(NHS Borders, Primary Care Division)

Practice Manager Kathleen Symonds

GP Harry John Christopher CROMBIE SMITH

Laurencekirk

Laurencekirk Medical Group
Blackiemuir Avenue, Laurencekirk AB30 1DX
Tel: 01561 377258 Fax: 01561 378270
(NHS Grampian, Primary Care Division)
Patient List Size: 4200

Practice Manager Marion Taylor

GP Neil James ANDERSON, Kerstin Margaret BOX, Patrick Declan MULCAHY

The Surgery
Netherton House, Auchenblae, Laurencekirk AB30 1XU
Tel: 01561 320202 Fax: 01561 320774
Email: administrator@auchenblae.grampian.scot.nhs.uk
(NHS Tayside, Primary Care Division)
Patient List Size: 1700

Practice Manager John Eddie

GP Keith PIRIE

Leven

The Health Centre
Victoria Road, Leven KY8 4ET
Tel: 01333 432555 Fax: 01333 422249
(NHS Fife, Primary Care Division)
Patient List Size: 3750

Practice Manager Ian Rennie

GP Ronald Mallis PAGE, June Ritchie CLARK, Mark McDONALD

The Health Centre
Victoria Road, Leven KY8 4ET
Tel: 01333 425656 Fax: 01333 422249
Email: levenhealthcentre1@doctor.com
Website: http://helloto/levenhealthcentre1
(NHS Fife, Primary Care Division)
Patient List Size: 3000

Practice Manager Elma Mathieson

GP James Douglas ROSS, David Maxwell SINCLAIR, Suguna NARAYANA

Kennoway Medical Group
Jordan Lane, Kennoway, Leven KY8 5JZ
Tel: 01333 350241 Fax: 01333 352884
Email: patricia.munro@gp20856.fife-hb.scot.nhs.uk
(NHS Fife, Primary Care Division)
Patient List Size: 3560

Practice Manager Patricia Munro

GP Howard Martin STEVENS, Sharon Elizabeth MULLAN, Fiona Elizabeth WOOLARD

Leven Health Centre
Victoria Road, Leven KY8 4ET
Tel: 01333 432588 Fax: 01333 422249
(NHS Fife, Primary Care Division)

Practice Manager Isabel Philp

GP Leslie George Moncrieff BISSET, Iain Nicolson CRUICKSHANK, Alison Laura HEAP, Jane Elizabeth HUNTER, Robert David KEIR, George Stuart McLAREN

Methilhaven Road Surgery
361 Methilhaven Road, Methil, Leven KY8 3HR
Tel: 01333 426913 Fax: 01333 422300
(NHS Fife, Primary Care Division)

Practice Manager Moira Kelly

GP Gordon Robert ALLAN, Paul Alan MacINTYRE, John Fraser MATHER, Lynn MILLER, Michael Joseph WARD

Muiredge Surgery
Merlin Crescent, Buckhaven, Leven KY8 1HJ
Tel: 01592 713299 Fax: 01592 715728
(NHS Fife, Primary Care Division)
Patient List Size: 7200

Practice Manager Maxine Jones

GP Lynne Catherine CHRISTIE, J D FERGUSON, Paul GUY, Swapan MUKHERJEE, Alasdair James Cameron SNEDDON

The Surgery
The Cannons, Fisher Street, Methil, Leven KY8 3HD
Tel: 01333 426083 Fax: 01333 421833
(NHS Fife, Primary Care Division)
Patient List Size: 5000

Practice Manager Christine Martin

GP Janice Anne DUNCAN, Jasbir Singh BUMBRA, Kenneth J THOMPSON

Linlithgow

Linlithgow Health Centre
288 High Street, Linlithgow EH49 7ER
Tel: 01506 670027 Fax: 01506 670548
(NHS Lothian, West Lothian Healthcare Division)

GP David Farquharson MacBeth COCHRAN

Linlithgow Health Centre
288 High Street, Linlithgow EH49 7ER
Tel: 01506 670027 Fax: 01506 670809
(NHS Lothian, West Lothian Healthcare Division)
Patient List Size: 13500

Practice Manager Lynn Chambers

GP Kenneth William MACKENZIE, Stewart A BOX, Michael Francis BOYLE, Angus CAMPBELL, Jean Mairi DAVIE, Neil JAMIESON, Louisa JOHNSTON, Hazel Elizabeth SMART

Livingston

Carmondean Medical Group
Carmondean Health Centre, Livingston EH54 8PY
Tel: 01506 430031 Fax: 01506 432775
(NHS Lothian, West Lothian Healthcare Division)
Patient List Size: 7202

Practice Manager Phyllis Carr

GP Mohamed Salim Ahmed PATEL, Nicola Margaret GIBSON, Colin Stewart MUSK, Jean Rosemary PRINGLE, David Alexander ROBERTSON

Carmondean Medical Group
Carmondean Health Centre, Livingston EH54 8PY
Tel: 01506 440050 Fax: 01506 433510
(NHS Lothian, West Lothian Healthcare Division)
Patient List Size: 1850

GP F H SHAH

Craigshill Health Centre
Craigshill Road, Livingston EH54 5DY
Tel: 01506 432621 Fax: 01506 430431
(NHS Lothian, West Lothian Healthcare Division)

Practice Manager Carole Robinson

GP John Edward HANDLEY, A M CAMPBELL, John Bell FERGUSON, Carolyn Margaret McCallum ROBERTSON, Edward Denham RUSSELL-SMITH, Richard Davidson SLOAN

Craigshill Health Centre
Craigshill Road, Craigshill, Livingston EH54 5DY
Tel: 01506 432621 Fax: 01506 430431
(NHS Lothian, West Lothian Healthcare Division)

GP Bharat Prasad TRIPATHI

Dedridge Health Centre
Nigel Rise, Livingston EH54 6QQ
Tel: 01506 414586 Fax: 01506 461806
(NHS Lothian, West Lothian Healthcare Division)

GP Robert Marshall FINNIE, William Donald GORMAN, Amanda Frances MacCOLL, Susan Jane PEPPER, Peter ROBERTSON, Sureshini SANDERS, Iain SMITH, Gillian Jane STEELE

Dr Forbes and Partners
East Calder Medical Practice, 147 Main Street, East Calder, Livingston EH53 0EW
Tel: 01506 882882 Fax: 01506 883630
(NHS Lothian, West Lothian Healthcare Division)
Patient List Size: 11500

Practice Manager M Ashcroft

GP Evelyn Joyce GOURLAY, Marian CAVES, Ian DEMPSTER, George MACKIE, Amanda Jennifer McEWAN, Iain Charles McLEOD, Suzanna Maria TYBULEWICZ, Kathryn Airlie WILD

East Calder Health Centre
147 Main Street, East Calder, Livingston EH53 0EW
Tel: 01506 880582 Fax: 01506 883630
(NHS Lothian, West Lothian Healthcare Division)

GP Evelyn GOURLAY, Marian CAVES, Ian DEMPSTER, George MACKIE, Amanda J McEWAN, S TYBULEWICZ, Kathryn A WILD

Howden Health Centre
Howden West, Livingston EH54 6TP
Tel: 01506 423800 Fax: 01506 460757
(NHS Lothian, West Lothian Healthcare Division)
Patient List Size: 11000

Practice Manager Jacqui Crosbie

GP Tim A BARNES, Assif ALI, Moray GRIGOR, Christina HENNESSEY, David MAXWELL, Alison MIDDLETON, Dr ZAW-HTET

Loanhead

Dick Place Surgery
15 Dick Place, Loanhead EH9 2JU
Tel: 0131 440 0593
(NHS Lothian, Primary and Community Division)

GP Stanley Augustine MOONSAWMY

Lochboisdale

South Uist Medical
Daliburgh, Lochboisdale HS8 5SS
Tel: 01878 700302 Fax: 01878 700909
Email: isobel.johnstone@gp90134.w.isles-hb.scot.nhs.uk
(NHS Western Isles)
Patient List Size: 1500

Practice Manager Isobel Johnstone

GP John BUCKMASTER

Lochgelly

Benarty Medical Practice
54-58 Lochleven Road, Lochore, Lochgelly KY5 8DA
Tel: 01592 860463 Fax: 01592 869628
(NHS Fife, Primary Care Division)
Patient List Size: 7100

Practice Manager Laura Adams

GP Peter Grant ROBSON, Eileen BROWN, Daniel Donald CARLIN, S MIDDLEMISS, M ROBERTSON

Cardenden Health Centre
Wallsgreen Road, Cardenden, Lochgelly KY5 0JF
Tel: 01592 722440 Fax: 01592 722955
(NHS Fife, Primary Care Division)
Patient List Size: 1790

Practice Manager Sarah Murdoch

GP Chhotalal Uttambhai MISTRY

The Health Centre
Wallsgreen Road, Cardenden, Lochgelly KY5 0JE
Tel: 01592 722441 Fax: 01592 722955
(NHS Fife, Primary Care Division)
Patient List Size: 1550

GP Bashier Ahmed Rashied Mousa OUDEH

Lochgelly Health Centre
David Street, Lochgelly KY5 9QZ
Tel: 01592 780277 Fax: 01592 784044
(NHS Fife, Primary Care Division)

Practice Manager Susan Davidson

GP Caroline Anne KIDD, Susan Jacqueline CATTANACH, Dr MARTINS DA SILVA

Lochgelly Health Centre
David Street, Lochgelly KY5 9QZ
Tel: 01592 780358 Fax: 01592 784139
(NHS Fife, Primary Care Division)

Lochgelly Health Centre
David Street, Lochgelly KY5 9QZ
Tel: 01592 782783 Fax: 01592 783874
(NHS Fife, Primary Care Division)
Patient List Size: 5500

Practice Manager Margaret Grey

GP Alan Alexander FARRELL, Diane CAMPBELL, John Robertson McKEAN

Lochgilphead

The Surgery
Lorne Street, Lochgilphead PA31 8LU
Tel: 01546 602921 Fax: 01546 606735
(NHS Argyll and Clyde, Lomond and Argyll Community Services Division)

Practice Manager Muriel Miller

GP Alistair Frank RANGER, Christopher DOWNS, Colin Skene MACKIE, Jeremy Keith PHILLIPS, Mark James SIMPSON, Richard SLOAN, Adrian Denis WARD

Lochmaddy

North Uist Medical Practice
Lochmaddy HS6 5AE
Tel: 01876 500333 Fax: 01876 500877
(NHS Western Isles)
Patient List Size: 1539

Practice Manager Helen MacLean

GP Peter KEILLER, Paul BRADLEY, Barbara PILKINGTON, Karen WILSON

Lochwinnoch

Lochwinnoch Surgery
31 Main Street, Lochwinnoch PA12 4AH
Tel: 01505 842200 Fax: 01505 843144
Email: administrator@gp87432.ac-hb.scot.nhs.uk
(NHS Argyll and Clyde, Renfrewshire and Inverclyde Community Services Division)

Practice Manager Rosemary H Scarff

GP Paul WATERSTON, Christine KIRK, Clare McCORMICK

Lockerbie

The Clinic
Main Road, Ecclefechan, Lockerbie DG11 3BT
Tel: 01576 300208 Fax: 01576 300694

The Clinic
Main Road, Ecclefechan, Lockerbie DG11 3BT
Tel: 01576 300208 Fax: 01576 300694
(NHS Dumfries and Galloway; NHS Dumfries and Galloway)
Patient List Size: 2100
Patient List Size: 2100

Practice Manager Mary Palmer, Mary Palmer, Mary Palmer, Mary Palmer

GP Roy Alan PALMER, Roy Alan PALMER, Craig PALMER, Craig PALMER

Lochmaben Medical Group
The Surgery, 42-44 High Street, Lochmaben, Lockerbie DG11 1NH
Tel: 01387 810252 Fax: 01387 811595
Email: administrator@y18377.dghb.scot.nhs.uk

Lochmaben Medical Group
The Surgery, 42-44 High Street, Lochmaben, Lockerbie DG11 1NH
Tel: 01387 810252 Fax: 01387 811595
Email: administrator@y18377.dghb.scot.nhs.uk
(NHS Dumfries and Galloway; NHS Dumfries and Galloway)
Patient List Size: 5100
Patient List Size: 5100

Practice Manager Joyce Roberts, Joyce Roberts, Joyce Roberts, Joyce Roberts

GP David FROST, David FROST, Craig A BROWN, Craig A BROWN, Fiona M JEFFORD, Fiona M JEFFORD, John Dawson SMITH, John Dawson SMITH

Lockerbie Medical Practice
Victoria Gardens, Lockerbie DG11 2BJ
Tel: 01576 203663 Fax: 01576 202773
Email: administrator@g18558.dghb.scot.nhs.uk

Lockerbie Medical Practice
Victoria Gardens, Lockerbie DG11 2BJ
Tel: 01576 203663 Fax: 01576 202773
Email: administrator@g18558.dghb.scot.nhs.uk
(NHS Dumfries and Galloway; NHS Dumfries and Galloway)
Patient List Size: 5300
Patient List Size: 5300

Practice Manager Halina Neil, Halina Neil, Halina Neil, Halina Neil

GP James John HILL, James John HILL, Alexa Clare CRAWFORD, Alexa Clare CRAWFORD, Colin Henry MALONE, Colin Henry MALONE, George Alexander PORTEOUS, George Alexander PORTEOUS, Nancy Dunlop RIGG, Nancy Dunlop RIGG

Lossiemouth

Laich Medical Practice
Clifton Road, Lossiemouth IV31 6DJ
Tel: 01343 812277 Fax: 01343 812396
Email: administrator@laich.grampian.scot.nhs.uk
(NHS Grampian, Primary Care Division)
Patient List Size: 8150

Practice Manager J Forman

GP Neil SABISTON, Sandy BARCLAY, Duncan GREEN, Ewen RIDDICK, Margaret SINCLAIR

Lybster

Althorpe Street Medical Centre
Althorpe Street, Lybster KW3 6BQ
Tel: 01593 721216 Fax: 01593 721344
Email: administrator@gp55094.highland-hb.scot.nhs.uk
(NHS Highland, Primary Care)
Patient List Size: 1000

Practice Manager P Hendry

Macduff

Macduff Medical Practice
100 Duff Street, Macduff AB44 1PR
Tel: 01261 833777 Fax: 01261 835100
(NHS Grampian, Primary Care Division)
Patient List Size: 2200

Practice Manager Murial Barclay

GP Iain Parkinson BROOKER, Alison Farquharson BARBOUR, Patricia HODDINOTT

Mallaig

Mallaig Heatlh Centre
Victoria Road, Mallaig PH41 4RN
Tel: 01687 462202 Fax: 01687 462410
(NHS Highland, Primary Care)
Patient List Size: 1200

Practice Manager Morven Weir

GP Anthony John WAITE

Mauchline

Ballochmyle Medical Group
Institute Avenue, Catrine, Mauchline KA5 6RU
Tel: 01290 551237 Fax: 01290 552784
(NHS Ayrshire and Arran, Community Health Division)
Patient List Size: 9000

Practice Manager Aileen Reid

GP John CLELAND, Katharine Mary MORRISON, David Andrew RICHARDSON, Walter Thomas CAMPBELL, Joyce Barbara MAY, Elizabeth McMILLAY

Maybole

Drs Scobie, Paton and Steele
6 High Street, Maybole KA19 7BY
Tel: 01655 882278 Fax: 01655 889616
(NHS Ayrshire and Arran, Community Health Division)
Patient List Size: 3700

Practice Manager Eleanor Scobie

GP Brian SCOBIE, Gerald PATON, Elizabeth Sandra STEELE

Maybole Health Centre
6 High Street, Maybole KA19 7BY
Tel: 01655 882708 Fax: 01655 882977
(NHS Ayrshire and Arran, Community Health Division)
Patient List Size: 4438

Practice Manager Tracey Barr

GP Charles LAU CHING HUNG, Jonathan Christopher SHEWARD, Eileen Cuthbertson WILSON

Melrose

Eildon Medical Practice
St Dunstan's Park, Melrose TD6 9RX
Tel: 01896 822161 Fax: 01896 820286
(NHS Borders, Primary Care Division)

Practice Manager Ian Duncan

GP Nicholas John McDONAGH, Roderick Duncan McDONALD, Geoffrey David WILSON

Millport

Dr James Bryson and Dr Elizabeth Bryson
10 Kelburn Street, Millport KA28 0DT
Tel: 01475 530329 Fax: 01475 530793
(NHS Ayrshire and Arran, Community Health Division)
Patient List Size: 1500

Practice Manager Heidi Harrison

GP Elizabeth Alice BRYSON, James Athol Mackenzie BRYSON, Prabhu RAVANGAVE

Moffat

Church Place Surgery
6 Church Place, Moffat DG10 9ES
Tel: 01683 220197
Email: administrator@gp18381.dghb.scot.nhs.uk

Church Place Surgery
6 Church Place, Moffat DG10 9ES
Tel: 01683 220197
Email: administrator@gp18381.dghb.scot.nhs.uk
(NHS Dumfries and Galloway; NHS Dumfries and Galloway)
Patient List Size: 2500
Patient List Size: 2500

Practice Manager Wendy Simpson, Wendy Simpson, Wendy Simpson, Wendy Simpson

GP Roderick GILLIES, Roderick GILLIES, Richard Robert CROSBY, Richard Robert CROSBY, Shona Ross GILLIES, Shona Ross GILLIES, Janet Anne ROBERTSON, Janet Anne ROBERTSON

The Surgery
High Street, Moffat DG10 9HL
Tel: 01683 220062 Fax: 01683 220453

The Surgery
High Street, Moffat DG10 9HL
Tel: 01683 220062 Fax: 01683 220453
(NHS Dumfries and Galloway; NHS Dumfries and Galloway)
Patient List Size: 3000
Patient List Size: 3000

Practice Manager Brenda Wallace, Brenda Wallace, Brenda Wallace, Brenda Wallace

GP Gordon Lawrence MacEWEN, Gordon Lawrence MacEWEN, Annie Sonia SHARKEY, Annie Sonia SHARKEY

Montrose

Annat Bank Practice
Links Health Centre, Marine Avenue, Montrose DD10 8TR
Tel: 01674 673400 Fax: 01674 672175
Email: administrator@annatbank.tayside.scot.nhs.uk
(NHS Tayside, Primary Care Division)
Patient List Size: 5500

Practice Manager Ann Falkowski

GP James Alexander GRANT, Margaret Joyce ANDERSON, Ruth Caldwell CRANSWICK, Monica IRELAND, Graham Andrew KRAMER, Richard Peter Burrington MARWOOD

Castlegait Surgery
Links Health Centre, Marine Avenue, Montrose DD10 8TR
Tel: 01674 672554 Fax: 01674 675025
(NHS Tayside, Primary Care Division)
Patient List Size: 4600

Practice Manager Gordon Reid

GP James George CALDER, Douglas Liddle CRAIG, Douglas Robert WALKER

Townhead Practice
Links Health Centre, Montrose DD10 8TY
Tel: 01674 676161 Fax: 01674 673151
Email: enquiries@townhead.tayside.scot.nhs.uk
(NHS Tayside, Primary Care Division)
Patient List Size: 6450

Practice Manager Vicki Brighton

GP John Morgan GRIFFITH, Alan Gordon BEGG, Andrew William ORR, Maureen J SIMPSON, Sally VOICE

Motherwell

Carfin Road Surgery
15 Carfin Road, Motherwell ML1 5AG
Tel: 01698 732501 Fax: 01698 733214
(NHS Lanarkshire, Primary Care Division)
Patient List Size: 2970

Practice Manager R Menon

GP Kollaikkal Vijaya Kumar MENON

MacInnes Medical Centre
60 High Street, Newarthill, Motherwell ML1 5JU
Tel: 01698 860246 Fax: 01698 861641
(NHS Lanarkshire, Primary Care Division)
Patient List Size: 5600

Practice Manager Margaret Carson

GP Wilma Jane HOGG, Arvind KOCHAR, Duncan Calum MacINNES, Pamela ROSS

Main Street Surgery
43-45 Main Street, Holytown, Motherwell ML1 4TH
Tel: 01698 732463
(NHS Lanarkshire, Primary Care Division)
Patient List Size: 3387

Practice Manager A F Kenn

GP Maddineni KOTESWARA RAO, S RAMAH

Modyrvale Medical Centre
Toll Street, Motherwell ML1 2PJ
(NHS Lanarkshire, Primary Care Division)

Motherwell Health Centre
138-144 Windmill Street, Motherwell ML1 1TB
Tel: 01698 266688 Fax: 01698 242621
(NHS Lanarkshire, Primary Care Division)
Patient List Size: 4000

Practice Manager N Nisbet

GP Alexander William GOUDIE, Marelle Margaret Ellen TILLEY

Motherwell Health Centre
138-144 Windmill Street, Motherwell ML1 1TB
Tel: 01698 264164
(NHS Lanarkshire, Primary Care Division)

Practice Manager Jean Slavin

GP Eileen Curran KERR, Gwen Boyd FISHER, Jacqueline KEENAN

Motherwell Health Centre
138-144 Windmill Street, Motherwell ML1 1TB
Tel: 01698 263288 Fax: 01698 251267
(NHS Lanarkshire, Primary Care Division)
Patient List Size: 3800

Practice Manager Janette Main

GP John Kerr LANDO, Kean BLAKE, Gillian KEMPSILL

Motherwell Health Centre
138-144 Windmill Street, Motherwell ML1 1TA
Tel: 01698 265193 Fax: 01698 253324
(NHS Lanarkshire, Primary Care Division)
Patient List Size: 5000

Practice Manager Isobel Cringles

GP Brian Walker McGILL, Helen Jeanne McKENZIE, James Liddell STURGEON

Motherwell Health Centre
138-144 Windmill Street, Motherwell ML1 1TB
Tel: 01698 265566
(NHS Lanarkshire, Primary Care Division)

GP Marcella Anne DUDDY, Robert David Sinclair LIDDLE, John David Richmond MORRISON, Aileen McKenzie PORTE, Musharaf SHAH

Motherwell Health Centre
138-144 Windmill Street, Motherwell ML1 1TB
Tel: 01698 266525 Fax: 01698 252427
(NHS Lanarkshire, Primary Care Division)

Practice Manager Aileen Martinus

GP Laurence BELL, Carolyn HYSLOP

Motherwell Health Centre
138-144 Windmill Hill Street, Motherwell ML1 1TB
Tel: 01698 275567 Fax: 01698 252147
(NHS Lanarkshire, Primary Care Division)
Patient List Size: 2335

Practice Manager Annette Brown

GP David F McBRIDE

Orchard Medical Centre
41 Ladywell Road, Motherwell ML1 3JX
Tel: 01698 242700 Fax: 01698 242720
(NHS Lanarkshire, Primary Care Division)
Patient List Size: 11500

Practice Manager Valerie Gilmore

GP Graeme Dick ROSE, David Matthew BARR, Carolyne CALDER, Brian Richard LOGIE, Amar N MISHRA

Muir of Ord

Guisachan
Black Isle Road, Muir of Ord IV6 7RR
(NHS Highland, Primary Care)

GP Alan Henry Girvin MUNRO

Munlochy

Brae Terrace Surgery
Brae Terrace, Munlochy IV8 8NG
Tel: 01463 811200 Fax: 01463 811383
Email: munlochy@ecosse.net
(NHS Highland, Primary Care)
Patient List Size: 1897

Practice Manager Gillian Kerr

GP David Adams WATSON, Colin David FETTES, Carol Joan MACDONALD

Musselburgh

East Wing
Esk Medical Centre, Ladywell Way, Musselburgh EH21 6AB
Tel: 0131 665 2267 Fax: 0131 653 2348
(NHS Lothian, Primary and Community Division)
Patient List Size: 8574

Practice Manager Anne Cunningham

GP Allan Bruce BLYTH, Karin Leonie BLAYMIRES, Nicola DUFFY, Robert Ernest James GEORGE, Isabel Jane MARSHALL, Monica MILNE

Eskbridge Medical Centre
8A Bridge Street, Musselburgh EH21 6AG
Tel: 0131 665 6821 Fax: 0131 665 5488
(NHS Lothian, Primary and Community Division)
Patient List Size: 7500

Practice Manager Margaret Marr

GP Alan Stuart CLUBB, Cathleen Alison BINNS, Kirsteen CARR, M Carmen COUPLAND, Lyn Marie MILLER, David G SELMAN, Johnstone SHAW

West Wing
Esk Medical Centre, Ladywell Way, Musselburgh EH21 6AB
Tel: 0131 665 2594 Fax: 0131 665 2428
Website: www.west-wing.co.uk
(NHS Lothian, Primary and Community Division)
Patient List Size: 8753

Practice Manager Lorna Johnston

GP Ian Stewart JOHNSTON, Alan J DOUGLAS, Murray Neil FISKEN, Janine Marie FREW, John HIND, Susan Lynn PEARSON

Nairn

Lodgehill Road Clinic
Lodgehill Road, Nairn IV12 4RF
Tel: 01667 452096 Fax: 01667 456785
(NHS Highland, Primary Care)

GP Alastair Lockington NOBLE, Alistair ADAM, A BAKER, Susan Christine HALLIDAY, Calum Zachary MACAULAY, Joan Lamont NOBLE, Alan Campbell STANFIELD

Newbridge

Baird Road Surgery
Baird Road, Ratho, Newbridge EH28 8RA
Tel: 0131 333 1062 Fax: 0131 333 1062
(NHS Lothian, Primary and Community Division)

GP A PANDOLFI

Newcastleton

Blair and Kennedy
The Surgery, 4 South Liddle Street, Newcastleton TD9 0RN
Tel: 01387 375202 Fax: 01387 375817
(NHS Borders, Primary Care Division)
Patient List Size: 1690

Practice Manager Gordon Blake

GP John Ferguson BLAIR, Howard William KENNEDY

Newton Stewart

Cairnsmore Medical Practice
Creebridge, Newton Stewart DG8 6NR
Tel: 01671 403609 Fax: 01671 404008

Cairnsmore Medical Practice
Creebridge, Newton Stewart DG8 6NR
Tel: 01671 403609 Fax: 01671 404008
(NHS Dumfries and Galloway; NHS Dumfries and Galloway)
Patient List Size: 3800
Patient List Size: 3800

Practice Manager S Binks, S Binks, S Binks, S Binks

GP David HANNAY, David HANNAY, Laura Marie JONES, Laura Marie JONES, Thomas Alan JONES, Thomas Alan JONES, Lesley Helen LITTLER, Lesley Helen LITTLER, Hannah McANDLISH, Hannah McANDLISH

Miscambell
Four Winds, Main Street, Glenluce, Newton Stewart DG8 0PU
Tel: 01581 300315 Fax: 01581 300502

Miscambell
Four Winds, Main Street, Glenluce, Newton Stewart DG8 0PU
Tel: 01581 300315 Fax: 01581 300502
(NHS Dumfries and Galloway; NHS Dumfries and Galloway)
Patient List Size: 1490
Patient List Size: 1490

Practice Manager Liz Miscampbell, Liz Miscampbell, Liz Miscampbell, Liz Miscampbell

GP Nigel Thomas MISCAMPBELL, Nigel Thomas MISCAMPBELL

The Surgery
3 St. John Street, Whithorn, Newton Stewart DG8 8PS
Tel: 01988 500218 Fax: 01988 500737

The Surgery
3 St. John Street, Whithorn, Newton Stewart DG8 8PS
Tel: 01988 500218 Fax: 01988 500737
(NHS Dumfries and Galloway; NHS Dumfries and Galloway)
Patient List Size: 3200
Patient List Size: 3200

Practice Manager Janice Bell, Janice Bell, Janice Bell, Janice Bell

GP Christopher John DUCKER, Christopher John DUCKER, Richard Arthur Edward GROVE, Richard Arthur Edward GROVE, Iain Cran McLEAN, Iain Cran McLEAN

The Surgery
St Couan Crescent, Kirkcowan, Newton Stewart DG8 0HH
Tel: 01671 830206 Fax: 01671 404163
Email: administrator@Y18165.dghb.scot.nhs.uk

The Surgery
St Couan Crescent, Kirkcowan, Newton Stewart DG8 0HH
Tel: 01671 830206 Fax: 01671 404163
Email: administrator@Y18165.dghb.scot.nhs.uk
(NHS Dumfries and Galloway; NHS Dumfries and Galloway)
Patient List Size: 2100
Patient List Size: 2100

Practice Manager Lesley Gillespie, Lesley Gillespie, Lesley Gillespie, Lesley Gillespie

GP Mary MARSHALL, Mary MARSHALL, David Macdonald BAIRD, David Macdonald BAIRD, Sandra Jane SUTHERLAND, Sandra Jane SUTHERLAND

Wigtown Medical Practice
High Vennel, Wigtown, Newton Stewart DG8 9JQ
Tel: 01988 402210 Fax: 01988 403482
Email: administrator@y18131.dehb.scot.nhs.uk

Wigtown Medical Practice
High Vennel, Wigtown, Newton Stewart DG8 9JQ
Tel: 01988 402210 Fax: 01988 403482
Email: administrator@y18131.dehb.scot.nhs.uk
(NHS Dumfries and Galloway; NHS Dumfries and Galloway)
Patient List Size: 2526
Patient List Size: 2526

Practice Manager Rosemary Cowan, Rosemary Cowan, Rosemary Cowan, Rosemary Cowan

GP John William Alexander MACDONALD, John William Alexander MACDONALD, James W M DUNN, James W M DUNN, Robert William MURPHIE, Robert William MURPHIE

Newtonmore

Gergask Surgery
Laggan, Newtonmore PH20 1AH
Tel: 01528 544225 Fax: 01528 544388
(NHS Highland, Primary Care)
Patient List Size: 500

Practice Manager David Massey

GP Karen MASSEY

North Berwick

North Berwick Health Centre
54 St Baldreds Road, North Berwick EH39 4PU
Tel: 01620 892169 Fax: 01620 892901
(NHS Lothian, Primary and Community Division)
Patient List Size: 7200

Practice Manager Norma McKay

GP Peter Alastair KEELING, Claire DOLDON, Morgan William FLYNN, Neil David JONES, Anne Therese MULRINE, Gabriele Umberto SALUCCI

Oban

Aline Park Surgery
Aline Park, Lochaline, Morvern, Oban PA34 5XT
Tel: 01967 421252 Fax: 01967 421303
(NHS Highland, Primary Care)
Patient List Size: 330

GP Susan TAYLOR

Finlaggan Surgery
Finlaggan, Clachan Seil, Easdale, Oban PA34 4TL
Tel: 01852 300223 Fax: 01852 300392
(NHS Argyll and Clyde, Lomond and Argyll Community Services Division)

GP George HANNAH, Fiona GRAHAM

Lorn Medical Centre
Soroba Road, Oban PA34 4HE
Tel: 01631 563175 Fax: 01631 562708
(NHS Argyll and Clyde, Lomond and Argyll Community Services Division)
Patient List Size: 10200

Practice Manager Mairi Dunnings, Sheena MacInnes

GP Angus Thomson CAMERON, Maureen Elizabeth CAMERON, Erik JESPERSEN, Ian Bruce LENNOX, Angus Gordon MURCHISON, Allyson May MURRAY, Colin Moffat WILSON

Orkney

Daisy Villa Surgery
Daisy Villa, West End, St. Margarets Hope, Orkney KW17 2SN
Tel: 01856 831206 Fax: 01856 831716
Patient List Size: 1250

Practice Manager Lorna Whyte

GP Catriona KEMP, Simon KEMP

Dounby Surgery
Dounby, Orkney KW17 2HT
Tel: 01856 771209 Fax: 01856 771320
Email: mailbox@dounbysurgery.co.uk
Website: www.dounbysurgery.co.uk
Patient List Size: 2136

Practice Manager Ony Tullock

GP James S FROST, Robert Vernon HAZLEHURST, Hazel V MASON

Elwick Bank Surgery
Elwick Bank, Shapinsay, Orkney KW17 2EA
Tel: 01856 711284 Fax: 01856 711348
Patient List Size: 301

GP Ceri Ann LE-MAR

Flebister House Surgery
Flebister House, Sanday, Orkney KW17 2BW
Tel: 01857 600221 Fax: 01857 600332
Patient List Size: 489

GP Anthony MILLS

Geramount
Geramount, Stronsay, Orkney KW17 2AE
Tel: 01857 616321 Fax: 01857 616294
Patient List Size: 360

GP Geogre McKAY

Greystones Surgery
Greystones, Evie, Orkney KW17 2PQ
Tel: 01856 751283 Fax: 01856 751452

Practice Manager Dorothy Scott

GP Elspeth Sarah LOGAN, Vidja Bhushan MALHOTRA

Heatherlea Surgery
Heatherlea, Eday, Orkney KW17 2AB
Tel: 01857 622243 Fax: 01857 622315
Email: louise.fortune@zetnet.co.uk
Patient List Size: 128

GP Louise Dorothy FORTUNE

Islands View Surgery
Rousay, Orkney KW17 2PU
Tel: 01856 821265 Fax: 01856 821348

GP Garry Stuart MEARNS

New Manse Surgery
Linklet House, North Ronaldsay, Orkney KW17 2BE
Tel: 01857 633226 Fax: 01857 633207

Practice Manager Alison Duncan

GP Kevin Francis WOODBRIDGE

Springbank Surgery
Springbank, Flotta, Orkney KW16 3NP
Tel: 01856 701246

GP George Franklyn DREVER

Trenabie House Surgery
Trenabie House, Westray, Orkney KW17 2DL
Tel: 01857 677209 Fax: 01857 617519
Patient List Size: 650

Practice Manager Ruth Bain

GP Karl GNATH, Pedro PONIZ, Wenner SLOKHANN

Paisley

Abbey Medical Centre
Lonend, Paisley PA1 1SU
Tel: 0141 889 4088 Fax: 0141 842 1169
(NHS Argyll and Clyde, Renfrewshire and Inverclyde Community Services Division)

GP Donald McARTHUR, Katherine CHAPMAN, John DALRYMPLE, William GIBSON, Sheila McARTHUR, Jacqueline McLOONE, Lesley SMITH

The Barony Practice
Northcroft Medical Centre, Paisley PA3 4AD
Tel: 0141 889 3732 Fax: 0141 889 7502
(NHS Argyll and Clyde, Renfrewshire and Inverclyde Community Services Division)

Practice Manager Bernadette Arthur

GP Christopher JOHNSTONE, Lorna CUFFIELD, Louise HALLAN, John HISLOP

Charleston Surgery
South Campbell Street, Paisley PA2 6LR
Tel: 0141 889 4373 Fax: 0141 848 0648
(NHS Argyll and Clyde, Renfrewshire and Inverclyde Community Services Division)
Patient List Size: 5850

Practice Manager Linda Winston

GP Colin REID, Fiona BALLANTYNE, Colin INNES, Catherine WILLS

The Consulting Rooms
21 Neilston Road, Paisley PA2 6LW
Tel: 0141 889 5277 Fax: 0141 848 5500
(NHS Argyll and Clyde, Renfrewshire and Inverclyde Community Services Division)

Practice Manager Polly Parkinson

GP Andrew BUCHANAN, Joan Carole BOAG, David Cunningham DAVIDSON, Alan Robert DOWNIE, Jack Leonard LEIGHTON

Feeney and Partners
Northcroft Medical Centre, Kelburn Practice, North Croft Street, Paisley PA3 4NX
Tel: 0141 889 3356 Fax: 0141 887 5526
(NHS Argyll and Clyde, Renfrewshire and Inverclyde Community Services Division)
Patient List Size: 4200

Practice Manager Elaine F Paul

GP Linda FEENEY, Kathryn CLARK, Fiona CRAMPSEY

Glenburn Surgery
36 Glenburn Road, Paisley PA2 8JG
Tel: 0141 884 7788 Fax: 0141 561 1090
(NHS Argyll and Clyde, Renfrewshire and Inverclyde Community Services Division)
Patient List Size: 2000

Practice Manager Freda C Elder

GP Colin Wylie BROWN, Sheeraza EJAZ

The Health Centre
Ardlamont Square, Linwood, Paisley PA3 3DE
Tel: 01505 321051 Fax: 01505 383302
(NHS Argyll and Clyde, Renfrewshire and Inverclyde Community Services Division)

GP Mark ANDERSON, Andrea COOPER, Timothy DUNLOP, Rhianne RICHMOND

Incle Street Surgery
8 Incle Street, Paisley PA1 1HP
Tel: 0141 889 8809 Fax: 0141 849 1474
(NHS Argyll and Clyde, Renfrewshire and Inverclyde Community Services Division)

GP Stewart McCORMICK, David BRYDIE, Colin HODGSON, Rhona McMILLAN, Michael REA

Love Street Medical Centre
40 Love Street, Paisley PA3 2DY
Tel: 0141 889 3355 Fax: 0141 889 4785
Email: lovestreet@dial.pipex.com
(NHS Argyll and Clyde, Renfrewshire and Inverclyde Community Services Division)
Patient List Size: 6060

Practice Manager Paula Gallagher

GP Daniel BRANDON, Julie CANNING, Jacqueline McKEON

St James Surgery
19 St James Street, Paisley PA3 2HQ
Tel: 0141 889 5505 Fax: 0141 848 9190
(NHS Argyll and Clyde, Renfrewshire and Inverclyde Community Services Division)

GP Ian HAMILTON, Ian MASON

The Surgery
15 King Street, Paisley PA1 2PR
Tel: 0141 889 3144 Fax: 0141 889 7134
(NHS Argyll and Clyde, Renfrewshire and Inverclyde Community Services Division)
Patient List Size: 10000

Practice Manager Margaret Banks

GP John IP, Wendy Susan KIRKWOOD, David McFADYEN, Christine Margaret MURRAY, Gavin Moffat WATSON, Winifred Isabella WEIR

The Surgery
3 Glasgow Road, Paisley PA1 3QS
Tel: 0141 889 2604 Fax: 0141 887 9039
(NHS Argyll and Clyde, Renfrewshire and Inverclyde Community Services Division)

GP Damian SCULLION, Geraldine HOUSTON, Anne KNOX, Kenneth LOWE, Thomas MACPHERSON, James WEIR

The Tannahill Centre
76 Blackstoun Road, Paisley PA3 1NT
Tel: 0141 889 7631 Fax: 0141 889 6819

(NHS Argyll and Clyde, Renfrewshire and Inverclyde Community Services Division)

GP Sabiha AL-JANABI, Abdul LATIF, Abid MAHMOOD

Pathhead

Pathhead Medical Centre
210 Main Street, Pathhead EH37 5PP
Tel: 01875 320302 Fax: 01875 320494
(NHS Lothian, Primary and Community Division)

Practice Manager Moira Grant

GP David Stewart DUMMER, Marleen MURRAY, Ian Alexander SUTHERLAND, Catherine Mary WILSON

Peebles

Hay Lodge Health Centre
Neidpath Road, Peebles EH45 8JG
Tel: 01721 720380 Fax: 01721 723430
(NHS Borders, Primary Care Division)

Practice Manager Margaret Mayer

GP Peter Timothy YOUNG, Maude BROEK, Declan Mary HEGARTY, Rachael Grace MILLER

Hay Lodge Health Centre
Neidpath Road, Peebles EH45 8JG
Tel: 01721 720380 Fax: 01721 723430
(NHS Borders, Primary Care Division)

Practice Manager Margaret Mayer

GP David Robert LOVE, Elizabeth CLYDE, George Ewan McINTOSH

Penicuik

Eastfield Medical Centre
Eastfield Drive, Penicuik EH26 8EY
Tel: 01968 675576 Fax: 01968 674395
(NHS Lothian, Primary and Community Division)
Patient List Size: 4300

Practice Manager Isabel Stenhosue

GP Ian Macleod FRASER, Ruth Margaret COLLINS, David Henry GILLESPIE, Karen E HAYCOCK, Kirsty E ZEALLEY

Penicuik Health Centre
37 Imrie Place, Penicuik EH26 8LF
Tel: 01968 672612 Fax: 01968 671543
(NHS Lothian, Primary and Community Division)
Patient List Size: 13248

Practice Manager Anne McCall

GP David Maldwyn BEGG, Alexander Drummond BEGG, Fiona CRUDEN, Carol LEVSTEIN, John MACLEAN, Anne C MARTIN, Hamish Andrew Harman REID, Agnes Pool WOOD

Perth

Carse Medical Practice
The Rowlands, High Street, Errol, Perth PH2 7QJ
Tel: 01821 642248 Fax: 01821 642922
(NHS Tayside, Primary Care Division)
Patient List Size: 2293

Practice Manager Susan Campbell

GP Lindsay James Crosbie EASTON

Glover Street Medical Centre
133 Glover Street, Perth PH2 0JB
Tel: 01738 639748 Fax: 01738 635133
(NHS Tayside, Primary Care Division)
Patient List Size: 9200

Practice Manager Mary Simpson

GP Ross Paterson REID, Duncan Stuart FOSTER, Elaine Elizabeth MATTHEWS, Neil Alexander McLEOD, Nicholas Ironside SHEPHERD, Alison Mavis SNEDDON

Glover Street Medical Centre
133 Glover Street, Perth PH2 0JB
Tel: 01738 621844 Fax: 01738 636070
(NHS Tayside, Primary Care Division)

Practice Manager Penelope MacGregor

GP James Humfrey Fairfax KYNASTON, David H McELNEA, George Alexander MELROSE, Gillian Margaret SCOTT

Marshall Place Surgery
1 Marshall Place, Perth PH2 8AJ
Tel: 01738 623463 Fax: 01738 580948
(NHS Tayside, Primary Care Division)

GP Isabelle Marie DONALD

Mauve Practice
Drumhar Health Centre, North Methven Street, Perth PH1 5PD
Tel: 01738 622421 Fax: 01738 444077
Email: mfairweather@drumhar1.tayside.scot.nhs.uk
(NHS Tayside, Primary Care Division)
Patient List Size: 3301

Practice Manager Marlen Fairweather

GP Lindsey Jane COMPSON, Jahangir A KHAN, Christine Macleod Campbell ROXBURGH

Medical Centre
Caledonian Road, Perth PH2 8HH
Tel: 01738 628234 Fax: 01738 624945
Email: dbruce@caledonian.finix.org.uk
(NHS Tayside, Primary Care Division)
Patient List Size: 9965

Practice Manager Donna Bruce

GP James Stuart RIPLEY, Paul CUNNINGHAM, Finlay Robert John CURRIE, Derek Scott DUNBAR, Aileen Anne GOURLEY, Sharon Elizabeth LEE

The Surgery
Main Street, Bridge of Earn, Perth PH2 9PL
Tel: 01738 812000 Fax: 01738 812333
Email: beena.raschkes@tpct.scot.nhs.uk
(NHS Tayside, Primary Care Division)
Patient List Size: 2700

GP David Watson KIRKWOOD, Beena RASCHKES

The Taymount Surgery
1 Taymount Terrace, Perth PH1 1NU
Tel: 01738 627117 Fax: 01738 444713
(NHS Tayside, Primary Care Division)

Practice Manager Hazel Kemp

GP Leonard D BURNETT, Alistair Fleming FALCONER, Kenneth Love McWILLIAM, David Alexander SHACKLES, Janet Isobel SINCLAIR, Christopher David STEWART

Whitefriars Surgery
Whitefriars Street, Perth PH1 1PP
Tel: 01738 625842 Fax: 01738 445030
(NHS Tayside, Primary Care Division)

Practice Manager Jean King

GP Alasdair Hugh DUTTON, John Maxwell AULD, Jane Helen REID, Bernard Martin Aloysius REILLY

Whitefriar's Surgery
Whitefriar's Street, Perth PH1 1PP
Tel: 01738 627912 Fax: 01738 643969
(NHS Tayside, Primary Care Division)
Patient List Size: 8500

Practice Manager Jacqui Dawson

GP Daniel Thomas CAREY, Steven A ELLIOTT, Julia Ruth HAMILTON, Samuel John HEWITT, Nora Anne MOLONEY, David Wood WRIGHT

Yellow Practice
Drumhar Health Centre, North Methven Street, Perth PH1 5PD
Tel: 01738 621726 Fax: 01738 643757
(NHS Tayside, Primary Care Division)
Patient List Size: 6133

Practice Manager Ann Adamson

GP Adrian John NAPPER, Yvonne D ALLAN, Eleanor Margaret CAVANAGH, Michael Robert MILNE

Peterculter

Peterculter Medical Practice
Coronation Road, Peterculter AB14 0RP
Tel: 01224 733535 Fax: 01224 739979
Email: administrator@peterculter.grampian.scot.nhs.uk
(NHS Grampian, Primary Care Division)

Practice Manager Alison Mackay

GP Stuart Henry Weir DUNCAN, Kathleen Jean DONALD, Douglas Cameron Mackay HARRIS, David Gavin MILLAR

Peterhead

Cruden Medical Group
The Surgery, Main St Hatton, Peterhead AB42 0QQ
Tel: 01779 841208 Fax: 01779 841239
Email: administrator@hatton.grampian.scot.nhs.uk
(NHS Grampian, Primary Care Division)
Patient List Size: 3500

GP James Meldrum SANDEMAN, Priscilla ARMSTRONG, George Graham FERGUSON

Mintlaw Group Practice
Newlands Road, Mintlaw, Peterhead AB42 5GP
Tel: 01771 623522 Fax: 01771 624349
Email: administrator@mintlaw.grampian.scot.nhs.uk
(NHS Grampian, Primary Care Division)
Patient List Size: 9000

Practice Manager Frances Smith

GP James Gordon MILLER, Alexander Riddell GAULD, Margaret Anne LESLIE, James Ross MACKAY, Russell McINNES, Douglas Robert Hamilton NICOL

Peterhead Group Practice
The Health Centre, Peterhead AB42 2XA
Tel: 01774 474841 Fax: 01774 474848
Email: administrator@peterhead.grampian.scot.nhs.uk
(NHS Grampian, Primary Care Division)
Patient List Size: 20000

Practice Manager Michelle Bibby

GP Greg BRUCE, Patricia Helen DONALDSON, Dale FENWICK, David John Grant KENNEDY, L D RITCHIE, Joyce Buchan ROBERTSON, Iain Robert SMALL, John Clark STOUT, Bruce STRACHAN, Graham STRACHAN, Kenneth Alexander Boyd STRACHAN

Pitlochry

Kinloch Rannoch Medical Practice
Kinloch Rannoch, Pitlochry PH16 5PR
Tel: 01882 632216 Fax: 01882 632772
Website: www.tayside.scot.nhs.uk/gpweb/t/13439
(NHS Tayside, Primary Care Division)
Patient List Size: 600

Practice Manager Helen Simmons

GP Roger SIMMONS, Kate FINLEY

Toberargan Surgery
27 Toberargan Road, Pitlochry PH16 5HG
Tel: 01796 472558 Fax: 01796 473775
(NHS Tayside, Primary Care Division)

GP David Alexander CRUIKSHANK, Douglas Samuel KENNEDY, David Paul LEAVER, James Iain Roderick MacHUGH, Graeme William McCRORY

Port Glasgow

Dr Ramanathan
The Health Centre, 2-4 Bay Street, Port Glasgow PA14 5EW
Tel: 01475 745321 Fax: 01475 745587
Email: administrator@gp86285.ac-hb.scot.nhs.uk
(NHS Argyll and Clyde, Renfrewshire and Inverclyde Community Services Division)
Patient List Size: 4000

Practice Manager Gwen Ramanathan

GP Gary R RAMANATHAN, Elizabeth FORBES, Hector MACDONALD

Medical Centre
4 Dubbs Place, Port Glasgow PA14 6HW
Tel: 01475 705604 Fax: 01475 701277
(NHS Argyll and Clyde, Renfrewshire and Inverclyde Community Services Division)
Patient List Size: 5200

GP Michael MUTCH, Joseph BOYCE, Jennifer DOOLEY, Lucy HOLMS

Port Glasgow Health Centre
2 Bay Street, Port Glasgow PA14 5ED
Tel: 01475 745321 Fax: 01475 744587
(NHS Argyll and Clyde, Renfrewshire and Inverclyde Community Services Division)

Practice Manager Maureen Havlin

GP George GOWLING, James FARRELL, David WILKIE

Port Glasgow Health Centre
2 Bay Street, Port Glasgow PA14 5ED
Tel: 01475 745321 Fax: 01475 744587
(NHS Argyll and Clyde, Renfrewshire and Inverclyde Community Services Division)
Patient List Size: 2424

Practice Manager Lorraine Grant

GP Joseph BOGAN, Zia HUSSAIN

Port Glasgow Health Centre
2 Bay Street, Port Glasgow PA14 5ED
Tel: 01475 745321 Fax: 01475 744587
Email: maureen.haulin@renver-pct.scot.nhs.uk
(NHS Argyll and Clyde, Renfrewshire and Inverclyde Community Services Division)
Patient List Size: 4026

GP Gordon JEFFERIES, Michael McCARTNEY, Maureen SMITH

Prestonpans

Cockenzie and Port Seton Health Centre
Avenue Road, Cockenzie, Prestonpans EH32 0JL
Tel: 01875 811501 Fax: 01875 814421
(NHS Lothian, Primary and Community Division)

Practice Manager Jane Johnston

GP William POLLOCK, Donald BREMNER, Susan CRAMMOND, Susan E MENZIES, Jonathan William TURVILL, Peter WOOD

Prestonpans Health Centre
Preston Road, Prestonpans EH32 9QS
Tel: 01875 810736 Fax: 01875 812979
(NHS Lothian, Primary and Community Division)
Patient List Size: 7630

Practice Manager Rosalynne Haig

GP John Lionel REEKS, Iain Stewart McNEILL, Graham Ramsay Herd SCOTT, Muriel Gwyneth SIMMONTE, Heather Mary THOMAS

Prestwick

Kirkhall Surgery
4 Alexandra Avenue, Prestwick KA9 1AW
Tel: 01292 476626 Fax: 01292 678022
Email: kirkhall.admin@aapct.scot.nhs.uk
(NHS Ayrshire and Arran, Community Health Division)
Patient List Size: 6900

Practice Manager Anne Caldwell

GP David Charles ROY, Robert PERCIVAL, Eleanor RAE, Anna Elizabeth Clark SMITH, Graham Fulton STEEL

Station Road Surgery
2 Station Road, Prestwick KA9 1AQ
Tel: 01292 671444 Fax: 01292 678023
(NHS Ayrshire and Arran, Community Health Division)
Patient List Size: 9800

Practice Manager Martin Shevlin

GP D J CATTANACH, J CURRANS, John Edward LINDSAY, John Good McCALL, T McLAUGHLIN, William Douglas PARK

Renfrew

The Health Centre
103 Paisley Road, Renfrew PA4 8LH
Tel: 0141 886 2012 Fax: 0141 886 2092
(NHS Argyll and Clyde, Renfrewshire and Inverclyde Community Services Division)
Patient List Size: 6200

Practice Manager Sandra Bryce

GP Alexander ANDERSON, Lorraine MURPHY

Renfrew Health Centre
103 Paisley Road, Renfrew PA4 8LL
Tel: 0141 886 2455 Fax: 0141 855 0457
(NHS Argyll and Clyde, Renfrewshire and Inverclyde Community Services Division)
Patient List Size: 7126

Practice Manager Jean Williams

GP Brian William SHAPIRO, J ANDERSON, Sarah Louise DAVIDSON, Alison Elizabeth RAMAGE

Renfrew Health Centre
103 Paisley Road, Renfrew PA4 8LL
Tel: 0141 886 3535 Fax: 0141 885 0098
Email: administrator@gp87714.ac-hb.scot.nhs.uk
(NHS Argyll and Clyde, Renfrewshire and Inverclyde Community Services Division)
Patient List Size: 6624

Practice Manager Evelyn Coyle

GP Kenneth George Blair LYONS, Christopher J COYLE, Anne SUNDERLAND

Roslin

Roslin Surgery
6 Main Street, Roslin EH25 9LE
Tel: 0131 440 2043 Fax: 0131 448 2558
(NHS Lothian, Primary and Community Division)
Patient List Size: 4500

Practice Manager Linda Wilson

GP Ludovic Grant McINTOSH, Louisa J MARTIN, Jacqueline McCrindle McDONALD

Rothesay

The Health Centre
High Street, Rothesay PA20 9JL
Tel: 01700 502290 Fax: 01700 505692
(NHS Argyll and Clyde, Lomond and Argyll Community Services Division)

GP David HERRIOT, Colin BOYD, Roger CLARK, Robert HAYES, Peter LEWIS-SMITH, John MORTON

Saltcoats

Saltcoats Group Practice
17-19 Raise Street, Saltcoats KA21 5LX
Tel: 01294 605141 Fax: 01294 462828
(NHS Ayrshire and Arran, Community Health Division)

GP Richard Lennox de COURCY, Kathryn J CAMERON, Alison CUNNINGHAM, David Simon Michael HALES, I HARDY, Richard JOHNSON, Paul B MONAGHAN

Sanquhar

Sanquhar Health Centre
Station Road, Sanquhar DG4 6BT
Tel: 01659 50221 Fax: 01659 58116

Sanquhar Health Centre
Station Road, Sanquhar DG4 6BT
Tel: 01659 50221 Fax: 01659 58116
(NHS Dumfries and Galloway; NHS Dumfries and Galloway)

Practice Manager M Weir, M Weir, M Weir, M Weir

GP Iain Richardson BAKER, Iain Richardson BAKER, Christopher David BURTON, Christopher David BURTON

Selkirk

Selkirk Health Centre
Viewfield Lane, Selkirk TD7 4LJ
Tel: 01750 21674 Fax: 01750 23176
(NHS Borders, Primary Care Division)
Patient List Size: 7500

Practice Manager William Roberts

GP Christopher James SHARPE, Jeffrey Graham CULLEN, Elizabeth Mary GILLIES, John Calum MacDonald GILLIES, Helen Jane WHITAKER, John Fairlie WILSON

Shetland

Bixter Health Centre
Langbiggin, Bixter, Shetland ZE2 9NA
Tel: 01595 810202 Fax: 01595 810493
Email: drmacfarlane@bixter.shetland.scot.nhs.uk
Website: www.bixter-surgery.shetland.co.uk
(NHS Shetland)
Patient List Size: 1060

GP David MACFARLANE, Andrew COOPER, Caroline HINTON

Brae Medical Centre
Brae, Shetland ZE2 9QJ
Tel: 01806 522543 Fax: 01806 522713
(NHS Shetland)

Practice Manager Helen Taylor

GP J THORNE, P SCOTT

Lerwick Health Centre
19 South Road, Lerwick, Shetland ZE1 0RB
Tel: 01595 693201 Fax: 01595 697113
Website: www.lerwickdoctors.co.uk
(NHS Shetland)
Patient List Size: 9600

Practice Manager Gordon Carle

GP Yvonne ANDERSON, Lynne BRANTHWAITE, Gill CLARKE, Elizabeth Helena Anne COUTTS, Martin KRUSCHE, Dylan MURPHY

Levenwick Medical Practice
Gord, Levenwick, Shetland ZE2 9HX
Tel: 01950 422240 Fax: 01950 422201
(NHS Shetland)
Patient List Size: 2637

Practice Manager Sheila Mann

GP Michael David HUNTER, Aileen BROWN, Amanda NICHOLLS

Scalloway Health Centre
Scalloway, Shetland ZE1 0UH
Tel: 01595 880219 Fax: 01595 880461
(NHS Shetland)
Patient List Size: 2750

GP Christine BEGG, Foster Bruce CLEMINSON, David MALCOLM

Unst Surgery
Bultasound, Unst, Shetland ZE2 9OY
Tel: 01957 711318 Fax: 01957 711479
(NHS Shetland)

GP Jacqueline Mary HOWELL

Walls Health Centre
Walls, Shetland ZE2 9PF
Tel: 01595 809352 Fax: 01595 809414
Email: walls.surgery@walls.shetland.scot.nhs.uk
(NHS Shetland)
Patient List Size: 687

GP Helen Mary WARD, Andrew COOPEr

West Ayre Surgery
West Ayre, Hillswick, Shetland ZE2 9RW
Tel: 01806 503277 Fax: 01806 503399
(NHS Shetland)
Patient List Size: 700

GP Susan Jacqueline BOWIE

Whalsay Health Centre
Symbister, Whalsay, Shetland ZE2 9AE
Tel: 01806 566219 Fax: 01806 566519
(NHS Shetland)

GP Brian MARSHALL

Yell Health Centre
Reafirth, Yell, Shetland ZE2 9BX
Tel: 01957 702127 Fax: 01957 702147
Email: surgery@yell.shetland.scot.nhs.uk
(NHS Shetland)
Patient List Size: 1022

Practice Manager Deborah Guthrie

GP Rosemary A BRISCOE, Mark P AQUILINA

Shotts

Harthill Health Centre
24-26 Victoria Street, Harthill, Shotts ML7 5QE
Tel: 01501 751795 Fax: 01501 751696
(NHS Lanarkshire, Primary Care Division)
Patient List Size: 4500

GP E L ECCLES, W R THOM

Shotts Health Centre
36 Station Road, Shotts ML7 5DS
Tel: 01501 821544
(NHS Lanarkshire, Primary Care Division)

GP Mecheril Itty GEORGE

Shotts Health Centre
36 Station Road, Shotts ML7 5DS
Tel: 01501 822099 Fax: 01501 826622
(NHS Lanarkshire, Primary Care Division)
Patient List Size: 5000

Practice Manager Mary Traynor

GP Colin Peter MACFARLANE, Valerie Alexandra MACFARLANE, Shaun William George MILLIKEN

Station Road Surgery
269 Station Road, Sykehead, Shotts ML7 4AQ
Tel: 01501 823490 Fax: 01501 825995
(NHS Lanarkshire, Primary Care Division)
Patient List Size: 2928

Practice Manager Margaret Russell

GP Sharadini WALIMBE

Skelmorlie

Skelmorlie Surgery
The Lane, Skelmorlie PA17 5AR
Tel: 01475 520248 Fax: 01475 520767
(NHS Ayrshire and Arran, Community Health Division)

GP Sudakar RAI, Daniel S C CHAN, B RAI

South Queensferry

South Queensferry Medical Practice
41 The Loan, South Queensferry EH30 9HA
Tel: 0131 331 1396 Fax: 0131 537 4433
(NHS Lothian, Primary and Community Division)

Practice Manager Ken Sinclair

GP James Douglas STUART, Colin George CACKETTE, Christopher J CREBER, Victor J JACK, Gordon John Matthews LECKIE, Alison MACARTNEY, Elizabeth J WILLIAMSON

St Andrews

The Health Centre
68 Pipeland Road, St Andrews KY16 8JZ
Tel: 01334 473441 Fax: 01334 466508
(NHS Fife, Primary Care Division)

Practice Manager Patricia Duff, Margaret Mackie

GP Elizabeth Mary RANDALL, John Richard BELL, A BOWMAN, K J RUSSELL, Alan John SCOTT

The Health Centre
68 Pipeland Road, St Andrews KY16 8JZ
Tel: 01334 477477 Fax: 01334 466512
(NHS Fife, Primary Care Division)

Practice Manager Morag Scott

GP Hubert Charles Talwin MORRIS, Jane CHURCH, Thomas James CLARK, Lesley HENDERSON, Louise LAMONT, Gerard SMYTH

The Surgery
11 Main Street, Leuchars, St Andrews KY16 0HB
Tel: 01334 839210 Fax: 01334 838770
(NHS Fife, Primary Care Division)
Patient List Size: 3000

Practice Manager Elizabeth Tough

GP Bryan William JOHNSTON, John Henry SALAMONSKI

Tait and Partners
68 Pipeland Road, St Andrews KY16 8JZ
Tel: 01334 476840 Fax: 01334 466516
(NHS Fife, Primary Care Division)
Patient List Size: 9000

Practice Manager Helen Smith

GP Hamish Adie TAIT, Gillian Anne Wilson BARCLAY, Karen GRAHAM, Ian Byrne MATHEWSON, Gillian Anne MILNE, Jonathan Mark NIXON

Stevenston

Drs McCallum, Martin and Convery
20 Main Street, Stevenston KA20 3BB
Tel: 01294 464141 Fax: 01294 466408
(NHS Ayrshire and Arran, Community Health Division)

GP Huntly Gill McCALLUM, C CONVERY, Clifford John MARTIN

Stevenson Group Practice
New Street, Stevenston KA20 3AA
Tel: 01294 464413 Fax: 01294 604234
(NHS Ayrshire and Arran, Community Health Division)
Patient List Size: 4286

GP Gilbert SCOLLAY, Arun Kumar DAS, Kiron GHOSH

Stirling

Aberfoyle Medical Centre
Main Street, Aberfoyle, Stirling FK8 3UX
Tel: 01877 382421 Fax: 01877 382718
Email: administrator@gp25629.forth-hb.scot.nhs.uk
(NHS Forth Valley, Primary Care Operating Division)
Patient List Size: 2300

Practice Manager Marilyn Dorrall

GP Anne LINDSAY, William Mowat POLLOK

Airthrey Park Medical Centre
Hermitage Road, Stirling University, Stirling FK9 4NJ
Tel: 01786 463831 Fax: 01786 447482
Email: administrator@gp25559.forth-hb.scot.nhs.uk
(NHS Forth Valley, Primary Care Operating Division)
Patient List Size: 6500

GP Caroline Joy Casse RENWICK, Aileen Margaret DOHERTY, Gregor John MURDOCH

Bannockburn Medical Practice
Bannockburn Health Centre, Firs Entry, Bannockburn, Stirling FK7 0HW
Tel: 01786 813435 Fax: 01786 817545
(NHS Forth Valley, Primary Care Operating Division)

Practice Manager Duncan Harris

GP James Gemmell McARTHUR, Diane BASQUILL, Michael Stephen BEYER, Douglas Baird Mackenzie KING, Mhairi Elizabeth McLEOD, John SCALES, Fiona J SPENS

Bridge of Allan Health Centre
Fountain Road, Bridge of Allan, Stirling FK9 4EU
Tel: 01786 833210
(NHS Forth Valley, Primary Care Operating Division)

Practice Manager Ann Taggart

GP Robert FAIRLEY, Fiona Margaret JOHNSTONE, Christopher MAIR, Alexander Barclay STUART

Fallin, Cowie and Airth Medical Practice
Stirling Road, Fallin, Stirling FK7 7JD
Tel: 01786 812412 Fax: 01786 817496
(NHS Forth Valley, Primary Care Operating Division)
Patient List Size: 5943

Practice Manager Louise ironside

GP William George FISHER, John Knox MACDONALD, Helen Jackson MacLARTY, Robert Arthur RODGER

Milliken and Young
The Surgery, Castlehill Loan, Kippen, Stirling FK8 3DZ
Tel: 01786 870369 Fax: 01786 870819
(NHS Forth Valley, Primary Care Operating Division)
Patient List Size: 2000

Practice Manager Amanda Stewart

GP Neil Kenneth Charles MILLIKEN, David Robertson YOUNG

New Allan Park Surgery
19 Allan Park, Stirling FK8 2QD
Tel: 01786 451375 Fax: 01786 448596
(NHS Forth Valley, Primary Care Operating Division)
Patient List Size: 2309

GP Mary Therese HIGGINS

Orchard House Health Centre
Union Street, Stirling FK8 1PH
Tel: 01786 450394 Fax: 01786 448284
Website: www.orchardhousehealthcentre.co.uk
(NHS Forth Valley, Primary Care Operating Division)
Patient List Size: 4500

Practice Manager Lesley Ferguson

GP Charles Clarke MULLEN, Rhoda Agnes ABEL, Neil William HAMILTON

Park Avenue Medical Centre
9 Park Avenue, Stirling FK8 2QR
Tel: 01786 473529
(NHS Forth Valley, Primary Care Operating Division)

GP Robert Ian HANLEY, Shona Mairi KENNEDY, Fiona Elizabeth LYLE, John Nestor Edgar RANKIN, Olga WALKINS, Ivan Richard Joseph WEIR

Park Terrace Surgery
7A Park Terrace, Stirling FK8 2JT
Tel: 01786 445888 Fax: 01786 449154
(NHS Forth Valley, Primary Care Operating Division)
Patient List Size: 6000

Practice Manager Christine Kelly

GP John Barclay LOUDON, Marie Therese BEATTIE, Ronald James Hamilton BROWN, Jane Helen GALLACHER, Simon RANDFIELD

Viewfield Medical Centre
3 Viewfield Place, Stirling FK8 1NJ
Tel: 01786 472028 Fax: 01786 463388
(NHS Forth Valley, Primary Care Operating Division)
Patient List Size: 9095

Practice Manager Elspeth Boyle

GP Justin BARNES, Thomas Wilson EVANS, Josefina de Unamuno ROBERTSON, Michael Charles William WHITELEY, Scott WILLIAMS, William David YOUNG

Wallace Medical Practice
Wallace House, Maxwell Place, Stirling FK8 1JU
Tel: 01786 448900 Fax: 01786 445276
(NHS Forth Valley, Primary Care Operating Division)
Patient List Size: 2330

Practice Manager Nan Bone

GP Ronald William PORTEOUS, William Campbell CONNOR

Stonehaven

Stonehaven Medical Group
Stonehaven Medical Centre, 32 Robert Street, Stonehaven AB39 2EL
Tel: 01569 762945 Fax: 01569 766552
(NHS Grampian, Primary Care Division)

Practice Manager Joan MacKenzie

GP Graham Henderson McINTOSH, Alfred George DOSSETT, James Michael Rodger HERD, David Michael HOWARD, Allison MACCUISH, Jane MACKENZIE, Fiona MACLEOD, Alastair Hamilton MORGAN, Stuart REARY, Alison Lesley STEWART

Stornoway

Archway Medical Practice
16 Francis Street, Stornoway HS1 2XB
Tel: 01851 703588 Fax: 01851 706338
(NHS Western Isles)

Practice Manager Murdeen MacLeod

GP Jonathan Neil DAVIS, R W HAMILTON, Anneniek M C KOK, Christine Rankin MacLENNAN

The Group Practice, Stornoway
Health Centre, Springfield Road, Stornoway HS1 2PS
Tel: 01851 703145 Fax: 01851 706138
Email: administrator@gp90031.w-isles-hb.scot.nhs.uk
(NHS Western Isles)
Patient List Size: 6754

Practice Manager Martin Palmer

GP Robert John DICKIE, Janice GILMOUR, Margaret Macdonald MACLEOD, Alistair Brian MICHIE, Shona MURRAY, Louise SCOTT, Antonio UCETA, Marten James WALKER

Springfield Medical Practice
Health Centre, Springfield Road, Stornoway HS1 2PS
Tel: 01851 704888 Fax: 01851 703005
Email: Administrator@gp90045.w-isles-hb.scot.nhs.uk
(NHS Western Isles)
Patient List Size: 3125

GP Margaret FERGUSON, Stewart Michael BRYDON, Ken MURRAY

Stranraer

The Clinic
Drummore, Stranraer DG9 9QQ
Tel: 01776 840205 Fax: 01776 840390

The Clinic
Drummore, Stranraer DG9 9QQ
Tel: 01776 840205 Fax: 01776 840390
(NHS Dumfries and Galloway; NHS Dumfries and Galloway)
Patient List Size: 800
Patient List Size: 800

Practice Manager W Ward, W Ward, W Ward, W Ward

GP Iris Margaret RITCHIE, Iris Margaret RITCHIE

Lochinch Practice
Waverley Medical Centre, Darlrymple Street, Stranraer DG9 7DW
Tel: 01776 706513 Fax: 01776704825

Lochinch Practice
Waverley Medical Centre, Darlrymple Street, Stranraer DG9 7DW
Tel: 01776 706513 Fax: 01776704825
(NHS Dumfries and Galloway; NHS Dumfries and Galloway)

Practice Manager Kerry Irving, Kerry Irving, Kerry Irving, Kerry Irving

GP Ranald John SPICER, Ranald John SPICER, Jonathan Niall Walton BALMER, Jonathan Niall Walton BALMER, Kieran George McANULTY, Kieran George McANULTY, Donna Athena VAUGHAN, Donna Athena VAUGHAN

Stranraer Health Centre
Edinburgh Road, Stranraer DG9 7HG
Tel: 01776 706566

Stranraer Health Centre
Edinburgh Road, Stranraer DG9 7HG
Tel: 01776 706566
(NHS Dumfries and Galloway; NHS Dumfries and Galloway)

GP Paul Albert CARNAGHAN, Paul Albert CARNAGHAN, Derek James WOOFF, Derek James WOOFF, Margaret Anne Rena YOUNG, Margaret Anne Rena YOUNG

Stranraer Health Centre
Edinburgh Road, Stranraer DG9 7HG
Tel: 01776 706566

Stranraer Health Centre
Edinburgh Road, Stranraer DG9 7HG
Tel: 01776 706566
(NHS Dumfries and Galloway; NHS Dumfries and Galloway)

GP Iain Drummond GORDON, Iain Drummond GORDON, Jane Fraser GALL, Jane Fraser GALL, Emer Mary LENNON, Emer Mary LENNON, John Christopher McTAGGART, John Christopher McTAGGART

Waverly Medical Centre
Dalrymple St, Stranraer DG9 7HG
Tel: 01776 706513 Fax: 017767 706566

Waverly Medical Centre
Dalrymple St, Stranraer DG9 7HG
Tel: 01776 706513 Fax: 017767 706566
(NHS Dumfries and Galloway; NHS Dumfries and Galloway)
Patient List Size: 5700
Patient List Size: 5700

GP Simon Charles Thomas REID, Simon Charles Thomas REID, Ann ADAMS, Ann ADAMS, Richard GARRAT, Richard GARRAT, R GRIEVE, R GRIEVE, Jennifer LEE, Jennifer LEE, Fiona Morrison McDOUGALL, Fiona Morrison McDOUGALL

White House Surgery
Sandhead, Stranraer DG9 9JA
Tel: 01776 830262 Fax: 01776 830440
Email: Agordonbaird@aol.com

White House Surgery
Sandhead, Stranraer DG9 9JA
Tel: 01776 830262 Fax: 01776 830440
Email: Agordonbaird@aol.com
(NHS Dumfries and Galloway; NHS Dumfries and Galloway)
Patient List Size: 1400
Patient List Size: 1400

GP Alastair Gordon BAIRD, Alastair Gordon BAIRD

Strathaven

Avondale Medical Practice
Strathaven Health Centre, The Ward, Strathaven ML10 6AS
Tel: 01357 529595 Fax: 01357 529494
Patient List Size: 5660

Practice Manager Yvonne Gilmour

GP Clifford Craig GODLEY, William Meldrum CAMPBELL, Irene PEPPERELL, Craig John SMITH

Strahaven Health Centre
The Ward, Strathaven ML10 6AS
Tel: 01357 522993 Fax: 01357 522714
Patient List Size: 6290

Practice Manager Margaret Dick

GP Carol Margaret Carmichael CAMPBELL, Christine Margaret HASSALL, Frank Norman SHAPIRO

Strathcarron

Ferguson Medical Centre
Lochcarron, Strathcarron IV54 8YQ
Tel: 01520 722215 Fax: 01520 722230
Email: administrator@gp55395.highland-hb.scot.nhs.uk
(NHS Highland, Primary Care)
Patient List Size: 950

GP David Barclay MURRAY, IAIN STRAITH

Milltown Surgery
Milltown, Applecross, Strathcarron IV54 8LS
Tel: 01520 744252 Fax: 01520 744344
(NHS Highland, Primary Care)

GP Janice Munro CARGILL

Strathdon

Strathdon Medical Centre
Newe, Strathdon AB36 8XB
Tel: 01975 651209

Practice Manager David Williams

GP Janet Lesley FITTON, Alan CARR

Strathpeffer

Strathpeffer Medical Practice
The Medical Centre, Strathpeffer IV14 9AG
Tel: 01997 421455 Fax: 01997 421172
Email: administrator@gp88412.highland-hb.scot.nhs.uk
(NHS Highland, Primary Care)
Patient List Size: 3470

Practice Manager Christine York

GP Howard Barton GATE, Thomas Stewart MACPHERSON, Alison Janet WOOD

Stromness

Hoy and Walls Health Centre
Longhope, Stromness KW16 3PA
Tel: 01856 701209 Fax: 01856 701309
Email: paul.kettle@nhs.net
Patient List Size: 375

Practice Manager Kathleen McFadyen

GP Paul Raymond KETTLE, Anthony Robert TRICKETT

The Surgery
77 John Street, Stromness KW16 3AD
Tel: 01856 850205 Fax: 01856 850868
Email: rats@stromenss.demon.co.uk
Patient List Size: 2900

Practice Manager Maureen Sinclair

GP Colin Kennedy RAE, Caroline SHEEHAN, Andrew TREVETT

Tain

Tain and District Medical Practice
The Health Centre, Scotsburn Road, Tain IV19 1PR
Tel: 01862 892203 Fax: 01862 892165
(NHS Highland, Primary Care)

GP Ian George COLVIN, Marion MACDONALD

Tain and Fearn Area Medical Practice
The Health Centre, Scotsburn Road, Tain IV19 1PR
Tel: 01862 892759 Fax: 01862 892579
(NHS Highland, Primary Care)
Patient List Size: 5200

Practice Manager Maureen Turnbull

GP Jenny ARMER, Martin ARMER, Andrew EVENNETT, Sandy Richard GORDON, Peter David GRAHAM, John Paul GREENWOOD, Kate SAVAGE

Tarbert

Muasdale Surgery
Greenhill, Muasdale, Tarbert PA29 6XD
Tel: 01583 421206 Fax: 01583 421220
Email: administrator@gp84472.ac.hb.scot.nhs.uk
(NHS Argyll and Clyde, Lomond and Argyll Community Services Division)
Patient List Size: 830

Practice Manager Dawn Kerr

GP Norman GOURLAY

North Harris Medical Practice
West Tarbert, Tarbert HS3 3BG
Tel: 01859 502421 Fax: 01859 502010
(NHS Western Isles)
Patient List Size: 1500

GP Jurgen TITTMAR, Angus McKELLAR, Kirsty McKELLAR

The Surgery
Tarbert PA29 6UL
Tel: 01880 820219 Fax: 01880 820104
(NHS Argyll and Clyde, Lomond and Argyll Community Services Division)

Practice Manager Mrs Inskip

GP John MAITLAND

Taynuilt

Taynuilt Medical Practice
Taynuilt PA35 1JE
Tel: 01866 822684 Fax: 01866 822363
(NHS Argyll and Clyde, Lomond and Argyll Community Services Division)
Patient List Size: 3900

Practice Manager Gail MacGregor

GP Katherine Mary Dickson ARMSTRONG, Neil Lachlan BENNETT, Allison Mochrie DAVIES, John Marechal LYON

Tayport

Tayview Medical Practice
21 Dougall Street, Tayport DD6 9JG
Tel: 01382 543251 Fax: 01382 552996
(NHS Fife, Primary Care Division)
Patient List Size: 10000

Practice Manager L De Villiers

GP David Martin HEPWORTH, Allan McKenzie COPLAND, Margaret Elizabeth INGLEDEW, Andrew Douglas KILPATRICK, Neil John MACKINTOSH, Nora Elizabeth Marjorie RICKETTS

Thornhill

Health Centre
Thornhill DG3 5AA
Tel: 01848 330208 Fax: 01848 330223

Health Centre
Thornhill DG3 5AA
Tel: 01848 330208 Fax: 01848 330223
(NHS Dumfries and Galloway; NHS Dumfries and Galloway)

Practice Manager Margaret Sword, Margaret Sword, Margaret Sword, Margaret Sword

GP Ian Macpherson BROWN, Ian Macpherson BROWN, Robert BRODIE, Robert BRODIE, Fiona Hyslop VERNON, Fiona Hyslop VERNON

Thurso

Armadale Medical Centre
Armadale, Thurso KW14 7SA
Tel: 01641 541212 Fax: 01641 541226
Email: administrator@gp55183.highland-hb.scot.nhs.uk
(NHS Highland, Primary Care)
Patient List Size: 1000

Practice Manager Isabel Moore

GP Rosemary Joyce LEE, Andreas Erich Wilhelm HERFURT

Castletown Medical Practice
Murrayfield, Castletown, Thurso KW14 8TY
Tel: 01847 821205 Fax: 01847 821540
(NHS Highland, Primary Care)

Patient List Size: 1862

Practice Manager Carol Mackenzie

GP Donald McNEILL, Wilma MACLEOD

Princes Street Surgery
69 Princes Street, Thurso KW14 7DH
Tel: 01847 893154 Fax: 01847 892113
(NHS Highland, Primary Care)

Practice Manager Christine Tait

GP Gavin Ramsay MacPherson BURNETT, Alison Graham BROOKS, Neil Lionel HARVEY, Morag L MACDONALD, J P Anthony PAGE

Riverbank Surgery
Riverbank, Janet Street, Thurso KW14 7AR
Tel: 01847 892027/892009 Fax: 01847 892690
(NHS Highland, Primary Care)
Patient List Size: 5980

GP John Duncan MORRISON, Stuart Robert FINDLAY, G J A MORRIS, A A H ROBERTSON

Tighnabruaich

Burnside Surgery
Tighnabruaich PA21 2BA
Tel: 01700 811207 Fax: 01700 811766
(NHS Argyll and Clyde, Lomond and Argyll Community Services Division)

GP George CARLE, Diane SINCLAIR

Tillicoultry

Tillicoultry Health Centre
Park Street, Tillicoultry FK13 6AG
Tel: 01259 750531 Fax: 01259 752818
(NHS Forth Valley, Primary Care Operating Division)
Patient List Size: 8000

Practice Manager J Macmillan

GP Joan Elizabeth BRODIE, Nicholas James EDMUNDS, James Adam KING, Andreas KOLLE, Jane Catherine MACPHIE, Alison ROBERTSON

Tranent

Tranent Medical Practice
Loch Road, Tranent EH33 2JX
Tel: 01875 610697 Fax: 01875 615046
(NHS Lothian, Primary and Community Division)
Patient List Size: 14000

Practice Manager Mary Gordon

GP Yvonne Elizabeth Barbara CRAWFORD, Andrew Doig DAVIES, Ian David DONALDSON, Jacqueline Claire HALLIDAY-PEGG, John Derek MACNAIR, Alison Margaret MACRAE, James MORRISON, Alan Iain REID

Troon

101 Medical Practice
101 Portland Street, Troon KA10 6QN
Tel: 01292 313593 Fax: 01292 312020
(NHS Ayrshire and Arran, Community Health Division)
Patient List Size: 6000

Practice Manager Barbara Sloan

GP Maureen Easton SCOTT, Christine Margaret AULD, Lesley SHEARER, Jill C SHENNAN

Portland Surgery
1 Dukes Road, Troon KA10 6QR
Tel: 01292 312489 Fax: 01292 317837
(NHS Ayrshire and Arran, Community Health Division)
Patient List Size: 3200

Practice Manager Margaret McKinlay

GP Adam Grant McHATTIE, J HOLLAND, A J McGREGOR

Templehill Surgery
23 Templehill, Troon KA10 6BQ
Tel: 01292 312012 Fax: 01292 317594
(NHS Ayrshire and Arran, Community Health Division)

Practice Manager Helen Clark

GP James McDonald BEATSON, Peter James BAIRD, John Martin MACPHERSON, Alasdair Duncan MORRISON, Joan Kathryn PITTAM

Turriff

Cuminestown Health Centre
Auchry Road, Cuminestown, Turriff AB53 5WJ
Tel: 01888 544232 Fax: 01888 544701
(NHS Grampian, Primary Care Division)
Patient List Size: 1350

Practice Manager M Fraser

GP Keith Gordon FRASER, Alan SINCLAIR

Fyvie Health Centre
Health Centre, 27 Parnassus Gardens, Fyvie, Turriff AB53 8QD
Tel: 01651 891205 Fax: 01651 891834
(NHS Grampian, Primary Care Division)

Practice Manager Sandra Yule

GP Ronald Macdonald WALLACE, David Garden CONNELL, Simon Bramwell ROBERTSON, Craig WATSON, Tanya D WILSON

Health Centre
Balmellie Road, Turriff AB53 4DQ
Tel: 01888 562323 Fax: 01888 564010
(NHS Grampian, Primary Care Division)

Practice Manager E. Shearer

GP Robert William LIDDELL, Katrina Evelyn Scott DUTHIE, Patricia Nell GUTHRIE, Steven Charles HENDERSON, Catriona LAWSON, Karen McLUCKIE

Ullapool

Ullapool Medical Practice
The Health Centre, North Road, Ullapool IV26 2XL
Tel: 01854 612015/612595 Fax: 01854 613025
Email: administrator@gp55451.highland-hb.scot.nhs.uk
(NHS Highland, Primary Care)
Patient List Size: 2600

Practice Manager Fiona Shaw

GP Alexander STEWART, Ishbel Mary HARTLEY, Colin McDOUGALL, Gerald Ian WATMOUGH, Richard D M WEEKES

West Calder

West Calder Medical Practice
Dickson Street, West Calder EH55 8HB
Tel: 01506 871403 Fax: 01506 873427
(NHS Lothian, West Lothian Healthcare Division)

Practice Manager Sue Brown

GP Cynthia Mary BROOK, Anne Morrison CAMPBELL, Steven John HAIGH, Michael John HEWITT, James MARPLE, James Loudon ROBERTSON, Carol SIMPSON

West Kilbride

West Kilbride Group Practice
107B Main Street, West Kilbride KA23 9AR
Tel: 01294 823607 Fax: 01294 829318
(NHS Ayrshire and Arran, Community Health Division)
Patient List Size: 5500

GP Kenneth George FEGAN, June Peterson CASKIE, Dr HOWIE, Hamish Donald SIMPSON

West Linton

Health Centre
Deanfoot Road, West Linton EH46 7EX
Tel: 01968 660808
(NHS Borders, Primary Care Division)
Patient List Size: 3270

Practice Manager Julie Downie

GP Alexander Chapman POLLOCK, John Sinclair HALCROW, Myra W POLLOCK

Westhill

Skene Medical Group
Westhill Drive, Westhill AB32 6FY
Tel: 01224 742213 Fax: 01224 748671
Patient List Size: 12800

GP Colin Calder HARRIS, Jennifer Edna BROWNHILL, Allan Wales BRUCE, Joanne M CURRIE, George G ELLIS, Elspeth C FRASER, Colin Moffat HUNTER, Kathleen E NIDOW, Robina Donaldson RITCHIE

Wick

Canisbay Surgery
Canisbay, Wick KW1 4YH
Tel: 01955 611205 Fax: 01955 611327
(NHS Highland, Primary Care)

GP Moray Ewen FRASER

Riverview Practice
Wick Medical Centre, Martha Terrace, Wick KW1 5EL
Tel: 01955 602355 Fax: 01955 605496
Website: www.riverviewpractice.co.uk
(NHS Highland, Primary Care)
Patient List Size: 5700

Practice Manager Geraldine Durrand, Carole Sinclair

GP Emily Jane COBB, Iain JOHNSTON, Carol LEEUWENBERG

Wick Medical Centre
Martha Terrace, Wick KW1 5EL
Tel: 01955 605885 Fax: 01955 602434
Email: mapwick@aol.com
(NHS Highland, Primary Care)

Practice Manager Pat Niwa

GP Maurice Robert PEARSON

Wick Medical Centre
Martha Terrace, Wick KW1 5EL
Tel: 01955 602595 Fax: 01955 602434
(NHS Highland, Primary Care)

Practice Manager Lesley Gunn

Wishaw

The Health Centre
Kenilworth Avenue, Wishaw ML2 7BQ
Tel: 01698 372201 Fax: 01698 371051
(NHS Lanarkshire, Primary Care Division)
Patient List Size: 9500

Practice Manager G Bell

GP Colin Maitland CLARK, Omer Nazir AHMED, Carol McLeod HOTCHKISS, Alexander John MILNE, Thomas Kyle WILSON

Newmains Health Centre
17 Manse Road, Newmains, Wishaw ML2 9AX
Tel: 01698 384482 Fax: 01698 387456
Email: administrator@sp62806.law.lanark-hb.scot.nhs.uk
(NHS Lanarkshire, Primary Care Division)
Patient List Size: 2133

Practice Manager Teresa O'Donnell

GP Nicolas Paul Matheson DEAR, Louise BEGG

Newmains Health Centre
18 Manse Road, Newmains, Wishaw ML2 9AX
Tel: 01698 383296 Fax: 01698 387157
(NHS Lanarkshire, Primary Care Division)

GP Soma Sudershan REDDY, Manusamy SETHU RAMAN

Newmains Health Centre
17 Manse Road, Newmains, Wishaw ML2 9AX
Tel: 01698 381074
(NHS Lanarkshire, Primary Care Division)
Patient List Size: 3100

Practice Manager Ann Ledgerwood

GP Abdullah A W MAJUMDAR, Ann SULLIVAN

Wishaw Health Centre
Kenilworth Avenue, Wishaw ML2 7BQ
Tel: 01698 357766 Fax: 01698 361384
(NHS Lanarkshire, Primary Care Division)
Patient List Size: 4750

Practice Manager G Docherty

GP Colette Mary MAULE, Elaine M CROSSAN, Antonette McCOACH

Wishaw Health Centre
Kenilworth Avenue, Wishaw ML2 7BQ
Tel: 01698 373341 Fax: 01698 373736
(NHS Lanarkshire, Primary Care Division)

Practice Manager Wilma Piling

GP Alastair Rowatt LOGAN, Alistair BELL, Janice CROFTS, Sheila DOBBIE, Alexander LOGAN, Robert PEARSALL, David Winterburn STEWART

Wishaw Health Centre
Kenilworth Avenue, Wishaw ML2 7BQ
Tel: 01698 365420
(NHS Lanarkshire, Primary Care Division)

GP Anne CONNELLY

Wishaw Health Centre
Kenilworth Avenue, Wishaw ML2 7BQ
Tel: 01698 372888 Fax: 01698 376289
(NHS Lanarkshire, Primary Care Division)
Patient List Size: 6000

Practice Manager Jacqueline Summers

GP James W MURPHY, Talib AL-KUREISHI, Julie Elizabeth CURRAN, Pauline KEEGANS

Wishaw Heath Centre
Kenilworth Avenue, Wishaw ML2 7BQ
Tel: 01698 361716 Fax: 01698 366086
(NHS Lanarkshire, Primary Care Division)

Practice Manager Donna McAleer

GP Kim Elizabeth Henderson McKAY, Susan Ann MURRAY, Sharon RITCHIE

Wales

Aberaeron

Oxford Street Surgery
Oxford Street, Aberaeron SA46 0JB
Tel: 01545 570273 Fax: 01545 571625
(Ceredigion Local Health Board)

GP Jonathan Christian PRICE-JONES, Dorothea Mary WILLIAMS

Tanyfron Surgery
7-9 Market Street, Aberaeron SA46 0AS
Tel: 01545 570271 Fax: 01545 570136
(Ceredigion Local Health Board)

Practice Manager Maria Siczowa

GP Margaret Helen HERBERT, David Owen EVANS, Richard Gerwyn THOMAS

Aberdare

Claypath Medical Practice
Glamorgan Street, Aberdare
Tel: 01685 872006 Fax: 01685 875380
(Rhondda Cynon Taff Local Health Board)

GP Indu B SAHAI, Shesh Nandan SAHAI

Cwmaman Surgery
6-14 Glanaman Road, Aberdare CF44 6HY
Tel: 01685 873002 Fax: 01685 872179
Email: enquiries@gp-w9506.wales.nhs.uk
(Rhondda Cynon Taff Local Health Board)
Patient List Size: 3183

Practice Manager Dawn M Jones

GP Syed A. ALI, Shaikh O RAHMAN

George Street Medical Centre
10 George Street, Aberaman, Aberdare CF44 6RY
Tel: 01685 874120 Fax: 01685 881581
(Rhondda Cynon Taff Local Health Board)

Practice Manager Mamata Chattopadhyay

GP Swapan K CHATTOPADHYAY

High Street Health Centre
High Street, Aberdare CF44 7DD
Tel: 01685 874614 Fax: 01685 877485
(Rhondda Cynon Taff Local Health Board)
Patient List Size: 3500

Practice Manager G Butler

GP Shah Mohammad IMTIAZ, Syed A. SHAH

High Street Health Centre
High Street, Aberdare CF44 7DD
Tel: 01685 874614 Fax: 01685 877485
(Rhondda Cynon Taff Local Health Board)
Patient List Size: 3500

Practice Manager G K Butler

GP Syed M S H ASHRAF

Hirwaun Health Centre
Hirwaun, Aberdare CF44 9NS
Tel: 01685 811999 Fax: 01685 814145
(Rhondda Cynon Taff Local Health Board)

GP A W ERHARDT, P K GEORGE

Maendy Place Medical Centre
1 Maendy Place, Weatherall Street, Aberdare CF44 7AY
Tel: 01685 872146 Fax: 01685 884767
(Rhondda Cynon Taff Local Health Board)

Practice Manager E Thomas

GP David Derek THOMAS, Rachel A HOOPER

Mill Street Health Centre
69 Mill Street, Trecynon, Aberdare CF44 8LY
Tel: 01685 872504 Fax: 01685 872504

Practice Manager C Parfitt

GP Mohammad Rafiq KHAN

Monk Street Health Centre
74 Monk Street, Aberdare CF44 7PA
Tel: 01685 875906 Fax: 01685 875906
(Rhondda Cynon Taff Local Health Board)
Patient List Size: 3600

GP Alan G WARDROP, T D DAVIES

The New Trap Surgery
5 Dean Street, Aberdare CF44 7BN
Tel: 01685 872045 Fax: 01685 870625
(Rhondda Cynon Taff Local Health Board)

GP Sultan MAHMUD

Pant Surgery
57 Aberdare Road, Cwmbach, Aberdare CF44 0HL
Tel: 01685 872434 Fax: 01685 878158
(Rhondda Cynon Taff Local Health Board)
Patient List Size: 2500

Practice Manager Shelia Stuckey

GP Indrajit MUKHERJEE

Park Surgery
Windsor Street, Trecynon, Aberdare CF44 8LL
Tel: 01685 872040 Fax: 01685 883696
(Rhondda Cynon Taff Local Health Board)
Patient List Size: 7100

Practice Manager Patricia Susan Shearn

GP Denis Joseph SLYNE, Jane Frances FLEMING, Mark Gregory FOSTER, Andrew SAMUELS

Abergavenny

Hereford Road Surgery
6 Hereford Road, Abergavenny NP7 5PR
Tel: 01873 855155 Fax: 01873 851075
(Monmouthshire Local Health Board)

GP H G WILLIAMS

Main Road Surgery
Main Road, Gilwern, Abergavenny NP7 0AS
Tel: 01873 830589 Fax: 01873 832161

Practice Manager Chris Stone

GP R J LEWIS, Aileen Baker THOMAS, Dr BARNES, Douglas Henry Hay PATON, Subhashish PODDAR, Catherine Jane STOKER

Old Station Surgery
39 Brecon Road, Abergavenny NP7 5UH
Tel: 01873 859000 Fax: 01873 850163
(Monmouthshire Local Health Board)
Patient List Size: 10600

Practice Manager Colin Jones

GP Nora Christine Joan KILLEEN, Jane MADDOCKS, Clare Alison WEEKES, Richard John WHEATLEY

Tudor Gate Surgery
Tudor Street, Abergavenny NP7 5DL
Tel: 01873 855991 Fax: 01873 850162
(Monmouthshire Local Health Board)

GP Elizabeth Claire EVANS, Robert Christopher Guy BRACCHI, Monica Anne CHIDGEY, Peter Llewelyn DAVIES, John Martin PLUMB

Abergele

Glasfryn Surgery
Glasfryn, Denbigh Rosd, Llanfairtalhaearn, Abergele LL22 8SN
Tel: 01745 720253
(Conwy Local Health Board)

GP Ahmed JAMIL

The Surgery
Kinmel Avenue, Abergele LL22 7LP
Tel: 01745 833158 Fax: 01745 822490
(Conwy Local Health Board)
Patient List Size: 13500

Practice Manager Avril Taylor

GP Humphrey Owen DAVIES, Nigel Charles CLARKSON, John Finbarr DROMEY, J D A EVANS, Jeremy Julian HONEYBUN, John Gerard McCORMACK

Abertillery

Aberbeeg Medical Centre
The Square, Aberbeeg, Abertillery NP13 2AB
Tel: 01495 320520 Fax: 01495 320084
(Blaenau Gwent Local Health Board)

GP Satish Kumar NARANG

The Blaina Surgery
Rear of High Street, (Portacabins), Blaina, Abertillery NP13 3AT
Tel: 01495 290325 Fax: 01495 292725
(Blaenau Gwent Local Health Board)

GP C GODWIN, S MAHESWARAN, George Keillor SKEA

The Bridge Centre
Foundry Bridge, Abertillery NP13 1BQ
Tel: 01495 322632 Fax: 01495 322621
(Blaenau Gwent Local Health Board)
Patient List Size: 2900

Practice Manager Katie Boud

GP C H ROY

The Bridge Street Centre
Foundry Bridge, Abertillery NP13 1BQ
Tel: 01495 322635
(Blaenau Gwent Local Health Board)

GP Chandra Has ROY

The Bridge Street Centre
Foundry Bridge, Abertillery NP13 1BQ
Tel: 01495 322682
(Blaenau Gwent Local Health Board)

GP Colin Geoffrey DEXTER, Andrew Joseph THORNTON, S J VENN

The Bridge Street Centre
Foundry Bridge, Abertillery NP13 1BQ
Tel: 01495 322750
(Blaenau Gwent Local Health Board)

GP K S SAYI

Llanhilleth Surgery
Llanhilleth Institute, Llanhilleth, Abertillery NP13 2JH
Tel: 01495 214255 Fax: 01495 320085
(Blaenau Gwent Local Health Board)

GP Balarami Reddy RAMPA

Six Bells Medical Centre
Eastville Road, Six Bells, Abertillery NP13 2PB
Tel: 01495 212128
(Blaenau Gwent Local Health Board)

GP B R AKHTAR, N HOSSAIN

Aberystwyth

Llanilar Health Centre
Llanilar, Aberystwyth SY23 4PA
Tel: 01974 241556 Fax: 01974 241579
(Ceredigion Local Health Board)
Patient List Size: 2800

Practice Manager Hazel Ellis

GP Patricia Michele Noelle GODFREY-GLYNN, Phoebe GARLAND, Dylan Wyn WILLIAMS

Meddygfa'r Llan
Church Surgery, Portland Street, Aberystwyth SY23 2DX
Tel: 01970 624855 Fax: 01970 625824
(Ceredigion Local Health Board)

GP Richard Bryn Llewelyn EDWARDS, John Alwyn JONES, Mark Gregson LORD, Heather NICHOLLS, Melinda Ann PRICE, Jonathan Wyn WILLIAMS

North Parade Surgery
26 North Parade, Aberystwyth SY23 2NF
Tel: 01970 624545 Fax: 01970 615612
(Ceredigion Local Health Board)

Practice Manager A Gee

GP Karen Sian PENRY, Richard EVANS, Nia MANNING, John ROBERTS, Felicity SMART, Mark STIELER

Ystwyth Medical Group
Ystwyth Primary Care Centre, Parc Y Llyn, Llanbadarn Fawr, Aberystwyth SY23 3TL
Tel: 01970 613500 Fax: 01970 613505
Website: www.ystwyth-medical.co.uk
(Ceredigion Local Health Board)
Patient List Size: 9100

Practice Manager Adrian Marfleet

GP D Rhoderi EVANS, Carole COLBOURN, Gail S DAVIES, Jonathan Adams DAVIES, Frances Elizabeth GERRARD, Shaun Wallace HUMPHREYS

Amlwch

Glannrafon Surgery
Glannrafon, Amlwch LL68 9AG
Tel: 01407 830235 Fax: 01407 832512
(Anglesey Local Health Board)
Patient List Size: 10500

Practice Manager Dilys J Roberts

GP Arthur THOMAS, Barbara Ann GRIFFITH, Adrian Howard KING, John Philip OWEN, Harry Robert Owen PRITCHARD

Ammanford

Brynteg Surgery
Brynmawr Avenue, Ammanford SA18 2DA
Tel: 01269 592058 Fax: 01269 596026
(Carmarthenshire Local Health Board)

Practice Manager David Pickering

GP David Edward MURFIN, Mark BARNARD, Sioned Ann JENKINS, Katherine PINKHAM, Darron Eufryn SMITH

Margaret Street Surgery
Margaret Street, Ammanford SA18 2PJ
Tel: 01269 592477 Fax: 01269 597326
Email: dawn.beynon@gp-W92040.wales.nhs.uk
(Carmarthenshire Local Health Board)
Patient List Size: 8100

GP Michael John GRIFFITHS, William Malcolm CAPPER, Helen Diane MORRIS, Paul MORRIS, K THEVAMANOHARAN

Station Road Medical Centre
53 Station Road, Brynamman, Ammanford SA18 1SH
Tel: 01269 823210

Practice Manager H Fender

GP Khandaker Masihur RAHMAN

Bala

Health Centre
Meddygfa, Canolfan Iechyd, Bala LL23 7BA
Tel: 01678 520308 Fax: 01678 520883
(Gwynedd Local Health Board)

GP Tecwyn JONES, David Henry LAZARUS, Dr DAVIES, Dr JONES

Bangor, Gwynedd

Bangor Medical Centre
Bryn Hydd, Holyhead Road, Bangor LL57 2EE
Tel: 01248 372373 Fax: 01248 372244
(Gwynedd Local Health Board)
Patient List Size: 1700

Practice Manager Karen Luton

GP Lindsay James Roscoe PRICE

Bodnant Surgery
Menai Avenue, Bangor LL57 2HH
Tel: 01248 364492 Fax: 01248 363789
(Gwynedd Local Health Board)
Patient List Size: 9600

Practice Manager Sally Lloyd-Davies

GP David Michael EVANS, Sally JONES, Jonathan Clifford MORGAN, Marilyn MOYSE, Rhodri Wyn OWEN, Christopher TILLSON

Bron Derw Medical Centre
Bron Derw, Glynne Road, Bangor LL57 1AH
Tel: 01248 370900 Fax: 01248 370652
Website: www.brondrew.co.uk
(Gwynedd Local Health Board)
Patient List Size: 7000

Practice Manager Carol Roberts

GP Antony Rathbone VAUGHAN, Elisabeth BOWEN, David Paul Ap Huw JONES, Lauren Margot-Alice KRAAIJEVELD, Lyndon MILES

Doctors Surgery
Glanfa, Orme Road, Bangor LL57 1AY
Tel: 01248 370540 Fax: 01248 370637
(Gwynedd Local Health Board)
Patient List Size: 3500

Practice Manager D Kalaji

GP Joan Alexandra MORTIMER, Karine OLDALE, Toeni ROBINSON

The Surgery
Glanfa, Orme Road, Bangor LL57 1AY
Tel: 01248 362055 Fax: 01248 372771
(Gwynedd Local Health Board)

GP G KURIAN

Victoria Place Surgery
11 Victoria Place, Bethesda, Bangor LL57 3AG
Tel: 01248 600212 Fax: 01248 602790
(Gwynedd Local Health Board)
Patient List Size: 5900

Practice Manager Jo Oliver

GP William John MITHAN, Nicoletta Ruth HEINERSDORFF, Gareth Lewes JONES, Paul Jeffrey NICKSON

Bargoed

Bargoed Hall Family Health Centre
Cardiff Road, Bargoed CF81 8NY
Tel: 01443 831211 Fax: 01443 821969
(Caerphilly Local Health Board)
Patient List Size: 4200

Practice Manager Sian Moore

GP R C RAMNANI, A J THOMAS

Bryntirion Surgery
Cardiff Road, Bargoed CF81 8NY
Tel: 01443 830796 Fax: 01443 835962
(Caerphilly Local Health Board)
Patient List Size: 8000

Practice Manager Jane Evans

GP Michael SHEEN, Philip Dudley BROWN, Gethin Thomas James PRIOR, J R WISBEY

Pant Street Health Clinic
Pant Street, Aberbargoed, Bargoed CF81 9BB
Tel: 01443 831185 Fax: 01443 839146
(Caerphilly Local Health Board)

GP Swadhin Kumar MAJUMDAR

South Street Surgery
South Street, Bargoed CF81 8SU
Tel: 01443 821255 Fax: 01443 875409
(Caerphilly Local Health Board)
Patient List Size: 3400

Practice Manager Janet Hagerty

GP Nishebita DAS, P B DAS

Barmouth

Minfor Surgery
Park Road, Barmouth LL42 1PL
Tel: 01341 280521 Fax: 01341 280912
Email: iansadore@gp-W94008.wales.nhs.uk
Website: www.primarycarebarmouth.co.uk
(Gwynedd Local Health Board)
Patient List Size: 5000

GP William Harold WHITEHEAD, Mary C S BRADLEY, Malcolm Scott HICKEY, Gawain O SHELFORD, Stephanie Patricia SHORT

Barry

Court Road Surgery
29 Court Road, Barry CF63 4YD
Tel: 01446 733181 Fax: 01446 420004
(Vale of Glamorgan Local Health Board)
Patient List Size: 7600

Practice Manager Joanne Bell

GP John Graham EVANS, Gareth George BROWN, S C CUNNINGHAM, Ceri Elizabeth DONAGHY, Anne HUGHES

High Street Family Centre
37-39 High Street, Barry CF62 7EB
Tel: 01446 733355 Fax: 01446 733489
(Vale of Glamorgan Local Health Board)
Patient List Size: 10761

Practice Manager Kirsten Jones

GP Simon Keith HOLGATE, S H CAMPBELL, Geoffrey Francis DAVIES, Stephen David JONES, Geraldine Fiona LAZARUS, Stephen James MATTHEWS

Holton Road Medical Centre
232 Holton Road, Barry CF63 4HS
Tel: 01446 420222 Fax: 01446 749003
(Vale of Glamorgan Local Health Board)

GP Ronald Dennis WILLIAMS

North Barry Medical Practice
98 Salisbury Road, Barry CF62 6PU
Tel: 01446 720049 Fax: 01446 733691
(Vale of Glamorgan Local Health Board)
Patient List Size: 6700

Practice Manager Karen Penney

GP A KUCZYNSKA, L NOURISH, Alan WEATHERUP, R D WILLIAMS

Porthceri Surgery
Park Crescent, Barry CF62 6HE
Tel: 01446 735365 Fax: 01446 700682
(Vale of Glamorgan Local Health Board)

Practice Manager T T Evans

GP Martin Albert Timothy COLEMAN

The Practice of Health
31 Barry Road, Barry CF63 1BA
Tel: 01446 700350 Fax: 01446 420795
(Vale of Glamorgan Local Health Board)

Practice Manager Cleona Jones

GP Marianne Antoinette Louise SULLIVAN, Hilary BUGLER, Alun James WILLIAMS

Ravenscourt Surgery
36-38 Tynewydd Road, Barry CF62 8AZ
Tel: 01446 733515/734744 Fax: 01446 701326
(Vale of Glamorgan Local Health Board)
Patient List Size: 7200

Practice Manager L Church

GP David Gordon TASKER, Elizabeth Jane DAVIES, Benjamin ROPER

Regional Medical Centre
Royal Air Force, St Athan, Barry CF62 4WA
Tel: 01446 797465 Fax: 01446 797459
Email: fsmed@stathan.raf.mod.uk
(Vale of Glamorgan Local Health Board)

Practice Manager Paul Rudd

GP Sqn Ldr ARORA, Dr WARNER, Dr WILLIAMS

The Towers Surgery
163 Holton Road, Barry CF63 4HP
Tel: 01446 734131 Fax: 01446 420002
(Vale of Glamorgan Local Health Board)
Patient List Size: 10518

Practice Manager Nicola Gilbert

GP Jonathan Roy CHAPMAN, Emyr James DAVIES, Nicholas Wynne DAVIES, Susan Helen DAVIES, Deborah Anne HARFOOT, Roderick MOORE, Joanna STROUD

Vale Family Practice
St Brides Way, Gibbonsdown, Barry CF63 1DU
Tel: 01446 744877 Fax: 01446 744900
(Vale of Glamorgan Local Health Board)
Patient List Size: 6200

Practice Manager Terry Evans

GP Akram BAIG

Beaumaris

Health Centre
New Street, Beaumaris LL58 8AL
Tel: 01248 810818 Fax: 01248 811589
(Anglesey Local Health Board)
Patient List Size: 5200

Practice Manager J Andreou, J Fisher

GP Gwen RICHARDS, Hywel Wyn JONES, Stephen MacVICAR, James Ernest VOUSDEN

Betws-y-Coed

Health Centre
Meddygfa, Betws-y-Coed LL24 0BB
Tel: 01690 710205 Fax: 01690 710051
(Conwy Local Health Board)

Practice Manager Pauline Pritchard

GP Michael Godfrey JEFFRIES, Jacqueline Ann MARSHALL

Blackwood

Ford Road Health Centre
Ford Road, Pengam, Blackwood NP12 3XS
Tel: 01443 834672 Fax: 01443 831365
(Caerphilly Local Health Board)
Patient List Size: 2700

Practice Manager Beverley Parry

GP M ALI

James Street Medical Centre
James Street, Markham, Blackwood NP12 0QN
Tel: 01495 224134 Fax: 01495 221449
(Caerphilly Local Health Board)
Patient List Size: 2100

Practice Manager Liz Waters

GP Birjees KHAN

Pengam Health Centre
Ford Road, Pengam, Blackwood NP12 3XS
Tel: 01443 831999 Fax: 01443 831365
(Caerphilly Local Health Board)

GP Kamla MAHTO

Pontllanfraith Health Centre
Off Blackwood Road, Pontllanfraith, Blackwood NP12 2YU
Tel: 01495 227156 Fax: 01495 220311
(Caerphilly Local Health Board)
Patient List Size: 10000

Practice Manager Ann Rutter

GP M A ALAM, M A HUSSAIN, J SWEETMAN

Pontllanfraith Health Centre
Off Blackwood Road, Pontllanfraith, Blackwood NP12 2YU
Tel: 01495 227131 Fax: 01495 220361
(Caerphilly Local Health Board)

GP S M U SUBZWARI, Abdul WAHEED

Sunnybank Health Centre
Bryn Road, Cefn Fforest, Blackwood NP12 1HT
Tel: 01443 875181 Fax: 01495 832156
Email: meryl.thomas@gp-w93014.wales.nhs.uk
(Caerphilly Local Health Board)
Patient List Size: 5000

GP S KUSATUASAN, Y NAVAMTNM, S NAVARATNAM

Blaenau Ffestiniog

Health Services Centre
Wynne Road, Blaenau Ffestiniog LL41 3DW
Tel: 01766 830205 Fax: 01766 831121
(Gwynedd Local Health Board)
Patient List Size: 5500

Practice Manager Gwen Burton

GP Owen Walter EVANS, D M JONES, Hugh Richard JONES, Tomos PARRY

Blaenavon

Carregwen Surgery
Church Road, Blaenavon NP4 9AF
Tel: 01495 790264 Fax: 01495 790334
(Torfaen Local Health Board)
Patient List Size: 5700

Practice Manager Maria Patter

GP Gareth John Gibson BUFFETT, David Paul GRANT, Sarah JONES, Teresa Lindsay LEWIS, Wayne LEWIS

Bodorgan

The Surgery
Parc Glas, Bodorgan LL62 5NW
Tel: 01407 840294 Fax: 01407 840997
(Anglesey Local Health Board)
Patient List Size: 4900

GP R W WILLIAMS, M WILLIAMS

Borth

Borth Surgery
High Street, Borth SY24 5JE
Tel: 01970 871475 Fax: 01970 871881
(Ceredigion Local Health Board)

GP I T HOSKER, John Tudor WILLIAMS

Brecon

Brecon Medical Group Practice
Ty Henry Vaughan, Bridge Street, Brecon LD3 8AH
Tel: 01874 622121 Fax: 01874 623742

Brecon Medical Group Practice
Ty Henry Vaughan, Bridge Street, Brecon LD3 8AH
Tel: 01874 622121 Fax: 01874 623742
(Powys Local Health Board; Powys Local Health Board)
Patient List Size: 15000
Patient List Size: 15000

Practice Manager Chris Johnson, Chris Johnson, Chris Johnson, Chris Johnson

GP John Arwyn Jones DAVIES, John Arwyn Jones DAVIES, Robert William BACON, Robert William BACON, Carolyn Diane DAVIES, Carolyn Diane DAVIES, Wafik Azer DIMYAN, Wafik Azer DIMYAN, Mark Bartholomew John HENEGHAN, Mark Bartholomew John HENEGHAN, David Barry JOHNSON, David Barry JOHNSON, P W METCALFE, P W METCALFE, Andrew Lester RICKETTS, Andrew Lester RICKETTS, Beryl Wyn WILLIAMS, Beryl Wyn WILLIAMS

Haygarth Doctors
The Medical Centre, Hay Road, Talgarth, Brecon LD3 0AW
Tel: 01874 713000 Fax: 01874 713016

Haygarth Doctors
The Medical Centre, Hay Road, Talgarth, Brecon LD3 0AW
Tel: 01874 713000 Fax: 01874 713016
(Powys Local Health Board; Powys Local Health Board)
Patient List Size: 7800
Patient List Size: 7800

Practice Manager R Gittoes, R Gittoes, R Gittoes, R Gittoes

GP Sean O'REILLY, Sean O'REILLY, Antonia BRADLEY, Antonia BRADLEY, Nansi EVANS, Nansi EVANS, Julie GRIGG, Julie GRIGG, Peter Alfred HORVATH-HOWARD, Peter Alfred HORVATH-HOWARD, Mary E ROTHWELL HUGHES, Mary E ROTHWELL HUGHES, James WRENCH, James WRENCH

Bridgend

Ashfield Surgery
Merthyr Mawr Road, Bridgend CF31 3NW
Tel: 01656 652774 Fax: 01656 661187
(Bridgend Local Health Board)
Patient List Size: 7500

Practice Manager S M R Tyndale-Biscoe

GP Philip David Rhodes WILLIAMS, Christopher Robert WILLIAMS, Michael Anthony WILLIAMS, Priscilla WILLIAMS

Heathbridge House
The Old Bridge, Kenfig Hill, Bridgend CF33 6BY
Tel: 01656 740359 Fax: 01656 745400
(Bridgend Local Health Board)

Practice Manager Ruth Richards

GP Keith THOMAS, Arfon Ieuan DAVIES, Christopher David EDWARDS, Philip Thornton JAGGER

Heol Fach Surgery
Heol Fach, North Cornelly, Bridgend CF33 4LD
Tel: 01656 740345 Fax: 01656 740872
(Bridgend Local Health Board)
Patient List Size: 3890

Practice Manager Jean Davies

GP Gareth WILLIAMS, Janet Beverley DAVIES, Seyed Kim Parviz MOHAJER, Rosser Ian THOMAS, Alan Robert WORKMAN

High Street Surgery
89 High Street, Ogmore Vale, Bridgend CF32 7AG
Tel: 01656 840750 Fax: 01656 842322
(Bridgend Local Health Board)

Practice Manager Winston Jones

GP K PALANIVEL

Nantymoel Surgery
Nantymoel, Bridgend CF32 7NA
Tel: 01656 840933 Fax: 01656 840030
(Bridgend Local Health Board)

Practice Manager Annette Williams

GP M VASU

New Street Surgery
3 New Street, Aberkenfig, Bridgend CF32 9BL
Tel: 01656 721268 Fax: 01656 724607
(Bridgend Local Health Board)
Patient List Size: 4300

Practice Manager Maureen Hodge

GP R W BEE, T A KHAN

New Surgery
Victoria Street, Pontycymer, Bridgend CF32 8NN
Tel: 01656 870237 Fax: 01656 870354
(Bridgend Local Health Board)

Practice Manager T Bibey, Julie Lewis

GP Alison MEREDITH-SMITH, Alison JONES, Alexandra F PORTER, Sean Patrick YOUNG

The New Surgery
Coychurch Road, Pencoed, Bridgend CF35 5LP
Tel: 01656 860343 Fax: 01656 864451
(Bridgend Local Health Board)

Practice Manager Margaret Robinson

GP Cerys Ashton MORGAN, C PHILIP

Newcastle Surgery
Llangewydd Road, Cefn Coed, Bridgend CF31 4XX
Tel: 01656 652721 Fax: 01656 662864
(Bridgend Local Health Board)
Patient List Size: 4500

GP Jaishankar Prasad BHARGAVA, Thomas Stephen LODWIG

Ogmore Vale Surgery
Commercial Street, Ogmore Vale, Bridgend CF32 7BL
Tel: 01656 840208 Fax: 01656 841227
(Bridgend Local Health Board)
Patient List Size: 4500

Practice Manager Diane Verghese

GP Subramaniam MURUGIAH, M YOGANATHAN

Oldcastle Surgery
South Street, Bridgend CF31 3ED
Tel: 01656 657131 Fax: 01656 657134
(Bridgend Local Health Board)
Patient List Size: 15100

Practice Manager Susan Leyshon

GP Stephen Karel MADELIN, John Ronald ANTHONY, Sarah-Ann CONNELLAN, Judith Patricia DAVIES, Jerome Geoffrey Francis DONAGH, Colin Huw MASON, Ian O'CONNOR

Pencoed and Llanharan Medical Centres
Heol-yr-Onnen, Pencoed, Bridgend CF35 5PF
Tel: 01656 860270 Fax: 01656 861228
Email: alan.davies@gp-w95018.wales.nhs.uk
(Bridgend Local Health Board)
Patient List Size: 10900

Practice Manager Alan Davies

GP Joseph Philip JONES, John Anthony CRANE, Geraint PREEST, Gail Victoria PRICE, Delyth Ann WARE

Riversdale Surgery
Riversdale House, Merthyrmawr Road, Bridgend CF31 3NL
Tel: 01656 766866 Fax: 01656 668659
(Bridgend Local Health Board)
Patient List Size: 16795

Practice Manager Elizabeth Davies

GP Robert John HADLEY, Alison CRAVEN, Justine C DAWKINS, Peter F N HARROP, Sian HUNT, Delyth JUDD, Richard John McCANN, Philip Denzil MORGAN, Christopher J OSBORNE, Jane Fiona SMILLIE

Tyn-y-Coed Surgery
20 Merfield Close, Bryncethin, Bridgend CF32 9SW
Tel: 01656 720334 Fax: 01656 721998
(Bridgend Local Health Board)

Practice Manager Jayne Rees

GP John MASON-WILLIAMS, Richard Michael BARRETT, S L JONES, Robert Owen MORGAN, S O REES, J A RICHARDS

Brynmawr

Aparajita Surgery
68 Worcester Street, Brynmawr NP23 4EY
Tel: 01495 310232/310266 Fax: 01495 310618
Email: practice.manager@gp-w93071.wales.nhs.uk
(Blaenau Gwent Local Health Board)
Patient List Size: 3300

GP A SINHA, S K DATTA

Blaina Road Surgery
Blaina Road, Brynmawr NP23 4PS
Tel: 01495 312909 Fax: 01495 310674
(Blaenau Gwent Local Health Board)

GP Nasim Ahmad MALIK

Essendene Surgery
3-4 Worcester Street, Brynmawr NP23 4DE
Tel: 01495 310217 Fax: 01495 312301
(Blaenau Gwent Local Health Board)
Patient List Size: 5100

Practice Manager Angela Graham

GP David Lawrence DAVIES, Cheryl Anne DENNIS

Nantyglo Medical Centre
Queen Street, Nantyglo, Brynmawr NP23 4LW
Tel: 01495 310381 Fax: 01495 310807
(Blaenau Gwent Local Health Board)

GP Kondru NOOKARAJU

Buckley

Buckley Health Centre
Padeswood Road, Buckley CH7 2JL
Tel: 01224 550536
(Flintshire Local Health Board)
Patient List Size: 6000

Practice Manager Helen Parsonage, Vanessa Williams

GP Geoffrey Ross HOGGINS, M DYMOCK, Karen HARRISON, E D McHUGH

The Marches Medical Practice
Mill Lane Surgery, 46 Mill Lane, Buckley CH7 3HB
Tel: 01224 550939 Fax: 01224 549592
(Flintshire Local Health Board)

GP M DONALDSON, Colin Wigmore SPENCER, Colin Simon BARNARD, Elizabeth Clare BOOTHROYD, Stephen Anthony BOTHAM, J M CHADWICK, Glenda Mai HILL, Susan Judith OWEN, Anthony Gerard TANSLEY

Roseneath Medical Practice
The Health Centre, Padeswood Road, Buckley CH7 2JL
Tel: 01224 550555 Fax: 01224 545712
(Flintshire Local Health Board)
Patient List Size: 9400

Practice Manager Claire Farr

GP Philip Frank SPEAKMAN, Robert Christopher ATTREE, Ann Christine BLAKE, James Patrick BOYD, Richard Michael LUCAS

Builth Wells

Builth Surgery
Glandwr Park, Builth Wells LD2 3TN
Tel: 01982 552207 Fax: 01982 553826
Email: enquiries@builthsurgery.co.uk
Website: www.builthsurgery.co.uk

Builth Surgery
Glandwr Park, Builth Wells LD2 3TN
Tel: 01982 552207 Fax: 01982 553826
Email: enquiries@builthsurgery.co.uk
Website: www.builthsurgery.co.uk
(Powys Local Health Board; Powys Local Health Board)

Practice Manager Lesley Grain, Lesley Grain, Lesley Grain, Lesley Grain

GP B BLERSCH, B BLERSCH, R GIBBINS, R GIBBINS, Martin RILEY, Martin RILEY, Thorsten STEIN, Thorsten STEIN, A WALLACE, A WALLACE, Richard Bryn WALTERS, Richard Bryn WALTERS

Burry Port

Meddygfa Tywyn Bach
Parc y Minos Street, Burry Port SA16 0BN
Tel: 01554 832240 Fax: 01554 836810
(Carmarthenshire Local Health Board)
Patient List Size: 5400

Practice Manager Eryl Jenkins

GP Stuart Michael WILLIAMS, Sally Claire HOLMES, David Gary HUGHES

Caernarfon

Bron Seiont Surgery
Bron Seiont, Segontium Terrace, Caernarfon LL55 2PH
Tel: 01286 672236 Fax: 01286 676404
(Gwynedd Local Health Board)

Practice Manager Bethan Jones

GP John Gwynfor EVANS, Henry Tudor HOLLAND, Nia Owain HUWS, Gareth Wyn OWENS, Gareth PARRY-JONES

Corwen House Surgery
Corwen House, Market Place, Penygroes, Caernarfon LL54 6NN
Tel: 01286 880336 Fax: 01286 881500
(Gwynedd Local Health Board)
Patient List Size: 1800

GP Edward Elwyn PARRY

Liverpool House Surgery
Liverpool House, Waunfawr, Caernarfon LL55 4YY
Tel: 01286 650223 Fax: 01286 650714
(Gwynedd Local Health Board)
Patient List Size: 4900

Practice Manager Laura Williams

GP R S WILLIAMS, Dr LLWYD, Dr ROBERTS

Llanberis Surgery
High Street, Llanberis, Caernarfon LL55 4SU
Tel: 01286 870634 Fax: 01286 871722
(Gwynedd Local Health Board)
Patient List Size: 5600

Practice Manager Brenda Parry

GP Robin PARRY, Sonia Elizabeth Louise MAXWELL, Alice Virtue ODDY, Alwyn Llewelyn PARRY, Aneurin Gwyn WILLIAMS

Llys Meddyg
Llys Meddyg, Victoria Road, Penygroes, Caernarfon LL54 6HD
Tel: 01286 880207 Fax: 01286 880859
(Gwynedd Local Health Board)

GP Paul Gary Egryn CRABTREE, Jonathan Stuart JONES

Market Street Surgery
3-5 Market Street, Caernarfon LL55 1RT
Tel: 01286 673224 Fax: 01286 676405
(Gwynedd Local Health Board)
Patient List Size: 5500

Practice Manager Valda Evans

GP D R DAVIES, Gwilym Miles EVANS, Mererid OWEN, Edwin WILLIAMS

The Surgery
Dolwenith, Snowden Street, Penygroes, Caernarfon LL54 6NG
Tel: 01286 880202 Fax: 01286 880093
(Gwynedd Local Health Board)

GP J M JONES

The Surgery
Bodnant, Water Street, Penygroes, Caernarfon LL54 6LU
Tel: 01286 880203 Fax: 01286 880629
(Gwynedd Local Health Board)
Patient List Size: 1700

GP J C B THOMPSON

Caerphilly

Bedwas Surgery
East Avenue, Bedwas, Caerphilly CF83 8AE
Tel: 029 2086 4989
(Caerphilly Local Health Board)

GP N RAJAN

Courthouse Practice Medical Centre
Heoh Bro Wen, Caerphilly CF83 3GH
Tel: 029 2088 7316 Fax: 029 2088 4445
(Caerphilly Local Health Board)
Patient List Size: 8600

Practice Manager Gaynor Miles

GP Patrick Joseph HARNEY, Julian BHOGAL, Peter Fraser COLES, Christopher John Charlton COX, Bernadette HARD, Judith JOHNSON

Lansbury Surgery
Wedgewood Court, Lansbury Park, Caerphilly CF83 1RD
Tel: 029 2086 1547 Fax: 029 2085 2220
Email: practice.manager@gp-w95636.wales.nhs.uk
(Caerphilly Local Health Board)
Patient List Size: 4885

Practice Manager Cathy Jones

GP Jennine TAYLOR, Dr CHIMEZIE, Olugbenga FAKANDE

Llan Aber Practice
Rear of Church Street, Llanbradach, Caerphilly CF83 3LS
Tel: 029 2086 2211 Fax: 029 2088 7009
(Caerphilly Local Health Board)

GP T C MAHANTY, S S MOHAN, P NARAIN

Market Street Practice
Ton-y-Felin Surgery, Bedwas Road, Caerphilly CF83 1PD
Tel: 029 2088 7831 Fax: 029 2086 9037
(Caerphilly Local Health Board)

Practice Manager Vicky Gray

GP Narendra Kumar CHAKRAVORTY, Michael David CHAPMAN, Malcolm Clive EDWARDS, J A T GALLETLY, Robert JONES, Jeffrey Wayne LEWIS, K LING, W RAHMAN

Morris and Partners
Ty Bryn Surgery, The Bryn, Trethomas, Caerphilly CF83 8GL
Tel: 029 2086 8011 Fax: 029 2086 9463
(Caerphilly Local Health Board)
Patient List Size: 11000

Practice Manager Jayne Billington

GP David Stephen BAILEY, Iwan Machreth MORRIS, Waseem Nayyar CHAUDHRY, Gwilym Pritchard DAVIES, Allin EDWARDS, Tina GORDON, David Maurice LEWIS

Nantgarw Road Surgery
9 Nantgarw Road, Caerphilly CF83 3FA
Tel: 029 2088 3174 Fax: 029 2086 6753
(Caerphilly Local Health Board)
Patient List Size: 5300

Practice Manager Shirley Turner

GP Susan Elisabeth EVANS, Michael GRIFFITHS, David Keith MINTON

St Cenydd Road Surgery
106 St. Cenydd Road, Trecenydd, Caerphilly CF83 2TE
Tel: 029 2088 8118 Fax: 029 2088 8604
(Caerphilly Local Health Board)
Patient List Size: 1979

Practice Manager Ann Muller

GP Rafiqul BASHAR, Nazma Ara BASHAR

Troed-y-Bryn Surgery
Troed-y-Bryn, Penyrheol, Caerphilly CF83 2PX
Tel: 029 2088 6501 Fax: 029 2088 8517
(Caerphilly Local Health Board)

GP Quamar DIN

The Village Surgery
2 Lewis Terrace, Llanbradach, Caerphilly CF83 3JZ
Tel: 0870 429 9679 Fax: 029 2088 9762
(Caerphilly Local Health Board)
Patient List Size: 2946

Practice Manager Alison Soos

GP Sneh L MATHUR

Cardiff

Albany Road Medical Centre
24 Albany Road, Roath, Cardiff CF24 3YY
Tel: 029 2048 6561 Fax: 029 2045 1403
(Cardiff Local Health Board)

GP Leslie David DINGLEY, Robert DOLBEN, A M C MACLAREN, Hugh Campbell McKIRDY

Ball Road Medical Centre
429 Ball Road, Llanrumney, Cardiff CF3 5NT
Tel: 029 2077 7515 Fax: 029 2079 4886

GP Derek James SADLER

Birchgrove Surgery
104 Caerphilly Road, Cardiff CF14 4AG
Tel: 029 2052 2344 Fax: 029 2052 2487
(Cardiff Local Health Board)
Patient List Size: 8000

Practice Manager Chris Price

GP Paul Richard HART, Jacqueline Anne GRAHAM, S M HART, Angus Charles Willard MACLEAN, Jonathan Edgar PRICHARD

Bishops Road Medical Centre
1 Bishops Road, Whitchurch, Cardiff CF14 1LT
Tel: 029 2052 2455
(Cardiff Local Health Board)

GP G LEWIS, D L JONES, G M REES

Bronllwyn Surgery
Bronllwyn, Pentyrch, Cardiff CF15 9GE
Tel: 029 2089 2670 Fax: 029 2089 2118
Email: canut.benedict@gp-W95626.wales.nhs.uk
(Cardiff Local Health Board)
Patient List Size: 1950

GP Canute BENEDICT

Brynderwen Surgery
Crickhowell Road, St. Mellons, Cardiff CF3 0EF
Tel: 029 2079 9921 Fax: 029 2083 9730
(Cardiff Local Health Board)
Patient List Size: 17400

Practice Manager Mari Thatcher

GP Richard Philip EDWARDS, Martyn Huw EVANS, Neil Richard JONES, Ieuan Winsey LLOYD, Helen Catherine Mary LYDON, John Gerard McWILLIAMS, R OWENS, Anthony Stephen PARSONS, Julie Anne SCHOLEY, Cecilia Elizabeth THOMAS

Butetown Health Centre
Loudoun Square, Butetown, Cardiff CF10 5UZ
Tel: 029 2048 3126 Fax: 029 2047 1879
Email: kay.saunders@gp-w97291.wales.nhs.uk
(Cardiff Local Health Board)
Patient List Size: 1700

Practice Manager Christine Read

GP Kay SAUNDERS

Butetown Health Centre
Loudoun Square, Cardiff CF10 5UZ
Tel: 029 2048 8027 Fax: 029 2034 3839
(Cardiff Local Health Board)

GP Dhanjibhi K MEGHANI

Butetown Health Centre
Loudown Square, Docks, Cardiff CF10 5UZ
Tel: 029 2046 2347 Fax: 029 2045 3080
(Cardiff Local Health Board)
Patient List Size: 2500

GP Ravindra TIWARI

Byways Surgery
Byways, 74 Pwllmelin Road, Llandaff, Cardiff CF5 2NH
Tel: 029 2056 2895 Fax: 029 2056 0702
(Cardiff Local Health Board)
Patient List Size: 3500

Practice Manager Lynne Mattey

GP John Victor ABEL, Helen DHARMASENA

Caerau Lane Surgery
Caerau Lane, Ely, Cardiff CF5 5XU
Tel: 029 2059 1855 Fax: 029 2059 9739
(Cardiff Local Health Board)

GP S K SHRIVASTAVA

Canton Health Centre
Wessex Street, Cardiff CF5 1XU
Tel: 029 2022 6016 Fax: 029 2023 8853
(Cardiff Local Health Board)

GP Peter MATTHEWS, Elizabeth Anne COOK, Andrew John Pittard DAVIES, Elizabeth IONS

Canton Health Centre
Wessex Street, Cardiff CF5 1XU
Tel: 029 2039 5115 Fax: 029 2039 4846
Email: practice.manager@gp-w97031.wales.nhs.uk
(Cardiff Local Health Board)
Patient List Size: 4400

Practice Manager T Skinner

GP Christopher John ROBINSON, Elizabeth Wynn COWELL, Warren HEYWOOD

Cardiff Road Medical Centre
31 Cardiff Road, Llandaff, Cardiff CF5 2DP
Tel: 029 2057 6675 Fax: 029 2057 5367
Email: pierry@aol.com
(Cardiff Local Health Board)
Patient List Size: 1996

Practice Manager Tracey Perriam

GP Adrian Arrau PIERRY

Cathays Surgery
137 Cathays Terrace, Cardiff CF24 4HU
Tel: 029 2022 0878 Fax: 029 2038 8771
Website: www.cathayssurgery.co.uk
(Cardiff Local Health Board)
Patient List Size: 6200

Practice Manager Susan Thomas

GP Nicola Kathryn BROWN, Patricia Jean HUNTER, Damian John Gallwey PATHY

City Road Surgery
187 City Road, Roath, Cardiff CF24 3WD
Tel: 029 2049 4250 Fax: 029 2049 1968
(Cardiff Local Health Board)
Patient List Size: 4100

Practice Manager Ron Ley

GP Om Parkash AGGARWAL, R AGGARWAL

Clare Street Surgery
6 Clare Street, Riverside, Cardiff CF11 6BB
Tel: 029 2066 4450 Fax: 029 2066 6466
(Cardiff Local Health Board)
Patient List Size: 2000

Practice Manager Yvette Herbert

GP Sudha VAID

Clifton Surgery
151-155 Newport Road, Roath, Cardiff CF24 1AG
Tel: 029 2049 4539 Fax: 029 2049 4657
Website: www.cliftonsurgery.co.uk
(Cardiff Local Health Board)
Patient List Size: 7600

Practice Manager Cheryl Smith

GP Susan Jane MORGAN, Charles Williamson ALLANBY, R EVANS, Joseph PEARSON, Susan Elizabeth Ellis TRIGG

Cloughmore Surgery
106 Splott Road, Splott, Cardiff CF24 2XY
Tel: 029 2046 2848 Fax: 029 20462034
(Cardiff Local Health Board)
Patient List Size: 6400

Practice Manager Ann Graham

GP John Gerard Donnelly FOY, David William Nathan COCKS, J M DAVIES, S PAWAR

Countisbury Surgery
152 Countisbury Avenue, Llanrumney, Cardiff CF3 5RS
Tel: 029 2079 2661 Fax: 029 2079 4537
(Cardiff Local Health Board)

GP Iorwerth Geraint HARRIES, Sian DAVIES, Albert William GUILLEM, Joanna Elizabeth LONGSTAFFE, Mary O'SULLIVAN, Daniel QUARRY, Mark THOMAS

Crwys Road Surgery
151 Crwys Road, Cathays, Cardiff CF24 4XT
Tel: 029 2039 6987 Fax: 029 2064 0523
(Cardiff Local Health Board)
Patient List Size: 8000

GP Martyn DAVIES, S F EVEREST, J A JOHNSON, D P QUARRY

Cyncoed Road Medical Centre
350 Cyncoed Road, Cardiff CF23 6XH
Tel: 029 2076 2514 Fax: 029 2076 4262
(Cardiff Local Health Board)
Patient List Size: 8400

Practice Manager Chris Wyatt

GP Peter John GROOM, John Alun Vaughan JONES, Manon KIRKWOOD, Anna MACLEAN, Guy Eland MARSHALL

Danescourt Surgery
4 Rachel Close, Danescourt, Cardiff CF5 2SH
Tel: 029 2057 8686 Fax: 029 2055 5001
Email: enquiries@gp-W97036.wales.nhs.uk
(Cardiff Local Health Board)

Practice Manager Carol Carter

GP P MATTHEWS, E A COOK, A J P DAVIES, E IONS, R P RICHARDS

Ely Bridge Surgery
23 Mill Road, Ely, Cardiff CF5 4AD
Tel: 029 2056 1808 Fax: 029 2057 8871
Email: elybridge@elybridge.co.uk
Website: www.elybridge.co.uk
(Cardiff Local Health Board)
Patient List Size: 12750

Practice Manager Nicola Gardner

GP Geoffrey Frank MORGAN, Huw Myrddin John CHARLES, Peter Howell EDWARDS, Jane EVANS, Helen Catherine LINDSEY, Karen Ann SANTOS, Trevor Henry Raymond THOMPSON

Fairwater Health Centre
Plasmawr Road, Fairwater, Cardiff CF5 3JT
Tel: 029 2056 6291 Fax: 029 2057 8870
(Cardiff Local Health Board)
Patient List Size: 9100

Practice Manager R Harrington

GP S BARFIELD, Andrew Michael COOPER, Martin David HARRISON, S PHILLIPS, N P R TRAVAGLIA

Four Elms Medical Centres
103 Newport Road, Cardiff CF24 0AF
Tel: 029 2048 5526 Fax: 029 2048 2871
(Cardiff Local Health Board)
Patient List Size: 9000

Practice Manager S Hopkins

GP Sarah Mary MORGAN, P BOSSI, Patricia DAVIES, Daniel FAGAN, Kamila HAWTHORNE, P SMITH

Grange Medical Practice
32 Corporation Road, Grangetown, Cardiff CF11 7XA
Tel: 029 2022 6057 Fax: 029 2064 0524
(Cardiff Local Health Board)
Patient List Size: 6200

Practice Manager C Wiggin

GP Stephen Graham LUSH, S R GRAY, S C ROBERTS, S SINHA

Grange Surgery
150 Clare Road, Grangetown, Cardiff CF11 6RW
Tel: 029 2023 1109 Fax: 029 2034 2122
Email: doctor.singh@gp-w97044.wales.nhs.uk
(Cardiff Local Health Board)
Patient List Size: 6000

Practice Manager Mary Kimberley

GP Hari B SINGH, Dhangibhai MEGHAWI, Mohamed Arfan NASEEM

Greenmount Surgery
25 Church Road, Ely, Cardiff CF5 5LQ
Tel: 029 2059 3003 Fax: 029 2059 1771
Website: www.greenmountsurgery.co.uk
(Cardiff Local Health Board)

Practice Manager Renu Sinha

GP Arun Kumar SINHA

Llandaff North Medical Centre
99 Station Road, Llandaff North, Cardiff CF14 2FD
Tel: 029 2056 7822 Fax: 029 2056 7814
(Cardiff Local Health Board)

Practice Manager Avril Calford

GP J J A BLACK, Kota S S DAYANANDA, Anne Catherine ROTHWELL, Susan Margaret ROWE

Llanedeyrn Health Centre
Maelfa, Llanedeyrn, Cardiff CF23 9PN
Tel: 029 2073 1671 Fax: 029 2054 0129
(Cardiff Local Health Board)
Patient List Size: 7000

Practice Manager S. Lockwood

GP Amanda FAULKNER, Paul KINNERSLEY, Roger Lloyd MORRIS, Penelope Anne OWEN, John Ignatius SHEWRING

Llanishen Court Surgery
Llanishen Court, Llanishen, Cardiff CF14 5YU
Tel: 029 2075 7025 Fax: 029 2074 7931
(Cardiff Local Health Board)
Patient List Size: 9500

Practice Manager Malcolm Davies

GP Erbin Hughes WILLIAMS, David Grenville EVANS, David Richard Llewelyn JENKINS, Ailwen Meinir OWEN, Jane STEINER

Llwynbedw Medical Centre
82/86 Caerphilly Road, Birchgrove, Cardiff CF14 4AG
Tel: 029 2052 1222 Fax: 029 2052 2873
Email: drj.harries-ptnrs@virgin.net
(Cardiff Local Health Board)

Practice Manager D McAdie

GP Jestyn HARRIES, Shonagh Helen Margaret MITCHELL, Martin John THOMAS, Mark Robert WATSON

Llwyncelyn Practice
Park RoadSurgery, Whitchurch, Cardiff CF14 7EZ
Tel: 029 2035 7602 Fax: 029 2061 7619
Website: www.llwyncelyn-gps.co.uk
(Cardiff Local Health Board)
Patient List Size: 3500

Practice Manager Carol Howells

GP Allan JONES, Catherine Ann HYETT, Maria JOHNSON

Meddygfa Canna Surgery
27 Wyndham Cresent, Canton, Cardiff CF11 9EE
Tel: 029 2039 0722 Fax: 029 2039 4433
Website: www.cannasurgery.co.uk
(Cardiff Local Health Board)
Patient List Size: 4778

Practice Manager Yvonne Proce

GP Alan Martin STONE, Siwan Gerallt EVANS, Phil GANDERTON, Bethan Angharad HERBERT

North Cardiff Medical Centre
Excalibur Drive, Thornhill, Cardiff CF14 9BB
Tel: 029 2075 0322 Fax: 029 2075 7705
Email: ncmc@gp-W97015.wales.nhs.uk
(Cardiff Local Health Board)
Patient List Size: 13000

Practice Manager Bev Davies

GP Michael Cupper BLOOMFIELD, Sion Meirion EDWARDS, Nick FRANCIS, Richard JONES, Haydn Guy MAYO, Jacqueline Noelle OGDEN, David SHELLING, Ann Iwan STEVENSON, Dr WOOLF

North Road Medical Practice
182 North Road, Cardiff CF14 3XQ
Tel: 029 2061 9188 Fax: 029 2061 3484
(Cardiff Local Health Board)

Practice Manager Barbara Luff

GP Jacqueline Mary GANTLEY, Trevor HOPKINS, Michelle Jayne McLEAN, David Charles MEADES, Nicholas Tudor YARR

Park Road Health Centre
Park Road, Radyr, Cardiff CF15 8DF
Tel: 029 2084 2767 Fax: 029 2084 2507
(Cardiff Local Health Board)
Patient List Size: 6400

Practice Manager Carol Atkins

GP Timothy David Owen JENKINS, Helen Lynne LAWTON, Margaret Mary PRICE, Samantha Jayne QUARRY

Penylan Road Surgery
74 Penylan Road, Cardiff CF23 5SY
Tel: 029 2049 8181 Fax: 029 2049 1507
(Cardiff Local Health Board)
Patient List Size: 10500

Practice Manager Alun Harris

GP Richard Gwilym BOWEN, Huw DAVIES, Alan Geoffrey LANE, Bethan Margaret REES, Kim Judith SCOLDING

Riverside Health Centre
Wellington Street, Canton, Cardiff CF11 9SH
Tel: 029 2064 5385
(Cardiff Local Health Board)

GP Abdulaziz Shariff JAMAL

Riverside Health Centre
Canton Court, Wellington Street, Cardiff CF11 9SH
Tel: 0870 890 2621 Fax: 029 2064 0349
(Cardiff Local Health Board)
Patient List Size: 4700

Practice Manager Margaret Letman

GP Roger Paul BENTLEY, Edmund Wyn DAVIES

Roath House Surgery
100 Penylan Road, Roath Park, Cardiff CF23 5RH
Tel: 029 2046 1100 Fax: 029 2045 1623
(Cardiff Local Health Board)
Patient List Size: 7500

Practice Manager J Corp

GP Lorna Maureen TAPPER-JONES, Siwan GWILYM, Philip Andrew Roach LLOYD, John David WESTLAKE

Roathwell Surgery
116 Newport Road, Roath, Cardiff CF24 1YT
Tel: 029 2049 4537 Fax: 029 2049 8086
(Cardiff Local Health Board)
Patient List Size: 6500

Practice Manager Pamela Jones

GP Sitaram Keshav KAMATH, Michelle DAVID, Andrew Richard DEARDEN, Uroosa KABEER, Susan Anne WILLIAMS

Rumney Medical Practice
840-842 Newport Road, Rumney, Cardiff CF3 4LH
Tel: 029 2079 7751 Fax: 029 2036 1971
(Cardiff Local Health Board)
Patient List Size: 7797

GP Joanne CORBETT, Armon Wyn DANIELS, Catriona Mary FINDLAY, David Arthur Harold GERSON, Nicholas Craig ROBERTSON

Saltmead Medical Centre
107 Clare Road, Grangetown, Cardiff CF11 6QQ
Tel: 029 2034 1103 Fax: 029 2064 4706
Email: enquiries@gp-w97029.wales.nhs.uk
(Cardiff Local Health Board)

Practice Manager Patricia Jones

GP Andrew Christopher JONES

Shirley Road Health Centre
20 Shirley Road, Cardiff CF23 5HN
Tel: 029 2049 6339
(Cardiff Local Health Board)

GP Rosentyl GRIFFITHS

St Davids Court Surgery
1 St. Davids Court, 68a Cowbridge Road East, Cardiff CF11 9DU
Tel: 029 2030 0266 Fax: 029 2030 0273
(Cardiff Local Health Board)
Patient List Size: 5100

Practice Manager Stephen Allen

GP Khalida HASAN, Abdul W SABIR

St Davids Medical Centre
Pentwyn Drive, Pentwyn, Cardiff CF23 7SD
Tel: 029 2073 3032 Fax: 029 2054 1392
(Cardiff Local Health Board)
Patient List Size: 7500

Practice Manager Anne Chugg

GP Jonathan EDWARDS, Sarah DAVIES, Ben ROBINSON, Jacqueline SCOTT

St Isan Road Surgery
46 St. Isan Road, Heath, Cardiff CF14 4LX
Tel: 029 2062 7518 Fax: 029 2052 2886
(Cardiff Local Health Board)
Patient List Size: 5800

Practice Manager A Beetham

GP Michael William WATSON, Noel Patrick Thomas McLOUGHLIN, Phillip Hywel SMITH

The Surgery
4 Corporation Road, Grangetown, Cardiff CF11 7AT
Tel: 029 2023 1259 Fax: 029 2064 0494
(Cardiff Local Health Board)
Patient List Size: 3900

Practice Manager Ann-Marie O'Hanlon

GP Aly M G E ANWAR, S S A SALEH

Taff Riverside Practice
Riverside Health Centre, Wellington Street, Canton, Cardiff CF11 9SH
Tel: 029 2080 3200 Fax: 029 2080 3209
Email: jane.griffiths@gp-w97016.wales.nhs.uk
(Cardiff Local Health Board)
Patient List Size: 4300

Practice Manager Jane Griffiths

GP Susanta Kumar CHAUDHURI, P S DANIEL, A K THAPAR

Taffs Wells Medical Centre
Taffs Well, Cardiff CF15 7YG
Tel: 029 2081 0260 Fax: 029 2081 3002
(Rhondda Cynon Taff Local Health Board)
Patient List Size: 6100

Practice Manager Paul Kelly

GP Allan Robertson CUTHILL, K HACKWELL, Christine MORGAN, I MORRIS

Wentloog Road Health Centre
98 Wentloog Road, Rumney, Cardiff CF3 3XE
Tel: 029 2079 7746 Fax: 029 2079 0231
(Cardiff Local Health Board)
Patient List Size: 8000

Practice Manager Cheryl Blake

GP Robert David JONES, Christopher Stuart DAVIES, Michael D LIVINGSTONE, Deborah Laura Jane VAUGHAN, Mary Clare WALSH

Westway Surgery
1 Wilson Road, Ely, Cardiff CF5 4LJ
Tel: 029 2059 2351 Fax: 029 2059 9956
(Cardiff Local Health Board)
Patient List Size: 7600

Practice Manager Lynette Williams

GP Sally Margaret WOOD, Lionel David JACOBSON, Gillian Ruth JAMES, John Rhys JENKINS, Judith Mary LEWIS

Whitchurch Road Medical Centre
210-212 Whitchurch Road, Heath, Cardiff CF14 3NB
Tel: 029 2062 1282 Fax: 029 2052 0210
(Cardiff Local Health Board)

Practice Manager Wendy Wallace

GP John David HUGHES, Dr LLOYD, Edwin Julian Mark WILTSHIRE

Whitchurch Village Practice
Park Road Surgery, Whitchurch, Cardiff CF14 7EZ
Tel: 029 2062 9602 Fax: 029 2062 3839
Email: pm@gp-w97294.wales.nhs.uk
Website: www.whitchurchvillagepractice.co.uk
(Cardiff Local Health Board)

Practice Manager Lynda Griffiths

GP G J HAYES, C DAVIES, N M McCONNELL

Willowbrook Surgery
Strathy Road, St Mellons, Cardiff CF3 0SH
Tel: 029 2036 0555 Fax: 029 2036 2120
(Cardiff Local Health Board)
Patient List Size: 3000

Practice Manager L Gibbs

GP Ann DISLEY, Rajiv Narain SAXENA

Woodlands Medical Centre
1 Greenfarm Road, Ely, Cardiff CF5 4RG
Tel: 029 2059 1444 Fax: 029 2059 9204
(Cardiff Local Health Board)
Patient List Size: 7500

Practice Manager Paul Harrison

GP Neil CUNNINGHAM, Debajit DAS, Christopher HEAVENS, Alison Jane McLAIN, Karen PASCOE

Cardigan

Ashleigh Surgery
Napier Street, Cardigan SA43 1ED
Tel: 01239 621227
(Ceredigion Local Health Board)

Practice Manager Anne Everitt

GP Dyfed William JAMES, Wendy Margaret JAMES, Simon Nicholas Kirkus KNIGHT, Shan Elizabeth Mary THOMAS

Feidrfair Health Centre
Feidrfair, Cardigan SA43 1EB
Tel: 01239 612021 Fax: 01239 613373
(Ceredigion Local Health Board)
Patient List Size: 7600

GP Brian Thomas RUSSELL, Joy Ann BULTER, David Roger COLE, Astrid Siobhan CUDDIGAN, Rhidian David THOMAS

Carmarthen

Coach and Horses Surgery
The Car Park, St. Clears, Carmarthen SA33 4AA
Tel: 01994 230379 Fax: 01994 231449
(Carmarthenshire Local Health Board)

Practice Manager Peter G Hughes

GP Gareth Walter Marsden DAVIES, Jason Robert EUSTACE, Elizabeth JONES, Gwen Eirian LEWIS, Huw Ioan WILDING

Furnace House Surgery
St Andrews Road, Carmarthen SA31 1EX
Tel: 01267 236616 Fax: 01267 222673
(Carmarthenshire Local Health Board)
Patient List Size: 13760

Practice Manager Sylvana Batkin-Woods

GP Gordon Howard LEWIS, Christopher Leighton JOHN, Carwyn JONES, Sarah Catherine JONES, Pravin Gulabbhai MISTRY, Charl NELL, Hilary Anne POTTER, Ruth Glyn WILLIAMS

Meddygfa Tywi
Nantgaredig, Station Road, Nantgaredig, Carmarthen SA32 7LG
Tel: 01267 290240 Fax: 01267 290062
(Carmarthenshire Local Health Board)

GP David Anthony DAVIES, Heather Aeronwen EVANS

Morfa Lane Surgery
2 Morfa Lane, Carmarthen SA31 3AX
Tel: 01267 234774 Fax: 01267 230628
(Carmarthenshire Local Health Board)

Practice Manager Janet Dooley

GP David Raymond BRENNAN

St Peters Surgery
St Peters Street, Carmarthen SA31 1AH
Tel: 01267 236241 Fax: 01267 234422
(Carmarthenshire Local Health Board)
Patient List Size: 6700

GP Michael Charles COLEMAN, Idris Paul GRAVELLE, Catherine Anne Meredith JONES, Gerald Brendan Francis WESTHOFF

Chepstow

Mount Pleasant Practice
Tempest Way, Chepstow NP16 5XR
Tel: 01291 636500 Fax: 01291 636518
(Monmouthshire Local Health Board)
Patient List Size: 6000

Practice Manager Adrian Hallworth

GP Paul HAWKINS, Robert John ALLISON, Matthew JONES, Judith OLDHAM, Ann Pia Mary PENDLETON

Town Gate Practice
Chepstow Community Hospital, Tempest Way, Chepstow NP16 5XP
Tel: 01291 636444 Fax: 01291 636465
(Monmouthshire Local Health Board)
Patient List Size: 8600

Practice Manager Jean Clement

GP Richard Harries JONES, Huw Lloyd DAVIES, Thomas John EDWARDS, Alison Elizabeth VAN BUREN

Vauxhall Surgery
Vauxhall Lane, Chepstow NP16 5PZ
Tel: 01291 623246 Fax: 01291 627975
(Monmouthshire Local Health Board)
Patient List Size: 8500

Practice Manager M Dale

GP Frances Jill PULLEN, Susanna Marie JACKS, Thomas Alasdair JACKS, Paul Philip MORTON, Charles S NICHOLLS

Wye Dean Practice
Tintern, Chepstow NP16 6TF
Tel: 01291 689355 Fax: 01291 689769
(Monmouthshire Local Health Board)
Patient List Size: 1840

GP Elizabeth F COLTER

Chester

The Marches Medical Practice
83 Main Road, Broughton, Chester CH4 0NR
Tel: 01244 520615 Fax: 01244 538203
Email: practice.manager@gp-w91021.wales.nhs.uk
(Flintshire Local Health Board)

Practice Manager Patrick Hughes

GP C S BARNARD, Elizabeth Clare BOOTHROYD, Stephen Anthony BOTHAM, Joanne Margaret CHADWICK, Neela CHATAKONDU, M DONALDSON, S J OWEN, C W SPENCER, Anthony Gerard TANSLEY, Richard James WYKES

Colwyn Bay

Cadwgan Surgery
11 Bodelwyddan Avenue, Old Colwyn, Colwyn Bay LL29 9NP
Tel: 01492 515410/ 515787 Fax: 01492 513270
(Conwy Local Health Board)
Patient List Size: 11600

Practice Manager Shelagh Hughes

GP David Huw Owen LLOYD, Marc EDWARDS, Sharon M FLANAGAN, Ann Wyn PARRY-WILLIAMS, Dylan C PARRY, Bryn ROBERTS, Jonathan Bevan SALISBURY

Rhoslan Surgery
4 Pwllycrochan Avenue, Colwyn Bay LL29 7DA
Tel: 01492 532125 Fax: 01492 530662
Email: rhoslansurgery@aol.com
(Conwy Local Health Board)
Patient List Size: 7700

Practice Manager G Jones

GP Geraint WYNNE-JONES, Connor CLOSE, Vincent McCANN, Mary Jean RATCLIFFE, Colin Peter THACKRAY

Rysseldene Surgery
98 Conway Road, Colwyn Bay LL29 7LE
Tel: 01492 532807 Fax: 01492 534846
(Conwy Local Health Board)

Practice Manager Diane Lewis

GP Gerald Vincent MURPHY, Keith OWEN, Michael Allan POWELL, Helen Margaret SISSONS

The Surgery
Tyn-Y-Coed, 61 Conway Road, Colwyn Bay LL29 7LG
Tel: 01492 533806 Fax: 01492 535385
(Conwy Local Health Board)

Practice Manager R Slater

GP Suriakant B K PATEL

Wynn Avenue Surgery
16 Wynn Avenue, Old Colwyn, Colwyn Bay LL29 9RF
Tel: 01492 515500 Fax: 01492 515559
(Conwy Local Health Board)
Patient List Size: 1700

Practice Manager Ruth Roberts

GP Uday Kumar BISARYA, Shakti BISARYA

Conwy

Bodreinallt Surgery
Bodreinallt, Conwy LL32 8AT
Tel: 01492 593385 Fax: 01492 573715
(Conwy Local Health Board)

Practice Manager Janet Roberts

GP Martin WILLIAMS, Alistair Hogg CRAWFORD, John REES, Jane SMITH

Drs Evans and Williams
Meddygfa Gyffin, Woodlands, Gyffin, Conwy LL32 8LT
Tel: 01492 596381 Fax: 01492 572708
Email: enquires@gp-w94046.wales.nhs.uk
(Conwy Local Health Board)
Patient List Size: 3900

Practice Manager Fiona Griffiths

GP John Gwynfor EVANS, Ian Peter WILLIAMS

Llys Meddyg Surgery
Llys Meddyg, 23 Castle Street, Conwy LL32 8AY
Tel: 01492 592424 Fax: 01492 593068
(Conwy Local Health Board)

Practice Manager Sue Turner

GP Philip GROUT, Dr GRIFFITHS, David George Edwin WOOD

Corwen

Health Centre
Green Lane, Corwen LL21 0DN
Tel: 01490 412362 Fax: 01490 412970
(Denbighshire Local Health Board)
Patient List Size: 4300

Practice Manager E Jones

GP Ian C M WILLIAMS, S J HESKETH

The Surgery
Meddygfa, Cerrigdrudion, Corwen LL21 9UB
Tel: 01490 420210 Fax: 01490 420 622
(Conwy Local Health Board)
Patient List Size: 2500

Practice Manager Enid Jones

GP Shelia DOBELL, Dermot Patrick NORTON

Cowbridge

Old Hall Grounds Health Centre
Old Hall Grounds, Cowbridge CF71 7AH
Tel: 01446 772237 Fax: 01446 775883
(Vale of Glamorgan Local Health Board)
Patient List Size: 6500

Practice Manager Rosemary P Smith

GP John Childs JEMMETT, Paul ARNOLD, Teresa Mary O'HANLON, Terence Michael STUART, Sian WILLIAMS

Old Hall Grounds Health Centre
Old Hall Grounds, Cowbridge CF71 7AH
Tel: 01446 772383 Fax: 01446 774022
(Vale of Glamorgan Local Health Board)
Patient List Size: 8657

Practice Manager Patricia Hold

GP Richard David JONES, Isabel GRAHAM, Dominic John Lloyd McGOVERN, Timothy Hugh PARDOE, Janet Margaret TAYLOR, Carole Dawn WILKINSON

Criccieth

Health Centre
Pwllheli Road, Criccieth LL52 0RR
Tel: 01766 523451 Fax: 01766 523453
(Gwynedd Local Health Board)

Practice Manager Catherine Ellen Williams

GP John Gilbert WEBB, J M EDWARDS

Crickhowell

Crickhowell Group Practice
War Memorial Health Centre, Beaufort Street, Crickhowell NP8 1AG
Tel: 01873 810255 Fax: 01873 813222

Crickhowell Group Practice
War Memorial Health Centre, Beaufort Street, Crickhowell NP8 1AG
Tel: 01873 810255 Fax: 01873 813222
(Powys Local Health Board; Powys Local Health Board)
Patient List Size: 8200
Patient List Size: 8200

Practice Manager Chris Stone, Chris Stone, Chris Stone, Chris Stone

GP Rollo James LEWIS, Rollo James LEWIS, M P BARNES, M P BARNES, Douglas Henry Hay PATON, Douglas Henry Hay PATON, Subhashish PODDAR, Subhashish PODDAR, Catherine Jane STOKER, Catherine Jane STOKER, Aileen B THOMAS, Aileen B THOMAS

Crymych

Crymych Surgery
Caerludd, Crymych SA41 3QE
Tel: 01239 831234 Fax: 01239 831234
(Pembrokeshire Local Health Board)

Practice Manager B S Virdi

GP Balbir S VIRDI

Cwmbran

Chestnut Green Surgery
27 Chestnut Green, Upper Cwmbran, Cwmbran NP44 5TH
Tel: 01633 482248 Fax: 01633 484228

GP Nalliah PARAMAGNANAM

Clark Avenue Surgery
Clark Avenue, Pontnewydd, Cwmbran NP44 1RY
Tel: 01633 482733 Fax: 01633 867758
Email: enquiries@gp-w93038.wales.nhs.uk
(Torfaen Local Health Board)
Patient List Size: 6500

Practice Manager Louise MacAlast

GP Bryan J HUGHES, John Lee KING, Gareth J OELMANN, Barbara Elsie THOMAS

Cwmbran Village Surgery
Victoria Street, Cwmbran NP44 3JS
Tel: 01633 871177 Fax: 01633 860234
(Torfaen Local Health Board)

GP Peter Julian ROWLANDS, Lucy Mary ALLEN, Christopher John PRICE

Fairwater Surgery
Fairwater, Cwmbran NP44 4TA
Tel: 01633 869544 Fax: 01633 483750
(Torfaen Local Health Board)

GP Divyabala Lalitkumar NIRMAL, R K SHARMA

Greenmeadow Surgery
Greenmeadow Way, Cwmbran NP44 3XQ
Tel: 01633 864110 Fax: 01633 483761
(Torfaen Local Health Board)
Patient List Size: 5900

Practice Manager Angela Lohfink

GP Robin Charles SKITT, Rosemary Anne DAVIES, Andrew Bernard LOHFINK, Jayne SPILLER

Llanyravon Way Surgery
Llanyravon Way, Llanyravon, Cwmbran NP44 8HW
Tel: 01633 483255 Fax: 01633 484130
(Torfaen Local Health Board)

Practice Manager Janet Busby

GP Hugh Ian BUSBY, A HUGHES

New Chapel Street Surgery
Harold Street, Pontnewydd, Cwmbran NP44 1DU
Tel: 01633 485155 Fax: 01633 484133
(Torfaen Local Health Board)

GP Hywel Selwyn EVANS, Jane Frances McEVOY, Nicola Anne MORGAN

Oak Street Surgery
Oak Street, Cwmbran NP44 3LT
Tel: 01633 866719 Fax: 01633 838208
(Torfaen Local Health Board)
Patient List Size: 9500

Practice Manager Lynne Bodman

GP Frederick Roger CRANFIELD, Sioned Seaton DAVIES, Gail Parnell HOLGATE, David John MILLAR-JONES, Elen WHARTON

Deeside

Chester Road East Surgery
17-21 Chester Road East, Shotton, Deeside CH5 1QA
Tel: 01244 831698 Fax: 01244 812847
(Flintshire Local Health Board)

GP Prabhat Kumar DAS, Colin Woodley JONES, Ranajit KAKATI

Doctors Surgery
Pierce Street, Queensferry, Deeside CH5 1SY
Tel: 01244 813340 Fax: 01244 822882
(Flintshire Local Health Board)

Practice Manager A Wareing

GP Timothy Martin Watkin JONES, Janette Frances FELLS, William Rees Stuart JONES

Fron Road Surgery
2 Fron Road, Connah's Quay, Deeside CH5 4PQ
Tel: 01244 814272 Fax: 01244 821204
(Flintshire Local Health Board)
Patient List Size: 6000

Practice Manager E Astles

GP Maqsood CHAUDHRY, Tim DAVIES, Mark Anthony John HARNEY

High Street Surgery
149 High Street, Connah's Quay, Deeside CH5 4DQ
Tel: 01244 812217 Fax: 01244 836166
(Flintshire Local Health Board)
Patient List Size: 2400

Practice Manager Norma Rapson

GP Amrit Lal GOYAL

New Hawarden Health Centre
27 Glynne Way, Harwarden, Deeside CH5 3PA
Tel: 01224 532223 Fax: 01224 520456
(Flintshire Local Health Board)

GP Ahmed Wagih Abdel Kader AMIN, Philip Cecil CARSON, Felicity Anne CHALLONER, Tanya Gail HUGHES, B J LANCHASHIRE

Rowleys Drive Clinic
Rowleys Drive, Shotton, Deeside CH5 1PU
Tel: 01244 830449
(Flintshire Local Health Board)

Practice Manager C Khamar

GP Guatam Chandulal KHAMAR

Shotton Lane Surgery
38 Shotton Lane, Shotton, Deeside CH5 1QW
Tel: 01244 812094 Fax: 01244 811728
(Flintshire Local Health Board)
Patient List Size: 7770

Practice Manager Kath Evans

GP Brendan Michael MARKEY, Rosa GIL-CANDON, Jose L OUTEIRAL, Hendrik Jan STIGGELBOUT

St Mark's Dee View Surgery
Church Street, Connah's Quay, Deeside CH5 4AD
Tel: 01244 812003 Fax: 01244 822609
(Flintshire Local Health Board)

Practice Manager K P Mayrick

GP David Evan MORRIS, David Frost ROBERTS, Alane SALT

Denbigh

Beech House Surgery
Beech House, 69 Vale Street, Denbigh LL16 3AU
Tel: 01745 812863 Fax: 01745 816574
Email: enquirie@gp-W91033.wales.nhs.uk
Website: www.beechhouse.org.uk
(Denbighshire Local Health Board)
Patient List Size: 9500

GP Peter Leonard HACKETT, Trevor OLDHAM, Peter ROMACHNEY, Ceri Alison SALUSBURY, Hywel WATKIN

Bronffynnon Surgery
24 Bridge Street, Denbigh LL16 3TH
Tel: 01745 814422 Fax: 01745 816763
(Denbighshire Local Health Board)

GP Timothy Roper PESKETT, Nicole BARRIE, Andrew HEATON, Laura Margaret JONES

Middle Lane Surgery
Middle Lane, Denbigh LL16 3UW
Tel: 01745 816481 Fax: 01745 816153
(Denbighshire Local Health Board)

GP Robert Watkin JONES, Matthew William DAVIES

Vale Street Surgery
24 Vale Street, Denbigh LL16 3BL
Tel: 01754 812689 Fax: 01754 812221
(Denbighshire Local Health Board)

GP David Gwyn JONES

Dinas Powys

Dinas Powys Health Centre
75 Cardiff Road, Dinas Powys CF64 4JT
Tel: 029 2051 2293 Fax: 029 2051 5318
(Vale of Glamorgan Local Health Board)

Practice Manager Roger Munkley

GP Susan THOMAS, Angharad COX, Rhian Jane REES, Huw REYNOLDS

Family Practice
75 Cardiff Road, Dinas Powys CF64 4JT
Tel: 029 2051 5455 Fax: 029 2051 5177
(Vale of Glamorgan Local Health Board)
Patient List Size: 2500

Practice Manager Anne Griffiths

GP Rhian LLEWELLYN, Ann Willoughby CHERRY

Dolgellau

Caer Ffynnon Surgery
Caer Ffynnon, Springfield Street, Dolgellau LL40 1LY
Tel: 01341 422431 Fax: 01341 423717
(Gwynedd Local Health Board)
Patient List Size: 4800

Practice Manager Caroline Vaughan

GP Joseph Nicholas BRADLEY, Juliet Jane EDWARDS, Jon P HOPKINS, Hazel May MARTIN

Ebbw Vale

Bridge Street Health Centre
Bridge Street, Ebbw Vale NP23 6EY
Tel: 01495 302268 Fax: 01495 305169
(Blaenau Gwent Local Health Board)

GP Sukhdev Singh SODHI

Cwm Health Centre
Canning Street, Cwm, Ebbw Vale NP23 7RW
Tel: 01495 370209 Fax: 01495 371697
(Blaenau Gwent Local Health Board)

GP A C MOHINDRU

Glanrhyd Surgery
Riverside, Beaufort, Ebbw Vale NP23 5NT
Tel: 01495 301210 Fax: 01633 350684
(Blaenau Gwent Local Health Board)
Patient List Size: 7400

Practice Manager L Noel

GP William David MORGAN, David Christopher Bruce BISSETT, David Meredith KATZ, Pamela SELWYN

Glyn Ebwy Surgery
James Street, Ebbw Vale NP23 6JG
Tel: 01495 302716 Fax: 01495 305166
(Blaenau Gwent Local Health Board)
Patient List Size: 6819

Practice Manager Sheila Brown

GP Mohamed YOUSU KUNJU, Sian Wyn DAVIES, M M HUSAIN, Mohammad WASIM

Rhys House Family Health Care
Rhys House, James St, Ebbw Vale NP23 6JG
Tel: 01495 307407
(Blaenau Gwent Local Health Board)
Patient List Size: 1759

Practice Manager Usha Varshney

GP Giriraj Kishore VARSHNEY

Ferndale

The Maerdy Ferndale Practice
Ferndale Medical Centre, 56-58 High Street, Ferndale CF43 4XX
Tel: 01443 730539
(Rhondda Cynon Taff Local Health Board)
Patient List Size: 8800

Practice Manager S Chamberlain

GP Kantimoy NATH, Ranadhir DUTTA, Opendea KUMAR, Anilk SHAH

Tylorstown Group Practice
Ferndale Road, Tylorstown, Ferndale CF43 3HB
Tel: 01443 730169 Fax: 01443 733788
(Rhondda Cynon Taff Local Health Board)
Patient List Size: 6500

Practice Manager Jan Lewis

GP Sakti Bhusan GUHANIYOGI, Probal BANERJEE, Nipun Tarunkumar RAIJIWALA

Ferryside

Mariners Surgery
Ferryside SA17 5SG
Tel: 01267 267239 Fax: 01267 267482
(Carmarthenshire Local Health Board)
Patient List Size: 1016

Practice Manager Alison Cotter

GP David Michael Graham JENKINS

Fishguard

Fishguard Health Centre
Ropewalk, Fishguard SA65 9BT
Tel: 01348 873041 Fax: 01348 874916
(Pembrokeshire Local Health Board)
Patient List Size: 5350

Practice Manager Chris Grosvenor

GP Bethan M EVANS, David Brian DAVIES, M MANN

Flint

Church Street Surgery
112 Church Street, Flint CH6 5AF
Tel: 01352 733194 Fax: 01352 763669
(Flintshire Local Health Board)

GP Zia-ur REHMAN, N SHAMAS

Davies and Kapoor
Alltgoch Medical Centre, Lon-y-Becwys, Flint CH6 5UZ
Tel: 01352 732207 Fax: 01352 730265
(Flintshire Local Health Board)

Practice Manager Shirley Parker

GP Christopher Paul DAVIES, Jagdish Chandra KAPOOR

The Laurels Surgery
73 Church Street, Flint CH6 5AF
Tel: 01352 732349 Fax: 01352 730678
(Flintshire Local Health Board)

GP James Nicholas FENNER, Paul DANIEL, Jane Elspeth MacKIRDY, Elizabeth Diana MATHEWS

Gaerwen

Meddygfa Star Surgery
Gaerwen LL60 6AH
Tel: 01248 714533 Fax: 01248 715824
(Anglesey Local Health Board)
Patient List Size: 1170

Practice Manager Margaret Alcock

GP Graham D THOMAS, Ben ALOFS

Goodwick

Meddygfa Wdig
Main Street, Goodwick SA64 0BN
Tel: 01348 872802 Fax: 01348 874717
Email: chris.vankempen@gp-w92061.wales.nhs.uk
(Pembrokeshire Local Health Board)
Patient List Size: 4082

Practice Manager Cilla Morgan

GP Christopher Edward VAN KEMPEN, Ingrid KAUSCHINGER, Elke KLUEBER, Kate READ

Haverfordwest

Solva Surgery
Cysgod-Yr-Eglwys, Solva, Haverfordwest SA62 6TW
Tel: 01437 721306 Fax: 01437 720046
(Pembrokeshire Local Health Board)
Patient List Size: 2650

Practice Manager Jayne Mowlam

GP Chittor Shadaksharam PREMKUMAR, V FLEMING, Kai Michael NEUMANN

St Davids Surgery
Eryl Mor, 36 New Street, St. Davids, Haverfordwest SA62 6SS
Tel: 01437 720303 Fax: 01437 721162
(Pembrokeshire Local Health Board)
Patient List Size: 2500

Practice Manager Anna Bennett

GP Gaylene DU PLESSIS, Sara Anne HAMILTON

St Thomas' Surgery
Rifleman Lane, St. Thomas' Green, Haverfordwest SA61 1QX
Tel: 01437 762162 Fax: 01437 776811
Email: linda.buttle@gp-w92002.wales.nhs.uk
(Pembrokeshire Local Health Board)
Patient List Size: 11400

Practice Manager Linda Buttle

GP Roger William BURNS, Vivek BUNTWAL, S C MORGAN, Alexander MacGregor PATERSON, Richard William Graham THOMPSON, Laurence Glyn WILLIAMS

Winch Lane Surgery
Winch Lane, Haverfordwest SA61 1RN
Tel: 01437 762333 Fax: 01437 766912
(Pembrokeshire Local Health Board)

Practice Manager Michael McManus

GP Andrew John WEAVER, Christopher Mark BATES, David Alun COOKE, David Huw DAVIES, Rhodri Wyn JONES, Arthur David RICHARDS, Ann Lynette Bartlett WEAVER

Hengoed

Gelligaer Surgery
Heol Penallta, Gelligaer, Hengoed CF82 8FA
Tel: 01443 875333 Fax: 01443 838247
(Caerphilly Local Health Board)
Patient List Size: 5100

Practice Manager Antonia Higgins

GP A M CUNNINGHAM, R GRAVELL, J HOLLAND, H HOUSTON, R SWAN

Scourfield and Partners
The Surgery, Oakfield Street, Ystrad Mynach, Hengoed CF82 7WX
Tel: 01443 813248 Fax: 01443 862283
Email: practice.manager@gp-W95065.wales.nhs.uk
(Caerphilly Local Health Board)
Patient List Size: 12740

Practice Manager Pam Williams

GP Alun James SCOURFIELD, Mir Mahmood ALI, Nicholas Frazer ELWOOD, J Alyson GRANT, William David GREVILLE, Heather Marie GRIFFITHS, Sarah Jane HENEGHAN, Alun J WALTERS

Holyhead

Cambria Surgery
Ucheldre Avenue, Holyhead LL65 1RA
Tel: 01407 762735/764239 Fax: 01407 766900
(Anglesey Local Health Board)
Patient List Size: 5230

Practice Manager Laraine McEnhill

GP Huw PARRY, Werner SPILL

The Surgery
Gwalchmai, Holyhead LL65 4RS
Tel: 01407 720202 Fax: 01407 720202
(Anglesey Local Health Board)

Practice Manager S Dawson

GP Richard LEAIINGE, Ingo Karl Heinz TORBOHM

The Surgery
Longford Road, Holyhead LL65 1TR
Tel: 01407 762341 Fax: 01407 761554
(Anglesey Local Health Board)

GP Dr BOWEN, Dr DAVIES, Dr ROBSON

Victoria Surgery
5 Victoria Road, Holyhead LL65 1UD
Tel: 01407 762713 Fax: 01407 765052
(Anglesey Local Health Board)
Patient List Size: 9500

Practice Manager Richard Bradshaw

GP Christopher Francis WALKER, Sharon Wyn BERTORELLI, Gareth FORD, Martyn Glyn David PETTY, David Thomas WILLIAMS

Holywell

Bodowen Surgery
Halkyn Road, Holywell CH8 7GA
Tel: 01352 710529 Fax: 01352 710784
(Flintshire Local Health Board)

Practice Manager Sian Hartley-Williams

GP Arthur ROBERTS, Nia BIBBY, Helen Margaret HARPER, Stephen Murray LLOYD, Rolf Gabor MAJOR

Panton House Surgery
Panton Place, Holywell CH8 7LD
Tel: 01352 712288 Fax: 01352 715299
(Flintshire Local Health Board)
Patient List Size: 3300

Practice Manager Dave Edwards

GP Atul Krishna SAHA, Parameswara Venugopal PRASAD

Pendre Surgery
Coleshill Street, Holywell CH8 7UP
Tel: 01352 712029 Fax: 01352 712751
(Flintshire Local Health Board)
Patient List Size: 10100

Practice Manager Wera Williams

GP Mark ROWLANDS, Patricia Anne BOISTON, Steven JONES, Iain REID, Christopher James WALLACE

Pennant Surgery
Off High Street, Holywell CH8 7TR
Tel: 01352 716766 Fax: 01352 716859
(Flintshire Local Health Board)
Patient List Size: 3100

Practice Manager A Hardwood

GP V JAYARAMAN, Y P KAPUR

Kidwelly

Derwendeg Medical Centre
19 Heol Llanelli, Trimsaran, Kidwelly SA17 4AG
Tel: 01554 810223 Fax: 01554 810752
(Carmarthenshire Local Health Board)
Patient List Size: 1750

Practice Manager Philip Hunt

GP Barrie WILLIAMS

Dundrow, Hopkins and Al-Abdullah
Meddygfa Minafon, Hillfield Villas, Kidwelly SA17 4UL
Tel: 01554 890234 Fax: 01554 891240
(Carmarthenshire Local Health Board)

Practice Manager Cynthia Frise

GP Jennifer Mary DUNDROW, Anees Farhan Ibraheem AL-ABDULLAH, Michael Patrick HOPKINS, Sally Jane JOHNSON

Meddygfa Minafon
Kidwelly SA17 4UL
Tel: 01554 890234 Fax: 01554 891240
(Carmarthenshire Local Health Board)

GP Jennifer Mary DUNDROW, Anees Farhan Ibraheem AL-ABDULLAH, Michael Patrick HOPKINS

Knighton

Erw Vane Surgery
Penybont Road, Knighton LD7 1HB
Tel: 01547 528330 Fax: 01547 520570
Email: gloria.hayman@nhs.net

Erw Vane Surgery
Penybont Road, Knighton LD7 1HB
Tel: 01547 528330 Fax: 01547 520570
Email: gloria.hayman@nhs.net
(Powys Local Health Board; Powys Local Health Board)
Patient List Size: 3100
Patient List Size: 3100

Practice Manager G J Hayman, G J Hayman, G J Hayman, G J Hayman

GP Kevin Michael HOWCROFT, Kevin Michael HOWCROFT, Roger D DAVIES, Roger D DAVIES, Jill Caroline Scott GRAY, Jill Caroline Scott GRAY

Wylewm Street Surgery
Wylewm Street, Knighton LD7 1AD
Tel: 01547 528523 Fax: 01547 529347

Wylewm Street Surgery
Wylewm Street, Knighton LD7 1AD
Tel: 01547 528523 Fax: 01547 529347
(Powys Local Health Board; Powys Local Health Board)

Practice Manager J Preece, J Preece, J Preece, J Preece

GP Martin Laurence KIFF, Martin Laurence KIFF, Maurice BETTS, Maurice BETTS, Adrian FINTER, Adrian FINTER, Anthony LEMPERT, Anthony LEMPERT

Lampeter

Taliesin Surgery
Taliesin, Lampeter SA48 7AA
Tel: 01570 422665 Fax: 01570 423810
(Ceredigion Local Health Board)

Practice Manager M R Jones

GP Tom Morgan Lloyd JONES, Aled Wyn DAVIES, Helen Maria HOWLEY, Emyr Wyn JONES, Rowena MATHEW

Llandeilo

Davies and Partners
Meddygfa Teilo, Crescent Road, Llandeilo SA19 6HL
Tel: 01558 823435 Fax: 01558 824045
(Carmarthenshire Local Health Board)
Patient List Size: 9270

Practice Manager Linda Whitehead

GP Terence Rees DAVIES, Rhodri Iwan GEORGE, Dafydd Huw JONES-EVANS, Robert Wynne LEWIS, Gillian TARR, Owain Aled WILLIAMS

Llandovery

Richards and Partners
Llanfair Surgery, Llanfair Road, Llandovery SA20 0HY
Tel: 01550 720648 Fax: 01550 721428
(Carmarthenshire Local Health Board)
Patient List Size: 5400

Practice Manager L Young

GP John Llewellyn RICHARDS, Mark Jeremy Michael BOULTER, Catherine Ruth BRISCOE, Mohan DE SILVA, Philip John REES, Robert William SALT

Llandrindod Wells

Spa Road Surgery
Spa Road East, Llandrindod Wells LD1 5ES
Tel: 01597 824291 / 842292 Fax: 01597 824503

Spa Road Surgery
Spa Road East, Llandrindod Wells LD1 5ES
Tel: 01597 824291 / 842292 Fax: 01597 824503
(Powys Local Health Board; Powys Local Health Board)

GP Simeon OVIS, Simeon OVIS, Gillian Mary ARKINSTALL, Gillian Mary ARKINSTALL, Ewart Ian HILSDEN, Ewart Ian HILSDEN, Jonathan Stuart MATSON, Jonathan Stuart MATSON, Toby TATTERSALL, Toby TATTERSALL, Michael John Sewell WARRICK, Michael John Sewell WARRICK, Stephanie Margaret WARRICK, Stephanie Margaret WARRICK

Llandudno

Craig y Don Medical Centre
Clarence Road, Llandudno LL30 1TA
Tel: 01492 864540 Fax: 01492 871480
(Conwy Local Health Board)
Patient List Size: 9000

Practice Manager Peter Smith

GP John Joseph GREEN, Mark Patrick CARRI, Paul Andrew EMMETT, Elaine HAMPTON, Philippa Anne MITCHELSON

The Medical Centre
Plas Penrhyn, Bae Penrhyn Bay, Llandudno LL30 3EU
Tel: 01492 549368 Fax: 01492 548103
(Conwy Local Health Board)

Practice Manager Dianne Windmill

GP Patrick Julien EDWARDS, Rodney GILMORE, Richard Alexander STUART, Ian Peter WILSON

Mostyn House Medical Practice
Mostyn Broadway, Llandudno LL30 1YL
Tel: 01492 860401 Fax: 01492 871479
(Conwy Local Health Board)

Practice Manager Karen Edwards

GP Dr FERRIS, Dr FLOOD, Dr HARVEY, Dr LUITHLE, Dr McCABE

West Shore Surgery
9 Bryniau Road, Llandudno LL30 2BL
Tel: 01492 872915 Fax: 01492 875581
(Conwy Local Health Board)

Practice Manager Joy Williams

GP G D KING

Llandudno Junction

The Surgery
Lonfa, Glyn y Marl Road, Llandudno Junction LL31 9NS
Tel: 01492 581172 Fax: 01492 593974
(Conwy Local Health Board)

Practice Manager Joan Green

GP Muddaiah JAYARAM

Llandysul

Llynyfran Surgery
Llynyfran Road, Llandysul SA44 4JX
Tel: 01559 364000 Fax: 01559 364001
Website: www.llynyfran.co.uk
(Ceredigion Local Health Board)
Patient List Size: 6000

Practice Manager Wendy Davies

GP Ian McDougall THOMAS, Richard John GARD, Nia LLEWELYN, S E ROOKE, Mark Stephen THOMAS

Meddygfa Teifi Surgery
New Road, Llandysul SA44 4QJ
Tel: 01559 362221 Fax: 01559 362080
(Ceredigion Local Health Board)

Practice Manager M Clarky

GP David A T ROBERTS, Katharine Jean GORDON, Ann Lilian JAY, David Thomas JONES

Llanelli

Adfer Medical Group
Llanelli Town Centre, Thomas Street, Llanelli SA15 3JH
Tel: 01554 775555 Fax: 01554 778868
(Carmarthenshire Local Health Board)
Patient List Size: 14600

Practice Manager Sue Morgan

GP A I HARRIES, Anthony Robin ASTON, D L GRAVELL, E W GRAVELL, Mervyn Thomas GREEN, K A KEIGHLEY, Mandy J REYNOLDS, Gwenyth THOMAS

Amman Valley Medical Practice
Cwmamman Road Surgery, Garnant, Llanelli SA18 1NH
Tel: 01269 823385
(Carmarthenshire Local Health Board)

GP D M WILLIAMS

Andrew Street Medical Centre
22 Andrew Street, Llanelli SA15 3YP
Tel: 01554 778017 Fax: 01554 778820
(Carmarthenshire Local Health Board)
Patient List Size: 3475

Practice Manager G Roberts

GP Prabodh DEVICHAND

Avenue Villa Surgery
Brynmor Road, Llanelli SA15 2TJ
Tel: 01554 774401 Fax: 01554 775229
(Carmarthenshire Local Health Board)

GP Edward Lyn ANTHONY, Liam Joseph CASSIDY, Bridget Mary GWYNNE, Mark Owen VAUGHAN

Camarthen Road Health Centre
Carmarthen Road, Cross Hands, Llanelli SA14 6SU
Tel: 01269 831091 Fax: 01269 832305
Email: practice.manager@gp-W92035.wales.nhs.uk
(Carmarthenshire Local Health Board)
Patient List Size: 7140

Practice Manager Jackie Jones

GP Goronwy Rhys JONES, Huw Eilian DAVIES, A A HILL, Gareth Lloyd JONES

Coalbrook Surgery
18 Coalbrook Road, Pontyberem, Llanelli SA15 5HU
Tel: 01269 870207 Fax: 01269 871314
(Carmarthenshire Local Health Board)
Patient List Size: 4000

Practice Manager Cynthia Fhso

GP Ewan John SCOURFIELD, Nicola FLOWER, Alan Edward SCOURFIELD

Fairfield Surgery
1 Park Crescent, Llanelli SA15 3AE
Tel: 01554 773133 Fax: 01554 777559
(Carmarthenshire Local Health Board)

GP Peter William FRANCIS, Alberto GONI SARRIGUREN, Alan John HOWARTH, Martin Hugh JOHN

LLwynhendy Health Centre
Llwynhendy, Llanelli SA14 9BN
Tel: 01554 772946 Fax: 01554 752570
(Carmarthenshire Local Health Board)

GP Delyth Lois GRAVELL, Emyr Wyn GRAVELL, Kay Alyson HUGHES

Meddygfa Penygroes
Heol y Bont, Penygroes, Llanelli SA14 7RP
Tel: 01269 831193 Fax: 01269 832116
(Carmarthenshire Local Health Board)
Patient List Size: 7500

Practice Manager Gloria Evans

GP Anthony Wayne GRIFFITHS, Heledd Ffion DANIELS, Gillian Wyn ELLIS-WILLIAMS, Gareth John JONES, J C KINNEAR

Meddygfa Twyn Bach
Par y Minos Street, Burry Port, Llanelli SA16 0BN
Tel: 01554 832240 Fax: 01554 836810
(Carmarthenshire Local Health Board)

Practice Manager Eryl Jenkins

GP S WILLIAMS, Dr HOLMES, Dr HUGHES

Meddygfa'r Sarn
Heol y Meinciau, Pontyates, Llanelli SA15 5TR
Tel: 01269 860348 Fax: 01269 860120
(Carmarthenshire Local Health Board)

GP Edwyn Carey Howell EDMUNDS, Huw Gruffudd OWEN

Meddygfa'r Tymbl
6 Heol y Bryn, Upper Tumble, Llanelli SA14 6DP
Tel: 01269 841289 Fax: 01269 841009
Email: practice.manager@gp-W92305.wales.nhs.uk
(Carmarthenshire Local Health Board)
Patient List Size: 7159

Practice Manager Jackie Jones

GP G R JONES, N E DAVIES, S L JONES, G T PRISMORE

Slader and Partners
The Surgery, Llangennech, Llanelli SA14 8TU
Tel: 01554 820287
(Carmarthenshire Local Health Board)

GP C J SLADER

Ty-Elli Group Practice
Ty Elli, Llanelli SA15 3BD
Tel: 01554 772678 / 773747 Fax: 01554 774476
(Carmarthenshire Local Health Board)

GP Benjamin Rees DAVIES, Kevin Eamonn JONES, Nicholas John LUPINI, Rhys Gwyn HUWS, Debbie Bevan THOMAS, Christopher James TREHARNE, Alan John WILLIAMS

Llanfairfechan

Health Centre
Village Road, Llanfairfechan LL33 0NH
Tel: 01248 680021 Fax: 01248 681711
(Conwy Local Health Board)

Practice Manager Jayne Westmoreland

GP Anne ELLIS, Clare Mary CAROLAN, Michael Dominic FLANNERY, Catherine Mair HUGHES, Richard Mark WALKER, Nefyn Howard WILLIAMS

Llanfairpwllgwyngyll

Health Centre
Llanfairpwllgwyngyll LL61 5YZ
Tel: 01248 714388 Fax: 01248 715826
(Anglesey Local Health Board)

Practice Manager Linda West

GP Gwynfor ROBERTS, Endaf AP IEUAN, Gudmundur Kjartan DAVIDSSON, Alun Gwyn Rhys GRIFFITHS, Nia Gwyn HOLLAND, Laura Miranda McEWAN

Penbryn Surgery
Dwyran, Ynys Mon, Llanfairpwllgwyngyll LL61 6YD
Tel: 01248 430253 Fax: 01248 430092
(Anglesey Local Health Board)
Patient List Size: 8100

Practice Manager Linda West

GP G ROBERTS, E AP IEUAN, D K DAVIDSON, A GRIFFITHS, N G HOLLAND, L McEWAN

Llanfyllin

Llanfyllin Medical Centre
High Street, Llanfyllin SY22 5DG
Tel: 01691 648054 Fax: 01691 648165

Llanfyllin Medical Centre
High Street, Llanfyllin SY22 5DG
Tel: 01691 648054 Fax: 01691 648165
(Powys Local Health Board; Powys Local Health Board)
Patient List Size: 8200
Patient List Size: 8200

Practice Manager Marilyn Shields, Marilyn Shields, Marilyn Shields, Marilyn Shields

GP Peter Nicholas Graham JONES, Peter Nicholas Graham JONES, Huw Charles EVANS, Huw Charles EVANS, Marcia Kay HANCORN, Marcia Kay HANCORN, A LOVELL, A LOVELL, M PLANT, M PLANT, J SHAW, J SHAW, Adrian Hugh Spencer WESTON, Adrian Hugh Spencer WESTON

Llangefni

Coed y Glyn Surgery
Coed y Glyn, Church Street, Llangefni LL77 7DU
Tel: 01248 722229 Fax: 01248 750551
(Anglesey Local Health Board)

Practice Manager Enid Griffiths

GP Gwylfa Wyn MORGAN, Barbara Anne HUGHES, Hugh Idris JONES, Ieuan Gwyned JONES

Llangollen

Llangollen Health Centre
Regent Street, Llangollen LL20 8HL
Tel: 01978 860625 Fax: 01978 860174
(Wrexham Local Health Board)
Patient List Size: 8600

Practice Manager W Penney

GP John Rhys Adams DAVIES, Ann Dilys EVANS, Alison HUGHES, Janet Rachel KNIGHT, Tim LYTHE, Robert Michael TANNER

Llanidloes

The Arwystili Medical Practice
Mount Lane, Llanidloes SY18 6EZ
Tel: 01686 412228 / 412322 Fax: 01686 413536

The Arwystili Medical Practice
Mount Lane, Llanidloes SY18 6EZ
Tel: 01686 412228 / 412322 Fax: 01686 413536
(Powys Local Health Board; Powys Local Health Board)

Practice Manager Margot Jones, Margot Jones, Margot Jones, Margot Jones

GP Nigel Huw JONES, Nigel Huw JONES, Martin William GREEN, Martin William GREEN, Stephen Mansfield LESLIE, Stephen Mansfield LESLIE, Hywel Spencer LLOYD, Hywel Spencer LLOYD,

Sara Melody Linda Buchanan SMITH, Sara Melody Linda Buchanan SMITH

Llanrwst

The Surgery

Scotland Street, Llanrwst LL26 0AL
Tel: 01492 640411 Fax: 01492 641402
(Conwy Local Health Board)

Practice Manager Enid Thomas

GP Peter Alwyn BRITT-COMPTON, Stevan JOHL, Roger Barrington RAMSAY

Llantwit Major

Eryl Surgery

Eryl, Station Road, Llantwit Major CF61 1ST
Tel: 01446 793444 Fax: 01446 793115
(Vale of Glamorgan Local Health Board)

GP William Robert Pendrice BEVINGTON, Geoffrey John CRIMMINS, Anna Jean FOREMAN, Rose KAVANAGH, James Martin MORRIS, Owen PEREGRINE

Llanybydder

Brynmeddyg Surgery

Llanybydder SA40 9RN
Tel: 01570 480244 Fax: 01570 481174
Email: enquiries:gp-W92045.wales.nhs.uk
(Ceredigion Local Health Board)
Patient List Size: 2350

Practice Manager Carol Cook

GP Stephen Gerent ROWLANDS

Lydney

Wye Valley Practice

Smithville Close, St Briavels, Lydney GL15 6SA
Tel: 01594 530334 Fax: 01594 530748
(Monmouthshire Local Health Board)

Practice Manager A. Calland

GP Anthony Lawson CALLAND, Jonathan Peter JENNINGS

Machynlleth

Drs Upadhyay, Church and Auf den Kamp

The Health Centre, Forge Road, Machynlleth SY20 8EQ
Tel: 01654 702224 Fax: 01654 703688

Drs Upadhyay, Church and Auf den Kamp

The Health Centre, Forge Road, Machynlleth SY20 8EQ
Tel: 01654 702224 Fax: 01654 703688
(Powys Local Health Board; Powys Local Health Board)
Patient List Size: 4500
Patient List Size: 4500

Practice Manager Jill Davies, Jill Davies, Jill Davies, Jill Davies

GP Mahendra UPADHYAY, Mahendra UPADHYAY, Marcel AUF DEN KAMP, Marcel AUF DEN KAMP, D CHURCH, D CHURCH

Glantwymryn Health Centre

Cemmaes Road, Machynlleth SY20 8LB
Tel: 01650 511227 Fax: 01650 511739

Glantwymryn Health Centre

Cemmaes Road, Machynlleth SY20 8LB
Tel: 01650 511227 Fax: 01650 511739
(Powys Local Health Board; Powys Local Health Board)
Patient List Size: 2050
Patient List Size: 2050

Practice Manager Cheryl Upadhyay, Cheryl Upadhyay, Cheryl Upadhyay, Cheryl Upadhyay

GP Raphael Andrew TEDDERS, Raphael Andrew TEDDERS, Simon Jonathan MORPETH, Simon Jonathan MORPETH

Maesteg

Bron-y-Garn Surgery

Station Street, Maesteg CF34 9AL
Tel: 01656 733262 Fax: 01656 735239
(Bridgend Local Health Board)
Patient List Size: 5000

Practice Manager Cherril Jones

GP Noel Bell THOMAS, Sarah MEDLICUTT, Ann MORGAN

High Street Surgery

77 High Street, Nantyffyllon, Maesteg CF34 0BT
Tel: 01656 732217 Fax: 01656 730119
(Bridgend Local Health Board)

Practice Manager Debby Rumph

GP Alok SHARMA, S P SINGH

Llynfi Surgery

Llynfi Road, Maesteg CF34 9DT
Tel: 01656 732115 Fax: 01656 737388
Email: enquiries@gp-w95009.wales.nhs.uk
Website: www.llynfisurgery.co.uk
(Bridgend Local Health Board)
Patient List Size: 9300

Practice Manager Paul Canham

GP Anthony David PEREGRINE, William H EDWARDS, Alan ROGERS, Michael Anthony ROGERS, Karen Anne STRATFORD

Woodlands Surgery

Woodlands Terrace, Caerau, Maesteg CF34 0SR
Tel: 01656 734203 Fax: 01656 734311
Email: joanne.carter@gp-w95012.wales.nhs.uk
(Bridgend Local Health Board)
Patient List Size: 6000

Practice Manager Joanne Carter

GP Geoffrey Leighton SMITH, M A JAVID, Catherine SAVAGE, Nagarajah THEVAMANOHARAN

Merthyr Tydfil

Brookside Medical Centre

Heol Afon Taf, Troedyrhiw, Merthyr Tydfil CF48 4DT
Tel: 01443 692647 Fax: 01443 690055
(Merthyr Tydfil Local Health Board)
Patient List Size: 1800

Practice Manager Cerys Lamb

GP Anil Kumar SRIVASTAVA

The Dowlais Medical Practice

Ivor Street, Dowlais, Merthyr Tydfil CF48 3LU
Tel: 01685 721400 Fax: 01685 375287
(Merthyr Tydfil Local Health Board)

GP Patel Duddappa Muppane MEGHARAJ, Venkatarama Raju GOTTUMUKKALA, Bhupendra T PATEL

Hollies Health Centre

Swan Street, Merthyr Tydfil CF47 8ET
Tel: 01685 721266 Fax: 01685 375787
(Merthyr Tydfil Local Health Board)

GP Vallathol S CHANDRAN

Hollies Health Centre

Swan Street, Merthyr Tydfil CF47 8ET
Tel: 01685 723363 Fax: 01685 350106
(Merthyr Tydfil Local Health Board)
Patient List Size: 9500

GP Balu R IYER, Nilima CHOUDHURY, Sadan CHOUDHURY, Subhas DAS, Neelakantan JAYARAMAN, Sudhir SAIGAL

Hollies Health Centre
Practice 6, Merthyr Tydfil CF47 8ET
Tel: 01685 722436 Fax: 01685 384286
(Merthyr Tydfil Local Health Board)
Patient List Size: 3350

GP Baguriah U JAYADEV, A JAYEDEV

Merthyr Tydfil Health Centre
Merthyr Tydfil CF47 0AY
Tel: 01685 350035 Fax: 01685 723345
(Merthyr Tydfil Local Health Board)

GP Abdur RAHIM

Merthyr Tydfil Health Centre
Merthyr Tydfil CF47 0AY
Tel: 01685 722884 Fax: 01685 370920
(Merthyr Tydfil Local Health Board)

GP Shalini S MURDESHWAR

Pantglas Surgery
Aberfan Community Centre, Aberfan, Merthyr Tydfil CF48 4QE
Tel: 01443 690382 Fax: 01443 690382
Email: pantglassurgery@merthyr.tydfil.co.uk
(Merthyr Tydfil Local Health Board)
Patient List Size: 1500

Practice Manager Janett Smart

GP Pankaj S SHAH

Pontcae Surgery
Dynevor Street, Georgetown, Merthyr Tydfil CF48 1YE
Tel: 01685 723931 Fax: 01685 377048
(Merthyr Tydfil Local Health Board)

GP Brian WOOKEY, Martyn John DAVIES, Hefin JONES, Gearoid A O'DWYER, Kevin Ross THOMAS

The Troedyrlin Surgery
66A Cardiff Road, Troedyrlin, Merthyr Tydfil CF48 4JZ
Tel: 01443 693250/249 Fax: 01443 693345
(Merthyr Tydfil Local Health Board)
Patient List Size: 1800

Practice Manager V Chillal

GP Balaji CHILLAL

Ty Morlais
Berry Square, Merthyr Tydfil CF48 3AL
Tel: 01685 722782 Fax: 0870 220 6765
Email: morlaismedicalpractice@yahoo.com
Website: www.morlaismedicalpractice.co.uk
(Merthyr Tydfil Local Health Board)
Patient List Size: 9000

Practice Manager Derek Burks

GP Jonathan Philip RICHARDS, Maria CRONJE, Sally Clare HOSEN, Melissa KIRKMAN, Sian NEWMAN, Christopher WAINWRIGHT

Yew Street Medical Centre
1 Yew Street, Troedyrhiw, Merthyr Tydfil CF47 8DY
Tel: 01443 690271 Fax: 01443 693066
(Merthyr Tydfil Local Health Board)

GP Satyendra N JHA, Ram S PRASAD

Milford Haven

Barlow House Surgery
22 Hamilton Terrace, Milford Haven SA73 3JJ
Tel: 01646 690674 Fax: 01646 690553
(Pembrokeshire Local Health Board)

Practice Manager P Smith

GP John G ROBERTS, Paul I CRAWFORD, Robert B DAVIES, Kevin J HILL, Catherine B MARTIN

Neyland Health Centre
Charles Street, Neyland, Milford Haven SA73 1SA
Tel: 01646 600268 Fax: 01646 602260
(Pembrokeshire Local Health Board)
Patient List Size: 2600

Practice Manager Lindsay Moran

GP D ZANGOURAS, R PHILLIPS

Robert Street Practice
140 Robert Street, Milford Haven SA73 2HS
Tel: 01646 690690 Fax: 01646 695305
(Pembrokeshire Local Health Board)
Patient List Size: 8300

GP John Finlay MACKINTOSH, Benjamin AUBREY, C DAVIES, C GARRETD, Joseph Martin MEAGHER

Mold

Bromfield Medical Centre
Sealmart House, Brynhilyn Lane, Mold CH7 1JY
Tel: 01352 700212 Fax: 01352 750721
(Flintshire Local Health Board)

GP Faulds Aliko Lydia Tom MWAMBINGU

Grosvenor Street Surgery
8 Grosvenor Street, Mold CH7 1EJ
Tel: 01352 756762 Fax: 01352 758631
(Flintshire Local Health Board)

GP Eric Ivor BECKETT

Pendre Surgery
Clayton Road, Mold CH7 1SS
Tel: 01352 759163 Fax: 01352 758255
(Flintshire Local Health Board)
Patient List Size: 12000

Practice Manager Alison Davies

GP Daniel Edmund MUCKLE-JONES, Marrion A CARSWELL, Martin James GRIFFITHS, Wendy SHILLITO

The Surgery
Queen Street, Leeswood, Mold CH7 4RQ
Tel: 01352 770212
(Flintshire Local Health Board)
Patient List Size: 2000

Practice Manager Irene Park

GP M ASOKAN

Monmouth

Chippenham Surgery
Monnow Street, Monmouth NP25 3EQ
Tel: 01600 713811 Fax: 01600 772652
Website: www.chippenhamsurgery.com
(Monmouthshire Local Health Board)
Patient List Size: 11200

GP Hubert Janusz MESSING, James Lewis ALLISON, Anne Rhys GRIFFITHS, Christine Joyce LENTON, John Halliday Rowland PAYNE, Stephen Hywel Dalzell SHAW

Dixton Surgery
Dixton Road, Monmouth NP25 3PL
Tel: 01600 712152 Fax: 01600 772634
(Monmouthshire Local Health Board)

GP Robert ALLIOTT, Brian David John HARRIES

Montgomery

Well Street Surgery
Well Street, Montgomery SY15 6PF
Tel: 01686 668217 Fax: 01686 668599

Well Street Surgery
Well Street, Montgomery SY15 6PF
Tel: 01686 668217 Fax: 01686 668599
(Powys Local Health Board; Powys Local Health Board)
Patient List Size: 7400
Patient List Size: 7400

GP John WYNN-JONES, John WYNN-JONES, Simon CURRIN, Simon CURRIN, Donna GRIFFITHS, Donna GRIFFITHS, Patricia Henrietta LINDSAY, Patricia Henrietta LINDSAY, Ainsley REID, Ainsley REID

Mountain Ash

Abercynon Health Centre
Abercynon, Mountain Ash CF45 4YB
Tel: 01443 740447 Fax: 01443 740228
(Rhondda Cynon Taff Local Health Board)
Patient List Size: 6400

GP Rajapsrka A M RAJAPAKSA, Jan KLOCKE, Jagjivan Valji SANGHANI, Neelam SANGHANI

Cardiff Road Surgery
8 Cardiff Road, Mountain Ash CF45 4EU
Tel: 01443 476505 Fax: 01443 473219
(Rhondda Cynon Taff Local Health Board)
Patient List Size: 2100

Practice Manager Sybil Neill

GP Eleanor BROWN

Hillcrest Medical Centre
Pryce Street, Mountain Ash CF45 3NT
Tel: 01443 473783
(Rhondda Cynon Taff Local Health Board)
Patient List Size: 2500

GP Joseph SKARIA

Miskin Surgery
215 Penrhiwceiber Road, Mountain Ash CF45 3UN
Tel: 01443 473218 Fax: 01443 477505
(Rhondda Cynon Taff Local Health Board)
Patient List Size: 2850

Practice Manager M Manjunath

GP M MANJUNATH

Rheola Street Medical Centre
50 Rheola Street, Penrhiwceiber, Mountain Ash CF45 3TB
Tel: 01443 473328 Fax: 01443 473796
Email: edi@gp-W95038.wales.nhs.uk
(Rhondda Cynon Taff Local Health Board)
Patient List Size: 3450

GP David Michael Trevor MORGAN

Rhos House Surgery
55 Oxford Street, Mountain Ash CF45 3HD
Tel: 01443 473214 Fax: 01443 473289
(Rhondda Cynon Taff Local Health Board)

Practice Manager Katrina Williams

GP Ramanthapur S S KRISHNAMURTHY

Narberth

Meddygfa Rhiannon
Northfield Road, Narberth SA67 7AA
Tel: 01834 860237 Fax: 01834 861625
(Pembrokeshire Local Health Board)
Patient List Size: 5800

Practice Manager Linda Phillips

GP Patricia Kathryn ALLEN, Rebecca Candia CADBURY, Eurig Wyn HARRIES, Martin MACKINTOSH

Northfield Health Centre
Northfield Road, Narberth SA67 7AA
Tel: 01834 860316 Fax: 01834 861394
(Pembrokeshire Local Health Board)

GP Stephanie Joan WOOD, Madeline EVANS

Neath

Briton Ferry Health Centre
Hunter Street, Briton Ferry, Neath SA11 2SF
Tel: 01639 812270 Fax: 01639 813019
(Neath Port Talbot Local Health Board)

GP Richard James AYERS, Andrew Menzies MUIR, Sian Eleri PHILLIPS, Heather Frances WILKES

Briton Ferry Health Centre
Hunter Street, Briton Ferry, Neath SA11 2SF
Tel: 01639 813272 Fax: 01639 820060
(Neath Port Talbot Local Health Board)
Patient List Size: 6200

Practice Manager Angela Worth

GP Ronald Bryn JOHN, Keatley Elizabeth JAMES, Julie LETHBRIDGE, Eamonn MURPHY

Castle Surgery
1 Prince of Wales Drive, Neath SA11 3EW
Tel: 01639 641444 Fax: 01639 636288
(Neath Port Talbot Local Health Board)

GP Rhidian Hywel LEWIS, Gloria Kachorn Staddon KAHAN, Alison Jean LILLEY, Huw MORGAN, Brendan David SHEEHAN

Dyfed Road Health Centre
Dyfed Road, Neath SA11 3AP
Tel: 01639 635331
(Neath Port Talbot Local Health Board)

GP Ann Edwards McMILLAN, Alistair Charles BENNETT, Anne C BOWEN, Alun Ap Gwilym HARRIS, Andrew David HOWE

Khan and Partners
Medical Centre, Church Road, Seven Sisters, Neath SA10 9DT
Tel: 01639 700203 Fax: 01639 700010
(Neath Port Talbot Local Health Board)
Patient List Size: 6500

Practice Manager Anne Hill

GP Sahib KHAN, Rebecca JONES, Naranjan Singh KHOSA, Clive Anthony ROSSER

Skewen Medical Centre
Queens Road, Skewen, Neath SA10 6UL
Tel: 01792 812316 Fax: 01792 323208
(Neath Port Talbot Local Health Board)
Patient List Size: 7600

Practice Manager Ann Howells

GP Brian Terry COOK, Dean Malcolm HARDIE, Gregory Christopher Thomas PAGE, Heather Christine POTTER

Tabernacle Street Surgery
4 Tabernacle Street, Skewen, Neath SA10 6UF
Tel: 01792 817009 / 817573 Fax: 01792 321029
Email: eleanormairwilliams@hotmail.com
(Neath Port Talbot Local Health Board)
Patient List Size: 4300

Practice Manager Rosalind Richards

GP Eleanor Mair WILLIAMS, William Emrys EVANS

The Vale of Neath Practice
Bodfeddyg, 102 High Street, Glynneath, Neath SA11 5AL
Tel: 01639 720311 Fax: 01639 722579
Website: www.valeofneathgps.co.uk
(Neath Port Talbot Local Health Board)
Patient List Size: 9600

Practice Manager Roy Miller

GP Mark Kevin DANIELS, Sianed BURROW, Patricia Rae DRYDEN, Steve HARROWING, John THOMAS, Paul Richard WESTWOOD

Victoria Gardens Health Centre
Victoria Gardens, Neath SA11 1HW
Tel: 01639 646888 Fax: 01639 633326
Email: george.john@gp-w98175.wlaes.nhs.uk
(Neath Port Talbot Local Health Board)
Patient List Size: 2800

Practice Manager Rhian Rooke

GP K G JOHN

Victoria Gardens Surgery
Victoria Gardens, Neath SA11 1HW
Tel: 01639 643786 Fax: 01639 640018
(Neath Port Talbot Local Health Board)
Patient List Size: 8400

Practice Manager Andrea Edwards

GP Gareth Rees THOMAS, C BOWDEN, L COPP, Pramod DEVICHAND, R ZIELINSKI

New Quay

Williams, O'Connor and Morgan
New Quay Surgery, Church Road, New Quay SA45 9PB
Tel: 01545 560203 Fax: 01545 560916
(Ceredigion Local Health Board)
Patient List Size: 5000

Practice Manager Pete Kemp

GP Dylan WILLIAMS, Robert David MORGAN, Leo Declan O'CONNOR

New Tredegar

Amery, Blythe-Wilkinson and Cecillia
White Rose Medical Centre, White Rose Way, New Tredegar NP24 6EE
Tel: 01443 878300 Fax: 01443 878302
(Caerphilly Local Health Board)

Practice Manager Karen Dyer

GP Justin AMERY, Debra BLYTHE-WILKINSON, Pyper CECILLIA

Newbridge

The Surgery
Crown Street, Crumlin, Newbridge NP11 4PQ
Tel: 0870 429 9642
(Caerphilly Local Health Board)
Patient List Size: 3400

Practice Manager Michelle Donavan

GP J S OJHA, K OJHA

Newcastle Emlyn

Meddygfa Emlyn
Lloyds Terrace, Newcastle Emlyn SA38 9NS
Tel: 01239 710479 Fax: 01239 711683
Email: name.surname@gp-W92018.wales.nhs.uk
(Ceredigion Local Health Board)
Patient List Size: 6500

Practice Manager Andrea Baker

GP Hedydd Parry JONES, Huw Owain EVANS, Andrew Owen LINDSAY, John Peter Llewelyn NOAKES, Alun John RISHKO

Newport, Dyfed

Newport Surgery
Long Street, Newport SA42 0TJ
Tel: 01239 820397 Fax: 01239 820056
(Pembrokeshire Local Health Board)
Patient List Size: 4200

Practice Manager Julie Evans

GP Leslie Samuel LEWIS, Catherine BURRELL, Richard JENKINS

Newport, Gwent

Allway Health Centre
18 Penkin Close, Alway, Newport NP19 9NT
Tel: 01633 277882 Fax: 01633 290627
(Newport Local Health Board)
Patient List Size: 1500

Practice Manager Annie Ispirian

GP Hayganoush ESPIRIAN, Peter JONES

Ashfield Road Surgery
Ashfield Road, Newbridge, Newport NP11 4RE
Tel: 01633 246531 Fax: 01633 249169
(Caerphilly Local Health Board)

GP Omprakash Vishindas LALLA

Beechwood Primary Care
371 Chepstow Road, Newport NP19 8HL
Tel: 01633 277771 Fax: 01633 290631
Website: www.beechwood.demon.co.uk
(Newport Local Health Board)
Patient List Size: 13 679

Practice Manager Angela Thompson

GP Adrian William Rowland CARR, Jacqueline ABBEY, M ECHEVESTE, Katherine Ursula GRIFFITHS, Eleri Wyn JONES, Joseph Marjan LAVRIC, Neil Anthony STRATHAM

Bellevue Surgery
Bellevue Terrace, Newport NP20 2WQ
Tel: 01633 256337 Fax: 01633 222856
(Newport Local Health Board)
Patient List Size: 12000

Practice Manager K Britten

GP Julian Paul COSTELLO, Pamela Elspeth CRIBB, John P CROSBIE, Rory Paul GLYNN, John HOLLAND, Tracey Elizabeth JAMES, Tony RILEY, Mark Andrew WELLS

Bryngwyn Surgery
4-6 Bryngwyn Road, Newport NP20 4JS
Tel: 01633 263463 Fax: 01633 221421
(Newport Local Health Board)

Practice Manager Sandra Bogue

GP Harmohan Singh NARULA, Surinder Kaur NARULA

Caldicot Medical Group
Gray Hill Surgery, Woodstock Way, Caldicot, Newport NP26 4DB
Tel: 01291 420282 Fax: 01291 425853
(Monmouthshire Local Health Board)
Patient List Size: 19340

GP P H JONES, Alison FERGUSON, John Keith GEDMAN, Andrew Richard GRAY, Ida HOUGHTON, N J JONES, Paul Martin McCARTHY, Elizabeth MOORE, Glyn OWEN, Jonathan Paul RACKHAM, Barbara SALT, Graham Black WILSON

Castell Clinic
Cwmfelinfach, Ynysddu, Newport NP1 7HB
Tel: 01495 200343 Fax: 01495 200847
(Newport Local Health Board)

GP Harcharan Singh SAHNI, Parmindar SAHNI

Central Surgery
North Street, Newport NP20 1HX
Tel: 01633 251228 Fax: 01633 221228
(Newport Local Health Board)
Patient List Size: 4450

Practice Manager Judith Davies

GP Milan Kumar BOSE, Lloyd J P GRANT, Eman MAHMOUD

Eveswell Surgery
254 Chepstow Road, Newport NP19 8NL
Tel: 01633 277494 Fax: 01633 290709
Email: gaynor.wheeler@gp-w93052.wales.nhs.uk
(Newport Local Health Board)
Patient List Size: 5640

Practice Manager Leigh Thomas

GP Clive William PHILLIPS, Alison Jane BURTON, Alwyn Lloyd DAVIES

Gaer Medical Centre
71 Gaer Road, Newport NP20 3GX
Tel: 01633 840827 Fax: 01633 221404
Email: practice.manager@gp-W93628.wales.nhs.uk
(Newport Local Health Board)
Patient List Size: 3000

Practice Manager Susila Velasami

GP Othimalaigounder VELUSAMI

The Grange Clinic
Westfield Avenue, Malpas, Newport NP20 6EY
Tel: 01633 855521 Fax: 01633 859490
(Newport Local Health Board)
Patient List Size: 7111

Practice Manager Julie Atyeo

GP David SWEENEY, Michael John REDMORE, Joanne Louise ROWE, Liam Paul Gerard TAYLOR

Isca Medical Centre
Cadoc House, High Street, Caerleon, Newport NP18 1AZ
Tel: 01633 423886 Fax: 01633 430153
(Newport Local Health Board)

Practice Manager G Pick

GP Samuel Jeffrey THOMAS, John Hamilton DIGGLE, Nigel John HOLGATE, Ann Elizabeth THOMAS

Kelvedon Clinic
5 Kelvedon Street, Newport NP19 0DW
Tel: 01633 258564 Fax: 01633 220781
(Newport Local Health Board)

GP Michael Robert THEAR-GRAHAM

Lliswerry Medical Centre
Fallowfield Drive, Lliswerry, Newport NP19 4TD
Tel: 01633 277333 Fax: 01633 290931
(Newport Local Health Board)
Patient List Size: 3500

Practice Manager S Watkins

GP Thomas Fook Wing LAU, Giovanna FARIELLO

Malpas Brook Health Centre
107 Malpas Road, Newport NP20 5PL
Tel: 01633 855808 Fax: 01633 859414
(Newport Local Health Board)
Patient List Size: 6100

Practice Manager M J George

GP Raymond DAVIES, Imke BARRETT, Susan JEAL, S N JONES

Malpas Medical Centre
535 Malpas Road, Newport NP20 6NA
Tel: 01633 850049 Fax: 01633 859749
(Newport Local Health Board)

GP Satish Karabhai JETHWA

Newbridge Medical Centre
High Street, Newbridge, Newport NP11 4FW
Tel: 01495 243409 Fax: 01495 243746
(Caerphilly Local Health Board)

GP Chandra Shaker SALVAJI

Padma Surgery
Willenhall Street, Off Corporation Road, Newport NP19 0GE
Tel: 01633 258073 Fax: 01633 221722
Email: practice.manager@gp-W93050.wales.nhs.uk
(Newport Local Health Board)

Practice Manager Karen Morgan

GP J Das MOHAPATRA, Maureen P GOLDEN

The Park Surgery
375 Chepstow Road, Newport NP19 8XR
Tel: 01633 277442 Fax: 01633 290708
Email: practice.manager@gp-w93040.wales.nhs.uk
(Newport Local Health Board)
Patient List Size: 6600

Practice Manager Catherine Kitson

GP John Buadoo DODOO, Dhurendre S KANDHAI, Roger Graham PAUL, Chitra S WEERAKKODY

Richmond Clinic
172 Caerleon Road, Newport NP19 7FY
Tel: 01633 259970 Fax: 01633 221210
Email: barbara.brown@gp-w93034.wales.nhs.uk
(Newport Local Health Board)
Patient List Size: 6750

Practice Manager Barbara Brown

GP Denis Mervyn MORGAN, Lydia JONES, Caroline STEELE

Risca Surgery
St Mary Street, Risca, Newport NP11 6YS
Tel: 01633 613131 Fax: 01633 615922
(Caerphilly Local Health Board)
Patient List Size: 16000

Practice Manager Gwyn Jones

GP Christopher James BEECH, Adam James BROWNHILL, Susan Clare EMERSON, Nigel Jeremy FARR, David Frederick OSMOND, Sophie Charlotte RUSSELL, Jonathan Carey STACEY, Rosemary Sian WILLIAMS

The Rogerstone Practice
Chapel Wood Primary Care Centre, Western Valley Road, Rogerstone, Newport NP10 9DU
Tel: 01633 890800 Fax: 01633 890810
(Newport Local Health Board)
Patient List Size: 9300

Practice Manager Roger Forbes

GP Roderic ASHTON, Thomas Bernard GALLAGHER, Vian HURLE, Richard PEMBERTON, Gareth Rhys PHILLIPS

The Rugby Surgery
1-5 Kelvedon Street, Newport NP19 0DW
Tel: 01633 258545 Fax: 01633 261907
Website: www.therugbysurgery.co.uk
(Newport Local Health Board)
Patient List Size: 3800

Practice Manager Rosemary Francis

GP Christopher James WHITE, John STANIFORTH, Nicola Jane WILLIAMS

St Brides Medical Centre
Tredegar House Drive, Duffryn, Newport NP10 8UX
Tel: 01633 815161 Fax: 01633 810900
Email: jasbir_mahapatra@yahoo.co.uk
(Newport Local Health Board)
Patient List Size: 2400

Practice Manager Molly E Jelley

GP Jasbir MAHAPATRA

St Davids Clinic
Bellevue Terrace, Newport NP20 2LB
Tel: 01633 251133 Fax: 01633 221096
Email: practice.manager@gp-w93054.wales.nhs.uk
(Newport Local Health Board)

Patient List Size: 13000

Practice Manager R Filkins

GP David William JOHN, Malcolm BRIGHT, Darren John CHANT, Edwin GREEN, Fiona Jane HAWKINS, Christopher Digby JOHN, Alina Phoebe McGARRIGLE, Hazel MILLS

St Julians Medical Centre
13A Stafford Road, Newport NP19 7DQ
Tel: 01633 251304 Fax: 01633 221977
Email: st-julians-medical-centre@ic24.net
(Newport Local Health Board)
Patient List Size: 11000

Practice Manager Ceri Kenvyn

GP Simon David PRICE, Malcolm Paul BROWN, Janet Frances EVANS, Amy HAMPTON, Raymond MONSELL, Sanna SALEH, Alexander Graeme YULE

St Lukes Surgery
Off Gwyddon Road, Abercarn, Newport NP11 5GX
Tel: 01495 244205 Fax: 01495 249189
(Caerphilly Local Health Board)

GP J MICHAEL, Nigel Francis BESWICK, J SWEETMAN, W THOMPSON

St Pauls Clinic
Palmyra Place, Keynsham Avenue, Newport NP20 4EJ
Tel: 01633 266140 Fax: 01633 221655
(Newport Local Health Board)
Patient List Size: 4300

Practice Manager J Lloyd

GP Chaman Lal BASSI, Asha Shabnam BASSI, G JOSEPH

Sullivan, Jones, Evans and Deignan
Ringland Health Centre, Ringland Circle, Newport NP19 9PS
Tel: 01633 274681 Fax: 01633 290706
Email: paul.sullivan@gp-w93047.nhs.co.uk
(Newport Local Health Board)
Patient List Size: 5700

Practice Manager Ann Oliver

GP Paul Andrew SULLIVAN, Eithne DEIGNAN, Gerald EVANS, Christopher JONES

Underwood Health Centre
81 Birch Grove, Underwood, Llanmartin, Newport NP18 2JB
Tel: 01633 413258 Fax: 01633 412462
Email: avril.fawsitt@gp-w93125.wales.nhs.uk
(Newport Local Health Board)
Patient List Size: 3575

Practice Manager Avril Fawsitt

GP James A LENEY, A CHURCH, P DAVIES

Wellspring Medical Centre
Park Road, Risca, Newport NP11 6BJ
Tel: 01633 612438 Fax: 01633 615958
(Caerphilly Local Health Board)
Patient List Size: 5500

Practice Manager Linda Beavis

GP David Andrew JOHNSON, Lynda BERRIDGE, Ann FROST, Stuart Winston THOMAS

Newtown

Newtown Surgery
Park Street, Newtown SY16 1EF
Tel: 01686 611611 Fax: 01686 611650
Email: enquiries@W86015.wales.nhs.uk

Newtown Surgery
Park Street, Newtown SY16 1EF
Tel: 01686 611611 Fax: 01686 611650
Email: enquiries@W86015.wales.nhs.uk
(Powys Local Health Board; Powys Local Health Board)

Practice Manager David J Roberts, David J Roberts, David J Roberts, David J Roberts

GP John David HARRIES, John David HARRIES, Stephen Piers JAMES, Stephen Piers JAMES, Margaret E JONES, Margaret E JONES, Timothy John McVEY, Timothy John McVEY, Christopher Gerald NEVILL, Christopher Gerald NEVILL, Alan PORTER, Alan PORTER, Jonathan THOMPSON, Jonathan THOMPSON, Michael St. George Kershaw WILSON, Michael St. George Kershaw WILSON

Pembroke

St Oswalds Surgery
The Parade, Pembroke SA71 4LD
Tel: 01646 682374 Fax: 01646 622424
(Pembrokeshire Local Health Board)

Practice Manager Phillip Rowe

GP Robert William HANNAFORD, Meredydd Owen COX, Darren Roger HUDSON, Stephanie Elisabeth RILEY, Hugh Vernon SHALLCROSS

Pembroke Dock

Dimond Street Surgery
Dimond Street East, Pembroke Dock SA72 6HA
Tel: 01646 682146 Fax: 01646 622414
(Pembrokeshire Local Health Board)
Patient List Size: 5950

Practice Manager Margaret Davies, Jane Gammon, Natalie Jones, Ceri Ralph

GP Andrew Neil EVANS, Richard Neil BURY

Law Street Surgery
49-51 Laws Street, Pembroke Dock SA72 6DJ
Tel: 01646 683113 / 682002 Fax: 01646 622273
(Pembrokeshire Local Health Board)
Patient List Size: 10525

GP John Victor DAVIES, Monica Mary COOPER, Paul GOODSON, Francis John POWER, Malcolm David THOMAS, Frank A TOBIN

Penarth

Albert Road Surgery
Albert Road, Penarth CF64 1BX
Tel: 029 2070 5884 Fax: 029 2071 1735
Email: steven.spear@gp-w97057.wales.nhs.uk
(Vale of Glamorgan Local Health Board)

GP Simon Andrew Bruce HARRIS, Deborah Elizabeth PARRY, Sara THOMAS

Redlands Surgery
Redlands Road, Penarth CF64 1WX
Tel: 029 2070 5013 Fax: 029 2071 2599
(Vale of Glamorgan Local Health Board)
Patient List Size: 6900

Practice Manager J A Jones

GP Peter Roydon William LEWIS, Michael Christopher DAVIES, S LINDSAY, J YAPP

Stanwell Surgery
Stanwell Road, Penarth CF64 3XE
Tel: 029 2070 3039 Fax: 029 20712047
(Vale of Glamorgan Local Health Board)
Patient List Size: 9000

Practice Manager Pauline Enson

GP Jonathan Gerwyn EVANS, Khan N KHAN, Eleanor Joan Robertson PEET, John Geraint THOMAS, Christine Anne WARREN

Station Road Surgery
15-16 Station Road, Penarth CF64 3EP
Tel: 029 2070 2301 Fax: 029 2071 2048
(Vale of Glamorgan Local Health Board)

Patient List Size: 5100

Practice Manager Philip Brooksby

GP Sian Angharad EDWARDS, Jonathan GRIFFIN, Stephen Richard WILLIAMS

Station Road Surgery
15-16 Station Road, Penarth CF64 2EP
(Vale of Glamorgan Local Health Board)

GP S A EDWARDS, N S SHAH, S R WILLIAMS

Sully Surgery
25 South Road, Sully, Penarth CF64 5TG
Tel: 029 2053 0255 Fax: 029 2053 0689
(Vale of Glamorgan Local Health Board)
Patient List Size: 3000

Practice Manager Kathy Stanton

GP Thomas Anthony ROBINSON, Beatriz FRANCO, Atual Jayantilal RAYANI

Penrhyndeudraeth

Bron Meirion Surgery
Castle Street, Penrhyndeudraeth LL48 6AL
Tel: 01766 779304 Fax: 01766 770705
(Gwynedd Local Health Board)
Patient List Size: 7100

Practice Manager Thelma Hughes

GP D W EVANS, Judith Heather CLARKE, Ian Richard DAPLYN, Owain EDWARDS, Ruth METCALFE

Pentre

St David's Street Surgery
St David's Street, Ton Pentre, Pentre CF41 7NE
Tel: 01443 435846 Fax: 01443 431480
(Rhondda Cynon Taff Local Health Board)

GP Hari N CHOUDHARY, Manorma CHOUDHARY, Syed Z A SAMI

Pontyclun

Newpark Surgery
Talbot Green, Pontyclun CF72 8AJ
Tel: 0870 890 2460 Fax: 01443 228319
Email: don.bell@gp-w95036.wales.nhs.uk
(Rhondda Cynon Taff Local Health Board)
Patient List Size: 11000

Practice Manager D E Bell

GP John Wynne JONES, Paul BEYNON, Colin Stephen JERRETT, Valerie Anne PARKER, David George WHITE

Old School Surgery
School Street, Pontyclun CF72 9AA
Tel: 01443 222567 Fax: 01443 229205
Email: practice.manager@gp-w95025.wales.nhs.uk
(Rhondda Cynon Taff Local Health Board)
Patient List Size: 10600

Practice Manager Alyson Berbillion

GP Christopher James Lewis MORGAN, Hywell DAVIES, Andrew DUFFIN-JONES, Mair HOPKIN, Ann PRICE, David Joseph ROBINSON, Paula VARMA

Pontypool

Abersychan Surgery
Old Road, Abersychan, Pontypool NP4 7BH
Tel: 01495 772239 Fax: 01495 773786
Website: www.abersychan.demon.co.uk
(Torfaen Local Health Board)
Patient List Size: 10500

Practice Manager R F Mills

GP Peter Albert DAVIES, Stephanie BALBOA, Douglas Rabindra DARE, Diane Edwards, deborah EVANS, Geraint JENKINS, Hasmukh Prataprai JOSHI, Francisco Roberto Da Silva MACHADO, E ROBERTS

Davies and Partners
Churchwood Surgery, Pontypool Meidical Centre, Pontypool NP4 6Dh
Tel: 01495 752444 Fax: 01495 767820
Email: enquiries@gp-W93056.wales.nhs.uk
(Torfaen Local Health Board)
Patient List Size: 5600

Practice Manager Derryn Morgan

GP Kerry DAVIES, David GRANT, Andrew Charles JEFFS, Deborah WATERS, Helen WEBBERLEY

Mill Road Surgery
Mill Road, Pontnewynydd, Pontypool NP4 6NG
Tel: 01495 757575 Fax: 01495 758402
Email: practice.manager@gp.w93621.wales.nhs.uk
(Torfaen Local Health Board)

Practice Manager Lisa Smith

GP Shirish Chunibhai PATEL

The Mount Surgery
Pontypool Medical Centre, town Bridge, Pontypool NP4 6DH
Tel: 01495 763141 Fax: 01495 767895
Email: practice.manager@w93058.wa;es.nhs.uk
(Torfaen Local Health Board)
Patient List Size: 10266

Practice Manager Lynne Jones, Louise Rosser

GP Derwyn Francis JONES, Jeremy Peter DAVIS, Rashid Iqbal HUSSAIN, William Sion JAMES, Diane TURNER

Panteg Health Centre
Kemys Street, Griffithstown, Pontypool NP4 5DJ
Tel: 01495 763608 Fax: 01495 753925
(Torfaen Local Health Board)
Patient List Size: 9400

Practice Manager Carol Gibbon

GP Nafis AHMAD, T AZIZ, Jeffrey TAYLOR

Trosnant Lodge Surgery
Trosnant Lodge, Trosnant Street, Pontypool NP4 8AT
Tel: 01495 762709 Fax: 01495 758177
Email: enquiries@gp-W93055.wales.nhs.uk
(Torfaen Local Health Board)
Patient List Size: 7000

Practice Manager Cliff James

GP Gregory Ian GRAHAM, Karen Tracey GRANT, Charles Edward Dumaresq GRANTHAM, Laura HOLLAND, David Gethin Hopcyn JONES

Pontypridd

The Ashgrove Surgery
Morgan Street, Pontypridd CF37 2DR
Tel: 01443 404444 Fax: 01443 490901
Email: ashgrove.surgery@gp-W95024.wales.nhs.uk
Website: www.ashgrove.uk.com
(Rhondda Cynon Taff Local Health Board)
Patient List Size: 15000

Practice Manager A Jones

GP David Roger JONES, Andrew David BLAIR, Paul COLQUHOUN, Karen Ann JONES, Christopher Barrie Anthony LLOYD-WILLIAMS, David Rhydian REES, Helen SHERWOOD, Barbara Lesley SIDDALL

Eglwysbach Surgery
Berw Road, Pontypridd CF37 2AA
Tel: 01443 406811 Fax: 01443 405457
Website: www.eglwysbachsurgery.com
(Rhondda Cynon Taff Local Health Board)
Patient List Size: 12500

Practice Manager Sybil P Neill

GP David Hugh WILLIAMS, Peter Timothy BROOKS, Mark Anthony BROWN, Nigel BROWN, Marian LEWIS, Philip Stephen LEWIS, Antonia Mary WIGLEY

The Park Canol Group Practice
Park Canol Surgery, Central Park, Church Village, Pontypridd CF38 1RJ
Tel: 01443 203414 Fax: 01443 218218
(Rhondda Cynon Taff Local Health Board)
Patient List Size: 16650

Practice Manager John Steward

GP Susan Elizabeth PIERREPOINT, Kurt Ivor BURKHARDT, Howel L W DAVIES, Patricia Jane HOWARTH, William Gavin MARSH, Thomas Philip O'LEARY, Badri Narayan PURBEY, Donald M YANG

Taff Vale Surgery
Duffryn Road, Rhydyfelin, Pontypridd CF37 5RW
Tel: 01443 400940 Fax: 01443 492900
(Rhondda Cynon Taff Local Health Board)

Practice Manager Teresa Bessington

GP Christopher David Vaughan JONES, Gail ALFORD, A CROSS, Timothy James DAVIES, Claire Lorraine EVELY, William Henry HARRIS, Geoffrey LLOYD, Mark John SAMUEL, Catherine Elizabeth TAYLOR, Alex Man Hien YEUNG

Ynysangharad Surgery
70 Ynysangharad Road, Pontypridd CF37 4DA
Tel: 01443 480521 Fax: 01443 400260
(Rhondda Cynon Taff Local Health Board)
Patient List Size: 2682

Practice Manager Pat Evans

GP Gail Elizabeth DAVIES, Neville Anthony ROBINSON

Ynysybwl Surgery
The Square, Robert Street, Ynysybwl, Pontypridd CF37 3HR
Tel: 01443 790360 Fax: 01443 791309
Email: r.g.menon@gp-w95619.wales.nhs.uk
(Rhondda Cynon Taff Local Health Board)
Patient List Size: 2500

GP Ramanpillai Gopinath MENON

Port Talbot

Commercial Road Surgery
37 Commercial Road, Taibach, Port Talbot SA13 1LN
Tel: 01639 899677
(Neath Port Talbot Local Health Board)

GP David Martin JENKINS

Cwmafan Health Centre
Cwmavon, Port Talbot SA12 9BA
Tel: 01639 871071
(Neath Port Talbot Local Health Board)

GP Huw Jones DAVIES, Huw BROWNING

Cwmavon Health Centre
Cwmavon, Port Talbot SA12 9PY
Tel: 01639 896244 Fax: 01639 895183
Email: richard.penney@gp-w98627.wales.nhs.uk
(Neath Port Talbot Local Health Board)
Patient List Size: 2440

Practice Manager J Rogers

GP Richard John PENNEY

Cymmer Surgery
Station Road, Cymmer, Port Talbot SA13 3HR
Tel: 01639 850543
(Neath Port Talbot Local Health Board)

GP M MUKERJEE, I SHARMA

Fairfield Medical Centre
Julian Terrace, Port Talbot SA12 6UQ
Tel: 01639 890916
(Neath Port Talbot Local Health Board)

GP Mark BENNETT, Michael COBBLEDICK, Gareth Bowen REES, Edward Morgan ROBERTS

Glyncorrwg Health Centre
Waun Avenue, Glyncorrwg, Port Talbot SA13 3DP
Tel: 01639 850407 Fax: 01639 850895
(Neath Port Talbot Local Health Board)
Patient List Size: 3400

Practice Manager Cath Edwards

GP Mark Jonathan GOODWIN, John HICKEY

Kings Surgery
Health Centre, Water Street, Port Talbot SA12 6HR
Tel: 01639 890983
(Neath Port Talbot Local Health Board)
Patient List Size: 5200

GP Craig Jeffrey DAVIES, Stephen Owen ROHMAN, Gordon Stirling SMITH

King's Surgery
28 Vivian Park Drive, Port Talbot SA12 6RT
Tel: 01639 890730
(Neath Port Talbot Local Health Board)

Practice Manager Deborah Picton

GP Gordon Stirling SMITH, Criag Jeffery DAVIES, Stephen Owen ROHMAN

Llysmeddyg Surgery
Dew Road, Sandfields Estate, Port Talbot SA12 7HE
Tel: 01639 871039 Fax: 01639 898616
Email: fanda.patel@gp-w98619.wales.nhs.uk
(Neath Port Talbot Local Health Board)
Patient List Size: 1914

Practice Manager Farida Patel

GP Yusuf Ahmed PATEL

Morrison Road Surgery
Morrison Road, Port Talbot SA12 6TH
Tel: 01639 887790 Fax: 01639 888093
(Neath Port Talbot Local Health Board)
Patient List Size: 4454

Practice Manager D Subbu

GP Venkata Subramanyam SUBBU, Huw Miles PERRY

New Mount Surgery
Margam Road, Port Talbot SA13 2BN
Tel: 01639 884111 Fax: 01639 871764
(Neath Port Talbot Local Health Board)
Patient List Size: 9435

Practice Manager Mari Carmichael

GP Gareth Emlyn GOWER, Jeffrey William BURRIDGE, Sarah Elizabeth ELLIOTT, Michael Howard LLEWELLYN

Riverside Surgery
Water Street, Port Talbot SA12 6LF
Tel: 01639 891376 Fax: 01639 870163
(Neath Port Talbot Local Health Board)
Patient List Size: 8300

Practice Manager J Larsen

GP Kevin Peter HUNT, Jonathan Christopher BARNES, Ian Philip COOMBS, Peter Michael TRACY

Porth

Gilfach Goch Health Centre
Gilfach Goch, Porth CF39 8TD
Tel: 01443 672622 Fax: 01443 672622

(Rhondda Cynon Taff Local Health Board)

GP Swadesranjan DAS

Gilfach Goch Health Centre
Gelliararel Road, Gilfach Goch, Porth CF39 8TD
Tel: 01443 672209 Fax: 01443 676556
(Rhondda Cynon Taff Local Health Board)

GP Raghumoni BAKSI

Greenfield Surgery
12 Porth Street, Porth CF39 9RP
Tel: 01443 682644 Fax: 01443 682291
(Rhondda Cynon Taff Local Health Board)

Practice Manager David C Morgan

GP Ved Parkash BALI, Visham BALI, Girija S CHOUDHURY

Parklane Surgery
Mill Street, Tonyrefail, Porth CF39 8AG
Tel: 01443 670567 Fax: 01443 674437
(Rhondda Cynon Taff Local Health Board)
Patient List Size: 8600

Practice Manager Jan Moss

GP Martin Stuart CARNE, Moses CHRISTIAN, Huw DAVIES

Porth Farm Surgery
Porth Street, Porth CF39 9RR
Tel: 01443 682579 Fax: 01443 683667
(Rhondda Cynon Taff Local Health Board)
Patient List Size: 5550

Practice Manager Janet Spencer

GP Ravindra D NARAYAN, Vijay L KAUSHAL, Motilal R POWAR

The Surgery
Tynybryn Park, Tonyrefail, Porth CF39 8EW
Tel: 01443 671068 Fax: 01443 674396
Patient List Size: 3400

Practice Manager Mrs Bishara

GP Samir A BISHARA

Porthcawl

Portway Surgery
1 The Portway, Porthcawl CF36 3XB
Tel: 01656 304204 Fax: 01656 772605
(Bridgend Local Health Board)

Practice Manager Ann Burtonwood

GP Pauline Elizabeth CROSSLAND, John Rhodri EVANS, Sharon GUEST, Richard Geraint JENKINS, John Arundel KIRKBY, Patricia Anne PARRY, George Geoffrey TINKLER, Colin Anthony WILLIAMS

Victoria Avenue Health Centre
36 Victoria Avenue, Porthcawl CF36 3HG
Tel: 01656 783349 Fax: 01656 783899
(Bridgend Local Health Board)

Practice Manager Gillian Crouch

GP Timothy David EALES

Porthmadog

Madoc Surgery
High Street, Porthmadog LL49 9HD
Tel: 01766 512284 Fax: 01766 514835
(Gwynedd Local Health Board)

GP Kenneth Patrick DONNELLY

Y Feddygfa Wen Surgery
Y Feddygfa Wen, Porthmadog LL49 9NU
Tel: 01766 514610 Fax: 01766 514828
(Gwynedd Local Health Board)
Patient List Size: 3000

GP Alison Janet NIESSER, A A NIESSER

Prestatyn

Pendyffryn Medical Group
Ffordd Pendyffryn, Prestatyn LL19 9DH
Tel: 01745 886444 Fax: 01745 889831
(Denbighshire Local Health Board)

Practice Manager Beth Roberts

GP Paul Trevor HOWES, Fraser CAMPBELL, Eamonn Dennis JESSUP, Clive Leonard MORRISON, Peter Rolleston PHILLIPS, Dhirendra POPAT, William Ashley SCRIVEN, Alastair Neil WARES, Paul Howard WILLIAMS

Priory Lane Surgery
Priory Lane, Prestatyn LL19 9DH
Tel: 01745 854496 Fax: 01745 854177
(Denbighshire Local Health Board)

GP A GOZZARD, H JONES, A SWINBURNE

Seabank Drive Surgery
Seabank Drive, Prestatyn LL19 7PP
Tel: 01745 852775 Fax: 01745 888659
(Denbighshire Local Health Board)
Patient List Size: 2015

Practice Manager S Murphy

GP D J BRADSHAW

Presteigne

Presteigne Medical Centre
Lugg View, Presteigne LD8 2RJ
Tel: 01544 267985 Fax: 01544 267682

Presteigne Medical Centre
Lugg View, Presteigne LD8 2RJ
Tel: 01544 267985 Fax: 01544 267682
(Powys Local Health Board; Powys Local Health Board)
Patient List Size: 2800
Patient List Size: 2800

Practice Manager Margaret Jones, Margaret Jones, Margaret Jones, Margaret Jones

GP Robert David Leslie SPRING, Robert David Leslie SPRING, Duncan JOHNSON, Duncan JOHNSON, Catherine Tracy WHITFIELD, Catherine Tracy WHITFIELD

Pwllheli

Isfryn Surgery
Isfryn, Ffordd Dewi Sant, Nefyn, Pwllheli LL53 6EA
Tel: 01758 720202 Fax: 01758 720083
(Gwynedd Local Health Board)

GP Richard Eryl JONES, Keith HARRIS, Arfon WILLIAMS

Meddygfa Surgery
Meddygfa Rhydbach, Botwnnog, Pwllheli LL53 8RE
Tel: 01758 730266 Fax: 01758 730307
(Gwynedd Local Health Board)
Patient List Size: 6000

Practice Manager Meryl Williams

GP Paul Roger LANGLEY, K EVANS, O G MORRIS, H J PARRY-SMITH, A SMITS

Treflan Surgery
Lower Cardiff Road, Pwllheli LL53 5NF
Tel: 01758 701458/701457 Fax: 01758 701209
Email: helen.roberts@gp-w94011.wales.nhs.uk
(Gwynedd Local Health Board)
Patient List Size: 7500

Practice Manager Helen Roberts

GP Dennis Kenneth WILLIAMS, J D GRIFFITHS, Branwen G JONES, David ROBYNS-OWEN, Robert Ian WILLIAMS

Rhayader

Rhayader Group Practice
Caeherbert Lane, Rhayader LD6 5ED
Tel: 01597 810231 Fax: 01597 811080

Rhayader Group Practice
Caeherbert Lane, Rhayader LD6 5ED
Tel: 01597 810231 Fax: 01597 811080
(Powys Local Health Board; Powys Local Health Board)
Patient List Size: 3400
Patient List Size: 3400

Practice Manager Jane Jones, Jane Jones, Jane Jones, Jane Jones

GP Barbara Karyn WYNNE EVANS, Barbara Karyn WYNNE EVANS, Paul William JOY, Paul William JOY, Mark A THOMPSON, Mark A THOMPSON

Rhyl

Clarence House
14 Russell Road, Rhyl LL18 3BY
Tel: 01745 350680 Fax: 01745 353293
(Denbighshire Local Health Board)
Patient List Size: 16100

Practice Manager K J Danes, P Stevens

GP Hugh Malcolm PRITCHARD, Murdo James ALEXANDER, Simon John DOBSON, Eilir Gilmour JONES, Martin Antony O'DONNELL, Gwyn PIERCE-WILLIAMS, J C STOCKPORT, L G WILLIAMS

Kings House
Kings Avenue, Rhyl LL18 1LT
Tel: 01745 344189 Fax: 01745 351150
(Denbighshire Local Health Board)
Patient List Size: 2900

Practice Manager Susan Dawson

GP Richard Antony LANDON

Kinmel Bay Medical Centre
The Square, Kinmel Bay, Rhyl LL18 5AU
Tel: 01745 338989 Fax: 01745 356407
(Conwy Local Health Board)
Patient List Size: 7200

Practice Manager Peter Dutton

GP Eric Richard COULTON, S H ANDERSON, J M HARDWAY, R J HARDWAY, G Z SPENCE, David Keith WHYLER

Lakeside Medical Centre
Wellington Road, Rhyl LL19 9DH
Tel: 01745 344680 Fax: 01745 344136
(Denbighshire Local Health Board)
Patient List Size: 3795

Practice Manager Nigel Ryland

GP Ranjit Singh DOGRA

Madryn House Surgery
6 Madryn Avenue, Rhyl LL18 4RS
Tel: 01745 342225 Fax: 01745 361739
(Denbighshire Local Health Board)
Patient List Size: 6000

Practice Manager Carol Davies

GP Gareth Wyn GOODWIN, Jane Louise BELLAMY, Stephen Jones ROBERTS

Rhymney

Victoria Road Health Centre
Victoria Road, Rhymney NP22 5NU
Tel: 01685 840627 Fax: 01685 843100
(Caerphilly Local Health Board)

Practice Manager Cheryl Patricia Merrick

GP A D EVANS, S D THOMAS

Victoria Surgery
Victoria Road, Rhymney NP22 5NU
Tel: 01685 840614 Fax: 01685 843770
(Caerphilly Local Health Board)
Patient List Size: 4100

Practice Manager Alyson Julie Jones

GP Timothy Marc POTTS, Robert Douglas WILSON

Ruthin

The Clinic
Mount Street, Ruthin LL15 1BG
Tel: 01824 703633 Fax: 01824 705503
(Denbighshire Local Health Board)
Patient List Size: 2800

GP Sion WILLIAMS, Peter LEATT, Catherine ROWLANDS

Plas Meddyg Surgery
Station Road, Ruthin LL15 1BP
Tel: 01824 702255 Fax: 01824 707221
(Denbighshire Local Health Board)

Practice Manager Julie Heath

GP Glyn Hywel ROBERTS, Adrian Richard BARRIE, Janet CAMERON, Karen Jane EVANS, Oliver Edmund PRYS-JONES, James Gideon Winstanley SEDDON, Siân WOODWARD

Saundersfoot

Saundersfoot Medical Centre
Westfield Road, Saundersfoot SA69 9JW
Tel: 01834 812407 Fax: 01834 811131
Email: sue.dooley@gp-w92033.wales.nhs.uk
(Pembrokeshire Local Health Board)

Practice Manager Susan Dooley

GP Kim O'DOHERTY, Roger Charles ALLAN, David Ebsworth CANTON, Huw Eirig DAVIES

St Asaph

Health Centre
Pen y Bont, The Roe, St Asaph LL17 0LU
Tel: 01745 583208 Fax: 01745 583748
(Denbighshire Local Health Board)
Patient List Size: 9800

GP Thomas Malcolm BARNSLEY, Huw Glynne JONES, David OLIVER, James Russell WAINWRIGHT

Swansea

Aberdybethi Street Surgery
89 Aberdybethi Street, Hafod, Swansea SA1 2NH
Tel: 01792 474994
(Swansea Local Health Board)

GP Jitendra Prasad ALLEY

Brunswick Health Centre
139-140 St. Helens Road, Swansea SA1 4DE
Tel: 01792 643001 / 643611 Fax: 01792 411391
(Swansea Local Health Board)
Patient List Size: 71020

Practice Manager Margaret Court

GP Robert Russell JONES, Sarah CRAVEN, Joanne EVANS, Cath HARRY, Gareth Owen JONES

Bryn Road Surgery
42 Bryn Road, Brynmill, Swansea SA2 0AP
Tel: 01792 456056

(Swansea Local Health Board)

GP Allan Kenneth Ivor HAWKINS

Brynhyfryd Surgery
Brynhyfryd Square, Brynhyfryd, Swansea SA5 9EB
Tel: 01792 655083 Fax: 01792 455739
(Swansea Local Health Board)
Patient List Size: 6200

Practice Manager Debra Beer

GP Arwel DAVIES, Ruydian JONES, Lynne REES, Owen THOMAS

Brynhyfryd Surgery
Llangyfelach Road, Brynhyfryd, Swansea SA5 9DS
Tel: 01792 655083
(Swansea Local Health Board)

GP Anthony Wyn DAVIES, Stephen Rhydian JONES, Lynne Justine REES, James Richard YORK

Cheriton Medical Centre
Cheriton Crescent, Portmead, Swansea SA5 5LB
Tel: 01792 561122 Fax: 01792 588792
(Swansea Local Health Board)
Patient List Size: 2666

Practice Manager Patricia Lewis

GP Anant Kumar SINHA

Clydach Health Centre
Sybil Street, Clydach, Swansea SA6 5EU
Tel: 01792 843831 Fax: 01792 844902
(Swansea Local Health Board)
Patient List Size: 11000

Practice Manager Anna Morgan

GP David John OSBORNE, Strephon Thomas Kingsley AMOS, Howard John BOWEN, Rhian Mererid FRANCIS, Terence John HAMMOND, Richard James TRISTHAM

Cwmfelin Medical Centre
298 Carmarthen Road, Swansea SA1 1HW
Tel: 01792 653941
(Swansea Local Health Board)

GP Michael John O'KANE, Charles Elwyn DANINO, David Henry DAVIES, Peter James DAVIES, Gillian SCOTT

Fforestfach Medical Centre
118 Ravenhill Road, Fforestfach, Swansea SA5 5AA
Tel: 01792 581666 Fax: 01792 585332
Email: mailforfmg@gp-w98007.wales.nhs.uk
Website: www.fforestfachmedicalcentre.co.uk
(Swansea Local Health Board)
Patient List Size: 7000

Practice Manager Cedric Williams

GP Ian M MILLINGTON, Keith RICHARDS, W Andrew BRADLEY, Sarah JARVIS, John Owen James POWELL, John W REES, Barbara Ann WEATHERILL, David John Siegmar WERNER

Gilbey
4 Gwilym Road, Cwmllynfell, Swansea SA9 2GH
Tel: 01639 844738
(Swansea Local Health Board)

Practice Manager J Davies

GP Andrew Graham GILBEY

Gower Medical Practice
Scurlage Surgery, Monksland Road, Scurlage, Swansea SA3 1AY
Tel: 01792 390413 Fax: 01792 391547
(Swansea Local Health Board)
Patient List Size: 6300

Practice Manager Sandra Mumby

GP John Stephen HILLIARD, Catherine WIGLEY, Stephen HAILEY, Philip Lyndon MATTHEWS, S E THOMAS

The Gowerton Medical Centre
Mill Street, Gowerton, Swansea SA4 3ED
Tel: 01792 872404 Fax: 01792 875170
(Swansea Local Health Board)
Patient List Size: 11300

Practice Manager Barry Matthews

GP Cyril Richard MORGAN, Richard ADAMS, Tracey Louise BRADY, Pauline Elizabeth CROSSLAND, Manisha RICKARDS, Neil UPTON

Grove Medical Centre
6 Uplands Terrace, Uplands, Swansea SA2 0GU
Tel: 01792 643000 Fax: 01792 472800
(Swansea Local Health Board)
Patient List Size: 6600

Practice Manager M O'Rourke

GP Anne NORTON, Julien Peter BELL, Pam BROWN, Margaret McArthur FERGUSON, Ashok Patel RAYANI

High Street Surgery
160 High Street, Swansea SA1 1NE
Tel: 01792 460015
(Swansea Local Health Board)

GP J B PATEL

Kings Road Surgery
2-6 Kings Road, Mumbles, Swansea SA3 4AJ
Tel: 01792 360933 Fax: 01792 368930
(Swansea Local Health Board)
Patient List Size: 4000

Practice Manager Carol Williamson

GP Mark Charles RIDGEWELL, Thomas MANSELL-WATKINS, Josephine SARTORI

Kingsway Surgery
37 The Kingsway, Swansea SA1 5LF
Tel: 01792 650716 Fax: 01792 456902
(Swansea Local Health Board)
Patient List Size: 9100

Practice Manager Karen Willett

GP Benjamin Sailen RAICHOUDHURY, Cathryn Jane BEVAN, Malcolm LEWIS, Lewis Bamford MORGAN, Robert John MORTIMER, B S SULLIVAN

Llwyn Brwydrau Surgery
3 Frederick Place, Llansamlet, Swansea SA7 9RY
Tel: 01792 771465
(Swansea Local Health Board)

GP Alun Lloyd FOULKES, Anna GAJEK, Michael John SULLIVAN, Jagdish Chand TANEJA, Elizabeth Ann WILKINS

Lon Teify Medical Centre
4 Lon Teify, Cockett, Swansea SA2 0YB
Tel: 01792 202700
(Swansea Local Health Board)
Patient List Size: 1900

Practice Manager E Garnett

GP John Clayson BEVAN

Manselton Surgery
Elgin Street, Manselton, Swansea SA5 8QE
Tel: 01792 653643 / 642459 Fax: 01792 645257
(Swansea Local Health Board)

Practice Manager C A England

GP Philip Powell WEBSTER, Eleni DAVIES, Robert John McHUGH, Andrew George Lloyd MORGAN

Mayhill Surgery
108 Pen-y-Graig Road, Mayhill, Swansea SA1 6JZ
Tel: 01792 655667
(Swansea Local Health Board)
Patient List Size: 4600

Practice Manager Julie Hayes

GP Christine HANCOCK, Melissa FORSYTH, Baljit Singh GHUMAN

Meddygfa Pengorof
Gorof Road, Ystradgynlais, Swansea SA9 1DS
Tel: 01639 843221 Fax: 01639 846920

Meddygfa Pengorof
Gorof Road, Ystradgynlais, Swansea SA9 1DS
Tel: 01639 843221 Fax: 01639 846920
(Powys Local Health Board; Powys Local Health Board)

Practice Manager K Lewis, K Lewis, K Lewis, K Lewis

GP Elwyn HUGHES, Elwyn HUGHES, Hermina Mary GRAY, Hermina Mary GRAY, Keith HUGHES, Keith HUGHES, Helen Ruth LONG, Helen Ruth LONG, Alun David REES, Alun David REES, Hefina J WEAVER, Hefina J WEAVER, Michael Wyn WILLIAMS, Michael Wyn WILLIAMS

The Mumbles Medical Practice
10 West Cross Avenue, Norton, Mumbles, Swansea SA3 5UA
Tel: 01792 403010 Fax: 01792 401934
(Swansea Local Health Board)

GP Adrian Phillip LLOYD, William Edward HILL, Kevin Simon HOCKRIDGE, Tracy Anne JONES, Neil Morgan Lloyd WHITE

Mynydd Garnlwyd Road Medical Centre
88 Mynydd Garnlwyd Road, Clase, Swansea SA6 7NZ
Tel: 01792 411166 Fax: 01792 411168
(Swansea Local Health Board)

GP Ramesh Dhanrajii BOHRA, Ghandi Jesudian NAVARATNASINGAM

New Cross Surgery
48 Sway Road, Morriston, Swansea SA6 6HR
Tel: 01792 771419
(Swansea Local Health Board)
Patient List Size: 6700

Practice Manager Lorraine Flower

GP Wynn BURKE, Conor Joseph GRIMES, Mary Marian OLDHAM, Hywel Wynn TOMOS

Nicholl Street Medical Centre
Nicholl Street, Swansea SA1 4HF
Tel: 01792 653548 Fax: 01792 653411
(Swansea Local Health Board)
Patient List Size: 5700

Practice Manager S D Simeone

GP David Howard EVANS, S P EVANS, J S SMITH

Penclawdd Health Centre
Penclawdd, Swansea SA4 3YN
Tel: 01792 850311
(Swansea Local Health Board)

GP George Barrington GUMBLEY

Pontardawe Health Centre
Pontardawe, Swansea SA8 4JU
Tel: 01792 863103 Fax: 01792 865400
(Neath Port Talbot Local Health Board)
Patient List Size: 10125

Practice Manager Patricia Davies

GP Trevor Vincent BARROW, Lettice Jane BIZBY, Mererid Jones DAVIES, Phillip Lionel DAVIS, John Albert HILL, Paul Gerard STUBBS

Port Tennant Surgery
125 Port Tennant Road, Port Tennant, Swansea SA1 8JN
Tel: 01792 654470 Fax: 01792 479870
Email: porttennant.surgery@gp-w98057.wales.nhs.uk
(Swansea Local Health Board)
Patient List Size: 5400

Practice Manager Jason Johns

GP Mahey Alam FAREEDI, Salar KASTO, Oluyele Adenike MAKINDE

Princess Street Surgery
Princess Street, Gorseinon, Swansea SA4 4US
Tel: 01792 895681 Fax: 01792 893051
Email: martin.collinson@gp-w98008.wales.nhs.uk
Website: www.drwillinsonandpartners.co.uk
(Swansea Local Health Board)
Patient List Size: 8600

Practice Manager Gaynor Walters

GP Martin Andrew COLLINSON, Nicola ENOCH, Ian Lyn MORGAN, Gail THOMAS, Rhian THOMAS

Sketty Surgery
De la Beche Road, Sketty, Swansea SA2 9EA
Tel: 01792 206862
(Swansea Local Health Board)
Patient List Size: 19000

Practice Manager Else Ulvi

GP D A O'KANE, Stephen David BASSETT, Christopher COSTELLO, David Eiddon DAVIES, John Moore HARKNESS, J J HILLARD, Christopher Julian Charles JOHNS, John Antony Rees LEWIS, S D LEWIS, Christopher Huw MELLOR, M SEAGER, Bethan WILLIAMS

St Helen's Medical Centre
151 St. Helens Road, Swansea SA1 4DF
Tel: 01792 476576 Fax: 01792 301136
(Swansea Local Health Board)

Practice Manager Lorna D Preece

GP David Colin HORSMAN, Paul CUMMINGS, Janik Josef Richard NOWAK, Laura STEENE

St Thomas Surgery
Ysyol Street, St Thomas, Swansea SA1 8LH
Tel: 01792 653992 Fax: 01792 457148
(Swansea Local Health Board)
Patient List Size: 8800

Practice Manager Linda Williams

GP David Putt HUGHES, Lisa J ADAMS, Mark P DAVIES, Francesca NEWMAN, W Ioan THOMAS, Kirsty H TRUMAN

Strawberry Place Surgery
5 Strawberry Place, Morriston, Swansea SA6 7AQ
Tel: 01792 522526 Fax: 01792 411020
(Swansea Local Health Board)

GP Catherine Sarah BAMBER, Paul HARRIS, Ann PRITCHARD, Stuart Morgan ROBERTS

Sway Road Surgery
65 Sway Road, Morriston, Swansea SA6 6JA
Tel: 01792 773150 / 771392 Fax: 01792 790880
(Swansea Local Health Board)
Patient List Size: 9100

Practice Manager Colin Morgan

GP Bruce LERVY, Richard Harold BAKER, Margot Elizabeth BUCK, Brendan Walsh LLOYD, Richard Glynne PINCOTT

Tal-y-Bont Surgery
Station Road, Pontardulais, Swansea SA4 1TL
Tel: 01792 882368
(Swansea Local Health Board)
Patient List Size: 7850

GP Ian DAVIES, Peter Arthen EDWARDS, Emma EVANS, T R GOWDA

Tawe Medical Centre
6 Thomas Street, St. Thomas, Swansea SA1 8AT
Tel: 01792 650400 Fax: 01792 464914
(Swansea Local Health Board)
Patient List Size: 4040

Practice Manager Dorothy Heyes

GP Yaduvansh Bahadur MATHUR, Gokul Maganlal PATEL

Ty'r Felin Surgery
Cecil Road, Gorseinon, Swansea SA4 4BY
Tel: 01792 898844
(Swansea Local Health Board)
Patient List Size: 10000

Practice Manager Joanne Lane

GP Elizabeth Corinne REES-JONES, Sheena H CLARK, Richard Gerwyn EVANS, Robert Byron EVANS, Russell Charles HARRIS, Stephen Robert PRITCHARD

University Health Centre
Fulton House, Singleton Park, Swansea SA2 8PR
Tel: 01792 295321 Fax: 01792 295854
Email: enquiries@gp-W98053.wales.nhs
(Swansea Local Health Board)
Patient List Size: 8225

Practice Manager Sian Howarth

GP Michael Arthur SANSBURY, R N DAVIES, Rachel Catherine LLOYD

Uplands Surgery
48 Sketty Road, Uplands, Swansea SA2 0LJ
Tel: 01792 298554 / 298555 Fax: 01792 280416
(Swansea Local Health Board)
Patient List Size: 8000

Practice Manager Simon Thomas

GP Thomas Wyn SAMUEL, Simon Anthony HELAN, Charlotte JONES, Ravindra MIDHA, Bethan MORGAN

Tenby

Tenby Surgery
The Norton, Tenby SA70 8AB
Tel: 01834 844161 Fax: 01834 844227
(Pembrokeshire Local Health Board)

Practice Manager Helen Roberts

GP John Robert BOWEN, Alun John GRIFFITHS, Iwan James GRIFFITHS, Damien Rex KELLY, Huw Gruffydd ROBERTS

Tonypandy

George Street Surgery
George Street, Penygraig, Tonypandy CF40 1JY
Tel: 01443 433125 Fax: 01443 422037
(Rhondda Cynon Taff Local Health Board)
Patient List Size: 7000

Practice Manager Bethan Dewdney

GP M P SRIVASTAVA, B KUMAR, Pothapragada VIJAYA BHASKAR

St Andrews Surgery
1 De Winton Street, Tonypandy CF40 2QZ
Tel: 01443 432243 Fax: 01443 442508
(Rhondda Cynon Taff Local Health Board)

GP Robert Thomas BARON, Ronald BARR, Rhiannon LLEWELLYN, Catherine ROBERT

Tonypandy Health Centre
Tonypandy CF40 2LE
Tel: 01443 432112 Fax: 01443 432803
(Rhondda Cynon Taff Local Health Board)
Patient List Size: 6500

Practice Manager Jean Evans

GP Derek Sidney JONES, Michael Andrew JENKINS, John Edward Peter REES

Tonypandy Health Centre
Winton Field, Tonypandy CF40 2LE
Tel: 01443 433284 Fax: 01443 436848
(Rhondda Cynon Taff Local Health Board)
Patient List Size: 4000

Practice Manager E Saear

GP Marada TIRUPATHI-RAO

Tyntyla Road Health Centre
150 Tyntyla Road, Llwynypia, Tonypandy CF40 2SX
Tel: 01443 432381 Fax: 01443 423099
(Rhondda Cynon Taff Local Health Board)

GP Hasmukhlal Vadilal SHAH

Tredegar

Glan Yr Afon Surgery
Shop Row, Tredegar, Tredegar NP22 4LB
Tel: 01495 722630/460 Fax: 01495 724410
(Blaenau Gwent Local Health Board)
Patient List Size: 7200

GP Syal KRISHAN GOPAL, Singh AJIT, Malcolm RIGLER, Subrata SINHA

Glan Yr Afon Surgery
Shop Row, Tredegar NP22 4LB
Tel: 01495 722460/630 Fax: 01495 724410
Website: www.w93065.wales.nhs.uk
(Blaenau Gwent Local Health Board)
Patient List Size: 7700

Practice Manager Leanne Light

GP K G SYAL, Ajit SINGH, Subrata SINHA

Park Row Health Centre
Park Row, Tredegar NP22 3XP
Tel: 01495 722530 Fax: 01495 726236
(Blaenau Gwent Local Health Board)
Patient List Size: 3800

Practice Manager Julie Price

GP A AHMED, A U KHAN

Tregaron

Tregaron Surgery
Salop House, Chapel Street, Tregaron SY25 6HA
Tel: 01974 298218 Fax: 01974 298207
(Ceredigion Local Health Board)
Patient List Size: 3400

Practice Manager Eileen Thomas

GP Keith Lewis THOMAS, Alyson ADAIR, Robert Carl LANGLEY

Treharris

Bryncelyn Clinic Premises
Bryncelyn, Nelson, Treharris CF46 6HL
Tel: 01443 450340 Fax: 01443 453127
(Caerphilly Local Health Board)
Patient List Size: 6300

Practice Manager Paulette Bridges

GP Dilip BHOWAL, M JEGASOTHY, J A WAKELING

Oaklands Surgery
13 Oakland Street, Bedlinog, Treharris CF46 6TE
Tel: 01443 710586 Fax: 01443 710786
(Merthyr Tydfil Local Health Board)

GP Nigel Ross WATKINS

Treharris Health Centre
Bargoed Terrace, Treharris CF46 5RB
Tel: 01443 410242 Fax: 01443 413312
(Merthyr Tydfil Local Health Board)
Patient List Size: 60005718

Practice Manager Caroline Scanlon

GP Mohan Lal NATH, Boyd Tilak BATUWITAGE, R KEJRIWAL

Treorchy

Bute Street Health Centre
34 Bute Street, Treorchy CF42 6BS
Tel: 01443 771728 Fax: 01443 772164
(Rhondda Cynon Taff Local Health Board)

GP Sudheer R SARNOBAT, Meenakshi S SARNOBAT

Calfaria Surgery
Regent Street, Treorchy CF42 6PR
Tel: 01443 773595 Fax: 01443 775067
(Rhondda Cynon Taff Local Health Board)
Patient List Size: 4050

Practice Manager Sarah Simpson

GP Hardev SINGH, E HENDERSON, W P SAUNDERS

Horeb Street Surgery
Horeb Street, Treorchy CF42 6RU
Tel: 01443 772185 Fax: 01443 773083
(Rhondda Cynon Taff Local Health Board)

GP Peddiraju GOPALA KRISHNA, Abdel Kader Kassem OBAJI

New Tynewydd Surgery
William Street, Tynewydd, Treherbert, Treorchy CF42 5LW
Tel: 01443 771557 Fax: 01443 775780
(Rhondda Cynon Taff Local Health Board)
Patient List Size: 7500

Practice Manager Susan Williams

GP Sankar DAS, Barrie Rosser DAVIES, Susan Irene REVILL

Tyn-y-Gongl

Gerafon Surgery
Benllech, Tyn-y-Gongl LL74 8TF
Tel: 01248 852122 Fax: 01248 853698
(Anglesey Local Health Board)

GP John David LEWIS, David Joseph LUPTON, J P MORGAN, D M ROBERTS, Ewan Llywelyn THOMAS

Tywyn

Health Centre
Pier Road, Tywyn LL36 0AT
Tel: 01654 710238 Fax: 01654 712143
(Gwynedd Local Health Board)
Patient List Size: 5700

Practice Manager Kim Richards

GP David CHURCH, David Llewelyn FARRELL, Michael FLANNERY, Terence Anthony TAYLOR

Usk

Monmouth House Medical Centre
Maryport Street, Usk NP15 1AB
Tel: 01291 672753
(Monmouthshire Local Health Board)

GP Alan Glyndwr JARRETT, Susan Alice JARRETT

Raglan Surgery
Chepstow Road, Raglan, Usk NP15 2EN
Tel: 01291 690222 Fax: 01291 690096
(Monmouthshire Local Health Board)
Patient List Size: 1965

Practice Manager Andrew Downing

GP Jane Ann DOWNING

The Surgery
James House, Maryport Street, Usk NP15 1AB
Tel: 01291 672633 Fax: 01291 672631
(Monmouthshire Local Health Board)
Patient List Size: 4100

Practice Manager Ruth Musker

GP Richard BODLEY SCOTT, Susan Jeanette FAIRWEATHER, Alison PARRY

Welshpool

Caereinion Medical Practice
Llanfair Caereinion, Welshpool SY21 0RT
Tel: 01938 810279 Fax: 01938 810955
Email: doctors/caereinionmeds@aol.com
Website: www.caereinionmeds.org

Caereinion Medical Practice
Llanfair Caereinion, Welshpool SY21 0RT
Tel: 01938 810279 Fax: 01938 810955
Email: doctors/caereinionmeds@aol.com
Website: www.caereinionmeds.org
(Powys Local Health Board; Powys Local Health Board)
Patient List Size: 4950
Patient List Size: 4950

Practice Manager Susan Hill, Susan Hill, Susan Hill, Susan Hill

GP Anthony Victor EVANS, Anthony Victor EVANS, Eleri Lloyd GITTINS, Eleri Lloyd GITTINS, R Alun JONES-EVANS, R Alun JONES-EVANS, Leslie Gordon MILNE, Leslie Gordon MILNE

Salop Road Medical Centre
Salop Road, Welshpool SY21 7ER
Tel: 01938 553118 Fax: 01938 553071

Salop Road Medical Centre
Salop Road, Welshpool SY21 7ER
Tel: 01938 553118 Fax: 01938 553071
(Powys Local Health Board; Powys Local Health Board)

Practice Manager Carol Jones, Carol Jones, Carol Jones, Carol Jones

GP Anthony Leopold SOLOMON, Anthony Leopold SOLOMON, Waseem ASLAM, Waseem ASLAM, James KIEL, James KIEL, Sara Katharine LAMBERT, Sara Katharine LAMBERT, Michael Reginald LEWIS, Michael Reginald LEWIS, Ian RUSSELL, Ian RUSSELL, Thomas Declan RYAN, Thomas Declan RYAN

Whitland

Meddygfa Taf
North Road, Whitland SA34 0AU
Tel: 01994 240195 Fax: 01994 241138
(Carmarthenshire Local Health Board)
Patient List Size: 6650

Practice Manager Jayne Jones

GP Christian Jacques Jules David L. ANTHONY, Paul CERVETTO, Helen Claire JENKINS, Rhian LASKEY, Donna Marie MAGUIRE, Byron David McNEIL

Wrexham

Beechley Medical Centre
73 Ruabon Road, Wrexham LL13 7PU
Tel: 01978 361279 Fax: 01978 350915
Email: beechleymedcen@tinyworld.co.uk
(Wrexham Local Health Board)
Patient List Size: 3500

Practice Manager Valerie Edwards

GP Thomas Gwyn ROBERTS, Clare WILKINSON

Borras Park Surgery
Borras Park Road, Wrexham LL12 7TH
Tel: 01978 352341 Fax: 01978 310294
(Wrexham Local Health Board)
Patient List Size: 5786

Practice Manager Linda M Rawlings

GP Helen WOOD, Gwyn CARNEY, Karen HARRISON

Bryn Darland Surgery
Bryn Darland, High Street, Coedpoeth, Wrexham LL11 3SA
Tel: 01978 720285 Fax: 01978 757871
(Wrexham Local Health Board)

GP Dyfrig Morris DAVIES, Debra Ann DAVIES

Castle Road
1 - 2 Castle Road, Chirk, Wrexham LL14 5BS
Tel: 01691 772434 Fax: 01691 773840
(Wrexham Local Health Board)
Patient List Size: 8750

Practice Manager Keith Benning

GP William Percival SEWARD, Judy GREAVES, Robert Corder GREAVES, Brian Gordon JOHNSON, Jane ROBERTS, Robert Malcolm Christie SMITH

Doctors Surgery
40 St. Georges Crescent, Wrexham LL13 8DD
Tel: 01978 290708 Fax: 01978 312030
(Wrexham Local Health Board)
Patient List Size: 6000

Practice Manager Nans Edwards

GP Phillip ALSTEAD, Jane Ann ALSTEAD, Tracey Elizabeth Jane WILLIAMS

Drs Saul, Botham and Kendall
The Health Centre, Beech Avenue, Rhosllanerchrugog, Wrexham LL14 1AA
Tel: 01978 845955 Fax: 01978 846757
Email: admin@rhosdoctors.co.uk
Website: www.rhosdoctors.co.uk
(Wrexham Local Health Board)
Patient List Size: 4060

Practice Manager Maria Hunt

GP Peter Damien SAUL, Lorraine BOTHAM, Nigel KENDALL

Forge Road Surgery
Forge Road, Southsea, Wrexham LL11 5RR
Tel: 01978 758311 Fax: 01978 752351
(Wrexham Local Health Board)

GP Denis Meyrick EDWARDS, Andrew BUKY, Patricia Elizabeth WALTERS

Gwalia Medical Centre
39-41 High Street, Caergwrle, Wrexham LL12 9LG
Tel: 01978 760413 Fax: 01978 760413
(Flintshire Local Health Board)

Practice Manager Elizabeth R Graves

GP Ashok Kumar MERWAH

Health Centre
Poplar Avenue, Gresford, Wrexham LL12 8EP
Tel: 01978 852208
(Wrexham Local Health Board)
Patient List Size: 11300

Practice Manager Susan Roberts

GP Adrian Paul TAFFINDER, Peter Gregory COLLIN, Jonathan David GRAHAM, Victoria Joy GUEST, Keith Gordon HALPIN, Ian Roy HAPPS, Gaenor Ann TAFFINDER

Health Centre
Prince Charles Road, Wrexham LL13 8TH
Tel: 01978 291129 Fax: 01978 351877
(Wrexham Local Health Board)

GP N Mukunda RAO

Health Centre
Beech Avenue, Rhosslanerchrugog, Wrexham LL14 1AA
Tel: 01978 840054 Fax: 01978 843344
(Wrexham Local Health Board)

GP Tamizuddin AHMAD, Syed AHMED

The Health Centre
Crane Street, Cefn Mawr, Wrexham LL14 3AB
Tel: 01978 822341 Fax: 01978 824660
(Wrexham Local Health Board)
Patient List Size: 3180

Practice Manager Seema Husain

GP Asfar HUSAIN

The Health Centre
Smithy Road, Coedpoeth, Wrexham LL11 3NS
Tel: 01978 720011 Fax: 01978 312523
(Wrexham Local Health Board)

GP Dulal Kumar BANERJEE, Sipra BANERJEE

The Health Centre
Crane Street, Cefn Mawr, Wrexham LL14 3AB
Tel: 01978 810844 Fax: 01978 810823
(Wrexham Local Health Board)

GP Muhammad Afzal SHAIKH, J PATEL

High Street Surgery
15 High Street, Overton, Wrexham LL13 0ED
Tel: 01978 710666 Fax: 01978 710494 (Call before faxing)
(Wrexham Local Health Board)
Patient List Size: 5000

GP Miles Paul MYRES, Silvanus Christopher BREESE, Jane Margaret McNEILL, Jawahar Babu VIBHISHANAN

Hill Crest Medical Centre
86 Holt Road, Wrexham LL13 8RG
Tel: 01978 262193 Fax: 01978 310193 (Call before faxing)
(Wrexham Local Health Board)
Patient List Size: 6200

Practice Manager Christine Hughes

GP Y SINGH, Kelvin Stewart DAVIES, Jayprakash Navalram NANKANI

Hope Family Medical Centre
Hawarden Road, Hope, Wrexham LL12 9NL
Tel: 01978 760468 Fax: 01978 760774
(Flintshire Local Health Board)
Patient List Size: 6991

Practice Manager Alan Gardner

GP Ewan David DEAS, N P BOOTH, Ann Margaret BOTTOMLEY, N WIGGS

Medical Centre
High Street, Ruabon, Wrexham LL14 6NH
Tel: 01978 823717 Fax: 01978 824142
(Wrexham Local Health Board)

GP Colin Charles JONES, David CLUETT, Philip Ivor DAVIES, Anthony David GARLAND, Mary Carmel PRENDERGAST

Nadra and Partners
The Surgery, Gardden Road, Rhosllanerchrugog, Wrexham LL14 2EN
Tel: 01978 840034 Fax: 01978 845782
(Wrexham Local Health Board)
Patient List Size: 8400

Practice Manager Maureen Bold

GP Asmat NADRA, Allen Edgar Brian COWARD, Mohamed Salah Eldin KHALIFA, Andrew McCADDON

Nightingale House Hospice
Chester Road, Wrexham LL11 2SJ
Tel: 01978 316800
(Wrexham Local Health Board)

GP Hilary A DUCKITT

Pen y Maes Health Centre
Beech Street, Summerhill, Wrexham LL11 4UF
Tel: 01978 756370 Fax: 01978 751870
(Wrexham Local Health Board)

GP Joseph TATTERSALL, G J BATES, Neil William BRAID, Mary Cecilia CUMMINS, Hilary Jane TATTERSALL

Plas y Bryn Surgery
Chapel Street, Wrexham LL13 7DD
Tel: 01978 351308 Fax: 01978 312324
(Wrexham Local Health Board)
Patient List Size: 11000

Practice Manager John Davenport

GP Richard Mark PICKLES, Paul Damian ATKIN, Alison HUGHES, Phillip Stuart KELLY, A M SHAHEIR

Sissons
12 High Street, Caergwrle, Wrexham LL12 9ET
Tel: 01978 760405
(Flintshire Local Health Board)

Practice Manager S Williams

GP David Ashley SISSONS

Strathmore Medical Practice
26-28 Chester Road, Wrexham LL11 2SA
Tel: 01978 352055 Fax: 01978 310689
(Wrexham Local Health Board)
Patient List Size: 16300

Practice Manager Dawn Jones

GP Abu BAKER, Ian Newton ASHWORTH, Alan MASON, Aye MAUNG, Richard David NEAL, Carol Anne Victoria OLIVER, Christopher David SHAW, Margaret VLIES, Kenneth William WILKINSON

Y Felinheli

Felinheli Terrace Surgery
1 Felinheli Terrace, Felinheli, Y Felinheli LL56 4JF
Tel: 01248 670423 Fax: 01248 670966
(Gwynedd Local Health Board)
Patient List Size: 5300

GP Philip Wayman WHITE, Tanya Carol GRAHAM, Peter Edward JONES, Dr McCANN

Northern Ireland

Antrim

Antrim Health Centre
Station Road, Antrim BT41 4BS
Tel: 028 9441 3940 Fax: 028 9441 3949
Email: gn.turk@p330.gp.n-i.nhs.uk
Patient List Size: 4000

Practice Manager M Casiddu

GP Gary Nicholas TURK, Michele McKENNA

Antrim Health Centre
Station Road, Antrim BT41 4BS
Tel: 028 9446 4937 Fax: 028 9446 4930

Practice Manager Mary Murray

GP William David HUTCHINSON, John Edward MOSS

Antrim Health Centre
Station Road, Antrim BT41 4BS
Tel: 028 9446 5667 Fax: 028 9446 4930

Practice Manager Elvina Carson

GP Alison KIDD

Antrim Health Centre
Station Road, Antrim BT41 4BS
Tel: 028 9446 4939 Fax: 028 9446 4930

GP Dr MAGEE, Dr McCUSKER

Antrim Health Centre
Station Road, Antrim BT41 4BS
Tel: 028 9446 4938 Fax: 028 9446 4930

GP William HOGG, Gary FIELD

Neillsbrook Road Surgery
5 Neillsbrook Road, Randalstown, Antrim BT41 3AE
Tel: 028 9447 2575 Fax: 028 9447 3653
Patient List Size: 9560

Practice Manager Sandra Bateo

GP Malcolm McCAUGHEY, R CURRIE, Brian Nevin FORD, Gordon Henry Corbett McILROY, Dr O'HANLON

Oriel Surgery
31 Oriel Road, Antrim BT41 4HR
Tel: 028 9446 4936 Fax: 028 9446 1316
Patient List Size: 5200

Practice Manager Mary Flannagan

GP Paul HUNTER, Davinder Kumar KAPUR, Dr PRAKASH

Armagh

Armagh Health Centre
Dobbin Lane, Armagh BT61 7QG
Tel: 028 3752 3165 Fax: 028 3752 2319

GP John Stephen GARVIN, Peter William Booth COLVIN, Catherine Claire GARVIN, Charles Waring Daniels KNIPE, Rosemary Elizabeth McELNAY

Dobbin Lane Health Centre
Dobbin Lane, Armagh BT61 7QG
Tel: 028 3752 3165

GP Noel Charles MARSHALL, Edmund Peter BECKETT, Katharine Mary MARSHALL, James Paul McCLUNG

Dorman, Dorman, Chambers, McCollum and Fearon
Willowbank Surgery, Crossmore Road, Keady, Armagh BT60 3RL
Tel: 028 3753 1248 Fax: 028 3753 1404
Patient List Size: 8300

Practice Manager Valerie Ferguson

GP David Eric DORMAN, Margaret Sarah CHAMBERS, Richard Hobart DORMAN, Eoghan Dwyer FEARON, Tinekea FEARON, William Robert Keith McCOLLUM

Friary Surgery
Dobbin Lane, Armagh BT61 7QG
Tel: 028 3752 1500 Fax: 028 3752 1514
Patient List Size: 8900

Practice Manager Sharon Clarke

GP Roisin O'REILLY, Edward FARNAN, Margaret Susan McNALLY, Frances T O'HAGAN, Garrett Vincent O'REILLY, Ruth Patricia REILLY

Market Street Surgery
18 Market Street, Keady, Armagh BT60 3RP
Tel: 028 3753 1215

GP Bernard Vincent WATTERS

Richhill Clinic
6 Greenview, Maynooth Road, Richhill, Armagh BT61 9PD
Tel: 028 38871701

Practice Manager L Williamson

GP Alan Manson TURTLE, Margaret Jacqueline LEETCH, Robert James LEETCH

Tynan Surgery
15 Dartan Ree, Tynan, Armagh BT60 4QT
Tel: 028 3756 8214 Fax: 028 3756 8837
Patient List Size: 4800

Practice Manager Nuala Mulligan

GP Robert Mark CARLILE, Valerie E GRANT, Sonniva McALINDEN, James Edward McMULLAN

Aughnacloy

Sydney Lane Surgery
2 Sydney Lane, Aughnacloy BT69 6AF
Tel: 028 8555 7234 Fax: 028 8555 7775
Patient List Size: 3550

Practice Manager Diane Singleton

GP William David George McCORD, Tania GRIBBEN

Ballycastle

Ballycastle Health Centre
Dalriada Hospital, 1A Coleraine Road, Ballycastle BT54 6BA
Tel: 028 2076 2684 Fax: 028 2076 9891
Patient List Size: 4544

Practice Manager Susan Gallagher

GP Ivan E BELL, F HASSON, Bernadette HEGARTY

Ballycastle Health Centre
Dalriada Hospital, 1A Coleraine Road, Ballycastle BT54 6BA
Tel: 028 2076 2684 Fax: 028 2076 9891
Patient List Size: 3844

Practice Manager Susan Gallagher

GP John McLAUGHLIN, Mary Suzanne McLISTER, Harold George RUSSELL

Ballyclare

Ballyclare Group Practice
Ballyclare Health Centre, George Avenue, Ballyclare BT39 9HL
Tel: 028 9332 2575 Fax: 028 9334 9897
Website: www.bgp.org.uk

Practice Manager Sean Quinn

GP Peter Ian MUNRO, Ian Paul CLARKSON, Louise HUGHES, James Hugh Craig Blair LOGAN, Charles Oscar McATEER, Dr RAFFERTY, Heather Eleanor Elizabeth SWINERTON

Templepatrick Surgery
80 Castleton, Templepatrick, Ballyclare BT39 0AZ
Tel: 028 9443 2202 Fax: 028 9443 3707
Email: surgery@dnet.co.uk
Website: www.tpsurgery.co.uk
Patient List Size: 8000

Practice Manager D A Bryson

GP Raymond George Hugh GREEN, John David CAMERON, Gillian Mary CROOKS, Timothy HUEY, Jonathan Agnew STIRLING

Ballymena

Ahoghill Health Centre
23 Portglenone Road, Ahoghill, Ballymena BT42 1LE
Tel: 028 2587 1200 Fax: 028 2587 8628
Patient List Size: 4500

GP Robert James KENNY, Audrey GILCHRIST

Antrim Coast Medical Practice
The Cloney, Glenarm, Ballymena BT44 0AB
Tel: 028 2884 1214 Fax: 028 2884 1202
Email: bd@gloverb.fsnet.co.uk

Practice Manager C Hunter

GP Benedict Daniel GLOVER

Ballymena Health Centre
Cushendall Road, Ballymena BT43 6HQ
Tel: 028 2564 2181 Fax: 028 2564 9138

GP Terence Desmond MAGOWAN, Mary Caroline MAGOWAN

Ballymena Health Centre
Cushendall Road, Ballymena BT43 6HQ
Tel: 028 2531 3110 Fax: 028 2565 8919
Email: mg.ohara@p315.gp.n-I.nhs.uk
Patient List Size: 3000

Practice Manager Jayne Service

GP Mary Geraldine O'HARA, Gladys Frances WRIGHT

Ballymena Health Centre
Cushendall Road, Ballymena BT43 6HQ
Tel: 028 2531 3030 Fax: 028 2565 8919
Email: pt.dick@p305.gpn-inhs.uk
Patient List Size: 4012

Practice Manager Jacquie Wilson

GP Charles Mark DICK, Colin DICK, Peter Thomas Holmes DICK, Joanne HARPER

Ballymena Health Centre
Cushendall Road, Ballymena BT43 6HQ
Tel: 028 2531 3070 Fax: 028 2565 8919

Practice Manager Sharon Maguire

GP Elizabeth Jill PURCE, Richard Ernest REA

Ballymena Health Centre
Cushendall Road, Ballymena BT43 6HQ
Fax: 028 2563 2380
Email: jd.mcquillan@p321.gp.n-i.nhs.uk
Patient List Size: 4000

Practice Manager McCrory Frances

GP James Dunlop McQUILLAN, Michael G ARMSTRONG

Ballymena Health Centre
Cushendall Road, Ballymena BT43 6HQ
Tel: 028 2564 2181 Fax: 028 2565 8919

GP Sidney Temple ARMSTRONG, John Robert Lithgow McFARLAND

Ballymena Health Centre
Cushendall Road, Ballymena BT43 6HQ
Tel: 028 2564 2181 Fax: 028 2565 8919

GP Denis Cormac DOYLE, Patrick Joseph FOX, Susan HUEY, Shobhna KHANNA

Broughshane Medical Practice
76 Main Street, Broughshane, Ballymena BT42 4JP
Tel: 028 2586 1214 Fax: 028 2586 2281
Email: p.butler@p317.gp.N-I.nhs.uk
Website: www.broughshanemedicalpractice.co.uk
Patient List Size: 5200

Practice Manager M E Butler

GP Robert Anthony Alexander REDMOND, Simon BAIRD, Laura BUNTING, Jan FERGUSON, Michael Robert REDMOND

Cloughmills Medical Practice
2 Main Street, Cloughmills, Ballymena BT44 9LG
Tel: 028 2763 8383 Fax: 028 2763 8364
Email: s.mccurdy@p367.gp.N-I.nhs.uk
Patient List Size: 3500

Practice Manager Peggy Butler

GP Steven J McCURDY, Hilary M ARMSTRONG, Amanda McCOLLUM

Cullybackey Health Centre
Tober Park, Cullybackey, Ballymena BT42 1NW
Tel: 028 2588 0505 Fax: 028 2588 2477
Email: jk.mckelvey@p310.gp.n-i.nhs.uk
Patient List Size: 7150

Practice Manager Janette McHenry

GP David James ALLEN, J Brian HUNTER, John McKELVEY, R David McKELVEY, Sharon SEYMOUR

The Gables Medical Centre
45 Waveney Road, Ballymena BT43 5BA
Tel: 028 2565 3237 Fax: 028 2564 0754
Patient List Size: 2550

Practice Manager Elaine McKay

GP Stephen George RUSSELL, Katharine Claire SIMMS

Glens of Antrim Medical Centre
Gortaclee Road, Cushendall, Ballymena BT44 0TE
Tel: 028 2177 1411

Practice Manager Christine McSparran

GP Alexander John McDonnell McSPARRAN, Dr BUCKLEY, Dr GRANT

Kells and Connor Medical Centre
31 Church Road, Kells, Ballymena BT42 3JU
Tel: 028 2589 1420 Fax: 028 2589 1557
Patient List Size: 3300

GP Richard BILL, William George SIMPSON, Susan BILL

Maine Medical Practice
Old Mill Park, Main Street, Cullybackey, Ballymena BT42 1GP
Tel: 028 2588 2222 Fax: 028 2588 3900
Patient List Size: 4100

Practice Manager J Stewart

GP David John JOHNSTON, Helen M'ATEER, Jean McCAUGHERN

Portglenone Health Centre
17 Townhill Road, Portglenone, Ballymena BT44 8AD
Tel: 028 2582 1551 Fax: 028 2582 2539

Practice Manager Cathy O'Neill

GP Brian George PATTERSON, Richard John BROWNE, Catriona McCRACKEN, Dorothy Patricia McCUSKER, William John Chesney WILSON

Rasharkin Health Centre
10 Moneyleck Road, Rasharkin, Ballymena BT44 8QB
Tel: 028 2557 1203 Fax: 028 2557 1709
Email: cp.young@P360.gp.n-i.nhs.uk
Patient List Size: 3400

Practice Manager J Adams

GP Robert Edwin HENDERSON, Catherine Rachel HENDERSON, Catherine Pamela YOUNG

Rockfield Medical Centre
Doury Road, Ballymena BT43 6JD
Tel: 028 2563 8800 Fax: 028 2563 3633
Email: j.crawford@p309.gp.N-I.nhs.uk
Patient List Size: 1500

Practice Manager Jean Crawford

GP Joseph WILSON

Smithfield Medical Centre
7 Smithfield Place, Ballymena BT43 5HB
Tel: 028 2565 2301 Fax: 028 2563 0869/028 2565 01193
Website: www.smithfieldmedicalcentre.co.uk
Patient List Size: 2500

Practice Manager Sally Fleming

GP Peter A E BROWN, John Derek SIMPSON

Ballymoney

Ballymoney Health Centre
Robinson Memorial Hospital, 21 Newal Road, Ballymoney BT53 6HG
Tel: 028 2766 0303 Fax: 028 2766 0321

Practice Manager E Milliken

GP Dr BOYD, Eileen Shauna FANNIN, Dr HUTCHINSON

Ballymoney Health Centre
Robinson Memorial Hospital, 21 Newal Road, Ballymoney BT53 6HG
Tel: 028 2766 0300 Fax: 028 2766 0321

Practice Manager E Milliken

GP John Edward JOHNSTON, Dr BURNS, John Gaston FLYNN, David W H JOHNSTON, Rory Norman Jonathan McCARTNEY, Oral Windsor Nelson MURDOCK

The Country Medical Centre
122 Ballinlea Road, Armoy, Ballymoney BT53 8TY
Tel: 028 2075 1266 Fax: 028 2075 1122
Email: mp.virapen@p349.gp.N-I.nhs.uk
Patient List Size: 5400

Practice Manager Iris Miskelly

GP Brian LYNCH, Ian HADDEN, Adrian Patrick STERNE

Ballynahinch

Montalto Medical Centre
2 Dromore Road, Ballynahinch BT24 8AY
Tel: 028 9756 2929

GP Carole Ann ASHTON-JENNINGS, John Waring BASSETT, Richard Watson FERGUSON, Richard Thomas Scott HARRISON, Patrick Joseph McGRATH, Fiona Mary SANDS, Ronald SCOTT

Saintfield Health Centre
Fairview, Saintfield, Ballynahinch BT24 7AD
Tel: 028 9751 0575 Fax: 028 9751 1895

Practice Manager Norma Agnew

GP Ronald William David ROSS, Michael William Donnachie CHRISTY, Sheila Catherine GUNN, Rosemary McCLINTOCK, Brian Robert WATTERSON

Banbridge

Banbridge Medical Group Centre
Linenhall Street, Banbridge BT32 3EG

Practice Manager Dorothy Kelly

GP Kieran CONNOLLY, Mary CULL, Cathal Gerard Patrick McNIFF

Banbridge Medical Group Centre
Linenhall Street, Banbridge BT32 3EG

GP Jacqueline Elizabeth AULD, James Henry MALLON, William McCANDLESS

Banbridge Medical Group Centre
Linenhall Street, Banbridge BT32 3EG

GP Barbara Anne MORROW, James Kenneth RAMSEY

Main Street Surgery
11 Main Street, Loughbrickland, Banbridge BT32 3NQ
Tel: 028 4066 2692 Fax: 028 4066 9517
Patient List Size: 7700

Practice Manager Maureen Cummins

GP Brian Barnett CUPPLES, Michael John HUEY, Ann Elizabeth McCREEDY

Scarva Street Surgery
60 Scarva Street, Loughbrickland, Banbridge BT32 3NH
Tel: 028 4062 2278 Fax: 028 4066 9182
Patient List Size: 2300

Practice Manager Stephanie Murray

GP Roisin Mary MULLAN, Marylou Anna Evelyn MURRAY

Bangor, County Down

Ashley Medical Centre
140 Groomsport Road, Bangor BT20 5PE
Tel: 028 9146 4444 Fax: 028 9127 2229

Patient List Size: 5000

Practice Manager Pearl Winters

GP Veronica CRAIG, R WILSON

Bangor Health Centre
Newtownards Road, Bangor BT20 4LD
Tel: 028 9151 5200 Fax: 028 9151 5296

Practice Manager Susan McGroupsey

GP William James Stewart BAIRD, Grace Ann Margretta CAMPBELL, Cathryn Patricia GILMORE, Richard David REID

Bangor Health Centre
Newtownards Road, Bangor BT20 4LD
Tel: 028 9146 9111

GP John Henry Edward DOUGLAS, Graeme Michael CRAWFORD, Grainne DORAN

Bangor Health Centre
Newtownards Road, Bangor BT20 4LD
Tel: 028 9151 5222 Fax: 028 91 515397
Patient List Size: 5143

Practice Manager L Wilkinson

GP Joanne Lesley DREW, Peter Alan NICOL

Bangor Health Centre
Newtownards Road, Bangor BT20 4LD
Tel: 028 9151 5300 Fax: 028 9151 5225
Patient List Size: 5000

Practice Manager June McMinn

GP Kenneth Robin THOMPSON, Nicola Jayne DOYLE, Stephen Alexander McMINN

Bangor Health Centre
Newtownards Road, Bangor BT20 4LD
Tel: 028 9146 9111

GP Henry Christie JOHNSTON, Timothy Hugh LYNAS, Julie Ann Hilda MILLIKEN

Bloomfield Surgery
95 Bloomfield Road, Bangor BT20 4XA
Tel: 028 9145 2426 Fax: 028 9127 2306
Patient List Size: 10500

Practice Manager Sharon Cherry

GP Timothy Peter LAIRD, Sheldon HINDS, Barbara Janet HOLMES, Charles McNUTT, Paul MEGARITY, Robert Alfred NEILL

Cleland Park Surgery
2 Cleland Park, Bangor BT20 3EB
Fax: 028 9146 8984

Practice Manager Anne O'Mahoney

GP David Kenneth McMANUS, Elizabeth Anne ABRAHAM, Timothy Greer COBAIN

Silverbirch Medical Practice
39A Silverbirch Road, Bangor BT19 6EU
Tel: 028 9145 5000

GP Nigel Tod MAJURY

Belfast

Albertbridge Road Surgery
189 Albertbridge Road, Belfast BT5 4PW
Tel: 028 9045 7109 Fax: 028 90225666
Patient List Size: 3000

Practice Manager Sharon Horner

GP Elizabeth Margaret CHRISTIE, Michael James JOHNSON

Albertville Surgery
16 McCandless Street, Crumlin Road, Belfast BT13 1RU
Tel: 028 9074 6308 Fax: 028 9074 9847
Patient List Size: 3500

Practice Manager Marian Williams

GP Stephnie Jane SAVAGE, Sigrun Karin WILLIAMSON

Antrim Road Surgery
515 Antrim Road, Belfast BT15 3BS
Tel: 028 9077 6600 Fax: 028 9077 3165
Patient List Size: 4800

Practice Manager Martin Devenney

GP Peter Joseph MacSORLEY, Michael Patrick MacSORLEY, Nuala McMAHON

Ardmore Medical Centre
485 Ormeau Road, Belfast BT7 3GR
Tel: 028 9064 1506 Fax: 028 9049 2617

Practice Manager Jean Osborne

GP Christopher Laurence CORKEY, David James Alexander BELL, George Martin CROMEY, Jane Catherine FLEMING

Ballygomartin Road Surgery
17 Ballygomartin Road, Belfast BT13 3BW
Tel: 028 9071 6333 Fax: 028 9072 1269
Patient List Size: 7200

Practice Manager Ruth Bruce

GP Paul Gilbert CONN, Simon Patrick HUTCHINSON, Noreen Mary McCAY, Thomas John Wyatt Alexander WRIGHT

Ballyowen Health Centre
179 Andersonstown Road, Belfast BT11 9EA
Tel: 028 9061 0611 Fax: 028 9043 1323

Practice Manager Sian McCaughey

GP Basudeb CHAKRAVARTY, Fiona Mary Elizabeth COLTON, Anneliese Gisela LAVERY

Ballyowen Health Centre
179 Andersonstown Road, Belfast BT11 9EA
Tel: 028 9061 0611 Fax: 028 9043 1323
Patient List Size: 5100

Practice Manager Georgina McGuigan

GP Kevin McFERRAN, Anthony James Gerard COX, Orla TREANOR

Ballysillan Group Practice
321 Ballysillan Road, Belfast BT14 6RD
Tel: 028 9071 3689/7843 Fax: 028 9071 0626
Patient List Size: 6000

Practice Manager Stephanie Ellison

GP Norman Alexander RAINEY, Jill MONTGOMERY, George Wesley RAINEY, Rosemary SMYTH

Balmoral Surgery
436 Lisburn Road, Belfast BT9 6GR
Tel: 028 9066 4595

Practice Manager Elizabeth Eagleton

GP John Stephen BOYD, Evelyn Alison HAMILTON

Bradbury Medical Practice
10-12 Lisburn Road, Belfast BT9 6AA
Tel: 028 9032 3035 Fax: 028 9024 8833
Patient List Size: 3200

Practice Manager Danna Cochrane

GP James Fredrick COLLIER, Richard Norman John THOMPSON

Bryson Street Surgery
115 Newtownards Road, Belfast BT4 1AB
Tel: 028 9045 8722 Fax: 028 9046 6766

Practice Manager Diane Gibson

GP Christine Mary HUNTER, Ellen Elizabeth CASSIDY, Richard Andrew CLEMENTS, Patricia JONES, Joanne Emily Mary KELLY

Carrick Hill Medical Centre
1 Carrick Hill, Belfast BT1 2JR
Tel: 028 9024 3973 Fax: 028 9032 8050
Patient List Size: 9561

Practice Manager T Fegan

GP Clare Mary CROSSIN, Una Mary CROSSIN, John Andrew HIGGINS, Philomena Marie McALEA, Siobhan McCARRON, Martin Joseph McMULLAN

Carrick Hill Medical Centre
1 Carrick Hill, Belfast BT1 2JR
Tel: 028 9043 973

GP Desmond Hugh CAMPBELL, John Oliver Plunket McHUGH, Peter Brendan McHUGH

Carryduff Surgery
Hillsborough Road, Carryduff, Belfast BT8 8HR
Tel: 028 9081 2211 Fax: 028 9081 4785
Email: gael.mejury@carryduffsurgery.gp.n-I.nhs.uk
Website: www.carryduffsurgery.co.uk
Patient List Size: 8500

Practice Manager Gael Mejury

GP Jonathan Norman BROWNE, Karen Elizabeth CLARKE, Ursula MASON, Cresson Caldwell Mark McIVOR, Andrea MURRAY, Patrick Joseph SHARKEY

Castlereagh Medical Centre
21 Ballygowan Road, Belfast BT5 7LH
Tel: 028 9079 8308 Fax: 028 9070 6939
Patient List Size: 4500

Practice Manager Diane Magrath

GP Andrew LEITCH, Ann Reid McKINSTRY, Deirdre Mary SAVAGE, Richard WHITESIDE

Castlereagh Road Surgery
50 Castlereagh Road, Belfast BT5 4NH

GP Charles Henry Wilson McKEE

Chapman and Partners
370-372 Cregagh Road, Belfast BT6 9EY
Tel: 028 9079 2214 Fax: 028 9070 5620
Patient List Size: 8020

Practice Manager Trish McComb

GP Robert George Clive McCONNELL, Colin James Daniel CHAPMAN, Valerie Susanna MORROW, Robert Stephen RAINEY

Cherryvalley Health Centre
Kings Square, Belfast BT5 7BP
Tel: 028 9040 1844 Fax: 028 9040 2069

Practice Manager Katharine Rogan

GP Shaun FINLAY, Neville McMULLAN, Evelyn Margaret MONCRIEFF, Alison Mary RAPHAEL, Peter RYAN

Cherryvalley Health Centre
Kings Square, Belfast BT5 7BP
Tel: 028 9040 1744 Fax: 028 9040 2069

GP Hugh Richard DUNLOP, Catherine HALLIDAY, Allison Mabel ROSS

Clifton Street Surgery
15-17 Clifton Street, Belfast BT13 1AD
Tel: 028 9032 2330 Fax: 028 9024 3673

Practice Manager Eilis Davis

GP John Edward DONNELLY, Martin Joseph DONNELLY, Monica D LAVERY, Dermot Francis MAGUIRE, Conor NEESON

Cliftonville Medical Practice
59/61 Cliftonville Road, Belfast BT14 6JN
Tel: 028 9074 7361 Fax: 028 90745995
Patient List Size: 6500

Practice Manager Geraldine Hamilton

GP Prabani SHARMA, Paul Gerard FLYNN, Martin David WELLS

Colgan
463 Falls Road, Belfast BT12 6DD
Tel: 028 9024 3593
Patient List Size: 2300

Practice Manager Linda Murphy

GP Brendan Joseph COLGAN

Cregagh Surgery
36 Montgomery Road, Belfast BT6 9HL
Tel: 028 9070 9079 Fax: 028 9070 4848
Website: www.surgeriesonline.com/cregaghsurgery
Patient List Size: 2500

Practice Manager B Roberts

GP Elaine Marie MURDOCK, Andrew FARRINGTON

Crumlin Road Health Centre
94-100 Crumlin Road, Belfast BT14 6AR
Tel: 028 9074 1188 Fax: 028 9075 8811

Practice Manager Dinah Corrie

GP Paul R CORRIE

Crumlin Road Health Centre
130-132 Crumlin Road, Belfast BT14 6AR
Tel: 028 9074 1188

GP Seamus Joseph Alphonsus McHUGH

Crumlin Road Health Centre
130-132 Crumlin Road, Belfast BT14 6AR

GP Damian Joseph O'KANE

Crumlin Road Surgery
130-132 Crumlin Road, Belfast BT14 6AR

GP Linda Marion KNOX, Amanda SHAW

Donegall Road Surgery
293 Donegall Road, Belfast BT12 5NB
Tel: 028 9032 3973

Practice Manager Damian Denver

GP Brendan Jude TOAL, Janet Patricia WATTERS

Dr Gilmer
Holywood Arches Health Centre, Westminster Avenue, Belfast BT4 1NS
Tel: 028 9056 3358 Fax: 028 9065 3257
Patient List Size: 3000

Practice Manager Debbie Nield

GP Samuel Owens GILMER

Dr Irwin
Holywood Arches Health Centre, Westminster Avenue, Belfast BT4 1NS
Tel: 028 9056 3360 Fax: 028 9056 3257
Patient List Size: 1320

Practice Manager Debbie Nield

GP David George IRWIN

Drumart Square Surgery
1B Drumart Square, Belvoir Estate, Belfast BT8 7EY
Patient List Size: 1900

Practice Manager Vanessa Reid

GP James Renton RUTHERFORD

Duncairn Gardens Surgery
36 Duncairn Gardens, Belfast BT15 2GH

GP Thomas George Frazer RYAN, Ronald SIMPSON

Duncairn Medical Practice
165 Duncairn Gardens, Belfast BT15 2GE
Tel: 028 9074 3416 Fax: 028 9074 3428
Email: ge.burns@duncairnmedical.gp.n-I.nhs.uk
Patient List Size: 2200

Practice Manager Nuala McErlane

GP Gearoid Eugene BURNS, Claire Marie LOUGHREY

Dundonald Medical Centre
16 Church Road, Dundonald, Belfast BT16 2LN
Tel: 028 9048 3100 Fax: 028 9041 3405
Patient List Size: 6100

Practice Manager Joy McGaughey

GP Maria Josephine CALLAGHAN, Juanita Lyn COOKE, Hubert James Majella CURRAN, Laurence John HASLAM

Dunluce Avenue Surgery
1-3 Dunluce Avenue, Belfast BT9 7AW
Tel: 028 9024 0884

Practice Manager Heather Coard

GP Robert Lawrence GUY, Alastair Charles Arthur GLASGOW, Sheila JOHNSTON, Maurice Glenn ROWAN, William Keith STEELE

Dunluce Health Centre
1 Dunluce Avenue, Belfast BT9 7HR

GP John Garvin CLEMENTS, William George Clements TRIMBLE, Jennifer Margaret FORBES, Andrew Edward William GILLILAND, Janet WILLIS

Eastside Surgery
56 Templemore Avenue, Belfast BT5 4FT
Tel: 028 9045 1000 Fax: 028 9073 2483
Email: ronnie-baird@lineone.net
Patient List Size: 2700

Practice Manager Helen Thorman

GP David James Ronald BAIRD, Rosemary Frances STEVENS

Falls Road Practice
181 Falls Road, Belfast BT12 6AF
Tel: 028 9032 0547 Fax: 028 9024 9674
Patient List Size: 1830

Practice Manager Sheila McClean

GP Michael McKENNA

Falls Road Surgery
186 Falls Road, Belfast BT12 6AG
Tel: 028 9032 3062
Patient List Size: 3200

Practice Manager Mary Toner

GP Philomena Josephine DIAMOND, Mark SALTERS

Finaghy Health Centre
13-25 Finaghy Road South, Belfast BT10 0BX
Tel: 028 9020 4444/5 Fax: 028 9020 4477
Patient List Size: 12000

Practice Manager Roisin Rafferty

GP Alan George Henry IRWIN, Alan William IRWIN, Eileen Margaret Jane McAULEY, Maria Bernadette MONAGHAN, James ROWNEY, Jean Alexandra WHITE, Susan Nicola YARR

Flax Centre
Ardoyne Avenue, Belfast BT14 7AD

GP Michael Chor Soon TAN

Grosvenor Road Surgery
216 Grosvenor Road, Belfast BT12 5LT
Tel: 028 9032 0777 Fax: 028 90325196
Patient List Size: 11200

GP Robert Edgar BUSBY, Marie Theresa GILLIGAN, Linda KELLY, James Peter LENFESTY, Michael Seamus McCLOSKEY, Mary Rose McCULLAGH

The Group Surgery
257 North Queen Street, Belfast BT15 1HS
Tel: 028 9074 8317 Fax: 028 9075 4438

Practice Manager Angela Mitchell

GP Basil John FARNAN, Arvind Kumar MAINI, Geraldine Lucy McKENNA

Hill Medical Group
The Hill, 192 Kingsway, Dunmurry, Belfast BT17 9AL
Tel: 028 9061 8211 Fax: 028 9060 3911
Email: Thehill@btinternet.com
Website: www.btinternet.com/~thehill
Patient List Size: 7700

Practice Manager Lesley Baxter

GP Denis Simpson WHITE, Andrew Gordon DICK, Sarah MONTGOMERY, John Bell WHITE

Hillhead Family Practice
33 Stewartstown Road, Belfast BT11 9FZ
Tel: 028 9028 6800 Fax: 028 9060 2944
Email: hillheadpractice@aol.com
Patient List Size: 6500

Practice Manager Paula McStravick

GP Grainne Elizabeth BONNAR, Domhnall Ciaran MACAULAY

Holywood Arches Health Centre
Westminster Avenue, Belfast BT4 1NS
Tel: 028 9056 3362 Fax: 028 9056 3327
Patient List Size: 3000

Practice Manager Karen Turner

GP Samuel John KYLE, Elaine COURTNEY

Holywood Arches Health Centre
Westminster Avenue, Belfast BT4 1NS
Tel: 028 9056 3354 Fax: 028 9065 3846

GP Helen Margaret BROWN, Andrew McCUTCHEON, Hugh Cameron RAMSEY, Rosemary Byers SMALL

Holywood Arches Health Centre
Westminster Avenue, Belfast BT4 1NS
Tel: 028 90563354 Fax: 028 9065 3846

GP Kee Sun TAN

Holywood Arches Health Centre
Westminster Avenue, Belfast BT4 1NS
Tel: 028 9056 3354 Fax: 028 9065 3846

Practice Manager Deborah Magill

GP John Millar BELL, Jennifer Doreen BELL, Terry PATTON

Holywood Arches Health Centre
Westminster Avenue, Belfast BT4 1NS
Tel: 028 9056 3354 Fax: 028 9065 3846

GP Samuel John KYLE

Holywood Arches Health Centre
Westminster Avenue, Belfast BT4 1QQ
Tel: 028 9056 3354 Fax: 028 9065 3846
Website: www.drsscottmercermarshall.co.uk
Patient List Size: 4400

GP Keith Wilson SCOTT, Barbara Ann MARSHALL, Colin Ian MERCER

Holywood Road Surgery
54 Holywood Road, Belfast BT4 1NT
Tel: 028 9065 4668 Fax: 028 9065 3071

Practice Manager Norma McQuitty

GP Susan Josephine McGARRITY, Andrea Jane CUMMINGS, Christopher Stanley GARDNER, Peter HAGAN

Kennedy Centre Surgery
568 Falls Road, Belfast BT11 9AE
Tel: 028 9061 1411

GP Francis McMULLAN, Maire Teresa O'DONNELL

Kensington Medical Centre
15A Donegall Road, Belfast BT12 5JJ
Tel: 028 9032 5679 Fax: 028 9024 4267

GP John Jackson ADAIR, Ian Samuel HAMILTON, Sarah Edith SINNAMON

Ligoniel Health Centre
74A Ligoniel Road, Belfast BT14 8BY
Tel: 028 9039 1690 Fax: 028 9071 6367
Email: gp.98@ligonielhc.gp.n-I.nhs.uk

Practice Manager Wendy McCullough

GP Peter James WILSON, Kathleen Anne McCLURE

Linen Court Surgery
336 Beersbridge Road, Belfast BT5 5DY
Tel: 028 9045 7677
Patient List Size: 2498

Practice Manager Anne Wallace

GP Bryan Edwin BURKE, Anne FAIR, Lorna Margaret Rosemary HOLMES

Lower Crescent Surgery
2 Lower Crescent, Belfast BT7 1NR
Tel: 028 90320919 Fax: 028 9024 6357

GP Maurice Enda CULLEN

McDonnell and Partners
139-141 Ormeau Road, Belfast BT7 1DA
Tel: 028 9032 6030

Practice Manager F Mawhinney

GP Alexander (Alasdair) McDONNELL, Mary Claire DIAMOND, Geraldine Anne McCREESH, Deirdre Mary O'HARE, Conn O'NEILL

McGlade, Holmes and Jones
1 Dunluce Avenue, Belfast BT9 7HR
Tel: 028 9024 0884

GP Stephanie Margaret HOLMES, David JONES, Kieran John McGLADE

Mount Oriel Medical Centre
2 Mount Oriel, Belfast BT8 7HR
Tel: 028 9070 1653 Fax: 028 9070 5572
Patient List Size: 5802

Practice Manager Roberta Walsh

GP John Brian PITT, Barbara Elizabeth CALLENDER, Sean Arthur HAIGNEY, David Samuel Porter McKEOWN

Mountain View Surgery
585A Crumlin Road, Belfast BT14 7GB
Tel: 028 9039 2392 Fax: 028 9039 2392
Email: rhmckee@p072.gp.n-i.nhs.uk

Practice Manager M McGlade

GP Robert Hastings McKEE

North Parade Surgery
6 North Parade, Belfast BT7 2GG

GP Daniel Robert DELARGY, Mary Philomena CASHELL, Michael CULLEN, Mary Teresa KEANE, Stephen Robert Edgar McCORMACK

North Queen Street Surgery
257 North Queen Street, Belfast BT15 1HS
Tel: 028 9074 8317 Fax: 028 9075 4438

Practice Manager Angela Mitchell

GP Jacqueline DOYLE, Andrew WILSON

Oldpark Road Surgery
460 Oldpark Road, Belfast BT14 6QG
Tel: 028 9074 6535 Fax: 028 9080 3033

Practice Manager Stella Woods

GP Kiran Behari SWAIN, Marion CONWAY, Denis SWEENEY

Ormeau Park Surgery
281 Ormeau Road, Belfast BT7 3GG
Tel: 028 9064 2914 Fax: 028 9064 3993
Patient List Size: 7500

Practice Manager Brenda Clingen

GP Brian Edwin DEAN, David Brian CHEYNE, Sharon Elizabeth GRACEY, Ian George ROWAN

Ravenbank Surgery
113 Ravenhill Road, Belfast BT6 8DR
Tel: 028 9045 7132 Fax: 028 9045 7132

GP Alan Terence DAWSON

Ross Road Surgery
21 Ross Road, Belfast BT12 4JR

GP Richard D. MURPHY, Joseph Fergus DONAGHY

Salisbury Medical Centre
474 Antrim Road, Belfast BT15 5GF
Tel: 028 9077 7905

GP James Niall Stevenson GREEN, John Carson Hamilton LOUGHRIDGE, Patrick Thomas McGEOUGH, Gillian Louise BROWN, Henry Colin BROWN, Dorothy J DAVIS, Paul Gabriel LOUGHREY, Norman Jan Piet WALKER

Shankill Health Centre
135 Shankill Parade, Belfast BT13 1SD
Tel: 028 9024 7181

GP Florence Jean COLLINS, William Peter CURRIE, Ruth DOGGART

Shankill Health Centre
135 Shankill Parade, Belfast BT13 1SD
Tel: 028 9024 7181 Fax: 028 9082 1664
Email: linda.brown@alcornrosspractice.co.uk
Patient List Size: 2270

Practice Manager Linda Brown

GP Ronald ALCORN, David ROSS, Valerie SHAW

Shankill Health Centre
135 Shankill Parade, Belfast BT13 1SD
Tel: 028 9024 7181

Practice Manager Elizabeth Wilson

GP Hilary Kathryn BUCHANAN, Peter Thomas Kirkwood BROWN, Clare Frances MAGENIS, Mark McCLEAN

Shankill Road Surgery
136-138 Shankill Road, Belfast BT13 2BD
Tel: 028 9031 6960 Fax: 028 9031 6969
Patient List Size: 2900

Practice Manager Jacqueline Kirk

GP Robin M CRAWFORD, Kenneth Andrew NELSON

Skegoneill Health Centre
195 Skegoneill Avenue, Belfast BT15 3LL
Tel: 028 9077 2471 Fax: 028 9077 2449

GP Hugh Donaldson Ferguson MINFORD, Jean Benson McCLUNE

Skegoneill Health Centre
195 Skegoneill Avenue, Belfast BT15 3LL
Tel: 028 9077 2471 Fax: 028 9077 2449
Email: William.Jackson@btinternet.com
Patient List Size: 5000

Practice Manager C Wilson

GP William Edward JACKSON, Pamela BRADLEY, Roger Swanston CROMEY, Sharon MORGAN

Skegoneill Health Centre
195 Skegoneill Avenue, Belfast BT15 3LL
Tel: 028 9077 2471 Fax: 028 9077 2449
Website: www.unidoctors.net
Patient List Size: 6500

Practice Manager Nicola Moore

GP Geoffery ALLEN, Victor John Richard DURKAN, Jennifer Margaret McAUGHEY

Springfield Medical Centre
44-46 Springfield Road, Belfast BT12 7AH
Tel: 028 9032 1454 Fax: 028 9020 1106

Patient List Size: 10000

Practice Manager Oonagh Toland

GP Claire GILES, Cyril Joseph GILES, Damien Joseph McGOWAN, Conor John McHUGH

Springfield Medical Practice
463 Springfield Road, Belfast BT12 7DP
Tel: 028 9032 7126 Fax: 028 9032 5976
Patient List Size: 6000

Practice Manager Anne Campbell

GP James Vevers Redman BARBOUR, Thomas Clement Flood KING, Anne Mary LEAVY, R O'KANE

Springfield Road Surgery
66-70 Springfield Road, Belfast BT12 7AH
Tel: 028 9032 3571 Fax: 028 9020 7707
Patient List Size: 8800

Practice Manager Mary Lambon

GP Kevin Aloysius BREADY, Kathleen Mary COLLINS, Marie-Louise LOGAN, George Dermot O'NEILL

Springfield Road Surgery
26 Springfield Road, Belfast BT12 7AG

GP Raymund Michael SHEARER, Maurice Enda CULLEN, Brendan Gerard DOWNEY, Bridget Anne MULHOLLAND, Kieran SHEARER

Stewartstown Health Centre
212 Stewartstown Road, Dunmurry, Belfast BT17 0FB
Tel: 028 9060 2931 Fax: 028 9060 5728

Practice Manager Mark Bradley

GP Terence BRADLEY, Margaret Elizabeth CUPPLES, Gerard Patrick Pancreas LUNDY, Michael Gerard MULHOLLAND, Gerard John James MURPHY

Templemore Avenue Health Centre
98A Templemore Avenue, Belfast BT5 4GR
Tel: 028 9020 4151 Fax: 028 9045 2640

Practice Manager Sharon Muldoon

GP M COOGAN, John Herdman DARRAGH, James Moffett WILSON

University Health Centre @ Queens
5 Lennoxvale, Belfast BT9 5BY
Tel: 028 9033 5551 Fax: 028 9033 5540
Email: cait.ashe@uhcq.gp.n-i.nhs.uk

Practice Manager Cait Ashe

GP Barbara Elizabeth FAIR, Denise Margaret DEASY

Whiterock Health Clinic
6 Whiterock Grove, Belfast BT12 7RQ
Tel: 028 9032 3153 Fax: 028 9061 9431
Email: cwasson@ireland.com
Website: http://doctor.medscape.com/CiaranWasson

Practice Manager M Wasson

GP Ciaran WASSON

Willowfield Surgery
50 Castlereagh Road, Belfast BT5 5FP
Tel: 028 9045 7862 Fax: 028 9045 9785
Patient List Size: 3943

Practice Manager Georgina Dickson

GP Edith Lindsay McILMOYLE, Katherine Anne RODDIE, William Neil WILSON

Woodstock Medical Centre
222 Woodstock Road, Belfast BT6 9DL
Tel: 028 9045 8103 Fax: 028 9073 9889
Email: drs_woodstoack@hotmail.com
Patient List Size: 4400

Practice Manager Ruth Crone

GP Robert Lewis MILLER, Margaret Ann LITTLE, Colin RODGERS

Yoong, Cummings and Donnelly
115-117 Falls Road, Belfast BT12 6AA
Tel: 028 9032 1009 Fax: 028 9023 8166
Patient List Size: 6600

Practice Manager Patricia Davidson

GP Hock Pin YOONG, Carl J CUMMINGS, Mark DONNELLY

Bushmills

Bushmills Medical Centre
6 Priestland Road, Bushmills BT57 8QP
Tel: 028 2073 1233 Fax: 028 2073 2810

Practice Manager A Douglas

GP Sian-Choong WEE, Tom BROWN

Carrickfergus

Castle Practice
Carrickfergus Health Centre, Taylors Avenue, Carrickfergus BT38 7HT
Tel: 028 9336 4193 Fax: 028 9331 5947
Email: l.buchanan@p390.gp.n-i.nhs.uk
Patient List Size: 13500

Practice Manager R Butler

GP Lorna Helen BOLTON, Shirley BRADLEY, Dr BUCHANAN, Jonathan George McALLISTER, Richard John Sydney REID, Robert Ian RYANS, John Ronald Andrew TURKINGTON

Old School Surgery
54 Station Road, Greenisland, Carrickfergus BT38 8TP
Tel: 028 9086 4455 Fax: 028 9036 5367

Practice Manager Dorothy Wright

GP Hall Stewart CAMPBELL, Elizabeth Dorothy CROTHERS, Norman David DIXON, Dr GAMBLE

Scotch Quarter Practice
Carrickfergus Health Centre, Carrickfergus BT38 7HT
Tel: 028 9331 5800 Fax: 028 9331 5911
Patient List Size: 7900

Practice Manager David J Anderton

GP James Rodney FERGUSON, Olive May BUCKLEY, Robert Nicholas HAGGAN, James J O McGRATH, Nigel MERCER-SMITH

Whitehead Health Centre
17B Edward Road, Whitehead, Carrickfergus BT38 9RU
Tel: 028 9335 3454 Fax: 028 9337 2625
Patient List Size: 9500

Practice Manager Frances McIlwinney

GP James Ronald Davis ESLER, Amelia Margaret Isobel CALWELL, Alan Kie Loong CHIN, Dermott Nigel DAVISON, Michele Patricia STONE

Castlederg

Castlederg Surgery
13A Lower Strabane Road, Castlederg BT81 7AZ
Tel: 028 8167 1211 Fax: 028 8167 9700

Practice Manager Susan Young

GP William A STEWART, Richard William Adam BAILIE, Linda KING, Brendan Joseph O'HARE, I P O'HARE

Castlewellan

BallywardSurgery
32 Station Road, Ballyward, Castlewellan BT31 9TU
Tel: 028 4065 0217 Fax: 028 4065 0437
Email: practice.manager@bwardsgy.gp.n-I.nhs.uk
Patient List Size: 2300

Practice Manager Alan Deane

GP John Alastair James CHESTNUTT

Coleraine

Coleraine Health Centre
Castlerock Road, Coleraine BT51 3HP
Tel: 028 7034 4833 Fax: 028 7032 8746
Email: www.drbeckandpartners.co.uk
Patient List Size: 4990

Practice Manager Celine Hill

GP Alan William BECK, Martin Cooke McCLENAHAN, Muriel R MOLES

Coleraine Health Centre
Castlerock Road, Coleraine BT51 3HP
Tel: 028 7034 4834 Fax: 028 7035 8914
Patient List Size: 4780

Practice Manager Beverley Goldsworthy

GP Aidan Francis John QUIERY, Hazel Elizabeth STEWART, Turlough John TRACEY

Garvagh Health Centre
110 Main Street, Garvagh, Coleraine BT51 5AE
Tel: 028 2955 8210 Fax: 028 2955 7089
Patient List Size: 5200

GP John Bernard Keith KERR, Brian William Desmond CONNOR, Louise DUNLOP, David Samuel Alexander ORR

Kilrea Medical Centre
36 Garvagh Road, Kilrea, Coleraine BT51 5QP
Tel: 028 2954 0231 Fax: 028 2954 0851
Email: rg.mcauley@P355.gp.n-i.nhs.uk
Patient List Size: 6000

Practice Manager Linda Porter

GP Grainne Maire McGURK, Reginald George McAULEY, John Paul McCORMACK

Liffock Surgery
69 Sea Road, Castlerock, Coleraine BT51 4TW
Tel: 028 7084 8206 Fax: 028 7084 9146

GP Desmond John Pattison NUTT, Hazel Margaret SIBERRY

Lodge Health
20 Lodge Manor, Coleraine BT52 1JX
Tel: 028 7034 4494 Fax: 028 7032 1759
Email: en.shannon@P346.gp.n-i.nhs.uk
Patient List Size: 9900

Practice Manager Lorna Fetherston

GP Ernest Nathaniel SHANNON, Richard William BURNS, Barry William MITCHELL, Sharon NESBITT, Michael Eakin NICHOLL, Walter Alan TOPPING, Siobhan WALLACE

Mountsandel Surgery
4 Mountsandel Road, Coleraine BT52 1JB
Tel: 028 7034 2650 Fax: 028 7032 1000

Practice Manager Linda Gowan

GP Thomas Blake TURNER, Brian Charles BONNAR, James Scott BROWN, C DOBBS, N McILMOYLE, Ian James McMASTER, Catherine Louise POLLOCK, Alan Frank ROWE

Cookstown

Cookstown Health Centre
52 Orritor Road, Cookstown BT80 8BN
Tel: 028 8676 2995 Fax: 028 7976 1383

Practice Manager Moira Doyle

GP Joseph Ernest SMYTH, Dr ACHARYA, Terry Christopher JOHNSTON, Dr WRAY

Fairhill Road Surgery
30C Fairhill Road, Cookstown BT80 8AG
Tel: 028 7976 2207

GP R GRAHAM

Loy Medical Centre
8 Loy Street, Cookstown BT80 8PE
Tel: 028 8676 3030 Fax: 028 8676 1400

Practice Manager Linda Mullan

GP Paul Patrick Joseph FLANIGAN, Gabrielle Teresa Mary McKEEVER

The Oaks Family Medical Centre
48 Orritor Road, Cookstown BT80 8BG
Tel: 028 8676 2249 Fax: 028 8676 6793
Email: john.o'kane@oaksfamilypracticegpn-I.nhs.uk
Website: www.oaksfamilymc.co.uk
Patient List Size: 6500

Practice Manager Moyra Lee

GP John Bernard O'KANE, Paul Berkeley IRWIN, John Brendan McBRIDE

Urbal Road Surgery
67 Urbal Road, Coagh, Cookstown BT80 0DP
Tel: 028 7973 7243 Fax: 028 7973 7602

GP Richard Cameron GILFILLAN, Margaret Carol DALZELL, Rachel Eileen FINCH

Craigavon

Adams Family Practice
The Health Centre, Tavanagh Avenue, Portadown, Craigavon BT62 3BU
Tel: 028 3835 1393 Fax: 028 3835 1246
Patient List Size: 2357

Practice Manager E Muldrew

GP John Drew ADAMS

Aghalee Dispensary
8A Lurgan Road, Aghalee, Craigavon BT67 0DD
Tel: 028 9265 1268 Fax: 028 9265 2665
Patient List Size: 3812

Practice Manager Eilish McNickle

GP James Allen BELL, Henry O'FRIEL, June WILSON

Blue Group Practice
The Health Centre, Tavanagh Avenue, Portadown, Craigavon BT62 3BU
Tel: 028 3835 1393 Fax: 028 3835 1246
Patient List Size: 9500

Practice Manager Christina McKeever

GP Gerard Francis ADAMS, Claire Diane EVANS, Mary Roberta Joan MORTON, Stephen William SHARPE, Ronald John WITHERS

Burnett and Burnett
The Health Centre, Tavanagh Avenue, Portadown, Craigavon BT62 3BU
Tel: 028 3835 0269

Practice Manager Joanne Cullough

GP Jonathan Alexander BURNETT, Ronald Alexander BURNETT, Tanya WINTER

Church Walk Surgery
28 Church Walk, Lurgan, Craigavon BT67 9AA
Tel: 028 3832 7834 Fax: 028 3834 9331
Patient List Size: 7600

Practice Manager Caroline Leathem

GP Catherine Mary ARMSTRONG, Jim HUNTER, Frederick James MacSORLEY, William Bruce THOMPSON, Christopher Sean WILSON

Gilford Health Centre
Castle Street, Gilford, Craigavon BT63 6JS
Tel: 028 3883 1225
Patient List Size: 4500

Practice Manager Brenda McConillie

GP Robert Alexander LOGAN, Victoria Elizabeth BLACK, Victor McMULLEN

Good and Conran
The Health Centre, Tavanagh Avenue, Portadown, Craigavon BT62 3BU
Tel: 028 3835 1497 Fax: 028 3835 1246
Patient List Size: 4000

Practice Manager Anne Todd

GP Brian GOOD, Thomas Martin CONRAN

Gray and Troughton
The Health Centre, Tavanagh Avenue, Portadown, Craigavon BT62 3BU
Tel: 028 3835 1393 Fax: 028 3839 9820

Practice Manager Wendy Stewart

GP Peter Lawrence GRAY, Alison Mary Josephine TROUGHTON

High Street Surgery
60 High Street, Lurgan, Craigavon BT66 8BA
Tel: 028 3832 4591 Fax: 028 3834 9000

Practice Manager Heather Little

GP Martin Ellison DAVIDSON, Michael Fergus CHAMBERS, John Maurice EAKIN, Owen John FITZPATRICK, Jill Kathryn WOODS

Hunter Family Practice
1 Legahory Centre, Legahory, Craigavon BT65 5BE
Tel: 028 3834 1431 Fax: 028 3834 5983

Practice Manager Lorraine Hughes

GP Denise Marie HUNTER, John Raymond HUNTER

Lakes Family Practice
Brownlow Health Centre, Legahory, Craigavon BT65 5BE
Tel: 028 3834 1431 Fax: 028 3834 5983
Patient List Size: 4995

Practice Manager Dympna Quinn

GP Sarah Christina Catherine CLARKE, Alan John EVANS, David RODGERS, Anne Marie WILKINSON

Lurgan Medical Practice
7 Moores Lane, Lurgan, Craigavon BT66 8DW
Tel: 028 3832 7626 Fax: 028 3834 9950
Patient List Size: 4600

Practice Manager Sally Betts

GP Michael D S WILSON, Maire Fionnuala DOYLE, Rodney PATTERSON

Main Street Surgery
60A Main Street, Donaghcloney, Craigavon BT66 7LR

GP Emer Mary LENNON, Keith Robert Graham MARTIN

Main Street Surgery
52 Main Street, Moira, Craigavon BT67 0LQ
Tel: 028 9261 1278 Fax: 028 9261 0909
Patient List Size: 7046

Practice Manager Carol Ritchie

GP Dr DAVIS, Dr PARKER, Dr SPENCE

McAnallen and McAnallen
Portadown H&SS Centre, Tavanagh Avenue, Portadown, Craigavon BT62 3BU
Tel: 028 3835 1347 Fax: 028 3835 1246

Practice Manager Evelyn McStravick

GP Cora McANALLEN, James Gerard McANALLEN

McConnell, Carson and Mathews
The Health Centre, Tavanagh Avenue, Portadown, Craigavon BT62 3BU
Tel: 028 3835 1145 Fax: 028 3839 2628
Email: orchard@familypractice.fsbusiness.co.uk
Website: www.orchardfamilypractice.com
Patient List Size: 4190

Practice Manager C Breen

GP John Paul McCONNELL, Patricia Elizabeth Rosemary CARSON, Colin Wallace MATHEWS

Moore and McAuley
Meadows Family Practice, Tavanagh Avenue, Portadown, Craigavon BT62 3BU
Tel: 028 3835 9909 Fax: 028 3835 1246
Patient List Size: 2400

Practice Manager Mandy Parks

GP J E M MOORE, Raymond T McAULEY

The Old School Medical Centre
1 Antrim Road, Lurgan, Craigavon BT67 9BW
Tel: 028 3831 1900 Fax: 028 3831 1904

GP James Desmond GORMLEY, Patricia McCLOSKEY

Tandragee Health Clinic
3 Montague Street, Tandragee, Craigavon BT62 2AN
Tel: 028 3884 0223

GP Peter Dudley GOOD, Dr GOOD

William Street Surgery
87 William Street, Lurgan, Craigavon BT66 6JB
Tel: 028 3832 2509 Fax: 028 3834 7673
Patient List Size: 3900

Practice Manager Nichola McGahey

GP Arthur Gerrard SOUTHWELL, Claire ZUBIER

Wynne Hill Surgery
51 Hill Street, Lurgan, Craigavon BT66 6BW
Tel: 028 3832 6333 Fax: 028 3834 7254
Patient List Size: 9800

Practice Manager U O'Kane

GP Julie Elizabeth BRONTE, Mary DOMMELLY, Alan John HAMILTON, Colin Michael McDONALD, Robert Harold RICE, Martin STEWART

Crumlin

Crumlin Medical Practice
5 Glenavy Road, Crumlin BT29 4LA
Tel: 028 9442 2209 Fax: 028 9442 2233

GP Robert Wilson HYNDMAN, Lawrence Edward THOMPSON, Joseph Howard THOMSON

Glenavy Family Practice
47 Main Street, Glenavy, Crumlin BT29 4LN
Tel: 028 9442 2287 Fax: 028 9442 2100
Patient List Size: 3700

Practice Manager Pauline Magee

GP Owen Thomas GALLAGHER, Hugh Joseph GALLAGHER

Donaghadee

Donaghadee Health Centre
3 Killaughey Road, Donaghadee BT21 0BU
Tel: 028 9188 2176 Fax: 028 9188 3090
Patient List Size: 8500

Practice Manager J Breadon

GP Joan MILLER, Heather Eileen BECKETT, Jennifer Anne Elizabeth McCLELLAND, John Hilton RUTHERFORD

Downpatrick

Downpatrick Road Surgery
14 Downpatrick Road, Killyleagh, Downpatrick BT30 9RG
Tel: 028 4482 8746 Fax: 028 4482 1458

GP John Ultan McGILL

Downpatrick Road Surgery
14 Downpatrick Road, Killyleagh, Downpatrick BT30 9RG
Tel: 028 4482 2812 Fax: 028 4482 2819

Practice Manager H Buchanan

GP Heather Yvonne McINTOSH

The Green Surgery
12 The Green, Irish Street, Downpatrick BT30 6BE
Tel: 028 4461 4421 Fax: 028 4461 7646
Patient List Size: 3000

Practice Manager Angela Brown

GP Margaret Mary MULHALL, Anne Patricia DEENY

Hannah and McGoldrick
Health Centre, Pound Lane, Downpatrick BT30 6HY
Tel: 028 4461 2962 Fax: 028 4461 7916

Practice Manager Joan Gilmore

GP Bernard Alexander HANNAH, Hugh Patrick Mary McGOLDRICK

James Street Practice
40 James Street, Crossgar, Downpatrick BT30 9JU
Tel: 028 4483 0230 Fax: 028 4483 0986
Patient List Size: 4500

GP Nuala Anne MacALEENAN, Martin Ronald PHILLIPS

Main Street Surgery
11 Main Street, Killough, Downpatrick BT30 7QA
Tel: 028 4484 1242

GP Malachy MURPHY

Pound Lane Health Centre
Pound Lane, Downpatrick BT30 6HY
Tel: 028 4461 3016 Fax: 028 4461 7915

Practice Manager Bridgeen Burns

GP Patrick Richard Joseph MOORE, Una Roisin SMALL

Stream Street Surgery
40 Stream Street, Downpatrick BT30 6DE
Tel: 028 4461 3029

GP Anne-Marie HARNEY, Edward James HARNEY

Dromore

Begney Hill Road Surgery
Begney Hill Road, Dromara, Dromore BT25 2AT
Tel: 028 9753 2217 Fax: 028 9753 3301

GP Neville Charles HICKS, Olwyn Ruth HILLIARD, Helen E KIRKPATRICK, Nigel RUDDELL, Edmund Mervyn SMITH, Michelle UREY

Gallows Street Surgery
50 Gallows Street, Dromore BT25 1BD
Tel: 028 9269 2758

GP Roy Archibald McNEICE, Eileen Maude ATCHISON, Colin Jordan KENNY, Jennifer Ann PAISLEY

Dungannon

Ardmore Medical Practice
57 Thomas Street, Dungannon BT70 1HW
Tel: 028 8772 2621 Fax: 028 2875 2526
Patient List Size: 5524

Practice Manager Bernardine McCaul

GP John Joseph McKAY, Maureen CRAWFORD, Una McLOUGHLIN

Barrack Street Medical Centre
Barrack Street, Coalisland, Dungannon BT71 4LS
Tel: 028 8774 7447

Practice Manager Dolores Murphy

GP Patrick Joseph HACKETT

Campbell Surgery
10 Quarry Road, Dungannon BT70 1QR
Tel: 028 8772 2751 Fax: 028 8772 2566

Practice Manager Elaine Bungard

GP Niaz AHMED, Pauline CARSON, Michael KENNEDY, Evangeline MILLAR, Peter SABHERWAL

Errigal Medical Centre
Old Dungannon Road, Ballygawley, Dungannon BT70 2EY

Practice Manager Gabrielle Nugent

GP Theodore Patrick Joseph NUGENT

Hillhead Health Centre
50 Hillhead, Stewartstown, Dungannon BT71 5HY
Tel: 028 8773 8648 Fax: 028 8773 8648
Patient List Size: 5200

Practice Manager Carmel Lyttle

GP Leonard Charles McCAMMON, Bernard Gerard MCCOY

Lineside Health Centre
10A Lineside, Coalisland, Dungannon BT71 4LP
Tel: 028 8774 8555 Fax: 028 8774 7001
Patient List Size: 2560

Practice Manager Paula Taggart

GP Patrick Hugh McKENNA

Moy Health Centre
40 Charlemont Street, Moy, Dungannon BT71 7SL

GP Lynn Averell HOBSON, Aine Marie McSHANE

Moy Health Centre
40 Charlemont Street, Moy, Dungannon BT71 7SL
Tel: 028 877 84551 Fax: 028 877 89711
Patient List Size: 2550

Practice Manager E Chambers

GP Dr MILLAR, Dr MULVENNA

Moy Health Centre
40 Charlemont Street, Moy, Dungannon BT71 7SL

GP Dr GHOSH

Northland Surgery
79 Cunninghams Lane, Dungannon BT71 6BX
Tel: 028 8772 2137 Fax: 028 8772 7696
Patient List Size: 6900

Practice Manager Anita McCreesh

GP Caroline Jane SANDS, Adrian CHURCH, Dr PAISLEY, Michael Robert THOMPSON

Parkview Surgery
14 Ballygawley Road, Dungannon BT70 1EL
Tel: 028 8772 2019 Fax: 028 8772 6616
Website: www.parkview-surgery.com

Practice Manager Michelle McGaul

GP Matthew GAFFNEY, John GARLAND, Michael Alfred O'LOUGHLIN

Thomas Street Practice
39 Thomas Street, Dungannon BT70 1HN
Tel: 028 8772 7235 Fax: 028 8772 7703

GP S R C MURTY

Enniskillen

Brookeborough Surgery
Tanyard Lane, Brookeborough, Enniskillen BT94 4AB
Tel: 028 8953 1225
Website: www.brookeboroughsurgery.com
Patient List Size: 2850

GP Michael Joseph SCOTT, William Neville CROMIE

Erne Health Centre
Cornagrade Road, Enniskillen BT74 6AY
Tel: 028 6632 2707

Practice Manager Helen Hazelton

GP Mark Edward Henry CATHCART, Elaine CONNOR, Simon William Henry FORSTER, C GRAHAM, R RICHEY

Erne Health Centre
Erne Road, Enniskillen BT74 6NN
Tel: 028 6632 7190 Fax: 028 6634 2486
Email: mleonard@atmelcnhc.pcwestni.nhs.uk
Patient List Size: 3600

Practice Manager Martha Leonard

GP James Davison ARMSTRONG, Lucia MAGUIRE, Patrick TOAL

Health Centre
Drumhaw, Lisnaskea, Enniskillen BT92 0FP
Tel: 028 6772 2913
Patient List Size: 1870

Practice Manager Maxine Leary

GP Robert Thomas LEARY

Irvinestown Health Centre
20 Church Street, Irvinestown, Enniskillen BT94 1EH
Tel: 028 6862 1212 Fax: 028 6862 8624
Patient List Size: 7700

GP Peter BLAKE, Margaret Elizabeth Lilian ELLIOTT, Alan Frederick HUTCHINSON, Colin John McCAW

Lakeside Medical Centre
Erne Road, Enniskillen BT74 6NN
Tel: 028 6632 7192 Fax: 028 6634 2457
Patient List Size: 6188

Practice Manager Catherine Gunn

GP Vincent DAVIDSON, G McGOVERN, James MEADE, Ann Bernadette WHITE

Lurganboy Surgery
Lurganboy, Clones Road, Newtownbulter, Enniskillen BT92 6JT
Tel: 028 6773 8203

GP Kevin Francis DEVLIN

Maguiresbridge Surgery
The Surgery, Maguiresbridge, Enniskillen BT94 4PB
Tel: 028 6772 1273 Fax: 028 6772 3303
Email: m.smyth@mgb.gp.n-i.nhs.uk
Website: www.gp4u.com
Patient List Size: 2102

Practice Manager Grainne O'Reilly-Smyth

GP Michael Gerard SMYTH

Main Street Surgery
75 Main Street, Derrylin, Enniskillen BT92 9LB
Tel: 028 6774 8250 Fax: 028 6774 8999
Patient List Size: 2300

GP John KIRBY, Aisling KIRBY

Main Street Surgery
32 Main Street, Derrygonnelly, Enniskillen BT93 6HW
Tel: 028 6864 1379 Fax: 028 6864 1832
Patient List Size: 2000

Practice Manager Jacqueline Pennock

GP Julia Caroline GROVES-RAINES

Maple Group Practice
Lisnaskea Health Centre, Drumhaw, Lisnaskea, Enniskillen BT92 0JB
Tel: 028 6772 1566 Fax: 028 6772 2526
Patient List Size: 8000

Practice Manager Maria Nugent-Murphy

GP Melapurethu George GEORGE, Miriam DOLAN, Patrick Norbert LYNCH, Barbara Ann McDERMOTT, John Patrick Joseph PORTEOUS

Rathmore Clinic
Cliff Road, Belleek, Enniskillen BT93 3FY
Tel: 028 6865 8382 Fax: 028 6865 8124
Patient List Size: 3600

Practice Manager Mary Catherine Deeny

GP Eugene Dominick Martin DEENY, Charlton Garth HERDMAN, Thomas Francis KIERNAN

Roslea Medical Practice
20 Upper Main Street, Roslea, Enniskillen BT92 7LT
Tel: 028 6775 1496 Fax: 028 6775 1872
Patient List Size: 1570

Practice Manager Dowres Clerkin

GP Donal COLLINS

The Surgery
1 Marble Arch Terrace, Florence Court, Enniskillen BT92 1EF
Tel: 028 6634 8275 Fax: 028 6634 8080
Patient List Size: 1600

Practice Manager Clarissa Willis

GP Julian Sinclair CAITHNESS, Enda CUNNINGHAM, Kathleen Mary Majella SWEENEY

The Surgery
Erne Drive, Ederney, Enniskillen BT93 0AR
Tel: 028 6863 1234 Fax: 028 6863 1721
Patient List Size: 1600

Practice Manager Fiona Colreavy

GP Michele MELLOTTE

The Surgery
Kinawley, Enniskillen BT92 4BU
Tel: 028 6774 8691 Fax: 028 6774 8949
Email: ksweeney@kinawley.pcwestni.nhs.uk
Patient List Size: 1236

Practice Manager Carmel Parkes

GP Kathleen M SWEENEY

Tempo Medical Centre
Main Street, Edenmore Tempo, Enniskillen BT94 3LU
Tel: 028 8954 1216

Practice Manager Regina Murphy

GP John Anthony McCUSKER, Maria Josephine MALLON, Joseph Martin McCONVILLE

Fivemiletown

The Valley Medical Centre
20 Cooneen Road, Fivemiletown BT75 0ND
Tel: 028 8952 1326
Email: walterboyd@nurchossey.freeserve.co.uk

GP Esther Mary RUTLEDGE, Walter BOYD, Charles McKIBBIN

Hillsborough

Hillsborough Medical Practice
Hillsborough Health Centre, Ballynahinch Street, Hillsborough BT26 6AW
Tel: 028 9268 2216 Fax: 028 9268 9721
Email: hillsboroughdocs@aol.com
Patient List Size: 6750

Practice Manager C Pielou

GP Ann SMYLIE, Michael C CRAWFORD, Jane Kathryn FLEMING, J Christopher HALL, Robert D McCREARY

Holywood

Brook Street Surgery
9 Brook Street, Holywood BT18 9DA
Tel: 028 9042 6984 Fax: 028 9042 6656
Website: www.brookstreetsurgery
Patient List Size: 7200

Practice Manager Elizabeth Carson

GP James Robert Boyd KANE, S GOLDRING, Joanna McCREERY, John Murdoch McGIMPSEY

Priory Surgery
26 High Street, Holywood BT18 9AD
Tel: 028 9042 6991 Fax: 028 9042 3643
Patient List Size: 15300

Practice Manager Hazel Gilliland

GP James Ronald COURTNEY, Thomas James Anthony EGERTON, James Tees LAVERY, Richard George LAWSON, Angela Catherine MACARI, Anthony Richard MILLER, Phyllis Sharon STEELE

Larne

Corran Surgery
Moyle Medical Centre, Old Glenarm Road, Larne BT40 1XH
Tel: 028 2826 1600 Fax: 028 2826 1603
Patient List Size: 5800

Practice Manager Wendy Kottenbelt

GP Alan James McILROY, Martin Patrick HOPKINS, Eileen MURPHY

Inver Surgery
Moyle Medical Centre, Old Glenarm Road, Larne BT40 1XH
Tel: 028 2826 1611 Fax: 028 2827 1614
Patient List Size: 4800

GP Dr DUNN, Dr KIRK, Dr SHEPHERD

Victoria Surgery
Moyle Medical Centre, Old Glenarm Road, Larne BT40 1XH
Tel: 028 2826 1620 Fax: 028 2826 1622
Email: gac.crory@victoriasurgey.gpn-i.nhs.uk
Patient List Size: 5458

Practice Manager Mary Murphy

GP George Albert Charles CRORY, Kathy FERGUSON, John Robert Willoughby WILSON

Limavady

Bovally Medical Centre
2 Rossair Road, Limavady BT49 0TE
Tel: 028 7776 6352 Fax: 028 7776 7592
Patient List Size: 5600

Practice Manager Hilary McGauock

GP William Paul FINLAY, Brendan Joseph McQUILLAN, Katherine Judith OLLERENSHAW

Drs McCleery, Devlin and Pratt
Boually Medical Centre, 2 Rossair Road, Limavady BT49 0TE
Tel: 028 7776 6354
Patient List Size: 6600

Practice Manager Georgina Davidson

GP William Finlay McCLEERY, David P DEVLIN, William Robert Mark PRATT

Limavady Health Centre
Scroggy Road, Limavady BT49 0NA
Tel: 028 777 61111 Fax: 028 7776 1102
Patient List Size: 6300

Practice Manager C Turley

GP Iain Keatley FARQUHARSON, Niall Vincent McKENNY, M QUINN

Limavady Health Centre
Scroggy Road, Limavady BT49 0NA
Tel: 028 7776 1112 Fax: 028 7776 1102
Patient List Size: 7000

Practice Manager Carmel Turley

GP Jill FULTON, Gregory Laurence HEANEY, Mark Edmund HENDERSON, William Houston Keith MAGEE

Lisburn

Lisburn Health Centre
Linenhall Street, Lisburn BT28 1LU
Tel: 028 9260 3333 Fax: 028 9250 1313
Patient List Size: 3600

Practice Manager Hazel Martin

GP Anona Elizabeth WALMSLEY, Michael Perry CARSON

Lisburn Health Centre
Linenhall Street, Lisburn BT28 1LU
Tel: 028 9260 3090 Fax: 028 9250 1310

GP Daphne Margaret GREENE, Nigel Stewart CAMPBELL, Michael Andrew RUDDELL, Sandra Louise SANDS, Wilson William John SHORTEN

Lisburn Health Centre
Linenhall Street, Lisburn BT28 1LU
Tel: 028 9260 3111

GP John Stewart Robert Lloyd HENRY, Patrick Dermott HUTCHINSON, Christine Marian RUSSELL

Lisburn Health Centre
Linenhall Street, Lisburn BT28 1LU
Tel: 028 9260 3203 Fax: 028 9250 1311
Patient List Size: 6800

Practice Manager May Armstrong

GP Mary Gertrude Bertha COWAN, Ivor Robert CAIRNS, Freda Mary TRIMBLE, Ian Kyle WARWICK

Lisburn Health Centre
Linenhall Street, Lisburn BT28 1LU

GP Harold Alexander JEFFERSON, Patricia Margaret CURRY, Derek Ian William HAMILL, Samuel MOORE, Bronagh Mary O'KANE, Ian Frederick Hall WALES

Lisburn Health Centre
Linenhall Street, Lisburn BT28 1LU
Tel: 028 9260 3133 Fax: 028 9250 1308
Patient List Size: 4000

GP Anthony FORDE, Patrick Thomas DOHERTY

Lisburn Health Centre
Linenhall Street, Lisburn BT28 1LU

GP Thomas Patrick DOHERTY

Lisburn Health Centre
Linenhall Street, Lisburn BT28 1LU
Tel: 028 9260 3177

GP C PATTERSON

Londonderry

Aberfoyle Terrace Surgery
3-5 Aberfoyle Terrace, Strand Road, Londonderry BT48 7NP
Tel: 028 7126 4868

GP Vincent Joseph CAVANAGH, Bronagh Mary MACMAHON, Martin Eugen McCLOSKEY, Patrick Joseph McEVOY, Thomas McGINLEY, John Kevin O'KELLY, Orla Gerrard QUIGLEY

Bayview Medical Centre
3 Bayview Terrace, Londonderry BT48 7EE
Tel: 028 7137 7027 Fax: 028 7136 4508
Patient List Size: 3011

Practice Manager Cheryl Hamilton

GP Aine ABBOT, Joseph Damian McEVOY, Heather WATSON

Bridge Street Medical Centre
30 Bridge Street, Londonderry BT48 6LA
Tel: 028 7126 1137

GP Maurice Robert MAGNIER, Keith Brian BANKHEAD, Judith Jane O'KANE

Clarendon Medical
35 Northland Avenue, Londonderry BT48 7JW
Tel: 028 7126 5391 Fax: 028 7126 5932
Email: Mon4298@aol.com
Patient List Size: 10500

Practice Manager Marelle O'Neill

GP Charles Keith MUNRO, Linda Elizabeth BOYD, Nagendrakumar Dalpatbhai CHAUHAN, Stephen LALSINGH, Robert Martin NAIRN, Iain Stuart PALIN

Clarendon Street Surgery
17 Clarendon Street, Londonderry BT48 7EP
Tel: 028 7126 1497

GP Patrick James DOHERTY

Claudy Health Centre
Irwin Crescent, Claudy, Londonderry BT47 4AB
Tel: 028 7133 8371

GP Ian Robert Oscar GORDON, Goay Meng KHOW, Brian TEDDERS

Dungiven Health Centre
1 Chapel Road, Dungiven, Londonderry BT47 4RS
Tel: 028 7774 3002 Fax: 028 7774 3017

Practice Manager A O'Neill

GP Francis Paul Damien JOHNSTON, Siobhan Marie MURPHY

Feeny Medical Centre
Main Street, Feeny, Londonderry BT47 4TD
Tel: 028 7778 1501 Fax: 028 7778 1925
Email: mariswamy@hotmail.com

Practice Manager Dolores Murphy

GP Saligrama Boranna MARISWAMY, Gerard Anthony BYRNE

Foyleside Family Practice
Bridge Street Medical Centre, 30 Bridge Street, Londonderry BT48 6LA
Tel: 028 7126 7847 Fax: 028 7137 0723
Website: www.foylesidefamilypractice.co.uk
Patient List Size: 5500

Practice Manager Anne Hutton

GP Thomas John Montgomery CRAIG, William Peter James LEESON, Andrew Finlay LINTON

Glendermott Medical
Waterside Health Centre, Glendermott Road, Londonderry BT47 6AU
Tel: 028 7132 0100 Fax: 028 7132 0117

Practice Manager Margaret Montgomery

GP Elma Margaret ASHENHURST, Noel Brian Joseph BOYLE, Nicola Mary HERRON, Kenneth Anthony O'FLAHERTY, John Edward SPENCE

Health Centre
Great James Street, Londonderry BT48 7DH
Tel: 028 7136 4016

GP Neil Raymond BRENNAN, Eamon Thomas Joseph BLACK, Colum Patrick FARRELLY, Brigid Teresa Mary SMITH

Health Centre
Great James Street, Londonderry BT48 7DH
Tel: 028 7137 8522

GP Michael Martin Anthony DEVLIN, Leo Joseph CASEY, Anne Mary DOHERTY, John Eamon Joseph DOOHAN, Jadhav Daniel SAMSON, Conor Vincent WHITE

Main Street Surgery
29 Main Street, Eglinton, Londonderry BT47 3AB
Tel: 028 7181 0252 Fax: 028 7181 1347
Patient List Size: 5150

Practice Manager Jean Stevenson

GP Charles Henry Ray HETHERINGTON, Helen Margaret KENNEDY, Richard William MANNING, David Robert PATTERSON

Park Medical
Great James Street Health Centre, Londonderry BT48 7DH
Tel: 028 7137 8500 Fax: 028 7137 8509
Email: anne.hutton@parkmedical.gp.n-I.nhs.uk
Patient List Size: 8100

Practice Manager Anne Hutton

GP Inder Pal SINGH, Heber Rory CANAVAN, John Martyn Mary HILL, Cora Mary MORRISON, John James Joseph O'DONNELL

Quayside Medical Practice
82-84 Strand Road, Londonderry BT48 7NN
Tel: 028 7126 2790 Fax: 028 7137 3729
Email: kcosgrove@quaysidemed.pcwestni.nhs.uk
Patient List Size: 12200

Practice Manager Katharine Friel

GP James Paul COSGROVE, Kevin Joseph COSGROVE, Michael Dominic Mary DURAND, William Thomas FOY, Margaret Bernadette GUNN, John REIDY, Ann Margaret Mary WARNOCK

Shantallow Health Centre
Racecourse Road, Londonderry BT48 8NL
Tel: 028 7135 3054

GP Zahir AHMED, Damien Michael DEANE, Michael John Bernard O'SULLIVAN

Shantallow Health Centre
Racecourse Road, Londonderry BT48 8NL
Tel: 028 7135 1323

GP Vincent John BRENNAN, Eileen Miriam DEVLIN, Mary Anne McCLOSKEY

Waterside Health Centre
Glenderercott Road, Londonderry BT47 6AU
Tel: 028 7132 0140 Fax: 028 7132 0127
Email: enquiries@drconnolly.com
Website: www.drconnolly.com

Practice Manager Majella Moore

GP Dermot Francis CONNOLLY, Caroline Ann Patricia DALY, Derval Mary DOLAN, Michael John HEALY, Ian Gerard McGINLEY, Brendan RODGERS

Waterside Health Centre
Glendermot Road, Londonderry BT47 6AU
Tel: 028 7132 0144 Fax: 028 7132 0107
Patient List Size: 9500

Practice Manager Maureen Carlin

GP James Ciaran STONE, Stephen CANAVON, Pauline COSGROVE, Nial Eugene McCALLION, Judith Elizabeth Jane McILWAINE, Leslie McNEILL

Maghera

Maghera Health Centre
3 Church Street, Maghera BT46 5EA
Tel: 028 7964 2579 Fax: 028 7964 3002
Patient List Size: 7500

Practice Manager Louise Murphy

GP John Simpson OVEREND, Dr COLLINS, Dr SHORTALL

Magherafelt

Castledawson Surgery
Station Road, Castledawson, Magherafelt BT45 8AZ
Tel: 028 7938 6237 Fax: 028 7946 9613
Patient List Size: 6000

Practice Manager Brenda Devlin

GP Denis BARKER, Michael Christopher HINDS, Christine Hilary WILSON

Diamond Medical Centre
Market Square, Magherafelt BT45 6ED
Tel: 028 7936 1000 Fax: 028 7936 1010

GP D G JOHNSTON

Garden Street Surgery
29 Garden Street, Magherafelt BT45 5DD
Tel: 028 7938 6237 Fax: 028 7930 1302

GP Bernard Patrick GLANCY, Elizabeth Ruth INGRAM, Dr SAYEE

High Street Medical Group Practice
29 High Street, Draperstown, Magherafelt BT45 7AB
Tel: 028 7962 8201 Fax: 028 7962 7523
Email: ca.harkin@p402.gp.n-i.nhs.uk
Patient List Size: 6800

Practice Manager Kathleen Kelly

GP Cyril Alexander HARKIN, Karen Anne HARKIN, J M LOGAN, Fionuala Ann WHITE

Magherafelt Health Centre
1 Fairhill Road, Magherafelt BT45 6BD
Tel: 028 7930 2904

GP Maura Alexandra CHARLTON

Magherafelt Medical Centre
1 Fairhill Road, Magherafelt BT45 6BD
Tel: 028 7930 2902
Patient List Size: 6000

GP John Gerard TOHILL, Dr NOBLE, Anne Genevieve O'KANE

Moneymore Medical Centre
Fairhill, Moneymore, Magherafelt BT45 7QX
Tel: 028 8674 8350 Fax: 028 8674 8684
Patient List Size: 3148

Practice Manager Aileen Nevin

GP Josef K KURIACOSE, Dawn HEARNSHAW, Mary F MILLER

Moneymore Medical Centre
Fairhill, Moneymore, Magherafelt BT45 7QX
Tel: 028 8674 8350 Fax: 028 8674 8684
Patient List Size: 1416

Practice Manager Aileen Nevin

GP Allen McKAY

Newcastle, County Down

Causeway Place Surgery
Causeway Place, Newcastle BT33 0DN

Practice Manager Fiona Savage

GP Stephen Colm HYLAND

Causeway Surgery
2 Causeway Place, Newcastle BT33 0DN
Tel: 028 4372 3438 Fax: 028 4372 6731
Patient List Size: 1800

Practice Manager Rene Blair

GP John Martin KYLE

Church View Surgery
14 Church View, Dundrum, Newcastle BT33 0NA

GP Alexander McConnell GREER, Alison Lindsay SMITH, Kieran Gerard WALSHE

Donard Group Practice
Branch Surgery, 4 Dublin Road, Castlewellan, Newcastle BT31 9AG
Tel: 028 4377 8260 Fax: 028 4377 0012
Patient List Size: 10300

GP Siobhan DEVLIN, W D BREADY, C D LEGGETT, N F O'CONNER, K E SHERRARD

Donard Group Practice
56 Main Street, Newcastle BT33 0AE
Tel: 028 4372 3221 Fax: 028 4372 3162
Email: donaldgroup@hotmail.com
Patient List Size: 10300

GP W D BREADY, S DEVLIN, C D LEGGETT, N F O'CONNER, K E SHERRARD

Dublin Road Surgery
4 Dublin Road, Castlewellan, Newcastle BT31 9AG
Tel: 028 4372 3221 Fax: 028 4372 3162

GP William Dominic BREADY, Siobhan DEVLIN, Christopher Denis LEGGETT, Niall Finbarr O'CONNOR, Kieran Edward SHERRARD, Patrick Martin WALSH

Newry

Clanrye Surgery
Newry Health Village, Monaghan Street, Newry BT35 6BW
Tel: 028 3026 7639 Fax: 028 3025 7414
Email: sdigney@shssb.n-i.nhs.uk
Patient List Size: 8271

Practice Manager Christine Hardy

GP Subir BANERJEE, John Marion Gerard DIGNEY, Michael Joseph FEARON, Clare SWEENEY

Cornmarket Surgery
Newry Health Village, Monaghan Street, Newry BT35 6BW
Tel: 028 3026 5838 Fax: 028 3026 6727

Practice Manager Pauline Clarke

GP Ian Charles HENRY, James McAREAVY, Mary Margaret QUINN

Cornmarket Surgery
6 Newry Health Village, Monaghan Street, Newry BT35 6BW
Tel: 028 3026 5838 Fax: 028 3026 6727

Practice Manager Martina Hanna

GP Mary Geraldine Elizabeth MACKLE, Richard Derek FLOOD, Gerard Aidan MULVANEY

Cornmarket Surgery
Newry Health Village, Monaghan Street, Newry BT35 6BW
Tel: 028 302 61236 Fax: 028 302 65549
Patient List Size: 5800

Practice Manager Jacinta O'Hara

GP Joseph M REYNOLDS, Patrick McKINLEY, Derval Maeve Martine O'REILLY

Crossmaglen Health Centre
McCormick Place, Crossmaglen, Newry BT35 9HD
Tel: 028 3086 1692

GP William John Anthony FARRELL, Dr GRIBBEN

Dundalk Street Surgery
53 Dundalk Street, Newtownhamilton, Newry BT35 0PB
Tel: 028 3087 8204 Fax: 028 3087 8196

Practice Manager Bernie McKenna

GP Thomas O'LEARY, Maeve Breige LAMBE, Mary Patricia LARKIN

Kilkeel Health Centre
Knockchree Avenue, Kilkeel, Newry BT34 4BS
Tel: 028 4176 0970 Fax: 028 4176 3774

Practice Manager A E McVeigh

GP Josephine Mary MERCER, Brian Aloysius DILLON, Kevin O'KANE

Kilkeel Health Centre
Knockchree Avenue, Kilkeel, Newry BT34 4BS
Tel: 028 4176 0950 Fax: 028 4176 3308
Website: www.drwoodsandchambers.co.uk
Patient List Size: 3615

Practice Manager Philomena Clarke

GP Margaret Rosemary Jane CHAMBERS, William Graham WOODS

Maphoner Surgery
Maphoner Road, Mullaghbawn, Newry BT35 9TR

Practice Manager Angela Smyth

GP Martin Gerard DEANE, Briegeen Mary MAGUIRE

Marina Surgery
15 Havelock Place, Warrenpoint, Newry BT34 3NE

GP Dr BONNER

McCann and Morgan
Rathfriland Health Centre, John Street, Rathfriland, Newry BT34 5QH
Tel: 028 4063 0666 Fax: 028 4063 1198
Patient List Size: 3411

Practice Manager Annie O'Hare

GP Brian McCANN

McDowell
Clanrye Surgery, Newry Health Village, Monaghan Street, Newry BT35 6BW
Tel: 028 3026 0949 Fax: 028 3025 7414
Patient List Size: 2392

Practice Manager A Hillis

GP William Arnold McDOWELL

McKnight
Clanrye Surgery, Newry Health Village, Monaghan Street, Newry BT35 6BW
Tel: 028 3026 0949 Fax: 028 3025 7414
Patient List Size: 2215

Practice Manager Fiona Burke

GP Michael McKNIGHT

McVerry, McEvoy Medical Centre
Newry Health Village, Monaghan Street, Newry BT35 6BW
Tel: 028 3026 1220/5853
Patient List Size: 9305

Practice Manager Christine Leneghan

GP P M McEVOY, Ian McVERRY, Mary McVERRY, Raymond McVERRY

Meadowlands Surgery
Newry Health Village, Monaghan Street, Newry BT35 6BW
Tel: 028 3026 7534

GP Myles Thomas SHORTALL, Mary Margaret O'NEILL, John Colin RADCLIFFE, John J TORNEY

Meigh Surgery
6 Dromintee Road, Meigh, Newry BT35 8SJ
Tel: 028 3084 8517 Fax: 028 3084 9006

Practice Manager Catriona Campbell

GP V V GEORGE, Giby G VETTIANKAL

Mourne Family Surgery
Mourne Hospital, Newry Street, Kilkeel, Newry BT34 4DN
Tel: 028 4176 5422 Fax: 028 4176 9137

Practice Manager Shirley Forsythe

GP Stephen Alan POOTS, Marie O'LOUGHLIN

Newtownhamilton Health Centre
2A Markethill Road, Newtownhamilton, Newry BT35 0BE
Tel: 028 3087 8202/8223 Fax: 028 3087 9043
Email: postmaster@newtownhamiltonhealthcentre.org
Website: www.newtownhamiltonhealthcentre.org
Patient List Size: 3200

Practice Manager Jennifer Reoney

GP Adrian Oliver MULHOLLAND, Ruadhri Paul QUINN

Old Forge Surgery
14 Kilkeel Road, Annalong, Newry BT34 4TH
Tel: 028 4376 8218

GP Jonathan Andrew Dale ALLEN, Adrienne KEOWN

O'Shaughnessy
Rathfriland Health Centre, John Street, Rathfriland, Newry BT34 5QH
Tel: 028 4063 0666 Fax: 028 4063 1198
Patient List Size: 2116

Practice Manager Annie O'Hare

GP Donal Michael Kevin O'SHAUGHNESSY

O'Tierney, Murphy and Ryan
Health Centre, Summerhill, Warrenpoint, Newry BT34 3JD
Tel: 028 4175 4100 Fax: 028 4175 4050

GP Donal Padraig O'TIERNEY, Mark Joseph MURPHY, Petrina Francis Maria RYAN

Rathfriland Surgery
9 Castlewellan Road, Rathfriland, Newry BT34 5LY
Tel: 028 4063 0034 Fax: 028 4063 1446

Practice Manager Judy Shortt

GP Rosemary SLOAN

Rathkeeland House
1 Castleblaney Road, Crossmaglen, Newry BT35 9AB
Patient List Size: 2100

GP Patrick Mary FEE

Shannon and Shannon
Rathfriland Health Centre, John Street, Rathfriland, Newry BT34 5QH
Tel: 028 4063 0666 Fax: 028 4063 1198
Patient List Size: 2820

Practice Manager Annie O'Hare

GP Elizabeth SHANNON, John SHANNON

Sweeney and Fee
Crossmaglen Health Centre, McCormick Place, Crossmaglen, Newry BT35 9HD
Tel: 028 3086 1226 Fax: 028 3086 8927
Patient List Size: 3000

Practice Manager Rosemary Garvey

GP Mark SWEENEY, Margaret FEE

Warrenpoint Health Centre
Summerhill, Warrenpoint, Newry BT34 3JD

GP David Hugh GAW, Anna Maria McGIVERN, Joseph McGIVERN, Dr McLAUGHLIN

Newtownabbey

Abbots Cross Medical Practice
92 Doagh Road, Newtownabbey BT37 9QW
Tel: 028 9036 4048 Fax: 028 9085 1804
Patient List Size: 6572

Practice Manager Liz Wilson

GP Dr FARRELL, Peter CUSICK, Mary Patricia HENDRON, Dr NAGLE

Rosehall Surgery
2 Mallusk Road, Newtownabbey BT36 4PP
Tel: 028 9083 2188 Fax: 028 9083 8820

Practice Manager Carol Read

GP William Derek McGIMPSEY, Paula Marie DAVISON, Elizabeth Anne FAIR, Michael Colin HEGAN, James Richard HOUSTON, Christopher James KYLE

Tramways Medical Centre
Farmley Road, Newtownabbey BT36 7XX
Tel: 028 9034 2131 Fax: 028 9083 9111
Patient List Size: 2100

GP George James BALMER

Tramways Medical Centre
Farmley Road, Newtownabbey BT36 7XX
Tel: 028 9034 2131 Fax: 028 9083 9111
Patient List Size: 2100

GP Colin Stanley SPENCE

Tramways Medical Centre
Farmley Road, Newtownabbey BT36 7XX
Tel: 028 9034 2131 Fax: 028 9083 9111
Patient List Size: 6100

GP Dermot M NEARY, Patricia K BEIRNE, John Gerard NEARY

Whiteabbey Health Centre
95 Doagh Road, Newtownabbey BT37 9QN
Tel: 028 9086 4341 Fax: 028 9086 0443

GP Patrick Joseph CROSBIE, Sarah Tracey CRUICKSHANKS, Rosemary KANE, Dr MEENAN, Dr STEVENSON

Whiteabbey Health Centre
95 Doagh Road, Newtownabbey BT37 9QN
Tel: 028 9080 8220
Email: chg.gould@p440.gp.n-I.nhs.uk

Practice Manager Anne McFall

GP Adrian James Jackson DARRAH, James Edward A MAGINNIS, Laura Louise SMALL, William James TOLAND, Mary Lorraine WHITESIDE

Newtownards

Ballywalter Health Centre
Fowler Way, Ballywalter, Newtownards BT22 2PY
Tel: 028 4275 8292 Fax: 028 4275 8540
Patient List Size: 2750

Practice Manager Phyllis Gilmore

GP Michael Alan STEELE, Daniel F HUGHES

Church Street Surgery
1 Church Street, Newtownards BT23 4FH
Tel: 028 9181 6333 Fax: 028 9181 8805

Practice Manager Sheila Currie

GP William Ian CLEMENTS, Gordon David KENNEDY, Janet Margaret McCANCE

Church Street Surgery
1 Church Street, Newtownards BT23 4FH
Tel: 028 9181 6333 Fax: 028 9181 8805

Practice Manager Sheila Currie

GP David Gibson McGAUGHEY, Peter HYLAND, Gillian LUNEY

Church Street Surgery
1 Church Street, Newtownards BT23 4FH
Tel: 028 9181 6333 Fax: 028 9181 8805

Practice Manager Sheila Currie

GP Michael Francis John ARMSTRONG, Dora Elizabeth STELFOX

Comber Health Centre
5 Newtownards Road, Comber, Newtownards BT23 5AU
Tel: 028 9187 8391 Fax: 028 9187 1396

GP Elizabeth Jane LEONARD, Millicent Iris McMILLAN

Comber Health Centre
5 Newtownards Road, Newtownards BT23 5BA

GP David Richard GIBSON, Deborah Karon SEMPLE

Lisbane Medical Centre
24 Lisbarnet Road, Comber, Newtownards BT23 6AW
Tel: 028 9754 1466 Fax: 028 9754 1734
Patient List Size: 4500

Practice Manager Anne Finlay

GP David John DONALDSON, George Iain David MOLES

Loughview Surgery
2 Main Street, Kircubbin, Newtownards BT22 2SP
Tel: 028 4273 8532 Fax: 028 4273 8070
Patient List Size: 5800

Practice Manager Carole Hill

GP Lorraine BAILIE, Robert James MAGEEAN, Herbert Desmond STEELE

MDP Practice
44 High Street, Portaferry, Newtownards BT22 1QT
Fax: 028 4272 9834
Patient List Size: 2872

Practice Manager Joan Kelly

GP Philip LAVERY, Michael Brendan DOYLE, David PEACOCK

Newtownards Health Centre
Frederick Street, Newtownards BT23 4LS
Tel: 028 9181 6880

GP John Stuart BURNHAM

Newtownards Health Centre
Frederick Street, Newtownards BT23 4LS

GP Kenneth Alfred STRONGE, Gillian Margaret LUNEY

Old Mill Surgery
Church Street, Newtownards BT23 4AS
Tel: 028 9181 7239 Fax: 028 9182 4742
Patient List Size: 10000

Practice Manager Miriam Millar

GP Thomas James QUAITE, Margaret Ruth BUCKLEY, Edgar John LEES, Gale Samuel John MOFFETT, John WINTER

Portaferry Health Centre
Ann Street, Portaferry, Newtownards BT22 1LX
Patient List Size: 3057

GP Desmond Michael COMPTON, Michael Brendan DOYLE

Regency Medical Centre
Frederick Street, Newtownards BT23 4LS
Tel: 028 9181 6880 Fax: 028 9181 1429
Patient List Size: 4300

GP Margaret Anne McCARTHY, Michael James WEBB

Regency Medical Centre
2A Frederick Street, Newtownards BT23 4LR
Tel: 028 9181 6880 Fax: 028 9181 1429
Patient List Size: 1990

Practice Manager Jenny Carson

GP Christopher David MATHISON

The Robert Henry Surgery
7A Newtownards Road, Comber, Newtownards BT23 5AU

GP James BISSETT

The Square Surgery
16A The Square, Comber, Newtownards BT23 5AP
Tel: 028 9187 8159

GP George Frederick Brian HORNER, Mary Ethel McKEOWN, Peter Jonathan MITCHELL

Omagh

Carrickmore Health Centre
Termon Road, Carrickmore, Omagh BT79 9JR
Tel: 028 8076 1242 Fax: 028 8076 1077

Practice Manager Sinead McGarrity

GP Charles Kieran Mary DEENY, Martin Joseph CORRY, Siobhan Mary DONAGHY, Michael Joseph HERRON

Drumragh Family Practice
Mountjoy Road, Omagh BT79 7BA
Tel: 028 8283 5570 Fax: 028 8283 5592
Patient List Size: 10300

Practice Manager C F McGrath

GP Paula Mary GALLAGHER, Desmond Gerard GORMLEY, Irfan-Ul HASSAN, Anne Louise HICKS, Michael Thomas Andrew KEMP, Michael McCAVERT

Fintona Medical Centre
33 Dromore Road, Fintona, Omagh BT78 2BB
Tel: 028 8284 1203 Fax: 028 8284 0545

Practice Manager Vincent McLaughlin

GP Lonan Gall Michel MAGFHOGARTAIGH, Kyran Francis MONAGHAN, Brian Edward SWEENEY

Grange Family Practice
Omagh Health Centre, Mountjoy Road, Omagh BT79 7BA
Tel: 028 8224 3521 Fax: 028 8283 5628
Email: rmckinney@drpllock.pcwestni.nhs.uk
Patient List Size: 5740

Practice Manager Rhonda McKinney

GP Nigel Charles POLLOCK, Deirdre CLEARY, Alyson NOONE, Patrick Henry Martin QUINN

Main Street Surgery
86 Main Street, Gortin, Omagh BT79 8PH
Tel: 028 8164 8216

Practice Manager Mary McKeown

GP Vakil SINGH, Kenny HICKS

Main Street Surgery
7-9 Main Street, Dromore, Omagh BT78 3AE
Tel: 028 8289 8137

GP Edward Joseph BURKE, Paul Hugh REILLY

Main Street Surgery
23 Omagh Road, Drumquin, Omagh BT78 4QY

Practice Manager Yvonne Little

GP Patrick Gerard SCULLY

Newtownstewart Medical Centre
5 Millbrook Street, Newtownstewart, Omagh BT78 4BW
Tel: 028 8166 1333 Fax: 028 8166 1883

Practice Manager Michelle McConomy

GP David Robert Peter THOMPSON, Siobhan GREENE

Omagh Health Centre
Mountjoy Road, Omagh BT79 7BA
Tel: 028 8224 3521

Practice Manager Patricia Rowan-Quinn

GP Paul Brendan BRADLEY, William McCALLION, Brendan Thomas McDONALD, Eamon Anthony McMULLAN, Ciara Anne O'NEILL

Omagh Road Surgery
12 Omagh Road, Drumquin, Omagh BT78 4QY
Tel: 028 8283 1275

GP Gordon Fraser GERVAIS

Strule Medical Practice
Omagh Health Centre, Mountjoy Road, Omagh BT79 7BA
Tel: 028 8224 3521/028 8283 5612 Fax: 028 8283 5629
Patient List Size: 3000

Practice Manager Lisa Stewart

GP Josephine Anne DEEHAN, Sandra ELLIOTT

Portrush

Portrush Medical Centre
Dunlace Avenue, Portrush BT56 8DW
Tel: 028 7082 3767 Fax: 028 7082 3413

Practice Manager Beth Graham

GP James Stephen BAILIE, Michael Craig GARDINER, Charlotte Pamela LOGUE, Michael David McCARTNEY

The Terrace Surgery
2 Dhu Varren Park, Portrush BT56 8EL
Tel: 028 7082 4637 Fax: 028 7082 4637

GP Owen Henry REA

Portstewart

Portstewart
Family Practice, 6 Lever Road, Portstewart BT55 7EF
Tel: 028 7083 2149 Fax: 028 7083 3223
Patient List Size: 2600

Practice Manager Celine Harley

GP James Bernard HARLEY, Dr DEARBHLA

Portstewart Medical Centre
Mill Road, Portstewart BT55 7SW
Tel: 028 7083 2600 Fax: 028 7083 6871

Practice Manager Claire Gibson

GP Paul Gerard Mary CARLIN, Philip Raymond O'LOAN

Strabane

Duncastle Road Surgery
275 Duncastle Road, Donermara, Strabane BT82 0LR
Tel: 028 7139 8226

GP Archibald Thomas FULLERTON

Mourneside Medical Centre
1A Ballycolman Avenue, Strabane BT82 9AF
Tel: 028 7138 3737 Fax: 028 7138 3979
Email: reception@mourneside.co.uk
Website: www.mourneside.co.uk
Patient List Size: 10600

Practice Manager Patricia Moron

GP James Gerard GILLESPIE, Joseph Gerard Anthony Jude McHALE, Martin Patrick O'Malley O'NEILL, Diane Patricia ROBINSON, Heather SMYTH

Riverside Practice
Upper Main Street, Strabane BT82 8AS
Tel: 028 7138 4100 Fax: 028 7138 4115

Practice Manager Jacqueline Barr

GP Brian Michael QUIGLEY, Eamonn Gerard KERR, C MULLAN, Gerard Martin O'FLAHERTY, Catherine Mary RAWDON

Strabane Health Centre
Upper Main Street, Strabane BT82 8AS
Tel: 028 7138 4118 Fax: 028 7138 4115

Practice Manager Siobhan Carey

GP Gerald Howard Vincent WATSON, Siobhan CAREY, Paul John CAVANAGH, John ETHERSON, P McIVOR, Aidan McMENAMIN

Channel Islands

Alderney

The Island Medical Centre
Sundial House, Les Rocquettes, Alderney GY9 3TF
Tel: 01481 822077 Fax: 01481 823900

GP Jonathan COOPER, Roxana SCHREIBER

Guernsey

Cobo Health Centre
Route de Carteret, Castel, Guernsey GY5 7HA
Tel: 01481 256404

Practice Manager Catherine Walter

GP Ian Bradshaw GEE, Duncan Stewart McKERRELL, James RAY, Philip SIMPSON, Catherine Ruth TABERNER

Eagle Medical Practice
Stefan House, Olivier St, Alderney, Guernsey GY9 3TD
Tel: 01481 822494 Fax: 01481 823892

Practice Manager Elizabeth Phelan

GP Rory LYONS, Richard SEYMOUR

L'Aumone Surgery
L'Aumone, Castel, Guernsey GY5 7RU
Tel: 01481 256517 Fax: 01481 251190
Email: enquires@health.gg
Website: www.islandhealth.co.uk
Patient List Size: 9850

Practice Manager Heather Gibbs

GP Timothy John SINNERTON, Nicholas William FAZAKERLEY, Robert George HANNA, Susan Jennifer HOLLWEY, Ruth Alison JONES, Joanne LE NOURY

Pier Steps Surgery
High Street, St. Peter Port, Guernsey GY1 2JT
Tel: 01481 711237 Fax: 01481 723991
Website: www.healthcaregroup.co.uk

GP Nicholas Anthony Fleetwood PALUCH, Eleanor Judith STEEL

Queens Road Medical Practice
The Grange, St. Peter Port, Guernsey GY1 1RH
Tel: 01481 724184/725121 Fax: 01481 716431
Email: admin@eqrmp.com
Website: www.eqrmp.com
Patient List Size: 20000

Practice Manager Chris Wakefield

GP Stephen WRAY, Maryse ASH, Richard William Francis BARKER, Michael Joseph BRERETON, Tony Siak Lam CHANKUN, John GIBBS, Hannah LAIDLOW, Antonia MACHIN, Maureen McGAVIGAN, Christopher Richard MONKHOUSE, Michael MOWBRAY, Janice PORRITT, Eric John SMITH, Ruth SWAINSTON, Jack WIELAND, Douglas WILSON, Susan Jane Vonda WILSON

Queen's Road Medical Practice
Le Longfrie Surgery, Rue de Longfrie, St. Pierre Du Bois, Guernsey GY7 9RZ
Tel: 01481 264185 Fax: 01481 264182
Email: admin@eqrmp.com

Practice Manager Tony Wills

GP Olaf CARSTENSEN, John Roger GIBBS, Maureen McGAVIGAN, Douglas Scott MacGregor WILSON

Rohais Health Centre
Rohais, St. Peter Port, Guernsey GY1 1FF
Tel: 01481 723322 Fax: 01481 725200
Email: admin@healthcare.gg
Patient List Size: 24539

Practice Manager Catherine Walter

GP Whitford ANDREWS, Simon Ernest BODKIN, David Sutherland BRAND, Mark Peter Richard DOWNING, Timothy Robert GILL, Brian Derek PARKIN, Louise PARKIN

St Martins Health Centre
La Grande Rue, St. Martins, Guernsey GY4 6RX
Tel: 01481 37757 Fax: 01481 395591

Practice Manager C Walter

GP Malcolm Robert CHAMBERLAIN, Nicholas Clive KING, Bruce Graham MACKAY, Michael McCARTHY, Anthony John O'DONNELL, Jennifer TURNER

St Sampson's Medical Centre
Grandes Maisons Road, St. Sampson, Guernsey GY2 4JS
Tel: 01481 245915 Fax: 01481 243179
Email: enquiries@health.gg
Website: www.islandhealth.co.uk
Patient List Size: 20166

Practice Manager Heather Gibbs

GP Stephen Michael BRENNAND ROPER, Elizabeth Margaret NORRIS, Jonathan Gale PEARCE, Graham David REILLY, Peter William RICHARDS, Stella Jane RICHARDS, Paul Graham WILLIAMS, Beverley Jane WORKMAN

Jersey

Clarendon Road Surgery
17 Clarendon Road, St Helier, Jersey JE2 3YW
Tel: 01534 23456

GP Nagy Fouad MICKHAEL

Cleveland Clinic
12 Cleveland Road, St Helier, Jersey JE1 4HD
Tel: 01534 722381/734121

Practice Manager Ronnie Jubb

GP Simon Michael Joseph BONN, Alex Michael BLAMPIED, Gordon Walter Robert CALLANDER, Innes Lorimer CAMERON, Jilesh CHOHAN, David Charles FRANK, Roderick Alfred HURRY, John Marshall MAXEY, Ian Richman SHENKIN, Eva Marie SLATER, Philippa Mary VENN

Clifden House Surgery
24 Vauxhall Street, St Helier, Jersey JE2 4TJ
Tel: 01534 726705 Fax: 01534 735082
Email: m8rv85@aol.com

GP Alison GROOM, Leonard Michael MIRVIS

Como Villa Surgery
7 Clarendon Road, St Helier, Jersey JE2 3YW
Tel: 01534 870151

GP David Geoffrey Boyd HAMILTON

Crahamel Medical Practice
Crahamel House, 1 Duhamel Place, St Helier, Jersey JE2 4TP
Tel: 01534 735742 Fax: 01534 735011

Practice Manager Ann Vautier

GP Roger Charles PORCHEROT, Christine BUDD, Michael CARPENTER, Peter Jeremy Haden GLYNN, James Edwin HUGH, Stephen Cameron KING, Jonathan NEWSTEAD, Robert PARRIS

David Place Medical Practice
56 David Place, St Helier, Jersey JE1 4HY
Tel: 01534 733322 Fax: 01534 731770
Email: scodavidplace@gpnet.je

Practice Manager Samantha Kezourec

GP Michael Francis MARKS, Michael John BELLAMY, Margaretta DE KLERK, Mark Edwin Nelson FULLERTON, Adam GARNETT, Michael Edward McBRIDE, Bryany PERCHARD, Steve PERCHARD, Swaz WATTS

David Place Surgery
7 David Place, St Helier, Jersey JE2 4TD
Tel: 01534 21261

GP William Ian McMath TAYLOR, Bryan HICKSON, Michael Bryan HOLMES

David Place Surgery
361/2 David Place, St Helier, Jersey JE2 4TE
Tel: 01534 619988

GP James DWYER

Elizabeth Place Surgery
8 Elizabeth Place, St Helier, Jersey JE2 3PN
Tel: 01534 25824 Fax: 01534 887443

GP Miriam Mary NOEL

Elizabeth Place Surgery
8 Elizabeth Place, St Helier, Jersey JE2 3PN
Tel: 01534 874095

GP Michel LAPASSET

Elizabeth Place Surgery
8 Elizabeth Place, St Helier, Jersey JE2 3PN
Tel: 01534 25824

GP David James BAILEY

Elizabeth Place Surgery
8 Elizabeth Place, St Helier, Jersey JE2 3PN
Tel: 01534 723718

GP James Edwin HUGH

Grosvenor Street Surgery
4 Grosvenor Street, St Helier, Jersey JE1 4HB
Tel: 01534 30541 Fax: 01534 887948

GP Gregory James INCE, David BAILEY, Dean Ivor BALBES, Richard Lawrence BROWN, John Barrie HOWELL, Robert Kenneth HURST, Roger Andrew MARSON-SMITH, Ben ROGERS, Philip Keith Dale TERRY

Grosvenor Street Surgery
5 Grosvenor Street, St Helier, Jersey JE2 3QR
Tel: 01534 20156

GP Mark Andrew EARLEY, Julie LE CORNU, Rhys Alan Bowen PERKINS

Halkett Place Surgery
84 Halkett Place, St Helier, Jersey JE1 4XL
Tel: 01534 36301 Fax: 01534 887793

GP Nicola Ann BAILHACHE, John Adrian COATES, Brendan Charles KELLETT, Jonathan Mark OSMONT, David Graham POPE, John STEWART-JONES

Ivy House Surgery
27 The Parade, St Helier, Jersey JE2 3QQ
Tel: 01534 728777 Fax: 01534 728977
Email: lecluse@itl.net
Patient List Size: 1600

GP Gareth HUGHES, Guy Stephen WILDY

La Route Du Fort Surgery
2 La Route Du Fort, St Helier, Jersey JE2 4PA
Tel: 01534 731421 Fax: 01534 280776
Email: laroutedufortsurgery@jerseymail.co.uk

Practice Manager S Le Bon

GP Margaret Joyce BAYES, William Eric Seaton BUIST, Pippa HARROLD, Sean RYAN, Peter Howard SMART, Sally Angela SPARROW

The Laurels Medical Practice
The Laurels, 28 Clarendon Road, Jersey JE2 3YS
Tel: 01534 733866 Fax: 01534 769597
Email: laurels@gpnet.je
Patient List Size: 6000

Practice Manager Janet Scholefield

GP Patrick HIGGINS, Penny LE BAS, Brendan LOANE, Nigel Anthony MINIHANE, Karen Elizabeth SINFIELD, Michael WINSPEAR

Le Ruisselet Surgery
c/o Mrs Stievenard, Le Ruisselet, Mount Rossignol, St Ouen, Jersey JE3 2LN
Tel: 01534 481215

GP Max Bray DEACON

Les Saisons Surgery
20 David Place, St Helier, Jersey JE2 4TD
Tel: 01534 720314 Fax: 01534 733205
Patient List Size: 5000

Practice Manager Elizabeth Lawrence

GP Simon Neil SLAFFER, Christopher COOK, Annabel NORMAN, Andrew Patrick VINCENT

Lister House Surgery
35 The Parade, St Helier, Jersey JE2 3QQ
Tel: 01534 736336 Fax: 01534 735304
Patient List Size: 12386

Practice Manager Sharon Louis

GP Richard Henry THACKER, Roelof EDELENBOS VALPY, John David JACKSON, Barbara Catto ROBERTSON, Michael John ROSSER, Malachy Gerard WILSON

St Peter Surgery
La Rue de L'Eglise, St Peter, Jersey JE3 7AG
Tel: 01534 484533 Fax: 01534 484531
Email: mbarrett@medhalth.co.uk

GP M BARRETT

Villa Surgery
7 Clarendon Road, St Helier, Jersey JE2 3YW
Tel: 01534 24256

GP Anthony Clare HALLIWELL

White Lodge Medical Centre
21 Grosvenor Street, St Helier, Jersey JE1 4HA
Tel: 01534 873786 Fax: 01534 601955
Patient List Size: 2500

Practice Manager Shelia McDonald

GP Michael VINCENT

White Lodge Practices
21 Grosvenor Street, St Helier, Jersey JE1 4HA
Tel: 01534 23892 Fax: 01534 601955

GP William Hugh FRANKLIN, Nola Jean WEBSTER

White Lodge Practices
21 Grosvenor Street, St Helier, Jersey JE1 4HA
Tel: 01534 723892 Fax: 01534 601955

Practice Manager Janet Jacques

GP Gail COCHRANE, Anne CURTIS, William FRANKLIN

Windsor Crescent Surgery
6 Windsor Crescent, Val Plaisant, St Helier, Jersey JE2 4TB
Tel: 01534 32341 Fax: 01534 870635

GP John Stanley LE GRESLEY, Anthony BALMER, Nigel Bradley STEVENS

Young, Ellis and Overton
41 David Place, St Helier, Jersey JE2 4TE
Tel: 01534 723318 Fax: 01534 611062
Patient List Size: 4500

Practice Manager Sandra Bouchere

GP Brian David ELLIS, Michael Andrew OVERTON, Michael John YOUNG

Sark

Sark Medical Centre
Sark, Sark GY9 0SF
Tel: 01481 832045 Fax: 01481 832496
Email: mbedford@sark.net
Patient List Size: 700

GP M C BEDFORD

Isle of Man

Ballasalla

Ballasalla Medical Centre
Main Road, Ballasalla IM9 2RQ
Tel: 01624 823243 Fax: 01624 822947
Patient List Size: 4000

Practice Manager Moira Pendlebury

GP Curphey Clague TAGGART, Alison Margaret BLACKMAN, Jane Elizabeth HOCKINGS

Castletown

Arbory Street Surgery
Arbory Street, Castletown IM9 1LN
Tel: 01624 823597 Fax: 01624 825245

GP John Edward BREWIS, Susanna Monica SWAINSON

Douglas

Hailwood Medical Centre
2 Hailwood Court, Governors Hill, Douglas IM2 7EA
Tel: 01624 675444 Fax: 01624 616290
Email: bert.hopkins@talk21.com
Website: www.hailwoodmc.co.uk
Patient List Size: 8000

Practice Manager R Alexander

GP Philip Alan HARRISON, E EVANS, Bert HOPKINSON, David JAMES

Kensington Group Practice
Kensington Health Centre, Westmoreland Road, Douglas IM1 4QA
Tel: 01624 676774 Fax: 01624 614668
Patient List Size: 12000

Practice Manager Andrea Castle

GP Neil Gow Sinclair GAVIN, Christopher Mark BLACKMAN, David Michael BULL, William James COWIE, Mark Christopher HARROP, Adrian Charles PILLING

Palatine Group Practice
Murray's Road, Douglas IM2 3TD
Tel: 01624 623931 Fax: 01624 611712
Email: palatineg.p.@manx.net
Patient List Size: 9500

Practice Manager Rosemary Kinrade

GP Frank William HARDING, Fiona Margaret BAKER, Julie Denise CRETNEY, John Keith DANIELS, Colin Neil GARVEY, John Douglas McDONALD

Promenade Medical Centre
46 Loch Promenade, Douglas IM1 2RX
Tel: 01624 675490
Patient List Size: 4000

Practice Manager Christine Dando

GP Vincent Paul BRADLEY, Clare HILLAS

Snaefell Surgery
Cushag Road, AnaghCoar, Douglas IM2 2BZ
Tel: 01624 676622 Fax: 01624 674515

Practice Manager Robin Hynes

GP David Hastings Kerr CHALMERS, Andrew Richard Sinclair VAUGHAN

Laxey

Laxey Medical Centre
New Road, Laxey IM4 7BF
Tel: 01624 861350 Fax: 01624 861469
Patient List Size: 6450

GP David Wallace YOUNG, Catriona FARRANT, James McALISTER, Alan Kenneth STONE

Peel

Peel Medical Centre
Derby Road, Peel IM5 1HP
Tel: 01624 843636 Fax: 01624 844543

Practice Manager Shirley Corrin

GP Keith Joseph JONES, John BLOOMER, Richard James HANKS, Andrew Bernard HUDSON

Port Erin

Southern Group Practice
Castletown Road, Port Erin IM9 6BD
Tel: 01624 832226 Fax: 01624 836759
Patient List Size: 7500

Practice Manager David Handscomibe

GP Craig Donald BLACKWELL, Veronica BREWS, Nigel MOUSLEY, Philip Harold SMITH, Deborah WIGNALL

Ramsey

Ramsey Group Practice Centre
Grove Mount South, Ramsey IM8 3EY
Tel: 01624 813881 Fax: 01624 811921
Patient List Size: 14000

Practice Manager Mandy Kelly

GP John Kirkpatrick BROWNSDON, Alex ALLINSON, James Keith ARMOUR, May Shiu CHAN, Hilary M CLARKE, Andrew Sean Charles KELSEY, Mariusz MASKA, Graham Martin WILSON

Health Authorities and Boards

England

Avon, Gloucestershire and Wiltshire Strategic Health Authority
Jenner House, Langley Park Estate, Chippenham SN15 1GG
Tel: 01249 858500 Fax: 01249 858501
Email: chief.executive@agwsha.nhs.uk
Website: www.agwsha.nhs.uk

Chair Anthea Millett
Chief Executive Trevor Jones

Bedfordshire and Hertfordshire Strategic Health Authority
Tonman House, 63-77 Victoria Street, St Albans AL1 3ER
Tel: 01727 812929 Fax: 01727 792800
Website: www.bhha.nhs.uk

Chair Ian White
Chief Executive John de Braux

Birmingham and the Black Country Strategic Health Authority
St Chad's Court, 213 Hagley Road, Edgbaston, Birmingham B16 9RG
Tel: 0121 695 2222 Fax: 0121 695 2233
Email: info@bbcha.nhs.uk
Website: www.bbcha.nhs.uk

Chair Elisabeth Buggins
Chief Executive David Nicholson

Cheshire and Merseyside Strategic Health Authority
Quayside, Wilderspool Park, Greenalls Avenue, Stockton Heath, Warrington WA4 6HL
Tel: 01925 406000 Fax: 01925 406001
Email: enquiries@cmha.nhs.uk
Website: www.cmha.nhs.uk

Chair Judith Greensmith
Chief Executive Christine Hannah

County Durham and Tees Valley Strategic Health Authority
Teesdale House, Westpoint Road, Thornaby, Stockton-on-Tees TS17 6BL
Tel: 01642 666700 Fax: 01642 666701

Chair Tony Waites
Chief Executive Ken Jarrold

Cumbria and Lancashire Strategic Health Authority
Preston Business Centre, Watling Street Road, Fulwood, Preston PR2 8DY
Tel: 01772 647000 Fax: 01772 220290
Website: www.clha.nhs.uk

Chair Kath Reade
Chief Executive Pearse Butler

Dorset and Somerset Strategic Health Authority
Wynford House, Lufton Way, Lufton, Yeovil BA22 8HR
Tel: 01935 384000 Fax: 01935 384079
Website: www.dorsetsomerset.nhs.uk

Chair Jane Barrie
Chief Executive Ian Carruthers

Essex Strategic Health Authority
Swift House, Hedgerows Business Park, Colchester Road, Chelmsford CM2 5PF
Tel: 01245 397600 Fax: 01245 397601
Email: enquiries@essexha.nhs.uk
Website: www.essex.nhs.uk

Chair Michael Brookes
Chief Executive Terry Hanafin

Greater Manchester Strategic Health Authority
Gateway House, Piccadilly South, Manchester M60 7LP
Tel: 0161 236 9456 Fax: 0161 237 2264
Email: claire.swithenbank@gmsha.nhs.uk
Website: www.gmsha.nhs.uk

Chair Philip Smith
Chief Executive Neil Goodwin

Hampshire and Isle of Wight Strategic Health Authority
Oakley Road, Southampton SO16 4GX
Tel: 023 8072 5400 Fax: 023 8072 5457
Email: communications@hiowha.nhs.uk, firstname.lastname@hiowha.nhs.uk
Website: www.hiow.nhs.uk

Chair Jonathan Montgomery
Chief Executive Gareth Cruddace

Kent and Medway Strategic Health Authority
Preston Hall, Royal British Legion Village, Aylesford ME20 7NJ
Tel: 01622 710161 Fax: 01622 719802
Email: general@kentmedway.nhs.uk
Website: www.kentmedway.nhs.uk

Chair Kate Lampard
Chief Executive Candy Morris

Leicestershire, Northamptonshire and Rutland Strategic Health Authority
Lakeside House, 4 Smith Way, Grove Park, Enderby, Leicester LE19 1SS
Tel: 0116 295 7500 Fax: 0116 295 7599
Email: enquiries@lnrsha.nhs.uk, firstname.surname@lnrsha.nhs.uk
Website: www.lnrsha.nhs.uk

Chair Richard Tilt
Chief Executive David Sissling

Norfolk, Suffolk and Cambridgeshire Strategic Health Authority
Victoria House, Capital Park, Fulbourn, Cambridge CB1 5XB
Tel: 01223 597500 Fax: 01223 597555
Email: firstname.lastname@nscstha.nhs.uk
Website: www.nscstha.nhs.uk

Chair Stewart Francis
Chief Executive Peter Houghton

North and East Yorkshire and Northern Lincolnshire Strategic Health Authority
St John's House, Innovation Way, York Science Park, Heslington, York YO10 5NY

Tel: 01904 724500 Fax: 01904 431765
Email: stcontact@neynlha.nhs.uk
Website: www.neynlsha.nhs.uk

Chair David Johns
Chief Executive David Johnson

North Central London Strategic Health Authority

Victory House, 170 Tottenham Court Road, London W1T 7HA
Tel: 020 7756 2500 Fax: 020 7756 2510
Email: firstname.lastname@nclha.nhs.uk
Website: www.nclha.nhs.uk

Chair Marcia Saunders
Chief Executive Mark Easton

North East London Strategic Health Authority

Aneurin Bevan House, 81 Commercial Road, London E1 1RD
Tel: 020 7655 6600 Fax: 020 7655 6666
Email: enquiries@nelondon.nhs.uk
Website: www.nelondon.nhs.uk

Chair Elaine Murphy
Chief Executive Carolyn Regan

North West London Strategic Health Authority

Victory House, 170 Tottenham Court Road, London W1T 7HA
Tel: 020 7756 2500 Fax: 020 7756 2502
Email: firstname.lastname@nwlha.nhs.uk
Website: www.nwlha.nhs.uk

Chair Caroline (Caro) Millington
Chief Executive Gareth Goodier

Northumberland, Tyne and Wear Strategic Health Authority

Riverside House, The Waterfront, Goldcrest Way, Newburn Riverside, Newcastle upon Tyne NE15 8NY
Tel: 0191 210 6400 Fax: 0191 210 6401
Website: www.ntwha.nhs.uk

Chair Peter Carr
Chief Executive David Flory

Shropshire and Staffordshire Strategic Health Authority

Mellor House, Corporation Street, Stafford ST16 3SR
Tel: 01785 252233 Fax: 01785 221111
Email: sasha@sasha.nhs.uk
Website: www.sasha.nhs.uk

Chair Michael Brereton
Chief Executive Bernard Crump

South East London Strategic Health Authority

1 Lower Marsh, London SE1 7NT
Tel: 020 7716 7000 Fax: 020 7716 7037
Email: communications@selondon.nhs.uk, firstname.lastname@selondon.nhs.uk
Website: www.selondon.nhs.uk

Chair Linda Smith
Chief Executive Michael Walsh

South West London Strategic Health Authority

41-47 Hartfield Road, Wimbledon, London SW19 3RG
Tel: 020 8545 6000 Fax: 020 8545 6001
Email: enquiries@swlha.nhs.uk
Website: www.swlha.nhs.uk

Chair James Cochrane
Chief Executive Julie Dent

South West Peninsula Strategic Health Authority

Peninsula House, Kingsmill Road, Tamar View Industrial Estate, Saltash PL12 6LE
Tel: 01752 315001 Fax: 01752 841696
Email: enquiries@swpsha.nhs.uk
Website: www.swpsha.nhs.uk

Chair Judith Leverton
Chief Executive Thelma Holland

South Yorkshire Strategic Health Authority

Fulwood House, Old Fulwood Road, Sheffield S10 3TH
Tel: 0114 271 1100 Fax: 0114 271 1101
Email: firstname.lastname@sysha.nhs.uk, information@sysha.nhs.uk
Website: www.southyorkshire.nhs.uk

Chair Kathryn Riddle
Chief Executive Mike Farrar

Surrey and Sussex Strategic Health Authority

York House, 18-20 Massetts Road, Horley RH6 7DE
Tel: 01293 778899 Fax: 01293 778888
Email: firstname.lastname@sysxha.nhs.uk, info@sysxha.nhs.uk
Website: www.surreysussexsha.nhs.uk

Chair Peter Bareau
Chief Executive Simon Robbins

Thames Valley Strategic Health Authority

Jubilee House, 5510 John Smith Drive, Oxford Business Park South, Cowley, Oxford OX4 2LH
Tel: 01865 337000 Fax: 01865 337099
Email: comms@tvha.nhs.uk
Website: www.tvsha.nhs.uk

Chair Bernard Williams
Chief Executive Nick Relph

Trent Strategic Health Authority

Octavia House, Interchange Business Park, Bostocks Lane, Sandiacre, Nottingham NG10 5QG
Tel: 0115 968 4444 Fax: 0115 968 4400
Website: www.tsha.nhs.uk

Chair Arthur Sandford
Chief Executive Alan Burns

West Midlands South Strategic Health Authority

Osprey House, Albert Street, Prospect Hill, Redditch B97 4DE
Tel: 01527 587500 Fax: 01527 587502
Website: www.wmssha.nhs.uk

Chair Charles Goody
Chief Executive Kevin Orford

West Yorkshire Strategic Health Authority

Blenheim House, West One, Duncombe Street, Leeds LS1 4PL
Tel: 0113 295 2000 Fax: 0113 295 2222
Email: sha.enquiries@westyorks.nhs.uk
Website: www.wysha.nhs.uk

Chair Linda Pollard
Chief Executive Richard Jeavons

Scotland

Golden Jubilee Hospital

Beardmore Street, Clydebank, Glasgow G81 4HX
Tel: 0141 951 5000
Website: www.show.scot.nhs.uk/gjnh/

Chair Lindsay Burley
Chief Executive Jill Young

NHS Argyll and Clyde
Ross House, Hawkhead Road, Paisley PA2 7BN
Tel: 0141 842 7200 Fax: 0141 848 1414
Email: public@achb.scot.nhs.uk
Website: www.nhsac.scot.nhs.uk

Chair John Mullin
Chief Executive Neil Campbell

NHS Ayrshire and Arran
Boswell House, 10 Arthur Street, Ayr KA7 1QJ
Tel: 01292 611040 Fax: 01292 286762
Website: www.nhsayrshireandarran.com

Chair George Irving
Chief Executive Wai-yin Hatton

NHS Borders
Newstead, Melrose TD6 9DB
Tel: 01896 825500 Fax: 01896 825580
Email: bordershb@borders.scot.nhs.uk
Website: www.nhsborders.org.uk

Chair Tony Taylor
Chief Executive John Glennie

NHS Dumfries and Galloway
Crichton Hall, Bankend Road, Dumfries DG1 4TG
Tel: 01387 246246 Fax: 01387 252375
Website: www.nhsdg.scot.nhs.uk

Chair John Ross
Chief Executive John Burns

NHS Fife
Hayfield House, Hayfield Road, Kirkcaldy KY2 5AH
Tel: 01592 643355 Fax: 01592 648142
Website: www.show.scot.nhs.uk/fhb

Chair James McGoldrick
Chief Executive George Brechin

NHS Forth Valley
33 Spittal Street, Stirling FK8 1DX
Tel: 01786 463031 Fax: 01786 471337
Email: email@fvhb.scot.nhs.uk
Website: www.show.scot.nhs.uk/nhsfv

Chair Ian Mullen
Chief Executive Fiona Mackenzie

NHS Grampian
Summerfield House, 2 Eday Road, Aberdeen AB15 6RE
Tel: 0845 456 6000
Website: www.nhsgrampian.org

Chair Jim Royan
Chief Executive Alex Smith

NHS Greater Glasgow
Dalian House, 350 St Vincent Street, Glasgow G3 8YZ
Tel: 0141 201 4444 Fax: 0141 201 4401
Website: www.nhsgg.org.uk

Chair John Arbuthnott
Chief Executive Tom Divers

NHS Highland
Assynt House, Beechwood Park, Inverness IV2 3HG
Tel: 01463 717123 Fax: 01463 235189
Email: nhsboardreception@hhb.scot.nhs.uk
Website: www.show.scot.nhs.uk/nhshighland

Chair Garry Coutts
Chief Executive Roger Gibbins

NHS Lanarkshire
14 Beckford Street, Hamilton ML3 0TA
Tel: 01698 281313 Fax: 01698 423134
Website: www.nhslanarkshire.co.uk

Chair Lex Gold
Chief Executive David Pigott

NHS Lothian
Deaconess House, 148 Pleasance, Edinburgh EH8 9RS
Tel: 0131 536 9000 Fax: 0131 536 9164
Website: www.nhslothian.scot.nhs.uk

Chair Brian Cavanagh
Chief Executive James Barbour

NHS Orkney
Garden House, New Scapa Road, Kirkwall KW15 1BQ
Tel: 01856 88800 Fax: 01856 888211
Email: name.surname@orkney-hb.scot.nhs.uk
Website: www.show.scot.nhs.uk/ohb

Chair Jenny Dewar
Chief Executive Steve Conway

NHS Shetland
Brevik House, South Road, Lerwick ZE1 0TG
Tel: 01595 696767 Fax: 01595 696727
Email: info@shb.shetland.scot.nhs.uk
Website: www.shetlandhealthboard.org

Chair Betty Fullerton
Chief Executive Sandra Laurenson

NHS Tayside
King's Cross, Clepington Road, Dundee DD3 8EA
Tel: 01382 818479 Fax: 01382 424003
Website: www.nhstayside.scot.nhs.uk

Chair Peter Bates
Chief Executive Tony Wells

NHS Western Isles
37 South Beach Street, Stornoway HS1 2BB
Tel: 01851 702997 Fax: 01851 704405
Email: ChiefExecutive@wihb.scot.nhs.uk
Website: www.show.scot.nhs.uk/wihb

Chair David Currie
Chief Executive Dick Manson

Scottish Ambulance Service
National Headquarters, Tipperlinn Road, Edinburgh EH10 5UU
Tel: 0131 446 7000 Fax: 0131 446 7001
Website: www.scottishambulance.com

Chair William Brackenridge
Chief Executive Adrian Lucas

State Hospitals Board for Scotland
The State Hospital, Carstairs, Lanark ML11 8RP
Tel: 01555 840293 Fax: 01555 840024
Email: info@tsh.scot.nhs.uk
Website: www.show.scot.nhs.uk/tsh

Chair Gordon Craig
Chief Executive Andreana Adamson

Wales

Mid and West Wales

Regional Office, St David's Hospital, 1st Floor, Jobswell Road, Carmarthen SA31 3YH

Tel: 01267 225250

Chief Executive Stuart Marples

Director of Public Health William Ritchie

Bridgend Local Health Board

North Court, David Street, Bridgend Industrial Estate, Bridgend CF31 3TP
Tel: 01656 754400 Fax: 01656 754497
Email: contact.us@bridgend-lhg.wales.nhs.uk
Website: www.bridgendlhb.wales.nhs.uk

Chair Colin Jones
Chief Executive Kay Howells

Carmarthenshire Local Health Board

Thyssen House, Heol y Bwlch, Bynea, Llanelli SA14 9SU
Tel: 01554 778593 Fax: 01554 780324
Email: mail@carmarthenlhb.wales.nhs.uk
Website: www.carmarthenlhb.wales.nhs.uk/

Chair Mark Vaughan
Chief Executive Alan Brace

Ceredigion Local Health Board

The Bryn, North Road, Lampeter SA48 7HA
Tel: 01570 424100 Fax: 01570 424102
Email: general.office@ceredigionlhb.wales.nhs.uk
Website: www.ceredigionlhb.wales.nhs.uk

Chair Mary Griffiths
Chief Executive Derrick Jones

Neath Port Talbot Local Health Board

Suite A, Britannic House, Llandarcy, Neath SA10 6JQ
Tel: 01792 326500 Fax: 01792 326501
Email: nptlhb@neathporttalbotlhb.wales.nhs.uk
Website: www.neathporttalbotlhb.wales.nhs.uk

Chair Edward Roberts
Chief Executive Katie Norton

Pembrokeshire Local Health Board

Unit 4 Merlin's Court, Winch Lane, Haverfordwest SA61 1SB
Tel: 01437 771220 Fax: 01437 771222
Email: firstname.surname@pembrokeshirelhb.wales.nhs.uk
Website: www.pembrokeshirelhb.wales.nhs.uk

Chair Chris Martin
Chief Executive Bernardine Rees

Powys Local Health Board

Mansion House, Bronllys, Brecon LD3 0LS
Tel: 01874 711661 Fax: 01874 711828
Email: firstname.lastname@powyslhb.wales.nhs.uk
Website: www.powyslhb.wales.nhs.uk

Chair Chris Mann
Chief Executive Andy Williams

Swansea Local Health Board

Kidwelly House, Charter Court, Phoenix Way, Llansamlet, Swansea SA7 9FS
Tel: 01792 784800 Fax: 01792 784855
Email: info@swansealhb.wales.nhs.uk
Website: www.swansealhb.wales.nhs.uk

Chair Susan Fox
Chief Executive Sue Heatherington

North Wales

Regional Office, Prestwylfa, Hendy Road, Mold CH7 1PZ
Tel: 01352 744040 Fax: 01352 755679

Director Derek Griffin
Director of Public Health Sandra Payne

Anglesey Local Health Board

17 High Street, Llangefni LL77 7LT
Tel: 01248 751229 Fax: 01248 751230
Email: angleseylhb@nwales-ha.wales.nhs.uk
Website: www.angleseylhb.wales.nhs.uk

Chair W H Roberts
Chief Executive Lynne Joannou

Conwy Local Health Board

Glyn Colwyn, Nant y Glyn Road, Colwyn Bay LL29 7PU
Tel: 01492 536586 Fax: 01492 536587
Website: www.conwylhb.wales.nhs.uk

Chair Alison Cowell
Chief Executive Wyn Thomas

Denbighshire Local Health Board

Ty Livingstone, H M Stanley Hospital, St Asaph LL17 0RS
Tel: 01745 589601 Fax: 01745 589685
Email: denbighshire.lhb@wales.nhs.uk
Website: www.denbighshirelhb.wales.nhs.uk

Chair Meirion Hughes
Chief Executive Alan Lawrie

Flintshire Local Health Board

Preswylfa, Hendy Road, Mold CH7 1PZ
Tel: 01352 700227 Fax: 01352 755006
Email: flintshire.lhb@flintshirelhb.wales.nhs.uk
Website: www.flintshirelhb.wales.nhs.uk

Chair Barry Harrison
Chief Executive Andrew Gunnion

Gwynedd Local Health Board

Eryldon, Campbell Road, Caernarfon LL55 1HU
Tel: 01286 672451 Fax: 01286 674197
Website: www.gwyneddlhb.wales.nhs.uk

Chair Lyndon Miles
Chief Executive Grace Lewis-Parry

Wrexham Local Health Board

Wrexham Technology Park, Rhyd Broughton Lane, Wrexham LL13 7YP
Tel: 01978 346500 Fax: 01978 346501
Email: wrexham.lhb@wrexhamlhb.wales.nhs.uk
Website: www.wrexhamlhb.wales.nhs.uk

Chair Gwyn Roberts
Chief Executive Geoff Lang

South East Wales

Regional Office, Temple of Peace and Health, Cathays Park, Cardiff CF10 3NW
Tel: 029 2040 2480 Fax: 029 2040 2504

Director Bob Hudson
Director of Infection and Communicable Diseases Tony Howard
Director of Public Health Paul Tromans

Blaenau Gwent Local Health Board

Station Hill, Abertillery NP13 1UJ
Tel: 01495 325400 Fax: 01495 325425
Email: enquiries@blaenaugwentlhb.wales.nhs.uk
Website: www.blaenaugwentlhb.wales.nhs.uk

Chair Marilyn Pitman
Chief Executive Joanne Absalom

Caerphilly Local Health Board
Ystrad Mynach Hospital, Caerphilly Road, Ystrad Mynach, Hengoed, Caerphilly CF82 7XU
Tel: 01443 862056 Fax: 01443 815103
Email: enquiry@caerphillylhb.wales.nhs.uk
Website: www.caerphillylhb.wales.nhs.uk

Chair Bob Mitchard
Chief Executive Judith Paget

Cardiff Local Health Board
Trenewydd, Fairwater Road, Llandaff, Cardiff CF5 2LD
Tel: 029 2055 2212 Fax: 029 2057 8032
Email: enquiries@cardifflhb.wales.nhs.uk
Website: www.cardifflhb.wales.nhs.uk

Chair Robert Jones
Chief Executive Siân Richards

Merthyr Tydfil Local Health Board
Units 2A & 4A Pentrebach Business Centre, Triangle Business Park, Pentrebach, Merthyr Tydfil CF48 4TQ
Tel: 01685 358500 Fax: 01685 358547
Email: contactus@merthyrtydfillhb.wales.nhs.uk
Website: www.merthyrtydfillhb.wales.nhs.uk

Chair Raymond Thomas
Chief Executive Ted Wilson

Monmouthshire Local Health Board
Chepstow Community Hospital, Tempest Way, Chepstow NP16 5YX
Tel: 01291 636400 Fax: 01291 636412
Email: enquiries@monmouthshirelhb.wales.nhs.uk
Website: www.monmouthshirelhb.wales.nhs.uk

Chair Sue Pritchard
Chief Executive Allan Coffey

Newport Local Health Board
Wentwood Suite, St Cadocs Hospital, Caerleon, Newport NP18 3XQ
Tel: 01633 436200 Fax: 01633 436229
Email: newport@gwent-ha.wales.nhs.uk
Website: www.newportlhb.wales.nhs.uk

Chair Susan Kent
Chief Executive Kate Watkins

Rhondda Cynon Taff Local Health Board
Unit 16-18 Centre Court, Treforest Industrial Estate, Pontypridd CF37 5YR
Tel: 01443 824400 Fax: 01443 824395
Email: enquiries@rhonddacynontafflhb.wales.nhs.uk
Website: www.rhonddacynontafflhb.wales.nhs.uk

Chair Christopher Jones
Chief Executive Mel Evans

Torfaen Local Health Board
Block C, Mamhilad House, Mamhilad Park Estate, Pontypool NP4 0YP
Tel: 01495 745868 Fax: 01495 765135
Email: enquiries@torfaenlhb.wales.nhs.uk
Website: www.torfaenlhb.wales.nhs.uk

Chair Doug Dare
Chief Executive John Skinner

Vale of Glamorgan Local Health Board
2 Stanwell Road, Penarth CF64 2AA
Tel: 029 2035 0600 Fax: 029 2035 0601
Email: enquiries@valeofglamorganlhb.wales.nhs.uk
Website: www.valeofglamorganlhb.wales.nhs.uk

Chair Michael Robinson
Chief Executive Abigail Harris

Northern Ireland

Eastern Health and Social Services Board
Champion House, 12-22 Linenhall Street, Belfast BT2 8BS
Tel: 028 9032 1313 Fax: 028 9055 3681
Email: enquiry@ehssb.n-i.nhs.uk
Website: www.ehssb.n-i.nhs.uk

Chair David Russell
Chief Executive Paula Kilbane

Northern Health and Social Services Board
County Hall, 182 Galgorm Road, Ballymena BT42 1QB
Tel: 028 2565 3333 Fax: 028 2566 2311
Email: info@nhssb.n-i.nhs.uk
Website: www.nhssb.n-i.nhs.uk

Chair Michael Wood
Chief Executive Stuart MacDonnell

Southern Health and Social Services Board
Tower Hill, Armagh BT61 9DR
Tel: 028 3741 0041 Fax: 028 3741 4550
Website: www.shssb.org

Chair Fionnuala Cook
Chief Executive Colm Donaghy

Western Health and Social Services Board
15 Gransha Park, Clooney Road, Londonderry BT47 6FN
Tel: 028 7186 0086 Fax: 028 7186 0311
Website: www.whssb.org

Chair Karen Meehan
Chief Executive Steven Lindsay

Channel Islands

States of Guernsey Board of Health
Corporate Headquarters, Le Vauquiedor, St Martin's, Guernsey GY4 6UU
Tel: 01481 725241 Fax: 01481 235341
Email: health@gov.gg
Website: www.health.gov.gg

Chief Executive D Hughes

States of Jersey Health and Social Services
4th Floor, Peter Crill House, Gloucester Street, St Helier, Jersey JE2 3QS
Tel: 01534 622291 Fax: 01534 622887
Email: health@gov.je
Website: www.health.gov.je

Chair Stuart Syvret
Chief Executive Mike Pollard

Isle of Man

Department of Health and Social Security, Health Services Division
Crookall House, Demesne Road, Douglas IM1 3QA
Tel: 01624 642608 Fax: 01624 642617
Email: healthservices@dhss.gov.im
Website: www.gov.im/dhss/health

Chief Executive Colin Brew

Independent Hospitals

England

Abbey Caldew Hospital
64 Dalston Road, Carlisle CA2 5NW
Tel: 01253 531713 Fax: 01228 590158
Email: caldew@abbeyhospitals.com
Website: www.abbeyhospitals.co.uk
Owners: Abbey Hospitals Ltd
Total Beds: 14

Manager S Harding

Abbey Gisburne Park Hospital
Gisburn, Clitheroe BB7 4HX
Tel: 01200 445693 Fax: 01200 445688
Email: gisburne@abbeyhospitals.com
Website: www.abbeyhospitals.co.uk
Owners: Abbey Hospitals Ltd
Total Beds: 35

Manager Liz Cousins

Abbey Park Hospital
Dalton Lane, Barrow-in-Furness LA14 4TP
Tel: 01229 813388 Fax: 01229 813366
Email: deborahbrown@abbeyhospitals.co.uk
Website: www.abbeyhospitals.co.uk
Owners: Covenant Healthcare
Total Beds: 12

Manager Deborah Brown, Deborah Brown

Dermatology P Harrison
ENT P Stoney
General Medicine J Keating, W Mitchell, C Sykes
General Surgery M C Ball, D G Nasmyth
Gynaecology V Bamigboye, I Y Hussein, P Misra, V Sharan
Ophthalmology E Khadem, B Moate
Orthopaedics A Baqai
Pain Management J Hodkinson
Psychotherapy R Harrington
Urology K Madhra, R Y Wilson

Abbey Sefton Hospital Sefton Suite
University Hospital Aintree, Lower Lane, Liverpool L9 7AL
Tel: 0151 257 6700 Fax: 0151 257 6719
Email: sefton@abbeyhospitals.co.uk
Website: www.abbeyhospitals.co.uk
Owners: Abbey Hospitals Ltd
Total Beds: 24

Manager Suzanne Greenwood

Cardiology A Amadi, G Davis, R S Hornung, E Rodrigues, P Wong
Dermatology R Parslew
ENT A Daud, S Jackson, T H J Lesser, V Nandapalan, N Roland, A Swift
Gastroenterology N Krasner, R Sturgess
General Medicine I F Casson, K Mohanty, A Sharma, M A Siddiqi, J Turner, C Warburton
General Surgery D J Cave-Bigley, J Dhorajiwala, J Joseph, D Kerrigan, L Martin, P McCulloch, M Scott, P Skaife, I Stevenson, A Wu
Gynaecology U Abdullah, P Bousfield, M Johnstone, D Parkinson, G Rowland, G Shaw, C Thom
Haematology A Olujohinobe, B Woodcock
Nephrology K A Abraham, C Gradden
Neurology N Fletcher, C A Young
Neurosurgery N Buxton
Ophthalmology D I Clark, A Kamal, S Kaye, M Khan, G M Kyle, I B Marsh
Oral and Maxillofacial Surgery J S Brown, C Jones, D Richardson, D Vaughan
Orthopaedics N Barton-Hanson, P Brownson, C Butcher, R A Evans, B Pennie, M H Thornloe, H P J Walsh
Pain Management T Nash, J Wiles
Plastic Surgery R Alvi, R Bryson, K Hancock
Psychiatry M Agarwal, J Mumford
Rheumatology R Moots, R N Thompson
Urology D Machin, S Vesey, E P M Williamson

All Hallows Hospital
Station Road, Ditchingham, Bungay NR35 2QL
Tel: 01986 892728 Fax: 01986 895063
Email: info@all-hallows.org.uk
Website: www.all-hallows.org.uk
Owners: Charity/Association
Total Beds: 30

Belvedere Private Clinic
Knee Hill, Abbey Wood, London SE2 0GD
Tel: 020 8310 8866 Fax: 020 8311 8249
Email: info@belvedereclinic.co.uk
Website: www.belvedereclinic.co.uk
Owners: Privately Owned
Total Beds: 8

Benenden Hospital
Goddards Green Road, Benenden, Cranbrook TN17 4AX
Tel: 01580 240333 Fax: 01580 241877
Owners: Benenden Healthcare Society Ltd
Total Beds: 145

Manager K J Hesketh

Birkdale Clinic (Rotherham) Ltd
Clifton Lane, Rotherham S65 2AJ
Tel: 01709 828928 Fax: 01709 828372
Email: reception@birkdale-clinic.com
Website: www.birkdaleclinic.com
Owners: Privately Owned
Total Beds: 22

Anaesthetics K Ahmed, P J Barrett, B B Bhala, S Bhandari, A Blackburn, M N Calhaem, K T Ch'Ng, R P Foo, I C Grant, J E Hunsley, P C Khandewal, A Mallick, B R Milne, R J Muirhead, Y Myint, D M Newby, C D Palmer, P Y A Poon, H H Raithatha, K Ruiz, R Shaikh, M M Shalaby, T P Sivagnanam, I P Whitehead, R Wveston
Cardiology R Muthusamy, L H Soo
Dental Surgery R Aggarwal, R K F Bird, C L Hemmington, K J Phelan
ENT L H Durham, P A Harkness, J M Lancer
General Practice P A Bardsley, P Basumani, P J A Willemse
General Surgery M M A Bassuini, I D Crate, R B Jones, N Kazzazi
Geriatric Medicine B K Mondal
Gynaecology D W Fenton, A Kumar, D Patel
Medico-Legal P A Bradley, M L Garrett, M Harding, P Majumdar, M S Sorefan
Ophthalmology M Atia, P Baranyovits, P K Bhatnagar, T K J Chan, A-S A Ibraheim, M Jabir, V V Kayarkar, K M Khan, A K Mishra, M D Saloojee, A A Zaidi
Oral and Maxillofacial Surgery D S Holt, P G McAndrew

Orthopaedics S H Ali, S Madan, A Mubashir, A J S Rees, M M Zaman
Physiotherapy A D Gleadall
Plastic Surgery C Adamo, H Antoniadou, H F Blaschke, S Ciaschi, M D'Arcangelo, M A Kelly, E Keramidas, M Marcellino, M Persico, A Rezai, B Sleiter
Psychiatry R T Abed, B M Mehta, A H Soliman
Urology A Q Khattak, B T Parys

Birmingham Central Daycare Unit

1sr Floor, Guildhall Buildings, Navigation Street, Birmingham B2 4BT
Tel: 08457 304030
Owners: BPAS (British Pregnancy Advisory Service)

Manager June Taylor

The Birmingham Nuffield Hospital

22 Somerset Road, Edgbaston, Birmingham B15 2QQ
Tel: 0121 456 2000 Fax: 0121 454 5293
Email: bir.enq@nuffieldhospitals.org.uk
Website: www.nuffieldhospitals.org.uk
Owners: Nuffield Hospitals
Total Beds: 60

Manager Juli Breakwell

Audiology S Burrell, H Cooper, S Hayes
Cardiology R Armad, N Buller, G Y Lip, R Watson
Dental J Hamburger, A McLaughlin, M J Shaw, A J Summerwill, K Warren
Dermatology A Abdullah, C J Paul, K Ryatt, D G Stewart, C Tan
Dietetics S Parkinson
ENT J B Campbell, P Dekker, E W Fisher, C R Jennings, A Johnson, M Kuo, D Morgan, D W Proops
Gastroenterology R Boulton, H Bradby, I Chesner, B T Cooper, T Iqbal, M Lewis, P Wilson
General Medicine A S Bates, D G Beevers, M Carmalt, P Davies, D McLeod, M Waite
General Surgery A Aukland, J Buckels, D J Campbell, I A Donovan, D England, J Fielding, T Ismail, H Khaira, M Lee, S Radley, S Shiralkar, S Silverman, S Smith, R Spychal, M Vairavan, R K Vohra
Genitourinary Medicine K Radcliffe
Gynaecology M Afnan, A S Arunkalaivanan, S Blunt, G Downey, J M Emens, J Gupta, D Luesley, C Mann, M H Mattar, M Shafi, P Toozs-Hobson, J Williamson
Haematology J Murray
Neurology C Clarke, M T Heafield, J Winer
Neurosurgery G Flint, A Jackowski, J Wasserberg, S C Zygmunt
Occupational Health L Wall
Oncology D Peake
Ophthalmology A Jacks, A T Murray, E O'Neill, T Reuser, R Scott, G Sutton
Oral and Maxillofacial Surgery S Dover, M Wake
Orthopaedics E K Alpar, K G Baloch, D Bowden, C F Bradish, G Brown, R Chakraverty, G S Chana, D Dunlop, S S Geeranavar, V Goswami, M Herron, J Kersley, D J McMinn, S Parekh, A Pimpalnerkar, J Plewes, K M Porter, H Rahman, B K Singh, A J Stirling, R Treacy, O N Tubbs
Paediatrics R G Buick, H Chandran, A Gatrad, P Gornall, D Kelly, S Murphy, K Nathavitharana, K Parashar, S Rose, A S Vathenen
Pain Management L Blaney, D Dubash, F Duncan, B Kumar, J Pooni
Plastic Surgery J Goldin, R Lester, H Nishikawa, H Peart, G Sterne, G Titley
Podiatry J Malik
Psychology D Muss, A Norris, F Zaw
Rheumatology S Bowman, K Grindulis, R Jubb, R Situnayake
Speech Therapy P O'Donnell, H Williams
Urology R Devarajan, A Doherty, D Farrar, P Ryan

Blackdown Clinic

Old Milverton Lane, Blackdown, Leamington Spa CV32 6RW
Tel: 08457 304030
Email: info@bpas.org
Website: www.bpas.org
Owners: BPAS (British Pregnancy Advisory Service)
Total Beds: 10

Manager Carol Gough

Blackheath Brain Injury Rehabilitation Centre

80-82 Blackheath Hill, London SE10 8AB
Tel: 020 8692 4007 Fax: 020 8694 8316
Email: blackheath@fshc.co.uk
Owners: The Huntercombe Hospitals

BMI The Alexandra Hospital

Mill Lane, Cheadle SK8 2PX
Tel: 0161 428 3656 Fax: 0161 491 3867
Email: alex@bmihealthcare.co.uk
Website: www.bmihealthcare.co.uk
Owners: BMI Healthcare
Total Beds: 170

Manager Geoff Williams

BMI The Alexandra Hospital, Victoria Park

108-112 Daisy Bank Road, Manchester M14 5QH
Tel: 0161 257 2233 Fax: 0161 256 3128
Email: gstone@bmihealthcare.co.uk
Website: www.bmihealthcare.co.uk
Owners: BMI Healthcare
Total Beds: 25

Manager Rob Thomas

BMI Bath Clinic

Claverton Down Road, Combe Down, Bath BA2 7BR
Tel: 01225 835555 Fax: 01225 835900
Email: bath@bmihealthcare.co.uk
Website: www.bmihealthcare.co.uk
Owners: BMI Healthcare
Total Beds: 75

Manager Robert Thomas

BMI The Beardwood Hospital

Preston New Road, Blackburn BB2 7AE
Tel: 01254 507607 Fax: 01254 507608
Email: beardwood@bmihealthcare.co.uk
Website: www.bmihealthcare.co.uk
Owners: BMI Healthcare
Total Beds: 31

Manager Mark Almond

BMI The Beaumont Hospital

Old Hall Clough, Chorley New Road, Lostock, Bolton BL6 4LA
Tel: 01204 404404 Fax: 01204 404488
Email: sjgreenhalgh@bmihealthcare.co.uk
Website: www.bmihealthcare.co.uk
Owners: BMI Healthcare
Total Beds: 34

Manager Kate Crewdson

BMI Bishops Wood Hospital

Rickmansworth Road, Northwood HA6 2JW
Tel: 01923 835814 Fax: 01923 835181
Email: bishopswood@bmihealthcare.co.uk
Website: www.bmihealthcare.co.uk
Owners: BMI Healthcare
Total Beds: 41

Manager Eileen Scrase

ENT Surgery V Cumberworth, R Farrell, A Kalan, J Marais
General Surgery E Babu, S Chadwcik, Mr Das, Mr Mitchenere, Y Mohsen, Mr Paes, Mr Sarin
Gynaecology V Cook, A Hextall, N Jackson, N S Nicholas, M L Padwick, V Robinson, N R Watson
Oncology K Ardeshna, R Ashford, Dr Fermont, Dr Glynne-Jones, Dr Harrison, Dr Makepeace, A Makris, P Nathan, Dr Ostler, Professor Rustin, N Shah
Ophthalmics Mr Bloom, Mr Kodati, Mr Lee, Mr Miller, Mr Tolia, Mr Townsend
Orthopaedics A Allardice, S Atrah, Mr Belham, Mr Bodey, R Coull, Mr Dooley, J Jessop, S Kamineni, R Kucheria, Mr Langstaff, Mr Mackenney, J Perez, Mr Reissis, Mr Thakkar
Plastic Surgery J Chana, Mr Cussons, Mr Gault, Mr Grobbelaar, Mr Harrison, N Kang, Mr Smith
Urology M Laniado, K J Ng, M Pancharatnam, A Pope

BMI The Blackheath Hospital

40-42 Lee Terrace, Blackheath, London SE3 9UD
Tel: 020 8318 7722 Fax: 020 8318 2542
Email: blackheath@bmihealthcare.co.uk
Website: www.bmihealthcare.co.uk
Owners: BMI Healthcare
Total Beds: 69

Manager Roger Skipp

BMI Chatsworth Suite

Chesterfield Royal Hospital, Calow, Chesterfield S44 5BL
Tel: 01246 544400 Fax: 01246 205703
Email: chatsworth@bmihealthcare.co.uk
Website: www.bmihealthcare.co.uk
Owners: BMI Healthcare
Total Beds: 18

Manager George Blanchard

BMI The Chaucer Hospital

Nackington Road, Canterbury CT4 7AR
Tel: 01227 825100 Fax: 01227 762733
Email: chaucer@bmihealthcare.co.uk
Website: www.bmihealthcare.co.uk
Owners: BMI Healthcare
Total Beds: 60

Manager Stephen Gough

Cardiology J Fisher, K Kamalvand, D Lythall, A Morgan, A Norris, A Owen
Dermatology D Goldin, M Hudson-Peacock, C Irvine, V Nield
ENT J Fairley, D Mitchell, N Padgham, P Robinson, H Sharp
Fertility Services J Davies, P Evans, N Rafla, L Shaw
Gastroenterology S Barton, A F Fuller, P Wheeler
General Medicine G Batty, M Flynn, A Heller, A Johnson, I Sturgess
General Surgery R Collins, R Heddle, D Jackson, G Tsavellas, N Wilson
Gynaecology J Davies, P Evans, H Hamoud, J Learmont, M Milligan, K Neales, A Nordin, N Rafla, L Shaw
Neurology N Moran, N Munro, S Pollock
Neurosurgery R Gullan, P Hamlyn
Oncology / Radiotherapy R Coltart, N Mithal, H Smedley
Ophthalmology N Andrew, R Darvell, R de Cock, R Edwards, M Fouladi, B Greaves, M Heravi, J McConnell, W Poon
Oral and Maxillofacial Surgery N Bradley, N Goodger, C Hendy, T J Storrs
Orthopaedic Surgery N Blackburn, J Casha, W Dunnet, P Housden, L Louette, R Shrivastava, R Wetherell, O Yanni, H Zahn
Paediatrics N Martin
Pain Management R Bhadresha, C Lamb, P Moskovits, N Senasinghe
Pathology G Evans, R Gale, C Pocock, M Winter
Plastic Surgery J Boorman, J Davison, R Norris
Radiology M Downws, P Elton, K Entwistle, S Moorhouse, I Morrison, V Soh
Rheumatology P Bull, A Leak, R Withrington
Urology W Choi, J W H Evans, K Murray, N Shrotri

BMI Chelsfield Park Hospital

Bucks Cross Road, Chelsfield, Orpington BR6 7RG
Tel: 01689 877855 Fax: 01689 837439
Email: chelsfield@bmihealthcare.co.uk
Website: www.bmihealthcare.co.uk
Owners: BMI Healthcare
Total Beds: 50

Manager Peter Harris

BMI The Chiltern Hospital

London Road, Great Missenden HP16 0EN
Tel: 01494 890890 Fax: 01494 890250
Email: chiltern@bmihealthcare.co.uk
Website: www.bmihealthcare.co.uk
Owners: BMI Healthcare
Total Beds: 75

Manager Roger Lye

BMI The Clementine Churchill Hospital

Sudbury Hill, Harrow HA1 3RX
Tel: 020 8872 3872 Fax: 020 8872 3871
Email: cch@bmihealthcare.co.uk
Website: www.bmihealthcare.co.uk/cch
Owners: BMI Healthcare
Total Beds: 141

Manager Michael Parsons

Allergies M Y Karim
Anaesthetics K Agyare, M Albin, M A Ali, L Allan, J Anadanesan, N Aravindhan, G Baker, J P Barcroft, S J Bates, M J Boscoe, B J Bracey, E Bradshaw, A Bristow, M D Brunner, A H Castello-Cortes, P Chakrabarti, M Chandra, R J Cohen, M A Cooper, C A Douglass, J P Downer, M D Esler, S Gautama, R A Griffin, S Guirguis, J W Harris, S J Harrison, M Hasan, M Hetreed, A M Hewlett, M Kadry, B S Kamath, K M Konieczko, T Kuwani, R S Laishley, A V Levison, S R Littler, D Lomax, B A Loughnan, D N Lucas, J Magner, P McGowan, M M Meurer-Laban, D C Mills, J Mukherjee, K N Nandakumar, D C Nathwani, M Nel, D Newton, C E Nightingale, B J Norman, A C O'Callaghan, S Papas, T Peachey, T M Peters, M W Platt, Z Qureshi, Y Rajakulendran, V Ramachandra, K V Ratnam, D R O Redman, M Renna, D Robinson, P N Robinson, A P Rubin, J S Ruston, G Rutter, M D Sacks, C L Sadler, J Salt, A Scurr, J Shah, R S Shanthakumar, R Sharpe, V S Sidhu, R S Simons, A M Skelly, J M B Smallman, M A Smith, I D Srikantharajah, T A Stambach, M E Stanford, M Stevens, E Stielow, S Sudunagunta, G Suntharalingam, D U Uzeirbegovic, D J A Vaughan, R K Verma, P M Ward, J Weinbren, E M Whitehead, A B Wijctillcka, A Wijetunge, R Woolf, M W Wrigley
Cardiology H W L Bethell, C M Dancy, S W Dubrey, M Z Farrag, J S Gill, R Greenbaum, R Grocott-Mason, D Hackett, C Isley, R R Kaprielian, A Kelion, J S Kooner, A Lahiri, I S Malik, G Mikhail, D J Patel, N S Peters, P Punjabi, R Senior, A Sethi, N G Stephens, A G Violaris
Chemical Pathology P Frost
Colorectal Surgery R K S Phillips
Dermatology S K Goolamali, C Hardman, A G L Lambiris, J N Leonard, L R Lever, J McFadden, F M Pope
Endocrinology J Burke, S McHardy-Young
ENT Surgery S Abramovich, R Auerbach, V L Cumberworth, N J Daly, R S Dhillon, R W Farrell, A Kalan, J Marais, A Narula, A Parikh, K S Patel, S H Paun, A C Robinson, R Ryan, P C Taylor, N S Tolley
Gastroenterology J D Arnold, D S Bansi, A V Emmanuel, G E Holdstock, M R Jacyna, D P Maudgal, N I McNeill, I C Mitchell, M C Pitcher, D Sherman, I F Trotman
General Medicine H M B Branley, D L Cohen, R N Davidson, P J Evans, M Harries, D D Lubel, V Mak, R Mathur, A Mir, D Ornadel, S W Roche, M Rudolf, K Steer, P R Studdy, M Sweatman

General Surgery D A M Al-Musawi, A Amin, R Anwar, M Burke, S Chadwick, A M Chopada, J N Crinnion, A Darzi, E Dinakara-Babu, P Forouhi, S Gould, N Hakim, T S Hussain, A Isla, C J Kelley, W Kmiot, P McDonald, P Mitchenere, Y M A Mohsen, A R Qureshi, S Ramesh, S C Renton, D P Sellu, B N Shah, D Sharma, H Singhal, J J Smith, R Vashisht
Genitourinary Medicine J John, M Kapembwa
Gynaecology Y Abrahams, S Banerjee, S Beski, O Braithwaite, L Fusi, A D Gordon, A D Haeri, K F Harrington, S Kerslake, R F Lamont, B V Lewis, O Louca, R Lyons, D E A Manning, N H Morris, M L Padwick, J Pitkin, S Porter, A R Priddy, F Raslan, P Sarhanis, P Sarkar, J A D Spencer, C S W Wright
Haematology Z Abboudi, G M Abrahamson, U Hegde, D MacDonald, N J Philpott
Histopathology E A Courtauld, G Dixon
Maxillofacial Surgery M G Gilhooly, N S Matthews
Nephrology A B D Palmer, M E Phillips, M M Yaqoob
Neurology M L P Gross, R Kapoor, O Malik, H Manji, D Peterson, R Shakir, P Sharma
Neuroradiology M C Patel
Neurosurgery J B Allibone
Oncology D C Fermont, R T Glynne-Jones, C Nutting, N Shah, C Vernon
Ophthalmology R Auplish, M Beaconsfield, P M H Cherry, W J Dinning, C F J Grindle, S Kheterpal, S M Kodati, A S Kosmin, N Lee, M H Miller, C K Patel, M Rahman, N J Young
Oral Surgery G Gardiner, G F Goubran, H Thuau
Orthopaedic Surgery G E Allardice, M Bartlett, J I Bayley, G J Belham, W Bodey, S Cannon, K Desai, J F Dooley, L Freedman, I F Fyfe, N A Hassan, L Heras, J Hollingdale, C J McCullough, J Murphy, S Nathan, R Pandit, M F Pearse, J Perez, N Reissis, E Saavedra, M Sala, R K Strachan, D H Thakkar, F H Thomas, T Zaman
Paediatrics W Hyer, G A Khakoo, C Kukendra-Raja, A F Massoud, K Sawhney, A R Shah, G Supramaniam
Physicians C Daniels, D F C Hopkins, S Rizvi
Plastic Surgery A Awwad, D Crawford, D Gault, A Grobbelaar, R Grover, D H Harrison, U Khan, P J Smith, V Vijh
Psychiatry (OP only) D Veale
Psychology D Shah-Armon
Radiology T Beale, B Gajjar, A L Hine, R J Kantor, D Katz, D Remedios, I M Shirley, W Te h, T Tran, B P Twomey, R Wilkins
Rheumatology A Al-Hussani, H Berry, C B Colaco, D M Davis, M Gumpel, M S Irani, R Keen, M Naughton, R Rees, G Room
Urology S Agarwal, M D Dinneen, J Elkabir, G A Fowlis, M J Gleeson, V Izegbu, M Laniado, A D Mee, S Minhas, H G Motiwala, K J Ng, N O'Donoghue, C W Ogden, A Pope, T P Rosenbaum, J Webster
Vascular Surgery S Das, G Geroulakos, D Greenstein, T Paes, S Sarin, S Selvakumar

BMI The Droitwich Spa Hospital

St Andrew's Road, Droitwich WR9 8DN
Tel: 01905 793333 Fax: 01905 773334
Email: droitwich@bmihealthcare.co.uk
Website: www.bmihealthcare.co.uk
Owners: BMI Healthcare
Total Beds: 46

Manager Michael Scott

BMI The Esperance Hospital

Hartington Place, Eastbourne BN21 3BG
Tel: 01323 411188 Fax: 01323 410626
Email: esperance@bmihealthcare.co.uk
Website: www.bmihealthcare.co.uk
Owners: BMI Healthcare
Total Beds: 50

Manager Sue Mulvey

Cardiology G Lloyd, N Sulke
Endocrinology J Bending
ENT G Manjaly, N Volaris
Gastroenterology A Dunk, D Neal
General Medicine C Arthulathmudali, J J Bending, D Maxwell, J Wilkinson
General Surgery A Aldridge, G Evans, P Rowe, M Saunders, B Stoodley
Gynaecology V Argent, K Ayers, D Chui, T M Malak, A Soyemi, J Zaidi
Nephrology S Holt
Neurology W Macleod
Oncology N Hodson, J Simpson
Ophthalmology D Garlick, J Hickman-Casey, A Plumb, M J Wearne
Oral and Maxillofacial Surgery K Altman, A Moody, M Williams
Orthopaedics A Armitage, A Bonnici, J D'Arcy, B Hinves, S James, K Rowe, J Sheppard, A Skyrme
Pain Management J McGowan
Plastic Surgery K Cullen, J Pereira
Rheumatology A Pool
Urology W Lawrence, R Plail, P Rimington, G Watson

BMI Fawkham Manor Hospital

Manor Lane, Fawkham, Longfield DA3 8ND
Tel: 01474 879900 Fax: 01474 879827
Email: marketing_fawkham@bmihealthcare.co.uk
Website: www.bmihealthcare.co.uk
Owners: BMI Healthcare
Total Beds: 39

Manager Sally Hill

Acupuncture/Pain Management S H Ahmad, B Lobo
Cardiology D Brennand-Roper, W Martin
Chest Medicine M Mushtaq
Clinical Haematology R Ezekwasili
Dermatology A Barkley, M Boss, A Shanks
ENT D A Bowdler, J P Davis, P Gluckman, A Hosny, S Surenthiran
Gastroenterology R Ede, W Melia
General Medicine S Ibrahim, P Ryan
General Surgery M Kerwat, O Khan, M J McIrvine, M C Parker, M Stewart, P Strauss, G Thomas, T K Walters, H Wegstapel
Microbiology A Shaw
Neurology P R J Barnes, I Zoukos
Obstetrics and Gynaecology I Jacobs, M H Jones, A Lesseps, R MacDermott, A Schreiner, R N J Smith
Ophthalmology M Gibbens, C Hugkulstone, O R Kamel, H Laganowski
Oral and Maxillofacial Surgery A Brown, C Howell
Orthopaedics A K L Addison, A A Bassily, K Borowsky, E Faddoul, M R Fraser, S Jain, B A Kamdar, A Leyshon, F S Moftah, S Purkayastha, M S Sait, D Thakkar
Paediatrics K Ogbuneke, H R Patel
Plastic Surgery P Chapman, A Hosny, A Khandwala, R W Smith
Psychiatry S Carman
Radiology Dr Al-Murrani, P D Holder, C Koo, M J Michell, N Sathananthan, S Sivathasan
Rheumatology El Medani, S Navaratnam, I Vadasz
Urology I K Dickinson, R Ravi, P M Thompson

BMI The Foscote Hospital

2 Foscote Rise, Banbury OX16 9XP
Tel: 01295 252281 Fax: 01295 272877
Email: foscote@bmihealthcare.co.uk
Website: www.bmihealthcare.co.uk
Owners: BMI Healthcare
Total Beds: 16

Manager Neil Webb

Adult Cardiology I Arnold
Anaesthesia A Bokhari, S Chamberlain, J Everatt, P Laurie, E Richards, C Wait, G Walker, D Willatts
Dental Surgery M Amsel
Gastroenterology A Ellis, J Marshall
General Surgery N Dehalvi, C Griffiths, R Marshall, J Perkins
Gynaecology S Canty, H Naoum, J Nicholls
Oncology E Sugden

Ophthalmology P Rosen
Oral/maxillofacial S Watt-Smith
Orthopaedics N Gillham, A Hughes, J Owen, B Shafighian
Plastic Surgery O Cassell
Radiology B Barry, K Choji, H D'Costa, P Haggett, F Macleod
Urology J Crew

BMI The Garden Hospital

46-50 Sunny Gardens Road, Hendon, London NW4 1RP
Tel: 020 8457 4500 Fax: 020 8457 4567
Email: garden@bmihealthcare.co.uk
Website: www.bmihealthcare.co.uk
Owners: BMI Healthcare
Total Beds: 30

Manager Elizabeth Sharp

Breast Surgery R Qureshi
Cardiology J Coghlan, J Davar, H Nouriel
Chest Medicine S Khan, H Makker
Dermatology R Aron, T Leslie, W Robles, Dr Rustin, Dr Stevens
Dietetics J Bernett
Endocrinology N Fand, Dr Jackson
ENT Surgery R Auerbach, E Douek, T Joseph, R Quiney, G Radcliffe, M Stearns
Gastroenterology G Bevan, O Epstein, M Hamilton, L Lovat, B Smith, R Vicary, V Wong
General Surgery D Baker, C Elton, R Le Roy Bird, A Loh, I Mitchell, K Waters
Geriatric Medicine D Levy, D Lubel
Gynaecology S Banerjee, L Bernhardt, M Broadbent, F Haddad, A Rodin
Haematology A Mehta, A Virchis
Neurology C Caplan, Dr Guiloff, P Jarman, Dr Rees
Neurophysiology Dr Youl
Ophthalmology T Fallon, J Forbes, M Harris, J Joseph, S Levy
Oral and Maxillofacial Surgery W Halfpenny, R Liversedge
Orthopaedics M Kurer, H Nwaboku, P Thomas, G Vardi
Paediatrics N Hasson, A Joffe, G Katz
Pain Management P McGowan, A Ordman
Plastic Surgery J Goldin
Radiology J Berger, L Berger, A Davies, J Festenstein, G Kaplan, K Lotzof, A Marcus, Dr Stein
Rheumatology H Beynon, F Girgis, N Hasson, J Rosenberg
Sports Medicine C Crosby
Urology T Briggs, J Gelister, F Mumtaz
Vascular Medicine D Baker, R Le Roy Bird, A Loh, K Waters

BMI Goring Hall Hospital

Bodiam Avenue, Goring-by-Sea, Worthing BN12 5AT
Tel: 01903 506699 Fax: 01903 242348
Website: www.bmihealthcare.co.uk
Owners: BMI Healthcare
Total Beds: 52

Manager Tim Walker

BMI The Hampshire Clinic

Basing Road, Old Basing, Basingstoke RG24 7AL
Tel: 01256 357111 Fax: 01256 329986
Email: hampshire@bmihealthcare.co.uk
Website: www.bmihealthcare.co.uk
Owners: BMI Healthcare
Total Beds: 65

Manager Jan Hale

Allergy Dr Turner
Chiropractic Mr Linscott
Dermatology Dr Crone, Dr Fawcett, Dr Powell
ENT Mr Blanshard, Mr Spraggs
General Medicine Dr Bishop, Dr Brookes, Dr Fowler, Dr Guy, Dr McKinlay, Dr Ramage, Dr Yek
General Surgery Mr Cecil, Mr Gold, Professor Heald, Mr John, Mr Moran, Mr Rees, Miss Stebbing
Gynaecology Miss Iffland, Mr Jardine Brown, Mr O'Sullivan, Mr Sayer
Haematology Dr Milne
Neurology Dr Lawton
Oncology Dr Sharpe, Dr Tinkler
Ophthalmology Mr Elliot, Mr Govan, Mr Keightley, Mr Morsman, Mr Moss, Mr Sandy
Oral and Maxillofacial Surgery C Kerawalla, Mr Ogus
Orthopaedics J Benfield, J Britton, R Browne, K Conn, J Hobby, G Stranks, N Thomas
Orthopaedics and Trauma B Elvin, H Simpson
Orthotics J Blair
Osteopathy I Harrison
Paediatrics I Primavesi
Pain Relief W Hamann, J Hurley
Plastic Surgery D Crawford, I Whitworth
Podiatry M Healey
Radiology D Bailey, I Green, H O'Neil, G O'Sullivan, D Peppercorn, G Plant, D Shelley, G Ubuyakar
Rheumatology P Prouse
Speech Therapy S Bell
Sports Medicine M Wotherspoon
Urology C Eden, H Mostafid
Varicose Vein Clinic S Tristram

BMI The Harbour Hospital

St Mary's Road, Poole BH15 2BH
Tel: 01202 244200 Fax: 01202 244201
Email: gtripp@bmihealthcare.co.uk
Website: www.bmihealthcare.co.uk
Owners: BMI Healthcare
Total Beds: 40

Manager Gill Tripp

Dermatology Dr Burden-Jones, C J Stevens
ENT H J Cox, D G John, S Rhys-Williams, P M Scott
General Medicine D Bruce, D Coppini, S Crowther, W Gatling, A McLeod, J Millar, N Sharer, J Snook, M Thomas
General Surgery N Bell, A Evans, S W Hosking, J Pain, R Talbot
Gynaecology J N T Edwards, R Henry, T Hillard, R Sawdy, J Scott, S Sullivan
Hand Surgery Mr O'Connor, J Southgate
Oncology P Crellin, D Goode, T Hickish, V Lawrence, R Osborne
Ophthalmology L Bray, Mr Morris, Mr Rowley, Mr Tadros
Oral and Maxillofacial Surgery V Lankovan, A Markus
Orthopaedics D Cain, J Dinley, M Farrar, R Hartley, A Harvey, R Middleton, L O'Hara
Plastic Surgery M Cadier, Mr Graham, J Hobby, E Tiernan
Rheumatology S Richards, P Thompson
Urology C Carter, J Rundle

BMI The Highfield Hospital

Manchester Road, Rochdale OL11 4LZ
Tel: 01706 655121 Fax: 01706 356759
Email: highfield@bmihealthcare.co.uk
Website: www.bmihealthcare.co.uk
Owners: BMI Healthcare
Total Beds: 57

Manager W Davies

Accident and Emergency K Ali, H Dardouri, S Derbyshire, Mr Duane, Dr Gorgees, J D Lewis, P K Luthra, M Saab, R Sohail, J Stuart
Anaesthetics Dr Abdelatti, Dr Aglan, A T Arasan, Dr Barrie, Dr Bhishma, Dr Boyd, Dr Brim, Dr Chadwick, Dr Cook, L Cook, P R Cook, Dr Deulkar, Dr Drake, Dr Eadsforth, N El Mikatti, T Eliathamby, Dr Eskander, Dr Gadiyar, Dr Gandhi, Dr Goldwater, N H Graveston, Dr Greenhalgh, Dr Gregory, Dr Gupta, Dr Hartopp, R Hockman, Dr Hussain, Dr Jena, Dr Jones, Dr Kapoor, Dr Kataria, J Kenworthy, J Kini, Dr Kotak, Dr Krishnan, Dr Kulkarni, Dr Longbottom, Dr Luthra, Dr Mc Geachie, Dr Madhavan, R M Mayall, J K Mazumder, Dr Middleton, S Mirza, Dr Mollah, Dr Ousta, Dr Pandya, Dr Petts, Dr Puddy, Dr Rehman, Dr Richards, Dr Ritto, Dr

Robson, A Sabri, K Sbrahan, Dr Shah, Dr Shaikh, A Shakir, Dr Simpson, Dr Sivagnanam, C Smith, Dr Stellar, Dr Stewart, K Sultan, A Swayamprakasam, Dr Tierney, Dr Vallance, S Varshney, Dr Watts, Y Y Youssef
Intensive Care Dr Graveston, Dr McGeachie, Dr Mazumder, Dr Middleton, Dr Mollah, Dr Richards, Dr Rittoo, Dr Swayamprakas, Dr Watts
Cardiology Dr Coupe, Dr Hargreaves, D S Horner, Dr Mushahwar, Dr Swan
Cardiothoracic Surgery Mr Grotte
Chest Diseases Dr Saboor
Colorectal Surgery Mr Carlson, Mr Kutiyanawala, A Rate, D Richards, H Sharif, Mr Siddiqui, Mr Wilson
Cytology Dr Butterworth
Cytopathology Dr El Terafi
Dermatology Dr Bhushan, Dr Fitzgerald, Dr Macdonald
Dietetics Mrs Jones
ENT Mr Brandrick, Mr Gordon, Mr Kobbe, Mr Mehta, P Morar, Mr Murthy, Mr Saha, P Sharma, V L Sharma, Mr Shehab, Mr Sheppard, H Tay, Mr Taylor
Gastroenterology Dr Babbs, P Conlong, Dr Foster, Dr George, Dr Goodman, C Grimley, Dr Haslam, Dr Rameh, Dr Whatley
General Medicine Dr Akintewe, Dr Babbs, B Bajaj, G L Bhan, M P Chopra, Dr Conlong, Dr Finlay, Dr Foster, Dr George, Dr Goodman, Dr Jegarajah, Dr Khanna, Dr Klimiuk, S Kouta, A Naraya, Dr Pattrick, R Prudham, Dr Rameh, A Robinson, Dr Savage, Dr Sharma, Dr Shreeve, Dr Smithard, Dr Sridharan, Dr Taylor, Dr Vedi, G Whatley
General Practice Dr Rajasansir
General Surgery Mr Akhtar, Mr Al-Khafaf, A Ben-Hamida, Mr Carlson, M Madan, Mr Siddiqui, Mr Wilson, Mr Afify, Mr DeSousa, Mr Ellenbogen, Mr Flook, M Hadfield, Mr Higham, Mr Hulton, Mr Kutiyanawala, Mr McIntosh, Mr Oshodi, Mr Pearson, A Rate, Mr Richards, S Salman, Mr Scott, Mr Sharif, Mr Tait, H J Vadegar, Mr Williams, M C Wilson, Mr Woodyer
Genitourinary Medicine Dr Ahmed
Geriatric Medicine Dr Bhan, Dr Khanna, A Narayan
Gynaecology Mr Ali, Mr Amu, Mr Atalla, Mr Aziz, Mr Boulos, Dr Dickson, Mr Edozien, Mr Ghobrial, Dr Haworth, Mr Hayden, Miss Jones, Mr MacFoy, Mr Mander, Dr Rahman, Dr Russell, A Smith, Dr Wake, Dr Watson, Dr Zaklama
Health Screening - Female Dr Michael, Dr Worsell
Health Screening - Male Dr Finlay, Dr Sharma
Homoeopathy Dr Demetriou
Neurology Dr Mottshead, Dr Sherrington
Neurophysiology Dr Alani, Dr Bangash
Neurosurgery Mr Sofat, Mr Victoratos
Oncology Dr Sykes, Mr Wylie
Ophthalmology Mr Chitkara, Mr Garston, Mrs Goodall, Mr Hashmi, N A Jacobs, K Kafle, Mr Khan, Mr Lipton, Miss Morrison, S Natha, Mr Nylander, I Pearce, Mr Suharwardy, Mr Wright
Oral and Maxillofacial Surgery Mr Addy, Mr Foster, Mr Langton, Mr White, Mr Woodwards
Orthopaedics Mr Ali, Mr Allcock, T Asumu, Mr Brewood, Mr Buch, Mr Clayson, Mr Devadoss, Mr Doyle, Mr Ebizie, Mr Elsworth, Mr Hegab, Mr Hodgkinson, B Ilango, Mr Jacobs, Mr Jago, E Jago, Mr Kay, A Kociailkauski, Mr Kolb, Mr McGivney, H Marynissen, Mr Muddu, Mr Obeid, Mr Pena, R Sarin, Mr Schmitgen, S Shafqat, Mr Sochart, Mr Sundar, Mr Walker, A Wojcik
Orthotics H Bowker, J Turner
Paediatrics Dr Blumenthal, B Padmakumar
Plastic Surgery Dr Whitby
Psychiatry Dr Deo, Dr Marshall, Dr Rahman
Psychology C Marklow, Mr Nightingale, Mr Pattinson, Dr Priestley
Radiology M Aird, N Desai, Dr Jeyagopal, Dr Khan, Mr Kumar, Dr Lee Cheong, N S Malik, Dr Panditaratne, Dr Raja, Dr Shah, Dr Singanayagam, N Thomas, K C Uzoka, Dr Whitecross, Dr Winarso
Rheumatology Dr Bowden, Dr Haynes, P Klimiuk, Dr Smith
Speech Therapy Mrs Taylor
Urology Mr Barnes, Mr Chow, Mr Chowdhury, Mr Costello, M Gupta, Mr Kourah, Mr Sharma

BMI The Kings Oak Hospital

Chase Farm (North Side), The Ridgeway, Enfield EN2 8SD
Tel: 020 8370 9500 Fax: 020 8370 9501
Email: kingsoak@bmihealthcare.co.uk
Website: www.bmihealthcare.co.uk
Owners: BMI Healthcare
Total Beds: 52

Manager Liz Sharp

BMI The London Independent Hospital

1 Beaumont Square, Stepney Green, London E1 4NL
Tel: 020 7780 2400 Fax: 020 7780 2401
Email: lih@bmihealthcare.co.uk
Website: www.bmihealthcare.co.uk/lih
Owners: BMI Healthcare
Total Beds: 80

Manager Timothy Hayes

BMI The Manor Hospital

Church End, Biddenham, Bedford MK40 4AW
Tel: 01234 364252 Fax: 01234 325001
Email: manor@bmihealthcare.co.uk
Website: www.bmihealthcare.co.uk
Owners: BMI Healthcare
Total Beds: 23

Manager Anne McGregor
Accident and Emergency S Shankar
Anaesthetics B Fahmy, J Hughes, R Kavan, D Liu, S Lua, J McNamara, D Niblett, J Sizer, S Snape, J Wilson
Cardiology I Cooper, J Cooper
Care of the Elderly K Nandi, N Thangarajah, R Trounson
Dermatology K Burova, B Monk
Endocrinology N Morrish
ENT R Arasaratnam, M Frampton, T Hoare
General Medicine M Azher, R Harvey, J Saunders, E Thomas
General Surgery M Callam, A Eldin, R Foley, P Omotoso, D Parsons, D Skipper, P Tisi
Gynaecology G Budden, E Neale, A Ogborn, D Patil, S Reynolds, R Wallace
Nephrology P Warwicker
Neurology M Manford
Oncology R Thomas
Ophthalmology F F Fisher, S Pieris, A Sharma
Oral and Maxillofacial Surgery C Chan, M Simpson
Orthodontics A Hewitt
Orthopaedics P Edge, R Gunn, C Handley, G Nel, R Rawlins, T Riley, M Sood
Plastic Surgery A Attwood, S Papanastasiou, F Schreuder
Radiology S Barter, A Booth, A Egan, P Hicks, R Moxon, R Oakley, C Onyekwuluje, M Shaikh
Rheumatology S Rae
Urology I Hussain, N Waterfall

BMI Meriden Wing

Walsgrave Hospital, Clifford Bridge Road, Walsgrave, Coventry CV2 2DX
Tel: 024 7660 2772 Fax: 024 7660 2329
Email: meriden@bmihealthcare.co.uk
Website: www.bmihealthcare.co.uk
Owners: BMI Healthcare
Total Beds: 9

Manager Kate Denham

BMI The Nuneaton Private Hospital

132 Coventry Road, Nuneaton CV10 7AD
Tel: 024 7635 7500 Fax: 024 7635 7520
Email: nuneaton@bmihealthcare.co.uk
Website: www.bmihealthcare.co.uk
Owners: BMI Healthcare
Total Beds: 24

Manager Anne McGregor

Anaesthetics Dr Atayi, Dr Chari, Dr Clayton, Dr Correa, Dr Dako, Dr Feaver, Dr Jayarantnasingam, Dr Krishnamoorty, Dr Lele, Dr Mead, Dr Mendonca, Dr Miller, Dr Murthy, Dr Pearson, Dr Radhakrishna, Dr Ramanchandran, Dr Roberts, Dr Shawket, Dr Srivastava, Dr Susarla, Dr Taggart, Dr Tripathy
Audiometry Mrs Hayes
Cardiology Dr Haider
Dermatology Dr Berth Jones
ENT Mr Dekker, P J Patel, Mr Rejali
General Medicine Dr Handslip, Dr Narayanan, V Patel, Dr Raman, Dr Wood
General Surgery Mr Barros D'sa, Mr Bullen, Mr Haynes, Mr Higman, Mr Imray, Mr Lam, Mr Lele, Mr Matthew, Mr Nangalia, Mr Parkianathan, Mr Zayyan
Gynaecology Dr Matts, Mrs Navaneetham, Mr Okojie, Mrs Wahab
Neurophysiology Dr Hedge
Neurosurgery Mr Choksey, Mr Saxena
Ophthalmology Mr Kumar, Mr Pagliarini
Oral and Maxillofacial Surgery Mr Fagan
Orthopaedics Mr Reddy, Mr Salam, Mr Sharif, Mr Steingold
Orthoptics H Simpson
Pain Management Dr Nithianandan
Plastic and Reconstruction Mr Eltigani, Mr Groves, Mr Matthews, Mr Park, Mr Srivastava, Mr Varma
Psychiatry Dr Javed
Psychology Dr Farrell
Radiology Dr Bera, Mr Palit, Dr Sinha, Dr Vallance
Urology Mr Apakama, Mr Blacklock, Mr Desai, Mr Prasad, Mr Sriram, Mr Wills

BMI The Paddocks Hospital

Aylesbury Road, Princes Risborough HP27 OJS
Tel: 01844 276000 Fax: 01844 344521
Email: paddocks@bmihealthcare.co.uk
Website: www.bmihealthcare.co.uk
Owners: BMI Healthcare
Total Beds: 28

Manager Roger Lye

BMI The Park Hospital

Sherwood Lodge Drive, Burntstump Country Park, Arnold, Nottingham NG5 8RX
Tel: 0115 967 0670 Fax: 0115 967 0381
Email: park@bmihealthcare.co.uk
Website: www.bmihealthcare.co.uk
Owners: BMI Healthcare
Total Beds: 69

Manager Terence Lees

BMI The Princess Margaret Hospital

Osborne Road, Windsor SL4 3SJ
Tel: 01753 743434 Fax: 01753 743435
Email: pmh@bmihealthcare.co.uk
Website: www.bmihealthcare.co.uk
Owners: BMI Healthcare
Total Beds: 80

Manager Rosie Faunch

Anaesthetics P Balakrishnan, P Barnardo, M Blackmore, E Bourov, D Bukht, P Dadarkar, M Davies, J Dawson, G Dhond, J Fernandes, J M G Foster, D Gatha, G Kadiwal, M Kadry, D Kruchek, M Kubli, R Laishley, A Lawson, L Leibler, A Levison, R Loveland, J Mackenzie, J Margary, A J May, G Nemeth, C Nightingale, S Papas, J Pattison, D Penney, A Qureshi, I Ranganathan, J Rangasami, J Restall, M Russell, C Siemaszko, T Silva, J Smallman, B L Smith, K Spelina, C Stapleton, E Taylor, K Thomson, E Umerah, G Vora, M Wattie, S White, R Woolf, J Wraight
Cardiology K Barakat, R Blackwood, A Chow, R Foale, K Fox, I Malik, V Markides, J Mayet, D Missouris, P Ramrakha, S Rex, R Schilling, N Spyrou, P Wilkinson
Cardiothoracic Surgery P Kallis, M Petrou
Clinical Biochemistry I Walker
Dermatology S Neill, S Parker, V Walkden
Dietetics B Bhumber, K Flemming, V Williams
ENT Surgery C Aldren, N Bleach, P Chapman, J Hadley, R Hehar, A Jefferis, G Sandhu, S Wood
Gastroenterology J Booth, G Holdstock, R Sarsam, J Thornton
General Medicine R Chauhan, D Dove, N Gunasekera, L Hart, J Jordaan, S Rao, R Russell, R Scott, M Smith, J Wiggins, A Winning
General Surgery G Barrett, S Baxter, P Bearn, N Browning, P Dawson, A Desai, J Gilbert, A Gordon, N Menezes, P Rutter, J Scurr, S Shrotria, B Soin
Haematology P Mackie
Histopathology S Ibrahim, H Sharif
Immunology L Hawk
Medical Microbiology M P A Lessing
Nephrology S Smith
Neurology M Johnson, R Lane, R Nicholas
Neurophysiology S M J Smith
Neuroradiology I Colquhoun
Neurosurgery N D Mendoza
Obstetrics and Gynaecology A Bahmaie, E Dimitry, A Elias, J Fairbank, D Hyatt, F Imoh-ita, S Kalla, F Raslan, P Reginald, P Sarkar, J Spring, N Wales, J Wright
Oncology R Ashford, M Hall, A Neal, H Thomas, H Wasan
Ophthalmology J Duvall-Young, A Gupta, S Kheterpal, J McAllister, J McGraw, R Packard, A Pearson, V Tanner, S-L Watson
Optometry B Holland
Oral and Maxillofacial Surgery M Amin, R Carr, C Yates
Orthodontics D Slattery
Orthopaedic Surgery R Allum, D Bickerstaff, M Bloomfield, C Busch, C Clark, B Cohen, R Dega, D Harrison, A Hassan, A Howard, J Jones, R Kucheria, M Maheson, I McDermott, M Moiz, N Morgan, R Pool, H Roushdi, E Schilders, G Singer, R Sinnerton, M Thomas, A Unwin, G Vardi, L Williams
Paediatric Medicine G Clark, Z Huma, J Pearce, R Richardson
Periodontology S Pritlove-Carson
Plastic Surgery A Armstrong, D Crawford, J Dickinson, D Evans, C Khoo, D Sammut
Podiatry M O'Neill
General Practice A Chauhan, B Gilfeather, I Kundu, U Sharma
Psychiatry G Andrews, G Bell, P Loughlin
Radiology L Bellamy, M Charig, S Colenso, S Davidson, R Davies, S Ghiacy, R Grant, D Grieve, A Hassan, I Liyanage, C Luck, D Maudgil, N Moore, M Moreland, S Patel, D Reiff, C Rogers
Rheumatology A Hall, S Liyanage, G Patel
Thoracic Surgery E Townsend
Urology W Dunsmuir, N Harvey-Hills, C Hudd, O Karim, R Kulkarni, M Laniado, H Motiwala

BMI The Priory Hospital

Priory Road, Edgbaston, Birmingham B5 7UG
Tel: 0121 440 2323 Fax: 0121 440 0804
Email: priory@bmihealthcare.co.uk
Website: www.bmihealthcare.co.uk/priory
Owners: BMI Healthcare
Total Beds: 113

Manager John Sharp

BMI The Ridgeway Hospital

Moormead Road, Wroughton, Swindon SN4 9DD
Tel: 01793 814848 Fax: 01793 814852
Email: ridgeway@bmihealthcare.co.uk
Website: www.bmihealthcare.co.uk
Owners: BMI Healthcare
Total Beds: 50

Manager Sheila Maslin

Anaesthetics G Baigel, C Beeby, A Bullough, N Campbell, R Craig, A Dale, M D Entwistle, J Griffiths, H Jones, N Jones, W B Maxwell, M O'Connor, S O'Kelly, A J Pickworth, I D Smith, J Stone, M Tattersall, J C Van Hamel, M Walters
Dermatology J P Ellis, L R Whittam

ENT S Chalstrey, J Donnelly, D Gupta, T Higazi, A Waddell
General Medicine Dr Ahmed, E Barnes, E Giallombardo, P J V Hanson, M D Hellier, D Howard, M Juniper, A J Leonard, W McCrea, D Mukherjee, P Price
General Psychiatry J W Eastgate, G J Turnbull, D A Veasey
General Surgery P Burgess, D R A Finch, M Galea, R E Glass, D Hocken, R N Lawrence, R Singh-Ranger
Gynaecology A P Bond, J Cullimore, P Forbes-Smith, D Griffiths, K Jones, D Majumdar
Haematology N Blesing, A Gray, S Green
Neurology S Wimalaratna
Oncology D J Cole
Ophthalmology P McCormack, J H Ramsey, T Yasen
Oral and Maxillofacial Surgery J Fieldhouse, R Greenwood
Orthopaedics A Brooks, S D Deo, A J-B Fogg, M Foy, G M N Holloway, J P Ivory, I M R Lowdon, M Rigby, D M Williamson, D A Woods
Paediatrics R Chinthapalli, H Price, S T Zengeya
Pathology C M Colley
Plastic Surgery D J Coleman, A Godfrey, J Hobby
Psychology I Burgess, R Lyle
Radiology A M Beale, S Blease, J-L Cook, T Cousins, J Henson, L Jackson, A M Jones, N Ridley, T Saunders, S Taylor, A Troughton
Rheumatology D Collins, E J Price, L Williamson
Urology R Beck, J Iacovou

BMI The Runnymede Hospital

Guildford Road, Ottershaw, Chertsey KT16 0RQ
Tel: 01932 877800 Fax: 01932 875433
Email: runnymede@bmihealthcare.co.uk
Website: www.bmihealthcare.co.uk
Owners: BMI Healthcare
Total Beds: 51

Manager Jenny Long

BMI The Sandringham Hospital

Gayton Road, King's Lynn PE30 4HJ
Tel: 01553 769770 Fax: 01553 767573
Email: sandringham@bmihealthcare.co.uk
Website: www.bmihealthcare.co.uk
Owners: BMI Healthcare
Total Beds: 35

Manager Peter Stratton

BMI Sarum Road Hospital

Sarum Road, Winchester SO22 5HA
Tel: 01962 844555 Fax: 01962 842620
Email: sarum@bmihealthcare.co.uk
Website: www.bmihealthcare.co.uk
Owners: BMI Healthcare
Total Beds: 44

Manager Martin Thomas

BMI The Saxon Clinic

Chadwick Drive, Saxon Street, Eaglestone, Milton Keynes MK6 5LR
Tel: 01908 665533 Fax: 01908 608112
Email: saxon@bmihealthcare.co.uk
Website: www.bmihealthcare.co.uk
Owners: BMI Healthcare
Total Beds: 40

Manager Maria Dimmock

BMI The Shelburne Hospital

Queen Alexandra Road, High Wycombe HP11 2TR
Tel: 01494 888700 Fax: 01494 888701
Email: shelburne@bmihealthcare.co.uk
Website: www.bmihealthcare.co.uk
Owners: BMI Healthcare
Total Beds: 31

Manager J Long

BMI Shirley Oaks Hospital

Poppy Lane, Shirley Oaks Village, Croydon CR9 8AB
Tel: 020 8655 5500 Fax: 020 8655 5555
Email: shirleyoaks@bmihealthcare.co.uk
Website: www.bmihealthcare.co.uk
Owners: BMI Healthcare
Total Beds: 49

Manager John Hare

BMI The Sloane Hospital

125 Albemarle Road, Beckenham BR3 5HS
Tel: 020 8466 4000, 020 8466 4002 Fax: 020 8466 4001
Email: sloane@bmihealthcare.co.uk
Website: www.bmihealthcare.co.uk
Owners: BMI Healthcare
Total Beds: 55

Manager G Strong

BMI The Somerfield Hospital

63-77 London Road, Maidstone ME16 0DU
Tel: 01622 208000 Fax: 01622 674706
Email: somerfield@bmihealthcare.co.uk
Website: www.bmihealthcare.co.uk
Owners: BMI Healthcare
Total Beds: 48

Manager Christine Ayton

BMI The South Cheshire Private Hospital

Leighton, Crewe CW1 4QP
Tel: 01270 500411 Fax: 01270 583297
Email: southcheshire@bmihealthcare.co.uk
Website: www.bmihealthcare.co.uk
Owners: BMI Healthcare
Total Beds: 32

Manager Sue Darbyshire

Cardiology R Butler, P A Dodds, A P S Mann
Cosmetic Surgery S Dhital, A Juma
Dermatology P J August, A Harris
ENT J E Davies, J A J Deans, A Dingle
Gastroenterology I J London, J S McKay
General Medicine R Kedia, V Lakshmi, C G Murugasu, M D Winson
General Surgery A Aluwihare, D Cade, D Corless, A J Guy, M Hanafy, J Slavin
Genitourinary Medicine M H Khan
Haematology M I Patterson
Obstetrics and Gynaecology R J Armatage, J E Felmingham, M Luckas, J W Meekins, G Scott, D Semple
Oncology P A Burt, J Logue
Ophthalmology L B Freeman, A Hubbard, B J Moriarty, A Needham, M A Neugebauer
Oral Surgery J R Cawood, E C H Huddy
Orthopaedic Surgery E N B Ahmed, S Barnes, I Dos Remedios, D Emery, R Gillies, N Hyder, V Jasani, R Krishnan, M O'Driscoll, D Pegg, T Redfern, D Rees, R Wade, C H Wynn-Jones
Pain Control F M Emery, R W Okell
Rheumatology A J Farrell
Urology P Irwin, P Javie

BMI Thornbury Hospital

312 Fulwood Road, Sheffield S10 3BR
Tel: 0114 266 1133 Fax: 0114 268 6913
Email: thornbury@bmihealthcare.co.uk
Website: www.bmihealthcare.co.uk
Owners: BMI Healthcare

Total Beds: 77

Manager John Lofthouse

BMI Three Shires Hospital

The Avenue, Cliftonville, Northampton NN1 5DR
Tel: 01604 620311 Fax: 01604 629066
Email: msheldon@bmihealthcare.co.uk
Website: www.bmihealthcare.co.uk
Owners: St Andrew's Hospital, BMI Healthcare
Total Beds: 54

Manager Michael Sheldon

BMI The Winterbourne Hospital

Herrington Road, Dorchester DT1 2DR
Tel: 01305 263252 Fax: 01305 265424
Email: winterbourne@bmihealthcare.co.uk
Website: www.bmihealthcare.co.uk
Owners: BMI Healthcare
Total Beds: 43

Manager Jane Bentley

The Bournemouth Nuffield Hospital

67 Lansdowne Road, Bournemouth BH1 1RW
Tel: 01202 291866 Fax: 01202 294612
Website: www.nuffieldhospitals.org.uk
Owners: Nuffield Hospitals
Total Beds: 75

Manager Bryn Jones

Brain Injury Services Elm Park

Elm Park, Station Road, Ardleigh, Colchester CO7 7RT
Tel: 01206 231055 Fax: 01206 231596
Email: info@partnershipsincare.co.uk
Owners: Partnerships in Care Ltd
Total Beds: 23

Manager Janet Luck

Brain Injury Services Northampton

Grafton Manor, Grafton Regis, Towcester NN12 7SS
Tel: 01908 543131 Fax: 01908 542644
Email: info@partnershipsincare.co.uk
Website: www.partnershipsincare.co.uk
Owners: Partnerships in Care Ltd
Total Beds: 28

Manager Moira Amos

The Bristol Nuffield Hospital at Chesterfield

Clifton Hill, Clifton, Bristol BS8 1BP
Tel: 0117 987 2727 Fax: 0117 925 4909
Website: www.nuffieldhospitals.org.uk
Owners: Nuffield Hospitals
Total Beds: 27

Manager Karen Miller

The Bristol Nuffield Hospital at St Mary's

Upper Byron Place, Clifton, Bristol BS8 1JU
Tel: 0117 987 2727 Fax: 0117 925 4909
Website: www.nuffieldhospitals.org.uk
Owners: Nuffield Hospitals
Total Beds: 36

Manager Karen Miller

British Home and Hospital for Incurables

Crown Lane, Streatham, London SW16 3JB
Tel: 020 8670 8261 Fax: 020 8766 6084
Owners: Charity/Association
Total Beds: 125

Manager Noelle Kelly

Broadway Lodge

Oldmixon Road, Weston Super Mare BS24 9NN
Tel: 01934 812319 Fax: 01934 815381
Email: mailbox@broadwaylodge.org.uk
Website: www.broadwaylodge.org.uk
Owners: Charity/Association
Total Beds: 33

BUPA Alexandra Hospital

Impton Lane, Walderslade, Chatham ME5 9PG
Tel: 01634 687166 Fax: 01634 686162
Email: cservice-al@bupa.com
Website: www.bupahospitals.co.uk/alexandra
Owners: BUPA Hospitals Ltd
Total Beds: 42

Manager Linda Dineen

Cardiology A Stewart
Chest Medicine I O'Brien
Dermatology J M Boss, S Halpern, L Shall
ENT J P Davis, P G Gluckman, R C Henry, M Oyarzabal, S S Surenthiran
Gastroenterology Dr Aga, G Bird, P Kitchen, P R Powell-Jackson, G Smith-Laing
General Medicine M Aldouri, B C Kundu, Dr Mamun, G Noble, P Ryan, I N Scobie, H J Taylor, Dr Thom
General Psychiatry S L Davenport, N Lockhart
General Surgery B Andrews, D I Beeby, C M Butler, J Coxon, R W Hoile, P Jones, O Khan, M Parker, P Strauss, P J Webb, H Wegstapel
Gynaecology A I H Ahmed, O Devaja, J R A Duckett, J D S Goodman, L M Hanson, D J Houghton, S Norman, D Penman, A Popadopoulos
Neurology M S Chong, K Citurel, B Moffat, R Selway
Ophthalmology F Ahfat, L Amaya, C F G Jenkins, C A Jones, A MacFarlane
Oral Surgery A Brown, K Lavery
Orthopaedics A Bassily, K Borowski, J P Fleetcroft, B Gopalji, A J Hammer, R Hay, S Jain, M Katchburian, S Purkayastha, C Rand, K J Ravikumar, S Sait, D Thakkar
Paediatrics B Bhaduri, B R Jani, R Merwaha, A Soe
Pain Management R K Buist
Plastic Surgery T Blair, P M Gilbert, G McKeever, R W Norris
Rheumatology G George, A Hammond, B K Sharma, P L Williams
Sports Medicine P Staker
Urology I Dickinson, G R Mufti, J Palmer, R Ravi, M Sheriff, Mr Wijesurendra

BUPA Cambridge Lea Hospital

30 New Road, Impington, Cambridge CB4 9EL
Tel: 01223 266900 Fax: 01223 233421
Email: cservice-cl@bupa.com
Website: www.bupahospitals.co.uk/cambridgelea
Owners: BUPA Hospitals Ltd
Total Beds: 68

Manager Charlotte Espie

Cardiology S Clarke, L Hughes, M C Petch, P Schofield, L Shapiro
Cardiothoracic D Jenkins, S Large, S Nashef, A Ritchie, S Tsui, J Wallwork, F C Wells
Dermatology N Burrows, P Norris, R Pye, P Todd
ENT P Axon, P Jani, D McKiernan
General Medicine J Bradley, R Dickinson, M Parkes, P Roberts, R Winter, J Woodward
General Surgery B Bekdash, J Boyle, P Forouhi, M Gaunt, N Hall, R Hardwick, R Praseedom, C Quick, J Reed
Geriatric Medicine D R Forsyth
Neurology C Allen, G Lennox, S Wroe

Neurosurgery H Fernandes, P Kirkpatrick, R Kirollos, R J C Laing, A Waters
Obstetrics and Gynaecology R Crawford, G Hackett, B Lim, A Prentice, M Slack
Ophthalmology L Allen, D Flanagan, D Newman, C Rene, N Sarkies, J Scott, M Snead, C Stephenson
Oral and Maxillofacial Surgery D Adlam
Orthopaedic Surgery J Chitnavis, D Edwards, G Keene, P J Owen, A Robinson, G Tytherleigh-Strong, R Villar
Pain Management D Hughes, R Munglani
Plastic Surgery T Ahmad, A Canal, P Hall, M Irwin, G Lamberty, C Malata
Radiology N Antoun, D S Appleton, N Carroll, R Coulden, C Cousins, C Hubbard, H Taylor
Rheumatology A Crisp, C Speed
Urology A Doble, J Kelly, W Turner

BUPA Dunedin Hospital

16 Bath Road, Reading RG1 6NB
Tel: 01189 587676 Fax: 01189 503847
Email: cservice-dn@bupa.com
Website: www.bupahospitals.co.uk/dunedin
Owners: BUPA Hospitals Ltd
Total Beds: 50

Manager Nicola Amery

Accident and Emergency Mr Soysa
Cardiology Dr Bell, Dr McKenna, Dr Orr
Clinical Pathology F M C Brito-Babapulle, Dr Grech
Dermatology Dr James
ENT Mr Marks
General Medicine Dr Davies, Dr Elsheikh, Dr Naik
General Surgery S P Courtney, Mr Faber, Mr Galland, Mr Magee, Mr Middleton, Mr Reece-Smith, Mr Umeh
Genitourinary Medicine Dr Tang
Gynaecology Mr Crystal, Mr Goswamy, Mr Greenhalf, Mr Williams
Oncology Dr Barrett, Dr Brown, Dr Charlton, Dr Freebairn, Dr Gildersleve, Dr Rogers
Ophthalmology Miss Bacon, Miss Billington, Mr Constable, Mr Leyland, Mr Pearson, Mr Richards, Mr Tanner, Miss Watson, Mr Welham
Oral and Maxillofacial Surgery Mr Patel, Mr Tomlins
Orthopaedics Mr Marshall, Mr Nugent, Mr O'Leary, Mr Tavares
Paediatrics Dr Newman
Pathology Dr Brito-Babapulle, Dr Challand, Dr Grech, Dr Horton, Dr Iyer, Dr Lewis, Dr Menai-Williams, Dr Saleem, Dr Stacey, Dr Williams
Plastic Surgery Mr Goodacre
Radiology Dr Archibald, Dr Bell, Dr Brown, Dr Derbyshire, Dr Elson, Dr Gibson, Dr Meanock, Dr Mills, Dr Rahim, Dr Robertson, Dr Stuart, Dr Torrie, Dr Walker

BUPA Fylde Coast Hospital

St Walburgas Road, Blackpool FY3 8BP
Tel: 01253 394188 Fax: 01253 397946
Website: www.bupahospitals.co.uk/fyldecoast
Owners: BUPA Hospitals Ltd
Total Beds: 37

Manager Chris Chadwick

Anaesthetics C Harle, N G Harper, G W Johnson
Cardiology M J Brack, A Chauhan, G K Goode, R More, D H Roberts, J E P Waktare
Cardiothoracic Surgery J Au, R J Millner
Dermatology W Bottomley
ENT A Keith, A Nigam
General Medicine A Baker Ahmed, P J Hayes, M T Hendrickse, P E T Isaacs, T C E Li Kam Wa, J D Mackay, M J O'Donnell, J F O'Reilly, K Raines, C J Shorrock, S Talab
General Surgery J Heath, H Osman, S Pettit, S Ravi, S Varadarajan
Neurology B Boothman, J Nixon
Neurosurgery N T Gurusinghe
Obstetrics and Gynaecology I D Arthur, N Bedford, S J Duthie, M R Steel, F L Wilcox
Oncology A Hindley, S Susnerwala
Ophthalmology J A Dunne, G Naylor, W S T Pollock, M F Raines
Oral and Maxillofacial Surgery S Akhtar
Orthopaedic Surgery I Guisasola, A Javed, S Mannion, G McLaughlan, S A C Sampath
Plastic Surgery A Juma, G Laitung
Radiology P K Bowyer, R W Bury, P Faux, G M Hoadley, C F Walshaw
Rheumatology S T M Jones
Urology N Rothwell

BUPA Gatwick Park Hospital

Povey Cross Road, Horley RH6 0BB
Tel: 01293 785511 Fax: 01293 774883
Email: cservice-gp@bupa.com
Website: www.bupahospitals.co.uk/gatwickpark
Owners: BUPA Hospitals Ltd
Total Beds: 64

Manager Matthew Dronsfield

Cardiology J Metcalfe
Care of the Elderly V Phongsathorn
Dermatology S Cliff
ENT K Bevan, G Warrington
General Medicine D Acharya, K J Foster, T Leigh, R Makadsi, C Prajapati, A G Vallon
General Surgery A B S Ball, N Gowland-Hopkins, J Grabham, R G Lightwood, T Loosemore, E Owen, A Stacey-Clear, A Yelland
Genitourinary Medicine T Peers
Haematology F Matthey, S Stern
Neurology M Gross, A Nisbet
Neurophysiology S Bajada
Neurosurgery J Akinwunmi
Obstetrics and Gynaecology S Butler-Manuel, A P Gordon-Wright, M Long, Z Nadim, J Penny, N G J Pipe, P T Townsend
Ophthalmology R Malhotra, F O'Sullivan, R S Wilson
Oral and Maxillofacial Surgery K Altman, J Tighe
Orthopaedic Surgery P Cheong-Leen, K J Drabu, M H Patterson, T Selvan, C D P Stone, G Tselentakis
Plastic Surgery J Davison, B Dheansa
Radiology T Bloomberg, C Good, R P McAvinchey, J Olney, J Vive
Urology P Miller, A Rane

BUPA Hartswood Hospital

Eagle Way, Brentwood CM13 3LE
Tel: 01277 232525 Fax: 01277 200128
Email: cservice-hw@bupa.com
Website: www.bupahospitals.co.uk/hartswood
Owners: BUPA Hospitals Ltd
Total Beds: 58

Anaesthetics M Ather, P Bawa, H Boralessa, S Chander Kapoor, G Chitra, B Emerson, S Fadheel, M Frost, S Gopinath, L Hoogsteden, J Lloyd, B Martin, M S May, R Mehta, S Oakey, D Parkhouse, V Punchihewa, B Robinson, S Sampathkumar, E Smithers, S Thomson, S F Tinloi, J Umo-Etuk, J Whitehead, R Wijesurenda, I Youkhana
Cardiology R K Aggarwal, J Hogan, H Kadr, T W Koh, J McEwan
Dermatology F Carabott, M Khorshid, S Matthews, R Mehta, W Robies
Endocrinology R Khan
ENT B Chopra, C Chowdhury, G Fayad, H Kaddour, B Kotecha, A Latif, T Owa, D Roy
General Medicine N Ahmad, M Apps, W Ashrah, E Bettany, R Burnham, I Fahal, W Fickling, D Gertner, D Hollanders, A S Jubber, E Marouf, K Metcalfe, E Osman, R M Pearson, J Subhani, R M Weatherstone, P Willoughby
General Surgery A Bhargava, T Cheatle, D G Collier, C Hepworth, R Inwang, W Ismail, T Jeddy, D Johnston, F H Kahn, D Khoo, K Lafferty, I Linehan, B Lovett, D Mukherjee, A Ogedegbe, A Ojo, M Saharay, A K Salih, S Shami, H Taylor
Haematology F Al-Refaie
Neurology R Capildeo, R De Silva, L Findley, C Hawkes

Neurosurgery R Aspoas, J Benjamin, K M David, J Kellerman
Obstetrics and Gynaecology P Bolton, S Burgess, Y Coker, J Emeagi, R Haloob, P Kollipara, M Ojutiku, I Opemuyi, U Rao, S Sathanandan, A Sharma, H Tebbutt, R Varma, C Welch
Oncology A Gershuny, E Sims
Ophthalmology J Chawla, C Claoue, G Dawidek, V Geh, N Karia, R V Pearson, J Pitts, S Ruben
Oral and Maxillofacial Surgery D Falconer, D Madan, J McKechnie, P Weller
Orthopaedic Surgery A Al-Sabti, A Ali, H Banan, R Carew, R Grewal, N Ker, S Kumar, A Lang-Stevenson, I Lennox, G MacLellan, T Peckham, K Ratnakumar, M Shoaib, H Singh Plaha, J Targett, J Wenger, J White
Paediatric Medicine S Jayakumar, T Matthews, R Ramanan, J Rawal, N Sharief, G Subramanian
Paediatric Surgery D Misra
Plastic Surgery M Gittos, F Iwuagwu, V Ramakrishnan, M Sood, C Walker
Podiatry G Michael
Psychiatry J Chaloner, F Dunne, C Murray, N Savla, J Taylor, A Winbow
Radiology M Alsewan, S Banyikidde, R Bessifi, T Chan, S Chawda, P Cory, M Farrugia, S Gademsetty, J Gutmann, T Sikdar, S R Srivatsa
Radiotherapy O Koriech
Rheumatology K Chakravarty, G Clarke, N Gendi, C Kelsey, J Palit, E Roussou
Urology J Barua, S Bhanot, P Ewah, S Gujral, J Hill, T Vandal, A Vohra

BUPA Hospital Bristol

The Glen, Redland Hill, Durdham Down, Bristol BS6 6UT
Tel: 0117 973 2562 Fax: 0117 974 3203
Email: cservice-br@bupa.com
Website: www.bupahospitals.co.uk/bristol
Owners: BUPA Hospitals Ltd
Total Beds: 72

Manager Sandie Foxall-Smith
Anaesthetics A Cohen, S Coniam, I Davies, M Milne, S Pryn, J Soar, A Wolf
Cardiology A Baumbach, P Boreham, T Cripps, H Joffe, K Karsch, A Skyrme-Jones, G Stuart, J Vann-Jones
Cardiothoracic Surgery G Angelini, R Ascione, A Bryan, F Ciuli, J Hutter, A Morgan
Dermatology C Archer, G Dunnill, C Kennedy
ENT M Birchall, P Robinson
General Medicine J Catterall, M Hetzel, C Horrocks, S Hughes, A Johnson, G McVie, M Plummeridge, R Przemioslo, J Smithson
General Surgery C Armstrong, A Baker, S Cawthorn, A Dixon, P Durdey, D Mitchell, J Morgan, A Sahu, F Smith, P Sylvester, M Thomas, M Thompson, Z Winters
Neurology I Ormerod
Neurosurgery R Nelson (Head), H Coakham, S Gill, R Nelson, R J Nelson, I Pople, D Porter
Obstetrics and Gynaecology S Glew, F McLeod, J Murdoch, P Smith, S Vyas
Oncology S Falk
Ophthalmology S Cook, J Diamond, M Greaney, J Luck, M Potts, D M Tole
Oral and Maxillofacial Surgery P Revington
Orthopaedic Surgery N Blewitt, T Chesser, J Hardy, W Harries, S Hepple, J Hutchinson, I Leslie, A Ward, J Webb, I Winson
Plastic Surgery J Kenealy
Psychiatry C Blacker
Radiology S Armstrong, M Callaway, M Darby, P Goddard, E Loveday, C Wakeley, P Wilde
Urology F Keeley, R Persad, T Whittlestone, M Wright

BUPA Hospital Bushey

Heathbourne Road, Bushey WD23 1RD
Tel: 020 8950 9090 Fax: 020 8950 7556
Email: cservice-bu@bupa.com
Website: www.bupahospitals.co.uk/bushey
Owners: BUPA Hospitals Ltd
Total Beds: 73

Manager Andrew Gore

Anaesthetics J S Berman, K Collins, P McGowan, V M Taylor
Cardiology E J Knight, D Lipkin, A W Nathan, M J Van Der Watt, W Wallis
Care of the Elderly A Sa'adu
Dermatology R Aron, H M Barnes, K Batta, H Bayoumi, S S Bleehen, T A Leslie, L R Lever, J Schofield, P Shahrad, H P Stevens
Endocrinology R Jackson
ENT R Auerbach, O P Chawla, V Cumberworth, M Dilkes, R Farrell, D F Johnston, A Kalan, R E Quiney, G Radcliffe, M Stearns
General Medicine G E Bevan, J Burke, M R Clements, D Cohen, D Evans, N R Farid, L J Farrow, J M Gumpel, A Leahy, D Levy, D D Lubel, B Macfarlane, D P Maudgal, G A Nelstrop, A Ogilvie, A Palmer, T Stamp
General Surgery M Al-Dubaisi, R Anwar, R W Awad, D M Baker, R Bird, M Chaudary, S J Cox, D Greenstein, R Harrison, J Livingston, A Loh, J Meyrick-Thomas, I C Mitchell, S Sarin, H Singhal, M Wallace
Haematology S Ardeman, D Cummins
Histopathology J El-Jabbour
Neurology G D Scott
Neurophysiology N Murray, B D Youl
Neurosurgery J Allibone
Obstetrics and Gynaecology N Bajekal, L Bernhardt, F A Boret, W Braithwaite, A Gordon, D Griffin, P F Haddad, A Hextall, L M Irvine, V Lewis, M Nadwick, C Naylor, M Nicholas, A Sanusi, R Sheridan
Oncology R F U Ashford, D C Fermont, R Glynne-Jones
Ophthalmology R Auplish, J Jones, S Kodati, A Kosmin, S G Levy, R Pearce
Oral and Maxillofacial Surgery G Bounds, R Liversedge, N A Nasser
Orthopaedic Surgery J Angel, R Bajekal, J S Blackburne, S R Canno, T Carlstedt, R Carrington, R Coull, B D Ferris, A Hashemi-Nejad, S Jayabalan, J Jessop, S Lambert, R P Mackenney, J P Murphy, H Nwaboku, J Perez, P Ray, N Reissis, D Rossouw, D Singh, M F Sullivan, B Taylor, P Thomas, L Wilson
Paediatric Medicine E Douek, M Eltumi, S Herman, S Roth, A Sharma, G Supramaniam
Plastic Surgery N Kang, R Sanders, P Smith
Podiatry J Livingstone
Radiology J Berger, D Boxer, N Damani, A Davies, T El-Sayed, J B Festenstein, B Gajjar, S G Johnson, G Kaplan, P Lai Chung Fong, K Lotzof, A J Marcus, M Patel, K Raza, K Rosenfeld, W Teh
Rheumatology S Bhalara, F Girgis, N A Pandit, J Rosenberg
Urology T Briggs, J C Crisp, G Fowlis, J Gelister, M Ruston, J Shah, A Thurston
Vascular Surgery H Hamilton

BUPA Hospital Clare Park

Clare Park, Crondall Lane, Crondall, Farnham GU10 5XX
Tel: 01252 850216 Fax: 01252 850228
Email: cservice-cp@bupa.com
Website: www.bupahospitals.co.uk/clarepark
Owners: BUPA Hospitals Ltd
Total Beds: 38

Manager Louise Bruce

Anaesthetics D Aldington, P Barnardo, M Blackmore, E Burov, R Cantelo, S Carroll, M Davies, C Edkins, W Fawcett, G Goddard, J Gudgeon, A Hendrickse, P Joshi, P Keeling, S Kilpatrick, A Landes, M Lucas, K Markham, T Pepall, L Shaikh, V Slade, N Taylor, D White
Care of the Elderly K Mundy, F Munim
ENT J Hern, A Hosni, D Jonathan, A McCombe

General Medicine R Bown, P Fabricius, R J Frankel, R Knight
General Surgery R Daoud, D Edwards, D Gerrard, M Gudgeon, I Laidlaw, P Leopold, F Massouh, I Paterson, S Singh
Genitourinary Medicine T Peers
Haematology J G Smith
Obstetrics and Gynaecology G Beynon, A Burnham, P Toplis
Oncology R Laing
Ophthalmology A Elliott, J Govan, T Poole, C Sandy
Oral and Maxillofacial Surgery M Danford, P Johnson, C Kerawala
Orthopaedic Surgery A Ashbrook, S Chatakondu, H Chissell, J Clasper, S Davies, D Dempster, P Hill, J Hull, A Perry, J Pike, A Quaile, A Sakellariou, M Solan, M Thomas
Pathology N Cumberland, P Denham, M Elmahallawy, C Smith, T Wang
Plastic Surgery D Martin
Psychiatry T Cantopher, A Gilham
Radiology S Ahmad, J Hall, A Hatrick, F Hearn, N Hughes, A Keightley, H Massouh
Rheumatology P Reilly
Urology B Montgomery, H Naerger, E Palfrey

BUPA Hospital Elland

Elland Lane, Elland, Halifax HX5 9EB
Tel: 01422 324000 Fax: 0800 138 8804
Email: cservice-el@bupa.com
Website: www.bupahospitals.co.uk/elland
Owners: BUPA Hospitals Ltd
Total Beds: 41

Manager Chris Harrison

Accident and Emergency A Mohammed, M Zahir
Anaesthetics N Alquisi, J Anathhanam, P Bamber, S Bhandari, S Cheema, K Ch'ng, J Esmond, B Ghoorun, P Goulden, P Hall, P Hutchings, K Ismail, F Jennings, R Johnson, P Knight, K Kyriakides, P Lesser, C Lok, M Nagar, C Nandakumar, J O'Riordan, T Riad, S Siddiqui, D Somerville, J Thomson, I Wilson
Cardiology S Grant, J Smyllie
Cardiothoracic Surgery A Thorpe
Care of the Elderly S Chandratre, J Sarin
Dermatology J Holder, M Shah
ENT D Boyd, G Kelly, D Martin-Hirsch, G Smelt, A Tucker
General Medicine V Bangar, D Currie, M Freeman, B Lalor, S Qureshi, P Rana, S Thomas, A Verma
General Surgery J Ajayi, M Aldoori, D Ali, M Basheer, W Case, B Dobbins, R Goodall, P Holdsworth, D Ilsley, P Lyndon, A Mahomed, V Modgill, N Sharma, A Subramanian, C White
Haematology A Steed
Neurology B Da Falla, L Loizou, S Omer
Neurophysiology S M Alani
Obstetrics and Gynaecology K Bhabra, J Campbell, C Choy, M Debono, K Fishwick, D Jones, S Kaufmann, P O'Donovan, B Onyeka, A Trehan
Oncology A Crellin, J Joffe
Ophthalmology N Anand, K Davey, C Hutchinson, T James, S Rehman, S Spencer
Oral and Maxillofacial Surgery J Jones
Orthopaedic Surgery P Angus, S Ankarath, C Chadwick, G Chakrabarty, A Chapman, B Flood, A George, L Koch, A Maarouf, P Muralikuttan, J Ridge, A Shenolikar, E Tolessa, M Walsh
Paediatric Medicine P Gorham, Y Oade
Plastic Surgery O Fenton, I Foo, D Sharpe
Radiology P Chennells, S Gurney, N Jain, P James, R Paes, L Sutton, A-M Wason
Rheumatology D McGonagle, R Reece
Urology M Ferro, M Murphy, K Rogawski, J Somerville, S K Sundaram

BUPA Hospital Harpenden

Ambrose Lane, Harpenden AL5 4BP
Tel: 01582 763191 Fax: 01582 712312
Email: cservice-hp@bupa.com
Website: www.bupahospitals.co.uk/harpenden
Owners: BUPA Hospitals Ltd
Total Beds: 62

Manager Steve Bird

Anaesthetics S Afolami, K Agyare, M A Alexander, G Baker, S Bates, J Binns, O W Boomers, A Borgese, S G Brosnan, M Carrington, M I Carter, M Chilvers, D Cranston, S J Eckersall, P G Edge, P Goldberg, S Gowrie-Moham, R P Griffin, M Henein, H M Hill, T V T Isitt, K Jani, N G Jeffs, T Kathirgamanathan, J Lalor, R Makker, A M Moxon, A R Moye, A Navapurkar, P B Patel, D U S Pathirana, M T Patten, S N Rahaj, A Rajah, W J K Rickford, C Roud-Mayne, N Royston, M Sair, K Sarang, M Sekar, P Sen-Gupta, R C Shah, Z P Shah, I Sockalingham, F Spiers, I Srikantharajah, S R Susay, J Thiagarajan, A Twigley, T J Walker, D A White, W A Yanny, B S Yogasakaran
Cardiology J F J Bayliss, M N Dubowitz, D Hackett, D K Jain, P I M Keir, C M Travill
Chest Medicine J W Cairn, R G Dent, I P Williams
Dermatology H M Barnes, V C Blackwell, P D L Maurice, A G Quinn, P Shahrad
Endocrinology N R Farid, C L W Johnston, P H Wincour
ENT H K Bail, O P Chawla, S Fahmy, A C Frosh, D F Johnston, G Mochloulis, J M Pickles, S J Quinn
Gastroenterology R J Aubrey, I G Barrison, S M Catnach, R S Graham, S M Greenfield, A E Griffiths, S R Jain, P B McIntyre, D Morris, D Rowlands
General Medicine R Banerjee, R Brenner, J J Day, D Evans, A A Gohil, P K Kanthapillai
General Surgery M C Aldridge, A Amin, T S Bhatti, K Brown, S Cheslyn-Curtis, P W Crane, A M Dalton, S Gupta, R I Hallan, V K Jain, M S Lennox, J C Nicholls, J R Novell, M C E Ormiston, M R Pittam, D Ravichandran, S P Raymond, N Reay-Jones, G R Sagor, S Selvakumar, S D Thompson
Genitourinary Medicine J John
Geriatric Medicine R R Farag, K Mylvaganam, S Puthrasingham, M Seevaratnam
Haematology J Kearney, J M Voke
Histopathology M S S Al-Izzi, A Fattah
Neurology A N Gale, R W Orrell, L M Parsons, P Watts
Obstetrics and Gynaecology R K Atalla, S Banerjee, F A Boret, S J Burrell, M Coker, N C Drew, E Y Hemaya, A Hextall, D H Horwell, D G McLintock, O J Owens, P C Reid, D R Salvesen, F A Sanusi, Y Tayob
Oncology A R Makepeace, N Shah
Ophthalmology J P Bolger, S H Campbell, T P Coker, F Goldin, J D Heath, D Michalik, A Parnaby-Price, S J P Pieris, J J Tolia, A Waldock, M K Wang
Oral and Maxillofacial Surgery G A Bounds, C-H Chan, A D Giles, M G Gilhooly, J A Sherman, M T Simpson, D P Von Arx
Orthopaedic Surgery D H Austwick, J P Beacon, B R D Bradnock, T W R Briggs, M Chatoo, N Davies, P Dyson, P G Hope, A S Irwin, J L Kitson, J Leitao, R Pandit, H Parmar, C J Read, J S Sarkar, J M Scott, R Sharma, M C Stallard, A H Waterfield, D J Williams
Paediatric Medicine M Arumugam, M J Chapple, A S Cohn, H M A El-Naggar, M Eltumi, E Rosenthal, A M L Shurz, P Sivakumar
Pain Management M H Fox, S A Guirguis, P S Hart
Pathology J W Dove, D Freedman, S Hill, D A S Lawrence, M Nayagam
Plastic Surgery A I Attwood, M G Dickson, N K James, N Kang, R Sanders, P J Smith
Podiatry J Bramhall
Psychiatry M D Beary, J J Hart, G Mathew, J McClure, C P Treves-Brown
Psychotherapy C McAllister
Radiology M S Alexander, S A Allen, S J Barter, A Divers, D Grimer, B Hartley, I P Hicks, G S Jutlla, S S Khan, A H Lynn, T K Mittal, K L Ng, A Platts, S Ramkumar, K M Rosenfield, D S Shetty, A Valentine, M J Warren, R Warwick, J N Wilkie, D J Wright
Rheumatology J M C Axon, D Fishman, M Stodell, M A Wajed, A Young
Urology A N Alam, G B Boustead, D C Hanbury, T A McNicholas, M Pancharatnam, A Thurston, J Vanwaeyenbergh

BUPA Hospital Hastings

The Ridge, St Leonards-on-Sea TN37 7RE
Tel: 01424 757400 Fax: 01424 757424
Email: bupahospitalhastings@bupa.com
Website: www.bupahospitals.co.uk/hastings
Owners: BUPA Hospitals Ltd
Total Beds: 29

Manager Sue Parsons

Cardiology Dr Walker, Dr Wray
Dermatology Dr Liddell, Dr von der Werth
ENT Mr Baer, Mr Meredith
Gastroenterology Dr Rademaker, M Whitehead
General Medicine Dr Bruce, Dr Clee, Dr Dennison, Dr Dyson, Dr Gorsuch, Dr McIntyre, Dr Rahmani
General Surgery Mr Khoury, Mr Lyttle, Mr Sandison, Miss Shah, S Whitehead
Gynaecology Mr Alaily, Mr Auld, Miss Sinha, Mr Zaidi
Hand Surgery Mr Underhill
Ophthalmics Mr Gregory, Mr Lloyd-Jones, Mr Merrick
Orthopaedics Mr Apthorp, Mr Buchanan, Mr Butler-Manuel, Mr Hinves, Mr Selmon, Mr Sheppard
Paediatrics Dr Scott, Dr Whincup
Plastic Surgery Mr Pickford
Radiology Dr Apthorp, Dr Foord, Dr Giles, Dr Guy, Dr Joarder
Rheumatology Dr Henderson
Urology Mr Plail

BUPA Hospital Hull and East Riding

Lowfield Road, Anlaby, Hull HU10 7AZ
Tel: 01482 659471 Fax: 01482 654033
Email: cservice-hl@bupa.com
Website: www.bupahospitals.co.uk/hull
Owners: BUPA Hospitals Ltd
Total Beds: 40

Manager Simon Harrison

Anaesthetics S Bennett, G Bwalya, A Coe, B Culbert, J M Donaldson, M El-Rakshy, P Evans, M Felgate, S Gower, I Locker, C Melville, B Mikl, R Owen-Smith, C Pollock, G Purdy, Z Rafique, S G Ram, C D Rigg, I Russell, A Saleh, M Shalaby, R Sharawi, C Smales, B Tandon, J Thind, J Thompson, J Waterland, T Williams, B S Withington
Cardiology M F Alamgir, J Caplin, J Cleland, J Dhawan, G Kaye, A Memon, M Nasir, R Oliver, J Sahu
Cardiothoracic Surgery A Cale, M Cowen, S Griffin, L Guvendik
Care of the Elderly A Farnsworth, J Knox
Dermatology A Butt, S Walton
Endocrinology S Atkin
ENT S Ell, J England, M Rogers, S Smith, N Stafford, E Whitehead
General Medicine V Anand, A Arnold, R Bain, S Bhandari, D Bhatia, M Dakkak, P Dore, S Khulusi, D McGivern, P Mysore, L Sellars, H K Thaker, H-H Tsai
General Surgery M Ahmad, P J Drew, G Duthie, J Fox, J Gunn, J E Hartley, A Kar, T Mahapatra, P McCollum, P McManus, J Monson, P Moore, C J O'Boyle, C Royston, P Sedman, J Tilsed, K Wedgwood, B Wilken, A Wilkinson
Genitourinary Medicine U Joshi, H McClean
Histopathology A Campbell, L Karsai, R Kumar, E D Long, N E New
Neurology F Ahmed, H H M Hamdalla, A Ming, M Rawson
Neurophysiology A Bajalan
Neurosurgery B Matthew, K Morris, D O'Brien, G O'Reilly
Obstetrics and Gynaecology J Ghandhi, R R Jha, S Killick, P Lesny, S Maguiness, W-L Noble, S Odukoya, K Phillips, S Sabharwal, E Speck, S Tyrrell, R Yeo
Oncology A Chaturvedi, M Holmes, M Lind, A Maraveyas
Ophthalmology Q Ali, A Babar, S Datta, J Innes, S Kotta, A Mathur, M Pande, O Stewart, N Zaman
Oral and Maxillofacial Surgery C Blackburn, M Cope, D Starr
Orthopaedic Surgery T Cain, F Howell, G V Johnson, G Kings, M Korab-Karpinski, A Mohsen, P Molitor, S Naima, A Nihal, S Shafqat, C Shaw, K Sherman, A Walker
Paediatric Medicine A M Azaz, I Beddis, M H El-Habbal
Paediatric Surgery S Besarovic, R D Daniel
Pathology P Burgess, D Crooks, A Macdonald, R Meigh, J Read, I Richmond, J Wilson
Plastic Surgery N Hart, A Platt, M Riaz, P Stanley
Podiatry S Coope
Psychiatry J Mullin, D Ryan
Radiology G Avery, R Bartlett, J Cast, P Clarke, A M Coady, A Early, D Ettles, M Finlay, C Hauf, D Horton, A Hubbard, S Mann, D Nag, N K [New Person], G Robinson, C Rowland-Hill, D Salvage, D Taylor
Rheumatology S Doherty, Y Patel, I Tomlinson
Urology D Almond, G Cooksey, L M Coombs, J Hetherington, S Kraus
Vascular Surgery A B Akomolafe, I Chetter, B Johnson, P Renwick

BUPA Hospital Leeds

Jackson Avenue, Roundhay, Leeds LS8 1NT
Tel: 0113 269 3939 Fax: 0113 268 1340
Email: cservice-ld@bupa.com
Website: www.bupahospitals.co.uk/leeds
Owners: BUPA Hospitals Ltd
Total Beds: 88

Manager Ros Mason

Accident and Emergency N Zoltie
Anaesthetics M Bellamy, A Bodenham, J L Brown, L Caldicott, A Cohen, M H Cross, R Cruickshank, N M Dearden, J Gibson, A Lumb, P McHugh, P Morgan, A Yates
Cardiology M Appleby, C Cowan, R Crook, E Grech, J Gunn, J McLenachan, J Perrins, M Pye, J West, G Williams, J Wilson
Cardiothoracic Surgery P Kaul, P Kay, J McGoldrick, U Nair, D O'Regan, A Thorpe
Dermatology R S Dare, M Goodfield, S M Wilkinson
Endocrinology P E Belchetz
ENT J D Fenwick, D Hanson, G Kelly, L Knight, Z Makura
General Medicine A Axon, R Baker, J Bodansky, N Breslin, G Davies, M Davies, M Denyer, M Elliott, S Everett, S Gilbey, M Henry, M Muers, C Pease, P Plant, G Sandle, H Vanharanta, P Wood
General Surgery S Ambrose, M Bello, D Berridge, I Botterill, T G Brennan, D Burke, S Dexter, R L Doig, P J Finan, M Gough, K Horgan, D Jayne, P Kent, R Kester, M Lansdown, P Lodge, A Mavor, K Menon, S Pollard, P M Sagar, A Sarela, D J A Scott, J I Spark, H Sue-Ling, G Toogood, P Turton
Genitourinary Medicine J Clarke
Haematology J A Child
Neurology J Bamford, P Goulding, M Johnson
Neurosurgery A A Da Costa, J Timothy, P Van Hille
Obstetrics and Gynaecology A Balen, T J Broadhead, J Buxton, J Campbell, S Duffy, M Griffith-Jones, R Hutson, G Jarvis, G Lane, L Rogerson, A Rutherford, V Sharma
Oncology T Perren, D Sebag-Montifiore
Ophthalmology O Backhouse, B Chang, T Dabbs, R M L Doran, J Hillman, A J Morrell, I Simmons
Oral and Maxillofacial Surgery R Loukota
Orthopaedic Surgery I Archer, S Calder, D Campbell, R Dunsmuir, M E Emerton, R Farnell, N Ghali, R Hackney, N Harris, J Lawton, D Macdonald, A Rao, M Stone
Paediatrics F M Campbell, S Conway, M Powis, R Squire
Pain Management A Bush, D Dickson, K Simpson
Pathology D Tompkins
Plastic Surgery A Batchelor, G Bourke, C Fenn, S Kay, S Knight, M Liddington, H Peach, W Saeed
Psychiatry J Nehaul
Radiology G Bonsor, B Carey, A Chalmers, A H Chapman, P Chennells, R Fowler, A Grainger, P O'Connor, J Rankine, P Robinson, M Weston
Urology I Eardley, A Joyce, S Lloyd, A Paul, S Prescott, P Weston, P Whelan

BUPA Hospital Leicester

Gartree Road, Oadby, Leicester LE2 2FF
Tel: 0116 272 0888 Fax: 0116 272 0666
Email: cservice-lc@bupa.com
Website: www.bupahospitals.co.uk/leicester
Owners: BUPA Hospitals Ltd
Total Beds: 76

Manager Keith Cunningham

Accident and Emergency G Bodiwala
Anaesthetics B Collett, C D Hanning, G Smith
Cardiology D Chin, M Galinanes, A H Gershlick, Y Haider, P J B Hubner, I Hudson, J Kovac, G A Ng, N J Samani, J D Skehan, P J Stafford
Cardiothoracic Surgery T Spyt
Care of the Elderly G Fancourt
Dermatology R Burd, R A C Graham-Brown, K Harman, G Johnston
ENT T Alun-Jones, A Banerjee, A A Moir, G E Murty, P Rea, R S A Thomas
General Medicine N J Brunskill, J S De Caestecker, T C N Lo, J F Mayberry, P McNally, B J Rathbone, R J Robinson, J Stewart, J M Wales, D A Waller, A C B Wicks, M Wiselka
General Surgery B Barrie, P Bell, D Berry, N Everson, A W Hall, D Hemingway, J Jameson, M J Kelly, D M Lloyd, N J London, M McCarthy, A Miller, R Naylor, M L Nicholson, G S M Robertson, R Sayers, A D N Scott, A Stotter, M Thomas, S Ubhi, P S Veitch
Genitourinary Medicine P Fisk
Haematology B Kennedy, J K Wood
Histopathology L J R Brown, P N Furness, C Richards
Neurology R Abbott, P H S Critchley, M C Lawden, S G Philip
Neurophysiology D S Holder
Neurosurgery R Ashpole, M Choksey, I Robertson
Obstetrics and Gynaecology F Al Azzawi, A C Davidson, Q Davies, J Emembolu, D Ireland, P Kirwan, C Mayne, R W Neuberg, C Oppenheimer
Oncology S Khanna, W P Steward, S Vasanthan
Ophthalmology D J Austin, K Bibby, R Chaudhuri, J Deane, J Prydal, P Richardson, R Sampath, G Woodruff
Oral and Maxillofacial Surgery C Avery, J Hayter, I W Ormiston
Orthopaedic Surgery M Allen, A Armstrong, B Bhowal, S Birtwistle, K Boyd, J J Dias, C Esler, S Godsiff, T Green, J M Jones, C Kershaw, M Newey, O O A Oni, R Pandey, R A Power, D Quinton, P J Sell, A Shair, S Tandon
Paediatrics A Elias-Jones, G K Ninan, R C Tamhne, R Walia
Pain Management M E Bone, S Tordoff
Pathology J Falconer Smith
Plastic Surgery H P Henderson, T M Milward, E O'Broin, S K Varma, D J Ward, N W Yii
Podiatry D Holland
Psychiatry T Friedman, D I Khoosal
Radiology J Entwisle, D Finlay, K Karup, R P Keal, N Messios, A B Rickett
Rheumatology W Hassan, F E Nichol, A K Samanta, P Sheldon
Urology P Butterworth, D P S Sandhu, T R Terry

BUPA Hospital Little Aston

Little Aston Hall Drive, Little Aston, Sutton Coldfield B74 3UP
Tel: 0121 353 2444 Fax: 0121 353 1592
Email: cservice-la@bupa.com
Website: www.bupahospitals.co.uk/littleaston
Owners: BUPA Hospitals Ltd
Total Beds: 70

Manager Anna Tchaikovsky

Anaesthetics R Alexander, M Ali, M Arif, O Babatola, M J Calhaem, F Duncan, M Elliot, J Hull, B Kumar, J W Martin, L L Mudie, K Nandi, C Newson, A Patel, R Patel, I Roberts, J Sheldrake, P Sinha, J Smith, M Suchak, D I Thomas, A Williamson, M Youssef
Cardiology R Ahmad, A R Cunnington, C Gibbs, F Leyva, M Payne, J Raj, R Smith
Chest Medicine J F Khalil-Marzou
Dermatology K Ryatt
ENT D East, E W Fisher, R M Irving, D Morgan, J Oates, P Pracy, T Rockley, A Thompson
Gastroenterology M A Cox, M Lewis, A Palejwala, S Singh
General Medicine V P Balagopal, S Dean, A J Fairfax, R Hawkes, P J Jordan, R C Joshi, D Mackay, D Mcleod, J J Milles, D A Robertson, M P Skander
General Surgery C Abrew, D Browse, M A S Chapman, S Dodds, K D Fortes Mayer, A J Jewkes, B G Jones, H Khaira, A H Khan, S Korsgen, T J Muscroft, I Paterson, J Stewart, M Vairavan, K Yoong
Genitourinary Medicine A Joseph
Haematology M S Hamilton
Histopathology Y L Hock, A M Light
Nephrology I Dasgupta
Neurology D A Francis, A Williams
Neurosurgery M Choksey, S Harland, J Wasserberg
Obstetrics and Gynaecology I Abukhalil, C Balachandar, R S V Cartmill, D Churchill, G Constantine, C Finn, A C Head, J Kabukoba, R Manivasagam, M H Mattar, J Pepper, R Reddy
Oncology I N Fernando, J Glaholm
Ophthalmology P Corridan, M Hope-Ross, P McDonnell, P Shah, G Shun-Shin, G A Sutton, M Tsaloumas, A Tyagi
Orthopaedic Surgery B Banerjee, G S Chana, J C Clothier, M M El-Safty, S S Geeranavar, A Khan, S L Khemka, I M Miller, T Sadique, K Sulaiman, M Taylor, K H A Wahab
Paediatric Medicine S Bennett-Britton
Pathology T Reynolds
Plastic Surgery H Goldin, C C Kat, A Khanna, R Lester, S Thomas
Podiatry D R Tollafield
Psychiatry G Tadros
Radiology E R Allan, D Chand, M Cleasby, C Holland, C Lee, E L Millar, A Parnell, M Thuse
Rheumatology T Price, T Sheeran
Urology B G Ferrie, M C Foster, S R Koneru, H Ojha

BUPA Hospital Manchester

Russell Road, Whalley Range, Manchester M16 8AJ
Tel: 0161 226 0112 Fax: 0161 227 9405
Email: cservice-mn@bupa.com
Website: www.bupahospitals.co.uk/manchester
Owners: BUPA Hospitals Ltd
Total Beds: 92

Manager David Pickering

Accident and Emergency A D Redmond
Anaesthetics M Allan, N R Anders, A Arasan, P Ashford, M S Ballin, J Benson, S M Berger, M Bewsher, C Carroll, I S Chadwick, M O Columb, P T Conroy, L Cook, A P Dobson, S Dolling, L A Doyle, N El-Mikatti, M E Eltoft, P Fernandez-Jimenez, M R Forrest, S D Ghandi, J Goodall, K M Grady, H S J Gray, D L Greenhaigh, S G Greenhough, B Greenwood, D G Greig, H A Hack, L Hartley, T K Howell, P Kirk, I Lieberman, R T Longbottom, W D Lord, A D Luthra, W R MacNab, M J McKavney, G H Meakin, P Nightingale, D Nolan, N O'Keeffe, M A Osborne, B Ousta, D Patel, H V Petts, A G Pocklington, B J Pollard, R H Rehman, G E W Robson, C M Rogers, J Rogers, A Shaw, M E Simpson, T Sivalingham, G J Smuthwaite, P H Steller, K Strahan, T I Strang, A N Thomas, C L Tolhurst-Cleaver, N A Uwubamwen, C Van Oldenbeek, R Vashisht, A Vohra, R W M Walker, R S Wheatly, D K Whitaker, N A Wisely
Cardiology W C Brownlee, S M Horner, R S Khattar
Care of the Elderly S N Laha
Dermatology P J August, J E Ferguson, L E Rhodes
Endocrinology D McDowell
ENT A R Birzgalis, A E Camilleri, A El-Kholy, W T Farrington, J Homer, A E R Kobbe, P Murthy, M P Rothera, S R Saeed, P D Sharma, P Sheehan, H Tay, D J Willatt, T Woolford, A P Zarod
General Medicine N K Ahluwalia, A Ahmed, J A Anandadas, C Babbs, F Ballardie, M P Chopra, P J Conlong, B A Enoch, B P Goorney, J Hebden, B G Issa, H J Klass, G R Lipscomb, A J Makin, X A McFarlane, J P Miller, S Musgrave, M G Pattrick, C R Payne, W Rees, A Robinson, C D Short, D R Shreeve, M Sood, S C Taggart, A G Thomas, E R E Van Ross, M C Venning, T Warnes, I Welch, G Whatley

General Surgery S E M Afify, A K R Al-Dabbagh, I M Aldean, I D Anderson, L Barr, M Borghol, N J Bundred, G J Byrne, B A Campbell, S Ellenbogen, L J Formela, S Galloway, G Gilling-Smith, C N Hall, J Hill, E M Hoare, E S Kiff, I Maclennan, M Madan, F X Mazarelo, H Michie, S T O'Dwyer, R C Pearson, Z A Saad, N Scott, P D Scott, P S Senapati, D Sherlock, K H Siddqui, A K Siriwardena, J V Smyth, W F Tait, D E F Tweedle, H J Vadeyar
Haematology R C Routledge
Histopathology J Coyne, N Y Haboubi, R S Reeve
Microbiology E Kaczmarksi
Neurology M Kellett, C E G Moore, A C Young
Neurophysiology S M Alani
Obstetrics and Gynaecology D Adegbite, A Ahluwalia, R Clayton, P Donnai, E Edi-Osagie, G F Falconer, A M Ferguson, R Howell, B A Liebermann, A Mander, M Maresh, A M Nysenbaum, D W Polson, M Quinn, R Slade
Oncology E Levine
Ophthalmology S M Ataullah, S J Charles, C L Dodd, S J Harper, B Hercules, K Ikram, B Leatherbarrow, C Lloyd, L H Morgan, J L Noble, A E A Ridgway, M Yodaiken
Oral and Maxillofacial Surgery S Clark, M E Foster, R Lloyd, R J Middlehurst, K J Sanders, P R White
Orthopaedic Surgery J G Andrew, T Asumu, J K Borrill, F Chan, A D Clayson, A O Ebizie, A J Fitzgerald, L Funk, C S B Galasko, R Goel, J F Haines, A I Hegab, A D Henry, B Ilango, A M Ismail, S Jari, A M Khan, M T Khan, A Kocialkowski, N Kurdy, B Maltby, H Maxwell, S McLoughlin, S Mohammad, B Muddu, L Muir, J Noble, E Obeid, J Pattison Hodgkinson, A S Paul, P J Rae, N Ramamohan, S V Shah, E R Smith Ross, B Sylvester, P G Turner, C Warren-Smith, M Webber, R A Wilkes, J B Williamson
Paediatric Medicine A K Akobeng, A Bianchi, J Bowen, R H A Campbell, A Dickson, D Gough
Pathology S Desai, H El-Teraifi
Plastic Surgery P J Davenport, C I Orton, D J Whitby, S Wilson
Podiatry S P Lyons
Psychiatry R E Ggoodman
Radiology R J Ashleigh, W Bhatti, R Bisset, C R Boggis, R Bramley, H C Burnett, N Desai, J E Gillespie, D G Hughes, P A Hulse, E Hurley, S J Jackson, A Jain, J P R Jenkins, J A L Lawrance, S H Lee, D F Martin, A T Mortimer, D A Nicholson, P S Norburn, S J O'Shea, S Rimmer, S A Russell, W St Clair-Forbes, S A Sukumar, P M Taylor, K Uzoka, R W Whitehouse, B P M Wilson, M Wilson
Rheumatology R Bernstein, M I V Jayson, P A Sanders, P Smith
Urology C D Betts, C B Costello, P Downey, N J R George, E W Lupton, R Napier-Hemy, K J O'Flynn, S R Payne, I Pearce, P N Roa
Vascular Surgery I Mohan

BUPA Hospital Norwich

Old Watton Road, Colney, Norwich NR4 7TD
Tel: 01603 456181 Fax: 01603 250968
Email: cservice-nw@bupa.com
Website: www.bupahospitals.co.uk/norwich
Owners: BUPA Hospitals Ltd
Total Beds: 67

Manager Paul Tempest

Anaesthetics G Barker, P Barker, B Fleming, S Fletcher, P Furniss, A Gray, P Hodgson, M Hudspith, P Hutchings, M Leadbeater, G Porter, B Poulton, L Rowe, J Valentine, N Woodall, C Woollam
Cardiology L Freeman, L Hughes, T Wistow
Cardiothoracic Surgery G Parry
Care of the Elderly R Fulcher, M Naguib
Dermatology J Garioch, R Graham, C Grattan, N Levell
Endocrinology R Greenwood
ENT A Bath, A Innes, P Montgomery, D Premachandra, P Prinsley, M Wickstead
General Medicine B Brett, I Fellows, D Hamilton, A Heaton, C Jamieson, H Kennedy, M Phillips, C Ramsey, R Tighe
General Surgery J Clarke, J Colin, S Kapur, M Lewis, D Ralphs, M Rhodes, S Scott, W Stebbings, J Studley, H Sturzaker
Haematology M T Jeha, G Turner, J Wimperis
Histopathology R Ball, L Igali, R Lonsdale, B McCann
Neurology J Cochius, D Dick, P Worth
Obstetrics and Gynaecology S Crocker, F De Boer, D Fraser, P Greenwood, F Harlow, E Morris, J Nieto, C Overton, T Overton, K Stanley, R Warren
Oncology H Baillie-Johnson, A Bulman, C Martin, M Ostrowski
Ophthalmology B Beigi, D Broadway, T Burton, P Davies, T Eke, A Glenn, C Jones
Oral and Maxillofacial Surgery S Hadinnapola, R Rees
Orthopaedic Surgery J Albert, D Calder, P Chapman, A Chojnowski, R Crawford, S Donell, P Gallagher, M Glasgow, P Hallam, C Mann, J Nolan, A Patel, H Phillips, A Rai, M Saleh, K Tucker, J Wimhurst
Paediatric Surgery A Mathur, T Tsang
Plastic Surgery A Bardsley, A Logan, M Meyer, T O'Neill, E Sassoon
Psychiatry B R Bhadrinath, R Devine, M Kitson
Radiology J Cockburn, E Denton, S Girling, T Marshall, J Saada, S Scott-Barrett, M Shaw, P Wilson
Rheumatology K Gaffney, P Merry, D Scott
Urology N Burgess, E Ho, S Irving, R Mills, K Sethia, R Webb

BUPA Hospital Portsmouth

Bartons Road, Havant PO9 5NP
Tel: 023 9245 6000 Fax: 023 9245 6100
Email: cservice-pt@bupa.com
Website: www.bupahospitals.co.uk/portsmouth
Owners: BUPA Hospitals Ltd
Total Beds: 49

Manager Heather Dob

Accident and Emergency P Wellington
Anaesthetics J Burden, N Campkin, A Conyers, S Dolin, J Eldridge, S Elliott, P McQuillan, J Nightingale, B Palmer, J Phipps, D Pounder, P Rogers, P Sadler, M Wood
Audiological Medicine H Thomas
Cardiology R Jones, J Watkins
Dermatology R Ashton, L J Cook, A Haworth, S Keohane, S Minor, H Smith
Endocrinology M Cummings
ENT A E Davis, I Johnstone, G Madden, E Nilssen, C Pearson, M B Pringle, A Resouly, J Skipper
General Medicine A Chauhan, S Drew, H Duncan, R Ellis, P Golding, D Meeking, E Neville, V Raman, K Shaw
General Surgery N Cripps, M Kelly, D O'Leary, S Payne, M Pemberton, S Sadek, A Senapati, G Sutton, M Terry, M R Thompson, S Toh, A M Waters, T Whitbread, M Wise, C Yiangou
Genitourinary Medicine E Foley
Neurology W Gibb
Obstetrics and Gynaecology A Clark, S Ewen, S Guirgis, C Guyer, P Hogston, M Jolly, M Salloum, R P Woolas
Oncology C Archer, D Boote, T Gulliford, G Khoury
Ophthalmology D Boase, R Butler, A Evans, D Farnworth, W Green, M Jeffrey, J Kirwan, H MacLean, Y F Yang
Oral and Maxillofacial Surgery P Baxter, P Brennan, T Mellor, G A Zaki
Orthopaedic Surgery H Clarke, D Dalton, G Evans, N Flynn, G Griffiths, M Grover, C Hand, G Harper, G Hill, C Hobbs, S Hodkinson, G Hussell, I Jeffrey, M Mclaren, G Pathak, S Phillips, D Prakash, R Richards
Plastic Surgery N Bennett, J Hurren, A Pandya, G Scerri
Psychiatry N Joughin, R Morgans, A N Wear
Radiology P Buxton, J Domjan, M Firth, P Gordon, L Jarvis, J Langham-Brown
Rheumatology R Hull, F McCrae, A L Thomas
Urology S Hall, V Harinda, S Holmes, S Keoghane, L Solomon, D Summerton, B H Walmsley

BUPA Hospital Southampton

Chalybeate Close, Southampton SO16 6UY
Tel: 023 8077 5544 Fax: 023 8070 1160
Email: cservice-cb@bupa.com
Website: www.bupahospitals.co.uk/southampton
Owners: BUPA Hospitals Ltd
Total Beds: 78

Manager Philip Housden

Cardiology C Barlow, S Biggart, A Calver, K Dawkins, T Edwards, H Gray, M Haw, R Jones, S Langley, S Livesey, A McLeod, J Monro, J Morgan, C Murphy, S Ohri, P Roberts, I Simpson, G Tsang, J Watkins, S Winterton
ENT N Haacke, P Harries, W Hellier, T Mitchell, C Randall
General Medicine R Dathan, A Frew, B Marshall, D Sandeman
General Surgery I Bailey, N Beck, F McGinn, M Midwinter, G Morris, P Nichols, K Nugent, J Primrose, D Rew, G Royle, J Smallwood, H Steer, M Van Den Bossche, N Wilson
Gynaecology I Boyd, P Gillibrand, G Masson, K Metcalf, J Miller, A Monga, A Moors, N Saunders, W Stones
Neurology N Brook, H Katifi, P Kennedy
Oncology K Gregory, C Hamilton, T Illindge, T Iveson
Ophthalmology C Canning, I Chisholm, P Hodgkins, A Luff, R Morris, R Newsom
Oral and Maxillofacial Surgery N Baker, B Evans
Orthopaedics D Barrett, N Clarke, A Cole, E Davies, D Dunlop, D Hargreaves, J Robertson, W Tice, M Uglow, D Warwick
Paediatrics P Malone, D Mervyn Griffiths, R Wheeler
Pathology B Addis, P Bass, A Bateman, N Carr, C Duboulay, G R Jones, A Lowes, H Millward-Sadler, I Moore, N O'Connell, S O'Connell, D O'Shaughnessey, N Singh, A Smith, J Theaker, V Walker
Plastic Surgery A Rossi
Radiology V Batty, S Birch, R Blaquiere, D Breen, M Briley, D Delaney, K Dewbury, A Ditchfield, J Fairhurst, N Hacking, C Houghton, A Odurny, B Ogilvie, C Peebles, C Rubin, M Sampson, J Smart, K Tung
Rheumatology R Armstrong, M Cawley, C Cooper, C Edwards
Urology B Birch, J Cumming, M Hayes, C Smart

BUPA Hospital Tunbridge Wells

Fordcombe Road, Fordcombe, Tunbridge Wells TN3 0RD
Tel: 01892 740047 Fax: 01892 740046
Email: cservice-tw@bupa.com
Website: www.bupahospitals.co.uk/tunbridgewells
Owners: BUPA Hospitals Ltd
Total Beds: 40

Manager Dominic Bath

Anaesthetics J Appleby, J Curran, H Hutchinson, S Thorp
Cardiology D Harrington
ENT J Shotton
General Medicine D Barnes, A Harris, J Hughes
General Surgery N Boyle, M Tyrrell
Neurology G Saldanha
Obstetrics and Gynaecology P Bamford, O Chappatte, D Garrioch, M Matthews
Ophthalmology J Bell
Oral and Maxillofacial Surgery K Lavery
Orthopaedics M Fordyce, P Skinner
Plastic Surgery H J Belcher, M Pickford, B Tanner
Psychiatry A Winbow
Radiology J Garrett, P Tallett
Rheumatology D MacFarlane
Urology M Cynk, J Lewis

BUPA Hospital Washington

Picktree Lane, Rickleton, Washington NE38 9JZ
Tel: 0191 415 1272 Fax: 0191 415 5541
Email: washington@bupa.com
Website: www.bupahospitals.co.uk/washington
Owners: BUPA Hospitals Ltd
Total Beds: 35

Manager Rod Mason

Anaesthetics Z Arfeen, S S Aslam, N Barham, P Barrow, R J Bray, M Bryson, R E Bullock, N Cardno, C M E Carr, J H Carter, M Checketts, A Choudhry, D J Comyn, D Crawford, P J Cudworth, S Dabner, S Deshpande, N Dhariwal, M P Down, S Dowson, A Espinet, J A Evans, R Goodwin, N M Heggie, I Herrema, S R Heynes, M Johnson, P Kalia, K P Karn, J P Khan, M S Kokri, B Lal, G Lear, B Lekhak, M Lothian, A R Mahroo, Z Masri, P Matthew, H A May, P E McAndrew, F McAuley, P A McBride, I McClintock, A McHutchon, R Meikle, A Mellor, M A Millar, U Misra, R W D Mitchell, H Mohan, A Morrison, C Muench, J Mullenheim, A Murray, O Olukoga, A S Orwin, J D Park, J Poltronieri, C Richmond, A I Roy, C S Roysam, U Saleh, L Sekhar, R K Singh, J H Smith, Q Smith, C Snowden, I Spencer, M A Stafford, S Stein, N Stratford, A Symon, A J Taylor, D G Thomas, C J Vallis, S Varma, J Watson, P R Wilkinson, R Will, D W Wood, P J Wood
Audiology G Holland
Cardiology J M Ahmed, M de Belder, M El-Harari, S Furniss, S Junejo, A Nasser, I Purcell, A Zaman
Cardiothoracic Surgery J Forty, C J Hilton, S Hunter, S Kendall, G Morritt, W A Owens, T M Pillay, J Wallis
Chemical Pathology Dr Dillon, S Smellie
Dermatology M Carr, J Langtry, S Natarajan, S A Sinclair
ENT M Hawthorne, J Heaton, T Leontsinis, L A Lindsey, M Morgan, M Reda El Badawey, P R Samuel, F Stafford, A Welch
General Medicine Dr Ahmed, M F Bone, T P Cassidy, H Clague, W R Ellis, M Hayat, S Kadis, T W I Lovel, H Mansy, D Nylander, K Oppong, J Painter, P Perros, J Silcock, I K Taylor
General Surgery H Y Ashour, S E A Attwood, I M Bain, V Bhattacharya, L Boobis, D Browell, K Clark, A Cook, J Corson, P Cullen, W Cunliffe, P Dunlop, S Green, S M Griffen, H Hashimi, I Hawthorn, C Hennessey, D W Herring, A Horgan, W Huizinga, B V Joypaul, D Lambert, T Layzell, T Lees, J Lennox, G R McLatchie, M Mercer-Jones, A Mudawi, H A Naqesh-Bandi, S R Preston, A J Rich, I Rogers, P Small, P Surtees, G J M Tervit, S Vetrivel, K Wynne
Genitourinary Medicine S Rashid
Haematology K Goff
Histopathology D J L Maloney
Mental Health R Marshall
Microbiology D Allison, G M Horne
Neurology P Cleland, P Dorman, A Goonetilleke, R E Jones, P Reading
Neurosurgery C Gerber, N Todd
Obstetrics and Gynaecology I Aird, M Dalton, M Das, Mr Gbolade, K A Godfrey, K Hinshaw, D Irons, R A K Jaiyesimi, A F Jones, A Jones, G MacNab, P Marsden, M Menabawey, G E Morgan, B Murray, A R M Sproston, C Steele
Oncology P J Atherton, A N Branson, F Y Coxon, W Dobrowsky, A Hughes, I D Pedley, T Roberts
Ophthalmology R Allchin, R W D Bell, M Birch, R Boyce, M Dang, J-P Danjoux, J P Deady, F C Figueiredo, S Fraser, S Morgan, P Phelan, R Robinson, D Steel, N Strong, S J Talks, P Tiffin, C Wood
Oral and Maxillofacial Surgery I Martin, J M Ryan, P J Thomson
Orthodontics I A Shaw
Orthopaedic Surgery J Buchanan, J Coorsh, A Cross, D J Deehan, G DeKiewiet, P K Dixon, B Dorani, J Du Fosse, H Epstein, D Fender, J Fraser, J Fraser, H W Fuchs, P J Gill, R J H Gregory, I Hugh, L Irwin, A Jennings, A M Nanu, S O'Brien, P Partington, G Prasad, S Roysam, N S Shankar, N Shaw, M Stewart, A Stirrat, I Talkhani, K Wright
Paediatric Surgery M Barrett
Paediatrics M Abu-harb, D R Smith
Pain Management S S Aslam, P Mathew, O Olukoga, P Wilkinson
Plastic Surgery B Berry, M Erdmann, S Jeffrey, N R McLean
Podiatry M Cummins, M Forster
Psychiatry A El-Sobky, S D Martin, K L Shrestha, C Tyrie
Psychology L H Cameron, J D McCarthy, W K Robertson
Radiology D Birchall, P Cadigan, J Connor, R C Cooper, J E M Cox, S Elliot, S J P England, T Featherstone, A Gholkar, L Lunt, S N E Marsden, R L Marsh, I Minty, A J Potterton, D Richardson, J Spratt, J B Wilsdon
Rheumatology T Daymond, C D Holland, D Wright
Urology T Armitage, P English, D Greene, T Hasan, P Johnson, C Roberts, B Satyavadanan, A Thorpe

BUPA Methley Park Hospital

Methley Lane, Methley, Leeds LS26 9HG
Tel: 01977 518518 Fax: 01977 519014
Email: cservice-mp@bupa.com
Website: www.bupahospitals.co.uk/methleypark

Owners: BUPA Hospitals Ltd
Total Beds: 29

Manager Gillian Bishop

Cardiology P Batin, P Brooksby, R Lewis, B Thanoon Saeed, J Wilson
Dermatology J Bothwell, B Pollock
ENT S Ajulo, S Clarke, R Henein, N Siddiqui, M Wickham
General Medicine Dr Ajaj, M Al-Bazzaz, K Kapur, D Nagi, P Sahay, A Soliman
General Surgery D Ali, S Anwar, M Basheer, P Curley, J Hossain, C Irvine, J Kenogbon, J Parmar, M Rogers, M H Shiwani, N R Womack, C-K Yeung
Neurology A Al-Din, M Lewis, L Loizou
Neurosurgery P Van Hille
Obstetrics and Gynaecology R Assassa, R Burr, G Hunter, J Jolly, V Kaul, C Kremer, P Macrow, R Raychaudhuri
Ophthalmology Mr Attia, P K Pauw, S Sharma, I Simmons, K Toor
Oral and Maxillofacial Surgery R Loukota
Orthopaedics Q Al-Dadah, P Bryant, P Deacon, M Gollapudi, M Hutson, B Ketzer, M Rawes, C Ruddlesdin, N Tulwa, C Tuson
Plastic Surgery O Austin, O Fenton, L Fourie, S Majumder, A Phipps, S Southern
Rheumatology A Harvey, S Jarrett
Urology A Browning, S Harrison, M Murphy, S K Sundaram, P Weston

BUPA Murrayfield Hospital - Wirral

Holmwood Drive, Thingwall, Wirral CH61 1AU
Tel: 0151 648 7000 Fax: 0151 648 7684
Email: cservice-wr@bupa.com
Website: www.bupahospitals.co.uk/murayfield
Owners: BUPA Hospitals Ltd
Total Beds: 63

Manager Margaret McNab

Accident and Emergency A Pannycook
Anaesthetics P Bapat, J Chambers, M Conway, J Dalton, J Devlin, D Eastwood, E Forrest, M Forrest, J Gannon, M R Goulden, B Guratsky, B Hedayarti, G Jefferies, A Leach, S Leith, J Moore, S M Mostafa, S H Pennefather, B Phillips, A Rao, H Romer, G Russell, M Smith, K Stevens
Cardiology P Currie, D Rittoo
Care of the Elderly J Barrett
Dermatology P Dufton, S Jones
ENT M Birchall, M McCormick, G O'Sullivan, I Sherman, V Srinivasan
General Medicine G Bell, D Bowen Jones, A V Crowe, J Dawson, J Delaney, R Faizallah, R Ferguson, D Galvani, I Gilmore, I Jones, D Lawrence, P McClelland, P Reid, J Silas, R Sturgess, J Vora
General Surgery J Anderson, D Berstock, S Blair, R Chandrasekar, G Gilling-Smith, M Greaney, M S Javed, D Kerrigan, C Makin, A Masteres, D Reilly, J Shennan, F Swe, C Walsh
Haematology T Deeble
Neurology P Humphrey, B Lecky
Neurosurgery G Findlay, C Mallucci
Obstetrics and Gynaecology B Alderman, P Bousfield, M Doyle, J Herod, A Murray, D Richmond, D Rowlands, J Sutherst, R Welch, I Williams
Oncology P Clark, D Errington, B Haylock, S Y Myint
Ophthalmology L Clearkin, B Damato, C Groenewald, A Kamal, P M Pennefather, S Prasad, M Watts, D Wong
Oral and Maxillofacial Surgery C Jones, D Richardson, G Wood
Orthopaedic Surgery V Bobic, P Brownson, N Donnachie, N Geary, I Harvey, R Harvey, M S Hennessy, J Kaye, A Morris, R Parkinson, D Smith, C Walker
Pathology A Clark, J Darroch, M Gillett, A Murray, K Sidky, H Zakhour
Plastic Surgery S Dhital, F S Fahmy, K Hancock, D McGeorge
Radiology J Curtis, K Das, A Garrett, C Garvey, K Grant, D Green, J Holemans, M Hughes, S Klenk, M Lipton, J Magennis, R G McWilliams, D Ritchie, C Romaniuk, P Rowlands, F Smethurst, S Vinjamuri, J Walsh, D White
Rheumatology R Bucknall, E George, T Kennedy, R Moots
Urology A Alawattegama, P Kutarski, N Parr, R Stephenson, A Woolfenden

BUPA North Cheshire Hospital

Fir Tree Close, Stretton, Warrington WA4 4LU
Tel: 01925 265000 Fax: 01925 215098
Email: cservice-nc@bupa.com
Website: www.bupahospitals.co.uk/northcheshire
Owners: BUPA Hospitals Ltd
Total Beds: 50

Manager Alison da Silva

Anaesthetics G Abdel-Salam, N Gbingie, R Ghaly, A Griffiths, A Higgs, A Hindle, S Jagadeesh, G Salem, K Strahan, J Tytler
ENT S Hampal, M Izzat, S Kent, N Kumar, K Reddy
General Medicine F Ballardie, S Bentley, A Khaleeli, B Linaker, W C Tan
General Surgery M Brett, D Cade, G Copeland, T Da Silva, M Hanafy, C Harding-Mackean, G Hutchinson, J Pollett, B Taylor, M Tighe
Genitourinary Medicine E Morgan
Neurology N Silver
Obstetrics and Gynaecology H Furniss, H Griffith, N Holland, E Kozman, J Langton, G Ramsden, G Rowland, R Slade
Ophthalmology M Halliwell, C Noonan, P Palimar, C Peckar, A Rowlands, M Wishart
Oral and Maxillofacial Surgery J Brown, J Stowell
Orthopaedic Surgery V Bobic, D Boot, H Casserly, M Hayton, E Jago, M Jones, S McLoughlin, M McNicholas, R Sanger, I Shackleford, P Sherry, M Webber
Paediatrics N Mir, N Wild
Pathology M Al-Jafari
Plastic Surgery V Kumar, D McGeorge
Radiology J Desmond, G Murphy, G Rosbotham-Williams
Radiotherapy D Errington
Rheumatology R Bernstein, R Mallya
Urology P Anandaram, R Ewing, P Jamieson, E Robinson

BUPA Parkway Hospital

1 Damson Parkway, Solihull B91 2PP
Tel: 0121 704 1451 Fax: 0121 711 7483
Email: cservice-pk@bupa.com
Website: www.bupahospitals.co.uk/solihull
Owners: BUPA Hospitals Ltd
Total Beds: 51

Manager Mary Hall

Accident and Emergency A Bleetman
Anaesthetics J Bleasdale, C Bonnici, D M Howes, C J Knickenberg, A C Marshall, T J Mcleod, R I Miller, B O'Connor, A Okubadejo, B Prasad, T D Priest, N Sherwood
Cardiology P F Ludman, M Payne, M Pitt
Cardiothoracic Surgery N Briffa, R Steyn
Care of the Elderly P Ramesh, P Ray
Dermatology T Finch, K Ryatt, I Zaki
ENT J Campbell, P Dekker, R M Irving, C Jennings, M Kuo, D Morgan, K Pearman, P Pracy
General Medicine J G Ayres, A S Bates, P Bright, I Chesner, P M Dodson, L Hill, J F Khalil-Marzou, C Nwokolo, S O'Hickey, R Palmer, R J Polson, M Sandler, D Stableforth, R Wears
General Surgery G Barsoum, A Bradbury, M Budhoo, D Burkitt, R Cobb, M Gannon, C Hendrickse, R Holl-Allen, I Paterson, P Super, R G Tudor
Genitourinary Medicine J Ross
Haematology R Johnson, D Milligan
Histopathology M Radojkovic
Neurology A Williams
Neurosurgery S Harland, J Wasserburg
Obstetrics and Gynaecology I Abukhalil, S Blunt, C Griffin, S Hall, S Irani, G Matharu, P Needham, R S Settatree, D Sturdee, G Sunanda
Oncology I Geh, T Latief, A Stockdale

Ophthalmology H Ahluwalia, M Benson, I Cunliffe, J Gibson, B Halliday, T Reuser, R Robinson, S Shah
Oral and Maxillofacial Surgery K Webster
Orthopaedic Surgery S Brooks, S Bryan, V Goswami, A W Hughes, S Hughes, T Lawrence, S Massoud, P C Moses, A Murray, I Nwachukwu, H Rahman, J Ramos, A Sambatakakis, M Shrivastava, R Tillman, P J F Wade
Paediatric Medicine K Nathavitharana, S Rose, R Sunderland
Plastic Surgery H Goldin, C C Kat, A Khanna, R Papini, C Rayner, B Richard
Podiatry S A Metcalfe
Radiology A Banerjee, P Crowe, J Henderson, V Kale, G Stewart
Rheumatology S Bowman, M Pugh, A Sinha
Urology Z Almallah, A Blacklock, R Devarajan, A Doherty, D Farrar, K Kadow, S R Koneru, S Morris
Vascular Surgery T Wilmink

BUPA Regency Hospital

West Street, Macclesfield SK11 8DW
Tel: 01625 501150 Fax: 01625 501505
Email: cservice-rc@bupa.com
Website: www.bupahospitals.co.uk/regency
Owners: BUPA Hospitals Ltd
Total Beds: 31

Manager John Cameron

Accident and Emergency N J Gathercole
Anaesthetics M Y Aglan, D Banks, P Board
Cardiology R Egdell
Dermatology J Ashworth, T Griffiths, J Lear
ENT J E Davies, J A J Deans, N J Kay, P Sheehan
General Medicine R Stead
General Surgery D Matheson, A Quayle, M Wilson
Genitourinary Medicine M Khan
Haematology J Hudson
Neurophysiology P Heath
Obstetrics and Gynaecology V Hall, V A Lether
Ophthalmology R Brown, A D Hubbard, A Moriarty, B J Moriarty, A Needham, M Neugebauer
Orthopaedics J M Auchincloss, K A Barnes, R Dalal, G Keys, M T Khan, P G Turner, C Warren-Smith, M Waseem
Plastic Surgery W Jaffe
Rheumatology S M Knight
Urology G Collins, D Holden, S Namisavayam

BUPA Roding Hospital

Roding Lane South, Ilford IG4 5PZ
Tel: 020 8551 1100 Fax: 020 8709 7804
Email: cservice-rd@bupa.com
Website: www.bupahospitals.co.uk/roding
Owners: BUPA Hospitals Ltd
Total Beds: 59

Manager Peter Lamond

Anaesthetics H Boralessa, J Lloyd, A G Morris, R Wijesurendra
Cardiology A Deaner, S Gupta, J Hogan, C Knight, A S Kurbaan, J Sayer, A Timmis
Care of the Elderly K Kafetz
Dermatology S Chopra, D G Paige
ENT A Bhattacharyya, B Chopra, C Chowdhury, M Dilkes, N Flower, N J Frootko, B Kotecha, G Morrison, M E Papesch, A Shaida
General Medicine N Ahmad, W Ashraf, R L Bagg, I Beasley, R Davison, S Grainger, R Greaves, V Kulhalli, J Mannakkara, K Niranjan, S Saboor, A Sawyerr, V L Sharman, R Storring, P Wright
General Surgery A Bhargava, A J Botha, S Brearley, J Crinnion, N Fieldman, S Jacob, G Lauffer, P N Luthra, K R Mannur, F Mihaimeed, A Ojo, D Shanahan, E Slater, S Snooks, P Thomas, J Wellwood
Genitourinary Medicine N Anand
Haematology C W M De Silva, I Grant
Neurology R Capildeo, J V Jestico
Neurophysiology B D Youl
Neurosurgery J Benjamin, K M David, J Kellerman
Obstetrics and Gynaecology Y Akinfenwa, M Al-Samarrai, H Annan, J Aquilina, G Cochrane, Y Coker, S K Ghatak, S Gupta, C Hargreaves, R J Howard, A R Jeyarajah, L McMillan, J F Odejinmi, I Opemuyi, P Rainsbury, J Swinhoe, D A Viniker
Oncology C Cottrill, N Davidson, A Gershuny
Ophthalmology K Barton, J Chawla, G Dawidek, N Kayali, S Ruben, H Towler
Oral and Maxillofacial Surgery J Evans, B Littler
Orthopaedic Surgery H Banan, M El-Zebdeh, Zahir Ghassem, B Goldie, G Iwegbu, S Kumar, A Lang-Stevenson, B Levack, T McAuliffe, W E Ogufere, B Okafor, G Robbins, S Tibrewal
Paediatrics J Allgrove, M Hameed, T Matthews, D Misra
Pain Management C Gauci
Plastic Surgery F Iwuagwu, M Sood, C Walker
Psychiatry A M Margo, N Savla
Radiology S Chawda, J Gutmann, C Padmanathan, N Reading
Rheumatology K Chakravarty, D Doyle, C Kelsey
Urology J Barua, S Bhanot, F Chinegwundoh, S Gujral, J Hines, A Hirsch, J Peters, T Philp, P Shridhar

BUPA St Saviour's Hospital

73 Seabrook Road, Hythe CT21 5BU
Tel: 01303 265581 Fax: 01303 261441
Email: cservice-ss@bupa.com
Website: www.bupahospitals.co.uk/stsaviours
Owners: BUPA Hospitals Ltd
Total Beds: 37

Manager Alan Park

Anaesthetics B Al-Shaikh, J Bulmer, M Hamer, C Lamb, C Lynch, M Mayall, C Miller Jones, J Morris, C Toner, P Venn, N Yardy
Cardiology K Kamalvand
Dermatology C Irvine
ENT J Fairley, G Kanegaonkar, P Robinson
General Medicine J Hossain, A Morris, D Smithard, M Vella, C Williams
General Surgery P Basnyat, T Bates, C Derry, R Insall, D Jackson, N Rao, N Wilson
Neurology N Munro
Obstetrics and Gynaecology J Learmont, J Seaton, B Wise
Ophthalmology N Andrew, M Heravi
Orthopaedics W Dunnet
Paediatrics V Shah
Psychiatry R Sammut
Radiology G Giancola, K Lashkari, S Moorhouse, D Rand, S Santhakumaran, W Webb
Urology A Deane

BUPA South Bank Hospital

139 Bath Road, Worcester WR5 3YB
Tel: 01905 350003 Fax: 01905 357765
Email: cservice-sb@bupa.com
Website: www.bupahospitals.co.uk/southbank
Owners: BUPA Hospitals Ltd
Total Beds: 41

Manager Ben Nicholson

Anaesthetics A Bennett, S Graystone, M Hardwick, J Lee, C Maile, D Phillips, J Prosser, N Rose, C Studd, H Williams
Cardiology D Pitcher, A Scriven
Dermatology F Lewis, W Tucker
ENT L Hollis, A Johnson, M Porter, M Smith, R Vaughan-Jones
General Medicine S Booth, N Hudson, R Lewis, M W [New Person], S O'Hickey
General Surgery M Corlett, R Downing, N Hickey, S Lake, S Radley, C Robertson, M Wadley
Neurophysiology A Blake
Obstetrics and Gynaecology P Moran, D Pickrell, J Watts
Oncology D Faruggia
Ophthalmology K Barber, P Chell
Oral and Maxillofacial Surgery P Earl, T Hall
Orthopaedic Surgery N Ahmed, J Davies, K O'Dwyer, P Ratcliffe, A Reading, D Robinson, E Rouholamin, M Trevett, P Turner

Paediatrics A Cole, K Nathavitharana
Palliative Medicine J Dale
Plastic Surgery C Rayner
Psychiatry S James
Radiology S Bailey, M Brown, P Holland, P Slaney, D South, U Udeshi, R Ward, B Wittkop
Rheumatology A Rai, I Rowe
Urology T Chen

BUPA Wellesley Hospital

Eastern Avenue, Southend-on-Sea SS2 4XH
Tel: 01702 462944 Fax: 01702 600160
Email: cservice-wl@bupa.com
Website: www.bupahospitals.co.uk/wellesley
Owners: BUPA Hospitals Ltd
Total Beds: 48

Manager Andy Wood

Accident and Emergency J Porter
Anaesthetics U Bopitna, I Ewart, J Kinnear, C Naylor, M J Woodham
Cardiology P A Kelly, A Khokhar
Care of the Elderly T O'Brien
Dermatology S Henderson, M Khorshid, R Mehta, W S Robles
ENT D J Gatland, N Warwick-Brown, G Watters
General Medicine J A Ahlquist, H Al-Saldar, G Bray, A Davison, J A Mellor, K Metcalfe, J D O'Brien
General Surgery A Brown, M Dworkin, E Gray, F Hughes, M Jakeways, N D Rothnie, M Salter
Genitourinary Medicine R Spitzer
Neurology A Hewazy, M Mavra, D M Park
Obstetrics and Gynaecology V P Aggarwal, P Hagan, D Jennings, C L Lee, K Lim, T J Pocock, N Tripathi, J Ward
Ophthalmology R Aggarwal, V Geh, N Karia
Oral and Maxillofacial Surgery D Madan, P Weller
Orthopaedic Surgery D A Boston, C Chauhan, R Khazim, G Packer, S Raza, S Sarkar, R A Sudlow, A White
Paediatrics A Shrivastava
Pathology M Chappell
Plastic Surgery D Elliot, M Gittos, L Kangesu
Psychiatry C Murray
Radiology M Aslam, M N Ibrahim, M D Lewars, S Perera, B D Shah, A B Tanqueray, T A Toma
Rheumatology B Dasgupta, T E Gordon
Urology A J Ball, T W Carr, R Lodge

BUPA Women's Health Centre Bristol

Wallace House, 116 Pembroke Road, Clifton, Bristol BS8 3EW
Tel: 0117 317 1300 Fax: 0117 317 1399
Email: cservice-br@bupa.com
Website: www.bupahospitals.co.uk/womenshealthbristol
Owners: BUPA Hospitals Ltd

Burrswood Hospital

Groombridge, Tunbridge Wells TN3 9PY
Tel: 01892 863637 Fax: 01892 863623
Owners: Charity/Association
Total Beds: 35

The Bury St Edmunds Nuffield Hospital

St Mary's Square, Bury St Edmunds IP33 2AA
Tel: 01284 701371 Fax: 01284 769998
Website: www.nuffieldhospitals.org.uk
Owners: Nuffield Hospitals
Total Beds: 40

Manager Jonathan Horrocks

Cardiology D Stone
Dermatology R Jenkins, T Sonnex
Dietetics J Rowlands
ENT P Axon, F Fahmy, B Fish, D McKiernan, R Skibsted
General Medicine I Aziz, J Clark, D O'Reilly, D Sharpstone, J Shneerson, S Whalley
General Surgery J Alberts, J Boyle, E Coveney, M Gaunt, T Justin, N Keeling, D Lawrence, D O'Riordan, O Ravisekar
Gynaecology R Giles, S Gull, D Ross, P Spencer
Neurology G Lennox, P Molyneux
Oncology H Ford, A Moody
Ophthalmology K Jordan, R Lamb, A Ramsay, A Vivian
Oral Surgery H Davies, R Tate
Orthopaedics A August, A Bedford, A Dunn, P Nicolai, M Porteous, W Schenk, S Sjolin, M Wood
Pain Management R Munglani
Plastic Surgery P Hall, M Irwin
Psychiatry M Mayall, Dr O'Flynn
Radiology R Bannon, R Darrah, R Godwin, M MacFarlane, H Taylor
Rheumatology P Johansen, D O'Reilly
Urology J Allan, C Kennedy, J McLoughlin

Capio Ashtead Hospital

The Warren, Ashtead KT21 2SB
Tel: 01372 221400 Fax: 01322 278704
Email: enquiries@ashtead-hospital.co.uk
Website: www.capio.co.uk
Owners: Capio Healthcare UK
Total Beds: 57

Manager Brett Powis

Audiology S J Robinson, L H Yeoh
Cardiology C Byrne, S Odemuyiwa, G Young
Cosmetic Surgery M Gardner
Dermatology S M Breathnach, S H Cliff, A Farrell, J N Leonard, J Rosbotham
ENT R Hehar, P J Robb, P Williamson
General Medicine P Andrews, S K F Chong, L G Darlington, S R Gould, G Knowles, A G Lim, P F Mitchell-Heggs, M Noble, S Rahman, D C Rangedara, G H Robb, M Simkins
General Practice W S Bellenger, Dr Houghton
General Surgery D Al-Musawi, W H Allum, A Halliday, M Kahn, TM Loosemore, R J McFarland, M Miller, D Nehra, S E P Pitt-Miller, M A K Raja, R S Taylor, P Thomas, P Toomey
Haematology L Jones, F Matthey, M J Semple
Health Screening W S Bellenger, F Z Henari, J A Houghton, J Pickin
Immunology A S Bansal
Neurology P Trend, S G Wilson
Neurophysiology M P Sheehy
Neurosurgery F G Johnston
Obstetrics and Gynaecology S Butler-Manuel, P M Coats, C E G Ellis, V Kakumani, M Katesmark, M G Long, J Penny, N G J Pipe, Mr Shehata, R W Worth
Ophthalmology R Coakes, S Daya, I Gillespie, R J Leitch, T J K Leonard, R J Marsh, S Shah, P G Ursell
Oral and Maxillofacial Surgery B M W Bailey, M H Danford, A J Lyons, M Partridge, M Preiss
Orthopaedics M Bircher, W Burgoyne, P Cheong-Leen, S Chockalingam, A G Cobb, R E Field, P Mitchell, D W H Mok, D W Parsons, V R Patel, M Proctor, M A Qureshi, R Twyman, G Wilson
Paediatrics G Baird, S N J Capps, S K F Chong, K Daly, K Holmes, J M Nicholls, J O'Connell, M R Ryalls
Pain Management C Pither
Plastic Surgery B W E Powell, P J Whitfield, G R Wilson
Psychiatry P Bailey, P G Mellet, R J Penrose, A J Winbow
Radiology J Britton, C D George, A Gregory, G Lamb, T Senbanjo, K B Stoner, W J Walker, K Younger
Radiotherapy J P Glees
Rheumatology J Etherington, S Patel, A S Torode
Sports Medicine W S Bellenger, J Etherington
Urology M J Bailey, C R Charig, H Ghaznavi, M R Gilbody, R Morley, A Rane
Vascular Medicine Miss Halliday, Mr McFarland, Mr Taylor, Mr Thomas

Capio The Berkshire Independent Hospital

Wensley Road, Coley Park, Reading RG1 6UZ
Tel: 0118 902 8000 Fax: 0118 902 8215
Website: www.capio.co.uk
Owners: Capio Healthcare UK
Total Beds: 61

Anaesthetics A Lawson
Audiology J Fisher, R Wills
Cardiology A Chow, N Spyrou
Dermatology L Fearfield, C Higgins
ENT W Colquhoun-Flannery, R Corbridge, R Herdman, N Mansell, J Smith
General Medicine J Booth, T Mee, M Myszor, S Packham, J Simmons, H Simpson, J Stratford, J Thomas
General Surgery M Booth, T Dehn, R Farouk
Genitourinary Medicine A Tang
Neurology J Adcock, R Gregory, N Hyman
Obstetrics and Gynaecology M Selinger, K Smith, P Street
Occupational Health J Walker
Orthopaedics A Andrade, H Brownlow, S Copeland, R Dodds, C Fergusson, O Levy, A Themen
Paediatrics A Boon, R Kumar, N Mann
Plastic Surgery A Armstrong, J Dickinson
Podiatry S Kriss
Psychiatry M Allsopp
Psychology T Powell, J Spinks
Rheumatology A Bradlow, J McNally
Urology D Fawcett, S Foley, A Jones, P Malone, H Whitfield

Capio Duchy Hospital

Penventinnie Lane, Treliske, Truro TR1 3UP
Tel: 01872 226100 Fax: 01872 226118
Website: www.capio.co.uk
Owners: Capio Healthcare UK
Total Beds: 39

Manager David Hillier

Cardiology S Evans, A Mourant, A Slade
Cosmetic Surgery J McDiarmid, R Morris
Dermatology D Gould, T W Lucke
ENT G Conrad, I Smith, D Whinney, A Wilde
General Surgery N Barwell, R Bourne, P Cox, J Davies, Mr Desmarowitz, E Lloyd-Davies, A Patterson, P Peyser, C Rickford, A Widdison, K Woodburn
Gynaecology S Bates, D Byrne, P Callen, S Grant, R Holmes, R Jones, Mr Oladipo
General Medicine I Coutts, H Dalton, H Hussaini, J Myers
Neurology B McLean
Ophthalmology W Carruthers, F Kumaravel, A Stockwell, W Westlake, N Wilson-Holt
Oral and Maxillofacial Surgery S Adcock, C Lansley
Orthopaedics D Bracey, D Fern, P Hutchins, R Kincaid, A Lee, M Norton, S Parsons, P Peace, M Regan, T Scott
Paediatrics G Taylor
Plastic Surgery J McDiarmid, R Morris
Psychology L Bowlby-West, J Noon
Rheumatology M Davies, A Woolf
Urology R Cox, J O'Rourke, R Willis

Capio Euxton Hall Hospital

Wigan Road, Euxton, Chorley PR7 6DY
Tel: 01257 276261 Fax: 01257 261882
Website: www.capio.co.uk
Owners: Capio Healthcare UK
Total Beds: 29

Manager C A Chadwick

Anaesthetics R G Ghaly, N J Manus
Cardiology A Chauhan, G K Davis
Dermatology M H Beck, D B Brookes
ENT J P De Charpentier, M Izzat, B N Kumar, V B Pothula, M S Small
General Medicine P W Bliss, I M Drake, R C Gupta, A Kumar, S I Madi, M M Mughal, I P M O'Connell, J B Ward
General Surgery A L Blower, P P George, R N L Harland, C A Harris, M Holbrook, W Jaffe, M Jameel, M M Mughal, Z Saidan, J B Ward
Haematology K Pendry
Neurology S Shaunak
Neurophysiology S M Alani
Neurosurgery A Golash
Obstetrics and Gynaecology K R Abdo, A J Bellis, R M El Gawly, R H Martin, S Prashar, S K Shah
Oncology E A Young
Ophthalmology D K Banerjee, A T N Ekdawy, C J Heaven, S Jain, J S Mars, S Natha
Orthopaedic Surgery R S Bale, A O Browne, A K Gambhir, A I Hassan, M J Hayton, P J Hughes, S Jari, A McEvoy, G J McLaughlan, A Mohammed, S R Murali, M L Porter, V Raut, D Redfern
Plastic Surgery W Jaffe, R p Jones
Podiatry C Parish
Psychology R Logie
Radiology S I Ali, S Desai, A Jain, J Lay, P J J Reston, D Sheals, B C Spinks, R C Stockwell, D Temperley
Urology J Husain, S S Matanhelia, A Thompson

Capio Fitzwilliam Hospital

Milton Way, South Bretton, Peterborough PE3 9AQ
Tel: 01733 261717 Fax: 01733 261119
Email: enquires@fitzwilliam-hospital.co.uk
Website: www.capio.co.uk
Owners: Capio Healthcare UK
Total Beds: 59

Manager Dominic Bath

Cardiology J N Porter, D Rowlands
Dermatology P Hudson, R B Mallett
ENT N Bhat, R H Cawood, Miss Horrocks, P Leong, A Pfeiderer
General Medicine M Dronfield, M A Khan, C Mistry, I Mungall, P Nair, S P Sahi
General Surgery T I Abdullah, F M Bajwa, A Choy, R J Guy, J H Hall, B Krijgsman, Mr Menon, J Thornton Holmes, D Valerio, R T Walker, A Wells
Gynaecology S Havenga, I Jelen, M Lumb, H Rai, B Ramsay, J Randall, A Sriemevan, S A Steel
Neurology J W Thorpe
Oncology R J Benson
Ophthalmology A W D Fitt, T Rimmer, S Vardy
Oral and Maxillofacial Surgery C E Moss, J M Robertson
Orthopaedic Surgery T P S Bhullar, A Doran, B Dutta, M Hutson, D L Johns, J W M Jones, A Kumar, S Lewis, Mr Massraff, Mr Pathak, G Pryor, M L Sutcliffe, G W Varley, S Venkatachalam
Pain Management E Erdmann, M Glavina, R Robertshaw
Plastic Surgery T Ahmad, B G H Lamberty, C M Malata
Psychology V Gardiner
Radiology J C Chadwick, A E Dux, H M Elmadbouh, J Marshall, B McKeown, B F Millet, R E Moshy, J N Perry, G Thorley
Rheumatology N J Sheehan, N E Williams
Urology H N Blackford, C Dawson, S D Sharma, A G Turner

Capio The Fotheringhay Suite

Lilford Floor, Kettering General Hospital, Rothwell Road, Kettering NN16 8UZ
Tel: 01536 492831 Fax: 01536 492830
Website: www.capio.co.uk
Owners: Capio Healthcare UK

Consultants see Capio Woodland Hospital

Capio Fulwood Hall Hospital

Midgery Lane, Fulwood, Preston PR2 9SZ
Tel: 01772 704111 Fax: 01772 795131
Website: www.capio.co.uk
Owners: Capio Healthcare UK

Total Beds: 29

Manager John Pickering

Anaesthetics P Bunting, N Hacking, A Lowrie
Cardiology A Chauhan, S Kahn
Dermatology W Bottomley, P Harrison
ENT J P De Charpentier, C Hartley, M Small
General Medicine A L Burton, S A Cairns, R A Coward, A A Lakhdar, J F McCann, M Munavvar, P Shields, L R Solomon, P Vice
General Surgery A Egun, P P George, A R Hearn, R Hughes, Z Saidan, D J Stewart, G J Thompson, J B Ward
Neurology J D Mitchell, J Nixon, S Shaunak, T Tidswell
Neurophysiology I H Bangash, G U Lekwuwu
Neurosurgery C H G Davis, A Golash, N Gurusinghe, G Roberts
Obstetrics and Gynaecology K R Abdo, P J Keating, S Prashar, I G Robertson
Oncology A Biswas, A C Hindley, M P Macheta, T Mughal, G Skailes, S Susnerwala, M Wise, E Young
Ophthalmology H P Adhikary, A Ekdawy, G A P Griffith, S Jain, E M Talbot
Oral and Maxillofacial Surgery S Akhtar, J Cornah
Orthopaedics R S Bale, J C Faux, P Hughes, S A Khan, A McEvoy, G J McLauchlan, A Mohammed, M L Porter, D R Redfern, S J Shaw, R B Smith, M R Wharton
Paediatrics A N Campbell
Plastic Surgery A J Howcroft, A Juma, J C Laitung
Psychology G S Lee
Radiology C Ali, C Coutinho, M J Dobson, S P D'Souza, S C Galletly, W J Gunawardena, I Harris, J C Hill, S Kearney, J P Y Lay
Rheumatology C Chattopadhyay
Urology S S Matanhelia, M E Watson

Capio Mount Stuart Hospital

St Vincent's Road, Torquay TQ1 4UP
Tel: 01803 313881 Fax: 01803 321698
Email: capio-mount-stuart-enquiries@capio.co.uk
Website: www.capio.co.uk
Owners: Capio Healthcare UK
Total Beds: 31

Manager Theresa Starling

Anaesthetics J Ackers, A Bainton, P Ballance, N Campbell, J Carlisle, S Fearnley, M Hearn, K Houghton, J Ingham, A Matthews, M Mercer, Dr Montgomery, I Norley, J Norman, J Pappin, D Snow, M Swart, R Tackley, J Thorn, A Varvinskiy
ENT S Hickey, F Houlihan, J Hutchison
General Medicine C Carey, R G Chadwick, L Dobson, R Dyer, C Edwards, D K George, J M Goldman, G Gribbin, J Gurrier-Adams, P Keeling, G Kendall, J Lowes, I Mahy, D G Sinclair, P Sleight, J Smith, R Teague
General Surgery I Currie, D DeFriend, P Donnelly, P W Houghton, R Hughes, N Johnson, M Kirollos, P Lewis, S MacDermott, R Mason, S Mitchell, R Pullan
Gynaecology J Barrington, M Leggott, R Ranjit, P Stannard
Maxillofacial Surgery D Cunliffe, P Douglas
Neurology P Sadler, S Weatherby
Neurosurgery T Germon
Occupational Health J Challenor
Oncology N Bailey, A Goodman
Ophthalmology A Frost, M Graham, C James, S Livesey, Y Osoba
Orthopaedics M Ashworth, P Birdsall, V Conboy, P Cox, J Davis, K Eyres, M Hockings, G B Irvine, R A Lofthouse, A G MacEachern, N Mackay, R Ramesh
Pain Management A Dashfield, F E Luscombe
Pathology L M Bower, J Bridger, D Day, M Garrido, A F Maggs, P Roberts, M G Ryley, N Rymes, S Smith, D Turner, P Turner
Plastic Surgery V S Devaraj, J Evans, A Fitton, J McDiarmid, R J Morris, P Saxby, B Tanner
Psychology M Fitzpatrick
Radiology D Buckley, R J Heafield, J Isaacs, P G Kember, E Morris, M Puckett, R Seymour, P White

Capio New Hall Hospital

Bodenham, Salisbury SP5 4EY
Tel: 01722 422333 Fax: 01722 435158
Email: kerry.warner@capio.co.uk
Website: www.capio.co.uk
Owners: Capio Healthcare UK
Total Beds: 34

Manager Julie Watkinson

Anaesthetics S Abbas, R Barrett, S Cockroft, C Cox, K Duggal, W Garrett, D Lintin, D McCallum, D Murray, J Onslow, R Scott, P Swayne, I Wright
Cardiology S Biggart
Dermatology R Meyrick-Thomas
ENT M Brockbank, M Collins, G Todd
Gastroenterology A Tanner
General Medicine A Jones, J Marigold, A Warley
General Surgery G Angell, N Carty, H Chave, J Cooke, D Finnis, C Ranaboldo
Gynaecology P Docherty, S Fountain, D McKenna
Neurology H Katifi
Oncology K Gregory, T Iveson
Ophthalmology R Collyer-Powell, R Humphry, A Tyers
Oral and Maxillofacial Surgery I Downie, T Flood
Orthopaedic Surgery A Beaumont, J Carvell, D Chapple, D Cox, G Rushforth, G Shergill
Paediatrics D Stratton
Plastic Surgery M Cadier, R Cole, J Hobby, N Horlock, R McDowell, D McNeill, A Rossi, E Tiernan, I Whitworth
Radiology J Annis, B Bentley, R Frost, S Hegarty, K Johnson, S McGee, A Morris
Rehabilitation A Soopramanien
Rheumatology M Cawley, R Ellis, J Robertson
Urology P Guy, G McIntosh

Capio Nightingale Day Hospital

1B Harewood Row, London NW1 6SE
Tel: 020 7725 9940 Fax: 020 7724 9092
Website: www.capionightingalehospitals.co.uk
Owners: Capio Nightingale Hospitals

Capio Nightingale Hospital

11-19 Lisson Grove, London NW1 6SH
Tel: 020 7535 7700 Fax: 020 7724 9440
Website: www.capionightingalehospitals.co.uk
Owners: Capio Nightingale Hospitals
Total Beds: 69

Manager Mary Kong

Capio Nightingale Hospital Chelsea

1-5 Radnor Walk, London SW3 4PB
Tel: 020 7349 3900 Fax: 020 7351 7098
Website: www.capionightingalehospitals.co.uk
Owners: Capio Nightingale Hospitals
Total Beds: 62

Manager Mary Kong

Capio Nightingale Hospital Liverpool

Park Road, Waterloo, Liverpool L22 3XE
Tel: 0151 257 6200 Fax: 0151 257 6215
Website: www.capionightingalehospitals.co.uk
Owners: Capio Nightingale Hospitals
Total Beds: 54

Manager Nick Ruffley

Capio North Downs Hospital

46 Tupwood Lane, Caterham CR3 6DP
Tel: 01883 348981 Fax: 01883 341163
Email: capio-north-downs-enquiries@capio.co.uk
Website: www.capio.co.uk

Owners: Capio Healthcare UK
Total Beds: 24

Manager Janene Madden

Cardiology R Allen, S P Joseph
Dermatology S H Cliff, N C Cowley, A Farrell, R Sarkany
ENT K Bevan, J D Brookes, L Hicklin, G Warrington
General Medicine D Acharya, A Mehta, M Mendall, V Phongsathorn, C Prajapati
General Surgery M Abulafi, J Derodra, M A Dissanayake, J Grabham, P Hurley, R G Lightwood, T Loosemore, R I Swift, M Williams
Neurology J Kimber
Obstetrics and Gynaecology M Booker, A P Gordon-Wright, R Hamid, M G Long, J Penny, A H Sultan, B R Thakar, P T Townsend
Ophthalmology R S Wilson
Oral and Maxillofacial Surgery A S Averill
Orthopaedics A J Campbell, K J Drabu, G D E Howell, A Iossifidis, G Marsh, H D Maurice, J Miller, T P Selvan, G Tselentakis
Paediatrics M H Jawad, I Lewis
Palliative Medicine J Kurian, M Nava
Plastic Surgery J Davison, P M Gilbert, A Khandwala, N S B Tanner
Psychiatry S McCluskey, J S McPherson, R Peermahomed, M Rowlands, Y Sokan, A Valmana, A Winbow
Radiology N Bees, H Blake, P D Byrne, C N O' Digges, R Evans, S Gwyther, C Hoskins, R P McAvinchey, D Mukasa, A P G Newman-Sanders, E A North, D I Sarma, N Sellars
Rheumatology A B Bhanji
Urology G Das, P D Miller, G Muir, P G S Raju, A Rane

Capio Oaklands Hospital

19 Lancaster Road, Salford M6 8AQ
Tel: 0161 787 7700 (Reception), 0161 789 4900 (Helpline)
Fax: 0161 787 8097
Email: enquiries@oaklands-hospitals.co.uk
Website: www.capio.co.uk
Owners: Capio Healthcare UK
Total Beds: 26

Manager James Mieszkowski

Anaesthetics Dr Kinsella
Cardiology P Barnes, A Cooper, A Fitchett
Dental Surgery Mr Ucer
Dermatology Dr Fitzgerald, J Yell
ENT M Rothera, Mr Saeed, Mr Willatt
General Medicine Dr Aziz, C Babbs, H Buckler, Dr Kalra, Dr New, Dr O'Donoghue, R O'Driscoll, W D W Rees, Dr Robinson
General Surgery I Anderson, S Attwood, G Carlson, Mr Madan, Z Saad, N Scott
Haematology Dr Garg
Neurology M Kellett
Neurosurgery Mr Safat
Obstetrics and Gynaecology G Falconer, T Kelly, D Polson, R Slade
Ophthalmology Mr Chitcara, B Mills, Mr Rosen
Oral and Maxillofacial Surgery R Lloyd, C Ucer
Orthopaedics Mr Andrew, L Funk, S Jari, H Maxwell, L Muir, D Sochart, R Wilkes
Paediatrics Mr Henry
Plastic Surgery G Byrne, S Dhital, W Jaffe, M Liddington
Podiatry F Webb
Respiratory Medicine Dr O'Driscoll
Rheumatology R Cooper, M Jayson
Urology C Betts, K O'Flynn

Capio Oaks Hospital

Oaks Place, Mile End Road, Colchester CO4 5XR
Tel: 01206 752121 Fax: 01206 852701
Website: www.capio.co.uk
Owners: Capio Healthcare UK
Total Beds: 57

Anaesthetics S Dixon, A G Eldridge, J P Harris, W Konarzewski, S MacDonnell, S Mackenzie, A Masters, M J McGinty, T McLoughlin, P Patient, D N Ranasinghe, D Thomas, G Timmins, G M Watling, A Masters
Cardiology P Mills, N M Robinson, J Stephens, K Tang
Care of the Elderly A Deb, P Dixon, V Paramsothy, P Rudra, T Shawis
Dermatology D Shuttleworth, D J Todd
ENT D McFerran, D McRae
General Medicine C Bodmer, N Chanarin, R Cowan, A J Handley, F MacNeill, S Marsh, S Nugent, D O'Riordan, D Read
General Surgery C Backhouse, F A MacNeill, S Marsh, A R L May, D Menzies, R W Motson
Neurology G Elrington
Obstetrics and Gynaecology J W Eddy, J C Evans-Jones, A Kadva, A M Lower, M K Oak, J Osborne, C K Partington, D Sanderson
Oncology P Murray, B Sizer, S Tahir
Ophthalmology N Ahmad, A Beckingsale, G Ghosh, P Gormley, J Sheldrick
Oral and Maxillofacial Surgery J Clarke, H Davies, G Walker
Orthodontics R Chate
Orthopaedics J Bradley, T Briggs, M Loeffler, D Moore, J Parker, S Shanker, J Stanton, T Thomas, J Tuite
Paediatrics S Mukerji, B S Sihra, J Symons
Plastic Surgery A F S Flemming, N Niranjan
Psychiatry C Andersson, N Coxhead, P Grahame, C Murray, E Youssif
Psychology S Lovett
Psychotherapy L Backhouse
Radiology M Al-Dabbagh, O Demuren, E Gannushkin, M Gould, N Lacey, N Sivananthan
Rheumatology P Byrne, S Daunt, T Walton
Sports Medicine P Marfleet
Urology C M Booth, J Corr, Mr Marfleet, T Tassadaq

Capio Park Hill Hospital

Thorne Road, Doncaster DN2 5TH
Tel: 01302 730300 Fax: 01302 322499
Email: lisa.stubbs@capio.co.uk
Website: www.capio.co.uk
Owners: Capio Healthcare UK
Total Beds: 21

Manager John Tounsend

Anaesthetics K Ahmed, A Blackburn, M N Calhaem, A Chaffe, J S Collins, N D Edwards, S M Enright, G A Francis, S Gill, D Graham, R W Harris, P S Hopton, T J Hughes, W U Karunaratne, T Kirkpatrick, P Matthews, B R Milne, N P Nagar, D M Newby, D Northwood, C Palmer, S Panjwani, H Raithatha, A J N Renshaw, K Ruiz, N Saquib, A Selim, P E Shannon, P Smith, A N Strachan, E Taylor, J J A Train, D J Wood
Cardiology M W Baig, G E Payne
Dermatology S B Bittiner
ENT R Capper, J M Dugar, L Durham, P Harkness, K B Hughes, J M Lancer, U D Masieh, M G Watson
General Medicine A N Alwail, R P Bolton, D K Chadha, E W Jones, R J E Leggett, R J Leigh, B K Mondal, A J Oates, A Rajathurai, T Rogers, J Sayer
General Surgery R Avill, J S Bagley, M M A Bassuini, A E O Coker, G B Coombes, I D Crate, G Jacob, R B Jones, A K Kar, N Kazzazi, K M Kolar, P Tan
Genitourinary Medicine T R Moss
Gynaecology M Alloub, G P Chandler, E Emovon, D W Fenton, H H Gergis, M R Heslip, F A Howard, P K Iqbal, M Mammo, M Michel, W K Moores, B C Rosenberg
Maxillofacial Surgery R K Lee, P G McAndrew, N S Peckitt
Neurology A Gibson
Oncology S Ramakrishnan
Ophthalmology V A Burton, S P Desai, M Jabir, D G Jayamanne, V V Kayarkar, L R Kolli, P J Noble, E Oji, A A Zaidi
Orthopaedics M Al-Khatib, S Ali, M S Bhamra, M S Binns, P S Fagg, M J Farthan, R Helm, B Ketzer, B Khuffash, K T Kumar, J G

Matthews, P J A Molitor, A Mubashir, K Ratnakumar, S O Shafquat, T S F Tadross, M Zaman, M Zeraati
Paediatrics S J Ahmad
Pathology S Beck, S Rogers, A Sheehan
Plastic Surgery O Fenton, P Jordan, J G Miller, D R Ralston
Psychiatry C L Kelly
Radiology J Y MacKinlay, A D Ward
Rheumatology J R Lambert
Urology J K Darrad, J Leveckis, B T Parys, I R Townend
Vascular Surgery R J Cuschieri, J V Psaila, S Singh

Capio Pinehill Hospital

Benslow Lane, Hitchin SG4 9QZ
Tel: 01462 422822 Fax: 01462 421968
Email: enquiries@pinehill-hospital.co.uk
Website: www.capio.co.uk
Owners: Capio Healthcare UK
Total Beds: 34

Manager Phil Curran

Anaesthetics S Bates, O Boomers, M Carrington, M Chilvers, S Eckersall, M Fox, P L Goldberg, S Gowrie-Mohan, M Henein, K Jani, S Jothilingham, J M Lalor, A Moye, A Rajah, S Rajah, W J K Rickford, K Sarang, P Sengupta, Z P Shah, I Sockalingam, S Susay, J Thiagarajan, B S Yogasakaran
Audiology F Bateson
Cardiology M Dubowitz, M Lynch
Dermatology H Bayoumi, C A Green, A Powles
ENT O Chalwa, A Frosh, G Mochloulis, S J Quinn
Gastroenterology S Greenfield, D Morris, I Sargeant
General Medicine L J Borthwick, S Chatfield, G Georgiou, S Graham, S A Khan, N N Stanley, T Tong
General Surgery S Gupta, T Holme, H H Thompson, J Wood
Geriatric M Ehsanullah, P Ghosh
Gynaecology R Atalla, S Banerjee, K El Farra, E Hemaya, D McLintock, D Salvesen, R Sattin, J B Webb
Haematology J Hanslip
Maxillofacial Surgery A D Giles, J A Sherman
Microbiology K M Alshafi
Nephrology K Farrington, P Warwicker
Neurology J Gibbs
Ophthalmology S H Campbell, T P Coker, M Toma
Orthopaedics M Chatoo, J H Dorrell, P Hope, P Kerr, J Kitson, J Leitao, R Pandit, H V parmar, D Powles, J Sarkar, R Sharma, G P Wilde
Paediatrics O Ahmed, J Reiser
Plastic Surgery M Dickson, N James, P Mahafrrey
Psychiatry M Clarke, B L Mason, A G Patel, G Rose, L Van Huyssteen
Psychology J Lillesater-Spendlove, J Neilson
Radiology F Alaeddin, D Amerasekera, P Brooks, S Kaniyur, C King, H Lee, I Mootoosamy, C Prendergast
Rheumatology A I Binder, S Ellis, M A Wajed
Specialist Services M Curtin, S Holland, M Hussein, G Webb
Urology G B Boustead, D C Hanbury, T A McNicholas
Vascular Surgery S Selvakumar, M T Simpson

Capio Reading Hospital

Swallows Croft, Wensley Road, Coley Park, Reading RG1 6UZ
Tel: 0118 902 8000 Fax: 0118 902 8125
Website: www.capio.co.uk
Owners: Capio Healthcare UK
Total Beds: 73

Manager Chris Wood

Orthopaedics A Andrade, H Brownlow, S Copeland, R Dodds, C Fergusson, O Levy, A Themen
Urology D Fawcett, S Foley, A Jones, P Malone, H Whitfield

Capio Renacres Hall Hospital

Renacres Lane, Halsall, Ormskirk L39 8SE
Tel: 01704 841133 Fax: 01704 842030
Email: enquiries@renacres-hall-hospital.co.uk
Website: www.capio.co.uk
Owners: Capio Healthcare UK
Total Beds: 32

Manager Chris Buckingham

Audiology J Brooks, P Zalewski
Cardiology J P Fox, J Mennim, E Rodrigues
Clinical Chemistry E Manning, C Van Heyninghen
Dermatology A Memon
ENT T Lesser, N Roland, A Swift
Gastroenterology G P Butcher, C F Kire
General Surgery R Anderson, D Artioukh, I D Harrison, Mr Jmor, D Jones, P F Mason, S E Meehan, I Stevenson, M R Zeiderman
Gynaecology M Davies, R P Edwards, G Foat, M N Iskander, S Jones, S Sharma
Neurology A Bowden, Dr Wieshman
Neurosurgery P R Eldridge, P May, T R K Varma
Oncology K Hayat, S Myint
Ophthalmology D K Chitkara, P W Joyce, S B Kaye, N O'Donnell, A P Watson
Oral and Maxillofacial Surgery M Boyle, S Rogers, D Vaughan
Orthopaedics R F Adam, M Ali, J Marshall, T J Menon, K H Suraliwala
Paediatrics M M Zbaeda
Pain Management A Head-Rapson, A J Zmyslowski
Pathology S Dundas, P Mansour, T Tagore
Physicians J Horsley, M Maciver, R Oelbaum, M J Serlin, J P Simmonds
Plastic Surgery R Alvi, K Graham, R Green
Psychiatry E S Hussain, M K Rahman
Psychology P Coll
Rheumatology K Binymin
Speech Therapy E Gilmartin
Urology M M Gammal, G Singh, S G Vesey

Capio The Rivers Hospital

High Wych Road, Sawbridgeworth CM21 0HH
Tel: 01279 600282 Fax: 01279 600212
Website: www.capio.co.uk
Owners: Capio Healthcare UK
Total Beds: 70

Manager Peter Curtis

Allergies V S Chakravarti
Anaesthetics R Khiroya
Audiology F Bateson
Cardiology J R Milne, J Sayer
Care of the Elderly G B Ambepitiya, R Morgan, J Tharakan, R Whale
Dermatology A H M Bayoumi, H Dodd
Diabetes S A Beshyah
ENT A A Amen, N Flower, A Frosh, D McKiernan, G Mochloulis
General Medicine S A Beshyah, R G Dent, I H Fahal, J R Milne, D M Preston, J Sayer, E Stoner, J Tadman, J F Waller, J P Warren
General Surgery H Bradpiece, M A Clifton, P W Crane, M Lennox, M W E Morgan, J L Peters, J Refson, S Selvakumar, S Vivek
Obstetrics and Gynaecology H Annan, R Atalla, K El Farra, R Hartwell, E Y Hemaya, P Kumaranayakan, D G McLintock, M A Samarrai, P Wilson
Haematology F N Al-Refaie
Neurology O C Cockerell, P Martin
Oncology N G P Davidson, J Singer
Ophthalmology S H Campbell, I M Fawcett, D Flaye, V M R Vempali
Oral and Maxillofacial Surgery K M Coghlan, F J H Evans, B Littler, J Sherman
Orthopaedics C H Aldam, P W Allen, A Amini, A A Hussein, J L Kitson, D S Nairn, H Parmar, R Sharma, A H Waterfield

Paediatrics V S Chakravarti, T N Hla, A M L Shurz, R St E Thambapillai, S F Zeidan
Plastic Surgery G E Alvarez-Parra, J D Frame
Podiatry M Hussein
Psychiatry S Abou-el-Fadl, O Daniels, J Jain, R Schapira, A K Upadhyaya
Psychotherapy L Harvey
Radiology C J Barber, A Chauhan, S Dimmock, J Kumaradevan, B Lan, J E Lockwood, M Long, A Lynn, S Redla, T Sikdar, D Wright
Rheumatology K Ahmed, J M C Axon, J Currey
Sexual Health G Crowe
Urology G Boustead, R Gilbody, B Potluri, R Samman, J Vanwaeyenbergh, J S Virdi

Capio Rowley Hospital

Rowley Park, Stafford ST17 9AQ
Tel: 01785 223203 Fax: 01785 249532
Email: enquiries@rowley-hall-hospital.co.uk
Website: www.capio.co.uk
Owners: Capio Healthcare UK
Total Beds: 15

Manager Alan Hufton

Anaesthetics Dr Johns
Audiology A Ridgeway
Cardiology Dr Mistry, Dr Woodmansey
Dental Surgery Mr Buglass
Dermatology Dr Hardwick, Dr Smith, K Ward
ENT Mr David, Mr Hughes, Mr Reddy
Gastroenterology Dr Gibson, Dr Hearing, Dr Singh
General Medicine Dr Daggett, Dr Fairfax, Dr Yeoh
General Surgery Mr Chaubey, Mr Crisp, Mr Durrans, Mr Gendy, Mr Gwynn, Mr Hutchinson, Mr Ravikumar
Gynaecology Mr Chin, Mr Dapash, Mr Elmardi
Ophthalmology Mr Manoi, Mr Price
Orthopaedics Mr Bhoora, Mr El-Fakhri, Mr Griffiths, Mr Hoyle, Mr Kathuria, Mr Loynes, D Remedios, P Shaylor, Mr Travlos
Plastic Surgery Mr Ali, Mr Davison, Mr Nishakawa, S Sterne
Psychology Dr Schwartz
Radiology Dr Steventon, Dr Suarez, Dr Willard
Urology Mr James, Mr Rao

Capio Springfield Hospital

Lawn Lane, Springfield, Chelmsford CM1 7GU
Tel: 01245 234000 Fax: 01245 234001
Email: capio-springfield-enquiries@capio.co.uk
Website: www.capio.co.uk
Owners: Capio Healthcare UK
Total Beds: 70

Manager Philip Tyler

Accident and Emergency V Gautam, A Mariathas, R B Zwink
Audiology B Mann
Cardiology G Clesham, J R Dawson, D Turner
Dermatology M Catterall, A Harrison, M Klaber, R Mehta
ENT A Pace-Balzan, D Roy, C Singh
General Medicine A Ali, A Blainey, D Cunnah, K L Hattotuwa, H Jenkins, A Jubber, C C Khin, H Rehman, S Saverymuttu, M Weston
General Surgery M Harvey, E R Inwang, S Kadirkamanathan, D Menzies, R Motson, P Pitt, N Richardson, A H M Ross, M Salter, P Sauven
Genitourinary Medicine S Ariyanayagam
Haematology V Chowdhury
Histopathology M Fallowfield
Nephrology A Ali
Neurology P Bradbury, I Zoukos
Neurosurgery R Aspoas, K David, A Kellerman
Obstetrics and Gynaecology C Goodfellow, J Onwude, C Partington, P Robarts, A Sharma, C Spencer
Oncology N Davidson, S Tahir
Ophthalmology R Aggarwal, P Andreou, T Bell, H Collette, S Hindi, H Kasaby, A Sinha, D Thoung
Oral and Maxillofacial Surgery G Walker
Orthopaedic Surgery G J Charnley, K Cheah, J Dowell, J Flanagan, H Lyall, A MacDowell, S Palmer, M Taylor, T Thomas, J Tuite, W Williams
Paediatrics S Chong, J Cyriac, S Jayakumar, A Lipscomb, R Mahesh Babu
Pain Management B Jegadish, C McCartney
Plastic Surgery P Dziewulski, D Elliot, S Flemming, J Frame, F Iwuagwu, T Kangesu, G Lennox, N Niranjan, V Ramakrishnan, J Scott, B Sommerlad
Radiology T Chan, G Harverson, P Lee, P G Pratt, H Punnyadasa, S Rao, R Whitney, P Wou
Rheumatology P G Davies, D Mukerjee, S Navaratnum, S Peskett, A Srinivasan
Sports Medicine T Crisp
Urology H Lewi, T Tassadaq, R Thilagarajah
Vascular Surgery T Browne, Y Panayiotopoulos

Capio West Midlands Hospital

Colman Hill, Halesowen B63 2AH
Tel: 01384 560123 Fax: 01384 411103
Email: csp.wmh@capio.co.uk
Website: www.capio.co.uk
Owners: Capio Healthcare UK
Total Beds: 33

Manager Tony Yates

Cardiology R Ahmad, C S Barr, J Flint, R Watson
Dermatology A Abdullah, C J Paul, D G Stewart, C Tan
ENT A Batch, P Glossop, M J Kuo, J Matthews, N C Molony, M O Oluwole, V V Raut, F Wilson
Gastroenterology N Fisher, B J M Jones
General Medicine R Ahmad, S M Athar, V Balagopal Pai, P De, J Delamere, M J Doherty, T Fiad, F H Khattak, G T Moleele
General Surgery R Blunt, A R Carmichael, J J Dmitrewski, D Ellis, D W England, R Grimley, F J Hoar, A Jayatunga, H S Kharia, M Lee, R Patel, A P Savage, S Shiralkar, M Vairavan, K F Yoong
Genitourinary Medicine P Sood
Haematology S Handa, M Labib
Neurology R Etti
Obstetrics and Gynaecology N Fitzgibbon, J Kabukoba, M Mattar, A Warwick, E A J Watson
Oncology D Ferry
Ophthalmology S Aggarwal, M Quinlan, S Shafquat, M Wevill
Oral and Maxillofacial Surgery N Whear
Orthopaedics M Ahmed, N Ahmed, M S Ali, T A Andrew, C E Bache, S Butt, S Deshmukh, S Geeranavar, J B Kersley, S N Massoud, R Mifsud, A Pimpalnerkar, I Sargeant, B K Singh, S K Sulaiman, N Tubbs
Paediatrics R G Buick, R Jayatunga
Plastic Surgery A Bracka, F Fatah, H Goldin, M D Humzah, C C Kat, K S A Mehboob Ali, N S Moiemen, J D Nancarrow, H Nishikawa, R Papini, F Peart, G Sterne, G Titley, R Waters, L H Yap
Podiatry C Heron, D Tollafield, J P Whiteing, H Williams
Radiology R Bhatt, J F Leahy, M Mantle, H Renny, A P Wolinski
Urology L Emtage, M Jones, A Rowse

Capio Winfield Hospital

Tewkesbury Road, Longford, Gloucester GL2 9WH
Tel: 01452 331111 Fax: 01452 331200
Email: capio-winfield-enquiries@capio.co.uk
Website: www.capio.co.uk
Owners: Capio Healthcare UK
Total Beds: 47

Anaesthetics P Clarke
Cardiology D Lindsay, M Petersen, N West
Care of the Elderly N Baldwin, M Banerjee, I Donald
Dermatology B Adriaans, T Millard, W Porter
ENT J Hamilton, M Hardingham, M Thomas, H Wheatley, R Youngs
General Medicine J Brown, R Butland, R Dedi, J Meecham Jones, J Prior, I Shaw, T Ulahannan, R Valori
General Surgery H Barr, T Cook, J Earnshaw, A Fowler, C Fowler, B Heather, M Lucarotti, M Vipond
Genitourinary Medicine Z Sulaiman

Health Screening G Rouse
Neurology G Fuller, R Martin, M Silva
Obstetrics and Gynaecology M James, D Mahendran, E Smith, G Swingler, M Whittaker
Oncology D Farrugia
Ophthalmology J Ferris, G Mackintosh, J Nairne
Oral and Maxillofacial Surgery S Thomas
Orthopaedics D Asante, R Close, J Craig, C Crawshaw, C Curwen, B Harcourt, M Henderson, C Knudsen, R Majkowski, V Takwale, T Tasker, M Tredgett
Paediatrics S Ackroyd
Plastic Surgery J McDiarmid, C Reid, G Sterne
Podiatry M Coates
Psychology P Allen, E Davis
Rheumatology D Collins
Sports Medicine D Asante, R Jaques
Urology D Jones, A Ritchie

Capio Woodland Hospital

Rothwell Road, Kettering NN16 8XF
Tel: 01536 414515 Fax: 01536 412155
Email: enquiries@woodland-hospital.co.uk
Website: www.capio.co.uk
Owners: Capio Healthcare UK
Total Beds: 39

Manager Brett Powis

Audiology M Eccles
Cardiology J Cullen
Dermatology W Branford, J Vorster
ENT M Latif, R Lee
General Medicine Dr Chilton, C Clifford, A Davidson, A Hussain, R Preston, A Steel, T Williams
General Surgery S Al Hamali, V Bahal, S Brar, J Dawson, S El Rabaa, R Jenner, M Rashed, R Stewart, M Taylor
Genetics S Prixce
Haematology E Craven, H Kelsey, M Lyttleton, Dr Wilson-Morkeh
Neurology M Lawden
Obstetrics and Gynaecology R Haughney, M Newman, R Smith, D Wilkin, P Wood
Oncology C Macmillan, R Mathew
Ophthalmology D Banerjee, P Baranyovits, T Blamires, J El Ghazali
Oral and Maxillofacial Surgery C Avery, C Harrop, W Smith
Orthodontics Mr O'Neill
Orthopaedics R Barrington, N Birch, S Biswas, D Bromage, P Latham, B Shah, B Shukla, D Stock, A Vince
Paediatrics H Bilolikar, T Biswas, C Nanyakkara
Palliative Care J Burnell, J Smith
Plastic Surgery E O'Broin, D Ward
Psychology J Regan, R Van Dyke
Radiology C Clark, G Goh, S Hamid, Dr Peterson, S Peterson, R Reeve, A Thompson, D Walter, D Woods
Rheumatology G Kallarackal, I Morris
Urology M Al Sudani, O Davison, M Lynch

Capio Yorkshire Clinic

Bradford Road, Bingley BD16 1TW
Tel: 01274 560311 Fax: 01274 551247
Website: www.capio.co.uk
Owners: Capio Healthcare UK
Total Beds: 71

Manager Michael Lord

Anaesthetics S Gupta, K Kyriakides, Dr McDowell, J Richardson, P Taylor
Cardiology S Lindsay, C Morley, P Silverton, A V Zezulka
Care of the Elderly J Tucker
Dermatology A Wright
ENT C Raine, I Smith, S Sood, D Strachan, A Tucker
General Medicine C Beckett, C Bradley, S Crawford, C Healey, R Jeffrey, L Juby, A Manning, D Newton, L Parapia, S Peacey, D Whitelaw
General Surgery R Antrum, J Ausobsky, J Davies, P Dewar, S Downey, J Griffith, I Hutchinson, C Kapadia, R Khan, J May, A Nejim, J Price, D Wilkinson
Genitourinary Medicine Dr Mohanty
Neurology M Busby, R Hakin, A Lansbury
Neurosurgery N Phillips
Obstetrics and Gynaecology I Beck, J Brash, P Brunskill, S Calvert, S Jones, P O'Donovan, N Samtaney, D Tufnell, J Wright
Oncology C Bradley, S Crawford
Ophthalmology A Atkins, P Atkinson, F Ghanchi, N James, N Litvin
Oral and Maxillofacial Surgery M Carroll, M Chan, V Joshi, S Worral
Orthopaedics D Beard, S Bollen, R Boome, A Faraj, K Jepson, W Kluge, S Ravindran, E Schilders, J Shanker, D Shaw, T Taggart, D Tang, A Watters, C Wray
Paediatrics D Crabbe, A Minford
Plastic Surgery I Foo, D Sharpe
Rheumatology R Melsom
Sports Medicine S Bollen, E Schilders
Urology G Flannigan, P Hamilton-Stewart, R Puri, T Shah, N Shaikh
Vascular Surgery N Shaper, P Vowden, D Wilkinson

Care Perspectives

St John's House Hospital, Lion Road, Palgrave, Diss IP22 1BA
Tel: 01379 643334 Fax: 01379 641455
Email: info@partnershipsincare.co.uk
Website: www.partnershipsincare.co.uk
Owners: Partnerships in Care Ltd
Total Beds: 89

Manager Rosario O'Connell

Central London Clinic

26-27 Bedford Square, London WC1B 2HB
Tel: 08457 304030
Owners: BPAS (British Pregnancy Advisory Service)

Manager Marguerite Bosticco

Chadwick Lodge

Chadwick Drive, Off Saxon Street, Eaglestone, Milton Keynes MK6 5LS
Tel: 01908 593000 Fax: 01908 593200
Email: chadwicklodge@blenheimhealth.com
Website: www.blenheim-forensics.co.uk
Owners: Priory Group
Total Beds: 92

Manager Tracy Harrison

Cheadle Royal Hospital

100 Wilmslow Road, Cheadle SK8 3DG
Tel: 0161 428 9511 Fax: 0161 428 1870
Email: info@affinityhealth.co.uk
Website: www.cheadleroyal.co.uk
Owners: Affinity Healthcare Ltd
Total Beds: 140

Manager Judy Douglass

Psychiatry K Callender, T Carnwath, L Faith, J Haslam, S McKeown, N Ring, M Spurrell, A Trumper, A Wood

The Cheltenham and Gloucester Nuffield Hospital

Hatherley Lane, Cheltenham GL51 6SY
Tel: 01242 246500 Fax: 01242 246501
Email: georgina.dikomite@nuffieldhospitals.org.uk
Website: www.nuffieldhospitals.org.uk
Owners: Nuffield Hospitals
Total Beds: 40

Manager Sheila Richards

Anaesthetics M V Copp, C M P Mather
Cardiology V Challenor, R F O Chamberlain-Webber
Dental Surgery R A Moore, J A Pritchard
Dermatology T Millard, J T Milne
ENT J Hamilton, M Hardingham, D M Thomas, A H Wheatley, R P Youngs
Gastroenterology J T Anderson, I R Crossley
General Medicine R J A Butland, A H Deering, I L Mortimore, A R L Penketh
General Surgery N Borley, J Bristol, H Chan, A Goodman, D Hewin, K Poskitt, J Wheeler, M Whyman
Neurology G N Fuller, M T Silva
Neurosurgery T Desjardins, N K R Patel
Obstetrics and Gynaecology R Gornall, D Griffiths, R G Hayman, D Holmes, M C James, K Jones, R Kerr-Wilson, M Pillai, K Reddy, M Whittaker
Oncology R Counsell, S Elyan, D Farrugia, P J Jenkins, R Owen
Ophthalmic R Caesar, J Ferris, R L Johnston, N Kirkpatrick, G I S Mackintosh, A McNaught, J Nairne, N Price
Oral and Maxillofacial Surgery D R P Godden, R Greenwood, J M Harrison, R Hensher
Orthopaedics D Ainscow, D Asante, P Birch, R Brown, J Craig, J Field, H S Gosal, G Holt, C J M Knudsen, J Mackinnon, R S Majkowski, G Rooker, M Tredgett, J Wand
Paediatrics R S Ackroyd
Plastic Surgery J McDiarmid, C Reid, P Townsend
Psychiatry C Batten, D Batten, D Kingham
Psychology L Horner-Baggs, H Koch, T Passenger, A Sedgwick-Taylor, C D Terrell
Rheumatology D Collins
Urology H Gilbert, D J Jones, R Kinder

The Chichester Nuffield Hospital

78 Broyle Road, Chichester PO19 6WB
Tel: 01243 530600 Fax: 01243 532244
Website: www.nuffieldhospitals.org.uk
Owners: Nuffield Hospitals
Total Beds: 40

Manager Vivienne Heckford

Anaesthetics N W Barnes, R J H Baylis, M R Bentley, A B Conyers, J G Dalgleish, D A B Desgrand, S J Dolin, R M F Hill, A P Kendall, M P Margarson, P F McDonald, S P McHale, R K Shankar, C Smith, A J Soppitt, G A Turner, J R Wace, J A Watt-Smith, M L B Wood
Cardiology C F Murphy, C J Reid, Y Wong
Dermatology P R Coburn, A V Levantine, S Minor
ENT A E Davis, C I Johnstone, G J Madden
General Medicine R A E Holman, K P Laji, G B Lee, B J Marien, I M Morrison, R D Simpson, A F M Stone
General Psychiatry N A Joughlin
General Surgery D R Allen, D K Beattie, R C Bowyer, N P J Cripps, H Hafez, G Harris, J N L Simson, G Slater, M H Wise
Gynaecology J L Beynon, J G Hooker, Z H Z Ibrahim, M C Jolly, A M Simons
Medical Microbiology M Greig
Neurology S R Hammans
Ophthalmology P D Fox, D A Hadley, C H Kon, T Niyadurupola, S M B Rassam, M Teimory, R Williams
Oral and Maxillofacial Surgery D W MacPherson, C A Pratt, J Townend, J L Williams, A Wilson
Orthopaedics S Burgert, S Cavanagh, H J Clarke, R Hill, M C Moss, N Sharma Kendall, L J Taylor
Paediatrics D C A Candy, M J Linney, T M Taylor
Pathology P C Bevan, J M Conroy, W P Stross, T Umar
Plastic Surgery N J Bennett, A N Pandya, N Parkhouse, G V Scerri
Radiology N S Ashford, B J Burns, A M Guilding, D N Kay, J B Murray, C M Young
Radiotherapy and Oncology G G S Khoury
Rheumatology S Menon, M G Ridley
Urology J P Britton, P G Carter, S N Venn

The Children's Trust

Tadworth Court, Tadworth KT20 5RU
Tel: 01737 365000 Fax: 01737 365084
Email: enquiries@thechildrenstrust.org.uk
Website: www.thechildrenstrust.org.uk
Owners: Charity/Association
Total Beds: 37

Claremont Hospital

401 Sandygate Road, Sheffield S10 5UB
Tel: 0114 263 0330 Fax: 0114 230 9388
Email: enquiries@claremont-hospital.com
Website: www.claremont-hospital.com
Owners: The Hospital Management Trust
Total Beds: 41

Manager Tony Barrett

The Cleveland Nuffield Hospital

Junction Road, Norton, Stockton-on-Tees TS20 1PX
Tel: 01642 360100 Fax: 01642 556535
Website: www.nuffieldhospitals.org.uk
Owners: Nuffield Hospitals
Total Beds: 30

Manager Debbie Dobbs

Anaesthetics K A Milligan
Cardiology J A Hall, A Shyam-Sundar, R A Wright
Dental Surgery B Avery
Dermatology D C Seukeran, W D Taylor
ENT D A Bosman, J Carlin, L M Flood, M R Hawthorne, F W Martin, R W Ruckley, R G Wight
General Medicine P A Cann, B K Chaudhury, A Davies, A D D Dwarakanath, J R Greenaway, A D Paterson, M D Rutter, J G Silcock, J D Vasani
General Surgery A K Agarwal, H N Bandi, R Brookstein, I A Cheema, D Clarke, A E Clason, W A Corbett, N B Corner, P J Cullen, P A Davis, P Durning, M Edwards, E L Gilliland, K Gunning, C Hennessy, D W Herring, M J Higgs, G G Kane, G R McLatchie, C Roberts, I L Rosenberg, E J Sinar, R D Strachan, M A Tabaqchali, Y K S Viswanath, C P L Wood
Neurosurgery S M Marks, F P Nath
Obstetrics and Gynaecology A S M Ali, S M Bailey, P Ballard, M Hatem, N Hebblethwaite, D J R Hutchon, J H Macaulay, I MacLeod, M Menabawey, K M Toop, S R Tosson, S M Walton
Ophthalmology D Ah Kine, P Chakraborty, J R Clarke, M S Dang, T C Dowd, D L Smerdon, R Stirling
Oral and Maxillofacial Surgery C J Edge, R J Langford
Orthopaedics A O Adedapo, K E G Allerton, N C Bayliss, H P Epstein, T S Friesem, A C W Hui, M Krishna, R Y L Liow, S S Maheswaran, A V F Nargol, A M F Port, A Rangan, J H Rutherford, M A Shaheen, M P M Stewart, C J Tulloch, L Van Niekerk, L Van Vuuren, I W Wallace
Paediatrics C K I Harikumar, J Jani
Plastic Surgery P E Baguley, H P Siddiqui
Radiology P Cadigan, K M A Clifford, I L Curzon, J R Dean, P Gill, T Hughes, J Latimer, G P Naisby, P J Raju, W D Thompson, M J Trewhella
Urology D J Chadwick, S Fulford, J R Hindmarsh, B S S Vadanan, J Whiteway
Vascular Surgery A D Parry

The Coach House

25 Brighton Road, Salfords, Redhill RH1 5DA
Tel: 01293 783004 Fax: 01293 771170
Email: coachhouse@prioryhealthcare.com
Website: www.prioryhealthcare.com
Owners: Priory Group
Total Beds: 11

Manager Brian Ballantyne

Cromwell Clinic

Cromwell House, 82 High Street, Huntingdon PE29 3DP
Tel: 01480 411411 Fax: 01480 422040
Email: info@cromwellclinic.co.uk
Website: www.cromwellclinic.co.uk
Owners: Privately Owned
Total Beds: 52

Manager Thelma Kimpton

Accupuncture S Ross
Cosmetic Surgery A Aslam, G Horn
Dermatology C Banfield
ENT R Gray, P Jani, P Leong
General Surgery B Bekdash, C Quick
Gynaecology M Al-Kurdi, G Das, B H Lim, M Slack
Oral and Maxillofacial Surgery L Cheng, J Robertson
Orthopaedics A Patel, Mr Sewell, Mr Southgate, T Vaughan-Lane, Mr Wojcik
Physiotherapy B A Kneeshaw
Podiatry R Roberts
Radiography R Barba
Urology C Dawson, G Williams
Vasectomy K Parwaiz

Cromwell Hospital

Cromwell Road, London SW5 0TU
Tel: 020 7460 2000 Fax: 020 7835 2444
Email: info@cromwellhospital.com
Website: www.cromwellhospital.com
Owners: Medical Services International
Total Beds: 150

Anaesthetics M Albin, P Amoroso, I Appleby, E Ashley, C Bailey, D Bamber, P Bras, A Carr, D Chisholm, S Cottam, M Cox, D Dob, P Doyle, P Evans, S George, C Gillbe, R Ginsburg, J Goldstone, T Goroszeniuk, E Grundy, M Gunning, K Haire, D Hall, L Harding, J Harris, M Harris, S Harrison, C J Irving, C Jooste, R Keays, R S Laishley, J B Liban, M Lim, C Mallinson, W Marchant, S Marshall, B Master, M Meurer-Laban, P Morrison, F Moulla, A Moustafa, M Naef, D Nathwani, B Norman, S Papas, R S Parsons, T Peters, A Petros, M Platt, M Plaza, J C Ponte, E J B Porter, Y Rajakulendran, M Renna, G Russell, M Sacks, J Salt, M Scallan, M Scott, A Scurr, J Sedgwick, J Shepherd, E Sherry, V S Sidhu, I P Slee, C Thoburn, P Ward, E Whitehead, J Wilson, P Wilton
Audiology B A Shihabi, L H Yeoh
Breast Surgery G P H Gui, J Lewis, N Roche, R Sainsbury, H D Sinnett
Cardiology F Akhras (Head), F Akhras, M Barbir, K J Beatt, C Brookes, P Clifford, C M Dancey, S Davies, S Jenkins, D Jewitt, P MacCarthy, G Mikhail, P Oldershaw, C Pumphrey, P J Richardson, E Rowland, P Stubbs
Cardiothoracic Surgery M Amrani, R Casula, A de Souza, G Dreyfus, A El-Gamel, M T Marrinan, M Petrou, P Punjabi, F P Shabbo, P Smith, C Young
Coloproctology P Dawson, W A Kmiot
Craniofacial Surgery M Kelly, N Kirkpatrick
Dental Surgery N Ahmad
Dermatology P M Dowd, J Leonard, S Mayou, R Russell-Jones
Elderly Medicine J Oram
Endocrine Surgery J Lynn
Endocrinolgy and Diabetes D C Brown, D Leslie, M Press
ENT G Alusi, P M Clarke, P R Evans, W E Grant, H B Holden, T Mugliston, K S Patel, H Saleh, G Sandhu, C Wallace
Gamma Knife Surgery D M C Forster
Gastroenterology M Anderson, J Arnold, D Bansi, J Devlin, B Gazzard, M Harbord, J Martin, N I McNeil, J Meenan, P Neild, A H Raimundo, D Sherman, D Westaby
General Medicine T G Allen-Mersh, S Clark, P Evans, W Fleming, N S Hakim, F I D Konotey-Ahulu, L Loughridge, H Minasian, J Scurr, B Shah, M Syada, J Thompson, R Vashisht
Genitourinary Medicine D Hawkins
GI (Upper) A M Isla, N A Theodorou
Gynaecology J S Bekir, R Forman, A D Gordon, T Ind, N Morris, C H Naylor, J C O'Sullivan, S Purkayastha, M Stafford, P van Geene
Haemato-oncology D Catovsky, A Pagliuca
Haematology Z Abboudi, R Arya, M Saary
Hepato-pancreato-biliary Surgery N D Heaton, M Rela
Histopathology S Blackie, E Courtauld
Infectious Diseases P Easterbrook
Intensive Care S Ashworth, M Palazzo
Invalid F Norman-Taylor
IVF K K Ahuja, N A Armar, P Bowen-Simpkins, A Gill, S Nair, A Priddy, E G Simons, T G Teoh
Liver Medicine M Heneghan, S Taylor-Robinson, R Williams
Microbiology G L Ridgway, G M Scott
Neurology P G Bain, T Britton, O Foster, R J Guiloff, M Hanna, A Kennedy, O Malik, R K B Pearce, G D Perkin, E H Reynolds, R A Shakir, B Turner, K Zilkha
Neuropathology P Lewis
Neurophysiology N Khalil (Head), N Khalil, I Mak, J Payan, S White
Neurosurgery C Adams, P Bullock, A Elsmore, N D Kitchen, C Lindquist, N D Mendoza, K O'Neill, D Peterson, D G T Thomas
Nuclear Medicine S Clarke (Head), S Clarke, I Fogelman
Oncology P N Plowman (Head), P N Plowman, R P Beaney, A Drury, P Ellis, M G Glaser, C Hamilton, I W F Hanham, M Harries, V Khoo, S M Lee, C Lewanski, C Lowdell, E A Macdonald, G Mikhaeel, C Nutting, S Partridge, R H Phillips, S Retsas, G Ross, P Ross
Ophthalmology W Dinning, G Duguid, K Gregory-Evans, N Joshi, P Kinnear, W Schulenburg
Oral and Maxillofacial Surgery D J Archer, S J Crean, K Hussain, H Thuau
Orthopaedics H B Al-Haddad, P Baird, M Beverly, R Coombs, K Desai, J Hucker, O Lahoti, J E Nixon, F W N Paterson, M A Qureshi, H G Zadeh, T Zaman
Paediatrics E Abrahamson, S Agarwal, I Balfour-Lynn, C Ball, N Barakat, M Barry, D Bentley, S Blaney, P Brooks, N Cavanagh, S Chong, G Clark, H Cox, K Daly, P Daubeney, M Davenport, H Daya, A Dhawan, D Dunaway, R El-Rifai, S El Abd, M Elsawi, M Eltumi, S Evans, J Fell, A Fleming, P Forrester, S Gautama, A Goodwin, M J Haddad, N Hadzic, D Hampson-Evans, J Harcourt, P Hargreaves, M Hariri, R Hayward, K Holmes, G Hosking, E Howard, A Hulme, M Kulkarni, J LaRovere, M Levinkind, E Maalouf, A Mackersie, N Madden, A Magee, M Markiewicz, A Martinez, A Massoud, D Misra, G Morrison, A Moss, I Mushtaq, V Novelli, J P O'Connell, B Okoye, K Patil, M Peters, K Rajput, M Rosenthal, E Shinebourne, J D Singer, M Thomas, V Thomas, M Thomson, R Trompeter, I Walker, P Wilson
Pain Management A D Lawson, A C O'Callaghan
Plastic Surgery A M Awwad, D Goldberg, L Ion, B Mayou, S Myers, R Ng, N Waterhouse
Radiology N K Barrett (Head), N K Barrett, C Blakeney, D Blunt, S Bradbrooke, R J S Chinn, I Colquhoun, S Comitis, T Cox, S Desai, W M Gedroyc, P Kane, J Karani, M King, D Kingsley, J MaCall, K Miszkiel, A J Molyneux, F Muncey, S Padley, Y Patel, M Phelan, P Shaw, P Sidhu, W Taylor, H Walters
Renal Medicine M A Mansell, A Palmer
Respiratory Medicine J Costello, W N Gardner, A Mier, B O'Connor
Rheumatology A S Al-Hussaini, S Allard, C Mackworth-Young, V Martin, G Room
Spinal Surgery - Orthopaedic J Lucas, C Natali, J O'Dowd, J K Webb
Urology C Anderson, K Anson, M Bailey, J Bellringer, M Dinneen, M Gleeson, R Kirby, J McDonald, A Mundy, C Ogden, N Watkin
Vascular Surgery C Bishop, D Black, A H Davies, I Franklin, D Nott, M Whiteley

Cygnet Clinic Beckton

23 Tunnan Leys, Beckton, London E6 6ZB
Tel: 020 7511 2299 Fax: 020 7511 3399
Owners: Cygnet Healthcare Ltd
Total Beds: 23

Psychiatry M Cozzolino, J Falkowski, N Lockhart, C Okocha, D White

Cygnet Hospital Ealing

22 Corfton Road, Ealing, London W5 2HT
Tel: 020 8991 6699 Fax: 020 8991 0440
Owners: Cygnet Healthcare Ltd
Total Beds: 29

Psychiatry T Soutzos, A Warren, N Yoganathan

Cygnet Hospital Wyke

Blankney Grange, Huddersfield Road, Lower Wyke, Bradford BD12 8LR
Tel: 01274 605500 Fax: 01274 604400
Owners: Cygnet Healthcare Ltd
Total Beds: 50

Psychiatry A F Duncan, R F Kehoe

Cygnet Wing Blackheath

80-82 Blackheath Hill, Blackheath, London SE10 8AB
Tel: 020 8694 2111 Fax: 020 8692 0570
Owners: Cygnet Healthcare Ltd
Total Beds: 21

Psychiatry M Baggaley, A Obuaya, W Onyeama

Danum Lodge Clinic

123 Thorne Road, Doncaster DN2 5BQ
Tel: 08457 304030
Owners: BPAS (British Pregnancy Advisory Service)
Total Beds: 11

Manager Tracy Lankenau

Dean Park Clinic

23-25 Ophir Road, Bournemouth BH8 8LS
Tel: 08457 304030
Email: info@bpas.org
Website: www.bpas.org
Owners: BPAS (British Pregnancy Advisory Service)
Total Beds: 11

Manager Cheryl Baillie

The Dene

Gatehouse Lane, Goddards Green, Hassocks BN6 9LE
Tel: 01444 231000 Fax: 01444 231086
Email: info@partnershipsincare.co.uk
Website: www.partnershipsincare.co.uk
Owners: Partnerships in Care Ltd
Total Beds: 50

Manager Doreen McCollin

Psychiatry W Busuttil, N Renton

The Diving Diseases Research Centre

The Hyperbaric Medical Centre, Tamar Science Park, Research Way, Plymouth PL6 8BU
Tel: 01752 209999 Fax: 01752 209115
Email: enquiries@ddrc.org
Website: www.ddrc.org
Owners: Charity/Association
Total Beds: 2

Drayton House Clinic

2 Lulworth Road, Birkdale, Southport PR8 2AT
Tel: 01704 563279 Fax: 01704 550057
Email: info@draytonhouseclinic.com
Website: www.draytonhouseclinic.com
Owners: Privately Owned

Anaesthetics J P Gannon, S E Leith, R McMillan, M W Smith
Ophthalmology T Akingbehin (Head), C Groenewald, N O'Donnell, S Prasad

Droitwich Knee Clinic

St Andrews Road, Droitwich WR9 8YX
Tel: 08702 412193 Fax: 01905 795916
Email: enquiries@droitwichkneeclinic.co.uk
Website: www.kneeclinics.co.uk, www.kneeguru.co.uk
Owners: Privately Owned

Manager D Bourne

Egerton Road

18 Egerton Road, Bexhill-on-Sea TN39 3HH
Tel: 01424 734464 Fax: 01424 734464
Email: egertonroad@prioryhealthcare.com
Website: www.prioryhealthcare.com
Owners: Priory Group
Total Beds: 10

Manager Carol Foord

The Essex Nuffield Hospital

Shenfield Road, Brentwood CM15 8EH
Tel: 01277 695695 Fax: 01277 201158
Website: www.nuffieldhospitals.org.uk
Owners: Nuffield Hospitals
Total Beds: 48

Manager Jose Perez

Anaesthetics M A Ather, M S May, S Thomson
Cardiology R Aggarwal, R Dawson, J McEwan, W Serino
Dermatology F Carabott, M Catterall, S M Khorshid, S Matthews, R Mehta
ENT B D Chopra, C R Chowdhury, G Fayad, B Kotecha, A Latif, A Owa, D Roy, A P Su, I Vanniasegaram
General Medicine I H Fahal, W Fickling, D Gertner, T Haider, A S Jubber, R Khan, A Lal, E Marouf, K Metcalfe, D K Mukherjee, E Osman, J Subhani, L S P Wicks, B Yung
General Psychiatry C Murray, A Winbow
General Surgery T R Cheatle, J Coker, D S Collier, C Hepworth, W Ismail, T Jeddy, F Kham, D Khoo, K Lafferty, I Linehan, B Lovett, K Ogedegbe, Y P Panayiotopoulos, B Ribeiro, M Saharay, A K Salih, S K Shami, H Taylor
Genitourinary Medicine S Ariyanayagam
Gynaecology J O Emeagi, A R Haloob, M A Ojutiku, C Paartington, S M Sathanandan, A Sharma, H Tebbutt, R Varma, C Welch
Nephrology I H Fahal, S Morgan
Neurology R Capildeo, R N de Silva, L Findley, C Hawkes
Neurosurgery J Benjamin, K David, N Garvan, J Kellerman
Ophthalmology R Aggarwal, J S Chawla, C Claoué, G M B Dawidek, N Karia, H Kasaby, R Pearson, S Ruben
Oral and Maxillofacial Surgery D T Falconer, D Madan, S V L Prasad, P Weller
Orthopaedics A Al-Sabti, A Ali, H Banan, G Charnley, K Cheah, R Grewal, N Ker, S Kumar, A Lang-Stevenson, I Lennox, G E MacLellan, A S Makar, T Peckham, H S Plaha, K Ratnakumar, M Shoaib, J Targett, R J J Wenger, J White
Plastic Surgery J D Frame, M J B Gittos, V V Ramakrishnan, B C Sommerlad, M Sood
Radiotherapy and Oncology N G P Davidson, A R Gershunny, E Sims
Rheumatology K Chakravarty, N S Gendi, J Palit
Urology S Bhanot, P Ewah, S Gujral, J T Hill, D Osborne, T Tassadaq, M T Vandal, A K Vohra

The Exeter Nuffield Hospital

Wonford Road, Exeter EX2 4UG
Tel: 01392 276591 Fax: 01392 425147
Website: www.nuffieldhospitals.org.uk
Owners: Nuffield Hospitals
Total Beds: 46

Manager Patricia Lee

Anaesthetics K Allman, P Ballard, L Barker, C Berry, W Boaden, D Conn, M Daugherty, C Day, P Dix, A Dow, A Grice, E Hammond, E

Hartsilver, P Marshall, P McIntyre, Q Milner, J Munn, J Pitman, J Purday, F Roberts, J Saddler, D Sanders, B Sandhar, A Teasdale, R Telford, P Thomas, I Wilson
Cardiology J Dean, M Gandhi, C Rinaldi, D Smith
Cardiothoracic Surgery M Dalrymple-Hay
Dermatology C Bower, T Downs
Endocrinology J Tooke
ENT A Brightwell, R Garth, S Hickey, M Hilton, J Hutchinson, G Weiner
General Medicine R Ayres, J Christie, T Daneshmend, M James, M Jeffreys, N Withers
General Surgery W B Campbell, M Cooper, A Cowan, J Dunn, A Gee, D Harvey, T Irvin, A Knox, J Thompson
Haematology M Joyner, M Pocock
Neurology C Gardner-Thorpe, N Gutowski
Obstetrics and Gynaecology N Acheson, N Colley, M E Dalton, S Eckford, N Liversedge, J Renninson, M Taylor, J West
Occupational Health R Cooke
Oncology A Goodman, A Hong, M Osborne
Ophthalmology D Byles, J Jacob, R Ling, A Quinn, P Simcock
Oral and Maxillofacial Surgery A Babajews, A McLennan
Orthopaedics T Bunker, D Chan, P Cox, K Eyres, G Gie, N Giles, J Howell, M Hubble, A MacEachern, N Mackay, A Omari, M Podmore, P Schranz, I Sharpe, A Timperley, C Weatherley
Pathology T Clarke, N Cope, D Day, C Keen, B Martin, C Mason, P McCullagh, M Morgan, P Sarsfield, R Simpson
Plastic Surgery V Deveraj, J Palmer, P Saxby, C Stone, A Watts
Psychiatry R Blacker, M Briscoe, L McClelland, M Upton
Psychology R Barker, N Booth
Radiology C Bayliss, J Coote, R Davies, L Gellet, C Hamilton-Wood, S Harries, J Harrington, R Heafield, D Kinsella, C Pinder, A Redfern, D Silver, A Spiers, R Thomas, A Watkinson
Renal R D'Souza
Respiratory Medicine D Halpin, C Sheldon, N Withers
Rheumatology H Averns, R Jacoby
Thoracic Surgery R Berrisford
Urology M Crundwell, R Pocock, M Stott

Fairfield Hospital

Crank, St Helens WA11 7RS
Tel: 01744 739311 Fax: 01744 453358
Email: er@fairfield.org.uk
Website: www.fairfield.org.uk
Owners: Charity/Association
Total Beds: 47

Cardiology R Charles, J Morris
Child Psychiatry J Ball, J Myler
Clinical Psychology R Rosser
Dermatology R Curley, J Yell
ENT M Birchall, A Daud, P Hardcastle, S Jackson, V Nandapalan, V Pothula
General Medicine D K Banerjee, J Corless, J Dawson, C Francis, E Haworth, J Hendry, K Leong, M Lynch, J McLindon, P Stockton, J A Tappin, J Vora
General Surgery R Audisio, A Blower, L Chagla, I Khan, R Kiff, D Maitra, T Nicholas, M Scott
Gynaecology S Burns, G Cawdell, J Davies, H Hamed, T Idama, P Morgan, N Nwosu
Neurology P Ray, M Steiger
Neurosurgery P May
Ophthalmology T Akingbehin, N Cota, M Hiranandani, P Joyce, S Kaye, I Marsh
Oral and Maxillofacial Surgery D Campbell, E Vaughan
Orthopaedics B Bolton-Maggs, A Gambhir, E R Jago, C Jaramillo, M Manning, P Rostron, S P Sirikonda, K Suraliwala, G Thomas
Paediatrics F Amagavie, A Dalzell
Pain Management E Ghadiali, J C D Wells
Plastic Surgery L Feldberg, K Graham, I James, S H Liew
Urology H Gana, A Massey, A Thompson

Farm Place

Stane Street, Ockley, Dorking RH5 5NG
Tel: 01306 627742 Fax: 01306 627756
Email: farmplace@prioryhealthcare.com
Website: www.prioryhealthcare.com
Owners: Priory Group
Total Beds: 24

Manager Andrew Vincent

Addictions M Rowlands

Farmfield

Farmfield Drive, Charlwood, Horley RH6 0BN
Tel: 020 8495 2700 Fax: 020 8495 2701
Email: farmfield@blenheimhealth.com
Website: www.blenheim-forensics.co.uk
Owners: Priory Group
Total Beds: 50

Manager Elaine Baigrie

Frenchay Brain Injury Rehabilitation Centre

Frenchay Hospital, Frenchay Park Road, Bristol BS16 1UU
Tel: 0117 956 2697 Fax: 0117 956 9941
Email: frenchay@fshc.co.uk
Owners: The Huntercombe Hospitals

Godden Green Clinic

Godden Green, Sevenoaks TN15 0JR
Tel: 01732 763491 Fax: 01732 763160
Owners: Cygnet Healthcare Ltd
Total Beds: 23

Manager Vicky McNally

Psychiatry M Baggaley, R Bearcroft, M H Best, M Bott, S Carman, N Clarke, M Cozzolino, S Davenport, R Gaind, H Garrett, G John, N Lockhart, S P C Maskey, J McPherson, C Okocha, W Onyeama, J Royds, R Sammut, A Winbow

The Grosvenor Nuffield Hospital

Wrexham Road, Chester CH4 7QP
Tel: 01244 680444 Fax: 01244 680812
Website: www.nuffieldhospitals.org.uk
Owners: Nuffield Hospitals
Total Beds: 36

Manager Liz Nerney

Anaesthetics S R W Bricker, D Childs, N V Fergusson, E T S Forrest, S Hill, P Jameson, J R Jamieson, A A Khalil, E W Moore, P M Mullen, R A Nelson, N M Robin, A St Clair Logan, G Salem, S Singh, M A Skues, S Q Tighe, A M Troy
Cardiology P G Reid, M Sedgewick, J D Somauroo
Dental Surgery R A Howell
Dermatology P A Dufton, J M Sowden
ENT N A Mackinnon, M G Spencer, R H Temple
General Medicine A V Crowe, D L Ewins, J P Finnerty, I M Keeping, I J London, P McClelland, J M Shennan, C F Sissons, T D Wardle
General Surgery G Foster, C E Harding-Mackean, G Hutchinson, M A Johnson, P J Marsh, D N Monk, T J D Pigott, J K Pye
Genitourinary Medicine C P O'Mahony
Haematology V J Clough, E S Lee, H M Leggat
Histopathology S A Hales
Neurology M D Boggild, A N Bowden, M Doran, N A Fletcher, N P Hinds, P R D Humphrey
Obstetrics and Gynaecology P J Banfield, J Davies-Humphreys, N Haddad, J A Hawe, M J McCormack, A Peattie, P G Toon, J H Williams
Oncology J Maguire
Ophthalmology S Armstrong, J M Butcher, D K Chitkara, M Hickey-Dwyer, M K Tutton
Oral and Maxillofacial Surgery J I Cawood, E C Huddy, C N Penfold, D Richardson

Orthopaedics J M Anderton, V Bobic, I J Braithwaite, D Campbell, I A Harvey, B N Livingstone, A Phillipson, M Porter, J Rao, I C Smith
Paediatrics D W Fielding
Pathology S A Bowles, B N A Hamid, R U Kahn, W E Kenyon, P T Mannion, P R M Steele
Plastic Surgery S K Dhital, F S Fahmy, D McGeorge
Podiatry A Williams
Psychiatry G R Wilkinson
Radiology G T Abbott, J M Curtis, G J Doyle, R J Etherington, J E Houghton, W J Pilbrow, C S Romaniuk, G R J Sissons, R A Sloka
Rheumatology D Y Bulgen, K Over
Urology P S Anandaram, A M Cliff, P A Jamieson, B A Petterson, C S Powell
Vascular Surgery L de Cossart, S Dimitri, P R Edwards, Y R Manesh

The Guildford Nuffield Hospital

Stirling Road, Guildford GU2 7RF
Tel: 01483 555800 Fax: 01483 555888
Website: www.nuffieldhospitals.org.uk
Owners: Nuffield Hospitals
Total Beds: 54

Manager Richard Dodds

Anaesthetics P Barnardo, M Blackmore, Y Buorov, R Cantelo, S Carroll, S Comara, M Davies, G Dhond, W Fawcett, J Fozard, T Gallagher, H Griffiths, A Hendrickse, G Jenkins, M Jordan, P Joshi, E Kershaw, J Leigh, A Lopez, M Lucas, J Margary, K Markham, N Payne, T Pepall, N Quiney, K Randall, P Saunders, M Scott, V Slade, J Stoneham, N Taylor, M Zuleika
Audiology V Jayarajan
Biochemistry T Wang
Cardiology T P Chua, T Foley, E Leatham, N Moat
Care of the Elderly H Powell, V Seth
Dental Surgery M Wardle
Dermatology E Wong
ENT P Chapman, P Hadfield, J Rowe-Jones, N Solomons, R Sudderick, D Wright
General Medicine P Andrews, G Ferns, W McAllister, D Russell-Jones, M Smith, J Stevenson
General Surgery M Bailey, N Karanjia, C Marks, N Menezes, T Rockall, J Stebbing, A Wan
Genitourinary Medicine A Beardall
Haematology I Douglas, G Robbins, J Shirley
Histopathology M Cook, S de Sanctis, P Jackson
Immunology S Deacock, H Griffiths
Neurology P Trend, G Warner
Neurophysiology P Sheehy
Obstetrics and Gynaecology S Butler-Manuel, E P Curtis, M Ford, R Hutt, R Irvine, A Kent, K Morton, C Sutton, A Tailor, S Whitcroft
Oncology S Essapen, R Laing, J Money-Kyrle, A Neal, H Thomas, C Topham, S Whitaker, W White
Ophthalmology A Gilvarry, J Keenan, C McLean
Oral and Maxillofacial Surgery M Danford, P Haers, A Hjort, P Johnson, C Newlands
Orthodontics G Wreakes
Orthopaedics N Bradley, H Chissell, C J Coates, M Flannery, P Halliwell, P Magnussen, G Paremain, A Quaile, J Rosson, A Sakellariou, M Solan
Paediatrics M Evans, E Nicholls, M Ryalls
Plastic Surgery M Kissin, G Layer, B Powell
Psychiatry M Bristow, N Clark, R Condon, A Gilham, G Hassan, M Illsley, C Kerawala, S Lieberman, K Newman, B Sekahawat, H Shoeb, R Sinnerton, P Valentine
Radiology C Bland, T Bloomberg, J Cooke, C Kirkpatrick, C Kissin, K Stoner, W Walker
Rheumatology A Behn, R Gray
Urology J Davies, S Langley, A Nigam
Vascular Surgery C McGuinness, B Price, M Whiteley

Guy's Nuffield House

Guy's & St Thomas's Hospital Trust, Newcomen Street, London SE1 1YR
Tel: 020 7955 4953 Fax: 020 7955 4476
Owners: Guy's and St Thomas' Hospital NHS Trust
Total Beds: 46

The Hand Clinic

Dedworth Road, Oakley Green, Windsor SL4 4LH
Tel: 01753 831333 Fax: 01753 832109
Email: mail@hand-clinic.co.uk
Website: www.hand-clinic.co.uk
Owners: Privately Owned

Manager David Evans, David Evans

Orthopaedics A Bremner-Smith, D M Evans, D P Sammut, D Warwick
Plastic Surgery D Evans (Head), A P Armstrong, D Evans, N Kang, C T K Khoo, D L Martin, D Sammut

The Harley Street Clinic

35 Weymouth Street, London W1G 8BJ
Tel: 020 7935 7700 Fax: 020 7487 4415
Email: info@harleystreetonline.hcahealthcare.co.uk
Website: www.theharleystreetclinic.com
Owners: HCA International Ltd
Total Beds: 105

Manager Rupert Cockcroft

Harrogate Clinic

23 Ripon Road, Harrogate HG1 2JL
Tel: 01423 500599 Fax: 01423 531074
Owners: Cygnet Healthcare Ltd
Total Beds: 19

Manager Alison Ireland

Psychiatry A Beaini, G Bridge, A Easton, C Kelly, S Konar, S Mahapatra, J Mumford, J Nehaul, S Shaw, C Taylor, G Vincenti, J Yeomans

The Heath Clinic

58 West Heath Drive, London NW11 7QH
Tel: 020 8458 4416 Fax: 020 8905 5274
Owners: Privately Owned
Total Beds: 10

Highgate Hospital Ltd

17-19 View Road, Highgate, London N6 4DJ
Tel: 020 8341 4182 Fax: 020 8341 4262
Email: highgate.privatehospital@lineone.net
Website: www.highgatehospital.co.uk
Owners: Aspen Healthcare Ltd
Total Beds: 33

Manager Shaun Stacey

ENT G Alusi, J Lavy, S Paun
General Surgery P Belsham, R Cohen, A Gordon, D Greenstein, G Horn, R Lock, A Oshowo, J Rennie, S Singh
Obstetrics and Gynaecology T Freeman-Wang, A Gadir, S Ghatak, A Kyei-Mensah
Ophthalmology R Daniel, P Rosen
Orthopaedics C Charlambides, M Jasani, P Thomas, G Vardi
Plastic Surgery R Grover, S Kahn
Podiatry S Kriss
Respiratory Medicine D Ornadel

Holly House Hospital

High Road, Buckhurst Hill IG9 5HX
Tel: 020 8505 3311 Fax: 020 8506 1013
Email: info@hollyhouse-hospital.co.uk
Website: www.hollyhouse-hospital.co.uk

Owners: Aspen Healthcare Ltd
Total Beds: 55

Manager Jackie Row

Holy Cross Hospital

Hindhead Road, Haslemere GU27 1NQ
Tel: 01428 643311 Fax: 01428 644007
Email: info@holycross.org.uk
Website: www.holycross.org.uk
Owners: Charity/Association
Total Beds: 40

Manager Christopher Hinton

The Horder Centre for Arthritis

St John's Road, Crowborough TN6 1XP
Tel: 01892 665577 Fax: 01892 662142
Email: arthritis@horder.co.uk
Website: www.hordercentre.co.uk
Owners: Charity/Association
Total Beds: 64

Manager Diane Thomas

Hospital of St John and St Elizabeth

60 Grove End Road, St Johns Wood, London NW8 9NH
Tel: 020 7806 4000 Fax: 020 7806 4001
Email: info@hje.org.uk
Website: www.hje.org.uk
Owners: Charity/Association
Total Beds: 155

Manager Christopher Board

Anaesthetics A Ordman, G Towlerton
Cardiology J Coghlan, R P Hayward, D Lipkin, S C Webb
Dermatology P Goldsmith, D Harris, T Leslie, J Ross, N P J Walker
ENT M Dilkes, A Parikh, S Paun, R E Quiney, N S Tolley
General Medicine H Beynon, J Croker, R A Jackson, M Johnson, N Johnson, R Lancaster, E Lever, D Lubel, M A Mansell, D P Maudgal, D J R Morgan, S Roche, D Suri, M Vanderpump, S C Webb, V S Wong
General Practice E Dan-Goor, J Eden, Y El Gazzar, S Foster
General Surgery R A M Al-Mufti, C Bishop, A Chang, C W K Choy, J Cochrane, M Ghilchik, S W T Gould, D Greenstein, M Hashemi, T S Hussain, A Lewis, R Lock, D M Melville, K Mokbel, H Mukhtar, S Parbhoo, J H Scurr, A J Wilson
Genitourinary Medicine P Kell, C Rodgers
Immunology J Brostoff
Neurology J Chataway, C Kaplan, D Kidd, N Legg
Obstetrics and Gynaecology O O Akinfenwa, J Aquilina, G Ayida, C Barnick, M L Bowen, J M Braithwaite, B Clausson, D Economides, Miss Freeman-Wang, Y Gordon, F Hadda, K Harrington, T Ind, Ms Kyei-Mensah, A Mahfouz, L McMillan, N Morris, T Shawaf, P Wilson, J S L Yoon
Ophthalmology C Davey, T J Fallon
Oral and Maxillofacial Surgery P Ayliffe, R L Livesedge
Orthodontics S Ash, M Levinkind
Orthopaedics P Ahrens, M Bankes, P Calvert, R Carrington, C Charalambides, C Cobiella, B Cohen, S Corbett, M Davies, G Dowd, P Dyson, R Eckersley, R J H Emery, N Garlick, N Goddard, F Haddad, A Hall, A Hashemi-Nejad, R A Hill, D M Hunt, R Marston, A Odgaard, M Solan, P Thomas, A L Wallace, J Witt, V Woolf
Plastic Surgery C Inglefield, A Karidis
Podiatry S Cox, A Kontos, S Kriss, J Olivelle, A A Raissi
Rheumatology H Beynon, V Martin, R Rees, M Seifert, R Stratton, C Tench, A White
Urology S Choong, N Christopher, P Dasgupta, J Elkabir, R Miller, S Minhas, R J Morgan, V H Nargund, D J Ralph

The Huddersfield Nuffield Hospital

Birkby Hall Road, Huddersfield HD2 2BL
Tel: 01484 533131 Fax: 01484 428396
Email: tracy.hampson@nuffieldhospitals.org.uk
Website: www.nuffieldhospitals.org.uk
Owners: Nuffield Hospitals
Total Beds: 29

Manager Tracy Hampson

Anaesthetics K Ahmed, N Al-Quisi, T Ammar, J K Anathhanam, K Bartholomew, S Bhandari, P Braithwaite, S R Bricker, K T Chng, P R Clarke, S Enright, J R Esmond, B S Ghoorun, S S Gill, P J Hall, R M Jackson, P M Jameson, F O Jennings, R V Johnson, K C Judkins, K K Kataria, A Krishnan, D R Lloyd, C Lok, A Mallick, M P Nagar, C G Nandakumar, H E Newbegin, J Nunez, H O'Beirne, J O'Riordan, R N N Shah, S A Siddiqui
Cardiology B T Saeed
Dermatology M J Cheesbrough
ENT D Boyd, D P Martin-Hirsh, C J R Newbegin, G Smelt
General Medicine A W Burrows, J B Halpern, S C Jones, M T N Knight, B C Laylor, O E A Mandour, P S Rana, I Shakir, N N Sivaramakrishnan, G M Sobala
General Surgery J D Ajayi, M I Aldoori, B M Dobbins, R J R Goodall, P J Holdsworth, S Iqbal, R C Macdonald, V K Modgill, I R Morris, K P Muralikuttan, J R Parmar, J J Price, J Salaman, N K Sharma, M H Shiwani, A Subramanian, E Tolessa, A K Tyagi
Haematology C Carter
Health Screening A K Aggarwal, H S Cheema, J A Gaunt, N U H Hasanie, C Isaac, J A Schembri
Histopathology M M Aslam, M A Kahn
Neurology D N Brooks, B E A Dafalla, B T Henderson
Neurosurgery A K Tyagi
Obstetrics and Gynaecology K Bhabra, J M Campbell, S J Kauffman, B A Onyeka, A Trehan
Oncology A M Crellin
Ophthalmology N Anand, K G Davey, C H Hutchinson, J C Pauw, R Rahman, S Rehman
Oral and Maxillofacial Surgery J Jones
Oral Surgery J Jones
Orthopaedics S Ankarath, P A Bryant, C J Chadwick, G Chakrabarty, J E Cleary, A F George, A M Kahn, B Ketzer, H Maxwell, N Mohan, K P Muralikuttan, R K Sharma, J G Shea, A Shenolikar, E Tolessa, G J Tudor
Paediatrics M G Miller, M A Sills
Pathology D Birkenhead, H Griffiths, G D H Thomas
Plastic Surgery O M B Austin, O M Fenton, L R Fourie, A R Phipps, S J Southern
Podiatry A Cast
Psychiatry M S Alexander, A Banymandhub, N H Booya, D J J Britto, N J Cooling, E W Gehlhaar, K J Gledhill, J Keen, R Kerry, J Royle, C M Spencer, G E P Vincenti
Psychotherapy B Pearson
Radiology A M Bowker, S Gurney, H Horsfall, N K Jain, P N E James, K Naik, A R Paes, F Roman, A M Wason
Respiratory Medicine R W Heaton
Rheumatology A Adebajo, A Harvey, R J Reece
Urology M A Ferro, J Harney, K Rogowski

The Huntercombe Maidenhead Hospital

Huntercombe Lane South, Taplow, Maidenhead SL6 0PQ
Tel: 01628 667881 Fax: 01628 666989
Email: huntercombe.maidenhead@fshc.co.uk
Website: www.huntercombehospitals.com
Total Beds: 55

Manager Isabel Archibald

Child and Adolescent Psychiatry M Clapham, S Davies, P Jonsson

The Huntercombe Roehampton Hospital

Holybourne Avenue, London SW15 4JL
Tel: 020 8780 6155 Fax: 020 8780 6156
Email: huntercombe.roehampton@fshc.co.uk
Website: www.huntercombehospitals.com
Owners: The Huntercombe Hospitals
Total Beds: 39

Manager Alan Watson

General Psychiatry P Hopley, P Matthiasson

The Huntercombe Stafford Hospital

Ivetsey Bank, Wheaton Aston, Stafford ST19 9QT
Tel: 01785 840000 Fax: 01785 842192
Email: huntercombe.stafford@fshc.co.uk
Website: www.huntercombehospitals.com
Owners: The Huntercombe Hospitals
Total Beds: 39

Manager Fiona Alcorn

Child and Adolescent Psychiatry A Ayton, A Leahy

Isham House

St Andrew's Group of Hospitals, Billing Road, Northampton NN1 5DG
Tel: 01604 616100 Fax: 01604 635571
Email: bronwenriordan@cygnethealth.co.uk
Owners: Cygnet Healthcare Ltd

Manager Bronwen Riordan

Psychiatry M Orr (Head), S Abu-Kmeil, R G Banhatti, H Baxter, I Coffey, A D Damle, C M Haw, T M Jukes, D G Nevison-Andrews, M Orr, C Staley, I R Wood, G Yorston, E Zapata-Bravo

Kemple View

Longsight Road, Langho, Blackburn BB6 8AD
Tel: 01254 248021 Fax: 01254 248023
Email: info@partnershipsincare.co.uk
Website: www.partnershipsincare.co.uk
Owners: Partnerships in Care Ltd
Total Beds: 64

Manager Peter Handy

King Edward VII Hospital

Midhurst GU29 0BL
Tel: 01730 812341 Fax: 01730 816333
Website: www.kingedwardhospital.co.uk
Owners: Charity/Association
Total Beds: 96

Anaesthetics S Dolin, N L Padfield
Cardiology C Barlow, W C Brownlee, M Connaughton, A de Souza, T G Farrell, C Foster, R A Jones, B J Kneale, E Leatham, N E Moat, R S More, C F Murphy, S Ohri, C J Reid, B Sethia, D F Shore, M Signy, M Thomas, U Trividi, J Watkins
Cardiothoracic Surgery G M K Tsang
Dermatology P Coburn, R H Felix, A V Levantine
ENT C I Johnstone, J Rowe-Jones
General Medicine H Duncan, R Ellis, P S G Eyers, P M Goggin, H M Hafez, R Holman, J A C Hopkirk, M Smith
General Surgery D R Allen, R C Bowyer, N Cripps, M J Payne, R M Pemberton, A Senapati, J N L Simson, S S Somers, G L J Sutton, S K C Toh
Hand Surgery I Winspur
Neurology S Hammans, P Trend, A Turner
Obstetrics and Gynaecology J L Beynon, P M Coats, S Ewen, A Kent, A Silverstone, A Simmons
Oncology R B Buchanan, V Hall, G G S Khoury, S J Whitaker, W F White
Ophthalmology D Farnworth, T J Ffytche, P D Fox, W Green, J Keenan, C Low, P Mann, S Rassam, M Teimory, R Williams
Oral and Maxillofacial Surgery P Haers, D McPherson, G Sockett, J L Williams
Orthopaedics S P Cavanagh, H J Clarke, M Flannery, J Goodall, G Harper, N Kendall, J D S McCutchan, M Moss, J Older, J Taylor
Pathology P Bevan, B French, P Stross, J Wright
Plastic Surgery L Kirwan, M Malyon, A Padya, N Parkhouse, P J Whitfield
Psychiatry N Joughin
Psychology B Marien
Radiology N S Ashford, S Barker, A Guilding, D N Kay, A J Lopez, J Murray
Rheumatology S Menon, M G Ridley, A S Torode
Urology J P Britton, P G Carter, J Davies, R Nigam, F A W Schweitzer, S Venn
Vascular Surgery B Price, M Whiteley

King Edward VII's Hospital Sister Agnes

Beaumont Street, London W1G 6AA
Tel: 020 7486 4411 Fax: 020 7467 4312
Email: info@kingedwardvii.co.uk
Website: www.kingedwardvii.co.uk
Owners: Charity/Association
Total Beds: 65

Anaesthetics G G Abbondati, D W L Davis, C Goldsack, C Greville, G H Hackett, W Harrop-Griffiths, P Howell, R M Langford, P Saunders, E Sherry, B Q Varley
Cardiology J Coltart, D Holdright, R Howard Swanton, P Mills, M Walker
Cardiothoracic Surgery P Magee, C W Pattison
Dental Surgery B D Glynn, N Sturridge
Dermatology C Bunker, J J H Gilkes, W A D Griffiths, R W Groves, M H A Rustin, R C D Staughton
Endocrinology G S Conway
ENT S P A Blaney, H Grant, I S Mackay, P H Rhys Evans, D N Roberts
General Medicine R Abraham, S Bloom, M G Britton, J R Croker, J Cunningham, R S Elkeles, D Empey, J George, A R W Hatfield, S Hurel, N Johnson, R Lancaster, C G Mackworth-Young, I M Murray-Lyon, B P Saunders, L H Sevitt, J Teare, H Thomas, R Thompson, S C Webb, C B Williams
General Practice J H Barretto, M Criswell, T Evans, M J Harding, H Rowbotham, P J Wheeler
General Surgery R Carpenter, A Darzi, T Davidson, S Dorudi, G Hamilton, M P Jenkins, T R Kurzawinski, J M A Northover, D M Nott, R C G Russell, R G Springall, H White, J H N Woolfe, A E Young
Geriatric Medicine J Oram
Infection Control J Holton, G Ridgeway, G Scott
Intensive Care G J Bellingan, J C Goldstone, M N E Harris, M Palazzo
Neurology O J Foster, J Gawler, R J Greenwood
Neurosurgery P Bullock, D Peterson, M P Powell
Obstetrics and Gynaecology J Bridges, A Cutner, A Farthing, Higham, A L Magos, R Marwood, P Mason, M Setchell, J H Shepherd, A Silverstone, C Spence-Jones
Ophthalmology D J Brazier, J R O Collin, V M G Ferguson, T J Ffytche, J T Jagger, B Little, M H Miller, D Spalton
Oral and Maxillofacial Surgery R Hensher, D R James, M McGurk, L Newman, H Thuau
Orthopaedics T M Bucknill, J P Cobb, M A Edgar, R J H Emery, A Jackson, J R Jackson, S Muirhead-Allwood, R Vickers, A L Wallace, J D Witt
Pain Management A Baranowski, J M G Foster, N L Padfield
Plastic Surgery D M Evans, J D Frame, R Grover, B M Jones, N Parkhouse, A E Searle, N Waterhouse
Psychiatry M Greenwood, G W Libby
Radiology Z Amin, C I Bartram, T J Beale, S Burnett, P Butler, M A Hall-Craggs, C W Heron, A L Hine, A M McLean, S McWilliams, I Nockler, N Perry, R Reznek, D Rickards, M B Rubens, K Walmsley
Radiotherapy and Oncology C A E Coulter, P Ellis, P G Harper, S Harris, M Leslie, P N Plowman
Rheumatology B Bourke, E C Huskisson, M Shipley

Urology D F Badenoch, S S-C Carter, R S Kirby, R W Lloyd Davis, R J Morgan, N O'Donoghue, J Shah, J A Vale, H N Whitfield

Kneesworth House Hospital

Bassingbourn-cum-Kneesworth, Royston SG8 5JP
Tel: 01763 255700 Fax: 01763 255718
Website: www.partnershipsincare.co.uk
Owners: Partnerships in Care Ltd
Total Beds: 145

Manager Frank Corr

The Lancaster and Lakeland Nuffield Hospital

Meadowside, Lancaster LA1 3RH
Tel: 01524 62345 Fax: 01524 844725
Website: www.nuffieldhospitals.org.uk/lancaster
Owners: Nuffield Hospitals
Total Beds: 27

Manager David Richardson

Anaesthetics A P Vickers
Audiology H Connor, K W Hamer
Dental Surgery J Tomlinson
Dermatology P Harrison, V Yates
ENT M E Baraka, C Bulman
General Medicine A Brodison, A Brown, C M Brown, P B M Clarkson, J P Halsey, A D Higham, J Keating
General Surgery J Abraham, R C Bollard, K Kalifeh, W P Morgan, P Wilson
Health Screening C Brennan, J Brice, J Frankland, A Matchett, H Pugh, D Roche
Immunology J Roberts
Neurology T Majeed
Neurophysiology G U Lekwuwa
Neurosurgery A Golash, N T Gurusinghe
Obstetrics and Gynaecology R Ghani, K Jones, R J Shepherd
Ophthalmology T O Akingbehin, G Griffith, R K Khana, G Ozuzu
Oral and Maxillofacial Surgery S Akhtar
Orthopaedics S K Garg, G Mclauchlan, S Radcliffe, D Redfern, B Rhodes, H Stewart
Plastic Surgery A J Howcroft, A Juma
Podiatry R Higton
Psychiatry W Radcliffe, J W Riach
Radiology P M Flanagan, J M Lavelle, J McGregor, L M Ness, D Sheals, A Taylor, W H J Wall
Urology P Duffy, K Madhra, C Rowbotham, W G Staff

The Leicester Nuffield Hospital

Scraptoft Lane, Leicester LE5 1HY
Tel: 0116 276 9401 Fax: 0116 246 1076
Email: leicester.enquiry@nuffieldhospitals.org.uk
Owners: Nuffield Hospitals
Total Beds: 46

Accident and Emergency P A Evans, D N Quinton
Biometry J Tanner, J Voller
Breast Surgery N Everson, J Jameson
Cardiology D Chin, J Davies, A H Gershlick, I Hudson, R Leanage, R K Pathmanathan, J Pohl, J D Skehan
Cardiothoracic Surgery R Firmin, M Galinanes, L Hadjinikolaou, M Hickey, J Leverment, A Sosnowski, T Spyt
Dermatology J Berth-Jones, R Burd, R Graham-Brown, K E Harman, G Johnston
ENT T Alun-Jones, A Banerjee, A A Moir, G Murty, P Rea, R S A Thomas
Gastroenterology J de Caestecker, I Lawrence, J Mayberry, B Rathbone, R Robinson, A Wicks
General Medicine G J Fancourt, R Gregory, S Jackson, N Lo, P McNally, J Wales, M Wiskela
General Surgery N Agrawal, D Andrew, W W Barrie, D Berry, M Dennis, A Dennison, N Everson, A Hall, D Hemmingway, J Jameson, M Kelly, D M Lloyd, N London, M J McCarthy, A Miller, A R Naylor, M Nicholson, G Robertson, R Sayers, S Scott, W M Thomas, S Ubhi, P Veitch, D Waller
Gynaecology F Al-Azzawi, P Bosio, A Davidson, Q Davies, R De Chazal, J Emembolu, D Ireland, P Kirwan, C Mayne, I Scudamore, J Waugh
Haematology S Pavord, H U R Qureshi, J A Snowden
Hand Surgery D Quinton
Homoeopathy S Miles
Maxillofacial Surgery C Avery, J Hayter, I Ormiston
Neurology R Abbott, P Critchley, M C Lawden
Neurophysiology D Holder
Neurosurgery R Ashpole
Obstetrics P M Bosio, C Oppenheimer, J Waugh
Oncology S Khanna
Ophthalmology D Austin, K Bibby, J M Cappin, J Deane, W Karawatowski, J Prydal, R Sampath, A Tekriwal, G Woodruff
Oral Surgery C Avery, J Hayter, I Ormiston
Orthopaedics M Allen, P Allen, A Armstrong, A Best, B Bhowal, S Birtwistle, K Boyd, J Davison, J J Dias, C Esler, A Furlong, S Godsiff, T Green, M L Harding, M A Hutson, C Kershaw, M L Newey, O O Oni, R Pandey, R Power, P Sell, B Shah, A Shair, P Singh, L A Spaine, S Tandon, G Taylor
Orthotics P Crocker
Paediatric Surgery N Everson, S Nour
Paediatrics A Elias-Jones, S Nichani, S Nour, S Sethi, R Tamhne, R Walia
Pain Management M Bone, B Collett, E Lin, S Tordoff
Plastic Surgery H Henderson, T Milward, E O'Broin, S Varma, D Ward, N W Yii
Podiatric Surgery D Holland, H Holmes, R Jogia, W Liggins
Psychiatry M Chawla, T Friedman, D Khoosal, M Shepherd
Psychology S Fraser, K Loumidis
Rheumatology W Hassan, F E Nichol, R Oldham, A Samanta
Speech Therapy P Barton
Thoracic Surgery D Waller
Urology P Butterworth, K Mellon, G Ninan, D Osborn, D Sandhu, T Terry

Leigham Clinic

76 Leigham Court Road, Streatham, London SW16 2QA
Tel: 08457 304030
Owners: BPAS (British Pregnancy Advisory Service)

The Lincoln Nuffield Hospital

Nettleham Road, Lincoln LN2 1QU
Tel: 01522 578000 Fax: 01522 514021
Email: firstname.surname@nuffieldhospitals.org.uk
Website: www.nuffieldhospitals.org.uk
Owners: Nuffield Hospitals
Total Beds: 40

Manager Edward Goldsmith

Cardiology R Andrews
Dermatology N C Hepburn
Diseases of the Breast O F Eremin
ENT M K Chaurasia, A A P Connolly, A R McRae, E Nouri
General Medicine H Maksoud, A K Mandal, J L W Parker, G M Spencer, M R Teli
General Surgery P K Agarwal, D R Andrew, A P Barlow, P K Basu, I M Hutton, J A Jibril, A J Lamerton, P G Reasbeck
Immunology W A C Sewell
Neurology J C Bowen, B Sharrack
Neurophysiology N S Mytheen
Obstetrics and Gynaecology A J Breeson, G W Gough, R P Husemeyer, M P Lamb, O Oteri, I D Vellacott
Oncology G A Read, T Sreenivasan
Ophthalmology A A Castillo, P M Drummond, E G Hale, B S Redmill
Oral and Maxillofacial Surgery S Layton
Orthopaedics M S C Feeney, D W Gale, A E G Halliday, I D Hyde, C T Lee, M Maqsood, E W Morris, S M O'Riordan, J M Wilkinson
Pain Management A D Reynolds
Plastic Surgery H P Henderson, T Milward, E S O'Broin, S K Varma, N W Yii

Radiology A L Griffiths, S G Hogg, M Kamal, C I Rothwell, S Stinchcombe, V R Thava, G W Thorpe, G T Vijaysimulhu, D C Wheatley
Rheumatology J E Carty, B P Hunt
Urology I R Mark
Vascular Surgery P G Dunning

Lindisfarne Suite

Newcastle Nuffield Hospital, Clayton Road, Jesmond, Newcastle upon Tyne NE2 1JP
Tel: 0191 281 4606 Fax: 0191 281 3157
Owners: Cygnet Healthcare Ltd
Total Beds: 13

Psychiatry M J Akhtar, D L Dunleavy, A El Sobky, D Hunsley, S R Merson, M R Parry, K L Shrestha, M J Tacchi, P J Tayler, C M Tyrie

The Lister Hospital

Chelsea Bridge Road, London SW1W 8RH
Tel: 020 7730 3417 Fax: 020 7824 8867
Email: info@lister.hcahealthcare.co.uk
Website: www.thelisterhospital.com
Owners: HCA International Ltd
Total Beds: 69

Manager Zorica Vujicic, Zorica Vujicic

Anaesthetics M Albin, J Allt-Graham, M Apthorp, P Arunasalam, E M C Ashley, B A Astley, E Aziz, C Bailey, D Bamber, R Bell, M Bloch, P Borra, P Bras, A Bristow, J Broadfield, G Browne, D Burt, A Carr, K Chandradeva, M Chapman, S Chieveley-Williams, C Chin, D Chisholm, A Choyce, S Clarke, M Cooper, M Cox, D Daniels, J Dasan, C Davies, D W L Davies, D Dob, M Dunstan, D Enderby, P J D Evans, W P Farquhar-Smith, J Filshie, P Forrester, P Found, S Gautama, A Girgis, J Goldstone, R Graham, C Greville, P Groves, E Grundy, D Guerin, M Hacking, K Haire, C Hamilton-Davies, D Hampson-Evans, M Harris, H Hartley, T Herbst, C Hill, W Howell, T Hunt, D Hunter, C J Irving, D James, P Jones, D Justins, R Keays, M B Kenny, B Keogh, M Kulkarni, M Lees, M Lim, C Mallinson, S Marshall, C B Martin, M Messent, C Morgan, A Morley, P Morrison, F Moscuzza, M M Naef, B J Norman, A Oliver, G O'Sullivan, N Padfield, W Pais, S Papas (Papasiopoulos), S Parsons, M Plaza, J Porter, A Powroznyk, S Rehor, D Robinson, A Rubin, J Salt, P Saunders, M Scallan, H Scott, A Scurr, N Seth, C Shannon, A Shariff, E Sherry, J Silver, V Skelton, I Slee, N Soni, G Stocks, N Stranix, G Towlerton, R Verma, A Visram, C Walker, P Ward, L Webb, M D Weston, S White, E Williams, J Williams, K N Williams, J Wilson, S Woods, M Wren, G Wright
Audiology B Borgstein
Breast Surgery G Gui, N Roche, N P M Sacks, D Sinnett, J M Thomas
Cardiology J Clague, L Corr, P V L Curry, S W Davies, S Kaddoura, C W Pumphrey, C Shakespeare
Cardiothoracic Surgery M Marrinan
Care of the Elderly P Kroker
Colorectal Surgery D Kumar, J G Payne
Dermatological Surgery A C Markey
Dermatology R J Barlow, T Basarab, S M Breathnach, P M Dowd, J J H Gilkes, E Higgins, H Kurwa, S C Mayou, L Ostlere, N M Roberts, B Sarkany, R C D Staughton, N P J Walker
Endocrinology R Abraham, R D G Leslie, N P M Sacks, J Smellie
ENT G A J Morrison, P H Rhys Evans, G Sandhu
Gastroenterology C Ainley, P J Ciclitira, J Martin, J Meenan, R Pollok, A H Raimundo, D Westaby, R Zeegen
General Medicine S Barton, J Collins, J Costello, R Davison, J Dawoodi, B Gibberd, M Green, A Jones, M Kinirons, P Kroker, R D G Leslie, J Martin, A Mier, D J R Morgan, B O'Connor, J J Oram, J Outhwaite, M D E Pelly, P Shah, S Singh, P K Thompson
General Surgery C Bishop, N S Hakim, A Hayes, M M Henry, D Kumar, D Nott, J G Payne, R J Reyes, J H Scurr, A Shankar, J Smellie, N Theodorou, J M Thomas, J N Thompson, R Vashisht
Gynaecology H I Abdalla, J Bidmead, J Bridges, H El-Rafaey, I L C Fergusson, M Fynes, T Ind, R Irvine, A Jeyarajah, C J Kelleher, Y Khalaf, R Marwood, D H Oram, R Richardson, J R Smith, M Stafford, S L Stanton, J Studd, J G Thorpe-Beeston
Haematology D Catovsky, C Costello, L A Kay
Microbiology G French, D Shanson
Nephrology J Pattison
Neurology A Al-Memar, O Foster, A M D Kennedy, M-H Marion, S Omer, B Turner
Neurophysiology I Mak
Neurosurgery P J Hamlyn
Obstetrics & Gynaecology O Akinfenwa, G Ayida, C Barnick, T Bourne, K Clifford, M Dooley, R Faris, A Gafar, E Horner, A Kenney, B Ogunyemi, J Parikh, H Shehata, M Y Thum, N M Wales, J Yoon
Oncology R Eeles, P Ellis, J Glees, T Ind, A Jeyarajah, C P Lowdell, C Nutting, R H Phillips, T Powles
Ophthalmology W Ayliffe, P Bloom, V Chong, M Corbett, G Duguid, N Joshi, S Mitchell, J Olver, G Thompson, T H Williamson
Oral and Maxillofacial Surgery R G D Burr, M Manisali
Orthopaedic Surgery P R E Baird, G J Belham, A Davies, M Davies, S C Evans, D Fahy, C Gibbons, A L Hulme, J R Lavelle, K Lehndorff, J Lucas, J E Nixon, W J P Radford, J Scott, J Sinha, M C P Wilkinson, A M Williams
Orthopaedics J Bliss, J Compson
Otolaryngology S Blaney, W Grant, J-P Jeannon, I S Mackay, V Moore-Gillon
Otorhinolaryngology T Mugliston, D Roberts, H Saleh
Paediatric Surgery E A Nicholls
Pain Management J Gallagher, C E Gillbe, T Goroszeniuk, A D Lawson
Palliative Medicine D Feuer
Plastic Surgery G Bantick, N P Haacke, P Harris, C Healy, N Joshi, M Kelly, U Khan, N Kirkpatrick, A Logan, D Martin, B J Mayou, S Myers, N Parkhouse, A E Searle, S Wood
Podiatry A Kontos
Psychiatry S Frank
Psychology S Barker
Radiology A Adam, C Blakeney, S Bose, G Brown, D Carr, R Chinn, S Connor, T Cox, S R Desai, D Elias, R Given-Wilson, J Healy, J Jarosz, P Kane, J Karani, M D King, S McWilliams, M J Michell, A Mitchell, C Morris, E Moskovic, S Padley, J Reidy, H L Walters, L Wilkinson
Rheumatology B Bourke, A Brand, G Hall, G Hughes, S A Kaye, A Keat, C Mackworth-Young
Uroandrology S Minhas, J P Pryor, D J Ralph
Urology S Agarwal, C Anderson, S Choong, M D Dinneen, M Feneley, D Hrouda, G Muir, C Ogden, J Poulsen, D J Ralph, J Ramsay, P M T Thompson, K Walsh, C R J Woodhouse
Vascular Surgery E Chaloner, S Ray, J H Scurr

London Bridge Hospital

27 Tooley Street, London SE1 2PR
Tel: 020 7407 3100 Fax: 020 7407 3162
Email: info@lbh.hcahealthcare.co.uk
Website: www.londonbridge-hospital.co.uk
Owners: HCA International Ltd
Total Beds: 119

Anaesthetics A Al-Kaisy, S Barker, T Goroszeniuk
Cardiac Surgery D R Anderson, C B Austin, W Awad, C I Blauth, J B Desai, A El-Gamel, P Kallis, S Kolvekar, K Lall, J O'Riordan, M Petrou, J C Roxburgh, F Shabbo, G H Venn, B T Williams, C P Young
Cardiology D A Brennand-Roper, C A Bucknall, J Clague, J Coltart, R Cooke, M Cooklin, L Corr, P V L Curry, J Foran, J S Gill, A Gupta, P M Holt, G Jackson, D E Jewett, K Kamalvand, E J Langford, C S Lawson, M Lowe, D Lythall, P MacCarthy, A Mathur, F A Murgatroyd, N Parchure, S R Redwood, N Robinson, R Schilling, A Shah, C Shakespeare, S Sharma, S Sporton, R Spurrell, M Webb-Peploe
Colorectal Surgery E Carapeti, M George, M H Jourdan, W A Kmiot, D Skidmore, A Williams
Dermatology J Barker, A S Barkley, D Creamer, E Higgins, C J O'Doherty
ENT S Blaney, D Bowdler, E B Chevretton, A F Fitzgerald-O'Connor, M Gleeson, N Haacke, J-P Jeannon, G Morrison, S Paun, D N Roberts

General Medicine I C Abbs, K Y Ahmed, J Allawi, A Anggiansah, I T Bjarnason, P J Ciclitira, M L Eilkinson, I Forgacs, S Hurel, C Macdougall, A McNair, J K Meenan, J W O'Donohue, J M Pattison, J Powrie, J D Sanderson, G Santis, C Streather, D Taube
General Psychiatry A H Fry, P Mallett
General Surgery S W Atkinson, N Beechey-Newman, S Bhattacharya, A Botha, J O Dalrymple, M El-Wahash, H Hamed, D I Heath, J G Hubbard, F Hughes, R Hutchins, M H Jourdan, W A Kmiot, L Lang-Lazdunski, S Papagrigoriadis, J A Rennie, J V Roberts, M Siddiqui, S D Singh
Genitourinary Medicine C Rodgers
Gynaecology J Aquilina, G H Barker, J P Bidmead, A Davies, O Devaja, G Grudzinskas, I Jacobs, Y Khalaf, A Kubba, F Lawton, C Leitch, L J Mascarenas, A Olaitan, D H Oram, A J Papadopoulos, S K Raju, M Savvas, G J Webb-Wilson
Hepatology G Foster, P Harrison
Intensive Care Medicine R J Beale, A Jones, P Roberts, R Weekes, D Wyncoll
Neurology T C Britton, E Silber, B Turner
Neurophysiology K Nagendran
Neurosurgery F Afshar, C Chandler, B Chitnavis, R Gullan, P Hamlyn, I Sabin, N Thomas, J Wadley
Occupational Health A Yardley-Jones
Oncology R P Beaney, P Ellis, P G Harper, M Leslie, G Mikhaeel, D W Miles, A Tutt
Oral and Maxillofacial Surgery R P Bentley, D Gibb, S Holmes, C Huppa, A J Lyons, M McGurk
Orthopaedics A R Adhikari, M Bankes, J Bliss, S Corbett, S Curry, G Holloway, A Iossifidis, O P Lahoti, J Lucas, C Natali, D Nunn, J O'Dowd, W W Ogufere, B Povslen, S G Rao, S Sakka, J Sinha, J D Spencer, D D M Spicer, A E Strover, G Vardi
Palliative Medicine T Bozek, D Feuer
Pathology P Fields, L Kay, M Kazmi, S A Schey
Plastic Surgery M Ho-Asjoe, C Inglefield, R Lip Hin Ng, D Ross, A R Rowsell, M Shibu
Radiology A Adam, K Britton, S Clarke, S Desai, J Donaldson, D Elias, I Fogelman, S Grubnic, J Jarosz, A Jones, P Kane, J Karani, E A MacDonald, M Maisey, M Mateen, S McWilliams, R Morgan, S Rankin, J Reidy, P Renton, G Rottenberg, T Sabharwal, R Salari, A Saunders, P Sidhu, A Timothy, H Walters, C Wilkins
Rheumatology D W Jones
Sports Medicine D Baron, I Beasley, S Motto
Transplantation N S Hakim, G Koffman
Urology N-P Bucholz, D Cahill, P Dasgupta, J Glass, T Greenwell, S Khan, A R Mundy, R Nauth-Misir, T O'Brien, R Popert, R Ravi, P M Thompson, R C Tiptaft
Vascular Surgery D Black, S Hussain, C McGuinness, A J McIrvine, B Price, H Rashid, P R Taylor, M Thompson, M Whiteley

The London Clinic

20 Devonshire Place, London W1G 6BW
Tel: 020 7935 4444 Fax: 020 7486 3782
Email: info@thelondonclinic.co.uk
Website: www.thelondonclinic.co.uk
Owners: Charity/Association
Total Beds: 191

Anaesthetics P Amoroso, G Belligan, A Bristow, R J Cohen, J Goldstone, M Harris, N Kellow, B M O'Donoghue, H Owen-Reece, S A White
Cardiology G J Davies, J R Dawson, R J C Hall, J R Muir, R Sutton
Cardiothoracic Surgery R Uppal
Care of the Elderly J P Keet
Dermatology R W Groves, C M E Rowland Payne
ENT G Alusi, L Badia, G B Brookes, D I Choa, D G Davies, C A East, J M Graham, J P Harcourt, G A J Morrison, M J Wareing, A Wright
General Medicine C C Ainley, G M Besser, A Blair, P-M G Bouloux, S-L Chew, J Devlin, D Empey, D F Evans, P Fairclough, N Farid, D Forecast, P S Freedman, J George, A R W Hatfield, S J Hurel, N Johnson, R Lancaster, J P Monson, I Murray-Lyon, S P Pereira, B P Saunders, L H Sevitt, R M Sheaves, J Teare, A V Thillainayagam, H Thomas, A J Williams, C B Williams
General Practice B Grimaldi, H D Rowbotham
General Surgery C A Akle, A Botha, P B Boulos, R Carpenter, C R G Cohen, T I Davidson, A B Gordon, G Gui, N Hakim, D Heath, R Hutchins, J S Kirkham, T Kurzawinski, S S Mudan, R J Nicholls, J M A Northover, R C G Russell, M N Siddiqui, R G Springall, A Steger, H White, A C J Windsor
Genitourinary Medicine F T K Lim
Gynaecology C C W Barnick, C Davis, D G Evans, A D Haeri, M Hatton, T Ind, A Lower, C Mellon, T Mould, M Setchell, J H Shepherd, C Spence-Jones, W J Walker
Haematology P Gravett, R M I Janmohamed, R Kaczmarski
Nephrology L R I Baker, J Cunningham, M Mansell, R Woolfson
Neurology P Bradbury, T Britton, O J Foster, J Gawler, P K P Harvey, P Jarman, M Rose
Neurophysiology G Badre, V P Misra, K Nagendran
Neurosurgery F Afshar, P Bullock, P Richardson
Ophthalmology J Brazier, R Daniel, J Dart, G Duguid, T J ffytche, D S Gartry, A M P Hamilton, P Hykin, J Jagger, D A H Laidlaw, T J K Leonard, D McHugh, C Migdal, P Riordan-Eva, E Schulenburg, G Vafidis
Oral and Maxillofacial Surgery R Burr, R Hensher, K Hussain, T W Lloyd
Orthopaedics K Bush, A Catterall, J P Cobb, P H P Dyson, M A Edgar, J Nixon, D Nunn, J P O'Brien, G Scott, M A Smith, D Spicer, J C Sutcliffe, R Vickers, J Witt, D H Yanni
Pathology R A S Blackie, E Calonje, R Goldin, D G Lowe, W J Marshall, A B Price, G Ridgway, G M Scott, I C Talbot, P A Trott, C Wells, A Wotherspoon
Plastic Surgery J E Bowen, D R Gateley, R Ng, D V Nield, N Parkhouse, D Ross
Radiology C Allen, Z Amin, P Armstrong, T Beale, S Bose, S Bradbrooke, J Brookes, P Butler, R Chaudhuri, R Chinn, M W Clarke, I Colquhoun, J Davis, S Desai, J Evanson, A Gillams, D Grant, S Grubnic, S Halligan, C Hare, J Hinton, J Husband, D MacVicar, M Matson, J McCall, A Mitchell, R Morgan, V Ng, I Nockler, A Padhani, S Padley, M Paley, M Patel, M Rafael, G Ralleigh, R Reznek, N Strickland, C Thakkar, J Tibballs, S Vinnicombe, A Waldman, A Watkinson, J Webb, A Wright
Radiotherapy and Oncology C Cottrill, M Glaser, D F H Gueret Wardle, P Harper, J Mackay, R T D Oliver, P N Plowman, M Powell, M L Slevin
Rheumatology H Fitz-Clarence, E Huskisson
Urology D F Badenoch, S S C Carter, S Chong, J Glass, R S Kirby, R J Morgan, V Nargund, S Nathan, N O'Donoghue, H Parkhouse, D Ralph, J W A Ramsay, J Vale, H N Whitfield
Vascular Surgery M Adiseshiah, C Bishop, F Cross, B J Pardy, M S Sobeh, J H N Wolfe

The London Knee Clinic

29 Tooley Street, London SE1 2PR
Tel: 020 7407 3069 Fax: 020 7407 3138
Email: londonkneeclinic@btconnect.com
Website: www.kneeclinics.co.uk
Owners: Privately Owned

Orthopaedics G Evans, A E Strover

The London Welbeck Hospital

27 Welbeck Street, London W1G 8EN
Tel: 020 7224 2242 Fax: 020 7224 2493
Website: www.londonwelbeckhospital.co.uk
Owners: Privately Owned

Lourdes Hospital

57 Greenbank Road, Liverpool L18 1HQ
Tel: 0151 733 7123 Fax: 0151 735 0446
Email: r.spalding@lourdeshospital.ord.uk
Owners: Charity/Association
Total Beds: 50

Lynden Hill Clinic

Linden Hill Lane, Kiln Green, near Twyford, Reading RG10 9XP
Tel: 0118 940 1234 Fax: 0118 940 1424
Email: enquiries@lynden-hill-clinic.co.uk
Website: www.lynden-hill-clinic.co.uk
Owners: Health Link, Isle of Man
Total Beds: 28

Manager Geraldine McHugh

The Manor Hospital, Oxford

Beech Road, Headington, Oxford OX3 7RP
Tel: 01865 307777 Fax: 01865 307788
Email: mel.maclean@nuffieldhospitals.org.uk
Website: www.nuffieldhospitals.org.uk
Owners: Nuffield Hospitals
Total Beds: 78

Acupuncture J Xu
Anaesthetics E V Addy, Q P Ainsworth, M T Ali, S W Benham, S J Berg, H S Bridge, G Burt, J M Chantler, D M Choi, M B Dobson, O J Dyar, C Edge, J M Evans, N Evans, R Evans, A D Farmery, C J Glynn, C S Grange, C R Grebenik, J Haldar, P R Hambly, H E Higham, E Hill, C F Kearns, J R Lehane, A B Loach, A G Marfin, D G Mason, C McGuiness, J M Millar, F Murray-Gibson, J J Pandit, T M Parry, D W Pigott, M T Popat, M J Quinlan, F M Ratcliffe, R Rogers, R M Russell, S Rutter, M C Sainsbury, J Salmon, N M Schofield, D Shlugman, J E Stevens, M D Stoneham, M E Ward, O Warner, J P Warwick, J L Westbrook, S Wheatley, D A Wilkinson, E M Williams, S Yarrow, J D Young
Audiology T M Tripp
Cardiac Surgery D Taggart
Cardiology A Banning, Y Bashir, H Becher, T Betts, K Channon, P Davey, C Forfar, A Kardos, I Mulligan, S Neubauer
Cardiothoracic Surgery R G Pillai, C P Ratnatunga
Clinical Psychology I Klimes, C Shackleton
Colorectal Surgery C Cunningham, I Lindsey
Dermatology N P J Walker
Dietetics J Dart, M O'Connor
Endocrinology H Turner, J A H Wass
ENT G J Bates, M J Burton, A P Freeland, C A Milford
Gastroenterology S P L Travis
General Medicine R C Armstrong, R W Chapman, A Darowski, A Edwards, D Edwards, R J Erin, D S Fairweather, J R Goves, P Kapff, M J Kenworthy-Browne, D Matthews, H Merriman, J S Meyrick, D Miller, P Sagar, J Sichel, C Tidy
General Surgery B J Britton, S J Cole, J Collin, N Dehalvi, N E Dudley, P J Friend, B D George, M J Greenall, A I Handa, N D Maynard, P McCulloch, N Mortensen, G P Sadler
Gynaecology F M L Charnock, T J Child, M D G Gillmer, S R Jackson, S Kehoe, A M Mander, J E McVeigh, H Naoum, J S Nicholls, V Rai
Haematology O I Atoyebi, C S R Hatton, A Peniket
Histopathology C Clelland, G Greywoode
Hypnotherapy R K Barden, A J Calleja
Neurology J Oxbury
Neuroradiology J V Byrne, W Kuker
Neurosurgery C B T Adams, T Z Aziz, T A D Cadoux-Hudson, S Cudlip, R S C Kerr, R Stacey
Oncology D J Cole, A C Jones, B A Lavery, M Middleton, A Protheroe, A Salisbury, E M Sugden, N J Warner, A Weaver
Ophthalmology S Downes, J S Elston, S Hague, C K Patel, P H Rosen, J F Salmon
Oral and Maxillofacial Surgery N R Saeed
Oral Surgery P F Caris, M G Hodge, S R Watt-Smith
Orthodontics G E Kidner, M McKnight, F G Nixon
Orthopaedic Surgery C J K Bulstrode, A J Carr, P H Cooke, C A F Dodd, J C T Fairbank, M Gibbons, R Gundle, R Jinnah, P D McLardy Smith, I McNab, D Murray, A Price, R J Sharp, T M Theologis, A Wainwright, J Wilson-Macdonald
Orthotics M Leonida
Paediatric Surgery H W Grant
Paediatrics E E Matthews
Pathology I D Buley, D R Davies, S Dhar, W Gray, K Hollowood, J Keenan, T J Littlewood, N Mahy, S Manek, M F Murphy, J Piris, I S D Roberts, D E Roskell, K Shah, B F Warren
Physiotherapy P J Booth
Plastic Surgery O Cassell, D J Coleman, P S Critchley, H P Giele, A M Godfrey, T E E Goodacre, A Pay, S A Wall
Psychiatry I D Coffey, P S Davison, H Fox, M Orr, P B Wilkinson, I R Wood, E Zapata-Bravo
Radiology R F Adams, P Anslow, M Betts, K Bradkey, H K M Bungay, N C Cowan, H D'Costa, R E English, C Ferret, F V Gleeson, D R M Lindsell, E G McNally, A J Molyneux, N R Moore, S J G Ostlere, J Phillips-Hughes, R Phillips, G Quaghebeur, J Teh, Z C Traill, R Uberoi, D J Wilson
Rehabilitation Medicine J M Outhwaite
Rheumatology M A Brown
Trauma and Orthopaedics G Kambouroglou, R I Keys
Urology K Bradley, D W Cranston, J P Crew, J G Noble, J Reynard, M Sullivan
Vascular Surgery C R Darby, J M T Perkins, J Walton

Marie Curie Centre, Bradford

Maudsley Street, Bradford BD3 9LH
Tel: 01274 337000 Fax: 01274 337094
Website: www.mariecurie.org.uk
Owners: Marie Curie Cancer Care

Manager Jane Edgeley

Marie Curie Centre, Edenhall

11 Lyndhurst Gardens, London NW3 5NS
Tel: 020 7853 3400 Fax: 020 7853 3437
Email: info@mariecurie.org.uk
Website: www.mariecurie.org.uk
Owners: Marie Curie Cancer Care
Total Beds: 32

Manager Kevin Keough

Marie Curie Centre, Liverpool

Speke Road, Woolton, Liverpool L25 8QA
Tel: 0151 801 1400 Fax: 0151 801 1458
Email: info@mariecurie.org.uk
Website: www.mariecurie.org.uk
Owners: Marie Curie Cancer Care
Total Beds: 30

Manager Elaine Rosser

Marie Curie Hospice, Caterham

Harestone Drive, Caterham CR3 6YQ
Tel: 01883 832600 Fax: 01883 832633
Website: www.mariecurie.org.uk
Owners: Marie Curie Cancer Care
Total Beds: 6

Manager Jane Eshelby

Marie Curie Hospice, Newcastle

Marie Curie Drive, Newcastle upon Tyne NE4 6SS
Tel: 0191 219 1000 Fax: 0191 219 1099
Email: pauline.lowes@mariecurie.org.uk
Website: www.mariecurie.org.uk
Owners: Marie Curie Cancer Care
Total Beds: 22

Manager Pauline Lowes

Marie Curie Hospice, Solihull

911-913 Warwick Road, Solihull B91 3ER
Tel: 0121 254 7800 Fax: 0121 254 7840
Email: elizabeth.cottier@mariecurie.org.uk
Website: www.mariecurie.org.uk
Owners: Marie Curie Cancer Care

Total Beds: 18

Manager Elizabeth Cottier

Marie Stopes Bristol
3 Great George Street, Clifton, Bristol BS1 5RR
Tel: 0117 900 5566, 0845 300 8090 Fax: 0117 900 5661
Owners: Marie Stopes International

Marie Stopes Central London
Marie Stopes House, 108 Whitfield Street, London W1T 5BE
Tel: 0845 300 8090 Fax: 020 7388 3409
Owners: Marie Stopes International
Total Beds: 4

Manager Elaine Teasdale

Marie Stopes Essex
88 Russell Road, Buckhurst Hill IG9 5QB
Tel: 020 8505 6358 Fax: 020 8498 9637
Owners: Marie Stopes International
Total Beds: 28

Marie Stopes Leeds
10 Queen Square, Leeds LS2 8AJ
Tel: 0845 300 8090 Fax: 0113 244 0685
Email: services@mariestopes.org.uk
Website: www.mariestopes.org.uk
Owners: Marie Stopes International

Manager C Lewis-Jones

Marie Stopes Maidstone
10 Brewer Street, Maidstone ME14 1RV
Tel: 0845 300 8090 Fax: 01622 620879
Owners: Marie Stopes International

Manager Julie Wilson

Marie Stopes Manchester
2 St John Street, Manchester M3 4DA
Tel: 0845 300 8090 Fax: 0161 834 4872
Owners: Marie Stopes International

Marie Stopes Reading
121 London Street, Reading RG1 4QA
Tel: 0845 300 8090 Fax: 0118 903 5073
Owners: Marie Stopes International

Marie Stopes South London
1A Raleigh Gardens, Brixton Hill, London SW2 6AB
Tel: 0845 300 8090 Fax: 020 8674 3173
Email: services@mariestopes.org.uk
Website: www.mariestopes.org.uk
Owners: Marie Stopes International
Total Beds: 16

Manager Danusia Bourdon

Marie Stopes West London
87 Mattock Lane, Ealing, London W5 5BJ
Tel: 0845 300 8090 Fax: 020 8567 3636
Website: www.mariestopes.org.uk
Owners: Marie Stopes International
Total Beds: 18

Manager S Baldock

McIndoe Surgical Centre
Holtye Road, East Grinstead RH19 3EB
Tel: 01342 330300 Fax: 01342 330301
Email: info@mcindoe-surgical.co.uk
Website: www.mcindoe-surgical.co.uk
Owners: Privately Owned

Anaesthetics P J Venn
ENT M O'Connell, R J Sergeant
Ophthalmology S M Daya, R Malhotra, M F O'Sullivan
Oral and Maxillofacial Surgery A E Brown, K M Lavery, < J Sneddon, J V R Tighe, P Ward Booth
Orthodontics A Cash, A Thom, L Winchester
Orthopaedics H J C Belcher
Paediatrics A J Allaway
Plastic Surgery P M Arnstein, J W Blair, J G Boorman, K W Cullen, J A Davison, B S Dheansa, P M Gilbert, N Parkhouse, J A Pereira, M A Pickford, R W Smith, T C Teo
Rheumatology and Rehabilitation R M N Makadsi
Urology P J Thomas

Merseyside Clinic
32 Parkfield Road, Liverpool L17 8UJ
Tel: 08457 304030
Owners: BPAS (British Pregnancy Advisory Service)
Total Beds: 30

Manager Kally Worthington

Middleton St George Hospital
Middleton St George, Darlington DL2 1TS
Tel: 01325 333192 Fax: 01325 333883
Email: info@affinityhealth.co.uk
Owners: Affinity Healthcare Ltd
Total Beds: 114

Manager Linda Stephens

Mount Alvernia Hospital
Harvey Road, Guildford GU1 3LX
Tel: 01483 570122 Fax: 01483 532554
Email: marketing@mount-alvernia.co.uk
Website: www.mount-alvernia.co.uk
Owners: Charity/Association
Total Beds: 90

Accident and Emergency A Wan
Anaesthetics P Barnado, S Carroll, S Comara, G Dhond, C Edkins, B W J Fawcett, J R Fozard, T Gallagher, G F Goddard, H B A Griffiths, G J Jenkins, M Jordan, P Joshi, E J Kershaw, J M Leigh, M A Lucas, K G Markham, N Payne, N Quiney, K Randall, J E J Saunders, M Scott, V Slade, J R Stoneham, A Zuleika
Audiology V Jayarajan
Biochemistry B Starkey, J Wright
Breast Surgery M W Kissin, G Layer
Cardiology T P Chua, T H Foley, E Leatham, E E J Smith, D E Ward
Dermatology R Felix, E Wong
ENT Surgery P Chapman, S Hehar, J Rowe-Jones, N Solomons, R Sudderick, N F Weir, D Wright
Gastroenterology N Karanjia, S Singh
General Surgery M E Bailey, C G Marks, I M Paterson, T Rockall, H J Scott, J Stebbing
Geriatric Medicine H J P Powell, V Seth
Gynaecology G H Barker, M Butler-Hauve, P M Coats, P P E Curtis, M Ford, R Hutt, A Kent, K Morton, A S Pooley, C J G Sutton, A Tailor, S Whitcroft
Haematology P Alton, A S M Rejman, G Robbins, J Shirley
Histopathology M G Cook, S de Sanctis, P A Jackson
Immunology S Deacock, H Griffiths
Microbiology R Y Cartwright, S Chambers
Nephrology P Andrews, M R Bending
Neurology H Foley, P Trend, G Warner
Oncology S Houston, M Illsley, R Laing, G Middleton, A Neal, H Thomas, C Topham, S J Whitaker, B W F White
Ophthalmology R Condon, S N Das, A Gilvarry, J A A Govan, J Keenan, C McLean, T Poole
Oral and Maxillofacial Surgery N R Attenborough, M Danford, P Haers, P A Johnson, C Newlands
Orthodontics N Taylor

Orthopaedics N Bradley, C J Coates, M Flannery, P J Halliwell, P A Magnussen, J Older, G Paremain, J W Rosson, P J Stiles
Paediatrics M Evans, F Howard, M Ryalls
Physicians B W A McAllister, D Russell-Jones, M G M Smith, M J Smith
Plastic Surgery P Whitfield
Psychiatry G Andrews, M Collins, B M Male
Radiology C J H Bland, T J Bloomberg, J Cooke, C Kissin, T A Lopez, W J Walker
Rheumatology A R Behn, R E S Gray
Thoracic Surgery R E Sayer
Urology J H Davies, S Langley, A K Nigam, R G Notley
Vascular Medicine K Dawson
Vascular Surgery K Dawson, C McGuiness, M Whiteley

New Victoria Hospital

184-188 Coombe Lane West, Kingston upon Thames KT2 7EG
Tel: 020 8949 9000 Fax: 020 8949 9099
Email: info@newvictoria.co.uk
Website: www.newvictoria.co.uk
Owners: Charity/Association
Total Beds: 37

The Newcastle Nuffield Hospital

Clayton Road, Newcastle upon Tyne NE2 1JP
Tel: 0191 281 6131 Fax: 0191 212 0163
Website: www.nuffieldhospitals.org.uk
Owners: Nuffield Hospitals
Total Beds: 40

Manager Caroline Griffiths

Cardiology J Ahmed, R S Bexton, J C Doig, S Junejo, J McComb, I Purcell, A Zaman
Care of the Elderly T P Cassidy
Dermatology M Dahl, C Lawrence, J McLelland, N J Reynolds, N Simpson
ENT S D Cameron, S Carrie, M El Badawey, J Hill, W J Issing, I J M Johnson, T Leontsinis, H Marshall, D Mathias, D Meikle, F Stafford, A Welch, J A Wilson, P Yates
General Medicine J Barton, I Cobden, M Hayat, M Hudson, R Kerr Thomson, S Louw, J Mackie, K Matthewson, K Oppong, P Perros, C Record, J Tapson, N Thompson
General Surgery S Attwood, I Bain, S Bawa, V Bhattachanpi, R Bliss, L Boobis, D Browell, M Carr, J Chamberlain, R Charnley, K Clark, M Clarke, P Cullen, W Cunliffe, H Gallagher, I Goulbourne, C Griffith, A B Griffiths, J Guest, P Hainsworth, J Hansen, I Hawthorn, N Hayes, M Higgs, A F Horgan, L F Horgan, W Huizinga, N A G Jones, S Kelly, T W J Lennard, D Manas, G R McLatchie, S Plusa, S Preston, G Stansby, I Taylor, J S Varma, S Vetrivel, R Weaver, M Wyatt
Haematology C W Tiplady
Neurology D Bates, N Cartilidge, P Cleland, P J Dorman, A Goonetilleke, D Turnbull, T Walls, T L Williams
Neurosurgery P Crawford, C Gerber, A Jenkins, A Mendelow, J Nissen, R Sengupta, N Todd
Obstetrics and Gynaecology I Aird, J Brady, M Das, J Davison, S Field, J P Forsey, P Franks, B Fulton, K Godfrey, M M H Guirguis, D Irons, R Jaiyesimi, T Lavin, M R Lawrence, A Lopes, M S A Mansour, G Morgan, M Roberts, A Sproston, C S Steele
Oncology P Atherton, T Branson, F Y Coxon, W Dobrowsky, A Hughes, C Kelly, I Pedley, J Roberts, M Verrill
Ophthalmology E Barnes, M Birch, R C Bosanquet, R Boyce, M Clarke, F C Figueiredo, C Neoh, N Ray-Chaudhuri, A E Shafiq, N Strong, S J Talks
Oral and Maxillofacial Surgery J Hawkesford, D Lovelock, K Postlethwaite
Orthopaedics S Asaad, N Brewster, P J Briggs, J Buchanan, J Coorsh, G De Kiewiet, D Deehan, B Dorani, J Du Fosse, K Emmerson, D Fender, A Gayner, C H Gerrand, C Gibbons, M Gibson, P Henman, J P Holland, R Hornby, A Innes, L Irwin, D Kramer, N E Moghal, P Partington, J Pooley, G Prasad, J Quinby, P Sanderson, M Scott, N Shankar, N Shaw, M Siddique, A Stirrat, P Stuart, D Weir, J Williams, K Wright
Paediatrics F Alexander, M A Barrett, M N de la Hunt, B Jaffray, C O'Brien
Plastic Surgery R Berry, N Collio, M Erdmann, P Hodgkinson, S Jeffery, N McLean, R Milner, J O'Donoghue, N Williams
Psychiatry M J Akhtar, D L F Dunleavy, D Hunsley, S R Merson, M R Parry, K L Shreshta, P J Tyalor, C Tyrie
Rheumatology T Daymond
Urology G Durkan, J G W Feggetter, D Greene, T Hasan, M Johnson, P Powell, P Ramsden, N Soomro, D Thomas, A Thorpe
Vascular Surgery D Lambert, T Lees

The North London Nuffield Hospital

Cavell Drive, Uplands Park Road, Enfield EN2 7PR
Tel: 020 8366 2122 Fax: 020 8367 8032
Website: www.nuffieldhospitals.org.uk
Owners: Nuffield Hospitals
Total Beds: 45

Cardiology S Banim, T Crake, R Davis, D Patel
Dermatology J Almeyda, H Bayoumi, A Lambiris, N Mann, W Robles, H Stevens
Dietetics A Holdsworth, S Shepherd
ENT B Djazaeri, M Farag, S Habashi, G Mochloulis, K Patel
Gastroenterology K Besherdas, D Maudgal, P Maxwell, A Millar, B Smith
General Medicine M Aziz, R Jackson, D Jain, B Kennedy, S Khan, S Lozewicz, R Luder, A Mahmood, H Makker, A Mier Mier, J Onwubalili, S Saboor, M Seervaratnam, S Shah, M Vanderpump
General Practice (Private) M Shah, V Singh
General Surgery M Al-Dubaisi, R Anwar, R Bird, J Bolton, R Croft, O Fafemi, H Hamilton, V Jaffe, M Klein, N Law, A Loh, L Meleagros, F Minasian, R Navaratnam, D Stoker, D Ward, J Wood
Gynaecology A Antoniou, R Atalla, N Bajekal, E Downes, F Evans, A Govind, P Hardiman, D McLintock, A Minchin, M Morcos, S Okolo, P Shah
Ophthalmology J Brazier, M Hulbert, L Kleanthous, G Palexas, J Raina, M Toma
Oral and Maxillofacial Surgery M Gaukroger, W Halfpenny, P McDermott, N Rosenbaum
Orthopaedics D Archibald, R A Bajekal, S Blackburne, T Bull, D Grace, R Kumar, J Neyt, H Nwaboku, H Parmar, P Ray, D Rossouw, R Sharma, D Singh, J Skinner, D Thakkar, S Trakru, H Ware, V Woolf
Paediatrics D Bentley, A Shah, O Wilkey, K Withana, B Yuksel
Plastic Surgery A Gaitanis, M Ho-Asjoe, M Shibu, C Tattari
Rheumatology M Grayson, A Jawad, G Panayi, M Persey
Urology P Copland, M Devereux, G Fowlis, H Godbole, L Kahn, J McDonald, F Mumtaz, M Pati, P Shridhar, G Webster

The North Staffordshire Nuffield Hospital

Clayton Road, Newcastle under Lyme ST5 4DB
Tel: 01782 625431 Fax: 01782 382509
Website: www.nuffieldhospitals.org.uk
Owners: Nuffield Hospitals
Total Beds: 33

Manager Andrew Lunt

Anaesthetics M N Calhaem, R Johns, C L Knight, F Lam, N Matthews, S G Seddon
Cardiology R Butler, J E Creamer, J A S Davis
Dermatology J P H Byrne, A G Smith, B B Tan
ENT V Carlin, R Courteney-Harris, P Wilson
General Medicine M Allen, J A Gibson, J Green, J Mucklow, J Scarpello, S Sen, A Walker, A Ward
General Psychiatry K Hussain
General Surgery J Adjogatse, S Caldwell, R Dawson, M Deakin, T J Duffy, J Elder, J Forrest, B R Gwynn, C Hall, G B Hopkinson, R Kirby, R H Morgan, K P Patel, A K M Walsh
Genitourinary Medicine A R Markos, G Singh
Gynaecology J C Cooper, V Menon, M Obhrai, P M S O'Brien
Histopathology M Stephens
Nephrology S J Davies
Neurology H G Boddie, M B Davies, S J Ellis
Neurosurgery P S Dias, J Singh

Ophthalmology M F Brown, R Brown, J Gillow, P A Shaw
Oral and Maxillofacial Surgery T Malins, M Perry
Orthopaedics E B Ahmed, J S M Dwyer, T El-Fakhri, D Emery, D Griffiths, V Jasani, N Maffulli, D McBride, I D M Remedios, J Travlos, R Wade, C Wynn-Jones
Paediatrics C Campbell, W Lenney
Plastic Surgery P M Davison, D Prinsloo, J O Roberts
Radiology S Bajwa, M Braithwaite, M Cowling, I Haq, N Haq, N Lane, P Richards, J Saklatvala, S Tebby, D West
Radiotherapy and Oncology F A Adab, A M Brunt
Rheumatology M F Shadforth, A B Ward

Nottingham Brain Injury Rehabilitation Centre

Hankin Street, Hucknall, Nottingham NG15 7RR
Tel: 0115 968 0202 Fax: 0115 964 2747
Email: nottingham@fshc.co.uk
Owners: The Huntercombe Hospitals
Total Beds: 71

Nottingham Brain Injury Rehabilitation Centre, Apsley Unit

Robins Wood Road, Apsley, Nottingham NG8 3LD
Tel: 0115 942 5153 Fax: 0115 942 5154
Email: nottingham@fshc.co.uk
Owners: The Huntercombe Hospitals
Total Beds: 32

The Nottingham Nuffield Hospital

748 Mansfield Road, Woodthorpe, Nottingham NG5 3FZ
Tel: 0115 920 9209 Fax: 0115 967 3005
Email: paul.pritchard@nuffieldhospitals.org.uk
Website: www.nuffieldhospitals.org.uk
Owners: Nuffield Hospitals
Total Beds: 41

Manager Rachel Bradbury

Audiology S Borucki, A Kayan
Cardiology A J Ahsan, K Baig, G K Morris
Care of the Elderly J D Morant
Dermatology B R Allen, J S C English, W Perkins, S Varma
ENT N Beasley, P J Bradley, K P Gibbin, N S Jones, J McGlashan, A Sama
General Medicine M K Al-Bazzaz, S P A Allison, D R Baldwin, T Bowling, R P Burden, I D A Johnston, R M Kupfer, R G Long, A E A Mahmoud, H Maksoud, T Masud, S D Ryder, D J Seddon
General Practice B Ahmed, N Ahmed, L Boruch, I Campbell, B P Collins, N Sarwar
General Surgery J Abercrombie, N C M Armitage, I J Beckingham, J B Bourke, B D B Braithwaite, K L Cheung, F A El-Sheikh, C Maxwell-Armstrong, S Parsons, M Robinson, J H Scholefield, G W Tennant, C S Ubhi, N T Welch, J Williams
Neurology D Annesley-Williams, N Bajaj, T Jaspan, R Lenthall, G V Sawle, A C Thomas, A M Whiteley
Neurophysiology P Choudhury, J Stocks
Neurosurgery R D Ashpole
Obstetrics and Gynaecology W Atiomo, C Bain, P T Edington, T N Fay, G Filshie, C Gie, R Hammond, J Hopkisson, D T Lui, M A Macpherson, D Nunns, M C Powell, S J Ward
Oncology D A L Morgan, M Sokal, S Sundar
Ophthalmology W M K Amoaku, L C Anderton, S Dhar-Munshi, H S Dua, A J E Foss, N R Galloway, R M C Gregson, A J W King, S Subramaniam, S A Vernon, A Watson, A Zaman
Oral and Maxillofacial Surgery I H McVicar, E J Rowson, A J Sidebottom
Orthopaedics G Ampat, A Broodryk, J Chell, E H Compton, T R C Davis, M G Dennison, S Dhar, N D Downing, I W Forster, R Gibson, M Grevitt, D M Hahn, B J Holdsworth, J B Hunter, P J James, S Jones, A R J Manktelow, H Mehdian, C G Moran, A Moultan, J A Oni, G M Orr, P J Radford, J M Rowles, S Royston, B Scammell, E P Szypryt, A Taylor, A Wallace
Plastic Surgery A Erian, M Henley, R D Macmillan, S McCulley, A G B Perks, I A Starley
Podiatry P Bewick
Psychiatry H Baxter, T Friedman, M S Gahir, P F Jamie, O Junaid, J C E Meikle
Psychology P Vessey
Radiology S S Amar, H C Burrell, E J Cornford, J S Dawson, R Dhingsa, A J Evans, K Fairbairn, D J Green, J J James, J C Jobling, R W Kerslake, K H Latief, A R Manhire, N McConachie, K Pointon, B J Preston, D H Rose, S C Whitaker, A R M Wilson
Respiratory Medicine S Wharton
Rheumatology P Lanyon
Sports Medicine M Batt, N Peirce
Urology M C Bishop, O Cole, M D Dunn, D Harriss, R J Lemburger
Vascular Surgery B R Hopkinson, S MacSweeney

Nuffield Hospital Cambridge

4 Trumpington Road, Cambridge CB2 2AF
Tel: 01223 303336 Fax: 01223 316068
Email: cambridge@nuffieldhospitals.org.uk
Website: www.nuffieldhospitals.org
Owners: Nuffield Hospitals
Total Beds: 52

Manager Colin Birse

Anaesthetics A Absalom, A R Bailey, J Bambar, S Bass, P M Benson, L Brennan, A M Brooks, Burnstein, R Campbell, F Falter, S Ghosh, F Gilder, C W Glazebrook, K Gunning, A Gupta, R Hall, I Hardy, M J Herrick, D R Hughes, N Jamali, R M Jones, D Kennedy, A Klein, J Klinck, J D Kneeshaw, R D Latimer, M J Lindop, J Mackay, I M J Mackenzie, B Matta, D K Menon, V Navapurkar, A Oduro, G R Park, R Rebbapragada, P Roe, D Sapsford, H Smith, R Tandon, D Tew, J M Turner
Cambridge ENT Consortium P R Axon, B M Fish, R F Gray, P Jani, D McKiernan
Cardiothoracic Surgery M C Petch, F C Wells
Dermatology N P Burrows, P Norris, R J Pye, P Todd
General Medicine R Miller (Head), G A Campbell, O M Edwards, D Forsyth, J O Hunter, S J Middleton, R Miller, M Parkes, J Woodward
General Surgery R Miller (Head), J R Boyle, P Forouti, M E Gaunt, N R Hall, R Hardwick, N V Jamieson, R Miller, K Varty, G Wishart
Genitourinary Medicine C Sonnex
Gynaecology R A F Crawford, G A Hackett, J Latimer, P J D Milton, M Shafi, M Slack, J G Williamson
Haematology T P Baglin, R E Marcus
Hand Surgery Mr Matthewson
Medico-Legal M Bowditch, P Caller, E H Compton, J C Evans, I Lillington, P M Scott, G Tyler
Neurology M Manford, E A Warburton
Neurosurgery P J Kirkpatrick, R J C Laing, R MacFarlane, A Waters
Occupational Medicine J Stevens
Oncology C Wilson (Head), R Benson, H M Earl, K M Fife, D Gilligan, S J Jeffries, R E Marcus, A M Moody, H Patterson, S Russell, L T Tan, R Thomas, M V Williams, C Wilson
Oral and Maxillofacial Surgery L Cheng
Oral Surgery K P Esplin, W Girgis, J C Martin, I Pearson, H Pritchard, G L Wickens
Orthopaedic Surgery J Chitnavis, D Conlan, C R Constant, D J Dandy, D Edwards, G Keene, M H Matthewson, P J Owen, A H N Robinson, G M Tytherleigh-Strong, A S Wojcik
Paediatrics R W Iles, A Parker
Pain Management I Hardy, D R Hughes, R Munglani, G R Park
Physiotherapy M Callingham, L Dawson, J Jones, S Lockley, A Melloy, P Smith
Plastic Surgery G Cormack (Head), T Ahmad, A Canal, G Cormack, M Irwin, C A Malata
Psychiatry R O'Flynn (Head), N Hunt, J McKeown, R O'Flynn
Radiology P Bearcroft, P D Britton, N R Carroll, J Cross, A H Freeman, J H Gillard, J P N Higgins, N Screaton, P Set, R Sinnatamby, A Tasker, H Taylor, A Warner
Renal Medicine J R Bradley
Respiratory Medicine S M Nasser, J Shneerson, R J D Winter
Rheumatology J R Jenner (Head), A J Crisp, B L Hazelman, J R Jenner

Urology K N Bullock (Head), K N Bullock, A Doble, J Kelly, N Shah, W Turner
Vascular Surgery K Varty (Head), J Boyle, M Gaunt, K Varty

Nuffield Hospital Derby

Rykneld Road, Littleover, Derby DE23 4SN
Tel: 01332 540100 Fax: 01332 540113
Website: www.nuffieldhospitals.org.uk
Owners: Nuffield Hospitals
Total Beds: 38

Anaesthetics A Ahmed, P Allsop, E Aly, M M Ankutse, R C E Bates, P Bavister, T Bhatti, A Boyd, D P Cartwright, N J Chesshire, A W A Crossley, M S Dawson, R Dua, R H Elliott, R J Erksine, R J Faleiro, P Gill, M Haldar, R T Hedge, B Ho, V Hodgkinson, P W Holgate, S Kiani, B T Langham, J H Low, J Martin, S Millar, N A Moore, D Mulvey, N Nandwani, S Piggott, S J Ralph, J Rayner-Klein, D Rogerson, Z A Sadiq, W E Scott, A E Searle, Z I Sheikh, C W Stenhouse, P Stewart, R K Tibble, R Verma, C A Webb, I P Whitehead
Dermatology T Bleiker, H Shahidullah
ENT M N Johnston, P K Lee, B Majumdar, S Mortimore, J Oates, D Parker, T J Rockley, J F Sharp, A C Thompson
General Medicine P M Amin, J H Baron, A Cole, R Fluck, J Freeman, A Goddard, H Maksoud, A J McCance, C McIntyre, M W Millar-Craig, K A Muhiddin, B Norton, A A Palejwala, I Wahedna, D Watmough
General Psychiatry K P Rao, M C Shepherd, M A Sherman
General Surgery T E Bucknall, K Callum, A El-Tahir, R I Hall, H W Holliday, S Y Iftikhar, R Lee, P C Leeder, M K Lingam, J N Lund, B S McIlroy, R Nash, J R Reynolds, C Rogers, D M Sibbering, A Sverrisdottir, G M Tierney, S A Vakis, Y Wahedna
Gynaecology J K Artley, R L K Chapman, V N Chilaka, M P Cust, F J Darne, A Fowlie, J Hollingworth, Y G Ibrahim, H Jenkins, K Lingam, A D G Roberts, I Scott
Neurology N Bajaj
Neurophysiology P P Choudhary
Ophthalmology S Chawdhary, H C Chen, P T C Docherty, I D Gardner, R Harrison, R Holden, A Rauf, H A M Salem, L Stevenson, T Worstmann
Oral and Maxillofacial Surgery A W Baker, A J Dickenson, P Doyle, K Jones
Orthopaedics L C Bainbridge, F Bindi, F D Burke, D Calthorpe, A O Cargill, J Chell, D I Clark, G G Geutjens, M R Hamlet, A P J Henry, C Heras-Palou, P W Howard, J Hutchinson, B C Karagkevrekis, S L Khemka, C Kitsis, P G Lunn, D M McDermott, R C Quinnell, D Quinton, J Rowles, A B Stephen, M E Wallace, T Wilton
Plastic Surgery J Daly, M Henley, I F Starley
Psychology A Lather, A D Levee
Radiology M J C Bagnall, D P Clarke, N Cozens, M de Nunzio, S Elliot, E L Loney, G Narborough, M Palaniappan, J Pallan, J G Pollock, D Smith, A Turnbull, G M Turner
Radiotherapy and Oncology P R Chakraborti
Urology C P Chilton, M J Henley, A M Peracha, D M Thomas, S A Thomas, J H Williams
Vascular Surgery K Callum, A El-Tahir, J W Quarmby

Nuffield Hospital Harrogate

Queens Road, Harrogate HG2 0HF
Tel: 01423 567136 Fax: 01423 524381
Website: www.nuffieldhospitals.org.uk
Owners: Nuffield Hospitals
Total Beds: 27

Manager Neil Berry

Anaesthetics J Berens, J Campbell, J Charlton, D Dickson, B Duncan, A Fale, R Frater, J Gasser, J Jones, E Moss, P Murphy, G Parkin, A Poon, A Quinn, M Simenacz, M Thompson
Cardiology M Appleby, H Larkin
Care of the Elderly S Brotheridge
Dermatology M Goodfield, A M Layton
ENT A Grace, A Nicolaides, G Reilly
General Medicine S Brotheridge, G Davies, P Hammond, J Ridpath
General Surgery G Dyke, J Harrison, R A Knox, D J Leinhardt
Gynaecology P Ballard, A Barnett, J Buxton, S Henalla
Neurology P Goulding, B Henderson, S Jamieson
Neurophysiology S Hasan
Neurosurgery P Chumas, P Marks, N Phillips, S Ross, A Tyagi
Ophthalmology T Metcalfe, R Taylor, G Walters
Oral and Maxillofacial Surgery M Telfer, P H Whitfield
Orthopaedics A Budjen, A Collier, N J London, J Mitchell, R Newman, G Sefton
Paediatrics P Chetcuti, D Gillies, M Rahman
Pathology G Bynoe, C Hall, M J Toop
Plastic Surgery S Kay
Radiology S Carradine, A Coral, R Mawhinney, H Moss, D Sapherson, D Scullion
Radiotherapy and Oncology D Bottomley, D Dodwell, A Melcher
Rheumatology A Gough, M Green, M Martin, C Pease
Urology S Prescott, P Singh

Nuffield Hospital Haywards Heath

Burrell Road, Haywards Heath RH16 1UD
Tel: 01444 456999 Fax: 01444 454111
Website: www.nuffieldhospitals.org.uk
Owners: Nuffield Hospitals
Total Beds: 42

Manager Deborah Muldoon

Anaesthetics H G Adams, J Andrews, F Baldwin, D J Bellis, D Campbell, L Campbell, C Carey, W Chappel, C Child, J Cooper, A K Daborn, A J Davey, C Fumagalli, D Gilman, M Harper, A Hill, R H A Hoyal, J Kunan, L S Lafreniere, I Littlejohn, M Lynch, D McDonald, C Osmer, M Parry, J Pateman, W A L Rawlinson, D H Read, J Rouse, J Sanders, M Street, S Sudan, C N Swaine, D Tayler, C Thompsett, S Thorp, M Twohig, S Ward, J Williams
Cardiology D Hildick-Smith, J M Metcalfe
Dentistry S Diu
Dermatology C Darley, R Emerson, A Woollons
ENT J A McGilligan, M O'Connell, R M D Tranter
Fertility I Craft
Gastroenterology S Cairns, T R Leigh, N Parnell
General Medicine A Gossage, K R Hinne, M Jackson, W Shattles, C Turton, T Wheatley
General Surgery C R R Corbett, P Farrands, N F Gowland-Hopkins, P Hale, M A Lavelle, D Manifold, E R T Owen, P C Ridings, M Uheba, A Yelland, C Zammit
Gynaecology T Bashir, K Boos, G Kalu, T Kelly, M Long, B McKenzie-Gray, O Ogueh
Haematology T J Corbett, J Duncan, P Hill, M Kenny
Medical Biochemistry S Iversen
Microbiology P A Donaldson
Neurology P J Hughes
Neuropsychology S Anderson
Neuroradiology C D Good, M A Jeffree, J S Olney
Neurosurgery J Akinwunmi, G P H Critchley, C Hardwidge, J S Norris
Oncology D Bloomfield, J Simpson, M Wilkins
Ophthalmology G P H Brittain, A G Casswell, M Eckstein, C Liu, B K McLeod
Oral and Maxillofacial Surgery J Herold
Orthopaedics S Bendall, I Bintcliffe, M A Cass, S I C Chauhan, C Hatrick, E Parnell, M Patterson, D Ricketts, C Williams
Paediatrics A J Allaway, I Lewis, A Mahomed
Pathology J Allen, P A Berresford, N Patel, G J Stockford, T Williams
Plastic Surgery K W Cullen, A Khandwala, N Parkhouse, M A Pickford, B Tanner, T C Teo
Psychiatry C Hindler, M M Venables
Radiology J Berry, J L Bush, R S Dossetor, R Evans, I Francis, A Hawrych, K Khan, J Richenberg, G Rubin, I J Runcie, C Sonksen, P Thompson
Rheumatology A Al-Husseini, G Papasavas, B M Stuart

Urology C Coker, M Fletcher, T Larner, P D Miller, J S Nawrocki, H Parkhouse, M Royle, P Thomas

Nuffield Hospital Hereford

Venns Lane, Hereford HR1 1DF
Tel: 01432 355131 Fax: 01432 274979
Website: www.nuffieldhospitals.org.uk
Owners: Nuffield Hospitals
Total Beds: 20

Manager Wendy Mawdesley

Anaesthetics N Bywater, C Day, R Dowling, J Harrad, J Hutchinson, W Moore, M Nicholls, N Salmon, C Studd, W Williams
Cardiology D Pitcher
ENT G Hanna, M Smith
General Medicine J Dalziel, J Glancy, M Hall, K Jobst, R Ransford, P Ryan
General Psychiatry C Thomas
General Surgery C Cheek, A Corder, A Corfield, E Grocott
Gynaecology M Cohn, R Smith, R Subak-Sharpe
Neurology N Davies
Ophthalmology J Deutsch, S Scotcher, A White
Oral and Maxillofacial Surgery T Hall
Orthopaedics M Oakley, I Reynolds, V Seal, P Shewell, F Sibly, R Walker, D Williams
Pathology L Robinson, S Willoughby
Plastic Surgery H Goldin, S Thomas, V Vijh
Radiology P Garwood, P Grech, G Rowe, P Wilson
Radiotherapy and Oncology S Elyan
Rheumatology D Rees, R Williams
Urology A Jha, G Sole
Vascular Surgery S Wilson

Nuffield Hospital Hull

Entrance 3, Castle Hill Hospital, Castle Road, Cottingham, Hull HU16 5FQ
Tel: 01482 623500 Fax: 01482 623510
Website: www.nuffieldhospitals.org.uk
Owners: Nuffield Hospitals
Total Beds: 38

Manager Tracy Hampson

Dermatology A Butt, S Walton
ENT S Ell, R England, M Rogers, S Smith, N Stafford
General Medicine V Anand, A Arnold, D Bhatia, M Dakkak, D Hepburn, S Khulusi, D McGivern, Y Patel, J Smithson, H Thaker, H Tsai
General Psychiatry V Iyer, J Mullin
General Surgery P Drew, G Duthie, J Fox, J Gunn, J Hartley, T Mahapatra, P McManus, J Monson, C O'Boyle, C Royston, P Sedman, J Tilsed, K Wedgwood
Genitourinary Medicine U Joshi
Gynaecology J Gandhi, S Killick, S Maguiness, W Noble, K Phillips, E Speck, S Tyrrell, R Yeo
Nephrology S Bhandari, D Eadington
Neurology F Ahmed, A Ming
Neurosurgery B Mathew, D O'Brien, G O'Reilly
Ophthalmology A Babar, S Datta, J Innes, A Mathur, M Pande, O Stewart, M Zaman
Orthopaedics J Bradley, T Cain, F Howell, G Johnson, K Karpinski, G Kings, A Mohsen, A Nihal, C Shaw, K Sherman
Paediatrics A Azaz, R Daniel, M El-Habbal
Plastic Surgery P O'Hare, A Platt, M Riaz, M Stanley
Radiotherapy and Oncology A Chaturvedi, M Holmes, M Lind, A Maraveyas
Urology D Almond, G Cooksey, J Hetherington, S Kraus
Vascular Surgery A Akomolafe, B Johnson, P McCollum, P Renwick

Nuffield Hospital Ipswich

Foxhall Road, Ipswich IP4 5SW
Tel: 01473 279100 Fax: 01473 279101
Email: jill.kettle@nuffieldhospitals.org.uk
Website: www.nuffieldhospitals.org.uk
Owners: Nuffield Hospitals
Total Beds: 60

Manager David Jowett

Anaesthetics M Bailey, J Broadway, J Brown, F Byrne, P Carroll, J Dixon, I Driver, M Garfield, I Hatcher, R Howard-Griffin, P Howell, A Jarvis, A Kong, N Lillywhite, M Mansfield, P Mills, A Nicholl, E Rush, J Skinner, M Smith, J Stevens
Cardiology R Chatoor, N Irvine
Dermatology T Cutler, S Gibbs
ENT A Hilger, M Salam, M Yung
General Medicine G Glancey, N Innes, Y Miao, G Rayman, D Seaton, P Williams, S Williams, R Wyke
General Surgery A Abu-Own, H Adair, T Archer, A Cameron, S Huddy, C Mortimer, I Osman, J Pitt, J Powell, D Rae, I Scott, M Sinclair
Geriatric Medicine M Grimmer, P Phillips
Gynaecology T Boto, B Johal, A Leather, P Mooney, C Spencer, G Thomas, D Vasey
Haematology J Ademokun
Neurology H Manji, S Wroe
Oncology J Le Vay, C Scrase
Ophthalmology Z Butt, C Edelsten, R Goble, S Hardman-Lea, R Lewis
Oral and Maxillofacial Surgery H Davies, R Tate
Orthopaedics R Baxandall, M Bowditch, J Hallett, J Hopkinson-Woolley, I Hudson, C Marx, M Shanahan, D Sharp
Pathology N Dodd
Plastic Surgery A Bardsley, A Logan, T O'Neill
Psychiatry M El-Gaddal
Radiology S Garber, P Jennings, K Karia, R Nightingale, G Picken, S Smith, P Whitear
Rheumatology G Clunie, R Watts
Urology G Banerjee, C Booth, P Donaldson, J Parry

Nuffield Hospital Leeds

2 Leighton Street, Leeds LS1 3EB
Tel: 0113 388 2000 Fax: 0113 388 2309
Email: anna.kennett@nuffieldhospitals.org.uk
Website: www.nuffieldhospitals.org.uk
Owners: Nuffield Hospitals
Total Beds: 88

Manager Karen Miller

Breast Surgery D Ali, K Horgan, M R J Lansdown
Cardiology M W Baig, P Brooksby, J Campbell Cowan, S C D Grant, R V Lewis, J McLenachan, C Pepper, E J Perrins, M Pye, R Sapsford, N P Silverton, U M Sivananthan, G Williams, I Wilson, A V Zezulka
Cardiothoracic Surgery P Kaul, P H Kay, J P McGoldrick, C M Munsch, U R Nair, D O'Regan, C Papagiannopolous, J A C Thorpe, K G Watterson
Care of the Elderly A Cameron, I Thompson
Chest Medicine M T Henry, M Muers
Dermatology W Cunliffe, V Goulden, R Sheehan-Dare, G Stables, M Wilkinson
Endocrinology P Belchetz, S G Gilbey, S M Orme, P Sheridan
ENT G Kelly, L Knight, Z Makura, S Sood
Gastroenterology A Axon, D Burke, M E Denyer, S Everett, M V Tobin
General Medicine H Bodansky, A Brownjohn
General Surgery R Antrum, J Ausobsky, D Burke, P Curley, S Dexter, R L Doig, P Finan, J P Lodge, M J McMahon, P Sagar, H Sue-Ling, G J Toogood
Genitourinary Medicine M Waugh
Gynaecology A Balen, T J Broadhead, E J Buxton, D Campbell, J Dwyer, M Glass, M D Griffiths-Jones, C C Kremer, C Landon, G Lane, K Peel, L J Rogerson, A Rutherford, J Tay

Haematology D Barnard, G Cook, P Hillmen, R J Johnson, G Morgan, R G Owen, G M Smith
Immunology P M Wood
Musculoskeletal S Brennan, M Brooke, T Crystal, T Hassan, M Hutson, J Sloan, J H V Vanharanta
Neurology J Bamford, M Johnson, L A Loizou
Neuropsychiatry and Neuropsychology A Coughlan
Neurosurgery P Chumas, P Marks, N Phillips, S Ross, G M Towns, A Tyagi, P T Van-Hille
Oncology D Ash, D Bottomley, A Crellin, D Dodwell, J K Joffe, T Perren
Ophthalmology T R Dabbs, R M L Doran, J S Hillman, A J Morrell, D O'Neill
Oral and Maxillofacial Surgery M F W Chan, D P Dyson, R Loukota, J L Russell, A G Smyth
Orthodontics D O Morris
Orthopaedic Surgery R Bale, S Bollen, S J Calder, M Emerton, R D Farnell, S M Gollapudi, R Hackney, C D R Lightowler, M Rawes, J Shanker, D Shaw, M H Stone, N Tulwa, M E Walsh, A Watters
Orthopaedics M Hutson
Paediatric Surgery D C G Crabbe, A Najmaldin
Paediatrics F M Campbell, S P Conway, C Ferrie
Pain Management D E Dickson
Pathology A P Boon, P J Carder, S A Lane, U Raja, C S Verbeke, M Wilcox
Plastic Surgery F S C Browning, C Fenn, M I Liddington, W Saeed
Psychiatry M S Alexander, A M Easton, J J Nehaul, D Yeomans
Radiology D Barron, A G Chalmers, A H Chapman, B J G Dall, M J Darby, R Dunham, R C Fowler, K S Gill, A J Grainger, J A Guthrie, K Harris, H C Irving, J C Liston, S McPherson, P O'Connor, G J S Parkin, J Rankine, R J H Robertson, P Robinson, J A Spencer, N J Spencer, J Straiton, S Swift, P J Turner, M J Weston
Rheumatology A Fraser, C T Pease
Urology J Cartledge, G Flannigan, A D Joyce, S N Lloyd, S Prescott, R Puri, S K Sundaram, P M T Weston
Vascular Surgery R L Doig, M J Gough, J F M Hossain, A I D Mavor

The Orchard Hospital

189 Fairlee Road, Newport PO30 2EP
Tel: 01983 520022 Fax: 01983 528788
Email: enquiries@theorchard.hospital.co.uk
Owners: Privately Owned
Total Beds: 30

Cardiology M Connaughton, D Price
Dental Surgery J Wickens
Dermatology M Hazell
ENT P Grimaldi, G S Weli
Gastroenterology C L Sheen
General Medicine A Baksi, A Demissie, E Hakim, A Hossenbocus, D Murphy, C Patel
General Surgery S Elsmore, V Mehmet, M Shinkfield, J Symes, T Walsh
Gynaecology A D McNeal, D Ridley, A Yoong
Neurology J P Frankel
Ophthalmology D K Dhingra, M Rhatigan
Oral Surgery P W Baxter, T Mellor
Orthopaedics N A Boyd, J Gardiner, N Hobbs, S E Nasra, N S Pradhan, E Rahall, P Wellington
Plastic Surgery M Cadier
Psychiatry S Lynch
Rheumatology T Mamoud, M T Pugh
Urology J Makunde

Parkside Hospital

49 Parkside, Wimbledon, London SW19 5NB
Tel: 020 8971 8000 Fax: 020 8971 8002
Email: info@parkside-hospital.co.uk
Website: www.aspen-healthcare.co.uk/parkside
Owners: Aspen Healthcare Ltd
Total Beds: 70

Oncology A Dalgleish, M Harries, R Huddart, V Khoo, F Lofts, C Lowdell, J Mansi, A Neal, C Nutting, M O'Brien, H Pandha, S Partridge, R Phillips, R Powles, T J Powles, G Ross, A Rostom, R Rubens, F Saran, I Smith, J Steele, P Stone, D Tait, S Whitaker

Parkside Oncology Clinic

49 Parkside, Wimbledon, London SW19 5NB
Tel: 020 8971 8000
Email: info@parkside-hospital.co.uk
Owners: Aspen Healthcare Ltd

Manager Sue Macleod

Oncology T Powles (Head), A Dalgleish, J Glees, M Harries, R Huddart, V Khoo, F Lofts, C Lowdell, J Mansi, A Neal, C Nutting, M O'Brien, H Pandha, S Partridge, R Phillips, R Powles, T Powles, G Ross, A Rostom, F Saran, I Smith, M Spittle, J Steele, P Stone, D Tait, S Whitaker

Parkview Private Clinic Limited

14 Seagry Road, Wanstead, London E11 2NG
Tel: 020 8518 8920 Fax: 020 8518 8307
Email: info@parkviewclinicltdwanstead.co.uk
Owners: Privately Owned

The Plymouth Nuffield Hospital

Derriford Road, Plymouth PL6 8BG
Tel: 01752 775861 Fax: 01752 768969
Owners: Nuffield Hospitals
Total Beds: 41

Manager Glenys Mansfield

Anaesthetics A Dashfield, F Luscombe, R Sawyer, M Taylor
Cardiology C Burrell, I Cox, G Haywood, A Marshall, J D Motwani
Cardiothoracic Surgery S Allen, J Kuo, T Lewis, A J Marchbank, M J Unsworth-White
Chest Medicine J Cowie, P Hughes, C McGavin
Dermatology M Davies, P Kersey
ENT M Bridger, S C Toynton, P Windle-Taylor
General Medicine C M Hayward, S J Lewis, T Wilkin, S J Wilkinson
General Psychiatry R Eastwood
General Surgery J Akoh, S Ashley, A J M Brodribb, M Coleman, E H Drabbie, B A Greenway, K B Hosie, W A Lambert, F C Oppong, J Shaw, A Walker, R Watkins, T Wheatly, D Wilkins
Genitourinary Medicine G Morrison
Gynaecology U Acharya, L Bombieri, A Falconer, J Frappell, R M Freeman, K R Greene, J Morsman, R Shrestha
Nephrology R McGonigle, P Rowe, W Y Tse
Neurology J Gibson, M Sadler, J Zajicek
Neurophysiology S Kodapala
Neurosurgery T Germon, J Palmer, P Whitfield
Ophthalmology A P Booth, N Evans, T Freegard, Mr Frimpong-Ansah, R Fuller, N Habib, V T Thaller
Oral and Maxillofacial Surgery D J Courtney, A Davies, G Jones
Orthopaedics H David, P Evans, S Fullilove, M Halawa, R Jeffery, J Keenan, P Loxdale, I Rawlings, D Stitson, W G Thomas
Paediatrics A Cade, P Gorham, T Perham
Plastic Surgery J Evans, A R Fitton, J G M McDiarmid, R J Morris
Psychology R Barker, A Carr, J McBrien
Radiology P A Dubbins, B Fox, S J Freeman, P Hughes, S A Jackson, N J Ring, C A Roobottom, J R Steel, I P Wells
Radiotherapy and Oncology F Daniel, P MacLeod, C Tyrrell, D Yiannakis
Rheumatology P Hickling, C Hutton
Thoracic Surgery J Rahamin
Urology A J Dickinson, J C Hammonds, P McInerney
Vascular Surgery S Ashley

The Portland Hospital for Women and Children

205-209 Great Portland Street, London W1W 5AH

Tel: 020 7580 4400 Fax: 020 7390 8012
Email: info@portland.hcahealthcare.co.uk
Website: www.theportlandhospital.com
Owners: HCA International Ltd
Total Beds: 106

Dermatology M Glover, J Harper
ENT D Albert, H Daya, B Hartley
Gynaecology P Carter, S Creighton, A Cutner, T Freeman-Wang, L McMillan, T Mould, A Naftalin, C Naylor, D Oram, J Osborne, N Pisal, A Robinson, E Saridogan, A Silverstone, A Singer, S Stanton, P Walker, M Whitehead
Neurology N Cavanagh, A Martinez, D Smyth
Obstetrics Y Akinfenwa, M Al-Samarrai, J Aquilina, P Armstrong, G Barker, C Barnick, T Beedham, S Beski, J Braithwaite, J Brooks, P Carter, P Cass, D Cowan, I Craft, C Davis, T Dutt, F Eben, D Economides, H El-Refaey, J Elias, K Erskine, R Forman, S George, S Ghatak, D Gibb, M Gillard, D Glyn-Evans, K Harrington, M Hatton, R Howell, R Irvine, J Iskaros, N Jackson, E Jauniaux, M Johnson, A Kenney, A Kyei-Mensah, C Leitch, U Lloyd, C B Lynch, R Marwood, P Mason, C Mellon, H Morgan, N Morris, A Naftalin, C Naylor, N Nicholas, B Obiekwe, P O'Brien, J Osborne, C Pavlou, J Price, M Setchell, C Spence-Jones, J Spencer, T G Teoh, G Thorpe-Beeston, N Wales, N Wathen, C Wright, J Yoon
Ophthalmology J Leigch, I Russell-Eggitt, D Taylor
Orthopaedics M Barry, R Hill, M Paterson
Paediatrics S Bignall, E Douek, J Fysh, I Hay, S Herman, S Hussain, G Katz, E Maalouf, A Massoud, S Rom, E Thambapillai, B Yuksel
Plastic Surgery D Gault
Radiology A Schneidau, S Vinnicombe
Rheumatology N Hasson
Urology P Cuckow, P Duffy, I Mushtaq, P Ransley

The Princess Grace Hospital

42-52 Nottingham Place, London W1U 5NY
Tel: 020 7486 1234 Fax: 020 7908 2492
Website: www.theprincessgracehospital.com
Owners: HCA International Ltd
Total Beds: 103

Manager Susan E Smith

The Priory Clinic Canterbury

92B Broad Street, Canterbury CT1 2LU
Tel: 01227 452171 Fax: 01227 452823
Email: canterbury@prioryhealthcare.com
Owners: Priory Group

Manager J M Overton

The Priory Clinic Nottingham

Ransom Road, Nottingham NG3 5GS
Tel: 0115 969 3388 Fax: 0115 969 3381
Email: nottingham@prioryhealthcare.com
Website: www.prioryhealthcare.com
Owners: Priory Group
Total Beds: 20

Priory Grange

Micklefield Lane, Rawdon, Leeds LS19 6BA
Tel: 0113 239 1999
Total Beds: 22

The Priory Grange

Tottingworth Park, Heathfield TN21 8UN
Tel: 01435 864545 Fax: 01435 869609
Email: grange@prioryhealthcare.com
Website: www.prioryhealthcare.com
Owners: Priory Group
Total Beds: 30

Manager Claudette Neville

Psychiatry J Almeida, G Bagley

Priory Grange Hemel Hempstead

Longcroft Lane, Felden, Hemel Hempstead HP3 0BN
Tel: 01442 255371 Fax: 01442 265630
Website: www.prioryhealthcare.com
Owners: Priory Group
Total Beds: 34

Manager Andy Worledge

Priory Highbank Rehabilitation Centre

Walmersley House, Walmersley Road, Bury BL9 5LX
Tel: 01706 829540 Fax: 01706 829534
Email: highbank@prioryhealthcare.com
Website: www.prioryhealthcare.com
Owners: Priory Group
Total Beds: 58

Manager Helen Molyneux

The Priory Hospital Altrincham

Rappax Road, Hale, Altrincham WA15 0NX
Tel: 0161 904 0050 Fax: 0161 980 4322
Email: altrincham@prioryhealthcare.com
Website: www.prioryhealthcare.com
Owners: Priory Group
Total Beds: 47

Manager Julie Stratton

Addictions B Hore, P Mbaya, J Pasterski
Psychiatry M H Al-Asady, A Bagadi, J S Bamrah, D Baynes, W Braude, A K Dey, A M El-Assra, C Findlay, T Garvey, J Gowrisunkur, P Haddad, J Haslam, B D Hore, A Kelly, P Mbaya, B Monteiro, A Oppenheim, L Pasterska, J K Pasterski, N Ring, S Serafi, S Soni, H Waring, M Yacoub

The Priory Hospital Bristol

Heath House Lane, Off Bell Hill, Bristol BS16 1EQ
Tel: 0117 952 5255 Fax: 0117 952 5552
Email: bristol@prioryhealthcare.com
Website: www.prioryhealthcare.com
Owners: Priory Group
Total Beds: 37

Manager Steve Conway

The Priory Hospital Chelmsford

Stump Lane, Springfield Green, Springfield, Chelmsford CM1 7SJ
Tel: 01245 345345 Fax: 01245 346177
Email: chelmsford@prioryhealthcare.com
Website: www.prioryhealthcare.com
Owners: Priory Group
Total Beds: 45

The Priory Hospital Hayes Grove

Prestons Road, Hayes, Bromley BR2 7AS
Tel: 020 8462 7722 Fax: 020 8462 5028
Email: hayesgrove@prioryhealthcare.co.uk
Website: www.prioryhealthcare.com
Owners: Priory Group
Total Beds: 47

Manager David Hill

The Priory Hospital Hove

14-18 New Church Road, Hove BN3 4FH
Tel: 01273 747464 Fax: 01273 727321
Email: hovehospital@prioryhealthcare.com
Website: www.prioryhealthcare.com
Owners: Priory Group
Total Beds: 34

Manager Ian Coldrick

Psychiatry D Angus, W Assin, G Berelowitz, R Bowskill, M Procopio

The Priory Hospital Lancashire

Rosemary Lane, Bartle, Preston PR4 0HB
Tel: 01772 691122 Fax: 01772 691246
Email: lancashire@prioryhealthcare.com
Website: www.prioryhealthcare.com
Owners: Priory Group
Total Beds: 18

Manager Pauline Wright

Psychiatry W Charles, S Chattree, A D'Souza, K C Gupta, D Kay, H Moosa, M K Rahman, P T Saleem

The Priory Hospital Marchwood

Hythe Road, Marchwood, Southampton SO40 4WU
Tel: 023 8084 0044 Fax: 023 8020 7554
Email: marchwood@prioryhealthcare.com
Website: www.prioryhealthcare.com
Owners: Priory Group
Total Beds: 46

Manager Philip Maliphant

Affective Disorders S Kelly
Alcohol and Substance Abuse A Tate (Head), N Choudry, A Tate, A Tate
Eating Disorders N Joughin, A Wear
General Psychiatry N Joughin, P Milln, I Plant, M Ramsey, A Wear
Psychiatry of Old Age A Barker

The Priory Hospital North London

Grovelands House, The Bourne, Southgate, London N14 6RA
Tel: 020 8882 8191 Fax: 020 8447 8138
Email: northlondon@prioryhealthcare.com
Website: www.prioryhealthcare.com
Owners: Priory Group
Total Beds: 58

Manager Lorraine Ahern

Adolescent, Mental Health Assessment Service R Graham
Alcohol and Substance Abuse N Brener
Behavioural and High Level Cognitive Problems N Brener
Psychiatry R Amin, M Beary, C Bernat, N Brener, C Clemente, R Finch, R Graham, K Hwang, G Ikkos, B Lipkin, G Lloyd, J Pfeffer, R Refaat, G Rose, N Savla, R Schapira, M Serfaty, L Sheldon, J Shipperheijn, D Sumners, N Trieman, D Veale, G Waldron, V Watkin, V Watts, J Wise

The Priory Hospital Roehampton

Priory Lane, Roehampton, London SW15 5JJ
Tel: 020 8876 8261 Fax: 020 8392 2632
Email: roehampton@prioryhealthcare.com
Website: www.prioryhealthcare.com
Owners: Priory Group
Total Beds: 112

Manager Peter Smith

The Priory Hospital Woking

Chobham Road, Knaphill, Woking GU21 2QF
Tel: 01483 489211 Fax: 01483 797053
Email: woking@prioryhealthcare.com
Website: www.prioryhealthcare.com
Owners: Priory Group
Total Beds: 26

Manager Michele Paley

Alcohol and Substance Abuse M Bristow, T Cantopher, M Rowlands
Eating Disorders A Key, S Lieberman
General Psychiatry A Gillham (Head), G Andrews, Dr Badrawy, Dr Boothby, M Bristow, Dr De Silva, I Drever, J Edwards, A Gillham, Dr Hawthorne, R Hennessy, A Key, S Khalaf, G Kidd, S Lieberman, P Loughlin, J Mugisha, J Perera, A Valmana, Dr Yousaf
Women's Health R Hennessy, A Key

The Priory Ticehurst House

Ticehurst, Wadhurst TN5 7HU
Tel: 01580 200391 Fax: 01580 201006
Email: ticehurst@prioryhealthcare.com
Website: www.prioryhealthcare.com
Owners: Priory Group
Total Beds: 51

Manager Belinda Malone

Child and Adolescent H Etkin, D Griffiths, J Ronder, H Steffen
Psychiatry P McLaren (Head), J Almeida, H Etkin, D Griffiths, R Rao, J Render, R Royston, H Steffen, G Turnbull

The Purey Cust Nuffield Hospital

Precentor's Court, York YO1 7EL
Tel: 01904 641571 Fax: 01904 643115
Website: www.nuffieldhospitals.org.uk
Owners: Nuffield Hospitals
Total Beds: 31

Manager Edmund Witkowski

Anaesthetics P A Hall, R C Johnson, H G W Paw, G S Priestley, I Woods
Cardiology R Crook, S G Megarry, M Pye
Dermatology A S Highnet, C C Lyon
ENT A Coatesworth, A R H Grace, A R Nicholaides, P G Reilly
General Medicine A M Hunter, P Jennings, A J Turnbull
General Surgery D Alexander, S G Brooks, S H Leveson, J B Mancey-Jones, A McLeary, G V Miller, S Nicholson, W Wong
Gynaecology A Evans, R W Hunter, S N Mitchell, D Pring
Haematology L R Bond, M R Howard
Homoeopathy H Khan
Neurology A Heald
Neurosurgery P Marks
Ophthalmology R Ellingham, M Hayward, P M Jacobs, T D Manners, R H Taylor
Oral and Maxillofacial Surgery J Taylor, M Telfer, P H Whitfield
Orthopaedics A Budgen, P Campbell, P de Boer, A J Gibbon, R Jain, C A N McLaren, I H Whitaker, H R Williams
Paediatrics S Rahman
Radiology A M B Bowker, R A Mannion, M Porte, N Warnock
Rheumatology M Green, J M Iveson
Urology K Seeni, P Singh, M J Stower, G Urwin

Redford Lodge Hospital

15 Church Street, Edmonton, London N9 9DY
Tel: 020 8956 1234 Fax: 020 8956 1233
Website: www.partnershipsincare.co.uk
Owners: Partnerships in Care Ltd
Total Beds: 61

Manager Chris Hird

The Retreat, York

107 Heslington Road, York YO10 5BN
Tel: 01904 412551 Fax: 01904 430828
Email: info@retreat-hospital.org
Website: www.retreat-hospital.org
Owners: Charity/Association
Total Beds: 135

Alcohol and Substance Abuse G Smith
Eating Disorders C Holman
Rehabilitation S Mitchell

Robert Clinic
162 Station Road, Kings Norton, Birmingham B30 1DB
Tel: 08457 304030
Owners: BPAS (British Pregnancy Advisory Service)
Total Beds: 14

Manager Barbara Owen

Rosslyn Clinic
15-17 Rosslyn Road, East Twickenham, Twickenham TW1 2AR
Tel: 08457 304030
Owners: BPAS (British Pregnancy Advisory Service)

Royal Hospital for Neuro-disability
West Hill, Putney, London SW15 3SW
Tel: 020 8780 4500 Fax: 020 8780 4501
Email: info@rhn.org.uk
Website: www.rhn.org.uk
Owners: Charity/Association
Total Beds: 260

Manager Pam Charteris

St Andrew's at Harrow (Bowden House Clinic)
London Road, Harrow-on-the-Hill, Harrow HA1 3JL
Tel: 020 8966 7000 Fax: 020 8864 6092
Email: nicky.runeckles.cygnethealth.co.uk
Website: www.cygnethealth.co.uk
Owners: Cygnet Healthcare Ltd
Total Beds: 72

Manager Nicky Runeckles

Alcohol and Substance Abuse Dr Alam
Behavioural and High Level Cognitive Problems Dr Broughton
Psychiatry R I Cohen (Head), A Al-Mousawi, F Alam, C Coghlan, R I Cohen, M Green, J Hart, Z Huq, Dr Jouhargy, J Lewin, A Lewis, G Matthew, M Millington, D Oyewole, R Pipe, L Rozewicz, R Sharma, A Shrivastava, I Singh, L Sireling, M Slater, T Soutzos, Dr Van Huyssteen, W Walsh, A Warren

St Andrew's Group of Hospitals
Billing Road, Northampton NN1 5DG
Tel: 01604 616000 Fax: 01604 232325
Email: admin@standrew.co.uk
Website: www.stah.org
Owners: Charity/Association
Total Beds: 625

Brain Injury J N Follansbee, B Moffatt, S Nagraj
Continuing Care I R Wood, G Yorston
General Psychiatry A D Damle, C Haw
Learning Disabilities L Duggan, Dr Grafton
Mental Health G N Brown, P D Leahy, F L Mason, S L Mitchell, T I Mutale, D G Nevison-Andrews, L Quinn, C Staley, P Sugarman

St Anthony's Hospital
London Road, North Cheam, Sutton SM3 9DW
Tel: 020 8337 6691 Fax: 020 8335 3325
Email: info@stanthonys.org.uk
Website: www.stanthonys.org.uk
Owners: Charity/Association
Total Beds: 92

Manager B M N Clarke

Audiology E Raglan, L H Yeoh
Breast Surgery D Banerjee, K Mokbel, G Querci della Rovere, A Sharma
Cardiac Surgery V Chandrasekaran, M Jahangiri, P Kallis, R Kanagasabay, M Sarsam, F Shabbo, E E J Smith
Cardiology S J D Brecker, R Canepa-Anson, T P Chua, P Clarkson, W Culling, J Foran, S Joseph, J Lyons, O Odemuyiwa, V Paul, C Pumphrey, S Redwood, R Roberts, A Vasudeva
Chest Medicine N Cooke, A Draper, B Madden, P Mitchell-Heggs, N Paramothayan, C Rayner
Colorectal Surgery M Abulafi, S Farhat, D Kumar, R Leicester, A Oshowo, M Raja
Dermatology S Cliff, C Harland, C A Holden
ENT R Hehar, A C John, T Odutoye, D Selvadurai, A Toma, P Williamson
General Medicine M Bending, M Benson, P Howard, S Hyer, J Kwan, C McIntosh, R Orchard, T Rahman, A Rodin, A Theodossi
General Surgery D Banerjee, N J Bett, M Chawdery, E Chemla, A S Chilvers, A Fiennes, A Halliday, T Loosemore, R McFarland, D Nehra, S Ray, K M Reddy, P Thomas, M Thompson
Geriatric Medicine M Cottee, S Samadian
Gynaecology M Booker, C Croucher, P M Gough, N A McWhinney, I Manyonda, Z Nadim, L Ross, P Shah, H Shehata, E Sherriff, G Welply
Hand Surgery N Citron, A Fleming, D Gateley
Immunology A Bansal
Nephrology P Andrews, M Bending, J Kwan
Neurology A Al-Memar, P Hart, R O McKeran, T Von Oertzen, S Wilson
Neurophysiology S Bajada, H Modarres
Ophthalmology W Ayliffe, P Fison, I Gillespie, J Leitch, A McElvanney, S Shah, P G Ursell
Oral and Maxillofacial Surgery M H Danford, A Stewart
Orthopaedics A Adhikari, S Bridle, P Cheong-Leen, M A Churchill, N Citron, R Field, T G Kavanagh, J Klosok, V Patel, R Shedden, T Tennent
Paediatrics C Burren, S N Capps, S K F Chong, R El-Ritai
Pain Management S Said
Plastic Surgery A Fleming, D Gateley, P Harris, P Meagher, M J Pohl, B W E Powell
Psychiatry E G Lucas, R S Stern
Rheumatology J Axford, L Darlington, O L Duke, S Patel
Thoracic Surgery V Chandrasekaran, R Kanagasabay, R E Sayer, E E J Smith
Urology P O Ewah, C R Jones, P Le Roux, P Raju, R Walker, N Watkin

St Hugh's Hospital
Peaks Lane, Grimsby DN32 9RP
Tel: 01472 251100 Fax: 01472 251130
Email: admin@sthughshospital.co.uk
Website: www.hmt-uk.org
Owners: The Hospital Management Trust
Total Beds: 31

St John of God Hospital
Scorton, Richmond DL10 6EB
Tel: 01748 811535 Fax: 01748 812345
Owners: Privately Owned
Total Beds: 92

St Luke's Hospital for the Clergy
14 Fitzroy Square, London W1T 6AH
Tel: 020 7388 4954 Fax: 020 7383 4812
Email: stluke@stlukeshospital.org.uk
Website: www.stlukeshospital.org.uk
Owners: Charity/Association
Total Beds: 22

St Michael's Hospital
4 Trelissick Road, Hayle TR27 4JA
Tel: 01736 753234
Owners: Privately Owned
Total Beds: 85

The Shropshire Nuffield Hospital
Longden Road, Shrewsbury SY3 9DP
Tel: 01743 282500 Fax: 01743 247575
Website: www.nuffieldhospitals.org.uk
Owners: Nuffield Hospitals

Total Beds: 34

Manager Michael Haffenden

Anaesthetics I Baguley, D Barton, H Brunner, R Carley, P Cartwright, D Christmas, G Corser, D Elcock, C Emmet, N Hadden, R Hatts, K Hickmott, R Hollands, E Hughes, S Jurai, D King, R Law, M Mehta, M Miller, G Phillips, S Ray, S Sanghera, G Thompson, A Windsor
Cardiology M Clarke, M Heber, D Mistry, D Wallbridge
Dermatology S Kelly, S Murdoch
ENT W Neil, A Prichard, D Skinner, S Thompson
General Medicine J Bateman, J Butterworth, J Dixey, L Hill, J Jones, Mr Khalil-Marzouk, A Macleod, D Maxton, P Moulik, W Perks, M Smith, G Townson, T Usman, T West
General Surgery R Diggory, R Duffield, A Fox, M Halliday, A Houghton, T Hunt, R Hurlow, M Prescott, J Quayle, A Schofield, A Sigurdsson
Gynaecology B Bentick, A Gornall, J Lane, D Redford, N Reed, A Tapp
Neurology S R Nightingale
Ophthalmology A Callear, E Craig, R Dapling, P Haigh, P Rao
Oral and Maxillofacial Surgery S Olley, J Smith
Orthodontics J Chadwick
Orthopaedics W Cool, T Crichlow, R Doddenhoff, S Eisenstein, D Ford, P Gregson, S Hay, S Hill, C Kelly, C McGeoch, P Moreau, J Patrick, R Perkins, J Richardson, R Spencer-Jones, J Trivedi, S White
Pathology N Capps
Plastic Surgery D Prinsloo
Radiology J Fielding, M Fryer, K Gill, R Groom, D Hinwood, R Jones, P Lowe, I McCall, R Miller, R Orme, V Pullicino, S Robbins, H Sansom, P Tyrell, H Watson
Radiotherapy and Oncology A N Abbasi, R K Agrawal, S Awwad
Rheumatology R Butler
Urology C Beacock, S Coppinger, A Elves

Sketchley Hall

Manor Way, Sketchley Village, Burbage, Hinckley LE10 3HT
Tel: 01455 890023 Fax: 01455 636282
Email: sketchleyreception@prioryhealthcare.com
Website: www.prioryhealthcare.com
Owners: Priory Group
Total Beds: 87

Manager Pamela Brown

The Somerset Nuffield Hospital

Staplegrove Elm, Taunton TA2 6AN
Tel: 01823 286991 Fax: 01823 338951
Website: www.nuffieldhospitals.org.uk
Owners: Nuffield Hospitals
Total Beds: 44

Manager Philip Eke

Dermatology J Boyle, D Pryce
ENT A J Drysdale, A Husband, S Sadek, S Wells
General Medicine M James, P Kist, C Laversuch, T MacConnell, D H MacIver, J Pepperall, S Pugh, T Solanki, R Stone, C Swinburn, P Thomas, S Walker, D Yates
General Surgery J F Chester, P Eyers, I Eyre-Brook, T Jobson, S Jones, A Klidjian, I Ramus, C Vickery, R Welbourn
Gynaecology G Fender, M Robson
Neurology E Fathers, P Heywood, S Lhatoo
Ophthalmology A K Bates, R Gray, K Hakin, S Rattigan, J Twomey
Oral and Maxillofacial Surgery M Davidson, L Fryer, J Hamlyn
Orthopaedics A Clarke, A Dunkley, A Kelly, P Madhavan, C Marsh, C Ogilvie, A Omari, B Squires, P Thorpe, P Webb
Urology A Cannon, T Porter, M Speakman

The Spencer Wing

Queen Elizabeth The Queen Mother Hospital, Ramsgate Road, Margate CT9 4BG
Tel: 01843 234555 Fax: 01843 296333
Owners: Privately Owned
Total Beds: 22

Manager Di Daw

Accident and Emergency R Freij
Anaesthetics K Adegoke, M Ashfaque, G K Ciccone, E Davies, J Ghazala, C K Guest, A MacDonald, W E Morcos, C Perrera, A E Proctor, P Teli, B Tofte, H J Wilton
Cardiology R Heppell
Colorectal Surgery H Benziger, E Sharp
Dermatology D Goldin, M J Hudson-Peacock, V Neild
Diabetes G Hamza, S Joseph
Endocrinology S Joseph
ENT J Chelladurai, D Mitchell, N D Padgham, P Robinson, H Sharp
Gastroenterology K Hills, A Piotrowicz
General Medicine N R Goldsack, K Hills, M L Jenkinson, S Joseph, A Marshall, A D Morgan, S B Mukherjee
General Surgery N Benziger, S Gibbs, D Jackson, D M Marzouk, P J Pheils, G Tsavellas, N Wilson
Geriatric Medicine M L Jenkinson, S B Mukherjee
Neurology W Howlett
Neurophysiology N Mullatti
Obstetrics and Gynaecology P Belguamkar, H Hammond, A J Nordin, N Rafla, G Ross, L M A Shaw, J Shervington
Oncology R D James, A J Nordin
Ophthalmology N Andrew, R H Darvell, R DeCock, M Fouladi, M Heravi, W Poon
Oral and Maxillofacial Surgery C Hendy
Orthopaedics F Kasiri
Paediatrics M Malik, E R Rfidah, A Sarmah
Pain Management A Al Kaisy, R Bhadresha, R N B Senasinghe
Radiology Dr Abdel-Hadi, P Barker, G Giancola, A M Greenhalgh
Rheumatology D De Lord, A M Leak
Trauma and Orthopaedics J Casha, M Cornell, S A Jain, L Louette, S S Rajan, D Saran, I B M Stephen, N Wilson
Urology J Shervington, N Shrotri
Vascular Surgery E Sharp, N Wilson

Stockton Hall Hospital

The Village, Stockton-on-the-Forest, York YO32 9UN
Tel: 01904 400500 Fax: 01904 400354
Email: info@partnershipsincare.co.uk
Website: www.partnershipsincare.co.uk
Owners: Partnerships in Care Ltd
Total Beds: 112

Manager David Ackroyd

Surgicare Hospital

Parkway House, Palatine Road, Northenden, Manchester M22 4DB
Tel: 0161 945 8688 Fax: 0161 945 8689
Email: info@surgicare.co.uk
Website: www.surgicare.co.uk
Owners: Privately Owned
Total Beds: 8

Manager Jillian Bird

Consultants A Marando, K G Rose, R Stones

The Sussex Nuffield Hospital

Warren Road, Woodingdean, Brighton BN2 6DX
Tel: 01273 624488 Fax: 01273 620101
Email: snhhelpline@nuffieldhospitals.org.uk
Website: www.nuffieldhospitals.org.uk
Owners: Nuffield Hospitals
Total Beds: 56

Manager Paul Cowling

Cardiology C Davidson, A de Belder, D Hildick-Smith, S Holmberg, S O'Nunain
Cardiothoracic Surgery A Cohen, A Forsyth, J Hyde, U Trivedi
Care of the Elderly G Mankikar, H O'Neal

Dermatology C Darley, R Emerson, A Woollons
ENT A Cheeseman, M Harries, A McGilligan, M O'Connell, J Topham, R Tranter, J Weighill
General Medicine S Cairns, J Hartley, A Ireland, M B Jackson, N Jackson, J Tibble, C Turton, N Vaughan
General Surgery M Brooks, G Bryant, R Corbett, P Farrands, R Gumpert, P Hale, P Hurst, M Lamah, D Manifold, C Strachan, S W Yusuf
Gynaecology K Boos, R Bradley, A Fish, D Holden, G Kalu, A Kelly, P Larsen-Disney, J Montgomery, O Ogueh
Nephrology L Goldberg, S Holt, J Kingswood
Neurology R Chalmers
Neurosurgery J Akinwunmi, D Campbell, G Critchley, J Norris
Ophthalmology P Brittain, A Casswell, M Eckstein, C Liu, B McLeod
Oral and Maxillofacial Surgery K Altman, J Herold
Orthopaedics I Bintcliffe, S Chauhan, C Hatrick, J D McCutchan, R Pattison, P Staniforth, T Turnbull, R Turner, C Williams
Paediatrics A Allaway, A Davidson, A Mohamed, S Nicholls, J Trounce, A Van der Avoirt
Pathology M Cubbon, J Duncan, A Iversen, M Kenny, N Kirkham, N Patel, A Williams
Plastic Surgery P Arnstein, K Cullen, M Pickford, B Tanner, T Teo, C Zammit
Radiology G Burkill, G Dodge, R Dossetor, T Doyle, R Evans, I Francis, T Good, I Kenney, J Olney, G Price, J Richenberg, G Rubin, C Sonksen, N Straiton
Radiotherapy and Oncology D Bloomfield, G Deutsch, N Hodson, S Mitra, J Simpson, A Webb, M Wilkins
Rheumatology L Fernandes, G Papasavvas, M Walters
Urology C Coker, M Fletcher, T Larner, J Nawrocki, P Thomas

Tetbury Hospital

Malmesbury Road, Tetbury GL8 8XB
Tel: 01666 502336 Fax: 01666 505719
Owners: Charity/Association

The Thames Valley Nuffield Hospital

Wexham Street, Wexham, Slough SL3 6NH
Tel: 01753 662241 Fax: 01753 662129
Website: www.nuffieldhospitals.org.uk
Owners: Nuffield Hospitals
Total Beds: 50

Manager Darren Burr

Anaesthetics N Allison, J Anandanesan, J Anderson, P Balakrishnan, A Bristow, P M Brodrick, M D G Bukht, P Dadarkar, S J Davies, D W L Davies, R Fernandes, D Gatha, S J Harrison, R Iyer, A B Knight-George, L Leibler, A Levison, D M Lomax, R Loveland, D N Lucas, J Mackenzie, J Margary, A J May, M R Nel, G Nemeth, C E Nightingale, S Papas, J Pattison, D J Penney, A Qureshi, J Rangasami, J Restall, D L Robinson, T S Silva, J M B Smallman, B Smith, M A S Smith, K R Spelina, E J Taylor, A Thorniley, J Weinbren, D A White, R Woolf, W J Wraight
Cardiology K Barakat, R A Blackwood, R A Foale, R Grocott-Mason, C Missouris, N Peters, S Rex
Dermatology J L M Hawk, R C Ratnavel, V Walkden
Dietetics B Bhumber, A Gates
ENT A Jefferis, G Sandhu
General Medicine R Chauhan, D S Dove, G E Holdstock, J Jordaan, A Lessing, S Levi, C G H Maidment, G A Mayadunne, R Russell, R Sarsam, J Wiggins
General Practice P Newman, K Saraogi
General Psychiatry G T Bell
General Surgery D Babu, S Baxter, N G Browning, D Cairns, P G Cassell, P Coleridge-Smith, S P Courtney, P M Dawson, A Desai, J M Gilbert, A M Gordon, S E Knight, T Paes, P Rutter, J Scurr, S Shrotria, B Soin, A R Taylor, H Umeh
Microbiology M McIntyre
Micropigmentation & Remedial Camouflage G Thompson
Neurology A Everitt, R Nicholas, J P H Wade
Obstetrics and Gynaecology S A Akinsola, E S Dimitry, A H Elias, J Fairbank, N V Jackson, S Kalla, L Mascarenhas, P Reginald, J E Spring, W R Tingey, N Watson
Ophthalmology J Duvall-Young, J J Kanski, S Kheterpal, C J McLean, K K Nischal, R B S Packard, A Pearson
Oral and Maxillofacial Surgery M Amin, A Babajews, M Issa, C Yates
Orthopaedics R L Allum, M Bloomfield, W N Bodey, C Clark, R K Dega, J Jones, R Kucheria, R Langstaff, M Moiz, G Singer, R Sinnerton, M Thomas
Orthoptics E Dawson, W Williams
Paediatrics L J Hawk
Pathology M H Ali, S Desai, C S R Hatton, P H Mackie, H Sharif, I Walker
Plastic Surgery A P Armstrong, D S Crawford, J Dickinson, D Gault, C T Khoo, D Sammut
Podiatry A Bhargava, B Francis, M P O'Neill
Radiology M Charig, M N Chetty, S Ghiacy, D Grieve, A Hassan, I Liyanage, C Luck, D Maudgil, M Moreland, S R Patel
Radiotherapy and Oncology R F U Ashford, R S D Brown, M Hall
Rheumatology A P Kirk, S Liyanage, A Steuer
Sexual & Relationship Therapy A Commins
Speech Therapy E Daniel
Urology C Hudd, O Karim, M Laniado, H Motiwala, J W A Ramsay

Thornford Park

Crookham Common, Thatcham RG19 8ET
Tel: 01635 860072 Fax: 01635 874580
Email: thornfordpark@blenheimhealth.com
Website: www.blenheim-forensics.co.uk
Owners: Priory Group
Total Beds: 86

Manager Tom Convery

The Tunbridge Wells Nuffield Hospital

Kingswood Road, Tunbridge Wells TN2 4UL
Tel: 01892 531111 Fax: 01892 515689
Website: www.nuffieldhospitals.org.uk
Owners: Nuffield Hospitals
Total Beds: 58

Manager Simon Monkman

Anaesthetics J Appleby, L Baldwin, C J Barham, H J Burdett, R A Chung, S M Fenlon, R H A Hoyal, H T Hutchinson, G Lawton, T Ludgrove, A Pyne, J Quaife, J J Sanders, P E Sigston, K M Sim, M Sinden, G P Sommerville, C H Taylor, P J H Venn, T N Vorster, D W Yates
Cardiology D W Harrington, C S Lawson
Dermatology J P McFadden, S Tharakaram
ENT R V Lloyd, R J Sergeant, J C Shotton
Gastroenterology A Harris, R Loke
General Medicine R A Banks, D J Barnes, M Chellappah, J A Hughes, D S J Maw, P J Reynolds, A D A Sikorski, P K H Tsang
General Surgery P G Bentley, N H Boyle, A J Cook, T G Williams
Gynaecology P N Bamford, O A Chappatte, A E Davies, O Devaja, S Flint, D B Garrioch, M A Hefni, M P Matthews, A J Papadopoulo, M Rimington, M Wilcox
Neurology T J Fowler, G Saldanha
Oncology D M Barrett, S H Beesley, M E Hill, R Jyothirmayi, F McKinna
Ophthalmology J A Bell, C A Jones, N Rowson
Oral and Maxillofacial Surgery A Brown, A C Hattingh, P Pavlovic
Orthopaedics P Gibb, J E Nicholl, P W Skinner, K W R Tuson
Paediatrics M F Robards
Pathology J P Allen, D S Gillett, R Liebmann, Y I Lolin, L Munthali, R S Pereira, G Russell, C G Taylor, D M Thomas
Plastic Surgery K W Cullen, M A Pickford, R W Smith, N S B Tanner, T C Teo
Psychiatry N A Clarke, P M McLaren, J S McPherson, T Raj-Manicka, H Steffen, A J Winbow, K K Zakrzewski

Radiology B G Conry, J J Flanagan, J P Garrett, P I Ignotus, S E M Kirwan, P R Tallett, C Wetton
Rheumatology S Dodman, D G Macfarlane
Urology M S Cynk, T F Ford, R A Isworth, J L Lewis
Vascular Surgery M R Tyrrell

Unsted Park Rehabilitation Hospital

Munstead Heath Road, Godalming GU7 1UW
Tel: 01483 892061 Fax: 01483 898858
Email: unsted@prioryhealthcare.com
Website: www.prioryhealthcare.com
Owners: Priory Group
Total Beds: 33

The Vines

Innhams Wood, Crowborough TN6 1TE
Tel: 01892 610414 Fax: 01892 610926
Email: thevines@prioryhealthcare.com
Website: www.prioryhealthcare.com
Owners: Priory Group

Manager Rob Bunting

The Warwickshire Nuffield Hospital

The Chase, Old Milverton Lane, Leamington Spa CV32 6RW
Tel: 01926 427971 Fax: 01926 428791
Owners: Nuffield Hospitals
Total Beds: 43

Manager Rachel Bradbury

Anaesthetics J M S Aulakh, N Bhasin, C Bonnici, E M Borman, D Bose, A J Brookes, S Chari, F Choksey, K C Clayton, R Correa, S A J Crighton, J A Dako, Dr Derbyshire, R J Elton, K R L Evans, S Evans, A Frost, G P Furlong, M C Holt, S Jayaratnasingam, R A Johnson, R N Joshi, P Kai, C Knickenberg, T M W Long, S P Mather, W J D McCulloch, M K Mead, C Mendonca, P L Mulrooney, B V R Murthy, T D Neal, S Nethisinghe, V Panek, J Parker, A A Phillips, J M Porter, S Radhakrishna, S Rasanayagram, D A Robinson, M Sebastian, M Srivastava, S J Thorpe, R Tripathy, R S Walker, D M Watson, E White, A Wright, M Wyse
Audiology R Hayes, R Stokes
Cardiology M Been, A Y Chaudhry, N Clarke, P Glennon, Y Haider, P King, N Qureshi, M F Shiu, H Singh, A Venkatarama
Cardiothoracic Surgery N Briffa, W R Dimitri, R Norton, R Patel, M D Rosin
Clinical Chemistry F E Wells
Cytopathology S R Ferryman, K M Newbold
Dermatology A Bedlow, R Charles-Holmes, S Charles-Holmes, A Heagerty, F Humphreys, A Ilchyshyn
Dietetics J Hughes
ENT R C Bickerton, H R Cable, J Diver, P Kander, P Patel, D E Phillips
Gastroenterology M Aldersley, J Eaden, J Eden, P C Hawker, L S Hill, D Loft, C U Nwokolo, J Shearman
General Medicine D A H Badwan, R Bell, P I Biggs, S Boardman, H N Desai, D P Dhillon, P G Ferry, S Fletcher, R Jones, C Marguerie, R Mattu, P Ray, M Sandler, F G Vaz, A K Viswan, Dr Wood
General Surgery P Baragwanath, A A J Barros D'Sa, P Blacklay, J Francombe, I A Fraser, I D L Fraser, S Harries, D J Higman, C H E Imray, A O B Johnston, F T Lam, V S Menon, P Murphy, R Nangalia, M Osbourne, P Roberts, N Williams, L S Wong
Genitourinary Medicine P G Natin, M Walzman
Gynaecology L Anyanwu, K Cietak, T B J Hughes, R Jackson, C R Kennedy, K J Nippani, K Olah, A D Parsons, M Pearson, L J Sant Cassia, O Sorinola
Haematology S Basu, P E Rose
Histopathology R A Carr, N Chachlani, K Chen, S Deen, S R Ferryman, Dr Guha, K J Holley, J C Macartney, K M Newbold, Dr Rollaston, S Sanders, F A Smew, D Snead
Imaging A Anbarasu, D Beale, S K Bera, J Chandy, D P Clarke, A Duncan, T Goodfellow, M Hughes, F C Millard, C Oliver, G Penter, S Rai, R Ramachandra, R Shatwell, K Sherlala, G Stewart, K Vallance, R Wellings, P Williams
Microbiology A Ghose, S J K, M Weinbren
Neurology A Shehu
Neurophysiology V Hegde, S Ponsford
Neuropsychology R S Dyal, A Pearson
Neurosurgery M S Choksey, M H Christie, A Saxena, P A Stanworth
Oncology R Grieve, D Jones
Ophthalmology H S Alhuwalia, M Benson, Mr Cunliffe, D David, F M Dean, Miss Hope-Ross, R D Kumar, G Mission, A O'Driscoll, S Pagliarini, R Robinson, G Smith
Oral / Dental Surgery J Fagan, J A Mander, J Moule, D Purnell
Orthopaedics M J Aldridge, P Binfield, M Blakemore, M S Butt, S N Deliyannis, S Drew, M R Gokhale, D Griffin, A Hughes, S Hughes, S Krikler, J M Kumar, M Margetts, D McCreadie, W F Merriam, I Nwachukwu, U Prakash, T Robertson, A Salaam, D Shakespeare, N Shergill, T Spalding, M J C Stanislas, R Steingold, M Taylor, S M Turner, P Wade, S K Young
Orthoptics D Davies
Paediatric Medicine N Coad, A Coe, V Datta, A Gatrad
Pain Management J H L Antrobus, S P Mather
Plastic Surgery T A Eltigani, A R Groves, S Liggins, R N Matthews, R Papini, A J Park, S Srivastava
Psychiatry A Aleniz, K Bluglass, S England, A Mahmood
Psychology G Bellamy
Psychotherapy A Aleniz, D Muss
Rheumatology J Coppock, C Marguerie, G Struthers
Speech Therapy P A O'Donnell
Thread Veins/Hair Removal S J Liggins
Urology A R E Blacklock, K M Desai, K Kadow, C Lewis, K K Prasad, R Sriram, J R Strachan, M Wills

The Wellington Hospital

Wellington Place, London NW8 9LE
Tel: 020 7586 5959 Fax: 020 7483 5030
Website: www.thewellingtonhospital.com
Owners: HCA International Ltd
Total Beds: 266

The Wessex Nuffield Hospital

Winchester Road, Chandlers Ford, Eastleigh SO53 2DW
Tel: 023 8026 6377 Fax: 023 8025 1525
Website: www.nuffieldhospitals.org.uk
Owners: Nuffield Hospitals
Total Beds: 54

Manager Robert Swindlehurst

Cardiology A Calver
Care of the Elderly C Gordon, N Sterling
Dermatology R Ashton, D H Jones, M Keefe, H Smith
ENT P Ashcroft, N Haacke, W Hellier, T Mitchell, S Nair, N Patel, C Randall
General Medicine A Brooks, J Chong, D Ellis, D Fine, R Holt, P Patel, J A Roberts
General Psychiatry P Courtney, J Grimshaw, M O'Connell, A Wear
General Surgery I Bailey, N Beck, J Byrne, P Gartell, A Gordon, C Johnson, M Midwinter, A Miles, G Morris, P Nichols, K Nugent, M Phillips, J Primrose, R Rainsbury, C Ranaboldo, D Rew, G Royle, C Shearman, J Smallwood, S Somers, H Steer, N Wilson
Genitourinary Medicine D Rowen
Gynaecology M Buckingham, S Crawford, M Heard, K Louden, K Metcalf, A Monga, A Moors, R W Stones
Neurology J Frankel, H Katifi, P Kennedy, N Lawton, A Turner
Neurosurgery N Brooke, W Gray
Ophthalmology D Anderson, C Canning, I Chisholm, W Green, P Hodgkins, A Lotery, A Luff, A Macleod, R Manners, C Morris, R Morris, R Newsom, J Watts
Oral and Maxillofacial Surgery N Baker, B Evans, T Mellor, A Webb
Orthopaedics D Barrett, N Boeree, G Bowyer, P Chapman-Sheath, A Cole, D Cox, E Davies, D Dunlop, N Flynn, A Foggitt, J Fowler, H Fox, E Gent, M Grover, D Hargreaves, J Harley, G Harper, S

Hodkinson, W Hook, J Latham, A W Samuel, J Shearer, G Taylor, N Thomas, W Tice, N Trimmings, D Warwick
Paediatrics M Griffiths, H Steinbrecher
Plastic Surgery N Bennett, J Hobby, J Hurren, G Scerri, I Whitworth
Radiology J Argent, S Barker, V Batty, S Birch, R Blaquiere, D Breen, M Briley, J Cheetham, K Dewbury, A Ditchfield, J Elford, J Fairhurst, M Gawne-Cain, N Hacking, C Hamilton, J Hogg, L King, J Laidlow, J Millar, A Odurny, A Page, C Peebles, C Rubin, M Sampson, J Smart, H Taylor, K Tung, O Wethered
Radiotherapy and Oncology V Hall, C Heath, T Iveson, A Last
Rheumatology N Arden, R Armstrong, N Buchanan, A Calogeras, C Edwards
Urology A Adamson, B Birch, J Cumming, M Harrison, M Hayes, C Smart

Wistons Clinic

138 Dyke Road, Brighton BN1 5PA
Tel: 08457 304030
Email: info@bpas.org
Website: www.bpas.org
Owners: BPAS (British Pregnancy Advisory Service)
Total Beds: 51

Manager Lin Pavey

The Woking Nuffield Hospital

Shores Road, Woking GU21 4BY
Tel: 01483 227800 Fax: 01483 227830
Email: info.woking@nuffieldhospitals.org.uk
Website: www.nuffieldhospitals.org.uk
Owners: Nuffield Hospitals
Total Beds: 47

Manager Chester Barnes

The Wolverhampton Nuffield Hospital

Wood Road, Tettenhall, Wolverhampton WV6 8LE
Tel: 01902 754177 Fax: 01902 793292
Website: www.nuffieldhospitals.org.uk
Owners: Nuffield Hospitals
Total Beds: 41

Manager Sue Gowers

Anaesthetics F Babatola, K Balachandar, G Bryan, R Carley, G Corser, S Fenner, R Giri, V Gnanadurai, K Hickmott, L Mudie, K Nandi, N Parekh, A Patel, D Perks, C Peters, A Philips, G Philips, J S Pooni, D Richmond, E Robson, G Simon
Cardiology M Bhabra, J Cotton, M Cusack, R C Horton, S Khogali, D K Mistry, M Norell, J W Pidgeon
Dermatology S Oliwiecki, D R Taylor
ENT R J Cullen, L P Glossop, J Mathews, N C Moloney, V Raut, R J Shortridge, M Wake, F Wilson
General Medicine H Buch, P Carmichael, S J Connellan, D F D'Costa, M A Jackson, S A Kapadia, J S Mann, B McKaig, J Odum, P B Rylance, B M Singh, E T Swarbrick, A M Veitch
General Psychiatry M Kurian
General Surgery L D Coen, F T Curran, T I M Gardecki, A W Garnham, B Isgar, J B Marczak, P Matey, S Sigurdsson, G Williams
Genitourinary Medicine J R Fernando
Gynaecology J H Adeghe, A J Browning, R Callender, C Cox, S Jenkinson, D Little, D J Murphy, J Pepper, R Reddy, J Samra, R Smith
Histopathology M Cooper, M Freeth, R Gama, A Patel, D Rowlands
Neurology H T S Ben Amer, R Hughes
Ophthalmology P Caruana, P Corridan, M Headon, B Manoj, N J Price, U Ramanthan, S Sandramouli, G A Shun-Shin, Y Yang
Oral and Maxillofacial Surgery N Grew, E B Larkin, B G Millar, N M Whear
Orthodontics M Hammond
Orthopaedics M Ahmed, G O Alo, M S Butt, S Chugh, E S Isbister, M Khan, N Kumar, A Marino, T Sadique, A W Simons, A P Thomas, O Thomas, R J Thomas
Paediatrics J M Anderson
Pathology S Basu, A Jacob, A M Patel
Plastic Surgery M D Humzah, N S Moiemen, J M Porter
Radiology J Blakeman, M Collins, C Deacon, R Fitzgerald, M Hale, M Mantle, M Qaiyum, P Strouhal
Radiotherapy and Oncology R Allerton, M J Churn, D Ferry
Rheumatology A W Al-Allaf, H A Ali, P Newton
Urology P Cooke, J A Inglis, N H Philp, T Wanas, B M Waymont

Women's Secure Services

Annesley House, Mansfield Road, Annesley NG15 0AR
Tel: 01623 727900 Fax: 01623 727942
Email: info@partnershipsincare.co.uk
Website: www.partnershipsincare.co.uk
Owners: Partnerships in Care Ltd
Total Beds: 58

Manager Dara Ni Ghadhra

Psychiatry Dr Connell-Jones, Dr Power-Smith, Dr Sreehari

Woodbourne Priory Hospital

21 Woodbourne Road, Edgbaston, Birmingham B17 8BY
Tel: 0121 434 4343 Fax: 0121 434 3270
Email: woodbourne@prioryhealthcare.com
Website: www.prioryhealthcare.com
Owners: Priory Group
Total Beds: 43

Manager Linda Archer

Addictions A Kahn, A Kahn
Adolescent Unit M Joseph, M Joseph
Eating Disorders A Villa
Psychiatry G Bates, K Bluglass, J J D Briscoe, L Brownell, S England, M Joseph, A Kahn, A Mahmood, V Murali, A Nasr, A Patel, A J Sheikh, M Shepherd, G Tadros, A Villa, A Villa, G Wainscott, A White

Woodlands Hospital

Morton Park, Darlington DL1 4PL
Tel: 01325 341700 Fax: 01325 341701
Email: enquiries@woodlandshealthcare.org
Website: www.woodlandshealthcare.org
Owners: Privately Owned
Total Beds: 38

Anaesthetics Dr Danjoux, Z A Daoud, R S Drummond, D Hamilton, Dr Khalia, H Khalil, C F Kotur, C Kumar, K C Macintosh, P A Mallinder, K Praveen, M A Quader, J J Rao, I Riddle, D K Saha, D K Sarma, C P Snowden, N S Suresh, W D Thompson, Dr Walton
Dermatology W D Taylor
ENT J Carlin, N Hawthorne, Mr Ruckby, C Watson
General Medicine E W Barnes, C K Connolly, S A Mitchell, Dr Murphy, D P S Spence
General Surgery R M Bryan, Mr Clayson, N Corner, P J Cullen, S A Debrah, M Edwards, K A Gunning, Mr Hawthorn, Mr Parry, Mr Viswanath
Neurosurgery E Sinar
Obstetrics and Gynaecology P Ballard, J Oghoetuoma
Oncology P J Hardman
Ophthalmology M S Dang, R J Stirling
Oral and Maxillofacial Surgery D Bryant, C Edge, Mr Martin
Orthopaedics Mr Assan, M Bawarish, Mr Escander, M Krishna, P Parker, A Port, J H Rutherford, Mr Shankaur, M Stewart, L Van Niekerk, L Van Vuuren, Mr Wallace
Plastic Surgery Mr Siddiqui, C Viva
Psychiatry Mr Burdett, Mr Carnworth, Professor Martin
Radiology J Anderson, N Bradey, P Cadigan, R S D Campbell, J Cox, I Curzon, E Dillon, T Featherstone, S Fitzgerald, N Grunshaw, R G Henderson, G P Naisby, J Spratt
Urology S Fulford, J Hindmarsh, C Roberts, B S Vadanan

Scotland

Abbey Carrick Glen Hospital

Dallmellington Road, Ayr KA6 6PG
Tel: 01292 288882 Fax: 01292 283315
Email: carrickglen@abbeyhospitals.com
Website: www.abbeyhospitals.co.uk
Owners: Covenant Healthcare
Total Beds: 22

Manager Alison Smith

Abbey King's Park Hospital

Polmaise Road, Stirling FK7 9PU
Tel: 01786 451669 Fax: 01786 465296
Email: kingspark@abbeyhospitals.com
Website: www.abbeyhospitals.co.uk
Owners: Abbey Hospitals Ltd
Total Beds: 19

Manager Beth Martin

BMI Albyn Hospital

21-24 Albyn Place, Aberdeen AB10 1RW
Tel: 01224 595993 Fax: 01224 589869
Email: info@albynhospital.co.uk
Website: www.bmihealthcare.co.uk/albyn
Owners: BMI Healthcare
Total Beds: 44

Manager Kenneth Hay

BMI Fernbrae Hospital

329 Perth Road, Dundee DD2 1LJ
Tel: 01382 667203 Fax: 01382 660155
Email: info-fernbrae@bmihealthcare.co.uk
Owners: BMI Healthcare
Total Beds: 20

Manager Peter Grant

BMI Ross Hall Hospital

221 Crookston Road, Glasgow G52 3NQ
Tel: 0141 810 3151 Fax: 0141 882 7439
Email: enquiry@rosshall.com
Website: www.rosshall.com
Owners: BMI Healthcare
Total Beds: 101

Manager David Tennent

BUPA Murrayfield Hospital - Edinburgh

122 Corstorphine Road, Edinburgh EH12 6UD
Tel: 0131 334 0363 Fax: 0131 334 7338
Email: cservice-ed@bupa.com
Website: www.bupahospitals.co.uk/edinburgh
Owners: BUPA Hospitals Ltd
Total Beds: 69

Manager Gair Stott

Accident and Emergency A Gray, D Steedman
Anaesthetics R Alston, P Andrews, P Armstrong, A S Buchan, D Burke, J Donnelly, M J Fried, D Henderson, J Jenkins, N Malcolm-Smith, J H McClure, A McCrae, D Mckeown, L Morrison, D Ray, L Rutledge, D H T Scott, C Sinclair, A Trench, T Walsh, D Watson
Cardiology N Boon, P A Broadhurst, A Flapan, A Jacob, T Shaw, I Starkey, N Uren
Cardiothoracic Surgery E Brackenbury, V Zamvar
Dermatology P Buxton, D Kemmett, O Schofield, M Tidman
ENT H Beg, D Cowan, A Kerr, R Mills, S Moralee, M Riad, R Sanderson, S Sheikh, D Sim, G Vernham
General Medicine W Alexander, D Farquhar, M Ford, B Frier, E Housley, A Jamieson, C Leen, A MacGilchrist, J McKnight, K Palmer, I Penman, C Stewart, K Trimble, J Walker, M Watson, A Williams
General Surgery M Akyol, D Bartolo, R Chalmers, U Chetty, A De Beaux, A M Jenkins, D Lee, I Macintyre, K Madhavan, J Mander, J Murie, G Neades, S Paterson-Brown, J Rainey, Z Raza, I Wallace
Genitourinary Medicine A Ghaly
Neurology R Aylward, R Davenport, C J Lueck, C Mumford, A Z J Zeman
Neurosurgery L Myles, T Russell, P Statham
Obstetrics and Gynaecology A D G Brown, D Farquharson, A Gebbie, W A Liston, H Macpherson, T Mahmood, A Milne, S Nicholson, J Thong
Oncology G C W Howard, I Kunkler, R H Macdougall, L Matheson, D McLaren
Ophthalmology A D Adams, H Bennett, B Dhillon, B Fleck, P Kearns, G Mcilwaine, A Mulvihill, J Singh, M Wright
Oral and Maxillofacial Surgery R D Brown, G Lello
Orthodontics J McDonald
Orthopaedics I H Annan, I Brown, R Burnett, J Campbell, C Court-Brown, J De Leeuw, J N A Gibson, H Gillies, W Hadden, C Howie, J F Keating, G Keenan, G M Lawson, R MacDonald, M Macnicol, J McBirnie, M McMaster, R Nutton, C Oliver, D Porter
Paediatric Surgery G A Mackinlay, J Orr
Pathology H Gilmour, K Grigor, P Rae, S Walker, A Williams, R Wiseman
Plastic Surgery M Butterworth, S Hamilton, J McGregor, A Quaba, K Stewart
Psychiatry J Mclennan, A Stewart
Radiology P Allan, J Brush, D Collie, M Errington, G Hendry, K McBride, S Moussa, D Patel, R Sellar, A J M Stevenson, J Walker, P White, A Wightman
Rheumatology N P Hurst, C M Lambert, R Luqmani, E McRorie
Urology P Bollina, T B Hargreave, J R Macfarlane, A McNeill, G Smith, L Stewart, D Tolley, D Tulloch

Central Scotland Brain Injury Rehabilitation Centre

Murdostoun Castle, Bonkle, Newmains, Wishaw ML2 7BY
Tel: 01698 384055 Fax: 01698 386099
Email: central.scotland@fshc.co.uk
Website: www.huntercombehospitals.com
Owners: The Huntercombe Hospitals
Total Beds: 20

Manager Ann Hunter

Erskine Hospital

Bishopton PA7 5PU
Tel: 0141 812 1100 Fax: 0141 812 3733
Email: enquiries@erskine.org.uk
Owners: Charity/Association
Total Beds: 254

The Glasgow Nuffield Hospital

25 Beaconsfield Road, Glasgow G12 0PJ
Tel: 0141 334 9441 Fax: 0141 339 1352
Website: www.nuffieldhospitals.org.uk
Owners: Nuffield Hospitals
Total Beds: 33

Manager David Whiteoak

Audiology P Darroch, B MacGillivray
Cardiology A Brady, F Dunn, H Eteiba, N E Goodfield, J McArthur, A Pell, A P Rae
Care of the Elderly W J Gilchrist
Dermatology D Burden, G Gupta, R Herd, R Kerr, J Thomson, N J Wainwright
ENT B Bingham, L Cooke, J Crowther, N K Geddes, J L Handa, A Kishore, F MacGregor, K Mackenzie, J Marshall, G W McGarry, S Morrissey, B O'Reilly, S Sheikh, D Simpson
Fertility Services D Conway, M Haxton, R Low, R Yates

General Medicine J G Allan, H Carmichael, S Dover, J H Forrest, R Fox, S Gallacher, F Johnston, J Mackenzie, E H McLaren, P Mills, A J Morris, R Seaton, A Stanley
General Surgery A Buter, D S Byrne, C R Carter, D Chong, D Deardon, J Ferguson, I Finlay, P Finn, G Fullarton, D Galloway, G Gillespie, J Goldring, D T Hansell, P Horgan, H Kasem, D Knight, A Lannigan, A MacDonald, I MacKenzie, A McKay, M McKirdy, R Molloy, A Nasser, J G Pollock, C Porteous, A Renwick, P N Rogers, R N Scott, I Smith, J S Smith, R P Teenan, M Tehrani, B W Williamson
Genitourinary Medicine R Nandwani
Haematology I Evans
Neurology W Durward, J Greene, R Metcalfe, C O'Leary, A Tyagi
Neurophysiology A Mann, A Weir
Neurosurgery W Taylor
Obstetrics and Gynaecology S Bjornsson, D Conway, J A Davis, M Deeny, T G B Dow, C Forrest, H Gordon, K Hanretty, R Hawthorn, R Low, H McEwan, M K Oak, P Owen, M Perera
Oncology J Graham, N Reed, D Ritchie, A G Robertson, G Wilson, H Yosef
Ophthalmology T Barrie, C Diaper, A Fern, M P Gavin, S Gupta, E Kemp, P Kyle, T E Lavy, D Montgomery, J Murdoch, S Murray, K A Ramaesh, M Virdi, L A Webb, W Wykes
Oral and Maxillofacial Surgery H A Critchlow, J Devine, D H Felix, J Gibson, N Hammersley, W S Hislop, D Koppel, G Wood
Orthopaedics G Bennet, S L Chitnis, S Ehrendorfer, U Fazzi, A Gray, M Hadidi, J Hay, M G Hullin, R Ingram, P J John, C S Kumar, W Leach, C Macleod, R D Meek, J S Moir, T Reece, D Sherlock, B Singh, E F Wheelwright
Paediatrics C Davis, P Galea, C Hajivassiliou, P McGrogan, S O'Toole, P Raine
Plastic Surgery D Dunaway, I Mackay, A Ray, J Scott, D Soutar, J Telfer, E Weiler-Mithoff
Podiatry J Black, R Sloss
Psychiatry S Groves, R Hunter, R Lindsay
Psychology E Campbell, J Doyle, V Gray Taylor, E Irvine, G Macpherson, D Markus, S McLaren, C Puckering, M Ross, G Tanner
Respiratory Medicine G Boyd, L G McAlpine, K Patel
Rheumatology M Gordon, J Hunter, D Marshall, P McGill
Sports Medicine M Watt
Urology M Aitchison, J Crooks, R F Deane, M Fraser, A James, G Jones, M Palmer, P Paterson, P Raju, J Sinclair, M Underwood, L Walker

The Huntercombe Edinburgh Hospital
Binny Estate, Ecclesmachan Road, Uphall, Broxburn EH52 6NL
Tel: 01506 856023 Fax: 01506 865270
Email: huntercombe.edinburgh@fhsc.co.uk
Website: www.huntercombehospitals.com
Total Beds: 22

Manager Diane Whiteoak

General Psychiatry J Duncan

Marie Curie Centre, Fairmile
Frogston Road West, Edinburgh EH10 7DR
Tel: 0131 470 2201 Fax: 0131 470 2200
Email: sandra.mcdonald@mariecurie.org.uk
Website: www.mariecurie.org.uk
Owners: Marie Curie Cancer Care
Total Beds: 32

Manager Sandra McDonald

Marie Curie Hospice, Glasgow
1 Belmont Road, Springburn, Glasgow G21 3AY
Tel: 0141 531 1300 Fax: 0141 531 1301
Email: info@mariecurie.org.uk
Website: www.mariecurie.org.uk
Owners: Marie Curie Cancer Care
Total Beds: 36

Manager Anna Grady, Anna Grady

Palliative Medicine J Adam, S McKay

The Priory Hospital Glasgow
38-40 Mansionhouse Road, Langside, Glasgow G41 3DW
Tel: 0141 636 6116 Fax: 0141 636 5151
Email: glasgow@prioryhealthcare.com
Website: www.prioryhealthcare.com
Owners: Priory Group
Total Beds: 42

Manager Neil Cruickshank

St Joseph's Service
72 Carnethie Street, Rosewell, Edinburgh EH24 9AR
Tel: 0131 440 7200 Fax: 0131 440 4556
Owners: Privately Owned
Total Beds: 120

Wales

BMI Werndale Hospital
Bancyfelin, Carmarthen SA33 5NE
Tel: 01267 211500 Fax: 01267 211511
Email: werndale@bmihealthcare.co.uk
Website: www.bmihealthcare.co.uk
Owners: BMI Healthcare
Total Beds: 28

Manager Chris Patching

Accident and Emergency G Evans, P Evans, J Williams
Anaesthetics J Bryant, R Cooke, J Dingley, M Esmail, A Laxton, C Loyden, H Maddock, S Mahon, G McFadyen, W McFadzean, A Mehta, L Middleton, A Nigam, B O'Donohoe, R Prasad, P Rimmel, D Thomas, M Turtle, B Yate
Biochemistry N Haboubi
Breast Surgery S Holt
Cardiology P Avery, A Raybould
Dermatology I Ralfs
Endocrinology T Williams
ENT B Davis, N Morgan, G Wiliiams
Gastroenterology I Salam
General Medicine C James
General Surgery A Locker, P Milewski, M Nutt, B O'Riordan, W Sheridan
Gynaecology T Bloomfield, W Clow, R Howells, G McSweeney
Haematology P Cumber
Ophthalmology D Jones, J Roberts-Harry
Oral and Maxillofacial Surgery D Patton, K Silvester
Orthopaedic Surgery J Black, S Chatterji, P Cnudde, P Kanse, R Morgan-Jones, G Phillips
Pathology R Denholm, J Murphy
Plastic Surgery M Cooper, M Murison
Psychiatry R Gill
Radiology J Al-Koteesh, K Bradshaw, D Khechane, I Martin, A Moalla, C Ngoma
Urology B Gana, M Taube

Brain Injury Services Beechwood House
Beechwood House, Penperlleni, Pontypool NP4 08H
Tel: 01873 881200 Fax: 01873 881201
Owners: Partnerships in Care Ltd
Total Beds: 18

Manager Trevor Irwin

BUPA Hospital Cardiff

Croescadarn Road, Pentwyn, Cardiff CF2 8XL
Tel: 029 2073 5515 Fax: 029 2073 5821
Email: cservice-cd@bupa.com
Website: www.bupahospitals.co.uk/cardiff
Owners: BUPA Hospitals Ltd
Total Beds: 64

Manager Rob Anderson

Anaesthetics I Bowler, M Cobley, D Cremin, R Davies, M Drage, D J Dye, D Evans, J Foy, N Groves, H Maddock, A Mehta, K Murrin, N Stallard, T Tipping, A Wagle, T G Watkins, P Woodsford
Cardiology M B Buchalter, P Groves, F L Lisawhee, N Masani, P O'Callaghan, W J Penny
Dermatology M Chowdhury, P Holt, A Knight, R Motley
ENT P Johnson, R Rivron, G Shone, V Singh, A Tomkinson, G Williams, H Williams
General Medicine R Alcolado, K Baboolal, I Campbell, B Davies, L George, B Hawthorne, R Moore, M Page, P Smith, G Thomas, J Thomas
General Surgery R Chavez, G W Clark, W T Davies, C Gateley, P Haray, J Harvey, T Havard, A Hedges, A Y izziden, S Karandikar, I Lane, M Lewis, R Mansel, I Monypenny, A G Radcliffe, B I Rees, D Scott-Coombes, H Sweetland, J Torkington, D Webster, M H Wheeler, R Williams, A Woodward
Haematology P Bentley, C H Poynton
Neurology J Heath, S Jayawant, G Llewelyn, I McQueen, P Smith
Neurosurgery R H Hatfield, B Simpson, J Vafidis
Obstetrics and Gynaecology J Arnold, B Beattie, N Davies, A Evans, J Evans, P Lindsay, N Myerson, R Penketh, D H Pugh, C J Richards, A Roberts, M Stone, S Vine
Oncology P Barrett-Lee, T Maughan
Ophthalmology E Ansari, A Feyi-Waboso, C Gorman, J Hunter, A H Khatib, C Lane, K Lowe, R McPherson, J Morgan, K Rajkumar, R Ram, R F Walters, P Watts
Oral and Maxillofacial Surgery M Fardy, M Hill
Orthopaedic Surgery J Davies, P Davies, C Dent, R O N Evans, J A Fairclough, G Graham, K Hariharan, S Hemmadi, J Howes, A John, M Maheson, R Morgan-Jones, D O'Doherty, T D Owen, D Pemberton, K Singhal, P Thomas, R Williams, C Wilson, G Zafiropoulos
Paediatric Medicine M Alfaham, I Hodges, H Jenkins
Paediatric Surgery S Huddart, K Hutton
Pathology P Williams
Radiology D Cochlin, M Crane, C Davies, S Davies, C Evans, D Foster, K Gower-Thomas, S Halpin, G Herdman, M Hourihan, D Lloyd, K Lyons, J Rees, A Roberts, A Wood
Rheumatology J Camillieri, J Jessop, S Jones
Urology S Datta, A Hart, B Jenkins, D Jones, H Kynaston, P Matthews, T P Stephenson

BUPA Yale Hospital

Wrexham Technology Park, Croesnewydd Road, Wrexham LL13 7YP
Tel: 01978 291306 Fax: 01978 291397
Email: cservice-yl@bupa.com
Website: www.bupahospitals.co.uk/yale
Owners: BUPA Hospitals Ltd
Total Beds: 27

Manager Rob Anderson

Anaesthetics V Scott-Knight, S Underhill
Cardiology R Cowell
Care of the Elderly I U Shah
Dermatology J Sowden
ENT A C Mohan, D Snow
General Medicine P Drew, C Sissons
General Surgery A Baker, P Billings, T Da Silva, P Marsh, J K Pye, M Scriven
Haematology J Duguid
Neurology M Moran, D Smith
Obstetrics and Gynaecology C Roseblade, W Taylor, R Vlies
Ophthalmology N Kaushik
Oral and Maxillofacial Surgery C Penfold
Orthopaedic Surgery S Eisenstein, G Evans, N Graham, A M Jamieson, P Laing, K Lewis, N Makwana, S Roberts, T Smith, J Wootton
Plastic Surgery S Dhital, F S Fahmy
Radiology C Laine, G Murray, D A Parker
Urology P Anandaram, B Petterson

Llanarth Court Hospital

Llanarth, Raglan NP15 2YD
Tel: 01873 840555 Fax: 01873 840591
Email: info@partnershipsincare.co.uk
Website: www.partnershipsincare.co.uk
Owners: Partnerships in Care Ltd
Total Beds: 81

Manager Barrie Crosbie

General Medicine P Feeney, C Foy, A Lillywhite, M Nelson-Owen, A Pantlin, J Sandford
Psychology D Fisher (Head), D Fisher

Marie Curie Hospice, Holme Tower

Bridgeman Road, Penarth CF64 3YR
Tel: 029 2042 6000 Fax: 029 2042 6036
Email: info@mariecurie.org.uk
Website: www.mariecurie.org.uk
Owners: Marie Curie Cancer Care
Total Beds: 30

Manager Viv Cooper

North Wales Medical Centre

Queen's Road, Craig-y-Don, Llandudno LL30 1UD
Tel: 01492 879031 Fax: 01492 876754
Owners: Bettercare Group
Total Beds: 32

Manager Lyn Williams

St Joseph's Private Hospital

Harding Avenue, Malpas, Newport NP9 6ZE
Tel: 01633 820300 Fax: 01633 858164
Email: saintjoseph@btclick.com
Owners: Privately Owned
Total Beds: 26

Manager Bernadette Marie Walsh

Cardiology N Brown, A Davies, S Hutchison, S Ikram
Clinical Microbiology E Kubiak
Dermatology A Anstey, C Matthews, C Mills, N Stone
ENT M Brown, M Clayton, D Ingrams, M Preece
Gastroenterology M Allison, P Neville, E Srivastava, T Yapp
General Medicine O Gibby, M Hack, M Llewelyn, J Thomas
General Surgery R Blackett, C Bransom, C Gateley, R Jones, W Lewis, A Shandall, K Shute, B Stephenson, K Vellacott
Gynaecology M Ashraf, A Dawson, G Edwards, R Gonsalves, W Jackson, I Stokes, M Stone, A Weerakkody, J Wiener
Neurology G Llewelyn
Ophthalmology E Ansari, C Blyth, A Feyi-Waboso, D Hughes, A Karseras, Y Khan, D O'Duffy
Orthopaedic Surgery P Alderman, H Davies, A Grant, S Hannaford-Youngs, K Hariharan, G Jones, R Kulkarni, W Mintowt-Czyz, A M Nada, Y Nathwarawala, P Roberts, R Savage, K Tayton, R Walker
Paediatrics I Bowler, P Buss
Pain Management T Ivanova-Stoilova, M Kocan, S Warton
Plastic Surgery W Dickson, H Laing, M Milling
Podiatry T Galloway
Psychiatry M M Jilani, P Ruth, U Sivagamasundari
Rheumatology A Borg, S Linton, P Williams
Therapeutic and Sports Massage C Spillane
Urology C Bates, W Bowsher, R Gower

Sancta Maria Hospital

Ffynone Road, Swansea SA1 6DF
Tel: 01792 479040 Fax: 01792 641452
Email: admin@hmt-sancta-maria.demon.co.uk
Website: www.hmt-uk.org
Owners: The Hospital Management Trust
Total Beds: 33

Manager Michael Davies

Northern Ireland

Marie Curie Centre, Belfast

Kensington Road, Belfast BT5 6NF
Tel: 028 9088 2000 Fax: 028 9088 2022
Email: info@mariecurie.org.uk
Website: www.mariecurie.org.uk
Owners: Marie Curie Cancer Care
Total Beds: 19

Manager Maeve Hully

North West Independent Hospital

Church Hill House, Ballykelly, Londonderry BT49 9HS
Tel: 028 7776 3090 Fax: 028 7776 8306
Website: www.nwindependent.co.uk
Owners: Privately Owned
Total Beds: 50

Manager Elizabeth Dallas

Anaesthetics K Anand, C Armstrong, I M Bali, N Beckeu, I Black, K P Bolleddula, N Chestnutt, A Chisakuta, M Coleman, F Connolly, P N Convery, R Cooper, E Devlin, G N Di Mascio, G Dobson, K T J Fitzpatrick, B Franklin, G Furness, P Glover, S M Gormley, D Grace, D J Grainger, S Irvine, A P Jain, G G Lavcry, P Lcyden, P Loan, J Lyons, D McAtamney, C P McCarroll, P McConaghy, K J McCourt, A W W McGowan, Dr McKaigue, D A McNamee, L McNichol, K Milligan, B Morrow, O Muldoon, B Mullan, G Nesbitt, J O'Hanlon, C V O'Hare, R A O'Hare, M O'Neill, K Pillow, D Qureshi, C Rafferty, A Rashid, T D E Sharpe, M Sheridan, J C Stanley, P C Stewart, J J M Symington, C Watters, J H Winn, D G Wright
Cardiology A McNeill, J A Purvis
Chemistry Dr O'Kane
Dermatology R Matthews
ENT J H A Black, J Cullen, T G Delap, Mr Harris, G McBride, C M Scally
Gastroenterology W Dickey, Dr O'Connor
General Surgery P Bateson, P Blair, M Brown, J S Dace, B Dane, S Dolan, B Harding, D W Harkin, M Hawe, Z Khan, K Khosraviani, A G McKinley, D G Mudd, F Mullan, K Panesar, R Thompson, A Varghese
Obstetrics and Gynaecology S Dobbs, G Dorman, S Fallows, Dr Marshall, R M McMillen, Dr Moohan, M Parker
Occupational Health W Jenkinson, P W McGucken
Ophthalmology P Hassett, S Kamalarajah, B Laccy, G McGinty, D Mulholland, J Sharkey
Oral Surgery M F Ryan
Orthopaedic Surgery J D Acton, P Charlwood, E A Cooke, D Deehan, M Eames, M P Foxworthy, J McCormack, S Simpson, D Swain, N Thompson, A Wilson
Paediatric Medicine F McCord, M Quinn
Paediatric Surgery S Brown, W A McCallion
Plastic Surgery K Khan
Psychiatry M Curran, Dr Leddy, D MacFarlane
Radiology A Adas, D Campbell, B Devlin, P Higgins, R Jackson, C M Morrison, M Reilly, A N Sharkey
Rheumatology P Gardiner, D Keegan, J McCarthy, D Raman
Urology R Kernohan, C Mulholland, F J Schattka

St John's House and Southern Area Hospice Services

Courtney Hill, Newry BT34 2EB
Tel: 028 3026 7711 Fax: 028 3026 8492
Owners: Privately Owned
Total Beds: 25

Ulster Independent Clinic

Stranmillis Road, Belfast BT9 5JH
Tel: 028 9066 1212 Fax: 028 9038 1704
Email: secretary@uic.org.uk
Website: www.ulsterindependentclinic.com
Owners: Ulster Independent Clinic
Total Beds: 48

Manager Diane Graham, Daine Graham

Educational Institutions

Universities and Medical Schools

England

University of Birmingham

Faculty of Medicine and Dentistry, Edgbaston, Birmingham B15 2TT
Tel: 0121 414 3858 Fax: 0121 414 4036
Website: www.bham.ac.uk

Vice-Chancellor and Principal M J H Sterling
Dean of Medicine William F Doe
Registrar and Secretary J Nichols
Director and Head of School of Dentistry P J Lumley
Head of the School of Health Sciences Pat Wrightson

Degrees and diplomas
MBChB, BDS, BMedSc, BNurs, BSc Physiotherapy, PhD, MD, DDS, MPhil, MSc, MPH

Recognised Clinical Institutions
Birmingham Children's Hospital NHS Trust, Birmingham Heartlands Hospital, Birmingham Women's Health Care NHS Trust, Burton Hospitals NHS Trust, Dudley Group of Hospitals NHS Trust, Good Hope Hospital, Heart of England NHS Foundation Trust, Hereford Hospitals NHS Trust, Northampton General Hospital NHS Trust, Royal Orthopaedic Hospital NHS Trust, Sandwell and West Birmingham Hospitals NHS Trust, Sandwell Mental Health NHS and Social Care Trust, University Hospital Birmingham NHS Foundation Trust, Walsall Hospitals NHS Trust, Worcestershire Acute Hospitals NHS Trust, Worcestershire Mental Health Partnership NHS Trust

Brighton and Sussex Medical School

BSMS Building, University of Sussex, Falmer, Brighton BN1 9PX
Tel: 01273 877575 Fax: 01273 877576
Website: www.bsms.ac.uk

Chair of Anatomy Diana Watt
Chair of Medicine Kevin Davies
Chair of Primary Care Helen Smith
Dean Jon Cohen
Associate Dean John Kay, Richard Vincent
Secretary Peter Dennis

University of Bristol

Faculty of Medicine and Dentistry, 69 St Michael's Hill, Bristol BS2 8DZ
Tel: 0117 331 1691 Fax: 0117 331 1687
Email: carolyn.donoghue@bristol.ac.uk
Website: www.bris.ac.uk

Vice-Chancellor Eric Thomas
Dean of Medicine and Dentistry Gareth Williams

Faculty of Medicine and Dentistry

Dean Gareth Williams
Faculty Administrator Sylvia Elliott
Faculty Operations Manager Carolyn Donoghue
Professor of Physics and Engineering in Medicine P N T Wells

Anatomy
Demonstrator M R E Harris, I G Sergides, C A Wong
Lecturer Z I Bashir, J F Burn, C J Fuller, M J Perry, A Sengupta, D J Tortonese
Lecturer in Equine Studies G R Colborne
Lecturer in Neuroscience E Molnar
Professor D S McNally
Professor of Anatomy and Cognitive Neuroscience M W Brown
Professor of Molecular Neuroscience J M Henley
Professor of Neuroscience J M Muller
Professor of Neuroscience in Anatomy G L Collingridge
Reader J B Wakerley
Research Associate in Anatomy A J Doherty
Research Fellow W W Anderson, J W Crabtree, A Terashima
Senior Lecturer M A Adams, P Dolan, J R T Greene, G K Wakley
Senior Lecturer in Anatomy G Clarke
Senior Lecturer in Anatomy (Oral Biology) J R Musgrave
Senior Research Fellow Z A Bortolotto
Teaching Fellow A M Roberts, J Townsend
Temporary Lecturer E C Warburton
Travelling Research Fellow S E Lauri

Biochemistry
Beit Memorial Research Fellow P J Lockyer
Lecturer M B Avison, P J Booth, S G Burston, C E Dempsey, J Frayne, K L Gaston, E J Griffiths, A T Hadfield, L M Henderson, M R Jones, D Meredith, S K Moule, N J Savery
Professor A R Clarke, R M Denton, A P Halestrap, S E Halford, J J Holbrook, M J A Tanner, J M Tavare
Professor of Molecular Genetics L Hall
Project Manager A Cameron
Reader G S Banting, R L Brady, P J Cullen, J D McGivan, A J Rivett, G A Rutter
Research Fellow G B Bloomberg, N A Gormley, P S Jayaraman, M A Jepson, W J Mawby, A H Mellor, R B Sessions, M D Szczelkun, A Varadi
Senior Lecturer P M Wood
Wellcome Trust International Prize Travelling Fellow M J Parker

Cardiac, Anaesthetic and Radiological Sciences
BHF Professor of Clinical Surgery and Director, Bristol Heart Institute G D Angelini
BHF Professor of Vascular Cell Biology A C Newby
Consultant Senior Lecturer R P Casula, A T Lovell, M A Oberhoff, M J Underwood
Consultant Senior Lecturer in Anaesthesia A M S Black, S J Howell
Lecturer, Vascular Cell Biology S J George
Lecturer in Cardiac Surgery C L Jackson
Professor of Cardiology K R Karsch
Professor of Clinical Radiology M R Rees
Reader in Cardiac Cellular Physiology M S Suleiman
Reader in Cardiology A Baumbach
Research Fellow in Cardiac Surgery R C Bush, G Sala-Newby
Senior Research Fellow J Y Jeremy

Care of the Elderly
Professor G K Wilcock
Research Associate in Medicine S H MacGowan

Centre for Ethics in Medicine

Lecturer S J L Edwards
Professor A V Campbell

Child Dental Health

Senior Research Fellow A J Sprod

Child Health

Head of Biological Collections R W Jones
Consultant Senior Lecturer J P Hamilton-Shield, A J W Henderson, M Saleem, O H Stanley
Lecturer in Neonatal Medicine D Harding
Medical Statistician in Child Health P S P Blair
Professor A G L Whitelaw
Professor of Infant Health and Developmental Physiology P J Fleming
Professor of Paediatric and Prenatal Epidemiology M J Golding
Research Assistant K North
Research Associate I S Cowan
Research Fellow J C Ingram
Senior Audiologist A J Hall
Senior Lecturer M Thoresen
Senior Lecturer in Medical Statistics L P Hunt
Senior Ophthalmologist C E M Williams
Senior Research Nutritionist P M Emmett

Dental Postgraduate Unit

Regional Adviser in General Dental Practice M E Green
Vocational Training Adviser M D Bruce, I Holloway

In-Vitro Centre for Reproductive Medicine

Clinical Co-ordinator in Reproductive Medicine C Kallasam

Laryngology, Rhinology and Otology

Clinical Lecturer C Dunning, M Hilton, K V Ravi, M Sauders, A Toma
Senior Clinical Lecturer D Baldwin, P G Bicknell, M V Griffiths, R K Mal, A R Maw, P J Robinson

Medical Postgraduate Division

Adviser D Kenny
GP Education Adviser P F Godfrey
Regional Adviser in General Practice R C W Hughes, A P Lewis

Medicine

Consultant Senior Lecturer R E Barry, A L Malizia, R M Smith
Consultant Senior Lecturer in Care of the Elderly and General Internal Manager L Dow
Consultant Senior Lecturer in Diabetic Medicine P J Bingley
Consultant Senior Lecturer in Medicine C S J Probert
Consultant Senior Lecturer in Neurology M E Hill
Consultant Senior Lecturer in Respiratory Medicine A B Millar
Lecturer K M Gillespie, S D Hearing
Lecturer in Medicine C H Bolton
Professor N J Scolding
Professor of Diabetic Medicine E A M Gale
Professor of Renal Medicine P W Mathieson
Research Fellow L Armstrong, A J Swan
Research Fellow in Medicine E C Smith
Senior Research Fellow in Medicine A P Corfield

Neuroendocrinology

Consultant Senior Lecturer C M Dayan, D Wynick
Professor S L Lightman, D Murphy
Reader in Medicine D Dawbarn, N C H Kerr, A Levy, C A McArdle, G G F Mason, J B Uney
Research Associate F M De Bree
Senior Lecturer in Medicine M S Harbuz, M R Norman
Senior Research Fellow D S Jessop
Sigmund Gestetner Research Fellow in Medicine S J Allen

Norah Fry Research Centre

Joseph Rowntree Research Fellow R J Townsley
Professor M Ward
Reader C E Robinson
Reader in Mental Health J A O Russell
Research Fellow J Rodgers
Senior Research Fellow K R Simons

Obstetrics and Gynaecology

Consultant Senior Clinical Lecturer in Reproductive Medicine and Surgery J M Jenkins
Consultant Senior Lecturer D J Cahill, D J Murphy
Consultant Senior Lecturer in Obstetrics and Gynaecology S S Glew
Consultant Senior Lecturer in Reproductive Medicine U D Gordon
Lecturer A J Hunter, L A Joels
Lecturer in Reproductive Immunology Beverley J Randle
Professor of Maternal and Foetal Medicine P W Soothill
Senior Lecturer A T A Thein
Senior Lecturer in Obstetrics and Gynaecology C H Holmes

Oncology

McAlpine Macmillan Consultant Senior Clinical Lecturer in Palliative Medicine A N T Davies
Professor of Palliative Medicine G W C Hanks
Research Fellow P Grainger

Ophthalmology

Consultant Senior Lecturer A J Churchill
Lecturer S Banerjee
Professor A D Dick
Research Fellow M S Berry, S M Nicholls, C Shimeld, V A Smith
Senior Research Fellow W J Armitage

Oral and Dental Science

Clinical Lecturer in Restorative Dentistry L M McNally, D J O'Sullivan
Clinical Research Fellow in Prosthodontics and Periodontology N C A Claydon
Clinical Research Lecturer S R Sheen
Consultant Senior Lecturer in Child Dental Health P J M Crawford
Consultant Senior Lecturer in Periodontology J M Moran
Consultant Senior Lecturer in Restorative Dentistry J S Rees
Lecturer Y E Y Aboush, H A Pontefract, S J Thavaraj
Lecturer in Cancer Studies A Hague, I C Paterson
Lecturer in Child Dental Health J P Mansell
Lecturer in Conservative Dentistry Susan M Hooper, K J Marshall
Lecturer in Dental Education S R Greenwood
Lecturer in Oral Microbiology D Dymock
Lecturer in Oral Pathology C M Robinson
Lecturer in Paediatric Dentistry K Duncan
Lecturer in Prosthetic Dentistry D R Williams
Lecturer in Restorative Dentistry G B Gray, N X West, R Yates
Locum Lecturer in Restorative Dentistry G M Boswell
Professor in Orthodontics C D Stephens
Professor in Periodontology M Addy
Professor of Dental Care of the Elderly Alan Harrison
Professor of Experimental Pathology S S Prime
Professor of Oral Microbiology H F Jenkinson
Professor of Oral Surgery J G Cowpe
Professor of Orthodontics J R Sandy
Reader in Oral Pathology J W Eveson
Senior Lecturer S J Thomas
Senior Lecturer in Dental Materials Science and Biomaterials K D Jandt
Senior Lecturer in Restorative Dentistry D C Jagger

Orthopaedic Surgery
Consultant Senior Lecturer in Orthopaedic Surgery J R W Hardy
Consultant Senior Lecturer in Orthopaedic Surgery and Pathology C P Case
Lecturer M J W Hubble
Professor of Orthopaedic Surgery I D Learmonth

Pathology and Microbiology
Clinical Fellow J M Bradshaw
Consultant Senior Lecturer C M P Collins, N J Goulden, R S Heyderman, M Moorghen, H J Porter, E A Sheffield, G R Standen, C G Steward, P C Turner
Lecturer P J Brown, A Herman, L J Moore, D J Morgan
Professor P J Berry, C J Elson, T R Hirst, C Paraskeva, M Pignatelli, M Virji, D C Wraith
Reader P M Bennett, W D Billington, F Carswell, M J Day, T J Hill, A J Morgan, G R Pearson
Research Assistant C I Westacott
Research Associate C M Richards
Research Fellow R J Birtles, D J E Elder, B Kenny, N M McKechnie, K T A Malik, G Mazza, S L Parry, A W Rowbottom, A D Wilson, N A P Wood
Senior Lecturer K W Brown, A M Pullen, N A Wiliams
Wellcome Senior Research Fellow in Clinical Science F S Wong

Pharmacology
Consultant Senior Lecturer C J C Roberts
Lecturer A W Poole, E S J Robinson
Professor G Henderson, P J Roberts
Reader R Z Kozlowski, N V Marrion
Research Assistant S J Culliford
Research Fellow D Shepherd
Senior Lecturer E P Kelly, P V Taberner, M M Usocwicz

Physiology
Professor D M Armstrong, P M Headley, S J W Lisney, B Matthews
Reader J C Hancox, M C Holley, R S G Jones, S N Lawson, R W Meech, K W Ranatunga
Research Associate D Davies, L Djouhri, G M Mutungi
Research Career Development Fellow H J Kennedy
Research Fellow D O Bates, C M N Rivolta
Senior Lecturer J R Harris, R M A P Ridge, D M Woolley
Senior Research Fellow R Apps, N Cooper, J F R Paton

Primary Care
Consultant Senior Lecturer C J Salisbury
Professor D J Sharp
Research Fellow C R Baxter
Senior Lecturer T P Fahey
Special Lecturer in Medical Education K A Feest

Psychiatry
Consultant Senior Lecturer J Evans, A R Lingford-Hughes
Lecturer S Argyropoulos, A Sipos
Locum Consultant Senior Lecturer J P Potokar
Norah Cooke Hurle Professor of Mental Health G L Harrison
Reader in Cross-cultural Psychiatry D B Mumford

Psycho-Pharmacology Unit
Professor D J Nutt
Research Fellow S J Wilson
Team Leader A L Hudson

Rheumatology Unit
Consultant Senior Lecturer J H Tobias
Professor A P Hollander
Reader J R Kirwan
Senior Research Fellow M E J Billingham, J M Rodgers

Social Medicine
Consultant Senior Lecturer Y Ben-Shlomo, M Egger, D J Gunnell, A Ness
Lecturer J Coast, Elise Whitley
Professor S B J Ebrahim, S J Frankel, G Davey Smith
Reader J L Donovan, T J Peters
Senior Lecturer J A C Sterne

Surgery
Consultant Senior Lecturer J M Blazeby, M Jackson, P A Lear, F C T Smith, M G Thomas
Professor D Alderson, J R Farndon, J M P Holly
Reader M A Birchall
Senior Clinical Lecturer R M Atkins, Z E Winters

Transplantation Sciences
Director B A Bradley
Professor J M Hows
Research Fellow P A Denning-Kendall, C Donaldson

Degrees and diplomas
BSc, MB ChB, PhD, MD, ChM, MSc, BDS, MCD, DDS

Recognised Clinical Institutions
Avon and Wiltshire Mental Health Partnership NHS Trust, North Bristol NHS Trust, United Bristol Healthcare NHS Trust

University of Cambridge

School of Clinical Medicine, Addenbrooke's Hospital, Hills Road, Cambridge CB2 2SP
Tel: 01223 336700 Fax: 01223 336709
Email: school-enquiries@medschl.cam.ac.uk
Website: www.cam.ac.uk

Vice-Chancellor Alison Richard
Clinical Dean D F Wood
Registrary T J Mead
Regius Professor of Physic D K Peters
Secretary General of the Faculties D A Livesey
Secretary of the Clinical School S M Pinnock

Degrees and diplomas
BA, MB, BChir, MChir, MSc, MEng, MBA, MD, MPhil, PhD, ScD

Recognised Clinical Institutions
Bedford Hospital NHS Trust, Cambridge University Hospitals NHS Foundation Trust, Hinchingbrooke Health Care NHS Trust, James Paget Healthcare NHS Trust, Luton and Dunstable Hospital NHS Trust, Milton Keynes General Hospital NHS Trust, Papworth Hospital NHS Foundation Trust, Peterborough and Stamford Hospitals NHS Foundation Trust, Queen Elizabeth Hospital King's Lynn NHS Trust, The Ipswich Hospital NHS Trust, West Suffolk Hospitals NHS Trust, Whipps Cross University Hospital NHS Trust

University of Durham

Queen's Campus Stockton, University Boulevard, Stockton-on-Tees TS17 6BH
Tel: 0191 334 0048
Email: dean.medicine@durham.ac.uk
Website: www.dur.ac.uk/phase1.medicine

Dean of Medicine Pali Hungin
Professor John Hamilton

Degrees and diplomas
Phase 1 Medicine

University of East Anglia

School of Medicine, Health Policy and Practice, Norwich NR4 7TJ
Tel: 01603 593061 Fax: 01603 593752
Website: www.med.uea.ac.uk

Dean Sam Leinster
Cell Biology Ian Beales
Chronic Illness Alex MacGregor
Clinical Oncology Anne Barrett
Clinical Psychology David Fowler, Shirley Reynolds
Epidemiology and Public Health Ian Harvey
Gastroenterology Andrew Hart
Health Economics Richard Cookson, Richard Fordham, Miranda Mugford, Richard Smith
Health Protection Paul Hunter
Healthcare Interfaces Max Bachmann
Medical Education Sam Leinster
Medical Statistics Lee Shepstone
Primary Care Amanda Howe

Hull York Medical School

University of York, Heslington, York YO10 5DD
Tel: 0870 124 5500 Fax: 01482 464705 (Hull), 01904 321696 (York)
Email: marilyn.balcombe@hyms.ac.uk
Website: www.hyms.ac.uk

University of Hull, East Riding Campus, Willerby, Hull HU10 6NS
Tel: 01482 466497 Fax: 01482 466931
Email: hull@hyms.ac.uk
Website: www.hyms.ac.uk

Dean W J Gillespie
Director of Medical Education John Cookson

Degrees and diplomas
MB BS

Imperial College Faculty of Medicine

Faculty Building, Imperial College Road, London SW7 2AZ
Tel: 020 7589 5111
Website: www.imperial.ac.uk/med

Principal Stephen Smith

Degrees and diplomas
MB BS BSc; MSc; MPhil; PhD; MD; MS

Recognised Clinical Institutions
Ashford and St Peter's Hospitals NHS Trust, Brent Teaching Primary Care Trust, Central and North West London Mental Health NHS Trust, Central Middlesex Hospital, Charing Cross Hospital, Chelsea and Westminster Hospital, Ealing Hospital, Ealing Primary Care Trust, Hammersmith and Fulham Primary Care Trust, Hammersmith Hospital, Harrow Primary Care Trust, Hillingdon Hospital, Hillingdon Primary Care Trust, Hounslow Primary Care Trust, Kensington and Chelsea Primary Care Trust, North West London Hospitals NHS Trust, Royal Brompton Hospital, St Mary's Hospital, West London Mental Health NHS Trust, Westminster Primary Care Trust

University of Keele

North Staffordshire Hospital, Thornburrow Drive, Hartshill, Stoke-on-Trent ST4 7QB
Tel: 01782 554047 Fax: 01782 747319
Website: www.keele.ac.uk

Head of Postgraduate Medicine Peter Crome
Emeritus Professor John Cox, James Elder, John Templeton
Hon. Clinical Lecturer Tarig Abdu, Peter Franklin, Janice Gerrard, David Pearson
Hon. Professor Warren Lenney, John Sanderson
Hon. Reader Andrew Spencer
Hon. Senior Lecturer Anthony Fryer
Lecturer S Cartmell, Do Kyung Kim, Paul Hoban, Jan Kuiper, Martyn Lewis, Andrew Neville, Tianshu Wang, Ying Yang
Professor Richard Clayton, Peter Croft, Ilana Crome, Simon Davies, Jon Dobson, Alicia El Haj, William Farrell, C Hawkins, Elaine Hay, Nicola Maffulli, Ian McCall, Shaughn O'Brien, James Richardson, David Smith, Richard Strange
Reader James Middleton, Sally Roberts
Senior Clinical Lecturer Brian Ashton, Johnathon Bache, Claire Barkley, Kenneth Barrett, Roger Bloor, Roderick Brooks, Peter Dawes, Waqih El-Masri, Simon Ellis, Stephen Field, Christopher Findlay, M J Y Fisher, Johnathon Green, David Griffiths, Khaled Ismail, Michael Jorsh, Fiona Macmillan, James Nolan, Barnabus Panayiotou, Charles Redman, Paula Richards, John Scarpello, Bruce Scheepers, Andrew Smith, Helen Thorley, A A Tomlinson, John Travlos, Anthony Ward
Senior Lecturer Stanley Acuda, H Arshad, Stephen Bridgman, Vincent Cooper, Mark Deakin, Andrew Hassell, Carole Henshaw, Simon Hill, Vinay Jasani, I Liu, Colin Melville, Patrick Naish, Charles Pantin, Brenda Roe, Christine Roffe, M Samuels, Ian Smith, Peter Thomas
SeniorClinical Lecturer Richard Hodgson

King's College London

James Clerk Maxwell Building, 57 Waterloo Road, London SE1 8WA
Tel: 020 7836 5454
Email: ceu@kcl.ac.uk
Website: www.kcl.ac.uk

Principal Rick Trainor
Vice-Principal and Dean G Catto
College Secretary and Registrar H T Musselwhite

Guy's, King's and St Thomas' Dental Institute

Guy's Tower, Guy's Hospital, London Bridge, London SE1 9RT
Tel: 020 7836 5454

Dean N H F Wilson

Craniofacial Development, Orthodontics and Microbiology
Head P T Sharpe

Dental Practice and Policy
Head S Dunne

Oral Medicine, Pathology, Immunology, Radiology and Human Disease
Head S J Challacombe

Restorative Dentistry
Head R M Palmer

Guy's, King's and St Thomas' School of Medicine

Management Suite, 1st Floor, Hodgkin Building, Guy's Campus, London SE1 9RT
Tel: 020 7848 6971 Fax: 020 7848 6969
Email: schoolofmedicine@kcl.ac.uk
Website: www.kcl.ac.uk/medicine/

Dean Robert Lechler
Dean of Research Ellen Solomon
Vice-Dean Anne Greenough
Vice-Dean of Research Pat Doherty
Postgraduate Dean, Guy's and St Thomas' Charles Twort
Postgraduate Dean, King's Denmark Hill Jan Welch

Asthma, Allergy and Respiratory Science
Head Tak Lee

Cardiology
Head Ajay Shah

Clinical Chemistry
Head Ramasamyiyer Swaminathan

Clinical Neurosciences
Head Richard Hughes

Clinical Pharmacology
Head Jim Ritter

Diabetes, Endocrinology and Internal Medicine
Head Alan McGregor

General Practice and Primary Care
Head Roger Jones

Haematology
Head Ghulam Mufti

Healthcare of the Elderly
Acting Head Stephen Jackson

Histopathology
Head Sebastian Lucas

Imaging
Acting Head Steven Williams

Immunobiology
Head Adrian Hayday

Infectious Diseases
Head Michael Malim

Liver Studies and Transplantation
Head Giorgina Mieli Vergani

Medical and Molecular Genetics
Head Ellen Solomon

Medical Education
Head John Rees

Medical Engineering and Physics
Acting Head Anne Greenough

Nephrology and Transplantation
Head Steve Sacks

Oncology
Head Henrik Moller

Paediatrics
Head Anne Greenough

Palliative Care and Policy
Head Irene Higginson

Public Health Sciences and Occupational Health
Head Peter Burney

Rheumatology
Head David Scott

Skin Sciences
Head Jonathan Barker

Surgery and Anaesthesia
Head Kevin Burnand

Women's Health
Head Peter Braude

University of Leeds

Leeds LS2 9JT
Tel: 0113 243 1751 Fax: 0113 244 3923
Email: enquiry@leeds.ac.uk
Website: www.leeds.ac.uk

Vice-Chancellor Alan Wilson
Secretary Roger Gair

Leicester Warwick Medical Schools

University of Leicester, Maurice Shock Medical Sciences Building, PO Box 138, University Road, Leicester LE1 9HN
Website: www.lwms.ac.uk

Dean I Lauder

Degrees and diplomas
MB ChB 5 year course (Leicester); MB ChB 4 year course (Warwick)

Recognised Clinical Institutions
Burton Hospitals NHS Trust, George Eliot Hospital NHS Trust, Kettering General Hospital NHS Trust, Leicestershire Partnership NHS Trust, Northampton General Hospital NHS Trust, Peterborough and Stamford Hospitals NHS Foundation Trust, South Warwickshire General Hospitals NHS Trust, United Lincolnshire Hospitals NHS Trust, University Hospitals Coventry and Warwickshire NHS Trust, University Hospitals of Leicester NHS Trust, Worcestershire Acute Hospitals NHS Trust

University of Leicester

Medical School, Maurice Shock Medical Sciences Building, PO Box 138, University Road, Leicester LE1 9HN

Vice-Chancellor R G Burgess
Dean, Faculty of Medicine and Biological Sciences I Lauder
Registrar K J Julian

Medical School

Maurice Shock Medical Sciences Building, PO Box 138, University Road, Leicester LE1 9HN
Tel: 0116 252 2522 Fax: 0116 252 3013
Website: www.le.ac.uk/medicine

Dean I Lauder
Sub-Dean A M Cashmore
Sub-Dean Graduate Studies P A Meacock
Vice Dean D J Taylor
Assistant Registrar (Medical School) A E Peppitt
Assistant Registrar (Personnel) L A Green
Accountant C A Burton
Assistant Faculty Secretary A L Collett
Secretary N P Siesage

Cancer Studies and Molecular Medicine
Professor of Oncology and Head of Department W P Steward
Hon. Professor of Oncology A J Gescher
Hon. Reader M Manson, I White
Professor of Forensic Pathology G Rutty
Professor of Haemato-Oncology M J Dyer
Professor of Histopathology and Deputy Head R A Walker
Professor of Medicine (Gastroenterology) J Jankowski

Professor of Obstetrics and Gynaecology J C Konje, D J Taylor
Professor of Reproductive Sciences S C Bell
Professor of Urology J K Mellon
Reader B Morgan, J H Pringle, R P Symonds
Senior Lecturer L M Al-Alousi, K Brown, M S Cooke, T L Griffiths, M Habiba, G D D Jones, G Saldanha, A Shaw, A L Thomas, D G Tincello

Cardiovascular Sciences

Professor of Cardiology and Head of Department N J Samani
Hon. Professor of Surgery A R Naylor
Professor of Accident and Emergency Medicine T Coats
Professor of Cardiac Surgery M Galinanes
Professor of Clinical Pharmacology D B Barnett
Professor of Medical Genetics R C Trembath
Professor of Medical Physics D H Evans
Professor of Medicine B Williams
Professor of Medicine and Deputy Head H Thurston
Professor of Medicine and Therapeutics L L Ng
Professor of Medicine for the Elderly J F Potter
Professor of Ophthalmology I Gottlob
Professor of Physiological Measurement R B Panerai
Professor of Radiology G R Cherryman
Professor of Surgery N J M London
Professor of Therapeutics K L Woods
Professor of Thrombosis and Haemostasis A H Goodall
Professor of Transplant Surgery M L Nicholson
Reader N P Brindle, M A Horsfield, D G Lambert
Senior Lecturer M A Aldred, M D Fotherby, K E Herbert, G A Ng, R I Norman, T G Robinson, I B Squire, J P Thompson, W D Toff

Clinical Divisions - Chairman

Anaesthesia, Critical Care and Pain Management D J Rowbotham
Child Health M Silverman
Epidemiology and Public Health R Hsu
General Practice and Primary Health Care R K McKinley
Medical Physics and Radiology D H Evans
Medicine H Thurston
Obstetrics and Gynaecology J Konje
Oncology W P Steward
Pathology R A Walker
Psychiatry J E B Lindesay
Surgery, Orthopaedic Surgery and Ophthalmology N J M London

Health Sciences

Professor of Quality in Healthcare and Head of Department R H Baker
Professor of Child and Adolescent Psychiatry P Vostanis
Professor of Criminological Psychology C R Hollin
Professor of Epidemiology C Jagger
Professor of Genetic Epidemiology P Burton
Professor of Medical Statistics K Abrams, D R Jones
Professor of Neonatal Medicine D J Field
Professor of Ophthalmic Epidemiology J R Thompson
Professor of Psychiatry M A Reveley
Professor of Psychiatry and Deputy Head T S Brugha
Professor of Psychiatry for the Elderly J E B Lindesay
Reader A D Wilson
Senior Clinical Research Fellow A Farooqui
Senior Lecturer M S Dennis, M M Dixon-Woods, N Dogra, K Khunti, C W McGrowther, R K McKinley, E J Palmer, R L Palmer, T N Stokes, A Sutton, M Tobin, A R Turrell, M Wailoo, P J Watson
University Fellow D Cameron

Infection, Immunity and Inflammation

Professor of Microbial Pathogenesis and Head of Department P W Andrew
Hon. Professor of Renal Medicine J Feehally
Hon. Professor of Renal Pathology P Furness
Hon. Reader I D Pavord
Professor of Child Health M Silverman
Professor of Clinical Microbiology and Deputy Head M R Barer
Professor of Dermatology R D R Camp
Professor of Environmental Microbiology W D Grant
Professor of Immunology W Schwaeble, H W L Zeigler-Heitbrock
Professor of Infectious Diseases K G Nicholson
Professor of Paediatrics C L P O'Callaghan
Professor of Respiratory Medicine A J Wardlaw
Reader P Bradding, K P G Harris, R F L James
Senior Clinical Research Fellow C E Brightling, P Topham
Senior Lecturer C S Beardsmore, M J Browning, N J Brunskill, J M Grigg, C D Ockleford, K Rajakumar, P J H Sheldon

Medical and Social Care Education

Professor of Medical Education and Head of Department S A Petersen
Senior Lecturer and Head of Professional Development Unit A I A Lennox
Senior Lecturer (Associate) and Head of School of Social Work G E Hurd
Phase 1 Co-ordinator J M Hales
Phase 2 Co-ordinator and Deputy Head D Henley
Reader K Owusu-Bempah
Senior Lecturer E S Anderson, A M Hastings, M Lakhanpaul, R O Law, W Montague
Senior Lecturer and Director of Human Morphology A P Gulamhusein
Senior Lecturer (Associate) L Howard

School of Biological Sciences

University Road, Leicester LE1 7RH

Director of Biological Studies J J A Scott
Head of School G C K Roberts

Biochemistry

Senior Lecturer and Head of Department T M Harrison
Professor C R Bagshaw, F Beck, W J Brammar, D R Critchley, E Cundliffe, I C Eperon, G C K Roberts, N S Scrutton
Reader M D Carr, A W Munro, M J Sutcliffe, A E Willis
Senior Lecturer P C E Moody

Biology

Professor and Head of Department G C Whitelam
Professor J S Heslop-Harrison, R H Smith, D Twell
Reader P J B Hart
Senior Lecturer R J Gornall, D M Harper, P M J Shelton

Cell Physiology and Phamacology

Professor and Head of Department S R Nahorski
Professor R A J Challis, I D Forsythe, N B Standen
Reader R J Evans, R E Fern, D G Lambert
Senior Lecturer N J Brunskill, B D Grubb, G B Willars

Genetics

Head of Department A M Cashmore
Professor Alec Jeffreys, J M Ketley, C P Kyriacou, E J Louis, R C Trembath, P H Williams
Reader R H Borts, Y E Dubrova, M A Jobling, P A Meacock
Senior Lecturer R W M Dalgleish, M A Plumb, N J Royle

School of Psychology

University Road, Leicester LE1 7RH

Professor and Head of School G M Davies
Professor A M Colley, A M Colman, M H Joseph, M A Stammers
Senior Lecturer J R Beech, J C Berryman, J C W Boon, R Gillett, A C North

Degrees and diplomas
MB ChB 4 & 5 year course, BSc in Biological Sciences, Biochemistry, Environmental Biology, Genetics, Microbiology, Physiology with Pharmacology, Zoology, Immunology, Medical Biochemistry, Medical Genetics, Psychology, Psychology with Biology, Psychology with Neuroscience, Psycholo, MD, PhD/MPhil, D Clin Psych, MSc Applied Forensic Psychology, MSc/Postgraduate Diploma in Assessment and Treatment of Sex Offenders, Bioinformatics, Child Welfare Studies, Forensic and legal Psychology, Forensic Psychology, Health Services Research, Medical Statistics, Molecular Genetics, Molecular Pathology and Tox, BMedSci, BSc Intercalated, Certificate in Community Care Contracting, Supervision and Mentorship, MA in Social Work

Recognised Clinical Institutions
Burton Hospitals NHS Trust, Charnwood and North West Leicestershire Primary Care Trust, Daventry and South Northamptonshire Primary Care Trust, Eastern Leicester Primary Care Trust, Hinckley and Bosworth Primary Care Trust, Kettering General Hospital, Leicester City West Primary Care Trust, Leicestershire Partnership NHS Trust, Melton, Rutland and Harborough Primary Care Trust, Northampton General Hospital NHS Trust, Northampton Primary Care Trust, Northamptonshire Heartlands Primary Care Trust, Peterborough and Stamford Hospitals NHS Foundation Trust, South Leicestershire Primary Care Trust, United Lincolnshire Hospitals NHS Trust, University Hospitals of Leicester NHS Trust

University of Warwick

Medical School, Coventry CV4 7AL

Vice-Chancellor D VandeLinde
Registrar J Baldwin

Medical School

Coventry CV4 7AL
Tel: 024 7657 3088 Fax: 024 7657 3079

Dean Y Carter
Associate Dean (Education) E Peile
Associate Dean (Research) S Thornton
School Secretary M Glover

Division of Clinical Sciences
Lecturer P McTernan, J T Powell
Professor D R Griffin, S Kumar, H Lehnert, S Murch, D R J Singer, D Spanswick, A Szczepura, S Thornton, V Zammit
Senior Clinical Lecturer K Matyka, H Randeva, M Vatish, D Zehnder

Division of Health in the Community
Associate Fellow C Moss
Lecturer A Adams, N Raymond, J Sturt
Professor J Dale, S Lamb, S Stewart-Brown, M Thorogood, S Weich
Reader J Barlow, M Cooke, H Hearnshaw, P Sidebottom
Senior Clinical Lecturer R Gadsby, F Griffiths, T Holt, J Powell, B Sheeham, D Simkiss
Senior Lecturer L Gill, C Meyer

Medical Education
Clinical Senior Lecturer C F MacDougall
GP Clinical Lecturer A Bhattacharya, M Garala, E Hopgood, C Humpherson, C Moss, J Piercy, R Prince, S Shannon, J Sihota, I Ward
Lecturer C Davies, G Grimshaw, A Stansbie, T Thornton
NHS Community Coordinator A Jackson
Non-Clinical Affiliate R A Baines, C Blackburn, R Bland, H Bradby, A Dolan, A K Green, M Hodgkin, G Hundt, J Hutton, K Lee, W A Markham, C Meyer, R Newton, P Squires, R Stanfield
Professor K W N Fulford, E Peile
Reader P O'Hare, V Patel
Senior Clinical Lecturer M Barnett, C Charlton, S Matthews, T Pawlikowska
Senior Lecturer C Rodgers
Senior Teaching Fellow E M Fleming, L Maxwell, A Rhodes

Non-Clinical
Lecturer R A Baines, R Bland, H Bradby, C Davies, A Dolan, A K Green, G M Grimshaw, M Hodgkin, W A Markham, C Meyer, R Newton, P Squires
Professor G Hundt, R Stanfield
Senior Lecturer C Blackburn, J Hutton, K Lee, D Spanswick

Warwick Diabetes Care
Director of Education D McAughey
Assistant Director of Education J Grant, M Mello
Senior Teaching Fellow Melanie Gray, Sakera Shaikh

School of Postgraduate Medical Education

Coventry CV4 7AL
Tel: 024 7657 3088 Fax: 024 7657 3079

Associate Teaching Fellow, Child Health J Rao, M A Sheikh
Associate Teaching Fellow, Obstetrics and Gynaecology F Smith
Associate Teaching Fellow, Public Health A Dale
Hon. Lecturer, Obstetrics and Gynaecology A D Parsons
Hon. Lecturer, Psychological Medicine C J Mace
Hon. Lecturer, Public Health L Gill, M Graveney
Lecturer, Epidemiology N Raymond
Professor, Child Health N J Spencer
Visiting Lecturer, Child Health M Hussain
Visiting Senior Clinical Lecturer, Child Health N Coad, C Essex, E Fleming, D Simkiss, A Stanton, A Williams
Visiting Senior Clinical Lecturer, Medicine R Cayton, J Cohen, H Desai, C Fox, V Patel, D A Robertson, J Rodgers, A J Smithers
Visiting Senior Clinical Lecturer, Obstetrics and Gynaecology L J Sant Cassia, M Walzman
Visiting Senior Clinical Lecturer, Psychological Medicine S Binyon, A P Winston
Visiting Senior Clinical Lecturer, Public Health J M Knight, K Millard, K Sidhu
Visiting Senior Clinical Lecturer, Surgery R Cherry, S Krikler, N Williams

Degrees and diplomas
MA/MSc Applied Health Studies in Diabetes Care, Emergency Care, Palliative Care, Primary Health Care, and Policy, Organisation and Primary Health Care, Post Graduate Award in Medical Education, MB ChB 4 year course, Diploma in Occupational Health, Certificate in Diabetes Care

University of Liverpool

Liverpool L69 3BX
Tel: 0151 794 2000 Fax: 0151 706 5667
Website: www.liv.ac.uk

Vice-Chancellor J D Bone
Dean of Faculty of Medicine J Caldwell
Postgraduate Dean D R Graham
Admissions Sub-Dean G S Vine
Registrar M D Carr
Academic Sub-Dean R C Richards

Degrees and diplomas
MBChB, BN, MD, ChM, MSc, MPhil, PhD, BSc, MChOrth, MCommH, MPH, MPsychMEd, DClinPsychol., MTropPaeds, MTropMed., MRad, BDS, MDS, MPhil (in Dentistry), MDentSci & PhD, DTM & H, DTCH, DMRD, MSc/Pg Dip/Pg Cert

Recognised Clinical Institutions
Aintree Hospitals NHS Trust, Ashworth Hospital, Clatterbridge Hospital, Countess of Chester Hospital, Glan Clwyd District General Hospital, Greaves Hall, Halton General Hospital, Leighton Hospital,

Liverpool Women's Hospital, Macclesfield Hospital, Ormskirk and District General Hospital, Royal Liverpool and Broadgreen University Hospitals NHS Trust, Royal Liverpool Children's NHS Trust, Royal Liverpool University Dental Hospital, Sefton General Hospital, Southport District General Hospital, The Cardiothoracic Centre Liverpool NHS Trust, University Hospital Aintree, Walton Centre for Neurology and Neurosurgery NHS Trust, Walton Hospital, West Cheshire NHS Trust, Whiston Hospital, Winwick Hospital, Wrexham Maelor Hospital

London School of Hygiene and Tropical Medicine

Keppel Street, London WC1E 7HT
Tel: 020 7636 8636 Fax: 020 7436 5389
Website: www.lshtm.ac.uk

Dean Andrew Haines
Press Office Lindsay Wright
Research Degrees Programme Director Donna Lamping, G Walt
Secretary and Registrar Wendy Surridge
Teaching Programme Director Martin Taylor

Epidemiology and Population Health

Head of Department Pat Doyle
Departmental Research Degrees Director Noreen Maconochie
Taught Course Director Lynda Clarke

Centre for Population Studies

Head of Unit Ian Timaeus
Professor of Demographic Gerontology Emily Grundy
Professor of Medical Demography John Cleland
Reader in Medical Demography Basia Zaba
Senior Lecturer Lynda Clarke

Medical Statistics Unit

Head of Unit Mike Kenward
Professor of Health Care Evaluation Diana Elbourne
Professor of Medical Statistics Stuart Pocock
Professor of Pharmacoepidemiology Stephen Evans
Reader in Biostatistics Bianca De Stavola
Reader in Medical Statistics Chris Frost
Senior Lecturer James Carpenter

Non-communicable Disease Epidemiology Unit

Head of Unit David Leon
Clinical Senior Lecturer Isabel dos Santos Silva
Emeritus Professor Tom Meade
Professor of Cancer Epidemiology Henrik Moller, Julian Peto
Professor of Epidemiology and Vital Statistics Michel Coleman
Senior Lecturer Elizabeth Breeze, Noreen Maconochie
Senior Lecturer in Clinical Epidemiology Liam Smeeth

Nutrition and Public Health Intervention Research Unit

Head of Unit Astrid Fletcher
Professor Betty Kirkwood, Ian Roberts
Professor of Community Nutrition Ann Ashworth Hill
Professor of International Nutrition Andrew Prentice
Professor of Public Health Nutrition Ricardo Uauy
Reader Simon Cousens, Sharon Huttly
Senior Lecturer Tom Marshall, Vikram Patel, Elizabeth M E Poskitt

Infectious and Tropical Diseases

Head of Department Hazel M Dockrell
Departmental Research Degrees Director Alero Thomas
Taught Course Director Quentin Bickle, John Porter

Clinical Research Unit

Head of Unit Diana Lockwood
Manson Professor of Tropical Medicine Brian Greenwood
Professor of Communicable Diseases David Mabey
Professor of International Eye Health Allen Foster
Reader Robin Bailey, Peter Godfrey-Faussett, John Porter
Senior Lecturer Ron Behrens, Elizabeth Corbett, Tom Doherty, Alison Elliott, Clare Gilbert, Alison Grant, Stephen Lawn, Philippe Mayaud, Chris Whitty, Richard Wormald

Disease Control and Vector Biology Unit

Head of Unit Clive Davies
Clinical Senior Lecturer Daniel Chandramohan, Hugh Reyburn
Professor David Bradley, Sandy Cairncross, Frank Cox, Chris Curtis
Professor of Immunology of Protozoal Diseases Geoffrey Targett
Senior Lecturer Robert Aunger, Valerie Curtis, Jo Lines, Mark Rowland, Joanna Schellenberg

Immunology Unit

Professor and Head of Unit Eleanor Riley
Professor Simon Croft, Martin Taylor
Reader Gregory Bancroft, Quentin Bickle
Senior Lecturer John Raynes
Senior Lecturer Clinical Alero Thomas
Teaching Staff Member P Kaye

Infectious Disease Epidemiology Unit

Head of Unit Laura Rodrigues
Professor of Communicable Disease Epidemiology Paul Fine
Professor of Epidemiology and International Health Richard Hayes
Professor of Infectious Disease Epidemiology Andy Hall
Professor of Public Health Norman Noah
Professor of Tropical Epidemiology Peter Smith
Reader in Epidemiology and International Health Heiner Grosskurth
Reader in Epidemiology and International Public Health David Ross
Reader in Medical Statistics and Epidemiology Paul Milligan
Senior Lecturer Neal Alexander, Oona Campbell, Mia Crampin, Katherine Fielding, Judith Glynn, Shabbar Jaffar, Punam Mangtani, Linda A Morison, Carine Ronsmans, David Schellenberg, Jim Todd, Helen Weiss

Pathologen Molecular Biology Unit

Head of Unit Brendan Wren
Professor John Ackers, Michael Miles, Polly Roy
Reader John Kelly
Senior Lecturer David Baker, Graham Clark, David Conway, Ursula Gompels

Public Health and Policy

Head of Department Gill Walt
Departmental Research Degrees Director Colin Sanderson
Taught Course Director Nicki Thorogood

Health Policy Unit

Head of Unit Ruairi Brugha
Emeritus Professor J Patrick Vaughan
Professor Anne Mills
Reader John Porter
Senior Lecturer Paul Wenzel Geissler, Kent Buse, Julia Fox-Rushby, Lucy Gilson, Stephen Jan, Barbara McPake, Robert Pool, Egbert Sondorp, Charlotte Watts

Health Services Research Unit

Head of Unit Judith Green
Professor Nick Black, John Cairns, Nicholas Mays, Martin McKee, Jenny Roberts
Reader Donna Lamping, Colin Sanderson
Senior Lecturer Stuart Anderson, Richard Coker, Naomi Fulop, Nick Goodwin, Rosalind Raine, Barney Reeves, Jan van der Meulen

Public and Environmental Health Research Unit

Head of Unit Paul Wilkinson
Professor Jack Dowie, Virginia Berridge, Susanne MacGregor, Kaye Wellings
Professor Emeritus Jerry Morris
Professorial Fellow Joy Townsend
Reader Ben Armstrong
Senior Lecturer Chris Bonell, Tony Fletcher, Martin Gorsky, Spencer Hagard, Kelley Lee, Kiran Nanchahal, Carolyn Stephens, Nicki Thorogood

University of Manchester

Oxford Road, Manchester M13 9PL
Tel: 0161 275 2000
Website: www.manchester.ac.uk

President and Vice Chancellor Alan Gilbert
Vice President and Dean, Faculty of Medicine and Human Sciences David Gordon

Faculty of Life Sciences

Stopford Building, Manchester M13 9PT
Tel: 0161 275 5632
Website: www.ls.manchester.ac.uk

Dean of Life Sciences Alan North
Professor Maynard Case, Terri Attwood, Richard Balment, Graham Barnes, Terry Broom, Neil Bulleid, Alan Crossman, Michael Dixon, Mark Duyne, Mark Ferguson, David Foster, David Garrod, Richard Grencis, Tim Hardingham, Stephen High, Martin Humphries, Ian Hutchinson, John Hyde, Karl Kadler, Risto Kauppinen, Cay Kielty, Andrew Loudon, John McCarthy, Allen Moore, Steve Oliver, John Pickstone, Leon Poller, Andy Prass, Ian Roberts, Nancy Rothwell, Andy Sharrocks, Colin Sibley, Colin Stirling, Charles Streuli, David Tomlinson, Simon Turner, Alex Verkhratsky, Michael Warboys, Arthur Weston, Anne White

Medical School

Stopford Building, Oxford Road, Manchester M13 9PT
Tel: 0161 275 5613 Fax: 0161 275 1702
Website: www.medicine.manchester.ac.uk

Dean Andrew Garner
Head of School Administration Caroline Lord

Cancer Studies

Chair of Oncology Nicholas Thatcher
Head of Division and Professor of Physiology Roger Green
Cancer Research Campaign Professor Robert Hawkins
Hon. Professor Terry Allen, Nic Jones, John Radford
Professor of Cancer Cell Biology Anthony Whetton
Professor of Cancer Epidemiology and Public Health Ciaran Woodman
Professor of Immunotherapy Tim Illidge
Professor of Oncology John Gallagher
Professor of Radiation Oncology Patricia Price

Cardiovascular and Endocrine Sciences

Chair of Medicine Ludwig Neyses
Head of Division and Professor of Medicine Anthony Heagerty
Hon. Professor Ramanlal Gokal, John Lui Yin, Michael Walker
Professor of Anaesthesia Brian Pollard
Professor of Cardiac Physiology David Eisner
Professor of Cardiology Clifford Garratt
Professor of Endocrine Sciences Anne White
Professor of Medicine Andrew Boulton, Julian Davis, Paul Durrington

Epidemiology

Head of Division and Professor of Epidemiology Gary Macfarlane
ARC Professor of Rheumatic Disease Epidemiology Alan Silman
Hon. Emeritus Professor Stuart Donnan
Hon. Professor John Newton
Professor of Biomedical Statistics Graham Dunn
Professor of Clinical and Occupational Rehabilitation Christopher Main
Professor of Epidemiological and Social Statistics Andrew Pickles
Professor of Health Services and Epidemiology Sarah O'Brien
Professor of Immunogenetics William Ollier
Professor of Occupational and Environmental Health Raymond Agius
Professor of Public Health Richard Heller
Professor of Rheumatological and Musculoskeletal Epidemiology Deborah Symmons

Human Development

Head of Division and Professor in Child Health and Paediatric Endocrinology Peter Clayton
Cancer Research UK Professorial Fellow Jillian Birch
CRC Professor of Paediatric Oncology Tim Eden
Hon. Professor Malcolm Chiswick, Gareth Evans
Hon. Professor of Ophthalmology Richard Abadi
Professor and Director of maternal and Fetal Health Research Centre Philip Baker
Professor of Child Health and Paediatrics Timothy David
Professor of Child Health and Physiology Colin Sibley
Professor of Genetics and Ophthalmology Graeme Black
Professor of Gynaecological Oncology Henry Kitchener
Professor of Human Molecular Genetics Dorothy Trump
Professor of Medical Genetics Dian Donnal
Professor of Ophthalmology David McLeod
Professor of Ophthalmology and Vision Science David Henson

Imaging Science and Biomedical Engineering

Chair in Molecular Imaging Terrence Jones
Chair of Imaging Science Stephen Williams
Chair of Medical Biophysics and Computer Science Christopher Taylor
Head of Division and Chair of Neuroradiology Alan Jackson
Emeritus Professor Ian Isherwood
Professor of Diagnostic Radiology Judith Adams

Laboratory and Regenerative Medicine

Head of Division and Professor of Osteoarticular Pathology Anthony Freemont
Hon. Professor Shant Kumar
Hon. Professor of Pulmonary Pathology Philip Hasleton
Professor of Infectious Diseases Ruth Matthews
Professor of Medical Microbiology James Burnie
Professor of Plastic and Reconstructive Surgery Duncan McGrouther
Professor of Tissue Giorgio Terenghi

Medicine and Neurosciences (Hope Hospital)

Head of Division and Professor of Gastroenterology David Thompson
Hon. Professor of Medicine David Neary
Professor of Dermatology Christopher Griffiths
Professor of Gastroenterology Qasim Aziz
Professor of Geriatric Medicine Michael Horan
Professor of Hand Surgery John Stanley
Professor of Neuropathology David Mann

Medicine and Surgery (South Manchester)

Head of Division and Professor of Thoracic Medicine Ashley Woodcock
Hon. Professor of Thoracic Medicine Anthony Webb
Professor of Medical Education Paul O'Neill
Professor of Medicine and Gastroenterology Peter Whorwell
Professor of Respiratory Medicine Jorgen Vestbo
Professor of Surgery Charles McCollum

Professor of Surgical Oncology Nigel Bundred
Professorial Research Fellow Adnan Custovic

Primary Care

Head of Division and Professor of General Practice Martin Marshall
Emeritus Professor Carl Whitehouse
Hon. Professor Caroline Glendinning, Hugh Gravelle
Hon. Professorial Fellow in General Practive Jacqueline Hayden
Professor of General Practice Martin Roland
Professor of Health Services Research Bonnie Sibbald
Professor of the Sociology of Health Care Anne Rogers

Psychiatry

Head of Division and Professor of Old Age Psychiatry Alistair Burns
Hon. Professor of Neuroscience Alan Cross
Hon. Professor of Psychiatry Robert Baldwin
Professor of Adult Psychiatry Shôn Lewis
Professor of Community Psychiatry Matthew Marshall
Professor of Psychiatric Social Work Michael Kerfoot
Professor of Psychiatric Social Work and Community Care David Challis
Professor of Psychiatry Loius Appleby, Bill Deakin

School of Dentistry

Higher Cambridge Street, Manchester M15 6FH
Tel: 0161 306 0220
Website: www.den.man.ac.uk

Head of School and Professor of Orthodentics K D O'Brien
Clinical Lecturer Alan Yeung
Clinical Lecturer in Orthodontics Nicola Mandall
Clinical Teacher Barbara Coyne, Hilary Firestone
Clinical Teacher in Oral and Maxillofacial Surgery Elizabeth McLean
Clinical Teacher in Oral Medicine Senathirajah Ariyaratnam
Clinical Teacher in Restorative Dentistry Amin Aminian, Alan Hopwood, Michael Horrocks, Mark Hunter, Clive Oldham, Richard Strange, Margaret Wilson
Hon. Clinical Lecturer Richard Middlehurst, Brian Musgrove, Robert Woodwards
Hon. Clinical Lecturer in Child Dental Health Fiona Blinkhorn, Collette Bridgman, Alex Crawford, Felicity Murray
Hon. Clinical Lecturer in Dental Health Promotion Michael Wanless
Hon. Clinical Lecturer in Dental Public Health Jacqueline Duxbury, Madeline Harding, Anthony Jenner, Gary Whittle
Hon. Clinical Lecturer in Oral Health Promotion Sabrina Fuller
Hon. Clinical Lecturer in Orthodontics David Lewis
Hon. Clinical Lecturer in Restorative Dentistry Martin Ashley, David Eldridge
Hon. Clinical Lecturer in Rheumatology and in Medicine for Dental Students Martin Pattrick
Hon. Clinical Lecturer in Surgery William Tait
Hon. Clinical Senior Lecturer in Dental Public Health Roger Elwood
Hon. Clinical Teacher R E Lloyd, Marie Morton, Gillian Nadin, Elizabeth Turbill
Hon. Clinical Teacher in Dental Public Health Keith Milsom
Hon. Clinical Teacher in Restorative Dentistry Craig Barcley
Hon. Lecturer in Oral Medicine Elizabeth Theaker
Hon. Senior Lecturer in Dental Medicine and Surgery Michael Pemberton
Lecturer in Dental Health Rebecca Craven
Lecturer in Dental Practice Stephen Davies
Lecturer in Dental Sciences Howard Carter
Lecturer in Dental Statistics Tatiana Macfarlane
Lecturer in Evidence Based Oral Health Care Anne-Marie Glenny
Lecturer in Oral and Maxillofacial Surgery Richard Oliver
Lecturer in Restorative Dentistry Julian Satterthwaite, Philip Smith
Lecturer on Orthodontics David Bearn
Professor Dental Genetics Michael Dixon
Professor Dental Health Services Research Elizabeth Kay
Professor Experimental Oral Pathology Philip Sloan
Professor in Clinical Dental Research Robin Davies
Professor of Dental Biomaterials David Watts
Professor of Maxillofacial Imaging Keith Horner
Professor of Oral and Maxillofacial Imaging Keith Horner
Professor of Oral Health A S Blinkhorn
Professor of Orthodontics and Dentofacial Development William Shaw
Professor of Restorative Care of the Elderly J F McCord
Reader in Dental Statistics Helen Worthington
Senior Clinical Teacher in Restorative Dentistry Nicholas Grey
Senior Lecture in Dental Public Health Martin Tickle
Senior Lecturer in Child Dental Health Iain Mackie, Ian Mackie
Senior Lecturer in Craniofacial Anomalies Gunvor Semb
Senior Lecturer in Dental and Maxillofacial Radiology Vivian Rushton
Senior Lecturer in Medical Genetics and Dental Medicine Nalin Thakkar
Senior Lecturer in Oral and Maxillofacial Surgery Paul Coulthard
Senior Lecturer in Periodontics Peter S Hull
Senior Lecturer In Primary Dental Care Anthony Mellor
Senior Lecturer in Restorative Dentistry Hugh Devlin, Alison Qualtrough
Specialist Registrar in Restorative Dentistry Derek Moore
Teacher in Child Dental Health Cheryl Rivkin
University Teacher in Restorative Dentistry C Potter

Recognised Clinical Institutions
Central Manchester and Manchester Children's University Hospitals NHS Trust, Christie Hospital, Manchester Mental Health and Social Care Trust, Salford Royal Hospitals NHS Trust, South Manchester University Hospitals NHS Trust

University of Newcastle upon Tyne

Faculty of Medical Sciences, Medical School/Dental School, Framlington Place, Newcastle upon Tyne NE2 4HH
Tel: 0191 222 7005 Fax: 0191 222 6521
Website: www.ncl.ac.uk

Dean of Clinical Medicine A D Burt
Dean of Development Michael Whittaker
Dean of Postgraduate Studies Barry Hurst
Dean of Research Tim Cawston
Dean of Undergraduate Studies Reginald Jordan
Cell and Molecular Biosciences M A Hughes
Clinical Medical Sciences C P Day
Dental Sciences R A Seymour
Medical Education Development G Hammond
Neurology, Neurobiology and Psychiatry I N Ferrier
Population and Health Sciences S Bond
Postgraduate Institute for Medicine and Dentistry P M Hill
Provost O F W James
Surgical and Reproductive Sciences T W J Lennard

Recognised Clinical Institutions
Newcastle upon Tyne Dental Hospital, University Hospital of North Durham

University of Nottingham

Medical School B Floor, Queen's Medical Centre, Nottingham NG7 2UH
Tel: 0115 970 9379 Fax: 0115 970 9922
Website: www.nottingham.ac.uk

Dean of the Faculty of Medicine and Health Sciences T Stephenson
Faculty Secretary Chris Farrell

Recognised Clinical Institutions
Derby City General Hospital, Derbyshire Children's Hospital, Derbyshire Royal Infirmary, King's Mill Hospital, Lincoln County Hospital, Nottingham City Hospital NHS Trust, Queen's Medical Centre, Nottingham University Hospital NHS Trust

University of Oxford

The Medical Sciences Office, John Radcliffe Hospital, Headington, Oxford OX3 9DU
Tel: 01865 221689 Fax: 01865 750750
Email: enquiries@medsci.ox.ac.uk
Website: www.medsci.ox.ac.uk

Director of Clinical Studies T Lancaster
Director of Clinical Studies (Deputy) P A Frith
Director of Graduate Entry Course P D Dennis
Director of Postgraduate Medical and Dental Education M J Bannon
Director of Pre-Clinical Studies S J Goss
Head of Division of Medical Sciences K A Fleming
Secretary of Faculties and Academic Registrar A P Weale
Secretary of the Medical Sciences Division D E H Bryan

Clinical Medicine

Anaesthetics
Head of Department C E W Hahn
Clinical Lecturer Vacancy
Clinical Reader J W Sear
Professor H J MacQuay

Cardiovascular Medicine
Head of Department H C Watkins
Clinical Lecturer R Choudhury, S G Myerson
Professor K M Channon, M Farrall, S Neubauer

Clinical Laboratory Sciences
Head of Department K C Gatter
Clinical Lecturer R A Malladi, N Meston, A Nemeth, G J Pillai, E J Soilleux, D H Wyllie
Clinical Reader S B Fox
Clinical Tutor J E Lortan
Professor D Y Mason, A O M Wilkie
University Lecturer R Callaghan, R J Gibbons

Clinical Medicine
Head of Department P J Ratcliffe
Clinical Lecturer A Frater, D Mole, K Owen
Clinical Tutor B J Angus
Professor M McCarthy, J O D McGee, C I Newbold, R Peto, R E Phillips, P Rorsman, D I Stuart, R V Thakker, A R M Townsend, D A Warrell
University Lecturer J M Gleadle, N R Moore

Clinical Neurology
Head of Department G C Ebers
Clinical Reader M J Donaghy
Professor M M Esiri, P Jezzard, A C Vincent
University Lecturer P M Rothwell

Clinical Pharmacology
Head of Department and Professor D J Kerr
Clinical Reader J K Aronson
University Lecturer L W Seymour

Geriatric Medicine
Professor A Buchan
University Lecturer D S Fairweather

Medical Oncology
Head of Department A L Harris

Molecular Medicine
Head of Department A J McMichael

Obstetrics and Gynaecology
Clinical Lecturer P T-Y Ayuk, D Tucker
Clinical Reader S H Kennedy, I Z Mackenzie
Professor S T Kehoe, H J Mardon, C W G Redman
University Lecturer P F Chamberlain, I L Sargent, K Turner

Ophthalmology
Professor N N Osborne
University Lecturer J M Tiffany

Orthopaedic Surgery
Head of Department R C G Russell
Clinical Lecturer A J Price
Clinical Reader M A Brown
Professor N A Athanasou, C J K Bulstrode, A J Carr
University Lecturer M J O Francis, J A D Loughlin

Paediatrics
Head of Department E R Moxon
Clinical Lecturer M A Herbert, S Segal
Professor A Harris, A R Wilkinson
University Lecturer J Hull, A Pollard, P B Sullivan

Psychiatry
Head of Department G M Goodwin
Clinical Lecturer Z H Bhagwagar, S M Carney, M Fazel
Clinical Tutor J Price
Professor A Bailey, T Burns, P J Harrison, R Jacoby, A Stein
University Lecturer R D Rogers

Public Health and Primary Health Care
Head of Department of Primary Health Care D Mant
Head of Department of Public Health H Jaffe
Clinical Lecturer E A Plugge, R Sharma, M Thompson
Clinical Reader P P Glasziou, T R Lancaster
Professor R A Hope
University Lecturer L M Carpenter, A R Harnden, A McPherson, H A W Neil, M Parker, P W Rose, K M Venables, P L N Yudkin

Rheumatology
Clinical Lecturer C Swales
Professor B P Wordsworth

Surgery
Head of Department J Meakins
Clinical Lecturer S Bach, A J McLaren, B Murphy
Clinical Reader L J Hands, P R V Johnson
Clinical Tutor A I Handa
Professor J M Austyn, P J Friend, D W R Gray, K J Wood
University Lecturer S J Golding

Physiological Sciences

Experimental Psychology
Head of Department O Braddick
Professor P E Bryant, A Cowey, M R C Hewstone, R M Martin, R E Passingham, K R Plunkett, J N P Rawlins, B J Rogers, E T Rolls
Reader A C de Ozorio Nobre
University Lecturer C Harmer, G B Henning, P D McLeod, K Nation, B Parkinson, C J Spence

Human Anatomy and Genetics
Head of Department K E Davies
Professor J F Morris, G M Morriss-Kay
Reader H M Charlton
University Lecturer C A R Boyd, H C Christian, T J Horder, Z Molnar, J S H Taylor, I M G Tracey, C Wilson, M J A Wood

Pathology

Head of Department H Waldman
Professor G G Brownlee, P R Cook, J Errington, S Gordon, N J Proudfoot
Reader G S MacPherson
University Lecturer S J Goss, D Greaves, S V Hunt, W James, C Norbury, Q Sattentau, D J T Vaux

Pharmacology

Head of Department E Sim
Professor A F Brading, A D Smith
Reader D A Terrar
University Lecturer G C Churchill, T C Cunnane, N J Emptage, A Galione, J Parrington

Physiology

Head of Department J C Ellory
Professor C C Ashley, J J B Jack, D Noble, A Parekh, A J Parker, D J Paterson, T Powell, P A Robbins, J F Stein, R D Vaughan-Jones
Reader S J Judge
University Lecturer K Buckler, K L Dorrington, P C G Nye, A B Parekh, O Paulsen, C Schnupp, I D Thompson, R J Wilkins

Degrees and diplomas

BM, BCh, DM, MCh, MSc, D.Phil

Recognised Clinical Institutions

Nuffield Orthopaedic Centre NHS Trust, Oxfordshire Mental Healthcare NHS Trust, Park Hospital for Children, Radcliffe Infirmary, The Churchill, The John Radcliffe, Warneford Hospital

Peninsula Medical School

Tamar Science Park, Research Way, Plymouth PL6 8BU
Tel: 01752 247444 Fax: 01752 517842
Website: www.pms.ac.uk

Chair of Exeter Locality Management Team Ken MacLeod
Dean John Tooke
Clinical Sub-Dean Adrian Copplestone, Paul Upton
Associate Dean John Bligh, Robert Sneyd
Associate Dean for Truro Tony Pinching
Director of Biomedical and Clinical Research Angela Shore
Director of Health and Social Care Research Stuart Logan
Community Sub-Dean for Cornwall Steve Watkins
Community Sub-Dean for Plymouth Neville Devonport
School Secretary Chris Lindsay

Royal Free and University College Medical School of University College London

Bloomsbury Campus, Gower Street, London WC1E 6BT
Tel: 020 7679 2000 Fax: 020 7383 2462
Website: www.ucl.ac.uk/medicalschool

Dean of the Faculty of Clinical Sciences L G Fine
Dean of the Faculty of Life Sciences P Mobbs
Vice-Dean and Director of Clinical Studies I Taylor
Vice-Dean and Campus Director (Whitt.) D I Patterson
Vice-Dean and Camputs Director (RF) H Hodgson
Vice-Dean (Curriculum) M Lloyd
Vice-Dean Primary Care P Wallace
Postgraduate Sub-Dean J Dooley
Faculty Sub-Dean D A Bender, J Dooley, G Hamilton
Sub-Dean and Assistant Faculty Tutor Archway Campus H Morgan
Sub-Dean and Assistant Faculty Tutor Hampstead Campus G Hamilton
Sub-Dean (Curriculum Innovation) J Cartledge, A Wagg
Sub-Dean (Quality Assurance) A Berlin
Sub-Dean (Student Support and Welfare) M Berelowitz, B Cross, D Jordan
Sub-Dean (Teaching) D A Bender, R Noble
Faculty Graduate Tutor, Clinical Sciences V Emery
Faculty Tutor, Clinical Sciences J Dacre
Faculty Tutor, Life Sciences B Cross
Vice-Provost Biomedicine and Dean of the Medical School K M Spyer

Archway Campus

Highgate Hill, London N19 5NF
Tel: 020 7272 3070

Vice-Dean and Campus Director D Patterson

Hampstead Campus

Rowland Hill Street, London NW3 2PF
Tel: 020 7794 0500
Vice-Dean and Campus Director H Hodgson

Division of Cancer Medicine

Divisional Chair D Linch

Haematology (Bloomsbury)

Clinical Lecturer R Benjamin, C Burton, P D Kottaridis, M Mansour, M Nash, M A Scully
Clinical Professor A Khwaja, D C Linch, S J Machin, J B Porter
Clinical Reader K L Yong
Clinical Senior Lecturer A Nathwani, K Peggs, T C P Somervaille
Reader R E Gale, I J Mackie

Haematology (Hampstead)

Clinical Lecturer D A Hughes
Clinical Professor S Mackinnon
Lecturer R J Anderson
Reader L Foroni, E Nacheva
Senior Lecturer M W Lowdell, R G Wickremasinghe

Histopathology (Bloomsbury)

Clinical Professor A Dogan, A M Flanagan, G H Williams
Clinical Senior Lecturer E Benjamin, G Kocjan
Lecturer C M Bacon, A Okorov, K Stoeber

Histopathology (Hampstead)

Clinical Lecturer S S El-Sheikh
Clinical Professor A P Dhillon, A Howie
Clinical Senior Lecturer J C Crow

Oncology (Bloomsbury)

Clinical Professor M I Saunders
Clinical Reader D Hochhauser, J A Ledermann
Clinical Senior Lecturer J A Bridgewater
Professor J A Hartley

Oncology (Hampstead)

Clinical Professor R H J Begent
Clinical Senior Lecturer T Myer
Reader K A Chester, R B Pedley
Senior Lecturer D Nagl

Division of Infection and Immunity

Divisional Chair M Collins

Immunology and Molecular Pathology (Bloomsbury)

Clinical Professor D R Katz, T W Rademacher, P M M Woo
Clinical Senior Lecturer M K Maini
Lecturer R S Coffin, S J Dawson
Professor B M Chain, M K L Collins, P M Lydyard, R A Weiss
Reader P J Delves, T Lund, N J Marshall, J T Roes
Senior Lecturer A Fassati, J S Skok, Y Takeuchi

Immunology and Molecular Pathology (Hampstead)
Clinical Professor G Janossy
Clinical Reader D P Mikhailidis
Professor A N Akbar
Senior Lecturer M R Dashwood

Infection (Bloomsbury)
Clinical Lecturer J W T Tang
Clinical Professor A M Emmerson, G A W Rook, R S Tedder, A Zumla
Clinical Reader J M Holton, D Pillay
Clinical Senior Lecturer J A Garson
Senior Lecturer H D Donoghue, P Kellam

Infection (Hampstead)
Clinical Professor S H Gillespie, P D Griffiths
Clinical Senior Lecturer J N Zuckerman
Lecturer D A Clark
Professor V C Emery
Senior Lecturer B M Charalambous, T D McHugh

Division of Medicine

Divisional Chair P Vallance

Clinical Neurosciences
Clinical Professor A H V Schapira
Clinical Reader T T Warner
Clinical Senior Lecturer D McCabe, R W Orrell, A Schrag
Lecturer J W Taanman
Senior Lecturer J M Cooper

Institute of Nuclear Medicine (Bloomsbury)
Clinical Professor P J Ell
Lecturer S Gacinovic
Professor B Hutton
Senior Lecturer I D Cullum

Medicine (Archway)
Clinical Professor J G Malone-Lee, J S Yudkin
Lecturer M Fader, V Mohamed Ali, J Patel
Senior Lecturer C Wu

Medicine (Bloomsbury)
Clinical Lecturer R A Breckenridge, R Jenkins, D Lambiase
Clinical Professor D J Betteridge, J C W Edwards, P C Hindmarsh, M A Horton, D A Isenberg, G J Laurent, R Littlewood, J F Martin, W McKenna, S Newman, A W Segal, M Singer, S G Spiro, G W Stewart, A Tinker, R J Unwin, P J T Vallance, R S Williams, D Withers, D M Yellon, A Zumla
Clinical Reader A A Bertoletti, A D Hingorani, R J MacAllister, J R McEwan, N V Naoumov
Clinical Senior Lecturer G J Bellingan, J Brown, S Dein, C Dollery, M R Ehrenstein, P M Elliott, A R Gillams, P A Glynne, R Jalan, Y C Lee, S P Pereira, G Prelevic, M A A Rahman
Lecturer S Behboudi, N A Davies, S Hodges, C Mauri
Professor J Godovac-Zimmermann, S E Humphries, G Scambler
Reader L H Clapp, P Higgs, R J McAnulty, P Talmud, I C Zachary
Senior Lecturer R C Chambers, S Jadhav, J M Leiper, L Myers, J T Norman, P Rabbits, C C T Smith, J Thompson, M Weale

Medicine (Hampstead)
Clinical Lecturer P Dupont, H B Goodman, S Kinloch, S Lala
Clinical Professor G M Dusheiko, P N Hawkins, H J F Hodgson, K P Moore, M B Pepys, R Pounder, S H Powis
Clinical Reader P M G Boulox, J S Dooley, M Y Morgan
Clinical Senior Lecturer S Al-Damluji, S Keshav, H J Lachmann, D Wheeler
Lecturer S Minogue, X Z Ruan
Professor J S Owen
Reader D J Abraham, T J Harrison, J J Hsuan
Senior Lecturer A C Selden, G A Tennent, A P Walker

Reta Lila Weston Institute of Neurological Studies (Bloomsbury)
Clinical Professor M J Harrison
Clinical Senior Lecturer D S Holder

Division of Population Health

Divisional Chair Michael Marmot

Epidemiology and Public Health (Bloomsbury)
Clinical Lecturer P Primatesta, G Tsakos
Clinical Professor M G Marmot, M McCarthy, J Y Nazroo
Clinical Reader M Bobak, H Hemingway, R G Watt
Clinical Senior Lecturer P A Batchelor
Lecturer A R Britton, Y J Kelly, V Marinho, H Pikhart
Professor M Bartley, A P A Steptoe, R J West
Reader J Adda, E J Brunner
Senior Lecturer E Breeze, T Chandola, J A Head, B Peter, M J Shipley

Mental Health Sciences (Archway/Bloomsbury)
Clinical Lecturer S Marwaha, N Perez-Achiaga
Clinical Professor P E Bebbington, H M Gurling, M W Orrell
Clinical Reader C Feinmann, G A Livingston
Clinical Senior Lecturer L C Bailly, P T Byrne, J E Carter, S L Dein, A Hassiotis, I S Johnson, J M Moncrieff, Z Walker

Mental Health Sciences (Hampstead)
Clinical Lecturer C W Ritchie
Clinical Professor M B King
Clinical Senior Lecturer M R Blanchard, H T Killaspy, K J Mckenzie, D P J Osborn, P W Raven, M A Serfaty
Senior Lecturer S M Wilkinson

MRC Clinical Trials Unit
Professor A J Nunn, M K B Parmar
Reader D M Gibb

Primary Care and Population Science (Archway and Hampstead)
Clinical Lecturer D J Bavin, P A Bryant, W G T Coppola, M M Jones, P S Salomon, A J Schamroth, A Selwyn, S Singh, D A Swinglehurst, G R Wong
Clinical Professor P M Greenhalgh, A M Johnson, M H Lloyd, I D Nazareth, L Sherr, P G Wallace
Clinical Reader S R Iliffe
Clinical Senior Lecturer A A P Berlin, M J Buszewicz, J A Cassell, A C Hayward, C G Helman, D L Kirklin, F Lefford, M H Leighton, R P Meakin, E Murray, G Rait, S Rogers, J J Rosenthal, J M Stephenson, N B D Towson
Lecturer J Barber, J Biddulph, P M Boynton, S Dinan, M A S Griffin, F C Lampe, P Lenihan, J Russell, F A Stevenson
Professor A Bowling, A N Phillips, C A Sabin
Reader R W Morris
Senior Lecturer V M Drennan, C M Goodman, A J Mocroft

Primary Care and Population Sciences (STDs Bloomsbury) Sexually Transmitted Diseases
Clinical Lecturer J E Richens
Clinical Professor I V D Weller
Clinical Reader R F Miller
Clinical Senior Lecturer F M Cowan, R J C Gilson, D E Mercey, G Williams
Lecturer A J Copas
Reader R M Power

Division of Surgical and Interventional Sciences

Institute of Orthopaedics and Musculoskeletal Science
Royal National Orthopaedic Hospital, Brockley Hill, Stanmore HA7 4LP
Tel: 020 8954 2300

Clinical Lecturer A Hart
Lecturer H L Birch, M J Coathup, J Hua, V Mudera
Professor G W Blunn, R A Brown, M W Ferguson-Pell, A E Goodship

Surgery (Archway)

Clinical Senior Lecturer M Hashemi, A Wilson

Surgery (Bloomsbury)

Clinical Lecturer J Winehouse
Clinical Professor P B Boulos, S G Bown, B Keogh, J M Ryan, I Taylor
Clinical Senior Lecturer S G E Barker, L M Bromley, M Douek, J A Hulf, A J Leathem, J R C Sainsbury, M R Sefaei Keshtgar
Lecturer S J Hollingsworth
Professor M J O'Hare
Reader A J MacRobert
Senior Lecturer J T Chowaniec, J Houghton, M C Loizidou

Surgery (Hampstead)

Clinical Lecturer Y Koak
Clinical Professor B R Davidson, M C Winslet
Clinical Senior Lecturer O A Ogunbiyi
Professor B J Fuller, A M Seifalian

Urology and Nephrology (Bloomsbury)

Clinical Professor A R Mundy
Clinical Reader C R J Woodhouse
Clinical Senior Lecturer M Emberton, M R Feneley, S J Harland, P J R Shah
Professor M D Craggs, C H Fry, J R W Masters

Division of Women's and Children's Health

Divisional Chair I Jacobs

Gynaecological Oncology

Clinical Lecturer A Rosenthal
Clinical Professor I Jacobs
Clinical Senior Lecturer U Menon
Senior Lecturer S A Gayther

Obstetrics and Gynaecology (Bloomsbury)

Clinical Lecturer F Shenfield, S M Whitten
Clinical Professor E R M Jauniaux, C H Rodeck
Clinical Reader D M Peebles
Clinical Senior Lecturer I Ozturk
Lecturer S Muttukrishna, S B Sengupta
Reader G Raivich
Senior Lecturer J Harper, R Noble

Obstetrics and Gynaecology (Hampstead)

Clinical Lecturer O A Oyawoye
Clinical Professor A B Maclean
Clinical Senior Lecturer P J J Hardiman
Senior Lecturer C W Perrett

Paediatrics and Child Health (Bloomsbury)

Clinical Lecturer T Austin, A Reece
Clinical Professor R M Gardiner, J S Wyatt
Clinical Senior Lecturer H M E Bantock, E M K Chung, N J Robertson, S C Roth
Lecturer F Capon
Senior Lecturer H M Mitchison, M Rees

Paediatrics and Child Health (Hampstead)

Clinical Lecturer I Banerjee, J M Ellis, A A O Fagbemi
Clinical Professor B W Taylor
Clinical Senior Lecturer R Senior, A G Sutcliffe

ACME (Academic Centre for Medical Education)

Clinical Professor J E Dacre
Clinical Senior Lecturer J D Cartledge, D Gill, J Kavanagh, C Moss
Lecturer L A Dunkley, P Washer
Reader J Radcliffe Richards
Senior Lecturer L Noble, J E Richardson

CHIME

Clinical Professor I C McManus
Clinical Senior Lecturer D Kalra
Lecturer H W Potts
Professor S P Bate, D Ingram
Senior Lecturer J Murphy, J Nicholls, P M Taylor

Ear Institute

Gray's Inn Road, London WC1X 8EE
Tel: 020 7837 8855

Clinical Professor V J Lund, A Wright
Clinical Senior Lecturer D J Howard
Lecturer G Al-Malky, S Casalotti, S Dawson
Professor J Ashmore, A Forge, D T Kemp, A Linney, D K Prasher
Reader D McAlpine
Senior Lecturer M Bitner-Glindzicz, H C Dodson

Eastman Dental Institute for Oral Health Care Science

256 Gray's Inn Road, London WC1X 8LD
Tel: 020 7915 1038 Fax: 020 7915 1012
Website: www.eastman.ucl.ac.uk

Dean and Director of Studies and Research C Scully

Biomaterials and Tissue Engineering

Lecturer F H Jones, S N Nazhat, V Salih, A M Young
Professor J C Knowles, I Olsen
Senior Lecturer M P Lewis

Biomedical Informatics

Professor P Hammond

Biostatistics

Senior Lecturer A Petrie

Conservative Dentistry

Clinical Lecturer G E Evans, R Kahan, Y L Ng, C J Tredwin
Clinical Senior Lecturer K Gulabivala, D J Setchell

Continuing Professional Development

Clinical Lecturer G R Finn, K Harper, G Lambourn, B Mizrahi, D Patel
Clinical Professor A Eder
Clinical Senior Lecturer A H Croysdill, M Faigenblum

Health Services Research

Clinical Senior Lecturer D R Moles

Implantology

Clinical Lecturer M C Haswell

Infection and Immunity

Lecturer E Allan, P M Brett, P Buxton, J R Pratten
Professor B Henderson, M Wilson
Reader S Meghji, P Mullany
Senior Lecturer S Nair, D Spratt

Oral and Maxillofacial Surgery

Clinical Lecturer M A El Maaytah

Clinical Senior Lecturer A W Evans, C Feinmann, C Hopper
Senior Lecturer A Bamber

Oral Medicine and Specialist Needs Dentistry

Clinical Professor S R Porter, C Scully

Oral Pathology

Clinical Lecturer J H Bennett

Orthodontics

Clinical Lecturer R Shah
Clinical Professor N P Hunt
Clinical Senior Lecturer S J Cunningham, P M Thomas

Paediatric Dentistry

Clinical Lecturer P F Ashley, M J Gelbier, S Parekh

Periodontology

Clinical Professor N Donos
Clinical Senior Lecturer G S Griffiths, I G Needleman

Prosthetic Dentistry

Clinical Professor J A Hobkirk
Clinical Senior Lecturer P G T Howell, J A Howlett

Radiology

Clinical Senior Lecturer J E Brown

Faculty of Life Sciences

Gower Street, London WC1E 6BT
Tel: 020 7679 2000

Anatomy and Developmental Biology

Lecturer D Becker, S Bhattacharya, J Linden, V Lo, S Price, D Whitmore, Y Yamamoto
Professor P N Anderson, J Browne, N Burgess, H Cook, R Cooter, T Cowan, S W Davies, M C Dean, S E Evans, M Fitzgerald, S Hunt, K Jessen, C J Lawrence, A R Lieberman, V Nutton, J O'Keefe, J G Parnavelas, F Spoor, C D Stern, A E Warner, S Wilson, C H Yeo
Reader T Arnett, L Dale, P Giese, A Hardy, P Salinas, E M Tansey, A Wear
Senior Lecturer J D W Clarke, J E Cook, B P Fulton, J Jacyna, I Johnson, J Lincoln, R Mayor, M Neve, J P Simons

Biochemistry and Molecular Pathology

Lecturer A Dingley, S Djordjevic, R E Drew, A Martin, S Naaby-Hansen, J F Timms, A Townsend-Nicholson
Professor J P Brockes, K R Bruckdorfer, A L Burlingame, M D Crompton, D C Cutler, P C Driscoll, I T Gout, A Hall, D T Jones, J E S Ladbury, M Marsh, C A Orengo, S J Perkins, A Ridley, E D Saggerson, E A Shephard, S K S Srai, J M Thornton, G Waksman, M D Waterfield
Reader B A Vanhaesebroeck, J M Ward, M Zvelebil
Senior Lecturer D A Bender, A E Michael, S Nagl, D J Williams

Biology

Lecturer D Gems, H J P Richards, H Smith, M Telford, A Wingler
Professor C Danpure, M C Evans, D B Goldstein, J S Jones, A M Lister, J Mallet, L Partridge, A Pomiankowski, M S Povey, P R Rich, W D Richardson, D M Swallow, J N Wood, R S Wotton, Z Yang
Reader K Fowler, G Hurst, S Purton, J Wolfe
Senior Lecturer J P Field, S E Mole, C W Mullineaux, J Pearson, T M Preston, A Ruiz-Linares, M Thomas

Human Communication Science

Lecturer S Beeke, S Bloch, C J Bruce, L J Cavalli, M Clarke, A L Constable, J Dankovicova, A S Edmundson, C Newton, R I Rees, S A Simpson, C Smith, M A Vance, J Wood
Professor R Campbell, J Maxim, H Van der Lely
Reader W Best, S Chiat
Senior Lecturer M Black, C Donlan, J Hald, M Kersner, M Mahon, A Parker, J Swettenham, R Wilkinson, J Wright

Pharmacology

Lecturer S Nurrish, J Pitcher, G Stephens, M Stocker, D Willis
Professor S G Cull-Candy, A H Dickenson, A C Dolphin, J C Foreman, J Garthwaite, T G Smart
Reader A J Gibb, N Millar, A G Ramage, R Schoepfer, T Sihra, S C Stanford
Senior Lecturer M Farrant, D G Haylett, G W J Moss, L Silvilotti

Physiology

Clinical Professor R J Unwin, D M Yellon
Lecturer S Casalotti, M J Mayston, G M H Thomas, R E A Tunwell
Professor J F Ashmore, D I Attwell, S Bolsover, S Cockcroft, M R Duchen, C H Fry, A R Gardner-Medwin, D Jordan, P G Mobbs, C D Richards, K M Spyer, J A Stephens
Reader J Carroll, E S Debnam, F A Edwards, M P Gilbey, B Lynn, D McAlpine, P Pedarzani, P E R Tatham
Senior Lecturer B A Cross, J P Fry, S D R Harridge, L M Harrison, P J Harrison, B F King, A Koffer, R Noble

Psychology

Lecturer R R Benedyk, S Blakemore, P Cairns, A Cox, L French, J Gilmore, C Harries, J Kaufman, O Mason, R Murphy, L Otten, G Pickup, J Rodd, K Scior, P Stenner
Professor J Atkinson, C Brewin, B L Butterworth, H V Curran, J S Driver, P Fonagy, N Frederickson, U Frith, A F Furnham, P Haggard, N J W Harvey, C Heyes, P Howell, A Johnston, N Lavie, I C McManus, H C Plotkin, T Shallice, D R Shanks
Reader P Burgess, S Channon, S Michie, G Vigliocco, J Ward, A Williams
Senior Lecturer C B Barker, A Blandford, S Butler, D F Einon, M Ennis, J Feigenbaum, D W Green, K Jeffery, H Joffe, P K Lunt, A G R McClelland, D A Oakley, N E Pistrang, R E Rawles, A Schlottmann, M Tallandini, M Target, J Wattam-Bell

Institute of Child Health

30 Guilford Street, London WC1N 1EH
Tel: 020 7242 9789 Fax: 020 7831 0488
Website: www.ich.ucl.ac.uk

Dean/Director A Copp
Vice-Dean P Scrambler

Biochemical and Nutritional Sciences

Professor B Winchester

Cancer

Reader H Brady

Cardiorespiratory Sciences

Professor M Mythen

Genes, Development and Disease

Professor P Scambler

Infection and Immunity

Professor C Kinnon

Neurosciences and Mental Health

Professor M Koltzenburg

Population Health Sciences

Professor A Tomkins

Institute of Neurology

Queen Square, London WC1N 3BG
Tel: 020 7837 3611
Website: www.ion.ucl.ac.uk

Clinical Sub-Dean S D Shorvon

Director R N Lemon
Secretary R P Walker

Clinical Neurology

Professor M M Brown, J Collinge, J S Duncan, D R Fish, C J Fowler, R S J Frackowiak, P J Goadsby, M Koltzenburg, D M Kullmann, A Lees, C J Mathias, D H Miller, P N Patsalos, N P Quinn, M N Rossor, J W A Sander, A H V Schapira, S D Shorvon, A J Thompson, N W Wood
Reader K Bhatia, P Brown, M Hanna
Senior Lecturer G Giovannoni, H Kaube, M Koepp, P D Limousin, E D Playford, G Rees, J Rees, M Reilly, M Richardson, S M Sisodiya, S J Tabrizi, D J Thomas, M Walker, N Ward

Miriam Marks Division of Neurochemistry

Lecturer J M Pocock
Professor J B Clark, E Fisher, L Lim, E J Thompson
Senior Lecturer C Hall, J M Land

Neuropathology

Lecturer M Groves
Professor T Revesz
Senior Lecturer J Holton, M Thom

Neuropsychiatry and Neuropsychology

Lecturer E Maguire
Professor R J Dolan, K J Friston, C D Frith, E Joyce, C J Price, M Ron
Reader M Jamanshahi

Neuroradiology and Neurophysics

Lecturer S Free
Professor P S Tofts, R Turner, T Yousry
Reader H-R Jaeger, L Lemieux

Neurosurgery

Lecturer T J Warr
Professor M Hariz, D G T Thomas
Senior Lecturer K ashkan, L D Watkins

Sobell Division of Neurophysiology

Lecturer L Greensmith
Professor H Bostock, R N Lemon, J Rothwell, D Wolpert
Reader P A Kirkwood
Senior Lecturer A H Pullen

Institute of Ophthalmology

11-43 Bath Street, London EC1V 9EL
Tel: 020 7608 6800
Website: www.ucl.ac.uk/ioo/

Director A M Sillito

Cell Biology

Clinical Lecturer T P Levine
Lecturer M Bailly, C E Futter
Professor S E Moss
Reader M S Balda, K Matter

Cellular Therapy

Lecturer P Turowski
Professor P Coffey, J Greenwood

Clinical Ophthalmology

Lecturer V Calder
Professor A C Bird, S L Lightman

Epidemiology and International Eye Health

Clinical Reader D Minassian
Clinical Senior Lecturer P Foster, I Murdoch, J S Rahi

Inherited Eye Disease

Clinical Lecturer A Webster
Professor A T Moore, J A Sahel

Molecular Genetics

Clinical Lecturer A Webster
Lecturer L Erskine
Professor S S Bhattacharya, D M Hunt
Senior Lecturer A J Hardcastle

Molecular Therapy

Professor R Ali

Ocular Immunology

Professor S J Ono

Pathology

Clinical Lecturer A Whitmore
Lecturer J Daniels
Professor P T Khaw, P J Luthert
Senior Lecturer M E Cheetham

Visual Rehabilitation

Professor G Rubin
Senior Lecturer P Bex

Visual Science

Lecturer R B Lotto
Professor J K Bowmaker, F Fitzke, T E Salt, A M Sillito, A Stockman
Senior Lecturer S C Dakin, G Jeffery

Wolfson Institute for Biomedical Research

Gower Street, London WC1E 6BT
Tel: 020 7679 6666

Lecturer K P Giese, H K Smith
Professor C Boshoff, I G Charles, J Garthwaite, M Hausser, S Moncada, W D Richardson
Reader J Erusalimsky, D Selwood
Senior Lecturer G Garthwaite, G Koentges, K Stoeber

Recognised Clinical Institutions

Barnet, Enfield and Haringey Mental Health NHS Trust, Barnet and Chase Farm Hospitals NHS Trust, Camden and Islington Community Health Services NHS Trust, Camden and Islington Mental Health and Social Care Trust, Great Ormond Street Hospital for Children NHS Trust Education Centre, Moorfields Eye Hospital NHS Foundation Trust, North East Essex Mental Health NHS Trust, North East London Mental Health NHS Trust, North Middlesex University Hospital NHS Trust, Royal Free Hampstead NHS Trust, Royal National Orthopaedic Hospital NHS Trust, Tavistock and Portman NHS Trust, The Eastman Dental Hospital, The National Hospital for Neurology and Neurosurgery, The Whittington Hospital NHS Trust, University College London Hospitals NHS Foundation Trust

St Bartholomew's and The Royal London School of Medicine and Dentistry

Turner Street, London E1 2AD
Tel: 020 7377 7611 Fax: 020 7377 7612
Website: www.mds.qmul.ac.uk

Dean for Education C G Fowler
Dean for Student Affairs B Colvin
Director of Research and Development T T Macdonald
Deputy Warden and Vice Principal - NHS Liaison P G Kopelman
Warden N A Wright

Recognised Clinical Institutions
Barking and Dagenham Primary Care Trust, Broomfield Hospital, Camden Primary Care Trust, Colchester General Hospital, East London and The City Mental Health NHS Trust, Havering Primary Care Trust, Homerton University Hospital, Islington Primary Care Trust, King George Hospital, Newham General Hospital, North East London Mental Health NHS Trust, Oldchurch Hospital, Princess Alexandra Hospital, Redbridge Primary Care Trust, Southend Hospital, St Bartholomew's Hospital, St Clements Hospital, The London Chest Hospital, The Royal London Hospital, Waltham Forest Primary Care Trust, Wellcome Trust, Whipps Cross University Hospital

St George's Hospital Medical School

Cranmer Terrace, Tooting, London SW17 0RE
Tel: 020 8672 9944 Fax: 020 8767 4696
Website: www.sghms.ac.uk

Principal Michael Farthing
Secretary Catherine Swarbrick

Recognised Clinical Institutions
Springfield Hospital, St George's Healthcare NHS Trust, St Helier Hospital

University of Southampton

Southampton SO17 1BJ
Tel: 023 8059 5000 Fax: 023 8059 4159
Email: medis@soton.ac.uk
Website: www.soton.ac.uk

Vice-Chancellor W Wakeham
Secretary and Registrar J F Lauwerys

School of Medicine

Head of School Iain Cameron

University of London

Senate House, London WC1E 7HU
Tel: 020 7862 8061 Fax: 020 7862 8052
Email: medinfo@lon.ac.uk
Website: www.lon.ac.uk

Vice-Chancellor Graeme Davies
Pro Vice-Chancellor for Medicine and Dentistry Graeme Catto
Secretary and Registrar for Medicine Kim Scrivener

Degrees and diplomas
MB, BS, MD, MS, BMedSci, BDS, MClinDent, MDS, MSc

Schools of the University
Imperial College Faculty of Medicine, Imperial College of Science, Technology and Medicine, Institute of Cancer Research, Royal Cancer Hospital, London School of Hygiene and Tropical Medicine, Queen Mary and Westfield College, School of Pharmacy, Royal Free and University College Medical School of University College London, St Bartholomew's and The Royal London School of Medicine and Dentistry

University of Sheffield

School of Medicine and Biomedical Sciences, Beech Hill Road, Sheffield S10 2RX
Tel: 0114 271 3349 Fax: 0114 271 3960
Website: www.shef.ac.uk/medicine

Dean A P Weetman
Postgraduate Dean S E Thomas
Sub-Dean for Admission A T Raftery
Director for Teaching N D S Bax
Administrative Officers C M Davison, K Dewsnap, J Harrison, K Kehtarnavaz, S Langridge, F Oldale, S L Watkinson
Associate Postgraduate Dean S E Ball, R Cuschieri, G Hood, P C Taylor
Emeritus Honorary Senior Clinical Lecturer A M Wilson
Honorary Clinical Lecturer I Ahmad, P R Beck, S J Bodden, M Boddy, D J Brooks, D T D Bulugahapitiya, J Burke, I Capriapa, C A Chambers, A K Chaudhary, A Chaudhuri, P C Corry, A J Coup, M Cruden, J Devlin, K Doran, A A Dorukhkar, I D Evans, A R W Forrest, S D R Green, D Haigh, A H Hamilton, J G Harris, L Harvey, M M Hassoon, C Haw, S M Herber, J P Hosker, D E Hughes, H M Inch, U Y Joshi, G T Lealman, J Lindsay, S MacDonald, M M Madlom, T Marsh, K McDonald, D M McKenna, B M Mehta, D Merrills, M G Miller, A M B Minford, B W Morris, H S Mulenga, S D Mullins, S O'Connor, H O'Sullivan, G E Parry, K V Phadke, C Pickstone, S Pownall, P M Preece, P J Pugh, E Purt, S A W Salfield, A K Samy, A Sharp, S Shekhar, M A Sills, C M L Smith, A Soliman, R D Start, D Taylor, J Thornton, L A Tierney, R M Tyler, N Ullrich, S Vadodaria, J Walmsley, G L Warren, L H P Williams, S M Wrigley, M N Zaman
Honorary Clinical Teacher F Ashby, K W Bennett, G C S Chow, S Coates, Z M Erza, A K Fletcher, S V Gandhi, S Girgis, P B Goodfellow, A D Hopper, P Hurlstone, S Majumdar, S Nagaraja, K Newton, C Padmakumar, A Rowlands, P Sterling, R Townsend, J M Wilkinson
Honorary Demonstrator I D Marsh
Honorary Lecturer R P Betts, R A D Bunning, J Conway, P R M Dobson, C P Dorries, C J Emery, G S Evans, G S Everson, L Frost, C Griffiths, P A Griffiths, B W Heller, S J Hodges, L Hughes, P M Ingleton, S Kitchen, R G Malia, A M Parfitt, J S Price, W I J Pryce, J Roch, J M Stamp, J C Stevens, W D Tindale, J Unsworth, L Walton, D J Watts, G Wild, C E Wilde, G Wilson, N Y J Woodhouse
Honorary Professor K D Bardham, A M El Nahas, D J Gawkrodger, S Mac Neil, R J Pollit, F E Preston, J T Reilly, M Saleh
Honorary Reader S J Ward
Honorary Research Contract Staff C Anthony, G Brown
Honorary Research Fellow H H Abo-Zenah, Y Al-Bazz, A K Al-Hadari, E Alboraey, K Bata, W H Brown, H Clayson, P Eglestone, M El Kossi, M Eneser, I E Erekosima, H O S Gabra, E George, A Hafiz, R Ireland, K Kosta, Y Kuan, R M Lalla, N Lekka, L L G McAllister, S S Mehta, M Nesbitt, G Parmakis, J L Schoffield, L A Scott, A K Siotia, P A Tate, D J A Thornton, S W Vietch, M Winslow, Y Zhao
Honorary Senior Clinical Lecturer R T Abed, R Ackroyd, N N Acladious, I J Adam, A O Adebajo, J A Adiotomre, N S Ahluwalia, M Akil, M K Al-Bazzaz, M A Al-Malik, F I Al-Modaris, A Al-Mohammad, W Al-Wali, J D Alderson, R B M Ali, L H Alison, A Allahabadia, S N O Amin, R S Amos, A J Anderson, J B Anderson, P B Anderson, J C Andrzejowski, S Anwar, D F J Appleton, T N Appleyard, R Atcheson, C A Austin, I R Ayllon, S Banerjee, F Barampouti, P A Bardsley, H F Barker, I Barker, N A Barrington, N M Barron, G S Basran, K K Basu, P Basumani, N D Bateman, C J Bates, R D E Battersby, D E Bax, A J Baxter, P S Baxter, J D Beard, A P G Beechey, J H Bell, M J Bell, N R Bennett, M C Berthoud, M S Bhamra, H D Bingham, R J S Birks, A Blakeborough, S C Blank, C M Blues, C M Blundell, I I Bolaji, J Bosma, S H Bostock, P Boston, R J Bowes, P C Braidley, A E Brand, C S Brand, D P Breen, J A G Bremner, J Brenchley, P O Brennan, S R Brennan, P Broadley, T M Brotherston, C B Brown, J N Brown, P W G Brown, S R Brown, V A Brown, D C Bryden, S C Buckley, M J Bull, P D Bull, D Burke, J P Burke, P C Bustani, U Butler, S L Caddick, C M Caddy, I C Cameron, S Campbell, I S Carey, T A Carroll, I Chakrabarti, N Chalhoub, D Chan-Lam, T K J Chan, J L Channer, K S Channer, J de l Chaplais, A L N Chapman, D F Chapman, C R Chapple, A K Chattopadyhay, V Chidambaram-Nathan, N Chiverton, L K L Chua, G P M Clark, P D Clark, S J Clark, T J Cleveland, C Clout, N R Coad, J W Coates, S E Cockayne, M C Cohen, A Cole, S C Coley, M Collins, D J A Connolly, M E Connor, J Cook, R C Coombs, A M Cooper, G J Cooper, J R Cooper, I D Crate, F M Creagh, A C Crosby, D R Cullen, Z Currie, P E Cutinha, D F da Costa, D Datta, A J Davidson, A G Davies, C H Davies, G K Davies, H A Davies, N P Davies, L M R Davis-Reynolds, P J de Ville McMullan, A R Dennis, M G Dennison, J Dhawan, G Dilke-Wing, P Dobbs, P M S Dobson,

P D F Dodd, M T Donnelly, T Dorman, D L Douglas, T W Downes, D F Doyle, A K Dube, D G Dujon, K S Dunn, D L Edbrooke, F P Edenborough, M P Edwards, N D Edwards, W Egner, A Eissa, K El-Ghariani, A E Eltrafi, L J Englert, L S Evans, M Evans, M L Everard, F M Fairlie, N J M Fardon, A G Farkas, T A Farrell, K M Feeley, D W Fenton, P A Fenton, C J Ferguson, J A Fernandes, N O J Fernandes, H J Filby, M E Finlay, P M Fisher, A Fitzgerald, M J Flowers, B Foran, D J Fothergill, G A Francis, E Freelander, R Freeman, D Furniss, P A Gaines, P D Gajjar, A Galimberti, S Gatscher, S Gentle, M P Gerrard, S P Gerrish, C J M Getty, H S Ghura, A Gibson, A T Gibson, R Gibson, A M Gillespie, G T Gillett, E Girgis, D C Gleeson, J Goddard, J R Goepel, M Gordon, S B Gordon, E A Y Gouta, S J Gowlett, C Gray, E D Grech, S T Green, R W Griffiths, E R Groves, R A D Grunewald, R Gupta, B Gurtl-Lackner, M Hadjivassiliou, J Hall, M Hamad, A J Hamer, D J Hamer, S Hancock, C A Hardisty, K A Harkness, C L Harper, V Harpin, B J Harrison, D A Harrison, N Harrison, K J Hastie, M Q F Hatton, S K Hawley, M J Heap, T J Hendra, J M Hill, M I Hobson, T J Hodgson, M E Holt, G Hood, D N Hopkinson, J Hornbuckle, A C Howard, S J L Howell, D Hughes, S R Hughes, J E Hunsley, L M Hunt, A Hunter, B J Hutchcroft, S P Hutchinson, A S Ibraheim, C E Ingram, A H M Ismaiel, M A Jabir, V James, S L Jankowski, J A Jarratt, S Jayamaha, D A Jellinek, S B Jenkins, R John, H Jones, S Jones, N Jordan, R H Kandler, J P Kankkunen, K Kapur, M S Karim, A Q Kattak, I A P Keitch, A A Kemeny, R H Keriakos, R M Kerry, M E Kesseler, A A Khan, D G Kiely, G R Kinghorn, P Kirkbride, V Kirkbridge, C Kirton, P E Kitsanta, P Knowles, S R Kohlhardt, A Kumar, S Kurian, O O Ladundoye, I M Lang, P J Lawson-Matthew, R A Lawson, F K T Lee, G Lepski, D P Levy, T C Li, B J Liddle, K Lingham, A Livesey, A J Lobo, T J Locke, S Longstaff, R Lonsdale, R Lord, E Lorenz, P I Macfarlane, C A MacKenzie, A Mackie, A D R Mackie, A E Mackinnon, R M Maclean, A W Majeed, I H Manifold, R Marks, J E Marr, S Marven, S Mason, N J A Massey, P Matthews, S Matthews, A-P T Mayer, M E McAlindon, M R McClelland, P H McCrea, A J G McDonagh, W S McKane, M W McKendrick, A G Messenger, S Michael, J G Miller, G H Mills, J Mohana Murali, A A Mohsini, C A Moore, D J Moore, S K Morcos, S Morley, F P Morris, G D Moss, H S Mudhar, J V B Mundy, I J Murphy, P Murray, R Muthusamy, Y Myint, A Mysore, R Nair, R A Nakielny, A A Naqvi, I Nasr, A H Nassef, V Natarajan, M E Nelson, J P Ng, P Norman, S H Noronha, S H Norris, G D G Oakley, N Oakley, S Odukoya, B Ola, S Orme, M S Osman, L O'Toole, R E Page, A J Parker, G Parker, M Parker, B T Parys, U J Patel, I G Paterson, M E L Paterson, R H Paton, J Peacock, H J Pearson, R G Pease, R J Peck, N F A Peel, I M Pepper, N Pereira, J Perring, S D Pledge, N P Plunkett, D Potter, D R Powell, M K D Prasad, K Price, S Price, A E Procter, M D Pullman, O P K Purohit, O Quarrell, M W R Radarz, S C Radley, D J Radstone, A T Raftery, D R Ralston, S Ramakrishnan, H M Ramsay, D G Rao, G Ravichandran, D S Ray-Chaudhuri, R K Raycjaidhuri, M Reuber, W E G Rhoden, M Richards, M Richmond, E J Ridgway, S A Riley, A Rimmer, D C Rittey, I Roberts, J Roberts, M J Robson, G Rocco, T K Rogers, K E Rogstad, C A J Romanowski, J G Rowe, S L Royston, P A Rundle, T S Z Saba, R A Sabroe, K M Sadler, B T Saeed, J Sahu, F Salim, N C Samaniego, D S Sanders, S Sanghera, S J Saunders, C J Scott, K F Selby, F M Shackley, B Sharrack, M Sharrard, I C Shaw, T C Shaw, R Shawis, R M Sheard, D B Shepherd, A S A Sherif, K M Sherry, M H Shiwani, A J Shorthouse, J R Shortland, B M Shrestha, N Sievewright, M Skelly, P P Skinner, J D Skull, D N Slater, A Smith, D J Smith, J A R Smith, J H F Smith, M F Smith, P D Smith, T W D Smith, M L Snaith, J Snape, J A Snowden, G J Sobey, A S G Soliman, S H Song, L H Soo, A Sprigg, C Stack, D Stanley, T J Stephenson, P Stewart, I Stockley, C J Stoddard, P M Sutton, S K Suvarna, J F Talbot, M D Talbot, D I Taylor, P C Taylor, S Tesfaye, B Tesfayohannes, A L Thomas, M G Thomas, S E Thomas, W E G Thomas, M Thomson, D Throssell, J A Tidy, S H Till, P R Tophill, O P Tungland, C S Tweed, B Vadodaria, G R Q Veall, G S Venables, A Vora, V Vora, J C Wadsley, J Walker, R E Waller, J Wardrope, C W Warren, G C Warren, S A Wasti, S J Webber, J Webster, V J Webster, J C Welch, E A Welchew, C L Welsh, J N F West, J N W West, N M Wheeldon, D J K White, S J Whittaker, J Wigfull, M E Wilkie, G A L Wilkinson, C Wilson, M J A Wilson, S Winder, D A Winfield, J Winfield, J S Witana, M R Withers, M L Wood, D K Woodward, I J Wrench, A M Wright, J G Wright, N P Wright, S R Wright, K Wylie, A Wyman, M P J Yardley, J Yassa, J B Zachary, P M Zadik

Honorary Senior Lecturer D Barnett, J R Bonham, A D Curran, A Harmer
Honorary Senior Research Fellow B L Petheram, S E Roulstone
Honorary Senior Tutor D Pratt
Honorary Teacher G Anderson, V A Binney, E Fitzpatrick, M Graham
Medical Admissions Officer A Berridge
Research Dean R Eastell
School Staffing Officer J Ginn
Secretary to the School of Medicine and Biomedical Sciences H A Shenton
SIFTR Liason Officer G Twelvetree
Undergraduate Dean R E Page, S Peters, J Walker
Visiting Lecturer S Bosjnak
Visiting Professor M Hassanzadeh-Khayyat, L Xiaodong, I R Young
Visiting Reader H S Christensen

Academic Unit of Medical Education

Academic Related S Cowley, M Hague, S M McGregor
Clinical Lecturer S Dubey
Emeritus Professor D I Newble
Honorary Associate Professor N D S Bax
Senior Lecturer C Roberts, P Stark
Senior Technical Staff A Milnes, A Self

Division of Clinical Sciences (North)

Director/Professor of Vascular Biology P G Hellewell, P G Hellewell
Deputy Director/Professor of Bone Metabolism E Eastell, E Eastell
Professor of Cardiology and Head of Section D C Crossman, D C Crossman
Professor of Endocrinology and Head of Section R J M Ross, R J M Ross
Professor of Social Gerontology and Head of Section A M Warnes, A M Warnes
Clinical Lecturer T J Chico, S Choksy, E Kiss-Toth, V Ridger, S B Williams
Clinical Research Fellow A Ahmed, B Ahmed, E Akowuah, S K Bal, P Choudhary, J A Clowes, F Dallas, M S Delbridge, C R Evans, H Fahmy-Ibrahim, A Gordan, A Hadarri, C Hernon, D A Hoad-Reddick, H Fahmy Ibrahim, S Jenkins, A Kamal, Y Kuan, R Lalla, A C Morton, K K Ray, A Salama, P J Sheridan, V Shrivastava, R Ulleggadi, J Walsh
Emeritus Professor D S Munro
Lecturer T N Johnson
National Kidney Research Fund Career Development Fellow A J Streets
Non Clinical Lecturer M E Barker, B M Corfe, C M Gott, K J McKee, C J Parker, E Williams, L Yang
Non Clinical Senior Lecturer J Haylor, P F Watson
Professor Associate J B Young
Professor of Health Care for Elderly People S G Parker, I Philp
Professor of Medicine A P Weetman
Professor of Nephrology A M El Nahas
Professor of Orthopaedic and Traumatic Surgery M Saleh
Professor of Tissue Engineering S MacNeil
Reader P Chan, R S Heller, A G Pockley, H J Powers, A M Ward
Research Associate G Basten, A J Bullock, H Chirakkal, P C Eves, L Ferrar, M Fisher, R A Hannon, L Heung, B Ingle, G Jiang, E H Kemp, M Maamra, E Nakano, K E Naylor, L J Newby, M A Paggiosi, E J Parker, A S Rinomhota, A Rogers, S Saha, L Smith-Thomas, C M Smith, S H Zarkesh-Esfahani
Senior Clinical Lecturer A Blumsohn, S E Francis, S E E Gariballa, J Gunn, M Jennings, J Newell-Price, C H Newman, K E Norman, A Ong, R F Storey
Senior Lecturer B Hocher, E V McCloskey

Cardiovascular Science

Professor of Cardiology and Head of Section D C Crossman
Chief Technician L Shepherd
Clinical Research Fellow S Smith, V Watt, M Wheatcroft
Lecturer E Kiss-Toth
Professor of Immunobiology A G Pockley
Professor of Vascular Biology P G Hellewell
Reader P Chan
Reseach Associate/Fellow J Chamberlain, D J Crosdale, K Jetha, H Judge, A Lawrie, M Marron, V Ridger, R D Walker
Reseach Associate/Fellows K Abbit
Senior Lecturer S E Francis, J Gunn, C H Newman, K E Norman, R F Storey

Human Metabolism

Chief Technician R A Metcalfe
Clinical Research Fellow A Ahmed, B Ahmed, M Y Chang, P Choudhary, J A Clowes, F Dallas, A Gordan, A Hadarri, H Fahmy Ibrahim, S Jenkins, A Kamal, Y Kuan, R Lalla, M P Revell, J Walsh
Emeritus Professor D S Munro
Lecturer M E Barker, B M Corfe, E Williams, L Yang
Professor of Bone Metabolism R Eastell
Professor of Medicine A P Weetman
Professor of Nephrology A M El Nahas
Professor of Nutritional Biochemistry H J Powers
Professor of Tissue Engineering S Mac Neil
Reader S R Heller
Research Administrator K Dobson
Research Associate A J Bullock, N R Bullock, H Chirakkal, P C Eves, L Ferrar, M Fisher, R A Hannon, L Huang, G Jiang, E H Kemp, S H Leech, M Maamra, D Moon, E Nakano, K E Naylor, L J Newby, M A Paggiosi, E Parker, A S Rinomhota, A Rogers, L Smith-Thomas, A J Streets, E L Stuart, S H Zarkesh-Esfahani
Senior Fellow T S Johnson
Senior Lecturer A Blumsohn, J Haylor, J Newell-Price, A C M Ong, P F Watson
Senior Nurse D Swindell

Division of Clinical Sciences (South)

Head of Technical Services J K Beresford
Deputy Non-Clinical Director L Lennard
Divisional Manager D Thwaites
Professor and Director of Division F C Hamdy
Professor and Deputy Clinical Director C S Reilly
Secretary to the Divisional Director and Academic Unit of Urology C Stenton
Technical Manager A Gregory, P D Henderson, C Nichols, J N Scaife

Academic Unit of Urology

Professor of Urology and Head of Unit F C Hamdy
Clinical Lecturer in Urology J W F Catto
Emeritus Professor of Medicine J D Ward
Emeritus Professor of Obstetrics and Gynaecology I D Cooke
Emeritus Professor of Surgery A G Johnson
Lecturer in Urology I Rehman
Research Staff R Bryant, N A Cross, D Yates
Senior Clinical Lecturer in Urology D J P Rosario
Senior Lecturer in Urological Sciences C L Eaton

Anaesthesia

Professor of Anaesthesia and Head of Unit C S Reilly
Lecturer in Anaesthesia and Microcirculation Z Brookes
Research Associate A Mansart
Senior Lecturer in Anaesthesia J Ross

Bone Biology

Professor of Bone Biology and Head of Unit P I Croucher
Research Fellow C H Buckle, K Still
Senior Research Scientist L Coulton

Child Health

Professor of Paediatric Bone Disease and Head of Unit N J Bishop
Clinical Lecturer in Paediatric Haematology R E Hough
Clinical Lecturer in Paediatrics L P Abbott
Clinical Research Fellow A Abdelhamid, P J Dimitri
Lecturer in Bone Biology P S Grabowski
Lecturer in Cell Biology R Muimo
Professor of Paediatric Gastroenterology C J Taylor
Professor of Paediatrics M S Tanner
Research Staff N J Beauchamp, L Hobson, J McGaw, S Y Ng
Senior Clinical Lecturer in Endocrinology J K H Wales
Senior Clinical Lecturer in Respiratory Medicine R A Primhak

Clinical Pharmacology

Professor of Molecular Pharmacology and Pharmacogenetics and Head of Unit G T Tucker
Lecturer S W Ellis, K Rowland-Yeo
Reader in Clinical Pharmacology and Therapeutics P R Jackson
Reader in Pharmacology G G S Collins, L Lennard, M S Lennard
Research Staff E A G Demoncheaux, E J Wallis
Senior Clinical Lecturer W W Yeo
Senior Lecturer in Pharmacology P T Peachell, A Rostami-Hodjegan

Medical Physics and Clinical Engineering

Professor and Head of Unit P D Griffiths
Lecturer J W Fenner
Professor of Medical Physics B H Brown
Professors Associate D C Barber, A T Barker
Research Staff R H Ireland, D M Jones, R Mehrem, P Milnes, A Narracott, J Van Der Meulen, D Walter, A Waterworth
Senior Lecturer D R Hopse, P V Lawford

Ophthalmology and Orthoptics

Professor of Opthalmology and Head of Unit I G Rennie
Lecturer in Opthalmology and Orthoptics R M Bhola, D Buckley, A Y Firth, H Griffiths, P D F Keating, C M Leach, K Sisley
Senior Clinical Lecturer in Opthalmic Pathology M A Parsons
Senior Lecturer in Orthoptics H Davis

Palliative Medicine

Professor of Palliative Medicine S H Ahmedzai
Research Staff N Ahmed
Senior Lecturer in Palliative Medicine T W Noble

Radiology

Professor of Academic Radiology and Head of Unit P D Griffiths
Lecturer in MR Physics K Lee
Professor of MR Physics M N J Paley
Reader in MR Physics I D Wilkinson
Senior Clinical Lecturer in Radiology S M Thomas, E Whitby
Senior Lecturer in MR Physics J M Wild

Reproductive and Developmental Medicine

Professor of Obstetrics and Gynaecology and Head of Unit W L Ledger
Clinical Fellow in Assisted Conception and Reproductive Surgery M McIlveen
Clinical Lecturer S Amer
Clinical Research Fellow G Ahmad
Lecturer A Fazeli, K Martin
Professor of Reproductive Biology H D M Moore
Reader R B Fraser
Senior Lecturer D O C Anumba, H Lashen
Senior Lecturer in Andrology A Pacey
Senior Secretary V Aram

Sports Medicine

Professor of Sports Medicine and Head of Unit C G Rolf
Senior Lecturer in Tissue Engineering A M Scutt

Surgical Oncology

Professor and Head of Academic Surgery and Head of Unit M W R Reed
Professor and Head of Microcirculation Research Group N J Brown
Clinical Lecturer in Surgical Oncology S P Balasubramanian
Lecturer D Mangnall
Lecturer in Surgical Oncology and Microcirculation Studies C A Staton
Lecturer in Surgical Sciences N C Bird
Research Staff L Burn, L J Caldon, S Hankin, D Wilde
Senior Clinical Lecturer in Surgical Oncology L Wyld
Senior Secretary A Duffes

Division of Genomic Medicine

Acting Divisional Superintendent K M Oxley
Deputy Superintendent K P Corke, C A Day
Divisional Superintendent J D Thomis
Professor of Clinical Oncology and Deputy Clinical Director of Division B W Hancock
Professor of Molecular Medicine and Director of Division G W Duff
Professor of Molecular Medicine and Deputy Non-Clinical Director of Division I R Peake
Senior Technical Staff S Bottomley, A Clegg, I Geary, L Goodwin, H Holden, I Newsome, A Platts, S Rodgers, H J Senior, R Stewart

Functional Genomics

Professor of Molecular Immunology and Head of Section S K Dower
Emeritus Professor in Medical Microbiology R Jennings
Lecturer F A Guesdon, S A Renshaw, J Shaw, A J Tunbridge
Professor I W Henderson, J R Sayers
Professor in Cell Bilology E E Qwarnström
Professor in Cell Signalling and Endocrinology B L Brown
Professor of Respiratory Medicine M K B Whyte
Reader D J Buttle, D Fishwick, A W Heath, I Sabroe
Research Assistant E Jones
Research Associate/Fellow L Bingle, J Carling-Wright, D T Y Chang, A Crawford, C D Ellis, P M Ingleton, D L Jack, R D Jones, H M Marriott, L C Parker, A C Pridmore, L Prince, S Vitovski, H L Wilson
Research Nurse S Naylor
Senior Lecturer C D Bingle, P R M Dobson, D Dockrell, A R Eley, M S Thomas

Genetics and Informatics

Professor of Academic Clinical Psychiatry and Head of Academic Clinical Psychiatry P W R Woodruff
Professor of Mathematics and Informatics and Head of Section C Cannings
Clinical Lecturer in Psychiatry P B Birkett, M Hunter, N Mir, T Y D Tsoi
Computer Systems Support Officer in Psychiatry M Brook
Honorary Professor of Dermatology D J Gawkrodger
Lecturer A J Grierson, N M Hunkin, J Kirby, D Mewar, P N Monk, J Nasir, R Tazi-Ahnini, M D Teare, K Walters, P R Winship, J D Wood
Lecturers in Psychiatry T F D Farrow, K Lee
Office Manager in Psychiatry B Nesbitt
Professor Associate in Haematology F E Preston
Professor of Molecular Medicine I R Peake
Professor of Neurology P J Shaw
Reader M J Cork, A C Goodeve, M Makris, A G Wilson
Reader in General Adult Psychiatry S A Spence
Research Assistant A Western
Research Associate/Fellow S Allen, M P Birch, S Blake, S Bond, A Brockington, V Ganesan, S Hague, P Heath, J Henderson, A Higginbottom, C J Hughes, J Shepherd, J Simpson, C Wood-Allum
Research Data Manager A Humphrey, R Le Grys
Research Nurse S Dawson, K Dobson, A Hinch, J McDermott, H Nixon, S Ryles, T Walsh
Senior Clinical Lecturer in Neuropsychology R Parks
Senior Lecturer O Bandmann, M E Daly, F S di Giovine, K K Hampton, M Nicklin
Senior Lecturer in Psychiatry/Undergraduate Clinical Tutor S Peters
Undergraduate Asministrator in Psychiatry S Turvey

Oncology and Pathology

Professor of Molecular and Cellular Pathology and Head of Section C E Lewis
Acting Research Network Co-ordinator L J Bruce
Cancer Research Centre Co-ordinator W Wilson
Clinical Trials Co-ordinator S Browne, R Burkinshaw, L Turner
Data Manager, Clinical Oncology R Bell, L Birch, J Bliss, M Cooper, R Else, C E Jones, T Khanna, J E Martindale, H Wood
Data Manager, Institute for Cancer Studies D Connley
Emeritus Professor J A Kanis
Lecturer M D Barker, J E Brown, J L Burton, J P Bury, C M Sanders, Y M Zhu
Professor of Cellular Genetics M Meuth
Professor of Clinical Chemistry A R W Forrest
Professor of Clinical Oncology B W Hancock
Professor of Forensic Pathology C M Milroy
Professor of Gynaecological Pathology M Wells
Professor of Medical Oncology R E Coleman, P J Woll
Professor of Neuropathology P Ince
Professor of Pathology J C E Underwood
Research Associate/Fellow O Al-Assar, S Bagstaff, J Coleman, K Dyker, L Elbarghati, S P Ellis, A Giannoudis, D Greenfield, S Gutcher, G Horsburgh, J Horsmann, E Katerinaki, J Lester, C Murdoch, H L Neville-Webbe, K Palmer, C Radstone, E Smith, C Wood
Research Nurse Manager F Armitage
Research Radiographers - Clinical Oncology C Anthony, G Brown, P Campbell, J Swinscoe, C Wilcock
Research Sister/Nurse H Beadle, J Bickerstaff, A Clarke, M Cooper-Dore, H Cramp, E Green, F Horwell, J Hutchinson, N M James, G A Jones, P Joyce, D Lucas, K Nicholson, L Reaney, V Spawton, D Stanton, G Tomlinson, M Trigg, S Turton, K Williams
Senior Lecturer A Cox, S S Cross, T Helleday, I Holen, M Marples, M H Robinson, S B Wharton

Scotland

University of Aberdeen

College of Life Sciences and Medicine, Polwarth Building, Foresterhill, Aberdeen AB25 2ZD
Tel: 01224 551249 Fax: 01224 550708
Email: infoclsm@abdn.ac.uk
Website: www.abdn.ac.uk/clsm

Head of College and Vice-Principal, College of Life Sciences and Medicine Neva Haites

University of Dundee

Faculty of Medicine, Dentistry & Nursing, Level 10, Ninewells Hospital & Medical School, Dundee DD1 9SY
Tel: 01382 632640 Fax: 01382 496391
Email: medschoff@dundee.ac.uk
Website: www.dundee.ac.uk/facmedden/meddemo.htm

Dean of Medicine Brian Burchell
Faculty Secretary W M Williamson

Biomedical Research Centre

Director C R Wolf
Lecturer D J Jamieson, B M McStay
Reader J D Hayes
Senior Lecturer T H Friedburg

Centre for Medical Education

Tay Park House, 484 Perth Road, Dundee DD2 1LR
Tel: 01382 631972 Fax: 01382 645748

Director R M Harden
Hon. Lecturer R Neil, R H Richardson
Lecturer Pauline Horton, Margaret Kindlen, J McAleer
Senior Lecturer M Davis, E C B Rogerson

Clinical Skills Centre

Director Jean Ker

Dental School and Hospital

Park Place, Dundee DD1 4HN

Hon. Lecturer A J Crighton, J Levitt, S Manton, A Neilson, C J Tilley
Hon. Senior Lecturer C J Allan, J D Clark, E Connor, C M Jones, I J McClure, M C W Merrett, A Shearer
Lecturer G Bateman, K Davey, J Foley, A Forgie, R V Hunter, P McGoldrick, M Macluskey, P Maillou, A G Mason, D N J Ricketts, S N Scrimgeour, F M J Stewart, C Tait
Professor D M Chisholm, G R Ogden, C Pine, N B Pitts, W P Saunders, S L Schor, D R Stirrups
Reader C H Lloyd, P A Mossey, N M Nuttall, A M Schor
Secretary to Dental School J D M Gray
Senior Lecturer S W Cadden, R G Chadwick, J E Clarkson, J R Drummond, R Duguid, D J P Evans, A D Gilbert, C Longbottom, J P Newton, J R Radford, E M Saunders, B J J Scott

Faculty of Medicine, Dentistry and Nursing

Level 10, Ninewells Hospital & Medical School, Dundee DD1 9SY
Tel: 01382 660111 ext: 2763 Fax: 01382 644267

Dean of Dentistry W P Saunders
Dean of Medicine Brian Burchell
Postgraduate Dean R Newton
Faculty Secretary W M Williamson

Anaesthesia

Hon. Senior Lecturer C W Allison, R H Allison, J Bannister, P A Coe, J Colvin, D M Coventry, S A Crofts, L Duncan, I G Gray, I G Grove-White, W F D Hamilton, A Houghton, T Houston, G L Hutchinson, W McClymont, N Mackenzie, W A Macrae, P R Manthri, M K Milne, A Ratcliff, A J Shearer, M F Thomson, E Wilson
Lecturer M R Checketts
Professor J A W Wildsmith
Senior Lecturer G A McLeod, F A Millar

Anatomy and Physiology

Head of Department M R Ward
Lecturer K N Christie, J R Elliott, A A Harper, J M Lucocq, P M Taylor, P W Watt
Professor E B Lane, C G Proud, M J Rennie, R R Sturrock, C A Tickle, J G Williams
Senior Lecturer A R Chipperfield, D L Dawson, G C Leslie, N J Part, C J Weiser
Senior Manager M R Ward

Biochemical Medicine

Hon. Assistant W A Bartlett, H G Clark, J Scott
Hon. Lecturer J B C Dick, J Evans, I Hanning, J P Moody, L M Nelson, K Tebbutt
Hon. Senior Lecturer C G Fraser, R Hume
Lecturer I J Holt
Professor B Burchell
Senior Lecturer J D Baty, M Cougtrie, C R Paterson

Biochemistry

Hon. Lecturer Elizabeth Carey, C Higgins, M A Kerr, M Lewis, G Warren
Lecturer G C Barr, M Ferguson, A J Flavell, S Homans, R Quinlan, M Stark, C Watts
Professor D H Boxer, P Cohen, C Downes, D Glover, D Lane, D Lilley, D Nicholls
Reader D Hardie
Senior Lecturer R Booth, P Cohen, J C Kernohan, D A Stansfield

Cardiovascular Epidemiology Unit

Director H Tunstall Pedoe
Hon. Lecturer S Somerville

Child Health

Hon. Lecturer S Dewar, P Fowlie, A Kurian, A McKinnon, J Mires, R A Wilkie
Hon. Senior Lecturer J S Forsyth, S A Greene, Valerie J Marrian, D C S Theodosiou, J A Young
Lecturer S Mukhopadhyay
Professor R Hume, R E Olver
Senior Lecturer J I Cater, H J McArdle, A Mehta

Dermatology

Hon. Senior Lecturer J Ferguson, C M Green, K J A Kenicer, J G Lowe, S Morley

Diagnostic Radiology

Hon. Lecturer N McConachie
Hon. Senior Lecturer J D Begg, W J A Gibson, K Hasan, A S McCulloch, J W McNab, R H S Murray, M Nimmo, J W Shaw, J Tainsh, A Thompson, C M Walker

Epidemiology and Public Health

Health Services Research Co-ordinator B Williams
Hon. Senior Lecturer K Adam, D Coid, M Kenicer, Z Mathewson, A J Tannahill
Lecturer S Ogston, F L R Williams
Professor I Crombie
Senior Lecturer P James

Forensic Medicine

Hon. Lecturer J A Dunbar, J A S Mitchell
Hon. Senior Lecturer D Marshall
Professor D J Pounder
Senior Lecturer D W Sadler

General Practice

Hon. Lecturer D Blaney, J Grant, R A Hendry, A D McKendrick, D H R Mowat, A Ramsay, A D Shaw
Hon. Senior Lecturer R F Scott
Professor D J G Bain, F Sullivan
Senior Lecturer D Snadden

Haematology

Hon. Senior Lecturer P G Cachia, A Heppleston
Professor M J Pippard
Senior Lecturer D T Bowen

Medical Microbiology

Hon. Sen. Clinical Teacher Paul G McIntyre
Hon. Senior Lecturer Gillian Valerie Orange, Gabby Phillips
Lecturer Bernard W Senior
Senior Registrar David A Hill
Senior Clinical Lecturer Jay Kavi

Medical Physics

Director of Medical Physics R A Lerski
Hon. Lecturer D K Harrison, N S J Kennedy, B W Millar, W W Stewart, D Sutton, F M Tulley
Hon. Senior Lecturer R A Lerski

Medicine
Hon. Assistant A Munishankarappa
Hon. Lecturer J Blair, B Dymock, U K Ghosh, M S R MacEwan, R J Swingler, C J A Thompson
Hon. Professor R T Jung, R W Newton
Hon. Senior Lecturer T S Callaghan, R A Clark, A A Connacher, D L W Davidson, D P Dhillon, A Forster, A J France, J D Fulton, W Gray, J L Hanslip, I S Henderson, J M Leiper, I M Lightbody, G P McNeill, R S McWalter, K D Morley, W J Mutch, D Nathwani, T H Pringle, T Pullar, D Shaw, A N Shepherd, P J Stephen, Joyce M Watson, J H Winter
Lecturer F G Inglis, M McLaren
Professor J J Belch, C D Forbes
Senior Lecturer M McMurdo, R C Roberts, P E Ross, H Tunstall-Pedoe

Molecular and Cellular Pathology
Head of Department Martin J Pippard
Hon. Senior Lecturer P G Cachia, A Heppleston
Senior Lecturer D T Bowen
Senior Manager Martin J Pippard

Neurosurgery
Head of Department M S Eljamel
Hon. Senior Lecturer M S Eljamel, Peter Mathew, T R K Varma

Obstetrics and Gynaecology
Hon. Lecturer J K Gupta, G J Mires
Hon. Senior Lecturer P Agustsson, R Allen, J A Mills, N K B Patel, W D P Phillips, R Smith, M A R Thomson
Lecturer C H Brierley
Professor A Burchell
Reader I D Duncan

Ophthalmology
Head C MacEwan
Clinical Research Fellow A D Brown
Hon. Senior Lecturer P S Baines, J A Coleiro, S T D Roxburgh, K H Weed, J D H Young
Lecturer J P Craig
Secretary Lynda Rose

Orthopaedics and Traumatic Surgery
Head of Department David I Rowley
Emeritus Professor G Murdoch
Hon. Lecturer G I Bardsley, C A Kirkwood, J R Linskell, C P U Stewart, D E Young
Hon. Senior Lecturer J R Buckley, D N Condie, A J Espley, W A Hadden, A S Jain, J E Scullion, M M Sharma, A J G Swanson, N W Valentine
Lecturer M J Dolan, G G McLeod
Professor D I Rowley
Senior Lecturer J Dent

Otolaryngology
Hon. Senior Lecturer R L Blair, J K Brennand, B C Davis, J Irwin, R P Mills, R Mountain, P S White

Pathology
Hon. Lecturer A Baird, M Boxer, K T Evans, B A Spruce, W W Stewart
Hon. Senior Lecturer D R Goudie, K Hussein, J Lang, S Lang, J B McCullough, B A Michie, S M Nicoll, A J Robertson
Lecturer J Woof
Professor S Fleming, D Levison
Reader D Hopwood, M A Kerr
Senior Lecturer M J W Faed, R A Kay

Pharmacology and Clinical Pharmacology
Hon. Lecturer G R Barclay, T R P Dodd, D A Johnston, A M MacConnachie, T A Moreland
Hon. Professor C Pennington
Hon. Senior Lecturer D MacLean, F E Murray
Hon. Tutor D M Shepherd
Lecturer K C Breen, B Lipworth, R J McFadyen, N M Wheeldon
Professor J Lambert, D G McDevitt, J McEwen, D G Nicholls, I H Stevenson, A D Struthers
Reader D J K Balfour, P Davey
Senior Lecturer G Lyles, T M McDonald, J Peters

Psychiatry
Head Ian C Reid
Emeritus Professor G W Fenton
Hon. Lecturer Joan Clark, M Guthrie, S E Hopwood, M M Semple, P Walker
Hon. Senior Lecturer Constance B Ballinger, S E Bonnar, I Clark, S Clark, P Connelly, P H Dick, M A Field, D J Findlay, B B Johnston, K M G Keddie, Anne M McHarg, A H Reid, P Rice, B M Shepherd, Anne H W Smith, C Smith, D Tait, L Treliving, P J Walker, A J Yellowlees
Lecturer D A Reid
Professor K Matthews, Ian C Reid
Senior Lecturer David Coghill, R C Durham, D R May, C de B White

Radiotherapy and Oncology
Hon. Senior Lecturer S Das, J A Dewar, P M Windsor

Surgery
Hon. Senior Lecturer K Baxby, D J Byrne, A I G Davidson, J C Forrester, A D Irving, M Lavelle-Jones, M H Lyall, P T McCollum, A M Morris, W J G Murray, J H Stevenson, P A Stonebridge, W H Townell, R A B Wood
Lecturer T G Frank, E L Newman, E L Newman
Professor A Cuschieri, D Lane, R J C Steele
Senior Lecturer S M Shimi, A M Thomson

Recognised Clinical Institutions
Monklands Hospital, Murray Royal Hospital, Ninewells Hospital, Perth Royal Infirmary, Queen Margaret Hospital, Raigmore Hospital, Royal Dundee Liff Hospital, St John's Hospital, St Luke's Hospital, Stirling Royal Infirmary, Stracathro Hospital, Stratheden Hospital, Sunnyside Royal Hospital, The James Cook University Hospital, West Cumberland Hospital

University of Edinburgh

College of Medicine and Veterinary Medicine, Research Institute, 47 Little France Crescent, Edinburgh EH16 4TJ
Tel: 0131 650 1000
Website: www.mvm.ed.ac.uk

Vice Principal and Head of College J S Savill
College Registrar L Golightley

Directorate of Undergraduate Learning and Teaching

Director/Senior Lecturer A D Cumming

Learning Technology
Director D G Dewhurst

Medical Teaching Organisation
Director H Cameron
Professor of Medical Ethics K M Boyd
Senior Lecturer P Warren

NHS Education Scotland
Postgraduate Dean S G Macpherson

School of Biomedical and Clinical Laboratory Sciences

Head of School D H Crawford

Division of Biomedical Sciences
Head of Division M J Shipston
Hon. Professor V van Heyningen
Hon. Senior Lecturer R R Meehan
Lecturer M W Simmen
Professor A Aitken, J B L Bard, M H Kaufman, G Leng, D J Price, J A Russell
Reader J A Davies, N R Spears
Senior Lecturer R H Ashley, M A Cousin, A Douglas, M B Dutia, D Ellis, G S Findlater, P W Flatman, G Gray, A C Hall, P Kind, M Ludwig, S K Maciver, N K MacLeod, J O Mason, I L Megson, I A Nimmo, N L Poyser, N H Wilson

Division of Medical Microbiology
Head of Division I R Poxton
Clinical Lecturer I Johannessen, O L Moncayo
Clinical Teacher M F Hanson
Hon. Clinical Senior Lecturer P Kalima, I F Laurenson, J Petrik, E Williamson
Hon. Senior Lecturer G R Barclay, S M Burns, H A Cubie, W Donachie, A P Gibb
Professor S G B Amyes, D H Crawford, P Ghazal, J R W Govan, P Simmonds
Reader S J Talbot
Senior Lecturer J Stewart

Division of Neuroscience
Head of Division A J Harmar
Lecturer P Larkman, P Skehel, E Wood, D Wyllie
Professor G W Arbuthnott, S.G.N. Grant, D S McQueen, J McCulloch, R G M Morris
Reader R R Ribchester
Senior Lecturer F Kristmundsdottir, H J Olverman
Wellcome Trust Lecturer K Horsburgh

School of Clinical Sciences and Community Health

Head of School O James Garden

Division of Clinical and Surgical Sciences, Accident and Emergency Medicine (Surgical Sciences Section)
Clinical Tutor P Freeland
Hon. Clinical Senior Lecturer A J Oglesby
Hon. Professor C Robertson
Hon. Senior Lecturer A J Gray, R G Mitchell, D J Steedman

Division of Clinical and Surgical Sciences, Anaesthesia, Critical Care and Pain Medicine (Surgical Sciences Section)
Clinical Teacher L M Alridge, I R Armstrong, F E Arnstein, D Beamish, G M R Bowler, D T Brown, A S Buchan, D Burke, V A Clark, T P Cripps, M J Cullen, J A Freeman, I S Grant, D J Henderson, I N Hudson, J Jenkins, G Jones, G M A Keenan, D G Littlewood, M R Logan, A F McCrae, J N Montgomery, A D Morley, C P J Morton, S M Nimmo, A J Pollok, G C Pugh, D A Rowney, M L C Rutledge, D H T Scott, G H Sharwood-Smith, E J Simon, D L Simpson, C J Sinclair, D Watson, K J Watson, D Weir, D J Wright, C H Young
Hon. Fellow R D F Forbes, N A Malcolm-Smith, W S Nimmo, B Tiplady
Hon. Senior Lecturer I T Foo, K P Kelly, A Lee, J H McClure, S J Mackenzie, D W McKeown, S Midgley, A F Nimmo, D C Ray, D Semple, A V G Stewart
Lecturer J A Wilson
Professor I Power
Pt. Reader P J D Andrews
Pt. Senior Lecturer R P Alston, L A Colvin, N J Maran, C Moores, D Swann, T S Walsh
Senior Lecturer G B Drummond

Division of Clinical and Surgical Sciences, Cardiac Surgery (Surgical Sciences Section)
Clinical Tutor E W J Cameron, C Campanella
Hon. Clinical Senior Lecturer E T Brackenbury
Hon. Senior Lecturer W S Walker
Pt. Senior Lecturer P Mankad

Division of Clinical and Surgical Sciences, Geriatric Medicine (Locomotor Sciences Section)
Clinical Teacher P J Beaugang, J Bishop-Miller, N C Chapman, A K Datta, J B Godfrey, A C Grant, D Grant, A D Jamieson, S B Kulkarni, R J Lenton, H MacMillan, P A Maguire, E Millar, P S Murdoch, C A Norris, S E Pound, G B Rhind, S J Smith, I C Stewart, J A Wilson
Hon. Senior Lecturer B J Chapman, N R Colledge, A T Elder, D L Farquhar, I F C Hay, D C Kennie, E MacDonald, L G Morrison, S G Ramsay, I J D Scougal
Professor A Young
Pt. Senior Lecturer P D Syme
Reader J M Starr
Senior Lecturer C T Currie
Senior lecturer G Mead

Division of Clinical and Surgical Sciences, Hepatology/Gastroenterology/Renal (Internal Medicine Section)
Head of Division A N Turner
Clinical Teacher D A S Jenkins, W S J Ruddell, J Wilson
Hon. Professor B M Frier
Hon. Senior Lecturer R W Crofton, J Goddard, A J MacGilchrist, J N Plevris, C P Swainson, K C Trimble, M L Watson, C E Whitworth, R Winney, S M Wood
Lecturer T E S Delahooke, J J Neary
Professor C D Gregory, P C Hayes, J S Savill
Professor, Renal A D Cumming
Pt. Senior Lecturer D B L McClelland, P L Yap
Senior Lecturer H Brash, D C Kluth, R G Phelps, K J Simpson

Division of Clinical and Surgical Sciences, Ophthalmology (Surgical Sciences Section)
Clinical Teacher A H Adams, G G McIlwaine
Hon. Fellow P A Aspinall
Hon. Senior Lecturer A Azuara-Blanco, B J Dhillon, B W Fleck, J Singh, M R Wright

Division of Clinical and Surgical Sciences, Orthopaedic Surgery (Locomotor Sciences Section)
Clinical Teacher I C Brenkel, T I S Brown, R Burnett, R A Buxton, G M Lawson, R J M MacDonald, J C McGregor, I G C Weir
Hon. Senior Lecturer I H Annan, J Christie, G Hooper, C R Howie, M J McMaster, R W Nutton, D Purdi, J Robb
Professor C M Court-Brown, A H R Simpson
Pt. Senior Lecturer S Breusch, J N A Gibson, J F Keating, M F MacNicol, M M McQueen, C W Oliver
Senior Lecturer D E Porter, C M Robinson

Division of Clinical and Surgical Sciences, Otolaryngology (Surgical Sciences Section)
Hon. Fellow M J O Clark, B A B Dale
Hon. Senior Lecturer David L Cowan, W E Grant, A I G Kerr, S Moralee, R J Sanderson, D W Sim
Pt. Senior Lecturer R P Mills

Division of Clinical and Surgical Sciences, Rehabilitation Medicine (Locomotor Sciences Section)
Pt. Senior Lecturer B Pentland, I C Todd

Division of Clinical and Surgical Sciences, Surgery (Surgical Sciences Section)
Clinical Teacher K C Ballantyne, G G P Browning, T Daniel, R Diggory, J M Gollock, R Halpin, M Hehir, M A Hosny, D Lee, J A E MacDonald, J S O'Neill, A A Quaba, R C Smith
Hon. Clinical Senior Lecturer D N Anderson, J Casey, T J Crofts, B R Tulloh
Hon. Fellow M Schindl

Hon. Senior Lecturer M Akyol, T J Crofts, A C De Beaux, J L R Forsythe, A Howd, K Madhaven, S Paterson-Brown, J B Rainey, J D Watson
Lecturer I Currie, A Tambyraja
Professor K C H Fearon, O J Garden, W R Miller
Reader J A Ross
Senior Lecturer L P Marson, R W Parks, S J Wigmore

Division of Clinical and Surgical Sciences, Vascular Surgery (Surgical Sciences Section)

Clinical Teacher W A Abdel-Razik, A D Al-Asadi, A A Milne
Hon. Senior Lecturer R T A Chalmers, S C A Fraser, J A Murie, Z Raza

Division of Community Health Sciences, General Practice Section

Head of Division D Weller
Clinical Teacher D Andrews, R Balfour, C B Bickler, Neil Black, A L M Currie, A Curtis, D W Ewart, D H Gillespie, W D Gorman, I S Johnston, M A Keith, G Leckie, F H Lossock, D Macaulay, I M McCulloch, P P McGavigan, L G McIntosh, I McKay, Helen F MacKinnon, J A McLaren, A P W McNutt, James M McCallum, C H Oliver, Dean G Pope, A G Reid, H J Rodgers, E D Russell-Smith, R Scott, D G Selman, I S M Smart, D Taylor, S A Tothill, W Treasure, M W Wilson, A P Wood
Hon. Senior Lecturer K J Boyd, A Brimelow, R I Dickson, J L Dunn, M J Ferguson, F O George, J Gillies, M A Grubb, A H McIntosh, A Mackay, G M McPartlin, L M Myskow, H E Ross, C J Sykes, R J Williams
Senior Lecturer K Fairhurst, S A Murray, A M D Porter, A A Sinclair, D Thomson

Division of Community Health Sciences, Public Health Sciences Section

Clinical Teacher A M A Bisset, T Cattermole, D R Gorman, S Payne, P Upton, A M Wallace
Clinical Tutor M J Douglas, L J C Graham
Hon. Fellow Leslie Alexander
Hon. Professor P Donnelly
Hon. Senior Lecturer M Bain, D M Brewster, L Burley, J W T Chalmers, G M Fletcher, A Mordue, H J T Ward, J G Wrench
Lecturer N Anderson, Angus Bancroft, N Hallowell, Jackie Price
Professor F E Alexander, R S Bhopal, H Campbell, F G R Fowkes, G D Murray, R J Prescott
Reader A Amos, S Cunningham-Burley
Senior Lecturer J F Forbes, P E Warner, S Wild

Division of Medical and Radiology Sciences, Cardiovascular Research Section

Head of Division K A A Fox
Hon. Senior Lecturer P Bloomfield, N Boon, A D Flapan, N Grubb, E H Horn, R J Kellett, D Northridge, T.R.D. Shaw, I R Starkey
Professor K A A Fox, C A Ludlam, J J Mullins
Pt. Senior Lecturer N G Uren
Senior Lecturer M A Denvir, D E Newby, R A Riemersma

Division of Medical and Radiology Sciences, Dermatology Section

Clinical Teacher R D Aldridge, V Doherty, G M Kavanagh, O M V Schofield
Hon. Fellow J A A Hunter
Hon. Senior Lecturer E C Benton
Professor J L Rees
Pt. Senior Lecturer M J Tidman
Senior Lecturer R P Weller

Division of Medical and Radiology Sciences, Medical Physics Section

Hon. Reader P R Hoeking
Hon. Senior Lecturer W J Hannan
Lecturer M E Bastin
Professor W Norman McDicken
Reader I Marshall

Division of Medical and Radiology Sciences, Medical Radiology Section

Clinical Teacher R D Adam, P S Bailey, I Beggs, S E Chambers, M E Chapman, M S Fleet, R J Gibson, D C Grieve, G M A Hendry, H L MacDonald, S Mackenzie, M McPhillips, H A McRitchie, S A Moussa, I Parker, J H Reid, L M Smart, A J M Stevenson, J S J Walsh
Hon. Senior Lecturer I N Gillespie, S Ingram, K.D.P. McBride, G McKillop, J T Murchison, D Patel, I Prossor, D Redhead, C M Turnbull, J Walker, A J A Wightman
Professor J J K Best
Pt. Senior Lecturer P L Allan, D A Collie, R J Sellar

Division of Medical and Radiology Sciences, Respiratory Medicine Section

Clinical Teacher J Gaddie, R S Gray, W G Middleton, D B Morrison
Hon. Professor J R Lamb
Hon. Senior Lecturer D Bell, P J Leslie, T Mackay, A W Patrick, A D Toft, J D Walker, S.C Wright, M J Young
Lecturer I Fairbairn
Professor N J Douglas, C Haslett, W MacNee, J Mullins, T J Sethi
Reader I B Dransfield
Senior Lecturer S Hart, N Hirani, A J B Simpson

Division of Reproductive and Developmental Sciences, Child Life and Health Section (Including Neonatology)

20 Sylvan Place, Edinburgh EH9 1UW
Tel: 0131 536 0690 Fax: 0131 536 0821
Clinical Teacher I A Abu-Arafeh, S B Ainsworth, M Aldoori, S Bloomfield, J W Cresswell, D E Goh, A M Grant, J Grigor, S E Ibhanesebhor, Lindsay Logie, M Loudon, U M Macfadyen, A C F Margerison, F D Munro, B Norton, J M Ritchie, L A Ross, C R Steer, J Stephen, L Stewart, D C S Theodosiou, R B Thomson, D E Valentine
Hon. Clinical Senior Lecturer P D Jackson
Hon. Senior Lecturer T F Beattie, D C Brown, J Burns, A J Burt, Z M Dunhill, P Eunson, F C M Forbes, Peter Gillett, H F Hammond, D A Johnson, A Lyon, D N Manders, T G Marshall, G Menon, J D Orr, R M Simpson, A Thomas
Lecturer A J Drake
Professor N McIntosh
Pt. Reader C J H Kelnar
Pt Senior Lecturer S Cunningham, I Laing, J Mok, A O'Hare, B J Stenson, W H Wallace, D Wilson-Storey
Senior Lecturer P Hoare, G A Mackinley, P Midgley, R A Minns, D C Wilson

Division of Reproductive and Developmental Sciences, Clinical Biochemistry Section

Clinical Teacher A C Don-Wanchope
Hon. Senior Lecturer J P Ashby, P W H Rae
Lecturer S D Morley, J E Roulston
Professor J I Mason
Reader G J Beckett
Senior Lecturer S W Walker

Division of Reproductive and Developmental Sciences, Genitourinary Medicine Section

Clinical Tutor D Clutterbuck
Hon. Senior Lecturer G R Scott, C Thompson
Pt. Senior Lecturer A McMillan

Division of Reproductive and Developmental Sciences, Obstetrics and Gynaecology Section

Head of Division A A Calder
Clinical Teacher T Cooper, M F Geals, I E Lowles, A M McCulloch, C K Tay
Hon. Clinical Lecturer T Anderson, J Simpson

Hon. Professor R W Kelly, A S McNeilly, R P Millar
Hon. Senior Lecturer R A Anderson, G J Beattie, P J Dewart, D I M Farquharson, Ailsa Gebbie, R G Hughes, D S Irvine, G Lello, W A Liston, T A Mahmood, J A Milne
Lecturer S Cameron, F Denison, G Zillywhite
Professor R Anderson, H O D Critchley, S G Hillier, I Wilmot
Pt. Senior Lecturer A F Glasier, K J Thong, C P West
Senior Lecturer T A Bramley, W C Duncan, S C Riley, J D West

Postgraduate Dental Institute

Professor and Head of Department R J Ibbetson
Hon. Clinical Lecturer T Anderson, J Simpson
Hon. Senior Clinical Lecturer L Chung, T Gillgrass, L McCaul, E Roebuck
Hon. Senior Lecturer P G Callis, C H Deery, J J Hammond, K E Harley, G Lello, J P McDonald, G H Moody, C Moran
Lecturer G Lillywhite
Research Assistant E Downie, Y Maidment, A Santini, T Simpson
Senior Lecturer M K Ross

School of Molecular and Clinical Medicine

Head of School J R Seckl
Honoarary Fellow Carrie E
Honorary Clinical Senior Lecturer C J Arango, G Kernbach-Wighton, H Monaghan, W A H Wallace
Honorary Fellow J Kyd, I Rahman
Honorary Senior Lecturer (Non-Clinical) G Entrican, I Tobbett, D Wielbo
Senior Lecturer (Non-Clinical) M Head

Division of Clinical Neurosciences

Head of Division P Sandercock
Hon. Clinical Senior Lecturer R E Cull, R Grant, G D Moran, C Mumford, P F X Statham
Hon. Professor M S Dennis, R G Will
Hon. Reader R S G Knight
Lecturer P Armitage
Professor P A G Sandercock, J M Wardlaw, Charles Warlow, I R Whittle
Pt. Hon. Clinical Senior Lecturer A Zeman
Reader M A Glasby, P A T Kelly
Senior Lecturer M Holmes

Division of Medical Sciences

Head of Division J R Seckl
Clinical Lecturer H Gillett, M Nyirenda
Clinical Senior Lecturer R Reynolds
Hon. Clinical Senior Lecturer I W Campbell, V B Dhillon, R J Fergusson, M J Ford, W Lam, J A McKnight, G R Nimmo, T R D Shaw, I R Starkey, M W J Strachan, P S Welsby
Hon. Clinical Tutor T F Benton, P D McSorley
Hon. Professor H Cooke, A P Greening, A F Wright
Hon. Reader D N Bateman, R P Brettle, P L Padfield, M E M Porteous
Hon. Senior Lecturer J Dorin, C J Kenyon, C M Lambert
Lecturer R Andrew, Y Kotelevtsev, J J Oliver, W G Waring
Professor D Porteous, J Satsangi, J R Seckl, B R Walker, D J Webb
Pt Senior Lecturer N P Hurst, C L S Leen, R Luqmani, I D Penman
Senior Lecturer C Abbot, R W Brown, R V Carlson, K E Chapman, M A Denvir, J A Innes, S Maxwell

Division of Oncology

Head of Division J Ansell
Hon. Clin. Senior Lecturer G Neades, D R Oxenham
Hon. Clinical Senior Lecturer D Brown, U Chetty, J M T Griffiths, G C W Howard, P R E Johnson, S P Langdon, M J Mackie, L Manson, M McKean, D Mclaren, C M McLean, A McNeill, H Roddie, S Rodgers, L Wall
Hon. Professor W R Miller
Hon Senior Clinical Lecturer A M Potter
Hon. Senior Lecturer A T Redpath, D I Thwaites
Lecturer D R Camidge, F Nussey
Professor J D Ansell, M G Dunlop, A Price, J F Smyth
Pt Senior Lecturer E D C Anderson, D A Cameron, I H Kunkler, S J Nixon
Reader F K Habib, D J Jodrell
Senior Lecturer J M Dixon, S C Erridge, M T Fallon, L Forrester, M L Turner

Division of Pathology

Head of Division D Harrison
Hon. Clinical Senior Lecturer C J Arango, H M Kamel, J W Keeling, G Kernbach-Wigton, A M Lessells, H Monaghan, J St J Thomas, W A H Wallace
Hon. Clinical Tutor C Anderson, R M Davie, K Kurian, K J Mckenzie, H Monaghan
Hon. Fellow E Carrie, J Kyd, I Rahman
Hon. Senior Lecturer G Entrican, I Tobbett, D Wielbo
Lecturer S Prost
Professor J E Bell, A Busuttil, D J Harrison, J W Ironside
Reader S E M Howie, D M Salter
Senior Lecturer A Al-Nafussi, C Bellamy, D Brownstein, E Duvall, P Finneron, H M Gilmour, K M Grigor, C Head, K M McLaren, W A Reid, C Smith, A R W Williams

Division of Psychiatry

Head of Division E Johnstone
Clinical Teacher S A Backett, A Beveridge, M S Bruce, J Craig, D Garbutt, S M Gilfillan, D J Hall, J D Hendry, R G McCreadie, S Machale, A R P Moffoot, T J C Murphy, W J R Riddle, C R Rodger, T D Rogers, S Roscrow, M Stewart, W A Tait, F E Watson
Hon. Clinical Senior Lecturer A J Carson, D Chiswick, A M Lodge, G Masterton, P McConville, D Morrison, P A Morrison, T J C Murphy, S Potts, A I F Scott, P Shah, K Slatford, J G Strachan, A Wells, K J Woodburn
Lecturer R Darjee, A M McIntosh, D MacIntyre, D M Semple
Professor JJK Best, D H Blackwood, K Ebmeier, E Johnstone, D G C Owens
Pt. Senior Lecturer A Carson, J Chick, C Freeman
Senior Lecturer P Hoare, W J Muir, M C Sharpe, L D G Thomson

University of Glasgow

Wolfson Medical School Building, University Avenue, Glasgow G12 8QQ
Tel: 0141 330 4979, 0141 330 5921 Fax: 0141 330 5440
Email: execdean@clinmed.gla.ac.uk
Website: www.gla.ac.uk

Deputy Dean I A Greer
Head of Undergraduate Medical School J H McKillop
Executive Dean D H Barlow

Degrees and diplomas
MB ChB, BDS, BN, BSc (Med Sci), PhD, D Clin Psy, MSc (Med Sci), MN, MPH, MD, DDS

University of St Andrews

Bute Medical School, Bute Building, St Andrews KY16 9TS
Tel: 01334 463597 Fax: 01334 463482
Email: medicine@st-and.ac.uk
Website: www.st-andrews.ac.uk

BUTE Medical School

Dean of Medicine R Hugh MacDougall
Director of Teaching S B Guild
Lecturer J Cecil, D Jackson, C J M Nicol
Professor C S Herrington, G M Humphris, A C Riches
Reader P E Bryant
Research Fellow Gozde Ozakinci
Senior Lecturer J F Aiton, R M Pitman, James Robb, D W Sinclair, S C Whiten

Teaching Fellow P Bjelogrlic, M Crosby, A Fleet, P R Nelson, Margaret Ritchie, E M Sinclair, G E Strugnell, Chris Von Wagner

Degrees and diplomas
BScMed.Sci (Hons), MSc, PhD, MD

Wales

University of Wales Aberystwyth

PO Box 2, King Street, Aberystwyth SY23 2AX
Tel: 01970 623111 Fax: 01970 611446
Website: www.aber.ac.uk

Dean of Science J Harries

Cardiff University

From 01 August 2004 merged with University of Wales College of Medicine.

PO Box 920, Cardiff CF10 3XP
Tel: 029 2087 4000 Fax: 029 2087 4457
Website: http://www.cardiff.ac.uk/medicine

Head of Cardiff School of Biosciences John Harwood
Head of Cardiff School of Optometry and Vision Sciences Michael Boulton
Head of Cardiff School of Psychology Dylan Jones
Head of Nursing and Dean, School of Nursing and Midwifery Studies Ann Tucker
Head of School and Dean, School of Dentistry Malcolm Jones
Head of School and Dean, School of Healthcare Studies Martyn Booy
Head of School and Dean, School of Postgraduate Medical and Dental Education Simon Smail
Head of School and Acting Dean, School of Medicine David Wynford-Thomas
Head of Welsh School of Pharmacy Stephen Denyer
Provost of the Wales College of Medicine, Biology, Life and Health Sciences Stephen Tomlinson

Department of Optometry and Vision Sciences
Redwood Building, King Edward VII Avenue, Cardiff CF10 3NB
Tel: 029 2087 6784 Fax: 029 2087 4859
Website: www.cardiff.ac.uk/optom/

Head of Department Mike Boulton
Professor (Acting Head of Department) John Wild
Lecturer Julie Albon, Jeremy Guggenheim, Pia Makela, Tom Margrain, Kola Oduwaiye, Andrew Quantock, Outi Ukkonen
Professor Neville Drasdo, Gerald Elliott, Stuart Hodson, Keith Meek, Jyrki Rovamo
Senior Lecturer Jon Erichsen, Paul Murphy, Rachel North, J M Woodhouse
Senior Professional Tutor Richard Earlam

Pure and Applied Biology
PO Box 915, Cardiff CF1 3TL
Tel: 029 2087 4000 Fax: 029 2087 4190

Director of Teaching D R Lees
Lecturer M J Bosley, J H Bourne, D W Bowker, R J Cowie, P J Evans, J D Hardege, A J Morgan, P F Randerson, H J Rogers, A J Weightman, T Wigham, J E Young
Professor L Boddy, I D Bowen, W T Coakley, J C Fry, T M G Gabriel, J Hemingway, D Lloyd, J H Slater, J W T Wimpenny
Reader M J Day, D Francis, N A C Kidd
Senior Lecturer B N Dancer, M S Davies, J R Dickinson, P N Ferns, M A Jervis, C J Mettam, S J Ormerod, D Pascoe, D J Stickler, D H Thomas, W A Venables

School of Biosciences
PO Box 911, Museum Avenue, Cardiff CF10 3US
Tel: 029 2087 4829 Fax: 029 2087 4116
Website: www.cardiff.ac.uk/biosi/

Experimental Officer J E Liddell
Fellow S Marshall
Lecturer Steve Barasi, J M Basford, J R Bedwani, Kelly Berube, R C Caswell, Alison Davies, D J R Evans, E J Evans, R C Hall, S K Hall, Alvin Kwan, D J Mason, A P Morby, Dipak Ramji, R M Rose, G E Sweeney, Tim Wells
Professor Charlie Archer, Bruce Caterson, Paul Chapman, Vincenzo Crunelli, Vic Duance, Ronald Eccles, Kevin Fox, John Harwood, Tim Jacob, Rob John, John Kay, Bernard Moxham, Roy Richards, M H T Roberts, D I Wallis
Reader Mike Benjamin, D A Carter, George Foster
Royal Society Fellow Colin Berry
School Administrator John Robertson
Senior Lecturer J G Jones, Peter Kille, Jim Ralphs, Rob Santer, A H D Watson, Graham White, Peter Winterburn, F S Wusteman

School of Psychology
PO Box 901, Cardiff
Tel: 029 2087 4007 Fax: 029 2087 4858
Website: www.cardiff.ac.uk/psych/

Head of School Dylan Jones
Emeritus Professor D E Blackman, K D Duncan
Hon. Associate Professional Tutor A Brooks, S A Ellis, P D G Harris, J Hill-Tout, R Jenkins, R T Kidd, M Thomson, S E Vivian-Byrne
Hon. Lecturer S V Austin, P D Bennett, A L Brazier, N J Frude, N Mills, J L Moses, J Onyett, J L Rose, F R Young
Hon. Professor Mansel Aylward, E W Farmer, R D P Griffiths, R D Hare, C M Judd, M E P Seligman, R F Westbrook
Hon. Research Fellow E A Gaffan, J E J Gallacher, S L Grand, D R Laws, P K H McKenna, T Mason, D S Owen, E M Pothos, S Tremblay
Lecturer John Aggleton, Todd Bailey, Simon Banbury, Jacky Boivin, Josie Briscoe, Marc Buehner, H C M Carroll, John Culling, Hadyn Ellis, Tom Freeman, Merideth Gattis, Nicola Gray, Geoffrey Haddock, Ulrike Hahn, Gordon Harold, Dale Hay, Rob Honey, Andrew Howes, Emma Laing, Michael Lewis, Bill Macken, Chris Miles, Janice Muir, John Patrick, John Pearce, Andy Smith, Geoff Thomas, Ulrich von Hecker, Ed Wilding, Patricia Wright, J E Young
Professional Tutor Diane Ellis, John Gameson, Gill Rhydderch
Professor Mike Oaksford, Stephen Payne, Robert Snowden
Professorial Research Fellow Peter Halligan
Reader Gregory Maio, Peter White
Research Assistant Melissa Allman, Phillip Barnes, Afia Begum, Vaughan Bell, Steve Belt, Andrea Chadwick, Rachel Dowling, Andrew Edmonds, Neil Ellis, Catrina Fraser, Adam Goody, Sarah Harrington, Mark Haselgrove, Sophie MacCulloch, Vanessa Marshall, Christopher McGowan, Nina Meikle, Hansjoerg Neth, Helen Phillips, Heather Watkins
Research Associate Gary Christopher, Bryany Cusens, Dominic Dwyer, James Futter, David George, Jane Herron, Robert Houghton, Robert Hughes, Anthony McGregor, Stuart McGregor, Rachel McNamara, Susanna Moss, Zoe Moss, Samantha Nabb, Nicholas Perham, Francis Rice, Helen Sharpe, David Sutherland, Seralynne Vann, Emma Wadsworth
Research Fellow Trisha Jenkins, Joselyn Sellen, Marie Thomas
Research Technician Eman Amin, Moira Davies, Gareth Lloyd, Heather Phillips, Heather Staal
Senior Lecturer Mark A Good
Senior Research Associate Christine Shaw, Jane Sumnall
Senior Research Fellow Simon Killcross, Mary McMurran

Welsh School of Pharmacy
Redwood Building, King Edward VII Avenue, Cathays Park, Cardiff CF10 3NB
Tel: 029 2087 4783 Fax: 029 2087 4149
Website: www.cardiff.ac.uk/phrmy/

Director - WCPPE David Temple

Head Welsh School of Pharmacy David Luscombe
Lecturer A S Cotterill, J R Furr, C Grout, Dai John, J Y Maillard, W J Pugh, R G Stevens
Professor K R Brain, Kenneth Broadley, Chris McGuigan, Paul Nicholls, Damaer Russell, R D Walker
Senior Lecturer Stephen Daniels, Ian Gilbert, R D E Sewell, Sam Shayegan-Salek, G Taylor, K Wann

Degrees and diplomas
BA, BSc, MA, MSc, BScEcon, MScEcon, MBA, DPhil, MPhil, PhD, MEng, Beng

University of Wales Swansea

The Clinical School, Swansea SA2 8PP
Tel: 01792 295149 Fax: 01792 513054
Website: www.medicine.swan.ac.uk

Head of School Julian Hopkin

Life Science Research

Chair, Cancer Studies R C F Leonard
Chair, Clinical Epidemiology D R R Williams
Chair, Developmental Medicine G Morgan
Chair, Genetics J M Parry, D O F Skibinski
Chair, Health Services Research J G Williams
Chair, Medical Microbiology & Infectious Disease D Mack
Chair, Medical Physics & Imaging H Griffiths
Chair, Medicine J M Hopkin
Chair, Microbial Genetics & Molecular Biology S L Kelly
Chair, Neurobiology M I Rees
Chair, Oncology J Wagstaff
Chair, Primary Care G Elwyn
Chair, Psychiatry J U V Thome
Chair, Psychological Medicine K R Lloyd
Chair, Public Health R Lyons
Chair, Reproductive Biology J O White
Chair, Surgery J N Baxter
Lecturer J Bishop, S Brophy, R S Conlan, A N Coogan, J T Cutmore, P Dyson, R Evans, D H Jones, J G L Mullins, S G Rees, M R Turner, C L Vogan, W Walker, S V Webster
Reader A G K Edwards, D Kelly, D C Lamb
Senior Lecturer S J Allen, J Beynon, W Cheung, A Delahunty, J Dingley, P Ebden, H Fielder, M B Gravenor, A P Griffiths, G J S Jenkins, J G C Kingham, B Lervy, K E Lewis, I Pallister, D W Patton, D E Price, I Sawhney, H A Snooks, A Sugar, H M Taylor, G A Thomas, C A Thornton, O M R Westwood

Medical Education

Reader P A Evans, C W Weston
Senior Clinical Tutor S A D Al-Ismail, M W Austin, M A Benton, S L W Blackford, T H Brown, S Browning, A Byrne, G V P Chamberlain, S P Closs, P J Davies, T G Davies, J Dawkins, P Donnelly, P Drew, A G K Edwards, M M Ellis, R G Evans, R M Evans, L Gibbs, A Gunneburg, W Harris, K N Harrison, S Hodder, D Hope, C Hudson, M James-Ellison, T Joannides, E Kevelighan, T M Lawson, M S Lewis, R Llewellyn, B W Mason, S H M Matthews, R Morgan, C J O'Brien, B Patel, H J Phillips, N Price, M W Ramsey, D Roberts, D L Roberts, C Samuel, L A Thomas, K C Vaughton, C M Wigley, A Williams, S Williams

Degrees and diplomas
MB BCh, MD/MCh, MSc, PhD

Northern Ireland

Queen's University of Belfast

Whitla Medical Building, 97 Lisburn Road, Belfast BT9 7BL
Tel: 028 9024 5133, 028 9027 2010, 028 9027 2186
Fax: 028 9033 0571
Email: k.copeland@qub.ac.uk
Website: www.qub.ac.uk

Head of Administration Karen Copeland

Faculty of Medicine and Health Sciences

Dean of Faculty R J Hay
Faculty Administrator Karen Copeland

Anaesthetics
Head J P H Fee
Professor R Mirakhur
Senior Lecturer J M Murray

Anatomy
Head D J Wilson
Lecturer A Al-Modhefer, S J McCullough, C B O'Reilly, J Smit

Child Health
Head D J Carson
Professor J M Savage
Senior Lecturer J Jenkins, M D Shields, Moira C Stewart

Clinical Biochemistry
Head Elisabeth Trimble
Lecturer W E Allen, L Powell, G Skibinski
Professor Madeline Ennis

Dental Education
Lecturer S Morison

Dental Public Health
Professor R E Freeman

Dental Surgery
Senior Lecturer C G Cowan

Epidemiology and Public Health
Head A E Evans
Lecturer G W Cran, M R Stevenson
Professor F E Kee
Reader N Donnelly, A Gavin, J W G Yarnell
Senior Lecturer P McCarron, L Murray, L J Murray, D O'Reilly, C C Patterson

General Practice
Head P M Reilly
Senior Lecturer M E Cupples, A E W Gilliland, K J McGlade, W K Steele

Geriatric Medicine
Head R W Stout
Lecturer D Craig, Vivienne Crawford, S P McIlroy
Senior Lecturer A P Passmore, I Maeve Rea

Haematology
Head T Lappin
Reader Mary F McMullin

Medical Education
Director J M Savage
Assistant Director K J McGlade

Lecturer M I Boohan
Senior Lecturer K Collins

Medical Genetics
Professor A P Maxwell
Reader Anne E Hughes
Senior Lecturer D A Savage

Medicine
Head D R McCluskey
Lecturer U Bayraktutan, G Cuskelly, A McGinty, M M T O'Hare, J V Woodside
Professor S Elborn, I S Young
Senior Lecturer A L Bell, S A Hawkins, L G Heaney, L McGarvey, P P Mckeown, M E Rooney, R G P Watson

Mental Health
Head S J Cooper
Professor R J McClelland
Senior Lecturer C C Mulholland, F A O'Neill

Microbiology and Immunology
Head J A Johnson
Professor L Cosby
Senior Lecturer M A Armstrong, M Gadina, S Patrick

Nursing Studies
Associate Head of School (Research & Development) A Lazenbatt
Professor/Head Jean A Orr
Lecturer A M Begley, B Blackwood, Kathy Rowe
Professor S Porter

Obstetrics and Gynaecology
Professor N McClure
Reader S E M Lewis
Senior Lecturer R Ayoub, I Cooke

Oncology
Head P G Johnston
Lecturer M Boland, D P Harkin, D J Waugh
Reader H van den Berg
Senior Lecturer J J A McAleer, S E H Russell, R Wilson

Ophthalmology
Head Giuiliana Silvestri
Lecturer T Curtis, T A Gardiner, D McDonald, O Simpson
Professor Usha Chakravarthy, A W Stitt
Senior Lecturer W J Curry

Oral Medicine
Lecturer F T Lundy
Professor P J Lamey
Senior Lecturer W A Coulter, J J Marley

Orthodontics
Head D J Burden
Senior Lecturer C D Johnson

Orthopaedic Surgery
Head D R Marsh
Lecturer G Jordan
Senior Lecturer G Li

Otorhinolaryngology
Head D A Adams

Pathology
Lecturer J Diamond, J Kirk, K M Williamson
Professor P Hall, W Hamilton
Senior Lecturer M D O'Hara

Physiology
Head J D Allen
Lecturer C Johnson
Professor N G McHale
Senior Lecturer Judith Allen, M A Hollywood, J G McGeown, C N Scholfield, K D Thornbury

Restorative Dentistry
Clinical Lecturer C A Burnett, S Killough
Professor G J Linden, E Lynch
Senior Lecturer T J Clifford, D L Hussey, C R Irwin, J G Kennedy, C A Mitchell, B H Mullally

Surgery
Head F C Campbell
Lecturer M El-Tanani, A McGinty
Senior Lecturer K Khosraviani

Therapeutics and Pharmacology
Head G D Johnston
Lecturer D Bell
Professor B J McDermott
Senior Lecturer G E McVeigh

Degrees and diplomas
MB, BCh, BAO, BMedSc, MD, MCh, MMedSc, BDS, BSc, MSc, MA

Recognised Clinical Institutions
Altnagelvin Area Hospital, Antrim Hospital, Arden Centre, Ards Community Hospital, Belfast City Hospital, Braid Valley Hospital, Causeway Hospital, Craigavon Area Hospital, Craigavon Psychiatric Unit, Daisy Hill Hospital, Downe Hospital, Downshire Hospital, Erne Hospital, Gransha Hospital, Holywell Hospital, Knockbracken Mental Health Services, Lagan Valley Hospital, Longstone Hospital, Lurgan Hospital, Massereene Hospital, Mater Hospital HSS Trust, Mater Infirmorum Hospital, Mid-Ulster Hospital, Muckamore Abbey Hospital, Musgrave Park Hospital, Royal Belfast Hospital for Sick Children, Royal Maternity Hospital, Royal Victoria Hospital, St Luke's Hospital, Stradreagh Hospital, The Ulster Hospital, Tyrone and Fermanagh Hospital, Tyrone County Hospital, University Dental Hospital, Whiteabbey Hospital

Postgraduate Medical Centres

England

Airedale NHS Trust, Department of Medical Education
Steeton, Keighley BD20 6TD
Tel: 01535 294414 Fax: 01535 292196
Email: anne.troth@anhst.nhs.uk
Website: www.airedale-trust.nhs.uk

Director Medical Education Janet Baker
Clinical Tutor (VTSO) J Hodgson, D Pearson, B Tones

The Avery Jones Postgraduate Medical Centre
Central Middlesex Hospital NHS Trust, Park Royal, London NW10 7NS
Tel: 020 8453 2501 Fax: 020 8453 2659

Centre Manager Irene Fernandez
Clinical Tutor D McCrea

Barnet Hospital Education and Information Centre
Barnet Hospital, Wellhouse Lane, Barnet EN5 3DJ
Tel: 020 8216 4514, 020 8216 4833 Fax: 020 8216 4678
Email: chris.clarke@barnet-chase-tr.nhs.uk
Website: www.barneteducationcentre.nhs.uk

Education Manager Chris Clarke

Barnsley Education Centre
Barnsley District Hospital NHS Trust, Gawber Road, Barnsley S75 2EP
Tel: 01226 730000 Ext: 2553 Fax: 01226 779319
Email: carol.youle@bdgh-tr.trent.nhs.uk

Clinical Tutor J P Ng
GP VTS Tutor & Course Organizer P Lane
Postgraduate Manager C Youle

Barrow Postgraduate Medical Centre
Furness General Hospital, Dalton Lane, Barrow-in-Furness LA14 4LE
Tel: 01229 491292

Clinical Tutor D E P Shapland
Specialty Tutor P K Misra, G Murray, L J Williams, R Y Wilson

Barts and The London NHS Trust
Royal London Hospital, 48 Ashfield Street, Whitechapel, London E1 2AJ
Tel: 020 7377 7760 Fax: 020 7377 7187

Director of Medical Education John Krapez
Assistant Director MDE Anita Kapoor

The Bateman Centre for Postgraduate Studies
The Education Centre, Rochdale Infirmary, Whitehall Street, Rochdale OL12 0NB
Tel: 01706 517057 Fax: 01706 517776
Email: lynda.hurst@pat.nhs.uk

Postgraduate Clinical Tutor R K Sharma
Specialist Tutor S Allcock, Dr Ariyawansa
Specialty Tutor Mr Akhtar, Dr Bradgate, C Datta, V Devadoss, Dr Gupta, Mr Hashmi, D Mackechnie, R Porter, Mr Read, Dr Sharma, Mr White, M Zaklama

Bedford Medical Institute
Bedford Hospital NHS Trust, South Wing, Ampthill Road, Bedford MK42 9DJ
Tel: 01234 792267 Fax: 01234 792127
Email: asa.mann@bedhos.anglox.nhs.uk
Website: www.bedfordhospital.org.uk

Director of Clinical Studies N B Waterfall
Clinical Tutor S Rae
Deputy Clinical Tutor D Liu
Postgraduate Centre Manager Åsa Mann
Specialty Tutor A B Hewitt, R D Mehta, S Reynolds, D Skipper, S Snape, R Zaman

Belmont Postgraduate Psychiatric Centre
Chiltern Wing, Sutton Hospital, Cotswold Road, Sutton SM2 5NF
Email: bpgpc@swlstg-tr.nhs.uk

College Tutor C Mathers

Blackburn Postgraduate Medical Centre
Royal Infirmary, Blackburn BB2 3LR
Tel: 01254 687242
Email: pgmc@mail.bhrv.nwest.nhs.uk

Director of Medical Education N A Roberts
Clinical Tutor - Surgery D Chang
Dental Tutor N Taylor
GP Tutor S Gunn
Royal College Tutor J W Benson, R S Emnott, E Martindale, A G E Nylander, R Prescott, M Rahman, S Ramhoolan, E Sultana

Blackpool Health Professional Education Centre
Blackpool Victoria Hospital, Whinney Heys Road, Blackpool FY3 8NR
Tel: 01253 303538
Email: communications@bfwhospitals.nhs.uk
Website: www.bfwhospitals.nhs.uk

Clinical Tutor P E T Isaacs
GP Tutor M Preskey
Specialty Tutor S J Aucott, G Dunkley, S J Duthie, P Flegg, L Hacking, A Javad, S Ravi, R Roberts, M Sedgwick, K S Vasudev

Booth Hall Postgraduate Medical Centre
Booth Hall Children's Hospital, Charlestown Road, Blackley, Manchester M9 7AA
Tel: 0161 220 5018 Fax: 0161 220 5579
Email: adrian.thomas@cmmc.nhs.uk

Clinical Tutor Adrian Thomas

Boston-Pilgrim Hospital Centre for Medical and Dental Education
United Lincolnshire Hospitals NHS Trust, Pilgrim Hospital, Sibsey Road, Boston PE21 9QS
Tel: 01205 364801 Fax: 01205 442150

Clinical Tutor D A Sagar
Dental Tutor (S. Lincs) D E H Glendinning
GP Tutor P J Woods
GPVTS Course Organiser C S Bull, N J C Humphrey, C Kelly
Manager K Skipp
Specialty Tutor - Anaesthetics A C Norton
Specialty Tutor - Medicine M Perry
Specialty Tutor - Obstetrics and Gynaecology S Ikhena
Specialty Tutor - Paediatrics M Pervez
Specialty Tutor - Radiology I Britton
Specialty Tutor - Surgery M Chaurasia

Bournemouth Postgraduate Medical Centre
Royal Bournemouth Hospital, Castle Lane East, Bournemouth BH7 7DW
Tel: 01202 704267 Fax: 01202 704489
Email: christine.hardwicke@rbch-tr.swest.nhs.uk

Associate Clinical Sub Dean Neil Hopkinson
Clinical Tutor Paul Winwood
Dental Tutor S Doman
GP Tutor P Blick
Postgraduate and Medical Personnel Manager Christine Hardwick

Bradbury Postgraduate Medical Centre
Epsom General Hospital, Dorking Road, Epsom KT18 7EG
Tel: 01372 735172/5/6 Fax: 01372 749502
Email: epsompgmc@aol.com
Website: www.epsompgmc.co.uk

Clinical Tutor Christopher George
District GP Tutor Azita Jones
GP VTS Course Organiser Richard Cowlard, Jane Moore, Alex Watson
Medical Education Manager Vivien Martin
Specialty Tutor (Anaesthetics) Joan Desborough
Specialty Tutor (Haematology) Margaret Semple
Specialty Tutor (Medicine) Mashkur Khan
Specialty Tutor (Obstetrics & Gynaecology) Richard Worth
Specialty Tutor (Orthopaedics) Will Burgoyne
Specialty Tutor (Paediatrics) Manil Katugampola
Specialty Tutor (Psychiatry) Farida Youssaf
Specialty Tutor (Radiology) Christopher George
Specialty Tutor (Surgery) Paul Toomey

Broomfield Hospital Medical Academic Unit
Broomfield Hospital, Broomfield, Chelmsford CM1 7ET
Tel: 01245 514731 Fax: 01245 514667
Email: kate.vann@meht.nhs.uk

Clinical Tutor D Turner
Specialty Tutor - Anaesthetics A Hassani
Specialty Tutor - General Surgery N Richardson
Specialty Tutor - Medicine G Clesham
Specialty Tutor - Obstetrics and Gynaecology A Sharma
Specialty Tutor - Orthopaedics G Charnley
Specialty Tutor - Paediatrics A Agrawal

Burnley Mackenzie Medical Centre
The Mackenzie Medical Centre, Casterton Avenue, Burnley BB10 2PQ
Tel: 01282 474723 Fax: 01282 474254

Associate Tutor for International Doctors S Bhattacharyya
Postgraduate Clinical Tutor R H Hyatt
PRHO Tutor J Iqbal
Specialty Tutor A A Al-Dawoud, H Al-Khaffaf, I H Brown, C E Calow, F Clarke, N M Craven, M Javeed, A G E Nylander, N H Taylor
Undergraduate Specialty Tutor F M Zaman

Burton Education Centre and Library
Queen's Hospital, Burton Hospitals NHS Trust, Belvedere Road, Burton-on-Trent DE13 0RB
Tel: 01283 566333 Fax: 01283 510347
Email: education.centre@burtonh-tr.wmids.nhs.uk
Website: www.burtonmedicaleducation.nhs.uk

Clinical Tutor A Manzoor

Bury Postgraduate Centre
Fairfield General Hospital, Rochdale Old Road, Bury BL9 7TD
Tel: 0161 778 2418 Fax: 0161 778 2419

Clinical Tutor A Narayan
Specialty Tutor V Gadiyar, D Gordon, B Hayden, K S Kotegaonkar, V Sanker
Undergraduate Tutor M Saab

Bury St Edmunds, Suffolk: Medical, Dental and AHP Office
Education Centre, West Suffolk Hospital NHS Trust, Hardwick Lane, Bury St Edmunds IP33 2QZ
Tel: 01284 713342 Fax: 01284 712598
Email: lynn.jones@wsh.nhs.uk
Website: www.wsufftrust.org.uk

Director of Postgraduate Medical Education S Edwards (Head)
Associate Director of Postgraduate Medical Education R Lakshman
Centre Manager L Jones
Clinical Tutor Psychiatry R Chipperfield
Dental Tutor J Barnet-Lamb
GP Tutor R West
Royal College Tutor Surgery N Keeling
Specialty Tutor J Buck, P Harris, R Lamb, J Majeed, P McKiernon, M Palmer, A Sauvage, H Taylor, M Wood
VTS Course Organiser P Lloyd Jones, D A Pearson, J Rutherford

Cambridge District Postgraduate Medical and Dental Education Centre
The Clinical School, Box 111, Addnebrooke's Hospital, Hills Road, Cambridge CB2 2SP
Tel: 01223 217105 Fax: 01223 217237
Email: maloool@medschl.cam.ac.uk

Director of Medical Education Arun Gupta (Head)
Assistant Director of Medical Education Pamela Todd
Dental Tutor Iain Robinson
GP Tutor Sarah Rann
Manager Mary Archibald
VTS Course Organiser Simon Brown, Tony Cole, Paul Sackin

Canterbury Centre for Health and Clinical Sciences
Kent & Canterbury Hospital, Ethelbert Road, Canterbury CT1 3NG
Tel: 01227 766877 Ext: 74361/74828/74200/74203/74667/74034, 01227 783135 Fax: 01227 864155
Email: june.toms@ekht.nhs.uk
Website: www.ekh.org.uk

Clinical Tutor N Wilson
College Tutor (Anaesthetics) M Mayall
College Tutor (Medicine) G Batty
College Tutor (Ophthalmology) R De Cock
College Tutor (Pathology) E Lamb
College Tutor (Radiology) I Morrison
College Tutor (Surgery) N Wilson
Dental Tutor G Manley
Dental Vocational Training Course Organiser / Regional Adviser H Winstone
Foundation Tutor M Mayall
GP Tutor P Biggs
GP Vocational Training Course Organiser P Livesey, K Stillman
Medical and Dental Education Manager June Toms

Central Manchester Postgraduate Health Sciences Centre
Manchester Royal Infirmary, Oxford Road, Manchester M13 9WL
Tel: 0161 276 4169 Fax: 0161 276 8012

Director of Postgraduate Medical Education M Cheshire
Course Manager K Stuart
GP Tutor A Danczak
Specialty Tutor I Dady, M Forrester, A Siriwardena, F Spencer, G Subramanian, S Vause, G Wilson

Centre for Medical and Dental Education Pilgrim Hospital United Lincolnshire Hospitals NHS Trust
Pilgrim Hospital, Sibsey Road, Boston PE21 9QS
Tel: 01205 364801 Fax: 01205 357494 (Centre Manager), 01205 442150 (Departmental)
Email: kate.skipp@ulh.nhs.uk

Centre Manager K A Skipp
Clinical Tutor Dr Sagar
Dental Tutor D E H Glendenning
GP Course Organiser N J C Humphry
GP Course Organiser/GP Adviser C Kelly
GP Tutor Dr Woods
Specialty Tutor I Britton, M Chaurasia, S Ikhena, Z Khan, A C Norton, M Perry, Dr Pervez

Charing Cross Hospital Postgraduate Medical Centre
Fulham Palace Road, London W6 8RF
Tel: 020 8846 7196 Fax: 020 8846 7704
Email: acheesman@hhnt.nhs.org

Clinical Tutor H Millington
GP/Dental Courses Administrator Sylvia Longman

Charles Hasting Postgraduate Medical Centre
Worcestershire Acute Hospitals NHS Trust, Newton Road, Worcester WR5 1HW
Tel: 01905 760600 Fax: 01905 767834

Clinical Tutor C Pycock

Chase Postgraduate Medical Centre
Chase Farm Hospital, The Ridgeway, Enfield EN2 8JL
Tel: 020 8375 1121 Fax: 020 8363 4662
Email: postgrad.reception@bcf.nhs.uk

Clinical Tutor C Baynes
Dental Tutor T Payne
GP Tutor R Hume
Medical Education Manager Z Khan
Undergraduate Tutor B Yuksel

Chelsea and Westminster Hospital Postgraduate Centre
369 Fulham Road, London SW10 9NH
Tel: 020 8746 5590, 020 8746 8310 Fax: 020 8746 8248
Email: r.wood@chelwest.nhs.uk

Clinical Tutor Kevin Shotliff
Postgraduate Centre Manager Rosamunde Wood

Cheltenham Postgraduate Medical Centre
2 College Lawn, Cheltenham GL53 7AG
Tel: 0845 422 3038 Fax: 0845 422 3242
Email: kate.bartlett@glos.nhs.uk

Clinical Tutor E Blundell, N J Morison
Royal College Tutor John Ferris, Tony Goodman, Michelle Hamilton Ayres, David Holmes, Garett McGann, Ted Rees, C E Robson, Mark Silva, Kelwyn Williams, Graham Wilson, Paul Wilson
Specialty Tutor John Anderson, Kim Benstead, Neil Borley, C C Burgess, Arnold Deering, W Foster, Hugh Gilbert, Harminder Gosal, Helen Gray, Mike Hardingham, John Harrison, Rob Jackson, R Mackay, D R Martin, William Porter, S Silver, Zubayr Sulaiman, Mark Whyman
Specialty Tutor (CGH) Ian Mortimore
Specialty Tutor (Delancey Hospital) Mick Bialas

Chesterfield Education Centre
Chesterfield and North Derbyshire Royal Hospital NHS Trust, Chesterfield S44 5BL
Tel: 01246 513041 Fax: 01246 512685
Email: val.johnson@chesterfieldroyal.nhs.uk
Website: www.chesterfieldroyal.nhs.uk

Clinical Tutor K Fairburn
Education Centre Manager V Johnson
Specialty Tutor J Glaves, D Hay, G Hutchison, K Kumar, P Medcalf, T Soe

Chichester Medical Education Centre
St Richards Hospital, Spitalfield Lane, Chichester PO19 4SE
Tel: 01243 788122 Fax: 01243 532576
Website: www.cmec.info

Clinical Tutor G Dewhurst
Dental Tutor D MacPherson
GP Education Manager B Smithers
GP Tutor A Copsey, J Price
Specialty Tutor D R Allen, F Barrett, A Carter, Dr Haigh, Mr Moss, Mr Simons, Dr Taylor
Undergraduate Tutor P Britton

Chiltern Medical Education Centre
Level 1 Phase 4, Wycombe Hospital, High Wycombe HP11 2TT
Tel: 01494 426382 Fax: 01494 426387

CDP Tutor (GP) B Neal
Clinical Tutor Go A Luzzi
Specialty Tutor A Bdesha, S Cox, D Eustace, A Fernandes, C Graham, A McIntyre, J Margo, J Maxmin, D Orton, D Potts, K Sawhney, R Stevens, H Thomson, M Turner

Chorley and Ribble Postgraduate Education Centre
Preston Road, Chorley PR7 1PP
Tel: 01257 245600

Clinical Tutor S Wallis
Specialty Tutor B Rambihar, I G Robertson, S Wallis

City Hospital NHS Trust Postgraduate Medical Centre
Dudley Road, Birmingham B18 7QH
Tel: 0121 507 4980 Fax: 0121 523 4562

Clinical Tutor D Dawkins
Manager J Collins

City Hospitals Sunderland, Postgraduate Medical Centre
Sunderland Royal Hospital, Kayll Road, Sunderland SR4 7TP
Tel: 0191 569 9634 Fax: 0191 569 9246
Email: pgmc@chs.northy.nhs.uk

Centre Manager Pat Wagner
Clinical Tutor C Steele
Specialty Tutor Dr Abu-Harb, Guiseppe Bignaroi, J Chapman, A Cross, S England, S Fraser, J Heaton, K Hinshaw, Gary Lear

Coastal Postgraduate Medical Centre
James Paget Hospital, Lowestoft Road, Gorleston, Great Yarmouth NR31 6LA
Tel: 01493 452466 Fax: 01493 452182
Email: irene.walker@jpaget.nhs.uk
Website: www.jpaget.co.uk

Clinical Tutor P Harrison
Dental Tutor J Lindsay
GP Tutor A Eastaugh, R Fleetcroft, P Quilliam, A Walker
Specialty Tutor A Amanat, T Cotter, Dr Hamelynck, M Hassanaien, C Johnson-Nurse, S Nirmal, D Peacock, P Prinsley, H Schneider, D Tupper-Carey
VTS Course Organiser A Bigg, N Statter

Colchester and North-East Essex Postgraduate Medical Centre
Colchester General Hospital, Turner Road, Colchester CO4 5JL
Tel: 01206 742149 Fax: 01206 851231
Email: penny.west@essexrivers.nhs.uk

Centre Manager P West
Clinical Tutor R A Elston
Secretary Marion Brown

Cornwall Postgraduate Medical Centre
Royal Cornwall Hospital, Truro TR1 3LJ
Tel: 01872 252613 Fax: 01872 278469
Email: johanna.gilbert@rcht.cornwall.nhs.uk

Clinical Tutor M Davis, G Edwards, R Farrow, R Marshall
Specialty Tutor S Adcock, L Barker, S Bates, C Cuff, H Dalton, D Fern, R Laugharne, J Mathew, P Munyard, B Padbury, C Ralph, T Sulkin, M Waldron, A Widdison, A Wilde, N Wilson-Holt, J Wyatt

County Durham and Darlington Acute Hospitals NHS Trust Education Centre

General Hospital, Bishop Auckland DL14 6AD
Tel: 01388 455657 Fax: 01388 455658
Email: ena.lawrence@cddah.nhs.uk

Clinical Tutor H Smith
Medical Staffing Manager W Oyston
Specialty Tutor P Blakeman, A Dhar, T Layzell, G Nyamugunduru, V Saleh

Crawley and Horsham Postgraduate Centre

Crawley Hospital, West Green Drive, Crawley RH11 7DH
Tel: 01293 600316 Fax: 01293 600387
Email: sharon.nunweek@sash.nhs.uk

Clinical Tutor Alan Vallon
GP Tutor E Hornung
Medical Education Co-ordinator Sharon Nunweek
PGEC Manager Linda Briant
Specialty Tutor D Acharya, W Chappell, I Lewis, E Owen, M Quenstedt
VTS Course Organiser T Conaty, P Stillman

Cripps Postgraduate Medical Centre

Northampton General Hospital, Northampton NN1 5BD
Tel: 01604 545448 Fax: 01604 545590
Email: pat.hawkins@ngh.nhs.uk

Associate Clinical Tutor G French
Directorate Manager Bob Butler, Chris Davison, Philip Mann, Peter Martin, Fiona Myers, Helen O'Connell
Associate Medical Director / Emergency Care and Workforce Planning A L Olgivie
Course Organiser Glynis Buckle
District Clinical Tutor A Jeffrey
District Tutor J O'Donnell
Educational Organiser P Gurr, C Harrop, C Pal, A Vince
Royal College Tutor Clive Aldridge, A Kerr, M Miller
Specialty Tutor F Ackland, J Anthony, P Davey, I Fearnley, J Hewertson, Dr Holloway, D C Hunter, G Kerr, D Ratliff, S Swart, F Thompson, R Webser, M Wilkinson, W Zaw
VTS Course Organiser A Craig, P Halstead

Darlington Postgraduate Medical Centre

Darlington Memorial Hospital, Hollyhurst Road, Darlington DL3 6HX
Tel: 01325 743232 Fax: 01325 743222

Clinical Tutor U Earl
Librarian C Houghton, C Masterman
Specialty Tutor A S M Ali, A Bawarish, J Carlin, N Corner, C F Kotur, N On Tin, R Stirling, A West, G William, C Williams

Department for NHS Postgraduate Medical and Dental Education (Yorkshire Deanery)

University of Leeds, Willow Terrace Road, Leeds LS2 9JT
Tel: 0113 343 1500 Fax: 0113 343 1530
Website: www.yorkshiredeanery.com

Dean of Postgraduate Medical Education William A Burr
Associate Dean for Medical Specialties J Ian Wilson
Associate Dean for North and East Yorkshire and North Lincolnshire Brian Johnson
Associate Dean for the Foundation Year Michael Harran
Associate Dean for the PRHO Year Stephen Gilbey
Associate Dean for the SHOs Alistair McGowan
Associate Dean for West Yorkshire and Overseas Doctors P Neligan
Associate Dean Training, Careers and Personal Development R Roden
Director of Postgraduate General Practice Education and Associate Dean George Taylor
Education Adviser Janice McMillan
Manager PGMDE Yorkshire Pat Kentley

Derby City General Hospital Medical Education Centre

Uttoxeter Road, Derby DE22 3NE
Tel: 01332 340131 Ext: 5189 Fax: 01332 207566

Clinical Tutor D Clarke

Derbyshire Royal Infirmary Postgraduate Medical Education Centre

Derbyshire Royal Infirmary, London Road, Derby DE1 2QY

Clinical Tutor D Clarke
Specialty Tutor J Bennett, Mr Chapman, H Holliday, B Langham, A R Lindop, C Mackaness, N Mylvahan, G Narborough, C Nelson, J Noble, M De Nunzio, P Pritty, D Young

Doncaster Postgraduate Medical Teaching Centre

Doncaster and Bassetlaw Hospitals NHS Foundation Trust, Armthorpe Road, Doncaster DN2 5LT
Tel: 01302 366666 Ext: 3583 Fax: 01302 320098
Email: lynn.hardy@dbh.nhs.uk
Website: www.dbh.nhs.uk

Director of Postgraduate Medical Education D K Chadha
GP CME Tutor M C Coleman
GP Dental Postgraduate Tutor K Woolass
Postgraduate Administrator Lynn Hardy
Royal College Tutor S J Ahmad, G P Chandler, A E O Coker, C L Kelly, T K Rogers, A Strachan
Specialty Tutor P Harkness, R Helm, A Holmes, D G R Jayamanne, J R Paskins
VTS Administrator J Morrison
VTS Course Organiser D R J Bunny, A Dexter, B Jackson, N M Sinclair, N Tupper

Douglas Pickup Postgraduate Medical Centre

Pontefract General Infirmary, Friarwood Lane, Pontefract WF8 1PL
Tel: 01977 606361 Fax: 01977 606361
Email: moira.fearnley@midyorks.nhs.uk

Director Postgraduate Medical Education A R Harvey
Medical Education Centre Manager S Hunt
Medical Education Development Manager D Mathews

Durham Postgraduate Medical Centre and Education Centre

University Hospital of North Durham, North Road, Durham DH1 5TW
Tel: 0191 333 2333, 0191 333 2485 Fax: 0191 333 2688
Email: anne.sewell@cddah.nhs.uk

Associate Clinical Tutor Surendra Pandey
Clinical Tutor Paul Barrett
Medical Education Manager Anne Sewell
Senior Lecturer Peter Cook
Undergraduate Tutor David Laird

Ealing Hospital NHS Trust Postgraduate Centre

Uxbridge Road, Southall UB1 3HW
Tel: 020 8967 5202 Fax: 020 8967 5008
Email: jacquire.speechley@eht.nhs.uk

Director of Medical Education and Training Hugh Mather
Clinical Tutor Jay Arnold
Deputy Clinical Tutor A Gordon, E Whitehead

East Cumbria Postgraduate Medical Centre

Cumberland Infirmary, Carlisle CA2 7HY
Tel: 01228 814883 Fax: 01228 814822
Email: margaret.tait@cumbria-acute.nhs.uk

Clinical Tutor R H Robson
GP Tutor C P Mitchell
Medical Education Manager Margaret Tait

Specialty Tutor M Bearn, J Fraser, R Lawley, C Lord, C E MacDonald, D Prosser, P Whitehead, M R Williams

East Riding Medical Education Centre

Hull Royal Infirmary, Anlaby Road, Hull HU3 2JZ
Tel: 01482 604313 Fax: 01482 586587
Email: ermec.reception@hey.nhs.uk, joanne.clemenson@hey.nhs.uk
Website: www.hey.nhs.uk

Director Colin Melville
Associate Royal College Tutor Surgery G V Johnson
Dental CME Tutor J Holguin
Deputy College Tutor Obstetrics and Gynaecology, HRI S Lindow
General Practice CME Tutor S Kapur, A Parkin
GP VTS Course Organiser P Davis, D Roper, S Towers
RCT Medicine G Anderson, D Lewis, H Thaker
RCT Obstetrics and Gynaecology K Phillips
RCT Ophthalmology O Stewart
RCT Oral and Maxillofacial Surgery M Cope
RCT Paediatrics A Azaz
RCT Pathology P Dore
RCT Psychiatry G Harkness
RCT Radiology CHH N Kennan
RCT Radiology HRI D Salvage
RCT Surgery P Rennick

East Surrey Hospital Postgraduate Medical Centre

Canada Avenue, Redhill RH1 5RH
Tel: 01737 231722 Fax: 01737 231723
Email: linda.briant@sash.nhs.uk
Website: www.surreyandsussex.nhs.uk

Director of Medical Education Alan Vallon
Associate Director of Medical Education Bruce Stewart
Anaesthetic Tutor Fred Sage
GP Education Convenor Chris Hughes
Library and Information Manager Rachel Cooke
Medical Education Manager Linda Briant
Medical Education Manager for Psychiatry Deborah Beisiegel-Lambert
Ophthalmology Tutor Fiona O'Sullivan
Orthopaedic Tutor G Tselentakis
Paediatric Tutor Ivor Lewis
Psychiatry Tutor Farida Yousaf
RCOG Tutor Zara Nadim
RCP Tutor D Acharya, Simon Stem
Royal College of Pathologists M Ameen
Surgical Tutor T Selvan
VTS Organiser Graham Carr, Terry Conaty, Paul Stillman

Eastbourne Postgraduate Medical and Dental Centre

District General Hospital, King's Drive, Eastbourne BN21 2UD
Tel: 01323 414967 Fax: 01323 414932
Email: liz.oliver-taylor@esht.nhs.uk

Centre Manager Liz Oliver-Taylor
Clinical Tutor Jeremy J Bending
GP Tutor I Adoki, P Williams
Specialty Tutor (Anaesthetics) M Lonsdale
Specialty Tutor (Dental) R Webster
Specialty Tutor (Obstetrics and Gynaecology) K Ayers
Specialty Tutor (Ophthalmology) M Wearne
Specialty Tutor (RCP) N Patel
Specialty Tutor (RCS) M Saunders
Vocational Training Scheme Tutor J M Cockburn, S Eyre

Eastern Deanery

Postgraduate Medical and Dental Education, Block 3, Ida Darwin Site, Fulbourn, Cambridge CB1 5EE
Tel: 01223 884848 Fax: 01223 884849
Website: www.easterndeanery.org

Postgraduate Dean D H Jones
Associate Dean (Flexible Training) C A Lawton
Associate Dean (Hospital Education) A M Burns, M Dronfield, A M Jennings, C A Lawton, J Waller
Associate Dean (Pre-Registration) A J Crisp, D R Hall
Director of Postgraduate Dental Education J M Heath
Director of Postgraduate General Practice A G Hibble

Edgware Postgraduate Centre

Edgware Community Hospital, Burnt Oak Broadway, Edgware HA8 0AD
Tel: 020 8952 9924 Fax: 020 8732 6626
Email: judy.maisner@barnet-pct.nhs.uk

Clinical Tutor George Ikkos
Postgraduate Centre Manager Judy Maisner

Education and Training Centre (East Cheshire NHS Trust)

East Cheshire NHS Trust, Victoria Road, Macclesfield SK10 3BL
Tel: 01625 661237 Fax: 01625 663145
Email: carol.eke@echeshire-tr.nwest.nhs.uk
Website: www.echeshire-tr.nwest.nhs.uk

Clinical Tutor H Waring
Course Organiser (VTSO) S Cocksedge, D Maxwell

The Education Centre

Tower Hamlets Primary Care Trust, Mile End Hospital, Bancroft Road, London E1 4DG
Tel: 020 7377 7000 Ext: 4436 Fax: 020 7377 7944
Email: ruth.caudwell@thpct.nhs.uk

Lead Clinician Ruth Caudwell

Education Service

Royal Liverpool and Broadgreen University Hospitals NHS Trust, Prescot Street, Liverpool L7 8XP
Tel: 0151 706 3752
Email: sarah.byrne@rlbuht.nhs.uk

Director of Education P Weston
Education Service Manager Sarah Byrne, Joanne Charing
Library Manager Angela Hall

Epsom and St Helier University Hospitals NHS Trust

St Helier Hospital, Wrythe Lane, Carshalton SM5 1AA
Tel: 020 8296 2000 Fax: 020 8641 4546
Website: www.epsom-sthelier.nhs.uk

Clinical Tutor O Duke
GPVTS Course Organisers B Ghoorbin, A Smith
Primary Care Tutor R Seyan
Specialty Tutor (Anaesthetics) A Hussein
Specialty Tutor (Medicine) J Kwan
Specialty Tutor (Obstetrics and Gynaecology) C Croucher
Specialty Tutor (Ophthalmology) A McElvanney
Specialty Tutor (Paediatrics) K Blewitt
Specialty Tutor (Pathology) J Merceica
Specialty Tutor (Radiology) V Cook
Specialty Tutor (Surgery) M Churchill

Exeter Postgraduate Education Centre

Royal Devon and Exeter NHS Foundation Trust, Barrack Road, Exeter EX2 5DW
Tel: 01392 403006 Fax: 01392 403007
Email: pgmc@rdehc-tr.swest.nhs.uk

Director of Medical Education Babinder Sandhar, Nick Withers
Clinical Tutor Richard D'Souza, Ed Hammond
College Tutor (Anaesthetics) David Conn
College Tutor (Haematology) Richard Lee
College Tutor (Medicine) Nick Withers
College Tutor (Obstetrics and Gynaecology) Rachel Sturley
College Tutor (Ophthalmology) Paeter Simcock

College Tutor (Orthopaedics) M Hubble
College Tutor (Paediatrics) Michael Quinn
College Tutor (Surgery) Andrew Cowan

Farnborough Education Centre

Farnborough Hospital, Farnborough Common, Orpington BR6 8ND
Tel: 01689 863000 Fax: 01689 864316
Email: lynne.archer@bromleyhospitals.nhs.uk
Website: www.bromleyhospitals.nhs.uk

Centre Manager Lynne Archer
Clinical Tutor Andrew Long
GP Tutor D Barker
Specialty Tutor M Ahmed, A Coumbe, M De Silva, G Ghosh, N Hill, E Langford, A Martin, I Stell, A Thomas
VTS Course Organiser C Bailey, D Masters, N Payne

Fieldhouse Teaching Centre

Bradford Royal Infirmary, Duckworth Lane, Bradford BD9 6RJ
Tel: 01274 364860 Fax: 01274 366920

Clinical Tutor D Wilkinson
CME Tutor J A Bibby
Medical Education Manager M Neary
VTS Course Organiser M Eisner, R Mehay, N Price

The Frank Rifkin Postgraduate Medical Education Centre

Hope Hospital, Stott Lane, Salford M6 8HD
Tel: 0161 206 5401 Fax: 0161 206 5408
Email: postgrad@srht.nhs.uk

Clinical Tutor T Johnson
GP Tutor W M Forman
Postgraduate Medical Education Manager Maggie Johnson
Specialty Tutor N Clarke, I Geraghty, A Jones, D Nicholson, A Robinson

Freeman Hospital Education Centre

Freeman Hospital, Newcastle upon Tyne NE7 7DN
Tel: 0191 223 1284 Fax: 0191 223 1247

Clinical Tutor S Murray
Specialty Tutor C Baudouin, K Beacham, C Hilton, R Pickard, V A Wadge

Frenchay Postgraduate Centre

Frenchay Hospital, Bristol BS16 1LE
Tel: 0117 975 3704 Fax: 0117 970 1691
Email: susan.nutland@north-bristol.swest.nhs.uk
Website: www.northbristol.nhs.uk

Director of Medical Education Joe Unsworth
Clinical Tutor J Kendall, P Younge
College Tutor N Baldwin, A Dixon, M Gregory, P Jardine, F McLeod, N Slack
Medical Education Administrator Elaine Monks, Heather Partridge
Receptionist Julie Vernon

Frimley Park Hospital Postgraduate Education Centre

Portsmouth Road, Frimley, Camberley GU16 7UJ
Tel: 01276 526388 Fax: 01276 604186
Email: pgecusers@fph-tr.nhs.uk
Website: www.frimleyparkpgec.org.uk

Administrator Linzi Hudson
Clinical Tutor/Director Alison Keightley, S Promachandean
GP Tutor Paula Roberts, Patrick Williams
Medical Education Manager Maureen Stephens
Specialty Tutor (Anaesthetics) Tim Pepall
Specialty Tutor (Medical) Mark Lloyd
Specialty Tutor (O&G) Ulrich Bartels
Specialty Tutor (Ophthamology) James Govan
Specialty Tutor (Orthopaedics) Anthony Sakellariou
Specialty Tutor (Paediatrics) Abous Mallik
Specialty Tutor (Radiology) Fiona Hearn
Specialty Tutor (Surgery) Raouf Daoud
VTS Course Organiser Brian Booth, Christine Marshall

Frognal Centre for Medical Studies

Queen Mary's Hospital, Sidcup DA14 6LT
Tel: 020 8308 3030 Fax: 020 8308 3058
Email: postgrad@qms.nhs.uk
Website: www.home.qms.com/postgrad

Specialty Tutor W Barry, K Hussain, R Kerwat, M Khan, D Lee, D Milne, S Morgan, K Pervaiz, E Richardson, M Rowntree, H Stoate, P Waterstone, G Yu

Gateshead Postgraduate Medical Centre

Queen Elizabeth Hospital, Gateshead NE9 6SX
Tel: 0191 482 0000 ext: 2107 Fax: 0191 482 3341

Clinical Tutor M Das
Education Centre Manager L Heppenstall
Specialty Tutor Dr Barker, Mr Beeby, Dr Beesley, John Gesse, Dr Harrison, J Henry, Dr May, Mr Mudawin, Dr Timmens

The George Pickering Postgraduate Centre

John Radcliffe Hospital, Headington, Oxford OX3 9DU

Associate Clinical Tutor C Conlon, H Jones, H Simpson
Associate GP Tutor H Merriman
Clinical Tutor M Burch
District Dental Tutor P Lawson
Specialty Tutor C Chubb, A P Freeland, M Gilmer, J Humphreys, J D Kay, N Mortensen, O O'Dayar, C Oppenheimer, S Ostlere, J Roblin, J Shakespeare, P Watts-Smith, P R Williams

Giving for Living Research and Postgraduate Centre

Royal Manchester Children's Hospital, Hospital Road, Pendlebury, Manchester M27 4HA
Tel: 0161 727 2155 Fax: 0161 727 2155
Email: dorothy.murphy@cmmc.nhs.uk
Website: www.cmmc.nhs.uk

College Tutor (Anaesthetics) R Perkins
College Tutor (Paediatrics) Guy Makin
College Tutor Pathology) John Grainger
College Tutor (Psychiatry) Leo Kroll
College Tutor (Radiology) Neville Wright
College Tutor (Surgery) John Day
Postgraduate Centre Manager Dorothy Murphy
Postgraduate Tutor Guy Makin

Gloucester Postgraduate Medical Centre

Gloucestershire Royal Hospital, Great Western Road, Gloucester GL1 3NN
Tel: 08454 226727 Fax: 08454 226734
Website: www.gloshospitals.org.uk/pgmec

Director of Medical Education E Spencer
Clinical Tutor T Mahajan, J McCarthy
Specialty Tutor B Adrianns, P A Birch, M D Read, A Rushforth, M Savidge, N A Shepherd, M Vipond
Sub-Specialty Tutor I Crabb, I Donald, G Fuller, S McCabe, R Majkowski, C Perkins, A Ritchie, J Ropner, M Thomas

Good Hope Education Centre and Library

Good Hope Hospital NHS Trust, Rectory Road, Sutton Coldfield B75 7RR
Tel: 0121 378 6038 Fax: 0121 378 6039
Email: sheila.hannington@goodhope.nhs.uk
Website: www.goodhope.org.uk

Clinical Tutor R S V Cartmill
GP Tutor A McDonald
Specialty Tutor (Accident and Emergency) M Gillett
Specialty Tutor (Anaesthetics) M Elliot

Specialty Tutor (General Surgery) A Jewkes
Specialty Tutor (Medicine) T Fletcher
Specialty Tutor (Obstetrics and Gynaecology) R Cartmill
Specialty Tutor (Paediatrics) N El-Shimy
Specialty Tutor (Trauma and Orthopaedics B Banerjee
Specialty Tutor (VTS) P Houlston

Gosport Postgraduate Medical Centre

The Royal Hospital Haslar, Gosport PO12 2AA
Tel: 023 9276 2446 Fax: 023 9276 2510

PGMC Manager Janis Richards

Grantham and District Hospital Postgraduate Medical Centre

United Lincolnshire Hospitals NHS Trust, Grantham & District Hospital, Manthorpe Road, Grantham NG31 8DG
Tel: 01476 565232
Email: grantham.postgrad@ulh.nhs.uk

Clinical Tutor J L Breckenridge
Postgraduate Administrator L Edwards
Specialty Tutor D Garrick, W Wijayawardhana

Great Ormond Street Hospital for Children NHS Trust Education Centre

Great Ormond Street, London WC1N 3JH
Tel: 020 7405 9200 Fax: 020 7813 8227
Email: info@gosh.nhs.uk
Website: www.gosh.nsh.uk

Vice-Dean for Training S Strobel
Director of Medical Education and Clinical Tutor H Cass (Head)
Medical Director D Drake
PGME Manager Rachel Moreton

Grimsby Postgraduate Medical Education Centre

Diana, Princess of Wales Hospital, Scartho Road, Grimsby DN33 2BA
Tel: 01472 875275 Fax: 01472 875329
Email: lynn.young@nlg.nhs.uk
Website: www.nlg.nhs.uk

Associate Director of Postgraduate Medical Education J A Adiotomre
Clinical Dental Tutor A P T Sims
Foundation Programme Director A A Naqvi
GP Tutor K Collett
Specialty Tutor P Bagga, I I Bolaji, T Gillott, S Herber, I McNeil, I Rehman, K Speed, M P Tilston
VTS Course Organiser J Potter

Guildford Postgraduate Medical Centre

Royal Surrey County Hospital, Guildford GU2 7XX
Tel: 01483 571122 ext: 4244 Fax: 01483 303691

Medical and Dental Education Manager Sue Cranham
Specialty Tutor S Chapman, P Curtis, S Deacock, A Gilvarry, H Griffiths, M Kissin, A Neal, H Powell, W Walker, M Whiteley

Gurney Postgraduate Centre

Hemel Hempstead General Hospital (Acute), Hillfield Road, Hemel Hempstead HP2 4AD
Tel: 01442 287666 Fax: 01442 287670
Email: hhghpostgrad@hotmail.com
Website: www.westhertshospitals.nhs.uk/pgmc

Director of Education I Barrison
Deputy Clinical Tutor S Hill
GP VTS Course Organiser B Covell, P Heatley
Specialty Tutor I Barrison, Mr Bhatti, S Catnach, R Gallow, S Hill, R Makker, M Padwick, A Young

Guy's and St Thomas' Hospital NHS Trust Centre for Postgraduate Professional Education

Ground Floor, Gassiot House, St Thomas' Hospital, Lambeth Palace Road, London SE1 7EH
Tel: 020 7928 9292 Fax: 020 7401 8591
Email: john.masih@kcl.ac.uk
Website: www.kcl.ac.uk

Postgraduate Dean C H C Twort
Postgraduate Sub-Dean S Mowle
Postgraduate Sub-Dean and Deputy Director Claire Mallinson
Conference and Events Co-ordinator I De Abreu
Education Co-ordinator S Young
Postgraduate Manager John Masih
Specialty Tutor D Goldsmith, B Lams

Guy's Department of Postgraduate Studies

Sherman Education Centre, Guy's Hospital, London SE1 9RT
Tel: 020 7955 4300/4301 Fax: 020 7955 4913

Postgraduate Dean Charles Twort
Postgraduate Sub-Dean Claire Mallinson, Steve Mowle

Halton Education Centre

North Cheshire Hospitals NHS Trust, Halton General Hospital, Hospital Way, Runcorn WA7 2DA
Tel: 01928 753318 Fax: 01928 753268

Clinical Sub-Dean A Moloney
Centre Manager D I Palmer
Clinical Tutor J N Johnson
GP Tutor P Johnson
Librarian L Chapelhow

Hammersmith Hospital Postgraduate Centre

Hammersmith Hospital, Du Cane Road, London W12 0HS
Tel: 020 8383 3462 Fax: 020 8383 3464
Email: mmcnamara@hhnt.org

Director of Postgraduate Education and Continuing Professional Development Jeremy Levy
Postgraduate Education Manager Maggie McNamara

Harefield Hospital Postgraduate Centre

Harefield Hospital, Hill End Road, Harefield UB9 6JU
Tel: 01895 828735 Fax: 01895 828735

Clinical Tutor D Cummins
Postgraduate Centre Manager Lesley Barker

Harold Wood Hospital Postgraduate Academic Centre

Gubbins Lane, Harold Wood, Romford RM3 0BE
Tel: 01708 345156 (Direct Line) Fax: 01708 345156

Director of Medical Education R Weatherstone
Associate Tutor A Aspoas
Contact Manager L Freegard
Specialty Tutor S Gibbs, H Haddock, M Saphandan, S Shami, M Smith, W White

Harperbury Horizon

Harperbury Hospital, Harperbury Lane, Shenley, Radlett WD7 9HQ
Tel: 01923 854861 Fax: 01923 859148

Clinical Tutor Iqbal Singh

Harrogate Postgraduate Medical Centre

Strayside Education Centre, Harrogate District Hospital, Lancaster Park Road, Harrogate HG2 7SX
Tel: 01423 553092 Fax: 01423 553094
Email: Strayside.Education@hhc-tr.northy.nhs.uk

Specialty Tutor J Brothwell, G Dyke, J Gasser, A Gough, C Gray, W Hulse, L Kidd, S Rahman, J Warren

Hartlepool Postgraduate Medical Centre

University Hospital of Hartlepool, Holdford Road, Hartlepool TS24 9AH
Tel: 01429 522343 Fax: 01429 522739

Clinical Tutor J Clancy
Postgraduate Medical Education Manager Suzanne Duncan
Specialty Tutor H Bandi, B K Chaudhury, J Frater, J Jani, A V Kidambi, H Mohan, A A Robertson

Hastings Postgraduate Medical Education Centre

The Education Centre, Conquest Hospital, The Ridge, St Leonards-on-Sea TN37 7RD
Tel: 01424 755255 Fax: 01424 758097
Email: sbruce@esht.nhs.uk
Website: www.esh.nhs.uk

Clinical Tutor S A Bruce
GP Tutor A Dunfield-Prayero
Specialty Tutor M Boxer, D Fitzpatrick, S Mansy, M Parsloe, P Sinha, M Whitehead

Hereford Hospitals NHS Trust Postgraduate Medical Centre

County Hospital, Hereford HR1 2ER
Tel: 01432 364025 Fax: 01432 355265
Email: pat.rossi@hhtr.nhs.uk
Website: www.herefordshire.nhs.uk

Associate Clinical Tutor P Ryan
Clinical Sub-Dean A Corder
Clinical Tutor C Byatt
Primary Care Medical Educator J Barnes, P Clayton, P Downey, S Hasan
Royal College Tutor A Butterfill, N Bywater, S Jones, P Ryan, S Scotcher, R B Smith, D H Williams

The Hertfordshire Partnership NHS Trust Postgraduate Centre

Harperbury Hospital, Harper Lane, Radlett WD7 9QH
Tel: 01923 427463 Fax: 01923 427370
Email: janet.gilfin@hpt.nhs.uk

Postgraduate Manager Janet Gilfin

Hexham Education Centre

General Hospital, Hexham NE46 1QJ
Tel: 01434 655655 Ext: 5719 Fax: 01434 655734
Email: kristina.mitchell@northumbria-healthcare.nhs.uk
Website: www.northumbria-healthcare.nhs.uk

Clinical Tutor P Sims
Postgraduate Centre Coordinator K Mitchell
Specialty Tutor M Mansour, J D O'Callaghan, A Wright

Hillingdon Hospital Postgraduate Centre

Pield Heath Road, Hillingdon, Uxbridge UB8 3NN
Tel: 01895 279799/279861 Fax: 01895 234150
Email: christine2.massey@thh.nhs.uk

Clinical Tutor Robin Kantor
Deputy Clinical Tutor Anthea Parry

Hinchingbrooke Postgraduate Medical Education Centre

Hinchingbrooke Hospital, Hinchingbrooke Park, Huntingdon PE29 6NT
Tel: 01480 416122 Ext: 6118
Email: phillipa.smith@hinchingbrooke.nhs.uk

Clinical Sub-Dean Liz Haslett
Specialty Tutor (Accident and Emergency) R K Das
Specialty Tutor (Anaesthetics) T Memon
Specialty Tutor (ENT) R Gray
Specialty Tutor (General Medicine) K J Walsh
Specialty Tutor (General Surgery) Basam Bekdash
Specialty Tutor (Haematology) K Rege
Specialty Tutor (Mental Health) Clare Hall
Specialty Tutor (Obstetrics and Gynaecology) S Hamilton
Specialty Tutor (Ophthalmology) Melanie Hingorani
Specialty Tutor (Orthopaedics and Trauma) S N Amarah
Specialty Tutor (Paediatrics) M Becker
Specialty Tutor (Pathology) S Lishman
Undergraduate Specialty Tutor (Anaesthesia) P Roberts
Undergraduate Specialty Tutor (Obstetrics and Gynaecology) B Lim
Undergraduate Specialty Tutor (Paediatrics) R N Miles
Undergraduate Specialty Tutor (Psychiatry) A Owen
Undergraduate Specialty Tutor (Surgery) J R Benson

Homerton University Hospital Postgraduate Education Centre

Homerton Hospital, Homerton Row, London E9 6SR
Tel: 020 8510 7747 Fax: 020 8510 7314
Website: www.homerton.nhs.uk

Clinical Tutor Helen Cugnoni

Huddersfield Medical Centre

Huddersfield Royal Infirmary, Lindley, Huddersfield HD3 3EA
Tel: 01484 342655 Fax: 01484 347052
Email: becky.jackson@cht.nhs.uk

Clinical Tutor G Chakrabarty
Clinical Tutor (VTSO) T D Swift
GP Tutor J Lord

Huntingdon District Postgraduate Medical Education Centre

Hinchingbrooke Hospital, Hinchingbrooke Park, Huntingdon PE18 8NT

Director Clinical Studies Kevin Walsh
Specialty Tutor S N Amarah, M G Becker, C Borland, R Das, S Forster, B Greenway, D S Hughes, R Latcham, D A Morris, J Oubridge, P Roberts, M Slack, I A Sweetenham, M Wright

Institute of Orthopaedics Postgraduate Medical Centre

Robert Jones & Agnes Hunt Orthopaedic and District Hospital NHS Trust, Oswestry SY10 7AG
Tel: 01691 404391 Fax: 01691 404071
Email: judith.harris@rjah.nhs.uk
Website: www.keele.ac.uk/depts/rjah/

Course Organiser Erica Wilkinson
Postgraduate Administrator Judy Harris
Programme Director R Spencer-Jones
Senior Clinical Lecturer B Ashton, M W J Davie, S M Eisenstein, W El Masri, G Evans, D C Jaffray, J Middleton, J H Patrick, V C Pullicino, J Richardson, A Roberts, S Roberts
West Midlands Specialty Adviser (T&O) D J Ford

Ipswich Hospital NHS Trust Postgraduate Centre

Ipswich Hospital, Heath Road, Ipswich IP4 5PD
Tel: 01473 702562 Fax: 01473 702503
Email: mary.bartlett@ipswichhospital.nhs.uk
Website: www.ipswichhospital.org.uk

Clinical Tutor R Howard-Griffin
Dental Tutor I Davies
Dental VTS Course Organiser J Stokes
GP VTS Course Organiser J Jesuthasan, K Rix, D Ward
Specialty Tutor G Banerjee, M Bowditch, H Davies, I Davies, Driver, J Gould, M Grimmer, S Hardman-Lea, D Hodgkinson, I Osman, M Salam, M Sule

Isle of Wight Healthcare NHS Trust Postgraduate Medical Education Centre
St Mary's Hospital, Newport PO30 5TG
Tel: 01983 534231 Fax: 01983 521963
Email: zorina.walsh@iow.nhs.uk
Website: www.iowht.org.uk

Associate Clinical Sub Dean P Close
Clinical Tutor M Pugh
Dental Tutor J Wickens
GP Tutor J Partridge
Medical Tutor D Murphy
PGMC Manager Zorina Walsh
Regional Adviser in Surgery (Wessex) T H Walsh
Specialty Tutor (Obstetrics and Gynaecology) P Vandekerckhove
Specialty Tutor (Paediatrics) P Rowlanoson
Surgical Tutor (Surgery) E Rahall

James Fawcett Education Centre
Barley Lane, Goodmayes, Ilford IG3 8YB
Tel: 020 8970 8017 Fax: 020 8970 8269
Email: barbara.hutton@bhrhospitals.nhs.uk

Director Postgraduate Education G Cochrane
Joint Associate Medical Director - Education M G W Cochrane

The John Fawcett Postgraduate Medical and Dental Education Centre
Peterborough District Hospital, Thorpe Road, Peterborough PE3 6DA
Tel: 01733 874660 Fax: 01733 875848
Email: barbara.petrie@pbh-tr.nhs.uk

Clinical Sub-Dean M Ninkovic
Director of Clinical Studies and Medicine Tutor P Nair
Clinical Tutor M Richardson
GP Tutor H Mistry, C Nnochiri
Specialty Tutor A Fitt, M Gervin, M Harris, S Havenga, S Lewis, C Moss, P Nair, V Reddy, M Stoker, A Wells
VTS Course Organiser A Bond, M L Denney, N Hume

John Lister Postgraduate Centre
Wexham Park Hospital, Slough SL2 4HL
Tel: 01753 634383 Fax: 01753 634385
Website: www.johnlister.ac.uk

Clinical Tutor P Sebire
Dental Tutor Ann Davidson
Primary Care CPD Tutor B Sainsbury
Specialty Tutor C Aldren, N Desmond, J Fairbank, A Gordon, S Kheterpal, C Khoo, C Litchfield, R Loveland, A Macaulay, V Mayadunne, H Motiwala, J Philpot, H Sharif, G Singer, B Soin
VTS Course Organiser M Kittel, B Sainsbury, M Uppal

Kendal Education Centre
Westmorland General Hospital, Burton Road, Kendal LA9 7RG
Tel: 01539 795230 Fax: 01539 795308

Associate Clinical Tutor Ian Chadwick
Clinical Education Manager Peter Benning
Specialty Tutor I M Huggett

Kidderminster Education Centre
Bewdley Road, Kidderminster DY11 6RJ
Tel: 01562 512343 Fax: 01562 825733
Email: sheenagh.gallagher@worcsacute.wmids.nhs.uk

Centre Manager Sheenagh Gallagher, Angela Haycock
Clinical Tutor P Newrick
GP Tutor C Prince
GP VTS Organiser C Wilkinson

King's Healthcare NHS Trust Postgraduate Medical Centre
Weston Education Centre, Cutcombe Road, London SE5 9RS
Tel: 020 7848 5525 Fax: 020 7848 5766
Email: joanne.hiley@kingsch.nhs.uk
Website: www.kingsch.nhs.uk

Director Postgraduate Medical Education / Postgraduate Dean Jan Welch
GP Tutor Niro Amin, Kishor Vasant
Librarian Rodney Amis
PGMDE Adviser / Manager Joanne Hiley
Postgraduate Dental Tutor Martin Kelleher

King's Lynn Postgraduate Medical and Dental Education Centre
The Queen Elizabeth Hospital, Gayton Road, King's Lynn PE30 4ET
Tel: 01553 613791 Fax: 01553 613903
Email: jane.dearling@qehkl.nhs.uk

Clinical Tutor E George
GP VTS Course Organiser H Lazarus, K Redhead
Specialty Tutor S Abukhalil, J Bottomley, Z Butt, A Chakrabarti, A Chan Seem, M Crowe, P Cullen, J Dossetor, A Douds, L Ho, H Hobbiger, A O'Neill

The Kings Mill Education Centre
Sherwood Forest Hospitals NHS Trust, Kings Mill Hospital, Sutton-in-Ashfield NG17 4JL
Fax: 01623 672374
Email: Margaret.Murray@kmc-tr.nhs.uk

Director of Postgraduate Education Mr Livesley (Head)
Course Organiser Mr Robertson, P Smith
Specialty Tutor R Weston-Price

Kingston Postgraduate Medical Centre
1 Galsworthy Road, Kingston upon Thames KT2 7QB
Tel: 020 8546 7711 Ext: 2579, 020 8934 2579
Fax: 020 8547 3960

Anaesthetics Tutor J Zwaal
Centre Manager Jeanne Browne
Clinical Tutor J Wilson
Dental Tutor M Preiss
GP Tutor M F D'Souza
GP VTS Joint Course Organiser I Johnson, D Tymens, M Vezterski
Ophthalmology Tutor C Roberts
Paediatrics and Child Health Tutor T Ayeni
Pathologists Tutor P McHugh
Physicians Tutor C Rodrigues
Specialty Tutor R Pearson, A Pooley
Surgery Tutor M Curtis

Kingsway Hospital Postgraduate Centre
Derbyshire Mental Health Services NHS Trust, Kingsway, Derby DE22 3LZ

Clinical Tutor J Tombs

Lancaster Postgraduate Medical Centre
Royal Lancaster Infirmary, Ashton Road, Lancaster LA1 4RR
Tel: 01524 583950 Fax: 01524 848289
Email: sue.newall@rli.mbnt.nhs.uk

Clinical Tutor and Specialty Tutor D Burgh
Dental Tutor C Hoyle
GP Tutor S Brear
Specialty Tutor R W Blewitt, M Bukhari, K Granger, W Morgan, A Napier, T Oldham, D Stacey

Learning and Development Centre
Calderdale Royal Hospital, Salterhebble, Halifax HX3 0PW
Tel: 01422 224385 Fax: 01422 224185
Email: Angela.Bottomley@calderdale.nhs.uk

Director Postgraduate Education S N Chater
Clinical Tutor (VTSO) T Swift

Librarian H Curtis, C Jackson
Manager A Bottomley

Leeds Infirmary Postgraduate Medical Centre

The General Infirmary, Great George Street, Leeds LS1 3EX
Tel: 0113 392 3965 Fax: 0113 392 3327
Email: mavisprice@leedsth-nhs.uk
Website: www.leedsteachinghospitals.com

Clinical Tutor O J Corrado
Clinical Tutor (PRHO) P A Templeton

Leicester Clinical Education Centre

University Hospitals of Leicester NHS Trust, Leicester Royal Infirmary, Leicester LE1 5WW
Tel: 0116 254 1414, 0116 258 6381 Fax: 0116 258 5679
Email: clinical.educationcentre@uhl-tr.nhs.uk

Director of Clinical Education T Alun-Jones
Centre Manager T Kissane
Clinical Tutor M Ardon
Specialty Tutor J Deane, F Dickenoan, W Hassan, J Konje, D Lloyd, D K Luyt, M Mushambi, S Vasanthan, D Ward, K P West

Leicestershire, Northamptonshire and Rutland Postgraduate Deanery

Lakeside House, 4 Smith Way, Grove Park, Enderby, Leicester LE19 1SS
Tel: 0116 295 7639 Fax: 0116 295 7640
Email: firstname.surname@lnrdeanery.nhs.uk
Website: www.inrdeanery.nhs.uk

Deanery Educational Adviser Susan Cavendish
Postgraduate Dean Derek Gallen (Head)
Director of Postgraduate General Practice Education Justin Allen
Deputy Director in General Practice Simon Gregory
Associate Postgraduate Dean Christina Faull, Robert Gregory
Associate Deputy Director in General Practice Roger Price, Aly Rashid
Business Manager Marcia Reid
Deputy Postgraduate Dean Davinder Sandhu
Medical Education Developer Richard Higgins

Lewisham Education Centre

Lewisham Hospital, High Street, London SE13 6LH
Tel: 020 8333 3000 Fax: 020 8333 3079

Clinical Tutor John Stroobant
Specialty Tutor Sarah Flint, F Majid, John Miell, D Misselbrook, John Pook, Gopal Rao, Richard Simo, Elizabeth Sleight, A Steger, H Tegner

Lincoln County Hospital Postgraduate Medical Centre

United Lincolnshire Hospitals NHS Trust, Sewell Road, Lincoln LN2 5QY
Tel: 01522 573866

Clinical Tutor D Stokoe
Senior Course Organiser C Campbell
Undergraduate Dental Tutor M A Coupland
VTS Course Organiser J Coffey, M Magee

Lister Hospital Postgraduate Centre

Coreys Mill Lane, Stevenage SG1 4AB
Tel: 01438 781076 Fax: 01438 781442
Email: postgradlister.enh-tr@nhs.net

Clinical Tutor S Khan
Dental Tutor J Chico
Deputy Medical Director K Farrington
Deputy Tutor I Sockalingham
GP Tutor R A S Christie, J Machen
Librarian Joan Lomas
Medical Director J McCue
Specialty Tutor S A Davies, M Ehsanullah, S Ellis, K Farrington, D Hanbury, T C Holme, N K James, P S Kerr, R Patel, C Prendergast, S J Quinn, R Sattin, I Sockalingham
VTS Course Organiser E Salik
VTS Course Organiser/GP Tutor M Hodgson

The London Chest Hospital Education Centre

Bonner Road, London E2 9JX
Tel: 020 8983 2342 Fax: 020 8983 2202

London Department of Postgraduate Medical and Dental Education

20 Guilford Street, London WC1N 1DZ
Tel: 020 7692 3232 Fax: 020 7692 3396
Website: www.londondeanery.ac.uk

Dean Director Elizabeth Paice (Head)
Dean of Postgraduate Dental Education Elizabeth Jones
Dean of Postgraduate General Practice Education Neal Jackson
Dean of Postgraduate Medical Education (North Central and North East) Wendy Reid
Dean of Postgraduate Medical Education (North West) Fiona Moss
Dean of Postgraduate Medical Education (South Thames) Ian Hastie
Deputy Dean Director Shelley Heard
Head of Human Resources and Central Services Tony Americano

Luton and Dunstable Hospital NHS Trust Medical Centre

Lewsey Road, Luton LU4 0DZ
Tel: 01582 497200 Fax: 01582 497389
Email: diana.hardy@ldh-tr.anglox.nhs.uk

Career and Counselling Tutor B Adler
Clinical Tutor J Day
Deputy Clinical Tutor T Isitt
GP Tutor A Sahdev
Medical Centre Manager D J Hardy
Medical Librarian D Johnson
Specialty Tutor D Freedman, L Hale, D Heath, D H Horwell, R Novell, D Peterson, J Pillai, J Scott, P Sivakumar
Tutor J Pickles, A Twigley
VTS Course Organiser R Khanchandani, J Marsden

Marsh-Jackson Education Centre

Yeovil District Hospital, Higher Kingston, Yeovil BA21 4AT
Tel: 01935 384476 Fax: 01935 384670
Email: botta@est.nhs.uk

Centre Manager Alison Bott
Clinical Tutor Dr Qadiri
Specialty Tutor N C G Bathurst, S Brooks, C Elsworth, P Heaton, M Niayesh, L Osoba, T G Palferman, T Porter, Dr Sinha, J Tricker
VTS Course Organiser M J O Minogue

Medical, Dental and AHP Office, Education Centre

West Suffolk Hospital, Hardwick Lane, Bury St Edmunds IP33 2QZ
Tel: 01284 713342 Fax: 01284 712598
Email: Lynn.Jones@wsh.nsh.uk
Website: www.wsufftrust.org.uk

Clinical Sub-Dean M Wood
Director of Postgraduate Medical Education S Edwards
Clinical Tutor R Chipperfield
Dental Tutor J Barnet-Lamb
GP Tutor R West
Medical Director/Director of Education R Bunnon
Royal College Tutor J Buck, A Burns, R Giles, S S Jolin, N Kealing, R Lamb, J Majeed, C Tremlett, L Watson
VTS Course Organiser P Lloyd-Jones, J Masters, D Pearson

Medway Postgraduate Medical Centre

Medway Maritime Hospital, Windmill Road, Gillingham ME7 5NY
Tel: 01634 830000 Fax: 01634 819425
Website: www.medwaymaritimehospital.nhs.uk

Clinical Tutor I N Scobie
Specialty Tutor S Day, P Green, H Wegstapel

Mersey Deanery

Hamilton House, 1st Floor, 24 Pall Mall, Liverpool L3 6AL
Tel: 0151 285 2093 Fax: 0151 236 5264
Email: firstname.surname@merseydeanery.nhs.uk
Website: www.merseydeanery.ac.uk

Associate Postgraduate Dean J Bache, M Bamforth, L de Cossart, R Gillies, J Higgins, B Shaw
Deputy Postgraduate Dean G Lamont
Head of Business Development and Strategy Diane Hart
Postgraduate Dental Dean B Grieveson
Postgraduate Medical Dean D R Graham
Regional Adviser for Postgraduate Medical and Dental Education D Bridgen

Mid Staffordshire Postgraduate Medical Centre

Staffordshire General Hospital, Weston Road, Stafford ST16 3SA
Tel: 01785 230634 Fax: 01785 230639
Email: postgraduatemedicalcentre@msgh-tr.wmids.nhs.uk
Website: www.postgrad.free-online.co.uk

Assistant Manager Barbara Alston
GDPVTS Course Organiser M J Gilmour
GPVTS Course Organiser D Palmer
Librarian Lynda Brain
Medical Education Director Bryan Gwynn
Postgraduate Services Manager Anne Herbert
Specialty Tutor (Anaesthetics) A Taylor
Specialty Tutor (Dental) S Suleman
Specialty Tutor (Medicine) D Mulherin
Specialty Tutor (Obs & Gynae) A Elmardi
Specialty Tutor (Paediatrics) A Gupta
Specialty Tutor (Pathology) L Yee
Specialty Tutor (Psychiatry) C K Dunn
Specialty Tutor (Surgery) V Kathuria
Undergraduate Secretary Elaine Weston

Mid-Sussex Postgraduate Medical Centre

Princess Royal Hospital, Lewes Road, Haywards Heath RH16 4EX
Tel: 01444 441881 Ext: 8459 Fax: 01444 451576
Email: eve.savage@bsuh.nhs.uk

Clinical Tutor David Read
Clinical Tutor (Psychiatry) Glen Berelowitz
Library Services Manager Amanda Lackey
Specialty Tutor (Accident and Emergency) Paul Ransom
Specialty Tutor (Anaesthetics) Lynne Lafreniere
Specialty Tutor (Dentistry) J Herold
Specialty Tutor (Gynaecology) Greg Kalu
Specialty Tutor (Histopathology) A Berresford
Specialty Tutor (Medicine) Martin Jones
Specialty Tutor (Neurology) P Hughes
Specialty Tutor (Neurosurgery) John Norris
Specialty Tutor (Orthopaedics) E Parnell
Specialty Tutor (Palliative Care) Cathy Gleeson
Specialty Tutor (Radiology) J Berry
Specialty Tutor (Surgery) Mike Lavelle
Specialty Tutor (Urology) J Nawrocki

Milton Keynes Postgraduate Education Centre

Milton Keynes Hospital, Standing Way, Eaglestone, Milton Keynes MK6 5LD
Tel: 01908 243178 Fax: 01908 234642
Email: marilyn.hopkins@mkgeneral.nhs.uk

Associate District Clinical Tutor E Miller, P Thomas
Centre Manager Marilyn Hopkins
CPO Tutor H Falcon
Dental Tutor G J Smart
District Clinical Tutor P Lakhari
Specialty Tutor A Assaf, P Evans, A Floyd, D G M Greig, D Gwilt, D Marchevsky, D Moir, R O'Hara, A Oomen, M Pandit, A Razzak
Tutor J Hall
VTS Course Organiser Dr Austin, Rosemary Walsh

Moorfields Eye Hospital NHS Trust Hospital Postgraduate Centre

City Road, London EC1V 2PD
Tel: 020 7566 2222 Fax: 020 7566 2223
Email: courses@moorfields.nsh.uk
Website:
www.moorfieldsco.uk/forhealthprofessionals/education/courses

Director of Medical Education John Lee (Head)

Mount Vernon Postgraduate Medical Centre

Mount Vernon Hospital, Rickmansworth Road, Northwood HA6 2RN
Tel: 01923 844237 Fax: 01923 827216
Email: lesley.barker@whht.nhs.uk

Clinical Tutor J Dickson
GP Tutor M Di Monaco
Postgraduate Centre Manager Lesley Barker
Specialty Tutor G Bounds, J Forsyth, A Grobbelaar, A Makris, T Paes, N Reissis

Newcastle General Hospital Postgraduate Medical Centre

Tomlinson Medical Centre, Department of Medical Education, Newcastle, North Tyneside and Northumberland Mental Health NHS Trust, Westgate Road, Newcastle upon Tyne NE4 6BE
Tel: 0191 256 3804 Fax: 0191 256 3264
Email: dee.smith@nmht.nhs.uk

Director of Medical Education Andrew Brittlebank
College Tutor Andrew Cole, Sylvia Dahabra, Dr Lambert, Dr Lyons
Education Support Officer Marilyn Lewis
Medical Director Andrew Fairbairn
Specialty Tutor Bob Barber

Newham General Hospital Education Centre

Glen Road, Plaistow, London E13 8SL
Tel: 020 7363 8144 Fax: 020 7363 9248
Email: acrb@newhamhealth.nhs.uk

Centre Manager Lesley Elias
Clinical Tutor A Naftalin

Norfolk and Norwich Institute of Medical Education

Norfolk and Norwich University Hospital, Colney Lane, Norwich NR4 7UY
Tel: 01603 286873 Fax: 01603 286779

Specialty Tutor T Daynes, H De Waal, P Hodgson, S Kapur, K Metcalf, M Meyer, E Morris, M Pasteur, A D Patel, Dr Ramakrishna, C Ramsay, C Ross, C Speakman, K Stanley, D Tewson, C Upton, K Walters

North Devon Postgraduate Medical Centre

North Devon District Hospital, Barnstaple EX31 4JB
Tel: 01271 311846 Fax: 01271 322374
Email: medical-education-centre@ndevon.swest.nhs.uk

Centre Manager Vicky Price
Clinical Tutor J Cox
GP Clinical Tutor J Wilson
Specialty Tutor Brian Attock, H Averns, J Cox, S Eckford, D Hurrell, M Menon, J Moore, S Nicholson, K Whittaker
Undergraduate Tutor M Dent
VTS Tutor T Bigge, K Brown, D York-Moore

North Hampshire Hospitals NHS Trust Department of PGME

Aldermaston Road, Basingstoke RG24 9NA
Tel: 01256 313380 Fax: 01256 313385
Email: laura.cullum@nhht.nhs.uk
Website: www.northhampshire.nhs.uk

Associate Clinical Sub-Dean H Simpson
Director of Medical Education D Gold
Dental Tutor C Kerawala
GP Tutor R Lorge
PGMC Assistant Manager Laura Cullum
Specialty Tutor A Haigh, K Harris, J Hobby, C Iffland, J Kitching, D Peppercorn, J Pleydell-Pearce, J Ramage, C Sandy, N Sorby, P Spraggs

North London Staff Development and Education Centre

St. Ann's Hospital, Tottenham, London N15 3TH
Tel: 020 8442 6000 Ext: 6492 Fax: 020 8442 6726
Email: jhansi.ramful@haringey.nhs.uk
Website: www.haringey.nhs.uk

Clinical Tutor Dr Bateman
Medical Director Dr Johnson-Sabine
Specialty Tutor Dr Shaw

North Manchester Postgraduate Medical Centre

North Manchester General Hospital, Delaunays Road, Crumpsall, Manchester M8 5RB
Tel: 0161 720 2720 Fax: 0161 720 2721
Email: gillian.webb@nmanhc-tr.nwest.nhs.uk

Clinical Tutor W F Tait
College Tutor S Chadwick, N Desai, V Khanna, D MacFoy, H Panigrahi, A Theodossiadis, G T Williams, R T M Woodwards
GP Tutor G O'Shea

North Middlesex Hospital Academic Centre

Sterling Way, Edmonton, London N18 1QX
Tel: 020 8887 2481 Fax: 020 8345 6809

Acting Postgraduate Education Manager Yasmin Michael

North Staffordshire Combined Healthcare NHS Trust Postgraduate Centre

The Clydesdale Centre, 167 Queen's Road, Penkhull ST4 7LF
Tel: 01782 427650 Fax: 01782 427659

Tutor H Thorley

North Tyneside HA Postgraduate Department

Education Centre, North Tyneside General Hospital, Rake Lane, North Shields NE29 8NH
Tel: 0191 293 4121 Fax: 0191 293 2762
Email: caroline.brown@northumbria-healthcare.nhs.uk
Website: nww.northumbria-healthcare.nhs.uk

Specialty Tutor Goulbourne, W Houlsby, R Jaiyesimi, Dave Morris, A Taylor, C Tiplady

North West Durham Postgraduate Medical Centre

General Hospital, Shotley Bridge, Consett DH8 0NB

Clinical Tutor S Dowson
Specialty Tutor P Robson, M Sekar, B S Sengupta, B Thalayasingham, P Watson

North Western Deanery

Department of Postgraduate Medicine and Dentistry, University of Manchester, Gateway House, Piccadilly South, Manchester M60 7LP
Tel: 0161 237 2045 Fax: 0161 237 2108
Email: j.hayden@gwh.pgmd.man.ac.uk
Website: www.pgmd.man.ac.uk

Dean of Postgraduate Medical Studies Jacky Hayden (Head)
Director of Postgraduate General Practice Education David McKinlay

Northallerton Postgraduate Medical Education Services

Academic Centre, South Tees Hospitals NHS Trust, Friarage Hospital, Northallerton DL6 1JG
Tel: 01609 764619 Fax: 01609 761126
Email: sue.fraser@stees.nhs.uk
Website: www.info4docs.org

Director Postgraduate Education Amanda Isdale
Course Organiser (VTSO) B H Davies, Roger Higson
Medical Education Tutor (CME) Peter Green
PGCM Sue Fraser

Northwick Park Hospital, Medical Education Department

Room 6V017, Watford Road, Harrow HA1 3UJ
Fax: 020 8869 2250

Director of Medical Education Clare Higgens
Medical Education Manager Sandy Thompson

Nottingham City Postgraduate Education Centre

Nottingham City Hospital NHS Trust, Hucknall Road, Nottingham NG5 1PB
Tel: 0115 962 7758, 0115 969 1169 Fax: 0115 962 7937
Website: www.ncht.org.uk

Director of Postgraduate Education David Baldwin
Specialty Tutor Dr Burrell, Mr Dhar, T Fay, Mr Henley, A E Jones, Dr McLachlan, Dr Marenah, S A Morgan, R Page, Dr Patel, Dr Pinder, Dr Skoyles, Dr Watkin

Oakwell Centre for Learning and Development

Dewsbury District Hospital, Halifax Road, Dewsbury WF13 4HS
Tel: 01924 816246 Fax: 01924 816081
Email: medical.education@dhc-tr.northy.nhs.uk

Director Postgraduate Medical Education J Brook, A Jackson
Clinical Tutor (VTSO) R J Adams

Oldham Medical and Dental Education Department

Royal Oldham Hospital, The Education Centre, Rochdale Road, Oldham OL1 2JH
Tel: 0161 627 8461 Fax: 0161 778 5628
Email: peter.nield@pat.nhs.uk

Clinical Tutor P R Cook
Medical and Dental Education Manager Peter Nield
PRHO Tutor M Hadfield
Royal College Tutor D Munro
Specialty Tutor (Adult Medicine) S Solomon
Specialty Tutor (Anaesthetics) I Brocklehurst
Specialty Tutor (Obstetrics and Gynaecology) A Boulos
Specialty Tutor (Ophthalmology) J Suharwardy
Specialty Tutor (Paediatrics) N Prakash
Specialty Tutor (Psychiatry) A Dey
Specialty Tutor (Radiology) N Jeyagopal
Specialty Tutor (Surgery) C Elsworth
Undergraduate Tutor E Odeka

Oliver Plunkett Postgraduate Centre

St Peters Hospital, Chertsey KT16 0PZ
Tel: 01932 722006
Email: angela.langwith-green@asph.nhs.uk
Website: www.ashfordstpeters.nhs.uk

College Tutor T Balakumar, D Flick, M Hall, S Newbold, D Robinson, H Scott, M Tappin
Deputy Head of Postgraduate Education A Khaleel

Education Centre and Business Manager Angela Langwith-Green
GP Tutor Olivia Kemp, Hugh Towie
Head of Postgraduate Medical Education Peter Martin
Librarian Sylvia Stafford

Ormskirk Clinical Education Centre

Ormskirk and District General Hospital, Wigan Road, Ormskirk L39 2AZ
Tel: 01695 656800 Fax: 01695 656704
Email: odette.bell@southportandormskirk.nhs.uk
Website: www.southportandormskirk.nhs.uk/clined/index.htm

Director of Medical Education M J Serlin
Clinical Tutor S Sharma
GP Tutor Dr Mullen
Manager of Medical Education Heather Ainscough
Specialty Tutor S Jmor, S Jones, M MacIver, M McKenzie, T Odedun
Trust Library Services Manager M Mason
Undergraduate Tutor Mr Anderson

Oxford Regional Postgraduate Medical

The Triangle, Roosevelt Drive, Headington, Oxford OX3 7XP
Tel: 01865 740600 Fax: 01865 740699
Email: pswan@oxford-pgmde.co.uk
Website: www.oxford-pgmde.co.uk

Director of General Practice S Phint
Director of Postgraduate Medical and Dental Education M Bannon (Head)
Associate Director Education and Training N Graham, A Jefferies
Associate Director Flexible Training B Thornley
Associate Director MMC A Edwards
Associate Director Overseas Doctors J Lourie

Peter Hodgkinson Centre

Lincoln Partnership NHS Trust, Postgraduate Centre, Greetwell Road, Lincoln LN2 5UA
Tel: 01522 573517 Fax: 01522 525327
Email: maria.blakesley@lht.nhs.uk
Website: www.lpt.nhs.uk

Clinical Director (CAHMS) S Nazir
Clinical Director (East) A Singh
Clinical Director (Local District) E Bonell
Clinical Director (Older Adults) J O Gonzalez
Clinical Director (South West) B Ferguson
Clinical Director (West) R Adeniran
Clinical Tutor T O'Grady
Medical Director M A Mohanna

The Philip Farrant Education Centre

Darent Valley Hospital, Dartford DA2 8DA
Tel: 01322 428542 Fax: 01322 428543
Email: sue.franklin@dag-tr.sthames.nhs.uk

Clinical Tutor M Stewart
Specialty Tutor M Mushtaq, M S Sait, A Schreiner, J Smith, P Strauss, P Thebie

Pinderfields Medical Education Centre

Mid Yorkshire Hospitals NHS Trust, Pinderfields General Hospital, Aberford Road, Wakefield WF1 4DG
Tel: 01924 212391 Fax: 01924 814546
Email: denise.matthews@panp-tr.northy.nhs.uk

Director of Postgraduate Education T Browning, D Nagi
Dental VTS Course Organiser S Bowen
Trust Medical Education Development Manager D A Matthews
VTS Course Organiser S Bullimore, T Gair

Plymouth Medical Centre

Derriford Hospital, Plymouth PL6 8DH
Tel: 01752 792715 Fax: 01752 792719
Email: mike.pengelly@phnt.swest.nhs.uk

Associate Director of Medical Education J Lovett
Clinical Tutor C Burrell, A Dashfield, J Morsman, T Nokes
GP Educationalist L Baxter
VTS Course Organiser A Eynon-Lewis, D Hopes, H Tulberg

Poole Postgraduate Medical Centre

Poole General Hospital, Longfleet Road, Poole BH15 2JB
Tel: 01202 442873 Fax: 01202 442368
Email: tim.battcock@poole.nhs.uk
Website: www.poolehos.org

Clinical Tutor T Battcock
PGMC Manager Gill Sibthorp
Specialty Tutor W Ashton, A Evans, W Gatling, R Henry, A McAulay

Portsmouth Hospitals NHS Trust

Department of Postgraduate Medical and Dental Education, Queen Alexandra's Hospital, Cosham, Portsmouth PO6 3LY
Tel: 023 9228 6000 Fax: 023 9228 6024
Email: michelle.lobo@porthosp.nhs.uk
Website: www.phtlearningzone.co.uk

Director of Postgraduate Medical and Dental Education Vicky Osgood
Associate Director of Medical and Dental Education Penelope Gordon
Associate Director of Medical And Dental Education Paul Sadler
Associate Director of Postgraduate General Practice Education Jane Bell
RCP Tutor K Mackay

Post Graduate Education Centre

South Rauceby, Sleaford NG34 8RB
Tel: 01592 416079

Preston Postgraduate Medical Centre

Watling Street Road West, Fulwood, Preston PR2 8DY
Tel: 01772 711234 Fax: 01772 774741

Clinical Tutor L R Solomon
Specialty Tutor P Bunting, A Davis, T A Flaherty, W J Gunawardena, M James, P McDonald, J McKenna, D A Mahmood, A Robb, R B Smith

Prince William Postgraduate Medical Education Centre

Kettering General Hospital, Kettering NN16 8UZ
Tel: 01536 492853 Fax: 01536 492856
Email: anne.gaunt@kgh.nhs.uk

Associate Tutor J O'Neill
Clinical Tutor A Steel
Specialty Tutor V Bahal, A Bilolikar, H Bilolikar, G Clifford, K El-Ghazali, J Hart, R Haughney, M A Latif, D Lawrence, S Mehra, J Mellor, V Sharma, R Thamizhavell, I Wilson-Morkeh
Undergraduate Tutor P Wood

Princess Alexandra Hospital Education Centre

Parndon Hall, Hamstel Road, Harlow CM20 1QX
Tel: 01279 827020 Fax: 01279 451263
Email: margaret.short@pah.nhs.uk
Website: www.paheducationcentre.org.uk

Clinical Skills Assessor Jonathan Kyffin
Clinical Tutor Keith Harvey
Education Centre Manager Margaret Short

Queen Elizabeth II Hospital Postgraduate Centre

Queen Elizabeth II Hospital, Howlands, Welwyn Garden City AL7 4HQ
Tel: 01707 265418 Fax: 01707 365421

Clinical Tutor Deepak Jain
Dental Tutor Kevin Jones
Deputy Medical Director Ken Farrington
GP Tutor (SE Herts PCT) Sue Greatrex, Janet Young
GP Tutor (Welwyn Hatfield PCT) Caroline Shaw
GP VTS Course Organiser A Drew, Alastair McGhee
Librarian Joan Lomas
Medical Director Jane McCue
Specialty Tutor Dr Ahmed, M Carrington, Ezzat Hemaya, Brian O'Rourke, Harish Parmar, Mark Tanner, Michael Toma

Queen Mary's Hospital Postgraduate Medical Centre

Roehampton Lane, London SW15 5PN
Tel: 020 8355 2405 Fax: 020 8355 2856
Email: shirley.webster@swlondon.nhs.uk

Clinical Tutor A F Neil
Primary Care Tutor Marek Jezeirski

Queen's Centre for Clinical Studies

East Kent Hospitals NHS Trust, Queen Elizabeth the Queen Mother Hospital, St Peters Road, Margate CT9 4AN
Tel: 01843 225544 Fax: 01843 296082
Email: jan.galbraith@ekht.nhs.uk
Website: www.eastkenthospitalstrust.nhs.uk

Clinical Tutor A M Leak

Queen's Medical Centre

Nottingham University Hospital NHS Trust, Nottingham NG7 2UH

Clinical Tutor R Stewart
Specialty Tutor L Kapila, S Karim, R Kupfer, A Lee, R Seth, M Varnam

The Robert Hardwick Postgraduate Centre

Maidstone Hospital, Hermitage Lane, Barming, Maidstone ME16 9QQ
Tel: 01622 729000 Fax: 01622 224141
Email: cheryl.vander@mtw-tr.nhs.uk

Clinical Tutor C Thom
GP Tutor T Jones
Manager C Vander
Specialty Tutor F Ahfat, S Andrews, B Bhaduri, A Henderson, R Leech

Romford Medical Academic Centre

Oldchurch Hospital, Romford RM7 0BE
Tel: 01708 746090

Specialty Tutor Mr Cheatle, T Ghosh, E Hawkins, Dr Jobber, G Subramanian, P Walter, J White

Rotherham General Hospitals NHS Trust Postgraduate Centre

Moorgate Road, Oakwood, Rotherham S60 2UD
Tel: 01709 304541 Fax: 01709 830740
Email: education.centre@rothgen.nhs.uk
Website: www.rotherhamhospital.trent.nhs.uk

Director of Public Health J Radford
Clinical Tutor A Cooper
Medical Education Manager E Webster
Specialty Tutor A Blackburn, P Harkness, S Muzulu, C Myers, S Rutter, S Suri, M G Thomas, A A Zaidi

The Royal Bolton Hospital Postgraduate Medical Education Centre

Bolton BL4 0JR
Tel: 01204 390426 Fax: 01204 527001
Email: carol.paisley@bolton-tr.nwest.nhs.uk

Clinical Tutor P Baker
GP Tutor M C Brown
Postgraduate Centre Manager C Paisley
Specialty Tutor K Bancroft, W Dougal, W Dougal, M Grey, S Hargreave, J J Henderson, C Inkster, J C Lowry, C Moulton, H Northover, N Smith, J Warner, G Yeung

Royal National Orthopaedic Hospital NHS Trust

Brockley Hill, Stanmore HA7 4LP
Tel: 020 8954 2300 Fax: 020 8954 9133
Email: enquiries@rnoh.nhs.uk
Website: www.rnoh.nhs.uk

Royal National Throat, Nose and Ear Hospital Postgraduate Centre

330 Gray's Inn Road, London WC1X 8EE
Tel: 020 7915 1514 Fax: 020 7837 9279

Clinical Tutor A Wright
Postgraduate Education Administrator C Overington

Royal Orthopaedic Hospital (Research and Teaching Centre)

The Woodlands, Northfield, Birmingham B31 2AP
Tel: 0121 685 4027 Fax: 0121 685 4030
Email: roh-postgrad@bham.ac.uk

Director Research and Teaching Centre P Pynsent
Clinical Tutor J Plewes
Manager Research and Teaching Centre A Weaver

Royal United Hospital Bath Postgraduate Centre

Combe Park, Bath BA1 3NG
Tel: 01225 824891 Fax: 01225 484926

PGMC Manager Lucy Motherwell

Royal Victoria Infirmary Education Centre

Queen Victoria Road, Newcastle upon Tyne NE1 4LP
Tel: 0191 282 4710 Fax: 0191 282 5464
Email: jane.brown@nuth.northy.nhs.uk

Clinical Tutor N M Girdler, U K Warmar
College Tutor R Milner
Royal College Tutor F Alexander, B Angus, R Bliss, M De La Hunt, G Enever, C Gerber, I Haq, D Neely, S Pedler, M Roberts, M Snow, H Spencer, J Talks, K Talks, D J Wilsden

St Albans City Hospital Postgraduate Centre

Floor 2 Moynihan Block, Waverley Road, St Albans AL3 5PN
Tel: 01727 897683 Fax: 01727 897246
Email: pgmc.sach@whht.nhs.uk

Deputy Clinical Tutor Sarah Hill
GP Tutor J Ferguson
Joint Associate Medical Director for Education and Training I Barrison
Postgraduate Centre Administrator C Roberts
Specialty Tutor B Covell

St Charles' Medical Centre

Exmoor Street, London W10 6DZ
Tel: 020 8969 2488

St David's Psychiatric Hospital Postgraduate Centre

Jobs Well Road, Carmarthen SA31 3HB

Tel: 01267 239650 Fax: 01267 237547
Email: mathew.sargeant@pdt-tr.wales.nhs.uk

St Helens and Knowsley Postgraduate Medical Centre

Whiston Hospital, Prescot L35 5DR
Tel: 0151 430 1759 Fax: 0151 430 1551
Website: www.merseyworld.com/skhealth

Director of Medical Education J McLindon
Clinical Tutor J Hendry

St James's Hospital Postgraduate Department

2nd Floor Ashley Wing, St James's University Hospital, Leeds LS9 7TF
Tel: 0113 206 4825 Fax: 0113 244 8575
Email: margaret.ward@leedsth.nhs.uk

Postgraduate Director Patrick Kent
Trust Medical Education Manager M M Ward

St Martin's Education Centre

St Martin's Hospital, Littlebourne Road, Canterbury CT1 1TD
Tel: 01227 812017 Fax: 01227 812005
Email: brigitte.frost@ekentc-tr.sthames.nhs.uk, education.centre@ekentc-tr.sthames.nhs.uk

Clinical Tutor B Plummer
CPD Co-ordinator R Harte
Education Centre Administrator Maureen Bryant
Education Centre Manager Brigitte Frost

St Mary's NHS Trust Postgraduate Centre

Postgraduate Centre, St Mary's Hospital, Praed Street, London W2 1NY
Tel: 020 7725 6151 Fax: 020 7725 6314
Website: www.st-marys.nhs.uk

Care of the Elderly Shane Roche
Centre Manager Gillian Brown
Chest Onn Min Kon
Clinical Tutor J Jones
Dermatology Jonathan Leonard
ENT Neil Tolley
Gastroenterology Julian Teare
General Manager, PGME and Research and Development R Abbott
General Surgery David Rosin
GP VTS Organiser P Kiernan
Haematology Barbara Bain
Heart and Lung Surgery Brian Glenville
HIV/GUM Paul Lamba
Hypertension Neil Chapman
Metabolic Medicine Jonathan Valabhji
Neurology Joanna Ball
Obstetrics and Gynaecology Katy Clifford
Oncology Simon Stewart
Ophthalmology Melanie Corbett
Orthopaedics Robert Marston
Paediatrics Mando Watson
Pathology Mary Thompson
Radiology Joanna Danin
Renal Andrew Palmer
Rheumatology Colin Tench
Specialist Medical Courses Organiser N Ognejenovic
Unit Director - A&E Ruth Brown
Unit Training Director - Anaesthetics Jevan Hood
Unit Training Director - Cardiology Jamil Mayet
Unit Training Director - General Medicine Colin Tench
Unit Training Director - Surgery Mike Jenkins
Urology Justin Vale
Vascular Surgery John Wolfe

Salisbury Education Centre

Salisbury District Hospital, Salisbury SP2 8BJ
Tel: 01722 336262 Ext: 4489 Fax: 01722 410942

Clinical Tutor C Fuller
Dental Tutor I Downie
GP Tutor P D Jenkins
GP VTS Course Organiser A Armstrong
Head of Learning J Osmond
Manager E Ormond
Undergraduate Tutor K Duggal

Sandwell and West Birmingham Hospitals NHS Trust Medical Education Centre

Sandwell General Hospital, Lyndon, West Bromwich B71 4HG
Tel: 0121 607 3436 Fax: 0121 607 3397
Email: jane.davies@swbh.nhs.uk
Website: www.swbh.nhs.uk

Clinical Sub-Dean K E Wheatley
Centre Manager Jane Davies
Clinical Tutor E Hughes
Specialty Tutor I Abukhalil, C Agwu, A Ahmed, A Khanna, C Sikka, S Singhal, P Stableforth, A Van Vuuren
VTS Course Organiser J Merron

Scarborough Postgraduate Medical Centre

Scarborough Hospital, Woodlands Drive, Scarborough YO12 6QL
Tel: 01723 342077 Fax: 01723 342018
Email: postgrad.scarborough@talk21.com
Website: www.scarboroughpostgrad.com

GP Tutor P Metcale
Postgraduate Clinical Tutor P Perry
VTS Course Organiser J Chadwick, E Powley

Scunthorpe Postgraduate Medical Centre

Scunthorpe General Hospital, Cliff Gardens, Scunthorpe DN15 7BH
Tel: 01724 290177 Fax: 01724 290090
Website: www.nlg.nhs.uk

Tutor O A Odukoya
VTS Course Organiser F Baker

Selly Oak Hospital Education Centre

Selly Oak Hospital, Birmingham B29 6JD
Tel: 0121 627 8748 Fax: 0121 627 8581

Clinical Tutor Kate Kane
Deputy Clinical Tutor Jason Goh

Sheffield Medical Education Centre

Northern General Hospital Campus, Sheffield Teaching Hospital Foundation Trust, Herries Road, Sheffield S5 7AU
Tel: 0114 2714076 Fax: 0114 2617533
Email: mac@nghospital.fsnet.co.uk

Director of PGME A Gibson
Deputy Director of PGME (Northern General Hospital) A D R Mackie
General Manager P Minton
Medical Education Manager (Northern General Hospital) L A Izzard
Medical Education Manager (Royal Hallamshire Hospital) L Laver

Sheila Sherlock Postgraduate Centre

Royal Free Hospital, Rowland Hill Street, London NW3 2PF
Tel: 020 7830 2182 Fax: 020 7830 2167

Director of Postgraduate Medical Education A Burns
Postgraduate Centre Administrator L Matthews

The Shrewsbury and Telford Hospital NHS Trust Postgraduate Medical Centre

Mytton Oak Road, Shrewsbury SY3 8XF

Tel: 01743 261079 Fax: 01743 261169
Email: violet@smirsh.demon.co.uk

Centre Manager V Redmond
Clinical Tutor D W Skinner
Librarian C Carr, Z Debenham

Somerset Postgraduate Centre

Taunton and Somerset Hospital, Musgrove Park, Taunton TA1 5DA
Tel: 01823 342430 Fax: 01823 342432
Email: postgrad.centre@tst.nhs.uk

Clinical Tutor D Pryce, R Welbourn
GP Tutor R Crabtree, A Wright
GP VTS Course Organiser P Hansford, I Kelham, R Rivett
Specialty Tutor G Bryce, D Cooke, S Cooper, A Dunkley, I Eyre-Brook, L Fryer, J Geraghty, S Johnson, J Phillips, D Stalker, J Twomey, D Wrede

South Cheshire Postgraduate Medical Centre

Leighton Hospital, Middlewich Road, Crewe CW1 4QJ
Tel: 01270 612015 Fax: 01270 250484
Email: leighton.postgrad@dialpipoex.com

Associate Postgraduate Clinical Tutor S Zaman
GP Tutor S Caesar
Postgraduate Clinical Tutor A P J Thomson
VTSO G Davenport

South Essex Postgraduate Medical Centre

Basildon Hospital, Nether Mayne, Basildon SS16 5NL
Tel: 01268 593360 Fax: 01268 598280
Email: jill.sharley@btuh.nhs.uk
Website: www.basildonandthurrock.nhs.uk

Director of Education and Training Keith Baggs
Director of Undergraduate Training A Lal, B F Ribeiro
Associate Directorate of Education and Training Jill Sharley
Acting Clinical Tutor I Barden
College Tutor R Haloob, A Lee, T Peckham, N Sharief, J Whitehead
Unit Training Director P Cory, I Gupta, R Haloob, M Imana, A Lee, B Lovett, J McKechnie, B O'Reilly, T Peckham, N Sharief, D Tullet, J Whitehead

South Tees Postgraduate Medical Centre

Academic Centre, The James Cook University Hospital, Marton Road, Middlesbrough TS4 3BW
Tel: 01642 854809 Fax: 01642 825337
Email: sue.fraser@stees.nhs.uk

Specialty Tutor (Anaesthesia) Sean Williamson
Specialty Tutor (Cardiology) Nick Linker
Specialty Tutor (Cardiothoracic Surgery) Simon Kendall
Specialty Tutor (ENT) D Bosman
Specialty Tutor (Medicine) Paul Cann, Adrian Davies
Specialty Tutor (Obstetrics and Gynaecology) Derek Cruickshank
Specialty Tutor (Ophthalmology) David Smerdon
Specialty Tutor (Paediatrics/Neonatology) Win Tin
Specialty Tutor (Radiology) J Dean, G Leen
Specialty Tutor (Radiotherapy) P D J Hardman
Specialty Tutor (Surgery) Pat Durning, Ian Wallace

South Tyneside Education Centre

South Shields District Hospital, Harton Lane, South Shields NE34 0PL
Tel: 0191 454 8888 Fax: 0191 427 0096
Email: nicola.whitelock@sthct.nhs.uk
Website: www.sthct.nhs.uk

Clinical Tutor H Fawzi
GP Tutor A Muchall
Specialty Tutor (Accident and Emergency) A Reece, R Singh
Specialty Tutor (Anaesthetics) S Stein
Specialty Tutor (General Medicine) S Soon
Specialty Tutor (General Surgery) K Wynne
Specialty Tutor (Obstetrics and Gynaecology) U Esen
Specialty Tutor (Orthopaedics) J Fraser
Specialty Tutor (Paediatrics) G Okugbeni
Specialty Tutor (Psychiatry) D Neill
Specialty Tutor (Radiology) R Cooper

South Western Deanery

Postgraduate Medical and Dental Education, Frenchay Hospital, 1st Floor, Academic Centre, Frenchay Park Road, Bristol BS16 1LE
Tel: 0117 975 7047 Fax: 0117 975 7060
Website: www.swndeanery.co.uk

Postgraduate Dean M N J Ruscoe
Course Organiser Philip Pemberton

South Yorkshire and South Humber Postgraduate Deanery

Centre for Postgraduate Medical and Dental Education, Don Valley House, Saville Street East, Sheffield S4 7UQ
Tel: 0114 226 4419 Fax: 0114 226 4442
Website: www.sypgme.nhs.uk

Postgraduate Dean S E Thomas
Director of Postgraduate General Practice Education Pat Lane
Regional Postgraduate Dental Dean C D Franklin

Southampton Postgraduate Medical Centre

South Academic Block, Mailpoint 10, General Hospital, Southampton SO16 6YD
Tel: 023 8079 4098 Fax: 023 8079 6816
Email: theresa.favell@suht.swest.nhs.uk
Website: www.suht.soton.ac.uk

Acting PGMC Manager Theresa Favell

Southend-on-Sea Medical Education Centre

Education Centre, Southend Hospital, Prittlewell Chase, Westcliff on Sea SS0 0RY
Tel: 01702 221070 Fax: 01702 221406
Email: education.centre@hospital.southend.nhs.uk, jsharpe@southend.nhs.uk

Clinical Tutor M Almond, A A Brown

Southmead Centre for Medical Education

Southmead Hospital, Westbury-on-Trym, Bristol BS10 5NB
Tel: 0117 959 5331 Fax: 0117 959 5332
Email: pat.hinton@nbt.nhs.uk

Director of Medical Education Joe Unsworth
Clinical Tutor Kathryn Holder, Desmond Nunez
Medical Education Administrator Julie Dennis
Receptionist Elizabeth Manning
Redeptionist Rebecca Attwood
Specialty Tutor D Bisson, M Brett, Fiona Donald, William Harries, P Jardine, A Johnson, David Mitchell, M Thornton
Study Leave Co-ordinator Donna Paddon

Southport and Ormskirk Hospital Clinical Education Centre

Southport and Formby District General Hospital, Town Lane, Southport PR8 6PN
Tel: 01704 704377 Fax: 01704 704452
Email: heather.ainscough@southportandormskirk.nhs.uk
Website: www.southportandormskirk.nhs.uk

Director of Medical Education M Serlin
GP Tutor R Patel
Librarian M Mason
Postgraduate Clinical Tutor S Sharma
Specialty Tutor Khalid Binymin, Ann Holden, Simon Jones, Tim McBride, Niall O'Donnell, Charles Scott, Pradip Sett, Mike Zeiderman

Stockport Postgraduate & Undergraduate Medical Education Centre

Pinewood House Education Centre, Stepping Hill Hospital, Poplar Grove, Stockport SK2 7JE
Tel: 0161 419 4684, 0161 419 4685 Fax: 0161 419 4686
Email: trish.sykes@stockport-tr.nwest.nhs.uk

Clinical Tutor S Southworth
Medical Education Manager T Sykes
Specialty Tutor (A&E) A J Gray
Specialty Tutor (Anaesthetics) A McCluskey
Specialty Tutor (Dental) L Petersen
Specialty Tutor (ENT) N J Kay
Specialty Tutor (Medicine) D Das
Specialty Tutor (Occupational Health) D Menzies
Specialty Tutor (O&G) C Candelier
Specialty Tutor (Ophthalmology) B Hercules
Specialty Tutor (Pathology) C R Hunt
Specialty Tutor (Psychiatry) P Joshi
Specialty Tutor (Radiology) C Keeling-Roberts
Specialty Tutor (Surgery) P Gallagher

Stoke Mandeville Hospital Postgraduate Medical Centre

Mandeville Road, Aylesbury HP21 8AL
Tel: 01296 315419 Fax: 01296 315437
Email: melita.smith@smh.nhs.uk

Specialty Tutor G Barton, Kimon Bizos, Ian Currie, Fadel Derry, S Edmonds, Marwan Farouk, Maria Forbes, Giles Kidner, Marion Lynch, Martin Paul, Marion Reid, Rajiv Sharma, Graham Smart, Richard Smith, Vippin Uthappa, Krishnan Ventakaraman, Chi Yau

Sussex Postgraduate Medical Centre

Brighton General Hospital, Elm Grove, Brighton BN2 3EW
Tel: 01273 696011 Fax: 01273 687338
Email: sue.hayes@bsuh.nhs.uk

Director of Medical Education J Montgomery
Clinical Tutor N Gainsborough
Course Organiser / Deputy Manager David Harrison
Dental Tutor Jim Herold
Dental VTS Advisor S Quelch
GP Tutor L Argent
GP VTS Organiser P Devlin, R McLintock
GPVTS Organiser Andrew Starkey
Postgraduate Centre Manager Sue Hayes
Specialty Tutor Christopher Aldridge, Philip Amess, Fiona Baldwin, David Bloomfield, Kelvin Boos, Paul Brittain, Charles Darley, Elizabeth Derrick, Peter Hale, Meredydd Harries, David Hildick-Smith, P Hildick-Smith, Mark Jackson, Shankar Kanumakala, Nigel Kirkham, Martin Parry, Paul Ransom, Camilla Sonksen, J Tibble, Tim Turnbull, Anouk Van der Avoirt, Deborah Williams, Syed Yusuf

Swindon Postgraduate Medical Centre

The Great Western Hospital, Marlborough Road, Swindon SN3 6BB
Tel: 01793 604416 Fax: 01793 604444
Email: swindon.education@smnhst.swest.nhs.uk

Clinical Tutor M O'Connor
PGMC Manager Siobhan Timms
Specialty Tutor A Beale, M Colley, S Deo, C Dukes, J Elliman, J Fieldhouse, S Green, I Kendall, P McCormack, D Majumdar, P O'Keeffe, S O'Kelly, S Wimalaratna, O Woods

Tameside Postgraduate Medical Centre

Tameside General Hospital, Ashton-under-Lyne OL6 9RW
Tel: 0161 331 6344 Fax: 0161 331 6345
Email: rosemary.hepburn@tgh.nhs.uk
Website: www.tamesidehospital.nhs.uk

Clinical Tutor B N Muddu
PRHO Clinical Tutor A Kulkarni
Specialty Tutor A Hameed, D Levy, T Mahmood, R H Rehman, C Shaw, K Siddiqui, V N H Tanna, P Unsworth

Terence Mortimer Postgraduate Education Centre

Horton Hospital, Banbury OX16 9AL
Tel: 01295 229314 Fax: 01295 254437
Email: liz.clarke-pgec@orh.nhs.uk

Clinical Tutor H D'Costa
Specialty Tutor I Arnold, D Chidwick, E Daniels, N Dehalvi, J Everatt, J Nicholls, N Thompson

Thomas Sydenham Educational Centre

Dorset County Hospital, Williams Avenue, Dorchester DT1 2JY
Tel: 01305 255258 Fax: 01305 255359
Email: educationcentre@wdgh.nhs.uk

Clinical Tutor A Blake
Dental Tutor H Bellis
Education and Development Manager Tina Jackson
GP Tutor N Lyons

Torbay Hospital Medical Education Department

Medical Centre, Lawes Bridge, Torquay TQ2 7AA
Tel: 01803 654708 Fax: 01803 616395

Director of Education J Lowes
Clinical Tutor N Campbell, N Viner
Specialty Tutor Rob Horvarth, Merven Leggott
Specialty Tutor (Anaesthetics) O Snow
Specialty Tutor (CCU) Jonathan Ingham
Specialty Tutor (ENT) David Aloerson
Specialty Tutor (Medicine) Keith George
Specialty Tutor (Ophthalmology) Andy Frost
Specialty Tutor (Surgery) O Defriend
Specialty Tutor (Trauma and Orthopaedics) A G MacEachern

Trafford Education Centre

Trafford General Hospital, Moorside Road, Davyhulme, Manchester M41 5SL
Tel: 0161 746 2036

Clinical Tutor R J Howell
Specialty Tutor P A Carrington, J Chilalia, W Fraser, J Helliwell, M Ishmail, H M Lewis, A Shaw

Trent Postgraduate Deanery

University of Nottingham, Floor 15 Tower Building, University Park, Nottingham NG7 2RD
Tel: 0115 846 7165 Fax: 0115 846 7107
Email: midtrentdeanery@nottingham.ac.uk
Website: www.trentdeanery.nottingham.ac.uk

Postgraduate Dean David Sowden
Head of Performance Development Kate Caulfield
Head of Professional Develpment Val Evans
Postgraduate Medical Dean Jas Bilkhu

Trust Education Centre

Royal Berkshire Hospital, London Road, Reading RG1 5AN
Tel: 0118 987 7832 Fax: 0118 987 7837

Associate Clinical Tutor Helen Allott
Director of Education Anthony Bradlow
Specialist Tutor Rogan Corbridge, Neil Derbyshire, Riduzan Farouk, Steve Foley, Alice Freebairn, Annette Goulden, Ravi Kumar, Charles Lewis, Martin Leyland, Jeremy McNally, Stephen Rear, Sue Ronay, Emma Vaux
Specialty Tutor R Dodds, James Gildersleve, Martin James, Sreenath Reddy, Jane Siddall, Christopher Tomlins

Tunbridge Wells Postgraduate Medical Centre

The Kent and Sussex Hospital, Mount Ephraim, Tunbridge Wells TN4 8AT
Tel: 01892 534477 Fax: 01892 517692
Email: pip.twpgc@ukgateway.net
Website: www.twpgc.com

Clinical Tutor D Yates
Course Organiser A Howitt, K Lay
Dental Tutor K Sneddon
GP Tutor C Dewing
Specialty Tutor L Baldwin, R Banks, W Bolsover, B Cowry, D Firth, S Flint, P Gibb, L Roberts, N Rowson, R Sergeant

UCL Hospitals Postgraduate Medical Education

48 Riding House Street, London W1W 7EY
Tel: 020 7679 9370 Fax: 020 7679 9248
Email: susan.harper@uclh.nhs.uk
Website: www.uclh.org/services/postgrad/uchmiddlesex/

Director Medical Education Lesley Bromley
Primary Care Tutor S Nazeer

United Bristol Healthcare NHS Trust Education Centre

Postgraduate Medical Education Department, Upper Maudlin Street, Bristol BS2 8AE
Tel: 0117 342 0054, 0117 342 0057 Fax: 0117 342 0055
Email: kay.collings@ubht.swest.nhs.uk

Clinical Tutor R Aspinall, S Bando, P Weir
Specialty Tutor M Aspinall, S Caine, Dr Callaway, K Hopkins, M Jackson, M Pignatelli, J Rooney, M Saunders, S Sellars, F Smith, D Tole, Dr Whaley

University Hospital NHS Trust Postgraduate Medical Centre

Queen Elizabeth Hospital, Metchley Park Road, Edgbaston, Birmingham B15 2TQ
Tel: 0121 627 2860 Fax: 0121 627 5798
Email: postgraduatecentre@uhb.nhs.uk

Director Robert Allan
Clinical Tutor Tom Gallacher
Manager Louise Atkins

University Hospital of North Staffordshire NHS Trust Postgraduate Medical Centre

Hartshill, Stoke-on-Trent ST4 7LN

Postgraduate Clinical Tutor C A Campbell

University Hospital of North Tees Postgraduate Department

Teaching Centre, Hardwick, Stockton-on-Tees TS19 8PE
Tel: 01642 624791 Fax: 01642 624918
Email: sue.grady@nth.nhs.uk

Director of Medical Education D Bruce (Head)
Assistant Director of Medical Education Julie Oakley
Clinical Tutor Z Maung
Postgraduate Medical Education Manager Sue Grady
RCA Tutor H Mohan
RCOG Tutor J Macaulay
RCPCH Tutor C Harikumar
RCS Tutor C Hennessy, P Mounter

University Hospitals Coventry and Warwickshire NHS Trust Postgraduate Medical Centre

Clifford Bridge Road, Walsgrave, Coventry CV2 2DX
Tel: 024 7653 8713 Fax: 024 7653 8802
Email: dan.higman@uhcw.nhs.uk

Business Manager Maureen Fern
Clinical Tutor D Higman

University of Newcastle Postgraduate Institute for Medicine and Dentistry

10-12 Framlington Place, Newcastle upon Tyne NE2 4AB
Tel: 0191 2222 6772 Fax: 0191 222 8620
Email: peter.hill@ncl.ac.uk
Website: www.campus.ncl.ac.uk/pimd

Postgraduate Dean Peter Hill

Walsall Hospitals NHS Trust Postgraduate Medical Centre

Manor Hospital, Moat Road, Walsall WS2 9PS
Tel: 01922 721172
Email: jane.flint@walsallhospitals.nhs.uk

Clinical Tutor A R Gatrad

Wansbeck Postgraduate Medical Centre

Woodhorn Lane, Ashington NE63 9JJ

Clinical Tutor P R Crook
Specialty Tutor P R Crook, L Edmondson, J L Sher, P R Sill

Wessex Deanery

Highcroft, Romsey Road, Winchester SO22 5DH
Tel: 01962 863511

Deanery Business Manager Jo Stevens
Director of Postgraduate General Practice Education F Smith
Postgraduate Dental Dean R T Reed
Postgraduate Medical Dean G Winyard

West Cheshire Postgraduate Medical Centre

Countess of Chester Hospital NHS Trust, Liverpool Road, Chester CH2 1UL
Tel: 01244 383676 Fax: 01244 364722
Email: barbara.kirkham@coch.nhs.uk

Clinical Tutor S Bowles, G Sissons
GP Tutor R Gleek
Librarian Samantha West

West Cumberland Postgraduate Medical Centre

West Cumberland Hospital, Hensingham, Whitehaven CA28 8JG
Tel: 01946 693181 Ext: 2538 Fax: 01946 591772
Email: bmusgrave@ncumbria-acute.nhs.uk
Website: www.northcumbriahealth.nhs

Clinical Tutor F J Local
College Tutor J Eldred, S Javaid, D Prosser, N S Rao

West Hertfordshire and Watford Postgraduate Medical Centre

Watford General Hospital, Vicarage Road, Watford WD1 0HB
Tel: 01923 217436 Fax: 01923 217910
Email: suzanne.watkins@whht.nhs.uk
Website: www.westhertshospitals.nhs.uk

Director of Medical Education Ian Barrison
Clinical Tutor Bruce MacFarlane
Deputy Clinical Tutor Ganesh Supramaniam
Postgraduate Manager Suzanne Watkins
Specialty Tutor R Awad, A Cohn, B Gajjar, J Jessop, A Kosmin, V Nanduri, S Rizvi, A Sanusi, M Soskin
Undergraduate Tutor A Ogilvie

West Hertfordshire Hospitals NHS Trust Postgraduate Medical Centre

Hemel Hempstead Hospital, Hillfield Road, Hemel Hempstead HP2 4AD
Tel: 01442 287666 Fax: 01442 287670
Email: pgmc.hemel@whht.nhs.uk

Deputy Clinical Tutor Sarah Hill
Medical Director for Education and Training Ian Barrison

West Midlands Board of Postgraduate Medical and Dental Education
The Medical School, The University of Birmingham, Edgbaston, Birmingham B15 2TT
Tel: 0121 414 6892 Fax: 0121 414 3155

Dean P Scriven
Consultant V Y Subhedar, A Whitehouse
Deputy Postgraduate Dean D W Wall
Regional Postgraduate Dean J G Temple (Head)

Weston General Hospital Postgraduate Medical Centre
Grange Road, Uphill, Weston Super Mare BS23 4TQ

Clinical Tutor M Lewis, P G P Stoddart
Specialty Tutor J Dixon, J H Dixon, A Gough, A Hinchliffe, M Lewis, E J Wakley

Wharfedale Medical Centre Department of Medical Education Postgraduate Centre
Wharfedale General Hospital, Newall Carr Road, Otley LS21 2LY
Tel: 0113 392 3010 Fax: 0113 392 7011
Email: Pat.Clark@leedsth.nhs.uk

Whipps Cross University Hospital Medical Education Centre
Whipps Cross Hospital, London E11 1NR
Tel: 020 8535 6419
Email: kim.lowe@whippsx.nhs.uk
Website: www.nthames.tprnde.ac.uk/ntrl/mec/index.htm

Clinical Tutor C M Roberts

Whittington Hospital Postgraduate Centre
Holborn Union Building, Archway Campus, Highgate Hill, London N19 5LW
Tel: 020 7288 5185 Fax: 020 7288 5625
Email: elena.power@whittington.nhs.uk
Website: www.whittington.nhs.uk/postgraduate

Director of Medical Education Jane Young
Bloomsbury RGM VTS A Dicker
Course Administrator George Borrie
Education Co-ordinator Elleni Ross
GP Tutor Simon Wiseman
GP VTS (RFH/Bloomsbury) Course Convenor Lenka Speight
GP VTS (Whittington) Course Convenor John Salinsky
Postgraduate Manager Elena Power

William Harvey Postgraduate Medical Centre
William Harvey Hospital, Kennington Road, Willesborough, Ashford TN24 0LZ
Tel: 01233 616055 Fax: 01233 613597

Clinical Tutor B Al-Shaikh
GP Tutor G Del Bianco
Specialty Tutor M Heravi, J Hossain, R Insall, R Lapworth, M Miller-Jones, M Milligan, M Rahman
VTS Course Organiser T Lister, A Lloyd-Smith

Wirral Postgraduate Medical Centre
Clatterbridge Hospital, Bebington, Wirral CH63 4JY
Tel: 0151 482 7848 Fax: 0151 334 6379

Director of Learning and Development D Bowen-Jones
Clinical Tutor R Morgan, J S Sprigge
Dental Course Organiser/IT Tutor M J R Williams
Dental Tutor M Woodhead
GP Tutor G G Francis
VT Course Organiser T Awan

Worthing Postgraduate Medical Centre
Park Avenue, Worthing BN11 2HR
Tel: 01903 285024 Fax: 01903 285125
Email: brenda.davies@wash.nhs.uk
Website: www.worthinghospital.nhs.uk

Associate Clinical Tutor Janice Bates
Director of Postgraduate Medical Education Gordon Caldwell
Centre Manager Brenda Davies
Undergraduate Sub-Dean John Southgate

Wrightington, Wigan and Leigh NHS Trust Medical Education Centre
Royal Albert Edward Infirmary, Wigan WN1 2NN
Tel: 01942 822507 Fax: 01942 822355
Email: postgrad@wwl.nhs.uk
Website: www.wwl.nhs.uk

Clinical Tutor J Marples
Education Department Manager Carol Hitchmough
Library Services Manager C Dagnall
PRHO Tutor S Arya
Specialty Tutor I Dhesi, R M Downes, B Duper, C Faris, B Hundle, G Kumar, S Madi, V Natha, P Wood

The Wynne Davies Postgraduate Medical Centre
Worcestershire Acute Hospitals NHS Trust, Alexandra Hospital, Woodrow Drive, Redditch B98 7UB
Tel: 01527 518490 Fax: 01527 518489
Email: pgmc@worcsacute.wmids.nhs.uk

Clinical Tutor K Nathavitharara
Royal College Tutor (RCOG) J Uhiara
Royal College Tutor (RCP) D Brockbank
Royal College Tutor (RCPCH) S Ghazi
Royal College Tutor (RCS) A Reading

Wythenshawe Hospital Postgraduate Medical Centre
Wythenshawe Hospital, Southmoor Road, Manchester M23 9LT
Tel: 0161 291 5765 Fax: 0161 291 5776
Email: postgrad@fs1.with.man.ac.uk

Accident and Emergency Tutor S Hawes
Dental Trainee Day Release Course Organiser M Milne
Deputy Manager Sara Kirkpatrick
Manager Teresa Gough
Overseas Tutor A Luthra, B Pal
Postgraduate Clinical Tutor S Hawes
RCA Tutor F Dodd, D Grieg
RCOG Tutor A Ahluwalia
RCP Tutor R Rowe, M Venning
RCPath Tutor P Bishop
RCPCH Tutor F Al-Zidgali
RCR Tutor S Sukumar
RCS Tutor S Galloway, A Nasim
Regional Adviser in Cardiothoracic Surgery G J Grötte
Specialty Tutor (General Practice) K Shearer
Specialty Tutor (PRHO) Dr Vernon

York Postgraduate Medical Centre
York Hospital, Wigginton Road, York YO31 8HE
Tel: 01904 726739 Fax: 01904 632811
Email: barbara.higginson@york.nhs.uk
Website: www.york.postgrad.clara.net

Associate PGMD A Corlett, A Garry, S H Leveson
GP Tutor J D Moroney
Postgraduate Medical Director J C Thow
VTS Course Organiser A S C Calder, J R Lloyd

Scotland

East of Scotland Regional Postgraduate Medical Centre

Level 7, Ninewells Hospital and Medical School, Dundee DD1 9SY
Tel: 01382 496516 Fax: 01382 632809

Postgraduate Dean Philip Cachia
Business Manager Donald Smith

Lister Postgraduate Institute

11 Hill Square, Edinburgh EH8 9DR
Tel: 0131 650 2609 Fax: 0131 662 0580
Website: www.lister-institute.ed.ac.uk

Dean of Postgraduate Medicine S G Macpherson
Postgraduate Dean S G Macpherson
Acting Personnel Manager I Wilson
Adviser to Women Doctors Jane Montgomery
Associate Postgraduate Dean D S Irvine, K R Palmer
Associate Postgraduate Dean (Flexible Training) Jane Montgomery
Associate Postgraduate Dean (General Practice) D Blaney
Postgraduate Dental Adviser R Ibbetson
Postgraduate Tutor A Gordon, D Henderson, A Jaap, P Mankad, A Mowbray, P Reid, P Roddam, A Thomas, J Walker

NHS Education for Scotland

Forest Grove House, Foresterhill Road, Aberdeen AB25 2ZP
Tel: 01224 554365 Fax: 01224 550670
Email: pgcentre.neast@nes.scot.nhs.uk
Website: www.nes.scot.nhs.uk

Postgraduate Dean Gillian Needham
Director of General Practice Education Michael Taylor
Associate Postgraduate Dean (North) Evelyn Dykes
Associate Postgraduate Dean (North East) Ken McHardy
Business Manager Pauline Browell-Hook
Education Director Kim Walker

North of Scotland Deanery

North of Scotland Institute of Postgraduate Medical Education, Raigmore Hospital, Inverness IV2 3UJ
Tel: 01463 704347, 01463 704348
Email: jane.jack@nes.scot.nhs.uk, roslyn.macdonald@nes.scot.nhs.uk, shirley.sturrock@nes.scot.nhs.uk, tina.bassindale@nes.scot.nhs.uk
Website: www.nes.nhs.uk

Assistant Director of Postgraduate Medical Education Ronald MacVicar
Associate Postgraduate Dean Evelyn Dykes
Associate Adviser in General Practice N Davis, R Dickie, C Higgott, I Johnston, J Nicholls, J O'Rourke, D Pinney, J Ramsey, R Spencer-Jones
Associate Advisor in General Practice A Sharma
Centre Manager T Bassindale
Postgraduate Tutor K N Achar, H M Fattah, R Rankin, P K Srivastava

University of Glasgow, Department of Postgraduate Medical Education/West of Scotland Region

NHS Education for Scotland, 3rd Floor, 2 Central Quay, 89 Hydepark Street, Glasgow G3 8BW
Tel: 0141 223 1400 Fax: 0141 223 1403
Website: www.show.scot.nhs.uk/scpmde

Postgraduate Dean K M Cochran
Director of Postgraduate General Practice Education T S Murray
Assistant Director (Accreditation and VT) M Kelly
Assistant Director (Audit) M Lough
Assistant Director (CPD) D Kelly
Administrative Officer E Watt
Associate Postgraduate Dean (Flexible Training) J Taylor
Associate Postgraduate Dean (Management Education) P Knight
Associate Postgraduate Dean (Poor Performance) B Williams
Associate Postgraduate Dean (PRHOs and Refugee Doctors) G Orr
Associate Postgraduate Dean (Research and Development) J McGregor
Associate Postgraduate Dean (SHOs) Colin Semple
Business Manager F Miller
CPD Officer E Duncan
Finance Officer M Paul
Head of Hospital Training J Allan
Officer Supervisor (GP) I Robertson
Postgraduate Tutor D Byrne, R Carachi, J Fox, S K Ghosh, I Gunn, A Henderson, S W Hislop, J Keaney, D McQueen, D Marshall, B Maule, R Milroy, H Neil, W Reid, I Ritchie, J Series, A Todd, A Wray
SHO Development Team Leader F Dorrian
Specialty Tutor M Aitchison, D B Allan, J G Allan, F Bryden, R Crawford, S Elder, D Galloway, N Gibson, B Irvine, J Kinsella, E Melrose, S Miller, J Murdoch, J Norman, D O'Reilly, R Rampling, J Reid, M Roberts, I R C Swan

Wales

Abergavenny Postgraduate Medical Centre

Education Centre, Nevill Hall Hospital, Abergavenny NP7 7EG
Tel: 01873 732660 Ext: 2660 Fax: 01873 732662
Email: roger.pritchard@gwent.wales.nhs.uk

Aberystwyth Postgraduate Medical Centre

Postgraduate Centre, Bronglais Hospital, Aberystwyth SY23 1ER
Tel: 01970 623131 Ext: 5619 Fax: 01970 635806

Bangor Postgraduate Medical Centre

Education Centre, Ysbyty Gwynedd, Penrhosgarnedd, Bangor LL57 2PW
Tel: 01248 385112 Fax: 01248 355819
Email: graham.whiteley@nww-tr.wales.nhs.uk

Bridgend Postgraduate Centre

Postgraduate Centre, Princess of Wales Hospital, Coity Road, Bridgend CF31 1RQ
Tel: 01656 752070 Fax: 01656 752086
Email: jackie.jones@bromor-tr.wales.nhs.uk
Website: www.bromor-tr.wales.nhs.uk

Centre Manager J A Jones
Medicine Tutor D Webb
Specialty Tutor A Allman, B Craddock, Dr Eggers, A Goodwin, R Hedges
VTS Specialty Tutor P Harrop, D Judd

Bronglais Hospital Postgraduate Medical Centre

Bronglais General Hospital, Aberystwyth SY23 1ER
Tel: 01970 635806 Fax: 01970 635806
Email: postgraduate-centre@ceredigion-tr.wales.nhs.uk

CPD Organiser Frances Gerrard
Hon. Senior Lecturer R Visvanathan
Postgraduate Organiser Karen Perry
Specialty Tutor (Medicine) G Boswell
Specialty Tutor (Obstetrics and Gynaecology) S A Awad
Specialty Tutor (Paediatrics) J Williams
Specialty Tutor (Surgery) R Visvanathan
VTS Organiser Roddy Evans

Caerphilly Postgraduate Medical Centre
Caerphilly District Miners' Hospital, Caerphilly CF83 2WW
Tel: 029 2080 7270 (Sec) Fax: 029 2080 7104
Email: mujtaba.hasan@gwent.wales.nhs.uk

Postgraduate Organiser Mujtaba Hasan

Cardiff Postgraduate Medical Centre
University Hospital of Wales, Heath Park, Cardiff CF14 4XW
Tel: 029 2074 2474 Fax: 029 2074 6239

Centre Manager C A Roberts
Postgraduate Organiser K Baboolal, M Stacey
Specialty Tutor G Clark, N Davies, J Grey, M Hourihan, C Poynton, A Turley, J T Waternaude
VTSO A Cooper

Carmarthen Postgraduate Medical Centre
Postgraduate Centre, West Wales General Hospital, Carmarthen SA31 2AF
Fax: 01267 223480

Cefn Coed Psychiatric Hospital Postgraduate Centre
Cefn Coed Hospital, Cockett, Swansea
Tel: 01792 516546 Fax: 01792 516516

Clwyd North Postgraduate Medical Centre
Glan Clwyd Hospital, Bodelwyddan, Rhyl LL18 5UJ
Tel: 01745 534516 Fax: 01745 584919
Email: john.williams@cd-tr.wales.nhs.uk

CME Tutor R Barrie
PA to Trust Chief Executive Joanne Wood
Specialty Tutor P Elliott, G J Green, D Hay, A P Lake, J G Thomas

Gwent Postgraduate Medical and Dental Centre
The Friars, Friars Road, Newport NP20 4EZ
Tel: 01633 238143 Fax: 01633 234929
Email: sandra.workman@gwent.wales.nhs.uk

Sub-Dean and Associate Medical Director H Jones
Associate Postgraduate Organiser J R Harding
Dental Adviser A Griffiths
Dental Postgraduate Organiser N Claydon
GPCPO Co-ordinator Sian Williams
Postgraduate Organiser F J Richardson
Specialty Tutor (Anaesthetics) R Walpole
Specialty Tutor (ENT) M Preece
Specialty Tutor (Maxillofacial and Oral Surgery) M Gregory
Specialty Tutor (Medicine) S Ikram
Specialty Tutor (Obstetrics and Gynaecology) A Weerakkody
Specialty Tutor (Ophthalmology) S Webber
Specialty Tutor (Orthopaedics) K Tayton
Specialty Tutor (Paediatrics) P Dale
Specialty Tutor (Pathology) M Penney
Specialty Tutor (Radiology) N Evans
Specialty Tutor (Surgery) P Holland
VTCO J Badger, J Keely, F Machado

Gwynedd Centre for Postgraduate Medical and Dental Education
Ysbyty Gwynedd, Penrhosgarnedd, Bangor LL57 2PW.
Tel: 01248 384621 Fax: 01248 355819
Email: postgrad@nww-tr.wales.nhs.uk

Events Co-ordinator D Lewis
Specialty Tutor D Crawford, J Horn, S Hunter, P Leach, A Roberts, A R Starczewski, C Tilson, P Tivy-Jones, A Valijan, C Walker

Haverfordwest Postgraduate Medical Centre
Withybush General Hospital, Haverfordwest SA61 2PZ
Tel: 01437 773726 Fax: 01437 773729
Email: jayne.noble@pdt-tr.wales.nhs.uk
Website: www.pdt-tr.wales.nhs.uk

Dental Tutor M Dodd
GP CPD Co-ordinator D Richards
Manager J Noble
Postgraduate Organiser I Martin
Royal College Tutor D Bryant, V Falcao, R Howells, C James, P Milewski
Specialty Tutor N Jowett, W A Maxwell
Undergraduate Organiser C James
VTSO R W Burns, R Davies

Llandough Postgraduate Medical Centre
Llandough Hospital, Penarth
Tel: 029 2071 6341 Fax: 029 2071 5631
Email: morrisS4@cardiff.ac.uk

Llanelli Postgraduate Medical Centre
Prince Philip Hospital, Llanelli SA14 8QF
Tel: 01554 756567 Ext: 3249 Fax: 01554 749962
Email: alison@llanpgmc.demon.co.uk

CME Associate N Flower
CPD Co-ordinator Carmarthenshire C Jones
Medical Tutor P Avery
Postgraduate Manager A Chapman
Postgraduate Organiser J Jaidev

Merthyr and Cynon Valley Postgraduate Centre
Prince Charles Hospital, Merthyr Tydfil CF47 9DT
Tel: 01685 721721 Ext: 8175, 01685 721721 Ext: 8412 (Sec)
Fax: 01685 721240
Email: elaine.thomas@nglam-tr.wales.uk

Specialty Tutor K A B Asaad, P Baynham, P Braithwaite, I B Davies, R J Evans, H Hawkes, A Y Izzidien, K Smart, M Winstone

Morriston Postgraduate Medical Centre
Morriston Hospital, Morriston, Swansea SA6 6NL.
Tel: 01792 703677 Fax: 01792 701007
Email: julie.ace@swansea-tr.wales.nhs.uk
Website: www.swansea-tr.wales.nhs.uk

Postgraduate Organiser T H Brown
Specialty Tutor (Accident and Emergency) H Allen
Specialty Tutor (Anaesthetics) J Morgan, T Wall
Specialty Tutor (Burns and Plastics) M A C Cooper
Specialty Tutor (Cardiac Centre) A Youhana
Specialty Tutor (General Medicine) U Dave
Specialty Tutor (General Surgery) L Fligelstone
Specialty Tutor (Neurosurgery) R Redfern
Specialty Tutor (Oral and Maxillofacial Surgery) D Patton
Specialty Tutor (Restorative Dentistry) K Silvester
Specialty Tutor (Trauma & Orthopaedics) N Price
Specialty Tutor (Urology) M G Lucas

Neath General Hospital Education Centre
Neath Port Talbot Hospital, Baglan Way, Port Talbot SA12 7BX
Tel: 01639 641161 Fax: 01639 639046
Email: amanda.hinkley@bromor-tr.wales.nhs.uk

Associate Postgraduate Organiser G M Jeremiah
Postgraduate Organiser Mercurius-Taylor
RCA Specialty Tutor G Thomas
RCOG Specialty Tutor Dossa
RCP Specialty Tutor S Lennor
Specialty Tutor Williams

Nevill Hall Education Centre
Nevill Hall Hospital, Abergavenny NP7 7EG
Tel: 01873 732660 Fax: 01873 732662
Website: www.gwent-tr.wales.nhs.uk

GP Tutor J Badger, J Keely, F Machado
Librarian Elizabeth Lewis
Overseas Representation Dr Bhonmurthy, Mr Yogesh
Postgraduate Centre Manager Lisa Cooper
Postgraduate Organiser Rachel Hargest, Roger Pickford
Specialty Tutor Anneli Allman, R L Blackett, H Habboush, N Jenkins, Huw Reed, Rachel Rouse, I M Stokes

Newport Postgraduate Medical Centre
The Friars, Friars Road, Newport NP20 4EZ
Tel: 01633 238125 Fax: 01633 234929
Email: sarah.still@gwent.wales.nhs.uk

Powys Postgraduate Medical Centre
Children's Centre, Brecon War Memorial Hospital, Brecon LD3 7NS
Tel: 01874 615671 Ext: 5671 Fax: 01874 615673
Email: chris.vulliamy@powyslhb.wales.nhs.uk

Postgraduate Organiser Chris Vulliamy

Royal Glamorgan Postgraduate Medical Centre
Postgraduate Centre, Royal Glamorgan Hospital, Ynysmaerdy, Llantrisant CF72 8XR
Tel: 01443 443571 Fax: 01443 443405
Email: postgrad@pr-tr.wales.nhs.uk

Associate Postgraduate Organiser Ahmed Kamal
Postgraduate Centre Manager Anne Cowell
Postgraduate Organiser M Foster
Specialty Tutor G Davies, P Fitzgerald, Dr Foo, S Jerrett, L Millar-Jones, N Nabi, D Pugh, Z Summers, E Vaughan-Williams, D H Williams, J Wynne Jones

St Cadoc's Psychiatric Hospital Postgraduate Centre
Lyndhurst, Eureka Place, Ebbw Vale NP23 6PN
Tel: 01495 353702 Fax: 01495 353737
Email: karl.rice@gwent.wales.nhs.uk

University of Wales Swansea Postgraduate Medical School
Singleton Park, Swansea SA2 8PP

Lecturer W Y Cheung, R Roberts
Professor (Cancer Studies) R Leonard
Professor (Experimental Medicine) J M Hopkin
Professor (General Surgery) J N Baxter
Professor (Health Services Research) J G Williams
Professor (Plastic and Reconstructive Surgery) A D McGregor
Senior Lecturer B Lervy, H A Snooks
Visiting Professor (Experimental Medicine) T Shirakawa

Welsh Deanery
School of Postgraduate Medical and Dental Education, Wales College of Medicine, Biology, Life and Health Sciences, Cardiff University, Heath Park, Cardiff CF 14 4XN
Tel: 029 2074 3927 Fax: 029 2075 4966
Email: pgdean@cf.ac.uk

Head of School and Dean Simon Smail

Welsh Rural Postgraduate Unit
Institute of Rural Health, Gregynog, Newtown SY16 3PW
Tel: 01686 650800 Fax: 01686 650300
Email: janers@irh.ac.uk
Website: www.irh.ac.uk

Chief Exexutive Jane Randall-Smith
CPD Co-ordinator John Wyn Jones
Training Manager Ann Whale

West Wales General Hospital Postgraduate Medical Centre
Francis Well, West Wales General Hospital, Carmarthen SA31 2AF
Tel: 01267 227505 Fax: 01267 223480
Email: sue@carmpostgrad.org.uk
Website: www.carmpostgrad.org.uk

CPD Co-ordinator C Jones
Manager's Assistant Angela Watts
Postgraduate Centre Manager S Harrison
Postgraduate Organiser P Cumber, C Llewellyn-Jones
VTS Course Organiser B McNeil, J Rees

Whitchurch Postgraduate Medical Centre
Whitchurch Hospital, Whitchurch, Cardiff CF14 7XB
Tel: 029 2061 0579 Fax: 029 2052 0170
Email: giselle.martinez@cardiffandvale.wales.nhs.uk

Postgraduate Organiser Giselle Martinez

Wrexham Medical Institute
Postgraduate Centre, Wrexham Medical Institute, Technology Park Centre, Croesnewydd Road, Wrexham LL13 7YP
Tel: 01978 727451 Fax: 01978 290346
Email: yvonne.smith@new-tr.wales.nhs.uk

Associate PGO C Edmondson
GP CME Tutor P Saul
GPVT Course Organiser B Tanner
GPVT Course Organisers I Happs
Postgraduate Centre Manager Yvonne Smith
Postgraduate Dental Tutor E E Roberts
Postgraduate Organiser C Roseblade
Undergraduate Tutor A Sen

Northern Ireland

Altnagelvin Hospital Postgraduate Medical Centre
Clinical Education Centre, Altnagelvin Hospitals HSS Trust, Altnagelvin Area Hospital, Londonderry BT47 6SB
Tel: 028 7134 5171 Fax: 028 7161 1272
Email: eobrien@alt.n-i.nhs.uk
Website: www.n-i.nhs.uk/trusts/altnagelvin

Clinical Tutor A Adas, P Bayliss, J A F Beirne, P Charlwood, W Dickey, R Gilliland, D F C Hughes, J F McCarthy, P McSorley, J Moohan, J Sinton
Consultant J G Daly, S E E Magee, A J McNeill, C Mulholland, M O'Kane, K J S Panesar, A R Wray
Posgraduate Clinical Tutor Neil Corrigan
VTSO D Dolan, P J McEvoy

Antrim Hospital Postgraduate Medical Centre
Antrim Hospital, 45 Bush Road, Antrim BT41 2RL
Tel: 028 9442 4275 Fax: 028 9442 4127
Email: viola.barker@uh.n-i.nhs.uk

Course Organiser (GP Registrars) Brian Bonnar, Michelle Stone
Course Organiser (GP SHOs) Jean McCaughern
Trust Clinical Tutor Calum MacLeod

Belfast Postgraduate Medical Centre
Belfast City Hospital, Lisburn Road, Belfast BT9 7AB

Clinical Tutor Patrick Morrison
VTSO J G Clements

Craigavon Area Hospital Medical Education Centre

Craigavon Area Hospital Group HSS Trust, 68 Lurgan Road, Craigavon BT63 5QQ
Tel: 028 3861 2399 Fax: 028 3861 2884
Email: pgc@cahgt.n-i.nhs.uk
Website: www.cahgt.org.uk

Clinical Tutor Colin Weir
Course Organiser (GP Registrars) Margaret Chambers
Course Organiser (GP SHOs) Aîne McShane
Librarian Hazel Neale

Northern Ireland Council for Postgraduate Medical and Dental Education

5 Annadale Avenue, Belfast BT7 3JH
Tel: 028 9049 2731 Fax: 028 9064 2279
Email: nicpmde@nicpmde.gov.uk
Website: www.nicpmde.com

Chair D A J Keegan
Vice-Chairman J G Jenkins
Chief Executive/Postgraduate Medical Dean J R McCluggage
Director of Postgraduate General Practice Education A McKnight
Administrative Director M Roberts
Postgraduate Dental Dean I D F Saunders

Channel Islands

Jersey Postgraduate Medical Centre

The General Hospital, Gloucester Road, St Helier, Jersey JE1 3QS
Tel: 01534 622742 Fax: 01534 622808
Email: p.gettens@gov.je
Website: www.gov.je

PGMC Manager Patricia Gettens

Isle of Man

DHSS Education and Training Centre

Strang IM4 4RH
Tel: 01624 651421 Fax: 01624 651429
Email: kate.thatcher@nobles.dhss.gov.im

Centre Manager Kate Thatcher
Clinical Tutor M J Divers
GP Tutor A M Blackman
Librarian C V Sugden

Royal Colleges and Faculties

Faculty of Accident and Emergency Medicine

35-43 Lincoln's Inn Fields, London WC2A 3PE
Tel: 020 7405 7071 Fax: 020 7405 0318
Email: faem@emergencymedicine.uk.net
Website: www.faem.org.uk

President-elect Jim Wardrope
President Alastair McGowan
Dean P Driscoll
Registrar R Brown
Treasurer Kevin Reynard

Faculty of Family Planning and Reproductive Health Care

27 Sussex Place, Regent's Park, London NW1 4RG
Tel: 020 7724 5534, 020 7724 5620 Fax: 020 7723 5333
Email: mail@ffprhc.org.uk
Website: www.ffprhc.org.uk

President Alison Bigrigg
Vice-President Christopher Wilkinson
Faculty Secretary Corin Jones
Hon. Secretary Christine Robinson
Hon. Treasurer Kate Guthrie

Faculty of Occupational Medicine of the Royal College of Physicians

6 St. Andrews Place, Regent's Park, London NW1 4LB
Tel: 020 7317 5890 Fax: 020 7317 5899
Email: fom@facoccmed.ac.uk
Website: www.facoccmed.ac.uk

President W J Gunnyeon
President Elect David Snashall
Chair, AFOM M R Dean
Chair, DAvMed A J Batchelor
Chair, DDAM T M Gibson
Chair, DOccMed S R Boorman
Registrar O H Carlton
Assistant Registrar K Holland-Elliott
Academic Dean John Harrison
Board Member R M Agius, L N Birrell, C Black, P S Burge, S E L Coomber, M F J Davidson, N F Davies, G Denman, G M Helliwell, R V Johnston, A M Leckie, J K Moore, D I M Skan
Chief Examiner D Ferriday
Conference Secretary R Thornton
CPD Director J S F Tamin
Interim Chief Executive Nicky Wilkins
Newsletter Editor C D Payton
Press Officer D Patel
Sponsorship Co-ordinator C Sharp
Training Dean Gordon Parker
Treasurer P Litchfield

Faculty of Pharmaceutical Medicine of the Royal Colleges of Physicians of the United Kingdom

1 St Andrew's Place, Regent's Park, London NW1 4LB
Tel: 020 7224 0343 Fax: 020 7224 5381
Email: fpm@fpm.org.uk
Website: www.fpm.org.uk

President Brian Gennery
Vice-President Stephen Hobbiger
Registrar Jane Barrett
Academic Registrar John Griffin
Treasurer Richard Tomiak

Faculty of Public Health Medicine of the Royal Colleges of Physicians of the United Kingdom

4 St Andrew's Place, Regent's Park, London NW1 4LB
Tel: 020 7935 0243 Fax: 020 7224 6973
Email: enquiries@fph.org.uk
Website: www.fph.org.uk

President Rod Griffiths
Vice-President Graham Winyard
Chief Executive Paul Scourfield
Registrar Selena Gray
Academic Registrar Steve George
Assistant Registrar Jean Chapple
Assistant Academic Registrar Sushma Acquilla
Treasurer Keith Williams

Elected Member James Connelly, Robert Cooper, Mary Corcoran, Paula Grey, Margaret Guy, Brian Keeble, John Kemm, Elizabeth Kernohan, Janet Little, Helen Maguire, Philip Monk, Kieran Morgan, Meradin Peachy, Rashmi Shukla, William Cairns Smith, Lillian Somervaille, Judy Thomas, Norman Vetter

Royal College of Anaesthetists

48-49 Russell Square, London WC1B 4JY
Tel: 020 7813 1900 Fax: 020 7813 1876
Email: info@rcoa.ac.uk
Website: www.rcoa.ac.uk

President Peter Simpson
Vice-President Griselda Cooper, David Saunders
Director of Professional Standards Charlie McLaughlan
Director of Training and Examinations David Bowman
College Secretary Kevin Storey

Council Member Paul Cartwright, Griselda Cooper, John Curran, Oliver Dearlove, Chris Dodds, Mark Garfield, Stephanie Glover, David Greaves, Michael Harmer, David Hatch, Christopher Heneghan, Judith Hulf, Sarah Hunt, Douglas Justins, Gavin Kenny, Alastair Lack, Andrew Lim, Anne May, Alastair McGowan, Rajinder Mirakhur, Andrew Mortimer, Keith Myerson, Peter Nightingale, Anna-Maria Rollin, Christopher Rowlands, Madeleine Wang, Anthony Wildsmith

Royal College of General Practitioners

14 Princes Gate, Hyde Park, London SW7 1PU
Tel: 020 7581 3232 Fax: 020 7225 3047
Email: info@rcgp.org.uk
Website: www.rcgp.org.uk

President Roger Neighbour
Chair of Education Network Stephen Field
Chair of Ethics Committee Clare Gerada
Chair of Examination Board Valerie Wass
Chair of International Committee John Howard
Chair of Northern Ireland Council Jennifer McAughey
Chair of Patient Partnership Group Joy Dale

Chair of Publishing Network Sunil Bhanot
Chair of Quality Network Theo Schofield
Chair of Research Group Nigel Mathers
Chair of Scottish Council Mairi Scott
Chair of Welsh Council Michael Jeffries
Chairman of Council Mayur Lakhani
Vice-Chair of Council Nigel Sparrow
Vice-Chair of Council and Chair of Clinical Network Graham Archard
Chief Executive Hilary De Lyon
Director of External Relations Jane Austin
Hon. Secretary Maureen Baker
Hon. Treasurer Colin Hunter

Council Member Justin Allen, Tina Ambury, Graham Archard, Ken Aswani, David Bailey, Maureen Baker, Stephen Bassett, Mike Bewick, Sunil Bhanot, Michael Boland, Scott Brown, Yvonne Carter, Robert Dickie, Anthony Downes, John Dracass, Steve Field, Richard Fieldhouse, Clare Gerada, Janet Hall, Simon Hambling, David Haslam, Jacky Hayden, Iona Heath, John Howard, Colin Hunter, Nigel Ineson, Indra Jayaweera, Michael Jeffries, Has Joshi, Brian Keighley, Jean Ker, Mayur Lakhani, Gordon Mackinnon, Nigel Mathers, Anthony Mathie, Helena McKeown, Geoffrey Morgan, Catti Moss, Orest Mulka, Chaand Nagpaul, Joe Neary, Roger Neighbour, Barbara Porter, Michael Pringle, Ken Prudhoe, Bashir Qureshi, Keith Richards, Geoff Roberts, James Rodger, Theo Schofield, Mairi Scott, Nigel Sparrow, Andrew Spooner, Vikram Tanna, Noel Tinker, John Toby, Nicola Toynton, Valerie Wass, Ruby Watt, David Whillier, Martin Wilkinson, David Wood, Nat Wright

Royal College of Midwives

15 Mansfield Street, London W1G 9NH
Tel: 020 7312 3535 Fax: 020 7312 3536
Email: info@rcm.org.uk
Website: www.rcm.org.uk

President Maggie Elliott
Chairman of Council Ruth Clarke
General Secretary Karlene Davis

Chairman Ruth Clarke
Deputy Chairman Claire Cutlan
Council Member Belinda Ackerman, Anna Agnew, Dorcas Akeju, Maria Brown, Kate Caldwell, Douglas Charlton, Margaret Chesney, Tracey Cooper, Fiona Dagge-Bell, Catherine Davis, Sarah Fox, Debby Gould, Jane Hervé, Kathleen Jones, Andrew Lingen-Stallard, Elizabeth Mackay, Marian McIvor, Sarah Montagu, Lorna Muirhead, Marlene Sinclair, Gill Skinner, Sharon Stafford, Mary Steen, Liz Stephens, Monica Thompson, Suzanne Truttero

Royal College of Nursing

20 Cavendish Square, London W1G 0RN
Tel: 020 7409 3333 Fax: 020 7355 1379
Website: www.rcn.org.uk

President Sylvia Denton
Chair of Council Eirlys Warrington
General Secretary Beverly Malone
Hon. Treasurer Jane McCready

Royal College of Obstetricians and Gynaecologists

27 Sussex Place, Regent's Park, London NW1 4RG
Tel: 020 7772 6200 Fax: 020 7723 0575
Email: coll.sec@rcog.org.uk
Website: www.rcog.org.uk

President Allan Templeton
Senior Vice-President James Connor Dornan
Hon. Secretary Richard Charles Warren
Hon. Treasurer Peter Bowen-Simpkins
Junior Vice-President Patrick Michael (Shaughn) O'Brien

Co-opted Member Melissa Whitten
Elected Fellow Sabaratnam Arulkumaran, Pamela Buck, John Philip Calvert, Linda Dolores Cardozo, Laura Jane Cassidy, Anthony Dale Falconer, Tahir Ahmed Mahmood, Roger Marwood, Michael Edward Lockhart Paterson, John Shepherd, Stuart Michael Walton, Julian Woolfson, Charles Stewart Weatherley Wright
Elected Fellow, England James Owen Drife
Elected Fellow, Ireland Colm O'Herlihy
Elected Fellow, Scotland David Ian Malcolm Farquharson
Elected Member Ian Currie, Keith Duncan, Mark James, Mark David Kilby, Justin Chi Konje, Mylvaganam Kumar Kumarendran, John Alexander Latimer, Philip Owen, Janice Rymer, Mourad Wahby Seif
Invited Member Valerie Alasia, Alison Bigrigg, Maggie Elliott

Royal College of Ophthalmologists

17 Cornwall Terrace, London NW1 4QW
Tel: 020 7935 0702 Fax: 020 7935 9838
Website: www.rcophth.ac.uk

President Nicholas Astbury
Senior Vice-President Stuart Roxburgh
Vice-President Stuart Cook, Harminder Dua
Chief Executive Margaret Hallendorff
Hon. Secretary Larry Benjamin
Hon. Treasurer John Talbot

Royal College of Paediatrics and Child Health

50 Hallam Street, London W1W 6DE
Tel: 020 7307 5600 Fax: 020 7307 5601
Email: enquiries@rcpch.ac.uk
Website: www.rcpch.ac.uk

President Alan Craft
Vice-President Patricia Hamilton, Simon Lenton, Neil McIntosh
Chairman Academic Board Chris Verity
Registrar Sheila Shribman
Hon. Treasurer Alun Elias-Jones

Royal College of Pathologists

2 Carlton House Terrace, London SW1Y 5AF
Tel: 020 7451 6700 Fax: 020 7451 6701
Email: info@rcpath.org
Website: www.rcpath.org

President James Underwood
Vice-President Graham Beastall, Clair du Boulay, Adrian Newland
Chief Executive Daniel Ross
Registrar Helen Williams
Assistant Registrar Stephen Bangert
Treasurer Tim Wreghitt

Council Member Jeffrey Barron, Andrew Boon, Christopher Catchpole, Jack Crane, John Crolla, Tony Elston, Gordon Ferns, Ian Franklin, Peter Furness, Trevor Gray, Andrew Hanby, Paul Kettle, Christopher Meehan, Lance Sandle, Robert Spencer, Tim Stephenson, Richard Tedder, Elisabeth Trimble, Isobel Walker, Tim Wallington, Geraint Williams, Chris Wright, Nicholas Wright

Royal College of Physicians

11 St Andrews Place, Regent's Park, London NW1 4LE
Tel: 020 7935 1174 Fax: 020 7487 5218
Email: info@rcplondon.ac.uk
Website: www.rcplondon.ac.uk

President Carol Black
Academic Vice-President Parveen Kumar
Chairman of MRCP(UK) Part 1 Examining Board J A Vale
Chief Executive Philip Masterton-Smith
Director, Health Informatics Unit John Williams
Director, Medical Workforce Unit R McIntyre
Director of Clinical Effectiveness and Evaluation Unit Michael Pearson
Director of Continuing Professional Development Ian Starke
Director of Professional Training Patrick Cadigan
Director of Publications Peter Watkins
Registrar Rodney Burnham
Academic Registrar Charles Pusey
Censor A M Brownjohn, B T Cooper, M Davies, T W Evans, P N Trewby, J A Vale
Clinical Vice-President Mary Armitage
Federation Director of Continuing Professional Development Mike Watson
Flexible Working Officer Anne Dornhorst
Harveian Librarian Leon Fine
Information Officer Julie Beckwith
Medical Director, Joint Committee on Higher Medical Training George Cowan
SpR Adviser Robert Coward
Treasurer Richard Thompson

Royal College of Physicians and Surgeons of Glasgow

232-242 St Vincent Street, Glasgow G2 5RJ
Tel: 0141 221 6072 Fax: 0141 221 1804
Email: registrar@rcpsg.ac.uk
Website: www.rcpsg.ac.uk

President Graham Teasdale
Vice-President (Dental) W M M Jenkins
Vice-President (Medical) D T Roberts
Vice-President (Surgical) J C Ferguson
Hon. Secretary P V Knight
Treasurer D J Galloway

Council Member I W R Anderson, J Bancewicz, H J G Burns, F C Campbell, R Carachi, J Connell, A Dunk, S Elgammal, J C Ferguson, D J Galloway, J R Hayes, W M M Jenkins, R W G Johnson, P V Knight, A Lannigan, J Long, L G McAlpine, J R McGregor, R Miller, P R Mills, C G Morran, J A Murie, W S Nimmo, W Reid, D T Roberts, M M Steven, R D Stevenson, R D Sturrock, A Zoma

Royal College of Physicians of Edinburgh

9 Queen Street, Edinburgh EH2 1JQ
Tel: 0131 225 7324 Fax: 0131 220 3939
Website: www.rcpe.ac.uk

President Neil Douglas
Vice-President Roger Smith
Dean Mike Watson
Registrar Andrew Elder
Assessor Douglas Mitchell
Convenor of Publications Anthony Busuttil
Deputy Editor John Kelly
Hon. Librarian Iain Donaldson
Secretary John Collins
Social Convener Martin Lees
Treasurer Derek Maclean

Council Member Patrick Bell, Christopher Birt, Anandapuram Dwarakanath, Grant Franklin, Brian Frier, David Jenkins, Alison Jones, Ian Laing, Steward Lambie, Joseph Legge, Thomas MacDonald, William MacNee, David Matthews, Denis McDevitt, Dorothy Moir, William Morrison, Angela Thomas

Royal College of Psychiatrists

17 Belgrave Square, London SW1X 8PG
Tel: 020 7235 2351 Fax: 020 7245 1231
Email: rcpsych@rcpsych.ac.uk
Website: www.rcpsych.ac.uk

President M Shooter
Vice-President S Hollins, A S Zigmond
Chief Executive Vanessa Cameron
Dean D K M Bhugra
Sub-Dean A S Bird, C J K Bouch, N S Brown, K Sivakumar
Registrar A F Fairbairn
Deputy Registrar J N Beezhold, S A Pidd
Head of Central Secretariat and HR Roberta Wheeler
Head of Examinations Services Lynn Bryson
Head of External Affairs Deborah Hart
Head of Facilities and Office Services Cathryn Freestone
Head of Financial Services Paul Taylor
Head of Postgraduate Education Gareth Holsgrove
Head of Publications Dave Jago
Editor J Tyrer
Immediate Past President John Cox
Librarian D H H Tait
Treasurer F E Subotsky

Council Member D N Anderson, S M Bailey, R A Baker, S Benbow, S Bhaumik, A P Boardman, T M Brown, F W A Browne, N Chada, D A Coia, I D Cormac, I B Crome, S Davenport, F M C Denman, K E M Ganter, E Gilvarry, N Greenberg, J C Gunn, G Ikkos, R Jenkins, R G Jones, J Knowles, G Lloyd, J V Lucey, I F Macllwain, C N Mayer, D McGovern, K J Mckenzie, R M Murray, S R Nimmagadda, M P Nowers, G O'Brien, R E O'Shea, R Ramsay, G Richardson, M M Robertson, P A Sugarman, P J Taylor, N J Warner, R J W Williams

Royal College of Radiologists

38 Portland Place, London W1B 1JQ
Tel: 020 7636 4432 Fax: 020 7323 3100
Email: enquiries@rcr.ac.uk
Website: www.rcr.ac.uk

President Janet Husband
Vice-President and Dean, Clinical Oncology R Hunter
Vice-President and Dean, Clinical Radiology P A Dubbins
Chief Executive A A Hall
Registrar, Clinical Oncology M Williams
Registrar, Clinical Radiology P Dawson
Treasurer H C Irving
Warden, Clinical Oncology F Calman
Warden, Clinical Radiology A K Dixon

Royal College of Speech and Language Therapists

2 White Hart Yard, London SE1 1NX
Tel: 020 7378 1200 Fax: 020 7403 7254
Email: postmaster@rcslt.org
Website: www.rcslt.org

Chair Sue Roulstone
Chief Executive Kamini Gadhok

Royal College of Surgeons of Edinburgh

Nicolson Street, Edinburgh EH8 9DW
Tel: 0131 527 1600 Fax: 0131 557 6406
Website: www.rcsed.ac.uk

President J A R Smith
Vice-President I M C Macintyre, J D Orr
Chief Executive J R C Foster
Dean and Convener of the Dental Council J P McDonald
Hon. Secretary P K Datta
Hon. Treasurer J R C Logie
PA to President Moira Stout
PA to Vice-Presidents Emma Cook

Council Member C J K Bulstrode, U Chetty, O Eremin, C M Evans, O J Garden, W S Hendry, M Khan, D Lee, S Nixon, C W Oliver, I K Ritchie, D I Rowley, A J W Steers, D A Tolley, W A Wallace

Royal College of Surgeons of England

35-43 Lincoln's Inn Fields, London WC2A 3PE
Tel: 020 7405 3474 Fax: 020 7831 9438
Website: www.rcseng.ac.uk

President Hugh Phillips
Vice-President Bernard Ribeiro, David Rosin
Chief Executive Craig Duncan

Council Member Brian Avery, John Black, Christopher Chilton, Richard Collins, David Dandy, Linda de Cossart, Anthony Giddings, David Jones, John Lowry, John Lumley, Valerie Lund, Peter May, Ian McDermott, Anne Moore, Anthony Mundy, Anthony Narula, David Neal, Dermot O'Riordan, Andrew Raftery, Brian Rees, Christopher Russell, Irving Taylor, William Thomas

Research Institutions

Bath Institute for Rheumatic Diseases

Allan Dixon Building, Trim Bridge, Bath BA1 1HD
Tel: 01225 448444 Fax: 01225 336809
Email: racheledwards@birdbath.org.uk

President Michael Gilbert
Chair N D Hall
Executive Director Rachel Edwards

Blond McIndoe Centre

Queen Victoria Hospital, East Grinstead RH19 3DZ
Tel: 01342 414295 Fax: 01342 414550
Email: enquiries@blondmcindoe.com
Website: www.blondmcindoe.com

Director Roger Smith
Operations Director Heather Shearer
Trust Chairman Vanora Marland

British Paediatric Surveillance Unit of the Royal College of Paediatrics and Child Health

50 Hallam Street, London W1W 6DE
Tel: 020 7307 5671 Fax: 020 7307 5694
Email: bpsu@rcpch.ac.uk
Website: www.bpsu.inopsu.com

Chairman of Executive Committee M Preece
Medical Adviser R Knowles, A Smith
Scientific Co-ordinator R Lynn

Cancer Research UK

National Office, PO Box 123, Lincoln's Inn Fields, London WC2A 3PX
Tel: 020 7242 0200 Fax: 020 7269 3100
Website: www.cancerresearchuk.org

Chair David Newbigging
Chief Executive Alex Markham

Institute for Ageing and Health

University of Newcastle upon Tyne, Newcastle General Hospital, Westgate Road, Newcastle upon Tyne NE4 6BE
Tel: 0191 256 3014 Fax: 0191 256 3011
Email: iah@ncl.ac.uk, L.patterson@ncl.ac.uk
Website: www.ncl.ac.uk/iah

Director J A Edwardson
Administrator Lynn Patterson

Institute of Cancer Research, Royal Cancer Hospital

123 Old Brompton Road, London SW7 3RP
Tel: 020 7352 8133 Fax: 020 7370 5261
Email: marjorie.kipling@icr.ac.uk
Website: www.icr.ac.uk

Chief Executive & Gene Function and Regulation P W J Rigby
Dean R J Ott
Biochemistry M Dowsett
Breakthrough Breast Cancer Toby Robins Research Centre A Ashworth
Cancer Genetics M Stratton
Cancer Research UK Centre for Cancer Therapeutics P Workman
Cancer Research UK Centre for Cell and Molecular Biology C J Marshall
Clinical Magnetic Resonance J E S Husband, M O Leach
Clinical Trials J Bliss
Epidemiology A Swerdlow
Haemato-oncology M Greaves
Head of Chester Beatty and Haddow Laboratories K R Willison
Head of Clinical Laboratories A Horwich
Leukemia Research Fund Centre M Greaves
Medical Oncology S B Kaye
Molecular Carcinogenesis C S Cooper
Paediatric Oncology A Pearson
Physics S Webb
Radiotherapy A Horwich
Secretary J M Kipling
Structural Biology D Barford, L Pearl

Institute of Occupational Medicine

Research Park North, Riccarton, Edinburgh EH14 4AP
Tel: 0870 850 5131 Fax: 0870 850 5132
Email: info@iomhq.org.uk
Website: www.iom-world.org

Chief Executive Philip Woodhead
Director of Research Fintan Hurley
Director of Research Development Robert Aitken
Director of Special Projects John Cherrie
Senior Consultant Richard Graveling

Ludwig Institute for Cancer Research

91 Riding House Street, London W1W 7BS
Tel: 020 7878 4000 Fax: 020 7878 4040
Website: www.licr.org

Director Xin Lu

Marie Curie Research Institute

The Chart, Oxted RH8 0TL
Tel: 01883 722306 Fax: 01883 714375
Website: www.mcri.ac.uk

Chair Nicholas Fenn
Chief Executive, Marie Curie Cancer Care Tom Hughes-Hallett
Director of Research Peter O'Hare
Hon. Treasurer Tony Doggart, David Gibson

Medical Research Council

20 Park Crescent, London W1B 1AL
Tel: 020 7636 5422 Fax: 020 7436 2665
Email: firstname.surname@headoffice.mrc.ac.uk
Website: www.mrc.ac.uk

Chairman Anthony Cleaver
Chief Executive Colin Blakemore
External Communications Administrator Heather Finch
Member D Armstrong, E M Armstrong, K Davies, Kay Davies, Carol Dezateux, P Fellner, D Flint, Ruth Hall, Andrew McMichael, Alan North, G Richardson, J Savill, Herb Sewell, Michael Wakelam

MRC Anatomical Neuropharmacology Unit

Mansfield Road, Oxford OX1 3TH
Tel: 01865 271865 Fax: 01865 271647
Website: www.mrcanu.pharm.ox.ac.uk
Director Peter Somogyi

MRC Biostatistics Unit
Institute of Public Health, University Forvie Site, Robinson Way, Cambridge CB2 2SR
Tel: 01223 330397 Fax: 01223 330388
Website: www.mrc-bsu.cam.ac.uk
Director Simon Thompson

MRC Cambridge Centre for Behavioural and Clinical Neuroscience
University of Cambridge, Department of Experimental Psychology, Downing Street, Cambridge CB2 3EB
Tel: 01223 333558 Fax: 01223 314547
Website: www.info.psychol.cam.ac.uk/~bcnc/
Director Trevor Robbins

MRC Cancer Cell Unit
Hutchison/MRC Research Centre, Department of Oncology, Hills Road, Cambridge CB2 2XZ
Tel: 01223 763240 Fax: 01223 763241
Website: www.hutchison-mrc.cam.ac.uk
Co-Director Ron Laskey

MRC Cell Biology Unit
University College London, Gower Street, London WC1E 6BT
Tel: 020 7679 7806 Fax: 020 7679 7805
Website: www.ucl.ac.uk/lmcb
Director Alan Hall

MRC Centre for Developmental Neurobiology
New Hunt's House, Guy's Campus, London SE1 1UL
Tel: 020 848 6521 Fax: 020 848 6550
Website: www.kcl.ac.uk/depsta/biomedical/mrcdevbiol/
Director Andrew Lumsden

MRC Centre for Protein Engineering
Department of Chemistry, University of Cambridge, Lensfield Road, Cambridge CB2 1EN
Tel: 01223 336341 Fax: 01223 336445
Website: www.mrc-cpe.cam.ac.uk
Director Alan Fersht

MRC Centre for Synaptic Plasticity
Department of Anatomy, University of Bristol, School of Medical Sciences, University Walk BS8 1TD
Tel: 0117 928 7402 Fax: 0117 929 1687
Website: www.bris.ac.uk/depts/synaptic/
Director G L Collingridge

MRC Clinical Sciences Centre
Imperial College Faculty of Medicine, Hammersmith Hospital Campus, Du Cane Road, London W12 0NN
Tel: 020 8383 8250 Fax: 020 8383 8337
Website: www.csc.mrc.ac.uk
Director Chris Higgins

MRC Clinical Trials Unit
222 Euston Road, London NW1 2DA
Tel: 020 7670 4700 Fax: 020 7670 4818
Website: www.ctu.mrc.ac.uk
Director J H Darbyshire

MRC Cognition and Brain Sciences Unit
15 Chaucer Road, Cambridge CB2 2EF
Tel: 01223 355294 Fax: 01223 359062
Website: www.mrc-cbu.cam.ac.uk
Director William Marslen-Wilson

MRC Dunn Human Nutrition Unit
The Wellcome Trust, MRC Building, Hills Road, Cambridge CB2 2XY
Tel: 01223 252700 Fax: 01223 252715
Website: www.mrc-dunn.cam.ac.uk
Director John Walker

MRC Epidemiology Resource Centre
Southampton General Hospital, Tremona Road, Southampton SO16 6YD
Tel: 023 8077 7624 Fax: 023 8070 4021
Director Cyrus Cooper

MRC Epidemiology Unit
Strangeways ResearchLaboratory, Worts Causeway, Cambridge CB1 8RN
Tel: 01223 330315 Fax: 01223 330316
Director Nick Wareham

MRC Functional Genetics Unit
University of Oxford, Department of Human Anatomy and Genetics, South Parks Road, Oxford OX1 3QX
Tel: 01865 272416 Fax: 01865 282651
Website: www.mrcfgu.ox.ac.uk
Director Kay Davies

MRC Health Services Research Collaboration
University of Bristol, Department of Social Medicine, Canynge Hall, Whiteladies Road, Bristol BS8 2PR
Tel: 0117 928 7343 Fax: 0117 928 7236
Website: www.hsrc.ac.uk
Director Paul Dieppe

MRC Human Genetics Unit
Western General Hospital, Crewe Road, Edinburgh EH4 2XU
Tel: 0131 322 2471 Fax: 0131 467 8456
Website: www.hgu.mrc.ac.uk
Director Nick Hastie

MRC Human Immunology Unit
Institute of Molecular Medicine, John Radcliffe Hospital, Headington, Oxford OX3 9DU
Tel: 01865 222336 Fax: 01865 222502
Website: www.imm.ox.ac.uk/groups/mrc-hiu/pages/home.htm
Hon. Director Andrew McMichael

MRC Human Reproductive Sciences Unit
Centre for Reproductive Biology, University of Edinburgh Chancellor's Building, 49 Little France Crescent, Edinburgh EH16 4SB
Tel: 0131 242 6200 Fax: 0131 242 6201
Website: www.hrsu.mrc.ac.uk
Director Robert Millar

MRC Immunochemistry Unit
University Department of Biochemistry, South Parks Road, Oxford OX1 3QU
Tel: 01865 275354 Fax: 01865 275729
Website: www.bioch.ox.ac.uk/immunoch
Director Kenneth Reid

MRC Institute for Environment and Health
University of Leicester, 94 Regent Road, Leicester LE1 7DD
Tel: 0116 223 1600 Fax: 0116 223 1601
Website: www.le.ac.uk/ieh
Director Paul Harrison

MRC Institute of Hearing Research
University of Nottingham, Clinical Section, Queens Medical Centre, Nottingham NG7 2RD
Tel: 0115 922 3431 Fax: 0115 951 8503
Website: www.ihr.mrc.ac.uk
Director Dave Moore

MRC Laboratory of Molecular Biology
Hills Road, Cambridge CB2 2QH
Tel: 01223 248011 Fax: 01223 213556
Website: www.mrc-lmb.cam.ac.uk
Director Richard Henderson

MRC Mammalian Genetics Unit and UK Mouse Genome Centre
Harwell, Didcot OX11 0RD
Tel: 01235 834393 Fax: 01235 834776
Website: www.mgu.har.mrc.ac.uk
Director of Mammalian Genetics Unit and UK Mouse Genome Centre Steve Brown

MRC Molecular Haematology Unit
The Weatherall Institute of Molecular Medicine, John Radcliffe Hospital, Headington, Oxford OX3 9DU
Tel: 01865 222398 Fax: 01865 222500, 01865 222501, 01865 222737
Website: www.imm.ox.ac.uk/groups/mrc_molhaem/
Director Doug Higgs

MRC Prion Unit
Institute of Neurology, Queen's Square, London WC1N 3BG
Tel: 020 7837 4888 Fax: 020 7837 8047
Website: www.prion.ucl.ac.uk
Director John Collinge

MRC Protein Phosphorylation Unit
School of Life Sciences, MSI/WTB Complex, University of Dundee, Dundee DD1 5EH
Tel: 01382 344241 Fax: 01382 223778
Website: www.dundee.ac.uk/lifesciences/mrcppu
Director Philip Cohen

MRC Radiation and Genome Stability Unit
Harwell, Didcot OX11 0RD
Tel: 01235 834393 Fax: 01235 834776
Website: www.ragsu.har.mrc.ac.uk/
Interim Director Peter O'Neill

MRC Resource Centre for Human Nutrition Research
Elsie Widdowson Laboratory, Fulbourne Road, Cambridge CB1 9NL
Tel: 01223 426356 Fax: 01223 437515
Website: www.mrc-hnr.cam.ac.uk
Director Ann Prentice

MRC Social, Genetic and Developmental Psychiatry Research Centre
Institute of Psychiatry, De Crespigny Park, Denmark Hill, London SE5 8AF
Tel: 020 7848 5341 Fax: 020 7848 0866
Website: www.iop.kcl.ac.uk
Director Peter McGuffin

MRC Social and Public Health Sciences Unit
4 Lilybank Gardens, Glasgow G12 8RZ
Tel: 0141 357 3949 Fax: 0141 337 2389
Website: www.msoc-mrc.gla.ac.uk
Director Sally Macintyre

MRC Toxicology Unit
Hodgkin Building, University of Leicester, PO Box 138 Lancaster Road, Leicester LE1 9HN
Tel: 0116 252 5544 Fax: 0116 252 5616
Website: www.le.ac.uk/cmht
Director Pierluigi Nicotera

MRC Virology Unit
Institute of Virology, University of Glasgow, Church Street, Glasgow G11 5JR
Tel: 0141 330 4017 Fax: 0141 337 2236
Website: www.vir.gla.ac.uk
Director Duncan McGeoch

MRC/University College London Centre Development for Medical Molecular Virology
Windeyer Institute of Medical Science, 46 Cleveland Street, London W1P 6DB
Tel: 020 7504 9343 Fax: 020 7387 3310
Website: www.ucl.ac.uk/medicalschool/infection-immunity/mrc-centre/mrc-centre.htm
Director Professor Griffiths

MRC/University of Birmingham Centre for Immune Regulation
University of Birmingham, Department of Immunology, Edgbaston, Birmingham B15 2TT
Tel: 0121 414 4068 Fax: 0121 414 3599
Website: www.bham.ac.uk/mrcbcir/home.htm

MRC/University of Edinburgh Centre for Inflammation Research
Edinburgh Royal Infirmary, Department of Clinical and Surgical Science, Lauriston Place, Edinburgh EH3 9YW
Tel: 0131 536 2238 Fax: 0131 536 2247
Website: www.mvm.ed.ac.uk/idg/inflamrs.htm
Director J Savill

MRC/University of Newcastle Development Grant in Clinical Brain Ageing
MRC Building, Newcastle General Hospital, Westgate Road, Newcastle upon Tyne NE4 6BE
Tel: 0191 273 5251 Fax: 0191 272 5291
Website: www.ncl.ac.uk/iah/cdcba.htm
Jim Edwardson

MRC/University of Sussex Centre Development in Genome Damage and Stability
University of Sussex, Falmer, Brighton BN1 9RR
Tel: 01273 678123 Fax: 01273 678121
Website: www.biols.susx.ac.uk/gdsc/frameset
Director Tony Carr

National Institute for Medical Research
The Ridgeway, Mill Hill, London NW7 1AA
Tel: 020 8959 3666 Fax: 020 8906 4477
Website: www.nimr.mrc.ac.uk
Director John Skehel

UK Human Genome Mapping Project Resource Centre
RC Rosalind Franklin Centre for Genomics Research, Hinxton, Cambridge CB10 1SB
Tel: 01223 494500 Fax: 01223 494512
Website: www.hgmp.mrc.ac.uk
Director Duncan Campbell

Novartis Foundation

41 Portland Place, London W1B 1BN
Tel: 020 7636 9456 Fax: 020 7436 2840
Email: dchadwick@novartisfound.org.uk
Website: www.novartisfound.org.uk

Director and Secretary to the Executive Council D J Chadwick
PA to Director Jane Dempster

Research Institute for the Care of the Elderly

St Martin's Hospital, Combe Down, Bath BA2 5RP
Tel: 01225 835866 Fax: 01225 840395
Email: r.w.jones@bath.ac.uk
Website: www.rice.org.uk

President Baroness Baroness Greengross

Chairman M Rowe
Director R W Jones
Office Administrator Jessica Kingscote

Royal College of Physicians, Clinical Effectiveness and Evaluation Unit

11 St Andrew's Place, Regent's Park, London NW1 4LE
Tel: 020 7935 1174 Ext: 500 Fax: 020 7487 3988
Email: ceeu@rcplondon.ac.uk
Website: www.rcplondon.ac.uk

Director Michael Pearson
Administrator Debbie Sears
Manager Jane Ingham

Tavistock Institute of Medical Psychology

Tavistock Centre, 120 Belsize Lane, London NW3 5BA
Tel: 020 7435 7111 Fax: 020 7435 1080
Email: admin@counselling4london.com, tccr@tccr.org.uk, timp@tccr.org.uk
Website: www.tccr.org.uk

Chair (TIMP Council) A Obholzer
Director (Tavistock Centre for Couple Relationships) C Clulow
Company Secretary D Obadina

Wellcome Trust

215 Euston Road, London NW1 2BE
Tel: 020 7611 8888 Fax: 020 7611 8545
Email: infoserve@wellcome.ac.uk
Website: www.wellcome.ac.uk

Chairman Dominic Cadbury
Director Mark Walport
PA to Head of Media Relations Sally Pearson

Government and Statutory Bodies

England

Army Medical Directorate

Former Army Staff College, Slim Road, Camberley GU15 4NP
Tel: 01276 412726 Fax: 01276 412737
Website: www.army.mod.uk/medical

Director General Louis Lillywhite

Charity Commission (for England and Wales)

Harmsworth House, 13-15 Bouverie Street, London EC4Y 8DP
Tel: 0870 333 0123 Fax: 020 7674 2300
Email: enquiries@charitycommission.gsi.gov.uk
Website: www.charitycommission.gov.uk

Chair Geraldine Peacock
Chief Executive Andrew Hind (Head)

Charity Commission - Liverpool

20 Kings Parade, Queens Dock, Liverpool L3 4DQ
Tel: 0870 333 0123 Fax: 0151 703 1555
Email: enquiries@charitycommission.gsi.gov.uk
Website: www.charitycommission.gov.uk

Charity Commission - Taunton

Woodfield House, Tangier, Taunton TA1 4BL
Tel: 0870 333 0123 Fax: 01823 345003
Email: enquiries@charitycommission.gsi.gov.uk
Website: www.charitycommission.gov.uk

Committee on Safety of Medicines

Market Towers, 1 Nine Elms Lane, London SW8 5NQ
Tel: 020 7084 2451 Fax: 020 7084 2493
Website: www.mhra.gov.uk

Chairman Gordon Duff (Head)
Chairman (Biologicals) Donald Jeffries
Chairman (Chemistry, Pharmacy and Standards) Graham Buckton
Chairman (Pharmacovigilance) Martin Kendall
Principal Assessor (Biologicals) Carole Penning
Principal Assessor (Chemistry, Pharmacy and Standards) Linda Anderson
Principal Assessor (Pharmacovigilance) Sarah Wark
Secretary Leslie R Whitbread

Department for Work and Pensions (Corporate Medical Group)

Office of the Chief Medical Adviser, Department for Work and Pensions, The Adelphi, 1-11 John Adam Street, London WC2N 6HT
Tel: 020 7962 8702 Ext: 28702 Fax: 020 7712 2330
Email: mansel.aylward@dwp.gsi.gov.uk
Website: www.dwp.gov.uk/medical

Principal Medical Adviser Moira Henderson, Philip Sawney
Medical Secretary/ Head Industrial Injuries Advisory Council Secretariat Paul Stidolph
Chief Medical Adviser Mansel Aylward (Head)
Medical Director Veterans Agency Paul Kitchen
Medical Policy Adviser Mark Allerton, Pam Ford, Nick Niven-Jenkins, Helen Porritt, Susan Reed, Kenneth Tremaine, Helen Watts
Medical Policy Manager (Disability and Carer Benefits) Roger Thomas
Medical Policy Manager (War Pensions) Anne Braidwood
National Expert in Respiratory Medicine Peter Wright
SPES to Chief Medical Adviser Tracy Straker

Department of Health

Richmond House, 79 Whitehall, London SW1A 2NS
Tel: 020 7210 4850 Fax: 020 7210 5661
Email: dhmail@doh.gsi.gov.uk
Website: www.dh.gov.uk

Chief Dental Officer Raman Bedi
Chief Health Professions Officer Kay East
Chief Medical Officer for England Liam Donaldson
Chief Medical Officer for Northern Ireland Henrietta Campbell
Chief Medical Officer for Scotland Mac Armstrong
Chief Medical Officer for Wales Ruth Hall
Chief Midwife Catherine McCormick
Chief Nursing Officer Christine Beasley
Chief Pharmaceutical Officer Jim Smith
Chief Scientific Officer Sue Hill
Deputy Chief Medical Officer Aidan Halligan
National Director for Emergency Access George Alberti
National Director for Heart Disease Roger Boyle
National Director for Mental Health in England Louis Appleby
National Director for Patients and the Public Harry Cayton
National Director of Older People's Services Ian Philp
National Clinical Director for Children Al Aynsley-Green
National Clinical Director for Diabetes Sue Roberts
National Clinical Director for Primary Care David Colin-Thome
National Cancer Director Mike Richards
NHS Chief Executive and Permanent Secretary Nigel Crisp

NHS Employment and Medical Services

Quarry House, Quarry Hill, Leeds LS2 7UE
Tel: 0113 254 5000

Social Care Group

Wellington House, 135-155 Waterloo Road, London SE1 8UG
Tel: 020 7210 3000

General Dental Council

37 Wimpole Street, London W1G 8DQ
Tel: 020 7887 3800 Fax: 020 7224 3294
Email: information@gdc-uk.org
Website: www.gdc-uk.org

President Hew Mathewson
Chief Executive and Registrar Antony Townsend

General Medical Council

Regent's Place, 350 Euston Road, London NW1 3JN
Tel: 0845 357 3456
Email: gmc@gmc-uk.org
Website: www.gmc-uk.org

President Graeme Catto
Chief Executive and Registrar of the Council Finlay Scott

Lay Members appointed by the Privy Council

Kevin Barron MP, Michael Buckley, Gillian Camm, Ruth Evans, Graham Forbes, Stuart Heatherington, Robin Macleod, Joan Martin, Arun Midha, Patricia Moberly, Robert Nicholls, Fiona Peel, Ann Robinson

Member appointed by the Academy of Medical Royal Colleges

Alan Craft

Member appointed by the Council of Heads of Medical Schools

Graeme Catto

Members elected by doctors in England, Scotland and Wales

Rachel Angus, Sathiyakeerthy Ariyanayagam, Edwin Borman, Stephen Brearley, Christopher Bulstrode, James Drife, Alexandra Freeman, John Jenkins, Brian Keighley, Krishna Korlipara, Malcolm Lewis, Mike Pringle, Rosalind Ranson, Wendy Savage, Robert Shaw, Robert Slack, Peter Terry, Nicola Toynton, Joan Trowell

General Optical Council

41 Harley Street, London W1G 8DJ
Tel: 020 7580 3898 Fax: 020 7436 3525
Email: goc@optical.org
Website: www.optical.org

Chairman of the Council R Varley
Registrar and Chief Executive Peter Coe
Deputy Chairman M Salmon
Hon. Treasurer M Black
Office Manager Catharine Perry
PA to Chief Executive / Registrar Allison Hughes

Health Professions Council

Park House, 184 Kennington Park Road, London SE11 4BU
Tel: 020 7582 0866 Fax: 020 7820 9684
Website: www.hpc-uk.org

President Norma Brook
Chief Executive Marc Searle

Health Protection Agency

11th Floor, The Adelphi, 1-11 John Adam Street, London WC2N 6HT
Tel: 020 7339 1300 Fax: 020 7339 1302
Email: webteam@hpa.org.uk
Website: www.hpa.org.uk

Chairman William Stewart
Chief Executive Pat Troop
Director, Specialist and Reference Microbiology and Director Research and Development Peter Borriello
Director Business Division Roger Gilmour
Director Chemical Hazards and Poisons Stephen Palmer
Director Communicable Disease Surveilllance Centre Angus Nicoll
Director Corporate Affairs Mike Harker
Director Emergency Response Division Nigel Lightfoot
Director Finance and Resources Tony Sannia
Director Human Resources John Phipps
Director Local and Regional Services Mary O'Mahony
Director National Radiological Protection Board Roger Cox
Diretor of Communications Lis Birrane

Health Service Commissioner (Ombudsman) for England

Millbank Tower, Millbank, London SW1P 4QP
Tel: 0845 015 4033 Fax: 020 7217 4940
Email: OHSC.Enquiries@ombudsman.gsi.gov.uk
Website: www.ombudsman.org.uk

Director Carole Auchterlonie, Linda Charlton, Valerie Harrison, Jack Kellett
Director of Clinical Advice Susan Lowson
Director of Strategy & Communications Sarah Sleet
Deputy Health Service Commissioner Trish Longdon
Health Service Commissioner Ann Abraham
Information Manager Suzanne Burge

Health Service Commissioner's Office - Wales

5th Floor, Capital Tower, Greyfriars Road, Cardiff CF10 3AG
Tel: 029 2039 4621, 0845 601 0987 Fax: 029 2022 6909
Email: WHSC.Enquiries@ombudsman.gsi.gov.uk
Website: www.ombudsman.org.uk

Senior Investigating Officer Suzanne Ryan

Healthcare Commission

Finsbury Tower, 103-105 Bunhill Row, London EC1Y 8TG
Tel: 020 7448 9200 Fax: 020 7448 9222
Email: feedback@healthcarecommission.org.uk
Website: www.healthcarecommission.org.uk

Chairman Ian Kennedy
Chief Executive Anna Walker
Head of Communications Stacey Adams
Head of Corporate Services Mick Linsell
Head of Information and Analysis Lorraine Foley
Head of Operations Simon Gillespie
Head of Strategy Jamie Rentoul

Human Fertilisation and Embryology Authority

21 Bloomsbury Street, London WC1B 3HF
Tel: 020 7291 8200 Fax: 020 7291 8201
Email: admin@hfea.gov.uk
Website: www.hfea.gov.uk

Chairman Suzi Leather (Head)
Chief Executive Angela McNab
Director of Policy and Communications Tim Whitaker
Head of HR Fiona Daffern
Head of IT David Moysen
Authority Member Hossam Abdullah, Tom Baldwin, David Barlow, Christopher Barratt, Ivor Brecker, Clare Brown, Iain Cameron, Neva Haites
authority Member Richard Harries
Authority Member Jennifer Hunt, Emily Jackson, Maybeth Jamieson, Simon Jenkins, Walter Merricks, Sara Nathan, Sharmila Nebhrajani

Medicines and Healthcare Products Regulatory Agency

Market Towers, 1 Nine Elms Lane, London SW8 5NQ
Tel: 020 7084 2000 Fax: 020 7084 2353
Email: info@mhra.gsi.gov.uk
Website: www.mca.gov.uk

Chairman Alasdair Breckenridge
Chief Executive Kent Woods

Medicines Commission

Market Towers, 1 Nine Elms Lane, London SW8 5NQ
Tel: 020 7084 2652 Fax: 020 7084 2121
Email: sue.jones@mhra.gsi.gov.uk

Chair Parveen Kumar
Secretary Sue Jones

Mental Health Act Commission

Maid Marian House, 56 Houndsgate, Nottingham NG1 6BG
Tel: 0115 943 7100 Fax: 0115 943 7101
Email: chiefexec@mhac.trent.nhs.uk
Website: www.mhac.trent.nhs.uk

Chairman Kamlesh Patel
Vice-Chair Deborah Jenkins
Chief Executive Christopher Heginbotham
Deputy Chief Executive (interim) Rachel Munton
Director of Corporate Services Martin Donohoe
Director of Strategy Gemma Pearce
Regional Director Suki Desai, Steve Klein, Sue McMillan, Philip Wales

National Blood Authority

Oak House, Reeds Crescent, Watford WD24 4QN
Tel: 01923 486800 Fax: 01923 486801
Website: www.blood.co.uk

Chairman Mike Fogden (Head)
Chief Executive Martin Gorham
Director of Finance Barry Savery
Director of Public and Customer Services Liz Reynolds
Medical Director Angela Robinson

Bio Products Laboratory

Dagger Lane, Elstree, Borehamwood WD6 3BX
Tel: 020 8258 2200 Fax: 020 8258 2601

Chief Executive Chris Hadfield

International Blood Group Reference Laboratory

Southmead Road, Bristol BS10 5ND
Tel: 0117 991 2103 Fax: 0117 959 1660

National Blood Service - Cambridge Centre

University of Cambridge, Long Road, Cambridge CB2 2PT
Tel: 01223 548000 Fax: 01223 458114

National Blood Service - Colindale Blood Centre

Colindale Avenue, Colindale, London NW9 5BG
Tel: 020 8258 2700 Fax: 020 8258 2970

National Blood Service - Tooting Blood Centre

75 Cranmer Terrace, Tooting, London SW17 0RB
Tel: 020 8258 8300 Fax: 020 8258 8453

National Blood Service - West Derby Blood Centre

West Derby Street, Liverpool L7 8TW
Tel: 0151 551 8800 Fax: 0151 551 8896

Consultant A J N Shepherd

National Blood Service - West End Donor Clinic

26 Margaret Street, London W1N 7LB
Tel: 020 7301 6900 Fax: 020 7301 6905

National Blood Service - Birmingham Blood Centre

Vincent Drive, Edgbaston, Birmingham B15 2SG
Tel: 0121 253 4000 Fax: 0121 253 4003

National Blood Service - Brentwood Blood Centre

Crescent Drive, Brentwood CM15 8DP
Tel: 01277 306000 Fax: 01277 306132

National Blood Service - Bristol Blood Centre

Southmead Road, Bristol BS10 5ND
Tel: 0117 991 2000 Fax: 0117 001 2002

National Blood Service - Lancaster Blood Centre

Ashfon Road, Royal Lancaster Infirmary, Lancaster LA1 3JP
Tel: 01524 306200 Fax: 01524 306273

National Blood Service - Leeds Blood Service

Bridle Path, Leeds LS15 7TW
Tel: 0113 214 8600 Fax: 0113 214 8737

National Blood Service - Manchester Blood Centre

Plymouth Grove, Manchester M13 9LL
Tel: 0161 251 4200 Fax: 0161 251 4331

National Blood Service - Newcastle Blood Centre

Holland Drive, Barrack Road, Newcastle upon Tyne NE2 4NQ
Tel: 0191 219 4400 Fax: 0191 219 4505

Operations Manager M E Ashford

National Blood Service - Oxford Blood Centre

John Radcliffe Hospital, Headington, Oxford OX3 9DU
Tel: 01865 447900 Fax: 01865 447915

National Blood Service - Plymouth Blood Centre

Derriford Hospital, Derriford Road, Plymouth PL6 8DH
Tel: 01752 61 7815 Fax: 01752 61 7806

National Blood Service - Southampton Blood Centre

Coxford Road, Southampton SO16 5AF
Tel: 023 8029 6700 Fax: 023 8029 6760

PTI Manager Mike Northcott

National Blood Service - Trent Blood Centre

Longley Lane, Sheffield S5 7JN
Tel: 0114 203 4800 Fax: 0114 203 4911

National Clinical Assessment Authority

Market Towers, 1 Nine Elms Lane, London SW8 5NQ
Tel: 020 7084 3850 Fax: 020 7084 3851
Email: ncaa@ncaa.nhs.uk
Website: www.ncaa.nhs.uk

Chairman Bob Nicholls
Medical Director Alastair Scotland

National Health Service Litigation Authority

Napier House, 24 High Holborn, London WC1V 6AZ
Tel: 020 7430 8700
Website: www.nhsla.com

Chairman R S Bradshaw
Chief Executive Stephen Walker

National Institute for Biological Standards and Control

Blanche Lane, South Mimms, Potters Bar EN6 3QG
Tel: 01707 641000 Fax: 01707 646730
Email: enquiries@nibsc.ac.uk
Website: www.nibsc.ac.uk

Director Stephen Inglis (Head)

National Institute for Health and Clinical Excellence

Formerly the National Institute for Clinical Excellence. From 01/04/2005 merged with the Health Development Agency to form the National Institute for Health and Clinical Excellence (NICE).

MidCity Place, 71 High Holborn, London WC1V 6NA
Tel: 020 7067 5800 Fax: 020 7067 5801
Email: nice@nice.nhs.uk
Website: www.nice.org.uk

Chairman Michael Rawlins
Chief Executive Andrew Dillon
Clinical and Public Health Director Peter Littlejohns
Implementation Systems Director Gillian Leng
Planning and Resources Director Andrea Sutcliffe

NHSU

88 Wood Street, London EC2V 7RS
Tel: 020 8528 1400 Fax: 020 8528 1301
Email: bob.fryer@nhsu.org.uk
Website: www.nhsu.nhs.uk

Chairman Barbara Stephens
Interim Chief Executive Philip Brown

Nursing and Midwifery Council

23 Portland Place, London W1B 1PZ
Tel: 020 7637 7181 Fax: 020 7436 2924
Email: communications@nmc-uk.org
Website: www.nmc-uk.org

President Jonathan Asbridge (Head)
Chief Executive Sarah Thewlis
Head of Communications Stuart Skyte

Office for National Statistics

London Office, 1 Drummond Gate, London SW1V 2QQ
Tel: 0845 601 3034 Fax: 01633 652747
Email: info@statistics.gov.uk
Website: www.statistics.gov.uk

Registrar General for England and Wales Len Cook
Chief Operating Officer Hilary Douglas

Pharmaceutical Services Negotiating Committee

59 Buckingham Street, Aylesbury HP20 2PJ
Tel: 01296 432823 Fax: 01296 438427
Email: psnc@psnc.org.uk
Website: www.psnc.org.uk

Chairman Barry Andrews
Chief Executive Sue Sharpe
Member Gerald Alexander, Penny Beck, Paul Bennett, Dhiren Bhatt, Peter Catee, Mark Collins, Ian Cowan, Ian Cubbin, Sid Dajani, Wally Dove, Steve Duncan, Digby Emson, John Evans, R Hazelhurst, Dilip Joshi, John Makepeace, Lisa Martin, Andrew Murdock, Gary Myers, Rakesh Panesar, Phil Parry, Bharat Patel, Indrajit Patel, Kalpesh Patel, Kirit Patel, Rajesh Patel, Umesh Patel, Ashak Soni, Allen Tweedie, Steven Williams

Postgraduate Medical Education and Training Board

5th Floor, 64 Wimpole Street, London W1G 8YS
Tel: 020 7563 6897 Fax: 020 7486 2527
Email: info@pmetb.org.uk
Website: www.pmetb.org.uk

Chief Executive Paul Streets (Head)
Director of Operations and Standards Isabel Nisbet
Acting Chairman Peter Simpson
Board Member Carol Black, Alan Craft, Stephen Field, Sian Griffiths, David Haslam, Peter Hill, John Jenkins, Hasmukh Joshi, Namita Kumar, Stuart MacPherson, David Neal, Trevor Pickersgill, Ewen Sim, Lesley Southgate, Anita Thomas
Lay Member Angela Coulter, Ian Cumming, Sue Fox, Frances Gawn, Janet Grant, Jane Reynolds, Susanne Roff, Finlay Scott

Royal Air Force Medical Services

Cranwell, Sleaford NG34 8GZ
Website: www.raf.mod.uk/ptc/medical.html

UK Transplant

Fox Den Road, Stoke Gifford, Bristol BS34 8RR
Tel: 0117 975 7575 Fax: 0117 975 7577
Email: enquiries@uktransplant.nhs.uk
Website: www.uktransplant.org.uk

Chair Gwynneth Flower
Chief Executive Sue Sutherland
Director of Communications Penny Hallett
Director of Donor Care and Co-ordination Sue Falvey
Director of Finance Martin Davis
Director of Information and Technology Management David Shute
Director of Statistics and Audit Dave Collett
Head of Information and Communications Technology Services Jon Ward
Medical Director Chris Rudge
Scientific Services Adviser Sue Fuggle

Unrelated Live Transplant Regulatory Authority

Room 415, Wellington House, 133-155 Waterloo Road, London SE1 8UG
Tel: 020 7972 4812 Fax: 020 7972 4790
Email: gladys.hall@dh.gsi.gov.uk
Website: www.advisorybodies.doh.gov.uk/ultra

Chair Roddy MacSween

Scotland

Blood Transfusion Service Scotland

Ellen's Glen Road, Edinburgh EH17 7QT
Tel: 0131 536 5700 Fax: 0131 536 5701
Website: www.show.scot.nhs.uk/snbts/

Acting Director of Finance Anne Marie Ingram
National Director Keith Thompson
National Medical and Scientific Director Ian Franklin
Personal Assistant Yvonne Todd
Quality Director Bruce Cuthbertson
Supply Chain Director Martin Bruce

Aberdeen and North East of Scotland Blood Transfusion Centre

Regional Transfusion Centre, Foresterhill Road, Foresterhill, Aberdeen AB25 2ZW
Tel: 01224 685685 Fax: 01224 695351

Director Henry Hambley

Diagnostics Scotland

21 Ellen's Glen Road, Edinburgh EH17 7QT
Tel: 0131 536 5700 Fax: 0131 536 5701

Director John Allan

East of Scotland Blood Transfusion Centre

Ninewells Hospital, Level 8, Dundee DD1 9SY
Tel: 01382 645166 Fax: 01382 642551

Director Sam Rawlinson

Edinburgh and South East Scotland Blood Transfusion Centre

Royal Infirmary of Edinburgh, 51 Little France Cresecent, Edinburgh EH16 4SA
Tel: 0131 536 5300 Fax: 0131 536 5352

Director Marc Turner

National Science Laboratory

21 Ellen's Glen Road, Edinburgh EH17 7QT
Tel: 0131 536 5700 Fax: 0131 536 5701

Director Chris Prowse

North of Scotland Blood Transfusion Centre

Raigmore Hospital, Inverness IV2 3UJ
Tel: 01463 705315 Fax: 01463 237020

Director Peter Forsyth

Protein Fractionation Centre

21 Ellen's Glen Road, Edinburgh EH17 7QT
Tel: 0131 536 5700 Fax: 0131 658 1624

Director Katherine Reid

West of Scotland Blood Transfusion Centre

Gartnavel General Hospital, 25 Shelly Road, Glasgow G12 0XB
Tel: 0141 357 7700 Fax: 0141 357 7701

Director Rachel Green

Common Services Agency for NHS Scotland

Also known as National Services Scotland.

Gyle Square, 1 South Gyle Crescent, Edinburgh EH12 9EB
Tel: 0131 275 6000 Fax: 0131 275 7500
Website: www.show.scot.nhs.uk/csa

Chairman David Campbell
Vice-Chair Alan Sibbald
Chief Executive Stuart Bain

Central Legal Office

Anderson House, Breadalbane Street, Bonnington Road, Edinburgh EH6 5JR
Tel: 0131 275 7800 Fax: 0131 275 7900
Website: www.show.scot.nhs.uk/clo

Legal Adviser Ranald Macdonald

Counter Fraud Services

Earlston House, Almondvale Business Park, Almondvale Way, Livingston EH54 6GA
Tel: 01506 705200 Fax: 08000 151628
Website: www.show.scot.nhs.uk/fiu

Director Neil Billing

Health Protection Scotland

Clifton House, Clifton Place, Glasgow G3 7LN
Tel: 0141 300 1100 Fax: 0141 300 1170
Website: www.show.scot.nhs.uk/hps

Director Tim Brett

Information Services

Gyle Square, 1 South Gyle Crescent, Edinburgh EH12 9EB
Tel: 0131 275 6000 Fax: 0131 275 7500
Website: www.show.scot.nhs.uk/isd

Director Richard Copland

National Services Division

Gyle Square, 1 South Gyle Crescent, Edinburgh EH12 9EB
Tel: 0131 275 6000 Fax: 0131 275 7500
Website: www.show.scot.nhs.uk/nsd

Director Deirdre Evans

Practitioner Services

Gyle Square, 1 South Gyle Crescent, Edinburgh EH12 9EB
Tel: 0131 275 6000 Fax: 0131 275 7500
Website: www.show.scot.nhs.uk/psd

Assistant Director Lorna Jackson

Scottish Health Service Centre

Crewe Road South, Edinburgh EH2 2LF
Tel: 0131 623 2500 Fax: 0131 315 2369
Website: www.show.scot.nhs.uk/shsc

Director Jan Lyell

Scottish Healthcare Supplies

Gyle Square, 1 South Gyle Crescent, Edinburgh EH12 9EB
Tel: 0131 275 6000 Fax: 0131 275 7500
Website: www.show.scot.nhs.uk/shs

Director Miles Moorhouse

Mental Welfare Commission for Scotland

K Floor, Argyle House, 3 Lady Lawson Street, Edinburgh EH3 9SH
Tel: 0131 222 6111 Fax: 0131 222 6112
Email: enquiries@mwcscot.co.uk
Website: www.mwcscot.org.uk

Chairman Ian J Miller
Director Donald Lyons
Head of Corporate Services Alison McRae

Medical Commissioner M Osborn
Nurse Commissioner Jamie Malcolm
Social Work Commissioner J Cheetham

MRC Technology Scotland

Crewe Road South, Edinburgh EH4 2LF
Tel: 0131 311 7010 Fax: 0131 311 7025

Director M Dalrymple

National Health Service Tribunal

40 Craiglockhart Road North, Edinburgh E14 1BT
Tel: 0131 443 2575 Fax: 0131 443 2575

Chairman Malcolm Thomson
Clerk to the NHS Tribunal W Bryden

NHS Education for Scotland

22 Queen Street, Edinburgh EH2 1NT
Tel: 0131 226 7371 Fax: 0131 225 9970
Website: www.nes.scot.nhs.uk

Chairman Ann Markham
Chief Executive Malcolm Wright
Head of Corporate Services Karen Stiven

NHS Health Scotland

Woodburn House, Canaan Lane, Edinburgh EH10 4SG
Tel: 0131 536 5500 Fax: 0131 536 5501
Website: www.healthscotland.com

Chair Lesley Hinds (Head)
Chief Executive Graham Robertson

Scottish Executive Health Department

St Andrews House, Regent Road, Edinburgh EH1 3DG
Tel: 0131 244 2410 Fax: 0131 244 2162
Email: ps.hd@scotland.gsi.gov.uk
Website: www.show.scot.nhs.uk/sehd

Chief Executive Trevor Jones

Chief Scientist's Office

Scottish Executive Health Department, St Andrews House, Regent Road, Edinburgh EH1 3DG
Tel: 0131 244 2248 Fax: 0131 244 2285
Website: www.show.scot.nhs.uk/cso

Director Alison M Spaull (Head)
Chief Scientist Roland Jung

Wales

Health Professions Wales

2nd Floor, Golate House, 101 St Mary Street, Cardiff CF10 1DX
Tel: 029 2026 1400 Fax: 029 2026 1499
Email: info@hpw.org.uk
Website: www.hpw.org.uk

Chief Executive Hilary Neagle
Director of Business Services Wendy Fawcus

National Public Health Service Wales

1 Charnwood Court, Heol Billingsley, Parc Nantgarw, Cardiff CF15 7QZ
Tel: 01443 824160 Fax: 01443 824161
Website: www.nphs.wales.nhs.uk

National Director Cerilan Rogers (Head)
PA to National Director Emma Morgan

Wales Centre for Health

14 Cathedral Road, Cardiff CF11 9LJ
Tel: 029 2022 7744 Fax: 029 2022 6749
Email: wch@velindre-tr.wales.nhs.uk

Chairman Mansel Aylward

Northern Ireland

Department of Health, Social Services and Public Safety

Castle Buildings, Stormont, Belfast BT4 3SJ
Tel: 028 9052 0500 Fax: 028 9052 0572
Website: www.dhsspsni.gov.uk

Chief Executive John Cole
Acting Chief Nursing Officer Francis Rice
Chief Dental Officer Doreen Wilson
Chief Inspector Social Services Inspectorate Paul Martin
Chief Medical Officer Henrietta Campbell
Chief Pharmaceutical Officer Norman Morrow
Permanent Secretary Clive Gowdy
Planning and Resources Don Hill
Primary, Secondary and Community Care Andrew Hamilton

Northern Ireland Blood Transfusion Service

Belfast City Hospital Complex, Lisburn Road, Belfast BT9 7TS
Tel: 028 9053 4646 Fax: 028 9043 9017
Website: www.nibts.org

Medical Director W M McClelland

Northern Ireland Central Services Agency for the Health and Social Services

25-27 Adelaide Street, Belfast BT2 8FH
Tel: 028 9032 4431 Fax: 028 9023 2304
Email: chiefexec@csa.n-i.nhs.uk
Website: www.centralservicesagency.com

Chair S Fulton
Chief Executive Stephen Hodkinson
Director of Family Practitioner Services Paula Sheils
Director of Finance Paul Gick
Director of Human Resources J Kennedy
Director of Legal Services Alfy Maginness
Director of NICARE Colin Sullivan
Operational Director of Research and Development M Neely
Regional Supplies Director Teresa Molloy

Northern Ireland Practice and Education Council for Nursing and Midwifery

Centre House, 79 Chichester Street, Belfast BT1 4JE
Tel: 028 9023 8152 Fax: 028 9033 3298
Email: enquiries@nipec.n-i.nhs.uk
Website: www.nipec.n-i.nhs.uk

Chief Executive Paddie Blaney
Head of Corporate Services Edmund Thom
Council Chair Maureen Griffith
Council Member Hazel Baird, Jennifer Boore, Thelma Byrne, Eleanor Hayes, Sara Magee, Brendan McCarthy, Dolores McCormick, Iain McGowan, Frances McMurray, Margaret O'Hagan, Maria O'Hare, Mary Patten, Michael Rea
Professional Officer Barbara Bradley
Senior Professional Officer Lesley Barrowman, Tanya McCance, Brendan McGrath

Coroners

England

The Royal Household
44 Ormond Avenue, Hampton TW12 2RX
Tel: 020 8979 6805 Fax: 020 8979 6805
Website: www.surreycoroner.info

Coroner M J C Burgess

Avon
Coroner's Court, Backfields, Bristol BS2 8QP
Tel: 0117 942 8322 Fax: 0117 944 5492

Coroner P E A Forrest

Bedfordshire and Luton
Coroner's Office, 15 Goldington Road, Bedford MK40 3JY
Tel: 01234 273011/2, 01234 273013 (Secretary)
Fax: 01234 273014

Coroner David S Morris

Berkshire
Yeomanry House, 131 Castle Hill, Reading RG1 7TA
Tel: 0118 901 5447 Fax: 0118 901 5448

Coroner Peter J Bedford

Berkshire, Reading District
Vane House, Nuffield, Henley-on-Thames RG9 5RT
Tel: 01491 641444
Email: coroner@reading.gov.uk

Coroner A J Pim

Berkshire, West District
The Old Rectory, Church Road, Shaw, Newbury RG14 2DR
Tel: 01635 40181

Coroner C Hoile

Blackburn, Hyndburn and Ribble Valley
7 Richmond Terrace, Blackburn BB1 7BB
Tel: 01254 263091 Fax: 01254 681442

Coroner Michael Singleton

Bournemouth, Poole and Eastern District
The Coronor's Court, Stafford Road, Bournemouth BHI IPA
Tel: 01202 310049 Fax: 01202 780423
Email: patrician@bournemouth.gov.uk

Coroner S Payne

Bracknell Forest, Slough, Windsor and Maidenhead, and Wokingham
Messrs Coleman, 27 Marlow Road, Maidenhead SL6 7AE
Tel: 01628 631051 Fax: 01628 622106

Coroner P J Bedford

Brighton and Hove District
Coroner's Office, Woodvale, Lewes Road, Brighton BN2 3QB
Tel: 01273 292046 Fax: 01273 292047

Coroner Veronica Hamilton-Deeley

Buckinghamshire District
Adelaide House, 17 High Street, Thame OX9 2BZ
Tel: 01844 214454 Fax: 01844 358186

Coroner Richard A Hulett

Cambridgeshire, North and East District
1 & 2 York Row, Wisbech PE13 1EA
Tel: 01945 461456 Fax: 01945 461364
Email: williammorris@dawbarnspearson.co.uk

Coroner W R Morris

Cambridgeshire, South and West District
Coroner's Office, Box Res 1407, Shire Hall Castle Hill, Cambridge CB3 0AP
Tel: 01223 718620 Fax: 01223 717586
Email: hmcoroners.cambridgeshire@cambridge.gov.uk

Coroner David Morris

Cheshire, Halton and Warrington
HM Coroner's Court, 57 Winmarleigh Street, Warrington WA1 1LE
Tel: 01925 444216 Fax: 01925 444219

Coroner Nichol Rheinberg

City of London District
Coroner's Court, Milton Court, Moor Lane, London EC2Y 2NJ
Tel: 020 7332 1598 Fax: 020 7601 2714
Email: paul.major@corpoflondon.gov.uk
Website: www.cityoflondon.gov.uk/corporation/our_services

Coroner Paul B Matthews

Cornwall, East District
14 Barrack Lane, Truro TR1 2DW
Tel: 01872 261612 Fax: 01872 262738

Coroner Emma Carlyon

Cornwall, Western District
14 Barrack Lane, Truro TR1 2DW
Tel: 01872 261612 Fax: 01872 262738

Coroner Emma Carlyon

County of Herefordshire
36-37 Bridge Street, Hereford HR4 9DJ
Tel: 01432 355301 Fax: 01432 356619
Email: herefordcoroner@lambecorner.co.uk

Coroner D Halpern

Cumbria, Furness District
Central Police Station, Market Street, Barrow-in-Furness LA14 2LE
Tel: 01229 848966 Fax: 01229 824705

Coroner I Smith

Cumbria, North Eastern District
Carlisle Police Station, Rickergate, Carlisle CA3 8QW
Tel: 01768 218344 Fax: 01768 218499
Email: john.grierson@cumbria.police.uk

Coroner Ian H Morton

Cumbria, Southern District
Central Police Station, Market Street, Barrow-in-Furness LA14 2LE
Tel: 01229 848966 Fax: 01229 848966

Coroner Ian Smith

Cumbria, Western District
38/42 Lowther Street, Whitehaven CA28 7JU
Tel: 01946 692461 Fax: 01946 692015

Coroner John Taylor

Darlington and South Durham
Post Office House, Elliott Street, Crook DH15 8QH
Tel: 01388 767770 Fax: 01388 766617

Coroner C E Penna

Derbyshire, Derby and South Derbyshire District
St Katherine's House, St Mary's Wharf, Mansfield Road, Derby DE1 1TQ
Tel: 01332 613014 Fax: 01332 294942

Coroner Peter Ashworth

Derbyshire, High Peak District
10 Buxton Road, Hazel Grove, Stockport SK7 6AD
Tel: 0161 419 9626 Fax: 0161 419 9604

Coroner C G Rushton

Derbyshire, Scarsdale District
69 Saltergate, Chesterfield S40 1JS
Tel: 01246 201391 Fax: 01246 273058

Coroner Thomas Kelly

Devon, South Devon and Torbay District
Coroner's Office, Cary Chambers, 1 Palk Street, Torquay TQ2 5EL
Tel: 01803 380705 Fax: 01803 380704
Email: h.m.coroner@torbay.gov.uk
Website: www.torbay.gov.uk/coroner

Coroner Ian Arrow

Devon, Plymouth and South West Devon District
3 The Crescent, Plymouth PL1 3AB
Tel: 01752 204636 Fax: 01752 313297

Coroner N S Meadows

Dorset, Western District
Outhays House, 2 The Plocks, Blandford Forum DT11 7QB
Tel: 01258 453733-5 Fax: 01258 455747

Coroner M C Johnston

Durham, Northern District
Post Office House, Elliott Street, Crook DH15 8QH
Tel: 01388 767770 Fax: 01388 766617
Email: hmcnorthdurham@btinternet.com

Coroner Andrew Tweddle

East Sussex District
28/29 Grande Parade, St Leonards on Sea TN37 6DR
Tel: 01424 200144 Fax: 01424 200145

Coroner A R Craze

Essex, No 1 District (inc Thurrock)
Essex County Council, County Hall, PO Box 11, Chelmsford CM1 1LX
Tel: 01245 430469 Fax: 01245 437142

Coroner C Beasley-Murray

Essex, No 2 District (inc Southend)
Rochford Police Station, South Street, Rochford SS4 1BL
Tel: 01702 530911 Fax: 01268 798179

Coroner Peter Dean

Exeter and Greater Devon District
Raleigh Hall, Fore Street, Topsham, Exeter EX3 0HY
Tel: 01392 876575 Fax: 01392 876574

Coroner Elizabeth A Earland

Gloucestershire, Cheltenham District
County Offices, 2nd Floor, St Georges Road, Cheltenham GL50 3PS
Tel: 01242 221064 Fax: 01242 226575

Coroner A L Maddrell

Greater London, Inner North London District
St Pancras Coroner's Court, Camley Street, London NW1 0PP
Tel: 020 7387 4882, 020 7387 4884 Fax: 020 7383 2485

Coroner Andrew Reid

Greater London, Eastern District
Coroner's Court, Queen's Road, Walthamstow, London E17 8QP
Tel: 020 8520 7245 Fax: 020 8521 0896

Coroner Elizabeth J E Stearns

Greater London, Inner South London District
Southwark & Lambeth Offices, Southwark Coroner's Court, Tennis Street, London SE1 1YD
Tel: 020 7407 5611 Fax: 020 7378 8401

Coroner John C Sampson

Greater London, Inner West London District
Westminster Coroner's Court, 65 Horseferry Road, London SW1P 2ED
Tel: 020 7802 4750 Fax: 020 7828 2837

Coroner Paul A Knapman

Greater London, Northern District
Hornsey Coroner's Court, Myddelton Road, Hornsey, London N8 7PY
Tel: 020 8348 4411 Fax: 020 8347 5229

Coroner William F G Dolman

Greater London, Southern District
Croydon Coroner's Court, Barclay Road, Croydon CR9 3NE
Tel: 020 8681 5019 Fax: 020 8686 3491
Email: hmc@southlondoncoroner.org

Coroner Roy N Palmer

Greater London, Western District
Coroner's Court, 25 Bagley's Lane, Fulham, London SW6 2QA
Tel: 020 8753 6800 Fax: 020 8753 6803

Coroner Alison M Thompson

Greater Manchester, West District
Paderborn House, Civic Centre, Howell Croft, Bolton BL1 1JW
Tel: 01204 338799 Fax: 01204 338798
Website: www.bolton.gov.uk

Coroner Jennifer Leeming

Greater Manchester, Manchester District
Fifth Floor, City Magistrate's Court, Crown Square, Manchester M60 1RP
Tel: 0161 819 5666 Fax: 0161 819 5330

Coroner L N Gorodkin

Greater Manchester, North District
Fourth Floor, Telegraph House, Baillie Street, Rochdale OL16 1QY
Tel: 0161 624 4971, 01706 649922 Fax: 01706 640720

Coroner Simon Nelson

Greater Manchester, South District
10 Greek Street, Stockport SK3 8AB
Tel: 0161 476 0971 Fax: 0161 476 0972

Coroner John S Pollard

Greater Suffolk District
2 Liitle Haylands, 99 High Road, Chigwell IG7 6QQ
Tel: 020 8502 6337 Fax: 020 8502 6337

Coroner P J Dean

Hampshire, Central District
19 St Peter Street, Winchester SO23 8BU
Tel: 01962 844440 Fax: 01962 842300

Coroner G A Short

Hampshire, North East District
76 Bounty Road, Basingstoke RG21 1BZ
Tel: 01256 322911 Fax: 01256 327811

Coroner Andrew M Bradley

Hampshire, Portsmouth and South East District
Room T20, The Guildhall, Guildhall Square, Portsmouth PO33 4DN
Tel: 02392 688327, 02392 688328, 02392 688329
Fax: 02392 688331

Coroner David C Horsley

Hampshire, Southampton and New Forest District
Civic Centre Police Station, Havelock Road, Southampton SO14 7LG
Tel: 023 8067 4266, 023 8067 4267 Fax: 023 8022 3631

Coroner Keith St John Wiseman

Hartlepool District
155 York Road, Hartlepool TS26 9EQ
Tel: 01429 274732 Fax: 01429 260199
Email: info@donnellyadamson.co.uk

Coroner C W M Donnelly

Herefordshire
36-37 Bridge Street, Hereford HR4 9DY
Tel: 01432 355301 Fax: 01432 356619

Coroner D Halpern

Hertfordshire District
The Old Courthouse, St Albans Road East, Hatfield AL10 0ES
Tel: 01707 897400 Fax: 01707 897398

Coroner Edward G Thomas

Isle of Wight District
The Coroner's Office, 3-9 Quay Street, Newport PO30 5BB
Tel: 01983 520697 Fax: 01983 520697

Coroner J A Mathews

Isles of Scilly District
20 Lelant Meadows, Lelant, St Ives TR26 3JS
Tel: 01736 756287

Coroner D W Pepperell

Kent, Central and South East District
The Police Station, Bouverie Road West, Folkestone CT20 4RW
Tel: 01303 289118 Fax: 01303 289164

Coroner H Rachel Redman

Kent, North East District
5 Lloyd Road, Broadstairs CT10 1HX
Tel: 01843 863260 Fax: 01843 603927

Coroner R M Cobb

Kent, North West District
The White House, 1 Hook Lane, Welling DA16 2DJ
Tel: 020 8306 2222 Fax: 020 8306 2221

Coroner R L Hatch

Kingston upon Hull and East Riding of Yorkshire District
Coroner's Court, Essex House, Manor Street, Kingston upon Hull HU1 1YU
Tel: 01482 613011 Fax: 01482 613020

Coroner Geoffrey M Saul

Lancashire, Blackburn, Hyndburn and Ribble Valley District
7 Richmond Terrace, Blackburn BB1 7BB
Tel: 01254 263091 Fax: 01254 274001

Coroner Michael J H Singleton

Lancashire, Preston and West Lancashire District
Coroner's Court, Lawson Street, Preston PR1 2QT
Tel: 01772 821788 Fax: 01772 828755

Coroner James R H Adeley

Lancashire, Blackpool and Fylde District
Phoenix House, 283 Church Street, Blackpool FY1 3PG
Fax: 01253 291915, 01253 625731

Coroner Anne V Hind

Lancashire, East District
6a Hargreaves Street, Burnley BB11 1ES
Tel: 01282 438446 Fax: 01282 446525
Email: burnley.coroners@btopenworld.com

Coroner Richard G Taylor

Leicestershire, Leicester City and South Leicestershire District
Room 6, Town Hall, Town Hall Square, Leicester LE1 9BG
Tel: 0116 225 2534/5 Fax: 0116 225 2537

Coroner J M Symington

Leicestershire, Rutland and North Leicestershire District
34 Woodgate, Loughborough LE11 2TY
Tel: 01509 268748 Fax: 01509 210744

Coroner T H Kirkman

Lincolnshire, Boston and Spalding District
c/o County Hall, Boston PE21 6LX
Tel: 01205 364342

Coroner M Taylor

Lincolnshire, Louth District
Thimbleby Fisher, Solicitors, Lindum House, 10 Queen Street, Spilsby PE23 5JE
Tel: 01790 752219 Fax: 01790 752427

Coroner S P G Fisher

Lincolnshire, North Lincolnshire and Grimsby District
Cleethorpes Town Hall, Knoll Street, Cleethorpes DN35 8LN
Tel: 01472 324005 Fax: 01472 324007

Coroner J S Atkinson

Lincolnshire, Spilsby District
Thimbleby Fisher, Solicitors, Lindum House, 10 Queen Street, Spilsby PE23 5JE
Tel: 01790 752219 Fax: 01790 752427

Coroner S P G Fisher

Lincolnshire, Stamford District
Lincolnshire Police Divisional HQ, St Catherine's Road, Grantham NG31 9DD
Tel: 01476 403217 Fax: 01476 567004

Coroner G S Ryall

Lincolnshire, West District
94 West Parade, Lincoln LN1 1JZ
Tel: 01522 530055 Fax: 01522 530055
Email: lincs@coroner.fsbusiness.co.uk

Coroner Roger D Atkinson

Merseyside, Knowsley, St Helens and Sefton District
County Coroner's Court, Gordon House, 3/5 Leicester Street, Southport PR9 0ER
Tel: 01704 531643 Fax: 01704 534321

Coroner C Sumner

Merseyside, Liverpool District
H M Coroner's Court, The Cotton Exchange, Old Hall Street, Liverpool L2 9UF
Tel: 0151 233 4701 Fax: 0151 233 4710

Coroner Andre J A Rebello

Merseyside, Wirral District
Midland Bank Buildings, Grange Road, West Kirby, Wirral L48 4EB
Tel: 0151 625 6414 Fax: 0151 625 7757

Coroner C W Johnson

Mid Kent and Medway District
The Coach House, Biddenden Road, Sissinghurst TN17 2JP
Tel: 01580 714182 Fax: 01580 174189

Coroner Roger Sykes

Milton Keynes
10 Market Square, Buckingham MK18 1NJ
Tel: 01280 822217 Fax: 01280 813269

Coroner R H G Corner

Newbury District
Vane House, Nuffield, Henley on Thames RG9 5RT
Tel: 01491 641444

Coroner D Pim

Norfolk, Great Yarmouth District
6 South Quay, Great Yarmouth NR30 2QJ
Tel: 01493 855555 Fax: 01493 330055

Coroner K M Dowding

Norfolk, King's Lynn District
Messrs Dawbarns, 1 York Row, Wisbech PE13 1EA
Tel: 01553 613613 (Queen Elizabeth Hospital Kings Lynn)
Fax: 01945 461364

Coroner W R Knowles

North Yorkshire, Western District
H M Coroner, Standard House, 48 High Street, Northallerton DL7 8EQ
Tel: 01609 766414 Fax: 01609 780970
Website: www.northyorks.gov.uk

Coroner Geoffrey Leonard Fell

North Yorkshire, Eastern District
4 Old Malton Gate, Malton YO17 0EQ
Tel: 01653 600070 Fax: 01653 600049

Coroner M D Oakley

Northamptonshire District
300 Wellingborough Road, Northampton NN1 4EP
Tel: 01604 624732 Fax: 01604 232282

Coroner A Pember

Northumberland, North District
c/o Northumbria Police, Ashington NE63 8HD
Tel: 01661 872555 Ext: 6165 Fax: 01661 861688

Coroner Ian G McCreath

Northumberland, South District
3 Stanley Street, Blyth NE24 2BS
Tel: 01670 354777 Fax: 01670 355951

Coroner E Armstrong

Norwich and Central Norfolk District
124 Barrack Street, Norwich NR3 1TL
Tel: 01603 663302 Fax: 01603 665511
Email: norwich@coroner.norfolk.gov.uk

Coroner William J Armstrong

Nottinghamshire District
50 Carrington Street, Nottingham NG1 7FG
Tel: 0115 941 2332 Fax: 0115 950 0141
Email: coroner@nottinghamcity.gov.uk

Coroner Nigel Chapman

Oxfordshire District
Southern House, 1 Cambridge Terrace, Oxford OX1 1RR
Tel: 01865 721451 Fax: 01865 251804

Coroner N G Gardiner

Peterborough District
10 Briggate Quay, Whittlesey, Peterborough PE7 1DH
Tel: 01733 203418 Fax: 01733 351141

Coroner G S Ryall

Shropshire, Mid and North West District
West Mercia Constabulary Police HQ, Clive Road, Monkmoor, Shrewsbury SY2 5RW
Tel: 01743 237445 Fax: 01743 264879

Coroner John P Ellery

Shropshire, South District
18 Broad Street, Ludlow SY8 1NG
Tel: 01584 873918/9 Fax: 01584 876787

Coroner A F T Sibcy

Somerset, Eastern District
Argyll House, Bath Street, Frome BA11 1DP
Tel: 01761 411030 Fax: 01761 416272
Email: info@hmcoroner.co.uk

Coroner Tony Williams

Somerset, Western District
Blackbrook Gate, Blackbrook Park Avenue, Taunton TA1 2PG
Tel: 01823 445372, 01823 666263 (24 hours) Fax: 01823 445800, 01823 445825

Coroner M R Rose

South Staffordshire District
15 Martin Street, Stafford ST16 2LX
Tel: 01785 276127 Fax: 01785 276128

Coroner A Haigh

South Yorkshire, East District
5 Union Street, Doncaster DN1 3AE
Tel: 01302 320844 Fax: 01302 364833
Email: hmcdoncaster@btconnect.com

Coroner E Stanley Hooper

South Yorkshire, West District
Medico-Legal Centre, Watery Street, Sheffield S3 7ES
Tel: 0114 273 8721 Fax: 0114 278 4909

Coroner C P Dorries

Stoke-on-Trent and North Staffordshire
Coroner's Chambers, 547 Hartshill Road, Stoke-on-Trent ST4 6HF
Tel: 01782 234777 Fax: 01782 234783

Coroner Ian S Smith

Suffolk, Lowestoft District
4 Halesworth Road, Reydon, Southwold IP18 6NH
Tel: 01502 726017 Fax: 01502 726048

Coroner A G L de Lacroix

Surrey District
H M Coroner's Court, Station Approach, Woking GU22 7AP
Tel: 01483 776138 Fax: 01483 765460

Coroner M J C Burgess

Teesside, Middlesbrough, Redcar and Cleveland and Stockton-on-Tees District
Newham House, 96-98 Borough Road, Middlesbrough TS1 2HJ
Tel: 01642 243221 Fax: 01642 248031

Coroner M J F Sheffield

Tyne and Wear, Gateshead and South Tyneside District
35 Station Road, Hebburn NE31 1LA
Tel: 0191 483 5422, 0191 483 8771 Fax: 0191 483 9761

Coroner T Carney

Tyne and Wear, Newcastle upon Tyne District
Coroner's Court, Bolbec Hall, Westgate Road, Newcastle upon Tyne NE1 1SE
Tel: 0191 261 2845 Fax: 0191 261 2952

Coroner David Mitford

Tyne and Wear, North Tyneside District
3 Stanley Street, Blyth NE24 2BS
Tel: 01670 354777 Fax: 01670 355951

Coroner E Armstrong

Tyne and Wear, Sunderland District
112 High Street West, Sunderland SR1 1TX
Tel: 0191 514 1001 Fax: 0191 514 8100

Coroner Derek Winter

Warwickshire District
Field Overall, Solicitors, 42 Warwick Street, Leamington Spa CV32 5JS
Tel: 01926 422101 Fax: 01926 450568

Coroner M F Coker

West Midlands, Birmingham District
Coroner's Court, 50 Newton Street, Birmingham B4 6NE
Tel: 0121 303 4274, 07970 312834 (Mobile) Fax: 0121 233 4841

Coroner Aidan Cotter

West Midlands, Coventry District
The Coroner's Office, Little Park Street, Coventry CV1 2JX
Tel: 024 7653 9018, 024 7653 9019 Fax: 024 7653 9804
Email: coventrycoroner@btopenworld.com

Coroner David R Sarginson

West Midlands, Dudley District
21 Dingle Road, Pedmore, Stourbridge DY9 0RS
Tel: 0121 626 8018, 01562 886177 (Home) Fax: 01384 354477

Coroner R Balmain

West Midlands, Sandwell District
The Register Office, Highfields, High Street, West Bromwich B70 8RJ
Tel: 0121 569 2472 Fax: 0121 569 2473

Coroner R Balmain

West Midlands, Walsall District
Addison, Cooper, Jesson & Co Solicitors, Kelvin House, 23 Lichfield Street, Walsall WS1 1UL
Tel: 01922 725515 Fax: 01922 643403

Coroner David Milne

West Midlands, Wolverhampton District
Underhill Langley & Wright, 7 Waterloo Road, Wolverhampton WV1 4DW
Tel: 01902 420261 Fax: 01902 426091

Coroner R J Allen

West Sussex District
50 Westgate, Chichester PO19 3HE
Tel: 01243 530388 Fax: 01243 530389
Email: hm.coroner@westsussex.gov.uk

Coroner Roger J Stone

West Yorkshire, Eastern District
71 Northgate, Wakefield WF1 3BS

West Yorkshire, Eastern District
Symonds House, Belgrave Street, Leeds LS2 8DD
Tel: 0113 243 2963, 01924 302180 Fax: 01113 244 8585, 01924 291603

Symonds House, Belgrave Street, Leeds LS2 8DD
Tel: 0113 243 2963 Fax: 0113 244 8585

Coroner D Hinchliff, D Hinchliff

West Yorkshire, Western District
Coroner's Court, The City Courts, The Tyrls, Bradford BD1 1LA
Tel: 01274 391362 Fax: 01274 721794

Coroner R L Whittaker

Wiltshire and Swindon District
Lloyds Bank Chambers, 6 Castle Street, Salisbury SP1 1BB
Tel: 01722 326870, 01722 337591 Fax: 01722 332223

Coroner D Masters

Worcester District
The Court House, Bewdley Road, Stourport-on-Severn DY13 8XE
Tel: 01905 331026
Email: coroner@worcestershire.gov.uk

Coroner Victor F Round

The Wrekin District
Edgbaston House, Walker Street, Wellington, Telford TF1 1HF
Tel: 01952 641651 Fax: 01952 247441

Coroner M T Gwynne

York District
Sentinel House, Peasholme Green, York YO1 7PP
Tel: 01904 716000 Fax: 01904 716000

Coroner W D F Coverdale

Wales

Bridgend and Glamorgan Valleys
3 Victoria Square, Aberdare CF47 7LA
Tel: 01685 881122 Fax: 01685 870322

Coroner P M Walters

Cardiff and Vale of Glamorgan
Coroner's Court, New Police Headquarters, Cathays Park, Cardiff CF1 3NN
Tel: 029 2023 3886 Fax: 029 2202 0638

Coroner L S Addicott

Carmarthenshire District
Solicitors, Corner House, Llandeilo SA19 6BN
Tel: 01558 822215 Fax: 01558 822933

Coroner W J Owen

Central North Wales District
Marble House, Overton Arcade, High Street, Wrexham LL13 8LL
Tel: 01978 357775 Fax: 01978 358000

Coroner J B Hughes

Ceredigion District
The Coroner's Office, 6 Upper Portland Street, Aberystwyth SY23 2DU
Tel: 01970 612567 Fax: 01970 615572

Coroner P L Brunton

Gwent District
Victoria Chambers, 11 Clytha Park Road, Newport NP9 4PB
Tel: 01633 264194 Fax: 01633 841146

Coroner D T Bowen

Neath and Port Talbot District
The Health Centre, Sybil Street, Clydach, Swansea SA6 5EU
Tel: 01792 845058/843821 Fax: 01792 844902

Coroner D J Osborne

North East Wales District
37 Castle Square, Caernarfon LL55 2NN
Tel: 01286 672804 Fax: 01286 675217
Email: coroner@pritchardjones.co.uk

Coroner John B Hughes, Dewi Pritchard Jones

North West Wales District
Evans Lane, Maes glas 37 y Maes, Caernarfon LL55 2NN
Tel: 01286 673387 Fax: 01286 672804

Coroner D Pritchard Jones

Pembrokeshire District
25 Hamilton Terrace, Milford Haven SA73 3JJ
Tel: 01646 698129 Fax: 01646 690607
Website: www.pembrokeshirecoroner.org

Coroner M S Howells

Powys District
4 Lion Street, Brecon LD3 7AU
Tel: 01874 622106 Fax: 01874 623702
Email: hmcpowys@ntlworld.com

Coroner Geraint U Williams

Swansea District
Calvert House, Calvert Terrace, Swansea SA1 6AP
Tel: 01792 655178, 10792 652272 Fax: 01792 467002

Coroner Phillip Rogers

Medical Associations and Societies

ABDO College of Education
The ABDO College, Godmersham Park, Canterbury CT4 7DT
Tel: 01227 738829 Fax: 01227 733900
Email: general@abdo.org.uk
Website: www.abdo.org.uk

Principal Jo Underwood

Action against Medical Accidents (AvMA)
44 High Street, Croydon CR0 1YB
Tel: 020 8688 9555 (Admin), 0845 123 2352 (Customer Helpline)
Fax: 020 8667 9065
Email: admin@avma.org.uk
Website: www.avma.org.uk

Action for Sick Children (National Association for the Welfare of Children in Hospital)
c/o National Children's Bureau, 8 Wakley Street, London EC1V 7QE
Tel: 0800 074 4519 Fax: 01455 845 593
Email: sue.langley@actionforsickchildren.org
Website: www.actionforsickchildren.org

Chairman Pamela Barnes
Senior Manager Sue Langley

Action Medical Research
Vincent House, North Parade, Horsham RH12 2DP
Tel: 01403 210406 Fax: 01403 210541
Email: info@action.org.uk
Website: www.action.org.uk

Chief Executive Simon Moore
Director of Research Tracy Swinfield

Action on Smoking and Health (ASH)
102 Clifton Street, London EC2A 4HW
Tel: 020 7739 5902 Fax: 020 7613 0531
Email: enquiries@ash.org.uk
Website: www.ash.org.uk

Director Deborah Arnott

Age Concern England (The National Council on Ageing)
Astral House, 1268 London Road, London SW16 4ER
Tel: 020 8765 7200 Fax: 020 8679 6069, 020 8765 7211
Email: ace@ace.org.uk, infodep@ageconcern.org.uk
Website: www.ace.org.uk

Director General Gordon Lishman

Agecare (Royal Surgical Aid Society)
47 Great Russell Street, London WC1B 3PB
Tel: 020 7637 4577 Fax: 020 7323 6878
Email: enquiries@agecare.org.uk
Website: www.agecare.org.uk

Chairman Martin Pavey
Chief Executive Ian McLintock

Alcohol Concern
Waterbridge House, 32-36 Loman Street, London SE1 0EE
Tel: 020 7928 7377 Fax: 020 7928 4644
Email: contact@alcoholconcern.org.uk
Website: www.alcoholconcern.org.uk

Director S Sen

Alzheimer's Society
Gordon House, 10 Greencoat Place, London SW1P 1PH
Tel: 020 7306 0606, 0845 300 0336 (Helpline)
Fax: 020 7306 0808
Email: info@alzheimers.org.uk
Website: www.alzheimers.org.uk

Director of Fundraising Stephanie Smith
Director of Research Clive Ballard
Assistant Chief Executive / Company Secretary Lindsay Sartori
Executive Director Neil Hunt
Information and Education Director Clive Evers
Interim Finance Director Joanne Knowles

Ambless - Accident Care and Support
Headquarters, Shalom House, Lower Celtic Park, Enniskillen BT74 6HP
Tel: 028 6632 0320, 028 6632 0321 (Accident Supportline)
Fax: 028 6632 0320

Chief Executive John Wood
Hon. President Rachel Wood

Anaesthetic Research Society
University Department of Anaesthesia and Intensive Care, Queen's Medical Centre, Nottingham NG7 2UH
Tel: 0115 970 9229 Fax: 0115 970 0739
Email: ravi.mahajan@nottingham.ac.uk
Website: www.ars.ac.uk

President C Reilly
Hon. Treasurer P Charters

Anatomical Society of Great Britain and Ireland
Department of Anatomy, University College, Cork
Tel: 00 353 21 490 2115, 00 353 21 490 2246
Fax: 00 353 21 427 3518
Email: j.fraher@ucc.ie
Website: www.anatsoc.org.uk

President B J Moxham
Assistant Secretary P Dockery
Secretary J P Fraher
Treasurer M Benjamin

Arthritis Research Campaign
Copeman House, St Mary's Court, St Mary's Gate, Chesterfield S41 7TD
Tel: 01246 558033 Fax: 01246 558007
Email: info@arc.org.uk
Website: www.arc.org.uk

Chief Executive Fergus Logan
Head of Finance and Administration Dominic Payne
Head of Research and Education Funding Mike Patnick
Marketing Manager Elaine Ingram
Press Officer Jane Tadman

Arts for Health
The Manchester Metropolitan University, All Saints, Oxford Road, Manchester M15 6BY
Tel: 0161 247 1091 Fax: 0161 247 6390
Email: p.senior@mmu.ac.uk
Website: www.mmu.ac.uk/artsforhealth

Director Peter Senior

Association for Cancer Surgery
Room 501 Royal College of Surgeons of England, 35-43 Lincoln's Inn Fields, London WC2A 3PE
Tel: 020 7405 5612 Fax: 020 7404 6574
Email: admin@baso.org.uk
Website: www.baso.org.uk

Hon. Secretary A Baildam

Association for Child and Adolescent Mental Health
St Saviour's House, 39-41 Union Street, London SE1 1SD
Tel: 020 7403 7458 Fax: 020 7403 7081
Website: www.acamh.org.uk

Senior Administrator Ingrid King

Association for Improvements in the Maternity Services (AIMS)
Tel: 0870 765 1433 (Helpline)
Website: www.aims.org.uk

Hon. Secretary Gina Lowdon

Association for Real Change
ARC House, Marsden Street, Chesterfield S40 1JY
Tel: 01246 555043 Fax: 01246 555045
Email: contact.us@arcuk.org.uk
Website: www.arcuk.org.uk

Chief Executive James Churchill

Association for Spina Bifida and Hydrocephalus (ASBAH)
ASBAH House, 42 Park Road, Peterborough PE1 2UQ
Tel: 01733 555988 Fax: 01733 555985
Email: info@asbah.org
Website: www.asbah.org

Executive Director A Russell
Senior Advisor - Health & Policy Issues R Batchelor

Association for the Study of Medical Education (ASME)
ASME Office, 12 Queen Street, Edinburgh EH2 1JE
Tel: 0131 225 9111 Fax: 0131 225 9444
Email: info@asme.org.uk
Website: www.asme.org.uk

President Kenneth Calman
Chairman Graham Buckley
Chief Executive Frank Smith
Journal Editor John Bligh
Treasurer Joe Herzberg

Association of Anaesthetists of Great Britain and Ireland
21 Portland Place, London W1B 1PY
Tel: 020 7631 1650 Fax: 020 7631 4352
Email: info@aagbi.org
Website: www.aagbi.org

President Mike Harmer
Hon. Secretary Alastair Chambers
Hon. Treasurer Richard Birks

Association of British Dispensing Opticians (ABDO)
199 Gloucester Terrace, London W2 6LD
Tel: 020 7298 5100 Fax: 020 7298 5111
Email: general@abdo.org.uk
Website: www.abdo.org.uk

General Secretary Anthony Garrett

Association of British Neurologists
Ormond House, 4th Floor, 27 Boswell Street, London WC1N 3JZ
Tel: 020 7405 4060 Fax: 020 7405 4070
Email: info@theabn.org
Website: www.abn.org.uk

Administrator Susan Tann
Hon. Secretary D E Bateman

Association of British Paediatric Nurses
Greenfield House, 9 Church Lane, South Gosland, Huddersfield HD4 7DB
Website: www.abpn.org.uk

General Secretary Pearl Matthews

Association of Clinical Biochemists
130-132 Tooley Street, London SE1 2TU
Tel: 020 7403 8001 Fax: 020 7403 8006
Email: admin@acb.org.uk
Website: www.acb.org.uk

President C Price
Chair J M Smith
Secretary G McCreanor

Association of Clinical Pathologists
189 Dyke Road, Hove BN3 1TL
Tel: 01273 775700 Fax: 01273 773303
Email: info@pathologists.org.uk
Website: www.pathologists.org.uk

Chairman Russell M Young
Hon. Secretary W A Telfer Brunton

Association of Forensic Physicians
1 Tennant Avenue, College Milton South, East Kilbride, Glasgow G74 5NA
Tel: 01355 244101 Fax: 01355 249959
Email: admin@afpweb.org.uk
Website: www.afpweb.org.uk

Hon. Secretary M Knight

Association of Medical Microbiologists
The Honorary Secretary, Royal London Hospital, Department of Microbiology, 37 Ashfield Street, London E1 1BB
Tel: 020 7377 7242 Fax: 020 7247 6750
Email: honsec@amm.co.uk
Website: www.amm.co.uk

President Tony Howard
Hon. Secretary A J Mifsud
Hon. Treasurer S T Chapman

Association of Medical Research Charities
61 Grays Inn Road, London WC1X 8TL
Tel: 020 7269 8820 Fax: 020 7269 8821
Email: info@amrc.org.uk

Chairman Bridget Ogilvie
Chief Executive Diana Garnham

Association of Operating Department Practitioners (AODP)
PO Box 1304, Wilmslow SK9 5WW
Tel: 0870 746 0984 Fax: 0870 746 0985
Email: info@aodp.org
Website: www.aodp.org

Chairman Martin Smith

Association of Optometrists
61 Southwark Street, London SE1 0HL
Tel: 020 7261 9661 Fax: 020 7261 0228
Email: postbox@aop.org.uk
Website: www.aop.ors.uk

Chief Executive Bob Hughes
Head of Communications David Craig

Association of Surgeons of Great Britain and Ireland

The Royal College of Surgeons, 35-43 Lincoln's Inn Fields, London WC2A 3PE
Tel: 020 7973 0300 Fax: 020 7430 9235
Email: admin@asgbi.org.uk
Website: www.asgbi.org.uk

Chief Executive N P Gair
Deputy Chief Executive Nechama Lewis
Hon. Secretary G T Layer

Assurance Medical Society, Lettsom House

11 Chandos Street, London W1G 9EB
Tel: 020 7636 6308 Fax: 020 7580 5793

Executive Secretary B A Smallwood
Hon. Secretary Ian Cox

Ataxia-UK

Winchester House, Kennington Park, Cranmer Road, London SW9 6EJ
Tel: 020 7582 1444, 0845 644 0606 (Helpline)
Fax: 020 7582 9444
Email: enquiries@ataxia.org.uk
Website: www.ataxia.org.uk

Director Alastair MacDougall

Backcare

16 Elmtree Road, Teddington TW11 8ST
Tel: 020 8977 5474, 08709 500275 (Helpline) Fax: 020 8943 5318
Email: info@backcare.org.uk
Website: www.backcare.org.uk

Chairman Frank Davies
Chief Executive Nia Taylor
Company Secretary Alistair Mackechnie

Bardhan Research and Education Trust of Rotherham Ltd

Modern House, Summer Lane, Barnsley S70 2NP
Tel: 01226 771226 Fax: 01226 771226

Barnardo's

Tanners Lane, Barkingside, Ilford IG6 1QG
Tel: 020 8550 8822 Fax: 020 8551 6870
Email: information@barnardos.org.uk
Website: www.barnardos.org.uk

Chief Executive Roger Singleton

Beit Memorial Fellowships for Medical Research

c/o Institute of Molecular Medicine, John Radcliffe Hospital, Headington, Oxford OX3 9DU
Tel: 01865 222679 Fax: 01865 222600
Email: beit.fellowships@hammer.immox.ac.uk

Administration Secretary M Goble

Biochemical Society

59 Portland Place, London W1B 1QW
Tel: 020 7580 5530 Fax: 020 7637 3626
Email: genadmin@biochemsoc.org
Website: www.biochemistry.org

Chairman Chris Leaver

Brain Research Trust

15 Southampton Place, London WC1A 2AJ
Tel: 020 7404 9982 Fax: 020 7404 9983
Email: thebrt@aol.com
Website: www.brt.org.uk

Administrator / Secretary Suzanne Gibbons

Breakthrough Breast Cancer

3rd Floor, Weston House, 246 High Holborn, London WC1V 7EX
Tel: 020 7025 2400 Fax: 020 7025 2401
Email: info@breakthrough.org.uk
Website: www.breakthrough.org.uk

Chief Executive Jeremy Hughes

British Academy of Forensic Sciences

Anaesthetic Department, The Royal London Hospital, Whitechapel, London E1 1BB
Tel: 020 7377 9201
Email: patricia.flynn@bartsandthelondon.nhs.uk, patricia.flynn@btconnect.com
Website: www.bafs.org.uk

British Association for Emergency Medicine

Royal College of Surgeons of England, 35-43 Lincoln's Inn Fields, London WC2A 3PE
Tel: 020 7832 9405 Fax: 020 7405 0318
Email: baem@emergencymedicine.uk.net
Website: www.baem.org.uk

President-Elect D W M Mackechnie
President M J Shalley
Administrator J Bloomfield
Deputy Administrator E Robinson
Hon. Secretary A P J Gammon
Hon. Treasurer A Sen

British Association for Paediatric Nephrology

Royal Hospital for Sick Children, York Hill NHS Trust, Dalnair Street, Glasgow G3 8SJ
Tel: 0141 201 0122
Website: www.bapa.uwcm.ac.uk

Hon. Secretary Heather Maxwell

British Association for Parenteral and Enteral Nutrition

BAPEN Office, Secure Hold Business Centre, Studley Road, Redditch B98 7LG
Tel: 01527 457850 Fax: 01527 458718
Email: bapen@sovereignconference.co.uk
Website: www.bapen.org.uk

Editor of 'In Touch' Vera Todorovic
Hon. Chairman Alastair Forbes
Hon. Secretary Penny Neild
Hon. Treasurer Niall Bowen
Press Officer Rhonda Smith

British Association for Psychopharmacology

BAP Office, 36 Cambridge Place, Hills Road, Cambridge CB2 1NS
Tel: 01223 358395 Fax: 01223 321268
Email: susan@bap.org.uk
Website: www.bap.org.uk

Executive Officer Susan Chandler
General Secretary Anne Lingford-Hughes

British Association for Service to the Elderly (BASE)

The Guildford Institute, Ward Street, Guildford GU1 4LH

Tel: 01483 451036 Fax: 01483 451034
Email: enquiries@base.org.uk
Website: www.base.org.uk

Chief Executive James Lewis

British Association for Sexual Health and HIV

Academic Department, c/o 1 Wimpole Street, London W1G 0AE
Tel: 020 7290 2968 Fax: 020 7290 2989
Email: bashh@rsm.ac.uk
Website: www.bashh.org

President A J Robinson
Vice-President S E Barton
BASHH Secretariat (Royal Society of Medicine) Muna Yahaya
Conference and Communication Secretary J Wilson
General Secretary K W Radcliffe
Secretariat / BASHH Secretariat Royal Society of Medicine Simon Croker
Treasurer J Clarke

British Association for Tissue Banking

20-22 Queensbury Place, London SW7 2DZ
Tel: 01707 338376
Email: stanjojo@aol.com
Website: www.batb.org.uk

President D G Galea
Secretariat Jo Staniforth
Vice President D C Womack

British Association of Day Surgery

35-43 Lincoln's Inn Fields, London WC2A 3PE
Tel: 020 7973 0308 Fax: 020 7973 0314
Email: bads@bads.co.uk
Website: www.bads.co.uk

President Jill Solly
President Elect Ian Jackson
Administration Manager Veronica Hall
Hon. Secretary Joe Cahill
Hon. Treasurer A Hart

British Association of Dermatologists

4 Fitzroy Square, London W1T 5HQ
Tel: 020 7383 0266 Fax: 020 7388 5263
Email: admin@bad.org.uk
Website: www.bad.org.uk

President Chris Griffiths
Chief Executive Marilyn Benham
Hon. Secretary Jane Sterling

British Association of Health Services in Higher Education (BAHSHE)

Cripps Health Centre, University Park, University of Nottingham, Nottingham NG7 2QW
Tel: 0115 925 8034 Fax: 0115 925 9943
Email: bahshe@nottingham.ac.uk
Website: www.bahshe.demon.co.uk

Hon. Secretary Angela White

British Association of Occupational Therapists and College of Occupational Therapists

The College of Occupational Therapists, 106-114 Borough High Street, London SE1 1LB
Tel: 020 7357 6480 Fax: 020 7450 2299
Email: cot@cot.co.uk
Website: www.cot.org.uk, www.baot.org.uk

Chairman Jenny Butler
Chief Executive Sheelagh Richards

British Association of Oral and Maxillofacial Surgeons

Royal College of Surgeons of England, 35-43 Lincolns Inn Fields, London WC2A 3PN
Tel: 020 7405 8074 Fax: 020 7430 9997
Email: office@baoms.org.uk
Website: www.baoms.org.uk

President B S Avery
President Elect P Wardbooth
Hon. Secretary S F Worrall
Hon. Treasurer M E Morton

British Association of Otorhinolaryngologists-Head and Neck Surgeons

The Royal College of Surgeons, 35-43 Lincoln's Inn Fields, London WC2A 3PE
Tel: 020 7404 8373 Fax: 020 7404 4200
Email: admin@entuk.org
Website: www.entuk.org

President David W Proops
Hon. Secretary Christopher A Milford

British Association of Paediatric Surgeons

Royal College of Surgeons of England, 35-43 Lincoln's Inn Fields, London WC2A 3PN
Tel: 020 7869 6915 Fax: 020 7869 6919
Email: president@baps.org.uk
Website: www.baps.org.uk

President Vic Boston

British Association of Perinatal Medicine

50 Hallam Street, London W1W 6DE
Tel: 020 7307 5627 Fax: 020 7307 5601
Email: bapm@rcpch.ac.uk
Website: www.bapm.org

President Malcolm Chiswick
Hon. Secretary Andrew Lyon
Hon. Treasurer Jagjit Ahluwalia

British Association of Plastic Surgeons

The Royal College of Surgeons, 35-43 Lincoln's Inn Fields, London WC2A 3PE
Tel: 020 7831 5161 Fax: 020 7831 4041
Email: secretariat@baps.co.uk
Website: www.baps.co.uk

Hon. Secretary J H E Laing
Senior Administrator H C Roberts

British Association of Psychotherapists

37 Mapesbury Road, London NW2 4HJ
Tel: 020 8452 9823 Fax: 020 8452 0310
Email: mail@bap-psychotherapy.org
Website: www.bap-psychotherapy.org

Chairman Helen Morgan
Chief Executive Elise Ormerod

British Association of Urological Surgeons

35-43 Lincoln's Inn Fields, London WC2A 3PE
Tel: 020 7869 6950 Fax: 020 7404 5048
Email: admin@baus.org.uk
Website: www.baus.org.uk

Chief Executive P M Neville

British Cardiac Society

9 Fitzroy Square, London W1T 5HW
Tel: 020 7383 3887 Fax: 020 7388 0903
Email: enquiries@bcs.com
Website: www.bcs.com

President H H Gray

Hon. Secretary M de Belder
Hon. Treasurer D W Davies

British Colostomy Association
15 Station Road, Reading RG1 1LG
Tel: 0118 939 1537 Fax: 0118 956 9095
Email: sue@bcass.org.uk
Website: www.bcass.org.uk

British Council for the Prevention of Blindness
29B Montague Street, London WC1 5BW
Tel: 020 7631 5100
Email: bcpb@btconnect.com

British Dental Association
64 Wimpole Street, London W1G 8YS
Tel: 020 7935 0875 Fax: 020 7487 5232
Email: enquiries@bda.org
Website: www.bda.org

Chief Executive Ian Wylie

British Dietetic Association
5th Floor, Charles House, 148-149 Great Charles Street, Queensway, Birmingham B3 3HT
Tel: 0121 200 8080 Fax: 0121 200 8081
Email: info@bda.uk.com
Website: www.bda.uk.com

Chief Executive Andy Burman
Hon. Chairman Susan Jones

British Eye Research Foundation
Ground Floor, 75 Westminster Bridge Road, London SE1 7HS
Tel: 020 7928 7743 Fax: 020 7928 7919
Email: info@berf.org.uk
Website: www.berf.org.uk

Chairman Faanya Rose
Executive Director Michael Roberts
Treasurer G M Powell

British Geriatrics Society
Marjory Warren House, 31 St John's Square, London EC1M 4DN
Tel: 020 7608 1369 Fax: 020 7608 1041
Email: info@bgs.org.uk
Website: www.bgs.org.uk

Chief Executive Alex Mair
Hon. Secretary K Kelleher

British Heart Foundation
14 Fitzhardinge Street, London W1H 6DH
Tel: 020 7935 0185 Fax: 020 7486 5820
Website: www.bhf.org.uk

Chairman of the Council Peter Morris
Director General Peter Hollis
Medical Director Peter Weissberg

British Homoeopathic Association
Hahnemann House, 29 Park Street West, Luton LU1 3BE
Tel: 0870 444 3950 Fax: 0870 444 3960
Email: info@trusthomeopathy.org
Website: www.trusthomeopathy.org

Chief Executive Sally Penrose

British Hypertension Society
Information Service, The Blood Pressure Unit, St George's Hospital Medical School, Cranmer Terrace, London SW17 0RE
Tel: 020 8725 3412 Fax: 020 8725 2959
Email: bhsis@sghms.ac.uk
Website: www.bhsoc.org

President N Poulter

Secretary F Potter
Treasurer M Caulfield

British Infection Society
Department of Infection and Tropical Medicine, Leicester Royal Infirmary, Leicester LE1 5WW
Tel: 0116 258 6952 Fax: 0116 258 5067
Email: martin.wiselka@uhl-tr.nhs.uk
Website: www.britishinfectionsociety.org

Hon. President N Beeching
Hon. Treasurer I M Gould
Membership Secretary Martin Wiselka

British Institute of Dental and Surgical Technologists
4 Thompson Green, Shipley BD17 7PR
Tel: 0845 644 3726
Website: www.bidst.org

Chair Mark Gilbert
Secretary Beryl Dawe
Treasurer Colin Dean

British Institute of Learning Disabilities (BILD)
Campion House, Green Street, Kidderminster DY10 1JL
Tel: 01562 723010 Fax: 01562 723029
Email: enquiries@bild.org.uk
Website: www.bild.org.uk

Chief Executive Keith Smith

British Institute of Musculoskeletal Medicine
34 The Avenue, Watford WD17 4AH
Tel: 01923 220999 Fax: 01923 249037
Email: info@bimm.org.uk
Website: www.bimm.org.uk

General Manager Deena Harris

British Institute of Radiology
36 Portland Place, London W1B 1AT
Tel: 020 7307 1400 Fax: 020 7307 1414
Email: admin@bir.org.uk
Website: www.bir.org.uk

Conference Manager Sarah McLellan
Facilities Manager Peter Coverdale
Finance Manager Ashok Dattani
General Secretary Tim Hogan
Hon. Secretary S Marchant
Hon. Treasurer A Budge
Publications Manager Louise Chantler

British Leprosy Relief Association (LEPRA)
Fairfax House, Causton Road, Colchester CO1 1PU
Tel: 01206 562286 Fax: 01206 762151
Email: lepra@lepra.org.uk
Website: www.lepra.org.uk

Chief Executive Terry Vasey
Director of Development Bernard Farmer

British Lung Foundation
73-75 Goswell Road, London EC1V 7ER
Tel: 020 7688 5555 Fax: 020 7688 5556
Email: enquiries@blf-uk.org
Website: www.lunguk.org

Chief Executive Helena Shovelton
Head of Finance Debbie Whatt
Head of Fundraising Catherine Lightfoot
Head of Public Affairs Sue Knight

British Medical Acupuncture Society
BMAS House, 3 Winnington Court, Northwich CW8 1AQ
Tel: 01606 786782 Fax: 01606 786783
Email: admin@medical-acupuncture.org.uk
Website: www.medical-acupuncture.co.uk

Chief Executive Julian Price

British Medical Association (BMA)
BMA House, Tavistock Square, London WC1H 9JP
Tel: 020 7387 4499 Fax: 020 7383 6400
Email: info.web@bma.org.uk
Website: www.bma.org.uk

President Charles George
Chair James Johnson
Secretary Tony Bourne

British Medical Ultrasound Society
36 Portland Place, London W1B 1LS
Tel: 020 7636 3714 Fax: 020 7323 2175
Email: secretariat@bmus.org
Website: www.bmus.org

President G M Baxter
President Elect K Martin
General Secretary E Brown
Hon. Secretary C Deane
Hon. Treasurer J M Walton

British Menopause Society
4-6 Eton Place, Marlow SL7 2QA
Tel: 01628 890199 Fax: 01628 474042
Email: director.bms@btconnect.com
Website: www.the-bms.org

Chairman J Pitkin
Deputy Director M A Upsdell
Executive Director F A Patterson
Hon. Treasurer A Mander

British Nuclear Medicine Society
Regent House, 291 Kirkdale, London SE26 4QD
Tel: 020 8676 7864 Fax: 020 8676 8417
Email: suehatchard@bnms.org.uk
Website: www.bnms.org.uk

Secretary Susan Hatchard

British Nutrition Foundation
High Holborn House, 52-54 High Holborn, London WC1V 6RQ
Tel: 020 7404 6504 Fax: 020 7404 6747
Email: postbox@nutrition.org.uk
Website: www.nutrition.org.uk

Director General Robert Pickard
Education Director Stephanie Valentine
Science Director Judith Buttriss

British Occupational Hygiene Society
Suite 2, Georgian House, Great Northern Road, Derby DE1 1LT
Tel: 01332 298101 Fax: 01332 298099
Email: admin@bohs.org
Website: www.bohs.org

Hon. Secretary H Jackson

British Orthodontic Society
291 Gray's Inn Road, London WC1X 8QJ
Tel: 020 7837 2193
Email: ann.wright@bos.org.uk
Website: www.bos.org.uk

Hon. Secretary David Tidy
Society Administrator Ann Wright

British Orthopaedic Association
35-43 Lincoln's Inn Fields, London WC2A 3PN
Tel: 020 7405 6507 Fax: 020 7831 2676
Email: ceo@boa.ac.uk
Website: www.boa.ac.uk

Hon. Secretary M J Bell

The British Pain Society
21 Portland Place, London W1B 1PY
Tel: 020 7631 8870 Fax: 020 7323 2015
Email: info@britishpainsociety.org
Website: www.britishpainsociety.org

President Beverly Collet
Hon. Secretary Cathy Stannard
Hon. Treasurer George Harrison

British Performing Arts Medicine Trust
196 Shaftesbury Avenue, London WC2H 8JL
Tel: 020 7240 4500, 0845 602 0235 Fax: 020 7240 3335
Email: bpamt@dial.pipex.com
Website: www.bpamt.co.uk

British Pharmacological Society
16 Angel Gate, City Road, London EC1V 2SG
Tel: 020 7417 0113 Fax: 020 7417 0114
Email: yn@bps.ac.uk
Website: www.bps.ac.uk

British Pharmacopoeia Commission
Market Towers, 1 Nine Elms Lane, London SW8 5NQ
Tel: 020 7084 2561 Fax: 020 7084 2566
Email: bpcom@mhra.gsi.gov.uk
Website: www.pharmacopoeia.org.uk

Secretary and Scientific Director Ged Lee

British Polio Fellowship
Ground Floor, Unit A, Eagle Office Centre, The Runway, Ruislip HA4 6SE
Tel: 0800 018 0586 Fax: 020 8842 0555
Email: info@britishpolio.org.uk
Website: www.britishpolio.org.uk

Chair Bryan Askew
Chief Executive Graham Ball
National Welfare Officer Dorothy Nattrass

British Pregnancy Advisory Service (BPAS)
Austy Manor, Stratford Road, Wootton Wawen, Henley in Arden B95 6BX
Tel: 01564 793225, 08457 304030 (Appts) Fax: 01564 794935
Email: info@bpas.org
Website: www.bpas.org

Chief Executive Ann Furodi

British Psychoanalytical Society
112A Shirland Road, London W9 2EQ
Tel: 020 7563 5000 Fax: 020 7563 5001
Website: www.psychoanalysis.org.uk

President Julia Fabricius
Institute Manager Nick Hall

British Psychological Society
St Andrews House, 48 Princess Road East, Leicester LE1 7DR
Tel: 0116 254 9568 Fax: 0116 247 0787
Email: mail@bps.org.uk, stewhi@bps.org.uk
Website: www.bps.org.uk

Directorate Manager Stephen White
Hon. General Secretary Ann Colley

British Red Cross Society
44 Moorfields, London EC2Y 9AL
Tel: 0870 170 7000 Fax: 020 7562 2000
Email: information@redcross.org.uk
Website: www.redcross.org.uk

Chief Executive Nicholas Young

British Retinitis Pigmentosa Society
PO Box 350, Buckingham MK18 1GZ
Tel: 01280 821334 (Office), 0845 123 2354 (Helpline)
Fax: 01280 815900
Email: info@brps.org.uk
Website: www.brps.org.uk

Secretary L Cantor

British Society for Haematology
100 White Lion Street, London N1 9PF
Tel: 020 8643 7305 Fax: 020 8770 0933
Email: jules.sleater@b-s-h.org.uk
Website: www.b-s-h.org.uk

President A G Prentice
Secretary Jennifer Duguid
Vice President S J Machin

British Society for Human Genetics
Clinical Genetics Unit Admin. Office, Birmingham Women's Hospital, Edgbaston, Birmingham B15 2TG
Tel: 0121 627 2634 Fax: 0121 623 6971
Email: bshg@bshg.org.uk
Website: www.bshg.org.uk

Executive Officer Ruth Cole
General Secretary Graham Taylor

British Society for Immunology
Triangle House, Broomhill Road, London SW18 4HX
Tel: 0870 833 2400
Email: bsi@immunology.org
Website: www.immunology.org

General Secretary Adrian Hayday

British Society for Music Therapy
61 Church Hill Road, East Barnet, Barnet EN4 8SY
Tel: 020 8441 6226 Fax: 020 8441 4118
Email: info@bsmt.org
Website: www.bsmt.org

Chair Claire Flower
Administrator Denize Christophers

British Society for Oral Medicine
Glasgow Dental Hospital and School, 378 Sauchiehall Street, Glasgow G2 3JZ
Tel: 0141 211 9600 Fax: 0141 353 2899
Email: enquiries@bsom.org.uk
Website: www.bsom.org.uk

Hon. General Secretary M A Lewis

British Society for Parasitology
BSP Secretariat, Logandale Financial Services, Covington Mains Farm, Covington, Biggar ML12 6NE
Tel: 01899 308886
Email: bsp@parasitology.org.uk
Website: www.mri.sari.ac.uk/bsp

Hon. General Secretary Fiona Tomley

British Society for Rheumatology
41 Eagle Street, London WC1R 4TL
Tel: 020 7242 3313 Fax: 020 7242 3277
Email: bsr@rheumatology.org.uk
Website: www.rheumatology.org.uk

President D Isenberg
Chief Executive Samantha Peters
Deputy Chief Executive Susan Murray Johnson
External Relations Manager Caroline Rattray
Hon. Secretary P Dawes
Hon. Treasurer T Price

British Society for Surgery of the Hand
The Royal College of Surgeons, 37-42 Lincoln's Inn Fields, London WC2A 3PE
Tel: 020 7831 5162 Fax: 020 7831 4041
Email: secretariat@bssh.ac.uk
Website: www.bssh.ac.uk

Hon. Secretary R Savage

British Society of Gastroenterology
3 St Andrews Place, Regent's Park, London NW1 4LB
Tel: 020 7387 3534 Fax: 020 7487 3734
Email: bsg@mailbox.ulcc.ac.uk
Website: www.bsg.org.uk

President E Elias
Hon. Secretary J de Caesteeker, A Harris

British Society of Gerontology
Department of Applied Social Science, Stirling FK9 4LA
Tel: 01786 467701 Fax: 01786 467689
Email: susan.tester@stir.ac.uk
Website: www.britishgerontology.org

Secretary Susan Tester

British Society of Medical and Dental Hypnosis
28 Dale Park Gardens, Cookridge, Leeds LS16 7PT
Tel: 07000 560309 Fax: 07000 560309
Email: natoffice@bsmdh.com
Website: www.bsmdh.com

National Office Secretary Angela Morris

British Society of Rehabilitation Medicine
c/o Royal College of Physicians, 11 St Andrews Place, London NW1 4LE
Tel: 01992 638865 Fax: 01992 638905
Email: admin@bsrm.co.uk
Website: www.bsrm.co.uk

Executive Secretary Sandy Weatherhead

British Thoracic Society
17 Doughty Street, London WC1N 2PL
Tel: 020 7831 8778 Fax: 020 7831 8766
Email: bts@brit-thoracic.org.uk
Website: www.brit-thoracic.org.uk

Chief Executive S Edwards

Cancer and Leukaemia in Childhood (CLIC)
Abbey Wood Business Park, Filton, Bristol BS34 7JU
Tel: 0845 301 0031 Fax: 0117 311 2649
Email: info@clic.org.uk
Website: www.clic.org.uk

Chief Executive David Ellis

CancerBacup
3 Bath Place, Rivington Street, London EC2A 3JR
Tel: 020 7696 9003, 0808 800 1234 (Freephone)
Fax: 020 7696 9002
Email: info@cancerbacup.org
Website: www.cancerbacup.org.uk

Chief Executive Joanne Rule

Central Council of Physical Recreation
Francis House, Francis Street, London SW1P 1DE
Tel: 020 7854 8500 Fax: 020 7854 8501
Email: admin@ccpr.org.uk
Website: www.ccpr.org.uk

Chief Executive Margaret Talbot
Head of Services Sallie Barker
Finance Director Jane Ollard

Centre for Policy on Ageing
25-31 Ironmonger Row, London EC1V 3QP
Tel: 020 7553 6500 Fax: 020 7553 6501
Email: cpa@cpa.org.uk
Website: www.cpa.org.uk

Deputy Director Gillian Crosby

Chartered Society of Physiotherapy
14 Bedford Row, London WC1R 4ED
Tel: 020 7306 6666 Fax: 020 7306 6611
Email: csp@csphysio.org.uk
Website: www.csp.org.uk

Chief Executive Phil Gray

Chest Heart and Stroke Scotland
65 North Castle Street, Edinburgh EH2 3LT
Tel: 0131 225 6963 Fax: 0131 220 6313
Email: admin@chss.org.uk
Website: www.chss.org.uk

Chief Executive D H Clark
Director of Public Relations Janet Buncle

Child Accident Prevention Trust
4th Floor, Clerks Court, 22-26 Farringdon Lane, London EC1R 3AJ
Tel: 020 7608 3828 Fax: 020 7608 3674
Email: safe@capt.org.uk
Website: www.capt.org.uk

Director Katrina Phillips
Projects Director M Hayes
Publicity Manager Amanda Pritchett

Child Growth Foundation (CGF)
2 Mayfield Avenue, Chiswick, London W4 1PW
Tel: 020 8995 0257 Fax: 020 8995 9075
Email: cgflondon@aol.com
Website: www.childgrowthfoundation.org

Hon. Chairman Tam Fry

Children's Liver Disease Foundation
36 Great Charles Street, Queensway, Birmingham B3 3JY
Tel: 0121 212 3839 Fax: 0121 212 4300
Email: info@childliverdisease.org
Website: www.childliverdisease.org

Chief Executive Catherine Arkley
Finance Manager Gill Bayliss
Office Manager Carol Fleet
Senior Family Support Officer Susan Davis

The Children's Trust
Tadworth Court, Tadworth KT20 5RU
Tel: 01737 365000 Fax: 01737 365084
Email: enquiries@thechildrenstrust.org.uk
Website: www.thechildrenstrust.org.uk

Chief Executive Andrew Ross
Director of Children's Services Sally Jenkinson
Financial Director John Grint
Service Development Manager Bob Butler

The College of Optometrists
42 Craven Street, London WC2N 5NG
Tel: 020 7839 6000 Fax: 020 7839 6800
Email: optometry@college-optometrists.org
Website: www.college-optometrists.org

Chief Executive B Pawinska

College of Pharmacy Practice
28 Warwick Row, Coventry CV1 1EY
Tel: 024 7622 1359 Fax: 024 7652 1110
Email: cpp@collpharm.org.uk
Website: www.collpharm.org.uk

Chief Executive Ian Simpson

The Commonwealth Nurses Federation
c/o Royal College of Nursing, 20 Cavendish Square, London W1G 0RN
Tel: 020 7647 3593 Fax: 020 7647 3413
Email: cnf@rcn.org.uk
Website: www.commonwealthnurses.org

Executive Secretary Michael Stubbings

Community and District Nursing Association
Walpole House, 18-22 Bond Street, Ealing, London W5 5AA
Tel: 020 8231 0180 Fax: 020 8231 0187
Email: cdna@tvu.ac.uk
Website: www.cdna.tvu.ac.uk

Director Anne Duffy

The Company Chemists' Association Ltd
Regus House, Fairbourne Drive, Atterbury, Milton Keynes MK10 9RG
Tel: 01908 487532 Fax: 01908 487501
Email: colin.baldwin@thecca.org.uk
Website: www.thecca.org.uk

Chairman A Digby Emson
Chief Executive Colin Baldwin

Conservative Medical Society
25 Victoria Street, London SW1H 0DL
Tel: 0870 749 0308

Chairman Anthony Clarke
Hon. Secretary William Cantello

Continuing Care at Home Association (CONCAH)
54 Glasshouse Street, Countess Wear, Exeter EX2 7BU

Coram Family
49 Mecklenburg Square, London WC1N 2QA
Tel: 020 7520 0300 Fax: 020 7520 0301
Website: www.coram.org.uk

Chairman David Goldstone
Chief Executive Gillian Pugh

CORE (Digestive Disorders Foundation)
3 St Andrews Place, London NW1 4LB
Tel: 020 7486 0341 Fax: 020 7224 2012
Email: info@corcharity.org.uk
Website: www.corecharity.org.uk

President John Bennet
Hon. Treasurer Clive Littler
Medical Director Alistair Forbes

Coronary Prevention Group
2 Taviton Street, London WC1H 0BT
Tel: 020 7927 2125 Fax: 020 7927 2127
Email: cpg@ishtm.ac.uk

President P James

Secretary A Dave
Treasurer T Mukherjee

Council for Awards in Children's Care and Education (CACHE)
8 Chequer Street, St Albans AL1 3XZ
Tel: 01727 847636 Fax: 01727 867609
Email: info@cache.org.uk
Website: www.cache.org.uk

Chief Executive Richard Dorrance
Marketing Manager Beth Peaker

Council for Music in Hospitals
74 Queens Road, Hersham, Walton-on-Thames KT12 5LW
Tel: 01932 252809, 01932 252811 Fax: 01932 252966
Email: info@music-in-hospitals.org.uk
Website: www.music-in-hospitals.org.uk

Chief Executive (England, Wales and Northern Ireland) Diana Greenman
Chief Executive (Scotland) Alison Frazer

Counsel and Care - Advice and help for older people
Twyman House, 16 Bonny Street, London NW1 9PG
Tel: 0845 300 7585 Fax: 020 7267 6877
Email: advice@counselandcare.org.uk
Website: www.counselandcare.org.uk

Chief Executive Stephen Burke

Cystic Fibrosis Trust
11 London Road, Bromley BR1 1BY
Tel: 020 8464 7211 Fax: 020 8313 0472
Email: enquiries@cftrust.org.uk
Website: www.cftrust.org.uk

Chairman J Littlewood
Chief Executive R Barnes
Communications Assistant M Heather
Life President R Luff

DEBRA
DEBRA House, 13 Wellington Business Park, Dukes Ride, Crowthorne RG45 6LS
Tel: 01344 771961 Fax: 01344 762661
Email: debra@debra.org.uk, john@debra.org.uk
Website: www.debra.org.uk

Director John Dart
Adult Nurse Specialist (North) Jacqueline Hitchin
Adult Nurse Specialist (South) Liz Pillay
Clinical Nurse Specialist (Paediatrics) Jacqueline Denyer
Social Work Manager Robert Snookes

Defeating Deafness (The Hearing Research Trust)
330-332 Gray's Inn Road, London WC1X 8EE
Tel: 020 7833 1733, 0808 808 2222 (Information Line)
Fax: 020 7278 0404
Email: info@defeatingdeafness.org
Website: www.defeatingdeafness.org

Chief Executive Vivienne Michael
Head of Information Geraldine Oliver
Fundraising Manager Anna Thompson

Diabetes UK
10 Parkway, London NW1 7AA
Tel: 020 7424 1000 Fax: 020 7424 1001
Email: info@diabetes.org.uk
Website: www.diabetes.org.uk

Chairman Board of Trustees Michael Hirst
Chief Executive Douglas Smallwood
Director of Research and Care Simon O'Neil

Disabled Drivers Association
National Headquarters, Ashwellthorpe, Norwich NR16 1EX
Tel: 0870 770 3333 Fax: 01508 488173
Email: hq@dda.org.uk
Website: www.dda.org.uk

Executive Director Douglas Campbell
Information Officer Theresa Border, Jim Rawlings

Disabled Living Foundation
380-384 Harrow Road, London W9 2HU
Tel: 020 7289 6111, 020 7432 8009 (Textphone), 0845 130 9177 (Helpline) Fax: 020 7266 2922
Email: info@dlf.org.uk
Website: www.dlf.org.uk

DrugScope
32-36 Loman Street, London SE1 0EE
Tel: 020 7928 1211 Fax: 020 7928 1771
Email: info@drugscope.org.uk
Website: www.drugscope.org.uk

Chief Executive Martin Barnes
Communications Officer Cara Macdowall

Emergency Bed Service
Fielden House, 28 London Bridge Street, London SE1 9SG
Tel: 020 7407 7181 Fax: 020 7357 6705

Manager Graham Hayter
Office Manager Leyla Strutt
Operations Manager Barry Khodabukus, Alison Oakes

Encephalitis Society
The Encephalitis Resource Centre, 7B Saville Street, Malton YO17 7LL
Tel: 01653 692583 (Admin line), 01653 699599 (Information line)
Fax: 01653 604369
Email: mail@encephalitis.info
Website: www.encephalitis.info

Children and Families Support Jon Ainley
Information Coordinator Elaine Dowell
Support Services Coordinator Ava Easton

Epilepsy Action
New Anstey House, Gate Way Drive, Yeadon, Leeds LS19 7XY
Tel: 0113 210 8800, 0808 800 5050 (Helpline)
Fax: 0113 391 0300, 0808 800 5555 (Fax Helpline)
Email: epilepsy@epilepsy.org.uk
Website: www.epilepsy.org.uk

Chief Executive Philip Lee
Press Officer Lucy Rollinson

Epilepsy Scotland
48 Govan Road, Glasgow G51 1JL
Tel: 0141 427 4911, 0808 800 2200 (Helpline)
Fax: 0141 419 1709
Email: enquiries@epilepsyscotland.org
Website: www.epilepsyscotland.org.uk

Chief Executive Hilary Mounfield
Policy and Development Manager Olivia Marks-Woldman

Family Welfare Association
501-505 Kingsland Road, Dalston, London E8 4AU
Tel: 020 7254 6251 Fax: 020 7249 5443
Email: fwaheadoffice@fwa.org.uk
Website: www.fwa.org.uk

Chief Executive Helen Dent
Secretary Damien Fallon

Federation of Independent Practitioner Organisations (FIPO)
14 Queen Anne's Gate, London SW1H 9AA
Tel: 020 7222 0975 Fax: 020 7222 4424
Email: info@fipo.org
Website: www.fipo.org

Chairman Geoffrey Glazer

Federation of Ophthalmic and Dispensing Opticians
199 Gloucester Terrace, London W2 6LD
Tel: 020 7298 5151 Fax: 020 7298 5111
Email: optics@fodo.com
Website: www.fodo.com

Chair Brian Collison

Fellowship of Postgraduate Medicine
12 Chandos Street, London W1G 9DR
Tel: 020 7636 6334 Fax: 020 7436 2535
Email: admin@fpm-uk.org

President Gordon C Cook
Hon. Secretary Alimuddin Zumla
Treasurer Michael W N Nicholls

Forensic Science Society
Clarke House, 18A Mount Parade, Harrogate HG1 1BX
Tel: 01423 506068 Fax: 01423 566391
Email: president@forensic-science-society.org.uk
Website: www.forensic-science-society.org.uk

Office Manager Tracey D'Alessandro-Rixon

Foundation for Liver Research (formerly Liver Research Trust)
Institute of Heptology, 69-75 Chenies Mews, London WC1E 6HX
Tel: 020 7679 6510, 020 7679 6511 Fax: 020 7380 0405
Email: roger.williams@ucl.ac.uk
Website: www.ac.uk/liver-research

Director R Williams
Assistant Director Nikolai V Naoumov

Foundation for the Study of Infant Deaths
Artillery House, 11-19 Artillery Row, London SW1P 1RT
Tel: 0870 787 0554 (Helpline 9am-11pm Mon-Fri, 6pm -11pm Sat-Sun), 0870 787 0885 Fax: 0870 787 0725
Email: fsid@sids.org.uk
Website: www.sids.org.uk/fsid

Chairman Colin Baker
Director Joyce Epstein
Editorial Enquiries Sarah Kenyon
Fundraising Manager Joanna Christophi
Information and Media Manager Sarah Kenyon
National Co-ordinator Ann Deri-Brown

FPA
2-12 Pentonville Road, London N1 9FP
Tel: 020 7837 5432, 0845 310 1334 (Helpline)
Fax: 020 7837 3042
Email: library&information@fpa.org.uk
Website: www.fpa.org.uk

Chief Executive Anne Weyman

Gay and Lesbian Association of Doctors and Dentists (GLADD)
PO Box 5606, London WC1N 3XX
Tel: 0870 765 5606
Email: secretary@gladd.org.uk
Website: www.gladd.org.uk

The Guide Dogs for the Blind Association
Hillfields, Burghfield Common, Reading RG7 3YG
Tel: 0118 983 5555 Fax: 0118 983 5433, 0118 983 5477
Email: guidedogs@guidedogs.org.uk
Website: www.guidedogs.org.uk

Chief Executive Bridget Warr

Guild of Catholic Doctors
Brampton House, Hospital of St John and St Elizabeth, 60 Grove End Road, London NW8 9NH
Tel: 020 7266 4246 Fax: 020 7266 4813
Email: enquiries@catholicdoctors.org.uk
Website: www.catholicdoctors.org.uk

Chaplain H MacKenzie
Hon. Registrar P Henshall
Hon. Secretary J Morewood
Master C Harrison

The Haemophilia Society
1st Floor, Petersham House, 57A Hatton Garden, London EC1N 8JG
Tel: 020 7831 1020, 0800 018 6068 (Helpline)
Fax: 020 7405 4824
Email: info@haemophilia.org.uk
Website: www.haemophilia.org.uk

Chief Executive Graham Whitehead
Information and Advice Worker Ruth Taylor

Harveian Society of London
11 Chandos Street, Cavendish Square, London W19 9EB
Tel: 020 7580 1043 Fax: 020 7580 5793
Email: medsoc@telinw.co.uk

Executive Secretary Richard Kinsella-Bevan

Headway - The Brain Injury Association
4 King Edward Court, King Edward Street, Nottingham NG1 1EW
Tel: 0115 924 0800, 0808 800 2244 (Helpline)
Fax: 0115 958 4446
Email: enquiries@headway.org.uk
Website: www.headway.org.uk

Chief Executive Peter McCabe
Communications Director Martin Wakeling
Fundraising Director Vicki Unwin
Group Support Manager Angela McFarlane

Help the Hospices
34-44 Britannia Street, London WC1X 9JG
Tel: 020 7520 8200 Fax: 020 7278 1021
Email: info@helpthehospices.org.uk
Website: www.helpthehospices.org.uk

Chairman Lord Newton of Braintree
Chief Executive David Praill

History of Anaesthesia Society
49 Howey Lane, Frodshay, Warrington WA6 6DD
Website: www.histansoc.org.uk

President Peter Morris
Hon. Editor P M S Drury
Hon. Secretary A M Florence
Membership Secretary and Treasurer J Pring

Hospital Chaplaincies Council (Church of England)
Church House, Great Smith Street, Westminster, London SW1P 3NZ
Tel: 020 7898 1894 Fax: 020 7898 1891
Email: edward.lewis@c-of-e.org.uk
Website: www.nhs-chaplaincy-spiritualcare.org.uk

Chief Executive and Director of Training Edward Lewis
Administrator Tim Battle

Hospital Consultants and Specialists Association (HCSA)

1 Kingsclere Road, Overton, Basingstoke RG25 3JA
Tel: 01256 771777
Email: conspec@hcsa.com

Chief Executive Stephen Campion
Advisory Sservice Manager John Brawley

Hunterian Society

Lettsom House, 11 Chandos Street, Cavendish Square, London W1G 9EB
Tel: 020 7436 7363
Email: mailbox@hunteriansociety.org.uk
Website: www.hunteriansociety.org.uk

Hon. Senior Secretary Neil Weir

IA (The Ileostomy and Internal Pouch Support Group)

Peverill House, 1-5 Mill Road, Ballyclare BT39 9DR
Tel: 028 9334 4043, 0800 018 4724 (Freephone)
Fax: 028 9332 4606
Email: info@the-ia.org.uk
Website: www.the-ia.org.uk

National Secretary Anne Demick

Independent Healthcare Association

Westminster Tower, 3 Albert Embankment, London SE1 7SP
Tel: 020 7220 9595 Fax: 020 7820 3738
Email: info@iha.org.uk

Chairman David T Ervine
Chief Executive Barry Hassell
Communications Manager Peter Fermoy
Executive Director Tim Evans, Ann Mackay

Institute of Biomedical Science

12 Coldbath Square, London EC1R 5HL
Tel: 020 7713 0214 Fax: 020 7436 4946
Email: mail@ibms.org
Website: www.ibms.org

Chief Executive Alan R Potter

Institute of Chiropodists and Podiatrists

27 Wright Street, Southport PR9 0TL
Tel: 01704 546141, 08700 110305 Fax: 01704 500477
Email: secretary@inst-chiropodist.org.uk
Website: www.inst-chiropodist.org.uk

Company Secretary Susan Mary Kirkham

Institute of Physics and Engineering in Medicine

Fairmount House, 230 Tadcaster Road, York YO24 1ES
Tel: 01904 610821 Fax: 01904 612279
Email: office@ipem.ac.uk
Website: www.ipem.ac.uk

Finance Ian Wolstencroft
General Secretary Robert W Neilson
Meetings and Exhibitions Eva Elsner

Institute of Psychosexual Medicine

12 Chandos Street, Cavendish Square, London W1G 9DR
Tel: 020 7580 0631 Fax: 020 7436 2768
Email: ipm@telinco.co.uk
Website: www.ipm.org.uk

Director of Training Jane Botell
Administrative Secretary Susan Beck

Institute of Sports Medicine

Department of Surgery, University College London, Charles Bell House, 67-73 Riding House Street, London W1W 7EJ
Tel: 020 7813 2832 Fax: 020 7813 2832
Email: m.hobsley@ucl.ac.uk

Chairman David Money-Coutts
Company Secretary D Meynell

International Glaucoma Association

PO Box 4993, London SE5 9XZ
Tel: 020 7737 3265 Fax: 020 7346 5929
Email: info@iga.org.uk
Website: www.iga.org.uk

President R Pitts Crick
Chairman M H Miller
Chief Executive D Wright
Director of Finance and Development T Berry
Information Services Manager J Eastick
Patient Support Secretary Valerie Greatorex

International Spinal Research Trust

Bramley Business Centre, Station Road, Bramley, Guildford GU5 0AZ
Tel: 01483 898786 Fax: 01483 898763
Email: info@spinal-research.org
Website: www.spinal-research.org

Chairman of Trustees Paul Sharpe
Chief Executive Jonathan Miall

King's Fund

11/13 Cavendish Square, London W1G 0AN
Tel: 020 7307 2400 Fax: 020 7307 2801
Website: www.kingsfund.org.uk

Chief Executive Niall Dickson
Director of Resources Frank Jackson

Leonard Cheshire Foundation

30 Millbank, London SW1P 4QD
Tel: 020 7802 8200 Fax: 020 7802 8250
Email: info@lc-uk.org.uk
Website: www.leonard-cheshire.org

Chair Charles Morland
Director General Bryan Dutton

Leukaemia Research Fund

Postal Address, 43 Great Ormond Street, London WC1N 3JJ
Tel: 020 7405 0101 Fax: 020 7405 3139
Email: info@lrf.org.uk
Website: www.lrf.org.uk

Chief Executive Douglas Osborne
Head of Communications Matthew Wall
Scientific Director David Grant

Limbless Association

Rehabilitation Centre, Roehampton Lane, London SW15 5PR
Tel: 020 8788 1777 Fax: 020 8788 3444
Email: enquiries@limbless-association.org
Website: www.limbless-association.org

Chairman Zafar Khan
Chief Executive Diana Morgan

Lincoln Clinic and Centre for Psychotherapy

19 Abbeville Mews, 88 Clapham Park Road, London SW4 7BX
Tel: 020 7498 7472, 020 7978 1545 Fax: 020 7720 4721
Email: info@lincoln-psychotherapy.org.uk
Website: www.lincoln-psychotherapy.org.uk

Director and Board Chair Michael Heavens
Professional Committee Chair Christine Smith

Listening Books
12 Lant Street, London SE1 1QH
Tel: 020 7407 9417 Fax: 020 7403 1377
Email: info@listening-books.org.uk
Website: www.listening-books.org.uk

Director Bill Dee

Lister Institute of Preventive Medicine
PO Box 1083, Bushey WD23 9AG
Tel: 01923 801886 Fax: 01923 801886
Email: secretary@lister-institute.org.uk
Website: www.lister-institute.org.uk

Chairman Bridget Ogilvie
Director Trevor Hince
Hon. Treasurer P W Allen

The Little Foundation
c/o Mac Keith Press, 30 Furnival Street, London EC4A 1JQ
Tel: 020 7831 4918 Fax: 020 7405 5365

Chairman A C Robinson
Hon. Scientific Director J-P Lin

London Clinic of Psycho-Analysis
Byron House, 112A Shirland Road, London W9 2EQ
Tel: 020 7563 5002 Fax: 020 7563 5003
Email: trudy.turner@iopa.org.uk
Website: www.iopa.org.uk

Clinic Director Marcus Johns-Acting
Clinical Administrator Trudy Turner

MACA (Mental After Care Association)
1st Floor, Lincoln House, 296-302 High Holborn, London WC1V 7JH
Tel: 020 7061 3400 Fax: 020 7061 3401
Email: info@maca.org.uk
Website: www.maca.org uk

Chief Executive Gil Hitchon
Head of Communications Mary Richardson

Macmillan Cancer Relief
89 Albert Embankment, London SE1 7UQ
Tel: 020 7840 7840 Fax: 020 7840 7841
Email: cancerline@macmillan.org.uk
Website: www.macmillan.org.uk

Chief Executive Peter Cardy

Marie Curie Cancer Care
89 Albert Embankment, London SE1 7TP
Tel: 020 7599 7777 Fax: 020 7599 7788
Email: info@mariecurie.org.uk
Website: www.mariecurie.org.uk

Chief Executive Thomas Hughes-Hallett

The Medical Council on Alcohol
3 St Andrew's Place, Regent's Park, London NW1 4LB
Tel: 020 7487 4445 Fax: 020 7935 4479
Email: mca@medicouncilalcol.demon.co.uk
Website: www.medicouncilalcol.demon.co.uk

Chair P B Brunt
Medical Director G E Ratcliffe

The Medical Foundation for the Care of Victims of Torture
111 Isleden Road, Islington, London N7 7JW
Tel: 020 7697 7777 Fax: 020 7697 7799
Email: mail@torturecare.org.uk
Website: www.torturecare.org.uk

Director Malcolm Smart
Director of External Affairs Sherman Carrol

Medical Protection Society
Granary Wharf House, Leeds LS11 5PY
Tel: 0113 243 6436 Fax: 0113 241 0500
Email: info@mps.org.uk
Website: www.medicalprotection.org

Chief Executive J Hickey
Communications and Policy Director G Panting
Company Secretary Simon Kayll
Marketing Manager David Gray

Medical Research Society
Dialysis Centre, Box 118 Addenbrooke's Hospital, Hills Road, Cambridge CB2 2QQ
Fax: 07092 388555
Email: mrs@dial.pipex.com
Website: www.medres.org

Chair C Haslett
Hon. Secretary Afzal Chaudhry
Membership Secretary Corinne Wade
Treasurer A Guz

The Medical Society of London
Lettsom House, 11 Chandos Street, London W1G 9EB
Tel: 020 7580 1043 Fax: 020 7580 5793
Email: medsoc@telinco.co.uk

Registrar Richard Kinsella-Bevan
Deputy Registrar B A Smallwood

Medical Women's Federation
Tavistock House North, Tavistock Square, London WC1H 9HX
Tel: 020 7387 7765 Fax: 020 7388 9216
Email: mwf@btconnect.com
Website: www.medicalwomensfederation.co.uk

President Selina Gray
Vice-President Bhu Sandhu

Medico-Legal Society
17 The Avenue, Radlett WD7 7DQ
Tel: 01923 330195
Email: jillcrombie@ntlworld.com
Website: www.medico-legalsociety.org.uk

Hon. Legal Secretary Jill Crombie
Hon. Treasurer Eloise Aspinall, Nathalie Richard

MENCAP
National Centre, 123 Golden Lane, London EC1Y 0RT
Tel: 020 7454 0454, 020 7608 3254
Email: information@mencap.org.uk
Website: www.mencap.org.uk

Chairman Brian Baldock
Chief Executive Jo Williams
Director - Community Support Neville Short
Director - Education and Employment Alison Sargent
Director - Housing and Support Jan Tregelles
Director - Human Resources Jill Tombs
Director of Communications and Fundraising Deborah Hamilton-Lewin
Director of Finance David Lawrence

Meningitis Trust
Fern House, Bath Road, Stroud GL5 3TJ
Tel: 01453 768000 Fax: 01453 768001
Email: info@meningitis-trust.org.uk
Website: www.meningitis-trust.org.uk

President Andrew Harvey
Chair Geoff Shaw
Chief Executive Philip Kirby

Mental Health Foundation
UK Office, 20 Upper Ground, London SE1 9QB
Tel: 020 7803 1100 Fax: 020 7803 1111
Email: mhf@mhf.org.uk
Website: www.mentalhealth.org.uk

Chief Executive Andrew McCulloch

Mental Health Matters
Avalon House, St Catherines Court, Sunderland SR5 3XJ
Tel: 0191 516 3500 Fax: 0191 549 7298
Email: rharris@mentalhealthmatters.co.uk
Website: www.mentalhealthmatters.com

Chief Executive Ian Grant

Mental Health Media
356 Holloway Road, London N7 6PA
Tel: 020 7700 8171 Fax: 020 7686 0959
Email: info@mhmedia.com
Website: www.mhmedia.com

Chief Executive David Crepaz-Keay

Migraine Action Association
Unit 6, Oakley Hay Lodge Business Park, Great Folds Road, Great Oakley NN18 9AS
Tel: 01536 461333 Fax: 01536 461444
Email: info@migraine.org.uk
Website: www.migraine.org.uk

Chief Executive Anita Few

Migraine Trust
2nd Floor, 55-56 Russell Square, London WC1B 4HP
Tel: 020 7436 1336 Fax: 020 7436 2880
Email: info@migrainetrust.org
Website: www.migrainetrust.org

Chief Executive Alan Bartle
Head of Fundraising Yvonne Lane
Education Officer Allinson Anthony, Elizabeth Rickarby
Support Services Manager Susan Haydon

MIND
15-19 Broadway, London E15 4BQ
Tel: 020 8519 2122, 0845 766 0163 (MIND Infoline)
Fax: 020 8522 1725
Email: contact@mind.org.uk
Website: www.mind.org.uk

Chief Executive Richard Brook

MMA HealthServe
Partnership House, 157 Waterloo Road, London SE1 8XN
Tel: 020 7928 4694 Fax: 020 7620 2453
Email: healthserve@cmf.org.uk
Website: www.healthserve.org

Director Steven Fouch
Administrator Laura Risdale
Medical Director Peter Armon

Motor Neurone Disease Association
PO Box 246, Northampton NN1 2PR
Tel: 08457 626262 Fax: 01604 624726
Email: enquiries@mndassociation.org
Website: www.mndassociation.org

Chair Alan Graham
Chief Executive G Levvy
Treasurer Alistair Johnston

Multiple Sclerosis Society of Great Britain and N. Ireland
MS National Centre, 372 Edgware Road, Staples Corner, London NW2 6ND
Tel: 020 8438 0700, 0808 800 8000 (Helpline)
Fax: 020 8438 0701
Email: info@mssociety.org.uk
Website: www.mssociety.org.uk

Chief Executive Mike O'Donovan

Muscular Dystrophy Campaign
7-11 Prescott Place, London SW4 6BS
Tel: 020 7720 8055 Fax: 020 7498 0670
Email: info@muscular-dystrophy.org
Website: www.muscular-dystrophy.org

Myasthenia Gravis Association
Business Office, 1st Floor, Southgate Business Centre, Normanton Road, Derby DE23 6UQ
Tel: 01332 290219 Fax: 01332 293641
Email: mg@mgauk.org.uk
Website: www.mgauk.org

Chief Executive Alasdair Nimmo

National Association for Medical Education Management (incorporating NAPMECA)
PO Box 375, York YO10 3WQ
Tel: 01904 414832
Email: ruth.bycroft@btinternet.com
Website: www.namem.org.uk

Chairman Judi Sharpe
Executive Secretary Ruth Bycroft
Executive Treasurer Andrea Thompson
Vice Chairman Andrina Hardcastle

National Association of Clinical Tutors
56 Queen Anne Street, London W1G 8LA
Tel: 020 7317 3109 Fax: 020 7317 3110
Email: office@nact.org.uk
Website: www.nact.org.uk

Chairman Andrew Long
Executive Manager Jane Litherland

National Association of GP Co-operatives
Regency House, 90-92 Otley Road, Leeds LS6 4BA
Tel: 0113 278 2381 Fax: 0113 278 3674
Email: manager@nagpc.org.uk
Website: www.nagpc.org.uk

Chair Mark Reynolds

The National Association of Primary Care
Lettsom House, 11 Chandos Street, Cavendish Square, London W1G 9DP
Tel: 020 7636 7228 Fax: 020 7636 1601
Email: napc@napc.co.uk
Website: www.napc.co.uk

Chief Executive Eric McCullough

National Asthma Campaign
Providence House, Providence Place, London N1 0NT
Tel: 020 7226 2260, 0845 701 0203 (Asthma Helpline)
Fax: 020 7704 0740
Website: www.asthma.org.uk

National Autistic Society
393 City Road, London EC1V 1NG
Tel: 020 7833 2299 Fax: 020 7833 9666
Email: nas@nas.org.uk
Website: www.nas.org.uk

Director of Services Neil McConachie

National Cancer Alliance
PO Box 579, Oxford OX4 1LB
Tel: 01865 793566 Fax: 01865 251050
Email: nationalcanceralliance@btinternet.com
Website: www.nationalcanceralliance.co.uk

Chair Rebecca Miles

The National Childbirth Trust
Alexandra House, Oldham Terrace, Acton, London W3 6NH
Tel: 0870 444 8707 (Enquiries),
0870 444 8708 (Breastfeeding Helpline),
0870 770 3236 (Administration), 0870 770 3238 (Press Office),
0870 990 8040 (Membership Hotline) Fax: 0870 770 3237
Email: enquiries@national-childbirth-trust.co.uk
Website: www.nctpregnancyandbabycare.com / www.ncts.co.uk

Chief Executive Belinda Phipps

National Children's Bureau
8 Wakley Street, London EC1V 7QE
Tel: 020 7843 6000 Fax: 020 7278 9512
Email: enquiries@ncb.org.uk
Website: www.ncb.org.uk

Chief Executive Paul Ennals

National Council for Palliative Care
1st Floor, 34-44 Britannia Street, London WC1X 9JG
Tel: 020 7520 8299 Fax: 020 7520 8298
Email: enquiries@ncpc.org.uk
Website: www.ncpc.org.uk

Chief Executive Eve Richardson

National Counselling Service for Sick Doctors
10 Carlton House Terrace, London SW1Y 5AH
Tel: 0870 321 1753
Email: contact@ncssd.org.uk
Website: www.ncssd.org.uk

Hon. Secretary Jolyon Oxley

The National Deaf Children's Society
National Office, 15 Dufferin Street, London EC1Y 8UR
Tel: 020 7490 8656, 0808 800 8880 (Helpline)
Fax: 020 7251 5020
Email: ndcs@ndcs.org.uk
Website: www.ndcs.org.uk

Chief Executive Susan Daniels

National Eczema Society
Hill House, Highgate Hill, London N19 5NA
Tel: 020 7281 3553, 0870 241 3604 (Helpline)
Fax: 020 7281 6395
Email: helpline@eczema.org
Website: www.eczema.org

Chief Executive Margaret Cox

The National Kidney Research Fund
Kings Chambers, Priestgate, Peterborough PE1 1FG
Tel: 01733 704650, 0845 300 1499 (Helpline) Fax: 01733 704699
Email: enquiries@nkrf.org.uk
Website: www.nkrf.org.uk

Chief Executive Charles Kernahan
Director of Finance C D Thomas
Director of Fundraising M Nation
Head of Marketing & Communications N Turkentine

The National League of the Blind and Disabled
NLBD / ISTC Division 8, Swinton House, 324 Gray's Inn Road, London WC1X 8DD
Tel: 020 7278 0436 Fax: 020 7278 0436
Website: www.istc-tu.org

General Secretary J P B Mann

National Library for the Blind
Far Cromwell Road, Bredbury, Stockport SK6 2SG
Tel: 0161 355 2000, 0161 355 2043 Minicom Fax: 0161 355 2098
Email: enquiries@nlbuk.org
Website: www.nlb-online.org

Acting Chief Executive Helen Brazier
Marketing Manager Mark Drury
Press and PR Officer Kirsti Frost

National Osteoporosis Society
Camerton, Bath BA2 0PJ
Tel: 01761 471771 Fax: 01761 471104
Email: info@nos.org.uk
Website: www.nos.org.uk

Chief Executive Terry Eccles
Communications and Fundraising Manager Trevor Reid

National Pharmaceutical Association
Mallinson House, 38-42 St Peter's Street, St Albans AL1 3NP
Tel: 01727 832161 Fax: 01727 840858
Email: npa@npa.co.uk
Website: www.npa.co.uk

Chief Executive John D'Arcy

National Society for Epilepsy
Chesham Lane, Chalfont St Peter SL9 0RJ
Tel: 01494 601300, 01494 601400 Helpline Fax: 01494 871927
Website: www.epilepsynse.org.uk

Chief Executive Graham Faulkner
Director of Development and Estates Tristram Reynolds
Director of External Relations David Josephs
Director of Finance Michael De Val
Director of Personnel and Training Carol Macham
Director of Services Karen Lane
Medical Director John Duncan
PA to Chief Executive Hilary Radburn, Liz Ward

National Society for the Prevention of Cruelty to Children (NSPCC)
Weston House, 42 Curtain Road, London EC2A 3NH
Tel: 020 7825 2500 Fax: 020 7825 2525
Email: info@nspcc.org.uk
Website: www.nspcc.org.uk

Chief Executive Mary Marsh
Deputy Librarian Joanne Wright

NCH
85 Highbury Park, London N5 1UD
Tel: 020 7704 7000 Fax: 020 7226 2537
Website: www.nch.org.uk

Chief Executive Clare Tickell

The Neuro-Disability Research Trust
Royal Hospital for Neuro-disability, West Hill, London SW15 3SW
Tel: 020 8780 4500 Fax: 020 8780 4501
Email: info@rhn.org.uk
Website: www.rhn.org.uk/nrt

Chairman Graham Gilchrist

NHS Confederation
29 Bressenden Place, London SW1E 5DD
Tel: 020 7074 3200, 020 7074 3201
Email: enquiries@nhsconfed.co.uk
Website: www.nhsconfed.org

Chief Executive Gillian Morgan

NHS Support Federation
Community Base, 113 Queens Road, Brighton BN1 3XG
Tel: 01273 234822 Fax: 01273 234820
Email: info@nhscampaign.org
Website: www.nhscampaign.org

President Harry Keen
Director Paul Evans

Nuffield Institute for Health
The University of Leeds, 71-75 Clarendon Road, Leeds LS2 9PL
Tel: 0113 343 6633 Fax: 0113 246 0899
Email: nuffield@leeds.ac.uk
Website: www.nuffield.leeds.ac.uk

Information and Admissions Co-ordinator Zeba Ahmed

Nuffield Trust
59 New Cavendish Street, London W1G 7LP
Tel: 020 7631 8450 Fax: 020 7631 8451
Email: mail@nuffieldtrust.org.uk
Website: www.nuffieldtrust.org.uk

Librarian Barbara Cohen
Secretary John Wyn Owen

Nutrition Society
10 Cambridge Court, 210 Shepherds Bush Road, London W6 7NJ
Tel: 020 7602 0228 Fax: 020 7602 1756
Email: office@nutsoc.org.uk
Website: www.nutritionsociety.org

President Ann Prentice
Hon. Secretary Judith Buttris

Obstetric Anaesthetists' Association
PO Box 3219, Barnes, London SW13 9XR
Tel: 020 8741 1311 Fax: 020 8741 0611
Email: secretariat@oaa-anaes.ac.uk
Website: www.oaa-anaes.ac.uk

President Gordon Lyons
Hon. Secretary Steve Yentis
Hon. Treasurer Roshan Fernando

Office of Health Economics
12 Whitehall, London SW1A 2DY
Tel: 020 7930 9203 Fax: 020 7747 1419
Email: ohegeneral@ohe.org
Website: www.ohe.org

Director Adrian Towse
Associate Director Jon Sussex

One Parent Families
255 Kentish Town Road, London NW5 2LX
Tel: 020 7428 5400, 0800 018 5026 (Helpline)
Fax: 020 7482 4851
Email: info@oneparentfamilies.org.uk
Website: www.oneparentfamilies.org.uk

Chief Executive Nicola Simpson

Parkinson's Disease Society
215 Vauxhall Bridge Road, London SW1V IEJ
Tel: 020 7931 8080, 0808 800 0303 Helpline (Freephone)
Fax: 020 7233 9908, 020 7963 9360
Email: enquiries@parkinsons.org.uk
Website: www.parkinsons.org.uk

Chief Executive Linda Kelly
Director of Community Services Peter Raymond
Director of Finance Lester Corp
Director of PCI Robert Meadowcroft
Director of Research & Development Kieran Breen
Head of PR Helen Garner
Information Adviser Anne Bridge

Pathological Society of Great Britain and Ireland
2 Carlton House Terrace, London SW1Y 5AF
Tel: 020 7976 1260 Fax: 020 7976 1267
Email: administrator@pathsoc.org.uk
Website: www.pathsoc.org.uk

President N A Wright
Administrator R A Pitts
General Secretary P A Hall
Meetings Secretary M Pignatelli
Treasurer A D Burt

The Patients Association
PO Box 935, Harrow HA1 3YJ
Tel: 020 8423 9111, 0845 608 4455 (Helpline)
Fax: 020 8423 9119
Email: mailbox@patients-association.com
Website: www.patients-association.com

President Claire Rayner
Director of Communication Katherine Murphy
Director of Policy Simon Williams
Vice President Phil Hammond, Angela Rippon

The Pituitary Foundation
PO Box 1944, Bristol BS99 2UB
Tel: 0870 450 0375 Fax: 0870 450 0376
Email: helpline@pituitary.org.uk
Website: www.pituitary.org.uk

Patient Support Manager Theresa O'Neill

Primary Immunodeficiency Association (PIA)
Alliance House, 12 Caxton Street, London SW1H 0QS
Tel: 020 7976 7640 Fax: 020 7976 7641
Email: info@pia.org.uk
Website: www.pia.org.uk

Chair Clare Tritton
Chief Executive Christopher Hugan
Treasurer Ray Dias

Psoriasis Association
7 Milton Street, Northampton NN2 7JG
Tel: 01604 711129, 08456 760076 (Helpline) Fax: 01604 792894
Email: mail@psoriasis.demon.co.uk
Website: www.psoriasis-association.org.uk

Chief Executive Gladys Edwards

Queen's Nursing Institute
3 Albemarle Way, Clerkenwell, London EC1V 4RQ
Tel: 020 7490 4227 Fax: 020 7490 1296
Email: mail@qni.org.uk
Website: www.qni.org.uk

Director Rosemary Cook
Admin Officer Catherine Brennan

QUIT
Ground Floor, 211 Old Street, London EC1V 9NR
Tel: 020 7251 1551, 0800 002200 (Helpline) Fax: 020 7251 1661
Email: info@quit.org.uk
Website: www.quit.org.uk

Chief Executive Steve Crone

Rainbow Trust Children's Charity
6 Cleeve Court, Cleeve Road, Leatherhead KT22 7UD
Tel: 01372 363438 Fax: 01372 363101
Email: enquiries@rainbowtrust.org.uk
Website: www.rainbowtrust.org.uk

Chief Executive Heather Wood

REMEDI For Relief of Disability
The Old Rectory, Stanton Prior, Bath BA2 9HT
Tel: 01761 472662 Fax: 01761 470662
Email: director.remedi@btinternet.com, fundraiser.remedi@btinternet.com
Website: www.remedi.org.uk

Chairman A K Clarke
Director P D Mesquita
Treasurer M A Hines

Research into Ageing
Help the Aged, 207-221 Pentonville Road, London N1 9UZ
Tel: 020 7278 1114, 0808 800 6565 (Helpline)
Fax: 020 7278 1116
Email: info@helptheaged.org.uk
Website: www.ageing.org

Director General Michael Lake

The Restoration of Appearance and Function Trust (RAFT)
Leopold Muller Building, Mount Vernon Hospital, Northwood HA6 2RN
Tel: 01923 835815 Fax: 01923 844031
Email: charity@raft.ac.uk
Website: www.raft.ac.uk

Director (Admin and Appeals) Hilary Bailey
Director of Research A O Grobbelaar
Accountant John Shepherd
Administrator Stephanie Easton
Board of Trustees Chairman David C T Pollock

Restricted Growth Association (RGA)
PO Box 4744, Dorchester DT2 9FA
Tel: 01308 898445 Fax: 01308 898445
Email: office@restrictedgrowth.co.uk
Website: www.restrictedgrowth.co.uk

Association Manager Sandy Marshall

Rethink Severe Mental Illness
28 Castle Street, Kingston upon Thames KT1 1SS
Tel: 0845 456 0455 Fax: 020 8547 3862
Email: info@rethink.org
Website: www.rethink.org

Chief Executive Cliff Prior

Richmond Fellowship
80 Holloway Road, Highbury, London N7 8JG
Tel: 020 7697 3300 Fax: 020 7697 3301
Website: www.richmondfellowship.org.uk

Chief Executive Maggie Hysel

Royal Association for Deaf People (RAD)
RAD Head Office, Walsingham Road, Colchester CO2 7BP
Tel: 01206 509509, 01206 711260 (Text) Fax: 01206 769755
Email: info@royaldeaf.org.uk
Website: www.royaldeaf.org.uk

Chief Executive Tom Fenton

Royal Association for Disability and Rehabilitation (RADAR)
12 City Forum, 250 City Road, London EC1V 8AF
Tel: 020 7250 3222 Fax: 020 7250 0212
Email: radar@radar.org.uk
Website: www.radar.org.uk

Director Kate Nash

The Royal British Legion
48 Pall Mall, London SW1Y 5JY
Tel: 0845 7725 725 Fax: 020 7973 7399
Email: info@britishlegion.org.uk
Website: www.britishlegion.org.uk

Secretary General I G Townsend

Royal British Nurses Association
River Bank House, Room 502, 5th Floor, 1 Putney Approach, London SW6 3JD
Tel: 020 7731 0550

Vice-President and Chairman of the Fund H M Campbell

Royal Institute of Public Health
28 Portland Place, London W1B 1DE
Tel: 020 7580 2731 Fax: 020 7580 6157
Email: marketing@riph.org.uk
Website: www.riph.org.uk

Communications Officer Julie Mulley
General Manager Wendy Moore

Royal Medical Benevolent Fund
24 King's Road, Wimbledon, London SW19 8QN
Tel: 020 8540 9194 Fax: 020 8542 0494
Email: info@rmbf.org
Website: www.rmbf.org

Chief Executive Michael Baber

The Royal Medical Foundation
College Road, Epsom KT17 4JQ
Tel: 01372 821010, 01372 821011 Fax: 01372 821013
Email: caseworker@royalmedicalfoundation.org
Website: www.royalmedicalfoundation.org

Administrator John H Higgs
Caseworker Nickie Colville

Royal Medical Society
Student Centre, 5/5 Bristo Square, Edinburgh EH8 9AL
Tel: 0131 650 2672 Fax: 0131 650 2672
Email: enquiries@royalmedical.co.uk
Website: www.royalmedical.co.uk

President Mayank Madhra, Stewart Pattman, Joanne Sells

Royal National Institute for Deaf People
19-23 Featherstone Street, London EC1Y 8SL
Tel: 020 7296 8000, 020 7296 8001 Fax: 020 7296 8199
Email: information@rnid.org.uk
Website: www.rnid.org.uk

Chairman James Strachan
Chief Executive John Low

Royal National Institute for the Blind (RNIB)
105 Judd Street, London WC1H 9NE
Tel: 020 7388 1266, 0800 515152 (Textphone via Typetalk), 0845 766 9999 (Helpline - UK callers only Monday to Friday 9am to 5pm) Fax: 020 7388 2034
Email: helpline@rnib.org.uk
Website: www.rnib.org.uk

Chairman Colin Low
Director General Lesley Anne Alexander
Hon. Treasurer David Gadbury

Royal Pharmaceutical Society of Great Britain
1 Lambeth High Street, London SE1 7JN
Tel: 020 7735 9141 Fax: 020 7735 7629
Email: enquiries@rpsgb.org
Website: www.rpsgb.org

President Nicholas Wood
Secretary and Registrar Ann Lewis

The Royal Society
6-9 Carlton House Terrace, London SW1Y 5AG
Tel: 020 7451 2500 Fax: 020 7451 2170
Email: info@royalsoc.ac.uk
Website: www.royalsoc.ac.uk

Executive Secretary Stephen Cox

Royal Society for the Prevention of Accidents (RoSPA)
Edgbaston Park, 353 Bristol Road, Birmingham B5 7ST
Tel: 0121 248 2000 Fax: 0121 248 2001
Email: help@rospa.com
Website: www.rospa.com

Chief Executive John D Hooper

The Royal Society for the Promotion of Health
38A St George's Drive, London SW1V 4BH
Tel: 020 7630 0121 Fax: 020 7976 6847
Email: rsph@rsph.org
Website: www.rsph.org

Executive Officer Amy Walton

The Royal Society of Medicine
1 Wimpole Street, London W1G 0AE
Tel: 020 7290 2900 Fax: 020 7290 2992
Email: membership@rsm.ac.uk
Website: www.rsm.ac.uk

Director of Communications and Marketing Janice Liverseidge
Director of Finance David Laughton
Director of Information Services Ian Snowley
Director of Membership Services Jo Parkinson, Joanna Parkinson
Director of Support Services John Tyrrell
Director of Symposia Marty Adair
Development Director Paul Summerfield
Executive Director Anne Grocock
Managing Director of RSM Press Peter Richardson

Royal Society of Tropical Medicine and Hygiene
50 Bedford Square, London WC1B 3DP
Tel: 020 7580 2127 Fax: 020 7436 1389
Email: mail@rstmh.org
Website: www.rstmh.org

Administrator Caryl Guest
Hon. Secretary Geoffrey Pasvol, Russell Stothard

The Sainsbury Centre for Mental Health
134-138 Borough High Street, London SE1 1LB
Tel: 020 7827 8300 Fax: 020 7403 9482
Website: www.scmh.org.uk

Chief Executive Angela Greatley

St Andrew's Ambulance Association
St Andrew's House, 48 Milton Street, Glasgow G4 0HR
Tel: 0141 332 4031 Fax: 0141 332 6582
Email: firstaid@staaa.org.uk
Website: www.firstaid.org.uk

Chief Executive Brendan Healy
Commercial Manager Tommy Dickson
Corps Support Manager Gordon Connell
Finance Manager Alan McQueen
Training Manager Jim Dorman

St Dunstan's (Caring for Blind Ex-Service Men and Women)
12-14 Harcourt Street, London W1H 4HD
Tel: 020 7723 5021 Fax: 020 7262 6199
Email: enquiries@st-dunstans.org.uk
Website: www.st-dunstans.org.uk

Chief Executive Robert Leader

St John Ambulance
27 St John's Lane, London EC1M 4BU
Tel: 0870 010 4950 Fax: 0870 010 4065
Email: chief-executive@nhq.sja.org.uk
Website: www.sja.org.uk

Chief Executive Roger Holmes

Stillbirth and Neonatal Death Society (SANDS)
28 Portland Place, London W1B 1LY
Tel: 020 7436 5881 (Helpline), 020 7436 7940 (Office)
Fax: 020 7436 3715
Email: support@uk-sands.org
Website: www.uk-sands.org

Chair Sue Annis Salter
Breavement Support Erica Stewart
Office Administrator Lesley Dewar

SANE/SANELINE
1st Floor, Cityside House, 40 Adler Street, London E1 1EE
Tel: 020 7375 1002, 0845 767 8000 (Helpline)
Fax: 020 7375 2162
Email: info@sane.org.uk
Website: www.sane.org.uk

Chief Executive Marjorie Wallace

Save the Children
1 St Johns Lane, London EC1M 4AR
Tel: 020 7012 6400 Fax: 020 7012 6962
Email: enquiries@scfuk.org.uk
Website: www.savethechildren.org.uk

Director General Michael Aaronson

Scope
Cerebral Palsy Helpline, PO Box 833, Milton Keynes MK12 5NY
Tel: 0808 800 3333 Fax: 01908 321051
Email: cphelpline@scope.org.uk
Website: www.scope.org.uk

Chairman Gerald McCarthy
Chief Executive Tony Manwaring
Executive Director John Adams, Richard Hall, Pauline Simpson, Jon Sparkes

Scottish Association for Mental Health
Cumbrae House, 15 Carlton Court, Glasgow G5 9JP
Tel: 0141 568 7000 Fax: 0141 568 7001
Email: enquire@samh.org.uk
Website: www.samh.org.uk

Chief Executive Shona M Neil

Scottish Committee of Optometrists
7 Queens Buildings, Queensferry Road, Rosyth, Dunfermline KY11 2RA
Tel: 01383 419444 Fax: 01383 416778
Email: scoptom@aol.com

Chairman Charles J MacKinnon
Secretary and Treasurer David S Hutton

Scottish Health Visitors' Association (UNISON)

Douglas House, 60 Belford Road, Edinburgh EH4 3UQ
Tel: 0870 777 7006 Fax: 0131 220 6389
Email: d.forbes@unison.co.uk
Website: www.unison-scotland.org.uk

General Administration Officer David F Forbes

Scottish Hospital Endowments Research Trust

Princes Exchange, 1 Earl Grey Street, Edinburgh EH3 9EE
Tel: 0131 659 8800 Fax: 0131 228 8118
Email: enquiries@shert.org.uk
Website: www.shert.org.uk

Chairman S Moira Brown
Trust Administrator Lesley More

The Scottish National Federation for the Welfare of the Blind

Redroofs, Balgavies, Forfar DD8 2TH
Tel: 01307 830265 Fax: 01307 830265
Email: snfwb@care4free.net

Hon. Treasurer John Duncan

Scottish Pharmaceutical General Council

42 Queen Street, Edinburgh EH2 3NH
Tel: 0131 467 7766 Fax: 0131 467 7767
Email: enquiries@spgc.org.uk
Website: www.spgc.org.uk

Secretary Colin Virden

Sesame Institute (UK)

27 Blackfriars Road, London SE1 8NY
Tel: 020 7633 9690
Email: info@seame-institute.org
Website: www.sesame-institute.org

Director Diana Cooper

Shaftesbury Society

16 Kingston Road, London SW19 1JZ
Tel: 0845 330 6033 Fax: 020 8239 5580
Email: info@shaftesburysoc.org.uk
Website: www.shaftesburysociety.org

Chief Executive Mary Bishop

Shape London

LVS Resource Centre, 356 Holloway Road, London N7 6PA
Tel: 020 7619 6160 Fax: 020 7619 6162
Email: info@shapearts.org.uk
Website: www.shapearts.org.uk

Chief Executive Steve Mannix

Sick Doctors Trust

36 Wick Crescent, Bristol BS4 4HG
Tel: 0870 444 5163 (Helpline) Fax: 0117 971 0505
Email: help@sick-dosctors-trust.co.uk
Website: www.sick-doctors-trust.co.uk

Chairman Jacqueline Chang
Secretary Jonathan Williams
Treasurer Robert Brown
Vice Chairman Alasdair Young

The Sigma Centre

29 Netherhall Gardens, London NW3 5RL
Tel: 020 7794 2445 Fax: 020 7431 3726
Email: info@thesigmacentre.plus.com

Chairman Warren Kinston
Managing Partner Verity Goitein

The Sir Jules Thorn Charitable Trust

24 Manchester Square, London W1U 3TH
Tel: 020 7487 5851 Fax: 020 7224 3976
Email: info@julesthorntrust.org.uk
Website: www.julesthorntrust.org.uk

Chairman Elizabeth Charal
Director David H Richings
Trust Secretary Marcia Howard
Trustee Bruce MacPhail, Ravinder N Maini, Nancy V Pearcey, Ann Rylands, Christopher H Sporborg, William H Sporborg, Nicholas Wilson

Smith and Nephew Foundation

15 Adam Street, London WC2N 6LA
Tel: 020 7960 2276
Email: barbara.foster@smith-nephew.com
Website: www.snfoundation.org.uk

Administrator Barbara Foster
Executive Secretary David Hawkins

The Society and the College of Radiographers

207 Providence Square, Mill Street, London SE1 2EW
Tel: 020 7740 7200 Fax: 020 7740 7204
Email: info@sor.org
Website: www.sor.org

Chief Executive Officer Richard Evans
Director of Finance Neil Williams
Director of Industrial Relations Warren Town
Director of Professional Policy Audrey Paterson

Society for Endocrinology

22 Apex Court, Woodlands, Bradley Stoke, Bristol BS32 4JT
Tel: 01454 642200 Fax: 01454 642222
Email: info@endocrinology.org
Website: www.endocrinology.org

Chair S R Bloom
Executive Director Sue Thorn
Secretary J A Wass

Society of Academic and Research Surgery (SARS)

Royal College of Surgeons of England, 35-43 Lincoln's Inn Fields, London WC2A 3PE
Tel: 020 7869 6640 Fax: 020 7869 6644
Email: sars@rcseng.ac.uk
Website: www.surgicalresearch.org.uk

President Irving Taylor
Hon. Secretary Michael Wyatt

Society of British Neurological Surgeons

Royal College of Surgeons, 35-43 Lincoln's Inn Fields, London WC2 3PE
Tel: 020 7869 6892 Fax: 020 7869 6890
Email: admin@sbns.freeserve.co.uk
Website: www.sbns.org.uk

President J Steers
Hon. Secretary P Van Hille
Treasurer B A Bell
Vice President D Hardy

Society of Cardiothoracic Surgeons of Great Britain and Ireland

Royal College of Surgeons of England, 35-43 Lincoln's Inn Fields, London WC2A 3PE
Tel: 020 7869 6893 Fax: 020 7869 6890
Email: sctsadmin@scts.org
Website: www.scts.org

President Pat Magee
Hon. Secretary James Roxburgh

The Society of Chiropodists and Podiatrists
1 Fellmongers Path, Tower Bridge Road, London SE1 3LY
Tel: 0845 450 3720, 0845 450 3721 Fax: 020 7234 8621
Email: enq@scpod.org
Website: www.feetforlife.org

Chief Executive Joanna Brown
Director of Education and Development David Ashcroft

Society of Occupational Medicine
6 St Andrew's Place, Regent's Park, London NW1 4LB
Tel: 020 7486 2641 Fax: 020 7486 0028
Email: admin@som.org.uk
Website: www.som.org.uk

Hon. Secretary D E S Macaulay

The Stroke Association
Stroke House, 240 City Road, London EC1V 2PR
Tel: 020 7251 9096 (Textphone), 020 7566 0300, 0845 303 3100 (Helpline) Fax: 020 7490 2686
Email: info@stroke.org.uk
Website: www.stroke.org.uk

Chief Executive Jon Barrick
Director of Public Relations Joe Korner
Secretary Richard Polson

Tavistock Institute
30 Tabernacle Street, London EC2A 4UE
Tel: 020 7417 0407 Fax: 020 7417 0567
Email: central.admin@tavinstitute.org
Website: www.tavinstitute.org/

Principal and Chair John Kelleher
Director Phil Swann
Institute Secretary Debbie Sorkin

Tenovus
43 The Parade, Cardiff CF24 3AB
Tel: 029 2048 2000 Fax: 029 2048 4199
Email: post@tenovus.com
Website: www.tenovus.com

Chairman Guy Clarke
Chief Executive Richard Walken
Director of Fundraising Sarah-Jayne Williams

Terrence Higgins Trust
52-54 Gray's Inn Road, London WC1X 8JU
Tel: 020 7831 0330 Fax: 020 7242 0121
Email: info@tht.org.uk
Website: www.tht.org.uk

Chief Executive Nick Partridge

TFC Frost Charitable Trust
Holmes & Co., 10 Torrington Road, Claygate, Esher KT10 0SA
Tel: 01372 465378 Fax: 01372 464539

Secretary J Holmes

Tuberous Sclerosis Association
PO Box 9644, Bromsgrove B61 0FP
Tel: 01527 871898 Fax: 01527 579452
Email: support@tuberous-sclerosis.org
Website: www.tuberous-sclerosis.org

Head of Appeals and Publicity Officer Anne Carter
Head of Support Services Janet Medcalf
Specialist Adviser Janet Bower, Hilary McCrlynn, Harriet Spencer

UK Centre for the Advancement of Interprofessional Education (CAIPE)
344-354 Gray's Inn Road, London WC1X 8BP
Tel: 020 7278 1083 Fax: 020 7278 6604
Email: admin@caipe.org.uk
Website: www.caipe.org.uk

Chief Executive Barbara Clague

UK Public Health Association (UKPHA)
7th Floor Holborn Gate, 330 High Holborn, London WC1V 7BA
Tel: 0870 010 1932 Fax: 020 7061 3393
Email: info@ukpha.org.uk
Website: www.ukpha.org.uk

Chair David Hunter
Chief Executive Angela Mawle

WellBeing
27 Sussex Place, Regent's Park, London NW1 4SP
Tel: 020 7772 6400 Fax: 020 7724 7725
Email: wellbeing@rcog.org.uk
Website: www.wellbeing.org.uk

Interim Director Shirley Farmer
PA to Director Nicola Retter

Wellbeing of Women
Wellbeing, 27 Sussex Place, Regent's Park, London NW1 4SP
Tel: 020 7772 6400 Fax: 020 7724 7725
Email: wellbeingofwomen@rcog.org.uk
Website: www.wellbeingofwomen.org.uk

Director Shirley Farmer

Wessex Medical Trust (Hope)
Allport House, Prince's Street, Southampton SO14 5RP
Tel: 023 8033 3366 Fax: 023 8033 3377
Email: info@hope.org.uk
Website: www.hope.org.uk

William Harvey Research Ltd (WHRL)
John Vane Science Centre, Charterhouse Square, London EC1M 6BQ
Tel: 020 7882 6120 Fax: 020 7882 6016
Website: www.williamharvey.co.uk

Chief Executive Chris Thiemermann

Women's Nationwide Cancer Control Campaign
1st Floor, Charity House, 14-15 Perseverance Works, London E2 8DD
Tel: 020 7729 4688 Fax: 020 7613 0771

The Worshipful Society of Apothecaries of London
Apothecaries Hall, Black Friars Lane, London EC4V 6EJ
Tel: 020 7236 1189 Fax: 020 7329 3177
Email: examoffice@apothecaries.org
Website: www.apothecaries.org

Registrar K E Edmunds
Beadle John Williams
Clerk A M Wallington-Smith

Yorkshire Cancer Research
39 East Parade, Harrogate HG1 5LQ
Tel: 01423 501269 Fax: 01423 527929
Email: hq@ycr.org.uk
Website: www.ycr.org.uk

Chairman B P Jackson
Chief Executive Elaine King
Scientific Advisory Committee Chair E A Dawes
Treasurer M R Harrison

Index by Organisation Name

Index of Hospitals by Town

Londonderry

Longfield

Louth

Lowestoft

Ludlow

Luton

Lydney

Lymington

Lytham St Annes